To borrow: send email to library@sharp.com with your *name, phone, email ba code of the book or CD*. You will have item for 4 weeks.

TEXTBOOK OF CRITICAL CARE

TEXTBOOK OF CRITICAL CARE

Sixth Edition

JEAN-LOUIS VINCENT, MD, PhD
Professor of Intensive Care Medicine
Université Libre de Bruxelles
Head, Department of Intensive Care
Erasme University Hospital
Brussels, Belgium

EDWARD ABRAHAM, MD
Professor and Chair
Spencer Chair in Medical Science Leadership
Department of Medicine
University of Alabama at Birmingham
School of Medicine
Birmingham, Alabama

FREDERICK A. MOORE, MD, FACS, FCCM
Professor of Surgery
Head, Acute Care Surgery
College of Medicine
University of Florida
Gainesville, Florida

PATRICK M. KOCHANEK, MD, FCCM
Professor and Vice Chairman
Department of Critical Care Medicine
Professor of Anesthesiology, Pediatrics, and Clinical and Translational Science
Director, Safar Center for Resuscitation Research
University of Pittsburgh School of Medicine
Pittsburgh, Pennsylvania

MITCHELL P. FINK, MD
Professor of Surgery and Anesthesiology
Vice Chair for Critical Care, Department of Surgery
David Geffen School of Medicine
University of California–Los Angeles
Los Angeles, California

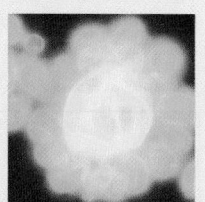
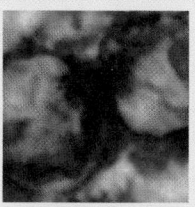
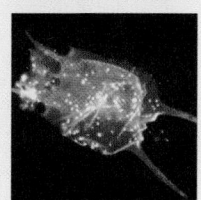

ELSEVIER
SAUNDERS

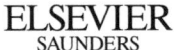

ELSEVIER
SAUNDERS

1600 John F. Kennedy Blvd.
Ste 1800
Philadelphia, PA 19103-2899

TEXTBOOK OF CRITICAL CARE   ISBN: 978-1-4377-1367-1

Notices

Library of Congress Cataloging-in-Publication Data

Textbook of critical care.—6th ed. / [edited by] Jean-Louis Vincent ... [et al.].
      p. ; cm.
   Includes bibliographical references and index.
   ISBN 978-1-4377-1367-1 (hardcover : alk. paper)   1. Critical care medicine.   I. Vincent, J. L.
   [DNLM: 1. Critical Care.   2. Intensive Care Unites.   WX 218]
   RC86.7.1453 2011
   616'.028—dc22

                                                                2011010767

Executive Publisher: Natasha Andjelkovic
Developmental Editor: Julia Bartz
Publishing Services Manager: Anne Altepeter
Project Manager: Cindy Thoms
Design Direction: Ellen Zanolle

Working together to grow
libraries in developing countries

www.elsevier.com | www.bookaid.org | www.sabre.org

ELSEVIER   BOOK AID International   Sabre Foundation

Printed in China

Last digit is the print number: 9 8 7 6 5 4 3 2 1

To Hac and Amélie, hoping for better care of the critically ill throughout the world — JEAN-LOUIS VINCENT

To Norma-May, my true love. To Claire and Erin, who bring me the greatest joy, and to my mother, Dale Abraham, for her support throughout my life — EDWARD ABRAHAM

To my father, Ernest E. Moore, who was a family practitioner for 50 years in Butler, Pennsylvania. He inspired me by his dedication to self education, humility, and service to his community — FREDERICK A. MOORE

To my parents, Stella and Julius Kochanek, for leading by example on the value of hard work; to my wife, Denise, and my children, Ashley, Stanton, and Jillian, for their many sacrifices; and to the late Dr. Peter Safar, for encouraging each of us to bring promising new therapies to the bedside of the critically ill — PATRICK M. KOCHANEK

To my two grown-up children, Emily and Matthew; may their lives be as professionally rewarding and personally satisfying as mine has been. To the memory of my parents, Walter and Betty, who taught me the virtues of honesty and hard work. And to Judy Rochlin, who I loved 40 years ago, and love again even more now — MITCHELL P. FINK

Edward Abraham, MD
Professor and Chair
Spencer Chair in Medical Science Leadership
Department of Medicine
University of Alabama at Birmingham
School of Medicine
Birmingham, Alabama

Peter Abrams, MD
Fellow in Abdominal Transplantation
Thomas E. Starzl Transplantation Institute
Department of Surgery
University of Pittsburgh School of Medicine
Pittsburgh, Pennsylvania

Kareem Abu-Elmagd, MD
Professor of Surgery
Director of Intestinal Rehabilitation and Transplant Center
Thomas E. Starzl Transplantation Institute
Department of Surgery
University of Pittsburgh School of Medicine
Pittsburgh, Pennsylvania

Yasir Abu-Omar, MBChB, DPhil, FRCS(C-Th)
Department of Cardiothoracic Surgery
Papworth Hospital
Cambridge, United Kingdom

Carlos Agustí, MD, PhD
Pneumology Department
Clinic Institute of Thorax (ICT)
Hospital Clinic of Barcelona-Institut d'Investigacions Biomèdiques
August Pi i Sunyer
University of Barcelona-Ciber de Enfermedades
Barcelona, Spain

William C. Aird, MD
Department of Medicine
Beth Israel Deaconess Medical Center and Harvard Medical School
Boston, Massachusetts

Philip Alapat, MD, DABSM, FCCP
Assistant Professor
Department of Pulmonary, Critical Care, and Sleep Medicine
Baylor College of Medicine
Ben Taub General Hospital
Houston, Texas

Ali H. Al-Khafaji, MD, MPH
Associate Professor and Consultant
Director
Transplant Intensive Care Unit
Department of Critical Care Medicine
University of Pittsburgh School of Medicine
Pittsburgh, Pennsylvania

Gustavo G. Angaramo, MD
Assistant Professor in Anesthesiology and Critical Care Medicine
Department of Anesthesiology
Former Instructor in Cardiothoracic Surgery
Department of Surgery
University of Massachusetts Medical School
Worcester, Massachusetts

Derek C. Angus, MD, MPH, FRCP
Chair, Department of Critical Care Medicine
The Mitchell P. Fink Endowed Chair in Critical Care Medicine
Professor of Critical Care Medicine, Medicine, Health Policy and
    Management, and Clinical and Translational Science
University of Pittsburgh School of Medicine and Graduate School
    of Public Health
Pittsburgh, Pennsylvania

Anastasia Antoniadou, MD, PhD
Assistant Professor of Internal Medicine and Infectious Diseases
Athens University Medical School
University General Hospital ATTIKON
Athens, Greece

Anupam Anupam, MBBS
Attending Physician, Department of Medicine
Advocate Illinois Masonic Medical Center
Chicago, Illinois

Andrew C. Argent, MBBCh (Wits), MMed (Paeds)(Wits), DCH (SA), FCPaeds (SA), FRCPCH(UK)
Professor, School of Child and Adolescent Health
University of Cape Town
Medical Director
Paediatric Intensive Care
Red Cross War Memorial Children's Hospital
Cape Town, Western Cape, South Africa

John H. Arnold, MD
Senior Associate
Department of Anesthesia
Medical Director of ECMO, Respiratory Care, and
    Biomedical Engineering
Children's Hospital Boston
Associate Professor of Anaesthesia and Pediatrics
Harvard Medical School
Boston, Massachusetts

Anna Arroyo, MD
Department of Medicine
Division of Hospital Medicine
Washington University School of Medicine
St Louis, Missouri

Stephen Ashwal, MD
Distinguished Professor of Pediatrics and Chief of the Division
    of Child Neurology
Department of Pediatrics
Loma Linda University School of Medicine
Loma Linda, California

Mark E. Astiz, MD
Chief, Division of Critical Care Medicine
Lenox Hill Hospital
New York, New York
Professor of Medicine
New York Medical College
Westchester County, New York

Elie Azoulay, MD, PhD
AP-HP, Hôpital Saint-Louis
Université Paris-7 Paris-Diderot
UFR de Médecine
Réanimation Médicale
Paris, France

Omer A. Bajwa, MD
Senior Fellow, Department of Critical Care Medicine
University of Pittsburgh
Allegheny General Hospital
Pittsburgh, Pennsylvania

Anthony Baldea, MD
Chief Resident
Department of Surgery
Loyola University Medical Center
Maywood, Illinois

Marie R. Baldisseri, MD, FCCM
Associate Professor of Critical Care Medicine
University of Pittsburgh Medical Center
Pittsburgh, Pennsylvania

Zsolt J. Balogh, MD, PhD, FRACS
Professor of Traumatology
Department of Traumatology
University of Newcastle
John Hunter Hospital
Newcastle, New South Wales, Australia

Rasheed Abiodun Balogun, MD
Associate Professor of Medicine
Division of Nephrology
Medical Director, Renal Unit and Extracorporeal Therapies
University of Virginia Health System
Charlottesville, Virginia

Arna Banerjee, MD
Assistant Professor of Anesthesiology
Assistant Professor of Surgery
Vanderbilt University School of Medicine
Nashville, Tennessee

Philip S. Barie, MD, MBA, FIDSA, FCCM, FACS
Professor of Surgery and Public Health
Weill Cornell Medical College
Chief, Preston A. Wade Acute Care Surgery Service
New York-Presbyterian Hospital/Weill Cornell Medical Center
New York, New York

Brendan Barrett, MB, MSc
Professor of Medicine
Division of Nephrology
Memorial University of Newfoundland
St. John's, Newfoundland, Canada

Robert Bartlett, MD
Professor of Surgery, Emeritus
University of Michigan
Ann Arbor, Michigan

John G. Bartlett, MD
Professor of Medicine
Division of Infectious Diseases
Johns Hopkins University School of Medicine
Baltimore, Maryland

Gianluigi Li Bassi, MD
Researcher
Respiratory Intensive Care Unit
Institut Clinic del Tòrax
Hospital Clinic of Barcelona
Institut d'investigacions Biomèdiques
August Pi i Sunyer
Centro de Investigación Biomedica en
    Red Enfermedades Respiratorias
Barcelona, Spain

Sarice L. Bassin, MD
Assistant Professor
Department of Neurology
Northwestern Memorial Hospital
Chicago, Illinois

Julie A. Bastarache, MD
Assistant Professor of Medicine
Division of Allergy, Pulmonary, and Critical Care Medicine
Department of Medicine
Vanderbilt University
Nashville, Tennessee

Colin Bauer, MD
Resident
Department of Anesthesiology
University of California–Los Angeles
Los Angeles, California

Daniel G. Bausch, MD, MPH&TM
Associate Professor
Department of Tropical Medicine and Section of
    Adult Infectious Diseases
Tulane University Health Science Center
New Orleans, Louisiana

Hülya Bayır, MD
Associate Professor
Department of Critical Care Medicine
Department of Environmental and Occupational Health
Director, Pediatric Critical Care Medicine Research
Associate Director
Center for Free Radical and Antioxidant Health
Safar Center for Resuscitation Research
Pittsburgh, Pennsylvania

David T. Bearden, PharmD
Clinical Associate Professor
Department of Pharmacy Practice
Oregon State University
Portland, Oregon

Gregory J. Beilman, MD
Professor and Vice Chair of Surgery
Chief of Critical Care/Acute Care Surgery
University of Minnesota
Minneapolis, Minnesota

Rinaldo Bellomo
Department of Intensive Care
Austin Hospital and University of Melbourne
Melbourne, Australia

E. David Bennett, MB, FRCP
Visiting Professor of Intensive Care
Kings College
Honorary Consultant Physician
Intensive Care Unit
St. Thomas' Hospital
London, United Kingdom

Gordon R. Bernard, MD
Professor of Medicine
Associate Vice Chancellor for Research
Vanderbilt University School of Medicine
Nashville, Tennessee

Jay K. Bhama, MD
Division of Cardiothoracic Surgery
University of Pittsburgh School of Medicine
Pittsburgh, Pennsylvania

Joost J.L.M. Bierens, MD
Anesthesiologist
Medical Commission International Life Saving Federation
Advising Governer Maatschappij tot Redding van Drenkelingen
The Netherlands

Walter L. Biffl, MD
Director of Surgery/Trauma Outreach
Assistant Director of Patient Safety and Quality
Denver Health Medical Center
Professor of Surgery
Associate Residency Program Director
University of Colorado
Denver, Colorado

Thomas P. Bleck, MD, FCCM
Professor of Neurological Sciences, Neurosurgery, Medicine,
  and Anesthesiology
Assistant Dean
Rush Medical College
Associate Chief Medical Officer for Critical Care
Rush University Medical Center
Chicago, Illinois

Thomas A. Bledsoe, MD
Clinical Assistant Professor
Brown University School of Medicine
Providence, Rhode Island

Karen C. Bloch, MD, MPH
Assistant Professor
Departments of Medicine (Infectious Diseases) and
  Preventive Medicine
Vanderbilt University Medical Center
Nashville, Tennessee

Frank Bloos, MD, PhD
Department of Anesthesiology and Intensive Care Medicine
Jena University Hospital
Jena, Germany

Desmond Bohn, MB, FRCPC
Chief
Department of Critical Care Medicine
The Hospital for Sick Children
Professor
Anesthesia and Pediatrics
University of Toronto
Toronto, Ontario, Canada

Nicole C. Bouchard, MD, FPCPC
Assistant Clinical Professor
Assistant Site Director
Director of Medical Toxicology
Emergency Medicine
New York-Presbyterian/Columbia University Medical Center
New York, New York

Arthur J. Boujoukos, MD
Professor, Department of Critical Care Medicine
University of Pittsburgh School of Medicine
Medical Director, Cardiothoracic Intensive Care Unit
University of Pittsburgh Medical Center
Pittsburgh, Pennsylvania

William J. Brady, MD
Professor
Department of Emergency Medicine and Medicine
University of Virginia
Operational Medical Director
Charlottesville-Albemarle Rescue and Albemarle County Fire-Rescue
Chair, Resuscitation Committee
University of Virginia
Charlottesville, Virginia

Serge Brimioulle, MD, PhD
Professor
Department of Intensive Care
Erasme Hospital
Free University of Brussels
Brussels, Belgium

Daniel E. Brooks, MD
Co-Medical Director
Banner Good Samaritan Poison and Drug Information Center
Department of Medical Toxicology
Banner Good Samaritan Medical Center
Phoenix, Arizona

Richard C. Brundage, PharmD, PhD
Distinguished University Teaching Professor
Experimental and Clinical Pharmacology
University of Minnesota
Minneapolis, Minnesota

Jeffrey P. Burns, MD, MPH
Chief
Division of Critical Care Medicine
Children's Hospital Boston
Associate Professor of Anaesthesia
Harvard Medical School
Boston, Massachusetts

Belén Cabello, MD
Unidad de Cuidados Intensivos
Hospital de Antequera
Antequera, Spain

Karen H. Calhoun, MD, FACS, FAAOA
Professor
Department of Otolaryngology, Head and Neck Surgery
The Ohio State University Medical Center
Columbus, Ohio

Clifton W. Callaway, MD, PhD
Associate Professor
Department of Emergency Medicine
Safar Center for Resuscitation Research
University of Pittsburgh
Pittsburgh, Pennsylvania

Peter M.A. Calverley, MBChB
Professor of Respiratory Medicine
School of Clinical Sciences
University of Liverpool
Liverpool, United Kingdom

John Camm, MD
Professor of Clinical Cardiology
St. George's University of London
Honorary Consultant Cardiologist
St. George's Healthcare Trust
London, United Kingdom

Diane M. Cappelletty, PharmD
Associate Professor
Pharmacy Practice
The University of Toledo
Toledo, Ohio

Joseph A. Carcillo, MD
Associate Professor of Critical Care Medicine and Pediatrics
Children's Hospital of Pittsburgh of UPMC
University of Pittsburgh School of Medicine
Pittsburgh, Pennsylvania

Anthony J. Carlese, DO, FCCP
Division of Critical Care Medicine
Montefiore Medical Center and the Albert Einstein College
  of Medicine
Bronx, New York

Juan Carlos-Puyana, MD
Department of Surgery
University of Pittsburgh
Pittsburgh, Pennsylvania

Franco A. Carnevale, RN, PhD
Associate Professor
School of Nursing
McGill University
Associate Member
Pediatric Critical Care
Montreal Children's Hospital
Montreal, Quebec, Canada

Edward D. Chan, MD
Associate Professor of Medicine
National Jewish Health
Staff Physician
Denver Veterans Affairs Medical Center
Denver, Colorado
Staff Physician
University of Colorado Denver
Anschutz Medical Center
Aurora, Colorado

Sanjay Chawla, MD, FCCP
Assistant Professor of Medicine
Weill Cornell Medical College
Assistant Attending Physician
Critical Care Medicine Service
Department of Anesthesiology and Critical Care Medicine
Memorial Sloan-Kettering Cancer Center
New York, New York

Lakshmipathi Chelluri, MD
Associate Professor
Departments of Critical Care Medicine and Medicine
University of Pittsburgh Medical Center
Pittsburgh, Pennsylvania

David C. Chen, MD
Assistant Clinical Professor
Department of Surgery
University of California–Los Angeles
Los Angeles, California

Annie S. Chevrier, RN, MScA
Clinical Nurse Specialist
Internal Medicine, Medical Mission
McGill University Health Centre
Montreal, Quebec, Canada

Su Min Cho, MD, MRCP(UK)
Division of Gastroenterology, Hepatology, and Nutrition
University of Pittsburgh School of Medicine
Pittsburgh, Pennsylvania

Robert S.B. Clark, MD
Professor and Chief, Division of Pediatric Critical Care Medicine
Children's Hospital of Pittsburgh of UPMC
Associate Director
Safar Center for Resuscitation Research
University of Pittsburgh
Pittsburgh, Pennsylvania

Michael A. Coady, MD
Attending Cardiac Surgeon
Heart and Vascular Institute
Stamford Hospital
Stamford, Connecticut

Stephen M. Cohn, MD, FACS
Witten B. Russ Professor of Surgery
University of Texas Health Science Center
San Antonio, Texas

Alan D. Cook, MD
Trauma Surgeon
Trauma Services
East Texas Medical Center
Tyler, Texas

Deborah J. Cook, MD, FRCPC, MSc(Epi)
Professor
Department of Medicine, Clinical Epidemiology, and Biostatistics
Academic Chair, Critical Care Medicine
McMaster University
Hamilton, Ontario, Canada

Robert N. Cooney, MD, FACS, FCCM
Professor of Surgery
Department of Surgery
SUNY Upstate Medical University
Syracuse, New York

Susan J. Corbridge, PhD, ACNP, AE-C, FAANP
Clinical Assistant Professor of Nursing
Clinical Assistant Professor of Medicine
Coordinator, Acute Care Nurse Practitioner Program
University of Illinois at Chicago
Chicago, Illinois

Thomas C. Corbridge, MD, FCCP
Professor of Medicine
Professor of Physical Medicine and Rehabilitation
Department of Medicine
Northwestern University Feinberg School of Medicine
Chicago, Illinois

Howard L. Corwin, MD
Professor of Medicine and Anesthesiology
Dartmouth Medical School
Hanover, New Hampshire

Mark A. Crowther, MD, MSc, FRCPC
Professor
Department of Medicine
McMaster University
St. Joseph's Hospital
Hamilton, Ontario, Canada

Burke A. Cunha, MD, MACP
Chief, Infectious Disease Division
Winthrop-University Hospital
Mineola, New York
Professor of Medicine
State University of New York School of Medicine
Stony Brook, New York

Cheston B. Cunha, MD
Department of Medicine
Brown University Alpert School of Medicine
Rhode Island Hospital and The Miriam Hospital
Providence, Rhode Island

J. Randall Curtis, MD, MPH
Professor of Medicine
Section Head, Pulmonary and Critical Care Medicine
Harborview Medical Center
University of Washington
Seattle, Washington

Vincenzo D'Intini, MD
Renal Medicine
Royal Brisbane and Women's Hospital
Brisbane, Queensland, Australia

Pirouz Daeihagh, MD
Associate Professor of Internal Medicine-Nephrology
Wake Forest University Baptist
Winston Salem, North Carolina

Joseph M. Darby, MD
Professor of Critical Care Medicine and Surgery
University of Pittsburgh School of Medicine
Medical Director, Trauma ICU
UPMC-Presbyterian Hospital
Pittsburgh, Pennsylvania

James M. Dargin, MD
Fellow
Critical Care Medicine
University of Pittsburgh Medical Center
Pittsburgh, Pennsylvania

Michaël Darmon, MD, PhD
Attending Physician
Medical-Surgical ICU
Saint-Etienne University Hospital
Jean Monnet University
Saint-Priest-en-Jarrez
France

Joseph F. Dasta, MSc, FCCM, FCCP
Professor Emeritus
The Ohio State University
College of Pharmacy
Columbus, Ohio

John D. Davies, MA, RRT, FAARC
Clinical Research Coordinator
Duke University Medical Center
Durham, North Carolina

Robert W. Derlet, MD
Professor
Emergency Medicine
University of California–Davis
Davis, California

Mark Dershwitz, MD, PhD
Professor and Vice Chair of Anesthesiology
Professor of Biochemistry and Molecular Pharmacology
University of Massachusetts
Worcester, Massachusetts

Anne Marie G.A. de Smet, MD, PhD
Department of Intensive Care
Onze Lieve Vrouwe Gasthuis
Amsterdam, The Netherlands

Monica Dhand, MD
Tulane University School of Medicine
New Orleans, Louisiana

Anahat Dhillon, MD
Assistant Clinical Professor
Department of Anesthesiology and Critical Care Medicine
University of California–Los Angeles
Los Angeles, California

Rajeev Dhupar, MD
Resident, General Surgery
University of Pittsburgh Medical Center
Pittsburgh, Pennsylvania

Michael N. Diringer, MD, FCCM, FAHA
Professor of Neurology, Neurosurgery, and Anesthesiology
Director, Neurology/Neurosurgery Intensive Care Unit
Washington University School of Medicine
St. Louis, Missouri

Peter Doelken, MD
Assistant Professor
Division of Pulmonology, Allergy, and Clinical Immunology
Medical University of South Carolina
Charleston, South Carolina

Michael Donahoe, MD
Associate Professor of Medicine
Division of Pulmonary, Allergy, and Critical Care Medicine
University of Pittsburgh School of Medicine
Pittsburgh, Pennsylvania

Timothy R. Donahue, MD
Assistant Professor
Departments of Surgery and Molecular and Medical Pharmacology
David Geffen School of Medicine
University of California–Los Angeles
Los Angeles, California

David J. Dries, MSE, MD
Assistant Medical Director of Surgical Care
HealthPartners Medical Group
Professor of Surgery and Anesthesiology
John F. Perry, Jr. Chair of Trauma Surgery
University of Minnesota
Minneapolis, Minnesota

Thomas D. DuBose Jr., MD
Tinsley R. Harrison Professor and Chair
Department of Internal Medicine
Wake Forest University School of Medicine
Winston-Salem, North Carolina

Susan Duthie, MD
Associate Medical Director
Pediatric Critical Care
UCSD-Rady Children's Hospital
San Diego, California

Randy Edwards, MD
Department of Surgery
Medical Director - Advanced Practitioners
Director - Outpatient Surgical Services
Surgical Critical Care
Hartford Hospital
Hartford, Connecticut

Philippe Eggimann, MD
Adult Critical Care
Centre Hospitalier Universitaire Vaudois
Lausanne, Switzerland

Waleed A. Elhassan, MD
Renal Fellow
University of Colorado Denver
Aurora, Colorado

E. Wesley Ely, MD, MPH
Professor of Medicine
Department of Allergy, Pulmonary, and Critical Care Medicine
Vanderbilt University Medical Center
Associate Director of Research GRECC
Tennessee Valley HealthCare System
Nashville, Tennessee

Guillaume Emeriaud, MD, PhD
Pediatric Intensivist
Assistant Clinical Professor
Department of Pediatrics
CHU Sainte-Justine
Université de Montréal
Montreal, Quebec, Canada

Gregory A. Eschenauer, PharmD, BCPS
Clinical Pharmacist, Infectious Diseases
Antibiotic Management Program
University of Pittsburgh Medical Center
Pittsburgh, Pennsylvania

Joel H. Ettinger
President and CEO
Category One Inc.
Pittsburgh, Pennsylvania

Joshua H. Ettinger, MBA
Executive Vice President
Category One, Inc.
Pittsburgh, Pennsylvania
President and CEO
The Magellan Institute, LLC
Louisville, Kentucky

David Clay Evans, MD
Clinical Instructor-Housestaff
Department of Surgery
The Ohio State University
Columbus, Ohio

Gregory T. Everson, MD
Professor of Medicine
School of Medicine
University of Colorado Denver
Director of Hepatology
Division of Gastroenterology and Hepatology
University of Colorado Denver
Aurora, Colorado

Derek V. Exner, MD, MPH, FRCPC, FACC, FHRS
Professor
Libin Cardiovascular Institute of Alberta
University of Calgary
Calgary, Alberta, Canada

Ronald J. Falk, MD
Doc J. Thurston Professor of Medicine
University of North Carolina
Director, UNC Kidney Center
Chief, Division of Nephrology and Hypertension
Chapel Hill, North Carolina

Jeremy Farrar, MBBS, FRCP, PhD
Clinical Reader University of Oxford
Director University of Oxford Research Unit
The Hospital of Tropical Diseases
Ho Chi Minh City, Vietnam

Alan P. Farwell, MD
Associate Professor of Medicine
Boston University School of Medicine
Director, Endocrine Clinics
Section of Endocrinology, Diabetes, and Nutrition
Boston Medical Center
Boston, Massachusetts

Kathryn Felmet, MD
Assistant Professor of Critical Care Medicine and Pediatrics
University of Pittsburgh School of Medicine
Medical Director
Critical Care Transport Team
Children's Hospital of Pittsburgh
Pittsburgh, Pennsylvania

Niall D. Ferguson, MD, MSc
Director, Critical Care Medicine
University Health Network and Mount Sinai Hospital
Assistant Professor
Interdepartmental Division of Critical Care Medicine
University of Toronto
Toronto, Ontario, Canada

Miguel Ferrer, MD, PhD
Assistant Professor of Medicine
University of Barcelona
Attending Physician
Respiratory Intensive Care Unit
Institut Clínic del Tòrax
Hospital Clínic, Barcelona, Spain
Institut D'investigacions Biomèdiques August Pi i Sunyer
Centro de Investigación Biomedica en Red
    Enfermedades Respiratorias
Barcelona, Spain

Mitchell P. Fink, MD
Professor of Surgery and Anesthesiology
Vice Chair for Critical Care
Department of Surgery
David Geffen School of Medicine
University of California–Los Angeles
Los Angeles, California

Ericka L. Fink, MD
Assistant Professor
Division of Pediatric Critical Care Medicine
Children's Hospital of Pittsburgh of UPMC
Pittsburgh, Pennsylvania

Douglas N. Fish, PharmD
Professor and Chair
Department of Clinical Pharmacy
University of Colorado Anschutz Medical Campus
Clinical Specialist in Critical Care/Infectious Diseases
Department of Pharmacy
University of Colorado Hospital
Aurora, Colorado

Diana F. Florescu, MD
Assistant Professor of Medicine
Department of Internal Medicine
University of Nebraska Medical Center
Omaha, Nebraska

Brett E. Fortune, MD
Gastroenterology/Hepatology Fellow
Division of Gastroenterology and Hepatology
University of Colorado Denver
Aurora, Colorado

Bradley D. Freeman, MD
Professor of Surgery
Washington University School of Medicine
St. Louis, Missouri

Blake Froberg, MD
Assistant Professor of Pediatrics and Emergency Medicine
Indiana University School of Medicine
Indianapolis, Indiana

John J. Fung, MD, PhD
Director, Cleveland Clinic Transplant Center
Chairman, Department of General Surgery
The Cleveland Clinic
Cleveland, Ohio

Brent Furbee, MD
Department of Emergency Medicine
Division of Medical Toxicology
Indiana University School of Medicine
Indianapolis, Indiana

Richard L. Gamelli, MD, FACS
Dean
Stritch School of Medicine
Loyola University Chicago
The Robert J. Freeark Professor of Surgery
Department of Surgery
Loyola University Medical Center
Chief, Burn Center
Department of Surgery
Loyola University Medical Center
Maywood, Illinois

Raúl J. Gazmuri, MD, PhD
Professor of Medicine
Associate Professor of Physiology and Biophysics
Director
Resuscitation Institute
Rosalind Franklin University of Medicine and Science
Section Chief
Department of Critical Care Medicine
Captain James Lovell Federal Health Care Center
North Chicago, Illinois

Robert H. Geelkerken, MD, PhD
Consultant Vascular Surgery
Medisch Spectrum Twente
Enschede, The Netherlands

Todd W.B. Gehr, MD
Professor of Medicine
Vice Chairman of Internal Medicine
Chairman, Division of Nephrology
Virginia Commonwealth University
Richmond, Virginia

Michael A. Gentile, RRT, FAARC, FCCM
Associate in Research
Division of Pulmonary and Critical Care Medicine
Duke University Medical Center
Durham, North Carolina

M. Patricia George, MD
Assistant Professor of Medicine
Department of Medicine (Pulmonary, Allergy, and
    Critical Care Medicine)
University of Pittsburgh
Pittsburgh, Pennsylvania

Herwig Gerlach, MD, PhD
Professor and Chairman
Department of Anesthesiology and Critical Care Medicine
Vivantes—Klinikum Neukoelln
Berlin, Germany

R. Mark Ghobrial, MD, PhD, FACS, FRCS (Ed)
Director, Center for Liver Disease and Transplantation
Director, Immunobiology Research Center
The Methodist Hospital
Houston, Texas
Professor of Surgery
Weill-Cornell Medical College
New York, New York

Helen Giamarellou, MD, PhD
Professor of Internal Medicine and Infectious Disease
Athens University Medical School
Head, 6th Department of Internal Medicine
Hygeia Hospital
Athens, Greece

Fredric Ginsberg, MD, FACC, FCCP
Assistant Professor of Medicine
Robert Wood Johnson Medical School at Camden
University of Medicine and Dentistry of New Jersey
Director, Nuclear Cardiology
Director, Heart Failure Program
Cooper University Hospital
Camden, New Jersey

Thomas G. Gleason, MD, MS
Associate Professor of Cardiothoracic Surgery
University of Pittsburgh School of Medicine
Pittsburgh, Pennsylvania

Jacques P. Goldstein, MD, PhD, FECTS
Principal Consultant
Cardio Gold Consulting
Bruxelles, Belgium

Hernando Gomez, MD
Instructor in Critical Care Medicine
University of Pittsburgh
Pittsburgh, Pennsylvania

Sherilyn Gordon Burroughs, MD, FACS
Department of Surgery
Weill Medical College of Cornell University, The Methodist Hospital
Methodist Transplant Center
Houston, Texas

Jeremy David Gradon, MD
Associate Professor of Medicine
The Johns Hopkins University School of Medicine
Attending Physician
Department of Medicine
Division of Infectious Diseases
Sinai Hospital of Baltimore
Baltimore, Maryland

Cornelia R. Graves, MD
Director of Perinatal Services
Obstetrics and Gynecology
Baptist Hospital
Medical Director
Tennessee Maternal Fetal Medicine
Clinical Professor
Obstetrics and Gynecology
Vanderbilt University
Nashville, Tennessee

Cesare Gregoretti, MD
Patient-Ventilator Interaction
DEA
CTO-M. Adelaide
Respiratory Mechanics
DEA
CTO-M. Adelaide
Torino, Italy

Jeffrey S. Groeger, MD
Chief, Urgent Care Service
Memorial Sloan Kettering Cancer Center
Professor of Medicine
Weill Medical College of Cornell University
New York, New York

R. Michael Grounds, MD
Reader in Intensive Care Medicine
St. George's Hospital
London, United Kingdom

Paul O. Gubbins, PharmD
Professor and Chair
Department of Pharmacy Practice
University of Arkansas for Medical Sciences College of Pharmacy
Little Rock, Arkansas

Kyle J. Gunnerson, MD
Associate Professor
Anesthesiology and Emergency Medicine
Associate Director, Center for Adult Critical Care
Director of Critical Care Anesthesiology
VCU Medical Center
Richmond, Virginia

Fahim A. Habib, MD FACS
Attending Trauma Surgeon
Ryder Trauma Center
Jackson Memorial Hospital
Director, Department of Critical Care
University of Miami Hospital
Assistant Professor of Surgery
DeWitt Daughtry Department of Surgery
University of Miami, Miller School of Medicine
Miami, Florida

Mitchell L. Halperin, MD, FRCPC, FRS
Department of Medicine
Division of Nephrology
St. Michaels Hospital
University of Toronto
Toronto, Ontario, Canada

Mary E. Hartman, MD, MPH
Pediatric Critical Care Medicine
Washington University
St. Louis, Missouri

Maurene A. Harvey, RN, MPH
Educator and consultant
Consultants in Critical Care Inc.
Glenbrook, Nevada

Moustafa A. Hassan, MD, FACS
Associate Professor of Surgery
SUNY Upstate Medical University
Syracuse, New York

Yoshiro Hayashi, MD, PhD
Department of Intensive Care Medicine
Royal Brisbane and Women's Hospital
University of Queensland Centre for Clinical Research
Brisbane, Australia

Jan A. Hazelzet, MD, PhD, FCCM
Assistant Professor
Pediatric Intensive Care
Erasmus MC
Rotterdam, The Netherlands

Stephen O. Heard, MD
Chairman
Department of Anesthesiology
Professor of Anesthesiology and Surgery
University of Massachusetts Medical School
Worcester, Massachusetts

Paul C. Hébert, MD
University of Ottawa Centre for Transfusion Research
Clinical Epidemiology Program of the Ottawa Health Research
    Institute
Department of Medicine
Ottawa Hospital
Ottawa, Ontario, Canada

Elizabeth D. Hermsen, PharmD, MBA, BCPS-ID
Antimicrobial Stewardship Program Coordinator
Pharmacy Relations and Clinical Decision Support
The Nebraska Medical Center
Adjunct Assistant Professor
Pharmacy Practice
University of Nebraska Medical Center, College of Pharmacy
Adjunct Assistant Professor
Department of Internal Medicine, Section of Infectious Diseases
University of Nebraska Medical Center, College of Medicine
Omaha, Nebraska

Daren K. Heyland, MD
Professor of Medicine
Queen's University
Director of Clinical Evaluation Research Unit
Kingston General Hospital
Kingston, Ontario, Canada

Jonathan R. Hiatt, MD
Professor and Chief
Division of General Surgery
Vice Chair for Education
Department of Surgery
David Geffen School of Medicine at UCLA
Los Angeles, California

Robert W. Hickey, MD
Emergency Department
Children's Hospital of Pittsburgh of UPMC
Pittsburgh, Pennsylvania

Tran Tinh Hien, MD
Professor
Hospital for Tropical Diseases
London, United Kingdom

Thomas L. Higgins, MD, MBA, FACP, FCCM
Interim Chairman
Department of Medicine
Baystate Medical Center
Springfield, Massachusetts
Professor of Medicine, Surgery, and Anesthesiology
Tufts University School of Medicine
Boston, Massachusetts

Nicholas S. Hill, MD
Chief
Division of Pulmonary, Critical Care, and Sleep Medicine
Tufts Medical Center
Professor of Medicine
Tufts University School of Medicine
Boston, Massachusetts

Horacio Hojman, MD, FACS
Associate Trauma Director
Department of Surgery
Tufts Medical Center
Assistant Professor
Department of Surgery
Tufts Medical School
Boston, Massachusetts

Steven M. Hollenberg, MD
Professor of Medicine
Robert Wood Johnson Medical School/UMDNJ
Director, Coronary Care Unit
Cooper University Hospital
Camden, New Jersey

J. Terrill Huggins, MD
Assistant Professor of Medicine
Department of Medicine
Division of Pulmonary, Critical Care, Allergy, and Sleep Medicine
Medical University of South Carolina
Charleston, South Carolina

David T. Huang, MD, MPH
Assistant Professor
Departments of Critical Care Medicine and Emergency Medicine
University of Pittsburgh
Attending Physician
University of Pittsburgh Medical Center
Pittsburgh, Pennsylvania

Christopher G. Hughes, MD
Assistant Professor of Anesthesiology
Vanderbilt University School of Medicine
Nashville, Tennessee

Russell D. Hull, MBBS, MSc, FRCPC, FACP, FCCP
Professor of Medicine, Hematology, and Internal Medicine
Director, Thrombosis Research Unit
University of Calgary
Calgary, Alberta, Canada

Margaret Isaac, MD
Acting Instructor
General Internal Medicine and Palliative Care
University of Washington/Harborview Medical Center
Seattle, Washington

James P. Isbister, MB, BS, BSc, FRACP, FRCPA
Clinical Professor of Medicine
Northern Clinical School
Royal North Shore Hospital
Sydney Medical School
St. Leonards, New South Wales, Australia

Connie Jastremski, RN, MS, MBA, FCCM
Network CNO/VP, Patient Care Services
Bassett Healthcare Network
Cooperstown, New York

Larry Jenkins, PhD
Associate Professor, Department of Neurosurgery
University of Pittsburgh School of Medicine
Pittsburgh, Pennsylvania

Paul Jodka, MD, FCCP
Baystate Health System
Springfield, Massachusetts
Intensivist, Adult Intensive Care Unit
Associate Professor of Medicine, Anesthesiology, and Surgery
Tufts University School of Medicine
Boston, Massachusetts

Robert G. Johnson, MD
C. Rollins Hanlon Professor and Chair
Department of Surgery
Saint Louis University
St. Louis, Missouri

Philippe G. Jorens, MD, PhD
Professor in Critical Care Medicine and Clinical
    Pharmacology/Toxicology
Department of Critical Care Medicine
Antwerp University Hospital (UZA)
University of Antwerp
Edegem, Belgium

Vern C. Juel, MD
Associate Professor of Medicine
Division of Neurology
Duke University School of Medicine
Durham, North Carolina

Rose Jung, PharmD, MPH, BCPS
Clinical Associate Professor
Department of Pharmacy Practice
The University of Toledo
Toledo, Ohio

Christina R. Kahl, MD, PhD
Fellow in Nephrology and Hypertension
UNC Kidney Center
University of North Carolina
Chapel Hill, North Carolina

Andre C. Kalil, MD
Associate Professor of Medicine
Department of Internal Medicine
University of Nebraska Medical Center
Omaha, Nebraska

Edo Kaluski, MD, FACC, FESC, FSCAI
Associate Professor of Medicine
University of Medicine and Dentistry of New Jersey
Director of Cardiac Catheterization Laboratories and
    Interventional Cardiology
University Hospital
Newark, New Jersey

Kamel S. Kamel, MBBCh
Division of Nephrology
St. Michael's Hospital
University of Toronto
Toronto, Canada

Sandra Kane-Gill, PharmD, MSc, FCCM, FCCP
Associate Professor
School of Pharmacy and Clinical Translational Science Institute
Center for Pharmacoinformatics and Outcomes Research
University of Pittsburgh
Critical Care Medication Safety Officer
Department of Pharmacy
University of Pittsburgh Medical Center
Pittsburgh, Pennsylvania

Jeffrey P. Kanne, MD
Associate Professor
Department of Radiology
University of Wisconsin School of Medicine and Public Health
Madison, Wisconsin

Lionel Karlin, MD
Department of Clinical Immunology
Hôpital Saint-Louis
Assistance Publique-Hôpitaux de Paris
Paris, France

Marinka Kartalija, MD
Infectious Diseases Research Fellow
University of Colorado Anschutz Medical Campus
Denver Veterans Affair Medical Center
Denver, Colorado

James Kasiewicz, MD
Surgeon
Lawnwood Regional Treasure Coast Trauma Center
Fort Pierce, Florida
University of Pittsburgh Medical Center
Pittsburgh, Pennsylvania

Kenneth D. Katz, MD, FAAEM, FACMT, ABMT
Chief, Division Medical Toxicology
Assistant Professor
UPMC Presbyterian Hospital
Medical Director
Pittsburgh Poison Center
Pittsburgh, Pennsylvania

David Kaufman, MD
Associate Professor
Department of Surgery, Anesthesiology, Medicine, Medical
    Humanities, Urology
University of Rochester
Rochester, New York

John A. Kellum, MD
Professor and Vice Chair
Critical Care Medicine
University of Pittsburgh
Pittsburgh, Pennsylvania

Rick Kingston, PharmD
President, Regulatory and Scientific Affairs
Senior Clinical Toxicologist
SafetyCall International Poison Center
Clinical Professor of Pharmacy
College of Pharmacy
University of Minnesota
Minneapolis, Minnesota

Orlando C. Kirton, MD, FACS, FCCM, FCCP
Professor of Surgery
Program Director
Integrated General Surgery Residency Program
Vice Chair
Department of Surgery
University of Connecticut School of Medicine
Farmington, Connecticut

Kurt Kleinschmidt, MD
Professor of Surgery
Division of Emergency Medicine
University of Texas Southwestern Medical Center
Section Chief and Program Director
Medical Toxicology
Dallas, Texas

Jason Knight, MD
Emergency Department Medical Director
Maricopa Medical Center
Phoenix, Arizona

Patrick M. Kochanek, MD, FCCM
Professor and Vice Chairman
Department of Critical Care Medicine
Professor of Anesthesiology, Pediatrics, and Clinical and
  Translational Science
Director
Safar Center for Resuscitation Research
University of Pittsburgh School of Medicine
Pittsburgh, Pennsylvania

W. Andrew Kofke, MD, MBA, FCCM
Professor, Director of Neuroanesthesia
Co-Director Neurocritical Care
Department of Anesthesiology and Critical Care
Department of Neurosurgery
University of Pennsylvania
Philadelphia, Pennsylvania

Jeroen J. Kolkman, MD, PhD
Gastroenterologist
Department of Gastroenterology
Medisch Spectrum Twente
Enschede, The Netherlands

Robert L. Kormos, MD, FRCS(C), FAHA
Director, Artificial Heart Program
Co-Director, Heart Transplantation
Medical Director, Vital Engineering
University of Pittsburgh Medical Center
Professor, Department of Surgery
University of Pittsburgh School of Medicine
Pittsburgh, Pennsylvania

Rosemary A. Kozar, MD, PhD
Professor of Surgery
Division of Acute Care Surgery
University of Texas—Houston
Houston, Texas

David J. Kramer, MD, FACP
Professor of Medicine
Mayo Clinic College of Medicine
Director, Transplant Critical Care Service
Mayo Clinic
Jacksonville, Florida

John W. Kreit, MD
Professor of Medicine
Division of Pulmonary, Allergy, and Critical Care Medicine
University of Pittsburgh School of Medicine
Pittsburgh, Pennsylvania

James A. Kruse, MD
Clinical Professor of Medicine
Columbia University College of Physicians and Surgeons
Chief, Critical Care Services
Bassett Medical Center
Cooperstown, New York

Anand Kumar, MD
Associate Professor of Medicine, Medical Microbiology, and
  Pharmacology/Therapeutics
University of Manitoba
Associate Professor of Medicine
University of Medicine and Dentistry of New Jersey
Newark, New Jersey

Vladimir Kvetan, MD, FCCM
Director, Jay B. Langner Critical Care System
Montefiore Medical Center
Director
Division of Critical Care Medicine
Department of Medicine
Professor of Anesthesiology and Clinical Medicine
Albert Einstein College of Medicine of Yeshiva University
Bronx, New York

Jacques Lacroix, MD, FRCPC, FAAP
Professor
Department of Pediatrics
Université de Montréal
Montréal, Québec, Canada

Gilles Lebuffe, MD, PhD
Professor
Department of Anesthesiology and Critical Care
University Hospital—Nord de France
Lille, France

Virginie Lemiale, MD
AP-HP, Hôpital Saint-Louis
Réanimation Médicale
1 Avenue Claude Vellefaux
Paris, France

Angela M. Leung, MD, MSc
Instructor of Medicine
Section of Endocrinology, Diabetes, and Nutrition
Boston University School of Medicine
Boston, Massachusetts

Sharon Leung, MD
Division of Critical Care Medicine
Montefiore Medical Center and the Albert Einstein College
  of Medicine
Bronx, New York

Allan D. Levi, MD, PhD, FACS
Professor of Neurosurgery
University of Miami, Miller School of Medicine
Chief of Neurosurgery
University of Miami Hospital
Miami, Florida

Phillip D. Levin, MA, MB, BChir
Attending Physician
Department of Anesthesiology and Critical Care Medicine
Hadassah Hebrew University Medical Center
Jerusalem, Israel

Mitchell M. Levy, MD
Professor of Medicine
Chief
Division of Pulmonary and Critical Care Medicine
Department of Medicine
Brown University
Director MICU
Rhode Island Hospital
Providence, Rhode Island

Mah Chou Liang, MD
Interdepartmental Division of Critical Care
University of Toronto
Toronto, Ontario, Canada
Department of Anaesthesia and Surgical Intensive Care Unit
Changi General Hospital
Singapore

Scott Liebman, MD, MPH
Assistant Professor of Medicine
Division of Nephrology
University of Rochester
Rochester, New York

Stuart L. Linas, MD
Professor of Medicine and Rocky Mountain Professor
  of Renal Research
University of Colorado Denver School of Medicine
Chief of Nephrology
Denver Health Medical Center
Denver, Colorado

Gregory Y.H. Lip, MD, FRCP, FESC, FACC
Professor of Cardiovascular Medicine
University of Birmingham
Visiting Professor of Haemostasis Thrombosis and Vascular Sciences
University of Aston
Centre for Cardiovascular Sciences
City Hospital
Birmingham, United Kingdom

Pamela A. Lipsett, MD
Professor of Surgery, Anesthesiology and Critical Care Medicine,
  and Nursing
Johns Hopkins University Schools of Medicine and Nursing
Co-Director, General Surgery Intensive Care Units
Program Director, General Surgery and Surgical Critical Care
Johns Hopkins
Baltimore, Maryland

Alan Lisbon, MD
Associate Professor of Anaesthesia
Harvard Medical School
Executive Vice Chair Anesthesia
Beth Israel Deaconess Medical Center
Boston, Massachusetts

Carmen Lucena, MD
Beca Josep Font. Hospital Clínic
Barcelona, Spain

Andrew I.R. Maas, MD, PhD
Professor and Chairman
University Hospital Antwerp
Antwerp, Belgium

Neil R. MacIntyre, MD
Professor of Medicine
Clinical Chief
Division of Pulmonary and Critical Care Medicine
Duke University
Durham, North Carolina

Duncan Macrae, MB ChB, FRCA, FRCPCH
Consultant Pediatric Intensivist
Royal Brompton and Harefield NHS Trust
London, United Kingdom

Bernhard Maisch, MD, FESC, FACC
Professor and Director
Department of Cardiology
Marburg Heart Center
Marburg, Germany

Amer M. Malik, MD, MBA
Vascular Neurology Fellow
UPMC Stroke Institute
University of Pittsburgh School of Medicine
Pittsburgh, Pennsylvania

Jordi Mancebo, MD
Director
Servei Medicina Intensiva
Hospital Sant Pau
Associate Professor of Medicine
Barcelona, Spain

Henry J. Mann, PharmD, FCCP, FCCM, FASHP
Dean and Professor
Leslie Dan Faculty of Pharmacy
University of Toronto
Toronto, Ontario, Canada

Sanjay Manocha, MD, FRCPC
Director
Division of Critical Care Medicine
Department of Medicine
Humber River Regional Hospital
Toronto, Ontario, Canada

Stéphane Manzo-Silberman, MD
Chief Resident
Interventional Cardiologist
Cardiology Department
Cochin Hospital
Paris Descartes University
Paris, France

Paul E. Marik, MD, FCP, FRCPC, FCCM, FCCP
Chief, Pulmonary and Critical Care Medicine
Eastern Virginia Medical School
Norfolk, Virginia

John J. Marini, MD
Director of Translational Research
HealthPartners Research Foundation
Professor of Medicine
University of Minnesota
Minneapolis, Minnesota

Donald W. Marion, MD, MS
Director of Clinical Affairs
The Defense and Veterans Brain Injury Center
Walter Reed Army Medical Center
Washington, DC

Steven J. Martin, PharmD, BCPS, FCCP, FCCM
Professor and Chairman
Department of Pharmacy Practice
The University of Toledo
Toledo, Ohio

Alvaro Martinez-Camacho, MD
Gastroenterology/Hepatology Fellow
University of Colorado Denver
Aurora, Colorado

Anne Marie Mattingly, MD
Fellow
Internal Medicine, Critical Care Division
University of Rochester
Rochester, New York

Gary R. Matzke, PharmD, FCP, FCCP, FASN, FNAP
Professor and Associate Dean for Clinical Research and Public Policy
Director ACCP/ASHP/VCU Congressional Health Care
    Policy Fellow Program
School of Pharmacy, Virginia Commonwealth
    University–MCV Campus
Richmond, Virginia

Adeline Max, MD
Medical ICU
Saint-Louis Hospital
Paris, France

George V. Mazariegos, MD
Chief Pediatric Transplantation
Hillman Center for Pediatric Transplantation
Children's Hospital of Pittsburgh of UPMC
Professor of Surgery and Critical Care Medicine
University of Pittsburgh Medical School
Pittsburgh, Pennsylvania

Joanne Mazzarelli, MD
Fellow, Cardiovascular Diseases
Cooper University Hospital
Camden, New Jersey

Stephen A. McClave, MD
Professor of Medicine
Director of Clinical Nutrition
Division of Gastroenterology, Hepatology, and Nutrition
University of Louisville School of Medicine
Louisville, Kentucky

Ryan M. McEnaney, MD
Division of Vascular Surgery
University of Pittsburgh Medical Center
Pittsburgh, Pennsylvania

John K. McIllwaine, DO
Section of Critical Care Medicine
Department of Anesthesiology
Dartmouth-Hitchcock Medical Center
Lebanon, New Hampshire

Michelle K. McNutt, MD
Assistant Professor of Surgery
Division of Acute Care Surgery
University of Texas Health Science Center at Houston
Houston, Texas

Sangeeta Mehta, MD
Associate Professor
Department of Medicine and Interdepartmental
Division of Critical Care
University of Toronto
Mount Sinai Hospital
Toronto, Ontario, Canada

Dieter Mesotten, MD, PhD
Professor of Medicine
Katholieke Universiteit Leuven
Department of Intensive Care Medicine
University Hospitals Leuven—Gasthuisberg
Leuven, Belgium

Kimberly S. Meyer, ACNP-BC, CNRN
Neurotrauma Nurse Practitioner
University of Louisville Hospital—Neurosurgery
Louisville, Kentucky
Neuroscience Clinician
Defense and Veterans Brain Injury Center
Washington, DC

David J. Michelson, MD
Assistant Professor
Department of Pediatrics, Division of Child Neurology
Loma Linda University School of Medicine
Loma Linda, California

Saar Minha, MD
Department of Cardiology
Assaf Harofeh Medical Center and Sackler School of Medicine
Tel Aviv University
Zerifin, Isreal

Marek A. Mirski, MD, PhD
Professor and Vice-Chair
Department of Anesthesiology and Critical Care Medicine
Professor of Neurology and Neurosurgery
Johns Hopkins University School of Medicine
Baltimore, Maryland

Rima A. Mohammad, PharmD, BCPS
Assistant Professor of Pharmacy and Therapeutics
Director, Internal Medicine Pharmacy Residency
School of Pharmacy, University of Pittsburgh
Pittsburgh, Pennsylvania

Xavier Monnet, MD, PhD
Professor of Critical Care Medicine
Medical Intensive Care Unit
Bicêtre University Hospital
Paris-South University
Paris, France

Frederick A. Moore, MD, FACS, FCCM
Professor of Surgery
Head, Acute Care Surgery
College of Medicine
University of Florida
Gainesville, Florida

Laura J. Moore, MD, FACS
Assistant Professor
Department of Surgery, Division of Acute Care Surgery
University of Texas
Health Science Center at Houston
Medical Director
Shock Trauma Intensive Care Unit
Memorial Hermann Hospital
Houston, Texas

Anne-Sophie Moreau
Service des Maladies du Sang
Hopital Huriez
CHRU Lille
Lille, France

Delphine Moreau, MD
Medical ICU
Saint Louis Teaching Hospital
Paris, France

Alison Morris, MD, MS
Associate Professor of Medicine, Immunology, and Clinical and
    Translational Research
Division of Pulmonary, Allergy, and Critical Care Medicine
University of Pittsburgh
Pittsburgh, Pennsylvania

Amy E. Morris, MD
Clinical Instructor
Pulmonary and Critical Care Medicine
University of Washington
Seattle, Washington

Bruno Mourvillier, MD
Assistant
Medical and Infectious Diseases Intensive Care
Bichat-Claude Bernard Hospital
Paris 7 University
Paris, France

Mark A. Munger, PharmD
Professor and Associate Dean for Academic Affairs
Pharmacotherapy and Internal Medicine
University of Utah
Salt Lake City, Utah

Raghavan Murugan, MD, MS, MRCP(UK)
Assistant Professor
Department of Critical Care Medicine
University of Pittsburgh School of Medicine
Pittsburgh, Pennsylvania

Claus-Martin Muth, MD, PhD
Associate Professor of Anesthesia
Department of Anesthesiology
University Hospital
Ulm University
Ulm, Germany

Kurt G. Naber, MD, PhD
Associate Professor
Technical University Munich
Munich, Germany

Lena M. Napolitano, MD
Professor and Associate Chair
Division Chief, Acute Care Surgery
Department of Surgery
Director, Trauma and Surgical Critical Care
University of Michigan Medical School
Ann Arbor, Michigan

Stanley A. Nasraway, MD, FCCM
Director
Surgical Intensive Care Units
Tufts Medical Center
Professor of Surgery, Medicine, and Anesthesia
Department of Surgery
Tufts University School of Medicine
Boston, Massachusetts

Jovany Cruz Navarro, MD
Baylor College of Medicine
Houston, Texas

Lewis S. Nelson, MD
Associate Professor of Emergency Medicine
Director, Fellowship in Medical Toxicology
New York University School of Medicine
New York, New York

Michael S. Niederman, MD
Chairman, Department of Medicine
Winthrop-University Hospital
Professor of Medicine
Vice-Chairman
Department of Medicine
SUNY at Stony Brook
New York, New York

Jessica C. Njoku, PharmD, BCPS
Infectious Diseases/Antimicrobial Stewardship Fellow
Nebraska Medical Center
Omaha, Nebraska

Scott Norwood, MD
Director, Trauma Services
Department of Surgery
East Texas Medical Center
Tyler, Texas

Juan B. Ochoa, MD
Department of Surgery and Critical Care Medicine
University of Pittsburgh Health System
Pittsburgh, Pennsylvania

Mark D. Okusa, MD
Chief, Division of Nephrology
John C. Buchanan Distinguished Professor of Medicine
University of Virginia
Charlottesville, Virginia

Keith M. Olsen, PharmD, FCCP, FCCM
Professor and Chair
Department of Pharmacy Practice
University of Nebraska Medical Center
Clinical Manager Education and Research
Department of Pharmaceutical and Nutrition Care
The Nebraska Medical Center
Omaha, Nebraska

Steven M. Opal, MD
Professor of Medicine
Warren Alpert Medical School of Brown University
Providence, Rhode Island
Chief, Infectious Disease Division
Memorial Hospital of Rhode Island
Pawtucket, Rhode Island

James P. Orlowski, MD, FAAP, FCCP, FCCM
Division of Pediatrics
Department of Pediatric Critical Care Medicine
University Community Hospital
Department of Pediatrics, Critical Care Medicine, and Medical Ethics
University of South Florida, Tampa
Tampa, Florida

Catherine M. Otto, MD
J. Ward Kennedy-Hamilton Endowed Chair of Medicine
Director, Training Programs in Cardiovascular Disease
University of Washington
Associate Director, Echocardiography
University of Washington Medical Center
Seattle, Washington

Heleen M. Oudemans-van Straaten, MD, PhD
Department of Intensive Care
Onze Lieve Vrouwe Gasthuis
Amsterdam, The Netherlands

Pratik P. Pandharipande, MD, MSCI
Associate Professor
Anesthesiology Service
Tennessee Valley Health Care System
Associate Professor
Anesthesiology and Critical Care
Vanderbilt University Medical Center
Nashville, Tennessee

Joseph E. Parrillo, MD
Professor of Medicine
Robert Wood Johnson Medical School
University of Medicine and Dentistry of New Jersey
Chief, Department of Medicine
Edward D. Viner MD Chair, Department of Medicine
Director, Cooper Heart Institute
Cooper University Hospital
Camden, New Jersey

David L. Paterson, MD
Professor of Medicine
University of Queensland Centre for Clinical Research
Royal Brisbane and Womens Hospital Campus
Brisbane, Australia

Frédéric L. Paulin, MD, FRCPC
Fellow, Cardiac Electrophysiology
Libin Cardiovascular Institute of Alberta
University of Calgary
Calgary, Alberta, Canada

Andrew B. Peitzman, MD
Mark M. Ravitch Professor and Vice-Chair
Chief, Division of General Surgery
University of Pittsburgh
Pittsburgh, Pennsylvania

Daleen Aragon Penoyer, PhD, RN, CCRP, FCCM
Director, Center for Nursing Research
Orlando Health
Orlando, Florida

Bradley Peterson, MD
Medical Director Critical Care
Associate Director Trauma
Department of Surgery, Anesthesia, and Critical Care
UCSD-Rady Children's Hospital
San Diego, California

Graham F. Pineo, MD
Professor of Medicine Emeritus
Department of Medicine
University of Calgary
Calgary, Alberta, Canada

Michael R. Pinsky, MD, Dr hc
Professor
Critical Care Medicine, Bioengineering, Cardiovascular Diseases,
  Anesthesiology, and Clinical & Translational Medicine
University of Pittsburgh
Pittsburgh, Pennsylvania

Greta Piper, MD
Assistant Professor
Department of Surgery
Yale University
New Haven, Connecticut

Didier Pittet, MD, MS
Director
Infection Control Programme and WHO Collaborating Centre
  on Patient Safety
University of Geneva Hospitals and Faculty of Medicine
Geneva, Switzerland

†Fred Plum, MD

Murray M. Pollack, MD, MBA
Chief Medical and Academic Officer
Phoenix Children's Hospital
Professor of Pediatrics
University of Arizona School of Medicine
Phoenix, Arizona

Lucido L. Ponce, MD
Department of Neurosurgery
Baylor College of Medicine
Houston, Texas

Robert Pousman, DO
Clinical Associate Professor
Anesthesiology
David Geffen School of Medicine at UCLA
Director, Surgical Intensive Care Unit
Anesthesiology
VA Greater Los Angeles Healthcare System
Los Angeles, California

Peter J. Pronovost, MD, PhD
Professor
Departments of Anesthesiology/Critical Care Medicine, Surgery,
School of Medicine, and Health Policy and Management
Bloomberg School of Public Health
Director, Quality and Safety Research Group
Johns Hopkins University
Baltimore, Maryland

Przemyslaw B. Radwański, PharmD, PhD
Post-Graduate Research Associate
Department of Physiology and Cell Biology
Davis Heart and Lung Research Institute
The Ohio State University
Columbus, Ohio

Thomas G. Rainey, MD, FCCM
President
CriticalMed, Inc.
Bethesda, Maryland

Thomas Rajan, MD
Fellow, Division of Pulmonary Critical Care and Sleep Medicine
Tufts-New England Medical Center
Tufts University School of Medicine
Boston, Massachusetts

Vito Marco Ranieri, MD
Chairman
Department of Anesthesia and Intensive Care Medicine
University of Turin
S. Giovanni Battista Molinette Hospital
Turin, Italy

Konrad Reinhart, MD
Professor
Director
Department of Anesthesiology and Intensive Care Medicine
University Hospital Jena
Jena, Germany

Jorge Reyes, MD
Chief of Pediatric Transplantation
Seattle Children's Hospital
Chief, Division of Transplant Surgery
University of Washington
Seattle, Washington

Andrew Rhodes, MD
Consultant in Intensive Care Medicine
St. George's Hospital
London, United Kingdom

Zaccaria Ricci, MD
Pediatric Intensive Care Unit
Department of Pediatric Cardiology and Cardiac Surgery
Ospedale Bambino Gesù
Rome, Italy

Christian Richard, MD
Professor of Critical Care Medicine
Medical Intensive Care Unit
Bicêtre University Hospital
Paris-South University
Paris, France

John R. Richards, MD
Professor
Emergency Medicine
UC Davis Medical Center
Sacramento, California

John Riordan, MD
Professor of Emergency Medicine
Department of Emergency Medicine
University of Virginia
Charlottesville, Virginia

---

†Deceased

Arsen D. Ristic, MD, PhD, FESC
Associate Professor of Internal Medicine—Cardiology
Belgrade University School of Medicine
Deputy Director, Polyclinic of the Clinical Center of Serbia
Chief, Interventional Pericardiology and Diseases
    of Pulmonary Circulation
Department of Cardiology
Clinical Center of Serbia
Belgrade, Serbia

Sandro Rizoli, MD, PhD
Associate Professor
Surgery and Critical Care Medicine
Sunnybrook Health Sciences Centre
University of Toronto
Toronto, Ontario, Canada

Claudia S. Robertson, MD
Professor
Department of Neurosurgery
Baylor College of Medicine
Houston, Texas

Emmanuel Robin, MD, PhD
Department of Anesthesiology and Critical Care
University Hospital—Nord de France
Lille, France

Ferran Roche-Campo, MD
Servei de Medicina Intensiva
Hospital Sant Pau
Barcelona, Spain

Paul Rogers, MD
Professor, Critical Care Medicine
Department of Critical Care
University of Pittsburgh
Pittsburgh, Pennsylvania

Claudio Ronco, MD
Professor of Medicine
Director
Department of Nephrology Dialysis and Transplantation
International Renal Research Institute
St. Bortolo Hospital
Vicenza, Italy

John C. Rotschafer, PharmD, FCCP
Professor
Department of Experimental and Clinical Pharmacology
College of Pharmacy
University of Minnesota
Minneapolis, Minnesota

Gordon D. Rubenfeld, MD, MSc
Professor of Medicine
University of Toronto
Chief, Program in Trauma, Emergency, and Critical Care
Sunnybrook Health Sciences Center
Toronto, Ontario, Canada

Lewis J. Rubin, MD, FACP, FRCP, FCCP, FAHA
Professor of Medicine, Emeritus
University of California San Diego
La Jolla, California

Randall A. Ruppel, MD
Department of Pediatrics
St. Vincent's Hospital
Indianapolis, Indiana

Laura T. Russo, RD, CSP, LDN
Senior PICU Dietitian
Children's Memorial Hospital
Chicago, Illinois

Daniel E. Rusyniak, MD
Associate Professor of Emergency Medicine, Pharmacology,
    and Toxicology
Adjuct Associate Clinical Professor of Neurology
Indiana University School of Medicine
Indianapolis, Indiana

Steven A. Sahn, BA, MD
Professor of Medicine and Director
Medicine, Division of Pulmonary, Critical Care, Allergy, and
    Sleep Medicine
Medical University of South Carolina
Charleston, South Carolina

Juan C. Salgado, MD
Pulmonary Transplant Medicine Fellow
Division of Pulmonary, Allergy, and Critical Care Medicine
University of Pittsburgh School of Medicine
Pittsburgh, Pennsylvania

Cristina Santonocito, MD
Anesthesia and Intensive Care Medicine
University Policlinico of Catania
Catania, Italy

Penny Lynn Sappington, MD
Assistant Professor
Department of Critical Care Medicine
University of Pittsburgh School of Medicine
Medical Director
Surgical Intensive Care Unit
University of Pittsburgh Medical Center
Pittsburgh, Pennsylvania

John Sarko, MD
Clinical Attending Physician
Emergency Medicine
Maricopa Medical Center
University of Arizona—Phoenix School of Medicine
Phoenix, Arizona

Richard H. Savel, MD, FCCM
Associate Professor of Clinical Medicine and Neurology
Division of Critical Care Medicine
Montefiore Medical Center and the Albert Einstein College
    of Medicine
Bronx, New York

Irina Savelieva, MD
St. George's Hospital Medical School
London, United Kingdom

Benoit Schlemmer, MD
Service de réanimation médicale, AP-HP
Hôpital Saint-Louis
Université Paris-7 Paris-Diderot
UFR de Médecine
Paris, France

Minka Schofield, MD
Assistant Professor
Department of Otolaryngology, Head and Neck Surgery
The Ohio State University Medical Center
Columbus, Ohio

Kristine S. Schonder, PharmD
Clinical Pharmacist
Thomas E. Starzl Transplantation Institute
Assistant Professor
University of Pittsburgh School of Pharmacy
Pittsburgh, Pennsylvania

Anton C. Schoolwerth, MD, MSHA
Professor of Medicine
Section of Hypertension/Nephrology
Dartmouth-Hitchcock Medical Center
Lebanon, New Hampshire

Robert W. Schrier, MD
Professor of Medicine
Department of Medicine
University of Colorado Denver
Aurora, Colorado

Carl Schulman
Director, Critical Care
University of Miami Hospital
Miami, Florida

Evan Schwarz, MD
Fellow in Medical Toxicology
Division of Emergency Medicine
University of Texas Southwestern Medical Center
Dallas, Texas

Aaron M. Scifres, MD
Assistant Professor of Surgery
University of Pittsburgh School of Medicine
Pittsburgh, Pennsylvania

Donna L. Seger, MD
Associate Professor of Medicine and Emergency Medicine
Department of Medicine
Vanderbilt University Medical Center
Medical Director
Tennessee Poison Center
Nashville, Tennessee

Amelie Seguin, MD
Intensive Care Unit
Hopital Saint Louis
Paris, France

Frank W. Sellke, MD, FACS
Karlson and Karlson Professor and Chief of Cardiothoracic Surgery
Alpert Medical School of Brown University
Providence, Rhode Island

Sajid Shahul, MD
Instructor in Anaesthesia
Harvard Medical School
Anesthetist
Beth Israel Deaconess Medical Center
Boston, Massachusetts

M. Khaled Shamseddin, MD, ABIM, FRCPC
Nephrology Fellow
Department of Medicine and Nephrology
Memorial University—Health Science Center
St. John's, Newfoundland, Canada

Erik S. Shank, MD
Assistant Professor of Anesthesia
Harvard Medical School
Boston, Massachusetts
Associate Chief of Pediatric Anesthesia,
Massachusetts General Hospital
Shriners Hospital for Children-Boston
Boston, Massachusetts

Eduard Shantsila
Postdoctoral Research Fellow
University of Birmingham Centre for Cardiovascular Sciences
City Hospital
Birmingham, United Kingdom

Kapil Sharma, MD
Assistant Professor
Division of Emergency Medicine
University of Texas Southwestern Medical Center
Dallas, Texas

Robert L. Sheridan, MD
Assistant Chief of Staff
Shriners Hospital for Children
Attending Surgeon
Burns and Trauma
Massachusetts General Hospital
Associate Professor of Surgery
Harvard Medical School
Boston, Massachusetts

Ariel L. Shiloh, MD
Division of Critical Care Medicine
Montefiore Medical Center and the Albert Einstein College
of Medicine
Bronx, New York

Debra J. Skaar, PharmD
Assistant Professor
Department of Experimental and Clinical Pharmacology
University of Minnesota College of Pharmacy
Minneapolis, Minnesota

Anthony D. Slonim, MD, DrPH
Professor, Internal Medicine and Pediatrics
Virginia Tech Carilion School of Medicine
Vice President, Medical Affairs and Pharmacy
Carilion Medical Center
Roanoke, Virginia

Teresa L. Smith Jacobs, MD
Clinical Assistant Professor
Western Michigan University College of Human Medicine
Neurointensivist
Bronson Memorial Hospital
Kalamazoo, Michigan

Jean-Louis Vincent, MD, PhD
Professor of Intensive Care Medicine
Université Libre de Bruxelles
Head, Department of Intensive Care
Erasme University Hospital
Brussels, Belgium

Elizabeth A. Vitarbo, MD
Assistant Professor
Department of Neurological Surgery and School of Medicine
University of Florida
Jacksonville, Florida

Louis Voigt, MD
Assistant Professor of Medicine
Weill Medical College of Cornell University
Assistant Attending Physician
Anesthesiology and Critical Care Medicine
Memorial Sloan Kettering Cancer Center
New York, New York

Florian M.E. Wagenlehner, MD, PhD
Professor of Urology
Clinic for Urology, Pediatric Urology, and Andrology
Justus-Liebig-University
Giessen, Germany

Christina J. Wai, MD
Chief Resident
Department of Surgery
Tufts Medical Center
Boston, Massachusetts

Keith R. Walley, MD
Professor of Medicine
Division of Critical Care Medicine
University of British Columbia
Vancouver, British Columbia, Canada

Nicholas S. Ward, MD
Assistant Professor, Department of Medicine
Brown University School of Medicine
Department of Pulmonary and Critical Care Medicine
Rhode Island Hospital
Providence, Rhode Island

Lorraine B. Ware, MD
Associate Professor of Medicine
Division of Allergy, Pulmonary, and Critical Care Medicine
Department of Medicine
Vanderbilt University
Nashville, Tennessee

Robert J. Weber, PharmD, MS, BCPS, FASHP
University of Pittsburgh School of Pharmacy
Thomas E. Starzl Transplantation Institute
University of Pittsburgh School of Medicine
Pittsburgh, Pennsylvania

Lawrence R. Wechsler, MD
Professor and Chief
Department of Neurology
Vice President for Telemedicine, PSD
University of Pittsburgh School of Medicine
Pittsburgh, Pennsylvania

David Weill, MD
Medical Director
Lung and Heart-Lung Transplant Program
Division of Pulmonary and Critical Care Medicine
Stanford University
Stanford, California

Craig R. Weinert, MD, MPH
Associate Professor of Medicine
Division of Pulmonary, Allergy, Critical Care, and Sleep Medicine
University of Minnesota
Minneapolis, Minnesota

Julia Wendon, MBChB, FRCP
Institute of Liver Studies
Kings College Hospital
London, United Kingdom

Michel Wolff, MD
Head
Medical and Infectious Diseases Intensive Care
Bichat-Claude Bernard Hospital
Paris 7 University
Paris, France

Benjamin Wrigley
University of Birmingham Centre for Cardiovascular Sciences
City Hospital
Birmingham, United Kingdom

Richard G. Wunderink, MD
Professor of Medicine
Pulmonary and Critical Care Division
Northwestern University Feinberg School of Medicine
Director, Medical Intensive Care Unit
Northwestern Memorial Hospital
Chicago, Illinois

Lam M. Yen
Director, Tetanus Unit
Hospital for Tropical Diseases
Ho Chi Minh City, Vietnam

Sergio L. Zanotti-Cavazzoni, MD, FCCM
Director, Fellowship Program
Division of Critical Care Medicine
Assistant Professor
Department of Medicine
Cooper University Hospital
Camden, New Jersey

Allyson R. Zazulia, MD
Associate Professor of Neurology and Radiology
Washington University
Saint Louis, Missouri

Janice Zimmerman, MD
Head of Critical Care Section
Department of Medicine
The Methodist Hospital
Professor of Clinical Medicine
Department of Medicine
Weill Cornell Medical College
Houston, Texas

Walter Zingg, MD
Infection Control Program
University of Geneva Hospitals
Geneva, Switzerland

CONTRIBUTORS, ONLINE CHAPTERS

Louis H. Alarcon, MD
Medical Director, Trauma Surgery
University of Pittsburgh Medical Center-PUH
Associate Professor of Surgery and Critical Care Medicine
University of Pittsburgh
Pittsburgh, Pennsylvania
W10 Paracentesis and Diagnostic Peritoneal Lavage (DPL)

Luke Aldo, MD
Hartford Hospital
Department of Anesthesiology and Critical Care Medicine
University of Connecticut School of Medicine
Farmington, Connecticut
W1 Difficult Airway Management for Intensivists

Massimo Antonelli, MD
Professor of Intensive Care and Anesthesiology
Director, General Intensive Care Unit
Policlinico Universitario
A. Gemelli, Università Cattolica del Sacro Cuore
Editor in Chief of Intensive Care Medicine
Rome, Italy
W13 Fiberoptic Bronchoscopy

Barbara L. Bass, MD
The Methodist Hospital
Weill Cornell Medical College
New York, New York
W23 Bedside Laparoscopy in the ICU

Sarice L. Bassin, MD
Assistant Professor of Neurology
Neurological Surgery and Anesthesiology
Program Director, Neurocritical Care Fellowship
Northwestern University
Feinberg School of Medicine
Chicago, Illinois
W18 Lumbar Puncture
W20 Intracranial Pressure Monitoring

Yanick Beaulieu, MD
Division of Cardiology and Critical Care Medicine
Hôpital Sacré Coeur de Montréal
Université de Montréal
Montreal, Québec, Canada
W2 Bedside Ultrasonography

Giuseppe Bello, MD
Assistant Professor of Intensive Care and Anesthesiology
General Intensive Care Unit
Policlinico Universitario
A Gemelli, Università Cattolica del Sacro Cuore
Rome, Italy
W13 Fiberoptic Bronchoscopy

Cherisse Berry, MD
Cedars Sinai Medical Center
Los Angeles, California
W15 Percutaneous Dilatational Tracheostomy

Thomas P. Bleck, MD, FCCM
Professor of Neurological Sciences, Neurosurgery, Medicine, and Anesthesiology
Assistant Dean, Rush Medical College
Associate Chief Medical Officer, Critical Care
Rush University Medical Center
Chicago, Illinois
W18 Lumbar Puncture
W20 Intracranial Pressure Monitoring

Jonathan D. Cohen, MD
Department of General Intensive Care
Rabin Medical Center
Beilinson Hospital
Kaplan St. Petah Tiqva, Israel
W21 Indirect Calorimetry

Gulnur Com, MD
Assistant Professor of Pediatrics
University of Arkansas for Medical Sciences
Arkansas Children's Hospital
Little Rock, Arkansas
W24 Pediatric Intensive Care Procedures

Jovany Cruz, MD
Baylor College of Medicine
Houston, Texas
W19 Jugular Venous and Brain Tissue Oxygen Tension Monitoring

Peter Doelken, MD
Associate Professor of Medicine
Medical University of South Carolina
Department of Medicine
Division of Pulmonary, Critical Care, Allergy, and Sleep Medicine
Charleston, South Carolina
W11 Thoracentesis

Howard R. Doyle, MD
Albert Einstein College of Medicine
Bronx, New York
W16 Esophageal Balloon Tamponade

Brian K. Eble, MD
Assistant Professor of Pediatrics
University of Arkansas for Medical Science
Arkansas Children's Hospital
Little Rock, Arkansas
W24 Pediatric Intensive Care Procedures

Lillian L. Emlet, MD, MS, FACEP
University of Pittsburgh Medical Center
Department of Critical Care Medicine
Department of Emergency Medicine
Pittsburgh, Pennsylvania
W14 Bronchoalveolar Lavage and Protected Specimen Bronchial Brushing

Raúl J. Gazmuri, MD, PhD, FCCM
Rosalind Franklin University of Medicine and Science and Captain
    James A. Lovell Federal Health Care Center
Chicago, Illinois
W6 Cardioversion and Defibrillation
W7 Transvenous and Transcutaneous Cardiac Pacing

Shankar Gopinath, MD
Baylor College of Medicine
Houston, Texas
W19 Jugular Venous and Brain Tissue Oxygen Tension Monitoring

John Gorcsan III, MD, FACC, FAHA, FACP, FASE
Professor of Medicine
Director of Echocardiography
University of Pittsburgh
Pittsburgh, Pennsylvania
W2 Bedside Ultrasonography

Y. Gozal, MD
Associate Professor of Anesthesiology
Hebrew University-Hadassah Medical School
Chair, Department of Anesthesiology, Perioperative Medicine, and
    Pain Treatment
Director, Operating Rooms
Shaare Zedek Medical Center
Jerusalem, Israel
W4 Arterial Cannulation and Invasive Blood Pressure Measurement

Brian G. Harbrecht, MD
Professor of Surgery
University of Louisville
Louisville, Kentucky
W12 Chest Tube Placement, Care, and Removal

J. Terrill Huggins, MD
Assistant Professor of Medicine
Medical University of South Carolina
Department of Medicine
Division of Pulmonary, Critical Care, Allergy, and Sleep Medicine
Charleston, South Carolina
W11 Thoracentesis

Robert L. Kormos, MD
University of Pittsburgh Physicians
Department of Cardiothoracic Surgery
Division of Cardiac Surgery
Pittsburgh, Pennsylvania
W8 Ventricular Assist Devices

Phillip D. Levin, MA, MB, BChir
Attending Physician
Anesthesia and Critical Care Medicine
Hadassah Hebrew University Medical Center
Jerusalem, Israel
W4 Arterial Cannulation and Invasive Blood Pressure Measurement

Stefano Maggiolini, MD
Cardiovascular Department
AO Ospedale di Lecco
Ospedale San Leopoldo Mandic
Merate (LC), Italy
W9 Pericardiocentesis

Daniel R. Margulies, MD
Cedars Sinai Medical Center
Los Angeles, California
W15 Percutaneous Dilatational Tracheostomy

Bartley Mitchell, MD
Baylor College of Medicine
Houston, Texas
W19 Jugular Venous and Brain Tissue Oxygen Tension Monitoring

Deepika Mohan, MD, MPH
Department of Critical Care Medicine
University of Pittsburgh
Pittsburgh, Pennsylvania
W17 Naso-Enteric Feeding Tube Insertion

Laura J. Moore, MD
The Methodist Hospital
Weill Cornell Medical College
New York, New York
W23 Bedside Laparoscopy in the ICU

Thomas C. Mort, MD
Senior Associate, Anesthesiology
Associate Director, Surgical Intensive Care Unit
Hartford Hospital
Associate Professor of Anesthesiology and Surgery
University of Connecticut
Hartford, Connecticut
W1 Difficult Airway Management for Intensivists

Michele Moss, MD
Professor and Vice Chair of Pediatrics
University of Arkansas for Medical Sciences
Arkansas Children's Hospital
Little Rock, Arkansas
W24 Pediatric Intensive Care Procedures

Judith Pepe, MD
Associate Professor of Surgery
University of Connecticut School of Medicine
Farmington, Connecticut
Associate Director
Surgical Critical Care
Hartford Hospital
Hartford, Connecticut
W3 Central Venous Catheterization

Lucido Ponce, MD
Baylor College of Medicine
Houston, Texas
W19 Jugular Venous and Brain Tissue Oxygen Tension Monitoring

Claudia S. Robertson, MD
Baylor College of Medicine
Houston, Texas
W19 Jugular Venous and Brain Tissue Oxygen Tension Monitoring

Santhosh Sadasivan, MD
Baylor College of Medicine
Houston, Texas
W19 Jugular Venous and Brain Tissue Oxygen Tension Monitoring

Steven A. Sahn, MD
Professor of Medicine and Division Director
Medical University of South Carolina
Department of Medicine
Division of Pulmonary, Critical Care, Allergy, and Sleep Medicine
Charleston, South Carolina
W11 Thoracentesis

Penny Lynn Sappington, MD
University of Pittsburgh Medical Center
Pittsburgh, Pennsylvania
W22 *Extracorpeal Membrane Oxygenation (ECMO) Cannuation*

Professor P. Singer, MD
Chairman, Department of Anesthesiology and Intensive Care
Sackler School of Medicine, Tel-Aviv University
Critical Care Medicine and
Institute for Nutrition Research
Rabin Medical Center
Beilinson Hospital
Petah Tikva, Israel
W21 *Indirect Calorimetry*

Joseph F. Sucher, MD
The Methodist Hospital
Weill Cornell Medical College
New York, New York
W23 *Bedside Laparoscopy in the ICU*

Fabio S. Taccone, MD
Erasme Hospital
Free University of Brussels
Brussels, Belgium
W20 *Intracranial Pressure Monitoring*

S. Rob Todd, MD
The Methodist Hospital
Weill Cornell Medical College
New York, New York
W23 *Bedside Laparoscopy in the ICU*

Jean-Louis Vincent, MD, PhD
Professor of Intensive Care Medicine
Université Libre de Bruxelles
Head, Department of Intensive Care
Erasme University Hospital
Brussels, Belgium
W5 *Bedside Pulmonary Artery Catheterization*
W20 *Intracranial Pressure Monitoring*

Giovanni Vitale, MD
Department of Anesthesia
Ospedale San Gerardo
Monza Italy
Felice Achilli
Cardiovascular Department
AO Ospedale di Lecco
Ospedale Alessandro Manzoni
Lecco, Italy
W9 *Pericardiocentesis*

Gregory A. Watson, MD
Assistant Professor of Surgery and Critical Care
University of Pittsburgh
Pittsburgh, Pennsylvania
W12 *Chest Tube Placement, Care, and Removal*

PREFACE

The sixth edition of *Textbook of Critical Care* continues the tradition of excellence established by earlier editions and builds on the success of new features and format changes that were introduced in the fifth edition. Several features of this new edition, such as that it is published in full color, deserve special emphasis. New color illustrations and clinical photographs offer outstanding visual guidance. A list of key points at the conclusion of each chapter will help readers remember the "take-home" messages for that topic.

The opening section comprises short chapters that provide a brief overview of clinical problems such as acute respiratory failure or diarrhea that are commonly encountered in the management of patients with critical illness.

The way this edition covers the basic science underlying the practice of critical care is also different from the previous edition, where it was contained in a separate section. Given the expanded volume of information that has necessitated increased depth related to the clinical practice of critical care, the editors have elected to integrate essential basic science information within the individual chapters rather than discuss it separately.

Because critical care medicine is now a mature specialty practiced all over the world, the experts selected to write chapters for the sixth edition are an international group. New pediatric coverage is also international in scope and addresses key topics within each area of pediatric critical care that are germane to our broader readership.

This edition still contains extensive citations to medical literature, but both the bulk and cost of the text have been decreased by providing extended reference lists on the companion website. The references are linked to Medline or directly to full-text articles where available, which will help expand your search capabilities. Each printed chapter still contains the most important references expanded by author annotation to point out their particular insights.

One of the most user-friendly and critically lauded features of the previous edition was the dedicated companion website. The premium website that accompanies the new edition has also been greatly enhanced. In addition to full text, references, and an index that are fully searchable, new features such as hyperlinked references, critical care calculators, and an image library are offered as well. All illustrations can be downloaded to PowerPoint to enhance your presentations or lectures. The most exciting feature of the website is a dedicated section on critical care procedures. All procedural chapters have been streamlined for online presentation, and most are accompanied by video clips to complement the text and offer visual guidance on how to perform a wide variety of procedures.

The sixth edition of this textbook would not have been possible without the enormous contributions made by the prior editors. We express our gratitude to Will Shoemaker, Steve Ayers, Ake Grenvik, and Peter Holbrook for the opportunity and great honor to follow in their footsteps.

We are indebted to numerous people, including our contributors, colleagues, and staff, who were instrumental in helping us assemble the text you are now holding in your hands.

Jean-Louis Vincent, MD, PhD

Edward Abraham, MD

Frederick A. Moore, MD, FACS, FCCM

Patrick M. Kochanek, MD, FCCM

Mitchell P. Fink, MD

CONTENTS

ONLINE CHAPTERS

Chapters and videos in this section can be found on the Expert Consult website accompanying this text.
You can access the site by activating the PIN code on the inside front cover of the book.

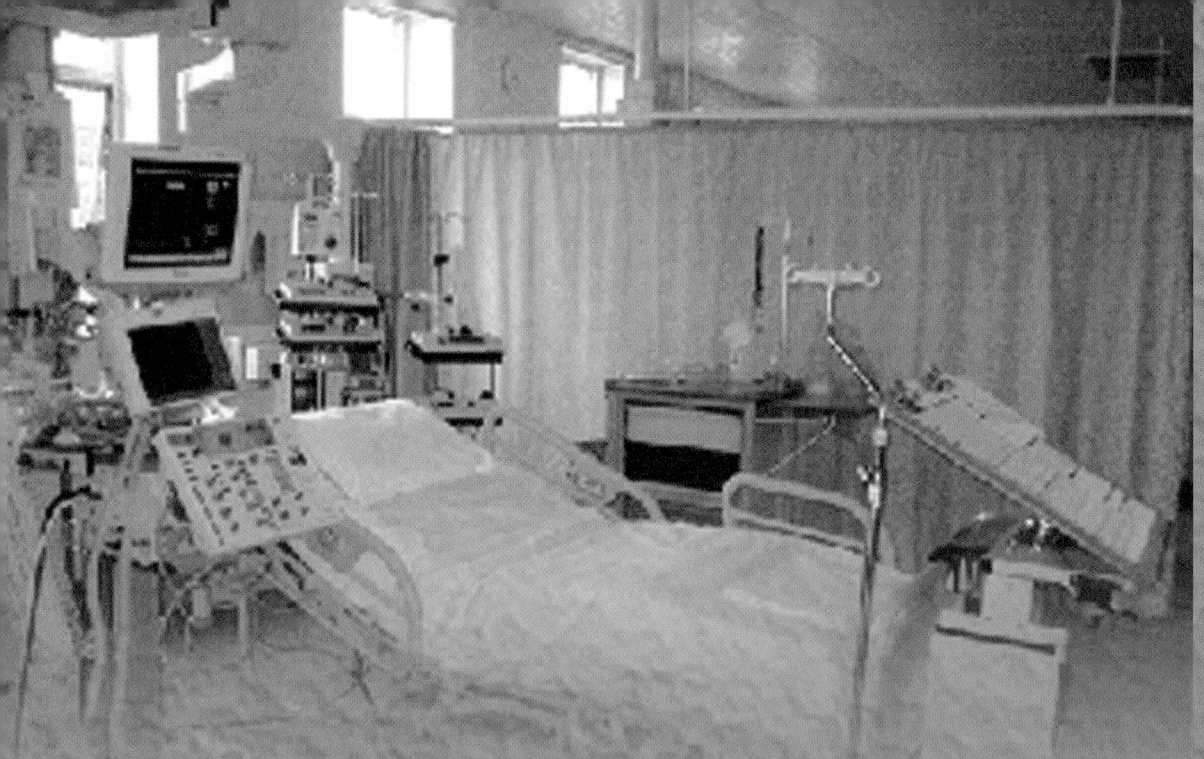

Common Problems in the ICU

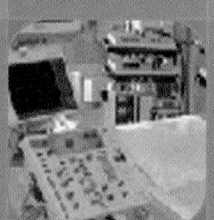

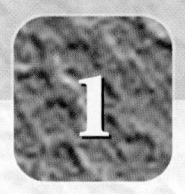

Sudden Deterioration in Neurologic Status

JOSEPH M. DARBY | ANUPAM ANUPAM

Patients admitted to the intensive care unit (ICU) with critical illness or injury are at risk for neurologic complications.[1-5] A sudden or unexpected change in the neurologic condition of a critically ill patient often heralds a complication that may cause direct injury to the central nervous system (CNS). Alternatively, such changes may simply be neurologic manifestations of the underlying critical illness or treatment that necessitated ICU admission (e.g., sepsis). These complications can occur in patients admitted to the ICU without neurologic disease and in those admitted for management of primary CNS problems (e.g., stroke). Neurologic complications also can occur as a result of invasive procedures and therapeutic interventions performed. Commonly, recognition of neurologic complications is delayed or missed entirely because ICU treatments (e.g., intubation, drugs) interfere with the physical examination or confound the clinical picture. In other cases, neurologic complications are not recognized because of a lack of sensitive methods to detect the problem (e.g., delirium). Morbidity and mortality are increased among patients who develop neurologic complications; therefore, the intensivist must be vigilant in evaluating all critically ill patients for changes in neurologic status.

Despite the importance of neurologic complications of critical illness, few studies have specifically assessed their incidence and impact on outcome among ICU patients. Available data are limited to medical ICU patients; data regarding neurologic complications in general surgical and other specialty ICU populations must be extracted from other sources. In studies of medical ICU patients, the incidence of neurologic complications is 12.3% to 33%.[1,2] Patients who develop neurologic complications have increased morbidity, mortality, and ICU length of stay. Sepsis is the most common problem associated with development of neurologic complications (sepsis-associated encephalopathy). In addition to encephalopathy, other common neurologic complications associated with critical illness include seizures and stroke. As the complexity of ICU care has increased, so has the risk of neurologic complications. Neuromuscular disorders are now recognized as a major source of morbidity in severely ill patients.[6] Recognized neurologic complications occurring in selected medical, surgical, and neurologic ICU populations are shown in Table 1-1.[7-41]

▨ Impairment in Consciousness

Global changes in CNS function, best described in terms of impairment in consciousness, are generally referred to as *encephalopathy* or *altered mental status*. An acute change in the level of consciousness undoubtedly is the most common neurologic complication that occurs after ICU admission. *Consciousness* is defined as a state of awareness (arousal or wakefulness) and the ability to respond appropriately to changes in environment.[42] For consciousness to be impaired, global hemispheric dysfunction or dysfunction of the brainstem reticular activating system must be present.[43] Altered consciousness may result in a sleeplike state (coma) or a state characterized by confusion and agitation (delirium). States of acutely altered consciousness seen in the critically ill are listed in Table 1-2.

When an acute change in consciousness is noted, the patient should be evaluated keeping in mind the patient's age, presence or absence of coexisting organ system dysfunction, metabolic status and medication list, and presence or absence of infection. In patients with a primary

CNS disorder, deterioration in the level of consciousness (e.g., from stupor to coma) frequently represents the development of brain edema, increasing intracranial pressure, new or worsening intracranial hemorrhage, hydrocephalus, CNS infection, or cerebral vasospasm. In patients without a primary CNS diagnosis, an acute change in consciousness is often due to the development of infectious complications (i.e., sepsis-associated encephalopathy), drug toxicities, or the development or exacerbation of organ system failure. Nonconvulsive status epilepticus is increasingly being recognized as a cause of impaired consciousness in critically ill patients (Box 1-1).[44-53]

States of altered consciousness manifesting as impairment in wakefulness or arousal (i.e., coma and stupor) and their causes are well defined.[42,43,54,55] Much confusion remains, however, regarding the diagnosis and management of delirium, perhaps the most common state of impaired CNS functioning in critically ill patients at large. When dedicated instruments are used, delirium can be diagnosed in more than 80% of critically ill patients, making this condition the most common neurologic complication of critical illness.[56-58] Much of the difficulty in establishing the diagnosis of delirium stems from the belief that delirium is a state characterized mainly by confusion and agitation and that such states are expected consequences of the unique environmental factors and sleep deprivation that characterize the ICU experience. Terms previously used to describe delirium in critically ill patients include *ICU psychosis, acute confusional state, encephalopathy,* and *postoperative psychosis.* It is now recognized that *ICU psychosis* is a misnomer; *delirium* is a more accurate term.[59]

Currently accepted criteria for the diagnosis of delirium include abrupt onset of impaired consciousness, disturbed cognitive function, fluctuating course, and presence of a medical condition that could impair brain function.[60] Subtypes of delirium include hyperactive (agitated) delirium and the more common hypoactive or quiet delirium.[58] Impaired consciousness may be apparent as a reduction in awareness, psychomotor retardation, agitation, or impairment in attention (increased distractibility or vigilance). Cognitive impairment can include disorientation, impaired memory, and perceptual aberrations (hallucinations or illusions).[61] Autonomic hyperactivity and sleep disturbances may be features of delirium in some patients (e.g., those with drug withdrawal syndromes, delirium tremens). Delirium in critically ill patients is associated with increased morbidity, mortality, and ICU length of stay.[62-64] In general, sepsis and medications should be the primary etiologic considerations in critically ill patients who develop delirium.

As has been noted, nonconvulsive status epilepticus is increasingly recognized as an important cause of impaired consciousness in critically ill patients. Although the general term can encompasses other entities, such as absence and partial complex seizures, in critically ill patients, *nonconvulsive status epilepticus* is often referred to as *status epilepticus of epileptic encephalopathy.*[53] It is characterized by alteration in consciousness or behavior associated with electroencephalographic evidence of continuous or periodic epileptiform activity without overt motor manifestations of seizures. In one study of comatose patients without overt seizure activity, nonconvulsive status epilepticus was evident in 8%.[51] Nonconvulsive status epilepticus can precede or follow an episode of generalized convulsive status epilepticus; it can also occur in patients with traumatic brain injury, subarachnoid hemorrhage, global brain

TABLE 1-1	Neurologic Complications in Selected Specialty Populations
Medical	
Bone marrow transplantation[7,8]	CNS infection, stroke, subdural hematoma, brainstem ischemia, hyperammonemia, Wernicke encephalopathy
Cancer[9]	Stroke, intracranial hemorrhage, CNS infection
Fulminant hepatic failure[10]	Encephalopathy, coma, brain edema, increased ICP
HIV/AIDS[11,12]	Opportunistic CNS infection, stroke, vasculitis, delirium, seizures, progressive multifocal leukoencephalopathy
Pregnancy[13,14]	Seizures, ischemic stroke, cerebral vasospasm, intracranial hemorrhage, cerebral venous thrombosis, hypertensive encephalopathy, pituitary apoplexy
Surgical	
Cardiac surgery[15-19]	Stroke, delirium, brachial plexus injury, phrenic nerve injury
Vascular surgery[20,21]:	
Carotid	Stroke, cranial nerve injuries (recurrent laryngeal, glossopharyngeal, hypoglossal, facial), seizures
Aortic	Stroke, paraplegia
Peripheral	Delirium
Transplantation[10,22-25]:	
Heart	Stroke
Liver	Encephalopathy, seizures, opportunistic CNS infection, intracranial hemorrhage, Guillain-Barré syndrome, central pontine myelinolysis
Renal	Stroke, opportunistic CNS infection, femoral neuropathy
Urologic surgery (TURP)[26]	Seizures and coma (hyponatremia)
Otolaryngologic surgery[27,28]	Recurrent laryngeal nerve injury, stroke, delirium
Orthopedic surgery[29]:	
Spine	Myelopathy, radiculopathy, epidural abscess, meningitis
Knee and hip replacement	Delirium (fat embolism)
Long-bone fracture/nailing	Delirium (fat embolism)
Neurologic	
Stroke[30-34]	Stroke progression or extension, reocclusion after thrombolysis, bleeding, seizures, delirium, brain edema, herniation
Intracranial surgery[35]	Bleeding, edema, seizures, CNS infection
Subarachnoid hemorrhage[32,36-38]	Rebleeding, vasospasm, hydrocephalus, seizures
Traumatic brain injury[32,39,40]	Intracranial hypertension, bleeding, seizures, stroke (cerebrovascular injury), CNS infection
Cervical spinal cord injury[41]	Ascension of injury, stroke (vertebral artery injury)

CNS, central nervous system; *HIV/AIDS*, human immunodeficiency virus/acquired immunodeficiency syndrome; *ICP*, intracranial pressure; *TURP*, transurethral prostatic resection.

ischemia or anoxia, sepsis, and multiple organ failure. Despite the general consensus that nonconvulsive status epilepticus is a unique entity responsible for impaired consciousness in some critically ill patients, there is no general consensus on the electroencephalographic criteria for its diagnosis or the optimal approach to treatment.[65]

Stroke and Other Focal Neurologic Deficits

The new onset of a major neurologic deficit that manifests as a focal impairment in motor or sensory function (e.g., hemiparesis) or results in seizures usually indicates a primary problem referable to the cerebrovascular circulation. In a study evaluating the value of computed tomography (CT) in medical ICU patients, ischemic stroke and intracranial bleeding were the most common abnormalities associated with the new onset of a neurologic deficit or seizures.[66] Overall, the frequency of new-onset stroke is between 1% and 4% in medical ICU patients.[1,2] Among general surgical patients, the frequency of perioperative stroke ranges from 0.3% to 3.5%.[67] Patients undergoing cardiac or vascular surgery and surgical patients with underlying cerebrovascular disease can be expected to have an increased risk of perioperative stroke.[19]

TABLE 1-2	States of Acutely Altered Consciousness	
State	**Description**	
Coma	Closed eyes, sleeplike state with no response to external stimuli (pain)	
Stupor	Responsive only to vigorous or painful stimuli	
Lethargy	Drowsy, arouses easily and appropriately to stimuli	
Delirium	Acute state of confusion with or without behavioral disturbance	
Catatonia	Eyes open, unblinking, unresponsive	

The frequency of new or worsening focal neurologic deficits in patients admitted with a primary neurologic or neurosurgical disorder varies. For example, as many as 30% of patients with aneurysmal subarachnoid hemorrhage develop delayed ischemic neurologic deficits.[36] Patients admitted with stroke often develop worsening or new symptoms as a result of stroke progression, bleeding, or reocclusion of vessels previously opened with interventional therapy. In patients who have undergone elective intracranial surgery, postsurgical bleeding or infectious complications are the main causes of new focal deficits. In trauma patients, unrecognized injuries to the cerebrovascular circulation can cause new deficits. Patients who have sustained spinal cord injuries, and those who have undergone surgery of the spine or of the thoracic or abdominal aorta, can develop worsening or new symptoms of spinal cord injury. Early deterioration of CNS function after spinal cord injury usually occurs as a consequence of medical interventions to stabilize the spine, whereas late deterioration is usually due to hypotension and impaired cord perfusion. Occasionally, focal weakness or sensory symptoms in the extremities occur as a result of occult brachial plexus injury or compression neuropathy. New cranial nerve deficits in patients without primary neurologic problems can occur after neck surgery or carotid endarterectomy.

Seizures

The new onset of motor seizures occurs in 0.8% to 4% of critically ill medical ICU patients.[1,2,68] The new onset of seizures in general medical-surgical ICU patients is typically caused by narcotic withdrawal, hyponatremia, drug toxicities, or previously unrecognized structural abnormalities.[3,68] New stroke, intracranial bleeding, and CNS infection are other potential causes of seizures after ICU admission. The frequency of seizures is higher in patients admitted to the ICU with a primary neurologic problem such as traumatic brain injury, aneurysmal subarachnoid hemorrhage, stroke, or CNS infection.[69] Because nonconvulsive status epilepticus may be more common than was previously appreciated, this problem should also be considered in the

Box 1-1

GENERAL CAUSES OF ACUTELY IMPAIRED CONSCIOUSNESS IN THE CRITICALLY ILL

Infection
Sepsis encephalopathy
CNS infection

Drugs
Narcotics
Benzodiazepines
Anticholinergics
Anticonvulsants
Tricyclic antidepressants
Selective serotonin uptake inhibitors
Phenothiazines
Steroids
Immunosuppressants (cyclosporine, FK506, OKT3)
Anesthetics

Electrolyte and Acid-Base Disturbances
Hyponatremia
Hypernatremia
Hypercalcemia
Hypermagnesemia
Severe acidemia and alkalemia

Organ System Failure
Shock
Renal failure
Hepatic failure
Pancreatitis
Respiratory failure (hypoxia, hypercapnia)

Endocrine Disorders
Hypoglycemia
Hyperglycemia
Hypothyroidism
Hyperthyroidism
Pituitary apoplexy

Drug Withdrawal
Alcohol
Opiates
Barbiturates
Benzodiazepines

Vascular Causes
Shock
Hypotension
Hypertensive encephalopathy
CNS vasculitis
Cerebral venous sinus thrombosis

CNS Disorders
Hemorrhage
Stroke
Brain edema
Hydrocephalus
Increased intracranial pressure
Meningitis
Ventriculitis
Brain abscess
Subdural empyema
Seizures
Vasculitis

Seizures
Convulsive and nonconvulsive status epilepticus

Miscellaneous
Fat embolism syndrome
Neuroleptic malignant syndrome
Thiamine deficiency (Wernicke encephalopathy)
Psychogenic unresponsiveness

CNS, central nervous system.

differential diagnosis of patients developing new, unexplained, or prolonged alterations in consciousness.

Generalized Weakness and Neuromuscular Disorders

Generalized muscle weakness often becomes apparent in ICU patients as previous impairments in arousal are resolving or sedative and neuromuscular blocking agents are being discontinued or tapered. Polyneuropathy and myopathy associated with critical illness are now well recognized as the principal causes of new-onset generalized weakness among ICU patients being treated for non-neuromuscular disorders.[5,70-73] These disorders also may be responsible for prolonged ventilator dependency in some patients. Patients at increased risk for these complications include those with sepsis, systemic inflammatory response syndrome, and multiple organ dysfunction syndrome, as well as those who require prolonged mechanical ventilation. Other risk factors include treatment with corticosteroids or neuromuscular blocking agents. In contrast to demyelinating neuropathies (e.g., Guillain-Barré syndrome), critical illness polyneuropathy is primarily an axonal condition. Critical illness polyneuropathy is diagnosed in a high percentage of patients undergoing careful evaluation for weakness acquired while in the ICU. Because primary myopathy coexists in a large number of patients with critical illness polyneuropathy, *ICU-acquired paresis*[72] or *critical illness neuromuscular abnormalities*[5] may be better terms to describe this problem. Although acute Guillain-Barré syndrome and myasthenia gravis are rare complications of critical illness, these diagnoses should also be considered in patients who develop generalized weakness in the ICU.

Neurologic Complications of Procedures and Treatments

Routine procedures performed in the ICU or in association with evaluation and treatment of critical illness can result in neurologic complications.[4] The most obvious neurologic complications are those associated with intracranial bleeding secondary to the treatment of stroke and other disorders with thrombolytic agents or anticoagulants. Other notable complications are listed in Table 1-3.

Evaluation of Sudden Neurologic Change

A new or sudden change in the neurologic condition of a critically ill patient necessitates a focused neurologic examination, review of the clinical course and medications administered before the change, a thorough laboratory assessment, and appropriate imaging or neurophysiologic studies when indicated. The type and extent of the evaluation depend on clinical context and the general category of neurologic change occurring. The history and physical examination should lead the clinician to the diagnostic approach best suited to the individual patient.

Essential elements of the neurologic examination include an assessment of the level and content of consciousness, pupillary size and reactivity, and motor function. Additional evaluation of the cranial nerves and peripheral reflexes and a sensory examination are conducted as indicated by the clinical circumstances. If the patient is comatose on initial evaluation, a more detailed coma examination should be performed to help differentiate structural from metabolic causes of coma.[43,55] When the evaluation reveals only a change in arousal without evidence of a localizing lesion in the CNS, a search for infection, discontinuation or modification of drug therapy, and a general metabolic evaluation may be indicated. Lumbar puncture to aid the diagnosis of CNS infection may be warranted in selected neurosurgical patients and immunocompromised individuals. Lumbar puncture to rule out nosocomially acquired meningitis in other patients is generally not rewarding.[74] Electroencephalography should

TABLE 1-3	Neurologic Complications Associated with ICU Procedures and Treatments	
Procedure	**Complication**	
Angiography	Cerebral cholesterol emboli syndrome	
Anticoagulants/antiplatelet agents	Intracranial bleeding	
Arterial catheterization	Cerebral embolism	
Bronchoscopy	Increased ICP	
Central venous catheterization	Cerebral air embolism, carotid dissection, Horner's syndrome, phrenic nerve injury, brachial plexus injury, cranial nerve injury	
DC cardioversion	Embolic stroke, seizures	
Dialysis	Seizures, increased ICP (dialysis disequilibrium syndrome)	
Endovascular procedures (CNS)	Vessel rupture, thrombosis, reperfusion bleeding	
Epidural catheter	Spinal epidural hematoma, epidural abscess	
ICP monitoring	CNS infection (ventriculitis), hemorrhage	
Intraaortic balloon pump	Lower-extremity paralysis	
Intubation	Spinal cord injury	
Left ventricular assist devices	Stroke, seizures	
Lumbar puncture or drain	Meningitis, herniation	
Mechanical ventilation	Cerebral air embolism, increased ICP (high PEEP and hypercapnia), seizures (hypocapnia)	
Nasogastric intubation	Intracranial placement	

CNS, central nervous system; *DC,* direct current; *ICP,* intracranial pressure; *ICU,* intensive care unit; *PEEP,* positive end-expiratory pressure.

be performed in patients with clear evidence of seizures, as well as when the diagnosis of nonconvulsive status epilepticus is being entertained. Continuous electroencephalography should be considered when the index of suspicion for nonconvulsive status epilepticus remains high and the initial electroencephalographic studies are unrevealing.

CT is indicated for non-neurologic patients with new focal deficits, seizures, or otherwise unexplained impairments in arousal.[66] In patients with primary neurologic disorders, CT is indicated if worsening brain edema, herniation, bleeding, and hydrocephalus are considerations when new deficits or worsening neurologic status occurs. In some cases, when the basis for a change in neurologic condition remains elusive, magnetic resonance imaging (MRI) may be helpful. In particular, the diffusion-weighted MRI technique can reveal structural abnormalities such as hypoxic brain injury, fat embolism, vasculitis, cerebral venous thrombosis, or multiple infarcts following cardiopulmonary bypass that are not apparent by standard CT or conventional MRI.[75-80] MRI may be the imaging modality of choice in patients with human immunodeficiency virus (HIV) and new CNS complications.[75] For patients who develop signs and symptoms of spinal cord injury complicating critical illness, MRI or somatosensory evoked potentials can be used to further delineate the nature and severity of the injury. For patients who develop generalized muscle weakness or unexplained ventilator dependency, electromyography and nerve conduction studies can confirm the presence of critical illness polyneuropathy or myopathy.

Monitoring for Neurologic Changes

The common occurrence of neurologic changes in critically ill patients emphasizes the need for vigilant monitoring. A variety of clinical techniques such as the Glasgow Coma Scale, National Institutes of Health Stroke Scale, Ramsay Sedation Scale, Richmond Agitation-Sedation Scale, and Confusion Assessment Method for the Intensive Care Unit (CAM-ICU) can be used to monitor clinical neurologic status.[57,58,81-86] Neurophysiologic methods such as the bispectral index may provide more objective neurologic monitoring in the future for patients admitted to the ICU with and without primary neurologic problems.[87-89] For patients admitted to the ICU with a primary neurologic disorder, a variety of monitoring techniques including measurements of intracranial pressure, near-infrared spectroscopy, brain tissue Po_2, transcranial Doppler, and electroencephalography are available.[90]

ANNOTATED REFERENCES

De Jonghe B, Sharshar T, Lefaucheur JP, et al. Paresis acquired in the intensive care unit. A prospective multicenter study. JAMA 2002;288:2859-67.

This prospective multicenter study of critically ill patients was the first to assess the clinical incidence, risk factors, and outcomes of mechanically ventilated patients developing ICU-acquired weakness, emphasizing a central role for corticosteroid use in its genesis and prolonged mechanical ventilation as a relevant ICU outcome.

Ely EW, Inouye SK, Bernard GR, et al. Delirium in mechanically ventilated patients. Validity and reliability of the Confusion Assessment Method for the Intensive Care Unit (CAM-ICU). JAMA 2001;286: 2703-10.

Recognizing that the diagnosis of delirium is often difficult in the critically ill patient receiving mechanical ventilation, the authors adapted a common method for assessing delirium using the Confusion Assessment Method to critically ill patients receiving mechanical ventilation. This prospective evaluation revealed high sensitivity, specificity, and inter-rater reliability in detecting delirium in 80% of the patient population they studied.

McGuire BE, Basten CJ, Ryan CJ, et al. Intensive care unit syndrome. A dangerous misnomer. Arch Intern Med 2000;160:906-9.

In an effort to dispel the myth that environmental conditions lead to "ICU psychosis," the authors of this article argue that ICU psychosis is more appropriately described as delirium. The etiology and management of delirium in critically ill patients are reviewed.

Naik-Tolani S, Oropello JM, Benjamin E. Neurologic complications in the intensive care unit. Clin Chest Med 1999;20:423-34.

The authors of this article present an overview of central nervous system (CNS) complications of critical illness and ICU procedures in critically ill patients without primary disorders of the CNS.

Sundgren PC, Reinstrup P, Romner B, et al. Value of conventional diffusion- and perfusion-weighted MRI in the management of patients with unclear cerebral pathology, admitted to the intensive care unit. Neuroradiology 2002;44:674-80.

This retrospective study of 21 critically ill patients undergoing MRI because of a disparity in clinical neurologic findings and CT imaging revealed that additional useful diagnostic and prognostic information can be obtained, especially when diffusion- and perfusion-weighted MR sequences are obtained.

REFERENCES

Access the complete reference list online at http://www.expertconsult.com.

Agitation and Delirium

ARNA BANERJEE | E. WESLEY ELY | PRATIK P. PANDHARIPANDE

Agitation and delirium are commonly encountered in the intensive care unit (ICU). They are more than just an inconvenience; these conditions can have deleterious effects on patient and staff safety and contribute to poor outcomes. It is therefore important for clinicians to be able to recognize agitation and delirium and to have an organized approach for its evaluation and management.

Agitation

Agitation is a psychomotor disturbance characterized by a marked increase in motor and psychological activity.[1] It is a state of extreme arousal, irritability, and motor restlessness that usually results from an internal sense of discomfort or tension and is characterized by repetitive, nonproductive movements that may appear purposeless, although careful observation of the patient sometimes reveals an underlying intent. In the ICU, agitation is frequently related to anxiety or delirium. Agitation may be caused by various factors: metabolic disorders (hypo- and hypernatremia), hyperthermia, hypoxia, hypotension, use of sedative drugs and/or analgesics, sepsis, alcohol withdrawal, and long-term psychoactive drug use to name a few.[2,3] It can also be caused by external factors such as noise, discomfort, and pain.[4] Associated with a longer length of stay in the ICU and higher costs,[2] agitation can be mild, characterized by increased movements and an apparent inability to get comfortable, or it can be severe. Severe agitation can be life threatening, leading to higher rates of self-extubation, self-removal of catheters and medical devices, nosocomial infections,[2] hypoxia, barotrauma, and/or hypotension due to patient/ventilator asynchrony. Indeed, recent studies have shown that agitation contributes to ventilator asynchrony, increased oxygen consumption, and increased production of CO_2 and lactic acid; these effects can lead to life-threatening respiratory and metabolic acidosis.[3]

Delirium

Delirium is an acute disturbance of consciousness accompanied by inattention, disorganized thinking, and perceptual disturbances that fluctuates over a short period of time (Figure 2-1).[5] Delirium is commonly underdiagnosed in the ICU and has a reported prevalence of 20% to 80%, depending on the severity of illness and the need for mechanical ventilation.[6-9] Recent investigations have shown that the presence of delirium is a strong predictor of longer hospital stay, higher costs, and increased risk of death.[10-12] Each additional day with delirium increases the risk of dying by 10%.[13] Longer periods of delirium are associated with greater degrees of cognitive decline when patients are evaluated after 1 year.[12] Thus, delirium can adversely affect the quality of life in survivors of critical illnesses and may serve as an intermediary recognizable step for targeting therapies to prevent poor outcomes in survivors of critical illness.[12,14]

Unfortunately, the true prevalence and magnitude of delirium has been poorly documented because myriad terms—*acute confusional state, ICU psychosis, acute brain dysfunction, encephalopathy*—have been used to describe this condition.[15] Delirium can be classified according to psychomotor behavior into hypoactive delirium or hyperactive delirium. Hypoactive delirium is characterized by decreased physical and mental activity and inattention. In contrast, hyperactive delirium is characterized by combativeness and agitation. Patients with both features have mixed delirium.[16-18] Hyperactive delirium puts both patients and caregivers at risk for serious injuries, but fortunately this form of delirium occurs in a minority of critically ill patients.[16-18] Hypoactive delirium actually may be associated with a worse prognosis.[19,20]

Although healthcare professionals realize the importance of recognizing delirium, it frequently goes unrecognized in the ICU.[21-28] Even when ICU delirium is recognized, most clinicians consider it an expected event that is often iatrogenic and without consequence,[21] though one needs to view this as a form of organic brain dysfunction that has consequences if left undiagnosed and untreated.

RISK FACTORS FOR DELIRIUM

The risk factors for agitation and delirium are many and overlap to a large extent (Table 2-1). Fortunately there are several mnemonics that can aid clinicians in recalling the list; two common ones are IWATCH-DEATH and DELIRIUM (Table 2-2). In practical terms, the risk factors can be divided into three categories: the acute illness itself, patient factors, and iatrogenic or environmental factors. Importantly, a number of medications that are commonly used in the ICU are associated with the development of agitation and delirium (Box 2-1). A thorough approach to the treatment and support of the acute illness (e.g., controlling sources of sepsis and giving appropriate antibiotics; correcting hypoxia, metabolic disturbances, dehydration, hyperthermia; normalizing sleep/wake cycle), as well as minimizing the iatrogenic factors (e.g., excessive sedation), can reduce the incidence or severity of delirium and its attendant complications.

Pathophysiology

The pathophysiology of delirium is poorly understood, although there are a number of hypotheses:

- **Neurotransmitter imbalance.** Multiple neurotransmitters have been implicated, including dopamine (excess), acetylcholine (relative depletion), γ-aminobutyric acid (GABA), serotonin, endorphins, norepinephrine, and glutamate.[29-32]
- **Inflammatory mediators.** Inflammatory mediators, such as tumor necrosis factor alpha (TNF-α), interleukin 1 (IL-1), and other cytokines and chemokines, have been implicated in the pathogenesis of endothelial damage, thrombin formation, and microvascular dysfunction in the central nervous system (CNS), contributing to delirium.[32]
- **Impaired oxidative metabolism.** According to this hypothesis, delirium is a result of cerebral insufficiency secondary to a global failure of oxidative metabolism.[33]
- **Large neutral amino acids.** Increased cerebral uptake of tryptophan and tyrosine can lead to elevated levels of serotonin, dopamine, and norepinephrine in the CNS. Altered availability of these amino acids is associated with increased risk of development of delirium.[34]

Assessment

Recently the Society of Critical Care Medicine (SCCM) published guidelines for the use of sedatives and analgesics in the ICU.[35] The SCCM recommended routine monitoring of pain, anxiety, and delirium and documentation of responses to therapy for these conditions.

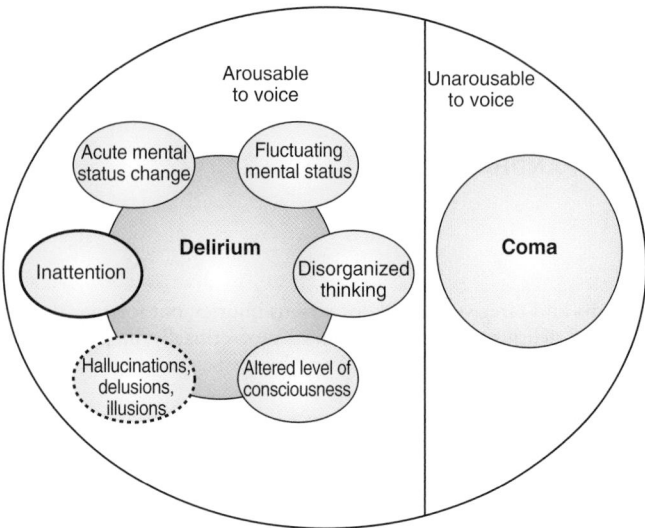

Figure 2-1 Acute brain dysfunction. Patients who are unresponsive to voice are considered to be in a coma. Those patients who respond to voice can be further evaluated for delirium using validated delirium monitoring instruments. Inattention is a cardinal feature of delirium. Other pivotal features include a change in mental status that fluctuates over hours to days, disorganized thinking, and altered level of consciousness. While hallucinations, delusions, and illusions may be part of the perceptual disturbances seen in delirium, they on their own are not synonymous with delirium and require the presence of inattention and the pivotal features outlined above. *(With permission from E. Wesley Ely and A. Morandi) (ww.icudelirium.org).*

There are many scales available for the assessment of agitation and sedation, including the Ramsay Scale,[36] the Riker Sedation-Agitation Scale (SAS),[37] the Motor Activity Assessment Scale (MAAS),[38] the Richmond Agitation-Sedation Scale (RASS),[39] the Adaptation to Intensive Care Environment (ATICE)[40] scale, and the Minnesota Sedation Assessment Tool (MSAT).[40] Most of these scales have good reliability and validity among adult ICU patients and can be used to set targets for goal-directed sedative administration. The SAS, which scores agitation and sedation using a 7-point system, has excellent inter-rater reliability (kappa = 0.92), and it is highly correlated (r^2 = 0.83 to 0.86) with other scales. The RASS (Table 2-3), however, is the only method

TABLE 2-1   Risk Factors for Agitation and Delirium

Age >70 years	BUN/creatinine ratio ≥18
Transfer from a nursing home	Renal failure, creatinine > 2.0 mg/dL
History of depression	Liver disease
History of dementia, stroke, or epilepsy	CHF
Alcohol abuse within past month	Cardiogenic or septic shock
Tobacco use	Myocardial infarction
Drug overdose or illicit drug use	Infection
HIV infection	CNS pathology
Psychoactive medications	Urinary retention or fecal impaction
Hypo- or hypernatremia	Tube feeding
Hypo- or hyperglycemia	Rectal or bladder catheters
Hypo- or hyperthyroidism	Physical restraints
Hypothermia or fever	Central line catheters
Hypertension	Malnutrition or vitamin deficiencies
Hypoxia	Procedural complications
Acidosis or alkalosis	Visual or hearing impairment
Pain	Sleep disruption
Fear and anxiety	

BUN, blood urea nitrogen; **CHF,** congestive heart failure; **CNS,** central nervous system; **HIV,** human immunodeficiency virus.

TABLE 2-2   Mnemonic for Risk Factors for Delirium and Agitation

IWATCHDEATH	*DELIRIUM*
Infection	Drugs
Withdrawal	Electrolyte and physiologic abnormalities
Acute metabolic	Lack of drugs (withdrawal)
Trauma/pain	Infection
Central nervous system pathology	Reduced sensory input (blindness, deafness)
Hypoxia	Intracranial problems (CVA, meningitis, seizure)
Deficiencies (vitamin B_{12}, thiamine)	Urinary retention and fecal impaction
Endocrinopathies (thyroid, adrenal)	Myocardial problems (MI, arrhythmia, CHF)
Acute vascular (hypertension, shock)	
Toxins/drugs	
Heavy metals	

CHF, congestive heart failure; **CVA,** cerebrovascular accident; **MI,** myocardial infarction.

shown to detect variations in the level of consciousness over time or in response to changes in sedative and analgesic drug use.[41] The 10-point RASS scale has discrete criteria to distinguish levels of agitation and sedation. The evaluation of patients consists of a 3-step process. First, the patient is observed to determine whether he or she is alert, restless, or agitated (0 to +4). Second, if the patient is not alert and does not show positive motoric characteristics, the patient's name is called and the sedation level is scored, depending on the duration of eye contact (−1 to −3). Third, if there is no eye opening with verbal stimulation, the shoulder is shaken or the sternum is rubbed, and the response is noted (−4 or −5). This assessment takes less than 20 seconds and correlates well with other measures of sedation (e.g., Glasgow Coma Scale [GCS], bispectral electroencephalography, neuropsychiatric ratings).[39]

Until recently, there was no valid and reliable way to assess delirium in critically ill patients, many of whom are nonverbal owing to sedation or mechanical ventilation. However, a number of tools have been developed recently to aid in the detection of delirium in the ICU. These tools have been validated for use in both intubated and nonintubated patients and measured against a "gold standard," the *Diagnostic and Statistical Manual of Mental Disorders* (DSM) criteria. The new tools are the Confusion Assessment Method for the ICU (CAM-ICU),[42-46] the Intensive Care Delirium Screening Checklist (ICDSC),[7] and the Neelon and Champagne (NEECHAM) Confusion Scale.[47,48]

The CAM-ICU (Figure 2-2) is a delirium measurement tool that was developed by a team of specialists in critical care, psychiatry, neurology, and geriatrics.[42,49] Administered by a nurse, the evaluation takes only 1 to 2 minutes to conduct and is 98% accurate for detecting delirium as compared with a full DSM-IV assessment by a geriatric psychiatrist.[42,43] To perform the CAM-ICU, patients are first evaluated for level of consciousness; patients who respond to verbal commands (a RASS score of −3 or higher level of arousal) can then be assessed for delirium. The CAM-ICU comprises four features: (1) a change in mental status

Box 2-1

COMMONLY USED DRUGS ASSOCIATED WITH DELIRIUM AND AGITATION

Benzodiazepines
Opiates (especially meperidine)
Anticholinergics
Antihistamines
H_2 blockers
Antibiotics
Corticosteroids
Metoclopramide

TABLE 2-3	Richmond Agitation-Sedation Scale	
+4	Combative	Combative, violent, immediate danger to staff
+3	Very agitated	Pulls or removes tube(s) or catheter(s); aggressive
+2	Agitated	Frequent nonpurposeful movement; fights ventilator
+1	Restless	Anxious, apprehensive, but movements not aggressive or vigorous
0	Alert and calm	
−1	Drowsy	Not fully alert but has sustained (>10 sec) awakening (eye opening/ contact) to voice
−2	Light sedation	Drowsy; briefly (<10 sec) awakens to voice or physical stimulation
−3	Moderate sedation	Movement or eye opening (but no eye contact) to voice
−4	Deep sedation	No response to voice, but movement or eye opening to physical stimulation
−5	Unarousable	No response to voice or physical stimulation

Procedure for Assessment

1. Observe patient. Is patient alert, restless, or agitated?   (Score 0 to +4)
2. If not alert, state patient's name and tell him or her to open eyes and look at speaker. Patient awakens, with sustained eye opening and eye contact.   (Score −1)

   Patient awakens, with eye opening and eye contact, but not sustained.   (Score −2)

   Patient does not awaken (no eye contact) but has eye opening or movement in response to voice.   (Score −3)

3. Physically stimulate patient by shaking shoulder and/or rubbing sternum. No response to voice, but response (movement) to physical stimulation.   (Score −4)
4. No response to voice or physical stimulation   (Score −5)

From Sessler CN, Gosnell MS, Grap MJ, et al. The Richmond Agitation-Sedation Scale: validity and reliability in adult intensive care unit patients. *Am J Respir Crit Care Med* 2002;166(10):1338-1344.

from baseline or a fluctuation in mental status, (2) inattention, (3) disorganized thinking, and (4) altered level of consciousness. Delirium is diagnosed if patients have features 1 and 2, and either 3 or 4 is positive (see Figure 2-2).

The ICDSC[7] (Table 2-4) is a checklist-based assessment tool that evaluates inattention, disorientation, hallucination, delusion or psychosis, psychomotor agitation or retardation, inappropriate speech or

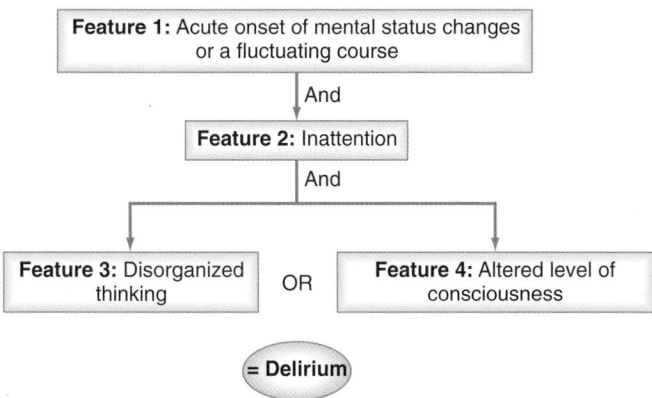

Figure 2-2 Confusion Assessment Method in the Intensive Care Unit (CAM-ICU).

TABLE 2-4	Intensive Care Delirium Screening Checklist	
Patient Evaluation		
Altered level of consciousness	(A–E)*	
Inattention	Difficulty in following a conversation or instructions. Easily distracted by external stimuli. Difficulty in shifting focus. Any of these scores 1 point.	
Disorientation	Any obvious mistake in time, place, or person scores 1 point.	
Hallucinations-delusions-psychosis	The unequivocal clinical manifestation of hallucination or behavior probably attributable to hallucination or delusion. Gross impairment in reality testing. Any of these scores 1 point.	
Psychomotor agitation or retardation	Hyperactivity requiring the use of additional sedative drugs or restraints to control potential danger to self or others. Hypoactivity or clinically noticeable psychomotor slowing.	
Inappropriate speech or mood	Inappropriate, disorganized, or incoherent speech. Inappropriate display of emotion related to events or situation. Any of these scores 1 point.	
Sleep/wake cycle disturbance	Sleeping less than 4 h or waking frequently at night (do not consider wakefulness initiated by medical staff or loud environment). Sleeping during most of the day. Any of these scores 1 point.	
Symptom fluctuation	Fluctuation of the manifestation of any item or symptom over 24h scores 1 point.	

Total Score (0-8)

*Level of consciousness:
A—No response: score 0.
B—Response to intense and repeated stimulation (loud voice and pain): score 0.
C—Response to mild or moderate stimulation: score 1.
D—Normal wakefulness: score 0.
E—Exaggerated response to normal stimulation: score 1.

mood, sleep/wake cycle disturbances, and fluctuation of these symptoms. Each of the eight items is scored as absent or present (0 or 1), respectively, and summed. A score of 4 or above indicates delirium, while 0 indicates no delirium. Patients with scores between 1 and 3 are considered to have subsyndromal delirium,[50] which has worse prognostic implications than absence of delirium but a better prognosis than clearly present delirium.

The NEECHAM scale[47,48] consists of nine items divided over three subscales. Each item consists of three to six descriptions. Subscale 1 (information processing) measures attention, processing of commands, and orientation; subscale 2 (behavior) measures appearance, motor behavior, and verbal behavior; subscale 3 (physiologic condition) measures vital function, oxygen saturation, and urinary continence. The overall score of the NEECHAM ranges from 0 to 30 points. The scale gives four grades of outcome: moderate to severe confusion and/or delirium (0-19 points), mild to early confusion and/or delirium (20-24 points), "not confused" but at high risk of confusion and/or delirium (25-26 points), and normal cognitive functioning—that is, absence of confusion and/or delirium (27-30 points). This instrument does not perform well in mechanically ventilated patients.

Management

The development of effective evidence-based strategies and protocols for prevention and treatment of delirium awaits data from ongoing randomized clinical trials of both nonpharmacologic and pharmacologic strategies. Refer to Chapter 205 for a detailed description of management strategies of delirium, including an empirical sedation and delirium protocol. A brief overview is provided here.

When agitation or delirium develops in a previously comfortable patient, a search for the underlying cause should be undertaken before attempting pharmacologic intervention. A rapid assessment should be performed, including assessment of vital signs and physical examination, to rule out life-threatening problems (e.g., hypoxia, self-extubation, pneumothorax, hypotension) or other acutely reversible physiologic causes (e.g., hypoglycemia, metabolic acidosis, stroke, seizure, pain). The previously mentioned IWATCHDEATH and DELIRIUM mnemonics can be particularly helpful for guiding this initial evaluation.

Once life-threatening causes are ruled out as possible etiologies, aspects of good patient care, such as reorienting patients, improving sleep and hygiene, providing visual and hearing aids if previously used, removing medications that can provoke delirium, and decreasing the use of invasive devices if not required (e.g., bladder catheters, restraints), should be undertaken.

A "liberation" and "animation" strategy provides a good framework to reduce the incidence and duration of delirium.[51] "Liberation" utilizes sedation protocols, linked spontaneous awakening and breathing trials, and proper sedation regimens to reduce the harmful effects of sedative exposure. Data from the Maximizing Efficacy of Targeted Sedation and Reducing Neurological Dysfunction (MENDS)[52] study and the Safety and Efficacy of Dexmedetomidine Compared to Midazolam (SEDCOM) trial[53] support the view that dexmedetomidine can decrease the duration and prevalence of delirium when compared to lorazepam or midazolam. "Animation" refers to early mobilization of ICU patients, which has been shown to reduce delirium and improve neurocognitive and functional outcomes.[54]

Pharmacologic therapy should be attempted only after correcting any contributing factors or underlying physiologic abnormalities. Although these agents are intended to improve cognition, they all have psychoactive effects that can further cloud the sensorium and promote a longer overall duration of cognitive impairment. Patients who manifest delirium should be treated with a traditional antipsychotic medication; the SCCM guidelines[35] recommend haloperidol as the drug of choice. A recommended starting dose is 2 to 5 mg every 6 to 12 hours (IV or PO); the maximal effective doses are usually around 20 mg/day. Newer "atypical" antipsychotic agents (e.g., risperidone, ziprasidone, quetiapine, olanzapine) also may prove helpful for the treatment of delirium.[55]

Benzodiazepines are not recommended for the management of delirium because they can paradoxically exacerbate delirium. These drugs also can promote oversedation and respiratory suppression. However, they remain the drugs of choice for the treatment of delirium tremens (and other withdrawal syndromes) and seizures.

At times, mechanical restraints may be needed to ensure the safety of patients and staff while waiting for medications to take effect. It is important to keep in mind, however, that restraints can increase agitation and delirium, and their use may have adverse consequences, including strangulation, nerve injury, skin breakdown, and other complications of immobilization.

Summary

Agitation and delirium are very common in the ICU, where their occurrence puts patients at risk for self-injury and poor clinical outcomes. Available sedation and delirium monitoring instruments allow clinicians to recognize these forms of brain dysfunction. Through a systematic approach, life-threatening problems and other acutely reversible physiologic causes can be rapidly identified and remedied. A strategy that focuses on early liberation from mechanical ventilation and early mobilization can help reduce the burden of delirium. Use of antipsychotics should be reserved for patients at imminent risk to themselves or staff.

ANNOTATED REFERENCES

Ely EW, Shintani A, Truman B, et al. Delirium as a predictor of mortality in mechanically ventilated patients in the intensive care unit. JAMA 2004;291(14):1753-1762.
  This large cohort study showed that delirium in the ICU was an independent risk factor for death at 6 months, and that each day with delirium increased the hazards of dying by 10%.
Bergeron N, Dubois MJ, Dumont M, Dial S, Skrobik Y. Intensive Care Delirium Screening Checklist evaluation of a new screening tool. Intensive Care Med 2001;27(5):859-864.
  The ICDSC provides healthcare providers with an easy to use bedside delirium monitoring instrument that can be incorporated in to the daily work flow of bedside nurses. It provides an ability to diagnose subsyndromal delirium.
Pisani M, Kong S, Kasl S, Murphy T, Araujo K, Van Ness P. Days of delirium are associated with 1-year mortality in an older intensive care unit population. Am J Respir Crit Care Med 2009;180(11):1092-1097.
  This cohort study demonstrated a dose-response curve between days of delirium and the risk of dying at 1 year.
Ely EW, Inouye SK, Bernard GR, et al. Delirium in mechanically ventilated patients: validity and reliability of the confusion assessment method for the intensive care unit (CAM-ICU). JAMA 2001;286(21):2703-2710.
  A landmark study validating for the first time an easy to use bedside delirium-monitoring instrument for nonverbal mechanically ventilated patients. Delirium monitoring with the CAM-ICU can be performed in less than 2 minutes and does not require a psychiatrist.
Schweickert W, Pohlman M, Pohlman A, et al. Early physical and occupational therapy in mechanically ventilated, critically ill patients: a randomised controlled trial. Lancet 2009;373(9678):1874-1882.
  This is the only interventional study that tested a nonpharmacologic intervention—early mobility—in ICU patients and showed a reduction in delirium and improvements in functional outcomes.

REFERENCES

Access the complete reference list online at http://www.expertconsult.com.

3

Management of Acute Pain in the Intensive Care Unit

GUSTAVO ANGARAMO | PAUL JODKA | STEPHEN O. HEARD

Critically ill patients frequently experience acute pain, but assessment rates for pain remain below 40% in mechanically ventilated patients.[1] Pain and discomfort can have multiple causes in the intensive care unit (ICU) setting, including surgical and posttraumatic wounds, the use of invasive monitoring devices and mechanical ventilators, prolonged immobilization, and routine nursing care (e.g., dressing changes, airway suctioning).[1-3] *Pain* is defined by the International Association for the Study of Pain (IASP-1979) as "an unpleasant sensory and emotional experience associated with actual or potential tissue damage."[4] The experience of pain differs among patients, but the physiologic sequelae of inadequately treated pain are relatively predictable and potentially deleterious. Some physiologic responses to acute pain and stress are mediated by neuroendocrine activation and increased sympathetic tone. As a consequence, patients develop tachycardia, increased myocardial oxygen consumption, immunosuppression, hypercoagulability, persistent catabolism, and numerous other metabolic alterations.[5] Additional morbidity may be incurred by pain-related functional limitations such as impaired pulmonary mechanics[6] or delayed ambulation.

Acute Pain Assessment

The past decade has seen an increase in the number of scales and assessment tools for the evaluation of sedation and analgesia in ICU patients. Several sedation scales—the Richmond Agitation Sedation Scale (RASS), Adaptation to the Intensive Care Environment (ATICE) tool, and the Minnesota Sedation Assessment Tool (MSAT)—as well as tools for assessment of analgesia in the ICU, such as the visual analog scale, the numeric rating scale, behavioral pain scale,[7,8] and critical care pain observation scale, have been developed (Figure 3-1). The actual percentage of ICUs implementing formal sedation and analgesia protocols is approximately 50% in the United States. Unfortunately, many ICU patients cannot provide full (or even partial) information regarding their pain. However, the inability of ventilated, sedated ICU patients to report pain should not preclude pain management and does not rule out the possibility that the patients are experiencing pain.[9] Caregivers sometimes must use signs of heightened sympathetic activity like hypertension, tachycardia, lacrimation, diaphoresis, and restlessness as surrogate indicators for the presence of pain. Trends in such signs provide a measure of the success of a given intervention.

Options for Acute Pain Therapy

Acute pain is triggered by stimulation of peripheral nociceptors in the skin or deeper structures and is a complex process involving multiple mediators at various levels of the neuraxis (Figure 3-2).[4] Different parts of the pain pathway can be targeted either individually or as part of a comprehensive strategy aimed at multiple sites for additive or synergistic effects. Thus, nociception can be influenced (1) peripherally by the use of nonsteroidal antiinflammatory drugs (NSAIDs) and nerve blocks, (2) at the spinal cord level by the use of epidural or intrathecal medications, and (3) centrally by the use of systemic medications.

NONSTEROIDAL ANTIINFLAMMATORY DRUGS

Drugs in this class inhibit cyclooxygenase (COX) enzymes, which are involved in synthesis of prostaglandins and related inflammatory mediators in response to injury. COX-1 is a constitutive enzyme that is present in most tissues and, through the production of prostaglandins E_2 and I_2, serves homeostatic and protective functions.[10] COX-2 is an inducible enzyme that is expressed in response to inflammation. NSAIDs are commonly used in conjunction with other agents such as opioids to take advantage of different side-effect profiles and possible synergistic efficacy. As a class, NSAIDs can cause adverse effects that include nausea, gastrointestinal (GI) bleeding, inhibition of platelet function, operative site bleeding, renal insufficiency, and bronchospasm in aspirin-sensitive patients (triad of asthma, nasal polyposis, and aspirin allergy).[2,4]

Ketorolac tromethamine (Toradol) is the only parenteral NSAID available in the United States. It has been shown to reduce postoperative opioid requirements and does not cause respiratory depression.[11] However, prolonged use has been associated with a significant incidence of the aforementioned side effects (primarily GI bleeding and renal failure)[12]; consequently, ketorolac therapy should be limited to a maximum of 5 days.[2] In addition, ketorolac should be used at decreased dosages or avoided altogether in patients at higher risk of such complications (e.g., advanced age, hypovolemia, preexisting renal insufficiency). This caution also applies to enterally administered NSAIDs.

Selective COX-2 inhibitors like celecoxib (Celebrex) are available for enteral administration, and injectable COX-2 agents are being studied primarily for the management of acute postoperative pain.[10] The main advantage of these agents over their nonselective relatives lies in the promise of decreased GI side effects.[10] A joint meeting of the U.S. Food and Drug Administration (FDA) Arthritis Advisory Committee and the Drug Safety and Risk Management Advisory Committee reaffirmed that COX-2 inhibitors are important treatment options for pain management and that the preponderance of data demonstrate that the cardiovascular risk associated with celecoxib is similar to that associated with commonly used older nonspecific NSAIDs.[13]

Acetaminophen is a paraaminophenol derivative with analgesic and antipyretic properties similar to those of aspirin. The mechanism of action of acetaminophen is still poorly defined. Recent evidence has suggested that it may selectively act as an inhibitor of prostaglandin synthesis in the central nervous system (CNS) rather than in the periphery. A meta-analysis of randomized controlled trials of acetaminophen for postoperative pain revealed that this analgesic induced a morphine-sparing effect of 20% (9 mg) over the first 24 hours postoperatively but did not reduce the incidence of morphine-related adverse effects.[14] It was concluded that acetaminophen may be a viable alternative to NSAIDs in high-risk patients because of the lower incidence of adverse effects. Therefore, it may be appropriate to administer acetaminophen with NSAIDs or COX-2 inhibitors, since the analgesics in these two classes may act additively or synergistically to improve analgesia.[15]

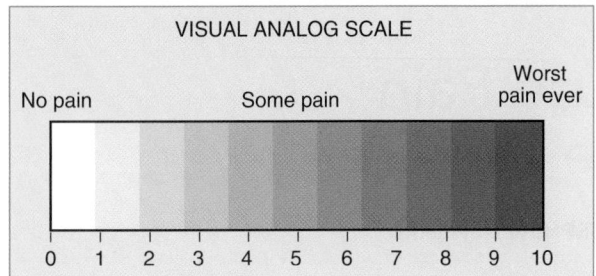

Figure 3-1 Visual analog scale. Pain can be rated between 0 (no pain) and 10 (extreme pain). Use of a graphic such as this allows an intubated patient to indicate his or her level of discomfort by pointing. Other scales use cartoon faces that are either smiling or frowning. (*From Higgins TL, Jodka PG, Farid A. Pharmacologic approaches to sedation, pain relief and neuromuscular blockade in the intensive care unit. Part II. Clin Intensive Care. 2003;14[3-4]:91-98.*)

OPIOID ANALGESICS

A number of opioids are available (Table 3-1), and this drug class remains the mainstay of ICU analgesia. Morphine, hydromorphone (Dilaudid), and fentanyl are commonly used in ICUs in the United States and have been recommended as first-line narcotic analgesics.[2] Opioids bind to a variable degree with opioid receptor subtypes (μ, δ, κ) located in the brain, spinal cord, and peripheral sites and modulate the transmission and processing of nociceptive signals.[4] The clinical and pharmacologic properties of opioids depend on several variables: chemical and solubility properties, dosing regimen, patient characteristics (Box 3-1), and presence of active metabolites. Drugs that are often thought of as short acting (e.g., fentanyl) actually have a

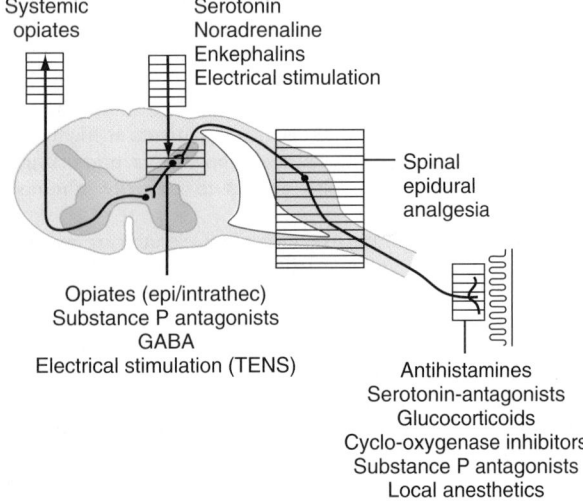

Figure 3-2 "Map" of the path of nociceptive information from periphery to central nervous system. Modification of information can occur at any point of information transfer. GABA, gamma-aminobutyric acid; TENS, transcutaneous electrical nerve stimulation. (*From Kehlet H. Modification of responses to surgery by neural blockade: clinical implications. In: Cousins MJ, Bridenbaugh PO, editors. Neural blockade in clinical anesthesia and pain management. 2nd ed. Philadelphia: Lippincott; 1988:145.*)

Box 3-1

FACTORS INFLUENCING NARCOTIC PHARMACOKINETICS

Age (increased sensitivity in elderly)
Acid-base status (increased arterial pH increases brain penetration)
Cardiopulmonary bypass (prolongs elimination half-life)
Liver disease
Renal disease (active metabolites may accumulate)
Other CNS depressants
Acute and chronic tolerance

markedly prolonged duration of action if given repeatedly or as an infusion (Figure 3-3).

Opioids are excellent analgesics, but they are not amnestic agents. As a class, opioids can suppress respiratory drive and promote sedation, GI symptoms (ileus, nausea and vomiting, constipation), urinary retention, pruritus, or hypotension. Morphine can cause hypotension by triggering the release of histamine and by the ablation of pain-mediated sympathetic stimulation. In actual practice, however, opioids are relatively neutral in their hemodynamic effects, so long as they are used judiciously in euvolemic patients.

Opioids are most commonly administered intravenously in critically ill patients and titrated to effect, either on a scheduled, intermittent basis or as a continuous infusion following a loading dose to achieve analgesia.[2] This strategy avoids concerns regarding unpredictable bioavailability associated with intramuscular, enteral, or transdermal administration and favors more stable analgesic drug concentrations. The benefits of administering analgesics (and sedatives) in such a fashion must be balanced against the possibility of unintentional excessive dosing, which may result in prolonged mechanical ventilation and longer hospital stays.[1] It has been reported, however, that scheduled daily interruption of sedative-analgesic drug infusions can help minimize this problem and may actually lead to a shorter duration of mechanical ventilation and a shorter ICU stay.[16,17]

Morphine is a naturally occurring narcotic analgesic.[2] It is metabolized mainly by the liver to an active compound (morphine-6-glucuronide) that can cause a prolonged drug effect in patients with renal insufficiency. Onset of action after intravenous (IV) administration is relatively slow (5-10 minutes) owing to low lipid solubility, and the duration of clinical effect is long enough to permit its use as either an intermittent injection or an infusion. Dosing requirements vary significantly from patient to patient and must be individualized (see Table 3-1).

Hydromorphone is a semisynthetic narcotic. Compared to morphine, hydromorphone has a similar duration of action, is a more potent analgesic, does not release histamine, and lacks an active metabolite. These properties make it an attractive alternative to morphine in patients with hemodynamic instability or significant renal impairment.[2] Hydromorphone is also best administered by either infusion or intermittent injection.

Fentanyl is a synthetic narcotic with a potency about 100 times that of morphine. Fentanyl has no active metabolites and generally has minimal effects on hemodynamics. It is very lipophilic, leading to a rapid onset of action. Fentanyl can accumulate in fat, giving rise to a prolonged drug effect, if it is given in very high doses or for a lengthy period, even in patients without significant renal or hepatic dysfunction.[2]

TABLE 3-1	Commonly Used Opioids			
Agent	*Intermittent Dose*	*Continuous Dose*	*Metabolism*	*Precautions*
Fentanyl	0.35-1.5 μg/kg IV q 0.5-1 h	0.7-10 μg/kg/h	Oxidation	Rigidity with high doses
Hydromorphone	10-30 μg/kg IV q 1-2 h	7-15 μg/kg/h	Glucuronidation	
Morphine	0.01-0.15 mg/kg IV q 1-2 h	0.07-0.5 mg/kg/h	Glucuronidation	Histamine release

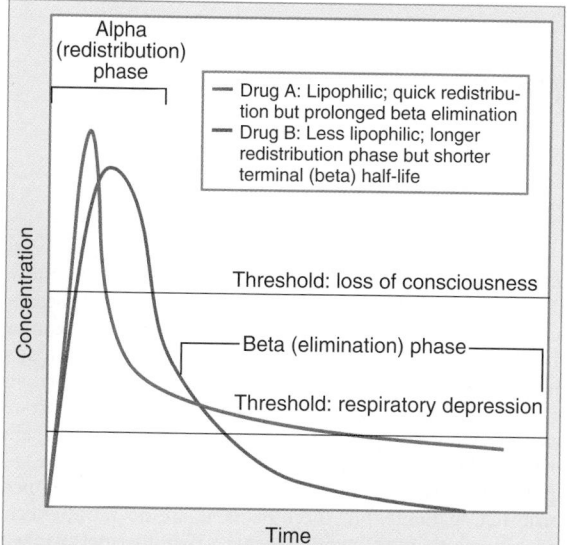

Figure 3-3 Pharmacokinetics. A lipophilic drug (drug A) may have a rapid onset and an initially quick distribution but a prolonged beta-elimination (metabolism) phase, resulting in respiratory depression with repeated doses or constant infusion. A less lipophilic drug (drug B) may take longer to redistribute, giving the impression of a prolonged initial duration of action, but it does not accumulate, owing to a shorter elimination half-life. Fentanyl is like drug A, whereas morphine is similar to drug B. *(From Higgins TL, Jodka PG, Farid A. Pharmacologic approaches to sedation, pain relief and neuromuscular blockade in the intensive care unit. Part II. Clin Intensive Care 2003;14[3-4]:91-98.)*

N-METHYL-D-ASPARTATE RECEPTOR ANTAGONIST

Ketamine has been a well-known general anesthetic and analgesic for the past 3 decades. With the discovery of the *N*-methyl-D-aspartate receptor (NMDAR) and its links to nociceptive pain transmission and central sensitization, there has been renewed interest in utilizing ketamine as a potential antihyperalgesic agent. Ketamine is a noncompetitive NMDAR antagonist. Although high doses (>2 mg/kg) of ketamine have been implicated in causing psychomimetic effects (excessive sedation, cognitive dysfunction, hallucinations, nightmares), subanesthetic or low doses (<1 mg/kg) of ketamine have demonstrated significant analgesic efficacy without these side effects. Furthermore, there is no evidence to indicate that low doses of ketamine exert any adverse pharmacologic effects related to respiration or cardiovascular function. Low doses of ketamine have not been associated with development of nausea, vomiting, urinary retention, or impaired intestinal motility.

Ketamine in combination with either parenteral or epidural opioids not only reduces postoperative opioid consumption but also prolongs and improves analgesia.[18,19,20] However, despite the opioid-sparing effect observed with the administration of ketamine, no reduction in opioid-related side effects has been documented.

ALPHA-2 ADRENERGIC AGONISTS

In addition to the opiate system, alpha-2 (α_2) adrenergic activation represents another inherent pain-control network in the CNS. The α_2-adrenergic receptor exists in the substantia gelatinosa of the dorsal horn, which is a primary site of action by which this class of drugs can inhibit somatic pain. This receptor system also exists in the brain, where stimulation of it can produce sedation. Cardiovascular depression from α_2-adrenergic agonists can occur at both brain and spinal cord sites. These side effects of sedation and sympathetic inhibition limit α_2-adrenergic agonists to only an adjuvant role as analgesics.

Clonidine was originally used to control blood pressure (BP) and heart rate. It binds to α_2-adrenergic and imidazole receptors in the CNS. It has been hypothesized that clonidine acts at α_2-adrenergic receptors in the spinal cord to stimulate acetylcholine release, which acts at both muscarinic and nicotinic receptor subtypes for postoperative pain relief. Clonidine can be administered by oral, IV, or transdermal routes.[21]

NEURAXIAL ANALGESIC TECHNIQUES

The administration of narcotics, local anesthetics, and other agents via intrathecal or epidural catheters targets the processing of pain signals at the level of the spinal cord or nerve root.[4] The use of epidural catheters for regional analgesia in ICU patients may be quite useful, assuming that the pain pattern is regionalized and that there are no contraindications to catheter placement (e.g., coagulopathy, uncontrolled infection, unstable spinal skeletal structures). In some patients, epidural analgesia may be preferable to intravenously administered medications, because this approach affords dense regional pain control[4,22] while largely avoiding the sedative and respiratory side effects of systemic medications.[22,23]

PERIPHERAL NERVE BLOCKS

Peripheral nerve blocks are an attractive method of providing postoperative analgesia for many orthopedic surgical procedures. Compared with general anesthesia, the use of peripheral nerve blocks achieved by either a single injection or by continuous infusion via a catheter for orthopedic anesthesia/analgesia has been associated with faster recovery times and decreased hospital readmission rates.[24]

On the basis of a recent meta-analysis,[25,26] continuous peripheral analgesic techniques provide superior analgesia, reduce opioid consumption, and reduce opioid-related side effects (nausea and vomiting, sedation, pruritus). This technique is not commonly used in the ICU setting, but it opens a wide range of possibilities for the future treatment of acute pain in critically ill patients.

ANNOTATED REFERENCES

Payen JF, Bosson JL, Chanques G, Mantz J, Labarere J for the DOLOREA investigators. Pain assessment is associated with decreased duration of mechanical ventilation in the intensive care unit. A post hoc analysis of the DOLOREA Study. Anesthesiology 2009;111(6):1187-8.

This is a prospective, multicenter, observational study of mechanically ventilated patients who received analgesia on day 2 of their ICU stay. Pain assessment in this ICU population was associated with a reduction in the duration of ventilator support and ICU stay. This might be related to higher concomitant rates of sedation assessments and a restricted use of hypnotic drugs when pain was assessed.

Kumar A, Brennan T. Pain assessment, sedation, and analgesic administration in the intensive care unit. Anesthesiology 2009;111(6):1308-16.

The author analyzes the recent DOLOREA study out of France and concludes that pain assessment seems to reduce sedative drug dosing, allowing for objective pain evaluation and analgesic drug dosing based on patient report, reducing ventilator days and duration of ICU stay.

Richman JM, Liu SS, Courpas G, et al. Does continuous peripheral nerve block provide superior pain control to opioids? A meta-analysis. Anesth Analg 2006;102(1):248-57.

The authors reviewed 236 articles, all of them randomized control trials that compared continuous peripheral nerve block (CPNB) analgesia with opioids for the management of postoperative pain. CPNB analgesia,

regardless of catheter location, provided superior postoperative analgesia and fewer opioid-related side effects when compared with opioid analgesia.

Gilron I, Milne B, Hong M. Cyclooxygenase-2 inhibitors in postoperative pain management: current evidence and future directions. Anesthesiology 2003;99(5):1198-208.

An up-to-date review of COX-2 inhibitors for analgesia in the postoperative period.

Jacobi J, Fraser GL, Coursin DB, et al. Clinical practice guidelines for the sustained use of sedatives and analgesics in the critically ill adult. Crit Care Med 2002;30(1):119-41.

A review of pain assessment and analgesic therapy in the critically ill patient, promulgated by a task force of the American College of Critical Care Medicine of the Society of Critical Care Medicine. Recommendations are made (and graded) based on a critical evaluation of the literature.

Kress JP, Pohlman AS, O'Connor MF, Hall JB. Daily interruption of sedative infusions in critically ill patients undergoing mechanical ventilation. N Engl J Med 2000;342(20):1471-7.

A classic study showing that the daily interruption of sedatives and analgesics can decrease the duration of mechanical ventilation.

REFERENCES

Access the complete reference list online at http://www.expertconsult.com.

4

Fever and Hypothermia

MITCHELL P. FINK

Fever is defined as an increase in body temperature. Normal body temperature is 36.8°C ± 0.4°C. Normally body temperature varies in a circadian fashion by about 0.6°C, being lowest in the morning and highest in the late afternoon or early evening. In 1998, the Society of Critical Care Medicine and Infectious Disease Society of America suggested that is "reasonable in many ICUs to consider all patients with temperatures ≥ 38.3°C to be febrile, warranting special attention to determine if infection is present."[1]

Fever is triggered by the release of various cytokines—notably, interleukin 1-beta (IL-1β), tumor necrosis factor (TNF), and interleukin 6 (IL-6)—that are capable of up-regulating expression of the enzyme cyclooxygenase (COX)-2 and thereby causing secretion of prostaglandin E_2 (PGE_2) in the hypothalamus.[2] PGE_2 binds to prostaglandin receptors located on a cluster of neurons in the preoptic region of the hypothalamus. Although there are four subtypes of PGE_2 receptors, only one, PGE_2 receptor 3 (EPR3), is required for the development of fever in response to IL-1β, lipopolysaccharide (LPS), or PGE_2.[2] Activation of EPR3 triggers a number of neurohumoral and physiologic changes that lead to increased body temperature. The antipyretic effects of various nonsteroidal antiinflammatory drugs (NSAIDs) such as aspirin and ibuprofen is due to inhibition of COX-2-dependent PGE_2 biosynthesis in the central nervous system (CNS). The mechanism whereby acetaminophen reduces fever is probably independent of COX-2 inhibition and remains controversial and poorly understood.[3,4]

Body temperature can be measured using an oral, axillary, or rectal mercury-filled glass thermometer. These traditional approaches, however, have been largely replaced by a variety of safer and more environmentally friendly methods that use thermistors located on catheters or probes situated in the pulmonary artery, distal esophagus, urinary bladder, or external ear canal.[3] Infrared detectors can also be used to measure tympanic membrane temperature. Forehead skin temperature can be measured using a temperature-sensitive patch.

Fever is a cardinal sign of infection. Accordingly, the new onset of fever should trigger a careful diagnostic evaluation, looking for a source of infection. The diagnostic evaluation should be thorough and tailored to the recent history of the patient. For example, the possibility of a CNS infection should receive greater attention in a patient with recent or ongoing CNS instrumentation. By the same token, if a patient recently underwent a gastrointestinal surgical procedure, the clinician should have a high index of suspicion for an intraabdominal source of infection. Key elements in the assessment of new-onset fever in the intensive care unit (ICU) are listed in Box 4-1. Common sources of infection in ICU patients are listed in Box 4-2.

Although fever in the ICU is most commonly due to infection, myriad noninfectious causes of systemic inflammation (Box 4-3) can also result in hyperthermia. Some authors claim that noninfectious causes of fever rarely result in a core temperature above 38.9°C[5,6] but rigorous data in support of this view are lacking. Still, infections are rarely if ever associated with core temperatures over 41.1°C. When the core temperature is this high, the clinician should suspect malignant hyperthermia, neuroleptic malignant syndrome, or heat stroke.

In general, fever should not be treated with antipyretics. This view is founded on data that suggest that hyperthermia is an adaptive response that enhances the host's ability to fight infection.[7,8] In addition, body temperature is an unreliable clinical parameter when patients are receiving antipyretic therapy. These considerations notwithstanding, antipyretic therapy should be administered to selected patients with fever, among them patients with acute coronary syndromes (i.e., myocardial infarction or unstable angina), because the tachycardia that usually accompanies the febrile response can exacerbate imbalances between myocardial oxygen delivery and demand. Febrile patients with head trauma, subarachnoid hemorrhage, or stroke should receive antipyretics to prevent temperature-related increases in cerebral oxygen utilization. Children with temperatures higher than 40°C or with a history of seizures should also be treated.

Hypothermia blankets are often used to lower the core temperature in febrile ICU patients, but these blankets are no more effective in cooling patients than antipyretic agents.[9] Hypothermia blankets can cause large temperature fluctuations and are associated with rebound hyperthermia when removed.[8] Additionally, external cooling can augment hypermetabolism and actually promote persistent fever. Lenhardt and colleagues demonstrated that active external cooling in volunteers with induced fever increased oxygen consumption by 35% to 40% and was associated with a significant increase in circulating epinephrine and norepinephrine concentrations.[10]

In view of those phenomena, when treatment of fever is warranted, administration of an antipyretic agent is the recommended approach. Commonly used antipyretics include isoform nonselective COX inhibitors, such as ibuprofen or aspirin, or acetaminophen. Because corticosteroids (hydrocortisone, methylprednisolone) are potent antiinflammatory agents, these drugs can suppress the febrile response to infection. Other antiinflammatory agents have a similar effect, so absence of fever should not be used to rule out infection, especially in patients receiving corticosteroids or other potent antiinflammatory drugs.

A reasonable approach for evaluating fever in ICU patients was described by Marik.[4] As depicted in Figure 4-1, blood cultures should be obtained whenever an ICU patient develops a new fever. The sensitivity of blood cultures for detecting bacteremia depends to a large extent on the volume of blood inoculated into culture media. Whenever possible, at least 10 to 15 mL of blood should be withdrawn and inoculated into 2 or 3 bottles or tubes at a ratio of 1 mL of blood per 5 mL of medium.[1]

A comprehensive physical examination should be carried out, and a chest x-ray obtained and reviewed. Noninfectious causes of fever should be excluded. In patients with an obvious focus of infection, a directed diagnostic evaluation is necessary. However, if there is no obvious source of infection and the patient is not deteriorating clinically, it is reasonable to obtain blood cultures and observe the patient for 48 hours before ordering additional diagnostic studies or starting empirical antibiotics. This approach is not reasonable, however, if new fever is accompanied by other signs of worsening clinical status such as arterial hypotension, oliguria, increasing confusion, rising serum lactate concentration, falling platelet count, or worsening coagulopathy. Nor is this approach reasonable if the core temperature is above 39°C but below 41.1°C. Patients in this category should receive empirical antimicrobial chemotherapy while aggressive attempts are made to diagnose the source of infection. All febrile neutropenic patients should receive broad-spectrum empirical antimicrobial chemotherapy after appropriate cultures are obtained.

Intravascular catheters are commonly suspected as a source of infection and fever in ICU patients; they can cause fever due to localized or systemic (bloodstream) infection. In patients with new-onset fever without other ominous signs (e.g., hypotension, profound thrombocytopenia, acute respiratory distress syndrome), it is unnecessary to

KEY ELEMENTS IN THE EVALUATION OF NEW-ONSET FEVER IN ICU PATIENTS

- Be familiar with the patient's history. Pay particular attention to possible predisposing causes of fever.
- Perform a careful physical examination. Pay particular attention to surgical wounds and vascular access sites. Look for evidence of pressure-induced skin ulceration. In patients with recent median sternotomy, evaluate the stability of the chest closure. Perform a careful abdominal examination.
- Obtain or review a recent chest x-ray, looking for evidence of new infiltrates or effusions.
- Obtain appropriate laboratory studies. At a minimum, these studies should include a peripheral white blood cell count and cultures of blood and urine. If the patient is endotracheally intubated or has a tracheotomy, obtain a sample of sputum for Gram stain. In some centers, sputum is routinely cultured. In other centers, bronchoalveolar lavage or bronchial brushing for quantitative microbiology is performed using blind or bronchoscopic methods.

- Central venous catheters that have been in place for longer than 96 hours should be removed. The tip should be submitted for semiquantitative microbiology.
- In patients receiving antibiotics for more than 3 days, a stool sample should be analyzed for the presence of *Clostridium difficile* toxin.
- More extensive diagnostic evaluation should be considered in a graded fashion based on history, physical examination findings, laboratory results, persistence of fever despite presumably appropriate antimicrobial chemotherapy, or clinical instability. These additional tests and procedures include diagnostic thoracentesis, paracentesis, and lumbar puncture. Imaging studies should be considered, including abdominal or cardiac ultrasonography and head, chest, or abdominal computed tomography.

COMMON INFECTIOUS CAUSES OF FEVER

Central Nervous System
Meningitis
Encephalitis
Brain abscess
Epidural abscess

Head and Neck
Acute suppurative parotitis
Acute sinusitis
Parapharyngeal and retropharyngeal space infections
Acute suppurative otitis media

Cardiovascular
Catheter-related infection
Endocarditis

Pulmonary and Mediastinal
Pneumonia
Empyema
Mediastinitis

Hepatobiliary and Gastrointestinal
Diverticulitis
Appendicitis
Peritonitis (spontaneous or secondary)
Intraperitoneal abscess
Perirectal abscess

Infected pancreatitis
Acute cholecystitis
Cholangitis
Hepatic abscess
Acute viral hepatitis

Genitourinary
Bacterial or fungal cystitis
Pyelonephritis
Perinephric abscess
Tubo-ovarian abscess
Endometritis
Prostatitis

Breast
Mastitis
Breast abscess

Cutaneous and Muscular
Cellulitis
Suppurative wound infection
Necrotizing fasciitis
Bacterial myositis or myonecrosis
Herpes zoster

Osseous
Osteomyelitis

NONINFECTIOUS CAUSES OF FEVER

Central Nervous System
Subarachnoid hemorrhage
Intracerebral hemorrhage
Infarction

Cardiac
Myocardial infarction
Pericarditis

Pulmonary
Atelectasis
Pulmonary embolism
Fibroproliferative phase of acute respiratory distress syndrome

Hepatobiliary and Gastrointestinal
Acalculous cholecystitis
Acute pancreatitis
Active Crohn's disease
Toxic megacolon
Alcoholic hepatitis

Rheumatologic Syndromes
Vasculitides (e.g., polyarteritis nodosa, temporal arteritis, Wegener's syndrome)

Systemic lupus erythematosus
Rheumatoid arthritis
Goodpasture's syndrome

Endocrine
Hyperthyroidism
Adrenal insufficiency
Pheochromocytoma

Other
Drug reactions ("drug fever")
Transfusion reactions
Neoplasms (especially lymphoma, hepatoma, renal cell carcinoma)
Malignant hyperthermia
Neuroleptic malignant syndrome
Serotonin syndrome
Opioid withdrawal syndrome
Ethanol withdrawal syndrome
Transient endotoxemia or bacteremia associated with procedures
Devitalized tissue secondary to trauma
Hematoma

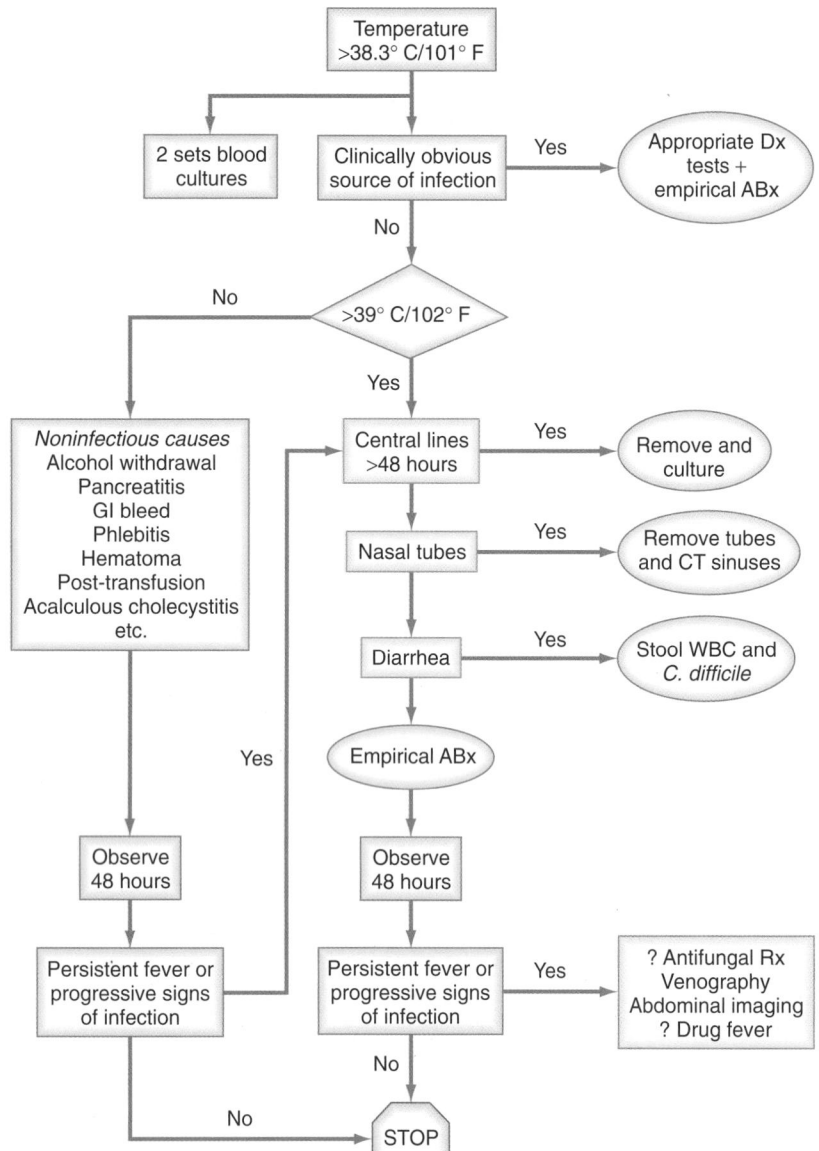

Figure 4-1 Approach to evaluating patients with fever in the intensive care unit. ABx, antibiotics; CT, computed tomography; Dx, diagnostic; GI, gastrointestinal; Rx, prescription; WBC, white blood cell. *(From Marik PE. Fever in the ICU. Chest. 2000;117(3):855-869.)*

remove all intravascular catheters. In contrast, if one or more of these (or other ominous) signs is present, the most prudent course of action is to remove all vascular access catheters, including tunneled and/or cuffed devices, and culture the tips using semiquantitative methods on solid media.[1]

Fever is a common feature of the systemic inflammatory response syndrome (SIRS), irrespective of whether the underlying cause is infectious or noninfectious.[11] Procalcitonin, a precursor of the polypeptide hormone, calcitonin, has been studied extensively as a circulating marker that can be used to differentiate infectious from noninfectious causes of SIRS in ICU or emergency department patients. Although enthusiasm for this approach for determining the presence of sepsis (i.e., SIRS plus infection) was initially high, one recent meta-analysis

suggested that the performance of this test is low, and that measurements of procalcitonin are unreliable for distinguishing infectious from noninfectious causes of SIRS in critically ill adult patients.[12] In contrast to these findings, another recent meta-analysis, which had looser criteria for the inclusion of studies, concluded that "procalcitonin represents a good biological diagnostic marker for sepsis, severe sepsis, or septic shock."[13] At present, therefore, it seems likely that measurements of procalcitonin might be a useful adjunct for the evaluation of fever in ICU patients, but this assay is not a replacement for other key diagnostic modalities: careful physical examination; chest x-ray; assessment of sputum Gram stain findings; and appropriate cultures of blood, urine, and sputum or bronchoalveolar lavage fluid.

REFERENCES

Access the complete reference list online at http://www.expertconsult.com.

5

Very High Systemic Arterial Blood Pressure

MICHAEL DONAHOE

The Joint National Committee (JNC) on Prevention, Detection, Evaluation, and Treatment of High Blood Pressure has defined two acute conditions of elevated systemic arterial pressure.[1] A *hypertensive emergency* is characterized by the presence of elevated systemic blood pressure (BP) and new or progressive end-organ damage, including but not limited to the cardiac, renal, and central nervous systems. A hypertensive emergency is an infrequent clinical situation that requires immediate BP reduction (not necessarily to normal ranges). Although the absolute BP elevation is not a criterion for the diagnosis, a hypertensive emergency is typically associated with a diastolic blood pressure (DBP) above 120 mm Hg. If unrecognized or left untreated, hypertensive emergencies can lead to acute myocardial infarction (MI), pulmonary edema from left ventricular (LV) dysfunction, hypertensive encephalopathy (HE), intracranial hemorrhage, microangiopathic hemolysis, and/or acute renal failure (Box 5-1).

In contrast, a critically elevated BP without evidence for acute and progressive dysfunction of target organs is termed a *hypertensive urgency*. In patients with hypertensive urgency, a more gradual reduction of BP over several hours to days is the goal, as there is no proven benefit to more rapid reduction of BP in asymptomatic patients. Furthermore, cerebral or myocardial ischemia is induced by aggressive antihypertensive therapy if the BP falls below a level needed for adequate tissue perfusion.

Using JNC definitions, hypertensive crises (urgency and emergency) account for more than 25% of all patient visits to a medical section of an emergency department (ED), with hypertensive emergencies accounting for one-third of the cases.[2] Central nervous system (CNS) complications are the most prevalent organ system dysfunction, followed by cardiovascular dysfunction. The incidence of the disorder has remained stable at 2 to 3 cases per 100,000 population over many decades, although the prognosis associated with aggressive medical management has improved significantly.[3] Most commonly, hypertensive emergencies occur in the setting of uncontrolled or unknown chronic hypertension. Hypertensive emergencies also may develop as secondary hypertension in association with such diverse etiologies as renal vascular disease, sleep apnea, hyperaldosteronism, pheochromocytoma, and pregnancy (preeclampsia).[4] Postoperative hypertension occurs most often following vascular surgery procedures in patients with a background history of hypertension. Untreated postoperative hypertension can contribute to postoperative bleeding in addition to the recognized complications of hypertensive emergencies.

Additional terms used by clinicians to describe very high systemic arterial BP include *accelerated hypertension*, which is a severely elevated BP associated with retinal findings of ocular hemorrhages and exudates. The term *malignant hypertension* includes severe hypertension with the presence of ocular hemorrhages and exudates with papilledema (grade IV Kimmelstiel-Wilson retinopathy). Vascular injury to the kidney in this setting is termed *malignant nephrosclerosis*. The term *hypertensive emergency* is preferred, as end-organ dysfunction can occur in the patient with hypertension in the absence of retinal findings.[5,6]

Pathophysiology

An acute elevation in systemic arterial BP most fundamentally involves an increase in systemic vascular resistance. This increase in vascular resistance is attributed to a complex interaction of circulating and local vascular mediators. Vasoconstriction is promoted by circulating catecholamines, angiotensin II (ATII), vasopressin, thromboxane (TxA_2), and/or endothelin 1 (ET1). In contrast, compensatory production of local counterregulatory vasodilators, including nitric oxide (NO) and prostacyclin (PGI_2), is inadequate to maintain homeostatic balance. This unregulated vasoconstriction promotes further endothelial dysfunction. A proinflammatory response, incorporating cytokine secretion, monocyte activation, and up-regulated expression of endothelial adhesion molecules, appears to occur in hypertensive emergencies, leading to promotion of endothelial hyperpermeability and activation of coagulation cascades.[7] This cascade of intravascular events leads to the characteristic pathologic findings of obliterative vascular lesions. These vascular changes, evident to the clinician by examination of the retina, are mirrored by changes in the kidney, leading to a proliferative arteritis, and in advanced stages of the process, fibrinoid necrosis. Relative ischemia results in affected organs, leading to end-organ dysfunction. Early control of elevated BP is critical to prevent progression to a more advanced stage of the disease process.

Aggressive control of elevated systemic arterial BP must be undertaken with caution, however. The potential adverse effects of aggressive BP control have been most carefully considered in the cerebral circulation. Normally, cerebrovascular arteriolar tone is adjusted over a range of cerebral perfusion pressures in order to maintain a constant cerebral blood flow (CBF). Increases in cerebral perfusion pressure (CPP) promote an increase in vascular resistance, whereas decreases in CPP act to vasodilate the cerebral vasculature. In normal individuals, constant flow is therefore maintained over a range of mean arterial pressure (MAP) from approximately 60 mm Hg to 150 mm Hg.[8] As MAP increases to values over 180 mm Hg, or the upper limit of autoregulation, cerebral hyperperfusion can occur, resulting in cerebral edema. Conversely, when CPP falls below the lower limit of autoregulation, CBF decreases, and tissue ischemia may occur. In patients with long-standing hypertension, a rightward shift of the CPP-CBF relationship occurs such that the lower limit of autoregulation occurs at a value higher than in normal subjects.[9] Comparative studies in hypertensive and normotensive patients suggest that the lower limit of autoregulation is about 20% below the resting MAP for both, although the absolute value is higher for hypertensive patients.[10] These data support the common recommendation for a maximum BP reduction in the acute setting of 20% to 25% of the MAP from the highest values, or a DBP goal typically in the 100 to 110 mm Hg range. This regulated level of BP reduction should maintain critical organ perfusion even for patients with long-standing hypertension.

Although the aggressiveness and timing of treatment are guided by the classification of hypertensive emergency versus urgency, the specific approach to the patient with hypertensive emergency is influenced significantly by the associated organ dysfunction. A few of the more common clinical examples will be reviewed.

Cerebrovascular Disease

HYPERTENSIVE ENCEPHALOPATHY

Acute elevations in systemic arterial BP can lead to HE, resulting from a failure of the upper level of cerebral vascular autoregulation. The most common clinical manifestations include headache, nausea and

---

HYPERTENSIVE EMERGENCIES

Cerebrovascular
Hypertensive encephalopathy
Acute ischemic stroke
Intracerebral hemorrhage

Cardiovascular
Acute coronary syndrome
Acute LV dysfunction
Acute aortic dissection

Renovascular Diseases
Acute glomerulonephritis
Renovascular hypertension
Scleroderma renal crisis
Post kidney transplantation

Endocrine Diseases
Pheochromocytoma
Cushing syndrome
Primary hyperaldosteronism

Drug Related
Cocaine
Amphetamine
MAOI-tyramine interaction
Antihypertensive withdrawal
Alpha—stimulant intoxication

Miscellaneous Conditions
Autonomic hyperactivity (Guillain-Barré syndrome)
Eclampsia/preeclampsia
Postoperative hypertension
Systemic vasculitis

LV, Left ventricular.

---

vomiting, visual disturbances, focal neurologic findings, or seizures. If left untreated, the condition can progress to coma and death. The majority of patients with HE will have a MAP significantly above the patient's baseline BP, although not always in the range typically associated with hypertensive emergency. Retinal findings including arteriolar spasm, exudates, hemorrhages, and papilledema are often present but are not required to establish the diagnosis. Magnetic resonance imaging (MRI) studies show a characteristic edema pattern involving the subcortical white matter of the parietooccipital regions; this finding is termed *posterior leukoencephalopathy*.[11] Best appreciated on T2-weighted images, posterior structures including the cerebellum, brainstem, and occasionally the cortex also can be affected. The findings typically are bilateral but can be asymmetric. The electroencephalogram (EEG) can show loss of the posterior dominant alpha rhythm, generalized slowing, and posterior epileptiform discharges, which resolve after appropriate therapy.[12]

In general, the neurologic symptoms of stroke or intracranial hemorrhage have a more acute onset than those associated with HE. The diagnosis of HE is confirmed by the absence of other conditions and the prompt resolution of symptoms and neuroimaging abnormalities with effective BP control. No improvement within 6 to 12 hours of BP reduction should prompt a search for an alternative cause of the mental status changes. In the majority of cases, the condition is entirely reversible with no observable adverse outcomes.

ACUTE STROKE

Hypertension is present in as many as 80% of patients with acute stroke, particularly in patients with preexisting hypertension. The incidence is higher among patients with primary intracerebral hemorrhage as compared to ischemic disorders.[13] The acute high systemic arterial BP most frequently declines to normal within 48 hours of presentation. The relationship between BP and mortality in patients with stroke may be "U-shaped." According to this notion, systolic BP

(SBP) values above or below 140 to 180 mm Hg are associated with increased mortality. In the International Stroke Trial, SBP above 200 mm Hg was associated with an increased risk of recurrent ischemic stroke (50% greater risk of recurrence), while low BP (particularly <120 mm Hg) was associated with an excess number of deaths from coronary heart disease.[14]

A number of important clinical features complicate the management of hypertension in acute stroke. First, during acute stroke, cerebral autoregulation may be compromised in ischemic tissue, and lowering of BP may further compromise CBF and extend ischemic injury. Second, medications used to treat hypertension can lead to cerebral vasodilation, augmenting CBF and leading to progression of cerebral edema.[15] Ideally a "correct" level of MAP should be maintained in each patient to maintain CPP without risking worsening cerebral edema or progression of the lesion, but the clinical determination of this "ideal" value is often difficult.

A Cochrane review of 12 trials comparing an active intervention to placebo/control with 1153 total participants concluded that insufficient evidence existed to favor altering BP in acute stroke.[16] Using available information, most consensus guidelines recommend that BP not be treated acutely in patients with ischemic stroke unless the hypertension is extreme (SBP >220 mm Hg or DBP >120 mm Hg) or the patient has active end-organ dysfunction in other organ systems.[17] When treatment is indicated, cautious lowering of BP by approximately 15% during the first 24 hours after stroke onset is suggested. Antihypertensive medications are restarted approximately 24 hours after stroke onset in patients with preexisting hypertension who are neurologically stable, unless a specific contraindication to restarting treatment exists. Requiring special consideration are patients with extracranial or intracranial arterial stenosis and candidates for thrombolytic therapy. The former group is dependent on perfusion pressure so BP therapy may be further delayed. In contrast, before lytic therapy is started, treatment is recommended so that SBP is 185 mm Hg or less and DBP is 110 mm Hg or less. Blood pressure should be stabilized and maintained below 180/105 mm Hg for at least 24 hours after intravenous lytic therapy.[17]

The natural history for stroke is for BP to begin falling shortly after the onset of the acute event and to stabilize within the first 24 hours. Agents that allow titration of therapy (i.e., intravenous (IV) medications) may be preferred over oral agents when treatment is necessary, provided the patient can be carefully monitored in a stroke unit.

Patients with hemorrhagic strokes provide an additional challenge. Severe elevations in BP may worsen intracranial hemorrhage by creating a continued force for bleeding. However, the increase in arterial pressure also may be necessary to maintain cerebral perfusion in this setting, and aggressive BP management could lead to worsening cerebral ischemia. Current guidelines advise aggressive BP reduction for patients with SBP above 200 mm Hg or MAP above 150 mm Hg, using IV titration of medications and continuous monitoring. For patients with suspected elevated intracranial pressure (ICP), ICP monitoring may be indicated to help maintain CPP during therapeutic interventions. For patients with SBP above 180 mm Hg or MAP above 130 mm Hg and no evidence or suspicion of elevated ICP, a more modest reduction of BP is suggested, using intermittent dosing or continuous infusion of IV medications.

Two recent clinical trials have suggested aggressive BP reduction limits hematoma expansion without clear benefit on mortality.[18,19]

SUBARACHNOID HEMORRHAGE

The patient with subarachnoid hemorrhage (SAH) provides the challenge of an acute neurologic syndrome secondary to an initial insult, followed by the ongoing risk of additional insults over time, including hydrocephalus, rebleeding, and vasospasm. The clinician faces the competing goals of lowering BP to minimize the rebleeding risk, and elevating BP to minimize the risk of cerebral vasospasm and infarction. In general, hypertension is not aggressively treated in this population for fear of precipitating cerebral ischemia. Treatment is guided by the neurologic condition. In the neurologically intact patient, small reductions in BP can be accomplished to minimize the risk of rebleeding. For the neurologically impaired patient, aggressive control of BP is avoided to maintain CPP.

Cardiovascular Disease

ACUTE CORONARY SYNDROME

Patients presenting with acute myocardial ischemia and/or infarction frequently suffer from elevated systemic arterial pressure. This increased afterload raises myocardial oxygen demand. A reduction in myocardial work, achieved by decreasing heart rate and BP, will favorably reduce myocardial oxygen demand and infarct size in these patients. However, a reduction of high systemic arterial pressure in this setting should be done cautiously. Excessive systemic vasodilation without coronary vasodilation can lead to a reduced coronary artery perfusion pressure and infarct extension. For this reason, nitroglycerin (NTG), a potent coronary vasodilator, is often the antihypertensive agent of choice in acute coronary syndromes. In combination with beta-blocker therapy, this approach can reduce cardiac workload significantly in the setting of ischemia. Careful monitoring of hemodynamic indices during treatment is paramount.

ACUTE LEFT VENTRICULAR DYSFUNCTION

The vast majority of patients presenting with acute heart failure are hypertensive on initial assessment.[20] Hypertension can be the inciting event, with secondary myocardial dysfunction; or alternatively, hypertension can be a secondary component of acute pulmonary edema due to the sympathoadrenal response to hypoxemia, increased work of breathing, and anxiety. Efforts to control elevated systemic arterial pressure in this setting are essential because high systemic arterial BP in the patient with acute pulmonary edema contributes to increased myocardial workload and diastolic dysfunction. In contrast, the use of vasodilators in patients with acute pulmonary edema and normal to low BP can have deleterious effects.[21,22] Similar to the patient with cerebrovascular disease, a U-shaped blood pressure/mortality relationship is expected.

For the hypertensive patient with acute heart failure, IV vasodilators such as NTG and sodium nitroprusside (SNP) permit rapid titration of BP and are preferred. Patients with acute pulmonary edema may be hypertensive secondary to high circulating catecholamine levels. With effective treatment or control of hypoxemia and anxiety, BP can decrease rapidly, especially in the setting of concomitant diuresis. Thus, longer-acting medications such as angiotensin-converting enzyme (ACE) inhibitors or angiotensin receptor blockers (ARBs) should be avoided early in the treatment period. Patients with hypertensive emergencies, in particular, may have undergone excessive natriuresis, resulting in elevated levels of renin production by the kidney and, hence, increased circulating levels of the potent endogenous vasoconstrictor, AT II. Further reduction in intravascular volume and renal perfusion can lead to a further increase in circulating AT II levels. Therefore, aggressive diuresis prior to BP control is generally not a good idea. Medications that increase cardiac work (e.g., hydralazine) or impair cardiac contractility (e.g., labetalol) are contraindicated as primary therapy for hypertension in the setting of acute LV dysfunction.

In addition to the more traditional IV vasodilators, IV calcium channel antagonists have demonstrated efficacy in the treatment of acute hypertension in the setting of LV dysfunction. The dihydropyridine calcium channel antagonists nicardipine and clevidipine can reduce systemic arterial pressure while preserving coronary blood flow.[23] Fenoldopam, a dopamine-1 receptor antagonist, also has been has been shown to preserve coronary blood flow during treatment to reduce systemic arterial pressure in this setting.[24] Despite their demonstrated efficacy in the treatment of hypertensive emergency, limited data exist with these newer agents to suggest superiority over NTG or nitroprusside. Agent selection should first be influenced by the adverse risk profile associated with the individual agents (Table 5-1). When not contraindicated by specific risk, the agents with a more favorable cost profile (i.e., NTG, nitroprusside) should be used based upon equivalent efficacy.

ACUTE AORTIC DISSECTION

Aortic dissection results from an intimal tear in the aortic wall. The primary morbidity and mortality results from extension of the tear. This extension is promoted by factors that increase the rate of change of aortic pressure (dp/dt), including elevation in BP, heart rate, and myocardial stroke volume. Blood pressure should be reduced promptly to near-normal levels. Aggressive control of BP with a vasodilator can trigger reflex tachycardia, leading to increased dp/dt. Combined

TABLE 5-1	Intravenous Antihypertensive Therapy			
Medication (Route)	*Pharmacology*	*Dosing*	*Indication*	*Contraindication*
Nitric Oxide Vasodilators				
Nitroprusside (IV infusion)	Onset: 2-3 min Duration: 2-3 min	Initial: 0.25 to 0.5 µg/kg/min Max: 10 µg/kg/min	Most hypertensive emergencies	Contraindicated in pregnancy. Caution with use in settings of cerebral edema, ACS, or azotemia.
Nitroglycerin (IV infusion)	Onset: 2-5 min Duration: 5-10 min	Initial: 5 µg/min Max: 200 µg/min	ACS	Contraindicated in pregnancy. Caution with use in a volume-contracted patient.
Calcium Channel Blockers				
Nicardipine (IV infusion)	Onset: 5-15 min Duration: 4-6 hours	Initial: 5 mg/h Max: 15 mg/h	Most hypertensive emergencies	Contraindicated in acute heart failure and caution with use in ACS.
Clevidipine (IV infusion)	Onset: 2-4 min Duration: 5-15 min	Initial: 1-2 mg/h Max: 32 mg/h	Most hypertensive emergencies	Contraindicated with allergy to soybean or egg products. Contraindicated with defective lipid metabolism.
Miscellaneous Medications				
Fenoldopam (IV infusion)	Onset: <5 min Duration: 30 min	Initial: 0.1 µg/kg/min Max: 1.6 µg/kg/min	Most hypertensive emergencies	Caution in patients with glaucoma and risk of increased CBF.
Labetalol (IV infusion, oral)	Onset: 2-5 min Duration: 2-4 hrs	Initial: IV bolus 20 mg Repeat bolus 20-80 mg every 10 min Infusion: 1 to 2 mg/min	Most hypertensive emergencies	Contraindicated in airflow obstruction, acute heart failure, or in patients intolerant of beta-blockers.
Phentolamine (IV infusion)	Onset: 1-2 min Duration: 10-30 min	5-10 mg every 5-15 min	Pheochromocytoma Catecholamine withdrawal Catecholamine excess	
Enalapril	Onset: 15 min Duration: 12-24 h	1.25-5 mg every 6 h	Scleroderma renal crisis	Caution with use in ACS. Not titratable.
Hydralazine (IV infusion, oral)	Onset: 10-20 min Duration: 2-4 h	Initial: 10 mg every 20 min Max: 20 mg every 4-6 h	Pregnancy	

ACS, acute coronary syndrome; *CBF*, cerebral blood flow; *IV*, intravenous; *NTG*, nitroglycerin.

modality therapy to promote vasodilation (SNP) and control cardiac contractility (beta-blocker) is advocated for this disorder.

Renovascular Disease

The kidney is both a source of mediators that promote hypertension (i.e., AT II) and a target of high systemic arterial pressure. Chronic hypertension is secondary only to diabetes mellitus as a primary cause of renal insufficiency. Elevated systemic arterial pressure should be regulated in patients with underlying renal insufficiency and a comprehensive workup initiated to determine the cause and effect relationship. Traditional vasodilator medications, such as labetalol and SNP, are preferred to ACE inhibitors in the acute setting, because ACE inhibitors can compromise renal function. The risk of ACE inhibitor–induced renal dysfunction is particularly great in patients with hyperkalemia and acute uremia.

SCLERODERMA RENAL CRISIS

Scleroderma renal crisis is characterized by the development of acute renal failure associated with moderate to severe hypertension and a normal to minimally abnormal urine sediment. The most significant risk factor for scleroderma renal crisis is the presence of diffuse skin involvement characteristic of the disease and recent treatment with high-dose corticosteroids.[25] The disorder results in marked activation of the renin-angiotensin system. Aggressive control of BP using ACE inhibitors, particularly early in the disease process, can control BP in up to 90% of patients and promote a greater rate of recovery in renal function.[26]

POST KIDNEY TRANSPLANTATION

Hypertension following renal transplantation occurs in the majority of patients.[27] In the immediate posttransplantation period, hypertension can be a manifestation of volume overload, graft rejection, ischemia, or toxic effects of calcineurin inhibitors used for immunosuppression. Treatment is directed primarily at the underlying mechanism. Renal artery stenosis can also complicate allograft function and should be evaluated in any patient with resistant hypertension. This complication can occur at any time within 1 month or up to 3 years after transplantation.[28] In the immediate posttransplant period, BP should be regulated at the upper limits of normal to preserve graft function. In the later postoperative period, more strict control of BP is favored.[29] Calcium channel blockers (CCBs) are frequently used to treat hypertension after renal transplantation, based upon their antagonism of cyclosporine-induced renal vasoconstriction. CCBs also have been studied extensively in renal transplant hypertension and are associated with preservation of allograft function in comparison to placebo.[29] ACE inhibitors have the potential to exacerbate renal dysfunction and augment hyperkalemia induced by calcineurin inhibitors.

Excess Catecholamine States

PHEOCHROMOCYTOMA

Pheochromocytoma can result in the production of circulating mediators, leading to catecholamine excess. These mediators result in hypertension, diaphoresis, tachycardia, and paresthesias of the hands and feet. These attacks can last from minutes to days and occur as frequently as several times a day or as infrequently as once a month.[30] Operative manipulation of the tumor can result in perioperative hypertension. The treatment of hypertension in this disorder must avoid the use of isolated therapy with a beta-blocker, a strategy that can lead to unopposed alpha-adrenergic stimulation, with the risk of further vasoconstriction and BP elevation. The preferred agent for treatment is phentolamine, a potent alpha-adrenergic antagonist. If needed, this medication can be combined with a beta-blocker, or a combined alpha/beta-blocker such as labetalol also can be used safely.

PHARMACOLOGICALLY MEDIATED

A broad range of medications have been associated with the development of hypertension or alternatively may limit the effectiveness of treatment for primary hypertension. A detailed medical history is required to evaluate patients with high systemic arterial BP. Attention should be paid to prescription medications as well as herbal supplements and substance abuse.[31] Both administration of exogenous substances and abrupt withdrawal of substances can be associated with hypertensive crises. As an example, clonidine withdrawal can mimic the crisis of pheochromocytoma. Clonidine is a centrally acting stimulant of alpha-adrenergic receptors that reduces peripheral adrenergic system activation. Rapid withdrawal or tapering of clonidine produces a hyperadrenergic state characterized by hypertension, diaphoresis, headache, and anxiety.[32] The syndrome is best treated by restarting treatment with clonidine. Extreme symptoms can be treated as outlined for the patient with pheochromocytoma. Hypertension also can occur during the withdrawal phase of alcohol abuse.

Monoamine oxidase (MAO) inhibitors are associated with marked elevations of systemic arterial BP if the patient consumes foods or medications containing tyramine or other sympathomimetic amines. Tyramine-containing foods include champagne, avocados, smoked or aged meats, and fermented cheeses. The MAO inhibitor interferes with degradation of tyramine in the intestine, leading to excess absorption of the amine and tyramine-induced catecholamine activity in the circulation.

Other medications, including metoclopramide, a dopamine agonist, the calcineurin inhibitors, cyclosporine and tacrolimus, and drugs of abuse such as cocaine, phenylpropanolamine, phencyclidine, and methamphetamine all must be considered as possible factors in the evaluation of elevated systemic arterial pressure.

Following spinal cord injury, hypertensive states may occur, particularly with stimulation of dermatomes and muscles below the level of the spinal cord injury. Patients with hypertension in this setting typically have lesions above the level of the thoracolumbar sympathetic neurons. The BP elevation is believed to result from excessive stimulation of sympathetic neurons. Hypertension is accompanied by bradycardia through stimulation of the baroreceptor reflex. Treatment is focused on minimizing stimulation and providing medical therapy as necessary. Patients with Guillain-Barré syndrome can present with a similar clinical picture.

Miscellaneous Conditions

PREECLAMPSIA/ECLAMPSIA

Preeclampsia/eclampsia remains the second most common cause of maternal death in the United States, following thromboembolic disease. Hypertension occurs as one manifestation of preeclampsia in the pregnant patient; the other key features are proteinuria and edema. Hypertension in pregnancy also can be seen secondary to chronic hypertension and transient or gestational hypertension. New onset of hypertension following 20 weeks of gestation is most characteristic of the patient with preeclampsia.

When possible, the optimal treatment of preeclampsia is delivery of the fetus, an approach that prevents progression to eclampsia. However, BP should be regulated to prevent end-organ damage. Hydralazine is considered the antihypertensive agent of choice in pregnant patients. SNP (fetal defects), ACE inhibitors (renal dysfunction in the fetus), and trimethaphan (meconium ileus) should be avoided in pregnant patients. Alternatives to hydralazine to control hypertension in pregnant patients include labetalol and nicardipine.

POSTOPERATIVE HYPERTENSION

Poorly controlled hypertension pre- and intraoperatively is associated with an increased rate of postoperative complications. Postoperative hypertension occurs in as many as 75% of patients, and the risk appears to be greater for vascular surgical procedures, including abdominal aortic aneurysm repair, carotid endarterectomy, and coronary artery revascularization. Postoperative hypertension in these patients can lead to complications including bleeding from suture lines, intracerebral hemorrhage, and LV dysfunction. Postoperative hypertension can be caused by elevated systemic vascular resistance in response to circulating stress hormones, renin-angiotensin-aldosterone system activation, or altered baroreceptor function.

Patients with postoperative hypertension must be thoroughly investigated to rule out reversible causes prior to the institution of drug therapy. Factors such as pain, anxiety, hypervolemia, hypoxemia, hypercarbia, and nausea can contribute to the disorder. Postoperative hypertension is often limited in duration (i.e., 2-12 hours), and aggressive attempts to acutely lower BP can lead to delayed hypotension.

Postoperative hypertension is typically treated with administration of vasodilators, including SNP and NTG or beta-blockers as needed.

Antihypertensive Medications

The goal of antihypertensive therapy in emergent situations is to lower BP to a safe range as quickly as possible. In general, IV medications are preferred, allowing titration of dosing to minimize the risk of excessive hypotension. As previously outlined, a commonly proposed goal is to lower the MAP by approximately 20% or to reduce DBP to 100 to 110 mm Hg. To carefully monitor the effect of antihypertensive therapy, these patients are best monitored in an intensive care unit (ICU). A gradual reduction to the patient's baseline "normal" BP with appropriate monitoring for signs or symptoms of organ ischemia is targeted over the initial 24 to 28 hours if the patient remains stable.

For hypertensive urgencies, oral therapy can be used to lower BP to safer levels over a 24-hour interval. These patients in general do not require monitoring in an ICU. A summary of the medications available for the treatment of hypertensive emergency is outlined in Table 5-2.

NITRIC OXIDE VASODILATORS

SNP is an NO donor that activates endovascular guanylyl cyclase, leading to the formation of the second messenger, cyclic guanosine monophosphate (cGMP) and ultimately smooth muscle relaxation. SNP has been the gold standard for the treatment of hypertensive emergencies, owing to its short duration of action, allowing careful titration. SNP acts as a direct vasodilator of arterioles and veins. The

BP response to SNP is rapid and mandates the use of this medication in a well-monitored environment. The infusion must be provided by a calibrated pump, with frequent BP recordings. Typically, intraarterial BP monitoring is preferred because of the need for rapid and frequent dosage adjustments, particularly during initial titration of the medication. However, an accurate noninvasive system may be sufficient in some cases.

SNP's arteriolar and venous vasodilating activity may not be uniform, however. Redistribution of oxygenated blood flow from unresponsive ischemic regions to vasodilated nonischemic coronary arteries can reduce coronary perfusion pressure, resulting in a "coronary steal" syndrome.[33] A similar "cerebral steal" syndrome has been suggested with SNP as a result of preferential vasodilation in systemic vascular beds versus cerebral vessels.[15] Additional concerns have been raised with the use of SNP in patients with increased ICP; dilatation of large-capacitance vessels by SNP can lead to an increase in CBF and ICP.[15]

In rare instances, SNP administration can lead to cyanide or thiocyanate toxicity. Cyanide intoxication is manifested by alterations in mental status, gastrointestinal (GI) complaints, arrhythmias, seizures, and/or lactic acidosis. The latter finding occurs in association with a reduced systemic oxygen uptake and a narrow arterial-venous oxygen gradient. Cyanide is liberated during the combination of nitroprusside with sulfhydryl groups in red cells and tissues. Cyanide is converted in the liver to thiocyanate, with subsequent excretion by the kidney.

Cyanide toxicity from SNP is uncommon and occurs primarily in patients receiving infusions for more than 24 to 48 hours, in the setting of underlying renal insufficiency, and/or the use of doses that exceed the capacity of the body to detoxify cyanide (>2 μg/kg/min). The treatment of cyanide intoxication involves the administration of sodium thiosulfate. Sodium thiosulfate donates its sulfane sulfur atom in a reaction catalyzed by the enzyme, rhodanese, to convert cyanide to the much less toxic thiocyanate ion, which is then excreted in the urine. For severe cases, sodium nitrite may also be administered. Sodium nitrite oxidizes hemoglobin (Hb) in the blood to methemoglobin, which binds cyanide with high affinity. Thus, methemoglobin competes with other cellular targets for cyanide, notably cytochrome a-a3 in mitochondria, and thereby decreases the toxic effects of cyanide ion. The onset of action of sodium nitrite is rapid, but the induction of methemoglobinemia decreases the oxygen-carrying capacity of blood and therefore can be harmful in patients with anemia or significant carboxyhemoglobinemia. Hydroxocobalamin (vitamin B_{12a}), is another safe and effective antidote for cyanide intoxication. Hydroxocobalamin administration does not affect the oxygen-carrying capacity of the blood, so this harmless agent may be preferable to sodium nitrite. Hydroxyocobalamin reacts with circulating cyanide to form cyanocobalamin, with subsequent urinary excretion. Hydroxocobalamin has been demonstrated to minimize the risk of cyanide accumulation during nitroprusside use in surgery.[34]

Thiocyanate toxicity in association with SNP infusion is also rare. The clinical manifestations include fatigue, GI complaints, and mental status changes. The symptoms most typically appear when plasma thiocyanate levels are over 5 to 10 ng/dL, and occur with higher-dose SNP infusion in the setting of renal impairment.

Nitroglycerin is a vasodilator known to promote coronary vascular dilation. The drug acts as a systemic venodilator, acting to reduce myocardial preload. It demonstrates arterial smooth muscle effects only at higher infusion rates. The drug is contraindicated in patients with significant volume depletion; venodilation in these patients will further lower preload, reduce cardiac output, and compromise overall systemic perfusion. When administered by the IV route, NTG has a relatively short duration of action. The drug has favorable effects for patients with acute coronary syndromes, including reducing myocardial oxygen demand via its effects on preload and afterload and augmenting myocardial oxygen delivery through its effects on the coronary circulation.

Headache is the most common adverse effect of NTG, and methemoglobinemia is a rare complication of prolonged NTG therapy.

TABLE 5-2	Suggested Therapy for Hypertensive Emergency	
Cerebrovascular Disease	
Acute ischemic stroke	Nicardipine, labetalol
Acute intracerebral hemorrhage	Nicardipine, labetalol
Cardiovascular Disease	
ACS	NTG
Acute LV dysfunction	NTG, nitroprusside
Acute aortic dissection	Beta-blocker followed by nitroprusside or nicardipine
Acute MI	Clevidipine, labetalol, nicardipine, NTG
Renovascular Disease	
Acute renal failure	Clevidipine, labetalol, nicardipine, nitroglycerin
Scleroderma renal crisis	ACE inhibitor
Endocrine Diseases	
Pheochromocytoma	Phentolamine, labetalol
Drug-Related Disorders	
Catecholamine toxicity	Phentolamine, labetalol
Perioperative hypertension	Clevidipine, nicardipine, NTG, nitroprusside
Preeclampsia or eclampsia	Hydralazine, labetalol

ACE, angiotensin-converting enzyme; *ACS*, acute coronary syndrome; *LV,* left ventricular; *MI*, myocardial infarction; *NTG*, nitroglycerin.

Tolerance to the medication is recognized and may limit the overall effectiveness in longer-term infusions.

CALCIUM CHANNEL BLOCKERS

Calcium channel blockers are a heterogenous class of medications used in the treatment of hypertension emergencies. A specific class of CCB called the *dihydropyridines* (e.g., nicardipine, clevidipine) are selective for vascular smooth muscle over the myocardium, having little if any activity on cardiac muscle or the sinoatrial node.[35] Because these drugs act to promote vascular smooth muscle relaxation without associated cardiac effects, they are attractive for the treatment of hypertensive emergencies. In contrast, CCBs from other pharmacologic classes, such as diltiazem and verapamil, affect the cardiac conduction system and myocardial calcium channels, making them less optimal choices for the treatment of hypertension.

Nicardipine hydrochloride is a dihydropyridine CCB that acts primarily as a systemic, cerebral, and coronary artery vasodilator. The greater water solubility of this drug, in comparison to other CCBs such as nifedipine, allows IV administration with a short onset and duration of action and therefore easy titration to therapeutic effect. The medication has no significant effect on cardiac inotropy and promotes afterload reduction. Nicardipine readily crosses the blood-brain barrier and relaxes vascular smooth muscle, especially in regions of ischemic tissue. The medication acts as a vasodilator of small-resistance cerebral arterioles but does not change intracranial volume or ICP; thus, cerebral oxygenation is preserved.[36]

Nicardipine has been studied as an alternative agent to SNP in the management of hypertension for patients with intracranial or subarachnoid hemorrhage. In comparison to SNP, nicardipine offers equal efficacy in terms of BP control. But nicardipine, avoiding problems related to the toxic metabolites of SNP, requires less frequent dose adjustments and carries less risk of increasing ICP.[37] Comparative investigations of nicardipine and nitroprusside in postoperative patients with hypertension suggest therapeutic equivalency.[38,39] Nicardipine is metabolized by the liver, and excretion can be impaired in patients with abnormal hepatic function.

Clevidipine is the first third-generation dihydropyridine CCB approved in the United States. It is supplied as a racemic mixture in a lipid emulsion for IV infusion. Clevidipine is an ultrafast arteriolar vasodilator that reduces afterload without affecting cardiac filling pressures or causing reflex tachycardia. Clevidipine has a rapid onset (~2-4 minutes) and offset of action (~5-15 minutes). It undergoes rapid ester hydrolysis by arterial blood esterases to form inactive metabolites, which makes clearance of this medication independent of renal or hepatic function.

Clevidipine has been most extensively investigated in adult patients (>18 years of age) with acute perioperative or postoperative hypertension in the setting of cardiac surgery. The antihypertensive efficacy of IV clevidipine was compared with that of SNP and NTG for perioperative hypertension, and with nicardipine for postoperative hypertension.[40] All agents were administered by IV infusion. The primary endpoint was the incidence of death, stroke, MI, or renal dysfunction from study drug initiation to 30 days after surgery. BP control was a secondary endpoint evaluated; using the area under the curve (AUC) of SBP excursions above or below predetermined limits (65-135 mm Hg, intraoperatively; 75-145 mm Hg, pre- and postoperatively).

There was no difference in the incidence of MI, stroke, or renal dysfunction for clevidipine-treated patients compared with the other treatment groups. There was no difference in mortality rates between the clevidipine, NTG, or nicardipine groups. Mortality was significantly higher, however, for SNP-treated patients compared with clevidipine-treated patients. Clevidipine was more effective compared with NTG (P <0.0006) or SNP (P <0.003) in maintaining BP within the prespecified BP range. Clevidipine was equivalent to nicardipine for keeping patients within a prespecified BP range; however, when the BP range was narrowed, clevidipine was associated with fewer BP excursions beyond these BP limits compared with nicardipine.

The antihypertensive efficacy of IV clevidipine in patients with acute severe hypertension has also been assessed in a large, noncomparative, open-label, multicenter, phase III study.[41] Clevidipine was administered as a non–weight-based dose of 2 mg per hour for patients with acute severe hypertension with or without end-organ injury. The medication provided rapid, predictable BP control, and the majority of patients reached the target BP within 30 minutes. Prolonged administration (>18 hours) was well tolerated.

Clevidipine is contraindicated in patients with allergies to soybeans, soy products, eggs, or egg products. Clevidipine is also contraindicated in patients with defective lipid metabolism. Owing to lipid-load restrictions, no more than 1000 mL or an average of 21 mg/h of clevidipine infusion is recommended per 24-hour period. Clinicians must account for the calories infused from the lipid emulsion and adjust the nutrition regimen as needed and monitor triglyceride levels during prolonged administration.

Miscellaneous Medications

Intravenous fenoldopam is a postsynaptic dopamine-1 receptor agonist with short-acting vasodilator properties. In contrast to SNP, fenoldopam administration is not associated with a risk of accumulation of toxic metabolites. Similar to SNP, fenoldopam lowers BP by decreasing peripheral vascular resistance. The medication causes a slight elevation of heart rate and an increase in renal blood flow. The preservation of renal blood flow is attributed to the drug's mechanism as a dopamine-1 receptor agonist.

The hemodynamic effects of fenoldopam and SNP were compared in a multicentric clinical trial that enrolled patients with acute hypertension. The researchers showed that fenoldopam was as effective as SNP for controlling acute systemic hypertension.[42] The average decreases in BP at 6 hours of infusion were similar in the two study groups. The average maintenance infusion rate for fenoldopam was 0.41 μg/kg/min (range, 0.1 to 1.62 μg/kg/min). The time required to reach the maintenance infusion rate was similar in the two groups. In a population subset, indices of renal function, including creatinine clearance, urinary output, and sodium excretion, were better in the group randomized to fenoldopam treatment. However, the study sample was too small to draw definitive conclusions. Both drugs were equally well tolerated.

The use of fenoldopam in patients with hypertensive emergencies was evaluated in 107 patients with DBP >120 mm Hg and clinical evidence of acute vasculopathy.[43] Infusion rates of 0.01, 0.03, 0.1, or 0.3 μg/kg/min for 24 hours were studied. Within this range of doses, fenoldopam was safe. Thus fenoldopam is an easily titrated drug that is effective when BP has to be reduced rapidly.

Dose-related tachycardia can occur with the administration of fenoldopam, especially at infusion rates exceeding 0.1 μg/kg/min. The drug should be used with caution in patients with angina, as reflux tachycardia could increase myocardial oxygen demand. Fenoldopam should also be used with caution in patients with open-angle glaucoma or intraocular hypertension. The drug has not been investigated in the setting of increased ICP and therefore should be used with caution in these patients.

Labetalol is an oral and parenteral agent that acts as an alpha- and nonselective beta-adrenergic blocker. The BP-lowering effect is produced through a reduction in systemic vascular resistance without a compensatory increase in heart rate. Labetalol has very little effect on the cerebral circulation and is thus not associated with an increase in ICP in the normal brain.[44] The drug has been used effectively in patients with end-organ dysfunction in the setting of acute neurologic injury, pheochromocytoma, cocaine intoxication, dissecting aneurysm, and eclampsia. The primary contraindication to the use of the medication relates to its nonselective beta-blocking properties. The drug should be used cautiously in patients with reactive airways disease, heart block, or decompensated LV failure.

Enalapril is an intravenously administered ACE inhibitor. The medication reduces renin-dependent vasopressor activity and blocks the conversion of angiotensin I to angiotensin II, a potent vasoconstrictor. Drugs in this class also block the degradation of bradykinin, a systemic vasodilator. Inhibition of bradykinin metabolism contributes to the antihypertensive effect of these medications. ACE inhibitors decrease systemic vascular resistance and cause minimal changes in heart rate, cardiac output, or LV filling pressures. Similar to other ACE inhibitors, enalapril is effective in patients with low to normal renin levels and hypertension. In contrast to the previously described medications for the treatment of hypertensive emergency/urgency, the peak effect of enalapril may not be seen for up to 4 hours, and the duration of action is 12 to 24 hours. These pharmacokinetic parameters limit the drug titration in the acute setting of hypertensive emergency. ACE inhibitors are contraindicated in the setting of renal artery stenosis and pregnancy.

Phentolamine is a rapid-acting alpha-adrenergic blocker. Phentolamine is the drug of choice for hypertensive emergencies secondary to pheochromocytoma, MAO-tyramine interactions, and clonidine rebound hypertension.

Summary

The treatment of high systemic arterial BP in the ICU must incorporate a comprehensive assessment of the patient. Clinical situations associated with progressive end-organ damage require urgent intervention, most frequently with a titratable medication and careful ongoing monitoring. In contrast, aggressive antihypertensive therapy in asymptomatic patients without immediate risk of organ dysfunction can be harmful. The intensivist is routinely challenged to recognize this distinction in the hypertensive ICU patient.

ANNOTATED REFERENCES

Aronson S, et al. The ECLIPSE trials: comparative studies of clevidipine to nitroglycerin, sodium nitroprusside, and nicardipine for acute hypertension treatment in cardiac surgery patients. Anesth Analg 2008;107(4):1110-21.
A summary of patient outcomes from prospective clinical trials of clevidipine use in cardiac surgery patients in comparison to more standard medications. The comparative trials suggest equal efficacy with a favorable safety profile in this population.

Lane DA, Lip GYH, Beevers DG. Improving survival of malignant hypertension patients over 40 years. Am J Hypertens 2009;22(11):1199-204.
A careful review of patient outcomes in a large cohort of patients with malignant hypertension seen over a 40-year interval. Provides a careful summary of underlying causes, clinical features, and outcome during that interval.

Geeganage C, Bath PM. Interventions for deliberately altering blood pressure in acute stroke. Cochrane Database Syst Rev 2008;(4):CD000039.
A Cochrane review updated now to include 12 clinical trials of antihypertensive therapy in acute stroke involving 1153 participants. The review concludes there is no evidence to support the effect of lowering blood pressure in acute stroke.

Grossman E, Messerli FH. Secondary hypertension: interfering substances. J Clin Hypertens (Greenwich) 2008;10(7):556-66.
A comprehensive review of prescription medications and chemical substances that must be considered in the patient with hypertensive emergency/urgency.

Immink RV, et al. Cerebral hemodynamics during treatment with sodium nitroprusside versus labetalol in malignant hypertension. Hypertension 2008;52(2):236-40.
A comparative clinical trial of sodium nitroprusside and labetalol in patients with malignant hypertension. The study highlights the variable effects of these medications on middle cerebral artery blood flow.

REFERENCES

Access the complete reference list online at http://www.expertconsult.com.

6

Low Systemic Arterial Blood Pressure

KYLE J. GUNNERSON

When initially assessing a critically ill patient, it is essential to perform a rapid, focused physical examination (the ABCs of resuscitation). After ensuring that the patient has a patent airway (A) and is effectively breathing (B), the next step is to assess the adequacy of the circulation (C).

Initial Evaluation

A clinician's initial evaluation should be a global assessment (Figure 6-1). When walking into a patient's room, you should think, "What do I see?" and quickly determine whether the patient is in distress or has problems related to the airway or breathing. Look for obvious signs of external hemorrhage, look for evidence of hypoperfusion, and assess the adequacy of intravenous (IV) access. Do not rely solely on blood pressure (BP) readings, as there is no "normal" BP for all patients, and a BP value in the "normal" range does not always equate with adequate tissue perfusion. A patient with a history of poorly controlled chronic hypertension may have signs of hypoperfusion even when the BP is within the normal range (for nonhypertensive patients). Conversely, a patient with cirrhosis may have adequate perfusion despite having a lower-than-normal BP. A quick bedside assessment of tissue perfusion should include evaluation of mental status, urine output, and skin findings (e.g., temperature, diaphoresis, mottling, and capillary refill). If any of these parameters are abnormal, a more urgent approach to treatment must be taken.

A focused cardiac and pulmonary examination is essential. Seek evidence of jugular venous distention, presence of an S_3 or S_4 heart sound, new or worsening murmurs, or muffled heart sounds. Check for the presence of crackles or rales, and note whether there are absent breath sounds, a finding suggestive of a pneumothorax.

During the initial evaluation, pay close attention to systolic (SBP) and diastolic (DBP) pressures in the context of pulse pressure (PP = SBP − DBP). Diastolic pressure is a reasonable surrogate for systemic vascular resistance (SVR). These basic physiology concepts will be useful in determining the cause and devising a treatment plan.

What Is the Cause?

To help focus the differential diagnosis of a hypotensive patient, it is important to review basic cardiovascular physiology. The first concept to remember is that *pressure = flow × resistance*, where flow is cardiac output, and resistance is SVR. Because cardiac output is determined by stroke volume (SV) × heart rate, the presence of hypotension means that at least one of these parameters (e.g., SV, SVR, or heart rate) is abnormal.[1] Disturbances in heart rate should be obvious by feeling the peripheral pulse, looking at the cardiac monitor, or evaluating a 12-lead electrocardiogram (ECG). The focus of this chapter is evaluating and treating conditions associated with decreased SV or SVR. By properly measuring pulse pressure and diastolic pressure, the clinician can determine whether the primary cause is a change in SVR or SV.

During systole, the SV is ejected into the proximal arterial conduits. Because more blood is being ejected than the peripheral circulation can accommodate in the arterioles, the arterial walls distend, increasing SBP in a way that is directly proportional to the SV and indirectly proportional to the capacitance (C) of the arterial wall. This relationship is represented by the formula[1]:

$$SBP = SV \div C$$

That is, for a fixed SV, if capacitance is higher, the SBP is lower.

During diastole, the portion of the SV that was "stored" by the distention of the arterial walls during systole fills the peripheral arterioles, leading to a progressive decrease in BP until the next systolic phase. This is the diastolic pressure, a parameter that is directly related to the SVR and capacitance (i.e., low diastolic pressure = low SVR and/or capacitance).[1] When using these basic cardiovascular principles to understand the cause of hypotension, it is important to remember the following: (1) capacitance does not change from heartbeat to heartbeat, and (2) SV depends on preload, afterload, and contractility.

Low SVR is characteristic of a number of pathologic conditions, including sepsis, adrenal insufficiency, vasodilating medications, neurogenic shock, post–cardiopulmonary bypass (CPB) vasoplegia, and severe liver dysfunction. Decreased SVR should be suspected in the presence of a widened pulse pressure and low diastolic pressure.[2,3]

Reduced SV can be due to decreased preload, decreased contractility, or increased afterload. The most common cause of inadequate preload is hypovolemia. Other causes of inadequate preload include increased intrathoracic pressure due to dynamic hyperinflation in mechanically ventilated patients[4,5] or tension pneumothorax, pulmonary embolism,[6] mitral valve stenosis,[7] cardiac tamponade,[8] and right ventricular failure.[9] Decreased contractility can be caused by myocardial ischemia or infarction, cardiomyopathy, myocarditis, negative inotropic drugs, myocardial stunning after CPB, and direct myocyte toxins, such as chemotherapeutic agents and inflammatory mediators (e.g., tumor necrosis factor [TNF] and interleukin 1-beta [IL-1β]).[10] A reduction in SV can be identified by decreased systolic BP and normal or narrow pulse pressure.

Treatment

Hypotension has been associated with higher morbidity and mortality in a variety of disease states, so until proved otherwise, hypotension should be considered synonymous with hypoperfusion and thus treated aggressively. This initial treatment includes monitoring *and* therapeutic measures. All patients should have adequate IV access, preferably two patent 18-gauge or larger catheters. The patient should be monitored using a standard ECG monitor and pulse oximetry. A 12-lead ECG should be performed to look for evidence of myocardial ischemia. Supplemental oxygen should be given as needed to keep oxygen saturation greater than 92%. A 1-L fluid bolus of an isotonic crystalloid solution should be infused as rapidly as possible while data are being gathered. The history, focused examination, and assessment of pulse pressure, systolic pressure, and diastolic pressure will aid in the formulation of a more specific treatment strategy.

There are several tools that aid in the workup of the hypotensive patient. One option is the use of ultrasound to evaluate inferior vena cava diameter variation during the inspiratory and expiratory phases of the respiratory cycle. Patients with a large variation (>50%) will most likely respond to additional volume.[11] Ultrasound, when used in a focused cardiac examination, can also identify the global quality of contractility, ventricular size and volume, obvious wall motion abnormalities, significant valvular abnormalities, and the presence of a pericardial effusion.[12]

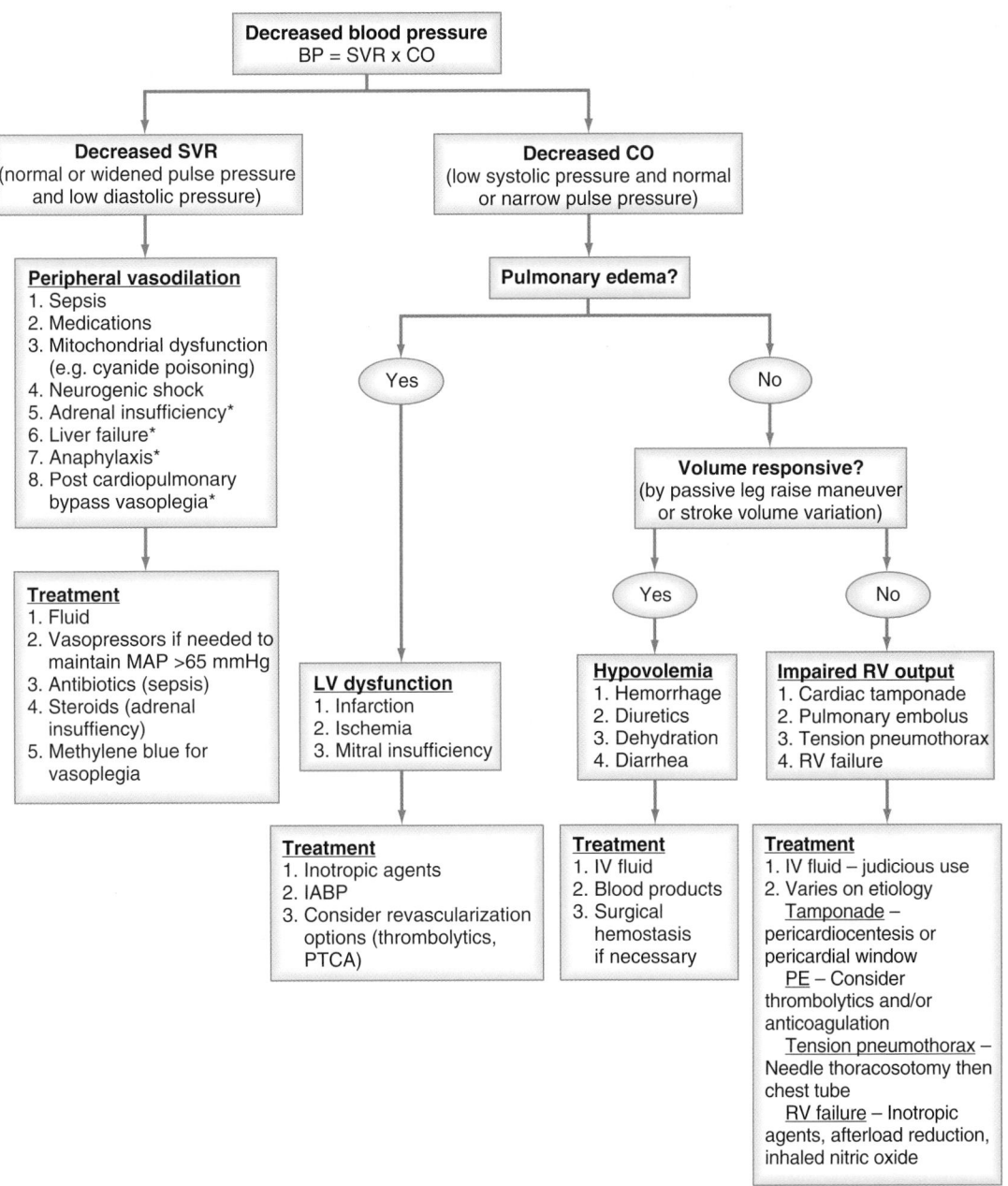

Figure 6-1 Initial approach to a patient with low systemic arterial blood pressure. *Adrenal insufficiency, liver failure, post–cardiopulmonary bypass vasoplegia, and anaphylaxis are commonly listed as vasodilatory shock; however, data are inconclusive, and components of other types of shock (hypovolemic, cardiogenic) may be also be present. *BP*, blood pressure; *CO*, cardiac output; *IABP*, intraaortic balloon pump; *IV*, intravenous; *LV*, left ventricle; *MAP*, mean arterial pressure; *PE*, pulmonary embolism; *PTCA*, percutaneous transluminal coronary angioplasty; *RV*, right ventricle; *SVR*, systemic vascular resistance.

An IV fluid bolus should be a first-line option in treating hypotension, but not every patient will have the desired response to fluid administration. The clinician can evaluate "volume responsiveness" by noninvasive or minimally invasive measures. In the nonintubated, supine patient, elevating the patient's legs in a 45-degree angle above the plane of the bed will cause a rapid temporary increase in venous return to the heart. If the patient's condition is dependent on additional volume, one will see an increase in SBP that also correlates to an increase in stroke volume. This maneuver increases pulse pressure in "responders." An increase in pulse pressure of more than 9% noted before and after the passive leg lifts will identify patients who are likely to respond to additional IV fluid administration.[13,14] A more invasive option is to measure pulse pressure or stroke volume variation in the intubated and mechanically

ventilated patient. In these patients, a decrease in stroke volume of 13% or more during the inspiratory cycle correlates with preload responsiveness of stroke volume (i.e., stroke volume and therefore cardiac output are likely to increase if intravascular volume is increased by infusing IV colloid or crystalloid solutions). This variation represents a decrease in venous return in conjunction with the increased intrathoracic pressure during the inspiratory phase of the ventilator. This measurement is only accurate when the heart rhythm is regular, so it is an unreliable index of preload responsiveness in patients with many kinds of arrhythmias, in the presence of an intraaortic balloon pump, or when there is loss of integrity in the arterial waveform. It is also only accurate in mechanically ventilated patients who are not experiencing large variations in intrathoracic pressures.[15,16]

In those patients where a low SVR is suspected as the primary cause of hypotension, the treatment is different. Large amounts of additional IV fluid will not adequately increase the BP to maintain tissue perfusion alone. Vasoconstrictor agents (e.g., norepinephrine, dopamine, phenylephrine, vasopressin) will be required in these patients. In certain specific cases, other pharmacologic adjuncts may be helpful.

Low-dose hydrocortisone in vasoconstrictor-resistant septic shock[17] and methylene blue in post CPB vasoplegia are two examples.[18]

Many occurrences of hypotension may have some qualities of both decreased SV and decreased SVR. However, by using a systematic approach, the clinician can rapidly start diagnostic and therapeutic measures needed to treat tissue hypoperfusion.

ANNOTATED REFERENCES

Kumar A, Haery C, Parrillo JE. Myocardial dysfunction in septic shock. Part I. Clinical manifestation of cardiovascular dysfunction. J Cardiothorac Vasc Anesth 2001;15:364-76.
   A superb review of myocardial dysfunction in sepsis from authors with extensive experience on the topic.
Landry DW, Oliver JA. The pathogenesis of vasodilatory shock. N Engl J Med 2001;345:588-95.
   An excellent basic science review of the physiology of vasodilatory shock.
Tapson VF. Acute pulmonary embolism. N Engl J Med 2008;358:1037-52.
   A very well-written and thorough review of acute pulmonary embolism by an authority in pulmonary thromboembolic disease.

Pinsky MR. Heart-lung interaction. Curr Opin Crit Care 2007;13:528-31.
   A timely, well-written review by an international expert in the field of heart-lung interactions, specifically discussing the hemodynamics of positive pressure ventilation.
Spodick DH. Acute cardiac tamponade. N Engl J Med 2003;349:684-90.
   A thorough review of cardiac tamponade that covers cause, diagnosis, and treatment.
Monett X, Teboul JL. Volume responsiveness. Curr Opin Crit Care 2007;13:549-53.
   An excellent current review of volume responsiveness as it applies to the critically ill patient; written by members of the pioneering group in this line of research.

REFERENCES

Access the complete reference list online at http://www.expertconsult.com.

7

Tachycardia and Bradycardia

PENNY LYNN SAPPINGTON

Cardiac arrhythmias, a common problem encountered in the intensive care unit (ICU), increase the length of stay and represent a major source of morbidity.[1] Clinical issues such as electrolyte derangements (particularly those related to potassium and magnesium ion concentrations), acidemia, hypoxia, cardiac ischemia or structural defects, and catecholamine excess (exogenous or endogenous) can play important roles in the cause of arrhythmias. Treatment of these arrhythmias depends most importantly on the cardiac physiology of the patient but also on the ventricular response rate and duration of the arrhythmia.

The two major categories of cardiac arrhythmias are defined by heart rate: bradycardia (heart rate <60 beats per minute [bpm]) and tachycardia (heart rate >100 bpm). Asymptomatic bradycardia does not carry a poor prognosis, and in general no therapy is indicated.[2] Bradycardia with or without hypotension should prompt a consideration of metabolic disturbances, hypoxemia, drug effects, and myocardial ischemia. Other causes of bradycardia are shown in Table 7-1.

The recommended initial therapy for bradycardia that is leading to inadequate cardiac output and organ perfusion is 1 mg atropine intravenously (IV). The underlying cause for bradycardia should be investigated; if it is of abrupt onset, hypoxemia or acidosis can be quickly excluded by obtaining an arterial blood gas measurement. If the patient is unresponsive, endotracheal intubation and mechanical ventilation are indicated and should be instituted promptly. If the patient is already intubated, disconnect the ventilator and manually ventilate the patient (using an Ambu bag) to ensure adequate ventilation and oxygenation. Mucous plugging of the endotracheal tube or airways should be excluded in an acutely hypoxemic patient. Once these conditions are excluded, evaluate the electrocardiogram (ECG) for evidence of second- or third-degree heart block or ischemic changes. Aminophylline (100 mg IV) has been reported to correct ischemic heart block.[3] Insertion of a temporary transvenous pacemaker may be indicated in the setting of ischemic heart block, because further deterioration can occur unpredictably.

Medications that can cause bradycardia include β-adrenergic blockers, Ca$^+$ channel blockers, clonidine, antiarrhythmics, digoxin, and propofol. Severe toxicity due to overdose with a β-adrenergic antagonist (leading to bradycardia, hypotension, shock) can be treated with glucagon (5 to 10 mg IV, followed by an infusion of 1 to 10 mg/h diluted in D$_5$W). Moderate drug-induced bradycardia (heart rate >40 bpm) can be observed until the offending drug is metabolized, so long as peripheral perfusion appears to be adequate. β-Adrenergic agonists, such as dopamine (3 µg/kg/min and titrated upward as needed), dobutamine, isoproterenol (2 µg/min and titrated upward as needed to increase heart rate and perfusion), or epinephrine, can be used to provide temporary support for bradycardic hypotensive patients. Bradycardia in the setting of preexisting shock and refractory acidosis is an ominous sign, and transcutaneous or transvenous pacing is generally futile.

The first step in evaluating the critically ill patient with tachycardia is to assess hemodynamic stability. It is critical to differentiate hypotension leading to tachycardia from hypotension caused by tachycardia. Examples of hypotension leading to tachycardia are the normal compensatory response to hypovolemic shock or atrial fibrillation with rapid ventricular response due to infusion of large doses of an arrhythmogenic agent (e.g., dopamine) to treat septic shock. An example of hypotension caused by tachycardia is the response to ventricular tachycardia (VT) after myocardial infarction (MI). In the former situation, intravascular volume loading or decreasing the dose of a β-adrenergic

agonist is indicated. In the latter circumstance, rapid conversion by electrical cardioversion should be performed unless pharmacologic treatment is immediately successful.

Sinus tachycardia is probably the most common dysrhythmia encountered in the ICU and often occurs as a response to a sympathetic stimulus (e.g., hypoxia, vasopressors, inotropes, pain, dehydration, or hyperthyroidism). The first step is to review the patient's medication list, including infusions, to exclude an iatrogenic etiology for the tachycardia. Treatment focuses on identifying and trying to correct the underlying cause. In trauma and postsurgical patients, tachycardia can be a sign of bleeding and hypovolemia. It is usually reasonable to administer an intravascular volume challenge (e.g., 500 mL of colloid solution in adults) and check the hemoglobin concentration. Sinus tachycardia and hypertension can be manifestations of opioid withdrawal, failure of a ventilator weaning trial, or inadequate sedation. Most patients at high risk for coronary disease warrant prophylactic treatment with a β-adrenergic blocker to prevent myocardial ischemia secondary to a high "rate-pressure product" and high myocardial oxygen demand.[4,5] In particular, perioperative patients with significant cardiac risk should have titrated therapy with a β-adrenergic blocker to maintain the heart rate at less than 80 bpm unless significant contraindications exist.[6]

Sustained regular tachycardia (heart rate >160 bpm) associated with a narrow QRS complex on the ECG often has a reentrant mechanism as the etiology. Reentrant narrow complex tachycardia is more prevalent in females and usually is not associated with structural heart disease. The key treatment is to block AV conduction.[1] These dysrhythmias can often be converted with carotid sinus massage. Adenosine can be administered (6 mg IV, followed by 12 mg IV if no response to the lower dose) if sequential carotid sinus massage fails to abort the dysrhythmia or is contraindicated. Patients presenting with reentrant supraventricular tachycardia in the ICU often have a past history of this dysrhythmia. β-Adrenergic blockers or calcium channel blockers are reasonable choices for both acute conversion and maintenance therapy. Specific β-adrenergic blockers include metoprolol (5 mg IV every 5 minutes until therapeutic effect is achieved) or esmolol (loading dose of 500 µg/kg over 1 minute, then 50 µg/kg/min infusion). Esmolol can be rebolused (500 µg/kg and the drip titrated to a maximum of 400 µg/kg/min). For diltiazem, use 5- or 10-mg boluses, using higher doses only after it is determined that administration of the agent does not lead to arterial hypotension.

The prevalence of atrial fibrillation (AF) in the general population increases exponentially with age, from 0.9% at 40 years to 5.9% in those older than 65.[7] The most important risk factors for development of AF in the general population are structural heart disease (70% in the Framingham study[8] over a 22-year follow-up), hypertension (50%),[8] valvular heart disease (34%),[9] and left ventricular hypertrophy. AF should be approached in the following manner: find the cause and try to fix it; if the underlying problem is not fixable, consider rate control and anticoagulation. AF with rapid ventricular response can cause significant hemodynamic instability requiring emergent electrical cardioversion (biphasic defibrillator). The initial attempt should be synchronized, using 50 J of energy. If unsuccessful, subsequent cardioversion attempts should use escalating energy levels (e.g., 100, 120, 150, 200 J). AF with rapid ventricular response in the absence of hemodynamic instability can be managed initially by using drugs or other interventions to provide rate control. The goal should be to reduce heart rate to less than 120 bpm. First, minimize adrenergic stimulation

TABLE 7-1	Common Causes of Bradycardia

Degeneration of heart tissue related to aging
Damage to heart tissues from heart disease or heart attack
High blood pressure (hypertension)
Heart disorder present at birth (congenital heart defect)
Infection of heart tissue (myocarditis)
Complication of heart surgery
Underactive thyroid gland (hypothyroidism)
Imbalance of electrolytes, mineral-related substances necessary for conducting electrical impulses
Obstructive sleep apnea, the repeated disruption of breathing during sleep
Inflammatory disease such as rheumatic fever or lupus
Hemochromatosis, the buildup of iron in organs
Medications, including some drugs for other heart rhythm disorders, high blood pressure, and psychosis

by instituting mechanical ventilation if high work of breathing and respiratory failure appear to be contributing factors. Reduce the rate of catecholamine (epinephrine, dobutamine, and/or dopamine) infusions if possible. If the patient is not currently receiving treatment with inotropes or vasopressors, consider β-adrenergic blockade as first-line therapy. Metoprolol (5 mg IV every 5 minutes) or esmolol (500 μg/kg over 1 minute, then 50 μg/kg/min infusion) are reasonable choices. A trial of diltiazem (5 to 10 mg IV bolus, followed by an infusion of 5 to 20 mg/h) also can be used. If the patient requires treatment with β-adrenergic inotropic agents to support cardiac output, amiodarone (150 mg IV bolus, followed by an infusion of 1 mg/min for 6 hours, followed by an infusion 0.5 mg/min) is a reasonable choice for both rate control and conversion therapy. Amiodarone can cause lung toxicity, even with short-term therapy, so caution is warranted when using this drug, particularly in critically ill patients with underlying lung pathology.[10] Digoxin is the least effective option acutely; it is relatively ineffective for controlling ventricular rate when endogenous or exogenous adrenergic tone is high.[11] With new-onset AF, conversion to sinus rhythm is desirable, especially for patients who are poor candidates for anticoagulation. Conversion to sinus rhythm is also beneficial for patients with profound left ventricular dysfunction, because coordinated atrial contraction can contribute substantially to cardiac output under these conditions. In other patients, the primary goal should be to achieve (ventricular) rate control.[12,13] Conversion is significantly more likely to occur during rate control with β-adrenergic blockers (e.g., esmolol) than diltiazem, but this observation actually may reflect a reduction in the spontaneous conversion rate when diltiazem is used.[14,15] Amiodarone, particularly in patients with impaired ventricular function, is generally the drug of choice to achieve conversion. Anticoagulation with IV heparin should be considered if AF persists for more than 48 hours. The stroke risk in unanticoagulated patients is approximately 2% per year (0.05% per day).

Regular narrow-complex tachycardia with a heart rate between 145 and 155 bpm is typically due to atrial flutter. Carotid sinus massage or adenosine can unmask this diagnosis if it is in doubt after inspection of the 12-lead ECG (Figure 7-1). Ventricular rate control is difficult to achieve pharmacologically when the dysrhythmia is atrial flutter; accordingly, conversion to sinus rhythm is the goal. Synchronized cardioversion should be tried starting at 50 J, using appropriate conscious sedation. If cardioversion converts the rhythm to AF, use synchronized electrical cardioversion again, starting with 100 J. If atrial fibrillation persists, treat with a rate-controlling agent and anticoagulation. If refractory or recurrent atrial flutter is the problem, attempt rate control with β-adrenergic blockers or diltiazem, as for AF.

Sustained tachycardia associated with hemodynamic instability (i.e., arterial hypotension) and a wide QRS complex on the ECG should be treated as ventricular tachycardia (Figure 7-2). Synchronized cardioversion with the biphasic defibrillator at 200 J should proceed expeditiously for VT with pulse, regardless of hemodynamics. For pulseless VT, unsynchronized cardioversion at 200 J should be performed. Sustained or nonsustained VT without hemodynamic instability typically occurs in patients with cardiomyopathy or acute MI. Initial interven-

NARROW COMPLEX TACHYCARDIA

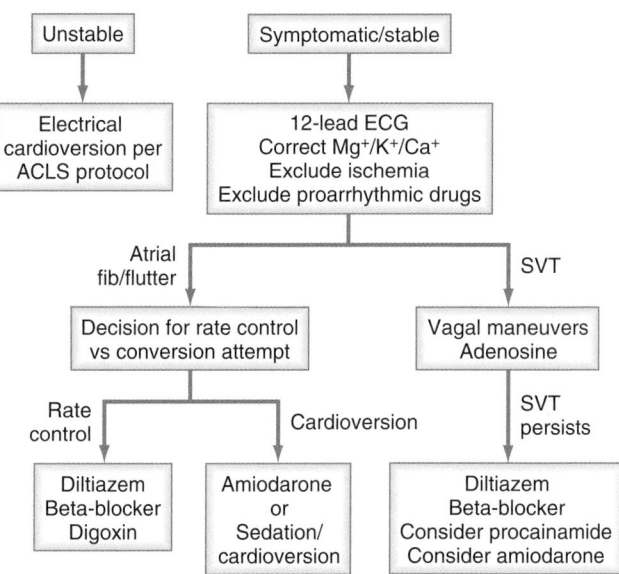

Figure 7-1 Algorithm for diagnosis and testing of narrow-complex tachycardia. ACLS, advanced cardiac life support; ECG, electrocardiogram; fib, fibrillation; SVT, supraventricular tachycardia.

tions should include correction of hypokalemia or hypomagnesemia (if present), reduction in the dose of β-adrenergic agonists (if being infused), and removal of physical stimuli such as pulmonary artery catheters. Amiodarone is the preferred pharmacologic therapy in this setting. Consider myocardial ischemia as the cause of monomorphic VT, and perform the appropriate diagnostic workup. The current American College of Cardiology/American Heart Association guidelines recommend implantation of an internal cardiac defibrillator (ICD) for nonsustained VT in patients with coronary disease, prior MI, left ventricular dysfunction, and inducible ventricular fibrillation (VF) or sustained VT (at the time of an electrophysiologic study) that is not suppressible by a class I antiarrhythmic drug.[16] Polymorphic VT should prompt a thorough evaluation of the medication list, searching for agents that prolong the QTc (Table 7-2).

TABLE 7-2	Common Medications That May Prolong the QTc

Antibiotics
Ciprofloxacin
Clarithromycin
Erythromycin
Ketoconazole
Itraconazole

Antiarrhythmics
Procainamide
Amiodarone
Sotalol
Ibutilide
Dofetilide
Quinidine
Flecainide
Propafenone

Psychiatric
Tricyclic antidepressants
Tetracyclic antidepressants
Ziprasidone
Droperidol
Haloperidol
Phenothiazines

Other
Methadone
Bepridil

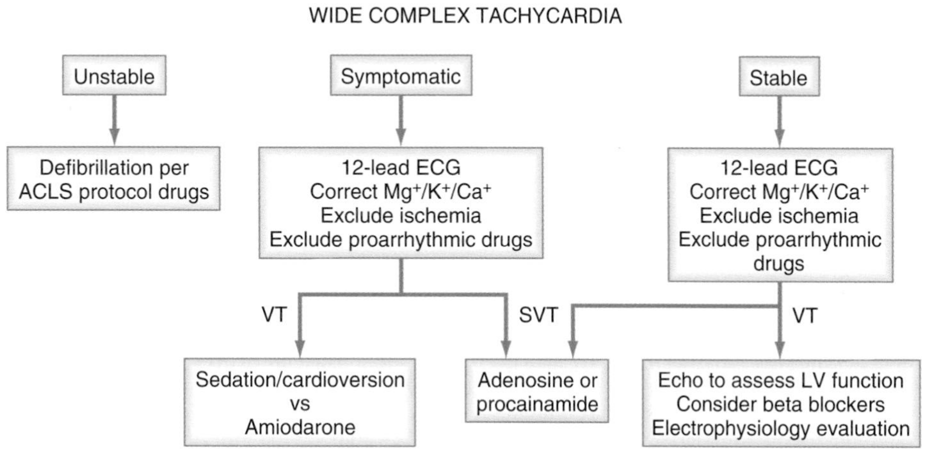

WIDE COMPLEX TACHYCARDIA

Unstable → Defibrillation per ACLS protocol drugs

Symptomatic → 12-lead ECG / Correct Mg+/K+/Ca+ / Exclude ischemia / Exclude proarrhythmic drugs

Stable → 12-lead ECG / Correct Mg+/K+/Ca+ / Exclude ischemia / Exclude proarrhythmic drugs

VT → Sedation/cardioversion vs Amiodarone

SVT → Adenosine or procainamide

VT → Echo to assess LV function / Consider beta blockers / Electrophysiology evaluation

Figure 7-2 Algorithm for diagnosis and testing of wide-complex tachycardia. ACLS, advanced cardiac life support; ECG, electrocardiogram; LV, left ventricle; SVT, supraventricular tachycardia; VT, ventricular tachycardia.

ANNOTATED REFERENCES

Tarditi DJ, Hollenberg SM. Cardiac arrhythmias in the intensive care unit. Semin Respir Crit Care Med 2006;27(3):221-9.
This is an excellent review that provides an update on current concepts of diagnosis and acute management of arrhythmias in the ICU and gives a systematic approach to diagnosis and evaluation of specific arrhythmias.

Gregoratos G, Cheitlin MD, Conill A, et al. ACC/AHA guidelines for implantation of cardiac pacemakers and antiarrhythmia devices: a report of the American College of Cardiology/American Heart Association Task Force on Practice Guidelines (Committee on Pacemaker Implantation). J Am Coll Cardiol 1998;31(5):1175-209.
This is an extensive review of the medical literature and related documents previously published by the American College of Cardiology, the American Heart Association, and the North American Society for Pacing and Electrophysiology, from which the writing committee members developed recommendations that are evidence based whenever possible.

Van Gelder IC, Hagens VE, Bosker HA, et al. A comparison of rate control and rhythm control in patients with recurrent persistent atrial fibrillation. N Engl J Med 2002;347(23):1834-40.
In this study, 522 patients who had persistent atrial fibrillation after a previous electrical cardioversion were assigned to receive treatment aimed at rate control or rhythm control. Patients in the rate-control group received oral anticoagulant drugs and rate-slowing medication. Patients in the rhythm-control group underwent serial cardioversions and received antiarrhythmic drugs and oral anticoagulant drugs. The endpoint was a composite of death from cardiovascular causes, heart failure, thromboembolic complications, bleeding, implantation of a pacemaker, and severe adverse effects of drugs.

Ashrafian H, Davey P. Is amiodarone an underrecognized cause of acute respiratory failure in the ICU? Chest 2001;120(1):275-82.
A review of the data and existing literature in which the authors concluded there is sufficient evidence of amiodarone's potentially serious side-effect profile in surgical ICU patients to advise continued caution in its use with this severely ill patient group. They suggest that amiodarone has a potentially important though underrecognized role in inducing an acute pulmonary toxicity in some patients, such as those undergoing cardiac surgery (a clinical scenario in which amiodarone is most commonly used).

Mooss AN, Wurdeman RL, Mohiuddin SM, et al. Esmolol versus diltiazem in the treatment of postoperative atrial fibrillation/atrial flutter after open heart surgery. Am Heart J 2000;140(1):176-80.
This is a randomized study designed to compare the safety and efficacy of intravenous diltiazem versus intravenous esmolol in patients with postoperative atrial fibrillation/atrial flutter (AF/AFL) after coronary bypass surgery and/or valve replacement surgery. A group of 30 patients received either esmolol (n=15) or diltiazem (n=15) for AF/AFL. This study showed that esmolol was not only more successful in chemical cardioversion but also more cost effective.

Polderman D, Boersma E, Bax JJ, et al. The effect of bisoprolol on perioperative mortality and myocardial infarction in high-risk patients undergoing vascular surgery. Dutch Echocardiographic Cardiac Risk Evaluation Applying Stress Echocardiography Study Group. N Engl J Med 1999;341(24):1789-94.
A randomized multicenter study that assessed the effect of perioperative β-blockade in high-risk vascular surgical patients in reducing nonfatal myocardial infarction and death from cardiac causes. They screened a total of 1351 patients, of which 846 were found to have one or more cardiac risk factors. Of these 846 patients, 173 had positive results on dobutamine echocardiography. Fifty-nine patients were randomly assigned to receive bisoprolol, and 53 to receive standard care. Fifty-three patients were excluded from randomization because they were already taking a beta-blocker, and eight were excluded because they had extensive wall-motion abnormalities either at rest or during stress testing. The study demonstrated that bisoprolol reduces the perioperative incidence of death from cardiac causes and nonfatal myocardial infarction in high-risk patients who are undergoing major vascular surgery.

REFERENCES

Access the complete reference list online at http://www.expertconsult.com.

Arterial Hypoxemia

PAUL ROGERS

Respiratory distress with hypoxemia is a common reason for patients to be admitted to the intensive care unit (ICU). Because a patient's arterial oxygen saturation can be monitored easily using a continuous pulse oximeter, nurses and physicians are alerted immediately to changes in a patient's oxygen saturation. For these reasons, it is important for healthcare providers to understand the meaning of this measurement, recognize its limitations, and outline a plan for diagnosing and managing patients with hypoxemia.

Arterial hypoxemia is defined as a partial pressure of oxygen in arterial blood (Pao_2) less than 80 mm Hg while breathing room air. The Pao_2 represents the amount of oxygen in physical solution, whereas the oxygen saturation represents the fractional amount of oxyhemoglobin relative to total hemoglobin concentration. Oxygen saturation varies with the Pao_2 in a nonlinear relationship and is affected by temperature, partial pressure of carbon dioxide in arterial blood ($Paco_2$), pH, and 2,3-diphosphoglycerate concentration (Figure 8-1).

Falsely low saturations can be recorded if there is a poor waveform or if light absorption is decreased by dark blue or black nail polish. Patients with methemoglobinemia can have a falsely low oxygen saturation, whereas patients with carboxyhemoglobinemia can have a falsely elevated oxygen saturation, because the pulse oximeter cannot differentiate carboxyhemoglobin from oxyhemoglobin.[1] Finally, because the oxygen-hemoglobin dissociation curve is affected by temperature, pH, partial pressure of carbon dioxide (Pco_2), and 2,3-diphosphoglycerate concentration, patients can have a higher or lower saturation for a given Pao_2.

Patients who have significant decreases in oxygen saturation attempt to maintain oxygen delivery by increasing cardiac output. Although patients with normal left ventricular function and normal coronary vasculature can tolerate lower oxygen saturation, patients with coronary artery disease or decreased myocardial contractility may not be able to tolerate the compensatory tachycardia. The decision to begin mechanical or noninvasive ventilation should be based on the patient's cardiopulmonary physiology and not the specific value for the oxygen saturation measurement. Pao_2 less than 40 mm Hg or oxygen saturation less than 75% results in tissue hypoxemia, however, despite compensatory increases in cardiac output. Generally, saturations in the low 90s on escalating levels of inspired oxygen concentration indicate impending respiratory failure, and invasive or noninvasive mechanical ventilation is necessary.

Etiologies for hypoxemia are best understood if approached from a physiologic point of view rather than by referring to a list of possible differential diagnoses. Simply stated, hypoxemia results from an imbalance between pulmonary ventilation and pulmonary capillary blood flow.[2]

Reduced Alveolar Oxygenation

Alveolar oxygenation is defined by the equation:

$$Palvo_2 = Fio_2(BP - BPH_2O) - Paco_2/RQ$$

where Fio_2 is the concentration of inspired oxygen, BP is the barometric pressure, BPH_2O is the partial pressure of water, and RQ is the respiratory quotient. The respiratory quotient represents the amount of oxygen consumed relative to the amount of carbon dioxide produced when nutrients are metabolized. RQ is generally assumed to be 0.8. Under normal conditions, where the Fio_2 is 21%, BP is 760 mm Hg, BPH_2O is 47 mm Hg, and $Paco_2$ is 40 mm Hg, the $Palvo_2 = 0.21(760 - 47) - 40/0.8 = 100$ mm Hg. According to the equation, several factors may contribute to lower alveolar oxygenation. One is a reduction in barometric pressure, causing hypobaric hypoxemia that affects those climbing at high altitudes.[3] The second factor is an increase in $Paco_2$, which can be explained by the relationship: $Paco_2 =$ carbon dioxide production/respiratory rate (tidal volume − dead space). Accordingly, the $Paco_2$ increases with either an increase in production or a decrease in alveolar ventilation. Alveolar ventilation represents that portion of the minute ventilation undergoing blood-gas exchange and is represented by the product of respiratory rate and tidal volume minus dead space. Medications such as narcotics and sedatives that reduce the respiratory rate, and processes such as neuromotor weakness that reduce tidal volume, are common causes of hypercarbia.

To summarize, if the alveolar oxygen tension is reduced, then arterial hypoxemia is due to factors responsible for the low alveolar oxygen tension. If alveolar oxygen tension is normal, then hypoxemia is the result of either a ventilation/perfusion imbalance or a diffusion abnormality.

Diffusion Abnormalities

Diffusion abnormalities are the least likely cause of hypoxemia in the ICU, but they can occur as a result of an increase in the thickness of the capillary membrane, a reduction in total alveolar surface area, or a reduction in the capillary transit time. Increases in sympathetic tone due to fever, anemia, work of breathing, or sepsis can increase cardiac output and heart rate, resulting in faster transpulmonary transit times. With less opportunity for alveolar oxygen to diffuse into red blood cells, diffusing capacity is reduced. When capillary transit time is faster, the mean capillary arterial oxygen partial pressure decreases, and the diffusing capacity is reduced.

Ventilation/Perfusion Mismatch

The most common cause of hypoxemia is ventilation/perfusion mismatch. When perfusion is reduced as a result of a decrease in cardiac output or obstruction from pulmonary emboli, the percent of alveoli with adequate blood flow is reduced, increasing functional dead space. If minute ventilation remains constant, the primary blood gas abnormality is an increase in carbon dioxide ($Pco_2 =$ carbon dioxide production/respiratory rate × tidal volume − dead space).

When ventilation is reduced relative to perfusion, alveolar oxygenation decreases and results in arterial hypoxemia. This problem occasionally occurs with bronchospasm or bronchitis. Patients with ventilation/perfusion abnormalities generally respond to increasing the Fio_2. When there is no ventilation (as opposed to reduced ventilation), increasing the Fio_2 is not beneficial.

The portion of cardiac output that does not participate in gas exchange is called the *shunt fraction*. The normal shunt fraction is approximately 3%, and this small amount of shunt is due to the bronchial arterial circulation. When alveoli are not ventilated, such as occurs with pulmonary edema, pneumonia, or atelectasis, the shunt

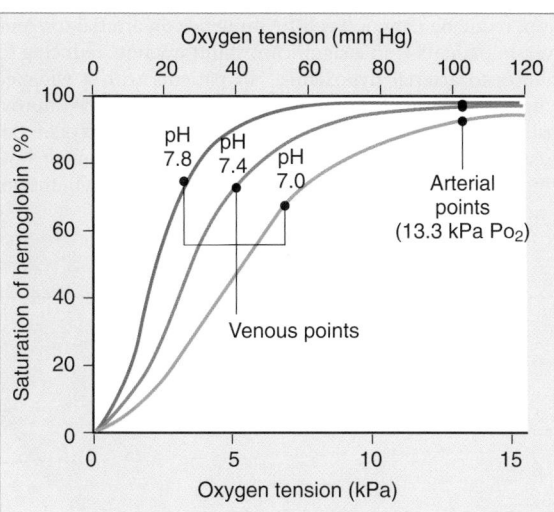

Figure 8-1 Oxygen saturation varies with the PaO_2 in a nonlinear relationship and is affected by temperature, $PaCO_2$, pH, and 2,3-diphosphoglycerate (2,3-DPG) concentration.

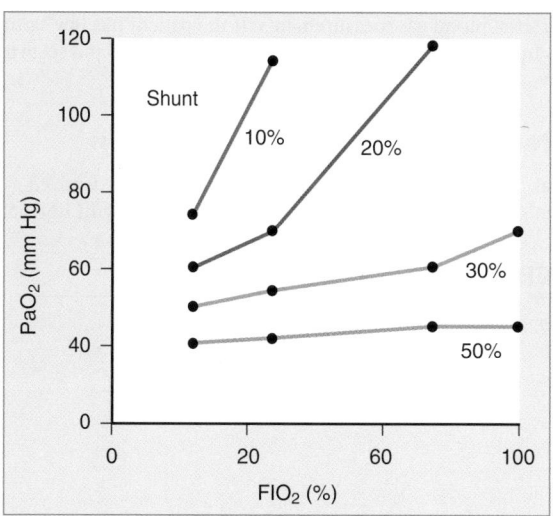

Figure 8-3 Blunted response to increasing the inspired oxygen concentration. A patient with a shunt greater than 50% has little response to increasing FIO_2.

fraction increases. As the shunt fraction increases, Pao_2 decreases (Figure 8-2), and there is a blunted response to increasing the FIO_2. When the shunt fraction is above 50%, there is little response to increasing FIO_2 (Figure 8-3).

Patients with refractory hypoxemia and a clear chest radiograph are often evaluated for a pulmonary embolus. In patients with otherwise previously normal lungs, pulmonary emboli are associated with modest decreases in arterial oxygenation; however, the major pathophysiology is an increase in dead space, which results in hypercarbia unless minute ventilation increases. The hypoxemia caused by pulmonary emboli is due to regional ventilation/perfusion abnormalities and responds to supplemental oxygen. If a patient with a pulmonary embolus has refractory hypoxemia unresponsive to supplemental oxygenation, an echocardiogram should be performed to rule out a patent foramen ovale, which creates a right-to-left intracardiac shunt in response to the acute increase in pulmonary artery pressure.

Other causes of refractory hypoxemia with a clear chest radiograph are intracardiac shunts and intrapulmonary shunts resulting from either arterial-venous malformations or end-stage liver disease. Often the cause of refractory hypoxemia without radiographic findings on the plain chest film is atelectasis, which is not seen on the typical anteroposterior portable study obtained in the ICU.

It also is relatively common for patients to develop significant hypoxemia when they are started on an intravenous vasodilator such as sodium nitroprusside. Infusion of sodium nitroprusside interferes with normal hypoxic vasoconstriction, leading to increased perfusion of poorly ventilated areas of the lung. As a result, shunt fraction increases.

Because calculating the shunt fraction, $QsCQ_t = Cco_2/Cco_2 - CVo_2$, requires arterial and mixed venous blood gases for calculation of $C_{Ca}O_2$ (arterial) and C_vo_2 (venous) oxygen contents, and because capillary oxygen cannot be directly measured, other indices have been used to estimate the extent of pulmonary gas exchange abnormality. These indices include the alveolar-to-arterial (A-a) Po_2 gradient and the arterial-to-alveolar Po_2 ratio.

Alveolar-Arterial Partial Pressure of Oxygen Gradient

The difference between the alveolar Po_2 and the arterial Po_2 (i.e., the A-a gradient) often is used to estimate the extent of pulmonary pathophysiology and to rule out hypoxemia due to low alveolar Po_2 as the cause of arterial hypoxemia.[4,5] A patient with a reduced alveolar Po_2 (e.g., secondary to breathing room air at high altitude) would have a normal A-a gradient, whereas a patient with ventilation/perfusion mismatching would have a widened A-a gradient. A patient with a Pao_2 of 48 mm Hg and a $Paco_2$ of 80 mm Hg would have an alveolar Po_2 on room air of 50 mm Hg; the normal A-a gradient of 2 mm Hg is consistent with reduced alveolar Po_2, and causes of hypercarbia need to be ruled out and reversed.

The A-a gradient increases with age or increasing FIO_2, making it an unreliable predictor of the degree of pulmonary dysfunction.[5,6] The Pao_2:FIO_2 ratio also correlates with shunt fraction but is influenced by increasing FIO_2.[4] The arterial-to-alveolar ratio is not influenced by FIO_2.[6]

These gradients and ratios are not a substitute for thorough bedside assessment. If a patient has low arterial oxygen saturation by pulse oximetry and is tolerating the reduced saturation without tachycardia or chest pain, adding supplemental oxygen and observing for an appropriate response is reasonable. If there is no increase in saturation, the patient has at least a 40% to 50% shunt and requires intubation or noninvasive ventilation to improve ventilation. Under these conditions, further increases in inspired oxygen concentration will not increase arterial saturation. If the saturation responds to increasing the FIO_2, then the patient has a shunt fraction less than 0.4 or ventilation/perfusion mismatching, and there is time to obtain a chest radiograph

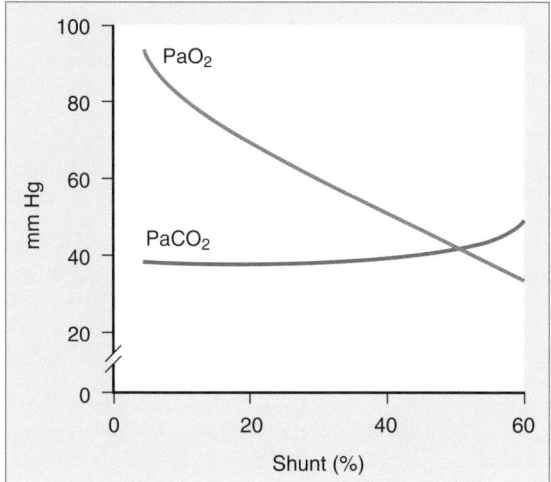

Figure 8-2 Decrease in PaO_2 with increasing shunt fraction.

and arterial blood gas measurements. If the patient has low saturation and is unstable, immediate bag-and-mask ventilation and securing the airway take precedence over establishing a diagnosis.

Reduced Mixed Venous Oxygen

A final contribution to hypoxemia may be a reduced mixed venous oxygen content (Cmv_{O_2}) or saturation. In patients with normal lung function, reducing Cmv_{O_2} has little influence on arterial oxygenation; however, in patients with a significant shunt fraction, reducing Cmv_{O_2} contributes to arterial hypoxemia.[7] In patients with a widened A-a gradient and abnormally low Cmv_{O_2}, oxygenation can be improved by increasing venous saturation either by increasing oxygen delivery (increased hemoglobin concentration or cardiac output or both) or reducing oxygen consumption (e.g., induction of hypothermia or using neuromuscular blocking agents).

REFERENCES

Access the complete reference list online at http://www.expertconsult.com.

9

Acute Respiratory Failure

LAKSHMIPATHI CHELLURI | ROBERT POUSMAN

Acute respiratory failure is one of the leading causes of admission to an intensive care unit (ICU). Behrendt et al. reported that the incidence of acute respiratory failure requiring hospitalization was 137 per 100,000 population in the United States, and the median age of the patients was 69 years.[1] More recently, Ray et al. reported that 29% of patients presenting to an emergency department (ED) with acute respiratory failure require admission to an ICU.[2]

Acute respiratory failure can be secondary to either a failure of oxygenation (hypoxic respiratory failure), a failure of elimination of carbon dioxide (hypercarbic respiratory [ventilatory] failure), or both problems simultaneously. Chronic obstructive pulmonary disease (COPD) with acute exacerbation is the most common cause of ventilatory failure requiring ICU admission.

Pathophysiology

The primary gas exchange functions of the lung are the transport of oxygen from inspired air (or some other gas mixture) to hemoglobin (Hb) in the bloodstream and elimination of carbon dioxide. Dysfunction of either function results in acute respiratory failure (or at least acute respiratory dysfunction).

Causes of Hypoxic Respiratory Failure

HYPOVENTILATION

The partial pressure of carbon dioxide in arterial blood ($Paco_2$) increases when minute ventilation decreases. An increase in $Paco_2$ decreases alveolar partial pressure of oxygen (Pao_2) because the carbon dioxide displaces oxygen in the alveoli. The relationship between Pao_2 and $Paco_2$ is described by the alveolar gas equation:

$$Pao_2 = Fio_2 \times (Patm - P_{H_2O}) - (Paco_2/0.8)$$

The causes of hypoventilation are discussed below.

VENTILATION/PERFUSION MISMATCH

Gas exchange is optimal when ventilation and perfusion in the lung are matched. A decrease in perfusion relative to ventilation (i.e., an increase in physiologic dead space) or a decrease in ventilation relative to perfusion (shunt) results in ventilation-perfusion ($\dot{V}/\dot{Q}$) mismatching. Hypoxia occurs as a result of $\dot{V}/\dot{Q}$ mismatching because of admixture of venous with arterial blood at the capillary level. $\dot{V}/\dot{Q}$ mismatching is the most common cause of hypoxia in hospitalized patients. In contrast to hypoxemia caused by an anatomic shunt, hypoxemia caused by $\dot{V}/\dot{Q}$ mismatching can be improved by administration of supplemental oxygen.

SHUNT

Right-to-left shunting refers to the process whereby deoxygenated venous blood bypasses functioning alveolar-pulmonary capillary units and then mixes with oxygenated arterial blood. Right-to-left shunts can be caused by anatomic derangements, such as certain congenital cardiac malformations (e.g., atrial septal defect), but they can also occur when $\dot{V}/\dot{Q}$ mismatching is so severe that a portion of pulmonary arterial blood flows through lung regions with essentially no ventilation. Potential causes of this sort of physiologic shunting include pneumonia, lung contusion, or severe congestive heart failure. Oxygenation cannot be improved with supplemental oxygen in patients with a true right-to-left shunt, irrespective of whether the shunt is caused by an anatomic or a functional derangement.

DIFFUSION IMPAIRMENT

Thickening of the alveolar endothelial/epithelial barrier or a decrease in transit time in the pulmonary capillary bed (due to very high cardiac output) can impair diffusion of oxygen from the alveoli into the blood.

HIGH ALTITUDE

Barometric pressure decreases with increasing altitude; as a result, the partial pressure of oxygen in the ambient atmosphere decreases as well. Consequently, unless supplemental oxygen is provided, hypoxia is an inevitable consequence of respiration at high altitude.

IMPAIRED TISSUE PERFUSION

When tissue perfusion is impaired, the cells attempt to maintain normal oxygen consumption by extracting more oxygen from the available blood supply. As a consequence, venous oxygen tension decreases. Unless the fractional pulmonary shunt flow is zero, the decrease in mixed venous oxygen tension inevitably leads to a decrease in arterial oxygen tension. Although low cardiac output or impaired blood flow to tissues can cause hypoxia, hypoperfusion per se is rarely a primary cause of clinically significant hypoxia. Nevertheless, hypoperfusion is a common factor that exacerbates the degree of hypoxia caused by other problems.

If the circulating concentration of carboxyhemoglobin or methemoglobin increases, the oxygen-carrying capacity of the blood decreases. Although arterial oxygen tension may be normal, arterial oxygen saturation is abnormally low because of the presence of Hb derivatives that are incapable of transporting oxygen.

Hypercarbic Respiratory Failure

$Paco_2$ is inversely proportional to alveolar ventilation; thus, $Paco_2$ increases when the elimination of carbon dioxide is decreased because of a decrease in minute ventilation. $Paco_2$ also increases if minute ventilation remains constant but carbon dioxide production increases. Primary pulmonary diseases are the most common cause of hypercarbia, although nonpulmonary causes contribute to hypoventilation, increased $Paco_2$, and the need for mechanical ventilatory support.

Minute ventilation can be decreased owing to pulmonary or nonpulmonary factors. Pulmonary causes of impaired minute ventilation include large airway obstruction (e.g., due to the presence of a foreign body or laryngeal spasm), small airway obstruction (e.g., bronchospasm), and destruction of lung parenchyma (e.g., emphysema). Extrapulmonary causes of hypercarbia include neurologic and muscular problems. Neurologic problems include depression of central respiratory drive due to the pharmacologic effects of narcotics or sedatives; depression of respiratory drive as a consequence of stroke, intracranial hemorrhage, or head trauma (i.e., central alveolar hypoventilation); and impaired neuromuscular transmission due to phrenic nerve injury or spinal cord injury (C5 or higher), Guillain-Barré syndrome, myasthenia gravis, or the polyneuropathy of critical illness. Muscular weakness or skeletal abnormalities can cause a decrease in tidal volume and minute ventilation. Causes of hypoventilation secondary to musculoskeletal abnormalities are prolonged use of neuromuscular blocking agents, malnutrition, hypomagnesemia, hypokalemia, hypophosphatemia, kyphoscoliosis, rib fractures, and flail chest, to name several.

In rare cases, hypercarbia can be secondary to increased carbon dioxide production and relative hypoventilation due to overfeeding, since fat synthesis increases the rate of carbon dioxide production relative to the rate of oxygen consumption (respiratory quotient >1.0). Hypermetabolism, such as occurs with high fever or thyrotoxicosis, also is associated with increased carbon dioxide production and (in the setting of already impaired minute ventilation) can exacerbate hypercarbia.

Clinical Presentation

Dyspnea is the most common symptom associated with acute respiratory failure. Dyspnea is usually associated with rapid shallow breathing and the use of accessory respiratory muscles. Active use of the accessory muscles of respiration during expiration is indicative of impaired airflow during exhalation, a common problem in patients with COPD.

The investigations to evaluate the causes of respiratory failure depend on the suspected mechanism of acute respiratory failure and the primary disease process. Pulse oximetry is a useful monitoring tool and should be carried out in all cases. Other worthwhile diagnostic studies include:
- *Analysis of arterial blood gases* – will permit diagnosis of a widened alveolar-arterial Po_2 gradient and/or hypercarbia.
- *Examination of the chest radiograph* – useful in almost all cases. If the chest film is clear, the differential diagnosis should include pulmonary embolism, anatomic right-to-left shunt, pneumothorax, cirrhosis, and COPD. If the chest radiograph shows unilateral infiltrates or effusion, the differential diagnosis should include pleural effusion, aspiration, lobar pneumonia, atelectasis, and infarction. If bilateral infiltrates are present, the differential diagnosis should include pulmonary edema (cardiac and noncardiac causes), pneumonia, and pulmonary hemorrhage.[3]

Other more specialized tests (e.g., computed tomography, cultures) are needed based on the differential diagnosis for the suspected primary disease.

Management

The goal is to maintain adequate oxygenation and ventilation and treat the primary cause of respiratory failure. For hypoxic respiratory failure, the primary goal is to improve arterial oxygenation. In most cases, a reasonable goal is to maintain Pao_2 above 65 to 70 mm Hg and arterial blood oxygen saturation (Sao_2) above 90%. In very severe cases of hypoxi respiratory failure, efforts to achieve these indices of arterial oxygenation will require interventions, namely very high airway pressures during mechanical ventilation and delivery of 100% oxygen in the inspired gas—interventions that can further damage the lung. Accordingly, in rare instances, it may be prudent to tolerate lower Sao_2 values rather than using ventilator settings that could exacerbate lung damage.

Administration of supplemental oxygen will improve oxygenation in most clinical situations except in the presence of a true shunt. Low-flow oxygen can be delivered using a nasal canula or a face mask. The maximum Fio_2 that can be delivered using these approaches is about 0.4. This level of oxygen supplementation is inadequate when the alveolar-arterial (A-a) Po_2 gradient is very wide. The Fio_2 in the inspired gas delivered using a nasal canula or face mask is a function of minute ventilation. When minute ventilation is high, the Fio_2 in the inspired gas delivered using a nasal canula or face mask is lower than when minute ventilation is lower. Accordingly, low-flow methods of providing supplemental oxygen should be used cautiously in patients

who are dependent on hypoxic drive or have very high minute ventilation. A higher Fio_2 can be provided if a face mask is combined with a reservoir bag, because contamination of the inspired gas mixture with room air is minimized.

Noninvasive positive pressure ventilation (NIPPV) and mechanical ventilation via an endotracheal tube are two approaches for providing supplemental oxygen and, at the same time, providing partial or total support for minute ventilation (i.e., decreasing the work of breathing). In hemodynamically stable patients with mild or moderate respiratory failure, NIPPV may decrease the need for intubation and mechanical ventilation and decrease the patient's length of stay in the ICU.[4,5] NIPPV should not be used in patients with altered mental status, who are unable to protect the airway, or for patients who are unable to clear secretions adequately. For some patients, tolerance for NIPPV can be improved by using a nasal mask and starting at a lower level of inspiratory pressure (5 cm H_2O).

In cases of hypercarbic respiratory failure, the primary goal of treatment is to maintain arterial pH above 7.32 with a $Paco_2$ appropriate for the pH.[6] In the absence of marked acidemia or hypoxemia, hypercarbia is well tolerated. Accordingly, it may be preferable under some circumstances to accept $Paco_2$ values that are abnormally high (e.g., >45 mm Hg) rather than risk damaging (or further damaging) the lungs with ventilator settings that promote excessive shear stress within the pulmonary parenchyma.

Bronchodilators can be delivered as metered dose inhalers or nebulizers. Patients with tachypnea and respiratory distress may not be able to use metered dose inhalers. The bronchodilating effects of β-adrenergic agonists and anticholinergic drugs are synergistic. Long-acting β-adrenergic agonists should not be used to treat acute exacerbations of chronic bronchospasm. Corticosteroids are often used to treat acute exacerbations of diseases associated with airway inflammation and bronchospasm (e.g., asthma, COPD). Intravenous methylprednisolone (40 mg IV every 12 hours to 125 mg IV every 6 hours) is often employed if the response is inadequate to initial efforts using bronchodilator treatments with β-adrenergic agonists and anticholinergic agents. Aerosolized steroids may not improve bronchospasm during the acute episode but are useful for maintenance treatment. Patients who experience changes in the nature of the sputum and signs of infection may benefit from a short course (7–10 days) of antibiotic therapy.

The use of NIPPV in hemodynamically stable patients with mild to moderate ventilatory failure may decrease the need for mechanical ventilatory support and length of stay. The precautions while using NIPPV are the same as listed previously.

INTUBATION AND MECHANICAL VENTILATION

The need for mechanical ventilatory support is a clinical decision based on increased work of breathing (i.e., respiratory rate >35/min, use of accessory muscles of ventilation) and inability to clear secretions, and maintain a patent, protected, adequate airway. The clinician has only two basic maneuvers for improving Pao_2 using mechanical ventilation. The first is to increase Fio_2. The second is to increase mean airway pressure. The latter goal can be achieved primarily in two ways: (1) application of positive end-expiratory pressure (PEEP) or (2) changing the duty cycle so that the duration of inspiration is longer (in the extreme, this maneuver is called *inverse ratio ventilation*). In patients with acute lung injury, tidal volume should be limited to 6 mL/kg (ideal body weight).[7] Prone positioning, high-frequency oscillatory ventilation, inhaled nitric oxide, differential lung ventilation, and transtracheal gas insufflation have been shown to improve arterial oxygenation in selected patients with profound hypoxemia due to acute lung injury, but none of these approaches has been shown to improve survival.

Ventilation should be adjusted to maintain pH and $Paco_2$ at levels that are appropriate for the patient, particularly in patients with COPD and chronic respiratory acidosis. Hyperventilation and excessive correction of $Paco_2$ in patients with chronic respiratory acidosis results in secondary metabolic alkalosis and delay in weaning from mechanical ventilation. Alveolar air trapping (so-called auto-positive end-expiratory pressure) and hypotension (due to impaired venous return) may develop in patients with inadequate exhalation time, and caution should be used when increasing minute ventilation by increasing either ventilator-delivered respiratory rate or tidal volume in patients with severe airway obstruction.

Prognosis

Mortality in patients with respiratory failure requiring positive pressure ventilatory support is dependent on the primary cause. The hospital mortality rate is 30% to 40%, and the 1-year mortality rate is 50% to 70%. Functional status deteriorates immediately after the illness and improves to baseline by 6 to 12 months in survivors.[8]

ANNOTATED REFERENCES

ARDSnet. Ventilation with lower tidal volumes as compared with traditional tidal volumes for acute lung injury and the acute respiratory distress syndrome. The Acute Respiratory Distress Syndrome Network. N Engl J Med 2000;342(18):1301-8.
  First ROCT to show outcome benefit in ventilation strategy in patients with ARDS.
Behrendt CE. Acute respiratory failure in the United States: incidence and 31-day survival. Chest 2000;118(4):1100-5.
  Provides excellent epidemiology data for acute respiratory failure in the United States.
Chelluri L. Critical illness in the elderly: review of pathophysiology of aging and outcome of intensive care. J Intensive Care Med 2001;16:114-27.
  Reviews specific factors affecting prognosis in the elderly.
Dakin J, Griffiths M. The pulmonary physician in critical care 1: pulmonary investigations for acute respiratory failure. Thorax 2002;57:79-85.
  Good review of bedside clinical evaluation tools in assessing etiology of acute respiratory failure.

Hill NS, Brennan J, Garpestad E, Nava S. Noninvasive ventilation in acute respiratory failure. Crit Care Med 2007;35(10):2402-7.
  Informative review of use of NIV for primarily medical causes of ARF.
Jaber S, Chanques G, Jung B. Postoperative noninvasive ventilation. Anesthesiology 2010;112(2):453-61.
  Discusses recent advances in use of NIPPV in postoperative patients with ARF.
MacIntyre N, Huang YC. Acute exacerbations and respiratory failure in chronic obstructive pulmonary disease. Proc Am Thorac Soc 2008;5(4):530-5.
  Reviews latest diagnostic, prognostic data and treatments for acute exacerbations of COPD.
Ray P, Birolleau S, Lefort Y, Becquemin MH, Beigelman C, Isnard R, et al. Acute respiratory failure in the elderly: etiology, emergency diagnosis and prognosis. Crit Care 2006;10(3):R82.
  Although a European study, sheds light on important factors influencing diagnosis and admission to ICU.

REFERENCES

Access the complete reference list online at http://www.expertconsult.com.

10

Polyuria

RAMESH VENKATARAMAN | JOHN A. KELLUM

Although polyuria in critically ill patients is less common than oliguria, it is an important manifestation of a number of important clinical conditions. Unless it is recognized and appropriately managed, polyuria can rapidly lead to the development of intravascular volume depletion and/or severe hypernatremia. Generally, urine flow varies depending on fluid intake, insensible losses (e.g., perspiration), and renal function. The average person excretes about 600 to 800 mOsm of solutes per day, and average urine output is about 1.5 to 2.5 L/day.

Polyuria has been defined variably in the literature. The most commonly used definition is based entirely upon absolute urine volume and arbitrarily defines polyuria as urine volume of more than 3 L/day. However, some authors prefer to define polyuria as "inappropriately high urine volume in relation to the prevailing pathophysiologic state," regardless of the actual volume of urine.[1,2]

Classification

Polyuria is broadly classified into *water diuresis* or *solute diuresis*, depending upon whether water or solute is the primary driving force for the increased urine output. However, some patients have a mixed water and solute diuresis.

WATER DIURESIS

Definition and Pathophysiology

If urine output is greater than 3 L/day and the urine is dilute (urine osmolality <250 mOsm/L), total solute excretion is relatively normal, and polyuria is due to excessive excretion of water. In general, diuresis is marked and urine osmolality (Uosm) is often less than 100 mOsm/L. Water diuresis is usually secondary to excess water intake (as in primary polydipsia) or inability of the renal tubules to reabsorb free water (as in central or nephrogenic diabetes insipidus). A good understanding of water homeostasis is critical for recognizing and managing water diuresis.

Normal plasma osmolality is 275 to 285 mOsm/L. To maintain this steady state, water intake must equal water excretion. The primary stimulus for water ingestion is thirst, mediated either by an increase in effective osmolality or a decrease in blood pressure (BP) or effective circulating volume. Under normal circumstances, water intake generally exceeds physiologic requirements.

Unlike water intake, water excretion is very tightly regulated by multiple factors. The most dominant regulating factor affecting water excretion is arginine vasopressin (AVP), a polypeptide synthesized in the hypothalamus and secreted by the posterior pituitary gland. Once released, AVP binds to vasopressin-2 (V2) receptors located on the basolateral membranes of renal epithelial cells lining the collecting ducts. Binding of AVP to V2 receptors initiates a sequence of cellular events, ultimately resulting in insertion of water channels into the luminal cell membrane. The presence of these water channels permits passive diffusion of water (hence its reabsorption) across the collecting duct. Any derangement in this process results in lack of or inadequate water reabsorption by the collecting duct, resulting in water diuresis. The major stimulus for AVP release is plasma hypertonicity. AVP release is also affected by other nonosmotic factors like effective circulating volume, hypoglycemia, and drugs. In summary, water diuresis occurs either because of excessive water intake sufficient enough to overwhelm the renal excretory capacity (primary polydipsia) or impairment of renal water reabsorption itself (central or nephrogenic diabetes insipidus). Impaired renal water reabsorptive capacity (leading to water diuresis) in turn can occur either as a result of failure of AVP release in response to normal physiologic stimuli (central or neurogenic diabetes insipidus) or failure of the kidney to respond to AVP (nephrogenic diabetes insipidus). In most patients, the degree of polyuria is primarily determined by the degree of AVP lack or resistance.

Primary Polydipsia

Primary polydipsia can be recognized clinically based on the history of the patient. Usually there is a history of psychiatric illness along with a history of excessive water intake. Many patients with chronic psychiatric illnesses have a moderate to marked increase in water intake (up to 40 L/day).[3,4] It is presumed that a central defect in thirst regulation plays an important role in the pathogenesis of primary polydipsia. In some cases, the osmotic threshold for thirst is reduced below the threshold for the release of AVP. The mechanism responsible for abnormal thirst regulation in this setting is unclear. There is evidence that these patients have other defects in central neurohumoral control as well.[5] Hyponatremia, when present, also points to the diagnosis of primary polydipsia. The diagnosis of primary polydipsia is usually evident from low urine and plasma osmolalities in the face of polyuria. Hypothalamic diseases such as sarcoidosis, trauma, and certain drugs like phenothiazines can lead to primary polydipsia (Table 10-1). There is no proven specific therapy for psychogenic polydipsia. Free water restriction is the mainstay of therapy.

Central Diabetes Insipidus

Inadequate secretion of AVP (central diabetes insipidus) can be caused by a large number of disorders that act at one or more of the sites involved in AVP secretion, interfering with the physiologic chain of events that lead to hormone release. However, the most common causes of central diabetes insipidus account for the vast majority of cases. These common causes include neurosurgery, head trauma, brain death, primary or secondary tumors of the hypothalamus, or infiltrative diseases such as Langerhans cell histiocytosis (see Table 10-1).

Nephrogenic Diabetes Insipidus

Nephrogenic diabetes insipidus refers to a decrease in urinary concentrating ability that results from renal resistance to the action of AVP. The collecting duct cells can fail to respond to the actions of AVP. Other factors that can cause renal resistance to AVP are problems that interfere with the renal countercurrent concentrating mechanism, such as medullary injury or decreased sodium chloride reabsorption in the medullary aspect of the thick ascending limb of the loop of Henle. In children, nephrogenic diabetes insipidus is usually hereditary. Congenital or hereditary nephrogenic diabetes insipidus is an X-linked recessive disorder resulting from mutations in the V2 AVP receptor gene.[6] The X-linked inheritance pattern means that males tend to have marked polyuria. Female carriers are usually asymptomatic but occasionally have severe polyuria. In addition, different mutations are associated with different degrees of AVP resistance. Nephrogenic diabetes insipidus also can be inherited as an autosomal recessive disorder due to mutations in the aquaporin gene that result in absent or defective water channels, thereby causing resistance to the action of AVP.[7]

TABLE 10-1	Causes of Polyuria

1. Polyuria secondary to water diuresis
   a. Excessive intake of water
      i. Psychogenic polydipsia
      ii. Drugs—anticholinergic drugs, thioridazine
      iii. Hypothalamic diseases—trauma, sarcoidosis
   b. Defective water reabsorption by the kidney
      i. Central diabetes insipidus (vasopressin deficiency)
      ii. Renal tubular resistance to AVP
2. Congenital nephrogenic diabetes insipidus
3. Acquired nephrogenic diabetes insipidus
   a. Hypercalcemia
   b. Hypokalemia
   c. Drugs—lithium, demeclocycline
   d. Chronic renal diseases—postobstructive diuresis, polyuric phase of ATN
   e. Other systemic diseases—amyloidosis, sickle cell anemia
4. Polyuria secondary to solute diuresis
   a. Electrolyte-induced solute diuresis
      i. Iatrogenic—excessive sodium chloride load, loop diuretic use
      ii. Salt-wasting nephropathy (rarely causes polyuria)
   b. Nonelectrolyte solute–induced diuresis
      i. Glucosuria—diabetic ketoacidosis, hyperosmolar coma
      ii. Urea diuresis—high-protein diet, ATN
      iii. Iatrogenic—mannitol

ATN, acute tubular necrosis; AVP, arginine vasopressin.

The most common cause of nephrogenic diabetes insipidus in adults is chronic lithium ingestion (see Table 10-1). Polyuria occurs in about 20% to 30% of patients on chronic lithium therapy. The impairment in the nephron's concentrating ability is thought to be due to decreased density of V2 receptors or to decreased expression of aquaporin-2, a water channel protein. Other secondary causes of nephrogenic diabetes insipidus include hypercalcemia, hypokalemia, sickle cell disease, and other drugs (see Table 10-1). A water diuresis also can follow relief of obstructive nephropathy. Hypercalcemia-induced nephrogenic diabetes insipidus occurs when the plasma calcium concentration is persistently above 11 mg/dL (2.75 mmol/L). This defect is generally reversible with correction of hypercalcemia. The mechanism(s) responsible for hypercalcemia-induced nephrogenic diabetes insipidus remain incompletely understood. Compared to hypercalcemia-induced diabetes insipidus, hypokalemia-induced nephrogenic diabetes insipidus is less severe and often asymptomatic. A rare form of nephrogenic diabetes insipidus can occur during the second half of pregnancy (gestational diabetes insipidus). This condition is thought to be caused by release of a vasopressinase from the placenta, leading to rapid degradation of endogenous or exogenous AVP.[8]

Approach to Hypotonic Polyuria (Water Diuresis)

The correct diagnosis is often suggested by the plasma sodium concentration and the history. When the problem is primary polydipsia, the plasma sodium concentration is usually low (dilutional), whereas when the problem is central or nephrogenic diabetes insipidus, the plasma sodium concentration typically is normal or high (due to loss of solute free water in excess of solutes). The rate of onset of polyuria can sometimes provide a clue about the diagnosis; when central diabetes insipidus is the problem, the onset of polyuria is generally abrupt, whereas when nephrogenic diabetes insipidus or primary polydipsia is the problem, the onset of polyuria tends to be more gradual. When the diagnosis of central versus nephrogenic diabetes insipidus is unclear, the diagnosis can be confirmed by determining the urinary response to an acute increase in plasma osmolality induced either by water restriction or, less commonly, by administration of hypertonic saline (Figure 10-1).

Comparing urinary osmolality after dehydration with that after vasopressin administration can help differentiate diabetes insipidus due to vasopressin deficiency from other causes of water diuresis (see Figure 10-1). In this test, fluids are withheld long enough to result in stable hourly urinary osmolalities (<30 mmol/kg rise in urine osmolality for 3 consecutive hours). Plasma osmolality and urine osmolality are measured at this time point, then the patient is given 5 units of

aqueous vasopressin intravenously (IV). The clinician then measures the osmolality of a urine sample collected during the interval from 30 to 60 minutes after administration of vasopressin. In subjects with normal pituitary function, urinary osmolality does not rise by more than 9% after vasopressin injection. However, in central diabetes insipidus, the increase in urine osmolality after vasopressin administration exceeds 9%. To ensure adequacy of dehydration, plasma osmolality prior to vasopressin administration should be greater than 288 mmol/kg. There is little or no increase in urine osmolality with dehydration in patients with nephrogenic diabetes insipidus, and there is no further change after vasopressin injection. In the future, a novel method to confirm the results of the water restriction test will be to measure the urinary excretion of aquaporin-2, the collecting tubule water channel that normally fuses with the luminal membrane of the collecting tubule cells under the influence of AVP. In one study, urinary aquaporin-2 excretion increased substantially and to a similar extent after the administration of vasopressin in normal subjects and those with central diabetes insipidus.[9] However, in patients with hereditary nephrogenic diabetes insipidus, urinary aquaporin-2 excretion was unchanged after vasopressin administration.

Treatment of Water Diuresis

Central diabetes insipidus can be treated by replacing AVP. The agent of choice is desmopressin, since it has prolonged antidiuretic activity and very minimal vasopressor effect. It is usually administered intranasally at doses of 10 to 20 µg once or twice a day. Patients with central diabetes insipidus with some residual releasable AVP can be treated with drugs such as carbamazepine (100-300 mg twice daily), clofibrate

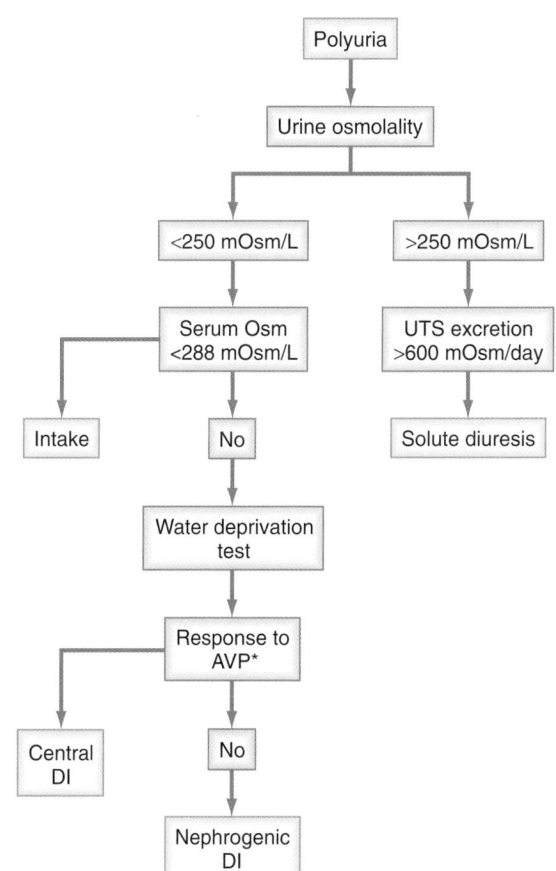

Figure 10-1 **Approach to polyuria.** *Response to AVP is defined as a greater than 9% increase in urine osmolality between 30 and 60 minutes after vasopressin administration (see text for details). *AVP,* arginine vasopressin; *DI,* diabetes insipidus; *UTS,* urine total solute concentration.

(500 mg every 6 hours), or chlorpropamide (125-250 mg once or twice a day) that stimulate AVP release.

Primary polydipsia can only be treated by eliminating the underlying problem. In patients with schizophrenia and polydipsia, clozapine has been shown to have a beneficial effect.

The mainstay of treatment of nephrogenic diabetes insipidus is solute restriction and diuretics. Thiazide diuretics in combination with a low-salt diet can diminish the degree of polyuria in patients with persistent and symptomatic nephrogenic diabetes insipidus. Thiazide diuretics (hydrochlorothiazide) act by inducing mild volume depletion. Hypovolemia induces an increase in proximal sodium and water reabsorption, thereby diminishing water delivery to the AVP-sensitive sites in the collecting tubules and reducing the urine output. The potassium-sparing diuretic, amiloride, also may be helpful.[10]

SOLUTE DIURESIS

Solute diuresis causing polyuria is due to solute excretion in excess of the usual excretory rate.[11] Daily urinary total solute excretion varies widely among different ethnicities, cultures, and dietary habits. The average urinary solute excretion in a healthy American adult is between 500 and 1000 mOsm/d. Solute diuresis can be very severe and can be caused by more than one solute concurrently. Solute diuresis is a relatively common clinical condition and one with important clinical implications. Unless there is adequate replacement of solute and water, a persistent solute diuresis contracts extracellular volume, leading to severe dehydration and hypernatremia. Although glucosuria is the major cause of an osmotic diuresis in outpatients, other conditions are often responsible when polyuria develops in the hospital. These conditions include administration of a high-protein diet, in which case urea acts as the osmotic agent, and volume expansion due to saline loading or the release of bilateral urinary tract obstruction. Multiplying urine osmolality by the 24-hour urine volume gives an estimate of total urine solute concentration. If urinary total solute concentration is abnormally large, a solute diuresis is present.

Solute diuresis can be due to either excessive electrolyte excretion or excessive nonelectrolyte solute excretion. If the total urinary electrolyte excretion exceeds 600 mOsm/d, then an electrolyte diuresis is present. The total urinary electrolyte excretion (in mOsm/d) can be estimated as $2 \times$ (urine $[Na^+]$ + urine $[K^+]$) $\times$ total urine volume.[1,12]

An electrolyte diuresis is usually driven by a sodium salt, usually sodium chloride (NaCl).[13] Common causes of NaCl-induced diureses are iatrogenic administration of excessive normal saline solution, excessive salt ingestion, and repetitive administration of loop diuretics. Most often, NaCl-induced diuresis is accompanied by water diuresis, causing a mixed solute-water diuresis. Also, more than one electrolyte may be responsible for the diuresis.

A clearly excessive value for urine nonelectrolyte excretion (i.e., >600 mOsm/d) implies that nonelectrolytes are the predominant solutes contributing to the diuresis. The urinary nonelectrolyte excretion can be calculated by subtracting urine electrolyte excretion from the total urine solute excretion. The urine osmolality in these disorders is usually above 300 mOsm/kg; the high osmolality contrasts with the dilute urine typically found with a water diuresis. Furthermore, total solute excretion (calculated as the product of urine osmolality and the urine output over a 24-hour urine collection period) is normal with a water diuresis (600 to 900 mOsm/d) but markedly increased with an osmotic diuresis. The most common nonelectrolyte solute causing excessive diuresis is glucose. Conditions associated with glucose-induced diuresis include diabetic ketoacidosis or hyperosmolar coma.[14] Excessive excretion of urea is another important cause of solute diuresis. This problem can occur as a consequence of enteral nutrition using a high-protein tube feeding formula or following relief of urinary tract obstruction or during recovery from acute tubular necrosis.[15] Mannitol administration (e.g., as a therapy for intracranial hypertension) also can lead to significant solute diuresis. This issue is pertinent because mannitol is often administered to patients with head trauma, who are at risk for development of nephrogenic diabetes insipidus. The correct diagnosis of solute diuresis depends on a clear systematic approach (see Figure 10-1). Management usually involves treatment of the underlying disorder and repletion of extracellular volume by hydration. Since solute diuresis is often accompanied by hypernatremia, and very rapid correction of hypernatremia can have disastrous consequences (e.g., cerebral herniation), it is crucial to carefully monitor serum $[Na^+]$. The serum $[Na^+]$ should not be permitted to decrease more than (0.5-1 mEq/L per hour).

REFERENCES

Access the complete reference list online at http://www.expertconsult.com.

11 Oliguria

SANJAY SUBRAMANIAN | RAMESH VENKATARMAN | JOHN A. KELLUM

Oliguria is an exceedingly common diagnostic problem faced on a daily basis by the critical care practitioner. The goal of this chapter is to provide a practical, physiology-based approach to diagnosing and treating oliguria.

Definitions and Epidemiology

A number of definitions for oliguria can be found in the literature. *Oliguria* is often defined as urine output less than 200 to 500 mL per 24 hours. In order to standardize the use of the term across different studies and populations, the Acute Dialysis Quality Initiative (ADQI) recently adopted a definition of oliguria as urine output of less than 0.3 mL/kg/h for at least 24 hrs (www.ADQI.net). For all practical purposes, however, urine output under 0.5 mL/kg/h is usually considered inadequate for most critically ill patients.

Given the lack of consensus over definitions, it has been difficult to determine the incidence of oliguria. Some studies have estimated that up to 18% of medical and surgical intensive care unit (ICU) patients with intact renal function exhibit episodes of oliguria.[1] Furthermore, 69% of ICU patients who develop acute kidney injury (AKI) are oliguric.[2] Overall, AKI in the ICU has a poor prognosis (mortality rates range from 30%-70%), and oliguric renal failure is associated with worse outcome compared to nonoliguric renal failure, although this distinction is less clear for AKI. It is essential to understand the physiologic derangements leading to this exceedingly common problem.

Pathophysiology

Urine output is a function of glomerular filtration, tubular secretion, and tubular reabsorption. Glomerular filtration is directly dependent on intravascular volume and renal perfusion. Renal perfusion in turn is a function of arterial pressure and renal vascular resistance. The intrarenal vasculature is capable of preserving glomerular filtration rate (GFR) in the face of varying systemic pressure through important neurohumoral autoregulating mechanisms that affect the afferent and efferent arterioles. The most important of these neurohumoral mechanisms is the renin-angiotensin-aldosterone system (Figure 11-1). Oliguria can be due to decreased GFR, increased tubular reabsorption of filtrate, or a combination of both. Oliguria also can be caused by mechanical obstruction to urine flow. In any case, oliguria is an insensitive clinical manifestation of AKI.

REDUCTION IN GLOMERULAR FILTRATION RATE

Oliguria secondary to a decrease in GFR is usually related to one of the following conditions:

1. Absolute decrease in intravascular volume, which can be due to myriad causes including trauma, hemorrhage, burns, diarrhea, excessive administration of diuretics, or sequestration of so-called third space fluid, as occurs in acute pancreatitis or abdominal surgery.
2. A relative decrease in blood volume in which the primary disturbance is an alteration in the capacitance of the vasculature due to vasodilation. This abnormality is commonly encountered in sepsis, hepatic failure, nephrotic syndrome, and use of vasodilatory drugs, including anesthetic agents.
3. Decreased renal perfusion due to various causes such as thromboembolism, atherosclerosis, aortic dissection, or inflammation

(vasculitis, especially scleroderma), affecting either the intra- or extrarenal circulation. Although renal arterial stenosis presents as subacute or chronic renal insufficiency, renal atheroembolic disease can present as AKI with acute oliguria. Renal atheroemboli (usually due to cholesterol emboli) usually affect older patients with a diffusive erosive atherosclerotic disease. The condition is most often seen after manipulation of the aorta or other large arteries, during arteriography, angioplasty, or surgery.[3] It also may occur spontaneously or after treatment with heparin, warfarin, or thrombolytic agents. Drugs such as cyclosporine, tacrolimus, and angiotensin-converting enzyme (ACE) inhibitors cause intrarenal vasoconstriction, resulting in reduced renal plasma flow and consequent oliguria. Decreased renal perfusion can also occur as a result an outflow problem, such as with abdominal compartment syndrome or (rarely) renal vein thrombosis.

4. Acute tubular necrosis (ATN). While this is often an end result of the listed factors, it may also be due to direct nephrotoxicity of agents such as antibiotics, heavy metals, solvents, contrast agents, crystals like uric acid or oxalate, or myoglobinuria.

MECHANICAL OBSTRUCTION

Oliguria secondary to mechanical obstruction can be further subclassified according to the anatomic site of the obstruction:

1. Tubular-ureteral obstruction may be caused by stones, papillary sloughing, crystals, or pigment.
2. Urethral or bladder neck obstruction, which is usually more common and typically due to prostatic hypertrophy or malignancy.
3. A malpositioned or obstructed urinary catheter.

Diagnostic Approach to Oliguria

Transient oliguria may not be an independent risk factor for morbidity and mortality in critically ill or injured patients, but sustained oliguria (>6 hrs) often indicates AKI and has been shown to be independently associated with hospital mortality. Oliguria can lead to fluid overload and tissue edema, which can cause a variety of adverse outcomes in critically ill patients. Merely reversing oliguria, particularly by the administration of diuretic agents, may confer some physiologic and clinical benefits. However, treating oliguria does not improve important clinical outcomes such as the need for renal replacement therapy, survival, or renal recovery. Thus, rapidly determining the cause of oliguria and correcting the underlying cause(s) is necessary to halt the progression kidney injury.

RULE OUT URINARY OBSTRUCTION

The first step in diagnosis is to rule out urinary obstruction. A prior history of prostatic hypertrophy may provide some clues to the presence of distal obstruction. However, in the ICU setting, distal obstruction presenting as oliguria is commonly due to obstruction of the urinary catheter (especially in male patients). Hence, in patients with new-onset oliguria, the urinary catheter must be flushed or changed in order to rule out obstruction. Although uncommon in the acute setting, complete or severe partial bilateral ureteral obstruction may also lead to acute, "acute on chronic," or chronic renal failure. Early

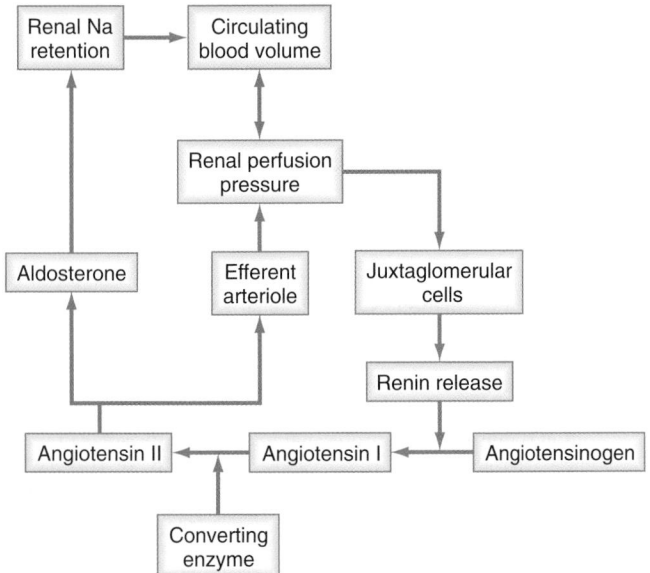

Figure 11-1 **Network of effects and feedback loop for the renin-angiotensin-aldosterone system.** As circulating blood volume or renal perfusion changes, renin is resulting in downstream effects that ultimately influence renal resistance and sodium handling by the kidney. Changes in urine output are a direct result of these changes.

diagnosis of urinary tract obstruction (UTO) is important, since many cases can be corrected, and a delay in therapy can lead to irreversible renal injury. Renal ultrasonography is usually the test of choice to exclude UTO.[4] It is noninvasive, can be performed by the bedside, and also carries the advantage of avoiding the potential allergic and toxic complications of radiocontrast media. In the majority of affected patients, ultrasonography can establish the diagnosis of hydronephrosis and often establish its cause. Ultrasonography also can be useful for detecting other causes of renal disease such as polycystic kidney disease. However, under some circumstances, renal ultrasound may not yield good results. For example, in early obstruction or obstruction associated with severe dehydration, hydronephrosis may not be seen on the initial ultrasound examination but may appear later in the course of the disease. Computed tomography (CT) scanning should be performed if the ultrasound results are equivocal or if the kidneys are not well visualized. CT also is indicated if the cause of the obstruction cannot be identified by ultrasonography.

LABORATORY INDICES

Although most authorities advocate examining the urine sediment, the yield of urine microscopy in the ICU is very low. Urine sediment is typically bland or reveals hyaline and fine granular casts in a prerenal state. By contrast, ATN is often associated with coarse granular casts and tubular epithelial casts. However, the discrimination of these findings is limited, and AKI may be present in the absence of changes in urinary sediment, particularly with sepsis-induced AKI. The main utility of examining the urine sediment is in the detection of red cell casts, which indicate primary glomerular disease. The urine sediment in postrenal failure is often very bland; casts or sediment typically are absent. Occasionally a few red cells and white cells may be seen. Eosinophilia, eosinophiluria, and hypocomplementemia, if present (although insensitive and nonspecific), point to the diagnosis of atheroembolic etiology of acute oliguria.[5]

Table 11-1 lists laboratory values that can be useful for distinguishing prerenal from intrarenal causes of oliguria. The fractional excretion of filtered sodium (FE_{Na}) is calculated according to the following formula:

$$FE_{Na} = [(\text{urine sodium} \times \text{plasma creatinine})] / (\text{plasma sodium} \times \text{urine creatinine}) \times 100$$

If the calculated FE_{Na} is less than 1%, a prerenal cause of oliguria should be suspected. Importantly, interpretation of the FE_{Na} is difficult or impossible if the patient has received diuretic or natriuretic agents (including dopamine and/or mannitol). Interpretation of the FE_{Na} also can be confounded by the presence of large amounts of endogenous osmotically active substances in the urine, such as glucose or urea. Drugs that interfere with the renin-angiotensin-aldosterone axis, such as ACE inhibitors or nonsteroidal antiinflammatory agents, also can confound the interpretation of FE_{Na}.

Several nephrotoxic factors, such as aminoglycosides, cyclosporine, and contrast media, are associated with FE_{Na} values below 1%, mimicking prerenal azotemia. Furthermore, sepsis may result in urine chemistries that resemble prerenal physiology even when renal blood flow is normal or increased.[6]

A low fractional excretion of urea (FE_{urea}) (<35%) has been proposed to be more sensitive and specific than FE_{Na} in differentiating between prerenal and renal causes of AKI, especially when diuretics have been administered.[7] The diagnostic accuracy of FE_{Na} versus FE_{urea} was recently compared in 99 patients hospitalized at a tertiary care center; study subjects had developed a 30% increase in SCr concentration from baseline within 1 week.[8] Patients were classified as having prerenal azotemia if the rise in SCr was transient and consistent with the clinical context. Each group also was subdivided according to exposure to diuretics. FE_{urea} of 35% or less and FE_{Na} of 1% or less were then analyzed for their ability to predict prerenal azotemia. Sensitivity, specificity, and receiver operating characteristic (ROC) curves were generated for each index. Sensitivity and specificity of FE_{urea} were 48% and 75%, respectively, in patients who did not receive diuretics, and 79% and 33%, respectively, in patients who received diuretics. Sensitivity and specificity of FE_{Na} were 78% and 75%, respectively, in patients not administered diuretics, and 58% and 81%, respectively, in those who received diuretics. ROC curves did not identify better diagnostic cutoff values for FE_{urea} or FE_{Na}. Unfortunately, the study did not examine the combination of these indices, so neither test provides a level of diagnostic accuracy that can be relied on in clinical practice.

CLINICAL PARAMETERS

Traditional indicators of fluid status and tissue perfusion—systemic arterial blood pressure, heart rate, body weight, presence of jugular-venous pulsations (JVP), and peripheral edema—can provide important clues about the etiology of oliguria. In the ICU, however, some of these indicators are less useful for a variety of reasons.

The presence or absence of JVP is not an accurate way to assess right ventricular or central venous pressures in the presence of positive pressure ventilation and positive end-expiratory pressure (PEEP). Similarly, peripheral edema is often due to coexistent hypoalbuminemia and decreased oncotic pressure in critically ill patients. Thus, patients

TABLE 11-1	Biochemical Indices Useful to Distinguish Prerenal from Intrarenal Acute Renal Failure		
		Prerenal	*Renal*
Osm u (mOsm/kg)		>500	<400
Na u (mmol/L or meq/L)		<20	>40
Urea/creatinine		>0.1	<0.05
U/S creatinine		>40	<20
U/S osmolality		>1.5	>1
FE$_{Na}$ (%)*		<1	>2
FE$_{urea}$ (%)		<25	>25

*((u Na / s Na) / (u creat / s creat)) × 100
ARF, acute renal failure; *S*, serum; *U*, urine.

can have an excessive volume of total body water and yet be intravascularly volume depleted. BP and heart rate are affected by numerous physiologic and treatment variables and are unreliable measures of volume status.

It is common to assume that one can obtain a more accurate assessment of preload by measuring the central venous pressure (CVP) or pulmonary capillary occlusion pressure (PAOP). However, these parameters do not provide reliable estimates of fluid responsiveness.[9] A cardiac index greater than 3.0 L/min/M² generally suggests *adequate* preload, but it may not reflect *optimal* preload.[10] The mixed venous oxygen saturation (Svo₂) can serve as a surrogate for cardiac output, but again does not define optimal filling. In patients on mechanical ventilation and without spontaneous triggering of the ventilator, an arterial pulse-pressure variation of more than 13% is strongly predictive of adequate (or more than adequate) preload.[11] In other cases, echocardiography may provide the only reliable evidence of fluid optimization (see Chapter 74).

ABDOMINAL COMPARTMENT SYNDROME

Another important and often overlooked reason for acute oliguria is abdominal compartment syndrome (ACS). *ACS* is defined as symptomatic organ dysfunction that results from an increase in intraabdominal pressure. Although this condition was initially described in trauma patients, ACS occurs in a wide variety of medical and surgical patients. ACS is sometimes seen after major abdominal surgeries requiring large-volume resuscitation, emergent laparotomies with tight abdominal wall closures, or abdominal wall burns with edema. ACS leads to AKI and acute oliguria mainly by directly increasing renal outflow pressure and thus reducing renal perfusion. Other mechanisms include direct parenchymal compression and arterial vasoconstriction mediated by stimulation of the sympathetic nervous and renin-angiotensin systems. Cardiac output also can be compromised by impaired venous return. These factors lead to decreased renal and glomerular perfusion and acute oliguria on this basis. Intraabdominal pressures over 15 mm Hg can lead to oliguria, and pressures over 30 mm Hg can cause anuria.[12]

ACS should be suspected in any patient with a tensely distended abdomen, progressive oliguria, and increased airway pressures (transmitted across the diaphragm). The mainstay of diagnosis is measurement of intraabdominal pressure, and the most common way to assess intraabdominal pressure is to measure pressure within the urinary bladder. Bladder pressure, obtained by transducing a fluid-filled Foley catheter, has been shown to correlate well with intraabdominal pressure over a wide range of pressures. Decompression of the abdomen with laparotomy, sometimes requiring that the abdomen be left open for a time, is the only definitive treatment for oliguria secondary to ACS.

Treatment of Oliguria

ENSURING ADEQUATE RENAL PERFUSION

The mainstay of treatment of oliguria is identification and correction of the precipitating factors. Instituting appropriate supportive measures, such as avoidance of nephrotoxic agents and adjustment of doses of renally excreted drugs, is also important. Efforts should be made to optimize renal perfusion by correcting hypotension and supporting appropriate intravascular volume expansion. However, volume overload can also compromise renal perfusion (see abdominal compartment syndrome earlier), so fluid should be carefully prescribed in patients with oliguria. Correction of hypotension is especially crucial, since in sepsis and ischemic AKI, some of the important autoregulating mechanisms that help preserve GFR in the face of fluctuating BP are disrupted. Vasoactive drugs may be necessary in the ICU setting to increase mean arterial pressures to more than usual values to maintain adequate renal perfusion pressure and adequate urine output.[13] In patients with chronic hypertension and renal vascular disease, the autoregulation curve can be shifted to the right, and higher than normal MAP may be required to ensure adequate renal perfusion. However, prior to initiation of treatment with vasoactive drugs, one must make sure the patient is adequately volume resuscitated. In many instances, the initial treatment consists of fluid challenges in the hope of correcting unrecognized volume depletion. Hemodynamic monitoring devices may provide important clues to the intravascular volume status that may enable a more streamlined, "goal-directed" approach to therapy.

ROLE OF DIURETIC AGENTS

The use of diuretic agents in oliguric renal failure is widespread despite the lack of convincing evidence supporting their efficacy. Traditionally, diuretics have been used in the early phases of oliguria to "jump start" the kidney and establish urine flow. Many clinicians believe that the absence of oliguria makes it easier to regulate intravascular volume status. Moreover, nonoliguric renal failure generally has a better prognosis than oliguric renal failure, and clinicians frequently use diuretics in an effort to avoid development of a low urine output state.[14] A study by Anderson et al. in 1977 claimed a reduction in mortality from 50% to 26% by using high doses of a loop diuretic to convert oliguric to nonoliguric renal failure.[15] This study excluded patients with shock and perioperative renal failure. More recent trials have failed to reproduce these results. A study in 1997 by Shilliday et al. examined the effect of loop diuretics on several outcomes in patients with AKI. While administration of loop diuretics increased average urine flow, there was no difference between the diuretic-treated and the placebo-treated groups with regard to the incidence of renal recovery, the need for renal replacement therapy, or death.[16] Two other randomized controlled clinical trials by Brown et al. and Kleinknecht et al. have failed to find any evidence of benefit on survival with the use of loop diuretics in oliguric renal failure.[17,18] The PICARD study group reported the results of a large cohort study of critically ill patients with AKI from 1989-1995.[19] The study showed that diuretic use was associated with an increased risk of death or non-recovery of renal function. Recently a large observational study (BEST kidney study) showed that use of diuretics has no beneficial effect on clinical outcomes.[20] Indeed, while not statistically significant, the odds ratio suggested that diuretic therapy might be harmful. Furthermore, high doses of loop diuretics can be associated with ototoxicity.

VASOACTIVE AGENTS

Other agents that have been used to treat oliguria include dopamine and related compounds. Because urine output often increases with the addition of low-dose dopamine, many intensivists assume that it has a beneficial effect. Indeed, low-dose dopamine has been advocated for nearly 30 years as therapy for oliguric renal failure on the basis of its action on DA1 receptors in doses of less than 5 µg/kg/min. However, there is abundant evidence that low-dose dopamine does not afford any renal protection in oliguria. Most evidence in favor of the treatment comes from uncontrolled trials or anecdotal studies. A comprehensive meta-analysis of dopamine in critically ill patients by Kellum et al. showed that dopamine did not prevent the onset of AKI, decrease mortality, or lessen the need for renal replacement therapy.[21]

Furthermore, there are important physiologic considerations that argue against a protective role for dopamine or any other dopamine receptor agonists (e.g., fenoldopam, dopexamine) in the oliguric state. First, the effect of dopamine agonists on urine output may be merely the natriuretic response mediated by inhibition of Na⁺/K⁺-ATPase at the tubular epithelial cell level.[22] In other words, dopamine increases urine output because it is a diuretic. Second, administration of dopaminergic antagonists (e.g., metoclopramide) has not been associated with loss of renal function. Third, the effect of dopamine may be counteracted by increased plasma renin activity in critically ill patients. Fourth, a significant hysteresis effect has been shown for the action of dopamine on renal blood flow. Finally, although dopamine increases renal blood flow, it does not increase medullary oxygenation.[23] Indeed, by increasing solute delivery to the distal tubule, dopamine agonists actually worsen medullary oxygen balance.[24] Despite claims to the contrary, newer dopaminergic agonists (e.g., fenoldopam, dopexamine) not only suffer from these limitations but also can induce hypotension and thereby further increase the risk of renal injury.

Conclusion

The presence of oliguria should alert the clinician to undertake a diligent search for any correctable underlying causes. The mainstay of treatment is to ensure adequate renal perfusion through optimization of cardiac output and intravascular volume status. The use of diuretics and vasoactive agents, while still fairly common, is not supported by the evidence, and emerging data actually suggest harm.

ANNOTATED REFERENCES

Bagshaw SM, Langenberg C, Bellomo R. Urinary biochemistry and microscopy in septic acute renal failure: a systematic review. Am J Kidney Dis 2006;48(5):695-705.
   A systematic review of studies examining urine chemistries in acute kidney injury in patients with sepsis. The authors conclude that urine chemistries are unreliable as a means to distinguish prerenal physiology from kidney damage.

Uchino S, Doig GS, Bellomo R, et al. Beginning and Ending Supportive Therapy for the Kidney (BEST Kidney) Investigators. Diuretics and mortality in acute renal failure. Crit Care Med 2004;32(8):1669-77.
   A large multicentered, multinational observational study examining the impact of diuretic therapy on outcomes in acute kidney injury. No clinical benefit could be demonstrated from the use of these agents.

REFERENCES

Access the complete reference list online at http://www.expertconsult.com.

Acid-Base Disorders

JOHN A. KELLUM

Conventional wisdom posits that acid-base disorders are more important for what they tell the clinician about the patient than for any harm that happens to the patient as a direct consequence of abnormal blood (or tissue) pH. This view is reasonable because most acid-base disorders are mild and well tolerated, but they allow the astute clinician to recognize underlying disorders that might be difficult to diagnose or even suspect otherwise. However, there are certain circumstances in which acid-base derangements are themselves dangerous, such as when the disorders are extreme (e.g., pH <7.0 or >7.7), especially when the acid-base derangement develops quickly. Such severe abnormalities can be the direct cause of organ dysfunction and can manifest as cerebral edema, seizures, decreased myocardial contractility, pulmonary vasoconstriction, and/or systemic vasodilation. Even less extreme derangements can produce harm because of the patient's response to the abnormality. For example, a spontaneously breathing patient with metabolic acidosis will attempt to compensate by increasing minute ventilation. The workload imposed by increasing minute ventilation can lead to respiratory muscle fatigue, with respiratory failure or diversion of blood flow from vital organs to the respiratory muscles, resulting in organ injury. Acidemia can promote the development of cardiac dysrhythmias in critically ill patients or increase myocardial oxygen demand in patients with myocardial ischemia. In such cases, one must treat the underlying disorder and also provide treatment for the acid-base disorder itself. Finally, emerging evidence suggests that changes in acid-base status influence immune effector cell function. Thus, avoiding acid-base derangements could influence outcome by modulating systemic inflammation and/or host defenses against infection.

General Principles

Three widely accepted methods are used to analyze and classify acid-base disorders, yielding mutually compatible results. The approaches differ only in assessment of the metabolic component (i.e., all three treat Pco_2 as an independent variable): (1) HCO_3^- concentration ($[HCO_3^-]$); (2) standard base-excess; (3) strong ion difference. All three yield virtually identical results when used to quantify the acid-base status of a given blood sample.[1-4] For the most part, the differences among these three approaches are conceptual; in other words, they differ in how they approach the understanding of mechanism.[5-7]

There are three mathematically independent determinants of blood pH:

1. The difference between the sum of the concentrations of strong cations (e.g., Na^+, K^+) and the sum of the concentrations of strong anions (e.g., Cl^-, lactate); this difference is called the *strong ion difference* (SID).
2. The total weak acid "buffers" concentration (A_{TOT}), which is mostly composed of the concentrations of albumin and phosphate.
3. Pco_2.

Only these three variables (SID, A_{TOT}, and Pco_2) can independently affect blood pH. $[H^+]$ and $[HCO_3^-]$ are dependent variables, being functions of SID, A_{TOT}, and Pco_2.

Changes in plasma $[H^+]$ result from dissociation of A_{TOT} and possibly water itself. The standard base-excess is mathematically equivalent to the change in SID required to restore pH to 7.4, given a Pco_2 of 40 mm Hg and the prevailing A_{TOT}. Thus, a standard base-excess of −10 mEq/L means that the SID is 10 mEq/L less than the SID that is associated with a pH of 7.4 when Pco_2 is 40 mm Hg.

Assessing Acid-Base Balance

Acid-base homeostasis is defined by the pH of blood plasma and by the conditions of the acid-base pairs that determine it. Because blood plasma is an aqueous solution containing both volatile (carbon dioxide) and fixed acids, its pH will be determined by the net effects of all these components. The determinants of blood pH can be grouped into two broad categories, respiratory and metabolic. Respiratory acid-base disorders are disorders of carbon dioxide (CO_2) tension, and metabolic acid-base disorders comprise all other conditions affecting the pH. This latter category includes disorders of both weak acids (often referred to as "buffers," although the term is imprecise) and strong acids and bases (including both organic and inorganic acids). Acid-base disorders can be recognized by any of the following:

1. An alteration in the pH of the arterial blood (normally 7.35-7.45). If the pH is <7.35, *acidemia* is said to be present; if the pH is >7.45, *alkalemia* is said to be present.
2. An arterial partial pressure of CO_2 ($Paco_2$) outside the normal range (35 to 45 mm Hg).
3. A plasma bicarbonate concentration outside the normal range (22-26 mEq/L).
4. An arterial standard base-excess of 3 or −3 mEq/L.

Although these criteria are useful in identifying an acid-base disorder, the absence of all four cannot exclude a mixed acid-base disorder—that is, alkalosis and acidosis that are completely matched. Fortunately, such conditions are quite rare.

Metabolic Acid-Base Disorders

Metabolic acid-base derangements are associated with a greater number of underlying conditions than are respiratory acid-base disorders and tend to be more difficult to treat. Metabolic acidosis is produced by a decrease in SID, which in turn generates an electrochemical force that increases $[H^+]$. The SID decreases when the concentration of organic anions (e.g., lactate, β-hydroxybutyrate) increases. The SID also decreases when there is a loss of sodium bicarbonate (e.g., due to diarrhea or renal tubular acidosis) or there is a gain of exogenous anions (e.g., iatrogenic acidosis, poisonings). Metabolic alkaloses occur when SID is inappropriately wide, although it need not be greater than the "normal" 40 to 42 mEq/L. Widening of SID can be brought about by the loss of strong anions in excess of strong cations (e.g., vomiting, diuretics), or (rarely) by administration of strong cations in excess of strong anions (e.g., transfusion of large volumes of banked blood containing sodium citrate).

Similarly, the treatment of metabolic acid-base disorders requires a change in SID. Metabolic acidoses are repaired by increasing plasma Na^+ concentration more than plasma Cl^- concentration (e.g., by infusing $NaHCO_3$), and metabolic alkaloses are repaired by replacing Cl^- as NaCl (large volumes), KCl, or even HCl. Note that so-called chloride-resistant metabolic alkaloses are resistant to chloride only because of ongoing renal losses that increase in response to increased Cl^- replacement (e.g., hyperaldosteronism).

PATHOPHYSIOLOGY OF METABOLIC ACID-BASE DISORDERS

Disorders of metabolic acid-base balance occur as a result of:

1. Dysfunction of the primary regulating organs.
2. Exogenous administration of drugs or fluids that alter the body's ability to maintain normal acid-base balance.
3. Abnormal metabolism that overwhelms the normal defense mechanisms.

The organs responsible for regulating SID in both health and disease are the kidneys and, to a lesser extent, the gastrointestinal (GI) tract.

The Kidneys

Normal plasma flow to the kidneys is approximately 600 mL/min in adults. The glomeruli filter the plasma to yield about 120 mL/min of filtrate. Normally, more than 99% of the filtrate is reabsorbed and returned to the plasma. Thus, the kidney can only excrete a very small amount of strong ions into the urine each minute, and several minutes to hours are required to achieve a significant impact on SID. The handling of strong ions by the kidney is extremely important because every Cl^- ion that is filtered but not reabsorbed decreases SID. Accordingly, "acid handling" by the kidney is generally mediated through changes in Cl^- balance. The purpose of renal ammoniagenesis is to allow the excretion of Cl^- without Na^+ or K^+. Viewed this way, renal tubular acidosis can be regarded as an abnormality of Cl^- handling rather than of H^+ or HCO_3^- handling.[3]

Renal-Hepatic Interaction

Ammonium ion (NH_4^+) is important to systemic acid-base balance not because it stores H^+ or has a direct action in the plasma (normal plasma NH_4^+ concentration is <0.01 mEq/L). NH_4^+ is important because it is "co-excreted" with Cl^-. Of course, NH_4^+ is not only produced in the kidney. Hepatic ammoniagenesis (and, as we shall see, glutaminogenesis) is also important for systemic acid-base balance and is tightly controlled by mechanisms sensitive to plasma pH.[8] This reinterpretation of the role of NH_4^+ in acid-base balance is supported by the evidence that hepatic glutaminogenesis is stimulated by acidosis.[9] Glutamine is used by the kidney to generate NH_4^+ and thus facilitates the excretion of Cl^-. The production of glutamine, therefore, can be seen as having an alkalinizing effect on plasma pH because of the way the kidney utilizes it.

The Gastrointestinal Tract

Different parts of the GI tract handle strong ions in distinct ways. In the stomach, Cl^- is pumped out of the plasma and into the lumen, thereby reducing the SID and pH of gastric juice. The pumping action of the gastric parietal cells increases SID of the plasma by promoting the loss of Cl^-; this effect produces the so-called alkaline tide at the beginning of a meal when gastric acid secretion is maximal.[10] In the duodenum, Cl^- is reabsorbed and the plasma pH is restored. Normally, only slight changes in plasma pH are evident because Cl^- is returned to the circulation almost as soon as it is removed. However, if gastric secretions are removed from the patient, either through a suction catheter or as a result of vomiting, Cl^- is lost and SID increases. It is important to realize that it is the Cl^- loss, not the H^+ loss, that is the cause for widening of the SID and the development of metabolic alkalosis. Although H^+ is "lost" as HCl, it is also lost with every molecule of water removed from the body.

In contrast to the stomach, the pancreas secretes fluid into the small intestine that has a SID much greater than that of plasma; the $[Cl^-]$ of pancreatic secretions is quite low. Thus, SID in the plasma perfusing the pancreas decreases, a phenomenon that peaks about an hour after a meal and helps counteract the alkaline tide. If large amounts of pancreatic fluid are lost, for example from surgical drainage, acidosis develops as a consequence of decreased plasma SID. Fluid in the lumen of the large intestine has a wide SID because most of the Cl^- has been removed in the small intestine, and the remaining electrolytes are mostly Na^+ and K^+ and HCO_3^-. The body normally reabsorbs much of

the water and electrolytes from this fluid, but when there is severe diarrhea, large amounts of this HCO_3^--rich and Cl^--poor fluid can be lost. If these losses are persistent, plasma SID decreases and acidosis results.

In addition, the small intestine may contribute strong ions to the plasma. This effect is most apparent when mesenteric blood flow is compromised and lactate is produced, sometimes in large quantities, by the tissues of the small intestine.

Metabolic Acidosis

Traditionally, metabolic acidoses are categorized according to the presence or absence of unmeasured anions. The presence of unmeasured anions is routinely inferred by measuring the concentrations of electrolytes in plasma and calculating the anion gap, as described later. The differential diagnosis for a positive–anion gap (AG) acidosis is shown in Box 12-1. Non–anion gap acidoses can be divided into three types: renal, GI, and iatrogenic (Figure 12-1). In the intensive care unit (ICU), the most common types of metabolic acidosis include lactic acidosis, ketoacidosis, iatrogenic acidosis, and acidosis secondary to toxins.

The potential effects of metabolic acidosis and alkalosis on vital organ function are shown in Table 12-1. Metabolic and respiratory acidosis may have different implications with respect to survival, an observation that suggests that the underlying disorder is perhaps more important than the absolute degree of acidemia.[11]

If metabolic acidemia is to be treated, consideration should be given to the likely duration of the disorder. If it is expected to be short lived (e.g., diabetic ketoacidosis), maximizing respiratory compensation is usually the safest approach. Once the disorder resolves, ventilation can be quickly reduced to normal, and there will be no lingering effects of therapy. However, if the disorder is likely to be more chronic (e.g., renal failure), therapy aimed at restoring SID is indicated. In all cases, the therapeutic target can be quite accurately determined from the standard base-excess. As discussed, the standard base-excess corresponds to the amount SID must change in order to restore the pH to 7.4, assuming a Pco_2 of 40 mm Hg. Thus, if the SID is 30 mEq/L and the

---

Box 12-1

CAUSES OF AN INCREASED ANION GAP (AG)

Common Causes
Alcoholism
Diabetes
Ethylene glycol
Ketoacidosis
Lactic acidosis
Metabolic errors
Methanol
Paraldehyde
Renal failure
Salicylates
Starvation
Toluene
Toxins

Rare Causes
Alkalemia
Carbenicillin (>30 g/day)
Decreased unmeasured cation
Dehydration
Hypocalcemia
Hypokalemia
Hypomagnesemia
Sodium acetate
Sodium citrate
Sodium lactate
Sodium PCN (>50 m units/day)
Sodium salts

URINE SID (Na⁺K⁻Cl)

```
            (+)                              (−)
     Renal tubular                     Nonrenal tubular
        acidosis                          acidosis
            │                                 │
            ▼                                 ▼
    Urine pH >5.5                            GI
    Distal (Type I)                       Diarrhea
            │                           Small bowel/
            ▼                          pancreatic drainage
    Urine pH <5.5                            │
    Low serum K⁺                             ▼
   Proximal (Type II)                    Iatrogenic
            │                       Parenteral nutrition
            ▼                             Saline
   High serum K⁺                   Anion exchange resins
  Aldosterone deficiency
      (Type IV)
```

Figure 12-1 **Differential diagnosis for a hyperchloremic metabolic acidosis.** *GI,* gastrointestinal; *SID,* Strong ion difference.

standard base-excess is −10 mEq/L, the target SID would be 40 mEq/L. Accordingly, the plasma Na⁺ concentration would have to increase by 10 mEq/L for NaHCO₃ administration to completely repair the acidosis. If increasing the plasma Na⁺ concentration is inadvisable for other reasons (e.g., hypernatremia), then NaHCO₃ administration is also inadvisable. Importantly, NaHCO₃ administration has not been shown to improve outcome in patients with lactic acidosis.[12]

TABLE 12-1	Potential Clinical Effects of Metabolic Acid-Base Disorders	
Metabolic Acidosis	*Metabolic Alkalosis*	
Cardiovascular	**Cardiovascular**	
Decreased inotropy	Decreased inotropy (Ca⁺⁺ entry)	
Conduction defects	Altered coronary blood flow*	
Arterial vasodilation	Digoxin toxicity	
Venous vasoconstriction		
Oxygen Delivery	**Neuromuscular**	
Decreased oxy-Hb binding	Neuromuscular excitability	
Decreased 2,3-DPG (late)	Encephalopathy seizures	
Neuromuscular	**Metabolic Effects**	
Respiratory depression	Hypokalemia	
Decreased sensorium	Hypocalcemia	
	Hypophosphatemia	
	Impaired enzyme function	
Metabolism	**Oxygen Delivery**	
Protein wasting	Increased oxy-Hb affinity	
Bone demineralization	Increased 2,3-DPG (delayed)	
Catecholamine, PTH, and aldosterone stimulation		
Insulin resistance		
Free radical formation		
Gastrointestinal		
Emesis		
Gut barrier dysfunction		
Electrolytes		
Hyperkalemia		
Hypercalcemia		
Hyperuricemia		

*Animal studies have shown both increased and decreased coronary artery blood flow.
2,3-DPG, 2,3-diphosphoglycerate; *oxy-Hb,* oxyhemoglobin; *PTH,* parathyroid hormone.

In addition, NaHCO₃ administration is associated with certain disadvantages. Large (hypertonic) doses given rapidly can lead to hypotension[13] and have the potential to cause a sudden marked increase in Paco₂.[14] Accordingly, it is important to assess the patient's ventilatory status before NaHCO₃ is administered, particularly in the absence of mechanical ventilation. NaHCO₃ infusion also affects circulating [K⁺] and [Ca⁺⁺] concentrations, which need to be monitored closely.

Tromethamine (Tris-buffer or Tham) is an organic buffer that readily penetrates cells.[15] It is a weak base (pK = 7.9) that does not alter SID and does not affect plasma [Na⁺]. Accordingly, it is often used when administration of NaHCO₃ is contraindicated because of hypernatremia. This agent has been available since the 1960s, but limited data are available on its use in humans with acid-base disorders. In small uncontrolled studies, tromethamine appears to be effective in reversing metabolic acidosis secondary to ketoacidosis or renal failure without obvious toxicity.[16] However, adverse reactions have been reported, including hypoglycemia, respiratory depression, and even fatal hepatic necrosis when concentrations exceeding 0.3 *M* are used. In Europe, a mixture of tromethamine, acetate, NaHCO₃, and disodium phosphate is available (Tribonate). This mixture seems to have fewer side effects than tromethamine alone, but experience with Tribonate is still quite limited.

ANION GAP AND STRONG ION GAP

For more than 30 years, AG has been used by clinicians, and it has evolved into a major tool to evaluate acid-base disorders.[17] AG is estimated from the differences between the routinely measured concentrations of serum cations (Na⁺ and K⁺) and anions (Cl⁻ and HCO₃⁻). Normally this difference, or "gap," is made up by albumin and, to a lesser extent, by phosphate. Sulfate and lactate also contribute a small amount, normally less than 2 mEq/L. However, there are also unmeasured cations, such as Ca⁺⁺ and Mg⁺⁺, and these tend to offset the effects of sulfate and lactate, except when the concentration of sulfate or lactate is abnormally increased (Figure 12-2). Plasma proteins other than albumin can be positively or negatively charged, but in the aggregate tend to be neutral except in rare cases of abnormal paraproteins, such as in cases of multiple myeloma.[18] In practice, AG is calculated as follows:

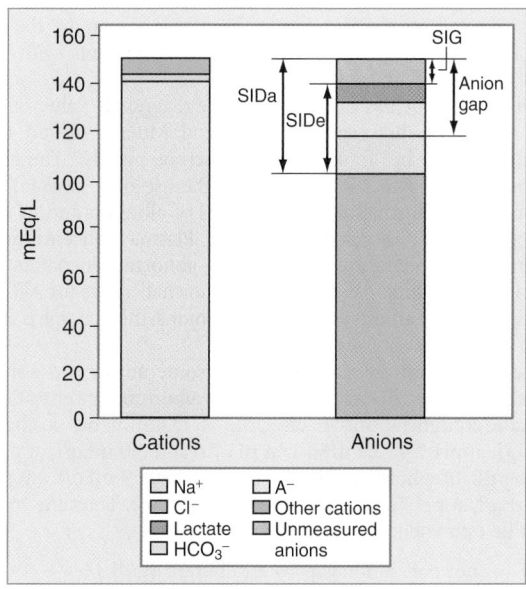

Figure 12-2 **Charge balance in blood plasma.** "Other cations" include Ca⁺⁺ and Mg⁺⁺. The strong ion difference (*SID*) is always positive (in plasma) and SID − *SIDe* (effective strong ion difference) must equal zero. Any difference between apparent SID (*SIDa*) and SIDe is the strong ion gap (*SIG*) and must represent unmeasured anions.

$$AG = ([Na^+] + [K^+]) - ([Cl^-] + [HCO_3^-])$$

Because of its low and narrow extracellular concentration range, K^+ is often omitted from the calculation. The normal value for AG is 12 ± 4 (if $[K^+]$ is considered) or 8 ± 4 mEq/L (if $[K^+]$ is not considered). The normal range has decreased in recent years following the introduction of more accurate methods for measuring Cl^- concentration.[19,20] However, the various measurement techniques available mandate that each institution reports its own expected "normal anion gap."

The AG is useful because this parameter can limit the differential diagnosis for patients with metabolic acidosis. If AG is increased, the explanation almost invariably will be found among five disorders: ketosis, lactic acidosis, poisoning, renal failure, or sepsis.[21] However, several conditions can alter the accuracy of AG estimation, and these conditions are particularly prevalent among patients with critical illness[22,23]:

- Dehydration can widen the apparent AG by increasing the concentration of all the ions used for the calculation.
- Hypoalbuminemia decreases AG, and it has been recommended to "correct" AG for changes in albumin concentration, because for every 1 g/dL decrease in serum albumin concentration, the apparent AG narrows by 2.5 to 3 mEq/L.[24]
- Respiratory and metabolic alkaloses are associated with an increase of up to 3 to 10 mEq/L in the apparent AG. The basis for this effect is enhanced lactate production (from stimulated phosphofructokinase enzymatic activity), reduction in the concentration of ionized weak acids (A^-), and possibly the additional effect of dehydration.

Other factors that can increase AG are low Mg^{++} concentration and administration of the sodium salts of poorly reabsorbable anions (e.g., beta-lactam antibiotics).[25] Certain parenteral nutrition formulations, such as those containing acetate, can increase AG. Citrate-based anticoagulants rarely can have the same effect after administration of multiple blood transfusions.[26] None of these rare causes, however, increases AG significantly,[27] and they are usually easily identified. In recent years, some additional causes of an increased AG have been reported. It is sometimes widened in patients with nonketotic hyperosmolar states induced by diabetes mellitus; the biochemical basis for this effect remains unexplained.[28] In recent years, unmeasured anions have been reported in the blood of patients with sepsis[29,30] and liver disease[31,32] and in experimental animals injected with endotoxin.[33] These anions may be the source of much of the unexplained acidosis seen in patients with critical illness.[34]

Additional doubt has been cast on the diagnostic value of AG in certain situations, however.[22,30] Salem and Mujais[22] found routine reliance on AG to be "fraught with numerous pitfalls." The primary problem with the AG is its reliance on the use of a "normal" range that depends on normal circulating levels of albumin and to a lesser extent phosphate, as discussed earlier. Plasma concentrations of albumin or phosphate are often grossly abnormal in patients with critical illness, leading to changes in the "normal" range for AG. Moreover, because these anions are not strong anions, their charge is affected by pH.

These considerations have prompted some authors to adjust the "normal range" for AG according to the albumin concentration[24] or phosphate concentration.[6] Each g/dL of albumin has a charge of 2.8 mEq/L at pH 7.4 (2.3 mEq/L at pH 7.0 and 3.0 mEq/L at pH 7.6). Each mg/dL of phosphate has a charge of 0.59 mEq/L at pH 7.4 (0.55 mEq/L at pH 7.0 and 0.61 mEq/L at pH 7.6). Thus, the "normal" AG can be estimated using this formula[6]:

$$\text{"normal" anion gap} = 2 \times [\text{albumin}](g/dL) + 0.5 \times [\text{phosphate}](mg/dL)$$

Or for international units:

$$\text{"normal" anion gap} = 0.2 \times [\text{albumin}](g/L) + 1.5 \times [\text{phosphate}](mmol/L)$$

These formulas only should be used when the pH is less than 7.35, and even then they are only accurate within 5 mEq/L. When more accuracy is needed, a slightly more complicated method of estimating $[A^-]$ is required.[31,35]

Another alternative to using the traditional AG is to use the SID. By definition, SID must be equal and opposite to the negative charges contributed by $[A^-]$ and total CO_2. The sum of the charges from $[A^-]$ and total CO_2 concentration has been termed the *effective strong ion difference* (SIDe).[18] The *apparent strong ion difference* (SIDa) is obtained by measurement of each individual ion. Both the SIDa and the SIDe should equal the true strong ion difference. If the SIDa and SIDe differ, unmeasured ions must exist. If the SIDa is greater than SIDe, these ions are anions; if the SIDa is less than SIDe, the unmeasured ions are cations. This difference has been termed the *strong ion gap* to distinguish it from AG.[31] Unlike the AG, the strong ion gap is normally zero and does not change with changes in pH or albumin concentration.

POSITIVE–ANION GAP ACIDOSES

Lactic Acidosis

In many forms of critical illness, lactate is the most important cause of metabolic acidosis.[36] Blood lactate concentration has been shown to correlate with outcome in patients with hemorrhagic[37] and septic shock.[38] Lactic acid has been viewed as the predominant source of metabolic acidosis due to sepsis.[39] In this view, lactic acid is released primarily from the musculature and the gut as a consequence of tissue hypoxia. Moreover, the amount of lactate produced is believed to correlate with the total oxygen debt, the magnitude of hypoperfusion, and the severity of shock.[36] In recent years, this view has been challenged by the observation that during sepsis, even with profound shock, resting muscle does not produce lactate. Indeed, studies by various investigators have shown that the musculature actually may consume lactate during endotoxemia.[40-42] Data concerning the gut are less clear. There is little question that underperfused gut can release lactate; however, it does not appear that the gut releases lactate during sepsis if mesenteric perfusion is maintained. Under such conditions, the mesenteric circulation can even become a net consumer of lactate.[40,41] Perfusion is likely to be a major determinant of mesenteric lactate metabolism. In a canine model of sepsis, gut lactate production could not be shown when flow was maintained with dopexamine hydrochloride.[42]

Studies in animals as well as humans have shown that the lung may be a prominent source of lactate in the setting of acute lung injury.[40,43-45] While studies such as these do not address the underlying pathophysiologic mechanisms of hyperlactatemia in sepsis, they suggest that using blood lactate concentration as evidence for tissue dysoxia is an oversimplification at best. Indeed, many investigators have begun to offer alternative interpretations of hyperlactatemia in this setting.[44-48] Box 12-2 lists several alternative sources of hyperlactatemia. In particular, pyruvate dehydrogenase, the enzyme responsible for moving pyruvate into the Krebs cycle, is inhibited by endotoxemia.[49] However, data from recent studies suggest that increased aerobic metabolism may be more important than metabolic defects or anaerobic metabolism.[50] Finally, administration of epinephrine promotes lactic acidosis, presumably by stimulating cellular metabolism (e.g., increased glycolysis in skeletal muscle).

Administration of epinephrine may be a common cause of lactic acidosis in patients with critical illness.[51,52] Interestingly, this phenomenon does not occur when dobutamine or norepinephrine is infused[53] and does not appear to be related to decreased tissue perfusion.

Although controversy exists as to the source and interpretation of lactic acidosis in critically ill patients, there is no question about the ability of lactate accumulation to produce acidemia. Lactate is a strong ion by virtue of the fact that at a pH within the physiologic range, it is almost completely dissociated; for instance, the pKa for lactic acid is 3.9. Thus, at pH 7.4, 3162 lactic acid molecules are dissociated for every one that is not. Because the body can produce and dispose of lactate rapidly, it functions as one of the most dynamic components of SID.

MECHANISMS ASSOCIATED WITH INCREASED SERUM LACTATE CONCENTRATION

Tissue Hypoxia
Hypodynamic shock
Organ ischemia

Hypermetabolism
Hematologic malignancies
Increased aerobic glycolysis
Increased protein catabolism

Decreased Clearance of Lactate
Liver failure
Shock

Inhibition of Pyruvate Dehydrogenase
Endotoxin?
Thiamine deficiency

Activation of Inflammatory Cells?

Plasma lactate concentration may be increased without an increase in $[H^+]$. There are two possible explanations for this phenomenon. First, if lactate is added to the plasma, not as lactic acid but rather as the salt of a strong acid (e.g., sodium lactate), there will be little change in the SID. The SID does not change because a strong cation (Na^+) is being added along with a strong anion. However, only if a very large amount of lactate is infused rapidly will there be an appreciable increase in the plasma lactate concentration. For example, the use of lactate-based hemofiltration fluid can result in hyperlactatemia with an *increased* plasma HCO_3^- concentration and pH.

A more important mechanism whereby hyperlactatemia exists without acidemia (or with less acidemia than expected) is when the SID is corrected by the elimination of another strong anion from the plasma.[54] In the setting of sustained lactic acidosis induced by lactic acid infusion, Cl^- moves out of the plasma space, thus normalizing pH. Under these conditions, hyperlactatemia may persist but base-excess may be normalized by compensatory mechanisms to restore the SID.

Traditionally, lactic acidosis is subdivided into type A, in which the mechanism is tissue hypoxia, and type B, in which there is no hypoxia.[55] However, this distinction may be artificial. Some disorders, such as sepsis, may be associated with lactic acidosis owing to a variety of mechanisms (see Box 12-2), some of the "A" type and some of the "B" type. A potentially useful method of distinguishing anaerobically produced lactate from other sources is to measure the blood pyruvate concentration. The normal lactate to pyruvate ratio is 10:1.[56] A lactate-to-pyruvate ratio greater than 25:1 is considered to be evidence of anaerobic metabolism.[48] This approach makes biochemical sense, because pyruvate is reduced to lactate during anaerobic metabolism, thereby increasing the lactate-to-pyruvate ratio. Unfortunately, pyruvate is very unstable in solution and, therefore, is difficult to measure accurately in the clinical setting, greatly reducing the clinical utility of lactate/pyruvate determinations.

Treatment of lactic acidosis remains controversial. The only non-controversial approach is to treat the underlying cause. The use of sodium bicarbonate ($NaHCO_3$) is equally controversial and remains of unproven value.[12]

Ketoacidosis

Another common cause of a metabolic acidosis with a positive AG is ketoacidosis. Ketones are formed by beta-oxidation of fatty acids, a process that is inhibited by insulin. In insulin-deficient states, ketone formation increases substantially. The accumulation of ketone bodies (acetone, β-hydroxybutyrate, and acetoacetate) in the plasma is exacerbated because elevated blood glucose concentrations promote an osmotic diuresis, leading to intravascular volume contraction. This state is associated with elevated circulating cortisol and catecholamine levels, which further stimulates free fatty acid production.[57] In addition, increased glucagon levels relative to insulin levels decreases intracellular concentrations of malonyl coenzyme A and increases the activity of carnitine palmitoyl acyl transferase, effects that promote ketogenesis.

Both acetoacetate and β-hydroxybutyrate are strong anions (pKa 3.8 and 4.8, respectively).[58] Thus, like lactate, the presence of these ions decreases the SID and increases $[H^+]$. Ketoacidosis may result from diabetes (diabetic ketoacidosis) or excessive alcohol consumption (alcoholic ketoacidosis). The diagnosis is established by measuring serum ketone levels. However, it is important to understand that the nitroprusside reaction only measures acetone and acetoacetate, and not β-hydroxybutyrate. Thus, the state of measured ketosis is dependent on the ratio of acetoacetate to β-hydroxybutyrate. This ratio is low when lactic acidosis coexists with ketoacidosis, because the reduced redox state of lactic acidosis favors production of β-hydroxybutyrate.[59] In this circumstance, the apparent level of ketosis is small relative to the amount of acidosis and the elevation of AG. There is also a risk of confusion during treatment of ketoacidosis, because ketones as measured by the nitroprusside reaction can increase despite resolving acidosis. This effect occurs as a result of rapid clearance of β-hydroxybutyrate, improving acid-base balance without changing the measured level of ketosis. Furthermore, circulating ketone levels can even appear to increase as β-hydroxybutyrate is converted to acetoacetate. Hence, it is better to monitor therapy by measuring blood pH and AG than by assaying levels of serum ketones.

Treatment of diabetic ketoacidosis includes infusing insulin and large amounts of fluid; 0.9% saline is usually recommended. Potassium replacement is often required as well. Fluid resuscitation reverses the hormonal stimuli for ketone body formation, as discussed earlier, and insulin promotes metabolism of ketones and glucose. Administration of $NaHCO_3$ may produce a more rapid rise in pH by increasing SID, but there is little evidence that this effect is desirable. Furthermore, because increasing the plasma Na^+ concentration increases the SID, the SID will be too high once the ketosis is cleared ("overshoot" alkalosis). In any case, administration of $NaHCO_3$ is rarely necessary and should be avoided except in extreme cases.[60]

A more common problem in the treatment of diabetic ketoacidosis is persistence of acidemia after resolution of ketosis. This hyperchloremic metabolic acidosis occurs as Cl^- replaces ketoacids, thus maintaining decreases in SID and pH. This effect appears to occur for two reasons. First, exogenous Cl^- is often provided in the form of 0.9% saline, which, if given in large enough quantities, results in a so-called dilutional acidosis (see later discussion). Second, renal Cl^- reabsorption increases as ketones are excreted in the urine. Increases in the tubular Na^+ load produce electrical-chemical forces favoring Cl^- reabsorption.[61]

The acidosis seen in patients with alcoholic ketoacidosis is usually less severe. Treatment consists of intravenous (IV) fluid administration and infusion of glucose instead of insulin, as would be the case with diabetic ketoacidosis.[62] Indeed, insulin is contraindicated because it may cause precipitous hypoglycemia.[63] Thiamine also must be given to avoid precipitating Wernicke encephalopathy.

Renal Failure

Renal failure, especially when chronic, leads to accumulation of sulfates and other acids, widening AG, although this increase usually is not large.[64] Similarly, uncomplicated renal failure rarely produces severe acidosis, except when it is accompanied by a high rate of acid generation, such as occurs during hypermetabolism.[65] In all cases, SID is decreased and remains so unless some therapy is provided. Hemodialysis removes sulfate and other ions and allows normal Na^+ and Cl^- balance to be restored, thus returning SID to normal (or near normal). However, patients not yet requiring dialysis and those who are between treatments often require some other therapy to increase SID. $NaHCO_3$ is used as long as the plasma Na^+ concentration is not already elevated.

Toxins

Metabolic acidosis with an increased AG is a major feature of various types of drug and substance intoxications (see Box 12-1).

Other and Unknown Causes

In the nonketotic hyperosmolar state associated with poorly controlled diabetes, AG widens for unexplained reasons.[28] Even when very careful methods are applied using the strong ion gap or similar strategies, unmeasured anions have been detected in the blood of patients with sepsis[29,30] and liver disease[31] and in experimental animals given endotoxin.[32] Furthermore, unknown cations also appear in the blood of some critically ill patients.[30] The significance of these findings remains to be determined.

NON–ANION GAP (HYPERCHLOREMIC) ACIDOSES

Hyperchloremic metabolic acidosis occurs as a result of either the increase in [Cl⁻] relative to strong cations, especially Na⁺, or the loss of cations with retention of Cl⁻. As seen in Figure 12-1, these disorders can be separated by history and by measurement of urinary Cl⁻ concentration. When acidosis occurs, the normal response by the kidney is to increase Cl⁻ excretion. If the kidney fails to increase Cl⁻ excretion appropriately, impaired renal function is at least part of the problem causing acidosis. Extrarenal causes of hyperchloremic acidosis are exogenous Cl⁻ loads (iatrogenic acidosis) or loss of cations from the lower GI tract without proportional losses of Cl⁻.

Renal Tubular Acidosis

Examination of the urine and plasma electrolytes and pH and calculation of the urine apparent SID allow one to correctly diagnose most cases of renal tubular acidosis (see Figure 12-1).[66] However, caution must be exercised when the plasma pH is greater than 7.35, because urinary Cl⁻ excretion is normally decreased when pH is this high. In such circumstances, it may be necessary to infuse sodium sulfate or furosemide. These agents stimulate Cl⁻ and K⁺ excretion and can be used to unmask the defect and probe K⁺ secretory capacity.

The defect in all types of renal tubular acidosis is an inability to excrete Cl⁻ in proportion to Na⁺, although the reasons vary by type. Treatment largely depends on whether the kidney responds to mineralocorticoid replacement or whether there are losses of Na⁺ that can be replaced as $NaHCO_3$.

Classic distal (type I) renal tubular acidosis responds to $NaHCO_3$ replacement; typically, only 50 to 100 mEq/day are required. Defects in K⁺ reabsorption are also common in this type of renal tubular acidosis, and K⁺ replacement is also required. A variant of the classic distal renal tubular acidosis is a hyperkalemic form that actually is more common than the classic type. The central defect here appears to be impaired Na⁺ transport in the cortical collecting duct. These patients also respond to $NaHCO_3$ replacement. Proximal (type II) renal tubular acidosis is characterized by both Na⁺ and K⁺ reabsorption defects. The disorder is uncommon and usually appears as a component of Fanconi syndrome, which also is characterized by defects in the reabsorption of glucose, phosphate, urate, and amino acids.

Treatment of this disorder with $NaHCO_3$ is ineffective because increased ion delivery merely results in increased excretion. Thiazide diuretics have been used to treat this disorder, with varying success.

Type IV renal tubular acidosis is caused by aldosterone deficiency or resistance. These disorders are diagnosed by the presence of high serum [K⁺] concentration and low urine pH (<5.5). Treatment is usually most effective if the cause can be removed; most commonly, drugs such as nonsteroidal antiinflammatory drugs (NSAIDs), heparin, or potassium-sparing diuretics are responsible. Occasionally, mineralocorticoid replacement is required.

Gastrointestinal Acidosis

Fluid secreted into the gut lumen contains higher amounts of Na⁺ than Cl⁻. Large losses of these fluids, particularly if volume is replaced with fluids containing equal amounts of Na⁺ and Cl⁻, results in a decrease in the plasma Na⁺ concentration relative to the Cl⁻ concentration and a decrease in SID. Such a scenario can be avoided if formulations such as lactated Ringer's solution are used instead of normal saline to replace GI losses.

Iatrogenic Acidosis

Two of the most common causes of a hyperchloremic metabolic acidosis are iatrogenic, and both are due to administration of Cl⁻. Modern parenteral nutrition formulas contain weak anions such as acetate in addition to Cl⁻. The proportions of each anion can be adjusted depending on the acid-base status of the patient. If an insufficient amount of weak anions is provided, the plasma Cl⁻ concentration increases, decreasing SID and resulting in acidosis. A similar condition can arise when normal saline is used for fluid resuscitation, resulting in the development of "dilutional acidosis." Dilutional acidosis was first described more than 40 years ago,[67,68] although some authors have argued that this problem is rarely clinically significant.[69] This view pertains because large doses of NaCl produce only minor degrees of hyperchloremic acidosis in healthy animals.[70] This line of reasoning cannot be applied to critically ill patients, who often require infusion of a very large volume of resuscitation fluid. Furthermore, acid-base balance is often already deranged in critically ill patients, and these patients may not be able to compensate normally by increasing ventilation or may have abnormal buffer capacity due to hypoalbuminemia. In ICU and surgical patients,[71-73] as well as in animals with experimental sepsis,[74] saline-induced acidosis clearly occurs.

Administration of normal saline causes acidosis because this solution contains equal amounts of Na⁺ and Cl⁻, whereas the normal Na⁺ concentration in plasma is 35 to 45 mEq/L greater than the normal Cl⁻ concentration. Administration of 0.9% saline increases the Cl⁻ concentration relatively more than the Na⁺ concentration. Many critically ill patients have a significantly lower SID than do healthy individuals, even when there is no evidence of a metabolic acid-base derangement.[75] The lower SID in critical illness is not surprising given that the positive charge of SID is balanced by the negative charges of A⁻ and total CO_2. Since many critically ill patients are hypoalbuminemic, A⁻ tends to be reduced. Because the body defends Pco_2 for other reasons, a reduction in A⁻ leads to a reduction in SID to maintain normal pH. Thus, a typical ICU patient might have a SID of 30 mEq/L rather than 40 to 42 mEq/L. If this same patient then develops a metabolic acidosis (e.g., lactic acidosis), SID decreases further. If the patient is resuscitated with a large volume of 0.9% saline, metabolic acidosis is exacerbated. This relationship is illustrated in Figure 12-3, which shows that a patient with a lower baseline SID is more susceptible to a subsequent acid load.

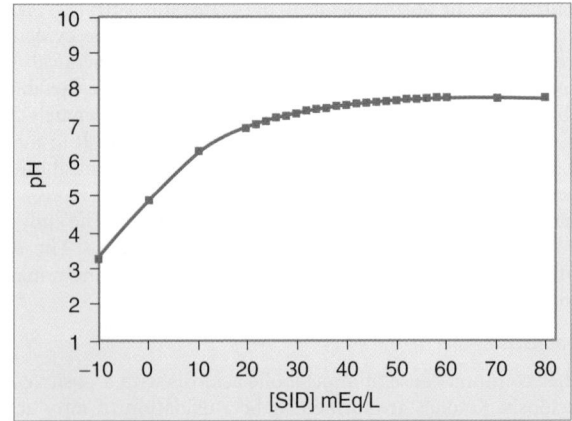

Figure 12-3 **Plot of pH versus strong ion difference (SID).** For this plot, A_{TOT} and Pco_2 were held constant at 18 mEq/L and 40 mm Hg, respectively. This plot assumes a water dissociation constant for blood of 4.4×10^{-14} (Eq/L). Note how steep the pH curve becomes at SID < 20 mEq/L.

One alternative to using normal saline to resuscitate patients is to use Ringer's lactate solution. This fluid contains a more physiologic difference between [Na⁺] and [Cl⁻], so its SID is closer to normal (28 mEq/L as compared to 0 mEq/L for normal saline). Morgan and colleagues recently showed that a solution with a SID of approximately 24 mEq/L results in a neutral effect on the pH as blood is progressively diluted.[76]

Unexplained Hyperchloremic Acidosis

Critically ill patients sometimes manifest hyperchloremic metabolic acidosis for unclear reasons. Often these patients have other coexisting types of metabolic acidosis, making the precise diagnosis difficult. Patients with sepsis and acidosis frequently have normal circulating lactate levels.[77] Often, unexplained anions are the cause,[29-31] but hyperchloremic acidosis also can be a contributing factor.

Metabolic Alkalosis

Metabolic alkalosis occurs as a result of an increase in SID or a decrease in A_{TOT}. These changes can occur secondary to the loss of anions (e.g., Cl⁻ from the stomach, albumin from the plasma) or the retention of cations (rare). Sometimes the loss of Cl⁻ is temporary and can be treated effectively by replacing the anion; metabolic alkalosis in this category is said to be "chloride responsive." In other cases, hormonal mechanisms produce ongoing losses of Cl⁻. Thus, at best, the Cl⁻ deficit can be offset only temporarily by Cl⁻ administration; this form of metabolic alkalosis is said to be "chloride resistant" (Box 12-3). Similar to hyperchloremic acidosis, these disorders can be distinguished by measurement of the urine Cl⁻ concentration.

CHLORIDE-RESPONSIVE DISORDERS

The chloride-responsive disorders usually occur as a result of Cl⁻ losses from the stomach, such as from vomiting or gastric drainage. The treatment is to replace the Cl⁻, which can be achieved slowly with NaCl

TABLE 12-2	Treatment of Metabolic Alkalosis
Condition	**Treatment**
Primary aldosteronism	Spironolactone or other agents that block distal tubular sodium reabsorption improve alkalosis, hypokalemia, and hypertension. Large doses may be necessary. Restriction of sodium intake and potassium supplementation may be necessary. When an adenoma can be identified, surgery is curative. When the cause is bilateral adrenal cortical hyperplasia, therapy is medical. Dexamethasone is effective in long-term therapy of familial dexamethasone-responsive aldosteronism.
Secondary aldosteronism	ACE inhibitors are usually effective. Repair of the underlying lesion, if feasible, may be required.
Cushing's syndrome	Due to pituitary oversecretion of ACTH: surgery or radiation. Due to adrenal adenoma or carcinoma: adrenalectomy. Due to secondary or ectopic ACTH production: address the underlying malignancy.
Liddle's syndrome	Triamterene may be effective.
Bartter's syndrome	Treatment often unsatisfactory long-term. Potassium-sparing diuretics, potassium and magnesium supplementation, ACE inhibitors, COX inhibitors are partially effective.
Exogenous corticoids	Discontinuation of the offending agent(s) and vigorous initial potassium replacement.
Severe potassium or magnesium depletion	Replacement of these electrolytes (may require very large amounts).

From Spital A, Garella S. Correction of acid-base derangments. In Ronco C, Bellomo R (eds) Critical Care Nephrology. Kluwer Academic Publishers, Dordrecht, The Netherlands, 1998; pp. 311-328. Used with permission.
ACE, Angiotensin-converting enzyme, *COX*, Cyclooxygenase.

Box 12-3

DIFFERENTIAL DIAGNOSIS OF METABOLIC ALKALOSIS (INCREASED STRONG ION DIFFERENCE)

Chloride Loss < Sodium
Chloride-responsive (urine Cl⁻ concentration <10 mmol/L)
GI losses
Vomiting
Gastric drainage
Chloride wasting diarrhea (villous adenoma)
Post diuretic use
Post hypercapnia
Chloride-unresponsive (urine Cl⁻ concentration >20 mmol/L)
Mineralocorticoid excess
Primary hyperaldosteronism (Conn's syndrome)
Secondary hyperaldosteronism
Cushing syndrome
Liddle syndrome
Bartter syndrome
Exogenous corticoids
Excessive licorice intake
Ongoing diuretic use

Exogenous Sodium Load (>Chloride)
Sodium salt administration (acetate, citrate)
Massive blood transfusions
Parenteral nutrition
Plasma volume expanders
Sodium lactate (Ringer's solution)

Other
Severe deficiency of intracellular cations
Magnesium, potassium

GI, Gastrointestinal.

or more rapidly with KCl or even HCl. Saline plus KCl is the treatment of choice because volume depletion and K⁺ usually coexist with the acid-base disturbance in patients with chloride-responsive metabolic alkalosis. Dehydration in turn stimulates aldosterone secretion, leading to increased tubular Na⁺ reabsorption and increased urinary losses of K⁺. Administration of normal saline is effective because the administration of equal amounts of Na⁺ and Cl⁻ result in larger relative increases in Cl⁻ concentration compared to Na⁺ concentration. In rare circumstances, when neither K⁺ nor intravascular volume depletion is a problem, it may be desirable to give back Cl⁻ as HCl.

Diuretics and other forms of volume contraction produce metabolic alkalosis predominantly by stimulating aldosterone secretion, as discussed earlier. However, diuretics also induce K⁺ and Cl⁻ excretion directly, further complicating the problem and inducing metabolic alkalosis more rapidly.

CHLORIDE-RESISTANT DISORDERS

The chloride-resistant disorders (see Box 12-3) are characterized by an increased urine Cl⁻ concentration (>20 mEq/L) and are said to be "chloride resistant" because of ongoing Cl⁻ losses. Most commonly, excessive chloride excretion occurs as a result of excessive mineralocorticoid activity. Treatment requires that the underlying disorder be addressed (Table 12-2).

OTHER CAUSES OF METABOLIC ALKALOSIS

Rarely, an increased SID and therefore metabolic alkalosis occurs secondary to cation administration rather than anion depletion. Examples of these disorders include milk-alkali syndrome and IV administration of strong cations without strong anions. The latter occurs with massive blood transfusion because Na⁺ is given with citrate (a weak anion) instead of Cl⁻. Similar results occur when parenteral nutrition formulations contain too much acetate and not enough Cl⁻ to balance the Na⁺ load.

⬛ Respiratory Acid-Base Disorders

Respiratory disorders are far easier to diagnose and treat than metabolic disorders because the mechanism is always the same, although the underlying disease process may vary. CO_2 is produced by cellular metabolism or by the titration of HCO_3^- by metabolic acids. Normally, alveolar ventilation is adjusted to maintain $Paco_2$ between 35 and 45 mm Hg. When alveolar ventilation is increased or decreased out of proportion to CO_2 production, a respiratory acid-base disorder exists.

PATHOPHYSIOLOGY OF RESPIRATORY ACID-BASE DISORDERS

Normal CO_2 production by the body (about 220 mL/min) is equivalent to 15,000 mM/day of carbonic acid.[78] This amount compares to less than 500 mM/day for all nonrespiratory acids that are handled by the kidney and gut. Pulmonary ventilation is adjusted by the respiratory center in response to changes in $Paco_2$, blood pH, and Pao_2 as well as other factors (e.g., exercise, anxiety, wakefulness). Normal $Paco_2$ (40 mm Hg) is maintained by precise matching of alveolar minute ventilation to metabolic CO_2 production. $Paco_2$ changes in compensation for alterations in arterial pH produced by metabolic acidosis or alkalosis in predictable ways (Table 12-3).

RESPIRATORY ACIDOSIS

When CO_2 elimination is inadequate relative to the rate of tissue production, $Paco_2$ increases to a new steady state determined by the new relationship between alveolar ventilation and CO_2 production. Acutely, the increase in $Paco_2$ increases both the $[H^+]$ and the $[HCO_3^-]$ in blood according to the carbonic acid equilibrium equation. Thus, the change in $[HCO_3^-]$ is mediated simply by the dissociation of H_2CO_3 into H^+ and HCO_3^-, not by an active physiologic adaptation response. Similarly, the increase in $[HCO_3^-]$ does not "buffer" the increase in $[H^+]$. There is no change in SID and hence no change in standard base-excess. Cellular acidosis always occurs in respiratory acidosis, since CO_2 builds up in the tissues. If the $Paco_2$ remains increased, active compensatory mechanisms are activated, and SID increases to restore $[H^+]$ toward normal.

Primarily, compensation is accomplished by removal of Cl^- from the plasma space. Since movement of Cl^- into the tissues or red blood cells results in intracellular acidosis, Cl^- must be removed from the body to achieve a lasting effect on the SID. The kidney is the primary organ for Cl^- removal, although the adaptive capacity of the GI tract for

Cl^- elimination has not been fully explored. Accordingly, patients with renal disease have a difficult time adapting to chronic respiratory acidosis. When renal function is intact, Cl^- is eliminated in the urine, and after a few days, the SID increases to the level necessary to return blood pH to about 7.35. It is unclear whether this amount of time is required by the physiologic constraints of the system or to avoid being overly sensitive to transient changes in alveolar ventilation. In any case, this adaptation results in an increased pH for any degree of hypercarbia. According to the Henderson-Hasselbalch equation, the increased pH will result in an increased $[HCO_3^-]$ for a given Pco_2. Thus, the "adaptive" increase in $[HCO_3^-]$ *results from* the increase in pH and is not the *cause for* the increase in pH.

Although the change in HCO_3^- concentration is a convenient and reliable marker for the metabolic compensation, it is not the mechanism. This point is more than semantic because only changes in the independent variables of acid base balance (Pco_2, A_{TOT}, SID) can affect the plasma $[H^+]$, and $[HCO_3^-]$ is not an independent variable.

Diseases of Ventilatory Impairment

As for virtually all acid-base disorders, treatment begins with addressing the underlying disorder. Acute respiratory acidosis can be caused by central nervous system (CNS) suppression, neuromuscular disease or impairment (e.g., myasthenia gravis, hypophosphatemia, hypokalemia), or airway and parenchymal lung disease (e.g., asthma, acute respiratory distress syndrome). This last category of conditions also produces primary hypoxia, not just alveolar hypoventilation. The two can be distinguished by the alveolar gas equation:

$$Pao_2 = Pio_2 - Paco_2/R$$

where R is the respiratory exchange coefficient (generally assumed to be 0.8), and Pio_2 is the inspired oxygen tension (room air is approximately 150). Thus, as $Paco_2$ increases, the Pao_2 will decrease in a predictable fashion. If the Pao_2 is reduced further, there is a defect in gas exchange.

Chronic respiratory acidosis is most often caused by chronic lung disease (e.g., chronic obstructive pulmonary disease) or chest wall disease (e.g., kyphoscoliosis). Rarely, its cause is central hypoventilation or chronic neuromuscular disease.

When and How to Treat

The primary threat to life in cases of respiratory acidosis comes not from acidosis but from hypoxemia. If the patient is breathing room air, $Paco_2$ cannot exceed 80 mm Hg before life-threatening hypoxemia results. Accordingly, supplemental oxygen is always required, although unfortunately, oxygen administration alone is almost never sufficient treatment, and the defect in ventilation must be addressed directly. When the underlying cause can be addressed quickly (e.g., reversal of narcotics with naloxone), it may be possible to avoid endotracheal intubation. More often, however, mechanical ventilation must be initiated. Mechanical support is indicated when the patient is unstable or at risk for instability or when CNS function deteriorates. Furthermore, in patients who are exhibiting signs of respiratory muscle fatigue, mechanical ventilation should be instituted before overt respiratory failure occurs. Thus, it is not the absolute $Paco_2$ value that is important but rather the clinical condition of the patient.

Chronic hypercapnia requires treatment when there is an acute deterioration. In this setting, it is important to recognize that the goal of therapy is not a normal value for $Paco_2$ (35-45 mm Hg) but rather restoration of the patient's baseline $Paco_2$ (if known). If the baseline $Paco_2$ is not known, a target $Paco_2$ of 60 mm Hg is reasonable. Overventilation has two undesirable consequences. First, life-threatening alkalemia can occur if the $Paco_2$ is rapidly normalized in a patient with chronic respiratory acidosis and an appropriately large SID. Second, even if the $Paco_2$ is corrected slowly, the patient will reduce the plasma SID over time, making it impossible to wean the patient from mechanical ventilation.

TABLE 12-3	Observational Acid-Base Patterns		
Disorder	*HCO_3^- (mEq/L)*	*Pco_2 (mm Hg)*	*SBE (mEq/L)*
Metabolic acidosis	<22	$= (1.5 \times HCO_3^-) + 8$ $= 40 + SBE$	< −5
Metabolic alkalosis	>26	$= (0.7 \times HCO_3^-) + 21$ $= 40 + (0.6 \times SBE)$	> +5
Acute respiratory acidosis	$= [(Pco_2 - 40)/10] + 24$	>45	= 0
Chronic respiratory acidosis	$= [(Pco_2 - 40)/3] + 24$	>45	$= 0.4 \times (Pco_2 - 40)$
Acute respiratory alkalosis	$= 24 - [(40 - Pco_2)/5]$	<35	= 0
Chronic respiratory alkalosis	$= 24 - [(40 - Pco_2)/2]$	<35	$= 0.4 \times (Pco_2 - 40)$

From Kellum JA, Elbers PWG, eds. Stewart's Textbook of Acid-Base. 2nd ed. Amsterdam: Acidbase.org; 2009. Used with permission.

Noninvasive ventilation is another treatment option that is useful in selected patients, particularly those with normal sensorium.[79] Rapid infusion of $NaHCO_3$ in patients with respiratory acidosis can induce acute respiratory failure if alveolar ventilation is not increased to adjust for the increased CO_2 load. Thus, if $NaHCO_3$ is used, it must be administered slowly and alveolar ventilation adjusted appropriately. Furthermore, as discussed previously, $NaHCO_3$ works by increasing the plasma $[Na^+]$. If this is not possible or not desirable, $NaHCO_3$ should be avoided.

Occasionally it is useful to reduce CO_2 production, which can be achieved by reducing the carbohydrate load in the nutritional support regimen, lowering the temperature in febrile patients, and providing adequate sedation for anxious or combative patients. Treatment of shivering in the postoperative period can reduce CO_2 production. However, it is unusual to control hypercarbia with these techniques alone.

PERMISSIVE HYPERCAPNIA

In recent years, there has been increased recognition of ventilator-associated lung injury. Accordingly, a strategy designed to reduce minute ventilation and hence increase $Paco_2$, so-called permissive hypercapnia or controlled hypoventilation, has been increasingly employed.[11] However, permissive hypercapnia is not without risks. Sedation is mandatory and the use of neuromuscular blocking agents is frequently required. Hypercapnia is associated with increased intracranial pressure and pulmonary hypertension, making this technique unusable in patients with brain injury or right ventricular dysfunction. Controversy exists as to how low to allow the pH to go. While some authors have reported good results with pH values less than 7.0,[11] most authors advocate more modest pH reductions (>7.25).

RESPIRATORY ALKALOSIS

Respiratory alkalosis may be the most frequently encountered acid-base disorder. It occurs in a number of pathologic conditions, including salicylate intoxication, early sepsis, hepatic failure, and hypoxic respiratory disorders. Respiratory alkalosis also occurs with pregnancy and with pain or anxiety. Hypocapnia appears to be a particularly bad prognostic indicator in patients with critical illness.[80] As in acute respiratory acidosis, acute respiratory alkalosis results in a small change in $[HCO_3^-]$ as dictated by the Henderson-Hasselbalch equation. If hypocapnia persists, the SID will begin to decrease as a result of renal Cl^- reabsorption. After 2 to 3 days, the SID assumes a new, lower steady state.[81] Severe alkalemia is unusual in patients with respiratory alkalosis, and management is therefore directed to the underlying cause. Typically, these mild acid-base changes are clinically more important for what they can alert the clinician to, in terms of underlying disease, than for any threat they pose to the patient. In rare cases, respiratory depression with narcotics is necessary.

PSEUDORESPIRATORY ALKALOSIS

The presence of arterial hypocapnia in patients with profound circulatory shock has been termed *pseudorespiratory alkalosis*.[82] This condition can be seen when alveolar ventilation is supported, but the circulation is grossly inadequate. In such conditions, the mixed venous Pco_2 is significantly elevated, but the arterial Pco_2 is normal or even decreased secondary to decreased CO_2 delivery to the lungs and increased pulmonary transit time. Overall CO_2 clearance is markedly decreased, and there is marked tissue acidosis, usually involving both metabolic and respiratory components. The metabolic component comes from tissue hypoperfusion and hyperlactatemia. Arterial oxygen saturation also may appear to be adequate despite tissue hypoxemia. This condition is rapidly fatal unless cardiac output is rapidly corrected.

Unified Approach to the Patient with Acid-Base Imbalance

CHARACTERIZING THE DISORDER

As described in greater detail in recent reviews,[6-7] the first step in the approach to a patient with an acid-base imbalance is to characterize the disorder. Acid-base imbalances are usually recognized by abnormalities in the venous plasma electrolyte concentrations, so it is useful to start there. Measurement of venous $[HCO_3^-]$ is the easiest way to screen for acid-base disorders. However, a normal $[HCO_3^-]$ does not exclude the possibility of an acid-base derangement, even a serious one. Therefore, if the history and physical examination findings lead one to suspect a disease process that results in an acid-base imbalance, more investigation is required. The normal $[HCO_3^-]$ is 22 to 26 mEq/L. Increases in $[HCO_3^-]$ occur with primary and compensatory metabolic alkaloses and decreases occur with primary or compensatory metabolic acidoses. Unfortunately, in mixed disorders, $[HCO_3^-]$ may be misleading, and the presence of any abnormality in $[HCO_3^-]$ requires further investigation. In addition to examining the $[HCO_3^-]$, venous blood can be used to calculate AG: $([Na^+] + [K^+]) - ([Cl^-] - [HCO_3^-])$. If $[HCO_3^-]$ or AG are abnormal or if there is clinical suspicion for a mixed disorder, arterial blood should be sampled for blood gas analysis. This test will provide information on the pH, $Paco_2$, and standard base-excess. Although simple disorders will conform to the equations presented in Table 12-3, "mixed" disorders are quite common.

In patients with acidemia, the next step is to examine AG. The AG should also be examined when there is suspicion of an occult metabolic acidosis, even in a patient with alkalemia. However, severe alkalemia will increase AG by 2 to 4 mEq/L, and hence wider "tolerance limits" should be used. If AG is calculated from an alkalemic blood sample, only significant abnormalities (>8-10 mEq/L above normal) should be considered important. More often, however, it is not excessive sensitivity but rather insensitivity that plagues AG calculation. The accuracy of AG can be improved easily by using a patient-specific normal range rather than a standard one. If unmeasured anions are detected, it is a good idea to compare their amounts to the abnormality in standard base-excess. For example, if the calculated AG is 5 mEq/L greater than expected and the standard base-excess is −15 mEq/L, a mixed metabolic acidosis is present. The unmeasured anions (e.g., ketones) are accounting for a standard base-excess of −5 mEq/L while some other process is responsible for another 10 mEq/L. This sort of abnormality can occur if very large amounts of 0.9% saline are used to treat a patient with diabetic ketoacidosis. As the ketosis resolves, the acidosis persists because SID has been decreased due to excessive Cl^- administration.

DETERMINING THE CAUSE

Once the disorder has been characterized, the clinician must integrate the information obtained from the history and physical examination to arrive at an accurate diagnosis. Mixed disorders continue to be problematic, as any acid-base disorder that fails to fit into the classification scheme shown in Table 12-2 can be considered a mixed disorder, but some mixed disorders appear to be simple disorders when first encountered. For example, a patient with chronic respiratory acidosis and a $Paco_2$ of 60 mm Hg would be expected to have a standard base-excess of +8 mEq/L (see Table 12-3). If this patient develops a metabolic acidosis, the standard base-excess will decrease and may be 0 mEq/L. At this point, it may appear that the patient has a pure acute respiratory acidosis rather than a mixed disorder. If the metabolic acidosis causes an increase in AG, this abnormality may provide a clue. Another useful method is to obtain at least two blood gas analyses to examine for trends. In general, however, it is only by careful attention to history and physical examination that the true diagnosis can be made.

ANNOTATED REFERENCES

Kellum JA, Elbers PWG, eds. Stewart's Textbook of Acid-Base. 2nd ed. Amsterdam: Acidbase.org; 2009.
  An expanded 2nd edition to Stewart's classic monograph. Additional chapter provided by leading experts covers clinical application.
Kellum JA. Disorders of acid-base balance. Crit Care Med 2007;35(11):2630-6.
  A case-based review of acid-base using modern methods.
Forsythe SM, Schmidt GA. Sodium bicarbonate for the treatment of lactic acidosis. Chest 2000;117(1):260-7.
  A systematic review of the evidence for and against use of sodium bicarbonate for lactic acidosis.

Morgan TJ, Venkatesh B, Hall J. Crystalloid strong ion difference determines metabolic acid-base change during in vitro hemodilution. Crit Care Med 2002;30(1):157-60.
  In vitro studies of hemodilution using different crystalloid solution. The authors demonstrate that the SID of the diluent is the decisive factor in determining final pH.

REFERENCES

Access the complete reference list online at http://www.expertconsult.com.

13

Hypernatremia and Hyponatremia

JOHN K. McILWAINE | HOWARD L. CORWIN

Disorders of plasma sodium concentration—that is, hypernatremia and hyponatremia—are among the most common clinical problems observed in the critically ill. These disorders are often asymptomatic, but in some patients, they may result in symptoms ranging from minor to life threatening. The approach to treating hyper- and hyponatremia in individual patients involves balancing the risks of treatment against the risks of the disorder.

Hypernatremia

Hypernatremia is a common clinical problem, observed in up to 2% of the general hospital population and 15% of patients admitted to the intensive care unit.[1-4] In the outpatient setting, hypernatremia is most prevalent in the geriatric patient population; in hospitalized patients, it is observed in all age groups.[1,5] Mortality rates in patients with hypernatremia can range as high as 70%.[1-6] Although the high mortality rate no doubt reflects the severity of underlying disease in these patients, there is significant morbidity related to hypernatremia itself. Neurologic sequelae from hypernatremia are common, particularly in the pediatric population.[6]

Maintaining a normal serum sodium concentration (135–145 mEq/L) is dependent on the balance between water intake and water excretion. Hypernatremia results from a deficit of free water that leads to an increase in serum tonicity. The usual mechanism underlying the development of hypernatremia is inadequate water intake and increased free water loss, but it can also result from the intake of hypertonic sodium solutions. Hypernatremia may be associated with volume depletion, euvolemia, or hypervolemia, depending on the balance of salt and water loss and intake. Sodium content is low, normal, or high, respectively, in each of these circumstances. Relative sodium and volume status has important implications for the treatment of hypernatremic patients.

The brain is particularly susceptible to the effects of hypernatremia. When the sodium concentration in plasma is higher than normal, water moves across cytosolic membranes (from the inside of cells to the outside of cells) to preserve osmotic equilibrium. As a consequence of intracellular dehydration, there is a net loss of brain volume, which in turn places mechanical stress on cerebral vessels, possibly resulting in bleeding.[6] With chronic hypernatremia, however, cellular adaptation occurs. Under these circumstances, so-called idiogenic osmoles accumulate in brain cells, minimizing cellular dehydration. Importantly, the presence of these idiogenic osmoles presents a risk for the development of cerebral edema during the treatment of hypernatremia.

The symptoms of hypernatremia are nonspecific and often difficult to separate from those of underlying illnesses in hospitalized patients. Central nervous system (CNS) abnormalities are most common and can include confusion, weakness, and lethargy in the early stages, progressing to seizures, coma, and death in later stages. The CNS symptoms result from the movement of water out of the brain cells rather than the hypernatremia per se. Neurologic deterioration can be seen during treatment as a result of the development of cerebral edema. Signs of volume depletion or volume overload may be present, depending on the cause of the hypernatremia.

The treatment of hypernatremia is water repletion (Box 13-1). Assuming total body water is 60%, the water deficit may be estimated as follows:

$$\text{Water deficit} = [0.6 \times \text{Total body weight}] \times [(\text{Serum sodium concentration}/140) - 1].$$

The percentage of water relative to total body weight is actually closer to 50% in women and about 50% in the elderly of both genders. Treatment should be instituted at a rate that balances the risk of hypernatremia with the risk of too rapid correction, particularly in cases of chronic hypernatremia. Half the calculated deficit should be replaced within the first 12 to 24 hours at a rate of sodium concentration correction not over 2 mEq/L per hour. The remainder of the water deficit can be replaced over the next 48 hours. The rapidity of replacement should be determined by the acuteness of onset and severity of symptoms.

Neurologic status has to be closely monitored during replacement for evidence of the development of cerebral edema. Ongoing replacement of fluid and electrolyte losses is also necessary during treatment. In patients with volume depletion and hemodynamic instability associated with hypernatremia, volume replacement with isotonic saline is initially indicated. Once hemodynamic stability is achieved, water replacement can be initiated. Hypotonic saline (e.g., 0.45% saline) may be preferable to water as the replacement fluid for these patients. If hypernatremia is associated with hypervolemia (e.g., as a consequence of treatment with hypertonic saline or hypertonic sodium bicarbonate solution), treatment should be directed toward reducing sodium intake while inducing sodium loss. In these patients, diuretics can be used along with free water (5% dextrose) infusion. Dialysis may be necessary if renal failure is present.

Hyponatremia

Hyponatremia is one of the most common electrolyte abnormalities seen in hospitalized patients. It occurs in 2% to 4% of hospitalized patients and up to 30% of patients in intensive care units.[7-10] Mortality for patients with acute hyponatremia is reportedly as high as 50%, whereas mortality for those with chronic hyponatremia is 10% to 20%.[7-11]

Hyponatremia is a water problem, not a sodium problem; there is always an excess of water relative to sodium when hyponatremia is present. In hyponatremia, water excretion by the kidney is impaired. Patients who are hyponatremic may be hypovolemic (water deficit and sodium deficit), euvolemic (water excess and normal sodium content), or hypervolemic (water excess and sodium excess). As is the case with hypernatremia, the patient's volume status has implications for the treatment of hyponatremia.

In the presence of hyponatremia, there is a decrease in extracellular tonicity relative to the intracellular space. The osmotic gap causes movement of water from the extracellular space into the intracellular space and results in cell swelling. In the CNS, cellular swelling manifests as cerebral edema and results in the symptoms associated with hyponatremia. The degree of cerebral cell swelling correlates with the severity of symptoms observed. The CNS adapts to hyponatremia in two ways. First, cerebral edema causes an increase in interstitial hydrostatic pressure and results in the movement of fluid from the interstitial space into the cerebrospinal fluid (CSF), leading to some amelioration of cerebral edema, assuming normal CSF production and resorption physiology. Second, solutes are lost from cells, resulting in a decrease in intracellular osmolarity and thus movement of water out of cells.

53

TREATMENT OF HYPERNATREMIA

Determine and treat the cause.
Calculate water deficit.
Replace half the deficit over 12–24 h.
Do not correct more rapidly than 2 mEq/L/h.
Replace the remaining deficit over 48 h.
If hemodynamic instability is present, give isotonic saline until
    stable before replacing water deficit with hypotonic saline.
If volume overload is present, treat with loop diuretic and 5%
    dextrose; consider adding thiazide.
Dialysis may be indicated if renal failure is present.
Ongoing fluid and electrolyte losses should be replaced.
Neurologic status should be closely monitored.

The solutes lost initially are sodium and potassium, followed by organic solutes over the next several days. Because of cerebral adaptation, the severity of neurologic symptoms is related to the acuity and magnitude of the hyponatremia. If hyponatremia develops gradually, brain cells can compensate by decreasing intracellular osmolarity through the loss of osmolytes, thereby limiting the degree of cerebral edema and resultant neurologic dysfunction. Importantly, during the correction of chronic hyponatremia, the regeneration of these osmolytes lags, and cerebral dehydration can occur with rapid correction.

In acute hyponatremia, nausea, vomiting, lethargy, and confusion can progress to coma, seizures, eventual cerebral herniation, and death.[11,12] The elderly and the young are more likely to be symptomatic from hyponatremia.[9] Menstruating women also tend to be more symptomatic and are at greater risk for neurologic complications from acute hyponatremia.[11] Early in the development of hyponatremia, the symptoms are difficult to separate from those related to the underlying disease process. Hyponatremic patients who have clinically significant space-occupying lesions in the CNS should be aggressively treated. Meanwhile, efforts should be made to determine the cause of hyponatremia by assessing intravascular volume status, measuring urine output, seeking the presence of exogenous sugars or sugar alcohols (e.g., mannitol), and determining urine sodium concentration and osmolarity.

Treatment of hyponatremia is dependent on the acuteness of the hyponatremia and the presence and severity of symptoms (Box 13-2). Acute (<48 hours) or chronic (>48 hours) symptomatic hyponatremia (e.g., seizures) requires immediate therapy. However, the optimal approach for the treatment of these patients is controversial.[12-14] The controversy results from reports of the occurrence of a central demyelination syndrome associated with the correction of hyponatremia in some patients.[15-22] This syndrome appears to be more common with chronic hyponatremia (>48 hours), overcorrection of hyponatremia, large corrections (>12 to 25 mEq/L per 24 hours), and rapid correction (>1 to 2 mEq/L per hour).[19-22]

The approach to the treatment of acute symptomatic hyponatremia is infusion of hypertonic saline (3%). Therapy is targeted toward resolution of symptoms or a 10% to 15% increase in serum sodium concentration. In patients with a high urine osmolarity, the addition of a loop diuretic facilitates correction of the hyponatremia by decreasing urine osmolarity. The rate of correction should be less than 2 mEq/L per hour and less than 15 mEq/L total over 24 hours. The amount of hypertonic saline necessary to correct the serum sodium concentration to a safe level (e.g., 120 mEq/L) can be estimated by calculating the sodium deficit:

$$\text{Sodium deficit} = 0.5 \times \text{Lean body weight} \times (120 - \text{Observed serum sodium concentration})$$

The amount of hypertonic saline required to replace the deficit is then infused at a rate that permits correction within the parameters noted earlier. Frequent checking of electrolytes is necessary to ensure that correction is not too rapid.

In treating patients with chronic (>48 hours or of unknown duration) symptomatic hyponatremia (seizures, coma, impending brain herniation), the higher risk of neurologic complications related to therapy mandates a more cautious approach. As with acute hyponatremia, neurologic symptoms predominate in the clinical presentation of these patients. Initial treatment with 3% sodium chloride should be directed toward the resolution of symptoms or a 10% increase in serum sodium concentration. The increase in serum sodium concentration should be at a rate less than 1.5 mEq/L per hour initially, and the total correction should not exceed 12 mEq/L per 24 hours. Close monitoring of serum electrolytes and neurologic status is mandatory. The resolution of symptoms allows for a decrease in the rate of correction. As noted earlier, calculation of sodium deficit can be used to estimate the volume of hypertonic saline necessary for correction.

Most patients with hyponatremia are asymptomatic. Aggressive correction of serum sodium in these patients is not indicated. Treatment in asymptomatic patients is based on the underlying cause of the hyponatremia and the patient's volume status: euvolemic, hypovolemic, or hypervolemic (edema).

The majority of chronic hyponatremic patients are euvolemic. In this group, the syndrome of inappropriate antidiuretic hormone (SIADH) is the most common diagnosis. The inappropriate (nonosmotic) presence of antidiuretic hormone impairs free water excretion by the kidney; impaired water excretion coupled with water intake results in hyponatremia. Water restriction is the mainstay of therapy for these patients. The amount of water restriction must be sufficient to achieve negative water balance (i.e., the difference between the total intake and excretion of water), or correction of hyponatremia will not occur. Therefore, all water losses (insensible losses, urinary losses, and gastrointestinal losses) must be considered when deciding on the degree of water restriction. If urine osmolarity is high, it may be necessary to decrease it to achieve a negative water balance. This can be achieved by adding a loop diuretic, but salt intake must be increased to correct for losses resulting from the increased natriuresis with diuresis. Less commonly, demeclocycline (300–600 mg twice a day), which interferes with the action of antidiuretic hormone, is used to decrease urine osmolarity. In patients with more pronounced hyponatremia,

---

TREATMENT OF HYPONATREMIA

Acute Symptomatic Hyponatremia
3% hypertonic saline with loop diuretic.
Correct no more than 2 mEq/L/h.
Correct no more than 12–15 mEq/L/h over the first 24 h.

Chronic Symptomatic Hyponatremia (>48 h or unknown duration)
3% hypertonic saline with loop diuretic.
Correct no more than 1.5 mEq/L/h initially.
Correct to resolution of symptoms or 10% correction of serum
    sodium.
Correct no more than 12 mEq/L/24 h.
Close monitoring of electrolytes and neurologic status.

Asymptomatic Hyponatremia
Euvolemia:
    Treat underlying cause.
    Water restriction.
    Occasionally loop diuretic or demeclocycline to lower urine
        osmolarity.
    Hypertonic saline rarely indicated.
Hypovolemia:
    Treat underlying cause of fluid loss.
    Normal saline until euvolemic.
Hypervolemia:
    Treat underlying cause of decreased effective circulating
        volume.
    Salt and water restriction.
    Loop diuretics for some patients.

the combination of normal saline and a loop diuretic can be used to correct hyponatremia. In asymptomatic patients, the use of hypertonic saline is rarely if ever indicated.

Two new Food and Drug Administration (FDA)-approved vasopressin receptor antagonists are now available in the United States. One of these agents, tolvaptan, is selective for the vasopressin 2 (V_2) receptor. The other agent, conivaptan, is less selective and binds to both V_{1A} and V_2 receptors. Both are indicated for treating euvolemic hyponatremia. Tolvaptan also is indicated for the treatment of hypervolemic hyponatremia. Neither drug has been extensively studied, and the effect of treatment with these agents on hard endpoints such as mortality have not been assessed. Both drugs, however, have been investigated for the adjunctive treatment of congestive heart failure, and neither has been shown to improve mortality or morbidity.[23,24] Given the paucity of clinically meaningful outcomes, we do not recommend the use of either of these antagonists for routine therapy of hyponatremia.

Hyponatremia associated with volume depletion is a result of the loss of both sodium and water, combined with the simultaneous intake of water or hypotonic fluids. The release of antidiuretic hormone stimulated by hypovolemia inhibits the kidney's ability to excrete water. The net result is positive water balance and hyponatremia. The treatment of hyponatremia in this setting is infusion of normal saline to correct the volume depletion. As volume status is corrected, antidiuretic hormone excretion is switched off, and the kidney excretes the excess water, correcting the serum sodium concentration. The cause of the initial sodium and water loss should also be identified and treated.

Hyponatremia associated with hypervolemia is very common and generally associated with low "effective" volume states such as (but not limited to) heart failure, cirrhosis, adrenal insufficiency, profound hypothyroidism, and nephrotic syndrome. The hallmark of these conditions is the presence of edema. The mechanism for the development of hyponatremia in these settings is diminished effective circulating volume, leading to sodium and water retention. The water retention is a result of nonosmotic antidiuretic hormone release impairing the kidney's ability to excrete water. In this respect, the mechanism is similar to that responsible for hyponatremia associated with volume depletion. Therapy is directed toward correcting the primary disease process responsible for the decrease in effective circulating volume. Specific treatment of the hyponatremia consists of sodium and water restriction. The use of loop diuretics may facilitate free water excretion and correction of the hyponatremia; notably, thiazide diuretics may exacerbate hyponatremia and should be avoided.

ANNOTATED REFERENCES

Ayus JC, Wheeler JM, Arieff AI. Postoperative hyponatremic encephalopathy in menstruant women. Ann Intern Med 1992;117(11):891-7.
This case-controlled and cohort study to determine the risk factors for hyponatremic encephalopathy and the clinical course of patients with encephalopathy found a correlation between poor neurologic outcomes and menstruant women in the setting of acute postoperative hyponatremia.

Karp BI, Laureno R. Pontine and extrapontine myelinolysis: a neurologic disorder following rapid correction of hyponatremia. Medicine (Baltimore) 1993;72(6):359-73.
In this retrospective study of patients who developed neurologic dysfunction after correction of hyponatremia, there appeared to be a correlation between the rate of sodium correction and neurologic dysfunction.

Palevsky PM, Bhagrath R, Greenberg A. Hypernatremia in hospitalized patients. Ann Intern Med 1996;124(2):197-203.
This well-done prospective cohort study identifying the epidemiology and causes of hypernatremia in a hospitalized patient population found that hospitalized patients of any age may develop hypernatremia.

Snyder NA, Feigal DW, Arieff AI. Hypernatremia in elderly patients: a heterogeneous, morbid, and iatrogenic entity. Ann Intern Med 1987;107(3):309-19.
These investigators followed a prospective cohort of hospitalized elderly patients (older than 60 years) and determined that hospitalized patients often develop hypernatremia secondary to inappropriate fluid management. These patients had a longer length of stay and slightly increased mortality, although there was no control for severity of illness.

Sterns RH, Cappuccio JD, Silver SM, et al. Neurologic sequelae after treatment of severe hyponatremia: a multicenter perspective. J Am Soc Nephrol 1994;4(8):1522-30.
This multicenter retrospective study evaluated the effect of correction rates of severe hyponatremia (<106 mEq/L) on outcome. Patients who were chronically hyponatremic and corrected to a normal serum sodium concentration at a rate of less than 12 mEq/day or 0.55 mEq/h did not develop postcorrection neurologic sequelae.

REFERENCES

Access the complete reference list online at http://www.expertconsult.com.

14

Hyperkalemia and Hypokalemia

SERGIO ZANOTTI-CAVAZZONI

Hyperkalemia and hypokalemia are the most common electrolyte abnormalities found in hospitalized patients.[1] The precise prevalence of potassium abnormalities in critically ill patients is unknown.[2] However, owing to comorbid conditions, critically ill patients are likely at a higher risk of developing complications from altered serum potassium levels. Therefore, timely recognition and intervention are essential for minimizing morbidity and mortality.

Hyperkalemia

Hyperkalemia is defined as a serum potassium concentration (serum [K+]) greater than 5.0 mEq/L. In critically ill patients, hyperkalemia is less frequent than hypokalemia but more likely to cause serious complications. Severe hyperkalemia requires rapid correction to prevent serious cardiovascular complications. The measured value for serum [K+] can be elevated as a result of in vitro phenomena, usually the release of K+ from cells during the clotting process. Pseudohyperkalemia should be recognized and considered in patients with marked elevations of white blood cell or platelet count.[3] Simultaneous measurements of plasma (unclotted) and serum (clotted) [K+] should identify this problem. A serum [K+] that is 0.2 to 0.3 mEq/L greater than plasma [K+] is indicative of pseudohyperkalemia. Pseudohyperkalemia also may result from hemolysis of a blood specimen after collection; this event is usually identified in the laboratory and reported.

True hyperkalemia occurs by two mechanisms: (1) impaired K+ excretion and (2) shifts in intracellular and extracellular K+ (Box 14-1). Renal insufficiency is the most common cause of altered K+ excretion. With acute oliguric renal failure, elevated potassium level, if not treated, is life threatening. In most patients with nonoliguric chronic renal failure, mild hyperkalemia is evident.[4] With some causes of chronic renal failure, such as diabetes mellitus and tubulointerstitial diseases, hyperkalemia is more pronounced and is probably related to low circulating renin and aldosterone levels.[5] Decreased aldosterone production promotes the development of hyperkalemia. Patients with acquired adrenal insufficiency develop hyperkalemia despite normal renal function. Various drugs used in the intensive care unit (ICU) can produce hyperkalemia by impairing K+ excretion.[6] Patients with abnormal renal function are more susceptible to drug-induced hyperkalemia, and potassium supplements are the most common cause. Potassium-sparing diuretics (spironolactone, amiloride, and triamterene) inhibit K+ excretion and can produce severe hyperkalemia.[7] Spironolactone is the most dangerous of these drugs with respect to impaired K+ excretion, and its effects can be persist even after discontinuation of the drug. Its use has increased significantly after reports of improved mortality in patients with congestive heart failure.[8] Angiotensin-converting enzyme (ACE) inhibitors reduce circulating aldosterone levels and are associated with hyperkalemia in patients with renal insufficiency.[9] Angiotensin receptor blockers (ARBs) have less impact on circulating aldosterone levels and are less likely to produce hyperkalemia.[9] Nonsteroidal antiinflammatory drugs (NSAIDs) and cyclooxygenase-2 (COX-2) inhibitors block prostaglandin synthesis, causing indirect suppression of renin release and aldosterone secretion. NSAIDs and COX-2 inhibitors also reduce renal blood flow and glomerular filtration rate, particularly in patients with prerenal azotemia (due to decreased intravascular volume or heart failure). These compounds may produce hyperkalemia by these mechanisms in patients with or without renal dysfunction.[10,11] Heparin inhibits aldosterone synthesis and can cause significant hyperkalemia in patients with altered renal function.[12-14] Other drugs that may cause hyperkalemia by decreasing glomerular filtration rate and aldosterone secretion include cyclosporine and tacrolimus.[15] Trimethoprim and pentamidine inhibit renal K+ excretion and can cause hyperkalemia in patients with renal insufficiency.[15] Hyperkalemia has also been described as one of the manifestations of the propofol infusion syndrome (PRIS), a rare but fatal complication of propofol infusion in critically ill patients.[16,17]

Alterations in the relationship between intracellular and extracellular [K+] may lead to severe hyperkalemia in critically ill patients, either by increased release of intracellular K+ or by inhibition of extracellular-to-intracellular K+ movement. The effects of acidosis on serum [K+] are complicated and not fully understood. The traditional teaching that acidosis produces a shift of K+ from the intracellular to the extracellular space, thus causing hyperkalemia, was based on observations of hyperkalemia in patients with diabetic ketoacidosis and renal failure.[18] This relationship has since been disproved, and changes in serum [K+] in relation to acid-base disorders are more complex than initially thought. Most forms of acute acidosis do not present with hyperkalemia. The most common forms of acute metabolic acidosis in critically ill patients, diabetic ketoacidosis and lactic acidosis, are not associated with shift K+ out of cells.[19] Hyperkalemia seen with diabetic ketoacidosis is most likely caused by increased release of intracellular K+ due to the breakdown of muscle cells.[20] Hypertonicity of the extracellular fluid causes water to exit cells, and K+ follows. Unless renal function is adequate to eliminate the excess K+, hyperkalemia develops. This situation may occur in patients with uncontrolled diabetes and can lead to severe hyperkalemia in the presence of renal failure and hypoaldosteronism.[20] Massive tissue breakdown can occur with trauma, burns, and rhabdomyolysis, leading to release of K+ into the extracellular space. If renal mechanisms for K+ excretion are impaired, severe hyperkalemia may develop. Drugs can affect the transmembrane balance of K+. β-Adrenergic blockers inhibit the entry of K+ into cells and, in combination with renal failure, can promote development of hyperkalemia.[21] Succinylcholine blocks normal reentry of K+ into cells after depolarization and causes a transitory increase in serum [K+].[22] In patients with severe burns or extensive trauma, the transient hyperkalemia induced by succinylcholine can be more prolonged and severe.[23] Digoxin impairs K+ entry into cells by inhibiting the cell membrane Na+/K+-ATPase.[24] It does not produce hyperkalemia in therapeutic doses, but may cause hyperkalemia with toxic levels.[24,25]

CLINICAL EFFECTS

Most of the clinical consequences of potassium abnormalities are related to the effect on the transmembrane resting cell potential. Cardiac and neuromuscular cells are particularly sensitive to changes in serum [K+]. Most often, hyperkalemia is asymptomatic. However, it affects the cardiac conduction system, as evidenced by characteristic changes in the electrocardiogram (ECG) that serve as indicators of potential life-threatening arrhythmias (Table 14-1). The first sign of increased serum [K+] is tenting of the T wave. Changes associated with progressive increases in serum [K+] include widening of the QRS

CAUSES OF HYPERKALEMIA

Impaired K$^+$ Excretion
Renal failure
Mineralocorticoid deficiency
Addison's disease
Renal tubular acidosis (type 4)
Heparin-induced inhibition of aldosterone synthesis
Hereditary enzyme deficiencies
Pseudohypoaldosteronism
Drugs: potassium-sparing diuretics, ACE inhibitors, NSAIDs, trimethoprim, cyclosporine, tacrolimus, pentamidine

Shifts of K$^+$ Out of Cells
Hypertonicity
Tissue breakdown: rhabdomyolysis, burns, trauma
Drugs: β-blockers, digoxin, succinylcholine, arginine, lysine
Familial hyperkalemic periodic paralysis
Insulin deficiency or resistance

ACE, Angiotensin-converting enzyme; *NSAIDs,* nonsteroidal antiinflammatory drugs.

TABLE 14-1	Electrocardiogram Changes Caused by Abnormal [K$^+$]	
Hyperkalemia	*Hypokalemia*
Peaked T waves	Broad, flat T waves
Loss of P waves	ST depression
Widening QRS complexes	U wave
Sine wave	QT interval prolongation
Ventricular arrhythmias	Ventricular arrhythmias
Asystole	

complex, progressive development of atrioventricular conduction blocks, slow idioventricular rhythm, an ECG tracing that looks like a sine wave, ventricular fibrillation, and finally asystole.[26] ECG changes are not always sensitive to changes in serum [K$^+$] levels. There is no absolute level of serum [K$^+$] associated with a particular ECG abnormality, but rapid rises seem to be more dangerous, particularly in patients without a history of chronic renal insufficiency.[27,28] However, normal ECGs have been described with extreme hyperkalemia, and in some cases the first manifestation of cardiac compromise from hyperkalemia may be ventricular fibrillation.[29,30] Hyperkalemia can cause paresthesias and weakness in the arms and legs, followed by a symmetrical flaccid paralysis of the extremities that ascends toward the trunk, finally involving the respiratory muscles. The cranial nerves are usually not affected by hyperkalemia.

TREATMENT

The primary goal of treating hyperkalemia is to prevent adverse cardiac complications. Treatment modalities are aimed at one of three mechanisms to prevent or decrease these complications: (1) direct antagonism of hyperkalemic effect on the cell membrane polarization, (2) movement of extracellular K$^+$ into the intracellular compartment, and (3) removal of K$^+$ from the body. Patients with a serum [K$^+$] greater than 6.5 mEq/L or ECG signs suggestive of hyperkalemia should be treated emergently.[31]

Direct Antagonism of Hyperkalemic Effect on Cell Membrane Polarization

The intravenous (IV) infusion of calcium gluconate antagonizes the effects of hyperkalemia on the heart. This effect occurs within minutes and lasts 30 to 60 minutes. If a salutary effect is noted, repeat doses may be used. The recommended dose is 10 mL of 10% calcium gluconate or chloride. Extreme caution must be used in patients with

hyperkalemia and digitalis toxicity, because the administration of ionized calcium may potentiate the effects of digoxin on the conduction system.[32] Calcium should be avoided in the setting of digoxin toxicity. Finally, IV hypertonic saline (3%) has been shown to reverse the ECG changes of hyperkalemia in patients with concomitant hyponatremia.[33] This effect is likely due to direct action on the cardiac cells and has not been demonstrated to be effective in patients with normal or elevated serum sodium levels.

Movement of Extracellular K$^+$ Into the Intracellular Compartment

Administration of insulin shifts K$^+$ into cells; this effect occurs in 15 to 30 minutes and lasts approximately 2 to 4 hours.[34] The recommended dose is 10 units of regular insulin IV; dextrose (50 g) should be added to avoid hypoglycemia. This dose will decrease serum [K$^+$] by 0.5 to 1.5 mEq/L. Patients without IV access can be treated with inhaled β$_2$-adrenergic agonists such as albuterol. Albuterol drives K$^+$ into cells by increasing Na$^+$/K$^+$-ATPase activity. Albuterol (10 to 20 mg in 4 mL of saline by nasal inhalation over 10 minutes) can lower the serum [K$^+$] by 0.5 to 1.5 mEq/L.[35] Sodium bicarbonate is much less effective than either insulin or albuterol but may produce shifting of [K$^+$] into cells.[36] The use of sodium bicarbonate should be limited to situations in which it is indicated for the treatment of concurrent acidosis.

Removal of K$^+$ from the Body

Removal of K$^+$ is necessary to prevent a recurrence of hyperkalemia once the effects of the preceding measures have waned. Loop diuretics can be helpful in patients with sufficient renal function (dosing depends on medication and renal function); however, most often, other measures are needed. Sodium polystyrene sulfonate (Kayexalate) binds to K$^+$ secreted in the colon. Each gram of resin removes 0.5 to 1 mEq of K$^+$. The usual dose of Kayexalate is 15 to 30 g orally. Because the resin causes constipation, sorbitol (15 mL of a 70% solution) should be administered to induce osmotic diarrhea. If oral administration is not feasible, Kayexalate can be given as a retention enema consisting of 30 to 50 g of the resin in 70% sorbitol solution. It is important, however, that the enema be retained for at least 30 to 60 minutes to obtain the desired therapeutic effect. The effects of Kayexalate on serum [K$^+$] occur in 4 to 6 hours when the agent is given orally and in 1 to 2 hours when it is given as an enema. Serious side effects of Kayexalate and sorbitol include bowel necrosis and perforation. These complications seem to be more likely in severely immunocompromised patients or shortly after surgery.[37,38] Kayexalate should be avoided in these circumstances. Both peritoneal dialysis and hemodialysis are very effective in removing K$^+$ from the body. In acute cases when serum [K$^+$] needs to be corrected rapidly, hemodialysis is preferred. Hemodialysis can quickly remove 50 to 125 mEq of K$^+$ and should be used as definitive treatment when other treatments fail. Peritoneal dialysis is also effective in removing K$^+$ from the body, but its effects are slower than those achieved with hemodialysis or cation exchange resins. In addition to the implementation of rapid treatment, the causes of hyperkalemia should be sought and corrected, and offending drugs should be discontinued when possible. Table 14-2 summarizes the treatment for hyperkalemia.

Hypokalemia

Hypokalemia is more common than hyperkalemia and is defined as serum [K$^+$] less than 3.6 mEq/L. Hypokalemia usually occurs as a consequence of K$^+$ depletion due to either increased excretion or inadequate intake. Shifts in extracellular and intracellular [K$^+$] also can cause hypokalemia (Box 14-2). Low serum [K$^+$] reflects an imbalance of normal K$^+$ homeostasis, with one rare exception. In patients with leukemia and markedly elevated white cell count, K$^+$ can be taken up by the abnormal cells in the test tube and produce pseudohypokalemia.[39] However, as noted earlier, in vitro changes in [K$^+$] more commonly produce pseudohyperkalemia.

TABLE 14-2	Treatment of Hyperkalemia			
Treatment	**Mechanism**	**Dosage/ Comment**	**Onset**	**Duration**
Calcium	Cardiac cell stabilizer	10 mL of 10% solution (calcium gluconate or calcium chloride)	Seconds	30-60 min
Insulin (regular)	Shifts K⁺ into cells	10 U IV + glucose (50 g)	15-30 min	2-4 h
Albuterol	Shifts K⁺ into cells	10-20 mg by inhaler over 10 min	20-30 min	2-3 h
Sodium bicarbonate	Shifts K⁺ into cells	In cases of acidosis	Delayed	—
Kayexalate with sorbitol	Removes K⁺ from body	Oral: 15-30 g	4-6 h	—
		Retention enema: 30-50 g	1 h	—
Loop diuretics	Removes K⁺ from body	Intravenous, varies by drug and renal function	1 h	—
Hemodialysis	Removes K⁺ from body	Preferred over peritoneal dialysis in acute cases	15-30 min	—

Box 14-2

CAUSES OF HYPOKALEMIA

Increased Excretion
Diarrhea, laxative, or enema abuse
Renal losses:
  Diuretics (loop and thiazides)
  Metabolic alkalosis
  Osmotic diuresis (uncontrolled hyperglycemia)
  Nonreabsorbable anions
  Mineralocorticoid excess:
    Primary hyperaldosteronism
    Congenital adrenal hyperplasia
    Glucocorticoid-responsive aldosteronism
  Other causes:
    Liddle's disease
    Enzyme deficiencies
    Bartter's syndrome
    Magnesium depletion
    High-dose glucocorticoids

Shifts of K⁺ into Cells
Drugs:
  β-Adrenergic agonists
  Insulin
  Theophylline
  Caffeine
Delirium tremens
Hyperthyroidism
Familial hypokalemic periodic paralysis
Barium poisoning

In critically ill patients, increased losses are more commonly responsible for K⁺ depletion than is inadequate ingestion. The use of diuretics is the most common cause of hypokalemia in hospitalized patients. Both loop and thiazide diuretics cause increased delivery of Na⁺ and Cl⁻ to the collecting duct, promoting the secretion of K⁺ and causing hypokalemia. Diuretics are often used in high doses or administered by continuous infusion in critically ill patients, increasing the risk of hypokalemia. K⁺ losses can also occur from increased stool output. Because K⁺ is secreted into the colon, patients with high outputs from ileal or jejunal ostomies do not develop hypokalemia. Causes of upper gastrointestinal (GI) losses, such as vomiting or nasogastric suctioning, usually do not promote depletion of K⁺ directly. However, upper GI losses are associated with hypochloremia and metabolic alkalosis, both of which may cause increased renal K⁺ excretion, exacerbating the resultant hypokalemia. Large doses of laxatives or repeated enemas lead to excessive K⁺ losses and hypokalemia. Magnesium depletion and some forms of renal tubular acidosis (type 1 and some forms of type 2) can cause renal K⁺ wasting.[40] Other drugs also can lead to hypokalemia. For example, fludrocortisone and hydrocortisone increase K⁺ excretion. Aminoglycosides, amphotericin B, cisplatin, and foscarnet cause magnesium depletion and increased K renal losses.[41] Penicillin and its synthetic derivatives, when given IV, cause increased Na⁺ delivery to the distal nephron, promoting K⁺ secretion and potentially causing hypokalemia.[41] Alkalosis can cause movement of K⁺ into cells. This effect is seen with both metabolic and respiratory alkalosis and occurs as a consequence of hydrogen ions leaving the cell to minimize changes in extracellular pH, and K⁺ moving into the cells to maintain electroneutrality. The direct effects of alkalosis on serum [K⁺] are small, and the hypokalemia seen with metabolic alkalosis is more often caused by chloride losses producing increased delivery of Na⁺ to the distal nephron, which stimulates K⁺ losses. A number of β₂-adrenergic agonist drugs, including bronchodilators, decongestants, and tocolytics, can cause K⁺ shifts into cells and transient hypokalemia.[42] Theophylline stimulates cell membrane Na⁺/K⁺-ATPase and promotes K⁺ entry into cells; hypokalemia is commonly seen with theophylline toxicity.[43] Barium can block the exit of K⁺ from cells and cause hypokalemia.[44] Thyroid hormone can stimulate Na⁺/K⁺-ATPase, and hypokalemia is sometimes seen with hyperthyroidism. Increased endogenous β-adrenergic stimulation occurs with delirium tremens, producing intracellular movement of K⁺ and hypokalemia.[45] Familial hypokalemic periodic paralysis, a rare hereditary disease, is associated with a mutation in cell membrane calcium channels and causes episodes of severe hypokalemia triggered by high sodium intake or exercise.[46] These patients can present with severe muscle weakness and respiratory failure from hypoventilation.

CLINICAL EFFECTS

It is estimated that approximately 20% of hospitalized patients have a serum [K⁺] less than 3.6 mEq/L; most are asymptomatic. As discussed earlier, the consequences of changes in serum [K⁺] occur as a result of alterations in the resting membrane potential, making cardiac and neuromuscular cells the most susceptible targets. The most serious and potentially fatal effects of hypokalemia are related to disturbances in cardiac electrical activity that can lead to cardiac arrest. However, cardiac arrest caused by hypokalemia occurs almost exclusively in patients with underlying cardiac disease or patients taking digitalis.[47] Hypokalemia is also associated with characteristic ECG changes (see Table 14-1). Progressive decreases in serum [K⁺] produce broad, flat T waves; ST depression; and the appearance of U waves, QT interval prolongation, and finally ventricular arrhythmias, leading to cardiac arrest.[26] When serum [K⁺] is less than 3.0 mEq/L, generalized weakness can develop. When serum [K⁺] decreases to less than 2.5 mEq/L, muscle necrosis and rhabdomyolysis can occur. With progression of hypokalemia, an ascending muscle paralysis develops, leading to respiratory failure and arrest.

TREATMENT

The immediate goal of treatment in hypokalemia is to prevent or correct cardiac electrical disturbances and serious neuromuscular weakness. The long-term goal of treatment is to achieve repletion of total body potassium to normal levels. Supplementation of [K⁺] is the principal treatment for hypokalemia and is achieved with the administration of potassium chloride or potassium phosphate. In general, plasma [K⁺] decreases by approximately 0.3 mEq/L for each 100 mEq decrease in total body K⁺. This relationship is more difficult to estimate when serum [K⁺] is less than 2 mEq/L.[42] K⁺ replacement should be given orally except when severe hypokalemia is associated with respiratory or cardiac instability, in which case the IV route is recommended. Intravenous administration of K⁺ should not exceed 20 mEq/h to minimize possible iatrogenic hyperkalemia. For infusion of K⁺, an infusion pump and continuous cardiac monitoring are mandatory. In the case of life-threatening arrhythmias due to severe hypokalemia, more rapid infusion into a central vein may be appropriate. In these rare circumstances, KCl should be diluted to 10 mEq per 100 mL of infusion fluid. In most cases, oral supplementation of K⁺ is preferred because this route is safer and produces a more gradual increase in serum [K⁺]. Because supplementation of K⁺ is usually not an emergency, it is best accomplished using moderate doses of KCl (20 to 40 mEq once or twice a day) over several days. Potassium phosphate is used when hypophosphatemia is also present (as in diabetic ketoacidosis); occasionally, potassium bicarbonate is used in the setting of metabolic acidosis and hypokalemia. However, for most cases of hypokalemia, KCl is the salt of choice for replacement of K⁺. Serum [K⁺] should be followed closely, especially when using IV or higher doses, to prevent the development of hyperkalemia. If magnesium levels are low, they should be corrected because hypomagnesemia promotes renal loss of K⁺, making correction of hypokalemia more difficult. Finally, prevention of further episodes should be addressed with proper K⁺ intake and supplementation in patients with a continuous cause for hypokalemia. Nurse-driven protocols for electrolyte (potassium) supplementation have been shown to be effective in preventing hypokalemia in patients admitted to the ICU.[48]

KEY POINTS

1. Hyperkalemia and hypokalemia are common electrolyte abnormalities found in ICU patients. Timely recognition and intervention are essential to prevent cardiovascular complications.

2. Hyperkalemia can cause severe cardiovascular manifestations. These are often preceded by progressive ECG changes such as peaking of T waves, loss of P waves, widening of the QRS complex, sine wave, and ventricular fibrillation.

3. Patients with hyperkalemia and ECG changes should receive calcium gluconate or chloride emergently to stabilize cardiac cell membranes. The recommended dose is 10 mL of 10% solution, which may be repeated as necessary.

4. Insulin and β-agonists are effective treatments to shift K⁺ into cells; this effect usually lasts 2 to 4 hours. Sodium bicarbonate is less effective and should be reserved for patients with an indication for its use in treating acidosis.

5. Removal of K⁺ from the body can be accomplished by the use of loop diuretics, sodium polystyrene sulfonate (Kayexalate), and dialysis. Hemodialysis is the definitive treatment for acute hyperkalemia not responsive to other measures.

6. Hypokalemia can cause muscular weakness and cardiac complications. Typical ECG changes caused by hypokalemia include: flattening of T wave, ST depression, QT interval prolongation, appearance of U waves, and various types of ventricular arrhythmias.

7. Treatment of hyperkalemia is based on administration of K⁺ with chloride- or phosphate-based salts. Correction of the underlying cause for hypokalemia is also essential.

8. Intravenous administration of K⁺ should be reserved for patients with severe hypokalemia and significant cardiovascular or neuromuscular complications. Intravenous administration of K⁺ requires continuous ECG monitoring and utilization of an infusion pump.

ANNOTATED REFERENCES

Weisberg LS, Weisberg LS. Management of severe hyperkalemia. Crit Care Med 2008;36: 3246-51.
Provides a practical review of the options for management of hyperkalemia in critically ill patients.
Buckley MS, Leblanc JM, Cawley MJ. Electrolyte disturbances associated with commonly prescribed medications in the intensive care unit. Crit Care Med 2010;38(Suppl):S253-64.
A recent article providing a comprehensive review of the spectrum of electrolyte disorders caused by commonly utilized drugs in the intensive care unit.
Adrogue HJ, Madias NE. Changes in plasma potassium concentration during acute acid-base disturbances. Am J Med 1981;71:456-67.
Classic paper that describes in detail the relationship of serum potassium concentrations to acute acid-base disturbances. The authors illustrate the complicated nature of serum potassium concentration and acidosis, refuting the concept that acidosis produces hyperkalemia.
Montague BT, Ouellette JR, Buller GK. Retrospective review of frequency of ECG changes in hyperkalemia. Clin J Am Soc Nephrol 2008;3:324-30.
A retrospective study describing the spectrum of electrocardiogram (ECG) changes seen in patients with hyperkalemia and demonstrating the poor sensitivity and specificity of ECG changes in relation to hyperkalemia. The authors suggest that management of hyperkalemia should be guided more by the clinical scenario and serial potassium measurements than by ECG changes.

REFERENCES

Access the complete reference list online at http://www.expertconsult.com.

Hypophosphatemia and Hyperphosphatemia

COLIN BAUER | ANAHAT DHILLON

Phosphate Homeostasis

Derangements in the metabolism of phosphate are common in the intensive care unit (ICU) and can be clinically significant. Phosphate serves a number of crucial functions. It is an essential component of the main energy "currency" of the cell, adenosine triphosphate; it is a component of phospholipids in cell membranes; it is a component of hydroxyapatite, the structural matrix of bone; and it serves as a buffer against acid-base derangements.

An important distinction must be made between low serum phosphate concentration, referred to as *hypophosphatemia*, and low total body phosphorus stores, referred to as *phosphate depletion*. Serum phosphate may not reflect total body phosphorus stores because: (1) the vast majority of total body phosphorus is in the form of hydroxyapatite; (2) phosphate is primarily intracellular, and extracellular phosphate accounts for only a small fraction of total body phosphorus stores; and (3) shifts between the intracellular and extracellular compartments occur. There is no common laboratory test to accurately measure total body phosphate stores.

Phosphate homeostasis is a function of bone metabolism, intestinal absorption, and kidney resorption. Bone metabolism is linked to calcium homeostasis. In the setting of hypocalcemia, increased parathyroid hormone levels cause phosphate and calcium to be released from the bone. Intestinal absorption of phosphate occurs in the small bowel, primarily in the jejunum. Vitamin D, produced by the kidney in increased amounts when serum phosphate levels are low, increases the intestinal absorption of both calcium and phosphate. Phosphate in the circulation is filtered by the kidneys, but most of the phosphate in the glomerular filtrate undergoes resorption in the proximal tubule. Parathyroid hormone increases phosphate excretion by inhibiting phosphate resorption in the kidney; resorption increases in the setting of phosphate deficiency. Newer research on phosphate homeostasis has focused on fibroblast growth factor 23 and klotho, which may result in new therapeutics for phosphate imbalances.[1]

Hypophosphatemia

Hypophosphatemia is typically classified as mild (serum phosphate concentration 2.5-3 mg/dL), moderate (1-2.5 mg/dL), or severe (<1 mg/dL). Although mild to moderate hypophosphatemia is often subclinical, severe hypophosphatemia can be associated with significant morbidity. All-cause mortality in patients with serum phosphate concentrations less than 1 mg/dL is as high as 30%.[2]

Common causes of hypophosphatemia are summarized in Table 15-1. Respiratory alkalosis (of any cause) can induce transcellular shifts of phosphate and cause hypophosphatemia. Renal losses of phosphate occur with osmotic diuresis or excessive diuretic therapy. Therapies instituted in the ICU, including overly aggressive renal replacement therapy[3] and erythropoietin therapy,[4] can increase the risk of hypophosphatemia. Hyperparathyroidism (either primary or secondary) causes hypophosphatemia by decreasing urinary resorption of phosphate. Proximal renal tubular disorders also can impair phosphate resorption and cause hypophosphatemia. Total body phosphate depletion also occurs in extreme catabolic states such as burns or sepsis.

Hypophosphatemia should be anticipated when nutritional support is initiated in chronically malnourished patients, such as those with a long history of alcohol abuse or elderly patients with oropharyngeal dysphagia,[5] who may already have low phosphate levels and are in a catabolic state. A carbohydrate load administered in the setting of chronic malnutrition rapidly switches the body to anabolism and causes a spike in insulin release. High circulating insulin levels promote cellular uptake of phosphate and can induce a precipitous decrease in serum phosphate concentration. This phenomenon has been termed the *refeeding syndrome*.[6] Profound hypophosphatemia in the refeeding syndrome can produce severe clinical manifestations including death. Concurrent hypokalemia and hypomagnesemia are common. In chronically malnourished patients, the refeeding syndrome can be avoided by cautiously ramping up nutritional support (especially administration of carbohydrates), careful monitoring of serum phosphorus levels, and appropriate phosphate supplementation when indicated.[6]

Patients with diabetic ketoacidosis often have phosphate depletion because hyperglycemia induces increased urinary losses of phosphate via osmotic diuresis. The serum phosphate concentration may be normal in the initial phase of therapy because severe acidosis causes a shift of phosphate into the extracellular space from the intracellular compartment. As acidosis is corrected, however, phosphate shifts back into the intracellular compartment, leading to a precipitous decrease in serum phosphate concentration.[7] Although common, the clinical significance of moderate hypophosphatemia in diabetic ketoacidosis is unclear. Therapy for hypophosphatemia in diabetic ketoacidosis is typically warranted only if the serum phosphate level is less than 1.0 mg/dL or if hypophosphatemia is associated with clinical manifestations such as central nervous system (CNS) or left ventricular (LV) dysfunction.[7]

Clinical manifestations due to hypophosphatemia are rare unless the serum phosphate concentration is below 1 mg/dL. The clinical findings are summarized in Table 15-2. Diffuse skeletal muscle weakness can be profound. Respiratory failure secondary to diaphragmatic weakness can occur.[8-10] Respiratory failure can be primary, or it can manifest as inability to liberate the patient from mechanical ventilation. CNS dysfunction can include confusion, lethargy, and gait disturbances. Hematologic manifestations, including acute hemolytic anemia and leukocyte dysfunction (impaired phagocytosis and chemotaxis), have been reported. Cardiovascular manifestations can include acute LV dysfunction and development of reversible dilated cardiomyopathy that typically responds only to phosphate repletion. Rhabdomyolysis also can occur.[11]

Hypophosphatemia also can cause disorders of oxygen transport. Profound hypophosphatemia can impair oxygen delivery to the tissues because of decreased production of 2,3-diphosphoglycerate, a key molecule found in erythrocytes that facilitates the release of oxygen from hemoglobin (hb). Decreased intracellular levels of 2,3-diphosphoglycerate cause a leftward shift of the oxyhemoglobin dissociation curve.

Because phosphate serves as a buffer against acid-base derangements, hypophosphatemia influences the interpretation of acid-base status. Phosphate and proteins (albumin) are measured anions. Unmeasured anions are accounted for in acid-base interpretation by calculation of the anion gap. Although there is no true "normal" value

TABLE 15-1	Common Causes of Hypophosphatemia

Transcellular shift:
    Refeeding syndrome
    Respiratory alkalosis
    Insulin administration
Renal losses:
    Diuretic therapy
    Osmotic diuresis
    Hyperparathyroidism (primary or secondary)
    Proximal renal tubular dysfunction:
        Fanconi syndrome
Insufficient intestinal absorption:
    Malnutrition
    Phosphate-binding antacids
    Vitamin D deficiency
    Chronic diarrhea
    Nasogastric suctioning
    Malabsorption syndromes
Extreme catabolic states:
    Burns
    Trauma
    Sepsis

TABLE 15-2	Clinical Manifestations of Severe Hypophosphatemia

Respiratory:
    Acute respiratory failure
    Ventilator dependence
Musculoskeletal:
    Muscle weakness
    Rhabdomyolysis
    Bone demineralization
Hematologic:
    Hemolysis
    Disorders of leukocyte phagocytosis or chemotaxis
Neurologic:
    Altered mental status
    Gait disturbance
    Paresthesias
Cardiovascular:
    Cardiomyopathy
    Decreased inotropy

for the anion gap, the value is typically lower for a patient with low measurable anions (i.e., either hypophosphatemia or hypoalbuminemia, or both). Therefore, the presence of a "normal" value for the calculated anion gap in the setting of profound hypophosphatemia can actually represent the presence of unmeasured anions (i.e., the presence of a wide anion gap). As a rule, the expected anion gap (in mEq/L) equals twice the serum albumin concentration (in g/dL) plus half the serum phosphate concentration (in mM/L). Thus, a patient with hypophosphatemia and hypoalbuminemia can have significant levels of unmeasured anions even if the measured anion gap is less than the commonly used threshold of 10 to 12.

Severe hypophosphatemia (phosphate concentration <1 mg/dL) mandates intravenous (IV) phosphate replacement. Phosphate should not be administered by the IV route to patients with renal failure; it should also be avoided in patients with hypercalcemia, because metastatic calcification can occur. For moderate hypophosphatemia (phosphate concentration 1-2.5 mg/dL), oral supplementation is adequate for patients who are able to take medications by mouth or via an enteral feeding tube. It is impossible to accurately predict the exact amount of phosphate supplementation required to replenish phosphate stores because most phosphate is intracellular.

TABLE 15-3	Common Causes of Hyperphosphatemia

Renal:
    Acute or chronic renal failure
    Increased renal resorption:
        Hypoparathyroidism
        Thyrotoxicosis
Cellular injury:
    Rhabdomyolysis
    Tumor lysis syndrome
    Hemolysis
Medication related:
    Abuse of phosphate-containing laxatives
    Excessive (iatrogenic) phosphate administration
    Bisphosphonate therapy

Hyperphosphatemia

Hyperphosphatemia is defined as a serum phosphate level above 4.5 mg/dL; it may be clinically significant at levels over 5 mg/dL. Causes of hyperphosphatemia are summarized in Table 15-3. The most common cause of hyperphosphatemia is renal failure. Renal insufficiency causes hyperphosphatemia because phosphate excretion by the kidneys is impaired; however, the serum phosphate level is usually normal until the creatinine clearance is less than 30 mL/min. Any insult causing extensive cell damage, including rhabdomyolysis, hemolysis, or tumor lysis syndrome,[12] can release phosphorus into the extracellular space. Hyperphosphatemia has been reported in patients using some bisphosphonate medications; the phosphate increase is due to decreased renal phosphate clearance.[13] There are numerous reports in the literature about hyperphosphatemia in patients using phosphate-containing laxatives or bowel preparations.[14]

The most frequent clinical findings in acute hyperphosphatemia are signs and symptoms of hypocalcemia. Hyperphosphatemia produces hypocalcemia by three mechanisms: (1) precipitation of calcium (formation of calcium-phosphorus complexes), (2) interference with parathyroid hormone–mediated resorption of bone, and (3) decreased vitamin D levels.[15] Clinical signs and symptoms of hypocalcemia such as muscle cramping, tetany, hyperreflexia, and seizures, as well as cardiovascular manifestations, can be evident.

Management of acute hyperphosphatemia includes limiting phosphate intake and enhancing urinary phosphate excretion. In the absence of end-stage renal disease, phosphate excretion can be optimized with saline infusion (volume diuresis) and diuretic administration. Diuretics that work in the proximal tubule (e.g., acetazolamide) are especially effective for enhancing phosphate excretion. Any patient with life-threatening hyperphosphatemia should be considered for dialysis.

Oral phosphate binders decrease the absorption of phosphate in the gut and are a mainstay for preventing and treating hyperphosphatemia in patients with chronic renal failure. Calcium and aluminum salts are widely used. However, calcium salts can produce hypercalcemia and metastatic calcification from a high calcium-phosphorus ($Ca \times PO_4$) product, and aluminum salts can be toxic. For patients requiring renal replacement therapy, chronic management of hyperphosphatemia with calcium-free phosphate binders (e.g., sevelamer hydrochloride [Renagel]) may reduce long-term mortality by preventing cardiovascular complications associated with a high $Ca \times PO_4$ product.[16] It should be noted that these investigations have been observational in nature, and to date, data are lacking to convincingly show that normalization of phosphate in chronic hyperphosphatemia decreases morbidity of chronic kidney disease. Sevelamer is highly effective for increasing fecal elimination of phosphate without producing hypercalcemia or aluminum toxicity.[17] In the acute management of patients with hyperphosphatemia accompanied by hypocalcemia, the likelihood (and clinical significance) of metastatic calcification with acute calcium administration is unclear.

ANNOTATED REFERNCES

Razzaque MS, Beate L. The emerging role of the fibroblast growth factor-23-Klotho axis in renal regulation of phosphate homeostasis: endocrine regulation of phosphate homeostasis. Nat Rev Endocrinol 2009;5(11):611-9.

A review of the role of fibroblast growth factor and Klotho in regulating phosphate homeostasis and how abnormal regulation may lead to pathology. The authors summarize experimental results that explain mechanisms of action of these endocrine factors. While this research is in its relative infancy, it gives readers a good understanding of newer regulatory factors they may not have studied previously.

The RENAL Replacement Therapy Study Investigators. Intensity of continuous renal-replacement therapy in critically ill patients. N Engl J Med 2009;361(17):1627-38.

A multicenter randomized trial to assess whether higher intensity of continuous renal replacement therapy would decrease all-cause mortality at 90 days. The study found no difference in the primary outcome of mortality, but did note significantly increased incidence of hypophosphatemia (65.1% versus 54%, P <

0.0001) in intensive renal replacement therapy. The study excluded patients who were already on hemodialysis for end-stage renal disease.

Fuentebella J, Kerner JA. Refeeding syndrome. Pediatr Clin North Am 2009;56(5):1201-10.

A recent review of the refeeding syndrome including risk factors, clinical management, and strategies to prevent it from occurring. Topics reviewed include the pathophysiology of starvation as well as the changes in metabolism that are responsible for the refeeding syndrome. It includes guidelines for replacement of potassium, magnesium, phosphate, and thiamine.

Knochel JP. Hypophosphatemia. West J Med 1981;134(1):15-26.

A comprehensive review of the clinical findings associated with hypophosphatemia, as well as mechanisms of pathophysiology. The paper is comprehensive in its scope, but does recognize areas of limited knowledge at the time of writing. More recent reviews focus on individual aspects of hypophosphatemia, without the broad overview of the pathophysiology presented in this article.

REFERENCES

Access the complete reference list online at http://www.expertconsult.com.

16

Hypomagnesemia

MOUSTAFA HASSAN | **ROBERT N. COONEY**

Magnesium is an important ion that participates in over 300 enzymatic reactions, especially those involving adenosine triphosphate (ATP) as a cofactor. Hypomagnesemia is common in critically ill patients and associated with increased mortality.[1] This chapter provides a brief overview of magnesium physiology and homeostasis, as well as potential etiologies, signs, and symptoms of magnesium deficiency and guidelines for treating hypomagnesemia in critically ill patients.

Cellular Physiology and Metabolism of Magnesium

Magnesium is a divalent cation (Mg^{++}) that is predominantly localized to the intracellular compartment (99%). It is the second most abundant intracellular cation after potassium and plays an important role in cellular metabolism and homeostasis. At the cellular level, Mg^{++} influences membrane function by regulating ion transport; Mg^{++} is required for sodium/potassium–adenosine triphosphatase (Na^+/K^+-ATPase) activity, which maintains transmembrane gradients for Na^+ and K^+.[2,3] Magnesium also regulates intracellular calcium (Ca^{++}) flux by competing for Ca^{++} binding sites and influencing intracellular Ca^{++} transport.[2,3] It is an essential cofactor for most ATP-requiring processes. Magnesium acts by neutralizing the negative charge on the phosphate anion of ATP to facilitate enzyme binding and hydrolysis of the phosphate moiety. Intracellular Mg^{++} is required for numerous critical biochemical processes, including DNA synthesis, activation of gene transcription, initiation of protein synthesis, and regulation of energy metabolism via glycolytic and tricarboxylic acid cycles.[2-5]

Total body magnesium (21-28 g) is distributed in bone (53%), muscle (27%), soft tissue (19%), and blood (0.8%).[2] The normal concentration of total magnesium in serum is 1.5 to 2.3 mg/dL. Approximately 19% of circulating magnesium is bound to protein (predominantly albumin), whereas 14% is complexed to serum anions (citrate, phosphate, and bicarbonate). The majority in serum exists in ionized form (67%), which represents the physiologically active species.[2,6] Consequently, measurements of total serum magnesium may not accurately reflect the relative abundance of circulating Mg^{++}.[1,2]

Magnesium homeostasis is maintained by the small intestine, kidney, and bone.[2,7] Average dietary intake is approximately 300 mg per day. Normally, only one-third of dietary Mg^{++} is absorbed.[7,8] However, intestinal Mg^{++} uptake may increase to compensate for dietary or total body Mg^{++} deficiency.[2,7,8] Unlike calcium, there are no hormonal mechanisms for regulating Mg^{++}. Consequently, normal renal filtration and reabsorption of Mg^{++} represent important regulatory mechanisms for Mg^{++} homeostasis.[2,7] Non–protein bound Mg^{++} is filtered by the glomerulus. Under normal conditions, up to 95% of filtered Mg^{++} is reabsorbed in either the proximal tubule (35%) or in the thick ascending loop of Henle (60%). Mg^{++} reabsorption in the loop of Henle is linked to sodium chloride (NaCl) transport and inversely related to flow. Consequently, diuretic use and other conditions associated with increased tubular flow result in decreased Mg^{++} reabsorption.[2,7] Under conditions of persistent Mg^{++} deficiency, mobilization of Mg^{++} from bone also represents a potential homeostatic mechanism.[2]

Prevalence and Etiology of Hypomagnesemia in Patients in the Intensive Care Unit

The reported prevalence of hypomagnesemia in adult intensive care unit (ICU) admissions ranges from 15 to 60, depending on whether total or ionized magnesium is measured.[1,9] A recent study identified severe ionized hypomagnesemia most commonly following liver transplantation and in patients with severe sepsis.[1] Magnesium deficiency in critically ill patients may be caused by inadequate Mg^{++} intake, increased renal or gastrointestinal (GI) losses, acute intracellular shifts of Mg^{++}, and other medical conditions (e.g., burn injury, massive blood transfusion, or cardiopulmonary bypass [CPB]). Increased renal losses of Mg^{++} are associated with alcohol abuse, diabetes, acute tubular necrosis (ATN), diuretics, aminoglycosides, amphotericin, cyclosporin, cisplatin, digoxin, and other medications.[1,2,7,10] Vomiting, diarrhea, nasogastric tube losses, and pancreatitis are associated with increased GI losses of Mg^{++}.[1,2,7,11] Acute intracellular shifts caused by refeeding with glucose or amino acids, insulin, catecholamines, or metabolic acidosis also may result in hypomagnesemia.[1,2,7,11] Hypoalbuminemia is associated with reductions in total Mg^{++} in plasma, but the ionized fraction may remain normal. The use of continuous renal replacement therapy causes significant loss of Mg^{++}, requiring more replacement than what is commonly prescribed in standard parenteral nutrition formulas.[12]

Critically ill patients are at increased risk for hypomagnesemia, and its development is associated with an increased risk of mortality.[1] Although the cause and effect of this association are unclear, the clinical effects of hypomagnesemia are significant from cardiovascular, metabolic, and neuromuscular standpoints.

Clinical Signs and Symptoms of Hypomagnesemia

Hypomagnesemia is frequently asymptomatic in critically ill patients and commonly identified through routine laboratory studies or when hypomagnesemia is clinically suspected.[7,9,10] However, the relationship between systemic and cytoplasmic hypomagnesemia is unclear, and whether changes in enzymatic function caused by cytoplasmic hypomagnesemia can subsequently lead to clinically significant problems is unknown. Hypomagnesemia is most commonly seen in conjunction with hypokalemia, hypocalcemia, and other electrolyte abnormalities. Consequently, determining the clinical consequences of isolated hypomagnesemia has been difficult. In most instances, symptoms were attributed to Mg^{++} deficiency only after other electrolyte abnormalities had been corrected.[2,7,9,10] As summarized in Table 16-1, the clinical sequelae of Mg^{++} deficiency are most commonly related to cardiovascular, metabolic, and neuromuscular systems.

Hypomagnesemia is associated with electrocardiogram (ECG) changes similar to those found in hypokalemia: flattened T-waves, U-waves, and prolonged QT interval. Magnesium is a cofactor for Na^+/K^+-ATPase in cardiac tissue.[2,7,9,10] Reductions in intracellular K^+ result in cellular depolarization and can lower the threshold for generation of an action potential as well as decrease the time for repolarization. Consequently, hypomagnesemia is associated with both atrial (premature atrial contractions, atrial fibrillation, multifocal atrial tachycardia), digoxin-related, and ventricular (ventricular tachycardia, torsades

TABLE 16-1	Clinical Signs and Symptoms of Magnesium Deficiency		
Cardiovascular	*Metabolic*	*Neurologic*	*Neuromuscular*
Atrial fibrillation, flutter	Hypokalemia	Seizures	Chvostek sign
Ventricular tachycardia, esp. torsades de pointes	Hypocalcemia	Nystagmus	Muscle cramps
Supraventricular tachycardia	Hypophosphatemia	Delirium	Carpopedal spasm
ECG changes (↑ PR, wide QRS, ↑ QT)	Insulin resistance	Coma	Muscle weakness
Hypertension		Athetoid movements	Muscle fasciculations
Risk of digitalis toxicity			

ECG, Electrocardiogram.

de pointes) dysryhthmias.[7,9,10] Magnesium is recommended as the initial therapy for torsades de pointes and as an adjunctive treatment for refractory ventricular dysrhythmias.[2,7,9,10] Magnesium administration during acute myocardial infarction was associated with reduced mortality in the second Leicester Intravenous Magnesium Intervention Trial (LIMIT-2).[11] Based on that study, there is some evidence that Mg[++] may be beneficial if given prior to coronary reperfusion.[13]

Hypomagnesemia is commonly associated with both hypokalemia and hypocalcemia.[7] These associations are related in part to the fact that medications and homeostatic changes that affect magnesium handling often affect K[+] handling as well. In addition, renal losses of potassium are increased under hypomagnesemic conditions and are refractory to supplementation unless the magnesium is replaced first.[2,7] A somewhat similar condition exists for hypocalcemia in that hypomagnesemia suppresses parathyroid hormone release and activity.[14] Consequently, hypocalcemia is refractory to Ca[++] replacement unless Mg[++] is replaced as well.[2,7]

Magnesium can have a depressant effect on the nervous system through its ability to cause presynaptic inhibition.[2,7,10] It may also depress the seizure threshold by its ability to competitively inhibit N-methyl-D-aspartate receptors.[2,7,9,10] The neurologic and neuromuscular manifestations of hypomagnesemia include coma, seizures, weakness, and signs of muscular irritability. Hypomagnesemic patients may have a positive Chvostek sign even when ionized calcium concentration is normal; they may develop nystagmus, tetany, or seizures

followed by rhabdomyolysis.[2,7,9,10] Serum Mg[++] deficit was also found to correlate with the severity of traumatic brain injury.[15] Consequently, Mg[++] replacement is indicated in this setting and is also commonly used in pregnant patients with preeclampsia (blood pressure >140/90 mm Hg with proteinuria) or eclampsia (associated seizures).[9,10]

Magnesium replacement has been used to treat bronchospasm in patients with asthma.[9,10] The proposed mechanism of action for the therapeutic benefit of Mg[++] in bronchospasm involves its relaxant effects on smooth muscle. Several studies have shown improved forced expiratory volume in the first second of expansion (FEV$_1$) following intravenous (IV) magnesium administration or improved peak flow rates with nebulized magnesium, while others have not.[10] Consequently, additional studies will be needed to adequately define the role of Mg[++] in patients with asthma.

Treatment of Hypomagnesemia

The initial step in managing hypomagnesemia is to identify and eliminate factors contributing to the development of Mg[++] deficiency. This may involve interventions to minimize GI losses or reevaluating the need for medications that cause renal Mg[++] wasting (e.g., aminoglycosides, diuretics). The severity of hypomagnesemia, urgency of clinical symptoms (e.g., dysrhythmias, muscle cramps), associated electrolyte abnormalities (K[+] and Ca[++]), and renal function should be assessed prior to initiating Mg[++] therapy.

In general, IV administration of Mg[++] is preferred in symptomatic critically ill patients. However, caution must be used with Mg[++] replacement when renal dysfunction is present, since severe hypermagnesemia may result. Current recommendations for Mg[++] replacement therapies are of somewhat limited value owing to the lack of adequately controlled studies. Magnesium may be administered IV as MgSO$_4$ (1 gm = 4 mmol) or MgCl$_2$ (1 gm = 4.5 mmol) and orally as magnesium gluconate (500 mg = 1.2 mmol) or magnesium oxide (400 mg = 6 mmol). When IV Mg[++] replacement is used, a bolus followed by continuous infusion or infusion alone are preferred, since renal filtration and excretion may limit Mg[++] retention. For torsades de pointes, 1 to 2 gm of IV MgSO$_4$ over 5 minutes is recommended. For urgent treatment of hypomagnesemia, an IV bolus of 8 to 12 mmol of Mg[++] (2-3 g MgSO$_4$) followed by an infusion of 40 mmol Mg[++] (10 g MgSO$_4$) over the next 5 hours should be considered. For routine treatment of hypomagnesemia, an infusion of 40 mmol Mg[++] can be given over a 24-hour period. For outpatients on diuretics with chronic Mg[++] losses, oral therapy with 2 to 3 gm (12-24 mmol) of magnesium per day is recommended; magnesium oxide is preferred because it is more easily absorbed than other formulations.

ANNOTATED REFERENCES

Soliman HM, Mercan D, Lobo SM, Melot C, Vincent JL. Development of ionized hypomagnesemia is associated with higher mortality rates. Crit Care Med 2003;31(4):1082-7.
A classic study demonstrating increased mortality in ICU patients with ionized hypomagnesemia.
Noronha JL, Matuschak GM. Magnesium in critical illness: metabolism, assessment, and treatment. Intensive Care Med 2002;28(6):667-79.
A comprehensive review summarizing the metabolic and physiologic roles of magnesium as well as its homeostasis.
Woods KI, Fletcher S, Roffe C, et al. Intravenous magnesium sulfate in suspected acute myocardial infarction: results of the second Leicester Intravenous Magnesium Intervention Trial. Lancet 1992;339(8809): 1553-8.

A landmark study demonstrating decreased mortality in patients with suspected acute myocardial infarction receiving magnesium supplementation.
Klein CJ, Moser-Veillon PB, Schweitzer A, et al. Magnesium, calcium, zinc and nitrogen loss in trauma patients during continuous renal replacement therapy. JPEN J Parenter Enteral Nutr 2002; 26(2):77-92.
This study examines magnesium losses in critically ill trauma patients requiring renal replacement therapy.

REFERENCES

Access the complete reference list online at http://www.expertconsult.com.

17

Hypercalcemia and Hypocalcemia

MOUSTAFA HASSAN | ROBERT N. COONEY

Abnormal serum calcium concentration is a common finding in critically ill patients. The prevalence of hypocalcemia in intensive care unit (ICU) patients ranges from 70% to 90% when total serum calcium is used and from 15% to 50% when ionized calcium is measured.[1] Hypercalcemia occurs less frequently, with a reported incidence of less than 15% in critically ill patients.[2] Hypocalcemia is associated with injury severity and mortality in critically ill patients,[1,3-5] but whether low serum calcium concentration is protective, harmful, or simply prognostic in critical illness is unclear. Therefore, in most instances, the management of hypocalcemia involves treating the underlying medical condition(s), except when patients are symptomatic or hemodynamically unstable. This chapter provides a brief overview of calcium physiology, the regulation of serum calcium concentration, potential etiologies and symptoms of hypocalcemia, conditions associated with hypocalcemia, and guidelines for treating hypo- and hypercalcemia in critically ill patients.

Calcium Physiology and Metabolism

Calcium is a divalent ion (Ca^{2+}) involved in critical biological processes like muscle contraction, blood coagulation, neuronal conduction, hormone secretion, and the activity of various enzymes.[3-5] Therefore, it is not surprising that intra- and extracellular calcium levels, like pH, are tightly regulated. A normal adult contains approximately 1 to 2 kg of total body calcium, which is located primarily in bone (99%) as hydroxyapatite.[1,3,5] Skeletal stores of calcium represent an unlimited reservoir that is regulated predominantly by extracellular Ca^{2+} concentration, parathyroid hormone (PTH), and calcitonin. Extracellular concentrations of Ca^{2+} are typically 10,000 times greater than cytoplasmic Ca^{2+} levels.[1,3] Similarly, the majority of intracellular calcium (>90%) is found in subcellular organelles (mitochondria, microsomes, endoplasmic or sarcoplasmic reticulum) as opposed to the cytoplasmic compartment. Ca^{2+}-mediated cell signaling involves rapid changes in cytoplasmic Ca^{2+} concentration, owing to release of the cation from both internal and external stores.[6,7] Cytoplasmic Ca^{2+} influx occurs through the cell membranes by receptor-activated, G protein–linked channels and the release of internal Ca^{2+} from endoplasmic or sarcoplasmic reticulum (ER/SR) by second messengers.[6] The efflux of cytoplasmic Ca^{2+} involves transport of Ca^{2+} across the cell membrane and into the ER/SR via specific transporters.[6-8] These tightly controlled pulsations of cytoplasmic Ca^{2+} thus regulate signal strength and frequency for calcium-mediated cellular functions. Alterations in Ca^{2+} signaling have been identified in muscle, hepatocytes, neutrophils, and T lymphocytes during sepsis and may contribute to the development of organ dysfunction during catabolic illnesses (for review see Ref. 7).

Extracellular calcium homeostasis is maintained by the coordinated actions of the gastrointestinal tract, kidneys, and bone.[1,3] Levels of extracellular Ca^{2+} are detected by calcium-sensing receptors on parathyroid cells.[8] In response to low serum Ca^{2+} concentration, the parathyroid gland secretes PTH, which reduces renal reabsorption of phosphate, increases renal calcium reabsorption, and stimulates renal hydroxylation of vitamin D.[1,3] PTH and 1,25-dihydroxy vitamin D (calcitriol) promote the release of calcium from bone by activating osteoclasts.[1,3] Calcitriol also stimulates intestinal absorption of dietary calcium and regulates PTH secretion by inhibiting PTH gene transcription. PTH secretion is also influenced by serum phosphate concentration, which stimulates PTH secretion by lowering extracellular Ca^{2+} concentration. Magnesium is required for the release of PTH from parathyroid cells and may explain the development of hypocalcemia in patients with magnesium deficiency. Calcitonin is a calcium-regulating hormone secreted by the parafollicular C cells of the parathyroid gland during hypercalcemia. Although calcitonin inhibits bone resorption and stimulates urinary excretion of calcium, its does not appear to play a major role calcium homeostasis in humans.[1,3]

The normal concentration of ionized calcium in the extracellular space (plasma and interstitium) is 1.2 mmol/L and represents 50% of the total extracellular calcium. The remaining 40% is bound to plasma proteins, and 10% is combined with citrate, phosphate, or other anions. Total serum calcium normally ranges from 9.4 to 10.0 mg/dL (2.4 mmol). The distribution of ionized and bound calcium may be altered in critically ill patients. Chelating substances like citrate and phosphate may influence the abundance of ionized Ca^{2+}. An increase in free fatty acids caused by lipolysis or parenteral nutrition results in increased binding of calcium to albumin.[9] Protein-bound calcium is also increased during alkalosis and reduced during acidosis.[1,3] Correcting total serum calcium for albumin and pH does not accurately estimate ionized Ca^{2+} concentration.[10,11] Therefore, direct measurement of ionized serum calcium concentration is more accurate and is the recommended assay when caring for critically ill patients.[12]

Hypocalcemia in Critically Ill Patients

Ionized hypocalcemia is frequently seen in critically ill patients with sepsis, acute pancreatitis, severe traumatic injuries, or following major surgery. The incidence of ionized hypocalcemia in ICU patients ranges from 15% to 50%.[3] The degree of hypocalcemia correlates with illness severity as measured by the APACHE II score (Acute Physiology and Chronic Health Evaluation) and is associated with increased mortality in critically ill patients.[4] In particular, the degree of systemic inflammation as measured by circulating cytokine (e.g., tumor necrosis factor [TNF]) or procalcitonin levels appears to correlate with the severity of hypocalcemia in ICU patients.[11] Potential etiologies for the hypocalcemia of critical illness include impaired PTH secretion or action, vitamin D deficiency or resistance, calcium sequestration or chelation, or impaired mobilization of Ca^{2+} from bone (Table 17-1).

Hypocalcemia in the ICU is rarely caused by primary hypoparathyroidism. However, sepsis and systemic inflammatory response syndrome (SIRS) are commonly associated with hypocalcemia, which is caused in part by impaired secretion and action of PTH and failure to synthesize calcitriol.[1,3,11] Hypomagnesemia may contribute to hypocalcemia during critical illness via inhibitory effects on PTH secretion and target organ responsiveness,[1,3,5] but the presence of hypomagnesemia only weakly correlates with hypocalcemia in ICU patients.[4]

In many instances, the hypocalcemia of critical illness is multifactorial in etiology. Elderly patients are at increased risk for vitamin D deficiency due to malnutrition, poor absorption, and hepatic or renal dysfunction.[3] Renal failure may precipitate hypocalcemia via decreased formation of calcitriol. Renal failure also can be associated with hyperphosphatemia, and phosphate anion can chelate ionized calcium.[1,3] The use of continuous renal replacement therapy in critically ill patients is associated with significant magnesium and calcium losses. These losses of divalent cations result in electrolyte replacement requirements that commonly exceed the calcium and magnesium supplementation provided in standard parenteral nutrition formulas.[13]

TABLE
17-1 **Causes of Hypocalcemia**

Impaired Parathyroid Hormone Secretion or Action

Primary hypoparathyroidism
Secondary hypoparathyroidism

Impaired Vitamin D Synthesis or Action

Poor intake
Malabsorption
Liver disease
Renal disease
Hypomagnesemia
Sepsis

Calcium Chelation/Precipitation

Hyperphosphatemia
Citrate
Pancreatitis
Rhabdomyolysis
Ethylene glycol

Decreased Bone Turnover

Hypothyroidism
Calcitonin
Cis-platinum
Diphosphonates
Mithramycin
Phosphates

Data from Zaloga GP. Hypocalcemia in critically ill patients. Crit Care Med. 1992;20(2):251-262.

Other potential causes of ionized hypocalcemia in critically ill patients include alkalosis (increased binding of Ca^{2+} to albumin), medications (anticonvulsants, antibiotics, diphosphonates, and radiocontrast agents), massive blood transfusion, sepsis, and pancreatitis.[1,3-5] More recently, propofol—particularly when given in large doses—has been shown to reduce circulating calcium concentrations by elevating serum PTH levels, but the physiologic significance of this pharmacologic side effect is unclear.[14]

Ionized hypocalcemia (<1.0 mmol/L) is associated with prehospital hypotension and represents a better predictor of mortality in severely injured patients than base deficit.[15] The exact reasons for the strong association between ionized hypocalcemia and mortality are unclear but potentially relate to head injury and/or the presence of hemorrhagic shock. Injured patients receiving blood transfusions may develop hypocalcemia as a consequence of Ca^{2+} chelation by citrate, which is used as an anticoagulant in banked blood.[16-18] The incidence of transfusion-related hypocalcemia is related to both the rate and volume of blood transfusion.[16,17] When blood transfusions are administered at a rate of 30 mL/kg/h (2 L/h in a 70-kg patient) and hemodynamic stability is maintained, ionized Ca^{2+} levels are preserved by physiologic compensatory mechanisms.[18] Transient hypocalcemia may be observed with rapid transfusion and can be prolonged or exacerbated by hypothermia as well as renal or hepatic failure.[16-18] Consequently, ionized calcium should be monitored and replaced when clinically indicated during massive transfusion.

Hypocalcemia in Sepsis and Pancreatitis

Hypocalcemia is especially common in critically ill patients with systemic infection and pancreatitis.[1,3,4,7,11] Animal models of sepsis demonstrate reductions in serum calcium concentration following endotoxin infusion.[7,11,19,20] When septic patients with hypocalcemia were compared with nonseptic controls, increased TNF and interleukin (IL)-6 levels correlated with ionized hypocalcemia.[21] Septic patients with hypocalcemia may demonstrate increased or decreased PTH levels, but urinary excretion of calcium and bone resorption appear to be preserved when compared to controls.[11,19] Procalcitonin levels appear to be increased during sepsis-induced hypocalcemia, but

mature calcitonin only exerts a weak and transient effect on calcium levels.[21,22] Collectively, the results suggest that hypocalcemia during severe infection is multifactorial in etiology but that inflammatory cytokines, impaired activation of vitamin D, and elevated procalcitonin levels are contributory.

It remains unclear whether sepsis-induced hypocalcemia is pathologic or protective. Calcium administration in experimental sepsis has been shown to increase or have no effect on mortality.[19,20] In fact, a recent Cochrane review found no evidence that parenteral calcium supplementation influences the outcome of critically ill patients.[23] Similarly, investigations of the effects of Ca^{2+} blockade on septic mortality demonstrate conflicting results.[21-24] Therefore, although sepsis-induced hypocalcemia is commonly seen in critically ill patients, neither routine replacement of calcium nor the use of calcium channel blockers are supported by the existing literature. As with most situations, sepsis-induced hypocalcemia should be treated if patients are symptomatic.

Pancreatitis represents another inflammatory condition associated with hypocalcemia in critically ill patients.[1,3,24,25] Saponification of retroperitoneal fat contributes to the development of hypocalcemia in this patient population.[3,24,25] In experimental pancreatitis, injection of free fatty acids into the peritoneum induced hypocalcemia in rats.[24] However, the amount of calcium chelated is relatively small compared to available calcium stores for exchange from the bone reservoir. Interestingly, elevated levels of PTH seen in pancreatitis, like sepsis, do not result in normalized ionized calcium levels.[24-26] Resistance of bone and kidney to PTH may be a factor, but it is likely that inflammatory pathways identical to those in sepsis are responsible. In pancreatitis, as in sepsis, hypocalcemia is an indicator of disease severity. As with most clinical conditions, calcium replacement during pancreatitis should be reserved for the symptomatic or hemodynamically unstable patient.

Signs and Symptoms of Hypocalcemia

Hypocalcemia is frequently asymptomatic, and attributable signs or symptoms may be difficult to elucidate in critically ill patients. In general, the signs and symptoms of hypocalcemia correlate with both the magnitude and rapidity of onset of the condition. Neurologic (paresthesias, seizures, dementia) and cardiovascular (hypotension, impaired cardiac contractility, dysrhythmias) signs may be seen with ionized hypocalcemia (Ca^{2+} <1.0 mmol/L).[3,5] Neuromuscular symptoms of hypocalcemia include muscle spasms and tetany when severe. Psychiatric disturbances (dementia, psychosis, depression) also may be due to hypocalcemia.[3,5]

Classic signs of hypocalcemia include the Chvostek and Trousseau signs, which test for latent tetany. The Chvostek sign is an involuntary twitching of facial muscles in response to light tapping of the facial nerve. It is nonspecific, present in 10% to 25% of normal adults, and may be completely absent in chronic hypocalcemia. Trousseau sign is carpopedal spasm induced by reduced blood flow to the hand in the presence of hypocalcemia; it is elicited by inflating a blood pressure (BP) cuff to a level 20 mm Hg higher than the systolic BP for 3 minutes. Trousseau sign is also nonspecific and may be absent in a third of patients with hypocalcemia.

Cardiac dysrhythmias such as ventricular tachycardia, prolonged QT interval, and heart block are more serious complications of hypocalcemia.[3,5] In addition, decreased cardiac output and hypotension, especially where refractory to inotropic agents and/or intravascular volume loading, should prompt calcium replacement when hypocalcemia is present.[3,5]

Treatment of Hypocalcemia

Critical thresholds for calcium replacement vary, but severe ionized hypocalcemia below 0.8 mmol/L and symptomatic hypocalcemia should be treated in critically ill patients.[1,3,5] Calcium treatment of asymptomatic ionized hypocalcemia above 0.8 mmol/L is usually unnecessary and potentially may be harmful in conditions like sepsis and cellular hypoxia.[1,3,5,26]

Treatment of hypocalcemia requires intravenous calcium replacement. The two solutions most commonly used are 10% calcium chloride and 10% calcium gluconate. Each solution contains 100 mg/mL of calcium salt and is provided in 10-mL ampules. 10% calcium chloride contains 27 mg of elemental calcium (1.36 mEq)/mL; 10% calcium gluconate contains 9 mg (0.46 mEq)/mL. Typically, 10 mL of 10% calcium gluconate solution is infused over 10 minutes. A total of 200 mg of elemental calcium may be necessary to raise the total serum calcium by 1 mg/dL. Since the effect of calcium infusion is usually brief, a continuous infusion may be necessary. Calcium chloride should not be infused peripherally if calcium gluconate is available, since the former can produce tissue necrosis and thrombophlebitis if extravasation occurs.

Hemodynamically unstable patients in the ICU who are hypocalcemic may show a transient increase in BP and/or cardiac output with calcium administration. This is probably due to increased cardiac performance.[26] However, in the presence of tissue hypoxia, calcium administration may aggravate the cellular injury.[9,22] Nonetheless, calcium administration is probably warranted in hypocalcemic, hemodynamically unstable patients, especially those requiring adrenergic support.

Hypercalcemia

Hypercalcemia is rare in critically ill patients, estimated to be present in between 1% and 15% of ICU patients.[2] Defined as an increase in serum calcium concentration to above 10.4 mg/dL (2.60 mmol/L), hypercalcemia usually is caused by excessive bone resorption. Hyperparathyroidism and humoral hypercalcemia of malignancy are the most common causes of hypercalcemia in hospitalized patients.[2,5,27] Less common causes of hypercalcemia include sarcoidosis, prolonged immobilization, and medications like thiazide diuretics.

Mild hypercalcemia is usually asymptomatic. However, patients with circulating Ca^{2+} levels above 12 mg/dL may manifest symptoms of confusion, delirium, psychosis, and coma.[2,5,27] Patients with hypercalcemia may also experience nausea, vomiting, constipation, abdominal pain, and ileus. Cardiovascular effects of hypercalcemia include hypotension, hypovolemia, and shortened QT interval. Profound skeletal muscle weakness may result. Seizures, however, are rare.

Treatment of hypercalcemia should be directed at the underlying medical condition. Saline infusion and diuresis is indicated in symptomatic patients and when the serum calcium level rises above 14 mg/dL (3.5 mmol/L). For patients with underlying malignancy, treatment with salmon calcitonin, pamidronate, or plicamycin may be necessary. These agents act to inhibit bone resorption. Hydrocortisone can also be used in combination with calcitonin to treat hypercalcemia associated with multiple myeloma.

ANNOTATED REFERENCES

Zaloga GP. Hypocalcemia in critically ill patients. Crit Care Med 1992;20(2):251-62.
Classic reference on the hypocalcemia of critical illness.
Berridge MJ, Bootman MD, Roderick HL. Calcium signaling: dynamics, homeostasis and remodeling. Nat Rev Mol Cell Biol 2003;4(7):517-29.
Excellent review of intracellular calcium signaling and homeostasis.
Sayeed MM. Signaling mechanisms of altered calcium responses in trauma, burn, and sepsis: role of Ca^{2+}. Arch Surg 2000;135(12):1432-42.
Summary of alterations in cellular calcium regulation and signaling during systemic inflammation.
Hofer AM, Brown EM. Extracellular calcium sensing and signaling. Nat Rev Mol Cell Biol 2003;4(7):530-8.
Overview of extracellular calcium sensing and signaling.

Zaloga GP. Ionized hypocalcemia during sepsis. Crit Care Med 2000;28(1):266-8.
Thoughtful review of physiology and clinical significance of hypocalcemia during sepsis.
Denlinger JK, Nahrwold ML, Gibbs PS, Lecky JH. Hypocalcemia during rapid blood transfusion in anaesthetized man. Br J Anaesth 1976;48(10):995-1000.
Classic study on blood transfusion and hypocalcemia.
Hotchkiss RS, Karl IE. Calcium: a regulator of the inflammatory response in endotoxemia and sepsis. New Horiz 1996;4(1):58-71.
A well-written review of calcium dyshomeostasis during sepsis.

REFERENCES

Access the complete reference list online at http://www.expertconsult.com.

Hypoglycemia

DIETER MESOTTEN | GREET VAN DEN BERGHE

Hypoglycemia is the most common endocrine emergency, the most frequent complication of insulin-requiring diabetes, and the principal factor limiting optimization of glycemic control in patients with diabetes mellitus and/or critical illness. When unrecognized and not treated appropriately, significant morbidity—including permanent neurologic deficits and death—may ensue.

The American Diabetes Association Workgroup on Hypoglycemia set the alert level for hypoglycemia at plasma glucose concentrations ≤70 mg/dL (3.9 mmol/L) in patients with diabetes mellitus. When the plasma glucose concentration is less than this threshold value, actions should be undertaken to prevent clinical/symptomatic hypoglycemia.[1] Clinical/symptomatic hypoglycemia is characterized by the Whipple triad: (1) symptoms of hypoglycemia, (2) simultaneous low blood glucose concentration, and (3) relief of symptoms with the administration of glucose. These symptoms may be neurogenic/autonomic or neuroglycopenic (Table 18-1). Symptoms of hypoglycemia are similar in type 1 and type 2 diabetes.[2] Elderly patients report fewer neurogenic/autonomic symptoms.[3] They and all other patients with "hypoglycemia unawareness" have a sevenfold increased risk of severe hypoglycemia. Episodes of hypoglycemia in these patients tend to be recurrent and unpredictable.[4] "Hypoglycemia unawareness" is the loss of autonomic warning symptoms of developing hypoglycemia. Likely pathogenic mechanisms for hypoglycemia unawareness include recurrent exposure to hypoglycemia, leading to increases in brain glucose uptake and possibly reduced β-adrenergic sensitivity.[5] Fortunately, scrupulous avoidance of hypoglycemia for a period of weeks to months restores hypoglycemia awareness.[6,7]

In critically ill patients, however, sedation strongly masks symptoms, so one can only rely on frequent and accurate blood glucose measurements to detect hypoglycemia. The most commonly used definition of hypoglycemia during critical illness is a plasma glucose concentration below 40 mg/dL (2.2 mmol/L) in the absence of symptoms.[8-10] Most reflectance blood glucose meters in home and hospital use have poor precision at low levels of blood glucose.[11] Capillary blood glucose testing may not be sufficiently reliable to guide management of blood glucose levels in critically ill patients.[12] The use of arterial blood samples for glucose measurements is recommended. However, anemia in critically ill patients can result in falsely elevated blood glucose measurements and mask hypoglycemia when using these blood glucose meters. Also, the recently developed continuous interstitial glucose monitoring system[13] and the noninvasive GlucoWatch Biographer[14] are less effective at detecting low blood glucose levels and can have a delayed response to low blood glucose concentrations. Therefore, for diabetes patients, the laboratory measurement of a low plasma glucose concentration in the presence of appropriate symptoms remains the most reliable way to diagnose severe hypoglycemia. In the ICU, measurements of arterial blood glucose concentration using modern blood gas analyzers approach the accuracy of conventional laboratory methods.[8,12]

Specific characteristics of the patient can also determine whether hypoglycemia will be symptomatic or increase the risk of hypoglycemia. For example, a precipitous fall from hyperglycemia to euglycemia in a patient with diabetes can produce hypoglycemic symptoms.[15] In contrast, hypoglycemia with glucose levels as low as 30 mg/dL (1.7 mmol/L) can occur asymptomatically during fasting in normal women and during pregnancy.[16] Some ICU patient populations, such as those with liver or renal failure and septic shock, are at higher risk

for hypoglycemia.[17] The characteristics of the hypoglycemia itself (absolute level, duration) and its treatment (avoiding overcorrection) also play a significant role (Table 18-2).

Incidence of Severe Hypoglycemia

A retrospective study of adults requiring hospitalization indicated that 0.4% of acute medical admissions per year are hypoglycemia related.[18] Severe hypoglycemia (i.e., with symptoms severe enough to require assistance) occurs commonly in patients with type 1 diabetes.[19] In type 2 diabetes, even with intensive therapy, the risk is probably 100-fold less. Over 6 years of observation in the United Kingdom Prospective Diabetes Study, severe hypoglycemia was reported in 2.4% of patients treated with metformin, 3.3% of those treated with a sulfonylurea, and 11.2% of those treated with insulin.[20] As insulin usage among patients with type 2 diabetes increases, it is inevitable that severe hypoglycemia will become more common in daily practice.

With the introduction of tight blood glucose control during ICU stay,[8] the incidence of blood glucose values below 40 mg/dL (2.2 mmol/L) has been reported to range from 5.1% to 18.7% of patients, depending on the targeted level of blood glucose control and the patient population under study.[8,9] With the use of accurate glycemia measurement methodologies and algorithms that advise frequent blood glucose measurements (i.e., every 1–4 hours), the incidence and impact of these brief episodes of hypoglycemia should be minimized.[17]

Physiologic Barriers Against Hypoglycemia

The central nervous system (CNS) relies primarily on glucose for the generation of cellular energy. Cells in the CNS have endogenous glucose reserves that are sufficient for only minutes if the supply of glucose from the bloodstream is inadequate. In addition, neurons are unable to synthesize glucose. Finally, the brain cannot use fuels other than glucose during acute hypoglycemia.[21] Hence, when the brain is acutely deprived of glucose, serious neurologic dysfunction occurs. Accordingly, the body has several mechanisms to maintain the plasma glucose concentration within the narrow range of 60 to 140 mg/dL (3.3–7.7 mmol/L) in both the fed and fasting states. When glucose use exceeds glucose production, the brain senses decreasing blood glucose levels and activates counterregulatory pathways.[22] The glucose threshold for activation of these mechanisms is approximately 67 mg/dL (3.6 mmol/L), but this setpoint can be altered by recent hyperglycemia or antecedent hypoglycemia. As glucose levels decline, the first counterregulatory mechanism activated is the suppression of endogenous insulin secretion.[23] Next in the hierarchy of responses is the release of two hormones, glucagon and epinephrine, that antagonize the action of insulin. These hormones activate glycogenolysis and gluconeogenesis and stimulate fatty acid oxidation and protein breakdown to provide substrates for gluconeogenesis. With more severe or prolonged hypoglycemia (>3 hours), increases in growth hormone and cortisol release raise blood glucose levels.

The physiologic responses to hypoglycemia and the glucose threshold at which they occur can be modulated. In type 1 diabetes, the glucagon response to hypoglycemia is lost within 3 years after diagnosis, rendering patients dependent on epinephrine-mediated counterregulation and making them more vulnerable to prolonged episodes of severe hypoglycemia. Exposure to antecedent hypoglycemia diminishes the counterregulatory response to a subsequent episode. The brain adapts to antecedent hypoglycemia by increasing glucose uptake so that a more profound hypoglycemic stimulus is required to trigger sympathoadrenal activation and autonomic symptoms.[24] The level of glycemic control also affects counterregulatory thresholds. With strict glycemic control, epinephrine release is not triggered until a lower glucose level is reached.[25,26] Conversely, diabetic patients with poor glycemic control can experience hypoglycemic symptoms when the blood glucose concentration decreases to lower values within the normal or even hyperglycemic range.[27]

Sequelae

Although severe hypoglycemia induces marked cognitive dysfunction, most patients recover rapidly and completely. The effect of repeated severe hypoglycemia on cognitive function in adults is controversial.[28,29] Although focal neurologic symptoms secondary to severe hypoglycemia occur occasionally, severe and permanent cognitive impairment is usually the result of protracted hypoglycemia, often in association with excessive alcohol consumption. The neuronal regions that are particularly vulnerable to hypoglycemia are the cerebral cortex, the substantia nigra, the basal ganglia, and the hippocampus.

The long-term neurologic effects of hypoglycemia during critical illness are poorly delineated.[17] It appears that brief episodes of hypoglycemia do not cause severe acute brain damage. A recent nested case-control study using more sophisticated neurocognitive tests showed that hypoglycemia mildly aggravated critical illness–induced neurocognitive dysfunction, notably the visuospatial domain.[30] This association, however, could not be dissociated from an effect of hyperglycemia or of glucose variability, as the patients who experienced hypoglycemia were also those with more severe hyperglycemia and greater glucose variability.

The overall mortality from severe hypoglycemia is unknown. The mortality rate from alcohol-induced hypoglycemia may be as high as 10% in adults.[31] About 2% to 4% of deaths in patients with type 1 diabetes have been attributed to hypoglycemia. Severe hypoglycemia is the cause of unexpected overnight deaths in young diabetic patients.[32] It may be explained by the impairment of hormonal responses to hypoglycemia during sleep, resulting in sudden cardiac arrhythmias.

The association of hypoglycemia and mortality during critical illness is very controversial.[33-35] Not only is hypoglycemia more frequent in the most severely ill patients (e.g., those with hepatic or renal failure or septic shock), these spontaneous hypoglycemic episodes also more strongly correlate with mortality risk than hypoglycemia induced by intensive insulin therapy. Nevertheless, as a quality-control measure, intensive insulin therapy in the ICU should be implemented with meticulous monitoring of the incidence of hypoglycemic episodes. The importance of careful monitoring of blood glucose concentration is further emphasized by the demonstration of a tight correlation between blood glucose variability and mortality.[36]

Differential Diagnosis

A clinical classification of hypoglycemic disorders separates patients who appear to be healthy (with or without coexistent disease) from those who appear to be ill (including those with a predisposing illness and those who are hospitalized). For otherwise healthy patients, the most important causes of fasting hypoglycemia are accidental or factitious drug ingestion and insulinoma. The differential diagnosis in ill or hospitalized patients includes predisposing illness, drug interactions, and other iatrogenic factors (Table 18-3).[37]

Insulin treatment of diabetes is the most common cause of hypoglycemia in adults. Risk factors for frequent severe hypoglycemia in type 1 diabetes include lower HbA_{1C} levels, higher daily insulin dose, longer duration of diabetes, absence of residual C peptide, hypoglycemia unawareness, and a prior history of severe hypoglycemia.[19] Insulin-treated type 2 diabetics are also vulnerable to severe hypoglycemia, especially if their disease is well controlled and they have been on insulin for many years.[2] Whether intensive insulin therapy increases

TABLE 18-1	Symptoms of Hypoglycemia	
Neurogenic		*Neuroglycopenic*
THE RESULT OF AN AUTONOMIC RESPONSE		THE RESULT OF BRAIN GLUCOSE DEPRIVATION
Blood glucose <55 mg/dL (3.7 mmol/L)		Blood glucose <45 mg/dL (2.5 mmol/L)
Cholinergic: hunger, sweating, paresthesias		Cognitive impairment Behavioral change
Adrenergic: tremor, palpitations, anxiety		Psychomotor abnormalities Seizure and coma

TABLE 18-2	Risk Factors Involved in Hypoglycemia	
Hypoglycemia		*Patient*
Level of hypoglycemia		Liver failure
Duration		Renal failure
(Over)correction of hypoglycemia		Sepsis or shock
Reperfusion damage		Prior history of diabetes mellitus

TABLE 18-3	Differential Diagnosis of Hypoglycemia			
	Increased Insulin Effect	*Hepatic Dysfunction*	*Decreased Substrate*	*Increased Glucose Consumption*
Drug/Toxin	Insulin overdose Sulfonylureas Rodenticide (Vacor) Pentamidine Quinine Angiotensin-converting enzyme inhibitors	Ethanol Nonselective β-blockers	Chronic renal insufficiency	Exercise
Fasting	Insulinoma Autoimmune disease Insulin-like growth factor II–secreting tumor	Congestive heart failure Septic shock Combined endocrine deficiencies	Uremia Severe wasting	Large tumors Prolonged exercise
Postprandial	Upper gastrointestinal surgery (e.g., Billroth II) Ethanol Noninsulinoma Pancreatogenous hypoglycemia	Unripe akee fruit *(Blighia sapida)* (hypoglycin)		

There are four pathophysiologic mechanisms capable of exceeding the body's counterregulatory capacity and causing severe hypoglycemia: (1) excessive insulin effect, (2) diffuse hepatic dysfunction, (3) limited substrate for gluconeogenesis, and rarely, (4) excessive glucose consumption. More than one mechanism can be operative in critically ill patients.

the incidence of severe hypoglycemia with sequelae is disputed.[38,39] Newer insulin analogs such as glargine and lispro, as well as continuous insulin delivery systems, may lessen the risk of fasting or postprandial severe hypoglycemia.[40,41]

Sulfonylureas are a common cause of severe hypoglycemia. The incidence is higher in the elderly, in patients with renal or liver insufficiency, and with the use of long-acting agents like glibenclamide.[42] Liver dysfunction prolongs the hypoglycemic activity of gliquidone and repaglinide. Renal insufficiency prolongs the activity of glyburide, chlorpropamide, and nateglinide.[43] A crude rate of serious hypoglycemia of 1.23 events per 100 person-years has been reported among elderly users of sulfonylureas.[44] Sulfonylurea-induced hypoglycemia can be prolonged (up to 27 days), and recurrences can occur after initial normalization of glucose levels.[45] Discovery of inadvertent or factitious sulfonylurea overdose can help avoid an exhaustive search for insulinoma in patients who present with hyperinsulinemic hypoglycemia.[46]

The metabolism of ethanol depletes hepatocellular levels of nicotinamide adenine dinucleotide, which is a cofactor critical for the entry of substrates into gluconeogenesis pathways.[47] Ethanol also inhibits cortisol and growth hormone responses and delays the epinephrine response to hypoglycemia.[48] However, ethanol does not inhibit glycogenolysis, so

ethanol-induced hypoglycemia does not occur until hepatic glycogen stores have been depleted (after 8–12 hours of fasting).[49] There is no correlation between blood ethanol levels (although alcohol is usually detected) and the degree of hypoglycemia. The incidence of alcohol-induced hypoglycemia is generally less than 1% in adults, but hypoglycemic coma is commonly related to ethanol ingestion.[50]

In the absence of a drug or toxic cause, adults with severe fasting hypoglycemia should be evaluated for insulinoma, insulin-secreting tumor of the islets of Langerhans,[51] or unusual causes such as excessive production of insulin-like growth factor II or rapid glucose consumption by tumors, diffuse hepatic dysfunction, septic shock, panhypopituitarism, polyglandular endocrine deficiency syndromes, and autoimmune hypoglycemia. The diagnosis of postprandial (reactive) hypoglycemia remains controversial.[52]

Evaluation

The first step in the evaluation of a patient with suspected hypoglycemia is documentation of low plasma glucose concentration in the presence of neuroglycopenic symptoms (Figure 18-1). Unless there is an obvious medication-related cause for severe hypoglycemia, blood should be drawn for the measurement of glucose, insulin, and C

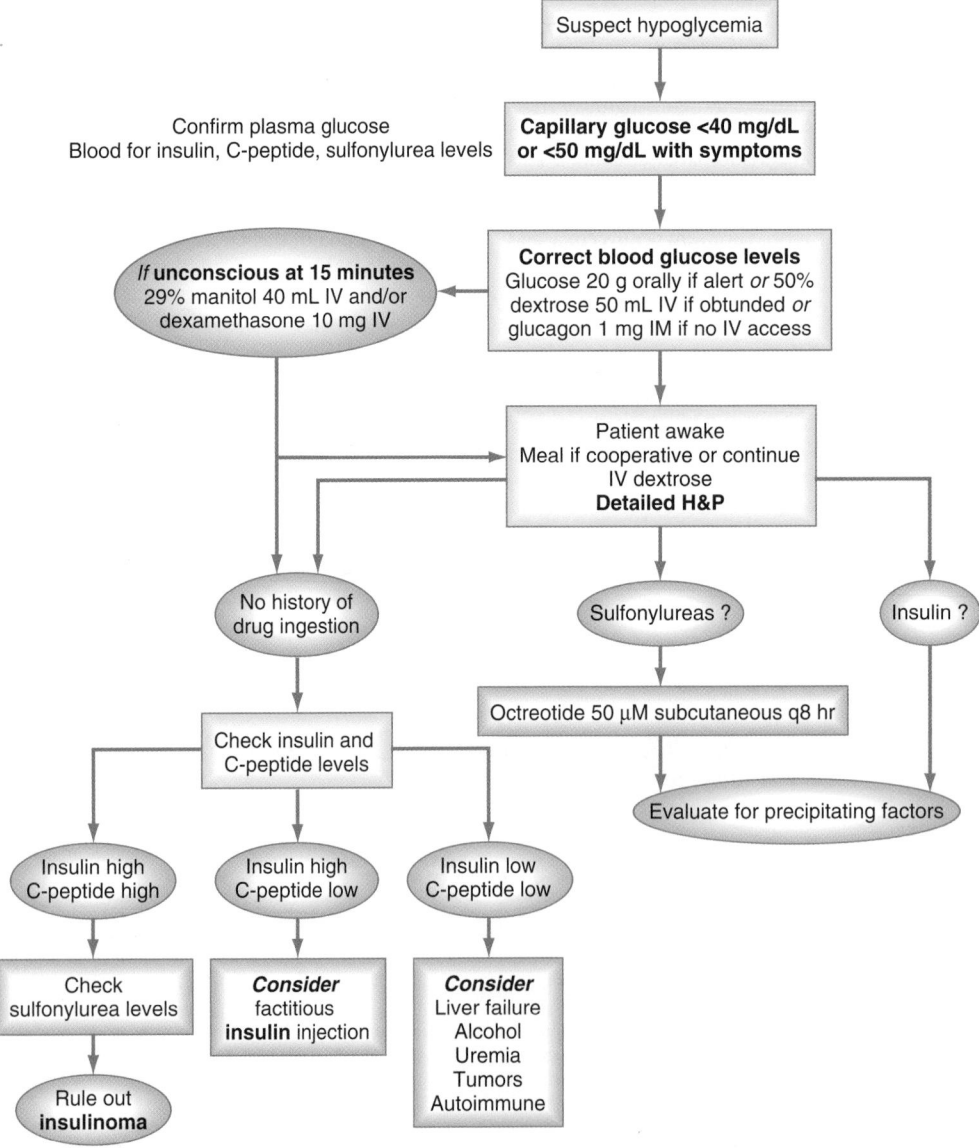

Figure 18-1 Decision tree for suspected hypoglycemia in adults.

peptide before the administration of glucose and, when indicated, for the workup of thyroid hormone and cortisol deficiency or uremia. In cases of fasting hypoglycemia, intentional, accidental, or surreptitious ingestion of glucose-lowering medications should be investigated to avoid the lengthy workup for insulinoma.[51] Sulfonylurea ingestion causes elevated insulin and C peptide levels, which mimics the findings associated with an insulinoma. Confirmation of the diagnosis of sulfonylurea ingestion can be made using high-pressure liquid chromatography or radioimmunoassay to detect sulfonylureas in blood or urine. The results of these tests are extremely important for further management.

Management

In all cases of suspected severe hypoglycemia, a patent airway and hemodynamic stability should be secured while a rapid bedside estimation of blood glucose concentration is performed. In cases of suspected overdose, emesis should not be induced in a hypoglycemic patient. When alcohol abuse is suspected, thiamine (100 mg IV or IM per day until the patient is consuming a complete diet) should be given to avoid acute Wernicke encephalopathy. Administration of glucose is the fundamental remedy. In awake patients with a protected airway, an initial oral dose of 20 g of glucose works. Examples of oral carbohydrates suitable for the correction of hypoglycemia are flavored glucose tablets and juices and sodas high in sugar content. A response should occur within 10 to 15 minutes and typically lasts 1 to 2 hours. Hence, a snack afterward is recommended to avoid recurrent hypoglycemia.

When patients are unwilling or unable to take oral carbohydrates, IV dextrose (glucose) should be given. The recommended initial dose of 50 mL of 50% dextrose provides 25 g dextrose; within 5 minutes, it produces a mean rise in blood glucose to 220 mg/dL (12.5 mmol/L) from nadir values as low as 20 mg/dL (1.1 mmol/L).[53] In ICU patients receiving insulin by continuous IV infusion and also receiving a baseline enteral or intravenous glucose load, a 10-g glucose bolus is usually sufficient to correct hypoglycemia, and the smaller glucose load avoids the need to greatly modify the insulin dosing regimen.[54] For prolonged hypoglycemia (e.g., caused by sulfonylurea overdose), prolonged dextrose infusion plus octreotide may be required.[55]

Parenteral glucagon directly stimulates hepatic glycogenolysis. Glucagon is effective in restoring consciousness if it is given soon after the onset of hypoglycemic coma. Glucagon is particularly effective in pancreatectomized patients but much less useful in type 2 diabetes, because it stimulates insulin secretion as well as glycogenolysis. Patients with depleted glycogen stores, such as those with alcohol-induced hypoglycemia, may not respond to glucagon. Adverse reactions to glucagon administration include nausea and vomiting, delaying carbohydrate ingestion.

In cases of sulfonylurea overdose, octreotide reverses hyperinsulinemia, reduces dextrose requirements, and prevents recurrent hypoglycemia.[55] The recommended dose of octreotide as an antidote for sulfonylurea overdose is 50 µg subcutaneously, repeated every 8 hours if necessary. Activated charcoal binds sulfonylureas and can be administered in cases of suspected overdose.

Cerebral edema can complicate severe hypoglycemia and should be suspected when unconsciousness lasts more than 30 minutes following normalization of blood glucose concentration. Treatment with IV mannitol (40 mL of a 20% solution) and glucocorticoids (10 mg of dexamethasone) in addition to IV dextrose is advised.

ANNOTATED REFERENCES

Cryer PE. The barrier of hypoglycemia in diabetes. Diabetes 2008;57(12):3169-76.
This paper gives a comprehensive overview of the incidence of hypoglycemia and the counterregulatory responses to it.

Diabetes Control and Complications Trial research group. Hypoglycemia in the Diabetes Control and Complications Trial. Diabetes 1997;46(2):271-86.
This paper reports on the incidence of hypoglycemia in a multicenter, randomized, controlled clinical trial (N = 1441) of intensive versus conventional diabetes therapy, with an average follow-up of 6.5 years.

Jacobson AM, Musen G, Ryan CM, et al. Long-term effect of diabetes and its treatment on cognitive function. N Engl J Med 2007;356(18):1842-52.
This paper reports on the long-term neurocognitive function of 1144 patients with type 1 diabetes as an 18-year follow-up of the DCCT study. Severe hypoglycemia appeared not to be worse than poor glycemic control for neurocognitive function.

Marks V, Teale JD. Drug-induced hypoglycemia. Endocrinol Metab Clin North Am 1999;28(3):555-77.
Therapeutically administered antidiabetic drugs—notably, insulin and sulfonylureas—are the most common causes of hypoglycemia in clinical practice. Nevertheless, an impressive list of other drugs can produce hypoglycemia, as discussed in this review paper.

Wang PH, Lau J, Chalmers TC. Meta-analysis of effects of intensive blood-glucose control on late complications of type 1 diabetes. Lancet 1993;341(8856):1306-9.
This paper reports the results of a meta-analysis of 16 randomized trials of intensive therapy to estimate its impact on the progression of diabetic retinopathy and nephropathy and the risk of severe hypoglycemia.

REFERENCES

Access the complete reference list online at http://www.expertconsult.com.

19

Anemia

FAHIM A. HABIB | CARL SCHULMAN | STEPHEN M. COHN

Anemia is a common clinical problem in critically ill patients. A large proportion of these patients are anemic on admission, and the majority of the remainder become anemic during their intensive care unit (ICU) stay. The likelihood of becoming anemic increases with the duration of stay in the ICU.

The traditional approach for the management of anemia in the ICU has been the administration of packed red blood cell (PRBC) transfusions. On average, about 40% of ICU patients are transfused (a mean of 5 units of PRBCs) in response to a mean pretransfusion hemoglobin (Hb) concentration of 8.5 g/dL.[1] Over the last decade, several studies have shown that PRBC transfusion is independently associated with worse clinical outcomes, independent of the degree of anemia or the severity of illness. Myriad complications resulting from PRBC transfusion are increasingly being recognized, and the scarcity of blood (expected annual shortfall of 4 million units by the year 2030[2]) and economic impact of PRBC transfusion (approximately $270 per unit transfused[3]) have prompted a paradigm change for managing anemia in the ICU.

Current approaches include recognition of absolute indications for PRBC transfusion, avoidance of transfusions based on "transfusion triggers" alone, prevention of anemia in critically ill patients, use of PRBCs that have been stored in the blood bank for shorter periods, and increasing acceptance of anemia. Many of these changes in approach are now evidence based.

Future directions focus on prevention of anemia, blood conservation, and the evaluation of blood substitutes.

Epidemiology

Anemia is defined as Hb level less than 13 g/dL for adult males and less than 12 g/dL for adult nonpregnant females.[4] Using this definition, more than 60% of all patients are anemic at admission, and the majority of those with normal Hb levels at admission become anemic while in the ICU.[5,6] Given enough time, virtually all patients will become anemic during their ICU stay. In the anemia and blood transfusion in critically ill patients study (the ABC trial), 63% of patients had Hb levels below 12 g/dL, and 29% had Hb levels below 10 g/dL.[5] Similarly, in the CRIT study, mean Hb level at baseline was 11 g/dL.[6]

The most frequent strategy for treatment of anemia is the transfusion of PRBC. As a consequence, more than 14 million units are transfused annually in the United States.[7] In patients with malignancy as their admission diagnosis, the prevalence and incidence of anemia are 68% and 47%, respectively.[8] Each day in the ICU increases the chance of being transfused by about 7%.[9]

Etiology

The etiology of anemia in the ICU is most often multifactorial, belonging to one or more of three major classes:
1. Hypoproliferative anemia due to marrow production defects
2. Ineffective erythropoiesis due to red cell maturation defects
3. Decreased survival of red cells secondary to blood loss, hemolysis, or both (Figure 19-1)

The most common causes of anemia include phlebotomy for diagnostic laboratory testing; acute hemorrhage due to trauma, gastrointestinal (GI) bleeding, or surgery—often exacerbated by the presence of coagulation abnormalities; treatment with chemotherapeutic agents; underlying chronic diseases such as renal and hepatic failure; reduced erythropoiesis; and shortened red cell survival.

Blood loss due to phlebotomy is an often unrecognized yet significant cause of anemia in the ICU, where patients are phlebotomized on average 4.6 times a day, with removal of 40 to 60 mL of blood daily.[5,6,10,11] The volume of blood removed varies with the test being ordered, but average volumes typically drawn are presented in Table 19-1. The presence of an arterial line further increases the phlebotomized blood volume.[11] Approximately half of all patients are transfused as a direct result of phlebotomy.[11]

Although rare since the advent of effective GI prophylaxis, GI bleeding can be a serious problem in the ICU. The overwhelming majority of critically ill patients demonstrate evidence of mucosal damage within the first 24 hours of admission. Overt anemia occurs in 5% of patients with stress-related GI bleeding, and clinically important bleeding necessitating transfusion is observed in 1% to 4% of critically ill patients.[12] Bleeding secondary to erosive gastritis is predominantly seen in patients on mechanical ventilation, patients with coagulopathy, patients with head injury, and/or patients receiving corticosteroids.[13]

Reduced erythropoietin production is a key feature of anemia of critical illness, a distinct clinical entity similar to anemia of chronic disease. This blunted erythropoietic response to low Hb concentration in the face of apparently adequate iron stores is due to a failure to produce appropriate levels of erythropoietin.[14,15] Blunted erythropoietin production in critically ill patients is probably mediated by proinflammatory cytokines such as tumor necrosis factor (TNF), interleukin (IL)-1, and IL-6, which down-regulate expression of the gene encoding erythropoietin.[16] IL-6 inhibits renal erythropoietin production.[17] Additional contributory effects of these proinflammatory cytokines include induction of a state of relative iron deficiency, vitamin deficiency, and altered iron metabolism in the bone marrow.[6,18] Anemia, therefore, is a result of both a blunted response to erythropoietin and abnormalities in iron metabolism.

Laboratory Evaluation of Anemia in the Intensive Care Unit

A comprehensive treatise on the evaluation of anemia is beyond the scope of this chapter. Discussion here is limited to pertinent iron studies that aid in the diagnosis of anemia of critical illness. A brief review of iron metabolism is essential to understanding the rationale behind the laboratory tests ordered.

Iron absorbed from food or released from stores circulates in plasma bound to transferrin, the iron transport protein. This iron-transferrin complex interacts with a specific transferrin receptor protein on the surface of early erythroid cells. This complex is then internalized and the iron released intracellularly. Within the erythroid cells, iron in excess of that needed for Hb synthesis binds to the storage protein, apoferritin, forming ferritin. Iron in the ferritin pool can be released and reused in the iron metabolism pathway. The levels of ferritin in serum correlate with total body iron stores and are therefore a suitable laboratory estimate of iron stores.[19] During maturation of reticulocytes to erythrocytes, the cells lose all activities of the Hb-synthesizing system, including surface expression of the transferrin receptors, which are released into the circulation.[20] Levels of transferrin receptor protein in the circulation provide a quantitative measure of total erythropoiesis and can be used to measure the expansion of

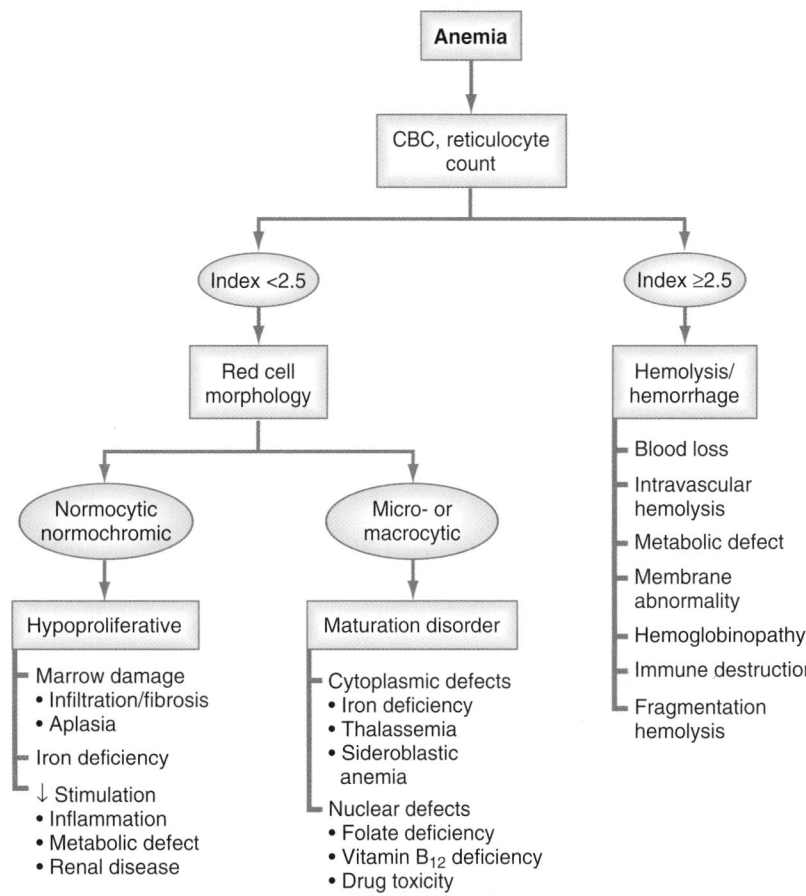

Figure 19-1 Physiologic Classification of Anemia.
CBC, complete blood count. (*Adapted from Fauci AS, Kasper DL, Braunwald E, et al, editors. The physiologic classification of anemia. In: Harrison's Principles of Internal Medicine, 17th ed., online: http://www.accessmedicine.com. Copyright © The McGraw-Hill Companies, Inc. All rights reserved.*)

the erythroid marrow in response to recombinant erythropoietin therapy. Serum iron levels represent the amount of circulating iron bound to transferrin. The total iron-binding capacity is an indirect measure of the circulating transferrin concentration.

Key tests necessary for establishing a diagnosis of anemia of critical illness include serum iron concentration, serum transferrin, transferrin receptor protein concentration, total iron-binding capacity, and serum ferritin concentration.

Anemia of critical illness is caused by impaired iron release, reduced production of erythropoietin, and a blunted response to erythropoietin, so this syndrome is characterized by a low serum iron concentration, low total iron-binding capacity, low transferrin saturation, normal transferrin-receptor protein levels, and a normal to high ferritin level. In contrast, iron-deficiency states are associated with transferrin saturation less than 18%. Consequently, critically ill patients may develop iron-deficiency anemia, anemia of chronic disease, or a combination of both.

Management

RED CELL TRANSFUSION

Transfusion of PRBCs remains the standard approach for the management of anemia in critically ill patients. Most transfusions are administered in response to a particular Hb level, the "transfusion trigger." Historically, transfusion was indicated for Hb concentrations below 10 g/dL. However, several considerations suggest a need to critically reevaluate this approach. First, scientific evidence suggests that most critically ill patients can safely tolerate lower Hb levels. Second, PRBC transfusions are associated with numerous potential complications. Third, blood is a scarce and costly resource that may not always be available,[21] hence its use must be limited to those most likely to benefit.

Finally, transfusions are associated with worse clinical outcomes. Transfusion of PRBCs must therefore be used for a physiologic indication and not in response to a transfusion trigger. The goals of these transfusions are to treat hemorrhage not responsive to fluid resuscitation and to correct hypoperfusion (as evidenced by blood lactate concentrations or base deficit measurements) not responsive to fluid resuscitation.

In recent years, evidence has begun to accumulate against the traditional liberal strategy of transfusion to achieve Hb concentration ≥10 g/dL. In the ABC trial, a prospective observational study of 3534 patients from 146 western European ICUs, 37% of all patients were transfused while in the ICU. The majority of transfusions were administered during the first week of ICU stay. Transfusion was more common in the elderly and in those with ICU stays longer than 1 week. Mortality, both in the ICU and overall, was significantly higher in the transfused group than for the group which avoided transfusion (18.5% versus 10.1%, $P<0.001$ for ICU death and 29.0% versus 14.9%, $P<0.001$ for overall mortality). The differences persisted even after the patients were matched for the degree of organ dysfunction.[5] In addition, transfused patients had longer lengths of stay and more severe degrees of

TABLE 19-1	Average Volumes of Blood Drawn for Diagnostic Testing[89]	
Arterial blood gas		2 mL
Chemistry		5 mL
Coagulation studies		4.5 mL
Complete blood counts		5 mL
Blood culture		10 mL
Drug levels		5 mL
Standard discard amount		2 mL

organ failure. The CRIT study was a prospective, multicenter, observational study of 284 ICUs in 213 hospitals in the United States. Overall, 44% of patients were transfused, most often within the first week of ICU admission; transfusion was independently associated with longer ICU and hospital stays and increased mortality.[6] Walsh and colleagues prospectively collected data on 1023 sequential admissions in 10 ICUs over 100 days in Scotland. Approximately 40% of patients were transfused, even with the application of evidence-based transfusion guidelines.[22] The multicenter trials group of the American Burn Association studied patients with ≥20% total body surface burns at 21 burn centers in the United States and Canada. Overall, they found that nearly 75% of patients were transfused during their hospital stay, receiving a mean of 14 units. The number of units transfused correlated significantly with the number of infections and mortality.[23] In a prospective observational study by the North Thames Blood Interest Group, 53% of patients were transfused for a mean pretransfusion Hb level of 8.5 g/dL. About two-thirds were transfused for low Hb levels and only 25% for hemorrhage. ICU mortality in the transfused patients was significantly higher than in the nontransfused patients (24.8% versus 17.7%, respectively).[24]

There is increasing recognition that anemia is well tolerated in critically ill patients. Much of clinical evidence in support of this approach comes from studies in Jehovah's Witness patients, who refuse to accept PRBC transfusions on religious grounds. Mortality increases significantly at Hb values below 5 g/dL, more so in individuals older than 50 years of age.[25] In conscious health volunteers, isovolemic dilution was performed to reduce the Hb concentration from 13.1 g/dL to 5 g/dL. Critical oxygen delivery was assessed by oxygen consumption, blood lactate concentration, and changes in the ST segment on the electrocardiogram. Oxygen consumption increased, but no increase in lactate concentration was found, suggesting that resting healthy humans can tolerate acute reductions in Hb to levels of 5 g/dL without the development of inadequate tissue perfusion.[26]

Clearly the risks of anemia must be balanced against the potentially deleterious effects of transfusion, especially since the efficacy of PRBC transfusions to augment oxygen delivery and the impact of this increase on tissue metabolism and clinical outcome remain unproven. In a recent meta-analysis, Marik and Corwin performed a systematic review of the literature and analyzed outcomes in 272,596 patients as reported in 45 studies. Blood transfusion was associated with an increased risk of death (pooled odds ratio 1.69, 95% confidence interval [CI] 1.46–1.92), increased risk of infectious complications (pooled odds ratio 2.5, 95% CI 1.52–2.44), and an increased risk of the development of acute respiratory distress syndrome (ARDS) (pooled odds ratio 1.88, 95% CI 1.66–3.34).[27]

The only absolute indication for PRBC transfusion is in the therapy of hemorrhagic shock.[28] However, only 20% of transfusions are used for this indication.

Most transfusions in the ICU are administered for the treatment of anemia. In the CRIT trial, over 90% of transfusions were given for this reason.[6] Perceived benefits of transfusion include increase in oxygen delivery to the tissues; increase in the cell mass and blood volume; alleviation of symptoms of anemia, including dyspnea, fatigue, and diminished exercise tolerance; and relief of cardiac effects. The optimal Hb concentration remains unknown and is likely influenced by the premorbid health status, disease process, and other unknown factors. Based on studies involving acute isovolemic reductions of blood Hb concentration, it has been demonstrated that reduction of the Hb concentration to levels of 5 g/dL does not produce evidence of inadequate systemic critical oxygen delivery as evidenced by blood lactate concentration[26]; significant cognitive changes were noted, however.[29] These effects were not seen when isovolemic dilution was performed to Hb levels of 7 g/dL. Clinical evidence of the validity of these findings is seen in the seminal Transfusion Requirements in Critical Care (TRICC) trial and has been instrumental in changing transfusion practices over the last decade.[30] In this study, 838 euvolemic critically ill patients with Hb levels less than 9 g/dL were enrolled. Of these, 418 patients were randomly assigned to a restrictive transfusion strategy,

where transfusion was provided if the Hb level fell below 7 g/dL, with a goal of maintaining circulating Hb concentration between 7 and 9 g/dL; and 420 patients were assigned to the liberal transfusion group and received transfusions for Hb levels of less than 10 g/dL, with transfusions provided to keep the Hb between 10 and 12 g/dL. Overall the 30-day mortality was similar between the two groups (18.7% versus 23.3%, $P=0.11$). However, a significantly lower mortality was seen with a restrictive transfusion strategy in those less severely ill who had APACHE II scores of ≤20 (8.7% versus 16.1%, $P=0.03$) and in those younger than 55 years of age (5.7% versus 13.0%, $P=0.02$). No difference in mortality was observed in those with stable, clinically significant cardiac disease (20.5% versus 22.9%, $P=0.69$). This strategy resulted in a 54% decrease in average number of units transfused and avoidance of transfusion in 33% of patients. Lowering of the transfusion threshold, therefore, is a simple and inexpensive strategy for improving outcome for critically ill patients. Caution must be used in applying this restrictive transfusion strategy to those patients with acute myocardial ischemia and unstable angina, as this group was excluded from the TRICC trial. Compensatory cardiac mechanisms in anemic patients include increases in blood flow during rest and a redistribution of blood away from the endocardium. In the presence of significant coronary artery disease, these adaptive changes are poorly tolerated, and anemic patients with myocardial infarction may have increased mortality.[31]

ADVERSE EFFECTS OF TRANSFUSION

A large proportion of ICU patients continue to receive PRBC transfusions for anemia, exposing them to serious risks, including transmission of infectious diseases, immune-mediated reactions (acute or delayed hemolytic reactions, febrile allergic reactions, anaphylaxis, and graft-versus-host disease), and non–immune related complications (fluid overload, hypothermia, electrolyte toxicity, and iron overload). Transfusion-related complications are encountered in approximately 4% of PRBC transfusions.[6] The risk of adverse outcomes increases incrementally with each unit of PRBCs transfused.[32,33] In an observational cohort study of 5814 patients undergoing coronary artery bypass grafting, each unit of PRBC transfused resulted in more than 100% odds of renal dysfunction, 79% odds for the need for mechanical ventilation for over 72 hours, 76% increase in odds for developing a serious postoperative infection, a 55% increase in odds for postoperative cardiac morbidity, and a 37% increase in odds for postoperative neurologic morbidity. Overall, there was a 73% increase in the odds of a major morbidity for each unit transfused (Table 19-2).[32]

With advances in screening and improvements in blood banking technology, transmission of infectious agents is less common. Current estimates of the risk of infection per unit of blood are approximately 1 in 2 million for human immunodeficiency virus (HIV), 1 in 1 million for hepatitis C virus, and 1 in 100,000 for hepatitis B virus.[34] The most common transfusion-related infections are secondary to bacterial contamination, which has an incidence of 12.6 events per 1 million units of allogeneic blood components transfused.[35] The risk of bacterial contamination is higher for PRBCs than for whole blood. Transfusion-related bacterial infections are most often caused by gram-positive organisms (e.g., staphylococcal spp., streptococcal spp., 58%) but also may be caused by gram-negative organisms (e.g., *Yersinia enterocolitica*, 32%). About 10% of these infections will result in a fatal outcome.[35] Increasing global travel has led to the emergence of infectious diseases not usually seen in the United States. Chagas disease, caused by *Trypanosoma cruzi*, is endemic in much of South and Central America. Immigrants from these endemic areas now form an increasing proportion of the blood donor pool. This issue is especially relevant in regions with high immigrant populations. In two such cities, Los Angeles and Miami, seropositive rates among donors were 1 in 7500 and 1 in 9000 and have been increasing.[36] Once acquired, the parasitemia persists long after acquisition of the infection.[37]

Major ABO mismatching is estimated to occur in 1 of 138,673 PRBC units transfused and results in 1 death per 2 million units transfused.[35]

TABLE 19-2	Potential Adverse Consequences Associated with Red Cell Transfusion[90]
Infectious Complications	
Human immunodeficiency virus infection	1 in 2.3 million
Human T-lymphotropic virus infection	1 in 2 million
Hepatitis C virus infection	1 in 1.8 million
Hepatitis B virus infection	1 in 350,000
Parvovirus B19 virus infection	1 in 10,000
Bacterial infections (*Staphylococcus*, streptococci, *Yersinia enterocolitica*, etc.)	1 in 250,000
Parasitic infections (Chagas disease)	1 in 29,000 donors seropositive
Noninfectious Complications	
Hemolytic transfusion reactions	1 in 10,000 to 1 in 50,000
Delayed hemolytic transfusion reaction	1 in 1500
Febrile nonhemolytic transfusion reactions	1 in 100 to 35 in 100
Major allergic reactions	1 in 20,000 to 1 in 50,000
ABO mismatching	1 in 14,000 to 1 in 38,000
Transfusion-related acute lung injury (TRALI)	1 in 5000
Transfusion-related immunomodulation (TRIM)	1 in 100
Transfusion-related immunomodulation (TRIM)	Observed once 2 blood volumes replaced
Transfusion-associated circulatory overload (TACO)	Observed after transfusion of 10 to 15 units
Coagulopathy	
Iron overload	
Hypothermia	
Hyperkalemia	
Thrombocytopenia	
Pulmonary hypertension	

Incompatibility also may result from antigens not routinely detected by current antibody assays. As a consequence, fatal acute hemolytic reactions still occur in 1 of every 250,000 to 1 million transfusions, and 1 patient per 1000 demonstrates the clinical manifestations of a delayed hemolytic transfusion reaction.[38]

Transfusion-related acute lung injury (TRALI) is a potentially serious pulmonary complication of transfusion. In severe cases, its clinical presentation is similar to that of the acute respiratory distress syndrome (ARDS).[39] Although initially described by Bernard in 1951[40] as noncardiogenic pulmonary edema related to transfusion, the term TRALI was coined by Papovsky et al.[41] TRALI presents with dyspnea and bilateral pulmonary edema during or within up to 6 hours of a transfusion, with no other risk factors to explain its development. It must be distinguished from pulmonary insufficiency due to circulatory overload, where the central venous pressure and pulmonary artery wedge pressure would be elevated. Hypoxemia, fever, hypotension, tachycardia, and cyanosis also may occur. Most often, symptoms appear within 1 or 2 hours following transfusion, but a delayed form with dyspnea appearing as late as 48 hours after transfusion has been reported. The chest x-ray shows bilateral infiltrates, which may progress and cause whiteout of the entire lung field. The criteria for clinical diagnosis of TRALI[42] include severe hypoxemia (with $Pao_2/Fio_2 < 300$ or O_2 saturation <90%), acute respiratory distress within 6 hours of a transfusion in the absence of evidence of circulatory overload, and x-ray evidence of bilateral pulmonary infiltrates. Differential diagnosis includes transfusion-associated circulatory overload, cardiac diseases, allergic and anaphylactic transfusion reactions, and bacterial contamination of the blood. Although the exact incidence is unknown, TRALI is estimated to occur in 1 of every 5000 transfusions[43] and has a mortality rate of 5% to 10%. Current evidence suggests two forms of TRALI: immune and nonimmune. Potential mediators include antileukocytic antibodies, products of lipid peroxidation, and other as yet unrecognized agents. The neutrophil is the key effector cell. Transfusions from multiparous female donors, owing to exposure to paternal leukocytes, are associated with the highest risk for the development of TRALI in the recipient.[44] Treatment is currently limited to supportive measures.

Transfusion-related immunomodulation (TRIM) results in an increased incidence of bacterial infections, cancer recurrence, and organ dysfunction.[45,46] Opelz and colleagues first suggested clinical evidence of transfusion-associated immunomodulation in 1973, when improved renal allograft survival was observed in patients transfused prior to transplantation.[47] Current evidence implicates transfusions in the development of nosocomial infections including wound infections, pneumonia, and sepsis. In a prospective observational study, Taylor et al. found a significant association between transfusion and development of nosocomial infections (14.3% versus 5.3%, $P<0.0001$). In addition, mortality and length of stay were increased in the transfused group. The risk of infection increases 9.7% for each unit of PRBC transfused.[48] Development of these infectious complications results not only in increased length of stay but in increased in-hospital deaths and increased costs as well.[49] These effects may be reduced by the use of prestorage leukocyte depletion.[50]

Other complications include transfusion-associated circulatory overload with the development of fluid overload and pulmonary edema, multisystem organ failure, systemic inflammatory response syndrome,[51,52] hypothermia, coagulopathy, thrombocytopenia, hyperkalemia, and pulmonary hypertension with an increase in pulmonary vascular resistance and decreased right ventricular ejection fraction.[53]

Finally, the transfusion of PRBCs may not augment the oxygen-carrying capacity of blood. This results from development of the "storage lesion" due to changes in red blood cells that occur during ex vivo storage. These changes are both structural and functional[54,55] and include reduced deformability impeding microvascular flow,[56] altered adhesiveness and aggregation,[57] reduced intracellular levels of 2,3-diphosphoglycerate (2,3-DPG, which shifts the oxyhemoglobin dissociation curve to the left and reduces oxygen delivery to the tissues), reduction in levels of nitric oxide and adenosine triphosphate,[58] and accumulation of bioactive compounds with proinflammatory activity.[59] The risk of complications increases with the duration of storage.[60,61] Although the U.S. Food and Drug Administration (FDA) approves storage of red cells for up to 42 days, transfusion of blood older than 2 weeks appears to be associated with a significantly worse outcome. Koch and colleagues examined data from 6002 patients undergoing coronary artery bypass grafting, heart valve surgery, or both. "Newer blood" stored for less than 14 days was administered to 2872 patients, while the remaining 3130 received "older blood" stored for ≥14 days. Patients given older blood had higher rates of in-hospital mortality (2.8% versus 1.7%, $P=0.004$), need for longer duration of intubation (9.7% versus 5.6%, $P<0.001$), higher incidence of acute renal failure (2.7% versus 1.6%, $P=0.003$), and higher incidence of sepsis (4.0% versus 2.8%, $P=0.001$). The difference in mortality persisted even at 1 year after transfusion (7.4% versus 11.0%; $P<0.001$).[62]

ROLE OF ERYTHROPOIETIN

Many factors contribute to the development of anemia in the critically ill, but inappropriately low endogenous levels of erythropoietin in response to anemia represents a key pathophysiologic issue. Further, there is a failure of circulating erythropoietin to induce a response commensurate with the degree of anemia.[63] Recognition of these considerations has prompted many clinicians to use pharmacologic doses of erythropoietin in an effort to reduce the need for and/or the amount of red cells transfused. While theoretically appealing, this approach has not been validated by scientific evidence. Corwin et al. conducted a prospective randomized, placebo-controlled trial (EPO3) that enrolled 1460 patients who were randomized to receive either 40,000 units of epoetin alfa or placebo weekly. Epoetin alfa therapy did not decrease the number of patients requiring a transfusion (46.0% versus 48.3%, relative risk 0.95, 95% CI 0.85–1.06, $P=0.34$), or the number of PRBC units transfused (mean 4.5 versus 4.3 units, $P=0.42$). No differences were seen in lengths of ICU or hospital stay, or time to weaning from mechanical ventilation. Although circulating Hb levels were significantly increased in the group receiving epoetin alfa, this effect did not translate into a survival benefit (adjusted hazard ratio 0.79, 95% CI 0.56–1.10). A significant increase in thrombotic events was noted (hazard ratio 1.41, 95% CI 1.06–1.86).[64] Based upon these data, a large number of patients would need to be treated with erythropoietin in order to avoid one transfusion-related adverse event.[65] As noted, treatment with erythropoietin also increases the risk for thrombotic complications. Accordingly, routine use of erythropoietin cannot be recommended. At our institutions, erythropoietin use is limited to patients with chronic renal failure and Jehovah's Witnesses.

CURRENT RECOMMENDATIONS

Transfusion of PRBCs should not be based on a transfusion trigger alone. The decision must be based instead on the patient's intravascular volume status, evidence of shock, duration and extent of anemia, and cardiopulmonary physiologic parameters.[1]

Transfusion is indicated for patients with hemorrhagic shock. In this instance, the number of units transfused is based not on a particular Hb level but on the physiologic state of the patient. Transfusion is also indicated in the presence of evidence of acute hemorrhage with either hemodynamic instability or evidence of inadequate oxygen delivery as demonstrated by elevated blood lactate levels or base deficit. Serial assessment of these parameters can be used to determine the efficacy of resuscitation.[66]

In hemodynamically stable patients with anemia, a restrictive strategy of transfusion can be employed. Transfusion with PRBCs should be instituted when the Hb level falls to less than 7 g/dL. For patients at risk for myocardial ischemia, a higher Hb concentration might be the appropriate transfusion trigger.

For patients with cardiac disease undergoing coronary artery bypass graft surgery, increased mortality is observed in patients with admission Hb levels below 8 g/dL. Reduction in mortality can be achieved by transfusing to a hematocrit of 30% to 33%. No mortality benefit is seen with hematocrits above 33%, and increased mortality is observed when hematocrits above 36% are achieved.[67-69]

Use of transfusions to wean patients from mechanical ventilation is not indicated. No benefit in the weaning process or difference in duration of mechanical ventilation has been observed.[70]

Transfusions should not be employed as the absolute method to improve tissue oxygen delivery in critically ill patients. In septic patients, PRBC transfusion increases oxygen delivery but not consumption.[71] Whereas increases in Hb levels are consistently seen following transfusion in septic patients, these increases do not translate to improvement in blood lactate levels or mixed venous oxygen saturation.[72] Transfusion may be indicated for failure to achieve an adequate mixed venous saturation after adequate fluid resuscitation.[73]

Transfusions can exacerbate acute lung injury and ARDS, and efforts must be made to avoid transfusions in this patient population.

The TRICC data fail to show any difference in outcome with a restrictive strategy in patients with traumatic brain injury, but the study was underpowered to detect differences in this subgroup of patients.[74] Others have shown transfusion-related improvement in brain tissue partial pressure of oxygen independent of cerebral perfusion pressure, arterial oxygen saturation, and F_{IO_2}.[75] Similar improvements have been observed in patients with subarachnoid hemorrhage who had higher initial and mean Hb values.[76] In other studies, an increased amount of angiographically confirmed vasospasm has been seen in patients receiving postoperative blood transfusions. Salim et al. retrospectively evaluated the effect of transfusion on outcome in 1150 patients with traumatic brain injury. On logistic regression, when both anemia and transfusion were included in the model, transfusion resulted in an increased mortality while anemia did not. When transfusion was removed from the model, anemia was a significant risk factor for mortality and for complications.[77] These confounding results preclude a definitive recommendation for patients with subarachnoid hemorrhage or brain trauma, and the decision to transfuse must be individualized. Recommendations are summarized in Table 19-3.

NOVEL STRATEGIES

It is evident that hemodynamically stable patients can tolerate marked degrees of anemia. Inasmuch as the transfusion of PRBCs is clearly deleterious, preventing the development and/or progression of anemia

TABLE 19-3	Summary of Current Recommendations[1]

1. Packed red blood cell (PRBC) transfusion is indicated in patients with hemorrhagic shock (Level 1).[91]
2. PRBC transfusion may be recommended for patients with acute hemorrhage after adequate fluid resuscitation if they have evidence of hemodynamic instability or evidence of inadequate systemic perfusion as demonstrated by elevated serum lactate or presence of a base deficit (Level 1).[66]
3. A restrictive strategy of transfusion for hemoglobin (Hb) levels <7 g/dL is recommended for hemodynamically stable critically ill patients, except for those with myocardial infarction or unstable angina.[92] This restrictive strategy is also recommended in critically ill trauma patients[93] and in those with stable cardiac disease (Level 1).[92]
4. Transfuse patients with acute coronary syndromes who have admission Hb levels of <8 g/dL. Achieve posttransfusion hematocrit (Hct) levels of 30% to 33% (Level 3).[68,69,94]
5. Do not transfuse based on a transfusion trigger alone. Instead, individualize the decision based on the patient's intravascular volume status, evidence of shock, duration and extent of anemia, and cardiopulmonary status.
6. Transfuse as single units (Level 5).[1]
7. Do not use transfusion as a means to wean patients off mechanical ventilation (Level 2).[6]
8. Do not use transfusion as a stand-alone strategy to improve tissue oxygen delivery (Level 2).[95]
9. In sepsis, transfusions are recommended as part of a strategy of early goal-directed therapy during the first 6 hours of resuscitation.[96] After this period, need for transfusion must be individualized, as the optimal level of Hb in sepsis remains unknown (Level 2).[72]
10. Avoid PRBC transfusion in patients with or at risk for acute lung injury (ALI) and acute respiratory distress syndrome (ARDS) (Level 2).[92]
11. Evidence for transfusion in patients with subarachnoid hemorrhage is lacking, and the decision must be individualized.[97] There appears to be no benefit of a liberal transfusion strategy in patients with mild to moderate traumatic brain injury (Level 3).[98]

is of paramount importance. Strategies to achieve this include retrieving and reusing blood shed during surgery,[78] limiting transfusions, using low-volume adult or pediatric sampling tubes to reduce phlebotomy volumes, reducing the number of laboratory tests ordered, using point-of-care microanalysis for laboratory tests, and using closed blood conservation devices (Venous Arterial Blood Management Protection [VAMP], Edward Lifesciences, Irvine, California). Use of the blood conservation device is associated with reduced red cell transfusion requirements and a smaller decrease in Hb levels in the ICU.[79]

Other approaches include the development of newer methods of blood storage that retard the development of storage-related changes,[80] use of advanced computing technologies to optimize the use of blood inventory,[81] and the development of blood substitutes.

Blood substitutes are being developed largely in response to concerns regarding the potential transmission of infectious agents and the impending shortage of blood in the face of increasing demands.[82] Blood substitutes offer the distinct advantages of better shelf life compared to banked blood, universal compatibility, clinically useful intravascular half-life (18–24 hours), and freedom from the risk of infectious disease transmission (possibly with the exception of prion-mediated diseases). Blood substitutes are also oncotically active and can increase blood volume by an amount in excess of the transfused volume.[83] Furthermore, blood substitutes can improve microcirculatory flow by reducing blood viscosity.[84] Most Hb-based oxygen carriers (HBOCs) scavenge nitric oxide and promote arteriolar vasoconstriction on this basis. Although nitric oxide scavenging was probably the cause of increased mortality in the trial of diaspirin cross-linked hemoglobin (DCLHb) for trauma victims,[85] nitric oxide scavenging might prove beneficial in patients with sepsis. In septic patients, inducible nitric oxide synthase expression is increased, leading to overproduction of nitric oxide and hypotension on this basis. HBOCs might overcome this distributive shock and restore blood pressure.[86]

McKenzie and colleagues recently described the outcome in 54 patients with severe life-threatening anemia (median Hb 4 g/dL) treated with the blood substitute, HBOC-201; 23 (41.8%) of 54 patients survived to discharge. Survival was significantly more likely when the blood substitute was administered earlier (3.2 days in survivors versus 4.4 days in non-survivors, P=0.027).[87]

While results from small individual studies, such as the one by McKenzie et al.[87] described earlier, have been promising, available data do not support the use of blood substitutes in their current form. In a meta-analysis of 16 trials involving 5 blood substitutes and over 3700

patients, Nathanson and colleagues[88] found a significantly increased risk of myocardial infarction (relative risk 2.71, 95% CI 1.67–4.40) and death (relative risk 1.30, 95% CI 1.30–1.61) among HBOC-treated patients. Poorer outcome was not related to the type of blood substitute employed or the clinical indication for its use. In light of this evidence, future phase 3 trials of these products are not warranted.

KEY POINTS

1. Anemia is exceedingly common in patients admitted to the ICU. Over 60% are anemic on admission, and 95% become anemic by day 3 of their ICU stay.

2. Anemia in the critically ill patient is multifactorial in etiology. Iron-deficiency anemia and anemia of critical illness are the most frequent causes.

3. Anemia of critical illness is cytokine-mediated and results from decreased production of erythropoietin, reduced response to erythropoietin, and altered iron metabolism.

4. Transfusion is clearly indicated for hemorrhagic shock and hemodynamic instability associated with blood loss after adequate fluid resuscitation.

5. Transfusion of packed red blood cells is still employed by the majority of clinicians as the mainstay of therapy for anemia in critical illness. However, the optimal Hb concentration essential to maintain ideal tissue oxygen delivery remains unknown.

6. The traditional approach of red cell transfusion to maintain hemoglobin concentration ≥10 g/dL has been refuted by current evidence.

7. Recent evidence supports a more restrictive transfusion strategy for critically ill, hemodynamically stable patients without evidence of cardiac ischemia. Based on class I data, transfusion in these patients is now recommended for a circulating Hb level below 7 g/dL.

8. Treatment with recombinant human erythropoietin initially showed promise as a strategy for reducing exposure to allogeneic blood. More recent evidence, however, refutes these findings, and points instead to an increase in thrombotic complications.

9. Transfusion-related acute lung injury is increasingly being recognized as a severe respiratory complication of transfusion.

10. Novel strategies to avoid the need for blood transfusion include use of blood conservation techniques, improved blood storage techniques, advanced inventory control, and evaluation of the efficacy of blood substitutes.

ANNOTATED REFERENCES

Weiskopf RB, Viele MK, Feiner J, et al. Human cardiovascular and metabolic response to acute, severe isovolemic anemia. JAMA 1998;279(3):217-21.
Acute isovolemic reduction of blood Hb concentration to 50 g/L in conscious, healthy, resting humans does not produce evidence of inadequate systemic oxygen delivery, as assessed by lack of change of VO2 and plasma lactate concentration. This important investigation established that significant anemia could be tolerated in healthy individuals.

Hébert PC, Wells G, Blajchman MA, et al. A multicenter randomized, controlled clinical trial of transfusion requirements in critical care. Transfusion Requirements in Critical Care Investigators, Canadian Critical Care Trials Group. N Engl J Med 1999;340(6):409-17.
Canadian study found no benefit of a liberal transfusion strategy when compared to a restrictive one when 838 anemic critically ill patients were compared for 30-day mortality or severity of organ dysfunction. This landmark trial demonstrated that a hemoglobin transfusion threshold of 7 was appropriate in critically ill patients without ongoing cardiac ischemia or GI bleeding.

Corwin HL, Gettinger A, Pearl RG, et al. The CRIT study: anemia and blood transfusion in the critically ill—current clinical practice in the United States. Crit Care Med 2004;32(1):39-52.
This prospective, multicenter, observational study described the transfusion experiences of ICU patients at 284 ICUs over a short time period in the United States. Among subjects enrolled, 44% were transfused a mean of 4.6 ± 4.9 units; average ICU stay was 21 days. This study examined red blood cell transfusion practices in the critically ill in the United States.

Koch CG, Li L, Duncan AI, et al. Morbidity and mortality risk associated with red cell and blood component transfusion in isolated coronary artery bypass grafting. Crit Care Med 2006;34(6):1608-16.
The study established the morbidity of transfusion in 11,963 patients who underwent isolated coronary artery bypass from 1995 through 2002, 5814 (48.6%) of whom were transfused. Transfusion of red blood

cells was associated with a risk-adjusted increased risk for every postoperative morbid event: mortality, renal failure, prolonged ventilatory support, serious infection, cardiac complications, and neurologic events.

Corwin HL, Gettinger A, Fabian TC, et al. Efficacy and safety of epoetin alfa in critically ill patients. N Engl J Med 2007;357(10):965-76.
In this prospective, randomized, placebo-controlled trial, 1460 anemic ICU patients received weekly recombinant human erythropoietin or placebo without benefit regarding 140-day mortality or transfusion requirements. EPO was associated with a significant increase in the incidence of thrombotic events. The purported benefits of EPO in the critically ill were clearly dispelled by this large multicenter trial.

Koch CG, Li L, Sessler DI, et al. Duration of red-cell storage and complications after cardiac surgery. N Engl J Med 2008;358(12):1229-39.
This study examined the relationship between serious complications and mortality after cardiac surgery and transfusions of "older blood." Transfusion of red cells stored for more than 2 weeks was associated with a significantly increased risk of postoperative complications as well as reduced survival. Findings supported the notion that blood stored for prolonged periods may be deleterious.

Natanson C, Kern SJ, Lurie P, Banks SM, Wolfe SM. Cell-free hemoglobin-based blood substitutes and risk of myocardial infarction and death: a meta-analysis. JAMA 2008;299(19):2304-12.
Definitive review of 16 trials involving 5 different oxygen therapeutic agents and 3711 patients in varied patient populations. Use of these blood substitutes was associated with a significantly increased risk of death and myocardial infarction.

Napolitano LM, Kurek S, Luchette FA, et al. Clinical practice guideline: red cell transfusion in adult trauma and critical care. J Trauma 2009;67(6):1439-42.
Recent comprehensive review of red cell transfusion practice produced by a combined task force of the Eastern Association for the Surgery of Trauma and the Society of Critical Care Medicine.

REFERENCES

Access the complete reference list online at http://www.expertconsult.com.

20 Thrombocytopenia

SANDRO RIZOLI | WILLIAM C. AIRD

Thrombocytopenia is the most common coagulation disorder in the intensive care unit (ICU). Classically defined as a platelet count less than 150×10^9/L, thrombocytopenia is frequently classified according to whether platelets are consumed, sequestered, or underproduced in the bone marrow. However, a more practical classification takes into account the clinical setting (Table 20-1). In the ICU, thrombocytopenia occurs in up to 20% of all medical and 35% of all surgical admissions.[1,2] It has many causes and results from the underlying disease plus the effects of medications that can impair platelet production and/or increase platelet consumption and destruction. The two most important causes of thrombocytopenia are sepsis and heparin-induced thrombocytopenia (HIT). Sepsis is associated with thrombocytopenia in 35% to 59% of cases, whereas HIT is the cause in approximately 25% of ICU patients.[1-5] The highest incidence of HIT is among patients on high doses of unfractionated heparin.[6] It is estimated that 2% of cardiac medical patients, 15% of orthopedic patients, and up to half of patients who undergo cardiac bypass surgery develop HIT antibodies against platelet factor 4 (heparin/PF4) following exposure to unfractionated heparin. However, most patients with heparin/PF4 antibodies do not develop thrombocytopenia, an important consideration when interpreting commonly available diagnostic tests that detect such antibodies.[7] The most important complication observed in patients with HIT is not bleeding but thrombosis, which occurs 30 times more frequently in patients with HIT than in the general population.[6]

Pathophysiology

A common cause of low platelet count is test tube clumping of platelets due to ethylenediamine-tetraacetic acid (EDTA)-dependent antibodies or insufficient anticoagulant.[8] When such "pseudothrombocytopenia" is considered as a possibility, the platelet count should be repeated in blood drawn into heparin- or citrate-containing tubes. Peripheral blood smears may help identify clumping platelets (Figures 20-1 and 20-2).

Immune mechanisms rarely contribute to sepsis-induced thrombocytopenia.[8] Nonspecific platelet-associated antibodies can be detected in up to 30% of ICU patients. In these cases, nonpathogenic immunoglobulin G (IgG) presumably binds to bacterial products on the surface of platelets, to an altered platelet surface, or as immune complexes. A subset of patients with platelet-associated antibodies has autoantibodies directed against the integrin glycoprotein IIb/IIIa. These antibodies have been implicated in the pathogenesis of immune thrombocytopenic purpura and, although not proved, may also play a role in mediating sepsis-induced thrombocytopenia. Besides sepsis, many drugs also have been implicated in the production of nonspecific platelet antibodies, which is relevant, considering that the thrombocytopenia may be reversed by stopping the offending medication.[9,10]

Nonimmune platelet destruction and/or consumption along with impaired production are the most important causes of thrombocytopenia in severe sepsis. There is increased binding of platelets to the activated endothelium, resulting in their sequestration, activation, and destruction. The inflammatory response to sepsis has been implicated directly in both impaired production and increased platelet destruction.[4,5] Bone marrow specimens from patients with sepsis and thrombocytopenia often demonstrate hematophagocytosis.[4,5] The degree to which this pathologic process is a cause or simply a marker of sepsis-related thrombocytopenia is unclear. Less commonly, thrombocytopenia is associated with underlying disseminated intravascular coagulation (DIC) and thrombotic microangiopathic disorders such as thrombotic thrombocytopenic purpura (TTP) and hemolysis-elevated liver enzymes and low platelet (HELLP) syndrome (Figure 20-3).[11]

HIT is a clinicopathologic syndrome diagnosed by the detection of circulating antibodies and thrombocytopenia with or without thrombosis.[5,6] Even though the platelet count commonly drops during the first days after starting heparin, HIT itself occurs 5 to 10 days later and in less than 5% of all patients treated with unfractionated heparin for up to 7 days.[5,6] An important exception to this rule is that patients who have been treated with heparin in the past 100 days are at risk for developing rapid-onset heparin-induced thrombocytopenia promptly on reexposure to any form of heparin, including flushes for IV lines.[8] Low-molecular-weight heparins are much less frequently associated with HIT.[5,12]

In addition to sepsis and heparin-related mechanisms, other causes of thrombocytopenia should be considered in critically ill patients: medications that cause platelet destruction and/or bone marrow suppression; dilutional thrombocytopenia, particularly following trauma, surgery and/or multiple transfusions[13]; acute folate deficiency; and other preexisting diseases such as cancer, hypersplenism, and immune thrombocytopenic purpura (ITP).[4,5,8]

Clinical Manifestations and Diagnosis

Patients with thrombocytopenia may develop petechiae, purpura, bruising, or frank bleeding. The diagnosis of thrombocytopenia is made from the complete blood count and it may be important to examine the peripheral blood smear to rule out platelet clumping. Peripheral blood smears also may provide additional information concerning the etiology (e.g., large platelets may indicate increased platelet turnover and adequate marrow production). If thrombocytopenia is associated with consumptive coagulopathy, any or all of the following laboratory tests may be abnormal: International Normalized Ratio (INR), partial thromboplastin time (PTT), thrombin time, circulating concentration of D-dimer, plasma fibrinogen level, concentration of thrombin-antithrombin complexes, plasma concentration of prothrombin fragment 1.2, and the peripheral smear (presence of schistocytes). Although patients with sepsis may have increased platelet-associated IgG, this test is nonspecific and does not help in guiding therapy. Platelet dysfunction associated with renal disease or the use of aspirin and/or other cyclooxygenase inhibitors should also be considered in patients with abnormal cutaneous or mucosal bleeding.[8]

It is important to emphasize that thrombocytopenia associated with sepsis or HIT can coexist with an underlying hypercoagulable state, and that thrombotic complications may occur with a "normal" platelet count.[5] Patients with HIT and thrombotic complications typically have mild to moderate reductions in platelet counts (median 60×10^9/L). Only 5% of cases are associated with platelet counts below 15×10^9/L.[6,14] Findings suggestive of the diagnosis of HIT in these patients include a 30% to 50% or greater fall in the platelet count within the normal range or the presence of erythematous or necrotic skin lesions at subcutaneous heparin injection sites.

TABLE 20-1	Differential Diagnosis of Thrombocytopenia

Outpatients

Pregnancy
Immune thrombocytopenic purpura
Myelodysplastic syndrome
Hypersplenism
Antiphospholipid antibody syndrome
Hereditary thrombocytopenia

Non-ICU and MICU Inpatients

Drugs, including heparin
Sepsis
Disseminated intravascular coagulation
Dilutional thrombocytopenia
Posttransfusion purpura
Folate deficiency

Coronary Care Unit Inpatients

Heparin
Glycoprotein IIb/IIIa antagonists
Adenosine diphosphate receptor antagonists
Coronary artery bypass surgery
Intraaortic balloon pump

Emergency Room Patients

Acute alcohol toxicity
Thrombocytopenic thrombotic purpura/hemolytic uremic syndrome
Immune thrombocytopenic purpura
Drugs

Prognosis

Thrombocytopenia is associated with longer ICU and hospital stays and is a predictor of mortality in ICU patients and patients with severe sepsis.[1,3,5,8] The degree and duration of thrombocytopenia, as well as the net change in the platelet count, are important determinants of survival.[1,3,5,8]

Treatment

Treatment of thrombocytopenia depends on the underlying cause. As a general rule, when thrombocytopenia is associated with an increased risk for bleeding and is not attributable to immune mechanisms, patients should be transfused with platelets to maintain a minimal platelet count. Although guidelines for prophylactic transfusions in patients with chemotherapy-induced thrombocytopenia have been established,[14] the threshold for transfusing ICU patients is not clear.[15] Thrombocytopenia is associated with increased risk of bleeding only when less than 50×10^9/L, when the risk increases four- to fivefold

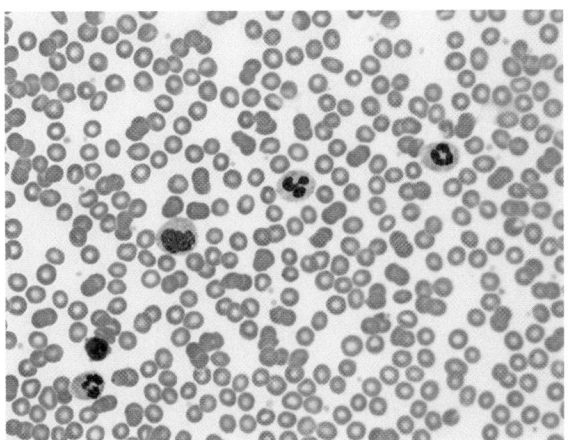

Figure 20-1 Normal peripheral blood film revealing normochromic normocytic red cells, morphologically unremarkable white cells, and adequate numbers of platelets. *(Courtesy Drs. David Good and Marciano Reis, Sunnybrook Health Sciences Centre, University of Toronto.)*

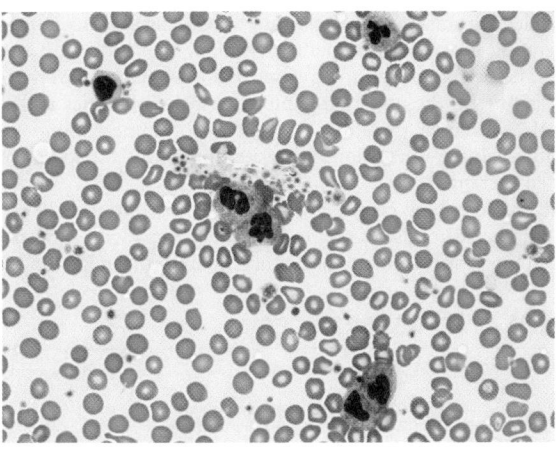

Figure 20-2 Peripheral blood film on a patient with sepsis. The neutrophils show toxic granulation and Döhle bodies, with more immature forms present (granulocytic left shift). Platelets are increased, with evidence of platelet clumping. *(Courtesy Drs. David Good and Marciano Reis, Sunnybrook Health Sciences Centre, University of Toronto.)*

compared to patients with higher counts.[5,8] Major surgeries and invasive procedures are not recommended when the platelet count is below 50×10^9/L. Spontaneous bleeding, particularly intracerebral, typically does not occur until the count drops to less than 20×10^9/L or (more likely) less than 10×10^9/L.[5,8,15-17] In the absence of evidence-based guidelines, most patients are transfused to achieve a platelet count of above 10×10^9/L. If the patient has a concomitant coagulopathy (e.g., due to DIC or liver disease), active bleeding, or platelet dysfunction (e.g., due to uremia), it may be prudent to employ a more liberal transfusion strategy with the goal of maintaining an even higher platelet count. It is important to consider that platelet transfusions have inherent risks, including infection transmission, transfusion-related acute lung injury (TRALI), and excessive clotting. Paradoxically, platelet transfusion may reduce endogenous platelet production by inactivating thrombopoietin.[15]

Patients with sepsis have an underlying shift in the hemostatic balance toward the procoagulant side. Indeed, platelets are activated in the setting of sepsis and likely contribute in important ways to the pathogenesis of the syndrome. When considering the cost-effectiveness

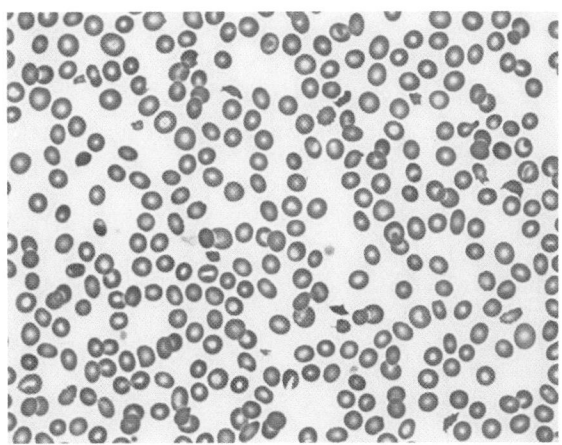

Figure 20-3 Peripheral blood film showing red blood cell fragmentation and decreased platelets. This picture may be seen in microangiopathic hemolytic processes including thrombotic thrombocytopenic purpura (TTP), hemolytic uremic syndrome (HUS), and in some cases of disseminated intravascular coagulation (DIC). *(Courtesy Drs. David Good and Marciano Reis, Sunnybrook Health Sciences Centre, University of Toronto.)*

of platelet transfusion, it is important to consider the theoretic risk of accelerating the underlying pathophysiology (i.e., "adding fuel to the fire"). The best approach for treating sepsis-associated thrombocytopenia is to treat the underlying infection with antibiotics and source control. Additional therapies may consist of some combination of low-tidal-volume ventilation,[18] activated protein C,[19] and early goal-directed therapy.[20]

The treatment of choice for HIT is to discontinue all heparin, including heparin flushes, and to institute therapy with an alternative rapid-acting anticoagulant that either inhibits thrombin or reduces thrombin generation. Warfarin, low-molecular-weight heparin, ε-aminocaproic acid (ancrod), and platelet transfusions should be avoided because they may exacerbate the underlying prothrombotic state. Two direct thrombin inhibitors, lepirudin and argatroban, have been evaluated and approved by the U.S. Food and Drug Administration for the treatment of heparin-induced thrombocytopenia-related thrombosis.[21] Selected patients with life- or limb-threatening thrombosis may benefit from adjuvant therapies, including thrombolytic drugs, surgical thromboembolectomy, intravenous gammaglobulin, plasmapheresis, and antiplatelet agents.

ANNOTATED REFERENCES

Rice TW, Wheeler AP. Coagulopathy in critically ill patients. Part 1: platelet disorders. Chest 2009;136(6):1622-30.
Overview of the most frequent causes of thrombocytopenia and their mechanisms.
Levi M, Opal S. Coagulation abnormalities in critically ill patients. Crit Care 2006;10(4):222-30.
Overview of coagulation disorders in ICU patients summarizing main differential diagnosis and the role of inflammation.
Aird WC. The hematologic system as a marker of organ dysfunction in sepsis. Mayo Clin Proc 2003;78(7):869-81.
This review places sepsis-associated thrombocytopenia in context with other hematologic changes and makes a distinction between adaptive and nonadaptive host responses.
Warkentin TE, Aird WC, Rand JH. Platelet-endothelial interactions: sepsis, HIT, and antiphospholipid syndrome. Hematology Am Soc Hematol Educ Program 2003;497-519.
This review summarizes both thrombocytopenia in sepsis and heparin-induced thrombocytopenia. Figure 5 in the article provides specific treatment recommendations for heparin-induced thrombocytopenia.

REFERENCES

Access the complete reference list online at http://www.expertconsult.com.

21

Coagulopathy

SANDRO RIZOLI | WILLIAM C. AIRD

Hemostasis is a dynamic and highly complex process typically divided into two components: primary and secondary. *Primary hemostasis* refers to the blood vessel and platelet response, whereas *secondary hemostasis* refers to the protein response (clotting cascade). In reality, both primary and secondary hemostasis are tightly interconnected, feed back on each other, and operate in unison. Nevertheless, from a conceptual standpoint, it is helpful to consider each limb of hemostasis separately. In this chapter, we review the clotting mechanism. The reader is referred to Chapter 20 for a discussion of the most common coagulation disorder in the ICU: thrombocytopenia.

General Principles

The blood clotting cascade is highly complex, consisting of a series of linked reactions. In each reaction, a serine protease, once activated, is capable of activating its downstream substrate. For the purposes of this chapter, the scheme will be simplified according to the following themes: (1) the final step in the clotting cascade is the conversion of fibrinogen to fibrin, a process mediated by thrombin; (2) fibrin is the "glue" that holds platelet plugs together and contributes to the host defense against pathogens; (3) there are two pathways—extrinsic and intrinsic—that converge to induce thrombin generation and fibrin formation; (4) blood coagulation is always initiated by the extrinsic pathway (via tissue factor) and amplified by the intrinsic pathway; (5) the prothrombin time (PT) measures the integrity of the extrinsic (and common) pathways, and the activated partial thromboplastin time (APTT) measures the integrity of the intrinsic (and common) pathways; and (6) every procoagulant step is balanced by a natural anticoagulant (antithrombin, protein C system, tissue factor pathway inhibitor). In the final analysis, hemostasis represents a balance between anticoagulant and procoagulant forces.[1-5]

Disorders in hemostasis occur when the hemostatic balance shifts toward one side or the other, resulting in one of two clinical phenotypes: bleeding or thrombosis. The myriad causes, diagnostic workup, and treatment of coagulation disorders are beyond the scope of this chapter. In the sections that follow, we consider the coagulopathy that occurs in patients with sepsis. The reasons for choosing sepsis as the case study are several-fold: (1) sepsis is common in the ICU and is responsible for most coagulation disorders; (2) a consideration of the mechanisms, diagnosis, and therapy of coagulopathy in this setting may be widely applicable to other conditions also associated with activation of the innate immune response (e.g., trauma, burns, postoperative systemic inflammatory response syndrome) and (3) recent therapeutic breakthroughs emphasize the importance of targeting the host response rather than the clotting cascade per se. In sepsis, hemostasis derangement is characterized by enhanced fibrin formation and dysfunction of the physiologic anticoagulant response, with depression of fibrinolysis and impaired fibrin removal.[2,4]

Incidence

Previous studies demonstrated that the coagulation system is activated in virtually all patients with severe sepsis.[2-4] In most such patients, activation may be minimal and detected only by test findings such as elevated circulating D-dimer levels,[6] low protein C levels, or antithrombin deficiency.[4,6] The activation also may be pronounced and characterized by the presence of thrombocytopenia or even disseminated intravascular coagulation (DIC), with evidence of both thrombosis and bleeding. It is estimated that DIC occurs in 15% to 30% of patients with severe sepsis or septic shock.[2,4,7,8]

Mechanisms

In sepsis, the clotting cascade is initiated by tissue factor (TF). When TF is exposed to blood, it binds to factor VII. The complex TF-FVIIa activates factor X, which in turn forms a prothrombinase complex, leading to the generation of thrombin. Finally, thrombin converts fibrinogen into fibrin. TF is exposed to blood through either endothelial disruption or expression on the surface of circulating monocytes, tissue macrophages, and even endothelial cells.[4,9,10]

At the same time, sepsis attenuates all three physiologic anticoagulant mechanisms: activated protein C (APC), antithrombin (AT) and tissue factor pathway inhibitor (TFPI). APC has a key role in sepsis; along with protein S and thrombomodulin, it degrades factors V and VIII by a process accelerated by endothelial protein C receptors (EPCR). In sepsis, APC, protein S, thrombomodulin, and EPCR are down-regulated, rendering the system ineffective.[11,12] AT is the main inhibitor of thrombin and factor Xa, whereas TFPI inhibits the TF-FVIIa complex. Levels of both AT and TFPI are markedly reduced in patients with sepsis.[4,13,14] Sepsis also inhibits fibrinolysis.[2,4] Together, these changes tilt the balance toward the procoagulant side, resulting in thrombin generation, fibrin deposition, and consumption of clotting factors and platelets. DIC represents the extreme case in this pathophysiologic continuum.[2-4]

Local activation of the coagulation system in sepsis is an integral component of the innate immune response and may play a protective role in walling off infection. However, in patients with severe sepsis, systemic activation of coagulation is harmful to the patient and associated with increased mortality.[15] Other common forms of coagulopathy in the ICU are associated with severe trauma, massive blood losses, and shock. Recent studies suggest that early trauma-associated coagulopathy is triggered mainly by shock, mediated by activated protein C, and exacerbated by dilution of plasma and hypothermia.[16,17] Interestingly, the early trauma-associated hypercoagulable state converts to a hypercoagulable one by 24 hours after trauma, carrying a higher risk of thrombotic complications.[18] Other common coagulopathies in the ICU are caused by liver dysfunction, heparin and other anticoagulant medications, and vitamin K deficiency (Figures 21-1 and 21-2).

Clinical Manifestations and Diagnosis

Severe sepsis is usually associated with a net procoagulant state, as evidenced by local or diffuse microvascular thrombi. These changes occasionally manifest as skin lesions, as occurs in purpura fulminans. More commonly, the coagulation cascade interacts with the inflammatory pathway to induce endothelial cell activation and secondary dysfunction of internal organs, including the liver, kidneys, lungs, and brain. Patients are at risk for bleeding when the consumption of clotting factors outstrips the production. Bleeding is more common when the coagulopathy is exacerbated by concomitant thrombocytopenia, liver disease, heparin use, and invasive procedures. In large prospective studies, the incidence of serious bleeding in patients with severe sepsis varies between 2% and 6%.[19] The most sensitive laboratory markers of sepsis-associated coagulopathy include reduced circulating protein C

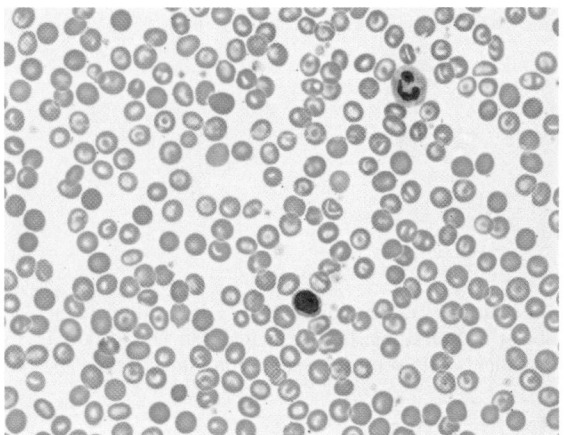

Figure 21-1 Normal peripheral blood film revealing normochromic normocytic red cells, morphologically unremarkable white cells, and adequate numbers of platelets. *(Courtesy Drs. David Good and Marciano Reis, Sunnybrook Health Sciences Centre, University of Toronto.)*

levels and increased circulating D-dimer levels. However, protein C levels are not routinely measured, and an elevated level of D-dimers is a nonspecific finding. In general, coagulation factor levels are inversely correlated with the severity of sepsis,[2] except for factor VIII, an acute-phase protein. Fibrinogen, another acute-phase protein, may be elevated in the early stages of sepsis but is reduced in up to 50% of patients with severe sepsis.[20]

Marked activation of coagulation and secondary consumption of clotting factors may lead to DIC. No single test is sufficiently sensitive or specific to make the diagnosis of DIC. Recently a scoring system was proposed that employs simple laboratory tests, including platelet count, elevated fibrin-related marker (e.g., soluble fibrin monomers, fibrin degradation products), prolonged PT, and fibrinogen level.[20,21] Other markers of coagulation activation such as thrombin-antithrombin complexes, fibrinopeptides, and prothrombin fragment 1.2 are considered investigational in this setting.

The PT or APTT may be elevated for reasons other than sepsis-associated consumption of clotting factors (Box 21-1). As a general rule, increased clotting times are caused by inhibitors against one or more clotting factors or a congenital or acquired deficiency state. In

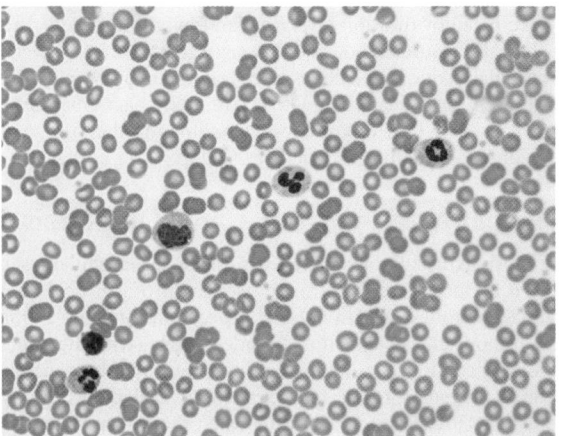

Figure 21-2 Peripheral blood film showing macrocytic red cells, numerous target cells, and slightly decreased platelets, indicative of liver failure. Thrombocytopenia is often accompanied by a coagulopathy, owing to dysfunctional platelets and decreased production of coagulation factors in the liver. *(Courtesy Drs. David Good and Marciano Reis, Sunnybrook Health Sciences Centre, University of Toronto.)*

Box 21-1

CAUSES OF INCREASED PROTHROMBIN TIME (PT) AND/OR ACTIVATED PARTIAL THROMBOPLASTIN TIME (APTT)

Increased PT—Defect in Extrinsic Pathway
Deficiency or inhibitor of factor VII
Early warfarin (Coumadin) therapy
Early liver disease

Increased APTT—Defect in Intrinsic Pathway
Deficiency or inhibitor of factors XII, XI, IX, or VIII
Heparin (though usually affects PT as well)
Liver disease (though usually affects PT as well)
Lupus anticoagulant (may affect PT as well)

Increased PT and APTT—Defect in Common Pathway or Combined Defect in Extrinsic and Intrinsic Pathways
Heparin (all serine proteases affected, especially II and X)
Disseminated intravascular coagulation (all factors, including pro- and anticoagulants, affected)
Liver disease (all factors except VIII affected)
Warfarin (factors II, VII, IX, and X affected)
Vitamin K deficiency (factors II, VII, IX, and X affected)
Direct thrombin inhibitors
Lupus anticoagulant

---

the ICU, prolongation of the PT or APTT is almost always related to an acquired deficiency state. An isolated increase in PT indicates factor VII (extrinsic pathway) deficiency and may be seen in early liver failure or during the initial stages of warfarin (Coumadin) therapy. An isolated increase in the APTT points to a defect in the intrinsic pathway—namely, factors XII, XI, IX, or VIII. An increase in both PT and APTT reflects an abnormality in the common pathway (factors X or V, prothrombin, or fibrinogen) or a combined deficiency in the extrinsic and intrinsic pathways. The latter occurs with heparin therapy, long-term warfarin treatment, vitamin K deficiency, advanced liver disease, DIC, or dilutional coagulopathy.[3,4]

Prognosis

Certain markers of coagulation activation have been correlated with negative outcome in patients with sepsis. For example, low antithrombin levels in patients with sepsis are predictive of poor survival.[7] Decreased protein C levels in severe sepsis have been shown to correlate with mortality, presence of shock, length of ICU stay, and ventilator dependence.[2,4] In clinical studies of multiple organ dysfunction, maximum PT and APTT were shown to be longer in nonsurvivors than in survivors.[15] DIC is an independent predictor for mortality in patients with sepsis.[22]

Treatment

The most important treatment for coagulopathy in septic patients in the ICU is to treat the underlying infection. Many patients, however, still require additional treatments directed at correcting either the hemostatic defect or the deficit of physiologic anticoagulants.

The consumption of clotting factors and platelets, with or without DIC, may result in bleeding diathesis in patients with sepsis. For such patients, transfusion therapy with platelets, fresh frozen plasma, or plasma components may be indicated if the patient is actively bleeding or if there is a high risk of bleeding (e.g., due to other types of coagulopathy, trauma, need for surgery, invasive procedures).[2,4,16]

In view of recent advances in our understanding of the underlying pathophysiology of sepsis, emphasis has shifted from procoagulant replacement to anticoagulant therapy. A variety of thrombin inhibitors have been tested in patients with sepsis, including antithrombin (AT), tissue factor pathway inhibitor (TFPI) and activated protein C (APC).

These drugs inhibit thrombin generation and fibrin formation and demonstrated promising results in animal and early-phase clinical studies.[23,24] One possible explanation for these results is that the natural anticoagulants have a dual function: inhibition of coagulation and suppression of inflammation. AT, TFI and APC each have been shown to modulate the inflammatory response under in vitro and in vivo conditions.[25]

However, in subsequent large, randomized controlled trials, infusions with AT and TFPI (tifacogin) failed to improve 28-day all-cause mortality in patients with severe sepsis.[7,26,27] In contrast, the PROWESS study, which was stopped ahead of time, demonstrated that recombinant human activated protein C had both anticoagulant and antiinflammatory properties and improved survival of patients with severe sepsis.[6] Recombinant APC is approved for use in the United States and most of the world; its use is an integral part of many guidelines for the treatment of sepsis.[28] Recombinant APC's role in sepsis, however, continues to be debated following publication of negative trials.[29,30] Furthermore, we do not know at present whether the different outcomes in the phase 3 trials of AT, TFPI, and APC can be explained by differences in study design or whether they reflect differences at the mechanistic level.

Conclusions

Most patients in the ICU have coagulation abnormalities and marked activation of the clotting cascade, which could be more apparent if these patients were routinely tested with assays such as protein C levels, markers of thrombin activation, or D-dimers. While the unrelenting coagulation activation leads to a prothrombotic state, it may also result in clotting factor consumption and bleeding diathesis. Important challenges for the intensivist are to (1) delineate and track a patient's position on the hemostatic scale (prothrombotic versus hemorrhagic), (2) understand that both phenotypes may occur concomitantly (e.g., microthrombi within internal organs and mucosal bleeding), and (3) target each component separately—that is, replenish the clotting factors in the face of bleeding (e.g., plasma products) while attenuating the underlying host response (e.g., low-tidal-volume ventilation, activated protein C, and early goal-directed therapy).

ANNOTATED REFERENCES

Aird WC. Vascular bed–specific hemostasis: Role of endothelium in sepsis pathogenesis. Crit Care Med 2001;29(Suppl. 7):S28-35.
This review emphasizes the notion of hemostasis as a balance between procoagulants and anticoagulants and the hemostatic changes in sepsis.
Bernard GR, Vincent JL, Laterre PF, et al. Efficacy and safety of recombinant human activated protein C for severe sepsis. N Engl J Med 2001;344(10):699-709.
This landmark study was the first to demonstrate a survival benefit of a drug in patients with severe sepsis.

Levi M, van der Poll T. Inflammation and coagulation. Crit Care Med 2010;38(Suppl):S26-34.
This is an excellent review of inflammation and coagulation, particularly in sepsis.
Taylor FB Jr, Toh CH, Hoots WK, et al. Towards definition, clinical and laboratory criteria, and a scoring system for disseminated intravascular coagulation. Thromb Haemost 2001;86(5):1327-30.
A remarkable paper introducing the definition and diagnostic criteria for DIC.

REFERENCES

Access the complete reference list online at http://www.expertconsult.com.

22

Jaundice

MITCHELL P. FINK

Bilirubin is a byproduct of heme metabolism. Heme, which is largely derived from the hemoglobin in senescent red blood cells, is oxidized in the spleen, liver, and other organs by two isoforms of the enzyme, heme oxygenase, in the presence of nicotinamide adenine dinucleotide phosphate (NADPH) and molecular oxygen, to form biliverdin, carbon monoxide, and iron.[1] Subsequently, biliverdin is converted into bilirubin by the phosphoprotein, biliverdin reductase, which also uses NADPH as a cofactor.

Bilirubin is lipophilic molecule. To be excreted, bilirubin that is produced in extrahepatic organs is bound to albumin and transported to the liver. The liver takes up the bilirubin-albumin complex through an albumin receptor. Bilirubin, but not albumin, is transferred across the hepatocyte membrane and transported through the cytoplasm to the smooth endoplasmic reticulum bound primarily to ligandin or Y protein, a member of the glutathione S-transferase gene family of proteins. Within hepatocytes, bilirubin is converted to water-soluble derivatives, bilirubin monoglucuronide, and bilirubin diglucuronide by the enzyme, uridine diphosphate-glucuronosyl transferase. These conjugated forms of bilirubin are secreted across the canalicular membrane into bile via an energy-dependent process. Conjugated bilirubin is excreted in the bile into the intestine, where it is broken down by gut flora to urobilinogen and stercobilin.

Total serum bilirubin consists of an unconjugated fraction and a conjugated fraction. The conjugated forms of bilirubin exist both free in the serum and bound covalently to albumin; the latter is known as *delta-bilirubin*.[2] Conjugated bilirubin is water soluble and reacts directly when certain dyes are added to the serum specimen. The unconjugated bilirubin does not react with the colorimetric reagents until a solvent is added. Accordingly, the conjugated and unconjugated forms of bilirubin are often referred to as "direct" and "indirect" bilirubin. The sum of these two measurements is "total" bilirubin. The normal total bilirubin concentration in adults is less than 18 μmol/L (1.0 mg/dL). Although any total bilirubin concentration higher than the upper limit of normal constitutes hyperbilirubinemia, jaundice (i.e., yellow discoloration of the sclerae, mucous membranes, and skin) is usually not clinically apparent unless the serum total bilirubin level is greater than 50 μmol/L (2.8 mg/dL). Unconjugated or indirect hyperbilirubinemia is present when the total serum bilirubin concentration is above the upper limit of normal, and less than 15% of the total is in the direct or conjugated form.

Differential Diagnosis

The long list of diagnoses depicted in Box 22-1 divides the causes of hyperbilirubinemia into two large groups according to whether the predominant abnormality is an increase in the circulating concentration of unconjugated (indirect) bilirubin or an increase in the concentration of conjugated (direct) bilirubin. Although this classification scheme is useful under some circumstances, many of the diagnoses listed in Box 22-1 are extremely rare and very unlikely to be encountered by the intensivist caring for critically ill (adult) patients. A more useful classification scheme is depicted in Box 22-2. In this scheme, the causes of jaundice are lumped into three primary categories: extrahepatic obstruction to bile flow, increased bilirubin production, or impaired excretion secondary to hepatocellular necrosis and/or intrahepatic cholestasis and/or hepatitis. Often multiple mechanisms are involved at once.

The incidence of hyperbilirubinemia among critically ill patients is quite variable. Jaundice is present in more than 50% of patients with intraabdominal sepsis, 33% of victims of severe polysystemic trauma, and from 3% to more than 20% of intensive care unit (ICU) patients recovering from cardiac surgery.[3-6] Determining the cause of hyperbilirubinemia of new onset is important when managing ICU patients because some problems can be corrected. Exclusion of a mechanical cause for jaundice (e.g., obstruction of the common bile duct due to choledocholithiasis or stricture) assumes the highest priority because failure to correct this sort of problem in a timely fashion can lead to serious morbidity or even mortality.

Iatrogenic injuries to the common bile duct are fortunately quite rare, although the incidence of this complication is greater after laparoscopic cholecystectomy than after open excision of the gallbladder.[7] Damage to the biliary tree, stricture of biliary anastomoses, or retained stones after cholecystectomy or common bile duct exploration present as hyperbilirubinemia and elevated circulating levels of alkaline phosphatase or gamma-glutamyl transpeptidase. Most often the diagnosis is made by detecting dilation of intrahepatic and extrahepatic bile ducts using ultrasonography.

By exceeding the capacity of the liver to conjugate and excrete bilirubin into the bile, hemolysis can produce jaundice. However, the liver can excrete about 300 mg/day of bilirubin,[8] so clinically significant hyperbilirubinemia is only apparent if the rate of hemolysis (i.e., number of red blood cells lysed per unit time) is fairly rapid. Approximately 10% of the erythrocytes in an appropriately crossmatched unit of packed red blood cells undergo rapid hemolysis, yielding about 250 mg of bilirubin.[9] Accordingly, transfusion of a single unit of packed red blood cells is not likely to increase serum total bilirubin concentration. However, transfusion of multiple units of blood over a short period almost inevitably leads to some degree of hyperbilirubinemia, particularly if hepatic function is already impaired. Other reasonably common causes of acute hemolysis in ICU patients include sickle cell disease, immune-mediated hemolytic anemia, and disseminated intravascular coagulation.

Any condition that leads to extensive hepatocellular damage will increase circulating total bilirubin concentration. Conditions in this category that are commonly encountered in ICU patients include viral hepatitis, "shock liver," alcoholic hepatitis, and hepatocellular injury induced by drugs, especially acetaminophen.[10] In most forms of jaundice due to hepatic inflammation or hepatocellular damage, circulating levels of transaminases are elevated to a greater extent than total bilirubin concentration. Making a diagnosis of acetaminophen overdose early is very important because specific therapy using N-acetylcysteine can be lifesaving.[10]

Two other conditions commonly associated with jaundice in ICU patients are sepsis and total parenteral nutrition (TPN). Both are associated with the development of intrahepatic cholestasis. Hyperbilirubinemia is a common occurrence in patients with extrahepatic infections leading to the development of severe sepsis.[11,12] Persistent hyperbilirubinemia in septic patients is associated with a significantly increased risk of mortality.[12] Efforts to understand the pathophysiologic mechanisms responsible for cholestatic jaundice due to sepsis have largely focused on lipopolysaccharide (LPS)-induced alterations in the function and expression of various bile acid transporters.[13-16] Nevertheless, another factor that probably contributes to the

Box 22-1

DIFFERENTIAL DIAGNOSIS OF HYPERBILIRUBINEMIA

A. Unconjugated hyperbilirubinemia
  1. Overproduction of bilirubin
    a. Hemolysis, intravascular: disseminated intravascular coagulation
    b. Hemolysis, extravascular
      i. Hemoglobinopathies
      ii. Enzyme deficiencies such as glucose-6-phosphate dehydrogenase deficiency
      iii. Autoimmune hemolytic anemias
    c. Ineffective erythropoiesis
    d. Resorption of hematoma
    e. Massive transfusion
  2. Hereditary unconjugated hyperbilirubinemia
    a. Gilbert's syndrome (autosomal dominant)
    b. Crigler-Najjar syndrome type I (autosomal recessive)
    c. Crigler-Najjar syndrome type II (autosomal dominant)
  3. Drugs
    a. Chloramphenicol: neonatal hyperbilirubinemia
    b. Vitamin K: neonatal hyperbilirubinemia
    c. 5β-Pregnane-3α, 20 α-diol: cause of breast milk jaundice
B. Conjugated hyperbilirubinemia
  1. Inherited disorders
    a. Dubin-Johnson syndrome (autosomal recessive)
    b. Rotor syndrome (autosomal recessive)
  2. Hepatocellular diseases and intrahepatic causes
    a. Viral hepatitis
    b. Alcoholic hepatitis
    c. Drug-induced hepatitis (e.g., due to isoniazid, nonsteroidal antiinflammatory drugs, zidovudine)
    d. Cirrhosis
    e. Drug-induced cholestasis (e.g., due to prochlorperazine, haloperidol [Haldol], estrogens)
    f. Sepsis
    g. Postoperative jaundice
    h. Infiltrative liver disease: tumor, abscesses (pyogenic, amebic), tuberculosis, parasites (e.g., *Toxoplasma*), *Pneumocystis jirovecii* pneumonia, *Echinococcus*
    i. Primary biliary cirrhosis
    j. Primary sclerosing cholangitis
  3. Extrahepatic causes
    a. Gallstone disease
    b. Pancreatitis-related stricture
    c. Pancreatic head tumor
    d. Cholangiocarcinoma
    e. Primary sclerosing cholangitis

Adapted from Bernstein MD. Hyperbilirubinemia. In: Rakel RE, editor. *Saunders Manual of Medical Practice*. Philadelphia: Saunders; 1996:371-373, with permission.

Box 22-2

CLASSIFICATION FOR ACUTE JAUNDICE ASSOCIATED WITH CRITICAL ILLNESS

I. Extrahepatic bile duct obstruction
  A. Choledocholithiasis
  B. Common bile duct stricture
  C. Traumatic or iatrogenic common bile duct injury
  D. Acute pancreatitis
  E. Malignancy (e.g., ampullary carcinoma)
II. Increased bilirubin production
  A. Massive transfusion
  B. Resorption of blood collections (e.g., hematomas, hemoperitoneum)
  C. Acute hemolysis
    1. Disseminated intravascular coagulation
    2. Immune-mediated
III. Impaired excretion due to hepatocellular dysfunction, hepatitis, or intrahepatic cholestasis
  A. Drug- or alcohol-induced hepatitis
  B. Drug-induced intrahepatic cholestasis
  C. Drug-induced hepatocellular necrosis
  D. Gilbert's syndrome
  E. Sepsis and other causes of systemic inflammation
  F. Total parenteral nutrition
  G. Viral hepatitis

development of intrahepatic cholestasis is back-leakage of bile from the canalicular spaces into the sinusoids.[17-19]

The basis for TPN-induced cholestasis is probably multifactorial. Prolonged bowel rest and ileus may promote bacterial overgrowth and increased translocation of LPS into the portal vein on this basis. Phytosterols are present in the lipid emulsions used for TPN and have been associated with cholestasis, especially in premature infants.[20] Results from two retrospective studies suggest that administration of more than 1 g/kg/day of lipid emulsion is associated with increased incidence of hepatocellular dysfunction.[21,22] These data, however, were derived by studying patients receiving TPN at home for very prolonged periods and may not be applicable to ICU patients. In any case, TPN is associated with the development of jaundice and hepatocellular damage. Accordingly, except in rare cases, most ICU patients are better served by receiving enteral rather than parenteral nutrition.

REFERENCES

Access the complete reference list online at http://www.expertconsult.com.

23

Management of Gastrointestinal Bleeding

NITIN DHAMIJA | ROBERT POUSMAN | OMER BAJWA | PAUL E. MARIK

The interdisciplinary management of gastrointestinal (GI) bleeding involves volume resuscitation, correction of coagulation disorders, and protection of the airway while initiating diagnostic procedures to determine the site of bleeding.

The incidence of upper GI bleeding is estimated to be 37 to 172 per 10,000 population per year. Upper GI bleeding is nearly twice as common in males as in females, and its incidence increases with age, a pattern that has been attributed to increased incidence of predisposing comorbid conditions.[1,2] The mortality rate for patients with upper GI bleeding has remained relatively stable over the past 40 years, ranging from 3% to 14%.[1] The risk of death depends on the patient's age, presence of shock, comorbid medical conditions, presence of recent hemorrhage, location of the onset of bleeding (inpatient versus outpatient), and underlying cause of the hemorrhage (Table 23-1). Scoring systems to predict mortality and risk of rebleeding are based on host factors, the patient's clinical course, and endoscopic findings.[1,2] Variceal hemorrhage is associated with a mortality rate of 15% to 20%, and the risk of recurrent bleeding is about 30%.[3,4]

Causes of Upper Gastrointestinal Bleeding

The source of upper GI bleeding can be anywhere proximal to the ligament of Treitz. Note that bleeding from the nose, oropharynx, mouth, or lungs can present with symptoms suggestive of upper GI bleeding (e.g., emesis of bloody gastric contents). Upper GI bleeding can be classified into several broad categories based on anatomic and pathophysiologic factors:

1. Erosive or ulcerative lesions in the mucosa
2. Portal hypertension
3. Arteriovenous malformation(s)
4. Traumatic or postsurgical causes
5. Tumors

Causes of Lower Gastrointestinal Bleeding

Lower GI bleeding that occurs from a site distal to the ligament of Treitz can be grouped into multiple etiologies:

1. Anatomic
2. Vascular
3. Inflammatory
4. Neoplastic

The most common cause of bleeding in patients younger than 50 years of age is hemorrhoids.[5]

Major Causes of Gastrointestinal Bleeding

PEPTIC ULCER DISEASE

Peptic ulcer disease accounts for as many as half of the cases of upper GI bleeding. It is also the most common cause of bleeding in patients with portal hypertension and varices.[1] Bleeding from mucosal ulceration adjacent to a vessel can result from a *Helicobacter pylori* infection,

use of nonsteroidal antiinflammatory drugs (NSAIDs), and/or critical illness. Concurrent aspirin and oral anticoagulation use further increases the risk of bleeding.[6-9] Acid suppression therapy (H_2-antagonists, proton pump inhibitors), however, has not affected the predominance of peptic ulcer bleeding as the cause of acute hemorrhage.[10]

STRESS ULCERS

Owing to aggressive resuscitation and early enteral nutrition, bleeding from stress-related gastric ulcers among hospitalized patients is now relatively uncommon.

ESOPHAGEAL VARICES

Gastroesophageal variceal hemorrhage is a major complication of portal hypertension from cirrhosis and accounts for 5% to 15% of all cases of bleeding from the upper GI tract.[11-14] The most common site of varices is the distal 2 to 5 cm of the esophagus. Superficial veins in this anatomic region lack support from surrounding tissues (Figure 23-1).[15] The dilation of distal esophageal varices depends on a threshold pressure gradient, most commonly measured by the hepatic venous pressure gradient, defined as the difference between the wedged, or occluded, hepatic venous pressure and the free hepatic venous pressure (normal gradient < 5 mm Hg). If the hepatic venous pressure gradient is below 12 mm Hg, varices do not form.[16,17] Varices do not invariably develop in patients with gradients ≥12 mm Hg, so this pressure gradient is necessary but may not be sufficient in and of itself for varix formation.[16,17] Gastroesophageal varices are present in 40% to 60% of patients with cirrhosis; their presence and size are related to the underlying cause, duration, and severity of cirrhosis.[18]

ESOPHAGITIS

Significant bleeding from esophagitis and erosive disease is the second most common cause of upper GI hemorrhage, often causing occult blood loss rather than acute bleeding.[6-9] Clinically obvious bleeding is most likely in patients with extensive ulcerative disease or with an underlying coagulopathy.

MALLORY-WEISS TEAR

Mallory-Weiss tears usually occur in gastric mucosa, although 10% to 20% occur in esophageal mucosa. They account for approximately 5% to 7% of cases of upper GI hemorrhage.[6-9] A history of retching is obtained in less than one third of patients.[19] Bleeding from Mallory-Weiss tears remits spontaneously in most patients; 5% experience rebleeding. Patients who experience rebleeding from a Mallory-Weiss tear usually have an underlying bleeding diathesis.[20,21]

ANGIODYSPLASIA

Angiodysplasia of the GI tract is a common source of bleeding that can occur anywhere from stomach to colon. The cause of these lesions is not clear. These lesions also occur in patients with Osler-Weber-Rendu syndrome.

TABLE 23-1	Risk Factors for Death After Hospital Admission for Acute Upper Gastrointestinal Hemorrhage

Advanced age
Shock on admission (pulse rate > 100 beats/min; systolic blood pressure < 100 mm Hg)
Comorbidity (particularly hepatic or renal failure and disseminated cancer)
Diagnosis (worst prognosis for advanced upper gastrointestinal malignancy)
Endoscopic findings (active, spurting hemorrhage from peptic ulcer; nonbleeding visible blood vessel; large varices with red spots)
Rebleeding (increases mortality 10-fold)

DIVERTICULOSIS

The prevalence of diverticular disease is age dependent, increasing from less than 5% at age 40 to 30% by age 60, to 65% by age 85. The high prevalence of the disease explains why diverticulosis is the most common cause of lower GI bleeding even though fewer than 15% of patients with diverticulosis develop significant diverticular bleeding. Diverticular bleeding typically occurs in the absence of diverticulitis, and the risk of bleeding is not further increased if diverticulitis is present.[22] Risk factors for diverticular bleeding include[23]:
1. Relative lack of dietary fiber
2. Aspirin and NSAID use
3. Advanced age
4. Constipation

COLITIS

Infectious, ischemic, and idiopathic colitis (inflammatory bowel disease) can all manifest initially with hematochezia. Mucosal inflammation (colitis) is the common response to acute or chronic injury, resulting in activation of the immune system and inflammatory cascades. Establishing a specific diagnosis is paramount in the treatment of acute colitis, since therapy is dependent on the underlying disease process. The diagnosis requires an interpretation of the histologic and gross findings within the clinical context.

NEOPLASMS

Colon cancer is a relatively less common but serious cause of hematochezia. Neoplasms are responsible for approximately 10% of cases of

rectal bleeding in patients older than 50 years, but neoplasms are rarely implicated as the etiology for GI bleeding in younger individuals.[24] Bleeding occurs as the result of erosion or ulceration of the overlying mucosa. The bleeding tends to be low grade and recurrent. Bright red blood suggests left-sided lesions; right-sided lesions can manifest with maroon blood or melena.

HEMORRHOIDS

Hemorrhoidal bleeding typically is painless, often presenting as bright red blood on stools, in the toilet, or on toilet paper. Hemorrhoids are dilated submucosal veins in the anus, located above (internal) or below (external) the dentate line.[25] They usually are asymptomatic but can manifest with hematochezia, thrombosis, strangulation, or pruritus. Hematochezia results from rupture of internal hemorrhoids that are supplied by the superior and middle hemorrhoidal arteries.

Initial Management of Gastrointestinal Bleeding

Bleeding stops spontaneously in most patients, but aggressive management is required when bleeding does not quickly resolve or when patients are at high risk for rebleeding. Priorities include achieving hemodynamic stability and preventing complications such as pulmonary aspiration.[26,27] The rate of bleeding dictates the urgency of management:
1. Patients with trace hemoccult test–positive stools and without severe anemia can be managed as outpatients.
2. Visible blood requires hospitalization and inpatient evaluation.
3. Persistent bleeding or rebleeding with hemodynamic instability necessitates admission to the intensive care unit (ICU).
4. Massive bleeding, defined as loss of 30% or more of estimated blood volume or bleeding requiring blood transfusion of 6 or more units in 24 hours, requires aggressive diagnostic and resuscitative methods in the ICU and the involvement of the intensivist, the gastroenterologist, and, frequently, the GI surgeon.

In patients with upper GI bleeding, the amount of blood loss can be estimated by measuring the return from a nasogastric tube. An approximate estimate of blood loss can be made by the hemodynamic response to a 2-L crystalloid fluid challenge:
1. If blood pressure returns to normal and stabilizes, blood loss of 15% to 30% has occurred.
2. If blood pressure rises but falls again, blood volume loss of 30% to 40% has occurred.
3. If blood pressure continues to fall, blood volume loss of greater than 40% has probably occurred.

The degree of blood loss also can be estimated clinically by an evaluation of the heart rate, blood pressure, respiratory rate, urine output, and mental status (Table 23-2). The clinical estimation of blood loss is somewhat more difficult in patients with cirrhosis who have

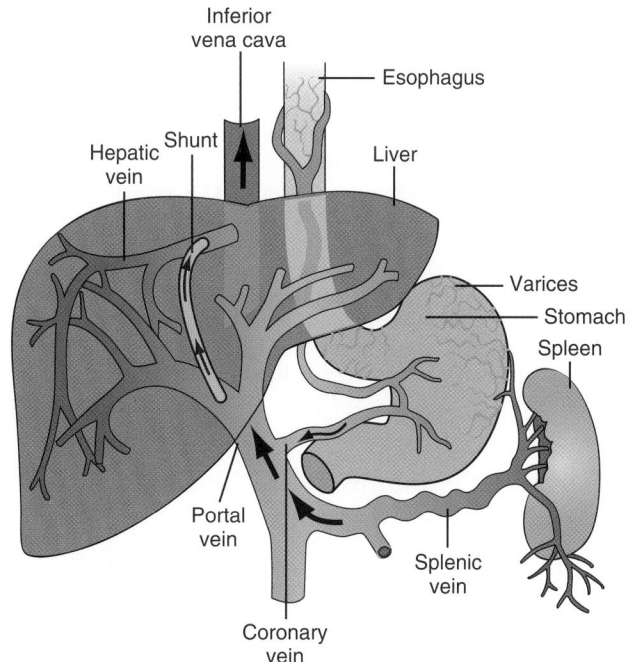

Figure 23-1 Transjugular intrahepatic portosystemic shunt (TIPS).

TABLE 23-2	Clinical Indicators as to Degree of Blood Loss			
Blood loss (mL)	<750	750-1500	1500-2000	>2000
Blood loss (% blood volume)	<15%	15%-30%	30%-40%	>40%
Blood pressure	Normal	Normal	Decreased	Decreased
Pulse pressure*	Normal	Decreased	Decreased	Decreased
Pulse rate	<100	>100	>120	>140
Respiratory rate	14-20	20-30	>30	>35
Urine output (mL/h)	>30	20-30	<20	<10
Mental status	Anxious	Anxious	Anxious and confused	Confused and lethargic
Fluid replacement	Crystalloid	Crystalloid	Crystalloid + blood	Crystalloid + blood

*Pulse pressure may be widened in patients with cirrhosis.

hyperdynamic circulation at baseline and a lower-than-normal systolic blood pressure and widened pulse pressure.

HISTORY AND EXAMINATION

Assessment of comorbidities, careful cardiopulmonary evaluation including measurement of blood pressure and postural changes, heart rate, chest auscultation, ability of the patient to protect his or her airway, and a digital rectal exam to evaluate stool quality and assess for mass, hemorrhoids, fissures, or fistula are essential.

The clinical features of the GI bleeding provide clues to the probable source of bleeding within the GI tract (Table 23-3). When small amounts of bright red blood are passed per rectum, the lower GI tract can be assumed to be the source. In patients with large-volume maroon stools, aspiration via a nasogastric tube should be performed to assess the possibility of upper GI bleeding. Examination of nasogastric aspirate has diagnostic value, although in approximately 15% of patients with upper GI bleeding, the nasogastric aspirate fails to reveals blood or "coffee ground" material.[26,27]

All patients with upper GI bleeding should have a nasogastric tube placed. Iced-saline lavage does not prevent or decrease upper GI bleeding.[28] Gastric lavage with lukewarm tap water offers an equally safe and cost-effective alternative.[29] Coffee-ground material or a frankly bloody gastric aspirate confirms an upper GI source of bleeding, whereas a nonbloody yellow-green nasogastric aspirate that contains duodenal secretions suggests the absence of bleeding proximal to the ligament of Treitz.[30] However, in up to 50% of patients with a bleeding duodenal ulcer, a nonbloody gastric aspirate is obtained,[29] possibly because of insufficient reflux of blood from the duodenum through the pylorus. Similarly, an intermittently bleeding upper GI lesion may result in a nonbloody gastric aspirate. The color of the gastric aspirate is of prognostic significance. Patients with coffee-ground or black gastric aspirates and whose stool is melanotic have a reported mortality rate of 9%.[30] However, patients who have bright red blood per gastric aspirate and red blood per rectum have a 30% mortality rate.[30] Red blood per rectum from an upper GI source usually signifies rapid bleeding.[31]

After the gastric contents have been aspirated, the nasogastric tube should be left in place to monitor ongoing bleeding and prevent pulmonary aspiration until there is no longer any evidence of bleeding. Maintaining this tube for a prolonged period, especially when the tube is attached to suction, may injure gastric mucosa and exacerbate GI hemorrhage.[32]

INITIAL RESUSCITATION

Volume resuscitation with crystalloids is the first priority in the management of any patient with GI bleeding. Two large-bore peripheral intravenous (IV) catheters should be inserted and/or a large-bore central line venous catheter should be established. Resuscitation should be initiated with crystalloid solutions, either normal saline (2 L) or lactated Ringer's solution. Large-volume resuscitation with normal saline alone may cause a hyperchloremic metabolic acidosis and is possibly associated with coagulation abnormalities. Colloidal solutions have no role in the management of patients with acute GI bleeding. A complete blood count including platelet count should be obtained.

Other key laboratory studies should include blood typing and cross-matching, prothrombin time (or international normalized ratio), activated partial thromboplastin time, blood chemistry panel, liver function panel. Transfusion of packed red blood cells should be initiated for patients with an estimated blood loss greater than 15%. Transfusion of fresh frozen plasma should be initiated for patients with preexisting coagulopathy (from liver disease or anticoagulation; see Table 23-2). Platelet transfusion is indicated if the platelet count is less than $50,000/\mu L$.

The endpoints of resuscitation include normalization of heart rate, blood pressure, and indices of end-organ perfusion. Vasopressor agents initially should be avoided because pressor-mediated vasoconstriction in a hypovolemic patient can cause severe end-organ ischemia.[33] Patients with a history of congestive heart failure, renal failure, or cirrhosis may require monitoring to assess cardiac parameters such as central venous pressure, cardiac output, stroke volume, and/or preload responsiveness. Although bedside pulmonary artery catheterization was widely used in the past for cardiac monitoring in the ICU, the recent trend in critical care medicine has been to use less invasive approaches such as bedside echocardiography or monitoring of pulse pressure variation.

Once venous access has been established, a nasogastric or orogastric tube should be placed to facilitate removal of particulate matter, fresh blood, and clots to facilitate endoscopy and decrease the risk of massive aspiration. Endotracheal intubation is recommended for patients with a high risk of aspiration, such as those with massive bleeding or altered mental status. In addition, endotracheal intubation facilitates endoscopy. While awaiting endoscopy or surgical intervention, octreotide infusion should be commenced in patients with severe upper GI bleeding.

TRIAGE: WHO TO ADMIT TO THE INTENSIVE CARE UNIT

Patients should be categorized as either low risk or high risk based upon prognostic scales that incorporate clinical, laboratory, and endoscopic data. Risk factors for rebleeding or mortality include age older than 65 years; shock; poor health status; comorbidities; low initial hemoglobin level; melena; need for transfusion; and fresh red blood on rectal examination, in emesis, or in nasogastric aspirate. Sepsis and elevated blood urea concentration, creatinine concentration, or serum aminotransferase level are additional risk factors. Endoscopic predictors include active bleeding, nonbleeding visible blood vessel, adherent clot, ulcer size greater than 2 cm, adverse ulcer location (posterior lesser gastric curvature or posterior duodenal wall), and adverse lesion type (ulcer, varices, or neoplasm).

The rate of rebleeding is approximately 3% in the low-risk group and 25% in the high-risk group. Patients in the low-risk group can be managed safely on a general medical floor. The decision regarding ICU admission should be individualized based on the patient's risk stratification, age, comorbid diseases, clinical presentation, and endoscopic findings. Patients with active bleeding and two or more comorbidities have a mortality rate above 10% and should be observed in an ICU.[34] Patients with coronary artery disease are best managed in an ICU because of the risk of myocardial ischemia secondary to hypovolemia and hypoperfusion.[45] Admission to an ICU should be considered when endoscopic stigmata of recent hemorrhage, particularly visible vessels, are noted.

▨ Further Management of Upper Gastrointestinal Bleeding

Endoscopy is the modality of choice for determining diagnosis, prognosis, and therapy for upper GI bleeding. Endoscopy should be performed after the patient has been adequately resuscitated and has achieved a degree of hemodynamic stability, but within 24 hours of presentation. In patients who have had relatively minor bleeding, endoscopy can be performed on a semielective basis.

TABLE 23-3	Clinical Indicators of Gastrointestinal Bleeding and the Probable Source Location Within the Gastrointestinal Tract		
Clinical Indicator	**Probability of Upper Gastrointestinal Source**	**Probability of Lower Gastrointestinal Source**	
Hematemesis	Almost certain	Rare	
Melena	Probable	Rare	
Hematochezia	Possible	Probable	
Blood-streaked stool	Rare	Almost certain	
Occult blood in stool	Possible	Possible	

NONVARICEAL BLEEDS

A meta-analysis of a large number of studies of nonvariceal bleeds demonstrated that endoscopic intervention decreased the mortality rate.[35] Multiple endoscopic therapies, including injection of epinephrine, injection of alcohol, injection of thrombin, injection of fibrin glue, thermal contact, or application of hemostatic clips, have been evaluated. Monotherapy with epinephrine provides suboptimal hemostasis. However, epinephrine plus a second method significantly reduces the risk of rebleeding, surgery, or mortality.

VARICEAL BLEEDING

Variceal bleeding stops spontaneously in more than half of patients; however, in those who continue to bleed, the mortality rate approaches 80%. Without treatment to obliterate the varices, there is a 60% to 70% risk of rebleeding. The risk for acute recurrent bleeding is highest within the first 72 hours of the initial bleed and decreases with time, similar to the case for peptic ulcer hemorrhage.[36,37] Another option is variceal band ligation[37,38]; advantages over injection sclerotherapy include fewer local and systemic complications, lower rebleeding rates, fewer endoscopic treatment sessions to obliterate varices, and lower mortality rate.[38-42]

The diagnostic and therapeutic value of endoscopy in patients with upper GI bleeding is often limited by the presence of residual blood or clots.[43] To avoid this problem, gastric lavage is usually performed with a large-diameter nasogastric tube just before endoscopy.[44] Erythromycin induces rapid gastric emptying in healthy subjects and in patients with diabetic gastroparesis.[44-46] Infusion of erythromycin (250 mg) just prior to endoscopy improves esophagogastroduodenal cleansing and enhances the quality of endoscopic findings.[45]

Further Management of Bleeding Peptic Ulcers

PHARMACOLOGIC THERAPY

Although gastric acid–suppressing agents such as histamine receptor 2 blockers (H_2 blockers) have long been available as treatment options for patients with peptic ulcer disease, in acutely bleeding patients, their use has not reduced the number of transfusions, episodes of further bleeding or rebleeding, or the need for surgery.[46]

Proton pump inhibitors (PPIs) are now widely used to suppress gastric acid secretion in patients with a variety of acid-related disorders.[47] Data from a number of studies[48-54] suggest that IV administration of a PPI reduces the risk of recurrent upper GI bleeding, but this therapy may not affect other outcome variables. Somatostatin is effective for controlling hemorrhage from esophageal varices,[55-57] but its efficacy in the setting of nonvariceal upper GI hemorrhage has not been demonstrated.[58]

ROLE OF SURGERY

Although surgical intervention for peptic ulcer bleeding is less common than in the past, the indications for operation remain unchanged, including severe hemorrhage unresponsive to initial resuscitative measures; unavailability or failure of endoscopic or other nonsurgical therapies to control persistent or recurrent bleeding; and a coexisting second indication for operation, such as perforation, obstruction, or suspicion of malignancy.[59,60]

In a clinical trial that enrolled patients with recurrent upper GI hemorrhage, patients who were randomized to receive endoscopic retreatment had significantly fewer complications and tended to have decreased transfusion requirements, 30-day mortality rate, and use of the ICU than patients who were randomized to surgery.[61] Nevertheless, 10% to 12% of patients with acute ulcer hemorrhage still require operative intervention for adequate hemostasis.[62]

Further Management of Esophageal Varices

PHARMACOLOGIC INTERVENTIONS

Vasopressin causes direct splanchnic and systemic vasoconstriction mediated via the V_1 receptor on vascular smooth muscle and thereby decreases portal venous flow and portal pressure.[63] Vasopressin can be administered either IV or directly into the superior mesenteric artery. As with other potent vasoconstrictors, vasopressin must be administered via a central venous line. Higher doses are associated with increased toxicity without further benefit. Vasopressin achieves hemostasis in about 55% of patients.[64] Systemic side effects, which occur in 20% to 30% of patients, can include myocardial ischemia, cerebral ischemia, acrocyanosis, congestive heart failure, cardiac arrhythmias, hyponatremia, hypertension, and phlebitis at the venous infusion site. Concomitant administration of nitroglycerin, either IV or sublingually, improves the safety and efficacy of vasopressin.[65] The combination of vasopressin and nitroglycerin more effectively controls bleeding and reduces toxicity but does not reduce mortality compared to vasopressin alone.[66] Terlipressin, a synthetic vasopressin analog, has been used instead of vasopressin to attempt to reduce the toxicity.[67] Terlipressin can be administered as intermittent boluses and has a better side-effect profile than vasopressin. A recent meta-analysis showed reduction in all-cause mortality with terlipressin compared to placebo. No statistical difference in outcome was noted among terlipressin and octreotide, vasopressin, or balloon tamponade. Terlipressin is not currently available for use in the United States.

Somatostatin causes splanchnic vasoconstriction, reduces azygos blood flow, reduces portal collateral circulation, and decreases portal pressure.[68] Somatostatin has been used successfully as an alternative to vasopressin to control variceal bleeding owing to its safer side-effect profile.[69] Octreotide, a synthetic somatostatin analog, is more commonly used than somatostatin and is the drug of choice in the United States. Somatostatin or octreotide therapy in addition to sclerotherapy is superior to either therapy alone in controlling bleeding and preventing rebleeding but has not been shown to improve long-term mortality. Likewise, the combination of somatostatin and endoscopic variceal ligation does not improve long-term mortality. Although both agents control acute bleeding and prevent rebleeding, neither somatostatin nor octreotide have a clearly demonstrated role in improving mortality.[70-74]

BALLOON TAMPONADE

Variceal hemorrhage that is unresponsive to combination therapy with octreotide and endoscopic therapy should be temporarily controlled by balloon tamponade, which initially can control hemorrhage in up to 90% of cases.[75,76] Rebleeding occurs in approximately 50% of cases after balloon deflation if balloon tamponade is used alone.[77] Endotracheal intubation and adequate sedation is essential before placement of the balloon.[78,79] Relative contraindications to balloon tamponade include esophageal stricture, recent caustic ingestion, recent esophageal surgery, large hiatal hernia, recent sclerotherapy, an unproven variceal source of bleeding, and an improperly trained support staff.[80,81] Esophageal rupture occurs in about 3% of cases. Other complications include pulmonary aspiration, alar necrosis, nasopharyngeal bleeding, and balloon impaction.[77,80,81]

TRANSJUGULAR INTRAHEPATIC PORTOSYSTEMIC SHUNT

Transjugular intrahepatic portosystemic shunt (TIPS) is an intrahepatic low-resistance shunt between the hepatic and portal veins created by angiographic methods (see Figure 23-1). The shunt is kept patent by a fenestrated metal stent and decompresses the portal vein, similar to a surgical side-to-side portacaval shunt, but avoids the need for laparotomy.

TABLE 23-4	Complications of Transjugular Intrahepatic Portosystemic Shunt (TIPS)		
Technique-Related Complications	**Complications Related to Portosystemic Shunting**	**Stent-Related Complications**
Neck hematoma	Hepatic encephalopathy	TIPS-associated
Cardiac arrhythmias	Increased risk of bacteremia	hemolysis
Perihepatic hematoma	Liver failure	Infection of stent
Extrahepatic puncture of portal vein		Stent stenosis or ruptured liver capsule malfunction

Approximately 10% to 20% of patients fail to stop bleeding with standard medical therapy. Others rebleed in the first few days after cessation of the index bleed. A second attempt at endoscopic hemostasis is sometimes effective and is generally recommended.[82] TIPS has been shown to achieve hemostasis in patients with refractory hemorrhage from varices. Among high-risk patients, placement of TIPS should be considered sooner rather than later, as significant improvement in mortality has been demonstrated in recent studies. TIPS also has been shown to improve long-term outcomes in patients who are poor candidates for surgery, such as those with sepsis, multiorgan failure, or cardiopulmonary compromise.[83-86] Principal complications of TIPS are listed in Table 23-4.

NONSELECTIVE BETA-BLOCKERS

Nonselective beta-blockers such as propranolol and nadolol have been used to prevent recurrent bleeding. Treatment with these agents can reduce the risk of recurrent bleeding and death from bleeding by about 40%. Sympathetic adrenergic activity regulates splanchnic arteriolar resistance.[87] Blockade of β-adrenergic receptors allows unrestricted α-adrenergic activity, producing splanchnic arteriolar vasoconstriction and decreasing portal venous inflow.

After an oral or IV dose of propranolol, portal pressure decreases by 9% to 31%.[88-95] It has been suggested that a decrease in heart rate and cardiac output also contributes to the decrease in portal venous inflow.[87-90] Findings suggest that the portal decompressive effect of propranolol is a specific splanchnic effect rather than a consequence of its systemic effects.[96] Nitrates such as isosorbide mononitrate have been shown to act synergistically with beta-blockers in reducing hepatic venous pressure gradient. The cumulative risk of hemorrhage was decreased from 29% among those who received nadolol alone to 12% among those who received the combination of nadolol and isosorbide mononitrate.[97] Nitrates, however, may worsen systemic arteriolar vasodilation due to cirrhosis and impair tissue oxygenation, presumably by dilation of arteriovenous channels in the peripheral circulation.

Nadolol has a longer half-life of biological activity[98,99] and can be administered once a day. It is more hydrophilic than propranolol; hydrophilicity limits intestinal absorption after oral administration as well as passage across the blood-brain barrier.[100,101] Propranolol is administered orally twice a day. The dose should be increased slowly until the heart rate decreases by 25% from baseline but remains above 55 beats per minute. Once a stable dose is achieved, propranolol can be changed to a once-a-day, sustained-release form[102] that is equally effective.[103-109]

Patients with a history of variceal bleeding should receive either combination pharmacologic therapy, including beta-blockers and nitrates, or a combination of endoscopic variceal ligation in addition to blood component therapy. The latter strategy has a significantly lower rate of bleeding, but it does not appear to affect survival rate. Combined use of endoscopic variceal ligation and nonselective beta-blockers is recommended for prevention of recurrent variceal bleeding. Combined drug therapy (beta-blockers and nitrates) should be reserved for patients who are not candidates for endoscopic variceal ligation.

SURGICAL MANAGEMENT

Surgery for bleeding esophagogastric varices continues to be the most reliable method to control acute hemorrhage and prevent its recurrence. Operative approaches generally consist of either (1) decompression of the high-pressure portal venous system into the low-pressure systemic venous system by creation of a shunt or (2) devascularization of the distal esophagus and proximal stomach with or without disconnection of the portal and azygous venous systems. In most instances, surgical procedures are used for prevention of recurrent hemorrhage rather than treatment of the initial bleeding episode. Because of the effectiveness of endoscopic therapies, emergency surgery for variceal hemorrhage in most centers is reserved for patients who have failed initial nonsurgical treatment and have reasonable hepatic function.[110]

ANTIBIOTICS IN VARICEAL BLEEDING

Bacterial infections are very common in patients with cirrhosis. Most common causes are urinary tract infections and spontaneous bacterial peritonitis (SBP). Mortality has been shown to be higher in patients with infections than in noninfected patients.[111,112] Infections also predispose patients to recurrent variceal hemorrhage.[113] A meta-analysis of five trials of short-term antibiotic prophylaxis in patients with variceal bleeding showed both a decrease in the number of infections in treated patients and improved survival.[114] Any patient with cirrhosis and GI bleeding should receive a short course of antibiotic therapy (oral norfloxacin, 400 mg twice a day; or IV ciprofloxacin, 1 g once a day).[115] The latter therapy may be appropriate in areas with high prevalence of fluoroquinolone-resistant organisms.

▣ Further Management of Lower Gastrointestinal Bleeding

Eliciting a medical history and identifying pertinent risk factors help in determining the cause of lower GI bleeding. Use of aspirin or NSAID use is strongly associated with diverticular bleeding. Bleeding associated with antecedent hypovolemia should raise the possibility of ischemic colitis, whereas prior radiation therapy for prostate or pelvic cancer suggests radiation proctitis, which can appear months or years after radiation. A history of severe constipation should raise the possibility of a stercoral ulcer, and a recent colonoscopic polypectomy suggests postpolypectomy bleeding.

A careful digital rectal examination and sigmoidoscopy should be done to exclude anorectal pathology and confirm the patient's description of the symptoms. Of rectal carcinomas diagnosed by proctoscopy, 40% are palpable on digital rectal examination.[116]

COLONOSCOPY

Colonoscopy is the mainstay of early and rapid diagnosis and treatment of lower GI bleeding. Colonoscopy has a very high diagnostic yield for patients presenting with lower GI bleeding.[117] In addition, endoscopic therapy is applied to lower GI bleeding for many cases. Modes of endoscopic therapy for acute lower GI bleeding, in particular for angiodysplasia and diverticular disease, include thermal contact probes, laser, monopolar electrocautery (hot biopsy forceps), injection sclerotherapy, and band ligation.

SCINTIGRAPHY AND ANGIOGRAPHY

If the source of bleeding is not detected on colonoscopy, a bleeding scan followed by angiography should be considered if bleeding is severe. Although not as precise in identifying the site of bleeding as angiography, scintigraphy is safe and more sensitive, detecting active bleeding reliably at rates less than 0.1 mL/min.[118,119] Angiographic demonstration of a tumor, neovascularization, or vascular lesions may identify a presumed source of bleeding in the absence of extravasation.

The specificity of this procedure is 100%, but sensitivity varies from 47% with acute bleeding to 30% with recurrent bleeding.

Angiography permits transcatheter administration of vasoconstrictors (vasopressin or terlipressin) for lower GI bleeding.[120] Although hemostasis is frequently achieved, rebleeding can occur in up to 50% of patients after cessation of therapy. Complications include abdominal pain, fluid retention, hyponatremia, transient hypertension, sinus bradycardia, premature ventricular contractions, and atrial fibrillation. Major complications have been reported and include pulmonary edema, serious arrhythmias, myocardial ischemia, and hypertension.[121]

Transcatheter embolization with various embolic agents (e.g., surgical gelatin sponges, microcoils, polyvinyl alcohol particles, detachable balloons) has been used with great success to control massive lower GI bleeding. Ischemic complications appear to be more common when embolization is performed for colonic rather than for upper GI hemorrhage because of the relatively sparse colonic collateral circulation. Embolic therapy may have utility in patients with coronary artery disease or in other situations where vasopressin therapy is relatively contraindicated or has failed. Embolization is an alternative to emergency surgery, primarily in non-neoplastic lesions and in high-risk patients.

SURGERY

Age, probably by association with increased comorbidity, is an important risk factor for postoperative mortality. The postoperative mortality rate in patients undergoing emergent colon surgery for colorectal cancer is 3.7% in patients aged 70 to 79 years, 9.8% in those aged 80 to 89 years, and 12.9% in those older than 90 years.[122] Surgery should be considered when a definite source of bleeding has been identified, but conservative measures have failed to achieve hemostasis. Accurate preoperative localization of the bleeding site is essential for successful segmental colonic resection. Blind segmental resection of the colon or segmental resection is associated with substantial risk of rebleeding and morbidity.[123]

ANNOTATED REFERENCES

van Leerdam ME, Vreeburg EM, Rauws EA, et al. Acute upper GI bleeding: did anything change? Time trend analysis of incidence and outcome of acute upper GI bleeding between 1993/1994 and 2000. Am J Gastroenterol 2003;98(7):1494-9.
This prospective study compared the incidence rate of acute upper GI bleeding as well as endpoints of rebleeding and mortality in a defined geographic area between 1993/1994 and 2000, noting a difference in incidence of bleeding, without substantial improvement in risk of rebleeding or mortality.
Chalasani N, Kahi C, Francois F, et al. Improved patient survival after acute variceal bleeding: a multicenter, cohort study. Am J Gastroenterol 2003;98(3):653-9.
This retrospective multicenter study defined outcomes in variceal bleeding between 1997 and 2000, focusing on several outcomes including in-hospital, 6-week, and overall mortality as well as rate of rebleeding, need for transfusion, and length of stay.
D'Amico G, Pietrosi G, Tarantino I, Pagliaro L, et al. Emergency sclerotherapy versus vasoactive drugs for variceal bleeding in cirrhosis: a Cochrane meta-analysis. Gastroenterology 2003;124(5):1277-91.
This meta-analysis evaluated 15 trials to compare efficacy of emergency sclerotherapy versus pharmacologic management as first-line therapy for variceal bleeding in cirrhotic patients.
Garcia-Pagán JC, Caca K, Bureau C, et al. An early decision for PTFE-TIPS improves survival in high risk cirrhotic patients admitted with an acute variceal bleeding: a multicenter RCT. Hepatology 2008;48(Suppl):373A-4A.
This multi-center randomized control trial evaluated treatment failure and mortality in high-risk variceal bleeders comparing medical/endoscopic therapy with early treatment with TIPS.
Bernard B, Grange JD, Khac EN, et al. Antibiotic prophylaxis for the prevention of bacterial infections in cirrhotic patients with GI bleeding: a meta-analysis. Hepatology 1999;29(6):1655-61.
This meta-analysis demonstrates the value of antibiotic prophylaxis in patients who have had a variceal bleeding episode.

REFERENCE

Access the complete reference list online at http://www.expertconsult.com.

24

Ileus

TIMOTHY R. DONAHUE | JONATHAN R. HIATT

Ileus is defined as disruption of coordinated physiologic bowel motility owing to a nonmechanical cause.[1] As a result, intestinal contents cannot progress through the gastrointestinal (GI) tract. The word *ileus* is derived from the Greek *eileos*, which means "twisting." An ileus can develop as a primary process or as a result of a separate process that is usually associated with inflammation. The diagnosis of ileus must be differentiated from the diagnosis of mechanical bowel obstruction, since the latter condition also blocks the normal aboral progression of bowel contents but is due to the presence of an extrinsic or intrinsic anatomic barrier. These two conditions are treated differently.

Pathophysiology

Physiologic bowel motility is a complex process that results from the interaction of various neural networks and neurohormonal mediators. During the fasting state, the coordinated contractions of the GI tract are referred to as *migrating motor complexes* (MMC). The contractions can be viewed as occurring in three phases: the resting phase, intermittent contractions of moderate amplitude, and high-pressure waves. When a food bolus is introduced into the intestine, the MMCs terminate, and the digested food, or chyme, is propelled through the GI tract via coordinated contractions of the smooth muscle in the intestinal wall, also referred to as *peristalsis*. This process is regulated primarily by the enteric nervous system (ENS), which is comprised of myenteric and submucosal sensory and motor nerve plexi and the interstitial cells of Cajal. The ENS transmits sensory information from the intestinal wall to the central nervous system (CNS) via a network of visceral sensory afferents in the vagus, splanchnic, and pelvic nerves. The ENS also connects the visceral motor efferents in these same nerves with the intestinal smooth muscle cells. The ENS and intestinal smooth muscle activity are inhibited by sympathetic signaling and stimulated by parasympathetic cholinergic signaling. Alternatively, the ENS can function independently of CNS control via the autonomic nervous system through secreted mediators that include substance P, vasoactive intestinal peptide, and nitric oxide.

Ileus can develop when physiologic neural signaling and neurohormonal networks are disrupted. Ileus can result from the presence of inhibitory neuroenteric signaling through increased sympathetic activity, inflammation of surrounding organs or the bowel wall itself, paracrine and endocrine activity of inhibitory gastrointestinal peptides or endogenous opioids, and the use of exogenous opioids for analgesia. The most common clinical situation associated with ileus is the immediate period following abdominal operations. In normal circumstances, physiologic small-bowel motility returns within the first 24 hours after the procedure, gastric motility returns within 24 to 48 hours, and colonic motility within 48 to 72 hours. If the return of normal GI function exceeds these time limits, or ileus develops that is independent of a recent operation, a cause for ileus should be sought.

Clinical Features and Diagnosis

Most patients with ileus exhibit abdominal distension, poorly localized bloating and pain, inability to tolerate oral intake, nausea and vomiting, and obstipation. The absence of bowel sounds on abdominal examination can help distinguish ileus from mechanical bowel obstruction; in the latter condition, high-pitched bowel sounds and/or borborygmi are often audible. Patients with severe and advanced cases of ileus can present with peritonitis due to intestinal ischemia or perforation from bowel dilatation, as well as abdominal compartment syndrome.

Radiographic studies are often obtained during the evaluation of patients with suspected ileus. Abdominal radiographs sometimes can be helpful for differentiating ileus from mechanical small bowel obstruction. The presence of gas in the stomach, small intestine, and colon (Figure 24-1) suggests ileus. In contrast, a paucity of gas within the abdomen, air/fluid levels within the small bowel, and absence of air within the colon suggest mechanical small bowel obstruction (Figure 24-2). A computed tomography (CT) scan with enteral contrast administration can better distinguish patients with ileus from those with mechanical bowel obstruction. Inspection of the abdominal CT scan often makes it possible to accurately localize a point of obstruction or a region of transition from dilated to decompressed bowel. If these findings are present, the diagnosis of mechanical bowel obstruction is established. Passage of oral contrast into the colon within 4 hours favors ileus over a bowel obstruction as the cause of intestinal dysmotility. The CT scan can also identify other intraabdominal inflammatory processes that can be the cause of ileus (e.g., appendicitis, pancreatitis, intraabdominal abscess).

Treatment and Outcome

Treatment is largely supportive until motility returns. Patients should be made nil per os (NPO) and given adequate intravenous fluids to replace insensible losses and sequestration of fluid ("third spacing") within the wall and lumen of the gut. Serum electrolyte levels should be measured and corrected as indicated. Electrolyte abnormalities, including hypokalemia, hyponatremia, hypo- and hypermagnesemia, and hypo- and hypercalcemia, can contribute to the development of ileus. Medications that can inhibit bowel motility—narcotics, phenothiazines, diltiazem, anticholinergics, and clozapine—should be discontinued if possible.

Nasogastric (NG) tube decompression is reserved for patients with abdominal distension, nausea, or vomiting. Several randomized clinical trials have shown that NG decompression does not shorten the duration of ileus in postoperative patients.[2] Moreover, presence of an NG tube can contribute to respiratory complications such as atelectasis and pneumonia.

Nonsteroidal antiinflammatory agents (NSAIDs) should be used for pain control where appropriate; NSAIDs have been shown to reduce postoperative nausea and vomiting as well as improve GI transit in several experimental and clinical studies.[3] NSAIDs not only reduce the need for high doses of narcotics but also can decrease inflammation in the intestinal wall.

A midthoracic epidural catheter should be considered for patients who are undergoing abdominal procedures. The level of the epidural catheter is important because low thoracic and lumbar catheters are less effective. Epidural administration of local anesthetics can reduce the incidence and degree of ileus by blocking afferent as well as efferent inhibitory reflexes, including inhibitory sympathetic efferent signals.[4] Total parenteral nutrition (TPN) should be considered when the duration of ileus exceeds 5 days, particularly for patients who are malnourished.

Most pharmacologic promotility agents that have been tested to hasten the resolution of ileus are ineffective. Metoclopramide

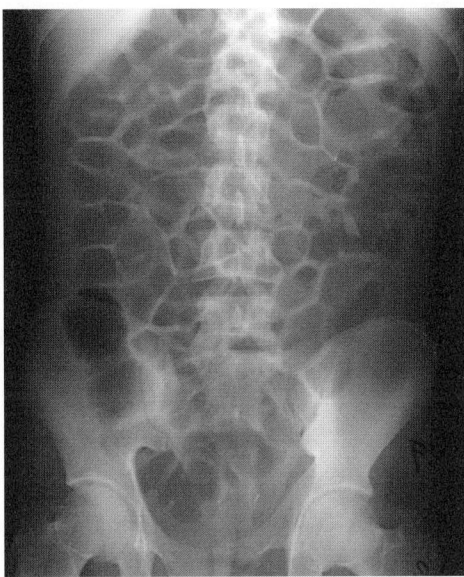

Figure 24-1 Ileus. Abdominal radiograph shows multiple air-filled dilated loops of small bowel as well as an air-filled colon and rectum.

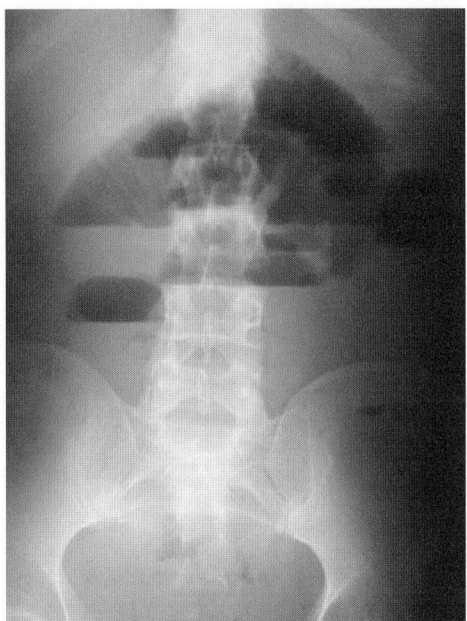

Figure 24-2 Small Bowel Obstruction. Abdominal radiograph shows dilated loops of small bowel and multiple air/fluid levels. Small bowel has a paucity of gas. No evidence of air within colon.

hydrochloride (Reglan), the most frequently used prokinetic agent, is a cholinergic agonist and dopamine antagonist. A number of randomized trials of metoclopramide have failed to demonstrate significant reduction of the duration of postoperative ileus.[5]

More recently, the mu opioid receptor antagonists, alvimopan[6] and methylnaltrexone,[7] have been evaluated in phase III randomized, controlled clinical trials. Because these agents do not cross the blood-brain barrier, they do not interrupt the analgesic effects of narcotics.

Unfortunately, results from studies of these newer agents have been mixed, and the trial designs used to evaluate them were less than optimal; neither are routinely used in clinical practice. Erythromycin is another prokinetic agent that binds to and stimulates the motilin receptor on small-intestinal smooth muscle cells. Two randomized trials examined the effects of erythromycin on the duration of postoperative ileus, and neither demonstrated a beneficial effect.[8]

ANNOTATED REFERENCES

Prasad M, Matthews JB. Deflating postoperative ileus. Gastroenterology 1999;117(2):489-92.
This review article summarizes the pathophysiology and various treatment strategies of postoperative ileus.
Nelson R, Edwards S, Tse B. Prophylactic nasogastric decompression after abdominal surgery. Cochrane Database Syst Rev 2007(3):CD004929.
This large meta-analysis of 33 randomized controlled trials encompassing 5240 patients showed that the routine use of nasogastric decompression did not reduce the incidence of postoperative complications, including return of bowel function.
Ferraz AA, Cowles VE, Condon RE, et al. Nonopioid analgesics shorten the duration of postoperative ileus. Am Surg 1995;61(12):1079-83.
This study showed that postoperative analgesia with the NSAID ketorolac resulted in faster resolution of ileus compared to morphine plus ketorolac by avoiding opioid-induced motor abnormalities in the colon.
Liu SS, Wu CL. Effect of postoperative analgesia on major postoperative complications: a systematic update of the evidence. Anesth Analg 2007;104(3):689-702.
This large meta-analysis identifies consistent evidence that epidural analgesia with local anesthetics is associated with faster resolution of postoperative ileus after major abdominal surgery.

Jepsen S, Klaerke A, Nielsen PH, Simonsen O. Negative effect of metoclopramide in postoperative adynamic ileus. A prospective, randomized, double blind study. Br J Surg 1986;73(4):290-1.
This randomized controlled study of 60 patients showed that metoclopramide did not hasten return of bowel function from the time of abdominal surgery but rather delayed it.
Traut U, Brugger L, Kunz R, et al. Systemic prokinetic pharmacologic treatment for postoperative adynamic ileus following abdominal surgery in adults. Cochrane Database Syst Rev 2008(1):CD004930.
This meta-analysis of 39 randomized controlled trials and 4615 patients showed that alvimopan may shorten the duration of postoperative ileus, whereas erythromycin showed a consistent absence of an effect.
Neyens R, Jackson KC, 2nd. Novel opioid antagonists for opioid-induced bowel dysfunction and postoperative ileus. J Pain Palliat Care Pharmacother 2007;21(2):27-33.
This review article summarizes the clinical trials that have examined the two new peripherally acting mu opioid receptor antagonists, methylnaltrexone and alvimopan.
Smith AJ, Nissan A, Lanouette NM, et al. Prokinetic effect of erythromycin after colorectal surgery: randomized, placebo-controlled, double-blind study. Dis Colon Rectum 2000;43(3):333-7.
This prospective, randomized, placebo-controlled trial enrolled 150 patients undergoing primary resection of colon or rectal cancer and showed that the routine use of erythromycin did not accelerate return of bowel function.

REFERENCES

Access the complete reference list online at http://www.expertconsult.com.

25

Diarrhea

RAJEEV DHUPAR | JUAN B. OCHOA

Diarrhea is one of the most common abnormal manifestations of gastrointestinal (GI) dysfunction in the intensive care unit (ICU); the reported incidence is between 2% and 63%.[1] *Diarrhea* is best defined as bowel movements that, owing to increased frequency, abnormal consistency, or increased volume, cause discomfort to the patient or the caregiver. This definition demonstrates the subjectivity in diagnosing diarrhea, a fact that complicates interpretation of the literature and limits applicability of guidelines. The impact of diarrhea on patient care in the ICU, including its cost in morbidity and mortality, is unknown. However, it is undeniable that diarrhea remains a persistent problem in many ICUs.

Criteria

Several criteria are used to diagnose diarrhea:
1. Abnormal frequency. Normal frequency is described as one or two bowel movements per day and is in part determined by the amount of fiber in the diet. Three or more bowel movements per day are considered abnormal.[1]
2. Abnormal consistency. Abnormal consistency is described as either nonformed stool or stool having excessive fluid content that causes "inconvenience" to the patient, nursing staff, or caregiver. Normal stool water content is 60% to 85% of the total weight.[1]
3. Abnormal amount. Stool amount and volume vary significantly with the amount and type of enteral intake. Insoluble fiber adds a significant amount of bulk volume. A "normal" amount is considered to be approximately 200 grams per day.[1] Abnormal amounts are considered to be greater than 300 grams/d, or volumes greater than 250 mL/d.[1,2]

To date, clinicians are lacking a consistent scale or index that allows a reliable and practical way of measuring stool volume, consistency, and frequency. In its absence, the bedside nurse remains the most reliable person to diagnose the presence of diarrhea.

Pathophysiology

Bowel movements with normal physiologic volume, consistency, and frequency are the result of a GI tract that integrates motility, secretion, and absorption of fluids and adapts to the quality of the food bolus given. The result is a fecal bolus that is produced once or twice every 24 hours and has consistency and fluidity within the boundaries of normal.

Diarrhea results when there is a disorder of GI physiology or when GI tract function is incapable of handling the food bolus. There are several classifications of diarrhea, suggesting that no classification is ideal at helping the clinician plan for patient care. Perhaps the most useful approach is to classify diarrhea according to alterations of physiologic events:
1. Increased fluid secretion that overwhelms absorption. On average, up to 9 liters of fluid is secreted into the GI lumen in addition to the normal oral intake. Less than 1% of that fluid is contained in stool, owing to the amazingly large absorptive capacity of the small and large bowel. Within the intestinal mucosa, passive and active transport of sodium determines the amount of water that is absorbed. Stimulation of the active secretion of fluids into the GI lumen occurs when intracellular levels of the second messenger, cyclic adenosine monophosphate

(cAMP), increase within enterocytes. Increased intracellular cAMP concentration promotes chloride secretion.[3] Thus, diarrhea caused by excessive secretion of fluids is called *secretory diarrhea*. Secretory diarrhea characteristically contains large amounts of fluid and is described as watery. Secretory diarrhea is observed in certain infectious diseases such as cholera or infections with rotavirus. Secretory diarrhea also can be observed in endocrine disturbances associated with carcinoid syndrome or vasoactive intestinal peptide (VIP)-secreting tumors.
2. Increased mucous secretion from the large bowel. Overproduction of mucus by the large bowel can lead to development of diarrhea. Excessive mucus secretion is observed in colonic infections such as *Clostridium difficile* colitis and amebiasis.[4] The incidence of infectious diarrhea in the ICU is unknown.
3. Contaminated food products. Of particular concern is the contamination of the food being given in the ICU. Contamination of enteral formulas can occur at multiple levels, including preparation of the enteral product, use of "open units," addition of modular dietary components, and contamination of the enteral access port (i.e., feeding tube, gastrostomy tube). The incidence of diarrhea due to contaminated feeding tubes is unknown.
4. Diarrhea due to increased osmotic load. Many substances that are taken orally and are not fully absorbed can exert a significant osmotic force, overwhelming the physiologic absorptive capacity of the GI tract. A significant number of patients with diarrhea in the ICU fall into this category.
   a. Osmotic diarrhea caused by medications. Sorbitol is frequently and inadvertently given to patients in the ICU as a means of preparing many medications for delivery via feeding tubes and is an often overlooked culprit causing diarrhea.[5] Other osmotic agents include Golytely and magnesium-containing medications.
   b. Incomplete digestion and malabsorption. The incidence of malabsorption in the ICU is unknown. However, there are many instances where malabsorption should be considered as a cause of diarrhea in the critically ill patient. These include:
      i. Incomplete protein digestion (azotorrhea). Protein digestion occurs mainly in the stomach by pepsin (only activated at low pH) and hydrochloric acid. In the ICU, virtually all patients receive medications to raise intragastric pH, such as histamine receptor type 2 (H_2) blockers or proton pump inhibitors.[6,7] In addition, feeding tubes frequently "bypass" the stomach, eliminating both gastric acid and gastric proteolytic digestion.
      ii. Undigested carbohydrates. In addition to sorbitol (see earlier discussion), excessive glucose, lactose, or fructose in tube-feeding formulas can overwhelm the absorptive capacity of the small bowel, causing an osmotic influx into the gut lumen.[8]
      iii. Undigested fats. Steatorrhea (diarrhea caused by undigested fats) is characteristically observed in patients with pancreatic insufficiency. Inadvertent lack of mixing pancreatic enzymes with the food bolus can occur in patients with intestinal bypass, pancreatic fistulas, or in patients who have undergone pancreatectomy. It is also observed in patients with incomplete bile production, such as patients who have a biliary diversion.

iv. Excessive dietary load. Diarrhea due to excessive load (overfeeding) of any of the main dietary components (protein, carbohydrate, or fat) can be observed in the ICU. Iatrogenic overfeeding occurs in up to 33% of patients in the ICU, and is a result of inappropriate estimations of caloric and protein needs or inadequate metabolic surveillance.[9] Excessive loads of protein, carbohydrate, or fat also occur with "specialized" formulas that contain altered amounts of one or more of these components. For example, certain diets may contain high amounts of fat, overwhelming digestive and absorptive processes.

v. Atrophy of the GI tract. Atrophy of the intestinal brush border is associated with decreased capacity of digestion and absorption. Atrophy is observed in malnourished patients; thus, diarrhea is observed commonly in patients with hypoalbuminemia. Atrophy also occurs when enteral intake is interrupted for more than a few days. This is a particular problem in surgical patients when prolonged "bowel rest" is ordered.

5. Abnormal motility. Intestinal dysmotility is a frequent problem in the ICU. The use of promotility agents (e.g., erythromycin) can inadvertently cause diarrhea in these patients.

6. Abnormal gut flora. Colonic flora is essential for normal absorption and function of the large bowel. Antibiotics create massive disruptions in colonic flora and can sometimes lead to nosocomial infections with resultant diarrhea. Currently, *C. difficile* is the leading cause of nosocomial diarrhea and accounts for 30% of patients with antibiotic-associated diarrhea.[10] The gut microflora can be modulated through the use of probiotic agents, but this topic is under intense investigation, and no current guidelines exist regarding their use to treat or prevent diarrhea in ICU patients.[11]

Clinical Consequences of Diarrhea

Untreated, diarrhea can lead to multiple problems. These include:

1. Wound breakdown and secondary soft-tissue infection. Diarrhea can cause a moist, contaminated environment; if left untreated, this can lead to skin breakdown and eventual soft-tissue infection. Particularly concerning are the presence of decubitus ulcers; diarrhea can be either a causative factor or worsen or complicate management.

2. Fluid and electrolyte disturbances are particularly frequent in patients with secretory diarrhea. In these patients, clinicians need to pay attention to fluid replacement and correct metabolic acidosis and/or hypokalemia.

3. Malnutrition. Inadequate nutrient absorption can lead to poor nutrient utilization.

4. Increased workload for nurses and caregivers. Diarrhea imposes a substantial burden on nurses and other caregivers. In addition, the presence of a soiled patient evokes a sense of poor quality of care. Maintaining a clean patient with diarrhea requires additional ICU personnel time and resources that could be better used.

Diagnosis

Careful and complete evaluation of diarrhea is necessary for good patient care. Unfortunately, diarrhea is often ignored or hastily "treated" while clinicians pay more attention to other organ systems. Diagnostic laboratory tests often do not exist, making it ever more difficult to identify and treat the patient. We propose the following approach:

1. Does the patient really have diarrhea? Clinicians rarely will question the diagnosis of diarrhea. Most diagnoses are probably made without a clear understanding of the definition of diarrhea. A concerted effort to diagnose diarrhea by all members of the ICU staff is essential. The creation of scales or indices could become particularly useful as a means of communication. These could also aid in following the effectiveness of treatment.

2. Can an iatrogenic cause explain the presence of diarrhea?
   a. Is the patient on prokinetic agents or stool softeners?
   b. Is the patient receiving medications with high concentrations of sorbitol?
   c. Is the patient being overfed?
   d. Is the patient intolerant to any of the components of the diet?
   e. Is a specialized diet providing an excessive amount of a substance (e.g., fat) that the patient is having difficulty digesting?
   f. Is bypassing the stomach or inhibiting acid secretion affecting the digestion of protein?
   g. Is the patient on any other medication that can cause diarrhea?

3. Assessing the patient's absorptive or digestive capacity.
   a. Does the patient have gut atrophy, as seen with prolonged bowel rest? Would this patient benefit from an intestinal rehabilitation strategy?
   b. Is the patient malnourished?
   c. Does the patient have a condition (e.g., pancreatitis) that alters the secretion of digestive enzymes?
   d. Does the patient have a chronic disease process (e.g., short gut syndrome) that alters absorption?

4. Does the patient have an infection?
   a. Is there any evidence of contamination of feeding tubes? Are you using a closed system? How often is it being changed?
   b. Is there cause for nosocomial bowel infection? Is the patient *C. difficile* toxin negative?
   c. Has colonic flora been altered significantly with antibiotics?

Treatment

Treatment is dependent on identification of the underlying cause. One or several reasons for the presence of diarrhea generally can be identified. Once identified, the causes of diarrhea should be eliminated, modified, or treated. In particular, iatrogenic causes of diarrhea should be identified and corrected whenever feasible. For example, prolonged courses of prophylactic antibiotics are no better than short courses for the prevention of surgical site infections; therefore, adherence to current guidelines to limit antibiotics is important.[12,13]

Modification of the diet may be important if the GI tract is being overwhelmed with high quantities of a particular nutrient. This is particularly important for patients receiving formulas that deliver excessive fat loads.

Digestive enzymes such as pancreatic enzymes or bile substitutes should be supplemented when the disease process (or treatment) is associated with decreased production of these enzymes.

Agents that inhibit GI motility, such as loperamide, should be used with caution. These drugs are often ordered empirically and may worsen underlying pathology, especially when the causative agent is infectious.

Bulk-forming agents are sometimes given to patients to improve the consistency of the fecal bolus. These agents have to be used in the appropriate amount, since they can also be a cause of diarrhea.[14]

Antibiotics to treat infectious diarrhea also should be used with caution. If the diarrhea is causing minimal discomfort and is of no physiologic consequence, waiting for arrival of results of tests for *C. difficile* may be advised.[15]

Restoring normal colonic flora has become an increasingly frequent practice in the ICU. Provision of prebiotics and probiotics in different presentations is now being suggested, but the implications of such therapies are not clear and require further investigation.[11,16] Soluble fiber may have a role in restoring normal colonic function and flora.

Stopping or decreasing the rate of enteral nutrition is often done; however, this is only advocated if the patient is being overfed or exhibits intolerance to the diet. Only under exceptional circumstances should stopping oral intake and giving total parenteral nutrition be advocated as a treatment for diarrhea.

Conclusions

Diarrhea is a poorly studied clinical manifestation of GI dysfunction in the ICU. The true incidence of diarrhea in ICU patients is unknown because of the lack of a universally accepted definition or a concerted effort to study the problem. Despite these limitations, when discovered, diarrhea can be effectively treated with careful clinical evaluation of the patient and easily implemented therapeutic measures.

ANNOTATED REFERENCES

Cunha BA. Nosocomial diarrhea. Crit Care Clin 1998;14:329–38.
  This article reviews both noninfectious and infectious causes of nosocomial diarrhea.
Dallal RM, Harbrecht BG, Boujoukas AJ, et al. Fulminant *Clostridium difficile*: an underappreciated and increasing cause of death and complications. Ann Surg 2002;235:363–72.
  This article is a single-institution review of the epidemiology and outcomes of patients with C. difficile colitis.
Nelson RL, Glenny AM, Song F. Antimicrobial prophylaxis for colorectal surgery. Cochrane Database Syst Rev 2009;1:CD001181.
  This reviews the evidence for the duration of antibiotics in the post-colorectal surgery patient and makes recommendations based on the most recent data.

Pilotto A, Franceshi M, Vitale D, Zaninelli A, DiMario F, Seripa D, et al; FIRI; SOFIA Project Investigators. The prevalence of diarrhea and its association with drug use in elderly outpatients: a multicenter study. Am J Gastroenterol 2008;103:2816–23.
  This is a multicenter study of the incidence of diarrhea in nonhospitalized elderly patients on different medication regimens including antibiotics and PPIs.
Wiesen P, van Gossum A, Presier JC. Diarrhoea in the critically ill. Curr Opin Crit Care 2006;12:149–54.
  This article reviews the causative factors, pathophysiology, and potential treatments of ICU-associated diarrhea.

REFERENCES

Access the complete reference list online at http://www.expertconsult.com.

26

Rashes and Fever

CHESTON B. CUNHA | BURKE A. CUNHA

Clinical Approach

The clinical diagnostic approach to rash and fever in the intensive care unit (ICU) depends on whether the rash and fever were community or nosocomially acquired. Community-acquired rash and fever is best approached by considering the distribution/characteristics of the rash.[1-5] Rashes are visible clues to infectious or noninfectious disorders. In addition to rash and fever, often associated findings such as history, physical examination, and laboratory abnormalities are keys to the correct diagnosis.[1,4,6-8]

Nosocomially acquired rashes have more limited differential diagnostic possibilities.[6] The clinician should determine whether the rash and fever represents the primary clinical problem or is a superimposed finding unrelated to another process—for example, ICU patients admitted for acute myocardial infarction can develop a drug rash from an antiarrhythmic medication, beta-blocker, diuretic, or sulfa-containing stool softener (Colace).[1,3]

Acutely ill patients with rash and fever in the ICU should have the benefit of an infectious disease consultation by an experienced infectious disease clinician.[1,3] Both community and nosocomial acquired rash/fever are best diagnosed using the clinical syndromic approach; associated clinical findings, not the appearance of the rash per se, are the main determinants of arriving at the correct diagnosis.[5,7]

COMMUNITY-ACQUIRED RASH AND FEVER

Patients admitted to the ICU from the community with rash/fever are best approached by the type/distribution of the rash.[2] The degree of fever relative to the pulse rate, and fever pattern are also important diagnostic considerations.[3,9]

Petechial/Purpuric Rashes and Fever

While petechial/purpuric rashes are common causes of community-acquired rash/fever, petechiae can accompany a variety of systemic infections as well as a variety of noninfectious disorders.[10-12] Rash/fever are often potentially life-threatening (e.g., meningococcemia [MC] with or without meningitis, Rocky Mountain spotted fever [RMSF], dengue fever [DF], and arboviral hemorrhagic fevers), and patients should have the benefit of a diagnostic evaluation by an experienced infectious disease consultant.[1,4,10,11]

The two most common infectious diseases presenting with a petechial/purpuric rash are MC and RMSF. RMSF should be suspected with a recent tick exposure history and/or a characteristic location/distribution of the rash. Importantly, RMSF is the only infectious exanthem that begins on the wrists and/or ankles.[13-15] In contrast, the rash of MC is asymmetrical with irregularly shaped painful petechial/purpuric lesions.[1,8,11]

Post-splenectomy sepsis (PSS) can resemble meningococcemia but only occurs in patients with impaired/absent splenic function.[1,4,11] Clinicians should be familiar with the disorders associated with diminished splenic function. A key clinical clue to impaired splenic function is the presence of Howell-Jolly bodies or "pocked/pitted" red blood cells in the peripheral smear. The number of Howell-Jolly bodies or "pocked/pitted" RBCs is inversely proportional to splenic function.[1,8]

High-grade/continuous Staphylococcus aureus bacteremias (methicillin sensitive/methicillin resistant [MSSA/MRSA]) from abscesses or acute bacterial endocarditis (ABE) are often accompanied by splinter hemorrhages and petechial/purpuric rashes on the distal extremities.[1,10,11]

Maculopapular Rashes and Fever

The most common maculopapular rashes/fever associated with serious systemic diseases are toxic shock syndrome (TSS) and systemic lupus erythematosus (SLE). SLE flares can mimic infectious diseases.[1,4,11] Thus, SLE pneumonitis can mimic community-acquired pneumonia (CAP), and SLE cerebritis can mimic acute bacterial meningitis (ABM). Laboratory studies can differentiate an SLE flare in the absence of infection from an SLE flare with infection. Typically, SLE flares without infection are accompanied by leukopenia, decreased complement levels, and elevated α_1/α_2 globulins on serum protein electrophoresis (SPEP).[1,8]

TSS can occur in any patient colonized/infected with a TSS-1-producing strain of S. aureus. TSS may not come to mind when there are no overt signs of clinical infection (e.g., staphylococcal colonization of the nares). TSS also may be due to group A streptococci or Clostridium sordelli.[2,4,11]

Vesicular/Bullous Rashes and Fever

Vesicular eruptions limit the diagnostic possibilities to chickenpox or herpes zoster (shingles) due to varicella zoster virus (VZV). Herpes zoster may be localized (dermatomal) or disseminated.[5-7] Before the appearance of the vesicular rash/fever, dermatomal herpes zoster, depending on dermatomal distribution, can be a difficult diagnostic problem, mimicking many disorders.[6] Herpes zoster involving the head and/or neck may be associated with VZV meningitis/encephalitis. Disseminated shingles can resemble chickenpox, but patients with herpes zoster have a prior history of chickenpox.[1,4,11]

Community-acquired bullous lesions in the ICU may be due to S. aureus soft-tissue infection, Vibrio vulnificus, or gas gangrene (clostridial myonecrosis). Except when due to S. aureus, all the causes of bullae/fever are painful and tense and accompanied by diarrhea. Clostridial myonecrosis, (i.e., gas gangrene) may be present after a crush injury or trauma. The commonest cause of bullae/fever is S. aureus cellulitis/pyoderma.[10-12]

The differential diagnostic features of community-acquired rash/fever are presented in tabular form in Tables 26-1 to 26-16.[1-19]

NOSOCOMIAL-ACQUIRED RASH AND FEVER

Petechial/Purpuric Rashes and Fever

Staphylococcal bacteremia (high-grade/continuous) is usually related to an intravascular/interventional procedure/device.[1,3] Staphylococcal bacteremias or ABE present initially with petechial/purpuric lesions that later can become hemorrhagic and/or gangrenous. The diagnosis is suggested by the peripheral location of the irregular painful petechial/purpuric lesions in the setting of high-grade and/or continuous staphylococcal bacteremia.[1,4,11]

An underrecognized but important cause of nosocomial rash/fever is cholesterol emboli syndrome (CES).[20] Cholesterol emboli may be released into the systemic circulation during or following cardiovascular procedures. CES presents as a petechial/purpuric rash with a livedo reticularis–like appearance.[1,8] The rash occurs on the trunk and/or extremities and may be accompanied by signs of cholesterol emboli to other organs such as the heart (myocardial infarction), pancreas (acute

TABLE 26-1 Community-Acquired Rash and Fever in the ICU

Petechial/Purpuric Rashes

Disorder	Central > Peripheral	Peripheral > Central	Palms and Soles Rash	Rash Details	Clinical Features	Other Features	Differential Diagnosis (Key DDx Points)
Meningococcemia (MC)		+	±	Rash appears 1-2 hours after fever Irregular/painful petechial lesions Early, spares palms/soles/face Late, may involve palms/soles Often appear in "crops," especially near pressure points Many petechial/purpuric lesions (vs. RMSF) Prognosis ~ number of petechiae	**Clinical Findings:** Headache, myalgias Hypotension (if Waterhouse-Friderichsen syndrome) Rapidly fatal (well at 1pm, dead at 3pm!) **Laboratory Findings:** Leukocytosis Thrombocytopenia SGOT/SGPT: WNL Early complement components ↓ (C_{1-3}) DIC (schistocytes and thrombocytopenia) common **Diagnosis:** Clinical appearance/presentation Blood cultures positive for Neisseria meningitidis Petechiae/purpura Gram stain/culture positive for N. meningitidis	History of recent upper respiratory tract infection Common in late winter–early spring May present alone or with meningococcal meningitis Digital gangrene (late)	**RMSF:** Tick exposure Common in early/late summer Relative brady-cardia Conjunctival suffusion Bilateral periorbital edema Petechial rash on wrists/ankles Edema of dorsum of hands/feet WBC count: WNL Elevated SGOT/SGPT Blood cultures negative for N. meningitidis Digital gangrene (late) **Enteroviruses:** Rash prominent on face/trunk Petechiae small/regularly shaped on face/extremities > trunk Loose stools/diarrhea common WBC/platelet counts: WNL Elevated enterovirus titers **Staphylococcus aureus bacteremia/SBE:** New/changing heart murmur PMH positive for valvular disease or recent intra-cardiac procedure/device High-grade bacteremia; blood cultures positive for (4/4–4/4) S. aureus (MSSA/MRSA) If ABE, TTE-positive vegetations **Postsplenectomy sepsis (PSS):** Underlying disorder associated with hyposplenic function (see PSS) No Howell-Jolly bodies and/or "pocked/pitted" RBCs No target cells or Pappenheimer bodies Blood cultures positive for Staphylococcus pneumoniae, Haemophilus influenzae, or Capnophagia canimorsus; (N. meningitidis) less likely **Henoch-Schönlein purpura (HSP):** Small-vessel vasculitis (more common in children) Often preceded by an upper respiratory viral infection, drugs, or immunizations Only extensive purpuric rash limited to below the waist Fevers < 102°F without chills Abdominal pain prominent ± Periarticular tenderness Palpable purpura below the waist with arthralgias, abdominal pain, or GMN should suggest HSP Blood cultures negative Urinalysis shows hematuria/RBC casts Skin biopsy shows leukoclastic vasculitis with IgA deposition in small vessel walls Kidney biopsy shows focal/segmental GMN

DIC, disseminated intravascular coagulation; GMN, glomerulonephritis; SGOT, serum glutamic-oxaloacetic transaminase; SGPT, serum glutamic-pyruvic transaminase.

TABLE 26-2	Community-Acquired Rash and Fever in the ICU

Petechial/Purpuric Rashes

Disorder	Central > Peripheral	Peripheral > Central	Palms and Soles Rash	Rash Details	Clinical Features	Other Features	Differential Diagnosis (Key DDx Points)
Rocky Mountain spotted fever (RMSF)		+	+	Rash appears 3–5 days after fever Begins on wrists/ankles Painless macular rash early Relatively few petechial/purpuric lesions (vs. meningococcemia)	**Clinical Findings:** Relative bradycardia Conjunctival suffusion Severe frontal headache Bilateral periorbital edema ±Splenomegaly ±Abdominal pain Edema of dorsum of hands/feet Hypotension late (due to excessive fluids/myocarditis) **Laboratory Findings:** WBC: WNL Thrombocytopenia Normal ESR Mildly Increased SGOT/SGPT CXR: No infiltrates **Diagnosis:** Clinical appearance/presentation Elevated Rickettsia rickettsii titers	Usually occurs in late spring/early fall History of recent tick exposure No infiltrates on CXR unless CHF (late)	**Meningococcemia (MC):** Not toxemic in appearance No relative bradycardia No periorbital edema No edema of hands/feet Doesn't start on wrists/ankles Leukocytosis Blood cultures/lesions positive for Neisseria meningitidis **Typhus:** Recent louse exposure (epidemic typhus) or flea exposure (murine typhus) Rash truncal (spares palms/soles) CNS symptoms (delirium, vertigo, tinnitus) common GI symptoms (nausea/vomiting) common Elevated Rickettsia prowazekii or Rickettsia typhi titers **Atypical measles:** Received killed measles vaccine (1963-1968) Nodular infiltrates on CXR with pleural effusions BHA on CXR Pneumonia predominant clinical finding (unlike RMSF) Maculopapular rash not petechial and does not begin on ankles/wrists Rash spreads centrally to trunk but does not spread above nipple line Dry cough frequent Myalgias and abdominal pain common Edema of hands/feet common Hepatosplenomegaly in some Leukopenia in some No thrombocytopenia Eosinophilia (late) Highly elevated measles titers **Enteroviruses:** Rash prominent on face/trunk Petechiae small/regularly shaped and relatively sparse Loose stools/diarrhea common WBC/platelet counts: WNL Elevated enteroviral titer **Henoch-Schönlein Purpura (HSP):** Small vessel vasculitis (more common in children) Often preceded by an upper respiratory viral infection, drugs, or immunizations Only extensive purpuric rash limited to below the waist Fevers <102°F without chills Abdominal pain prominent ±Periarticular tenderness Urinalysis shows hematuria/RBC casts Palpable purpura below the waist with arthralgias, abdominal pain, or GMN should suggest HSP Skin biopsy shows leukoclastic vasculitis with IgA deposition in small vessel walls Kidney biopsy shows focal/segmental GMN Blood cultures negative

BHA, bilateral hilar adenopathy; CHF, congestive heart failure; CXR, chest x-ray; ESR, erythrocyte sedimentation rate; SGOT, serum glutamic-oxaloacetic transaminase; SGPT, serum glutamic-pyruvic transaminase.

TABLE 26-3	Community-Acquired Rash and Fever in the ICU						
Petechial/Purpuric Rashes							
Disorder	Central > Peripheral	Peripheral > Central	Palms and Soles Rash	Rash Details	Clinical Features	Other Features	Differential Diagnosis (Key DDx Points)
Staphylococcus aureus high-grade continuous bacteremia/ABE		+	+	Rash appears days after fever Irregular painful petechial/gangrenous lesions on distal extremities	**Clinical Findings:** Fever >102°F Shaking chills New/changing heart murmur if ABE Clinical focus/source of bacteremia (e.g., abscess) usually apparent **Laboratory Findings:** Leukocytosis ±Thrombo-cytopenia Increased ESR/CRP SGOT/SGPT: WNL **Diagnosis:** Clinical appearance/presentation Petechial/purpuric lesions Gram stain/culture positive for S. aureus (MSSA/MRSA) Continuous/high-grade (3/4-4/4) MSSA/MRSA bacteremia TTE: if ABE, positive for vegetation	Recent history of S. aureus (MSSA/MRSA) skin/soft-tissue infections Recent S. aureus (MRSA/MSSA) abscesses	**RMSF:** Tick exposure Common in early/late summer Relative bradycardia Conjunctival suffusion Bilateral periorbital edema Petechial rash on wrists/ankles Edema of dorsum of hands/feet WBC count: WNL Elevated SGOT/SGPT Blood cultures negative for S. aureus (MSSA/MRSA) Digital gangrene (late) **Vasculitis:** No heart murmur No chills Blood cultures negative for MSSA/MRSA TTE: no cardiac vegetations ANA, p-ANCA/c-ANCA positive

ANA, antinuclear antibody; ANCA, antineutrophil cytoplasmic autoantibody; CRP, C-reactive protein; ESR, erythrocyte sedimentation rate; SGOT, serum glutamic-oxaloacetic transaminase; SGPT, serum glutamic-pyruvic transaminase; TTE, transthoracic echocardiography.

TABLE 26-4	Community-Acquired Rash and Fever in the ICU

Petechial/Purpuric Rashes

Disorder	Central > Peripheral	Peripheral > Central	Palms and Soles Rash	Rash Details	Clinical Features	Other Features	Differential Diagnosis (Key DDx Points)
Postsplenectomy sepsis (PSS)	+		−	Rash appears 1-2 days after fever	**Clinical Findings:** Diffuse *asymmetrical purpuric lesions* Fulminant *hypo-tension/shock* **Laboratory Findings:** *Leukopenia Thrombocytopenia Howell-Jolly bodies"pocked/ pitted" RBCs Pappenheimer bodies* and/or *target cells* **Diagnosis:** Clinical appearance/ presentation in *patients with splenectomy scar or disorders associated with hyposplenism** Blood cultures *positive for Streptococcus pneumoniae, Haemophilus influenzae, Neisseria meningitidis,* or *Capnophagia canimorsus* (DF-2)	No seasonal incidence Occurs *in asplenics* (e.g., trauma, staging procedures for lymphoma, congenital asplenia) Also occurs *in patients with disorders that impair splenic function**	**Meningococcemia (MC):** *Not toxemic* in appearance *No relative bradycardia No periorbital edema No edema of hands/feet Doesn't start on wrists/ankles* Blood cultures/lesions *positive* for *Neisseria meningitidis* **Toxic shock syndrome (TSS)** ***Staphylococcus aureus:*** *Hypotension* common *Scarlatiniform rash Conjunctival suffusion Bilateral periorbital edema Mucosal hyperemia Edema dorsum of hands/feet Elevated SGOT/SGPT Elevated CPK Colonization/infection* with *S. aureus* TSS-I producing strain **Henoch-Schönlein Purpura (HSP):** *Small* vessel vasculitis (more common in children *Often preceded by an upper respiratory viral infection, drugs, or immunizations Only extensive purpuric rash limited to below the waist* Fevers <102°F *without chills Abdominal pain prominent ±Periarticular tenderness Palpable purpura below the waist* with arthralgias, abdominal pain, or GMN should suggest HSP Urinalysis shows *hematuria/RBC casts* Skin biopsy shows *leukoclastic vasculitis with IgA deposition in small vessel walls* Kidney biopsy shows *focal/segmental GMN Blood cultures negative*

*Sickle cell trait/disease, cirrhosis, rheumatoid arthritis, SLE, systemic necrotizing vasculitis, amyloidosis, celiac disease, chronic active hepatitis, Fanconi's syndrome, IgA deficiency, intestinal lymphangiectasia, intravenous gamma-globulin therapy, myeloproliferative disorders, non-Hodgkin's lymphoma, regional enteritis, ulcerative colitis, Sézary syndrome, splenic infarcts/malignancies, steroid therapy, systemic mastocytosis, thyroiditis, infiltrative diseases of spleen, mechanical compression of splenic artery/spleen, Waldenström's macroglobulinemia, hyposplenism of old age, congenital absence of spleen.

DIC, disseminated intravascular coagulation; *CPK*, creatine phosphokinase; *SGOT*, serum glutamic-oxaloacetic transaminase; *SGPT*, serum glutamic-pyruvic transaminase; *TSS*, toxic shock syndrome.

pancreatitis), kidneys (acute renal failure), or central nervous system (stroke). Excluding drug rash/fever, cholesterol emboli syndrome is the only acute rash in the ICU associated with peripheral eosinophilia.[8,20]

Drug rashes are drug hypersensitivity reactions with rash/fever. Most patients who develop drug rashes do so after receiving new medications in the hospital, but some develop drug rash/fever years after being on sensitizing chronic medications. Drug rashes are generalized, maculopapular/petechial, and may be pruritic. Fever is usually present and may be high (>102°F); it is regularly accompanied by relative bradycardia.[8,9] Mild increases of serum transaminase levels and eosinophiles in the blood smear are common findings.[8] The clinical difficulty with drug rash/fever is distinguishing it from underlying medical disorders. Even after discontinuing the sensitizing drug, rash/fever may take days/weeks to resolve.[1,3,4,9]

Maculopapular Rashes and Fever

Maculopapular rash due to surgical TSS is uncommon. Typical surgical TSS occurs from wound infection several days after surgery. A key clinical clue is that drainage from the wound is serosanguineous rather than purulent.[5,7,11,12]

Vesicular/Bullous Rashes and Fever

Particularly following distant extremity trauma or distal abdominal surgery, gas gangrene should be considered in the differential diagno-

sis.[3,6] In patients with gas gangrene (i.e., clostridial myonecrosis), the vesicular/bullous eruptions spread rapidly (over minutes/hours). The skin near the bullous lesions is tense and extremely tender, and the fluid in the lesions is not foul smelling. Patients with gas gangrene are afebrile or have only a low-grade fever, but these patients often have watery diarrhea.[1,3] A key clinical clue to gas gangrene is rapidly progressive hemolytic anemia due to lysis of red blood cells by clostridial lethicinases.[1,4,11] On physical examination, gas in tissues is not clinically detectable or obvious and is not a feature of gas gangrene. On computed tomography (CT) scan, small gas bubbles may be visible along muscle planes.[1,3] Large collections of gas in the soft tissues on imaging studies should suggest a mixed aerobic-anaerobic infection by nonclostridial gas-producing organisms. Mixed aerobic-anaerobic soft-tissue infections are most common in diabetics and do not involve muscle (myonecrosis).[1,3,10]

Fever is usually prominent with mixed aerobic/anaerobic soft-tissue infections, but clostridial gas gangrene characteristically is associated with little or no fever. The differential diagnosis of nosocomial rashes/fever is presented in Tables 26-17 to 26-22.[1,4,10,11]

The diagnostic approach to rash/fever depends on correctly correlating the location/characteristic of the rash with associated non-dermatologic features such as physical examination findings or laboratory findings, or both, to arrive at a clinical syndromic diagnosis (Tables 26-23 and 26-24).[1-20]

TABLE 26-5	Community-Acquired Rash and Fever in the ICU

Petechial/Purpuric Rashes

Disorder	Central > Peripheral	Peripheral > Central	Palms and Soles Rash	Rash Details	Clinical Features	Other Features	Differential Diagnosis (Key DDx Points)
Dengue fever (DF), Dengue shock syndrome (DSS), Dengue hemorrhagic fever (DHF)	+		–	Rash appears *2-6 days after fever* Rash *begins on thorax* *Scarlatiniform truncal rash with palpable "pinpoint petechiae" (feels like sandpaper)* *Facial flushing*	**Clinical Findings:** Fevers <103°F and are *continuous, not spiking* *"Camel back" fever pattern* *Severe frontal headache and myalgias* *Retro-ocular pain* *Pain on eye movement* *Conjunctival suffusion* *Generalized lymphadenopathy* DSS → same as DF *plus hypotension* DHF → same as DF *plus hemorrhagic manifestations* **Laboratory Findings:** *Leukopenia* *Relative lymphocytosis* late Hemoconcentration (increased Hct >20%) Increased SGOT/SGPT **Diagnosis:** Clinical presentation/ appearance *Increased IgM Dengue virus titers*	Recent travel history to Caribbean, Latin America, or Asia Recurrent *mosquito exposure*	**Chikungunya fever (CK):** *Not endemic* in Caribbean, Latin America *Relative bradycardia* *Polyarthralgias* prominent *Arthralgias* > myalgias *Rash pruritic* *No pinpoint palpable petechiae* Meningoencephalitis *uncommon* *Conjunctival suffusion* Generalized *adenopathy uncommon* Leukocytosis (not leukopenia) *No hemoconcentration* *Elevated* SGOT/SGPT *Elevated* Chikungunya fever titers

DHF, Dengue hemorrhagic fever; *DSS,* Dengue shock syndrome; *Hct,* hematocrit; *SGOT,* serum glutamic-oxaloacetic transaminase; *SGPT,* serum glutamic-pyruvic transaminase.

TABLE 26-6	Community-Acquired Rash and Fever in the ICU

Petechial/Purpuric Rashes

Disorder	Central > Peripheral	Peripheral > Central	Palms and Soles Rash	Rash Details	Clinical Features	Other Features	Differential Diagnosis (Key DDx Points)
Arboviral hemorrhagic fevers (yellow fever, Lassa fever, Ebola fever, Omsk hemorrhagic fever, Marburg virus)	+		±	Rash appears *5-7 hours after fever* Maculopapular rash day # 5 *(early)* *Hemorrhagic manifestations prominent* (epistaxis *late)* *Jaundice early with yellow fever*	**Clinical Findings:** *Hyperacute onset* *Relative bradycardia* Severe headache *Conjunctival suffusion* *Facial flushing/edema* *Severe myalgias/back pain* *Dry cough* *Severe prostration* Sore throat ±*Encephalopathy* ±*Generalized adenopathy* ±*Cervical adenopathy* *(Lassa fever)* **Laboratory Findings:** *Leukopenia* *Thrombocytopenia* Hematuria *Elevated* SGOT/SGPT **Diagnosis:** Clinical appearance/ presentation CDC ELISA RT-PCR (CDC) *positive* for *arboviruses*	History of *recent travel to Africa, Latin America, Asia* *Rapidly fatal*	**RMSF:** *Subacute onset* *Tick exposure* Common in *early/late summer* *Relative bradycardia* Conjunctival suffusion Bilateral *periorbital edema* Petechial rash on *wrists/ ankles* *Edema of dorsum of hands/feet* WBC count: WNL Elevated SGOT/SGPT Blood cultures *negative* Digital gangrene (late) **Meningococcemia (MC):** *Not toxemic* in appearance *No relative bradycardia* *No periorbital edema* *No edema of hands/feet* *Doesn't start on wrists/ankles* Blood cultures/lesions *positive* for *Neisseria meningitidis* **Smallpox (hemorrhagic):** Petechial/purpuric rash in *"swimming trunks"* distribution *Toxemic appearance* *Delirium common* No dry cough *Rapidly fatal early, before vesicles* appear Myalgias *not* prominent

CDC, Centers for Disease Control and Prevention; *DIC,* disseminated intravascular coagulation; *SGOT,* serum glutamic-oxaloacetic transaminase; *SGPT,* serum glutamic-pyruvic transaminase.

TABLE 26-7	Community-Acquired Rash and Fever in the ICU

Petechial/Purpuric Rashes

Disorder	Central > Peripheral	Peripheral > Central	Palms and Soles Rash	Rash Details	Clinical Features	Other Features	Differential Diagnosis (Key DDx Points)
Smallpox (hemorrhagic/ toxic)* **Types:** Hemorrhages *before* rash (**"purpura variolosa"**) Hemorrhages *after* rash (**"variola pustulosa hemorrhagica"**)	+		+	Rash appears *with the* fever *Petechial/hemorrhagic rash in a "swimming trunk" distribution* Petechiae appear *early on inner thighs (Simon's crural triangle) and groin* Petechia in *lateral line from thorax along rib margins to navel* Generalized erythroderma (*"scarlatiniform" rash*) by 2nd day in some Those with "scarlatiniform" rash develop *dark purple velvet skin color by 4th day*	**Clinical Findings:*** *Severe headache and backache precede rash* *Profound toxemia and restlessness* Profound *prostration* Conjunctival *hemorrhages early* Epistaxis *Fetid breath* *Chest heaviness/pain* common Hematuria **Laboratory Findings:** *Leukopenia* *Relative lymphocytosis* *Monocytosis* Normoblasts with basophilic stippling *Thrombocytopenia* SGOT/SGPT: WNL **Diagnosis:** Clinical appearance/ presentation	Patients may expire *before* vesicular lesions develop *Sudden death* on 6th day fever from pulmonary edema *not* hemorrhages *Suspect bioterrorism*	**Toxic shock syndrome (TSS)** ***Staphylococcus aureus:*** *Hypotension* common *Scarlatiniform rash* *Conjunctival suffusion* Bilateral *periorbital edema* *Mucosal hyperemia* *Edema dorsum of hands/feet* *Elevated SGOT/ SGPT* *Elevated CPK* *Colonization/infection* with *S. aureus* TSS-I producing strain **Typhus:** Recent *louse exposure* (epidemic typhus) or *flea exposure* (murine typhus) Rash truncal (*spares palms/soles*) CNS symptoms (delirium, vertigo, tinnitus) *common* GI symptom (nausea/vomiting) *common* Elevated *Rickettsia prowazekii* or *Rickettsia typhi* titers **Postsplenectomy sepsis (PSS):** *Underlying disorder associated with hyposplenic function (see PSS)* No *Howell-Jolly bodies* and/or *"pocked/pitted" RBCs* No *target cells* or *Pappenheimer bodies* *Blood cultures positive* for *Streptococcus pneumoniae, Haemophilus influenzae,* or *Capnophagia canimorsus (N. meningitidis) less likely* **Meningococcemia (MC):** *Not toxemic* in appearance *No relative bradycardia* *No periorbital edema* *Diffuse* (irregularly shaped) *painful petechiae* Petechiae not in a "*swimming trunks*" distribution *No edema of hands/feet* *Doesn't start on wrists/ankles* *Leukocytosis* (not leukopenia) Blood cultures/lesions *positive* for *Neisseria meningitidis*

*Refers to early hemorrhagic smallpox
DIC, disseminated intravascular coagulation; *SGOT,* serum glutamic-oxaloacetic transaminase; *SGPT,* serum glutamic-pyruvic transaminase.

TABLE 26-8	Community-Acquired Rash and Fever in the ICU

Maculopapular Rashes

Disorder	Central > Peripheral	Peripheral > Central	Palms and Soles Rash	Rash Details	Clinical Features	Other Features	Differential Diagnosis (Key DDx Points)
Systemic lupus erythematous (SLE)	+			Rash may appear *with flare* *Periorbital rash* (common) *Vasculitic rash* (±*painful*) *on extremities* not uncommon	**Clinical Findings:** High-spiking fevers, ±chills *No* relative bradycardia Fevers may be due to *SLE flare* ±*Abdominal pain* **Laboratory Findings:** *Leukopenia* *Relative lymphopenia* ±*Thrombo-cytopenia* *Elevated ESR* SGOT/SGPT: WNL SPEP Elevated α_2-globulins with SLE flare but *not with infection* In SLE, *if* elevated SGOT/SGPT or *atypical lymphocytes present*, test for elevated CMV IgM titer/CMV PCR **Diagnosis:** Clinical appearance/presentation *Leukopenia* + *ANA* + *ds-DNA* *Decreased* CH50 *Negative* blood cultures *With SLE flare, positive* CMV or Parvo B_{19} titers	*PMH: SLE* SLE *flare common during/after steroid taper* CMV *may induce SLE flare* Associated with SLE *flare are: cerebritis, pneumonitis, peritonitis, or serositis* *Migratory pulmonary infiltrates with effusions characteristic of SLE pneumonitis* Rule out infection and *diagnose SLE flare* Bacterial infections common in SLE, but *not during SLE flare*	**Drug rash:** *Often atopic* PMH Cause of drug fever *usually not an antibiotic* Patient looks "relatively well" (*not septic*" for degree of fever 102°F-106°F *Relative bradycardia* (if temperature >102°F and not on β-blockers, diltiazem, or verapamil) *Pruritus common* Rash *usually due to chronic drugs, not new drugs* *Rash always generalized*, not localized *Leukocytosis* common (with left shift) *Eosinophils common* (eosinophilia less frequent) Elevated ESR Mildly elevated SGOT/SGPT After sensitizing medication stopped, *fevers may persist for days or weeks* **Adult Kawasaki's disease:** *High fevers* (>102°F) >5 days *No relative bradycardia* *Conjunctival suffusion* Mild *anterior uveitis* (in most) *Nonexudative pharyngitis* *Mucosal hyperemia* *Bilateral cervical adenopathy* Scarlatiniform rash Erythema multiforme–like rash (in some) Diarrhea/abdominal pain common *Carditis* (nonspecific) ST/T wave abnormalities) ±*Splenomegaly* *Perianal hyperemia* *Edema of dorsum of hands/feet* *Leukocytosis* *Thrombocytopenia* (1st week) *Thrombocytosis* (2nd-3rd week) *Highly/persistently elevated ESR* *Mildly elevated* SGOT/SGPT *Highly elevated ferritin levels* *Sterile pyuria*

ANA, antinuclear antibodies; *CH*, total hemolytic complement; *CMV*, cytomegalovirus; *ds-DNA*, double-stranded DNA; *ESR*, erythrocyte sedimentation rate; *SGOT*, serum glutamic-oxaloacetic transaminase; *SGPT*, serum glutamic-pyruvic transaminase; *SPEP*, serum protein electrophoresis.

TABLE 26-9	Community-Acquired Rash and Fever in the ICU

Maculopapular Rashes

Disorder	Central > Peripheral	Peripheral > Central	Palms and Soles Rash	Rash Details	Clinical Features	Other Features	Differential Diagnosis (Key DDx Points)
Drug rash	+		+	*Rash appears hours-days after fever* Rash often *pruritic* *Drug rash is generalized, not localized* (chest, back, or only extremities)	**Clinical Findings:** Patient *appears "relatively well"* *Relative bradycardia* constant finding if patient has temperature >102°F and is not on β-blockers, diltiazem, or verapamil **Laboratory Findings:** *Leukocytosis* (with left shift) *Eosinophils common in CBC* (eosinophilia *less frequent*) ±Thrombo-cytopenia Elevated ESR *Mildly elevated SGOT/SGPT* *Elevated IgE levels* **Diagnosis:** Clinical appearance/ presentation Blood cultures *negative excluding contaminants* (unless underlying infection) After stopping sensitizing medication rash may *continue for days* *Fevers may also for continue weeks*	Patient on a "sensitizing" medication* Drug rashes often due to chronic medications (*not usually new medications*) *Pruritus is* common May have an infectious disease *plus* a drug rash	**Contact dermatitis:** *Pruritus common* *Limited to one area of the body* *No eosinophilia* *SGOT/SGPT: WNL* Due to *local contact* with tape, topical medications, gowns/bedding **Toxic shock syndrome (TSS)** *Staphylococcus aureus:* *Hypotension* common *Scarlatiniform rash* *Conjunctival suffusion* Bilateral *periorbital edema* *Mucosal hyperemia* *Edema dorsum of hands/feet* *Elevated SGOT/SGPT* *Elevated CPK* *Colonization/infection* with S. aureus TSS-I producing strain **Scarlet fever:** Not atopic; *not on sensitizing medications* *No relative bradycardia* Most common in *children and young adults* <30 years Sore throat with *bilateral anterior cervical adenopathy* Rash *prominent early on face/trunk* Rash *spreads rapidly* to rest of body *Rash blanches on pressure* and has "sandpaper texture" *Mucosal hyperemia* ("strawberry tongue") *Circumoral pallor* *Pastia's lines* in axilla/antecubital fossa *Only bacterial infection with eosinophilia* SGOT/SGPT=WNL *Throat culture positive* for Group A streptococci *Elevated ASO titer* **Adult Kawasaki's disease:** *High fevers* (>102°F) >5 days *No relative bradycardia* *Conjunctival suffusion* Mild *anterior uveitis* (in most) *Nonexudative pharyngitis* *Mucosal hyperemia* *Bilateral cervical adenopathy* *Scarlatiniform rash* *E. multiforme*-like rash (in some) Diarrhea/abdominal pain common *Carditis* (nonspecific) ST/T wave abnormalities) ±Splenomegaly *Perianal hyperemia* *Edema of dorsum of hands/feet* Leukocytosis *Thrombocytopenia* (1st week) *Thrombocytosis* (2nd-3rd week) *Highly/persistently elevated ESR* *Mildly elevated SGOT/SGPT* *Highly elevated ferritin levels* *Sterile pyuria*

*Common causes (sensitizing medications) of drug fever/drug rash including allopurinol, sulfa containing drugs e.g., Colace, Lasix, narcotics, antihypertensives, sleep medications, some antibiotics (e.g., β-lactams and TMP-SMX).

ASO, antistreptolysin O; *CPK,* creatine phosphokinase; *ESR,* erythrocyte sedimentation rate; *SGOT,* serum glutamic-oxaloacetic transaminase; *SGPT,* serum glutamic-pyruvic transaminase, *TSS,* toxic shock syndrome.

TABLE 26-10	Community-Acquired Rash and Fever in the ICU

Maculopapular Rashes

Disorder	Central > Peripheral	Peripheral > Central	Palms and Soles Rash	Rash Details	Clinical Features	Other Features	Differential Diagnosis (Key DDx Points)
Measles	+		−	Rash appears *4 days after fever* Rash *begins at hairline and behind ears on head/face* Rash *blanches* on pressure Rash *blotchy/mottled on trunk* Rash *rapidly becomes confluent first on face* Rash *spreads from head to feet in 3 days*	**Clinical Findings:** *Dry cough, runny nose, and sore throat* prominent Laryngitis common *Conjunctivitis* *Tender anterior cervical adenopathy* common **Laboratory Findings:** *Leukopenia* *Relative lymphopenia* ±Thrombo-cytopenia **Diagnosis:** Clinical appearance/presentation *Elevated* IgM measles titers	Mild upper respiratory tract infection *precedes* rash Common in *spring* Toxemic early, but toxemic appearance fades as rash reaches feet *Koplik's spots* ("grains of salt" appearance) on dark red buccal mucosa opposite lower 2nd molar appear 1-2 days before rash (*not* Fordyce aphthae on *pale* buccal mucosa) *May later develop "giant cell" measles pneumonia or later bacterial pneumonia* (rare) In some, abdominal pain (*pseudo-appendicitis*) *Fever peaks day 2 or 3 of rash* then falls Encephalitis (rare) Hemorrhagic measles (mucosal/skin); measles with hemorrhages rare but *often fatal*	**Rubella:** Also occurs in spring Fever <102°F (short duration) Patient *not toxemic* *No URI* symptoms *No conjunctivitis* *No enanthem* Bilateral *posterior cervical adenopathy* *Forchheimer's spots (petechiae) on soft palate* Rash transient and *not confluent* Rash *spreads in 1 day* and *rapidly fades* Rash *doesn't spread from head → feet* WBC count *usually WNL* (mild leukopenia in some) *Elevated* rubella titers **Adult Kawasaki's disease:** *High fevers* (>102°F) >5 days *No relative bradycardia* *Conjunctival suffusion* Mild *anterior uveitis* (in most) *Nonexudative pharyngitis* *Mucosal hyperemia* *Bilateral cervical adenopathy* Scarlatiniform rash Erythema multiforme–like rash (in some) Diarrhea/abdominal pain common *Carditis* (nonspecific (ST/T wave abnormalities) ±Splenomegaly *Perianal hyperemia* *Edema of dorsum of hands/feet* *Leukocytosis* *Thrombocytopenia* (1st week) *Thrombocytosis* (2nd-3rd week) *Highly/persistently elevated ESR* *Mildly elevated* SGOT/SGPT *Highly elevated ferritin levels* *Sterile pyuria* **Epstein-Barr virus (EBV) infectious mononucleosis:** High fevers with *prominent fatigue* Rash has "*sprinkled paprika*" appearance *Bilateral upper eyelid edema* early (Hoaglund's sign) Exudative/nonexudative *pharyngitis* *Palatal petechiae* *Bilateral posterior cervical adenopathy* Splenomegaly (*late*) *Leukopenia* ±Thrombocytopenia Lymphocytosis/atypical lymphocytes (2nd week) Highly elevated ESR 30% have *positive Group A streptococci throat cultures* *Mildly elevated* SGOT/SGPT *Elevated* Epstein-Barr virus VCA IgM titers

IgM, immunoglobulin M; *SGOT*, serum glutamic-oxaloacetic transaminase; *SGPT*, serum glutamic-pyruvic transaminase, *URI*, upper respiratory infection; *VCA*, viral capsid antigen.

TABLE 26-11	Community-Acquired Rash and Fever in the ICU

Maculopapular Rashes

Disorder	Central > Peripheral	Peripheral > Central	Palms and Soles Rash	Rash Details	Clinical Features	Other Features	Differential Diagnosis (Key DDx Points)
Chikungunya fever (CK)		+	±	*Rash appears 3 days after fever* Rash *spares face, palms, soles* Rash *not petechial* "Stocking glove" rash *in some*	**Clinical Findings:** Fever/malaise *initial* manifestations Headache and sore throat *Meningoencephalitis common Severe arthralgias (symmetrical) of distal joints typical Joint tenderness/tenosynovitis* common *Generalized adenopathy common; regional adenopathy (cervical)* uncommon **Laboratory Findings:** *Leukopenia Relative lymphopenia Thrombocytopenia Elevated* SGOT/SGPT **Diagnosis:** Clinical appearance/ presentation *Recent exposure* to chikungunya virus *Elevated chikungunya virus IgM titers*	History of recent travel to *Indian Ocean region or West Africa* Recent *mosquito exposure* Most *common in warmest months*	**Dengue fever:** Recent *travel to Caribbean, Latin America, or Asia Scarlatiniform truncal rash* with palpable "*pinpoint petechiae*" (feels like sandpaper) *Severe* frontal *headache Retro-ocular pain Pain on eye movement Conjunctival suffusion Generalized lymph-adenopathy is tender* Rash begins on *thorax Facial flushing Myalgias* > arthralgias **Typhus:** Recent *louse exposure* (epidemic typhus) or *flea exposure* (murine typhus) *Rash truncal (spares palms/soles) CNS symptoms* (delirium, vertigo, tinnitus) *common GI symptoms* (nausea/vomiting) *common* Elevated *Rickettsia prowazekii* or *Rickettsia typhi* titers

CNS, central nervous system; *GI*, gastrointestinal; *SGOT*, serum glutamic-oxaloacetic transaminase; *SGPT*, serum glutamic-pyruvic transaminase.

TABLE 26-12	Community-Acquired Rash and Fever in the ICU

Vesicular Rashes

Disorder	Central > Peripheral	Peripheral > Central	Palms and Soles Rash	Rash Details	Clinical Features	Other Features	Differential Diagnosis (Key DDx Points)
Disseminated herpes zoster (shingles) VZV	+		±	Rash appears *3-4 hours after fever* Vesicles are *painful* Vesicles *may be pruritic* Early, *spares palms and soles* Vesicles *irregular in shape and not deep in dermis* Vesicles *often hemorrhagic* Vesicles *become pustules (but are not infected with bacteria*	**Clinical Findings:** Rash extends to > *dermatomes* Associated *aseptic* (viral) *meningitis* with VZV of *head/neck* Vesicles on *nose tip* predicts *ocular involvement* (Hutchinson's sign) **Laboratory Findings:** CBC count: WNL *No basophilia* Platelet count: WNL SGOT/SGPT: WNL **Diagnosis:** Clinical appearance/ presentation	Usually occurs in *older adults* History of severe *stress or recent immunosuppression* Underlying *immunosuppression or malignancy (decreased CMI)* May present *alone or may follow dermatomal zoster (<3 dermatomes) that* disseminates	**Chickenpox:** Patients *not toxemic* Vesicles primarily on *trunk > extremities/face* (hands/feet *relatively spared*) Vesicles appear in "*successive crops*" from day 1 to day 3 *Vesicles in different stages of* development *Vesicles superficial* not deep in dermis ("*dew drop*" on rose petal *appearance*) ±*Basophilia Tzanck test positive* Vesicle *fluid DFA positive* for VZV **Hand-foot-mouth disease (HFM):** *Fevers <102°F and prolonged Not toxemic (appear relatively well) Oral vesicles (fragile) appear early (if mouth involved) Any combination* of vesicles/pustules possible (*not always* HFM) Vesicles/pustules surrounded by "*red halos*" *Vesicles oval* in shape and *oriented along skin lines* Vesicles often on *lateral aspects of fingers/toes Elevated coxsackie A/B titers*

CMI, cell-mediated immunity; *SGOT*, serum glutamic-oxaloacetic transaminase; *SGPT*, serum glutamic-pyruvic transaminase.

TABLE 26-13	Community-Acquired Rash and Fever in the ICU

Vesicular Rashes

Disorder	Central > Peripheral	Peripheral > Central	Palms and Soles Rash	Rash Details	Clinical Features	Other Features	Differential Diagnosis (Key DDx Points)
Smallpox (ordinary) Subtypes: Confluent Semi-confluent Discrete	+		±	Rash appears *2-4 days after fever decreases* Macular lesions ("*herald spots*") *appear at hairline* (followed by *papules*) *Exanthem on hard palate*, soft palate, and tongue *early when macules appear* On 3rd day of rash, *papules become vesicular* *Vesicles/pustules rapidly cover the face and upper extremities* Relative *sparing of the trunk* Rash on *palms/ soles appear last* *Umbilication of pustules begins on 5th day*. All vesicles become pustules by 6th day. *Umbilicated pustules are deep in the dermis* Rash is *pruritic* Usually skin lesions are in *same stage of development in each anatomic region* but *stage of rash differs from region to region* *All pustules in same stage of development by 7th day* Rarely, lesions may appear as a "*single crop*" and then present with all lesions in same stage Lesions on extremities (*distal > proximal, extensor* surfaces > flexor surfaces *convexities > concavities*) *Apex of axilla free of lesions* (Rickett's sign) On 9th day, *pustules reach maximum size and begin to flatten* Pustular *scabbing begins on 13th day*	**Clinical Findings:** Prodrome: 10-14 days Patient *appears toxic* *Patient feels better when fever decreases on 3rd day and rash begins* *Abdominal pain common* (pseudo-appendicitis if in RLQ). *Severe headache/backache before rash* Dry cough common Nausea, vomiting or diarrhea in some *Delirium is some* Fever reappears on 7th or on 8th day **Laboratory Findings:** *Leukocytosis* Relative *lymphocytosis* ±*Basophilia* Platelet count: WNL SGOT/SGPT: WNL **Diagnosis:** Clinical appearance/ presentation *Tzanck test negative*	*Suspect bioterrorism* *Exanthem source of airborne viral spread during coughing*	**Chickenpox:** Patients *not toxemic* Vesicles primarily on *trunk > extremities/face* (hands/feet *relatively spared*) Vesicles appear in "*successive crops*" from day 1 to day 3 *Vesicles in different stages of development* *Vesicles superficial not deep in dermis* ("*dew drop on rose petal*" *appearance*) ±*Basophilia* *Tzanck test positive* Vesicle *fluid DFA positive for VZV* **Monkeypox:** Endemic in *West Africa* Exposure to *cats, prairie dogs or West African rodents* Patients *not toxemic* Usually *fewer lesions than smallpox* *Painful regional adenopathy*

DFA, direct fluorescent antibody; *RLQ*, right lower quadrant; *SGOT*, serum glutamic-oxaloacetic transaminase; *SGPT*, serum glutamic-pyruvic transaminase.

TABLE 26-14	Community-Acquired Rash and Fever in the ICU

Vesicular Rashes

Disorder	Central > Peripheral	Peripheral > Central	Palms and Soles Rash	Rash Details	Clinical Features	Other Features	Differential Diagnosis (Key DDx Points)
Chickenpox (VZV)		−	±	Rash appears *with the fever* Lesions *appear in crops for 3 days* then abruptly stop. Vesicles are *at different stages of development* Vesicles lying on skin surface have "*dew drop on rose petal*" appearance *Vesicles surrounded by "red halo"* Vesicles are *pruritic* Vesicles become pustules (but are *not infected with bacteria*) Early, *spares palms and soles*	**Clinical Findings:** Prodrome: 0-2 days Patient does *not appear toxic* Vesicular lesions *not deep in dermis* Vesicles may also be in eye, nose, mouth, vagina, urethra, rectum May develop *chickenpox pneumonia* **Laboratory Findings:** WBC count: WNL ±*Basophilia* Platelet count: WNL ±Increased SGOT/ SGPT **Diagnosis:** Clinical appearance/ presentation *Tzanck test positive*	*Recent close contact with case* Common in *late winter–early spring*	**Smallpox (ordinary):** Patients *toxemic* Vesicles primarily *face, trunk*, and lastly hands/feet Vesicles appear on face *Vesicles in same stages* of development (late) Vesicles transient and *rapidly become pustules* *Vesicles deep in dermis* ±*Basophilia* *Tzanck test negative* Vesicle *fluid DFA positive* for VZV **Monkeypox:** Endemic in *West Africa* Exposure to *cats, prairie dogs or West African rodents* Usually *fewer lesions than smallpox* *Painful regional adenopathy* Patients *not toxemic* **Disseminated herpes zoster (shingles) VZV:** Vesicles *irregular* in shape and *not deep in dermis* Usually occurs in *older adults* History of severe *stress or recent immunosuppression* Underlying *immunosuppression or malignancy* (decreased CMI) May present *alone or may follow dermatomal zoster* (< 3 dermatomes) that disseminates Vesicles become pustules (but are *not infected with bacteria*) Vesicles *often hemorrhagic* Vesicles fluid DFA positive for VZV

SGOT, serum glutamic-oxaloacetic transaminase; *SGPT*, serum glutamic-pyruvic transaminase.

TABLE 26-15	Community-Acquired Rash and Fever in the ICU

Bullous Rashes

Disorder	Central > Peripheral	Peripheral > Central	Palms and Soles Rash	Rash Details	Clinical Features	Other Features	Differential Diagnosis (Key DDx Points)
Vibrio vulnificus	+		−	Rash appears *hours-days after fever* Painful bullous lesions *usually on buttocks*	**Clinical Findings:** Fever/chills *Watery diarrhea prominent* ±*Abdominal pain* **Laboratory Findings:** *Leukocytosis* SGOT/SGPT: WNL **Diagnosis:** Clinical appearance/ presentation Blood/stool/wound cultures *positive* for *V. vulnificus*	Ingestion of *water contaminated with "halophilic vibrios"* Recent exposure of *wound* with water contaminated *with "halophilic vibrios"*	**Gas gangrene:** No recent *colon/pelvic surgery* No exposure to *"halophilic vibrios"* No *fever/chills* No *muscle involvement (myonecrosis)* Culture of bullae *negative* for *Vibrio vulnificus* **Diabetic cSSSIs:** Diabetes may develop bullae (*without infection*) but are *not toxemic* Diabetes with mixed aerobic/anaerobic infections are *febrile but have no muscle* involvement (myonecrosis) Diabetes with mixed aerobic/anaerobic with cSSSIs have *crepitus/abundant gas on soft-tissue x-rays* No *acute hemolytic anemia* No *watery diarrhea* Bullous fluid *foul smelling* Bullous fluid/soft-tissue cultures positive for aerobes/anaerobes (*not clostridia*)

SGOT, serum glutamic-oxaloacetic transaminase; *SGPT*, serum glutamic-pyruvic transaminase.

TABLE 26-16	Community-Acquired Rash and Fever in the ICU

Bullous Rashes

Disorder	Central > Peripheral	Peripheral > Central	Palms and Soles Rash	Rash Details	Clinical Features	Other Features	Differential Diagnosis (Key DDx Points)
Gas gangrene (clostridial myonecrosis)	+		−	Rash appears *suddenly* and *advances in minutes to hours* *Very painful bullae (fluid not foul smelling)* *Skin discolored (orange/black)* and *tense*	**Clinical Findings:** *Low grade/no fevers* *Relative tachycardia* No *crepitus!* Odor of bullous fluid sweetish (*not foul*) **Laboratory Findings:** Leukocytosis *Acute/profound hemolytic anemia* ↑↑↑ LDH *Little/no gas on soft tissue x-rays* **Diagnosis:** Clinical appearance/ presentation Blood or wound cultures *positive* for *clostridial sp.*	*Recent soil related trauma* *Watery diarrhea common* Patient appears *extremely toxemic* *Rapidly fatal without prompt adequate débridement*	**Vibrio vulnificus:** Recent exposure to "halophilic vibrios" *Fever/chills* Watery diarrhea *prominent* *No acute hemolytic anemia* *No myonecrosis* Culture of blood/bullae *positive* for *V. vulnificus* **Diabetic cSSSIs:** Diabetes may develop bullae (*without infection*) but are *not toxemic* Diabetes with mixed aerobic/anaerobic infections are *febrile but have no muscle* involvement (myonecrosis) Diabetes with mixed aerobic/anaerobic with cSSSIs have *crepitus/abundant gas on soft tissue x-rays* *No acute hemolytic anemia* *No watery diarrhea* Bullous fluid *foul smelling* Bullous fluid/soft tissue culture positive for aerobes/anaerobes (*not clostridia*)

cSSSI, complicated skin/skin structures infections; *LDH*, L-lactate dehydrogenase.

TABLE 26-17	Hospital-Acquired Rash and Fever in the ICU

Petechial/Purpuric Rashes

Disorder	Central > Peripheral	Peripheral > Central	Palms and Soles Rash	Rash Details	Clinical Features	Other Features	Differential Diagnosis (Key DDx Points)
Staphylococcus aureus **high-grade continuous bacteremia/ABE**		+	+	Rash appears *3-5 hours after fever* *Irregular painful petechial/gangrenous lesions* on distal extremities	**Clinical Findings:** Fever > 102°F Shaking *chills* *New/changing heart murmur if ABE* *Source of bacteremia* (abscess, CVC, etc.) *usually clinically apparent* **Laboratory Findings:** *Leukocytosis* *±Thrombo-cytopenia* Increased ESR/CRP SGOT/SGPT: WNL **Diagnosis:** Clinical appearance/ presentation Petechial/purpuric lesions Gram stain/culture *positive* for *S. aureus (MSSA/MRSA)* *Continuous/high-grade bacteremia* 3/4-4/4 blood cultures positive for MSSA/ MRSA TTE: If ABE, positive for *vegetation*	Recent history of *intracardiac procedure, CVC, pacemaker/ defibrillator, vascular grafts/ shunts* Recent *post-op MSSA/MRSA skin/soft-tissue infection or abscesses*	**Drug Rash:** *Often atopic* PMH Cause of drug fever *usually not an antibiotic* Patient looks "relatively well" (*not septic*" for degree of fever 102°F-106°F *Relative bradycardia* (if temperature >102°F and not on β-blockers, diltiazem, or verapamil) *Pruritus common* Rash *usually due to chronic drugs, not new drugs* *Rash always generalized*, not localized *Leukocytosis* common (with left shift) *Eosinophils common* (eosinophilia less frequent) Elevated ESR Mildly elevated SGOT/SGPT After sensitizing medication stopped, *fevers may persist for days or weeks* **Cholesterol emboli syndrome:** History of *recent carotid surgery, cardiac catheterization, coronary angioplasty, anticoagulation*, or *open heart surgery* day before rash *Leg pain prominent* Otherwise unexplained, *acute renal failure* typical *GI bleed* common *Normal* peripheral pulses *Toes often purple and painful* **Vasculitis:** *No heart murmur* No chills Blood cultures *negative* for MSSA/MRSA TTE: No cardiac vegetations ANA, p-ANCA/c-ANCA *positive*

ABE, acute bacterial endocarditis; *ANA*, antinuclear antibody; *ANCA*, antineutrophil cytoplasmic autoantibody; *CRP*, C-reactive protein; *CVC*, central venous catheter; *ESR*, erythrocyte sedimentation rate; *MRSA*, methicillin-resistant *Staphylococcus aureus*; *MSSA*, methicillin-sensitive *S. aureus*; *TTE*, transthoracic echocardiography.

TABLE 26-18	Hospital-Acquired Rash and Fever in the ICU

Petechial/Purpuric Rashes

Disorder	Central > Peripheral	Peripheral > Central	Palms and Soles Rash	Rash Details	Clinical Features	Other Features	Differential Diagnosis (Key DDx Points)
Cholesterol emboli syndrome	+	±		Rash appears *hours to days after fever* *Livedo reticularis* extremity rash	**Clinical Findings:** *Signs/symptoms of emboli to various organs may dominate the clinical presentation,* such as heart (acute MI), GI tract (mesenteric ischemia), CNS (CVA), pancreas (pancreatitis), kidneys (renal failure) **Laboratory Findings:** *Leukocytosis* *Eosinophilia* Platelet count: WNL SGOT/SGPT: WNL Other abnormal tests *depending on embolic organ involvement* **Diagnosis:** Clinical appearance/ presentation Blood cultures *negative* for pathogens Petechial/purpuric lesions Gram stain/culture *negative* for pathogens	History of *recent carotid surgery, cardiac catheterization, coronary angioplasty, anticoagulation,* or *open heart surgery* day before rash *Livedo reticularis* extremity rash *Leg pain prominent* *Toes often purple and painful* Otherwise unexplained, *acute renal failure* typical *Eosinophilia* Platelet count: WNL	**SLE:** PMH of SLE ±Heart murmur *Leukopenic* *No eosinophilia* No chills Elevated ESR SGOT/SGPT: WNL Blood cultures *negative* TTE: ±cardiac vegetations Elevated ANA and ds-DNA elevated **Drug rash:** *Often atopic* PMH Cause of drug fever *usually not an antibiotic* Patient looks "relatively well" (*not septic*" for degree of fever 102°F-106°F *Relative bradycardia* (if temperature >102°F and not on β-blockers, diltiazem, or verapamil) *Pruritus common* Rash *usually due to chronic drugs, not new drugs* *Rash always generalized*, not localized *Leukocytosis* common (with left shift) *Eosinophils common* (eosinophilia less frequent) Elevated ESR Mildly elevated SGOT/SGPT After "sensitizing medication" stopped, *fevers may persist for days or weeks* (see drug rash) **Vasculitis:** *No heart murmur* No chills Blood cultures *negative* for MSSA/MRSA TTE: No cardiac vegetations *Positive ANA, p-ANCA/c-ANCA* **S. aureus bacteremia/ABE:** *New/changing heart murmur* PMH positive for valvular disease or *recent intra-cardiac procedure/device* High-grade/bacteremia blood cultures *positive* for (4/4-4/4) *S. aureus* (MSSA/MRSA) TTE: If ABE, *positive* vegetation

ABE, acute bacterial endocarditis; *ANCA,* antineutrophil cytoplasmic autoantibody; *CVA,* cerebrovascular accident; *GI,* gastrointestinal; *MI,* myocardial infarction; *MRSA,* methicillin-resistant *Staphylococcus aureus*; *MSSA,* methicillin-sensitive *S. aureus*; *PMH,* past medical history; *SGOT,* serum glutamic-oxaloacetic transaminase; *SGPT,* serum glutamic-pyruvic transaminase; *SLE,* systemic lupus erythematosus; *TTE,* transthoracic echocardiography.

TABLE 26-19 — Hospital-Acquired Rash and Fever in the ICU

Maculopapular Rashes

Disorder	Central > Peripheral	Peripheral > Central	Palms and Soles Rash	Rash Details	Clinical Features	Other Features	Differential Diagnosis (Key DDx Points)
Surgical toxic shock syndrome (TSS)	+		±	*Diffuse erythroderma* *Erythema intense around wound* *Generalized erythroderma (in some)* *Severe back pain* Wound pain *disproportionate to appearance of wound* *Diffuse erythroderma* *Local wound edema*	**Staphylococcus aureus:** **Clinical Findings:** *Abrupt-onset* fever, rash, and hypotension *Mucosal hyperemia* Edema of *dorsum of hands/feet* Leukocytosis but *not eosinophilia* *Wound discharge serosanguineous (not purulent)* **Diagnosis:** *Blood cultures for S. aureus negative* *Wound cultures for S. aureus positive* **Group A streptococci** **Clinical Findings:** *Often associated with necrotizing fasciitis* *Purple bullae/edema at site (necrotizing fascitis)* *Acute onset hypotension and renal failure in most* **Laboratory Findings:** WBC count: WNL/leukocytosis (*but left shift*) Platelet count: WNL Increased SGOT/SGPT **Diagnosis:** *Blood cultures positive for group A streptococci* *Wound culture positive for group A streptococci* **Clostridium sordellii:** **Clinical Findings:** Acute onset of hypotension, fever and *weakness* Nausea/vomiting common **Laboratory Findings:** ↑↑↑ WBC count: (*leukemoid reactions common* with WBC counts >50 K/mm³) *Thrombocytopenia* Increased SGOT/SGPT **Diagnosis:** Cultures negative for all other pathogens Culture of blood/wound *positive* for C. sordellii	Often nausea, vomiting or diarrhea *Delirium* common History of *recent surgery* Some on *NSAIDs* Cellulitis *Varicella (VZV) infection* Recent *childbirth* *Burn wounds* Associated with *necrotizing soft-tissue infections* Associated with *trauma or cadaveric musculoskeletal grafts* Associated with *recent childbirth or abortion* Associated with *black tar heroin use*	**Drug rash:** *Often atopic* PMH Cause of drug fever *usually not an antibiotic* Patient looks "relatively well" (*not septic*) for degree of fever 102°F–106°F *Relative bradycardia (if temperature >102°F and not on β-blockers, diltiazem, or verapamil)* *Pruritus common* Rash *usually due to chronic drugs, not new drugs* Rash *always generalized*, not localized *Leukocytosis common (with left shift)* *Eosinophils common (eosinophilia less frequent)* Elevated ESR Mildly elevated SGOT/SGPT After sensitizing medication stopped, *fevers may persist for days or weeks*

SGOT, serum glutamic-oxaloacetic transaminase; *SGPT*, serum glutamic-pyruvic transaminase; *VZV*, varicella zoster virus.

TABLE 26-20 — Hospital-Acquired Rash and Fever in the ICU

Maculopapular Rashes

Disorder	Central > Peripheral	Peripheral > Central	Palms and Soles Rash	Rash Details	Clinical Features	Other Features	Differential Diagnosis (Key DDx Points)
Surgical scarlet fever (group A streptococci)	+		±	Rash appears *1-3 days after fever* Scarlatiniform *rash (not pruritic)* *Circumoral pallor* *Mucosal hyperemia* Pastia's *lines in antecubital fossae*	**Clinical Findings:** *Not critically ill* *Not hypotensive* *Conjunctival suffusion* *Wound discharge serosanguineous (not purulent)* **Laboratory Findings:** *Leukocytosis* *Eosinophilia* Platelet count: WNL SGOT/SGPT: WNL **Diagnosis:** Clinical appearance/ presentation Blood/wound cultures *positive* for group A streptococci	History of *recent surgery*	**Surgical TSS:** **Staphylococcus aureus:** Abrupt-onset *fever, rash, and hypotension* *Diffuse erythroderma* *Mucosal hyperemia* Nausea, vomiting, or diarrhea common *Delirium* common *Edema of dorsum of hands/feet* *Erythema intense around wound* *Wound discharge serosanguineous* (not purulent) Leukocytosis but not *eosinophilia* Blood cultures for *S. aureus negative* Wound cultures *positive* for *S. aureus* **Surgical TSS:** **Group A streptococci:** History of *recent surgery* Associated with *NSAIDs* Associated with *cellulitis* Associated with varicella (VZV) *infection* Associated with *recent childbirth* Associated with *burn wounds* *Generalized erythroderma* in some *Severe local pain disproportionate to appearance of wound* *Often associated with necrotizing fasciitis* *Purple bullae/edema at site (necrotizing fascitis)* Acute onset of *hypotension and renal failure in most* *Blood cultures positive* for group A streptococci *Wound culture positive* for group A streptococci

NSAIDs, nonsteroidal antiinflammatory drugs; *SGOT*, serum glutamic-oxaloacetic transaminase; *SGPT*, serum glutamic-pyruvic transaminase; *VZV*, varicella zoster virus.

TABLE 26-21	Hospital-Acquired Rash and Fever in the ICU

Maculopapular Rashes

Disorder	Central > Peripheral	Peripheral > Central	Palms and Soles Rash	Rash Details	Clinical Features	Other Features	Differential Diagnosis (Key DDx Points)
Drug rash	+		+	Rash appears hours-days after fever Rash often pruritic Drug rash is generalized, not localized (chest, back, or only extremities)	**Clinical Findings:** Patient appears "relatively well" Relative bradycardia constant finding if patient has temperature >102°F and is not on β-blockers, diltiazem, or verapamil **Laboratory Findings:** Leukocytosis (with left shift) Eosinophils common in CBC (eosinophilia less frequent) ±Thrombocytopenia Increased ESR Mildly increased SGOT/SGPT Increased IgE levels **Diagnosis:** Clinical appearance/ presentation Blood cultures negative excluding contaminants (unless underlying infection) After stopping sensitizing medication, rash may continue for days Fevers may also continue for weeks	Patient on a "sensitizing" medication Drug rashes most often due to chronic medications (not usually new medications) Sulfa-containing medications common cause of drug fever/rash (e.g., Colace, Lasix) Other common causes of hospital-acquired drug rashes are allopurinol, opiates, and β-lactam antibiotics Pruritus is common May have an infectious disease plus a drug rash	**Contact dermatitis:** Pruritus common Limited to one area of the body No eosinophilia SGOT/SGPT: WNL Due to local contact with tape, topical medications, gowns/ bedding **Toxic Shock Syndrome (TSS)** **S. aureus:** Hypotension common Scarlatiniform rash Conjunctival suffusion Bilateral periorbital edema Mucosal hyperemia Edema dorsum of hands/feet Elevated SGOT/SGPT Elevated CPK Colonization/infection with S. aureus TSS-I producing strain

CPK, creatinine phosphokinase; SGOT, serum glutamic-oxaloacetic transaminase; SGPT, serum glutamic-pyruvic transaminase; TSS, toxic shock syndrome.

TABLE 26-22	Hospital-Acquired Rash and Fever in the ICU

Bullous Rashes

Disorder	Central > Peripheral	Peripheral > Central	Palms and Soles Rash	Rash Details	Clinical Features	Other Features	Differential Diagnosis (Key DDx Points)
Gas gangrene (clostridial myonecrosis)	+		−	*Initial rash appears suddenly and advances in minutes to hours* *Extremely painful bullae (fluid not foul smelling)* *Skin discolored (orange/black) painful and tense*	**Clinical Findings:** *Low grade/no fevers* *Relative tachycardia* *No crepitus!* Odor of bullous fluid sweetish *(not foul)* **Laboratory Findings:** Leukocytosis *Acute/profound hemolytic anemia* ↑↑↑ LDH *Little/no gas on soft-tissue x-rays* **Diagnosis:** Clinical appearance/ presentation Wound Gram stain *positive* from gram-*positive* bacilli (*with few PMNs*) Blood or wound cultures *positive* for *clostridial sp.*	*Recent trauma* Recent *colon/ pelvic surgery* Patient appears *extremely toxemic* *Rapidly fatal without prompt adequate débridement* *Watery diarrhea common*	**Diabetic cSSSIs:** Diabetes may develop bullae (*without infection*) but are *not toxemic* Diabetes with mixed aerobic/ anaerobic infections are *febrile but have no muscle involvement (myonecrosis)* Diabetes with mixed aerobic/ anaerobic with cSSSIs *have crepitus/abundant gas on soft-tissue x-rays* *No acute hemolytic anemia* *No watery diarrhea* Bullous fluid *foul smelling* Bullous fluid/soft-tissue culture *positive for aerobes/anaerobes (not clostridia)*

cSSSI, complicated skin/skin structures infection; LDH, lactate dehydrogenase.

TABLE 26-23	Differential Diagnostic Clinical Features of Fever and Rash in the ICU	
	Infectious Causes	*Noninfectious Causes*
Rash with Shock	TSS MC PSS Overwhelming *Staphylococcus aureus* bacteremia/ABE Arboviral hemorrhagic fevers Hemorrhagic smallpox *Vibrio vulnificus* Gas gangrene Dengue fever	SLE (on steroids)
Rash with Mental Changes	RMSF MC (with meningitis) *S. aureus* ABE (with CNS bleeding) Chikungunya fever Typhus	SLE
Rash with Conjunctival Suffusion	RMSF Dengue fever Arboviral hemorrhagic fevers TSS	Adult Kawasaki's disease
Rash with Relative Bradycardia	RMSF Typhus Dengue fever Typhoid Arboviral hemorrhagic fevers	Drug rash
Rash with Abdominal Pain	*V. vulnificus* Gas gangrene *Clostridium sordelli* Scarlet Fever	Cholesterol emboli syndrome SLE
Rash on Palms and Soles	RMSF TSS Chickenpox Smallpox Monkeypox Scarlet fever	Drug rash
Rash with Diarrhea	*V. vulnificus* Gas gangrene TSS Dengue fever Arboviral hemorrhagic fevers	None
Rash with Edema of Dorsum of Hands/Feet	RMSF TSS	Adult Kawasaki's disease
Rash with Bullae	*V. vulnificus* *S. aureus* cSSSI Gas gangrene	None
Rash with Heart Murmur	ABE	SLE
Rash with Gangrene of Nose Tip	*S. aureus* ABE	SLE Vasculitis
Rash with CVA	Cholesterol emboli syndrome *S. aureus* ABE	None
Rash with Splenomegaly	RMSF Typhus	SLE Adult Kawasaki's disease
Rash with Deafness	RMSF Typhus Meningococcal meningitis	None
Rash with Hepato splenomegaly	RMSF Typhus	Atypical measles
Rash with Hepatomegaly	Typhus	None

ABE, acute bacterial endocarditis; *cSSSI*, complicated skin/skin structure infection; *CVA*, cerebrovascular accident; *DF*, dengue fever; *MC*, meningococcemia; *PSS*, postsplenectomy sepsis; *RMSF*, Rocky Mountain spotted fever; *SLE*, systemic lupus erythematosus; *TSS*, toxic shock syndrome.

TABLE 26-24	Differential Diagnostic Laboratory Features of Fever and Rash in the ICU	
	Infectious Causes	*Noninfectious Causes*
Rash with Elevated SGOT/SGPT	RMSF PSS Arboviral hemorrhagic fevers TSS Dengue fever	Drug rash Adult Kawasaki's disease
Rash with Relative Lymphopenia	RMSF Chikungunya fever Dengue fever	SLE Adult Kawasaki's disease
Rash with Leukocytosis	RMSF ABE (*Staphylococcus aureus*) MC Chikungunya fever	Drug rash
Rash with Eosinophilia	Scarlet fever	Cholesterol emboli syndrome Drug rash
Rash with Leukopenia	TSS PSS Dengue fever Smallpox Arboviral hemorrhagic fevers	SLE Atypical measles
Rash with Generalized Adenopathy	Arboviral hemorrhagic fevers Dengue fever Scarlet fever Measles Rubella	SLE Adult Still's disease

ABE, acute bacterial endocarditis; *DF*, dengue fever; *MC*, meningococcemia; *RMSF*, Rocky Mountain spotted fever; *SLE*, systemic lupus erythematosus; *TSS*, toxic shock syndrome.

ANNOTATED REFERENCES

Cunha BA, editor. Infectious diseases in critical care medicine. 3rd ed. New York: Informa; 2010.
  The only text on infectious diseases in critical care, this book presents a clinical diagnostic and therapeutic approach to infectious and noninfectious disorders with fever and rash in the ICU.
Cunha BA. The diagnostic approach to rash and fever in the critical care unit. Crit Care Clin 1998;8:35–54.
  The classic clinical syndromic approach for clinicians for rash and fever encountered in the ICU.
Schlossberg D. Fever and rash. Infect Dis Clin North Am 1996;10:101–10.
  Classic review on the clinical approach to rash and fever.
Schneiderman PI, Grossman ME, editors. A clinician's guide to dermatologic differential diagnosis. New York: Informa; 2006.
  Two-volume tome on dermatologic differential diagnosis. This is the definitive reference work in the field and should be consulted for the most difficult rash/fever problems.
Lopez FA, Sanders CV. Rash and fever. In: Cunha BA, editor. Educational review manual in infectious disease. 4th ed. New York: Castle Connolly; 2009, p. 15–72.
  Intended for infectious fellow board review, the chapter on rash and fever is excellent and reviews the rash/fever from a clinician's standpoint.
Cunha CB. Differential diagnosis in infectious diseases. In: Cunha BA, editor. Antibiotic essentials. 9th ed. Sudbury, MA: Jones & Bartlett; 2010.
  The best source on differential diagnosis of infectious diseases and their mimics by physical findings and laboratory abnormalities.

REFERENCES

Access the complete reference list online at http://www.expertconsult.com

27

Chest Pain

JAMES M. DARGIN | DAVID T. HUANG

Chest pain in the intensive care unit (ICU) is a somewhat different entity from chest pain seen in the office, inpatient ward, or emergency department. The keys to management of chest pain in the ICU are rapid assessment and treatment of immediately life-threatening conditions, careful consideration of the differential diagnosis, a logical evaluation plan, and empirical treatment while pursuing a definitive diagnosis.

Initial Approach

Several life-threatening conditions can cause chest pain in the critically ill, and the initial approach should focus on prompt evaluation and resuscitation of the airway, breathing, and circulation. Assess the patient's level of consciousness, palpate the pulse, and listen to the breath sounds and heart. Obtain vital signs, including oxygen saturation by pulse oximetry, and ensure that the patient is on a cardiac monitor and has adequate intravenous (IV) access. Adhering to this algorithmic approach (Figure 27-1) in patients with chest pain will ensure that critical conditions such as hypoxemia, hypotension, tension pneumothorax, and unstable ventricular arrhythmias are quickly identified and treated. These conditions, as well as the life-threatening causes of chest pain discussed below, are covered in greater detail in other chapters in this textbook.

History

After the initial evaluation and stabilization, obtain a more detailed history. If the patient can communicate, start with an open-ended question like "What's going on, Mr. Jones?" Physicians typically interrupt patients within 23 seconds, but one should resist this temptation and allow the patient to describe their symptoms.[1] Physicians often neglect to ask even basic questions about the quality of chest pain in patients with aortic dissection, and this omission is associated with a delay in diagnosis.[2] The mnemonic *OLDCAAR* can help avoid this mistake (Table 27-1). Ask the bedside nurse about recent changes in the patient's condition (e.g., changes in mental status, respiratory pattern, or recent medications). Lastly, a quick "chart dissection" should be performed, focusing on the findings noted on initial presentation, reason for ICU admission, past history, and recent progress notes.

Physical Examination

Inspect the chest for asymmetrical excursions, rashes, or obvious sources of pain, such as chest tubes. Palpate the chest and neck for crepitus, which can result from a pneumothorax or pneumomediastinum. Check for pulsus paradoxus and jugular venous distention. Assess for asymmetry in the carotid, femoral, or radial pulses, which can be a sign of aortic dissection. If the breath sounds are asymmetrical, hyperresonance to percussion may confirm a pneumothorax. Cardiac auscultation may reveal a friction rub from pericarditis, "crunching" sounds from mediastinal emphysema, a systolic murmur of aortic stenosis, or an aortic insufficiency murmur from a proximal aortic dissection. A focused examination also should include the abdomen to avoid missing an abdominal catastrophe masquerading as chest pain. Unfortunately, the physical examination has its limitations, and further diagnostic testing is often necessary.

Diagnostic Adjuncts

In the absence of an obvious cause of chest pain (e.g., shingles), a portable chest x-ray (CXR) and electrocardiogram (ECG) should be obtained. Serial cardiac enzymes should be strongly considered to exclude a myocardial infarction (MI). The ECG is often nonspecific but occasionally will show evidence of acute coronary syndromes (ACS), pericarditis, or pulmonary embolism (PE). The CXR is a useful screening tool for life-threatening causes of chest pain, including aortic dissection, pneumothorax, and esophageal rupture. Both the ECG and CXR should be compared with those performed prior to the onset of pain. Although the ECG or CXR may be suggestive of a diagnosis, other confirmatory studies may be necessary.

An IV contrast-enhanced computed tomography (CT) scan can help diagnose a number of causes of chest pain, including PE, aortic dissection, esophageal rupture, pneumothorax, and pneumonia. The benefits of CT scanning, however, must be weighed against the risks of transporting a critically ill patient out of the ICU and the potential for causing contrast nephropathy. Ultrasound can be rapidly performed with minimal risk to the patient and does not require transport out of the ICU. Pericarditis with associated effusion, wall motion abnormality from MI, aortic stenosis, aortic dissection, and pneumothorax are all within the diagnostic realm of ultrasound. Ultrasound has the added benefit of providing information about cardiac function.

Differential Diagnoses

Two rules to live by:
1. Do not assume the admission diagnosis is correct or all inclusive. "Premature closure," or failing to consider alternative diagnoses after a diagnosis has been made is a common cause of medical error.[3] Premature closure likely contributes to the delay in diagnosis described in hospitalized patients with aortic dissection.[4]
2. Do not be biased by the type of ICU to which the patient is admitted. Aortic dissection can present as a stroke, prompting admission to a neurologic ICU; an acute abdomen can develop in a medical ICU patient. Indeed, a review of abdominal catastrophes concluded that "delays in surgical evaluation and intervention are critical contributions to mortality rate in patients who develop acute abdominal complications in a medical ICU."[5]

POTENTIALLY LIFE-THREATENING CAUSES OF CHEST PAIN

Acute Coronary Syndromes

ACS include unstable angina and ST-segment and non–ST-segment elevation MI. The "classic" symptoms of ACS include chest pressure radiating to the left arm, nausea, and diaphoresis, but the history has several limitations with regard to the diagnosis of ACS. Although certain features (pain radiating down the right arm or both arms) are associated with a higher likelihood of ACS, and other characteristics (pleuritic, positional, or sharp pain) with a lesser likelihood, none of these can reliably confirm or exclude the diagnosis.[6,7] Further complicating matters, diabetes, smoking, dyslipidemia, hypertension, and a family history predict the development of heart disease over years in asymptomatic patients but may be less useful in predicting ACS in patients with acute chest pain.[8] Reduction in pain after the

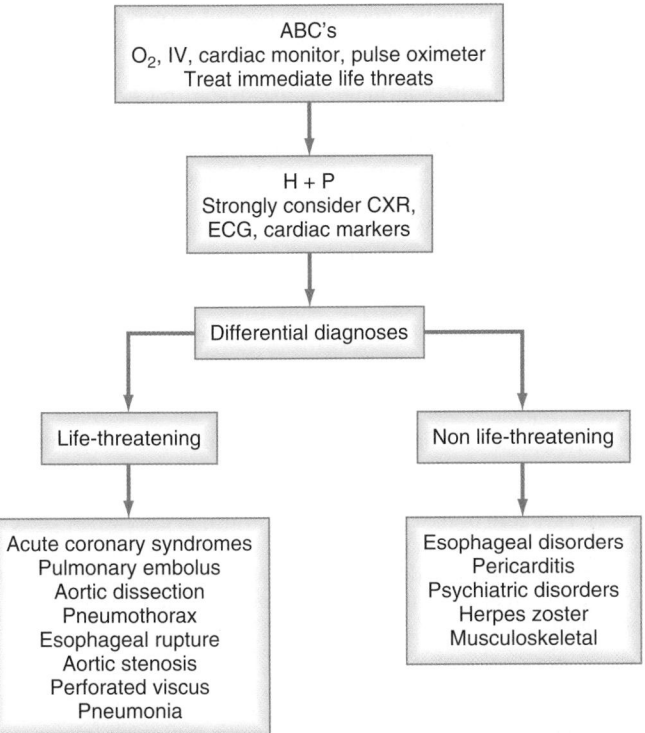

ABC's
O₂, IV, cardiac monitor, pulse oximeter
Treat immediate life threats

↓

H + P
Strongly consider CXR,
ECG, cardiac markers

↓

Differential diagnoses

Life-threatening | Non life-threatening

Life-threatening
Acute coronary syndromes
Pulmonary embolus
Aortic dissection
Pneumothorax
Esophageal rupture
Aortic stenosis
Perforated viscus
Pneumonia

Non life-threatening
Esophageal disorders
Pericarditis
Psychiatric disorders
Herpes zoster
Musculoskeletal

Figure 27-1 Approach to chest pain in the ICU. ABC, airway, breathing, circulation; CXR, chest x-ray; ECG, electrocardiogram; H + P, history and physical examination; IV, intravenous access.

administration of nitroglycerin is also not a reliable indicator of cardiac chest pain.[9] Thus, ACS should almost never be excluded as a cause of chest pain based on the history alone.

Physical examination findings in patients with ACS include signs of left ventricular dysfunction, such as hypotension, jugular venous distention (JVD), and an S_3 heart sound. The ECG should be examined for ST-segment elevation or depression, Q waves, and T wave inversions. The ECG has a low sensitivity for diagnosing MI, but yield increases with serial ECGs. Given the limitations of the ECG and history and examination findings, cardiac enzymes should be measured in most ICU patients with chest pain.

All patients suspected of having ACS should be placed on oxygen and, if not contraindicated, treated with aspirin (or clopidogrel in the setting of aspirin allergy). Sublingual nitroglycerin and IV morphine should be used to relieve pain if the systolic pressure is above 90 mm Hg. Further treatment of ACS is primarily dictated by ECG findings and may include emergency percutaneous intervention or fibrinolysis in the setting of ST-segment elevation.

TABLE 27-1	OLDCAAR Mnemonic for Evaluating Pain
Domain	*Suggested Questions*
Onset	Sudden or gradual? Maximal pain at onset?
Location	Generalized or localized? Can you point with one finger to where it hurts?
Duration	When did it start? Just now, or did the pain occur earlier, but you didn't want to bother anyone? Is it constant or intermittent? If intermittent, is there a trigger, or is it random?
Character	Sharp? Dull? Ache? Indigestion? Pressure? Tearing? Ripping?
Associated symptoms	"Dizzy"—vertiginous or presyncopal? Diaphoresis? Palpitations? Dyspnea? Nausea or vomiting?
Alleviating/aggravating	Position? Belching? Exertion? Deep breathing? Coughing?
Radiation	To the back? Jaw? Throat? Arm? Neck? Abdomen?

Pulmonary Embolism

Approximately 1% to 2% of ICU patients develop deep vein thrombosis (DVT) or PE, but the true incidence is probably higher.[10] Unrecognized PE carries a high mortality, but survival improves dramatically with prompt diagnosis and treatment. Chest pain due to PE is usually pleuritic and often associated with dyspnea, hemoptysis, cough, or syncope.[11] ICU patients usually have risk factors for PE including immobility, advanced age, recent surgery or trauma, malignancy, and central venous catheterization. Do not be deterred from working up PE in patients receiving subcutaneous heparin, as two-thirds of those with DVT and PE are receiving prophylaxis at the time of diagnosis.[10]

Physical examination findings are generally nonspecific in PE. Unexplained tachypnea or tachycardia may be the only diagnostic clues. Hypoxia is often present but is not a universal finding, and its absence cannot exclude PE. A large PE may present as hypotension or cardiovascular collapse. Signs of pulmonary hypertension and right heart failure, such as a loud second heart sound (P_2), JVD, or an S_4 heart sound may be present. Lung examination may reveal crackles, decreased breath sounds, wheezing, rhonchi, or a pleural friction rub.

An elevated arterial-alveolar gradient may be noted on blood gas analysis, but this is a nonspecific finding in the critically ill. The ECG is often normal, but it may show sinus tachycardia, nonspecific ST-segment and T-wave changes, or a right bundle branch block.[12] The CXR can be normal but more commonly reveals nonspecific findings such as pleural effusion, infiltrates, or atelectasis.[13] Although D-dimer testing has been used to rule out venothromboembolic disease in outpatients with a low likelihood of this diagnosis, the D-dimer assay does not appear to be a particularly useful diagnostic tool in the ICU setting.[14] The sensitivity of transthoracic echocardiography (TTE) for PE varies considerably, but the test can be useful in patients who have larger clots that are of hemodynamic significance.[15] In such cases, TTE can be performed rapidly at the bedside when patients are unsafe for transport out of the ICU. TTE has the added benefit of assessing the response to thrombolytics by evaluating right heart function and changes in pulmonary artery pressure.[15] A ventilation/perfusion scan can be time consuming and difficult to perform in mechanically ventilated patients; its interpretation may be obscured by other lung pathology.[16] An IV contrast-enhanced CT of the chest can be performed rapidly, and newer scanners have high sensitivity and specificity, making this the diagnostic study of choice in most ICU patients.

Initial treatment of patients with confirmed PE involves anticoagulation with subcutaneous low-molecular-weight heparin or IV unfractionated heparin. Patients with hemodynamic instability due to PE may require thrombolysis or surgical embolectomy.[17]

Thoracic Aortic Dissection

Aortic dissection results from a tear in the aortic intima, allowing blood to dissect between the intima and adventitia. The Stanford system classifies dissections as type A (involving the ascending aorta) or type B (not involving the ascending aorta). Risk factors include hypertension, advanced age, atherosclerosis, cocaine use, intraaortic catheterization, Ehlers-Danlos syndrome, Turner syndrome, and giant cell arteritis.[18] Patients younger than 40 years are more likely to have Marfan syndrome, bicuspid aortic valve, prior aortic surgery, or aortic aneurysm.[19] The mortality rate is as high as 1% to 2% per hour from symptom onset, and the history remains critical to early diagnosis.[19] Clinicians correctly suspect aortic dissection in more than 90% of cases when questions about quality, radiation, and intensity of the pain are asked. If one or more of these questions is omitted, the correct diagnosis is missed in over half of cases.[2] Many patients complain of sudden onset of chest pain that radiates to the back or abdomen. Contrary to popular belief, patients more commonly describe their pain as sharp, rather than "tearing."[19] Dissection can extend into any of the major aortic branches, causing a multitude of clinical presentations owing to ischemia of the brain, heart, kidney, spinal cord, or gut.

Certain physical examination findings should raise the suspicion of aortic dissection. About one third of patients have pulse deficits in the carotid, radial, or femoral arteries, and some have focal neurologic deficits related to cerebral or spinal cord ischemia.[18] Hypotension often occurs with type A dissection, whereas hypertension is more commonly seen in type B dissection.[20] A significant difference in systolic blood pressure (>20 mm Hg) between the upper extremities may be seen with dissection, but this is not a pathognomonic finding. A diastolic murmur of aortic insufficiency can result from retrograde dissection into the aortic valve.

The ECG may be normal or show nonspecific ST-segment or T-wave changes or left ventricular hypertrophy (LVH) from hypertension. Rarely, the ECG reveals evidence of an MI from dissection into a coronary artery. Over 90% of patients will have some abnormality on CXR, such as widening of the mediastinum, an abnormal aortic contour, pleural effusion, or displacement of intimal aortic calcification from the outer border of the aortic knob.[21] Therefore, it behooves the clinician to scour the CXR for these findings when considering aortic dissection as a cause of chest pain. The diagnosis can be confirmed with CT, magnetic resonance imaging (MRI), or transesophageal echocardiography, all of which have high sensitivity and specificity. The choice of diagnostic study will depend on physician preference and the risks involved. Initial management should focus on blood pressure control, usually with beta-blockers and a potent vasodilator such as nitroprusside.[20]

Pneumothorax

Pneumothorax is caused by air entry from the alveolar space or the atmosphere into the potential space between the parietal and visceral pleura. Pneumothorax in the ICU is often iatrogenic and results from mechanical ventilation (particularly with acute respiratory distress syndrome), attempts at central venous catheterization, thoracentesis, tracheostomy, or bronchoscopy.[22] Virtually any lung pathology can contribute to a pneumothorax, but a ruptured bleb from chronic obstructive pulmonary disease is the most common culprit. Patients with pneumothorax typically complain of sudden onset of ipsilateral pleuritic chest pain with associated dyspnea.

Chest examination may reveal palpable crepitus, decreased breath sounds, decreased chest wall excursion, or hyperresonance to percussion on the affected side. Vital signs may be significant for tachycardia, hypoxia, or tachypnea. Patients with a tension pneumothorax classically have tracheal deviation, JVD, and hypotension. Patients on mechanical ventilation can have increased peak inspiratory airway pressures. The signs of pneumothorax are nonspecific, and any significant deterioration in a patient on a ventilator should prompt a diagnostic evaluation for pneumothorax.

CXRs are often performed in the semiupright or supine position in the ICU, and the classic finding of a visceral pleural line is often seen only on upright CXR. In supine patients, a deep sulcus sign may be seen where the costophrenic angle extends more inferiorly than normal as air collects in this space. Alternatively, a sharp delineation of the cardiac silhouette from the lucency of an anteromedial pneumothorax may be seen. In an experienced operator's hands, ultrasound can effectively rule out a pneumothorax in seconds.[23]

Because of a high rate of conversion to tension pneumothorax in patients on mechanical ventilation, prompt diagnosis and treatment are critical. Treatment involves evacuation of air from the pleural space, usually through tube thoracostomy. In patients with hemodynamic compromise from a suspected tension pneumothorax, treatment with immediate needle thoracostomy, followed by tube thoracostomy, should not be delayed while waiting for a CXR.

Esophageal Rupture

A full-thickness tear of the esophagus carries high mortality, owing to the intense inflammatory response to gastric contents in the mediastinum, secondary bacterial infection, and subsequent sepsis and multisystem organ failure. Most cases of esophageal perforation are caused by upper gastrointestinal tract endoscopy.[24] The risk of esophageal injury from a diagnostic endoscopy is low but increases dramatically when interventions such as dilation or stent placement are performed. Esophageal rupture may be caused by other procedures commonly performed in the ICU, including nasogastric or tracheal intubation. Spontaneous rupture of the esophagus (Boerhaave syndrome) occurs from a sudden increase in intraluminal pressure, usually from vomiting or retching. Patients with esophageal disease such as cancer, Barrett's esophagus, strictures, prior radiation, and varices are particularly vulnerable to rupture. With thoracic perforations, the pain localizes to the substernal or epigastric area, but it may occur in the neck with cervical perforations. Other associated symptoms include dysphagia, odynophagia, and dyspnea.

The patient is often febrile. Crepitus can be felt in the neck with perforation of the cervical esophagus. Mediastinal emphysema can sometimes be detected by a crunching sound on cardiac auscultation, termed *Hamman's sign*. A CXR often reveals subcutaneous emphysema, pneumomediastinum, pneumothorax, or pleural effusion. The CXR is abnormal in almost 90% of cases but may be normal early after the perforation occurs.[24] A water-soluble contrast study of the esophagus or a CT scan of the chest can be performed in cases where there is a high clinical suspicion and the CXR is nondiagnostic.

Treatment may involve operative repair, endoscopic therapies, or conservative management with broad-spectrum antibiotics and close observation.

Aortic Stenosis

Aortic stenosis causes left ventricular outflow obstruction, which leads to left ventricular hypertrophy. Aortic stenosis may result from a congenitally abnormal (bicuspid) valve or rheumatic heart disease in young adults or from valvular calcification in the elderly. Clinical manifestations of aortic stenosis, including angina, congestive heart failure, and syncope, occur when the hypertrophied left ventricle can no longer overcome the valvular stenosis, or when the hypertrophy itself causes diastolic dysfunction or excessive myocardial oxygen demand.

Physical examination features of aortic stenosis include narrow pulse pressure, slow rise of the carotid pulse, a systolic murmur at the right second intercostal space, and an S_4 heart sound. CXR and ECG may show signs left ventricular hypertrophy, but the diagnostic study of choice is a Doppler echocardiogram.

Definitive therapy involves valve replacement. Temporizing management focuses on cautiously decreasing afterload with vasodilators. Angina and congestive heart failure are treated with oxygen and the careful administration of nitrates, morphine, and diuretics. Close hemodynamic monitoring is essential with vasodilators because of the risk of hypotension.

Miscellaneous

Other causes of potentially life-threatening chest pain in the ICU include pneumonia and acute abdominal processes. Pneumonia is often accompanied by pleuritic chest pain or shoulder pain referred from diaphragmatic irritation. A perforated ulcer can sometimes present as a chest pain, and the diagnosis is often made when free air is incidentally discovered under the diaphragm on an upright CXR.

NON–LIFE THREATENING CAUSES OF CHEST PAIN

The following causes of chest pain should be considered only after life-threatening causes have been excluded.

Esophageal Disorders

In patients with noncardiac chest pain, gastroesophageal reflux disorder and esophageal motility disorders (e.g., esophageal spasm) are common. Esophageal disease is associated with pain precipitated by lying flat, postprandial pain, heartburn, or dysphagia. Owing to the shared innervation of the heart and esophagus, visceral pain originating from these two organs can be similar in character. Relief of symptoms after a "GI cocktail" cannot be relied upon to identify chest pain as noncardiac in origin.[25] Confirmatory tests including esophageal manometry and esophageal pH monitoring can be performed, but a trial of a proton pump inhibitor may be a more practical diagnostic approach.[26] Lastly, a nasogastric tube with the distal tip in the esophagus can produce chest pain; this is easily remedied by advancing the tube distally into the stomach.

Musculoskeletal Disorders

The chest wall is a common source of pain in patients without a cardiorespiratory etiology of their symptoms. Pain from costochondritis is often reproduced with palpation or with arm movement. Up to 15% of patients with MI also have chest wall tenderness, so this finding does not exclude ACS.[27] Most cases of costochondritis are self-limiting and treated with nonsteroidal antiinflammatory drugs (NSAIDs). ICU patients may have other causes of chest wall pain, including rib fractures, chest tubes, postoperative pain after cardiothoracic surgery, or an intercostal muscle strain from coughing.

Pericarditis

Pericarditis is a relatively rare cause of chest pain in the inpatient setting.[28] The condition most commonly results from viral or idiopathic causes, but other etiologies include bacterial infections, malignancy, tuberculosis, uremia, autoimmune diseases, transmural MI, and cardiac surgery. Chest pain from pericarditis is typically pleuritic, sharp, retrosternal, and radiates to the back, neck, or arms. The pain is often relieved by sitting forward and exacerbated by lying flat. Although uncomplicated pericarditis is not generally life threatening, pericardial inflammation can lead to pericardial effusion and cardiac tamponade if the effusion is large or acute.

A pericardial friction rub is highly specific for pericarditis and is present in the majority of cases. A pericardial rub sounds similar to hair being rubbed together and is best heard with the diaphragm of the stethoscope over the left sternal border, with the patient sitting forward. Beck's triad (JVD, hypotension, muffled heart tones) is the classic description of pericardial tamponade, but unexplained tachycardia and tachypnea may be early signs. Pulsus paradoxus, or a fall in systolic blood pressure by more than 10 mm Hg with inspiration, is often seen in tamponade but is nonspecific.

ECG findings can clinch the diagnosis of pericarditis. Both MI and pericarditis may result in ST-segment elevation, but with pericarditis, ST-segment depression is typically absent in the reciprocal leads. Absence of Q waves, concave ST-segment elevation, and PR depression strongly favor pericarditis.[28] Careful ECG review, auscultation, and history are key to distinguishing ACS from pericarditis and avoiding the potentially fatal complication of administering thrombolytics to a patient with pericarditis and precipitating hemotamponade. Electrical alternans and low voltage on the ECG, coupled with cardiomegaly on CXR, strongly favor pericardial effusion. Although the ECG and CXR findings of pericardial effusion can be useful, echocardiography should be performed to confirm the diagnosis.

Treatment is aimed at the underlying etiology. NSAIDs relieve pain and inflammation in cases of viral or idiopathic pericarditis. Pericardiocentesis is performed for therapeutic purposes in the case of tamponade and for diagnostic purposes if tuberculosis, bacterial infection, or malignancy is suspected. An IV fluid challenge may be a helpful temporizing measure in hypovolemic patients with tamponade.

Psychiatric Disorders

A significant number of patients with noncardiac chest pain suffer from panic disorder.[29] In addition to chest pain, panic attacks can cause other symptoms that mimic MI, including diaphoresis, dyspnea, palpitations, and a sense of impending doom. A self-report of anxiety helps clue into the diagnosis of underlying panic disorder. Severe illness and its treatment with invasive procedures in the ICU can provoke profound psychological distress. The development of posttraumatic stress disorder is well described in ICU survivors, particularly in patients who experience episodes of extreme fear.[30] Thus, the diagnosis of chest pain due to panic attack may not be acutely life threatening, but this condition should not be considered benign and must be treated. Benzodiazepines are helpful in this regard. Psychiatric patients with cardiac or pulmonary disease can be especially challenging to diagnose, and a thorough, empathetic history is essential.

Herpes Zoster

Reactivation of the varicella-zoster virus from thoracic sensory ganglia causes a painful, dermatomal rash across the chest. The pain of shingles may precede the rash by several days, which can delay the diagnosis. The rash is characterized by vesicles that crust over after approximately one week. Oral acyclovir reduces the duration of herpetic neuralgia. Immunocompromised hosts are at high risk of complications from zoster infections and often require more aggressive treatment with IV acyclovir.

Conclusion

Attention to immediate life-threatening conditions and a thorough history and physical examination after initial stabilization are fundamental to managing chest pain in the ICU. A CXR, ECG, and serial cardiac enzymes should be ordered liberally but intelligently. A high index of suspicion for occult disease is necessary for complex ICU patients.

ANNOTATED REFERENCES

Gajic O, Urrutia LE, Sewani H, et al. Acute abdomen in the medical intensive care unit. Crit Care Med 2002;30(6):1187-90.
  In this retrospective study, delays in surgical evaluation and intervention were independent correlates of mortality. Risk factors for surgical delay included opioid use, mechanical ventilation, no peritoneal signs, antibiotics, and altered mental state. A heightened index of suspicion for an acute abdomen is necessary in ICU patients with these risk factors.
Graber ML, Franklin N, Gordon R. Diagnostic error in internal medicine. Arch Intern Med 2005;165(13):1493-9.
  An analysis of 100 cases identified "premature closure," or failing to consider alternatives once an initial diagnosis was made, as the most common cause of diagnostic error by internists. This study underscores the importance of not assuming that the admission diagnosis is necessarily correct or inclusive.
Hagan PG, Nienaber CA, Isselbacher EM, et al. The International Registry of Acute Aortic Dissection (IRAAD): new insights into an old disease. JAMA 2000;283(7):897-903.
  The IRAAD is composed of 12 international referral centers, from which 3 years of data and 464 patients were analyzed. A key finding was that classic presentations such as tearing or ripping chest pain (50.6%),
aortic regurgitation (31.6%), and pulse deficit (15.1%) were frequently absent, leading the authors to urge clinicians to maintain a high index of suspicion.
Han JH, Lindsell CJ, Storrow AB, et al. The role of cardiac risk factor burden in diagnosing acute coronary syndromes in the emergency department setting. Ann Emerg Med 2007;49(2):145-52, 52 e1.
  This post hoc analysis of more than 10,000 emergency department patients suspected of having ACS suggests that clinicians should not use cardiac risk factor burden to determine whether or not chest pain is cardiac in nature for patients older than 40. Interestingly, for patients younger than 40, the odds of ACS increased dramatically as the total number of cardiac risk factors increased.
Marvel MK, Epstein RM, Flowers K, Beckman HB. Soliciting the patient's agenda: have we improved? JAMA 1999;281(3):283-7.
  Although this study was conducted in primary care offices and not in an ICU, it emphasizes the importance of the basic history-taking process and listening to patients. It found that physicians interrupted their patients after a mean of only 23.1 seconds and that late-arising patient concerns were more common when physicians did not solicit questions during the interview.

REFERENCES

Access the complete reference list online at http://www.expertconsult.com.

28

Biochemical or Electrocardiographic Evidence of Acute Myocardial Injury

JUSTIN SZAWLEWICZ | STEVEN M. HOLLENBERG

The identification of myocardial injury is an important problem in the critical care setting. The development of more sensitive serologic techniques, while allowing the clinician to detect smaller amounts of myocardial necrosis, can pose several interpretive challenges. What constitutes significant myocardial damage? How should evidence of myocardial necrosis be interpreted in the absence of classical clinical criteria for myocardial infarction? In response to some of these challenges, a task force was organized to formulate a universal definition of myocardial infarction, and what emerged from the collaboration was a clinical classification of different types of myocardial infarction (Table 28-1).[1] Of the five types, the most pertinent in the critical care setting are type I (plaque rupture) and type II (demand ischemia leading to infarction). These definitions rely on both electrocardiographic and biochemical information.[1] As previously, diagnosis of type I infarction requires a compatible clinical scenario and either biochemical or electrocardiographic evidence.

Electrocardiographic Evidence

Acute coronary syndromes are classified by the initial electrocardiogram (ECG), and patients are divided into three groups: those with ST-elevation myocardial infarction (STEMI), those without ST elevation but with enzyme evidence of myocardial damage (non–ST-elevation myocardial infarction, or NSTEMI), and those with unstable angina. Classification according to the presenting ECG coincides with current treatment strategies, since patients presenting with ST elevation benefit from immediate reperfusion. An ECG in patients with suspected acute coronary syndrome (ACS) should be obtained and interpreted within 10 minutes of presentation.[2]

Criteria for the diagnosis of STEMI include[1-3]:

- New ST elevation greater than 2 mm at the J point in at least two contiguous leads V_1 to V_3.
- New ST elevation greater than 1 mm at the J point in at least two contiguous leads (II, III, aVF) or (V_5, V_6, I, aVL).
- New left bundle branch block (LBBB).
- New horizontal or downsloping ST depression V_1 to V_3 with a positive terminal T wave and prominent R wave or R/S ratio greater than 1 (posterior MI).

A number of potential pitfalls can contribute to misinterpretation of the ECG. Many conditions can mimic STEMI and lead to false positives. An early repolarization pattern with ≤ 3 mm ST elevation in leads V_1 to V_3 can be seen in healthy individuals, usually young men. Preexcitation, bundle branch block, pericarditis, pulmonary embolism, subarachnoid hemorrhage, metabolic disturbances such as hyperkalemia, hypothermia, and left ventricular (LV) aneurysm can be associated with ST elevation in the absence of acute myocardial ischemia. On the other hand, some conditions can lead to false negatives, including prior myocardial infarction (MI), paced rhythm, and LBBB when acute ischemia is not recognized. These pitfalls are common in the real world and in large clinical trials. For example, when ECGs from the GUSTO IIB trial were reviewed by expert readers at a core laboratory, 15% of patients with STEMI were found to have been misclassified as NSTEMI, and these patients had a 21% higher mortality rate.[4]

"Nondiagnostic" ECGs are common in the setting of acute MI. Up to 18% of patients subsequently determined to have MI have a normal ECG, and an additional 25% have nonspecific changes. These nondiagnostic ECG findings may be due to occlusion of small vessels only or to insensitivity of the 12-lead ECG to ischemia in the lateral or posterior LV territory. Visualization in the horizontal plane can be extended laterally and posteriorly by the addition of leads V_7 to V_9 and rightward by the addition of V_{4R} and V_{5R}. Systematic 15-lead ECG to include V_{4R}, V_8, and V_9 has been suggested to increase the sensitivity of diagnosing ST elevation from 47% to 59% without decreasing specificity.[5] In fact, an 80-lead body surface mapping system has been shown to increase sensitivity and specificity of ECG diagnosis of ischemia, but challenges with rapid application at the bedside remain.[6] If ischemia is strongly suspected, but changes are not seen on standard leads, obtaining an ECG with additional leads should be considered.[3]

ST-segment depression on ECG identifies patients with ACS at high risk. In the TIMI risk score, which has been shown to predict the likelihood of death and ischemic events, ST-segment changes, along with advanced age and prior coronary artery disease, show the strongest association with severe epicardial disease.[7]

The significance of T-wave changes is directly related to the pretest probability of disease. Large studies in asymptomatic patients show that most T-wave changes are nonspecific. In the coronary care unit, however, 87% of patients with only T-wave inversions across the precordium will have a significant left anterior descending (LAD) coronary artery stenosis by angiography. Among patients presenting to the emergency department with ACS, those with isolated T-wave changes have lower risk than those with ST depression but higher risk than those with a normal ECG.[8]

Cardiac Biomarkers

With cardiac cell death, proteins are released into the blood, and detection of these proteins has played a key role in establishing the diagnosis of ACS, risk stratification, and prediction of outcome. Beginning early in the 1970s, creatine kinase (CK) and its isoenzyme, MB, became the biomarkers of choice to establish myocardial injury and infarction. The sensitivity of CK-MB for diagnosis of MI at 6 hours is 91%, but at 2 and 4 hours, sensitivity is only 21% and 46%.[9] The poor performance of CK-MB early in the course of MI led to the continued search for biomarkers that could diagnose MI early. Myoglobin was a contender for just such a role, because serum levels increase earlier than CK-MB, but the degree to which early sensitivity is increased is uncertain, and myoglobin lacks specificity.[10]

These biomarkers have now been superseded by troponin T and I, parts of the troponin-tropomyosin complex in cardiac myocytes. Troponin elevations are highly specific for myocardial cellular injury, except for infrequent false positives due to fibrin interference or cross-reacting antibodies.[11] Troponin is also much more sensitive than CK-MB because of its higher concentration in cardiac muscle; minor cardiac injury can elevate levels.[11] Even small increases in circulating troponin values correlate with adverse outcomes in the short and long term.[11] In non–ST-elevation ACS, elevated troponin levels not only predict increased risk but also identify the patients most likely to benefit from more aggressive antiplatelet strategies using IIb/IIIa inhibitors, use of low-molecular-weight heparin, and an early invasive strategy with coronary angiography and revascularization when appropriate.[3]

TABLE 28-1	Clinical Classification of Different Types of Myocardial Infarction

Type 1

Spontaneous myocardial infarction related to ischemia due to a primary coronary event such as plaque erosion and/or rupture, fissuring, or dissection

Type 2

Myocardial infarction secondary to ischemia due to either increased oxygen demand or decreased supply (e.g., coronary artery spasm, coronary embolism, anemia, arrhythmias, hypertension, hypotension)

Type 3

Sudden unexpected cardiac death including cardiac arrest, often with symptoms suggestive of myocardial ischemia, accompanied by presumably new ST elevation, new left bundle branch block, or evidence of fresh coronary thrombus by angiography or autopsy

Type 4a

Myocardial infarction associated with percutaneous coronary intervention

Type 4b

Myocardial infarction associated with stent thrombosis as documented by angiography or at autopsy

Type 5

Myocardial infarction associated with coronary artery bypass grafting

From Thygesen K, Alpert JS, White HD, et al. Universal definition of myocardial infarction. Circulation. 2007;116(22):2634-2653.

The challenge for the clinician, and in particular the intensivist, is that while elevation of serum troponin concentration is highly specific for myocardial cell damage, not all of that damage is a consequence of rupture of an atherosclerotic plaque. Other causes of elevated troponin, many of which are common in the intensive care unit (ICU), are listed in Table 28-2.

Troponin release in critically ill patients may not always represent myocardial cell death. Endotoxin, cytokines, and other inflammatory mediators, along with catecholamines and conditions such as hypotension, therapy with inotrope agents, or hypoxia, can cause the breakdown of cytoplasmic troponin into smaller fragments that can pass through endothelial monolayers and subsequently be detected by sensitive assays for troponin.[12] Thus, detectable circulating troponin levels, although they usually emanate from myocardial cells, may not always represent either irreversible cell death or myocardial ischemia. Renal dysfunction is another factor associated with elevated circulating troponin levels, and both the sensitivity and specificity of this biomarker is decreased in this population.

Regardless of cause, it is clear that elevation of serum troponin levels is associated with worsened outcomes, both in and out of the ICU, even after adjustment for severity of disease.[13] What is less clear is whether myocardial dysfunction represents the proximate cause of the worsened prognosis. It is often difficult to exclude ischemia in critically ill patients, but in a study of patients with septic shock, troponin predicted mortality, even among patients without flow-limiting coronary lesions (as assessed by stress echocardiography or autopsy).[14]

A further difficulty in the ICU is that patients may not experience classic symptoms of ischemia or may be unable to report them. Despite this potentially confounding factor, it is useful for the clinician to recall

TABLE 28-2	Nonischemic Conditions Commonly Associated with Elevated Cardiac Troponin

Myocarditis
Aortic dissection
Pulmonary embolism
CHF
Renal failure
Sepsis
Burns
Extreme exertion
Stress cardiomyopathy

that MI is diagnosed when sensitive and specific biomarkers are elevated in the right clinical setting.[1] A characteristic rise and fall should be seen, as an initially elevated troponin may not result from ischemia.[15] Troponin levels should be repeated at 6-hour intervals to define the clinical course.

Other Biomarkers

A number of novel cardiac biomarkers are being studied actively, including ischemia-modified albumin, high-sensitivity C-reactive protein (CRP), B-type natriuretic peptide (BNP), and others. In general, these markers detect conditions other than MI, and few currently have a well-recognized use in patients with ACS or those who are critically ill.

The theory behind ischemia-modified albumin is that ischemia changes the ability of the amino terminus of albumin to bind cobalt, and that this modified form can be measured in serum. Validation of this marker has been limited by lack of a gold standard for ischemia.[15] Pregnancy-associated plasma protein-A is associated with neovascularization and is thus thought to be a potential marker for plaque rupture. Choline is released into the blood when phospholipids are cleaved, and thus might be a marker of ischemia and/or necrosis. None of these markers have been validated in the clinical setting, and none have been shown to add prognostic information to currently available techniques.

CRP is an acute-phase reactant synthesized in the liver and is a marker of inflammation. Levels of CRP have been used for detection and prevention of cardiac disease in ambulatory populations, and a recent study suggests that elevated circulating levels of CRP—measured using a high-sensitivity assay—may identify patients with normal low-density lipoprotein (LDL) levels who can benefit from therapy with statin.[16] In critically ill patients, however, the value of measuring CRP is much less certain. Circulating concentrations of CRP may indicate the degree of inflammation, but how measurement of this analyte would impact management has not been defined in this context.

B-type natriuretic peptide is released by atrial and ventricular myocytes in response to increases in wall stress. BNP has been shown to facilitate the differential diagnosis of patients presenting with dyspnea, and to confer prognostic information in patients with heart failure.[17]

BNP is also released by ischemic myocardium. Circulating BNP levels are higher in patients with three-vessel coronary artery disease, tighter stenoses, and LAD disease. Higher BNP levels in ACS patients correlate with an increased risk of subsequent death, and BNP appears to confer information independent of other clinical markers. For example, in a study of 449 ACS patients, those with a high GRACE Risk Score and high serum BNP level were more likely to die than those with a high GRACE Risk Score and low serum BNP level.[18] Interpretation of BNP levels can be complicated by the fact that women and older individuals have higher values, so age and gender-specific cutoffs may be needed. Obese individuals have lower values, but renal dysfunction increases BNP levels, sometimes dramatically. BNP levels also can be increased in the setting of right ventricular (RV) strain, including patients with pulmonary embolism, in whom both elevated circulating BNP and troponin levels predict worsened prognosis.[19] BNP remains a good indicator of ventricular dysfunction myocardial wall stress, but what cutoff levels should be used in the ICU and what the clinician should do when serum BNP levels exceed those cutoff values remains unclear.

Conclusion

The ECG remains a valuable tool to diagnose myocardial injury. The clinician needs to remain aware of the myocardial injury imposters as well as methods to increase the sensitivity of the ECG in diagnosing myocardial injury. Biochemical markers, particularly troponin, are useful tools to confirm an ECG diagnosis as well as to predict prognosis in ACS patients and critically ill patients. In all settings, but especially in the ICU, these markers must be interpreted in the clinical context.

ANNOTATED REFERENCES

Thygesen K, Alpert JS, White HD, et al. Universal definition of myocardial infarction. Circulation 2007;116(22):2634-53.

Consensus conference presenting updated guidelines for diagnosis of myocardial infarction.

Goodman SG, Fu Y, Langer A, et al. The prognostic value of the admission and predischarge electrocardiogram in acute coronary syndromes: the GUSTO-IIb ECG Core Laboratory experience. Am Heart J 2006;152(2):277-84.

Analysis of data from a large randomized clinical trial by the ECG Core Laboratory. Misclassification of the initial ECG was associated with a 21% increase in mortality.

Saenger AK, Jaffe AS. Requiem for a heavyweight: the demise of creatine kinase-MB. Circulation 2008;118(21):2200-6.

Excellent review of utility and potential pitfalls with use of troponin in the diagnosis of acute coronary syndromes.

Babuin L, Vasile VC, Rio Perez JA, et al. Elevated cardiac troponin is an independent risk factor for short- and long-term mortality in medical intensive care unit patients. Crit Care Med 2008;36(3):759-65.

In a cohort of ICU patients, elevated serum troponin levels were associated with worsened outcomes, even after adjustment for severity of disease.

Jaffe AS, Babuin L, Apple FS. Biomarkers in acute cardiac disease: the present and the future. J Am Coll Cardiol 2006;48(1):1-11.

Comprehensive review of current status of various biomarkers.

Maisel A, Hollander JE, Guss D, et al. Primary results of the Rapid Emergency Department Heart Failure Outpatient Trial (REDHOT). A multicenter study of B-type natriuretic peptide levels, emergency department decision making, and outcomes in patients presenting with shortness of breath. J Am Coll Cardiol 2004;44(6):1328-33.

In patients presenting to the emergency department with dyspnea, measurement of BNP was useful to make clinical decisions, and elevations had prognostic value in patients with heart failure.

REFERENCES

Access the complete reference list online at http://www.expertconsult.com.

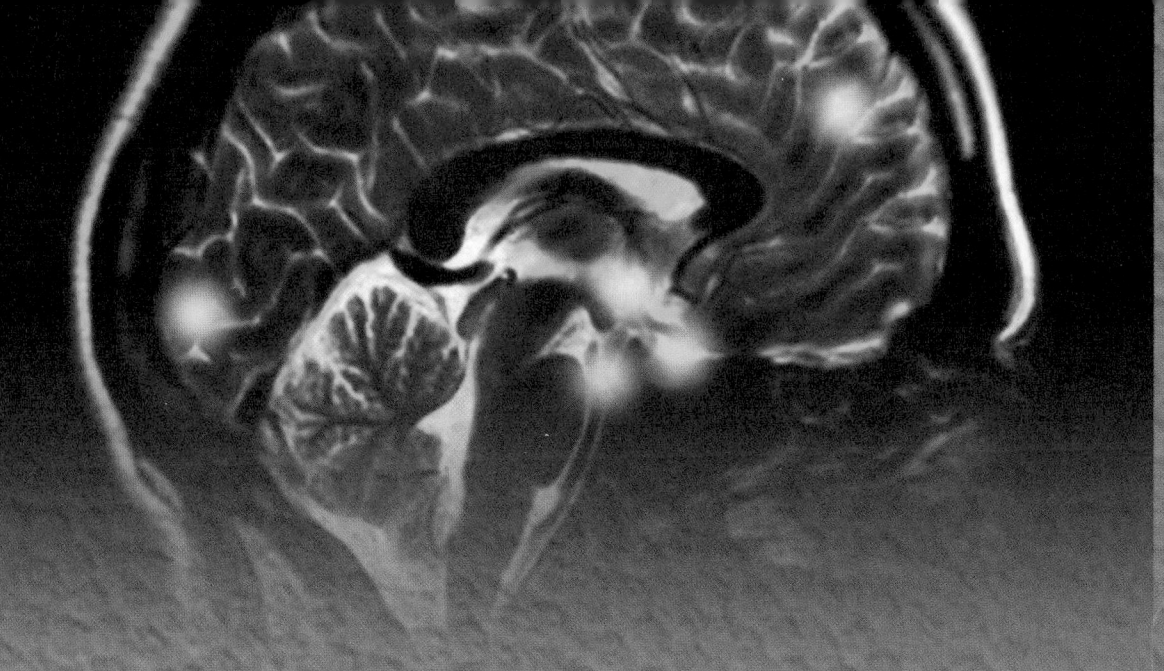

Central Nervous System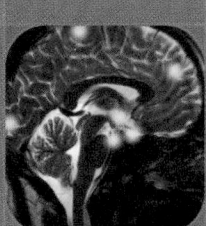

29

Biochemical, Cellular, and Molecular Mechanisms of Neuronal Death and Secondary Brain Injury in Critical Care

ROBERT S.B. CLARK | LARRY JENKINS | HÜLYA BAYIR | PATRICK M. KOCHANEK

In this chapter, we provide a general discussion of the biochemical, cellular, and molecular mechanisms of neuronal death and secondary brain injury that are germane to the central nervous system (CNS) insults that require neurointensive care, highlighting the important shared mechanisms in these conditions. In Chapter 30, Dr. Kofke builds upon the biochemical and molecular mechanisms to address general pathophysiologic principles in neurointensive care, focusing on intracranial dynamics and the cerebral circulation. Chapters 31 through 42 of Part 2 address other important facets of neurointensive care, such as monitoring and coma, along with the specific pathophysiology and treatment of the key disease processes central to neurointensive care in both adults and children. This includes traumatic brain injury (TBI), cardiopulmonary arrest, stroke, subarachnoid hemorrhage (SAH), and seizures, among other insults.

A thumbnail sketch of the most important mechanisms of secondary injury involved in the brain after a traumatic or ischemic insult is provided in Figure 29-1. Central to all brain insults relevant to neurointensive care is the occurrence of cerebral ischemia and/or cerebral energy failure. The principal consequence of ischemic injury and/or energy failure is neuronal death. The two principal forms of ischemia in neurointensive care are global and focal, as seen in cases of cardiopulmonary arrest and stroke, respectively.

In cases of TBI, direct parenchymal or vascular disruption or vasospasm often leads to cerebral ischemia, although tissue deformation such as axonal and vascular stretching and shearing along with hemorrhage and dendritic injury also are involved. In cases of SAH, hemorrhage is often followed by delayed vasospasm, with subsequent secondary cerebral ischemia. Finally, seizures and hypoglycemia can lead to neuronal death and represent situations in which relative ischemia is produced, either from enhanced metabolic demands that are greater than supply or from reduced substrate delivery. Energy failure ensues, and if the insult is sufficient in duration, cellular injury or death can occur. Clearly, ischemia and energy failure are key culprits in producing the pathophysiology of neurointensive care insults.

Global Cerebral Ischemia

In patients with global cerebral ischemia, insults are dense and often square-wave in nature.[1] The classic example of a global cerebral ischemic insult in neurointensive care is ventricular fibrillation cardiopulmonary arrest (see Chapter 33). Using conventional approaches, patients can be successfully resuscitated from these insults only if they are brief—that is, circulation must be restored in 5 to 12 minutes, although the maximal duration compatible with intact neurologic outcome can depend on a variety of factors, such as temperature. In cases of complete global cerebral ischemia, adenosine triphosphate (ATP) and phosphocreatine levels in brain are depleted in less than 2 minutes.[2,3] Membrane failure ensues, with loss of ion homeostasis that includes cellular release of K^+ and uptake of Ca^{++}, Na^+, and Cl^-.[2,3] Upon reperfusion, a complex sequence of events is set into motion that depends on the duration of the insult. Disturbances in lipid metabolism such as free fatty acid release and DNA damage result, along with

a series of deleterious cascades including oxidative and nitrosative stress, excitotoxicity, poly-ADP-ribose polymerase (PARP) activation, mitochondrial and endoplasmic reticulum (ER) dysfunction, and a host of cell-signaling abnormalities. A number of endogenous neuroprotectant responses are also initiated. The specific biochemical, cellular, and molecular events are discussed later. The aforementioned increases in intracellular calcium level are believed to play a critical role in initiating many of these events. In situations where the patient is potentially salvageable, such as with threshold insults, reperfusion results in transient hyperemia (minutes) followed by delayed hypoperfusion (hours).[1,4,5] The pattern of neuronal damage seen after global cerebral ischemia is classically termed *selective vulnerability*. This is often delayed and primarily neuronal in nature, and it is believed to result from complex biological cascades involving some features of programmed cell death (discussed later).

A number of brain regions are specifically vulnerable to ischemia, including the CA1 region of the hippocampus, cortical layers 3 and 5, portions of the amygdaloid nucleus, and cerebellar Purkinje cells, among others.[2,3,5] Global ischemic insults from cardiopulmonary arrest from which there is some potential for recovery are generally believed to be devoid of important increases in intracranial pressure, since, based on studies in animal models, it has been shown that the threshold for producing poor outcome in patients with global ischemic insults is less than that needed to generate clinically significant intracranial hypertension.[6] Thus, brain edema and vascular injury are not believed to represent important therapeutic targets after global cerebral ischemia. Two relevant but atypical global insults in neurointensive care are asphyxial cardiopulmonary arrest (particularly important in children and discussed in Chapter 42), and near-hanging episodes. In the latter, obstruction of cerebral venous drainage during the asphyxial insult compounds the ischemic insult.

Focal Cerebral Ischemia

Focal ischemic insults in neurointensive care are produced by thrombotic or embolic events and generally produce a dense ischemic focus that is surrounded by a periischemic penumbral region with intermediate cerebral blood flow (CBF) values.[2] The ischemic focus is generally believed to be unsalvageable unless reperfused almost immediately. In contrast, the ischemic penumbra is a region with some collateral flow and represents a therapeutic target for reperfusion with thrombolytics and/or pharmacologic therapy. In cases of focal cerebral ischemia, a hierarchy of CBF thresholds has been demonstrated in experimental studies, with inhibition of protein synthesis being the most sensitive to CBF reductions, followed by loss of electrical activity (evoked potentials and electroencephalogram), and eventually membrane failure.[7-8] Unlike the selective vulnerability seen in global ischemic insults, focal cerebral ischemia produces pan-necrosis of the vasculature and astrocytes, resulting in infarction. However, cell death in the penumbra can demonstrate necrotic, apoptotic, and mixed phenotypes. Again, however, classic apoptosis is not seen. Astrocyte swelling and blood-brain barrier injury with focal cerebral edema can play important roles.

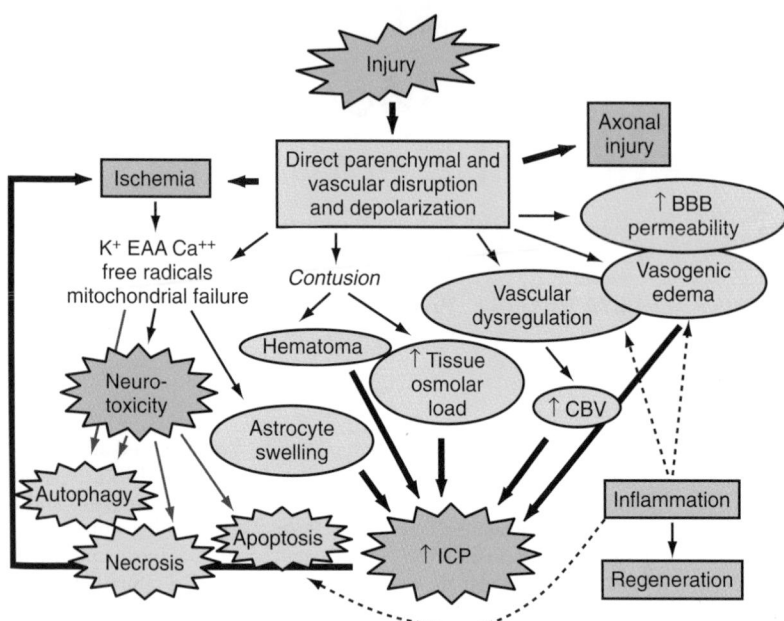

Figure 29-1 Categories of biochemical, cellular, and molecular mechanisms proposed to be involved in the evolution of secondary damage after ischemic or traumatic brain injury. Three major categories for these secondary mechanisms include (1) ischemia, excitotoxicity, energy failure, and cell death cascades; (2) cerebral swelling; and (3) axonal injury. A fourth category, inflammation and regeneration, influences each of these cascades.

In the penumbra, spreading depression waves resulting in depolarization can enhance excitotoxic damage with expansion of the lesion core. Reperfusion can occur spontaneously or with the administration of thrombolytics and can produce a microcosm of the aforementioned oxidative and nitrosative stress, mitochondrial and ER damage, and cell signaling abnormalities seen in global cerebral ischemia. In patients with focal cerebral ischemia with large infarcts, brain swelling can be substantial enough that secondary ischemia can result from intracranial hypertension. Dr. Kofke discusses these concepts in greater detail in Chapter 30. Focal cerebral ischemia from delayed vasospasm is also the most common critical complication of SAH and is discussed in Chapter 35.

Traumatic Brain Injury

In cases of severe TBI, the biochemical and molecular mechanisms involved depend on the specific type of injury. In cases of focal contusion, direct disruption of parenchyma with local necrosis and hemorrhage results in superimposed vascular disruption, blood-brain barrier permeability, and local ischemia. This sets the stage for excitotoxicity and necrotizing cascades in the contusion penumbra, including oxidative and nitrosative stress, and calpain-mediated proteolysis, among other mechanisms.[9,10] Local axonal injury is also seen in patients with contusions. Focal contusions are commonly complicated by marked local swelling and often by intracranial hypertension, with the potential for secondary focal or global ischemic insults or herniation syndromes. In contrast in diffuse injury, a constellation of diffuse axonal and vascular disruption can be seen, with characteristic findings of petechial hemorrhages in the white matter.[11] This insult can be devastating even in the absence of intracranial hypertension.[12] The biochemical and molecular events involved in axonal injury are discussed later. In cases of severe TBI, combined insults that include both multiple contusions and diffuse injury are also common. Finally, in addition to secondary compression ischemia from refractory intracranial hypertension, secondary extracerebral insults such as hypotension and hypoxemia can also negatively affect outcome and, importantly, complicate the biochemical and molecular response to severe TBI, markedly enhancing delayed neuronal death in brain regions that might otherwise have recovered.[13,14]

Key Biochemical and Molecular Mechanisms of Neuronal Secondary Damage

A number of pathologic cascades are shared by these important insults in neurointensive care, including excitotoxicity, programmed cell death, axonal injury, and inflammation, along with a spectrum of endogenous neuroprotectant responses.

EXCITOTOXICITY

Excitotoxicity describes the process by which glutamate and other excitatory amino acids cause neuronal damage. Lucas and Newhouse[15] first described the toxicity of glutamate. Olney[16] subsequently reported that intraperitoneal administration of glutamate produces brain injury in experimental animals. Although glutamate is the most abundant neurotransmitter in the brain, exposure to toxic levels produces neuronal death.[17] Glutamate exposure produces neuronal injury in two phases. Minutes after exposure, sodium-dependent neuronal swelling occurs.[18] This is followed by delayed calcium-dependent degeneration. These effects are mediated through both ionophore-linked receptors, labeled according to specific agonists (N-methyl-D-aspartate [NMDA], kainite, and α-amino-3-hydroxy-5-methyl-4-isoxazolepropionic acid [AMPA]), and receptors linked to second messenger systems, called metabotropic receptors. Activation of these receptors leads to calcium influx through receptor-gated or voltage-gated channels, or through the release of intracellular calcium stores. Increased intracellular calcium concentration is the trigger for a number of processes that can lead to cellular injury or death (Figure 29-2). One mechanism involves activation of neuronal nitric oxide synthase (nNOS), leading to nitric oxide (NO) production, peroxynitrite formation, and resultant DNA damage. PARP is an enzyme normally operative in DNA repair. In the face of overwhelming DNA damage, PARP overactivation leads to depletion of NAD^+ and ATP, metabolic failure, and cell death.[19-21] PARP may also impair ATP production directly via posttranslational modification of electron transport chain proteins.[22] This may be important, since PARP knockout mice exhibit improved outcome versus controls after experimental stroke or TBI.[20,23]

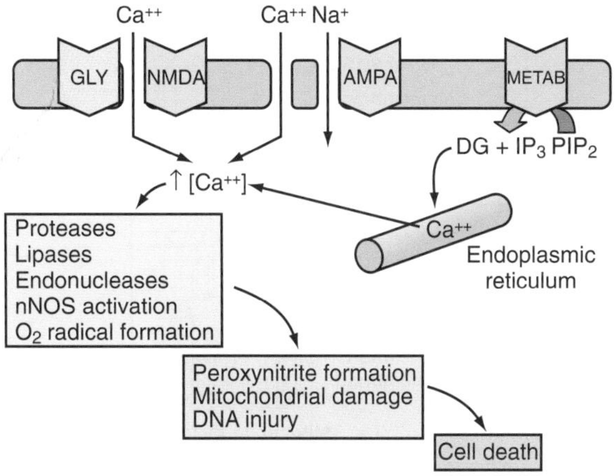

Figure 29-2 Mechanisms involved in excitotoxicity. Glutamate causes an increase in intracellular calcium concentration through stimulation of (1) the NMDA receptor with opening of the receptor-linked calcium iono-phore, (2) the AMPA receptor with opening of the voltage-gated calcium channels, and (3) the metabotropic receptor, with the release of intracel-lular calcium stores via the second messengers, inositol triphosphate and diacylglycerol. Increased intracellular calcium concentration leads to activation of proteases, lipases, and endonucleases along with neuronal NOS (nNOS) stimulation and production of oxygen radicals. This results in peroxynitrite formation, mitochondrial damage, and DNA injury, with subsequent cellular injury and death. AMPA, a-amino-3-hydroxy-5-methylisoxazole-4-propionic acid receptor; DG, diacylglycerol; GLY, glycine co-agonist site; IP_3, inositol triphosphate; METAB, glutamate metabotropic receptor; NMDA, N-methyl-D-aspartate receptor; NOS, nitric oxide synthase; PIP_2, phosphoinositide.

There is considerable evidence in experimental laboratory models supporting an important contribution of excitotoxicity to the evolu-tion of secondary damage in cases of global and focal cerebral isch-emia, severe TBI, SAH, and status epilepticus.[24-31] Evidence supporting an important role for excitotoxicity in humans has similarly been provided in cases of severe TBI, stroke, and SAH. Persson and Hill-ered[32] reported increases in brain interstitial levels of glutamate in a patient with SAH as early as 1992. Palmer et al.[33] first demonstrated increased concentrations of excitatory amino acids in ventricular cere-brospinal fluid (CSF) from adult patients with TBI. Glutamate con-centrations were about fivefold greater than in control patients (up to 7 µM)—levels sufficient to cause neuronal death in cell culture.[34] Bullock et al.[35] characterized patterns of glutamate release by measur-ing excitatory amino acids by microdialysis in patients after TBI. Patients with a normal head computed tomography (CT) scan and no secondary ischemic events had interstitial concentrations of glutamate that were increased early in their course then returned to normal. In contrast, patients with a progressively rising level of glutamate died. Similarly, in cases of human stroke, Bullock et al.[36] also reported massive increases in the excitatory amino acids, glutamate and aspar-tate, in a patient who required decompressive craniectomy to prevent brainstem herniation.

Despite these and many other clinical reports, clinical trials with anti-excitotoxic therapies have been unsuccessful in patients with either stroke or TBI. This may be due to problems with patient selec-tion, side effects of the anti-excitotoxic agents that were tested, and the likelihood that treatment was initiated too late.[37] Inhibition of plastic-ity by anti-excitotoxic therapies may also limit their efficacy, especially at the interface between the acute and subacute periods after injury.[38]

PROGRAMMED CELL DEATH CASCADES

It is now increasingly clear from experimental models and human data that cells dying after global or focal cerebral ischemia or TBI can be categorized on a morphologic continuum ranging from necrosis to apoptosis.[39,40] Recently, additional phenotypic definitions have been included within this continuum: those of autophagic degeneration, programmed necrosis, and "parthanatos."[41-43] Apoptosis is a morpho-logic description of cell death defined by cell shrinkage and nuclear condensation, internucleosomal DNA fragmentation, and the forma-tion of apoptotic bodies.[44] In contrast, cells dying of necrosis display cellular and nuclear swelling with dissolution of membranes. Apopto-sis requires a cascade of intracellular events for completion of cell death; thus, the term *apoptosis* was previously used synonymously with *programmed cell death*.[45] Because other types of cell death have now been characterized that can also be considered "programmed," *apop-tosis* now refers primarily to the phenotypic definition as classically defined by Kerr et al.[44] In diseases with complex and multiple mecha-nisms, such as stroke and TBI, it is typically the rule rather than the exception to detect dying cells with many or all currently defined cell-death phenotypes.[46] For example, some cells may display DNA frag-mentation and activation of proteases involved in apoptosis, despite having nuclear and cellular swelling. Dying cells with mixed pheno-types may represent particularly difficult therapeutic targets.

Biochemical Pathways in Delayed Neuronal Death

Apoptosis is an evolutionarily conserved process required for selective cell elimination during development, and it occurs in all tissues, including brain. Execution of apoptosis requires novel gene expression and protein synthesis.[47-49] Apoptosis is an intricate and critical mecha-nism for balancing cell proliferation, remodeling of tissues during development, and maintenance of tissues with a high rate of cell turnover. Apoptosis can be thought of as "molecular débridement," delicately eliminating unwanted cells, with minimal disturbance of neighboring cells. Apoptosis is cybernetic and may occur via multiple pathways that can be independent (Figure 29-3); however, cross-talk between these (and other nonapoptotic) pathways also may occur.[50,51] At present, neuronal apoptosis can be segregated into two pathways, one involving the activation of a family of cysteine proteases termed *caspases*, and one that is caspase independent.[52]

Caspase family proteases include 14 currently identified members that are synthesized as proenzymes, which for the most part are pro-teolytically activated.[50] Initiator caspases, including caspase 8, 9, and 10, are activated by autocleavage and aggregation. Executioner cas-pases, including caspase 3, 6, and 7, are cleaved and activated by initia-tor caspases. The proteolytic cleavage of caspase substrates produces the phenotypic changes characteristic of apoptosis, including cytoskel-etal disintegration, DNA fragmentation, and disruption of cellular and DNA repair processes (Figure 29-4). Cytoskeletal caspase targets include spectrin and nuclear lamin[53]; in addition, caspase 3 activates the enzyme, gelsolin, which cleaves actin.[54] Active caspase 3 can also cleave the inhibitor of caspase-dependent deoxyribonuclease, permit-ting caspase-dependent deoxyribonuclease to digest DNA into small oligonucleosomal fragments.[55] These small DNA fragments (multiples of approximately 180 base pairs) can be seen on a DNA gel as a ladder and are a hallmark of caspase-dependent apoptosis. Caspase 3 also inhibits DNA repair by proteolytically inactivating many DNA repair proteins, including PARP.[56-58] This combination of features—silencing of the genome and incapacitation of DNA repair processes, and destruction of key cytoskeletal components, all with surgical-like pre-cision and ultimately leading to cell death—illustrates why apoptosis has been referred to as "cell suicide."

Extrinsic Pathways of Apoptosis and Programmed Necrosis

Programmed cell death can be initiated by extrinsic or intrinsic signals. Extrinsic signals include cell surface death receptor-ligand interactions and cell signaling pathways. The most prominent cell death receptor family is the tumor necrosis factor (TNF) receptor superfamily, which includes TNF-α and Fas.[59] The coupling of cell surface TNF or Fas receptors with extracellular TNF-α or Fas ligand induces trimerization of the receptors that leads to the formation of submembrane com-plexes with intracellular death domain–signaling molecules. This death-inducing signaling complex then activates caspase 8[60] or 10.[61]

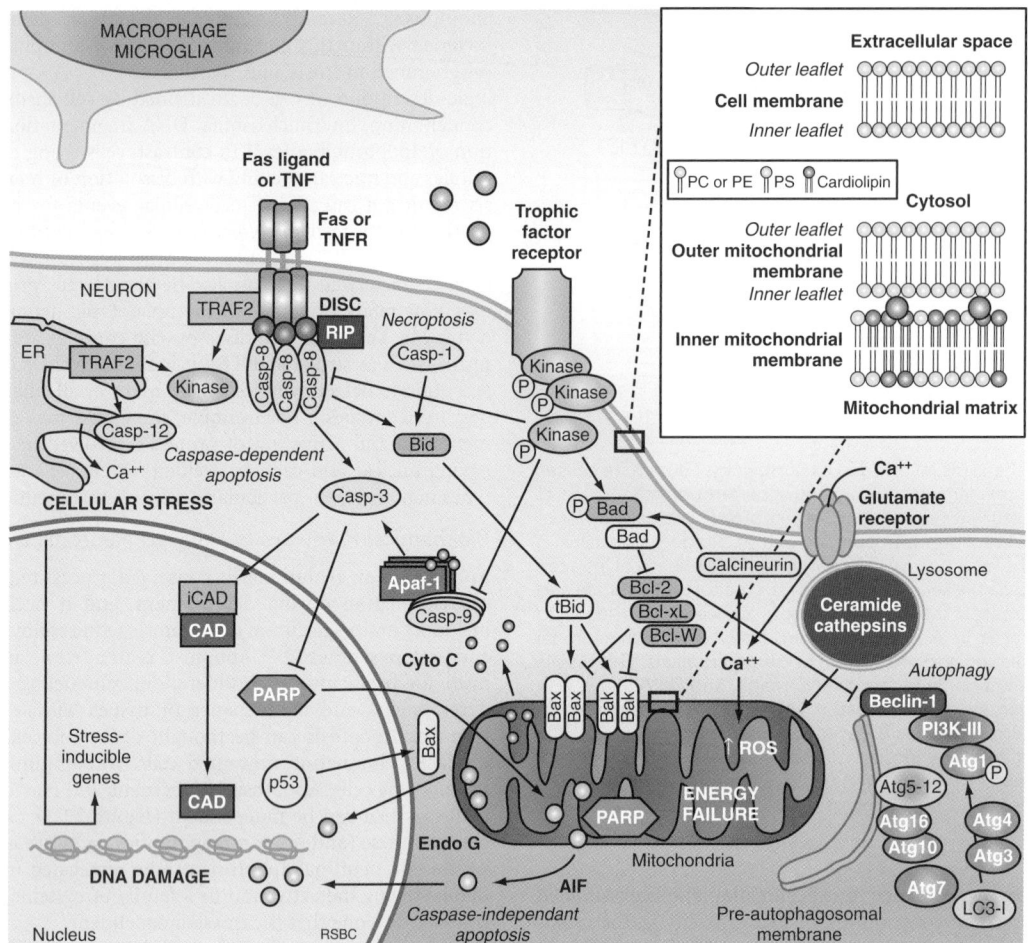

Figure 29-3 A simplified schematic representation of the initiation and regulation of neuronal programmed cell death after brain injury. Pathologic mechanisms triggering programmed cell death after brain injury include ischemia, oxidative stress, energy failure, excitotoxicity (primarily excess glutamate), axonal injury, trophic factor withdrawal, ER stress, and death receptor–ligand binding (e.g., TNF, Fas). Regulation of programmed cell death occurs via multiple pathways, including kinase-dependent intracellular signaling pathways and Bcl-2 family proteins. AIF, apoptosis-inducing factor; Apaf-1, apoptotic protease–activating factor 1; Atg, autophagy-related protein; Bcl, B-cell lymphoma; CAD, caspase-activated deoxyribonuclease; Casp, caspase; Cyto C, cytochrome C; DISC, death-inducing signaling complex; Endo G, endonuclease G; ER, endoplasmic reticulum; iCAD, inhibitor of CAD; PARP, poly(ADP-ribose) polymerase; PC, phosphatidylcholine; PE, phosphatidylethanolamine; PI3K-III, class III phosphoinositide-3 kinase; PS, phosphatidylserine; RIP, receptor interacting protein; ROS, reactive oxygen species; tBid, truncated Bid; TNF, tumor necrosis factor; TNFR, TNF receptor; TRAF2, TNF receptor. associated factor.

Caspase 3 is then cleaved and activated, perpetuating the cascade. The extrinsic pathway can also be regulated by multiple intracellular signal transduction pathways that are initiated by G-protein coupled cell surface receptors, which can be either activated by neurotransmitters (e.g., cyclic nucleotides) or inactivated by interruption of trophic factors (e.g., nerve growth factor) after injury.[62] Perturbations in neurotransmitters and trophic factors controlling these pathways occur after ischemia and TBI. Multiple interrelated pro-death or pro-survival kinase pathways have been identified, including those involving mitogen-activated protein kinases, and protein kinase B and protein kinase C.[63,64] Caspase 8 and 3 cleavage consistent with activation has been demonstrated in humans after TBI.[39,65]

More recently, programmed cell death with phenotypic characteristics of necrosis (programmed necrosis) or shared characteristics of apoptosis and necrosis (necroptosis) have been described.[66] Programmed necrosis occurs through TNF receptor signaling involving receptor interacting protein 1 (RIP-1) and TNF receptor-associated factors (TRAFs) and regulation by protein ubiquitination and phosphorylation.[66] Effector mechanisms of programmed necrosis are thought to involve caspase 8 but may also occur via direct effects on mitochondrial permeability transition. Thus, caspase 8 activation may reflect either extrinsic apoptosis or programmed necrosis, or both.

Intrinsic Pathways of Apoptosis

The intrinsic pathway of apoptosis is triggered by stress on cellular organelles, notably mitochondria and ER. Mitochondrial stress can lead to caspase-dependent apoptosis via mitochondrial release of cytochrome C induced upon mitochondrial membrane depolarization. Egress of cytochrome C into the cytosol enables interaction with apoptotic protease activating factor-1 (Apaf-1), dATP, and procaspase 9 to form a complex termed an *apoptosome*. Apaf-1 activates caspase 9 and subsequently caspase 3.[67] Several mitochondrial proteins are capable of inducing apoptosis without direct activation of the caspase cascade, thus exemplifying pathways that are caspase independent. Apoptosis-inducing factor (AIF) within the mitochondria serves as an antioxidant[68]; however, upon mitochondrial membrane depolarization, it can translocate from the mitochondria to the nucleus, where it is sufficient to induce apoptosis.[69] Translocation of AIF into the nuclei induces the formation of large-scale DNA fragmentation (>50 kilobase pairs), in contrast to cytochrome C-mediated, caspase-dependent apoptosis, which leads to oligonucleosomal DNA fragmentation (180-1200 base pairs). AIF-mediated apoptosis occurs in neurons under conditions of experimental TBI[52] and cerebral ischemia.[70] It is now accepted that PARP-1 overactivation mediates AIF-translocation and subsequent cell

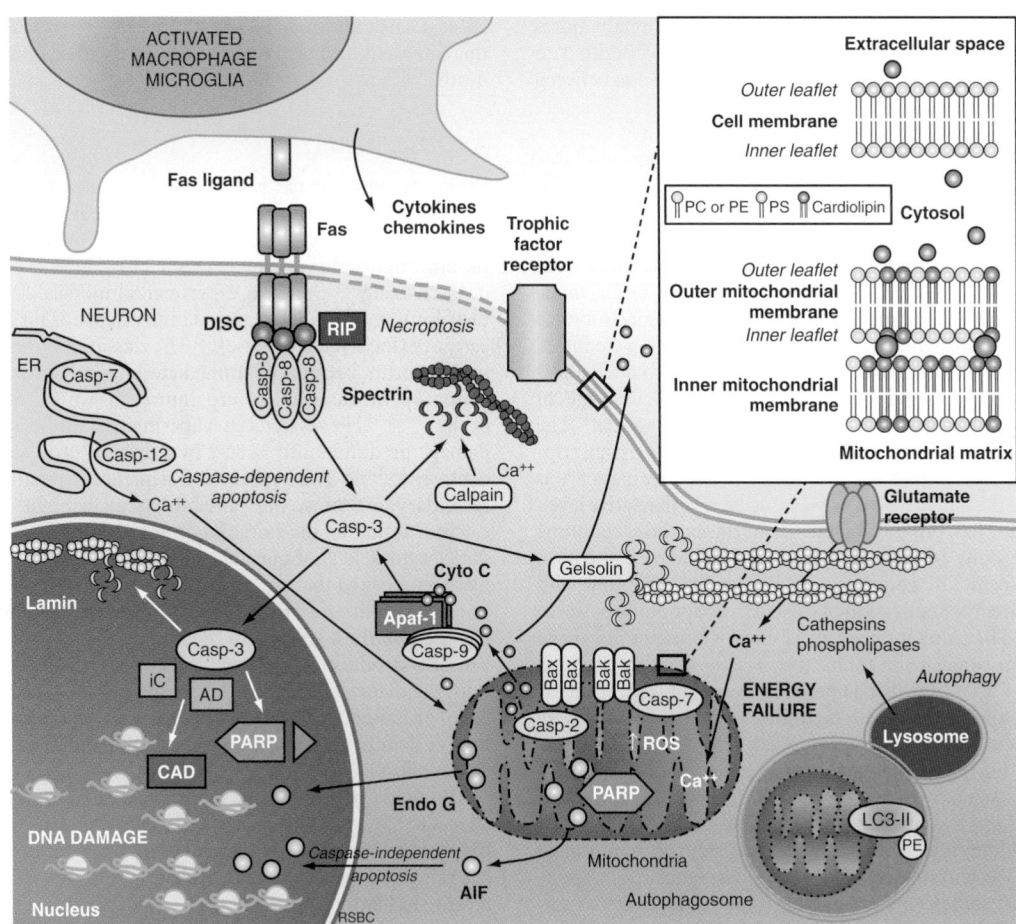

Figure 29-4 A simplified schematic representation of the execution of neuronal programmed cell death after brain injury. Execution of programmed cell death involves the caspase cascade and/or release of apoptogenic factors from organelles such as mitochondria. Ultimately, DNA fragmentation, cytoskeletal disintegration, and externalization of membrane phosphatidyl serine occur, signaling macrophages and microglia to engulf cellular debris. AIF, apoptosis-inducing factor; Apaf-1, apoptotic protease activating factor 1; Bcl, B-cell lymphoma; CAD, caspase-activated deoxyribonuclease; Casp, caspase; Cyto C, cytochrome C; DISC, death-inducing signaling complex; Endo G, endonuclease G; ER, endoplasmic reticulum; iCAD, inhibitor of CAD; PARP, poly(ADP-ribose) polymerase; PC, phosphatidylcholine; PE, phosphatidylethanolamine; PI3K-III, class III phosphoinositide-3 kinase; PS, phosphatidylserine; RIP, receptor interacting protein; ROS, reactive oxygen species.

death.[19,71] As noted earlier, "parthanatos" was recently coined to describe poly(ADP-ribose)-related cell death (from the Greek *thanatos*, referring to the personification of death).[42]

Other mitochondrial proteins related to programmed cell death include endonuclease G,[72] Htr2A/Omi,[73] and Smac/Diablo[74]; however, their roles in neuronal death after brain injury remain unexplored. Disruption of ER calcium homeostasis and/or accumulation of excess proteins can lead to ER stress, which in turn can trigger programmed cell death via activation of ER-localized caspase 12, an upstream initiator caspase. ER stress-related activation of caspase 12 has been detected in experimental models of cerebral ischemia[75] and TBI.[76]

Autophagic Neurodegeneration

Autophagy is a homeostatic physiologic process important for recycling amino acids by digestion of proteins and organelles. Literally meaning "eating oneself," this is an important response to nutrient deprivation in every organism. Like apoptosis, disrupted autophagy results in disease, in this case resulting in accumulation of intracellular proteins and aged organelles.[77] Possibly like apoptosis, too much autophagy may also contribute to disease, depending upon the insult, organ, and cell type involved. For example, even under conditions of starvation, inhibition of autophagy protects neurons, whereas it exacerbates cell death in fibroblasts.[78] Although there is considerable controversy regarding its role, increased autophagy has been demonstrated in models of cerebral ischemia[79] and TBI[80] and in brain tissue from humans with critical illness.[81] The controversy arises in terms of whether or not inhibition or promotion of autophagy is beneficial after brain injury, insofar as both of these divergent strategies have been shown to be protective in various experimental models.[80,82-84] There is also cross-talk between autophagy and apoptosis, perhaps at the level of the Bcl-2 protein family.[51,85]

Regulation of Programmed Cell Death by the Bcl-2 Protein Family

Caspase-dependent and caspase-independent apoptosis, as well as autophagy, are regulated by the B-cell lymphoma-2 (Bcl-2) family of proteins. The Bcl-2 family contains both pro-death and pro-survival members.[86] Bcl-2 family proteins regulate changes in permeability of the mitochondrial outer membrane independent of permeability transition pore formation. Bcl-2 family proteins contain highly conserved Bcl-2 homology domains (BH1-BH4) essential for homo- and heterocomplex formation.[87] Complexes formed between proteins containing BH3 domains such as Bax, truncated Bid, and Bad can facilitate mitochondrial cytochrome C release.[88,89] The antiapoptotic members Bcl-2, Bcl-xL, and Mcl-1L prevent the release of mitochondrial proteins by inhibiting the pore formation.[90] Bax expression is associated with neuronal cell death after cardiac arrest in dogs.[91] Transgenic mice overexpressing Bcl-2 are partially protected from the neuropathologic sequelae of TBI versus wild-type mice,[92] and overexpression of Bcl-xL also inhibits neuronal cell death after focal cerebral ischemia.[93] The

Bcl-2 interacting partner Beclin 1 contains a BH3-only domain and is required for autophagy.[94] It is postulated that binding of Beclin 1 to Bcl-2 or Bcl-xL via the BH3 domain is how cross-talk occurs between apoptosis and autophagy.[85]

Programmed Cell Death in Human Brain Injury

Phenotypic descriptions of programmed cell death occurring after brain injury in humans date back to the 1940s.[95,96] However, biochemical evidence of programmed cell death after brain injury in humans has been reported only within the last decade and has now been reported after TBI,[39,65,81,97,98] stroke,[99] and epilepsy.[100] Brain tissue samples from TBI patients requiring decompressive craniectomy for the treatment of life-threatening intracranial hypertension were found to have evidence of DNA fragmentation by terminal deoxynucleotidyl transferase–mediated nick-end labeling (TUNEL) and cleavage of caspase 1 and 3, suggesting activation of the apoptotic cascade.[39] The up-regulation of caspase-8 in human brain after TBI at both transcriptional and translational levels has also been reported.[65] Caspase 8 was found predominantly in neurons and was associated with relative levels of the death receptor Fas, providing evidence of the extrinsic apoptotic pathway within neurons. Increases in Fas and Fas ligand have also been reported in CSF from TBI patients, with Fas levels correlating with intracranial pressure.[101,102] Activation of the intrinsic apoptotic pathway also occurs after TBI. Alteration of Bcl-2-family proteins has been reported in human brain from adults and in CSF from infants and children after TBI.[39,97,103] In pediatric patients, lower concentrations of Bcl-2 were detected in patients who died than in those who survived, supporting a pro-survival role for Bcl-2.[97] After TBI in adults, the presence of pro-death Bcl-2 family protein Bax in patients in whom Bcl-2 was also detectable represented a more favorable outcome as compared with patients in whom Bax but not Bcl-2 was detectable.[104] In contrast to TBI patients, patients after stroke demonstrate reductions in soluble Bcl-2 and soluble Fas within CSF,[99] suggesting dysregulation of apoptosis after stroke. In adolescents and young adults with refractory seizures, increases in Bcl-2 and Bcl-xL, as well as increases in expression and proteolysis of caspase 1 and 3, occur in resected temporal lobe.[100] These patients have had medically refractory seizures for several years, implying both protracted and acute apoptosis within the brain. Protracted programmed cell death after TBI also occurs. Cells with apoptotic morphologies and DNA damage detected by TUNEL have been reported in autopsy specimens from patients dying up to 12 months after injury,[105] perhaps implying that a relatively wide therapeutic window exists for the administration of treatments aimed at reducing programmed cell death.

Many of these clinical observational studies suggest potential sex differences in cell death mechanisms operative after brain injury. For example, CSF levels of cytochrome C are associated with female gender after TBI in children,[106] and CSF levels of the biochemical footprint of PARP activation are associated with male gender after TBI in both children[107] and adults.[108] These studies are strikingly consistent with experimental studies of neuronal death in vitro[109] and in vivo.[110,111]

Several notes of caution are in order. First, it is unclear what the quantitative contribution of programmed cell death, particularly apoptosis, is in clinical cases of cerebral ischemia or TBI. It is likely that dying cells demonstrate some biochemical and phenotypic features of programmed cell death, but that the actual deathblow to the cell is not dependent on an active process.[112] Even if programmed cell death mechanisms do play a key role, it is unclear whether inhibiting neuronal death after injury is entirely beneficial, since apoptosis is a vital mechanism for biological systems to eliminate abnormal or aging cells, and autophagy is important for protein and organelle turnover. In other words, quiet elimination via "cell suicide" of damaged or dysfunctional cells and/or organelles may lead to overall benefit to the patient, in essence "molecular débridement." Only clinical trials of novel therapies targeting individual programmed cell death cascades will be able to determine whether these mechanisms, alone or in combination, represent important targets in neurointensive care. Recent studies of the efficacy of mild hypothermia after experimental and clinical cardiopulmonary arrest, however, suggest that the success of this intervention may be derived from its effects on programmed cell death.[113-115]

AXONAL INJURY

White matter damage is important in infarction that results from stroke but probably plays only a limited role in the pathology of reversible global cerebral ischemia. In contrast, axonal injury is of paramount importance in patients with TBI. This has been demonstrated both clinically[116,117] and in experimental models.[118-120] The extent and distribution of traumatic axonal injury depends on injury severity and category (focal versus diffuse).[121] The classic view that traumatic axonal injury occurs because of immediate physical shearing is represented primarily in cases of severe injury in which frank axonal tears occur.[116,122,123] However, recent experimental studies suggest that axonal damage predominantly occurs by a delayed process termed *secondary axotomy*.[118,124,125] Two hypothetical sequences have attempted to explain secondary axotomy, one attributing axolemmal permeability and calcium influx as the initiating event (Figure 29-5), and the other a direct cytoskeletal abnormality impairing axoplasmic flow.[118,125,126] It has been posited that both forms of reactive axonal swelling take place but in different proportions depending on the severity of injury. Superimposed on these theories is the finding that hypoxic/ischemic insults can also produce axonal swelling.[127] As a result, differing as well as unifying theories for axonal injuries in patients with brain injury have been proposed.[128] Common mechanistic features include focal ion flux, calcium dysregulation, and mitochondrial and cytoskeletal dysfunction.

Traumatic axonal injury contributes to morbidity and mortality after TBI.[118,121,122] Until recently, the contributions of axonal injury to morbidity have remained speculative, since traumatic axonal injury has remained refractory to treatment even in the laboratory. However, recent studies in experimental TBI models have shown that hypothermia or cyclosporin-A can both reduce white matter damage.[129,130] These therapeutic advances should help determine more definitively the contributions of traumatic axonal injury to secondary damage. Recent application of magnetic resonance imaging (MRI) to the study of traumatic axonal injury and axonal connectivity may improve our understanding of both this injury mechanism and axonal regeneration.[131,132]

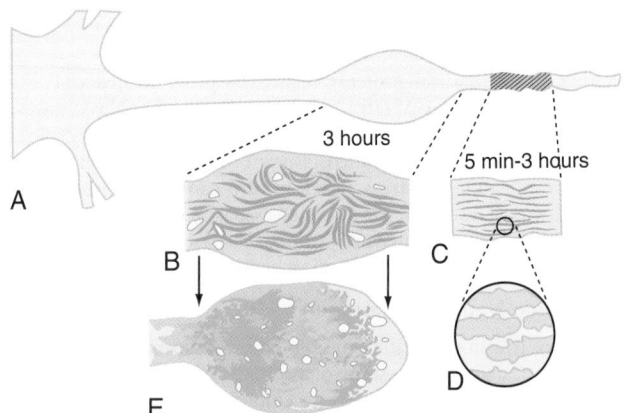

Figure 29-5 Reactive axonal swellings have been proposed to result from focal axolemmal disruption, ionic shifts, and neurofilamentous compaction. One or all of these events at site *A* results in a reactive swelling at site *B* in an upstream region of the axon. At the site of ionic influx, neurofilamentous compaction and mitochondrial swelling is seen (*C*). Neurofilament compaction is associated with neurofilament sidearm loss (*D*). Obstructed axonal transport results in upstream axonal enlargement, neurofilament misalignment, organelle accumulation, and formation of the typical reactive axonal swelling (*E*).

CEREBRAL SWELLING

In addition to cascades of neuronal death and axonal damage, brain swelling is a hallmark finding in cases of focal cerebral ischemia, severe TBI, and severe global cerebral ischemia from prolonged cardiopulmonary arrest. Brain swelling often results in the development of intracranial hypertension. Cerebral swelling and accompanying intracranial hypertension contribute to secondary damage in two ways. Intracranial hypertension can compromise cerebral perfusion, leading to secondary ischemia. It can also produce the devastating consequences of brain deformation and vascular compression through herniation syndromes. Intracranial hypertension results from increases in intracranial volume from a variety of sources, outlined in Figure 29-1. In some cases of TBI or spontaneous intracranial hemorrhage, such as with epidural, subdural, or parenchymal hematoma formation, an extraaxial or parenchymal blood collection is the key culprit and can be addressed by surgical evacuation.[133] However, there are several important mechanisms more uniformly involved in the development of intracranial hypertension. These are related to either brain swelling from vasogenic edema, astrocyte swelling, and an increase in tissue osmolar load, or vascular dysregulation with swelling secondary to an increase in cerebral blood volume (CBV).

Most of the mechanistic work in this area has come from studies in the field of TBI. Recent data suggest that brain swelling after severe TBI results from edema rather than increased CBV. Marmarou and colleagues[134] measured both CBV and brain water in adults with TBI. Using a dye indicator technique (coupled to CT) to measure CBV and MRI to quantify brain water, increases in brain water were commonly observed but were generally associated with reduced (not increased) CBV (Figure 29-6).

Thus, edema rather than increased CBV appears to be the predominant contributor to cerebral swelling after TBI. Both cytotoxic and vasogenic edema may play important roles in cerebral swelling, but the biochemical and molecular pathways involved in our traditional concept of cytotoxic and vasogenic edema are evolving. There appear to be four putative mechanisms for edema formation in the injured brain. First, vasogenic edema may form in the extracellular space as a result of disruption of the blood-brain barrier. Second, cellular swelling can be produced in two ways. Astrocyte swelling can occur as part of the homeostatic uptake of substances such as glutamate. Glutamate uptake is coupled to glucose utilization via a sodium/potassium ATPase, with sodium and water accumulation in astrocytes. Astrocyte swelling appears to be importantly linked to water movement through the aquaporin-4 channel found in the astrocyte foot processes near capillaries.[135-137] Studies have demonstrated reduced cerebral edema in

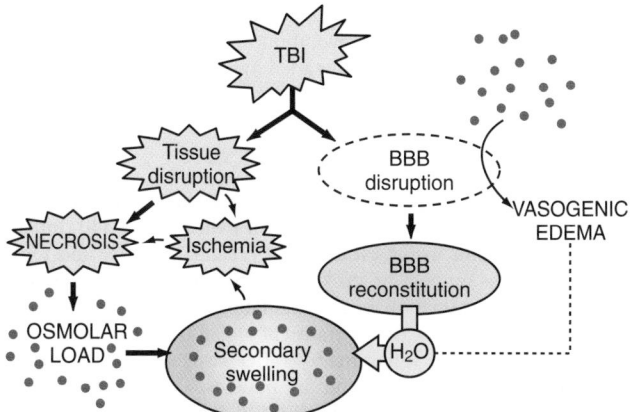

Figure 29-7 Schematic based on hypothesis of Katayama et al.,[141] suggesting that as osmolar load increases (breakdown of macromolecules in the region of contusion necrosis), a considerable driving force develops for the accumulation of water, resulting in the secondary swelling so often seen in and around cerebral contusions.

mice genetically deficient in this channel.[138] Swelling of both neurons and other cells in the neuropil can also result from ischemia- or trauma-induced ionic pump failure. This can be important in the penumbral regions of focal cerebral ischemia and around cerebral contusions. Finally, osmolar swelling may also contribute to edema formation in the extracellular space, particularly in maturing cerebral contusions. Osmolar swelling, however, is actually dependent on an intact blood-brain barrier or an alternative solute barrier.

In both cerebral ischemia and TBI, cellular swelling may be of greatest importance. Using a model of diffuse TBI in rats, Barzo and colleagues[139] applied diffusion-weighted MRI to localize the increase in brain water. A decrease in the apparent diffuse coefficient after injury suggested predominantly cellular swelling rather than vasogenic edema in the development of intracranial hypertension. Cellular swelling may be of even greater importance in the setting of TBI with a secondary hypoxemic-ischemic insult.[140] Katayama et al.[141] also suggested that the role of the blood-brain barrier in the development of posttraumatic edema might have been overstated, even in the setting of cerebral contusion. One intriguing possibility is that as macromolecules are degraded within injured brain regions, the osmolar load in the contused tissue or infarcts increases. As the blood-brain barrier reconstitutes (or as other osmolar barriers are formed), a considerable osmolar driving force for the local accumulation of water develops, resulting in the marked swelling so often seen in and around cerebral contusions (Figure 29-7). This has been supported by recent clinical studies of human cerebral contusion.[142]

In some cases, increases in CBV can be seen after TBI and contribute to intracranial hypertension. When an increase in CBV is seen, it may result from local increases in cerebral glycolysis, "hyperglycolysis" as described by Bergsneider and colleagues.[143] In regions with increases in glutamate levels, such as in contusions, increases in glycolysis are observed because astrocyte uptake of glutamate is coupled to glycolysis rather than oxidative metabolism. Recall that oxidative metabolism is generally depressed by approximately 50% in comatose victims of severe TBI in the intensive care unit.[144] Hyperglycolysis results in a marked local increase in cerebral glucose utilization, with a coupled increase in CBF and CBV and resultant local brain swelling. That said, the contribution of hyperglycolysis to the pathogenesis of TBI remains unclear, and there have been few recent reports focusing on hyperglycolysis after brain injury.

A detailed discussion of this topic is beyond the scope of this chapter, but an expanded discussion of intracranial dynamics and vascular dysregulation in neurointensive care is provided in the next chapter. As MRI and magnetic resonance spectroscopic methods continue to develop and become applied to critically ill patients,[132] our knowledge of the mechanisms involved in cerebral swelling should greatly advance.

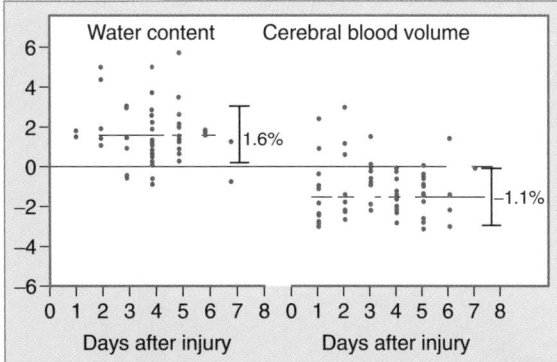

Figure 29-6 The percentage of change in brain water content as assessed by magnetic resonance imaging, and cerebral blood volume (CBV) as measured by computed tomography and indicatory dilution technique in 109 studies of adults with traumatic brain injury (TBI). Brain water is increased and CBV is reduced in adults with severe TBI. *(From Marmarou A, Barzo P, Fatouros P, et al. Traumatic brain swelling in head injured patients: brain edema or vascular engorgement? Acta Neurochir Suppl. 1997;70:68-70.)*

It must be remembered that although neuronal and axonal injury are key downstream events in the evolution of damage after severe TBI, brain swelling and resultant intracranial hypertension is still the principal target for titration of therapy in the intensive care unit.

INFLAMMATION AND REGENERATION

There appear to be both acute detrimental and subacute/chronic beneficial aspects of inflammation in cerebral ischemia and TBI. Inflammatory mechanisms in the evolution of secondary injury and repair have the greatest support in stroke and TBI, although some support for a role of inflammation in the regulation of neuronal death has been suggested even in cases of transient global ischemic insults.[145-149] There is robust acute inflammation after stroke and TBI in both experimental models[146,150,151] and in patients.[152-155] Nuclear factor-κB,[156] TNF-α,[99,157-160] interleukin (IL)-1β,[161,162] eicosanoids,[163] neutrophils,[164,165] and macrophages[166,167] contribute to both secondary damage and repair.

Markers of inflammation after TBI have been assessed in humans using two general strategies, (1) examination of inflammation in contused brain tissue or cerebral infarcts resected from patients with refractory intracranial hypertension, and (2) study of mediator levels in CSF. Consistent with a role for IL-1β in the evolution of tissue damage in cases of human TBI, Clark et al.[39] performed western blot analysis of brain samples resected from adults with refractory intracranial hypertension secondary to severe contusion. Interleukin-1-converting enzyme (ICE), also known as *caspase 1*, was activated, as evidenced by specific cleavage in patients with TBI. ICE activation is critical to the production of IL-1β. ICE activation was not detected in patients who died of non-CNS causes (Figure 29-8). This supports the production of IL-1β, a pivotal proinflammatory mediator, in the traumatically injured brain in humans. Similar support for increases in a variety of inflammatory mediators exists in human stroke.[99,155,159,160,164]

Studies of CSF further support a role for inflammation in TBI. Marion and associates[154] demonstrated increases in IL-1β in CSF after severe TBI in adults. These increases were attenuated by the use of moderate therapeutic hypothermia. Satchell et al.[106] demonstrated increases in ICE that were followed by a reduction in pro-IL-1β and an increase in IL-1β in CSF after severe TBI in children. Similarly, there are increases of a number of cytokines in CSF after severe TBI and stroke, including IL-6 and IL-8.[159,168] Contusion and local tissue necrosis appear to be important to trigger neutrophil influx, with resultant secondary tissue damage.[169] Neutrophil influx is accompanied by increases in inducible nitric oxide synthase (iNOS) in brain[155,170] and is followed by macrophage infiltration, which peaks between 24 and 72 hours after injury.[171] Macrophage infiltration and the differentiation of endogenous microglia into resident macrophages may signal the link between inflammation and regeneration with elaboration of a number of trophic factors (i.e., nerve growth factor [NGF], nitrosothiols, vascular endothelial growth factor).[161,168,172,173] Kossmann et al.[168]

reported a link between IL-6 production and the production of neurotrophins such as NGF in human head injury. Cultured astrocytes treated with either IL-6 or IL-8 in CSF from brain-injured adults produced NGF. Cytokine production after cerebral ischemia and TBI may be important to neuronal plasticity and repair, as discussed later.

Studies in models of TBI suggest early detrimental effects of a number of inflammatory mediators but beneficial effects of inflammation on long-term outcome.[157,174] Mice deficient in TNF-α exhibit improved functional outcome (versus wild-type) early after TBI. However, the long-term consequences of TNF-α deficiency on outcome are detrimental.[157] Similarly, despite a detrimental role for iNOS in the initial 72 hours after trauma,[175] iNOS-deficient mice demonstrated impaired long-term outcome versus controls[176]; iNOS is important in wound healing, and iNOS-derived nitrosylation of proteins may play a role.[172] Regeneration and plasticity play important roles in mediating beneficial long-term effects on recovery, and these responses are linked to inflammation. Analogs of these beneficial consequences of inflammation are anticipated in humans but remain to be demonstrated.

The contribution of the inflammatory response to cerebral ischemia and TBI remains to be determined. Although there are a few promising reports in models of the use of antiinflammatory therapies in TBI and ischemia (targeting IL-1β, ICE/caspase 1, and TNF-α), it is unclear whether antiinflammatory therapies will improve outcome after stroke or TBI in humans. Initial trials have not been promising.[164] Finally, the consequences of antiinflammatory therapies on the incidence of sepsis or secondary infectious complications must also be considered.[177] Similarly, the potential CNS consequences of novel immunostimulatory therapies (such as GCSF or GMCSF) for the treatment of sepsis and multiple organ failure must also be carefully considered when these agents are used in patients with multisystem disease that includes CNS injury.[177]

ENDOGENOUS NEUROPROTECTANTS

Ischemia, excitotoxicity, or their combination, are key facets of secondary injury. These mechanisms are linked to calcium overload, oxidative stress, and mitochondrial failure. There is, however, a coupled endogenous retaliatory response to these ischemic and excitotoxic insults. Two important components of this cascade are adenosine and heat shock protein 70 (Hsp70). Adenosine is an endogenous neuroprotectant produced in response to both ischemia and excitotoxicity. It antagonizes a number of events thought to mediate neuronal death.[178] Breakdown of ATP leads to formation of adenosine, a purine nucleoside that decreases neuronal metabolism and increases CBF among other mechanisms. Adenosine binding to A1 receptors decreases metabolism by increasing K^+ and Cl^- and decreasing Ca^{++} conductances in the neuronal membrane. A1 receptors bind adenosine with high affinity and are located on neurons in brain regions that are susceptible to injury and are spatially associated with NMDA receptors.[179] Thus, locally released adenosine minimizes excitotoxicity. Binding of adenosine to lower-affinity A2 receptors (on

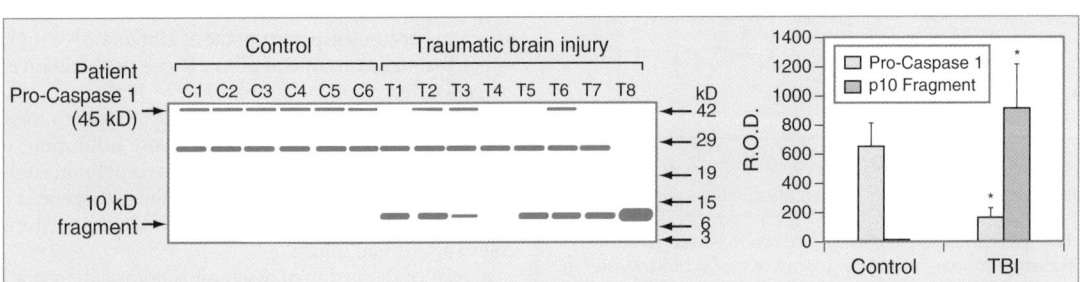

Figure 29-8 Evidence for interleukin 1β–converting enzyme (ICE/caspase 1) activation in cerebral contusions resected from adult patients with severe traumatic brain injury (TBI) and refractory intracranial hypertension. Western blot analysis demonstrating cleavage of the intact 45-kD pro-caspase 1 to the 10-kD fragment in each of 8 victims of severe TBI but in none of 6 control brain samples from patients who died of non–central nervous system causes. *(From Clark RS, Kochanek PM, Chen M, et al. Increases in Bcl-2 and cleavage of caspase-1 and caspase-3 in human brain after head injury. FASEB J. 1999;13(8):813-821.)*

cerebrovascular smooth muscle) causes vasodilation, although binding to A2a receptors on neurons may be detrimental. Brain interstitial levels of adenosine are increased 50- to 100-fold early after experimental cerebral ischemia or TBI.[180-183]

In clinical studies, marked increases in brain interstitial levels of adenosine in adults with TBI were seen during episodes of jugular venous desaturation (secondary insults), supporting a role of adenosine as a "retaliatory" defense metabolite.[184] Surprisingly, increases in CSF levels of the commonly consumed adenosine receptor antagonist, caffeine, were associated with favorable outcome after severe TBI in humans, a finding that may be explained by up-regulation of A1 receptors by chronic caffeine exposure.[185,186] Another endogenous neuroprotectant that plays a role after cerebral ischemia, severe TBI, and SAH is Hsp70. Hsp70 optimizes protein folding as a molecular chaperone. It also inhibits proinflammatory signaling.[187] Hsp70 is induced as part of the preconditioning response in brain and has been shown to be increased in both CSF and brain tissue after severe TBI in humans.[103,188,189] Thus, the brain mounts an important endogenous defense response to TBI. Therapies designed to augment these pathways have not been examined adequately.

Summary

Biochemical, cellular, and molecular mechanisms involved in the evolution of secondary brain injury after global and focal ischemia and TBI have been reviewed with particular attention to clinical studies relevant to neurointensive care. Our understanding of the biochemical, cellular, and molecular responses has progressed, particularly with the application of molecular biology methods to human materials. Future investigation should integrate these findings with bedside physiology and an improved assessment of outcome. Finally, novel imaging and diagnostic methods—particularly MRI, magnetic resonance spectroscopy, and positron emission tomography—must be coupled with biochemical and molecular methods to clarify the mechanisms involved in secondary damage and the local effects of novel therapies, including the study of brain pharmacodynamics.

KEY POINTS

1. Many of the biochemical, cellular, and molecular mechanisms that are important to the evolution of secondary brain damage after insults in neurointensive care, including cardiopulmonary arrest, stroke, traumatic brain injury, subarachnoid hemorrhage, status epilepticus, and hypoglycemia, share cerebral ischemia and/or energy failure as a critical initiator of damage.

2. Global cerebral ischemic insults, such as those that result from cardiopulmonary arrest, are generally brief in cases of patients who can be resuscitated successfully. The pathobiological condition that results is characterized by delayed neuronal death in selectively vulnerable brain regions, and the biochemical and molecular cascades in these cases involve components of programmed cell death.

3. Focal cerebral ischemic insults, such as those that result from stroke and subarachnoid hemorrhage, generally include an ischemic focus surrounded by periischemic penumbral regions. The biochemical and molecular cascades involve necrosis and/or infarct expansion into the penumbra. Cell death in the penumbra can include phenotypes that span the continuum from necrosis to apoptosis.

4. In cases of traumatic brain injury, the biochemical and molecular mechanisms involved depend on the specific type of insult, ranging from focal contusion (in which local osmolar swelling and excitotoxicity predominate) to diffuse axonal injury (in which secondary axotomy from proteolysis predominates).

5. Excitotoxicity, resulting from increases in brain interstitial concentrations of a number of excitatory amino acids, is a common mediator of secondary injury across insults.

6. Apoptosis involves several distinct pathways, including an extrinsic pathway triggered by external cell signals such as death receptor–ligand interaction, an intrinsic pathway triggered by signals from mitochondrial or endoplasmic reticulum, and a caspase-independent pathway involving mitochondrial dysfunction. However, delayed neuronal death in patients with critical central nervous system insults in the intensive care unit does not demonstrate classic apoptotic features but rather commonly exhibits a mixed phenotype.

7. Cerebral swelling can result from a variety of cellular mechanisms, including vasogenic edema, astrocyte swelling, increased tissue osmolar load, or vascular dysregulation with increased cerebral blood volume.

8. Inflammation appears to have a dichotomous role after cerebral ischemia or traumatic brain injury, including early exacerbation of damage by inflammatory mediators but secondary benefit through the link between inflammation and regeneration.

9. Autophagic neurodegeneration is observed after acute brain injury from trauma or ischemia; however, whether autophagy (cellular self-consumption) contributes to or protects from neuronal death or is merely an epiphenomenon remains to be determined.

ANNOTATED REFERENCES

Barone FC, Feuerstein GZ. Inflammatory mediators and stroke: new opportunities for novel therapeutics. J Cereb Blood Flow Metab 1999;19(8):819-34.
A superb review article describing the molecular components and temporal sequence of events in the inflammatory cascade set into motion in cases of ischemic brain injury.
Bullock R, Zauner A, Woodward JJ, et al. Factors affecting excitatory amino acid release following severe human head injury. J Neurosurg 1998;89(4):507-18.
A superb clinical report on excitotoxicity that used cerebral microdialysis to assess levels of glutamate in 80 consecutive severely head-injured patients. Four patterns of brain interstitial levels of excitatory amino acids were described, and increases in glutamate were as much as 50 times normal in 30% of the patients. This manuscript raises the important point that mechanisms such as excitotoxicity appear to vary greatly depending on the type of traumatic injury, time after injury, and presence of secondary insults such as hypoxemia or intracranial hypertension.
Clark RS, Kochanek PM, Chen M, et al. Increases in Bcl-2 and cleavage of caspase-1 and caspase-3 in human brain after head injury. FASEB J 1999;13(8):813-21.
This is a bench-to-bedside study of a number of key molecular events in cases of secondary damage in human cerebral contusions, including activation of caspase 1 and caspase 3. These two processes are central to inflammation and programmed cell death. This was the first report of caspase activation in either ischemic or traumatic brain injury in humans.
Povlishock JT. Traumatically induced axonal injury: pathogenesis and pathobiological implications. Brain Pathol 1992;2(1):1-12.

This is an outstanding review on the biochemical and molecular events involved in the evolution of axonal damage after severe traumatic brain injury. This article discusses evidence supporting the now accepted concept of secondary axotomy and its consequences.
Siesjo BK. Cell damage in the brain: a speculative synthesis. J Cereb Blood Flow Metab 1981;1(2):155-85.
Highly quoted classic reference discussing a number of speculative biochemical mechanisms involved in the evolution of secondary damage after cerebral ischemia, epilepsy, and hypoglycemia. Despite being written before the molecular explosion, many of these hypotheses have shown merit as research in this area has progressed over the subsequent 25 years.
Siesjö BK, Katsura K, Zhao Q, et al. Mechanisms of secondary brain damage in global and focal ischemia: a speculative synthesis. J Neurotrauma 1995;12(5):943-56.
This is an outstanding review article that contrasts the biochemical and molecular alterations seen in focal versus global cerebral ischemia. The discussion is based on studies done in experimental models but is germane to the clinical conditions of cardiopulmonary arrest and stroke.
Snyder JV, Nemoto EM, Carroll RG, Safar P. Global ischemia in dogs: intracranial pressures, brain blood flow and metabolism. Stroke 1975;6(1):21-7.
Experimental animal study that constituted the first description of the development of early postischemic hypoperfusion after complete global cerebral ischemia, a fundamental finding in cardiopulmonary arrest and resuscitation that has withstood the test of time.

REFERENCES

Access the complete reference list online at http://www.expertconsult.com.

Critical Neuropathophysiology

W. ANDREW KOFKE

Neural function is essential to human existence. Thus, loss of any neural element in the course of a critical illness represents a major loss to a given individual. Neurons or supporting elements can be lost in a small, virtually unnoticeable manner, or there can be widespread selective neuronal loss or tissue infarction. Based on the notion that neural function is the essence of acceptable survival from critical illness, it is crucial for critical care management to include considerations of neural viability and the impact and interactions of the primary diseases and therapeutics on the nervous system.

There are numerous clinical scenarios in which a critically ill patient may present with a primary neurologic illness. In a general sense, these scenarios often involve ischemia, trauma, or neuroexcitation. Each of these may include a period of decreased cerebral perfusion pressure (CPP), usually due to elevated intracranial pressure (ICP), eventually compromising cerebral blood flow (CBF) sufficiently to produce permanent neuronal loss, infarction, and possibly brain death. In this chapter, we review the physiologic factors and ICP considerations critical to contemporary neurointensive care.

▨ Elevated Intracranial Pressure

PHYSIOLOGY OF INTRACRANIAL PRESSURE AND CEREBRAL BLOOD FLOW

The brain, spinal cord, cerebrospinal fluid (CSF), and blood are encased in the protecting but noncompliant skull and vertebral canal, constituting a nearly incompressible system (Figure 30-1). In a totally incompressible system, pressure would rise linearly with increased volume. However, there is capacitance in the system, thought to be provided by the intervertebral spaces. Once this capacitance is exhausted, the ICP increases dramatically with increased intracranial volume.

Based on the following relationship:

$$CBF = (MAP - ICP)/CVR$$

the concern is raised mathematically that increasing ICP is associated with decrements in CBF. However, the effect of increasing ICP on CBF is not straightforward, as mean arterial pressure (MAP) may increase with ICP elevations,[1] and cerebral vascular resistance (CVR) adjusts with decreasing CPP (increasing cerebral vessel diameter) to maintain CBF until maximal vasodilatation occurs.[2,3] This results in an increase in cerebral blood volume (CBV). This is thought to occur at a CPP less than 50 mm Hg, although considerable individual heterogeneity in this value exists with good reasons to believe that the lower limit of autoregulation (LLA) may be higher.[4] Thus, increasing ICP initially is often associated with vasodilatation and/or increasing MAP to maintain CBF without a nutritive decrement.

Normal ICP is less than 10 mm Hg. ICP greater than 20 mm Hg is generally treated with ICP-reducing agents,[5] but this is an epidemiologically derived action. Head trauma studies have indicated that patients with ICP over 20 mm Hg generally do poorly,[5,6] although simply elevating ICP to above 20 mm Hg (in experimental animals) is not necessarily associated with decrements in CBF or permanent sequelae, provided the above-noted compensatory mechanisms occur,[7,8] and venous ICP-related venous outflow obstruction with positive-feedback exacerbation of ICP does not occur.[9]

Nonetheless, increasing ICP due to mass lesions or obstruction of CSF outflow can exhaust compensatory mechanisms, with compromise of CBF. Initially, distal runoff of the cerebral circulation increases. As the process continues, the normally continuous (through systole and diastole) cerebral perfusion becomes discontinuous (systolic perfusion only) (Figure 30-2).[10] Further compromise of CPP results in further oxygen extraction progressing to anaerobic metabolism, exacerbation of edema, and ultimately intracranial circulatory arrest.[10] Thus, when ICP increases, early recognition is important to determine whether a deleterious sequence of events is starting.

Traditional notions of cerebral autoregulation, with CBF constant over a CPP range of approximately 50 to 150 mm Hg, has not gone without challenge.[4] Drummond argues that this common notion derives from a figure in a review article by Lassen,[11] which itself was an estimate based on data published by McCall in 1953[12] from pregnant volunteers undergoing blood pressure (BP) alteration with hydralazine and *Veratrum viride*. Despite the use of potentially cerebral vasoactive drugs, these observations remained unconfirmed in humans. Drummond suggests that most human data published since 1953 support an LLA of 70 mm Hg, with one investigator suggesting the onset of cerebral ischemia symptoms in normal humans to arise at a MAP of 55 mm Hg.[13] Moreover, his closer review of published data suggests large interindividual variation in LLA. Drummond suggests that the only safe approach to an individual patient is to assume that no less than 75% of his/her resting MAP should be assumed to be the LLA. Symptoms of cerebral hypoperfusion tend to arise when MAP falls to about 50% of the resting value. These assertions of the need to individualize are increasingly being supported in the context of head injury with recent studies of the use of dynamic autoregulation assessment to determine optimal BP for a given patient.[6,14-16]

It is also of interest that LLA, based on CPP (MAP − ICP), may vary with ICP and with jugular venous pressure. McPherson et al., in a canine model, noted LLA was higher with elevated jugular venous pressure. This may, however, actually reflect the lack of knowledge regarding the proper definition for CPP, and that it may vary depending on the influence of the venous Starling resistor.[8,17] Brady et al.,[18] in an atraumatic immature piglet model of intracranial hypertension, found that LLA had a positive correlation with ICP. That is, LLA CPP was higher with higher levels of ICP. They suggest the possibility that compensating for an increase in ICP with an equivalent increase in arterial blood pressure (ABP) may not be sufficient to prevent a decrement in CBF and cerebral ischemia. Further studies in adults will be needed. Nonetheless, Brady et al.[18] point out that Cremer et al.[19] observed an LLA elevation in adult trauma patients with intracranial hypertension. The overall suggestion is that there is a need for individualized dynamic autoregulation assessment to determine each patient's optimal CPP.[6,14-16] Indeed, this may be only one component of a battery of multimodal monitoring, so-called integrative neuromonitoring, that is increasingly being advocated.[20]

Another approach to characterizing cerebral autoregulation has been espoused by Dewey et al.,[21] Early et al.,[22] and Burton et al.[23] Using observations in pacemaker-dependent dogs and a beat-to-beat measure of brain blood flow, they observed that abrupt cessation of cardiac activity produced zero CBF well above the generally accepted LLA. Indeed, they reported that this critical closing pressure varied with the resting MAP, generally being about 40 to 50 mm Hg below MAP. They concluded that the normal cerebral circulation assumes a tonic state of contraction that varies with MAP and ICP, more tone at higher BP or lower ICP, less at lower BP or higher ICP, such that the true dynamic cerebral perfusion pressure is MAP − CCP,

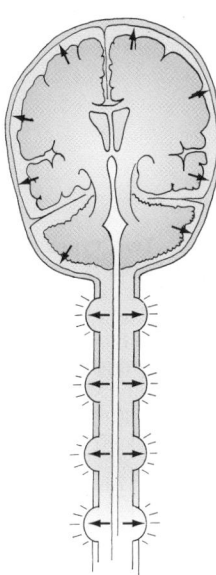

Figure 30-1 The brain, spinal cord, and blood are encased in the skull and vertebral canal, thus constituting a nearly incompressible system. System capacitance is thought to be provided via intervertebral spaces. *(From Kofke W, et al. Neurologic intensive care. In: Albin M, editor. Textbook of Neuroanesthesia. New York: McGraw-Hill; 1997: 1272.)*

with CBF = (MAP − CCP)/CVR. Burton's model can be use to describe CCP as: CCP = ICP + tension of arterial walls.[21] The CCP is presumed to be altered by various drugs and disease states to thereby produce variations in CBF, despite otherwise unchanged traditional CPP (MAP − ICP). Thus the true definition and measurement of CPP may be a good deal more dynamic and complex than is understood at this time.

CCP was further studied more recently by Czosnyka et al.[24] in humans with traumatic brain injury (TBI). If autoregulation is relatively intact, CCP-ICP remains high, but with injury sufficient to produce dysautoregulation, CCP-ICP decreases, indicating decreased tension in arterial walls.

CONTRIBUTORS TO INTRACRANIAL HYPERTENSION

Brain

The brain normally occupies about 80% of the contents of the skull, but its volume can be increased by edema. There are two types of edema, *cytotoxic* and *vasogenic*, referring to swelling produced by cellular or vascular processes, respectively.[25] Any edema can increase ICP.

It can be heterogeneously distributed such that pressure gradients occur, leading to a variety of herniation syndromes.

Cerebrospinal Fluid

CSF is generated in the choroid plexus and absorbed in the arachnoid villi. An equilibrium normally exists between production and absorption. Disruption of this equilibrium can lead to increased ICP with hydrocephalus, the condition wherein there is an excess of fluid in all or part of the CSF in the brain. Hydrocephalus is generally categorized as communicating or noncommunicating. In communicating hydrocephalus, the CSF circulation between the site of CSF production and absorption is intact. However, abnormally decreased absorption or increased production results in increased CSF accumulation. In noncommunicating hydrocephalus, the pathways are blocked such that CSF cannot circulate to the convexity of the brain to be absorbed. This results in accumulation of CSF in the ventricles, producing distension.[26]

Blood

CBV is an important contributor to variations in ICP, in part due to the wide variations in CBV that can occur with normal physiologic homeostasis and with the effects of drugs and disordered physiology. When CBV increases due to increased CBF, this can produce a dramatic increase in ICP if intracranial compliance is abnormal. However, unlike ICP elevation due to increased CSF volume, edema, or a tumor—in which decreased CBF is expected—this variety of ICP increase is often produced by increased CBF, making the significance of the ICP elevation unclear. This is discussed later.

Another mechanism of increased CBV occurs with obstruction of venous outflow. This results in brain engorgement and edema and CBV-mediated increased ICP, but without increased CBF[27]; this too is discussed in more detail later.

Masses

The fourth cause of increased ICP is pathologic masses. These can be in the form of hematoma or neoplastic tumors. In both cases, the faster the onset of the mass effect, the more acute the rise in ICP. Evidently there are compensatory mechanisms in intracranial compliance that can allow quite large slow-growing masses to arise in the brain without elevated ICP. On the other hand, similarly sized masses arising acutely are associated with symptomatic increases in ICP.

Venous Pathology

Venous pathology also plays a role in the genesis and propagation of intracranial hypertension. Blood coursing through the brain runs through arteries, capillaries, veins, sagittal and other dural sinuses, and then on to the internal jugular and other extracranial veins. In the context of a closed intracranial space, the relationship of these vessels to the tissue and CSF surrounding them becomes important. Notably, several investigators, in laboratory preparations, have observed a distinct drop off in intraluminal pressure in going from cerebral cortical

Figure 30-2 Progression of transcranial Doppler waveforms with decreasing cerebral perfusion pressure after head injury. Progression is apparent from a normal-appearing transcranial Doppler waveform to intracranial hypertension sufficient to induce intracerebral circulatory arrest. *(From Hassler W, Steinmetz H, Gawlowski J. Transcranial Doppler ultrasonography in raised intracranial pressure and in intracranial circulatory arrest. J Neurosurg 1988; 68[5]:745-751.)*

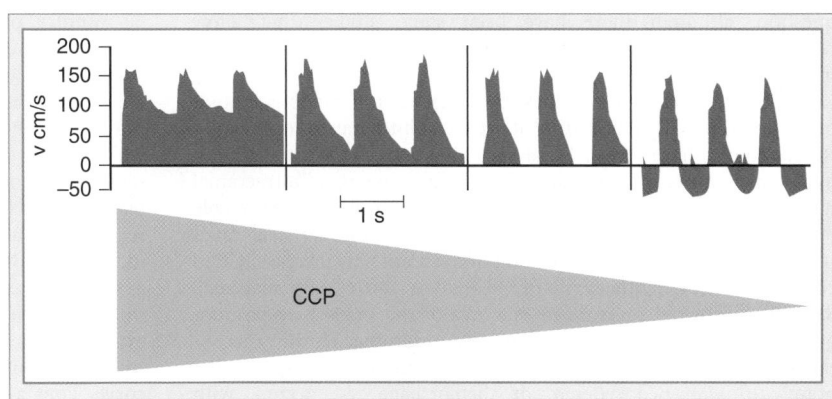

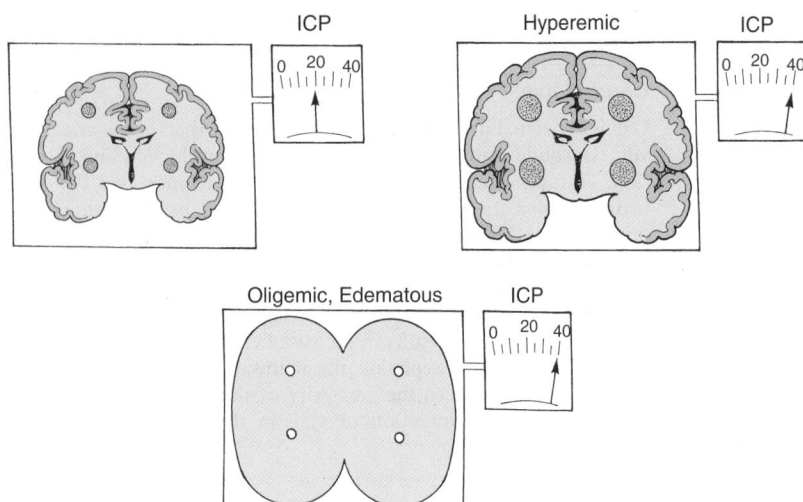

Figure 30-3 Two types of intracranial hypertension. From a baseline condition, intracranial pressure (ICP) can increase in two ways: (1) an increase in cerebral blood volume associated with reflex vasodilation due to moderate blood pressure decreases and (2) via malignant brain edema or other expanding masses encroaching on the vascular bed to produce intracranial ischemia. Stippled circles in each coronal brain section represent cerebral vasculature/blood volume. (From Kofke W, et al. Neurologic intensive care. In: Albin M, editor. Textbook of Neuroanesthesia. New York: McGraw-Hill; 1997: 1274.)

veins to the sagittal sinus. This is most evident when ICP is elevated and indicates the presence of a vascular waterfall at a point just proximal to the sagittal sinus as the extraluminal high-pressure CSF acts to impede flow from cortical veins to the sagittal sinus.[8,9,28,29] In fact, Nemoto[9] and Nakagawa et al.[28] have further observed that the cerebral venous pressure tends to be consistently higher than the ICP. The implications of these observations are that elevated ICP begets increased cerebral venous pressure. The increased cerebral venous pressure promotes and exacerbates brain edema, which may have been the initial cause of the intracranial hypertension. This then leads to a positive-feedback cycle wherein increased ICP increases cerebral venous pressure which then increases ICP.[9,30] Thus any other factors that may promote brain edema or otherwise increase ICP in this tenuous situation (e.g., high extraventricular drain, systemic hypertension,[31] hypoosmolarity) may initiate such a positive-feedback process.

TYPES OF INTRACRANIAL HYPERTENSION

There are two types of intracranial hypertension, categorized according to CBF as hyperemic or oligemic (Figure 30-3).[6] In the normal state, increases in CBF are not associated with increased ICP, because capacitive mechanisms compensate for the CBV-mediated increased intracranial volume. However, in the situation of disturbed intracranial compliance, small increases in intracranial volume produce significant increases in ICP.[2,3]

This suggests an important issue: raised ICP has traditionally been considered a concern because it indicates that cerebral perfusion might be jeopardized. It is unclear whether it is appropriate to be concerned about the potential for ICP-induced intracranial oligemia when the cause of the high ICP is intracranial hyperemia with associated increased CBV. There have been no detailed examinations of this question, although there have been some studies that allow reasonable inferences about the significance of hyperemic intracranial hypertension.

For many years it has been known that abrupt noxious stimuli briefly increase ICP in the setting of decreased intracranial compliance. Recent studies have revealed that such situations are associated with hyperemia, strongly suggesting that brief hyperemic intracranial hypertension is not a dangerous situation.[32] However, it is reasonable to be concerned about such hyperemia for four reasons. First, elevated ICP due to hyperemia in one portion of the brain may increase ICP to compromise CBF in other areas of the brain in which CBF is marginal. Secondly, increased pressure in one area of the brain may produce gradients that might lead to a herniation syndrome. Thirdly, there is theoretical concern that inappropriate hyperemia predisposes the brain to worsened edema or hemorrhage as occurs with

hyperperfusion syndromes. And fourthly, there is increasing evidence that increased ICP obstructs venous outflow to further exacerbate brain edema in a positive-feedback manner.[9,30] Thus hyperemic intracranial hypertension has a theoretical potential to be deleterious, although this has yet to be demonstrated in a systematic fashion. For brief periods, as may occur during intubation or other limited exposure to noxious stimuli, it is suggested (but not proven) that it may not be problematic.[33] An example of this conundrum is illustrated in Figure 30-4.

In contrast, oligemic intracranial hypertension is associated with compromised cerebral perfusion and is clearly deleterious.[6,10] This is supported by the high mortality rate observed in head trauma patients in whom ICP rises due to brain edema with decrements in CBF.[10,34] Transcranial Doppler echography and CBF studies on these patients have demonstrated that CBF is low and perfusion is discontinuous during the cardiac cycle (see Figure 30-2).[10,35] Moreover, jugular venous bulb data indicate that oxygen extraction is markedly increased, suggesting loss of reserve with occurrence of anaerobic metabolism.[35] In this setting, noxious stimuli can further increase the ICP, producing the situation of hyperemic added to oligemic intracranial hypertension. Presumably, in this setting the hyperemic rise in ICP acts to further reduce regional CBF in compromised areas with brain edema and may contribute to vasogenic edema.

BLOOD PRESSURE EFFECTS ON INTRACRANIAL PRESSURE: PLATEAU WAVES

Lundberg, in a pioneering 1960 study,[34] monitored ICP in hundreds of patients, identifying characteristic pressure waves. One category of these waves has been identified as *plateau waves*, which are known to be associated with increased CBV (Figure 30-5).[2] Such waves occur when the ICP abruptly increases to systemic BP levels for about 15 to 30 minutes, occasionally accompanied by neurologic deterioration. Rosner[3] synthesized the data and convincingly suggests that intracranial blood volume dysautoregulation is responsible for plateau waves. He induced mild head trauma in cats and subsequently intensively monitored the animals after the insult. With normal fluctuations in BP, while in the normal range, he observed that mild BP decrements to a mean of approximately 70 to 80 mm Hg preceded the development of plateau waves (Figure 30-6). Cerebral blood volume in normally autoregulating brain tissue increases with decreasing BP. However, the increase in CBV is nonlinear. There is an exponential increase in CBV as CPP decreases to levels of 80 mm Hg and below (Figure 30-7).[3] A small decrease in BP, although in the normotensive range, produces exponential increases in CBV in a setting of abnormal intracranial compliance with the ICP at the elbow of the ICP-intracranial volume curve. Thus a small decrease in BP introduces an exponential CBV

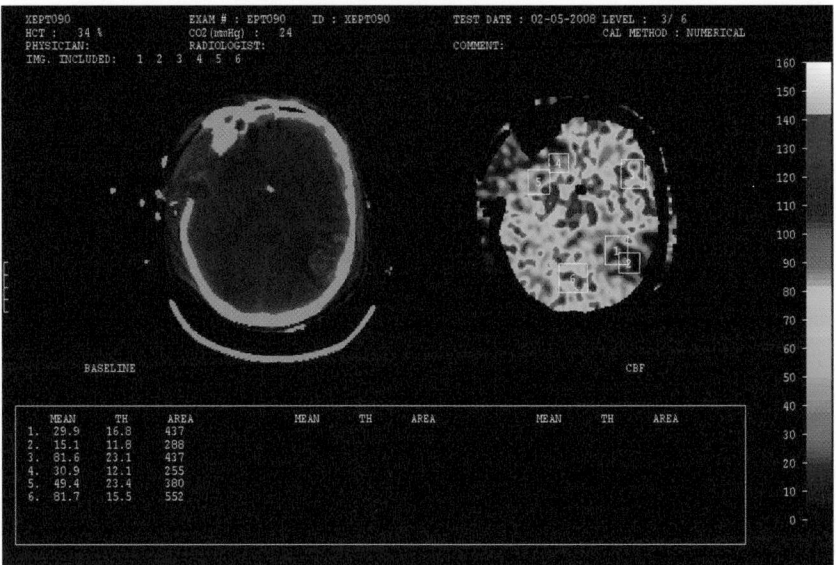

Figure 30-4 Computed tomography scan of a head-injury patient 5 days after admission and surgery for epidural and subdural hematomas with an intracranial pressure (ICP) of 20-30 mm Hg, jugular bulb saturation 90%, brain tissue PO_2 35-50 mm Hg (FIO_2 0.5 with PaO_2 192) showing oligemic to normal to hyperemic cerebral blood flows. Depicted regions of interest show cerebral blood flows (mL/100 gm/min) of 29.2 (ROI 1), 15.1 (ROI 2), 81.6 (ROI 3), 30.9 (ROI 4), 49.4 (ROI 5), and 81.7 (ROI 6). There is an overall pattern of significant hyperemia but with areas at risk of ischemia. Some cerebral blood flow artifact is evident in the area of the craniectomy.

change upon an exponential ICP relationship such that ICP will increase abruptly and to a significant extent. Cremer et al.'s observations of ICP increases with deliberate ABP decreases in TBI patients provide further support that these concepts are relevant to clinical practice.[19]

Plateau waves spontaneously resolve with a hypertensive response or with hyperventilation that will act to oppose the increase in CBV. Clearly, to develop a plateau wave there must be a portion of the brain with normally reactive vasculature in the presence of other brain areas with a mass effect and raised ICP, a situation of *heterogeneous autoregulation*. In addition to preventing and treating plateau waves, data indicate that it is probably important to maintain MAP in the 80 to 100 mm Hg range in patients with high ICP.

Conversely, hypertension can also increase ICP, with animal models showing increased brain water with dopamine-induced increased blood pressure.[31,36] Typically, within the normal autoregulatory range, changes in BP have no effect on ICP. However, with brain injury and associated vasoparalysis, BP increases mechanically to produce cerebral vasodilatation, increasing ICP (Figure 30-8).[6,15,16,37-40]

It appears that both increasing and decreasing BP can increase ICP, suggesting the presence of a CPP optimum for ICP—based on Rosner's observations,[3,6,41,42] probably about 80 to 100 mm Hg, although this has not been definitively determined experimentally (Figures 30-9 and 30-10). An alternate view that lower BP should be employed has been argued as the so-called Lund approach by Grände et al.,[30] with much of its rationale based on the earlier discussion of the role of venous obstruction in intracranial hypertension. Indeed, recent studies are increasingly supporting the notion that the CPP optimum is highly variable and should be individually determined with emerging technologies.[6,15,16]

BLOOD PRESSURE, BRAIN INJURY, AND INTRACRANIAL HYPERTENSION—BEYOND PLATEAU WAVES

Recent advances in transcranial Doppler (TCD) ultrasonography have allowed insights into dynamic, nearly instantaneous assessment of cerebral autoregulation in critically ill patients. Such technology has permitted the aforementioned observations of CCP in head-injured

Figure 30-5 Plateau waves. Simultaneous recordings of regional cerebral blood volume (rCBV) and ventricular fluid pressure (VFP) during three consecutive plateau waves. The rCBV was measured in eight regions over the left hemisphere. Mean changes in the eight regions are shown in the uppermost curve of the rCBV diagram. Note that rCBV and VFP curves show a very similar course during the three waves. *(From Risberg J, Lundberg N, Ingvar DH. Regional cerebral blood volume during acute transient rises in the intracranial pressure (plateau waves). J Neurosurg 1969;31(3):303-310.)*

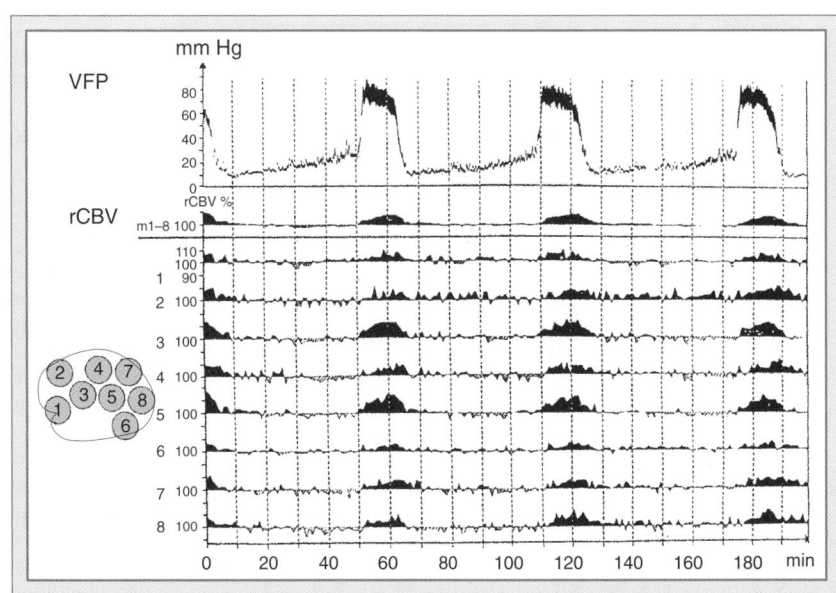

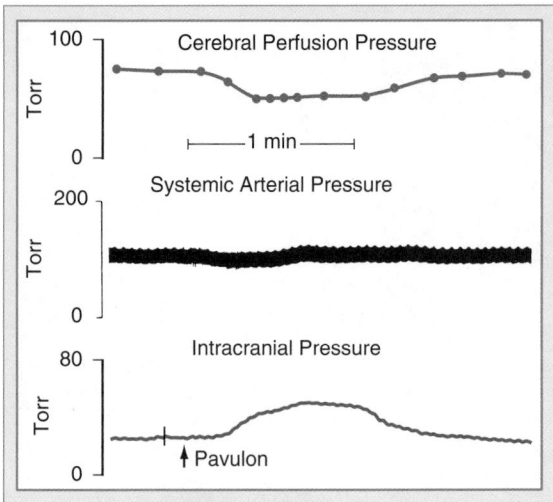

Figure 30-6 In an animal head-trauma model, a trivial-appearing and transient decrease in systemic arterial blood pressure in the setting of borderline cerebral perfusion pressure precipitates sufficient cerebral vasodilatation to markedly increase intracranial pressure. Restoration of cerebral perfusion pressure is associated with abolition of the plateau wave. *(From Rosner MJ, Becker DP: Origin and evolution of plateau waves. Experimental observations and a theoretical model. J Neurosurg 1984;60(2):312-324.)*

humans[24] and the report of apparent diminution in arterial wall tension in patients with cerebral dysautoregulation. Moreover, Czosnyka et al.[14] observed in TBI patients a U-shaped curvilinear relationship in flow velocity versus ABP, with worse autoregulation with ABP lower than 75 mm Hg and ABP higher than 125 mm Hg. They also noted increasing ABP to also increase ICP, further indicating a marker of dysautoregulation, the so-called PRx[6,15,16] (see following paragraph). Dynamic time domain analysis of cerebrovascular autoregulation using near-infrared spectroscopy (NIRS) or TCD is a current topic of

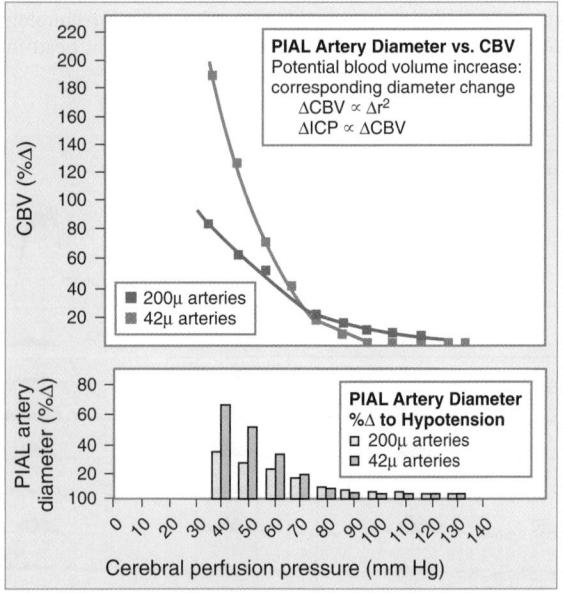

Figure 30-7 Cerebral vasodilatation occurs exponentially as cerebral perfusion pressure is reduced. *(From Rosner MJ, Becker DP. The etiology of plateau waves: a theoretical model and experimental observations. In: Ishii S, Nagai H, Brock M, editors. Intracranial Pressure V. New York: Springer-Verlag; 1983:301.)*

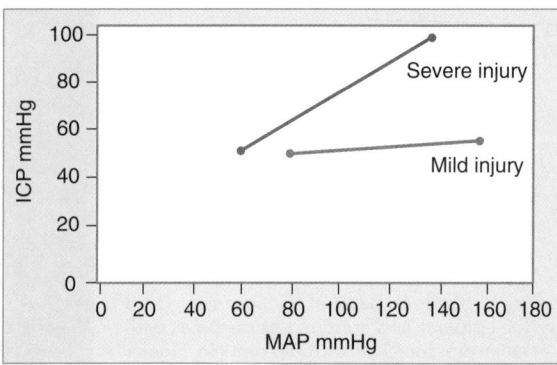

Figure 30-8 Blood pressure changes within the normal autoregulatory range have no effect on intracranial pressure (ICP). However, with brain injury, increases in mean arterial pressure (MAP) produce increases in ICP, with this effect more pronounced with more severe injury. Presumably, this effect is due to distention of vasoparalyzed blood vessels, with a consequent increase in cerebral blood volume. *(From Kofke W, et al. Neurologic intensive care. In: Albin M, editor. Textbook of Neuroanesthesia. New York: McGraw-Hill; 1997: 1276.)*

investigation with promising reports of potential efficacious and valid bedside use.[15,39,43-45]

The ICP pressure-reactivity index (PRx) is a more recently described quantitation of the earlier description of abnormal dynamic correlation of ICP changes with ABP changes and is another means to dynamically evaluate autoregulation,[6,15,16,40] with reports indicating that PRx correlates well with other autoregulation indices.[6,16,38,46] Steiner et al.[15] reported on the use of PRx monitoring in TBI patients to determine the optimal CPP. Patients with better autoregulation as defined by PRx had better outcomes. Moreover, patients with dysautoregulation related to higher ABP with corresponding ICP elevation also had worse outcomes, suggesting that autoregulation monitoring to ensure adherence to an individual's optimal CPP may be an outcome-altering intensive care unit (ICU) measure. Zweifel et al.[6] report congruent observations. Notably, PRx, as with TCD-based autoregulation studies, also appears to undergo a U-shaped curvilinear relationship with variations in CPP, with it being abnormally high (i.e., ICP varies with ABP) at low (ischemic) and high (hyperemic) CPP in TBI patients. Further complementing this are observations of abnormally high oxygen extraction fraction (OEF) and low OEF at these respective ABP extremes. This is underscored by several reports of a significant ischemic burden in TBI patients,[47-50] suggesting a delicate balance between hypotension-associated hypoperfusion and hypertension-associated edema exacerbation, both of which will worsen regional ischemia. Taken altogether, these autoregulation studies introduce the hypothesis that there is an individualized ABP optimum in TBI patients[6] that should be a therapeutic goal.

POSITIVE END-EXPIRATORY PRESSURE AND INTRACRANIAL HYPERTENSION

Positive end-expiratory pressure (PEEP) can increase ICP in two ways. The first is through impedance of venous return, increasing cerebral venous pressure and ICP. The second is through decreased BP and reflex increase of CBV, increasing ICP (Figure 30-11). The latter is likely the most common mechanism. Huseby's data[51] suggest that cerebral venous effects only occur with very high PEEP, a notion theoretically supported by the earlier discussion on the role of the veins in autoregulation of CBF and genesis of intracranial hypertension.

Shapiro and colleagues[52] demonstrated increases in ICP in head-injured humans during intracranial hypertension with application of PEEP (Figure 30-12). Examination of their data suggests that the most profound decreases in CPP occurred in patients with PEEP-induced decrements in MAP. This is consistent with the view put forth by

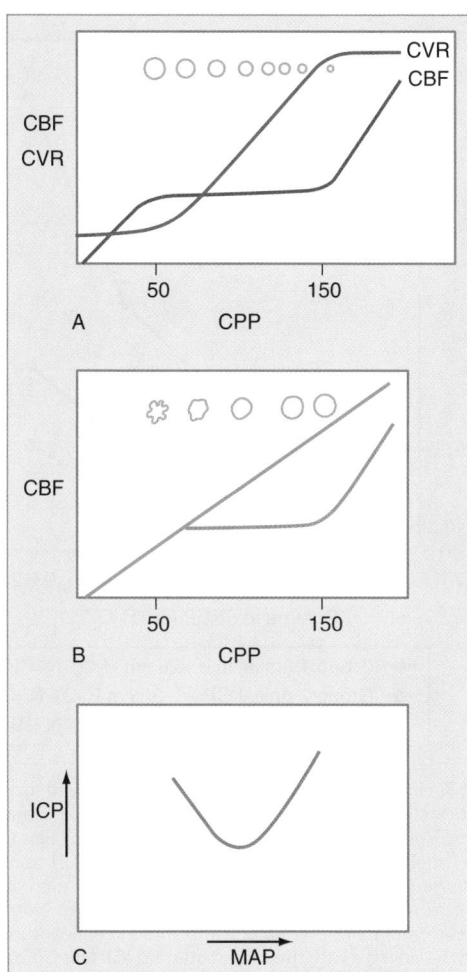

Figure 30-9 Cerebral perfusion pressure (CPP) versus cerebral blood flow (CBF) and cerebrovascular resistance (CVR). A, Blood flow is normally maintained constant through changes in CVR, depicted as changes in vascular diameter (and therefore cerebral blood volume [CBV]) in the figure. CBV varies inversely with CPP. **B,** With vasoparalysis due to injury, CVR does not change with CPP variations, such that CBF and CBV vary directly with CPP. **C,** In the situation of decreased intracranial compliance, both factors illustrated in **A** and **B** may interact to increase ICP. Normally autoregulating tissue **(A)** will predispose to CBV-mediated ICP elevation with decreasing blood pressure, whereas vasoparalyzed tissue **(B)** will predispose to CBV-mediated ICP elevations with increasing blood pressure, leading to the notion of an ICP optima (probably approximately 80 to 100 mm Hg) with varying CPP. *(From Kofke W, et al. Neurologic intensive care. In: Albin M, editor. Textbook of Neuroanesthesia. New York: McGraw-Hill; 1997: 1277.)*

Figure 30-10 In the setting of heterogeneous autoregulation in the brain, conditions may predispose to cerebral blood volume–mediated increases in intracranial pressure (ICP) with both increases or decreases in blood pressure. Stippled circles in each coronal brain section represent cerebral vasculature/blood volume. *(From Albin M, ed: Textbook of Neuroanesthesia. New York: McGraw-Hill; 1997: 1277.)*

Rosner[3] that decreases in BP increase CBV and ICP. Aidinis and colleagues,[53] in studies on cats, confirmed these observations in a more controlled setting. In addition, they assessed the role of pulmonary compliance, finding that decreased pulmonary compliance induced by oleic acid injections results in less effect of PEEP to increase ICP. In situations in which PEEP is likely to be needed, with decrements in pulmonary compliance, such observations indicate that any adverse effects on ICP are less likely to be manifest. This may be related to observations that hemodynamic effects of PEEP are less apparent with noncompliant lungs,[53,54] such that hypotensive-mediated increases in CBV do not occur.

The intuitive notion that PEEP increases cerebral venous pressure to increase ICP is not as straightforward as it initially may seem. For PEEP to increase cerebral venous pressure to levels that will increase ICP, the cerebral venous pressure must at least equal the ICP, which affects the Starling resistor just proximal to the sagittal sinus.[28] Thus the higher the ICP, the higher PEEP must be to have such a direct hydraulic effect on ICP. This concept was nicely proved by Huseby and colleagues[51] in dog studies in which PEEP was increased progressively, with different starting levels of ICP (Figure 30-13). It is important to note that they prevented PEEP-induced decrements in BP, thus avoiding any reflex increases in CBV. They suggested a hydraulic model to better conceptualize this (Figure 30-14). For example, if all of a 10 cm H_2O PEEP application were transmitted to the cerebral vasculature—which is unlikely given the decreased pulmonary compliance associated with the need for such PEEP—ICP will only be affected if it is less than 10 cm H_2O (7.7 mm Hg), increasing to a level no higher than the applied PEEP. This presupposes no PEEP-induced arterial pressure decrement.

ANTIHYPERTENSIVE THERAPY EFFECTS ON INTRACRANIAL PRESSURE

Intracranial pressure can also be influenced by antihypertensive drugs. In general, vasodilator drugs such as nitroprusside,[55,56] nitroglycerin,[57] and nifedipine[58] can be expected to increase ICP. Conversely, nonvasodilator antihypertensive drugs, generally sympatholytic drugs such as trimethaphan or beta-adrenergic blocking drugs such as esmolol or labetalol,[59] can be expected to have little or no effect on ICP. These observations suggest that the rise in ICP due to vasodilators is caused by increased CBF with an attendant increase in CBV. Also, decreases in BP, as an indirect consequence, may produce vasodilation in autoregulation brain areas, with increased CBV and ICP as discussed earlier for plateau wave physiology. The increase in ICP by these direct and indirect mechanisms thus does not threaten ischemia directly, although herniation and hyperperfusion syndromes and the aforementioned issues with venous outflow obstruction may occur and might be problematic. There has been a report of neurologic deterioration with nitroprusside use despite no change in BP.[56] Another consideration in the use of vasodilators is the propensity to reflexively increase

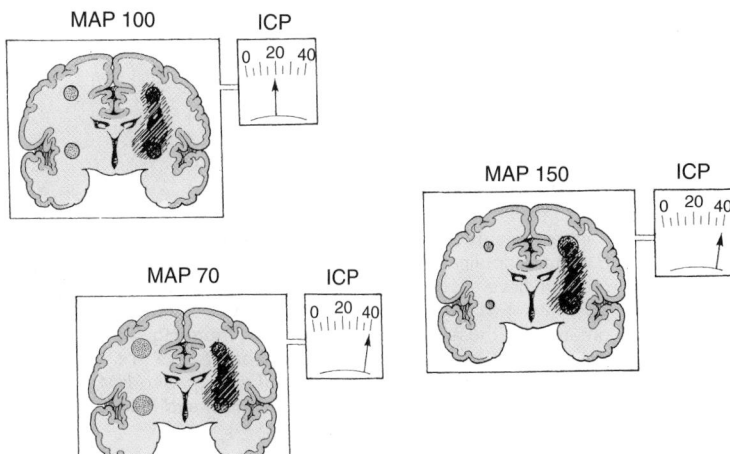

```
Low PEEP → ↓CO → ↓BP → ↑CBV → ↑ICP

High PEEP → ↑CVP → ↑Pss > ICP → ↑ICP
```

Figure 30-11 **Two mechanisms of positive end-expiratory pressure (PEEP)-mediated increases in intracranial pressure (ICP).** The addition of PEEP decreases cardiac output (CO) and blood pressure (BP), leading to a reflex increase in cerebral blood volume (CBV). If cerebral perfusion pressure is marginal with heterogeneous autoregulation, this can lead to further increases in ICP. Conversely, to increase sagittal sinus pressure to an extent sufficient to further increase ICP, which is already elevated, PEEP levels at or greater than the ICP must be applied. P_{ss}, sagittal sinus pressure.

endogenous plasma catecholamine concentrations.[60] Such increases in plasma catecholamines may be deleterious to the marginally perfused injured brain.[61-63]

Hyperperfusion Syndromes

In a variety of clinical situations, CBF may be inappropriately increased for a given BP. In the extreme case of such situations, vasoparalysis is present, and CBF becomes more or less a linear function of BP as described in recent dynamic autoregulation studies in TBI.[6,14,15,38] Such hyperperfusion syndromes may occur early in cases of severe hepatic encephalopathy,[64,65] 2 to 3 days after severe head injury,[35] after resection of large arteriovenous malformations (AVMs),[66-68] after carotid

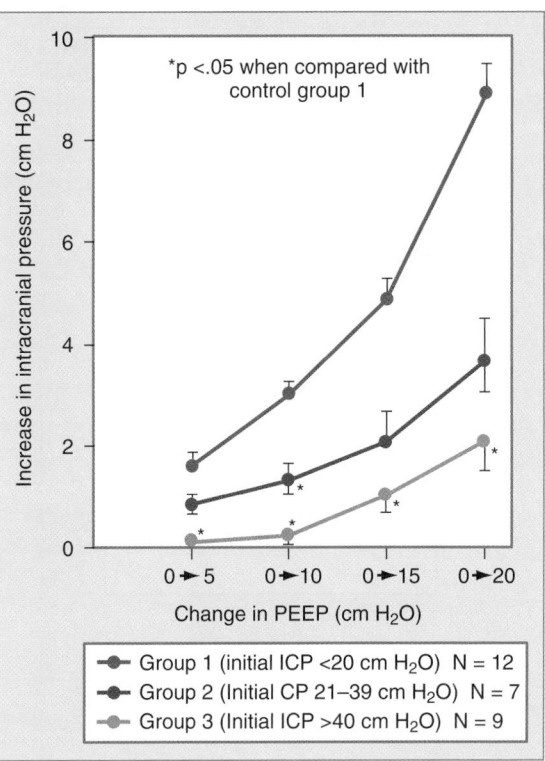

Figure 30-13 Increases in intracranial pressure (ICP) with positive end-expiratory pressure (PEEP) in dogs. Values are mean ± standard error of the mean. Group 1 included 12 animals with initial ICP less than 20 cm H_2O; group 2 included seven animals with initial ICP of 21 to 39 cm H_2O; group 3 included nine animals with initial ICP greater than 40 cm H_2O. Blood pressure was maintained constant in all animals. Note that with blood pressure maintained constant, the most significant increases in ICP occur in the animals with the lowest starting ICP level. *(From Huseby JS, Luce JM, Cary JM, et al. Effects of positive end-expiratory pressure on intracranial pressure in dogs with intracranial hypertension. J Neurosurg 1981;55(5):704-705.)*

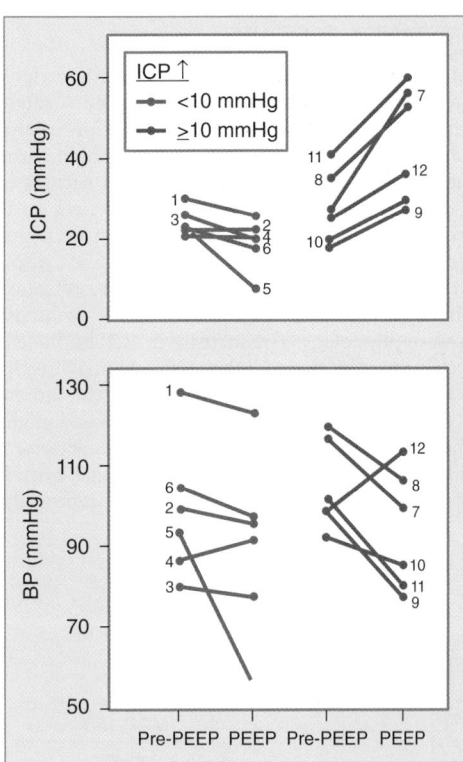

Figure 30-12 Intracranial pressure (ICP) and arterial blood pressure (BP) before and with the application of positive end-expiratory pressure (PEEP) (4-8 cm H_2O) in severely head-injured patients. The patients are arbitrarily divided into two groups: those with an ICP increase of 10 mm Hg or greater and those with ICP gains below 10 mm Hg. Note that PEEP-induced blood pressure decreases appear to be more marked in patients sustaining larger ICP increases. *(From Shapiro HM, Marshall LF. Intracranial pressure responses to PEEP in head-injured patients. J Trauma 1978;18(4):254-256.)*

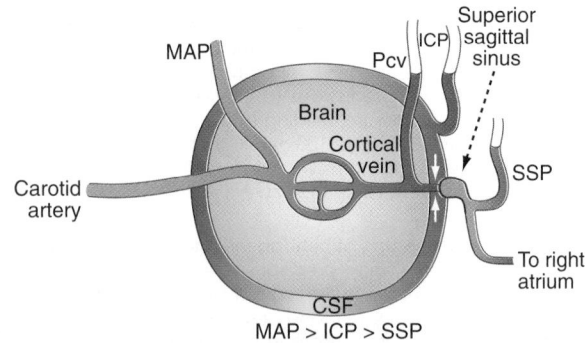

Figure 30-14 Schematic illustration of the intracranial space during raised intracranial pressure (ICP). Arrows indicate position of the hypothesized Starling resistor. Here, mean arterial pressure (MAP) is greater than ICP, which is greater than sagittal sinus pressure (SSP). Cortical vein pressure (Pcv) cannot fall below ICP, so flow is dependent on MAP minus ICP and independent of small changes in SSP. *(From Huseby JS, Luce JM, Cary JM, et al. Effects of positive end-expiratory pressure on intracranial pressure in dogs with intracranial hypertension. J Neurosurg 1981;55(5):704-705.)*

endarterectomy of severely stenotic lesions with poor collaterals,[69,70] after cerebral arterial thrombolysis,[71] and possibly during administration of cerebral vasodilators at high systemic BP.

Fulminant hepatic failure produces widespread physiologic changes, including altered cerebral physiology.[64,65] Aggarwal and coworkers[64,65] systematically examined cerebral hemodynamics and metabolism in severe hepatic encephalopathy and during recovery after hepatic transplantation. They have identified phases that are traversed in the course of going from normal cerebral physiology to brain death. Patients initially demonstrate elevated CBF at normotension. This is usually followed by hyperemic (high CBF and/or CBV) intracranial hypertension, then edema with oligemic intracranial hypertension, and finally intracranial circulatory arrest and brain death. The data clearly suggest that the hyperemia may be deleterious, possibly contributing to the development of subsequent cerebral edema. This is supported by observations that the cerebral edema seems to be prevented through the use of barbiturates and hyperventilation during the hyperemic phase.

Several investigators, in the course of examining cerebrovascular physiology after head trauma, have observed that patients with severe head injury initially have normal or low CBF. This is followed a few days later by increased CBF, which is associated with intracranial hypertension.[34] This may contribute to subsequent oligemic intracranial hypertension. This concept has been challenged by Marmarou et al. in a clinical study which did not reveal delayed hyperemia in most patients.[72]

The concept of normal perfusion pressure breakthrough indicates hyperperfusion at normal BP, such as after resection of a large AVM, when the remaining blood vessels lack the ability to constrict normally and regulate blood flow, resulting in abnormally high regional CBF. The pathogenesis is thought to be related to chronic arterial hypotension proximal to the AVM. The larger the AVM, the lower the intracranial BP to which the patient is acclimated (i.e., the cerebral vasculature locally down-regulates the CBF-MAP autoregulatory relationship). Removing the AVM abruptly exposes the cerebral arterial vessels and arterioles to pressure never before experienced.[67] Thus despite the BP being within normal limits, the pressure-naïve vasculature is unable to autoregulate, and the physiology of malignant hypertension may ensue to cause cerebral edema and/or hemorrhage. This is an attractive hypothesis that makes physiologic sense. However, Young and coworkers[68] report that autoregulation of the vascular bed after AVM resection is generally intact, indicating that vasoparalysis due to chronic hypotension may not be the most important contributor to normal perfusion pressure breakthrough.

One cause of neurologic deterioration after carotid endarterectomy is cerebral edema and/or hemorrhage. This is rather unusual, but the presence postoperatively of a unilateral throbbing headache suggests that it may be present. Blood flow studies reveal such patients to have cerebral hyperemia associated with removal of a large proximal obstruction. While normotension is usually well tolerated, hypertension probably increases the risk of hemorrhage, especially if there was a preoperative cerebral infarction. Similar to the AVM situation described earlier, vasculature that has acclimated to low proximal pressure now is presented with arterial pressure that is much higher, although within the epidemiologic norm.[69]

After thrombolysis of a cerebral artery, one important source of morbidity is edema or hemorrhage of the reperfused territory. With reperfusion of the ischemic tissue, hyperemia and dysautoregulation occurs for a period of time.[71] If sustained, this suggests that irreversible endothelial damage has occurred, and the patient is at risk for secondary edema or hemorrhage, particularly if the depth of ischemia is sufficient to produce early changes on a computed tomography scan.[73]

Vasodilators such as nitroprusside are frequently used in patients with severe arterial hypertension. When CBF is measured, it is noted that nitroprusside has minimal CBF effect with induced hypotension.[74] However, data are not available on its CBF-CBV effects with treatment of hypertension. Such vasodilators are known to cause an increase in ICP,[56,75] suggesting an element of cerebral hyperemia. This is supported by reports of cerebral dysautoregulation induced by nitroprusside.[76] This ICP elevation and hyperemia[74,77] appear to decrease as BP is lowered. This notion is supported by observations during neurosurgery with cerebral swelling present when nitroprusside is administered.[78] With its use for induced hypotension during neurosurgery, the brain is noted to be flaccid with no hyperemia evident. Thus cerebral vasodilators can produce a cerebral dysautoregulation/hyperperfusion syndrome, the extent of which is likely dependent on BP. Their use has not yet been reported to be associated with exacerbation of cerebral edema/hemorrhage.

All of the above syndromes describe a clinical course in humans consisting of inappropriate hyperemia for a given BP, followed by cerebral edema or hemorrhage. This suggests that the failure to autoregulate at normal pressure results in exposure of arterioles and capillaries to unacceptably high pressure. This then results in disruption of the blood-brain barrier, with consequent transudation of fluid or frank bleeding. The recent PRx data in humans with TBI and hyperemia with higher BPs in dysautoregulating brain[6] further supports these concepts.

Hyperthermia

Temperature management can be critical in neurointensive care. In animal models, hyperthermia has been shown to have deleterious effects on outcome after cerebral ischemia,[79] head trauma,[79] and seizure.[80] Nonrandomized human studies in stroke, TBI, and spinal cord injury strongly suggest a negative effect of hyperthermia on outcome,[81-86] with protective effects when induced normothermia is employed in TBI.[84] Conversely, mild hypothermia has been shown to have potential for neuroprotection.[87-94] The extent of hypothermia required to produce protection is modest (32°C to 36°C). The extent of protection is not adequately explained by reduction in cerebral metabolic rate,[95] suggesting that hypothermia has additional beneficial effects such as decreased free radical production or reduction in neurotransmitter neurotoxicity.[96]

Preliminary reports from a single-center trial of head trauma patients indicated that moderate hypothermia confers cerebral protection when applied within 6 hours of insult and maintained for 24 to 48 hours.[97] This observation was not confirmed in a subsequent multi-institutional trial, although head-injured patients who presented with hypothermia had a better outcome.[98] In addition, two recent single-center reports of hypothermia after cardiac arrest provide strong support for the notion that mild hypothermia is protective after cerebral ischemia.[99,100] Based on these reports, the American Heart Association has adopted hypothermia as a recommended therapy after resuscitation from cardiopulmonary arrest.[101] Reports on its use in TBI are conflicting, but nonetheless the Brain Trauma Foundation suggests selective and cautious application of prophylactic moderate hypothermia to 32°C to 35°C for 48 hours may be useful.[102]

Further complicating the role of hypothermia, however, are the recent results of the IHAST trial[103] showing no protection from mild hypothermia (used for all patients regardless of whether focal ischemia arose) during cerebral aneurysm surgery.

Gas Exchange

Cerebrovascular reserve is compromised in many intracranial pathologic processes. Normally, the brain compensates for decrements in supply of oxygen and substrates by vasodilating to maintain or increase flow.[104] Animal experiments indicate that it is possible to produce a condition in which cerebrovascular reserve is compromised with increased tendency to cerebral infarction. For example, occlusion of one carotid artery or inducing moderate hypoxemia does not produce symptoms as cerebral vasodilatation occurs to compensate. Indeed, some investigators contend that arterial hypoxemia occurring with normal cerebral vascular compensatory mechanisms does not cause brain damage. Of course, one contributing factor to this view is that hypoxic myocardial dysfunction produces circulatory collapse and death such that isolated posthypoxic (without ischemia) neuronal injury cannot occur. However, if hypoxemia is added to carotid occlusion, or vice versa, a stroke can occur because compensatory mechanisms, already fully utilized, cannot accommodate the further decrease in oxygen supply.[105,106] Examples of variants of this situation abound clinically.[107] Such examples of attenuated cerebrovascular reserve include cerebral edema, hypoxemia, carotid artery stenosis, peri-infarct penumbra, and anemia. Menon et al.,[50] using perilesional OEF data, report impaired reserve around contusions in TBI patients, raising the notion of heterogeneous distribution of cerebrovascular reserve after TBI in humans. This further supports their observations in other reports of an increased ischemic burden with TBI.[48,49] In each of these situations, although not easy to quantify, it is clear that added situations of compromised oxygen supply to the brain will risk neuronal injury.

Changes in $Paco_2$ have a profound impact on CBF. Normally, CBF varies linearly with $Paco_2$ between 20 and 60 mm Hg.[107] $Paco_2$-mediated changes in CBF occur with corresponding changes in CBV. In situations of abnormal intracranial compliance in which small changes in intracranial volume have large ICP effects, decreasing $Paco_2$ reduces ICP, and increasing $Paco_2$ raises ICP.

The primary concern with raised ICP is that it may be associated with cerebral oligemia, so these effects of $Paco_2$ on ICP are paradoxical. That is, decreasing $Paco_2$ reduces ICP but at the expense of CBF (Figure 30-15).[108] Minhas and colleagues[109] report that mild hyperventilation in brain-injured patients produces dangerous perilesional CBF decrements. However, Gupta and colleagues,[110] using tissue measures of brain-injured humans, reported sequential increases in $Ptio_2$ with decreasing $Paco_2$, with an optimum at 26 to 30 mm Hg. Nonetheless, data from head-trauma studies indicate that routine use of hyperventilation can worsen outcome.[111] Conversely, allowing hypercapnia to occur, although leading to increased ICP, is associated with increased CBF. These observations pertain to normally autoregulating tissue. The CBF effects in injured brain tissue can be unpredictable. For example, allowing $Paco_2$ to increase CBF in autoregulating brain areas by increasing ICP may compromise flow or produce venous outflow obstruction in other injured, already fully vasodilated regions.

Related to these concerns is the growing practice of permissive hypercapnia in some types of respiratory failure, performed to reduce the risk of ventilator-mediated lung injury. Reports are somewhat conflicting regarding its safety in the brain-injured patient. In a non-trauma porcine model, van Huls and colleagues[112] found that hypercapnia to 90 mm Hg increased tissue Po_2 while increasing ICP

from 20 to 30 mm Hg. Zhou et al.[113] in a rodent ischemia model demonstrated neuroprotection with modest hypercapnia. These reports and those of others suggest no direct neurotoxic harmful effects, but theoretically it seems hyperemia-mediated increased ICP still might introduce a risk of hyperemia-mediated herniation or inducement of a positive-feedback cycle through venous outflow obstruction and worsened edema[9] as discussed earlier. A recent report by Tasker and Peters,[114] however, suggests that the negative hyperemic effects associated with hypercapnia resolve over a day or so such that the pulmonary benefits of the hypercapnia can be gained as the adverse neurologic effects subside. This does raise the possibility of an unacceptable respiratory alkalosis on cessation of the permissive hypercapnia. Moreover, in neonates, hypercapnia increases CBF[115] that may lead to cerebral edema, increased ICP, and intraventricular hemorrhage.[116-119] Concerns are also raised by a pediatric case report of nonaneurysmal subarachnoid hemorrhage associated with and seemingly caused by permissive hypercapnia.[120]

The possibility of a neuroprotective effect of respiratory acidosis has also been reported.[113,121] Brain homogenates develop far fewer free radicals and less lipid peroxidation when pH is lowered by carbon dioxide than when it is lowered by hydrochloric acid,[122] and greater inhibition of tissue lactate production occurs when lowered pH is due to carbon dioxide than when it is due to hydrochloric acid.[123] Vanucci et al.[124] report a protective effect of modest hypercapnia in an in vivo model of neuronal hypoxia. In trauma patients with multiple organ dysfunction, Gentilello and colleagues[125] found permissive hypercapnia to increase ICP but adjusted the level of hypercapnia if ICP rises occurred. Similar problematic ICP increases were also observed in two head-injured patients by Levy et al.,[126] which they managed using tracheal gas insufflation, which may be a compromise solution in this conundrum of conflicting physiology and no outcome data. In summary, the data are not conclusive regarding the safety of permissive hypercapnia in the presence of brain injury. It seems that the optimal approach would be to cautiously apply it and adjust according to the ICP response. If unacceptable ICP elevations arise, the options would include abandoning permissive hypercapnia, treating the ICP to allow normalization of the CBF response to the CO_2 elevation over a few days, and possibly adding tracheal insufflation to the ventilator strategy to control $Paco_2$.

Hyperglycemia

Hyperglycemia has been associated with exacerbation of brain damage with both head trauma and cerebral ischemia,[127-129] but it is not a straightforward issue. Clearly, neuronal damage after global cerebral

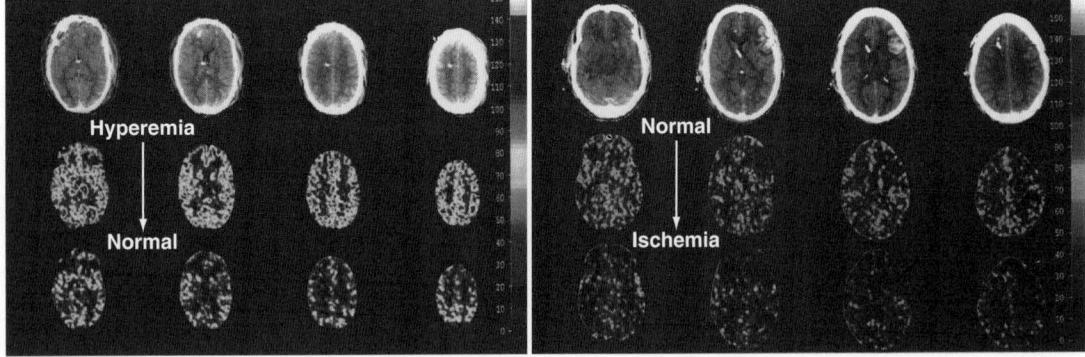

Figure 30-15 **Effects of $Paco_2$ changes on cerebral blood flow (CBF).** Two examples of disparate effects of hyperventilation on CBF. Both figures are stable xenon CBF scans in head trauma patients with and without hyperventilation. CBF scale is indicated on the right in mL/100 g/min, and Pco_2 is indicated above each study. Computed tomography images are indicated in the upper figures and CBF maps in the lower figures. In the left figure, $Paco_2$ was decreased from 40 to 30 mm Hg. Baseline scan shows hyperemia, and hyperventilated scan shows CBFs of approximately 60 to 70 mL/100 g/min, probably acceptable flows. In the right figure, $Paco_2$ was decreased from 38 to 30 mm Hg. Baseline CBFs were acceptable. The effect of this modest extent of hyperventilation was to produce widespread areas of CBF less than 20 mL/100 g/min, probably unacceptable flows. (See color section in this text.) *(Courtesy Howard Yonas, University of Pittsburgh.)*

ischemia is exacerbated by hyperglycemia.[130] Some studies have suggested that a blood glucose level over 120 mg% is deleterious in stroke patients.[127] However, subsequent studies with subhuman primates subjected to global ischemia have suggested a threshold of around 180 mg%.[112] Clearly, a blood glucose concentration greater than 400 mg% causes striking worsening of neurologic outcome with global ischemia.[128,131] The issue is further clouded by observations from brain microdialysis in human TBI patients of increased lactate/pyruvate ratio with aggressive control of blood glucose.[132]

With focal cerebral ischemia, the situation is less clear. There have been animal and human studies showing that brain damage is worsened, not affected, or lessened with hyperglycemia.[133-137] One report by Prado and colleagues[137] in rats suggested that the discriminating factor regarding worsened brain damage with hyperglycemia is whether there is collateral flow. Areas of the brain with minimal or absent collateral vessels were not affected or were improved with hyperglycemia. Brain areas with a continued trickle of flow sustained worse damage. Presumably, the continued substrate supply in anaerobic/oligemic (not ischemic) areas allowed greater accumulation of organic acids in the cells, leading to worsening brain damage.[133,138] Unfortunately, these observations are difficult to apply clinically to individual patients with focal ischemia.

Hyperglycemia has not been shown to have either deleterious or protective effects in two animal models of status epilepticus.[139,140] The model used in Swan's report[140] produced limbic system damage, whereas Kofke and colleagues[139] used a model producing substantia nigra damage. Seizure-induced nigral damage in rats is associated with hypermetabolic lactic acidosis[141] that was not exacerbated by hyperglycemia. The fact that nigral damage was not exacerbated with hyperglycemia suggests that metabolic acidosis may not be the sole factor in the development of brain damage after seizure.

Sepsis

In animal models, sepsis is known to decrease CBF while inducing neuroinflammation[142] with altered cerebral metabolic rate (up or down), mitochondrial disfunction,[143-145] metabolomic and proteomic disturbances,[146] and disruption of the blood-brain barrier (BBB).[147-149] These alterations and others undoubtedly underlie the clinical syndrome of septic encephalopathy with associated cognitive impairment.[150-152] In addition, it can decrease BP in a manner that may not be well tolerated by the brain with abnormal cerebrovascular reserve. Sepsis-induced decreases in BP can turn an area of cerebral oligemia into an area of ischemic cerebral infarction.

Sodium

HYPERNATREMIA

Hypernatremia can occur in neurologic ICU patients because of nonketotic diabetic coma, dehydration from lack of fluid intake or diuretic use, hypertonic fluid administration, diabetes insipidus, or panhypopituitarism.[153] It can be associated with thirst, irritability, seizures, intracranial hemorrhage, or coma, although the rate of increase in sodium concentration is thought to be an important factor in the clinical presentation. For example, a sodium level of 170 mEq/L can be associated with little neurologic symptomatology if the rise occurs over a prolonged period. Indeed, hypertonic saline is occasionally used as a primary therapy for raised ICP,[154-157] in which case the elevation in sodium should be considered desirable, with desirable ICP, vasoregulatory, and neurochemical effects. Moreover, treating it could precipitate a rebound increase in ICP.

Diabetes insipidus can occur when disease processes affect the pituitary gland or its vascular supply. It should be suspected when urine output is inappropriately increased. Typically, urine output can increase abruptly to greater than 1 L per hour and be associated with severe hypernatremia and hypovolemic hypotension. Diagnosis of diabetes insipidus is based on continued output of dilute urine in the context of hypertonic serum. The specific gravity of urine will be close to 1.001, with osmolarity less than 200 mOsm/L despite serum osmolarity that may be greater than 320 mOsm/L.[158]

HYPONATREMIA

Hyponatremia can occur because of the syndrome of inappropriate secretion of antidiuretic hormone, so-called cerebral salt wasting, or excessive free water administration. Syndrome of inappropriate secretion of antidiuretic hormone is generally associated with hypervolemia and cerebral salt wasting with hypovolemia. Both syndromes can be associated with elevated urinary sodium concentrations, making differentiation between the two difficult in routine clinical practice.[159] Rapidly increasing the sodium concentration can produce permanent neurologic damage due to central pontine myelinolysis.[160] When the sodium level achieved with such overcorrection is extreme (i.e., 168 to 195 mmol/L), extrapontine myelinolysis has also been reported.[161]

Catecholamines

Subarachnoid hemorrhage is an entity particularly notable for catecholamine effects, some of which are described elsewhere in this book. However, catecholamine effects also occur with increased ICP, stroke, head trauma, or any situation of compromised midbrain-hindbrain oxygen delivery. Notably, intraarterial catecholamine infusions into human cerebral arteries without evident BBB disruption has little effect on CBF and CMR.[162] However, subhuman primate studies in which BBB was disrupted indicate that such disruption followed by norepinephrine infusion produces significant increases in CBF and CMR,[163] indicating apparent neuroactivation by intravenous catecholamines.

Johnston et al.[164] evaluated a small group of patients for neurochemical effects of dopamine versus norepinephrine in brain-injured humans. Norepinephrine, but not dopamine, was associated with decreased arterial-venous oxygen differences and increased brain tissue oxygen but without differences in microdialysis indicators of anaerobiasis. In another report, dopamine increased ICP without having an impact on blood flow velocity or Sjvo2 compared to norepinephrine in humans with TBI.[165] Nonetheless, catecholamine-based vasopressor therapy is extremely common, although there remain significant knowledge gaps regarding the effects of these drugs, which basically are intravenous (IV) neurotransmitters, by and large, on the brain. A review specifically of their interaction in SAH illustrates many of these issues.

The dramatic increase in serum catecholamine levels after SAH peak at the same time as the peak incidence of post-SAH vasospasm, with symptom development corresponding to serum catecholamine levels.[166-170] This leads to the notion that hypothalamic injury with excess catecholamine release may be an important factor in the genesis of post-SAH spasm and stroke.[167] Several lines of evidence further support this hypothesis:

1. The cerebral vasculature is invested somewhat with adrenergic nerves. With SAH, the adrenergic receptors in the cerebral vessels decrease in quantity.[170,171] This suggests that denervation hypersensitivity may be occurring such that the increase in humoral catecholamines with SAH produces spasm in hyperreacting vessels.
2. Catecholamine release after SAH is sufficient to produce electrocardiographic changes[166,168,172,173] with ventricular wall motion abnormalities[174] and myocardial injury.[175,176] Notably, the left insular area of the brain has been associated with myocardial injury.[177-179]
3. Treatment of humans with SAH with beta- and alpha-adrenergic antagonists is associated with an improvement in neurologic outcome (Figure 30-16)[62] and electrocardiographic abnormalities.[173] Catecholamine infusion to induce hypertension can have unpredictable effects on CBF.[180]

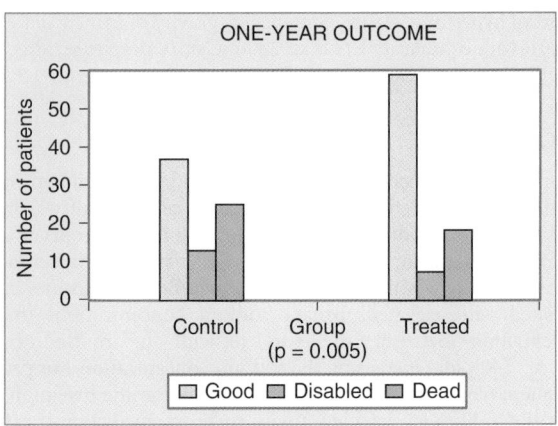

Figure 30-16 Subarachnoid hemorrhage patients were randomly treated with propranolol or placebo. Neurologic outcome was better in patients undergoing beta-blockade. *(Data from Neil-Dwyer G, Walter P, Cruickshank JM. Beta-blockade benefits patients following a subarachnoid hemorrhage. Eur J Clin Pharmacol 1985;28[Suppl]: 25-29.)*

4. In animal models, selective destruction of hindbrain adrenergic nuclei with cephalad projections prevents the development of vasospasm.[176] Moreover, laboratory studies indicate an important role for vasopressin in cases of vasospasm, because vasospasm cannot be produced in vasopressin-deficient rats.[181]

5. Studies in cerebral ischemia models provide strong support for the idea that catecholamines can exacerbate ischemic injury. Compared with hemorrhage-induced hypotension, ischemic damage was decreased with hypotension induced through the use of ganglionic blockade with hexamethonium,[61] central adrenergic blockade with alpha$_2$-agonists,[63] and angiotensin-converting enzyme inhibition.[182] Hemorrhaged control rats were noted to sustain an increase in exogenous catecholamine concentrations. To test the hypothesis that these catecholamines contributed to brain damage, some of the animals treated with hexamethonium also received IV catecholamine infusions. Reversal of the hexamethonium brain-protective effect was observed in these animals (Figure 30-17).[61]

6. Brain protection has been observed in laboratory studies with preischemic[183] and preseizure[184] treatment using reserpine, a drug that depletes presynaptic catecholamine stores.

7. Application of catecholamines directly to nonischemic cortical tissue has also been observed to have neurotoxic potential.[185] In addition, IV administration can exacerbate brain swelling after head trauma, although this is most likely a direct effect of BP on a dysautoregulating brain (see Figure 30-8)[14] rather than a manifestation of biochemical neurotoxicity.[36]

Summary

Brain damage can arise from a variety of seemingly disparate neurologic disease states. Such conditions, discussed in subsequent chapters, include ischemia, seizures, trauma, or other adverse processes. Raised ICP typically occurs as these types of conditions progress. When episodes of intracranial hypertension occur, it is important to distinguish hyperemic (with high CBV) from oligemic causes and any possible role of venous outflow obstruction in its genesis and its continuation. Any brain injury is significantly impaired by the extracranial environment. Such extracranial factors include temperature, gas exchange, glucose, sepsis, sodium, and catecholamines. Optimal physiology-guided therapy is essential to optimize outcomes in neurointensive care.

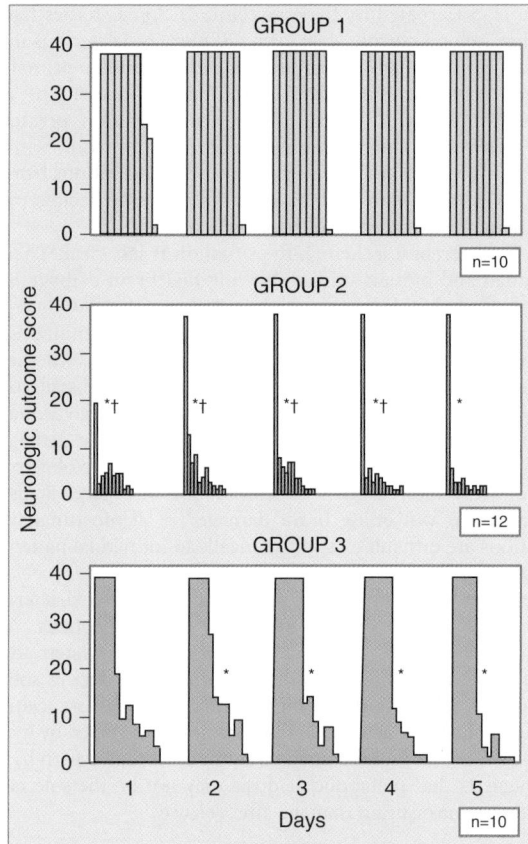

Figure 30-17 Neurologic deficit scores after incomplete focal cerebral ischemia in rats over a 5-day examination period. Each bar represents the neurologic score for each rat (*$P < .05$ vs. group 1; †$P < .05$ vs. group 3). Rats are ranked according to total outcome score in descending order (0 = normal). Cerebral ischemia was induced with occlusion of one carotid artery with hemorrhagic hypotension. Group 1 rats received no vasoactive drugs, group 2 rats received preischemic hexamethonium, and group 3 rats received hexamethonium plus intravenous epinephrine and norepinephrine. Protection was conferred by hexamethonium in a catecholamine-reversible manner. *(From Werner C, Hoffman WE, Thomas C, et al. Ganglionic blockade improves neurologic outcome from incomplete ischemia in rats: partial reversal by exogenous catecholamines. Anesthesiology 1990;73(5):923-929.)*

KEY POINTS

1. The contributors to intracranial hypertension are defined by the contents of the brain: brain tissue, cerebrospinal fluid, blood, and masses. Brain tissue becomes important in the presence of edema, cerebrospinal fluid in the presence of hydrocephalus, blood volume in the presence of vasodilating or vasoconstricting conditions, and masses when of an unacceptable size. In clinical practice, physiologic and pharmacologic manipulations have the most impact on blood volume.

2. There are two types of intracranial hypertension, categorized according to cerebral blood flow as hyperemic or oligemic. Abrupt noxious stimuli briefly increase intracranial pressure (ICP) in the setting of decreased intracranial compliance. Such situations are associated with hyperemia, strongly suggesting that brief hyperemic intracranial hypertension is not a dangerous situation. However, it is reasonable to be concerned about such hyperemia related to herniation risk. In contrast, oligemic intracranial hypertension is associated with compromised cerebral perfusion and is clearly deleterious. Venous outflow obstruction may be an important contributor to the genesis and exacerbation of intracranial hypertension.

3. One category of pressure waves has been identified as plateau waves, which are known to be associated with increased cerebral blood volume (CBV). CBV increases exponentially as perfusion pressure decreases to levels of 80 mm Hg and below. A small decrease in BP produces exponential increases in CBV in a setting of abnormal intracranial compliance with the ICP at the elbow of the ICP-intracranial volume curve. Correlation of changes in ICP with changes in BP correlates with worse outcome.

4. Positive end-expiratory pressure can increase ICP in two ways. The first is through impedance of venous return, increasing cerebral venous pressure and ICP. The second is through decreased BP and reflex increase of CBV, increasing ICP.

5. Intracranial pressure can also be influenced by antihypertensive drugs. In general, vasodilator drugs such as nitroprusside, nitroglycerin, and nifedipine can be expected to increase ICP. Conversely, nonvasodilator antihypertensive drugs, generally sympatholytic drugs such as beta-adrenergic blocking drugs, can be expected to have little or no effect on ICP.

6. Temperature management can be critical in neurointensive care. In animal models and some clinical reports, hyperthermia has been shown to have deleterious effects on outcome after cerebral ischemia, head trauma, and seizure. Conversely, mild hypothermia (32°C to 36°C) has been shown to be protective.

7. Cerebrovascular reserve is compromised in many intracranial pathologic processes. Normally the brain compensates for decrements in supply of oxygen and substrates by vasodilating to maintain or increase flow. Clinical examples of attenuated cerebrovascular reserve include cerebral edema, hypoxemia, carotid artery stenosis, peri-infarct and pericontusion penumbra, and anemia. In each of these situations, although not easy to quantitate, it is clear that added situations of compromised O_2 supply to the brain will risk neuronal injury.

8. Hyperglycemia is clearly deleterious in the context of global cerebral ischemia. Clinical studies suggest a deleterious effect in head trauma and stroke. It seems most appropriate to prevent severe hyperglycemia; however, the optimal target blood glucose level remains to be determined in patients with brain injury. A blood glucose of 180 mg% seems reasonable at this time.

9. Ample laboratory and clinical evidence supports the notion that endogenous and exogenously administered catecholamines can be deleterious with compromised cerebral perfusion.

ANNOTATED REFERENCES

Grände PO, Asgeirsson B, Nordström CH. Volume-targeted therapy of increased intracranial pressure: the Lund concept unifies surgical and non-surgical treatments. Acta Anaesth Scand 2002;46(8):929-41.
This paper presents the physiologic rationale for the Lund approach to managing intracranial hypertension.
Huseby JS, Luce JM, Cary JM, et al. Effects of positive end-expiratory pressure on intracranial pressure in dogs with intracranial hypertension. J Neurosurg 1981;55(5):704-5.
This study in dogs identified the role of hydraulic issues in the genesis of PEEP-induced increases, or lack of increases, in the presence of varying levels of ICP. The authors nicely showed, while maintaining MAP constant, that the higher the ICP was, the less likely it was for PEEP to increase sagittal sinus pressure to an extent sufficient to increase ICP.
Levine S. Anoxic-ischemic encephalopathy in rats. Am J Pathol 1960;36:1-17.
This article demonstrated the importance of cerebrovascular reserve. Rodents exposed to either hypoxia or carotid ligation sustained no deficits. However, induction of both insults reproducibly caused a stroke.
Lundberg N. Continuous recording and control of ventricular fluid pressure in neurosurgical practice. Acta Psychiatr Scand Suppl 1960;36(149):1-193.
This is the original paper, now a classic, describing plateau waves in a large number of patients. Lundberg placed ICP monitors in patients with nontraumatic intracranial hypertension and recorded his observations, identifying three types of plateau waves.
Nakagawa Y, Tsuru M, Yada K. Site and mechanism for compression of the venous system during experimental intracranial hypertension. J Neurosurg 1974;41(4):427-34.
This paper presents experimental evidence for the existence of a venous vascular waterfall in the context of intracranial hypertension.
Neil-Dwyer G, Walter P, Cruickshank JM. Beta-blockade benefits patients following a subarachnoid hemorrhage. Eur J Clin Pharmacol 1985;28(Suppl):25-9.
This paper in humans with SAH showed an improvement in neurologic outcome when sympatholytic drugs were employed.

Nemoto EM. Dynamics of cerebral venous and intracranial pressures. Acta Neurochir Suppl 2006;96:435-7.
The author presents the notion of cerebral venous outflow obstruction due to intracranial hypertension exacerbating brain edema to thus constitute a positive-feedback cycle for the continuation and exacerbation of elevated ICP.
Rosner MJ, Becker DP. Origin and evolution of plateau waves. Experimental observations and a theoretical model. J Neurosurg 1984;60(2):312-24.
This important paper identified the relationship between blood pressure variations and plateau waves, and then synthesized it with work of others to suggest an important role for changes in cerebral blood volume in still autoregulating brain to produce plateau waves.
Steiner LA, Czosnyka M, Piechnik SK, et al. Continuous monitoring of cerebrovascular pressure reactivity allows determination of optimal cerebral perfusion pressure in patients with traumatic brain injury. Crit Care Med 2002;30(4):733-8.
The authors describe the use of pressure reactivity index (PRx) monitoring in TBI patients, observe improved outcome in a retrospective patient analysis, and suggest that PRx monitoring may have an important role in the management of TBI.
Werner C, Hoffman WE, Thomas C, et al. Ganglionic blockade improves neurologic outcome from incomplete ischemia in rats: partial reversal by exogenous catecholamines. Anesthesiology 1990;73(5):923-9.
This paper (and that of Hoffman et al.[63]) on rodents provides excellent support for the notion that catecholamines can worsen the results of brain ischemia.
Zweifel C, Lavinio A, Steiner LA, et al. Continuous monitoring of cerebrovascular pressure reactivity in patients with head injury. Neurosurg Focus 2008;25(4):E2.
The authors of this paper evaluated a group of TBI patients with PRx- and TCD-based dynamic autoregulation techniques, finding that the methods were in agreement, that there was an apparent CPP optimum, and that patients not at a CPP optimum had worse outcomes.

REFERENCES

Access the complete reference list online at http://www.expertconsult.com.

31

Advanced Bedside Neuromonitoring

LUCIDO L. PONCE | JOVANY CRUZ NAVARRO | CLAUDIA S. ROBERTSON

Currently, little can be done to reverse the primary brain damage caused by an insult; however, one of the major factors influencing outcome in patients with acute brain injury is the additional brain damage that occurs from secondary injury processes. Intracranial hypertension and cerebral ischemia are the most significant secondary injury processes that can be monitored and treated in the intensive care unit (ICU). In addition, secondary ischemic insults of extracerebral origin (e.g., arterial hypotension, hypoxia) can be prevented or treated before they become severe enough to injure the brain. The purpose of advanced monitoring of the brain in the ICU is to detect these secondary insults, allowing for a more informed, individualized approach to treatment.

Monitoring Neurologic Status

The analytical approach to a patient with a neurologic problem is a process that requires the physician to have a specialized anatomic and physiologic knowledge of the nervous system. Daily evaluation of neurologic and mental status should be included in the neuromonitoring protocol. Function of pyramidal and extrapyramidal systems, status of cranial nerves, function of cerebellum and spinal cord whenever possible, and any trend in change of neurologic status should be recorded for every patient as part of neuromonitoring. In critically ill patients, however, such a complete neurologic evaluation can sometimes be unreliable or impossible owing to the use of sedatives and the need for intubation and ventilatory support as part of the medical treatment of the neurologic problem. Along with the neurologic examination, information about vital signs and key laboratory values should be available at the bedside in a 24-hour record sheet. A handheld pupillometer (ForSite NeurOptics Automated Infrared Pupillometer, NeurOptics Inc., Irvine, California) is a new technology that may reduce observer variability in the neurologic examination. Infrared quantitative pupillometry can produce accurate, reproducible pupillary measurements which are clearly superior to those obtained manually at the patient's bedside by even an experienced nurse or physician.[1] An important limitation of this device is that assessment is quite challenging in patients with altered mental status, in patients with periorbital or scleral edema, and in uncooperative patients. Ambient light and physiologic factors may also affect the measured pupillary characteristics.[2] A recent study using this device reported good reliability when correlating the pupillary constriction velocity as a predictor of intracranial pressure (ICP) elevation in neurosurgical patients. More clinical experience is needed before including the pupillometer as a standard of care.[3]

The Glasgow Coma Scale (GCS) is used as a standardized scale for recording neurologic status in the ICU. The Glasgow outcome scale has been the standard outcome tool for neurocritical care. New tools such as the Neurological Outcome Scale for TBI (NOS-TBI) have been adapted for traumatic brain injury (TBI) patients from the National Institutes of Health Stroke Scale (NIHSS) and potentially could serve as a tool for initial stratification of injury severity and prediction of long-term outcome.[4]

Intracranial Pressure and Cerebral Perfusion Pressure

Normal resting ICP in an adult is less than 10 mm Hg. A sustained ICP value greater than 20 mm Hg is considered clearly abnormal. Mild to moderate intracranial hypertension is considered to be present when ICP is between 20 and 40 mm Hg, and values greater than 40 mm Hg are considered severe, life-threatening intracranial hypertension. In the 2007 Guidelines for the Management of Severe TBI, an ICP threshold above 20 to 25 mm Hg was adopted as a level III recommendation to initiate treatment to reduce ICP in patients with severe life-threatening head injury.[5]

Cerebral perfusion pressure (CPP) is the difference between the mean arterial blood pressure (MAP) and ICP. Under normal physiologic conditions, a MAP of 80 to 100 mm Hg and an ICP of 5 to 10 mm Hg generate a CPP of 70 to 85 mm Hg.[6]

Cerebral blood flow (CBF) is determined by both CPP and cerebrovascular resistance (CVR) as shown in the following formula:

$$CBF = CPP/CVR$$

Under normal circumstances, the brain is able to maintain a relatively constant CBF of approximately 50 mL per 100 g/min over a wide range of CPP (60 to 150 mm Hg).[7] This process called *pressure autoregulation* is a complex regulatory mechanism involving both myogenic and metabolic components. Following injury, the ability of the brain to pressure autoregulate can be impaired, and CBF is often dependent on CPP.

The indications and thresholds for monitoring of CPP remain controversial. The current recommendation in TBI is to target CPP values within the range of 50 to 70 mm Hg.[8] CPP values less than 50 mm Hg increase the risk of cerebral ischemia and hypoperfusion, while therapies required to maintain CPP values greater than 70 mm Hg have been associated with an increased risk of acute respiratory distress syndrome (ARDS).[9] Some recent evidence suggests that the status of cerebral autoregulation should play a role in therapeutic decisions. If pressure autoregulation is intact, a CPP-directed therapy may be used with a greater chance for a favorable outcome. However, if pressure autoregulation is impaired, ICP-guided therapy may be of more benefit.[10] The on-line correlation between ICP and MAP (pressure reactivity index [PRx]) or between middle cerebral artery blood flow velocity and MAP (Mx) is used to assess the status of pressure autoregulation and direct management in some critical care units.[11,12]

INTRACRANIAL PRESSURE MONITORING DEVICES

The current gold standard for ICP monitoring is the ventriculostomy catheter or external ventricular drain (EVD), which is a catheter inserted in the lateral ventricle, usually via a small right frontal burr hole. This ventricular catheter is connected to a standard pressure transducer via fluid-filled tubing. The external transducer must be maintained at a specific level. The reference point for ICP is the foramen of Monro, although in practical terms, the external auditory meatus is often used as a landmark. EVDs measure global ICP and have some useful advantages over other ICP monitors, including the ability to perform periodic in vivo external calibration and therapeutic CSF drainage and CSF sampling. When intracranial mass lesions or ventricular effacement due to swelling are present, EVD placement may be difficult even for the most experienced neurosurgeon. Intraventricular catheters are also associated with the highest rate of infection among the ICP monitors. Several microtransducer-tipped ICP monitors are now available on the market for clinical use (e.g., Camino ICP monitor, Codman microsensor, and Neurovent-P ICP monitor). These microtransducers can be inserted in the subdural space or directly into the brain parenchyma. Neurovent microsensors incorporating three monitoring variables (ICP, brain tissue oxygen partial pressure, and temperature) are now available; however, current clinical data with this device are limited.[13] Although there are fewer risks of infection and intracranial hemorrhage with these catheters, the main disadvantage is that none can be calibrated in vivo; after preinsertion calibration, they may exhibit zero drift (degree of difference relative to zero atmospheres) over time.[14]

The Spiegelberg ICP monitor, which incorporates pneumatic technology, has been recently introduced. This device uses a small air pouch balloon at the end of a catheter to sense changes in pressure and automatically does in vivo calibration. A novel "lab-on-a-tube" intraventricular catheter was recently developed for multimodal neuromonitoring in patients with TBI; it provides real-time ICP, glucose, oxygen, and temperature monitoring and in situ therapeutic CSF drainage.[15]

Noninvasive ICP monitoring methods have been developed with the aim to reduce the risks associated with invasive monitors. Displacement of the tympanic membrane has been used to determine temporal changes in ICP.[16] Recent data suggest that optical detection of cerebral edema using either broadband halogen illumination or a single-wavelength near-infrared (NIR) laser diode may allow earlier detection of cerebral edema compared with the traditional ICP monitors.[17] Transcranial Doppler (TCD) pulsatility index and magnetic resonance imaging (MRI) of the optic nerve sheath have been used to provide a noninvasive estimate of ICP.[18-21] Measurement of peripapillary retinal nerve fiber layer thickness with optical coherence tomography is a noninvasive quantitative technique to monitor evolution of papilledema as a predictor of intracranial hypertension.[22] So far, none of these methods have provided accuracy sufficient to replace invasive ICP monitors.

ICP Waveforms

Typically, the normal ICP waveform consists of three arterial components superimposed on the respiratory rhythm. The first arterial wave is the percussion wave, which reflects the ejection of blood from the heart transmitted through the choroid plexus in the ventricles. The second wave is the tidal wave, which reflects brain compliance; and finally, the third wave is the dicrotic wave that reflects aortic valve closure. Under physiologic conditions, the percussion wave is the tallest, with the tidal and dicrotic waves having progressively smaller amplitudes. When intracranial hypertension is present, cerebral compliance is diminished. This is reflected by an increase in the peak of the tidal and dicrotic waves exceeding that of the percussion wave (Figure 31-1).

Complications

Among the complications related to ICP monitoring, intracranial hemorrhage and infections are the most common. Less frequent complications are malfunction, malposition, and obstruction. Although these complications generally do not produce long-term morbidity in patients, they can cause inaccurate ICP readings and could increase hospitalization costs by requiring replacement of the monitor.

The incidence of infection for ICP devices is reported to be 1% to 27%,[23] depending on the type of ICP monitoring device. A recent study investigated the complications with use of an ICP fiberoptic device (Camino) alone and in combination with an external ventricular drain

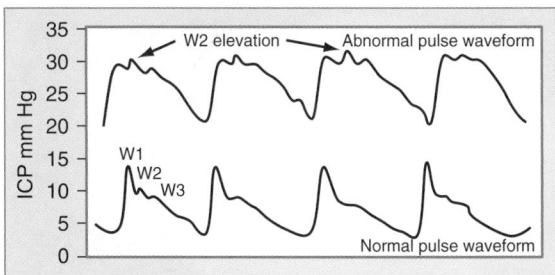

Figure 31-1 **(Upper tracing)** Normal intracranial pressure (ICP) waveform and its components, W1 (percussion wave), W2 (tidal wave), and W3 (dicrotic wave). **(Bottom tracing)** As ICP increases, distinctive waveform changes occur (e.g., elevation of the second pulse wave and "rounding" in the ICP wave form).

(EVD) catheter; the infection rate was 1.8% and 7.9%, respectively.[24] Several other factors have been identified that may affect the risk of EVD infection: use of prophylactic parenteral antibiotics; presence of other concurrent systemic infections; presence of intraventricular or subarachnoid hemorrhage; duration of monitoring; open skull fracture, including basilar skull fractures with CSF leak; leakage around the ventriculostomy catheter; and repeated flushing of the EVD. Routine exchange of ventricular catheters and prophylactic antibiotic use for EVD placement is not recommended to reduce infection rate.[25] However, placement of ICP monitors should be done under the most sterile possible conditions, minimizing excessive manipulation and flushing. Although there is evidence that antibiotic-impregnated catheters may decrease rates of infection, more trials should be conducted to evaluate the beneficial effect on clinical outcome.[26]

The second most common complication related to ICP monitoring is intracerebral hemorrhage; the risk is very low, with an average incidence of 1.1%, but it is an important complication to recognize and treat whenever possible.

Jugular Venous Oxygen Saturation

Placement of a jugular venous oxygen saturation (Sjvo₂) catheter involves retrograde insertion into the internal jugular vein of a catheter equipped with an oxygen sensor at the tip. The internal jugular vein catheter is similar to the type used for CVP monitoring but is directed cephalad into the jugular bulb.[27] The tip of the catheter must be placed above the C1-C2 vertebral bodies to avoid contamination with blood coming from the facial vein. Correct positioning of the catheter can be confirmed with a lateral skull x-ray (Figure 31-2). The incidence of complications related to the Sjvo₂ catheter is low but includes carotid artery puncture, hematoma formation, infection, thrombosis, and increase in ICP that may arise during catheter insertion or due to prolonged monitoring.

The development of in vivo reflectance oximetry using fiberoptic catheters has allowed continuous monitoring of Sjvo₂ without the need of continuous blood sampling, except for calibration purposes.[28] Changes in Sjvo₂ should be confirmed by measuring the oxygen saturation in a blood sample withdrawn from the jugular venous catheter, and the catheter should be recalibrated if the difference is more than 4% to increase the duration of good-quality records.[27,29] Risks of intravascular catheters and possible contamination with noncerebral blood being monitored might be eliminated in the future with a promising noninvasive technique of monitoring the superior sagittal sinus. The technique detects ultrasound waves generated in tissue as pulsed NIR radiation is absorbed, resulting in thermoelastic expansion of the irradiated volume.[30]

SIDE OF JUGULAR CATHETERIZATION

The choice of side for jugular bulb monitoring remains a debate.[31,32] The jugular venous catheter can be placed on the side with the worst

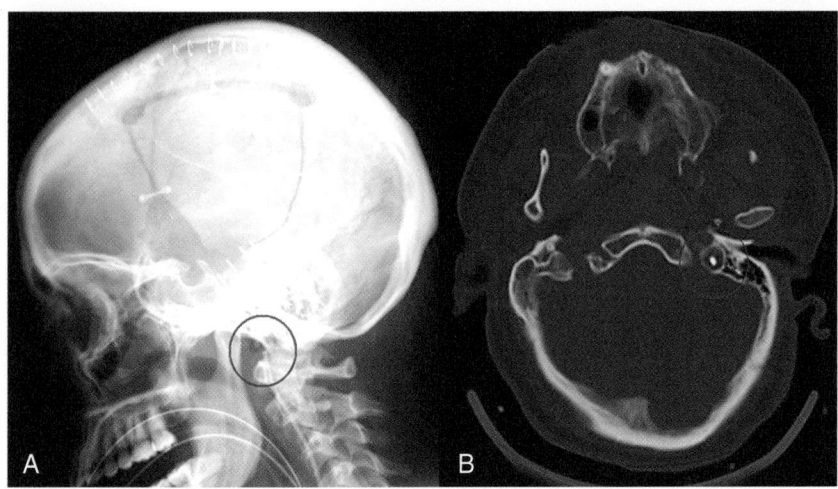

Figure 31-2 A, Lateral skull x-ray confirming adequate $SjvO_2$ catheter placement at C1-C2 level. **B,** Head CT scan showing the catheter tip correctly placed at the jugular venous bulb level.

pathology or the side where the internal jugular vein circulation is dominant. The dominant internal jugular vein is the side with the largest vein by ultrasound imaging or by ICP response to venous compression. If the strategy is to use $SjvO_2$ as a monitor of global oxygenation, then cannulating the dominant jugular vein is logical because it is most representative of the whole brain. However, if the strategy is to identify the most abnormal oxygen saturation, then the side with the most severe injury should be cannulated.[33]

NORMAL JUGULAR VENOUS OXYGEN SATURATION

$SjvO_2$ reflects the global balance between cerebral oxygen delivery (supply) and the cerebral metabolic rate of oxygen (demand). When arterial oxygen saturation, hemoglobin concentration, and the hemoglobin dissociation curve remain stable, $SjvO_2$ generally parallels changes in CBF. Values defining the normal range of $SjvO_2$ are still debated but are usually considered to be 50% to 54% for the lower range and 75% for the upper range.[28,34,35] Multiple pathologic clinical scenarios may cause an increase or decrease in $SjvO_2$ values (Table 31-1). A large number of studies have assessed the role of jugular venous saturation monitoring in patients with severe TBI. In 1992, Sheinberg et al. demonstrated that single or multiple episodes of jugular venous desaturation were associated with a higher mortality rate.[36] However, high $SjvO_2$ values indicating low cerebral oxygen extraction have also been associated with poor outcome,[35] and an elevated mean arteriojugular oxygen content difference has been associated with a better outcome.[37] This apparent discrepancy where increased cerebral oxygen extraction is both associated with a higher mortality rate and a better neurologic outcome can probably be explained by specific circumstances in individual patients. Greater cerebral oxygen extraction means a higher cerebral metabolic rate (and better prognosis) so long as cerebral metabolic requirements are met.[38] According to the most recent consensus for brain oxygen monitoring and thresholds, evidence supports a level III ($SjvO_2$ <50%) recommendation for use of jugular venous oxygen saturation, in addition to the standard ICP monitors in the management of patients with TBI.[39] Because $SjvO_2$ provides only information of a global state of cerebral oxygenation, focal ischemic areas are not evaluated with this technique.

Local or Regional Monitoring

TRANSCRANIAL DOPPLER FLOW VELOCITY AND FLOW VOLUME

TCD ultrasonography is a noninvasive monitor that measures blood flow velocity in one of the major arteries at the base of the brain. A 2-MHz pulsed ultrasound signal is transmitted through the skull (usually through the temporal bone) and, using the shift principle, measures red cell flow velocity. Flow volume is directly proportional to flow velocity and can be calculated by multiplying the velocity by the cross-sectional area of the vessel insonated.

Cerebral vasospasm is a major cause of disability after subarachnoid hemorrhage (SAH) and TBI, with similar incidence in both groups.[40] The incidence of critical regional CBF reductions due to vasospasm are seen progressively when flow velocities above 120 cm/sec are present by TCD examination.[41] Angiography remains the gold standard for diagnosing cerebral vasospasm, but TCD ultrasonography gives a noninvasive alternative for daily bedside monitoring of the CBF dynamics. The Lindegaard ratio (middle cerebral artery-to-extracranial internal carotid artery flow velocity ratio) helps in differentiating vasospasm from hyperemia; vasospasm is considered to be present if the Lindegaard index is greater than 3:1.[42] In hyperemia, flow velocity for both intracranial and extracranial vessels increases, whereas in vasospasm, high flow velocity is seen only in intracranial vessels, resulting in a high ratio.

Vasospasm following TBI or SAH has an impact on morbidity and mortality. Frequently the first clinical sign is a deterioration in the neurologic examination, which may be too late to reverse the process. TCD ultrasonography may identify changes in flow velocity that can precede these clinical findings and may lead to further diagnostic assessment and therapy. The major drawback of TCD ultrasonography is that it is operator dependent, though color-coded TCD provides improved accuracy of measurement.

TCD studies have high specificity for the confirmation of brain death. Brief systolic forward flow spikes with reversed or absent diastolic flow found bilaterally or in three different arteries are accepted TCD criteria for supporting the diagnosis of brain death.[43]

BRAIN TISSUE OXYGEN PARTIAL PRESSURE

A major limitation of $SjvO_2$ technology as a monitor of CBF adequacy is that regional ischemia cannot be identified. Following TBI and other

TABLE 31-1	Clinical Conditions Associated with Alterations in $SjvO_2$ Values
Increased $SjvO_2$	Restricted oxygen diffusion or extraction due to neuronal infarction or inflammation Decreased cerebral metabolism Increased systemic oxygen supply due to hyperoxia Hyperemia
Decreased $SjvO_2$	Local or systemic hypoperfusion (e.g., intracranial hypertension, shock or prolonged hypotension, vasospasm) Decreased systemic oxygen supply (e.g., low PaO_2) Increased cerebral metabolism or oxygen extraction (e.g., seizures, fever)

neurosurgical conditions, regional differences in CBF occur commonly, giving brain tissue oxygen partial pressure ($Pbto_2$), which measures Po_2 in the local area of brain surrounding the catheter, an important advantage in monitoring cerebral oxygenation.

With recent technological advances, two commercially available sensors have been produced. One sensor measures only $Pbto_2$, using a polarographic Clark-type electrode; the other multiparameter sensor measures $Pbto_2$, carbon dioxide, and pH, using fiberoptic technology. Both of these methods have the ability to measure brain temperature using a thermocouple. Both sensors are approximately 0.5 mm in diameter and can be inserted intraoperatively at the time of a craniotomy or through a specially designed bolt that allows insertion and fixation to the skull in the ICU. The Clark electrode polarographic probe has a semipermeable membrane covering two electrodes. In the presence of dissolved oxygen crossing the membrane, an electric current is generated then transferred to a monitor for interpretation. Temperature is also needed to calculate the oxygen tension. Brain temperature rather than core temperature is preferred for this purpose.[44]

Normal values for $Pbto_2$ are 20 to 40 mm Hg, and critical levels are 8 to 10 mm Hg. The likelihood of death following a severe TBI increases the longer the $Pbto_2$ remains below 15 mm Hg and with any occurrence of $Pbto_2$ below 6 mm Hg.[45] Attempts to identify specific Po_2 thresholds for ischemia have been made by different authors using different approaches. Although this threshold is as yet not clearly defined with relation to outcome, there are some reports indicating that $Pbto_2$ values less than 8 to 10 mm Hg represent a high risk of ischemia, although others suggest higher threshold values. Other parameters ($PbtH < 7.0$ and $Pbtco_2 > 60$ mm Hg) have been proposed as an increased risk for vasospasm and mortality in stroke and TBI, respectively.

Correct probe placement into the region of interest and probe depth are key for successful monitoring of $Pbto_2$. Two general strategies have been used for placement of the Po_2 probe. Some recommend placement of the probe into relatively normal brain tissue so that the Po_2 values reflect global brain oxygenation. Changes in $Pbto_2$ correlate well with changes in $Sjvo_2$ when the sensor is inserted into noncontused areas of the brain. Others recommend placement of the probe into penumbra tissue so that Po_2 values reflect oxygenation in the most vulnerable areas of the brain. Regardless of the strategy used, the Po_2 values must be interpreted with the understanding that the values measure only the local tissue surrounding the catheter.

For TBI patients, $Pbto_2$ monitoring has been incorporated into an overall management strategy, along with ICP and other standard monitoring. Decreased mortality in TBI patients managed using a $Pbto_2$-targeted management strategy (maintaining $Pbto_2 > 25$ mm Hg) has been reported.[46] Narotam et al. also reported an improved 6-month clinical outcome over the standard ICP/CPP-directed therapy when aggressive treatment of cerebral hypoxia with a $Pbto_2$-directed protocol (>20 mm Hg).[47]

Treating a reduced $Pbto_2$ should be first directed to any underlying causes of inadequate cerebral oxygen delivery. Such corrections might include increasing CPP (reducing ICP, increasing MAP), improving arterial oxygenation, transfusions for a low hemoglobin concentration, reducing fever, or treating subclinical seizures. If an underlying cause for the low $Pbto_2$ is not found, or if $Pbto_2$ remains low after optimizing oxygen delivery, obtaining a follow-up CT scan of the head might be considered to assess whether a delayed hematoma or hemorrhagic contusion has developed. A sustained (>30 min) $Pbto_2$ of 0 mm Hg and unresponsive to oxygen challenge is consistent with brain death,[48] although care related to interpretation in this regard is needed depending on the location of the probe or malfunction of the probe.

NEAR-INFRARED SPECTROSCOPY

The principle of near-infrared spectroscopy (NIRS) is based on the fact that light in the near-infrared range (700 to 1000 nm) can pass through skin, bone, and other tissues relatively easily. Oxygenated hemoglobin,

deoxygenated hemoglobin, and cytochrome $aa3$ have different absorption spectra. Changes in the absorbance of near-infrared light as it passes through these compounds can be quantified using a modified Beer-Lambert law, which describes optical attenuation. The main advantage of NIRS is that it is a noninvasive method of estimating regional changes in cerebral oxygenation. However, its clinical use is limited by an inability to differentiate between intracranial and extracranial changes in blood flow and oxygenation. This shortcoming adversely affects the reliability of the readings[47] and results in an inconsistent impact for monitoring of decreased oxygenation on neurologic outcome.[49]

ELECTROENCEPHALOGRAM

An electroencephalogram (EEG) represents spontaneous electrical activity of the cerebral cortex and is generated mainly by the summation of excitatory and inhibitory postsynaptic potentials of cortical neurons. EEG does not reflect activity in subcortical levels, cranial nerves, or the spinal cord. The electrical signal is amplified, filtered, and then displayed as either 2 (monitoring) or 16 channels (diagnostic) to give a representation of electrical activity of the cortex. EEG activity is usually interpreted in terms of frequency, amplitude, pattern, and symmetry. Indications for continuous EEG (cEEG) include detection of nonconvulsive electrographic seizures (NCSZs); periodic epileptiform discharges (PEDs) or status epilepticus (NCSE) in patients with unexplained fluctuating mental status; better characterization of suspicious tremors, nystagmus, or clonus and inexplicable changes in blood pressure and heart rate; evaluation of level of coma during sedation and burst-suppression management in drug-induced coma (Figure 31-3); uncovering ischemia due to vasospasm or during neurovascular procedures; and for prognostication.

Compressed displays of EEG frequency spectra (such as compressed spectral array [CSA]) can facilitate interpretation of continuous EEG by allowing the reader to observe patterns evolving over many minutes or hours on a single screen. Frequency analysis takes the raw EEG waves, mathematically analyzes them into their component frequencies (using fast Fourier transform [FFT]). The CSA "stacks" each spectrum one below the other at fixed intervals (usually 2 s). Seizures show a typical activity in crescendo pattern on the CSA display; in burst-suppression pattern, the bursts appear as isolated segments of activity bounded by flat lines (suppression) on CSA; ischemia results in progressive appearance of slower frequencies.

To facilitate continuous EEG monitoring, several other automated EEG processing systems have been developed. Quantitative cEEG (qEEG) allows for evaluation of a large amount of data over long periods of time (raw EEG waveforms) in the form of a summary, many of which were found to correlate with poor prognosis. A recent study confirmed a long-held (but previously unsupported) premise that electrographic seizures are deleterious for TBI patients, resulting in delayed and prolonged increase in ICP and lactate/pyruvate ratio.[50] Decreased relative alpha variability may detect the onset of vasospasm up to 2 days before clinical symptoms.[51] In patients with acute intracranial hemorrhage, NCSZ was associated with midline shift increase, early hematoma enlargement, and a trend toward poor outcome.[52]

EEG recordings using depth electrodes are much less frequently contaminated by shivering artifact during induced hypothermia. Studies suggest that epileptiform activity registered with the mini-depth electrode was more sensitive in detecting metabolic crisis confirmed by microdialysis.[53] Intracortical EEG can provide high-fidelity intracranial EEG in an ICU setting, can detect ictal discharges not readily obvious on scalp EEG, and can recognize early changes in brain activity caused by secondary neurologic complications.[54]

The difficulties with implementing cEEG in the ICU setting include easy artifact generation and high costs for EEG equipment and human resources, including EEG technicians to preserve high-quality recordings, electroencephalographers to review the studies, and the need for training nursing and medical staff to recognize basic EEG patterns.

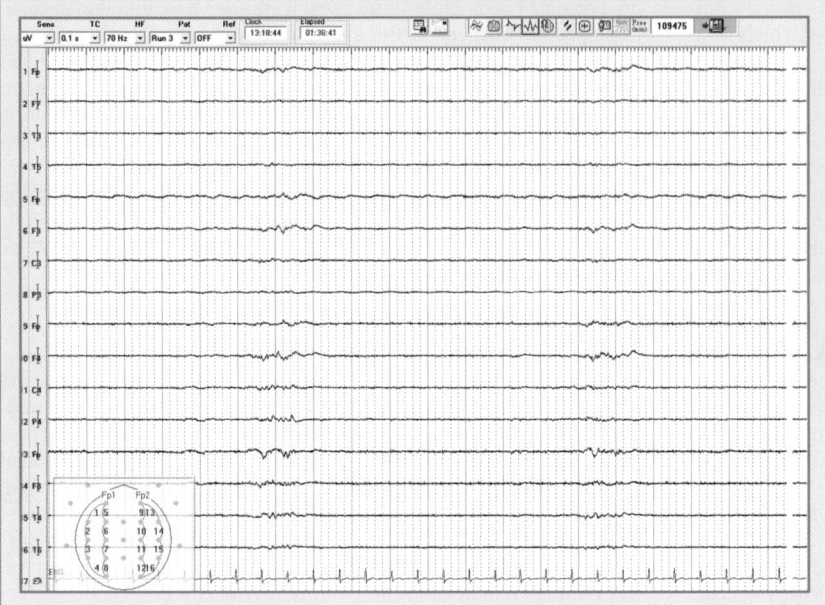

Figure 31-3 A 20-second EEG sample demonstrating burst-suppression pattern in a patient with refractory elevated ICP requiring pentobarbital-induced coma.

Randomized clinical trials comparing EEG-guided therapy with standard medical therapy are warranted, with predetermined endpoints such as neurologic outcomes, ICU and hospital length of stay, and cost-effectiveness.[55]

MICRODIALYSIS

Microdialysis is a technique of sampling the extracellular space of a tissue. It is based on the diffusion of water-soluble substances through a semipermeable membrane. Small molecules (<20,000 D) from the extracellular fluid can diffuse across the membrane and enter the perfusate. Conversely, substances that have been added to the perfusate can diffuse across the membrane to gain entry to the tissue. The degree of permeability of the membrane determines the molecular weight of the substances that cross it. The concentration of substances in the dialysate depends on the flow rate and chemical composition of the perfusate, the length of the dialysis membrane, the type of dialysis membrane, and the diffusion coefficient of the tissue.

The technique of cerebral microdialysis allows continuous and on-line monitoring of changes in brain tissue chemistry. As with brain tissue oxygenation monitoring, microdialysis involves inserting a fine catheter (diameter 0.62 mm) into the brain. The catheter has a polyamide dialysis membrane at the tip and is perfused with a physiologic solution (Ringer's solution) at an ultra-low flow rate using a precision pump. This allows measurement of the concentration of chemicals in the extracellular space of the brain. Molecules below the cutoff size of the semipermeable membrane (20 kD and 100 kD) diffuse from the extracellular space into the perfusion fluid, which is collected in vials that are changed every 10 to 60 minutes and analyzed by enzyme spectrophotometry or high-performance liquid chromatography at the bedside.

In theory, any substance small enough to diffuse through the dialysis membrane can be measured, but the typical key substances can be categorized as follows:

1. Energy-related metabolites (glucose, lactate, pyruvate, adenosine, xanthine)
2. Neurotransmitters (glutamate, aspartate)
3. Markers of tissue damage and inflammation (glycerol)
4. Exogenous substances (administered drugs)

The recovery of a particular substance is defined as the concentration in the dialysate divided by the concentration in the interstitial fluid. If the membrane is long enough and the flow rate slow enough, the concentration in the perfusate will be the same as that in the interstitial fluid (i.e., 100%). The parameters that are commonly used in clinical studies (i.e., 10-mm membrane, perfusion with Ringer's solution, flow rate of 0.3 μL/min) provide an in vivo recovery rate (extrapolation to zero flow method) of approximately 70%.

Continuous on-line measurements of glucose, lactate, pyruvate, glutamate, and glycerol can be achieved using a bedside CMA600 microdialysis analyzer (CMA Microdialysis, Stockholm, Sweden). In 2002, CMA/Microdialysis received U.S. Food and Drug Administration (FDA) approval for the application of cerebral microdialysis for bedside clinical monitoring.

Cerebral microdialysis has been applied to patients in many different clinical situations, including those with TBI, SAH, epilepsy, ischemic stroke, and tumor, as well as during neurosurgery and cardiac surgery. A high lactate/pyruvate ratio (LPR >40) has been classically linked to ischemia/hypoxia and poor prognosis.[56] Isolated "nonischemic" elevated LPR due to diminished pyruvate has also been associated with cerebral metabolic derangement.[57] Newer semipermeable membranes with a higher limit in size (up to 300 kD) also allow for the passage of polypeptides and proteins from the extracellular space (e.g., cytokines,[58] antibiotics, free phenytoin in experimental research).

As with Po$_2$ probes, the location of the microdialysis catheter is critical for interpretation of measurements. The catheter can be inserted into areas at risk of ischemia, such as the vascular territory most likely affected by vasospasm or brain regions surrounding a mass lesion, or in a standardized location such as the right frontal lobe in diffuse brain injury. Different patterns of energy substrates have been described at different levels of hypoxia, which could be helpful clinically in assessing effects of treatment and providing prognosis.[59] Specific patterns of energy substrates may warn of evolving brain injury after evacuation of subdural hematomas (Figure 31-4).[60] Providing nutritional amino acids intravenously in neurointensive care patients does not increase cerebral glutamate.[61] Glycerol has also been validated as a marker of cell membrane damage.[62] Glutamate levels have been correlated with mortality rate and 6-month functional outcome after severe TBI.[63] In patients with SAH where CSF cell count is not helpful, microdialysis may serve as an adjunct criterion for early diagnosis of meningitis (fever + low glucose in microdialysate).[64] A new, yet-to-be-characterized small peptide m/z (mass/charge) ≈ 5000 found in the microdialysate after TBI might represent a novel biomarker of metabolic distress.[65] Interstitial T-tau levels were higher in microdialysate

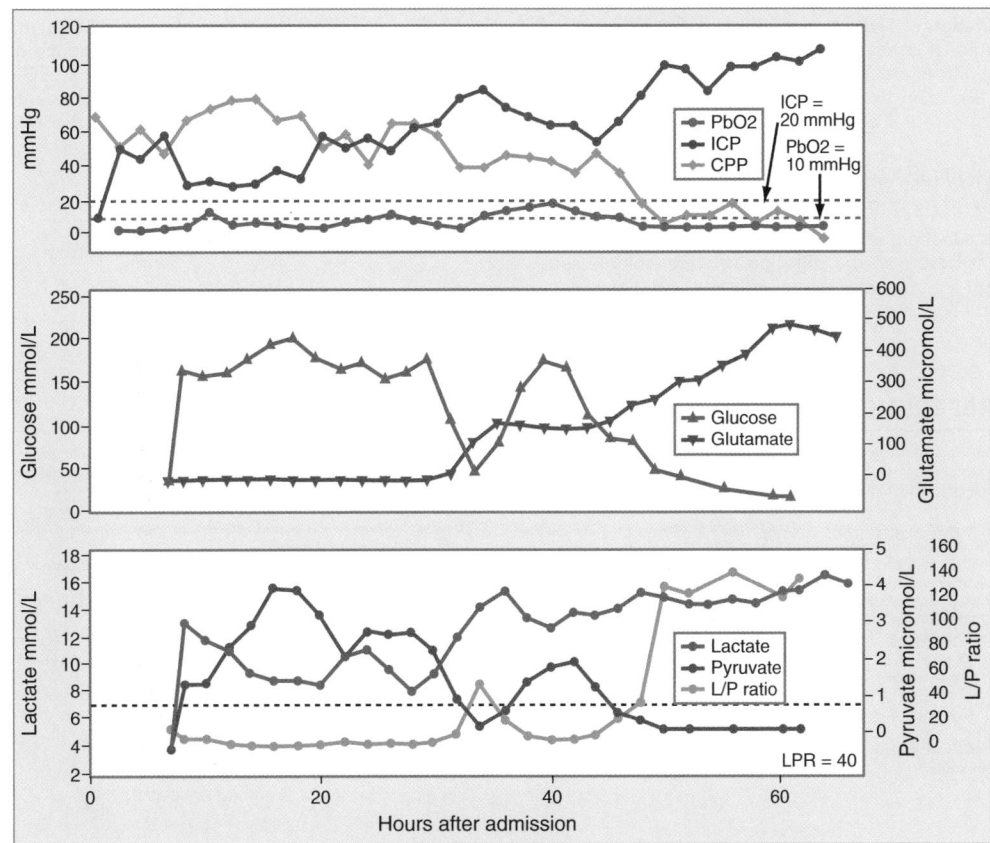

Figure 31-4 A patient with traumatic subdural hematoma was brought in 7 hours after the injury. He underwent evacuation of the hematoma and decompressive craniectomy, but he had refractory increased intracranial pressure, low brain tissue oxygen partial pressure, and high lactate concentrations in the microdialysate. Thirty hours after admission to the NICU, glucose and pyruvate became depleted, lactate/pyruvate ratio increased above 40, and glutamate level became strikingly elevated. The clinical examination was consistent with brain death and was confirmed by a nuclear medicine perfusion test.

of TBI patients with mass lesions, whereas Aβ42 levels were found to be higher in TBI patients with diffuse axonal injury.[66]

Inserting single or multiple microdialysis catheters by using a percutaneous technique has a low complication rate (infection 0%, hemorrhage 3%), but the incidence of technical problems with malfunctioning catheters is high (15%) because of membrane fragility, especially during patient transport.[67] In addition, medical staffs find maintaining microdialysis to be cumbersome. High sample storage volume and questionable accuracy of further off-line analysis, owing to thawing/evaporation, are its major disadvantages. Microdialysis may be further innovated by coupling capillary and microchip electrophoresis.[68] Currently, microdialysis can only be fruitfully used in combination with other monitoring methods. Evidence of its usefulness is growing, although studies targeting threshold values for metabolites and neurotransmitters are needed.

ACKNOWLEDGEMENT

This chapter is dedicated to our wonderful colleague, Dr. Roman Hlatky, co-author of this chapter in the previous edition.

KEY POINTS

1. Evaluation of neurologic and mental status should be included in the monitoring protocol whenever possible.

2. The ventriculostomy catheter remains the preferred device for monitoring intracranial pressure (ICP) and is the standard against which all new monitors are compared.

3. The two major complications of ICP monitoring are ventriculitis and intracranial hemorrhage.

4. Normal resting ICP is less than 10 mm Hg. Transient elevations of ICP occur normally with straining, coughing, or the Trendelenburg position. A sustained ICP greater than 20 mm Hg is clearly abnormal. An ICP greater than 40 mm Hg represents severe, usually life-threatening, intracranial hypertension.

5. The simplest measure of cerebral perfusion is cerebral perfusion pressure (CPP). For equivalent levels of CPP, cerebral perfusion is impaired more by reductions in blood pressure than by increases in ICP.

6. In head-injured patients, the average jugular venous oxygen saturation (SjvO₂) is higher than normal (55% to 75%), higher and lower ranges correlate with poor outcome, and the range for SjvO₂ is considerably wider than it is in normal subjects. If the strategy is to use SjvO₂ as a monitor of global oxygenation, cannulating the dominant jugular vein is logical because it is most representative of the whole brain.

7. Transcranial Doppler (TCD) ultrasonography is a noninvasive monitor that provides indirect information about cerebral blood flow (CBF) in one of the major arteries at the base of the brain. In the absence of vessel stenosis or vasospasm or changes in arterial blood pressure or blood rheology, the pulsatility reflects the distal cerebrovascular resistance.

8. The Lindegaard (hemispheric) index is a ratio of flow velocity in the middle cerebral artery and internal carotid artery. The mean hemispheric index in normal individuals is 1.76 ± 0.1, and pathologic values suggestive of vasospasm are generally above 3.

9. The major limitation of $SjvO_2$ as a monitor of the adequacy of CBF is that regional ischemia is not identified. In situations in which regional differences in CBF may occur, such as traumatic brain injury (TBI), brain tissue oxygen partial pressure ($PbtO_2$) as a monitor of cerebral oxygenation may have an important advantage.

10. Normal values for $PbtO_2$ are 20 to 40 mm Hg, and critical reductions are below 10 mm Hg.

11. Microdialysis is a technique for sampling the extracellular space of a tissue. It is based on the diffusion of water-soluble substances through a semipermeable membrane and allows continuous and on-line monitoring of changes in brain tissue chemistry.

12. The use of electroencephalograms (EEGs) in the ICU to detect early subclinical seizures may help reduce mortality and morbidity in status epilepticus. Continuous EEG monitoring is also useful in detecting ischemic cerebral events, including vasospasm following subarachnoid hemorrhage (SAH) and intracranial hypertension after TBI.

ANNOTATED REFERENCES

Brain Trauma Foundation; American Association of Neurological Surgeons; Congress of Neurological Surgeons; Joint Section on Neurotrauma and Critical Care, AANS/CNSJ. Guidelines for the management of severe traumatic brain injury. IX. Cerebral perfusion thresholds. Neurotrauma 2007;24(Suppl 1):S59-64.
These guidelines summarize the current clinical applications of CPP-based therapy.
Brady KM, Shaffner DH, Lee JK, et al. Continuous monitoring of cerebrovascular pressure reactivity after traumatic brain injury in children. Pediatrics 2009;124(6):e1205-12.
These authors report the important role of cerebral autoregulation in the management of patients with TBI.
Andrews PJ, Citerio G, Longhi L, Polderman K, Sahuquillo J, Vajkoczy P; Neuro-Intensive Care and Emergency Medicine (NICEM) Section of the European Society of Intensive Care Medicine. NICEM consensus on neurological monitoring in acute neurological disease. Intensive Care Med 2008;34(8):1362-70. Epub 2008 Apr 9.
The most recent consensus in neuromonitoring. This report includes recommendations for ICP monitoring, Pbto2, and microdialysis.
Wartenberg KE, Schmidt JM, Mayer SA. Multimodality monitoring in neurocritical care. Crit Care Clin 2007;23(3):507-38.
An excellent review of neuromonitoring which covers most of the technological equipment and medical procedures used in critical care units.

Vespa PM, Miller C, McArthur D, et al. Nonconvulsive electrographic seizures after traumatic brain injury result in a delayed, prolonged increase in intracranial pressure and metabolic crisis. Crit Care Med 2007;35(12):2830-6.
Patients with TBI and seizures were compared with a matched cohort with TBI without seizures. Posttraumatic seizures were associated with episodic and long-lasting increases in ICP and lactate/pyruvate ratio, measured by microdialysis.
Claassen J, Jetté N, Chum F, et al. Electrographic seizures and periodic discharges after intracerebral hemorrhage. Neurology 2007;69(13):1356-65.
This study demonstrates that enlarging hemorrhage size and midline shift is associated with electrographic seizures after ICH.
Marcoux J, McArthur DA, Miller C, et al. Persistent metabolic crisis as measured by elevated cerebral microdialysis lactate-pyruvate ratio predicts chronic frontal lobe brain atrophy after traumatic brain injury. Crit Care Med 2008;36(10):2871-7.
These authors demonstrate that elevated L/P ratio acutely is associated with increased frontal lobe brain atrophy chronically after TBI.

REFERENCES

Access the complete reference list online at http://www.expertconsult.com.

Coma

JOERG-PATRICK STÜBGEN | FRED PLUM | PATRICK KOCHANEK

Altered states of consciousness are a common reason for visits to the emergency room and admission to intensive care units (ICUs). Few problems are more difficult to manage than the unconscious patient, because there are many potential causes of an altered mental status, and the time for diagnosis and effective intervention is short. *Consciousness* is defined as the state of awareness of the self and the environment. The phenomenon of consciousness requires two intact and interdependent physiologic and anatomic components: (1) arousal (or wakefulness) and its underlying neural substrate, the ascending reticular activating system (ARAS) and diencephalon, and (2) awareness, which requires the functioning cerebral cortex of both hemispheres. Most disorders that acutely disturb consciousness are in fact impairments of arousal that create circumstances under which the brain's capacity for consciousness cannot be accurately assessed; in other words, failure of arousal renders it impossible to test awareness.

Alterations of arousal may be transient, lasting only several seconds or minutes (following seizures, syncope, and cardiac dysrhythmia) or sustained, lasting hours or longer. Four terms describe disturbed arousal of a patient: *Alert* refers to a normal state of arousal. *Stupor* describes a state of unarousability in which strong external stimuli can transiently restore wakefulness. Stupor implies at least a limited degree of cognitive activity accompanies the arousal, even if transient. *Coma* is characterized by an uninterrupted loss of the capacity for arousal. The eyes are closed, sleep/wake cycles disappear, and even vigorous stimulation elicits at best only reflex responses. *Lethargy* describes a range of behavior between arousal and stupor. Only the terms *alert* and *coma* have enough precision to be used without further qualification; possibly, coma has gradations in depth, but this cannot be accurately assessed once the patient no longer responds to external stimuli. Stupor and coma imply an acute or subacute brain insult. Cerebral reserve capacity is large, so altered consciousness reflects either diffuse and bilateral cerebral dysfunction, failure of the brainstem-thalamic ARAS, or both. All alterations in arousal should be regarded as acute and potentially life-threatening emergencies.

Evaluation of a comatose patient demands a systematic approach with appropriate directed diagnostic and therapeutic endeavors; time should not be wasted on irrelevant considerations. Urgent steps are required to prevent or minimize permanent brain damage from reversible causes. Patient evaluation and treatment must necessarily occur simultaneously. Such a systematic approach demands an understanding of the pathophysiology of consciousness and mechanisms by which it may be deranged.

Anatomy, Pathology, Pathophysiology

Consciousness depends upon an intact ARAS in the brainstem and adjacent thalamus, which acts as the alerting or awakening element of consciousness, together with a functioning cerebral cortex of both hemispheres, which determines the content of that consciousness.[1,2] The ARAS lies within a more or less isodendritic core that extends from the medulla through the tegmentum of the pons to the midbrain and median thalamus. The system is continuous caudally with the intermediate gray matter of the spinal cord and rostrally with the thalamus, hypothalamus, anterior thalamus, and basal forebrain. The ARAS itself arises within the rostral pontine tegmentum and ends across the mesencephalic tegmentum and its adjacent thalamic nuclei. ARAS functions and interconnections are

considerable and likely contribute more than only a cortical arousal system. The specific role of the various links from the reticular formation to the thalamus has yet to be fully identified.[4] Furthermore, the cortex feeds back on the thalamic nuclei to contribute an important loop that amplifies arousal mechanisms.[5,6]

The ascending arousal system contains cholinergic, monoaminergic, and γ-amino butyric acid (GABA) systems, none of which has been identified as the arousal neurotransmitter.[2,7,8] Acute structural damage to, or metabolic/chemical disturbance of, either the ascending brainstem-thalamic activating system or the thalamocorticothalamic loop can alter the aroused attentive state. Consciousness depends on continuous interaction between the mechanisms that provide arousal and awareness. The brainstem and thalamus provide the activating mechanism, and the cerebrum provides full cognition and self-excitation. Content of consciousness is best regarded as the amalgam and integration of all cognitive function that resides in the thalamo-cortical circuits of both hemispheres. Altered awareness is due to disruption of this cortical activity by diffuse pathology. Focal lesions of the cerebrum can produce profound deficits such as aphasia, alexia, amnesia, and hemianopsia, but only diffuse bilateral damage sparing the ARAS and diencephalon can lead to wakeful unawareness. Thus there are two kinds of altered consciousness: (1) altered arousal due to dysfunction of the ARAS-diencephalon and (2) altered awareness due to bilateral diffuse cerebral hemisphere dysfunction.

Four major pathologic processes can cause such severe global, acute reductions of consciousness.[1,9] (1) In the presence of diffuse or extensive multifocal bilateral dysfunction of the cerebral cortex, the cortical gray matter is diffusely and acutely depressed or destroyed. Concurrently, cortical-subcortical physiologic feedback excitatory loops are impaired, with the result that brainstem autonomic mechanisms become temporarily profoundly inhibited, producing the equivalent of acute "reticular shock" below the level of the lesion. (2) Direct damage to a paramedian upper brainstem and posterior-inferior diencephalic ascending arousal system blocks normal cortical activation. (3) Widespread disconnection between the cortex and subcortical activating mechanisms acts to produce effects similar to both conditions 1 and 2. (4) Diffuse disorders, usually metabolic in origin, concurrently affect both the cortical and subcortical arousal mechanisms, although to a different degree according to the cause.

STRUCTURAL LESIONS CAUSING COMA

Intracranial mass lesions that cause coma may be located in the supratentorial or infratentorial compartments. From either location, impaired arousal or coma is caused by compression of the brainstem-hypothalamic activating mechanisms secondary to swelling and displacement of deep-lying intracranial contents; the ultimate event occurs either by halting axoplasmic flow or by sustained neuronal depolarization due to ischemia or hemorrhage. Factors important to the degree of loss of arousal are rate of development, location, and ultimate size of the lesion. Cerebral mass lesions distort the intracranial anatomy and thereby alter the cerebrospinal fluid (CSF) circulation and brain blood supply. These changes result in increased bulk of the injured tissue and a reduction in intracranial compliance. Intercompartmental pressure gradients result in herniation syndromes that are not necessarily associated with large increases in intracranial pressure (ICP). Recently sustained or evolving mass lesions can disturb cerebral vascular autoregulation, which results in abrupt, briefly lasting vasodilatation. This in turn causes recurrent increases in ICP (pressure waves), with additional compromise of cerebral blood supply to injured regions.

Two herniation syndromes demonstrate the mechanism by which supratentorial lesions produce coma. The rate of evolution of a mass dictates whether the anatomic distortion precedes (in slowly evolving lesions) or parallels the patient's deterioration of wakefulness. *Transtentorial herniation* can be central or predominantly unilateral. Central herniation results from caudal displacement by deep midline supratentorial masses, large space-occupying hemisphere lesions, or large uni- or bilateral compressive extraaxial lesions with compression of the ARAS. The progressive rostral-caudal pathologic and clinical stages of this herniation syndrome were outlined.[1] Pathologically, bilateral symmetric displacement of the supratentorial contents occurs through the tentorial notch into the posterior fossa. Alertness is impaired early, pupils become small (to 3 mm) and reactive, and bilateral upper motor neuron signs develop. Cheyne-Stokes breathing, grasp reflexes, roving eye movements, or depressed escape of oculocephalic reflexes are the clinical manifestations. In the absence of effective therapy at this diencephalic stage, herniation progresses caudally to compress the midbrain, leading to a deep coma and fixed midposition (3-5 mm) pupils, signifying both sympathetic and parasympathetic interruption. Spontaneous eye movements cease, and oculovestibular and oculocephalic reflexes become difficult to elicit. Spontaneous extensor posturing may occur. Once this stage is reached, full recovery becomes unlikely. As the caudal compression-ischemia process advances, pontine and medullary function becomes destroyed, with variable breathing patterns and absent reflex eye movements. Finally, autonomic cardiovascular and respiratory functions cease as medullary centers fail.

Uncus herniation results from laterally placed hemisphere lesions, particularly of the temporal lobes, that cause side-to-side cerebral displacement as well as transtentorial herniation. Focal hemisphere dysfunction (hemiparesis, aphasia, seizures) precedes unilateral (usually ipsilateral) compression paralysis of the third cranial nerve. An early sign of uncus herniation is an ipsilateral (rarely contralateral) enlarged pupil that responds sluggishly to light, followed by a fixed, dilated pupil and an oculomotor palsy (eye turned downward and outward).[1] The ipsilateral posterior cerebral artery can become compressed as it crosses the tentorium and causes ipsilateral occipital lobe ischemia. Progressively, the temporal lobe compresses the midbrain, with loss of arousal and bilateral or contralateral extensor posturing. Ipsilateral to the intracranial lesion, a hemiparesis may develop if the opposite cerebral peduncle becomes compressed against the contralateral tentorial edge (Kernohan notch). Abnormal brainstem signs become symmetric, and herniation proceeds in the same pattern seen with central herniation as rostrocaudal brainstem displacement progresses.

Infratentorial lesions cause coma by displacement, compression, or direct destruction of the pontomesencephalic tegmental activating system. Displacement of the medulla downward sufficient to push the brainstem and cerebellar tonsils into the foramen magnum causes cardiorespiratory collapse. Acute intrinsic lesions of the brainstem, usually hemorrhagic or ischemic, cause abrupt onset of coma and are associated with abnormal neuro-ophthalmologic findings. Pupils are pinpoint due to disruption of pontine sympathetic pathways, or are dilated due to destruction of the third cranial nerve nuclei or intraaxial exiting fibers. Disconjugate eye movements and nystagmus occur, while vertical eye movements are relatively spared. Ocular bobbing signifies pontine damage. Upper motor neuron signs develop, and patients can become quadriplegic; flaccidity in the upper extremities and flexor withdrawal responses in the lower extremities often accompany midbrain-pontine damage.

Pathologically, basilar artery occlusion leads to asymmetric ischemia of the brainstem, with involvement of the ARAS, the neighboring densely packed neuropil, as well as the descending and ascending motor and sensory tracts. Thrombosis of the rostral basilar artery leads to infarction of the midline thalamic nuclei and brief coma without other obvious brainstem signs. Hemorrhage into the ventral pons sometimes spares consciousness but produces neuro-ophthalmologic signs and motor dysfunction. Extension of hemorrhage into the rostral pontine tegmentum results in stupor, coma, or death. Basilar artery migraine can produce altered consciousness, possibly by interfering with arterial blood flow in the basilar artery system. Rapidly developing extensive central pontine myelinolysis may cause coma by extension into the pontine tegmentum. Other intrinsic brainstem lesions (e.g., tumor, abscess, granuloma, demyelination) tend to progress slowly and usually spare arousal mechanisms; however, they may reduce attention and other cognitive functions, leading to severe psychomotor retardation.

Extraaxial posterior fossa lesions cause coma by direct compression of the ARAS in the brainstem, and in the diencephalon by upward transtentorial herniation. Compression of the pons may be difficult to distinguish from intrinsic lesions but is often accompanied by headache, vomiting, and hypertension due to a Cushing reflex. Upward herniation at the midbrain level is initially characterized by coma, reactive miotic pupils, asymmetrical or absent caloric eye responses, and decerebrate posturing; caudal-rostral brainstem dysfunction then occurs, with midbrain failure and midposition fixed pupils.[10] Causes of brainstem compression include cerebellar hemorrhage, infarction and abscess, rapidly expanding cerebellar or fourth-ventricle tumors, or less commonly, infratentorial epidural or subdural hematomas. Drainage of the lateral ventricles to relieve obstructive hydrocephalus due to posterior fossa masses can potentially precipitate acute upward transtentorial herniation.[11,12]

Downward herniation of the cerebellar tonsils through the foramen magnum causes acute medullary dysfunction and abrupt respiratory and circulatory collapse. Less severe impaction of the tonsils in the foramen magnum can lead to obstructive hydrocephalus and consequent bihemispheric dysfunction with altered arousal. Clinical manifestations include headache, nausea, vomiting, lower cranial nerve signs, vertical nystagmus, ataxia, and irregular breathing. Lumbar puncture in this setting carries a risk of catastrophic consequences.[11]

NONSTRUCTURAL CAUSES OF COMA

Nonstructural disorders such as metabolic or toxic disturbances produce coma by diffusely depressing the function of the brainstem and cerebral arousal mechanisms. The anatomic locus of metabolic brain diseases has not been clearly defined. Onset of coma can be abrupt, as with toxic drug ingestion, general anesthesia, or cardiac arrest, or it may evolve slowly after a period of confusion and inattention. The chief manifestations of metabolic encephalopathy are disturbances in arousal and cognitive function. Other findings include abnormalities of the sleep/wake cycle, autonomic disturbances, and abnormal breathing variations.

A helpful distinguishing clinical feature of diffuse encephalopathy is preservation of the pupillary light response; the only exceptions are overdose of anticholinergic agents, near-fatal anoxia, or self-initiated malingering. Usually, lack of pupillary reactivity requires a search for an underlying structural lesion. Neurologic examination shows a decreased level of arousal and widespread cognitive decline. Deeply comatose patients without brainstem or hemisphere function and known cause for coma must be assumed to have suffered accidental or intentional poisoning. Metabolic disturbances of arousal and cognition particularly affect elderly patients who suffer serious medical illnesses or have undergone complicated surgery.

Metabolic encephalopathy is clinically characterized by CNS dysfunction. At onset, abnormalities in cognition may be as severe as the disturbance of arousal. Misperceptions, hallucinations, concentration and memory deficits, or hypervigilance may progress to profound alterations in the patient's level of arousal and consciousness on serial examinations. Motor abnormalities, if present, tend to be and bilateral. Patients often suffer tremor, asterixis, or myoclonus. Spontaneous motor activity may be decreased (in cases of sedating drug or endogenous

hyperactivity (after drug withdrawal or overdose of stimulants such as cocaine and phencyclidine). Seizures occasionally occur, particularly after alcohol or drug withdrawal, and in patients with established cortical pathology. Focal seizures may occur even without structural disease during hypoglycemia, hepatic encephalopathy, uremia, abnormal calcium levels, or toxin ingestion. Autonomic dysfunction can manifest as hypothermia with hypoglycemia, myxedema, or sedative drug overdose. Hyperthermia can occur in withdrawal states, particularly delirium tremens, anticholinergic drug overdose, infection, neuroleptic malignant syndrome, or malignant hyperthermia.

The metabolic need of the brain largely depends on oxidation of glucose to carbon dioxide and water. Certain fatty acids and ketone bodies can supply part of the metabolic needs in emergency circumstances, but these alternate fuels never provide an entirely sufficient substrate to meet all energy requirements. Normal cerebral blood flow (CBF) is around 55 mL/100 g tissue/min. At CBF less than 20 mL/100 g/min, oxygen delivery becomes insufficient for normal levels of oxidative metabolism, and cerebral glycolytic rate increases. Patients lose consciousness, and the electroencephalogram (EEG) is suppressed secondary to synaptic failure at CBF levels between 16 and 20 mL/100 g/min. The cortical evoked response is abolished below about 15 mL/100 g/min. At CBF around 8 mL/100 g/min, the energy-dependent membrane pump fails, and the membrane potential collapses. Unless CBF is restored promptly, irreversible neuronal injury will ensue. However, the threshold for ischemic neuronal injury is time dependent. Complete cessation of CBF leads to loss of consciousness in 8 seconds, and EEG suppression occurs at 10 to 12 seconds. ATP exhaustion and ionic pump failure occurs in 120 seconds. Selective neuronal damage starts after periods as brief as 5 minutes, and severe neuronal damage occurs after 20 to 30 minutes. Brain necrosis or infarction starts in 1 to 2 hours.

Under physiologic conditions, glucose is the brain's only substrate and crosses the blood-brain barrier by facilitated transport. The normal brain uses about 55 mg glucose/100 g/min. Hypoglycemia—in adults, a blood glucose concentration below 40 mg/dL—produces signs and symptoms of encephalopathy resulting from dysfunction of the cerebral cortex, before the brainstem. Neurologic presentation of hypoglycemia can vary from focal motor or sensory deficits to coma. Acute symptoms of hypoglycemia are better correlated with the rate at which blood glucose levels decrease than with the degree of hypoglycemia. The blood glucose level at which cerebral metabolism fails and symptoms develop varies among individuals, but in general, confusion occurs at levels below 30 mg/dL and coma below 10 mg/dL. The brain stores about 2 g of glucose and glycogen, so a patient in hypoglycemic coma may survive 90 minutes without suffering irreversible brain damage. The pathophysiology of coma from hypoglycemia is not well understood. The disorder cannot solely be attributed to glucose starvation of neurons. Rather than such an internal catabolic death, evidence suggests that neurons are killed from without. Around the time the EEG becomes isoelectric, endogenous neurotoxins are produced and released by the brain into tissue and CSF. The distribution of necrotic neurons is unlike that of ischemia and is related to white matter and CSF pathways. The toxins act by first disrupting dendritic trees, sparing the intermediate axons, an indication of excitotoxic neuronal injury. The exact mechanism of excitotoxic neuronal necrosis is now becoming clear and involves hyperexcitation and culminates in cell membrane rupture. Also during hypoglycemia, synthesis of amino acids such as GABA, glutamate, glutamine, and alanine, as well as acetylcholine, is suppressed. Whether reduction of these molecules or alteration in nerve synaptic transmission significantly contributes to the onset of coma associated with severe hypoglycemia is not established.

The pathophysiology of other metabolic encephalopathies is less well established and is extensively discussed elsewhere.[1] Hepatic encephalopathy is caused not merely by ammonia intoxication but likely also involves accumulation of neurotoxins such as short-chain and medium-chain fatty acids, mercaptans, and phenols. Altered neurotransmission may play a role with accumulation of benzodiazepine-like substances, imbalance of serotonergic and glutaminergic neurotransmission, and accumulation of false neurotransmitters. The identity of the neurotoxin in uremic encephalopathy is uncertain and includes urea itself, guanidine and related compounds, phenols, aromatic hydroxyacids, amines, various peptide "middle molecules," myoinositol, parathormone, and amino acid imbalance. The cause of the dysequilibrium syndrome may entail more than osmotic water shifts from plasma into brain cells, and reduction is reported in cortical potassium, with intracellular acidosis due to increased production of organic acids in the brain. The pathogenesis of pancreatic encephalopathy may involve patchy demyelination of brain white matter due to liberated enzymes from a damaged pancreas, disseminated intravascular coagulation, or fat embolism.

The mechanism of action of exogenous toxins or drugs depends partly on the structure and partly on the dose. As well as can be determined, none of the sedatives taken acutely produces permanent damage to the nervous system, making prompt diagnosis and effective treatment particularly important.

Differential Diagnosis

Several different behavioral states appear similar to, and can be confused with, coma. Differentiation of such states from true coma has important diagnostic, therapeutic, and prognostic implications. Moreover, coma is not a permanent state; patients who survive initial coma may evolve through and into these altered behavioral states. All patients who survive beyond the stage of acute systemic complications reawaken and either proceed to recovery (with none or varying degrees of disability) or remain in a vegetative state.

The *vegetative state* can be defined as wakefulness without awareness and is the consequence of various diffuse brain insults.[1,13] It may be a transient phase through which patients in coma pass as the cerebral cortex recovers more slowly than the brainstem. Clinically, vegetative patients appear to be awake and to have cyclical sleep patterns; however, such individuals do not show evidence of cognitive function or learned behavioral responses to external stimuli. Vegetative patients may exhibit spontaneous eye opening, eye movements, and stereotypic facial and limb movements, but they are unable to demonstrate speech or comprehension, and they lack purposeful activity. Vegetative patients generate normal body temperature and usually have normally functioning cardiovascular, respiratory, and digestive systems, but they are doubly incontinent. The vegetative state should be termed *persistent* at 1 month after injury and *permanent* at 3 months after nontraumatic injury or 12 months after traumatic injury.[14,15] Extended observation of the patient is required to assess behavioral responses to external stimulation and demonstrate cognitive unawareness. The EEG is never isoelectric but shows various patterns of rhythm and amplitude, inconsistent from one patient to the next. Normal EEG sleep/wake patterns are absent.

In the *locked-in syndrome*, patients retain or regain arousability and self-awareness, but because of extensive bilateral paralysis (i.e., de-efferentation) can no longer communicate except in severely limited ways. Such patients suffer bilateral ventral pontine lesions with quadriplegia, horizontal gaze palsies, and lower cranial nerve palsies. Voluntarily they are capable only of vertical eye movements and/or blinking.[1] Sleep may be abnormal, with marked reduction in non-REM and REM sleep phases. The most common etiology is pontine infarction due to basilar artery thrombosis, but others are pontine hemorrhage, central pontine myelinolysis, and brainstem mass lesions. Neuromuscular causes of locked-in syndrome include severe acute inflammatory demyelinating polyradiculoneuropathies, myasthenia gravis, botulism, and neuromuscular blocking agents. In these peripheral disorders, upward gaze is not selectively spared.

Akinetic mutism describes a rare subacute or chronic state of altered behavior in which an alert-appearing patient is both silent and immobile but not paralyzed.[16] External evidence of mental activity is unobtainable. The patient usually lies with eyes opened and retains cycles of self-sustained arousal, giving the appearance of vigilance. Skeletal muscle tone can be normal or hypertonic but usually not spastic.

Movements are rudimentary even in response to unpleasant stimuli. Affected patients are usually doubly incontinent. Lesions that cause akinetic mutism may vary widely. One pattern consists of bilateral damage to the frontal lobe or limbic-cortical integration with relative sparing of motor pathways. Vulnerable areas involve both basal medial frontal areas. Somewhat similar behavior also can follow incomplete lesions of the deep gray matter (paramedian reticular formation of the posterior diencephalon and adjacent midbrain), but such patients usually suffer double hemiplegia and act slowly yet are not completely akinetic or noncommunicative.

Catatonia is a symptom complex associated most often with psychiatric disease. This behavioral disturbance is characterized by stupor or excitement and variable mutism, posturing, rigidity, grimacing, and catalepsy. Catatonia can be caused by a variety of illnesses, both psychiatric (affective more than psychotic) disorders and structural or metabolic diseases (e.g., toxic and drug-induced psychosis, encephalitis, alcoholic degeneration). Psychiatric catatonia may be difficult to distinguish from organic disease, because patients often appear lethargic or stuporous rather than totally unresponsive. Such patients also may have a variety of endocrine or autonomic abnormalities. Patients in catatonic stupor do not move spontaneously and appear unresponsive to the environment despite what appears to be a normal level of arousal and consciousness. This impression is supported by a normal neurologic examination and subsequent recall of most events that took place during the unresponsive period. Patients usually lie with eyes opened, may not blink to visual threat, but one can usually elicit optokinetic responses. The pupils are semidilated and reactive to light, oculocephalic reflexes are absent, and vestibulo-ocular testing evokes normal nystagmus. Patients may hypersalivate and be doubly incontinent. Passive movement of the limbs meets with waxy flexibility, and catalepsy is seen in 30% of patients. Choreiform jerks of the extremities and facial grimaces are common. The EEG, both of catatonic excitement and stupor, most often shows a reactive, low voltage, fast-normal record rather than the slow record of a comatose patient.

Approach to Coma

The initial approach to stupor and coma is based on the principle that all alterations in arousal are acute, life-threatening emergencies. Urgent steps are required to prevent or minimize permanent brain damage from reversible causes, often before the cause of coma is definitely established. Patient evaluation and treatment must necessarily occur simultaneously. Serial examinations are needed, with accurate documentation, to determine a change in state of the patient. Accordingly, management decisions (therapeutic and diagnostic) must be made. The clinical approach to an unconscious patient logically entails the following steps: (1) emergency treatment, (2) history (from relatives, friends, and emergency medical personnel), (3) general physical examination, (4) neurologic profile, the key to categorizing the nature of coma, and (5) specific management.

EMERGENCY MANAGEMENT

Initial assessment must focus on the vital signs to determine the appropriate resuscitation measures; the diagnostic process begins later. Urgent, and sometimes empirical, therapy must be given to avoid additional brain insult.

Oxygenation must be ensured by establishing an airway and ventilating the lungs. The threshold for intubation should be low in the comatose patient, even if respiratory function is sufficient for proper ventilation and oxygenation: the level of consciousness may deteriorate, and breathing may decompensate suddenly and unexpectedly. An open airway must be maintained and protected from aspiration of vomitus and blood. While preparing for intubation, maximal oxygenation can be ensured by suctioning the upper airway, gently extending the neck, elevating the jaw, and manually ventilating with oxygen using a mask and bag. Bag-valve mask ventilation with 100% oxygen and 1 mg of intravenous (IV) atropine helps prevent cardiac dysrhythmias.

If a severe neck injury is a possibility or has not been excluded, intubation should be performed by the most skilled practitioner available, with cervical spine precautions. A brief neurologic examination is mandatory prior to sedation required for intubation.

The key points of the *rapid neurologic exam* are: hand drop from over the head (to assess for malingering or hysterical loss of consciousness); pupillary size and response to light; abnormal eye movements (active disconjugate, unilaterally paralytic, passively induced, or absent); grimacing/withdrawal from noxious stimulation; and abnormal plantar response (unilateral or bilateral Babinski sign).[17] Assisted ventilation should continue during the examination if necessary. Neuromuscular blockade required for patient management and care should be deferred if possible until the neurologic examination is completed (3-5 minutes). Signs of arousal or inadequate sedation include dilated reactive pupils, copious tears, diaphoresis, tachycardia, systemic hypertension, and increased pulmonary artery pressure. Thereafter, monitoring patients neurologically may require head computed tomography (CT) more frequently.

Evaluate respiratory excursions: Arterial blood gas measurement is the only certain method to determine adequate ventilation and oxygenation. Pulse oximetry is useful, however, because it provides immediate, continuous information regarding arterial oxygen saturation. The comatose patient ideally should maintain a Pao_2 greater than 100 mm Hg and a $Paco_2$ between 34 and 37 mm Hg. Hyperventilation ($Paco_2 < 35$ mm Hg) should be avoided unless herniation is suspected. PEEP should be avoided if increased ICP is suspected, unless hypoxemia is not responsive to supplemental oxygen. Place a nasogastric tube to facilitate gastric lavage and prevent regurgitation.

Maintain circulation to assure adequate cerebral perfusion. Appropriate resuscitation fluid is lactated Ringer's solution; normal saline is also used when intracranial hypertension is suspected. A mean arterial pressure around 100 mm Hg is adequate and safe for most patients. While obtaining venous access, collect blood samples for anticipated tests (Box 32-1). Treat hypotension by replacing any blood volume loss, and use vasoactive agents. Judiciously manage systemic hypertension with hypotensive agents that do not substantially raise ICP by their vasodilating effect (labetalol, hydralazine, or a titrated nitroprusside infusion are the favored agents for managing uncontrollable hypertension). For most situations, systolic blood pressure should not be treated unless it is above 160 mm Hg. Maintain urine output at least 0.5 mL/kg/h; accurate measurement requires bladder catheterization.

Glucose and thiamine: Hypoglycemia is a frequent cause of altered consciousness; administer glucose (25 g as a 50% solution, IV) immediately after drawing blood for baseline values. Empirical glucose treatment will prevent hypoglycemic brain damage and outweighs the theoretical risks of additional harm to the brain in hyperglycemic, hyperosmolar, or anoxic coma. Thiamine (100 mg) must be given with the glucose infusion to prevent precipitation of Wernicke encephalopathy in malnourished, thiamine-depleted patients. Rarely, an established thiamine deficiency can cause coma.

Repeated generalized seizures damage the brain and *must be stopped.* Initial treatment should include IV benzodiazepines, lorazepam (2-4 mg), or diazepam (5-10 mg). Seizure control can be maintained with phenytoin (18 mg/kg IV at a rate of 25 mg/min). Seizure breakthrough requires additional benzodiazepines.

Careful and mild sedation should be given to the agitated, hyperactive patient to prevent self-injury. Sedation facilitates ventilator support and diagnostic procedures. Small doses of IV benzodiazepines, intramuscular haloperidol (1 mg as often as hourly until desired effect), or morphine (2-4 mg IV) are appropriate.

Consider specific antidotes: Drug overdose is the largest single cause (30%) of coma in the emergency room. Most drug overdose can be treated by supportive measures alone. However, certain antagonists specifically reverse the effects of coma-producing drugs. Naloxone (0.4-2 mg, IV) is the antidote for opiate coma. The reversal of narcotic effect, however, may precipitate acute withdrawal in an opiate addict. In suspected opiate coma, the minimum amount of naloxone should be administered to establish the diagnosis by pupillary dilation and

EMERGENCY LABORATORY TESTS OF METABOLIC COMA

Immediate Tests
Venous blood:
  Glucose
  Electrolytes (Na, K, Cl, CO_2, PO_4)
  Urea and creatinine
  Osmolality
Arterial blood (check color):
  pH
  Po_2
  Pco_2
  HCO_3
  HbCO (if available)
Cerebrospinal fluid:
  Gram stain
  Cell count
  Glucose
Electrocardiogram

Deferred Tests (Initial Sample, Process Later)
Venous blood:
  Sedative and toxic drugs
  Liver function tests
  Coagulation studies
  Thyroid and adrenal function
  Blood cultures
  Viral titers
Urine:
  Sedative and toxic drugs
  Culture
Cerebrospinal fluid:
  Protein
  Culture
  Viral and fungal titers

to reverse respiratory depression and coma. Do not attempt to reverse completely all drug effects with the first dose. IV flumazenil reverses all benzodiazepine-induced coma. Coma unresponsive to 5 mg flumazenil in divided doses given over 5 minutes is not due to benzodiazepine overdose. Recurrent sedation can be prevented with flumazenil (1 mg IV) every 20 minutes.[18] The sedative effects of drugs with anticholinergic properties, particularly tricyclic antidepressants, can be reversed with physostigmine (1-2 mg IV). Pretreatment with 0.5 mg atropine will prevent bradycardia. Only full awakening is characteristic of an anticholinergic drug overdose, as physostigmine has nonspecific arousal properties. Physostigmine has a short duration of action (45-60 minutes), and doses may have to be repeated.

Adjust body temperature: hyperthermia is dangerous because it increases brain metabolic demand and, at extreme levels, denatures brain proteins.[19] Hyperthermia greater than 40°C requires nonspecific cooling measures even before the underlying etiology is determined and treated. Hyperthermia most often indicates infection but may be due to intracranial hemorrhage, anticholinergic drug intoxication, or heat exposure. A body temperature of less than 34°C should be *slowly* increased to above 35°C to prevent cardiac dysrhythmia. Hypothermia accompanies profound sepsis, sedative-hypnotic drug overdose, drowning, hypoglycemia, or Wernicke encephalopathy.

HISTORY

Once vital functions have been protected and the patient's condition is stable, clues to the cause of coma must be sought by interviewing relatives, friends, bystanders, or medical personnel who may have observed the patient before or during the decline in consciousness. The history should include:

- Witnessed events: Head injury, seizure, details of a motor vehicle accident, circumstances under which the patient was found.
- Evolution of coma: Abrupt or gradual, headache, progressive or recurrent weakness, vertigo, nausea and vomiting.
- Recent medical history: Surgical procedures, infections, current medication.
- Past medical history: Epilepsy, head injury, drug or alcohol abuse, stroke, hypertension, diabetes, heart disease, cancer, uremia.
- Previous psychiatric history: Depression, suicide attempts, social stresses.
- Access to drugs: Sedatives, psychotropic drugs, narcotics, illicit drugs, drug paraphernalia, empty medicine bottles.

GENERAL PHYSICAL EXAMINATION

A systematic, detailed examination is helpful and necessary in the approach to the comatose patient, who is in no condition to describe prior or current medical problems. This examination is an extension of the initial rapid evaluation and should look for:

- Efficacy of resuscitation measures, determined by repeated assessment of vital signs.
- External evidence of trauma.
- Evidence of acute or chronic medical illnesses.
- Evidence of ingestion or self-administration of drugs (needle marks, alcohol on breath).
- Evidence of nuchal rigidity. Caution is required if severe neck injury is possible or has not been excluded. Nuchal rigidity may disappear in deeply comatose patients with meningeal infection/inflammation.

NEUROLOGIC PROFILE

Establishing the nature of coma is critical for appropriate management and requires:

- Correct interpretation of neurologic signs that reflect either the integrity or impairment of various functional levels of the brain.
- Determining whether the pattern and evolution of these signs are best explained by a supratentorial or infratentorial structural lesion, a metabolic-toxic encephalopathy, or a psychiatric cause (Box 32-2 and Table 32-1).

The clinical neurologic functions that provide the most useful information in making a categorical diagnosis are outlined in (Box 32-3). These indices are easily and quickly obtained. Furthermore, they have a high degree of interexaminer consistency, and when applied serially, they accurately reflect the patient's clinical course. Once the cause of coma can be assigned to one of these categories, specific radiographic, electrophysiologic, or chemical laboratory studies can be used to make a disease-specific diagnosis and detect existing or potential complications.

SPECIFIC MANAGEMENT

Supratentorial Mass Lesions

If the cause of coma is a presumed supratentorial mass, determine the severity and rate of evolution of signs. A stabilized patient next requires an emergency head CT or magnetic resonance imaging (MRI) scan. Carotid angiography is considerably less informative; a skull x-ray is a waste of time. The priority in deep coma or established/threatening transtentorial herniation is to successfully apply medical treatment of intracranial hypertension. Brief hyperventilation to a $Paco_2$ between 25 and 30 mm Hg is the most rapid method to reduce intracranial hypertension. This is achieved by adjusting the ventilation rate to 10 to 16 per minute and tidal volume to 12 to 14 mL/kg. An osmotic agent must be administered concurrently. The preferred osmotic agent is a 20% mannitol solution as a 1g/kg body weight IV bolus. Maximum ICP reduction occurs within 20 to 60 minutes, and the effect of a single bolus lasts about 6 hours. Corticosteroids are not indicated in emergent empirical management of increased ICP, as full effects are observed

---

NEUROLOGIC PROFILE (MODIFIED GLASGOW COMA SCALE)

Verbal Response
Oriented speech
Confused conversation
Inappropriate speech
Incomprehensible speech
No speech

Eye Opening
Spontaneous
Response to verbal stimuli
Response to noxious stimuli
None

Motor Response
Obeys
Localizes
Withdraws (flexion)
Abnormal flexion
Abnormal extension
None

Pupillary Reaction
Present
Absent

Spontaneous Eye Movement
Orienting
Roving conjugate
Roving disconjugate
Miscellaneous abnormal movements
None

Oculocephalic Response
Normal (unpredictable)
Full
Minimal
None

Oculovestibular Response
Normal (nystagmus)
Tonic conjugate
Minimal or disconjugate
None

Deep Tendon Reflexes
Normal
Increased
Absent

---

of a ventriculostomy into the lateral ventricle. The ventriculostomy allows accurate measurement of intraventricular ICP and provides a method for CSF drainage if necessary. The placement of a ventriculostomy allows calculation of CPP (mean systemic arterial pressure minus ICP), a critical determinant of CBF and therefore of oxygen and substrate delivery. Monitoring ICP also allows adjustment of therapeutic intervention before clinical deterioration occurs in patients with diminished intracranial compliance. Drainage of CSF aims to relieve raised ICP to maintain CPP (>60 mm Hg) and improve intracranial compliance. After increased ICP has responded to emergency management and the patient's condition has stabilized, definitive treatment of the mass lesion is required as deemed appropriate.

Infratentorial Lesions

The evolution of neurologic symptoms and signs, and the neurologic examination, generally give sufficient information to localize the lesion to the posterior fossa; the lesions themselves may be intrinsic or extrinsic to the brainstem.

Rapid neurologic deterioration of a patient suspected of harboring an infratentorial lesion sometimes demands emergency treatment before a head CT scan is performed. Treatment of a presumed extrinsic compressive lesion of the brainstem entails measures that decrease ICP as outlined earlier. Patients in stupor or showing signs of progressive brainstem compression from a cerebellar hemorrhage or infarction require urgent evacuation. Intrinsic brainstem lesions are best treated conservatively; an incomplete stroke may benefit from thrombolysis and/or heparin anticoagulation. Posterior fossa tumors are managed initially with osmotic agents and steroids; definitive treatment includes surgery and/or radiation. Placement of a ventricular catheter for acute hydrocephalus must be considered cautiously and in consultation with a neurosurgeon; the danger exists of potentially fatal upward transtentorial herniation.[12]

Metabolic Toxic Coma

The task of the physician in first contact with the patient in metabolic coma is to preserve and protect the brain from permanent damage.

---

only after a few hours. Furthermore, since steroids are effective only for certain lesions (e.g., edema around a brain tumor or abscess), use can be delayed until a diagnosis has been made by head CT. Following such initial ICP management, a head CT or MRI is required. The scan will demonstrate the nature of the supratentorial lesion and associated mass effect. Arrangements must be made to promptly evacuate an epidural or subdural hematoma. Intraparenchymal masses that acutely produce deep stupor or coma initially are best managed nonsurgically. When steroids are indicated for severe vasogenic edema, a dexamethasone bolus should be given (up to 100 mg IV), followed by 6 to 24 mg every 6 hours. Once signs of herniation have abated, the ventilator rate should be carefully reduced to achieve a $Paco_2$ of 34 to 37 mm Hg.

The patient's vital signs and neurologic condition require repeated examination. The head should be kept slightly elevated (15 degrees). Mannitol may be repeated if necessary every 4 to 6 hours; serum electrolytes and fluid balance must be monitored.

When patients with presumed increased ICP do not respond clinically as expected to medical management, or when obstructive hydrocephalus complicates a supratentorial mass lesion, we favor placement

---

CHARACTERISTICS OF CATEGORIES OF COMA

Supratentorial Mass Lesion Affecting Diencephalon/ Brainstem
Initial focal cerebral dysfunction
Dysfunction progresses rostral to caudal
Signs reflect dysfunction at one level
Signs often asymmetrical

Subtentorial Structural Lesion
Symptoms of brainstem dysfunction or sudden-onset coma
Brainstem signs precede/accompany coma
Cranial nerve and oculovestibular dysfunction
Early onset of abnormal respiratory patterns

Metabolic-Toxic Coma
Confusion/stupor precede motor signs
Motor signs usually symmetrical
Pupil responses generally preserved
Myoclonus, asterixis, tremulousness, and generalized seizures common
Acid-base imbalance common, with compensatory ventilatory changes

Psychogenic Coma
Eyelids squeezed shut
Pupils reactive or dilated, unreactive (cycloplegics)
Oculocephalic reflex unpredictable, nystagmus on caloric tests
Motor tone normal or inconsistent
No pathologic reflexes
(Awake-pattern EEG)

TABLE 32-1	Correlation Between Levels of Brain Function and Clinical Signs	
Structure	*Function*	*Clinical Sign*
Cerebral cortex	Conscious behavior	Speech (including any sounds) Purposeful movement: Spontaneous To command To pain
Brainstem activating and sensory pathways (reticular activating system)	Sleep/wake cycle	Eye opening: Spontaneous To command To pain
Brainstem motor pathways	Reflex limb movements	Flexor posturing (decorticate) Extensor posturing (decerebrate)
Midbrain CN III	Innervation of ciliary muscle and certain extraocular muscles	Pupillary reactivity
Pontomesencephalic MLF	Connects pontine gaze center with CN III nucleus	Internuclear ophthalmoplegia
Upper pons: CN V CN VII	Facial and corneal Facial muscle innervation	Corneal reflex-sensory Corneal reflex-motor response: Blink Grimace
Lower pons: CN VIII (vestibular portion) connects by brainstem pathways with CN III, IV, VI	Reflex eye movements	Doll's eyes Caloric responses
Ponto-medullary junction	Spontaneous breathing Maintained BP	Breathing and BP do not require mechanical or chemical support
Spinal cord	Primitive protective responses	Deep tendon reflexes Babinski response

BP, Blood pressure; *CN*, cranial nerve.

Metabolic and toxicologic studies must be performed on the first blood drawn (see Box 32-1). Treatable conditions that quickly, irreversibly damage the brain include:

Hypoglycemia. As noted previously, glucose (50 mL of a 50% solution IV) should be administered during emergency treatment before blood results return. Prolonged hypoglycemic coma that has considerably damaged the brain will not be reversed by a glucose load; a glucose bolus may transiently worsen hyperglycemic hyperosmolar coma. In contrast, the osmolar load of IV glucose may transiently decrease elevated ICP and lighten non-hypoglycemic coma. A glucose infusion is needed to prevent recurrent hypoglycemia.

Acid-Base Imbalance. The hyperventilating comatose patient with acute severe metabolic acidosis and threatening cardiovascular collapse requires emergency treatment. For accurate assessment, an arterial blood gas is mandatory. Administration of $NaHCO_3$ (1 mEq/kg body weight IV) can be life saving. Simultaneously, a search for and specific treatment of the cause must be conducted.

Hypoxia. Carbon monoxide poisoning requires hyperoxygenation with 100% oxygen to facilitate excretion of this toxin. Closely monitor and correct blood pressure and cardiac rhythm abnormalities. Idiopathic and drug-induced methemoglobinemia is treated with methylene blue (1-2 mg/kg IV over a few minutes; repeat dose after 1 hour if needed). Anemia alone does not cause coma but exacerbates other forms of hypoxemia. Transfusion of packed red cells is appropriate for severe anemia (hematocrit < 25%). Cyanide poisoning causes histotoxic hypoxia of the brain. Treatment entails amyl nitrite (vapor or crushed ampule inhaled every minute), sodium nitrite (300 mg IV), followed by sodium thiosulfate (12.5 g IV).

Acute Bacterial Meningitis. A lumbar puncture must be considered in any unconscious patient with fever and/or signs of meningeal irritation. If possible, an emergency head CT should be performed before lumbar puncture on a comatose patient to rule out unexpected mass lesions. Increased ICP is present in all cases of bacterial meningitis, but a lumbar puncture is not contraindicated when this diagnosis is suspected. Cerebral herniation seldom, if ever, occurs except in small

children.[20] Clinical correlates of impending herniation demanding a more cautious approach to lumbar puncture include coma or rapidly deteriorating level of arousal, focal neurologic signs, and tonic or prolonged seizures. Papilledema is rare in acute bacterial meningitis. Should unexpected herniation occur after lumbar puncture, treatment with hyperventilation and IV mannitol is indicated. Appropriate antibiotic treatment can usually await the results of spinal fluid Gram stain. If the Gram stain is negative, yet a bacterial etiology is suspected, empirical broad-spectrum antibiotic treatment with a third-generation cephalosporin and vancomycin is appropriate.

Drug Overdose. Certain general principles apply to all patients suspected of having ingested sedative drugs.[21,22] Most drug overdose is treated by emergent and supportive measures (Table 32-2). Once vital signs are stable, attempts should be made to remove, neutralize, or reverse the effects of the drug. Patients in coma from recent drug ingestion require gastric lavage after otracheal intubation. A large (preferably double-lumen) gastric tube must be placed orally. Lavage is performed in the head-down position on the left side, using a 200- to 300-mL bolus of tap water or 0.45% saline and continued until the return is clear. After lavage, 1 or 2 tablespoons of activated charcoal are passed down the lavage tube. With meticulous supportive measures, patients with uncomplicated drug-induced coma should recover without neurologic deficit. The recovery from coma due to massive doses of barbiturates or glutethimide can be hastened by hemodialysis.

Constant vigilance and attention to the patient's condition, with timely and appropriate diagnostic and therapeutic evaluation, assures the best possible outcome of metabolic coma. Effective care demands meticulous attention to maintenance of tissue perfusion and oxygenation, documentation and anticipation of acute neurologic events (particularly diminished cerebral perfusion, herniation, or seizures), aggressive, rapid treatment of initial or subsequent infections, and prevention of agitation. Deep venous thrombosis can be prevented with either subcutaneous heparin (5000 units every 12 hours) or full-length leg pneumatic compression boots. Enteral or parenteral feeding within 36 to 48 hours is required to satisfy nutritional needs. Corneal injury can be prevented by protecting the eyes with lubricants and taping the lids shut.

TABLE 32-2	Neurologic Manifestations of Common Drug Poisoning		
Drug	*Signs & Symptoms*	*Diagnostic Test*	*Treatment*
Carbon monoxide	Confusion, agitation, headache, convulsions, coma, respiratory failure, cardiovascular collapse	History Carboxyhemoglobin level	Remove patient from area, 100% oxygen until carboxyhemoglobin levels fall to <5% Hyperbaric oxygen if central nervous system affected Treat cerebral edema with hyperventilation, diuretics, and cerebrospinal fluid drainage if necessary
Salicylate	Tinnitus, hyperpnea, confusion, convulsions, coma, hyperthermia	Blood	Supportive care, gastric lavage, charcoal, systemic alkalinization, hemodialysis for coma or seizures
Cyanide	Agitation, confusion, headache, vertigo, hypertension, hypotension, seizures, paralysis, apnea, coma	Blood	Amyl nitrate, sodium nitrate, sodium thiosulfate, 100% oxygen, hyperbaric oxygen for refractory signs Vitamin B_{12} injection
Anticonvulsants			
Phenytoin Carbamazepine Phenobarbital (see barbiturates) Valproic acid Primidone Ethosuximide Felbamate Clonazepam (see benzodiazepines)	Drowsiness, ataxia, nystagmus, tremulousness, coma Dysrhythmias with carbamazepine or phenytoin overdose	Blood Ammonia level in patients taking valproic acid	Supportive care, gastric lavage, charcoal Watch for withdrawal seizures
Sedative Hypnotics			
Benzodiazepines Barbiturates Chloral hydrate Meprobamate Ethchlorvynol	Confusion, lethargy, ataxia, nystagmus, hypothermia, dysarthria, respiratory depression, coma Pupillary reactions preserved except in instances of deep barbiturate coma Possible withdrawal seizures	Blood	Supportive care, gastric lavage, flumazenil for benzodiazepine overdose, hemoperfusion for extreme barbiturate intoxication
Methaqualone	Agitation, hypertonic hyperreflexia, ataxia, hallucinations, convulsions	Blood	As above
Ethanol	Confusion, agitation, delirium, ataxia, nystagmus, dysarthria, coma	Blood, breath	Supportive care, lavage if within 1 hour of ingestion, thiamine, glucose
Opioids	Lethargy, small reactive pupils, hypothermia, hypotension, urinary retention, shallow irregular respirations, convulsions	Urine Response to naloxone	Naloxone, 0.4 mg IV or IM; continuous naloxone infusion if necessary Supportive care with intubation as necessary Lavage if overdose is by ingestion
Stimulants			
Amphetamine Methylphenidate Cocaine	Hypervigilance, paranoia, violent behavior, tremulousness, dilated pupils, hyperthermia, tachycardia or arrhythmia, focal neurologic signs secondary to CNS stroke or hemorrhage, seizures	Blood, urine	Supportive care, sedation with benzodiazepines Treat hypertensive crisis with sodium nitroprusside or labetalol Watch for rhabdomyolysis
Psychedelics (LSD, mescaline, phencyclidine)	Delirium, delusions, marked agitation, hallucinations, hyperactivity, dilated pupils, hyperreflexia, nystagmus	Blood Measure phencyclidine levels in gastric juice	Gastric lavage, charcoal Benzodiazepines and haloperidol for sedation
Antidepressants			
Tricyclic antidepressants	Anticholinergic effects: dry mouth, agitation, restlessness, ataxia, tachycardia or arrhythmias, hyperthermia, hysteria, convulsions, mydriasis	Blood, urine	Cardiac monitoring, gastric lavage, charcoal, mild systemic alkalinization Physostigmine for refractory arrhythmias Anticonvulsants for seizures
Monoamine oxidase inhibitors	Drowsiness, ataxia, seizures, hypertensive crisis Hypotension with severe overdose		Symptomatic care, gastric lavage, avoid narcotics
Neuroleptics	Dystonia, drowsiness, coma, convulsions, hypotension, miosis, tremor, hypothermia, neuroleptic malignant syndrome	Urine	Gastric lavage Treat extrapyramidal signs with diphenhydramine or benztropine mesylate Treat neuroleptic malignant syndrome with dantrolene or bromocriptine
Lithium	Lethargy, tremulousness, weakness, polyuria, polydipsia, ataxia, seizures, coma	Blood	Hemodialysis for delirium, seizures, or coma
Methanol, ethylene glycol	Drunkenness, hyperventilation, stupor, convulsions, coma Blindness with methanol use	Blood	Symptomatic care, gastric lavage, ethanol infusion, hemodialysis For methanol intoxication, 4-methylpyrazole under investigation
Antihistamines	Anticholinergic effects: dry mucosa, flushed skin, hyperthermia, dilated pupils, delirium, hallucinations, seizures, coma		Supportive care, gastric lavage, control of seizures with benzodiazepines, physostigmine for life-threatening anticholinergic effects
Organophosphates	Cholinergic crisis: cramps, excessive secretions, diarrhea, bronchoconstriction Later: tremulousness, fasciculations, weakness, convulsions, hypertension, tachycardia, confusion, anxiety, coma	RBC cholinesterase level	Symptomatic care, decontamination, atropine, pralidoxime

The Role of Special Investigations

NEURODIAGNOSTIC IMAGING

Once the patient with altered mental status is appropriately resuscitated and stabilized, further investigation may be necessary to document the location and type of the lesion and provide guidance for therapeutic intervention. CT and MRI provide an anatomic and/or functional assessment of the CNS and helpful information for defining the localization of lesions that produce coma. Details on the use of these modalities in neurointensive care are provided in Chapter 31.

Cranial CT scan is currently the most expedient imaging technique for evaluating the comatose patient and gives the most rapid information about possible structural lesions with the least risk. The value of CT in demonstrating mass lesions, hemorrhage, and hydrocephalus is well established. The CT scan shows tissue shifts due to intracranial intercompartmental pressure gradients but compared to MRI may underestimate the anatomy of herniation.[11] Certain lesions such as early infarction (less than 12 hours duration), encephalitis, and isodense subdural hemorrhage may be difficult to visualize. Posterior fossa pathology may be somewhat obscured by bone artifact inherent

in the CT technique. Raised ICP is suggested by effacement of cortical sulci, a narrow third ventricle, and obliteration of the suprasellar or quadrigeminal cisterns but cannot be otherwise quantified.

MRI can be performed depending on the clinical setting and stability of the patient's condition. The use of MRI is limited in the urgent setting of coma evaluation because of the length of time required to perform the imaging, image degradation by even a slight movement of the patient, and the relative inaccessibility of the patient for emergencies that may occur during the imaging process. Nevertheless, MRI provides superb visualization of posterior fossa structures, which is useful when intrinsic brainstem lesions are suspected as the cause of coma.[11] MRI images anatomic lesions such as those resulting from acute stroke, encephalitis, central pontine myelinolysis, and traumatic shear injury, with greater resolution and at an earlier time than CT scanning. Injection of the paramagnetic substance, gadolinium, helps delineate areas of blood-brain barrier breakdown and may augment the sensitivity of this scanning technique. Diffusion imaging can demonstrate ischemic brain virtually immediately. Sagittal MRI views are particularly useful in documenting the degree of supratentorial or infratentorial herniations and may enable intervention before clinical deterioration (Figure 32-1).[11] Newer MRI techniques allow functional

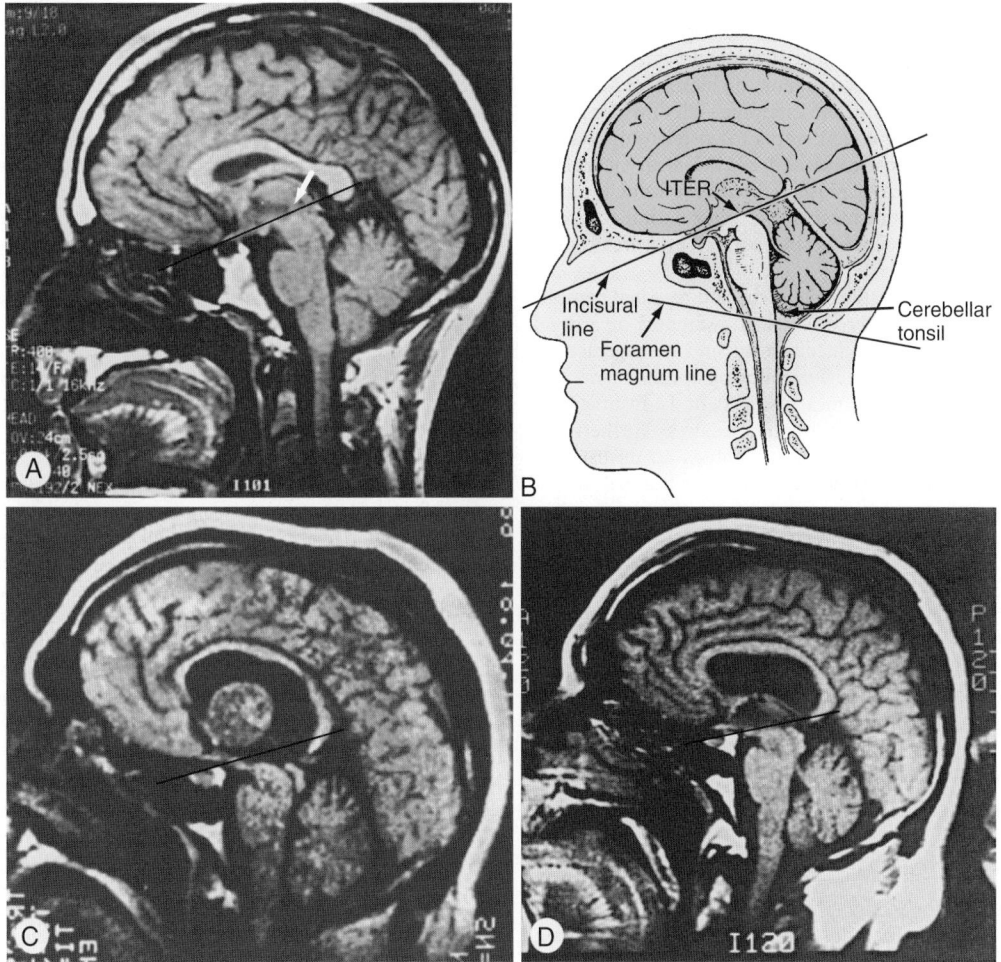

Figure 32-1 **Midsagittal magnetic resonance imaging (MRI) views of a normal adult brain and a brain with reversible downward transtentorial herniation. A,** MRI view of normal adult male brain. **B,** Schematic representation. Opening of tentorium of cerebellum or anterior cerebellar notch lies along a line (incisural line) defined anteriorly by anterior tubercle of sella turcica and posteriorly by junction of Galen's vein, inferior sagittal sinus, and confluence of straight sinus. Proximal opening of aqueduct of Sylvius, the iter ad infundibulum (*top arrow*), lies within 2 mm of incisural line. Foramen magnum line is defined between inferior tip of clivus anteriorly and bony base of posterior lip of foramen magnum. **C,** A 47-year-old man who experienced 1 week of headache, nausea, vomiting, and gait ataxia presented with abrupt-onset coma, palsy of cranial nerve III, hyperreflexia, and bilateral extensor plantar responses. MRI revealed third-ventricular mass, obstructive hydrocephalus, and displacement of iter ad infundibulum inferiorly by 6.5 mm. Cerebellar tonsils were not displaced. **D,** Subsequent MRI view in same patient 2 weeks after surgical removal of a colloid cyst. Iter ad infundibulum is 1.2 mm below incisural line. Patient had full neurologic recovery. (*A, C, and D From Reich JB, Sierra J, Camp W, et al. Magnetic resonance imaging measurements and clinical changes accompanying transtentorial and foramen magnum brain herniation. Ann Neurol 1993;33:159-70.*)

imaging of the CNS by measurement of CBF to a particular region. Future application of this technique may allow rapid determination of diminished CBF, such as occurs in stroke or vasospasm, and will probably be useful in assessing the effect of therapeutic interventions.

ELECTROENCEPHALOGRAM

The EEG can sometimes give useful additional information in the evaluation of the unresponsive patient. With metabolic and toxic disorders, EEG changes generally reflect the degree and severity of altered arousal or delirium, characterized by decreased frequency of the background rhythm and appearance of diffuse slow activity in the theta (4-7 Hz) and/or delta (1-3 Hz) range. Bilaterally synchronous and symmetric medium- to high-voltage broad triphasic waves are seen in various metabolic encephalopathies, most often in hepatic coma. Rapid beta activity (>13 Hz) in a comatose patient suggests ingestion of sedative hypnotics such as barbiturates and benzodiazepines. Acute focally destructive lesions show focal slow activity. When periodic lateralized epileptiform discharges appear acutely in one or both temporal lobes, herpes simplex encephalitis must be strongly considered. A nonreactive diffuse alpha pattern in a comatose patient usually implies a poor prognosis and is most often seen after anoxic insults to the brain or after acute destructive pontine tegmentum damage.[23,24] A normally reactive EEG in an unresponsive patient suggests psychiatric disease, but a relatively normal EEG can accompany the locked-in syndrome, some examples of akinetic mutism, and catatonia—all of which can be caused by structural brain lesions. Attempts to correlate the pattern and frequency spectra of post-resuscitative EEG with neurologic outcome have been unsatisfactory, since its predictive value is at best 88% accurate.[25] At present, the most useful information regarding patient prognosis is still obtained by the correct interpretation of physical signs.

Nonconvulsive generalized status epilepticus and repeated complex partial seizures may produce altered levels of awareness or arousal; the EEG is an indispensable tool in diagnosis and management of both these disorders. Continuous EEG monitoring optimizes management of status epilepticus, as clinical assessment is insufficiently sensitive to detect continued electrographic seizures. Furthermore, continuous EEG monitoring in the ICU has shown an unsuspected high incidence of electrographic seizure activity in critically ill neurologic patients.[26,27]

JUGULAR VENOUS OXIMETRY

Changes in jugular venous oxygen saturation measure the relationship between cerebral metabolic rate and CBF, and this monitoring tool is discussed in Chapter 31.[28] This form of monitoring offers the potential to minimize secondary insults after traumatic brain injury (TBI) by providing warning of cerebral ischemia. It should be considered in comatose patients in conjunction with ICP monitoring (discussed later) to provide a logical approach to the treatment of brain injury.

TRANSCRANIAL DOPPLER ULTRASONOGRAPHY

Transcranial Doppler ultrasonography (discussed in Chapter 31) allows noninvasive measurement of blood flow velocity in basal cerebral arteries.[29] The high dynamic resolution provided and confirmed correlation with other hemodynamic modalities encourages increasing numbers of neurointensivists to adopt the technique. Its importance in coma is in early detection of vasospasm in subarachnoid hemorrhage and at the time of brain death,[30] where an oscillating reverberatory movement has been noted in flow-velocity waveforms. The diagnosis is suspected based on the finding of the reflux phenomenon during late systole following anterograde injection of blood into the vascular tree.

EVOKED POTENTIALS

Evoked potentials (EPs) are used to follow the level of CNS function in comatose patients.[31] Clinical use of brainstem auditory evoked potential (BAEP) and short latency somatosensory evoked potential (SEP) responses stem from the correlation between EP waveform and presumed generators within certain CNS structures. The SEP shows special promise in the ICU field, because EP components generated supratentorially in the thalamus and primary sensory cortex can be identified and followed over time. Shifts of intracranial structures that lead to herniation syndromes are reflected in abnormalities in SEPs, whereas BAEPs are generated entirely at or below the lower midbrain and are less often affected. EPs are less affected than EEG readings by sedative medications and septic or metabolic encephalopathies, factors that frequently confound interpretations in comatose patients. Anatomic specificity and physiologic and metabolic immutability are the basis of clinical utility of EPs. Abnormal test results, however, are etiologically nonspecific and must be carefully integrated into the clinical situation by a physician familiar with their clinical use. Caution is needed in the interpretation of SEPs to insure that absent responses are not due to technical problems. Repeat SEPs are useful in following patients' progress. A progressive decline in response amplitude appears to be associated with worsening prognosis. Studies have shown that all patients with anoxic coma and bilaterally absent SEPs had died or remained in persistent vegetative state.[32] In traumatic coma, absent SEPs may be a less definitive prognostic indicator, as recovery of consciousness has been reported in some patients.[33] Furthermore, comatose patients, especially those with motor response of flexor posture or better, with an initial poor prognostic EEG pattern but normal SEPs, may have the potential for recovery and should be supported until their condition has changed to a more prognostically definitive category.[34] BAEPs and median SEPs obtained within 24 hours of coma onset had a 3-month predictive outcome (compared to Glasgow Outcome Scale [GOS]) in patients with head injury, brain hemorrhage, or neoplasm.[35] Diagnostic sensitivity for an unfavorable outcome was low for both parameters, though specificity and positive predictive value was equally high for abnormal wave VI of BAEPs and median SEPs.

INTRACRANIAL PRESSURE MONITORING

ICP monitoring in neurointensive care is discussed in detail in Chapters 30 and 31. A review of published randomized controlled studies of real-time ICP monitoring by invasive or semi-invasive means in acute coma (traumatic or nontraumatic etiology) versus no ICP monitoring (i.e., clinical assessment of ICP) looked at outcome measures of all-cause mortality and severe disability at the end of a given follow-up period.[36] The conclusion drawn is that there are insufficient data to clarify the role of routine ICP monitoring in all severe cases of acute coma. However, it is of value in TBI and should be considered on a case-by-case basis in other cases of coma.

POSITRON EMISSION TOMOGRAPHY

Recent studies comparing patients in a minimally conscious state and controls, using oxygen-15 positron emission tomography (PET), revealed activation patterns in key brain regions linked to pain processing that were distinguishable from patterns in patients in a persistent vegetative state. These observations suggest the need for analgesic treatment in the minimally conscious state but not for patients in the persistent vegetative state.[37] Additional use of brain PET as a research tool to study patients in comatose states will provide important further insight into this condition.

Prognosis

A complete evaluation of the comatose patient must include an estimate of prognosis. The outcome in a given comatose patient cannot be predicted with absolute certainty. Available serial data are not sufficiently specific or selective to help in establishing the prognosis in an individual patient. Guidelines on the outcome of coma have been compiled based on serial examinations. Although the status of the comatose patient on admission is valuable in providing early informed discussion with relatives of patients and medical colleagues, that moment in most instances does not provide sufficient information to withhold immediate therapy. However, early establishment of a highly probable poor outcome ideally should be made within 24 hours after hospital admission to ration intensive care services and protect families from false hope in futile cases. A logical and sensible approach to prognostication includes an etiological subcategorization into medical, drug-induced, and traumatic coma.

Numerous descriptive scoring systems, both pre- and in-hospital, are used to attempt to assess severity of illness and predict patient outcome. A 2-year prospective study compared severity-of-illness scoring systems (Acute Physiology and Chronic Health Evaluation [APACHE] II and Mainz Emergency Evaluation System [MEES]) to mental status measurement (Glasgow Coma Scale [GCS]) in predicting outcome of 286 consecutive adult patients hospitalized for nontraumatic coma.[38] There were no statistically significant differences among the scoring systems to correctly predict outcome. APACHE II and MEES should not replace GCS. For prediction of mortality, GCS score also provides the best indicator in nontraumatic comatose patients (simple, less time consuming, and accurate in an emergency situation). Useful factors in determining the outcome of medical coma include cause, depth, and duration of coma. Clinical signs reflecting brainstem, motor, and verbal function are the most helpful and best validated predictors (confidence interval 0.95).[39-42] Overall, only 15% of patients in established medical coma for 6 hours will make a good or moderate recovery; others will die (61%), remain vegetative (12%), or become permanently dependent on others for daily living (11%). Prognosis depends on etiology of medical coma. Patients in coma due to a stroke, subarachnoid hemorrhage, or cardiorespiratory arrest have only about a 10% chance of achieving independent function. Some 35% of patients will achieve moderate to good recovery if coma is due to other metabolic reasons including infection, organ failure, and biochemical disturbances. As noted earlier, almost all patients who reach the hospital after sedative overdose or other exogenous agents will recover moderately or completely. Depth of coma affects individual prognosis. Patients who open their eyes in response to noxious stimuli after 6 hours of coma have a 20% chance of making a good recovery, versus 10% if eyes remain closed. The longer coma persists, the less likely the chances for recovery; 15% of patients in coma for 6 hours make a good or moderate recovery compared with only 3% who remain unconscious at 1 week.[39,40] Coma following head trauma has a somewhat better prognosis (see later discussion).

The severity of signs of brainstem dysfunction on admission inversely correlates with the chance of good recovery in medical coma. Absent pupillary responses at any time after onset and, except in barbiturate or phenytoin poisoning, absent caloric-vestibular reflexes 1 day after onset indicate a poor prognosis (<2% recovery). Except for sedative drug poisoning, no patient with absent pupillary light reflexes, corneal reflexes, oculocephalic or caloric responses, or lack of a motor response to noxious stimulation at 3 days after onset is likely to ever regain independent function. In a prospective study of 500 patients in medical coma, a uniform group of 210 patients suffered anoxic injury: 52 of these had no pupillary reflex at 24 hours, all of whom died. By the third day, 70 were left with a motor response worse than withdrawal and all died. By the seventh day, the absence of roving eye movements was seen in 16 patients, all of whom died.[39,40]

Patients likely to recover to functional independence will within 1 to 3 days speak words, open their eyes to noise, show nystagmus on caloric testing, or have spontaneous eye movements. More than 25% of patients with anoxic injury who show roving conjugate eye movements within 6 hours of the onset of coma, or who show withdrawal responses to pain or eye opening to pain, will recover independence

and make a moderate or good recovery. The use of combinations of clinical signs helps improve the accuracy of prognosis: at 24 hours, the absence of a corneal response, pupillary light reaction, or caloric or doll's-eye response is not compatible with recovery to independence.

Postanoxic convulsive status epilepticus and/or myoclonic status epilepticus reflect a poor prognosis. Occasional patients recover consciousness but remain vegetative.[43,44] Most die or become vegetative. Associated clinical findings such as loss of brainstem reflexes or eye opening at the onset of myoclonic jerks, and sinister EEG patterns such as suppression or burst-suppression, confirm a grim neurologic outcome in this group. Autopsy studies show that cerebral and cerebellar damage can be ascribed to the initial ischemic hypoxic event; there is no evidence that status epilepticus further contributes to this damage. We initially treat patients with an IV loading dose of a major anticonvulsant (phenytoin, 13-18 mg/kg at 25 mg/min; and/or phenobarbital, 20 mg/kg at 50 mg/min). Myoclonic status epilepticus is generally resistant to therapy; we give intermittent doses of benzodiazepines (lorazepam, 2-4 mg; or clonazepam, 0.5 mg IV) as needed to suppress particularly severe myoclonus that interferes with ventilatory support. Anesthetic agents are rarely indicated and are unlikely to alter outcome.

A meta-analysis of prognostic studies in anoxic-ischemic coma examined the value of biochemical markers of brain damage in CSF or serum.[45] Only concentrations of CSF markers (creatine kinase brain isoenzyme, neuron-specific enolase, lactate dehydrogenase, and glutamate oxaloacetate) reached 0% false-positive rate. Because of small numbers of patients involved in studies (wide confidence levels) and methodological limitations of studies, the results available are not sufficiently accurate to provide a solid basis for management decisions of patients in coma.

The most accurate prediction of outcome in a patient in medical coma is obtained from the use of a combination of clinical signs, and there is little to be added by more sophisticated testing, other than identifying the cause of the coma.[39,40] Within the first week, it is hard to justify the withdrawal of therapy from patients in medical coma unless they are already brain dead or lack all signs of brainstem function. After that, the probability of being able to predict the quality of life increases steadily. A multi-society task force of neurologists and neurosurgeons obtained a large number of data concerning the persistent vegetative state that provides guidelines to outcomes in patients remaining vegetative 1 month following severe head trauma or coma-producing medical illness (mostly anoxic).[15]

The recent and widespread application of mild therapeutic hypothermia after cardiac arrest has raised concern about reduced or altered ability to prognosticate outcome. Clinical variables such as brainstem reflex recovery, myoclonus, and absent motor response to pain showed higher false-positive mortality predictions in comatose survivors of cardiac arrest compared to predictions by the American Academy of Neurology guidelines at 72 hours.[46] Greater use of higher doses of sedatives related to hypothermia therapy or direct effects of hypothermia may play a role.[47,48] Therefore, caution in prognostication is advised until a better understanding of the effects of this important new therapy emerges.

Among adults with head trauma who were in a vegetative state at 1 month (n = 434), 33% died, 15% remained vegetative, and 28% suffered severe disability at 1 year. Among children vegetative for 1 month post trauma (n = 106), 9% died, 29% remained in a persistent vegetative state, and 35% were severely disabled at 1 year; only 27% attained moderate/good recovery.

Nontraumatic (medical) coma results were even worse. Among 169 adults with nontraumatic brain injury and vegetative at 1 month, 53% died within one year, 32% remained vegetative, and only 14% made a moderate/good recovery. Outcome of 45 children in similar circumstances showed 22% dead, 65% still vegetative, and only 6% made a moderate/good recovery at 1 year.

It is possible in a fraction of patients to predict within the first week those who will recover, those who will die in coma or enter a vegetative state, and those who will survive with severe disability. It is well established that patients in anoxic coma who are in a vegetative state at 1 month will never recover their full preanoxic physical or cognitive function.

Patients in coma due to exogenous agents (except carbon monoxide poisoning) carry an overall good prognosis, provided that circulation and respiration are protected by avoiding or correcting cardiac dysrhythmia, aspiration pneumonia, and respiratory arrest. Despite absent brainstem reflexes (electrocerebral silence on EEG), patients with deep sedative drug intoxication have the potential for complete recovery. Therefore, in the emergent situation, patients in coma of uncertain etiology should be supported vigorously until the precise cause of coma has been fully established.

The outcome of traumatic coma is generally better than medical coma, and prognostic criteria are somewhat different.[15,33,49] Many patients with head injury are young; prolonged posttraumatic unconsciousness of up to several months does not always preclude a satisfactory outcome; and compared to the initial degree of neurologic abnormality, patients in traumatic coma improve more than patients in medical coma. Patients in coma for longer than 6 hours after TBI have a 40% chance to recover to moderate disability or better at 6 months. The most reliable predictors of outcome at 6 months are:

1. Patient age (worse outcome especially after 60 years).
2. Depth and duration of coma (an inverse correlation with GCS).
3. Pupil reaction and eye movements (absence at 24 hours predicts death or a vegetative state in 90%).
4. Motor response in the first week of injury (Table 32-3).

An independent poor prognostic indicator is sustained, uncontrollably increased ICP (>20 mm Hg). Additional factors play a role in the eventual outcome from traumatic coma. Specific lesions such as subdural hematoma that result in coma can have less than 10% recovery rate.[50] In studies with blunt trauma, comatose patients with increased plasma glucose, hypokalemia, or elevated blood leukocyte counts were associated with lower GCS scores and increased probability of death.[51] There are some reports of patients who have suffered coma as a result of TBI in whom an improvement from the vegetative state has been recognized after months, but these anecdotal cases of recovery are difficult to validate. It seems possible that such patients were not truly

vegetative but rather in a state of profound disability with minimal cognition at the beginning of observation.[52] In a recent case report, however, patient recovery from a 19-year-duration TBI-induced minimally conscious state was associated with improvements in white matter tracts, demonstrated with MRI diffusion tensor technique.[53] Novel MRI technology may thus aid in explaining these unusual recoveries; additional studies are warranted.

A systematic review of trials reporting on multisensory stimulation programs in TBI patients in coma or the vegetative state found no reliable evidence of the effectiveness of such techniques when compared to standard rehabilitation.[54] Outcome measures included duration of unconsciousness (time between injury and response to verbal commands), level of consciousness (GCS), level of cognitive functioning, functional outcomes (GOS), or by disability rating scale. The overall methodological quality was poor, and studies differed widely in design and conduct. Owing to the diversity in reporting of outcome measures, a meta-analysis was not possible. Recently, continuous subcutaneous apomorphine infusion (to stimulate dopaminergic neurotransmission) has been suggested to facilitate awakening, specifically in traumatic coma.[55] Similarly, recent work has suggested possible arousal effects from either prolonged coma or minimally conscious state with zolpidem administration.[56] However, larger series are required to confirm or refute these findings.[57]

Prognostic guidelines for medical and traumatic coma should be applied with care. One must be sure evaluation and interpretation of clinical signs are correct. The prognostic signs, however, predict general outcomes in large patient groups and cannot be applied with absolute precision to every individual comatose patient. In addition, one must selectively exclude the effects of anticholinergic agents (used during resuscitation) on pupillary reactivity and paralytic agents on motor response.

The ability to predict prognosis following coma can benefit the patient, family, and physician. Families can be spared both the emotional and financial burdens of caring for individuals with an insignificant chance of independent function and quality of life. Physicians can then properly allocate limited resources to patients with the potential to benefit from advanced medical care.

There are recognized difficulties in interpreting outcome studies of coma prognosis: lack of prospective studies, failure to state confidence intervals, and the fact that patients in coma may die of a nonneurological disease. The self-fulfilling nature of poor prognoses is difficult to eliminate: the care of a patient will reflect the treating physicians' impressions and opinions on patient outcome. Ideally, prognostic studies should only be performed on patients who will receive maximal life support for as long as possible, but this is inconsistent with humane and sensitive management of patients and their relatives.

Analysis of the SUPPORT (Study to Understand the Prognoses and Preferences for Outcomes and Risks of Treatments) trial was used to estimate the cost-effectiveness of aggressive care for patients in nontraumatic coma.[58,59] Patients with reversible metabolic causes of coma were excluded. The incremental cost-effectiveness was calculated for aggressive care versus withholding cardiopulmonary resuscitation and ventilatory support after day 3 of coma. The incremental cost-effectiveness of the more aggressive strategy was $140,000 (1998 dollars) per quality-adjusted life year for high-risk patients and $87,000 per quality-adjusted life year for low-risk patients (five risk factors were age older than 70 years, absent verbal response, absent withdrawal to pain, abnormal brainstem response, and serum creatinine >1.5 mg/ dL). From a purely economic standpoint, making earlier decisions to withhold life-sustaining treatments for patients with very poor prognoses may yield considerable cost savings. On moral and ethical grounds, however, many physicians object to having to consider the cost factor when it comes to making treatment decisions for more or less sick patients. But growing financial constraints now imposed on the medical community from the top down by politicians and the business culture may no longer afford such luxury, even in a country like the United States.

TABLE 32-3	Trauma Scale	
Glasgow Coma Scale Total		
14-15		5
11-13		4
8-10		3
5-7		2
3-4		1
Respiratory Rate		
10-24/min		4
25-35/min		3
>35/min		2
1-9/min		1
None		0
Respiratory Expansion		
Normal		1
None		0
Systolic Blood Pressure		
>89 mm Hg		4
70-89 mm Hg		3
50-69 mm Hg		2
0-49 mm Hg		1
No pulse		0
Peripheral Perfusion (Capillary Refill)		
Normal		2
Delayed		1
None		0
Total Trauma Score (Sum of Individual Scores)*:		

*Scores < 10 represent < 60% chance of survival.

KEY POINTS

1. Altered arousal is due to an acute or subacute brain insult and reflects either diffuse and bilateral cerebral dysfunction, failure of the brainstem-thalamic ascending reticular activating system, or both.

2. Coma is not a permanent state. Patients who survive evolve through and into altered behavioral states that reflect various degrees of recovery.

3. Urgent steps are required to minimize additional brain damage, often before the cause of coma is definitely established.

4. Initial assessment must focus on vital signs to determine the appropriate resuscitation measures (Airway-Breathing-Circulation).

5. When the patient is stable, clues to the cause of coma must be sought from informative sources.

6. A systematic, detailed examination is necessary for the comatose patient, who is in no condition to describe past or current medical history.

7. To determine the cause and evolution of coma, correct interpretation of neurologic signs that reflect the integrity or impairment of brain functional levels is required.

8. Categorization of coma (supra- or infratentorial structural lesions, metabolic-toxic encephalopathy, or psychogenic unresponsiveness) is important in deciding the sequence of diagnostic and therapeutic steps that ensure the best possible patient outcome.

9. The CT scan is the most expedient imaging technique to give rapid information about a brain structural lesion and its consequences.

10. Although the outcome of a comatose patient cannot be absolutely predicted, a highly probable poor prognosis should ideally be made with 24 hours after admission to ration intensive care services and protect families from false hope.

11. As a rule, patients in coma due to exogenous agents carry a favorable prognosis, and patients in posttraumatic coma fare better than medical coma.

12. With the recent advent of mild hypothermia therapy after cardiac arrest, caution in prognostication is advised because compared to present published guidelines, clinical variables at 72 hours after arrest can show higher false-positive mortality predictors in treated comatose survivors.

ANNOTATED REFERENCES

Plum F, Posner JB. The Diagnosis of Stupor and Coma. Philadelphia: FA Davis; 1980.
This book is a convenient "one-stop" reference to stupor/coma. It is an excellent source of information about the pathophysiology and etiology of altered consciousness.

Hund EF, Lehman-Horn F. Life-threatening hyperthermic syndromes. In: Hacke W, editor. Neurocritical Care. Berlin: Springer-Verlag; 1994. p. 888-96.
This textbook on neurocritical care gives concise access to causes and treatment of medical and neurologic coma. Easy-to-access topics are discussed in short, easy-to-read chapters with a short list of references.

Synek VM. Prognostically important EEG coma patterns in diffuse anoxic and traumatic encephalopathies in adults. J Clin Neurophysiol 1988;5:161-74.
The EEG is often used by clinicians (and requested by family) to help establish cause and prognosis of stupor and coma. This article usefully categorized EEG patterns according to a severity scale that can be incorporated into the bedside evaluation of a patient with altered consciousness.

Levy DE, Bates D, Caronna JJ, et al. Prognosis in non-traumatic coma. Ann Intern Med 1981;94:293-301.

Levy DE, Caronna JJ, Singer BH, et al. Predicting outcome from hypoxic-ischemic coma. JAMA 1985;253:1420-6.
These two articles recognize the value/importance of the bedside evaluation in predicting outcome of medical (hypoxic-ischemic) coma. This bedside knowledge helps clinicians orient patient care in an increasingly high-tech hospital environment.

Jennett B, Teasdale G, Braakman R, et al. Prognosis of patients with severe head injury. Neurosurgery 1979;4:283-301.
This article helps guide physicians to focus on the important clinical prognostic factors when managing severely head-injured patients. Because the prognosis of traumatic coma is better than medical coma, these guidelines potentially minimize management errors in patients with other severe injuries.

Rossetti AO, Oddo M, Logroscino G, Kaplan PW. Prognostication after cardiac arrest and hypothermia: a prospective study. Ann Neurol 2010;67:301-7.
This article discusses the need to exercise caution when prognosticating in comatose patients treated with mild therapeutic hypothermia after cardiac arrest.

REFERENCES

Access the complete reference list online at http://www.expertconsult.com.

33

Cardiopulmonary Cerebral Resuscitation

CLIFTON W. CALLAWAY

Cardiopulmonary arrest may occur as the endpoint or consequence of many diseases. Examples include acute dysrhythmias, cardiac pump failure, hypoxemia, sepsis, hemorrhage, drug toxicity, and metabolic disturbances. Often the mechanism is unknown when treatment is initiated, and an algorithmic approach titrated to real-time monitoring (ECG, capnometry, oximetry, blood pressure) is used. When the cause is known or suspected, therapy may be individualized and directed at that cause. In all cases, management has two priorities: (1) rapid restoration of cardiopulmonary function and (2) minimization of ischemic damage to end organs, especially the brain. Restoration of circulation is comprised largely of mechanical and electrical treatment. In contrast, treatment of brain and other organ injury involves primarily prevention of secondary cellular and molecular events using specific and detailed intensive care. Meaningful survival is unlikely without attention to both heart and brain.

Between 1960—when closed-chest compressions were first introduced—and 2000, there was little or no change in long-term survival after cardiac arrest.[1,2] However, regional efforts to improve resuscitation practices at multiple levels, including the emergency response and the post–cardiac arrest care, have resulted in significant improvements in meaningful survival over time.[3,4] There is accumulating evidence about which aspects of post–cardiac arrest management influence final outcomes,[5,6] and specific patterns of physiologic changes after cardiac arrest have been described.[7] Improving outcome will require an integrated approach to immediate resuscitation and subsequent intensive care management. This chapter will review the epidemiology of cardiac arrest, the initial approach for reversing cardiopulmonary arrest, modifications of this approach appropriate for specific disease states, and post–cardiac arrest care designed to minimize brain injury.

Epidemiology

In industrialized countries, heart disease is the overall leading cause of death. Estimates of the incidence of cardiopulmonary arrest outside the hospital vary from 55 to 100 to 120 events per 100,000 people per year,[8,9,10] with one large sample estimating a median incidence of 52.1 per 100,000 people per year.[11] Likewise, median survival after out-of-hospital cardiac arrest is estimated at 8.4%,[11] but the range varies from several large U.S. cities that reported survival rates less than 2%[12,13] to exemplary systems with survival over 16%.[11] The incidence of cardiac arrest in the hospital is about 0.17 events per hospital bed per year.[14] For inpatients experiencing cardiac arrest, survival to hospital discharge is estimated at 17%. Less than half of cardiac arrests occur in an intensive care unit (ICU) setting, and survival does not appear to be related to the location of collapse.[15] As many as 17% of episodes of respiratory compromise in the hospital may progress to cardiac arrest.[16]

Demographic features of sudden cardiac death are similar to the characteristics of cardiovascular disease. Sudden cardiac death is more common in males than females both outside the hospital[10] and in the hospital.[14] However, the incidence of cardiac arrest is higher in women (6%) than in men (4.4%) who are admitted to the hospital for acute myocardial infarction (MI).[17] Cardiac arrest outside the hospital affects blacks more than whites or Asians.[10,12] In addition, cardiac arrest is more common in areas with lower socioeconomic status,[18] and survival may be worse for individuals in regions with lower property values.[19]

While sudden death can affect patients of all ages, the mean age for sudden cardiac arrest is between 65 and 70 years in most studies.[10,11,14]

Two temporally and mechanistically separate processes contribute to mortality: cardiopulmonary collapse and neurologic injury. In evidence of the first process, only one-third of patients who collapse outside of the hospital have restoration of circulation long enough to be admitted to the hospital. Likewise, only 44% of patients who collapse in the hospital have return of circulation.[14] In evidence of the second process, two-thirds of patients admitted to the hospital after out-of-hospital collapse[20] and 60% of patients resuscitated from cardiac arrest in the hospital[14] die prior to discharge from the hospital. The most common reason for death among patients admitted to the ICU after out-of-hospital cardiac arrest is postischemic brain injury, whereas multiple organ failure is more common for patients after in-hospital cardiac arrest.[21] Failure to awaken contributes to withdrawal of care and in-hospital death for as many as 44% to 68% of patients after initial restoration of circulation.[14,22]

Restoring Circulation

Acute treatment of cardiac arrest consists of two concurrent, goal-directed activities: (1) artificial circulation (usually chest compressions augmented by peripheral vasoconstrictors) to circulate oxygenated blood to heart and brain and (2) electric shock to terminate ventricular fibrillation (VF) and unstable tachyarrhythmias. There is increasing recognition that continuous, uninterrupted chest compressions are critically important for restoring circulation.[23] Electrical rescue shocks are used only when appropriate. Rescue shock is the only procedure for which interruption of artificial circulation is absolutely necessary and justified.

Continuous reassessment of the patient can be reduced to constant awareness of two parameters (Figure 33-1). The organization of the electrocardiogram (ECG) and the presence of pulses will prompt appropriate selection of therapy. The recommended division of time and prioritization of activities to accomplish these goals is depicted in Figure 33-2. All other activities, including medications and advanced airway maneuvers, are designed to supplement these two core activities. Optimization of resuscitation requires that any interruption in the two core activities, especially artificial circulation, be minimized.

The American Heart Association and European Resuscitation Council provide consensus scientific statements about the acute management of cardiac arrest.[24] Those guidelines have detailed review of specific drugs and procedures. The following section provides an overview of airway management, circulation support, rescue shock for defibrillation, and drug therapy during cardiac arrest.

AIRWAY AND VENTILATION

Obstruction of the airway can occur in any patient with impaired consciousness including cardiac arrest.[25] If uncorrected, this obstruction prevents oxygenation and ventilation, leading to or perpetuating cardiopulmonary collapse. In patients who are comatose because of primary cardiac arrest, the airway usually is not patent. Animal models typically do not mimic ventilation through the human airway, because the most common research animals (dogs and swine) have straight oral-tracheal passages.

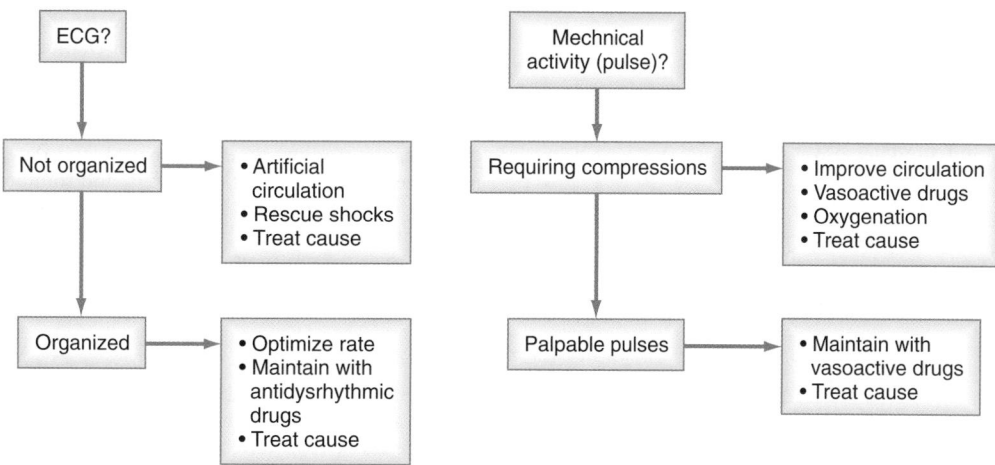

Figure 33-1 Continuous reassessment of the patient during cardiac resuscitation relies on the ECG and on the presence of cardiac mechanical activity (pulses). If an organized ECG is not present, interventions should be undertaken to restore an organized ECG. If mechanical cardiac activity is not present, interventions should be undertaken to improve mechanical cardiac activity. Achieving both goals results in return of circulation.

Agonal respirations occur after acute cardiac arrest for an additional 1 to 2 minutes.[26] These respirations may confuse lay people, delaying recognition of cardiac arrest. It is unclear whether agonal respirations can generate sufficient ventilation to support life. The presence of gasping is associated with survival, but it also may be a surrogate marker for brief collapse-to-resuscitation intervals.[27] Regardless, the amplitude and frequency of agonal respirations declines over 1 to 2 minutes, necessitating artificial ventilation for all patients requiring more than momentary resuscitation efforts.

Simple maneuvers can open the human airway. Extension of the neck (head tilt) and forward displacement of the mandible (chin lift) straightens and opens the pharynx. The tongue can be displaced from the posterior pharynx by insertion of an oropharyngeal airway. With these steps, positive-pressure ventilation can be provided using mouth-to-mouth or bag-valve-mask ventilation. A positive-pressure breath of as little as 400 mL in adults (6-7 mL/kg) delivered over 2 to 3 seconds will cause the chest to rise.[28] Recent studies have indicated that hyperventilation or hyperexpansion of the chest can impair venous return and decrease circulation during resuscitation.[29] In addition, minute ventilations that are smaller than those required for long-term support probably provide adequate gas exchange during cardiac arrest.

The optimal rate and timing for positive-pressure breathes during resuscitation in humans has not been established. The need for gas exchange must be balanced against the fact that interrupting chest compressions even for a few seconds can reduce coronary perfusion pressure (Figure 33-3).[30] In swine, comparison of different ratios of chest compressions to ventilation suggests that 2 breaths per 50 chest compressions or more may be optimal for resuscitation.[31] An extreme point of view is that chest compressions without any artificial ventilation may be sufficient to accomplish resuscitation in certain individuals.[32] This position is contrary to early work demonstrating that the human airway collapses in most unconscious subjects, and that compressions alone are unable to provide ventilation.[25] Recent studies in humans indicate that chest compressions generate tidal volumes that are likely less than the physiologic dead space.[33] Nevertheless, passive insufflation of oxygen without positive-pressure ventilation has been reported to be beneficial in humans.[34] As a compromise, some medical systems employ continuous chest compressions without pauses for positive-pressure ventilation. In these systems, positive-pressure breathes are delivered asynchronously by bag-mask during chest compressions, and the actual minute ventilation achieved is unknown. Therefore, the most recent guidelines recommend a ratio of 30 chest compressions to 2 ventilations, but even higher ratios or asynchronous ventilation may be optimal. Certainly, the duration of any pauses to deliver breaths must be minimized.

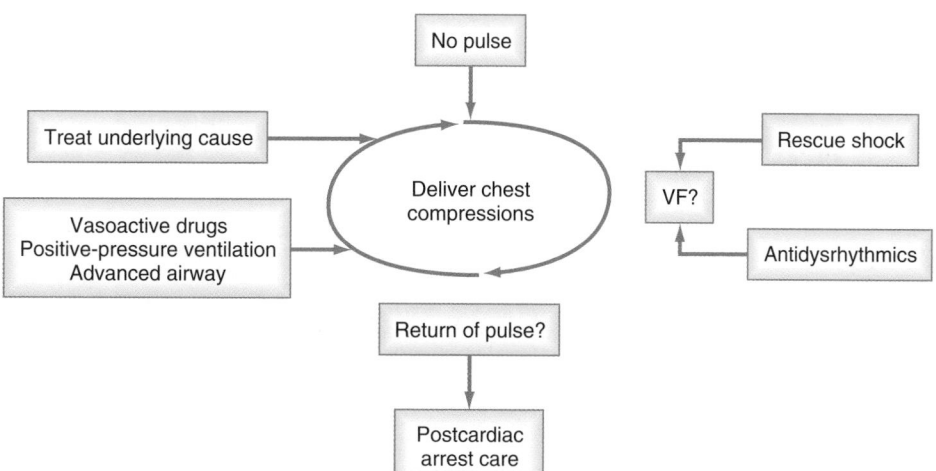

Figure 33-2 Prioritization of activities must occur during cardiac resuscitation. Central circle emphasizes that core activity of chest compression should be interrupted only to provide rescue shocks when appropriate or when restoration of circulation occurs. All drugs, airway devices, and other interventions are designed to augment either artificial circulation or defibrillation. None of these adjuncts should interrupt or detract from providing artificial circulation. VF, ventricular fibrillation.

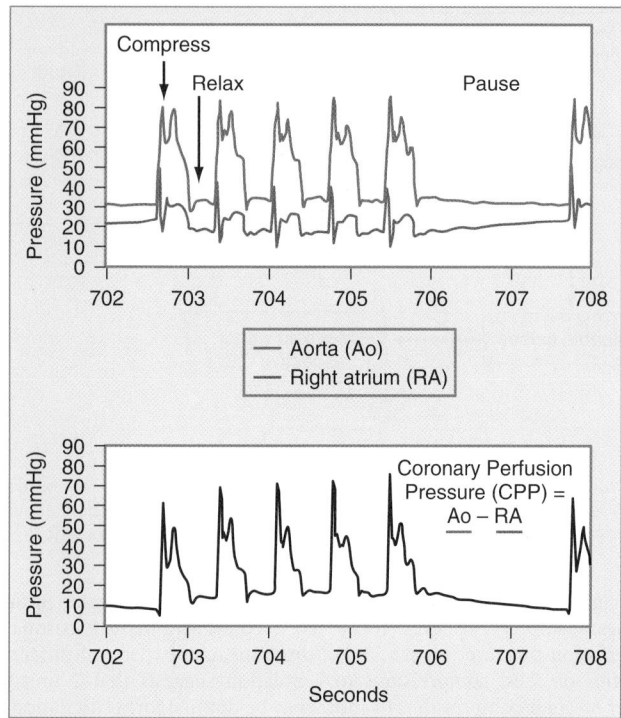

Figure 33-3 Chest compressions provide coronary perfusion by creating a pressure gradient between aorta (Ao) and inside of ventricles (approximated by right atrium [RA]). Gradient between sites is the coronary perfusion pressure (CPP). During chest compression, pressure increases in both Ao and RA. During relaxation, pressure persists in Ao more than RA. Thus, myocardial blood flow is most related to CPP during relaxation phase of chest compressions. Note that CPP declines within 1 to 2 seconds when compressions pause for ventilation. (Unpublished laboratory data.)

Waveform capnography is an extremely useful monitor during resuscitation, both for confirming ventilation and for monitoring adequacy of circulation. During cardiac arrest, end-tidal CO_2 measurement is related to cardiac output and pulmonary blood flow.[35] Therefore, CO_2 levels may be very low (<10 mm Hg) at the onset of resuscitation. Adequate artificial circulation will cause CO_2 levels to increase, and these levels may be used as a feedback to improve or modify chest compressions. Data from emergency department patients

suggest that an end-tidal CO_2 level greater than 15 to 16 mm Hg is associated with successful cardiac resuscitation.[36,37] Conversely, end-tidal CO_2 less than 10 mm Hg after 20 minutes of resuscitative efforts appears to confirm failure of resuscitation.[38] However, drugs commonly used during resuscitation can disrupt the association between capnography readings and pulmonary blood flow. For example, epinephrine infusion reduces CO_2 levels, and sodium bicarbonate infusion produces a transient but profound elevation of CO_2 levels. An abrupt increase in end-tidal CO_2 levels, usually to levels over 35 mm Hg, accompanies the return of spontaneous circulation. This finding may be useful for recognizing return of circulation, thereby minimizing any interruptions of chest compressions for pulse checks (Figure 33-4).

Airway Devices

The most common ventilation device used by rescue personnel, paramedics, and other healthcare providers is a self-inflating bag attached to a face mask (bag-valve-mask [BVM]), which has several pitfalls. First, it is difficult to maintain an airtight seal between the mask and the face of the patient, particularly when simultaneously performing head-tilt, chin-lift maneuvers. Adequate training and practice increases ventilation success by a single provider, but two providers achieve more reliable airway management. One provider squeezes the bag, while the second provider uses two hands to hold the mask on the face and position the head.

A second difficulty with BVM ventilation is insufflation of the stomach.[39] Excessive air in the stomach can promote emesis, and the abdominal distension may impair venous return and lung compliance.[40] The esophagus prevents air entry into the stomach unless upper airway pressures exceed 15 to 20 cm H_2O.[41] However, esophageal muscle tone declines during cardiac arrest, allowing air to enter the stomach with upper airway pressures over 5 to 8 cm H_2O.[42] If the upper airway is not patent, providers may try to ventilate with increased pressure to achieve chest rise. Furthermore, rapid squeezing of the bag during the excitement of the situation results in too-high upper airway pressures. To avoid these problems, rescuers should emphasize gentle and well-paced inflation of the lungs during resuscitation.

Tracheal intubation can secure the airway definitively. A cuffed tracheal tube protects from emesis and maintains airway patency. However, laryngoscopy requires an interruption in chest compressions, and the tracheal tube by itself does not correct cardiac arrest. Observations of paramedics have documented extremely long interruption of chest compressions during "uncomplicated" tracheal intubation.[43] Therefore, consideration should be made to delay tracheal intubation during initial resuscitation to reduce delays or interruptions of other life-saving interventions. After restoration of circulation, patients with

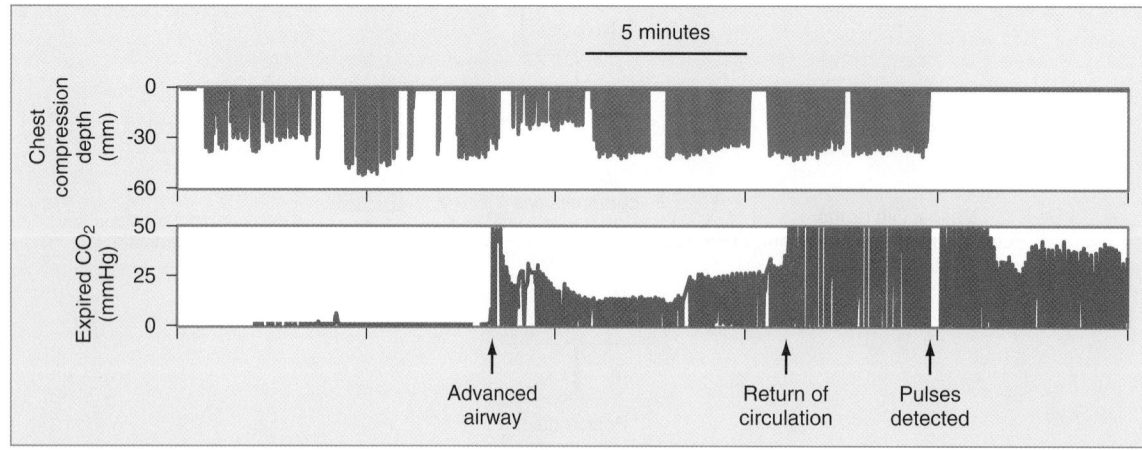

Figure 33-4 End-tidal CO_2 changes during resuscitation. Tracings from monitor-defibrillator with an accelerometer to measure chest compression depth (*top trace*) and waveform capnography to measure exhaled CO_2 (*bottom trace*). Exhaled CO_2 confirms correct placement of an advanced airway. Note frequent interruptions in chest compressions prior to placing advanced airway. More continuous chest compressions are followed by an abrupt rise in exhaled CO_2, corresponding to return of circulation, including pulmonary circulation. Chest compressions continue for 2 to 3 minutes until providers detect a palpable pulse.

coma or continued respiratory failure will require tracheal intubation.

Alternative supraglottic airway adjuncts such as double-lumen combination tracheal-esophageal tubes (e.g., Combi-tube), laryngeal tubes (e.g., King-LT), or laryngeal mask airways (LMA) can be used to temporarily manage the airway during resuscitation.[44,45] These devices have the advantage that they can be inserted blindly in seconds without laryngoscopy and without interruption of chest compressions.[39] The degree to which these devices can protect from aspiration is debated, but it is clear that they can allow adequate control of the airway to achieve resuscitation during cardiac arrest. Clinicians should strongly consider using these supraglottic airways as the first advanced airway during resuscitation because of the advantage of these devices for reducing interruptions in chest compressions.

ARTIFICIAL CIRCULATION

In the patient without pulses, circulation of blood can be accomplished by mechanical compression of the heart and chest. The critical parameter for restoring spontaneous circulation is the development of adequate coronary perfusion pressure (CPP). CPP is quantified by the pressure gradient between the aorta and the inside of the ventricles (usually approximated by the pressure in the right atrium or the central venous pressure [CVP]). Measurement of CPP in clinical practice is difficult unless the patient has invasive monitoring prior to cardiopulmonary collapse. CVP can be estimated from a central line, and peripheral arterial pressures developed approximate aortic pressures. In the spontaneously beating heart, most blood flows through the ventricular walls during diastole, when the ventricular pressure is lowest. With mechanical compression of the heart and chest during resuscitation, the primary perfusion of the heart occurs during the relaxation phase (see Figure 33-3). Therefore, CPP is usually measured at the end of the relaxation phase. CPP is highly correlated with myocardial perfusion, and consequently with the likelihood of resuscitation.[46] In humans, return of circulation requires that the developed CPP exceed 15 to 20 mm Hg. It is likely that with CPP less than 15 mm Hg, perfusion is inadequate to replete the energy state of the myocardium during cardiac arrest.

Even brief interruptions in chest compressions can result in decreased CPP. This fact has clinical importance, as evidenced by the fact that more uninterrupted chest compression are highly associated with restoring circulation and survival.[23] When chest compressions are measured during actual resuscitations by paramedics or hospital providers, interruptions and pauses are frequent.[47,48] These observations have prompted the development of monitor-defibrillators with features to measure and record chest compressions, and even to provide real-time feedback to providers.[49] These devices often employ an accelerometer in the defibrillation pads or in a separate attachment that is placed on the sternum of the patient. It is unknown if real-time feedback can improve resuscitation success, but it is clear that the continuity and quality of chest compressions are important parameters to maximize for resuscitation to succeed. Recent literature has used the chest-compression fraction to quantify this parameter (Figure 33-5).

It is important to recognize that peak arterial pressure or palpable pulses measured during chest compressions do not necessarily represent CPP, because ventricular pressures are simultaneously elevated. Consequently, palpation of pulses developed by chest compressions and systolic pressures developed by chest compressions may be misleading. It is most useful to follow the "diastolic" or relaxation-phase arterial pressure. If unable to follow any of these pressures, the clinician must rely on indirect evidence of myocardial perfusion, such as improved electrical and mechanical activity or increased pulmonary CO_2 excretion.

Direct cardiac compression via a thoracotomy is more effective than external chest compressions, producing roughly threefold increases in CPP.[50,51] This approach also allows recognition of cardiac tamponade and treatment by pericardiotomy. Mechanical activity and fibrillation are immediately visible, and electrical rescue shocks or pacing can be applied directly to the heart. In the setting of cardiopulmonary collapse due to exsanguination, thoracotomy also allows aortic compression to shunt blood to heart and brain, as well as direct control of intrathoracic bleeding. Until the 1960s, thoracotomy was the standard approach for treatment of sudden cardiac arrest, but this procedure has now been supplanted by closed-chest compressions. Cases series describe how this technique continues to be successful, and its use should be considered when closed-chest compressions are ineffective.[50]

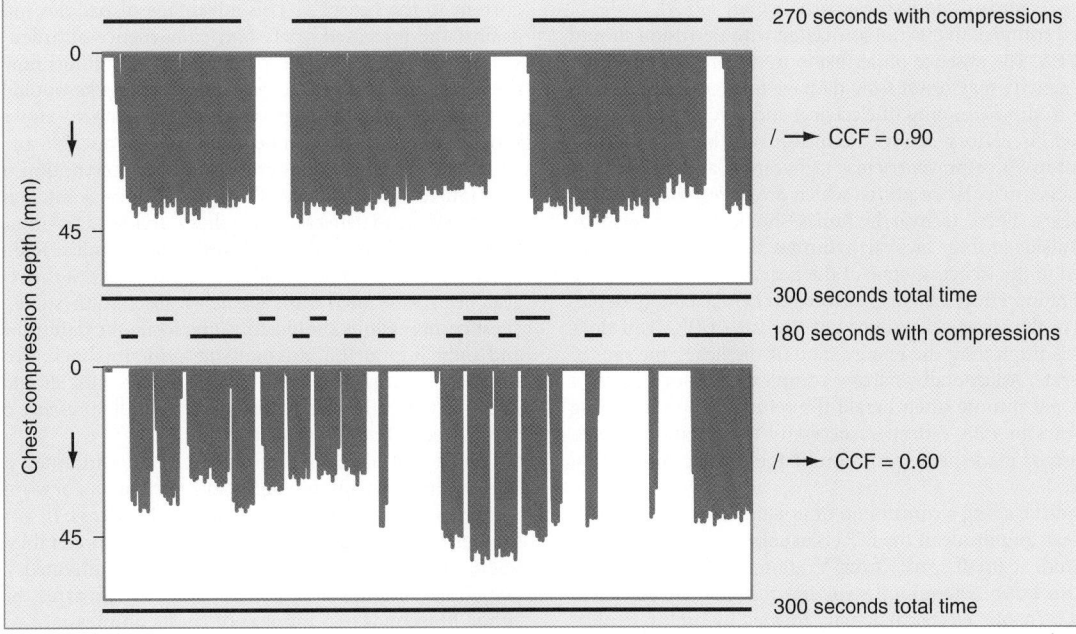

Figure 33-5 Chest compression fraction (CCF) describes the continuity of chest compressions during resuscitation. Tracings of chest compressions detected by the accelerometer of a monitor-defibrillator can be used to calculate the proportion of time when chest compressions are occurring. In top tracing, there are few pauses, and CCF is 0.90. In lower tracing, frequent interruptions for breaths or procedures results in CCF of 0.60.

Open-chest cardiac massage is most likely to succeed if initiated early during resuscitation.[52]

Delivery of chest compressions is often inadequate, and uninterrupted chest compressions are critical for restoration of circulation.[23,30,53,54] A variety of mechanical devices have been developed to provide more consistent and continuous chest compressions.[55] Some of these devices exploit circumferential compression or active compression/decompression of the chest to increase the efficiency of artificial circulation. Clinical trials comparing these devices have not demonstrated any benefit versus manual chest compressions, and one trial found a trend towards worse neurologic outcome.[56] While no current device is poised to solve this challenge, the constant attention of industry to this area illustrates the need for strategies to improve delivery of chest compressions.

Extracorporeal perfusion for restoration of circulation is highly effective and can be used to resuscitate subjects for whom chest compressions have failed.[57,58,59] With extracorporeal support, more time becomes available to address the primary cause for cardiac arrest. However, this approach requires specialized technical skill and has increased cost and risk. Logistical issues include limited availability of perfusion equipment, setup time for circuit priming, and delays in establishing adequate venous and arterial access. Development of portable cardiopulmonary bypass devices that can be primed quickly, along with improved techniques for rapid vascular access, could broaden the use of this technology. At present, this approach is used only in specialized centers that have devoted institutional resources to set up a dedicated program.

ECG MONITORING

Continuous three-lead ECG monitoring is essential for guiding resuscitation. A practical division of the ECG is to divide rhythms into organized and not organized. Organized rhythms include supraventricular rhythms or ventricular tachycardia (VT). Not-organized rhythms include ventricular fibrillation (VF) and asystole. Not-organized rhythms cannot support the pumping of blood, regardless of volume status, cardiac muscle state, and vascular integrity. Therefore, restoring cardiac electrical activity to an organized rhythm is an essential step in resuscitation. Organized rhythms can support pumping of blood unless they are too slow (<30-40 complexes/min) or too fast (>170-180 complexes/min). An organized rhythm in the absence of pulses is termed *pulseless electrical activity* (PEA).

Any organized complex that is not associated with perfusion should be considered PEA. The absence of perfusion in the presence of organized electrical activity may result from damage to heart muscle (as in massive MI) or from uncoupling of electrical and mechanical activity (as in prolonged circulatory arrest). Perfusion may be so poor that pulses are absent in VT, supraventricular tachycardia, and atrial fibrillation with rapid ventricular response, which are unresponsive to the filling of the heart. These tachyarrhythmias should be corrected by rescue shock. Outside of these tachyarrhythmias, the rate of complexes in PEA is related to the ischemic state of the heart and may be used to monitor resuscitation efforts. With increasing ischemia, energy depletion will occur in the electrical system, and the rate of PEA will slow. If resuscitation is improving the energy state of the heart, the rate of PEA will accelerate. Anecdotally, narrow complexes reaching rates of 80 to 100 beats per minute often herald the return of pulses. Falling rates of complexes in PEA reflect unsuccessful resuscitation efforts, probably because of inadequate perfusion of the cardiac conduction system.

VF and asystole lie along a continuum of not-organized ECG. Arbitrary peak-to-peak amplitude of the ECG is usually used to distinguish asystole (amplitude < 0.1-0.2 mV) from VF (amplitude > 0.2 mV).[60] However, VF also exhibits temporal structure that may be absent in asystole.[61] VF is a chaotic electrical activity formed by multiple interacting waves of activation within the heart.[62] VF emerges from broken wavefronts that result from an area of ischemia (as in MI), an area of prolonged refractoriness (as in drug-induced or inherited prolonged

QT intervals), or too-rapid succession of activation potentials (as in tachycardia or an "R on T" premature beat). As the organization and amplitude of these waves decline, because of ischemia or hypoxemia, the amplitude of the ECG also declines. Reperfusion of the heart in asystole may restore VF. Furthermore, the amplitude and organization of the VF increase with reperfusion, providing a marker of adequate artificial perfusion.

RATIONAL USE OF RESCUE SHOCKS FOR DEFIBRILLATION

Delivery of immediate transthoracic electric (rescue) shocks to patients in VF can convert VF into an organized cardiac rhythm. Rescue shocks are highly effective when VF is of very brief duration (<1-2 minutes). These shocks may work by depolarizing the heart, canceling the original wavefronts, or by prolonging the refractory periods.[62] Although rescue shocks can successfully restore an organized rhythm, repeated shocks may directly damage the myocardium. The precise magnitude of this damage is still unclear.[63] Nevertheless, optimal therapy should provide rescue shocks at the lowest effective energy while minimizing the number of unsuccessful rescue shocks.

Rescue shocks are more likely to fail when cardiac arrest has lasted more than a few minutes. In the out-of-hospital setting when the collapse is not witnessed by the paramedic, only 9% to 12% of rescue shocks restore an organized ECG.[64,65] Furthermore, resuscitation is less likely after rescue shocks that convert VF into asystole.[66] In one model for defibrillation, a "critical mass" of the heart must be depolarized by a rescue shock to ensure that VF activation potentials are extinguished.[62] If a critical mass is not defibrillated, chaotic activity in the remaining regions will spread throughout the heart, rekindling VF. However, even when the entire heart is depolarized by the shock, VF may recur, perhaps because of heterogeneous areas of refractoriness or persistent foci.[67] Regardless, shocks must be of sufficient intensity to deliver depolarizing current to the majority of the heart.

Several maneuvers can facilitate electrical defibrillation. Multiphasic shock waveforms that produce more effective depolarization of individual myocytes (biphasic waveforms, for example) tend to accomplish defibrillation with less energy than monophasic waveforms.[62] Consequently, most defibrillators available now deliver biphasic waveforms. Increased pressure of paddles from 0.5 to 8 kg on the chest will decrease transthoracic impedance by as much as 14%, increasing delivery of current to the heart.[68,69] This advantage of paddles must be weighed against the increased safety and convenience afforded by hands-free self-adhesive defibrillation pads, and most settings now have adopted the hands-free pads. In the past, multiple shocks would be delivered in rapid succession to decrease chest impedance. However, repetitive shocks decrease chest impedance only about 8% or less in actual patients,[68,70,71] which does not justify the interruption of artificial circulation to deliver "stacked" shocks. Minimal interruption of chest compressions to deliver a single shock, followed by immediate resumption of chest compressions, is now recommended. Reducing the delay from the last chest compression to the delivery of the rescue shock has also been associated with greater resuscitation success.[72] Therefore, chest compressions should continue while the defibrillator is charging and only stop at the last moment prior to shock. Rescue shocks of sufficient energy with multiphasic waveforms should be delivered singly to the patient in VF using firm paddle pressure on the chest or hands-free self-adherent pads.

For VF that has lasted more than a 3 to 4 minutes, preclinical data suggest that delaying rescue shocks until after a few minutes of chest compressions will improve rescue shock success. In animals, reperfusion prior to rescue shocks appears to be preferable to immediate rescue shock after more than 5 minutes of untreated VF.[73-76] To date, two clinical studies in out-of-hospital cardiac arrest have found that either 90 seconds or 3 minutes of chest compressions prior to delivery of the initial rescue shock improved resuscitation rates for subjects with VF outside the hospital, particularly when rescuer response intervals are longer than 4 minutes.[2,77] However, a third study found no difference in outcomes with 5 minutes of chest compressions prior to shock,[78] while a fourth study found no difference in outcomes with 3 minutes of chest compressions prior to shock.[79] Finally, a large multicenter trial comparing immediate rescue shock to 3 minutes of chest compressions prior to rescue shock recently stopped enrollment, reportedly finding no difference between groups.[80] Taken together, the clinical data suggest that the first rescue shock for VF should be delivered as soon as possible within 3 to 5 minutes as long as chest compressions are started immediately, but that there is no reason to intentionally delay the rescue shock.

Quantitative analysis of the VF waveform can distinguish early VF from late VF and may be useful for estimating the likelihood of rescue shock success.[81] Larger amplitude of VF suggests early VF and is associated with more successful resuscitation.[82] However, amplitude can be affected by body habitus and other recording conditions. Frequency-based measures, as well as nonlinear dynamical measures, also can be used to quantify VF and estimate the probability of rescue shock success and are less dependent on recording conditions.[83-86] All these measures, or some combination of these measures, are likely to be implemented in future generations of defibrillators. These devices may provide real-time, semiquantitative estimates of the probability that a rescue shock will succeed in restoring an organized rhythm. Using this information, the clinician will be able to choose to shock VF when the probability of shock success is high, or to concentrate on improving the situation with artificial perfusion when the probability of shock success is low.

DRUG THERAPY

All drug therapy in cardiac arrest can be divided into three categories: pressors, antidysrhythmics, and metabolic drugs. There is good evidence that pressors improve artificial circulation, making restoration of pulses more likely. However, recent data in out-of-hospital cardiac arrest accentuate the point that no drug therapy has been demonstrated to improve long-term survival.[87] Antidysrhythmic drugs are effective for preventing dysrhythmias and therefore have a role in stabilizing the heart once circulation is restored. The value of antidysrhythmic drugs for terminating VF or reversing asystole is less clear. Metabolic drugs, primarily bicarbonate, can be used to reverse acidosis or other electrolyte problems when they are recognized. However, there are no data to support routine use of these drugs for all patients.

Pressors used during resuscitation include epinephrine and vasopressin. Both of these drugs can increase CPP via actions on α-adrenergic (epinephrine) or vasopressin receptors (Figure 33-6).[88,89] Epinephrine is usually administered in 1-mg (~0.015 mg/kg) increments. In laboratory studies, the pressor effects of epinephrine during cardiac arrest are brief (~5 minute). Vasopressin has been administered as 40-unit boluses (~0.5 units/kg) and produces a longer-lasting increase in CPP (~10 minutes). Both drugs should be titrated to improvement in clinical indicators (ECG waveform, mechanical activity, changes in end-tidal CO_2 or CPP). Direct comparisons between vasopressin and epinephrine have failed to demonstrate a clear superiority of one drug over the other or of the combination of the two over either alone.[90-93]

The 1-mg dose of epinephrine may be too small to restore pulses after circulatory arrest lasting more than a few minutes. However, trials in out-of-hospital patients comparing higher initial boluses of epinephrine (15 mg versus 1 mg) found a higher rate of restoration of pulses (13% versus 8%) and admission to the hospital (18% versus 10%),[94] but overall survival was not different. Comparison of a lower dose (7 mg versus 1 mg) of epinephrine in both in-hospital and out-of-hospital cardiac arrest found no change in restoration of pulses or survival.[95] Likewise, comparison of 0.02 mg/kg versus 0.2 mg/kg epinephrine found no change in restoration of pulses, or survival.[96]

It is possible that the β-adrenergic effect of these higher doses of epinephrine produces toxicity that limits long-term survival. Postarrest impairment of cardiac index and oxygen delivery has been related to epinephrine dose.[97] Likewise, neurologic impairment has been related to epinephrine dose.[98] No trial has completed a direct comparison of epinephrine with more selective α-adrenergic agents such as phenylephrine. However, one trial found no advantage from administration of 11 mg of norepinephrine.[94]

Vasopressin can increase CPP without complicating β-adrenergic effects. Resuscitation rates and survival are identical for patients resuscitated with vasopressin and standard doses of epinephrine after in-hospital[90] or out-of-hospital cardiac arrest.[91] However, post hoc analyses suggest vasopressin may be superior for resuscitation and survival of patients whose first ECG rhythm is asystole and for those subjects requiring multiple doses of vasopressors.[91] Subsequent studies examined the combination of epinephrine with vasopressin versus epinephrine alone for treatment of cardiac arrest.[92,93] These studies found no difference in outcomes with the combination of drugs. Therefore, use of either vasopressin or epinephrine is justified in the setting of cardiac arrest. None of the studies on these pressors standardized post–cardiac arrest care, and therefore all are limited for assessing drug effects on neurologic recovery.

Although preclinical and existing clinical data support the conclusion that vasoactive drugs during CPR can increase the probability of

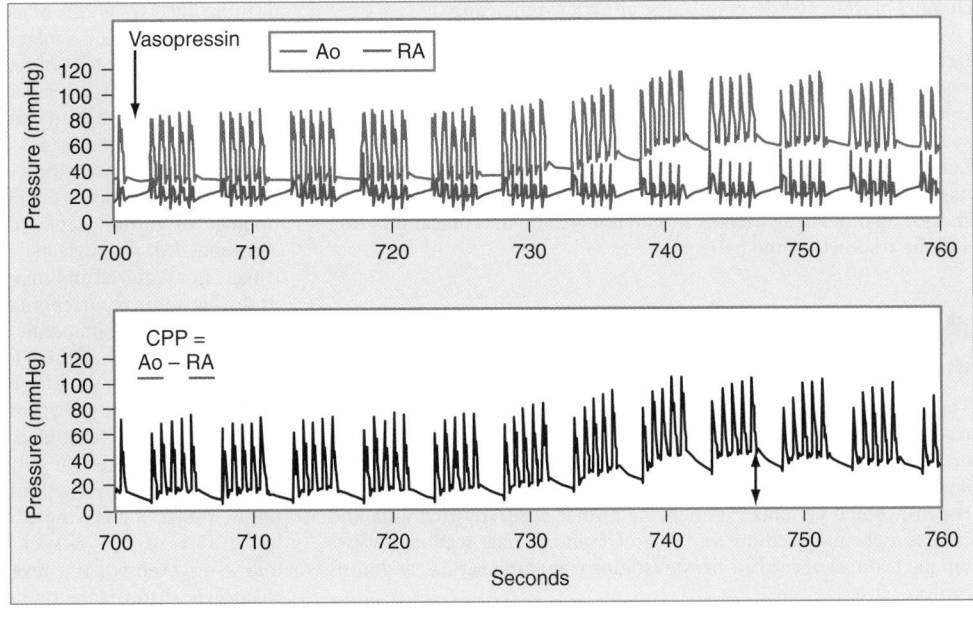

Figure 33-6 Administration of a vasoactive drug, in this case vasopressin, can increase coronary perfusion pressure (CPP) produced by chest compressions. Note that CPP generated by chest compressions alone is below the 15 to 20 mm Hg believed necessary for restoration of circulation. However, aortic pressure (Ao) and thus CPP increases above this threshold 40 to 60 seconds after drug administration *(arrow)*, while right atrial (RA) pressure remains unchanged. When treating cardiac arrest, it is reasonable to expect vasoactive drug will act after 60 more seconds of chest compressions. (Unpublished laboratory data.)

restoring spontaneous circulation, it is unclear whether these drugs actually improve overall survival. A recent trial in out-of-hospital cardiac arrest compared resuscitation without intravenous (IV) drugs to resuscitation with IV drugs.[87] In this study, which accounted for many aspects of post–cardiac arrest care, IV drugs clearly increased the rate of restoration of pulses (32% versus 21%), but the rate of neurologically good survival did not differ (9.8% versus 8.1%). It is possible the study was underpowered to detect differences in long-term outcomes. However, the data raise the worrisome possibilities that when IV drugs are required to restore cardiac activity, severe brain injury has already occurred, or even that the drugs used add to brain injury.[98]

The role of antidysrhythmic drugs during cardiac arrest is equivocal.[99,100] Atropine may relieve bradycardia when it is vagally mediated. However, nervous system influences on the heart are largely eliminated after more than 1 to 2 minutes of circulatory arrest. Therefore, there is little expectation that atropine will improve resuscitation from asystole or PEA. Lidocaine, procainamide, and bretylium have a long history of use in the treatment of VF. The basis for this use is principally the observation that these drugs can suppress dysrhythmias prior to cardiac arrest. Once VF is established, lidocaine can actually increase the electrical energy required to defibrillate by more than 50%.[101] This effect is not true for agents that are less potent, as sodium channel antagonists. For example, administration of amiodarone (5 mg/kg) is superior to placebo[102] and to lidocaine[103] for restoration of pulses to out-of-hospital patients with VF that is not terminated by three rescue shocks. These studies did not control subsequent critical care and are thus not designed to determine any effect on long-term survival. In summary, antidysrhythmic drugs are commonly used during resuscitation, but only amiodarone use has supporting human data.

Empirical treatments of metabolic disturbances during cardiac arrest are not supported by prospective human data. Bicarbonate or other buffers may improve acidemia resulting from ischemia, and systems with increased use of bicarbonate report higher rates of successful resuscitation.[104] However, no trial has demonstrated that sodium bicarbonate administration improves outcome.[105,106] Aminophylline has been proposed as an antagonist of adenosine released during ischemia. Adenosine is hypothesized to suppress cardiac electrical activity. Two prospective studies of aminophylline administration to subjects with PEA or asystole failed to demonstrate any improvement in resuscitation.[107,108] Use of dextrose-containing fluids versus dextrose-free fluids did not alter outcome for out-of-hospital cardiac arrest.[109] Other metabolic therapies including calcium and magnesium also lack supporting data.[110,111] However, it is appropriate to consider specific use of these agents to correct known abnormalities that are contributing to cardiac arrest, such as known hyperkalemia, calcium channel blocker overdose, torsades, or hypomagnesemia.

Taken together, data support a simple pharmacologic approach to treatment of cardiac arrest. First, the vasopressors epinephrine and vasopressin are useful for augmenting CPP generated during chest compressions. Other vasopressors should also be useful but lack prospective data. Second, antidysrhythmic drugs may be useful for maintaining organized rhythms but not for terminating VF. Only amiodarone has clinical data supporting its use during VF that persists after rescue shocks. All other drug therapy should be based on the clinical situation and the response of the patient.

▓ Aspects of Cardiac Arrest in Specific Situations

The original etiology of cardiac arrest may not be known during acute resuscitation. However, if this information is available, treatment and prognosis can be individualized to the specific patient. Among out-of-hospital patients, as many as 66% have primary cardiac disturbances.[112] For in-hospital patients experiencing cardiac arrest, dysrhythmia and cardiac ischemia account for 59% of events.[14] This section reviews unique features of cardiac arrest resulting from both cardiac and non-cardiac causes.

PRIMARY CARDIAC EVENTS

Cardiac arrest is most commonly attributable to cardiac disease. A primary dysrhythmia or cardiogenic shock is the most common proximate cause of cardiac arrest.[112,113] Patients undergoing angioplasty have 1.3% incidence of cardiac arrest, and survival in these patients resembles survival in other populations.[114] Among patients admitted to the hospital with acute MI, cardiac arrest occurs in 4.8%.[17] Dysrhythmias are common during the hours after reperfusion therapy,[114] although reperfusion therapy reduces the overall risk of cardiac arrest.[115] During acute MI, cardiac arrest is most likely in patients with lower serum potassium levels, more than 20 mm of total ST elevation, and a prolonged QTc interval during the first 2 hours of their event.[115] With a mean follow up of 43 months, 3.3% of subjects surviving acute MI suffered sudden cardiac death.[116] Abnormalities of the heart are present in most cases of cardiac arrest, with coronary artery disease present in at least 65% of autopsies.[117] Taken together, these data suggest that most patients with cardiac arrest will have contributing cardiovascular disease.

An acute coronary syndrome is present in more than half of patients presenting with primary cardiac arrest outside of the hospital. When angiography was performed on consecutive patients resuscitated from cardiac arrest, coronary artery occlusion was identified in 48%.[118] Similarly, 51% of initially resuscitated outpatients exhibited cardiac enzyme elevation or ECG evidence of acute MI.[119] In one series, troponin T was elevated in 40% of out-of-hospital patients undergoing CPR, regardless of whether circulation was restored.[120] The direct myocardial injury from defibrillation and CPR may cause spurious elevations of creatine kinase that are unrelated to cardiovascular disease.[121] However, cardiac troponin elevations are believed to reflect acute MI rather than injury from electric shocks.[122] Thus the 40% of subjects undergoing CPR with elevated troponin probably suffered myocardial injury prior to collapse.

The high likelihood of an acute coronary syndrome in the patient suffering cardiac arrest should prompt consideration of antiplatelet therapy, anticoagulation, beta-blockade, and nitrates during the post–cardiac arrest care. Unless a clearly noncardiac etiology for cardiac arrest is evident, acute coronary angiography may reveal an indication for angioplasty, thrombolysis, or other reperfusion therapy. Early angioplasty or reperfusion therapy is associated with improved survival and outcome.[17,118,123,124] Primary angioplasty is safe in comatose patients undergoing hypothermia treatment, and good outcomes have been reported.[125,126] Therefore, coma and its treatment should not delay emergent treatment of acute coronary syndromes if they are suspected.

Primary ventricular tachyarrhythmias are rapidly reversible and may be more likely than PEA or asystole for patients with a primary cardiac cause of collapse. Ventricular tachyarrhythmias are the initially recorded rhythm in 23% to 41% of out-of-hospital cardiac arrests[10,11,127] and in 25% of in-hospital cardiac arrests.[14] Because VF is rapidly reversible, patients with this rhythm comprise the majority of survivors of cardiac arrest. Data collected over 3 decades in one city noted that the prevalence of VF in out-of-hospital cardiac arrest has declined since 1978.[10] This trend may reflect a change in preventive medicine or in the epidemiology of cardiovascular disease over time. Once defibrillation is accomplished, prophylactic treatment of ventricular dysrhythmias is usually not required and may be harmful, given the side effects of most drugs. However, recurrent malignant dysrhythmias may be treated with infusions of lidocaine, amiodarone, procainamide, or other antidysrhythmics while searching for and treating the underlying etiology. Current practice most often employs amiodarone or lidocaine.

Long-term antidysrhythmia treatment should be considered for patients who survive sudden cardiac arrest. At a minimum, treatment should be considered for patients with decreased left ventricular function or primary dysrhythmia without a reversible cause.[128] Importantly, subjects surviving a life-threatening ventricular dysrhythmia had a 15% to 20% risk of death during a mean of 16 months of follow-up, even when a reversible cause of the dysrhythmia such as electrolyte disturbance or hypoxia can be identified.[129] Implantable defibrillators have been found to be superior to antidysrhythmic drugs for reducing the risk of subsequent death.[130] This benefit is primarily in subjects with a left ventricular ejection fraction (LVEF) less than 0.35.[131] Implantable defibrillators were not better than antidysrhythmic drugs in a European trial that enrolled subjects resuscitated from cardiac arrest secondary to ventricular dysrhythmia without regard to LVEF.[132] Nevertheless, these devices offer significant hope of preventing sudden cardiac death, and identification of patients they may benefit is an active area of research. At present, implantable defibrillators should be discussed for patients who recover from coma with LVEF less than 0.35 or survive a ventricular arrhythmia in the absence of clearly reversible causes.

ASPHYXIA

Asphyxia-induced cardiac arrest can result from drowning, choking, asthma, progressive respiratory failure with hypoxemia, or traumatic coma with hypoventilation. Acute asphyxia causes transient tachycardia and hypertension, followed by bradycardia and hypotension, progressing to PEA or asystole. This period of blood flow with severe hypoxemia prior to cardiac arrest may make asphyxiation a more severe injury than VF or other rapid causes of circulatory arrest.[133] Brain edema is more common on CT scans after resuscitation when cardiac arrest was caused by pulmonary rather than cardiac etiologies.[134]

During cardiac arrest, pulmonary edema develops from redistribution of blood into the pulmonary vasculature.[135] Thus, oxygenation is only worsened in the asphyxiated patient. Attention to the primary cause of asphyxia, as well as to maneuvers that will increase oxygenation (e.g., increased end-expiratory pressure or increased inspiration to expiration time ratios), may be necessary.

PULMONARY EMBOLISM

Pulmonary emboli may occur in the postsurgical patient, as well as in medical patients with impaired mobility.[136] In one series, pulmonary emboli were present in 10% of in-hospital deaths,[137] and the prevalence among out-of-hospital deaths was similar.[138] Pulmonary emboli can result in rapid cardiopulmonary collapse and should be considered as a possible etiology of cardiac arrest in the proper clinical setting or when collapse is preceded by sudden shortness of breath, hypoxemia and/or pleuritic chest pain.

Physiologically, pulmonary emboli can result in cardiac arrest if a large thrombus obstructs right ventricular outflow into the pulmonary arteries. This situation results in a dilated, distended right ventricle and an empty left ventricle. Right ventricular dilation is sufficiently profound that it can be seen on transthoracic echocardiogram. Circulation cannot be restored unless this obstruction is relieved. Because the primary disturbance is hypoxemia and decreased cardiac output, cardiac arrest from pulmonary embolism should present with an initial rhythm of PEA or asystole.

Administration of bolus fibrinolytic drugs (tissue plasminogen activator, streptokinase, or urokinase) has been speculated to help acutely during resuscitation of a patient with a suspected pulmonary embolism. Smaller pulmonary emboli can lead to cardiac arrest due to hypoxemia, and resuscitation may be possible prior to fibrinolysis if adequate oxygen exchange can be restored. Tenecteplase has been used with reported success in non-randomized trials during resuscitation of undifferentiated patients,[139] but it failed to demonstrate benefit in a larger randomized trial of undifferentiated patients in cardiac arrest.[140] Likewise, a randomized trial of tissue plasminogen activator to patients with out-of-hospital cardiac arrest and an initial rhythm of PEA failed to demonstrate any benefit, although drug administration was late during resuscitation.[141] There are few data about treatment of cardiac arrest resulting from massive pulmonary emboli, and certainly the overall prognosis in this setting is dismal. Individual decisions to use fibrinolytics in this setting must be tempered by the low probability of success.

ELECTROLYTE DISTURBANCES

Potassium disturbances are the most likely electrolyte disturbance to result in cardiac arrest. In cardiac patients, hypokalemia has been linked to the incidence of VF after MI.[115,142] Hypokalemia also may account for the increased incidence of sudden death in patients taking large doses of diuretics. VF is rare in patients where serum potassium is maintained over 4.5 mEq/L. Conversely, hyperkalemia can prolong repolarization increasing the likelihood of VF initiation. Hyperkalemia may also suppress automaticity in the myocardial electrical system, leading to bradycardic PEA or asystole. Interestingly, cardiac arrest occurring during hemodialysis is not associated with high or low potassium levels but is more common when patients are dialyzed against a low (0 or 1 mEq/L) potassium dialysate.[143] These data suggest that rapid changes in potassium rather than the absolute value are important triggers of cardiac arrest in this population. Derangements of calcium and magnesium may produce similar or synergistic changes in cardiac conduction.

The clinical setting of cardiac arrest may suggest a primary electrolyte disturbance. Heavy diuretic use or intestinal fluid loss, for example, suggests potassium depletion. Suspected hypokalemia will not change acute resuscitation, but it must be addressed promptly in the post–cardiac arrest stabilization of the patient. Cardiac arrest in a patient with renal failure or during potassium infusion suggests hyperkalemia. Widened ventricular complexes with repolarization abnormalities on ECG would heighten this suspicion. If hyperkalemia is suspected, the usual acute resuscitation maneuvers can be supplemented by bolus injection of calcium carbonate (1 mg), bicarbonate (1 mEq/kg), and perhaps insulin (0.1 units/kg) with glucose (0.5-1 gm/kg). These drugs may improve cardiac electrical stability, facilitating restoration of circulation.

POISONING

Cardiac arrest can result from drug overdose. Therapy does not change except when specific antidotes or countermeasures to the poison are available. For example, calcium channel blocker overdose may be countered by administration of IV calcium.[144] Beta-blocker toxicity may require large doses of inotropic agents[145] or may respond to glucagon.[146] Digoxin overdose may respond to digoxin-binding antibodies.[147] In the case of narcotic-induced respiratory depression, subsequent cardiac arrest usually is a specific case of asphyxia rather than specific cardiotoxic effects. Case reports have suggested treating local anesthetic toxicity with 1 to 3 mL/kg of Intralipid.[148] This intervention is likely to be explored for other lipid-soluble poisonings.[149] One principle of poisonings is that the patient was often healthy prior to the event, and may recover well once the poison is eliminated. This potential for a better outcome may justify longer and more aggressive efforts at resuscitation.

SEPSIS

Cardiac arrest can develop from sepsis for several reasons. Direct myocardial depression occurs, probably due to humoral factors.[150,151] Vasodilation results in apparent hypovolemia. Finally, impaired oxygen extraction, shunting, and mitochondrial depression can produce cellular hypoxia. Because pump and vascular failure are the principle physiologic derangements, the most common initial ECG rhythm would be expected to be a rapid PEA that slows to asystole with ischemia. When these processes have progressed to cardiac arrest, large doses of inotropes, vasoconstrictors, and volume may be needed to restore circulation. Acute volume resuscitation may require 100 mL/kg of isotonic fluids or more and must be titrated to physiologic endpoints (for example, central venous oxygen saturation, CVP, or urine output) rather than according to recipe. Because the underlying sepsis physiology will still be present if pulses are restored, these patients may prove exceedingly unstable during the subacute recovery period and have a reduced chance for survival.[27,152-154]

TRAUMA/HEMORRHAGE

Hypovolemic cardiac arrest occurs after severe trauma, gastrointestinal hemorrhage, or other blood loss. Absence of venous return results in an empty heart that cannot produce cardiac output despite normal inotropic state and normal vascular tone. As with sepsis, this situation would most likely present with a rapid PEA that slows to asystole, but VF can develop in response to the global ischemia. Because cardiac function and vascular function are initially normal, inotropes and vasoconstrictors are unlikely to benefit hypovolemic cardiac arrest. Rapid replacement of volume with crystalloid infusion is indicated. Colloid or blood infusion should correct the situation more rapidly.[155] After restoration of circulation, patients with hemorrhagic cardiac arrest are likely to develop multisystem organ failure.[155]

During hypovolemic cardiac arrest, the empty cardiac ventricles render external chest compressions ineffective. If blood loss is ongoing or if massive volume replacement cannot be instituted rapidly, thoracotomy allows clamping or compression of the aorta, perhaps retaining sufficient blood in the proximal aorta to perfuse the coronary and cerebral arteries. This procedure has reported success in the treatment of penetrating traumatic injuries,[156] but not in blunt trauma.[157] Survival is better if thoracotomy occurs in the operating room after brief loss of pulses, and best if the penetrating injury has created cardiac tamponade that is directly relieved by pericardotomy. Clearly, restoration of circulation must be accompanied by repair of the site of hemorrhage.

HYPOTHERMIA

Hypothermia represents an important situation where prolonged resuscitative efforts are justified. If hypothermia develops prior to circulatory arrest, the tolerance of the heart and brain to ischemia is greatly prolonged. Survival with favorable neurologic recovery has been reported after cold-water submersion or exposure with cardiac arrest and resuscitation efforts lasting several hours.[158,159] Although all data are retrospective, subjects in whom circulatory arrest occurs because of hypothermia appear to be more salvageable than subject who asphyxiate or have circulatory arrest prior to becoming cold.[160]

Treatment should be based upon the initial temperature of the patient. Between 32°C and 37°C, no change in drug or electrical treatment is required, and this level of hypothermia may be beneficial for resuscitation of both brain and heart.[161,162] Between 29°C and 32°C, cardiac activity may be preserved, and external warming (warm air, heating lights, warm blankets) and warm IV fluids should accompany usual resuscitation efforts. The likelihood of generating sufficient perfusion to rewarm the body declines as temperature decreases from 32°C to 29°C, and more invasive warming should be considered if there is not a rapid response with external warming. More invasive and aggressive treatment will almost certainly be required for cooler patients, because both mechanical and electrical activity of the heart is disrupted at temperatures below 28°C. Patients below this temperature may exhibit PEA, VF that is refractory to defibrillation attempts, or asystole. Repetitive rescue shocks in such patients are not justified and may be detrimental. Efficacy of most resuscitation drugs may be impaired.

Several techniques for active rewarming during resuscitation of victims of severe hypothermia are available. Given the potentially prolonged tolerance of the cold patient to ischemia, there may be sufficient time to establish arterial and venous access for partial or complete cardiopulmonary bypass. Extracorporeal circulation is particularly useful in these subjects because it can provide artificial circulation at the same time as rewarming.[160,163,164] In the absence of extracorporeal circulation, placement of thoracostomy tubes and lavage of the chest with warm fluids is an option.[165] Thoracostomy is intuitively preferable to peritoneal lavage because the heart can be directly warmed. Warm air forced over the body surface can rewarm a patient, although this technique may provide the least heat exchange.[166] In any case, it is difficult to determine whether or not circulation can be reestablished in the profoundly hypothermic patient until near physiologic core temperatures (33°C-37°C) are restored.

OTHER MEDICAL CONDITIONS

Comorbidities have a tremendous influence on the outcome from cardiac arrest.[113,167,168] In some cases, cardiac arrest may be an expected progression of the patient's disease, but guidelines about limiting resuscitation were not set out. For example, no survivors were reported among cancer patients with expected cardiac arrest.[168] Therefore, it may be appropriate to set limits on resuscitation efforts in certain medical conditions prior to cardiopulmonary collapse. Ideally, discussion about the expectations for resuscitative efforts should be held with the patient, their family, or the patient's representatives prior to cardiac arrest. If those discussions did not occur prior to the first cardiac arrest, they should follow promptly any initially successful resuscitation.

▣ Post–Cardiac Arrest Care to Minimize Brain Injury

Management of the patient after restoration of circulation affects ultimate outcome. For example, long-term survival differed for comparable patients treated by a single ambulance service but delivered to separate hospitals.[5,6] Institutional differences in in-hospital management were identified, particularly the permitted frequency of hyperthermia and hyperglycemia, that may have accounted for these differences. Despite the apparent importance of post–cardiac arrest critical care, there are few guidelines for treatment.

Brain injury appears not to be acute neuronal necrosis during ischemia, but instead to be an active process that develops over hours to days after resuscitation. Multiple cellular and molecular mechanisms contribute to neurologic injury after global brain ischemia.[169] During brain ischemia and immediately after reperfusion, studies have detected increased release of excitatory amino acids, free radicals, and energy failure. Protein synthesis is inhibited at the level of translation initiation for several hours.[170] There are focal disturbances of cerebral blood flow.[171] Specific intracellular and extracellular signaling pathways are activated for several hours after brain ischemia,[172,173] which may lead to specific changes in gene transcription. Finally, activation of specific proteases between 24 and 72 hours after reperfusion is associated with appearance of histologic signs of neuronal death.[174] The relative contribution of each of these processes to neuronal injury is unknown, and all may contribute synergistically to brain injury. All represent potential targets for therapeutic intervention.

Despite detailed knowledge of the mechanisms involved with brain ischemia, drugs that target specific pathways provide modest effects in laboratory studies, and no drug to date has demonstrated clear benefit in human trials. Randomized trials have examined thiopental, the calcium channel blocker lidoflazine, magnesium, and diazepam.[175-177] One explanation for this failure is that multiple mechanisms contribute simultaneously to the process of ischemic neuronal death. Antagonizing one pathway leading to neuronal death may leave other backup mechanisms unaffected. Less-specific therapies or multifaceted therapies that affect multiple pathways may prove more effective.

In support of this idea, prospective randomized clinical trials confirm that induction of mild hypothermia (32°C-34°C) for 12 to 24 hours after resuscitation improves survival and neurologic recovery.[161,178] Observational data also support avoidance of fever, hypotension, and hyperglycemia.[5,179-181] Therefore, systematic brain-oriented intensive care rather than a single therapeutic drug or intervention is required to improve outcome (Table 33-1).

TEMPERATURE CONTROL

Meticulous avoidance of fever is important during the first 24 to 48 hours after ischemic brain injury. Temperature control after cardiac arrest may be confounded by the fact that bacteremia and spontaneous

TABLE 33-1	Post–Cardiac Arrest Intensive Care
Temperature	Avoid fever for 48 hours. Induced mild hypothermia 32°C-34°C for 12-24 hours Rewarm slowly (<0.25°C/h).
Cardiovascular	Mean arterial pressure 80-100 mm Hg for first day (inotropic and vasopressor support as needed; invasive monitoring as needed). Suppress dysrhythmias. Reperfusion therapy for acute myocardial infarction, regardless of concurrent coma or treatment with hypothermia. Medical management for acute coronary syndromes (antiplatelet drugs, anticoagulation).
Pulmonary	Usual care. Avoid hyperventilation. Avoid hypoxia or hyperoxia. Pneumonitis is common.
Gastrointestinal	Usual care. Consider early refeeding (after hypothermia) to reduce translocation.
Fluids/Electrolytes	Monitor CVP and urine output with hypothermia/rewarming. Monitor potassium/electrolytes during temperature changes. Keep potassium ≥ 4.5 mEq/L. Monitor glucose frequently, avoid hyperglycemia > 180 mg/dL.
Infection	Bacteremia and pneumonia are common. Prophylactic antibiotics are of unproven benefit. Antipyretics are reasonable.
Neurologic	CT scan to exclude intracranial lesions. Sedation and muscle relaxation as needed for hypothermia induction. Monitor for seizures with EEG if available. Serial clinical examinations for prognosis. Examinations may change dramatically over first 72 hours (or longer with hypothermia treatment). EEG, SSEP, and MRI with DWI may supplement clinical examination for prognosis in selected patients.

CT, computed tomography; *CVP,* central venous pressure; *DWI,* diffusion-weighted imaging; *EEG,* electroencephalogram; *MRI,* magnetic resonance imaging; *SSEP,* somatosensory evoked potential.

fever is common in the resuscitated patient.[182,183] The benefit of lower temperatures for injured brain has been demonstrated after traumatic brain injury, stroke, and cardiac arrest.[179,184,185] Mechanistically, temperature probably affects more than brain metabolic rate. For example, manipulations of temperature that improve neurologic recovery in laboratory studies produce no effect on jugular venous lactate or oxygen uptake.[186] Recent laboratory investigations suggest that a variety of signaling pathways and cellular responses are sensitive to relatively small (1°C-2°C) changes in brain temperature.[172,173]

Induction of mild hypothermia for resuscitated patients produces a 24% to 30% relative risk reduction for death or poor neurologic outcome.[187] Mild hypothermia (32°C-34°C) maintained for 12 or 24 hours significantly improved the odds of survival and good neurologic outcome for subjects resuscitated from VF cardiac arrest.[161,178] There is no biological basis to believe that this neurologic benefit of induced hypothermia is specific to patients with one type of cardiac rhythm, and use in all patients who remain comatose after cardiac arrest seems reasonable. Multiple case series report successful application of therapeutic hypothermia for patients after out-of-hospital and in-hospital cardiac arrest with all initial rhythms.[3,188,189] At the time of resuscitation, many patients are already mildly hypothermic, with core temperatures between 35°C and 35.5°C.[161,178,190] This spontaneous cooling may result from equilibration of core and peripheral blood compartments during circulatory arrest. Subsequent to restoration of circulation, patients will rewarm within a few hours unless specific interventions are instituted.[179,191]

The optimal duration of cooling, the maximum delay in achieving target temperatures, the optimal target temperature, and the preferred rate of rewarming are unknown. Laboratory studies suggest that cooling to between 32°C and 35°C for 12 to 24 hours is beneficial, particularly if cooling is achieved within 6 hours after resuscitation. These studies also suggest that temperature is less important more than 48 hours after resuscitation, but that rewarming should be performed slowly (<0.25°C/hour). Clinical data to answer these practical questions are likely to become available over the next few years as therapeutic hypothermia becomes widespread.

After cardiac arrest, mild hypothermia can be induced and maintained by a variety of techniques including surface cooling and endovascular devices.[162] Surface cooling with ice packs and cooling blankets is tolerated by the comatose patient.[178,192] Initial studies using surface cooling alone suggested that it is slow and may require 4 to 6 hours to reach 34°C.[161,184,193] However, neuromuscular blockade and sedation can help prevent shivering or other compensatory responses and thereby greatly facilitate surface cooling. Recent reports indicated that core temperature can be reduced below 34°C for the majority of patients within 4 hours with surface cooling.[194] There are few direct comparisons of surface cooling and endovascular cooling. What data exist suggest that endovascular devices are no faster than water-circulating surface devices, but that endovascular catheters provide more stable control of temperature over time.[195,196] Local cooling of the head is unlikely to produce brain hypothermia when there is adequate perfusion by warm core blood,[190] although the head can be an effective site for removing heat from the body.[197]

Additional maneuvers are available to accelerate cooling after cardiac arrest. For example, rapid infusion of 30 mL/kg cold (4°C) crystalloid produces a rapid decrease in core temperature and is tolerated by the post–cardiac arrest patient.[191,198-200] Effective use of cold fluid boluses requires that they are administered quickly into the central circulation (via central line or under pressure infusion via peripheral line). The volume required may limit this intervention to those patients without renal failure or pulmonary edema. Gastric or bladder lavage are labor intensive and less effective than cold fluid administration. It is also critical to appreciate that cold IV fluids only produce a transient decrease in core temperature, requiring that a maintenance technique (endovascular or surface cooling device) be in place after the infusion.[191,200] Taken together, these data support the rapid induction of mild hypothermia by bolus infusion of cold IV fluids (unless contraindicated), followed by maintenance of hypothermia by surface or endovascular cooling, neuromuscular paralysis, and sedation. One additional precaution that must be considered if neuromuscular blockade is required is the high incidence of seizures after cardiac arrest. Neurophysiologic monitoring should be in place if the patient is paralyzed.

Fluid and electrolyte shifts are the primary management concerns during induction of hypothermia. Induction of cooling can result in peripheral vasoconstriction, with an apparent reduction in vascular volume.[201] CVP will rise, followed by diuresis. Conversely, at the time of rewarming, vessels will dilate, CVP will fall, and the patient may appear relatively hypovolemic. Volume status should be followed closely, and a need for additional volume infusion to maintain blood pressure and urine output should be anticipated at the time of rewarming. Inattention to this fluid shift was cited as a pitfall in trials of therapeutic hypothermia for traumatic brain injury.[201] The initial diuresis, along with shifts between intracellular and extracellular compartments, can result in hypokalemia, hypophosphatemia, and hypomagnesemia at cooling, followed by hyperkalemia at rewarming.[202,203] Frequent monitoring and correction of electrolytes during these transitions is warranted.

When indicated, primary angioplasty can be conducted in patients undergoing hypothermia treatment.[125,126] Conscious patients undergoing angioplasty for acute MI tolerate mild hypothermia.[162] In these patients, cooling did not interfere with defibrillation when it was required. Cardiovascular complications of hypothermia are rare with temperatures greater than 30°C. Cooling from 37°C to 31°C actually has a positive inotropic effect, increasing stroke volume to a greater extent than it decreases heart rate.[204] Systemic vascular resistance does not appear to change greatly. Clinical data report a transient 18% decline in cardiac index with cooling to 33°C.[205]

Other complications of mild hypothermia are few when the cooling period lasts less than 24 hours. Infections become more common if cooling is prolonged for more than 24 hours. There is a suggestion that infections were slightly more common in post–cardiac arrest patients cooled for 24 hours,[161] but not in those cooled for 12 hours.[178] Although mild hypothermia can inhibit platelet function and coagulation,[206] these changes are of small magnitude, leading to few bleeding complications in studies to date. These studies included subjects with concurrent trauma or administration of heparinoids and glycoprotein IIb/IIIa inhibitors.[162,184] There are reports of infrequent but increased bleeding in post–cardiac arrest patients treated with hypothermia and cardiac catheterization (6.2% of patients).[207] Elevations of pancreatic enzymes have been reported in cooled patients, but these changes resolve with rewarming.[161,205] Creatinine clearance and platelet count may fall during cooling, but both parameters normalize with rewarming.[205]

BLOOD PRESSURE AND CEREBRAL BLOOD FLOW

After cardiac arrest, the heart experiences a reversible period of decreased mechanical function.[208] The biochemical basis for this dysfunction is an active area of study. Moreover, reperfusion at the time of resuscitation includes oxidative stress or other triggers that can lead to myocyte death over time.[209] From a clinical standpoint, some vasoactive drug support is necessary in a large proportion of patients resuscitated from cardiac arrest lasting more than 3 or 4 minutes. This dependence on vasoactive drugs should decline over the subsequent 24 to 48 hours.

Autoregulation of cerebral blood flow is disturbed after cardiac arrest. Although rarely used clinically, measurement of oxygen saturation in the jugular bulb venous blood allows calculation of brain oxygen extraction. Furthermore, cerebral blood flow can be estimated using transcranial Doppler ultrasound or nuclear imaging. During the first day after resuscitation from cardiac arrest, patients exhibit increased cerebral vascular resistance[210] and impaired cerebral autoregulation.[211,212] When autoregulation is present, it is right shifted such that brain perfusion declines when mean arterial pressure (MAP) declines below 80 to 120 mm Hg. When blood pressure is maintained, clinical positron emission tomography (PET) studies suggest that regional perfusion remains matched to metabolic activity after cardiac arrest.[213,214] Thus, available data indicate that normal perfusion of the brain requires a higher MAP than normal during the first few hours after cardiac arrest. Periods of hypotension after restoration of pulses may add significant secondary ischemic brain injury.

If tolerated by the heart, relative hypertension (MAP of 80–100 mm Hg) should be maintained to prevent brain hypoperfusion. Maintaining this level of hypertension often requires infusions of inotropes and/or pressors. In support of this recommendation, hypotension during the first 2 hours after resuscitation is associated with poor neurologic recovery in patients admitted to the hospital after cardiac arrest.[180] No specific choice of pressors has been demonstrated to be superior. Dopamine 5 to 20 µg/kg/min, norepinephrine (0.01-1 µg/kg/min) and/or epinephrine (0.01-1 µg/min) are all potential agents. In addition, the doses of these agents must be titrated, and patient requirements may be very dynamic in the early period after cardiac arrest.

GLUCOSE CONTROL

Elevated serum glucose is associated with poor outcome after cardiac arrest[109] and may be a marker of prolonged or difficult resuscitation. Both epinephrine and physiologic stress can elevate serum glucose. However, multivariate models that accounted for resuscitation time and medication usage still show an effect of serum glucose on admission and during the first 48 hours of intensive care on long-term outcome.[5,215] Despite this association, both studies noted that monitoring of glucose in nondiabetic patients was infrequent.

It has not been established whether any specific strategy to control hyperglycemia will improve outcome after cardiac arrest. Intensive glycemic control with a low target range (72-108 mg/dL, 4-6 mmol/L) is quite controversial outside of the surgical population where it was first studied[216] and has not proven beneficial and may be harmful in medical intensive care.[217,218] After cardiac arrest, there was no difference in outcome when a moderate glucose was targeted (108-144 mg/dL; 6-8 mmol/L) versus a strict lower range (72-108 mg/dL; 4-6 mmol/L).[219] However, the incidence of hypoglycemic events was higher in the strict versus moderate control group (18% versus 2% of patients). Given the available data, control of glucose levels above 180 mg/dL (10 mmol/L) seems reasonable, and 144 to 180 mg/dL (8-10 mmol/L) would be a safe target range. However, lower ranges (72-108 mg/dL; 4-6 mmol/L) have risk of complication without benefit and should be avoided.

HEMATOLOGIC CHANGES

Cardiac arrest is associated with activation of coagulation that is not balanced by fibrinolysis. This hematologic profile is reminiscent of disseminated intravascular coagulation and may contribute to subsequent end-organ dysfunction. Markers of thrombogenesis that have been reported include increased thrombin-antithrombin complexes and fibrinopeptide A.[220,221] These increases are not balanced by fibrinolytic factors for at least 24 hours. The etiology of these changes is unknown and may be related to ischemic injury to the endothelium.

At present, use of anticoagulation is variable, and there are no prospective trials evaluating the effect of anticoagulation after resuscitation. Anticoagulation and even fibrinolytic drugs are safe after cardiopulmonary resuscitation.[140,221-223] A retrospective series noted a univariate relationship between anticoagulation and 6-month survival that was not significant in a multivariate model.[215] Given the hematologic evidence of active thrombogenesis, these data suggest that at least anticoagulation should be considered immediately after resuscitation.

INFECTION

The physiology of the post–cardiac arrest patient resembles the systemic inflammatory response syndrome, and post–cardiac arrest infections are common. Bacteremia has been noted in 39% of patients during the first 12 hours after resuscitation.[182] Fever is common in patients within 48 hours after resuscitation from cardiac arrest if active temperature control is not in place. Potential causes include contamination during emergent line placement, aspiration or transient bacteremia during airway management, and mesenteric ischemia contributing to bacterial translocation from the gut. Endotoxin and various cytokines are elevated in serum after resuscitation.[224] While an intestinal origin of endotoxin was suspected, pulmonary infections were more common than bacteremia. Pneumonitis is evident in 33% to 41% of patients after cardiac arrest,[161,207] although microbiological confirmation of pneumonia is often lacking. Severe infections may contribute to overall mortality.[183] Despite these observations, the role of routine antibiotics and antipyretics has not been examined.

Predicting Neurologic Recovery

The goal of clinical practice always is to restore the patient to full consciousness and function.[225] All subjects with circulatory arrest of more than 1 or 2 minutes will be comatose at initial presentation, but some of these same patients can recover and awaken. Therefore, signs of neurologic activity immediately after restoration of circulation are good, but their absence does not preclude eventual recovery. Unfortunately, many cardiac arrest survivors fail to completely awaken and may meet criteria for a persistent vegetative state.[226,227] The status of patients who do not quite meet these criteria but are not awake has been described as a minimally conscious state.[228]

Determining the neurologic prognosis of patients resuscitated from cardiac arrest has been the subject of multiple reviews.[229,230] At this time, there are limited data about whether the traditional findings associated with universally poor outcome[231-233] are still valid in the setting of modern ICU care and treatment with therapeutic hypothermia (targeted temperature management). In fact, good survival has been reported after some situations previously believed to have universally poor outcome such as post–cardiac arrest status myoclonus and seizures[234] or the absence of cortical responses on evoked potentials.[235] In general, there is agreement that the neurologic examination continues to evolve over a longer time period than the 1 to 3 days recommended in historical publications,[229,230] suggesting that longer periods of support and observation may be appropriate for some patients. There is also belief that a multimodal approach to determining prognosis that includes imaging and neurophysiologic studies may be useful to sort out difficult cases in which the physical examination is equivocal.[234] Unfortunately, the published case series from modern ICU care are too small to provide tight confidence intervals for determining when further support is futile. The intensivist can assist families and proxy decision makers by interpreting available data in terms of the probabilities of meaningful survival, and by revising the likelihood of meaningful survival based on the progress of the patient from day to day.

Several clinical signs have been used to assess and predict neurologic recovery after cardiac arrest. A classic case series found that pupillary reaction to light, corneal reflexes, and motor activity can change over the first 72 hours after resuscitation.[233] By 72 hours, absence of eye reflexes and failure to have a localizing response to pain were highly predictive of permanent coma. A systematic review of literature since that initial report confirms the value of these clinical findings.[231] These classic series show how specific clinical signs can provide quantitative estimates of the probability of awakening, but the actual benchmarks and timing of examinations proposed in these studies were derived from data in the 1980s.

Only a few modern case series have reported the sensitivity and specificity of clinical signs for determining poor outcome.[234,236,237] These studies tend to support the finding that persistent absence of one or more brainstem reflexes for more than 3 days portends poor outcome, but the prediction is not perfect, and the small number of patients observed with absent brainstem reflexes results in wide confidence intervals. A significant difference in these studies is the less robust predictive value of motor examination after 3 days. Specifically, motor response less than flexion at 3 days was reported to have a false-positive rate ([FPR] percentage where test predicts poor outcome, but patients have good outcome) of 14% (95% CI 3%-44%)[236] or 8% (FPR 8%, 95% CI 2%-25%).[234] Therefore, the modern case series suggest that improvement in the clinical examination can occur over a more protracted time course than previously believed.

NEUROPHYSIOLOGY

It is common for an electroencephalogram (EEG) to be obtained for prognostic purposes. However, the prognostic value of EEG after resuscitation from cardiac arrest is limited by its nonspecific nature and by the dynamic changes in EEG over time.[238] Perhaps the greatest utility of the EEG is to diagnose seizures and exclude nonconvulsive seizures as an etiology of unresponsiveness. Seizures are diagnosed clinically in 5% to 20% of comatose patients after cardiac arrest,[161,239] and the true incidence of nonconvulsive electrographic seizures may be higher. Termination of seizures, if possible, is essential to allow untainted assessment of the neurologic examination. Aside from seizures, certain malignant EEG patterns have a strong albeit imperfect association with poor outcome. Specifically, generalized suppression ($<20\ \mu V$), burst-suppression pattern associated with generalized epileptic activity, or diffuse periodic complexes on a flat background during the first week after resuscitation are associated with poor neurologic outcome.[231] Thus EEG cannot be used by itself to determine prognosis, but the information provided by EEG can exclude confounders (seizures) and can be integrated into the total clinical picture used to assess prognosis.

Electrophysiologic response to stimuli also can be used to assess whether the patient is neurologically intact. Recovery of longer-latency event-related potentials is associated with awakening.[238,240,241] Conversely, absence of a cortical response to somatosensory evoked potentials (SSEPs) is very specific for poor neurologic outcome.[230,231] Cortical response is usually assessed as the N20 response to electrical stimulation of the median nerve. Like EEG, SSEP responses vary with the elapsed time since resuscitation.[238] Recent data suggest that the use of therapeutic hypothermia may increase the time-dependent changes in SSEP. One case series reported two patients treated with hypothermia who had absent N20 responses at 3 days after cardiac arrest but recovered cognition.[235] Therefore, it may be reasonable to repeat SSEPs that show absent N20s several days apart in order to avoid false-negative tests.

BLOOD MARKERS

Several neuronal peptides appear in the blood after injury to the brain, including neuron-specific enolase (NSE) and the glia-derived protein, S-100B. After cardiac arrest, NSE reaches a maximum level in serum at 72 hours. High NSE levels at 48 to 72 hours after resuscitation are associated with poor outcome.[241-243] Serial NSE levels that continue to rise over the first 72 hours also are associated with poor outcome.[243] In contrast to NSE, peak levels of S-100B in serum occur during the first 24 hours after resuscitation.[242] Higher S-100B levels are also associated with poor neurologic outcome.[242,244] Hypothermia treatment appears to alter serum NSE levels.[245] Use of NSE or S-100B to determine prognosis is limited by the absence of a clear cutoff value that is unsurvivable. In addition, laboratory assays are not sufficiently standardized to be certain that cutoff values derived in one location are relevant to another, and at least NSE can be released by non-brain injury.[246] These neuronal markers might be considered a tool for following brain injury, analogous to troponin levels for following myocardial injury, but lack the specificity or clarity required to guide therapeutic decisions.

IMAGING STUDIES

Imaging of the brain is important to exclude injury incurred at the time of collapse and to exclude intracranial causes of collapse. A noncontrast cranial computed tomography (CT) scan to exclude hemorrhage may be prudent in the comatose patient after cardiac arrest prior to anticoagulation or fibrinolytic therapy. Several series have reported a reasonable yield of clinical information from CT scans after cardiac arrest.[247,248] In general, noncontrast CT scan is insufficiently sensitive to determine prognosis after cardiac arrest unless severe changes are present. For example, severe generalized edema is often associated with loss of brainstem reflexes and may progress to herniation and brain death (Figure 33-7).

Magnetic resonance imaging (MRI) has a capacity to visualize more subtle changes in brain after cardiac arrest. For example, increased cortical signals on diffusion-weighted images (DWI) or fluid-attenuated inversion recovery (FLAIR) are associated with poor neurologic outcome.[249] For patients who remain comatose for several days and in whom clinical or electrophysiologic testing is indeterminate, MRI may be considered as an adjunct to assess the extent of brain injury. Expectations and enthusiasm for long-term support may be reduced if extensive cortical lesions are present, whereas persistence may be justified if injury is limited. In the long term, cognitive deficits are associated with global brain volume loss after cardiac arrest.[250] An important caveat with interpretation of all brain imaging after global ischemia is the differing clinical impact of lesions in different brain regions. The anatomic complexity of the brain precludes any simple quantitative relationship between the number or size of lesions and outcome. At present, the role of MRI as an adjunct for assessing post–cardiac arrest brain damage is evolving, and its interpretation should be considered in combination with neurologic or neuroradiologic expertise.

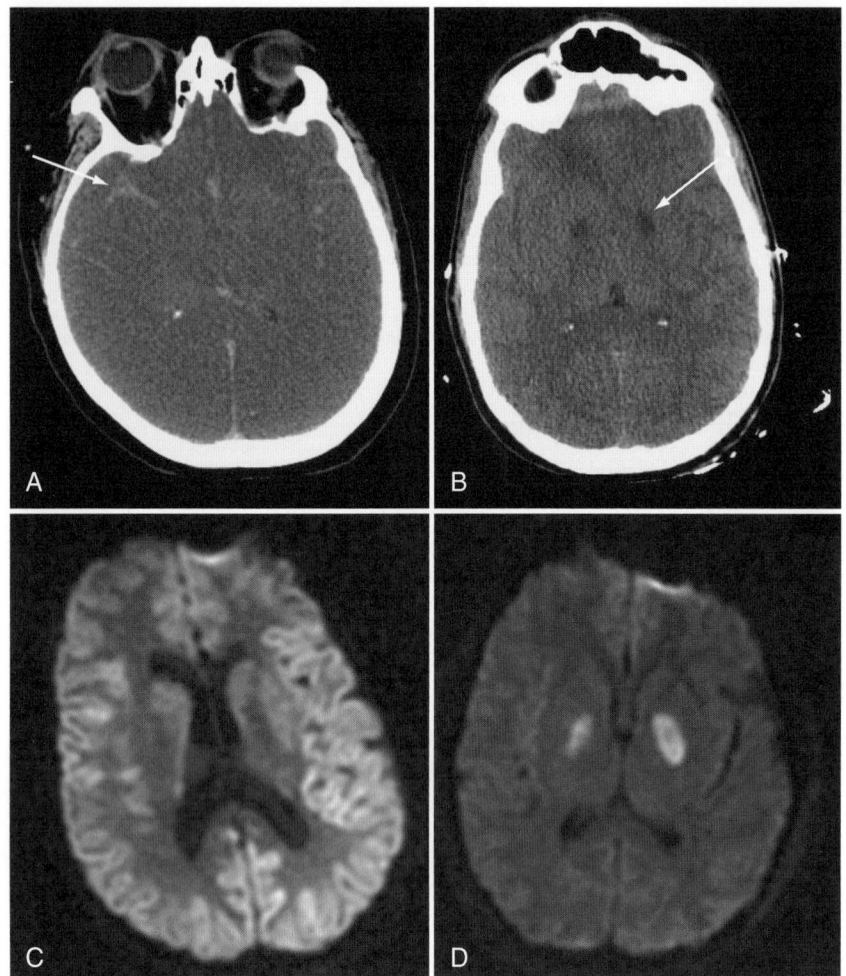

Figure 33-7   Imaging of the brain after cardiac arrest. A, Severe cerebral ischemia appears as sulcal effacement, with loss of contrast between gray matter and white matter. Congestion of blood in meninges (pseudo-subarachnoid hemorrhage [arrow]) sometimes is evident. This pattern on early computed tomography (CT) scan often progresses to herniation and brain death. **B,** Less severe early changes show edema (hypodensity) restricted to basal ganglia (arrow), with sparing of cortex. **C,** Increased magnetic resonance imaging (MRI) signal from extensive areas of cortex on diffusion-weighted images (DWI) of this patient correspond to devastating brain injury with persistent coma. This patient showed no improvement in coma. **D,** DWI for same patient in **B** illustrates high-intensity signal from damaged subcortical areas. In this case, cortex and other structures are normal. After 5 days of coma, this patient awoke, completed rehabilitation, and recovered completely.

In summary, the determination of neurologic prognosis after cardiac arrest varies from patient to patient. Changes in the clinical examination are the cornerstone of prognostication. While the patient is recovering, hypothermia and supportive care may increase the likelihood of recovery. However, electrophysiologic and imaging techniques can add additional useful information to help guide clinicians and families. The approximate timing for each of these studies is depicted in Figure 33-8.

Rehabilitation

The role of rehabilitation or other therapy in recovery from neurologic impairment after cardiac arrest is relatively unstudied. It is clear that both patients and their caregivers have complex needs if neurologic injury is severe.[251] Older data suggest that long-term improvement is less common when neurologic devastation follows a medical cause like

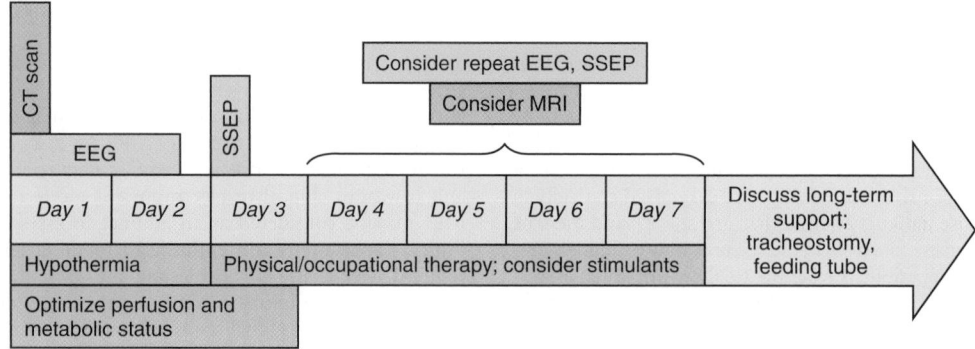

Figure 33-8   Rational approach to neurologic treatment, monitoring, and testing after cardiac arrest. For patients remaining in coma, hypothermia treatment followed by therapy and stimulation may improve recovery. Early electroencephalogram (EEG) monitoring is recommended not for prognosis but to allow detection and treatment of seizures. Absence of cortical response on somatosensory evoked potential (SSEP) or malignant EEG patterns after hypothermia treatment may help identify subsets of patients unlikely to ever show improvement. When those tests are indeterminate, and there is no sign of clinical improvement, magnetic resonance imaging (MRI) of the brain may help quantify extent and location of injury, which in turn assists in decisions about continuing long-term support. Most tests are not required when patients exhibit clear clinical improvement. Conversely, patients who progress to brain death should undergo brain death testing once toxicologic confounds, metabolic abnormalities, and shock have been corrected.

cardiac arrest than when it results from traumatic brain injury.[227] More recent work suggests that rehabilitation can produce similar improvements after global brain ischemia.[252,253] Nevertheless, early consideration of rehabilitative services including physical therapy and occupational therapy may help promote recovery, just as in acute stroke.[254] Physical stimulation and maintenance of muscle tone could conceivably promote awakening. When arousal or level of consciousness is impaired after traumatic brain injury, stimulants such as methylphenidate or amantadine have been employed with reduction in total ICU stay or improved final status.[255,256] While these data are few and indirect, addition of stimulants for post–cardiac arrest patients who linger in intermediate coma might be considered if medically tolerated.

Withdrawal of Support

For adults who are neurologically devastated after cardiac arrest in North America, it is more common to die in the hospital than to receive long-term care. An estimated 44% of patients who are initially resuscitated from cardiac arrest in the hospital have withdrawal of care later during their hospitalization.[14] For patients resuscitated from out-of-hospital cardiac arrest, 68% have do-not-resuscitate (DNR) status established in the hospital, perhaps representing a comparable outcome.[22] These decisions are often based on the neurologic prognosis of the patient,[21] and such decisions limit the number of neurologically impaired individuals who are discharged from the hospital. Consequently, quality of life for those patients who do leave the hospital is generally high.[20,257,258] Popular reports of awakening after long coma may cause inappropriate optimism for families of patients or surrogate decision makers. Partial awakening of the patient into a persistent vegetative state or minimally conscious state can further confuse their expectations. Decision makers should receive information about these syndromes, realistic expectations of recovery, and any specific considerations for the individual patient. Religious, cultural, and personal beliefs will contribute to decisions, and appropriate social service and pastoral support should be provided.

Summary

Improvement in outcome after cardiac arrest will require attention both to the reversal of cardiopulmonary arrest and to restoration of consciousness. Isolated attention to only the heart or only the brain is unlikely to improve outcomes for many patients. Appropriate prioritization of the various tools for cardiac resuscitation, along with emphasis on the basic mechanics of artificial circulation, may increase the number of individuals reaching the ICU. Induction of mild hypothermia, management of blood pressure and ventilation, along with proper treatment of the root cause of the cardiac arrest may increase the number of initially comatose patients who awaken. Constant reassessment of the likelihood of meaningful recovery, based on clinical examination and ancillary testing, can guarantee that continued care and interventions are appropriate.

KEY POINTS

1. Improvement in outcome after cardiac arrest requires attention both to immediate reversal of cardiopulmonary arrest and to promoting recovery of brain function through subsequent intensive care unit (ICU) interventions. Isolated attention to only the heart or only the brain is unlikely to improve outcomes for many patients (see Figure 33-8).

2. Increased emphasis on the basic mechanics of artificial circulation, specifically uninterrupted vigorous chest compressions, may increase the number of individuals reaching the ICU.

3. It is necessary to prioritize the various adjunct tools for cardiac resuscitation. For example, time devoted to tracheal intubation may delay drug therapy and interrupt chest compressions without altering overall hemodynamics.

4. The cornerstone of drug therapy during resuscitation attempts is the administration of vasoactive drugs that will increase coronary perfusion pressure developed by chest compressions.

5. Induction of mild hypothermia, optimal management of blood pressure, and proper treatment of the root cause of the cardiac arrest may increase the number of initially comatose patients who awaken.

6. Neurologic prognosis is determined using serial clinical examinations supplemented by neurophysiologic or imaging tests. Clinical examination continues to change for many days after cardiac arrest, and even longer periods of observation may be required for patients treated with hypothermia. Constant reassessment of the likelihood of meaningful recovery can guarantee that continued care and interventions are appropriate.

ANNOTATED REFERENCES

Aufderheide TP, Sigurdsson G, Pirrallo RG, Yannopoulos D, McKnite S, von Briesen C, et al. Hyperventilation-induced hypotension during cardiopulmonary resuscitation. Circulation 2004;109:1960-5.
This study noted the high incidence of unintentional hyperventilation when manual bagging was used during actual resuscitations. This common practice has adverse hemodynamic effects that can reduce survival, and training is proposed to prevent hyperventilation.

Bobrow BJ, Ewy GA, Clark L, Chikani V, Berg RA, Sanders AB, et al. Passive oxygen insufflation is superior to bag-valve-mask ventilation for witnessed ventricular fibrillation out-of-hospital cardiac arrest. Ann Emerg Med 2009;54:656-62.
This paper discusses not using positive-pressure ventilation at all during the initial resuscitation, and reports higher neurologically intact survival when passive insufflation of oxygen was chosen over bag-valve-mask ventilation.

Christenson J, Andrusiek D, Everson-Stewart S, Kudenchuk P, Hostler D, Powell J, et al; Resuscitation Outcomes Consortium Investigators. Chest compression fraction determines survival in patients with out-of-hospital ventricular fibrillation. Circulation 2009;120:1241-7.
This study monitored the performance of chest compressions in out-of-hospital VF. There is a strong association between survival and the proportion of time when chest compressions are performed (chest-compression fraction).

Don CW, Longstreth Jr WT, Maynard C, Olsufka M, Nichol G, Ray T, et al. Active surface cooling protocol to induce mild therapeutic hypothermia after out-of-hospital cardiac arrest: a retrospective before-and-after comparison in a single hospital. Crit Care Med 2009;37:3062-9.

Results are presented of implementing a therapeutic hypothermia treatment program that included both VF and other cardiac rhythms. Improved survival was robustly evident in the VF cohort.

Kim F, Olsufka M, Longstreth Jr WT, Maynard C, Carlbom D, Deem S, et al. Pilot randomized clinical trial of prehospital induction of mild hypothermia in out-of-hospital cardiac arrest patients with a rapid infusion of 4°C normal saline. Circulation 2007;115:3064-70.
This feasibility study confirmed the safety of infusing up to 2 liters of cold saline to patients immediately after cardiac arrest. This intervention was well tolerated and is the fastest mechanism to achieve therapeutic hypothermia.

Olasveengen TM, Sunde K, Brunborg C, Thowsen J, Steen PA, Wik L. Intravenous drug administration during out-of-hospital cardiac arrest: a randomized trial. JAMA 2009;302:2222-9.
This study compared resuscitation of patients with out-of-hospital cardiac arrest with and without IV drugs in a mature and well-monitored system, with attention to post–cardiac arrest care. Although IV drugs improved the rate of restoration of circulation, there was no difference in long-term outcome, challenging the current role of IV drugs during resuscitation.

Sunde K, Pytte M, Jacobsen D, Mangschau A, Jensen LP, Smedsrud C, et al. Implementation of a standardised treatment protocol for post resuscitation care after out-of-hospital cardiac arrest. Resuscitation 2007;73:29-39.
This report described the implementation of multiple changes in a system of care, from ambulance destination to implementation of specific goals in the ICU. This system-wide change resulted in significant improvements in long-term survival.

REFERENCES

Access the complete reference list online at http://www.expertconsult.com.

34

Management of Acute Ischemic Stroke

AMER M. MALIK | LAWRENCE R. WECHSLER

Stroke is currently recognized as the third most common cause of death and the leading cause of adult morbidity in the United States, affecting nearly 795,000 people annually.[1] Acute ischemic stroke is a true medical emergency and must be treated in a swift yet pragmatic approach. The rationale for acute ischemic stroke treatment is based on the concept of the *ischemic penumbra*. When an arterial occlusion occurs, an area of irreversibly infarcted brain (i.e., core infarct) is surrounded by a region that has reduced blood flow impairing function (i.e., ischemic penumbra), although not of sufficient severity to result in irreversible infarction. If adequate blood flow can be restored within a critical time frame, this area of at-risk tissue may be salvageable and return to normal function. Experimental models of stroke indicate that lower levels of blood flow are tolerated for brief periods, whereas slightly higher blood flow can be maintained for several hours without developing infarction.[2,3] The precise relationships between blood flow levels and duration for human stroke are still being elucidated, but the prevailing concept is that the more quickly restoration of blood flow occurs, the greater the probability that the salvageable tissue will be spared from permanent damage.

In 1995, the National Institute of Neurological Disorders and Stroke (NINDS) rt-PA Stroke Study Group showed for the first time an improvement in ischemic stroke outcome with acute treatment.[4] At present, intravenous (IV) recombinant tissue plasminogen activator (tPA) is the only treatment that has been approved by the U.S. Food and Drug Administration (FDA) for acute ischemic stroke patients presenting within 3 hours of symptom onset. Other treatments for acute ischemic stroke—intraarterial thrombolysis, devices for mechanical clot disruption, and neuroprotective agents—continue to be investigated.

Emergent Stroke Evaluation

For patients in the field who develop symptoms concerning for acute ischemic stroke, once emergency medical services (EMS) are activated, a rapid neurologic assessment is performed by these personnel using one of several prehospital stroke scales. These quick screening tools allow uniformity in assessing stroke deficits that clarifies communication of the patient's status to the receiving emergency department. It is helpful if prehospital personnel are able to firmly establish with family or bystanders who witnessed the patient's symptom onset at what time exactly the patient was last seen normal. Upon arrival, or more ideally, prior to arrival in the emergency department, a "brain attack code" or "stroke code" is disseminated to members of the stroke team.

A stroke team typically consists of individuals from multiple disciplines with specialized knowledge and interest in acute stroke care and often includes a vascular neurologist, nursing coordinator, and where available, a neurointerventionalist. A neurologist performs a National Institutes of Health Stroke Scale (NIHSS) (Table 34-1) assessment as an additional rapid neurologic assessment tool to better localize and ascertain the degree of clinical deficit. The score may impact which therapies may be available to patients. For patients presenting with stroke-like symptoms while already hospitalized in an intensive care unit (ICU) or other hospital floor, the algorithm should be identical.

Ischemic strokes generally are classified as large artery atherosclerosis, small vessel occlusion, cardioembolism, stroke of other determined etiology, or stroke of undetermined etiology.[5] In the first few minutes to hours after ischemic stroke, identification of stroke mechanisms may be difficult or impossible. Emergent diagnosis is enhanced significantly by imaging modalities, including computed tomography (CT) and magnetic resonance imaging (MRI).

Imaging of Acute Stroke

It is necessary to differentiate ischemic from hemorrhagic stroke before deciding on thrombolytic administration, and imaging obviously plays a key role in this regard. However, imaging may provide much more information. At most stroke centers, time from symptom onset (i.e., time when patient was last confirmed to be seen at normal baseline) is a major determining factor in whether a patient may be a candidate for IV thrombolysis (i.e., up to 3 hours) or intraarterial therapy (i.e., 3 to 6 hours). One emerging concept gaining more acceptance is that physiology rather than time should be used to decide on eligibility for treatment.[6] For example, some patients within the 3-hour time window may already have established infarction that would not reverse with thrombolysis and may result in hemorrhage due to reperfusion of infarcted brain. Conversely, some patients may have salvageable brain tissue despite presentation well after the 3-hour time window. A physiologic estimate of tissue viability would be preferable to a fixed time interval if a study were found that reliably predicted viability of brain after stroke. CT and MRI have the potential to provide this measurement.[7]

COMPUTED TOMOGRAPHY

A noncontrast head CT is the initial imaging modality of choice for patients with suspected stroke for two main reasons. The foremost is the expediency with which one can obtain a CT scan because of its widespread availability, and the second is the ability of CT to exclude intracranial hemorrhage. However, in addition to differentiating ischemic stroke from hemorrhage, CT may demonstrate subtle parenchymal abnormalities indicative of early edema or infarction. It was previously believed that these changes did not occur on CT for at least 6 hours after ischemic stroke. More recent studies indicate, however, that early changes of ischemia frequently occur within a few hours of stroke onset and have been seen as soon as 1 hour after stroke.[8] These changes include reduced attenuation in the basal ganglia,[2] loss of gray-white differentiation particularly in the insular region,[9] low density in the cortex and subcortical white matter, and loss of sulcal markings, suggesting early mass effect and edema (Figure 34-1, *A* and *B*).[10]

A hyperdense middle cerebral artery occurs in 20% to 37% of cases,[11] indicating acute thrombus within the artery. It rarely occurs without at least one other early CT abnormality. Hyperdensity in the basilar artery associated with thrombosis also has been reported.[12] In 100 patients studied within 14 hours (mean 6.4 hours) of stroke onset, multiple early CT abnormalities correlated with size of subsequent infarct and poor outcome.[11] In the ECASS I trial of tPA for acute stroke, early CT changes correlated with larger subsequent infarct volume and a greater likelihood of hemorrhagic conversion after tPA.[13] Quantitative assessment of CT changes using the Alberta Stroke Program Early CT Score (ASPECTS) scale in patients treated with IV tPA also showed a relationship between early CT hypodensity (ASPECTS < 8) and hemorrhage (Table 34-2).[14,15] Based on these results, some experts recommend withholding thrombolytic therapy in patients with extensive early CT changes, particularly in patients later in the thrombolytic time window,[16] although this practice is somewhat controversial. For

TABLE 34-1	National Institutes of Health Stroke Scale	

1A. Level of Consciousness (LOC)	**1B. LOC Questions**	**1C. LOC Commands**
0 = Alert 1 = Not alert, but arousable 2 = Not alert, obtunded 3 = Coma	Ask the month and his/her age. 0 = Answers both correctly 1 = Answers one correctly 2 = Answers neither correctly	Open and close the eyes. Open and close the non-paretic hand. 0 = Performs both tasks correctly 1 = Performs one task correctly 2 = Performs neither task correctly

2. Best Gaze (Horizontal)	**3. Visual Fields**	**4. Facial Palsy**
0 = Normal 1 = Partial gaze palsy 2 = Forced deviation or total gaze paresis	0 = No visual loss 1 = Partial hemianopia 2 = Complete hemianopia 3 = Bilateral hemianopia	0 = Normal 1 = Minor paralysis 2 = Partial paralysis (total or near total paralysis of lower face) 3 = Complete paralysis of upper and lower face

5. Motor Arm	**6. Motor Leg**	**7. Limb Ataxia**
Right Arm extended with palms down 90 degrees (if sitting) or 45 degrees (if supine) for 10 seconds 0 = No drift 1 = Drift; limb drifts down from position and does not hit bed or support in 10 sec 2 = Some effort against gravity 3 = No effort against gravity 4 = No movement *Left*	*Right* Leg extended at 30 degrees, always tested supine for 5 seconds 0 = No drift 1 = Drift; limb drifts down from position and does not hit bed or support in 5 sec 2 = Some effort against gravity 3 = No effort against gravity 4 = No movement *Left*	The finger-nose-finger and heel-shin tests 0 = Absent 1 = Present in one limb 2 = Present in two limbs

8. Sensory	**9. Best Language**	**10. Dysarthria**
To pinprick or noxious stimuli 0 = Normal 1 = Mild to moderate sensory loss 2 = Severe to total sensory loss	0 = No aphasia, normal 1 = Mild to moderate aphasia 2 = Severe aphasia 3 = Mute, global aphasia, coma	0 = Normal 1 = Mild to moderate 2 = Severe (including mute/anarthric due to aphasia) Do not score if intubated.

11. Extinction and Inattention		
0 = No abnormality 1 = Present 2 = Profound (2 modalities)	**TOTAL SCORE:**	

Figure 34-1 A, Normal computed tomography (CT) scan of brain 2 hours after onset of aphasia and left hemiparesis. **B,** Repeat CT scan at 5 hours after stroke onset shows early CT changes, including basal ganglia hypodensity, loss of the insular ribbon, and slight effacement of the sulci on the left. **C,** CT angiogram at 5 hours after stroke onset shows complete occlusion of the left middle cerebral artery. **D,** Rapid reconstruction of the CT angiogram again shows occlusion of the left middle cerebral artery.

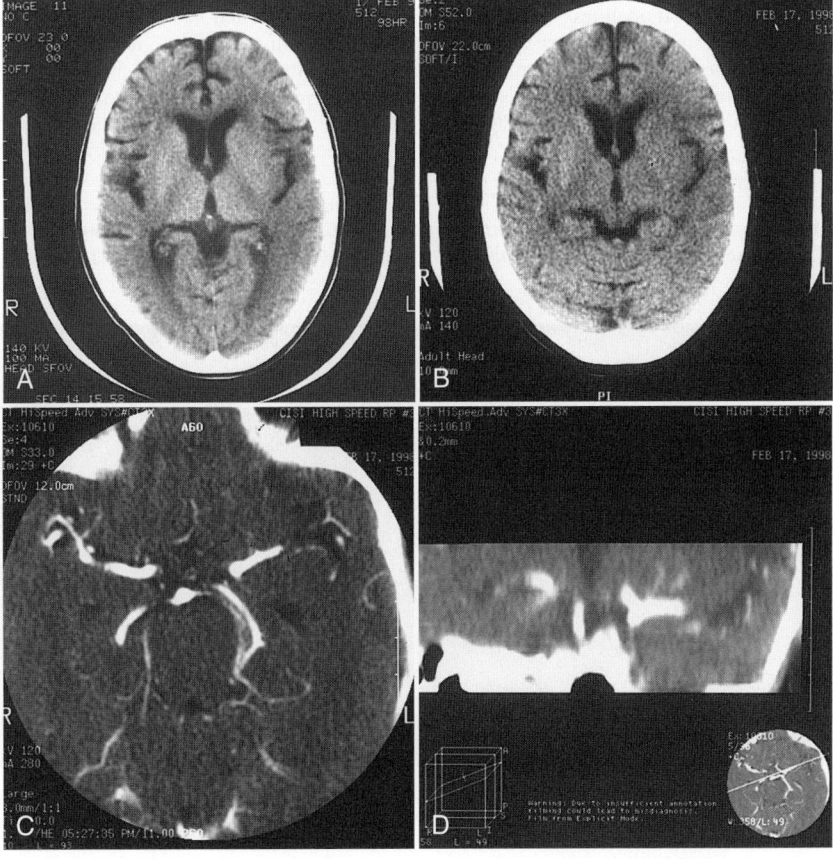

TABLE 34-2	ASPECTS Measurement Tool for Early Changes on Computed Tomography
10 Regions of Interest*:	
At the Level of the Basal Ganglia and Thalamus	*At the Level Just Rostral to Deep Nuclei*
Anterior middle cerebral artery (MCA) cortex	Superior to anterior MCA cortex
MCA cortex lateral to insula	Superior to MCA cortex lateral to insula
Posterior MCA cortex	Superior to posterior MCA cortex
Caudate	
Lentiform nucleus Internal capsule Insular ribbon	**1 point is subtracted for each defined area of early ischemic change, such as focal swelling or parenchymal hypoattenuation. Score varies from 0 to 10.

*One point is subtracted for each defined area of early ischemic change, such as focal swelling or parenchymal hypoattenuation. Score varies from 0-10.

Adapted from Pexman JH, Barber PA, Hill MD, et al. Use of the Alberta Stroke Program Early CT Score (ASPECTS) for assessing CT scans in patients with acute stroke. *AJNR Am J Neuroradiol.* 2001;22(8):1534-1542.

example, subsequent analysis of the NINDS rt-PA trial data discovered that early ischemic changes did not predict symptomatic hemorrhage or response to treatment,[17] and more recent evidence reports no association between early ischemic CT changes and outcome.[18]

COMPUTED TOMOGRAPHY ANGIOGRAPHY

CT angiography (CTA) can be performed using spiral CT technology, allowing for imaging of the intracranial and extracranial circulation. Optimally, CTA of the neck should include visualization of the aortic arch as well. The typical single bolus of iodine contrast material is approximately 70 mL of iodine. Owing to this injection, CTA is of limited use in patients with renal failure or contrast hypersensitivity. In acute stroke, CTA of the head and neck has been shown to be highly reliable for diagnosis of intracranial occlusions and correlates with other imaging modalities.[19,20] Three-dimensional reconstruction images can also be created using this technology and can provide additional views and information about the carotid bifurcation and carotid lesions, showing eccentric lesions or ulceration not visualized by conventional angiography (see Figure 34-1, *C* and *D*).

COMPUTED TOMOGRAPHY PERFUSION

In addition to imaging the brain parenchyma with a noncontrast head CT and the cerebral vasculature with CTA, CT perfusion (CTP) adds

assessment of cerebral blood volume (CBV) and cerebral blood flow (CBF). Using a helical scanner during a bolus of IV contrast, the time-dependent concentration curve of contrast in each pixel can be acquired. Mean transit time (MTT) and subsequently CBF can be calculated (Figure 34-2). In patients with acute stroke, CTP has been correlated with final infarct size and outcome, particularly after recanalization.[21] CTP maps combining CBV and CBF information identify brain tissue that progresses to infarction if not reperfused, consistent with ischemic penumbra.[22] Recent evidence suggests that the inclusion of CTP in a stroke imaging protocol increases diagnostic performance.[21,23,24]

Whereas CTP serves as a qualitative measure of blood flow, there have been recent investigations into using xenon CT as a quantitative measure of blood flow.[25] Stable xenon is an inert gas inhaled as a mixture of 27% xenon and 73% oxygen. During inhalation over a few minutes, rapid scanning is performed and pixel-by-pixel blood flow values are calculated at different brain levels (Figure 34-3). In a series of patients with middle cerebral artery (MCA) occlusion studied with xenon CT, areas of penumbra were present in all patients, and the percentage of MCA territory in the penumbral range (i.e., cerebral blood flow 8 to 20 mL/100 g/min) remained relatively constant across the group. In contrast, the percentage of MCA territory with CBF values representing infarcted tissue (i.e., cerebral blood flow <8 mL/100 g/min) varied greatly. Outcome was highly correlated with the area of infarcted MCA territory, not the amount of ischemic penumbra. These results suggest that after the first few hours, the size of the core infarcted tissue, not the amount of penumbral tissue, may be the most important imaging parameter to determine suitability for acute stroke therapy.[26]

MAGNETIC RESONANCE IMAGING

Compared to CT modalities, MRI brain imaging is advantageous because it is more sensitive to cerebral infarction, especially in the brainstem and deep white matter. Typical sequences included in a MRI stroke protocol include diffusion-weighted imaging (DWI) and apparent diffusion coefficient (ADC) to evaluate for potential acute ischemia, multiplanar gradient-recalled (MPGR) or gradient recalled echo (GRE) to evaluate for hemorrhage, and fluid attenuated inversion recovery (FLAIR) to evaluate for important signs in both hyperacute and acute stages of stroke (i.e., assessment for absence of flow void in major cerebral arteries, which suggests occlusion or slow flow in that artery). Perfusion-weighted imaging (PWI) is also a sequence often used to determine abnormal tissue perfusion based on transit times for contrast material through brain parenchyma (Figure 34-4).

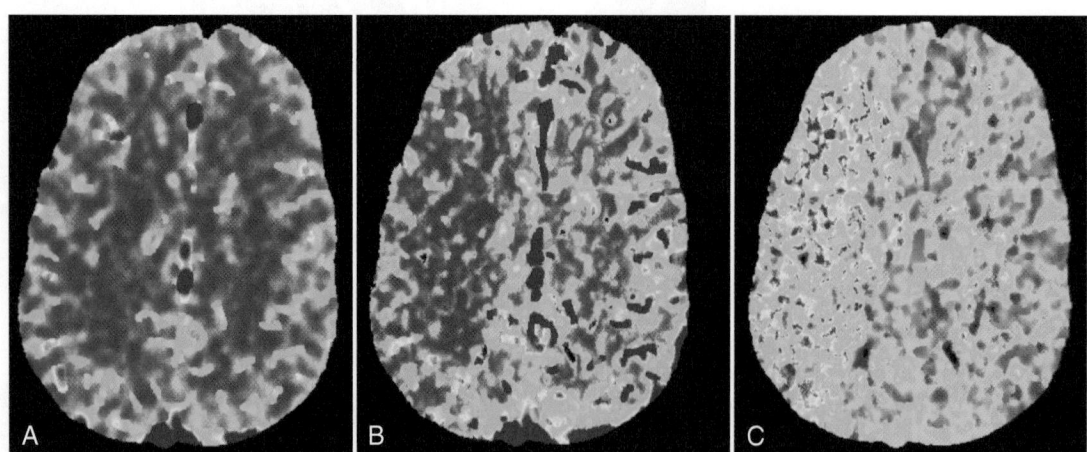

Figure 34-2 Computed tomography brain perfusion scan with sequencing maps. **A,** Cerebral blood volume (CBV) showing no clear evidence of core infarct. **B,** Cerebral blood flow (CBF) showing a decrease in the right middle cerebral artery (MCA) territory. **C,** Mean transit time (MTT) showing delayed perfusion in the right MCA territory. These sequences together indicate a large ischemic penumbra in the right MCA territory.

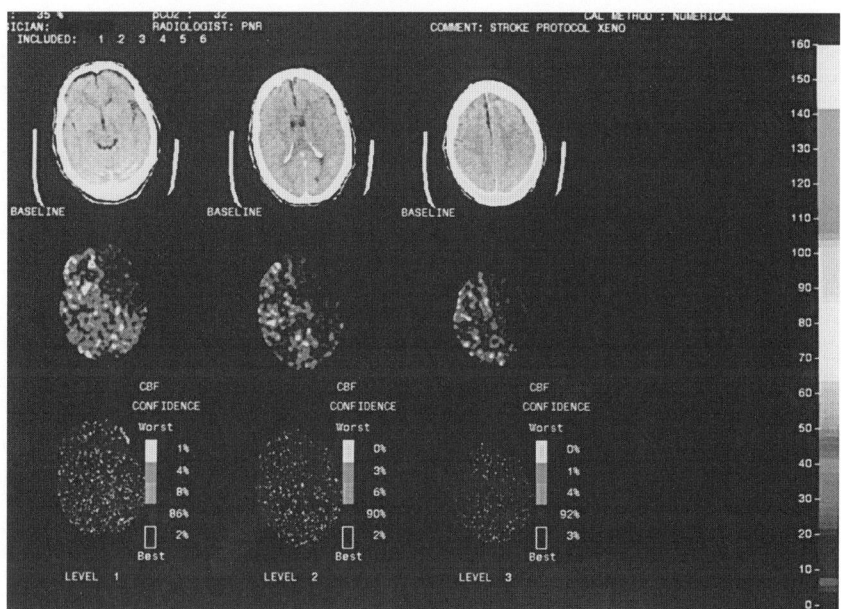

Figure 34-3 Xenon computed tomography blood flow study from a patient with large left hemisphere stroke 3 hours after onset of symptoms. Flow is nearly absent throughout the middle cerebral artery territory on the left.

DWI shows parenchymal abnormalities earlier than conventional T2-weighted images in patients with acute stroke.[27] DWI detects the diffusion of water in the brain and shows hyperintensity in areas of reduced diffusion (see Figure 34-4). As water moves from the extracellular to the intracellular space, there is less movement of water and loss of signal, resulting in hyperintensity.[28] DWI provides advantages in the evaluation of acute stroke. Early detection of lesions helps differentiate cerebral ischemia from other conditions that mimic stroke, such as seizures or toxic metabolic states. Additionally, combining DWI with PWI may identify reversibly ischemic tissue. If there is a large area of PWI abnormality indicating reduced blood flow but limited established infarction as evidenced by DWI abnormality, penumbral tissue is likely present, indicating areas of impaired flow at risk of undergoing infarction.

In stroke patients, the size of the DWI lesion and the growth of these abnormal DWI regions are strong predictors of outcome. In acute stroke, a marker of tissue viability is needed, and some investigators have suggested that the extent of mismatch between lesions on DWI and PWI could serve as this marker. The concept of DWI/PWI mismatch has been used as an inclusion criterion in several clinical trials (i.e., DIAS, DIAS-2, DEDAS, DEFUSE, EPITHET) assessing

thrombolytic agents and is being employed more frequently to select patients that may ultimately benefit from reperfusion therapy.[29-34] Patients with mismatch might be more likely to respond to reperfusion therapy.[35] Patients with large areas of DWI abnormality or large severe PWI abnormalities may in fact be at greater risk for hemorrhage if reperfusion therapy is pursued.[36]

MAGNETIC RESONANCE ANGIOGRAPHY

Magnetic resonance angiography (MRA) of the head and neck offers a noninvasive method of imaging the intracranial and extracranial vasculature. MRA typically uses gadolinium contrast in appropriate patients, but important information can be obtained based on time-of-flight techniques not utilizing contrast.[37,38] Detection of dissection or occlusion in the circle of Willis and the extracranial vertebral and carotid arteries can be examined with MRA, but occlusions of small peripheral branch arteries may not be detected. Artifact may also wreak havoc in some cases by obscuring proper identification of arterial pathology. Signal dropout may occur at the site of arterial stenosis, owing to the effects of turbulent flow. If an artery is tortuous, it may extend out of the imaging section and appear occluded. MRI tends to

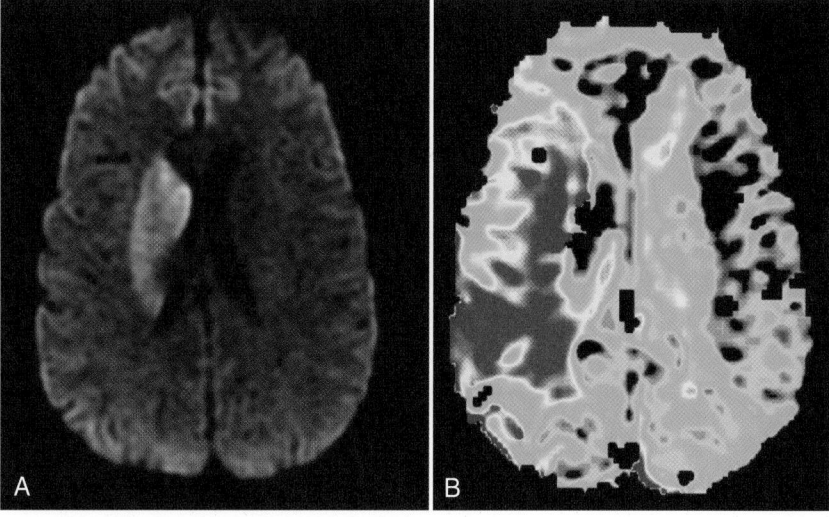

Figure 34-4 Magnetic resonance imaging of the same patient in Figure 34-2. **A,** Diffusion-weighted imaging (DWI) showing right basal ganglia stroke. **B,** Perfusion-weighted imaging (PWI) showing enhanced mean time to enhancement. These sequences together suggest a large ischemic penumbra in the right MCA territory.

overestimate the severity of stenosis, and evidence of severe stenosis should be confirmed with another modality. MRA is better for localizing the site of stenotic lesions than determining severity of stenosis. Similarly, differentiation between severe stenosis and occlusion is unreliable with MRI, and apparent occlusions by MRA should also be confirmed with angiography.

Treatment of Acute Stroke

INTRAVENOUS THROMBOLYSIS

Acute stroke trials using IV thrombolytic agents date back to the early 1960s with use of streptokinase,[39] fibrinolysin,[40] and urokinase,[41] showing either no benefit or a higher mortality in patients treated with thrombolysis. These studies preceded CT imaging, so patients with hemorrhage were not excluded. The discouraging results hindered the development of more acute stroke trials until the 1980s, when several case reports showed favorable outcomes with intraarterial thrombolytic therapy within a few hours of stroke onset.[42,43] These reports resulted in small randomized trials and feasibility studies of IV thrombolytics[44,45] which ultimately gave rise to the pivotal NINDS rt-PA trial that showed for the first time a beneficial effect of thrombolytic therapy for acute stroke treatment when administered within 3 hours of symptom onset.[4]

Tissue Plasminogen Activator Within 3 Hours

The NINDS trial included more than 600 patients with acute ischemic stroke. All patients were treated within 3 hours, and half of them were treated within 90 minutes. Patients were randomly assigned to receive either IV tPA at a dose of 0.9 mg/kg to a maximum of 90 mg, or IV placebo. Primary outcome measures were favorable outcomes at 90 days measured by the NIHSS, Barthel Index, Glasgow Outcome Scale, and modified Rankin Scale (mRS). By all four measures, significantly more patients had a favorable outcome at 90 days in the tPA group compared with placebo. Treatment with tPA resulted in an 11% to 13% absolute increase in good outcomes and a minor, non-significant decrease in mortality at 3 months. The benefit was sustained at 12 months.[46] Intracerebral hemorrhage with clinical deterioration occurred in 6.4% of patients treated with tPA as compared to only 0.6% of placebo patients. Despite the increased hemorrhage rate, there was no significant increase in mortality or severe disability in the tPA group compared with placebo. When strokes were classified according to initial impression of stroke subtype, all types of strokes had more favorable outcomes with tPA. There were no clear factors that predicted response to tPA.[47] Patients with large strokes as measured by NIHSS score higher than 20 and evidence of early low density or edema on CT had a higher rate of hemorrhage after tPA.[48]

On the strength of these results, in June 1996 the FDA approved IV tPA for treatment of stroke within 3 hours of onset. This recommendation was supported by the results of an analysis of patients treated within 3 hours of onset in the ATLANTIS trial.[49] A subsequent pooled analysis of NINDS rt-PA, ECASS, and ATLANTIS data showed that clinical benefit with tPA is greatest when given early, especially if started within 90 minutes (Table 34-3).[50] It was noted that not all

TABLE 34-3	Odds Ratios for Modified Rankin Score 0-1 in the Combined tPA Analysis		
Time	*N*	*Odds Ratio*	*95% CI*
0-90	311	2.83	1.77, 4.53
91-180	618	1.53	1.11, 2.11
181-270	801	1.40	1.06, 1.85
271-360	1046	1.16	0.91, 1.49

CI, confidence interval; tPA, tissue plasminogen activator.
Data from The ATLANTIS, ECASS, and NINDS rt-PA Study Group Investigators. Association of outcome with early stroke treatment: pooled analysis of ATLANTIS, ECASS and NINDS rt-PA stroke trials. *Lancet.* 2004;363(9411):768-774.

TABLE 34-4	Inclusion and Exclusion Criteria for Intravenous tPA

Inclusion Criteria:
1. Ischemic stroke onset within 3 hours of drug administration.
2. Measurable deficit on NIH Stroke Scale examination.
3. Patient's CT does not show hemorrhage or non-stroke cause of deficit.
4. Patient's age is >18 years old.

Exclusion Criteria (Absolute):
1. Patient's symptoms are minor or rapidly improving.
2. Patient had seizure at onset of stroke.
3. Patient has had another stroke or serious head trauma within the past 3 months.
4. Patient had major surgery within the last 14 days.
5. Patient has known history of intracranial hemorrhage.
6. Patient has sustained systolic blood pressure >185 mm Hg.
7. Patient has sustained diastolic blood pressure >110 mm Hg.
8. Aggressive treatment is necessary to lower the patient's blood pressure.
9. Patient has symptoms suggestive of subarachnoid hemorrhage.
10. Patient has had gastrointestinal or urinary tract hemorrhage within the last 21 days.
11. Patient has had arterial puncture at noncompressible site within the last 7 days.
12. Patient has received heparin with the last 48 hours and has elevated PTT.
13. Patient's PT is >15 seconds.
14. Patient's platelet count is <100,000 μL.
15. Patient's serum glucose is <50 mg/dL or >400 mg/dL.

Exclusion Criteria (Relative):
1. Patient has a large stroke with NIH Stroke Scale score >22.
2. Patient's CT shows evidence of large MCA territory infarction (i.e., sulcal effacement or blurring of gray-white junction in greater than 1/3 of MCA territory).

CT, computed tomography; MCA, middle cerebral artery; NIH, National Institutes of Health; PT, prothrombin time; PTT, partial thromboplastin time; tPA, tissue plasminogen activator.

patients recanalize with IV tPA. In a dose escalation trial of IV tPA, angiography was performed before thrombolysis in all patients, documenting the site of arterial occlusion and repeated 2 hours later. Proximal occlusions in the MCA opened less frequently than distal branch occlusions, and only 8% of carotid occlusions recanalized.[51]

Tissue Plasminogen Activator Beyond 3 Hours

Several subsequent tPA trials attempted to extend the window for treatment beyond 3 hours. The ECASS I and II trials and the ATLANTIS trial treated patients with IV tPA up to 6 hours after stroke onset but failed to show a significant benefit compared with placebo.[52-54] Pooled analysis of NINDS rt-PA, ECASS, and ATLANTIS data suggested a potential benefit beyond 3 hours. The ECASS III trial recently revealed that IV alteplase administered between 3 and 4.5 hours after symptom onset significantly improved clinical outcomes in patients with acute ischemic stroke, thereby potentially extending the therapeutic window in which patients may receive IV tPA. In addition to standard IV tPA exclusion criteria (Table 34-4), ECASS III exclusion criteria includes combination of previous stroke and diabetes, NIHSS score greater than 25, oral anticoagulant treatment, or age older than 80 years.[55] Whether patients in this time window with these exclusions also benefit from IV tPA is unknown.

Other Thrombolytic Options

Desmoteplase (i.e., *Desmodus rotundus* salivary plasminogen activator) is a recombinant form of vampire bat saliva that is more potent than tPA. Desmoteplase possesses high fibrin selectivity, allowing it to dissolve a clot locally with less effect on the blood coagulation system. This property is thought to potentially reduce the risk of intracranial and systemic bleeding as compared to less fibrin-specific plasminogen activators like tPA. Desmoteplase was investigated in multiple trials to determine whether it could extend the treatment window for IV thrombolysis up to 9 hours.[30,32] Unfortunately, no benefit of desmoteplase was realized between 3 and 9 hours after stroke symptom onset.[31]

Tenecteplase is a modified form of human tPA designed to achieve more effective thrombolysis. The half-life of tenecteplase is significantly longer, allowing administration as a single bolus. Similar to desmoteplase, tenecteplase has greater fibrin specificity and less fibrinogen depletion than tPA.[56] A pilot safety study of tenecteplase for acute ischemic stroke was initiated but was recently discontinued due to slow enrollment; therefore no convincing conclusions at this time can be made about the promise of future study of tenecteplase in acute stroke.[57,58]

Reteplase is another recombinant form of human tPA that has been shown to be effective in the treatment of acute myocardial infarction.[59] Reteplase also possesses a longer half-life compared to tPA, and a small case series found that in patients treated 9 hours after stroke onset with intraarterial reteplase, 88% completely recanalized and 44% achieved clinical improvement at 24 hours.[60] Intraarterial reteplase has also been studied in conjunction with IV abciximab, a glycoprotein IIb/IIIa inhibitor, in a phase 1 study administering the combination therapy to stroke patients presenting between 3 and 6 hours.[61] Abciximab may direct its effect through powerful antiplatelet effects or by direct thrombolysis. Abciximab monotherapy as emergent stroke treatment has also been evaluated in a phase 2 trial, with improved clinical outcome at 3 months in patients with mild to moderate strokes.[62] Subsequently, a phase 3 trial was initiated but stopped prematurely due to an unfavorable benefit-risk profile.[63]

Sonothrombolysis is also currently being evaluated as an advantageous strategy for improving acute thrombolytic efficacy. The CLOTBUST trial indicated that continuous 2-MHz transcranial Doppler enhances tPA-induced arterial recanalization with a trend towards increased recovery from stroke.[64] More recently, the TUCSON trial evaluated whether the addition of microspheres MRX-801 (ImaRx Therapeutics Inc., Round Rock, Texas) may further enhance the process of recanalization. Microspheres are a blend of phospholipids encapsulating a mixture of air and octafluoropropane gas (C_3F_8) that has the property of cavitation (i.e., rapid expansion and collapse) when exposed to ultrasound waves. The microspheres are administered IV, and when they reach intracranial occlusions, they transmit energy momentum from an ultrasound wave to residual flow and therefore promote recanalization. In TUCSON, it was concluded that microspheres could be safely combined with systemic tPA and ultrasound at a dose of 1.4 mL; however, there were safety concerns in the second dose tier of 2.8 mL that resulted in early termination of the trial. In both dose tiers, sonothrombolysis with microspheres and tPA showed a trend toward higher rates of early recanalization and clinical recovery compared to standard IV tPA therapy.[65]

INTRAARTERIAL THERAPY

Intraarterial Thrombolysis

An alternative approach to IV thrombolysis is direct delivery of thrombolytic agents by a microcatheter embedded in the clot (Figure 34-5). The advantage of the intraarterial approach is direct visualization of the occluded artery and knowledge of the recanalization status as thrombolysis proceeds. Theoretically, delivery of the thrombolytic agent to the site of the clot should be more effective than IV infusion. The disadvantage is the additional time needed to bring the patient to the angiography suite, prepare the groin, catheterize the femoral artery, and guide the catheter from the femoral artery to the intracranial circulation before the thrombolytic agent can be administered.

Urokinase was used in early studies of intraarterial thrombolysis but is no longer available.[66] Recombinant prourokinase was evaluated formally in clinical trials,[67-69] and the PROACT II study was the first acute stroke trial to show a statistically significant improvement in clinical outcome when administered within 6 hours of stroke symptom onset. The median time to treatment was 5.5 hours, and most patients were treated after 5 hours.[68] The clinical benefit was apparent despite this late time to treatment, and possibly a greater benefit would have been found had patients been treated earlier or mechanical manipulation also been allowed. Symptomatic hemorrhage occurred in 10% of patients treated with recombinant prourokinase and in 2% of controls.

Although the hemorrhage rate was higher than previous IV thrombolytic studies, the median NIHSS score of 17 indicates that the patients in the PROACT II study had more severe strokes treated at a later time interval. A higher hemorrhage rate would be expected in these scenarios. Based on factors predicting outcome in this group of patients, the treatment and control groups can be stratified according to risk. There was no differential effect of recombinant prourokinase across risk strata, indicating that all patients, regardless of risk, benefit equally from recombinant prourokinase.[69] Despite these results, prourokinase has not been FDA approved to date, and tPA tends to be more often used in cases of intraarterial thrombolysis. The exact dose, efficacy, and safety profile of intraarterial tPA is limited, but recent studies have suggested doses up to 40 mg are reasonably safe for use.[70]

Mechanical Devices

Although most thrombolytic studies concentrate on time to treatment, the most important factor for clinical outcome is probably time to recanalization of an occluded vessel. When infusion of thrombolytic agents often requires 1 to 2 hours for complete thrombus dissolution, time to recanalization can be quite long. Mechanical devices offer the

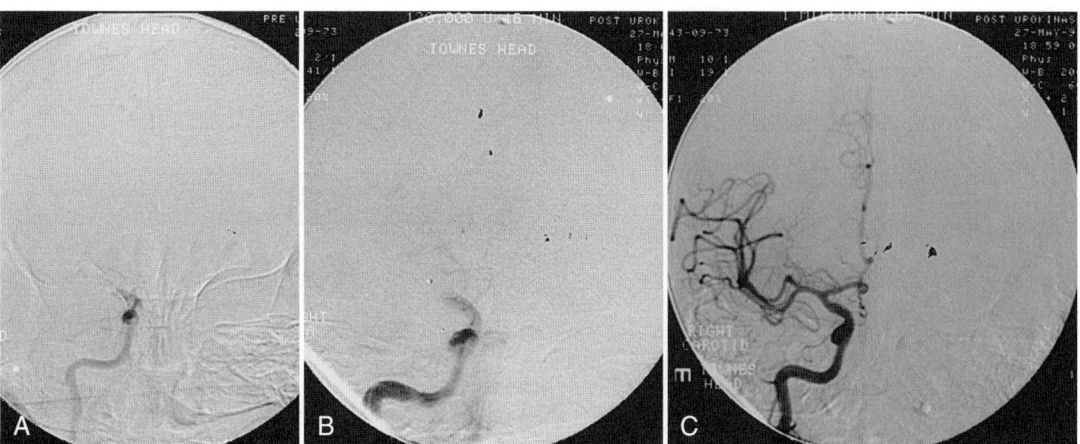

Figure 34-5 **A,** Right carotid angiogram from a patient with embolic occlusion of the right middle cerebral artery (MCA) 4 hours after onset of symptoms. **B,** Angiogram from the same patient after placement of a microcatheter into the MCA clot and infusion of 120,000 U of urokinase. There is no recanalization. **C,** Angiogram after infusion of 1 million U of urokinase directly into the clot, showing complete recanalization of the MCA.

possibility of considerably shortening time to recanalization. In contrast to thrombolytic infusions, devices may be able to clear thrombus from large arteries within a few minutes. Thrombolytic agents may not have to be used, possibly reducing the rate of intracranial hemorrhage.

The revolutionary Merci Retriever clot retrieval device (Concentric Medical Inc., Mountain View, California) received FDA approval for the removal of blood clots from the brain in patients experiencing an ischemic stroke after it was shown to be effective in restoring vascular patency in patients within 8 hours of symptom onset and could serve as an alternative therapy for patients who are otherwise ineligible for thrombolytic administration.[71] The Merci device is a flexible nickel titanium (i.e., nitinol) wire that obtains a helical shape once it is passed through the tip of the guidance catheter. In practice, the catheter/wire is passed distal to the thrombus, the catheter is removed, and a helical configuration is assumed by the wire. The clot is then trapped in the helix and withdrawn from the vasculature. Second-generation Merci devices (e.g., L5 Retriever) have been developed and recently studied for recanalization efficacy. These new devices were associated with higher rates of recanalization, although these differences did not achieve statistical significance. They were also noted to produce lower mortality and a higher proportion of good clinical outcomes.[72] An even newer generation of devices known as *retrievable stents*, specifically the Trevo System (Concentric Medical Inc., Mountain View, California) and Solitaire FR Revascularization System (ev3 Neurovascular, Irvine, California), have been developed and have been used in Europe, with very promising results.

Mechanical embolectomy using an aspiration platform was the basis for the creation of the Penumbra System (Penumbra Inc., Alameda, California). This device uses a microcatheter and separator-based debulking approach that allows for continuous aspiration of thrombus. A recent trial found that the Penumbra System resulted in safe and effective revascularization in patients who present with large-vessel occlusive disease within 8 hours of stroke onset, as 81.6% of patients achieved a Thrombolysis In Myocardial Infarction (TIMI) grade of 2 or 3.[73]

Angioplasty and stent placement without the use of thrombolytics have become routine modalities for treatment of acute coronary syndromes, with the intent to achieve timely reperfusion. The same principle could be applied to acute ischemic stroke therapy and might decrease hemorrhagic complications. One recent study found that this approach could be safely performed and improved neurologic status in patients without the use of thrombolysis. TIMI grade 3 was achieved in 88.9% of patients, and the mean 30-day NIHSS score improvement was 15.5 ± 5.6.[74]

MULTIMODAL APPROACH

Many stroke investigators believe that a combined approach of IV thrombolysis and intraarterial thrombolysis may prove to be more beneficial for acute ischemic stroke patients with severe deficits and persistent arterial occlusion who present within 3 hours from symptom onset. Two initial studies demonstrated that a combined IV and intraarterial approach to recanalization may be more effective than standard IV rt-PA alone.[75,76] The ongoing IMS III trial is a phase 3 study to formally evaluate this strategy. Patients are randomized into either an IV rt-PA only group treated with the standard 0.9 mg/kg dose, or IV/intraarterial therapy with a lower IV tPA dose of 0.6 mg/kg followed by intraarterial therapy. In the combined IV-IA group, patients may receive intraarterial tPA or one of the two FDA-approved devices, the Merci clot retriever or Penumbra device. The trial is using an mRS score of 0 to 2 at 3 months as its primary outcome measure, and mortality at 3 months and symptomatic intracerebral hemorrhage within 24 hours of randomization as its primary safety measures.[77]

NEUROPROTECTION

The extent of ischemic injury in the brain depends on the level of cerebral blood flow in the affected territory. Cerebral blood flows less than 10 mL/100 g/min are probably tolerated only for minutes, whereas intermediate levels of blood flow of 20 to 30 mL/100 g/min may be tolerated for several hours before irreversible changes occur.[78] During ischemia, there is insufficient energy for maintenance of normal membrane pump activity. Sodium diffuses into the cell across its gradient, causing neuronal depolarization and impairing the ability of the neuron to generate an action potential. In addition, there is an outpouring of excitatory neurotransmitters, particularly glutamate. Glutamate activates *N*-methyl-D-aspartate and non–*N*-methyl-D-aspartate receptors, causing influx of calcium into neurons.[79] This influx results in production of toxic products including nitric oxide, free radicals, and activation of phospholipases. The duration of reversibility of ischemia is uncertain, but animal models of focal stroke suggest it is only a few hours.[2]

Neuroprotective therapy is designed to interfere with the cascade of cellular events which results in cell death. Blocking any of the events involved in ischemic cell death may preserve function or prolong the time window for restoration of blood flow by other means, such as thrombolysis or reperfusion modalities. Current neuroprotective agents under investigation are from a variety of categories that include interventions related to nitric oxide inhibitors, free radical scavengers, neuronal metabolism suppressors, anticytokine and antiinflammatory agents, neurotrophic agents, inhibitors of calcium entry, inhibitors of excitotoxic neurotransmission, and promoters of membrane repair.

In animal models of stroke, many drugs have shown promise in reducing infarct size and improving function.[80] Unfortunately, attempts to extrapolate these findings to human stroke in phase 3 trials have largely failed to provide any evidence of efficacy. One prominent example studied in recent years was NXY-059, a nitrone spin-trap agent that showed improved outcomes in nonhuman models of acute stroke. The SAINT I and SAINT II trials assessed the efficacy of IV NXY-059 within 6 hours of stroke onset. A pooled analysis showed that NXY-059 was ineffective for treatment of stroke patients within 6 hours, and this finding applied to all subgroups.[81,82] Despite this negative result, as well as those for other neuroprotection agents (Table 34-5), there has been no deterrence to the continued investment in investigating neuroprotection agents for their efficacy in stroke.

Albumin

Albumin is the protein of highest concentration in plasma. Albumin transports many small molecules in blood and is of prime importance in keeping the fluid from blood from leaking out into the tissues. Albumin thus may help to minimize damage related to ischemia. The ALIAS trial is an ongoing trial evaluating whether high-dose serum albumin (2 g/kg, administered over 2 hours) given to patients within 5 hours of stroke onset improves clinical outcome at 3 months.[83,84] The mechanism by which albumin provides neuroprotection is unclear. Although albumin causes hemodilution and increased cerebral blood flow, it also has many other effects, including reduction of cerebral edema and diminished platelet aggregation. In addition, albumin may act as an oxygen radical scavenger and antioxidant.

TABLE 34-5	Failed Neuroprotective Trials		
Study	*Type*	*Time to Treatment (h)*	*Results*
Lubeluzole	Phase 3	8	No benefit
Cerestat	Phase 3	6	No benefit
Selfotel	Phase 3	6	No benefit
Enlimomab	Phase 3	6	Treatment worse
Cervene	Phase 3	6	No benefit
GM1 ganglioside	Phase 3	12	No benefit
Nimodipine	Phase 3	24	No benefit
Fosphenytoin	Phase 3	6	No benefit
NXY-059	Phase 3	6	No benefit
GV150526	Phase 3	6	No benefit

Magnesium

Within in vitro models, magnesium has been shown to relax vascular smooth muscle and result in vasodilation of vascular beds and increased cerebral blood flow, replete an ischemia-induced magnesium-deficient state, inhibit excitatory neurotransmitters from presynaptic vesicles, and block the NMDA receptor, among its intrinsic properties. The IMAGES trial evaluated whether IV magnesium given within 12 hours of stroke onset could significantly reduce the chances of death or disability. Unfortunately, these outcome measures were not realized, although a benefit in lacunar strokes was suggested.[85] The ongoing FAST-MAG trial is looking at whether hyperacute paramedic-initiated IV magnesium sulfate administration improves long-term functional outcome. Half of the participants randomized to magnesium therapy will receive treatment within 1 hour of stroke onset with a 4-g bolus dose over 15 minutes, followed by an in-hospital infusion of 16 g over 24 hours. The other half of the randomized treatment group will be treated within 1 to 2 hours.[86]

Minocycline

Minocycline is a semisynthetic tetracycline that has antibacterial and antiinflammatory effects. There is strong preclinical data that minocycline can effectively reduce infarct size and improve functional outcome in animal stroke models.[87-90] Minocycline also inhibits matrix metalloproteinase 9 (MMP-9), which helps mediate tissue injury during human ischemic stroke and is also associated with intracranial hemorrhage after tPA. Once the efficacy of IV doses (i.e., 3 mg/kg) of minocycline tolerable to the human body was established,[91] subsequent human clinical trials using minocycline were initiated. A trial of oral minocycline within 6 to 24 hours of symptom onset improved outcome at 7, 30, and 90 days after stroke.[92] The MINO trial is an early-phase trial underway to determine the safety of 4 escalating doses (i.e., 3 mg/kg to 10 mg/kg) of minocycline in acute ischemic stroke patients.

Hypothermia

Hypothermia has been recognized to reduce cerebral edema and intracranial pressure in patients with traumatic brain injury (TBI), and its efficacy for improving outcome in patients with post cardiac arrest hypoxic-ischemic brain injury is well documented.[93-96] Mild to moderate hypothermia (i.e., core temperature > 32.0°C) appears to be the most accepted therapeutic range for focal or global ischemia. Adverse systemic effects at this therapeutic range are limited to confusion, shivering, catecholamine release, peripheral vasoconstriction, and cold-induced diuresis.[97]

There have been a few small pilot studies evaluating hypothermia as a treatment for acute ischemic stroke. The COOL-AID feasibility trial of endovascular cooling randomized acute ischemic stroke patients within 12 hours from symptom onset between a hypothermia group and a placebo group. An endovascular cooling device was inserted into the inferior vena cava of those patients randomized to hypothermia. A core body temperature of 33.0°C was targeted for 24 hours. Induced moderate hypothermia was found to be feasible in most patients with acute ischemic stroke.[98] The ICTuS-L study recently confirmed that endovascular hypothermia after stroke can be safely combined with IV tPA in patients within 6 hours from stroke onset, but it was noted that pneumonia occurred more frequently after hypothermia treatment.[99] There are also two currently ongoing international parallel studies (i.e., CHIL and CHILI) examining whether mild hypothermia administered either by systemic or local head cooling attenuates infarct expansion and salvages penumbral brain tissue, using imaging outcome parameters. Hypothermia is also being studied in both animal models and human clinical trials in combination with minocycline and magnesium.[89,100]

NEURORESTORATION

Neurorestoration therapies are neuroplasticity-enhancing therapies that aim to facilitate brain repair and improve long-term functional outcomes after ischemic stroke. When the best time to exactly initiate treatment remains unclear; some agents under investigation are given very acutely (i.e., within 24 hours), whereas others are administered during the subacute period.

Citicoline

Citicoline is an exogenous choline precursor that once ingested is converted to choline in the body. Choline fosters the maintenance, repair, and de novo formation of cell membrane phospholipids as well as acetylcholine and dopamine.[101,102] In a meta-analysis of hemorrhagic or ischemic stroke trials using citicoline over extended periods of treatment, there was a statistically significant reduction in the rate of death or dependency at long-term follow-up.[101] Citicoline has also been shown to have a significant impact on reducing lesion volume growth in ischemic stroke, based on MRI outcome measures from baseline to week 12 of treatment.[103] The ICTUS trial in Europe is ongoing and involves administering 1000 mg of citicoline IV every 12 hours during the first 3 days and orally from day 4 until the end of the 6-week treatment period.[104] The results of this trial will be highly anticipated when available.

Stem Cell Therapy

Stem cells are present to a limited extent in adult tissue and may offer a new frontier into neurorestorative stroke therapy if their pluripotency can be harnessed. Many different cell types are available, ranging from embryonic stem cells to neural progenitor cells and immortalized tumor cells. Potential sources of stem cells include bone marrow, umbilical cord blood, and embryonic sources. Cells can now be reengineered to return to a more primitive pluripotent state and later differentiate into neuronal cell types. In animal models of stroke, stem cells stereotactically injected into the area of stroke reduce infarct size and improve function.[105-107] Rodent studies in TBI models have shown that stem cells remain in tissues 2 weeks after being incorporated, with improvement in motor function tests.[108] Several small human safety studies have been completed. Using immortalized tumor cells injected into the basal ganglia, Kondziolka et al. found no significant cell-related complications and a suggestion of clinical improvement in some patients.[109,110] A study of five patients treated with porcine xenografts was halted because of two complications causing transient neurologic worsening.[111] Another small trial of IV bone marrow stem cells also demonstrated safety.[112] A study examining children with acute TBI treated with autologous stem cells is completed, with results pending. Drawing from these findings, there is a current trial assessing the safety and feasibility of autologous mononuclear bone marrow stem cell treatment in adult ischemic stroke patients. The study design calls for bone marrow aspiration and subsequent infusion of autologous stem cells in patients who have recently (i.e., 24 to 72 hours) suffered an acute ischemic stroke. Many important questions regarding cell therapy for stroke remain, including the optimal cell type, route of administration, timing of treatment, adjuvant therapies, number of cells, and selection of patients.

SURGICAL OPTIONS

Cerebral edema and herniation is a frequent cause of death from stroke in the first few days after massive infarction. Cerebral edema gradually increases and peaks 2 to 3 days after stroke onset.

Steroids do not effectively reduce edema due to stroke, and antiedema measures such as mannitol or hyperventilation are of limited benefit. Control of intracranial pressure is associated with improved outcome, but whether intracranial pressure monitoring is helpful to guide therapy remains unclear. Surgical decompression of large hemispheric infarcts causing edema and increased intracranial pressure is a logical method of treatment because the edema is usually self-limited. If herniation can be avoided, recovery may occur similar to stroke without severe edema. Several different approaches to decompression have been proposed.

Hemicraniectomy is the first and most commonly performed procedure. It involves removal of a generous bone flap ipsilateral to the side of the infarction. Often a durotomy is performed in order to allow outward herniation of the brain to decrease ICP and prevent downward herniation. For large MCA infarctions, timing of surgery, side of lesion, presence of signs of herniation prior to surgery, and involvement of other vascular territories were analyzed but were found to not significantly affect outcome.[113] This analysis was obtained from uncontrolled, retrospective data; therefore, no formal meta-analysis could be completed.

The optimal timing of hemicraniectomy in patients with malignant MCA infarction is unclear. If herniation is already in progress, irreversible brainstem damage may occur, thereby limiting the benefit of the operation. More recent evidence suggests that surgical intervention should occur early regardless of whether signs of herniation are present. Three concurrent European trials (i.e., DECIMAL, DESTINY, HAMLET) including patients undergoing hemicraniectomy for malignant MCA infarction were combined in a pooled analysis. The three trials had similar inclusion/exclusion criteria, except for time from stroke onset to surgery. The time from stroke onset to surgery was 30 hours, 36 hours, and 99 hours in DECIMAL, DESTINY, and HAMLET, respectively.[114-116] In the pooled analysis, thresholds were established for 45 hours to randomization and 48 hours to surgery from stroke onset. The combined results showed that decompressive surgery undertaken within 48 hours of stroke onset significantly decreased mortality and increased the number of patients with a favorable functional outcome.[117]

There has been a report of four patients with cerebral edema after stroke with impending herniation who experienced a "strokectomy" based on results of xenon CT CBF studies indicating areas of nearly absent flow.[118] The imaging studies help guide surgical removal by providing information to avoid areas of intact cortex. This procedure prevents fatal herniation, but whether long-term outcome is truly improved must be determined by future randomized clinical trials.

Surgical decompression for hemispheric infarction should be considered for younger patients with a greater potential for recovery from massive stroke or patients with large non-dominant hemispheric strokes. Cerebellar infarction is a special case that clearly requires urgent surgical intervention.[119] Compression of the brainstem and fourth ventricle leading to hydrocephalus or severe pontomedullary compromise can be reversed by rapid surgical decompression of the infarcted cerebellum.

OTHER MEDICAL THERAPIES

Anticoagulation

The use of anticoagulants in acute stroke is controversial, although several randomized clinical trials provide information regarding its efficacy. Retrospective data previously suggested a significant incidence of early recurrences after ischemic stroke, with reported rates of 20%. These studies also suggested that anticoagulation with heparin reduced recurrences. Hemorrhagic complications were acceptably low, particularly when patients with large strokes and

uncontrolled hypertension were excluded from treatment. The results of recent randomized clinical trials have challenged these findings and call into question the value of anticoagulation for treatment of acute stroke.[120] However, more recent studies indicate that for cardioembolic stroke, warfarin can be safely started shortly after stroke without bridging therapy with heparin or enoxaparin.[121] The major results of these studies are summarized in Table 34-6.

The studies do not support a reduced recurrence rate or improved outcome with anticoagulation when administered within 24 to 48 hours of stroke onset. Hemorrhage rates ranged from 1% to 2.5%. The results suggest that there is little value in anticoagulation for all patients with acute stroke, but it remains possible that some subgroups benefit. The TOAST study suggested that patients with large vessel disease may achieve better functional outcome with anticoagulation.[122] The relatively high hemorrhage rate in some studies also may have obscured some benefit. In the International Stroke Trial (IST), a significant reduction in recurrent strokes from 3.8% in the control group to 2.9% in patients treated with subcutaneous heparin ($P < 0.01$) was offset by an increase in hemorrhagic stroke from 0.4% in controls to 1.2% in patients receiving heparin ($P < 0.00001$).[123] Even in patients with atrial fibrillation, the value of early anticoagulation is uncertain, with some studies showing benefit and others showing lack of benefit in reducing recurrent stroke.[120] If anticoagulation is to be started, it should only be given more than 24 hours after IV thrombolysis and following imaging confirmation that no hemorrhagic transformation of the ischemic stroke has occurred. The roles of newer anticoagulant drugs in development (e.g., rivaroxaban, apixaban, dabigatran) in the acute stroke setting will need to be addressed as they become available.

Antiplatelet Therapy

There is less uncertainty about the benefit of aspirin in acute stroke. Two large randomized controlled trials, CAST[124] and IST,[123] showed a small but significant improvement in outcome in patients treated with aspirin. In IST, patients received 300 mg of aspirin daily for 14 days. There was a significant reduction in stroke recurrence within 14 days in the aspirin group (2.8%) versus nonaspirin groups (3.9%) and a significant decrease in the risk of death or nonfatal recurrent stroke in the aspirin group (11.3%) versus nonaspirin groups (12.4%). In CAST, 160 mg of aspirin was given per day for 4 weeks or until hospital discharge. In the aspirin group, there was a significant reduction in death within 4 weeks (3.3%) versus placebo (3.9%) and a significant reduction in death or nonfatal stroke during hospitalization. There also was a significant reduction in recurrent ischemic strokes in the aspirin group (1.6%) versus placebo (2.1%), which was offset only by a nonsignificant trend of excess hemorrhagic strokes (aspirin 1.1% versus placebo 0.9%).

CAST and IST were designed to be considered together and include more than 40,000 patients. Combining the results of both studies shows a significant reduction in recurrent stroke of 7 per 1000 ($P < 0.000001$) and reduction of death or dependency of 12 per 1000 ($P = 0.01$).[125] The risk of aspirin in the absence of thrombolytics is minimal, and the small but significant benefit argues in favor of routine treatment, but only after 24 hours if IV thrombolysis has been used and there is confirmation that there is no hemorrhagic transformation.

TABLE 34-6	Randomized Trials of Anticoagulation in Acute Stroke					
Study	*Treatment*	*Patients*	*Recurrence: Treatment Versus Control*	*Favorable Outcome: Treatment Versus Control*	*Hemorrhage: Treatment Versus Control*
FISS	Nadroparin	308	1% vs. 4.7%	48% vs. 35%	0% vs. 1%
IST	Subcutaneous heparin	19,435	1.6% vs. 2.2%	17% vs. 17%	1.8% vs. 0.3%
TOAST	Danaparoid	1281	1.1% vs. 1.1%	49% vs. 47%	2.9% vs. 0.9%
HAEST	Dalteparin	449	8.5% vs. 7.5%	23% vs. 21%	2.8% vs. 1.8%
TAIST	Tinzaparin	1486	3.3% vs. 3.1%	38% vs. 43%	1.4% vs. 0.2%

Statin Therapy

Statins have been shown to reduce the incidence of strokes among patients who are at increased risk for cardiovascular disease. However, whether statins reduce the risk of stroke after a recent stroke or TIA was not firmly established until the SPARCL trial was completed. In SPARCL, patients who had a stroke or TIA within 1 to 6 months prior to randomization, had LDL of 100 to 190, and had no known coronary artery disease were randomized to receive 80 mg of atorvastatin or placebo. The primary endpoint was a first nonfatal or fatal stroke. In the cohort receiving high-dose atorvastatin, the overall incidence of strokes and cardiovascular events was significantly reduced. These findings argue that high-dose atorvastatin should be administered in the setting of acute ischemic stroke.[126]

Special ICU Management Considerations

GENERAL ASSESSMENT

In patients with acute stroke, initial concerns include assessment of respiratory function, cardiovascular stability, and level of consciousness. An adequate airway must be established to ensure proper ventilation, particularly in obtunded or comatose patients. Aspiration is a serious concern that often results in pneumonia and serves as a major cause of morbidity and mortality during hospitalization. Supplemental oxygen is often administered, but the benefit is uncertain when oxygenation is already adequate. Hypoxemia should be corrected immediately, however, and its source aggressively investigated. Arrhythmias are common in acute stroke, and bradycardia may signal underlying increased intracranial pressure or cardiac ischemia. Atrial fibrillation associated with rapid ventricular response often impairs cardiac output, requiring immediate treatment; it may also be an embolic source of stroke. Ventricular tachycardia or fibrillation rarely occurs with stroke and when present usually is due to coexistent myocardial infarction. Hypotension should be corrected with IV fluids. Seizures should be controlled with anticonvulsants. Fever should be treated aggressively with antipyretics.

Blood Pressure

Hypertension commonly accompanies ischemic stroke, and in most cases abrupt lowering of blood pressure (BP) is not advised because of the risk of causing further impairment of perfusion in the ischemic region.[127] When a systemic or cardiac reason for reducing BP is present, such as aortic dissection or acute myocardial infarction, the relative importance of the systemic and neurologic issues must be considered. Hypertensive encephalopathy is a syndrome of extreme hypertension, papilledema, altered mental status, microangiopathic hemolytic anemia, and renal insufficiency that responds to lowering BP. In the absence of papilledema or systemic features, it is unlikely that acute neurologic deficits are due to hypertensive encephalopathy, and acutely lowering BP is more likely to worsen deficits rather than improve them.

When thrombolytic therapy is considered, reducing BP within the prescribed limits is necessary. Before thrombolytic therapy is administered, systolic BP should be less than 185 mm Hg and diastolic less than 110 mm Hg.[16] Labetalol typically is administered in increasing doses every 5 to 10 minutes to control BP. If beta-blockers cannot be used, enalapril is a reasonable alternative. Sublingual nifedipine should be avoided because of the potential to lower BP precipitously. If these agents do not provide adequate control, a nicardipine drip could be considered, although such patients may not be good candidates for thrombolysis. Following thrombolysis, BP should be aggressively controlled, keeping systolic BP below 185 mm Hg and diastolic below 110 mm Hg for the first 24 hours.

Fluids

Most patients with acute stroke are volume depleted, and IV fluids should be repleted with either normal saline or lactated Ringer's solution. In patients with large strokes in danger of developing brain edema, fluid administration should be titrated carefully, and free water must be limited. Mild hyponatremia need not be treated acutely, but more severe hyponatremia should be corrected slowly and usually reverses with infusion of normal saline.

There has been some literature on the role of hypertonic saline, ranging from 3% to 23% concentration, in TBI patients. However, its role in the treatment of acute ischemic stroke and its ability to minimize cerebral edema remains controversial. Those who oppose its use cite that it can lead to rebound parenchymal swelling once it is weaned off. Proponents will usually use a goal serum sodium range of 145 to 150 mEq/L and a serum osmolality goal of 315 to 320 mOsm/L. Serum sodium and osmolality levels are usually checked every 6 hours.[128, 129]

Glucose

Evidence from animal models of stroke suggests that hyperglycemia increases the severity of ischemic injury.[130] Increased glucose concentration in the area of ischemia causes higher lactate concentrations and local acidosis, which increases free radical formation and thus damages neurons. Hyperglycemia also may increase ischemic edema, release excitatory amino acid neurotransmitters, and damage blood vessels in the ischemic area.

Studies of stroke in humans show an inconsistent association between stroke outcome and initial blood glucose; however, admission glucose concentration correlates with initial stroke severity. Initial hyperglycemia also has been associated with higher mortality rates after stroke.[131] Some authors have suggested that hyperglycemia in acute stroke is a stress reaction, but the relationship between initial blood glucose concentration and outcome is independent of initial stroke severity, arguing against a stress phenomenon.

The GIST-UK trial investigated whether treatment with a glucose-potassium-insulin (GKI) infusion to maintain euglycemia immediately after the acute stroke event had an impact on mortality at 90 days. This trial was stopped due to slow enrollment but concluded that GKI infusions significantly reduced plasma glucose concentrations and BP, but treatment within the trial protocol was not associated with significant clinical benefit. It is notable that the study was underpowered, and alternative results should not be dismissed.[132] The GRASP pilot trial found that insulin infusion for patients with acute ischemic stroke is feasible and safe. In this trial, three treatment arms were used utilizing tight control (70 to 110 mg/dL), loose control (70 to 200 mg/dL), and usual control (70 to 300 mg/dL).[133] Additional comparative studies are being pursued, and results from these trials should help clarify future treatment regimens in an effort to improve functional outcomes.

Summary

The availability of effective treatment to alter outcome within the first few hours after stroke onset is rapidly evolving. Patients with symptoms suggesting cerebral ischemia must be treated emergently, and imaging must be performed rapidly and in a high-quality manner. Therapy for acute stroke includes much more than thrombolysis, and understanding the benefits and hazards of thrombolysis continues to evolve with greater experience and additional clinical trials. Newer-generation mechanical devices are being developed, and neuroprotection and neurorestoration hold great promise as synergistic complements to stroke reperfusion therapies. Appropriate management of BP, glucose, and IV fluids all contribute to the overall outcome from acute stroke. At present, only a small percentage (i.e., less than 5%) of patients with stroke arrive at an emergency department in time for acute stroke therapy. Development of new acute stroke therapies and expected improvements in outcome with lower hemorrhage rates should encourage the medical system to further support the framework for a seamless and integrated stroke system of care to ensure that all stroke patients receive the optimal available therapy in the shortest time possible.

KEY POINTS

1. When an arterial occlusion occurs, an area of irreversibly infarcted brain (i.e., core infarct) is surrounded by a region of reduced blood flow impairing function (i.e., ischemic penumbra) that is not yet severe enough to result in irreversible infarction. If adequate blood flow can be restored within a critical time frame, this area of at-risk tissue may be salvageable and return to normal function.

2. The most important historical question in acute ischemic stroke is "When was the patient last witnessed to be normal?"

3. Acute ischemic stroke imaging ideally involves some combination of noncontrast head computed tomography (CT), CT angiography (CTA) of the head and neck, CT brain perfusion, magnetic resonance imaging (MRI) of the brain, MR angiography (MRA) of the head and neck, or MR brain perfusion.

4. The only FDA-approved therapy for acute ischemic stroke presenting within 3 hours of symptom onset is intravenous tissue plasminogen activator (IV tPA).

5. There is recent evidence based on the ECASS III trial that the therapeutic window for IV tPA may be extended to 4.5 hours in selected patients.

6. Intraarterial therapy is not FDA approved for the treatment of acute ischemic stroke. The MERCI and Penumbra devices are FDA approved for removal of thrombus from intracranial arteries in patients with stroke but have not been shown to improve outcomes.

7. Combination IV and intraarterial therapy for acute ischemic stroke presenting within 3 hours is currently under investigation in the IMS III study.

8. Several potential neuroprotective agents (e.g., albumin, magnesium, minocycline) and modalities (e.g., hypothermia) and neurorestorative agents (e.g., citicoline, stem cells) look very promising for improving functional outcome in acute ischemic stroke.

9. Surgical decompression for large infarctions is recommended to be completed within 48 hours from symptom onset in appropriately selected patients.

10. In patients receiving IV thrombolysis, no anticoagulation or antiplatelet agents should be administered in the first 24 hours until hemorrhagic transformation can be excluded. After that time, anticoagulation can be started in appropriate patients. If anticoagulation is not used, antiplatelet agents should always be started.

11. High-dose statin therapy can be administered acutely after ischemic stroke in patients with prior stroke or transient ischemic attack (TIA) and without history of coronary artery disease.

12. Hyperglycemia should be treated aggressively because it has been associated with higher mortality in acute ischemic stroke patients.

13. It is unclear whether hypertonic saline has a clearly defined role in acute stroke management.

ANNOTATED REFERENCES

Chen ZM, Sandercock P, Pan HC, et al. Indications for early aspirin use in acute ischemic stroke: a combined analysis of 40,000 randomized patients from the Chinese Acute Stroke Trial and the International Stroke Trial. On behalf of the CAST and IST collaborative groups. Stroke 2000;31:1240-9.
This article represents a combined analysis of two clinical trials, each with 20,000 patients, showing a significant reduction of recurrent stroke and death with aspirin treatment. There was a highly significant reduction of 7 per 1000 in recurrent ischemic stroke in patients treated with aspirin versus control, and a significant reduction of 4 per 1000 in death with aspirin treatment. The authors concluded that early aspirin treatment is of benefit for a wide range of patients, and its prompt use should be widely considered for all patients with suspected acute ischemic stroke to reduce the risk of early occurrence.

Smith WS, Sung G, Starkman S, et al. Safety and efficacy of mechanical embolectomy in acute ischemic stroke: results of the MERCI trial. Stroke 2005;36(7):1432-8.
This prospective, non-randomized, multicenter trial evaluated the alternative strategy of mechanical embolectomy for opening intracranial vessels during stroke. Patients who were ineligible for IV tPA and found to have occluded intracranial large vessels within 8 hours of stroke symptom onset received this therapy. The strategy was deemed both safe and efficacious and was the primary support for the FDA approval of the Merci Retriever device.

Furlan A, Higashida R, Wechsler L, et al. Intra-arterial prourokinase for acute ischemic stroke. The PROACT II study: a randomized controlled trial. JAMA 1999;282(21):2003-11.
A randomized controlled clinical trial of the use of intraarterial thrombolytics in 180 patients at 50 centers, showing significant improvement in outcome with treatment given up to 6 hours from stroke onset. Patients were randomized to receive 9 mg of IA r-pro UK plus heparin (n = 121) or heparin only (n = 59). The primary outcome was based on the proportion of patients with slight or no neurologic disability at 90 days as defined by a modified Rankin score of 2 or less.

Amarenco P, Bogousslavsky J, Callahan A, 3rd, et al. High-dose atorvastatin after stroke or transient ischemic attack. N Engl J Med 2006;355(6):549-59.
This randomized, double-blinded controlled trial evaluated whether statins reduced the risk of stroke in patients who experienced a recent stroke or TIA and were not known to have coronary artery disease. Over 4700 patients were randomized to receiving 80 mg atorvastatin per day or placebo. High-dose statin therapy reduced the overall incidence of strokes and cardiovascular events, despite a small increase in the hemorrhage rate.

Vahedi K, Hofmeijer J, Juettler E, et al. Early decompressive surgery in malignant infarction of the middle cerebral artery: a pooled analysis of three randomised controlled trials. Lancet Neurol 2007;6(3):215-22.
Pooled analysis of three concurrent European randomized controlled trials (i.e., DECIMAL, DESTINY, HAMLET) evaluating decompressive surgery for patients with large MCA hemispheric infarctions in terms of mortality and functional outcome. The analysis included 93 patients between the ages of 18 and 60 years who were either treated within 48 hours after stroke onset or randomized to a control group. Early decompressive surgery was found to reduce mortality and increase the likelihood of favorable outcome.

Hacke W, Kaste M, Bluhmki E, et al. Thrombolysis with alteplase 3 to 4.5 hours after acute ischemic stroke. N Engl J Med 2008;359(13):1317-29.
This is the first randomized controlled trial confirming the efficacy and safety of alteplase administered between 3 and 4.5 hours after the onset of a stroke. There are some exclusion criteria in addition to the normal contraindications for administration of IV tPA for this extended therapeutic window. Intravenous alteplase administered between 3 and 4.5 hours significantly improved clinical outcomes in patients with acute ischemic stroke, but it was also more frequently associated with symptomatic intracranial hemorrhage when compared to placebo.

The ATLANTIS, ECASS and NINDS rt-PA Study Group Investigators. Association of outcome with early stroke treatment: pooled analysis of ATLANTIS, ECASS and NINDS rt-PA stroke trials. Lancet 2004;363(9411):768-74.
This article represents a combined analysis of five clinical studies in 2775 patients randomly allocated to rt-PA or placebo. The study addresses the use of IV rt-PA and provides specific insight into its use beyond 3 hours of the onset of stroke. The authors concluded that the sooner rt-PA is given to stroke patients, the greater the benefit, especially if started within 90 minutes. Their findings also suggested a potential benefit from this therapy applied beyond 3 hours, but this potential might come with some risks.

The National Institute of Neurological Disorders and Stroke rt-PA Stroke Study Group. Tissue plasminogen activator for acute ischemic stroke. N Engl J Med 1995;333(24):1581-7.
A key clinical report in the field of stroke that showed for the first time in a randomized controlled trial a reduction in stroke morbidity with acute treatment. In June 1996, the FDA approved IV tPA for the treatment of stroke within 3 hours of onset.

REFERENCES

Access the complete reference list online at http://www.expertconsult.com.

35

Nontraumatic Intracerebral and Subarachnoid Hemorrhage

ALLYSON R. ZAZULIA | MICHAEL N. DIRINGER

Intracerebral Hemorrhage

Spontaneous (nontraumatic) intracerebral hemorrhage (ICH) accounts for approximately 10% of all strokes in North America and about 20% to 30% in East Asia. It is associated with greater mortality and more severe neurologic deficits than any other stroke subtype.[1-3] Nearly half of all patients die within the first 30 days; survivors often have significant residual disability.[4]

PATHOPHYSIOLOGY

The pathophysiologic mechanisms of brain injury due to ICH are complex. The primary injury is one of local tissue destruction as rupture of a cerebral blood vessel introduces a sudden stream of blood into the brain parenchyma. In over one third of patients, continued bleeding or rebleeding results in hematoma enlargement and further mechanical injury within the first few hours after onset.[5] The mass of the hematoma produces tissue shifts within the intracranial cavity.

In addition to the primary mechanical injury, further damage is believed to occur after the bleeding stops. The mechanisms underlying this secondary injury are unknown, but ischemia, edema, and toxic effects of parenchymal blood have been implicated. While each of these processes has been demonstrated in animal models, the clinical importance of any of them remains unsettled.

Experimental models of ICH consistently suggest that ischemia is an important part of the pathophysiology of ICH.[6,7] In clinical studies, peri-clot and ipsilateral hemispheric hypoperfusion have been demonstrated,[8-10] but the hypoperfusion does not appear to represent ischemia.[11,12] Positron emission tomography (PET) studies in humans performed 5 to 22 hours after symptom onset showed that perihematomal cerebral metabolism was reduced to a greater degree than cerebral blood flow (CBF), suggesting that the hypoperfusion reflects reduced metabolic demand of the damaged tissue surrounding the hematoma rather than ongoing ischemia.[12] Magnetic resonance imaging (MRI) studies within 6 hours after symptom onset demonstrate hypoperfusion without restricted diffusion, findings that are inconsistent with ischemia.[13]

Cerebral edema has been demonstrated to occur within hours of experimental ICH, variably thought to result from the toxic effects of blood-derived enzymes, from increased osmotic pressure exerted by clot-derived serum proteins, or from ischemia.[14-16] The presence, time course, and importance of edema formation in humans are debated, however. Signal changes on radiographic studies after ICH indicate increased water content in the area surrounding the clot, but the clinical and pathophysiologic significance of this is not known. Edema does not appear to contribute to early increases in mass effect[17] and is not associated with worsened functional outcome or increased mortality.[18,19]

Hemostasis after hemorrhage is initially achieved at the site of vascular injury by the formation of a platelet-fibrin plug. After several days, red blood cells within the clot begin to lyse, cellular infiltrates appear, and the process of reabsorption begins. Months later, a residual collapsed cavity is all that remains.

CAUSES AND RISK FACTORS

The leading risk factor for ICH, occurring in over half of all cases, is chronic hypertension.[20] Long-term adequate treatment of chronic hypertension significantly reduces this risk.[21] Increasing age is another risk factor, with a doubling of the rate of hemorrhage with each decade of life until age 80, when the incidence plateaus at nearly 25 times that of the previous decade.[22] In the United States, ICH is 2 to 3 times more common in African Americans and Hispanics than in Caucasians (incidence rates of 32, 35, and 10 to 15 per 100,000 population, respectively).[23,24] The incidence in Asian countries is considerably greater (61 per 100,000 population).[25]

Low serum cholesterol has been implicated in a number of studies,[26] and use of high-dose statins appears to increase the risk of ICH, particularly in those with prior history of ICH.[27] The impact of smoking,[28] alcohol abuse,[29,30] and diabetes[31,32] on the risk of ICH is disputed.

Hypertensive Hemorrhage

Hypertensive ICH predominantly occurs deep in the cerebral hemispheres, most often in the putamen[33] (Figure 35-1). Other frequently involved sites include the thalamus, lobar white matter, cerebellum, and pons. The common link between these sites is that they are all supplied by small penetrating arteries,[34] perpendicular branches directly off major arteries that are subject to high sheer stress and that have no collaterals. These features make them vulnerable to the effects of increased blood pressure. Chronic hypertension damages the tunica media, resulting in lipohyalinosis, fibrinoid necrosis, and microaneurysms (Charcot-Bouchard aneurysms). Although Charcot-Bouchard aneurysms have been demonstrated in the weakened vessel walls of patients with ICH, their pathogenetic role in vascular rupture is uncertain.[35] The occurrence of ICH in an atypical location, in multiple locations, or in association with subarachnoid hemorrhage raises the suspicion of a non-hypertensive etiology, such as a cerebral vascular anomaly, blood dyscrasia, or trauma.

Intracranial Aneurysms and Vascular Malformations

Although aneurysmal rupture is most commonly associated with hemorrhage in the subarachnoid space, the blood may also be directed into the substance of the brain if the aneurysm is adherent to the brain parenchyma. Rarely, aneurysms located at the middle cerebral artery bifurcation can produce hemorrhages that appear identical to hypertensive hemorrhage into the basal ganglia, and anterior communicating artery aneurysms can produce flame-shaped hemorrhages in the base of the frontal lobes.

Approximately half of intracranial AVMs in adults present with hemorrhage.[36] In 60% of cases, the hemorrhage is parenchymal, involving virtually any location within the cerebrum, brainstem, or cerebellum.[37] The majority of AVMs become symptomatic by age 40; thus hemorrhage due to AVM occurs in a younger population than that due to aneurysms or hypertension. Multiple calcified vascular channels may be seen within the hematoma on CT scan, suggesting the presence of an AVM. MRI and four-vessel cerebral angiography are useful adjuncts in the diagnosis of these lesions.

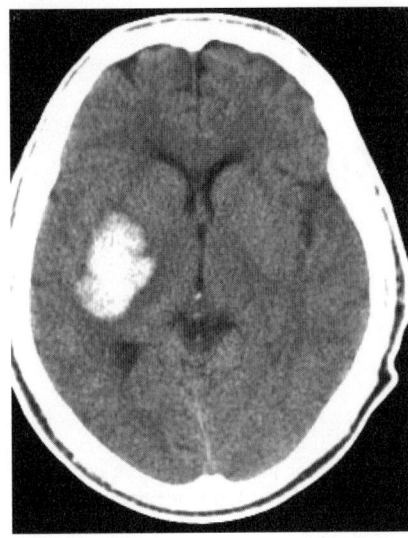

Figure 35-1   Typical moderate-sized putamenal hemorrhage.

Other Causes

Cerebral amyloid angiopathy (CAA) is an important cause of predominantly lobar, often recurrent, ICH in the elderly. Histopathologic studies in CAA demonstrate the deposition of beta-amyloid protein in the media and adventitia of small meningeal and cortical vessels; deposition in the typical sites for hypertensive hemorrhage is rare but has been reported in the cerebellum.[38] The prevalence of amyloid in cerebral vessels increases dramatically with age[39,40] and may partially account for the exponential rise in the risk for ICH with increasing age. There is an overrepresentation of the apolipoprotein E ε2 and ε4 genotypes in CAA-related hemorrhage, and these alleles are associated with an earlier age of onset of first hemorrhage and a higher risk of early recurrence.[41,42] Although neuropathologic examination remains the only means of definitively diagnosing CAA, the presence of multiple or recurrent lobar ICH (including asymptomatic microhemorrhages detected on gradient-echo MRI) in individuals 55 years or older without other known causes of hemorrhage strongly suggests the diagnosis.[43] Recent PET studies with ^{11}C-Pittsburgh compound B (PIB) suggest an occipital predominant increase in amyloid in such patients.[44] Neuropathologic correlation remains to be demonstrated, but PIB-PET appears to be a promising tool for in vivo diagnosis of CAA.

Hematologic causes of ICH include the use of antithrombotic and thrombolytic agents as well as systemic disease (e.g., thrombocytopenia, leukemia, and hepatic and renal failure) and congenital or acquired factor deficiencies. The incidence of oral anticoagulant (OAC)-associated ICH has been increasing in parallel with the increased use of warfarin following pivotal trials in atrial fibrillation in the 1990s. A recent population-based study in the greater Cincinnati area identified a fivefold increased incidence of OAC-associated ICH between 1988 and 1999, such that this condition now accounts for 17% of all ICH cases.[45] The incidence is anticipated to rise further in the coming years as the population ages. Although the risk of ICH is greater in the setting of very elevated international normalized ratio (INR), a significant number of hemorrhages occur when the INR is within the therapeutic range.[46] Hematoma expansion may be more common in OAC-associated ICH and occur over a longer time frame because of persistent coagulopathy, contributing to the doubling of mortality rate compared to spontaneous ICH.[47]

The relationship between antiplatelet agent use and hematoma size, hematoma expansion, and outcome in ICH are active areas of investigation. Most studies suggest that antiplatelet use at ICH onset is not associated with larger hematoma size, hematoma growth, or poor clinical outcome[48]; however, an association has been demonstrated between reduced platelet activity and hematoma growth and poor

outcome.[49] Whether platelet transfusion is beneficial in this situation is unknown.

Hemorrhage from an underlying neoplasm is rare but occasionally occurs with malignant primary CNS tumors such as glioblastoma multiforme and lymphoma and with metastatic tumors such as melanoma, choriocarcinoma, renal cell carcinoma, and bronchogenic carcinoma.[50] Benign tumors are almost never associated with ICH.

ICH may also occur in association with infection (e.g., infiltration of vessel wall by fungal organisms,[51] necrotizing hemorrhagic encephalitis with herpes simplex,[52] vasculitis,[53] venous sinus occlusion,[54] in a delayed fashion after head trauma,[55] following reperfusion (e.g., after carotid endarterectomy or acute thrombolysis),[56] and with the use of various drugs, particularly sympathomimetics (e.g., cocaine, amphetamines, pseudoephedrine, and phenylpropanolamine).[57] Finally, some degree of hemorrhagic transformation of acute cerebral infarcts is common,[58] though symptomatic ICH in this setting is rare in the absence of anticoagulation or thrombolytic therapy.

CLINICAL FEATURES

The clinical presentation of ICH is often indistinguishable from that of ischemic stroke but more commonly includes altered level of consciousness, headache, and vomiting, reflecting the presence of increased intracranial pressure (ICP).[33] Blood pressure is elevated in the majority of patients (see later discussion). Seizures occur in nearly one-third of patients at onset or within the first few days, particularly in those with lobar hemorrhages or underlying vascular or neoplastic lesions, and may be purely electrographic.[59] Symptoms are maximal at onset or develop over minutes to hours. Neurologic deterioration within 48 hours after hospital admission has been reported to occur in 22% of patients with ICH.[60] The cause for clinical worsening is not always evident, but it is predicted by clinical and biological markers of inflammation on admission and commonly associated with increased hematoma size and intraventricular bleeding.

DIAGNOSTIC STUDIES

Noncontrast computed tomography (CT) scanning has been the traditional gold standard for diagnosis of acute ICH. The typical CT appearance of an acute hematoma consists of a well-defined area of increased density surrounded by a rim of decreased density. Over time, the borders of both the high- and low-attenuation regions become increasingly indistinct such that the hematoma is isodense with adjacent brain parenchyma by 2 to 6 weeks.[61] Peripheral contrast enhancement can often be seen at this time.[62] By 2 to 6 months, there may be no CT evidence of previous hemorrhage or there may be an area of hypodensity or a slit-like scar.[63]

Recent studies have suggested that MRI has high sensitivity and specificity for the diagnosis of acute ICH.[64-66] These studies have been criticized, however, for major methodological limitations including the basing of sensitivity estimates on only a small fraction of patients investigated, lack of CT comparator in many patients, and both incorporation and spectrum bias (highly selected patient sample) that may have overestimated diagnostic accuracy of MRI.[67] In addition, MRI may not be feasible in a substantial number of patients with acute ICH because of impaired consciousness, hemodynamic compromise, or vomiting.[68] The benefits of MRI over CT are its superior performance in the identification of associated vascular malformations, greater accuracy in determining the approximate age of a hematoma (because each hemoglobin oxidation state during evolution of the hematoma produces a predictable pattern of MR signal intensity),[69] and its utility in demonstrating the iron-containing deposits of previous asymptomatic hemorrhages.[70]

Angiography is useful in evaluating the cause of ICH if an underlying aneurysm or vascular malformation is suspected, but the yield of such studies is extremely low when the patient has chronic hypertension and the hemorrhage is in one of the typical sites associated with hypertensive hemorrhage.[71] Multidetector CT angiography is evolving as an alternative to conventional angiography. In a retrospective review of 623 patients, multidetector CT angiography identified a vascular etiology for ICH in 91 (15%), with a sensitivity of 96% and a specificity of 99%. The yield was higher in patients who were younger than 46 (47%), had lobar (20%) or infratentorial (16%) ICH locations, had lobar hemorrhages with intraventricular extension (25%), and had neither hypertension nor impaired coagulation (33%).[72] In another study of 78 patients, CT angiography identified all but one of the 22 lesions seen on conventional angiography, with a sensitivity of 96% and a specificity of 100%.[73]

Multidetector CT angiography can also be used to identify the presence of active contrast extravasation into the hematoma, an indicator of active hemorrhage. Termed the "spot sign," these foci of intralesional enhancement are seen in up to one third of patients with acute ICH[74] and are associated with an increased risk of hematoma expansion, in-hospital mortality, and poor outcome in survivors.[75]

TREATMENT

Initial Stabilization

Acute ICH is a medical emergency requiring considerable attention to airway and respiratory management, hemodynamic status, and correction of any underlying coagulopathy. As many as half of all patients with ICH undergo mechanical ventilation.[76] Blood pressure is often elevated at presentation, sometimes markedly so. Finally, given the frequency of hematoma enlargement over the first few hours, aggressive correction of coagulopathies might be helpful.

Airway and Respiratory Management

Airway difficulty in ICH may occur for two reasons. First, with diminished consciousness, the pharyngeal and tongue musculature relax, and cough and gag reflexes are inhibited. In ICH involving the posterior fossa, there may be complete loss of pharyngeal tone, resulting in early obstruction of the upper airway.

Initial airway management includes proper positioning, frequent suctioning, and placement of an oral or nasal airway. Frequent assessments for sonorous respiration, inability to manage oral secretions, or decreased oxygen saturation are necessary. If conservative measures are ineffective, intubation may be necessary. Intubation of patients with ICH requires adequate sedation and jaw relaxation as well as prevention of elevation of ICP. Several factors may conspire to raise ICP during intubation: hypoxia, hypercarbia, and direct tracheal stimulation causing systemic and intracranial hypertension. Intravenous (IV) lidocaine (1-1.5 mg/kg) has been recommended to block this response,[77] although data supporting its use are lacking.[78] Short-acting IV anesthetic agents (thiopental, 1-5 mg/kg; or etomidate, 0.1-0.5 mg/kg) also block this response[79] and additionally suppress brain metabolic rate,[80] theoretically improving tolerance of a transient fall in cerebral perfusion pressure (CPP) should it occur. Etomidate is generally preferred over thiopental, since it is less likely to lower blood pressure. Paralytic agents are usually unnecessary but, if needed, short-acting agents should be used.

Noninvasive ventilation offers a potential alternative to intubation; it can be used to overcome mild upper airway obstruction and support oxygenation but may compromise management of secretions. It is difficult to provide adequate suctioning when a mask is present.

Hemodynamics

Arterial blood pressure is elevated on admission in the majority of patients with ICH, even in the absence of a history of hypertension.[33] Mean arterial pressure (MAP) is greater than 120 mm Hg in over two-thirds of patients and greater than 140 mm Hg in over one-third.[81] Although this acute increase in blood pressure is often implicated as the cause of the hemorrhage, it may simply be a reflection of chronic hypertension, the brain's attempt to maintain CPP in response to the sudden increase in ICP, pain and anxiety, and sympathetic activation. Even without pharmacologic intervention, blood pressure tends to decline to premorbid levels during the first 7 to 10 days after hemorrhage.[82]

There is substantial controversy over if and when to lower blood pressure after acute ICH and how aggressive any intervention should be.[83] Proponents of rapid treatment of acute hypertension argue that high blood pressure may predispose to hematoma enlargement and may exacerbate vasogenic edema by increasing capillary hydrostatic pressure, especially in areas with a damaged blood-brain barrier. Yet, an association between hypertension and edema has never been demonstrated, and data on the effect of hypertension on hematoma enlargement have been inconsistent.[84,85] Another potential reason to lower blood pressure is that hypertension during the acute phase of ICH has been shown to correlate with a poor prognosis in some studies.[86,87] One compelling reason to consider lowering blood pressure in ICH patients with moderate to severe hypertension is the potential for end-organ damage. Such patients are at risk for systemic complications of elevated blood pressure, including myocardial ischemia, congestive heart failure, and acute renal failure.

The major argument against the treatment of elevated blood pressure is that lowering blood pressure might exacerbate ischemic damage in the tissue surrounding the hematoma by impairing blood flow.[88] Chronic hypertension shifts the cerebral autoregulatory curve to the right such that a higher CPP is required to maintain adequate CBF.[89,90] Lowering the blood pressure to "normal" levels in these patients might thus lead to inadequate CBF. Similarly, since CPP is equal to the difference between MAP and ICP, lowering blood pressure may reduce CPP below the autoregulatory limit in patients in whom ICP is elevated due to a large space-occupying clot or hydrocephalus.

Seeking to address the issue of whether lowering blood pressure produces cerebral ischemia in acute ICH, several studies of CBF autoregulation in patients with recent ICH and elevated blood pressure (MAP > 130-140 mm Hg) have been carried out.[91-93] Taken together, these studies demonstrate that regional and global autoregulation are preserved after ICH down to a lower MAP limit that averages 110 mm Hg or about 80% of the admission MAP.

These observations set the stage for the INTERACT trial,[94] a prospective trial of blood pressure management beginning within 6 hours of symptom onset in 404 patients with spontaneous ICH and elevated systolic blood pressure (150-220 mm Hg). Patients were randomized to an early intensive blood pressure–lowering strategy that targeted a reduction in systolic blood pressure to below 140 mm Hg within 1 hour, or control, with a target systolic pressure of less than 180 mm Hg. The primary efficacy endpoint was hematoma growth at 24 hours. After the first hour of treatment, mean blood pressure was 13.3 mm Hg lower (95% confidence interval [CI] 8.9-17.6 mm Hg; $P < 0.0001$) in the intensive blood pressure–lowering group. Hematoma growth at 24 hours was 36.3% in the control group and 13.7% in the intensive treatment group, a 22.6% difference (95% CI 0.6%-44.5%; $P=0.04$). After adjusting for initial hematoma volume and time from onset to CT, median hematoma growth at 24 hours differed by 1.7 mL (95% CI 0.5-3.9, $P=0.13$). Intensive blood pressure–lowering treatment did not increase the risk of adverse events or improve 90-day clinical outcome. A much larger follow-on trial is currently underway.

If the decision is made to treat hypertension in acute ICH, the most appropriate antihypertensive agent would have a short half-life and minimal cerebrovascular effects and would be administered in such a way as to avoid sudden large reductions in blood pressure. Vasodilators, especially those that dilate veins, can raise ICP by increasing cerebral blood volume and hence should be avoided. Sodium nitroprusside and nitroglycerin increase ICP and lower CBF in patients with reduced intracranial compliance. Ganglionic blockers may also lower CBF. Calcium channel blockers, beta-blockers, and angiotensin-converting enzyme (ACE) inhibitors have minimal effect on CBF within the autoregulatory range of MAP and do not alter ICP. Therefore, popular treatment options in the setting of acute ICH include intermittent boluses of labetalol, enalapril, and/or hydralazine or continuous infusion of nicardipine.

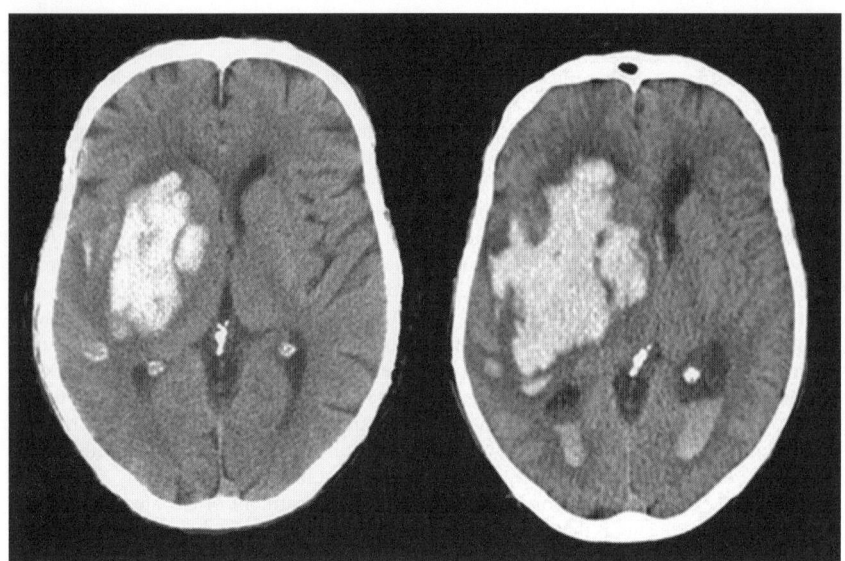

Figure 35-2 Example of hematoma enlargement. Computed tomography (CT) on left was obtained 2 hours after onset of left hemiparesis and shows right putamenal hemorrhage. CT on right was obtained 1 hour later when patient acutely deteriorated and shows expansion of hematoma, with intraventricular extension, midline shift, and enlarging ventricles.

Prevention of Hemorrhage Extension

Because hemorrhage extension occurs within the first few hours after symptom onset in about one-third of patients (Figure 35-2), it seems appropriate that any coagulopathy should be corrected as rapidly as possible. Patients taking warfarin should receive IV vitamin K and enough fresh frozen plasma (FFP) to normalize the coagulation profile. Prothrombin complex concentrate may be a useful alternative. Care must be taken not to precipitate congestive heart failure, however, and diuretics may be required. Additionally there is risk of transfusion-related acute lung injury with the administration of fresh frozen plasma, which can complicate the process considerably. Correcting coagulopathy associated with thrombolytic-induced ICH is discussed later.

Even in those patients without coagulopathy, promoting early hemostasis might limit ongoing bleeding and decrease hematoma volume. Factor VIIa is a coagulation factor that interacts with tissue factor exposed in the wall of a damaged blood vessel to drive a burst of thrombin that initiates platelet aggregation and accelerates formation of a stable fibrin clot. A phase IIb placebo-controlled dose-ranging proof-of-concept study found that treatment with recombinant factor VIIa (rFVIIa) given as a single IV bolus within 4 hours of ICH onset decreased hematoma growth and improved clinical outcome despite a small increase in thromboembolic events. A much larger phase III trial comparing placebo to 20 and 80 μg/kg of rFVIIa followed. This study confirmed the ability of rFVIIa to reduce hematoma growth; however, at 90 days there was no difference in clinical outcome.[95] A post hoc exploratory analysis suggested that a subgroup of younger patients who present earlier and have no significant intraventricular hemorrhage might benefit from rFVIIa, but this has not been tested.[96]

INTRAVENTRICULAR HEMORRHAGE AND HYDROCEPHALUS

In approximately 40% of patients with ICH, blood extends into the ventricular system (intraventricular hemorrhage [IVH]).[97] Mortality in these patients is high.[98,99] IVH may contribute to poor outcome by blocking cerebrospinal fluid (CSF) pathways, with resultant hydrocephalus and increased ICP. In addition, intraventricular blood and/or its breakdown products may exert direct chemical irritative effects on periventricular structures. Hydrocephalus may develop after ICH either in association with IVH or because of direct mass effect on a ventricle (e.g., on the third ventricle with a thalamic hemorrhage) (Figure 35-3). External ventricular drainage (ventriculostomy) is frequently used to treat hydrocephalus and IVH, but its efficacy has never been established. Ventriculostomy in the setting of IVH is difficult to manage because the catheter frequently becomes obstructed with thrombus, interrupting drainage and raising ICP. Flushing the system helps remove thrombus from the catheter but increases the risk of ventriculitis. Recently, investigators have attempted to facilitate removal of blood from the ventricles via direct intraventricular administration of thrombolytic agents. Preliminary studies have been promising,[100] and a multicenter randomized trial is currently underway.

INTRACRANIAL HYPERTENSION

The incidence, impact, and appropriate management of intracranial hypertension in ICH are not well understood. Factors likely to contribute to elevated ICP in this population include large hematoma size, minimal degree of underlying cerebral atrophy, hydrocephalus, and edema, but the true incidence of intracranial hypertension is unclear, since routine ICP monitoring is not performed. Because the hematoma is localized and the increase in volume it produces can be compensated for to some degree by reduction in the size of the ventricles and subarachnoid space, a global increase in ICP may not be seen unless the

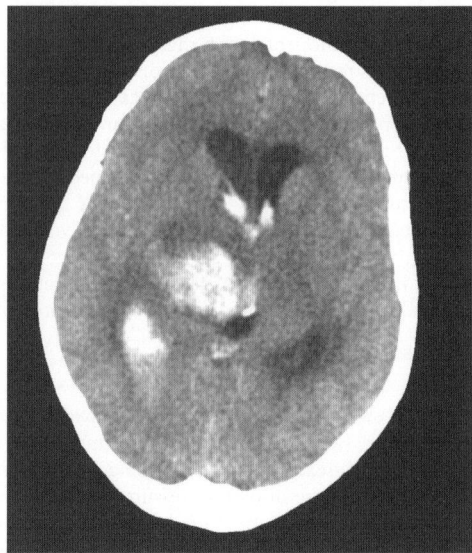

Figure 35-3 Example of a small thalamic hemorrhage with blood obstructing the foramen of Monro, causing hydrocephalus.

hemorrhage is very large or is associated with marked hydrocephalus. However, mass effect from the hematoma and local tissue shifts can compress the brainstem or result in herniation in the absence of a global increase in ICP.[101,102] Thus the utility of ICP monitoring has never been established.

Invasive ICP monitoring devices with implantable transducers can be placed in extradural, subdural, intraparenchymal, and intraventricular locations, but external ventricular drains (EVD) have the added capacity to remove CSF and thus lower ICP. The appropriate time to use an EVD is uncertain; however, patients who have progressive deterioration in level of consciousness and enlarging ventricles on serial imaging are most likely to benefit. Those with very large parenchymal hematomas are least likely to benefit, and overdrainage of the contralateral ventricle could worsen tissue shifts and lead to deterioration.

Elevated ICP is often treated with osmotic agents (mannitol, hypertonic saline) and, if the ventricles are enlarged, CSF drainage. A recent case series suggested that rapid reversal of clinical transtentorial herniation (decreased level of consciousness and dilated pupil) with hyperventilation and osmotic agents improved long-term outcome.[103] There are only a few small clinical trials of osmotic agents in ICH, which do not provide sufficient data to support their routine use.[104] The best available data on corticosteroids in ICH indicate that they do not provide any benefit and increase the rate of complications.[105]

SURGICAL EVACUATION

The rationale for surgical evacuation of a hematoma is that reducing mass effect and removing neurotoxic clot constituents should minimize injury to adjacent brain tissue and hence improve outcome. Unfortunately, several randomized controlled trials of surgery for supratentorial ICH dating back to 1961 have all failed to show a benefit of the intervention.[106-109] A meta-analysis of three of these trials reported that patients undergoing surgical evacuation via open craniotomy had a higher rate of death or dependency at 6 months compared to those managed medically (83% versus 70%).[110] Criticisms of these trials are that the surgical techniques used were outdated, patient selection was inadequate, and surgery was delayed too long.

Because open craniotomy is complicated by tissue damage sustained during the approach to the hematoma, a variety of new techniques for clot removal have been proposed, including an Archimedes screw, ultrasonic aspirator, modified endoscope, modified nucleotome, double track aspirator, intraoperative CT monitoring, and instillation of thrombolytics. However, the recurrence of bleeding due to the loss of tamponade effect on adjacent tissue that occurs in 10% of patients treated with open craniotomy remains an issue with the newer techniques. In addition, because the newer techniques involve limited surgical exposure, concern exists that rebleeding will be more difficult to control than with open craniotomy. One study comparing endoscopic aspiration to medical management found a better outcome in the surgical group (74% death or disability compared to 90%), but the benefit was limited to patients with lobar hematomas.[111] Three studies addressed the feasibility of early craniotomy for ICH. In one,[112] 34 patients were treated within 12 hours of ICH. Mortality was 18% in the surgical group and 23% in the medical group. In another study,[113] 20 patients were randomized, with a median time to surgery of 8.5 hours from onset. Good outcome (Glasgow Outcome Scale score > 3) was 56% with surgery and 36% in the medically treated group (P = NS). The third, a study of ultra-early surgery (<4 hours), found a disturbingly high rate of postoperative rebleeding.[114]

A lack of benefit of surgery in ICH was also shown in a recently completed multicenter trial in which 1033 patients were randomized within 72 hours of ICH onset to surgical hematoma evacuation (open craniotomy or stereotactic aspiration, at surgeon's discretion) or initial conservative management. Favorable outcome occurred in 26.1% in the surgery group and 23.8% in the initial conservative treatment group, a nonsignificant difference (odds ratio 0.89; 95% CI 0.66-1.19). There was also no difference in mortality (surgery 62.6% versus

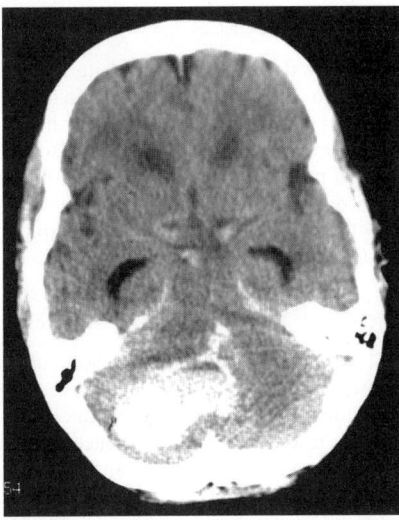

Figure 35-4 Typical cerebellar hemorrhage with effacement of basal cisterns and early hydrocephalus manifest by enlargement of temporal horns of lateral ventricles.

conservative treatment 63.7%). Subgroup analysis suggested a possible benefit of surgery in patients with superficial hematomas (less than 1 cm from cortical surface).[115] A trial comparing surgical and medical management of superficial hematomas is currently underway.

Cerebellar hemorrhages were excluded from the randomized trials of surgery, but nonrandomized case series report good outcomes for surgically treated patients with cerebellar hemorrhages that are large or associated with brainstem compression or obstruction of the fourth ventricle. Recommended criteria for when to evacuate a cerebellar hematoma have thus included diminished level of consciousness, large size of the hematoma (>3 cm^3), midline location, compression of basal cisterns and/or brainstem, and presence of hydrocephalus (Figure 35-4).[116-118] Patient selection is important as many patients with smaller hemorrhages do well with medical management.[119]

MANAGEMENT OF THROMBOLYTIC-INDUCED ICH

Associated with considerable morbidity and mortality, symptomatic ICH is a feared complication of thrombolytic therapy. Symptomatic ICH occurs after thrombolytic treatment of acute ischemic stroke in approximately 6% of patients.[120] It is substantially less common after thrombolytic treatment of extracerebral thrombosis (myocardial infarction, pulmonary embolism, deep venous thrombosis, and arterial and graft occlusion)[121] but results in a similarly poor outcome.[122] Factors that increase the risk of symptomatic ICH include intraarterial versus IV route of administration, early ischemic changes on pretreatment CT, greater symptom severity, and elevated serum glucose or history of diabetes mellitus.[123,124]

In the setting of thrombolytic therapy, any new neurologic deficit, especially with a decline in consciousness, should be assumed to be due to hemorrhage. Management of a suspected ICH should begin with stopping the thrombolytic infusion, reassessing the patient's airway, and obtaining an emergent CT scan. Blood studies (prothrombin time, partial thromboplastin time, thrombin, and fibrinogen levels) should be performed to assess fibrinolytic state. Preparations for giving FFP, cryoprecipitate, and platelets should be initiated at the first suspicion of hemorrhage so that they will be ready if needed; however, no reliable data are available to guide the choice of blood product. The NINDS rt-PA study[125] stipulated 6 to 8 units of cryoprecipitate or FFP and 6 to 8 units of platelets, but only rarely was this amount of blood product given to an individual patient during the study. Although neurosurgical consultation was frequently obtained in patients with symptomatic ICH in the NINDS trial, only one patient in the study underwent surgery, and that patient died.

MANAGEMENT OF SEIZURES

Although seizures may theoretically exacerbate ICH, they have not been demonstrated to alter outcome. Prophylactic anticonvulsants may reduce the risk of early seizures in patients with lobar ICH but do not affect the risk of developing epilepsy.[126] Thus reasonable approaches include either a brief period of prophylaxis or treating only if seizures occur. As for any hospitalized patient, the treatment of clinical seizures typically begins with an IV benzodiazepine such as lorazepam followed by an IV agent such as fosphenytoin.

SUPPORTIVE CARE

Patients with ICH are prone to the same medical complications seen in patients with ischemic stroke, including fever, deep venous thrombosis (DVT), pulmonary embolism, and pneumonia.[127,128] Given the association between fever and worsened outcome in experimental models of brain injury, it is reasonable for antipyretic medications to be administered in febrile patients with ICH. The use of pneumatic sequential compression devices and elastic stockings has been shown to significantly decrease the incidence of DVT in patients with acute ICH relative to elastic stockings alone.[129] Subcutaneous heparin at a dose of 5000 U three times daily when initiated on day 2 after hemorrhage has been shown to significantly reduce the frequency of DVT relative to treatment begun on day 4 or 10, with no concomitant increase in hematoma expansion.[130] In another study, subcutaneous enoxaparin (40 mg daily) initiated at 48 hours after ICH was also safe. A benefit of enoxaparin over compression stockings could not been detected because of the low incidence of DVT in both treatment groups.[131]

Similar to patients with ischemic stroke, ICH patients should not be fed orally until swallowing is evaluated. If aspiration is detected or the patient is not alert enough to eat safely, nasogastric tube feeding should be begun promptly. Patients should be monitored for signs of aspiration pneumonia, whether taking food orally or via nasogastric tube.

Early mobilization and rehabilitation are generally recommended for clinically stable patients with ICH.

PROGNOSTIC FACTORS AND CAUSES OF MORTALITY

Mortality following ICH is high (25%-50%), with over half of the deaths occurring in the first 48 hours. Although patients who have small hemorrhages and mild deficits may recover completely, the majority of ICH survivors have significant residual disability.[4,132,133] A variety of clinical, laboratory, and radiographic predictors of poor outcome have been identified, the most consistent being impaired level of consciousness and large hematoma size on admission. Other predictive clinical features variably include increasing age, elevated admission blood pressure on admission, rapid decline in blood pressure over the first 24 hours, history of diabetes, antecedent OAC use, male gender, and in-hospital neurologic deterioration. Laboratory parameters identified in at least one study include hyperglycemia, elevated troponin level, elevated plasma S100B level, elevated plasma D-dimer level, elevated INR, low serum cholesterol and triglyceride levels, and apolipoprotein E ε2 or ε4 allele. Radiographic features include infratentorial hematoma location, intraventricular spread of blood, midline shift, hydrocephalus, hematoma growth, and presence of the spot sign on CT angiography. A number of prognostic models of varying complexity have been developed to allow risk stratification upon presentation with ICH. One easy to use model is the ICH score,[134] which is based on point assignments for Glasgow Coma Scale score, ICH volume, presence of intraventricular hemorrhage, infratentorial location, and patient age and has been validated to accurately predict 30-day mortality. It has been demonstrated, however, that withdrawal of support in patients felt likely to have a poor outcome biases predictive models in ICH and negates the predictive value of all other variables.[135] Thus, the most frequent cause of death after ICH is withdrawal of care, followed by early (within 48 hours) transtentorial herniation with progression

to brain death. Medical complications of immobility (pulmonary embolism, pneumonia, sepsis) account for most of the other deaths.[133] For survivors of ICH, the risk of recurrent stroke is approximately 4% per year. Recurrent ICH occurs about twice as often as ischemic stroke, especially in those with previous lobar hemorrhage.[136]

Subarachnoid Hemorrhage

Although it is the least common form of stroke, subarachnoid hemorrhage (SAH) has great impact on its sufferers. One-quarter of patients die before reaching medical attention,[137] and because of the consequences of secondary insults—rebleeding, hydrocephalus, and delayed ischemia due to vasospasm—more than half of those that reach medical attention either die or are left with neurologic deficits.

PATHOPHYSIOLOGY

In SAH, the primary site of bleeding is within the subarachnoid space, but may also involve hemorrhage into the brain parenchyma, ventricular system, or subdural space. Rupture of an intracranial saccular aneurysm (Figure 35-5) is by far the most common cause of spontaneous SAH. Saccular or berry aneurysms are small, rounded protrusions of the arterial wall occurring predominantly at bifurcations of the large arteries of the circle of Willis at the base of the brain. The most common sites of ruptured aneurysms are the distal internal carotid artery and its posterior communicating artery junction (41%); anterior communicating artery/anterior cerebral artery (34%); middle cerebral artery (20%); and vertebrobasilar arteries (4%).[138] About 20% of patients have multiple aneurysms.

The pathogenesis of aneurysms remains controversial, especially in regard to the relative important of developmental versus acquired factors. Proponents of the congenital theory suggest that aneurysms arise at sites of faulty fusion between muscular segments within the arterial wall. Supporters of the acquired-degenerative theory focus on the role of vascular damage caused by hemodynamic stress.[139] The third possibility is that aneurysms develop at sites harboring congenital defects with superimposed degenerative changes.

What leads to aneurysmal growth and rupture is also debated. Hemodynamic stress and other factors intrinsic to the involved vessels may play a role. The time course over which aneurysms grow and subsequently rupture is unknown, although some aneurysms appear to grow rapidly over weeks, whereas others grow slowly over years.

Most aneurysms rupture at the dome, where the wall may be as thin as 0.3 mm. Tension on the aneurysm wall is determined by the radius of the aneurysm and the pressure gradient across the wall (law of La

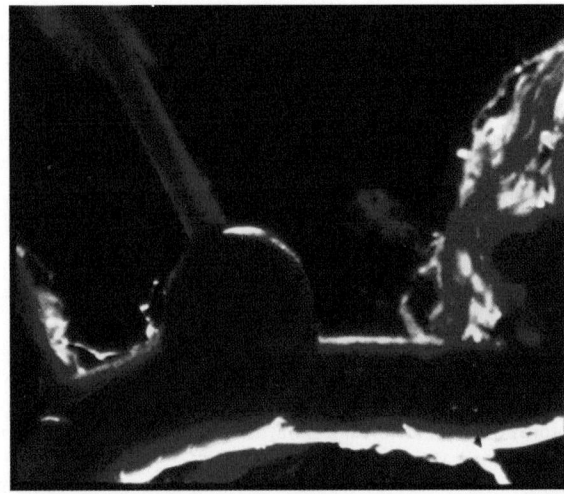

Figure 35-5 Autopsy specimen of intracranial aneurysm filled with pressurized blood to simulate subarachnoid hemorrhage.

Place). The probability of rupture is related to size; aneurysms less than 5 millimeters in diameter have a very low rate of rupture. Aneurysm rupture causes local tissue damage due to the jet of blood under high pressure, as well as a transient increase in ICP.

CAUSES AND RISK FACTORS

Genetic conditions that predispose to aneurysm formation include polycystic kidney disease, connective tissue disorders, and coarctation of the aorta. Recently it has become clear that in some patient populations, genetic factors play a role in aneurysm formation, without other associated conditions.[140] There is a familial form as well.[141] Other types of aneurysms that less commonly cause SAH include atherosclerotic, mycotic, and traumatic aneurysms.

Trauma is the most common cause of non-aneurysmal SAH. Arteriovenous malformations, cocaine and stimulant abuse, neoplasia, and vasculitis account for the bulk of the remainder. Bleeding into the subarachnoid space may accompany ICH, particularly in the setting of CAA. In 10% to 15% of cases of SAH, no source of bleeding is identified.

The risk of SAH increases with age, peaking at 55 to 60 years. There is a slight male predominance in younger age groups and a slight female predominance among older patients.[142] Potentially reversible risk factors for SAH include cigarette smoking, oral contraceptive use, alcohol abuse, and hypertension.[143] Prospective cohort studies have reported a relative risk of SAH as high as 5.7 for female and 4.7 for male smokers,[144] but no increased risk in former smokers. Oral contraceptive use, in addition to being an independent risk factor for SAH, dramatically increases the risk among smokers.[145] A dose-response relationship exists between alcohol consumption and incidence of SAH.

CLINICAL FEATURES

Presentation

The most common initial symptom of SAH, occurring in over 90% of patients, is a sudden severe headache. Less severe warning ("sentinel") headaches[146] may precede the presenting event in as many as half and are thought to represent minor leaks. In about half of patients, loss of consciousness accompanies the headache.[147] The mechanisms thought to be responsible for the loss of consciousness are the sudden surge in ICP at the moment of hemorrhage or cardiac arrhythmias. Vomiting can be a prominent symptom. Seizure activity may be reported,[148] but it is unclear whether this represents true epileptic seizures or reflex posturing related to the sudden rise in ICP. Focal deficits at the onset of hemorrhage occur in less than 10% of cases. After a few hours, a stiff neck can develop, reflecting the sterile meningeal inflammation induced by the presence of blood in the subarachnoid space.

Complications

A worsening of neurologic status often indicates one of the three major complications of SAH: rebleeding, hydrocephalus, or vasospasm. An understanding of the timing and nature of the deterioration facilitates rapid diagnosis and treatment. It must be emphasized that systemic perturbations such as infection, hyponatremia, fever, hypoxia, and hypotension may produce similar symptoms and should be sought and corrected as part of the evaluation process.

Early Complications

Rebleeding. Rebleeding is heralded by a sudden worsening of headache, vomiting, blood pressure elevation, development of a new neurologic deficit, or arrhythmia. It occurs in up to one-third of patients and is often fatal. The risk of rebleeding is greatest during the first 24 hours, declining rapidly over the next 2 weeks.[149] Rates of rebleeding are highest in women, those who are a poor clinical grade, those in poor medical condition, and those with elevated systolic blood pressure.

Hydrocephalus. Hydrocephalus occurs after SAH because of disturbances of CSF flow or reabsorption: subarachnoid blood may impair CSF reabsorption at the arachnoid granulations, and ventricular blood may obstruct its flow. Acute hydrocephalus can develops within hours of SAH,[150] often in the absence of intraventricular blood. It usually manifests as a gradual decline in level of consciousness and can easily be treated by placement of an external ventricular drain. Delayed hydrocephalus may also develop gradually days to weeks later. Hydrocephalus must be distinguished from metabolic derangements, infection, and vasospasm. CT scan is essential in making the diagnosis. The natural history of untreated acute hydrocephalus is that about one third of patients progress, one-third spontaneously improve, and one third remain static.[151]

Delayed Complications

Vasospasm. The term *vasospasm* refers to complex changes in intracerebral vessels, with segmental or diffuse narrowing of the lumen due to arterial wall thickening, vasoconstriction, and impaired relaxation that reduce CBF. If the reduction in flow is severe enough, ischemia and infarction follow. The term *delayed cerebral ischemia* (DCI) describes the clinical situation where these and other factors conspire to produce ischemia. Other factors that may contribute to DCI include impaired autoregulation, hypovolemia, and microthrombosis.[152] DCI is a leading cause of morbidity and mortality following SAH.

Arterial narrowing can be detected angiographically (Figure 35-6) in up to 70% of patients,[153] of whom almost half become symptomatic. The pathogenesis of arterial vasospasm is complex and not fully understood, but sustained exposure of vessels to extraluminal blood constituents and catecholamines is thought to play a role. It involves structural changes in the vessel walls and in adrenergic nerve fibers. The onset of vasospasm is delayed, most commonly developing 5 to

Figure 35-6 Baseline angiogram obtained shortly after subarachnoid hemorrhage (*left*) and repeat angiogram obtained 7 days later (*right*) showing severe vasospasm of basilar artery, with reduced distal flow.

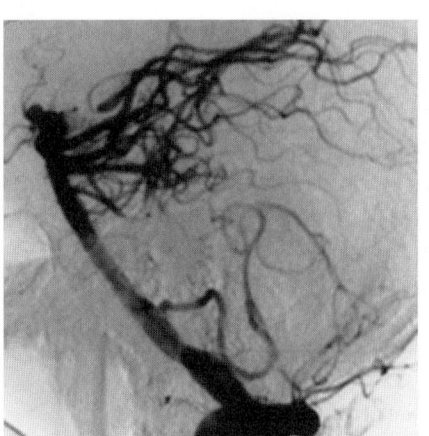
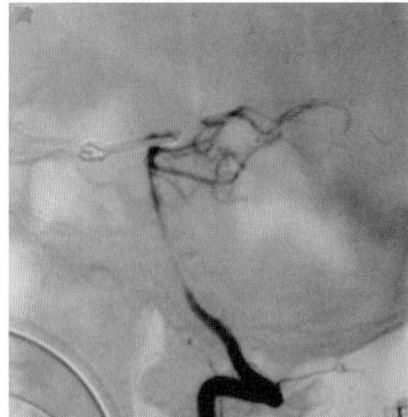

TABLE 35-1	Fisher Grade of Subarachnoid Hemorrhage on Initial Computed Tomography

1 No blood detected
2 Diffuse or vertical layers <1 mm thick
3 Localized subarachnoid clot and/or vertical layers ≥1 mm thick
4 Intraparenchymal or intraventricular clot with diffuse or no SAH

Modified Fisher CT Rating Scale

1 Minimal or diffuse thin SAH without IVH
2 Minimal or thin SAH with IVH
3 Thick cisternal clot without IVH
4 Thick cisternal clot with IVH

CT, computed tomography; IVH, intraventricular hemorrhage; SAH, subarachnoid hemorrhage.

10 days after initial hemorrhage, and may persist for up to 3 weeks. The strongest predictor of vasospasm is the amount of subarachnoid blood on the initial CT scan, with the greatest risk occurring in those having thick subarachnoid clots and intraventricular blood (graded using Fisher Scale and modified Fisher Scale; Table 35-1).[154,155] Focal neurologic deficits resulting from vasospasm may appear abruptly or gradually and may fluctuate, exacerbated by hypovolemia or hypotension. If untreated, infarction may occur.

Medical Complications. Blood pressure is often elevated after SAH and is associated with a greater risk of rebleeding and vasospasm as well as higher mortality. Multiple factors may underlie the rise in blood pressure, including increased sympathetic outflow, agitation, and pain. Early on, blood pressure management focuses on preventing re-rupture of the aneurysm. Following repair of the aneurysm, the risk of rebleeding is virtually eliminated, and spontaneous elevations in blood pressure should be allowed to occur without intervention, since now the risk of vasospasm is the primary concern.

Disturbances in sodium and water balance occur in approximately one-third of patients, and hyponatremia and volume depletion after SAH are correlated with an increased risk of symptomatic vasospasm and poor outcome.[156] Although hyponatremia was previously attributed to inappropriate secretion of antidiuretic hormone (SIADH) and was therefore treated with fluid restriction, later evidence suggested that both sodium and water are lost. In fact, when administered normal "maintenance" volumes of fluid (2-3 L/day), as many as half of patients develop intravascular volume contraction.[157]

Cardiac abnormalities are common in the first 48 hours after SAH. Electrocardiographic (ECG) changes (Figure 35-7) including tall peaked T waves ("cerebral T waves"), diffuse T-wave inversion, ST-segment depression, and prolonged QT segments[158] occur frequently and have been linked to elevated levels of circulating catecholamines. It appears that these changes usually do not represent myocardial ischemia, as the myocardial lesions reported are pathologically distinct from ischemia. Cardiac enzymes may be mildly elevated.[159] Cardiac rhythm disturbances occur in about 30% to 40% of patients, especially on the day of hemorrhage or in the postoperative period. Arrhythmias are typically benign but can be life threatening in about 5%.[160,161] In rare cases, "stunned myocardium" may occur, with impairment of myocardial contractility leading to a fall in cardiac output, hypotension, and pulmonary edema.[162] This phenomenon can be dramatic but is transient, usually lasting 2 to 3 days, after which cardiac function returns to baseline.[163] Management is the same as with other causes of cardiogenic shock.[164] During hemodynamic treatment for vasospasm, pulmonary edema may occur in up to one-quarter of patients,[165] though its incidence is lower with careful monitoring.[166]

In a review of over 450 patients with SAH, Solenski et al.[167] reported some degree of hepatic dysfunction in 24%. The majority had only mild abnormalities of hepatic enzymes without clinical accompaniment, but severe hepatic dysfunction occurred in 4%. Thrombocytopenia was found in 4% of patients, usually occurring in the setting of systemic sepsis. Renal dysfunction occurred in 7% of patients.

Fever, anemia, hyperglycemia, pneumonia, and hypertension occur frequently after SAH. Potential treatments include maintaining normothermia with antipyretics and possibly systemic cooling devices, administration of erythropoietin to prevent anemia, and preserving normoglycemia.[168]

DIAGNOSTIC STUDIES

CT is the imaging modality of choice in screening for SAH, having a sensitivity of better than 90%.[169] Blood appears as high attenuation within the perimesencephalic and interpeduncular cisterns surrounding the brainstem (the basal cisterns), Sylvian fissure, and sulci (Figure 35-8).

CT may fail to demonstrate SAH if the volume of blood is very small, if the hemorrhage occurred several days prior to the CT scan, or if the hematocrit is extremely low.[170] Lumbar puncture for CSF analysis is indicated if CT is negative and clinical suspicion is high. Red blood cells in the CSF are indicative of SAH but can also be seen with traumatic puncture. The common technique of comparing cell counts in the first and last tubes collected is not reliable; however, the presence of yellow pigment (xanthochromia), resulting from red cell breakdown, can be helpful in distinguishing between the two.[171] Xanthochromia develops 2 to 6 hours after hemorrhage and persists for 1 to 4 weeks. It can also be seen in the setting of high protein levels due to diabetes, renal failure or infection, in which case spectrophotometric analysis to identify hemoglobin breakdown products improves diagnostic accuracy.[172]

Once SAH has been diagnosed, cerebral angiography should be performed as soon as possible to identify the responsible vascular

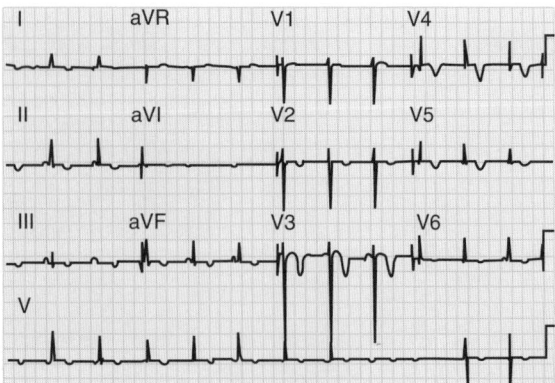

Figure 35-7 Electrocardiogram in a patient with acute subarachnoid hemorrhage, demonstrating diffuse T-wave inversions.

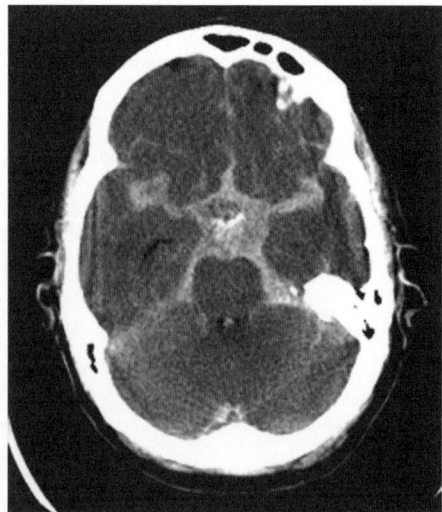

Figure 35-8 Computed tomography scan of acute subarachnoid hemorrhage, with a thick layer of hyperdense blood filling basal cisterns.

TABLE 35-2	Hunt & Hess Clinical Classification of Subarachnoid Hemorrhage
I	Asymptomatic or mild headache and neck stiffness
II	Moderate to severe headache and neck stiffness ± cranial nerve palsy
III	Mild focal deficit, lethargy, or confusion
IV	Stupor, moderate to severe hemiparesis
V	Deep coma, extensor posturing

lesion, search for other lesions (multiple aneurysms are found in 20% to 30% of patients with aneurysmal SAH), and assist in operative management. Angiography does not identify a source of bleeding in 10% to 15% of patients with nontraumatic SAH. In some cases, this may be due to vasospasm or inadequate views to detect a subtle aneurysm, especially in the region of the anterior communicating artery or in the posterior circulation. Repeat angiography in about one week is recommended.[173] There is a subset of patients in whom the blood on CT is localized to the perimesencephalic cisterns. In these cases, angiography is usually negative, and the bleeding is thought to be venous in origin; the prognosis is excellent, and repeat angiography is almost always negative.[174]

With its wide availability, ease of use, and safety profile, CT angiography is increasingly being used as the initial diagnostic tool in the investigation of SAH. Overall sensitivity is 90% or greater compared to conventional angiography but is notably lower for aneurysms smaller than 5 mm[175]; thus, a negative CT angiogram should be followed by conventional catheter angiography. A negative CT angiogram alone may be sufficient in the case of perimesencephalic SAH.[174] Magnetic resonance angiography (MRA) has good sensitivity for detecting medium and large aneurysms, but sensitivity falls to less than 40% for small aneurysms. In addition, MRA is impractical for many acutely ill patients with SAH because of logistics, movement artifact, need for sedation, and difficulty in monitoring clinical status in the scanner.

MRA and CT angiography may also be of assistance in planning surgical or endovascular approaches to aneurysm treatment.

TREATMENT

Initial Stabilization

The initial steps in the evaluation of a patient with suspected SAH should include assessment of airway, hemodynamic status, and the level of neurologic function. The Hunt and Hess Scale[176] and the World Federation of Neurological Surgeons Scale[177] provide standardized measures of the patient's clinical condition (Tables 35-2 and 35-3).

As in ICH, some patients with SAH may be unable to protect their airway because of diminished consciousness. If the patient is lethargic or agitated, elective intubation should be considered prior to angiography. This is because sedation is often necessary for angiography and may result in unrecognized hypoventilation or airway obstruction.

Routine Care and Monitoring

The routine monitoring of all patients with acute SAH should include serial neurologic examinations, continuous ECG monitoring, and frequent determinations of blood pressure, electrolytes, body weight, and fluid balance. The role of prophylactic anticonvulsants in patients who have not had a seizure is controversial. Initial use of anticonvulsants is generally recommended; however, the duration of administration should be limited to several days during the periprocedural period.[178]

TABLE 35-3	World Federation of Neurologic Surgeons Clinical Classification of Subarachnoid Hemorrhage	
Grade	Glasgow Coma Scale	Motor Deficits
I	15	Absent
II	13-14	Absent
III	13-14	Present
IV	7-12	Present or absent
V	3-6	Present or absent

Recent retrospective studies have suggested that routine use of anticonvulsants for a longer duration is associated with worse neurologic outcome.[179] Dexamethasone is widely used to reduce meningeal irritation and intra- and postoperative edema, but there is no convincing evidence documenting its efficacy.

Fluid Management. A stable intravascular volume should be maintained by hydration with isotonic saline and daily monitoring of fluid balance, body weight, and hematocrit. Monitoring of fluid balance alone may not be adequate to prevent hypovolemia, and combining multiple clinical indicators of volume status are needed.[180,181] In some patients with severe cerebral salt wasting, large volumes of fluid are required to prevent intravascular volume contraction.[182] Hyponatremia can often be managed with restriction of *free* water by administering only isotonic IV fluids, minimizing oral liquids, and using concentrated enteral feedings. It is important to adjust the *tonicity* of the fluid, not the *volume* of fluids administered. Fludrocortisone is of marginal benefit in treating salt wasting[183,184]; however, one study suggested that hydrocortisone may be helpful.[185] Persistent hyponatremia can be treated by using mildly hypertonic solutions (1.25%-2% saline) as the sole IV fluid. There may be a role for ADH antagonists such as conivaptan, but since they increase urine volume, extreme caution must be exercised to avoid hypovolemia.[186]

Hypertension. Initial attempts to treat hypertension should consist of analgesics and nimodipine; other antihypertensive agents should follow if needed. Useful medications include intermittent doses of beta-blockers and vasodilators. If a continuous infusion is needed, nicardipine is the preferred agent. When significant hydrocephalus is present, hypertension should not be treated until after the hydrocephalus is addressed. This is because the hypertension may be acting to maintain adequate cerebral perfusion in the face of elevated ICP.

Magnesium Sulfate. Magnesium antagonizes calcium and thus could reduce vasospasm. Almost 40% of patients with SAH have low serum magnesium levels on presentation, leading to speculation that the administration of magnesium may improve outcome of SAH patients. Advantages of magnesium include ease of administration, low cost, and favorable safety profile.[187] Several studies have suggested benefit,[188,189] but controlled trials have been inconclusive.[190,191] A large phase III randomized controlled international trial is currently underway.

Statins. Statins may be beneficial in SAH through their ability to induce nitric oxide synthetase, leading to dilation of cerebral vessels, or through their antiinflammatory effects. Some preliminary studies have suggested that they may reduce vasospasm and improve outcome,[192,193] while others have not.[194-196] A multicenter placebo-controlled double-blinded phase III trial is underway.

Management of Secondary Complications

Rebleeding. Multiple clinical trials have demonstrated that antifibrinolytic agents such as epsilon aminocaproic acid and tranexamic acid reduce the risk of rebleeding, but this benefit is offset by an increased incidence of vasospasm and hydrocephalus.[197,198] With the advent of early surgery and now endovascular treatment of aneurysms, the use of these agents has declined dramatically. More recently, there has been interest in a shorter course of antifibrinolytic therapy while awaiting surgery or endovascular treatment. Tranexamic acid begun immediately upon SAH diagnosis and continued only until the aneurysm was secured (always within 72 hours) reduced the risk of rebleeding from 10.8% to 2.4% and did not increase risk of DCI.[199]

Other measures directed at prevention of rebleeding include avoiding situations that produce sudden changes in the transmural pressure across the wall of the aneurysm (i.e., sudden increases in arterial or venous pressure or decreases in ICP). Patients are placed on bed rest with minimal stimulation. In the agitated patient, sedation is indicated, though care must be taken to preserve the ability to assess the patient's responsiveness to stimulation. Opiates are a good choice for sedation, since they also provide analgesia for treating headache. Because of the

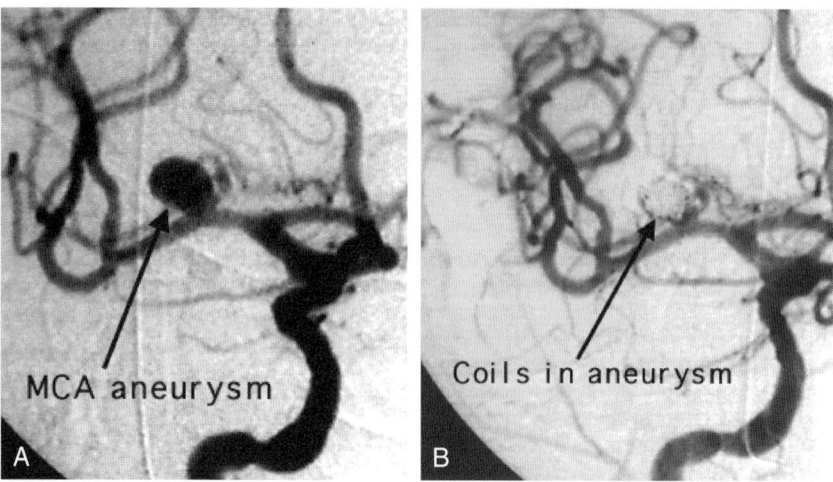

Figure 35-9   Angiogram demonstrating middle cerebral artery aneurysm before **(A)** and after placement of detachable coils to thrombose the aneurysm **(B)**.

risk of impairing the ability to evaluate for clinical deterioration, long-acting sedative agents such as phenobarbital should be avoided. Measures should be taken to minimize cough and Valsalva maneuvers. In intubated patients, frequent coughing should be suppressed prior to aneurysm repair. Stool softeners are administered to avoid straining. If lumbar puncture or ventriculostomy is performed, rapid drainage of a large volume of CSF should be avoided so as not to induce sudden changes in the transmural pressure and rebleeding.

The definitive way to prevent rebleeding is to repair the aneurysm by surgical or endovascular means. Endovascular techniques involving electrolytically detachable platinum coils that thrombose the aneurysm are now routinely used to repair acutely ruptured aneurysms (Figure 35-9).

The International Subarachnoid Aneurysm Trial was a multinational, prospective, randomized trial that compared surgical clipping with endovascular coiling of acutely ruptured intracranial aneurysms. Participating centers were required to treat at least 60 SAH patients per year and offer both treatment modalities. Patients were eligible to be enrolled only if there was clinical equipoise regarding the best method to repair the aneurysm. Initial results favored endovascular coiling, with 23.7% dead or dependent at 1 year compared to 30.6% in the surgery group.[200] Long-term follow-up indicated an increased risk of recurrent bleeding from a coiled aneurysm compared with a clipped aneurysm. At 5 years, the risk of death remained significantly lower in the coiled group than in the clipped group, but the proportion of survivors who were independent did not differ between the two groups.[201]

Hydrocephalus. The decision to treat hydrocephalus is usually based on the CT appearance of enlarging ventricles in a patient whose level of consciousness is deteriorating. During placement of an external ventricular drain, the CSF pressure must be reduced slowly to lessen risk of aneurysmal re-rupture. CSF drainage may be needed for many days to clear intraventricular blood before it can be determined if a permanent shunt is required.

Vasospasm. Monitoring for vasospasm involves serial neurologic exams, serial transcranial Doppler (TCD) measurement of blood flow velocities,[202,203] and catheter angiography. Neurologic signs may be vague, such as a global decline in responsiveness, or consist of focal deficits such as hemiparesis or language disturbance. Symptoms may wax and wane, being exacerbated by hypovolemia or hypotension. Vasospasm can be identified on TCD by an increase in linear blood flow velocity (LBFV): mild (>120 cm/sec), moderate (>160 cm/sec), or severe (>200 cm/sec) vasospasm.[204] Alternatively, the rate of rise in the LBFV is used to define the onset of vasospasm. The sensitivity of TCD in detecting vasospasm is about 80% when compared to angiography, at least partly because TCD samples only a small segment of the vasculature.[205] It has a very high negative predictive value, and the presence of normal velocities usually indicates the absence of vasospasm. Newer CT and MRI techniques including angiography and perfusion may have a role in assessing for delayed ischemia in the future.

When making a clinical diagnosis of vasospasm, alternative causes of neurologic changes such as sedatives, rebleeding, hydrocephalus, cerebral edema, metabolic derangements and infections should be promptly excluded using radiographic, clinical and laboratory assessments. Detection of clinical signs of vasospasm is particularly difficult in poor grade patients because of the limited exam that is possible.

Prevention. Routine measures taken to prevent or ameliorate the effects of vasospasm include mechanical removal of subarachnoid blood at the time of aneurysm surgery or by CSF drainage, administration of the centrally acting calcium channel antagonist nimodipine, and avoidance of intravascular volume contraction (see earlier) and hypotension. Nimodipine (60 mg orally every 4 hours) for 3 weeks after SAH reduces the impact of symptomatic vasospasm and improves outcome.[206,207] It is not clear whether this beneficial effect is due to action on the cerebral vessels or to prevention of calcium influx into ischemic neurons. Any hypotension developing with nimodipine administration can usually be managed with fluids or adjusting the dosage schedule to 30 mg every 2 hours. In patients receiving hemodynamic augmentation for symptomatic vasospasm, nimodipine may have to be discontinued if it interferes with maintenance of blood pressure goals.

While there is general agreement that hypovolemia must be avoided, the use of prophylactic hypervolemia is more controversial.[208-210] In a prospective controlled study, prophylactic volume expansion with albumin failed to reduce the incidence of clinical or TCD-defined vasospasm, did not improve CBF, and had no effect on outcome.[211] Costs and complications may be higher with the use of prophylactic hypervolemia.

Prophylactic use of transluminal balloon angioplasty has recently been evaluated.[212] Although it reduced the need for therapeutic angioplasty and reduced ischemic deficits, these benefits were offset by procedure-related vessel complications.

Treatment of Delayed Ischemic Deficits. The trigger for instituting more aggressive interventions varies widely. Some centers actively intervene in the setting of rising TCD velocities[213] or angiographic vasospasm in asymptomatic patients,[214] whereas others institute aggressive measures in the setting of clinical deterioration. Aggressive measures include both hemodynamic and endovascular manipulations.[215-217] The goal is to improve CBF in ischemic regions. Since patients with SAH tend to become hypovolemic and lose pressure autoregulation,[218] it has been inferred that hypervolemia, induced hypertension, and augmentation of cardiac output would accomplish that goal.

Hemodynamic Augmentation. Hemodynamic manipulations aiming to improve cerebral perfusion include hypervolemia, hypertension, and hemodilution, or "triple-H therapy." Because of the risk of rebleeding with hemodynamic augmentation, triple-H therapy is reserved for patients who have had repair of the ruptured aneurysm. The presence of other small untreated aneurysms does not exclude use of this therapy. Support for the benefit of hemodynamic augmentation is based on case series. The relative contribution of each component is debated.

Data supporting the use of hypervolemia are scant. As described earlier, prophylactic hypervolemia had no impact on CBF, vasospasm, or outcome.[211] In one study of patients with symptomatic vasospasm, hypervolemia was reported to improve CBF, but a proper control group was not used.[219] Other studies question whether hypervolemia adds further benefit beyond correction of hypovolemia and report that the impact of volume expansion on CBF is modest compared to induced hypertension.[220]

Hemodilution is perhaps the least understood component of triple-H therapy. The rationale is to augment CBF by reducing blood viscosity. The tradeoff is that oxygen-carrying capacity is reduced, reducing oxygen delivery. It has been suggested that a hematocrit of 30% provides the optimal balance between oxygen-carrying capacity and viscosity; however, one study found that despite a rise in CBF, oxygen delivery fell with hemodilution.[221]

Blood pressure augmentation may be the most effective hemodynamic intervention. Studies have demonstrated a consistent rise in CBF in response to blood pressure elevation with dopamine and phenylephrine, although the optimal target has not yet been identified.[220] Under normal conditions, cardiac output does not influence CBF; however, with cerebral ischemia or impaired autoregulation, changes in cardiac output may alter CBF. Dobutamine or milrinone may be effective in improving cardiac output and CBF in some patients.

The initial step is to rapidly correct any possible hypovolemia with isotonic crystalloid or colloid fluids. If there is no immediate response to fluid administration, vasoactive agents are instituted—vasopressors (phenylephrine, norepinephrine) or, alternatively, inotropes (dobutamine, milrinone).

Recently there has been a decline in the use of Swan-Ganz catheters to manage hemodynamic augmentation. The arbitrary pulmonary capillary wedge pressure goals used in the past have largely been abandoned. If alternative means of monitoring cardiac output are available, fluid administration should be adjusted to optimize cardiac output. Goals for blood pressure should be defined as a percent change from baseline (beginning with an approximately 15% change) rather than prespecified levels. While defining such goals is useful to guide therapy, the degree of hemodynamic augmentation should be titrated continuously to the patient's neurologic status; thus, if a goal is reached but there is no neurologic improvement, the goal should be modified. Once the optimal goals have been reached, they are usually maintained for 2 to 3 days. Hemodynamic augmentation is then weaned gradually over several days, guided by neurologic status. If neurologic deterioration occurs during weaning of therapy, the blood pressure goals should be returned to higher levels, and attempts to wean therapy should be delayed for 1 or 2 days.

Endovascular Treatments. The endovascular approach to vasospasm involves treatment of constricted vessels with either balloon angioplasty or intraarterial infusion of vasodilating agents.[180,222] Angioplasty on the proximal segments of vasospastic cerebral vessels yields impressive angiographic changes (Figure 35-10) that appear to be long lasting.[223,224] Vasoconstriction in more distal vessels usually cannot be reached by angioplasty catheters and can be treated with intraarterial infusion of vasodilators.

Intraarterial papaverine has an immediate and dramatic effect on blood vessels, but reversal of clinical deficits is inconsistent.[225-227] The use of papaverine has largely been abandoned because of its short-lived effect and complications including increased ICP, apnea, worsening of vasospasm, neurologic deterioration and seizures.[228] It has been replaced by nicardipine, verapamil, nimodipine, and milrinone.[229-231]

The timing of when to initiate endovascular therapy is debated. It is generally used if after a few hours, the response to hemodynamic augmentation is inadequate, but it may be the initial therapy in patients

Figure 35-10 Example of severe distal internal carotid and proximal middle cerebral artery vasospasm *(arrows)* before **(A)** and after **(B)** angioplasty.

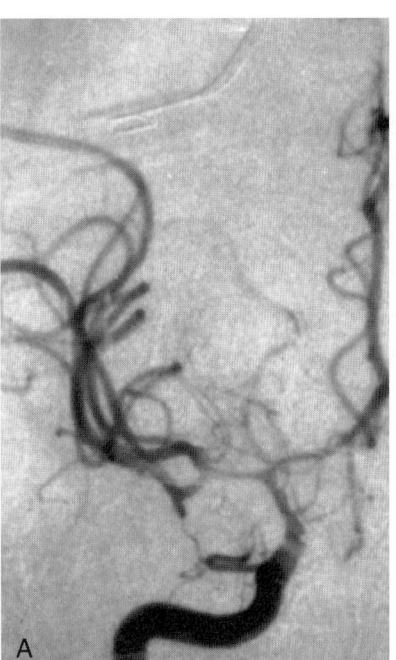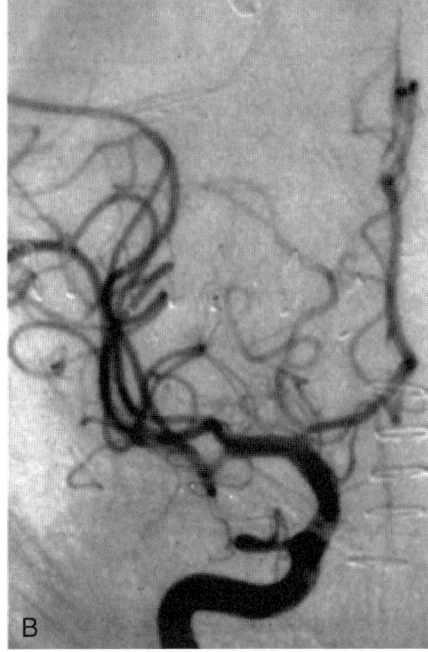

with poor cardiac function who are at high risk of complications of hemodynamic augmentation.[232]

Endothelin-1 Antagonists. Endothelin-1 (ET-1) is a 21–amino acid peptide found on vascular smooth muscle cells and mediates vasoconstriction. It appears to reduce angiographic vasospasm[233-234] and tends to reduce vasospasm-related morbidity/mortality. Trials in patients with SAH are underway.

PROGNOSTIC FACTORS AND CAUSES OF MORTALITY

Untreated aneurysmal SAH carries a poor prognosis, with an estimated mortality rate of approximately 50%. Of those who make it to medical attention, mortality is 20% to 40%. Causes of death are about equally distributed among direct effects of the initial hemorrhage, rebleeding, vasospasm, and medical complications. Overall, less than one-third of patients achieve good neurologic recovery. Predictors of poor prognosis include loss of consciousness or poor neurologic condition (i.e., high Hunt & Hess grade) on admission, older age, hypertension, preexisting medical illness, ≥1 mm thickness of subarachnoid blood on CT (Fisher grade 3), seizures, cerebral edema, aneurysm location in the basilar artery, and symptomatic vasospasm.[235-239] Scales quantifying degree of physiologic illness are also predictive of outcome in patients with SAH.[240] Long-term survivors of the initial hemorrhage continue to suffer a 3% annual risk of re-hemorrhage.

KEY POINTS

INTRACEREBRAL HEMORRHAGE

1. Intracerebral hemorrhage (ICH) primarily injures the brain through direct mechanical compression. Ischemia does not appear to contribute to secondary injury in the acute period.

2. Hematoma expansion occurs within the first few hours after symptom onset in over one third of patients and is the primary cause of early neurologic deterioration. While the use of recombinant activated Factor VII reduces hematoma growth, it did not improve outcome in a large randomized trial.

3. The impact of lowering blood pressure on hematoma growth is currently under investigation.

4. Randomized trials of surgical hematoma evacuation and corticosteroid treatment have failed to show a consistent benefit in the management of ICH. The efficacy of osmotic agents has not been evaluated in a randomized trial.

5. The most common cause of death after ICH is withdrawal of care, followed by transtentorial herniation and medical complications of immobility.

SUBARACHNOID HEMORRHAGE

1. Subarachnoid hemorrhage (SAH) typically presents as the sudden onset of a severe headache, often associated with nausea, vomiting, and syncope. Focal neurologic deficits are uncommon.

2. Rebleeding, which is often fatal, occurs most commonly within the first 24 hours and is heralded by a sudden worsening of headache, new neurologic deficit, or arrhythmia. It can be prevented by early surgical or endovascular repair of the aneurysm.

3. Hydrocephalus may develop acutely within hours of SAH or gradually up to weeks later and usually manifests as an insidious decline in mental status.

4. Delayed arterial vasospasm seen on angiography occurs in more than two-thirds of patients, especially those with large amounts of subarachnoid blood. About one third of patients develop delayed cerebral ischemia, which can cause focal neurologic deficits and infarction. Management options include nimodipine, hemodynamic augmentation, and endovascular maneuvers.

5. Management of SAH-associated "cerebral salt wasting" often requires the administration of large volumes of isotonic saline to prevent intravascular volume contraction and restriction of free water to treat hyponatremia.

6. Cardiac abnormalities, including electrocardiographic changes, mildly elevated cardiac enzymes, and arrhythmias, are common after SAH and are thought to be related to elevated catecholamine levels rather than myocardial ischemia. Rarely a more extreme form of cardiac dysfunction occurs at the time of hemorrhage with cardiomyopathy, hypotension, and pulmonary edema.

ACKNOWLEDGMENTS

This work was supported by grants from the National Institutes of Health (NS35966 and NS044885).

ANNOTATED REFERENCES

Frontera JA, Claassen J, Schmidt JM, Wartenberg KE, Temes R, Connolly ES Jr, et al. Prediction of symptomatic vasospasm after subarachnoid hemorrhage: the modified Fisher scale. Neurosurgery 2006;59:21-7.
 This paper describes an important modification to the Fisher scale that improves its ability to predict which patients are likely to develop delayed cerebral ischemia following SAH.
Macdonald RL, Pluta RM, Zhang JH. Cerebral vasospasm after subarachnoid hemorrhage: the emerging revolution. Nat Clin Pract Neurol 2007;3:256-63.
 Advances in diagnosis and treatment have improved the prospects for patients with SAH, but outcomes remain disappointing. This review proposes alternative causes of neurologic deterioration and poor outcome after SAH, including delayed effects of global cerebral ischemia, thromboembolism, microcirculatory dysfunction, and cortical spreading depression.
Mayer SA, Brun NC, Begtrup K, Broderick J, Davis S, Diringer MN, et al. Efficacy and safety of recombinant activated factor VII for acute intracerebral hemorrhage. N Engl J Med 2008;358:2127-37.
 This phase III randomized controlled trial of recombinant activated factor VII (rFVIIa) in acute spontaneous ICH found that, as in the preceding phase II trial, rFVIIa reduces hematoma growth when administered within 4 hours after ICH. That finding did not, however, translate into a clinical benefit, as had been suggested by the prior study.
Suarez JI, Tarr RW, Selman WR. Aneurysmal subarachnoid hemorrhage. N Engl J Med 2006;354:387-96.
 This paper provides a comprehensive review of aneurysmal SAH.

Treggiari MM, Deem S. Which H is the most important in triple-H therapy for cerebral vasospasm? Curr Opin Crit Care 2009;15:83-6.
 This paper summarizes the available literature on the various components of "triple-H" therapy in the management of delayed cerebral ischemia following SAH.
Vergouwen MD, de Haan RJ, Vermeulen M, Roos YB. Effect of statin treatment on vasospasm, delayed cerebral ischemia, and functional outcome in patients with aneurysmal subarachnoid hemorrhage: a systematic review and meta-analysis update. Stroke 2010;41:e47-52.
 This recent meta-analysis included all randomized, placebo-controlled trials on the efficacy of statin treatment in patients with aneurysmal SAH. The results do not lend support to the finding of a beneficial effect of statins reported in a previous meta-analysis.
Anderson CS, Huang Y, Wang JG, Arima H, Neal B, Peng B, et al. Intensive blood pressure reduction in acute cerebral haemorrhage trial (INTERACT): a randomised pilot trial. Lancet Neurol 2008;7:391-9.
 This pilot study investigated the impact of acute blood pressure reduction in hypertensive ICH. There was a trend toward reduction in hematoma growth but no impact on clinical outcome.
Prasad K, Mendelow AD, Gregson B. Surgery for primary supratentorial intracerebral haemorrhage. Cochrane Database Syst Rev 2008;CD000200.
 This analysis included studies in the Cochrane Stroke Group Trials Register, Current Opinion in Neurology and Neurosurgery, Neurosurgical Clinics of North America (1991 to July 1993), and three monographs. It concluded that in patients with supratentorial ICH, surgery marginally reduces the odds of being dead or dependent compared with medical management alone.

REFERENCE

Access the complete reference list online at http://www.expertconsult.com.

36

Seizures in the Critically Ill

SARICE L. BASSIN | THOMAS P. BLECK

Seizures complicate the course of about 3% of adult intensive care unit (ICU) patients admitted for non-neurologic conditions.[1] The medical and economic impact of these seizures confers importance on them out of proportion to their incidence. A seizure is often the first indication of a central nervous system (CNS) complication, and delay in recognition and treatment of seizure is associated with an increased risk of mortality[2]; thus, rapid diagnosis of this disorder is mandatory. In addition, since epilepsy affects 2% of the population, patients with preexisting seizures occasionally enter the ICU for treatment of other problems. Because initial treatment of these patients is the province of the intensivist, he or she must be familiar with seizure management as it affects the critically ill patient. Patients developing status epilepticus often require a critical care specialist in addition to a neurologist.

Seizures have been recognized at least since Hippocratic times, but their relatively high rate of occurrence in critically ill patients has only recently been appreciated. Seizures complicating critical care treatments (e.g., lidocaine use) are also a recent phenomenon. Early attempts at treatment included bromides[3] and morphine as well as ice applications. Barbiturates were first employed in 1912, and phenytoin in 1937.[4] Paraldehyde was popular in the next 2 decades.[5] More recently, emphasis has shifted to the benzodiazepines, which were pioneered in the 1960s.[6] Newer agents for treatment of seizures in critically ill patients include the phenytoin prodrug, fosphenytoin; the anesthetic agent, propofol; and the water-soluble benzodiazepine, midazolam.

Status epilepticus refers to prolonged seizure episodes; it may be the primary indication for admission to the ICU, or it may occur in any ICU patient with CNS disease. The definitions employed in studies of status epilepticus have varied substantially. Although conventional definitions of status epilepticus have used a cutoff of 30 or 60 minutes of sustained seizure duration, or discrete seizures without recovery, clinicians should recognize that most seizures terminate spontaneously within a few minutes. Recent data suggest that in only half of patients with seizure episodes lasting 10 to 29 minutes will the seizure self-terminate.[7] Therefore, seizures that persist longer than 5 to 7 minutes should probably be treated as status epilepticus.[8]

Epidemiology

Limited data are available on the epidemiology of seizures in the ICU. A 10-year retrospective study of all ICU patients with seizures at the Mayo Clinic revealed that 7 patients had seizures per 1000 ICU admissions.[9] Our 2-year prospective study of medical ICU patients identified 35 with seizures per 1000 admissions.[1] These two studies are not exactly comparable, as the patient populations and methods of detection differed. A recent series found 8% of comatose patients without clinical signs of seizure activity to be in electrographic status epilepticus.[10]

Up to 34% of hospital in-patients experiencing a seizure die during their hospitalization.[1] Our prospective study of neurologic complications in medical ICU patients showed that having even one seizure while in the ICU for a non-neurologic reason doubled in-hospital mortality.[10] Incidence estimates for generalized convulsive status epilepticus in the United States vary from 50,000 cases per year[11] to 195,000 cases per year.[12] Some portion of this difference can be accounted for by different definitions; however, the latter estimate represents the only population-based data available and may be more accurate. Mortality estimates similarly vary from 1% to 2% in the

former study to 22% in the latter. This disagreement follows from a conceptual discordance: the smaller number describes mortality the authors directly attribute to status epilepticus, whereas the larger figure estimates the overall mortality rate, even though death was frequently caused by the underlying disease rather than by status epilepticus itself. The elderly have an incidence of status epilepticus almost twice that of the general population and the highest associated mortality rate of any age group at 38%.[13]

Table 36-1 summarizes the most common causes of status epilepticus in adults in the community. Almost 50% of the cases were attributed to cerebral vascular disease.[11] Garzon and colleagues[14] found antiepileptic drug noncompliance as the main cause of status epilepticus in patients with a prior history of epilepsy, and CNS infection, stroke, and metabolic disturbances predominated in the group without previous seizures.

Three major factors determine outcome in patients with status epilepticus: the type of status epilepticus, its cause, and its duration. Generalized convulsive status epilepticus has the worst prognosis for neurologic recovery; myoclonic status epilepticus following an anoxic episode carries a very poor prognosis for survival. Complex partial status epilepticus can produce limbic system damage, usually manifested as a memory disturbance. Causes associated with increased mortality included anoxia, intracranial hemorrhages, tumors, infections, and trauma. The mortality of patients with nonconvulsive status epilepticus has been reported as high as 33%[15] and correlates with the underlying cause, severe impairment of mental status, and the development of acute complications, especially respiratory failure and infection.[16] Data strongly suggest that prolonged seizure duration is a negative prognostic factor. A study of 253 adult status epilepticus patients demonstrated a 30-day mortality rate of 2.7% in patients with seizures lasting 30 to 59 minutes, compared with 32% in those with seizures of 60 minutes or longer.[17]

Limited data are available concerning the functional abilities of generalized convulsive status epilepticus survivors, and no data reliably permit a distinction between the effects of status epilepticus and effects of its causes. One review concluded that intellectual ability declined as a consequence of status epilepticus.[18] Survivors of status epilepticus frequently seem to have memory and behavioral disorders out of proportion to the structural damage produced by the cause of their seizures. Case reports of severe memory deficits following prolonged complex partial status epilepticus have been published.[19] Conversely, one prospective study of 180 children with febrile status epilepticus demonstrated no deaths and no cases of new cognitive or motor handicap.[20] Experimental animal[21] and human epidemiologic[22] studies suggest that status epilepticus may be a risk factor in the development of future seizures. Whether treatment of prolonged seizures reduces the risk of subsequent epilepsy remains uncertain.

Classification

The most frequently used classification scheme is that of the International League Against Epilepsy (Box 36-1).[23] This scheme allows classification on clinical criteria without inferring cause. *Simple partial seizures* start focally in the cerebral cortex without invading other structures. The patient is aware throughout the episode and appears otherwise unchanged. Bilateral limbic dysfunction produces a *complex partial seizure;* awareness and ability to interact are diminished (but

TABLE 36-1	Causes of Status Epilepticus in Adults Presenting from the Community	
Prior Seizures		*No Prior Seizures*
Common		
Subtherapeutic anticonvulsant		Ethanol-related
Ethanol-related		Drug toxicity
Intractable epilepsy		CNS infection
		Head trauma
		CNS tumor
Less Common		
CNS infection		Metabolic aberration
Metabolic aberration		Stroke
Drug toxicity		
Stroke		
CNS tumor		
Head trauma		

CNS, central nervous system.

may not be completely abolished). *Automatisms* (movements a patient makes without awareness) may occur. *Secondary generalization* results from invasion by epileptic electrical activity of the other hemisphere or subcortical structures.

Primary generalized seizures arise from the cerebral cortex and diencephalon at the same time; no focal phenomena are visible, and consciousness is lost at the onset. *Absence seizures* are frequently confined to childhood; they consist of the abrupt onset of a blank stare that usually lasts 5 to 15 seconds, after which the patient abruptly returns to normal. *Atypical absence seizures* occur in children with the Lennox-Gastaut syndrome. *Myoclonic seizures* start with brief synchronous jerks without alteration of consciousness, initially followed by a generalized convulsion. They frequently occur in patients with genetic epilepsy; in the ICU, they commonly follow anoxia or metabolic

---

Box 36-1

INTERNATIONAL CLASSIFICATION OF EPILEPTIC SEIZURES

1. Partial seizures (seizures beginning locally)
   A. Simple partial seizures (consciousness not impaired; simple partial seizures)
      i. With motor symptoms
      ii. With somatosensory or special sensory symptoms
      iii. With autonomic symptoms
      iv. With psychic symptoms
   B. Complex partial seizures (with impairment of consciousness; complex partial seizures)
      i. Beginning as simple partial seizures and progressing to impairment of consciousness
         a. Without automatisms
         b. With automatisms
      ii. With impairment of consciousness at onset
         a. With no other features
         b. With features of simple partial seizures
         c. With automatisms
   C. Partial seizures (simple or complex), secondarily generalized
2. Primary generalized seizures (bilaterally symmetric, without localized onset)
   A. Absence seizures
      i. True absence ("petit mal")
      ii. Atypical absence
   B. Myoclonic seizures
   C. Clonic seizures
   D. Tonic seizures
   E. Tonic-clonic seizures ("grand mal")
   F. Atonic seizures
3. Unclassified seizures

Adapted from Bleck TP. Status epilepticus. In: Klawans HL, Goetz CG, Tanner CM, editors. Textbook of clinical neuropharmacology. 2nd ed. New York: Raven Press; 1992, p. 65-73.

Box 36-2

CLINICAL CLASSIFICATION OF STATUS EPILEPTICUS

1. Generalized seizures
   A. Generalized convulsive status epilepticus
      i. Primary generalized status epilepticus
         a. Tonic-clonic status epilepticus
         b. Myoclonic status epilepticus
         c. Clonic-tonic-clonic status epilepticus
      ii. Secondarily generalized status epilepticus
         a. Partial seizure with secondary generalization
         b. Tonic status epilepticus
   B. Nonconvulsive status epilepticus
      i. Absence status epilepticus (petit mal status)
      ii. A typical absence status epilepticus (e.g., in the Lennox-Gastaut syndrome)
      iii. Atonic status epilepticus
      iv. Nonconvulsive status epilepticus as a sequel of partially treated generalized convulsive status epilepticus
2. Partial status epilepticus
   A. Simple partial status epilepticus
      i. Typical
      ii. Epilepsia partialis continua
   B. Complex partial status epilepticus
3. Neonatal status epilepticus

Adapted from Lothman EW. The biochemical basis and pathophysiology of status epilepticus. Neurology 1990;40:13-23.

disturbances.[24] *Tonic-clonic seizures* start with tonic extension, evolve to bilaterally synchronous clonus, and conclude with a postictal phase. Clinical judgment is required to apply this system in the ICU. In patients in whom consciousness has already been altered by drugs, hypotension, sepsis, or intracranial pathologic lesion, the nature of partial seizures may be difficult to classify.

Status epilepticus is classified by a similar system that has been altered to match observable clinical phenomena (Box 36-2).[25] Generalized convulsive status epilepticus is the most common type encountered in the ICU and poses the greatest risk to the patient. It may either be primarily generalized, as in the drug-intoxicated patient, or secondarily generalized, as in the brain abscess patient who develops generalized convulsive status epilepticus. *Nonconvulsive status epilepticus* in the ICU frequently follows partially treated generalized convulsive status epilepticus. Some practitioners use the term for all cases of status epilepticus that involve altered consciousness without convulsive movements; this blurs the distinctions among absence status epilepticus, partially treated generalized convulsive status epilepticus, and complex partial status epilepticus, which have different causes and treatments. *Epilepsia partialis continua* (a special form of partial status epilepticus in which repetitive movements affect a small area of the body) sometimes continues for months or years.

The International League Against Epilepsy continues to work toward revising and updating the current classification system. The goal is a multi-axis diagnostic scheme that incorporates anatomic, etiologic, therapeutic, and prognostic implications. For the most recent information regarding this ongoing project, refer to www.epilepsy.org.[26]

Pathogenesis and Pathophysiology

The causes and effects of status epilepticus at the cellular, brain, and systemic levels are interrelated, but their individual analysis is useful for understanding them and their therapeutic implications. The ionic events of a seizure follow the opening of ion channels coupled to excitatory amino acid receptors. From the standpoint of the intensivist, three channels are particularly important, because their activation may raise intracellular free calcium to toxic concentrations: alpha-amino-3-hydroxy-5-methyl-4-isoxazole propionic acid (AMPA), *N*-methyl-D-aspartate (NMDA), and metabotropic channels. These excitatory amino acid systems are crucial for learning and memory. Many drugs that block these systems are available but are too toxic for chronic use. Counter-regulatory ionic events are triggered by the epileptiform discharge as well, such as the activation of inhibitory interneurons which suppress excited neurons via $GABA_A$ synapses.

The cellular effects of excessive excitatory amino acid channel activity include (1) generation of toxic concentrations of intracellular free calcium; (2) activation of autolytic enzyme systems; (3) production of oxygen free radicals; (4) generation of nitric oxide, which both enhances subsequent excitation and serves as a toxin; (5) phosphorylation of enzyme and receptor systems, making seizures more likely; and (6) an increase in intracellular osmolality, which produces neuronal swelling. If adenosine triphosphate production fails, membrane ion exchange ceases, and neurons swell further. These events produce the neuronal damage associated with status epilepticus. Longer status epilepticus duration produces more profound alterations and an increasing likelihood of permanence and of becoming refractory to treatment.[27] The processes involved in a single seizure and the transition to status epilepticus have been reviewed.[28]

Many other biophysical and biochemical alterations occur during and after status epilepticus. The intense neuronal activity activates immediate-early genes and produces heat shock proteins, providing indications of the deleterious effects of status epilepticus and insight into the mechanisms of neuronal protection.[29] The mechanisms by which status epilepticus damages the nervous system have been reviewed.[30] Absence status epilepticus is an exception among these conditions; it consists of rhythmically increased inhibition and does not produce clinical or pathologic abnormalities.

The electrical phenomena of status epilepticus at the whole brain level, as seen in the scalp electroencephalogram (EEG), reflect the seizure type that initiates status epilepticus (e.g., absence status epilepticus begins with a 3-Hz wave-and-spike pattern). During status epilepticus, this rhythm slows, but the wave-and-spike characteristic remains. Generalized convulsive status epilepticus goes through a sequence of electrographic changes (Table 36-2).[31] The initial discharge becomes less well formed, implying that neuronal firing loses synchrony. The sustained depolarizations that characterize status epilepticus alter the extracellular milieu, most importantly by raising extracellular potassium. The excess potassium ejected during status epilepticus exceeds the buffering ability of astrocytes.

The increased cellular activity of status epilepticus elevates demand for oxygen and glucose, and cerebral blood flow initially increases. After approximately 20 minutes, however, energy supplies are exhausted, causing local catabolism to support ion pumps (in an attempt to restore the internal milieu); this is a major cause of epileptic brain damage. In addition to damaging the CNS, generalized convulsive status epilepticus produces life-threatening systemic effects.[32] Excess secretion of epinephrine and cortisol cause systemic and pulmonary arterial pressures to rise dramatically at seizure onset and also produce hyperglycemia. Muscular work raises blood lactate levels. Both airway obstruction and abnormal diaphragmatic contractions impair respiration. Carbon dioxide excretion falls while its production increases markedly. Muscular work accelerates heat production, raising core body temperature.

The combined respiratory and metabolic acidoses frequently reduce the arterial blood pH to 6.9 or lower. The acidemia may produce hyperkalemia; in addition to its deleterious effects on cardiac electrophysiology, the elevated extracellular potassium level helps propagate seizure activity. Coupled with hypoxemia and the elevation of circulating catecholamine concentrations, these conditions rarely can produce cardiac arrest. This sequence probably accounts for some cases of epileptic sudden death; neurogenic pulmonary edema is the likely cause of many others. The severity of the acidosis may prompt consideration of bicarbonate administration. When this is attempted, however, the likelihood of the occurrence of pulmonary edema is inordinately high. Rapid termination of seizure activity is the most appropriate treatment; the restitution of ventilation and the metabolism of lactate quickly restore a normal pH.

After approximately 30 minutes of continuous convulsions, motor activity may diminish while electrographic seizures persist. Hypotension and hyperthermia ensue, and gluconeogenesis can fail, resulting in hypoglycemia. Generalized convulsive status epilepticus patients often aspirate oral or gastric contents, producing chemical pneumonitis or bacterial pneumonia. Rhabdomyolysis is common and may lead to renal failure. Compression fractures, joint dislocations, and tendon avulsions are other serious sequelae.

The mechanisms that terminate seizure activity are poorly understood. The leading candidates are inhibitory mechanisms, primarily GABA-ergic interneurons and inhibitory thalamic neurons.

Clinical Manifestations

Three problems complicate seizure recognition: (1) the occurrence of complex partial seizures in the setting of impaired awareness, (2) the occurrence of seizures in patients receiving pharmacologically induced paralysis and/or sedation, and (3) misinterpretation of other abnormal movements as seizures. ICU patients often have depressed consciousness in the absence of seizures owing to their disease, its complications (such as hepatic[33] or septic[34] encephalopathy), or drug administration. A further decline in alertness may reflect a seizure; an EEG is required to confirm that one has occurred.

Patients receiving neuromuscular junction blocking agents do not manifest the usual signs of seizures. Patients with increased intracranial pressure (ICP) from primary brain injury, hepatic encephalopathy, or other critical illnesses may be both paralyzed and sedated, making identification of seizures particularly challenging. Tachycardia, tachypnea, and hypertension are signs of seizure that can be misinterpreted as evidence of inadequate sedation. Continuous EEG monitoring is warranted in this population if seizures are suspected.

Patients with metabolic disturbances, anoxia, and other types of nervous system injury may demonstrate abnormal movements that can be confused with seizure. Asterixis is a brief asynchronous loss of tone at the wrist or hip joints that can appear in the setting of hepatic dysfunction. Stimulus-sensitive massive myoclonus after anoxia can be dramatic but usually self-abates in a few days. Controversy exists as to the epileptic origin of this disorder, and postanoxic myoclonus has been reported in the presence of almost total cortical suppression.[35] Brain-injured patients may manifest paroxysmal episodes of sympathetic hyperactivity and associated rigidity or decerebrate posturing. These "hypothalamic seizures" can sometimes be distinguished from epileptic seizures with observation. Patients with tetanus are awake during their spasms and flex rather than extend their arms as seizure

TABLE 36-2	Electrographic-Clinical Correlations in Generalized Convulsive Status Epilepticus	
Stage	Typical Clinical Manifestations*	Electroencephalographic Features
1	Tonic-clonic convulsions; hypertension and hyperglycemia common	Discrete seizures with interictal slowing
2	Low or medium amplitude clonic activity, with rare convulsions	Waxing and waning of ictal discharges
3	Slight but frequent clonic activity, often confined to the eyes, face, or hands	Continuous ictal discharges
4	Rare episodes of slight clonic activity; hypotension and hypoglycemia become manifest	Continuous ictal discharges punctuated by flat periods
5	Coma without other manifestations of seizure activity	Periodic epileptiform discharges on a flat background

Data from Treiman DM. Generalized convulsive status epilepticus in the adult. Epilepsia 1993;34: S2-11.
*Clinical manifestations may vary considerably depending on the underlying neuropathophysiologic process (and its anatomy), systemic diseases, and medications. In particular, stages of the electrographic progression may be sufficiently brief to be overlooked. Partially treating status epilepticus may dissociate the clinical and electrographic features.

patients do. Psychiatric disturbances in the ICU occasionally resemble complex partial seizures. If doubt about the nature of abnormal movements persists, an EEG should be obtained.

The manifestations of status epilepticus depend on the type and, for partial status epilepticus, the cortical area of abnormality. Box 36-2 presents the types of status epilepticus encountered and focuses on those seen most frequently in the ICU.

Primary generalized convulsive status epilepticus begins as tonic extension of the trunk and extremities without preceding focal activity. No aura is reported, and consciousness is immediately lost. After several seconds of tonic extension, the extremities start to vibrate; clonic (rhythmic) extension of the extremities quickly follows. This phase wanes in intensity over a few minutes. The patient may then repeat the cycle of tonus followed by clonic movements or continue to have intermittent bursts of clonic activity without recovery. *Myoclonic status epilepticus* (bursts of myoclonic jerks that increase in intensity and lead to a generalized convulsion) is a less common form of generalized convulsive status epilepticus usually associated with anoxic coma.

Secondarily generalized status epilepticus begins with a partial seizure and progresses to a convulsive activity. The initial focal clinical activity may be overlooked. This seizure type implies a structural lesion, so care must be taken to elicit evidence of lateralized movements.

Of the several forms of generalized nonconvulsive status epilepticus, the one of greatest importance to intensivists is nonconvulsive status epilepticus as a sequela of inadequately treated generalized convulsive status epilepticus. When a patient with generalized convulsive status epilepticus is treated with anticonvulsants in inadequate doses, visible convulsive activity may stop, but the electrochemical seizure continues. Patients begin to awaken within 15 to 20 minutes after the successful termination of status epilepticus; many regain consciousness much faster. Patients who do not start to awaken after 20 minutes should be assumed to have entered nonconvulsive status epilepticus. Careful observation may disclose slight clonic activity. Nonconvulsive status epilepticus is an extremely dangerous problem because the destructive effects of status epilepticus continue even without obvious motor activity. Nonconvulsive status epilepticus demands emergency treatment guided by EEG monitoring to prevent further cerebral damage, since there are no clinical criteria to indicate whether therapy is effective.

Failure to recognize nonconvulsive status epilepticus is common in patients presenting with nonspecific neurobehavioral abnormalities such as delirium, lethargy, bizarre behavior, cataplexy, or mutism.[36] Patients may present in nonconvulsive status epilepticus without an inciting episode of generalized convulsive status epilepticus. A high suspicion for this disorder should be maintained in patients with unexplained alteration in level of consciousness or cognition admitted to the ICU.

Partial status epilepticus in ICU patients often follows a stroke or occurs with the rapid expansion of brain masses. Clonic motor activity is most easily recognized, but the seizure takes on the characteristics of adjacent functional tissue. Therefore, somatosensory or special sensory manifestations occur, and the ICU patient may be unable to report such symptoms. *Aphasic status epilepticus* occurs when a seizure begins in a language area and may resemble a stroke. *Epilepsia partialis continua* involves repetitive movements confined to a small region of the body. It may be seen with nonketotic hyperglycemia[37] or with focal brain disease; anticonvulsant treatment is seldom useful. *Complex partial status epilepticus* manifests with diminished awareness. The diagnosis often comes as a surprise when an EEG is obtained.

Diagnostic Approach

When an ICU patient has a seizure, one has a natural tendency to try to stop the event. This leads to both diagnostic obscuration and iatrogenic complications. Beyond protecting the patient from harm, very little can be done rapidly to influence the course of the seizure. Padded tongue blades, or similar items, should not be placed in the mouth; they are more likely to obstruct the airway than to preserve it. The seizures of most patients stop before any medication can reach the brain in an effective concentration.

Observation is the most important activity to perform when a patient has a single seizure. This is the time to collect evidence of a partial onset to implicate structural brain disease. The postictal examination is similarly valuable; language, motor, sensory, or reflex abnormalities after an apparently generalized seizure are evidence of focal pathology.

Seizures in ICU patients have several potential causes that must be investigated. Drugs are a major cause of ICU seizures, especially in the setting of diminished renal or hepatic function or when the blood-brain barrier is breached. Theophylline frequently produces seizures or status epilepticus if it has been rapidly loaded or if high concentrations of the drug occur; occasionally, however, these complications arise at "therapeutic" levels. Imipenem-cilastatin[38] and fluoroquinolones[39] have substantial potential to lower the seizure threshold, especially in patients with renal dysfunction. They should be avoided if possible in patients already at risk for seizure. Other antibiotics, especially β-lactams, are occasionally implicated.[40] Sevoflurane, a volatile anesthetic agent, is dose-dependently epileptogenic in patients with no predisposition to seizures.[41]

Recreational drugs are frequently overlooked offenders in patients presenting to the ICU. Acute cocaine or methamphetamine intoxication is characterized by a state of hypersympathetic activity followed by seizures.[42] Although ethanol withdrawal is a common cause of seizures, discontinuing any hypnosedative agent may prompt convulsions 1 to 3 days later. One report suggests that narcotic withdrawal may produce seizures in the critically ill.[1] In the absence of other clear causes for seizure, complete toxicologic screening should be performed.

Serum glucose, electrolyte concentrations, and serum osmolality should also be measured. Nonketotic hyperglycemia[43,44] and hyponatremia can precipitate both focal and generalized seizures. Seizure activity may infrequently be the first presenting sign of diabetes mellitus. However, hypocalcemia rarely causes seizures beyond the neonatal period; its identification on analysis must *not* signal the end of the diagnostic workup. Hypomagnesemia has an equally unwarranted reputation as the cause of seizures in malnourished alcoholic patients.

The physical examination should emphasize assessment for both global and focal abnormalities of the CNS. Evidence of cardiovascular disease or systemic infection should be sought and the skin and fundi examined closely.

The need for imaging studies in these patients has been an area of uncertainty. A prospective study of neurologic complications in medical ICU patients determined that 38 of 61 patients (62%) had a vascular, infectious, or neoplastic explanation for their seizures.[45] Hence, head computed tomography (CT) or magnetic resonance imaging (MRI) should be performed on ICU patients with new seizures. With current technology, there are almost no patients who cannot undergo CT scanning, and MRI is particularly helpful in detecting evidence of acute ischemic stroke and encephalitis. MRI cannot be performed on patients with pacemakers. Many ICP monitor catheters are compatible with MRI provided the device is not coiled when it is secured to the scalp. Patients who need cerebrospinal fluid analysis always require imaging of the brain first. When CNS infection is suspected, empirical antibiotic treatment should be started while these studies are being performed.

Electroencephalography is a vital diagnostic tool for evaluating the seizure patient. Partial seizures usually show EEG abnormalities that begin in the area of cortex that produces seizures. Primary generalized seizures appear to start over the entire cortex simultaneously. Postictal slowing or depressed amplitude provides clues as to the focal cause of the seizures, and epileptiform activity helps classify the type of seizure and guide treatment. An emergency EEG is necessary to exclude nonconvulsive status epilepticus in those patients who do not begin to awaken soon after seizures have apparently been controlled (Figure 36-1).

In contrast to the patient with a single or a few seizures, the status epilepticus patient requires concomitant diagnostic and therapeutic

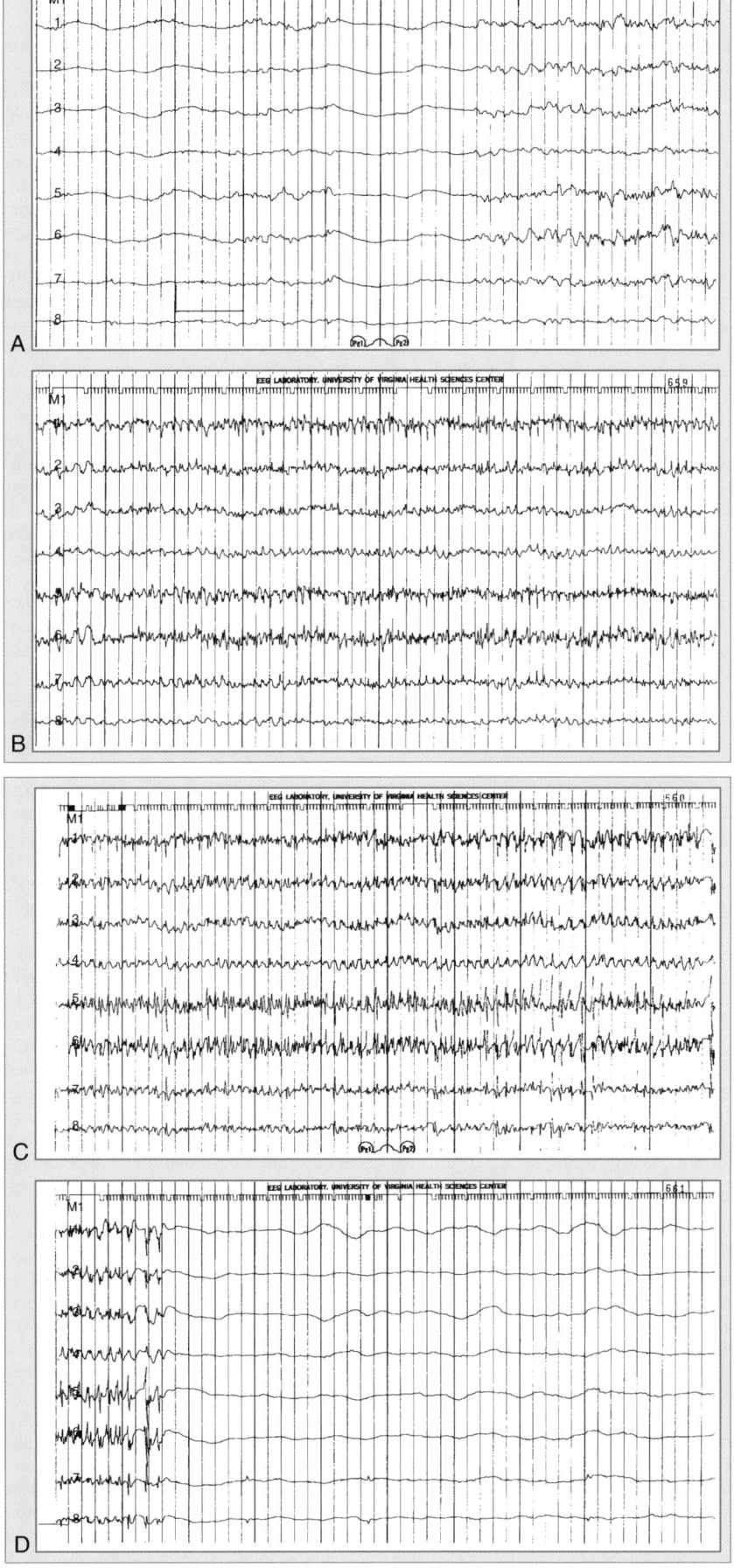

Figure 36-1 Electroencephalographic recording during status epilepticus. First panel illustrates onset of seizure; subsequent panels show its evolution. Montage: longitudinal bipolar; channels 1-4, left temporal, and channels 5-8, left parasagittal. Calibration: vertical, 50 μV; horizontal, 1 sec.

efforts. Although 30 minutes of continuous or recurrent seizure activity usually define status epilepticus, one should not stand by waiting for this period to pass to start treatment. Since most seizures in critically ill patients stop within 2 to 3 minutes, it is reasonable to start treatment after 5 minutes of continuous seizure activity or after the second or third seizure occurs without recovery between the spells.

Treatment for status epilepticus should not be delayed to obtain an EEG. However, a prospective evaluation of 164 patients demonstrated that nearly half manifested persistent electrographic seizures in the 24 hours after clinical control of convulsive status epilepticus.[46] These data suggest that EEG monitoring after control of convulsive status epilepticus can be essential in directing the course of treatment. A variety of findings may be present on the EEG, depending on the type of status epilepticus and its duration (see Table 36-2). Complex partial status epilepticus patients are often without such organized discharges of generalized convulsive status epilepticus; instead, they have waxing and waning rhythmic activity in one or several brain regions. A diagnostic trial of intravenous (IV) benzodiazepine therapy is often necessary to diagnose complex partial status epilepticus. Patients developing refractory status epilepticus or having seizures during neuromuscular junction blockade require continuous EEG monitoring.

The availability of continuous paperless EEG monitoring allows for detection of seizure activity over a long period.[47] Subclinical seizures have been observed to occur in patients receiving aggressive treatment for status epilepticus and even in patients treated with barbiturates to a burst-suppression EEG pattern. The clinical significance of these subclinical seizures, and their effect on prognosis, remains uncertain.

Management Approach

TREATING ISOLATED SEIZURES

Making the decision to administer anticonvulsants to an ICU patient who experiences one or a few seizures requires consideration of a provisional cause, estimation of the likelihood of recurrence, and recognition of the utility and limitations of anticonvulsants. For example, the occurrence of seizures during ethanol withdrawal does not indicate the need for chronic treatment, and giving phenytoin does not prevent further withdrawal convulsions. The patient may need prophylaxis against delirium tremens, but the few seizures themselves seldom require treatment. Patients with convulsions during barbiturate or benzodiazepine withdrawal, in contrast, should usually receive short-term treatment with lorazepam to prevent status epilepticus. Prolonged or frequent seizures caused by metabolic disturbances can be treated temporarily with benzodiazepines while the abnormality is being corrected. Seizures in these settings are notoriously resistant to treatment with phenytoin. In particular, treatment of patients with partial seizures related to nonketotic hyperglycemia should be directed at correction of the hyperglycemia and hypovolemia rather than anticonvulsant therapy.[44]

The ICU patient with CNS disease who has even one seizure should be given chronic anticonvulsant therapy, and this approach should be reviewed before the patient is discharged. Initiating this treatment after the first *unprovoked* seizure may help prevent subsequent epilepsy,[48] although there is considerable difference of opinion regarding this concept.[49] Starting therapy after the first seizure in a critically ill patient at risk for seizure recurrence may be even more important, especially if the patient's condition would be seriously complicated by a convulsion.

In the ICU setting, phenytoin is frequently selected for prophylaxis or prevention of subsequent seizures, owing to its ease of administration and lack of sedative effects. Hypotension and arrhythmias may complicate IV administration and can usually be prevented by slowing the infusion to less than 25 mg/min. Because of the rare occurrence of third-degree atrioventricular block, an external cardiac pacemaker should be available when patients with conduction abnormalities receive IV phenytoin. The parenteral formulation of phenytoin is very alkaline, and this contributes to pain, burning, and redness at the injection site.[50]

The phenytoin prodrug, fosphenytoin, is water soluble, and its vehicle does not contain propylene glycol. Local adverse effects are less common with fosphenytoin than with IV administration of phenytoin, although cardiovascular complications are just as frequent.[51,52] Fosphenytoin is dosed by phenytoin-equivalent units; therefore, no dosage adjustments are needed when converting patients from phenytoin to fosphenytoin. Fosphenytoin can be administered by intramuscular injection or by IV infusion at a rate of up to 150 mg phenytoin equivalents/min. Fosphenytoin is rapidly converted to phenytoin in vivo, and free phenytoin levels after fosphenytoin administration are not markedly different compared with phenytoin.

Whether phenytoin or fosphenytoin is used, the serum phenytoin concentration should be kept in the "therapeutic" range of 10 to 20 µg/mL (corresponding to an unbound or "free" concentration of 1 to 2 µg/mL) unless further seizures occur; the level can then be increased until signs of toxicity occur. Failure to prevent seizures at a concentration of 25 µg/mL is usually an indication to add phenobarbital to the regimen. When fosphenytoin is administered, phenytoin concentrations should not be measured until the biological conversion to phenytoin is complete: 2 hours after an IV infusion or 4 hours after an intramuscular injection of fosphenytoin.

Phenytoin is approximately 90% protein bound in normal hosts. Patients with renal dysfunction have lower total phenytoin levels at a given dose because the drug is displaced from binding sites, but the unbound level is not affected. Thus renal failure patients, and perhaps others who are receiving highly protein-bound drugs (which compete for binding), may benefit from determination of free phenytoin level. Only the free fraction is metabolized, so the dose is not altered with changes in renal function. The clearance half-time with normal liver function varies from about 12 to 20 hours (IV form) to more than 24 hours (extended-release capsules), so a new steady-state serum concentration occurs in 3 to 6 days. Phenytoin need not be given more frequently than every 12 hours. Hepatic dysfunction mandates a decrease in the maintenance dose. Hypersensitivity is the major adverse effect of concern to the intensivist. This may manifest itself solely as fever but may include rash and eosinophilia. Adverse reactions to phenytoin and other anticonvulsants have been reviewed elsewhere.[53] Levetiracetam and lacosamide are newer anticonvulsants available for IV use. The appropriate loading and maintenonce doses in critically ill patients remain to be determined.

Phenobarbital remains a useful anticonvulsant for patients who are intolerant to phenytoin or have persistent seizures after adequate phenytoin administration. The target for phenobarbital in the ICU should be a serum concentration of 20 to 40 µg/mL. Hepatic and renal dysfunction alter phenobarbital metabolism. Since its usual clearance half-time is about 96 hours, maintenance doses of this agent should be given once a day. A steady-state level takes about 3 weeks to become established. Sedation is the major adverse effect; allergy to the drug occurs rarely.

TREATING STATUS EPILEPTICUS

Generalized convulsive status epilepticus obviously constitutes a medical emergency; however, nonconvulsive status epilepticus and complex partial status epilepticus are also emergencies but are more difficult to recognize. In each circumstance, one must act quickly to prevent additional cerebral damage. Figure 36-2 shows a management algorithm for status epilepticus and Box 36-3 presents a sample management protocol for drug administration.[54] Patients with simple partial status epilepticus or epilepsia partialis continua are at less risk for the development of widespread cerebral damage and are also less likely to respond to the aggressive approach outlined in Box 36-3. In these patients, correcting underlying problems such as nonketotic hyperosmolar hyperglycemia is crucial. Errors in terminating status epilepticus include inadequate dosing of effective drugs and continued use of drugs that are ineffective in the patient being treated.

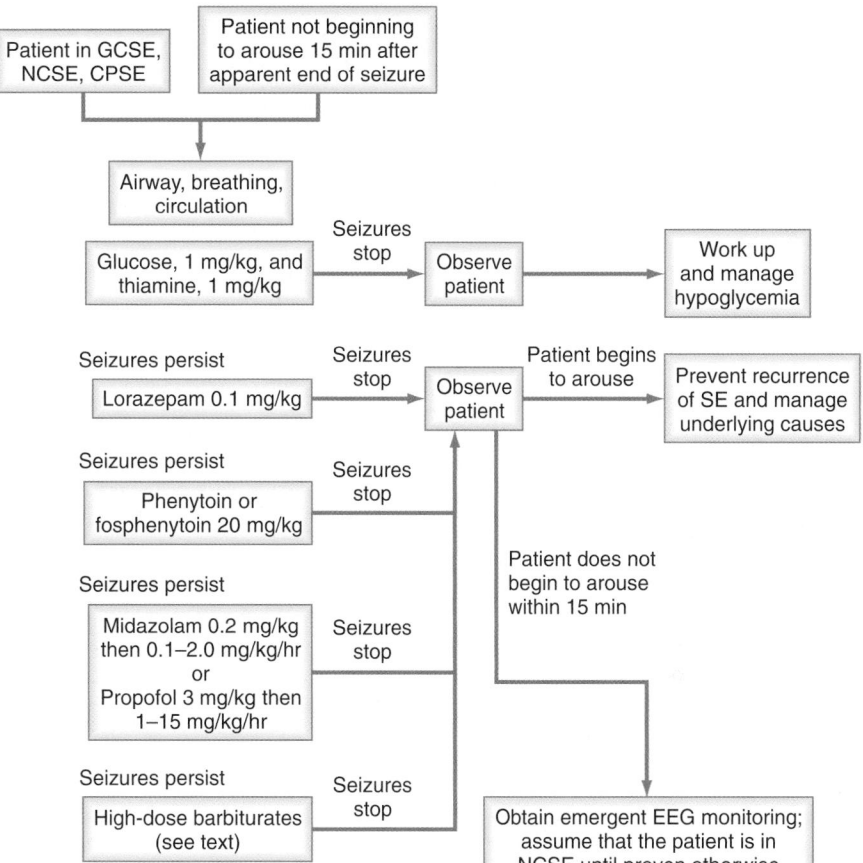

Figure 36-2 Management algorithm for status epilepticus. CPSE, complex partial status epilepticus; GSCE, generalized convulsive status epilepticus; NCSE, nonconvulsive status epilepticus; SE, status epilepticus.

The conventional agents used as first-line treatment of status epilepticus are the benzodiazepines (especially lorazepam, diazepam, and midazolam), phenytoin, and phenobarbital. Status epilepticus that is refractory to the traditional agents is treated with continuous infusions of the short-acting barbiturates, midazolam, or propofol. A major multicenter clinical trial[55] that compared lorazepam alone, phenytoin alone, diazepam followed by phenytoin, and phenobarbital alone as initial drug treatment for generalized convulsive status epilepticus showed that the highest rate of successful treatment of "overt" generalized convulsive status epilepticus was achieved with lorazepam. There was no demonstrable difference among these four drug regimens in the initial treatment of "subtle" generalized convulsive status epilepticus. Lorazepam has been our agent of first choice for terminating status epilepticus for many years and remains so with support from this study.

Advantages of lorazepam over diazepam are its duration of action against status epilepticus (4 to 14 hours as opposed to 20 minutes) and its higher initial response rate. European practitioners often use midazolam or clonazepam initially. In patients in whom IV access is difficult to attain, 0.2 mg/kg of midazolam administered intramuscularly will be rapidly and reliably absorbed. The use of midazolam in refractory status will be discussed later. Respiratory depression is the major adverse effect of the benzodiazepines, especially when they are given together with barbiturates or paraldehyde.

Phenytoin is a less effective agent in the treatment of status epilepticus; in addition, the constraint on the rate of IV administration is of concern. Phenytoin has a long duration of action when an adequate dose is given (a 20 mg/kg dose produces a serum level above 20 μg/mL for 24 hours). Adding 5 mg/kg if the first 20 mg/kg load fails to stop status epilepticus may be useful. Fosphenytoin can be administered by a more rapid IV infusion, but the brain concentration of the phenytoin derived from it does not appear to rise faster than with the native drug. Free phenytoin levels reach a therapeutic range 10 to 20 minutes after

an infusion of fosphenytoin is started.[56,57] Intramuscular injection of fosphenytoin in patients with status epilepticus should not be considered acceptable therapy and should be reserved for only those rare circumstances in which IV access cannot be obtained.

Some practitioners advocate the use of phenobarbital as a first-line drug,[58] but it has typically been used as a third-line agent after administration of a benzodiazepine and phenytoin.[59] Although this approach has been widely accepted by the neurologic community, we rarely use phenobarbital for two reasons. First, only a small percentage of patients who have failed treatment with the first anticonvulsant drug respond to a second or third conventional agent[60]; second, at least an additional 20 minutes are required to obtain control in the few patients who do respond. Phenobarbital remains an important drug in the management of simple partial status epilepticus and for those patients who are being weaned from high-dose midazolam or anesthetic barbiturates.

Pentobarbital and thiopental infusions are usually reserved for refractory status epilepticus.[56] Although these drugs are effective in sufficiently large doses, their side effects can limit their use and may be fatal.[61] However, they are important when other modalities have failed (see Box 36-3). Endotracheal intubation and mechanical ventilation are mandatory when high-dose barbiturates are used, and both continuous EEG and invasive hemodynamic monitoring are highly recommended. Severe hypotension is the most frequent side effect of pentobarbital therapy, and its occurrence is associated with increased mortality.[62] An increased occurrence of nosocomial respiratory tract infection has been reported in patients treated with pentobarbital infusion.[63] An inhibitory effect on leukocyte chemotaxis and paralysis of respiratory cilia by the barbiturates have been postulated. Despite these side effects, barbiturate anesthesia should not be rapidly discontinued if it is successful in terminating refractory status epilepticus; rather, continuing therapy for at least 48 hours, gradual tapering of the infusion dose, and the administration of phenobarbital during the drug taper are recommended.[64]

Box 36-3

SUGGESTED PROTOCOL FOR TREATING STATUS EPILEPTICUS

1. Establish an airway, provide oxygen, and ensure ventilation. If neuromuscular junction blockade is required for intubation, use a short-acting agent (e.g., succinylcholine or vecuronium).
2. Determine blood pressure. If the patient is hypotensive, begin volume replacement or administration of vasoactive agents (or both), as indicated. Generalized convulsive status epilepticus patients who present with hypotension will usually require admission to a critical care unit. Hypertension should not be treated until status epilepticus is controlled, since terminating status epilepticus usually substantially corrects it, and many of the agents used to terminate status epilepticus can produce hypotension.
3. Unless the patient is known to be normo- or hyperglycemic, administer dextrose (1 g/kg) and thiamine (1 mg/kg).
4. Terminate status epilepticus. The following sequence is recommended (see text for details); be cognizant of the potential of these drugs to eliminate the visible convulsive movements of generalized convulsive status epilepticus when leaving the patient in nonconvulsive status epilepticus. Patients who do not begin to respond to external stimuli 15 minutes after the apparent termination of generalized convulsive status epilepticus should be considered at risk for nonconvulsive status epilepticus and should undergo emergent EEG monitoring.
   A. Give lorazepam, 0.1 mg/kg, at a rate of 0.04 mg/kg/min. This drug should be diluted in an equal volume of the solution being used for intravenous infusion, as it is quite viscous. Most adult patients who respond do so by a total administered dose of 8 mg. The latency of effect is debated, but lack of response after 5 minutes should indicate failure.
   B. If status epilepticus persists after lorazepam administration, consider phenytoin at up to 50 mg/min; or fosphenytoin, 20 mg/kg, at up to 150 mg/min (dosed by phenytoin equivalent). Many investigators believe an additional 5 mg/kg dose of phenytoin equivalent should be administered before the next line of therapy is attempted. However, this step may have more value for preventing status epilepticus recurrence than for its initial control.
   C. If status epilepticus persists, administer midazolam, 0.2 mg/kg as a bolus, followed by an infusion of 0.1-2 mg/kg/h to achieve seizure control (as determined by EEG monitoring). Intubate the patient at this stage if this has not already been accomplished. A patient reaching this stage should be treated in a critical care unit.
   D. Should the patient's condition not be controlled with midazolam, administer propofol or pentobarbital. Propofol is given as a continuous infusion at a rate of 1-15 mg/kg/h

to achieve seizure control (as determined by EEG monitoring). A bolus dose of propofol (3 mg/kg) is often given but may increase the occurrence of hypotension. Pentobarbital is given as a bolus dose of 12 mg/kg at a rate of 0.2-0.4 mg/kg/min as tolerated, followed by an infusion of 0.25-2 mg/kg/h, as determined by EEG monitoring (with an initial goal of burst-suppression; in some cases, an isoelectric electroencephalogram may be required to eliminate all electrical seizures). Most patients require systemic and pulmonary arterial catheterization, with fluid and vasoactive drug therapy as indicated to maintain blood pressure. Other complications of this treatment are discussed in the text.

5. Prevent recurrence of status epilepticus. The choice of drugs depends greatly on the cause of status epilepticus and the patient's medical and social situation. In general, patients not previously receiving anticonvulsants whose status epilepticus is easily controlled often respond well to chronic treatment with phenytoin or carbamazepine. In contrast, others (e.g., patients with acute encephalitis) will require two or three anticonvulsants at "toxic" levels (e.g., phenobarbital at greater than 100 µg/mL) to be weaned from midazolam or pentobarbital and may still have occasional seizures.
6. Treat complications.
   A. Rhabdomyolysis should be treated with a vigorous saline diuresis to prevent acute renal failure; urinary alkalinization may be a useful adjunct. If definitive treatment of generalized convulsive status epilepticus takes longer than expected because of hypotension or arrhythmias, neuromuscular junction blockade under EEG monitoring might be considered.
   B. Hyperthermia usually remits rapidly after termination of status epilepticus. External cooling usually suffices if the core temperature remains elevated. In rare instances, cool peritoneal lavage or extracorporeal blood cooling may be required. High-dose pentobarbital generally produces poikilothermia.
   C. Treatment of cerebral edema occurring secondary to status epilepticus has not been well studied. When substantial edema is present, one should suspect that status epilepticus and cerebral edema are both manifestations of the same underlying condition. Mannitol and mild hyperventilation may be valuable if edema is life threatening. If substantial cerebral edema is present, ICP monitoring should be strongly considered. Edema due to status epilepticus is vasogenic in origin; thus, steroids may be useful as well, but they have not been studied in this setting.

Midazolam is a water-soluble benzodiazepine that has demonstrated high efficacy in refractory status in adults and children.[65,66] At our institution, this agent is used as a second-line drug after lorazepam has failed to control status epilepticus. Clinically significant hypotension is rare even at very high doses that are often required to address tachyphylaxis. Respiratory depression is uncommon after a loading dose but should be anticipated with infusions of any duration. Sedation is quickly reversed after short-term infusions are discontinued. However, terminal half-lives of three to eight times normal have been reported with extended administration.[67] In addition, prolonged elimination times have been associated with critical illness and hepatorenal dysfunction. Others have recently discussed its use in this setting.[68]

Isoflurane, an inhaled anesthetic, controls refractory status epilepticus; however, it is difficult to deliver such a gas outside of the operating suite or the recovery area. It has no known advantage over IV anticonvulsants and can raise ICP.

Propofol has been reported to be effective in the treatment of refractory status epilepticus, but direct comparisons with other agents have shown mixed results.[69,70] It may offer a lower risk of ventilatory depression and promote more rapid awakening compared with other drugs when it is discontinued. Early fears of a possible proconvulsant effect

appear to be unfounded, although withdrawal convulsions may occur if the drug is abruptly terminated. A dosage range of 1 to 15 mg/kg/h has been studied,[71] although the actual upper limit is not known. Acidosis and oxygenation difficulties have been reported in children.[72] Mortality with its use appears to be greater than with midazolam.[70] Careful monitoring of creatine kinase and oxygen saturation would be prudent.[73]

Levetiracetam is emerging as a very commonly used IV and enteral antiseizure drug in critical care. Unfortunately, no organized dose-finding has been undertaken in critically ill patients; published series have included loading doses between 1 and 6 grams, with a wide range of maintenance doses.[74] Levetiracetam has been used for prophylaxis after head trauma, but the higher mortality in the patients receiving this drug in comparison to those receiving phenytoin argues for some caution.[75]

IV valproate has emerged as an important drug for the treatment of several forms of status epilepticus.[76] IV lacosamide is also available, but information about its use in status is limited. Topiramate may also be useful for refractory status epilepticus[77] but lacks an IV form. Levetiracetam (1 gm loading dose, 1-9 gm/d maintenance) or lacosamide (300-400 mg loading dose, 300-400 mg/d maintenance) may also be useful.

KEY POINTS

1. Although conventional definitions of status epilepticus have used a cutoff of 30 or 60 minutes of sustained seizure duration, or discrete seizures without recovery, clinicians should recognize that most seizures will terminate spontaneously within a few minutes. Therefore, seizures that persist longer than 5 to 7 minutes should probably be treated as status epilepticus.

2. Patients begin to awaken within 15 to 20 minutes after the successful termination of status epilepticus; many regain consciousness much faster. Patients who do not start to awaken after 20 minutes should be assumed to have entered nonconvulsive status epilepticus. Nonconvulsive status epilepticus demands emergency treatment guided by electroencephalographic monitoring to prevent further cerebral damage, since there are no clinical criteria to indicate whether therapy is effective.

3. Observation is the most important activity to perform when a patient has a single seizure. This is the time to collect evidence of a partial onset to implicate structural brain disease. The post-ictal examination is similarly valuable; language, motor, sensory, or reflex abnormalities after an apparently generalized seizure are evidence of focal pathology.

4. In contrast to the patient with a single or a few seizures, the status epilepticus patient requires concomitant diagnostic and therapeutic efforts. Although 30 minutes of continuous or recurrent seizure activity usually define status epilepticus, one should not stand by waiting for this period to pass to start treatment. Since most seizures in critically ill patients stop within 2 to 3 minutes, it is reasonable to start treatment after 5 minutes of continuous seizure activity or after the second or third seizure occurs without recovery between the spells.

5. Electroencephalographic monitoring after control of convulsive status epilepticus can be essential in directing the course of treatment.

6. The ICU patient with central nervous system disease who has even one seizure should usually be given chronic anticonvulsant therapy, and this approach should be reviewed before the patient is discharged. Initiating this treatment after the first unprovoked seizure may help prevent subsequent epilepsy. In the ICU setting, phenytoin is frequently selected because of its ease of administration and lack of sedative effects.

7. The conventional agents used in the first-line of treatment of status epilepticus are the benzodiazepines (especially lorazepam, diazepam, and midazolam), phenytoin, and phenobarbital. Status epilepticus that is refractory to the traditional agents is treated with continuous infusions of the short-acting barbiturates, midazolam, or propofol.

ANNOTATED REFERENCES

Bleck TP. Critical care of the patient in status epilepticus. In: Wasterlain C, Treiman D, editors. Status epilepticus. Boston: MIT Press; 2006. p. 607-13.
A comprehensive review of ICU management of status epilepticus.

Fountain NB, Adams RE. Midazolam treatment of acute and refractory status epilepticus. Clin Neuropharmacol 1999;22:261-7.
This thorough review discusses both the pharmacology of and the data supporting midazolam use in patients with status epilepticus. Practical clinical hints are conveyed regarding specific advantages and potential disadvantages of midazolam.

Lothman E. The biochemical basis and pathophysiology of status epilepticus. Neurology 1990;40 (suppl 2):13-23.
A classic, comprehensive summary of clinical and experimental evidence explaining the alterations in systemic physiology and brain metabolism that occur during prolonged seizures.

Shneker BF, Fountain NB. Assessment of acute morbidity and mortality in nonconvulsive status epilepticus. Neurology 1996;47:83-9.
A retrospective review of 100 patients with nonconvulsive status epilepticus found a mortality rate of 18% that correlated with the underlying cause, severe impairment of mental status, and development of acute complications. Generalized spike-and-wave discharges did not correlate with mortality. This is the largest series to date.

Towne AR, Waterhouse EJ, Boggs JG, Garnett LK, Brown AJ, Smith Jr JR, et al. Prevalence of nonconvulsive status epilepticus in comatose patients. Neurology 2000;54:340-5.
A retrospective review of the EEG recordings of 236 comatose ICU patients without clinical signs of status epilepticus found that nonconvulsive status epilepticus occurred in 18%. These findings suggest that EEG is an essential part of the coma evaluation.

Treiman DM, Meyers PD, Walton NY, Collins JF, Colling C, Rowan AJ, et al. A comparison of four treatments for generalized convulsive status epilepticus. N Engl J Med 1998;339:792-8.
This 5-year randomized, double-blind, multicenter trial of four IV regimens in the first-line treatment of generalized convulsive status epilepticus demonstrated that lorazepam is more effective than phenytoin. Although lorazepam was not found to be more efficacious than phenobarbital or diazepam and phenytoin, it was easier to use and therefore recommended for initial IV treatment. There were no significant differences in side effects among the four treatment groups.

REFERENCES

Access the complete reference list online at http://www.expertconsult.com.

Neuromuscular Disorders in the ICU

VERN C. JUEL | THOMAS P. BLECK

Abnormal neuromuscular function may precipitate a patient's admission to an intensive care unit (ICU) or may develop as a consequence of another critical illness and its treatment. This chapter focuses primarily on respiratory failure due to neuromuscular disease but also addresses autonomic dysfunction occurring in this setting. To facilitate understanding of the concepts involved, a brief review of the motor unit and its physiology is provided and specific muscles critical to ventilation are identified.

The Motor Unit and Its Physiology

Central nervous system activity designated for motor output is ultimately conducted to lower motor neurons, also known as *alpha motor neurons*. A motor unit is composed of a lower motor neuron and its distal ramifications, its neuromuscular junctions, and the muscle fibers it innervates. The cell bodies of the lower motor neurons are located in the brainstem for cranial musculature and in the anterior horn of the spinal cord for somatic muscles. At the level of the brainstem or spinal cord, the motor neurons receive various excitatory and inhibitory inputs. Motor axons project through the subarachnoid space and penetrate the dura mater as nerve roots. They may join with other motor axons and with sensory and autonomic fibers in a plexus and then travel in peripheral nerves to the muscles they innervate. Alpha motor neurons are myelinated, a feature that accelerates nerve impulse propagation. The multiple terminal ramifications of the motor neuron synapse on individual muscle fibers.

The motor axon communicates with muscle via a specialized area termed the *neuromuscular junction*. On the presynaptic side of the neuromuscular junction, the neurotransmitter acetylcholine is synthesized, packaged in vesicles, and stored for release. Depolarization of the axon opens presynaptic voltage-gated calcium channels, which activate the molecular machinery responsible for drawing the vesicles to the presynaptic membrane. The vesicles then fuse with the membrane and release acetylcholine into the synaptic cleft. Acetylcholine molecules bind to receptors on the postsynaptic membrane and cause an influx of sodium, which in turn increases the muscle end-plate potential. When the end-plate potential exceeds the threshold level, the muscle membrane becomes depolarized. This depolarization releases calcium ions from the sarcoplasmic reticulum, and muscle contraction occurs through a process known as *excitation-contraction coupling*. After activating the acetylcholine receptor complex, the acetylcholine molecule is degraded by cholinesterase; the choline released by this reaction is then recycled by the presynaptic neuron.

Muscles of Respiration

Three muscle groups may be defined based on their importance for respiration (Figure 37-1):[1]
1. *Upper airway muscles:* palatal, pharyngeal, laryngeal, and lingual
2. *Inspiratory muscles:* sternomastoid, diaphragm, scalenes, and parasternal intercostals
3. *Expiratory muscles:* internal intercostal muscles (except for parasternals) and abdominal muscles

The upper airway muscles receive their innervation from the lower cranial nerves. Sternomastoid innervation arrives predominantly from cranial nerve XI, with a small contribution from C2. The phrenic nerve originates from cell bodies located between C3 and C5, with a maximum contribution from C4, and innervates the diaphragm. Innervation to the scalenes arises from C4 to C8, whereas that of the parasternal intercostals is from T1 to T7. The intercostal muscles receive innervation from T1 to T12, and the abdominal musculature receives it from T7 to L1. Reference to this innervation scheme is important in understanding the effects of spinal cord and nerve root injuries on respiration and for the differential diagnosis of disorders producing apparently diffuse weakness.

CLINICAL PRESENTATION OF NEUROMUSCULAR RESPIRATORY FAILURE

Patients experiencing respiratory dysfunction due to neuromuscular disease typically present with a combination of upper airway dysfunction and diminished tidal volume (VT). Difficulty with swallowing liquids, including respiratory secretions, is the most typical presentation of pharyngeal weakness, although some patients have an equal or greater degree of difficulty with solid food. A hoarse or nasal voice may also signal problems with the upper airway. These conditions are noted in patients who are at risk for aspiration and present with difficulty with attempts at negative-pressure ventilation (cuirass or iron lung), because the weakened muscles may not be able to keep the airway open as the pressure falls.[2] Paradoxical abdominal movement (inward movement of the abdomen during inspiration) is an important sign of diaphragmatic weakness.[3]

Loss of VT occurs most dramatically with diaphragmatic weakness but also follows insults that affect the ability of the parasternal intercostals to keep the chest wall expanded against negative intrapleural pressure. This is most apparent in lower cervical spinal cord injuries where atelectasis commonly develops despite preserved phrenic nerve function. This problem usually diminishes over weeks as the parasternal intercostal muscles develop spasticity.

Patients with progressive generalized weakness (e.g., Guillain-Barré syndrome) commonly begin to lose VT before developing upper airway weakness. To maintain minute ventilation, and therefore carbon dioxide excretion, a patient's respiratory rate increases. Respiratory rate is thus one of the most important clinical parameters to monitor. As the vital capacity falls from the norm of about 65 to 30 mL/kg, a patient's cough weakens, and clearing secretions becomes difficult. A further decrease of vital capacity to 20 to 25 mL/kg results in an impaired ability to sigh with progressive atelectasis. At this point, hypoxemia may be present because of ventilation-perfusion mismatching and because an increasing percentage of VT is used to ventilate dead space. Before the vital capacity reaches 18 mL/kg, a patient should be in an ICU, because respiratory failure is imminent and endotracheal intubation should be considered. The precise point at which mechanical ventilation is necessary varies with the patient, the underlying condition, and especially with the likelihood of a rapid response to treatment.

Regardless of the vital capacity, however, indications for intubation and mechanical ventilation include evidence of fatigue, hypoxemia despite supplemental oxygen administration, difficulty with secretions, and a rising Paco$_2$. In the absence of hypercapnia, occasional patients (e.g., those with myasthenia gravis) can be managed under very close observation in an ICU with less invasive techniques (e.g., bilevel positive airway pressure [BiPAP]).[4]

In addition to vital capacity, trended measurements of the maximum inspiratory pressure (PImax, more typically recorded as negative

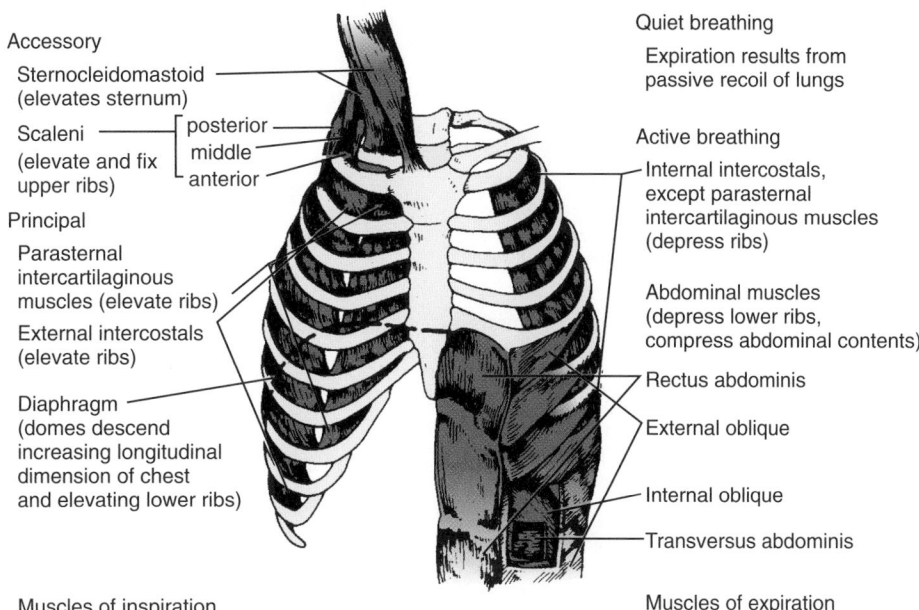

Figure 37-1 **Major respiratory muscles.** Inspiratory muscles are indicated on the left and expiratory muscles are indicated on the right. *(From Garrity ER. Respiratory failure due to disorders of the chest wall and respiratory muscles. In: MacDonnell KF, Fahey PJ, Segal MS, editors. Respiratory Intensive Care. Boston: Little, Brown; 1987, p. 313.)*

inspiratory force [NIF]), are useful indicators of ventilatory capacity. Inability to maintain a PImax greater than 20 to 25 cm H_2O usually indicates a need for mechanical ventilation. Although the maximum expiratory pressure (PEmax) is a more sensitive indicator of weakness,[5] it has not proved to be as useful as an indicator of the need for mechanical ventilation. A more detailed discussion of these variables and their use may be found elsewhere.[6,7]

Because a patient with neuromuscular respiratory failure has intact ventilatory drive,[8] the fall in V_T is initially matched by an increase in respiratory rate, keeping the $Paco_2$ normal or low until the vital capacity becomes dangerously reduced. Many patients initially maintain their $Paco_2$ in the range of 35 mm Hg because of either (1) a subjective sense of dyspnea at low V_T or (2) hypoxia from atelectasis and increasing dead space. When the $Paco_2$ begins to rise in this circumstance, abrupt respiratory failure may be imminent.

The modest degree of hypoxia in most of these patients worsens when the $Paco_2$ begins to rise, displacing more oxygen from the alveolar gas. However, aspiration pneumonia and pulmonary embolism are also frequent causes of hypoxia in these patients. To determine the relative contributions of these conditions to a patient's hypoxemia, one can use a simplified version of the alveolar gas equation as follows (derived elsewhere)[6,7]:

$$PAO_2 = PIO_2 - (PaCO_2/R)$$

where PAO_2 is the alveolar partial pressure of oxygen, PIO_2 is the partial pressure of inspired oxygen (in room air, 150 mm Hg), and R is the respiratory quotient (on most diets, about 0.8). This allows estimation of the alveolar-arterial oxygen difference ($PAO_2 - PaO_2$). Under ideal circumstances in young people breathing room air, this value is about 10 mm Hg, but it rises to about 100 mm Hg when the fraction of inspired oxygen (FIO_2) is 1.0. The alveolar air equation allows one to factor out the contribution of hypercarbia to the decrease in arterial partial pressure of oxygen (PaO_2); it should be used to determine whether there is a cause of significant hypoxemia in addition to the displacement of oxygen by carbon dioxide.

Patients with orbicularis oris weakness may have artifactually low vital capacity and NIF measurements because they cannot form a tight seal around the spirometer mouthpiece. The need for nursing and respiratory therapy personnel who are experienced in the care of these patients is thus underscored. It is also important for physicians to observe these patients directly rather than relying solely on reported measurements. The physical findings associated with neuromuscular respiratory failure are reviewed elsewhere.[6,7] Among the most important findings are rapid, shallow breathing,[9] the recruitment of accessory muscles, and paradoxical movement of the abdomen during the respiratory cycle. Fluoroscopy of the diaphragm is occasionally valuable for the diagnosis of diaphragmatic dysfunction.[10]

Autonomic dysfunction commonly accompanies some of the neuromuscular disorders requiring critical care, such as Guillain-Barré syndrome, botulism, and porphyria (Table 37-1). In Guillain-Barré syndrome (discussed later) dysautonomia is common and may arise in parallel with weakness or may follow the onset of the motor disorder after one week or more.

Neuromuscular Disorders

Many chronic neuromuscular disorders and other central nervous system conditions affecting the suprasegmental innervation and control of respiratory muscles eventually compromise ventilation. In this chapter, however, we emphasize the more common acute and subacute neuromuscular disorders that precipitate or prolong critical illness due to ventilatory failure and autonomic dysfunction. A more complete listing of neuromuscular diseases appears in Table 37-1; reviews of this subject[11,12] or the references listed in Table 37-1 may be consulted for details of the more rare disorders. Some of the diseases listed (e.g., Lambert-Eaton myasthenic syndrome) rarely cause respiratory failure in isolation but may be contributing causes in the presence of other conditions[13] such as neuromuscular junction blockade intended only for the duration of a surgical procedure.[14]

NEUROMUSCULAR DISEASES PRECIPITATING CRITICAL ILLNESS

Guillain-Barré Syndrome

Guillain-Barré syndrome, or acute inflammatory demyelinating polyradiculoneuropathy, is typically a motor greater than sensory peripheral neuropathy with subacute onset, monophasic course, and nadir within 4 weeks. Although the precise etiology is unknown, Guillain-Barré syndrome is immune mediated and related to antibodies directed against peripheral nerve components. Approximately 1.7 cases occur

TABLE 37-1	Neuromuscular Causes of Acute Respiratory Failure	
Location	**Disorder**	**Associated Autonomic Dysfunction?**
Spinal cord	Tetanus[112]	Frequent
Anterior horn cell	Amyotrophic lateral sclerosis[113]	No
	Poliomyelitis	No
	Rabies	Frequent
	West Nile virus flaccid paralysis	No
Peripheral nerve	Guillain-Barré syndrome	Frequent
	Critical illness polyneuropathy	No
	Diphtheria	No, but cardiomyopathy and arrhythmias may occur
	Porphyria	Occasional
	Ciguatoxin (ciguatera poisoning)	Occasional
	Saxitoxin (paralytic shellfish poisoning)	No
	Tetrodotoxin (pufferfish poisoning)	No
	Thallium intoxication	No
	Arsenic intoxication[114,115]	No
	Lead intoxication	No
	Buckthorn neuropathy	No
Neuromuscular junction	Myasthenia gravis	No
	Botulism[116]	Frequent
	Lambert-Eaton myasthenic syndrome[117]	Yes, frequent dry mouth and postural hypotension
	Hypermagnesemia[118]	No
	Organophosphate poisoning	No
	Tick paralysis	No
	Snake bite	No
Muscle	Polymyositis/dermatomyositis	No
	Acute quadriplegic myopathy	No
	Eosinophilia-myalgia syndrome[119]	No
	Muscular dystrophies[120]	No, but cardiac rhythm disturbances may occur
	Carnitine palmitoyl transferase deficiency	No
	Nemaline myopathy[121]	No
	Acid maltase deficiency[122]	No
	Mitochondrial myopathy[123]	No
	Acute hypokalemic paralysis	No
	Stonefish myotoxin poisoning	No
	Rhabdomyolysis	No
	Hypophosphatemia[124]	No

per 100,000 population per year.[15] Most patients suffer a demyelinating neuropathy, but in about 5% of cases the condition is a primary axonopathy.[16] Numerous antecedents have been implicated[17]; the more frequent ones are listed in Box 37-1. The association with antecedent infections suggests that certain agents may elicit immune responses involving antibodies that cross-react with peripheral nerve gangliosides. In particular, the development of ganglioside antibodies has been observed in Guillain-Barré syndrome after *Campylobacter jejuni* infections, such as GM_1 antibodies in axonal forms of Guillain-Barré syndrome[18] and GQ_{1b} antibodies in the Miller-Fisher variant of Guillain-Barré syndrome.[19]

The initial findings of patients with Guillain-Barré syndrome are subacute and progressive weakness, usually most marked in the legs, associated with sensory complaints but without objective signs of sensory dysfunction.[20] Deep tendon reflexes are often significantly reduced or absent at presentation, though this finding may take several days to develop. The cerebrospinal fluid (CSF) typically reveals an albuminocytologic dissociation or elevated protein content without pleocytosis; this may not evolve until the second week of illness. The major reason to examine the CSF is to preclude other diagnoses. Although mild CSF lymphocytic pleocytosis (10-20 cells/mm³) may suggest the possibility of associated human immunodeficiency virus (HIV) infection, in most patients, the nucleated cell count is less than 10 cells/mm³.[21] Although they may be normal initially, results of electrodiagnostic studies (motor and sensory nerve conduction studies and needle electromyography) often reflect segmental nerve demyelination with multifocal conduction blocks, temporally dispersed compound muscle action potentials, slowed conduction velocity, and prolonged or absent F waves.[22] Differential diagnostic considerations for patients with suspected Guillain-Barré syndrome are primarily those listed in the "Peripheral Nerve" section of Table 37-1.

The components of treatment for patients with Guillain-Barré syndrome are as follows:

- Management of ventilatory failure
- Management of autonomic dysfunction
- Meticulous nursing care
- Psychological support
- Physical and occupational therapy
- Prevention of deep venous thrombosis
- Nutritional support
- Early planning for rehabilitation
- Immunotherapy for the underlying autoimmune process

Patients with Guillain-Barré syndrome with evolving respiratory failure should generally be intubated when the vital capacity falls to about 15 mL/kg or when difficulty with secretions begins, because the response to treatment is slow. If a patient has been immobile for several days before intubation and neuromuscular junction blockade is needed, a nondepolarizing agent should be used to avoid transient hyperkalemia. Oral intubation is again being viewed as preferable to the nasal route, because the endotracheal tube is frequently required for a week or longer, raising the risk of sinusitis with nasal intubation.

Many patients are too weak to trigger the ventilator; in such cases, the assist/control or intermittent mandatory ventilation mode is initiated. Weaning patients with Guillain-Barré syndrome from mechanical ventilation must wait for adequate improvement in strength. We usually shift to pressure support ventilation for weaning, although evidence of its superiority over intermittent mandatory ventilation or synchronized intermittent mandatory ventilation modes is only anecdotal. Although the majority of patients require mechanical ventilation for less than 4 weeks, as many as one-fifth need 2 or more months of support before they can breathe without assistance. Improvement in vital capacity to greater than 15 mL/kg and in NIF to greater than

MAJOR ANTECEDENTS OF GUILLAIN-BARRÉ SYNDROME

Frequent

Upper respiratory tract infections
Campylobacter jejuni enteritis
Cytomegalovirus (CMV) infection
Epstein-Barr virus (EBV) infection
Hepatitis A infection
Hepatitis B infection
Hepatitis C infection
Human immunodeficiency virus (HIV) infection

Infrequent

Mycoplasma pneumoniae infection
Haemophilus influenzae infection
Leptospira icterohaemorrhagiae infection
Salmonellosis
Rabies vaccine
Tetanus toxoid
Bacille Calmette-Guérin immunization
Sarcoidosis
Systemic lupus erythematosus
Lymphoma
Trauma
Surgery

Questionable

Hepatitis B vaccine
Influenza vaccine
Hyperthermia
Epidural anesthesia

---

25 cm H_2O suggests that a patient has improved enough to begin weaning from the ventilator. A formula using a combination of ventilatory and gas exchange variables may allow more accurate determination of a patient's ability to be weaned.[23]

Autonomic dysfunction related to Guillain-Barré syndrome most typically presents as a hypersympathetic state and is often heralded by unexplained sinus tachycardia. The blood pressure may fluctuate wildly. Patients may rarely experience bradycardic episodes, which may require temporary pacing. Autonomic surges during tracheal suctioning or due to a distended viscus may be very dramatic and should be minimized. Autonomic failure and pulmonary embolism are now the major causes of mortality in Guillain-Barré syndrome.

Nursing care for patients with Guillain-Barré syndrome is similar to that for other paralyzed and mechanically ventilated patients, but special care must be taken to remember that patients with Guillain-Barré syndrome are completely lucid. In addition to explaining any procedures carefully, arranging for distractions during the daytime (e.g., television, movies, conversation, visitors) and adequate sleep at night is very important. For the most severely affected patients, sedation should be considered. In concert with physical and occupational therapists, passive exercise should be performed frequently throughout the day.

Deep venous thrombosis is a significant danger for patients with Guillain-Barré syndrome. Episodic arterial desaturation is a common event, presumably owing to transient mucus plugging; submassive pulmonary emboli may therefore be overlooked. Adjusted-dose heparin (to slightly prolong the partial thromboplastin time) should be given, and sequential compression devices should be used on the legs; therapeutic anticoagulation may be considered. The risk of fatal pulmonary embolism extends through the initial period of improvement until patients are ambulatory.

Nutritional support should begin as soon as a patient is admitted, with appropriate concern for the risk of aspiration.[24] Most mechanically ventilated patients with Guillain-Barré syndrome can be fed via soft, small-caliber feeding tubes; autonomic dysfunction affecting the gut occasionally requires total parenteral nutrition.

Immunotherapy for Guillain-Barré syndrome includes removal of autoantibodies with plasma exchange or immune modulation with high-dose intravenous immunoglobulin (IVIg). The efficacy of plasma exchange has been evaluated in a Cochrane systematic review of six class II trials comparing plasma exchange alone with supportive care.[25] Most of the trials employed up to 5 plasma exchanges of 50 mL/kg over 2 weeks. In a large North American trial,[25] the time needed to improve one clinical grade (being weaned from the ventilator or being able to walk) was reduced by 50% in the plasma exchange group by comparison with the control group. There was no significant benefit when plasma exchange was begun later than 2 weeks after symptom onset. A meta-analysis demonstrated more rapid recovery in ventilated patients treated with plasma exchange within 4 weeks of onset.[26] The optimal number of plasma exchanges has been assessed in patients with mild (unable to run), moderate (unable to stand without assistance), and severe (requiring mechanical ventilation) Guillain-Barré syndrome by the French Cooperative Group.[27] On the basis of this trial, two exchanges are better than none in mild Guillain-Barré syndrome; four are better than two in moderate Guillain-Barré syndrome; and six are no better than four in severe Guillain-Barré syndrome. Albumin is the preferred replacement solution.[28] Treatment with IVIg for Guillain-Barré syndrome has also been examined in a Cochrane systematic review. Three randomized controlled trials demonstrated class I evidence that IVIg (2 g/kg over 2-5 days) is as effective as plasma exchange in Guillain-Barré syndrome patients with impaired walking.[29] Complication rates were somewhat higher in the plasma exchange groups. A large international multicenter randomized trial compared plasma exchange (50 mL/kg × 5 exchanges over 8-13 days), IVIg (0.4 g/kg × 5 days), and plasma exchange followed by IVIg.[30] No significant outcome differences between these therapies were found with respect to functional improvement at 4 weeks or at 48 weeks.

Evidence-based guidelines for Guillain-Barré syndrome immunotherapy have been published by the Quality Standards Subcommittee of the American Academy of Neurology.[31] Plasma exchange is recommended for adult patients who cannot walk within 4 weeks of symptom onset. IVIg is recommended in these patients within 2 or possibly 4 weeks of symptom onset. Both treatments are deemed equivalent in efficacy, and combining treatment with plasma exchange and IVIg confers no additional benefit. In light of their therapeutic equivalence, the decision whether to employ plasma exchange or IVIg in treating acute Guillain-Barré syndrome may be determined by resource availability and by avoiding potential side effects related to a patient's medical comorbidities. Patients with heart disease, renal insufficiency or failure, hyperviscosity, or IgA deficiency may be more susceptible to complications of treatment with IVIg, whereas plasma exchange may be complicated in patients with labile blood pressure, septicemia, and significant venous access problems.

Despite the autoimmune pathophysiology of Guillain-Barré syndrome and the efficacy of corticosteroids in more chronic forms of inflammatory neuropathy, corticosteroids have not demonstrated effectiveness in Guillain-Barré syndrome and are therefore not recommended for Guillain-Barré syndrome treatment.[31] A large multicenter trial failed to demonstrate efficacy of high-dose intravenous methylprednisolone,[32] and another large multicenter trial demonstrated no added clinical benefit in combined treatment with IVIg and methylprednisolone.[33]

West Nile Virus Acute Flaccid Paralysis Syndrome

The large outbreak of West Nile virus encephalitis in the summer of 1999 in New York City marked the emergence of a relatively new cause for neuromuscular weakness with the potential for neuromuscular respiratory compromise. West Nile virus is a flavivirus transmitted between birds and mosquitoes. Humans may acquire West Nile virus from the bite of an infected *Culex* species mosquito, and a corresponding peak in human disease occurs in the late summer and fall. West Nile virus may also be transmitted to humans by organ transplantation,[34] blood and blood product transfusion,[35] transplacental exposure,[36] breast feeding,[37] and percutaneous laboratory injuries.[38] About 20% of humans experience a mild flulike illness lasting 3 to 6 days, and about 1 in 150 develop central nervous system disease, which usually presents as meningoencephalitis.[39]

In the initial North American outbreak of West Nile virus, about 10% of infected patients experienced flaccid weakness with clinical features resembling Guillain-Barré syndrome.[40] In one report from the original outbreak, a patient developed electromyographic evidence for segmental demyelination compatible with Guillain-Barré syndrome.[41] Although patients with West Nile virus infection exhibit a spectrum of clinical weakness,[42] the most prominent and distinctive syndrome documented in several subsequent reports of West Nile virus infection is an acute "poliomyelitis-like" or acute flaccid paralysis syndrome with pathology localizing to the ventral horns of the spinal cord and/or ventral roots.[43-49] These patients developed acute, asymmetrical, flaccid weakness in the absence of sensory abnormalities, diffuse areflexia, or bowel/bladder dysfunction. Some of the patients experienced concurrent meningoencephalitis, and a few required mechanical ventilation.[44,45] West Nile virus acute flaccid paralysis syndrome may occur in the absence of overt encephalitic signs (e.g., fever, confusion) or meningismus. Although the risk for West Nile virus encephalitis is significantly increased with age,[50] West Nile virus acute flaccid paralysis syndrome occurs in relatively younger patients.[43-49]

Electrodiagnostic studies in patients with West Nile virus acute flaccid paralysis syndrome demonstrate normal sensory potentials, the absence of findings suggesting segmental demyelination (e.g., motor conduction block, reduced conduction velocities, prolonged distal and F-wave latencies), low-amplitude compound muscle action potentials in affected regions, and marked denervation changes in affected limb and in corresponding paraspinal muscles on needle electromyography. Corresponding magnetic resonance imaging (MRI) findings are sometimes observed and include abnormal signal in the spinal cord on T2-weighted images[47,48] and abnormal enhancement of the nerve roots and cauda equina.[46,47] CSF analysis usually demonstrates mild pleocytosis with lymphocytic predominance, mild to moderate protein elevation, and normal glucose.[51] Prognosis for recovery of strength in these patients appears poor.[52]

West Nile virus infection may be diagnosed by demonstrating West Nile virus RNA in serum, CSF, or other tissues by reverse-transcriptase polymerase chain reaction, although this is insensitive.[53] More commonly, a diagnosis is made by demonstration of West Nile virus IgM in CSF or serum by antibody-capture enzyme-linked immunosorbent assay. When serum West Nile virus IgM is present, diagnosis is confirmed by a fourfold increase in West Nile virus IgG titers between acute and convalescent sera obtained 4 weeks apart. Positive IgM and IgG antibody titers should be confirmed by plaque-reduction viral neutralization assay to exclude false-positive results related to other flaviviral infections such as St. Louis encephalitis. Serology may not become positive until 8 days after symptom onset.[39]

Particularly in the absence of a more typical encephalitic presentation of West Nile virus infection, a high index of clinical suspicion is needed to make a diagnosis of West Nile virus acute flaccid paralysis syndrome and to distinguish such cases from Guillain-Barré syndrome in patients presenting with acute weakness in the late summer or fall. Electrodiagnostic studies may help localize the pathology to the ventral horns of the spinal cord or ventral roots in West Nile virus cases and to exclude findings of segmental demyelination suggesting Guillain-Barré syndrome. CSF should also be evaluated to help discriminate between the albuminocytologic dissociation of Guillain-Barré syndrome and the lymphocytic pleocytosis observed in West Nile virus infection.

Although there is currently no specific treatment for West Nile virus acute flaccid paralysis syndrome, a multicenter study to evaluate the efficacy of Israeli IVIg in patients with West Nile virus meningoencephalitis or weakness began in the summer of 2003. The IVIg for this study contains high levels of West Nile virus antibodies because it was prepared from sera obtained after an Israeli West Nile virus epidemic in 2000.[54] Two candidate vaccines against West Nile virus are also being evaluated.[51]

Myasthenia Gravis

Myasthenia gravis is a consequence of autoimmune attack on the acetylcholine receptor complex at the postsynaptic membrane of the neuromuscular junction. This process results in clinical weakness with a fluctuating pattern that is most marked after prolonged muscle exertion. Myasthenia gravis occurs at a higher rate in early adulthood in women, but in later life the incidence rates for men and women become nearly equal. The reported prevalence is 14.2 cases per 100,000 population.[55] Myasthenia gravis typically involves ocular muscle weakness producing ptosis and diplopia, as well as bulbar muscle weakness resulting in dysphagia and dysarthria. This diagnosis should be considered in patients who have acute respiratory failure with these cranial nerve findings. A clinical diagnosis of myasthenia gravis may be supported by edrophonium testing, by electrophysiologic studies including repetitive nerve stimulation studies and single-fiber electromyography, and by acetylcholine receptor and muscle-specific receptor tyrosine kinase (MuSK) antibody testing.

Approximately 20% of patients with myasthenia gravis develop myasthenic crisis with respiratory failure requiring mechanical ventilation.[56] Intensivists may also encounter myasthenic patients for management of complications of immunomodulating treatment or for postoperative care after thymectomy The most common precipitating factors for myasthenic crisis include bronchopulmonary infections (29%) and aspiration (10%).[57] Other precipitating factors include sepsis, surgical procedures, rapid tapering of immune modulation, beginning treatment with corticosteroids, pregnancy, and exposure to drugs that may increase myasthenic weakness (Box 37-2).[58] Patients with myasthenia gravis are exceptionally sensitive to nondepolarizing neuromuscular blocking agents but are resistant to depolarizing agents.[59] Thymomas are associated with more fulminant disease and have been identified in about one third of patients in myasthenic crisis.[57]

Although sometimes less appreciated than respiratory muscle weakness, upper airway muscle weakness is a common mechanism leading to myasthenic crisis.[60] Oropharyngeal and laryngeal muscle weakness may result in upper airway collapse with obstruction, along with inability to swallow secretions that may also obstruct the airway and become aspirated. Because direct assessment of oropharyngeal muscle strength is impractical, a focused history and examination to assess surrogate muscles in the head and neck region is important. Findings of bulbar myasthenia associated with upper airway compromise include flaccid dysarthria with hypernasal, staccato, or hoarse speech, dysphagia (sometimes associated with nasal regurgitation), and chewing fatigue. Patients may exhibit facial weakness with difficulty holding air within the cheeks. Jaw closure is often weak and cannot be maintained against resistance. Patients with myasthenic tongue weakness may be unable to protrude the tongue into either cheek. Although

---

Box 37-2

DRUGS THAT MAY INCREASE WEAKNESS IN MYASTHENIA GRAVIS

Neuromuscular blocking agents
Selected antibiotics:
   Aminoglycosides, particularly gentamycin
   Macrolides, particularly erythromycin and azithromycin
Selected cardiovascular agents:
   Beta-blockers
   Calcium channel blockers
   Procainamide
Quinidine
Quinine
Corticosteroids
Magnesium salts:
   Antacids, laxatives, intravenous tocolytics
Iodinated contrast agents
D-Penicillamine

neck flexors are often weaker, a dropped head syndrome due to neck extensor weakness may occur. Vocal cord abductor paralysis may produce laryngeal obstruction with associated stridor.[61,62]

Patients with features of impending myasthenic crisis including severe bulbar weakness, marginal vital capacity (less than 20 to 25 mL/kg), weak cough with difficulty clearing secretions from the airway, or paradoxical breathing while supine should be admitted to an ICU and made NPO to prevent aspiration.[63] Serial vital capacity and NIF measurements may be used to monitor ventilatory function in impending myasthenic crisis. However, with significant bulbar weakness, these measurements are often inaccurate if the patient has difficulty sealing the lips around the spirometer mouthpiece or is unable to seal the nasopharynx. Vital capacity measurements may not reliably predict respiratory failure in myasthenia gravis, owing to the fluctuating nature of myasthenic weakness.[64] The criteria for intubation and mechanical ventilation are similar to those discussed earlier for Guillain-Barré syndrome. If the upper airway is competent and there is no difficulty handling secretions or gross hypercapnia ($Paco_2 > 50$ mm Hg), intermittent nasal BiPAP may be a useful temporizing measure.[4] The majority of patients who develop hypercapnia in myasthenic crisis require intubation, as do those who are becoming fatigued.

Plasma exchange is an effective short-term immunomodulating treatment for myasthenic crisis and for surgical preparation in symptomatic myasthenic patients. Significant strength improvement in myasthenic crisis is well documented in several series,[65-69] although there have been no controlled clinical trials. We perform a series of five to six exchanges of 2 to 3 L every other day. Onset of improved strength is variable but generally occurs after two to three exchanges.

IVIg may represent an alternative short-term treatment for myasthenic exacerbations or crises in patients who are poor candidates for plasma exchange because of difficult vascular access or septicemia. Comparable efficacy for plasma exchange and IVIg was demonstrated in myasthenic exacerbations and crises in a relatively small randomized controlled trial of IVIg at 1.2 and 2 g/kg over 2 to 5 days.[70] However, in a retrospective multicenter study of myasthenic crisis, plasma exchange proved more effective than IVIg in ability to extubate at 2 weeks and in 1-month functional outcome.[69] Treatment failures to IVIg subsequently responding to plasma exchange have also been reported.[71] Recent experience with preoperative IVIg for thymectomy in myasthenia gravis suggests that the time course of maximal response may be considerably delayed in some patients.[72]

Corticosteroids (e.g., prednisone, 1 mg/kg/day) are occasionally used in prolonged myasthenic crises that fail to respond to treatment with plasma exchange or IVIg. If begun early in the course of myasthenic crisis, the transient increase in myasthenic weakness associated with initiating corticosteroids may prolong mechanical ventilation. When preceded by unequivocal improvement in strength after plasma exchange or IVIg treatment, long-term treatment with corticosteroids may begin, with reduced risk for corticosteroid-related exacerbations.

In the context of myasthenic crisis, excessive dosing of cholinesterase inhibitors may superimpose a cholinergic crisis due to depolarization blockade and result in increased weakness. Other symptoms of cholinergic crisis include muscle fasciculations and prominent muscarinic symptoms including miosis, excessive lacrimation and salivation, abdominal cramping, nausea, vomiting, diarrhea, thick bronchial secretions, diaphoresis, and bradycardia. Cholinergic crisis is rare in contemporary series of myasthenic crisis,[57] and it is now common practice to avoid repeated dose escalations of cholinesterase inhibitors in impending myasthenic crisis and to discontinue the use of cholinesterase inhibitors after intubation to reduce muscarinic complications. When there is a question of cholinergic excess contributing to respiratory insufficiency, it is most prudent to discontinue all cholinesterase inhibitors, protect the airway, and support respiration as necessary.

Thymectomy may result in long-term improvement in patients with a suspected thymoma or with a life expectancy of more than 10 years.

However, a patient in acute respiratory failure is generally considered a poor operative risk, and thymectomy is generally delayed until the patient's condition has improved.[73] Post-thymectomy pain control and ventilatory function may be improved by postoperative administration of epidural morphine.[74]

NEUROMUSCULAR DISEASES SECONDARY TO CRITICAL ILLNESS AND ITS TREATMENT

Critical Illness Polyneuropathy

Critical illness polyneuropathy is a widespread axonal peripheral neuropathy that develops in the context of multiple organ failure and sepsis. This entity was recognized by several investigators in 1983[75-77] and has been further characterized in large part by Bolton and colleagues.[78,79] In a prospective series of 43 consecutive patients with sepsis and multiorgan failure, 70% developed electrophysiologic evidence of a sensorimotor axonal neuropathy, and 15 patients developed difficulty weaning from mechanical ventilation as a consequence of the neuropathy.[80] Critical illness polyneuropathy is possibly the most common neuromuscular cause of prolonged ventilator dependency in patients without prior known neuromuscular disease.[81] Given the limitations to detailed clinical motor and sensory examinations in the setting of critical illness, the clinical features of critical illness polyneuropathy (extremity muscle weakness and wasting, distal sensory loss, and paresthesias) may not be recognized. Deep tendon reflexes are generally reduced or absent. In the setting of superimposed central nervous system insult with pyramidal tract dysfunction, however, deep tendon reflexes may be normal or increased.[82]

Electrodiagnostic studies are important in establishing a diagnosis of critical illness polyneuropathy, because the clinical findings may be unobtainable or indeterminate in this setting.[82] Nerve conduction findings include normal or near-normal conduction velocity and latency values and significantly reduced compound muscle action potential and sensory nerve action potential amplitudes. Needle electrode examination reveals denervation changes that are most marked in distal muscles, including fibrillation potentials, positive sharp waves, and reduced recruitment of motor unit potentials.[83] With recovery over time, the denervation potentials abate, and the motor unit potentials become polyphasic and enlarged. Peripheral nerve histopathology has revealed widespread primary axonal degeneration in distal motor and sensory fibers, and skeletal muscle has exhibited fiber-type grouping.[79]

Although the clinical history is usually adequate to distinguish between critical illness polyneuropathy and Guillain-Barré syndrome, the latter has developed in the context of recent surgery complicated by infection.[84] In some such instances, it may be necessary to differentiate between these two peripheral neuropathic disorders in a patient with extremity weakness and inability to wean from mechanical ventilation. Although only a few severe cases of critical illness polyneuropathy have been associated with facial weakness,[85] facial and oropharyngeal weakness are common in Guillain-Barré syndrome.[84] Dysautonomia and occasionally external ophthalmoplegia are also observed in Guillain-Barré syndrome but have virtually never been attributed to critical illness polyneuropathy.[85]

Electrophysiologic findings are also helpful in distinguishing these two disorders. Features of segmental demyelination may be observed in Guillain-Barré syndrome on nerve conduction studies (e.g., reduced conduction velocity, prolonged distal and F-wave latencies, conduction block, and temporal dispersion of compound muscle action potentials); these findings are not observed in critical illness polyneuropathy. Needle electromyographic findings may differ in that relatively less spontaneous activity is observed in clinically weak muscles within the first few days in Guillain-Barré syndrome.[83] Although electrophysiologic studies are quite helpful in demonstrating the classic demyelinating form of Guillain-Barré syndrome, an electrophysiologic distinction between axonal forms of Guillain-Barré syndrome and critical illness polyneuropathy may not be reliable. The mean CSF protein level in Guillain-Barré syndrome is significantly higher than in critical illness polyneuropathy, although there is overlap between these populations.[83] Peripheral nerve histopathology may also distinguish between these two groups, because segmental demyelination and inflammatory changes may be observed in Guillain-Barré syndrome and are not seen in critical illness polyneuropathy.[79]

Although overall prognosis in critical illness polyneuropathy is dependent on recovery from the underlying critical illness, most patients who survive experience a functional recovery from the neuropathy within several months.[79] Critical illness polyneuropathy may prolong ventilator dependence, but it does not worsen long-term prognosis.[82] Proper positioning and padding are important to prevent compression neuropathies, because prognosis from superimposed compression neuropathies in the context of critical illness polyneuropathy is less favorable.[82]

The pathophysiology of critical illness polyneuropathy is unknown. No clear metabolic, drug, nutritional, or toxic factors have been identified,[79] although the severity of critical illness polyneuropathy has been correlated with the amount of time in the ICU, the number of invasive procedures, an increased glucose level, a reduced albumin level,[80] and the severity of multiple organ failure.[86] Given the common antecedents of multiple organ failure and sepsis in which significant release of various cytokines occurs, increased microvascular permeability has been postulated to ultimately result in axonal hypoxia and degeneration as a consequence of endoneurial edema.[87]

Prolonged Effects of Neuromuscular Blocking Agents

Prolonged neuromuscular blockade may occur with most depolarizing and nondepolarizing agents, particularly when hepatic or renal function is impaired.[88] In one study, administration of vecuronium for 2 or more consecutive days resulted in prolonged neuromuscular blockade and paralysis lasting from 6 hours to 7 days.[89] Although vecuronium is hepatically metabolized, patients with renal failure were susceptible to prolonged effects due to delayed excretion of the active 3-desacetyl metabolite. Acidosis and elevated serum magnesium levels were also associated with prolonged paralytic effects of vecuronium. A peripheral nerve stimulator may be used to monitor muscle twitch responses to a train-of-four stimulus during use of neuromuscular blocking agents. Drug dosage should be titrated to preserve one or two twitches to avoid overdosing. Two- to 3-hertz repetitive nerve stimulation studies may also be used to confirm neuromuscular blockade when it is suspected. Since atracurium and cisatracurium do not require organ metabolism for clearance, they are rarely associated with this problem.

Acute Quadriplegic Myopathy

The syndrome known as *acute quadriplegic myopathy*[90] or *acute myopathy of intensive care*[91] was originally described in 1977 in a young woman who developed severe myopathy after treatment of status asthmaticus with high doses of corticosteroids and pancuronium.[92] Subsequent to that report, there have been numerous citations of an acute myopathy developing in critically ill patients without preexisting neuromuscular disease. Acute quadriplegic myopathy has developed most frequently in the setting of severe pulmonary disorders in which neuromuscular blockade is used to facilitate mechanical ventilation, and high doses of corticosteroids are concurrently administered. In a majority of reported cases, myopathy developed when nondepolarizing neuromuscular blocking agents were used for more than 2 days.[90-100] The development of acute, necrotizing myopathy with myosin loss also occurs in patients receiving high doses of corticosteroids and hypnotic doses of propofol and benzodiazepines to induce paralysis.[101] This observation highlights the significance of high-dose corticosteroid exposure in the development of this syndrome and suggests that paralyzed muscles may be generally susceptible to the toxic effects of corticosteroids. The mechanism of this myosin abnormality appears to lie at the level of transcriptional regulation of protein synthesis.[102] The occurrence of acute quadriplegic myopathy after organ transplantation may be caused by the use of high doses of corticosteroids to prevent graft rejection, along with perioperative exposure to neuromuscular blocking agents.[103]

Although most cases of acute quadriplegic myopathy have been associated with critical illness, high doses of corticosteroids, and paralytic agents, acute quadriplegic myopathy has developed after isolated corticosteroid exposure,[90,104-107] isolated nondepolarizing neuromuscular blocking agent use,[100,104,108] or neither.[109] Factors that may impair neuromuscular transmission (e.g., hypermagnesemia, aminoglycoside exposure), factors that may slow the elimination of nondepolarizing neuromuscular blocking agents (e.g., hepatic or renal failure), and factors associated with critical illness (e.g., sepsis and acidosis) have also been associated with acute quadriplegic myopathy.[93]

In typical cases, a diffuse flaccid quadriparesis with involvement of respiratory muscles and muscle wasting evolves after several days of induced paralysis. External ophthalmoparesis has rarely been noted.[110] Sensation remains intact, but deep tendon reflexes are reduced or absent. The creatine kinase level is commonly elevated, but this may not be observed if creatine kinase is measured well after the myopathy has developed. Although the paralysis may be quite severe and may necessitate or prolong mechanical ventilation, the prognosis from the myopathy itself is good, with functional recovery over several weeks to months.[95] Electromyographic findings include reduced amplitude of compound motor action potentials with normal sensory nerve action potentials and normal nerve conduction velocities. M-wave amplitude improvement accompanies clinical recovery.[100] Repetitive nerve stimulation studies may yield significant decremental responses while residual effects of nondepolarizing neuromuscular blocking agents or their active metabolites persist.[93,100] Needle electromyography often reveals small, low-amplitude, polyphasic motor unit potentials exhibiting early recruitment, sometimes along with positive sharp waves and fibrillation potentials.

A spectrum of muscle histologic changes may be observed, ranging from type II fiber atrophy and loss of adenosine triphosphatase (ATPase) reactivity in atrophic fibers to fiber necrosis in severe cases. However, the distinctive finding in most cases of acute quadriplegic myopathy is an extensive loss of thick filaments corresponding to myosin loss.[90,94,99,104,109] This finding may be demonstrated with immunohistochemical staining or electron microscopy. The increased expression of steroid receptors in denervated and immobilized muscle[111] may render these muscles susceptible to toxic catabolic effects of steroids.[90] Given the growing recognition of acute quadriplegic myopathy, the use of high doses of corticosteroids should be avoided if possible when neuromuscular blockade or induced paralysis is required.

KEY POINTS

1. Respiratory dysfunction due to neuromuscular disease typically presents with a combination of upper airway dysfunction and diminished tidal volume (V_T).

2. Along with vital capacity, trended measurement of the maximum inspiratory pressure (PImax or negative inspiratory force [NIF]) is a useful index of ventilatory capacity. Inability to maintain a PImax greater than 20 to 25 cm H_2O usually indicates a need for mechanical ventilatory assistance.

3. Autonomic failure and pulmonary embolism are now the major causes of mortality in Guillain-Barré syndrome.

4. Evidence-based guidelines for Guillain-Barré syndrome immunotherapy have been published by the Quality Standards Subcommittee of the American Academy of Neurology. Plasma exchange is recommended for adult patients who cannot walk within 4 weeks of symptom onset. Intravenous immune globulin (IVIg) is recommended in these patients within 2 or possibly 4 weeks of symptom onset. Plasma exchange and IVIg are considered equivalent in efficacy, and no additional benefit is conferred by combining these treatments. In light of the therapeutic equivalence, the decision whether to employ plasma exchange or IVIg in treating acute Guillain-Barré syndrome may be determined by resource availability and by avoiding potential side effects related to a patient's medical comorbidities.

5. In the initial North American outbreak of West Nile virus, about 10% of infected patients experienced flaccid weakness with clinical features resembling Guillain-Barré syndrome.

6. Approximately 20% of patients with myasthenia gravis develop myasthenic crisis with respiratory failure requiring mechanical ventilation.

7. Critical illness polyneuropathy is a widespread axonal peripheral neuropathy that develops in the context of multiple organ failure and sepsis. Critical illness polyneuropathy is possibly the most common neuromuscular cause of prolonged ventilator dependency in patients without prior known neuromuscular disease.

8. Acute quadriplegic myopathy has developed most frequently in the setting of severe pulmonary disorders in which neuromuscular blockade is used to facilitate mechanical ventilation, and high-dose corticosteroids are concurrently administered. Given the growing recognition of acute quadriplegic myopathy, the use of high-dose corticosteroids should be avoided if possible when neuromuscular blockade is required.

ANNOTATED REFERENCES

Hughes RA, Swan AV, Raphaël JC, Annane D, van Koningsveld R, van Doorn PA. Immunotherapy for Guillain-Barré syndrome: a systematic review. Brain 2007;130:2245-5.
This contemporary report derives evidence-based guidelines for immunotherapy (plasma exchange, IVIg, corticosteroids) in Guillain-Barré syndrome based on a review of available literature.

Chawla J, Gruener G. Management of critical illness polyneuropathy and myopathy. Neurol Clin 2010;28:961-77.
An excellent comprehensive review of this difficult management problem.

Sejvar JJ, Haddad MB, Tierney BC, et al. Neurologic manifestations and outcome of West Nile virus infection. JAMA 2003;290:511-5.
This community-based prospective case series of patients with suspected West Nile virus infection in Louisiana documents a spectrum of neurologic presentations of acute West Nile virus infection, including a poliomyelitis-like syndrome of irreversible flaccid paralysis.

Thomas CE, Mayer SA, Gungor Y, et al. Myasthenic crisis: clinical features, mortality, complications, and risk factors for prolonged intubation. Neurology 1997;48:1253-60.
This large series provides a contemporary review of myasthenic crisis, including its antecedents, course, complications, and outcome subsequent to the widespread use of immunotherapy in myasthenia gravis.

Witt NJ, Zochodne DW, Bolton CF, et al. Peripheral nerve function in sepsis and multiple organ failure. Chest 1991;99:176-84.
This prospective series identified a 70% incidence of polyneuropathy developing in patients with multiorgan failure and sepsis.

REFERENCES

Access the complete reference list online at http://www.expertconsult.com.

38

Traumatic Brain Injury

KIMBERLY S. MEYER | DONALD W. MARION

It is estimated that 3.2 million people are living with long-term disability related to traumatic brain injury (TBI).[1] In addition to the personal toll, the direct and indirect costs of these disabilities are estimated to exceed $60 billion annually.[2] Americans sustain an estimated 1.6 million TBIs each year. Approximately 290,000 require hospitalization, and 51,000 die of their injuries.[3] However, the true incidence of TBI is unknown because current surveillance methodologies do not capture those treated in non-hospital settings (e.g., primary care office) or those who do not seek treatment at all.

TBI is the leading cause of morbidity and mortality for Americans between the ages of 1 and 45 years. Teenagers and the elderly are most at risk, although the primary causes vary demographically. Motor vehicle crashes are the main cause of head injuries in those 5 to 64 years old, whereas falls are most common in people aged 65 years and older. The primary cause of penetrating head injury is gunshot wounds. Males have twice the risk of sustaining TBI as females across all age groups and are three times more likely to die as a result of their injury.

TBI death rates in the United States fell during the 1980s. A substantial decline in motor vehicle–related fatalities was primarily responsible. At the same time, the incidence of gunshot wounds to the head rose, and in 1990, firearms surpassed motor vehicle crashes as the single largest cause of death due to TBI in some urban areas. However, in-hospital mortality rose to 8% during the last decade, presumably because of the increase in hospitalization rates of severe and moderate TBI.[4]

Pathophysiology

Trauma to the head causes primary injury such as skull fracture, cerebral contusion, and hemorrhage that is a direct physical consequence of the impact. Hours or days after the traumatic incident, secondary injury usually occurs and may be a major determinant of the patient's ultimate neurologic outcome.

PRIMARY INJURY

Injury to the brain is caused by external forces to the head that strain the tissue beyond its structural tolerance.[5] These forces can be classified as contact or inertial.[6] Contact forces typically produce focal injuries such as skull fractures, contusions, and epidural or subdural hematomas. Inertial forces result from the brain undergoing acceleration or deceleration (translational, rotational, or both) and can occur without head impact. Inertial forces can cause focal or diffuse brain injuries: pure translational acceleration leads to focal injuries such as contrecoup contusions, intracerebral hematomas, and subdural hematomas, whereas rotational or angular acceleration, common with high-speed motor vehicle crashes, usually causes diffuse injuries. Although external signs of head injury such as scalp abrasions, lacerations, and hematomas are common with blunt-force trauma, the brain can also be severely injured solely by inertial forces, without evidence of scalp or facial injuries.

Skull fracture results from a contact force to the head that is usually severe enough to cause at least brief loss of consciousness. Linear fractures are the most common type of skull fracture and typically occur over the lateral convexities of the skull. Most often, they are nondisplaced cracks in the skull (linear fractures), but a particularly intense impact can cause a gap (diastasis) between the edges of the fracture. A depressed skull fracture, in which skull fragments are pushed into the cranial vault, usually results from blunt force by an object with a relatively small surface area, such as a hammer (Figure 38-1). The base of the skull can be fractured by severe blunt trauma to the forehead or the occiput. Basilar skull fractures are most common in the anterior skull base and often involve the cribriform plate, disrupting the olfactory nerves (Figure 38-2). Posterior basilar skull fractures may extend through the petrous bone and internal auditory canal, thereby damaging the acoustic and the facial nerves.

Skull fractures per se are less detrimental than the associated damage to underlying tissues or vessels. For example, linear skull fractures that involve the squamous portion of the temporal bone are frequently accompanied by a tear of the middle meningeal artery, causing an epidural hematoma. They may also cause facial nerve injury, exhibited as facial asymmetry that can present immediately or in a delayed fashion. Treatment may require steroids or in severe cases, surgical decompression of the facial nerve. Depressed skull fractures are often associated with contusions of the underlying brain tissue, and a scalp laceration overlying a depressed skull fragment can contaminate the fragment with bacteria from the scalp and hair. With a basilar skull fracture, the dura underlying the fracture is often disrupted, resulting in a cerebrospinal fluid (CSF) fistula and leakage of CSF from the nose or ear. Such fistulas allow bacteria to enter the intracranial space from the normally colonized nose, paranasal sinuses, or external auditory canal.

Common posttraumatic intracranial lesions are hemorrhage (epidural, subdural, and intraparenchymal), contusion, and diffuse brain injury. Subdural hematomas are seen in 20% to 25% of all comatose victims of TBI (Figure 38-3). They develop between the surface of the brain and the inner surface of the dura and are believed to result from the tearing of bridging veins over the cortical surface or from disruption of major venous sinuses or their tributaries. The hematoma typically spreads over most of the cerebral convexity; the dural reflections of the falx cerebri prevent expansion to the contralateral hemisphere. Swelling of the cerebral hemisphere is common in those with subdural hematomas, given the associated damage to underlying brain tissue. Underlying cerebral contusions were found in 67% of patients with subdural hematomas in one series.[7] Subdural hematomas are classified as acute, subacute, or chronic, each having a characteristic appearance on computed tomography (CT): acute hematomas are bright white, subacute lesions are isodense with brain tissue and are therefore often overlooked, and chronic hematomas are hypodense relative to the brain.

Epidural hematomas develop between the inner table of the skull and the dura, usually when the middle meningeal artery or one of its branches is torn by a skull fracture. They occur in 8% to 10% of those rendered comatose by TBI.[8,9] The majority of epidural hematomas are located in the temporal or parietal regions, but they can also occur over the frontal or occipital lobes and (rarely) in the posterior fossa. They appear as hyperdense mass lesions on CT. Unlike subdural hematomas, their spread is limited by the suture lines of the skull, where the dura is very adherent. Because an epidural space normally does not exist, the clot must strip the dura from the inner table of the skull as it enlarges, resulting in its classic biconvex or lenticular shape (Figure 38-4). Epidural hematomas are uncommon in infants and toddlers, presumably because their skulls are more deformable and less likely to fracture, and in TBI victims older than 60 years, because the dura is extremely adherent to the skull.

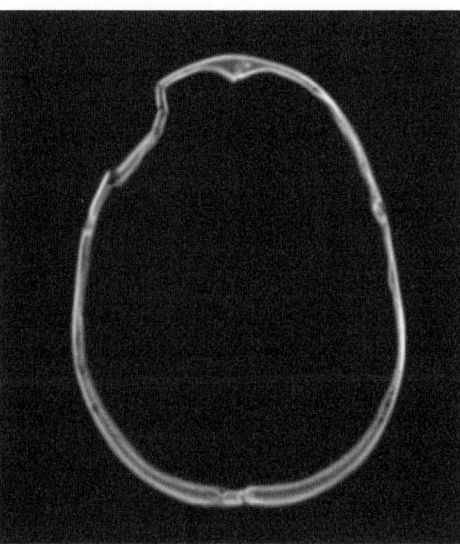

Figure 38-1   Right frontal depressed skull fracture caused by an assault with a hammer (axial CT scan, bone window).

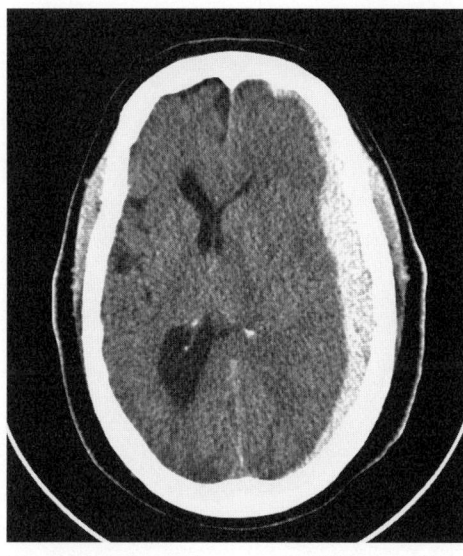

Figure 38-3   Acute subdural hematomas (SDH) typically spread over entire surface of the hemisphere. Occasionally, mixed-density SDH is seen, indicative of injuries occurring at different times.

An intraparenchymal hematoma is a hemorrhage within the brain substance that occurs after a very severe TBI. It is usually associated with contusions of the surrounding tissue. Duret's hemorrhage, or hemorrhage into the base of the pons or midbrain, is thought to result from disruption of the perforating arteries at the time of uncal herniation. Such brainstem hemorrhage almost always leads to death or minimally responsive survival.

Traumatic subarachnoid hemorrhage often results from tearing of the corticomeningeal vessels. Though common after severe TBI, subarachnoid hemorrhage does not produce a hematoma or mass effect.[10] However, it may be associated with an increased risk for posttraumatic vasospasm, which may adversely affect clinical outcome.[11]

Contusions are heterogeneous lesions comprising punctate hemorrhage, edema, and necrosis and are often associated with other intracranial lesions. One or more contusions occur in 20% to 25% of patients with severe TBI. Because they evolve over time, contusions

may not be evident on the initial CT scan or may appear as small areas of punctate hyperdensities (hemorrhages) with surrounding hypodensity (edema) (Figure 38-5). Local neuronal damage and hemorrhage lead to edema that may expand over the next 24 to 48 hours. With time, contusions may coalesce and look more like intracerebral hematomas. Depending on their size and location, they may cause significant mass effect, resulting in midline shift, subfalcine herniation, or transtentorial herniation. Contusions are most common in the inferior frontal cortex and the anterior temporal lobes,[12] where the surface of the inner table of the skull is very irregular; they result from shifting of the brain over this irregular surface at the time of impact. Direct blunt-force trauma to the head can produce a contusion in the tissue underlying the point of impact (coup contusion). If the head was in motion upon collision with a rigid surface, a contusion may occur in the brain contralateral to the point of impact (contrecoup contusion).

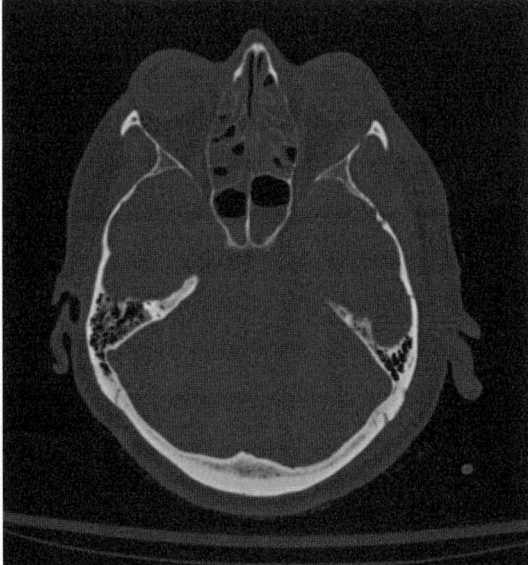

Figure 38-2   Basilar skull fractures through the anterior skull base typically cause cerebrospinal fluid rhinorrhea and tears in adjacent dura. CT scans through the base of the skull may not show the fracture itself but often show fluid in the sphenoid sinus or other paranasal sinuses (axial CT scan, bone window).

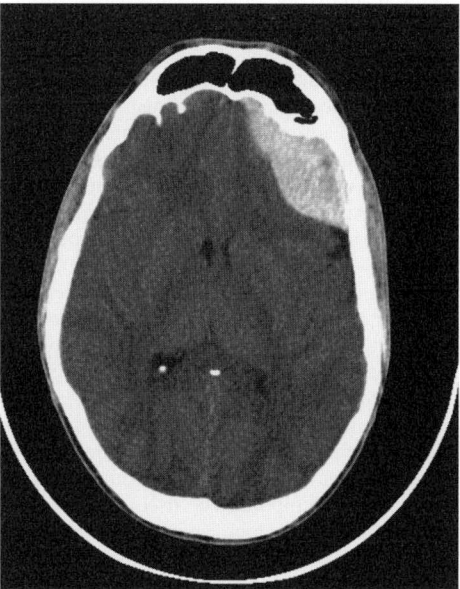

Figure 38-4   Epidural hematomas have a lens shape and smooth inner border because they strip the dura from the inner table of the skull as they enlarge (axial CT scan).

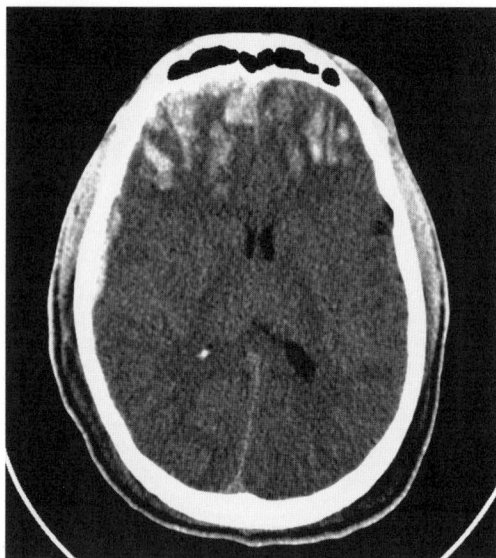

Figure 38-5 Contusions are most common in the inferior temporal and frontal lobes. In the first few hours after injury, they appear only as areas of hemorrhage mixed with edematous brain. Within 24 to 48 hours after injury, further hemorrhage may occur, causing significant enlargement of the contusion and hematoma (axial CT scan).

Diffuse axonal injury refers to lacerations or punctate contusions at the interface between the gray and white matter. Such punctate contusions are thought to result from the disparate densities of the gray and white matter and the consequent difference in centripetal force associated with a rotational vector of injury.[13] Thus, diffuse axonal injury most often occurs after a high-speed motor vehicle crash, during which severe angular and rotational forces are applied to the head. Diffuse axonal injury was once thought to result solely from mechanical disruption at the time of impact; however, more recent research has identified cases in which the histologic footprints of diffuse axonal injury, such as fragmentation of axons and axonal swelling, do not appear until 24 to 48 hours after the incident, suggesting that some cases are a secondary manifestation of trauma.[14,15] Diffuse axonal injury is present in almost half of all patients with severe TBI and in a third of those who die, and it is a common cause of persistent vegetative or minimally conscious state.

Posttraumatic intracranial lesions cause neurologic dysfunction via direct and in some cases indirect mechanisms. By destroying brain tissue, contusions and intraparenchymal hemorrhage cause deficits directly related to the function of the damaged tissue. Uncal herniation is also an important mechanism of temporary or permanent neurologic deficits.[16,17] Semirigid dural reflections divide the intracranial contents into compartments. The tentorium cerebelli separates the anterior and middle cranial fossae from the posterior cranial fossa. The brainstem, specifically the midbrain, traverses an opening, the tentorial foramen, in the anterior central portion of this partition. The medial portion of the temporal lobe, the uncus, lies on both sides of the tentorial foramen. Because the most common TBIs, such as hematomas and contusions, are usually located over the lateral surfaces of the brain, and because the brain's extreme lateral surface is the rigid skull, such lesions tend to depress the brain medially. Therefore, a subdural hematoma over the surface of the temporal lobe or a hemorrhagic contusion of the temporal lobe itself is likely to displace the medial portion of the temporal lobe (uncus) into the tentorial foramen (i.e., uncal herniation). Such displacement compresses the midbrain, which contains neurons that are part of the reticular activating system. At the base of the midbrain is the crus cerebri, which contains pyramidal fibers from the cortex, and the third cranial nerve, which exits the midbrain through the interpeduncular cistern. Midbrain

compression due to uncal herniation damages the reticular activating system, causing loss of consciousness; stretches the third cranial nerve and its associated parasympathetic fibers, causing pupil dilatation and loss of the light reflex; and injures the pyramidal fibers in the crus cerebri, causing abnormal posturing responses in the contralateral arm and leg.

Medial displacement of a cerebral hemisphere resulting from hemispheric swelling or a subdural or epidural hematoma also can cause herniation of the cingulate gyrus under the falx cerebri. Permanent neurologic dysfunction usually does not result, however.

Intracranial hypertension is a major cause of posttraumatic neurologic morbidity and mortality.[18] The intracranial pressure (ICP) is defined by the volume of CSF, blood, and brain tissue in the cranial vault. The volume of these components is dynamic, and the brain can accommodate moderate changes in any of the three. For example, the blood volume can rise or fall by as much as 30% to 40%, CSF absorption can increase to reduce the size of the ventricles by up to 90%, and brain tissue itself is compressible. Thus, the intracranial volume can gain 100 to 150 mL, equivalent to a moderate-sized subdural hematoma, without the ICP increasing significantly. When these buffering mechanisms have been exhausted, however, even a small increase in the size of a hematoma will cause a rapid rise in ICP. If appropriate treatment is delayed, the ICP may approach the mean arterial pressure (MAP), causing a hydrostatic block of blood flow to the brain and brain death. Intracranial hypertension, particularly if refractory to medical or surgical treatment, is the most common cause of death after severe TBI.

SECONDARY INJURY

Posttraumatic ischemia initiates a cascade of metabolic events that lead to the surplus production of oxygen free radicals,[19-21] excitatory amino acids,[22,23] cytokines,[24,25] and other inflammatory agents.[26] Glutamate and aspartate are the excitatory amino acids most commonly implicated in excitotoxic injury,[27] which is mediated by activation of N-methyl-D-aspartate, α-amino-3-hydroxy-5-methylisoazole-4-proprionic acid, or kainic acid receptors.[23] Overactivation of these receptors causes an excessive influx of ionized calcium into the cytosol, and elevated amounts of ionized intracellular calcium play a key role in neurodegeneration after injury to the central nervous system (CNS).[28,29] In addition, posttraumatic nonischemic events such as an increase in intracellular free Ca^{++} via receptor-gated or voltage-dependent ion channels induce the release of oxygen free radicals from mitochondria.[30] Excessive levels of highly reactive oxygen free radicals cause lipid peroxidation of cell membranes, oxidation of intracellular proteins and nucleic acids, and activation of phospholipases A_2 and C, which hydrolyze membrane phospholipids, thereby releasing arachidonic acid. The liberation of arachidonic acid triggers the generation of free fatty acids, leukotrienes, and thromboxane B_2, all of which are associated with neurodegeneration and poor outcome after experimental TBI.[31-33] Inflammatory cytokines, particularly interleukin (IL)-1, IL-6, and tumor necrosis factor, also are overproduced after TBI.[34-36] In animal models, posttraumatic activation of microglia is a principal source of these cytokines.[25] IL-1 and IL-6 provoke an exuberant cellular inflammatory response believed to be responsible for astrogliosis, edema, and tissue destruction.[26,37]

TBI also increases extracellular potassium levels,[38] leading to an imbalance of intracellular and extracellular K^+, disruption of the Na^+/K^+-ATPase cell membrane regulatory mechanisms, and subsequent cell swelling.[39,40] Astrocyte swelling has been attributed to the clearance of excessive extracellular K^+.[41] High levels of extracellular K^+ have also been implicated as the cause of widespread neuronal depolarization and spreading depression seen after experimental TBI.[27,38,42] Moreover, potassium stimulates increased oxygen uptake in glial cells, potentially depriving adjacent neurons of oxygen.[43,44] Severe TBI also causes a substantial decrease in extracellular magnesium (Mg^{++}) levels, thereby impairing normal glycolysis, cellular respiration, oxidative phosphorylation, and the biosyntheses of DNA, RNA, and protein.[45-47] Because

Mg^{++} competes with Ca^{++} at voltage-gated cell membrane–associated Ca^{++} channels, reduced levels of Mg^{++} will result in an abnormal influx of Ca^{++} into the cell.

Prehospital Care

The acutely injured brain is vulnerable to further damage from systemic hypotension, cerebral hypoperfusion, hypercarbia, hypoxemia, and elevated ICP. Preventing these physiologic insults is crucial to limiting secondary brain injury. Care of the TBI victim always should begin with evaluating and securing a patent airway and restoring normal breathing and circulation. Early endotracheal intubation usually benefits comatose patients. Securing and maintaining an airway are essential to optimal oxygenation and ventilation, and early intubation has been found to reduce mortality after severe TBI.[48]

The airway is usually most easily and safely secured by orotracheal intubation, a method in which most emergency medical personnel are trained and experienced. Patients with severe maxillofacial trauma may require nasotracheal intubation, but this is less desirable because it is a relatively blind procedure. The nasal passageways can be irritated, causing blood pressure (BP) and ICP to surge, and in those with severe anterior skull base fractures, the tube can inadvertently be passed into the brain. A third alternative for securing the airway is the laryngeal mask airway, an easily learned and rapidly applied device that has undergone successful field trials.[49] However, it does not protect against aspiration and cannot be used to achieve high airway pressures. A surgical airway (cricothyroidotomy) should be performed only after other attempts to secure an airway have failed, and only by an experienced provider.

The patient should be sedated and pharmacologically paralyzed before intubation, because irritation of the oropharynx typically causes transient hypertension, tachycardia, increased ICP, and agitation that can interfere with the procedure. Fentanyl, a short-acting opioid agonist that produces analgesia and sedation, is the most commonly used sedative. The usual dose is 3 to 5 µg/kg body weight, administered intravenously (IV) 3 minutes before intubation. Etomidate, an alternative to opioids, provides adequate sedation and is less likely to cause hypotension. Some prefer thiopental because it is an ultra-short-acting barbiturate and is thus less likely to conceal the neurologic status when the patient reaches the trauma center; however, it is more likely than other agents to cause hypotension. Neuromuscular blocking agents commonly used for tracheal intubation include succinylcholine (1.5 mg/kg IV), which has the advantages of rapid onset, complete reliability, and very short duration of action. This last attribute is particularly important in the prehospital setting, where attempts at intubation sometimes fail. Vecuronium (0.01 mg/kg IV) is an alternative that offers the theoretical advantage of being a nondepolarizing muscle relaxant. Because it has a relatively long duration of action (1 to 2 hours), it is less forgiving of failed intubation attempts. Table 38-1 shows a recommended rapid-sequence intubation pathway.

Supplemental oxygen should be provided before and immediately after intubation. Ventilatory rates of 10 to 12 breaths per minute for adults, 20 breaths per minute for children, and 25 breaths per minute

for infants should supply adequate oxygenation. Therapeutic hyperventilation is inadvisable unless neurologic deterioration is clearly evident during evaluation and transport. Aggressive hyperventilation can cause cerebral vasoconstriction, reducing already low cerebral blood flow (CBF) and potentially causing or exacerbating cerebral ischemia.

Rapid fluid resuscitation and restoration of a normal BP are critical in the prehospital setting, because hypotension has been associated with doubling of the mortality rate after severe TBI.[50] The most likely cause of hypotension is hemorrhage, usually in the abdomen or chest; therefore, hypovolemia should be assumed. Lactated Ringer's or normal saline solutions should be infused through a large-bore IV catheter as quickly as possible until normotension is achieved. Although preclinical studies suggest that hypertonic saline may be more effective than isotonic solutions for rapid volume resuscitation,[51,52] results of several small clinical trials have not been convincing.[53,54]

In all cases of severe TBI, defined as a Glasgow Coma Scale (GCS) score of 3 to 8 and an inability to follow commands, patients should be treated as if they have a spinal fracture until an adequate examination of the spine proves otherwise. Among those who survive long enough to reach the emergency department, the likelihood of a cervical spine fracture is 2% to 7%. More troubling, however, is that an estimated 10% to 25% of all posttraumatic spinal cord injuries are iatrogenic, occurring during transport to the hospital.[55] After respiratory and hemodynamic stabilization, the patient should be placed in a neutral position on a flat, hard surface. If the patient requires immediate tracheal intubation, it should be performed while another person provides in-line cervical spine immobilization. A rigid cervical spine collar should be placed as soon as possible. Next, the patient should be placed on a backboard; the cervical spine can then be further immobilized with a buttress of foam or towels placed on both sides of the head. To prevent any movement during transport, the patient should be strapped to the board in several locations.

The organization of emergency medical services and regional trauma programs has improved outcomes for victims of trauma, particularly those with severe TBI.[56] A very large prospective study of the cost and outcomes associated with trauma center designation found more than a 25% reduction in in-hospital mortality for those with severe TBI who were initially treated at a level I trauma center compared to similarly injured patients treated at hospitals of similar size that were not designated trauma centers.[57] This is likely because designation as a level I or II trauma center by the American College of Surgeons Committee on Trauma or a state health department ensures the availability of immediate neurosurgical care when the patient arrives. Therefore, every effort should be made to transport severely injured patients directly to a designated trauma center. Nonetheless, if an adequate airway or venous access cannot be obtained in the field, some patients may need to undergo respiratory or hemodynamic stabilization at a nearby emergency department en route to the trauma center. Once hemodynamic and airway stability is achieved, immediate transport to a designated trauma center should occur without delays for imaging or secondary surveys.

Emergency Department Care

Upon arrival at the trauma center, the emergency medical personnel should concisely report their prehospital assessment and management, including mechanism of injury, stabilizing maneuvers, medications given, initial vital signs, GCS score, and hemodynamic stability during transport. A thorough physical and radiographic examination to identify all life-threatening injuries should then be performed. Most trauma centers follow the Advanced Trauma Life Support protocol, a comprehensive routine that has proved successful in quickly detecting all major injuries.[58] First the airway is reassessed, and the need for tracheal intubation is carefully reconsidered. For patients intubated in the field, proper placement of the tracheal tube is verified both clinically and radiographically. When the airway is secure and adequate oxygenation is confirmed using a percutaneous oxygen saturation monitor or

TABLE 38-1	Recommended Rapid-Sequence Induction for Severely Head-Injured Patients

1. **Preoxygenation**
   100% oxygen for 5 min or four vital capacity breaths
2. **Pretreatment**
   Fentanyl (3 to 5 µg/kg IV)
3. **Wait 2 to 3 min if possible**
   Continue preoxygenation
4. **Neuromuscular blockade and sedation**
   Succinylcholine (1.5 mg/kg IV)
5. **Intubation with in-line cervical spine immobilization**
   Positive-pressure ventilation and possibly reparalysis with vecuronium if prolonged transport time is anticipated

TABLE 38-2	Glasgow Coma Scale[59]	
Response		*Points*
Speech		
Alert, oriented, and conversant		5
Confused, disoriented, but conversant		4
Intelligible words, not conversant		3
Unintelligible sounds		2
No verbalization, even with painful stimulus		1
Eye Opening		
Spontaneous		4
To verbal stimuli		3
To painful stimuli		2
None, even with painful stimuli		1
Motor		
Follows commands		6
Localizes painful stimulus		5
Withdraws from painful stimulus		4
Flexor posturing with central pain		3
Extensor posturing with central pain		2
No response to painful stimulus		1

Data from Teasdale G, Jennett B. Assessment of coma and impaired consciousness: a practical scale. Lancet. 1974;2(7872):81-84.

arterial blood gas analysis, two large-bore IV catheters are inserted to provide sufficient venous access for high-volume fluid resuscitation. An isotonic saline solution is infused to continue volume replacement, which probably began at the scene. Any life-threatening injuries such as overt hemorrhage, tension pneumothorax, or cardiac tamponade should be treated immediately upon discovery. A brief neurologic examination is performed, including assessment of the GCS score (Table 38-2), pupillary size and reaction to light, and symmetry and extent of extremity movements. The head is palpated to detect fractures, lacerations, or penetrating wounds, and lacerations are probed gently to ascertain the presence of a depressed skull fracture or foreign body. Large lacerations are compressed with pressure dressings or temporarily sutured to prevent further hemorrhage. Careful inspection of the head should reveal hemotympanum, periorbital or mastoid ecchymosis, and CSF rhinorrhea or otorrhea.

Oxygen saturation is monitored continually, and BP is measured frequently during this primary examination. A Foley catheter is placed to help monitor the fluid status, and an orogastric tube is inserted and connected to suction to decompress the stomach. Blood specimens are obtained and analyzed for glucose, electrolytes, complete blood count, platelets, prothrombin and partial thromboplastin times, and International Normalized Ratio (INR). Type and crossmatch of a blood specimen should be considered, and an arterial blood gas obtained. Serum and urine toxicology screens are advisable if alcohol or substance abuse is suspected, and women of child-bearing age should undergo a pregnancy test.

Coagulopathy resulting from TBI is thought to occur when hypoperfusion causes activation of the protein C pathway, thereby inducing alterations in the clotting cascade.[60] It is also commonly seen as a result of therapeutic anticoagulation with warfarin, especially in the geriatric population. Rapid identification and correction of coagulopathy is critical to prevent expansion of intracranial hematomas and allow surgical intervention. Fresh frozen plasma and cryoprecipitate can be used to correct the INR to 1.3 or less. Recombinant factor VIIa has been shown to decrease blood product requirements and costs associated with correction of coagulopathy.[61] Other studies demonstrate more rapid correction times compared to blood product administration, although differences in outcomes have not been significant. Product expense and concern for thromboembolic complications have limited the routine use of recombinant factor VIIa.

The initial x-ray evaluation is usually performed in the trauma bay during the primary survey and includes chest, pelvis, and lateral cervical spine films. If the lower cervical spine is not visible on the lateral cervical spine film, a swimmer's view can be obtained, or this area can be imaged with axial CT.

After all life-threatening injuries have been identified and stabilized, the immediate concern is whether the patient requires a craniotomy to evacuate an intracranial mass lesion. A CT scan of the head should be performed at intervals of 10 mm or less from the C2 vertebra to the vertex. In addition to posttraumatic intracranial lesions, the scan should be examined for brain swelling, patency of the basal cisterns, and other characteristics that will guide subsequent treatment. If no surgical intracranial mass lesion is evident on the scan of the head, CT scans of the chest and abdomen can be performed to detect occult hemorrhage in these cavities. If a surgical mass lesion is seen on the head CT scan, however, it should be evacuated immediately, postponing any other imaging studies. Diagnostic peritoneal lavage is often performed during the craniotomy to detect abdominal bleeding. Conversely, if hemodynamic instability necessitates an emergent laparotomy or thoracotomy before a head CT scan can be obtained, several diagnostic procedures can be performed in the operating room to confirm a suspected intracranial injury. These procedures include an air ventriculogram or diagnostic burr holes and are most appropriate if the patient has lateralizing neurologic deficits, particularly a unilateral fixed and dilated pupil.

Definitive Treatment

Critical to determining the severity of the brain injury and appropriate treatment are CT findings combined with a reliable postresuscitation GCS score and assessment of pupil size and reactivity. In the case of an acute subdural hematoma, for example, a patient with a moderate-sized lesion who has normal pupil size and reactivity and is able to follow commands might safely be treated nonoperatively. Conversely, surgery is unlikely to benefit an elderly patient with fixed and dilated pupils and a GCS score of 3 or 4, regardless of the CT findings. Other determining factors include size and location of the hematoma, presence and extent of an underlying contusion or brain swelling, and results of the neurologic examination. Neurologic deterioration, particularly a decline in mental status, suggests enlargement of the hematoma, and a new CT scan should be obtained promptly. Hematomas less than 10 mm thick that cause a midline shift of less than 5 mm can usually be observed, especially if they do not involve the middle cranial fossa.[62] If nonoperative management is chosen for an intracranial hematoma, the patient should be monitored with frequent neurologic assessments in the intensive care unit (ICU). If the patient cannot follow commands, ICP monitoring is recommended.

The classic presentation of a patient with an epidural hematoma is a period of unconsciousness immediately after impact to the head, followed by a so-called lucid interval in which consciousness returns for a few minutes to an hour or more before the patient lapses into a coma. This lucid interval actually occurs in less than a third of patients with epidural hematomas, however; most either remain conscious after the injury (smaller clots) or remain comatose.

A hematoma that compresses the temporal lobe is particularly ominous and can rapidly cause uncal herniation with minimal enlargement. Thus, such lesions warrant a lower threshold for evacuation compared with hematomas in other locations. If the clot is small enough to not require evacuation, it should be monitored with frequent CT scans during the first several days after injury. Enlarging middle fossa hematomas, even those large enough to cause herniation, do not always cause an increase in the ICP; therefore, ICP monitoring should not be relied on to follow their status.

The initial signs and symptoms of contusions vary greatly, depending on their size and location and the presence of other associated lesions. A small contusion may cause only a headache or no symptoms at all. If located in an eloquent area of the brain, such as the speech or motor areas, it may cause focal neurologic symptoms. Larger contusions, especially those involving the frontal or temporal lobes, typically cause elevated ICP and coma. Patients with small or

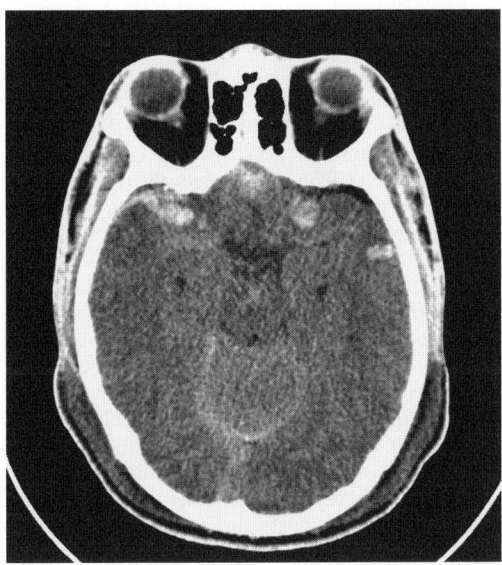

Figure 38-6 Temporal lobe contusions must be monitored closely because even a slight enlargement can cause uncal herniation, often without an increase in intracranial pressure (ICP) (axial CT scan).

deep-seated contusions without mass effect initially can be managed nonoperatively. The contusion should be followed closely with serial CT scans, however, because there is a 20% to 30% risk that the contusion will enlarge during the next 24 to 48 hours. The ICP should be monitored if the patient cannot follow commands. As with hematomas in the middle cranial fossa, contusions of the temporal lobes should be closely watched with CT scans. A temporal contusion can enlarge to the point of uncal herniation without a significant rise in ICP, so the threshold for evacuation of these lesions should be low (Figure 38-6). Unilateral frontal or temporal lobectomies are usually well tolerated and do not cause measurable neurologic deficits, while allowing space for further brain swelling.

In the ICU, the primary goal is to prevent cerebral ischemia and thereby limit secondary brain injury. The most common preventable causes of cerebral ischemia are hypotension, hypoxemia, and intracranial hypertension. Comprehensive physiologic monitoring should be performed so that these physiologic insults can be detected and treated promptly.

PHYSIOLOGIC MONITORING

Continual monitoring of the end-tidal partial pressure of carbon dioxide (Pco_2) and frequent analyses of arterial blood gases enable the early detection of deteriorating ventilatory status, which should prompt appropriate ventilator adjustments. Oxygen saturation should also be monitored continually with pulse oximetry. BP monitoring is best accomplished with an indwelling arterial catheter coupled to a pressure transducer. The catheter is usually inserted into the radial artery and can also be used to obtain arterial blood samples for blood gas analysis. Hypovolemia is a common cause of posttraumatic hypotension. It can result from overt hemorrhage, usually detected soon after injury; from occult hemorrhage, which may not be recognized for several hours or days; or from soft-tissue inflammation and swelling. Consequently, central venous pressure (CVP) monitoring should be considered for patients with severe TBI, particularly those with significant non-CNS injuries. Indwelling subclavian or internal jugular venous catheters are used, coupled to pressure transducers. In elderly patients or those with severe pulmonary contusions, intravascular volume may be more accurately assessed by pulmonary artery catheterization with a Swan-Ganz catheter. Monitoring urine output with an indwelling Foley catheter is essential for determining the patient's fluid status.

Continuous ICP monitoring is essential for all patients who have severe TBI and abnormal CT findings, because intracranial hypertension develops in 53% to 63% of such patients.[63] ICP monitoring is also recommended for comatose patients who are older than 40 years and have unilateral or bilateral motor posturing or a systolic blood pressure (SBP) less than 90 mm Hg, even if no abnormalities are seen on the initial CT scan.[64] The gold standard for ICP monitors is the ventricular catheter coupled to an external strain-gauge transducer.[65] It is accurate, reliable, and far less expensive than newer self-contained pressure-sensing devices. In addition, ventricular pressure is considered more reflective of global ICP than is subdural, subarachnoid, or epidural pressure. Catheters placed in these extracerebral spaces are more prone to occlusion and, owing to the effects of compartmentalization, typically record a pressure that is lower than the global ICP. Other advantages of the ventriculostomy method of ICP monitoring are that the system can be re-zeroed after insertion—not possible with most of the newer self-contained devices—and CSF can be withdrawn to treat intracranial hypertension. The overall complication rate for ventricular ICP monitoring is 7.7% (infection, 6.3%; hemorrhage, 1.4%),[63] and some studies indicate that the infection rate increases significantly when a catheter remains in place for more than 5 days.[66]

Alternatives to the ventriculostomy technique have been developed that provide relatively accurate measurements of global ICP, are easier to insert, and may cause fewer complications. They include devices that contain a pressure-sensing transducer (either strain-gauge or fiber-optic technology) within the tip of the catheter.[65] These pressure sensors provide reliable ICP measurements even if they are inserted into the white matter and are often used when a ventricular catheter is difficult to insert because of small or collapsed ventricles. The primary disadvantage is that CSF drainage is not possible. In addition, these devices can be calibrated only once, before insertion, and with some of them, measurement drift is as much as 1 to 2 mm Hg per day.

The cerebral perfusion pressure (CPP), defined as the difference between MAP and ICP, is a calculated physiologic measurement that is used to describe actual cerebral perfusion. Some have suggested that maintaining the CPP above a certain threshold is more important than any particular MAP or ICP.[67]

Devices that monitor the oxygen partial pressure of oxygen (Po_2) of brain tissue can be used to determine whether cerebral oxygenation is adequate. These monitors continually measure the tissue Po_2 in the small region of brain into which they are inserted. Studies suggest that mortality may be decreased in those undergoing oxygen directed therapy.[68] Although no methods are available for continuously monitoring global CBF, transcranial Doppler insonation of the middle cerebral arteries can provide indirect information. Positron emission tomography (PET) or CBF measurements with xenon, either as a radiolabeled agent or as a CT contrast medium, can provide periodic snapshots of the blood flow.

MEDICAL TREATMENT

Hypoxemia is best avoided with the use of tracheal intubation and mechanical ventilation. The fraction of inspired oxygen should be titrated to provide an arterial Po_2 of 100 mm Hg. Maintaining an arterial Pco_2 of approximately 35 mm Hg is advised to avoid the cerebral vasoconstriction associated with aggressive hyperventilation. A form of acute respiratory distress syndrome (ARDS) can develop in patients with severe chest injuries. In such cases, adequate oxygenation requires the use of positive end-expiratory pressure (PEEP). Concern has been raised that the use of PEEP in patients with TBI may increase the ICP. However, clinical studies have shown that in the presence of ARDS, up to 14 to 15 cm H_2O of PEEP can be used without measurable changes in ICP, most likely because ARDS significantly reduces pulmonary compliance.

Hypotension, defined as a MAP of less than 90 mm Hg, should be treated aggressively. Normovolemia should be restored by infusing isotonic saline as needed to achieve a central venous pressure of 7 to 12 cm H_2O. Hypotonic intravenous solutions can exacerbate cerebral edema and should be avoided. If the patient is anemic, packed red blood cells should be transfused to restore the hematocrit to at least 30%. If hypotension is refractory to volume resuscitation, the patient should be given a continuous IV infusion of a vasopressor medication, with the dose titrated to raise the MAP above 90 mm Hg. Norepinephrine has been shown to be most efficacious at maintaining MAP and CPP without deleteriously affecting ICP.[69]

Although some advocate the used of induced hypertension to raise the CPP above 70 mm Hg, particularly if the ICP is elevated and difficult to reduce,[70] others do not support this practice. A prospective, randomized clinical trial of patients with TBI compared a group whose CPP was kept above 70 mm Hg via induced hypertension with a group whose CPP was allowed to drift to 60 mm Hg.[71] Six-month clinical outcomes did not differ between the two groups. Moreover, the group whose CPP was kept above 70 mm Hg required more vasopressor agents and had a significantly higher incidence of ARDS and other pulmonary complications. Others have found that the brain tissue Po_2 in patients with TBI typically does not fall until the CPP drops below 60 mm Hg.[72] Based on these findings, the current recommendation is to maintain a CPP above 60 mm Hg.

Intracranial hypertension is defined as sustained ICP greater than 20 mm Hg. Several clinical studies have found that mortality and morbidity increase significantly when the ICP persistently remains above this threshold.[73] Based on this association and the widely accepted premise that elevated ICP can compromise cerebral perfusion and cause ischemia, the aggressive treatment of intracranial hypertension is almost uniformly endorsed. Before beginning therapy for intracranial hypertension, however, medical or physiologic conditions that can increase ICP should be considered and, if present, treated. These include seizures, fever, jugular venous outflow obstruction (e.g., poorly fitting cervical collars), and agitation.

Several medical and surgical options are available to reduce ICP. Depending on the type of brain injury, some may be more effective than others, and each is associated with potential adverse effects. A stepwise approach is usually followed, with the least toxic therapies utilized first and more toxic therapies added only if the initial treatment is unsuccessful. Sedation and neuromuscular blockade are often an effective first treatment, particularly if the patient is agitated or posturing. Narcotics (e.g., morphine, fentanyl), short-acting benzodiazepines (e.g., midazolam), or hypnotic agents such as propofol can be used for sedation, and vecuronium bromide as the paralytic agent. Narcotic-induced hypotension can be averted by using relatively low doses and ensuring the patient is normovolemic before treatment. Because the ability to obtain an accurate GCS score is lost during this treatment, the pupil status, ICP, and CT scans must be closely monitored.

If intracranial hypertension is refractory to sedation and neuromuscular blockade, intermittent ventricular CSF drainage is used. Intermittent rather than continuous drainage enables reliable measurement of the ICP. If these measures fail to reduce the ICP, a bolus administration of mannitol is recommended (0.25 to 1 g/kg every 3 to 4 hours as needed). This osmotic diuretic lowers ICP and increases CPP by expanding the blood volume, reducing the blood viscosity, and increasing CBF and oxygen delivery to the tissues within a few minutes of infusion. Its duration of effect averages 3 to 5 hours. Continuous infusion is less desirable than bolus infusion, because the former is more likely to lead to extravasation of the drug into brain tissue, causing a reverse osmotic gradient and increased edema and ICP.[74] The serum osmolarity and sodium level should be monitored frequently during mannitol administration. The drug should be discontinued if the serum sodium level exceeds 160 mg/dL or the osmolarity exceeds 320 mOsm in order to minimize the risk of acute tubular necrosis and renal failure. The intravascular volume should also be closely monitored to prevent dehydration. Recent studies have shown that hypertonic saline may also be effective at reducing ICP. Hypertonic saline appears to create osmotic mobilization of water across the blood-brain barrier.

Concentrations ranging from 3% to 23.4% have been used to decrease ICP.[75]

If despite these measures the ICP remains above 20 mm Hg, the ventilatory rate can be adjusted to reduce the arterial Pco_2 to 30 mm Hg. Hyperventilation should be used cautiously during the first 24 to 48 hours after injury, however, because it will cause cerebral vasoconstriction at a time when CBF is already critically reduced. Evidence also suggests that even brief periods of hyperventilation can lead to secondary brain injury by causing an increase in extracellular lactate and glutamate levels.[76] Prophylactic hyperventilation is always contraindicated in the absence of elevated ICP.[77] If hyperventilation is used, the brain tissue Po_2 or jugular venous oxygen saturation should be monitored to detect any cerebral ischemia that the treatment might cause. The risk of tissue ischemia and poor outcome may increase if the brain tissue Po_2 falls below 10 mm Hg.[72]

If intracranial hypertension persists despite all these treatments, particularly if the ICP rises rapidly or if the patient's initial CT scan showed a small contusion or hematoma, another CT scan should be obtained immediately to determine whether there is a new mass lesion or a preexisting lesion has enlarged. Even if the lesion has enlarged only slightly, an emergent craniotomy and evacuation of the contusion or hematoma may be the best way to reduce the ICP quickly and effectively.

If the CT scan does not reveal an intracranial mass lesion requiring surgery, the next recommended treatment for intracranial hypertension is high-dose barbiturates. Barbiturates are thought to be effective by reducing cerebral metabolic demand and blood flow, and preclinical studies suggest significant cerebral protective effects.[78] Pentobarbital is the most commonly used drug for this purpose and is administered as an IV loading dose of 10 to 15 mg/kg over 1 to 2 hours, followed by a maintenance infusion of 1 to 2 mg/kg per hour. The dose can be increased until intracranial hypertension subsides or MAP begins to fall. Continuous electroencephalographic monitoring is recommended while increasing the dose until a burst suppression pattern is observed. Hypotension, the most common adverse effect of barbiturates, can usually be averted by ensuring a normal intravascular volume before administering the drug.

Only a few options remain when intracranial hypertension is recalcitrant to all these measures, and they are controversial and not uniformly embraced. Therapeutic moderate hypothermia has been used in several clinical trials over the past decade. The body temperature is lowered to 32°C to 33°C as soon as possible after injury and kept at that temperature for 24 to 48 hours using surface cooling techniques. Although some clinical trials have not found that this treatment improves neurologic outcome compared with normothermia, they have consistently shown that hypothermia significantly reduces ICP.[79,80] Moreover, hypothermia does not cause significant medical complications when used for no longer than 48 hours.

Some advocate the use of decompressive craniectomies, such as large lateral or bifrontal bone flaps, with or without a generous temporal or frontal lobectomy In one study of patients with severe TBI, 6-month outcomes were similar for a group that had large decompressive craniectomies and a group that did not, even though the craniectomy group had lower initial GCS scores and more severe radiographic injuries.[81] Importantly, the craniectomy group did not have a higher incidence of persistent vegetative state. Two studies reported good outcomes in 56% to 58% of patients whose refractory intracranial hypertension was treated with decompressive craniectomy as a last resort,[82,83] and another study suggested that decompressive temporal lobectomy, when performed soon after injury, improves the outcome for young patients.[84] However, others found that decompressive craniectomy does not improve ICP, CPP, or mortality rates.[85] The decision to perform decompressive surgery should take into account the patient's ultimate prognosis. Because age has such a profound impact on the likelihood of a meaningful recovery, these therapies are recommended only for patients who are younger than 40 years old.

Failure to control intracranial hypertension may result in brain death, the irreversible cessation of cerebral function. Clinically, this is manifested by loss of motor function and brainstem reflexes including pupillary response, corneal reflex, cough reflex, and oculovestibular reflexes. Once these criteria are met, confirmatory testing such as apnea testing or nuclear medicine perfusion studies can be performed. Federal law requires notification of the local organ procurement office prior to formal brain death testing. However, medical staff should avoid mentioning organ donation to family members to minimize the appearance of conflict of interest; this is best left to designated requestors after decoupling has occurred.

Patients who have TBI, particularly those who are comatose or have significant non-CNS injuries, are at high risk for pneumonia and other infections, fever, malnutrition, seizures, deep venous thrombosis (DVT), pulmonary embolism, and other maladies endemic to the ICU. Most of these complications cause secondary brain injury and should be diagnosed and treated without delay. Fever is very common in the ICU and occurs in more than 79% of patients within the first week following injury.[86] Preclinical studies have found that there is a log increase in neuronal death in ischemic brain regions for every degree of brain temperature above 39°C,[87] and this effect is observed for 24 hours or more after injury.[88] Clinical studies of TBI patients have shown that the brain temperature is often 1°C to 2°C higher than body temperature,[89] though the effect of hyperthermia on ICP is less clear.[90,91] Consequently, the body temperature should be kept below 37°C at all times, and infectious or other causes of fever should be aggressively sought and treated.

Patients who are comatose, those being maintained on neuromuscular blocking agents, and those with pelvic or long-bone fractures are at high risk for deep venous thrombosis and pulmonary embolism. They should receive early prophylaxis, which typically includes the use of lower extremity sequential compression devices as well as subcutaneous heparin or enoxaparin. The early (2 to 3 days after injury) use of minidose heparin or low-molecular-weight heparin is safe and has not been found to cause or worsen intracranial hemorrhage after TBI.[92,93] DVT is prevalent in TBI patients despite early use of prophylaxis.[94]

Malnutrition is also common after severe TBI. The resting metabolic expenditure typically increases by 140% in a non-paralyzed patient with severe TBI.[95] Branched-chain amino acids from muscle protein are used preferentially for energy metabolism, potentially compromising the effectiveness of physical therapy. Nitrogen wasting is also increased, with excretion of as much as 9 to 12 g/day. Thus, early enteral or parenteral feeding is advisable, with the aim of providing at least 140% of the daily basal metabolic caloric requirements by the third or fourth day after injury.[96] A normal-sized adult patient usually needs 2000 to 3000 kcal/day. Because parenteral feeding increases the risk of infection, continuous enteral administration is preferable. For a patient expected to be in a prolonged coma, a percutaneous gastrostomy or surgical jejunostomy provides a convenient and well-tolerated route to administer tube feeding. Hyperglycemia is associated with TBI and is associated with prolonged hospital stays and increased mortality.[97] Aggressive management of hyperglycemia has been shown to decrease complications and improve long-term outcome,[98] but the optimal blood glucose range in patients with severe TBI remains controversial, and tight glucose control may be problematic.[99,100]

Posttraumatic contusions and subdural hematomas are well-known causes of generalized seizures which can precipitate secondary injury. Anticonvulsant prophylaxis, usually with phenytoin, is therefore recommended for patients with these lesions. The drug should be given for the first 7 days after injury; a prospective clinical trial found no advantage to longer prophylactic treatment.[101] A common side effect of phenytoin is fever; this should be considered if infectious causes of fever have been ruled out. If a patient has seizures, especially if they are prolonged, the associated cerebral hypermetabolism will cause secondary brain injury. Seizures should thus be treated aggressively, up to and including the use of general anesthesia if necessary. Subclinical seizures may occur in up to 33% of patients in the first week following TBI.[102] Therefore, EEG should be considered for those with unexplained depressed mental status, abruptly deteriorating cerebral

oxygenation, or a sudden increase in ICP; however, enlarging intracranial mass lesions remain the most likely cause.

Physical Therapy and Rehabilitation

The number of survivors of TBI is increasing because of greater success in understanding and treating the disease and improved motor vehicle safety devices. Accordingly, the demand for high-quality, well-organized TBI rehabilitation programs is also increasing. The primary goal of these programs is to reintegrate patients into their communities by either restoring normal or near-normal ability to function or teaching them alternative strategies to function well despite their disabilities. Such programs should involve a multidisciplinary team of physical, occupational, and speech therapists, neuropsychologists, and social workers, ideally coordinated by a physiatrist or a neurologist with special training in physical medicine and rehabilitation. The team should be experienced in TBI rehabilitation and thoroughly understand the special needs of these patients. Programs that focus exclusively on TBI rehabilitation are far preferable to those that mix patients with TBI, stroke, neurodegenerative diseases, and tumors, because the typical age groups are very different, as are their rehabilitative needs.

Rehabilitation of TBI patients should begin in the ICU during the first few days after injury, in consultation with a physiatrist, and include passive range-of-motion exercises and functional splinting of the extremities. Mobilization helps prevent DVT, and studies indicate that early sitting of comatose patients may hasten the return of consciousness. Supplementing physical therapy with central neurostimulant medications is being investigated for those with more severe injuries and minimal responsiveness.[103] Rehabilitation after TBI entails many other factors that are critical to optimizing outcome, but a thorough review is beyond the scope of this chapter.

Penetrating Injuries

Gunshot wounds to the head, the predominant cause of penetrating head injury, usually cause massive destruction of brain tissue, severe brain swelling, and if transcranial trajectory, death. The wounding potential of a bullet depends primarily on its velocity at impact and its mass, although the shape of the bullet and its lateral movements also play a role. The relationship of bullet mass and velocity to the energy imparted to the head is described by the equation $KE = 1/2MV^2$, where *KE* is kinetic energy, *M* is the mass of the bullet, and *V* is the impact velocity of the bullet. According to this equation, the impact velocity is by far the most important determinant of a bullet's wounding potential. Consequently, high-velocity rifle wounds to the head are invariably fatal, whereas low-velocity open-chambered handgun wounds often are not. When a bullet enters the skull, it creates a variety of pressure waves within the brain, some of which can cause tissue pressures of nearly 100 atmospheres, resulting in further tissue injury. In addition to forward velocity, the bullet's lateral motion before and after impact affects the severity of tissue destruction. Such motion is described as *yaw*, or the angle between the bullet's path of flight and its long axis, and *precession* and *nutation*, which are circular rotations of the bullet around the center of its mass. These movements increase the bullet's relative surface area at the point of impact and enable it to pass more of its kinetic energy to the surrounding tissue. They increase the size of the entrance wound and cause greater cavitational injury. Bullets often fragment after they strike the skull, fracturing a portion of the skull into multiple fragments. Both the bullet and the bone fragments then become numerous secondary missiles that cause additional tissue damage.

Low-velocity missile wounds, such as those from knives, ice picks, or arrows, do not cause the massive brain injuries seen with bullets, as might be predicted by the kinetic energy equation. Usually, only the tissue in the immediate path of the missile is damaged, and patients often have a complete neurologic recovery after the missile is surgically extracted. Rarely, a missile injures a major intracranial artery or venous sinus, and these vascular injuries can result in large intracranial hematomas. Nonetheless, vascular injuries are always possible with high- or low-velocity missile injuries to the head, especially those in or near the skull base or the sylvian fissures.

The initial assessment and resuscitation of patients with penetrating head injuries are the same as for those with closed head injuries, as detailed earlier in this chapter. Prompt and aggressive cardiopulmonary resuscitation is critical. Knives or other missiles protruding from the head should never be removed in the field or emergency department; if they are tamponading a damaged intracranial vessel, removal could lead to massive intracranial hemorrhage. Wounds with active bleeding should be sutured immediately, as this is a source of ongoing blood loss and can contribute to hemodynamic instability. When a patient has a gunshot wound to the head, the neck, chest, and abdomen should be inspected carefully for other gunshot wounds, because wounds to the heart or great vessels in the chest or abdomen may be even more life threatening. A postresuscitation GCS score should be obtained as soon as possible to guide future therapeutic decision making. A CT scan of the head defines the intracranial path of the missile and related skull and tissue damage. More importantly, it identifies any large intracranial hematomas or contusions that may significantly affect outcome. If the missile trajectory is in or near the skull base or sylvian fissures and the patient is deemed salvageable, cerebral angiography should be performed because this injury pattern is associated with development of pseudoaneurysm.

Most patients who are expected to survive a penetrating head injury require at least limited operative treatment. Large intracranial hematomas should be evacuated promptly. A craniotomy is required for low-velocity missile wounds in which the object is still protruding from the head. After removing a segment of skull containing the missile and large enough to allow for intracerebral exploration, the surgeon can seek and immediately repair or occlude any vascular injuries caused by the missile. For gunshot wounds to the head, the surgeon should perform a limited débridement of the scalp and skull wound, removing scalp, bone, and bullet fragments penetrating the brain only if they lie near the surface. Easily accessible necrotic brain should be débrided and meticulous hemostasis achieved. Dural closure is important because it reduces the risk of CSF leak and infection, but it usually requires a pericranial graft. Artificial dural substitutes and allografts increase the risk of infection and therefore are not recommended.

Subsequent medical management of penetrating injuries is as described previously for closed head injuries. In addition, patients should receive prophylactic antibiotics for at least 14 days, because the missile usually carries skin and hair into the brain. Because a penetrating TBI by definition disrupts and contuses brain tissue, all patients with these injuries should also receive anticonvulsants for at least 7 days.

Mild and Moderate Injury

A mild TBI or concussion is defined by an initial GCS score of 14 or 15; a moderate TBI by a GCS score of 9 to 13. These injuries typically involve a brief loss of consciousness or alteration of consciousness at the time of impact to the head and some degree of retrograde or posttraumatic amnesia; however, patients with such injuries can follow commands. They usually do not have the complex intracranial pathology associated with severe TBI and therefore are unlikely to die from the injury; mortality rates are near zero for those with mild TBI and approximately 4% for those with moderate TBI. Nonetheless, these injuries can cause long-term cognitive and neuropsychological impairment. As many as 10% of those with mild injuries and 66% of those with moderate injuries suffer prolonged or permanent disabilities that prevent them from returning to work or school.

Rotational, acceleration, and deceleration forces are common causes of these injuries, particularly those that result in loss of consciousness. The impact usually is not intense enough to cause intracranial hematoma, cerebral contusion, skull fracture, or brain swelling. Although a small amount of subarachnoid hemorrhage may be present, usually in

the sulci over the frontal or temporal lobes, CT findings are usually normal. Abnormal magnetic resonance imaging (MRI) findings have been reported in as many as 30% of these patients, most commonly diffuse hyperdense lesions on T2-weighted images. These lesions are thought to represent focal or punctate contusions.[104,105] Functional MRI often shows abnormal activation patterns, particularly if the patient has lost consciousness or is symptomatic at the time of the study.[105]

Several factors determine the appropriate level of medical evaluation and treatment after mild or moderate TBI. Any loss of consciousness at the time of impact or retrograde or antegrade amnesia of at least several minutes warrants a thorough medical assessment, as do persistent headache, confusion, dizziness, diplopia, blurry vision, weakness, or numbness. A formal examination in the emergency department is generally advisable. Patients who are neurologically normal and asymptomatic after at least one hour of observation and serial evaluations can usually be safely discharged, with clear instructions to return immediately if symptoms or signs of TBI develop. Ideally, these instructions are given to both the patient and a responsible companion.

A patient with persistent symptoms or neurologic deficits should have a CT scan of the head and be admitted to the hospital for observation. This is particularly important for those with GCS scores of 13 or less, because the risk of an intracranial hematoma or contusion large enough to require emergent craniotomy increases as the GCS score decreases among patients whose initial GCS scores are 9 to 13. As many as 40% have CT abnormalities, and 8% require neurosurgical intervention.[106]

Athletes—especially those involved in contact sports such as boxing, football, soccer, wrestling, and field hockey—are at high risk for mild and moderate TBI. One report found that 47% of high school football players sustained a concussion, with 35% sustaining multiple concussions.[107] Multiple concussions are much more likely to cause prolonged or permanent neurologic disability than a single concussion, particularly if they occur over a short time span. Second impact syndrome is a rare but potentially lethal problem first noted in athletes in 1973 and later implicated as the cause of sudden death in several high school football players.[108]

Because sports-related concussions are associated with such disabling and potentially life-threatening consequences, coaches and athletic trainers must carefully consider whether an athlete should be advised to return to play or retire from athletic competition after a concussion. Several groups have devised concussion grading scales to evaluate concussion severity and developed guidelines to determine when an athlete can safely resume play. The most widely adopted scales are those developed by Kelly and colleagues at the University of Colorado,[109] Cantu,[110] and the American Academy of Neurology[111] (Tables 38-3 and 38-4). Most authorities recommend that athletes abstain from play for at least one season if, during that season, they sustain three or more grade I or II concussions or two grade III concussions.[112] In addition, many athletic organizations at the high school, college, and professional levels have adopted neuropsychological testing as a

TABLE 38-3	Grading Scales for Concussion		
	Grade of Concussion		
Scale	*I*	*II*	*III*
Colorado[96]	Confusion; no LOC; PTA <30 min	LOC <5 min; confusion; PTA >30 min	LOC >5 min; PTA >24 h
Cantu[97]	PTA <30 min; no LOC	LOC <5 min; PTA 30 min to 24 h	LOC >5 min; PTA >24 h
AAN[98]	Transient confusion; symptoms <15 min; no LOC	No LOC; transient confusion; symptoms >15 min	Any LOC

AAN, American Academy of Neurology; *LOC*, loss of consciousness; *PTA*, posttraumatic amnesia.

TABLE 38-4	Recommendations for Return to Play		
Concussion Grade	Colorado Guidelines[96]	Cantu Guidelines[97]	AAN Guidelines[98]
I	Return after 20 min if normal examination	Return same day if normal at rest and exertion	Return same day if normal at rest and exertion
II	Return after 7 days if asymptomatic	Return after 2 wk if asymptomatic at rest and exertion for 7 days	Return after 7 days if asymptomatic
III	Evaluation by neurologist or neurosurgeon; return after 2 wk if asymptomatic and cleared by specialist	Return after 1 mo if asymptomatic at rest and exertion for 7 days	Evaluation by neurologist or neurosurgeon; return after 2 wk if neurologically cleared

AAN, American Academy of Neurology.

means of objectively evaluating the cognitive and neuropsychological consequences of each concussion.[113] Comparison of postinjury and preseason scores is a powerful tool for guiding return-to-play decisions.

A common sequela of mild or moderate TBI is postconcussion syndrome, a constellation of symptoms that can be disabling for weeks or even months. The most common symptoms are headache, irritability, dizziness, tinnitus, lethargy, and sleep disturbance. One or more of these symptoms develop in approximately 30% of patients 1 week after a mild or moderate TBI, but they usually subside within 3 months.[114] After 1 year, only 7% of patients report residual symptoms, most commonly persistent headache. Postconcussion syndrome is best treated by a primary care physician or neuropsychologist who thoroughly understands the disorder. Cognitive testing is recommended for patients whose symptoms last more than a few weeks, because symptoms such as frustration and irritability are often linked to an inability to resume normal daily activities. Neuropsychological testing often indicates deficits in attention and concentration rather than memory. If such testing identifies specific deficits, cognitive rehabilitation is recommended.[115] Persistent headaches, dizziness, and tinnitus should be treated symptomatically after a CT scan of the head establishes the absence of intracranial lesions. Posttraumatic disturbances of the ossicles of the inner ear semicircular canals can cause severe positional vertigo which can be immediately improved with canalith repositioning. In other cases, dizziness is more complex and may result from problems with the vestibular-ocular reflex, so patients with vertigo or tinnitus may benefit from evaluation by an otolaryngologist. Factors associated with an adverse long-term outcome after a concussion include old age, prolonged posttraumatic amnesia, and a below-normal premorbid intellectual capacity.[114]

Prognosis

Predicting outcome soon after a TBI can help guide acute and chronic care and help prepare family members for the typically protracted recovery process. Equally important is that further treatment may be deemed futile, and expensive critical care or surgery can be reserved for those who are likely to benefit. Of course, early prognostication must be reliable, especially when withdrawal of life support is a consideration.

Several clinical and radiographic characteristics have proved useful for outcome prediction, but they must be used in concert.[116] Moreover, these criteria are more reliable for predicting death or vegetative survival than for accurately predicting mild or no dysfunction and a complete return to normalcy. The most powerful outcome predictors are age, initial GCS score (particularly the motor component), pupil size and reaction to light, ICP, and the nature and extent of intracranial injuries.

Old age correlates most consistently with a poor outcome after TBI. In the Traumatic Coma Data Bank study of more than 700 patients with severe TBI, the incidence of death, persistent vegetative state, or severe disability was 92% for those older than 60 years, 86% for those older than 56 years, and 50% for younger patients.[117] The older groups had a higher incidence of traumatic intracranial mass lesions, midline shift, and subarachnoid hemorrhage, and the presence of these insults correlated strongly with poor outcome. Subsequent studies confirmed the low probability of a good recovery for patients older than 60 years whose initial GCS scores are 8 or less.[118]

The second most important predictor of outcome is the initial postresuscitation GCS score. Among patients with severe closed head injuries in the Traumatic Coma Data Bank study, good outcomes occurred in 4.1% of those with an initial GCS score of 3, in 6.3% whose score was 4, and in 12.2% whose score was 5. Again, later clinical studies corroborated the strong direct correlation between initial GCS score and outcome.[119]

Unilaterally or bilaterally dilated pupils that are unreactive to light usually reflect uncal herniation and significant brainstem compression and damage, so this sign is ominous. Several large clinical studies found that patients with bilaterally fixed and dilated pupils had a greater than 90% likelihood of death or vegetative survival.[120,121] Also, intracranial hypertension refractory to medication is associated with a 43% mortality rate and 0% chance of a functional outcome.[122]

Various studies have analyzed the effect of the type and size of posttraumatic intracranial lesions on outcome in terms of both the specific lesions and the CT-defined characteristics of their mass effect. Subdural hematomas are associated with the worst prognosis. One study found that only 26% of patients with these clots had a functional recovery.[123] However, the prognosis for patients with subdural hematomas is also related to how soon after injury the clot is evacuated, with the best outcomes in those who have surgery within 2 hours.[7]

Epidural hematomas pose a much lower risk of mortality because, unlike subdural hematomas, they usually are not associated with underlying cerebral contusions or swelling. If left untreated, however, epidural hematomas can cause uncal herniation and death. One report noted an increase in mortality from 17% to 65% if an epidural hematoma was not evacuated within 2 hours after the onset of coma.[8]

The presence of traumatic subarachnoid hemorrhage is associated with a 50% greater risk of death.[10] The link between traumatic subarachnoid hemorrhage and worse outcomes is controversial, however. Many believe that this condition merely indicates a more severe TBI and has no direct association with outcome.

Marshall and colleagues devised a CT-based classification scheme that proved prognostically useful when applied to the patients in the Traumatic Coma Data Bank study (Tables 38-5 and 38-6).[124] The classification emphasizes the mass effect of posttraumatic intracranial lesions. Not surprisingly, these investigators found the worst outcomes among patients with large intracranial mass lesions and uncal herniation.

Based on these studies, one can say with certainty that an 80-year-old patient who presents with bilaterally fixed and dilated pupils, a GCS score of 3 or 4, and a large subdural hematoma will not have a

TABLE 38-5	Computed Tomographic Classification of Traumatic Brain Injury
Category	Definition
Diffuse injury I	No visible intracranial pathology
Diffuse injury II	Cisterns present, with midline shift 0 to 5 mm; no high-density lesion >25 mL
Diffuse injury III (swelling)	Cisterns compressed or absent, with midline shift 0 to 5 mm; no high-density lesion >25 mL
Diffuse injury IV (shift)	Midline shift >5 mm; no high-density lesion >25 mL
Evacuated mass lesion	Any lesion surgically evacuated
Nonevacuated mass lesion	High-density lesion >25 mL; not surgically evacuated

Data from Marshall LF, Marshall SB, Klauber MR, Clark M. A new classification of head injury based on computerized tomography. J Neurosurg. 1991;75(Suppl):S14-S20.

TABLE 38-6	Relationship of Computed Tomographic Classification to Outcome at Discharge		
Category	*No. of Patients*	*Unfavorable Outcome* (%)	*Favorable Outcome† (%)*
Diffuse injury I	52	38	62
Diffuse injury II	177	65	35
Diffuse injury III	153	84	16
Diffuse injury IV	32	94	6
Evacuated mass	276	77	23
Nonevacuated mass	36	89	11

Data from Marshall LF, Marshall SB, Klauber MR, Clark M. A new classification of head injury based on computerized tomography. J Neurosurg. 1991;75(Suppl):S14-S20.
*Death, persistent vegetative state, or severe disability.
†Moderate disability or good recovery.

functional outcome regardless of treatment. However, the prognosis is much better for young patients with higher GCS scores, and aggressive surgical and medical management is usually warranted.

The patient's salvageability and prognosis after a penetrating injury are far clearer than for those with closed head injuries. Most victims of gunshot wounds to the head die before or shortly after hospital admission. Among 314 patients with civilian craniocerebral gunshot wounds, 92% died; 73% of them were pronounced dead at the scene of the injury, and 12% died within 3 hours of injury.[125] In the Traumatic Coma Data Bank study, the mortality rate was 88% for the 151 patients with gunshot wounds to the head.[126] No patient with an initial GCS score of 8 or less regained normal neurologic function, and only three recovered to the level of moderate disability, suggesting that the initial GCS score is an even more powerful predictor of outcome for these patients than for those with closed TBI. A meta-analysis of recent clinical studies examining civilian gunshot wounds to the head found that favorable outcomes (Glasgow Outcome Scale scores of 4 or 5) occurred in only 5 of 490 patients with initial GCS scores of 3 to 5.[127] Mortality rates ranged from 51% to 87% for patients with scores of 8 or less. In contrast, those whose initial GCS scores were 13 to 15 all survived and had favorable outcomes. Other clinical signs associated with death or a poor outcome are fixed and dilated pupils, intracranial hypertension, and hypotension. Also, a gunshot wound is more likely to be lethal if self-inflicted.

The CT-defined extent of intracranial injury caused by the missile also has prognostic significance. Hyperdense lesions with a volume greater than 15 mL, midline shift of more than 3 mm, compressed or absent basal cisterns, subarachnoid hemorrhage, and intraventricular hemorrhage are all associated with mortality rates of 80% to 90%, as is a bullet trajectory that traverses both hemispheres, the basal ganglia, or the posterior fossa.[126,128]

KEY POINTS

1. Severe traumatic brain injuries are the leading cause of morbidity and mortality for Americans between the ages of 1 and 45 years.

2. Outcome following traumatic brain injury is determined not only by the primary injury, such as skull fracture and subdural hematoma, but also by secondary injuries initiated by post-traumatic ischemia.

3. Secondary brain injuries are primarily responsible for the development of delayed intracranial hypertension.

4. The goal of critical care management of patients with severe traumatic brain injury is to enhance cerebral perfusion and avoid therapy that may cause regional cerebral ischemia.

5. Early assessment and triage of patients with severe traumatic brain injury should use the advanced trauma life support protocol prescribed by the American College of Surgeons Committee on Trauma.

6. Patients with severe traumatic brain injury are best managed at a level I trauma center with immediate neurosurgical availability.

7. All patients with contusions or hematomas visible on head computed tomography scans, and Glasgow Coma Scale scores of 8 or less, benefit from intracranial pressure monitoring.

8. A ventricular catheter coupled to an external strain-gauge transducer is the optimal means of monitoring intracranial pressure, because it provides accurate measurements and allows for CSF drainage—the most benign way of treating elevated intracranial pressure.

9. Prophylactic hyperventilation therapy, particularly when the intracranial pressure is less than 20 mm Hg, should be avoided.

10. Patients with subdural hematomas or contusions benefit from anticonvulsive prophylaxis for 7 days after injury.

11. Early evaluation of brain-injured patients by a physical therapist and rehabilitation specialist is highly recommended to prevent immobility-related complications and facilitate rapid mobility.

12. Patients with mild or moderate brain injuries, particularly those with sports-related concussions, benefit from careful neuropsychological evaluation before returning to contact sports.

13. Athletes who have persistent headaches and focal neurologic deficits should not be allowed to return to play until these symptoms have subsided.

ANNOTATED REFERENCES

Chestnut RM, Marshall SB, Piek J, et al. Early and late systemic hypotension as a frequent and fundamental source of cerebral ischemia following severe brain injury in the Traumatic Coma Data Bank. Acta Neurochir Suppl (Wien) 1993;59:121-5.
The authors reviewed blood pressure readings in a group of several hundred patients admitted to the Traumatic Coma Data Bank. They found that hypotension (systolic blood pressure <90 mm Hg) was associated with a twofold increase in the mortality rate compared with head-injury patients who did not have hypotension.
Haas B, Jurkovich GJ, Wang J, Rivara FP, Mackenzie EJ, Nathens AB. Survival advantage in trauma centers: expeditious intervention or experience? J Am Coll Surg 2009;208(1):28-36.
In a multicenter prospective cohort study of 1331 adult trauma patients cared for in trauma centers (TC) and nondesignated centers (NTC), times from admission to relevant interventions were assessed, as were relative risks of in-hospital death. The relative risk of death was 0.61 (95% CI, 0.43–0.86) among patients managed at TC compared with those admitted to NTC. This survival advantage was greatest among patients with penetrating trauma, though the relative risk of death at a TC among patients in the TBI group

was 0.72 (95% CI, 0.50–1.0). These outcomes were not a result of more rapid assessment and intervention alone and emphasize the complex factors that contribute to the survival benefit of trauma center care.
Narayan RK, Kishore PR, Becker DP, et al. Intracranial pressure: to monitor or not to monitor? A review of our experience with severe head injury. J Neurosurg 1982;56(5):650-9.
The authors reviewed their experience with more than 100 patients with severe TBI and identified indications for ICP monitoring. They found that patients who had GCS scores of 8 or less and abnormal CT scans were very likely to have problems with intracranial hypertension and would benefit from ICP monitoring.
Temkin NR, Dikmen SS, Wilensky AJ, et al. A randomized, double-blind study of phenytoin for the prevention of posttraumatic seizures. N Engl J Med 1990;323(8):497-502.
In this randomized, controlled, double-blind study of the benefit of prophylactic anticonvulsant therapy for patients with TBI, the authors found a significant reduction in the incidence of posttraumatic seizures during the first week of therapy, but no subsequent benefit was observed when therapy was continued longer than 7 days. This study has led most to discontinue the use of anticonvulsants 1 week after TBI, regardless of the nature of the injury.

REFERENCES

Access the complete reference list online at http://www.expertconsult.com.

39

Spinal Cord Injury

ELIZABETH A. VITARBO | ALLAN D. LEVI

Despite substantial improvements in emergency, diagnostic, and surgical care, spinal trauma continues to present a challenging spectrum of diseases for the neurosurgeon to manage. When spinal trauma results in a spinal cord injury (SCI), the emotional and financial toll inflicted on individuals and their families is enormous. Improvements in the quality of care delivered over the past few decades are partially reflected in the recognition that centers of excellence that focus on acute treatment and rehabilitation of the SCI patient are best equipped to deal with the magnitude of services these patients require.

Epidemiology

Spinal cord injury typically occurs in males at the peak of their productive lives. The incidence of traumatic SCI is approximately 11,000 new cases each year in the United States,[1] with a prevalence of 191,000. The prevalence of SCI patients is increasing steadily owing to improved survival in both the acute and chronic stages of the disease. The amount spent on the treatment of spinal cord injuries in the United States is approximately 5.6 billion dollars each year and rising annually.[2] The cost of caring for the individual spinal cord–injured patient is directly related to the injury level of the spinal cord and to the patient's age, with the highest costs associated with older quadriplegic patients who are dependent on a ventilator.[2]

Etiology

Most spinal injuries result from high-speed motor vehicle accidents (Figure 39-1). Falls and work-related injuries are other important contributors. Spinal cord injury that is due to violence is on a dramatic rise secondary to increased incidence of assaults. These injuries include both blunt and penetrating injuries, such as gun and knife wounds. Sports-related injuries, which include football, horseback riding, and hockey injuries, are relatively rare but have received recent media attention.[3-4] Finally, recreational injuries from jet skis, snowmobiles, snow skiing, snowboarding, and parachuting, to name but a few, appear to be on the rise as "extreme sports" become more prevalent.

Initial Management

Suspected SCI alters the basics of the "ABCs" of resuscitation in several important ways. With respect to airway management, suspected SCI dictates in-line immobilization of the spine at all times, so hyperextension of the neck is contraindicated. A jaw thrust must be used to open the airway, and required intubation must be done with the head/neck in a neutral position. This is an important point to remember because patients with a high SCI will have diminished or absent respiratory capacity and frequently require emergent intubation.

Aggressive resuscitation of SCI patients proceeds as with all trauma patients. As indicated earlier, however, upper SCI may be associated with neurogenic shock, requiring large-volume fluid replacement. Although pressors are likely to be required in the setting of neurogenic shock, field management is commonly limited to fluid resuscitation. High incidence of associated head injury often requires use of colloid solutions in addition to normal saline/lactated Ringer's solution in an effort to adequately resuscitate the patient while minimizing exacerbation of cerebral edema.

Immobilization and Diagnostic Evaluation

Rigid immobilization is indicated if there is any doubt about the presence of SCI. Presence of altered mental status in any way dictates the use of "spinal cord precautions." These include use of in-line immobilization, maintenance of neutral position, cervical immobilization with a rigid collar, and use of backboards for transport.

After initial resuscitative efforts, diagnostic studies are undertaken. Fine-cut helical computed tomography (CT) scan with coronal and sagittal reconstructions have supplanted plain radiographs in most trauma centers as an initial evaluation in detecting spine fractures. Additional spine studies may be obtained after the patient has been stabilized and more emergent diagnostic studies have been undertaken. During this time, rigid cervical collar and backboard immobilization must be continued.

Further diagnostic studies will be dictated by the findings of the initial and secondary surveys as well as findings of initial diagnostic studies. Several points are important to keep in mind. First, important information can be obtained from studies performed for other reasons. For example, routine chest and abdominal radiographs may provide important information regarding the presence of significant thoracic/lumbar spine injury. Although these do not replace subsequent "formal" spine studies, they are often obtained as part of the routine trauma workup and provide early clues to the presence of spine trauma and may help prioritize subsequent imaging studies (Figure 39-2). Radiographs and particularly the CT are the most sensitive tools in detecting a fracture of the spine, but occasionally it is difficult to clear the spine—even in the absence of a fracture—because an unstable ligamentous injury without fracture may exist.

Patients with a suspected spinal column injury who are unconscious, uncooperative, or intoxicated or who have associated traumatic injuries that distract from their assessment will often require further radiographic study of the cervical spine before the discontinuation of cervical spine immobilization. Several options exist and include (1) maintenance of the collar and/or spine precautions until the patient becomes coherent and responsive, (2) dynamic imaging of the spine with physician monitoring, and (3) magnetic resonance imaging (MRI) of the spine to rule out a purely ligamentous injury. Of the three options, we frequently use MRI to clear the spine because a completely negative MR image in the setting of trauma indicates that there is no instability of the cervical spine (Figure 39-3). Malalignment and evidence of spine trauma on these imaging studies frequently determines subsequent management and diagnostic decision making. Cervical subluxations often require the use of traction and/or manual reduction of the fracture-dislocation. Diazepam (Valium) or lorazepam (Ativan), along with careful neurologic monitoring, often in the intensive care unit (ICU) setting, is required because application of traction can realign the spine but can also result in neurologic deterioration.

Pediatric Spinal Cord Injury

Pediatric spine trauma is relatively uncommon, representing approximately 5% of all spinal cord injuries.[5] For a specific discussion of pediatric SCI, please see Chapter 210. In addition, guidelines have been published on this topic.[6]

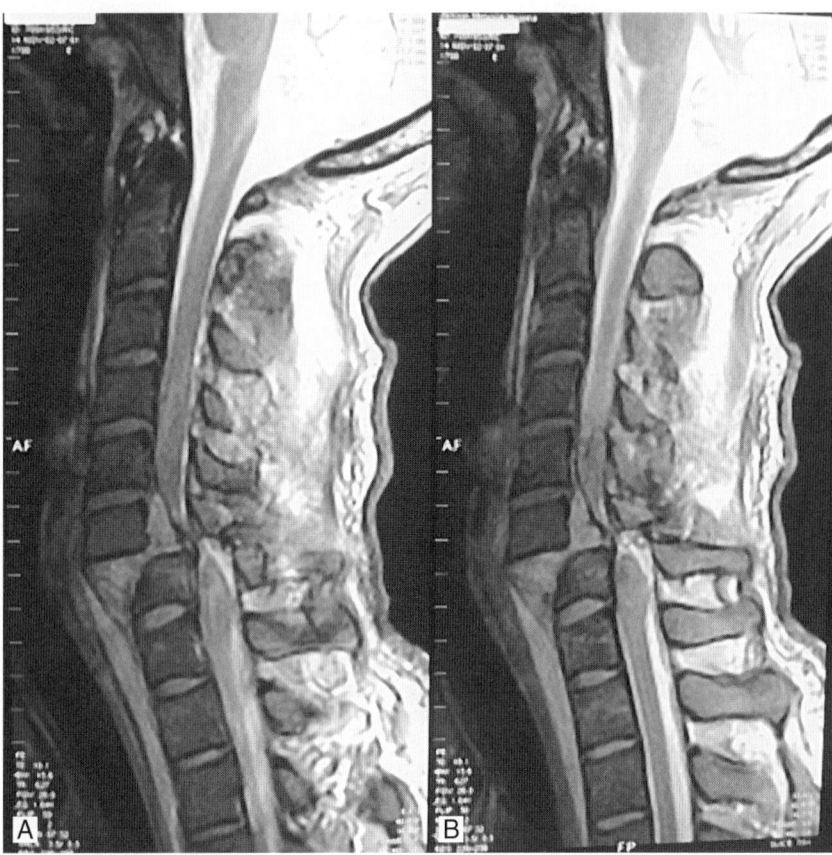

Figure 39-1 **A,** Sagittal T2-weighted MRI demonstrates a C6-C7 fracture-dislocation with severe cord compression in a patient who presented with complete C6 quadriplegia-ASIA. **B,** Patient was treated surgically to realign the spine and gained significant root recovery without any recovery of hand or lower extremity function.

Pharmacotherapy

The concepts of primary and secondary SCI are important principles in understanding the pathophysiology and the role of pharmacotherapeutic agents in emergent treatment. The primary injury mechanism results from a mechanical insult that occurs at the time of impact and includes acute compression, impaction, distraction, laceration, and shear.[7] Secondary injuries occur after the initial injury and account for some of the progressive pathologic changes associated with SCI.[7] A number of drugs have been tested in the laboratory, but only a few of these agents have progressed to clinical trials to evaluate their efficacy. Five randomized controlled trials of pharmacotherapy for acute SCI have been conducted, focusing on the therapeutic effect of either corticosteroids or gangliosides.

CORTICOSTEROIDS

A number of studies have shown improved neurologic recovery in animals with spinal cord injuries that have received either dexamethasone or methylprednisolone.[8-12] Corticosteroid treatment initially held promise as a potential therapeutic agent for its putative role in reducing white matter edema and inflammation. Current evidence, however, suggests that the major mechanism of action is reduction of the effects of secondary injury—in particular, the destructive effects of lipid peroxidation on cell membranes.[2] Other actions include improving spinal cord blood flow, enhancing the postinjury activity of Na^+/K^+-ATPase, and facilitating the recovery of extracellular calcium ion.[8,13]

The first NASCIS trial (NASCIS I) examined low- (100 mg) and high- (1000 mg) dose methylprednisolone given for 10 days. Unfortunately, this trial had no control group, and no significant difference in outcome was found except for an increased number of wound infections among patients in the high-dose group.[14] The second NASCIS trial (NASCIS II) was a prospective, randomized, double-blind, multicenter trial that demonstrated improved neurologic outcomes after 6 weeks, 6 months, and 1 year in patients with nonpenetrating SCI who had received a regimen of methylprednisolone, which included a bolus dose of 30 mg/kg.[15] Improvement in motor and sensory scores associated with administration of methylprednisolone was only observed if the drug was given within 8 hours of injury when compared with naloxone or a placebo. Results of this study have been criticized.[16,17] Some of the criticisms relate to difficulties in randomization, reporting methods, analysis of benefit limited to small subgroups within the larger study, and lack of replication of results by a completely independent group of investigators, among others. However, the administration of methylprednisolone is believed to reduce the amount of secondary injury that occurs after SCI and has become an important tool in the treatment of SCI in most North American centers. The results of NASCIS III have been published and compared the dosage of methylprednisolone used in the NASCIS II protocol with a longer dosing regimen (48 hours) as well as with a 21-aminosteroid. The 21-aminosteroids (lazaroids), a new class of steroids that are potent inhibitors of lipid peroxidation, lack much of the glucocorticoid activity of many of the traditional steroid compounds. Results of the study suggested that when patients are seen within 3 hours of their injury, they should receive a bolus dose of methylprednisolone (30 mg/kg intravenously [IV]) followed by 23 hours of treatment (5.4 mg/kg/h IV). Patients seen between 3 and 8 hours should receive the same bolus followed by a longer dosing regimen (48 hours). Complications from 48 hours of treatment included a significant increase in severe sepsis and pneumonia.[18] Neurosurgical guidelines for management of spine trauma recommend methylprednisolone as a treatment option, recognizing that the risks of use have been more clearly demonstrated than benefit.[19,20]

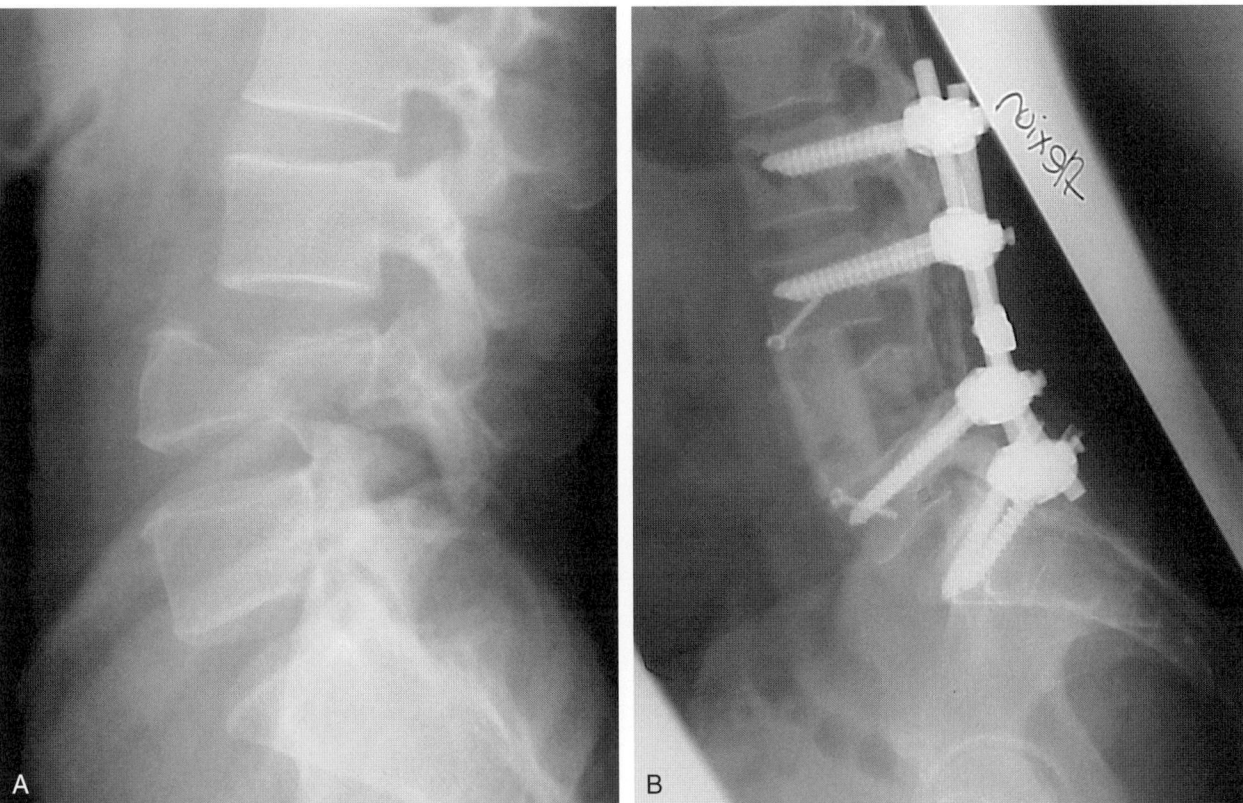

Figure 39-2 This 45-year-old man sustained **(A)** an L4 fracture-dislocation and presented with a dense footdrop. He underwent **(B)** anteroposterior reconstruction with instrumentation.

GANGLIOSIDES

Gangliosides are complex sialic acid–containing glycosphingolipids which are present in high concentrations in neural membranes. These compounds are involved in a variety of cell-surface phenomena such as cell-substrate binding and receptor functions.[21] Basic research in the past 15 years has demonstrated that these compounds can (1) promote the survival of neurons in cell culture; (2) increase the number, length, and branching of neuronal processes in cell culture; and (3) improve functional recovery after a variety of traumatic and ischemic insults to the peripheral and central nervous system. A limited number of animal studies have examined the role of gangliosides after SCI and have shown only a modest effect on the regeneration of serotonergic neurons.[22] A recent prospective, randomized, double-blind, single-center study found a beneficial effect in functional neurologic outcomes when the ganglioside GM[1] was administered within 72 hours of human SCI.[23] However, a multicenter trial demonstrated no statistically significant benefit with administration of this agent at 26 and 52 weeks after injury.[24]

Hypothermia

Two recent studies were published on the safety and feasibility of mild to moderate intravascular cooling for SCI. Levi et al. reported on a series of 14 patients with American Spinal Injury Association (ASIA) classification A complete cervical cord injuries who underwent a protocol to achieve temperatures of 33.5°C via a closed-loop delivery system. Researchers found good correlation between intravascular and intrathecal cerebrospinal fluid temperature.[25] Average time between inductions of hypothermia was 9.17 ± 2.24 hours (mean ± SEM); time to target temperature was 2.72 ± 0.42 hours; duration of cooling at

target was 47.6 ± 3.1 hours; and average total length of time of cooling was 93.6 ± 4 hours. A subsequent paper summarized the complications and neurologic outcomes seen in the SCI patients treated with hypothermia and compared them to age- and injury-matched controls. The hypothermia group ASIA conversion rate to a higher grade was approximately 42%, with a similar frequency of complications to institutional controls.[26] This pilot study suggested that systemic intravascular cooling can be accomplished with minimal variations in temperature and few adverse events, and may pave the way for larger multicenter SCI trials to test the efficacy of mild to moderate hypothermia in SCI.[27]

Intensive Care Unit Management

Spinal cord injury is associated with profound effects on all vital systemic functions. Through primarily class III medical evidence, numerous reports indicate lower morbidity and mortality rates in patients with SCI managed with ICU monitoring and aggressive medical management of these changes.[28-36] At the least, these studies taken together indicate that a systematic approach must be taken to evaluate and treat each of the potential complications. Early and late complications will be seen, and the degree of involvement of each system is usually correlated with the level and severity of injury.

RESPIRATORY SYSTEM

Respiratory complications are a major source of morbidity and mortality after SCI, with an 18% to 30% mortality rate reported in patients with tetraplegia.[32,37] In a study by Hachen and associates,[28,30] most early deaths were related to pulmonary complications, with the likelihood

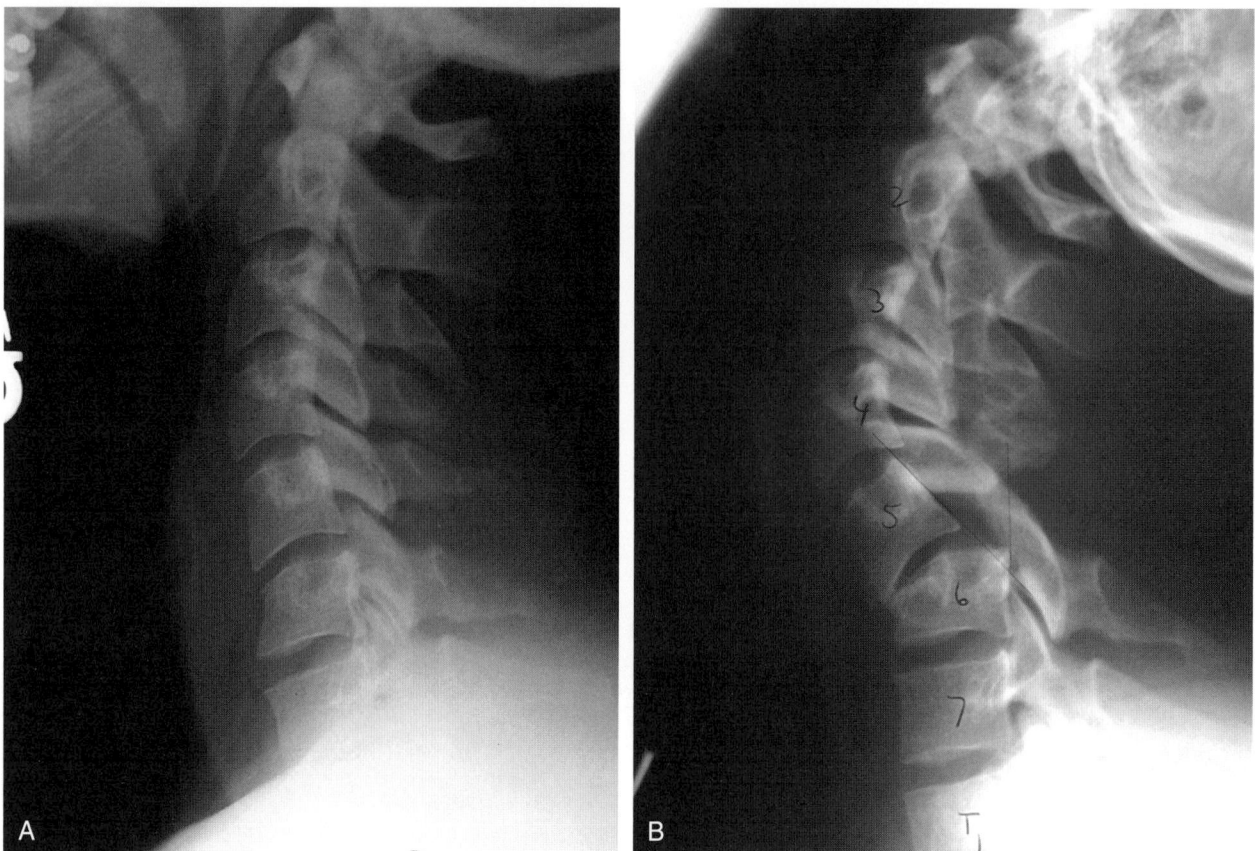

Figure 39-3   **A,** Admission lateral radiograph of a 31-year-old man who was "cleared" in the emergency department after cervical spine series and CT failed to demonstrate a fracture. Patient had a Glasgow Coma Scale score of 11 on admission and significant facial fractures. **B,** He presented 1 year post admission with increasing neck pain and was diagnosed with a severe cervical kyphotic deformity with bilateral perched facets at C5-C6. MRI (gradient-echo sequence) done on admission in this obtunded patient would have easily demonstrated the posterior ligamentous injury between the C5 and C6 spinous process, which is relatively subtle on the admission lateral cervical spine radiograph seen in **A.**

of severe insufficiency related to SCI severity. Whereas most cervical spinal cord injuries occur below C4, with the phrenic nerves continuing to innervate the diaphragm, the respiratory system is frequently severely affected, particularly after cervical spinal cord injuries. Specifically, marked reductions in (forced) vital capacity, inspiratory capacity, and expiratory flow rates frequently result in hypoxemia.[28,32,38-41] These changes may be attributed to variable paralysis of the intercostal muscles and accessory muscles of respiration. Loss of abdominal muscle tone and ileus also reduce the mechanical efficiency of breathing.

In general, there is a period of grace in which the patient with a cervical SCI will maintain his or her respiratory status. However, respiratory failure can ensue 24 to 48 hours after admission. Additional injuries such as rib fractures, hemothorax, and so on can accelerate this respiratory deterioration. Preparation for such events should be undertaken early so that if intubation is required, it can be done with stabilization using in-line traction, often supplemented by fiberoptic technique using a bronchoscope. Measurements of arterial blood gases, negative inspiratory force, and forced vital capacity may provide a method of early detection of respiratory failure.

The most common respiratory complications include atelectasis, pneumonia, pulmonary embolus, pulmonary edema, and acute respiratory distress syndrome. In addition to difficulty with taking deep breaths and coughing, patients are often unable to clear airway secretions. Accumulation of secretions and/or mucus plugs can result in respiratory failure. Prevention includes respiratory treatment with bronchodilators, frequent pulmonary toilet, chest physiotherapy, increasing airway humidity, intubation, and mechanical ventilation including the use of continuous positive airway pressure. The use of the RotoRest bed significantly decreases pulmonary complications associated with SCI[32,42] because it improves pulmonary blood flow and reduces the incidence of pulmonary emboli.

Pulmonary infections frequently complicate spinal cord injuries. Within days of admission, the normal flora of the oral cavity will contain increasing numbers of nosocomial organisms. Hospital-acquired pulmonary infections are heralded by fever, increased white blood cells both in the sputum and in the peripheral blood, and changes on the chest radiograph. After obtaining appropriate cultures, commencement of broad-spectrum antibiotics should be instituted.

Most patients can be discontinued or weaned from the ventilator after they have been medically stabilized, which usually means treatment of pulmonary infections, reestablishment of euvolemia, enhancement of respiratory muscle function, and nutritional supplementation to offset the high caloric requirements of the trauma. Initially, weaning the intermittent mandatory ventilation rate is followed by weaning of the positive airway pressure (either continuous or end-expiratory). With prolonged periods of ventilation (>2 weeks), and/or multiple failed extubations, one should consider a tracheostomy. The likelihood of requiring a tracheostomy increases after a high SCI, preexisting pulmonary disease, and the age of the patient. Tracheostomy effectively reduces the physiologic dead space. Northrup and colleagues[43] have demonstrated that a tracheostomy can be performed before anterior cervical instrumentation of the spine, with a low risk of infection; but in our patient population, early surgery for stabilization is advocated, and consequently, few patients undergo tracheostomy before anterior cervical stabilization surgery.

CARDIOVASCULAR SYSTEM

Significant confusion arises when the term *spinal shock* is used after SCI. The misunderstanding regarding its use stems from multiple causes. First, many physicians use the terms *spinal shock* and *neurogenic shock* interchangeably. *Neurogenic shock*, however, refers to a condition characterized by hypotension and bradycardia resulting from interruption of the sympathetic nervous system pathways within the spinal cord. The incidence of significant neurogenic shock increases with injuries above the T6 level, because unopposed vagal tone slows the heart and reduces systemic vascular resistance, resulting in venous pooling. The condition responds to administration of fluids and/or colloids and occasionally requires the use of pressors. Neurogenic shock is distinct from hypovolemic shock, which may occasionally occur concomitantly in the multitrauma patient with SCI who has evidence of either external or internal bleeding. Whereas isolated hypovolemic shock is characterized by hypotension with tachycardia, relative bradycardia (for a given degree of hypotension) is to be expected in the setting of multitrauma with SCI.

Spinal shock encompasses a number of different neurologic manifestations of SCI with varying time courses. Traumatic injuries to the spinal cord interrupt and/or temporarily damage a number of descending and ascending pathways. The most common initial presentation of a complete SCI with respect to reflex and autonomic function is a period of areflexia and flaccidity that is gradually replaced by hypertonia, exaggerated reflexes, and (in many cases) spasticity. The transition period may last from days to weeks. The immediate onset of hyperreflexia and spasticity is uncommon; when it occurs, it is a bad prognostic sign. The period of transition in reflex and autonomic function is often referred to as *spinal shock*. Concomitant changes in motor and sensory function are also common.

Animal studies indicate that ischemia underlies many of the secondary mechanisms of post SCI, often dictating the resultant deficits.[28,44-46] Human studies suggest a direct correlation between the severity of SCI and the incidence and severity of cardiovascular problems.[28,47] Together, this suggests that reducing the magnitude of secondary injury should be at the forefront of medical management of SCI.

The typical patient with SCI without associated vascular or visceral injury presents to the emergency department with a mean arterial blood pressure of 80 mm Hg and a heart rate of 65 beats/min.[35] Persistent bradycardia is a frequent finding and is often profound enough to produce hemodynamic compromise.[28,48] The patient's blood pressure may respond to volume resuscitation, but often these patients require low-dose pressors. Aggressive medical management, including volume expansion and maintenance of mean arterial blood pressure greater than 85 mm Hg, is believed to potentially enhance neurologic outcome by maximizing spinal cord perfusion at the injury site and thus reducing the likelihood of secondary injury.[7] Invasive hemodynamic monitoring will demonstrate a normal cardiac index with a low systemic vascular resistance. In the elderly patient with SCI, careful attention to volume replacement is required so as not to precipitate heart failure.

GASTROINTESTINAL SYSTEM

Hypoactive bowel sounds and impaired peristalsis are a common accompaniment after SCI, owing to the lack of sympathetic modulation. To avoid gastric and small-bowel dilatation, it is wise to delay enteral feeding. In any patient in whom gastric distention impairs respiratory function, a nasogastric tube is indicated. Most cervical cord injuries require nasogastric suction because of impaired bowel motility, air swallowing producing gastric distention, and respiratory compromise due to paralysis of intercostal muscles.

Patients with spinal cord injuries are at high risk of developing gastric and duodenal stress ulcers. Use of steroids compounds the risk of developing significant gastrointestinal hemorrhage. All patients with spinal cord injuries should receive at minimum an H_2 blocker to prevent this dreaded complication. The reported risk of gastrointestinal hemorrhage in NASCIS II for the control group was 3% and for the methylprednisolone group, 4.5%.[15]

URINARY SYSTEM

During the period of spinal shock after a cervical or thoracic SCI, the urinary bladder is atonic and flaccid. Over time it becomes an upper motor neuron bladder with small capacity. An indwelling Foley catheter is initially placed. After 3 to 4 days this is switched to intermittent bladder catheterization to maintain urinary volumes below 500 mL. Urinary tract infections are common, and if any fevers occur, urine cultures must be obtained and antibiotics selected based on culture sensitivities. Patients with spinal injuries above T6 may also develop autonomic dysreflexia if the bladder becomes overdistended or sometimes with catheterization; sympathetic overactivity and thus headaches, hypertension, sweating, and reduced body temperature result. Long-term complications include chronic infections, obstructive uropathy, and renal calculi; if left untreated, renal failure may develop.

INTEGUMENT

The SCI patient is extremely susceptible to developing decubiti. Frequent log rolling is invaluable in preventing skin breakdown. Specialized beds to turn SCI patients (e.g., RotoRest[42] [KCI,]) can reduce the incidence of skin breakdown by preventing pressure on a single area. Early intervention for skin breakdown frequently involves application of the DuoDERM patch (ConvaTec, Princeton, New Jersey) to prevent progression.

THROMBOEMBOLIC COMPLICATIONS

Patients with SCI are at high risk of lower-extremity venous thromboembolism, which may manifest as deep vein thrombosis (DVT) in the lower or upper extremities and lead to leg swelling and/or pulmonary embolism. Depending on injury severity, age, and diagnostic methods, incidence of thromboembolic events ranges from 7% to 100%.[49] The majority of these events occur within the first 3 months after injury, except in patients who are elderly, obese, or who have had prior thromboembolic events.[49]

Numerous studies have addressed the issue of preventive measures for DVT. Prevention has traditionally included the administration of low doses of heparin (5000 units subcutaneously) twice daily or more. However, meta-analysis of available literature suggests that better alternatives include the combination of pneumatic compression stockings with low-molecular-weight heparin (Lovenox) or adjusted-dose heparin.[49]

Current recommendations for evaluation of suspected thromboemboli include use of Doppler ultrasound for suspected DVT and venography if a strong clinical suspicion exists for DVT despite a negative ultrasound or if pulmonary embolism is suspected.[49,50] Treatment of pulmonary emboli or above-knee DVT requires heparinization. Should there be a contraindication to heparinization, an inferior vena cava filter should be placed. Prophylactic placement of inferior vena cava filters has been advocated,[27,49,51,52] but these procedures are not without risk, and no study thus far compares success rates to the aforementioned conservative prevention modalities.[49,53]

Prognostic Factors for Recovery

The clinician uses the neurologic examination, patient age, and appearance of the spinal cord on MRI as well as other clinical data to guide the patient and his or her family on the expected outcome for a specific injury. In any traumatic SCI, it is important to ascertain whether the patient has a functionally complete or incomplete neurologic deficit. The distinction is important because the prognosis for neurologic recovery differs for these two conditions. Patients with no evidence of motor or sensory function below their spinal column injury are considered to have functionally complete injuries. Patients with no voluntary motor control and only slight sensory preservation in their lowest sacral dermatomes or some anal tone are still considered to have incomplete injuries. Functionally, patients with complete cervical spinal cord injuries who remain complete within the first 24 hours of admission are unlikely to regain significant ambulatory function (1% to 3%).[54,55] However, most patients who enter the hospital with an incomplete neurologic injury obtain some degree of recovery. The level and degree of an incomplete injury also provides important prognostic information. Cervical injuries have a higher potential for recovery when compared with thoracic and/or thoracolumbar injuries. The less severe the SCI, the more likely the patient will recover.[56]

The majority of injuries occur in males, with well over half the injuries occurring in the 16- to 30-year-old age group. Prognosis for recovery is inextricably linked to age, with younger patients fairing much better than their older counterparts for regaining neurologic function after SCI.[57,58] The two most important potential neurologic explanations are the capacity of the "young" spinal cord to function with major deficiencies in the neural circuitry and the possibility of some spontaneous regeneration of the CNS after injury.[59] The reverse also appears to be true. It is well recognized that patients with stable incomplete injuries who age may lose function, and this may simply be the result of the loss of the last few functioning neurons or axons within the damaged region of spinal cord.[60] Neuronal loss is a normal part of the aging process for both the brain and spinal cord, and the clinical deterioration observed after SCI may be likened to the postpolio syndrome.

MRI after SCI allows visualization of the spinal cord in a noninvasive manner. The images provide immediate feedback to the surgeon about the degree of spinal cord compression, as well as information regarding the stability of the spinal column through an assessment of the integrity of the ligaments, disks, and surrounding soft tissues. In addition, intramedullary hemorrhage may be easily discerned, providing important prognostic information. Intramedullary hemorrhage is more commonly observed after neurologically complete injuries, and hemorrhage signifies a worse neurologic and functional outcome.[61,62] MRI of SCI is discussed in greater detail in Chapter 40.

Research

Spinal cord injury research is an absolute priority of the National Institutes of Health. Models of SCI, mechanisms of secondary injury, treatment of the acute phase of SCI, and development of transplantation strategies to repair a damaged spinal cord are ongoing across North America and around the world. The treatment arms of research can be divided into two categories: (1) agents that can be given during the acute phase of injury to limit secondary injury mechanisms or (2) strategies to promote regeneration. Two of the most promising drugs, methylprednisolone and ganglioside GM,[1] have only yielded modest results. Methylprednisolone, which is used in almost all major SCI centers, is coming under closer scrutiny as to its effectiveness.[17] Drugs of the future include neurotrophins, which can promote survival and regeneration of injured nerve cells, drugs that prevent the inflammatory response to SCI,[63] and drugs that prevent apoptotic cell death.[64] In the transplantation arena, cellular therapies to treat chronic injury are important. Cells of interest include Schwann cells, olfactory ensheathing glia, embryonic spinal cord, and neural progenitor cells. Antibodies that neutralize inhibitory proteins within myelin have also demonstrated promise. Strategies that combine a number of the aforementioned treatments are most likely to have a beneficial effect in the future.

Conclusion

It appears that despite enormous advancements in the diagnosis and treatment of spinal fractures over the past 3 decades, there exist a number of unanswered questions regarding the most appropriate management of patients with traumatic spinal fractures. Although only a few aspects of the surgical management of spine trauma are raised in this chapter, it is clear a number of issues remain unresolved.

Technologic advancements in spinal instrumentation and pharmacotherapeutics will continue in the 21st century. It will be critical that both neurosurgeons and orthopedic surgeons work together to test both the efficacy and cost-effectiveness of some of the newer treatment modalities, because both the best possible treatment and cost containment will be part of the management equation in the future. Outcome assessment should be at the forefront of all new ideas. Only through a critical and open-minded analysis of our treatment strategies will we be able to provide the best care for those patients who will often be changed for the remainder of their lives by their injuries and the rapid sequence of events that revolve around their acute hospitalization.

KEY POINTS

1. Most spinal injuries result from high-speed motor vehicle accidents.

2. The primary injury mechanism results from a mechanical insult that occurs at the time of impact and includes acute compression, impaction, distraction, laceration, and shear. Secondary injuries occur after the initial injury and account for some of the progressive pathologic changes associated with spinal cord injury (SCI).

3. Respiratory complications are a major source of morbidity and mortality after SCI.

4. In the elderly patient with SCI, careful attention to volume replacement is required so as not to precipitate heart failure.

5. The prognosis for recovery and survival from SCI is inextricably linked to age, with younger patients fairing much better than their older counterparts for survival.

ANNOTATED REFERENCES

Deep venous thrombosis and thromboembolism in patients with cervical spinal cord injuries. Neurosurgery 2002;50(3 Suppl):S73-80.
Recommendations of the recent (2002) guidelines for the management of acute cervical spine and spinal cord injuries that are pertinent to prophylaxis for prevention of deep venous thrombosis.

Northrup BE, Vaccaro AR, Rosen JE, et al. Occurrence of infection in anterior cervical fusion for spinal cord injury after tracheostomy. Spine (Phila Pa 1976) 1995;20(22):2449-53.
A small clinical study in 11 patients found that tracheostomy was not associated with an increased infection risk in subsequent anterior cervical surgery in adults with cervical spine injury.

Schaefer DM, Flanders AE, Osterholm JL, et al. Prognostic significance of magnetic resonance imaging in the acute phase of cervical spine injury. J Neurosurg 1992;76(2):218-23.
Clinical study of 57 patients that suggests that the MR imaging pattern observed in the acutely injured human spinal cord has a prognostic significance in the final outcome of the motor system.

Tator CH, Fehlings MG. Review of the secondary injury theory of acute spinal cord trauma with emphasis on vascular mechanisms. J Neurosurg 1991;75(1):15-26.
Review article by two respected authorities in clinical SCI on the mechanisms involved in the evolution of secondary damage.

Vale FL, Burns J, Jackson AB, et al. Combined medical and surgical treatment after acute spinal cord injury: results of a prospective pilot study to assess the merits of aggressive medical resuscitation and blood pressure management. J Neurosurg 1997;87(2):239-46.
Clinical trial in 77 patients with acute SCI in which aggressive ICU care, including optimized volume expansion and pressor support, was associated with favorable outcome.

REFERENCES

Access the complete reference list online at http://www.expertconsult.com.

40 Neuroimaging

DAVID J. MICHELSON | STEPHEN ASHWAL

Methods

PLAIN RADIOGRAPHS

Plain radiographs can be acquired rapidly and inexpensively but are of limited value in studying patients with suspected central nervous system (CNS) pathology. In the initial evaluation of patients with traumatic injuries, plain radiography of the head and neck may be useful when a surgical or unstable injury such as a depressed skull fracture, vertebral fracture, or subluxation is identified. Because plain radiographic studies are unable to identify intracranial injuries or exclude spinal injuries, CT is required whenever aspects of the clinical presentation suggest the presence of significant injury. Retrospective studies suggest that when patients have such minor trauma or symptoms that cervical spine plain radiography is ordered, instead of CT, the images are of little clinical benefit.[1]

COMPUTED TOMOGRAPHY

Computed tomography (CT) is the most widely used imaging modality for evaluating critically ill patients. CT is widely available, rapid, and accurate and has virtually no contraindications in the acute setting. The utility of CT is increased by multiple modifications, including the use of contrast, windowing techniques, and image-reconstruction techniques. Iodinated contrast agents given intravenously (IV) visualize lesions that disrupt the blood-brain barrier as well as normal and abnormal vascular structures. Varying the grayscale "window level" improves the evaluation of osseous and soft-tissue structures. Concerns about the long-term risks of malignancy from CT radiation exposure need to be considered in young patients and those likely to require repeated neuroimaging studies.[2]

Spiral or helical CT scanners allow rapid imaging through a large volume of the body, usually with a single breath hold, making sedation for imaging unnecessary in most children. Rapid thin-section axial images can be acquired with little artifact, merged, and reconstructed for display along any plane. CT angiography (CTA) uses tracking of a contrast bolus and the subtraction of background tissue to visualize blood vessels.

Xenon CT tracks the diffusion of inhaled xenon gas to measure cerebral perfusion. Rapid CT scanning has also led to the development of CT perfusion studies that track IV contrast, providing estimates of cerebral blood volume (CBV), cerebral blood flow (CBF), and mean transit time. Although bolus tracking techniques are less quantitative than nuclear medicine studies such as xenon CT, positron emission tomography, and single-photon emission computed tomography (SPECT), they are more widely available. Perfusion studies are increasingly used to evaluate vascular injuries[3] and may have applications in the study of other diseases.

MAGNETIC RESONANCE IMAGING

Magnetic resonance imaging (MRI) uses an intense magnetic field and radiofrequency pulses to produce images without the use of ionizing radiation. There are numerous MRI "sequences" for which imaging parameters are varied to highlight different tissue characteristics, identifying both anatomic and physiologic variations from normal. The availability of increasingly powerful MRI magnets and more refined methods for signal collection and processing have reduced imaging times and increased image clarity, sensitivity, and specificity.[4]

Gadolinium-based, noniodinated IV contrast agents are used to assess vascular integrity. Arterial spin labeling and contrast bolus tracking methods can be used to create MR angiography (MRA) and MR perfusion-weighted images (PWI).

Functional MRI (fMRI) can detect changes in blood flow and map the performance of cognitive tasks to areas of increased or decreased brain activity, but its use outside of research is limited to the presurgical workup of patients with tumors or focal epilepsy. Diffusion-weighted imaging (DWI) evaluates the directional movement of water molecules to assess tissues for increased diffusion, as occurs with decreased cell density (encephalomalacia) or increased extracellular water content (vasogenic edema), or decreased or restricted diffusion, as occurs with increased water content within injured cells (cytotoxic edema) or between layers of injured myelin. DWI is very useful for early identification of acute ischemic stroke, for the differentiation of necrotic tumor from pyogenic abscess, and in evaluation of the cellularity and grade of tumors.[5-7] PWI studies are used to look for an ischemic penumbra around an area of infarction that might remain viable and respond to reperfusion or neuroprotection. Patients with an area of poor perfusion much larger than their area of diffusion restriction (DWI/PWI mismatch) are more likely to respond favorably to interventional thrombectomy,[8] but there is still little agreement as to how to measure core and penumbral tissues.[9]

Magnetic resonance spectroscopy (MRS) can noninvasively measure brain metabolites in a small volume (voxel) of tissue. Carbon and phosphorous spectroscopy have shown promising applications in research, but proton spectroscopy is more commonly used. Current applications include assessing the severity of traumatic and ischemic injuries, characterizing tumors and differentiating them from infections, demyelination, and postradiation injury, and evaluating patients with metabolic disorders.[10,11] Diffusion tensor imaging (DTI), which measures the diffusion of water molecules along a higher number of planes than conventional DWI in order to assess the directionality of fiber tracts, is an emerging technology for visualizing the relationship between mass lesions and large, projecting fiber tracts, such as the visual and corticospinal tracts, and for monitoring the severity and evolution of axonal injuries.[12]

The disadvantages of performing MRI on critical care patients include the need for preprocedural preparation and screening. Patients must be screened carefully for the presence of implanted devices and ferromagnetic metal fragments or prostheses that may preclude their exposure to the powerful magnetic field used in MRI.[13] The website www.MRIsafety.com is a useful resource for checking the MRI compatibility of particular medical devices. Respirators and physiologic monitors must also be MRI compatible. Only oxygen and nitrogen tanks composed of aluminum can enter the magnet suite. All these precautions and modifications can significantly delay imaging. There are protocols to rapidly evaluate patients with suspected acute stroke, but most routine MRI studies take approximately 45 minutes to perform, and studies of the entire neuroaxis with and without contrast can require more than 90 minutes. Critically ill patients are often unable to tolerate MRI until they are more hemodynamically stable.

NUCLEAR MEDICINE STUDIES

Nuclear medicine techniques provide somewhat quantitative physiologic imaging of the brain. PET measures the distribution of radioisotope-containing compounds (e.g., 8F-fluorodeoxyglucose

[FDG]) that are given IV and can study cerebral perfusion as well as cerebral energy metabolism. SPECT can study the distribution of isotopes incorporated into other biologically active compounds, allowing measurement of other aspects of tissue metabolism.[14] PET studies provide higher-resolution images that can more easily be co-registered with MRI, but PET can only be done in hospitals with their own cyclotrons, as the isotopes used have shorter half-lives than those used for SPECT. The most common application of PET is in the diagnosis, staging, and monitoring of tumors, although other applications are undergoing evaluation.[15,16] SPECT using technetium-99m hexamethylpropyleneamine oxime (^{99m}Tc-HMPAO) is often used to assess overall CBF as a confirmatory test in the determination of brain death.[17]

ANGIOGRAPHY

Percutaneous transfemoral catheterization is used to evaluate cerebral and spinal vascular anatomy. It is an invasive procedure but has a fairly low rate of complications in experienced centers, with most complications being minor and transient, such as groin hematoma, asymptomatic femoral artery or carotid artery dissections, and minor allergic reactions.[18] Permanent neurologic complications such as cerebral infarction due to thromboembolism are rare with diagnostic procedures but occur more often in older patients, with prolonged study times, and when angiography is used for interventional procedures such as intraarterial thrombolysis or thrombectomy, balloon angioplasty for patients with subarachnoid hemorrhage–associated vasospasm, and occlusion of aneurysms and arteriovenous malformations.[19]

Although noninvasive imaging tests of the cerebral vasculature including transcranial Doppler (TCD) ultrasonography, CTA, and MRA are useful in evaluating large- and medium-sized vessels, catheter angiography is still considered necessary for evaluating individuals with suspected vascular malformations or small-vessel vasculitis.

Brain

PATTERNS OF DISEASE

Edema

Cerebral edema is an abnormal accumulation of water within brain tissue that can be localized or diffuse. Three types of edema have been described:

1. Vasogenic edema, an accumulation of water in the interstitial spaces related to increased capillary permeability, is most prominent within white matter and is often seen with traumatic, neoplastic, infectious, and inflammatory diseases but can also be seen with toxic, ischemic, and hemorrhagic injuries.
2. Cytotoxic edema, an accumulation of intracellular water related to altered ion and water homeostasis, can involve gray and white matter equally and is often seen with ischemic injuries but also can be seen with severe diffuse axonal injury (DAI).
3. Interstitial edema, an accumulation of water in the interstitial areas of the subependymal white matter, is caused by transependymal migration of ventricular cerebrospinal fluid (CSF) and is associated with obstructive hydrocephalus.

Except for location, the CT and MRI appearance of all types of edema is similar. Increased water content appears dark on CT because of hypodensity. It also appears dark on T1-weighted imaging (T1WI) but bright on T2-weighted imaging (T2WI) sequences, including fluid-attenuated inversion recovery (FLAIR) studies in which CSF in the ventricles, cisterns, and arachnoid spaces is made to appear dark. Vasogenic edema within the white matter extends along fiber tracts, creating "fingers" that extend toward the cortical gray matter (Figure 40-1). This pattern has a nonvascular distribution and is associated with mass effect. Cytotoxic edema can involve gray and white matter, follows a vascular distribution when associated with ischemic injury, and produces less mass effect for its size (Figure 40-2). DWI can distinguish between the increased diffusivity of vasogenic edema and the restricted diffusivity of cytotoxic edema. Interstitial edema may be limited to a narrow rim that abuts the ventricular wall and fades gradually into the surrounding white matter and is best seen on MRI, particularly with FLAIR sequences.[20] Engorgement caused by increased arterial or venous CBV, often localized when associated with an arteriovenous dural fistula, can mimic edema on routine imaging studies but is apparent on cerebral perfusion studies.[21]

Hemorrhage

Intracranial hemorrhage may be parenchymal or extraaxial (epidural, subdural, or subarachnoid) in location. Parenchymal hemorrhage can be traumatic in origin but in adults is more likely nontraumatic, associated with an underlying lesion such as a tumor or vascular malformation, a vasculopathy such as vasculitis or cerebral amyloid angiopathy, or a systemic disease such as hypertension. Extraaxial hemorrhages are most often due to trauma, but subarachnoid hemorrhage also is commonly seen with aneurysm rupture.

The imaging appearance of hemorrhage depends on the stage of clot formation and lysis, location, and the degree to which it is mixed with other fluids. On CT, hemorrhage may be isodense to brain parenchyma and difficult to visualize in the hyperacute stage, but it typically becomes hyperdense within several hours (Figure 40-3, A) before again becoming isodense over days to weeks and then hypodense over several weeks (Table 40-1). Acute hematomas may continue to appear isodense in the acute stage in anemic patients with a hemoglobin (Hb) below 8 to 10 g/dL or in patients with a coagulopathy who fail to produce clot retraction.[22,23] The final CT appearance of resolved hemorrhage may show no residual abnormality or demonstrate a focus of low attenuation or calcification.

On MRI, the evolving appearance of a hemorrhage is largely explained by Hb having different paramagnetic properties as it is deoxygenated and metabolized. In the hyperacute to acute stages, diamagnetic oxyhemoglobin is predominant and appears slightly hypo- to isointense on T1WI and iso- to hyperintense on T2WI. As Hb becomes deoxygenated, it becomes paramagnetic and very hypointense on T2WI. In the subacute stage, Hb breakdown to methemoglobin begins peripherally and advances toward the center of the clot. Intracellular methemoglobin appears hyperintense on T1WI and hypointense on T2WI. As red blood cells lyse and release methemoglobin into the extracellular space, its signal becomes hyperintense on T1WI and T2WI. In the chronic stage, beginning within 2 weeks and lasting for years, methemoglobin undergoes phagocytic degradation to hemosiderin, which appears hypointense on T1WI and T2WI.[7] The evolution of a hematoma is influenced by many factors, and there may be simultaneous overlap of two or more of these stages (see Figure 40-3, B and C). The widespread use of the gradient-recalled echo (GRE) sequence, and the increasing use of susceptibility-weighted imaging (SWI) sequences, has greatly increased the sensitivity of MRI for extravasated blood.[24]

Most intraparenchymal hematomas are associated with a surrounding area of vasogenic edema and evolve somewhat more quickly (owing to higher tissue thromboplastin concentration and lower oxygen tension) than extraaxial blood collections. Intraparenchymal hematomas expand significantly, usually within 3 hours from onset, in about one-third of patients,[25] and contrast extravasation into the hematoma on CT is predictive of expansion.[26] Vasogenic edema surrounding an intraparenchymal hematoma can also expand over several days, causing a significant increase in mass effect.

Mass Effect, Shift, and Herniation

Cerebral lesions may lead to brain herniation, either as a direct result of lesion growth, as with tumor growth or hematoma expansion, or secondary to intralesional cytotoxic edema, perilesional vasogenic edema, or obstructive hydrocephalus.[27] Two relatively fixed dural partitions are present within the skull and create compartments across which the brain may herniate. The falx cerebri separates the cerebral hemispheres, and the tentorium cerebelli separates the cerebral hemispheres from the posterior fossa structures. Herniation is described in terms of location.

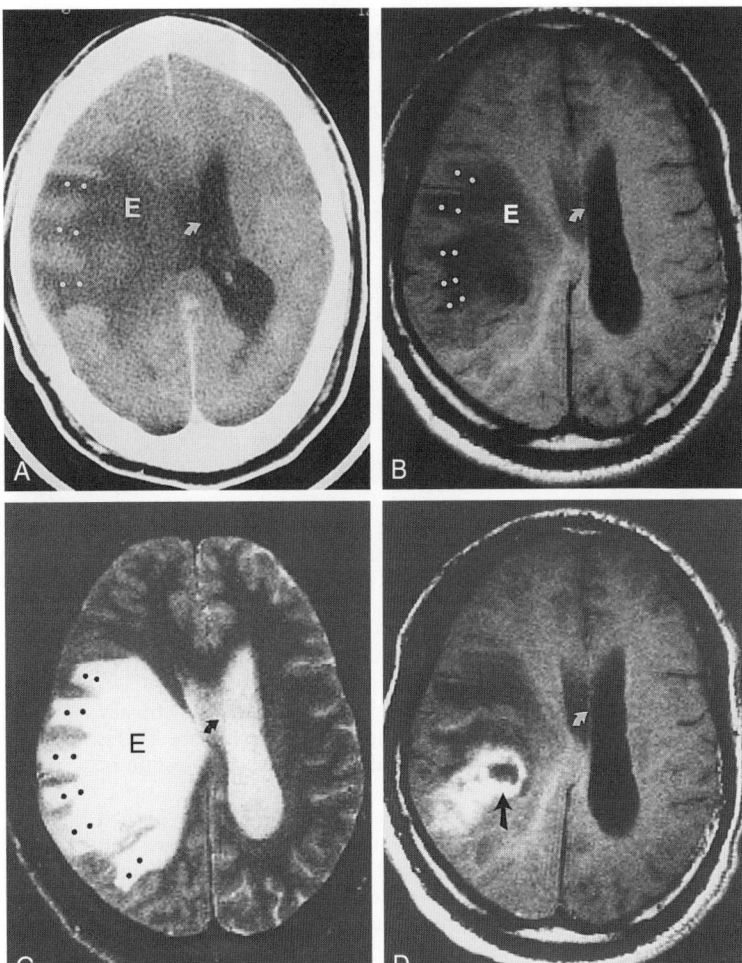

Figure 40-1 Vasogenic edema in glioblastoma. Non-contrast-enhanced axial CT scan **(A)**, axial T1-weighted MRI scan **(B)**, and axial T2-weighted MRI scan **(C)** all demonstrate an area of edema (E). Edema extends along white matter fibers *(dots)*, with normal gray matter interposed. Axial T1-weighted MRI scan following contrast enhancement **(D)** demonstrates the enhancing tumor nidus *(arrow)*, distinct from surrounding edema. Subfalcine herniation is also demonstrated on these images by displacement of the falx *(curved arrows)*.

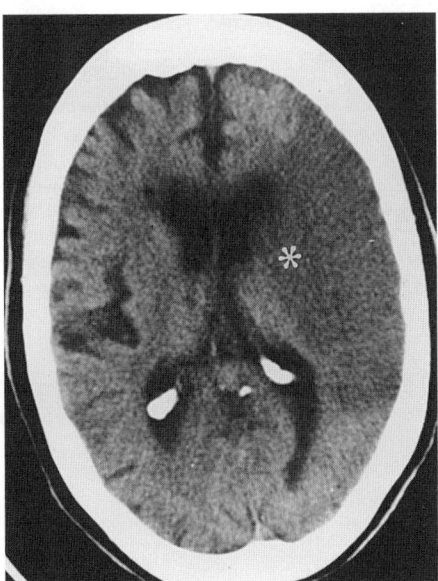

Figure 40-2 Cytotoxic edema and acute infarct. Axial non-contrast-enhanced CT scan demonstrates an area of decreased density *(asterisk)* involving the left middle cerebral artery territory. Gray and white matter structures are involved, and there is little mass effect.

Subfalcine herniation occurs when the medial surface of a hemisphere, usually the cingulate or supracingulate gyrus, is compressed against and displaced beneath the falx. With CT or MRI, early signs may appear as compression or distortion of the lateral ventricles (see Figure 40-1). Later stages are recognized by deviation of the falx, identification of the hemispheric structures that are crossing the midline, and ischemia from compression of the anterior cerebral artery.

Transalar herniation occurs when a mass displaces brain tissue across the ridge of the greater sphenoid wing. *Ascending transalar herniation* refers to a large temporal lobe mass displacing brain above the sphenoid ridge and into the anterior cranial fossa. *Descending transalar herniation* refers to a large frontal lobe mass displacing brain below the sphenoid ridge and into the middle cranial fossa. Imaging studies may identify displacement of the sylvian portion of the middle cerebral artery (MCA), which may lead to ischemia and infarction within the MCA territory.

Masses arising on either side of the tentorium can result in transtentorial herniation. Descending transtentorial herniation involves a supratentorial mass pushing the medial temporal lobe through the incisura. On CT or MRI, the herniated brain pushes against and rotates the brainstem. This produces widening of the ipsilateral brainstem cistern and effacement of the contralateral cistern (Figure 40-4). Associated findings may include dilatation of the contralateral temporal horn secondary to ventricular trapping. Ascending transtentorial herniation is caused by an infratentorial mass displacing the pons, vermis, and adjacent portions of the cerebellar hemispheres upward through

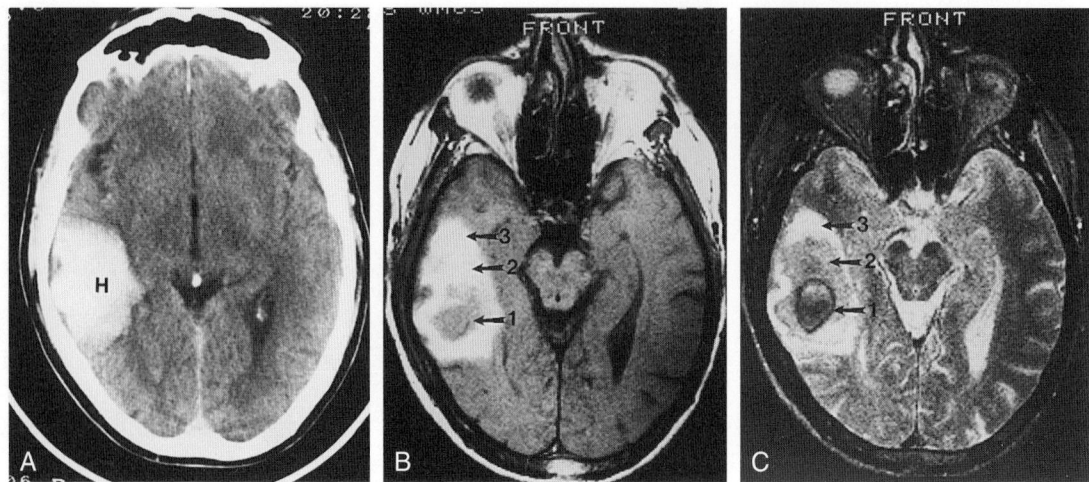

Figure 40-3 **Hemorrhage.** Axial CT image **(A)** demonstrates a large area of acute hemorrhage (H) in right temporal lobe. T1-weighted **(B)** and T2-weighted **(C)** MRI scans demonstrate the hemorrhage in various stages of breakdown. Center of lesion is dark on T1- and T2-weighted images, indicating oxyhemoglobin (1). Intermediate zone is bright on T1-weighted image and gray on T2-weighted image, indicating intracellular methemoglobin (2). Outer rim is bright on both T1-and T2-weighted images, indicating extracellular methemoglobin (3).

the incisura. On CT and MRI, the brainstem cisterns are symmetrically effaced as the cerebellar vermis bulges up through the incisura. This is often associated with acute hydrocephalus caused by compression of the cerebral aqueduct.

Tonsillar herniation occurs when the cerebellar tonsils are pushed through the foramen magnum. This results in medullary compression and dysfunction of vital respiratory and cardiac control centers. Sagittal MRI is the preferred modality for demonstrating tonsillar herniation and the secondary effects on the brainstem.

SPECIFIC DISEASE PROCESSES

Traumatic Brain Injury

Noncontrast head CT continues to be the primary modality for the initial evaluation of patients with traumatic brain injury (TBI).[28] Its advantages include fast examination time, wide availability, fracture detection, lack of contraindications, and high accuracy. Although MRI is more sensitive in detecting intracranial injuries, it is limited by longer examination times, need for sedation in uncooperative patients, and difficulties with monitoring potentially hemodynamically unstable patients. Once patients have been stabilized, MRI becomes the modality of choice for fully elucidating the nature and extent of the injury and for informing prognosis.[29]

Injury to brain parenchyma may result in contusion, axonal (shear) injury, or hematoma. Contusions are caused by the direct impact of parenchyma against bone and are most common along the gyral

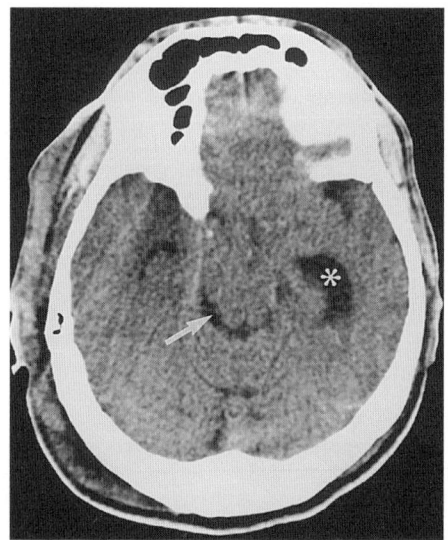

Figure 40-4 **Right descending transtentorial herniation in patient with large right parietal subdural hematoma.** Axial non-contrast-enhanced CT scan of head at level of midbrain shows that ipsilateral subarachnoid cistern is widened (*arrow*), and contralateral subarachnoid cistern is obliterated because of brainstem rotation. Left temporal horn is also dilated (*asterisk*), indicating trapping of left lateral ventricle.

TABLE 40-1	**Evolution of Computed Tomography and Magnetic Resonance Imaging Appearance of Hemorrhage**				
Stage	*Time Period*	*Blood Product*	*CT**	*T1WI†*	*T2WI†*
Hyperacute	<12 hours	Oxyhemoglobin	↔ or ↑	↓ or ↔	↑
Acute	1-3 days	Deoxyhemoglobin	↑	↓ or ↔	↓↓
Early subacute	3-14 days	Intracellular methemoglobin	↔	↑	↓↓
Late subacute	2-4 weeks	Extracellular methemoglobin	↔	↑↑	↑
Chronic	>2 weeks	Hemosiderin	↓	↔	↓↓
		Nonparamagnetic hemichromes	↓	↓	↑
		Calcification	↑↑	↓	↓

*Density relative to brain parenchyma
†Intensity relative to brain parenchyma

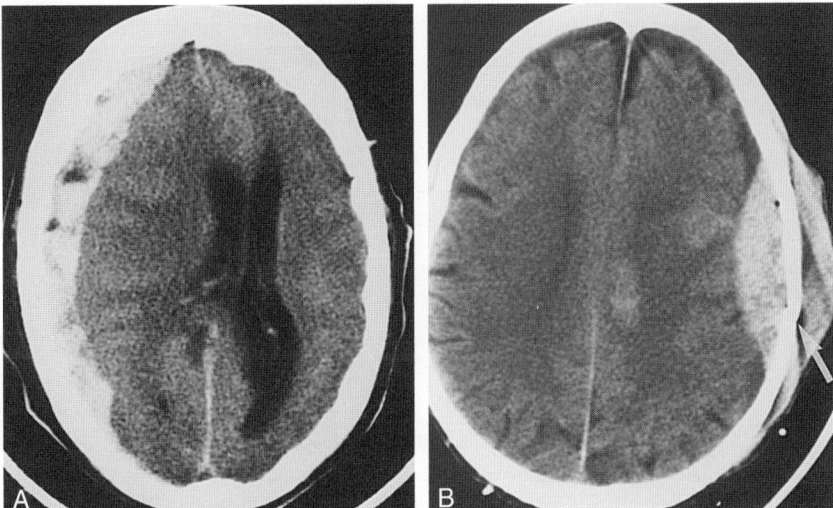

Figure 40-5 Subdural and epidural hematoma. A, Axial CT scan of head demonstrates a mixed-density subdural hematoma along right frontoparietal lobes. Mixed-density appearance is most likely due to presence of unretracted semiliquid clot. **B,** Axial CT scan of head demonstrates a left biconvex hyperdense collection that is classic for epidural hematoma. A fracture *(arrow)* can also be identified.

surface of the frontal and temporal lobes. Larger contusions may contain petechial hemorrhage and appear as ill-defined heterogeneous lesions with little or no mass effect. Edema and mass effect may increase in the first 48 hours after TBI, making these lesions more evident on imaging studies.

Shear injuries are secondary to rotational forces that produce tears in axonal fibers and are most common within the white matter (subcortical white matter, corpus callosum, internal capsule, and brainstem). Except for location, the imaging characteristics of non-hemorrhagic contusions and shear injuries are similar. Initial studies may be normal or demonstrate small foci of edema. Shear injuries may be apparent on MRI, particularly with the use of (1) susceptibility-weighted imaging (SWI), which is exquisitely sensitive to the microhemorrhages associated with moderate shear injuries; (2) DWI, which may show cytotoxic edema from more severe shear injuries; and (3) MRS, which may show elevations of choline (Cho) and myoinositol (mI) and decreases in N-acetylaspartate (NAA) proportional to injury severity.

Damage to the brain coverings may lead to hemorrhage into the epidural, subdural, and subarachnoid (and, by extension, intraventricular) spaces. On CT, intraventricular and subarachnoid hemorrhage is identified by replacement of the normal low-density CSF by high-density blood. When subtle, subarachnoid hemorrhage can be mistaken for generalized edema, with loss of the basal cisterns. Subdural hematomas typically appear as crescentic mixed or hyperdense collections that cross suture lines but not dural attachments (Figure 40-5, *A*). Epidural hematomas typically appear as biconvex hyperdense collections that cross dural attachments but not suture lines (see Figure 40-5, *B*). With rapid accumulation of blood, unretracted semiliquid clot may be present. In this situation, CT demonstrates hypodense areas within the hyperdense hematoma, the so-called swirl sign.[30] Distinction between epidural and subdural hematomas is important, because epidural hematomas often have an arterial source, expand rapidly, and require emergent drainage to avoid herniation.[31]

Abusive head trauma (AHT) is a significant cause of neurodevelopmental morbidity and mortality in children younger than 2 years old.[32] Mechanisms that have been proposed include blunt trauma, axonal shearing from shaking, and secondary ischemic injury from strangulation, arterial dissection, suffocation, or brainstem injury leading to respiratory arrest. Intracranial injuries commonly encountered include skull fracture, subdural hematoma, subarachnoid hemorrhage, and shear injuries. Subdural hematoma is regarded as one of the most characteristic CNS lesions encountered in the "shaken baby" syndrome. In fact, subdural hematomas in young children are more often associated with AHT than with accidental trauma.[32] The CT appearance of AHT in children is similar to that in adults. However, subdural

hematoma is more common along the posterior interhemispheric fissure and appears as increased attenuation along the falx. Other common locations include the anterior interhemispheric, tentorial, and parieto-occipital regions. MRI can determine the age of the blood products and provide an estimate of when the hemorrhage occurred, as discussed earlier. Coexistence of blood products of different ages (Figure 40-6) is suggestive of recurrent bleeding and repeated abuse but must be interpreted with great caution.[7]

Vascular Lesions

Ischemia, Hypoxia, and Infarct. Although CT demonstrates only about half of infarcts within the first 48 hours, it remains the imaging modality of choice in the acute evaluation of patients with transient or persistent focal neurologic deficits that may be associated with cerebral ischemia, because rapid exclusion of a hemorrhagic etiology is critical in determining whether a patient can be treated with thrombolytic agents.[33] CT can in some cases confirm the thromboembolic etiology of an ischemic stroke by showing subtle cerebral edema in a vascular distribution or by showing hyperdense clot within a thrombosed artery. It can also be immediately helpful in demonstrating mass lesions such as tumors, infections, and vascular lesions that can produce symptoms that mimic stroke and may require emergent

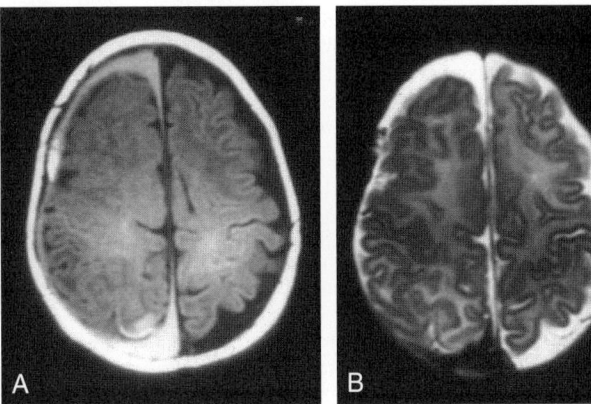

Figure 40-6 Abusive head trauma. Axial T1- **(A)** and T2-weighted **(B)** MRI scans of an infant reveal bilateral subdural blood collections of different ages. Right collection shows blood in the late subacute phase (2–4 weeks old), and left shows blood in the chronic phase (>1 month). This finding is almost proof positive of repeated abuse.

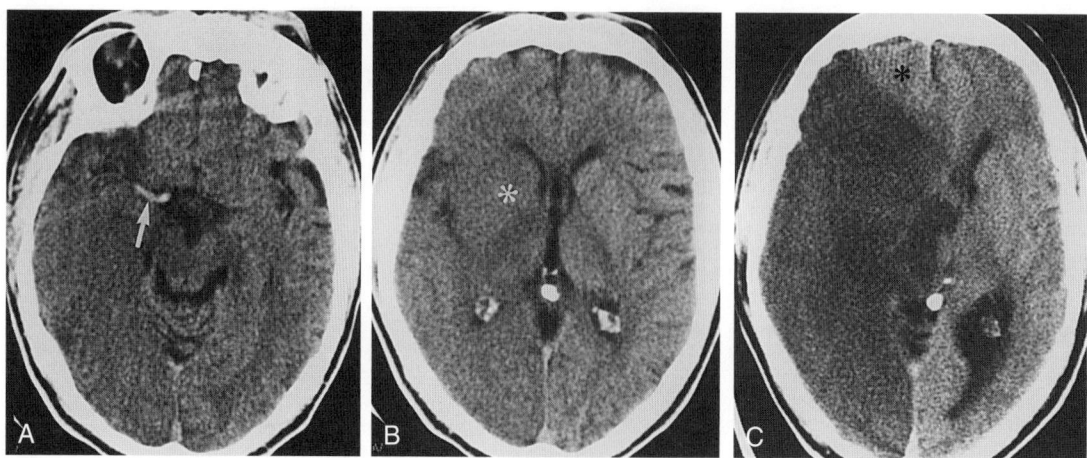

Figure 40-7   Acute infarct. Axial non-contrast-enhanced CT images obtained at level of temporal lobe **(A)** and through level of basal ganglia **(B)** demonstrate area of low density involving gray and white matter of right hemisphere. There is loss of gray-white matter differentiation, especially noticeable in region of basal ganglia *(asterisk, B)*. Compare right and left sides. High density is identified within right middle cerebral artery *(arrow, A)*, representing clot. Axial non-contrast-enhanced CT scan obtained 48 hours later **(C)** demonstrates marked edema involving territories of right, middle, and posterior cerebral arteries. Note sparing of right anterior cerebral artery territory *(asterisk, C)*.

surgical treatment.[5] Small lacunar infarcts and infratentorial strokes are more difficult to visualize by CT.[34]

The CT appearance of an ischemic injury evolves over time. In the hyperacute stage (first 24 hours), the CT scan may be normal or demonstrate a subtle decrease in density and loss of gray-white differentiation (Figure 40-7). An artery obstructed by thromboembolism may appear hyperdense. During the acute stage (within the first week), the infarct becomes more pronounced owing to the mass effect and decreased density related to cytotoxic edema (see Figure 40-2). The infarct is better defined, involves gray and white matter, and corresponds to a known vascular territory. During the subacute stage (1–3 weeks), the edema and mass effect begin to resolve. Chronic infarcts demonstrate parenchymal replacement, with well-defined, sharply marginated zones of cystic encephalomalacia and gliosis. The infarct behaves like a contracting rather than an expanding mass.

The MRI appearance of an ischemic infarct also evolves in a predictable fashion (Figure 40-8). Nonhemorrhagic infarcts begin with subtle increased signal intensity on T2WI and minimal changes on T1WI. Subtle findings include stagnation of blood flow (arterial enhancement) and swelling of the involved gyri. DWI (Figure 40-9) can show cytotoxic edema within minutes of the onset of a stroke, and the intensity of the abnormal signal is typically maximal at 3 to 5 days and then gradually fades over another 1 to 2 weeks. Because DWI shows directionally restricted water movement as a bright signal but also shows bright signal in areas that are bright on T2WI (T2 shine through), the presence of cytotoxic edema is best evaluated by the apparent diffusion coefficient (ADC) map, in which brain regions with fully restricted water diffusion appear darker than surrounding brain.

CT and MRI perfusion techniques can demonstrate diminished blood perfusion within minutes of an insult. When MRI perfusion studies are coupled with diffusion images, a penumbra can be identified as a zone of decreased perfusion surrounding an area of absent perfusion (Figure 40-10). Only the central area shows the diffusion restriction. The penumbra represents viable tissue at risk for infarction, which may still be salvageable.[9]

Imaging protocols that use a number of MRI sequences for acute evaluation of a suspected stroke may provide the ideal combination of information about regional anatomy (standard MRI), presence of blood (GRE or SWI), extent of infarction (DWI), vascular anatomy (MRA), blood flow (PWI), and metabolic alterations (MRS) (see Figure 40-10). The feasibility of using such protocols continues to be studied.[35]

Hypertensive encephalopathy is a syndrome that occurs in patients with elevated blood pressure of any cause. Severe preeclampsia and

eclampsia of pregnancy are the most common causes, and CNS involvement is common. MRI findings include symmetric vasogenic edema in the subcortical white matter, primarily in the occipital and parietal lobes but occasionally extending into the frontal lobes. Radiologically similar lesions, referred to as *posterior reversible encephalopathy syndrome* (PRES), have been seen in association with a number of other conditions, including thrombotic thrombocytopenic purpura, sepsis, glomerulonephritis, and exposure to the immunosuppressants, cyclosporine and tacrolimus. The association with hypertension led to the presumption that edema was secondary to hyperemia and blood-brain barrier breakdown, but nearly half of patients with PRES lack a history of even moderate hypertension, and most perfusion studies have shown decreased perfusion in the areas of edema, rather than hyperemia, and the typical watershed distribution of the lesions is consistent with hypoperfusion contributing somewhat to the pathophysiology.[36] In 15% to 25% of cases, cytotoxic edema and hemorrhage are also seen, and these patients are less likely to show the typical reversibility of the associated clinical symptoms.[37] Brief episodes of severe hypotension, hypoxia, and hypoglycemia will typically result in infarction within a similar watershed distribution, whereas more prolonged episodes will cause progressively more severe injuries to the basal ganglia, thalami, hippocampi, cerebellum, and brainstem.[38]

Venous infarction can occur in isolation and is associated with thrombosis of a dural sinus or large draining vein. In contrast to arterial infarctions, venous infarctions are typically hemorrhagic and primarily affect the white matter. Pregnancy, dehydration, sepsis, and other acquired hypercoagulable states are common risk factors. CT can demonstrate the hemorrhagic infarct as well as the high-density clot in the venous sinus. MRI is very sensitive in detecting the hemorrhage and edema as well as the thrombosis of the venous sinus. Magnetic resonance venography can also be helpful in identifying the occlusion.

Imaging of newborns and children with cerebrovascular disease must take into account the imaging changes that occur with development. In general, the brain of a term infant has its greatest myelination and metabolic activity in the brainstem, basal ganglia, cerebellum, and perirolandic cortex. Global hypoxic-ischemic injuries in term neonates are most commonly seen in these areas, particularly in the specific regions with the highest expression of excitatory NMDA receptors, including the putamina, ventrolateral thalamic nuclei, lateral geniculate bodies, dorsal brainstem nuclei, hippocampi, and perirolandic cortex.[39] Because of the greater propensity for the injured cells of neonates to undergo apoptosis, the full extent of an ischemic injury

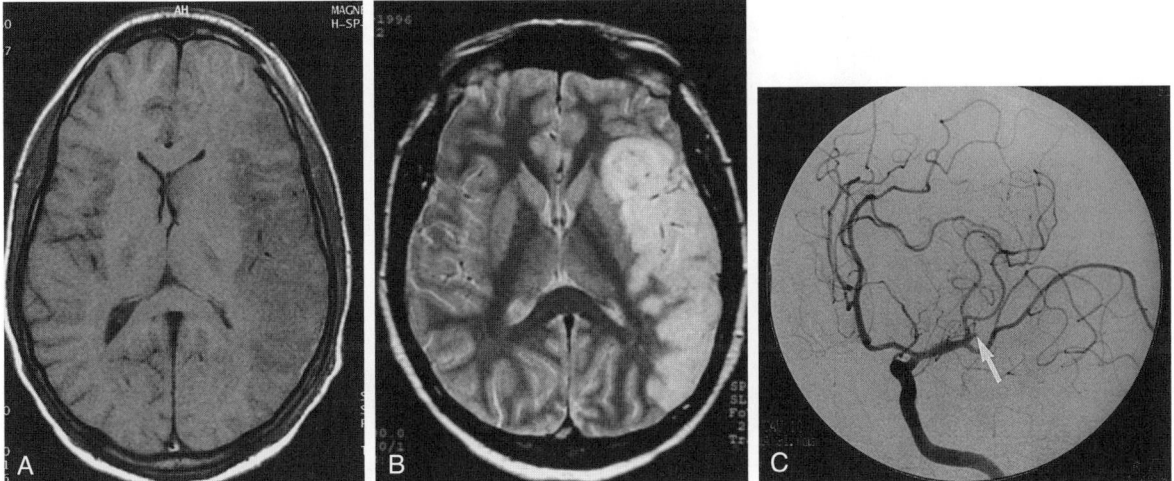

Figure 40-8 Infarct. Axial T1-weighted **(A)** and T2-weighted **(B)** MRI scans of patient being evaluated for stroke. Initial CT scan (not shown) was normal. MRI demonstrates an area of cytotoxic edema involving distal left middle cerebral artery territory. Edema is hypointense to brain on T1-weighted image and hyperintense to brain on T2-weighted image. Left internal carotid artery angiogram **(C)** demonstrates occluded branch of left middle cerebral artery *(arrow)*. Within the proper time frame, intraarterial thrombolysis would be a method of management for this patient.

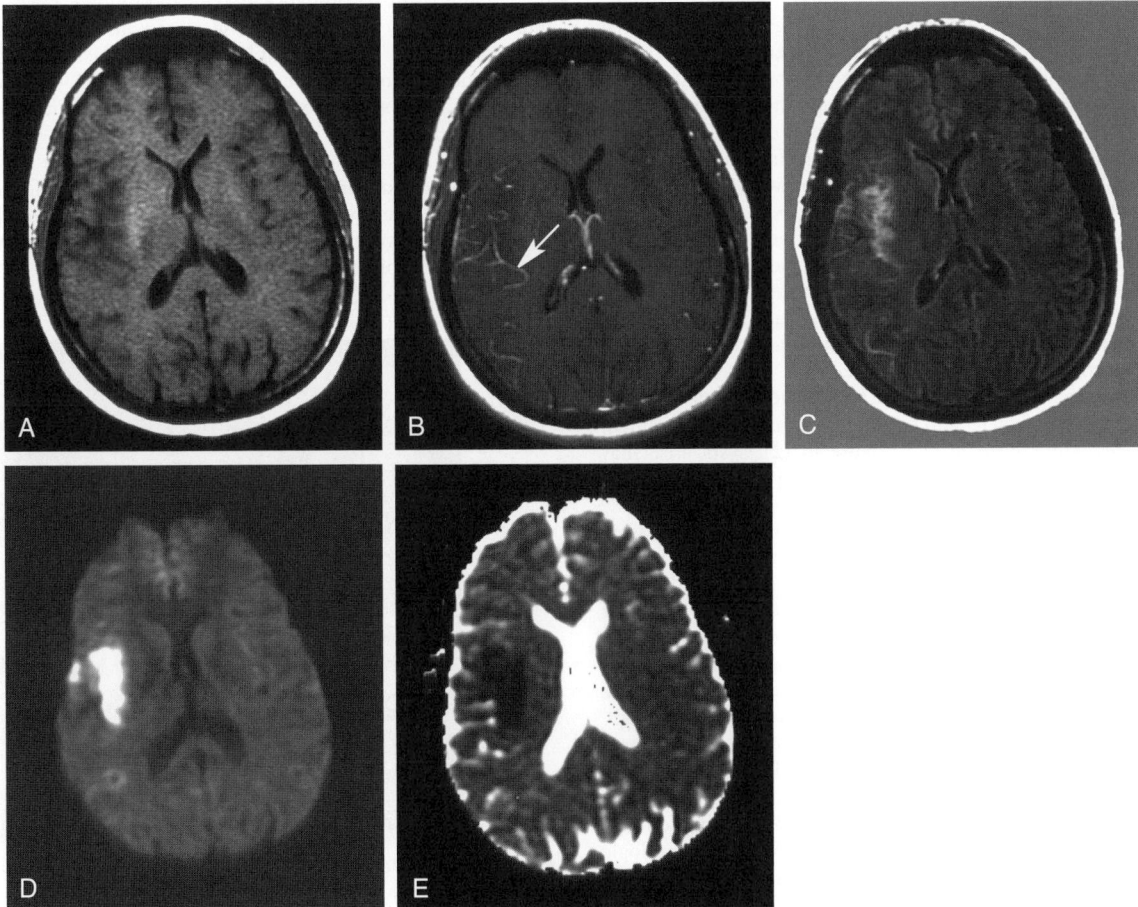

Figure 40-9 Hyperacute infarct. Axial T1-weighted image before **(A)** and after **(B)** contrast administration reveal subtle low intensity and arterial enhancement *(arrow)* in right insular cortex. Fluid-attenuated inversion recovery (FLAIR) sequence **(C)** helps define area of involvement. Diffusion-weighted sequence **(D)** shows infarct to best advantage. Acute phase is confirmed by low signal on apparent diffusion coefficient map **(E)**.

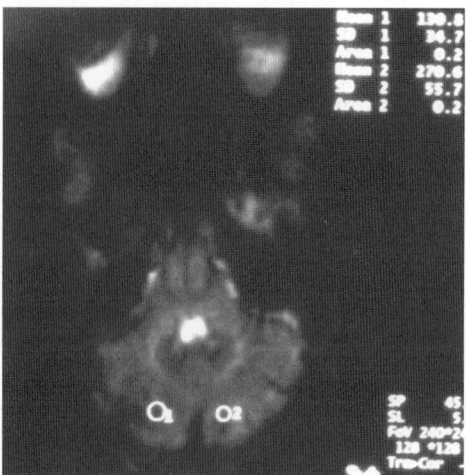

Figure 40-10 Perfusion deficit. MRI perfusion study shows hypoperfusion in right posterior inferior cerebellar artery territory. Normal left side measured 270.6, and abnormal right side measured 130.8.

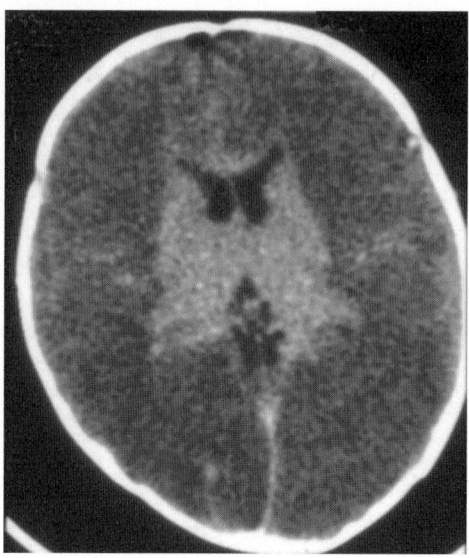

Figure 40-11 Global anoxic injury. Axial CT scan of a child following cardiac arrest. There is diffuse low density in cerebral hemispheres and compression of ventricles and sulci, reflecting increased water accumulation (edema) and resultant mass effect. Basal ganglia and thalami appear bright, showing the "reversal" sign of global anoxia.

may not be apparent on MRI for at least 72 hours. During a child's first year, as cerebral myelination proceeds from inferior to superior and posterior to anterior, the patterns of injury seen from vascular insults become more similar to those seen in older children and adults, with selective vulnerability seen in the striatum, lateral geniculate bodies, hippocampi, and frontal and parieto-occipital cortex, with sparing in moderate injuries of the thalami and perirolandic cortex.[38] The relative sparing of the cerebellum, even with severe global hypoxic-ischemic injury of the cerebral hemispheres, can result in a "cerebellar reversal" sign on CT (Figure 40-11) in which the supratentorial structures all appear hypodense in comparison to the cerebellum.[40]

In the preterm brain, early imaging findings after an anoxic event include germinal matrix hemorrhage, periventricular venous infarction, and periventricular leukomalacia. The germinal matrix is a rich vascular stroma in the subependymal caudothalamic groove that is very vulnerable to hemorrhage. When an insult occurs, the germinal matrix bursts, and blood leaks into the ventricles or parenchyma. Ultrasonography is used to stage the degree of hemorrhage. Venous infarctions are similar to those discussed earlier but occur in the periventricular region. These focal hemorrhages are readily seen with MRI and are frequently seen with CT. Periventricular leukomalacia represents areas of coagulation necrosis of the white matter, leading to reduction of the central white matter. CT and MRI demonstrate loss of white matter in the parietal and occipital regions, and enlargement of the ventricles, with ragged borders (Figure 40-12). Cystic areas may be present, and the sulci may extend almost to the ventricles.[38]

Congenital Aneurysm and Subarachnoid Hemorrhage. Evaluation of a patient with suspected subarachnoid hemorrhage should begin with a noncontrast head CT (Figure 40-13). If subarachnoid blood is confirmed by CT or lumbar puncture, a conventional angiographic study is done to assess the patient for the presence of cerebral aneurysms (see Figure 40-13). MRA and CTA may be helpful in the evaluation of patients suspected of having unruptured aneurysms but are insufficiently sensitive to exclude an aneurysmal source of bleeding.[41] In addition, when one or more aneurysms are present, conventional angiography provides the superior anatomic detail needed for planning endovascular occlusion or surgical treatment.

From 10% to 30% of patients with aneurysmal subarachnoid hemorrhage will develop morbidity from a delayed ischemic neurologic deficit from vasospasm, but many such patients are obtunded or sedated and are clinically difficult to assess for new deficits. A combination of imaging modalities may be best for identifying patients with vasospasm and ischemia.[42] Angiographic studies show vasospasm in most patients and do not clearly differentiate between patients

with symptomatic and asymptomatic narrowing. TCD is commonly used to identify vessels with increased blood flow velocity from narrowing, but comparison between TCD and xenon CT has shown that increased velocity is commonly associated with increased rather than decreased flow.[43] Transluminal balloon angioplasty and intraarterial papaverine infusion improve outcomes for patients with symptomatic vasospasm, and several other interventional techniques are under investigation.[44,45]

Vascular Malformations. Four types of vascular malformations are described: (1) arteriovenous malformation (AVM), (2) capillary telangiectasia, (3) cavernous angioma, and (4) developmental venous anomaly (DVA) or venous angioma.

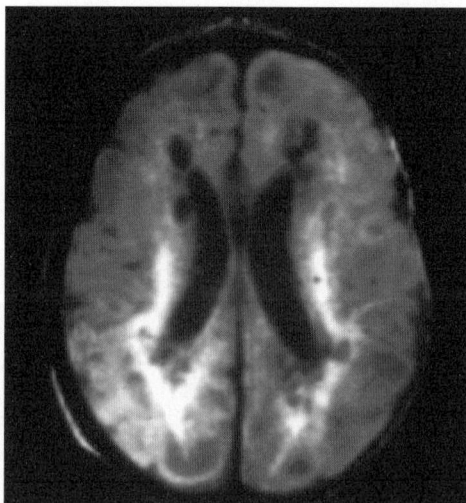

Figure 40-12 Periventricular leukomalacia. Axial fluid-attenuated inversion recovery (FLAIR) image obtained on a child with spastic diplegia and a history of prematurity and hypoxic episodes. Multifocal white matter hyperintensities, reduced white matter volume, irregular ventricular contours, and cystic changes are typical findings of periventricular leukomalacia.

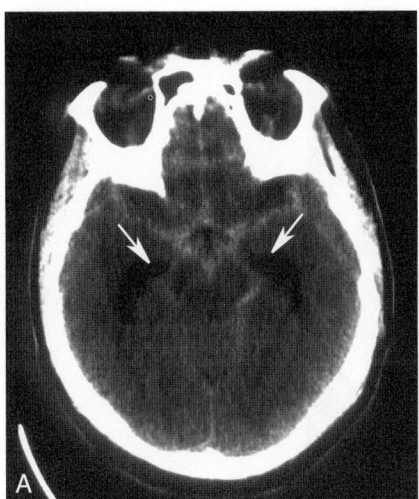 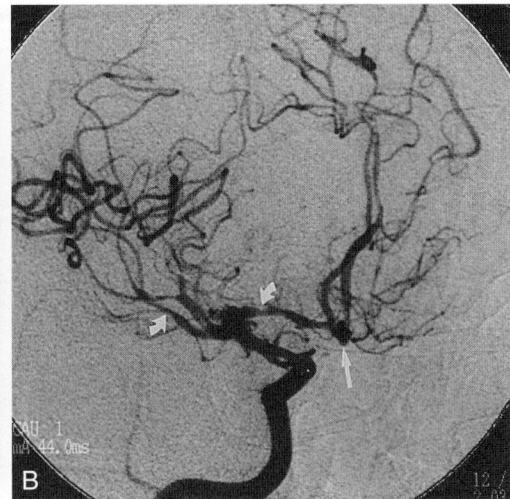

Figure 40-13 **Subarachnoid hemorrhage and aneurysm. A,** Axial non-contrast-enhanced CT scan of head reveals high density (blood) replacing normal low density of CSF within suprasellar cistern and subarachnoid spaces. This indicates subarachnoid hemorrhage. Also note dilated temporal horns (arrows), indicating acute hydrocephalus. **B,** Right internal carotid artery angiogram demonstrates presence of congenital anterior communicating artery aneurysm (arrow), as well as vasospasm (curved arrows).

AVMs are the most common type. The vessels of an unruptured AVM may be apparent on CT as tubular structures that become hyperdense with contrast administration. On MRI, the abnormal vessels may appear hypointense due to blood flow. Conventional angiography is preferred for the evaluation of suspected AVMs to differentiate them from arteriovenous fistulas, identify associated aneurysms, and provide a detailed assessment of the number, size, and location of feeding arteries and draining veins (Figure 40-14).[46] The interventional radiologist may be able to embolize some or all of the arterial feeders, making surgery either less complex or unneccesary.[47]

Capillary telangiectasia and cavernous angioma are best evaluated by MRI, because angiography is typically normal and CT is insensitive. The MRI signal characteristics vary based on the presence or absence of associated hemorrhage.

DVAs are composed of a large draining vein surrounded by a caput medusae of small feeding veins. The veins are typically inapparent on non-contrast-enhanced CT but enhance with contrast and can be seen on conventional MRI as flow voids. DVAs are rarely symptomatic other than when associated with a cavernous angioma or AVM, and conventional angiography is recommended only when an apparently simple DVA is associated with hemorrhage or edema that cannot be explained by thrombosis of the draining vein.[48]

Neoplasms

Neoplasms are typically grouped according to location. Knowledge of the imaging characteristics of specific tumors, age and gender of the patient, clinical presentation, and lesion location can narrow the differential diagnosis further and often provides a specific diagnosis. On CT, low-grade gliomas may appear as subtle nonenhancing masses, but higher-grade gliomas often demonstrate heterogeneous enhancement, with large areas of necrosis and vasogenic edema (see Figure 40-1). Metastatic lesions may be low-density and enhancing masses, as seen with lung or breast carcinoma, or they may have high density secondary to hemorrhagic components, as seen with melanomas and thyroid or renal cell carcinomas (Figure 40-15). Cystic tumors such as cystic astrocytomas may be composed of large cysts with the density of CSF (Figure 40-16). Epidermoid and dermoid tumors frequently contain areas of fat density that appear hypodense to CSF.

MRI has high sensitivity but low specificity in the evaluation of neoplasms, because most tumors appear similar. Tumors are typically of low intensity on T1WI and high intensity on T2WI (see Figure 40-1), although there are a few exceptions. Advanced imaging

techniques have many applications in the study of brain tumors.[15] DWI and MRS are helpful in presurgical grading, selection of optimal biopsy sites, determining the extent of subtle dissemination, and monitoring the response to therapy.[49] DTI and fMRI have proven useful in visualizing the relation between eloquent cortex and critical white matter tracts around tumors, which can aid in defining and minimizing risk of morbidity from resection.[50] MRS and DWI can help in distinguishing delayed treatment effects like postradiation ischemic necrosis from tumor recurrence, which can both show contrast-enhancing hyperintensity on conventional T2WI.[10] PET studies show CBF, glucose consumption, and oxygen metabolism to be increased in recurrent tumor and decreased in necrosis.[51]

Infection and Inflammation

Parenchymal Infection. Parenchymal infections include encephalitis and pyogenic abscess. Encephalitis, a diffuse inflammation of the brain, is often viral or toxic in origin. Conventional CT and MRI may initially appear normal but later show areas of cortical edema or hemorrhage. DWI is often able to show areas of diffusion restriction early in the disease, making it important to include in the evaluation of patients with suspected encephalitis.[6] The herpes simplex virus (HSV) shows a strong predilection for the temporal, insular, and cingulate regions in older children and adults but a more variable degree of involvement of cortex and deep grey matter in neonates.[52] Acute disseminated encephalomyelitis (ADEM) is an immune-mediated encephalitis that typically occurs in response to a previous viral infection or vaccination but which may also be the initial presentation of a patient with multiple sclerosis. MRI with contrast is considerably more sensitive than CT for detecting the demyelination and edema most often seen in the bilateral deep white matter but may in some cases primarily affect the deep gray matter or present with a single mass-like (tumefactive) lesion. The combined information from conventional MRI, DWI, MRS, and perfusion studies may allow for the noninvasive discrimination of tumefactive demyelination from other mass lesions such as lymphoma, metastatic tumor, primary brain tumor, or pyogenic abscess.[53]

Cerebral abscess results from liquefactive necrosis, producing a localized collection of pus or caseous material in a cavity surrounded by a fibrous capsule. On CT, the abscess cavity demonstrates central hypodensity (necrotic cavity), a thin isodense wall (capsule), and surrounding low density (edema). Following contrast administration, there is enhancement of the capsule. Unlike the shaggy irregular walls

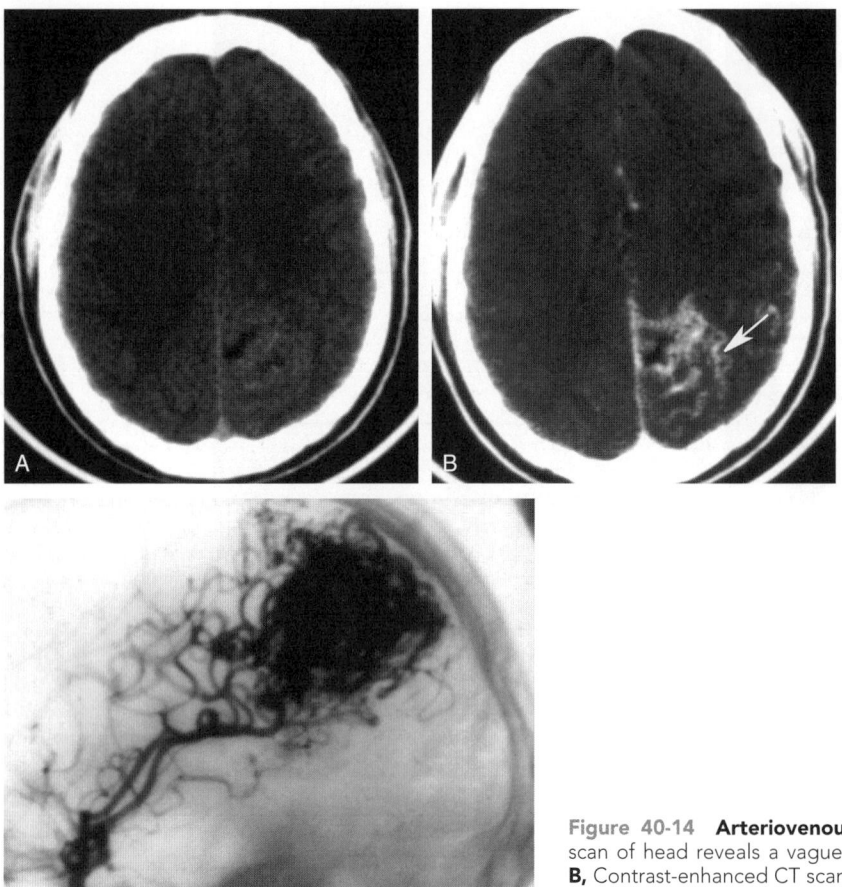

Figure 40-14 Arteriovenous malformation. A, Axial non-contrast-enhanced CT scan of head reveals a vague area of hyperdensity in posterior left parietal region. **B,** Contrast-enhanced CT scan demonstrates serpiginous enhancement of this lesion *(arrow).* **C,** Internal carotid artery angiogram demonstrates arteriovenous malformation being fed by middle cerebral artery.

of a tumor, the walls of an abscess are typically smooth, well defined, and uniform in thickness; these are important differential features. MRI findings are similar to CT findings. The central cavity has variable signal characteristics, depending on its contents. The capsule is iso- to hyperintense on T1WI, hypointense on T2WI, and enhances after contrast administration. Pyogenic abscess almost always shows

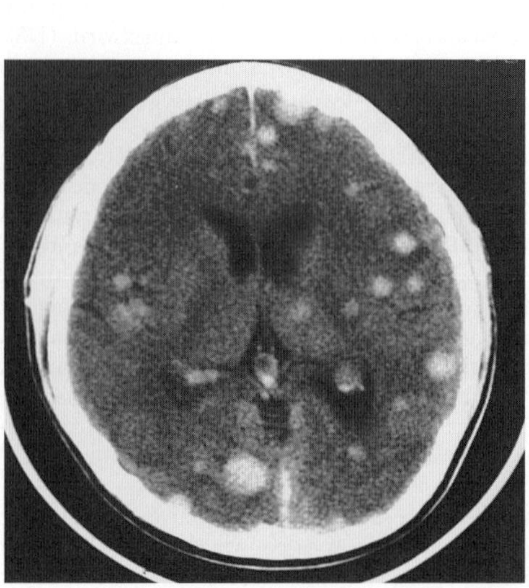

hyperintensity on DWI, differentiating it from most nonpyogenic lesions, but MR spectroscopy can also be used to investigate lesions of uncertain significance.[6]

Extraaxial Infection. Extraaxial infections include meningitis, ventriculitis, and subdural and epidural empyemas. A contrast-enhanced CT is sufficient for the initial evaluation of suspected meningitis, but a contrast-enhanced MRI is better able to demonstrate other extraaxial infections. In meningitis, CT and MRI may be normal or demonstrate diffuse meningeal contrast enhancement. The diagnosis of meningitis can be based on clinical signs and supportive CSF studies, but imaging is still indicated to exclude an associated abscess or empyema and to evaluate for nonpyogenic complications such as hydrocephalus and arterial or venous thrombosis. Ventriculitis is characterized by contrast enhancement on CT or MRI of the involved ventricular walls. Subdural and epidural empyemas most often occur as complications of meningitis, sinusitis, otitis, surgery, or trauma. On CT, the purulent collections frequently have a density intermediate between CSF and acute blood. On MRI, the collections are typically hypointense to brain on T1WI and hyperintense on T2WI.

WHITE MATTER AND METABOLIC DISEASES

Most white matter diseases can be classified as dysmyelinating (myelin is improperly formed or maintained) or demyelinating (myelin is destroyed after being properly formed). Dysmyelinating disorders include the leukodystrophies and storage diseases. Demyelinating disorders can be auto-immune (ADEM and multiple sclerosis), infectious (progressive multifocal leukoencephalopathy, subacute sclerosing

Figure 40-15 Intracranial metastatic disease. Axial contrast-enhanced CT scan of head reveals multiple enhancing nodules throughout gray and white matter structures, consistent with metastatic disease.

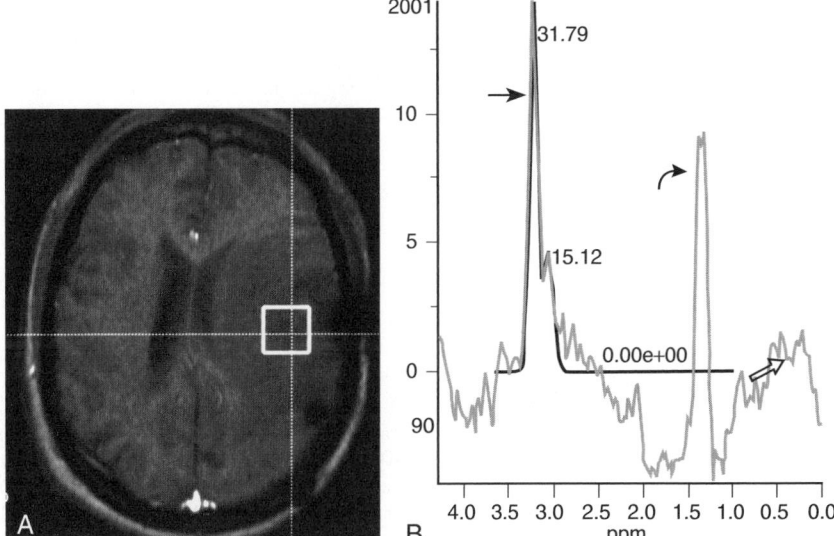

Figure 40-16 Recurrent high-grade astrocytoma. Study performed after radiation therapy (not shown) showed increased edema and mass effect; differential diagnosis included recurrent tumor and radiation necrosis. **A,** Axial MRI scan shows volume of tissue *(box)* selected for spectroscopy. **B,** Proton spectroscopy reveals increase in choline peak *(arrow)*, decrease in *N*-acetyl aspartate peak *(curved arrow)*, and appearance of a lactate peak *(open arrow)*. This appearance is consistent with recurrent tumor, which was verified with repeat surgery and biopsy.

panencephalitis), toxic-degenerative, or vascular. MRI is much more sensitive than CT and is the study of choice for determining the presence and extent of white matter disease (Figure 40-17). These lesions appear hypointense on T1WI and hyperintense on standard T2WI and on FLAIR sequences, which increase the conspicuity of subependymal white matter lesions. The majority of white matter diseases appear similar on imaging studies.

White matter diseases seldom present with acute encephalopathy, other than when there are exacerbations and complications during their usually slowly progressive course. When the presentation is acute, toxic and vascular causes of encephalopathy deserve primary consideration.[54] Carbon monoxide poisoning causes hypoxic injury, visible early on as cytotoxic edema on DWI, with selective vulnerability in adults in the putamina, thalami, caudate heads, cerebellum, and cerebral white matter. Spectroscopy can show hypoxic demyelination in the white matter, with elevated Cho and decreased NAA.[55] Severe and chronic malnutrition with thiamine deficiency, often associated in developed societies with alcoholism but also seen with hyperemesis gravidarum, gastric bypass surgery, or chronic renal failure, can lead to Wernicke encephalopathy. The classic clinical triad of ophthalmoplegia, cerebellar ataxia, and confusion is not always present or recognized. MRI can show evidence of vasogenic edema, cytotoxic edema, or hemorrhage within the thalami, hypothalamus, periaqueductal dorsal midbrain, mamillary bodies, and medullary tectum.[56] Methanol ingestion causes contrast-enhancing hemorrhagic necrosis of the bilateral caudate heads, putamina, pons, optic nerves, and subcortical white matter, which can lead to intraventricular hemorrhage and diffuse cerebral edema.[57]

Several immunosuppressive medications have been associated with PRES, as previously described. A number of chemotherapeutic agents have the potential to cause toxic demyelination. Intrathecally administered methotrexate has a particularly well-known risk of acute, subacute, and chronic forms of toxicity, typically seen as hyperintensity on T2WI in the periventricular and deep white matter but sometimes involving the cerebellar white matter and thalami.[10] Osmotic myelinolysis occurs with rapid correction of a hypoosmolar state, commonly hyponatremia in alcoholic, malnourished, or dehydrated patients. MRI shows hyperintensity on T2WI, with or without diffusion restriction on DWI, involving the central pons but sparing the periphery. Extrapontine structures, including the thalami, basal ganglia, and deep white matter, can also be involved.[58] Encephalopathy occurs with many types of chronic liver disease, such as alcoholic cirrhosis, hepatitis, and portal

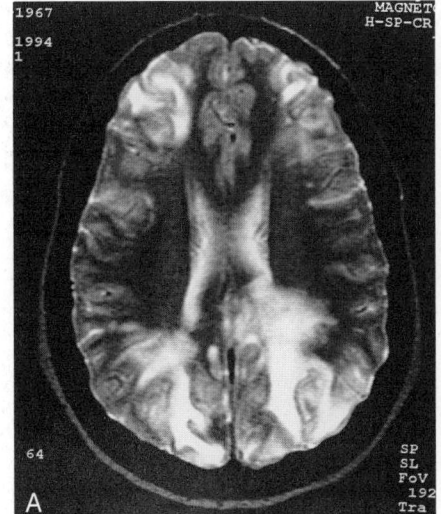
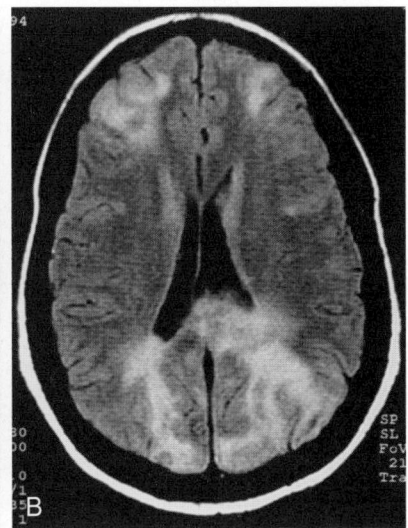

Figure 40-17 Progressive multifocal leukoencephalopathy. Axial T2-weighted **(A)** and fluid-attenuated inversion recovery (FLAIR) **(B)** images in patient with human immunodeficiency virus (HIV). Multiple areas of white matter disease are identified; FLAIR image increases their conspicuity. These findings in an HIV-positive patient indicate a postinfectious demyelinating process: progressive multifocal leukoencephalopathy.

systemic shunts. MRI frequently demonstrates hyperintensity on T1WI in the basal ganglia, particularly the globus pallidi and subthalamic nuclei and in the midbrain. Hyperintensity on T2WI may be seen diffusely in the cortex, although there often is sparing of the perirolandic and occipital regions. MRI shows evidence of hypoosmolarity, with decreased Cho and mI peaks, but also shows an increase in signal from glutamine and glutamate.[59]

Spine

PATTERNS OF DISEASE

It is often useful to classify spinal canal pathology according to the three spinal compartments, or spaces: intramedullary, extramedullary-intradural, and extradural (Figure 40-18). Certain pathologic lesions occur with greater frequency in specific spaces; therefore, diagnostic considerations can be significantly narrowed if a lesion can be localized. In most instances, MRI is the modality of choice in evaluating spinal pathology. The high degree of tissue contrast and spatial resolution can localize most lesions to a specific compartment, determine the extent of disease, and suggest a differential diagnosis.[60] The only exception is acute trauma, in which case bony alignment and stability are better demonstrated by plain radiography and CT.

Intramedullary lesions expand the spinal cord as they enlarge, compressing the subarachnoid space, usually symmetrically (see Figure 40-18, *A*). If of sufficient size and chronicity, the intramedullary expansion may produce changes in the bony spinal canal, including posterior scalloping of the vertebral bodies, flattening of the spinous processes, widening of the interpeduncular distance, and overall widening of the canal. Intramedullary disease is usually neoplastic, and the most common tumors are gliomas (ependymoma, astrocytoma, glioblastoma), although other tumors (dermoid cysts, sarcomas, hemangioblastomas, and intramedullary metastases) can be seen. In the acute setting, intramedullary infectious (tuberculosis, bacterial abscess), inflammatory (sarcoidosis, transverse myelitis), and vascular insults must be considered.

Extramedullary-intradural lesions displace the arachnoid layer of the meninges but leave the dura in place such that the subarachnoid CSF flares out to form a "cap" at its interface with the lesion (see Figure 40-18, *B*). Meningiomas, nerve sheath tumors (neurofibromas and schwannomas), and other benign tumors (lipomas, dermoid and epidermoid tumors) account for the majority of lesions in this space, while more aggressive tumors (hemangiopericytomas), metastatic tumors, inflammatory disorders (arachnoiditis and sarcoidosis), vascular lesions (spinal-dural arteriovenous fistulas), and cystic lesions (perineural and arachnoid) are less commonly seen.[61]

Extradural lesions typically produce a more gradual displacement of the subarachnoid space and spinal cord (see Figure 40-18, *C*). Excluding disc disease, the most common extradural pathology is metastatic disease with epidural extension. Pathologic fractures of the involved vertebrae occur frequently and are often associated with spinal cord compression. Primary tumors of the spine and direct extension from paraspinal neoplasms make up the other malignant lesions of the extradural compartment; these include lymphomas, plasmacytomas, sarcomas, neuroblastomas and vertebral body chordomas. Benign lesions are uncommon in this compartment. Discitis and osteomyelitis with epidural abscess is an additional consideration.

SPECIFIC DISEASE PROCESSES

Spinal Cord Injury

The sequence of performing the various imaging studies to evaluate spine injury remains controversial and is usually based on their availability at the particular trauma center. Initial evaluation usually involves a series of plain x-rays, which are able to identify most unstable injuries. Lateral and anteroposterior studies are sufficient for most thoracic and lumbar injuries, although oblique views are sometimes added for clarification; lateral, oblique, and odontoid views are typically ordered for cervical injuries. However, some vertebral fractures and misalignments are missed on these screening studies (Figure 40-19, *A*). CT with axial, coronal, and sagittal reconstructions should be considered whenever fractures are seen or suspected because of the severity of trauma or if the patient's examination is unreliable owing to altered mental status or a distracting injury.[62]

MRI is recommended when the patient has neurologic deficits, an unstable injury by prior imaging, or symptoms of an unstable injury despite a normal CT. MRI will rarely identify spinal injuries that require surgical stabilization in patients with no apparent neurologic deficits and a normal CT,[63] but most studies suggest that spinal MRI is unnecessary even in obtunded and comatose trauma patients.[64] MRI is the only imaging modality that can directly visualize intrinsic spinal cord and soft-tissue injuries. It can identify and distinguish between hemorrhagic (hematoma) and edematous (contusion) cord injuries. Cord hematoma has a poor prognosis and indicates a complete lesion, whereas localized edema has a better prognosis for functional recovery. Traumatic disc herniations can be readily identified. A disc herniation with cord compression can change management from nonsurgical to surgical or change a posterior stabilization approach to a combined anterior and posterior approach. MRI is also useful in detecting ligamentous injury by showing edematous changes or discontinuity in the ligaments. Although these findings are usually secondary, detection of isolated ligamentous injury may identify patients at risk for delayed instability. Epidural hematomas and the extent to which they compress the cord are also identified with MRI. Finally, although fractures are difficult to detect with MRI, the effect of bony fragment displacement and alignment abnormalities on the cord or nerve roots is elegantly seen with this modality (see Figure 40-19, *D*).

Spinal Infection

Infections involving the spine may involve the vertebral bodies (spondylitis), intervertebral discs (discitis), epidural and subdural spaces, or the spinal cord (myelitis, pyogenic cord abscess). In the management

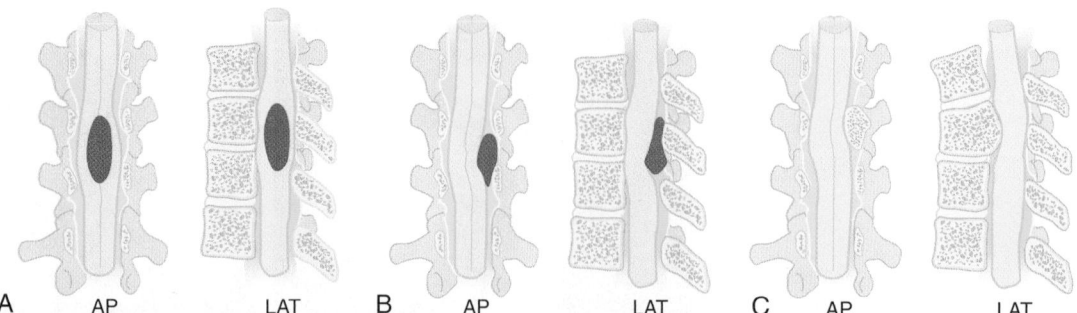

Figure 40-18   Spinal compartments. Anteroposterior (AP) and lateral (LAT) views of spinal cord and canal demonstrate appearance of an intramedullary lesion **(A)**, extramedullary intradural lesion **(B)**, and extradural lesion **(C)**.

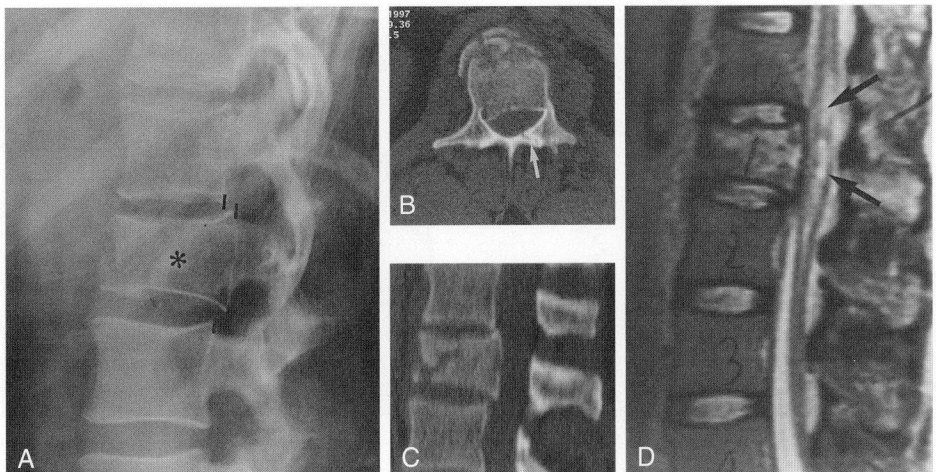

Figure 40-19 **Post-traumatic vertebral body compression fracture. A,** Lateral plain film of thoracolumbar junction reveals a compression fracture involving L1 vertebral body *(asterisk)*. Decreased height of vertebral body and inferior anterior corner fracture are well seen. Retropulsed body can also be seen when outline of adjacent vertebral bodies *(lines)* are compared. Axial **(B)** and sagittal reconstructed **(C)** CT scans of same patient add substantial detail to degree of canal narrowing secondary to retropulsed fragment. Left laminar fracture *(arrow, B)* is also seen—not apparent on the plain film. **D,** Sagittal T2-weighted MRI demonstrates compression fracture of L1 and retropulsed posterior body, as well as contusion and swelling of conus *(arrows)* as a direct result of compression fracture.

of spinal infections, delayed treatment can lead to increased morbidity and mortality, making early diagnosis critical. MRI is the primary imaging modality in all types of spinal infection because of its higher sensitivity and ability to detect changes earlier than plain films and CT.[65]

In spondylitis, involvement is seen in at least one entire spinal segment composed of two consecutive vertebrae and the intervening disc. Characteristic MRI findings include narrowing of the disc space, contrast enhancement, hypointensity on T1WI in the vertebral bodies, and hyperintensity on T2WI in the vertebral bodies and disc (Figure 40-20). These findings may not be present early, however, and can be mimicked by noninfectious processes. Skip lesions and associated large

paraspinal abscesses are very suggestive of mycobacterial infection. Nuclear medicine studies such as FDG PET may be particularly useful in evaluating patients suspected of having chronic spondylitis or infected surgical hardware.[66] Although MRI is sensitive in defining areas of myelitis, the findings are nonspecific and resemble those of other noninfectious and demyelinating disorders. Typically, focal or diffuse areas of hyperintensity are seen on T2WI with variable contrast enhancement.[67]

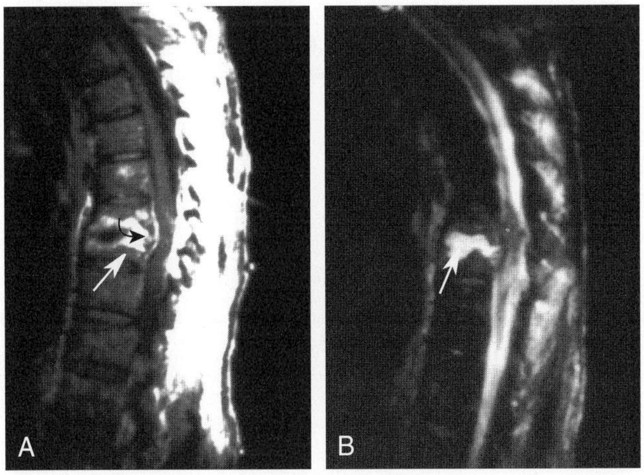

Neoplasm

Neoplasms involving the spinal axis typically present with progressive symptoms of myelopathy or cord compression. MRI is the primary modality for the evaluation of any suspected spinal tumor. It can demonstrate the location, extent, and nature of most tumors, regardless of the compartment of origin. Primary tumors of the bony elements and direct extension from paraspinal neoplasms are also easily identified with MRI.[68]

The spinal column is among the most common sites of tumor metastasis, third only to the lungs and liver. The most common primary tumor sites responsible for spinal metastasis are breast, prostate, thyroid, lung, and kidney. Plain radiographs can suggest the presence of spinal metastasis, with a blurred outline or generally moth-eaten appearance of a vertebral body suggesting diffuse cortical destruction. Focal bone loss that involves the posterior wall of the vertebral body is fairly indicative of neoplasia. Vertebral collapse is more likely to be due to neoplasia than degenerative disease when there is unilateral bone destruction, irregular or angular distortion of the vertebral endplates, involvement of the upper thoracic spine, a soft-tissue mass, or pedicle destruction.[69] CT is more sensitive than plain radiography for many of these features, and MRI is yet more sensitive, particularly for epidural and paraspinous soft-tissue involvement and cord compression. The bone marrow of vertebral bodies with neoplastic infiltration appears hypointense on T1WI and hyperintense on T2WI (Figure 40-21). The bone marrow of vertebral fractures with benign fractures has normal imaging characteristics (Figure 40-22).

ACKNOWLEDGEMENT

Portions of this chapter, including some of the images used as examples, appeared in the previous edition of this book and were authored by Dr. Fred J. Laine.

Figure 40-20 **Discitis with epidural abscess.** Sagittal postcontrast T1-weighted **(A)** and T2-weighted **(B)** MRI scans demonstrate features of discitis and adjacent osteomyelitis. Vertebral bodies and disc space are of low signal intensity on T1-weighted image and of bright signal intensity on T2-weighted image *(straight arrows)*. Epidural abscess surrounding and compressing cord is also identified *(curved arrow)*.

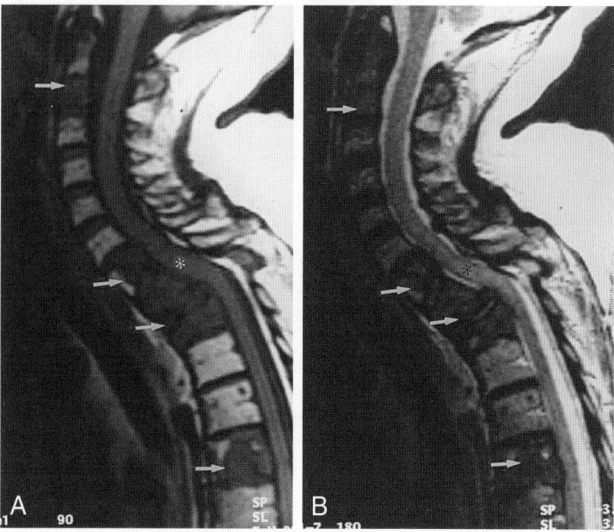

Figure 40-21 Metastatic disease. Sagittal T1-weighted **(A)** and T2-weighted **(B)** MRI scans of spine show metastatic lesions (arrows) as low intensity on T1-weighted image, replacing normal bright marrow. High signal within uninvolved vertebral bodies represents postradiation changes. Hypointense lesions on T2-weighted image (in contrast to more typical hyperintensity) reflect posttreatment appearance. Multiple compression fractures are identified within upper thoracic spine, with collapse, retropulsed fragments, and cord compression. Edematous changes within cord secondary to compression (asterisk) are also identified.

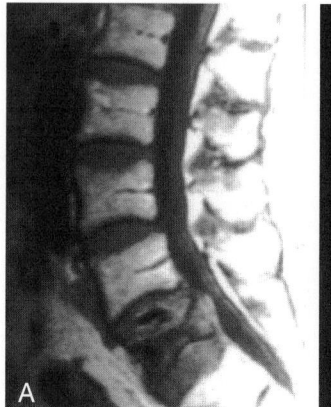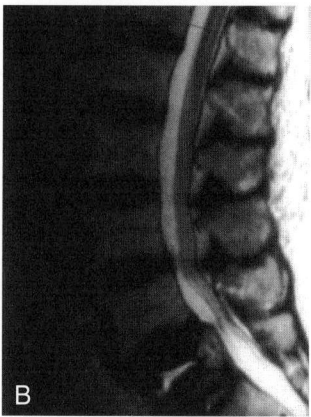

Figure 40-22 Benign compression fracture. Sagittal T1-weighted **(A)** and T2-weighted **(B)** MRI scans demonstrate compression fracture of L5. Compare signal characteristics of remaining bony elements and pedicles with signal of normal bony structures.

KEY POINTS

Methods

1. Computed tomography (CT) is useful in acute settings, as it can be acquired quickly with few contraindications.

2. Magnetic resonance imaging (MRI) is useful in most situations in which greater detail is needed regarding brain and spinal cord lesions, but it requires longer acquisition times and is contraindicated in some patients.

3. Newer applications of CT (e.g., angiography and perfusion) and MRI (e.g., angiography, perfusion, spectroscopy, diffusion, and diffusion tensor imaging) are providing increasingly detailed, noninvasive evaluations of brain lesions.

Brain

1. The location and radiographic appearance of lesions on CT and MRI help differentiate underlying traumatic, infectious, inflammatory, neoplastic, and vascular pathologies.

2. Infarctions and intracranial hemorrhages change in appearance over time on CT and MRI, helping determine the evolution of vascular injuries.

3. A patient's need for acute surgical intervention due to subarachnoid hemorrhage, obstructive hydrocephalus, or a mass lesion causing or threatening herniation can be evaluated well by CT.

4. CT is currently used to exclude hemorrhage in the initial evaluation of patients with suspected acute ischemic infarction when intravenous thrombolysis is being considered. Other imaging modalities, including MRI and conventional angiography, are frequently used in evaluating patients with vascular injuries.

5. Multiple imaging modalities can be used presurgically to determine the location, histology, and grade of tumors and can aid in the differentiation of radiation necrosis from tumor recurrence.

Spine

1. CT is useful for identifying patients with spinal trauma who have unstable lesions requiring neck stabilization or surgical intervention because of vertebral fractures and subluxations. MRI is more sensitive for surrounding soft-tissue injuries and is the only modality capable of visualizing spinal cord contusion, compression, or infarction.

2. MRI is the modality of choice for evaluating patients with suspected neoplastic, infectious, and inflammatory diseases of the spinal cord.

ANNOTATED REFERENCES

Vezina G. Assessment of the nature and age of subdural collections in nonaccidental head injury with CT and MRI. Pediatr Radiol 2009;39(6):586-90.
The appearance of blood on CT and MRI is described in such detail as to provide the reader with an understanding of the typical evolution of an intracranial hematoma, but the article also offers useful insights into the complexities of interpreting individual studies.

Wardlaw JM. Neuroimaging in acute ischaemic stroke: insights into unanswered questions of pathophysiology. J Intern Med 2010;267(2):172-90.
This paper begins with an excellent explanation of how different imaging modalities are used for evaluating acute stroke. The discussion of how diffusion-weighted imaging and perfusion imaging are used to identify an ischemic penumbra is particularly well written.

Huang BY, Castillo M. Hypoxic-ischemic brain injury: imaging findings from birth to adulthood. Radiographics 2008;28(2):417-39.
This paper explains why hypoxic-ischemic brain injury causes age-dependent patterns of injury. The selective vulnerability of different brain regions in premature infants, term neonates, infants, older children, and adults is described and illustrated.

Arora A, Neema M, Stankiewicz J, et al. Neuroimaging of toxic and metabolic disorders. Semin Neurol 2008;28(4):495-510.
This paper provides numerous detailed examples of how neuroimaging, particularly MRI, is able to demonstrate the patterns by which various toxic and metabolic disorders affect the central nervous system.

Menaker J, Philp A, Boswell S, Scalea TM. Computed tomography alone for cervical spine clearance in the unreliable patient—are we there yet? J Trauma 2008;64(4):898-903.
The authors compare their experience in the use of CT and MRI for evaluating traumatic cervical spine injury in unreliable patients to previously published reports on the false-negative rate of CT studies in these diagnostically challenging patients. They also review landmark studies and current practice guidelines for evaluation of the spinal cord in trauma patients.

REFERENCES

Access the complete reference list online at http://www.expertconsult.com.

41

Intensive Care After Neurosurgery

ANDREW I.R. MAAS | PHILIPPE G. JORENS | NINO STOCCHETTI

Overview

Appropriate neurocritical care is fundamental to the success of neurosurgical interventions to the brain and spinal cord. Great technical advances in operative procedures have made lesions previously considered inoperable now treatable, and advances in anesthesia have led to an increased number of operative procedures in both elderly and critically ill patients. Consequently, the number of patients requiring postoperative intensive care has increased.

Successful care for the neurosurgical patient requires close collaboration between various specialists: neurosurgeons, intensivists, and neuroradiologists. The result of a technically perfect operation can be ruined by inadequate postoperative care. A complex operative procedure requires expert intensive care to correct abnormalities in homeostatic mechanisms, ensure adequate cerebral perfusion and oxygenation, and promote recovery of brain function. The complex interaction between the central nervous system (CNS) and systemic functioning requires intimate knowledge of both general intensive care and cerebral and spinal pathophysiology. Anticipation and early response prior to the full-blown development of complications are hallmarks of good neurocritical care. For example, when plasma sodium levels are slowly decreasing, correction should be implemented before hyponatremia develops, as this may lead to increased brain edema. The best care for neurosurgical patients can be provided by dedicated specialists with knowledge of both fields and a great deal of experience treating such patients.

The benefit of concentration of care in units with sufficient case volume has been well established in different fields of intensive care medicine including trauma,[1] neonatology, and specifically neurointensive care.[2,3]

Treatment of patients with spontaneous intracerebral hemorrhage in a neurointensive care unit is associated with reduced mortality when compared with patients admitted to a general intensive care unit (ICU).[4,5] Mortality following aneurysmal subarachnoid hemorrhage (SAH) is lower in centers with a higher case volume.[6] Patel and colleagues[7] unequivocally showed a 2.15 times increase in the odds of death (adjusted for case mix) for patients with severe traumatic brain injury (TBI) treated in non-neurosurgical centers versus neurosurgical centers. Their report makes a strong case for transferring and treating all patients with severe head injury in a setting with 24-hour neurosurgical facilities. Protocol-driven approaches also improve results.[8-10]

The admission policy for postoperative neurosurgical ICU care varies widely between countries and centers and even within centers. In some centers, all patients are admitted for a 24-hour observation period following intracranial procedures. This practice is motivated by the observation that some patients, although fully alert and neurologically intact initially, may develop complications such as a postoperative hematoma with rapid neurologic deterioration, necessitating prompt intervention.

In other centers, patients are only admitted to the ICU after intracranial complications have been detected. Some hospitals have dedicated neuro-ICUs; in others, patients are admitted to a general intensive care, sometimes even to different ICUs within one hospital. In general, the scarcity of intensive care beds has led to a more restrictive admission policy for postoperative neurosurgical care. The institution of high-care units, sometimes termed *step-down units*, may permit more rational allocation of scarce intensive care resources and at the same time afford sufficient guarantees for adequate postoperative monitoring. Here again, however, care should be provided by personnel well experienced in the care of such patients, thus permitting early detection of possible deterioration and prevention of secondary complications.

Priorities and Goals of Postoperative Neurosurgical Care

The principal goal of postoperative neurosurgical intensive care is early detection and treatment of postsurgical complications. The next is preventing second insults that may initiate or exacerbate secondary damage in a vulnerable CNS.

Consequently, priorities are to ensure adequate monitoring facilities, which may in the sedated and ventilated patient require further invasive monitoring of the intracranial system, and to ensure adequate oxygenation and perfusion of the brain.

Postoperative complications may be systemic or neurosurgical (Table 41-1).

Prevention and Management of Systemic Complications After Neurosurgery

GENERAL PRINCIPLES AND SECOND INSULTS

The prevention and management of systemic complications after neurosurgical procedures follows general principles of "intensive care" medicine. It is, however, important to realize that systemic complications and second insults may initiate or aggravate cerebral damage. Aggressive treatment aimed at preventing and limiting second insults is of paramount importance. The main second insults, their causes, and adverse effects on brain homeostasis and function are summarized in Table 41-2, further illustrating the complex interactions between systemic events and CNS function.

Conversely, CNS events may induce systemic derangement. For example, in response to raised intracranial pressure (ICP), mean arterial blood pressure (MABP) may increase as a compensatory mechanism to ensure adequate cerebral perfusion (Cushing response). In such situations, treatment of hypertension is contraindicated, as this may exacerbate cerebral ischemia. In other situations, however, arterial hypertension may aggravate the occurrence of cerebral edema and/or increase the risk of intracranial bleeding. Surgeons may request prevention of any episode of high blood pressure (BP) in situations where adequate hemostasis was difficult, or conversely may wish to maintain BP at relatively high levels when cerebral vasospasm may be a problem, for example after cerebral aneurysm surgery. The clinical dilemma is to balance the necessity of limiting edema formation and the risk of postoperative hemorrhage with the goal of maintaining adequate perfusion. Knowledge of the operative findings and close interaction with the surgeon are of paramount importance.

Many drugs routinely used in neurosurgical patients (e.g., steroids, antiepileptic agents) may cause complications or side effects; awareness of potential side effects is essential. CNS damage, particularly to the hypothalamic region, brainstem, and cervical spinal cord may lead to disturbance in temperature control, causing hypo- or hyperthermia. In patients with spinal cord injury, loss of autonomic sympathetic

TABLE 41-1	Postoperative Complications	
Systemic Complications	**Neurosurgical Complications**
Coagulation disorders: blood loss, disseminated intravascular coagulation, drug induced	Postoperative hematoma: subgaleal, epidural, subdural, intraparenchymal
Thromboembolic: DVT, pulmonary embolism, myocardial infarction	Cerebral ischemia: subarachnoid hemorrhage, vasospasm, vessel occlusion
Pulmonary: atelectasis, pneumothorax	Brain swelling: edema, vasodilation
Hypovolemia: insufficient pre- and perioperative hydration, blood loss	Infection: meningitis, subdural empyema, cerebral abscess
Infection: pneumonia, urinary tract infection, catheter sepsis	Seizures: infection, depressed compound skull fracture, cortical lesions
Metabolic: hyperglycemia [steroid induced], diabetes insipidus, hyponatremia	Hydrocephalus: obstruction/resorption
	Tension pneumocephalus
Air embolism: sitting position, opening of large cerebral veins during surgery	CSF fistula
	Inverse cerebellar herniation
	Cranial nerve lesions
Pressure sores and decubitus ulcers: intraoperative positioning, cervical traction, paraplegia	

CSF, cerebrospinal fluid; *DVT,* deep venous thrombosis.

function may further lead to peripheral vasodilation and low BP. In the absence of beta-blocking agents, hypotension in combination with bradycardia is strongly suggestive of damage to the spinal cord.

CARDIAC DYSFUNCTION

Electrocardiographic (ECG) abnormalities, usually diffuse ST-segment changes mimicking cardiac ischemia and cardiac arrhythmias, may be caused by SAH, TBI, or raised ICP. The devastating effects of a sudden catecholamine release following acute intracranial bleeding have recently received further attention. The left ventricle suffers a typical bulging (indicating ischemic changes and functional impairment) which has been awarded the term *Takotsubo syndrome,* with reference to the shape of a pot used by ancient Japanese fishermen for catching octopus. The extent of left ventricular dysfunction is variable, but it may lead to extreme cardiac failure and pulmonary edema.[11,12]

NEUROGENIC PULMONARY EDEMA

The development of neurogenic pulmonary edema has been described early in the postoperative period after a variety of neurosurgical procedures, including brain tumors (particularly those resected in the posterior fossa), cysts, hydrocephalus, intracranial hemorrhages, and brainstem lesions.[13-16] Although an infrequent event, this is potentially life threatening and requires rapid evaluation and emergent therapy in the ICU. A 9% mortality rate directly attributable to neurogenic pulmonary edema has been reported in a recent review of this condition. Generally this complication appears in the initial 4 hours after the neurologic event and is more common in women than in men, possibly related to the preponderance of cases in patients with SAH.[16] The mechanisms underlying this condition are unclear; a sudden central sympathetic discharge may trigger pulmonary venoconstriction, systemic arterial hypertension, increased left ventricle afterload, increased capillary permeability in the pulmonary vascular bed, and simultaneously cause cardiac ischemia and ventricular failure.[12,17] Because of these multiple mechanisms, neurogenic pulmonary edema can be interpreted as noncardiogenic or, at least in part, as cardiogenic.[18] Both low and high protein content have been reported in the edema fluid.[16,19] It is commonly associated with raised ICP, so in addition to therapies directed at intracranial hypertension, therapeutic measures are mostly supportive. To attenuate the massive sympathetic discharge, opioids and sedatives are used. Supplemental oxygen is uniformly required, and tracheal intubation with mechanical ventilation and application of positive end-expiratory pressure (PEEP) has been reported in about

75% of patients.[16] Diuretics have been used, provided volume status is adequate, but diuresis causes less effect than in cardiac edema. Most patients require vasoactive drugs.[19]

HYPERCOAGULOPATHY AND THROMBOSIS PROPHYLAXIS

Release of factors from damaged brain tissue may induce local and systemic hypercoagulopathy.[20-22] Various studies have confirmed a transient hypercoagulopathy syndrome both in the immediate postoperative phase after brain surgery and in patients with TBI.[20,23-25] In patients with a subdural hematoma, consumption of clotting factors may lead to coagulopathy in up to 22% of the patients.[26]

Deep venous thrombosis (DVT) has been reported to occur in 18% to 50% of neurosurgical cases[27] and pulmonary embolism (PE) in 0% to 25%. DVT and PE incidence is particularly high in brain tumor patients. Nevertheless, neurosurgeons tend to underestimate the risk of DVT and PE[28] and are sometimes reluctant to routinely prescribe anticoagulant prophylaxis for fear of increasing the risk of postoperative bleeding.[29] Options for prevention of thrombosis prophylaxis in neurosurgical patients include both mechanical (graduated

TABLE 41-2	Systemic Second Insults	
Event	**Main Causes**	**Adverse Effects**
Hypoxemia	Hypoventilation Aspiration atelectasis Pneumothorax Pneumonia Anemia	Decrease in oxygen delivery and increased risk of ischemic damage
Hypotension	Hypovolemia	Decreased CPP, decrease in CBF, increased risk of ischemia
	Cardiac failure	
	Sepsis, spinal cord injury	
Anemia	Blood loss	Decrease in oxygen transport and delivery and increased risk of ischemic damage
Hypercapnia	Respiratory depression	Increased CBV, raised ICP
Hypocapnia	Hyperventilation, spontaneous or induced	Cerebral vasoconstriction with increased risk of ischemic damage
Hyperthermia	Hypermetabolism, stress response, infection	Metabolic requirements may exceed substrate delivery, resulting in energy depletion
	Central dysregulation	
Hypothermia	Exposure, central dysregulation	May be neuroprotective but can cause significant coagulopathy and electrolyte disturbances
Hyperglycemia	IV infusion of dextrose, steroids, stress response	Acidosis, electrolyte disturbances
Hypoglycemia	Inadequate nutrition, insulin overdose, pituitary insufficiency	Energy depletion in the brain, seizures
Hyponatremia	Inadequate salt intake (hypotonic fluids) Excessive sodium loss (cerebral salt wasting/CSF drainage) Syndrome of inappropriate ADH	Increased edema, seizures
Hypernatremia	Diabetes insipidus Osmotic agents (mannitol, hypertonic saline)	Lethargy, coma

ADH, antidiuretic hormone; *CBF,* cerebral blood flow; *CBV,* cerebral blood volume; *CPP,* cerebral perfusion pressure; *CSF,* cerebrospinal fluid; *ICP,* intracranial pressure; *IV* intravenous.

compression stockings, intermittent pneumatic compression stockings) and pharmacologic (low dose of classic heparin and low-molecular-weight heparin) therapies. Intuitively, mechanical therapies carry less associated risk, but pharmacologic approaches are more effective in preventing thrombotic complications. Various studies have indeed shown a higher incidence of postoperative hemorrhagic complications,[30] but not all are clinically relevant.

Overall, existing evidence, however, shows that the beneficial effects in reducing DVT and in particular PE[31,32] outweigh a slightly increased risk of clinically significant hemorrhagic complications with anticoagulant prophylaxis.

These data support the administration of antithrombotic prophylaxis to patients undergoing neurosurgical procedures,[33] including those with intracranial hemorrhagic lesions,[34] closed TBI,[35,36] or high-risk trauma patients.[37,38] It has been recommended to remove catheters or drainage tubes in the postoperative phase when anticoagulant effects are low (e.g., just prior to administration of next dose).[39]

Uncertainty exists on the preferred choice of medication, optimal dosing regimen, and time of initiation of thrombosis prophylaxis, particularly in patients with higher risk for bleeding. Any decision regarding the use of thrombosis prophylaxis must weigh efficacy against harm from the proposed intervention. In addition, early mobilization in the postoperative phase, whenever possible, is recommended. More consensus exists concerning routine administration of anticoagulant therapy in patients with spinal cord injuries.

Prevention and Management of Neurosurgical Postoperative Complications

SUPRATENTORIAL PROCEDURES

Postoperative Subgaleal Hematoma

Postoperative subgaleal hematoma may occur in up to 11% of procedures. These hematomas generally result from inadvertent damage of the superficial temporal artery, inadequate hemostasis, or hemorrhage from the temporal muscle. If the superficial temporal artery is damaged during the operation, ligation is preferred over coagulation. The occurrence of subgaleal hematomas can be minimized by routine use of postoperative wound drainage for 24 hours. Reoperation for subgaleal hematomas is seldom necessary unless there is a communication with the intracranial compartment, with secondary compression of the brain.[40]

Intracranial Hemorrhage

Intracranial postoperative hemorrhage occurs in approximately 1% of procedures and mainly concerns intraparenchymal hematomas (43%-60%), epidural hematomas (28%-33%) and subdural hematomas (5%-7%).

After every supratentorial procedure, some blood may accumulate in the epidural space. Appropriate surgical techniques aim to minimize this epidural space by circumferentially suturing the dura to the bone, periosteum, or galea. Inadequate hemostasis of meningeal arteries, blood loss from the temporal muscle, or blood loss from the bone may, however, induce a larger postoperative epidural hematoma. In cases of neurologic deterioration considered due to the postoperative epidural hematoma, surgical evacuation is indicated. Postoperative subdural hematomas occur less frequently and may result with some delay owing to later rupture of bridging veins following a large intracerebral decompression. On occasion, such subdural hematomas may occur distant from the primary site of operation.

Parenchymal hemorrhages are the most frequent cause of postoperative hematomas following supratentorial procedures and generally occur at the site of operation, particularly following partial tumor resection. An increase in systemic BP at the end of surgery may increase the risk of parenchymal hemorrhage. In rare cases, the hematoma may be located distant from the primary site of operation, and cerebellar hematomas have even been described after supratentorial surgery.[41,42]

The possibility of a postoperative hematoma should be considered in all patients who are not fully alert post anesthesia, as well as in those who exhibit secondary deterioration.

Postoperative Brain Swelling

Modern neuroanesthesiology techniques have diminished the incidence of peri- and postoperative brain swelling. Nevertheless, significant swelling may sometimes occur, causing surgical difficulties and possibly critical problems in the ICU. Predisposing factors are hypercapnia, arterial hypertension, hyponatremia, obstruction of venous drainage, and silent or overt seizures during surgery or in the immediate postoperative phase. Further significant brain swelling after uneventful surgery has been attributed to intracranial hypotension caused by subgaleal suction.[42,43] In any patient with brain swelling during the surgical procedure, the possibility of a deep hematoma should be considered, and an urgent computed tomography (CT) scan should be performed. Brain swelling due to vasodilation can be corrected by hyperventilation and barbiturate administration; brain swelling due to cerebral edema should preferentially be treated by mild hyperventilation and osmotic agents.

Tension Pneumocephalus

Some air collection is generally observed on postoperative CT scans.[44] In rare circumstances, the rewarming of air in the intracranial compartment postoperatively or continuous air leakage due to a cerebrospinal fluid (CSF) fistula of the skull base may lead to a tension pneumocephalus, with clinical symptomatology including decreasing level of consciousness, signs of raised ICP, and occasionally seizures. Generally, postoperative air accumulations are self-limiting and do not require specific treatment.

Seizures

An epileptic seizure in the direct postoperative phase should be considered a serious complication that may cause significant deterioration secondary to vasodilation, increased cerebral oxygen consumption, and increased brain edema. Occult seizure activity can occur in 15% to 18% of patients with moderate and severe TBI.[45] The benefits of prophylactic antiseizure medication should be balanced against risks. In some centers, routine prophylaxis is prescribed in all patients undergoing supratentorial brain surgery. In others, the indications are restricted to patients with a higher risk:

- Cerebrovascular surgery (arteriovenous malformation, aneurysm)
- Cerebral abscess and subdural empyema
- Convexity and parafalcial meningiomas
- Penetrating brain injury
- Compound depressed skull fracture

Opinions vary on the duration of prophylactic antiseizure therapy, some centers recommending a treatment duration of 2 weeks and others continuing for at least 3 months. In any case of unexplained neurologic deterioration or delayed awakening from anesthesia, the possibility of seizures should be considered.

INFRATENTORIAL PROCEDURES

The care for patients in the direct postoperative phase following infratentorial procedures poses specific problems. Postoperative complications in the posterior fossa can lead to rapid deterioration because of the relatively small infratentorial volume reserve and the immediate compression of the brainstem, resulting in respiratory insufficiency and acute herniation. Irritation of the brainstem may induce large swings in arterial BP, enhancing the risk of postoperative hemorrhage during hypertensive episodes. Cranial nerves are more susceptible to damage due to surgical manipulation than peripheral nerves.[46] Lesions of the lower cranial nerves may lead to a diminished gag reflex, with increased risk of aspiration and pneumonia. After surgery in the cerebellopontine angle, specific attention should be paid to the function of the trigeminal and facial nerves and prophylactic measures to prevent damage of the cornea taken.

After any infratentorial procedure, the risk of acute hydrocephalus due to obstruction at the level of the fourth ventricle is present. Increased pressure in the infratentorial compartment may, in rare cases in which supratentorial CSF drainage is performed, cause upward (inverse) herniation.

These specific aspects warrant routine admission of all patients who have undergone posterior fossa surgery to the ICU for careful observation and monitoring. Particular attention should be paid to the presence of the gag reflex before extubation and in the early stages after extubation, and frequent monitoring of the respiratory status and adequacy of respiration is imperative.

After posterior fossa surgery, some patients may develop a syndrome of aseptic meningitis.[47] This is characterized by meningeal symptoms, headaches, and an inflammatory response of the CSF in the absence of evidence for infection. The origin of this syndrome has not been fully clarified, but symptoms may resolve sooner with intermittent CSF drainage.

An infrequent transitory complication observed after resection of large midline posterior fossa tumors is cerebellar mutism.[47] The exact cause is poorly understood, but a vascular phenomenon has been hypothesized.[48]

CEREBROVASCULAR PROCEDURES

Postoperative care for patients undergoing cerebrovascular surgery poses specific challenges in neurointensive care. In patients operated for arteriovenous malformations, the risk of seizures is particularly high, and focal deficits may occur secondary to changes in cerebral hemodynamics. Following treatment for a cerebral aneurysm, medical and cerebral complications can occur either related to the disease or to treatment (surgical clipping or endovascular coiling). Medical complications specifically linked to SAH are neurogenic pulmonary edema, cardiac arrhythmias, and ventricular failure.[11] Electrolyte disturbances, in particular hyponatremia, are also frequently observed.[49]

The main cerebral complications are:
1. Rebleeding
2. Delayed cerebral ischemia
3. Hydrocephalus

Rebleeding occurs mainly in the first weeks after the aneurysmal rupture, and current approaches are to prevent rebleeding by early surgical clipping or endovascular obliteration of the aneurysmal sack. Delayed cerebral ischemia, often due to vasospasm is—besides rebleeding—the most common cause of death and disability due to SAH. The reported incidence of this complication varies widely, but angiographic vasospasm is seen with angiography in over 67% of untreated patients at the time of maximum spasm around the end of the first week.[50]

Delayed cerebral ischemia (DCI) is considered to be caused by vasospasm. However, not all patients with DCI have vasospasm. Inversely, not all patients with vasospasm develop clinical symptoms and signs of DCI. Recent studies show that DCI cannot always be attributed to vasospasm but more to the occurrence of microthrombosis.[51,52] DCI is associated with an activation of the coagulation cascade within a few days after SAH, preceding the time window during which vasospasm occurs. Furthermore, both impaired fibrinolytic activity and inflammatory and endothelium-related processes may lead to the formation of microthrombi, further promoting the development of DCI.

Clinically evident delayed ischemic deficits (DID) affect approximately one third of patients. Various studies have shown a beneficial effect of the administration of oral calcium antagonists in preventing DID.[53,54] Beneficial effects of intravenous administration of nimodipine remain unproven.

Following evidence that patients with SAH had reduced blood volume, plasma volume, and erythrocyte mass, triple-H therapy (hypervolemia, hypertension, and hemodilution) was proposed for both prophylaxis and treatment of DID after SAH. Various studies have shown a reduction of DID with triple-H prophylaxis,[55] but some debate remains.[56,57]

The usefulness of triple-H treatment is generally accepted, but it has never been unequivocally demonstrated by a randomized controlled trial to be superior to simple moderate fluid loading. The relative importance of the three components of triple-H therapy is uncertain.[58,59] Adequate fluid loading should be considered the most important aspect of early treatment and prophylaxis of DID, but it may be considered reasonable to reserve the more vigorous loading and induced hypertension for situations in which there is clinical evidence of delayed ischemia.[59-61]

Progressive signs of DID may require more aggressive approaches including angioplasty.[62] Transluminal balloon angioplasty is generally recommended, but this requires special equipment and a highly skilled and experienced interventional neuroradiology team. Alternatively, "chemical angioplasty" in which the angiography catheter is used to instill papaverine or nimodipine may be considered.[63]

Chemical angioplasty often has to be repeated within hours or days and carries complications including pupillary changes, seizures, or respiratory arrest with vertebral artery injection. Alternatively, possibilities of cisternal therapy should be considered, injecting recombinant tissue plasminogen activator (tPA) or urokinase in the basal cisterns to break down the accumulated blood,[64] or even nitric oxide donors to improve vascular tone.

Various studies have shown clinical benefit of this approach, with the added benefit of reducing the incidence of hydrocephalus. Acute hydrocephalus after SAH is not uncommon. The reported frequency depends on the criteria used for the diagnosis and ranges from 9%[65] up to 67%.[66] Spontaneous improvement of hydrocephalus has been reported in approximately half of patients with acute hydrocephalus and impaired consciousness on admission, but it may be difficult to predict spontaneous improvement, because treatment is generally instituted. Evidence exists that in the absence of a hematoma with mass effect or an obstructive element, serial lumbar punctures may be the initial optimal method of treatment, reserving continuous CSF drainage procedures for patients in whom the hydrocephalus does not resolve over time.

Admission Examination and Monitoring in the Intensive Care Unit

Specific care and monitoring of the postoperative neurosurgical patient requires accurate knowledge of the preoperative situation and the intraoperative procedure, including the surgery, anesthesiology, and any surgical complications or difficulties. Pertinent aspects are summarized in Table 41-3.

TABLE 41-3	Postoperative Intake After Neurosurgical Operations
Preoperative situation	Neurologic deficit (level of consciousness, focal paresis, cranial nerve lesions, hormonal deficits) Preexisting disease (especially pulmonary and cardiac) Preoperative medication History of seizures Allergy
Intraoperative details (anesthesia)	Narcotic agents and antagonists Blood loss and substitution Intraoperative laboratory values Intraoperative second insults, diabetes insipidus, etc.
Intraoperative course (surgical)	Indication, approach, and duration of surgery Surgical position Surgical difficulties and complications (brain swelling, difficult hemostasis, temporary or definite vascular occlusion, opening of air sinus) Immobilization/positioning of patient
Postoperative instructions (surgeon and anesthetist)	Postoperative medication (e.g., anticonvulsants, antibiotics, steroids, mannitol, antithrombosis prophylaxis) Instructions for postoperative care and monitoring Instructions for removal of drainage, tubes, and stitches Preferred duration of postoperative artificial ventilation Instructions for follow-up CT or MRI examination (if indicated)

On admission, a full examination of the patient is required; wherever possible, this includes assessment of level of consciousness and neurologic functioning. Medical care for the patient should be provided in joint collaboration between the intensivist and neurosurgeon. Intensive care monitoring includes clinical surveillance, technical monitoring, and follow-up CT or magnetic resonance imaging (MRI). Various approaches to monitoring are summarized in Table 41-4.

CLINICAL SURVEILLANCE

Even in this era of sophisticated monitoring procedures, routine clinical examinations are essential. The clinical assessment has the purpose of disclosing major life-threatening complications early after surgery and of assessing and tracking neurologic deficits in the hours to days that follow.

EARLY EVALUATION

A simple check of consciousness, pupils, and the development of focal (mostly motor) deficits remains the most important method for assessing patients in the neurosurgical ICU. Neurologic assessment should be repeated at regular intervals throughout the ICU course; change in examination findings is the most sensitive method for detecting neurologic deterioration.

The level of consciousness should be assessed by the Glasgow Coma Scale (GCS).[67] In this scale, standardized assessment of three aspects of responsiveness is performed: the eye, motor and verbal reaction (Table 41-5).

When administration of painful stimuli is necessary to assess the level of responsiveness, standardized administration is required: pressure on the nail bed and supraorbital pressure to test the localizing response of the motor scale (Figure 41-1).

Accurate determination of the full GCS is not always possible because of sedation and paralysis, but when possible, at least the best motor score should be recorded. Approaches to daily interruption of sedation that allow intermittent wake up in ventilated patients not only help care providers to monitor neurologic status but also have been shown to result in better outcome.[68] Some authors advocate imputing the eye and verbal scores from the motor score in sedated and/or ventilated patients.[69]

We would prefer an approach in which only the motor score is assessed at times when the level of sedation permits, as this is an important parameter of neurologic function and the main predictor of outcome in unconscious patients. The development of pupillary abnormalities is a sensitive indicator for pressure on the midbrain (tentorial herniation). Pupillary reaction to light is mediated through parasympathetic fibers of the third cranial nerve (oculomotor nerve). Afferent light perception, conducted through the second cranial nerve (optic nerve) connects at the level of the internal eye muscle nuclei to the oculomotor nerve supplying parasympathetic fibers to the sphincter pupillae muscle via the ciliary ganglia.

Pressure on the oculomotor nerve leads to a loss of function of the parasympathetic fibers, causing a diminished pupillary response or absent pupillary reactivity, generally initially on the side of a lesion (Figure 41-2). With progressive increase in pressure, both pupils become dilated and unresponsive to light. In patients with a lesion of the optic nerve, the consensual light reflex—contraction of the pupil when a light is shone into the opposite eye—remains intact.

FURTHER EVALUATION

When major complications have been ruled out, it remains necessary to evaluate the persistence of previous deficits, their improvement after surgery, or the appearance of new signs attributable to surgery. It is expected, for example, that following the surgical removal of an eighth nerve neurinoma, some degree of damage of cranial nerve VII can occur. After surgical intervention on structures located in or close to the brainstem, deficits of the lower cranial nerves can occur as well. A careful, complete neurologic examination is required at this stage, since the simple check proposed in the previous section is not meant to fully evaluate cranial nerve function. This evaluation is important, since cranial nerve deficits can require immediate treatment—for example, protection of the ocular bulb to prevent keratitis, or avoidance of oral feeding if swallowing is impaired.

TABLE 41-5	Glasgow Coma Scale		
Eyes		**Motor**	**Verbal**
1. None	1. None		1. None
2. To pain	2. Abnormal extension		2. Incomprehensible (groaning)
3. To speech	3. Abnormal flexion		3. Inappropriate
4. Spontaneous	4. Flexion (withdrawal)		4. Disoriented, confused
	5. Localizing		5. Oriented
	6. Obeying commands		

NOTES: The best score for each response should be documented and communicated in the format described above. Assessment of the best motor score is based on the best response of the arms. For use in individual patients, separate description of the three components of the Glasgow Coma Scale (GCS) is strongly recommended. For purposes of classification, the total GCS can be calculated by adding the best score obtained in each category. The GCS should be annotated to indicate confounding factors: *T* signifies an intubated patient; *S*, sedation; *P*, neuromuscular blockade.

TABLE 41-4	Postoperative Monitoring After Intracranial Procedures
Clinical surveillance	Level of consciousness (Glasgow Coma Scale), pupillary reactivity, focal deficits, cranial nerve lesions
Systemic monitoring	Electrocardiogram and heart rate, respiration, pulse oximetry, end-tidal CO_2, blood pressure (invasive, noninvasive), temperature, central venous pressure, Swan Ganz catheter
Brain-specific monitoring	Intracranial pressure and cerebral perfusion pressure, jugular oximetry, brain oxygen tension monitoring, microdialysis, transcranial Doppler, electroencephalogram, evoked potentials
Accesses	Central or peripheral venous catheter, arterial catheter, urinary catheter, gastric tube
Laboratory examinations	Blood gases, hematology, electrolytes, glucose and on indication coagulation status
Imaging examinations	Chest radiograph (ventilated patients and after lung procedures) Computed tomography or magnetic resonance imaging follow-up (as required)

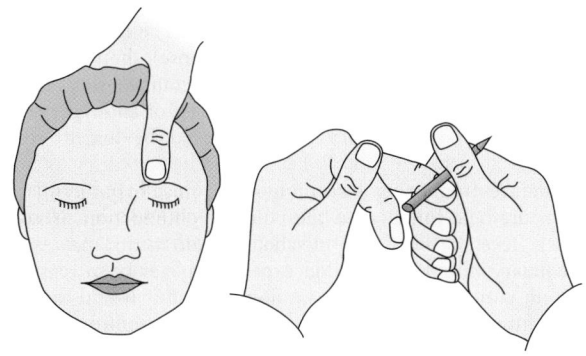

Figure 41-1 Supraorbital and nailbed pressure for assessment according to the Glasgow Coma Scale.

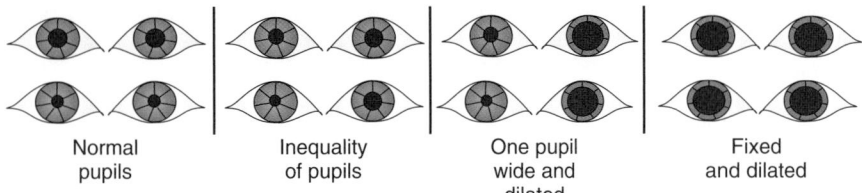

Normal pupils   Inequality of pupils   One pupil wide and dilated   Fixed and dilated

Figure 41-2   Pupillary reactivity and size.

Systemic Monitoring: Cardiopulmonary, Respiratory Status, and Temperature

The goal of cardiopulmonary and respiratory monitoring is to ensure accurate control of systemic hemodynamic and respiratory function, essential for optimization of cerebral oxygenation. Invasive arterial BP monitoring is recommended, with the reference point set at the same level as ICP measurement to allow accurate calculation of cerebral perfusion pressure (CPP).

Hypovolemic shock is most common in the setting of multisystem injury or intraoperative blood loss with inadequate replacement. It is important to recognize that tachycardia and signs of peripheral vasoconstriction such as skin pallor and poor capillary refill may precede a drop in BP. Treatment is rapid fluid resuscitation employing isotonic crystalloid fluids, volume expanders, small-volume resuscitation (hypertonic saline), and blood transfusions. Central venous pressure monitoring, or preferably pulmonary artery catheterization, can guide the use of intravenous fluids and vasopressor therapy, aiming for a pulmonary artery wedge pressure of 12 to 14 mm Hg to optimize organ perfusion. After initial volume resuscitation, we suggest a hematocrit of approximately 30% to 33% as optimal in the acute postoperative period in patients in the neurosurgical ICU. Although debate still exists, available evidence suggests that restrictive blood transfusion strategies may be less appropriate in neurointensive care.[70-74]

After intracranial or spinal cord procedures, we would advocate a more liberal use of blood transfusions than generally recommended in intensive care medicine, aiming at a hemoglobin of at least 5.5 to 6.0 mmol/L (9-10 mg/dL) in order to promote adequate oxygenation of the CNS. This corresponds to the recommendations proposed by Goodnough et al.[75] in case of ischemia.

Cardiogenic shock due to primary loss of cardiac function is less common in neurosurgical patients, but it can occur, particularly in the elderly patient with secondary cardiac ischemia/arrhythmias or in case of Takotsubo syndrome. These patients may require sequential echocardiographic follow-up and/or the use of a pulmonary artery catheter to optimize volume status and cardiac output. Large pulmonary emboli, sepsis, or spinal paraplegia should also be considered in patients with systemic hypotension. In patients with spinal distributive shock, typically the hypotension is associated with bradycardia, with a pulse in the range of 35 to 50. These patients should not be managed with excessive volume resuscitation but rather with vasopressors to restore α-adrenergic peripheral vasomotor tone. The combination of hypertension and bradycardia (Cushing response) should alert the physician to the potential of an expanding intracranial lesion and risk of brainstem herniation. In this situation, the use of antihypertensive agents is contraindicated, and therapy should be aimed at the raised ICP.

Temperature monitoring is also important, since hypothermia can depress neurologic function to the point of obtundation or coma. Conversely, fever, by increasing metabolic requirements, may exacerbate secondary injury. Mean energy expenditure may be increased up to 200% in patients following brain injury,[76] and it would therefore appear appropriate not to risk increasing metabolic requirements even further. Consequently, we recommend that core temperature should be kept lower than 38.0°C, using medications (e.g., acetaminophen, paracetamol, diclofenac) and surface or intravascular cooling.

Hypothermia may be due to adrenal or pituitary insufficiency, hypothalamic disorders, hypoglycemia, or intraoperative exposure. Deliberate hypothermia is sometimes used in complicated cerebrovascular procedures and as second-tier therapy in patients with TBI to reduce ICP. For the indication TBI, hypothermia has been shown to effectively reduce ICP, but uncertainty still exists whether this may translate into an improvement of functional outcome.[77,78]

Various approaches to cooling have been adopted, but the most frequently used employ surface cooling or gastric lavage with cold fluids. Marion[79] reported favorable results with the use of devices for intravascular cooling, and this technique can be expected to become standard for induction of hypothermia in the near future.

Hypothermia has been associated with several complications including cardiovascular instability (mainly arrhythmias), coagulopathy, electrolyte shifts, fluid overload, and increased risk of infection and shivering.[80,81] The management of a patient treated with hypothermia over longer periods of time for control of raised ICP can be much more complex than the use of short-term hypothermia post cardiac arrest. Ideally, normothermia could represent the best tradeoff between the dangers of hyperthermia and the complexities and side effects of hypothermia. In practice, a recent trial in neurointensive care comparing conventional treatments with prophylactic normothermia has failed to show benefit.[82]

BIOCHEMICAL PARAMETERS: ELECTROLYTES, OSMOLARITY, AND BLOOD GLUCOSE

A major focus for neurointensive care is to prevent and limit brain damage and provide the best conditions for natural brain recovery from surgery or injury by ensuring optimal oxygenation, perfusion, ionic homeostasis, glycemic control, and temperature management. Keeping biochemical parameters within physiologic ranges is obviously desirable, but this apparently simple goal may require a lot of work. Repeated determinations are necessary for early detection of derangements and to prevent overcorrection. Patients with comorbidities (diabetes, cardiac failure, etc.) and concomitant medications are especially at risk.

ELECTROLYTES AND OSMOLARITY

A direct link exists between plasma osmolarity and water flux into and out of brain cells[83,84]; if the blood-brain barrier is intact, any decrease in plasma osmolarity will cause an increase of intracellular water in the brain, with potential increase in intracranial pressure, alteration of the transmembrane potential, and so on.[85] It is important to prevent the development of hyponatremia, because it may exacerbate the development of brain edema in the postoperative setting. Particularly in pediatric patients undergoing external CSF drainage, replacement of drained CSF by physiologic saline should be considered.

Various factors may contribute to the high risk of electrolyte disorders in neurointensive care:

- The use of osmotically active drugs (e.g., mannitol, hypertonic saline, other diuretics) for the treatment of raised ICP. These may induce electrolyte derangements or increase serum osmolarity to levels that kidney function may be compromised. Careful and frequent monitoring is therefore required. General recommendation is that serum osmolarity should be kept below 320 mOsm.
- The common use of steroids in brain surgery to prevent cerebral edema. These may increase blood glucose to levels that exceed the

maximum renal capabilities for glucose transport. If glycosuria follows, it causes osmotic diuresis.

- When surgery or injury impacts neurohypophyseal function, causing a deficit in the release of antidiuretic hormone (ADH), sudden episodes of diabetes insipidus are likely.[86] Large urinary volumes have to be replaced with appropriate solutions to preserve euvolemia and osmolarity, in addition to the administration of ADH.
- Cerebral salt waisting. This disorder is still poorly understood,[87] and it is often difficult to differentiate from an inappropriate ADH syndrome. Fluid restriction for correction should generally be avoided; it is often better to administer hypertonic saline.

GLUCOSE

Glucose is an essential substrate for brain metabolism, and every effort should be made to ensure adequate delivery to the nervous tissue. In general intensive care, tight glycemic control has been advocated based on the knowledge that outcome is poorer in the presence of hyperglycemia and following the results of the study by van den Berghe et al.,[88] showing reduced mortality in surgical intensive care by keeping glycemia within narrow limits (80-110 mg/dL). These promising findings have, however, been challenged by a more recent trial.[89]

Although in neurointensive care as well, various studies have demonstrated an association between elevated glucose levels and poorer outcome,[90-93] the question whether this association may be causal or simply a marker has remained unanswered. In neurointensive care, the concern is that the injured brain cannot tolerate hypoglycemia, which might result as an adverse event from overenthusiastic glycemic control. There is a strict relationship between the increased use of insulin (for tight glycemic control) and the occurrence of hypoglycemia.[94,95]

Moreover, lowering blood glucose to "normal" levels may result in unacceptably low levels of glucose in the brain, depriving the most complex organ in the human body of its most essential metabolic substrate. That this concern is real has been demonstrated in microdialysis studies.[96-98]

Such observations illustrate the complex interactions between systemic and cerebral parameters and highlight that correction of biochemical parameters in the blood may not always be good for the brain, in particular when recovering from surgery or injury. In our opinion, the currently available evidence would not support the use of tight glucose control in neurointensive care.

Brain Monitoring and Specific Therapeutic Approaches

In comparison to the setting in cardiac intensive care, the possibilities for brain monitoring are still relatively limited.[99] In cardiac care, routinely measured parameters include a multitude of pressure indices and a number of different serum markers (e.g., creatine kinase fractions, troponin) to determine if the heart is at risk for further injury. Physiologically, the heart is monitored by electrocardiography and intermittently with echocardiography. In contrast, routine monitoring of the brain is restricted in most centers to ICP and CPP monitoring, but the field is rapidly evolving. Monitoring of cerebral oxygenation is now being increasingly implemented in clinical practice[100-102] and continuous EEG performed in some centers.[103-105] Magnetic resonance spectroscopy now offers opportunities to noninvasively assess brain metabolism.[106,107] Advances in the field of biomarkers are encouraging and offer hope that detection and tracking of pathophysiologic processes in the brain may now be within reach.[108,109]

As noted, current approaches to brain-specific monitoring include measurements of ICP, cerebral oxygenation, cerebral blood flow (CBF), electrical monitoring, and metabolic monitoring. These specific modalities are discussed in detail in Chapter 31. Here we focus on essential aspects regarding interpretation of monitoring results and therapeutic implications.

INTRACRANIAL PRESSURE AND CEREBRAL PERFUSION PRESSURE

ICP monitoring is most commonly performed in trauma patients and indicated in those with severe brain injury (GCS < 8) with abnormalities on the initial CT scan, and further in patients with a normal admission CT scan if two or more of the following features are present: age older than 40 years, unilateral or bilateral motor posturing, systolic BP less than 90 mm Hg.

Routine ICP monitoring is not generally indicated in patients with mild or moderate TBI but may be considered when other severe extracranial injuries are present, necessitating anesthesia for surgery, or when the initial CT shows traumatic lesions with space-occupying effects.[110] ICP monitoring is further indicated in poor-grade patients with aneurysmal SAH.[111-113] Further, it may be considered in patients with other intracranial disorders who are sedated and ventilated and in whom the risk of raised ICP is considered present (postoperative swelling, stroke, Reye syndrome).

ICP monitoring carries a 0.5% risk of hemorrhage and a 2% risk of infection.[114] Intracranial hemorrhages are a rare complication of ICP monitoring and are usually caused by multiple punctures in the presence of coagulopathies. The risk of infection is higher in the case of ventricular monitoring, and the rate of infection is proportional to the duration of monitoring.[115] Intraventricular catheters are preferable because they are accurate, can be recalibrated, and allow drainage of CSF. Intraparenchymal probes are user friendly and accurate. Less accurate data are provided by subdural catheters,[116] and epidural probes are unreliable.[117,118] The accuracy of ICP monitoring can be enhanced by use of computer-supported systems.[119] Attempts to monitor ICP noninvasively have been unsatisfactory.[120,121]

Relatively few data exist on routine ICP monitoring in the postoperative situation. In a series of 30 patients after severe TBI and elective craniectomy, 156 instances of raised ICP and/or reduced CPP were recorded.[122] These instances were only accompanied by clinical deterioration in 15 cases. Telemetric ICP control has been proposed after posterior fossa surgery.[123] In a series of 514 patients after supra- and infratentorial surgery, Constantini et al.[124] described raised ICP in 13% and 18% of cases, respectively. Neurologic deterioration occurred in approximately half of the patients suffering ICP rise and was always preceded by the ICP increase. In a large series of 780 patients submitted to routine ICP monitoring after intracranial surgery, 47% required ICP-directed therapy.[125] In a report concerning 850 cases, Bullock and associates[126] concluded that ICP monitoring allows earlier identification of recurrent hematomas. These data would support a more routine application of ICP monitoring after intracranial surgery, particularly in more complex cases. In some institutions, ICP is routinely measured as part of postoperative surveillance after major neurosurgical procedures, especially when risk of postoperative bleeding exists. Figure 41-3 illustrates a case in which a substantial ICP rise was detected in the first postoperative hours. An enlarging hemorrhage was responsible and required reintervention.

Normal values for ICP are up to 15 mm Hg in adults, and consensus supports maintaining ICP below 20 mm Hg, but the absolute value of ICP measured should never be viewed in isolation. More important is the trend over time and the relation to the arterial BP. Cerebral perfusion pressure is calculated as:

$$MABP - ICP = CPP$$

It is important to recognize that physiologic and nonphysiologic wave forms may occur. Technical artifacts and systemic causes should be excluded before specific diagnostic procedures are instituted or ICP-directed therapy initiated or intensified (Table 41-6).

In some patients, the normal pressure autoregulatory mechanisms are disturbed, and the risk exists that increased CPP may worsen cerebral edema. Careful observation of the change in ICP with respect to arterial BP changes is required to determine whether autoregulation is disturbed or intact. For continuous evaluation of the autoregulatory status, it has been proposed to calculate the pressure-reactivity index

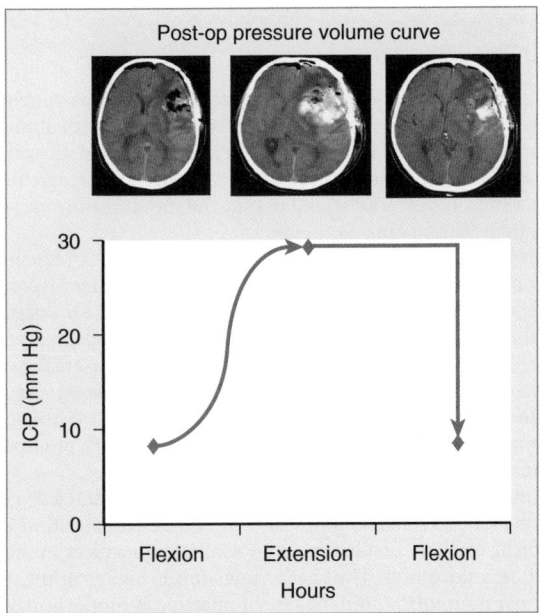

Figure 41-3 Raised intracranial pressure (ICP) as the first indication of a developing postoperative hematoma.

TABLE 41-6	Remediable Extracranial Causes of Intracranial Hypertension

Calibration errors
Airway obstruction (kinked endotracheal tube, tongue, sputum retention, pneumothorax)
Hypoxia (low FiO₂, lung disease/collapse)
Hypercapnia (hypoventilation)
Hypertension (pain, sedation, coughing/straining)
Hypotension (hypovolemia, sedation, cardiac)
Posture (Trendelenburg position, neck rotation)
Hyperpyrexia
Seizures
Hypo-osmolality (sodium, protein)

(PRx) as the moving correlation coefficient between MABP and ICP.[127-129] The added value of this approach, however, still requires confirmation.

TREATMENT OF CEREBRAL HERNIATION AND ELEVATED ICP

The development of cerebral herniation (tentorial herniation/cerebellar tonsillar herniation) constitutes a neurosurgical emergency. Rapid intervention is required prior to further investigations to determine the cause. According to the concept of the pressure volume curve (Figure 41-4), a small reduction in intracranial volume will already significantly decrease raised ICP and reverse herniation. The emergency measures to be taken include:
- Ventricular CSF drainage (if access available)*
- Bolus administration of high-dose hyperosmolar agents: mannitol: 1 to 1.5 g/kg bodyweight; hypertonic saline (HTS) 1 to 2 mL/kg body weight 7.5% saline infused over 5 minutes
- Rapid-sequence intubation and moderate hyperventilation

Following these emergency procedures, emergency head CT scan should be performed to detect the cause of raised ICP and permit targeted treatment, such as evacuation of a postoperative clot or further treatment of an acute obstructive hydrocephalus.

The main intracranial causes of raised ICP are:
- Mass lesions (hematoma)
- Edema (vasogenic, cytotoxic, osmotic, hydrostatic)
- Increased cerebral blood volume (vasodilation)
- Disturbance of CSF flow (hydrocephalus, benign intracranial hypertension)

In the absence of an acute cerebral herniation, elevated ICP is addressed first by ruling out treatable intracranial mass lesions and remediable extracranial causes or monitor malfunction (see Table 41-6).

Where appropriate, surgical intervention is indicated. Conservative therapy of elevated ICP includes:
- Sedation, analgesia, and mild to moderate hyperventilation (Paco₂ 4-4.5 kPa; 30-35 mm Hg)

---

*Lumbar CSF drainage should never be attempted in this situation, as this may increase the degree of herniation.

- Osmotic therapy: preferably mannitol given in bolus infusions (dose: 0.25-0.5 g/kg bodyweight, or as indicated by monitoring). Alternatively, HTS may be considered. Effective doses as bolus infusion range between 1 and 2 mL/kg of 7.5% saline. Effective doses as a continuous infusion of 3% range between 75 and 150 mL/h. Comparison of effectiveness of mannitol versus HTS is confounded by the wide variability in concentrations and doses used for HTS. Table 41-7 presents an overview of osmolarity and electrolyte concentration of different commercially available hypertonic solutions used for treating raised ICP. Serum osmolarity should be maintained below 320 mOsm/L. Particular vigilance is warranted when mannitol and HTS are given concomitantly. If osmotherapy has insufficient effect, furosemide can be given additionally.
- CSF fluid drainage
- Volume expansion and inotropes or vasopressors when arterial BP is insufficient to maintain CPP and CBF in a normovolemic patient

If these methods fail, second-tier therapies for raised ICP include:
- Mild or moderate hypothermia
- Decompressive surgery
- Administration of barbiturates
- More intensive hyperventilation (which should be used with monitoring of cerebral oxygenation to detect cerebral ischemia)

CEREBRAL BLOOD FLOW

Recent years have seen great advances in approaches to monitoring CBF and CBF-related variables, particularly in the field of neuroimaging. Both CT and MRI techniques have been developed for perfusion

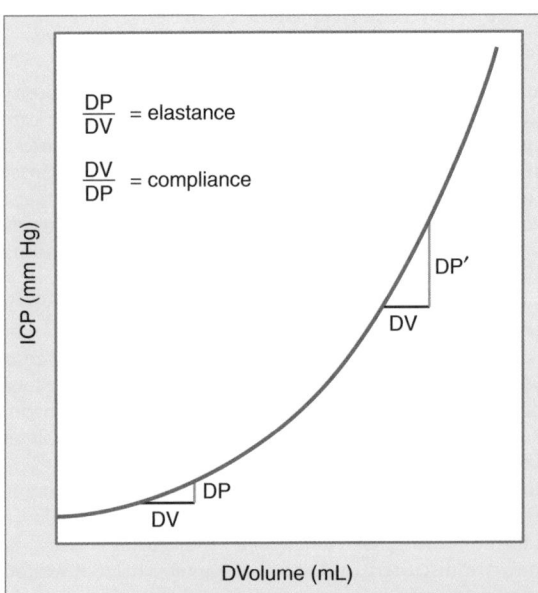

Figure 41-4 Intracranial pressure (ICP) volume curve.

TABLE 41-7	Composition of Different Commercially Available Hypertonic Solutions Used for Treatment of Raised Intracranial Pressure			
Drug	**Osmolality**	**Sodium**	**Chloride**	**Colloid**
20% Mannitol	1098 mmol/L	—	—	—
40% Sorbitol	2200 mmol/L	—	—	—
10% Glycerol	1379 mmol/L	77 mmol/L	77 mmol/L	—
Ringer's Lactate	277 mmol/L	130 mmol/L	112 mmol/L	—
0.9% NaCl	309 mmol/L	154 mmol/L	154 mmol/L	—
1.7% NaCl	598 mmol/L	268 mmol/L	268 mmol/L	—
3% NaCl	1030 mmol/L	515 mmol/L	515 mmol/L	—
5.85% NaCl	2000 mmol/L	1000 mmol/L	1000 mmol/L	—
20% NaCl	6800 mmol/L	3400 mmol/L	3400 mmol/L	—
23.8% NaCl	8200 mmol/L	4100 mmol/L	4100 mmol/L	—
7.5% NaCl/6% dextran 70	2567 mmol/L	1283 mmol/L	1283 mmol/L	Dextran
7.2% NaCl/6% HES 200	2264 mmol/L	1132 mmol/L	1132 mmol/L	HES

imaging and angiography, and possibilities for determining areas of the brain at risk for ischemia are now routinely available to the clinician. These approaches have replaced measurements of CBF with stable xenon CT scanning. Positron emission tomography (PET) studies for CBF and metabolic studies of the brain have largely remained in the domain of research. Thermal diffusion flowmetry has been introduced as a bedside technique for continuously monitoring CBF, but experience is as yet limited.[116,130,131] A major drawback of this sensor is that it is not MRI compatible. Transcranial Doppler (TCD) provides a noninvasive assessment of blood flow velocity through the basal cerebral arteries. TCD is widely used for the detection and tracking of cerebral vasospasm,[132] but various studies have shown a disappointing correlation when measured flow velocities are compared with direct measurements of CBF.[133,134] In patients with stroke, detection of emboli is possible with most current TCD devices.[135]

Vasopressor therapy may be needed in the postoperative care of patients in the neuro-ICU. Vasopressors are often required in the treatment of SAH and severe TBI (see Chapters 35 and 38). It is important to realize that the pathophysiologic mechanism in these disorders is different, and that commonly employed approaches for treatment of delayed ischemic deficits following aneurysmal SAH cannot be directly translated to the situation of TBI.

In analogy to the laws of electricity, in which the current (ampere) is dependent on voltage and resistance according the formula: I = V/R, the CBF is dependent on the driving pressure (CPP) and cerebrovascular resistance (CVR): CBF = CPP/CVR. With reference to the Hagen Poiseuille equation, the CVR is determined by the radius and length of the blood vessel and blood viscosity according to the formula:

$$\frac{8 \eta l}{k \times \pi r4}$$

where k = a constant, r = radius of the blood vessel, l = the length of the blood vessel (practically constant), and η = dynamic blood viscosity. The most powerful factor in this equation is the vessel radius.

The concept of triple-H and CPP therapy is that if CVR is increased, a high driving pressure is required to overcome the increased resistance. In patients with delayed ischemia following SAH, the primary pathophysiologic event is vasoconstriction, and to maintain CBF within normal limits, a considerable increase of CPP is required to maintain CBF. In patients with TBI, in contrast, the diameter of the major basal cerebral arteries is not clearly constricted in the acute phase, and it is still uncertain whether observed reductions of CBF in the acute phase after injury are caused by a vasoconstriction of the microcirculatory circulation or secondary to decreased metabolic requirements, possibly due to mitochondrial dysfunction, or both. Furthermore, in these patients the normal pressure autoregulatory

mechanisms may be disturbed, and the risk exists that increased CPP may worsen cerebral edema.

The vasopressors most frequently used in the care of the postoperative neurosurgical patients are listed in Table 41-8. Dose ranges are provided, but in general it is recommended to titrate the required dose versus the desired BP or CPP.

CEREBRAL OXYGENATION AND METABOLISM

Three approaches to monitoring cerebral oxygenation are available to the clinician: jugular bulb oximetry ($Sjvo_2$), noninvasive cerebral oximetry (i.e., near-infrared spectroscopy [NIRS], rSo_2, somanetics; or tissue index of oxygenation, Hamamatsu), and cerebral parenchymal oximetry monitors (LICOX [$Pbro_2$]).

Global cerebral oxygenation may be assessed using jugular oximetry, which is discussed in Chapter 31. When hemoglobin concentration and arterial hemoglobin saturation remain constant, $AJDo_2$ may be estimated by simply recording $Sjvo_2$. A decrease in $Sjvo_2$ indicates that the brain is extracting more oxygen, suggesting that the oxygen supply is inadequate for metabolic demands. Values below 55% indicate an increased oxygen extraction relative to perfusion and suggest the presence of ischemia.[136,137]

Interpretation of results of jugular oximetry requires that both systemic information (e.g., hemoglobin concentration and arterial saturation) and intracranial data (e.g., CPP) be combined. The technique has limitations: first, continuous monitoring of $Sjvo_2$ with fiberoptic devices is prone to artifact; and second, under conditions of anemia or arterio venous shunting, hypoxia may be present at the tissue level despite normal values of jugular saturation.[138] Moreover, $Sjvo_2$ is a measure of global cerebral oxygenation and does not reflect disturbances due to focal lesions, thus potentially failing to detect ischemia in relevant portions of brain tissue.[139]

NIRS is a noninvasive technique that permits estimation of oxyhemoglobin (Hbo_2), deoxyhemoglobin (Hb), and oxidized cytochrome oxidase (CytOx) over the combined arterial, capillary, and venous compartments.[140] Various assumptions are made in the calculation algorithm of cerebral oxygen saturation with NIRS that may not always be valid, and uncertainty exists whether NIRS, as claimed, mainly measures the intracranial compartment or that recorded values are "contaminated" by the extracranial compartment.[141] The main clinical applications are in neonatology and in coronary or carotid artery surgery.[142,143] Recent intracranial surgery and subcutaneous swelling or wounds to the scalp, common in patients with TBI, preclude application of this technique. We do not consider it suitable for routine use in monitoring oxygenation in patients undergoing neurosurgical operations; yet, a noninvasive technique to assess cerebral oxygenation is attractive, and further clinical research should be encouraged.

Monitoring of $Pbro_2$ is possible by inserting an oxygen-sensitive electrode into the cerebral cortex or white matter. By definition, this concerns a regional technique, and there is still considerable debate whether this technique should be employed in relatively undamaged parts of the brain—and as such be considered representative of more global oxygenation and metabolism—or preferably be employed in the penumbra zone of lesions, the aim being to limit secondary damage in potential viable regions.

TABLE 41-8	Vasopressors Commonly Used in the Neurocritical Care Unit	
Agent	**Adrenergic Effect**	**Doses ($\mu g/kg/min$) in Adults**
Norepinephrine	Mixed α and β ($\alpha \ggg \beta$)	0.02-1.5
Phenylephrine	Pure α	0.1-9.0
Adrenaline	Mixed α and β ($\alpha > \beta$)	0.1-1

NOTE: The use of dopamine, a precursor of norepinephrine, has mainly been abandoned because of its interference with hormone secretion. α, alpha-adrenergic effect; β, beta-adrenergic effect.

Brain tissue oxygen tension indicates the balance between oxygen delivered to the tissue and its consumption in a specific area and can indicate regional hypoxia if it falls below 15 to 20 mm Hg.[144,145] The diameter of microvascular vessels and diffusion barriers might also influence recorded values.[146,147] In TBI, low values of Pbro$_2$ occur in over 50% of patients during the first 24 hours, and depth and duration are related to outcome. Increased hyperventilation has further been shown to reduce Pbro$_2$.[139,146] Experimental and clinical evidence suggests that CPP therapy may be targeted towards appropriate levels, based on results of tissue Pbro$_2$ monitoring.[148] Non-randomized studies have indicated benefit of an oxygen-targeted treatment protocol.[149-151]

MICRODIALYSIS

The technique of microdialysis allows for measurement of substrate and metabolites (glucose, lactate, pyruvate), amino acids (glutamate), as well as indicators of cerebral damage (glycerol or other proteins as tau and beta amyloid) in the extracellular fluid of the brain.[152,153] Dialysate fluid obtained after infusing saline through a semipermeable membrane reflects the composition of the extracellular fluid around the probe. Microdialysis is employed in various specialized neurointensive care units, mainly for research purposes. Technical and logistic considerations, as well as delays in obtaining real-time values, have inhibited the routine application of results toward individualized targeted treatment. The availability of microdialysis catheters with a high cutoff membrane now permit detection of larger molecules and may offer opportunities for tracking the inflammatory response.[154-158]

ELECTRICAL MONITORING

Continuous EEG (cEEG) monitoring has the potential for detecting nonconvulsive status epilepticus in ICU patients. As a primary monitor of brain function, cEEG can be used to titrate continuous infusion of sedative agents, and the technique can further alert the physician to development of focal or global ischemia.[159,160] The sensitivity for detecting ischemia and hypoxia is high, but the specificity is low owing to effects of sedative medications. Continuous EEG may permit detection and treatment of such adverse events at an early stage, with a potential positive effect on outcome.[161] Electroencephalographic bispectral analysis (BIS) may be useful in assessing the level of sedation in neurocritical care patients.[162]

In the research setting, interest exists in monitoring cortical spreading depression. Traumatically damaged neurons decrease their firing rates substantially in the early postinjury period. Waves of depolarization result in ionic flux and loss of resting membrane potential, which worsens neurochemical dysregulation and places extra metabolic demands on damaged tissue.[163-166] Measurement of evoked potentials,[167] assessing the integrity of sensory and motor pathways, may provide diagnostic and prognostic information, but because of the complexity of the technique, it is not recommended for general use.

▓ Neuroprotection

The original concept of neuroprotection depended upon the initiation of treatment before the onset of an event leading to brain damage, and the methods employed aimed to minimize the intensity of an insult or its immediate effects upon the brain.

Over the past decades, the concept of neuroprotection has been extended to include treatment started after the onset of an insult, reflecting our increased understanding of progressive pathophysiologic mechanisms causing and/or enhancing secondary brain damage. In neuroprotection, four main approaches can be discerned (Table 41-9).

TABLE 41-9	Main Approaches in Neuroprotection

Strategies aimed at improving metabolism and microenvironment:
- For example hypothermia and mannitol

Agents acting on specific mechanisms:
- Examples: antiinflammatory agents, apoptosis inhibitors, calcium channel antagonists, neurotransmitter-targeted agents, free radical scavengers, and inhibitors of lipid peroxidation

Pluripotent agents affecting various mechanisms (so called "dirty drugs")

Combination therapies (including sequential administration)

Strategies promoting cell survival and regeneration (cellular replacement, gene therapy, and neurotrophic factors)

STRATEGIES AIMED AT IMPROVING METABOLISM AND MICROENVIRONMENT

Methods for improving metabolism and microenvironment include hypothermia to minimize the effects of energy failure and hyperosmolar therapy to reduce ICP and improve CBF. Hypothermia decreases cerebral blood flow by approximately 5.2% per degree of reduction in body temperature. The cerebral metabolic rate for oxygen (CMRO$_2$) and the arterial jugular venous oxygen difference (AVDO$_2$) fall after the institution of moderate hypothermia. This reflects a reduction in energy requirement and hence less energy loss in the injured brain. Many other effects of hypothermia, such as stabilization of the cell membrane[168] and reduction of neurotransmitter turnover, may also contribute to the benefit seen in models of ischemia.[169] Consequently, hypothermia is currently seen more as a neuroprotective approach than as a metabolic depressant. The use of hypothermia is therefore not without risks and requires high-level neurointensive care.

Hyperosmolar therapy is widely used in neurosurgery to treat raised ICP and to decrease brain bulk during intracranial operations and to treat cerebral ischemia. Hypertonic fluids are considered to exert beneficial effects by two mechanisms:

1. An immediate plasma-expanding effect, reducing hematocrit and blood viscosity and consequently increasing CBF and cerebral oxygen delivery
2. An osmotic effect; this effect is delayed for 15 to 30 minutes while gradients are established between plasma and cells. Hypertonic solutions may be given in acute emergency situations such as cerebral herniation or as part of a conservative approach to treatment of raised ICP.

AGENTS ACTING ON SPECIFIC MECHANISMS

Increased understanding of the existence of progressive pathophysiologic mechanisms causing or enhancing secondary brain damage has led to the development of a large range of specifically targeted neuroprotective agents aimed at ameliorating such mechanisms, often showing marked beneficial effect in experimental studies.[170] Unfortunately, in various fields of neurointensive care, promising experimental results have not translated into clinical efficacy. In addition to the heterogeneity of patient populations, the lack of clinical parameters for effectively identifying mechanistic targets has contributed to these failures. The emerging field of biomarkers and advanced neuroimaging offer hope for the future.

PLURIPOTENT AGENTS AND COMBINATIONAL THERAPIES

The realization that various pathophysiologic mechanisms are often concurrently or sequentially active has increased interest in the use of agents with multiple mechanisms; for such agents, the term "dirty drugs" has been coined.[171]

Corticosteroids, barbiturates, and magnesium are examples of pluripotent neuroprotective agents. Despite their efficacy in treating vasogenic edema, as encountered in brain tumors, corticosteroids are not efficacious in improving cytotoxic edema, as seen after TBI or SAH.

Various studies support a neuroprotective effect of magnesium in patients with SAH.[172,173] A recent randomized controlled trial, however, could not confirm benefit.[174] In TBI, greater mortality and poorer outcome was found in a randomized clinical trial investigating the efficacy of magnesium.[175]

Erythropoietin (EPO), cyclosporine, and progesterone are agents with neuroprotective potential currently undergoing further clinical evaluation. Rather than seeking a single "silver bullet" agent targeting multiple mechanisms, it may be better to consider combining agents with complementary targets and effects.[176] Fundamental to this approach, and in fact to any neuroprotective strategy, would be the accurate detection and tracking of pathophysiologic processes occurring in individual patients, which would provide better evidence for combining or sequential administration of neuroprotective agents.[170]

▧ Strategies Promoting Cell Survival and Regeneration

Strategies to promote cell survival and regeneration include cellular replacement, gene therapy, and administration of trophic factors. These approaches are aimed at promoting regeneration and neuroplasticity and may ultimately lead to improved functional recovery.[177,178] The potential of these novel approaches is strengthened by promising experimental and clinical results obtained in neurodegenerative diseases including Parkinson's disease, Huntington's disease, and stroke.[178-181] Promoting cell survival and regeneration is currently the focus of large research efforts that may provide possibilities for further improving outcome in the subacute and chronic phases.

KEY POINTS

1. Successful care for the neurosurgical patient requires excellent collaboration between neurosurgeon and intensivist. The result of a technically perfect operation can be ruined by inadequate postoperative care, and a complex operative procedure requires expert intensive care to correct abnormalities in homeostatic mechanisms, ensure adequate cerebral perfusion and oxygenation, and promote recovery of brain function.

2. The principal goal of postoperative neurosurgical intensive care is early detection and treatment of postsurgery complications. The second goal is to prevent second insults, which may initiate or exacerbate secondary damage in a vulnerable central nervous system.

3. Specific care and monitoring of the postoperative neurosurgical patient requires accurate knowledge of the preoperative situation and the intraoperative procedure, including the surgery, anesthesiology, and any surgical complications or difficulties.

4. The goal of cardiopulmonary and respiratory monitoring is to ensure adequate hemodynamic and respiratory function, essential for optimization of cerebral oxygenation. The driving force here should be formed by cerebral parameters, rather than simply keeping systemic parameters within normal ranges. Invasive arterial blood pressure monitoring is recommended, with the reference point set at the same level as intracranial pressure measurement to allow accurate calculation of cerebral perfusion pressure.

5. The development of cerebral herniation (tentorial herniation/cerebellar tonsillar herniation) constitutes a neurosurgical emergency. Rapid intervention is required prior to further investigations to determine the cause.

ANNOTATED REFERENCES

Heros RC. Case volume and mortality. J Neurosurg 2003;99(5):805-6.
This editorial comment on a manuscript by Cross and Dacey discusses the various confounders and implications with regard to the relation between case volume and mortality. The manuscript by Cross and Dacey had shown that after controlling for important predictors, the mortality rate is significantly higher in hospitals that admit a low volume of patients with SAH compared with higher-volume hospitals. This review concludes that only well-controlled studies, including data on initial clinical severity and detailed outcome information, can definitively demonstrate the advantages of centralized care.

Dubey A, Sung WS, Shaya M, et al. Complications of posterior cranial fossa surgery–an institutional experience of 500 patients. Surg Neurol 2009 Oct;72(4):369-75.
Retrospective study of 500 patients undergoing posterior fossa surgery in a single center. The overall complication rate was 31.8%. Cerebrospinal fluid leaks were the most frequently encountered complications, followed by infections and cranial nerve palsies. The authors conclude that posterior fossa surgery involves greater morbidity and mortality and has a wider variety of complications than surgery in the supratentorial compartment. The necessity for careful perioperative planning and the importance of surgical techniques is emphasized.

Dankbaar JW, Slooter AJ, Rinkel GJ, Schaaf IC. Effect of different components of triple-H therapy on cerebral perfusion in patients with aneurysmal subarachnoid haemorrhage: a systematic review. Crit Care 2010;14(1):R23.
Systematic review of the literature on the effect of triple-H components on cerebral perfusion in SAH patients; 11 studies were included in the review. The large heterogeneity in interventions and study populations prohibited meta-analysis. The authors conclude that there is no good evidence from controlled studies for a positive effect of triple H or its separate components on CBF in SAH patients. In uncontrolled studies, hypertension seems to be more effective in increasing CBF than hemodilution or hypervolemia.

Sen J, Belli A, Alborn H, Morgan L, Petzold A, Kitchen N. Triple-H therapy in the management of aneurysmal subarachnoid hemorrhage. Lancet Neurol 2003;2(10):614-21.
Review manuscript discussing the rationale and clinical studies on the use of triple-H therapy in the management of delayed ischemic deficits after aneurysmal subarachnoid hemorrhage. New insights into the pathogenesis of delayed cerebral ischemia are discussed, as well as the potential of biomarkers, advanced monitoring, and neuroimaging to better detect and track the development of vasospasm and ischemia. A flow chart example for approaches to treatment is presented.

Leal-Noval SR, Munoz-Gomez M, Murillo-Cabezas F. Optimal hemoglobin concentration in patients with subarachnoid hemorrhage, acute ischemic stroke and traumatic brain injury. Curr Opin Crit Care 2008;14(2):156-62.
Non-systematic review of clinical and experimental studies supporting blood transfusion strategies in neurocritical care patients, with a specific focus on identifying optimal hemoglobin concentration. Available

evidence in the field of subarachnoid hemorrhage, acute ischemic stroke, and TBI is reviewed. Both severe anemia and red blood cell transfusion are associated with poor clinical outcome in neurocritical care patients. Red blood cell transfusion may improve cerebral oxygenation and brain microcirculation but has not been shown to improve clinical outcome. However, higher hemoglobin levels result in improved clinical outcome. Parameters for cerebral oxygenation have potential as transfusion triggers in the near future.

Oddo M, Schmidt JM, Carrera E, et al. Impact of tight glycemic control on cerebral glucose metabolism after severe brain injury: a microdialysis study. Crit Care Med 2008;36(12):3233-8.
Observational prospective cohort of 20 neurocritical care patients monitored with cerebral microdialysis; 2131 cerebral microdialysis samples were analyzed. Tight systemic glucose levels were associated with lower cerebral microdialysis glucose levels and increased episodes of brain energy crises. This correlates with increased mortality. The authors conclude that intensive insulin therapy may impair cerebral glucose metabolism after severe brain injury.

Bhatia A, Gupta AK. Neuromonitoring in the intensive care unit. Intracranial pressure and cerebral blood flow monitoring. Intensive Care Med 2007;33(7):1263-71.
Combination of ICP monitoring (including analysis of ICP waveform) with techniques of CBF assessment (including TCD ultrasonography, laser Doppler and thermal diffusion flowmetry) increase our capabilities, provided limitations inherent to each method are acknowledged.

Broessner G, Beer R, Lackner P, et al. Prophylactic, endovascularly based, long-term normothermia in ICU patients with severe cerebrovascular disease: bicenter prospective, randomized trial. Stroke 2009;40(12):657-65.
Prospective, randomized, controlled trial with a blinded neurologic outcome evaluation comparison between prophylactic catheter-based normothermia (51 patients) and conventional stepwise fever management with antiinflammatory drugs and surface cooling (51 cases). Prophylactic normothermia did not lead to an increase of major adverse events, but neither was a significant difference in outcome found.

Margulies S, Hicks R. The Combination Therapies for Traumatic Brain Injury Workshop Leaders. Combination therapies for traumatic brain injury: prospective considerations. J Neurotrauma 2009;26(6):925-39.
This manuscript reports the proceedings of an interagency workshop coordinated by NIH-NINDS to discuss the opportunities and challenges of testing combination therapies for TBI. Potential was seen for combining agents with complementary targets and effects, rather than focusing on a single target with multiple agents. Standardization of data collection, data sharing, collaboration, and development of clinically relevant biomarkers and outcome measures were seen as necessary ingredients for the development of successful combination therapies for TBI.

REFERENCES

Access the complete reference list online at http://www.expertconsult.com.

42

Key Issues in Pediatric Neurointensive Care

PATRICK M. KOCHANEK | **ROBERT W. HICKEY** | **HÜLYA BAYIR** | **ERICKA L. FINK** | **RANDALL A. RUPPEL** | **ROBERT S.B. CLARK**

In this chapter we outline the epidemiology, presentation, course, and management of key disorders in pediatric neurointensive care. Critically ill infants and children with a compromised central nervous system (CNS) are complex patients and are often highly vulnerable to secondary brain injury. Minimizing physiologic derangements and optimizing therapy are essential from the scene through the pediatric intensive care unit (ICU). In most cases, transport to a specialized pediatric facility is desirable. Trained specialists in pediatric critical care medicine, pediatric neurologic surgery, and child neurology should deliver the ICU care to these infants and children, with appropriate pediatric ancillary support. The information provided in this chapter is germane to practitioners involved in stabilization, emergency treatment, and transport, and to pediatric subspecialists at the tertiary care centers. Recommendations in the areas of pediatric trauma (head and spinal cord injury), procedures, and monitoring are addressed in Chapters 30, W24 (Pediatric Intensive Care Procedures), and 210. Neurointensive care issues relevant to the field of neonatology are outside the scope of this chapter; specialized textbooks and/or reviews in this area should be sought for information in that field.

■ Issues Unique to Pediatrics

Two key factors contribute to the unique nature of the practice of pediatric neurointensive care: differences in the specific insults to the CNS in infants and children versus adults and age-related differences in the response to these insults.

CENTRAL NERVOUS SYSTEM INSULTS IN INFANTS AND CHILDREN

Unlike in adults, atherosclerotic vascular disease resulting in stroke, intracerebral hemorrhage, and cardiopulmonary arrest plays little role in pediatric neurointensive care. For example, cardiopulmonary arrest in infants and children results primarily from asphyxia rather than myocardial infarction. Similarly, traumatic brain injury (TBI) in infants younger than 2 years of age is largely the result of abusive head trauma (shaken baby syndrome, child abuse). Unique issues in victims of child abuse, such as chronic injury or delay in presentation, contribute to important differences in diagnosis, treatment, and outcome. The specific CNS insults relevant to pediatric neurointensive care include TBI and spinal cord injury, cardiopulmonary arrest, status epilepticus, stroke, critical CNS infections, postoperative neurosurgical conditions, and several other less common disorders; traumatic brain and spinal cord injury are addressed in Chapters 38 and 39.

AGE-RELATED DIFFERENCES IN THE RESPONSE TO CENTRAL NERVOUS SYSTEM INSULTS

Brain Water and Blood-Brain Barrier

Many biochemical, physiologic, and physical factors exhibit large fluctuations during brain development. Although the magnitude of these changes are most dramatic during prenatal development, they may contribute to age-related differences in response to critical CNS disorders.[1,2] Large decreases in brain water content occur during postnatal development into adult life.[3-5] These changes are global and correlate with the amount of myelination. The impact of these changes on edema formation after brain injury is unclear; however, the rapid and diffuse cerebral swelling phenomenon described in many CNS insults in infants and children may be related to this high water content in the immature brain. This is suggested by studies showing that parenchymal injection of glutamate into the immature (but not adult) rat brain rapidly produces a large area of edema.[6] The rapidity of development and the great magnitude of edema may result in part from rapid diffusion of glutamate and other mediators through the immature brain. In contrast to the changes in brain water during development, there is little evidence to support similar changes in blood-brain barrier permeability.[7,8] However, studies in experimental models suggest that the immature blood-brain barrier is highly vulnerable to injury.[9-11] Blood-brain barrier permeability after CNS insults has received little study in pediatric patients.

Cerebral Blood Flow and Energy Metabolism

Postnatal changes in cerebral blood flow (CBF) and energy metabolism have been reported in numerous mammalian species including humans.[12-19] In all cases, CBF is quite low both before birth and during infancy, rapidly increases to a peak during childhood, and then decreases to a plateau with a gradual decline with increasing age during adulthood. In a study of 42 normal infants and children, cortical CBF in newborns was between 30 and 45 mL/100 g/min—lower than that reported in adults. In contrast, cortical flow in children between the ages of 5 and 6 years was between 50% and 85% higher than in adults. CBF decreased to adult values by about age 15 years (Figure 42-1).[20,21] Increased CBF in children (versus either adults or infants) corresponds to the period of maximal postnatal "brain growth," specifically, maximal increases in the number of synapses.[22-24] Similarly, cerebral metabolic rate for glucose is maximal in children between the ages of 3 and 9 years.[17] The impact of these factors in CNS injury is poorly understood. Hyperemia after injury has been implicated as an important facet of the pathophysiology of pediatric CNS injury. Because the level of CBF in the normal child is greater than in adults, the frequency of hyperemia in children is probably lower than has been suggested. Hyperemia in most gray matter structures in children between the ages of 3 and 10 years should probably be based on a flow value greater than about 70 mL/100 g/min[19-21,24] rather than the value of about 45 mL/100 g/min suggested for adults.[25] Alterations in metabolic demands after injury must also be considered.

Cerebral Perfusion Pressure

Cerebral perfusion pressure (CPP; mean arterial blood pressure–intracranial pressure [ICP]) is a critical determinant of CBF outside the limits of autoregulation or when autoregulation of blood pressure (BP) is disturbed. In adults, the normal range for CPP is generally accepted to be between 60 and 150 mm Hg.[26,27] Based on studies in normal immature animals, the lower limit for BP autoregulation of CBF is directly related to age.[28-30] This is anticipated, since CPP is a function of arterial blood pressure, which is dependent on age. Unfortunately, few data are available on normal values for CPP in infants and children. A mean value of 37.5 ± 4.9 mm Hg ($\pm$SD) was

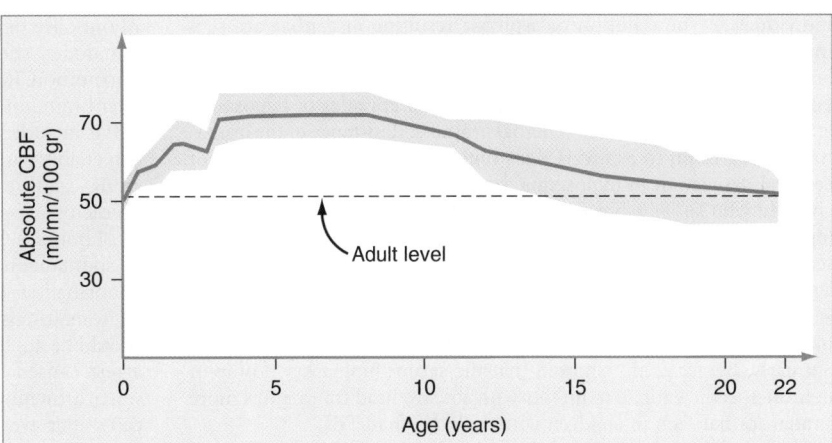

Figure 42-1 Mean *(the curve)* and ±1 SD *(hatched area)* for normal cerebral blood flow in 42 children from 2 days to 19 years of age, compared with adult values *(dotted line)*. Compared with adult values, cerebral blood flow is lower in infancy, but thereafter values throughout childhood exceed those of adults. *(From Chiron C, Raynaud C, Maziere B et al. Changes in regional cerebral blood flow during brain maturation in children and adolescents. J Nucl Med 1992;33:696–703. Reprinted by permission of the Society of Nuclear Medicine.)*

reported in normal preterm infants.[31] The lower limit of BP autoregulation was not determined. There are also limited data available on the lower limit of BP autoregulation of CBF in brain-injured infants and children. A study carried out in 1983 in 17 infants and children with meningitis and encephalitis showed a critical threshold for CPP of about 30 mm Hg.[32] However, survival, not CBF, was the outcome variable in that study. Muizelaar and coworkers[20,21] and Sharples and colleagues[33] examined CBF autoregulation after TBI in children; however, values for BP autoregulation of CBF for infants and children were not determined. Recently, Vavilala et al.[34] studied CBF autoregulation in 53 healthy infants and children. Surprisingly, the lower limit of autoregulation was between 50 and 60 mm Hg across the age groups of younger than 2 years, 2 to 5 years, 6 to 9 years, and 10 to 14 years. This important study suggests that there is substantially less autoregulatory reserve (the difference between baseline MAP and the lower limit of autoregulation) in infants and young children than in older children or adults. It would suggest that modest BP reductions in infants with severe TBI could compromise CBF. This may help explain the important deleterious effects of hypotension as a side effect in recent RCTs in pediatric TBI.[35] It also suggests that the lower limit for CPP in brain injured infants and young children of ~50 mm Hg might be wise. Two recent studies also suggest that the presence of mild hypertension after severe TBI is associated with improved outcome in infants and children.[36,37] However, the impact of inducing mild hypertension in this setting on outcome remains to be studied.

Myelination

In humans, considerable myelination occurs during postnatal life.[23] The impact of this process on the age-related response in pediatric CNS injury is not known but has been suggested by many to contribute to enhanced plasticity in the pediatric brain.

Excitotoxicity

Increases in brain interstitial concentrations of excitatory amino acids such as glutamate are part of a fundamental response to CNS insults across all ages.[38-47] Excitotoxicity-mediated damage after brain injury has been reported in laboratory models in mature and immature animals and is suggested in clinical reports in children.[39,43-47] There are, however, important age-dependent facets of excitotoxicity. At several periods in development, large numbers of excitatory amino acid receptors are produced, and these periods correlate temporally with increased synaptic plasticity.[40-43] Experimental data strongly suggest that the immature brain is at great risk for excitotoxicity.[39-41] In hypoxia-ischemia models, studies in immature animals (particularly those modeling the newborn) suggest that glutamate receptor antagonists such as MK-801 are potent neuroprotectants.[40,41,43] The results of clinical trials in adults of agents targeting this receptor may not predict their effectiveness in infants or children with critical CNS insults. Further study in children is warranted.

Apoptosis

Experimental models and human data have made it increasingly clear that cells dying after CNS insults can be categorized on a morphologic continuum from necrosis to apoptosis.[48-50] The event involved in the cascades of neuronal death after CNS insults is discussed in detail in Chapter 29. The importance of balanced apoptosis (or programmed cell death) in embryogenesis and recent reports examining apoptosis in experimental TBI suggest that there may be important age-related differences in the cell death cascades in response to traumatic or ischemic brain injury.[51] For example, neurons in developing animals appear to be more vulnerable to apoptosis than in mature animals.[48,51] There are also data supporting the concept that physiologic levels of excitatory amino acids are necessary for neuronal survival in the developing brain.[52] The implications on these data in experimental animals must be assessed with caution, but they raise concern about the ability of therapies such as barbiturates or inhibitors of excitatory amino acid receptors to actually induce neuronal death during development. The fetal alcohol syndrome is the prototypical condition cited in this regard.[53] What remains unclear, however, is if this enhanced apoptotic response to CNS injury is limited to prenatal development or if it is important during treatment of infants and children in the pediatric ICU. Nevertheless, an important role for apoptosis in pediatric brain injury is suggested by the fact that analysis of cerebrospinal fluid (CSF) in infants and children with severe TBI has provided some of the most compelling molecular data for the participation of these pathways in humans.[2] These data include participation of death effectors such as cytochrome-c and Fas receptor/ligand interactions and failure of antiapoptotic pathways in infants and children with poor outcome after severe brain injury.[2,54-57] How these findings will influence our therapies remains to be determined, but they suggest that apoptotic neuronal death may represent a particularly important therapeutic target in pediatric neurointensive care.

Extracerebral Factors

Many "extracerebral" factors play a role in the age-related differences in the response to critical CNS disorders, including age-related differences in (1) the response to hypoxemia-ischemia and hypotension, (2) atherosclerosis and other risk factors for stroke, and (3) acute and chronic ethanol consumption. These are rarely discussed in this context.

Hypotension and hypoxemia are the two most important secondary insults in patients with critical CNS disorders. Hypotension is the most important extracerebral factor associated with poor outcome after severe TBI.[58] This may contribute to the high mortality rate (62%) in this condition in children younger than age 4 years.[59] Nearly 50% of these children present with shock, versus only 30% of adults.[59] The limited blood volume of infants and young children make relatively small amounts of blood loss from scalp lacerations or other foci important. In contrast, the immature brain and cardiovascular systems are resistant to hypoxic-ischemic insults compared with mature individuals.[60] The duration of asphyxia resulting in cardiac arrest is inversely related to age.[61-64] Resistance to asphyxia-induced cardiac arrest in the immature individual, however, could have complex effects. For example, children may survive protracted episodes of hypoxemia and hypotension that would be lethal in adults. Resistance of the immature myocardium to asphyxia does not preclude the development of cerebral damage from hypoxemia, because between 25% and 56% of children who suffer asphyxia without cardiac arrest have poor neurologic outcome.[65] This might also explain some of the severe pathology seen in infants after abusive head trauma, in which apnea, seizures, and agonal states occur.[66] Recently Ichord et al.[67] showed that a hypoxic-ischemic injury pattern was commonly seen on diffusion-weighted magnetic resonance imaging (MRI) in victims of abusive head trauma. Similarly, Berger et al.[68] showed that the serum biomarker profile of neuron-specific enolase in infants with abusive head trauma was more similar to that seen in children with asphyxia than TBI.

Unlike adults, atherosclerotic vascular changes are largely absent in children. This influences pathophysiology. Although normal aging produces a gradual decline in CBF, this decline is accentuated in adults by the presence of risk factors for stroke (e.g., diabetes, cigarette smoking, hypertension), which enhance incipient cerebrovascular disease.[69] Atherosclerosis also limits the ability of cerebral circulation to respond to a metabolic challenge.[70-73] Some adults may even have maximally dilated cerebral vessels in the resting state. The potential of these factors to unfavorably affect outcome in adults (versus children) is obvious. Ethanol consumption is associated with severe TBI in adults, with as high as 50% of patients having positive blood alcohol levels.[74-77] Chronic and acute alcohol consumption can have either detrimental or beneficial effects on brain injury.[77] Ethanol use or intoxication is uncommon in pediatric TBI, particularly in infants and young children.

■ Specific Diseases or Conditions

CARDIOPULMONARY ARREST

Cardiopulmonary arrest in adults is addressed in detail in Chapter 33. Although some of that chapter is germane to pediatric patients, the importance of asphyxia as the etiology in children mandates a separate discussion.

Epidemiology

The causes of cardiopulmonary arrest in childhood are heterogeneous. Causes of arrest in the prehospital setting include trauma, sudden infant death syndrome, poisoning, and respiratory distress secondary to drowning, choking, severe asthma, or pneumonia.[78] Traumatic arrest secondary to exsanguination, massive head injury, or airway compromise is the leading cause of death in childhood and young adulthood. Nontraumatic arrest typically occurs as a consequence of hypoxemia and hypercarbia, leading to respiratory arrest, bradycardia, and ultimately asystole or pulseless electrical activity.[78-80] Ventricular tachycardia or fibrillation occurs less commonly in children than adults, but it is not rare; 5% to 15% of children with prehospital arrest have these rhythms.[81-83] The majority of arrests in the prehospital setting occur in previously healthy patients, whereas most in-hospital arrests occur in children with preexisting medical conditions.[84] Children with special healthcare needs are especially vulnerable to acute deterioration.

Outcome

The rate of survival from pediatric cardiopulmonary arrest is about 13%, with survival from in-hospital arrest greater than that from prehospital arrest (24% versus 9%).[80] Asystolic patients have the lowest rate of survival (~5%), whereas patients with ventricular fibrillation or ventricular tachycardia have higher rates of survival (~30%). Patients presenting with isolated respiratory arrest have the highest rate of survival (~75%).[85,86] Witnessed arrest and bystander cardiopulmonary resuscitation (CPR) are associated with survival, whereas CPR of greater than 30 minutes and administration of more than two doses of epinephrine are associated with poor outcome.[78,81,87,88]

About 60% of survivors will have good neurologic outcome, with the remainder showing severe disabilities. Intermediate outcomes are uncommon. Reported mortality rates for children remaining comatose after brain injury range between 34% and 73% dependent on whether TBI is included.[89-94] Accurate prediction of poor outcome in this group can enable withdrawal of support and decrease the possibility of "rescuing" children to survival in a neurologically devastated state.[95,96] Predictors of poor outcome in children include remaining comatose at 24 hours, a Glasgow Coma Scale (GCS) score of less than 5, absence of spontaneous respirations, absence of pupillary reflex, and specific abnormalities found on electroencephalography (EEG) or after testing of somatosensory evoked potentials. Predictors of poor outcome should be applied with caution to children suffering cardiopulmonary arrest caused by drug overdose or hypothermic exposure (ice-cold water drowning) in which good outcomes have been reported in some cases after even prolonged durations of arrest.

Treatment

The optimal treatment of pediatric cardiopulmonary arrest is prevention. The use of child restraints in motor vehicles, bicycle helmets, pool fences, and fire alarms has contributed to important reductions in morbidity and mortality. Also, the number of cases of sudden infant death syndrome has decreased in the United States from 4900 infants in 1992 to 2600 infants in 1999 in association with the recognition that placing infants on their backs during sleep lowers the risk of this condition. For health care providers, the key to prevention is recognizing and treating *early* signs of cardiopulmonary compromise (tachycardia and increased work of breathing).

If cardiopulmonary arrest occurs, the most important first step is to provide immediate CPR. Many infants and children, especially in the prehospital setting, will be rescued solely by the administration of CPR.[78] Important differences are emerging in resuscitation of adults versus children with cardiac arrest. Although there has been a general movement toward bystander compression-only CPR in adults, recently Kitamura et al.[97] compared conventional versus compression-only CPR in over 5000 children in Japan. In arrests of noncardiac origin, both survival and favorable neurologic outcomes were better in children given conventional CPR. In addition, outcomes were similar in the setting of arrests of cardiac origin. This study strongly suggests that the lay public should be taught conventional CPR for all children who suffer cardiac arrest. In addition the technique for compressions in children is different than in adults. Only one hand is used to deliver chest compressions to children younger than age 8 years. Two methods are approved for delivering chest compressions to infants. When two or more rescuers are available, one rescuer provides chest compressions by encircling the chest with two hands and depressing the sternum with both thumbs while the other rescuer provides ventilation (Figure 42-2). When only one rescuer is present, two fingers from one hand are used to provide chest compressions and the other hand is used to maintain the head-tilt. Providing adequate ventilation is especially important for children, because most pediatric arrests are

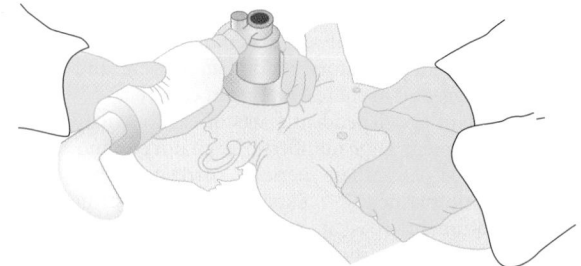

Figure 42-2   Two-person technique for cardiopulmonary resuscitation in infants and young children. *(Reprinted from Pediatric Basic Life Support. Guidelines 2000 for Cardiopulmonary and Emergency Cardiovascular Care: International Consensus on Science. Circulation 2000;102(Suppl):I253–90.)*

TABLE 42-1	Drugs Commonly Used in Arrest or Peri-Arrest Conditions		
Drug	*Dose*	*Maximum Single Dose*	*Route*
Adenosine*	0.1 mg/kg Repeat dose: 0.2 mg/kg	12 mg	IV (rapid push)
Atropine	0.2 mg/kg (0.1 mg/min)	Children: 0.5 mg Adolescents: 1 mg	IV, IO, T
Amiodarone	5 mg/kg	300 mg	IV, IO (bolus in pulseless arrest, otherwise give slowly)
Calcium chloride (10%)	20 mg/kg	500 mg	IV, IO (slowly)
Dextrose	0.5-1 mg/kg	N/A	IV, IO
Epinephrine	0.01 mg/kg (0.1 mg/kg if given ET)	5 mg	IV, IO, T
Lidocaine	1 mg/kg	100 mg	IV, IO, T
Narcan	0.1 mg/kg	2 mg	IV, IO, T
Magnesium	25-50 mg/kg	2 g	IV, IO
Sodium bicarbonate (8.4%)	1 mEq/kg	N/A	IV, IO

*For supraventricular tachycardia.
IO, intraosseous; *IV*, intravenous; *T*, tracheal.

secondary to airway compromise. In contrast, adults frequently suffer from cardiac causes of arrest and require intensified efforts at providing chest compressions and early defibrillation. Thus, the recommended ratio of chest compressions to ventilations for young children is 5:1, compared with a ratio of 15:2 for older children and adults. Once the patient is intubated, ventilations should be asynchronous. Although ventricular fibrillation and ventricular tachycardia are uncommon in children, survival with this rhythm is high (about 30%), so cardiac rhythm should be ascertained as early as possible.[80] Automated external defibrillators that can deliver a 50-J dose are now available and are appropriate for use in children aged 1 to 8 years.[98]

Intubation of pediatric patients is a difficult task for inexperienced providers. Furthermore, the short length of the trachea combined with patient movement during transport and patient care can easily result in displacement of the endotracheal tube.[99] Secondary confirmation of tracheal tube placement is critical. End-tidal CO_2 detection is the method most commonly utilized for secondary confirmation of endotracheal tube placement in children. However, a false-negative reading can occur when circulatory collapse is so severe that CO_2 is not delivered to the alveolar space. If CO_2 is not detected during CPR, tube placement can be confirmed by visualizing the airway with a laryngoscope. Although no single confirmation technique is 100% reliable in all circumstances, some effort of secondary confirmation of tube placement can be helpful.

Patients are initially resuscitated using 100% oxygen. The rationale is that hypoxia often causes or contributes to the development of cardiac arrest, and an oxygen debt accumulates during cardiac arrest. However, there is increasing awareness that oxygen might contribute to reperfusion injury, and thus *prolonged* delivery of *unnecessarily* high concentrations of oxygen should be avoided.[100,101]

Adults resuscitated from cardiac arrest demonstrate intact cerebrovascular reactivity with evidence of hyperventilation-associated ischemia.[102] Although there is evidence that injured brain has diminished metabolism, which may offset the decrease in blood flow, it seems prudent to avoid decreasing CBF to injured brain. Therefore, hyperventilation should be reserved for patients with signs of cerebral herniation syndrome or suspected pulmonary hypertension. In addition to avoiding purposeful hyperventilation, it is prudent to guard against inadvertent hyperventilation during patient transport.[103] Increased use of quantitative continuous CO_2 monitors throughout the health care system would decrease the occurrence of inadvertent hyperventilation.

Establishing vascular access in children can be challenging. Fortunately, intraosseous access can be achieved within 30 to 60 seconds and provides a route for drug and fluid administration when intravascular access cannot be readily achieved. Drugs including lidocaine, epinephrine, atropine, and naloxone (mnemonic "LEAN") can be administered through the tracheal tube. Optimal doses for drugs given via the tracheal tube are not established, but the recommended dose of epinephrine is 0.1 mg/kg (10 times the intravenous [IV] dose). A

bedside glucose measurement should be obtained, and if hypoglycemia is present, it should be treated with 0.5 to 1 g/kg of glucose given IV. There is experimental evidence that hyperglycemia exacerbates ischemic injury in mature brain, and hypoglycemia exacerbates ischemic injury in immature brain. Thus, euglycemia is desirable. Initial resuscitation fluids should be limited to isotonic crystalloid solutions such as normal saline or lactated Ringer's solution.

The most commonly used drugs in pediatric resuscitation are epinephrine, atropine, and sodium bicarbonate (Table 42-1). Magnesium and calcium are reserved for specific indications such as torsades de pointes, hypocalcemia, and calcium channel blockade. Amiodarone has recently been added to the American Heart Association (AHA) pediatric algorithms, based on extrapolation from adult experience.[104] Adults with ventricular fibrillation or ventricular tachycardia in the prehospital setting are more likely to be successfully defibrillated after IV administration of amiodarone compared with lidocaine.[105] Accordingly, amiodarone (5 mg/kg bolus) is a therapeutic option for children with pulseless arrest. Amiodarone (5 mg/kg infused over 20 to 60 min) is also an option for ventricular tachycardia with a pulse but should be used with extreme caution because of the risk for profound hypotension. Vasopressin has been added to the AHA adult algorithms as an alternative to epinephrine on the basis of its improved myocardial and CBF effects. However, subsequent clinical data in adults have not consistently yielded positive results, and pediatric data are limited to small case series.[106,107] The optimal vasopressor for hemodynamic support after return of circulation in children is not known.

Extracorporeal membrane oxygenation (ECMO) has been used to successfully resuscitate children from selected causes of in-hospital cardiac arrest.[108-112] ECMO-CPR provides greater cerebral and myocardial blood flow than either closed- or open-chest CPR and facilitates titration of temperature, blood flow, and oxygen-carrying capacity. Good outcomes have been documented with the use of ECMO even when initiated after durations of conventional CPR typically associated with poor outcome. It is best reserved for patients with reversible conditions or as a bridge to cardiac transplantation.

Post-Resuscitative Care

Temperature control is a priority for patients who remain comatose after cardiac arrest. Adults cooled to 32°C to 34°C for 12 to 24 hours after resuscitation from ventricular fibrillation demonstrate improved survival and neurologic outcome.[113,114] In contrast, fever worsens outcome in experimental models of brain injury and has been associated with worse clinical outcome in adults with ischemic brain injury. Children resuscitated from cardiac arrest often develop mild hypothermia followed by delayed fever.[115] There is a consensus that initial hypothermia, if tolerated, should be permitted to continue and fever should be vigilantly avoided. The practice of inducing hypothermia in normothermic children is more controversial. Experimental models using either pediatric mechanisms of injury (asphyxia, hypovolemic shock) or examining the immature brain suggest a beneficial effect of induced hypothermia. However, clinical data are limited and there is a concern about hypothermia-impaired immune function and risk of pneumonia/sepsis.[116,117] Clinical trials of induced hypothermia for neonatal asphyxia have been remarkably positive,[118-120] and important data in newborns with asphyxia indicate that even one degree of hyperthermia after the insult is associated with neurologic morbidity.[121] This supports the need for targeted temperature management after cardiac arrest.

During recovery from global ischemia there may be a period of prolonged, multifocal, decreased CBF. Hypotension and hypoxia should be avoided during this period to prevent development of a secondary brain injury. As previously mentioned, the optimal regimen of oxygen and pressor therapy is not known and requires further study.

Sustained elevation of ICP may be more common after asphyxial arrests versus arrests of cardiac origin[122] and is a poor prognostic sign in children with drowning. ICP monitoring fell out of favor in the 1980s when it was found to not influence outcome in small case series.[123] However, studies using contemporary ICP-directed therapy (perhaps including induced hypothermia) deserve reevaluation.

Miscellaneous

Most pediatric victims of cardiopulmonary arrest will not be successfully resuscitated. The difficulty of accepting this reality often results in prolonged attempts at resuscitation. The AHA guidelines state, "In the absence of recurring or refractory ventricular fibrillation or ventricular tachycardia, history of a toxic drug exposure, or a primary hypothermic insult, resuscitative efforts may be discontinued if there is no return of spontaneous circulation despite advanced life support. In general, this requires no more than 30 minutes."[104] This acknowledges the futility of prolonged resuscitative efforts and empowers clinicians to feel *permitted to stop* resuscitative efforts. The guideline does not mandate stopping at a specific duration of CPR, but clinicians should recognize that the chance of survival with lifelong severe disabilities correlates with the duration of CPR.

Surveys indicate that most family members would like to be present during resuscitation attempts of a loved one[124-127]; presence during resuscitation can help family members adjust to the death.[128,129] Although allowing family presence during resuscitation requires planning and additional resources, when done properly it is worth the effort. Perhaps one of the most disheartening statistics in resuscitation research is the high divorce rate (up to 90%) of parents after the death of a child. Thus, pastoral and social services can be integral components of care during both the acute resuscitation event and long-term follow-up.

STATUS EPILEPTICUS

Status epilepticus is a pediatric emergency traditionally defined as either a continuous seizure of at least 30 minutes or more than two discrete seizures without complete recovery of consciousness. *Refractory status epilepticus* is defined as failure of two first-line antiepileptic medications to treat this condition for greater than 60 minutes. Many children with refractory status epilepticus have new or established CNS lesions.[130]

Epidemiology and Etiology

The incidence of pediatric status epilepticus from a prospective study is 40 cases/100,000 per year. Infants younger than 1 year of age have the highest incidence at 150 cases/100,000 per year.[131] More than 90% of cases are convulsive status epilepticus. The first episode of status epilepticus occurs at a mean age of 4.2 years.[132] There is a slight male predominance in status epilepticus.[131,133]

There are five etiologic categories of status epilepticus that have bearing on treatment and prognosis. A child with *idiopathic or cryptogenic* status epilepticus has no prior history of seizures and no known risk factors. *Atypical febrile* status epilepticus occurs during fever in children with no prior history of seizures without fever. Children with *acute symptomatic* status epilepticus have new CNS lesions such as encephalitis, trauma, tumor, stroke, or anoxia. Children with *remote symptomatic* status epilepticus have preexisting CNS lesions and

---

Box 42-1

ETIOLOGY OF STATUS EPILEPTICUS

Idiopathic/cryptogenic (24%)
Atypical febrile (24%):
   Previously normal
   Previously abnormal
Acute symptomatic (23%):
   CNS infection
   Anoxia
   Trauma
   Stroke/hemorrhage
   Intoxication
   Metabolic
   Anticonvulsant withdrawal
Remote symptomatic (23%)
Progressive encephalopathy (6%):
   Neurocutaneous syndrome
   Neoplasm
   Genetic/metabolic

---

therefore a lowered seizure threshold. In these children, status epilepticus can occur without provocation, sometimes even years after the initial insult. Finally some children have status epilepticus resulting from *progressive encephalopathy*, including neurodegenerative diseases, malignancies, and neurocutaneous syndromes (Box 42-1).[131,133,134]

In one study, status epilepticus accounted for 1.6% of total pediatric ICU admissions, and etiology varied with age. In children younger than 2 years of age, *acute symptomatic* status epilepticus from meningitis and encephalitis accounted for 51% of cases, whereas *remote symptomatic* status epilepticus in children with a prior diagnosis of epilepsy was seen in 16% of children. Older children were more likely than younger children to have a history of epilepsy.[133] Mortality rates for status epilepticus in children are between 3% and 6%.[131,134] Mortality is dependent on etiology, age, and duration of status epilepticus. Mortality rates of 0% and 12.5% were seen when patients were divided into either unprovoked/febrile status epilepticus or acute CNS insult/progressive encephalopathy groups, respectively.[133] Morbidity risk varies from between 11% and 25%. Infants are at great risk for morbidity because the etiology in this group is commonly *acute symptomatic* status epilepticus. Neurologic sequelae of status epilepticus include epilepsy, recurrence, mental retardation, and motor disorders. However, many of the morbidities can be attributed to the underlying disease and not status epilepticus per se. Risk of recurrence in the category of *idiopathic* status epilepticus is less than 5%. In contrast, recurrence of status epilepticus in children in the *acute symptomatic* groups can be as high as 60%.[131,135] Systemic complications occur with increasing frequency in proportion to the duration of status epilepticus, the most important being respiratory failure and cardiovascular compromise and autonomic and metabolic disturbances.[136]

Diagnosis

Status epilepticus can be convulsive or nonconvulsive when comparing clinical events with electrographic information. Convulsive seizures either begin as generalized seizures or progress from partial seizures. Nonconvulsive seizures are characterized as having subtle clinical signs such as nystagmus, irregular clonic twitches along with decreased consciousness, and/or ictal discharges on EEG. Included under the subheading of nonconvulsive seizures are complex and simple partial and absence seizures.[137]

Treatment

The goals in treating status epilepticus are to provide respiratory and cardiovascular support, terminate clinical and electrical seizure activity, identify and treat precipitating factors, and prevent systemic complications.[137] Recognizing that a prolonged duration of seizure increases the risk of morbidity and mortality, the Epilepsy Foundation of America published a consensus view to initiate antiepileptic drugs for

TABLE 42-2	Suggested Timetable for Emergency Diagnosis and Treatment of Status Epilepticus	
Time	*Exam/Intervention*	*Testing*
Initial presentation: 0 min	Airway, breathing, circulation, IV access, monitoring	Glucose, oxygenation via pulse oximetry ± blood gas analysis
Primary survey: 5 min	Neurologic exam Administer antiepileptic drugs Lorazepam, 0.1 mg/kg IV Phenobarbital, 20 mg/kg IV Normal saline maintenance IV Reduce fever	Electrolytes, renal and liver function, ammonia, anticonvulsant levels, toxicology, complete blood cell count, urinalysis
Secondary survey: 15-30 min	Evaluate treatment results Second-line antiepileptic drug if seizure persists Fosphenytoin, 20 mg/kg IV; or phenytoin, 20 mg/kg IV	Patient-specific: cranial imaging (CT vs MRI), lumbar puncture, EEG, ECG
Status epilepticus: >30 min	Intubation and mechanical ventilation	
Refractory status epilepticus: >60 min	Titrate antiepileptic drug to burst suppression Pentobarbital, 10 mg/kg IV given over 30 min, then 5 mg/kg every hour for 3 doses, then 1 mg/kg/h; titrate to effect Midazolam, 0.15 mg/kg IV, then 1-2 μg/kg/min, titrate to effect Phenobarbital, 5-10 mg/kg IV every 20 minutes to achieve burst suppression, then every 12 hours Evaluate need for vasopressors	Continuous EEG Neurologic consultation Consider anesthesia consultation for treatment with inhaled anesthetic

CT, computed tomography; *ECG,* electrocardiogram; *EEG,* electroencephalogram; *IV,* intravenous; *MRI,* magnetic resonance imaging.

treatment 10 minutes after the onset of an episode of status epilepticus.[138] A timetable for treatment of status epilepticus in children is provided in Table 42-2.

History of present and past illness may be useful in determining the cause of status epilepticus and in choosing therapy but it should not delay resuscitation efforts. Initial treatment includes basic life support—airway, breathing, and circulation (ABCs). Prevention of hypoxemia and hypotension, which exacerbate neuronal injury, is important. The airway should be kept open with simple maneuvers and 100% oxygen applied to the patient with a nonrebreathing mask. The airway should also be kept clear of airway secretions. Efficacy of oxygenation efforts should be monitored by pulse oximeter. Ventilation efforts are assessed clinically or by arterial blood gas determinations. If the patient is unable to maintain adequate oxygenation or ventilation, tracheal intubation using rapid sequence intubation technique is indicated. Circulation is monitored by assessment of ECG, BP, and perfusion. Ideally, a large-bore peripheral IV catheter should be placed for fluid and drug administration. A bedside blood glucose determination should be obtained. Serum electrolyte levels, renal and liver functions, and anticonvulsant levels should be assessed. Serum and urine toxicology screen should be obtained. Fever and hypoglycemia should be treated as quickly as possible to prevent CNS injury. The neurologic examination follows, focusing on GCS score, signs of raised ICP, focal deficits, and pupil size. In patients receiving neuromuscular blockade, electrical seizure activity should be monitored with continuous EEG. The ABCs should be reassessed throughout the resuscitation.

First-line antiepileptic drugs for pediatric status epilepticus include benzodiazepines, phenytoin or fosphenytoin, and phenobarbital. Drug choice depends on the route available (IV is preferred), the patient's maintenance anticonvulsants (a different class is recommended), and patient characteristics. Evidence-based studies of anticonvulsants in children are rare. Recommendations are extrapolated from studies in adults. The optimal first-line treatment of status epilepticus in children is controversial.

Phenytoin/Fosphenytoin. In a study in adults comparing lorazepam, phenytoin, phenobarbital, and diazepam, phenytoin had the highest success rate in stopping status epilepticus.[139] Phenytoin is not commonly associated with respiratory depression and has less of an effect on the impairment of consciousness than either benzodiazepines or barbiturates. Fosphenytoin has the advantage of having a faster infusion rate, shorter onset of action, and less cardiovascular side effects than phenytoin but is more expensive.

Lorazepam. In the same study in adults, lorazepam had the second highest success rate in stopping status epilepticus.[139] Lorazepam can be administered rapidly, has a long duration of effect, and is effective even when administered rectally. Lorazepam produced less respiratory failure requiring intubation than diazepam in retrospective[140] and prospective studies.[141] Incidence of respiratory depression in these studies varied widely—between 3% and 76%. Support for selection of Lorazepam over diazepam was also shown in a recent Cochrane review.[142]

Diazepam. Although the onset of action of diazepam is rapid (between 1 and 3 minutes after IV administration), it has a large volume of distribution; therefore, its duration of action is only 15 to 30 minutes. Thus, concomitant maintenance antiepileptic drugs are generally needed. Rectal diazepam has gained attention recently through its use as a first-line outpatient drug for use by parents or emergency services.

Phenobarbital. Phenobarbital is a very effective anticonvulsant, but it is often not the first choice in the treatment of status epilepticus because of side effects of respiratory depression and cardiovascular disorders, especially when it is used in combination with benzodiazepines. Infants metabolize phenobarbital more rapidly than older children and often require higher doses adjusted for body weight. Nevertheless, the pharmacokinetics of phenobarbital are more predictable than those of phenytoin in infants.

Additional Diagnostic Workup

Lumbar puncture is best performed early after presentation, but not in unstable patients or those who may have increased ICP. The decision to perform lumbar puncture should be guided by head CT. Otherwise, the type of neuroimaging used in infants and children with status epilepticus should be individualized, depending on history and physical findings. Both electrocardiography (ECG) and EEG are useful to investigate cause of status epilepticus (i.e., long QT syndrome or identifiable EEG patterns). EEG is also useful in titrating therapy (see later discussion).[137]

Drug Treatment for Refractory Status Epilepticus

Initiation of treatment for refractory status epilepticus should occur by 60 minutes, usually with neurologic consultation and with appropriate monitoring in a pediatric ICU or intermediate unit. These patients are mechanically ventilated, and seizures are typically treated with a variety of therapies, generally to induce burst suppression on continuous EEG. Most commonly, pentobarbital is used as a continuous infusion to treat refractory status epilepticus. Pentobarbital is given initially as a slow IV loading dose of 5 to 15 mg/kg, followed by an infusion rate of 1 mg/kg/h titrated to effect. There are differing opinions on when to begin to wean therapy, but it is generally recommended that about 12 hours of seizure cessation be attained before

---

Box 42-2

MOST COMMON RISK FACTORS FOR CHILDHOOD ISCHEMIC STROKE

Vascular
Arteriopathies
  Transient cerebral arteriopathy of childhood
  Postvaricella angiopathy
  Fibromuscular dysplasia
  Moyamoya syndrome
  Postradiation vasculopathy
Vasospastic Disorders
  Migraine
  Ergot poisoning
  Vasospasm with systemic arterial hypertension
Vasculitis
  Meningitis
  Systemic lupus erythematosus
  Polyarteritis nodosa
  Granulomatous angiitis
  Takayasu arteritis
  Dermatomyositis
  Inflammatory bowel disease
  Drug abuse (cocaine, amphetamines)
Systemic Vascular Disease
  Early atherosclerosis
  Diabetes
  Ehlers-Danlos syndrome
  Pseudoxanthoma elasticum
  Homocystinuria
  Fabry disease
Trauma
  Brain herniation and arterial compression
  Posttraumatic dissection
  Intraoral trauma
  Carotid ligation (e.g., extracorporeal membrane oxygenation)
  Arteriography

Intravascular
Hematologic Disorders
  Hemoglobinopathies (sickle cell anemia)
  Thrombocytosis
  Polycythemia
  Leukemia or other hematologic neoplasms

Acquired Prothrombotic States
  Prothrombotic medications
  Pregnancy and the postpartum period
  Lupus anticoagulant
  Anticardiolipin antibodies
  Lipoprotein abnormalities
  Hyperhomocysteinemia
Congenital Prothrombotic States
  Antithrombin deficiency
  Protein S deficiency
  Protein C deficiency
  Plasminogen deficiency
  Factor V Leiden
  Prothrombin gene mutation
  Methylenetetrahydrofolate reductase
Metabolic Disorders
  Hyperhomocysteinemia
  Hyperlipidemia

Embolic
Congenital Heart Disease
  Complex congenital heart defect
  Ventricular/atrial septal defect
  Coarctation of the aorta
  Patent foramen ovale
  Patent ductus arteriosus
Acquired Heart Disease
  Rheumatic heart disease
  Prosthetic heart valve
  Bacterial endocarditis
  Cardiomyopathy and myocarditis
  Atrial myxoma
  Cardiac rhabdomyoma
  Cardiac arrhythmia
Trauma
  Amniotic fluid or placental embolism
  Fat or air embolism
  Foreign body embolism
  Cardiac catheterization

---

weaning the infusion.[143] In children, placement of either a central venous pressure or pulmonary artery catheter is indicated to titrate fluid, inotropic, and/or pressor support. Pentobarbital use often requires the addition of inotropes or pressors. As an alternative to continuous barbiturate infusion, phenobarbital can be administered every 20 minutes (5-10 mg/kg IV) to achieve burst suppression, and then as a chronic therapy every 12 hours. A midazolam infusion has also been shown to be effective in refractory status epilepticus in some children (0.15 mg/kg IV bolus followed by infusion of 1-2 µg/kg/min). The infusion can be increased every 15 minutes if seizures are still present on continuous EEG or if burst suppression is not achieved. With this approach in one series, inotropic support was not required.[144]

STROKE

Epidemiology

Stroke in children is becoming increasingly recognized and now exceeds an incidence of 8 cases per 100,000 children per year.[145] Substantial advances in our knowledge of this condition in children have resulted from the work of the Canadian Pediatric Ischemic Stroke Registry. Neonates account for about 25% of these cases. The increasing incidence is believed to result from improvements in diagnostic tools (MRI, computed tomography [CT], magnetic resonance angiography [MRA]) applied to the pediatric population and to increasing survival rates in infants and children with stroke risk factors (e.g., complex congenital heart disease, malignancies).

Etiology

As discussed, atherosclerosis is a key risk factor for stroke in adults. In pediatric and neonatal stroke, extracerebral risk factors contribute to about 75% of cases; however, the spectrum of risk factors differs from those seen in adults. DeVeber[145] grouped the most common risk factors for childhood ischemic stroke into vascular, intravascular, and embolic categories (Box 42-2). The most common vascular risk factor has been reported to be transient cerebral arteriopathy.[146] Post-varicella arteriopathy, migraine, traumatic carotid dissection, and vasculitis, such as moyamoya, are also important examples in this category. In the intravascular category, sickle cell anemia, sinus thrombosis, leukemias, and both acquired and congenital prothrombotic states are important examples. Dehydration and intravascular volume depletion increase stroke risk in these settings, which are of special importance in the pediatric ICU. There is an 84% incidence of an acute systemic illness and a 30% incidence of dehydration in cerebral sinovenous thrombosis in infants and children.[147] Congenital and acquired heart disease in infants and children are the most important underlying causes of embolic stroke.[145] The risk of stroke in children after surgery for congenital heart disease is about 1 in 250 cases.[148]

Diagnosis

The clinical presentation of stroke in infants and children is age related. Infants present typically with seizures and lethargy, whereas older children may present with acute focal neurologic deficits or diffuse symptoms (headache, lethargy, or seizures).[145,149] In some cases, the duration of neurologic deficits in pediatric stroke may be shorter than the 24-hour deficits classically required to differentiate stroke from transient ischemic attack in adults.[150] It is often difficult to differentiate migraine, Todd paralysis, and stroke in children. Complicating this problem, CT may be normal within the initial 12 hours.[145] MRI is a more sensitive technique for diagnosing stroke, and advanced MRI modalities such as perfusion, diffusion, and MRA are important adjuncts to making the diagnosis. These methods are discussed in Chapter 31. Because of the impact of making specific vascular diagnoses on the management strategy, angiography is often recommended in children with idiopathic stroke.[145]

In addition to the importance of echocardiography in the diagnostic work of stroke after cardiac surgery or catheterization, endocarditis, cardiomyopathy, and other occult cardiac abnormalities are also important risk factors for embolic stroke, thus recognizing the importance of echocardiography and the general diagnostic workup for stroke in children.[151,152] A general diagnostic approach to pediatric stroke is presented in Box 42-3.

Treatment

In the acute setting, antithrombotic therapy has been used increasingly in the therapy for pediatric stroke. Strater and colleagues[153] compared treatment with low-molecular-weight heparin versus aspirin in 135 children across a variety of causes (including idiopathic, cardiac, vascular, and infectious) and suggested safety when used to prevent stroke recurrence. This is a controversial area for which there is a lack of systematic study.[154] DeVeber[145] recommends that neonates do not require antithrombotic treatment because of negligible recurrence risk, whereas older children require aspirin (2-3 mg/kg/d).[155] In dissection,

---

Box 42-3

DIAGNOSTIC WORKUP IN PEDIATRIC STROKE

There are no published consensus guidelines on the evaluation of stroke in children, but several systematic approaches have been recommended. The evaluation should include:
1. History of head trauma, neck trauma, recent infection, illness, unexplained fever or malaise, drug ingestion, developmental delay, family history of bleeding problems, and associated headache
2. Family history, with special attention to premature vascular disease, hematologic disease, and mental retardation
3. Physical examination including head circumference, skin abnormalities, cardiac evaluation, and carotid artery examination
4. MRI and MRA (CT if MR unavailable)

If the MRI and MRA reveal an infarct with vascular distribution, then consider:
1. Echocardiogram, electrocardiogram
2. Blood studies including complete blood cell count, erythrocyte sedimentation rate, hemoglobin electrophoresis, protein S, protein C, antithrombin III, factor V Leiden, anticardiolipin antibodies, lupus anticoagulant, homocysteine, cholesterol, and varicella titer
3. Lumbar puncture
4. Transcranial Doppler with bubble study
5. Radiograph of cervical spine (posterior infarctions)

If the MRI and MRA reveal an infarct with nonvascular distribution, then consider:
1. Cerebrospinal fluid lactate levels
2. Plasma ammonia and amino acids
3. Urine organic acids

If the MRI and MRA reveal a hemorrhage, then consider:
1. Coagulation studies
2. Conventional angiography

If the MRA is normal, then consider conventional angiography.

CT, Computed tomography; *MRA,* magnetic resonance angiography; *MRI,* magnetic resonance imaging.
Adapted from the Children's Hemiplegia and Stroke Association. Website: http://www.chasa.org/diagnosis.htm

---

high-grade stenosis, or severe prothrombotic state, low-molecular-weight heparin or warfarin (Coumadin) is recommended for several months. In endocarditis, anticoagulation is not recommended because of the risk of rupture of occult mycotic aneurysms. Thrombolytic therapy has been subjected to very limited study in children. Cases describing the use of tissue plasminogen activator and cerebral balloon angioplasty in acute stroke in children with dramatic results are being reported.[156] Table 42-3 compares key management issues across three recent guidelines documents in acute ischemic stroke, as summarized by DeVeber and Kirkham.[157]

Supportive Care in the Pediatric Intensive Care Unit (ICU)

An evidence-based approach for care in the pediatric ICU of children with stroke is lacking. Nevertheless, intensive care for the child with stroke must be at a level commensurate with that provided for other critical pediatric neurologic disorders such as severe TBI[158] and ruptured arteriovenous malformation.[159]

Careful attention to the ABCs with a neurointensive care approach is essential. If the GCS score is 8 or less and/or the airway or ventilation is compromised, intubation is indicated and should be performed using a neuroprotective rapid-sequence approach. Normal values for both $Paco_2$ and Pao_2 should be ensured.

Arterial blood pressure must be adequate to optimize cerebral perfusion. The management of systemic hypertension in the setting of pediatric stroke can be complicated by the variety of underlying disorders (i.e., status post cardiac surgery, underlying hypertension) and the presence or absence of hemorrhage. In adults with thrombotic or hemorrhagic stroke and systemic hypertension, it is generally recommended that mean arterial blood pressure not be aggressively reduced below 130 mm Hg.[160] Age-appropriate guidelines for this question are not available for children. In the pediatric ICU, for acute stroke, it is a reasonable first approach to extrapolate from the adult recommendations.

In infants and children with severe stroke with infarction and cerebral swelling, signs and symptoms of raised ICP can develop. Standard protocols for monitoring ICP and treatment of raised ICP in stroke in infants and children have not been developed. Nevertheless, intracranial hypertension can develop; and even in the absence of controlled trials on the beneficial effects of ICP-directed therapy in severe pediatric stroke, ICP monitoring and ICP-directed therapy should be considered if signs and symptoms of intracranial hypertension develop. Anecdotal reports of successful treatment with a variety of therapies including mild hypothermia and decompressive craniectomy have been reported.[161,162] Plasticity in the pediatric brain, particularly in the recovery from focal lesions, should prompt the consideration of an aggressive approach.[163-165] However, long-term morbidity remains substantial after stroke in childhood.[166]

Other aspects of contemporary pediatric neurointensive care should include maintenance of euglycemia and careful fluid management to maintain both a euvolemic state and avoid hyponatremia. In children, normal saline or 5% dextrose in normal saline should be used in the initial 24 hours, carefully following blood glucose concentration, followed by the addition of dextrose or initiation of hyperalimentation after 24 hours. In infants, either 5% or 10% dextrose in normal saline should be used, with insulin titrated to treat hyperglycemia. The specific glucose level associated with the exacerbation of secondary damage in infants and children has not been determined. A value of 200 mg/dL is a reasonable threshold in the absence of clear-cut evidence. Appropriate nutritional support should also be instituted as soon as possible. Rehabilitation services should be consulted during the pediatric ICU admission.

Critical Central Nervous System Infections

Any microbe may cause CNS infections; age and immune status of the host and epidemiology of the pathogen give evidence to the specific

TABLE 42-3	Comparison of Guidelines for Acute Management of Ischemic Stroke in Children by Subtype*							
	UK Guidelines: 2004 Recommendation	**G**	**S**	**Chest Guidelines: 2008 Recommendation**	**G**	**S**	**American Heart Association: 2008 Recommendation**	**G**	**S**
General	Aspirin 5 mg/kg	WPC	1	UFH or LMWH or aspirin 1-5 mg/kg/d until cardioembolic and dissection subtypes excluded	1B	1	UFH or LMWH (1 mg/kg q 12 h) up to 1 week until cause determined	2B-C	3
Sickle cell disease	Exchange transfusion to HbS <30%	WPC	1	Intravenous hydration and exchange transfusion to HbS <30%	1B	1	Optimal hydration, correction of hypoxemia and hypotension	1C	1
							Exchange transfusion to HbS <30%	2A-B	2
Cardiac	Anticoagulation should be discussed by senior pediatric neurologist and pediatric cardiologist	WPC	1	LMWH for over 6 weeks	2C	3	Therapy for heart problem	1C	1
Dissection of neck vessels	Anticoagulation for extracranial with no hemorrhage	WPC	1	LMWH for over 6 weeks	2C	3	UFH or LMWH as a bridge to oral anticoagulation	2A-C	3
Alteplase in children	Not recommended	—	1	Not recommended	1B	1	Not recommended	3C	1
Alteplase in teenagers	Not addressed	—	—	Not addressed	—	—	No consensus on use	—	3
Cerebral sinovenous thrombosis	Anticoagulation until recanalization for up to 6 months	—	C3	Initial UFH or LMWH, then LMWH for 3 months plus another 3 months if not fully recanalized	1B	1	Initial UFH or LMWH followed by warfarin for 3-6 months	2A-C	3

From DeVeber G, Kirkham F. Guidelines for the treatment and prevention of stroke in children. Lancet 2008;7:983–5. Reproduced with permission.
G, Grade of evidence or recommendation; *HbS*, sickled hemoglobin; *LMWH*, low-molecular-weight heparin; *S*, strength of evidence or recommendation; *UFH*, unfractionated heparin; *WPC*, working party consensus.
Childhood is defined as 28 days to 18 years (*Chest*) or 1 month to 16 years (UK). Comparison of guidelines for acute management of ischemic stroke in children by subtype of stroke.

pathogens. Regardless of the etiology, most children with CNS infection present with nonspecific symptoms including fever, headache, nausea, vomiting, anorexia, and irritability. Photophobia, neck pain and rigidity, seizures, mental status change, and focal neurologic deficits are common signs that are determined by the specific pathogen and area of CNS infected.

BACTERIAL MENINGITIS

Epidemiology

The etiology of bacterial meningitis and its treatment differ in neonates (0–28 days of life) versus older infants and children. During the first 2 months of life, the bacteria that cause meningitis in normal infants reflect the maternal flora and the environment to which the infant is exposed. The most common pathogens include groups B and D streptococci, gram-negative enteric bacilli, and *Listeria monocytogenes*. Occasionally, *Haemophilus influenzae* (both type B and nonencapsulated strains) and other pathogens—more typically found in older patients—can be the etiologic agent. Bacterial meningitis in children between 2 months and 12 years of age is usually caused by *Streptococcus pneumoniae*, *Neisseria meningitides*, or *H. influenzae* type B. After the implementation of immunization against *H. influenzae*, the incidence of *H. influenzae* meningitis decreased rapidly. Subsequent to the universal recommendation for the use of conjugated pneumococcal vaccine at 2 months of age in 2000, the incidence of meningitis caused by this pathogen is also decreasing. Anatomic abnormalities, surgical procedures, neurotrauma, or immune deficiency often underlie meningitis caused by other agents.[167]

Bacterial meningitis most commonly results from hematogenous dissemination of microorganisms from a distant site of infection; bacteremia usually precedes meningitis or occurs concomitantly. Colonization of the nasopharynx with a pathogenic microorganism is the usual source of bacteremia. Bacteria gain entry to the CSF through the choroid plexus of the lateral ventricles and the meninges and then circulate to the extracerebral CSF and the subarachnoid space. Bacterial cell wall lipopolysaccharide of gram-negative bacteria and pneumococcal cell wall components stimulate a marked inflammatory response, with local production of tumor necrosis factor alpha, interleukin-1β, prostaglandin E, and other mediators, leading to neutrophil infiltration, increased vascular permeability, and thrombosis. Inflammation of spinal nerves and roots produces meningeal signs, and inflammation of the cranial nerves produces optic, oculomotor, facial, and auditory neuropathies. Intracranial hypertension can produce oculomotor and abducens nerve palsy. Intracranial hypertension in meningitis is believed to result from a combination of cell death (cytotoxic cerebral edema), cytokine-induced increased capillary vascular permeability (vasogenic edema), and increased hydrostatic pressure after obstruction of CSF reabsorption and/or flow. Rarely, meningitis may follow bacterial invasion from a contiguous focus of infection such as paranasal sinusitis, otitis media, mastoiditis, orbital cellulites, or cranial or vertebral osteomyelitis or may occur after introduction of bacteria via penetrating head trauma or meningomyelocele.[168]

Diagnosis

The clinical presentation may be as fulminant as rapidly progressing shock, purpura, disseminated intravascular coagulation, and altered consciousness, frequently resulting in death within 24 hours. More often, however, children present with several days of fever with upper respiratory tract or gastrointestinal symptoms, followed by nonspecific signs of CNS infection such as lethargy and irritability. The presence of headache, emesis, bulging fontanelle, widening of the sutures, oculomotor or abducens nerve paralysis, hypertension with bradycardia, apnea, or hyperventilation suggests intracranial hypertension. Papilledema is uncommon in uncomplicated meningitis and suggests a more chronic process, such as intracranial abscess, sinus thrombosis, or subdural empyema. Seizures can result from cerebritis, infarction, or electrolyte abnormalities and occur in between 20% and 30% of children with meningitis. Seizures that occur at presentation or within first 4 days of onset are usually of no prognostic significance. Seizures that persist beyond the fourth day of illness and those that are difficult to treat are associated with poor prognosis.[169]

The diagnosis of acute bacterial meningitis is confirmed by analysis of CSF. Contraindications for an immediate lumbar puncture are (1) evidence of increased ICP (other than bulging fontanelle), (2) presence of severe cardiopulmonary compromise or likelihood that positioning for the procedure would significantly compromise cardiopulmonary function, (3) infection of the skin overlying the needle insertion site, and (4) coagulopathy. If lumbar puncture is delayed, empirical antibiotic treatment should be started after a blood culture is obtained. Blood culture reveals the susceptible bacteria in 80% to 90% of cases of meningitis. The need for a cranial CT scan, for signs and symptoms of increased ICP or brain abscess, should not delay therapy. Table 42-4 summarizes the CSF findings in CNS infections. Pleocytosis with lymphocyte predominance may be seen early in bacterial meningitis;

TABLE 42-4	Cerebrospinal Fluid Findings in Central Nervous System Infections			
Type of Infection	Pressure (cm H$_2$O)	Leukocytes (mm^3)	Protein (mg/dL)	Glucose (mg/dL)
Normal	5-8	<5, ≥75% lymphocytes <30 for neonates	20-45 Up to 180 for neonates	>50 (or 75% serum glucose)
Acute bacterial	↑ (10-30)	300-2000 PMNs predominate	100-500	↓ (<40 or <50% serum glucose)
Partially treated bacterial meningitis	Normal or ↑	5-10,000 Usually PMNs	100-500	Normal or ↓
Viral meningitis or meningoencephalitis	Normal or slightly ↑ (8-15)	Rarely >1000 PMNs early, then mononuclear cells	50-200	Normal (decreased in some mumps cases)
Tuberculous meningitis	↑	10-500 PMNs early, lymphocytes predominate through most of the course	100-3000	<50
Fungal meningitis	↑	5-500 PMNs early, lymphocytes predominate through most of the course	25-500	<50
Syphilis	↑	50-500 Lymphocytes predominate	50-200	Normal
Amebic (*Naegleria*) meningoencephalitis	↑	1000-10,000 or more PMNs predominate	50-500	Normal or slightly ↓

conversely, neutrophilic pleocytosis may be present in patients during the early stages of acute viral meningitis. The shift to lymphocytic-monocytic predominance in viral meningitis invariably occurs within 8 to 24 hours. A traumatic lumbar puncture complicates the diagnosis of meningitis. If the CSF is bloody, it should be collected in three or more tubes. If the CSF clears in successive tubes, it suggests a traumatic lumbar puncture. Blood that does not clear is more suggestive of intracranial bleeding. The CSF leukocyte to erythrocyte ratio in CSF from a traumatic lumbar puncture is generally similar to that in a concurrently obtained peripheral blood sample (usually 1:500 to 1:1000).[170]

The mortality rate of bacterial meningitis after the neonatal period is less than 10%, owing to appropriate recognition, prompt antibiotic treatment, and supportive care. Severe neurodevelopmental sequelae occur in between 10% and 20% of pediatric patients. The most common sequelae include hearing loss, mental retardation, epilepsy, delay in language acquisition, visual impairment, and behavioral problems. Sensorineural hearing loss occurs in 30%, 10%, and 5% to 10% of patients with pneumococcal, meningococcal, and *H. influenzae* type B meningitis, respectively.[171]

Treatment

The initial (empirical) choice of antibiotic treatment in immunocompetent infants and children is primarily determined by the antibiotic susceptibilities of *S. pneumoniae*. In the United States, between 25% and 50% of strains of *S. pneumoniae* are currently resistant to penicillin, and up to 25% of isolates are resistant to cefotaxime or ceftriaxone. Based on this, empirical therapy is with vancomycin (60 mg/kg/24 h, divided q 6 h) and cefotaxime (200 mg/kg/24 h, divided q 6 h) or ceftriaxone (100 mg/kg/24 h, given either as a single daily dose or divided q 12 h). Patients allergic to beta-lactam antibiotics can be treated with chloramphenicol (100 mg/kg/24 h, divided q 6 h). If *L. monocytogenes* infection is suspected, as in infants between 1 and 2 months of age or patients with T-lymphocyte deficiency, ampicillin (200 mg/kg/24 h, divided q 6 h) should be administered with either cefotaxime or ceftriaxone. If a patient is immunocompromised and gram-negative bacterial meningitis is suspected, ceftazidime and an aminoglycoside may be used as initial therapy. The duration of treatment should be either 10 or 14 days, depending on the bacteria; gram-negative bacillary meningitis should be treated for 3 weeks or for at least 2 weeks after sterilization of CSF. Repeat lumbar puncture may be indicated in some neonates and in children with gram-negative or beta-lactam–resistant meningitis caused by *S. pneumoniae*. Of the adjunctive treatments that might limit CNS inflammation, only corticosteroids have been properly assessed in clinical trials. Adjuvant corticosteroid use was associated with lower case fatality and lower rates

of both severe hearing loss and long-term neurologic sequelae in acute bacterial meningitis. Corticosteroids administered either before or with the first dose of antibiotic reduced severe hearing loss in bacterial meningitis caused by *H. influenzae* as well as in meningitis caused by *S. pneumoniae*.[172] The recommended dose of dexamethasone is 0.6 mg/kg/24 h, divided every 6 hours for 4 days.[168] A recent meta-analysis of individual patient data from five randomized, double-blind, placebo-controlled trials (two of them including pediatric patients from 2 months to 16 years of age) of dexamethasone published since 2001 did not show benefit of adjunctive dexamethasone on mortality or neurologic disability.[172] Therefore the role of dexamethasone in prevention of death or neurologic sequelae needs reevaluation. There are no data about the role of corticosteroids in newborns or in patients with nosocomial or CSF shunt–associated meningitis.

Peltola et al.[173] reported improved outcomes in 654 children with meningitis with oral glycerol therapy (6 mL/kg/d divided in 4 doses; maximum 25 mL/dose). However, a more recent study did not demonstrate benefit from oral glycerol on hearing impairment in pediatric meningitis.[174] Nevertheless, glycerol was recommended in pediatric meningitis in two recent reviews, albeit not at a guidelines level.[175,176] Patients who (1) manifest signs of poor perfusion, cutaneous manifestations of disseminated intravascular coagulation (purpura, petechiae), irregular respiratory pattern, altered mental status, cranial nerve involvement, and other signs potentially indicative of raised ICP and patients who (2) have rapid clinical presentation, significant metabolic acidosis, hypoxemia, hypercapnia, neutropenia, hyponatremia, anemia, and abnormal liver or renal function should be admitted to the pediatric ICU—at least until the course of illness can be determined, the first several doses of antibiotics are administered, and a tentative bacteriologic diagnosis is made. Early recognition of complications such as shock or raised ICP and initiation of treatments in a timely fashion may improve outcome in cases of fulminate meningitis.

Acute CNS complications during the treatment of meningitis include seizures, intracranial hypertension, cranial nerve palsies, stroke, herniation, and thrombosis of the dural venous sinuses.[177] Subdural effusions develop in between 10% and 30% of pediatric patients and are more common in infants. They are asymptomatic in between 85% and 90% of cases. Aspiration of subdural effusions is indicated in the presence of raised ICP; fever alone is not an indication for aspiration. The syndrome of inappropriate secretion of antidiuretic hormone (SIADH) with hyponatremia and reduced serum osmolality occurs in between 30% and 50% of children. Cerebral salt wasting can also be seen. Attention to maintaining a normal serum sodium concentration using either normal saline or judicious titration of hypertonic saline is important to preventing exacerbation of brain edema. Prolonged fever (>10 days) occurs in 10% of the patients. It is usually due to intercurrent viral infection, secondary or nosocomial bacterial infection, thrombophlebitis, drug reaction, pericarditis, or arthritis. Thrombocytosis, eosinophilia, or anemia may also develop during treatment.[169]

Supportive Care in the Pediatric ICU

The issues in ICU care for infants and children with bacterial meningitis are similar to ones mentioned under encephalitis. The reader is referred to the following section for details.

VIRAL ENCEPHALITIS

Epidemiology

Enteroviruses are the most common etiologic agent for encephalitis in children. The severity of the disease ranges from mild illness to severe encephalitis with death or long-term morbidity. Enterovirus infections spread directly from person to person, with an incubation period of between 4 and 6 days. Most cases occur in summer and fall in temperate climates. Arboviruses are responsible for some cases of encephalitis in children. The most common arboviruses responsible for CNS infection in the United States are St. Louis and California encephalitis and the West Nile virus.[178]

Several members of the herpesvirus family can cause encephalitis. Herpes simplex virus (HSV) type 1 is an important cause of severe encephalitis in children and adults. The cerebral cortex, especially the temporal lobe, is often severely affected by HSV. Neonatal herpes infections are usually caused by HSV type 2 contracted at delivery via vertical transmission. Three forms of the disease develop in neonates: (1) skin, eye, mouth disease (seen in 45% of cases), (2) encephalitis (seen in 35% of cases), and (3) disseminated intravascular coagulation (seen in 20% of cases). The transmission rate from mother to infant is between 30% and 40% when genital infection is primary and 3% for reactivated herpes infection. The mean age at onset of cutaneous or systemic disease is 6 days after birth. In contrast, the mean age at onset of encephalitis is 11 days after birth. The diagnosis of HSV infection in neonates can be difficult to make unless skin lesions are present. Cultures of conjunctiva, nasopharynx, and rectum at between 48 hours and 72 hours of age may identify early infection. In neonates, the mortality rates are approximately 50% and 14% for HSV disseminated disease and encephalitis, respectively.[178]

A number of other viral causes are important in pediatric encephalitis. Varicella-zoster may cause CNS infection in close proximity to chickenpox. The most common manifestation of CNS infection by varicella-zoster is cerebellar ataxia. Cytomegalovirus infection of the CNS may be either part of congenital infection or disseminated disease in an immunocompromised host. CNS diseases caused by Epstein-Barr virus may present as perceptual distortions of sizes, shapes, and spatial relationships known as "Alice in Wonderland syndrome." There may be meningitis, seizures, ataxia, facial palsy, transverse myelitis, and encephalitis.[178] Influenza A (H1N1) has taken on considerable significance during the pandemic and a recent report by Baltagi et al.[179] demonstrated important neurologic sequelae of this infection in children including altered mental status, seizures, and encephalopathy. Notably, these findings were seen in children without significant respiratory symptomatology.

Infectious agents can enter the brain via a hematogenous route or by neuronal tracts. Many hematogenous pathogens cause direct endothelial damage to arteries, arterioles, and capillaries, resulting in vasculitis, hemorrhage, and thrombosis. Postinfectious encephalitis is an autoimmune process characterized by a perivenulitis with demyelination. It is uncommon in children younger than 1 year of age.[180] The mortality rate in untreated cases of HSV encephalitis is 70%, and fewer than 3% return to normal function. Early treatment with acyclovir reduces the mortality rate to 20% to 30%, but there is still substantial morbidity.[181]

Diagnosis

The onset of illness is generally acute and often preceded by a nonspecific febrile illness of few days' duration. The manifestations of viral encephalitis in older children are headache and hyperesthesia, whereas in infants, irritability and lethargy predominate. Adolescents frequently complain of retrobulbar pain. Fever, nausea, vomiting, photophobia, and pain in the legs, back, and neck are common. Exanthems often precede or accompany the CNS signs. Seizures occur in 60% of the cases during the course of HSV encephalitis. The diagnosis of viral encephalitis is usually made on the basis of clinical presentation of nonspecific prodrome followed by progressive CNS symptoms. The CSF usually shows a mild mononuclear predominance. In the diagnostic workup, the CSF should be cultured for viruses, bacteria, fungi, and mycobacteria.[182] Detection of viral DNA or RNA by polymerase chain reaction is useful for diagnosis of HSV, varicella-zoster, cytomegalovirus, Epstein-Barr virus, and enteroviral meningoencephalitis. Polymerase chain reaction of CSF is 100% specific and more than 90% sensitive for HSV.[183] About 50% of patients with HSV encephalitis have focal abnormalities on nonenhanced CT. MRI is the imaging modality of choice and should ideally be the first step after initial clinical examination. The EEG is abnormal in almost all cases of HSV encephalitis and may show periodic lateralized epileptiform discharges (Figure 42-3).[184]

Treatment

Antiviral therapy with acyclovir is indicated for HSV encephalitis. Acyclovir has a relatively short half-life in plasma, and more than 80% is excreted unchanged in the urine, so renal impairment can exacerbate toxicity. The standard dose of acyclovir for HSV encephalitis is 30 mg/kg/24 h, divided every 8 hours for 14 days. The dose in neonates is 60 mg/kg/d. The duration of treatment is 21 days for immunocompromised patients. Acyclovir is effective in encephalitis due to HSV types 1 and 2 and varicella-zoster. The dose of acyclovir for varicella-zoster encephalitis is similar to that for herpes simplex encephalitis.[182] Antiviral therapy with oseltamivir is indicated in H1N1 encephalopathy.[179]

Supportive Care in the Pediatric Intensive Care Unit

A substantial body of data supporting an evidence-based approach to care in the pediatric ICU of children with meningitis and encephalitis is lacking. Careful attention to the ABCs with a neurointensive care approach is essential. If the GCS score is less than 8 and/or the airway or ventilation is compromised, intubation is indicated and should be performed using a neuroprotective rapid-sequence approach. Normal values for both $Paco_2$ and Pao_2 should be ensured. Bacterial meningitis and encephalitis can be associated with severe septic shock that should be approached and treated according to published guidelines.[185] Arterial blood pressure must be adequate to optimize cerebral perfusion.

In infants and children with meningitis and encephalitis, increased ICP may develop. The most important morbidity and mortality of CNS infections is herniation of brain tissue secondary to intracranial hypertension. No randomized controlled trial has been conducted to evaluate the effect ICP monitoring has on outcome in meningitis or encephalitis in children or adults. However, evidence supports the association of intracranial hypertension and poor neurologic outcome in infants and children.[186-188] In addition, ICP monitoring and aggressive treatment of intracranial hypertension showed reductions in the expected mortality rate in pediatric and adult patients with meningitis and encephalitis.[189-192] ICP monitoring and ICP-directed therapy should be considered if signs and symptoms of intracranial hypertension develop in children with meningitis and encephalitis. ICP monitoring in patients with known or suspected CNS infection with a GCS score less than 8 may be considered at the discretion of the physician. An external ventricular drain is the preferred route of ICP monitoring if there is hydrocephalus or CSF is required for therapeutic or diagnostic drainage. Likely benefit derived from oral glycerol, as previously discussed, is mediated via an osmolar effect.

Other aspects of contemporary pediatric neurointensive care should be included in the treatment regimen, including maintenance of euglycemia and careful fluid management to maintain both a euvolemic

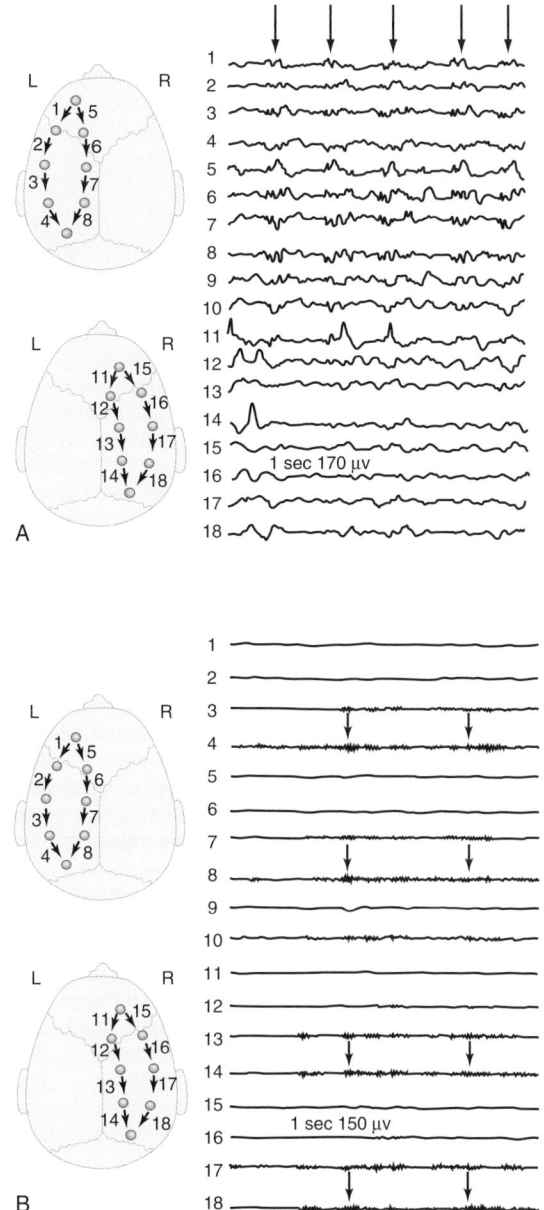

Figure 42-3 **A,** Electroencephalogram showing periodic lateralized epileptiform discharges (PLEDS) in a child with herpes simplex encephalitis. Discharges are seen diffusely in left hemisphere (leads 1 to 10), occurring at intervals at about 2.5 seconds (*arrows*). **B,** Normal background activity in an awake subject for comparison. Arrows show normal alpha rhythm in posterior leads bilaterally. (*From Watenberg N, Morton LD. Images in clinical medicine. Periodic lateralized epileptiform discharges. N Engl J Med 1996;334:634.*)

state and avoid hyponatremia. This is particularly important because SIADH is common in these conditions. Appropriate nutritional support as outlined in Chapter 95 should also be instituted as soon as possible.

BRAIN ABSCESS

Epidemiology and Diagnosis

Brain abscesses are most common in children between the ages of 4 and 8 years. The underlying causes of brain abscess include chronic otitis media and sinusitis, orbital cellulitis, dental infections, penetrating head injury, infection of ventriculoperitoneal shunts, immunodeficiency states, embolization due to congenital heart disease with left-to-right shunts, and meningitis. About 80% of brain abscesses in children occur in frontotemporal and parietal lobes, and 30% have multiple sites of involvement. Table 42-5 summarizes the relationships between predisposing conditions and site of brain abscess, likely pathogens, and suggested initial empirical treatment. In the early stages, the clinical presentation of brain abscess includes low-grade fever, headache, and lethargy. Vomiting, papilledema, focal neurologic signs, and seizures may develop as the inflammation proceeds. Nystagmus, ipsilateral ataxia and dysmetria, headache, and vomiting are characteristic signs of cerebellar brain abscess. If the abscess ruptures into the ventricular cavity, severe shock may rapidly develop and death may result.[193]

Contrast medium–enhanced head CT and MRI are the most reliable methods of identifying brain abscess. An abscess cavity shows a ring-enhancing lesion with enhanced CT. MRI with gadolinium administration may reveal a capsule. Blood cultures are positive in roughly 10% of cases. Lumbar puncture should not be undertaken in a patient with suspected brain abscess because examination of CSF is seldom useful and this procedure may precipitate herniation.

Treatment

Treatment is initiated with an antibiotic regimen that is based on the probable pathogenesis and most likely organism. An encapsulated abscess should be treated by antibiotics and aspiration, which is also the most likely diagnostic approach. Surgery is indicated when the abscess (1) is larger than 2.5 cm in diameter, (2) contains gas, (3) is multiloculated, (4) is located in the posterior fossa, or (5) when fungus is identified. The duration of treatment depends on the organism and response but usually ranges between 4 and 6 weeks. Other aspects of neurointensive care in the pediatric ICU for infants and children with brain abscess should mirror those presented previously for meningitis and encephalitis.[194]

■ Postoperative Neurosurgical Cases

EPIDEMIOLOGY

Neurosurgical procedures for children vary widely in all aspects and include elective and emergent operations in all ages of children for a variety of illnesses, most commonly brain tumors, hydrocephalus, and arteriovenous malformations.

TABLE 42-5	Predisposing Conditions, Etiologic Agents, and Empirical Treatment in Brain Abscess		
Predisposing Condition	**Site of Abscess**	**Etiologic Agents**	**Treatment**
Sinusitis Orbital cellulitis Dental infection	Frontal lobe	Streptococci *Bacteroides* Enterobacteriaceae *Staphylococcus aureus* *Haemophilus* spp.	Vancomycin + third-generation cephalosporin + metronidazole
Otitis media Mastoiditis	Temporal lobe/ cerebellum	Streptococci *Bacteroides* Enterobacteriaceae *S. aureus* *Haemophilus* spp. *Pseudomonas aeruginosa*	Vancomycin + third-generation cephalosporin + metronidazole
Head trauma Postsurgical infection	Site of injury or surgery	*S. aureus* Streptococci Enterobacteriaceae *Clostridium*	Vancomycin + third-generation cephalosporin + metronidazole
Congenital cyanotic heart disease	Middle cerebral artery distribution	*Streptococcus viridans* Anaerobic and microphilic streptococci	Penicillin + metronidazole
Ventriculoperitoneal shunt	Site of shunt	*P. aeruginosa* Streptococci Enterobacteriaceae	Vancomycin + ceftazidime

DIAGNOSIS

The need for admission to a pediatric ICU is largely determined by the potential complications associated with the specific surgery involved. The most common complications that require intensive monitoring after neurosurgical procedures include hydrocephalus, airway compromise, bleeding, vascular complications, fluid and electrolyte abnormalities, and seizures. Hydrocephalus is an obvious concern in patients undergoing procedures for the treatment of hydrocephalus, either with shunting, ventriculostomy, or a decompressive procedure. Patients with congenital hydrocephalus require ICU monitoring depending largely on their preoperative status. A child with slowly progressive hydrocephalus with few clinical symptoms may not require admission to the pediatric ICU, whereas preoperative symptoms that raise a concern of potential herniation will require close observation and monitoring. Patients with Chiari malformations, tumors impinging on CSF drainage, or ventricular hemorrhages all carry a significant risk of developing postoperative hydrocephalus.

Airway compromise is a potentially life-threatening complication that is of particular concern after neurosurgical procedures involving the brainstem, because vocal cord paralysis or cranial nerve damage is possible. Patients with congenital facial abnormalities are also at risk for respiratory compromise. A third scenario that predisposes neurosurgical patients to airway problems is a procedure requiring prone positioning during surgery, because significant facial swelling can result.

Although the potential for bleeding is always a concern after surgical procedures, there are certain diseases that carry more than the typical risk for hemorrhage. In particular, surgical resection of a vascular malformation is of concern for bleeding if complete resection is incomplete or impossible. However, all procedures carry a risk for postoperative bleeding, including procedures that do not involve a craniotomy.

Surgical procedures near major arteries can cause vasospasm with resultant cerebral ischemia or infarct. Subarachnoid hemorrhage from aneurysmal or vascular malformation rupture is another well-known cause of vasospasm.

Electrolyte abnormalities can result from three disturbances in normal regulatory mechanisms: diabetes insipidus, SIADH, and cerebral salt wasting (see later discussion for management). Other complications from neurosurgical procedures include CSF leak, aseptic meningitis, and pseudomeningocele.

PHYSICAL EXAMINATION

The immediate examination should include an evaluation of the ABCs. Specific to neurosurgical patients, however, a rapid neurologic examination is important to evaluate for baseline deficits after surgery. This is essential for evaluation of changes in neurologic status. For example, unequal pupillary size may be a result of surgical intervention and would be present immediately after the surgery. However, development of unequal pupils in a patient who previously had equal pupillary size may be the first sign of impending herniation. The initial neurologic examination should include a gross evaluation of mental status. Patients routinely have a depressed level of consciousness after anesthesia, but repeated examinations are necessary to ensure that mental status continues to improve. Measurement of the GCS score is one means of objectively quantifying a child's level of consciousness. Cranial nerve examination is limited by the child's ability to cooperate but should include pupillary response (cranial nerve II), observation of extraocular movements (cranial nerves III, IV, and VI), jaw deviation during sucking in an infant (cranial nerve V), facial asymmetry while crying or laughing (cranial nerve VII), gag reflex (cranial nerves IX and X), and shoulder droop (cranial nerve XI). The motor examination relies heavily on careful observation of movements, because few patients will be able to cooperate with a formal examination early after surgery. Similarly, the sensory examination involves observing gross responses to stimuli. A full evaluation of deep tendon reflexes is usually possible. Neurologic evaluation should be repeated frequently during the first 24 hours, evaluating for new or progressing neurologic deficits.

TREATMENT

All patients in the pediatric ICU should have cardiorespiratory monitoring. Respiratory monitoring should be designed to warn of impending airway compromise, including measurement of respiratory rate, pulse oximetry, and repeated examinations evaluating work of breathing, air entry, and evidence of stridor. Hemodynamic monitoring is useful for evaluating both hemodynamic and neurologic status. Increases in heart rate and BP can be an indication of pain or of seizure activity. Increased BP with a low heart rate is worrisome for raised ICP and impending herniation, although herniation is not always signaled by Cushing's triad in children. Tachycardia with prolonged capillary refill or hypotension may indicate excessive fluid losses, either from bleeding, third space losses, or excessive urine output. Tachycardia and hypotension can also result from loss of vasomotor tone, either from infection, medications, or loss of neurologic regulation after spinal surgery. Invasive BP monitoring is necessary when patients are at high risk for any of the complications listed earlier. Strict measurement of fluid intake and output is essential to monitor fluid balance and interpret disturbances in fluid and electrolyte regulation. When the surgical procedure carries a high risk of a complicating fluid regulation abnormality, as in craniopharyngioma resections, serum and urine electrolytes should be tested every 4 to 6 hours, along with continuous urine measurement and central venous pressure monitoring.

Temperature control is important after neurosurgical procedures and should therefore be monitored closely. Aggressive measures to prevent hyperthermia are warranted because neurologic injury may be exacerbated by high brain temperature.

Fluid management for the postoperative neurosurgical patient differs from other postoperative patients in a few key ways. Although maintenance of circulating volume is important, it is important to avoid excessive hydration to prevent exacerbating cerebral edema. In general, neurosurgical procedures do not result in the large third-space losses seen with other surgeries. Once adequate volume status is achieved to maintain perfusion, fluid requirements will usually be met with a maintenance fluid rate.

Euglycemia is important after neurologic surgery, because both hypoglycemia and hyperglycemia can exacerbate neurologic injury. Based on recommendations in adults, initial IV fluids in older children should generally be normal saline or 5% dextrose in normal saline, and serum glucose levels should be monitored closely. The duration for the dextrose restriction in older children is controversial because ketosis develops even with euglycemia. Generally this is maintained for the initial 24 hours. Hyperglycemia, however, should probably be avoided throughout the entire acute period after CNS insults. Infants, on the other hand, do not have the same capacity for maintaining serum glucose levels if maintained with no source of carbohydrate intake. Initial dextrose concentration in the infant with a CNS insult should probably be 5% (in normal saline). When higher dextrose concentrations are used, such as with hyperalimentation, hyperglycemia should be carefully managed with insulin infusion. It must be recognized that the risk of exacerbation of brain injury by hyperglycemia in infants and children is likely but somewhat theoretical. In contrast, it is clear that hypoglycemia can be harmful to the injured brain and should be avoided.

Hyponatremia is of particular concern in neurosurgical patients, because the osmotic effects can result in increasing cerebral edema. The incidence is as high as 31% at 48 hours in pediatric surgical patients,[195] and the use of isotonic fluid in the pediatric ICU can reduce iatrogenic hyponatremia.[196] Thus, normal saline is the preferred IV fluid to avoid this complication. When hyponatremia occurs in conjunction with a decreasing urine output, a high specific gravity, and a high sodium concentration in the urine, it is likely a result of SIADH.

In this case, fluid restriction is indicated. Neurosurgical patients also have two unique possible sources for excessive sodium loss: CSF losses from extraventricular drainage and urine losses from cerebral salt wasting. Both require correction of sodium losses.

Mild hypernatremia is generally not detrimental and is usually a result of excessive sodium intake or osmotic diuresis. A progressively increasing serum sodium concentration in the presence of increasing volume of hypo-osmolar urine, however, suggests diabetes insipidus. This complication is unusual except with surgeries that have the potential for pituitary injury. Management of diabetes insipidus requires careful titration of fluids, with a maintenance rate to cover insensible losses (300 mL/m^2/d) plus total replacement of urine output with a fluid that matches the urine electrolyte concentrations. Vasopressin or desmopressin therapy may be required to control the free water loss.

A few medications should be considered for every neurosurgical patient. First, antiemetics are important to prevent postanesthesia nausea and vomiting, because vomiting can cause a dramatic increase in intracranial pressure. Ondansetron and droperidol are good choices for antiemetic therapy because they are minimally sedating.[197] Postoperative seizures can have serious consequences. Antiepileptics should be considered in all patients at risk for postoperative seizures. Typically, phenytoin is the least sedating drug for seizure prophylaxis. Patients on chronic anticonvulsants should have their usual regimen started as soon as possible after the surgery. Dexamethasone is used to reduce edema formation around brain tumors and reduce tumor size.[198] The use of corticosteroids is controversial in most other settings. However, patients who received corticosteroids preoperatively may require stress-dose corticosteroids during the postoperative period. Prophylaxis with H$_2$ blockers may reduce gastrointestinal hemorrhage in critically ill patients[199] but may also increase the risk of nosocomial infections.[200] Gastrointestinal bleeding is more common after resection of a posterior fossa tumor, and use of prophylaxis has been advocated in these patients.[201]

EMERGENCY INTERVENTION

The postoperative problem of most concern, and sometimes the most difficult to evaluate in a child, is an altered mental status. Although anesthetics or narcotics can produce an altered sensorium, emergent evaluation is indicated if reversal of these medications does not yield a reassuring examination. If the patient's GCS score is less than 8, intubation should be performed before any transport or testing. If an extraventricular drain is in place, it should be opened and low enough to allow CSF drainage. Mannitol should be given if signs of impending herniation exist and transient hyperventilation begun until a definitive surgical intervention is carried out. An emergent head CT should then be performed. Further action will be guided by the CT findings.

Other Critical Central Nervous System Disorders in Infants and Children

There are other critical CNS disorders in infants and children, including hepatic encephalopathy, hypertensive encephalopathy, and Reye syndrome. Discussion of these less common disorders is beyond the scope of this chapter, and the reader is referred to the appropriate primary references or other textbooks focused on pediatric critical care medicine. Reye syndrome was once a key disorder in the field of pediatric neurointensive care—reaching a peak of 555 cases in the United States in 1980. In the past decade, fewer than 2 cases per year have been reported.[202]

KEY POINTS

1. There are important age-related differences in both CNS insults and the response to these insults in infants and children.

2. Neurointensive care for infants and children should focus on preventing secondary extracerebral insults and optimizing brain-directed therapies. Optimization of cardiopulmonary physiology, maintenance of euglycemia, and prevention of hyperthermia and hyponatremia are important to best outcomes.

3. Cardiopulmonary arrest in infants and children results from asphyxia in the majority of cases.

4. The goals of treating status epilepticus are to provide respiratory and cardiovascular support, terminate seizure activity, identify and treat the precipitating factors, and prevent systemic complications.

5. Congenital and acquired heart disease are the most important underlying causes of embolic stroke in infants and children.

6. The etiology and treatment of bacterial meningitis differ between neonates and older infants and children.

7. Herpes simplex virus is an important cause of severe encephalitis in children.

8. Treatment of impending herniation includes immediate airway control, mannitol or hypertonic saline administration, hyperventilation, cerebrospinal fluid drainage (if available), and emergent CT evaluation.

ANNOTATED REFERENCES

Chiron C, Raynaud C, Maziere B, et al. Changes in regional cerebral blood flow during brain maturation in children and adolescents. J Nucl Med 1992;33:696-703.
The most comprehensive study of normal CBF in infants and children.

DeVeber G, Kirkham F. Guidelines for the treatment and prevention of stroke in children. Lancet 2008; 7:983-5.
Outstanding review and comparison of the three recently published guidelines for acute management of ischemic stroke in children.

Kitamura T, Iwami T, Kawamura T, Nagao K, Tanaka H, Nadkarni VM, et al. implementation working group for All-Japan Utstein Registry of the Fire and Disaster Management Agency. Conventional and chest-compression-only cardiopulmonary resuscitation by bystanders for children who have out-of-hospital cardiac arrests: a prospective, nationwide, population-based cohort study. Lancet 2010;375:1347-54.
Landmark study in over 5000 children in Japan, showing benefits of conventional versus compression-only CPR in children.

Kochanek PM, Tasker RC. Pediatric neurointensive care: 2008 update for the Rogers' textbook of pediatric intensive care. Pediatr Crit Care Med 2009;10:517-23.
Contemporary review of key new developments in the emerging field of pediatric neurocritical care.

Lacroix J, Deal C, Gauthier M, et al. Admissions to a pediatric intensive care unit for status epilepticus: a 10-year experience. Crit Care Med 1994;22:827-32.
Classic case series on status epilepticus in 147 children, covering the spectrum of etiologies from the perspective of the PICU.

Laptook A, Tyson J, Shankaran S, McDonald S, Ehrenkranz R, Fanaroff A, et al. National Institute of Child Health and Human Development Neonatal Research Network. Elevated temperature after hypoxic-ischemic encephalopathy: risk factor for adverse outcomes. Pediatrics 2008;122:491-9.

Secondary evaluation in the aforementioned randomized controlled trial of hypothermia versus normothermia in perinatal asphyxia, which showed that even a single degree of hyperthermia in the postinsult period is associated with deleterious consequences.

Peltola H, Roine I, Fernández J, Zavala I, Ayala SG, Mata AG, et al. Adjuvant glycerol and/or dexamethasone to improve the outcomes of childhood bacterial meningitis: a prospective, randomized, double-blind, placebo-controlled trial. Clin Infect Dis 2007;45:1277-86.
Randomized controlled trial showing benefit of oral glycerol in the management of pediatric meningitis.

Shankaran S, Laptook AR, Ehrenkranz RA, Tyson JE, McDonald SA, Donovan EF, et al. National Institute of Child Health and Human Development Neonatal Research Network. Whole-body hypothermia for neonates with hypoxic-ischemic encephalopathy. N Engl J Med 2005;353:1574-84.
Important multicenter randomized controlled trial showing beneficial effect of mild hypothermia in perinatal asphyxia.

Topjian AA, Berg RA, Nadkarni VM. Pediatric cardiopulmonary resuscitation: advances in science, techniques, and outcomes. Pediatrics 2008;122:1086-98.
Comprehensive review of the pathobiology and treatment of pediatric cardiac arrest.

Vavilala MS, Lee LA, Lam AM. The lower limit of autoregulation in children during sevoflurane anesthesia. J Neurosurg Anesthesiol 2003;15:307-12.
Important study that shows that the lower limit of CBF autoregulation in infants and young children is similar to that in older children—indicating enhanced vulnerability of the brain of infants and young children to hypotension, given the reduced autoregulatory reserve (difference between mean arterial pressure and the lower limit of autoregulation).

REFERENCES

Access the complete reference list online at http://www.expertconsult.com.

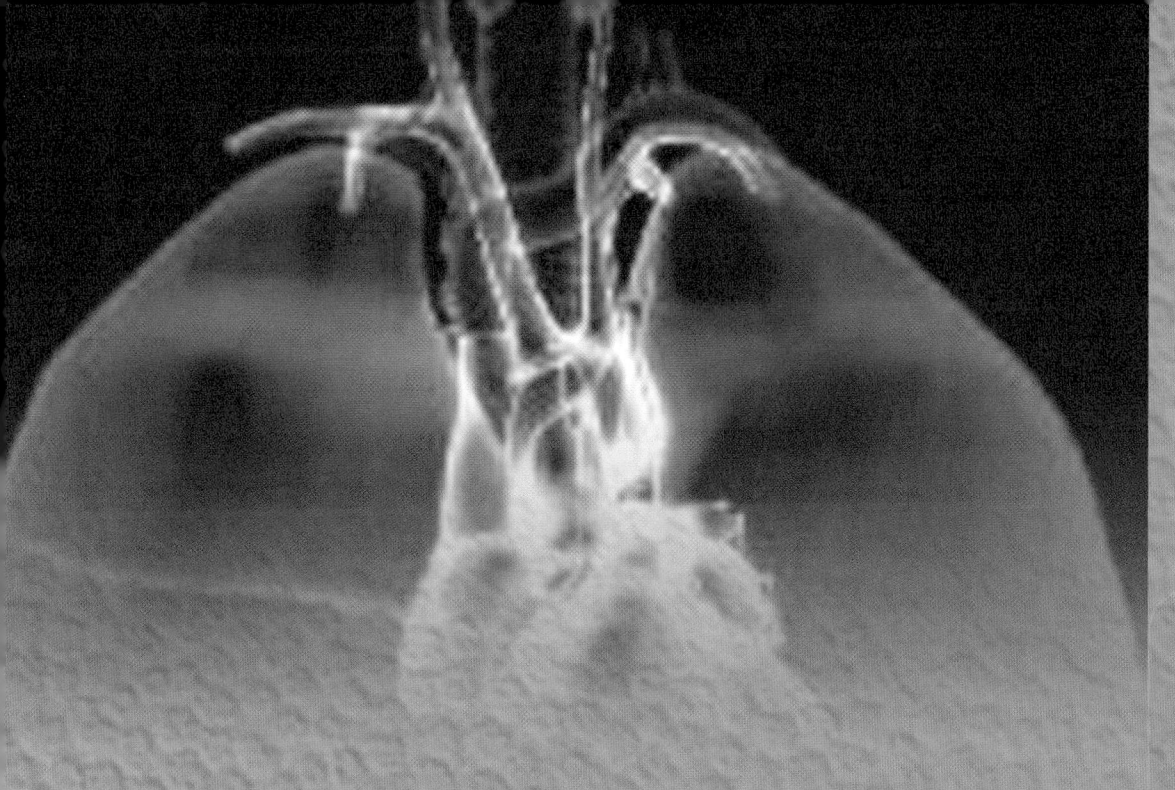

PART 3

Pulmonary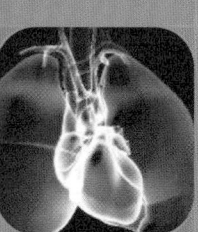

43

Bedside Monitoring of Pulmonary Function

MICHAEL A. GENTILE | JOHN D. DAVIES

The safe and effective management of patients with acute respiratory failure requires accurate bedside monitoring of pulmonary function. This chapter focuses on the more common noninvasive techniques for monitoring pulmonary gas exchange, respiratory system mechanics, and breathing pattern. These techniques may lead to rapid assessment of patient respiratory function and appropriate clinical action.

Pulse Oximetry

Pulse oximetry is a microprocessor-based instrument that incorporates both oximetry and plethysmography to provide continuous noninvasive monitoring of the oxygen saturation of arterial blood (SpO_2). Often considered the "fifth vital sign," it is one of the most important technologic advances for monitoring patients during anesthesia, in the intensive care unit (ICU), on the general ward, in the emergency department, and during a wide variety of procedures.[1-3] The pulse oximeter probe is embedded into either a clip or an adhesive wrap and consists of two light-emitting diodes on one side, with a light-detecting photodiode on the opposite side. Either a finger or an earlobe serves as the sample "cuvette." The tissue bed is transilluminated, and the forward-scattered light is measured. Pulse oximetry targets the signal arising from the arterial bed as light absorbance fluctuates with changing blood volume. Arterial blood flow causes signal changes in light absorption (the pulsatile component called *photoplethysmography*) that can be distinguished from venous and capillary blood in the surrounding tissues (the baseline, or direct current, component; Figure 43-1).

Oximetry uses spectrophotometry to determine SaO_2. According to the Beer-Lambert law, the concentration of a substance can be determined by its ability to transmit light.[4] Oxygenated hemoglobin (HbO_2) and deoxygenated or "reduced" hemoglobin (HbR) species absorb light differently, so that the ratio of their absorbencies can be used to calculate saturation. In addition, there are two minor hemoglobin (Hb) species: carboxyhemoglobin (COHb) and methemoglobin (MetHb). Fractional SaO_2 is the proportion of oxygenated hemoglobin relative to the four hemoglobin species:

$$HbO_2 + HbR + COHb + MetHb$$

Measuring fractional hemoglobin requires a co-oximeter that incorporates four wavelengths to distinguish each species (Figure 43-2). In contrast, oxygen saturation as determined by pulse oximeter (SpO_2) uses two wavelengths, so that it measures functional SaO_2:

$$HbO_2 + HbR$$

ACCURACY AND PRECISION

Because pulse oximeters themselves cannot be calibrated, their accuracy is highly variable and dependent on both the calibration curve programmed into the monitor and the quality of signal processing.[5,6] The ratio of absorbencies is calibrated empirically against SaO_2 measured by co-oximetry in normal volunteers subjected to various levels of oxygenation. Pulse oximeters are calibrated against measured SaO_2 down to 70% (saturations below this level are determined by

extrapolation).[5] The resulting calibration curve is stored in the monitor's microprocessor to calculate SpO_2.[6]

The accuracy of the calibration curve depends on laboratory testing conditions (co-oximeter used, range of oxygenation studied, and characteristics of sample subjects). Most manufacturers report an accuracy of ±2% at an SaO_2 greater than 70% and ±3% when the SaO_2 is 50% to 70%.[2] In normal subjects tested at an SaO_2 between 99% and 83%, pulse oximetry has a bias and precision that are within 3% of co-oximetry.[7] However, under hypoxic conditions (SaO_2 78% to 55%), when the monitor must rely on extrapolated values, bias increases (8%) and precision deteriorates (5%).[7] Likewise, in critically ill patients, pulse oximeters historically perform well when the SaO_2 is greater than 90% (bias of 1.7%; precision of ±1.2%), but accuracy diminishes at an SaO_2 below 90% (bias of 5.1%; precision of ±2.7%)[8] (Figure 43-3). Technologic advances over the past decade have apparently improved this performance; a recent study comparing pulse oximetry to co-oximetry reported a bias of 0.19% and a precision of ±2.22% over an SaO_2 range of 60% to 100%.[9]

DYNAMIC RESPONSE

Because pulse oximeters detect very small optical signals (and must reject a variety of artifacts), data must be averaged over several seconds, thus affecting response time.[5] Pulse oximeters may register a near-normal SpO_2 when the actual SaO_2 is less than 70%.[5] A prolonged lag time is more common with finger probes than ear probes[5,10,11] and is attributed to hypoxia-related peripheral vasoconstriction.[5] Bradycardia also is associated with a prolonged response time.[11]

SOURCES OF ERROR

Motion artifact and low perfusion are the most common sources of SpO_2 inaccuracies, because the photoplethysmographic pulse signal is very low in these settings compared with the total absorption signal.[12,13] The combination of motion artifact and low perfusion substantially lowers SpO_2 accuracy compared with either artifact alone.[14] Causes of motion artifact include shivering, twitching, agitation, intraaortic balloon pump assistance, and patient transport.[15,16] Signs of motion artifact include a false or erratic pulse rate reading or an abnormal plethysmographic waveform. Peripheral hypoperfusion from hypothermia, low cardiac output, or vasoconstrictive drugs may increase bias, reduce precision, and prolong the detection time for a hypoxic event.[16] Newer technologies have helped reduce the incidence of these problems but they have not been eliminated as a source of error. Relocation of the probe may be required to obtain a more accurate signal.

Despite recent technologic advances, there still are a number of factors that may affect the accuracy of the pulse oximeter. Table 43-1 lists the most common factors.

Dyshemoglobins and Vascular Dyes

Significant amounts of COHb or MetHb can cause errors in SpO_2. Carboxyhemoglobin and HbO_2 absorb equivalent amounts of red light, so carbon monoxide poisoning results in a falsely elevated SpO_2 because the pulse oximeter reports total Hb saturation not just HbO_2

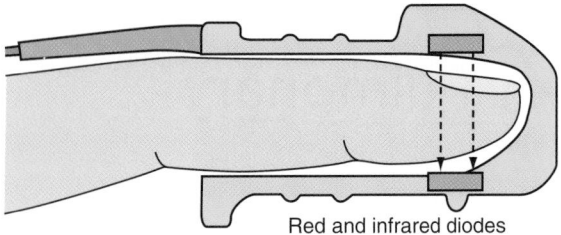

Figure 43-1 Schematic depiction of the pulse oximeter light absorption signal. (*Adapted with permission from Phillips Medical Systems, Carlsbad, California.*)

saturation. In the setting of carbon monoxide poisoning, the amount of COHb is elevated, resulting in a falsely high Spo_2. The patient, however, could be experiencing profound hypoxemia. In contrast, MetHb causes substantial absorption of both red and infrared light, so the ratio approaches 1 (estimated Spo_2 of 85%).[4] Significant MetHb causes falsely low Spo_2 values when the actual Sao_2 is greater than 85% and falsely high values when the Sao_2 is less than 85%.[4] Administration of methylene blue or indocyanine green dyes for diagnostic tests causes a false, transient (1- to 2-minute) drop in Spo_2 to as low as 65%.[17,18]

Nail Polish and Skin Pigmentation

Both dark skin pigmentation and dark nail polish interfere with absorption of the wavelengths used by pulse oximetry. Pulse oximeters thus have greater bias and less precision in black patients.[8] Whereas an Spo_2 of 92% is sufficient to predict adequate oxygenation in white patients, a saturation of 95% is required in black patients.[8] Dark nail polish can falsely lower Spo_2, whereas red polish tends not to affect accuracy.[19] However, with newer technology, the negative effects of nail polish are lessened. A recent study showed that there was an effect of dark nail polish on the pulse oximetry reading, but it was not clinically relevant.[20] When nail polish cannot be removed, mounting the oximeter probe sideways on the finger yields an accurate reading.[21]

Ambient Light, Anemia, and Hyperbilirubinemia

Although pulse oximeters compensate for the presence of ambient light, the sensor should be shielded from intense light sources with an opaque material. Falsely low Spo_2 readings occur when even minor gaps exist between the probe and skin, allowing reflected light off the skin surface to "shunt" directly to the photodiode.[22] Xenon surgical

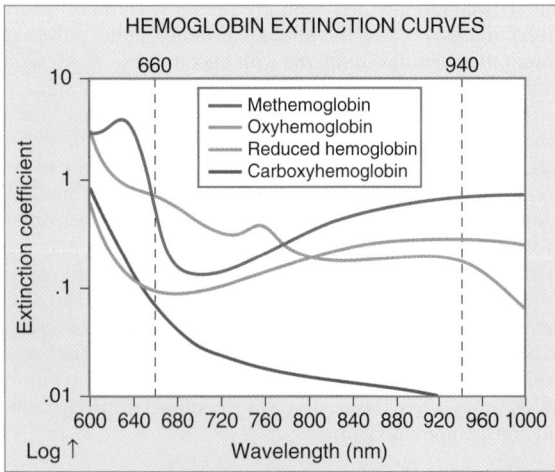

Figure 43-2 Extinction coefficients of the four types of hemoglobin at the red and infrared wavelengths. Methemoglobin absorbs light at both wavelengths to an equal extent; absorption of red light by carboxyhemoglobin is similar to oxyhemoglobin. (*From Tremper KK, Barker SJ. Pulse oximetry. Anesthesiology 1989;70:98-108.*)

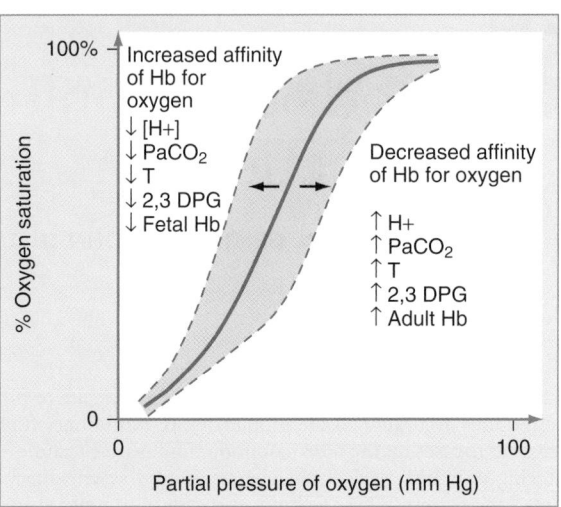

Figure 43-3 Oxyhemoglobin dissociation curve relates oxygen saturation and partial pressure of oxygen in the blood, and is affected by many variables. (*Courtesy Phillips Medical Systems, Carlsbad, California.*)

lamps and fluorescent lighting can cause a falsely low Spo_2.[23] Under conditions of anemia (Hb 8 g/dL) and severe hypoxia (Sao_2 54%), Spo_2 bias is markedly increased (−14%).[24] Hyperbilirubinemia does not affect Spo_2 directly.[25] However, carbon monoxide is a byproduct of heme metabolism, and icteric patients tend to have higher levels of COHb,[25] so Spo_2 may be falsely elevated.

REFLECTANCE PULSE OXIMETRY

Reflectance pulse oximetry was designed to counter signal-detection problems associated with finger probes during hypoperfusion. The reflectance sensor is designed for placement on the forehead just above

TABLE 43-1	Common Factors Affecting Pulse Oximetry Measurements
Factor	**Effect**
Carboxyhemoglobin (COHb)	Slight reduction of the assessment of oxygen saturation (Sao_2) by pulse oximetry (Spo_2) (i.e., overestimates the fraction of hemoglobin available for O_2 transport)
Methemoglobin (MetHb)	At high levels of MetHb, Spo_2 approaches 85%, independent of actual Sao_2
Methylene blue	Transient, marked decrease in Spo_2 lasting up to several minutes; possible secondary effects as a result of effects on hemodynamics
Anemia	If Sao_2 is normal, no effect; during hypoxemia with Hb values less than 14.5 g/dL, progressive underestimation of actual Sao_2
Ambient light interference	Bright light, particularly if flicker frequency is close to a harmonic of the light-emitting diode switching frequency, can falsely elevate the Spo_2 reading
Blood flow	Reduced amplitude of pulsations can hinder obtaining a reading or cause a falsely low reading
Motion	Movement, especially shivering, may depress the Spo_2 reading
Nail polish	Slight decrease in Spo_2 reading, with greatest effect using blue nail polish, or no change
Sensor contact	"Optical shunting" of light from source to detector directly or by reflection from skin results in falsely low Spo_2 reading
Skin pigmentation	Small errors or no significant effect reported; deep pigmentation can result in reduced signal
Tape	Transparent tape between sensor and skin has little effect; falsely low Spo_2 has been reported when smeared adhesive is in the optical path
Vasodilation	Slight decrease
Venous pulsation	Artifactual decrease in Spo_2

the orbital area, where superficial blood flow is abundant and less susceptible to vasconstriction.[26] Whereas traditional probes work by transilluminating a tissue bed and measuring the forward-scattered light on the opposite side of the finger or earlobe, reflectance probes are constructed with the light-emitting diodes and the photodetector located on the same side. The photodetector measures the back-scattered light from the skin.[26] In addition, more liberal placement sites for reflectance pulse oximetry has allowed fetal monitoring during labor.[27] Intraesophageal SpO_2 monitoring is currently under investigation.[28] Anasarca, excessive head movement, and difficulty in securing the probe site are some of the problems encountered with reflectance pulse oximetry.[29] Light "shunting" from poor skin contact and direct sensor placement over a superficial artery are associated with artifacts.[30] Reflectance pulse oximetry is also limited by poor signal-to-noise ratio and variability among sites in the arrangement of blood vessels and tissue blood volume.[30] However, recent studies have shown reflectance pulse oximetry to be as effective as finger sensors in many situations.[31-34]

TECHNOLOGIC ADVANCES

Recent advances in signal analysis and processing have markedly improved SpO_2 accuracy during low perfusion and reduced the problem of motion artifact.[16,35] According to recent independent testing, these advances occur with pulse oximeters made by several manufacturers.[36] Durban and Rostow reported that new pulse oximeter technology can accurately detect SaO_2 in 92% of the cases in which traditional SpO_2 monitoring failed owing to low perfusion and motion artifact[37] (Box 43-1).

Capnometry

Capnometry consists of the measurement and numeric display of expired carbon dioxide (CO_2) at the patient's airway opening.[38] When a waveform plotting CO_2 against time or volume is also displayed, it is referred to as *capnography*, and the waveform is referred to as a *capnogram*.[38] Capnometry is most commonly used on patients receiving mechanical ventilation and works by passing infrared light through a sample chamber to a detector on the opposite side. CO_2 absorbs infrared light at a peak wavelength of approximately 4.27 μm.[38,39] More infrared light passing through the sample chamber (i.e., less CO_2) causes a larger signal in the detector relative to the infrared light passing through a reference cell. The sample chamber is either connected directly to the Y-adapter of the ventilator circuit (mainstream), or by a sampling line at the Y-adapter that continuously aspirates gas into a sampling chamber located inside the monitor (sidestream).

CLINICAL APPLICATIONS

Capnometric determination of the partial pressure of CO_2 in end-tidal exhaled gas ($PetCO_2$) is used as a surrogate for the partial pressure of CO_2 in arterial blood ($PaCO_2$) during mechanical ventilation[40,41] (Figure 43-4). Although widely available today, the utilization of $PetCO_2$ to represent $PaCO_2$ in ICUs remains unclear. While perhaps not an exact match for $PaCO_2$, $PetCO_2$ does provide a valuable trending tool. Also, with newer technologies, the accuracy of $PetCO_2$ measurements is improving. In a recent study, McSwain et al. showed strong correlations between $PetCO_2$ and $PaCO_2$ across a wide range of dead-space conditions.[42] Capnometry is used for a variety of purposes, such as the diagnosis of pulmonary embolism, determination of lung recruitment response to positive end-expiratory pressure (PEEP), detection of intrinsic PEEP, evaluation of weaning, indirect marker of elevated dead-space ventilation, assessment of cardiopulmonary resuscitation, indirect determination of cardiac output through partial CO_2 rebreathing, verification of endotracheal cannulation, detection of airway accidents, and even determination of feeding tube placement.[43-55] Guidelines for the use of capnometry/capnography are outlined by the American Association for Respiratory Care (Box 43-2).

$PaCO_2$-$PetCO_2$ GRADIENT

Normal subjects have a $PaCO_2$-$PetCO_2$ gradient of 4 to 5 mm Hg.[40,43,47,56-60] In critically ill patients, the $PaCO_2$-$PetCO_2$ gradient can be markedly elevated, with a tendency toward wider gradients in obstructive lung diseases (7-16 mm Hg) than in acute lung injury or cardiogenic pulmonary edema (4-12 mm Hg).[46,47,61-63] A strong correlation between $\Delta PetCO_2$ and $\Delta PaCO_2$ ($r = 0.82$), along with minor bias and reasonable precision between $PetCO_2$ and $PaCO_2$, suggests that arterial blood gas monitoring may not be needed to assess ventilation unless the $\Delta PetCO_2$ exceeds 5 mm Hg.[48] Yet several studies found that the $\Delta PetCO_2$ often falsely predicts the degree and direction of $\Delta PaCO_2$.[58-60,63] Therefore, despite $PetCO_2$ monitoring, routine arterial blood gas analysis is still required in critically ill patients.

Several factors determine the $PaCO_2$-$PetCO_2$ gradient. Whereas $PaCO_2$ reflects the mean partial pressure of CO_2 in alveolar gas ($PaCO_2$), $PetCO_2$ approximates the peak $PaCO_2$.[64] During expiration, lung regions

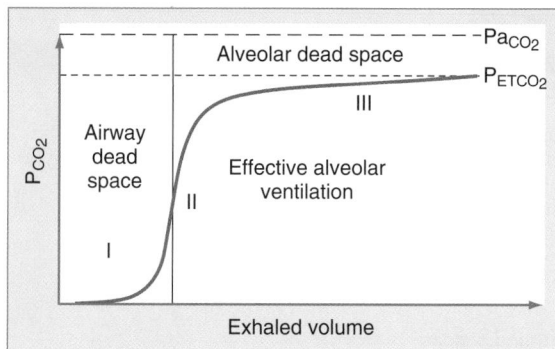

Figure 43-4 Single-breath carbon dioxide waveform depicts carbon dioxide elimination as a function of the volume of gas exhaled. Phase 1 represents gas exhaled from upper airways. Phase 2 is the transitional phase from upper to lower airway ventilation and tends to depict changes in perfusion. Phase 3 is the area of alveolar gas exchange and represents changes in gas distribution. P_{ETCO_2}, partial pressure of end-tidal carbon dioxide.

with high ventilation-to-perfusion ratios dilute the mixed CO_2 concentration so that P_{ETCO_2} is usually lower than Pa_{CO_2}.[65] However, when CO_2 production is elevated (or expiration is prolonged), P_{ETCO_2} more closely resembles mixed venous P_{CO_2}, as a higher amount of CO_2 diffuses into a progressively smaller lung volume.[64] Thus, the Pa_{CO_2}-P_{ETCO_2} gradient can be affected by changes in respiratory rate and tidal volume (VT) due to alterations in expiratory time and by

CO_2 production and mixed venous CO_2 content.[64] In fact, it is not uncommon for P_{ETCO_2} to exceed Pa_{CO_2}.[65] Inotropic or vasoactive drugs may affect the Pa_{CO_2}-P_{ETCO_2} gradient in an unpredictable manner, either by increasing cardiac output and pulmonary perfusion (thereby reducing alveolar dead space) or by reducing pulmonary vascular resistance and magnifying intrapulmonary shunt by countering hypoxic pulmonary vasoconstriction.[58]

Mechanical factors can cause either inconsistencies or inaccuracies in P_{ETCO_2}. The sample tubing length and aspirating flow rates used in sidestream capnometers affect the time required to measure changes in tidal CO_2 concentration.[66] At respiratory frequencies above 30, capnometers tend to underreport the true P_{ETCO_2}.[67] This may occur because of gas mixing between adjacent breaths during transport down the sampling line and in the analysis chamber.[67] This problem can be avoided with mainstream analyzers, which provide near-instantaneous CO_2 measurement (<250 msec).[68]

Pa_{CO_2}-P_{ETCO_2} GRADIENT, POSITIVE END-EXPIRATORY PRESSURE, AND LUNG RECRUITMENT

PEEP recruits collapsed alveoli, improves ventilation-perfusion matching, and reduces alveolar dead space, although excessive levels cause overdistention and increased alveolar dead space.[69] Because the Pa_{CO_2}-P_{ETCO_2} gradient correlates strongly with the physiologic dead space–to–tidal volume ratio (VD/VT), it may be useful in titrating PEEP in patients with acute lung injury (ALI) or acute respiratory distress syndrome (ARDS).[49,50] An animal model of ARDS found that the stepwise application of PEEP progressively reduced the Pa_{CO_2}-P_{ETCO_2} gradient and coincided with maximal or near-maximal improvements in

Box 43-2

AARC CLINICAL PRACTICE GUIDELINE: CAPNOGRAPHY/CAPNOMETRY DURING MECHANICAL VENTILATION

Indications
- Capnography should not be mandated for all patients receiving mechanical ventilatory support, but it may be indicated for:
  - Evaluation of the exhaled CO_2, especially end-tidal CO_2 (P_{ETCO_2}).
  - Monitoring severity of pulmonary disease and evaluating response to therapy, especially therapy intended to improve the ratio of dead space to tidal volume (VD/VT) and the matching of ventilation to perfusion (V/Q) and, possibly, to increase coronary blood flow.
  - Use as an adjunct to determine that tracheal rather than esophageal intubation has taken place.
  - Continued monitoring of the integrity of the ventilatory circuit, including the artificial airway.
  - Evaluation of the efficiency of mechanical ventilatory support by determination of the difference between Pa_{CO_2} and P_{ETCO_2}.
  - Monitoring adequacy of pulmonary, systemic, and coronary blood flow.
  - Estimation of effective (nonshunted) pulmonary capillary blood flow by a partial rebreathing method.
  - Use as an adjunctive tool to screen for pulmonary embolism.
  - Monitoring inspired CO_2 when CO_2 gas is being therapeutically administered.
  - Graphic evaluation of the ventilator-patient interface.
  - Measurement of the volume of CO_2 elimination to assess metabolic rate and/or alveolar ventilation.

Contraindications
- There are no absolute contraindications to capnography in mechanically ventilated patients, provided the data obtained are evaluated with consideration given to the patient's clinical condition.

Precautions and Possible Complications
- With mainstream analyzers, the use of too large a sampling window may introduce an excessive amount of dead space into the ventilator circuit.
- Care must be taken to minimize the amount of additional weight placed on the artificial airway by the addition of the sampling window or, in the case of a sidestream analyzer, the sampling line.

Assessment of Need
- Capnography is considered a standard of care during anesthesia. The American Society of Anesthesiologists has suggested that capnography be available for patients with acute ventilatory failure on mechanical ventilatory support. The American College of Emergency Physicians recommends capnography as an adjunctive method to ensure proper endotracheal tube position.
- Assessment of the need to use capnography with a specific patient should be guided by the clinical situation. The patient's primary cause of respiratory failure and the acuteness of his or her condition should be considered.

Assessment of Outcome
- Results should reflect the patient's condition and should validate the basis for ordering the monitoring.
- Documentation of results (along with all ventilatory and hemodynamic variables available), therapeutic interventions, and/or clinical decisions made based on the capnogram should be included in the patient's chart.

Monitoring
- During capnography, the following should be considered and monitored:
  - Ventilatory variables: tidal volume, respiratory rate, positive end-expiratory pressure, inspiratory-to-expiratory time ratio (I:E), peak airway pressure, and concentrations of respiratory gas mixture.
  - Hemodynamic variables: systemic and pulmonary blood pressures, cardiac output, shunt, and ventilation-perfusion imbalances.

From AARC clinical practice guideline: capnography/capnometry during mechanical ventilation. Respir Care 2003;48:534-9.

oxygenation.[61] However, PEEP applied beyond the lowest $Paco_2$-$Petco_2$ gradient caused a secondary rise in the gradient, along with decreased cardiac output. Although a subsequent trial was unable to reproduce these findings in humans, another study found that the $Paco_2$-$Petco_2$ gradient narrowed (14 to 8 mm Hg) and oxygenation improved when PEEP was set at the lower inflection point of the pressure-volume curve.[45,62] When PEEP was set 5 cm H_2O above the lower inflection point, the $Paco_2$-$Petco_2$ gradient rose to 11 mm Hg, and cardiac output trended downward. In patients without a lower inflection point, the $Paco_2$-$Petco_2$ gradient did not change in response to PEEP. Thus, in a subset of ARDS patients, the $Paco_2$-$Petco_2$ gradient may be an effective way to titrate PEEP.

$Petco_2$ MONITORING DURING CARDIOPULMONARY RESUSCITATION

Monitoring end-tidal CO_2 concentration is a reliable method for evaluating the effectiveness of cardiopulmonary resuscitation.[70] In animal models, $Petco_2$ is strongly correlated with coronary perfusion pressure and successful resuscitation,[71] whereas in humans, changes in $Petco_2$ are directly proportional to changes in cardiac output.[72] $Petco_2$ during precordial compressions can distinguish successful from unsuccessful resuscitation, with values greater than 10 mm Hg[73] or greater than 16 mm Hg[74] associated with successful resuscitation.

MEASUREMENT OF DEAD-SPACE VENTILATION

Ventilation-perfusion abnormalities are the primary physiologic disturbance in nearly all pulmonary diseases and the principal mechanism for elevated $Paco_2$.[75] Dead-space ventilation (V_D), the portion of V_T that does not encounter perfused alveoli, directly impacts CO_2 excretion and is used as an indirect measure of ventilation-perfusion abnormalities. Physiologic V_D represents the summation of anatomic-conducting airway) and nonperfused alveolar components.

Physiologic V_D/V_T has historically been measured during a 3- to 5-minute exhaled gas collection into a 30- to 60-L Douglas bag. An arterial blood gas reading is obtained during the midpoint of the collection. V_D/V_T is calculated using the Enghoff modification of the Bohr equation, whereby the difference between $Paco_2$ (a surrogate for the mean $Paco_2$) and mean expired CO_2 tension ($Peco_2$) is divided by $Paco_2$:

$$\frac{V_D}{V_T} = \frac{Paco_2 - Peco_2}{Paco_2}$$

The dead-space volume per breath or per minute can be determined by multiplying V_D/V_T by the simultaneously measured average V_T or minute ventilation ($\dot{V}_E$)[76]:

$$V_D = \frac{(Paco_2 - Peco_2)}{Paco_2} \times V_T \text{ or } V_D = \frac{(Paco_2 - Peco_2)}{Paco_2} \times \dot{V}_E$$

By subtracting the physiologic V_D per minute from the $\dot{V}_E$, the alveolar minute ventilation ($\dot{V}_E$) is obtained ($\dot{V}_A = \dot{V}_E - \dot{V}_D$). $\dot{V}_A$ also can be calculated as the volume production of CO_2 per minute ($\dot{V}CO_2$) divided by the $Paco_2$[76]:

$$\dot{V}_A = \frac{\dot{V}CO_2}{Paco_2} \times 0.863$$

Expired gas collection with a Douglas bag is the classic method for measuring V_D/V_T. However, the gas collection system requires additional valving and connectors, making the procedure time consuming and awkward. Metabolic monitors produce equally accurate, reliable results and are less cumbersome.[77,78] The Douglas bag method and metabolic monitors, however, do share a limitation when used on a mechanically ventilated patient. During mechanical ventilation, gas is compressed in the circuit, which dilutes the fractional expired carbon dioxide concentration.[79] A correction factor can be used to offset mathematical effects of gas compression. Volumetric capnography is an alternative method of measuring $Peco_2$ and V_D/V_T and has the

advantage of being measured at the patient, thus eliminating the effects of compression volume contamination and the need to apply a correction factor.[80] In patients with ARDS, it has been shown that measurements of V_D/V_T using volumetric capnography is as accurate as those obtained through the use of a metabolic monitor.[81] In addition, newer monitors incorporating capnography and pneumotachygraphy provide accurate single-breath determinations of V_D/V_T.[82]

A significant source of measurement error for V_D/V_T is the contamination of expired gas with circuit compression volume.[83] During positive-pressure ventilation, part of the V_T is compressed in the circuit, and during expiration, this gas mixes with CO_2-laden gas from the lungs. The dilution of the expired CO_2 results in a falsely elevated V_D/V_T that is directly proportional to the peak inspiratory pressure and circuit compliance. Clinically, correcting V_D/V_T for compression volume is done by multiplying the measured $Peco_2$ by the ratio of the ventilator-set V_T to the V_T delivered to the patient.[84] This requires determination of the ventilator circuit compliance.

Clinically, V_D/V_T may assist in the management of pulmonary disease in terms of both ventilator adjustments and diagnostic testing. Suter and colleagues found that V_D/V_T decreased as the lung was recruited but increased with lung overdistention during PEEP titration in ARDS.[69] A more recent study involving the use of dead-space calculations in ARDS showed that increased dead space is associated with a higher mortality in the early and intermediate phases of ARDS.[85] Fletcher and Jonson used V_D/V_T to optimize V_T and inspiratory time settings during general anesthesia.[86] Measuring V_D/V_T may assist in identifying patients who can be removed from mechanical ventilation. Hubble and coworkers found that values less than 0.50 predicted successful extubation, and values greater than 0.65 identified patients at risk for post-extubation respiratory failure.[82]

One of the main clinical uses of V_D/V_T is to aid in the diagnosis of acute pulmonary embolism. V_D/V_T is comparable to radioisotopic lung scanning in detecting acute pulmonary embolism, with a value less than 0.40 suggesting that a significant embolus is improbable.[87] Single-breath estimates of alveolar V_D are also capable of identifying patients with pulmonary embolus.[88] Increased physiologic V_D/V_T (>0.60) was found to be significantly associated with mortality in patients with ARDS and in neonates with congenital diaphragmatic hernia.[89,90] In particular, the findings that V_D/V_T is elevated early in the course of ARDS and is associated with increased mortality may be particularly useful. The efficacy of new therapies for ARDS may be judged, in part, by their ability to reduce V_D/V_T.

TRANSCUTANEOUS MONITORING

Transcutaneous blood gas monitoring involves the use of a surface skin sensor to provide continuous noninvasive estimates of arterial Po_2 and Pco_2 (Tco_2 and $Tcco_2$, respectively). The sensor warms the skin to promote arterialization as well as to increase the permeability of the skin to oxygen and carbon dioxide (Figure 43-5). Elements of the sensor include a heating element, O_2 electrode, and a CO_2 electrode. The electrodes measure the gas tensions in an electrolyte gel located between the sensor and the skin. Similar to end-tidal CO_2 and pulse oximetry, transcutaneous monitoring has the potential advantages over direct arterial blood gas sampling of reducing the amount of blood drawn, time spent for analysis, and associated costs. $Tcco_2$ tends to be more reliable, most likely because of the greater diffusion capacity of CO_2 through the skin and the skin's own oxygen consumption.[91] $Tcco_2$ has historically been used more frequently in the neonatal and pediatric population, but recent technologic advances have led to increased utilization in adults, despite the effects of a thicker epidermis. Its use in neonates in particular has been shown to be the most accurate because of their thin, poorly keratinized skin, which has fewer diffusion barriers to capillary gases.[92]

The gradient between $TcPco_2$ and $Paco_2$ is influenced by skin perfusion and skin temperature. Thus, factors affecting cutaneous vasoconstriction could potentially influence $Tcco_2$ measurement (vasopressors, cardiac output, and cutaneous vascular resistance). Technical factors

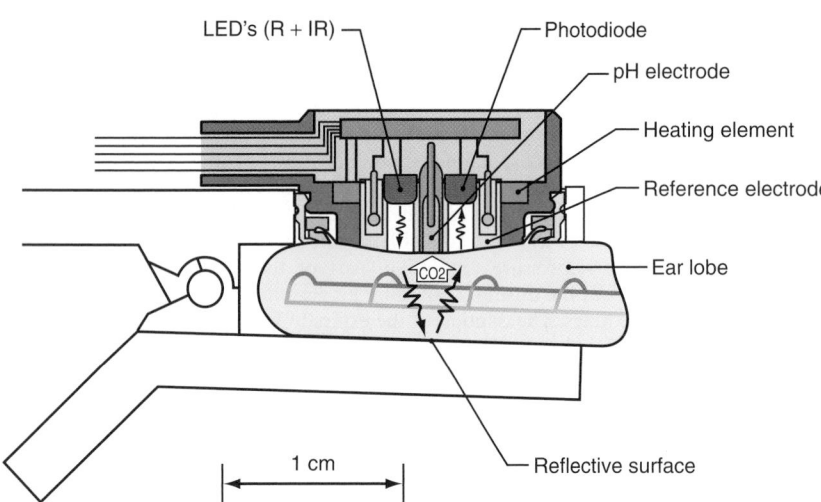

LED's (R + IR) — Photodiode
— pH electrode
— Heating element
— Reference electrode
— Ear lobe
1 cm
— Reflective surface

Figure 43-5 A combined SpO_2/$TcPCO_2$ sensor at the ear lobe. *(From Eberhard P. The design, use, and results of transcutaneous carbon dioxide analysis: current and future directions. Anesth Analg 2007;105:S48-52.)*

that can affect the accuracy of $Tcco_2$ measurements are similar to $ETCO_2$ and center around the inevitable gradient with $Paco_2$.

The accuracy of transcutaneous arterial blood gas measurement in adults remains a point of debate. A number of studies have shown that $Tcco_2$ monitoring is accurate in adult patients with respiratory disorders.[93-96] Some studies even suggest that $Tcco_2$ monitoring may be more accurate than $ETCO_2$ monitoring owing in part to elimination of dead space.[97-99] Conversely, some reports suggest that $TcPO_2$ is not accurate enough to be used clinically in the adult population or even with preterm infants.[100,101]

The use of transcutaneous arterial blood gas measurement is increasing, but it should not take the place of invasive arterial blood gas measurement; it may have a place in trending oxygenation and carbon dioxide levels. However, care must be taken to ensure that variables that could affect the readings have been eliminated and that the unit is calibrated per manufacturer specifications and when erroneous readings are suspected.

Assessment of Pulmonary Mechanics

Assessment of basic pulmonary mechanics is crucial to monitoring pulmonary function during mechanical ventilation. It requires the measurement of V_T, peak inspiratory flow rate, and four pressures: peak airway pressure, end-inspiratory plateau pressure, end-expiratory pressure in the circuit, and if intrinsic PEEP is suspected, end-expiratory pressure measured during an end-expiratory pause maneuver. From these variables, the compliance and resistance of the respiratory system are determined.

COMPLIANCE

Under conditions of passive mechanical ventilation, peak airway pressure denotes the total force necessary to overcome the resistive and elastic recoil properties of the respiratory system (i.e., both lungs and chest wall). Compliance is expressed as the ratio of volume added to pressure applied. Dynamic compliance is ratio of volume added to the peak airway pressure (Paw) and includes the resistive forces in the tracheobronchial tree. A more useful measurement is that of static compliance. Static compliance requires the use of an end-inspiratory hold.[102] During an end-inspiratory pause, peak airway pressure dissipates down to a stable plateau pressure. At the end of the inspiratory hold maneuver, "static" conditions usually exist (resistive forces have been eliminated), and the corresponding "plateau pressure" represents the elastic recoil pressure.

Dividing the V_T by the plateau pressure (Pplat) minus the PEEP yields the static compliance of the respiratory system (Crs-stat).[103] Even at moderate levels of $\dot{V}_E$ (>10 L/min), dynamic gas trapping can occur (intrinsic PEEP) and, if suspected, Crs-stat must be calculated using

total PEEP (PEEPtot) measured during an end-expiratory pause rather than the PEEP applied at the airway[104]:

$$Crs\text{-}stat = \frac{V_T}{Pplat - PEEPtot}$$

During patient-triggered ventilation, the assessment of pulmonary mechanics becomes more difficult because of the patient's spontaneous contributions, which may falsely raise or lower the plateau pressure. Obtaining an accurate measurement requires that the clinician perform the inspiratory hold when spontaneous efforts are absent and the pause will most likely be of a shorter duration.

RESISTANCE

Respiratory system resistance (Rrs) is the ratio of driving pressure to flow.[105] It is calculated as the difference between Paw and Pplat divided by the preocclusion peak inspiratory flow rate ($\dot{V}_I$) and expressed as cm H_2O/L per second[106]:

$$Rrs = \frac{Paw - Pplat}{\dot{V}_I}$$

Resistance is flow dependent because the driving pressure necessary to overcome resistance increases disproportionately to changes in $\dot{V}_I$ (due to increased turbulence).[107] Therefore, respiratory system resistance can be accurately determined only with a constant inspiratory flow (square wave) pattern.[106]

COMPLIANCE AND RESISTANCE IN NORMAL AND PATHOLOGIC CONDITIONS

In mechanically ventilated normal patients, compliance is 57 to 85 mL/cm H_2O, and resistance is 1 to 8 cm H_2O/L per second.[108-110] Abnormalities in compliance and resistance in patients with acute respiratory failure are dependent on both the cause and severity of the disease. Patients with ARDS or cardiogenic pulmonary edema tend to have a low compliance (35 or 44 mL/cm H_2O, respectively) and an elevated resistance (12 or 15 cm H_2O/L per second, respectively).[111] In contrast, patients with chronic airway obstruction tend to have both a higher compliance (66 mL/cm H_2O) and a higher resistance (26 cm H_2O/L per second).[111]

DYNAMIC GAS TRAPPING AND INTRINSIC POSITIVE END-EXPIRATORY PRESSURE

At end expiration, if the respiratory system remains above its relaxed position, gas gets trapped and the elastic recoil pressure in the lungs remains above baseline and is considered positive. This phenomenon is referred to as *intrinsic PEEP* (PEEPi).[112] PEEPi can be measured by an end-expiratory circuit occlusion whereby, after a normal expiratory time elapses, both the inspiratory and expiratory ventilator valves close for 3 to 5 seconds, allowing alveolar pressure to equilibrate with airway pressure (see Figure 43-3).[113,114] This pressure represents an average PEEPi throughout the lungs.[113,115] However, it is important to keep in mind that different degrees of intrinsic PEEP may coexist in the lungs because of regional variations in time constants from underlying pathology.[114,115] Intrinsic PEEP is more common in mechanically ventilated patients with chronic obstructive lung diseases (where dynamic hyperinflation slows elastic recoil) and patients who require high respiratory rates (where there is inadequate time for complete exhalation).

PRESSURE-VOLUME CURVES

The static pressure-volume relationship can be used to analyze the elastic properties of the respiratory system and help guide mechanical ventilation.[116] Pressure-volume (P-V) curves usually have a sigmoidal shape (Figure 43-6). When inflation begins below functional residual capacity (FRC), there is relatively little volume change as transpulmonary pressure increases. This is referred to as the *starting compliance* and corresponds to the first 250 mL of volume change.[117] It reflects either the relatively high pressure required to overcome small airway closure in the dependent lung zones or the relatively small area of aerated lung tissue as inflation commences.[117,118] Typically this low compliance segment in the P-V curve is followed by an abrupt slope change with a concave appearance that is termed the *lower inflection point*,[100] or "Pflex."[101] A common interpretation of the lower inflection point is that it signifies an abrupt reopening of collapsed peripheral

airways and alveoli.[116,118-120] Above the lower inflection point, the P-V curve becomes linear and is referred to as the *inflation compliance*.[121] As the total lung capacity is approached, compliance decreases and the P-V curve becomes convex (bow shaped). This is referred to as *end compliance*[121] and is thought to signify the loss of distensibility at maximal inflation.[118] This point is termed the *upper inflection point*.[121] As the lung is deflated, the linear portion of the curve is referred to as the *deflation compliance*, or *true physiologic compliance*, as it represents the elastic properties of the lung after full recruitment.[122] As lung deflation proceeds below FRC, an inflection point often occurs on the deflation limb that represents small-airway closure.[122] This airway closure tends to occur at a lower pressure than the lower inflection point on the inflation limb because the minimal force necessary to maintain patent airways is less than the pressure needed to recruit collapsed ones.[123]

Constructing a Pressure-Volume Curve

There are three general approaches for determining the P-V curve: the supersyringe method, constant flow method, and multiple occlusion method.[121,124,125] The supersyringe method involves the use of a large syringe that can accommodate up to 2 liters of volume. At exhalation, insufflated volume and the resulting pressures are recorded (after a 2-3 second pause at each point to eliminate the resistive forces) in a stepwise fashion (usually 100-mL increments).[125] Usually, when airway pressure reaches the 40 cm H_2O range, inflation is stopped and deflation is performed the same way. Volume steps are plotted against the corresponding static pressure points on graph paper to obtain the curve. Respiratory system compliance is the slope of the inflation and deflation curves between volumes of 0.5 and 1 L.[119] The disadvantage

Figure 43-6 Pressure-volume curves of the respiratory system of patients in various phases of acute respiratory distress syndrome. **A,** Decreased compliance and little hysteresis (early fibroproliferative phase). **B,** Almost normal compliance with large hysteresis (early exudative phase). **C,** Decreased compliance with large hysteresis (later exudative phase). **D,** Low compliance and little hysteresis (late fibroproliferative phase). *(From Bigatello LM, Davignon KR, Stelfox HT. Respiratory mechanics and ventilator waveforms in the patient with acute lung injury. Respir Care 2005;50:235-45.)*

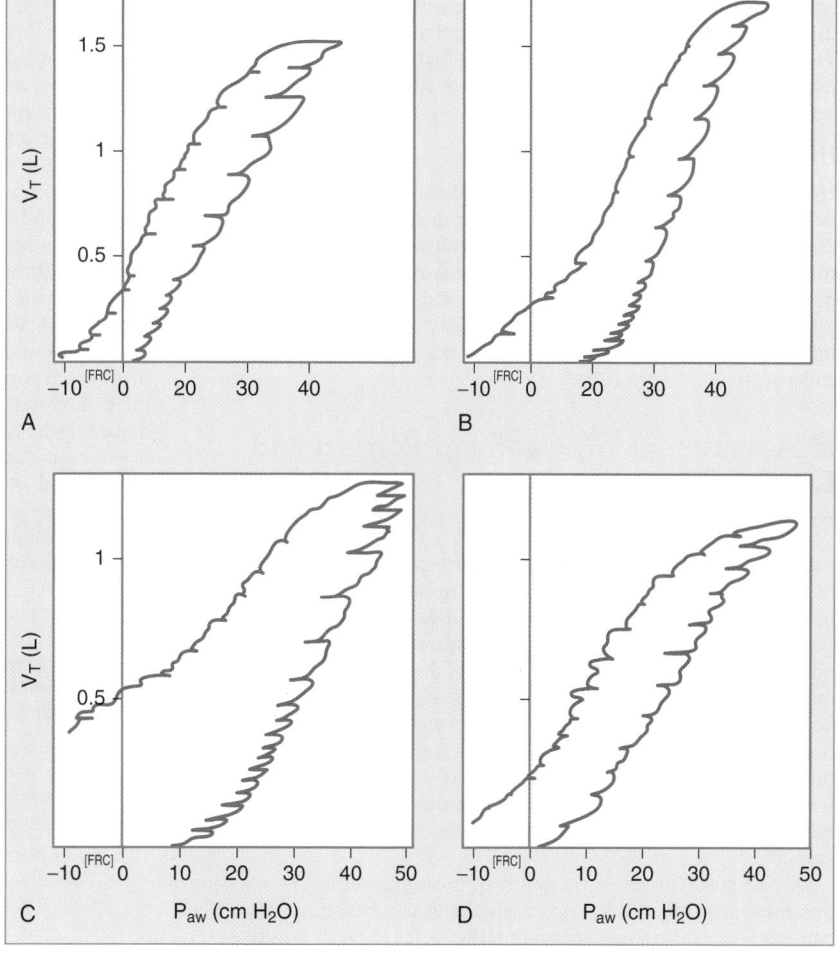

to the supersyringe method is that it requires additional equipment, the patient has to be disconnected from the ventilator, and patient paralysis is required. The constant flow method is available on some ventilators and involves the use of very low inspiratory and expiratory flows. The ventilator will then display the pressure-volume plot. Higher flows, though, will allow the viscoelastic properties of the lung to shift the curve to the right. Disadvantages to this method include the fact that some ventilators cannot control expiratory flow (the deflation limb would be inaccurate) and, in most instances, the patient will require additional sedation so as not to contribute any spontaneous efforts.

The multiple occlusion method is also done with the ventilator. It involves periodically interrupting tidal breathing at different lung volumes to obtain each pressure-volume point. The ventilator, as was the case with the constant flow method, then displays the pressure-volume plot. The advantage of this method is that both the inflation and deflation limbs are obtained, and the patient does not have to be disconnected from the ventilator. Sedation and/or paralysis is still required with this method to prevent spontaneous efforts.

Determination of Lower and Upper Inflection Points

In clinical practice, the lower inflection point of the inflation limb is usually determined by the graphic technique.[97] First, a tangent is drawn extending the slope of the starting compliance. Another tangent is drawn extending the slope of the inflation compliance down toward the horizontal axis. Where the two tangents intersect, a third tangent is drawn down to the horizontal axis, and this point is considered the lower inflection point. The same technique can be used to determine the upper inflection point on the inflation limb, as well as the deflation limb's lower inflection point. Typically, PEEP is set 2 cm H_2O above the lower inflection point to ensure optimal lung recruitment, and V_T is set below the upper inflection point to prevent lung injury from excessive stretch.[116,126] Pressure-volume curves obtained through the use of a ventilator require visual interpretation of the inflection points. The problem with visual interpretation is that the inflection points are not always completely evident. This can lead to differing interpretations among clinicians.

Hysteresis

Hysteresis refers to the difference in compliance during inflation versus deflation. Compliance tends to be higher during deflation than inflation because higher pressures may be required during inspiration to recruit collapsed alveoli. This "extra" pressure is not required during deflation to prevent derecruitment. Ultimately then, the deflation limb may be more important for setting PEEP, since the deflation limb inflection point represents the point at which the alveoli will collapse.[127]

🖼 Assessment of Breathing Pattern and Central Drive

RATE AND TIDAL VOLUME

Basic assessment of the respiratory pattern includes the measurement of respiratory rate and V_T. A normal respiratory rate is 12 to 24 breaths/min, and mechanical ventilation is generally indicated when it exceeds 35.[128] A V_T of 5 mL/kg is considered sufficient to maintain unassisted breathing.[129] Tachypnea is often the earliest sign of impending respiratory failure, even when arterial blood gases remain within normal limits.[130] This may reflect the fact that muscle fatigue (which results from a mechanical workload that exceeds the power capacity of the ventilatory muscles) occurs before overt ventilatory pump failure.[131] If untreated, a rapid-shallow breathing pattern can develop that will be progressively ineffective in maintaining acceptable arterial blood gases.[132] Of particular interest is the utility of breathing pattern in assessing the feasibility of weaning from mechanical ventilation. Typically, patients who fail to wean are more tachypneic (respiratory rate > 32)

and have an abnormally low V_T (<200 mL).[133] The respiratory rate–V_T ratio (rapid shallow breathing index [RSBI]) is a method that helps in evaluating readiness to wean. The RSBI is thought to be an accurate predictor of breathing effort.[134,135] A RSBI threshold of less than 105 has both a high positive predictive value (0.78) and negative predictive value (0.95) for the ability to maintain unassisted breathing.[136] Although the utility of RSBI has support from various studies,[137,138] the original negative predictive value, at a cutoff greater than 105, may be too low according to some.[138,139] While not an absolute predictor in and of itself, RSBI can be a valuable tool in helping to predict readiness to wean.

CENTRAL VENTILATORY DRIVE

In some situations, clinicians may want to assess the central ventilatory drive. A heightened drive will increase the patient's work of breathing during mechanical ventilation.[140] Measuring the respiratory rate will give the clinician an indication of the central ventilatory drive but not the depth of the drive. Depth of the drive can be measured by a brief (100 msec) inspiratory occlusion after the onset of an effort, called $P_{0.1}$. Briefly occluding the airway at the onset of inspiratory effort results in isometric contraction of the inspiratory muscles, so $P_{0.1}$ is independent of respiratory system mechanics.[141] Measuring airway pressure at 100 msec indirectly reflects efferent motor neuron output. An increasing stimulus to the inspiratory muscles causes a more forceful contraction, with a proportional increase in pressure development. The selection of 100 msec is based on the fact that conscious or nonconscious perception of (and response to) sudden load changes requires approximately 250 msec.[142] It is convenient that during mechanical ventilation, the lag associated with the trigger phase provides sufficient time to measure $P_{0.1}$.[143] Some ventilators[144] and pulmonary mechanics monitors[145] now measure P_{01}. Experimentally, $P_{0.1}$ has been used for closed-loop control of pressure support levels during weaning from mechanical ventilation.[146]

At rest, $P_{0.1}$ is normally 0.8 cm H_2O, whereas in patients with respiratory failure, it can range from 2 to 6 cm H_2O, depending on the level of ventilatory support.[143,145,147-150] $P_{0.1}$ correlates highly with patient work of breathing, and changes in $P_{0.1}$ (which occur with ventilator adjustments) show a high degree of sensitivity and specificity for corresponding changes in patient work.[151,152] $P_{0.1}$ has been used to predict weaning and extubation success in patients recovering from acute respiratory failure. Levels exceeding 6 cm H_2O may predict weaning failure in chronic obstructive lung disease, whereas a $P_{0.1}$ greater than 4 cm H_2O may presage failure in ARDS.[153,154]

During brief trials of unassisted breathing, a $P_{0.1}$ greater than 7 cm H_2O tends to describe patients requiring total ventilatory support and has been reported as a cutoff level in patients who ultimately fail a trial of extubation.[155] $P_{0.1}$ values between 4 and 7 cm H_2O may indicate patients who can be managed with partial ventilatory support, whereas a value less than 4 cm H_2O may indicate patients no longer in need of mechanical assistance.[154]

A limitation of $P_{0.1}$ is that it dissociates from ventilatory drive when muscle weakness is present or hyperinflation alters the force-length relationship of the inspiratory muscles.

KEY POINTS

Pulse Oximetry

1. Because pulse oximeters cannot be calibrated, their accuracy is highly variable and dependent on both the calibration curve programmed into the monitor and the quality of signal processing.

2. Carboxyhemoglobin and oxyhemoglobin absorb equivalent amounts of red light, so carbon monoxide poisoning can result in falsely elevated oxygen saturation as measured by pulse oximeter (SpO_2).

3. Motion artifact and low perfusion are the most common sources of SpO_2 inaccuracies.

4. Falsely low SpO_2 readings occur when even minor gaps exist between the probe and skin.

5. Pulse oximeters have greater bias and less precision in patients with dark pigmentation.

Capnometry

1. In normal subjects, the gradient of partial pressure of carbon dioxide in arterial blood to partial pressure of carbon dioxide in end-tidal exhaled gas ($PaCO_2$-$PETCO_2$ gradient) is 4 to 5 mm Hg, whereas in critically ill patients, the $PaCO_2$-$PETCO_2$ gradient can be markedly elevated and inconsistent, particularly in those with obstructive lung diseases (7 to 16 mm Hg).

2. The $PaCO_2$-$PETCO_2$ gradient is affected by changes in respiratory rate, tidal volume, CO_2 production, and mixed venous CO_2 content.

3. At respiratory frequencies above 30, capnometers tend to underreport the true $PETCO_2$

4. In some patients with acute respiratory distress syndrome, the $PaCO_2$-$PETCO_2$ gradient may be an effective way to titrate positive end-expiratory pressure (PEEP).

5. During pericardial compressions, $PETCO_2$ can distinguish between successful and unsuccessful resuscitation, with values greater than 10 mm Hg associated with successful resuscitation.

Assessment of Pulmonary Mechanics

1. Distinguishing resistive from elastic recoil-related pressures in the lungs requires the introduction of an end-inspiratory circuit occlusion after tidal volume delivery.

2. In clinical practice, the pause time used for an end-inspiratory circuit occlusion is set at 0.5 to 1 second to limit any potential artifact from spontaneous breathing efforts that may falsely raise or lower the end-inspiratory plateau pressure.

3. The driving pressure necessary to overcome resistance increases disproportionately to changes in gas flow, so resistance can be determined accurately only with a constant inspiratory flow (square wave) pattern.

4. Intrinsic PEEP is measured by occluding both limbs of the ventilator circuit for 3 to 5 seconds at end-expiration, thus allowing alveolar pressure to equilibrate with airway pressure. This pressure represents the average intrinsic PEEP throughout the lungs.

5. When using the pressure-volume curve of the respiratory system for lung-protective ventilation in patients with acute respiratory distress syndrome, PEEP is set 2 cm H_2O above the lower inflection point to ensure optimal lung recruitment, and tidal volume is set below the upper inflection point to prevent lung injury from excessive stretch.

Assessment of Breathing Pattern, Strength, and Central Drive

1. A threshold value of less than 105 for the respiratory rate/tidal volume ratio has both a high positive predictive value (0.78) and negative predictive value (0.95) for the ability to maintain unassisted breathing.

2. During brief trials of unassisted breathing, an inspiratory occlusion pressure 100 msec after the onset of effort ($P_{0.1}$) greater than 7 cm H_2O tends to describe patients requiring total ventilatory support and has been reported as a cutoff level in patients who ultimately fail a trial of extubation.

ANNOTATED REFERENCES

Alberti A, Gallo F, Fongaro A, et al. $P_{0.1}$ is a useful parameter in setting the level of pressure support ventilation. Intensive Care Med 1995;21:547-53.
This paper describes the potential use of $P_{0.1}$, an indirect measurement of central respiratory drive and inspiratory effort, as a simple method for both titrating the level of mechanical ventilatory support and assessing weaning tolerance.

Falk JL, Rackow EC, Weil MH. End-tidal carbon dioxide concentration during cardiopulmonary resuscitation. N Engl J Med 1988;318:607-11.
This landmark paper introduced one of most important clinical applications of capnography: the monitoring of spontaneous circulation and the effectiveness of precordial compressions in the setting of cardiac arrest. A sudden rise in end-tidal CO_2 concentration from approximately 1% to 3% (7 to 20 mm Hg) coincides with the return of spontaneous circulation.

Nuckton TJ, Alonso JA, Kallet RH, et al. Pulmonary dead-space fraction as a risk factor for death in acute respiratory distress syndrome. N Engl J Med 2002;346:1281-6.

This study provides the first evidence that a pulmonary-specific variable can independently predict the risk of death in patients with ARDS. Dead-space fraction may prove to be a useful measurement by which to judge the efficacy of future therapies for ARDS.

Pepe PE, Marini JJ. Occult positive end-expiratory pressure in mechanically ventilated patients with airflow obstruction. Am Rev Respir Dis 1982;126:166-70.
This case series report introduced one of the most crucial concepts and monitoring imperatives of invasive mechanical ventilation. This description of the mechanics and clinical implications of dynamic hyperinflation remains one of the most lucid in the critical care and pulmonary literature.

Tremper KK, Barker SJ. Pulse oximetry. Anesthesiology 1989;70:98-108.
This paper remains one of the best written on the subject of pulse oximetry. It provides clinicians with an elegant discussion of the history, physics, engineering, and clinical aspects of this technology.

REFERENCES

Access the complete reference list online at http://www.expertconsult.com.

Principles of Gas Exchange

JOHN J. MARINI | DAVID J. DRIES

The primary purpose of the lung is to allow the respiratory gases, oxygen (O_2), and carbon dioxide (CO_2) to exchange freely between gas and blood. Unless otherwise compensated by adjustments of blood flow and cardiac output, failure to maintain arterial values of O_2 and CO_2 within tolerated physiologic limits interferes with effective cellular energy production, upsets the body's chemical balance, and when severe, may be the proximate cause of lasting disability or death.

Oxygen Exchange

Most oxygen carried in the blood is bound reversibly to hemoglobin (Hb), with only a small quantity dissolved in plasma. Whereas O_2 binding by hemoglobin is essentially complete at a partial pressure (Pao_2) less than 150 mm Hg (depending on pH, temperature, and innate hemoglobin affinity), the dissolved fraction continues to rise linearly with increasing Pao_2. The equation relating blood oxygen content, expressed as milliliters per deciliter (dL), to hemoglobin concentration (grams per dL), O_2 saturation (a decimal fraction), and to the partial pressure of oxygen is:

$$Cao_2 = 1.31 \times [Hb] \, Sao_2 + 0.0031 \times Pao_2$$

Except in extreme conditions under which Hb is unable to bind O_2 (e.g., carbon monoxide intoxication, methemoglobinemia) or under which very severe anemia limits the amount of O_2 that can bind to Hb, dissolved O_2 accounts for a very small percentage of the total.[1] In fact, Hb is such an effective carrier for O_2 that the quest to develop an effective blood substitute for clinical use has been only partially successful. Intravascularly delivered products based on stroma-free Hb (an avid oxygen binder) and perfluorocarbon (an efficient dissolver of oxygen) are potentially effective but have encountered problems with stability, toxicity, and cost.[2] For the present, blood substitutes must be considered impractical for the clinical setting.

OXYGEN DELIVERY

Metabolizing tissues require an adequate supply of oxygen to efficiently produce the energy needed for cellular function. The quantity of oxygen loaded onto the arterial bloodstream per unit time (O_2 delivery) is the product of the cardiac output and the oxygen contained within each milliliter of blood. Therefore, a deficiency of either cofactor can be partially offset by a compensatory increase of the other. Conversely, sluggish blood flow, whether caused by low cardiac output or high resistance through the tissues, can limit the O_2 actually delivered to the cell. Increased blood viscosity impedes the transit of erythrocytes through the capillary bed, tending to limit oxygen consumption (Vo_2).[3] For this reason, paraproteinemia, extreme leukocytosis, and polycythemia can pose life-threatening challenges to O_2 consumption that are independent of any impact on cardiac output.[3] Studies performed in animal models demonstrate that hematocrit (Hct), a primary determinant of viscosity, bears a nonlinear relationship to oxygen delivery that varies somewhat with circulating blood volume.[4] At low values of Hct, a rising Hb concentration predictably adds to O_2 content and delivery. Above a Hct of 30% to 34%, however, it is difficult to demonstrate in critically ill patients an increase in oxygen consumption or an outcome benefit that derive from increases of O_2

content arising from further increments of Hb.[5] At an Hct of around 55% to 57%, O_2 delivery reaches its maximum in normal subjects, falling sharply with each further rise in Hct (Figure 44-1). Above an Hct of approximately 65%, phlebotomy may be required to avert a hemodynamic crisis, as vital tissues may be deprived of delivered oxygen. Viscosity, and therefore tolerance for higher Hct, is partially determined by the circulating blood volume; the polycythemia associated with intravascular volume contraction is much less well tolerated than that of polycythemia vera, a condition in which circulating blood volume is expanded.[3] As might be expected, patients with vascular disease are less tolerant to the adverse rheologic effects of high Hct.

At the mitochondrial level, oxygen acts as the terminal acceptor in a chain of organic electron donors known as *cytochromes*. The Po_2 within the mitochondrion needed to sustain this process is very low—estimated to be much less than 1 mm Hg.[6] To provide that needed level of mitochondrial oxygen tension, an appropriate oxygen diffusion gradient must be established from the arterial blood, across tissue and cellular boundaries, and into the cellular organelles. At sea level, normal levels of mitochondrial O_2 are achieved at a Pao_2 of about 95 mm Hg. The actual Po_2 within the mitochondrion, however, is affected by many factors other than arterial Po_2: tissue metabolic rate, microvascular control, tissue properties, and blood flow. Over time, varying degrees of accommodation to subnormal Pao_2 occur by adjustments of the cardiovascular system, Hb concentration, capillary system, and mitochondrial density.[7] Although this adaptive phenomenon is commonly observed in patients with chronic lung diseases, the extent to which gradual accommodation to hypoxemia can occur and should be encouraged in patients who are critically ill is a provocative and largely unexplored question.

OXYGEN TRANSFER ACROSS THE LUNG

Oxygen is driven from the airspace to the pulmonary capillary by a diffusion gradient determined by the Po_2 difference between them and the resistance to diffusion presented by the intervening tissues and fluids. To keep the alveolar O_2 tension adequate, the oxygen supplied to the alveolus must be replaced at a rate equal to or greater than that at which the oxygen is removed by the passing capillary blood. Classically, six mechanisms can account for hypoxemia:

1. Low Fio_2
2. Hypoventilation
3. Impaired diffusion capacity
4. Ventilation-perfusion imbalance
5. Shunt
6. Desaturation of pulmonary arterial (mixed venous) blood

Low Fio_2 is an important mechanism of hypoxemia occurring at altitude and in fires that occur in confined spaces. Although the relationship is not a strictly linear function, as a rough estimate, inspired O_2 declines approximately 15 mm Hg for each 1000 meters of altitude above sea level.[8] For practical purposes, however, a reduced concentration of inspired oxygen does not account for hypoxemia that occurs in the setting of critical illness. Hypoventilation alters the alveolar oxygen tension (Pao_2) in proportion to the rise of $Paco_2$ (and $Paco_2$) and becomes an important factor when it occurs during breathing of room air (as in narcotic overdose) or of relatively low inspired concentrations of supplemental oxygen (e.g., via nasal cannulae). The importance of impaired diffusion as a hypoxemic mechanism is sometimes

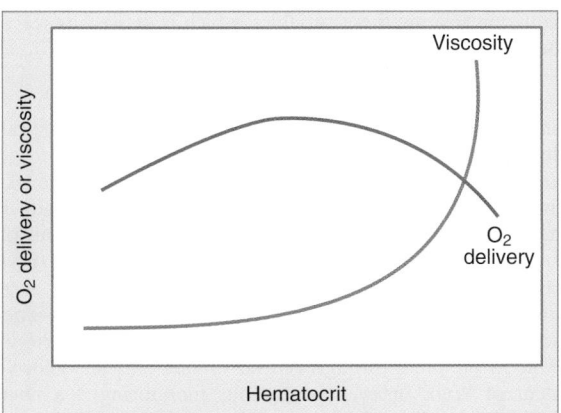

Figure 44-1 **Effect of hematocrit on viscosity and oxygen delivery.** Raising hematocrit simultaneously increases oxygen content and viscosity, which adversely affects blood rheology. Consequently, oxygen delivery reaches a maximum at hematocrit values in the upper midrange.

debated, since the transfer of O_2 from alveolus to Hb usually requires only a brief time for completion—somewhat less than the normal transit time of the erythrocyte through the capillary.[9] Yet under many conditions that are commonly encountered, fewer capillaries are available to accept the cardiac output, so the rate at which blood flows through the lung is accelerated. Simultaneously, diffusion distances are lengthened, and the driving gradient is reduced by disease. For this reason, impaired diffusion is likely to contribute to hypoxemia occurring in the stressed patient with critical illness who receives near-normal FIO_2.

Not only is ventilation perfusion (V/Q) imbalance the most common contributor to clinical hypoxemia but it is also the mechanism least well understood among practitioners. It is the relative *distribution* of ventilation and perfusion that is critical to effective oxygenation. Ventilation must take place where perfusion does, or else the same levels of each that normally allow oxygenation and alveolar ventilation may produce both hypoxemia and wasted ventilation (ventilatory dead space). With respect to impaired oxygenation, this concept is perhaps best understood by considering the fall in alveolar oxygen tension that occurs as a result of regional alveolar hypoventilation. Owing to the sigmoidal shape of the oxyhemoglobin dissociation curve, excess ventilation of normal alveoli cannot fully compensate for regional desaturation elsewhere, so the net PaO_2 declines after blood from these two types of unit admix in the pulmonary veins. Like hypoxemia due to low FIO_2, hypoventilation, and diffusion impairment, hypoxemia resulting from V/Q imbalance responds to supplementation of inspired oxygen. Poor ventilation of a given lung unit can be compensated by raising the O_2 concentration of the inspired gas it receives.

Whereas the relationship of FIO_2 to PaO_2 is more or less linear for the first three oxygen-responsive mechanisms already covered, the response to oxygen supplementation for V/Q imbalance depends on the distribution of abnormal V/Q units contributing to the problem.[10] Hypoxemia due to a relatively small number of lung units with very low V/Q characteristics may not respond noticeably to supplemental oxygen unless a very high FIO_2 is employed. Conversely, a lung comprised predominantly of lung units with mild V/Q impairment tends to respond in more linear fashion (Figure 44-2). It is also possible to convert very poorly ventilated lung units into airless, unventilated units with inspired gas having a very high FIO_2, owing to replacement of unabsorbable nitrogen with diffusible oxygen, leading to the unit's contraction and eventual collapse as this process continues below the closing volume of the compromised region (absorption atelectasis).[11] Unless compensation by hypoxic vasoconstriction is complete, raising FIO_2 can paradoxically increase shunt even as it improves O_2 transfer in units that remain patent.

Given the importance of matching blood flow to ventilation, it is not surprising that several mechanisms have developed to effect pulmonary microvascular regulation. Autonomic control, although less prominent and less precise than in the peripheral vasculature, is important nonetheless. Severe head injury, for example, can cause dysregulation and hypoxemia via this mechanism.[12] Local acidosis, such as that existing in poorly ventilated areas, tends to vasoconstrict the pulmonary arterial microvessels. The strength of this reflex, however, pales before that of hypoxic pulmonary vasoconstriction, which for most individuals is a well-developed protection against the consequences of perfusing underventilated areas.[13] These mechanisms may be overpowered by pathologic processes or by pharmacologic interventions. For example, local release of inflammatory mediators or use of certain vasoactive drugs (e.g., nitroprusside) may counter these protective reflexes,[14] and an abrupt rise of pulmonary artery pressure may overwhelm them.

Shunting occurs when systemic venous blood is not brought into close proximity with the inspired gas. Shunt can originate in the heart (e.g., through a patent communication at the atrial or ventricular level). Rarely, direct venous-to-arterial transfer occurs through micro- or macrovascular defects known as *pulmonary arteriovenous fistulae.* Such communications are encountered in relatively common diseases such as hepatic cirrhosis as well as in other settings, exemplified by the heritable Osler-Weber-Rendu abnormality. Diseases that affect the lung parenchyma are much more common causes of shunt than these cardiovascular disorders. Filling of the airspaces with fluid (e.g., edema) or cellular infiltrate (e.g., pneumonia) prevents effective gas-blood interchange. Inflammatory conditions may inhibit hypoxic vasoconstriction, worsening arterial hypoxemia, as does hypocapnic alkalosis.[15] Collapse of lung units may occur on any anatomic scale, resulting in shunt through the affected regions. Causes for collapse vary from compression (e.g., by a pleural effusion), to disease-induced surfactant depletion or inactivation, to airway plugging, such as by retained secretions or a misplaced endotracheal tube. Sustained reversal of atelectasis requires attention to the inciting cause as well as recruitment of the problem area by deep lung expansion. Pure oxygen breathing will not improve hypoxemia due to shunting. Conversely, reduction of FIO_2 will not cause shunt-related hypoxemia to worsen and may spare ventilated areas the exposure to potentially toxic concentrations of inspired O_2 (Figure 44-3).

In the clinical setting, shunting due to collapse of unstable alveolar units can be addressed by increasing transpulmonary pressure after

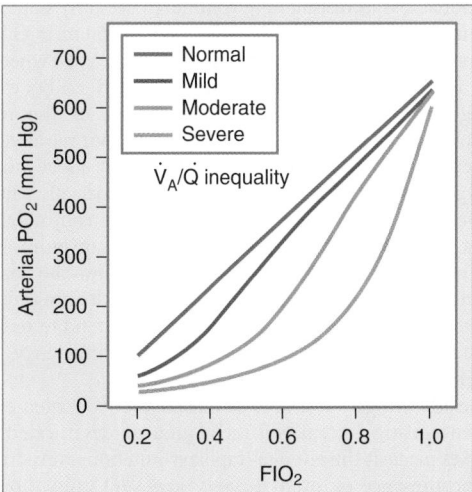

Figure 44-2 **Influence of severity of ventilation/perfusion inequality on the FIO_2/arterial PO_2 relationship.** Arterial PO_2 rises linearly in normal and mildly affected lungs, whereas very high inspired oxygen fractions may be necessary to raise arterial PO_2 when the V/Q abnormality is severe.

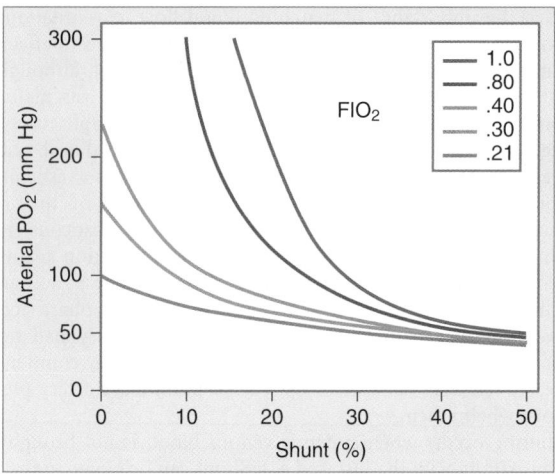

Figure 44-3 **Effect of shunt percentage on arterial Po₂ for a range of Fio₂.** When shunt percentage exceeds 35% to 40%, variations of Fio₂ only modestly affect arterial Po₂. Moreover, because the risk of oxygen toxicity rises hyperbolically with inspired oxygen concentration, reductions of Fio₂ from 1.0 to 0.8 may yield benefit with only marginal impact on arterial oxygenation.

they are reopened. Raising mean alveolar pressure by elevating end-expiratory airway pressure (positive end-expiratory pressure [PEEP]), extending the inspiratory time fraction or changing body position can be effective once the collapsible alveoli are reopened (recruited) to become part of the communicating airspace. Available evidence does not clearly indicate the best method to select PEEP in patients with hypoxemic respiratory failure. If recruitment potential is low, an increase in PEEP will have marginal effects on shunt and arterial oxygen tension. Simultaneously, higher PEEP may contribute to over-distention of open alveoli, increasing the risk of ventilator-induced lung injury (VILI) and dead-space formation as pulmonary blood flow is redirected to less well-ventilated regions. PEEP may adversely affect arterial oxygen tension in the presence of unilateral or asymmetric lung disease or when PEEP impairs venous return, limits oxygen delivery, and obligates oxygen extraction.

While the benefit of PEEP in patients with refractory hypoxemia depends on the potential for alveolar recruitment, not providing PEEP to a recumbent patient is usually inappropriate because of the associated positional loss of resting lung volume. In the early stage of hypoxemic respiratory failure, a PEEP setting of 8 to 15 cm H₂O is suitable for most patients. Higher levels of PEEP should be used when a greater potential for recruitment can be demonstrated to be effective in improving oxygen delivery and/or compliance of the respiratory system; however, PEEP above 24 cm H₂O is seldom required.

Modification of body position may dramatically affect shunting and blood oxygenation when the lungs are injured, especially when disease is asymmetrically distributed. Prone positioning routinely improves oxygen exchange by altering the distribution of transpulmonary pressure as it modifies chest wall compliance and allows the heart to sink to a dependent position that does not compress the lungs. The dorsal lung zones, which are generally the best perfused, tend to reopen when prone. Drainage of secretions and lymphatic efficiency may also improve (Figure 44-4).

With healthy lungs, variations in mixed venous oxygen content do not influence Pao₂ perceptibly; recharging of desaturated Hb with oxygen takes place at the alveolar-capillary junction, even during exercise. In the presence of shunt or very low V/Q units, however, the influence of mixed venous oxygen content may be profound because of its admixture with well-oxygenated pulmonary venous blood. Because mixed venous O₂ content is influenced primarily by the ratio of oxygen consumption to oxygen delivery, hypoxemia may be at least partially alleviated by reducing O₂ demand or improving O₂ delivery.

The equation relating these variables, which is derived by rearrangement of the Fick equation for oxygen, is:

$$S\overline{v}o_2 \approx Sao_2 - Vo_2/([Hb][Sao_2] \times Q)$$

On-line measurements of $S\overline{v}o_2$ with a fiberoptic Swan-Ganz catheter enable venous desaturation to be detected and monitored.

Venous oxygen saturation is a clinical tool to evaluate the relationship between oxygen uptake and delivery for the whole body. In the absence of pulmonary artery catheter–derived mixed venous oxygen saturation ($S\overline{v}o_2$), the central venous oxygen saturation ($Scvo_2$) is increasingly being used as an imprecise but convenient surrogate measure. Central venous catheters are simpler to insert, less expensive, and associated with fewer complications than pulmonary artery catheters. Blood sampling through central venous catheters allows measurement of $Scvo_2$ or even continuous monitoring if a fiberoptic oximetric catheter is used. The normal range for $S\overline{v}o_2$ is 68% to 77%, and $Scvo_2$ is considered to be approximately 5% above these values.[16,17]

A decrease in Hb is associated with a decrease in oxygen delivery when cardiac output remains unchanged, since oxygen delivery is the product of cardiac output and arterial oxygen content. A decrease in Hb is one of four determinants responsible for a decrease in $S\overline{v}o_2$ (or $Scvo_2$). Anemia can act alone or in combination with hypoxemia, increased oxygen consumption, or reduced cardiac output. When oxygen delivery decreases, oxygen consumption is maintained (at least initially) by an increase in oxygen extraction (O_2ER). O_2ER and $S\overline{v}o_2$ are linked by a simple equation:

$$O_2ER \approx (Sao_2 - S\overline{v}o_2)/Sao_2, \text{ or even simpler:}$$

$$O_2ER \approx 1 - S\overline{v}o_2 \text{ if we assume that } Sao_2 \text{ approximates unity}$$

In human studies, dysoxia is usually present when $S\overline{v}o_2$ falls below 45%. Tissue oxygen privation may occur at higher levels of $S\overline{v}o_2$ when oxygen extraction is impaired. Ideally, efforts to boost cardiac output (by intravenous fluids or inotropes), Hb, and/or arterial oxygen saturation return $S\overline{v}o_2$ to levels above 65% (or $Scvo_2$ to ≥70%).[16,18]

Relationship of Po₂ to Blood O₂ Content

Even though the oxyhemoglobin dissociation relationship is implicitly used for clinical decision making, there are important nuances (Figure 44-5). Over the clinically relevant range, the oxyhemoglobin dissociation curve is highly nonlinear, so that a drop of a few percentage points in Sao₂ over the 95% to 100% interval reflects a much larger change

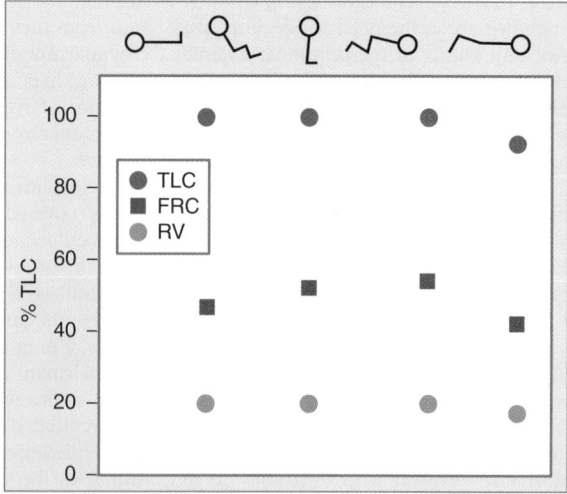

Figure 44-4 **Lung volumes in various body positions.** Compression by the abdominal viscera compresses the dependent (dorsal) lung in the supine position, decreasing the functional residual capacity (FRC). Changing body position modifies both chest wall compliance and resting lung volume. RV, residual volume; TLC, total lung capacity.

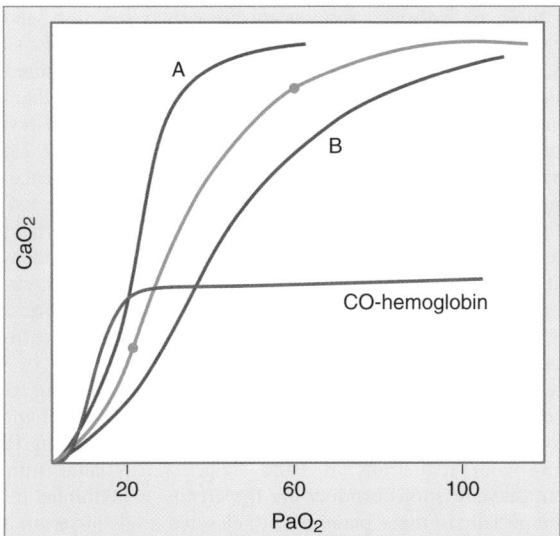

Figure 44-5 **Relationship of Pa_{O_2} to blood oxygen content (Ca_{O_2}).** The oxyhemoglobin dissociation curve normally plateaus at a P_{O_2} of approximately 100 mm Hg *(upper solid line)*. Alkalosis and hyperthermia (A) shift the relationship up and to the left, whereas acidosis and hyperthermia (B) shift it downward to the right. Carbon monoxide causes tighter binding of oxygen to hemoglobin (Hb) but reduces the capacity of Hb to bind oxygen.

in Pa_{O_2} than does a similar decrement that occurs over the 80% to 85% interval. Pulse oximeters record the relative absorption of light by oxyhemoglobin and deoxyhemoglobin. For a fixed value of Hb, the O_2 saturation parallels its relative O_2 content, but a high saturation guarantees neither its total O_2 content nor the adequacy of tissue O_2 delivery. For example, a patient may have a "full" Sa_{O_2} after inhaling a high concentration of carbon monoxide, and yet directly measuring arterial oxygen *content* per deciliter of blood (e.g., using a co-oximeter) may demonstrate profound arterial O_2 depletion (see Figure 44-5). Moreover, a patient in circulatory shock may maintain a perfectly normal Sa_{O_2} despite serious O_2 privation. Because cyanide blocks the uptake of oxygen by the tissues, O_2 consumption is low in cyanide poisoning, even though arterial and mixed venous saturations are normal or increased. It is occasionally forgotten that arterial oxygen saturation bears no direct relationship to the adequacy of ventilation; a patient breathing a high inspired concentration of oxygen will maintain a nearly normal Sa_{O_2} for a brief period in the face of a full respiratory arrest.

Controversy has surrounded the concept of supply dependency of oxygen consumption for patients who have sustained trauma, massive surgery, or sepsis. Prognosis in these conditions is somewhat better for critically ill patients in whom higher oxygen delivery is manifest. By inference, it has been suggested that in these settings, supranormal oxygen delivery is needed to satisfy the oxygen demands of key vital organs. There is little doubt that prompt and vigorous resuscitation must be carried out, or that patients who do not spontaneously generate sufficient oxygen delivery or who cannot extract oxygen effectively have a worse prognosis than other patients undergoing the same stress who do. But it is inappropriate to sustain oxygen delivery at supranormal values in critically ill patients. Some data even suggest potential harm.[18]

A multicenter Italian trial demonstrated that aggressive fluid administration toward supranormal values for oxygen delivery conferred no routine benefit for patients in the medical/critical care unit.[19] For nonmoribund patients with sepsis and/or acute respiratory distress syndrome (ARDS), supply dependency may not, in fact, exist. Therefore, without better evidence, maximizing oxygen delivery cannot be accepted as a goal for circulatory support in patients admitted to the

ICU. An often cited study of patients in septic shock provides strong evidence in support of aggressive, early resuscitation in improvement of outcome. This trial was directed at early normalization of central venous oxygen saturation rather than a supranormal physiologic response.[20]

Two studies emanating from a large National Institutes of Health (NIH)-sponsored multicenter trial provide additional data in regard to fluid resuscitation and end-organ function. In the first, fluid management protocols compared the impact of central venous versus pulmonary artery catheter monitoring in patients sustaining acute lung injury.[17] Mortality in the first 60 days was similar in patients whose fluid management was guided by data from central venous and pulmonary arterial catheters. Pulmonary artery catheter–guided therapy did not improve outcomes for patients in shock at the time of enrollment in the study. There were no differences between groups in renal or pulmonary function or the use of other end-organ support. Patients receiving pulmonary artery catheterization experienced approximately twice as many catheter-related complications (mainly arrhythmias). In the second article from this seminal study, conservative and liberal strategies for fluid management were compared in patients with acute lung injury. In this trial, the difference in fluid administration was approximately 7 liters over 7 days. The rate of death at 60 days was comparable between patients receiving a conservative fluid administration strategy and a more liberal fluid administration strategy. Conservative fluid management was associated with improved pulmonary function, reduced duration of mechanical ventilation, and shorter ICU stay. These outcomes were achieved without increasing the incidence or severity of nonpulmonary organ failure.[21]

ASSESSING THE EFFICIENCY OF OXYGEN EXCHANGE

Mean alveolar oxygen tension (PA_{O_2}) must first be computed to judge the efficiency of gas exchange across the lung. The ideal PA_{O_2} is obtained from the modified alveolar gas equation:

$$PA_{O_2} = PI_{O_2} - (Pa_{CO_2}/R) + [(Pa_{CO_2} \times FI_{O_2} \times (1-R)/R)]$$

where R is the respiratory exchange ratio, and PI_{O_2} is the inspired oxygen tension adjusted for FI_{O_2} and water vapor pressure at body temperature (47 mm Hg at 37°C). Therefore,

$$PI_{O_2} = (\text{barometric pressure} - 47) \times FI_{O_2}$$

Under steady-state conditions, R normally varies from around 0.7 to 1.0, depending on the mix of metabolic fuels (see later discussion). When the same patient is monitored over time, R generally is assumed to be 0.8 or neglected entirely. Under most clinical conditions, the alveolar gas equation can be simplified to:

$$PA_{O_2} = PI_{O_2} - (1.25 \times Pa_{CO_2})$$

For example, at sea level with a normally ventilated patient breathing room air:

$$PA_{O_2} = 0.21 \times (760 - 47) - 1.25 \times (Pa_{CO_2}) = 150 - (1.25 \times 40)$$
$$\cong 100 \text{ to } 110 \text{ mm Hg}$$

Alveolar-Arterial Oxygen Tension Difference P(A-a)O₂

The difference between alveolar and arterial oxygen tensions, $P(A-a)_{O_2}$, takes account of alveolar CO_2 tension, thereby eliminating hypoventilation and hypercapnia from consideration as the sole cause of hypoxemia. However, a single value of $P(A-a)_{O_2}$ does not characterize the efficiency of gas exchange across all FI_{O_2} values—even in normal subjects. The $P(A-a)_{O_2}$ normally ranges from approximately 10 mm Hg (on room air) to approximately 100 mm Hg (on an FI_{O_2} of 1.0). Moreover, PA_{O_2} changes nonlinearly with respect to FI_{O_2} as the extent of V/Q mismatch increases. Thus, when the V/Q abnormality is severe and nonhomogeneously distributed among gas exchanging units, the PA_{O_2} may vary little with FI_{O_2} until high fractions of inspired oxygen are given (see Figure 44-2). Finally, the $P(A-a)_{O_2}$ may be influenced by fluctuations in *venous* oxygen content.

Simplified Measures of Oxygen Exchange

Several pragmatic approaches have been taken to simplify bedside assessment of O_2 exchange efficiency. The first is to quantitate $P(A\text{-}a)O_2$ during the administration of pure O_2. After a suitable wash-in time (5-15 minutes depending on the severity of the disease), shunt (uncontaminated by V/Q mismatch) accounts for the entire $P(A\text{-}a)O_2$. Furthermore, if Hb is fully saturated with O_2, dividing the $P(A\text{-}a)O_2$ by 20 approximates shunt percentage (at $FIO_2 = 1$). As pure O_2 replaces alveolar nitrogen, some patent but poorly ventilated units may collapse—the process of absorption atelectasis.[11] Moreover, because shunt percentage is affected by changes in cardiac output and mixed venous O_2 saturation, these simplified measures may give a misleading impression of changes within the lung itself.

The Pao_2/FIO_2 (or "P/F") ratio is a convenient and widely used bedside index of oxygen exchange that attempts to adjust for fluctuating FIO_2. However, although simple to calculate, this ratio is affected by changes in PEEP and variations in $S\bar{v}O_2$ and does not remain equally sensitive across the entire range of FIO_2—especially when shunt is the major cause for admixture. Another easily calculated index of oxygen exchange properties, the Pao_2/PAo_2 (or "a/A") ratio, offers similar advantages and disadvantages as FIO_2 is varied. Like the P/F ratio, it is a useful bedside index that does not require blood sampling from the central circulation but loses reliability in proportion to the degree of shunting. Furthermore, in common with all measures that calculate an "ideal" PAo_2, even the a/A ratio can be misleading when fluctuations occur in the primary determinants of $S\bar{v}O_2$ (Hb and the balance between oxygen consumption and delivery).

None of the indices discussed thus far account for changes in the functional status of the lung that result from alterations in PEEP, auto-PEEP, or other techniques for adjusting average lung volume (e.g., inverse ratio ventilation, lateral or prone positioning). If the objective is to categorize the severity of disease or to track the true O_2 exchange status of the lung in the face of such interventions, the P/F ratio falls short. The oxygenation index (OI):

$$OI = (FIO_2 \times \text{mean Paw})/Pao_2$$

takes mean airway pressure (mean Paw) resulting from PEEP and inspiratory time fraction into account. This calculation has gained popularity in neonatal and pediatric practice but has yet to be widely used in adult critical care. Although preferable to the unadjusted P/F ratio, this index too is imperfect; mean airway pressure and FIO_2 bear complex and nonlinear relationships to Pao_2 when considered across their entire ranges.

Carbon Dioxide Exchange

PHYSIOLOGIC EFFECTS OF CO2

Carbon dioxide, the major waste product of oxidative metabolism, is a relatively well-tolerated gas. Apart from its key role in regulation of ventilation, the clinically important effects of CO_2 relate to changes in cerebral blood flow, pH, and adrenergic tone. Hypercapnia dilates the cerebral vessels and hypocapnia constricts them—a point of importance for patients with raised intracranial pressure. Acute increases in CO_2 depress consciousness, probably as the result of intraneuronal acidosis. Slowly developing increases in CO_2 can be easily endured, presumably because buffering has time to occur. Nonetheless, a higher $Paco_2$ signifies alveolar hypoventilation which tends to cause associated decreases in alveolar and arterial Po_2. With hypoxemia and acidosis compensated by supplemental oxygen and compensatory retention of bicarbonate, some outpatients with $Paco_2$ levels that chronically exceed 90 mm Hg continue to lead active lives. Conversely, patients with renal insufficiency lack the ability to buffer carbonic acid and tolerate hypercapnia poorly.

The adrenergic stimulation that accompanies acute hypercapnia causes cardiac output to rise and peripheral vascular resistance to increase. During acute respiratory acidosis, these effects may partially offset those of hydrogen ion on cardiovascular function, allowing better tolerance of lower pH than with metabolic acidosis of a similar degree. Constriction of glomerular arterioles also occurs by adrenergic stimulation, producing oliguria in some patients. Plethora, diaphoresis, muscular twitching, asterixis, and seizures may be observed at extreme levels of hypercapnia in patients made susceptible by electrolyte or neural disorders. Prompted by a favorable experience with "permissive hypercapnia" on important clinical outcomes of life-threatening asthma[22] and ARDS,[23] considerable attention has been directed toward the beneficial actions of CO_2 as an antioxidant and antiinflammatory agent.[24,25] It is conceivable that in selected circumstances, hypercapnia may not only be acceptable but desirable.

The major cardiovascular effects of acute hypocapnia relate to alkalosis and diminished cerebral blood flow.[26] Abrupt lowering of $Paco_2$ reduces cerebral blood flow and raises neuronal pH, altering cortical and peripheral nerve function. Lightheadedness, circumoral and fingertip paresthesia, and muscular tetany can result in this setting. Rarely, sudden major reductions of $Paco_2$ (e.g., shortly after initiating mechanical ventilation) produce life-threatening arrhythmias and seizures, especially in those patients with elevated levels of serum bicarbonate. Because of the importance of adrenergic compensation for the vasodilatory effects of hypercapnic acidosis, hemodynamic manifestations of acute hypercapnia are more profound in the presence of β- and/or α-adrenergic blockade.

CO2 PRODUCTION AND STORAGE

The quantity of CO_2 produced is a function of oxygen consumption and any CO_2 that is liberated in the buffering of hydrogen ion. The metabolic exchange ratio, R, varies with the mix of metabolic fuels, with carbohydrate, protein, and fat associated with ratios of 1.0, 0.7, and 0.6 respectively. CO_2 is both more diffusible and more soluble than O_2, and most CO_2 carried in the blood is in dissolved form. A smaller but very significant proportion of CO_2 is bound within the erythrocyte as bicarbonate through the action of carbonic anhydrase.

As reflected by the relatively small difference between systemic venous (45 mm Hg) and arterial (40 mm Hg) concentrations, only about one-eighth of circulating CO_2 is discharged as blood passes through the lungs. Yet, because the amount dissolved CO_2 is a linear function of its partial pressure (Pco_2), large quantities of CO_2 can be efficiently extracted from relatively small quantities of blood through a gas-permeable membrane purged on its opposite side by fresh gas. This is the principle behind passive and active extrapulmonary CO_2 removal devices now commonly deployed in critical care. The ability of these devices to extract CO_2 is comparatively great relative to their capacity for oxygen loading, as the latter can only work with a potential Hb saturation difference between 25% and 50%. (As already noted, $S\bar{v}O_2$ usually ranges between 50 and 75%).

Body stores of carbon dioxide are far greater than those of oxygen. When breathing room air, only about 1.5 L of O_2 are stored (much of it in the lungs), and some of this stored O_2 remains unavailable for release until life-threatening hypoxemia is underway. Although breathing pure O_2 can fill the alveolar compartment with an additional 2 to 3 L of oxygen (a safety factor during apnea or asphyxia), these O_2 reserves are still much less than the 120 L or so of CO_2 normally stored in body tissues. Because of limited oxygen reserves, Pao_2 and tissue Po_2 change rapidly during apnea at a rate that is highly dependent on FIO_2.

Carbon dioxide stores are held in several forms (dissolved, bound to protein, fixed as bicarbonate) and distributed in compartments that differ in their volumetric capacity and ability to exchange CO_2 rapidly with the blood.[27] Well-perfused organs constitute a small reservoir for CO_2 that is capable of quick turnover; skeletal muscle is a larger compartment with sluggish exchange, and bone and fat are high capacity chambers with very slow filling and release. From a practical point of view, the existence of large CO_2 reservoirs with different capacities and time constants of filling and emptying means that equilibration to a new steady-state $Paco_2$ after a step change in ventilation (assuming a constant rate of CO_2 production, VCO_2) takes longer than generally

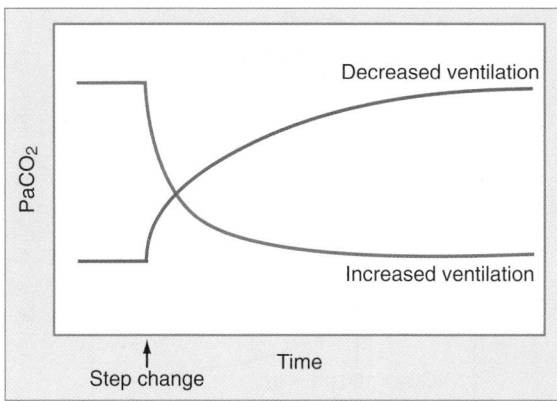

Figure 44-6 Effect of step changes of ventilation on $Paco_2$. A stepped increase in ventilation will cause $Paco_2$ to fall in approximately exponential fashion. A stepped decrease in ventilation will cause $Paco_2$ to approach equilibrium exponentially at a slower rate that is influenced by the magnitude of CO_2 storage capacity and CO_2 production.

appreciated—especially for step *reductions* in alveolar ventilation (Figure 44-6). With such a large capacity and only a modest rate of metabolic CO_2 production, the CO_2 reservoir fills rather slowly, so that $Paco_2$ rises only 6 to 9 mm Hg during the first minute of apnea and 3 to 6 mm Hg each minute thereafter. Depletion of this reservoir can occur at a considerably faster rate.

Measurement of CO_2 excretion is valuable for metabolic studies, computations of dead-space ventilation, and evaluation of hyperpnea. Estimates of CO_2 production are representative when the sample is collected carefully in the steady state over adequate time. The rate of CO_2 elimination is a product of minute ventilation ($\dot{V}E$) and the expired fraction of CO_2 in the expelled gas. If gas collection is timed accurately and the sample is adequately mixed and analyzed, an accurate value for excreted CO_2 can be obtained. However, whether this value faithfully represents metabolic CO_2 production depends on the stability of the patient during the period of gas collection—not only with regard to VO_2, but also in terms of acid-base fluctuations, perfusion constancy, and ventilation status with respect to metabolic needs. During acute hyperventilation or rapidly developing metabolic acidosis, for example, the rate of CO_2 excretion overestimates metabolic rate until surplus body stores of CO_2 are washed out or bicarbonate stores reach equilibrium. The opposite situation occurs during abrupt hypoventilation or transient reduction in cardiac output.

EFFICIENCY OF CO_2 EXCHANGE

The volume of CO_2 produced by the body tissues varies with metabolic rate (and is affected by conditions such as fever, pain, agitation, and sepsis). In the mechanically ventilated patient, many vagaries of CO_2 flux can be eliminated by controlling ventilation and quieting muscle activity with deep sedation with or without paralysis. $Paco_2$ must be interpreted in conjunction with the $\dot{V}E$. For example, the gas exchanging ability of the lung may be unimpaired even though $Paco_2$ rises when reduced alveolar ventilation is the result of diminished respiratory drive or marked neuromuscular weakness. As already noted, alveolar and arterial CO_2 concentrations respond quasi-exponentially after step changes in ventilation, with a half-time of about 3 minutes during hyperventilation, but a slower half-time (16 minutes) during hypoventilation.[28] These differing time courses should be taken into account when sampling blood gases after making ventilator adjustments.

Dead Space

The *physiologic dead space* (VD) refers to the "wasted" portion of the tidal breath that fails to participate in CO_2 exchange. A breath can fail to accomplish CO_2 elimination either because fresh (CO_2-free) gas is

not brought to the alveoli or because fresh gas fails to contact systemic venous blood. Thus, tidal ventilation is wasted whenever CO_2-laden gas is recycled to the alveoli with the next tidal breath. Alternatively, a portion of the tidal volume is wasted if fresh gas distributes to inadequately perfused alveoli so that CO_2-poor gas is exhausted during exhalation (Figure 44-7). If this concept is understood, it becomes clear why VD should not be considered as a composite of physical volumes. Nonetheless, wasted ventilation traditionally is characterized as the sum of the "anatomic" (or "series") dead space, and the "alveolar" dead space. Because the airways fill with CO_2-containing alveolar gas at the end of the tidal breath, the physical volume of the airways corresponds rather closely to their contribution to wasted ventilation (the series or "anatomic" dead space) provided that mixed alveolar gas is similar in composition to the gas within a well-perfused alveolus. This is almost true for a quietly breathing normal subject in whom the alveolar dead space (poorly perfused alveolar volume) is very small. When the lung parenchyma is well aerated and well perfused, the anatomic dead space is relatively fixed at approximately 1 mL per pound (0.4 kg) of body weight.[29] Of note, patients with endotracheal tubes and tracheostomies have less series dead space, while those with attached breathing apparatus may have more.

Anatomic dead space becomes an important concern at very low tidal volumes. For patients with lung disease that affects the lung parenchyma, and those ventilated at pressures that overinflate some lung units, alveolar dead space predominates. In these settings, the lung is composed of well-perfused and poorly perfused units, so the *mixed* alveolar gas within the airways at end exhalation has a CO_2 concentration lower than that of pulmonary arterial blood.

For normal subjects, dead space increases with advancing age and body size and is reduced modestly by recumbency, extended breath holding, and decelerating inspiratory gas flow patterns. External

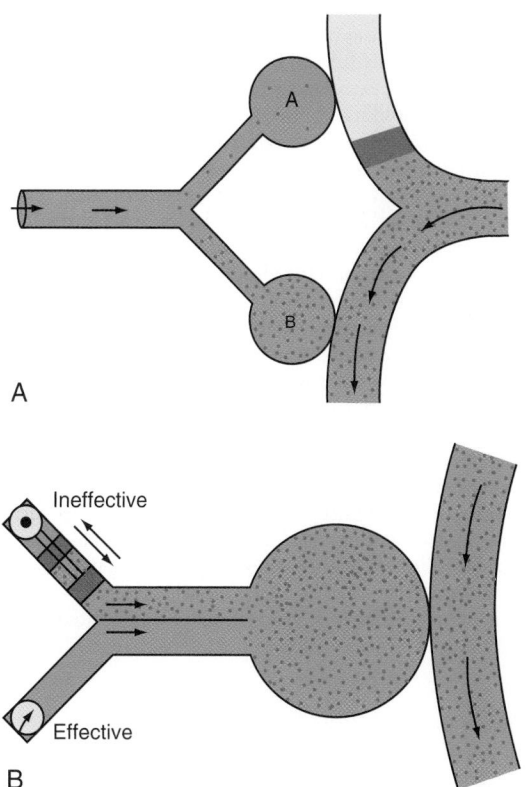

Figure 44-7 Concept of ventilatory dead space. A, Wasted ventilation (dead space) develops as the result of inadequate perfusion (alveolar compartment A, upper panel) or **B,** from the failure of ventilation to eliminate carbon dioxide from the conducting airways (lower panel). In both instances efforts expended in ventilation do not result in effective CO_2 elimination from the affected lung units.

apparatus attached to the airway that remains unflushed by fresh gas may add to the series dead space, whereas tracheostomy reduces it. The supine position reduces dead space by decreasing the average size of the lung and by increasing the number of well-perfused lung units.

Numerous diseases increase V_D. Destruction of alveolar septae, low-output circulatory failure, pulmonary embolism, pulmonary vasoconstriction or vascular compression, and mechanical ventilation with high tidal volumes or PEEP are common mechanisms that often act in combination to increase V_D.

Dead-Space Fraction

In the setting of parenchymal lung disease, dead space varies in proportion to tidal volume over a remarkably wide range. Series dead space tends to remain fixed but generally constitutes a small percentage of the total physiologic V_D, and is overwhelmed by the alveolar dead space component. Therefore, except at very small tidal volumes or when extensive tidal recruitment of collapsed units occurs, the *fraction* of wasted ventilation (V_D/V_T) tends to remain relatively constant as the depth of the breath varies. The dead-space fraction can be estimated from analyzed specimens of arterial blood and mixed expired (P_{ECO_2}) gas:

$$(V_D/V_T) = (Pa_{CO_2} - P_{ECO_2})/Pa_{CO_2}$$

where P_{ECO_2} is the CO_2 concentration in mixed expired gas. (This expression is known as the *Enghoff-modified Bohr equation*.) As already noted, P_{ECO_2} can be determined on a breath-by-breath basis if exhaled volume is measured simultaneously. Alternatively, exhaled gas can be collected over a defined period. The P_{CO_2} of gas exiting a mixing chamber attached to the expiratory line provides a continuous "rolling average" value. In collecting the expired gas sample during pressurized ventilator cycles, an adjustment should be made for the volume of any sampled gas stored in the compressible portions of the ventilator circuit.

In healthy persons, the normal V_D/V_T during spontaneous breathing varies from roughly 0.35 to 0.15, depending on the factors noted earlier (e.g., position, exercise, age, tidal volume, pulmonary capillary distention, breath holding). In the setting of critical illness, however, it is not uncommon for V_D/V_T to rise to values that exceed 0.7. Indeed, increased dead-space ventilation usually accounts for most of the increase in the $\dot{V}_E$ requirement and CO_2 retention that occur in the terminal phase of acute hypoxemic respiratory failure. High and increasing dead-space values may portend an adverse outcome in ARDS.[30] Conversely, improving dead space has been reported as a propitious sign in prone positioning.[31] In addition to pathologic processes that increase dead space, changes in V_D/V_T occur during periods of hypovolemia or overdistention by high airway pressures. This phenomenon often is apparent when progressive levels of PEEP are applied to support oxygenation. Conversely, recruitment of functioning lung tissue tends to reduce the dead-space fraction. Examination of the airway pressure tracing under conditions of controlled, constant inspiratory flow ventilation may demonstrate concavity or a clear point of upward inflection, indicating overdistention, accelerated dead-space formation, and escalating risk of barotrauma. Small reductions in PEEP or tidal volume may then dramatically reduce peak cycling pressure and V_D/V_T.

Pa_{CO_2} is influenced by CO_2 production, minute ventilation, and the ventilatory dead space according to the following equation:

$$Pa_{CO_2} = (\dot{V}_{CO_2}/V_A) \times 0.863$$

In a different form:

$$Pa_{CO_2} = P_B \times \dot{V}_{CO_2}/[\dot{V}_E(1 - V_D/V_T)]$$

Here Pa_{CO_2}, V_A and P_B refer to alveolar P_{CO_2}, alveolar ventilation, and barometric pressure, respectively. In view of the hyperbolic relationship of Pa_{CO_2} to alveolar ventilation (Figure 44-8), it can be understood that relatively small changes of effective ventilation can profoundly influence Pa_{CO_2} and pH when alveolar ventilation is low and Pa_{CO_2} is high. Once Pa_{CO_2} has climbed to approximately double

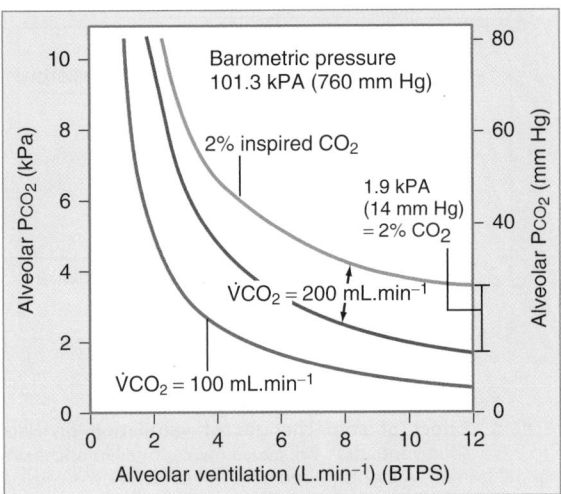

Figure 44-8 **Relationship of alveolar ventilation and alveolar CO_2.** Despite the varying conditions depicted, the hyperbolic function relating alveolar ventilation implies that small changes of effective ventilation translate into marked changes of alveolar P_{CO_2} and consequently of Pa_{CO_2} and pH.

its normal value, fluctuations of pH and Pa_{CO_2}, with their attendant adverse effects on hemodynamics and pulmonary artery pressure, place the critically ill patient at increased risk. Moreover, ventilatory drive is blunted when Pa_{CO_2} values are increased, while small changes in ventilation may cause Pa_{CO_2} to plummet. In the context of increased Pa_{CO_2}, it is interesting to consider tracheal gas insufflation (TGI), a novel technique in which fresh gas is injected near the carina so as to wash the proximal airway free of carbon dioxide during exhalation and thereby improve ventilation efficiency with little effect in inspiratory airway pressure.[32] In the setting of extreme hypercapnia, the ordinarily small improvement in alveolar ventilation that TGI affords proves valuable in reducing Pa_{CO_2} and its attendant consequences.

MONITORING OF EXHALED GAS

Capnography analyzes the CO_2 concentration of the expiratory air stream, plotting CO_2 concentration against time or, more usefully, against exhaled volume. Although most capnometers in clinical use currently display P_{CO_2} as a function of time, much of the attention will focus on the CO_2 versus volume plot because it provides more information of clinical value. After anatomic dead space has been cleared, the CO_2 tension rises progressively to its maximal value at end exhalation, a number that reflects the CO_2 tension of mixed alveolar gas. For normal subjects, the transition between phases of the capnogram is sharp, and once achieved, the alveolar plateau rises only gently. Furthermore, when ventilation and perfusion are evenly distributed, as they are in healthy subjects, end-tidal P_{CO_2} (P_{ETCO_2}) closely approximates Pa_{CO_2}, with P_{ETCO_2} normally underestimating Pa_{CO_2} by 1 to 3 mm Hg. The difference between P_{ETCO_2} and Pa_{CO_2} widens when ventilation and perfusion are matched suboptimally, so that alveolar dead-space gas admixes with CO_2-rich gas from well-perfused alveoli.

When plotted against a *volume* axis, as opposed to the more commonly encountered time axis, the capnogram offers data of considerable clinical value. Inspection of such tracings can yield estimates for the "anatomic" (Fowler) dead space, as well as for the end-tidal and mixed expired CO_2 concentrations (Figure 44-9). Knowing the barometric pressure, the mixed expired value can be expressed as a percentage of the exhaled volume, which is also immediately available from the tracing. If the V_T remains constant, the product of the P_{ECO_2}:P_B ratio and $\dot{V}_E$ is the $\dot{V}_{CO_2}$, and the mixed expired CO_2 concentration can be used in the Enghoff-modified Bohr equation to estimate the physiologic dead-space fraction.

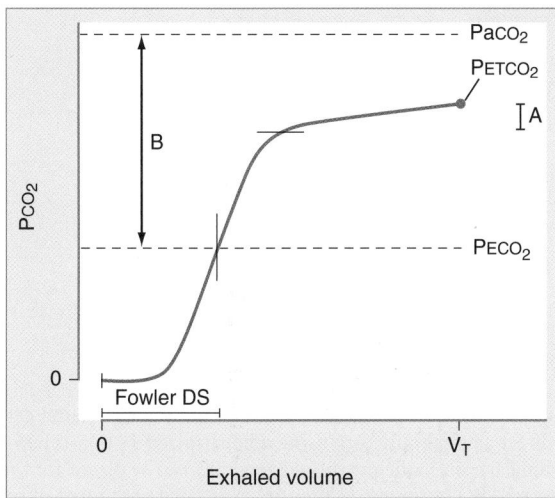

Figure 44-9 **Capnogram with expired P_{CO_2} plotted against exhaled volume.** Important data can be derived from the expired capnogram obtained under steady-state passive conditions: anatomic or "Fowler" dead-space; physiologic dead space (the difference [B] between Pa_{CO_2} and mixed expired CO_2, $P\bar{E}_{CO_2}$, expressed as a fraction of Pa_{CO_2}); slope of the "alveolar plateau" (A), an indicator of the heterogeneity of ventilation; and an estimate of CO_2 production (obtained from the product of mixed expired CO_2 referenced to total barometric pressure and exhaled volume).

As with other monitoring techniques, exhaled CO_2 values must be interpreted cautiously. The normal capnogram comprises an ascending portion, a plateau, a descending portion, and a baseline. In disease, the sharp distinctions between phases of the capnogram as well as the slopes of the composite segments are blurred. Moreover, failure of the airway gas to equilibrate with gas from well-perfused alveoli invalidates $P_{ET}_{CO_2}$ as a reflection of Pa_{CO_2}, especially as respiratory frequency fluctuates; the $P\bar{E}_{CO_2}$ per cycle, however, remains valid under these conditions. End-tidal P_{CO_2} gives a low range estimate of Pa_{CO_2} in virtually all clinical circumstances, so that a high $P_{ET}_{CO_2}$ strongly suggests hypoventilation. Abrupt changes in $P_{ET}_{CO_2}$ may reflect such acute processes as aspiration or pulmonary embolism if the $\dot{V}_E$ and breathing pattern (f, V_T, and I:E ratio) remain unchanged. Although breath-to-breath fluctuations in $P_{ET}_{CO_2}$ can be extreme, the trend of $P_{ET}_{CO_2}$ over time helps identify underlying changes in CO_2 exchange.

KEY POINTS

1. The quantity of oxygen loaded onto the arterial bloodstream per unit time (O_2 delivery) is the product of the cardiac output and the oxygen contained within each milliliter of blood. Thus, a deficiency of either cofactor can be partially offset by a compensatory increase of the other.

2. Hypoxemia due to a relatively small number of lung units with very low V/Q characteristics may not respond noticeably to oxygen therapy unless a very high F_{IO_2} is employed; however, it is possible to convert very poorly ventilated lung units into airless, unventilated units with inspired gas having a very high F_{IO_2}, owing to replacement of unabsorbable nitrogen with absorbable oxygen (absorption atelectasis).

3. In the presence of shunt or very low V/Q units, however, the influence of mixed venous oxygen content may be profound because of its admixture with well-oxygenated pulmonary venous blood.

4. Because of the hyperbolic relationship of Pa_{CO_2} to alveolar ventilation, relatively small changes of effective ventilation can profoundly influence Pa_{CO_2} and pH when alveolar ventilation is low and Pa_{CO_2} is high. Once Pa_{CO_2} has climbed to approximately double its normal value, fluctuations of pH and Pa_{CO_2}, with their attendant adverse effects on hemodynamics and pulmonary artery pressure, place the critically ill patient at risk and blunt ventilatory drive.

5. The expiratory capnogram offers data of considerable clinical value when P_{CO_2} is plotted along a volume axis: estimates for the "anatomic" (Fowler) dead space, as well as for the mixed expired CO_2 concentration used in calculations of dead-space fraction and CO_2 production.

ANNOTATED REFERENCES

Pontoppidan H, Geffin B, Lowenstein E. Acute respiratory failure in the adult. Parts 1-3. N Engl J Med 1972;287:690-8; 743-52; 799-806.
An ageless comprehensive review of physiologic principles that guide management of acute respiratory failure.
West JB. State of the art: ventilation-perfusion relationships. Am Rev Respir Dis 1977;116:919-43.
An instructive overview of the complex interrelationships between the blood and gas flows to the lung.
Gattinoni L, Brazzi L, Pelosi P, et al. A trial of goal-oriented hemodynamic therapy in critically ill patients. $S\bar{v}o_2$ Collaborative Group. N Engl J Med 1995;333:1025-32.
Increasing cardiac output toward greater than customary targeted values did not improve outcome. Many patients could not reach the therapeutic targets despite aggressive intravascular volume expansion and vasoactive drugs.

Rivers E, Nguyen B, Havstad S, et al. Early goal-directed therapy in the treatment of severe sepsis and septic shock. N Engl J Med 2001;345:1368-77.
An influential clinical trial that demonstrated the value of quickly reversing the hemodynamic compromise associated with sepsis.
Laffey JG. Protective effects of acidosis. Anaesthesia 2001;56:1013-14.
This provocative commentary reviews the experimental evidence and argues the benefit of hypercarbic acidosis on inflammation.
Nuckton TJ, Alonso JA, Kallet RH, et al. Pulmonary dead-space fraction as a risk factor for death in the acute respiratory distress syndrome. N Eng J Med 2002;346:1281-6.
High levels of ventilatory dead space were associated with greater risk for adverse or fatal outcomes.

REFERENCES

Access the complete reference list online at http://www.expertconsult.com.

45

Arterial Blood Gas Interpretation

PAUL E. MARIK

Arterial blood gas (ABG) analysis plays a pivotal role in the management of critically ill patients. Although no randomized controlled study has ever been performed evaluating the benefit of ABG analysis in the intensive care unit (ICU), it is likely this technology stands alone as the diagnostic test which has had the greatest impact on the management of critically ill patients; this has likely been translated into improved outcomes. Prior to the 1960s, clinicians were unable to detect hypoxemia until clinical cyanosis developed. ABG analysis became available in the late 1950s when techniques developed by Clark, Stow and coworkers, and Severinghaus and Bradley permitted measurement of the partial pressures of oxygen (Pao_2) and carbon dioxide ($Paco_2$) in arterial blood.[1-3] The ABG remains the definitive method to diagnose, categorize, and quantitate respiratory failure. In addition, ABG analysis is the only clinically applicable method of assessing a patient's acid-base status. ABGs are the most frequently ordered test in the ICU and have become essential to the management of critically ill patients.[4] Indeed, a defining requirement of an ICU is that a clinical laboratory should be available on a 24-hour basis to provide blood gas analysis.[5]

Indications for Arterial Blood Gas Sampling

ABGs are reported to be the most frequently performed test in the ICU.[4] There are, however, no published guidelines and few clinical studies that provide guidance as to the indications for ABG sampling.[6] It is likely that many ABGs are performed unnecessarily. Muakkassa and coworkers studied the relationship between the presence of an arterial line and ABG sampling.[7] These authors demonstrated that patients with an arterial line had more ABGs drawn than those who did not, regardless of the value of the Pao_2, $Paco_2$, the Acute Physiology and Chronic Health Evaluation (APACHE) II score, or the use of a ventilator. In that study, multivariate analysis demonstrated that the presence of an arterial line was the most powerful predictor of the number of ABGs drawn per patient independent of all other measures of the patient's clinical status. Roberts and Ostryznuik demonstrated that with use of a protocol they were able to reduce the number of ABGs by 44%, with no negative effects on patient outcomes.[4]

The ubiquitous use of pulse oximetry in the ICU has made the need for frequent ABG sampling to monitor arterial oxygenation unnecessary. Furthermore (as discussed later), venous blood gas analysis can be used to estimate arterial pH and bicarbonate (HCO_3^-) but not arterial carbon dioxide tension ($Paco_2$). Previously, ABGs were drawn after every ventilator change and with each step of the weaning process; such an approach is no longer recommended.

The indications for ABG analysis should be guided by clinical circumstances. However, as a "general rule" all patients should have an ABG performed on admission to the ICU and/or following (10-15 minutes) endotracheal intubation. Patients with respiratory failure should have an ABG performed at least every 24 to 48 hours. Patients with type II respiratory failure (see definitions later in this chapter) will require more frequent ABG sampling than those with type I respiratory failure. Furthermore, patients with complex acid-base disorders and patients undergoing permissive hypoventilation will require more frequent ABG sampling.

Arterial Blood Gas Sampling

ABG specimens may be obtained from an indwelling arterial catheter or by direct arterial puncture using a heparinized 1- to 5-mL syringe. Indwelling arterial catheters should generally not be placed for the sole purpose of ABG sampling, as they are associated with rare but serious complications. Arterial puncture is usually performed at the radial site. When a radial pulse is not palpable, the brachial or femoral arteries are suitable alternatives. Serious complications from arterial puncture are uncommon; the most common include pain and hematoma formation at the puncture site. Laceration of the artery (with bleeding), thrombosis, and aneurismal formation are rare but serious complications.[8,9]

ABG analysis is typically performed on whole blood. The partial pressure of oxygen (Pao_2), partial pressure of carbon dioxide ($Paco_2$), and pH are directly measured with standard electrodes and digital analyzers; oxygen saturation is calculated from standard O_2 dissociation curves and may be directly measured with a co-oximeter. The bicarbonate (HCO_3^-) concentration is calculated using the Henderson-Hasselbalch equation:

$$pH = pK_A + \log\{[HCO_3^-]/[CO_2]\}$$

where pK_A is the negative logarithm of the dissociation constant of carbonic acid. The *base excess* is defined as the quantity of strong acid required to titrate blood to pH 7.40 with a $Paco_2$ of 40 mm Hg at 37°C. In practice, acid is not titrated as suggested but calculated using a variety of established formulae or normograms. The base excess thus "removes" the respiratory element of acid-base disturbance and identifies the metabolic contribution to interpret with pH and [H+]. The standard bicarbonate is broadly similar and is the calculated [HCO_3^-] at a $Paco_2$ of 40 mm Hg. Although the base excess and standard bicarbonate allow for a metabolic acidosis to be diagnosed, they provide few clues as to the pathophysiology or underlying diagnosis.

As with any diagnostic test, it is important that the specimen for an ABG measurement be collected and processed correctly and that quality assurance methods exist to ensure the accuracy of the measurements. Aside from interlaboratory variation, errors in calibration and electrode contamination with protein or other fluids may alter results. Heparin is usually added to the blood to prevent coagulation, and dilution with older liquid solutions previously caused spuriously low $Paco_2$. Sample preparation is important because air bubbles falsely elevate Pao_2.

To avoid errors in blood gas interpretation, the following points must be considered before obtaining the sample:

1. *Steady state*: Blood sampling must be done during steady state following the initiation or change in oxygen therapy or changes in ventilatory parameters in patients on mechanical ventilation. In most ICU patients, a steady state is reached between 3 and 10 minutes and in about 20 to 30 minutes in patients with chronic airway obstruction.[10]
2. *Anticoagulants*: Excess of heparin may affect the pH. Only 0.05 mL is required to anticoagulate 1 mL of blood. The dead space volume of a standard 5-mL syringe with 1-inch, 22-gauge needle is 0.02 mL; filling the syringe dead space with heparin provides sufficient volume to anticoagulate a 5-mL blood sample.

Today, calibrated volumes of dry (sodium or lithium) heparin are used in ABG kits, minimizing this problem.

3. *Delay in processing of the sample*: Because blood is a living tissue, O_2 is being consumed and CO_2 is produced in the blood sample. Red blood cell glycolysis may generate lactic acid and change pH. Significant increases in $Paco_2$ and decreases in pH occur when samples are stored at room temperature for more than 20 minutes. In circumstances when a delay in excess of 20 minutes is anticipated, the sample should be placed in ice; iced samples can be processed up to 2 hours after collection without affecting the blood gas values.

4. *Venous sampling*: Arterial blood provides more information than venous blood with regard to acid-base and oxygenation status (see later discussion). At times it may be difficult to distinguish arterial from venous blood. The following points may help in recognizing inadvertent venous sampling:
   - Failure to observe a flash of blood on entry into vessel or pulsation during syringe filling
   - Incompatibility of values with clinical condition
   - Low Pao_2 and high $Paco_2$
   - Spo_2 by pulse oximetry more than Sao_2 by ABG analysis
   When in doubt, simultaneous sampling of arterial and venous blood should help solve this problem.

5. *Collection equipment and technique*: Increased dead space in the syringe lowers $Paco_2$ content. Needle size rarely causes variability; however, a smaller (25 g) needle is recommended. In patients with an indwelling arterial line, a discard volume of at least twice the dead space (priming volume from sample port to catheter tip) is required to prevent sample dilution.[11]

6. *Hypotension*: Severe hypotension may require forceful aspiration, and results—particularly for Pao_2—may be falsely low.

7. *Hyperventilation*: Hyperventilation resulting from anxiety and/or pain may acutely alter results from baseline values.

8. *Leukocytosis*: Leukocytosis accelerates the decline of Pao_2 and pH and elevation of $Paco_2$ within a stored sample. This Pao_2 decrease is more pronounced at higher Pao_2 levels, is attributable to cellular oxygen consumption, and may be attenuated when samples are stored at colder temperatures.

9. *Hypothermia*: Blood gas values are temperature dependent, and if blood samples are warmed to 37°C before analysis (as is common in most laboratories), Po_2 and Pco_2 will be overestimated and pH underestimated in hypothermic patients. The following correction formulas can be used:
   - Subtract 5 mm Hg Po_2 per 1°C that the patient's temperature is less than 37°C.
   - Subtract 2 mm Hg Pco_2 per 1°C that the patient's temperature is less than 37°C.
   - Add 0.012 pH units per 1°C that the patient's temperature is less than 37°C.

Arterial Blood Gas Analysis

An ABG provides a rapid and accurate assessment of oxygenation, ventilation, and acid-base status. These three processes are closely interrelated with each other, and an alteration in one process will affect the other two. However, for the sake of simplicity and ease of understanding, each will be discussed separately.

ALVEOLAR VENTILATION

The arterial CO_2 content as reflected by arterial CO_2 tension ($Paco_2$) at any given moment depends on the quantity of CO_2 produced and its excretion through alveolar ventilation (VA) and can be expressed by the equation, $Paco_2 \sim CO_2/VA$. The alveolar ventilation is that portion of total ventilation that participates in gas exchange with pulmonary blood. If it is assumed that CO_2 production is constant, then CO_2 homeostasis can be simplified to $1/VA \sim Paco_2$. Thus $Paco_2$ becomes very useful for the assessment of alveolar ventilation. High

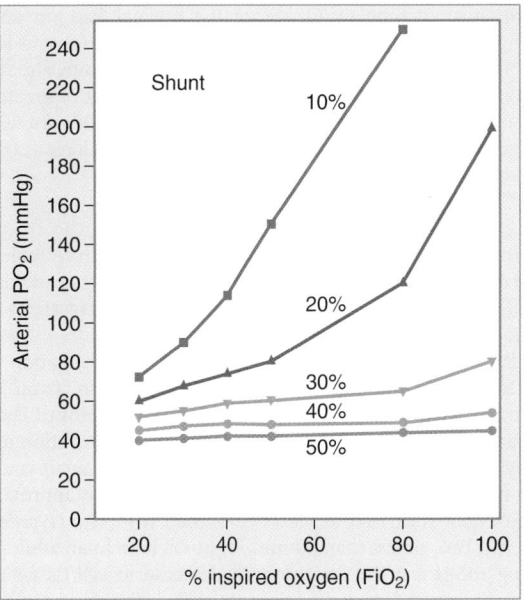

Figure 45-1 The effect on Pao_2 of increasing Fio_2 according to shunt fraction.

$Paco_2$ (>45 mm Hg) indicates alveolar hypoventilation, and low $Paco_2$ (<35 mm Hg) implies alveolar hyperventilation.

OXYGENATION

The ultimate aim of the cardiorespiratory system is to provide adequate delivery of oxygen to the tissues. This is largely dependent upon cardiac output, hemoglobin (Hb) concentration, and Hb saturation. The Pao_2 is a measure of the oxygen tension in plasma; while the dissolved fraction makes a negligible contribution to oxygen delivery (<2%), it is a major factor affecting Hb saturation. In turn, the Pao_2 is dependent on the concentration of oxygen in the inspired air (Fio_2), oxygen exchange in the lung (V/Q mismatching), and the venous oxygen saturation ($Smvo_2$). The Pao_2 must always be interpreted in conjunction with the Fio_2 and age.

Relation Between Pao_2 and Fio_2

The Pao_2 alone provides little information regarding the efficiency of oxygen loading into the pulmonary capillary blood. The Pao_2 is determined largely by the Fio_2 and the degree of intrapulmonary shunting (Figure 45-1). The Pao_2 must therefore *always* be interpreted in conjunction with the Fio_2. The Pao_2 alone does not quantitate the degree of intrapulmonary shunt, which is required for assessing the severity of the underlying lung disease and in guiding the approach to oxygen therapy and respiratory support. There are various formulas for calculating the intrapulmonary shunt, including the classic "shunt equation," which is the gold standard but requires mixed venous sampling through a pulmonary artery catheter, and the alveolar-arterial oxygen gradient equation (Table 45-1). Clinically the Pao_2-to-Fio_2 ratio (Pao_2/Fio_2) is most commonly used to quantitate the degree of ventilation/

TABLE 45-1	Formulas for Evaluating Patients in Respiratory Failure

Age-predicted Pao_2 = Expected Pao_2 − 0.3(age − 25) [expected Pao_2 at sea level is 100 mg/Hg]
As a rough rule of thumb: Expected $Pao_2 \approx Fio_2$ (%) × 5
$AaDO_2 = (Fio_2 \times [BP^* - 47]) - (Pao_2 + Paco_2)$, where BP = barometric pressure
Pao_2/Fio_2 ratio
Oxygenation index = [(mean airway pressure × Fio_2)/Pao_2] × 100
$Vd/Vt = (Paco_2 - PEco_2)/Paco_2$ (N = 0.2-0.4)

perfusion mismatching (V/Q). Since the normal Pao_2 in an adult breathing room air with an Fio_2 of 0.21 is 80 to 100 mm Hg, the normal value for Pao_2/Fio_2 is between 400 and 500 mm Hg. A Pao_2/Fio_2 ratio of less than 200 most often indicates a shunt of greater than 20%. A notable limitation of the Pao_2/Fio_2 is that it does not take into account changes in $Paco_2$ at a low Fio_2, which tends to have a considerable effect on the ratio.

Age

The normal arterial oxygen tension decreases with age (see Table 45-1). The normal Pao_2 at sea level and breathing room air is approximately 85 to 90 mm Hg at the age of 60 and 80 to 85 mm Hg at the age of 80 years.

The Pao_2 is primarily used for assessment of oxygenation status, since Pao_2 accurately assesses arterial oxygenation from 30 to 200 mm Hg, whereas Sao_2 is normally a reliable predictor of Pao_2 only in the range of 30 to 60 mm Hg. However, oxygen saturation as measured by pulse oximetry (Spo_2) or by ABG analysis (Sao_2) is a better indicator of arterial oxygen content than Pao_2, since approximately 98% of oxygen is carried in blood combined with Hb. *Hypoxemia* is defined as a Pao_2 of less than 80 mm Hg at sea level in an adult patient breathing room air; the concomitant decrease in cell/tissue oxygen tension is known as *hypoxia* (or tissue hypoxia). The degree of hypoxia in patients with hypoxemia depends on the severity of the hypoxemia and the ability of the cardiovascular system to compensate. Hypoxia is unlikely in mild hypoxemia ($Pao_2 = 60$-79 mm Hg). Moderate hypoxemia ($Pao_2 = 45$-59 mm Hg) may be associated with hypoxia in patients with anemia or cardiovascular dysfunction. Hypoxia is almost always (but with a few exceptions) associated with severe hypoxemia (Pao_2 <45 mm Hg). However, it must be recognized that the human body has an extraordinary capacity to adapt to hypoxemia. Indeed, patients with cyanotic heart disease do not have evidence of tissue hypoxia at rest. Most remarkably, at the top of Mount Everest (29,028 ft; 253 torr) and without supplemental oxygen, experienced mountain climbers have been reported to have a mean Pao_2 of between *24 and 28* mm Hg in the absence of tissue hypoxia.[12,13]

Acute respiratory failure occurs when the pulmonary system is no longer able to meet the metabolic demands of the body. Respiratory failure is classically divided into two types:

- Type I, hypoxemic respiratory failure: $Pao_2 \leq 60$ mm Hg when breathing room air (sea level).
- Type II, hypercapnic respiratory failure: $Paco_2 \geq 50$ mm Hg.

ACID-BASE BALANCE

The normal diet generates volatile acid (CO_2), primarily from carbohydrate metabolism, and nonvolatile acid (hydrogen ion, H^+) from protein metabolism. The aim of the body's homeostatic system is to maintain pH within a narrow range, and pH homeostasis is accomplished through the interaction of the lungs, kidneys, and blood buffers. Alveolar ventilation allows for excretion of CO_2. The kidneys must reclaim filtered bicarbonate (HCO_3^-), because any urinary loss leads to gain of H^+. In addition, the kidney must excrete the daily acid load generated from dietary protein intake. Less than half of this acid load is excreted as titratable acids (i.e., phosphoric and sulfuric acids); the remaining acid load is excreted as ammonium. The blood pH is determined by the occurrence of these physiologic processes and by the buffer systems present in the body.

The history of assessing the acid-base equilibrium and associated disorders is intertwined with the evolution of the definition of an acid. In the 1950s, clinical chemists combined the Henderson-Hasselbalch equation and the Brønsted-Lowry definition of an acid to produce the current *bicarbonate ion*–centered approach to metabolic acid-base disorders.[14] Stewart repackaged pre-1950 ideas of acid-base in the late 1970s, including the Van Slyke definition of an acid.[15] Stewart also used laws of physical chemistry to produce a new acid-base approach.[14] This approach, using the strong ion difference (SID) and the concentration of weak acids (particularly albumin), pushes bicarbonate into a

minor role as an acid-base indicator rather than as an important mechanism:

$$SID = ([Na^+] + [K^+] + [Ca^{2+}] + [Mg^{2+}]) - [Cl^-] + [lactate])$$

The SID is not identical to anion gap (AG) and contains [lactate], although it does share a number of parameters, and the trends will often be close. The normal SID has not been well established, but the quoted range is 40 to 42 mEq/L.

As the SID approaches zero, anions "accumulate" and acidity increases. This approach provides a physicochemical model for "hyperchloremic acidosis" following 0.9% saline administration,[21] and the systemic alkalosis of hypoalbuminemia (regarded as a weak acid).

Most clinicians use the bicarbonate ion–centered approach for the diagnosis and management of acid-base disorders; this approach is easier to understand and more practical. Furthermore, there are no clinical data to suggest that the Steward approach has any advantages over the classic (bicarbonate) approach.[16] The Henderson-Hasselbalch equation describes the fixed interrelationship between $Paco_2$, pH, and HCO_3^- being described as *pH = pK_c log HCO_3^-/dissCO_2*. If all the constants are removed, the equation can be simplified to $pH = HCO_3^-/Paco_2$ (~Kidney/Lung). The HCO_3^- is controlled mainly by the kidney and blood buffers. The lungs control the level of $Paco_2$ by regulating the level of volatile acid, carbonic acid, in the blood. Buffer systems can act within a fraction of a second to prevent excessive change in pH. The respiratory system takes about 1 to 15 minutes and kidneys many minutes to days to readjust H^+ ion concentration.

The Anion Gap

Following the principle of electrochemical neutrality, total [cations] must equal total [anions], and so in considering the commonly measured cations and anions and subtracting them, a fixed number should be derived. The measured cations are in excess; mathematically this "gap" is filled with unmeasured anions ensuring electrochemical neutrality. There is never a "real" AG, in line with the law of electrochemical neutrality; it is rather an index of nonroutinely measured anions. The anion gap is calculated using the following formula[17]:

$$AG = [Na] - ([Cl] + [HCO_3^-]): Normal\ 10 \pm 2\ meq/L$$

Critical illness is typically associated with a rapid fall in the plasma albumin concentration. Albumin is an important contributor of the "normal" AG. Therefore, as the albumin concentration falls, it tends to reduce the size of the AG, or have an alkalinizing effect. Various corrections are available; however, Figge's AG correction (AGcorr) is most commonly used[17]:

$$Albumin\ gap = 40 - apparent\ albumin\ (normal\ albumin = 40\ g/L)$$

$$AGcorr = AG + (albumin\ gap/4)$$

A STEPWISE APPROACH TO ACID-BASE DISORDERS

Step 1: Do a Comprehensive History and Physical Exam

A comprehensive history and physical examination can often give clues as to the underlying acid-base disorder (Table 45-2). For example, patients who present with gastroenteritis manifested as diarrhea typically have a non–anion gap metabolic acidosis from loss of fluid containing HCO_3^-. Patients who present with chronic obstructive lung disease usually have underlying chronic respiratory acidosis from retention of CO_2.

Step 2: Order Simultaneous Arterial Blood Gas Measurement and Chemistry Profile

Step 3: Check the Consistency and Validity of the Results

Normal ABG results are provided in Table 45-3.

Step 4: Identify the Primary Disturbance

The next step is to determine whether the patient is acidemic (pH <7.35) or alkalemic (pH >7.45) and whether the primary process is

TABLE 45-2	Common Clinical States and Associated Acid-Base Disorders
Clinical State	*Acid-Base Disorder*
Pulmonary embolus	Respiratory alkalosis
Hypotension/shock	Metabolic acidosis (lactic acidosis)
Severe sepsis	Metabolic acidosis, respiratory alkalosis
Vomiting	Metabolic alkalosis
Severe diarrhea	Metabolic acidosis
Renal failure	Metabolic acidosis
Cirrhosis	Respiratory alkalosis
Pregnancy	Respiratory alkalosis
Diuretic use	Metabolic alkalosis
COPD	Respiratory acidosis
Diabetes	Metabolic acidosis (ketoacidosis)
Ethylene glycol poisoning	Metabolic acidosis
Post normal saline resuscitation	Metabolic acidosis (non–anion gap)

TABLE 45-4	Acid-Base Disorders	
Acid-Base Disorder	*Criteria*	
Respiratory acidosis	$Paco_2$ >45 mm Hg	
Respiratory alkalosis	$Paco_2$ <35 mm Hg	
Acute respiratory failure	$Paco_2$ >45 mm Hg; pH < 7.35	
Chronic respiratory failure	$Paco_2$ >45 mm Hg; pH 7.36-7.44	
Acute respiratory alkalosis	$Paco_2$ <35 mm Hg; pH > 7.45	
Chronic respiratory alkalosis	$Paco_2$ <35 mm Hg; pH 7.36-7.44	
Acidemia	pH <7.35	
Alkalemia	pH >7.45	
Acidosis	HCO_3 <22 mEq/L	
Alkalosis	HCO_3 >26 mEq/L	

metabolic (initiated by change in HCO_3^-) or respiratory (initiated by a change in $Paco_2$) (Table 45-4).

Step 5: Calculate the Expected Compensation

Any alteration in acid-base equilibrium sets into motion a compensatory response by either the lungs or the kidneys. The compensatory response attempts to return the ratio between $Paco_2$ and HCO_3^- to normal and thereby normalize the pH. Compensation is predictable; the adaptive responses for the simple acid-base disorders have been quantified experimentally[18] (Table 45-5). Determine whether the compensatory response is of the magnitude expected—that is, is there a secondary (uncompensated) acid-base disturbance?

Step 6. Calculate the "Gaps"

Calculate the Anion Gap. In high-AG metabolic acidosis, acid dissociates into H^+ and an unmeasured anion. H^+ is buffered by HCO_3^-, and the unmeasured anion accumulates in the serum, resulting in an increase in AG. In non–AG metabolic acidosis, H^+ is accompanied by Cl^- (a measured anion); therefore, there is no change in AG. Acid-base disorders may present as two or three coexisting disorders. It is possible for a patient to have an acid-base disorder with normal pH, Pco_2, and HCO_3^-, the only clue to an acid-base disorder being an increased AG. If the AG is increased by more than 5 meq/L (i.e., an AG > 15 meq/L), the patient most likely has a metabolic acidosis. Compare the fall in plasma HCO_3^- (25 − HCO_3^-) with the increase in the plasma AG (ΔAG); these should be of similar magnitude. If there is a gross discrepancy (>5 meq/L), then a mixed disturbance is present:

- If increase in AG > fall in HCO_3^-: suggests that a component of the metabolic acidosis is due to HCO_3^- loss.
- If increase in AG < fall in HCO_3^-: suggests coexistent metabolic alkalosis.

Osmolar Gap. Calculate the osmolar gap in patients with an unexplained AG metabolic acidosis to exclude ethylene glycol or methanol toxicity (Table 45-6):

$$Estimated\ serum\ osmolality = 2 \times [Na] + [glucose]/18 + [BUN]/2.8$$

$$Normal \approx 290\ mOsm/kg\ H_2O$$

$$Osmolal\ gap = Osm\ (measured) - Osm\ (calculated)$$

$$Normal < 10$$

COMMON ACID BASE DISTURBANCES IN THE ICU

Metabolic Acidosis

The clinical manifestations of a metabolic acidosis are largely dependent on the underlying cause and the rapidity with which the condition develops. An acute, severe metabolic acidosis results in myocardial depression with a reduction in cardiac output, decreased blood pressure, and decreased hepatic and renal blood flow. Reentrant arrhythmias and a reduction in the ventricular fibrillation threshold can occur. Brain metabolism becomes impaired, with progressive obtundation and coma.

A metabolic acidosis in the critically ill patient is an ominous sign and warrants an aggressive approach to the diagnosis and management of the cause(s) of the disorder (Figure 45-2 and Table 45-7). In the vast majority of patients the cause(s) of the metabolic acidosis are usually clinically obvious, with lactic acidosis (from tissue hypoxia/hypermetabolism), ketoacidosis, and renal failure being the most common causes. In patients with an unexplained AG, metabolic acidosis methanol or ethylene-glycol toxicity should always be considered.[19] Accumulation of 5-oxoproline related to the use of acetaminophen is a rare cause of an anion-gap metabolic acidosis.[20] Prolonged high-dose administration of lorazepam can result in the accumulation of the vehicle, propylene glycol, resulting in worsening renal function, metabolic acidosis, and altered mental status.[21,22] Toxicity is typically observed after prolonged (>7 days), high-dose (average 14 mg/h), continuous lorazepam infusion and can be recognized by an increased osmolal gap.[23] Similarly, prolonged high-dose propofol (>100 μg/kg/min) is rarely associated with the "propofol infusion syndrome" characterized by rhabdomyolysis, metabolic acidosis, and renal and cardiac failure.[24]

The prognosis is related to the underlying disorder causing the acidosis. In almost all circumstances, the treatment of a metabolic acidosis involves treatment of the underlying disorder. Except in specific circumstances (outlined later), there is no scientific evidence to support treating a metabolic or respiratory acidosis with sodium bicarbonate.[25] Furthermore, it is the intracellular pH which is of importance in determining cellular function. The intracellular buffering system is much more effective in restoring pH to normal than the extracellular buffers. Consequently, patients have tolerated a pH as low as 7.0 during

TABLE 45-3	Normal Acid-Base Values		
	Mean	*1 SD*	*2 SD*
$Paco_2$ (mm Hg)	40	38-42	35-45
pH	7.4	7.38-7.42	7.35-7.45
HCO_3 (meq/L)	24	23-25	22-26

TABLE 45-5	Compensation Formulas for Simple Acid-Base Disorders
Acid-Base Disorder	*Compensation Formula*
Metabolic acidosis	Change in $Paco_2$ = 1.2 × change in HCO_3^-
Metabolic alkalosis	Change in $Paco_2$ = 0.6 × change in HCO_3^-
Acute respiratory acidosis	Change in HCO_3^- = 0.1 × change in $Paco_2$
Chronic respiratory acidosis	Change in HCO_3^- = 0.35 × change in $Paco_2$
Acute respiratory alkalosis	Change in HCO_3^- = 0.2 × change in $Paco_2$
Chronic respiratory alkalosis	Change in HCO_3^- = 0.5 × change in $Paco_2$

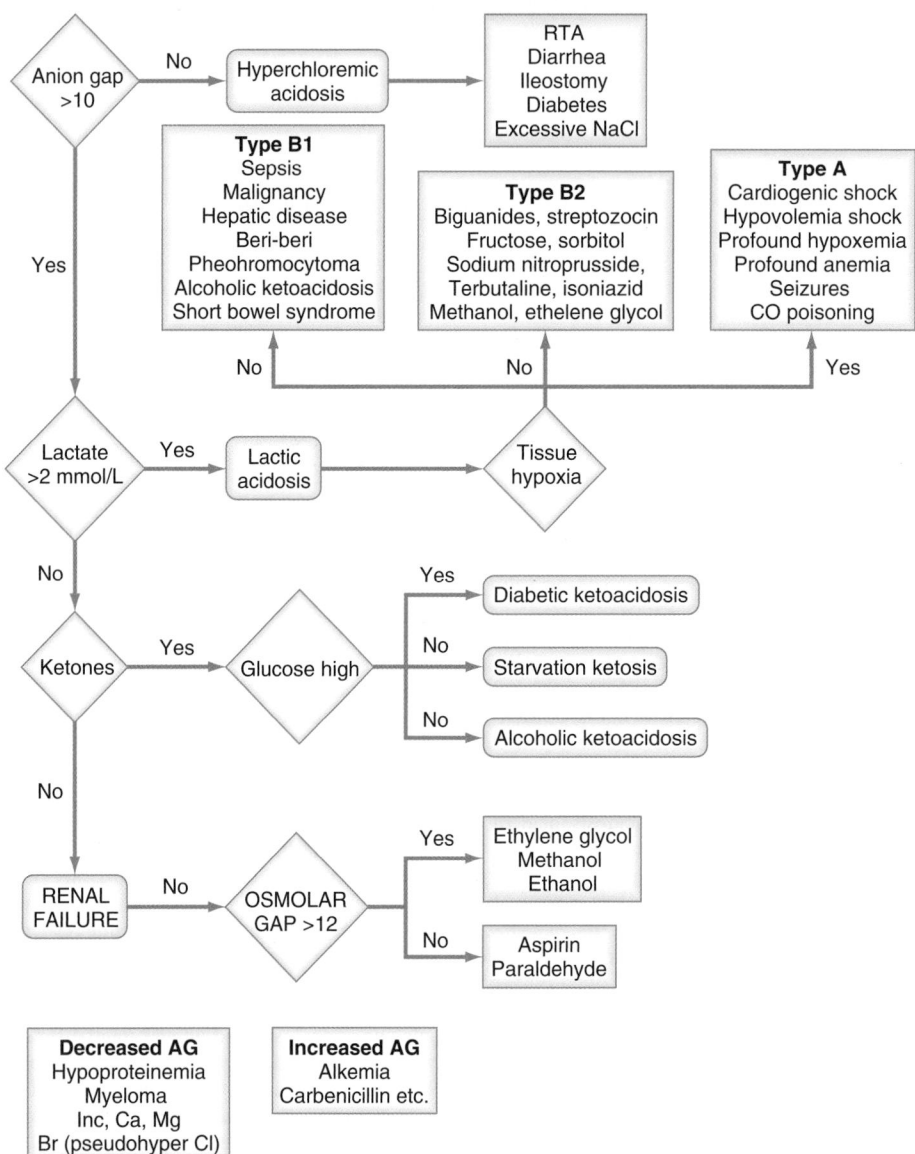

Figure 45-2 Diagnostic approach to metabolic acidosis.

sustained hypercapnia, without obvious adverse effects. Paradoxically, sodium bicarbonate can decrease intracellular pH (in circumstances where CO_2 elimination is fixed). The infusion of bicarbonate can lead to a variety of problems in patients with acidosis, including fluid overload, a postrecovery metabolic alkalosis, and hypernatremia. Furthermore, studies in both animals and humans suggest that alkali therapy may only transiently raise the plasma bicarbonate concentration. This

TABLE 45-6	Causes of an Increased Osmolal Gap

Ethylene glycol
Alcohol (ethanol)
Methanol
Isopropyl alcohol (does not cause an anion gap nor an acidosis)
Mannitol
Sorbitol
Paraldehyde
Acetone

finding appears to be related in part to CO_2 generated as the administered bicarbonate buffers excess hydrogen ions. Unless the minute ventilation is increased (in ventilated patients), CO_2 elimination will not be increased, and this will paradoxically worsen the intracellular acidosis. Currently, there are no data to support the use of bicarbonate in patients with lactic acidosis.[25,26]

Bicarbonate is frequently administered to "correct the acidosis" in patients with diabetic ketoacidosis (DKA). However, paradoxically, bicarbonate has been demonstrated to increase ketone and lactate production. Studies have demonstrated an increase in acetoacetate levels during alkali administration, followed by an increase in 3-hydroxybutyrate levels after its completion.[27,28] In pediatric patients, treatment with bicarbonate has been demonstrated to prolong hospitalization.[29] In addition, bicarbonate may decrease CSF pH, as increased CO_2 produced by buffering acid crosses the blood-brain barrier, combines with H_2O, and regenerates H^+. It is generally believed that adjunctive bicarbonate is unnecessary and potentially disadvantageous in severe DKA.[30]

TABLE 45-7	Causes of Metabolic Acidosis

Elevated Anion Gap

Renal failure
Rhabdomyolysis
Ketoacidosis:
- Diabetes mellitus
- Starvation
- Alcohol associated
- Defects in gluconeogenesis

Lactic acidosis:
- Hypermetabolism
- Tissue ischemia
- Sepsis
- Drugs
- Liver failure

Toxins/drugs:
- Ethylene glycol
- Methanol
- Salicylates
- Paraldehyde
- Lorazepam
- Propofol
- Metformin

5-Oxoproline
Beri-beri

Normal Anion Gap

Hypokalemic acidosis
- Renal tubular acidosis
- Diarrhea
- Posthypocapnic acidosis
- Carbonic anhydrase inhibitors
- Ureteral diversions

Normal to hyperkalemic acidosis
- Early renal failure
- Excessive 0.9% NaCl
- Hydronephrosis
- Addition of HCl
- Sulfur toxicity

Bicarbonate is considered "life saving" in patients with severe ethylene glycol and methanol toxicity. In hyperchloremic acidosis, endogenous regeneration of bicarbonate cannot occur (bicarbonate has been lost rather than buffered). Therefore, even if the cause of the acidosis can be reversed, exogenous alkali is often required for prompt attenuation of *severe acidemia*. Bicarbonate therapy is therefore indicated in patients with severe hyperchloremic acidosis when the pH is less than 7.2; this includes patients with severe diarrhea, high-output fistulas, and renal tubular acidosis. To prevent sodium overload, we suggest that 2×50 mL ampules of $NaHCO_3^-$ (each containing 50 mmol of $NaHCO_3^-$) be added to 1 L of 5% D/W and infused at a rate of 100 to 200 mL/h.

Lactic Acidosis. Lactic acid, like most substances with a pKa of less than 4 (pKa 3.78), circulates almost entirely as the freely dissociated anion, lactate (i.e., it releases its proton), at physiological pH—strongly favoring the right of the equation below:

$$CH_3CHOCOOH \leftrightarrow CH_3CHOCOO^- + H^+$$

Hyperlactatemia refers to an elevated plasma concentration of lactate anions. In clinical practice, *lactic acidemia* is defined as a pH less than 7.35 with a lactate concentration greater than 4 mmol/L. Lactic acidemia typically develops as a result of endogenously produced lactic acid, with lactate being measured as the dissociated base. During critical illness, the source of lactate is often believed to be ischemic anaerobically metabolizing tissues, such as the gut and muscle. However, lactate metabolism in critical illness is complex and often does not indicate ischemic tissues.[31] The anatomic source of lactate in critical illness is not consistent and may be dependent on the disease process and timing. Furthermore, it should be noted that both the pH and AG are insensitive markers of an elevated lactate; patients with an elevated lactate may have a normal pH and AG.[32]

D-Lactic Acidosis. Certain bacteria in the GI tract may convert carbohydrate into organic acids. The two factors that make this possible are slow GI transit (blind loops, obstruction) and change of the normal flora (usually with antibiotic therapy). The most prevalent organic acid is D-lactic acid. Since humans metabolize this isomer more slowly than L-lactate, and production rates can be very rapid, life-threatening acidosis can be produced.[33] The usual laboratory test for lactate is specific for the L-lactate isomer. Therefore, to confirm the diagnosis, the plasma D-lactate must be measured.

Metabolic Alkalosis

Metabolic alkalosis is a common acid-base disturbance in ICU patients, characterized by an elevated serum pH (>7.45) secondary to plasma bicarbonate (HCO_3^-) retention. Metabolic alkalosis is usually the result of several therapeutic interventions in the critically ill patient (Table 45-8). Nasogastric drainage, diuretic-induced intravascular volume depletion, hypokalemia, and the use of corticosteroids are common causes of metabolic alkalosis in these patients. In addition, citrate in transfused blood is metabolized to bicarbonate, which may compound the metabolic alkalosis. Overventilation in patients with type II respiratory failure may result in a posthypercapnic metabolic alkalosis. In many patients, the events that generated the metabolic alkalosis may not be present at the time of diagnosis.

Metabolic alkalosis may have adverse effects on cardiovascular, pulmonary, and metabolic function. It can decrease cardiac output, depress central ventilation, shift the oxyhemoglobin saturation curve to the left, worsen hypokalemia and hypophosphatemia, and negatively affect the ability to wean patients from mechanical ventilation. Increasing serum pH has been shown to correlate with ICU mortality. Correction of metabolic alkalosis has been shown to increase minute ventilation, increase arterial oxygen tension and mixed venous oxygen tension, and decrease oxygen consumption. It is therefore important to correct metabolic alkalosis in all critically ill patients.

The first therapeutic maneuver in patients with a metabolic alkalosis is to replace any fluid deficit with normal saline and correct electrolyte deficits. Aggressive potassium supplementation is warranted to achieve a K^+ above 4.5 mEq/L. If these interventions fail, ammonium chloride, hydrochloric acid, or arginine hydrochloride may be given. The disadvantage of these solutions is that they are difficult to use and require the administration of a large volume of hypotonic fluid. Extravasation of hydrochloric acid may result in severe tissue necrosis, mandating administration through a well-functioning central line. Acetazolamide is a carbonic anhydrase inhibitor that promotes the renal excretion of bicarbonate and has been demonstrated to be effective in treating metabolic alkalosis in ICU patients. A single dose of 500 mg is recommended. The onset of action is within 1.5 hours, with duration of approximately 24 hours.[34-37] Repeat doses may be required as necessary.

TABLE 45-8	Causes of Metabolic Alkalosis

Low Urine Chloride (Volume or Saline Responsive)

Gastric volume loss
Diuretics
Post hypercapnia
Villous adenoma (uncommon)
Cystic fibrosis (if there has been excessive sweating)

High Urine Chloride with Hypertension

Primary and secondary hyperaldosteronism
Apparent mineralocorticoid excess
Liddle's syndrome
Conn's syndrome
Cushing disease

High Urine Chloride without Hypertension

Bartter syndrome
Gitelman syndrome
Excess bicarbonate administration

Venous Blood Gas Analysis

Studies performed in the emergency room have demonstrated a strong correlation between arterial and venous blood pH and HCO_3^- levels in patients with DKA and uremia.[36,37] In these studies, the difference between arterial and venous pH varied from 0.04 to 0.05, and the difference in bicarbonate levels varied from −1.72 to 1.88. However, as one would anticipate, the correlation between arterial and venous Pco_2 was poor. These observations have been confirmed in a cohort of unselected emergency room patients[38] and patients with tricyclic antidepressant poisoning.[39] Similarly, an excellent correlation has been demonstrated between mixed venous pH and HCO_3^- with arterial pH and HCO_3^- in ICU patients.[40,41] The association between arterial and venous pH, HCO_3^- and Pco_2 is, however, not valid in patients with shock. In a now classic study, Weil and coauthors reported that during cardiopulmonary resuscitation, the arterial blood pH averaged 7.41, whereas the average mixed venous blood pH was 7.15.[42] Similarly, the $Paco_2$ was 32 mm Hg, whereas the mixed venous Pco_2 was 74 mm Hg. Androgue and colleagues have reported similar findings in patients with circulatory failure.[43]

In hemodynamically stable (and resuscitated patients) without known hypercarbia, ABG analysis may not be required; pulse oximetry and venous blood gas analysis should suffice in most circumstances. Furthermore, a venous blood gas can be useful to screen for arterial hypercarbia, with a venous Pco_2 level > 45 mm Hg being highly predictive of arterial hypercarbia (sensitivity and negative predictive value of 100%).[44] In hemodynamically unstable patients and those with complex acid-base disorders, a venous blood gas cannot be substituted for an ABG analysis. In these situations, both arterial and mixed venous/central venous blood gas analysis provides useful information (see later discussion).

MIXED VENOUS/CENTRAL VENOUS OXYGEN SATURATION

Monitoring of the mixed venous oxygen saturation ($Smvo_2$) has been used as a surrogate for the balance between systemic oxygen delivery and consumption during the treatment of critically ill patients. Generally an Svo_2 of less than 65% is indicative of inadequate oxygen delivery. Measurement of Svo_2 involves placement of a pulmonary artery catheter (PAC); this is an invasive device that has not been shown to improve patient outcome, so its use has fallen out of favor. However, since most critically ill patients have a central venous catheter in situ, the central venous oxygen saturation ($Scvo_2$) has been used as an alternative to the $Smvo_2$.

Regional variations in the balance between DO_2 and VO_2 result in differences in the Hb saturation of blood in the superior and inferior venae cavae. Streaming of caval blood continues within the right atrium and ventricle, and complete mixing only occurs during ventricular contraction. The drainage of myocardial venous blood directly into the right atrium via the coronary sinus and cardiac chambers via the thebesian veins results in further discrepancies.[45,46] Consequently, $Smvo_2$ reflects the balance between oxygen supply and demand averaged across the entire body, but $Scvo_2$ is affected disproportionately by changes in the upper body. In healthy individuals, $Scvo_2$ is usually 2% to 5% less than Svo_2, largely because of the high oxygen content of effluent venous blood from the kidneys.[47] This relationship changes during periods of hemodynamic instability, because blood is redistributed to the upper body at the expense of the splanchnic and renal circulations. In shock states, therefore, the observed relationship between $Scvo_2$ and Svo_2 may reverse, and the absolute value of $Scvo_2$ may exceed that of Svo_2 by up to 20%.[48] This lack of numerical equivalence has been demonstrated in various groups of critically ill patients, including those with cardiogenic, septic, and hemorrhagic shock. Based on these data, the Surviving Sepsis Campaign has recommended achieving an $Smvo_2$ level of 65% or a $Scvo_2$ level of 70% in patients with severe sepsis and septic shock.[49] Although trends in $Scvo_2$ may reflect those of $Smvo_2$, the absolute values differ, and the variables cannot be used interchangeably.[48,50-52] In addition to guiding resuscitation, $Scvo_2$ may have prognostic significance, with low values during the first 24 hours of hospitalization or in the postoperative period being predictive of a worse outcome.[53-55]

In patients with sepsis and liver failure, a low $Scvo_2$/$Smvo_2$ is usually indicative of decreased cardiac output (oxygen delivery)[56]; however, normal values do not exclude adequate resuscitation or tissue hypoxia.[57,58] The presence of functional and/or anatomic shunting results in "arterialization" of venous blood. In addition, cytopathic hypoxia may further decrease oxygen uptake and result in a "spuriously high" $Scvo_2$.[59] Indeed, patients dying of both sepsis and liver failure usually have a high $Scvo_2$/$Smvo_2$. In an intriguing study, Pope and colleagues demonstrated that in patients with sepsis, a high $Scvo_2$ (90%-100%) at any time during hospitalization was an independent predictor of mortality, whereas a low $Scvo_2$ (<70%) was only predictive of mortality if this value remained low following resuscitation.[60] It is noteworthy that in a recent goal-directed sepsis study, the mean $Scvo_2$ was 74% at enrollment, and less than 10% of patients required specific interventions to achieve $Scvo_2$ above 70%.[61]

Experimental models have demonstrated that a high mixed venous–to-arterial Pco_2 gradient is a reliable marker of decreased cardiac output and global tissue ischemia.[62,63] This observation has been confirmed by Weil et al. and Androgue et al., who demonstrated that a high mixed venous–to-arterial Pco_2 gradient is a sensitive marker of global tissue ischemia during cardiopulmonary resuscitation and in patients with circulatory failure.[43,64,65] In patients with septic shock, Bakker and colleagues demonstrated that the venous-to-arterial Pco_2 gradient was directly related to cardiac output.[66] In resuscitated patients ($Scvo_2$ > 70%) with septic shock, Vallee and coworkers demonstrated that a widened central venous-to-arterial Pco_2 gradient (>6 mm Hg) identified patients with a low cardiac index who were inadequately resuscitated.[58] The central venous-to-arterial Pco_2 gradient may prove to be a better endpoint for resuscitation of septic patients than the $Scvo_2$.

KEY POINTS

1. Arterial blood gas (ABG) analysis is the gold standard for the assessment of oxygenation, ventilation, and acid-base status.

2. Pulse oximetry provides a surrogate measure of arterial oxygen tension (Pao_2). Venous pH and bicarbonate (HCO_3^-) allow for the estimation of arterial pH and HCO_3^- in hemodynamically stable patients. Venous carbon dioxide tension is a poor proxy of arterial Pco_2. Venous blood gas analysis can be useful to screen for arterial hypercarbia, with a venous Pco_2 level above 45 mm Hg being highly predictive of arterial hypercarbia.

3. The indications for ABG sampling have not been well defined; however, an ABG should generally be performed on admission to the ICU, following endotracheal intubation, and as clinical circumstances dictate.

4. ABG sampling does not have to be performed after each ventilator change or after each step in the weaning process.

5. Metabolic acidosis is a serious medical disorder, the etiology of which must always be determined.

6. In most clinical situations, sodium bicarbonate ($NaHCO_3^-$) is useless therapy for metabolic acidosis.

7. In patients with a metabolic alkalosis, correct the volume and potassium deficit first.

8. The central venous oxygen saturation ($Scvo_2$) and the central venous-to-arterial Pco_2 gap have utility in assessing the adequacy of resuscitation and oxygen delivery.

REFERENCES

Access the complete reference list online at http://www.expertconsult.com.

46

Respiratory System Mechanics and Respiratory Muscle Function

CESARE GREGORETTI | VITO MARCO RANIERI

In its simplest form, the respiratory system can be modeled as a balloon connected to a tube. The balloon represents the elastic element (lungs and chest wall), and the tube represents the resistive element (conducting airways). To serve the purpose of ventilation, the respiratory pump (or a mechanical ventilator) must generate sufficient pressure to overcome both the elastic and flow-resistive properties of the respiratory system.

Classic respiratory mechanics are based on Newtonian physics, as expressed in the equation of motion. The respiratory system model is derived from an elementary monodimensional system, as depicted by a block with an attached spring, acted on by a unidirectional force (Figure 46-1, A).[1,2] Upon application of force, the response of the system can be characterized in terms of displacement, velocity, and acceleration of a block with a mass of M. The balance of forces acting on the block can be expressed as follows:

$$F_{appl(t)} = F_{el(t)} + F_{res(t)} + F_{in(t)} \qquad \text{(Equation 1)}$$

where the total force applied to the system (F_{appl}) at a given time (t) is equal to the sum of the elastic (F_{el}), resistive (F_{res}), and inertial (F_{in}) forces.

The equation of motion for a three-dimensional pneumatic system may be written as:

$$P_{(t)} = E(V_{(t)}) + R\dot{V}_{(t)} + I\ddot{V}_{(t)} \qquad \text{(Equation 2)}$$

where $P_{(t)}$ is the pressure exerted on the system at a given time; E is the elastance (the reciprocal of compliance, i.e., 1/C), which relates pressure to volume (V), and R is the resistance constant, relating pressure to flow. The third term of the equation describes the pressure required to accelerate tissue and gas in the airway, which is an important factor under certain circumstances such as coughing or high-frequency oscillatory ventilation. The inertance constant (I) relates pressure to linear acceleration ($\ddot{V}$). However, the third term is usually omitted in this model of the respiratory system, because inertive forces are negligible during quiet breathing and most forms of mechanical ventilation.[3] Thus, in most applications, the respiratory system derivative of the equation of motion considers only the elastic and flow-resistive elements that oppose an applied pressure at time (t):

$$P_{(t)} = E(V)_{(t)} + R\dot{V}_{(t)} \qquad \text{(Equation 3)}$$

which may also be expressed as:

$$P_{(t)} = 1/C(V)_{(t)} + R\dot{V}_{(t)} \qquad \text{(Equation 4)}$$

In this model, any force applied to the respiratory system is either stored as elastic energy or dissipated as resistive energy. Figure 46-1, B shows a three-dimensional model of the respiratory system as it relates to the equation of motion.

This simple model of respiratory system mechanics is useful because, in the normal operating range, the relationships among airway pressure, volume, and flow can be approximated by straight lines. Linear one-compartment analogs are particularly well suited for modeling mechanical ventilation because the pressure applied to lungs and chest wall can be readily measured and displayed. In turn, departures from linearity provide useful clues about concurrent respiratory muscle activity, alert the healthcare provider to the presence of lung disease,

or serve as a warning that the lungs are being ventilated at inappropriately high or low volumes.

Static Behavior of the Respiratory System

Static behavior of the respiratory system defines a condition in the absence of flow. Under such conditions, and in accordance with the model described in the preceding section, a pressure applied to the respiratory system is opposed by elastic forces (P_{el}). During flow, this pressure can be approximated by alveolar pressure (P_{alv}) which, upon interruption of airflow, equilibrates with airway opening pressure (P_{ao}):

$$P_{el} = P_{ao} = P_{alv} \qquad \text{(Equation 5)}$$

The elastic element of the respiratory system (rs) consists of two component structures, the chest wall (w)—functionally, the thoracic cage and abdomen—and the lungs (l). The forces that act on these two structures can be summed, because the lungs and chest wall behave like springs in series:

$$P_{el,rs} = P_{el,w} + P_{el,l} \qquad \text{(Equation 6)}$$

The net distending pressure applied to the lung by contraction of the inspiratory muscles or by positive-pressure ventilation is represented by transmural forces, termed the *transpulmonary pressure* (P_L), is determined by the difference between alveolar pressure (P_{alv}) and pleural pressure (P_{pl}):

$$P_L = P_{alv} - P_{pl} \qquad \text{(Equation 7)}$$

The pressure across the chest wall (transthoracic pressure, P_w) is determined by the difference between pleural pressure and atmospheric pressure (P_{pbs}):

$$P_w = P_{pl} - P_{bs} \qquad \text{(Equation 8)}$$

Because it is used as a reference to all other measured pressures, atmospheric pressure is considered to be zero, thus:

$$P_w = P_{pl} \qquad \text{(Equation 9)}$$

An esophageal balloon catheter can be used to approximate pleural pressure, keeping in mind that pleural pressure is nonuniform and that topographic gradients in pleural pressure vary with posture.[4] In the recumbent posture, there is no site in the esophagus at which local pressure approximates average lung surface pressure (i.e., average pleural pressure). However, at least in normal lungs, the average change in surface or pleural pressure can be inferred using esophageal manometry.

The static pressure across the entire respiratory system in the absence of flow and assuming the pressure at the airway opening (P_{ao}) equals alveolar pressure can be summarized as follows:

$$P_{rs} = P_L + P_w = (P_{ao} - P_{pl}) + (P_{pl} - P_{bs}) = P_{ao} \qquad \text{(Equation 10)}$$

By assuming that P_{bs} is considered to be zero:

$$P_{rs} = P_L + P_w = P_{ao} \qquad \text{(Equation 11)}$$

303

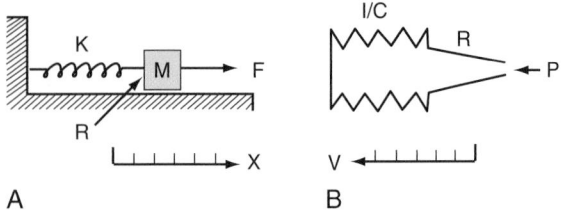

Figure 46-1 Mechanical analogs of the equation of motion. **A,** System with unidirectional motion. **B,** Three-dimensional system. *(From Rodarte JR, Rehder K. Dynamics of respiration. In: Macklem PT, Mead J, editors. Handbook of Physiology. Baltimore: Williams & Wilkins; 1986:131-144.)*

The static respiratory system pressure-volume (P-V) curve is often measured in intubated, mechanically ventilated patients to make inferences about the mechanical properties of the lungs. Although the utility of P-V measurements in clinical decision making remains to be established, the determinants of the P-V relationship should nevertheless be understood. The P-V curve is generated by inflating and deflating the relaxed respiratory system in a stepwise fashion between residual volume and total lung capacity. The airway occlusion pressure at each volume defines the corresponding elastic recoil pressures of the lungs and chest wall. Because the inflation and deflation relationships differ from each other, the resulting curve is often referred to as a *P-V loop*. The respiratory system P-V loop is the summation of individual lung and chest wall P-V loops, termed a *Rahn diagram* (Figure 46-2). Because during normal tidal volume breathing (30% to 70% vital capacity), the relationship between elastic pressure and volume is essentially linear, the system's elastic properties can be defined by a constant, namely *elastance*. The term *compliance* is more frequently used and is simply the inverse of elastance, defined as the change in volume per unit change in applied pressure. Static respiratory system compliance can be determined by the slope of the P-V curve. In the quiet breathing range, the normal respiratory system elastance averages 8 to10 cm H_2O/L, corresponding to a static respiratory system compliance of 0.12 to 0.1 L/cm H_2O.

Figure 46-2 shows the P-V curves of the respiratory system's component structures, the lung and chest wall. At high lung volumes, the total respiratory system compliance is reduced (the P-V curve is concave to the pressure axis), primarily because the lung reaches total capacity, its structural limit. In contrast, the P-V curve of the chest wall remains linear at high volumes (i.e., the chest wall offers much less resistance to further lung expansion).

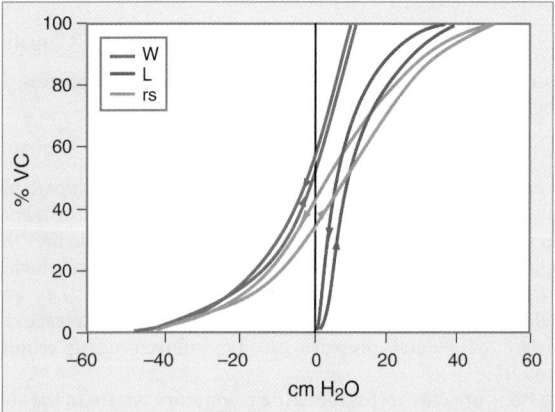

Figure 46-2 Pressure-volume (P-V) loop (Rahn diagram) of the respiratory system (rs), and summation of individual chest wall (W) and lung (L) loops. During normal tidal volume breathing (30%–70% vital capacity), the relationship between elastic pressure and volume is essentially linear. VC, vital capacity. *(From Agostoni E, Hyatt RE. Static behavior of the respiratory system. In: Fishman AP, editor. Handbook of Physiology. Baltimore: Williams & Wilkins; 1986:113-130.)*

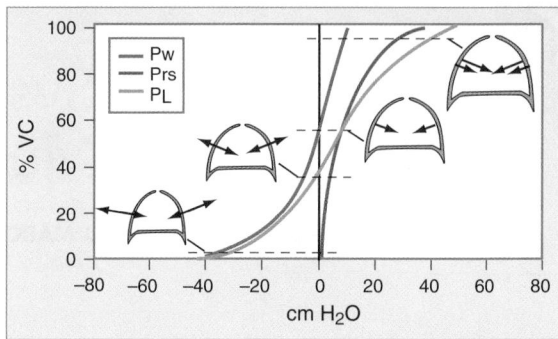

Figure 46-3 Static pressure-volume curves of the chest wall (P_w), lungs (P_L), and respiratory system (P_{rs}). Drawings of the thorax *(left to right)* at residual volume, functional residual capacity, resting position (no force exerted by the chest wall), and total lung capacity. Arrows indicate direction of elastic recoil. VC, vital capacity. *(From Agostoni E, Hyatt RE. Static behavior of the respiratory system. In: Fishman AP, editor. Handbook of Physiology. Baltimore: Williams & Wilkins; 1986:113-130.)*

At low lung volumes, a decrease in chest wall compliance is the major contributor to low respiratory system compliance. At relaxation volume (functional residual capacity), the inward recoil of the lung is equal to the outward recoil of the chest wall, so that alveolar pressure is atmospheric. At a volume of 60% of vital capacity, the chest wall reaches a "resting" position, that is, it exerts no force on the lungs, and the pleural pressure is atmospheric. In the normal tidal breathing range, the slopes of the lung and chest wall P-V curves are similar (i.e., lung and chest wall contribute about equally to overall respiratory system compliance). Figure 46-3 shows the volume dependence of the inwardly and outwardly directed forces of the respiratory system during inflation.[4]

Lung recoil is the collapsing force of the lung; it is in equilibrium with the transpulmonary distending pressure originating from the chest wall and inspiratory muscles and generated by:
1. Tension carried by lung parenchyma, including the collagen network that extends from the alveolar septae to the visceral pleura
2. Surface forces originating from air-liquid interfaces in distal lung units[5]

Surface forces (i.e., surface tension) are generated because liquid molecules in contact with air attempt to conserve energy by decreasing the area available for interaction. In the lung, the resulting force acts parallel to the alveolar septa and balances a helical fiber network that supports alveolar ducts and forms alveolar entrance rings.[6]

As demonstrated in Figure 46-4, the elimination of surface tension has two important consequences on lung mechanics[7]:
1. There is an approximately 50% reduction in recoil pressure at all lung volumes.
2. The difference in isovolume recoil pressure between inflation and deflation (hysteresis) is largely abolished.

Findings indicate not only that surface tension is an important source of lung elastic recoil but also that recoil pressure varies with volume, volume history, and time.

In the normal lung, hysteresis is caused by volume- and time-dependent changes in the molecular composition and hence the biophysical properties of surfactant. *Surfactant* is a protein-enriched lipid film that coats air-liquid interfaces in distal lung units and lowers surface tension. *Hysteresis* implies that energy added to the system during inflation is not fully recovered during deflation. The hysteretic loss of energy does not scale with frequency and flow the way a Newtonian viscous resistance does, underscoring one of the many limitations of linear resistance-compliance circuits in modeling lung mechanics.[8] Whereas interfacial phenomena are the primary source of hysteresis in the normal lung, alveolar recruitment and derecruitment are important sources of hysteresis in disease.

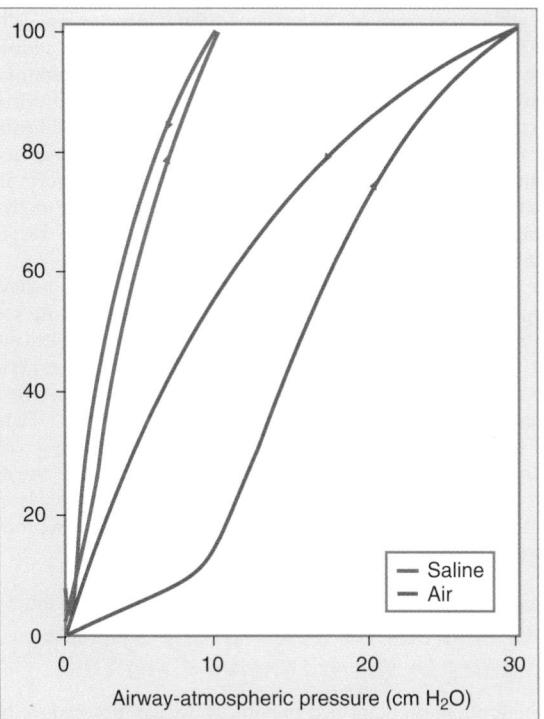

Figure 46-4 Plot of airway–atmospheric pressure gradient for an isolated lung inflated with air (*purple line*) and saline (*red line*). Reduction in surface tension in the saline-filled lung results in increased compliance. (*From Taylor A, Rehder K, Hyatt R, et al. Mechanics of breathing: static. In: Taylor AE, editor.* Clinical Respiratory Physiology. *Philadelphia: Saunders; 1989:89-105.*)

According to the law of Laplace, the pressure (P) required to inflate a bubble is directly related to the surface tension (T) and is inversely proportional to the radius of curvature (r):

$$P = 4T/r \qquad \text{(Equation 12)}$$

Applied to the lung, this means that changes in alveolar dimensions at low lung volumes would promote alveolar collapse were it not for surfactant's surface tension–lowering properties. A surfactant-depleted lung exhibits alveolar instability and collapse in the tidal breathing range. In normal pigs, high-tidal-volume ventilation does not alter alveolar mechanics in the normal lung; however, in the surfactant-deactivated lung, it causes alveolar overdistension and exacerbates alveolar instability.[9] Figure 46-5 shows a pressure-volume loop of a normal lung and a surfactant-depleted lung. As a consequence of surfactant depletion, larger than normal transpulmonary pressures are required to keep the surfactant-depleted lung inflated.

Dynamic Behavior of the Respiratory System

The transpulmonary pressure generated by the respiratory pump must overcome the resistive forces related to gas flow in order to generate a given volume in a given time. The *respiratory system resistance constant* scales resistive pressure and flow in the equation of motion discussed previously. The reciprocal of resistance is *conductance*, which is proportional to lung volume as the airways, tethered to the entire connective tissue network, are pulled open with larger inflation volumes.

According to Ohm's law, resistance (R) can be calculated by dividing the driving pressure by flow:

$$R = (P_{alv} - P_{ao})/\dot{V} \qquad \text{(Equation 13)}$$

Total pulmonary resistance reflects the gas flow–dependent pressure dissipation in the conducting airways (airway resistance) and the

frequency-dependent loss of energy associated with parenchymal deformation (tissue resistance). Originally considered only a minor component of total pulmonary resistance, it is now appreciated that the so-called tissue resistance dominates the measurement, at least at low frequencies.[10] As outlined by Fredberg and Stamenovic,[8] tissue resistance and tissue hysteretic properties are model-specific descriptors of energy loss, the structural and molecular basis of which remains uncertain.[11]

The physical laws governing fluid flow in tubes can be applied to gas flow in the airways. According to fluid mechanics, tube length and geometry and gas velocity and physical properties (i.e., density and viscosity) determine whether flow is *laminar* or *turbulent.*

These determinants can be captured by *Reynold's number*, a quantity that represents the ratio of inertial forces to viscous forces.[12] A low Reynold's number (<50) corresponds to laminar flow, and a Reynold's number greater than 2300 is associated with turbulent flow. Accordingly, the low gas velocity in peripheral airways favors laminar flow, and the acceleration associated with the decrease in total cross-sectional area in central airways promotes turbulence.

In the presence of laminar flow, frictional pressure losses are linearly related to flow and viscosity and inversely proportional to tube radius to the fourth power (Poiseuille's equation):

$$\Delta P = 8\mu LQ/\pi r^4 \qquad \text{(Equation 14)}$$

where ΔP is the pressure drop, L is the length of pipe, μ is the dynamic viscosity, Q is the volumetric flow rate, r is the radius, and π is the mathematical constant (approximately 3.141592654). In contrast, turbulent flow is associated with nonlinear pressure-flow relationships that are gas-density dependent. The density dependence of turbulent flow is occasionally exploited in the medical use of heliox, a low-density helium-oxygen mixture given to patients with central airway lesions or asthma.[13] However, the available clinical data on inhaled He/O_2 mixtures are insufficient to prove that this therapy has benefit with respect to outcome variables.[14]

The flow-dependent shift from laminar to turbulent flow is captured in the *Rohrer equation:*

$$P = K_1 \dot{V} + K_2 \dot{V} \qquad \text{(Equation 15)}$$

where K_1 and K_2 are constants that scale frictional pressure dissipation associated with laminar and turbulent flow, respectively.

A second mechanism of pressure loss during gas flow is related to the *Bernoulli principle*, which describes convective pressure dissipation. That is, as a gas flows from a large cross-sectional area to a smaller area, velocity must increase to maintain flow. This results in energy

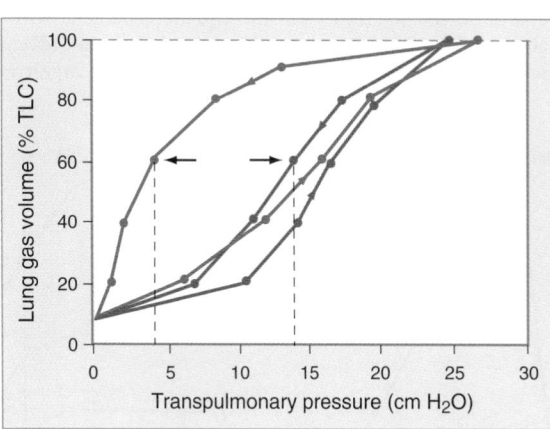

Figure 46-5 Pressure-volume loop of a normal lung (*solid line*) and a surfactant-depleted lung (*dashed line*). Larger than normal transpulmonary pressures are required to keep the surfactant-depleted lung inflated. TLC, total lung capacity. (*From Taylor A, Rehder K, Hyatt R, et al. Mechanics of breathing: static. In: Taylor AE, editor.* Clinical Respiratory Physiology. *Philadelphia: Saunders; 1989:89-105.*)

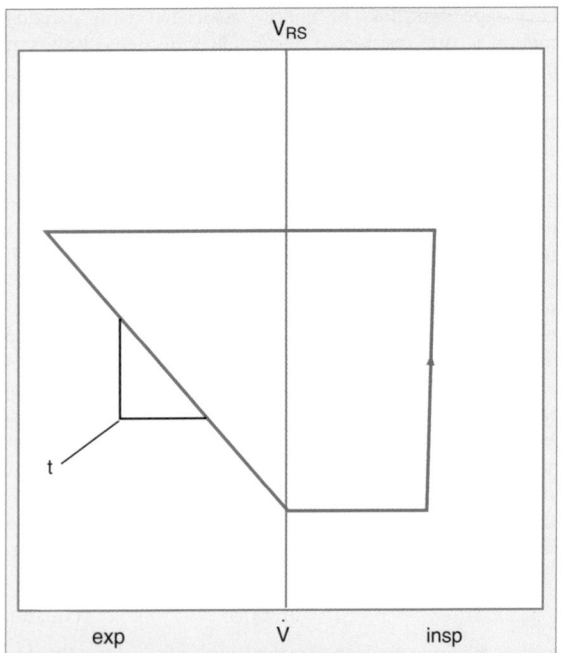

Figure 46-6 Flow-volume curve. The expiratory time constant (τ) is equal to the slope of the expiratory limb. V̇ flow; V$_{RS}$, volume of respiratory system. (*From Loring SH. Mechanics of the lung and chest wall. In: Marini JJ, Slutsky AS, editors.* Physiological Basis of Ventilatory Support. *New York: Marcel Dekker; 1998:177-205.*)

dissipation and a drop in pressure and correlates to expiratory flow of gas from the bronchioles to the central airways. As mentioned previously, *ohmic resistance* can be computed by dividing resistive pressure by inspiratory flow (see Equation 13).

The respiratory time constant (τ) is the time required for the lung to fill or passively discharge approximately 63% of its contents. It can be determined from the slope of the passive expiratory flow-volume curve (Figure 46-6) or calculated directly by the equation:

$$\tau = R_{rs} / E_{rs} = R_{rs} \times C_{rs} \qquad \text{(Equation 16)}$$

where τ is usually measured in seconds because respiratory system resistance (R$_{rs}$) is expressed in units of pressure × time × volume^{-1}, and respiratory system compliance (C$_{rs}$) is expressed in units of volume × pressure^{-1}.

The value of τ for a normal respiratory system is approximately 0.3 second.[3] As can be inferred from the equation, patients with high respiratory system resistance or compliance, such as those with chronic obstructive lung disease (COPD), have correspondingly large τ values.

The added resistance of the artificial tubing in a mechanically ventilated patient may increase τ to 1 second or more. In addition, in patients with even minimally elevated τ values, the expiratory time (depending on the preset inspiratory time in time cycled ventilatory support or from the expiratory threshold in a flow cycled ventilatory mode[15]) may not be enough to fully empty the lungs during mechanical ventilation. Consequently, the demand for expiratory flow is not met as the lungs near relaxation volume, resulting in dynamic hyperinflation even in healthy lungs at high rates of respiratory frequency.

Another important concept that explains the dynamic behavior of the respiratory system is shown in Figure 46-7. Higher lung volumes (curve A) yield higher expiratory flow rates compared with the flow seen at lower lung volumes (curve C). In a classic set of experiments performed on normal subjects, Fry and Hyatt demonstrated that maximal expiratory flow is determined by lung volume.[16] They concluded that on the basis of volume-related dynamic airway collapse, expiratory flow plateau cannot be exceeded irrespective of the magnitude of subject effort or applied transpulmonary pressure. Herein lies the value of the forced vital capacity maneuver as a reproducible measure of maximal expiratory flow.

Assessment of Respiratory System Mechanics in the Intensive Care Unit

With the foundation described previously, we can proceed to the correlation of mechanics with clinical conditions encountered in the intensive care unit (ICU). To examine basic concepts, we use the example of expected waveforms generated by a volume-preset mechanical ventilator in a relaxed or paralyzed patient with otherwise normal respiratory system mechanics.

Assuming constant flow in a relaxed or paralyzed patient without respiratory muscle contribution, pressure at the ventilator inlet increases linearly with time and volume to a peak. A typical simplified waveform output is demonstrated by Figure 46-8, with a model of the system represented on the right. Pressures are measured at the ventilator inlet or at the airway opening at the level of the "Y" connection. Assuming inflation onset with a constant (square wave) flow, an initial step change in driving pressure is recorded, which precedes alveolar filling and corresponds to resistive pressure related to gas flow in the airways (see Figure 46-8, *dotted arrow*). When making an end-inspiration airway occlusion after a rapid initial step-off in resistive pressure drop (Pmax–P1), there is then a gradual decrease in pressure to a plateau value (P2) (see Figure 46-8, *full thick arrows*). This pressure, usually reached after 3 seconds of end-inspiratory occlusion, indicates the true static end-inspiratory elastic recoil pressure of the total respiratory system (P$_{st,rs}$)[17-18] and represents the static summation of elastic recoil forces corresponding to the applied tidal volume.

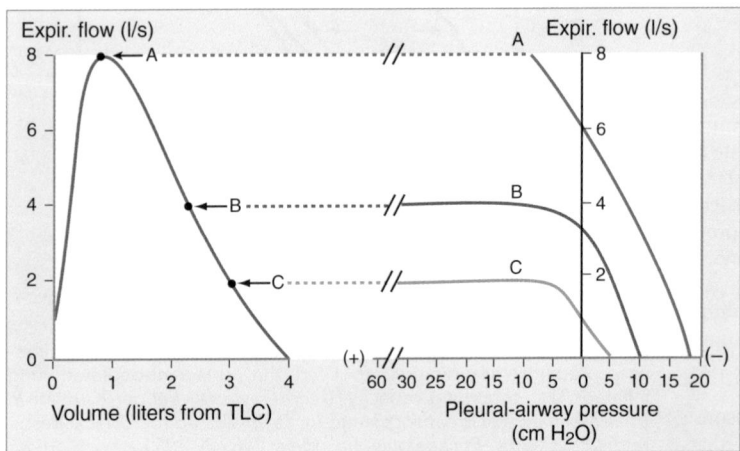

Figure 46-7 *Left,* maximal expiratory flow-volume curve. *Right,* three isovolume pressure-flow curves at different lung volumes (A, B, C). Left side of figure shows an expiratory flow-volume plot for a normal subject, similar to that generated by a forced vital capacity maneuver in the pulmonary function lab. Right side of figure shows three driving pressure-flow curves at progressively smaller lung volumes from A to C. Curves are nonlinear, and each has a driving pressure–dependent and –independent limb separated by the critical driving pressure. Note flow limitation associated with submaximal lung volumes B and C. TLC, total lung capacity. (*From Hyatt RE. Forced expiration. In: Macklem PT, Mead J, editors.* Handbook of Physiology. *Baltimore: Williams & Wilkins; 1986:295-314.*)

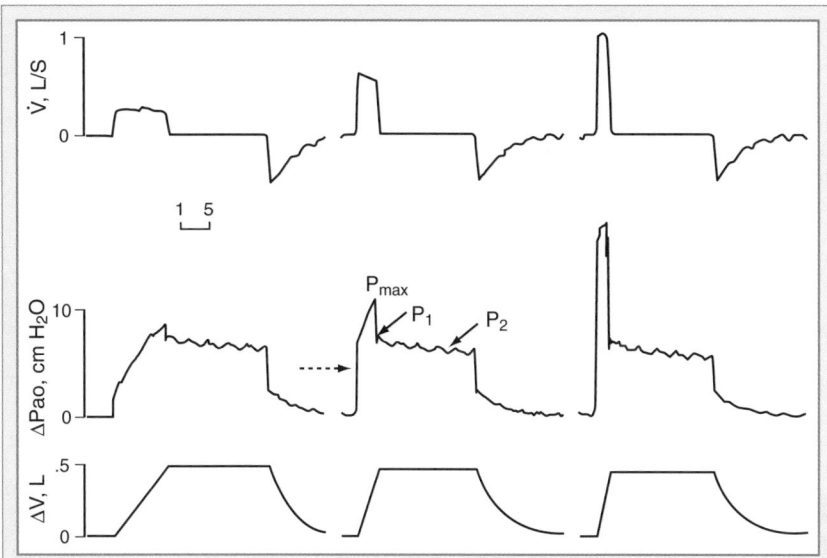

Figure 46-8 Airway pressure and flow wave patterns during volume-preset mechanical ventilation. After an end-inspiratory airway occlusion, there is an immediate drop in pressure from Pmax to P1, followed by a slow decay to a plateau value (P2) that represents static elastic recoil pressure (Pst$_{rs}$) at end-inspiratory lung volume. Increasing inspiratory flow also determines an increase in Pmax to P1; difference due to an increase in "ohmic "airway resistance (R$_{min,rs}$). *(Modified from D'Angelo E, Calderini E, Torri G, et al. Respiratory mechanics in anesthetized paralyzed humans: effects of flow, volume, and time. J Appl Physiol. 1989;67[6]:2556-64.)*

During this period, the contribution in reduction in pressure due to volume loss by continuing gas exchange should be negligible.

The initial drop in Pmax, namely P1 divided by the preceding steady flow, provides the so-called ohmic resistances (Rmin,rs). Rmin,rs increases linearly with flow according to the Rohrer equation. The slow decrease of pressure (P1 − P2) divided by the preceding steady flow yields the effective additional resistance (ΔRs) due to the viscoelastic properties of the thoracic tissues and time constant inequalities within the lung and the chest wall (so-called pendelluft).[19] The sum of Rmin,rs and ΔRs is defined as *Rmax.rs*.[20] In a mechanically ventilated patient, where endotracheal tube resistance dominates measured total respiratory system resistance, the derived value of respiratory resistance must be interpreted with caution.

Artificial tubing is not a truly ohmic resistor, and estimates of resistance are highly dependent on inspiratory flow rates. Even after correction for tube size, high inspiratory resistance may be confounded by inspissated secretions or "tube biting."

When using inspiratory flow settings of less than 1 L/sec with an endotracheal tube larger than 7 mm in internal diameter, resistive pressure (Rmin,rs) is usually less than 10 cm H$_2$O. When peak airway pressure deviates from the inspiratory occlusion pressure (P1) by more than 10 cm H$_2$O in a healthy subject, an increase in airway resistance should be suspected. In the absence of obvious intrinsic airway disease (acute or chronic), a ventilator hardware problem, tube kinking, or sputum retention should be suspected. However, more than the absolute value of the drop of pressure from peak to P1 deviation from the difference (Pmax − P1) in baseline value from the institution of mechanical ventilation may identify an airway resistive problem. It should also be kept in mind that a normal inspiratory resistance does not preclude the presence of expiratory resistance in severe airflow obstruction, as seen in COPD patients.

As previously mentioned, the elastic properties of the respiratory system can be determined from the slope of the P-V curve. Provided there is no contribution from respiratory muscles (as shown by a perfectly linear inspiratory P-V curve), the elastance (E$_{rs}$), or reciprocal of compliance, can be derived from time-based curves with the following equation:

$$E_{rs} = \Delta P_{el}/\Delta vol = dP/dt \times dt/dV = dP/dt \times 1/V \quad \text{(Equation 17)}$$

where *dP* = change in pressure; *dt* = change in time; and *dV* = change in volume.

Elastance (E$_{rs}$) can be measured at bedside during constant flow volume–preset mechanical ventilation. Pst,rs (P2 divided by ΔV) provides the static elastance of the total respiratory system (Est,rs):

$$E_{rs} = P_{st,rs} - (\text{PEEP-PEEPi})/\Delta vol \quad \text{(Equation 18)}$$

where *PEEP* is the set end-expiratory positive pressure and *PEEPi* the intrinsic PEEP (see below).

As mentioned previously, during mechanical ventilation, the pressure applied to the respiratory system (P$_{rs}$) overcomes PEEPi, flow resistance, and elastance of the respiratory system (E$_{rs}$). Assuming a linear pressure volume curve, the total E$_{rs}$ (=1/compliance) equals the sum of the elastance of the chest wall (E$_{cw}$) and the lung (E$_L$), which are mechanically in series:

$$E_{rs} = E_{cw} + E_L \quad \text{(Equation 19)}$$

Neglecting intrinsic PEEP and flow resistance, P$_{rs}$ is the sum of the pressures required to distend the chest wall (P$_{cw}$) and to inflate the lung (P$_L$). The fractions E$_L$/E$_{rs}$ and E$_{cw}$/E$_{rs}$ determine how P$_{rs}$ is partitioned between the lung:

$$P_L = P_{rs} \times E_L/E_{rs} \quad \text{(Equation 20)}$$

and the chest wall:

$$P_{cw} = P_{rs} \times E_{cw}/E_{rs} \quad \text{(Equation 21)}$$

For example, if the elastance of the chest wall is twice that of the lung, then two-thirds of P$_{rs}$ is used to distend the chest wall and only one-third to inflate the lung.[21] Of note, the chest wall in this context comprises not only the thoracic rib cage but also the abdomen.

Compliance of the respiratory system can be also measured by the super syringe method. This method for static P-V curve recordings has been associated with spurious changes in lung volume because of gas absorption during measurement.[22] There are also issues related to user interpretation (e.g., difficulties in defining morphologic characteristics of the curve), and interobserver variability is often high.[23,24] Some have advocated inductive machine learning in an attempt to standardize interpretation.[25]

Passive expiration of the respiratory system is driven by elastic recoil, as manifested by alveolar pressure at a corresponding lung volume. Expiratory flow is a function of the elastance and resistance and is derived from the following relationship:

$$\dot{V}_{exp(t)} = P_{el(t)}/R_{rs} \quad \text{(Equation 22)}$$

Because the elastic pressure is determined by elastance and the corresponding lung volume, the equation may be rewritten as:

$$V_{exp(t)} = [E \times V_{(t)}]/R = V_{(t)}/(\tau) \quad \text{(Equation 23)}$$

As noted previously, τ is the product of resistance and compliance. It is possible to overwhelm the expiratory function of either a normal or a diseased lung during mechanical ventilation with a combination of relatively large tidal volume and relatively short expiratory time, leading to intrinsic PEEP. The volume of trapped gas that corresponds to the inadvertent PEEP can be calculated by the formula:

$$V_{trapped} = V_{(t)}/(e^{Te/\tau}-1) \qquad \text{(Equation 24)}$$

where *Te* is the expiratory time.

Intrinsic PEEP can occur in any mechanically ventilated patient once a certain threshold of ventilation is reached. As noted earlier, PEEPi may even be present when ventilating healthy lungs with high respiratory rates and too short an expiratory time. In patients with deranged respiratory system mechanics, particularly obstructive lung disease (with abnormally large τ values), the propensity to develop intrinsic PEEP is increased.

Respiratory Mechanics and Lung Diseases

ACUTE LUNG INJURY AND ACUTE RESPIRATORY DISTRESS SYNDROME

Acute lung injury (ALI) and acute respiratory distress syndrome (ARDS) are associated with impaired lung barrier function. Because respiratory system elastance scales with lung size, injured lungs appear stiff.[26-28] Total respiratory system resistance is also increased, particularly in the dependent regions of the lungs.[28,29] In ARDS, a significant increase in the value of viscoelastic constants is found.[28] Whether abnormal lung mechanics reflect the collapse of dependent units or are the consequence of alveolar flooding remains controversial.[30]

There is clear evidence that the injured lung is susceptible to further injury related to mechanical ventilation, termed *ventilator-associated lung injury*.[31] An understanding of respiratory mechanics provides some insight into the possible pathogenetic mechanisms of this injury. First, the number of recruitable alveoli capable of expanding during inspiration is reduced. This results in what has been termed the "baby lung," where gas flow is directed to aerated low-impedance units.[27] Thus tidal volumes are distributed to fewer lung units and produce a greater local deformation.

Second, the heterogeneous distribution of liquid and associated surface tension in distal airspaces results in adjacent units with vastly different mechanical properties (e.g., opening pressure). This invokes the theory of injury related to interdependence, whereby during the opening of a flooded unit juxtaposed with an open unit, a shear stress across the tissue attachment results in pressures that are substantially higher than the average transpulmonary pressure.[32]

Mechanical ventilation induces a pulmonary and systemic cytokine response that can minimized by limiting recruitment or derecruitment and overdistention.[33] ARDS patients ventilated with pressure-volume curve analysis to titrate PEEP and tidal volume values show attenuation of the inflammatory response if compared to patients ventilated with a strategy based only on obtaining normal values of arterial carbon dioxide tension and producing the greatest improvement in arterial oxygenation.[33]

Much attention has been focused on the pressure-volume relationship in injured lungs as a means to improve gas exchange and prevent ventilator-associated lung injury in predisposed lungs. Compared with the static P-V curve shown in Figure 46-2, the P-V curve measured with the super syringe method in ARDS and ALI (Figure 46-9) has a number of distinguishing features. These include:
1. Sigmoidal shape with two "knees"—the upper and lower inflection points
2. Increased recoil pressure at all lung volumes
3. Reduced compliance defined by the slope of the inflation curve between the lower and upper inflection points

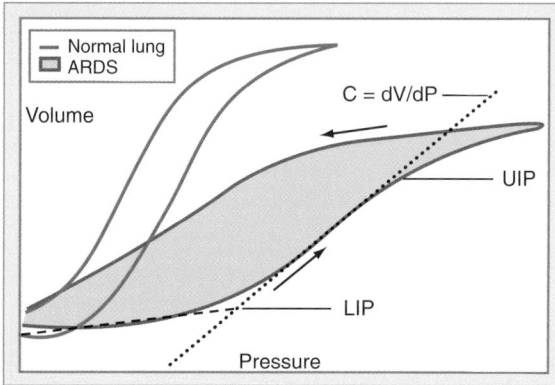

Figure 46-9 Pressure-volume curve in acute respiratory distress syndrome (ARDS) compared with the normal respiratory system. C, compliance; dV/dP, change in volume/change in pressure; LIP, lower inflection point; UIP, upper inflection point. *(From de Chazal I, Hubmayr RD. Novel aspects of pulmonary mechanics in intensive care. Br J Anaesth. 2003;91[1]:81-91.)*

Traditionally, the lower inflection point (LIP) has been interpreted as the pressure at which underventilated or collapsed airways or alveoli are recruited (the average critical opening pressure above which alveolar units start to reopen), corresponding to the pressure at which "best PEEP" should be set. Similarly, the upper inflection point (UIP) where the inflation curve loses its linearity is thought to be the pressure at which no further increases in lung recruitment occur, thereby representing the highest airway pressure that can be safely administered before stretching and overdistention occurs. If these assumptions are correct, ventilator settings should be adjusted until lung expansion is restricted to the linear midrange of the inflation P-V curve.

Characteristics of the P-V curve have been examined in animal models and in patients with ALI[34-36] to study mechanisms responsible for pulmonary injury due to mechanical ventilation (ventilator-induced lung injury: VILI).[37] These studies have demonstrated that tidal inflation starting below the LIP on the P-V curve (leading to tidal recruitment/derecruitment of previously collapsed alveoli) and/or tidal ventilation occurring above the UIP (pulmonary overstretching) could potentially cause a spectrum of pulmonary and systemic lesions including air leaks, alterations in lung fluid balance, increases in endothelial and epithelial permeability, severe tissue damage, and pulmonary and systemic production of inflammatory mediators that could potentially initiate a cascade leading to lung injury and a systemic inflammatory response.[38]

Mead and co-workers,[39] in a classic study, examined the distribution of pressure during tidal inflation in a model of a heterogeneous lung. They found that atelectatic regions in a non-homogeneously inflated lung could be exposed to stresses up to about 140 cm H_2O when the transpulmonary pressure was only 30 cm H_2O. These stresses are generated by shear forces due to (1) recruitment of atelectatic areas surrounded by normal alveoli and (2) overdistension of alveoli adjacent to atelectatic zones or to the pleura. These findings led to the concept that recruitment/derecruitment of previously collapsed alveoli and/or pulmonary overstretching were potential mechanisms responsible for VILI.[33]

Use of the P-V curve in clinical decision making, however, has been the subject of much controversy.[30,34] Critical appraisal of the P-V curve has revealed that there are technical limitations related to the numerous methods used to generate a P-V curve and low specificity for some derived parameters. Attention has also been refocused on edema, airway liquid, and interfacial phenomena as causes of higher opening pressures and increased lung impedance.[30] The lower inflection point may originate in the chest wall rather than the lung in some patients, particularly in those with low end-expired thoracic volumes (recall that the P-V curve of the chest wall is nonlinear at low lung volumes; see Figure 46-2).[40]

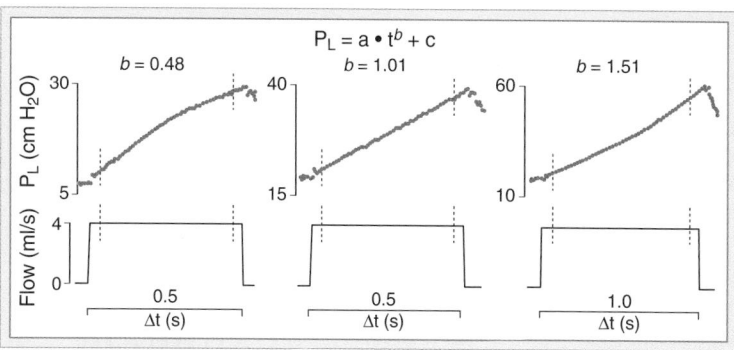

Figure 46-10 Dynamic pressure-time relationships during constant flow. During constant flow, the P-time relation can be described by a power equation where a, b, and c are constants; *a* represents the slope of the P-t relation at time = 1 s, *b* is a dimensionless number that describes the shape of the P-t curve, *c* is the pressure at t = 0. Analysis of P-time profile can unmask tidal volume ongoing recruitment or overdistension. *(From Ranieri VM, Zhang H, Mascia L, et al. Pressure-time curve predicts minimally injurious ventilatory strategy in an isolated rat lung model. Anesthesiology. 2000;93[5]:1320-1328.)*

It is clear that adjustments in PEEP are helpful in optimizing gas exchange, with improvements noted in the ratio of arterial oxygen pressure to inspired oxygen fraction (Pao_2:Fio_2). However, PEEP adjustments via P-V loop guidance do not necessarily translate into improvements in outcome or survival. As previously mentioned, if the assumptions on the lower and upper inflection point are true, ventilator settings should be adjusted until lung expansion is restricted to the linear midrange of the inflation P-V curve. This hypothesis finds application in stress index monitoring,[41-42] which allows for breath-by-breath assessment of adherence to this treatment target.

Ranieri et al. showed that the shape of the dynamic inspiratory P-t profile during constant flow inflation allows prediction of a ventilatory strategy that minimizes the occurrence of VILI in an isolated lung model of ALI. Figure 46-10 shows the behavior of the dynamic pressure-time (P-t) curve under such conditions. In addition, the shape of the Paw-t curve detects tidal recruitment and tidal hyperinflation.[43]

Evidence of alveolar hyperinflation was found in patients with focal ARDS ventilated with the ARDSNet protocol. Individual positive end-expiratory pressure titration based on "stress index" monitoring reduced the risk of alveolar hyperinflation.[44] However, patients characterized by a larger amount of collapsed lung may be exposed to VILI despite tidal volume and pressure limitation. As suggested by the study of Terragni et al., plateau pressure should be limited to 28 cm H_2O to guarantee lung protection.[45]

In the ARDSNet trial, early improvements in arterial oxygenation were noted in patients who were ventilated with higher tidal volumes, but such patients turned out to have increased mortality.[31] A subsequent study by the same group showed no difference in mortality between ARDS patients randomized to higher "optimal" PEEP and "conventional" PEEP.[46]

It was suggested that patients with ARDS ventilated at relatively high respiratory rates develop greater PEEPi than when ventilated at lower rates, even for the same minute volume (V). This mechanism may produce decreased lung injury secondary to recruitment/derecruitment, and hence provides a plausible explanation for some of the decreased mortality observed in the ARDSNet trial in the 6 mL/kg ideal body weight (IBW) group.[47]

Many clinicians have advocated using the upper inflection point as an analog of plateau pressure (end-inspiratory occlusion pressure), and recommendations not to exceed 30 to 35 cm H_2O have been advanced. Although some regions of the lungs may approach their maximal volume at pressures near the upper inflection point, the evidence is circumstantial that ventilating patients near this airway pressure (with relatively low tidal volume) causes injury.

Because of concerns about chest wall–related P-V artifacts, esophageal manometry has been used to guide the ventilatory management of patients with injured lungs. Ranieri et al.[48] showed that interpretation of the mechanical properties of the respiratory system requires assessment of both lung and chest wall mechanics and may vary with the underlying disease responsible for ARDS. In patients with medical ARDS, the inspiratory P-V curve of the respiratory system and lung showed a progressive reduction in elastance with inflating volume because of alveolar recruitment. In patients in whom ARDS followed major abdominal surgery, abdominal distension, with increased values for chest wall elastance, were observed. When abdominal pressure was normalized by surgical reexploration, improvement of the mechanical properties of the respiratory system, lung, and chest wall was observed. This study suggests that the flattening of the P-V curve at high pressures observed in some patients with ARDS may be due to increase in chest wall elastance related to abdominal distension. These results may also have importance for the optimal ventilatory management of critically ill patients with ARDS with respect to the selection of best PEEP and VT levels to minimize ventilator-induced lung injury. However, data from esophageal catheters may be misleading because derecruited dependent lung units that appose the esophageal probe may fail to generate local pressure swings, thereby biasing the measurement.[49]

In conclusion, over the past few years, we have learned that the application of a ventilatory strategy that minimizes VILI can decrease mortality rate in patients with ALI and ARDS.[31] The key elements of such a lung-protective strategy are minimization of overdistension (volutrauma) and the use of sufficient positive end-expiratory pressure (PEEP) to prevent cyclic alveolar collapse (atelectrauma). The most common approach of trying to ensure a lung-protective strategy makes use of measurements at the airway opening of the pressure applied to he respiratory system. It thus appears that respiratory mechanics in patients with injured lungs are helpful in identifying those at greatest risk for ventilator-associated lung injury, and reassessment of the ventilation strategy limiting tidal volume to 6 mL/kg IBW and plateau pressure to 28 to 30 cm H_2O may protect the lungs of patients with acute respiratory distress syndrome from VILI. However, although prevention of ventilator-induced lung injury is primarily based on recognizing the "harmful" threshold for pressure and volume (28-30 cm H_2O airway plateau pressure (Pel,rs) and 6 mL/kg VT IBW), VT IBW and airway plateau pressure may be inadequate surrogates for lung stress and strain. Specific elastance (Espec) may play a major role in determining stress and strain.[50]

Last but not least, the effects of high PEEP strictly depend on lung recruitability, which widely varies during ARDS. Unfortunately, increasing PEEP may lead to opposing effects on two main factors potentially worsening the lung injury: alveolar strain and intratidal opening and closing, being detrimental (increasing the former) or beneficial (decreasing the latter). It has been found that especially in ARDS patients with higher lung recruitability, the beneficial impact of reducing intratidal alveolar opening and closing by increasing PEEP overcomes the effects of increasing alveolar strain.[51]

OBSTRUCTIVE PULMONARY DISEASE

A hallmark finding of all patients with obstructive lung disease is the inability to generate normal expiratory flows which, in a mechanically ventilated patient, leads to dynamic hyperinflation. One of the most readily available means to detect hyperinflation is the measurement of intrinsic PEEP by the end-expiratory airway occlusion method. *Intrinsic PEEP* is defined as total PEEP minus applied or extrinsic PEEP, and it reflects the elastic recoil of the respiratory system at end-expiration.[52]

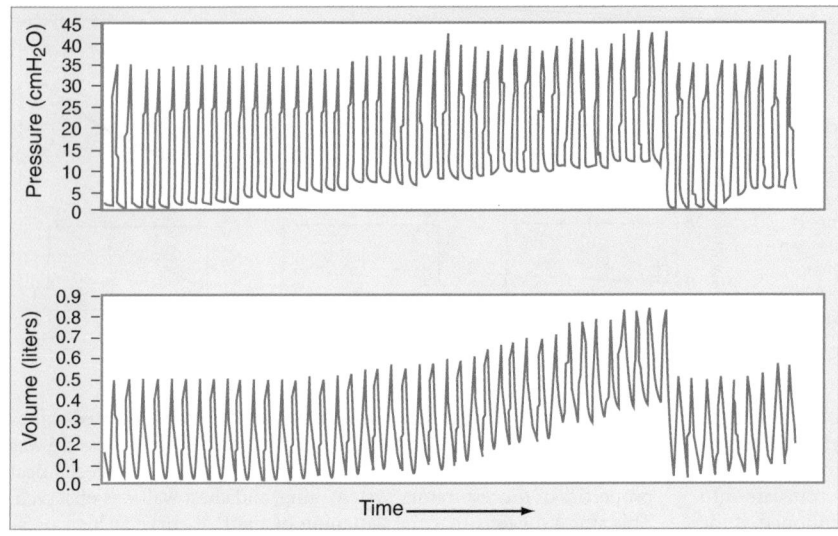

Figure 46-11 Response of airway pressure and volume to extrinsic positive end-expiratory pressure in a dynamically hyperinflated, mechanically ventilated patient with chronic obstructive pulmonary disease. *(From Gay PC, Rodarte JR, Hubmayr RD. The effects of positive expiratory pressure on isovolume flow and dynamic hyperinflation in patients receiving mechanical ventilation. Am Rev Respir Dis. 1989;139[3]:621-626.)*

It should be noted, however, that intrinsic PEEP is not a specific marker of airway obstruction. Patients with "normal" lungs can hyperinflate above a critical minute ventilation, as explained by Equation 23; the presence of intrinsic PEEP and dynamic hyperinflation does not necessarily indicate an absolute increase in end-expiratory volume. For example, on the basis of mass loading of the chest wall in the recumbent position, many patients with ascites or obesity breathe at lung volumes near residual volume.[53] It should also be noted that the reliability of the end-expiratory occlusion method is dependent on complete respiratory muscle inactivity and therefore may not be reliable in a patient who assists the ventilator.

In assessing for the presence of airflow limitation, the expiratory time constant, τ, can be determined by the slope of the flow-volume curve (see Figure 46-6) or by the product of resistance and compliance (see Equation 23). However, a more readily available tool for detecting an in increase in resistive or threshold load is simple pattern recognition of ventilator-generated waveforms during a constant flow breath. Recall from Figure 46-8 that the initial step change in airway pressure during lung inflation should be equal to the recovery of pressure at the end of the tidal volume—that is, the difference between peak and plateau or airway occlusion pressure. The early step change is determined by any load that must be overcome to commence lung inflation. This includes resistive pressure as well as intrinsic PEEP, which drives expiratory flow. Thus, dynamic hyperinflation should be considered when the initial pressure step change significantly exceeds the terminal pressure recovery. This concept is also demonstrated in Figure 46-11, which shows an example of typical volume, airway pressure, and flow curves in an obstructed, dynamically hyperinflated patient.[54] This method of assessing for hyperinflation has the added advantage of being less susceptible to patient effort, because thoracic neuromechanical feedback mechanisms tend to blunt effort at end-inspiration.

In the normal lung, expiratory driving pressure is determined by the difference between alveolar pressure and airway opening pressure. In the relaxed or paralyzed state, this driving pressure is the respiratory system recoil pressure at end-inspiratory lung volume. In normal lungs, the net driving pressure may be reduced by the application of extrinsic PEEP, which serves as a load that must be overcome before volume can be expired. Consequently, in a volume-preset ventilatory mode, this would result in reduced expiratory flow, hyperinflation, and elevated peak airway pressures over subsequent breaths. As explained in Figure 47-7, if extrinsic PEEP does not affect expiratory flow, flow limitation is present. In other words, in patients with severe airway obstruction who are breathing in the tidal volume range, end-inspiratory recoil pressure far exceeds that required for maximal expiratory flow. These patients would not exhibit reductions in expiratory

flow in response to the application of small levels of extrinsic PEEP.[55] Accordingly, as shown in Figure 46-11, the application of up to 5 cm H_2O of extrinsic PEEP in an obstructed patient fails to raise volume or peak pressure.

Respiratory Muscle Function in Healthy Lungs and in Pathologic Conditions

The primary task of the respiratory muscles is to drive the respiratory pump. To do so, they must generate forces necessary to overcome the elastic and resistive load of the respiratory system described in the preceding sections.

The chest wall collectively includes the thoracic cage and the abdominal compartment, which compose a parallel circuit. The respiratory muscles are striated in nature and thus subscribe to Starling's law regarding length-tension relationships. As such, inspiratory muscles that act to expand the chest wall exert their greatest forces at low lung volumes (Figure 46-12). Conversely, expiratory muscles, working to actively deflate the lungs, are most efficient at high lung volumes.[4]

The muscles of respiration perform in a complex integrated fashion to maximize breathing efficiency. Although the diaphragm is the primary muscle of respiration, it is known that muscles previously

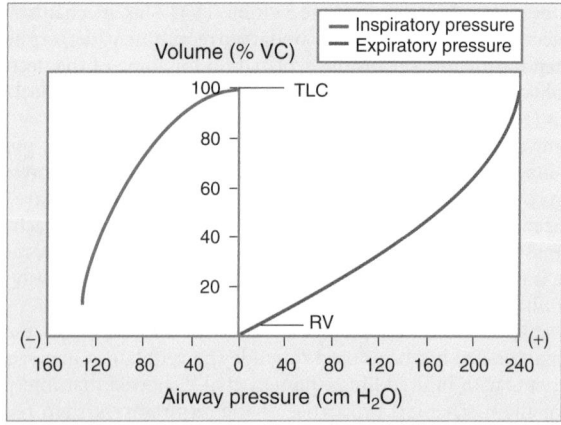

Figure 46-12 Plot of inspiratory and expiratory pressures as a function of lung volume. Note higher pressures generated by expiratory muscles. TLC, total lung capacity; VC, vital capacity. *(From Taylor A, Rehder K, Hyatt R, et al. Mechanics of breathing: static. In: Taylor AE, editor. Clinical Respiratory Physiology. Philadelphia: Saunders; 1989:89-105.)*

thought to have only an accessory role in breathing, including the intercostal and scalene muscles, are actively taking part in quiet respiration to aid in movement of the chest wall.[56] Relaxation allows passive recoil of the respiratory system to its resting functional residual capacity position. During exercise, phasic contraction of expiratory muscles drives the respiratory system below its resting position. Subsequent relaxation at end-expiration increases lung volume, thereby reducing the load on the inspiratory muscles for the next respiratory cycle.[3]

The rib cage is the most extensive portion of the chest wall and therefore contributes most to thoracic displacement during breathing. The ribs are situated ventrally during rest, with a downward slope. Because of their articulations with the sternum and spinal transverse processes, they are confined and move in a stereotypical manner during breathing. During inspiration, the ribs are displaced cranially to become more horizontal so that both the anteroposterior and transverse diameters of the rib cage increase.

The intercostal muscles, innervated by the intercostal nerves, act directly on the ribs to effect movement. Three different intercostal muscle groups have varying effects on respiration, depending on their origin and insertion points, which dictate orientation. The parasternal and external intercostals serve as primary inspiratory muscles by raising the ribs during contraction. In contrast, the internal intercostal muscles, which run at right angles to the externals, serve an expiratory function by contracting during expiration to induce caudal motion of the lower ribs.

The most important inspiratory muscle is the dome-shaped diaphragm. It is composed of muscle fibers that radiate from the central tendon to attach to the lower rib cage. The crural portion inserts on the anterior portions of lumbar vertebrae 1 through 3, and the costal portion inserts on the xiphoid process and the upper inner margins of the lower six ribs. The majority of the muscular portion of the diaphragm lies directly beside the lower rib cage, referred to as the *zone of apposition* (Figure 46-13). The zone of apposition is 6 to 9 cm in height and occupies 25% to 30% of the total interior surface of the rib cage.[56]

The diaphragm exerts two types of forces upon contraction. First, there is an insertional force during contraction, related to the shortening of muscle fibers, to displace the dome caudally. This increases intraabdominal pressure, which causes ventral displacement of the anterior abdominal wall. The net effect is the lowering of pleural pressure to effect lung expansion. In other words, diaphragmatic contraction increases transdiaphragmatic pressure (P_{di}), which is partially dependent on abdominal pressure (P_{ab}), as shown in the equation:

$$P_{di} = P_{ab} - P_{pl} = P_{ga} - P_{es} \qquad \text{(Equation 25)}$$

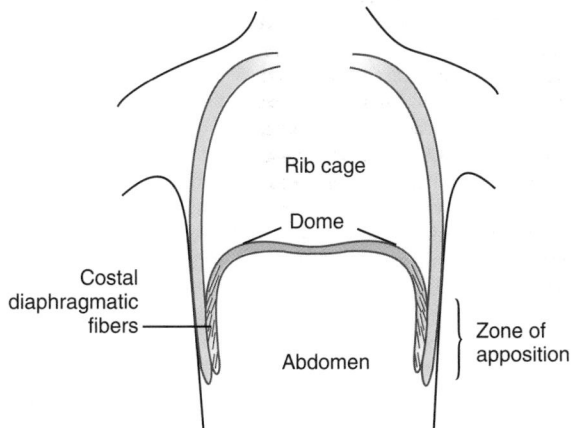

Figure 46-13 Chest wall, frontal section, at end-expiration. Costal diaphragmatic fibers are cranially oriented, resulting in apposition to lower rib cage. *(From De Troyer A. Respiratory muscle function. In: Pinsky MR, editor.* Textbook of Critical Care. *Philadelphia: Saunders; 2000:1172-1184.)*

where P_{ga} is gastric pressure, and P_{es} is esophageal pressure. Second, the contracting diaphragm exerts what is termed an *appositional force*. This is related to the configuration of the muscle fibers in the zone of apposition which, in contrast to fibers in the dome, have a much larger radius of curvature (i.e., less of a curve). In accordance with the law of Laplace, less pressure is therefore generated to move the diaphragm. Instead, the pleural space in the zone of apposition is exposed to approximate abdominal pressure, thereby acting directly to push the lower rib cage in an outward direction.[57] Thus the rise in abdominal pressure caused by descent of the diaphragmatic dome is transmitted through the appositional portion of the diaphragm to expand the lower rib cage.[58] Accordingly, pressure in the pleural recess between the apposed diaphragm and the rib cage actually *increases* during inspiration.

It should be noted that diaphragmatic contraction can have inspiratory *or* expiratory effects on the thoracic cage, depending on several factors.[3] For example, mechanical properties of the abdominal compartment have a marked influence on diaphragmatic function. Low compliance (or high elastance) of the total respiratory system, as in tense ascites, results in reduced dome excursion and decreased insertional force, whereas decrements in abdominal resistance (evisceration) cause loss of the zone of apposition, with resultant expiratory actions on the lower rib cage.[56] There are also important effects related to lung volume. The area of apposition increases as the lungs approach residual volume, causing a greater inspiratory effect on the lower rib cage. Conversely, near total lung capacity, the zone of apposition is nearly absent, resulting in an expiratory force. Studies of diaphragmatic contraction in subjects with cervical spinal cord transection have demonstrated expiratory effects on the upper rib cage and inspiratory effects on the lower rib cage.[59,60]

The scalene muscles, considered primary muscles of respiration, originate at the cervical spine transverse processes and insert on the first two ribs anteriorly. Their contraction aids inspiration by expanding the rib cage. A number of muscles serve an accessory role, facilitating the primary muscles' role during periods of increased effort (exercise, fatigue). These muscles include the sternocleidomastoids, pectoralis minor, and erector spinae, all of which elevate the ribs during contraction.[3]

The respiratory muscles of the abdominal wall, including the obliques, rectus abdominis, and transversus abdominis, are primarily expiratory in function by virtue of the increase in abdominal pressure upon contraction. This becomes important when flow demands are not met by passive elastic recoil. As mentioned previously, the abdominal musculature aids in unloading the inspiratory muscles during times of stress by their effects on lung volume. In addition, the tonic contraction of the abdominal muscles to help maintain posture in the upright position elongates the diaphragm, thus improving its length-tension relationship.

Expiratory muscles are also involved in generating cough.[56] In tetraplegic subjects, the clavicular portion of the pectoralis major plays a major role during coughing. Its contraction causes a reduction in the size of the upper part of the rib cage and a rise in intrathoracic pressure; this pressure rise results secondarily in an outward (paradoxical) motion of the abdomen and the lower rib cage.[61] Measurement of peak cough maximal expiratory flow rate (PCEF) is a simple and reproducible intervention to assess capability of coughing in spontaneous breathing patients. Values below 3.5 to 4L/sec have been associated with poor coughing.[62-63] Measurement of peak flow rate (PEF) during induced cough also seems to improve predictability of successful decannulation or extubation in critical care patients.[64-67]

The abdomen plays a major role in respiratory mechanics. The abdomen, with the exception of the diaphragm superiorly and the anterior abdominal wall (and small amounts of gas in the gastrointestinal tract), is an essentially incompressible compartment with fixed boundaries. As such, the movement of the diaphragm and thoracic cage is coupled with movement of the anterior abdominal wall. This is a clinically important relationship that should be assessed during a physical examination, because asynchronous and paradoxical motion of the rib cage and abdomen has been associated with increased respiratory drive[68] and possible risk of ventilatory failure.[69]

Pressure measurements across the chest wall can be readily obtained to assess the ability of the respiratory muscles to perform the work of breathing. As mentioned earlier with regard to the respiratory system, the chest wall can be studied during static as well as dynamic maneuvers to obtain important information about function. It should be noted that although these functional tests are of interest to physiologists and researchers, their clinical application is limited.

The Rahn diagram is a graphic representation of the relaxed respiratory system's P-V characteristics (see Figure 46-2). It provides information on the passive elastic properties of the components of the respiratory system. For accurate chest wall measurements, complete respiratory muscle relaxation is required. The function of the active chest wall can be assessed with the Campbell diagram,[70] which plots changes in lung volume against pleural pressure.

Because use of this methodology is difficult in mechanically ventilated patients, simple ventilator waveform analysis can be helpful. For example, deviation of the inspiratory flow waveform from the relaxed tracing indicates active patient effort as a result of flow deprivation—that is, the patient's demands are not being met by the set inspiratory flow.[71] Maximal inspiratory pressure is a commonly used measurement in the ICU, particularly in weaning protocols. High generated pressures probably correlate with adequate muscle strength, but low values may be related to volitional factors. Moreover, standardized testing has shown poor reproducibility.[72]

Impairment or failure of the respiratory pump can occur at any of several levels. Dysfunctional central respiratory control, such as during coma or intoxication, alters neural output to the respiratory muscles. Neuromuscular diseases such as myasthenia gravis or muscular dystrophy result in primary muscle weakness, whereas metabolic abnormalities (malnutrition, thyroid disease) affect the muscle tension-generating machinery. Lung hyperinflation, such as occurs in COPD or asthma, puts the chest wall at a mechanical disadvantage because of alterations in the length-tension relationship.

Much attention has been given to the concept of respiratory muscle fatigue,[73] both in acute respiratory failure and in relation to chronic lung disease. *Muscle fatigue* is defined as a condition associated with loss of the capacity for developing force, velocity, or both resulting from muscle activity, which is reversible by rest.[74] This contrasts with the definition of *muscle weakness*, in which the rested muscle remains impaired. Fatigue can be induced in striated muscle when working against an increased load. This has been reproduced in normal human respiratory muscles forced to work against high inspiratory airflow resistance.[75] Fatigue can be classified as central fatigue, peripheral high-frequency fatigue, or peripheral low-frequency fatigue.[76,77] It is likely that all three play a role in respiratory muscle fatigue at any given time.

There is no single measurement of force that can adequately measure respiratory muscle fatigue. Rather, fatigue is implied by the deterioration of force during serial measurements over time. The factors important in respiratory muscle fatigue—magnitude and duration of contraction—are incorporated into the calculation of the pressure-time index of the diaphragm (PT_{di}):

$$PT_{di} = (P_{di}/P_{di,max})(T_i/T_{tot}) \qquad \text{(Equation 26)}$$

where P_{di} denotes transdiaphragmatic pressure (a measure of magnitude), T_i is inspiratory time, and T_{tot} is total breath time. When breathing is accomplished primarily by diaphragmatic function, a critical pressure-time index is reached at values of 0.15 to 0.18, above which functional failure readily occurs.[51] Similar ranges have been obtained for rib cage muscles as well.[78] Unfortunately, because these values were experimentally obtained in normal subjects breathing against imposed loads, the true values that apply to patients with impending respiratory failure, in whom other factors (hypoxemia, hemodynamic instability) are in play, is not known. In addition, when respiration is accomplished only by the diaphragm without the contribution of the other respiratory muscles, as in quadriplegic patients, the fatigue threshold is lower than previously reported.[79]

The inability of the respiratory pump to meet metabolic demands, resulting in acute respiratory failure, is a result of either increase in the ventilatory load above a critical level or inability of the respiratory muscles to generate sufficient force. Assessment of the breathing pattern may be helpful in patients with impending respiratory failure. For example, tachypnea and paradoxical motion of the thorax and abdomen are frequently encountered in this setting, but they are not specific or diagnostic of muscle fatigue.

Work of breathing is a global measure of respiratory pump activity and reflects the imposed respiratory load, which is often a result of abnormalities in respiratory mechanics. Most of the work of breathing, in both health and disease states, occurs during inspiration (W_i) and is related to the static elastance (E_{st}) of the respiratory system[80]:

$$W_{i,st} = 0.5\, E_{st} \times \Delta V \qquad \text{(Equation 27)}$$

A linear relationship is assumed between elastance and the volumes measured.

The contribution of dynamic factors to work of breathing, such as increases in airway resistance in COPD or asthma resulting in dynamic hyperinflation, must also be accounted for. In such cases, the equation becomes:

$$W_{i,st} = 0.5\, E_{st} \times \Delta V + PEEP_i \times \Delta V \qquad \text{(Equation 28)}$$

Patients with acute respiratory failure related to COPD have been found to have increased inspiratory resistance, increased dynamic elastance, and up to twice the level of intrinsic $PEEP_i$ compared with COPD patients not in acute respiratory failure.[81] Dynamic hyperinflation has secondary deleterious effects on respiratory muscle function related primarily to Starling's law (suboptimal coupling of the tension-generating components of the muscle fibers).[82] Thus the increased work of breathing and subsequent respiratory muscle fatigue due to disruption of the optimal length-tension relationships of respiratory muscles[83] could precipitate acute respiratory failure in patients with "compensated" COPD. Although impairment of inspiratory muscle function related to dynamic hyperinflation is classically associated with COPD, a number of other disorders seen in critical illness have been associated with reduced respiratory muscle force generation. Sepsis, even in the absence of direct lung involvement, can cause respiratory failure related to increased metabolic demands as well as respiratory muscle dysfunction.[84] Direct effects on muscle function have been related to failure of neuromuscular contraction, derangements in excitation-contraction coupling, and direct cytotoxic effects.[84]

Critical illness polyneuropathy, associated with varying degrees of weakness and axonal degeneration on electromyography and denervation atrophy on muscle biopsy, has a reported incidence as high as 25%.[85] The causative role of critical illness polyneuropathy in respiratory failure is controversial because it is often associated with other conditions that affect global muscle function, such as sepsis and multiorgan system failure.[86] Critical illness polyneuropathy has, however, been documented in cases of respiratory failure independent of these risk factors.[87] Critical illness myopathy, which can coexist with polyneuropathy, is most commonly reported in cases of severe asthma and may be related to glucocorticoid and neuromuscular blocking agent administration.[88] Finally, there is increasing animal model data showing that mechanical ventilation has direct harmful effects on diaphragmatic structure and function.[89,90] Putative mechanisms include atrophy related to disuse (particularly with prolonged mechanical ventilation), tonic effects of PEEP, and confounding effects of anesthesia and neuromuscular blocking agents.

Weaning from Mechanical Ventilation

Clinical assessment alone is insufficient to predict successful weaning from mechanical ventilation,[91] and respiratory muscle function is only one determinant of weaning ability. Unfortunately, the incorporation of many objective methods into weaning paradigms has not proved particularly useful. The shortcomings of breathing pattern assessment were mentioned earlier, and measurements of maximal inspiratory pressures are not easily reproduced. Measurement of pressure-time indices has not been readily adopted in ICU practice, and work-of-breathing determinations are cumbersome and seemingly restricted to the research setting.

The most widely adopted and useful predictor of weaning success is the ratio of breathing frequency to tidal volume, as first reported by Yang and Tobin.[92] This involves the simple use of a spirometer attached to the endotracheal tube during a spontaneous breathing trial. A ratio of 105 breaths/min/L provides the best separation between subjects who will succeed or who will fail at weaning.

KEY POINTS

1. Pressures applied to the respiratory system are either stored as a function of elasticity or dissipated as resistive energy. A basic understanding of the mechanics from pressures and flow derived from mechanical ventilator output is useful during the bedside assessment of ICU patients.

2. Information about respiratory system mechanics derived from the pressure-volume curve can be helpful in identifying patients at risk for ventilator-associated lung injury.

3. Determining respiratory muscle function is important in the clinical setting. Current methods of quantifying muscle fatigue, beyond patient clinical examination, are limited by their low specificity.

4. The movement of the diaphragm and thoracic cage is coupled with movement of the anterior abdominal wall. This clinically important relationship should be assessed during physical examination, because asynchronous and paradoxical motion of the rib cage and abdomen have been associated with risk of respiratory failure.

5. Critical illness polyneuropathy and myopathy, as well as mechanical ventilation itself, are important causes of respiratory muscle dysfunction in the ICU and are associated with modifiable risk factors, including the use of neuromuscular blocking agents.

ANNOTATED REFERENCES

Fredberg JJ, Stamenovic D. On the imperfect elasticity of lung tissue. J Appl Physiol 1989;67(6):2408-19.
An elegant exploration of energy losses related to tissue resistance and hysteresis and the coupling of changes in elastic energy storage and dissipative energy loss, which appear to reside within the same stress-bearing element of the lung.

Fry DL, Hyatt RE. Pulmonary mechanics: a unified analysis of the relationship between pressure, volume and gas flow in the lungs of normal and diseased human subjects. Am J Med 1960;29:672-89.
Report of a classic set of human experiments that forms the physiologic basis of the forced vital capacity maneuver in modern pulmonary function testing.

Hubmayr RD. Perspective on lung injury and recruitment: a skeptical look at the opening and collapse story. Am J Respir Crit Care Med 2002;165(12):1647-53.
A discussion of current controversies about ventilation strategies, emphasizing the uncertainties of physiologic changes at the acinar level. The theory of alveolar collapse in derecruitment is questioned, and the interpretation of the P-V curve and the best PEEP is argued.

Laghi F, Tobin M. Disorders of the respiratory muscles. Am J Respir Crit Care Med 2003;168(1):10-48.
A wide-ranging discussion of various diseases of respiratory muscles, including an explanation of the molecular mechanisms of clinically applicable disorders encountered in the ICU.

Loring S. Mechanics of the lung and chest wall. In: Marini JJ, editor. Physiological Basis of Ventilatory Support. New York: Marcel Dekker; 1998:177-205.
A comprehensive review of the physiologic basis of classic respiratory system mechanics. Discusses lung and chest wall mechanical properties, as well as assessment of respiratory muscle function.

Ranieri VM, Zhang H, Mascia L, et al. Pressure-time curve predicts minimally injurious ventilatory strategy in an isolated rat lung model. Anesthesiology 2000;93(5):1320-8.
A very interesting study testing the hypothesis that the pressure-time (P-t) curve during constant flow ventilation can be used to set a noninjurious ventilatory strategy. The predictive power of coefficient b to predict noninjurious ventilatory strategy in a model of acute lung injury was high.

de Durante G, del Turco M, Rustichini L, et al. ARDSNet lower tidal volume ventilatory strategy may generate intrinsic positive end-expiratory pressure in patients with acute respiratory distress syndrome. Am J Respir Crit Care Med 2002;165(9):1271-4.
The challenging findings of this study suggest that patients with ARDS ventilated at relatively high respiratory rates develop greater PEEPi than when ventilated at lower rates, even for the same minute volume. This mechanism may produce decreased lung injury secondary to recruitment-derecruitment and hence provides a plausible explanation for some of the decreased mortality observed in the ARDSNet trial in the 6 mL/kg group.

Terragni PP, Rosboch G, Tealdi A, et al. Tidal hyperinflation during low tidal volume ventilation in acute respiratory distress syndrome. Am J Respir Crit Care Med 2007;175(2):160-6.
An interesting study evaluating whether limiting tidal volume to 6 mL/kg and plateau pressure to 30 cm H2O protect the lungs of patients with acute respiratory distress syndrome from ventilator-induced lung injury (VILI). The authors found that patients characterized by a larger amount of collapsed lung may be exposed to VILI despite tidal volume and pressure limitation; plateau pressure should be limited to 28 cm H2O to guarantee lung protection.

Chiumello D, Carlesso E, Cadringher, et al. Lung stress and strain during mechanical ventilation for acute respiratory distress syndrome. Am J Respir Crit Care Med 2008;178(4):346-55.
Another challenging study analyzing whether lung stress and strain and their surrogates, airway pressure and tidal volume per weight (VT IBW), are the primary determinants of ventilator-induced lung injury. The authors demonstrated that VT IBW and airway plateau pressure may be inadequate surrogates for lung stress and strain.

REFERENCES

Access the complete reference list online at http://www.expertconsult.com.

47

Heart-Lung Interactions

MICHAEL R. PINSKY | HERNANDO GOMEZ

Ventilation can profoundly alter cardiovascular function. The boundaries of the cardiovascular unit's responsiveness are defined by both cardiovascular and pulmonary factors. These limitations include myocardial reserve, circulating blood volume, blood flow distribution, autonomic tone, endocrinological responses, lung volume, intrathoracic pressure (ITP) and surrounding pressures for the remainder of the circulation. That positive-pressure ventilation may influence cardiovascular function in ways not seen during spontaneous ventilation was appreciated when positive-pressure ventilation was first introduced over 50 years ago[1] and still results in new perspectives today.[2]

The final response to ventilatory stress is dependent on the baseline cardiovascular state of the subject. In the most extreme of examples, maximal exercise tolerance in young healthy subjects is primarily limited only by muscle strength, endurance, and coordination, rather than by minute ventilation or cardiac output. However, in the same subject following a disease process that compromises cardiovascular or respiratory function—such as may occur following trauma, sepsis, and acute lung injury (ALI)—even simple tasks like breathing spontaneously or sitting up in bed may be outside their realm of possibilities. At the opposite end of this spectrum, artificial ventilation may introduce dynamic and complex changes to cardiopulmonary interactions that neither nature nor evolution could foresee. Thus, normal adaptive autonomic reflexes may not be appropriate in the setting of artificial ventilation.

First we shall address the basic mechanisms underlying the cardiopulmonary interactions, and then using these constructs, we shall examine recent clinical trials of established and novel ventilatory therapies relative to their observed hemodynamic effects.

Airway Pressure, Intrathoracic Pressure, and Lung Volume Relationships

Since positive-pressure ventilation was introduced, the concept of relating hemodynamic consequences to airway pressure was widely accepted.[3,4] This oversimplification has been the source of much of the confusion in the clinical literature. A major source of such confusion rests in equating changes in airway pressure (Paw) with changes in both pleural pressure (Ppl) and lung volume. Physicians often equate Paw with the hemodynamic effects seen because (1) Paw can be measured easily at the bedside in patients receiving mechanical ventilation, (2) mean Paw reflects mean alveolar pressure, and (3) increases in Paw qualitatively reflect increases in both lung volume and Ppl. However, the association between Paw and other hemodynamically relevant factors (1) is highly variable as ventilatory patterns, airway resistance, and lung compliance change, (2) does not accurately reflect changes in pericardial pressure (Ppc), which is a primary determinant of transmural left ventricular (LV) pressure, and (3) may mislead the caregiver at the bedside into altering therapy based on these wrong assumptions. Numerous studies have demonstrated that the primary determinants of hemodynamic responses to ventilation are due to changes in intrathoracic pressure and lung volume, and not Paw.[5] Thus, prior to examining heart-lung interactions, we shall address the relation between Paw, Ppl, Ppc, and lung volume. To simplify the discussion, we shall use the term *intrathoracic pressure* (ITP) to refer to nonspecific intrathoracic surface pressure. When specific intrapleural surface pressures are identified, they will be referred to either as the *lateral chest wall, diaphragm, and juxtacardiac pleural pressures* or *pericardial pressure* where appropriate.

AIRWAY PRESSURE, LUNG VOLUME, AND REGIONAL PLEURAL PRESSURES

During positive-pressure inspiration, increases in Paw parallel increases in lung volume. In the sedated and paralyzed patient at end-inspiration, only lung and thoracic compliance determine the relationship between Paw and lung volume. However, if ventilated patients actively resist lung inflation or sustain expiratory muscle activity at end-inspiration, then end-inspiratory Paw will exceed resting Paw for that lung volume. Similarly, if patient activity prevents full exhalation by expiratory braking, then for the same end-expiratory airway pressure (often measured as positive end-expiratory pressure [PEEP]), lung volume may be higher than predicted from end-expiratory Paw values alone. Finally, even if inspiration is passive and no increased airway resistance is present, Paw may rapidly increase as chest wall compliance decreases, especially as chest wall compliance includes diaphragmatic dissention. If intraabdominal pressure were to increase then end-expiratory Paw must also increase for a constant tidal volume. In acute respiratory distress syndrome (ARDS), increases in intraabdominal pressure can occur with gut wall swelling (third-spacing) and gut distention.[6]

During inspiration, Paw increases as a function of both total thoracic compliance and airway resistance. Thus, in subjects with marked bronchospasm, such as asthmatics, peak Paw will greatly exceed end-inspiratory plateau Paw. Accordingly, changes in Paw are related to changes in lung volume through the interaction of airway resistance and both lung and chest compliances, as manifested by the relative increase in ITP during inspiration. Several common clinical examples serve to support this statement. If either lung or chest wall compliance changes, then Paw may change without an actual change in the tidal breath. The two common clinical scenarios of this phenomenon are mucus plugging and fighting the ventilator. Similarly, if spontaneous breaths cause ITP to decrease during positive-pressure inspiration, then both peak and mean Paw will decrease, whereas if bronchospasm cause airway resistance to increase, then for a constant volume tidal breath, both peak and mean Paw will increase.

As the lung expands, it pushes on surrounding structures, distorting them and causing their surface pressures to increase. Thus lung expansion induces an increase in lateral wall, diaphragmatic, and juxtacardiac Ppl as well as Ppc. The degree of increase in each of these surface pressures will be a function of the compliance and inertance of their opposing structures. These interactions were described by Novak et al.,[6] who demonstrated that changes in Ppl induced by positive-pressure ventilation are not similar in all regions of the thorax and increase differently as inspiratory flow rate and frequency increase. Pleural pressure on the diaphragm increases least during inspiration, and juxtacardiac Ppl increases most. Since the diaphragm is very compliant, it seems reasonable that diaphragmatic ITP should increase less than lateral chest wall Ppl to sudden increases in lung volume. However, if abdominal distention develops, as commonly occurs in the setting of sepsis, the diaphragm will become relatively noncompliant because of the increase in abdominal pressure. Under these conditions, ITP

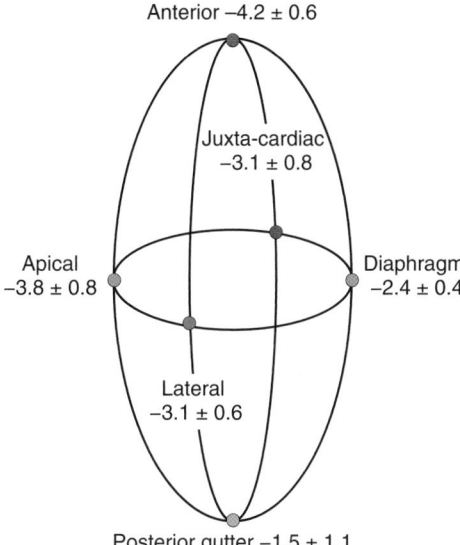

Figure 47-1 Apneic pleural pressure (Ppl) (mean ± SE) in Torr for six pleural regions of the right hemothorax of an intact supine canine model. Ellipses represent regional measurements defining three orthogonal planes. (*Reproduced with permission from Novak, et al. J Appl Physiol 1995;65:1314-1323.*)

PLEURAL PRESSURE AND LUNG VOLUME IN ACUTE LUNG INJURY

The interaction of Paw, lung volume, and ITP in the setting of lung disease is complex and can be different for the same pathologic setting depending on the tidal volume, inspiratory flow rate, ventilatory frequency, and body position. The presence of parenchymal disease, airflow obstruction, and extrapulmonary processes that directly alter chest wall–diaphragmatic contraction also profoundly alter these interactions. Static lung expansion occurs as Paw increases because the transpulmonary pressure (Paw relative to ITP) increases. If lung injury induces alveolar flooding or increased pulmonary parenchyma stiffness, greater increases in Paw will be required to distend the lungs to a constant end-inspiratory volume. Romand et al.[8] demonstrated that Paw increased more during ALI than in control conditions for a constant tidal volume, whereas lateral chest wall Ppl and Ppc increased similarly between both conditions if tidal volume was held constant (Figure 47-2). These data agree with the studies of O'Quinn et al.[9] that the primary determinant of the increase in Ppl and Ppc during positive-pressure ventilation is lung volume change, not Paw change. Data from Romand et al.[8] demonstrated that the increase in ITP during sustained increases in lung volume is greater than the increase in Ppc. Presumably, Ppc does not increase as much as ITP because increasing lung volume also reduces filling of the ventricles, thereby reducing their size inside the cardiac fossa. To summarize, for a constant increase in lung volume, ITP will increase similarly despite drastic changes in lung compliance and airway resistance.

tends to increase similarly across the thorax, so one may incorrectly assume with abdominal distention that the lung is injured and becoming stiffer. In fact, lung compliance may be normal, but chest wall compliance is restricting expansion.[6] This distinction is important because increasing Paw to overcome chest wall stiffness should increase ITP more with greater hemodynamic consequences but should not improve gas exchange, since the alveoli are not damaged. If lung compliance is reduced, as in ALI, similar increases in Paw should not increase ITP as much but should also recruit collapsed and injured alveolar units, improving gas exchange but having smaller hemodynamic effects.

A hydrostatic pressure gradient exists in the pleural space. Dependent regions have a higher baseline pressure than nondependent regions in proportion to their height above or below the heart in centimeters and equate to an equal cm H_2O pressure difference. In the supine subject, steady state apneic Ppl along the horizontal plane from the apex of the lung to the diaphragm are similar, whereas anterior Ppl is less, and posterior gutter Ppl is greater (Figure 47-1).

Care must be taken to determine not only what types of ventilation are being compared but also how and where estimates of Ppl and Ppc are made. For example, if estimates of transpulmonary pressure are needed to define lung compliance and its change with recruitment maneuvers, lateral chest wall Ppl appears to more accurately reflect the pressure volume characteristics of the intact lung.[6] Similarly, if diaphragmatic work is to be monitored, either esophageal or diaphragmatic Ppl should be used. Finally, if heart-lung interactions are being examined, juxtacardiac Ppl is the most accurate measure of Ppl, and increases during positive-pressure inspiration will be underestimated by esophageal pressure. Since the heart is fixed within the cardiac fossa, juxtacardiac Ppl increases more than lateral chest wall or diaphragmatic Ppl. Pinsky and Guimond[7] demonstrated that heart failure was associated with a greater increase in Ppc than juxtacardiac Ppl, presumably because of pericardial restraint. Importantly, with progressive increases in PEEP, juxtacardiac Ppl increased toward levels of Ppc found without PEEP, whereas Ppc initially remained constant. Once these two surface pressures became equal, further increases in PEEP increased both juxtacardiac Ppl and Ppc in parallel. If pericardial volume restraint exists, juxtacardiac Ppl will underestimate Ppc, but with sustained lung compression of the heart overriding tamponade, juxtacardiac Ppl and Ppc will become similar.

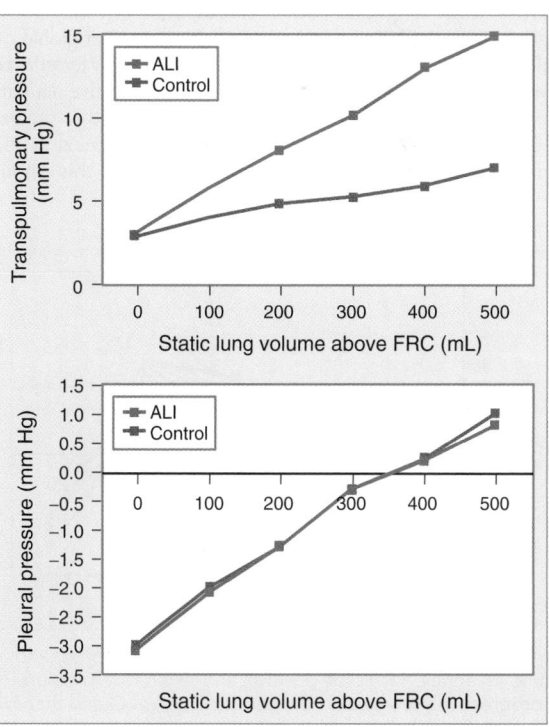

Figure 47-2 Relation between airway pressure (Paw) and tidal volume (VT) and between pleural pressure (Ppl) and VT in control and oleic acid–induced acute lung injury (ALI) conditions in a canine model. Note that despite greater increases in Paw for the same VT during ALI as compared to control conditions, Ppl and Ppc increase similarly during both control and ALI conditions for the same increase in VT. (*Reproduced with permission from Romand JA, Shi W, Pinsky MR. Cardiopulmonary effects of positive pressure ventilation during acute lung injury. Chest 1995;108:(4)1041-1048.*)

RELATION BETWEEN AIRWAY, PLEURAL, AND PERICARDIAL PRESSURES

Since the distribution of alveolar collapse and alterations in lung compliance in ARDS and ALI is non-homogeneous, lung distention during positive-pressure ventilation must reflect overdistention of some regions of the lung at the expense of noncompliant or poorly compliant regions. Accordingly, Paw will reflect distention of lung units that were aerated prior to inspiration but may not reflect the degree of lung inflation of nonaerated lung units. Pressure-limited ventilation assumes this is the case and aims to limit Paw in ALI so as to prevent overdistention of aerated lung units, with the understanding that tidal volume, and thus minute ventilation, must decrease. Therefore, pressure-limited ventilation will hypoventilate the lungs, leading to "permissive" hypercapnia. It is not surprising that in an animal model of ALI in which tidal volume was either kept constant at pre-injury levels or reduced to match pre-injury plateau Paw (pressure-limited ventilation), both Ppl and Ppc increased less compared to both pre–lung injury states or in ALI when tidal volume remained at pre-injury levels.[8] These points underlie the fundamental hemodynamic differences seen when different modes of mechanical ventilatory support are compared to each other.

Because ALI is often non-homogeneous, with aerated areas of the lung displaying normal compliance, large increases in Paw can overdistend aerated lung units.[10] Vascular structures that are distended will have a greater increase in their surrounding pressure than collapsible structures that do not distend.[11] However, Romand et al.[8] and Scharf and Ingram[12] demonstrated that despite this non-homogeneous pattern of alveolar distention, if tidal volume is kept constant, Ppl increases in a homogeneous manner independent of the mechanical properties of the lung. Under constant tidal volume conditions, changes in peak and mean Paw will reflect changes in the mechanical properties of the lungs and patient coordination but may not reflect changes in ITP. Similarly, changes in Paw may not alter global cardiovascular dynamics. Underscoring this limitation of Paw to reflect either ITP or Ppc, Pinsky et al.[13] demonstrated in postoperative patients that the percentage of Paw increase that will be transmitted to the pericardial surface is not constant from one subject to the next as PEEP is increased (Figure 47-3). Thus, one cannot predict the amount of increase in Ppc or Ppl that will occur in patients as PEEP is increased. Accordingly, assuming some constant fraction of Paw transmission to the pleural surface as a means of calculating the effect of increasing Paw on Ppl is inaccurate and potentially dangerous to patient management.

Although it may be difficult to know the actual Ppl, it is possible to determine the ventilation-induced change in Ppl. Since during airway occlusion maneuvers lung volume does not change, transpulmonary pressure is also constant so that the change in ITP is equal to the change in Paw.[14] Accordingly, an increase in Paw of 20 mm Hg during a Valsalva maneuver will reflect an increase in ITP of 20 mm Hg, and a decrease in Paw to −20 mm Hg during a Mueller maneuver will reflect a decrease in ITP of 20 mm Hg below atmospheric pressure.

Clinically, esophageal pressure is often used as a surrogate for Ppc and ITP. Two limitations to the use of esophageal pressure (Pes) in estimating Ppc and ITP exist. First, Ppc and ITP may not be similar nor increase by similar amounts with the application of positive Paw if the pericardium becomes a limiting membrane.[15,16] Operationally, this equates to Ppc exceeding juxtacardiac Ppl by the degree to which the pericardium limits biventricular dilation. Thus, estimates of Ppc made by using ITP measures may underestimate Ppc and overestimate the increase in Ppc as Paw is increased. Second, although esophageal pressure is often used clinically to estimate swings in both Ppl and Ppc so as to calculate the work cost of breathing, esophageal pressure is only accurate at reflecting negative swings in Ppl during spontaneous inspiration in upright seated individuals[3] and in recumbent dogs in the left lateral position.[17] Esophageal pressure changes underestimate both the positive swings in Ppl and the mean increase in Ppl seen with increases in lung volume during positive-pressure ventilation. During Mueller and Valsalva maneuvers, however, because lung volume does not change, swings in esophageal pressure will accurately reflect swings in ITP.[3] In fact, documenting that airway and esophageal pressure swings are identical in magnitude is how esophageal manometers are validated at the bedside.

Hemodynamic Effects of Ventilation

Lung volume increases during both spontaneous and positive-pressure ventilation, but ITP decreases during spontaneous inspiration and increases during positive-pressure inspiration. Changes in ITP and the metabolic demand needed to create these changes represent the primary determinants of the hemodynamic differences between spontaneous and positive-pressure ventilation.[18,19]

The circulation can alter ventilation, and ventilation can alter the circulation. These heart-lung interactions can be broadly grouped into interactions that involve three basic interrelationships that usually coexist in the clinical setting. First, spontaneous ventilatory efforts are exercise and require O_2 and blood flow, thus placing demands on cardiac output and producing CO_2, adding additional ventilatory stress on CO_2 excretion. Second, inspiration increases lung volume above resting end-expiratory volume, so some of the hemodynamic effects of ventilation may be due to changes in lung volume and chest wall expansion. Third, spontaneous inspiration decreases ITP, whereas positive-pressure ventilation increases ITP, so the differences between spontaneous ventilation and positive-pressure ventilation primarily reflect differences in ITP swings and the energy necessary to produce them.

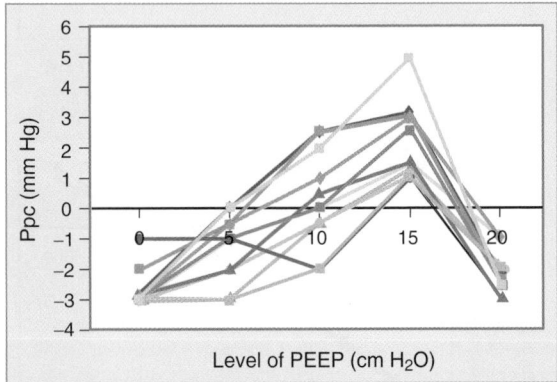

Figure 47-3 Relation between pericardial pressure (Ppc) and airway pressure as apneic levels of positive end-expiratory pressure (PEEP) were progressively increased from zero to 15 cm H_2O and then back to zero in 5 cm H_2O increments in patients immediately following open heart surgery. Note that although Ppc increases in all subjects as PEEP is increased from 0 to 15 cm H_2O, the initial Ppc value and the proportional change in Ppc among incremental increases in PEEP are quite different among subjects, such that no specific proportion of airway pressure transmission to the pericardial surface can be assumed to occur in all patients. *(Reproduced with permission from Pinsky MR, Vincent JL, DeSmet JM. Estimating left ventricular filling pressure during positive end-expiratory pressure in humans. Am Rev Respir Dis. 1991;143[1]:25-31.)*

VENTILATION AS EXERCISE

Spontaneous ventilatory efforts are produced by respiratory muscle contraction. Blood flow to these muscles is derived from several arterial circuits whose absolute flow is believed to exceed the highest metabolic demand of maximally exercising skeletal muscle.[20] Thus, under normal cardiovascular conditions, blood flow is not the limiting factor determining maximal ventilatory effort. Although ventilation normally requires less than 5% of total O_2 delivery to meet its demand,[20] in lung disease states where the work of breathing is increased (e.g., pulmonary edema, bronchospasm), the work cost of breathing can increase metabolic demand for O_2 to 25% or 30% of total O_2 delivery.[20-23] Furthermore, if cardiac output is limited, blood flow to other organs and to the respiratory muscles may be compromised, inducing both tissue hypoperfusion and lactic acidosis.[24-27] Starting mechanical ventilation may reduce metabolic demand, increasing Svo_2 for a constant cardiac output and Cao_2. Intubation and mechanical ventilation, when adjusted to the metabolic demands of the patient, may dramatically decrease the work of breathing, resulting in increased O_2 delivery to other vital organs and decreased serum lactic acid levels. These cardiovascular benefits can also be realized with effective use of noninvasive ventilation mask continuous positive airway pressure (CPAP).[28] The obligatory increase in Svo_2 will result in an increase in the Pao_2 if fixed right-to-left shunts exist, even if mechanical ventilation does not alter the ratio of shunt blood flow to cardiac output. Finally, if cardiac output is severely limited, respiratory muscle failure develops despite high central neuronal drive such that many heart failure patients experience respiratory arrest prior to cardiovascular standstill.[29]

Ventilator-dependent patients who fail to wean from mechanical ventilation may occasionally have impaired baseline cardiovascular performance[30] but routinely develop overt signs of heart failure during weaning, including pulmonary edema,[30,31] myocardial ischemia,[32-35] tachycardia, and gut ischemia.[36] Jubran et al.[37] demonstrated that although all subjects increase their cardiac outputs in response to a weaning trial, those who subsequently fail to wean demonstrate a reduction in mixed venous O_2 saturation, consistent with a failing cardiovascular response to increased metabolic demand. Importantly, the increased work of breathing may come from endotracheal tube flow resistance.[38] Thus, weaning from mechanical ventilatory support can be considered a cardiovascular stress test. Again, investigators have documented weaning-associated ECG and thallium cardiac blood flow scan-related signs of ischemia in subjects with known coronary artery disease[32] and in otherwise normal patients.[34,35] Placing patients with severe heart failure and/or ischemia on ventilatory support by either intubation and ventilation[39] or noninvasive CPAP[40] can reverse myocardial ischemia.

HEMODYNAMIC EFFECTS OF CHANGES IN LUNG VOLUME

Changing lung volume alters autonomic tone and pulmonary vascular resistance; at high lung volumes, the enlarged lungs compress the heart in the cardiac fossa, limiting absolute cardiac volumes in a fashion analogous to tamponade. But unlike tamponade, where Ppc selectively increases, with hyperinflation, juxtacardiac Ppl and Ppc increase together.

Autonomic Tone

The lungs are richly enervated with integrated somatic and autonomic fibers that originate, traverse through, and end in the thorax. These neuronal networks mediate multiple homeostatic processes through the autonomic nervous system that alter both instantaneous cardiovascular function (e.g., respiratory sinus arrhythmia) and steady state cardiovascular status (e.g., ADH-induced fluid retention). Numerous cardiovascular reflexes are centered within this network. Inflation induces immediate changes in autonomic output. The most commonly described inflation-chronotropic responses act through vagal-mediated reflex arcs.[41,42] Lung inflation to normal tidal volumes (<10 mL/kg) increases heart rate via parasympathetic tone withdrawal. Inspiration-associated cardioacceleration is referred to as *respiratory sinus arrhythmia* (RSA)[43] and denotes normal autonomic tone.[44] Loss of RSA is associated with dysautonomia, and its reappearance precedes the return of peripheral autonomic control in diabetics with peripheral neuropathy.[45] However, some degree of respiratory-associated heart rate change is intrinsic to the heart itself. For example, in denervated human hearts (transplants), a small degree of ventilation-associated changes in heart rate persists,[46] suggesting that mechanoreceptors in

the right atrium can alter sinoatrial tone. Bernardi et al.[46] demonstrated that this heart rate variability in cardiac transplant recipients had a periodicity twice that of the ventilatory cycle, suggesting that both increases and decreases in venous return and ventricular loading impart some RSA. In support of this concept, Pinna et al. documented that most of the heart rate and arterial pressure changes seen during breathing in patients with severe congestive heart failure (CHF) are more reflective of changes in intrathoracic blood volume than of alterations in autonomic input.[47]

Lung inflation to larger tidal volumes (>15 mL/kg) decreases heart rate. Pulmonary vasoconstriction may occur through vagal reflex arcs[48] but does not appear to induce significant hemodynamic effects. Reflex arterial vasodilatation can also occur with lung hyperinflation.[41,49-53] This inflation-vasodilatation response appears to be mediated by afferent vagal fibers, because it is abolished by selective vagotomy. Interestingly, blocking sympathetic afferent fibers also blocks this reflex,[51,54] presumably by withdrawing central sympathetic tone. Although this inflation-vasodilatation response induces expiration-associated reductions in LV contractility in healthy volunteers[55] and in ventilator-dependent patients with the initiation of high-frequency ventilation[41] or hyperinflation,[51] its clinical significance in other patient groups is unknown. Since patients with ALI often ventilate only a relatively small amount of their lungs, the potential exists that these patients may experience regional hyperinflation and may develop reflex cardiovascular depression. Interestingly, several studies comparing larger tidal volume ventilation with pressure-limited ventilation document better hemodynamic status with pressure-limited ventilation. Similarly, although humoral factors (including compounds whose production is dependent on cyclooxygenase activation[56]) released from pulmonary endothelial cells during lung inflation may also induce this depressor response,[57-59] these interactions do not appear to grossly alter cardiovascular status.[60] In fact, unilateral lung hyperinflation (unilateral PEEP) does not appear to influence systemic hemodynamics.[61] Interestingly, increased levels of nitric oxide (NO) in the exhaled gas of rabbits ventilated at increasing tidal volumes have been reported.[48] Importantly, for the same decrease in cardiac output, heart rate increases less with the application of PEEP than with hemorrhage.[48] The reasons for this difference are unknown but may reflect PEEP-induced sympatholytic actions and increased arterial pressure minimizing baroreceptor stimulation.

Both positive-pressure ventilation and sustained hyperinflation stimulate endocrinological responses that induce fluid retention via right atrial stretch receptors. Plasma norepinephrine, plasma renin activity,[62,63] and atrial natriuretic peptide (ANP)[64] increase during positive-pressure ventilation with or without PEEP. Interestingly, when subjects with CHF are given nasal CPAP, plasma ANP activity decreases in parallel with improvements in blood flow.[65,66]

Determinants of Pulmonary Vascular Resistance

Changes in lung volume are caused by changes in transpulmonary distending pressure, the pressure difference between alveolar pressure and ITP. Since pulmonary tissue pressure and ITP are nearly identical, increasing lung volume increases the difference between alveolar and tissue pressures, making pulmonary vascular resistance increase independent of any effect of volume change on humoral or autonomic responses.[18,67-72]

Lung inflation primarily affects cardiac function and cardiac output by altering right ventricle (RV) preload and afterload.[72] RV afterload is the maximal RV systolic wall stress during contraction[73] which, by Laplace's law, equals the product of the RV radius of curvature (a function of end-diastolic volume) and transmural pressure (a function of systolic RV pressure).[74] Changes in ITP that occur without changes in lung volume, as may occur with obstructive inspiratory efforts, will not alter the pressure gradient between the RV and pulmonary artery nor result in change of pulmonary vascular resistance. Thus, neither straining at stools (Valsalva maneuver) nor obstructive inspiratory efforts (Mueller maneuver) primarily affect RV afterload. Although obstructive inspiratory efforts are usually associated with increased RV afterload, the reason for this effect is backward LV failure and reactive hypoxic pulmonary vasoconstriction.[75,76]

Systolic RV pressure approximates transmural systolic pulmonary artery pressure (Ppa) when no pulmonary stenosis is present. Transmural Ppa can increase by one of two mechanisms: (1) an increase in pulmonary arterial pressure without change in pulmonary vasomotor tone, as occurs with increases in blood flow (exercise) or passive increases in outflow pressure (LV failure), or (2) an increase in pulmonary vascular resistance. Usually any increase in transmural Ppa during positive-pressure ventilation is due to an increase in pulmonary vascular resistance, because neither instantaneous cardiac output[77] nor LV filling[14] changes. Increases in transmural Ppa impedes RV ejection,[78] decreasing RV stroke volume[79] and causing RV dilation and passive obstruction to venous return,[56,58] which may rapidly progress to acute cor pulmonale.[80] If RV dilation and pressure overload persist, RV free wall ischemia and infarction can develop.[81] Importantly, rapid fluid challenges in the setting of acute cor pulmonale can precipitate profound cardiovascular collapse due to excessive RV dilation, RV ischemia, and compromised LV filling through the process of ventricular interdependence. During normal end-inspiration, mild hypoxemia ($Pao_2 > 65$ mm Hg) and low levels of PEEP (<7.5 cm H_2O) should minimally increase transmural Ppa. If slight increases in transmural Ppa are sustained, however, fluid retention occurs, either by intrinsic humoral mechanisms (increased ANP secretion) or by therapeutic intravascular volume infusion,[82] resulting in an increase in RV end-diastolic volume maintaining cardiac output.[74,83]

The mechanism by which ventilation alters pulmonary vasomotor tone is complex. If regional alveolar Po_2 (Pao_2) decreases below 60 mm Hg, local pulmonary vasomotor tone increases, reducing local blood flow.[84] This process of hypoxic pulmonary vasoconstriction is mediated in part by variations in the synthesis and release of NO by pulmonary vascular endothelial cells. The pulmonary endothelium normally synthesizes a basal low amount of NO, a potent vasodilator, using endothelial nitric oxide synthase. This basal NO release is highly regulated and dependent on O_2 and is inhibited by both hypoxia and acidosis. If O_2 becomes scarce, NO is not made, and pulmonary vasomotor tone increases to the level that would exist if no NO were present.

Many pulmonary pathologic processes are associated with regional reductions in Pao_2, such as atelectasis, airway obstruction, and ventilation/perfusion mismatching. Hypoxic pulmonary vasoconstriction, by reducing pulmonary blood flow to those hypoxic regions, optimizes ventilation/perfusion matching. However, if alveolar hypoxia occurs throughout the lungs, overall pulmonary vasomotor tone increases, raising pulmonary vascular resistance and impeding RV ejection.[73] At low lung volumes, alveoli spontaneously collapse as a result of loss of interstitial traction and closure of the terminal airways, causing alveolar hypoxia. Patients with acute hypoxemic respiratory failure have small lung volumes.[85,86] Therefore, pulmonary vascular resistance is often increased in these patients owing to alveolar collapse and resultant hypoxic pulmonary vasoconstriction.

Mechanical Ventilation-Induced Changes in Pulmonary Vascular Resistance

Mechanical ventilation may reduce active pulmonary vasomotor tone by one of several related processes. Hypoxic pulmonary vasoconstrictor tone may be decreased by increasing global Pao_2 by enriching alveolar gas O_2,[87-90] reexpansion of collapsed alveolar units thereby increasing Pao_2 in those local alveoli,[5,91-93] increased alveolar ventilation and reversal of acute respiratory acidosis,[90] or merely through decreasing central sympathetic output by allowing the patient in ALI to not fight for every breath.[94,95] Similarly, these effects need not require positive-pressure breaths as much as expansion of collapsed alveoli.[96] Such recruitment of lung units is usually accomplished by the addition of PEEP or CPAP. Thus, if PEEP opens collapsed lung units and replenishes alveolar gas with O_2, hypoxic pulmonary vasoconstriction will be reduced, pulmonary vascular resistance will decrease, and RV ejection will improve.

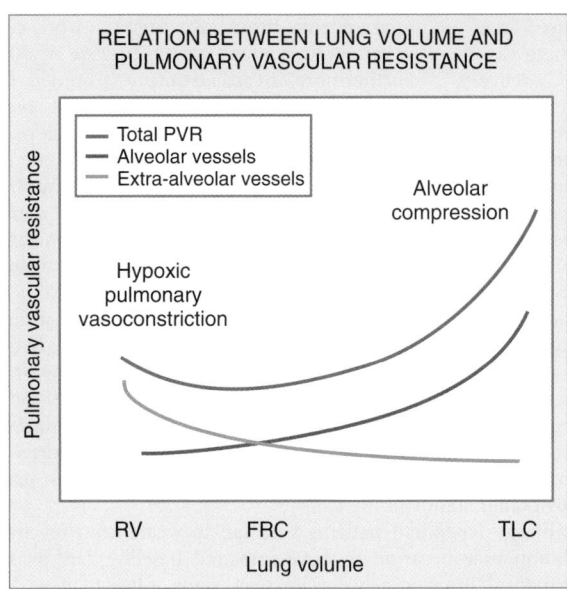

Figure 47-4 Schematic diagram of the relation between changes in lung volume and pulmonary vascular resistance, where the extraalveolar and alveolar vascular components are separated. Note that pulmonary vascular resistance is minimal at resting lung volume or functional residual capacity (FRC). As lung volume increases toward total lung capacity (TLC) or decreases toward residual volume (RV), pulmonary vascular resistance also increases. However, the increase in resistance with hyperinflation is due to increased alveolar vascular resistance, whereas the increase in resistance with lung collapse is due to increased extraalveolar vessel tone.

Changes in lung volume can also profoundly alter pulmonary vasomotor tone by passively compressing the alveolar vessels.[85,92,93] Pulmonary circulation can be separated into two groups of blood vessels depending on what pressure surrounds them[92] (Figure 47-4). The small pulmonary arterioles, venules, and alveolar capillaries sense alveolar pressure as their surrounding pressure and are referred to as *alveolar vessels*. The large pulmonary arteries and veins, as well as the heart and intrathoracic great vessels of the systemic circulation, sense interstitial pressure or ITP as their surrounding pressure and can be called *extraalveolar vessels*. Alveolar pressure minus ITP is the transpulmonary pressure. Increasing lung volume requires a rise in transpulmonary pressure, so the extravascular pressure gradient between alveolar and extraalveolar vessels varies proportionally with changes in lung volume. Importantly, the radial interstitial forces of the lung that keep the airways patent[91,97,98] also act upon the extraalveolar vessels. As lung volume increases, the radial interstitial forces increase, increasing the diameter of both extraalveolar vessels and airways and resulting in a reduction in airway resistance at higher lung volumes, as well as increased extraalveolar vessel diameter and capacitance.[99] This tethering effect is lost with lung deflation, thereby increasing pulmonary vascular resistance.[88,91] The collapse of small airways also induces alveolar hypoxia. Thus, at small lung volumes, pulmonary vascular resistance is increased owing to the combined effect of hypoxic pulmonary vasoconstriction and extraalveolar vessel collapse.

Increases in lung volume progressively raise alveolar vessel resistance, becoming noticeable above resting lung volume or functional residual capacity (FRC).[88,100] There are two causes of the increased alveolar vessel resistance. First, the heart and extraalveolar vessels sense ITP as their surrounding pressure, whereas the alveolar vessels sense alveolar pressure as their surrounding pressure, so an extralumenal transpulmonary pressure gradient exists between extraalveolar and alveolar vessels. As lung volume increases, the extralumenal pressure difference increases as well. If transpulmonary pressure increases enough to exceed intralumenal vascular pressure, the pulmonary

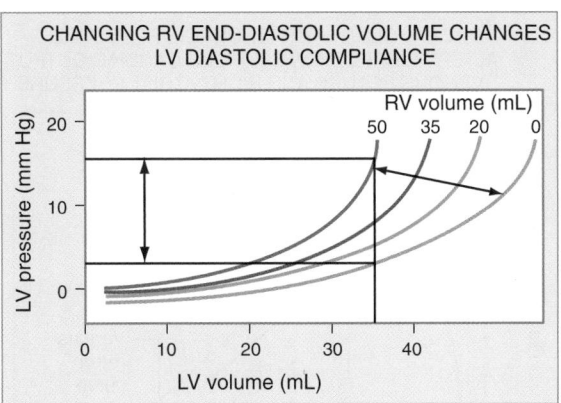

Figure 47-5 Schematic diagram of the effect of increasing right ventricular (RV) volumes on the left ventricular (LV) diastolic pressure-volume (filling) relationship. Note that increasing RV volumes decrease LV diastolic compliance such that a higher filling pressure is required to generate a constant end-diastolic volume. *(After Taylor RR, Covell JW, Sonnenblick EH, Ross J Jr. Dependence of ventricular distensibility on filling of the opposite ventricle. Am J Physiol 1967;213[3]:711-718.)*

vasculature will collapse where extraalveolar vessels pass into alveolar loci, reducing the vasculature cross-sectional area and increasing pulmonary vascular resistance. Similarly, increasing lung volume by stretching and distending the alveolar septa may also compress alveolar capillaries, although this mechanism is less well substantiated. Hyperinflation can create significant pulmonary hypertension and may precipitate acute RV failure (acute cor pulmonale)[101] and RV ischemia.[81] Thus PEEP may increase pulmonary vascular resistance if it induces overdistention of the lung above its normal FRC. Recently the effect of inflation on RV input impedance was validated in humans, using echocardiographic techniques.[102] Similarly, if lung volumes are reduced, then increasing lung volume back to baseline levels by the use of PEEP will decrease pulmonary vascular resistance by reversing hypoxic pulmonary vasoconstriction.[103]

Ventricular Interdependence

Changes in RV output must invariably alter LV filling because the two ventricles are serially linked through the pulmonary vasculature. However, LV preload can also be directly altered by changes in RV end-diastolic volume.[104] If RV volume increases, LV diastolic compliance will decrease by the mechanism of ventricular interdependence.[105] Ventricular interdependence functions through two separate processes. First, increasing RV end-diastolic volume will induce a shift of the intraventricular septum into the LV, thereby decreasing LV diastolic compliance[106] (Figure 47-5). For the same LV filling pressure, RV dilation will decrease LV end-diastolic volume and therefore cardiac output. This interaction is believed to be the major determinant of the phasic changes in arterial pulse pressure and stroke volume seen in tamponade, referred to as *pulsus paradoxus*. Spontaneous inspiration increases venous return, causing RV dilation and decreasing LV end-diastolic compliance. Maintaining a relatively constant rate of venous return, either by volume resuscitation[107] or vasopressor infusion,[4] will minimize this effect. Thus, the presence of pulse paradoxus can be used as a marker of functional hypovolemia, even if actual intravascular volume status is not reduced.

Mechanical Heart-Lung Interactions

With hyperinflation, the heart may be compressed between the two expanding lungs,[108] increasing juxtacardiac ITP. The chest wall and diaphragm can move away from the expanding lungs, whereas the heart is trapped within its cardiac fossa, so juxtacardiac ITP may increase more than lateral chest wall or diaphragmatic ITP.[6,16] This compressive effect of the inflated lung can be seen with either spontaneous[109] or positive pressure–induced hyperinflation.[97,98] This decrease

in "apparent" LV diastolic compliance[106] was previously misinterpreted as impaired LV contractility, because LV stroke work for a given LV end-diastolic pressure or pulmonary artery occlusion pressure is decreased.[110,111] However, numerous studies have shown that when patients are fluid resuscitated to return LV end-diastolic volume to its original level, both LV stroke work and cardiac output also returned to their original levels[69,107] despite the continued application of PEEP.[112]

Takata et al.[113] proposed a novel approach to understanding tamponade that lends itself to mechanical heart-lung interactions. Hyperinflation directly alters biventricular filling, whereas inspiration primarily alters RV filling and only indirectly affects LV volumes through changes in diastolic compliance. Thus, hyperinflation—as occurs in severe asthma and with the use of excessive amounts of PEEP—would produce a clinical picture indistinguishable from tamponade. Indeed, Rebuck and Read[114] made this same observation in their analysis of the hemodynamic effects of severe asthma over 30 years ago, although they did not postulate a specific mechanism to explain this phenomenon. Presumably, the shift from "uncoupled" to "coupled" cardiac fossal restraint would occur as absolute lung volume increased, biventricular volume increased, or both. If cardiac volumes are small, and lung inflation does not overdistend the chest, RV filling will be primarily impeded. In contrast, in CHF states and with marked lung overdistention, both RV and LV filling may be compromised by ventilation.

HEMODYNAMIC EFFECTS OF CHANGES IN INTRATHORACIC PRESSURE

The heart within the thorax is a pressure chamber within a pressure chamber. Therefore, changes in ITP will affect the pressure gradients for both systemic venous return to the RV and systemic outflow from the LV, independent of the heart itself (Figure 47-6). Increases in ITP, by increasing right atrial pressure and decreasing transmural LV systolic pressure, will reduce the pressure gradients for venous return and LV ejection, thereby decreasing intrathoracic blood volume. Using the same argument, decreases in ITP will augment venous return and impede LV ejection and increase intrathoracic blood volume.

Systemic Venous Return

Blood flows back to the heart from the periphery through low-pressure, low-resistance venous conduits. Guyton et al. characterized venous flow from the venous reservoirs into the right atrium.[115] As downstream right atrial pressure varies, as occurs with ventilation, the rate of venous return inversely changes. Pressure in the upstream venous reservoirs is called *mean systemic pressure*. Mean systemic pressure is a function of blood volume, peripheral vasomotor tone, and the distribution of blood within the vasculature.[116] Mean systemic pressure does not change rapidly during the ventilatory cycle, whereas right atrial pressure does owing to concomitant changes in ITP. Accordingly, variations in right atrial pressure represent the major factor determining

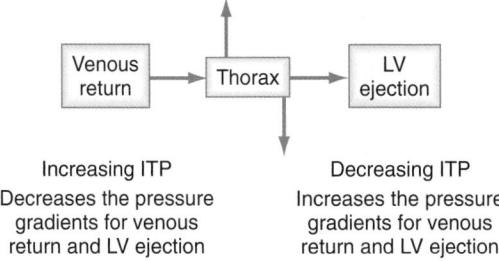

Figure 47-6 Schematic diagram of the effect of increasing or decreasing intrathoracic pressure on left ventricular (LV) filling (venous return) and ejection pressures.

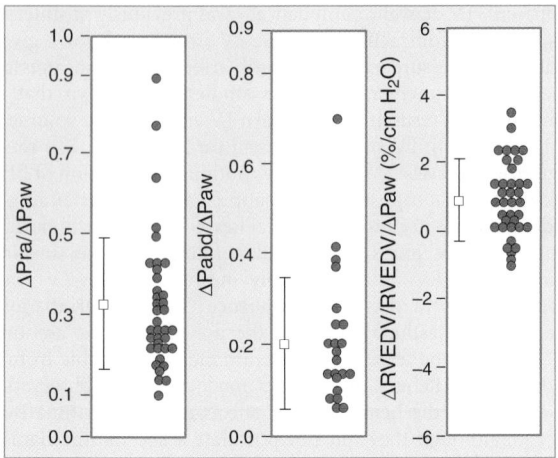

Figure 47-7 Effect of increasing levels of CPAP on the relations between increasing airway pressure and right atrial pressure (left graph), airway pressure and intraabdominal pressure (center graph), and airway pressure and changes in RV end-diastolic volume in 43 postoperative fluid-resuscitated cardiac surgery patients. *(Derived from data in Van den Berg P, Jansen JRC, Pinsky MR. The effect of positive-pressure inspiration on venous return in volume loaded post-operative surgical patients. J Appl Physiol 2002;92[3]:1223-1231.)*

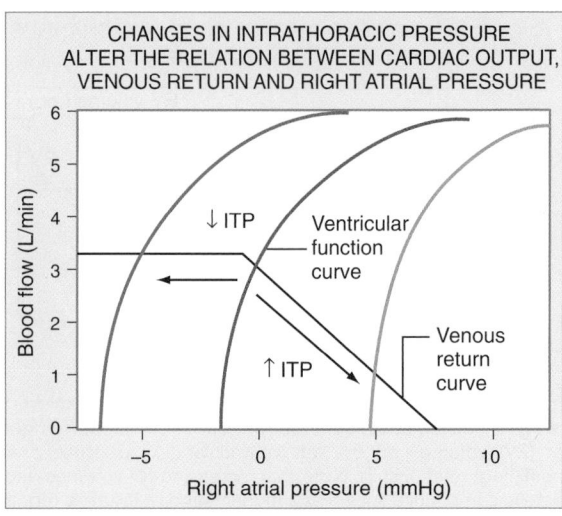

Figure 47-8 Schematic representation of the effects of increasing or decreasing intrathoracic pressure (ITP) on steady state venous return. Note that decreases in ITP which decrease right atrial pressure to below zero relative to atmospheric pressure will only increase venous return by a limited amount, whereas increases in ITP will progressively decrease venous return to a complete circulatory standstill.

the fluctuation in pressure gradient for systemic venous return during ventilation.[77,117] Positive-pressure inspiration increases ITP and right atrial pressure, decreasing the pressure gradient for venous return and RV filling,[79] and consequently, RV stroke volume.[77,79,118-125] These physiologic effects have recently been validated in humans, using minimally invasive echocardiographic techniques wherein vena caval flow varies with the phase of the ventilatory cycle[25,126] (Figure 47-7). During normal spontaneous inspiration, the converse occurs: with decreases in ITP, right atrial pressure decreases, accelerating venous blood flow and increasing RV filling and RV stroke volume* (Figure 47-8).

The decrease in venous return during positive-pressure ventilation is often lower than one might expect based on the increase in right atrial pressure. Fessler et al.[129] and Takata and Robotham[130] demonstrated in dogs that PEEP increases intraabdominal pressure by causing the diaphragm to descend, thereby increasing the pressure surrounding the intraabdominal vasculature. Because a large proportion of venous blood is in the abdomen, the net effect of PEEP is to increase mean systemic pressure and right atrial pressure. Accordingly, the pressure gradient for venous return may not be reduced by PEEP, especially in patients with hypervolemia. In fact, abdominal pressurization by diaphragmatic descent may be the major mechanism by which the decrease in venous return is minimized during positive-pressure ventilation.[131-135] Furthermore, Matuschak et al.[131] found that although PEEP decreased blood flow to the liver in proportion to the induced decrease in cardiac output in normovolemic dogs, the liver's ability to clear hepatocytic-specific compounds, such as indocyanine green, was unaltered. Finally, when cardiac output is restored to pre-PEEP levels by fluid resuscitation[131,136] while PEEP is maintained, liver clearance mechanisms increase above pre-PEEP levels.[136-139] These data are consistent with a PEEP-induced alteration in intrahepatic blood flow distribution. Thus, ventilation may have less of an effect on venous return than originally postulated, but the effect may be more complicated than we have imagined. Van den Berg et al.[140] examined the effects of varying levels of CPAP on right atrial pressure, intraabdominal pressure, and cardiac output in 42 postoperative cardiac surgery patients. Up to 20 cm H_2O CPAP did not significantly decrease cardiac output, as measured 30 seconds into an inspiratory hold maneuver. The reason for this apparent paradoxical effect became obvious when they compared the associated changes in right atrial pressure, abdominal

pressure, and RV end-diastolic volume (Figure 47-9). What they documented was that only 30% of the increased airway pressure was transmitted to the right atrium. Perhaps more importantly, most of the increase in right atrial pressure was also realized by an increase in intraabdominal pressure, so it was not surprising that RV end-diastolic volume fell by less than 8% from pre-CPAP values. These data demonstrate that in the fluid-resuscitated patient, institution of positive-pressure ventilation may not result in a decrease in blood flow. However, if intraabdominal pressure is allowed to decrease, as would occur with an open laparotomy and decompression of tense ascites, a marked preload-responsive effect of positive-pressure ventilation can occur.

With exaggerated swings in ITP, as occur with obstructed inspiratory efforts, venous return behaves as if abdominal pressure is additive to mean systemic pressure in defining total venous blood flow.[141-144] Recent interest in inverse ratio ventilation has raised questions as to its hemodynamic effect because its application includes a large component of hyperinflation. However, Mang et al.[145] demonstrated in an animal model of ALI that if total PEEP (intrinsic PEEP plus extra extrinsic PEEP) was similar, no hemodynamic difference between conventional ventilation and inverse ratio ventilation was seen.

Right Ventricular Filling

Under normal conditions, it is difficult to document any relation between RV filling pressure and volume. When RV filling pressure, defined as right atrial pressure minus Ppc, was directly measured in patients undergoing open chest operations, RV filling pressure was unaltered by acute volume loading.[146] Although right atrial pressure increased, Ppc also increased such that RV filling pressure remained unchanged. Similar data were seen when RV volumes are reduced by the application of PEEP in postoperative cardiac patients.[147] These findings suggest that under normal conditions, RV diastolic compliance is very high, and most of the increase in right atrial pressure seen during volume loading reflects pericardial compliance and cardiac fossa stiffness, more than changes in RV distending pressure. These data also imply that with RV filling, right heart sarcomere length remains constant. Presumably, conformational changes in the RV more than wall stretch are responsible for RV enlargement.[15] Accordingly, changes in right atrial pressure do not follow changes in RV end-diastolic volume. When cardiac contractility is reduced and intravascular volume is expanded, RV filling pressure increases as a result of

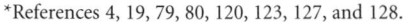

*References 4, 19, 79, 80, 120, 123, 127, and 128.

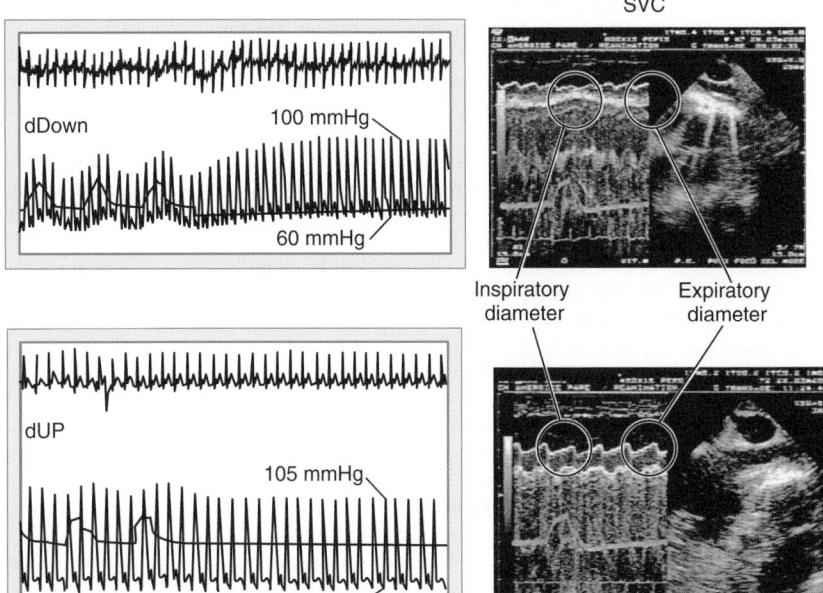

Figure 47-9 Echocardiographic and pulse Doppler images of superior vena caval flow patterns during positive-pressure ventilation. Note the inspiratory phase-dependent decrease in venous flow. *(Reproduced with permission from Jardin F, Vieillard-Baron A. Right ventricular function and positive-pressure ventilation in clinical practice: from hemodynamic subsets to respirator settings. Intensive Care Med. 2003;29[9]:1426-1434.)*

decreased RV diastolic compliance, increased pericardial compliance, increased end-diastolic volume, or a combination of all three. In support of this hypothesis, RV filling pressure does not increase until RV volume exceeds a certain threshold value.[105] Furthermore, in dogs with acute ventricular failure, volume loading increases Ppc more than ITP, consistent with pericardial rather than cardiac fossal restraint. If PEEP is increased in this setting, ITP but not Ppc selectively increases until ITP equals Ppc, then both ITP and Ppc increase equally if PEEP is increased further.[7] In postoperative cardiac surgery patients,[13,22,148] PEEP—and by extension lung expansion—compresses the heart within the cardiac fossa in a fashion analogous to pericardial tamponade.

Venous return is the primary determinant of cardiac output.[116] Since right atrial pressure is the backpressure to venous return, venous return is maintained near maximal levels at rest[51,125,126] because RV filling occurs with minimal changes in filling pressure.[148] The closer right atrial pressure remains to zero relative to atmospheric pressure, the greater the pressure gradient for systemic venous blood flow.[115,121] For this mechanism to operate efficiently, RV output must equal venous return, otherwise sustained increases in venous blood flow would overdistend the RV, increasing right atrial pressure. Fortunately, under normal conditions of spontaneous ventilation, the increase in venous return is in phase with inspiration, decreasing again during expiration as ITP increases.[77] Likewise, the pulmonary arterial inflow circuit is highly compliant and can accept large increases in RV stroke volume without changing pressure.[79,83] Thus, any increase in venous return is proportionally delivered to the pulmonary circuit without forcing the RV to increase its force of contraction or myocardial oxygen demand. Importantly, this compensatory system will rapidly become dysfunctional if RV diastolic compliance decreases or if right atrial pressure increases independent of changes in RV end-diastolic volume. An example of decreased RV diastolic compliance is acute RV dilation or cor pulmonale (pulmonary embolism, hyperinflation, and RV infarction) that induce profound decreases in cardiac output not responsive to fluid resuscitation. Dissociation between right atrial pressure and RV end-diastolic volume occurs during either tamponade or positive-pressure ventilation, because right atrial pressure is artificially increased by the increasing ITP. Accordingly, positive-pressure ventilation impairs normal circulatory adaptive processes. Furthermore, even if one restores the coupling of right atrial pressure and RV volume by using partial ventilatory support modes of ventilation,

cardiac output will increase only if the RV can transduce the associated increase in venous return to forward blood flow. Thus, during weaning from mechanical ventilation, occult RV failure may be exposed and will manifest as a rapid rise in right atrial pressure and a fall in cardiac output. Since the primary effect of any form of ventilation on cardiovascular function in normal subjects is to alter RV preload via altering venous blood flow, the detrimental effect of positive-pressure ventilation on cardiac output can be minimized by either fluid resuscitation to increase mean systemic pressure[4,118,140,141] or by keeping both mean ITP and swings in lung volume as low as possible. Accordingly, prolonging expiratory time, decreasing tidal volume, and avoiding PEEP all minimize the decrease in systemic venous return to the RV.[1,21,77,120-124,149]

Since spontaneous inspiratory efforts increase lung volume by decreasing ITP, one sees an increase in venous return with spontaneous inspiration owing to the fall in right atrial pressure.[19,67,121-123] However, this augmentation of venous return is limited[142,143] because if ITP decreases below atmospheric pressure, venous return becomes flow-limited as the large systemic veins collapse as they enter the thorax.[115] This flow limitation is a safety valve for the heart because ITP can decrease greatly with obstructive inspiratory efforts,[52] and if not flow-limited, the RV could become overdistended and fail[150] (see Figure 47-8). Still, in patients with decreased RV compliance, negative swings in ITP can augment RV filling. Interestingly, negative pressure ventilation, by augmenting venous return, was shown to increase cardiac output by 39% in intubated children following repair of tetralogy of Fallot.[151] In this condition, impaired RV filling secondary to RV hypertrophy and reduced RV chamber size are the primary factors limiting cardiac output.

Left Ventricular Preload and Ventricular Interdependence

Changes in venous return must eventually result in directionally similar changes in LV preload, because the two ventricles are linked in series. For example, during a Valsalva maneuver, initially RV filling is reduced, but LV filling is unaltered.[14] Then, as the strain is sustained, LV filling and cardiac output both begin to decrease.[108,152] This phase delay in changes from the RV to the LV is exaggerated if tidal volume or respiratory rate are increased and in the setting of hypovolemia.* Independent of this series interaction, direct ventricular

---

*References 1, 21, 70, 71, 107, 110, 111, 125, and 153-157.

interdependence can also occur and be clinically significant. Increasing RV volume shifts the intraventricular septum into the LV and simultaneously decreases LV diastolic compliance. During positive-pressure ventilation, RV volumes are usually decreased, minimizing ventricular interdependence.[105,155-158] Echocardiographic studies document that although PEEP results in some degree of right-to-left intraventricular septal shift, the shift is small.[69,70] In fact, increases in lung volume during positive-pressure ventilation primarily compress the two ventricles into each other, decreasing biventricular volumes.[159] The decrease in cardiac output commonly seen during PEEP is due to a decrease in LV end-diastolic volume; in this setting, both LV end-diastolic volume and cardiac output are restored by fluid resuscitation[160,161] without any measurable change in LV diastolic compliance.[106]

During spontaneous inspiration, RV volumes increase transiently, shifting the intraventricular septum into the LV,[106] decreasing LV diastolic compliance and LV end-diastolic volume.[103,158,162] This transient RV dilation–induced septal shift is the primary cause of inspiration-associated decreases in arterial pulse pressure; if greater than 10 mm Hg or 10% of the mean pulse pressure, the phenomenon is referred to as *pulsus paradoxus*.[19] Since spontaneous inspiratory efforts can occur during positive-pressure ventilation and especially during partial ventilatory assist modalities, pulsus paradoxus can also be seen in mechanically ventilated patients.

Left Ventricular Afterload

Left ventricular afterload can be equated to systolic wall tension which, by the Laplace equation, is proportional to the product of transmural LV pressure and the radius of curvature of the LV, which itself is proportional to LV volume. Maximal LV wall tension normally occurs at the end of isometric contraction, reflecting both a maximal product of the LV radius of curvature (end-diastolic volume) and aortic pressure (diastolic pressure). Under normal conditions during LV ejection, LV afterload progressively decreases because LV volumes decrease markedly despite the small increase in ejection pressure. Importantly, when LV dilation exists, as in CHF, maximal LV wall stress occurs during LV ejection, since the maximal product of these two variables occurs at this time. Accordingly, LV afterload varies on the baseline level of cardiac contractility, arterial pressure, and intravascular volume. LV ejection pressure is the transmural LV systolic pressure, which can be approximated as transmural arterial pressure. Since normal baroreceptor mechanisms located in the carotid body tend to maintain arterial pressure constant with respect to atmosphere, if arterial pressure were to remain constant as ITP increased, LV wall tension would decrease as well. Similarly, if transmural arterial pressure were to remain constant as ITP increased, but LV end-diastolic volume decreased because of the increased ITP-induced decrease in systemic venous return, LV wall tension would also decrease.[163] Thus, by either mechanism, increases in ITP decrease LV afterload. Similarly, decreases in ITP with a constant arterial pressure will increase LV transmural pressure, increasing LV afterload.[14,164]

Any process associated with marked decreases in ITP must also be associated with increased LV afterload and myocardial O₂ consumption (MVO₂). In fact, decreasing ITP, a common occurrence during spontaneous inspiratory efforts with bronchospasm and obstructive breathing, reflects an important cardiac stress inducing CHF. Furthermore, since weaning from positive-pressure ventilation to spontaneous ventilation may reflect dramatic changes in ITP swings and the energy requirements of the respiratory muscles, weaning from mechanical ventilation is a cardiovascular stress test.[163,165,166] Interestingly, Jabran et al.[37] demonstrated that all ventilator-dependent patients increased their cardiac outputs during weaning, but in those that failed to be liberated from mechanical ventilation, Svo₂ decreased, consistent with cardiovascular compromise. A similar argument can be given for the observed improvement in LV systolic function in patients with severe LV failure when placed on mechanical ventilation.[166] Interestingly, similar "auto-EPAP" effects of expiratory grunting have been reported in infants during crying[71] and in an adult with severe LV failure.[167] It

may well be that our failure to define specific physiologic parameters to describe subjects who may successfully be liberated from mechanical ventilation is because we do not include in these analyses measures of cardiovascular reserve.

Pulsus paradoxus occurs during spontaneous inspiration under conditions of marked pericardial restraint. This may occur because of pericardial limitations such as tamponade or constrictive pericarditis, as well as during loaded spontaneous ventilatory efforts when RV volumes swell and ITP decreases. In both cases, LV stroke volume decreases.[168-172] Perhaps the most prominent mechanism creating an inspiratory decrease in both LV stroke volume and systolic arterial pressure is the increased venous return–induced transient decrease in LV diastolic compliance that then results in decreased LV end-diastolic volume. The negative swings in ITP also increase LV ejection pressure (LV pressure minus ITP), increasing LV end-systolic volume.[14] Other influences on LV systolic function can also occur during loaded inspiratory efforts, such as with obstructive sleep apnea. These include an increase in aortic input impedance,[173] altered synchrony of contraction of the global LV myocardium,[174] and hypoxemia-induced decreased contractility.[175] Hypoxia has the added detriment of also directly reducing LV diastolic compliance as well as decreasing myocardial contractile function.[176]

Experimental repetitive periodic airway obstructions induce pulmonary edema in normal animals.[75,76] Furthermore, removing the negative swings in ITP by applying nasal CPAP results in improved global LV performance in patients with combined obstructive sleep apnea and CHF.[176]

If ITP were to increase rapidly, as during a cough, arterial pressure would also increase by a similar amount such that both arterial pressure relative to ITP (transmural arterial pressure or LV ejection pressure)[14,177] and aortic blood flow[108] would remain constant. However, sustained increases in ITP must eventually decrease aortic blood flow and arterial pressure as a result of the associated decrease in venous return.[14] Since normal baroreceptor-based homeostatic mechanisms tend to sustain a constant arterial pressure so as to maintain organ perfusion constant,[51] if ITP increased arterial pressure without changing transmural arterial pressure, the periphery would reflexively vasodilate to maintain a constant extrathoracic arterial pressure-flow relation.[153] Since coronary perfusion pressure reflects the intrathoracic pressure gradient for blood flow, it is not increased by ITP-induced increases in arterial pressure. However, compression of the coronaries by the expanding lungs may obstruct coronary blood flow. Thus, the combined decrease in coronary blood flow may induce myocardial ischemia.[178-180]

The effect of removing large negative levels of ITP is not similar to adding positive ITP on venous return. Relative increases in ITP from very negative values to zero, relative to atmosphere, will minimally alter venous return, whereas increases in ITP above atmosphere will impede venous return by increasing right atrial pressure. Once right atrial pressure becomes negative, venous return becomes flow limited. Very negative swings in ITP, as seen during vigorous inspiratory efforts in the setting of airway obstruction (asthma, upper airway obstruction, vocal cord paralysis) or stiff lungs (interstitial lung disease, pulmonary edema, and ALI), will selectively increase LV afterload. Such spontaneous inspiratory efforts may be the cause of LV failure and pulmonary edema that is often seen in these conditions,[18,52,75,76] especially if LV systolic function is already compromised[30,181] (see Figure 47-8). Similarly, removing large negative swings in ITP by either bypassing upper airway obstruction (endotracheal intubation) or through the institution of mechanical ventilation or PEEP-induced loss of spontaneous inspiratory efforts should selectively reduce LV afterload without significantly decreasing either venous return or cardiac output.* Reversing this argument, weaning from mechanical ventilation, with its associated increase in both metabolic demand and LV afterload, is a form of cardiac stress testing.

---

*References 4, 40, 83, 115, 152, 179, and 182.

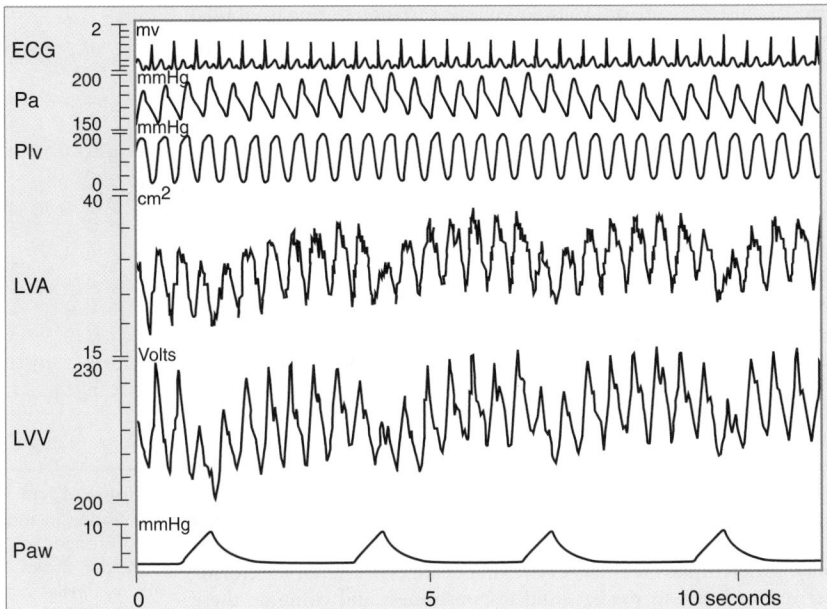

Figure 47-10   Effect of positive-pressure ventilation on LV volumes and related hemodynamic measures in a perioperative intact patient. *(Reproduced with permission from Denault AY, Gasior TA, Gorcsan J III, Mandarino WA, Deneault LG, Pinsky MR. Determinants of aortic pressure variation during positive-pressure ventilation in man. Chest 1999;116[1]: 176-186.)*

Using Changes in Intrathoracic Pressure to Define Cardiovascular Performance

Renewed interest in using the cardiovascular response to either spontaneous or positive-pressure ventilation as a means to diagnose cardiovascular responsiveness has recently occurred. However, sustained increases in airway pressure can also be used to measure cardiac contractility, as defined by the end-systolic pressure-volume relation (ESPVR).[183] Traditionally, LV ESPVR is generated by rapidly reducing LV preload by transient inferior vena caval occlusion. In the preload-dependent patient, passive inspiratory hold maneuvers that increase airway pressure by 5 to 10 cm H_2O (e.g., CPAP) will selectively decrease venous return without substantially altering either pulmonary vascular resistance or LV afterload, because the changes in lung volume and ITP are relatively small. Using this approach, Haney et al.[184,185] generated LV ESPVR similar to that created by transient inferior vena caval occlusion in a canine model. Since it is much easier to give 5 to 10 cm H_2O CPAP to patients than to pass an intravascular balloon into the inferior vena cava to induce transient vascular obstruction, this technique has promise as a means of selectively altering venous return in the bedside assessment of LV contractility. Denault et al., using the same logic, documented in mechanically ventilated patients during cardiac surgery that LV performance could be measured during ventilation using combined estimates of LV volume and ejection pressure.[186] As shown in Figure 47-10, ventilation induces profound dynamic changes in LV volumes consistent with rapidly varying changes in LV filling.

Clinical Application of Heart-Lung Interaction Physiologic Concepts: Predicting Preload Responsiveness

One of the fundamental uses of hemodynamic monitoring is to access intravascular volume status and predict the cardiac output response to volume loading.[187] Regrettably, measures of ventricular filling pressure and volumes, though useful in assessing cardiac performance, are very poor predictors of volume responsiveness.[188] Traditionally, the bedside clinician simply gave a rapid infusion of volume (e.g., 500 mL saline over 15 minutes) and noted whether cardiac output increased or not. Although effective at defining volume responsiveness, a volume challenge is time consuming and may delay appropriate treatment if there is no increase in cardiac output in response to this fluid challenge. Importantly, fully 50% of all hemodynamically unstable patients are not volume responsive[188]; thus giving volume to all unstable patients will

not benefit half. Consequently, interest in using the responses of the cardiovascular system to ventilation as a surrogate for a transient volume challenge emerged. Based on the previously described physiologic principles of heart-lung interaction, we know that positive-pressure inspiration will decrease venous return to the right ventricle, which will decrease filling of the left ventricle in 2 to 3 beats, resulting in a decrease in LV stroke volume if both ventricles are volume responsive. Under such conditions, LV stroke volume will decrease from apneic baseline values proportional to the IPPV-induced decrease in venous return and the slope of the LV function curve. Since arterial pulse pressure (diastolic to systolic arterial pressure) changes directly with LV stroke volume, one can use either stroke volume or pulse pressure variation to define volume responsiveness. Analysis of the arterial pressure waveform and its phase relationship to inspiration yield powerful tools to understanding the stroke volume and pulse pressure variations with inspiration. These variations are the basis for the prediction of preload responsiveness, and thus the application of the previously described physiologic considerations to the practical management of ventilator-dependent patients. A pulse pressure variation more than 13% or a stroke volume variation more than 10% on positive-pressure ventilation is highly predictive of volume responsiveness.[189]

One of the most central aspects of cardiovascular homeostasis is the preload-dependent nature of LV performance. Documenting that LV EDV is above some minimal value, despite cardiac output and stroke work both being depressed, is essential for the diagnosis of cardiac pump dysfunction. Similarly, demonstrating that LV EDV is decreasing in the setting of hemodynamic instability presumes the diagnosis of inadequate circulating blood volume as the most likely cause of the hemodynamic instability, even though other etiologies (e.g., tamponade, cor pulmonale, restrictive cardiomyopathies) can coexist and require different treatments. However, knowing absolute LV EDV does not predict whether LV stroke volume will increase in response to volume loading.[188] Knowing the preload of a patient is not the same as knowing if the patient will be preload responsive. In addition, being preload responsive is not necessarily indicative of fluid requirement. Just knowing that a patient is volume responsive does not equate to the need for fluid resuscitation. One must also presume or document that inadequate blood flow exists, because normal subjects who are otherwise healthy may also be volume responsive but do not need fluid resuscitation.

Three techniques presently exist for defining preload responsiveness: (1) the traditional volume challenge, (2) noting the magnitude of the arterial pulse pressure or LV stroke volume variation during fixed tidal volume positive-pressure ventilation, and (3) determining the change in mean cardiac output in response to a passive leg-raising maneuver. The second of these three techniques is central to the clinical use of heart-lung interactions to diagnose and treat cardiovascular insufficiency.

Assessing Fluid Responsiveness During Positive-Pressure Ventilation

For either pulse pressure variation (PPV, ratio of maximal minus minimal pulse pressure to mean pulse pressure over 5 or more breaths) or stroke volume variation (SVV, ratio of maximal minus minimal stroke volume to mean stroke volume over 5 or more breaths) to reflect preload responsiveness, the tidal volume must be fixed, the sequential R-R intervals must be constant (i.e., no arrhythmias), and both parameters should be measured during unassisted positive-pressure breathing with a tidal volume (VT) of 8 mL/kg or more. Several studies have been conducted to assess the reliability of this technique in the assessment of volume responsiveness. Marik et al. summarized the published data in the last 10 years in a systematic review of the literature specifically "to determine the ability of dynamic changes in arterial waveform-derived variables to predict fluid responsiveness and compare these with static indices of fluid responsiveness."[190] Twenty-nine studies, which enrolled 685 patients, were selected. The authors concluded that PPV, SVV, and systolic pressure variation (SPV) consistently predicted increments in stroke volume with fluid challenges. They also reported that the threshold values for such prediction of volume responsiveness were remarkably consistent throughout the studies and pointed to being between 11% and 13%. The diagnostic accuracy of these variables, as judged by area under the curve, was excellent (PPV 0.94, SPV 0.86, and SVV 0.84), with PPV significantly better than either SVV or SPV ($P < 0.001$). The efficacy of using either SVV or PPV metrics to predict fluid responsiveness has been validated in different clinical scenarios and populations, such as cardiac surgery,[191] orthotopic liver transplantation,[192] sepsis,[193] ARDS,[194-197] and critically ill children.[198]

Effect of Tidal Volume on Pulse Pressure Variation and Stroke Volume Variation

Changes in tidal volume also alter the phasic swings in ITP and thus the dynamic changes in venous return. The greater the tidal volume, the greater the cycle-specific changes in venous return augmenting PPV and SVV at the same volume status. This is not surprising given that PPV is generated by the pressure transmitted from the airways to the pleural and pericardial spaces and thus will theoretically be decreased with low tidal volume ventilation and low pulmonary compliance. These interactions were reported by three separate groups of investigators. DeBacker et al.,[199] in a simple and elegant clinical description of the impact of changing tidal volume on PPV, showed that PPV varied directly with tidal volume. Renner et al.[200] demonstrated that SVV also varied directly with tidal volume. Finally, Kim and Pinsky[201] showed that in anesthetized ventilated dogs, PPV decreased from 20.1 ± 10.8 to 9.5 ± 5.4% when tidal volume was decreased from 20 to 5 mL/kg. This can be conceptually described as the change in intrathoracic blood volume on a beat-to-beat basis as the difference between SV_{RV} and SV_{IV} associated with increasing tidal volume during intermittent positive-pressure ventilation. The greater the tidal volume the greater dynamic change in intrathoracic blood volume (Figure 47-11).

PPV is generated by the pressure transmitted from the airways to the pleural and pericardial spaces, and thus will theoretically be decreased with low tidal volume ventilation and low pulmonary compliance. In addition, Muller et al.[202] showed that PPV failed to predict fluid responsiveness (defined as an increase of stroke index > 15%) after a fluid challenge (normal saline or hydroxy-ethyl-starch 6% 500 mL) in patients with low airway driving pressure (PPlat – PEEP < 20 cm H_2O). In that study, PPV over 13% or even over 7% was highly

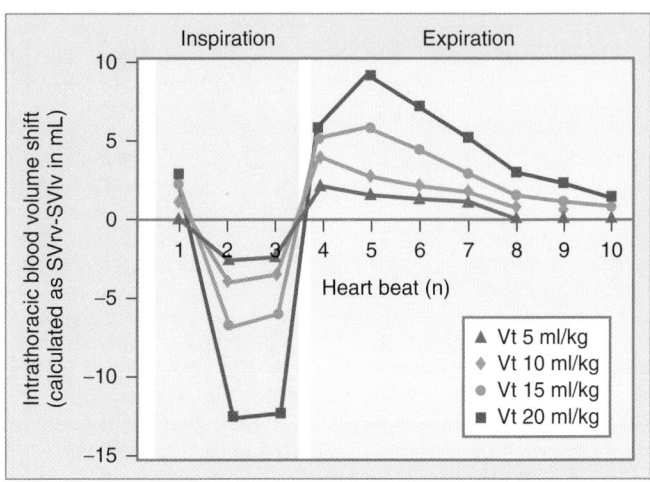

Figure 47-11 Effect of different tidal volumes (Vt) on the dynamic changes in intrathoracic blood volume (ITBV) as calculated from the differences in paired right ventricular stroke volume (SV_{RV}) to left ventricular stroke volume (SV_{LV}) for a single breath. *(Data from Mesquida, Kim, Pinsky in abstract form at the National Spanish Critical Care Medicine, 2010.)*

predictive of fluid responsiveness, but fluid responsiveness could not be ruled out in patients with lower PPV values.

Vistisen et al. have suggested that PPV should be indexed to tidal volume.[203] In their study, they showed that PPV increased significantly with increments in tidal volume in three different states: hypovolemia, normovolemia, and hypervolemia. This approach is appealing because as Romand et al. previously showed,[8] it is the change in lung volume, not in airway pressure, that determines the ITP change during positive-pressure breathing, and changes in ITP create the changes in venous return.

Effect of Positive End-Expiratory Pressure on Pulse Pressure Variation and Stroke Volume Variation

Since the primary effect of PEEP is to distend the lungs and increase ITP, PEEP normally reduces venous return and creates a functional hypovolemic state. Accordingly, Kubitz et al.[204] showed in a porcine model that increasing PEEP levels increased both PPV and SVV. Interestingly, they also saw that this effect persisted in an open chest condition, albeit to a lesser degree. Potentially one could use the emergence of an increasing PPV during positive-pressure ventilation as a sign that lung recruitment has occurred and may have started to create hyperinflation.

Limits on the Ability of Arterial Pulse Contour to Assess Stroke Volume Variation

DeCastro et al.[205,206] validated the finding that stroke volume calculated by the PiCCO arterial pulse contour technique closely tracks steady state arterial pressure but does not track dynamic SVV. These data agree with a canine study by Gunn et al.[207] that examined how accurately this same device tracked SVV as vasomotor tone was pharmacologically varied. These findings are important because they illustrate that the technique and device used to estimate SVV will have limitations minimizing its clinical utility. To reduce this inherent measurement bias across monitoring devices, clinicians should use only one minimally invasive device for the continuous measuring of SVV in the same patient over time.

Fluid Responsiveness Assessment During Spontaneous Ventilation

In spontaneously breathing patients and those with arrhythmias, the mean increase in flow 20 seconds after passive leg raising to 30 to 45 degrees gives a predictive value similar to PPV/SVV during positive-pressure ventilation. However, in this setting, the variable to measure is not PPV/SVV but the change in flow of greater than 10%. Passive leg raising (PLR) is a suitable test, given that it induces a gravitational transfer of blood from the periphery to the central circulatory compartment sufficient to significantly modify the preload of the LV and cause a change in flow or cardiac output.[208]

The best hemodynamic marker of passive leg raising as a predictor of volume responsiveness is a change in stroke volume, given that the test is transient in nature. Monnet et al.[209] demonstrated that a change in descending aortic blood flow (measured by esophageal Doppler) more than 10% after passive leg raising was predictive of volume responsiveness in spontaneously breathing patients, with or without arrhythmia, and in sedated patients with sinus rhythm. Furthermore, Lamia et al.,[210] using transthoracic echocardiography, studied the stroke volume response to passive leg raising in patients breathing spontaneously. They showed that an increment in stroke volume over 12.5% was predictive of fluid responsiveness, with a sensitivity of 77% and a specificity of 100%.

Hemodynamic Effects of Ventilation Based on Cardiopulmonary Status

Spontaneous and positive-pressure ventilation may have profound hemodynamic consequences. Furthermore, the same ventilatory maneuver (initiation or withdrawal from mechanical ventilation) can have the opposite effects on cardiovascular stability in differing patient populations. Schematic examples of how increasing or decreasing ITP will alter the LV pressure-volume relation are depicted for conditions in which LV function is normal (Figure 47-12) and depressed (Figure 47-13). Since the hemodynamic responses to ventilation are highly dependent on existing cardiovascular state, specific responses to defined ventilatory maneuvers not only define the baseline cardiovascular state but also allow for accurate predictions about what hemodynamic effects will occur.

In patients with cardiovascular insufficiency due to impaired LV ejection and/or volume overload, the institution of mechanical ventilatory support can be lifesaving because of its ability to support the cardiovascular system while decreasing global O_2 demand. In patients who are predominately preload dependent or hypovolemic (hemorrhagic shock, loss of vasomotor tone) and those who may develop RV

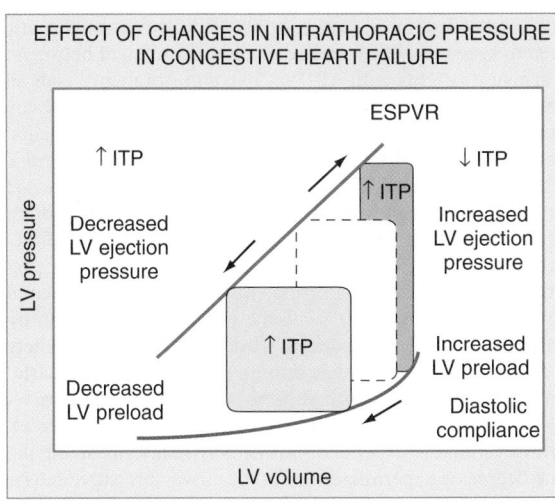

Figure 47-13 Schematic representation of the effects of changes in intrathoracic pressure (ITP) on left ventricular (LV) pressure-volume relations when cardiac contractility is impaired and intravascular volume status is expanded. ESPVR, end-systolic pressure-volume relation.

failure with hyperinflation (anterior chest trauma, spinal cord shock, severe obstructive lung disease), the institution of positive-pressure ventilation must be done with caution; profound cardiovascular insufficiency may rapidly develop during the course of intubation and initiation of mechanical ventilation. Similarly, withdrawal of ventilatory support can be considered an exercise stress test such that if patients have limited cardiovascular reserve, they may not be weaned even if their traditional weaning parameter values are acceptable.[30,181]

MECHANICAL VENTILATION

The hemodynamic differences between different modes of total mechanical ventilation at a constant airway pressure and PEEP can be explained by their differential effects on lung volume and ITP.[211] Importantly, when two different modes of total or partial ventilatory support have similar changes in ITP and ventilatory effort, their hemodynamic effects are also similar despite markedly different airway waveforms. Partial ventilatory support with either intermittent mandatory ventilation or pressure support ventilation gives similar hemodynamic responses when matched for similar tidal volumes.[212] Sternberg and Sahebjami[213] demonstrated similar tissue oxygenation in stable ventilator-dependent patients when they were switched from assist-control intermittent mandatory ventilation to pressure-support ventilation with matched tidal volumes. Finally, high-frequency jet ventilation delivered at low levels results in a constant cardiac output in patients with heart failure as compared to conventional.[214]

ACUTE LUNG INJURY

Patients with ALI often require PEEP to maintain alveolar distention and arterial oxygenation. Positive-pressure ventilation decreases intrathoracic blood volume,[121] and PEEP decreases it even more[146,147] without altering LV contractile function.[215] However, increases in airway pressure may not reflect increases in ITP because patients with ALI have varying degrees of increased lung stiffness and decreased chest wall compliance. Furthermore, it is the increase in lung volume, not airway pressure, that defines the degree of increase of ITP during positive-pressure ventilation.[8] Lessard et al.[216] saw no significant hemodynamic differences between volume-controlled,

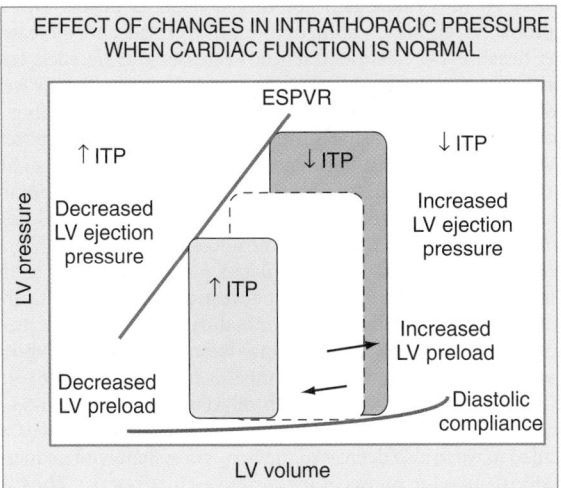

Figure 47-12 Schematic representation of the effects of changes in intrathoracic pressure (ITP) on left ventricular (LV) pressure-volume relations when cardiac contractility is normal. ESPVR, end-systolic pressure-volume relation.

pressure-controlled, and pressure-controlled inverse-ratio ventilation adjusted to keep total PEEP and tidal volume consistent between treatment arms in patients with ARDS. Chan and Abraham[217] saw similar results in patients with ARDS matched for comparable tidal volumes and total PEEP. However, when pressure control with a smaller tidal volume was compared to volume control, both Abraham and Yoshihara[218] and Poelaert et al.[219] found that pressure control was associated with a higher cardiac output. Davis et al.[220] studied the hemodynamic effects of volume control versus pressure-controlled ventilation in 25 patients with ALI. When matched for the same mean airway pressure, both methods gave the same cardiac outputs. However, when airway pressure was increased during volume-controlled ventilation by sign wave to square wave flow pattern, cardiac output fell. Furthermore, Kiehl et al.[221] found that cardiac output was better with biphasic positive airway pressure than with volume-controlled ventilation, leading to an increased Svo2 and indirectly increasing Pao2. Singer et al.[222] showed in ventilator-dependent but hemodynamically stable patients that the degree of hyperinflation, not the airway pressure, determined the decrease in cardiac output. Different modes of mechanical ventilation will affect cardiac output to a similar extent for similar increases in lung volume.[134,217,223] Most of the decrement in cardiac output can be reversed by fluid resuscitation that restores intrathoracic blood volume to pre-PEEP levels, as assessed by noninvasive blood pool scanning[215] or echocardiography[224-226]; in addition, cardiac output also returned to its basal level despite the continued application of PEEP. That the PEEP-induced decrease in cardiac output was due to a decreased pressure gradient for venous return was elegantly shown by Gunter et al.,[227] who minimized the decrease in cardiac output in ventilator-dependent septic patients by lowering body compression. Importantly, if cardiac output does not increase with fluid resuscitation, then other processes (e.g., cor pulmonale, increased pulmonary vascular resistance, cardiac compression) may also be inducing this cardiovascular depression.[228]

CONGESTIVE HEART FAILURE

Increases in cardiac output with increases in airway pressure suggest the presence of CHF.[40,229] Grace and Greenbaum[230] noted that adding PEEP to patients with heart failure did not decrease cardiac output, and actually increased cardiac output if pulmonary artery occlusion pressure exceeded 18 mm Hg. Similarly, Calvin et al.[231] noted that patients with cardiogenic pulmonary edema had no decrease in cardiac output when given PEEP.[232] Unfortunately, PEEP may be detrimental in patients with combined heart failure and ALI. PEEP can result in increased leukocyte retention in human lungs.[233] Rasanen et al. documented that decreasing levels of ventilatory support in patients with myocardial ischemia and acute LV failure worsened ischemia[40,233] and could be minimized by preventing spontaneous inspiratory effort–induced negative swings in ITP.[39] Since weaning from mechanical ventilatory support is a form of exercise stress test, withdrawal of ventilatory support can unmask cardiac failure in otherwise stable patients with acute respiratory failure.[30] Such patients may not be "weanable" from mechanical ventilatory support unless supplemented by positive inotropes.[181]

The cardiovascular benefits of positive airway pressure can be seen by withdrawing negative swings in ITP by using increasing levels of CPAP.[234,235] Even CPAP levels as low as 5 cm H2O can increase cardiac output in CHF patients, whereas cardiac output decreases with similar levels of CPAP in both normal subjects and in heart failure patients without volume overload; these hemodynamic effects of increased airway pressure do not require endotracheal intubation. Patients with CHF, but in whom forced diuresis has induced a relative hypovolemic state (as manifested by a pulmonary artery occlusion pressure ≤12 mm Hg), decreased their cardiac outputs equally whether they received CPAP or BiPAP at the same mean airway pressure.[236] Nasal CPAP can also accomplish the same results in patients with obstructive sleep apnea and heart failure,[237] although the benefits do not appear to

be related to changes in the obstructive breathing pattern.[238] Prolonged nighttime nasal CPAP can selectively improve respiratory muscle strength as well as LV contractile function in patients with preexistent heart failure.[239,240] These benefits are associated with reductions of serum catecholamine levels.[241]

If positive airway pressure augments LV ejection in heart failure states, systolic arterial pressure should not decrease but actually increase during inspiration, so-called reverse pulsus paradoxus. This was what Abel et al.[207] found in post–cardiac surgery patients. Perel et al.[242-244] suggested that the relation between ventilatory efforts and systolic arterial pressure may be used to identify which patients may benefit from cardiac assist maneuvers. Patients who increase their systolic arterial pressure during ventilation relative to an apneic baseline tend to have a greater degree of volume overload[243] and heart failure,[242] whereas those subjects in whom systolic arterial pressure decreases tend to be volume responsive. This logic has been recently taken to be used as a hemodynamic test, and arterial pulse pressure substituted for systolic pressure. Michard et al.[245] found in a series of ventilator-dependent septic patients that the greater the degree of arterial pulse pressure variation during positive-pressure ventilation, the greater the subsequent increase in cardiac output in response to volume expansion therapy.

CHRONIC OBSTRUCTIVE PULMONARY DISEASE

The primary hemodynamic problem seen in patients with COPD is related to hyperinflation, either due to bronchospasm, loss of lung parenchyma, or dynamic hyperinflation. In each case, the lungs expand, compressing the heart, increasing pulmonary vascular resistance, and impeding RV filling. Dynamic hyperinflation is also referred to as *intrinsic PEEP*. Intrinsic PEEP will alter hemodynamic function in patients in a fashion similar to extrinsic PEEP. Matching intrinsic PEEP with externally applied PEEP has no measurable detrimental hemodynamic effect,[246-248] although such matching decreases the work cost of spontaneous breathing. Furthermore, CPAP, like PEEP, has little detrimental effect in these patients when delivered below the intrinsic PEEP level.[249] There is little hemodynamic difference between increasing airway pressure to generate a breath and decreasing extrathoracic pressure (as with iron lung negative-pressure ventilation). Ambrosino et al.[250] used negative-pressure ventilation to augment ventilation in COPD patients and found no differences in hemodynamic response with similar levels of tidal volume.

Weaning of patients with COPD will tax the cardiovascular system. Patients with severe COPD but adequate ventilatory weaning parameters may go into cardiogenic pulmonary edema during weaning.[30] This probably reflects combined volume overload and increased LV failure, because LV ejection fraction decreases during such trials[251]; following diuresis, many of these patients can be subsequently weaned. The difficulty bedside clinicians have in predicting weaning from mechanical ventilation using simple measures of ventilatory reserve, airflow, and gas exchange parameters may reflect lack of insight into the patient's cardiovascular reserve and the exercise load spontaneous breathing places on the rest of the circulation. Mohsenifar et al. assessed the effect of weaning on gastric intramucosal pH (pHi), as a marker of splanchnic blood flow, in ventilated patients deemed ready for weaning.[36] Patients who could not be weaned demonstrated substantially reduced gastric pHi, from 7.36 during intermittent positive-pressure ventilation to 7.09 during weaning. Patients who were successfully weaned showed no change in pHi (7.45 to 7.46). Jabran et al.[37] demonstrated that although all ventilator-dependent COPD patients increased their cardiac outputs during weaning trials, those who failed to wean also decreased the Svo2, consistent with an increased metabolic demand in excess of the cardiovascular reserve. Thus, occult cardiovascular insufficiency may play a major role in the development of failure to wean in critically ill patients.[252] However, this assumption, though attractive, has not been proven conclusively, only suggested by this one clinical trial.

ANNOTATED REFERENCES

VENTILATION AND VENOUS RETURN

Holt JP. The effect of positive and negative intrathoracic pressure on cardiac output and venous return in the dog. Am J Physiol 1944;142(4):594-603.
One of the original papers showing the reciprocal and changing effects of cyclic breathing on venous return. They attributed all the hemodynamic effects to changes in venous return.

Sharpey-Schaffer EP. Effects of Valsalva's manoeuver on the normal and failing circulation. Br Med J 1955;1(4915):693-9.
This classic article described the arterial pressure response to a Valsalva maneuver in patients with either normal cardiac function or heart failure. Sharpey-Schaffer was the first to describe the "square wave" arterial pressure response of heart failure, now used as a diagnostic tool.

Marini JJ, Culver BN, Butler J. Mechanical effect of lung distention with positive pressure on cardiac function. Am Rev Respir Dis 1980;124(4):382-6.
This study alerted clinicians to the cardiac-depressive effects of hyperinflation and auto-PEEP in impeding both venous return and cardiac filling.

Jardin F, Farcot JC, Boisante L, et al. Influence of positive end-expiratory pressure on left ventricular performance. N Engl J Med 1981;304(7):387-92.
The authors documented for the first time in humans that the cardiac-depressive effects of PEEP were due to decreased venous return, because when they restored left ventricular volumes, cardiac output returned to baseline despite continuing PEEP. This stopped the search for the PEEP-induced cardiac depressant.

Van den Berg P, Jansen JRC, Pinsky MR. The effect of positive-pressure inspiration on venous return in volume loaded post-operative cardiac surgical patients. J Appl Physiol 2002;92(3):1223-31.
The first study in humans to show that positive-pressure inspiration does not reduce the pressure gradient for venous return because it simultaneously increases intraabdominal pressure, this article offers a good discussion of heart-lung interactions.

Jardin F, Vieillard-Baron A. Right ventricular function and positive-pressure ventilation in clinical practice: from hemodynamic subsets to respirator settings. Intensive Care Med 2003;29(9):1426-34.
This was the first study in humans to show dynamic and cycle-specific changes in venous return and right ventricular stroke volume during positive-pressure ventilation, as predicted by earlier studies in animals. Although not new information, the article includes elegant illustrations and web-based video.

VENTILATION AND LEFT VENTRICULAR PERFORMANCE

Buda AJ, Pinsky MR, Ingels NB, et al. Effect of intrathoracic pressure on left ventricular performance. N Engl J Med 1979;301(9):453-9.
The study that marked the first demonstration in humans that swings in intrathoracic pressure inversely alter left ventricular afterload independent of any changes in venous return.

Calvin JE, Driedger AA, Sibbald WJ. Positive end-expiratory pressure (PEEP) does not depress left ventricular function in patients with pulmonary edema. Am Rev Respir Dis 1981;124(2):121-8.
This was the first study to report in humans improved left ventricular function with the use of PEEP in patients with congestive heart failure.

Rasanen J, Nikki P, Heikkila J. Acute myocardial infarction complicated by respiratory failure. The effects of mechanical ventilation. Chest 1984;85(1):21-8.
First study to report in humans the association between negative swings in intrathoracic pressure, left ventricular afterload, and myocardial ischemia and reversal of ischemia with removal of negative swings

in intrathoracic pressure. This concept altered the management of cardiogenic pulmonary edema in the setting of on-going ischemia.

Pinsky MR, Matuschak GM, Klain M. Determinants of cardiac augmentation by increases in intrathoracic pressure. J Appl Physiol 1985;58(4):1189-98.
The definitive physiological study of the dynamic effects of positive-pressure ventilation on venous return and left ventricular afterload, this article offers an excellent discussion of ventriculo-arterial coupling.

Lemaire F, Teboul JL, Cinoti L, et al. Acute left ventricular dysfunction during unsuccessful weaning from mechanical ventilation. Anesthesiology 1988;69(2):171-9.
This was the first study in humans to show that weaning to spontaneous ventilation could induce immediate and severe left ventricular failure and pulmonary edema.

Denault AY, Gorcsan 3rd J, Pinsky MR. Dynamic effects of positive-pressure ventilation on canine left ventricular pressure-volume relations. J Appl Physiol 2001;91(1):298-308.
The definitive physiologic study showing the dynamic effects of ventilation on instantaneous left ventricular pressure-volume relations, this study defined the interactions between preload, ventricular interdependence, and left ventricular afterload on left ventricular performance.

Kaneko Y, Floras JS, Usui K, et al. Cardiovascular effects of continuous positive airway pressure in patients with heart failure and obstructive sleep apnea. N Engl J Med 2003;348(13):1233-41.
Good clinical trial documenting the sustained improvement in left ventricular function in patients with heart failure and obstructive sleep apnea given nighttime CPAP to relieve the repetitive negative swings in intrathoracic pressure and presumably left ventricular afterload. Good discussion on the mechanisms of interaction in this very large outpatient population.

Kim HK, Pinsky MR. Effect of tidal volume, sampling duration and cardiac contractility on pulse pressure and stroke volume variation during positive-pressure ventilation. Crit Care Med 2008;36(10):2858-62.
Animal study documenting that in anesthetized ventilated dogs, PPV decreased from 20.1 ± 10.8 to 9.5 ± 5.4% when tidal volume was decreased from 20 to 5 mL/kg.

Monnet X, Rienzo M, Osman D, et al. Passive leg raising predicts fluid responsiveness in the critically ill. Crit Care Med 2006;34(5):1402-7.
Clinical study showing that a change in descending aortic blood flow (measured by esophageal Doppler) more than 10% after PLR was predictive of volume responsiveness in spontaneously breathing patients and/ or having arrhythmia, and in sedated patients with sinus rhythm.

Pinsky MR. Hemodynamic evaluation and monitoring in the ICU. Chest 2007;132(6):2020-9.
Good review of the literature and state of the art as of 2007, of the clinical utility of SVV and PPV in the assessment of fluid responsiveness, and most importantly, of the limitations of this approach.

Marik PE, Cavallazzi R, Vasu T, Hirani A. Dynamic changes in arterial waveform derived variables and fluid responsiveness in mechanically ventilated patients: a systematic review of the literature. Crit Care Med. 2009;37(9):2642-7.
This complete systematic review of the literature sought "to determine the ability of dynamic changes in arterial waveform-derived variables to predict fluid responsiveness and compare these with static indices of fluid responsiveness." The review showed, in 29 studies that included 685 patients, that PPV, SVV, and systolic pressure variation (SPV) very consistently predicted increments in stroke volume with fluid challenges. The authors also reported that threshold values for such prediction of volume responsiveness were remarkably consistent throughout the studies: between 11% and 13%, with a diagnostic accuracy (area under the curve or AUC) above 0.84 for PPV, SPV and SVV.

Kubitz JC, Annecke T, Kemming GI, et al.
This animal study showed the impact of increasing PEEP levels in PPV and SVV. The authors were able to show that increasing PEEP will increase both PPV and SVV; this effect persisted even during open chest conditions, albeit to a lesser degree.

REFERENCES

Access the complete reference list online at http://www.expertconsult.com.

48

Mechanical Ventilation

NEIL R. MACINTYRE

Positive-pressure mechanical ventilatory support provides pressure and flow to the airways to effect oxygen (O_2) and carbon dioxide (CO_2) transport between the environment and the pulmonary capillary bed. The goal is to maintain appropriate levels of partial pressure of O_2 and CO_2 in arterial blood while unloading the ventilatory muscles. Conceptually, mechanical ventilatory support can be either total or partial. With total support, the mechanical device is designed to provide virtually all the work of breathing. Although patient effort may be present and may trigger ventilator breaths or even provide a small number of spontaneous breaths, total support should provide virtually all needed minute ventilation, with minimal patient contributions. In contrast, with partial support, the mechanical device is designed to only partially unload ventilatory muscles, requiring the patient to provide the remainder of the work of breathing. In general, total support is used in acute respiratory failure when the patient's muscles are overloaded or fatigued or when gas exchange is very unstable or unreliable. Partial support is generally used in less severe forms of respiratory failure (especially during the recovery or weaning phase). Partial support issues are discussed in Chapters 49 and 50. This chapter focuses on positive-pressure ventilation designed to provide total support.

Device Design Features for Total Ventilatory Support

POSITIVE-PRESSURE BREATH CONTROLLER

Most modern ventilators use piston-bellows systems or high-pressure gas sources to drive gas flow.[1,2] Tidal breaths are generated by this gas flow and can be classified in terms of what initiates the breath (trigger variable), what controls gas delivery during the breath (target or limit variable), and what terminates the breath (cycle variable).[3] During total support, breaths can be initiated (triggered) by patient effort (assisted breaths) or by the machine timer (controlled breaths). Target or limit variables are generally either a set flow or a set inspiratory pressure. With flow targeting, the ventilator adjusts pressure to maintain a clinician-determined flow pattern; with pressure targeting, the ventilator adjusts flow to maintain a clinician-determined inspiratory pressure. Cycle variables are generally a set volume or a set inspiratory time. Breaths can also be cycled if pressure limits are exceeded. The four common breath types supplied by modern mechanical ventilators to provide total support are volume control (VC), volume assist (VA), pressure control (PC), and pressure assist (PA).[3] These breaths are classified by their trigger, target, and cycle features in Figure 48-1.

MODE CONTROLLER

The availability and delivery logic of different breath types define the mode of mechanical ventilatory support.[3] The mode controller is an electronic, pneumatic, or microprocessor-based system designed to provide the proper combination of breaths according to set algorithms and feedback data (conditional variables). For total support, the most commonly used modes are volume assist-control and pressure assist-control. Synchronized intermittent mandatory ventilation (SIMV) can provide VA and VC or PA and PC breaths interspersed with either unsupported or partially supported spontaneous breaths (volume-targeted SIMV and pressure-targeted SIMV, respectively). When the SIMV machine breath rate is set sufficiently high, the bulk of the work required for the desired delivered minute ventilation is borne by the

ventilator such that these modes can be considered to provide virtual total support. A variation on the SIMV approach is to use a pressure-targeted mode with a long inspiratory time/short expiratory time pattern and allow spontaneous breaths to occur during the long inflation phase. This approach goes by a variety of proprietary names but is most commonly referred to as *airway pressure release ventilation* (APRV).[4] These modes are summarized according to available breath types in Table 48-1.

New ventilator designs incorporate advanced monitoring and feedback functions into these controllers to allow continuous adjustments in mode algorithms as the patient's condition changes.[5] The most common of these new feedback designs is the addition of a volume target backup to pressure assist-control, termed *pressure-regulated volume control* (PRVC). This feature adjusts the inspiratory pressure level above or below the clinician-set target to achieve the volume target. A more sophisticated feedback system for pressure-targeted breaths calculates a frequency–tidal volume combination that requires the least ventilator work for the desired minute ventilation. Known as *adaptive support ventilation* (ASV), this mode also incorporates a calculation of the expiratory time constant to assure that an expiratory time to minimize air trapping is also present.[6] Finally, two new modes that are driven entirely by patient effort can be set to provide virtually all the work of breathing and thus could be considered forms of total support. One is *proportional assist ventilation* (PAV), which drives ventilator gas flow as a proportion of patient flow demand; the other is *neurally adjusted ventilator assistance* (NAVA), which drives ventilator gas flow as a proportion of the diaphragmatic electromyogram signal.[6-8] These two interactive modes are discussed in more detail in Chapter 49.

OTHER DEVICE FEATURES SUPPORTING MECHANICAL VENTILATION

Effort sensors are pressure and/or flow transducers in the ventilator circuitry that detect patient breathing efforts and are characterized by their sensitivity and responsiveness.[9] *Blenders* mix air and O_2 to produce a delivered inspired O_2 fraction (F_{IO_2}) from 0.21 to 1.0. On newer systems, blenders are also available for other gases such as heliox, nitric oxide, and anesthetic agents. *Humidifiers* adjust blended gas mixtures to approximate body conditions using either passive heat-moisture exchangers in the circuitry or active systems that add heat and moisture directly. *Positive end-expiratory pressure (PEEP)* is usually applied by regulating pressure in the expiratory valve of the ventilator system, but a continuous flow of source gas during the expiratory phase can produce a similar effect. The *gas delivery circuit* consists of flexible tubing that often has pressure or flow sensors and an exhalation valve. It is important to remember that this tubing has measurable compliance (generally 1-4 mL/cm H_2O), and significant amounts of delivered gas may only distend this circuitry rather than enter the patient's lungs when high airway pressures are encountered.

Physiologic Effects of Positive-Pressure Mechanical Ventilation

EQUATION OF MOTION

Lung inflation during mechanical ventilation occurs when pressure and flow are applied at the airway opening. These applied forces interact with respiratory system compliance (both lung and chest wall

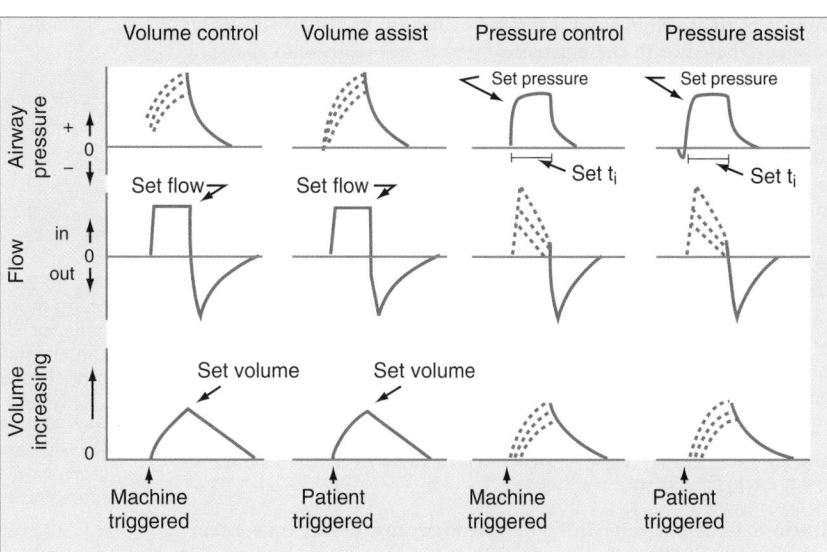

Figure 48-1 Airway pressure, flow, and volume tracings over time depicting the four basic breaths available for assist-control ventilation on most modern mechanical ventilators. Breaths are classified by their trigger, target or limit, and cycle variables. Patient-triggered assisted breaths are identified by the small drop in airway pressure before pressure and flow delivery; machine-triggered controlled breaths have no such drop. The target or limit is a clinician-set flow or inspiratory pressure. On most modern ventilators, flow-targeted assist-control breaths are volume cycled; pressure-targeted assist-control breaths are time (t_i) cycled. *(Modified from Habashi NM. Other approaches to open-lung ventilation: airway pressure release ventilation. Crit Care Med. 2005;33(3 Suppl):S228-240.)*

components), airway resistance, and to a lesser extent, respiratory system inertance and lung tissue resistance to effect gas flow.[10,11] For simplicity's sake, because inertance and tissue resistance are relatively small, they can be ignored, and the interactions of pressure, flow, and volume with respiratory system mechanics can be expressed by the simplified equation of motion:

$$\text{Driving pressure} = (\text{Flow} \times \text{Resistance}) + (\text{Volume}/\text{System compliance})$$

In a mechanically ventilated patient, this relationship is expressed as:

$$dPAO = (V' \times R) + V_T/CRS$$

where *dPAO* is the change in pressure above baseline at the airway opening; *V'* is the flow into the patient's lungs; *R* is the resistance of the circuit, artificial airway, and natural airways; *V_T* is the tidal volume; and *CRS* is the respiratory system compliance.

By performing an inspiratory hold at end-inspiration (i.e., no-flow conditions: V' = 0), the components of dPAO required for flow and for respiratory system distention can be separated. Specifically, when V' = 0 at end-inspiration, dPAO is referred to as a "plateau" pressure and reflects the static respiratory system compliance (CRS = V_T/dPAOplateau). Adding dPAO to the baseline pressure gives the total respiratory system distending pressure at end-inspiration (dPAOplateau + baseline pressure = PAOplateau). Calculating the difference in dPAO during flow and during no-flow (the "peak to plateau difference") allows the calculation of inspiratory airway resistance (R = dPAOpeak − dPAOplateau/V').

Separating chest wall and lung compliance (CCW and CL, respectively) during a passive, machine-controlled positive-pressure breath requires an esophageal pressure measurement (Pes) to approximate pleural pressure. With this measurement, the inspiratory change in

Pes (dPes) can be used in the following calculations: CCW = V_T/dPes, and CL = V_T/(dPAO − dPes). In clinical practice, because CCW is usually quite high and dPes is thus quite low, dPAOplateau and PAOplateau are often taken as an approximation of lung distending pressure. However, in situations in which CCW is reduced (e.g., obesity, anasarca, ascites, surgical dressings), the stiff chest wall can have a significant effect on dPAOplateau and PAOplateau and must therefore be considered when using these measurements to assess lung stretch.[12]

PATIENT-VENTILATOR INTERACTIONS AND SYNCHRONY

During the assisted breaths of assist-control ventilation, patients interact with all three phases of breath delivery: trigger, target, and cycle.[13] As noted, breath triggering occurs when patient effort is sensed by the ventilator and flow delivery is initiated. Breath triggering is characterized by sensitivity (the amount of effort required to trigger the breath) and responsiveness (the time required to have flow delivery meet the target value). Once flow delivery is initiated, ventilator flow delivery interacts with patient flow demand. Flow synchronized to demand is characterized by an airway pressure profile that is similar in shape to a controlled breath. Ventilator breath cycling that is synchronous to patient effort is characterized by a smooth transition in the airway pressure and flow graphic from inspiration to expiration.

RESPIRATORY SYSTEM MECHANICS AND BREATH DESIGN FEATURES

As noted earlier, there are two basic approaches to delivering positive-pressure breaths during assist-control ventilation: pressure targeting–time cycling and flow targeting–volume cycling. Although similar

TABLE 48-1	NIH ARDS Network PEEP-F$_{IO_2}$ Tables															
Conservative PEEP Approach																
F$_{IO_2}$	30	40	40	50	50	60	70	70	70	80	90	90	90	1.0	1.0	1.0	1.0
PEEP	5	5	8	8	10	10	10	12	14	14	14	16	18	18	20	22	24
Liberal PEEP Approach																
F$_{IO_2}$	30	30	40	40	50	50	60	60	70	80	80	90	1.0	1.0			
PEEP	12	14	14	16	16	18	18	20	20	20	22	22	22	24			

Data from Lellouche F, Brochard L. Advanced closed loops during mechanical ventilation (PAV, NAVA, ASV, SmartCare). *Best Pract Res Clin Anaesthesiol.* 2009;23(1):81-93.
Targets: Po₂ 55-80, Spo₂ 88%-95%. Move up one step if below target, down one step if above target. F$_{IO_2}$, fraction of inspired oxygen; PEEP, positive end-expiratory pressure (cm H₂O).

ranges of tidal volume and inspiratory time are available with either strategy, these breath characteristics interact differently with changing respiratory system mechanics and patient effort.[10,11] Changes in compliance or resistance cause a change in tidal volume (but not in pressure at the airway opening) with a pressure-targeted breath. In contrast, similar changes in compliance or resistance cause a change in pressure at the airway opening (but not in flow or volume) with a flow-targeted breath. Patient effort during a pressure-assist breath causes the ventilator to augment flow (and thus volume) to maintain the inspiratory pressure target; this same effort during a volume-assist breath does not affect delivered flow or volume but instead causes a fall in the measured circuit pressure. The hybrid breath design pressure-regulated volume control described earlier has basic features of pressure targeting but also has a volume feedback feature that adjusts the pressure target to maintain a clinician set volume.

INTRINSIC POSITIVE END-EXPIRATORY PRESSURE AND THE VENTILATORY PATTERN

Intrinsic PEEP develops within the alveoli because of inadequate expiratory time or collapsed airways during expiration (or both). Intrinsic PEEP depends on three factors: minute ventilation, the expiratory time fraction, and the respiratory system's expiratory time constant (the product of resistance and compliance).[14] As minute ventilation increases, expiratory time fraction decreases, or time constant lengthens (i.e., higher resistance or compliance values), the potential for intrinsic PEEP to develop increases.

The development of intrinsic PEEP has different effects on volume assist-control and pressure assist-control ventilation. In volume assist-control, the constant delivered tidal volume (and thus the change in pressure at the airway opening) in the setting of a rising intrinsic PEEP increases both the peak airway opening pressure and the end-inspiratory plateau airway opening pressure. In contrast, in pressure assist-control, the limit on airway opening pressure coupled with a rising intrinsic PEEP level decreases the delta pressure at the airway opening and thus the delivered tidal volume (and minute ventilation).

In a passive patient, intrinsic PEEP can be assessed in two ways. First, when an inadequate expiratory time is producing intrinsic PEEP, analysis of the flow graphic will show that expiratory flow has not returned to zero before the next breath is given. Second, intrinsic PEEP in alveolar units with patent airways can be quantified during an expiratory hold maneuver that permits equilibration of the intrinsic PEEP throughout the ventilator circuitry.

DISTRIBUTION OF VENTILATION

A positive-pressure tidal breath must distribute itself among the millions of alveolar units in the lung.[15,16] Factors affecting this distribution include regional resistances, compliances, and functional residual capacities and the delivered flow pattern (including inspiratory pause). In general, positive-pressure breaths tend to distribute more to units with high compliance and low resistance and away from obstructed or stiff units (Figure 48-2). This creates the potential for regional overdistention of healthier lung units, even in the face of "normal-sized" tidal volumes.

It should be noted that a more uniform ventilation distribution does not necessarily mean better ventilation-perfusion ($\dot{V}/\dot{Q}$) matching (e.g., a more uniform ventilation distribution may actually worsen ($\dot{V}/\dot{Q}$) matching in a lung with inhomogeneous perfusion). Because of all these considerations, predicting which flow pattern will optimize $\dot{V}/\dot{Q}$ matching is difficult and often an empirical trial-and-error exercise.

◼ Alveolar Recruitment

Infiltrative lung disease produces severe ($\dot{V}/\dot{Q}$) mismatching through alveolar flooding and collapse.[17] In many (but not all) of these disease processes, the collapsed alveoli can be recruited during a

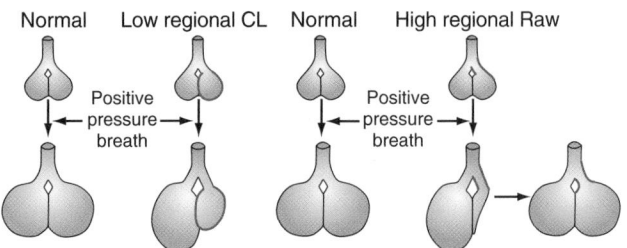

Figure 48-2 Schematic effects of the distribution of ventilation in two-unit lung models with homogeneous mechanical properties, abnormal compliance distribution, and abnormal resistance distribution. Note that in situations involving inhomogeneous lung mechanics, positive-pressure breaths are preferentially distributed to "healthier" regions of the lung and can produce regional overdistention—even when a normal-sized global tidal volume is delivered. CL, lung compliance; Raw, airway resistance. (Adapted from MacIntyre NR. Mechanical ventilatory support. In: Dantzker D, MacIntyre NR, Bakow E, editors. Comprehensive Respiratory Care. Philadelphia: Saunders; 1995.)

positive-pressure ventilatory cycle.[18,19] Three specific techniques to optimize recruitment are the application of PEEP, use of recruitment maneuvers, and prolongation of inspiratory time.

PEEP is defined as an elevation of transpulmonary pressures at the end of expiration.[18-20] As discussed, PEEP can be produced either by expiratory circuit valves (applied PEEP) or as a consequence of ventilator settings interacting with respiratory system mechanics (intrinsic PEEP). Note that expiratory muscle contraction can also raise intrathoracic pressures at end-expiration; this should not be considered PEEP, however, because it is not a transpulmonary pressure (i.e., alveolar-pleural pressure).

Alveoli that are prevented from "derecruiting" by PEEP provide several potential benefits. First, recruited alveoli improve ($\dot{V}/\dot{Q}$) matching and gas exchange.[18-21] Second, as discussed in more detail later, patent alveoli throughout the ventilatory cycle are not exposed to the risk of injury from the shear stress of repeated opening and closing.[22] Third, PEEP prevents surfactant breakdown in collapsing alveoli and thus improves lung compliance.[23]

PEEP can also be detrimental. Because the tidal breath is delivered on top of the baseline PEEP, end-inspiratory pressures are raised by PEEP application.[24] This must be considered if the lung is at risk for stretch injury (see Ventilator-Induced Lung Injury). Moreover, because alveolar injury is often quite heterogeneous, appropriate PEEP in one region may be suboptimal in another region and excessive in another. Optimizing PEEP is thus a balance between recruiting the recruitable alveoli in diseased regions without overdistending already recruited alveoli in healthier regions. Another potential detrimental effect of PEEP is that it raises mean intrathoracic pressure. This can compromise cardiac filling in susceptible patients (see Cardiac Effects).

Recruitment maneuvers are based on the concept that alveolar recruitment occurs throughout a positive-pressure inflation—all the way to total lung capacity.[25] In practice, recruitment maneuvers are performed using sustained inflations (e.g., 30 to 40 cm H_2O for up to 2 minutes).[25-27] An alternative approach is to use frequent "sigh breaths" that briefly take the lung to near total capacity on a frequent basis.[28] It must be pointed out that recruitment maneuvers provide only initial alveolar recruitment; the duration of recruitment almost certainly depends on an appropriate setting of PEEP to prevent subsequent derecruitment.[27]

Prolonging the inspiratory time (generally by adding a pause), often used in conjunction with a rapid-decelerating flow (i.e., pressure-targeted) breath, has several physiologic effects.[29,30] First, the longer inflation period may lead to the opening of more slowly recruitable alveoli. Second, increased gas mixing time may improve ($\dot{V}/\dot{Q}$) matching in infiltrative lung disease. Third, the development of intrinsic PEEP can have similar effects to that of applied PEEP (see earlier). Indeed, much of the improvement in gas exchange associated with long inspiratory time strategies may be merely a PEEP phenomenon.[30] It should be noted, however, that the distribution of intrinsic PEEP (most pronounced in lung units with long time constants) may be different from that of applied PEEP; thus, ($\dot{V}/\dot{Q}$) effects may also be different.[31] Fourth, because these long inspiratory times significantly increase total intrathoracic pressures, cardiac output may be affected (see Cardiac Effects). Finally, inspiratory-expiratory ratios that exceed 1:1 (so-called inverse ratio ventilation [IRV]) are uncomfortable, and patient sedation or paralysis is often required unless a relief mechanism allows spontaneous breathing during the inflation period (airway pressure release ventilation; see later).

Adverse Effects of Positive-Pressure Ventilation

VENTILATOR-INDUCED LUNG INJURY

The lung can be injured when it is stretched excessively by positive-pressure ventilation. The most well-recognized injury is alveolar rupture, presenting as extraalveolar air in the mediastinum (pneumomediastinum), pericardium (pneumopericardium), subcutaneous tissue (subcutaneous emphysema), pleura (pneumothorax), and vasculature (air emboli).[3] The risk for extraalveolar air increases as a function of the magnitude and duration of alveolar overdistention. Thus, interactions of respiratory system mechanics and mechanical ventilation strategies (high regional tidal volume and PEEP—both applied and intrinsic) that produce regions of excessive alveolar stretch (i.e., transpulmonary distending pressures in excess of 40 cm H_2O) for prolonged periods create alveolar units that are at risk for rupture.

A parenchymal lung injury not associated with extraalveolar air can also be produced by mechanical ventilation strategies that stretch the lungs beyond the normal maximum (i.e., transpulmonary distending pressures > 30 to 35 cm H_2O).[32-35] Pathologically, this manifests as diffuse alveolar damage and is associated with cytokine release[36] and bacterial translocation.[37]

In addition to being caused by simple overstretching of the lung, ventilator-induced lung injury (VILI) may have other determinants. Among these may be excessive tidal stretch (i.e., repetitive cycling of the lungs with tidal volumes larger than the normal 4-8 mL/kg ideal body weight)[38] and a shear stress phenomenon that occurs when injured alveoli are repetitively opened and collapsed during the ventilatory cycle.[22,35,39,40] VILI may also be worsened by increasing the frequency of excessive lung tidal stretch and from acceleration forces associated with rapid initial gas flow into the lung.[41]

VILI occurs clinically when low-resistance/high-compliance units receive a disproportionately high regional tidal volume in the setting of high alveolar distending pressures (see Figure 48-2). Concern about overdistention injury is the rationale for using "lung-protective" ventilator strategies that accept less than normal values for pH and O_2 partial pressure in exchange for lower (and safer) distending pressures.

CARDIAC EFFECTS

In addition to affecting ventilation and ventilation distribution, intrathoracic pressure changes resulting from positive-pressure ventilation can affect cardiovascular function.[42] In general, as mean intrathoracic pressure is increased, right ventricular filling is decreased. This is the rationale for using volume repletion to maintain cardiac output in the setting of high intrathoracic pressure. Conversely, elevations in intrathoracic pressure can actually improve left ventricular function because of an effective reduction in afterload.[43] Indeed, a sudden release of intrathoracic pressure (e.g., during a ventilator disconnect or spontaneous breathing trial) can sometimes precipitate flash pulmonary edema because of the acute increase in afterload coupled with increased venous return.[44]

Intrathoracic pressures can influence the distribution of perfusion. The relationship of alveolar pressures to perfusion pressures in the three-zone lung model can help explain this.[45] Specifically, the supine human lung is generally in a zone 3 (distention) state. As intraalveolar pressures rise, however, zone 2 and zone 1 regions can appear, creating high $\dot{V}/\dot{Q}$ units. Indeed, increases in dead space (i.e., zone 1 lung) can be a consequence of ventilatory strategies using high ventilatory pressures (e.g., IRV).

Positive-pressure mechanical ventilation can affect other aspects of cardiovascular function. Specifically, dyspnea, anxiety, and discomfort from inadequate ventilatory support can lead to stress-related catechol release, with subsequent increases in myocardial O_2 demands and risk of dysrhythmias. In addition, coronary blood vessel O_2 delivery can be compromised by inadequate gas exchange from lung injury, coupled with low mixed venous O_2 partial pressure due to high O_2 consumption demands by the ventilatory muscles.

PATIENT-VENTILATOR DYSSYNCHRONY

As mentioned, patients can interact with all three phases of an assisted breath: trigger, target, and cycle. Patients dyssynchronous with any of these phases will have unnecessary loads placed on their respiratory muscles, thereby increasing the risk of muscle fatigue. Moreover, dyssynchronous interactions produce discomfort and a sense of dyspnea. When severe, patients are often noted to be "fighting the ventilator." This leads to unnecessary sedation and a consequent prolongation of the need for ventilatory support.[46]

INTRINSIC PEEP/AIR TRAPPING

The development of intrinsic PEEP can produce significant adverse events. In flow- and volume-targeted ventilation, all intrathoracic pressures are increased, which can lead to risk of VILI and reduction in cardiac filling. In pressure-targeted ventilation, buildup of intrinsic PEEP results in loss of tidal volume and minute ventilation. Intrinsic PEEP can also create a significant triggering load in patients, since inspiratory muscles must first overcome intrinsic PEEP before airway and circuit pressures and flows change sufficiently to initiate the assisted breath.[47]

OTHER ADVERSE EFFECTS

Oxygen concentrations approaching 100% are known to cause oxidant injury to airways and lung parenchyma.[48] Many of the data supporting this concept, however, have come from animal studies, and animals and humans often have different O_2 tolerances. It is unclear what the "safe" O_2 concentration or duration of exposure is in sick humans. Most consensus groups have argued that F_{IO_2} values less than 0.4 are safe for prolonged periods, and F_{IO_2} values greater than 0.8 should be avoided if possible.

Mechanically ventilated patients are at risk for pulmonary infections for several reasons.[49,50] First, the natural protective mechanism of glottic closure is compromised by an endotracheal tube. This permits continuous seepage of oropharyngeal material into the airways. Second, the endotracheal tube itself impairs the cough reflex and serves as a potential portal for pathogens to enter the lungs. This is particularly important if the circuit is contaminated. Third, airway and parenchymal injury from both the underlying disease and management complications make the lung prone to infections. Fourth, the intensive care unit (ICU) environment itself, with its heavy antibiotic use and the presence of very sick patients in close proximity, poses a risk for a variety of infections.

Preventing ventilator-associated pneumonias is critical because length of stay and mortality are heavily influenced by their development.[49,50] Handwashing and carefully chosen antibiotic regimens for other infections can have important beneficial effects. Management strategies that avoid breaking the integrity of the circuit (e.g., circuit changes only when visibly contaminated) also appear to be helpful. Finally, continuous drainage of subglottic secretions may be a simple way of reducing lung contamination with oropharyngeal material.

Applying Assist-Control Mechanical Ventilation

TRADEOFFS

To provide adequate support but minimize VILI, mechanical ventilation goals must involve tradeoffs. Specifically, the need for potentially injurious pressures, volumes, and supplemental O_2 must be weighed against the benefits of gas exchange support. To this end, a rethinking of gas exchange goals has occurred over the last decade; pH goals as low as 7.15 to 7.20, and O_2 partial-pressure goals as low as 55 mm Hg, are now considered acceptable if the lung can be protected from VILI.[51,52] Ventilator settings are thus selected to provide at least this level of gas exchange support while at the same time meeting two mechanical goals: (1) provision of enough PEEP to enlist the recruitable alveoli and (2) avoidance of a PEEP–tidal volume combination that unnecessarily overdistends lung regions at end-inspiration. These goals embody the concept of a "lung-protective" mechanical ventilatory strategy, and these principles guide current recommendations for the specific management of parenchymal and obstructive lung disease.

MANAGING PARENCHYMAL LUNG INJURY

Parenchymal lung injury describes disease processes that involve the air spaces and interstitium of the lung. In general, parenchymal injury produces stiff lungs and reduced lung volumes.[17] Functional residual capacity is thus reduced, and the compliance curve is shifted to the right. It is important to realize, however, that in all but the most diffuse diseases (e.g., diffuse cardiogenic edema), there are often marked regional differences in the degree of inflammation present and thus the degree of mechanical abnormalities that exist. This heterogeneity can have a significant impact on the effects of a particular mechanical ventilation strategy. This is because delivered gases will preferentially go to the regions with the highest compliance and lowest resistance (i.e., the more normal regions) rather than to sicker regions with low compliance (see Figure 48-2). A "normal-sized" tidal volume may thus be distributed preferentially to the healthier regions, resulting in a much higher regional tidal volume and the potential for regional overdistention injury.

Parenchymal injury can also affect the airways, especially the bronchioles and alveolar ducts.[17] These narrowed and collapsible small airways can contribute to reduced regional ventilation to injured lung units. This can also lead to air trapping, and it may be a factor in subsequent cyst formation during the healing phase after lung injury.

Gas exchange abnormalities in parenchymal lung injury are a consequence of alveolar flooding or collapse coupled with a maldistribution of ventilation that results in $\dot{V}/\dot{Q}$ mismatching and shunts. Because dead space ($\dot{V}/\dot{Q} = \infty$) is not a major manifestation of parenchymal lung disease unless there is severe or end-stage injury, hypoxemia tends to be a greater problem than CO_2 clearance.

Frequency–tidal volume settings for supporting a patient with parenchymal lung injury must focus on limiting end-inspiratory stretch. The importance of this limitation in improving outcome has been suggested by several recent clinical trials,[53,54] but it was most convincingly demonstrated by the NIH ARDS Network trial, which showed a 10% absolute reduction in mortality with a ventilator strategy using a tidal volume calculated on ideal body weight of 6 mL/kg compared with 12 mL/kg.[55] Because of this, initial tidal volume settings should start at 6 mL/kg ideal body weight. Moreover, strong consideration should be given to further reducing this setting if end-inspiratory plateau pressures, adjusted for any effects of excessive chest wall stiffness, exceed 30 cm H_2O. Increases in tidal volume settings might be considered if there is marked patient discomfort or suboptimal gas exchange, provided the subsequent plateau pressures do not exceed 30 cm H_2O. Respiratory rate settings are then adjusted to control pH. Unlike in obstructive diseases (see later), the potential for air trapping in parenchymal lung injury is low if the breathing frequency is less than 35 breaths per minute and may not develop even at frequencies exceeding 50 breaths per minute.

The choice of pressure-targeted or volume-targeted breaths often depends more on clinician familiarity with the two modes than on important clinical differences between them. As noted earlier, both modes provide a comparable range of tidal volumes and inspiratory times. In general, pressure-targeted breaths are preferable when an absolute pressure limit is desired in the circuit or when patient effort is very active, with variable flow demands. In contrast, volume-targeted breaths are preferable when it is critical to maintain a certain level of minute ventilation.

Setting the inspiratory time and the inspiratory-expiratory ratio in parenchymal injury involves several considerations. The normal ratio is roughly 1:2 to 1:4; such ratios produce the most comfort and are the usual initial ventilator setting. Assessment of the flow graphic should also be done to ensure that an adequate expiratory time is present to avoid air trapping. As noted earlier, inspiratory-expiratory prolongation beyond the physiologic range of 1:1 (IRV) can be used as an alternative to increasing PEEP to improve $\dot{V}/\dot{Q}$ matching in severe respiratory failure.[29,30] A variation on IRV is airway pressure release ventilation (also known as *biphasic* or *bilevel ventilation*).[4] Airway pressure release ventilation incorporates the ability to spontaneously breathe during the long inflation period of a pressure-controlled breath—a feature that may enhance recruitment and comfort.[4,56]

IRV strategies are generally reserved for patients in whom the plateau pressure from the PEEP–tidal volume combination exceeds 30 cm H_2O, and potentially toxic concentrations of FIO_2 are being used without meeting arterial O_2 saturation or O_2 delivery goals. It must be emphasized, however, that although IRV strategies have physiologic appeal, good outcome studies supporting their use do not exist.

There are both mechanical and gas exchange approaches to setting the PEEP-FIO_2 combination to support oxygenation. Mechanical approaches often use either a static pressure-volume plot to set the PEEP–tidal volume combination between the upper and lower inflection points[57] or step increases in PEEP to determine the PEEP level that gives the best compliance.[58,59] A simpler mechanical approach involves analyzing the airway pressure waveform during a set constant flow breath (the "stress index").[60] If the pressure waveform shows a steady rise, this implies that no derecruitment or overdistension is occurring during the breath. In contrast, if the pressure waveform is concave upward, it suggests overdistension is occurring; if the pressure waveform is concave downward, it implies derecruitment occurred during the previous exhalation. With any of these approaches, a recruitment maneuver could be used to recruit the maximal number of recruitable alveoli before setting the PEEP. FIO_2 adjustments are then set as low as clinically acceptable.

Because these mechanical approaches are time consuming and technically challenging, gas exchange criteria are often used to guide PEEP and FIO_2 settings. These generally involve algorithms designed to provide adequate values for arterial partial pressure of O_2 while minimizing FIO_2 (see Table 48-1).[61,62] Note that constructing a PEEP-FIO_2 algorithm is usually an empirical exercise in balancing arterial O_2 saturation with FIO_2 and depends on the clinician's perception of the relative "toxicities" of high thoracic pressures, high FIO_2, and low arterial O_2 saturation. Of note, however, is that recent meta-analyses of three large trials comparing conservative versus aggressive PEEP-FIO_2 tables (mean PEEP of 7–9 cm H_2O versus mean PEEP of 14–16 cm H_2O) suggested benefit to the more aggressive strategies in patients with more severe lung injury.[62]

OBSTRUCTIVE AIRWAY DISEASE

Respiratory failure from airflow obstruction is a direct consequence of increases in airway resistance. Airway narrowing and increased resistance lead to two important mechanical changes. First, the increased pressures required for airflow may overload ventilatory muscles, producing a "ventilatory pump failure," with spontaneous minute ventilation inadequate for gas exchange. Second, the narrowed airways create regions in the lungs that cannot properly empty and return to their normal resting volume, and intrinsic PEEP is produced.[14] These regions of overinflation create dead space and put inspiratory muscles at a substantial mechanical disadvantage, which further worsens muscle function. Overinflated regions may also compress healthier regions of the lung, impairing $\dot{V}/\dot{Q}$ matching. Regions of air trapping and intrinsic PEEP also function as a threshold load to trigger mechanical breaths.[47,63]

Several gas exchange abnormalities can accompany worsening airflow obstruction. First, although there may be transient hyperventilation due to dyspnea in patients with asthma, worsening respiratory failure in those with obstructive lung disease is generally characterized by falling minute ventilation as respiratory muscles become fatigued in the face of airflow obstruction. The result of this clinical situation is termed *hypercapnic respiratory failure*. Second, as noted earlier, regional lung compression and regional hypoventilation produce $\dot{V}/\dot{Q}$ mismatch, which results in progressive hypoxemia. Alveolar inflammation and flooding, however, are not characteristic features of respiratory failure due to pure airflow obstruction; thus, shunts are less of an issue than in parenchymal lung injury. Third, overdistended regions of the lungs, coupled with underlying emphysematous changes in some patients, result in capillary loss and increasing dead space. This wasted ventilation further compromises the inspiratory muscles' ability to supply adequate ventilation for alveolar gas exchange. Emphysematous regions also have reduced recoil properties that can worsen air trapping. Fourth, hypoxemic pulmonary vasoconstriction, coupled with chronic pulmonary vascular changes in some airway diseases, overloads the right ventricle, further decreasing blood flow to the lung and making dead space worse.

Setting the frequency–tidal volume pattern in obstructive lung disease involves many considerations that are similar to those in parenchymal lung injury. Specifically, tidal volumes should be sufficiently low (e.g., 6 mL/kg ideal body weight) to ensure that plateau pressure is less than 30 cm H_2O. In obstructive disease, however, clinicians should be aware that high *peak* airway pressures, even in the presence of acceptable values for plateau pressure, may transiently subject regions of the lung to overdistention injury due to a pendelluft effect (see Figure 48-2). As with parenchymal lung injury, tidal volume reductions should be considered to meet plateau pressure goals. Tidal volume increases can be considered for comfort or gas exchange, provided plateau pressure values do not exceed 30 cm H_2O. The set rate is used to control pH. Unlike parenchymal disease, however, the elevated airway resistance and often low recoil pressures of emphysema greatly increase the potential for air trapping, and this limits the range of breath rates available.

The inspiratory-expiratory ratio in obstructive lung disease is generally set as low as possible to minimize the development of air trapping. For the same reason, approaches using IRV strategies are almost always contraindicated.

Because alveolar recruitment is less of an issue in obstructive lung disease than in parenchymal lung injury, the PEEP-F_IO_2 steps in Table 48-1 should probably be shifted to emphasize F_IO_2 for oxygenation support. A specific role for PEEP in an obstructed patient occurs when intrinsic PEEP serves as an inspiratory threshold load on the patient's attempting to trigger a breath. Under these conditions, judicious application of circuit PEEP (up to 75% to 85% of intrinsic PEEP) can "balance" expiratory pressure throughout the ventilator circuitry to reduce this triggering load and facilitate the triggering process.[47,63]

In severe airflow obstruction, use of low-density helium can facilitate ventilator settings. Helium is available as 80:20, 70:30, or 60:40 helium-oxygen breathing gas mixtures and can both reduce patient inspiratory work and facilitate lung emptying (recall that driving pressure decreases and flow increases through a tube as gas density decreases).[64] If using a helium-oxygen gas mixture, it must be remembered that many flow sensors must be recalibrated to account for the change in gas density.

NEUROMUSCULAR RESPIRATORY FAILURE

The risk of VILI is generally less in a patient with neuromuscular failure, because lung mechanics are often near normal, making regional overdistention less likely. More "generous" tidal volumes can thus be used to improve comfort, maintain recruitment, and prevent atelectasis. At the same time, however, maximal distending pressures should be monitored and kept as low as possible while still being compatible with the other goals noted earlier. Certainly, plateau pressure should always be kept well below 30 cm H_2O. Low levels of PEEP are often beneficial in preventing derecruitment (atelectasis) in these patients, who are often supine and incapable of secretion clearance or spontaneous sigh breaths.

RECOVERING RESPIRATORY FAILURE— THE VENTILATOR WITHDRAWAL PROCESS

Once the cause of respiratory failure stabilizes and begins to reverse, attention turns to the ventilator withdrawal process. Numerous evidence-based guidelines have focused on the pivotal role of spontaneous breathing trials (SBTs) in determining the need for continued mechanical ventilatory support.[65] In patients failing SBTs, comfortable forms of interactive ventilatory support should be provided until the next attempt at an SBT. Although the pressure-support mode is often used for this purpose, pressure assist-control can also fill this role. When using pressure assist-control, the control rate is generally set quite low (or even to zero), and the inspiratory pressure is titrated to comfort. Like pressure support, this approach is patient triggered and pressure targeted but is time cycled as opposed to the flow cycling of pressure support. Weaning and the use of partial support modes are discussed in more detail in Chapters 49 and 50.

Conclusion

Mechanical ventilatory support is a critical component in the management of patients with respiratory failure. It must be remembered, however, that this technology is supportive, not therapeutic; it cannot cure lung injury. Indeed, the best we can hope for is to "buy time" by supporting gas exchange without harming the lungs.

Assist-control ventilation is designed to provide substantial levels of respiratory support. The major goals of assist-control ventilation are to substantially unload ventilatory muscles, provide the bulk of required minute ventilation, and optimize ventilation-perfusion matching to ensure adequate oxygenation. Important complications include ventilator-induced lung injury, cardiac compromise, and patient discomfort. Applying assist-control ventilation requires tradeoffs as clinicians attempt to balance gas exchange needs with the risk of these complications. Future innovations cannot focus simply on physiologic endpoints. Rather, innovations need to show benefits in clinically relevant factors such as mortality, ventilator-free days, barotrauma, and costs. Only then can we properly assess the sometimes bewildering array of new approaches to this vital life-support technology.

KEY POINTS

1. Ventilator breath delivery is characterized by the trigger, target, and cycle variables.

2. The interaction of a positive-pressure breath and respiratory system mechanics is summarized by the equation of motion:

   Driving pressure = (Flow × Resistance) + (Volume/System compliance)

3. The goal of assist-control ventilation is to provide adequate gas exchange while protecting the lung from overdistention and recruitment-derecruitment injury.

4. Assist-control ventilation in obstructive lung disease poses the additional risk of producing overdistention from air trapping.

5. High-frequency ventilation shows promise as a better lung-protective strategy in parenchymal lung injury.

ANNOTATED REFERENCES

Tremblay LN, Slutsky AS. Ventilator-induced lung injury: from the bench to the bedside. Intensive Care Med 2006;32(1):24-33.

An excellent review attempting to link important data from animal studies of ventilator-induced lung injury to the clinical setting, with an emphasis on how ventilator strategies can produce both lung and systemic injury.

NIH ARDS Network. Ventilation with lower tidal volumes as compared with traditional tidal volumes for acute lung injury and the acute respiratory distress syndrome. N Engl J Med 2000;342(18):1301-8.

This landmark study clearly established the link between excessive lung stretch during mechanical ventilation and worse survival in patients with acute lung injury. The message from this paper is very clear: even though large tidal volumes may improve gas exchange, they ultimately cause harm by overstretching healthier regions of the lung.

Pinsky MR, Guimond JG. The effects of positive end-expiratory pressure on heart-lung interactions. J Crit Care 1991;6(1):1-15.

An excellent overview of the complex interactions of intrathoracic positive pressure and cardiac function. The fact that the twin effects of decreased right heart filling and decreased left ventricular afterload can have both positive and negative effects is carefully explained.

Slutsky AS. ACCP consensus conference: mechanical ventilation. Chest 1993;104:1833-59.

An excellent review of the application of mechanical ventilation, stressing the balance between providing respiratory support and not harming the patient.

, Truwit JD, Marini JJ. Evaluation of thoracic mechanics in the ventilated patient. Part I. Primary measurements. J Crit Care. 1988;3:133-50; Part II. Applied mechanics. *J Crit Care*. 1988;3:192-213.

This two-part report comprehensively reviews all aspects of respiratory system mechanics as they apply to mechanical ventilation. Both theory and practical applicability are provided.

Briel M, Meade M, Mercat A, et al. Higher vs lower positive end-expiratory pressure in patients with acute lung injury and acute respiratory distress syndrome: systematic review and meta-analysis. JAMA 2010;303(9):865-73.

This is a meta-analysis of the three large trials conducted in the last decade examining high versus low PEEP strategies in the setting of low-V_T ventilation. The results show that in ARDS patients, a high PEEP strategy offers a mortality benefit. However, in the less severe ALI patients, a high PEEP strategy trended towards a worse mortality.

REFERENCES

Access the complete reference list online at http://www.expertconsult.com.

49

Patient-Ventilator Interaction

V. MARCO RANIERI | CESARE GREGORETTI | VINCENZO SQUADRONE

The clinical management of patients with acute respiratory failure is based on the assumption that significant abnormalities in respiratory mechanics, respiratory muscle performance, and control of breathing are the underlying mechanisms responsible for acute respiratory failure.[1] The effects of mechanical ventilation on gas exchange, respiratory muscle load, and dyspnea depend on the matching between the ventilator settings and the patient's respiratory physiology. However, mechanical ventilation is rarely optimized, which would require that ventilator settings be based on accurate and reproducible measurements of lung and chest wall mechanics, respiratory muscle function, and respiratory drive.[2-5]

Respiratory Physiology

The goal of the intrinsic ventilatory control system is to integrate the timing and intensity of the phrenic nerve signal, inputs from chemoreceptors and pulmonary stretch receptors, and variations in metabolic demands. Contraction of the respiratory muscles leads to the generation of flow and volume to provide adequate alveolar ventilation with minimal work of breathing.[6] During spontaneous breathing,[7] the respiratory muscles generate pressure (Pmus) to generate flow against the resistive properties (Rrs) and volume against the elastic properties (E_{RS}) of the respiratory system to eventually overcome intrinsic positive end-expiratory pressure (PEEPi). Under these circumstances, the act of spontaneous breathing can be described at any instant as follows:

$$Pmus = Pres + Pel + PEEPi \qquad \text{(Equation 1)}$$

where *Pres* represents the resistive pressure and is a function of flow (Pres = Flow × Rrs), and *Pel* represents the elastic recoil pressure and is a function of volume (Pel = Volume × Ers). Assuming that R_{RS} and E_{RS} are linear, the equation becomes:

$$Pmus = PEEPi + (Flow \times R_{RS}) + (Volume \times E_{RS}) \qquad \text{(Equation 2)}$$

In patients with acute respiratory failure requiring ventilatory support, pressure generated by the ventilator (Pappl) is added to the pressure generated by the contraction of the respiratory muscles according to the following equation:

$$Pmus + Pappl = PEEPi + (Flow \times R_{RS}) + (Volume \times E_{RS}) \qquad \text{(Equation 3)}$$

The complex interaction among all the variables in equation 3 can be summarized by the concept of neuroventilatory coupling (Figure 49-1).[8] Under normal conditions, as well as at the onset of acute respiratory failure, the spontaneous contraction of the respiratory muscles suddenly generates flow and volume; the slope of the relationship between effort and ventilatory output is conditioned by the contractile properties of the respiratory muscles and the impedance of the respiratory system. When positive pressure is applied to assist the action of breathing in most common modes of mechanical ventilation (pressure-support or pressure-assist mandatory ventilation), the coupling between effort and output is compromised. During assist-control ventilation, flow and volume remain constant despite changes in muscle contraction; during pressure-support ventilation, despite coupling between inspiratory effort and ventilatory output, any increase in respiratory impedance decreases the amount of delivered flow and volume.[8] During noninvasive ventilation (NIV), air leaks may further compromise the coupling between patient effort and ventilatory output.[9]

Patient and Ventilator Variables

PATIENT VARIABLES

The patient interacts with the ventilator based on three physiologic variables[2,10,11]:
1. Ventilatory drive, or when inspiration starts[12]
2. Ventilatory requirements, or how much flow and volume are necessary to satisfy metabolic demands[5]
3. Timing of the integrated circuits generating the respiratory rhythm, as measured by the duration and ratio of inspiratory time to total breath cycle duration[10]

VENTILATOR VARIABLES

Three phase variables define inspiration[13,14]:
- The trigger that begins inspiration (pressure, volume, flow, and time dependent)
- The limit that cannot be exceeded during inspiration (pressure, volume, and flow)
- The cycling-off criteria

In other words the ventilator interfaces with the patient's physiology based on three technologic variables:
1. The inspiratory trigger, or when the ventilator starts to deliver flow, volume, and pressure[15,16]
2. The delivery mechanisms—that is, the algorithm used by the ventilator to assist ventilation through the delivery of flow, volume, or pressure[17-22]
3. The cycling-off criteria, or when the ventilator stops assisting inspiratory effort and lets the patient exhale spontaneously[20,21]

Features of ventilators such as blowers and inspiratory, expiratory, and positive end-expiratory pressure (PEEP) valves are also important in determining the interaction between patient and ventilator.[23-26]

To unload the respiratory muscles, restore sufficient gas exchange, and relieve the patient from dyspnea, the healthcare team must establish an interface between patient and ventilator. To do so, there are two options: total ventilator-controlled mechanical support or partial patient-controlled support.

TOTAL VENTILATOR-CONTROLLED MECHANICAL SUPPORT

In this mode, the patient's breathing pattern is totally controlled by the ventilator. The pressure generated by the respiratory muscles is abolished by paralysis or sedation. Flow, volume, and pressure are imposed by the ventilator, and the patient's breathing pattern is totally replaced by that of the ventilator. The risk of patient-ventilator asynchrony is therefore abolished, but there are potential risks associated with sedation and paralysis,[27] respiratory muscle atrophy,[28] lung damage due to overdistention,[29] patient discomfort,[30] and difficulty weaning after prolonged controlled mechanical ventilation.[1]

PARTIAL PATIENT-CONTROLLED MECHANICAL SUPPORT

With this mode, spontaneous breathing activity is partially preserved.[31] The need for sedation and paralysis may be reduced, disuse atrophy of the respiratory muscles may be minimized, and the weaning process may be accelerated, provided the patient's ventilatory demand and

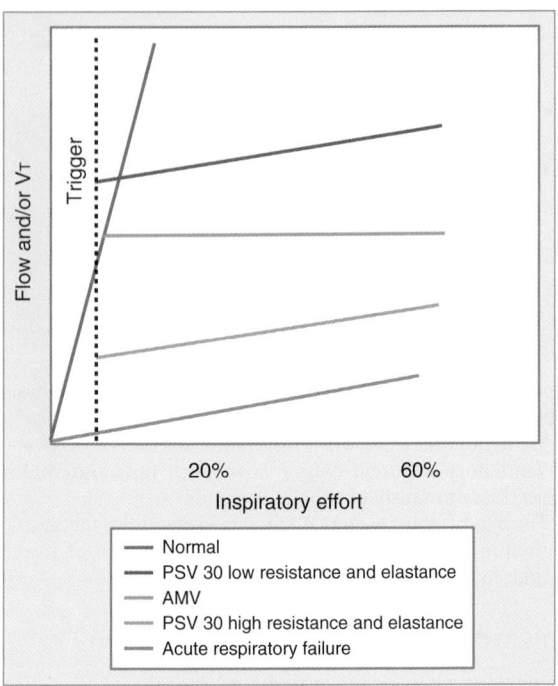

Figure 49-1 Neuroventilatory coupling. Under normal conditions, as well as at onset of acute respiratory failure, spontaneous contraction of respiratory muscles suddenly generates flow and volume. The slope of the relationship between effort and ventilatory output is conditioned by the contractile properties of the respiratory muscles and impedance of the respiratory system. When positive pressure is applied to assist the action of breathing in most common modes of mechanical ventilation, the coupling between effort and output is compromised. During assisted mandatory ventilation (AMV), flow and volume remain constant despite changes in muscle contraction. During pressure-support ventilation (PSV), despite a sort of coupling between inspiratory effort and ventilatory output, any increase in respiratory impedance decreases the amount of delivered flow and volume. VT, tidal volume.

ventilator settings are synchronized.[32] The ability to restore gas exchange, unload respiratory muscles, and relieve patient dyspnea with partial patient-controlled mechanical support therefore depends on the absence of patient-ventilator asynchrony.[33]

Although there are no well-accepted definitions, patient-ventilator asynchrony is common; it is often unrecognized, underestimated, and inappropriately treated.[3-5,22,33-35] The cause of patient-ventilator asynchrony can be described as occurring because of a mismatch between the three physiologic variables characterizing spontaneous breathing (ventilatory drive, ventilatory requirements, and duration and ratio of inspiratory time to total breath cycle duration) and the three technologic variables characterizing ventilator function (trigger function, gas delivery algorithm, and cycling criteria).

Respiratory Drive–Ventilator Trigger Asynchrony

During partial ventilatory assistance (assisted breath), the inspiratory synchronization system (inspiratory trigger) detects any patient inspiratory effort and activates a mechanical act. Therefore, inspiratory effort is tracked in order to couple the patient's effort with the delivery of pressure, flow, or volume. The goal of a good inspiratory trigger is to reduce as much as possible the duration and intensity of the muscular effort that comes before mechanical support, while avoiding autotrigger effects.[36] *Auto-triggering* can be defined as a mandatory breath not following a patient's inspiratory effort.

It has been suggested that a trigger (independently of its algorithm) must have a response time less than 100 ms. However, the inspiratory

effort necessary to trigger a breath may be a significant part of the total inspiratory effort, representing 17% and 12% of the total inspiratory effort during pressure and flow triggering, respectively.[15-23,34,35] Aslanian and coworkers found that even though the time required for triggering was 43% shorter, and effort during the time of triggering was 62% less with flow triggering than with pressure triggering, effort during the post-triggering phase was equivalent for both pressure and flow triggering.[37] The clinical benefit of flow triggering therefore appears to be much less relevant than commonly stated.[3]

Inspiratory phase asynchrony may be due to problems with inspiratory triggering, and this can be correlated with respiratory drive. Phase lag quantifies the delay between the commencement of inspiratory muscle activity and the beginning of mechanical inflation (Figure 49-2).[3,10,11] The presence of a threshold load, such as dynamic intrinsic PEEP, may further complicate patient-ventilator interaction during the triggering phase.[15] Giuliani et al. suggested that effort during triggering determines patient effort during the remaining portion of inspiration.[38] Leung and coworkers demonstrated that the higher the level of ventilator-applied pressure, the lower the respiratory drive, but the longer the time required to trigger the ventilator. As a result, respiratory muscles generate smaller inspiratory swings in intrathoracic pressure but over a longer inspiratory time.[2] Another problem is related to the fact that pressure is mostly detected inside the ventilator; therefore, any resistive load (e.g., endotracheal tube or upper airways during noninvasive ventilation) reduces the responsiveness of the gas delivered by the ventilator in response to patient effort.[22]

Ineffective triggering is due to the ventilator's inability to detect the patient's "request" for an assisted breath despite substantial inspiratory effort (Figure 49-3). This phenomenon usually occurs with high levels of ventilator assistance and short expiratory times. Mechanical characteristics that may induce ineffective triggering include low elastance, high resistance, and intrinsic PEEP; ineffective triggering is not correlated to an increase in the patient's inspiratory effort.[2] The application of external PEEP below the intrinsic PEEP level can reduce the inspiratory effort required to trigger the ventilator.[39] Parthasarathy and coworkers demonstrated that prolonging mechanical inflation into neural expiration reduces the time available for unopposed exhalation, resulting in the need for a greater inspiratory effort to trigger

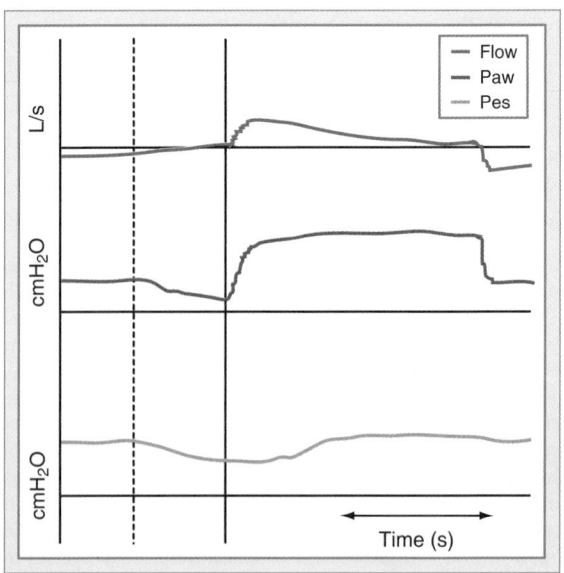

Figure 49-2 Representative tracings show interaction between patient effort and triggering of ventilator. Delay between beginning of inspiratory muscle activity (*dotted line*) and beginning of mechanical inflation (*solid line*) can cause an inspiratory phase asynchrony. Flow, flow generated at airway opening; Paw, pressure applied at airway opening; Pes, esophageal pressure.

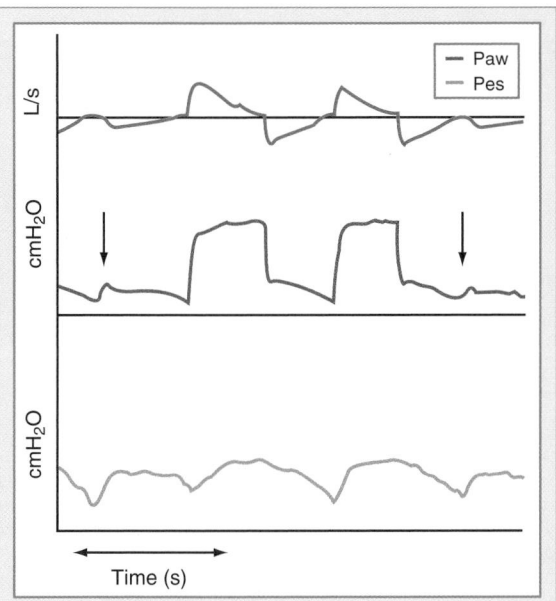

Figure 49-3 Representative tracings show ineffective triggering due to ventilator's inability to detect patient's "request" for an assisted breath. A substantial inspiratory effort *(arrows)* generates only a bump in the flow and pressure tracings instead of a mandatory assisted breath. Flow, flow generated at airway opening; Paw, pressure applied at airway opening; Pes, esophageal pressure.

the ventilator.[40] Younes and colleagues found that ineffective triggering in ventilator-dependent patients exacerbates dynamic hyperinflation.[41]

New trigger algorithms aim at improving patient-ventilator interaction during sudden changes in flow or respiratory rate or in the presence of air leaks during NIV. This can be achieved with volume triggers, triggers linked to flow waveform algorithms, combining pressure and flow signals in the same trigger algorithm, or using both pressure and flow triggers. However, all inspiratory trigger drawbacks may be overcome by using a neural trigger obtained by means of a dedicated nasogastric tube with a multiple array of electrodes placed in the distal esophageal portion.[8,42,43]

Ventilatory Requirement–Gas Delivery Asynchrony

Gas delivery asynchrony occurs when ventilator-delivered flow, volume, and pressure are insufficient to meet the patient's ventilatory demand. Ward and coworkers demonstrated that increasing the flow rate could be used as a means of reducing the patient's respiratory drive and active respiratory muscle work,[17] although doing so may exert an excitatory effect on respiratory rate and on the rate of rise of inspiratory muscle activity.[3,20,21,44-50] Laghi and colleagues demonstrated that the imposed inspiratory time during mechanical ventilation determines respiratory frequency independent of inspiratory flow and tidal volume.[20] Pressure-targeted breaths may better match the patient's ventilatory requirements, because flow is the dependent variable during constant pressure delivery. In addition, rapid pressurization of the airways is coupled with high inspiratory flow only at the beginning of inspiration, thus reproducing the physiologic flow profile.[51] However, during a pressure-targeted breath, the pressure-rise time setting—the time taken to reach the pressure set on the ventilator—may influence patient-ventilator interaction because its modification determines the dependent flow output.[13,14]

Inspiratory Time–Ventilator Cycling Asynchrony

A breath can be pressure-, time-, volume-, or flow-cycled.[14] Ventilator-patient asynchrony occurs when the patient is trying to exhale, but the ventilator is still delivering gas.[37,40,52] In patients ventilated with a time-cycled breath, expiratory phase asynchrony takes place when the patient's neural inspiratory time is shorter or longer than the ventilator inflation time. For proper cycling off the ventilator and optimal patient-ventilator synchrony, the patient's inspiratory flow and ratio of inspiratory time–to–total breath cycle duration must be tracked.

During flow-cycled breaths, inspiratory time is determined exclusively by the time taken for the exponentially declining flow to reach the flow threshold value (when cycling between inspiration and expiration occurs).[34,53] As a consequence, a flow-cycled ventilation mode (e.g., pressure-support ventilation [PSV]) is cycled when inspiratory flow decay reaches a given threshold value. The inspiratory flow threshold value, also called *expiratory trigger*, thus controls the inspiration-to-expiration switch in these modalities.[13,54] The aim is to detect the very end of patient inspiration through inspiratory flow measurement. The goal of these ventilatory modes is to optimize synchronization between spontaneous patient inspiratory time and ventilator inspiratory time. However, for proper cycling off and optimal patient-ventilator synchrony, the ventilator always has to track the patient's inspiratory flow.[40,55,56]

Patient-Ventilator Asynchrony During Pressure-Support Ventilation

Three phases may influence patient-ventilator interaction during PSV: the threshold value of inspiratory flow decay (expiratory trigger), the pressure ramp (pressure slope), and the level of PSV.

(1) The expiratory trigger sensitivity can be fixed (default at 25% of peak flow) or can vary from 5% to 90% or from 5 to 25 L/min (Figure 49-4).[57] It can also be linked to algorithms where there is a ranking logic of expiratory cycling criteria that links cycling to expiration. Setting the expiratory trigger at a higher percentage of peak inspiratory flow (i.e., 50% to 70% of decay of peak inspiratory flow) in patients with obstructive pulmonary disease improves patient-ventilator synchrony and reduces inspiratory muscle effort.[58]

In addition, the modification of cycling-off criteria may have a beneficial effect on reducing the dynamic hyperinflation and inspiratory effort in chronic obstructive pulmonary disease patients, especially at low levels of pressure support.[59]

The proper adjustment of expiratory trigger threshold may be also important in improving patient-ventilator synchrony and in decreasing the work of breathing during acute lung injury. Unlike in obstructive pulmonary disease, setting the lower threshold at 5% of the peak inspiratory flow might be the optimal value for patients with acute respiratory distress syndrome or acute lung injury.[60]

Chiumello et al. found in patients recovering from acute lung injury during PSV at 15 cm H_2O, the lowest cycling-off criteria reduced the respiratory rate and increased the tidal volume without modifying the work of breathing.[61]

The expiratory sensitivity setting is crucial when ventilators are used to deliver NIV, because air leaks may cause an abnormal prolongation of the inspiratory time; during this time, the patient may make efforts to exhale against the machine or to inhale, without receiving any ventilatory support (inspiratory hang-up) (Figure 49-5).[62-66] In addition, leak-compensating capabilities differ markedly between ventilators.[56,67]

(2) The setting of the pressure-rise time (pressure slope) can also affect the expiratory threshold by modifying the dependent inspiratory flow.[61,68-71] Although there is some evidence that rapid pressure-rise times might reduce a patient's work of breathing,[69] a fast pressure increase may lead to particularly high peak inspiratory flow, which may

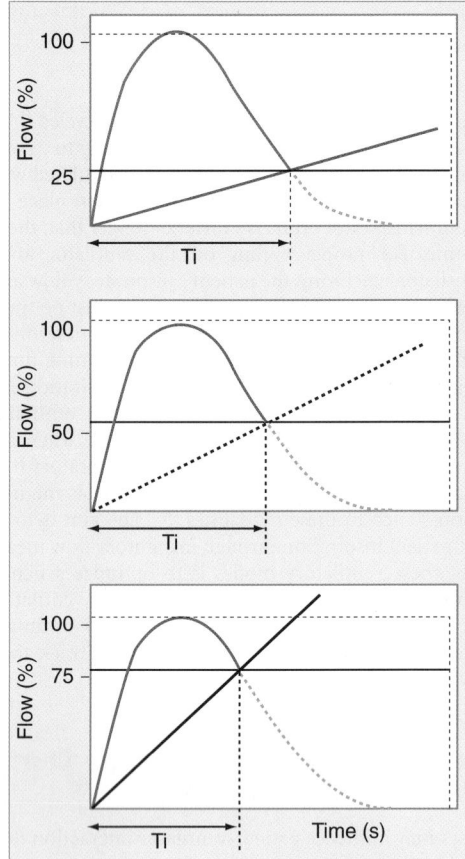

Figure 49-4   Representative tracings show different settings for expiratory trigger sensitivity on a flow-time plot. *Top to bottom,* Expiratory trigger set at 25%, 50%, and 75% of peak flow. Ventilator inspiratory time is influenced by preset flow expiratory trigger sensitivity, at which point the ventilator switches to expiration.

cause premature termination of inspiration when the fixed percentage criterion for expiratory cycling is reached (Figure 49-6).[22,59,71]

Prinianakis et al. assessed the effects of varying the rate of pressure change during noninvasive PSV on the breathing pattern of patients with COPD, as well as inspiratory effort, arterial blood gases, tolerance to ventilation, and amount of air leakage. No significant changes were observed in breathing pattern and arterial blood gases between the differing amounts of pressure change. The pressure-time product of the diaphragm, an estimate of its metabolic consumption, was significantly lower with all rates of pressure change than with spontaneous breathing, but it was significantly lower with the fastest rate. Interestingly, air leak—assessed by the ratio between expired and inspired tidal

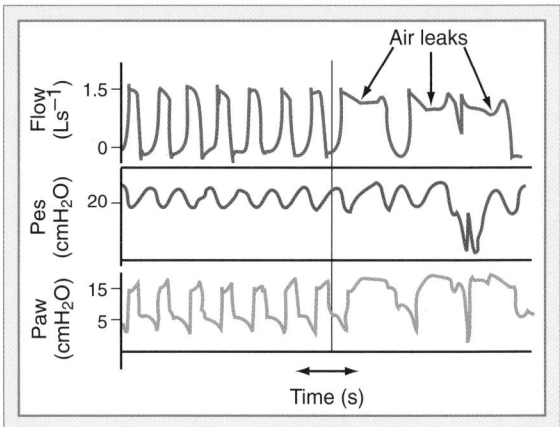

Figure 49-5   Representative record of air leaks during noninvasive face mask pressure-support ventilation. Presence of air leaks causes prolonged ventilator inspiratory time *(arrows)*. Flow, flow generated at airway opening; Paw, pressure applied at airway opening; Pes, esophageal pressure.

volumes—increased, and the patients' tolerance of ventilation, measured using a standardized scale, was significantly poorer with the fastest rate of pressure change.[72] In invasively ventilated patients recovering from acute lung injury, Chiumello et al. found that the shortest inspiratory rise time reduced the work of breathing.[61]

(3) The pressure-support level also determines the dependent flow output. During NIV, patient-ventilator asynchrony is a common occurrence, mainly owing to air leaks.[9,63] Because air leaks may determine modification in flow output, reducing PSV level even by 1 or 2 cm H_2O may reduce air leaks, thus improving patient-ventilator asynchrony.[9]

In conclusion, modifications of inspiratory rise time and cycling-off criteria must be carefully adjusted during PSV, as well as the level of PSV. Dyssynchrony at the termination of a PSV breath can be corrected by varying the cycling-off criteria (e.g., the expiratory trigger threshold) or modulating inspiratory flow (e.g., modifying the pressure slope or varying the set pressure level).[9] Automated modes designed to achieve an optimal expiratory cycling during PSV may deserve further investigation.[73-74]

Total Patient-Controlled Mechanical Support

Optimization of patient-ventilator interactions can be obtained only by continuous matching between the triggering, flow delivery, and cycling functions of the ventilator and the patient's ventilatory drive, spontaneous inspiratory flow demand, and ratio of inspiratory time to

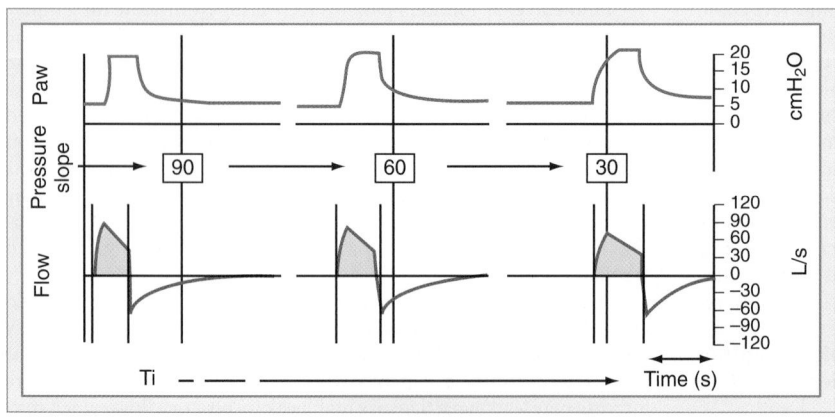

Figure 49-6   Representative tracings show different pressure-rise time sensitivities on a flow-time plot. *Left to right,* Pressure-rise time set at 90%, 60%, and 30% of maximal pressurization time. Ventilator inspiratory time *(shaded area)* is influenced by preset pressure-slope sensitivity that generates a different peak inspiratory flow. Paw, pressure applied at airway opening; Flow, flow generated at airway opening.

total breath cycle. This implies continuous measurement of physiologic variables and continuous adaptation of the ventilator to the spontaneous variations in these variables. Future development in ventilator technology should be oriented toward systems with the capability to automatically interface between physiologic parameters and ventilator output. Such technology will be based on closed-loop algorithms able to achieve total patient-controlled mechanical support.[4]

The design features of an automatic control system in a mechanical ventilator include (1) what activates the system (the input), (2) what the system produces (the output), and (3) the protocol used to link input and output (the controlling algorithm). In a closed-loop system, the output will activate and condition the input. When changes in output are opposite to changes in input, the closed loop is said to be negative. The closed loop is positive when variations in output mirror variations in input. The most common example of a negative closed-loop control system in the clinical setting is the ventilator humidifier. In this case, the input is the temperature inside the chamber, and the output is the temperature of the gas being delivered to the patient. The controlling algorithm is designed to keep the latter constantly above a value set by the operator. If the output (i.e., the temperature of gas delivered to the patient) is lower than the preset level, the algorithm will increase the input (i.e., the temperature in the chamber); if the output is higher than the preset level, the algorithm will decrease the input. Closed-loop systems are hence able to stabilize and limit the performance of a mechanical system.

In the case of acute respiratory failure, the patient is unable to provide sufficient output (i.e., minute ventilation). The ventilator should therefore be able to detect the input from the patient and continuously adapt the output. If the input is increasing (i.e., ventilatory requirements are increasing), the ventilator will increase the output (i.e., apply more positive pressure); if the input is decreasing (i.e., ventilatory requirements are decreasing), the ventilator will decrease the output (i.e., apply less positive pressure). The controlling closed loop eventually applied by the ventilator must therefore be positive. Positive closed-loop control systems are inherently unstable in the sense that they tend to (1) "run away" with ventilatory assistance—if the pressure generated by the ventilator is higher than the pressure required to offset the passive properties of the respiratory system, the ventilator will continue to deliver flow and volume while the patient stops his or her inspiratory effort and tries to initiate expiration; and (2) "extinguish" ventilatory assistance—if the patient does not produce any inspiratory effort, the ventilator will not produce any ventilatory support.

Based on closed-loop algorithms, new modes of mechanical ventilation have been proposed. Such approaches represent modifications of PSV and are characterized by the patient's ability to control the amount of assistance provided by the ventilator. They are differentiated by the patient-related variable used to close the loop.

Proportional Assisted Ventilation (PAV), Proportional Pressure Support (PPS), and Proportional Assisted Ventilation Plus (PAV+)

During proportional assisted ventilation (PAV) and proportional pressure support (PPS), the ventilator generates pressure in proportion to patient-generated flow and volume[75,76]; the ventilator amplifies patient effort without imposing any ventilatory or pressure targets. Ventilator-generated pressure rises as long as inspiratory muscle effort is produced by the patient. During PAV or PPS, the preset parameter is therefore not a pressure target. During these modes of mechanical support, the clinician adjusts the percentage of flow-assisted or volume-assisted ventilation after determining the patient's resistance and elastance. In other words, the physician must determine how much to reduce the load imposed by the patient's elastance[77] and resistance.[78,79]

Despite the exciting potential of these techniques,[79-82] applied either invasively or noninvasively,[73-89] no large-scale studies have demonstrated an improvement in patient outcome compared with other modes of ventilation. PAV+ provides continuous measurement of the value of elastance and resistance of the patients according to the method described by Younes and coworkers.[77-79,89,90] This option requires that the physician sets only a given percentage level of gain. During invasive ventilation, PAV+ seems to considerably reduce the incidence of patient-ventilator asynchronies compared to proportional ventilation with the manual adjustment of the percentage of flow-assisted or volume-assisted ventilation according to patient's respiratory mechanics[90] (Figure 49-7). As compared to PSV, PAV+ also was able to reduce the time for ventilatory settings and changes in sedative doses.[91]

Neural-Adjusted Ventilatory Assistance

With neural-adjusted ventilatory assistance (NAVA), electrical activity of the diaphragm is measured by means of an electrode array inserted into a nasogastric tube and placed in the lower esophagus; this information is then used to control the ventilator to generate flow, volume, and pressure.[8,42,43,92] Unlike with the proportional mode described earlier, estimates of respiratory mechanics are not needed; with NAVA, the patient's respiratory center controls the assisted positive breaths in all phases of the ventilation cycle, from triggering to cycling off of

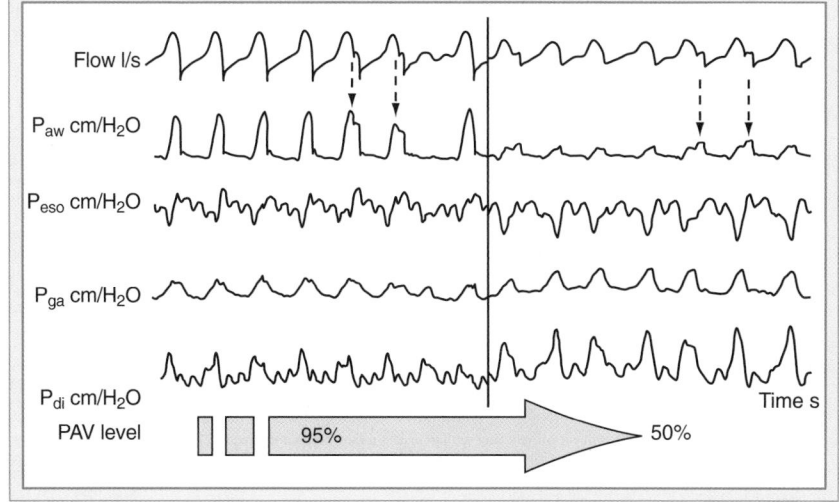

Figure 49-7 Representative tracing of flow (Flow), airway pressure (P$_{aw}$), esophageal pressure (P$_{eso}$), gastric pressure (P$_{ga}$) and transdiaphragmatic pressure (P$_{di}$) during PAV+ ventilation. Directional arrow *(bottom)* going from left to right shows the gain is reduced from 95% to 50% with subsequently increased inspiratory effort. Dotted arrows *(top)* indicate the measurement of respiratory mechanics automatically computed by the ventilator.

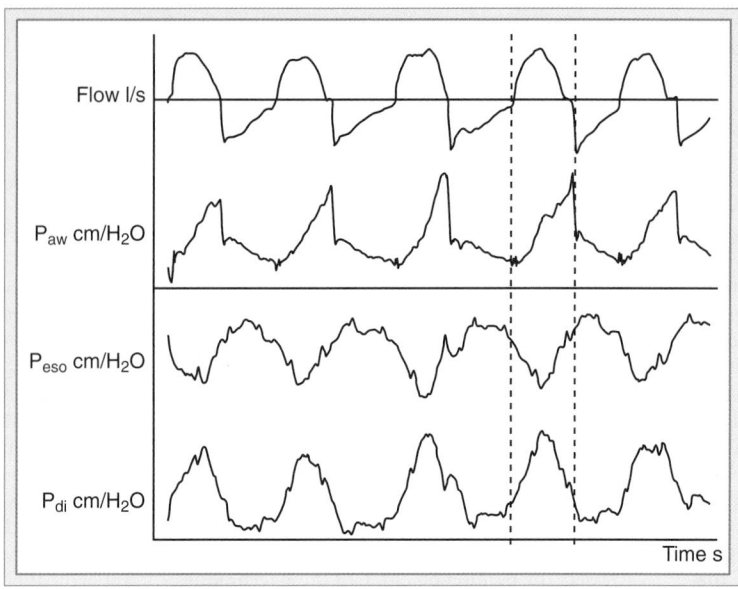

Flow l/s

P_{aw} cm/H_2O

P_{eso} cm/H_2O

P_{di} cm/H_2O

Time s

Figure 49-8 Representative tracing of flow (Flow), airway pressure (P_{aw}), esophageal pressure (P_{eso}), and transdiaphragmatic pressure (P_{di}) during NAVA ventilation. The two dotted lines define the beginning and end of patient's inspiratory effort.

inspiration. Any change in patient ventilatory output is matched breath by breath by the ventilator, even in the presence of variations in respiratory mechanics. A NAVA level equal to 1 corresponds to a support of 1 cm H_2O for 1 µV of electrical diaphragm activity (EAdi). A representative tracing of NAVA is shown in Figure 49-8.

Adaptive-Support Ventilation

Adaptive-support ventilation is an assist time–limited, pressure-targeted mode of ventilation (pressure-controlled ventilation) that relies on a negative closed-loop system of regulating ventilator settings in response to changes in both respiratory impedance (elastance and resistance) and the patient's spontaneous efforts.[93] The basic principle relies on the work of Otis and coworkers[94] and Mead,[6] demonstrating that for a given level of minute alveolar ventilation, there is a respiratory rate that is least costly in terms of respiratory work. With adaptive support ventilation, the operator enters the patient's body weight and sets the desired percentage of minute ventilation. The expiratory time constant is determined by analysis of the expiratory flow-volume curve,[95] adjusting inspiratory pressure, inspiratory-expiratory time ratio, and respiratory rate to obtain the prescribed minute ventilation. Adaptive support ventilation thus adjusts inspiratory pressure, inspiratory-expiratory time ratio, and mandatory respiratory rate to maintain the target minute ventilation and respiratory rate within a framework designed to avoid both rapid, shallow breathing and excessive inflation volumes. Spontaneous breathing triggers either a pressure-controlled or a spontaneous breath with inspiratory pressure support, the level of which is adjusted to meet the target respiratory rate–tidal volume combination.

KEY POINTS

1. Patient-ventilator asynchrony is common during mechanical ventilatory support. It is often unrecognized, underestimated, and inappropriately treated in the clinical setting.

2. Patient-ventilator asynchrony takes place when the three physiologic variables of the patient's breathing pattern—ventilatory drive, ventilatory requirements, and duration and ratio of inspiratory time to total breath cycle duration—do not match ventilator trigger, ventilator-delivered flow, and ventilator cycling criteria.

3. Clinical optimization of patient-ventilator interactions can be obtained only by continuously matching the triggering, flow delivering, and cycling functions of the ventilator with the patient's physiologic variables.

4. Optimization of patient-ventilator interactions during invasive or noninvasive ventilation implies continuous measurement of physiologic variables and continuous adaptation of the ventilator to the spontaneous variations in these physiologic variables.

5. Future developments in ventilator technology should be oriented toward a system with the capability to automatically interface between physiologic parameters and ventilator outputs. Such technology will be based on closed-loop algorithms able to achieve total patient-controlled mechanical support.

ANNOTATED REFERENCES

Appendini L, Purro A, Gudjonsdottir M, et al. Physiologic response of ventilator-dependent patients with chronic obstructive pulmonary disease to proportional assist ventilation and continuous positive airway pressure. Am J Respir Crit Care Med 1999;159(5):1510-7.
This study found that in difficult-to-wean patients with chronic obstructive pulmonary disease, proportional assisted ventilation (PAV) improves ventilation and decreases inspiratory muscle effort. It also found that the combination of PAV and continuous positive airway pressure can unload the inspiratory muscles to values close to those in normal subjects.

Beck J, Sinderby C, Lindström L. Effects of lung volume on diaphragm EMG signal strength during voluntary contractions. J Appl Physiol 1998;85(3):1123-34.
These authors found that variations in end-expiratory lung volume between breaths can affect the transformation of respiratory muscle activation into mechanical output (neuromechanical coupling).

Calderini E, Confalonieri M, Puccio PG, et al. Patient-ventilator asynchrony during noninvasive ventilation: the role of the expiratory trigger. Intensive Care Med 1999;25(7):662-7.
This article describes the loose patient-ventilator synchrony in the presence of air leaks and noninvasive pressure-support ventilation.

Laghi F, Karamchandani K, Tobin MJ. Influence of ventilator settings in determining respiratory frequency during mechanical ventilation. Am J Respir Crit Care Med 1999;160(5):1766-70.
These authors found that during assist-control mode, ventilator inspiratory time can determine respiratory frequency independently of inspiratory flow and tidal volume.

Leung P, Jubran A, Tobin MJ. Comparison of assisted ventilator modes on triggering, patients' effort, and dyspnea. Am J Respir Crit Care Med 1997;155(6):1940-8.
This study found that when receiving assist-control ventilation or high levels of pressure support, one-quarter to one-third of a patient's inspiratory efforts may fail to open the inspiratory valve triggering the machine. The number of ineffective triggering attempts increases in proportion to the level of ventilatory assistance and is not correlated to the magnitude of inspiratory effort at a given level of assistance.

Parthasarathy S, Jubran A, Tobin MJ. Cycling of inspiratory and expiratory muscle groups with the ventilator in airflow limitation. Am J Respir Crit Care Med 1998;158(5):1471-8.
These authors found that the continuation of a mechanical mandatory breath into neural expiration is associated with a waste of inspiratory effort, defined as failure of the subsequent inspiratory attempt to trigger the ventilator.

Parthasarathy S, Tobin JM. Effect of ventilator mode on sleep quality in critically ill patients. Am J Respir Crit Care Med 2002;166(11):1423-9.
These authors found that inspiratory assistance during pressure support causes hypocapnia, which combined with lack of a backup rate and wakefulness drive can lead to central apneas and sleep fragmentation, especially in patients with heart failure. A backup rate, as during assist-control volume-targeted ventilation, prevents the development of apneas and perhaps decreases arousals.

Sinderby C, Navalesi P, Beck J, et al. Neural control of mechanical ventilation in respiratory failure. Nat Med 1999;5(12):1433-6.

This article describes a completely new mode of detecting inspiratory effort, based on the measurement of electrical activity of the diaphragm by means of an electrode array inserted into a nasogastric tube and placed in the lower esophagus. Output generated from the electrodes, filtered out for, is used to control the ventilator that finally generates the respiratory output.

Tobert DG, Simon PM, Stroetz RW, Hubmayr RD. The determinants of respiratory rate during mechanical ventilation. Am J Respir Crit Care Med 1997;155(2):485-92.

The authors examined the rate response of eight normal volunteers during both quiet wakefulness and non-rapid-eye-movement (non-REM) sleep in the setting of mechanical ventilation through a nasal mask in an assist-control mode with a machine backup rate of 2 breaths per minute. They found that both tidal volume and inspiratory flow settings affect the respiratory rate and can affect carbon dioxide homeostasis. During non-REM sleep, hypocapnia resulted in wasted ventilator trigger efforts. Thus, ventilator settings appropriate for wakefulness may cause ventilatory instability during sleep.

Younes M, Webster K, Kun J, et al. A method for measuring passive elastance during proportional assist ventilation. Am J Respir Crit Care Med 2001;164(1):50-60.

A noninvasive method to continuously measure elastance of the respiratory system during proportional assisted ventilation is described.

REFERENCES

Access the complete reference list online at http://www.expertconsult.com.

50 Weaning from Mechanical Ventilation

BELÉN CABELLO | FERRAN ROCHE-CAMPO | JORDI MANCEBO

The Concept of Liberation and Extubation

Weaning from mechanical ventilation represents the period of transition from total ventilatory support to spontaneous breathing. About 70% of intubated mechanically ventilated patients are extubated on the first spontaneous breathing trial (SBT) attempt, whether by disconnection from the ventilator or after breathing at low levels of pressure support for short periods of time, such as 30 to 120 minutes.[1,2] This pattern has recently been categorized as "simple weaning," and the prognosis for such patients is good. The remaining patients, about 30%, need progressive withdrawal from artificial ventilatory support. These patients can be classified either as "difficult weaning" when they require up to three SBTs to achieve successful weaning, or "prolonged weaning" if they fail at least three weaning attempts or require more than 7 days of ventilatory support from the first SBT. The mortality rate for patients not simple/easy to wean is approximately 25%.[3]

Early liberation from mechanical ventilation and removal of the endotracheal tube is clinically important. Unnecessary prolongation of mechanical ventilation increases the risks of complications including infections (particularly of bronchopulmonary origin), barotrauma, cardiovascular compromise, tracheal injuries, and muscle deconditioning. To optimize patient outcomes, clinicians should hasten the process that ultimately leads to removal of the endotracheal tube.[4]

Liberation and extubation are different issues.[5] *Liberation* refers to weaning from mechanical ventilation and means that a patient no longer requires ventilatory support. When this step is achieved, the clinician has to consider a different question: Is the patient able to breathe spontaneously without the endotracheal tube? Removal of the endotracheal tube is referred to as *extubation*. In terms of magnitude, the extubation failure rate—that is, the need to replace the endotracheal tube and reinstitute mechanical ventilation—is variable and ranges from 5% to 20% of extubated patients.[1,6-8]

Mechanisms Explaining Liberation Failure

RESPIRATORY PUMP FAILURE

The most common reason for weaning failure is respiratory pump insufficiency due to an imbalance between the patient's capabilities and respiratory demands.[9-11] During spontaneous breathing, the inspiratory muscles must generate sufficient force to overcome the elastance of the lungs and chest wall (lung and chest wall elastic loads) as well as the airway and tissue resistances (resistive load). This requires signal generation in the respiratory centers of the brainstem, anatomic and functional integrity of nerves that conduct the signal, unimpaired neuromuscular transmission, and adequate muscle strength (the aggregate term is *neuromuscular competence*). The ability of the respiratory muscles to sustain these loads without fatiguing is called *endurance* and is determined by the balance between energy supply and energy demand.

Jubran and Tobin[12] investigated the progression of respiratory mechanics during SBT in patients with chronic obstructive pulmonary disease (COPD). At the very beginning of the trials, patients who subsequently failed had a slightly higher airway resistance, respiratory system elastance, and intrinsic positive end-expiratory pressure (PEEP) compared to those who succeeded. However, during the course of the trials, respiratory mechanics progressively worsened in patients who

failed to be liberated from the ventilator. Subjects who failed developed rapid, shallow breathing, and most developed an increase in Paco₂. Together these abnormalities resulted in increased inspiratory muscle effort which, in some patients, was probably close to the threshold of muscle fatigue.

The issue of fatigue has been revisited by Laghi et al.[13] The authors studied 19 intubated patients during weaning from mechanical ventilation. Eleven patients failed and eight succeeded. Several physiologic indices were measured before and 30 minutes after SBT. The transdiaphragmatic twitch pressure, elicited by magnetic bilateral phrenic stimulation, did not differ before the SBT between the patients that failed or succeeded at ventilator liberation, and this variable did not decrease after the trial in either group. A fall in transdiaphragmatic twitch pressure is a physiologic index of low-frequency fatigue. Patients failing the SBT were reconnected to the ventilator because of clinical signs of intolerance. These alterations, together with the reinstitution of mechanical ventilation, are mechanisms that might defend against the development of low-frequency fatigue. It was concluded that weaning failure was not accompanied by low-frequency diaphragmatic fatigue, although weaning-failure patients exhibited severe diaphragmatic weakness, since twitch pressures were always low.

COMMON DISORDERS THAT ALTER THE BALANCE OF CAPACITY AND LOAD IN CRITICAL ILLNESS

Reduced Neuromuscular Capacity

Reduced output of the respiratory control centers may occur following administration of sedatives, narcotics, and anesthetic agents. Phrenic nerve dysfunction can occur after traumatic injuries (e.g., high cervical spine lesions) and is also common after cardiac surgery.[14] Diaphragmatic dysfunction may occur following upper abdominal surgery,[15] and an elegant study has shown atrophy of diaphragm fibers after only 18 hours of mechanical ventilation and complete diaphragmatic inactivity.[16] Critical illness polyneuropathy and myopathy, which are frequent complications of sepsis and multiple organ system failure, may also impede weaning.[17,18] Finally, neuromuscular blocking agents (with or without concomitant corticosteroids) and aminoglycosides may contribute to weaning failure.[19-24] In addition, malnutrition and deconditioning due to prolonged bed rest/mechanical ventilation can induce severe muscle dysfunction.[25]

In a multicenter study by De Jonghe et al., a high incidence of intensive care unit (ICU)-acquired neuromuscular dysfunction was reported in patients without preexisting neuromuscular disorders who underwent mechanical ventilation for at least 7 days.[18] In this group of 95 patients, 25% were diagnosed with acquired paresis. The duration of mechanical ventilation after the removal of sedation was significantly longer in patients with paresis compared to those who without paresis (18 vs. 8 days; P = 0.03). In this investigation, the independent predictors of ICU-acquired paresis were female sex, number of days with dysfunction of two or more organs, duration of mechanical ventilation before awakening, and administration of corticosteroids. The same group also found that respiratory muscle weakness was associated with delayed extubation.[26]

Increased Muscle Loads

Increased work of breathing results from increased mechanical loads (elastic and/or resistive) and processes that require higher minute ventilation. Increased ventilatory requirements are common in critically ill patients, particularly during periods of hyperthermia, overfeeding, and hyperventilation (related to anxiety and/or pain). An increase in the dead space/tidal volume ratio is another source of increased ventilatory need.

Increased elastic workloads occur when lung and/or chest wall compliance is reduced (e.g., pulmonary edema, extreme hyperinflation during an acute asthmatic attack, pulmonary fibrosis, abdominal distension, obesity, trauma, or thoracic deformities).[13] The presence of intrinsic PEEP is another example of increased elastic workload and is a relatively common phenomenon, especially in patients with COPD.[27,28] Dynamic pulmonary hyperinflation, apart from generating an elastic threshold load, places the diaphragm at a mechanically disadvantageous position in which its capacity to generate pressure decreases.

Resistive work of breathing during critical illness may increase because of bronchospasm, excessive secretions, endotracheal tube resistance (which augments with kinking and deposition of secretions), and ventilator valves/circuits and humidifiers, especially when conditioning of inspired gases is provided with heat and moisture exchangers. The latter also increase the instrumental dead space.

Cardiovascular Dysfunction

The presence of cardiovascular dysfunction can contribute to weaning failure by augmenting loads on the respiratory system and by reducing neuromuscular capacity.[29,30] A study by Epstein[31] showed that as many as one third of weaning failures resulted solely or in part from congestive heart failure (CHF), although other studies found that fewer episodes of weaning failure (14%) were due to cardiovascular reasons.[32] Cardiovascular dysfunction may result from physiologic changes that occur during the resumption of spontaneous unassisted breathing.[33] When spontaneous breathing resumes, intrathoracic pressure swings during inspiration are negative, a situation that results in increased left ventricular preload and afterload. A significant decrease in left ventricular ejection fraction has been described during spontaneous breathing trials in COPD patients without coronary artery disease.[34]

Increased myocardial loading may be sufficient, especially when coupled with left ventricular noncompliance, to precipitate CHF (which stiffens the lungs and further increases respiratory muscle load). Moreover, increased heart loads augment myocardial oxygen demand and may precipitate myocardial ischemia in patients with coronary artery disease.[35] Myocardial ischemia causes left ventricular dysfunction that may induce acute pulmonary edema and arterial hypoxemia.

Jubran et al.[36] examined hemodynamics and mixed venous saturations in patients during weaning trials. Successfully weaned patients demonstrated increases in cardiac index and oxygen transport compared to values during mechanical ventilation. Patients who failed weaning did not increase oxygen delivery to the tissues owing in part to elevated right- and left-ventricular afterloads. Consequently, these abnormalities can jeopardize respiratory muscle function.

In ICU patients, CHF may be diagnosed for the first time or worsen in patients with this condition as a consequence of increase in venous return, volume overload, or catecholamine release induced by physiologic stress, such as weaning.[33,37,38] These factors have negative effects on cardiac function, and together with hypoxemia can result in the development of acute pulmonary edema.[33,36,37] Impairment of cardiovascular function can be magnified in the setting of positive fluid balance.[39,40]

It has been recently shown that performing an SBT in difficult-to-wean patients with a T-tube (instead of pressure support and PEEP) elicits a totally different cardiovascular response and, as expected, as long as support is added (in the form of pressure support and PEEP) the respiratory and cardiovascular function both improve.[41]

In the ICU there are new noninvasive tools available that help physicians make the diagnosis of cardiovascular dysfunction, such as echocardiography and measurement of plasma B-type natriuretic peptide (BNP).One study found that patients exhibiting weaning failure had higher BNP values than patients who were successfully weaned.

Patients who failed weaning were treated with diuretics, and this was accompanied by successful extubation and a decrease in BNP levels.[42] Another study compared the use of echocardiography in diagnosing pulmonary edema induced by weaning. The authors showed that an increase in the value of the pulmonary artery occlusion pressure (PAOP) was correlated with echocardiographic signs of increase in left-ventricular filling pressures.[43]

Mechanisms Explaining Extubation Failure

Extubation failure can be defined as reinstitution of ventilatory assistance within 24 to 48 hours of extubation. Consequently, the extubation failure rate is the number of patients requiring reinstitution of mechanical ventilation divided by the total number of extubated patients.

The reintubation rate may differ according to the etiology of respiratory failure. For instance, in a study that included 217 medical and surgical patients, Vallverdú et al.[8] noted that the overall reintubation rate was 15% and ranged from 36% (15 of 42) in neurologic patients to 0% (zero of 13) in COPD patients. The reintubation rate in patients who had acute respiratory failure of other etiologies was 9% (8 of 93). Data by Esteban et al.[6,44] indicate that the reintubation rate is about 13% to 19%.

Mechanisms explaining extubation failure include impending abnormalities not diagnosed at the time extubation is performed (e.g., pneumonia, ongoing cardiac failure) and the inability to keep the tracheobronchial tree free of copious secretions.[8,45] Intubation can result in laryngotracheal injury, which tends to occur more frequently with increasing duration of intubation and in women, which could explain some episodes of extubation failure.[46]

Extubation failure results in a marked increase in the duration of mechanical ventilation, ICU and hospital stay, need for tracheostomy, and hospital mortality.[6,8,44,47-49] The etiology of extubation failure also influences outcome. Interestingly, patients requiring reintubation because of respiratory failure had a mortality rate of 30%, whereas mortality in patients needing reintubation because of upper airway obstruction was only 7%.[49,50] In one study,[42] the time to reintubation was found to be an independent predictor of outcome.

Indices to Predict Weaning Outcome

Many indices have been proposed in an attempt to predict weaning outcome and have used assessment of: (1) simple ventilatory parameters, (2) oxygenation, (3) respiratory muscle strength, (4) central respiratory drive, (5) respiratory muscle reserve, (6) work of breathing, (7) different variables of respiratory function, and (8) the pattern of spontaneous breathing in terms of tidal volume (V_T) and respiratory rate (f) or f/V_T.

Yang and Tobin[51] studied the predictive power of several weaning indices and showed that the rapid, shallow breathing index (f/V_T) had the best predictive value. In their study, 95% of patients with a ratio f/V_T greater than 105 failed during a test of spontaneous breathing. In general, except for f/V_T, these indices exhibit relatively poor positive and negative predictive values. In addition, the performance of these indices is affected by a number of factors, such as selection bias, outcome misclassification, and confounding variables.[52]

The rapid, shallow breathing index appears to be the most useful bedside method for screening a patient for readiness for liberation. If the value is less than 105, 30 to 120 minutes of an SBT should be used as confirmation of the patient's capability of breathing spontaneously without assistance. Screening tests are typically performed when the pretest probability of a condition is low. High-sensitivity tests (as is the case with f/V_T) are very useful for screening: weaning success is high among patients in whom the test is positive (f/V_T <105) and low among those in whom the test is negative (f/V_T >105). However, since f/V_T has low specificity (a relatively large proportion of weaning-failure subjects in whom the test is positive), the f/Vᴛ alone is insufficient to predict weaning failure. For this reason, clinicians utilize additional testing (i.e., 30-120 minutes of SBT).[53] From a practical point of view, the information conveyed by weaning indices and clinical judgment should be considered together in making clinically important decisions about extubation.[43]

Indices to Predict Extubation Failure

The frequency of reintubation and the adverse impact it has on survival indicate that accurate prediction of extubation outcome is important. Most clinicians assess patient readiness for both liberation and extubation by conducting an SBT of variable duration. The crucial importance of performing an SBT before deciding on extubation has been highlighted by Zeggwagh et al.[54] These authors proceeded directly to extubation (without performing an SBT) after medical ICU patients had demonstrated clinical improvement. Of the 119 episodes of extubation, 44 (37%) subsequently required reintubation. This rate is much higher than that reported for patients who were extubated after passing an SBT.

Patients incapable of protecting their airway and clearing secretions with an effective cough are at increased risk for extubation failure. Traditional assessment has consisted in demonstrating a cough reflex when the airways are stimulated with a suction catheter and by the absence of excessive secretions, but these criteria have not been standardized. In mechanically ventilated subjects, a "sawtooth" pattern on the flow-volume curve indicates the presence of excess airway secretions but does not provide quantitative information.[55]

Although tolerance of an SBT up to 120 minutes is a good predictor of successful extubation, Vallverdú et al.[8] noted that a high percentage (36%) of neurologic patients who successfully passed a 2-hour SBT and were extubated needed subsequent reintubation. Coplin et al.[56] have studied extubation in brain-injured patients. Their data provide no justification for delaying extubation in patients whose only indication for prolonged intubation is a depressed level of consciousness. This study found that timely extubation of patients who met standard weaning criteria appeared to be safe, with no increased risk of reintubation or subsequent tracheotomy, potentially beneficial (associated with a lower incidence of pneumonia), and less expensive (shorter ICU and hospital cost). In that study, the reintubation rate was 18% (24 of 136 patients). Only two components of a semiquantitative assessment of need for airway care were associated with successful extubation: spontaneous cough ($P = 0.01$) and suctioning frequency ($P = 0.001$).

Smina et al.[57] studied a group of 95 patients admitted to a medical ICU who passed an SBT and were ready to be extubated. They found that patients with peak expiratory flows equal to or below 60 L/min were five times as likely to have an unsuccessful extubation as patients with expiratory flows greater than 60 L/min. These data emphasize the notion that patients incapable of protecting the airways and clearing secretions are at increased risk for unsuccessful extubation.

Progressive Withdrawal of Mechanical Ventilation

Weaning from mechanical ventilation represents the period of transition from total ventilatory support to spontaneous breathing. The most common techniques used to withdraw mechanical ventilation in patients who failed an initial weaning trial are pressure-support ventilation (PSV) and breathing through a T-piece. Two prospective multicenter randomized clinical trials have shown that the use of synchronized intermittent mandatory ventilation (SIMV) is less efficacious than the other techniques.[1,2]

ROLE OF PROTOCOLS

Various studies have shown that weaning protocols administered by nursing and respiratory care staff can shorten the duration of

mechanical ventilation.[7,58-60] The methodological approach is nearly always the same and primarily consists of daily checking of the patient's ability to breathe spontaneously. This simple approach is associated with faster extubation and a shorter ICU stay, without any increase in the reintubation rate.

An important study revealed that abrupt daily interruption of sedation significantly reduced the duration of mechanical ventilation.[61] More recently, a no-sedation strategy has shown better results than daily interruption of sedation.[62] However, because this was a single-center study with several limitations, the findings must be confirmed before this strategy becomes more generalized. Because sedation and weaning from mechanical ventilation cannot be separated from one another, when these two strategies are combined (i.e., daily interruption of sedation and systematic use of SBTs to hasten liberation from the ventilator), the results are better than if the two strategies are used separately.[63]

The impact of protocols in hastening the weaning process has been questioned. In a prospective controlled trial, Krishnan et al.[64] compared protocol-based weaning to usual physician-directed weaning in a closed medical ICU with high physician staffing levels and structured system-based rounds. The authors could not document any improvement in clinical outcomes with protocols. These results have stimulated debate regarding the use of protocols and especially about what is understood by control groups and usual care.[65]

PRESSURE-SUPPORT VENTILATION

Pressure-support ventilation allows patients to retain relative control over respiratory rate and timing, inspiratory flow rate, and tidal volume. During weaning, the PSV levels are decreased according to the patient's clinical tolerance, usually by steps of 2 to 4 cm H_2O at least twice a day. In general, clinical tolerance to a level of PSV of about 8 cm H_2O without PEEP is required before performing extubation, although this level may vary according to a given patient's overall clinical status.

Clinical experience[1,2] and data coming from clinical trials[66,67] suggest that "optimal" initial levels for PSV are those that provide respiratory rates between 25 and 30 breaths/min. In this scenario it is particularly important to rule out the existence of asynchronous breathing or ineffective respiratory effort, respiratory events that are especially prevalent in COPD patients. Ineffective effort occurs when the patient initiates inspiration that does not trigger the ventilator. A study[68] has shown that high pressure-support levels, large tidal volumes, and increase in serum bicarbonate level with alkalosis were associated with ineffective triggering. Therefore, a ventilator setting with a high level of pressure support can be the cause of patient-ventilator asynchrony. The patients who showed ineffective triggering exhibited a longer time on mechanical ventilation, and tracheostomy was more frequent in these patients. The same group of authors performed a second study[69] in difficult-to-wean patients who exhibited ineffective efforts while being ventilated with PSV. The study found a decrease in the number of ineffective efforts—without changes in the work of breathing and without modifications in the respiratory rate—when pressure support levels were reduced. These studies[68,69] show that some patients are receiving excessive levels of mechanical ventilation during the weaning process. This situation can result in delaying the moment of performing an SBT if the patient is unnecessarily ventilated with a high level of pressure support.

The level of external PEEP used in patients with clinically suspected dynamic hyperinflation and dynamic airway collapse should be adjusted with great caution, since measurement of dynamic intrinsic PEEP in spontaneously breathing patients is not easily performed. To that end, it has been suggested that external PEEP can be titrated according to the changes in airway occlusion pressure.[70]

SPONTANEOUS BREATHING WITH T-TUBE

Tolerance to breathing through a T-tube represents a good test to evaluate patients' capacity to maintain autonomous spontaneous breathing.[71] The optimal duration of a T-tube trial is at least 30 minutes and no more than 120 minutes.

The main disadvantage of the T-piece trial is related to the absence of a connection to a mechanical ventilator. Since the patients are not monitored by the alarms on the ventilator, they need to be closely supervised, and this is highly demanding for the nursing staff. Additionally, the transition between periods of muscular rest and periods of spontaneous unassisted breathing with a T-tube can be excessively abrupt for some patients, especially for those who have panic reactions after disconnecting from the ventilator and those with latent left-ventricular failure and myocardial ischemia.

NONINVASIVE VENTILATION

We must distinguish three scenarios:

1. When noninvasive ventilation (NIV) is used as a substitute for invasive ventilation in patients with chronic respiratory failure who do not meet extubation criteria. This situation is found in patients with chronic respiratory failure who present with difficult weaning and high risk for a tracheotomy. In studies examining the use of NIV in this setting, in the control group, patients were extubated only after having passed the weaning test, while patients in the intervention group were extubated despite having failed the test but were immediately given intensive NIV. Of the three published studies, two showed a higher percentage of successful weaning with lower mortality rates in the NIV group,[72,73] while one found no differences.[74]

2. Preventive NIV in patients at high risk of reintubation. In this situation, the weaning test is passed, and all criteria for extubation are present. The endotracheal tube is then removed, but the patient is considered an a priori high-risk candidate for reintubation. Examples of such patients include those who present hypercapnia at the end of the weaning test, patients older than 65 years with a history of heart problems, and patients whose weaning was difficult. Of the three studies that have been carried out, one showed a reduction in the reintubation rate when NIV was used post extubation,[75] while the other showed, in addition to the reduced reintubation, a decrease in the mortality rate.[76]

3. NIV for "de novo" respiratory failure after extubation. A Canadian study examined the use of NIV for respiratory failure after extubation but found no difference, either in terms of reintubation or mortality.[77] In 2004, a study was published questioning the use of NIV for de novo postextubation respiratory failure.[78] The patients were randomized to receive treatment with oxygen and usual care versus NIV treatment and intubation if needed. Although the rate of reintubation was similar to the Canadian study, the group treated initially with NIV had a higher mortality rate. The authors concluded that NIV could delay reintubation in certain patients, leading to a worse outcome. However, the data from this study are difficult to interpret, since a subgroup of patients who failed usual treatment were given an NIV trial before intubation. These individuals fared much better than those who received NIV from study entry. These results have put an end to the indiscriminate use of NIV, so that NIV is only recommended in specific populations, including those with chronic respiratory problems[79] and postoperative patients.[80,81]

NEW MODALITIES

Several novel weaning modalities have been examined, including those using closed-loop PSV[82,83] providing continuous adaptation of ventilator assistance to patients' needs 24 hours a day.[84] A recent study examined this modality in two groups of patients during the weaning period.[85] In the "usual weaning group," weaning was performed as usual based on written weaning guidelines. In the "study group," weaning was carried out using a computer-driven weaning protocol. Weaning time was reduced in the study group in comparison to the usual weaning group (3 days versus 5 days, respectively). Reduction in

weaning time was associated with a decrease in both total duration of mechanical ventilation and ICU length of stay. A study performed in Australia by Rose et al.[86] showed different results. In that study, the authors compared an automated weaning system group with a usual care control group, and no differences were found in weaning time between groups.

ROLE OF TRACHEOTOMY

With the introduction of percutaneous techniques performed at the bedside, tracheotomy has become an increasingly common intervention in ICUs. Tracheotomy can facilitate weaning by reducing dead space and decreasing airway resistance, improving clearance of secretions, reducing the need for sedation, and decreasing the risk of aspiration. Nevertheless, the results from different studies are controversial.[87-90]

A randomized controlled trial[91] examined the hypothesis that tracheotomy performed after 6 to 8 days of endotracheal intubation compared with tracheostomy performed after 13 to 15 days would reduce the incidence of ventilator-associated pneumonia. The duration of mechanical ventilation, length of stay, and mortality were analyzed as secondary outcomes. No differences were found between the two groups in terms of incidence of ventilator-associated pneumonia. Although the numbers of ventilator-free days and ICU-free days were greater in the early tracheotomy group, there were no 28-day survival differences between the groups. Given these results, at the present time tracheostomy should not be performed earlier than after 15 days of endotracheal intubation except in selected populations.

Unplanned Extubation During Weaning

Removal of the endotracheal tube under unexpected conditions is defined as unplanned extubation. It may be deliberate (induced by the patient) as a result of patient agitation or lack of cooperation, or accidental, due to rupture of the endotracheal cuff, nursing procedures, coughing, or other events. Endotracheal unplanned/unexpected extubation (EUE) is estimated to occur in approximately 10% of intubated mechanically ventilated patients.[92-98]

In a prospective study[96] carried out during a 32-month period, 59 episodes of EUE were observed in 55 (frequency 7%) out of 750 patients who required mechanical intubation for more than 48 hours. EUE was deliberate in 78% and accidental in 22% of cases. Twenty-seven episodes (46%) occurred in patients on full mechanical ventilatory support and 32 (54%) during the weaning period from mechanical ventilation. Patients with EUE during weaning required significantly fewer reintubations than those who were not undergoing weaning (odds ratio 6.6). Only 16% of EUE patients who were undergoing weaning from mechanical ventilation (5/32) needed reintubation, whereas reintubation was required in 82% of EUE patients (22/27) receiving full mechanical ventilatory support ($P < 0.01$).

Epstein et al.[97] performed a case-control study involving 75 patients with EUE and 150 controls matched for APACHE II score, presence of comorbid conditions, age, indication for mechanical ventilation, and gender. They found that EUE was not associated with increased mortality when compared to matched controls, although they noted an increased total duration of mechanical ventilation, ICU and hospital stay, and need for chronic care in the EUE group. Mortality was increased in the group that needed reintubation as compared to the group that did not. Reintubation rates were lower among patients who had an EUE during weaning trials as compared to those who had an EUE during full ventilatory support (44% in the former and 76% in the latter).

Summary

The vast majority of intubated mechanically ventilated patients can be successfully liberated from the ventilator after passing a short SBT. The best strategy to shorten the total time of mechanical ventilation is based on a simple daily clinical approach that evaluates the ability of patients to tolerate spontaneous unassisted breathing. This approach requires that a screening test be performed as early as possible and, if positive, the patient is continued on a confirmatory SBT of 30 to 120 minutes of duration. When patients fail SBTs, techniques for progressive withdrawal of mechanical ventilation (PSV and volume-assisted mechanical ventilation with daily SBTs) seem to be equivalent. Automated systems seem to perform as well as usual care. NIV may be useful to hasten weaning in some selected populations. Extubation failure is poorly understood and portends a high mortality rate.

KEY POINTS

1. Making the distinction between liberation and extubation during withdrawal from mechanical ventilation has opened a new understanding in the concept of weaning. These are different processes with different pathophysiologic mechanisms that may lead to failure in weaning or extubation.

2. One important mechanism explaining liberation failure is cardiovascular dysfunction. It may complicate ventilator weaning in a significant number of patients during the switch from positive intrathoracic pressure to spontaneous breathing and the consequent increase in preload and afterload.

3. Mechanisms explaining extubation failure are still poorly understood, and much research is needed in this area. Patients with extubation failure have an increased mortality rate that varies depending on the specific cause of the failure.

4. The implementation of a weaning strategy based on solid clinical and pathophysiologic knowledge improves outcomes in terms of duration of mechanical ventilation and length of stay in the ICU. This effect can be attributed mostly to the fact that patients are screened daily for the capability to maintain spontaneous breathing.

5. Noninvasive ventilation (NIV) is used to facilitate weaning and extubation but with some reservations. Patients should be carefully selected, and NIV administration should be tailored on a patient-by-patient basis.

ANNOTATED REFERENCES

Brochard L, Rauss A, Benito S, et al. Comparison of three methods of gradual withdrawal from ventilatory support during weaning from mechanical ventilation. Am J Respir Crit Care Med 1994; 150(4):896-903.

This is the first randomized trial comparing three different methods of weaning. The authors conclude that outcome of weaning is influenced by the modality chosen during this period. The weaning duration was shorter with pressure support than with SIMV or T-piece when pooled together.

Esteban A, Frutos F, Tobin MJ, et al. A comparison of four methods of weaning patients from mechanical ventilation. N Engl J Med 1995;332(6):345-50.

This is a randomized multicenter study comparing four different methods of weaning. Results showed that weaning after a once-daily spontaneous breathing trial occurred twice as fast as with pressure support and three times more quickly than SIMV. Multiple trials of spontaneous breathing did not reduce the time of weaning compared with a once-daily trial.

Jubran A, Tobin MJ. Pathophysiologic basis of acute respiratory distress in patients who fail a trial of weaning from mechanical ventilation. Am J Respir Crit Care Med 1997;155(3):906-15.

This physiologic study to determine the mechanisms of acute respiratory distress showed that COPD patients who failed a spontaneous breathing trial developed rapid, shallow breathing with worsening of pulmonary mechanics, which caused an increased $Paco_2$.

Boles JM, Bion J, Connors A, et al. Weaning from mechanical ventilation. Eur Respir J 2007; 29(5):1033-56.

Recommendation of an international multisociety consensus conference on weaning.

Girard TD, Kress JP, Fuchs BD, et al. Efficacy and safety of a paired sedation and ventilator weaning protocol for mechanically ventilated patients in intensive care (awakening and breathing controlled trial): a randomised controlled trial. Lancet 2008;371(9607):126-34.

Randomized controlled trial demonstrating that a strategy combining cessation of sedation followed by spontaneous breathing shortens the duration of mechanical ventilation and improves outcome.

REFERENCES

Access the complete reference list online at http://www.expertconsult.com.

Noninvasive Positive-Pressure Ventilation

THOMAS RAJAN | NICHOLAS S. HILL

Noninvasive ventilation is defined as the provision of ventilatory assistance to the lungs without an invasive artificial airway. Noninvasive ventilators consist of a variety of devices, including negative- and positive-pressure ventilators. Until the early 1960s, negative-pressure ventilation in the form of tank ventilators was the most common type of mechanical ventilation outside the anesthesia suite.[1] However, during the Copenhagen polio epidemic of 1952, it was observed that the survival rate improved when patients with respiratory paralysis were treated with invasive positive-pressure anesthesia devices. After that, invasive positive-pressure mechanical ventilation gradually became the preferred means of treating acute respiratory failure.[2] Negative-pressure and other so-called body ventilators were the mainstay of ventilatory support for patients with chronic respiratory failure until the mid-1980s.[1]

With improving mask and ventilator technology and the many advantages over negative-pressure ventilation,[1] noninvasive positive-pressure ventilation (NIPPV) displaced negative-pressure ventilation as the treatment of choice for chronic respiratory failure in patients with neuromuscular and chest wall deformities.[3] Over the past 15 years, noninvasive ventilation has moved from the outpatient to the inpatient setting, where it is used to treat acute respiratory failure. A 1997 survey of medical intensive care units (ICUs) in France, Switzerland, and Spain demonstrated that noninvasive ventilation was used in 16% of cases in which mechanical ventilation was required for respiratory failure, and a follow-up survey found that this rate was up to 23% in 2001.[4] More recent surveys suggest that rates continue to increase over these levels.[5] This chapter discusses the rationale for the increasing use of NIPPV in critical care, as well as appropriate indications, practical applications, and monitoring.

Rationale

The most important advantage of noninvasive ventilation is the avoidance of complications associated with invasive mechanical ventilation. These include complications related to direct upper-airway trauma, bypass of the upper-airway defense mechanisms, increased risk of nosocomial pneumonia, and interference with upper-airway functions, including the ability to eat and communicate normally.[6] By averting airway intubation, noninvasive ventilation leaves the upper airway intact, preserves airway defenses, and allows patients to eat orally, vocalize normally, and expectorate secretions. Compared with invasive mechanical ventilation, noninvasive ventilation reduces infectious complications including pneumonia, sinusitis, and sepsis.[7-9] Strengthening the rationale for its use is evidence accumulated over the past decade that noninvasive ventilation lowers morbidity and mortality rates of selected patients with acute respiratory failure and may shorten hospital length of stay or avoid hospitalization altogether,[10] thus reducing costs.

The main indication for mechanical ventilatory assistance is to treat respiratory failure, either type 1 (hypoxemic), type 2 (hypercapnic), or both. Figure 51-1 shows that airspace collapse, surfactant abnormalities, and airway narrowing and closure contribute to ventilation-perfusion abnormalities and shunt, which cause hypoxemia. By opening collapsed airspaces and narrowed airways, positive airway pressure reduces shunt and improves ventilation-perfusion relationships, ameliorating hypoxemia. In addition, positive airway pressure can reduce the work of breathing by improving lung compliance as a

consequence of opening collapsed airspaces. Another potential benefit of positive airway pressure is enhanced cardiovascular function via the afterload-reducing effect of increased intrathoracic pressure. Conversely, deleterious cardiovascular effects may occur if the preload-reducing effect outweighs the afterload-reducing effect, as may be seen in patients with reduced intravascular fluid volume.

Mechanisms of Action

Figure 51-2 shows the pathophysiologic mechanisms that contribute to ventilatory failure. Increased airway resistance, reduced respiratory system compliance, and intrinsic positive end-expiratory pressure (PEEP) contribute to increased work of breathing, predisposing to respiratory muscle fatigue. In patients with chronic obstructive pulmonary disease (COPD), the increased radius of the diaphragmatic curvature, which increases muscle tension and thereby increases impedance to blood flow, exacerbates the situation. By counterbalancing intrinsic PEEP with extrinsic PEEP and by augmenting tidal volume with intermittent positive-pressure ventilation, NIPPV reduces the work of breathing and averts the vicious circle leading to respiratory failure. Work of breathing measurements, including transdiaphragmatic pressure, diaphragmatic pressure-time product, and diaphragmatic electromyographic amplitude, are all decreased when NIPPV is delivered to patients with exacerbations of COPD. In such patients, continuous positive airway pressure (CPAP) and pressure-support ventilation (PSV) both reduce the work of breathing, but the combination of the two (PSV + PEEP) is more effective than either alone.[11]

Indications

A number of causes of acute respiratory failure are now considered appropriate for noninvasive ventilation therapy and are listed in Box 51-1. Evidence supporting these indications is rated and briefly discussed here; guidelines for patient selection are discussed later.

AIRWAY OBSTRUCTION

Chronic Obstructive Pulmonary Disease

A number of randomized controlled trials[12,13] and meta-analyses[14] have consistently shown that compared with conventional therapy, NIPPV improves vital signs, gas exchange, and dyspnea scores; reduces the rates of intubation, morbidity, and mortality; and shortens hospital length of stay in patients with moderate to severe exacerbations of COPD. Thus NIPPV is considered the ventilatory mode of choice in selected patients with acute exacerbations of COPD. Some studies suggest that the addition of heliox to NIPPV further improves the work of breathing and gas exchange during COPD exacerbations,[15] but a subsequent multicenter trial found no improvement in other outcomes compared with noninvasive ventilation alone.[16]

Asthma

Uncontrolled studies have reported improvements in gas exchange and low rates of intubation after the initiation of NIPPV in patients with severe asthma attacks. Two controlled trials have demonstrated a more rapid improvement in expiratory flow rates with NIPPV,[17,18] and one showed a decreased hospitalization rate in acute asthma patients

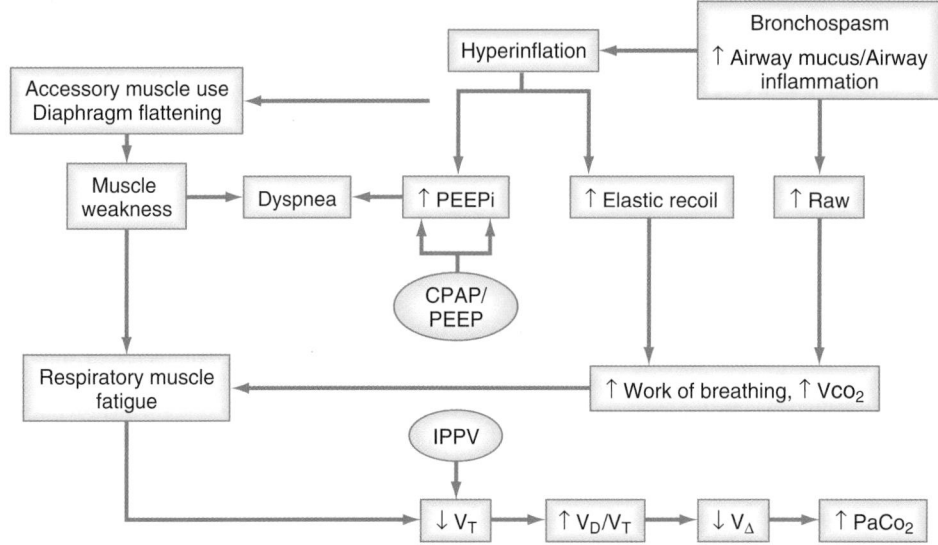

Figure 51-1 Pathophysiology of acute hypoxemic respiratory failure and points where positive-pressure and oxygen supplementation interrupt the process. Low ventilation-perfusion ratios, shunt, and alveolar hypoventilation cause hypoxemia. Hypoxemia is treated by increasing inspired oxygen fraction (FiO_2) (limited benefit with shunt) and applying positive pressure (continuous positive airway pressure [CPAP] or positive end-expiratory pressure [PEEP]) to increase functional residual capacity, open collapsed alveoli and narrowed airways, and enhance compliance. An additional beneficial effect of CPAP may occur in patients with cardiogenic pulmonary edema, because it reduces both venous return and left ventricular afterload, which may enhance cardiovascular performance in patients with dilated, hypocontractile left ventricles.

treated with noninvasive ventilation compared with a sham mask.[18] Neither study was powered adequately to assess intubation or mortality rates. Nonetheless, these data support a trial of NIPPV in asthmatics responding poorly to initial bronchodilator therapy. Noninvasive ventilation can be combined with continuous nebulization and heliox, although the added value of these latter therapies has not been established in controlled trials.

Cystic Fibrosis

Uncontrolled studies indicate that noninvasive ventilation is useful to stabilize gas exchange in the treatment of acute episodes of respiratory

failure in end-stage cystic fibrosis patients and can serve as a bridge to transplantation.[19]

Upper Airway Obstruction

Anecdotally, noninvasive ventilation can be used to treat patients with upper airway obstruction such as that caused by glottic edema following extubation. In this situation, noninvasive ventilation can be combined with aerosolized medications or heliox, but no controlled trials have demonstrated the efficacy of this approach. If therapy with noninvasive ventilation is considered, patients should be selected with great caution and monitored closely, because upper airway obstruction

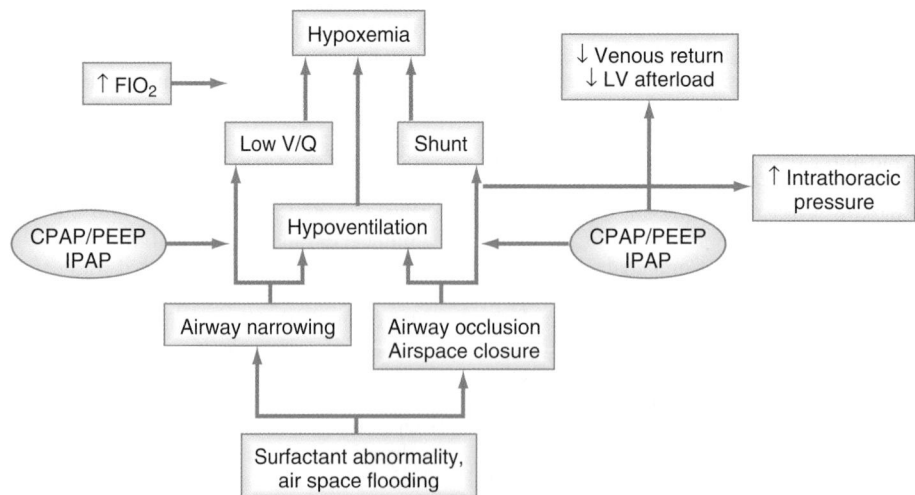

Figure 51-2 Pathophysiology of acute hypercapnia and points where continuous positive airway pressure (CPAP), positive end-expiratory pressure (PEEP), and pressure support (PS) interrupt the process *(large arrows)*. Hypercapnia (increased partial pressure of carbon dioxide in arterial blood [$PaCO_2$]) occurs when respiratory muscles fail to adequately ventilate alveoli to maintain homeostasis with carbon dioxide production. Respiratory muscle failure occurs when work of breathing is normal (e.g., acute or chronic neuromuscular disease) or increased (e.g., patients with chronic obstructive pulmonary disease, asthma, or obesity hypoventilation syndrome), and presumably because of inadequate oxygen delivery to respiratory muscles (e.g., ~ a third of patients presenting with cardiogenic pulmonary edema). Strategies to counter these pathophysiologic mechanisms include applying CPAP or PEEP to counterbalance intrinsic PEEP (PEEPi), increasing alveolar ventilation by augmenting tidal volume (V_T), using intermittent positive-pressure ventilation (IPPV), and reducing CO_2 production by decreasing the work of breathing.

INDICATIONS FOR USE OF NONINVASIVE VENTILATION IN THE ACUTE CARE SETTING

Airway Obstruction
COPD (A)*
Asthma (B)
Cystic fibrosis (C)
Obstructive sleep apnea or obesity hypoventilation (C)
Upper airway obstruction (C)
Facilitation of weaning in COPD (A)
Extubation failure in COPD (B)

Hypoxemic Respiratory Failure
ARDS (C)
Pneumonia (C)
Trauma or burns (C)
Acute pulmonary edema (use of CPAP) (A)
Immunocompromised patients (A)
Restrictive thoracic disorders (C)
Postoperative patients (B)
Do-not-intubate patients (C)
During bronchoscopy (C)

*Letters in parentheses indicate the level of evidence supporting use of noninvasive ventilation: A, multiple randomized, controlled trials—recommended; B, at least one randomized, controlled trial—weaker recommendation; C, case series or reports—can be tried, but with close monitoring.
ARDS, acute respiratory distress syndrome; *COPD*, chronic obstructive pulmonary disease; *CPAP*, continuous positive airway pressure.

can lead to precipitous deterioration. The use of noninvasive ventilation in patients with tight, fixed upper-airway obstruction is inappropriate because it delays the institution of definitive therapy.

HYPOXEMIC RESPIRATORY FAILURE

Hypoxemic respiratory failure is defined as severe hypoxemia (arterial oxygen partial pressure-inspired oxygen fraction ratio <200) combined with a respiratory rate above 35 breaths per minute and a non-COPD diagnosis including acute pneumonia, acute lung injury (ALI), acute respiratory distress syndrome (ARDS), pulmonary edema, or trauma. Controlled trials of noninvasive ventilation to treat patients with acute hypoxemic respiratory failure have shown statistically significant reductions in the rate of intubation, length of hospital stay, incidence of infectious complications,[8,20] and in one study, ICU mortality.[20] However, because of the heterogeneity of causes, these studies fail to demonstrate that all patient subgroups with hypoxemic respiratory failure benefit equally from noninvasive ventilation. Further, when patients are stratified according to acuity of illness, patients with a simplified acute physiologic score (SAPS II) less than 35 fare considerably better with NIPPV than do those with higher scores.[21] Thus the selection of patients with less severe disease is likely to enhance the success of NIPPV in treating hypoxemic respiratory failure, and studies that examine individual subgroups within the larger category are likely to be more useful clinically.

Pneumonia

One controlled trial showed that noninvasive ventilation in patients with severe community-acquired pneumonia lowers the rate of endotracheal intubation and shortens the length of ICU stay compared with conventional therapy; however, a subgroup analysis revealed that the benefits occurred only in patients with underlying COPD.[22] No benefit was apparent in the non-COPD patients with severe pneumonia. A subsequent uncontrolled trial in non-COPD patients with severe pneumonia found that two-thirds of such patients treated with noninvasive ventilation eventually required intubation.[23] Although the latter authors deemed a trial of noninvasive ventilation in non-COPD

patients with severe pneumonia to be a reasonable approach, controlled data to support such a recommendation are currently lacking.

Immunocompromised States

The dismal prognosis of invasively ventilated immunocompromised patients makes noninvasive ventilation an appealing ventilatory mode, with its demonstrated ability to decrease the rate of nosocomial infection.[7] In a study of 51 patients undergoing solid organ transplantation who developed acute hypoxemic respiratory failure within 3 weeks, noninvasive ventilation reduced the rate of intubation, frequency of invasive procedures, rate of nosocomial infection, duration of ICU stay, and ICU mortality (but not hospital mortality) compared with conventional therapy.[24] In a subsequent randomized trial of neutropenic patients with pulmonary infiltrates and acute hypoxemic respiratory failure (most of whom had hematologic malignancies), noninvasive ventilation lowered the intubation rate, occurrence of nosocomial infections, and ICU and hospital mortality rates (the latter from 80% to 46%).[25] More recently, noninvasive ventilation has been reported to yield similar benefits in acquired immunodeficiency syndrome (AIDS) patients with *Pneumocystis carinii* pneumonia versus invasive mechanical ventilation in physiologically and demographically matched patients.[26] Thus, whenever possible, noninvasive ventilation should be tried first in immunocompromised patients with hypoxemic respiratory failure because of the potential to avoid the high morbidity and mortality rates associated with invasive mechanical ventilation in these patients.

Acute Respiratory Distress Syndrome

A small retrospective study reported that NIPPV averted intubation in 50% of patients during the early phase of acute lung injury or ARDS.[27] However, for ARDS patients with severe oxygenation defects and multiple organ system dysfunction, invasive ventilation remains the preferred modality. A prospective cohort study[28] using noninvasive ventilation as a "first-line" intervention for ARDS found that ventilator associated pneumonia and mortality were much reduced when patients succeeded rather than failed noninvasive ventilation, and a simplified acute physiology score of 34 or less and PaO_2/FiO_2 above 175 within the first hour predicted noninvasive ventilation success. Thus, noninvasive ventilation could be considered in ARDS patients meeting these criteria, but such patients must be monitored closely to avoid any delay in intubation if deterioration occurs.

Acute Cardiogenic Pulmonary Edema

Meta-analyses of randomized, controlled trials demonstrated that compared with oxygen therapy, CPAP (though not a true mode of ventilatory support) is highly effective at relieving respiratory distress, improving gas exchange, and averting intubation when used to treat patients with acute cardiogenic edema.[29,30] Inspiratory assistance combined with expiratory pressure can reduce the work of breathing and alleviate respiratory distress more effectively than CPAP alone, and several uncontrolled trials and two controlled trials found that noninvasive ventilation and CPAP are equally effective in improving vital signs and avoiding intubation. The current recommendation is to use CPAP alone or noninvasive ventilation as initial therapy; if CPAP is used initially, inspiratory pressure support should be added if the patient has persistent hypercapnia or dyspnea.[31]

Postoperative Respiratory Failure

NIPPV and CPAP alone have been studied in postoperative patients who develop respiratory failure after various kinds of surgery. It reduces extravascular lung water and improves lung mechanics and gas exchange after coronary artery bypass surgery.[32] Controlled trials show that CPAP averts postoperative complications compared to oxygen supplementation after high risk procedures like thoracoabdominal aortic procedures.[33] Noninvasive ventilation improves oxygenation, reduces the need for re-intubation, lowers the mortality rate after lung resectional surgery,[34] and enhances pulmonary function after gastroplasty.[35] Thus noninvasive ventilation should be considered in selected postoperative patients at high risk of pulmonary complications or with frank respiratory failure, especially in the setting of underlying COPD or pulmonary edema.

Trauma and Burns

Trauma patients develop respiratory failure for a multitude of reasons, but some have chest wall injuries such as flail chest or mild acute lung injury that might respond favorably to NIPPV. In a retrospective survey of 46 trauma patients with respiratory insufficiency that had been treated with NIPPV, Beltrame and coworkers found rapid improvements in gas exchange and a 72% success rate; however, patients with burns responded poorly.[36] More recently, a randomized trial of NIPPV versus high-flow oxygen in thoracic trauma patients with P_{AO_2}/F_{IO_2} less than 200 was stopped early after enrollment of 50 patients because of significant reductions in intubation rate (12% versus 40%) and hospital length of stay (14 versus 21 days) in the NIPPV group.[37] These promising results justify a cautious trial of NIPPV in carefully selected and monitored thoracic trauma patients, but data are too limited to draw firm conclusions.

Restrictive Lung Disease

The use of noninvasive ventilation in patients with underlying restrictive disease and acute deterioration of respiratory status has not been studied extensively because they constitute only a small portion of patients admitted to acute care hospitals. Patients with restriction related to an underlying neuromuscular disease and superimposed acute respiratory failure may benefit from a trial of NIPPV. Small case series have reported that using NIPPV in patients with myasthenic crises may avoid intubation.[38] In contrast, patients with end-stage pulmonary fibrosis in respiratory extremis have been reported to do poorly with mechanical ventilation.[39]

Do-Not-Intubate Patients

Although controversial, noninvasive ventilation may be a useful tool in patients with acute respiratory failure who do not wish to be intubated. There are several reports of good outcomes (>50% survival to discharge) with noninvasive ventilation in this subset of patients, especially those with COPD and congestive heart failure.[40] Noninvasive ventilation may also be used as a palliative technique to reduce dyspnea, preserve patient autonomy, and provide time for finalization of affairs for some terminal patients.[41] However, there is concern that this may merely prolong the dying process, and patients and their families must be informed that noninvasive ventilation is being used as a form of life support in this setting and should be given the option to refuse it.

Facilitation of Weaning and Extubation

Patients who require invasive mechanical ventilation initially and fail to wean promptly are potential candidates for noninvasive ventilation to facilitate extubation, thus reducing the complications related to prolonged intubation. Several randomized controlled trials have demonstrated that noninvasive ventilation significantly shortens the duration of invasive mechanical ventilation, reduces the length of ICU stay, and improves survival compared with patients weaned in the routine fashion.[42-44] Another potential application of noninvasive ventilation in the weaning process is to avoid reintubation in patients with extubation failure, a complication of invasive mechanical ventilation associated with a high mortality rate. Earlier studies looking at the role of NIPPV in this situation showed promise, but one randomized trial found that NIPPV may delay needed intubation in this setting, resulting in an increased ICU mortality rate.[45] More recent studies have demonstrated that patients at high risk for extubation failure,[46] especially those with hypercapnia,[47] have reduced need for intubation and mortality if treated with noninvasive ventilation as opposed to oxygen supplementation alone. Thus, although the use of noninvasive ventilation to facilitate weaning and extubation appears to benefit hypercapnic patients with COPD or congestive heart failure, its overzealous application could lead to increased extubation failure rates and other adverse consequences.

Bronchoscopy

Both CPAP and NIPPV have been studied as ways of supporting oxygenation and ventilation during bronchoscopy. Using a specially designed open CPAP system during bronchoscopy in patients with marginal oxygenation, Maitre et al. observed maintenance of adequate gas exchange and avoidance of respiratory failure.[48] In a controlled trial, Antonelli et al. demonstrated equivalent oxygenation and complication rates in patients undergoing bronchoscopy and supported with either noninvasive or invasive mechanical ventilation.[47] Thus NIPPV is an effective way of providing ventilatory support in patients undergoing bronchoscopy.[49]

▣ Practical Application

PATIENT SELECTION

Noninvasive ventilation should be viewed as a "crutch" that assists patients through a period of acute respiratory failure while reversible factors are being treated, helping them avoid invasive mechanical ventilation and its attendant complications. To optimize the chance of success, noninvasive ventilation should be used early, when patients first develop signs of incipient respiratory failure. In addition, predictors of success are useful in identifying patients most likely to benefit (Box 51-2). The selection process might be viewed as taking advantage of a "window of opportunity": the window opens when the patient first needs ventilatory assistance and closes when the patient becomes too unstable.

Based on the predictors of success and criteria used in prior controlled trials, we recommend the following three-step selection process. First, the patient should have an etiology of respiratory failure likely to respond favorably to noninvasive ventilation. The second step is to identify patients in need of ventilatory assistance by using clinical and blood gas criteria. Patients with mild respiratory distress and no more than mild gas exchange derangement are likely to do well without ventilatory assistance and should not be considered. Good candidates are those with moderate to severe dyspnea, tachypnea, and impending respiratory muscle fatigue, as indicated by the use of accessory muscles of breathing or abdominal paradox. The level of tachypnea used as a criterion depends on the underlying diagnosis. Those with COPD are considered candidates for noninvasive ventilation when the respiratory rate exceeds 24 breaths per minute; with hypoxemic respiratory failure, higher respiratory rates are used, in the range of 30 to 35 breaths per minute. The third step is to exclude patients for whom noninvasive ventilation would be unsafe. Those with frank or imminent respiratory arrest should be promptly intubated because the successful initiation of noninvasive ventilation requires some time for adaptation. Patients who are medically unstable with hypotensive shock, uncontrolled upper gastrointestinal bleeding, unstable arrhythmias, or life-threatening ischemia are better managed with invasive mechanical ventilation. Additionally, noninvasive ventilation should not be used

---

Box 51-2

PREDICTORS OF NONINVASIVE VENTILATION SUCCESS IN PATIENTS WITH ACUTE RESPIRATORY FAILURE

Lower acuity of illness (Acute Physiology and Chronic Health Evaluation [APACHE] score)
Ability to cooperate; better neurologic score
Ability to coordinate breathing with ventilator
Less air leakage; intact dentition
Hypercarbia, but not too severe ($PaCO_2$ between 45 and 92 mm Hg)
Acidemia, but not too severe (pH between 7.1 and 7.35)
Improvements in gas exchange and heart and respiratory rates within first 2 hours

for patients who are uncooperative, unable to adequately protect their upper airway or clear secretions, or intolerant of masks, or for recipients of recent upper gastrointestinal or airway surgery.

INITIATION OF NONINVASIVE VENTILATION

Once an appropriate candidate for noninvasive ventilation has been selected, a ventilator and interface must be chosen, initial settings must be selected, and the patient must be monitored closely in an appropriate location until stabilized. The roles of physicians, respiratory therapists, and nurses are of paramount importance in explaining the process to and gaining the confidence of the patient. Noninvasive ventilation can be initiated wherever the patient presents with acute respiratory distress, but he or she should be transferred to a location with sufficient monitoring (usually an ICU or step-down unit) until stabilized. During transfers, ventilatory assistance and monitoring should be continued.

VENTILATOR SELECTION

Selection of a ventilator is based largely on availability, practitioner experience, and patient comfort. Pressure-limited modes, including pressure support and pressure control, are available on most critical care ventilators. Pressure-control ventilation delivers time-cycled, preset inspiratory and expiratory pressures with adjustable inspiratory/expiratory ratios at a controlled rate. Most such modes also permit patient triggering and selection of a backup rate. PSV delivers preset inspiratory and expiratory pressures to assist spontaneous breathing efforts. Nomenclature and the specific characteristics of these modes may differ among ventilators, and this must be taken into account to avoid errors. For example, with some ventilators, pressure support is the amount of inspiratory assistance added to the preset expiratory pressure. Others require independent selection of inspiratory and expiratory positive airway pressures, with the difference between the two determining the level of pressure support.

PSV is a flow-triggered and flow-cycled mode, and patient effort determines tidal volume and duration of inspiration. Pressure-support modes have the potential to match breathing pattern quite closely, and they have been rated by patients as more comfortable for NIPPV than volume-limited ventilation.[50] However, leaks during noninvasive ventilation can interfere with the detection of reduced inspiratory flow at the termination of inspiration, causing expiratory asynchrony. Noninvasive pressure-limited modes of ventilation are usually administered using either standard critical care ventilators or portable bilevel ventilators.

Traditional bilevel devices designed for home use have limited pressure-generating capability (≤ 30 cm H_2O) and lack oxygen blenders or sophisticated alarm or battery backup systems, precluding their use in patients who require high oxygen concentrations or inflation pressures. Newer versions designed for the acute setting are equipped with sophisticated alarm and monitoring capabilities, graphic displays, and oxygen blenders. These devices are capable of enhancing synchrony by offering ways to limit inspiratory duration and an adjustable "rise time"—the time to reach the targeted inspiratory pressure. Many critical care ventilators now include an "NIV" mode that enhances leak compensation capabilities and silences "nuisance" alarms, but many of these have difficulty maintaining performance in the face of variable air leaks.[51] If desired, volume-limited ventilation can be delivered using critical care ventilators, but a higher tidal volume than that commonly used for invasive mechanical ventilation is recommended to compensate for air leakage.

Initial ventilator pressure settings are usually low to facilitate patient acceptance, but they can be set higher if necessary to alleviate respiratory distress. Typical starting pressures are an inspiratory positive airway pressure of 10 to 12 cm H_2O and a PEEP (or expiratory positive airway pressure) of 4 to 5 cm H_2O. L'Her et al.[52] demonstrated that increases in inspiratory pressure are helpful to alleviate dyspnea, whereas increases in expiratory pressure are better to improve

oxygenation. For volume ventilation, initial tidal volumes range from 6 to 7 mL/kg. The ventilator is set in a spontaneously triggered mode, with or without a backup rate. Pressures commonly used to deliver CPAP in patients with acute respiratory distress range from 5 to 12.5 cm H_2O. CPAP can be applied using compressed air with a regulator system, blower-based CPAP devices, bilevel devices, or critical care ventilators.

INTERFACES

The major difference between invasive and noninvasive ventilation is that with the latter, pressurized gas is delivered to the airway via a mask rather than via an invasive conduit. The open breathing circuit of noninvasive ventilation permits air leaks around the mask or through the mouth, rendering the success of noninvasive ventilation dependent on ventilators designed to deal effectively with air leaks and to optimize patient comfort and acceptance. Interfaces—the devices that connect the ventilator tubing to the nose, mouth, or both—enable pressurized gas to enter the upper airway during noninvasive ventilation. Commonly used interfaces in the acute setting include nasal masks and full face (or oronasal) masks.

Nasal masks are widely used for the administration of CPAP or NIPPV, particularly for chronic applications. Nasal masks are usually better tolerated than full face masks for long-term applications, because they cause less claustrophobia and discomfort and allow eating, conversation, and expectoration. The standard nasal mask is a triangular or cone-shaped clear plastic device that fits over the nose and uses a soft cuff that forms an air seal over the skin. The mask exerts pressure over the nasal bridge, often causing skin irritation and redness and occasionally ulceration. Many modifications are available to avoid complications, such as the use of forehead spacers or masks with ultra-thin silicon seals or heat-sensitive gels that minimize skin trauma.

Full facemasks cover both the nose and the mouth (Figure 51-3) and are preferable to nasal masks in the acute setting. The efficacy of both nasal and oronasal masks in lowering $Paco_2$ and avoiding intubation is similar in the acute setting, but a randomized controlled trial[53] observed better patient tolerance with full facemasks because of reduced air leakage through the mouth. More recently, a "total" facemask has become available; it seals around the perimeter of the face and resembles a hockey goalie's mask. Made of optical-grade plastic, it is easy to apply and causes no more claustrophobia than standard facemasks. Mouthpieces are seldom used to administer noninvasive

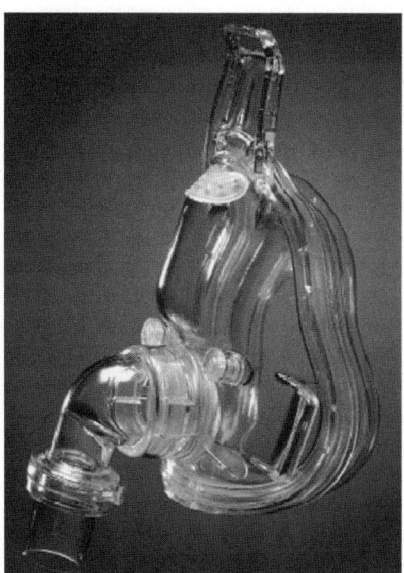

Figure 51-3   Full facemask with soft silicon seal to minimize pressure on nasal bridge. A disposable version of this mask is widely used in the acute care setting.

ventilation in the acute setting but are occasionally used during initiation, when the patient holds the mouthpiece in place to adapt to the sensation of positive-pressure ventilation.

Selection of a comfortable mask that fits properly is key to the success of noninvasive ventilation. The full facemask should be tried first in the acute setting, and if possible, the patient should be allowed to hold the mask in place initially. The mask straps are then tightened with the least tension necessary to avoid excessive air leakage. Some leaking is acceptable and even obligatory with bilevel ventilators, because of the need to flush carbon dioxide from the single-channel ventilator circuit. Bilevel ventilators compensate for air leakage better than critical care ventilators do, but excessive air leakage can lead to noninvasive ventilation failure with any ventilator.

Head straps hold the mask in place and are important for patient comfort. Straps attach at two to five points, depending on the type of mask. More points of attachment add to stability.

OXYGENATION AND HUMIDIFICATION

Oxygen is titrated to achieve a desired oxygen saturation, usually greater than 90% to 92%, either by using oxygen blenders on critical care and some bilevel ventilators or by adjusting liter flow (up to 15 L/min, as per manufacturer's recommendations) delivered via oxygen tubing connected directly to the mask or ventilator circuit. Bilevel ventilators have limited oxygenation capabilities (maximal inspired oxygen fraction, 0.45-0.5), so ventilators with oxygen blenders should be used for patients with hypoxemic respiratory failure. A heated humidifier should be used to prevent drying of the nasal passage and oropharynx when the duration of application is anticipated to be more than a few hours.

MONITORING

Once noninvasive ventilation is initiated, patients should be closely monitored in a critical care or step-down unit until they are sufficiently stable to be moved to a regular medical floor. The aim of monitoring is to determine whether the main goals are being achieved, including relief of symptoms, reduced work of breathing, improved or stable gas exchange, good patient-ventilator synchrony, and patient comfort (Box 51-3). A drop in the respiratory rate with improved oxygen saturation or improving pH with a lower $Paco_2$ within the first 1 to 2 hours portends a successful outcome.[54] Abdominal paradox, if present initially, subsides, and the heart rate usually falls. The absence of these propitious signs indicates a poor response to noninvasive ventilation

and the need to make further adjustments. Leaks should be sought and corrected, patient-ventilator synchrony should be optimized, and pressures may have to be adjusted upward to relieve respiratory distress and achieve a reduction in $Paco_2$. If these adjustments fail to improve the response within a few hours, noninvasive ventilation should be considered a failure, and the patient should be promptly intubated if it is still clinically indicated. Excessive delay in intubation may precipitate a respiratory crisis and add to morbidity and mortality.

Adverse Effects and Complications

When applied by experienced caregivers to appropriately selected patients, noninvasive ventilation is usually well tolerated and is associated with minimal complications. The most frequent adverse effects and complications are related to the mask, ventilator airflow or pressure, patient-ventilator interaction, or airway secretions.

Common adverse effects related to the mask include discomfort and erythema or skin ulcers, usually on the nasal bridge, related to pressure from the mask seal. Proper fitting and attachment, consistent use of artificial skin over the nose, and newer masks with softer silicone seals help minimize these problems. Adverse effects related to airflow or pressure include conjunctival irritation caused by air leakage under the mask into the eyes and sinus, or ear pain related to excessive pressure. Refitting the mask or lowering inspiratory pressure may ameliorate these problems. Nasal or oral dryness caused by high airflow is usually indicative of air leaking through the mouth. Measures to minimize leakage may be useful, but nasal saline or emollients and heated humidifiers are often necessary to relieve these complaints. Nasal congestion and discharge are also frequent complaints and can be treated with topical decongestants or steroids and oral antihistamine-decongestant combinations. Gastric insufflation occurs commonly, may respond to simethicone, and is usually tolerated.

Patient-ventilator asynchrony is a common occurrence during NIPPV. Failure to adequately synchronize compromises the ventilator's ability to reduce the work of breathing and may contribute to NIPPV failure. The asynchrony may be related to patient agitation, which can be treated with the judicious use of sedatives. Failure to synchronize can also result from inadequate ventilator triggering or inability to sense the onset of patient expiration because of air leakage. This can be corrected by minimizing air leaks and using ventilator modes that permit limitation of maximal inspiratory duration. Even with the best efforts to optimize settings and comfort, a minority of patients still fail. This may be partly due to progression of the underlying disease process or the patient's inability to tolerate NIPPV, but every effort should be made to ascertain that it is not due to technologic problems that could be corrected by mask or ventilator adjustments. Once again, intubation should not be delayed if improvement is not apparent within a few hours.

Box 51-3

MONITORING OF PATIENTS RECEIVING NONINVASIVE VENTILATION IN ACUTE CARE SETTINGS

Location:
  Critical care or step-down unit
  Medical or surgical ward if able to breathe unassisted for
    >20-30 min
"Eyeball" test:
  Dyspnea
  Comfort (mask, air pressure)
  Anxiety
  Asynchrony
  Leaks
Vital signs:
  Respiratory and heart rates
  Blood pressure
  Continuous electrocardiography
Gas exchange:
  Continuous oximetry
  Arterial blood gases (baseline, after 1-2 h, and as clinically
    indicated)

KEY POINTS

1. The use of noninvasive positive-pressure ventilation (NIPPV) in patients with certain forms of acute respiratory failure is becoming established, mainly because of increasing evidence for efficacy and advances in noninvasive interfaces and ventilators.

2. NIPPV delivered by nasal or oronasal mask reduces the need for endotracheal intubation, decreases the length of stay in the ICU and hospital, and reduces mortality when used in selected patients with exacerbations of chronic obstructive pulmonary disease (COPD).

3. The efficacy of NIPPV has been demonstrated for acute pulmonary edema, for respiratory failure in immunocompromised patients, and to facilitate extubation in COPD patients.

4. Patients who develop respiratory failure and who refuse intubation are potentially good candidates for NIPPV, but all patients must be selected carefully.

5. Several factors are vital to the success of NIPPV: careful patient selection; properly timed initiation; comfortable, well-fitting interface; coaching and encouragement; and careful monitoring.

6. Noninvasive ventilation should be used to avert endotracheal intubation rather than as an alternative to it. One should not persist in the use of NIPPV if it will lead to a delay in necessary intubation.

7. A trial of noninvasive ventilation should be instituted in properly selected patients with acute respiratory failure before respiratory arrest is imminent, to provide ventilatory assistance while the factors responsible for the respiratory failure are aggressively treated.

8. Noninvasive ventilation is an important addition to the methods available to assist patients with acute respiratory failure and, if properly applied, improves patient outcome in the critical care setting.

ANNOTATED REFERENCES

Antonelli M, Conti G, Esquinas A, et al. A multiple-center survey on the use in clinical practice of noninvasive ventilation as a first-line intervention for acute respiratory distress syndrome. Crit Care Med 2007;35:18-25.
A multicenter survey of over 400 ARDS patients, two-thirds of whom were already intubated before they were admitted to the ICU. The remaining patients were treated with noninvasive ventilation when they reached the ICU, and outcomes were assessed. Intubation was avoided in 54% of these patients (one-sixth of the total), and outcomes of these successes were much better than in the failures.

Demoule A, Girou E, Richard JC, Taillé S, Brochard L. Increased use of noninvasive ventilation in French intensive care units. Intensive Care Med 2006;32:1747-55.
Follow-up survey of mainly French ICUs, demonstrating an increase in the use of noninvasive ventilation between 1997 and 2002, mainly in patients with hypercapnic respiratory failure.

Farha S, Ghamra ZW, Hoisington ER, Butler RS, Stoller JK. Use of noninvasive positive-pressure ventilation on the regular hospital ward: experience and correlates of success. Respir Care 2006;51:1237-43.
This prospective cohort examined the outcomes of 76 patients with respiratory failure treated with noninvasive ventilation on a medical ward. Of these, 31% required intubation and were transferred to an ICU. The authors considered this intubation rate comparable to that encountered in ICUs and opined that noninvasive ventilation could be safely administered on a regular floor.

Ferrer M, Sellares J, Valencia M, et al. Non-invasive ventilation after extubation in hypercapnic patients with chronic respiratory disorders: randomised controlled trial. Lancet 2009;374:1082-8.
This randomized trial on patients with postextubation respiratory failure identified hypercapnic patients as those likely to benefit form noninvasive ventilation.

Maheshwari V, Paioli D, Rothaar R, Hill NS. Utilization of noninvasive ventilation in acute care hospitals: a regional survey. Chest 2006;129:1226-33.
This survey of respiratory therapy directors at acute care hospitals in Massachusetts and Rhode Island found a large disparity in noninvasive ventilation rates between different institutions. Lack of experience or knowledge and inadequate equipment were identified as barriers to use.

Winck JC, Azevedo LF, Costa-Pereira A, Antonelli M, Wyatt JC. Efficacy and safety of non-invasive ventilation in the treatment of acute cardiogenic pulmonary edema—a systematic review and meta-analysis. Crit Care 2006;10:R69.
One of a number of meta-analyses showing benefits of CPAP and noninvasive ventilation in patients with cardiogenic pulmonary edema. Intubation, mortality, and myocardial infarction rates were improved by both modalities but did not differ between them. The authors concluded that CPAP or noninvasive ventilation were becoming "mandatory" to treat cardiogenic pulmonary edema patients.

REFERENCES

Access the complete reference list online at http://www.expertconsult.com.

High-Frequency Ventilation

MAH CHOU LIANG | NIALL D. FERGUSON | THOMAS E. STEWART | SANGEETA MEHTA

High-frequency ventilation is a collection of ventilator modes in which small tidal volumes are delivered at supra-physiologic frequencies. Various types of high-frequency ventilation have been developed over the last 3 decades, including high-frequency positive-pressure ventilation, high-frequency percussive ventilation, high-frequency jet ventilation, and the most commonly employed mode, high-frequency oscillatory ventilation. Initially, high-frequency ventilation was used mainly in neonates with respiratory distress syndrome (RDS); however, there has been increased interest in its use in adults with acute lung injury (ALI) and acute respiratory distress syndrome (ARDS), given its potential for lung protection.

Over the last 30 years, our understanding of the potential harm of mechanical ventilation has evolved, and it has been clearly demonstrated that lung injury may occur through injurious mechanical forces generated during mechanical ventilation. Potential causes of lung injury include gross air leaks (barotrauma), diffuse alveolar injury due to overdistension (volutrauma), injury due to repeated cycles of recruitment and derecruitment (atelectrauma), and injury due to the release of mediators from the lung (biotrauma).[1,2] Importantly, volutrauma and atelectrauma lead to biotrauma, which affects not only the lung but may also contribute to multiple organ dysfunction, the major cause of death in patients with ARDS. Lung-protective mechanical ventilation strategies aim to reduce these injurious forces and subsequent lung damage while providing adequate ventilation and oxygenation. The mechanics of high-frequency ventilation, particularly high-frequency oscillatory ventilation (HFOV), make it particularly well suited to protect the lung, and there is growing clinical experience with the use of high-frequency ventilation as an alternative to conventional mechanical ventilation or as salvage therapy in patients failing conventional ventilation strategies.

Description and Classification

HIGH-FREQUENCY POSITIVE-PRESSURE VENTILATION

High-frequency positive-pressure ventilation (HFPPV) delivers small volumes (approximately 3-4 mL/kg) of conditioned gas at high frequencies (60-100 breaths/minute) using a conventional mechanical ventilator. Valves in the inspiratory and expiratory limbs of the ventilator circuit allow control of the generally high inspiratory flow rate and positive end-expiratory pressure (PEEP), respectively. Expiration is passive and relies on the elastic recoil of the patient's respiratory system. The clinician controls the respiratory rate, inspiratory flow rate, driving pressure, and PEEP. Because high respiratory rates leave little time for passive expiration, there is a risk of gas trapping, with hyperinflation and resultant overdistension injury.

HFPPV was first described in 1969 as an experimental technique[3] and has subsequently found only limited clinical use in specialized upper-airway surgical procedures and bronchoscopy.[4] Published clinical experience with HFPPV is largely limited to neonatal populations. One meta-analysis in newborn infants found that synchronized mechanical ventilation delivered as HFPPV was associated with reduced barotrauma and shorter hospital stay compared with conventional mechanical ventilation (CMV),[5] but the effect on mortality and chronic oxygen dependency was unclear. In adult patients,

HFPPV has been used only in specialized applications in the field of anaesthesia.[6-8]

HIGH-FREQUENCY PERCUSSIVE VENTILATION

High-frequency percussive ventilation (HFPV) is a hybrid mode that combines the principles of high frequency and CMV using a proprietary mechanical ventilator.[9] A conventional ventilation circuit is fitted with a gas-driven piston at the end of the endotracheal tube. The reciprocating piston generates pressure oscillations at 3 to 15 Hz, with short expiratory times that are superimposed on the conventional inspiratory-expiratory pressure waves. The high-frequency beats are delivered in bursts to generate auto-PEEP through breath stacking, and then are interrupted to allow alveolar pressure to return to baseline. It has been hypothesized that the auto-PEEP generated improves alveolar recruitment without exposing the alveoli to the high peak airway pressures that would be generated with comparable CMV. Although the high-frequency pressure oscillations are driven actively in both directions, the bulk of exhalation is passive, from the underlying CMV breaths. The high-frequency percussion also provides some internal mucokinesis, potentially improving pulmonary toilet and reducing endotracheal suctioning requirements.[10] Indeed, it may be because of this property that HFPV has been most commonly used in adult patients with inhalational injury, burns, and trauma.

HIGH-FREQUENCY JET VENTILATION

High-frequency jet ventilation (HFJV) employs a small-aperture nozzle inserted into the endotracheal tube in order to direct a high-pressure stream of gas into the lung (Figure 52-1). During inspiration, a high-pressure jet streams into the proximal airways, entraining air from the circuit, and tidal volume is therefore largely dependent on the Venturi and Coanda effects. The parameters controlled by the clinician are frequency, inspiratory time, jet drive pressure, and PEEP applied through the ventilator circuit. Tidal volumes are determined by the jet driving pressure and inspiratory time (i.e., larger tidal volumes can be delivered by increasing jet drive pressure and inspiratory time). Tidal volumes will also be augmented by using a larger jet catheter and a larger endotracheal tube, which increase the amount of jet flow and gas entrainment, respectively. Because expiration is passive, gas trapping may occur at higher frequencies with progressively shorter expiratory times.

A complication specific to HFJV is traumatic upper airway injury. The high-velocity inspiratory jet may cause direct trauma to the proximal airways, and necrotizing tracheobronchitis is a recognized complication of HFJV in both infants and adults.[11,12] Gas conditioning during HFJV, particularly humidification and warming, is also problematic. Although the gas entrained from the proximal circuit is warmed and humidified, the gas injected from the jet nozzle expands and cools, compromising the overall conditioning of the inspired gas. It has also been hypothesized that high gas flow rates and rapid increases in lung volume could cause lung injury through the generation of shear forces at the interface of adjacent compliant and atelectatic lung units.[13]

The clinical utility of HFJV is specific to certain clinical settings such as pulmonary air leak syndromes, when the ability to achieve adequate gas exchange with lower peak airway pressures may be advantageous.[14]

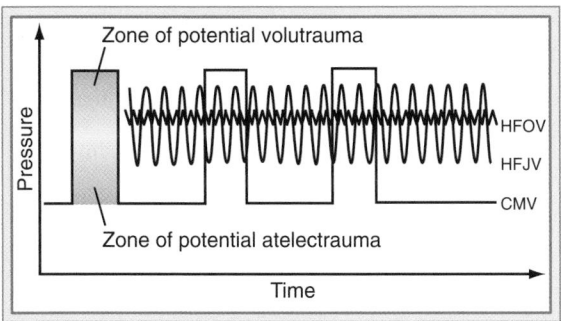

Figure 52-1 Theoretic comparison of the alveolar pressure swings seen with high-frequency ventilation versus conventional mechanical ventilation.

In addition, the decreased reliance on bulk flow with HFJV may improve gas distribution and gas exchange in the presence of large air leaks, although this theoretical advantage has not been borne out in clinical studies.[15]

The published clinical experience with HFJV in acute respiratory failure remains small, and to date, the greatest clinical experience is in the neonatal and pediatric populations and in anesthesia for airway stability during respiratory tract surgery. There is limited research in its utility in adult respiratory failure, although many intensive care units (ICUs) have sizable anecdotal experience. Comparative clinical trials have shown that high-frequency jet ventilation is safe and offers improved oxygenation and ventilation compared with CMV, while improving respiratory parameters and decreasing required peak pressures.[16-18] None of these trials, however, demonstrated a significant survival advantage.

HIGH-FREQUENCY OSCILLATORY VENTILATION

During HFOV, a piston pump oscillates a diaphragm at frequencies between 3 and 15 Hz (180-900 breaths/min) to create pressure waves in the ventilator circuit (see Figure 52-1). Because the diaphragm is actively driven in both directions, the ventilator creates both inspiratory and expiratory pressure waves, meaning that expiration is also active. The use of active expiration distinguishes HFOV from other forms of high-frequency ventilation, in which expiration is passive and dependent on the elastic recoil of the respiratory system. Active expiration may be advantageous in controlling CO_2 and preventing hyperinflation. Indeed, HFOV has been shown to be associated with less gas trapping than other forms of high-frequency ventilation.[19] The mean airway pressure is maintained by a resistance valve in the circuit, together with the inspiratory bias flow. Changes in alveolar pressure are kept low by small excursions of the piston. Humidification is achieved by passing the bias flow of gas through a humidifier.[20]

It is this ability to deliver very small tidal volumes at a relatively constant mean airway pressure that makes HFOV theoretically ideal for minimizing ventilator-induced lung injury (VILI) in addition to being an effective mode for oxygenation in severe ARDS. In view of these unique features of HFOV, recent research has focused on this particular mode of high-frequency ventilation in the management of adult patients with ARDS.

Mechanisms of Gas Transport with High-Frequency Oscillatory Ventilation

During CMV, gas exchange is largely related to bulk flow of gas to the alveoli. However, since the tidal volumes generated during HFOV may be smaller than the anatomic dead space, ventilation relies on alternative gas exchange mechanisms related largely to enhanced gas mixing within the lung. These gas exchange mechanisms are summarized in Table 52-1[21] and Figure 52-2. Experimental models suggest that in contrast to CMV, CO_2 elimination is a product of the frequency and the square of the tidal volume ($Vco_2 \alpha = f \times V_T^2$)[22] such that adequate

TABLE 52-1	Mechanisms of Gas Exchange During High-Frequency Oscillatory Ventilation
Site	*Proposed Mechanism*
Proximal airway	**Bulk flow**—remains an important mechanism of gas transport in proximal airways
Mid-airway	**Pendelluft**—phenomenon of regional gas movement that occurs as a result of heterogeneity in alveolar filling and emptying rates. Adjacent lung units with different time constants may fill at different rates during inspiration. Following inspiration, there is redistribution of inspired gas from full, fast-filling units to slower-filling units, augmenting gas exchange.[9] **Taylor dispersion**—enhanced diffusion augmented by radial transport mechanisms **Asymmetrical velocity profiles**—results in a net convective transport of material, especially at airway bifurcations. Fresh gas streams toward alveoli along inner airway walls, while "alveolar" gas streams cranially along outer airway wall.
Distal airway	**Cardiogenic mixing**—rhythmic contraction of heart promotes peripheral gas mixing by generating flow within neighboring parenchymal regions **Collateral ventilation**—gas exchange between noncommunicating neighboring alveoli via collateral channels

From Chang HK. Mechanisms of gas transport during ventilation by high-frequency oscillation. J Appl Physiol. 1984;56(3):553-563.

CO_2 elimination may become problematic as tidal volumes decrease, unless accompanied by proportionately larger increases in frequency. Regardless, clinical experience has demonstrated that adequate gas exchange can be achieved in adults with HFOV using frequencies in the 8- to 10-Hz range, delivering tidal volumes that are less than anatomic dead space.[23]

Rationale for High-Frequency Oscillatory Ventilation

In the last few decades, there has been an enormous increase in understanding of the effects of mechanical ventilation on the lung and elucidation of VILI and its pathophysiology, namely volutrauma, atelectrauma, and biotrauma. Furthermore, the clinical relevance of VILI was solidified by a landmark study published by the ARDS Network in 2000 that demonstrated a 9% absolute mortality reduction in patients with ARDS ventilated with tidal volumes of 6 mL/kg ideal body weight compared with 12 mL/kg.[24]

HFOV would appear to be the ideal lung-protective ventilation strategy in patients with ALI/ARDS because of two principal properties: (1) prevention of VILI by delivery of small tidal volumes with limitation

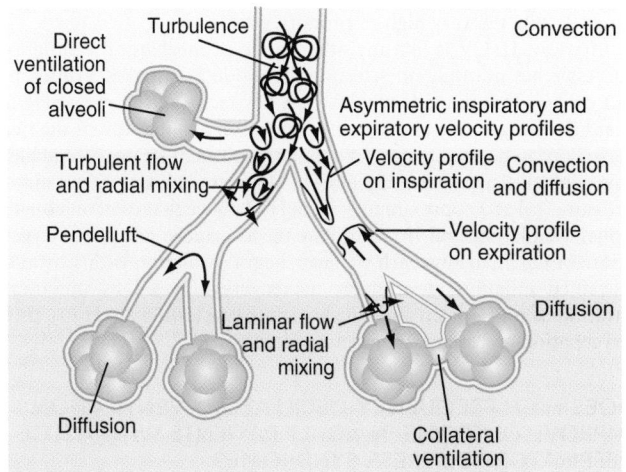

Figure 52-2 Mechanism of gas exchange during high-frequency oscillatory ventilation (HFOV). *(From Slutsky AS, Drazen JM. Ventilation with small tidal volumes. N Engl J Med. 2002;347:630-631.)*

of alveolar overdistension and (2) promotion of alveolar recruitment through application of a higher mean airway pressure than can be safely applied with CMV, promoting more alveolar recruitment and avoiding cyclic opening and closing of alveolar units throughout the respiratory cycle. Indeed, there is a wealth of preclinical animal data demonstrating that compared with both injurious and lung-protective conventional ventilation, HFOV is advantageous in terms of gas exchange, markers of inflammation, and lung pathology scores.[25]

DOES HIGH-FREQUENCY OSCILLATORY VENTILATION TRULY DELIVER SMALL TIDAL VOLUMES?

Although tidal volumes are not measured directly on the oscillator that is commercially available in the United States, several investigators have measured delivered tidal volumes. In a sheep saline-lavage model of ALI, Sedeek et al. measured delivered tidal volumes with a pneumotachograph[26] and found that HFOV applied with a frequency of 4 Hz and pressure amplitude of 60 cm H_2O resulted in tidal volumes of 4 mL/kg—not large, but not as small as had been anticipated. More recently, however, Hager and colleagues measured tidal volumes in adults with ARDS receiving HFO using a hot-wire anemometer, which may provide more accurate measurements. These investigators found that usual tidal volumes delivered during adult HFOV were indeed small, in the 1 to 2 mL/kg range, and that frequency[27] rather than pressure amplitude was the dominant determinant of tidal volume in adults with ARDS. These authors emphasized that while low tidal volumes can be delivered during HFO, at low frequencies, tidal volumes may be larger than anticipated. This suggests that a strategy that achieves acceptable CO_2 clearance while employing the highest tolerated frequency is likely to be most lung protective. To practically achieve these goals, we generally use a relatively high power set to achieve a pressure amplitude (delta P [ΔP]) of 90 cm H_2O, and then adjust frequency as high as tolerated to achieve an adequate pH (>7.25), at times using a partial leak around the endotracheal tube cuff to facilitate CO_2 clearance and higher frequency tolerance.

DOES HIGH-FREQUENCY OSCILLATORY VENTILATION PROMOTE ALVEOLAR RECRUITMENT?

Alveolar recruitment refers to the dynamic process of reopening unstable collapsed alveoli. Easley et al. performed a study in healthy dogs, using computer tomographic imaging to look at the distribution of lung volume.[28] They matched the mean airway pressure with conventional CPAP and noted small decreases in total and regional lung volume with HFOV, especially at lower mean airway pressure and accompanying lower frequency. These authors concluded that there was low risk of occult regional overdistension during HFOV in healthy lungs despite the very high respiratory rates.

In a way, HFOV is like any other mode of mechanical ventilation: success relies not only on selecting the mode that makes a difference but on *how* that mode is employed. A key factor in the use of HFOV that has emerged from both animal and neonatal literature is the need for HFOV to be used as part of a lung recruitment strategy. To achieve this goal, clinicians generally either (1) select a starting mean airway pressure (mPaw) approximately 5 cm H_2O above that used on conventional ventilation and titrate mPaw up to achieve adequate oxygenation; or (2) in an approach we favor, begin oscillation with 1 or more sustained inflation recruitment maneuvers followed by downward titration of mPaw from a relatively high mPaw (30-35 cm H_2O), using oxygenation as a surrogate for lung recruitment.[29]

DOES HIGH-FREQUENCY OSCILLATORY VENTILATION IMPROVE OUTCOME IN ADULT PATIENTS WITH ACUTE RESPIRATORY DISTRESS SYNDROME?

HFOV in principle fulfils the criteria for lung-protective ventilation and can achieve effective ventilation despite very small tidal volumes. However, it is not yet clear whether this ventilatory mode impacts the outcome of adult patients with ARDS. The clinical trials and systematic reviews evaluating HFOV in adults are summarized in Tables 52-2 and 52-3, respectively. Based on the current evidence presented in these two tables, we can conclude the following regarding the use of HFOV in adults with ARDS:

1. Most studies utilized HFOV as rescue therapy in patients with severe ARDS.
2. The use of HFOV was associated with improvements in oxygenation.
3. The use of HFOV was well tolerated and not associated with harm.
4. All of the previous randomized controlled trials have been underpowered to detect a mortality benefit with HFOV; however, a recent meta-analysis did show significant reduction in mortality (risk ratio [RR] 0.77 with 95% confidence interval [CI] of 0.46-0.99), but this conclusion is still based on a relatively small number of patients.
5. Many of the studies on HFOV are confounded by a comparison with CMV that would not be considered optimally lung protective with current practice guidelines.

Thus, despite the increasing number of studies on HFOV, no large prospective randomized controlled trials have yet been completed to evaluate the efficacy of HFOV against the best conventional lung protective ventilation, and the question about any survival benefit due to the use of HFOV remains unanswered.

Current High-Frequency Oscillatory Ventilation Practices in Patients with Acute Respiratory Distress Syndrome

High-frequency ventilation has been in use for at least 3 decades, and the clinical application has evolved over the years. For a detailed discussion of specific recommendations regarding HFOV settings and monitoring, readers are referred to a recent roundtable report on HFOV use.[30]

FREQUENCY

In adults, HFOV frequency is most commonly 5 to 7 Hz, while higher frequencies are used in neonates (8-15 Hz).[31] If there is a need for greater CO_2 clearance, the most common approach is to decrease the frequency to less than 5 Hz after ΔP has been optimized. This approach, however, results in delivery of larger tidal volumes and may not optimize the potential of HFOV to deliver small tidal volumes. A recent study in adults[23] demonstrated that frequencies greater than 6 Hz (with 1 patient reaching 15 Hz) can maintain adequate gas exchange. In that study, an endotracheal cuff leak was applied in 30% of patients to aid CO_2 clearance. The rationale for exploring higher frequencies during HFOV is the ability to achieve smaller tidal volumes and attenuate potential overdistension injury.

TIMING OF HIGH-FREQUENCY OSCILLATORY VENTILATION

In early studies, HFOV was initiated approximately 5 days following the start of CMV.[32] However, several observational studies have suggested better outcomes if HFOV is initiated earlier.[32,33] David et al.[34] observed that mortality was reduced when HFOV was initiated within 3 days following the start of CMV, compared to after 3 days (20% versus 64%, respectively). Thus in recent years, investigators have initiated HFOV earlier: 1.9 days in the trial by Derdak et al.[35] and 1.8 days in the trial by Bollen et al.[36] Nonetheless, a meta-analysis evaluating determinants of mortality with HFOV in adults with ARDS did not find a relationship between late initiation of HFOV and higher mortality.[36]

RECRUITMENT MANEUVERS

The use of recruitment maneuvers has gathered intense interest in the management of adults with ARDS and has been incorporated by some

TABLE 52-2	Clinical Trials Evaluating High-Frequency Oscillatory Ventilation in Adults		
Publication Trial Design	**Number of Patients**	**Study Summary/Major Findings**	**Adverse Effects**
Fort et al., 1997[32] Prospective clinical study	17 ARDS	13 pts showed improved gas exchange with HFOV Hemodynamically well tolerated More CMV days prior to HFOV, and OI >47 associated with higher mortality	3 pts (17.6%) had hypotension 1 pt had bilateral pneumothorax 30-day survival: 47%
Claridge et al., 1999[47] Case series	5 Trauma patients	HFOV used as rescue therapy for refractory hypoxemia P/F improved significantly in all patients with HFOV	No complications reported Mortality: 20% (1 of 5)
Mehta et al., 2001[33] Prospective clinical study	24 ARDS	HFOV used in pts with refractory hypoxemia HFOV: significant increase in P/F, reduction in F_{IO_2} Hemodynamics: HFOV associated with increases in PAOP and CVP; decrease in CO, but no change in BP More CMV days prior to HFOV associated with death	2 (8.3%) pts with pneumothorax 30-day mortality: 66%
Cartotto et al., 2001[48] Retrospective study	6 Burn patients	All pts had rapid and significant improvements in P/F and OI by 12 hours ($P =0.02$) HFOV used in the operating room, permitting surgery in 4 pts who were otherwise too unstable	No complications reported Mortality: 5 out of 6 pts (83%), but not from oxygenation failure
Derdak et al., 2002[35] Prospective, 13-center, randomized controlled trial	148 ARDS	HFOV group: early improvement in P/F, but no difference beyond 24 hours No differences in hemodynamics, oxygenation/ventilation failure, barotrauma, or mucous plugging between groups Fewer CMV days prior to HFOV was a predictor of survival	No difference in complications 30 day mortality: 37% HFOV vs. 52% CV ($P =0.102$)
Andersen et al., 2002[49] Retrospective study	16 ARDS	HFOV associated with significant increase in P/F and no hemodynamic compromise	1 (6.3%) pt had pneumothorax Mortality: 31% (5 of 16)
Mehta et al., 2003[50] Prospective observational study	23 ARDS	83% pts had significant increase in P/F with the addition of iNO (5 to 20 ppm) during HFOV	5 (21.7%) pts had pneumothorax; Mortality: 61%
David et al., 2003[34] Prospective observational study	42 ARDS	HFOV associated with significant increase in P/F. More CMV days and failure to improve oxygenation within 24 h of HFOV associated with greater mortality	1 (2.4%) pt had pneumothorax, Mortality 43% (18 of 42)
Mehta et al., 2004[37] Retrospective study	156 ARDS	P/F ratios and OI improved significantly with HFOV Independent predictors of death: older age, higher APACHE II, lower pH, more CMV days prior to HFOV	HFOV discontinued in 19 pts (12%) for oxygenation, ventilation, or hemodynamics Pneumothorax: 34 pts (21.8%) Mortality: 61.7%
Ferguson et al., 2005[29] Prospective (pilot) clinical study	25 ARDS	Pilot study demonstrating safety and efficacy of combining RM with HFOV for rapid and sustained improvement in O_2	Barotrauma in 8%, RM aborted in 3.3% for hypotension Mortality: 44%
Papazian et al., 2005[51] Prospective comparative randomized study	39 ARDS	Evaluated HFOV, prone, or the combination Prone: improved oxygenation, reduced lung inflammation Prone-HFOV: improved oxygenation, higher BALF indexes of inflammation Supine-HFOV: did not improve gas exchange and associated with enhanced lung inflammation	1 (2.5%) pt had mucous plugging requiring change of ETT
Bollen et al., 2005[36] Prospective, four-center, randomized controlled trial	61 ARDS	Trial prematurely stopped for low enrollment HFOV group: OI response higher than CMV group between first and second day	No difference in therapy failure or barotrauma Mortality: 43% HFOV, 33% CMV
Pachl et al., 2006[52] Prospective clinical study	30 ARDS	HFOV more effective at alveolar recruitment in extrapulmonary vs. pulmonary ARDS	Complications not reported No difference in mortality
Finkielman et al., 2006[53] Retrospective study	14 ARDS	HFOV used as rescue therapy in pts with hypoxemia P/F ratios and OI improved significantly with HFOV	1pt had hypotension No barotrauma Mortality: 57%
Demory D et al., 2007[54] Prospective randomized comparative study	43 ARDS	HFOV maintained improvement in oxygenation related to prone positioning when ARDS patients returned to supine position	No pulmonary or cardiovascular complications
Mentzelopoulos et al., 2007[55] Prospective, randomized, physiologic, crossover study	14 ARDS	Evaluated acute effects of HFOV combined with tracheal gas insufflation (TGI) Short-term, HFO-TGI improved oxygenation relative to HFOV and ARDS network CMV	None reported
Fessler et al., 2008[23] Observational study	30 ARDS	A study evaluating very high frequency ventilation Most patients maintain adequate gas exchange using f > 5-6 Hz	Pneumothorax occurred in 6 (20%) 13 (43%) pts required paralysis Mortality: 63%
Mentzelopoulos et al., 2010[56] Prospective, randomized, physiologic crossover study	22 ARDS	HFOV combined with TGI compared with HFOV at two different mean airway pressures, an equivalent pressure, and a pressure 3 cm H_2O higher than preceding CMV HFOV combined with TGI produced superior gas exchange than HFOV alone	None reported

ARDS, Acute respiratory distress syndrome; *BALF,* bronchoalveolar lavage fluid; *BP,* blood pressure; *CMV,* conventional mechanical ventilation; *CVP,* central venous pressure; *ETT,* endotracheal tube; *HFOV,* high-frequency oscillatory ventilation; *iNO,* inhaled nitric oxide; *OI,* oxygenation index; *PAOP,* pulmonary artery occlusion pressure; *P/F,* partial pressure of oxygen/fractional inspired oxygen ratio; *ppm,* parts per million; *Pt(s),* patient(s); *RM,* recruitment maneuver; *TGI,* tracheal gas insufflation.

TABLE 52-3	Systematic Reviews Evaluating High-Frequency Oscillatory Ventilation in Adults with Acute Respiratory Distress Syndrome	
Publication	**Number of Studies/Patients**	**Study Summary/Major Findings**
Bollen et al., 2005[57] Systematic review	ARDS 2 RCT 7 Observational studies	Systematic review of determinants of mortality in HFOV in ARDS Prolonged CMV prior to HFOV did not relate to mortality OI associated with mortality independently of other disease markers and could be important for selecting ARDS pt that could benefit from HFOV
Wunsch et al., 2004[58] Cochrane Systematic Review [Abstract]	ARDS 2 RCTs Children, N=58 Adult, N=148	Systematic review comparing HFOV and CMV Inadequate evidence to conclude whether HFOV reduces morbidity or mortality in pts with ALI or ARDS
Sud et al., 2010[44] Systematic review and meta-analysis	ARDS 8 RCTs N=419	HFOV may improve survival; unlikely to cause harm Reduced mortality (RR 0.77, 95% CI 0.61-0.98) and treatment failure (refractory hypoxemia, hypercapnia, hypotension, barotrauma, RR 0.67, 95% CI 0.46-0.99)

ARDS, Acute respiratory distress syndrome; *CI*, confidence interval; *CMV*, conventional mechanical ventilation; *HFOV*, high-frequency oscillatory ventilation; *OI*, oxygenation index; *Pt(s)*, patient(s); *RCT*, randomized controlled trial; *RR*, risk ratio.

intensivists with the use of high-frequency ventilation. A pilot study by Ferguson et al. found that the combination of recruitment maneuvers and HFOV can be safely applied and results in rapid and sustained improvement in oxygenation.[29]

Complications of High-Frequency Oscillatory Ventilation

HFOV has generally been shown to be safe if applied appropriately. However, as with all modes of mechanical ventilation, there are potential complications.

BAROTRAUMA

Given the higher mean airway pressures applied during HFOV, there is a concern regarding the risk of barotrauma. The incidence of pneumothorax with the use of HFOV in observational studies varies from 2.4%[34] to 21.8%[37]; however, HFOV was generally applied as rescue therapy in patients with severe ARDS, who are likely to already be at greater baseline risk of developing barotrauma. In two published randomized controlled trials[35,36] comparing HFOV with CMV, there was no difference in the incidence of pneumothorax between CMV and HFOV groups.

HEMODYNAMIC INSTABILITY

Another potential effect of a high mean airway pressure, regardless of mode of ventilation, is a reduction in venous return secondary to increased intrathoracic pressure. Thus it is important to consider the patient's volume status prior to and during the transition from CV to HFOV, and consider judicious volume administration to ensure adequate intravascular volume.[20,38]

INADEQUATE HUMIDIFICATION

Inadequate humidification of inspired gas may lead to desiccation of secretions, potentially mucous inspissation and obstruction of the endotracheal tube. This is uncommon during HFOV,[32,33] as adequate humidification can usually be achieved by passing the bias flow of gas through a humidifier.[39] However, problems with endotracheal tube obstruction may occasionally arise and can be indicated by a sudden rise in generated pressure amplitude for a given power setting.

SEDATION AND PARALYSIS

Unlike neonates, the majority of adults require suppression of their respiratory efforts during HFOV so their inspiratory flow rate does not outstrip the provided bias flow. Heavy sedation and occasionally paralysis are required in the majority of patients[37]; patient selection is therefore important to ensure that the severity of illness is sufficiently high to justify the use of sedation and paralysis, given the adverse effects of these agents.[40,41] In contrast to previous literature associating neuromuscular blockade with the development of critical illness polyneuropathy,[42] the early short-term use of paralytic agents has recently been reported to improve survival in patients with ARDS.[43]

The Future of High-Frequency Oscillatory Ventilation

After several decades of research regarding the physiologic principles and clinical application of HFOV (and high-frequency ventilation in general), many questions have been addressed, but other important issues remain unresolved, particularly regarding the utility of HFOV as a primary mode for reducing mortality in adults with ARDS. The optimal settings to maximize lung protection, lung recruitment, and gas exchange are unclear for many modes of high-frequency ventilation. Nonetheless, advances have been made with the use of HFOV, with evidence demonstrating that targeting lung recruitment and delivering low tidal volumes may be the optimal strategy to reduce the risk of overdistention injury and cyclic alveolar collapse, utilizing alternative gas transport mechanisms.

One of the most important questions regarding HFOV is whether it truly improves mortality when compared to lung-protective conventional ventilation. To date, several small studies[35,36] and a meta-analysis[44] suggest that HFOV may be beneficial, but there are issues with many of these studies which used antiquated strategies for both CMV and HFOV. For the definitive answer to this question, we will need to await the results of two large phase 3 studies comparing HFOV with best current conventional ventilation.[45,46]

Conclusion

All high-frequency ventilation modes are characterized by small tidal volumes delivered at high frequencies, which utilize alternative mechanisms to achieve adequate gas exchange. Evolving understanding of VILI has prompted clinicians to apply mechanical ventilators in a way that minimizes such injury—so-called lung-protective ventilation. The mechanical characteristics of high-frequency ventilation make it well suited for use in the injured lung, because it may reduce volutrauma-type injury while achieving higher mean airway pressures and maintaining end-expiratory lung volume, thus reducing cyclic collapse. Clinical experience with high-frequency ventilation, particularly high-frequency oscillatory ventilation, has found it to be a safe and effective mode for improving oxygenation in neonatal and adult populations failing conventional mechanical ventilation. It may also be advantageous to apply HFOV early in the course of ARDS to avoid VILI related to aggressive conventional mechanical ventilator settings. Despite these initial promising results, however, we await the results of ongoing large clinical trials to determine the optimal place for HFOV in clinical ARDS management—either as rescue therapy for patients failing conventional ventilation or potentially as primary therapy to reduce mortality.

KEY POINTS

1. High-frequency ventilation is a method of mechanical ventilation that uses very small tidal volumes at high frequencies. The most commonly used modes include high-frequency jet ventilation and high-frequency oscillatory ventilation.

2. Ventilator-induced lung injury can be a clinically important consequence of mechanical ventilation in patients with respiratory failure, particularly those with underlying acute lung injury. Volutrauma from high transpulmonary pressures, atelectrauma, and oxygen toxicity may all contribute to lung injury, and mechanical ventilation strategies should attempt to mitigate these injurious forces.

3. Despite the recent clinical success of conventional lung-protective ventilation strategies, they do not completely prevent lung injury and may be associated with other clinical problems such as respiratory acidosis.

4. Experimental models suggest that high-frequency ventilation may mitigate ventilator-induced lung injury.

5. In adults, high-frequency oscillatory ventilation has been shown to be safe and effective as salvage therapy for patients with hypoxic respiratory failure deemed to be failing conventional mechanical ventilation.

6. Despite recent clinical validation of high-frequency ventilation in adults with respiratory distress, significant research remains to be done to determine the best application of high-frequency ventilation modes.

ANNOTATED REFERENCES

Derdak S, Mehta S, Stewart TE, et al. High-frequency oscillatory ventilation for acute respiratory distress syndrome in adults: a randomized, controlled trial. Am J Respir Crit Care Med 2002;166(6):801-8.
This trial represents the first prospective, randomized clinical trial comparing conventional mechanical ventilation and high-frequency oscillatory ventilation (HFOV) early in the course of ARDS. It found HFOV to be effective and safe, with a trend toward decreased mortality in patients randomized to receive it. Of note, pre-enrollment conventional ventilation for more than 5 days was predictive of mortality.

Easley RB, Lancaster CT, Fuld MK, et al. Total and regional lung volume changes during high-frequency oscillatory ventilation of the normal lung. Respir Physiol Neurobiol 2009;165(1):54-60.
This animal study used computer tomographic imaging to quantify lung volumes. The authors demonstrated that HFOV resulted in no major regional differences in lung volume distribution, suggesting that occult lung overdistention is not a significant risk.

Fessler HE, Hager DN, Brower RG. Feasibility of very high-frequency ventilation in adults with acute respiratory distress syndrome. Crit Care Med 2008;36(4):1043-8.
This clinical study showed that adequate gas exchange can be maintained on the high-frequency ventilator in adults at frequencies well above 5 to 6 Hz. The authors also suggested that higher frequencies should minimize tidal volumes, and it may be speculated that it has a role in reducing ventilatory-induced lung injury.

Hager DN, Fessler HE, Kaczka DW, et al. Tidal volume delivery during high-frequency oscillatory ventilation in adults with acute respiratory distress syndrome. Crit Care Med 2007;35(6):1522-9.
This laboratory (utilizing a test lung) and clinical study (on ARDS patients) demonstrated that HFOV did deliver small but not uniform low tidal volume (23.1-225.3 ml and 0.8-3.3 mL/kg, respectively). This study also demonstrated that tidal volumes decrease with increasing frequency, increase with pressure amplitude, and that endotracheal internal diameter is an important determinant of tidal volume.

Mehta S, Lapinsky SE, Hallett DC, et al. Prospective trial of high-frequency oscillation in adults with acute respiratory distress syndrome. Crit Care Med 2001;29(7):1360-9.
This prospective clinical study established the safety and efficacy of HFOV as salvage therapy in adults with ARDS failing conventional mechanical ventilation. HFOV was safe and effective at improving oxygenation, and prolonged conventional ventilation before switching to the high-frequency mode was predictive of death, suggesting the need for further investigation into the timing of high-frequency ventilation.

Sud S, Sud M, Friedrich JO, et al. High frequency oscillation in patients with acute lung injury and acute respiratory distress syndrome (ARDS): systematic review and meta-analysis. BMJ 2010;340:c2327.
This is the latest systemic review and meta-analysis, which suggests that high-frequency oscillation might improve survival and is unlikely to cause harm.

REFERENCES

Access the complete reference list online at http://www.expertconsult.com.

53

Extracorporeal Life Support for Cardiopulmonary Failure

ROBERT H. BARTLETT

Extracorporeal life support (ECLS) or extracorporeal membrane oxygenation (ECMO) involve the use of mechanical devices during life-threatening cardiac or pulmonary failure. ECMO can provide partial or total support, is temporary, and requires systemic anticoagulation. ECMO is not a treatment; it is a life-support system that allows time for evaluation, diagnosis, and treatment of the condition which caused heart or lung failure. The indication for ECMO is high risk of mortality despite and after optimal treatment.

ECMO controls gas exchange and perfusion, stabilizes the patient physiologically, decreases the risk of ongoing ventilator- or vasopressor-induced iatrogenic injury, and allows ample time for diagnosis, treatment, and recovery from the primary injury or disease. Right atrial venous blood is drained through a large cannula, pumped through an artificial lung and back into the patient, either into the aorta (venoarterial [VA]) or into the right atrium (venovenous [VV] mode). VA access puts the artificial lung in parallel with the native lungs and substitutes for both heart and lung function. VV access puts the artificial lung in series with the native lung. These modes of access are shown in Figures 53-1 and 53-2. For respiratory failure, VV access is preferred because normal hemodynamics are maintained, and there is little risk of systemic embolism. For total support in either mode, the blood flow required is 60 to 100 mL/kg/min (the entire cardiac output); large-bore, low-resistance cannulas are required to achieve this amount of flow. The flow is limited by resistance in the venous access catheter. For vascular access, the cannulas are placed via the large vessels in the neck or groin. Cannulas can be placed by direct cutdown access to these vessels or, more commonly, via percutaneous placement over a guide-wire. After cannulas are placed, the circuit primed with crystalloid solution is attached, heparin is given for anticoagulation, and extracorporeal flow is established at 50 to 100 mL/kg/min. The membrane lung is ventilated with 100% oxygen.

When adequate extracorporeal flow and gas exchange are achieved, the ventilator is turned down to resting settings (typically F_{IO_2} 0.3, pressure 20/10, rate 4). In many cases, the patient can be extubated, and the extracorporeal circuit takes over all respiratory and cardiac function. As the native heart and lungs improve, the extracorporeal flow is decreased proportionately, and when heart and lung function are fully restored, the patient is weaned from extracorporeal support, and cannulas are removed.

The major complication associated with ECMO is bleeding, which occurs in 10% to 30% of patients. Bleeding is managed by reducing or discontinuing the heparin infusion, optimizing the native coagulation status, and direct surgical control. Failure of the membrane lung or pump occurs in less than 5% of patients and is managed by replacing the device. Other uncommon complications are related to cannulation, systemic air embolism, thromboembolism, and infection.

ECMO is used in a variety of clinical circumstances, and results depend on the primary indication. ECMO provides life support, but it is not treatment. The clinical outcome depends on the response to treatment for the primary condition. Because ECMO is a life-support technique, the primary outcome variable is survival. Survival outcome for nine categories of patients is shown in Figure 53-3. Survival ranges from 30% in extracorporeal cardiopulmonary resuscitation (ECPR) to 95% for neonatal meconium aspiration syndrome.

The devices for extracorporeal support used in the past carried a significant risk of blowout, air embolism or thromboembolism, and device failure. The current generation of devices are much simpler and inherently safer. The major change is in the membrane lung. The Kolobow spiral coil membrane lung[1] has been reliably used for ECMO for over 30 years. This membrane lung works well for weeks at a time but has an affinity for platelets, causing thrombocytopenia, and has high blood flow resistance, requiring high pressure generated by the pump for high blood flow. When centrifugal pumps are used to generate high pressure, hemolysis and thrombosis can occur, so most of the experience with ECMO has been with modified roller pumps.

The new membrane lungs from Maquet, Novalung, Medos, and Dideco are nonporous hollow fiber devices with low blood flow resistance, allowing safe use of the centrifugal pumps designed for prolonged use (e.g., Maquet Rotaflow, Levitronix Centrimag). The polymethylpentene fibers in these lungs, combined with nonthrombogenic coatings, decrease the need for platelet transfusion and for continuous heparin infusion in some cases. New vascular access devices have wire-reinforced walls, allowing very thin cannula walls to minimize blood flow resistance.

The major use of ECLS has gone from neonatal respiratory failure to many causes of cardiorespiratory failure in all age groups. The Extracorporeal Life Support Organization (ELSO; elso@med.umich.edu) is an international consortium of medical centers with major ECMO programs. ELSO maintains a registry of ECMO cases. The types of cases represented in the ELSO Registry are shown in Figure 53-3. The indications, practice management, and outcome are quite different in each of these patient groups.

Neonatal Respiratory Failure

The major application of ECMO began with neonatal respiratory failure. The first successful case was reported in 1975, and ECMO became standard treatment in major neonatal centers.[2] In retrospect, the reason for this success was that regardless of primary diagnosis, the major pathophysiology in neonatal respiratory failure is persistent fetal circulation (PFC), a condition that is almost always reversible in a few days. In the early 1980s, PFC was treated by hyperventilation to induce alkalosis, which is damaging to the neonatal lung. ECMO eliminated this iatrogenic injury and allowed time for PFC to resolve. Neonatal ECMO was proven effective and beneficial in four prospective randomized trials, an effect that was confirmed in a Cochrane meta-analysis.[3-7] A major lesson learned from the neonatal experience was the advantage of resting the native lungs by extracorporeal support.

Inhaled nitric oxide administered with high-frequency oscillation was shown to be effective treatment for PFC in the 1990s.[8,9] The need for extracorporeal support thereafter decreased significantly. The exception is PFC combined with lung hypoplasia in congenital diaphragmatic hernia patients. This condition is now the primary indication for ECMO in newborn infants. Vascular access in neonates is always gained via the neck vessels, usually by placement of a double-lumen catheter into the right atrium via the jugular vein.

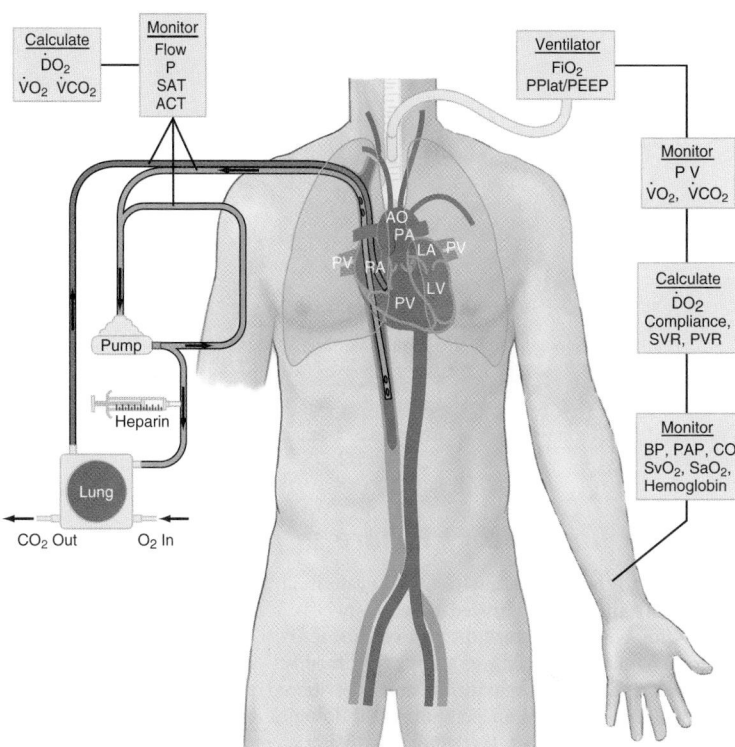

Figure 53-1 Venovenous (VV) access via a double-lumen cannula in the right atrium. Extracorporeal blood flow mixes with native venous return in the right atrium and ventricle. If there is no native lung function, systemic arterial saturation is 75% to 85%. Parameters in the boxes are measured and used to control the system.

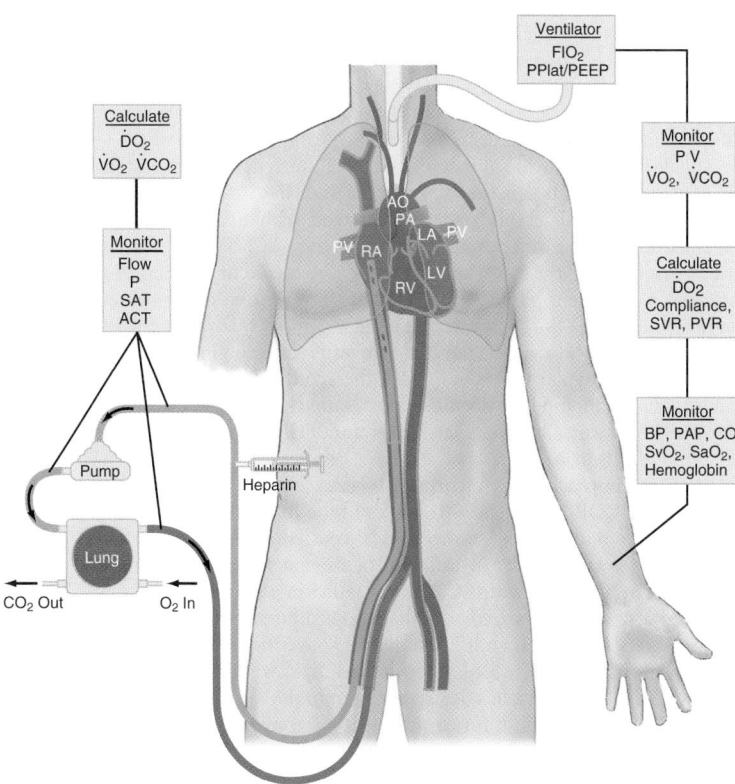

Figure 53-2 Venoarterial (VA) access via the femoral vessels. Extracorporeal blood flow in the aorta is retrograde and mixes with native blood flow in the proximal aorta. Parameters in the boxes are measured and used to control the system.

Pediatric Respiratory Failure

Severe respiratory failure in children arises from a wide range of conditions including viral infections in infants and trauma in 18-year-olds. The indication for ECMO is failure to respond to optimal ventilator and supportive care. Vascular access is venovenous, usually with a double-lumen catheter placed via the jugular vein. Green demonstrated the efficacy of ECMO in pediatric respiratory failure in a matched-pairs analysis using a large multicenter database.[10] In that analysis, survival with ECMO was 75% compared to 50% with conventional management.[10]

ELSO Registry Data		July 2010			
	Total Patients	Survived ECLS		Survived to DC	
Neonatal					
Respiratory	24,017	20,346	85%	18,044	75%
Cardiac	4,103	2,474	60%	1,603	39%
ECPR	586	373	64%	224	38%
Pediatric					
Respiratory	4,635	3,002	65%	2,575	56%
Cardiac	5,026	3,179	63%	2,386	47%
ECPR	1,128	594	53%	442	39%
Adult					
Respiratory	2,121	1,319	62%	1,124	53%
Cardiac	1,238	598	48%	424	34%
ECPR	476	179	38%	137	29%
Total	43,330	32,064	74%	26,959	62%

Figure 53-3   Summary of cases in the ELSO registry in 2010 (elso.med.umich.edu).

Adult Respiratory Failure

Hill reported the first successful ECMO case in an adult with respiratory failure in 1972.[11] This led to a prospective randomized trial of ECMO in acute respiratory distress syndrome (ARDS) in 1975-1978. After 90 patients, the trial was stopped for futility.[12] In retrospect, this study was undertaken prematurely in inexperienced centers using conventional and ECMO management methodologies that would not be used today. Nonetheless, the report of this trial essentially stopped research on ECMO for ARDS for many years. Over the ensuing decades, a few centers reported 50% survival in severe ARDS.[13] A second prospective randomized trail was conducted in the United Kingdom from 2004-2007, within which the best conventional care in many intensive care units (ICUs) was compared to protocolized care including ECMO in a single center.[14] Twenty-eight day survival was 76% in protocolized care compared to 50% with conventional care. Six-month survival free of disability was 63% versus 47%.

The H1N1 worldwide flu epidemic in 2009 renewed interest in ECMO for ARDS. Investigators in Australia and New Zealand reported 78% survival in 68 H1N1 patients managed with ECMO.[15] In the recent studies suggesting benefit with ECMO, new ECMO devices were used, emphasizing the safety and simplicity of the second generation of ECMO. At present, vascular access is gained by a large double-lumen catheter placed via the right internal jugular vein, or by drainage from the inferior vena cava via the femoral vein and reinfusion into the right atrium via the jugular vein. On ECMO, the ventilator is set at rest settings to avoid ongoing iatrogenic injury. Native lung function usually becomes even worse before it gets better and, ECLS support is usually required for 10 to 20 days.

Another approach to extracorporeal gas exchange is selective CO_2 removal (ECCOR).[16] In ECCOR, a membrane lung is used with low blood flow to remove CO_2, so mechanical ventilation is not necessary, and oxygen is supplied by insufflation of the native lungs. Gattinoni reported 56% survival with ECCOR in ARDS in 1986.[17] Morris later reported a small randomized trial that showed no survival difference between patients treated with ECCOR and conventional therapy.[18]

ECCOR has been studied and refined by Zwischenberger and others.[19] ECCOR using a low-resistance membrane lung perfused by a femoral arterial venous shunt or pumped VV access is being studied in the management of ARDS in Europe. ECCOR is ideal for CO_2 retention syndromes like status asthmaticus but does not provide sufficient oxygenation for full respiratory support.

Lung transplantation has been very successful in the management of end-stage lung disease but is rarely considered in intubated ventilated patients because nosocomial pneumonia and multiple organ failure usually occur before a donor is found. ECMO is rarely used as a bridge to transplant for the same reason.[20] In addition, many patients with respiratory failure awaiting lung transplant have right ventricular failure requiring venoarterial access.[21] Recently, some centers have reported success with ECMO as a bridge to lung transplantation, using an implantable (paracorporeal) membrane lung allowing extubation, ambulation, and rehabilitation while bridging to lung transplantation.[22]

Cardiac Failure in Children

The major application of ECMO today is to support children with profound cardiac failure.[23] Most of these patients are infants who show cardiovascular deterioration immediately after operations for congenital heart disease. Support with VA ECLS is used as a bridge to recovery from myocardial stunning, and if recovery does not occur, as a bridge to a cardiac-assist device and perhaps transplantation.[24] Other applications for ECMO include myocarditis and myocardiopathy. Venoarterial access is required via the neck vessels or using direct cardiac cannulas if the chest is already open.

Cardiac Failure in Adults

Unlike the pediatric population, the major application of ECLS in adult cardiac failure is cardiogenic shock following myocardial infarction, myocardiopathy, myocarditis, or inability to come off cardiopulmonary bypass following cardiac operation.[25-27] Venoarterial access is required in these settings. The femoral vessels are used in almost all cases because of a 10% to 15% incidence of stroke when the carotid artery is used in patients with profound shock or cardiac arrest. Vascular access is usually percutaneous, although direct cutdown access is the most reliable in patients with profound cardiogenic shock. Centers in Paris[28] and Taiwan[29] have reported a large experience in cardiogenic shock using ECMO to stabilize hemodynamics while proceeding to cardiac catheterization and revascularization of the myocardium if needed, followed by cardiac recovery or bridging to a ventricular assist device and perhaps transplantation.

Extracorporeal Support During Cardiopulmonary Resuscitation

Extracorporeal support during cardiopulmonary resuscitation (ECPR) is the extension of VA support in cardiogenic shock to patients in overt cardiac arrest.[30,31] Venoarterial access is used, usually by direct vessel exposure. The neck vessels are used for children up to the age of 5 or 6, and the femoral vessels for older children and adults. The use of ECPR requires having a primed circuit and a cannulation team immediately available. With the new simplified devices, and with appropriate training of emergency room physicians, the use of ECPR is increasing in major academic hospitals.

Other Applications of ECMO

ECMO is being investigated for applications to other conditions where perfusion and gas-exchange support is needed. Controlled warming after accidental hypothermia has been reported with ECMO.[32] A major advantage for ECMO compared to conventional techniques is to avoid or treat the cardiac arrhythmias that often occur during rewarming. Maclaren and others from Australia have reported the use of ECMO in profound septic shock in children.[33] They found that very high blood flow achieved with direct cardiac vascular access led to 75% survival in profound septic shock. When the team and circuit can be quickly assembled in the setting of massive pulmonary embolism, the results are very good.[34] The management of prematurity using ECMO as an artificial placenta to avoid intubation and mechanical ventilation is being studied in the laboratory.

The major limitation to organ transplantation is availability of donors. The largest potential source of donors is donation after cardiac death (DCD). However, this technique is rarely used because of poor organ function and long periods of lung ischemia. Several centers are using VA ECMO after cardiac death to resuscitate abdominal organs[35] and lungs to transplantable status.[36] Organs resuscitated in this fashion function as well or better than those obtained from conventional brain-dead donors.

Extracorporeal Life Support in the Future

The first generation of membrane lungs and pumps was expensive, cumbersome, difficult to manage, and limited to specialized teams in dedicated centers, primarily in children's hospitals. The next generation of equipment and access devices makes ECLS much simpler, safer, less complicated, and easier to manage in any ICU. With these devices, the major limitation to widespread application is the need for anticoagulation and the associated bleeding complications. With the new devices, bleeding still occurs but is rarely a fatal complication. Research on nonthrombogenic surfaces holds the promise of prolonged extracorporeal circulation without anticoagulation and without bleeding.

ANNOTATED REFERENCES

Hill JD, O'Brien TG, Murray JJ, et al. Prolonged extracorporeal oxygenation for acute post-traumatic respiratory failure (shock-lung syndrome). Use of the Bramson membrane lung. N Engl J Med 1972;286(12):629-34.
The first successful case of ECLS in adult respiratory failure.
Bartlett RH, Gazzaniga AB, Jefferies MR, Huxtable RF, Haiduc NJ, Fong SW. Extracorporeal membrane oxygenation (ECMO) cardiopulmonary support in infancy. Trans Am Soc Artif Intern Organs 1976;22:80-93.
The first successful cases of cardiac and neonatal ECLS.
Bartlett RH, Roloff DW, Cornell RG, Andrews AF, Dillon PW, Zwischenberger JB. Extracorporeal circulation in neonatal respiratory failure: a prospective randomized study. Pediatrics 1985;76(4):479-87.
The prospective randomized trial of ECMO in neonatal respiratory failure.

Gattinoni L, Pesenti A, Mascheroni D, et al. Low-frequency positive-pressure ventilation with extracorporeal CO$_2$ removal in severe acute respiratory failure. JAMA 1986;256(7):881-6.
The first case series of ECCOR in ARDS.
Peek GJ, Mugford M, Tiruvoipati R, et al. Efficacy and economic assessment of conventional ventilatory support versus extracorporeal membrane oxygenation for severe adult respiratory failure (CESAR): a multicentre randomised controlled trial. Lancet 2009;374(9698):1351-63.
The randomized trial of protocol care including ECMO in ARDS.
Combes A, Leprince P, Luyt CE, et al. Outcomes and long-term quality-of-life of patients supported by extracorporeal membrane oxygenation for refractory cardiogenic shock. Crit Care Med 2008;36(5):1404-11.
The major series of ECMO in adult cardiogenic shock.

REFERENCES

Access the complete reference list online at http://www.expertconsult.com.

54

Adjunctive Respiratory Therapy

SANJAY MANOCHA | KEITH R. WALLEY

Many critically ill patients are unable to effectively clear secretions that accumulate in the central and peripheral airways. This can be due to factors such as increased secretion production, impaired cough reflex, weakness, and pain. The presence of an endotracheal tube prevents closure of the glottis to generate the high expiratory pressures necessary for an effective cough, thereby promoting the retention of secretions. In addition, in critically ill patients, cilia in the pulmonary tree are impaired in function and reduced in number.[1,2] This leads to an increased risk of aspiration, atelectasis, and pneumonia, which are all detrimental in the critically ill patient.

Adjunctive respiratory therapy is able to prevent and treat respiratory complications that are encountered in the critically ill patient. As highlighted in Table 54-1, measures available range from those that are simple to institute, such as proper body positioning and suctioning, to more complex interventions such as chest physiotherapy, bronchoscopy, and use of aerosolized/inhaled medications that act directly on the pulmonary system.

Methods to Improve Pulmonary Mucociliary Clearance

PERCUSSION

Percussion of the chest can aid in secretion clearance. It is performed by clapping cupped hands over the thorax in a rhythmic fashion or using mechanical devices that mimic the same action. The energy of the force generated by the cupped hands is transmitted through the thorax to dislodge secretions. When used in conjunction with postural drainage, this is an effective method to mobilize secretions from the pulmonary tract. It is a technique often used in the daily management of cystic fibrosis patients[3] and those with severe bronchiectasis.

HIGH-FREQUENCY CHEST COMPRESSION

High-frequency chest compression (HFCC) relies on rapid pressure changes to the respiratory system during expiration to enhance movement of mucus from the peripheral airways to the central airways for clearance. This method employs an automated vest device worn by the patient. The vest is attached to an air-pulse generator, and small volumes of gas are introduced into it at a rapid rate ranging from 5 to 25 Hz, producing pressures up to 50 cm H_2O. This technique, mainly used in cystic fibrosis patients, is equivalent to conventional chest physiotherapy techniques of percussion and postural drainage.[4-6] One study examined the use of HFCC in nine long-term mechanically ventilated patients.[7] In this small observational study, HFCC was compared to percussion and postural drainage. No difference was seen in the amount of sputum production, oxygen saturation, or patient comfort between the two methods, but HFCC was determined to be safe and felt to save staff time. It is difficult to apply this technique to most critically ill patients because of the size of the vest; covering the thorax may prevent adequate monitoring.

MANUAL HYPERINFLATION

Manual hyperinflation with an inflation bag and using high tidal volumes involves disconnecting the patient from the ventilator. Typically the lungs are inflated slowly to 1.5 to 2 times the tidal volume or

to peak airway pressures of 40 cm H_2O (as measured by a manometer) and then at end inspiration with an inspiratory pause to allow for filling of alveoli with slow time constants. This is followed by a quick release to allow for rapid expiration. The goal of manual hyperinflation is to recruit atelectatic lung regions to improve oxygenation and improve clearance of secretions. Similar to recruitment maneuvers described with mechanical ventilators, manual hyperinflation leads to only transient improvements in oxygenation, without any long-term clinically significant improvement in outcomes.[8-12] It also has the disadvantage of requiring a ventilator disconnect, and this method can be mimicked by a mechanical ventilator.[13]

Contraindications to manual hyperinflation include hemodynamic compromise and elevated intracranial pressure. There is also a risk of barotrauma due to preferential inflation of open lung regions that are highly compliant compared to collapsed regions.

POSITIONING AND MOBILIZATION

Mobilization of patients in the intensive care unit (ICU) either through active or passive limb exercises may improve overall patient well being and, in the long term, may lead to better patient outcomes. In a recent randomized controlled trial of ventilated patients, the addition of early physiotherapy and occupational therapy to daily interruption of sedation resulted in slightly more ventilator-free days and improved functional capacity.[14]

Positioning also plays an important role in improving physiology and outcome in critically ill patients. Position of the patient with the head of the bed elevated at least 30 degrees significantly reduces the risk of aspiration and ventilator-associated pneumonia.[15] Upright positioning of patients in whom there is no contraindication improves lung volumes and therefore gas exchange and work of breathing, especially in those where the supine or semirecumbent position leads to increased work of breathing. In some individuals with unilateral lung disease, positioning with the affected side up can lead to improved ventilation/perfusion ($\dot{V}/\dot{Q}$) matching by increasing perfusion to the dependent "good" side.[16,17] If atelectasis secondary to retained secretions is the cause, having the affected side up leads to improved postural drainage.

Postural drainage involves positioning the body to allow gravity to assist in the movement of secretions and is indicated in patients with sputum production of more than 25 to 30 mL/day who have difficulty clearing their secretions.[18] In cystic fibrosis, postural drainage with percussion is an effective method to clear pulmonary secretions and is associated with improved lung function.[19,20]

TRACHEAL SUCTION

Used in conjunction with other techniques to mobilize secretions from the peripheral to the central airways, suctioning is an effective way of removing secretions to improve bronchial hygiene. It can be performed using open methods where the patient is disconnected from the ventilator and a disposable suction catheter is placed. The closed system involves a suction catheter placed in a protective sheath and directly connected to the ventilator circuit. No disconnect is required, and the risk of environmental cross-contamination is reduced. Routine changes of in-line suction catheters are not required and are cost-effective.[21,22] Overall, the risk of nosocomial pneumonia between the two systems is not different.[23-25]

TABLE 54-1	Adjunctive Respiratory Therapies

Methods to Improve Pulmonary Mucociliary Clearance

Chest physiotherapy:
- Percussion
- Postural drainage
- Chest vibration

Suctioning:
- Oropharyngeal suctioning
- Nasopharyngeal suctioning
- Endotracheal suctioning

Continuous lateral rotation
Positive expiratory pressure devices
Forced expiration
Closed chest oscillation
Bronchoscopy
Manual hyperinflation
Bronchodilators
Mucoactive agents

Methods to Improve Lung Expansion

Deep breathing
Incentive spirometry
Intermittent positive ventilation
Optimum body position

Methods to Improve Oxygenation and Ventilation

Inhaled vasodilators:
- Nitric oxide
- Prostaglandins

Helium-oxygen (heliox)

Because of the anatomic arrangement of the large central airways, most often a suction catheter enters the right main bronchus over the left side. Specially designed curved-tipped "left sided" suction catheters increase the likelihood of suctioning from the left mainstem bronchus.

Nasotracheal suctioning has fallen out of favor over direct tracheal suctioning and should only be considered in patients who are able to protect their airway and in conjunction with assisted coughs and other forms of chest physiotherapy.

Complications with suctioning include hypoxemia, especially in the setting of a ventilator disconnect, increased intracranial pressure with vigorous stimulation of the airways, mechanical trauma to the trachea, bronchospasm, and bacterial contamination of the airways. All patients should be preoxygenated with 100% oxygen for 1 or 2 minutes prior to suctioning. To reduce the risk of agitation, the patient should be informed before tracheal suctioning is performed. The suctioning should be limited to 15 to 20 seconds, and the suction port on the catheter should be opened and closed intermittently but not closed for more than 5 seconds at a time.

CONTINUOUS ROTATION THERAPY

Continuous rotational or kinetic therapy extends the practice of regular 2-hourly repositioning of patients from one side to the other by placing the patient on a bed that moves to preprogrammed angles on a more frequent basis or through the use of air mattresses that deflate alternatively from side to side to provide postural position changes. Most studies demonstrate a lower incidence of nosocomial pneumonia or atelectasis.[26-32] Only one small randomized trial found a reduction in duration of mechanical ventilation and length of stay, which was not confirmed in other prior studies.[33]

ASSISTED COUGHING

Assisted coughing is often required in spontaneously breathing patients who have an ineffective cough. Techniques include "huffing" in the setting of an open glottis, where in expiration the patient forcibly exhales quickly several times. Other maneuvers include abdominal or thoracic compression on expiration to generate high intrathoracic pressures mimicking a cough.

POSITIVE EXPIRATORY PRESSURE THERAPY

Positive expiratory pressure therapy (PEP) involves use of a facemask or mouthpiece that provides resistance to airflow of 10 to 20 cm H_2O on expiration. After repeating this maneuver a number of times, mucus in the peripheral airways is mobilized and moved toward the larger airways to be coughed or expelled with other techniques. The use of PEP in critically ill patients who are spontaneously breathing is likely limited because of the coordination involved for slow expirations. Other methods to aid in secretion clearance may be easier to perform in this patient population.

BRONCHOSCOPY

Fiberoptic bronchoscopy has the advantage of providing direct visualization of the airways and permits suctioning of specific segments where secretions may be retained, causing problems such as atelectasis. The role of bronchoscopy in the ICU is reviewed elsewhere, but it can be considered an adjunctive therapy for the treatment of atelectasis or removal of secretions. As a recent review highlighted,[29,34] bronchoscopy is a moderately effective technique for the treatment of atelectasis in the critically ill patient, with success rates ranging from 19% to 89% depending on the extent of atelectasis (lobar atelectasis responds better than subsegmental atelectasis). When compared with aggressive multimodal chest physiotherapy in the only randomized trial, no difference in the rate of resolution was seen between the two methods.[35] Because bronchoscopy is an invasive procedure, it is not without associated risks and complications: sedation required for the procedure, transient increases in intracranial pressure, hypoxemia, and hemodynamic consequences/arrhythmias. Therefore bronchoscopy cannot be recommended as first-line therapy except in situations such as extensive unilateral atelectasis leading to significant difficulties in oxygenating or ventilating that have not resolved with other methods such as suctioning.

CHEST PHYSIOTHERAPY

Chest physiotherapy is a multimodal therapy with the goals of improving pulmonary function (gas exchange, improved lung compliance, and improved pulmonary mucus clearance). Techniques include percussive therapies (manual or mechanical chest percussion), postural drainage, chest vibration, manual hyperinflation, mobilization, suctioning, and rotational therapy. Overall, chest physiotherapy provides transient improvements in oxygenation and lung compliance, likely secondary to airway clearance and recruitment of atelectatic regions. In specific situations, it may improve outcome and clinical course, such as preventing ventilator-associated pneumonia[36] or acute lobar atelectasis.[37]

Aerosol Therapies

AEROSOLIZATION

Aerosolization of medications is an effective method for drug delivery directly to lungs. The theoretical advantage of this form of therapy includes direct delivery and activity at the site of pathology and the ability to deliver high concentrations with minimal systemic absorption and toxicity. The most common aerosolized therapy is administration of bronchodilators. Other medications that can be administered directly to the lungs include corticosteroids, antibiotics, antifungal agents, surfactant, mucolytic agents, and saline.

The two most common methods of delivery by aerosolization are via nebulization or metered-dose inhalers. *Nebulization* is the process of using a high flow of gas (usually 6–8 L/min) to produce small particles of the liquid medium with the medication of interest. The most common nebulizer uses a pneumatic jet. In the spontaneously breathing patient, approximately 50% of the nebulized liquid is in the respirable range, with a mass median aerodynamic diameter (MMAD) of

1 to 5 μm; approximately 10% reaches the lower respiratory tract/small airways. In mechanically ventilated patients, 1% to 15% of the nebulized liquid and medication is delivered to the lower respiratory tract. Ultrasonic nebulization uses high-frequency ultrasonic waves on the surface of the liquid medium to generate respirable particles. Its use is limited by the expense of the equipment involved.

Metered-dose inhalers (MDI) are pressurized canisters with the drug suspended as a mix of propellants, preservatives, and surfactants. On activation, particles ranging in size from 1 to 2 μm are produced. An MDI used in conjunction with a chamber/spacer device significantly increases drug delivery in both spontaneously breathing patients and when attached to the ventilator circuit—either directly to the endotracheal tube or as part of an in-line device in the inspiratory limb of the Y-piece.

Factors that influence the efficacy of aerosol delivery in the mechanically ventilated patient include[38]:

1. Position of administration in the circuit: an MDI should be closer to the endotracheal tube at the Y-piece and used with a spacer; a pneumatic nebulizer should be at least 30 cm from the Y-piece.
2. Humidification: can decrease aerosol delivery to the respiratory tract because of greater deposition in the ventilator circuit. Higher doses may be required to achieve the desired effect.
3. Timing of delivery: should be delivered during the inspiratory phase to maximize drug delivery.
4. Flow rates: slower inspiratory flow rates (and therefore longer inspiratory time) increase delivery of nebulized medications. A decelerating flow pattern can also increase delivery to the lower airways.
5. Tidal volumes: larger tidal volumes (greater than 500 mL) ensure optimal delivery.
6. Endotracheal tube size: tube sizes less than 7 mm reduce delivery.
7. Density of inhaled gas: low-density gases such as helium-oxygen mixtures increase deposition to the lower airways by increasing laminar flow and producing smaller respirable particle size.

BRONCHODILATORS

Bronchodilators are the most frequently administered aerosolized therapy in critically ill patients. Inhaled β₂-agonists, such as albuterol or fenoterol, are generally well tolerated in the critically ill patient and are known to improve lung mechanics in patients with and without airflow obstruction. In acute lung injury, β₂-agonists may improve lung edema clearance and have additional antiinflammatory properties, although the clinical significance of such therapy has yet to be established.[39-42] Adverse effects (e.g., arrhythmias, hypokalemia) can occur in patients receiving excessive doses where significant systemic absorption is likely. Other bronchodilators including ipratropium bromide can also be effective in patients with increased airway reactivity, especially when used in conjunction with a β₂-agonist. Bronchodilators administered via MDI are equally as effective as a nebulizer in spontaneously breathing patients.[38] In mechanically ventilated patients, the use of nebulization is either equally as good as[43] or less effective[44,45] than an MDI with a spacer. MDI administration has the advantage of easier use without the risk of bacterial contamination and need for adjustment of flow rates.[38]

ANTIBIOTICS

Aerosolization of antibiotics as a form of topical treatment for pulmonary infections has been studied for over 20 years. Theoretical advantages of aerosolized antibiotics include direct therapy to the site of infection at higher concentrations, with a lower risk of systemic absorption and side effects. In chronic pulmonary infective states such as cystic fibrosis and severe bronchiectasis,[46-48] aerosolized antibiotics have a role in reducing bacterial concentrations in the sputum, but they have only be shown to provide clinical long-term benefit in cystic

fibrosis.[48] In the acute infective state, aerosolized antibiotics have no additional benefit compared to parenteral antibiotics.[49-51]

In the intubated or tracheostomized patient, the risk of colonization of the airway is high, with a significant increase in the risk for nosocomial pneumonia. In an observational study of six chronically ventilated patients, aerosolized aminoglycosides (tobramycin or amikacin) eradicated the colonizing bacteria 67% of the time and significantly reduced the levels of inflammatory markers in the sputum.[52] As a preventive measure, a recent meta-analysis of prospective clinical trials of aerosolized aminoglycosides suggested a significant reduction in the development of ventilator-associated pneumonia but no difference in overall mortality.[53] As an adjunct for treatment of ventilator-associated pneumonia, a meta-analysis of five randomized controlled trials suggested a significant improvement in the clinical resolution of pneumonia.[54] Despite the findings, limitations of these analyses must be considered, given the heterogeneity of the trials. In addition, concerns of bacterial resistance must also be considered. Side effects reported in spontaneously breathing patients treated with inhaled tobramycin include increased cough, dyspnea, and chest pain.[46]

The role for aerosolized or instilled (via the endotracheal tube) antibiotics as adjuvants for prevention or treatment of pulmonary infections in the ICU remains to be defined with adequately powered future clinical studies.

MUCOACTIVE AGENTS

In chronic inflammatory lung conditions such as chronic obstructive pulmonary disease (COPD), cystic fibrosis, bronchiectasis, and intubation/tracheostomy, overproduction of mucus and impaired clearance results in complications such as airflow obstruction, atelectasis, and infection. Mucus is primarily composed of water, mucin glycoprotein, cellular debris, neutrophil-derived filamentous actin and DNA, and bacteria.[55] Mucoactive agents can help improve the clearance of mucus secretions.

Expectorant methods such as simple hydration together with oral expectorant medications (e.g., guaifenesin, bromhexine) that act via the vagal-mediated increase in airway secretion to decrease mucus viscosity have not been shown to be effective methods of clearing secretions.[56,57] Oral iodine preparations (e.g., saturated solution of potassium iodide), although described as mucoactive agents, are similarly ineffective and may be associated with significant side effects such as hypothyroidism or hyperkalemia.[55]

Mucolytic agents reduce the viscosity of mucus by breaking down the mucin glycoprotein network or free DNA strands, thereby improving mucus rheology to improve clearance. Aerosolized N-acetylcysteine (NAC) breaks down the disulfide bonds of the mucin glycoprotein network and is associated with improved mucus clearance. However, because of increased incidence of bronchospasm with its use, therapy with NAC is not frequently initiated but may be used in conjunction with an inhaled bronchodilator.[55] Free DNA can significantly increase the viscosity of mucus and therefore impede clearance from the airways. Recombinant human DNase (rhDNase, dornase alpha) improves pulmonary function in the chronic management of cystic fibrosis patients but has no significant effect in acute exacerbations of cystic fibrosis.[58,59] In bronchiectasis not due to cystic fibrosis, rhDNase is not effective and may potentially be harmful.[60]

OTHER AEROSOL THERAPIES

Additional aerosol therapies include racemic epinephrine (for acute upper airway obstruction due to inflammation), corticosteroids, and surfactant.

▨ Methods to Improve Lung Expansion

Atelectasis is a common complication encountered in the critically ill patient and is often due to prolonged supine body position and retained secretions obstructing airways. Lung expansion techniques that mimic normal sigh maneuvers may help reverse and prevent atelectasis. These techniques are often used in postoperative patients at high risk for pulmonary complications, such as those undergoing thoracic and upper abdominal surgery, and patients with neuromuscular or chest wall disorders.

Deep breathing and incentive spirometry involve coached inspiratory maneuvers to voluntarily increase lung volumes to greater than the vital capacity of the patient. These techniques require an awake, cooperative patient who is able to tolerate the maneuver. The only advantage of using an incentive spirometer is that it provides visual feedback and a reminder to the patient to continue these maneuvers. Incentive spirometry and deep breathing are equally effective in reducing postoperative pulmonary complications compared to chest physiotherapy.[61,62]

Intermittent positive-pressure breathing to improve lung expansion has fallen out of favor as a preventive measure in postoperative patients because of its expense, lack of difference in outcomes compared to deep breathing or incentive spirometry, and complications such as abdominal distension.[62,63]

Methods to Improve Oxygenation and Ventilation

NITRIC OXIDE

Nitric oxide (NO) was first described as a vascular-derived relaxing factor that caused vasodilation via vascular smooth muscle relaxation. It is a highly lipid-soluble gas that allows for rapid diffusion through the alveolar-blood barrier into the pulmonary circulation and smooth muscle cells of the vasculature. The main action of NO is mediated by activating guanylate cyclase, increasing intracellular cyclic guanylate monophosphate (cGMP), thereby causing smooth muscle and subsequent vasomotor relaxation.[64] The beneficial effects observed with inhaled NO are mediated primarily through its actions on pulmonary vascular smooth muscle. A reduction in pulmonary vascular resistance from arteriolar and venous vasodilation leads to reduced intravascular pressure at the level of the capillaries, with the potential benefit of reduced fluid leak into the alveoli. Additional benefits observed include a reduction in platelet aggregation and neutrophil adhesion/sequestration in the lungs.[65-67] NO is rapidly inactivated by binding to the heme moiety of hemoglobin. Because of its short half-life, NO does not enter the systemic circulation, making it an ideal selective pulmonary vasodilator.

The most common use of NO in the ICU is in the setting of acute lung injury (ALI) and acute respiratory distress syndrome (ARDS). Numerous clinical observational studies in ALI/ARDS have demonstrated improvements in oxygenation by improving $\dot{V}/\dot{Q}$ mismatch as demonstrated by a 10% to 20% increase in $Pao_2:Fio_2$ ratio and a reduction in pulmonary vascular resistance and mean pulmonary arterial pressures by at least 5 to 8 mm Hg.[68] These physiologic benefits in both animal and clinical observational studies suggested that the use of NO in critically ill patients could be beneficial. Randomized control trials of varying sample size and design had similar findings[69-72] and showed that NO improved the Pao_2 and $PaO_2:Fio_2$ ratios acutely, but by 24 to 72 hours, those in the control group achieved the same level of improvement. Similarly, a reduction in mean pulmonary artery pressure was also observed in these trials with the use of NO. Only 60% of ALI/ARDS patients had a response with improved oxygenation after institution of inhaled NO.[69] However, the improvement in oxygenation did not translate into clinically meaningful outcomes such as decrease in mortality, reduction in organ failure, or increased numbers of days free of mechanical ventilation. A trend towards a benefit was seen in a post hoc analysis in one trial in the more severe forms of ARDS, but further studies are needed.[69] In fact, a meta-analysis of twelve randomized controlled trials did not support the routine use of inhaled NO in ALI and even suggested a possible increase in renal dysfunction.[73]

No clear predictors of what patient will respond to NO exist. Given that doses below 40 ppm were safe without any significant adverse

TABLE 54-2	Clinical Conditions Where Inhaled Nitric Oxide May Be Used

Acute respiratory distress syndrome
Severe primary and secondary pulmonary hypertension[95]
Congenital cardiac syndromes[96,97]
Right ventricular failure in acute pulmonary embolism or after cardiac surgery[98-100]
Pulmonary ischemic-reperfusion injury after a heart-lung or lung transplant[76,101]
Sickle cell crisis[102,103]

effects, NO can be considered a "rescue" therapy to possibly allow for the institution of more protective forms of ventilation, with decreases in Fio_2 and mean airway pressures to maintain acceptable oxygenation. It might also be used in situations where secondary pulmonary hypertension leads to compromised hemodynamic function from right ventricular failure.

Almitrine bismesylate enhances pulmonary vasoconstriction in areas of hypoxic vasoconstriction, thereby enhancing redistribution of blood flow from shunt areas to lung units with normal $\dot{V}/\dot{Q}$ ratios.[74,75] This effect of almitrine therefore potentates the effects of inhaled NO on gas exchange. Almitrine is not readily available in North America and requires further study to define its role in combination with NO.

In addition to ALI/ARDS, other clinical conditions where NO use may be beneficial are listed in Table 54-2. Inhaled NO has been used post heart and lung transplants as a method to reduce right ventricular afterload in the setting of elevated pulmonary artery pressures.[76] In lung transplants, NO has been described to reduce the risk of ischemia-reperfusion injury. But this effect was not supported by a recent randomized clinical trial in which NO was instituted early after lung transplantation.[77]

Inhaled NO is typically started at low doses ranging from 1 to 2 ppm and gradually increased until the desired effect is achieved. One method recommended in the United Kingdom, based on American-European Consensus Conference on ALI/ARDS guidelines, is to perform a dose/response test starting at 20 ppm and reducing the concentrations to 10, 5, and 0 ppm to find the lowest effective dose.[78] A significant response should be considered a 20% increase in the $Pao_2:Fio_2$ ratio or at least a 5 mm Hg decrease in mean pulmonary artery pressure (PAP). Improvements in gas exchange are usually seen at lower doses than are reductions in PAP. The usual dose of inhaled NO ranges from 10 to 40 ppm. Doses greater than 80 ppm are associated with a higher risk for adverse effects. From the clinical trials, longer administration is generally safe with no evidence of the effect diminishing. However, inhaled NO should be weaned as soon as possible as a patient's condition improves.

Adverse effects of NO include the formation of methemoglobin and spontaneous oxidation to nitrogen dioxide (NO_2). NO_2 is known to be toxic to the respiratory system with maximum exposure limited to 5 ppm. Complications from NO_2 exposure include airway irritation and hyperreactivity with levels as low as 1.5 ppm and pulmonary edema and pulmonary fibrosis developing after exposure to higher levels. Despite these adverse effects, the development of methemoglobinemia or other toxicities related to NO_2 during acute or prolonged NO inhalation has been unusual, especially when NO has been administered at concentrations less than 80 ppm.[79]

To reduce the risk of exposure to NO_2, NO should be stored at concentrations no higher than 1000 ppm in a pure nitrogen environment and only exposed to oxygen at the time of administration. NO should be delivered into the ventilator circuit as close to the patient as possible. NO and NO_2 levels should be monitored closely on the inspiratory side of the Y-piece when using doses above 2 ppm. Care should be taken to prevent abrupt discontinuation of NO. Rebound pulmonary vasoconstriction can occur with sudden discontinuation, leading to rapid worsening of $\dot{V}/\dot{Q}$ mismatch and pulmonary hypertension with significant hemodynamic collapse.[80] Backup supplies of NO and delivery systems should be readily available.

An absolute contraindication to NO therapy is methemoglobinemia reductase deficiency (congenital or acquired). Relative contraindications include bleeding diathesis (secondary to reports of altered platelet function and bleeding time with iNO), intracranial hemorrhage, and severe left ventricular failure (NHA grade III or IV).[78]

INHALED PROSTAGLANDINS

Inhaled prostaglandins I2 (PGI2) and E1 (PGE1) have similar effects to inhaled nitric oxide, with minimal systemic effects. For PGI2, doses ranging from 1 to 50 ng/kg/min are favorably tolerated and reduce pulmonary artery pressures and improve oxygenation similar to iNO.[81-83] PGE1 has the advantage of a more rapid degradation by pulmonary endothelial cells, providing a selective advantage over PGI2 at higher doses.[84] Additional studies are required to define a role for these agents, but they can be considered as alternatives for rescue therapy when used for conditions similar to those treated with iNO. As with iNO, care must be taken to avoid abrupt discontinuation of PGI2 or PGE1, because rebound pulmonary hypertension and cardiovascular collapse can result.

HELIOX

Helium is an inert gas with significantly lower density than room air (1.42 g/L for oxygen versus 0.17 g/L for helium). By substituting helium for nitrogen in the helium-oxygen mix (heliox), the degree of reduction in density of the gas is directly proportional to the fraction of the inspired oxygen concentration in the mix. Heliox reduces the Reynolds number, permitting more laminar flow and reducing airflow resistance and the work of breathing and dynamic hyperinflation associated with high airway resistance. Clinical situations where heliox may be used include conditions with high airflow resistance such as severe acute asthma or COPD exacerbations, bronchiolitis, bronchopulmonary dysplasia, and extrathoracic or tracheal obstruction. Heliox has been used to improve lung compliance during noninvasive ventilation in COPD patients, to reduce the work of breathing, to avoid intubation,[85,86] and to improve aerosolized drug delivery.[87] In the management of moderate to severe asthma exacerbations, routine use of heliox is not supported by systematic reviews of the literature but can be considered as an adjuvant in severe cases.[88-90] In COPD exacerbation, two multicentered trials found no difference in intubation rate or length of stay in the ICU when heliox was added to noninvasive ventilation.[91,92] However, there appeared to be a cost benefit resulting from a shorter overall hospital length of stay associated with the use of heliox.[91] Heliox is generally well tolerated and produces no significant adverse effects. Disadvantages of its use in critically ill patients include cost of therapy and the high concentrations of helium required. Most studies utilize helium/oxygen mixes of 80:20 or 70:30 to achieve therapeutic benefit. At higher concentrations of oxygen, the effect of helium declines, and therefore heliox is limited in use to patients who are not severely hypoxemic. When used in conjunction with nebulized medications, higher flows of heliox may be required to ensure adequate delivery of the medication, though this may be offset by the smaller particle size generated in a heliox mixture.[87,93] Ventilators also require recalibration for measured F_{IO_2}, flows, and tidal volumes when using heliox.[94]

Summary

Pulmonary disease and complications are common in the critically ill patient, especially those undergoing mechanical ventilation. It is important for the clinician to recognize these potential complications and the many forms of adjunctive respiratory therapies available to prevent further morbidity. Simple therapies such as chest physiotherapy, suctioning, and positioning should be utilized in most patients, with more advanced procedures and therapies used on a selective basis based on the underlying clinical condition.

KEY POINTS

1. Inability to effectively clear secretions is common in critically ill patients, increasing the risk of aspiration, atelectasis, and pneumonia.

2. Chest physiotherapy, positional therapy, and early mobilization should be considered in all critically ill patients.

3. Other adjunctive forms of respiratory therapy should be considered on an individual basis based on the underlying clinical condition.

4. Aerosolization of medications is an effective way of direct delivery to the lungs.

5. Metered-dose inhalers (MDI) are preferred over nebulization for the delivery of bronchodilators in both the spontaneously breathing and mechanically ventilated patient.

6. With proper monitoring, inhaled nitric oxide can be safely administered in the critically ill patient.

7. Inhaled nitric oxide is associated with improved pulmonary and cardiac physiologic parameters when administered in a variety of clinical conditions encountered in the ICU.

ANNOTATED REFERENCES

Kollef MH, Prentice D, Shapiro SD, et al. Mechanical ventilation with or without daily changes of in-line suction catheters. Am J Respir Crit Care Med 1997;156(2 Pt 1):466-72.
A randomized trial comparing daily versus as-needed in-line suction catheter change. This study demonstrated that the rate of ventilator-associated pneumonia and hospital mortality was not different between the two groups and that an "as-needed" approach was highly cost effective. This provides good evidence that routine changes of in-line suction catheters is not necessary.

Ntoumenopoulos G, Presneill JJ, McElholum M, Cade JF. Chest physiotherapy for the prevention of ventilator-associated pneumonia. Intensive Care Med 2002;28(7):850-6.
A small prospective clinical trial that examined the benefit of a common adjunctive respiratory therapy—chest physiotherapy—on a common clinical complication of mechanical ventilation—ventilator associated pneumonia (VAP). In this study, routine twice-daily chest physiotherapy was associated with a lower occurrence of VAP compared to standard therapy, supporting its role as a simple preventive measure for VAP.

Dellinger RP, Zimmerman JL, Taylor RW, et al. Effects of inhaled nitric oxide in patients with acute respiratory distress syndrome: results of a randomized phase II trial. Inhaled Nitric Oxide in ARDS Study Group. Crit Care Med 1998;26(1):15-23.
A multicentered, randomized, blinded, controlled trial of 177 patients within 72 hours of developing ARDS. In this patient population, inhaled nitric oxide was associated with a transient improvement in oxygenation and mean pulmonary artery pressures, but this did not translate into differences in 28-day mortality or days alive and free of mechanical ventilation.

Meade MO, Granton JT, Matte-Martyn A, et al. A randomized trial of inhaled nitric oxide to prevent ischemia-reperfusion injury after lung transplantation. Am J Respir Crit Care Med 2003;167 (11):1483-9.
A small randomized, placebo-controlled trial that did not demonstrate a protective effect of inhaled nitric oxide therapy on the risk of developing ischemia-reperfusion injury after a lung transplantation when given soon after reperfusion of the transplanted lung.

Maggiore SM, Richard JC, Abroug F, et al. A multicenter, randomized trial of noninvasive ventilation with helium-oxygen mixture in exacerbations of chronic obstructive lung disease. Crit Care Med 2010;38(1):145-51.
In this well-conducted randomized multicenter study, the addition of heliox to noninvasive positive-pressure ventilation in patients with acute exacerbations of COPD did not demonstrate a beneficial effect with respect to intubation rate, ICU length of stay, or mortality.

Schweickert WD, Pohlman MC, Pohlman AS, et al. Early physical and occupational therapy in mechanically ventilated, critically ill patients: a randomised controlled trial. Lancet 2009;373(9678): 1874-82.
This randomized controlled trial looking at the addition of early, aggressive rehabilitation therapy to daily sedation interruption found a significant increase in the return to independent functional capacity and ventilator-free days compared to standard care, without any significant adverse events.

REFERENCES

Access the complete reference list online at http://www.expertconsult.com.

55

Indications for and Management of Tracheostomy

BRADLEY D. FREEMAN

Tracheostomy is one of the most commonly performed surgical procedures in critically ill patients who require prolonged mechanical ventilation.[1] A large body of literature describes the potential benefits, risks, and technical aspects of this procedure, but there is little guidance as to what constitutes optimal tracheostomy practice in the critically ill patient.[2,3] This chapter reviews basic aspects of tracheostomy management, focusing in particular on indications, timing, technique, and postprocedure care.

Indications for Tracheostomy

The presence of a "difficult airway" in a patient requiring prolonged mechanical ventilatory support constitutes an absolute indication for tracheostomy. Patients with so-called difficult airways include those with conditions such as significant maxillofacial trauma, angioedema, obstructing upper-airway tumors, or other anatomic characteristics that would render translaryngeal intubation technically difficult to perform in the event of inadvertent airway loss. Patients with difficult airways represent a small fraction of all individuals undergoing tracheostomy. More commonly, patients undergo this procedure for subjective indications (e.g., to facilitate ventilator weaning, to promote oral hygiene and pulmonary toilet, or to enhance comfort).[4] Tracheostomy is most commonly performed in an elective fashion; accordingly, patients should be clinically optimized to minimize risk (e.g., minimal ventilatory support [$Fio_2 \leq 50\%$, $PEEP \leq 7.5$ cm H_2O], hemodynamically stable, metabolic and hemostatic derangements corrected). Because many of the benefits of tracheostomy relative to prolonged translaryngeal intubation are unproven, unambiguous criteria for selecting patients for tracheostomy are lacking.[3]

Timing of Tracheostomy in Acute Respiratory Failure

In the early years of critical care medicine, endotracheal tubes (ETTs) were composed of rigid materials and incorporated a low-volume, high-pressure pneumatic cuff. During this era, it became common practice to perform tracheostomy early—within 48 hours of initiating mechanical ventilation—in an effort to minimize laryngeal and tracheal injury associated with endotracheal intubation.[5] With advances in ETT design, the trauma associated with prolonged translaryngeal intubation lessened.[5] Further, a prospective study examining risks associated with tracheostomy suggested that this procedure was accompanied by high rates of morbidity and mortality.[6] Accordingly, enthusiasm for the routine performance of tracheostomy waned. With refinement in techniques, perioperative complication rates associated with tracheostomy diminished. In addition, subsequent studies attempting to establish the relationship between prolonged translaryngeal intubation, prolonged tracheostomy, and laryngeotracheal damage produced conflicting findings.[5] At present, no data clearly establish that translaryngeal intubation should be limited to any specific duration or that tracheostomy should be performed at any specific point in a patient's course in an effort either to limit chronic laryngeal dysfunction or minimize tracheal injury.

Recent investigations examining timing of tracheostomy have focused on duration of mechanical ventilation and related measures of resource expenditure. Rodriguez et al. assigned 106 patients who developed acute respiratory failure following major trauma to either undergo tracheostomy within 7 days of intensive care unit (ICU) admission ("early" tracheostomy) or to tracheostomy at least 8 days following ICU admission ("late" tracheostomy). Compared to patients undergoing late tracheostomy, patients in the early tracheostomy group had a trend toward a lower incidence of pneumonia, as well as significant reductions in duration of mechanical ventilation, ICU length of stay, and hospital length of stay.[7] Likewise, Lesnik et al. reported a retrospective analysis of 101 patients who developed acute respiratory failure following blunt trauma, comparing patients who underwent early tracheostomy (within 4 days of ICU admission) to late tracheostomy (>4 days following ICU admission). Compared to patients undergoing late tracheostomy, patients in whom tracheostomy was established early had a significantly shorter duration of mechanical ventilation and lower incidence of pneumonia.[8] Others have likewise reported a benefit of early tracheostomy.[9,10] In contrast, Blot et al. reported that neutropenic patients developing acute respiratory failure who underwent early tracheostomy (within 48 hours of intubation) had longer duration of mechanical ventilation and longer hospital length of stay than did patients who either underwent tracheostomy formation after 7 days or not at all.[11] Given the conflicting results, variability in study quality, heterogeneity in populations enrolled, and inconsistency in endpoints studied, it is difficult to draw on the conclusions of these and similar studies to ascertain the optimal timing of tracheostomy creation. As a consequence, tracheostomy practice varies substantially.[1]

There are several reasons why tracheostomy may facilitate weaning from mechanical ventilation.[5] Resistance to airflow in an artificial airway is proportional to air turbulence, tube diameter, and tube length. Air turbulence is increased in the presence of extrinsic compression and inspissated secretions.[12] Airflow resistance and associated work of breathing should theoretically be less with tracheostomies than with ETTs because of an ETT's rigid design, shorter length, and removable inner cannula (to allow for evacuation of secretions).[12] Further, the presence of a tracheostomy may allow clinicians to be more aggressive in weaning patients from mechanical ventilation. Specifically, if a patient with a tracheostomy tube in place does not tolerate liberation from ventilatory support, he or she may be simply reconnected to the ventilator. In contrast, if a patient who is translaryngeally intubated does not tolerate extubation, he or she must be sedated and reintubated. This might represent a potential barrier to extubation in patients who are of marginal pulmonary status. Finally, patients with tracheostomies may receive less sedation than individuals with translaryngeal airways.[13] Reduction in sedation may be accompanied by increases in mobility, differences in approaches to and success of weaning, and other factors that may shorten duration of ventilatory support.

TECHNICAL CONSIDERATIONS

Traditionally, tracheostomies have been performed in the operating room using standard surgical principles.[14] In 1985, Ciaglia et al. described percutaneous dilational tracheostomy (PDT) in which tracheostomy is accomplished via a modified Seldinger technique, typically with the aid of bronchoscopy.[15] PDT has subsequently gained wide acceptance and has become the predominate method of tracheostomy creation in many centers.[16-18]

There are several potential advantages of PDT relative to surgically created tracheostomies (SCT). PDT may be performed at the bedside, avoiding the inconvenience and risk of transporting a critically ill patient, as well as the expense of utilizing operating room resources. In a prospective randomized study comparing PDT and SCT, Freeman et al. found that PDT was associated with a reduction of approximately $1500 in patient charges per procedure.[19] Other investigators have reported comparable findings.[20] In addition, a meta-analysis of prospective trials comparing PDT with SCT suggests that PDT may be associated with fewer complications, specifically postprocedure bleeding and peristomal infection.[21] The reduction in these complications may reflect that there is minimal dead space between the tracheostomy tube and adjacent pretracheal tissues following PDT, which may have a tamponading effect on minor bleeding and serve as a barrier to infection.[21] Finally, PDT is relatively simple to learn. Individuals who have not received formal surgical training may become facile with this procedure and perform it safely and effectively.[17,22]

Patient selection is essential to achieving satisfactory results with PDT. Candidates for PDT should be on low levels of ventilatory support (i.e., $FiO_2 \leq 50\%$, $PEEP \leq 7.5$ cm H_2O), have an intact coagulation system (international normalized ratio and platelet counts correctable to <1.3 and >100,000/mm³, respectively), and suitable neck anatomy such that external landmarks (cricoid cartilage, trachea, and sternal notch) are easily palpable with the neck positioned in moderate extension. In the author's opinion, PDT is contraindicated in patients who are so obese as to obscure these anatomic landmarks, as well as in patients with unstable cervical spines that preclude neck extension. Likewise, PDT is contraindicated in patients with "difficult airways," such as patients with maxillofacial trauma, glottic edema, poorly visualized vocal cords, or any condition that would make it difficult to reestablish translaryngeal intubation in the event of airway loss. Finally, PDT is an elective procedure and should not be used to establish an emergent airway.

While there are many potential advantages of PDT, this procedure has been associated with a number of highly morbid complications, many of which (e.g., pretracheal insertion, tracheal laceration, esophageal perforation, pneumothorax, loss of airway) are unusual in surgically created tracheostomies.[23-28] Accordingly, whereas PDT may be performed competently by those not trained in surgical techniques, persons who are expert at surgical airway management should be immediately available in the event complications arise.[22]

Selection, Maintenance, and Care of Tracheostomy Tubes

TRACHEOSTOMY TUBE SELECTION

A detailed discussion of the various types and designs of tracheostomy tubes is beyond the scope of this text, but a working knowledge of tracheostomy tube features is essential to the competent care of patients who have undergone placement of these devices (Figure 55-1). Briefly, most tracheostomy tubes are manufactured from polyvinyl chloride, silicone, a combination of these materials, or metal. They are available in either single-lumen (no removable inner cannula) or dual-lumen (removable inner cannula) configurations. The purpose of the removable inner cannula is to facilitate cleaning of inspissated secretions that may lead to tube occlusion. Because silicone is relatively secretion resistant, tubes manufactured from this material frequently do not have an inner cannula. Tracheostomy tubes are available with and without pneumatic cuffs. The purpose of the cuff is to maintain a seal between the tube and the tracheal mucosa sufficient to prevent escape of air from around the tracheostomy tube during mechanical ventilation (i.e., cuff leak). Further, the cuff minimizes but does not prevent aspiration. Tracheostomy tubes with foam cuffs conform to a patient's trachea and remain consistently inflated at low pressure. These tubes are indicated in patients who have sustained damage from excessive cuff pressure (e.g., tracheomalacia). Once a cuffed tracheostomy tube is no longer required—that is, the patient no longer requires mechanical ventilatory support and is not considered an aspiration risk—the cuffed tube is exchanged for a cuffless tube. Tracheostomy caps are generally provided with tracheostomy tubes for use in the decannulation process (see later discussion). Fenestrated tubes are used to promote speech and are generally used in individuals who tolerate liberation from mechanical ventilation for varying periods of time. Fenestrated tubes have an opening on their superior aspect such that when the inner cannula is removed, the cuff deflated, and the external orifice occluded (such as with a Passey-Muir type valve), air can pass the vocal cords, allowing phonation.

EXCHANGING TRACHEOSTOMY TUBES

Tracheostomy tubes should be changed due to malfunction (e.g., pilot balloon rupture), inspissated secretions compromising luminal diameter, or when another tracheostomy tube design is desired. The author is of the opinion that "routine" changing of a tracheostomy tube (e.g., every 7 days) is neither indicated nor supported by available literature. Changing a tracheostomy tube is not a benign procedure, is frequently uncomfortable for the patient, and may be complicated by the inability to insert the replacement tube or insertion of the replacement tube into a false passage in the pretracheal space. If indicated, it is desirable to postpone the initial tracheostomy tube exchange for at least 1 week following creation of the tracheostomy to allow the surgical tract to sufficiently mature.

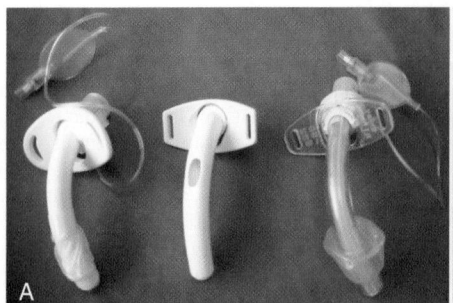 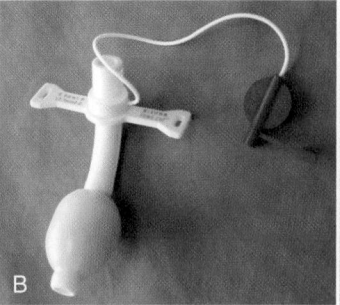 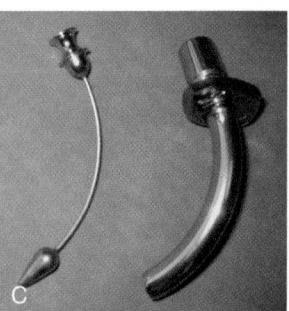

Figure 55-1 **Standard tracheostomy tube designs. A,** *Left to right,* standard cuffed tracheostomy tube, cuffless fenestrated tube, and cuffed tracheostomy tube with elongated "limbs" (portion of tube proximal and distal to curvature) to accommodate patients with variant neck anatomy. **B,** Tracheostomy tube with foam cuff; designed to provide a large-volume, low-pressure cuff and particularly suited to patients with tracheomalacia or patients who have sustained complications from tracheostomy tube or endotracheal tube cuffs. **C,** Cuffless metal tracheostomy tube (shown with obturator *[left]*); useful for decannulation or in patients who require a tracheostomy but have no need for a cuff.

To accomplish tracheostomy tube exchange, the replacement tube should have the pilot balloon tested to insure that there are no leaks. The tube should be lubricated with either sterile water or a small amount of water-soluble lubricant and inserted over a semirigid rubber catheter (such as a Robnel) or a suctioning catheter to lessen the likelihood that the tracheostomy tube is inserted into a false passage. Gentle dilation of the tracheostomy tract may be useful when exchanging a tracheostomy that has been placed by percutaneous technique.

MONITORING CUFF INFLATION PRESSURE

Tracheostomy tube pneumatic cuffs require monitoring to maintain an inflation pressure of approximately 20 to 25 mm Hg. Assuming a tracheostomy tube is of appropriate size, an insufficiently inflated cuff may both result in a sizable amount of air leaking around the cuff ("cuff leak"), rendering mechanical ventilation difficult, and provide poor protection against aspiration. Alternatively, excessive cuff pressures (exceeding 25 mm Hg) may result in compression of mucosal capillaries, giving rise to mucosal ischemia and attendant complications such as tracheomalacia and tracheal stenosis. The most reliable method of monitoring cuff inflation pressure is through direct measurement. Maneuvers such as pilot balloon palpation to estimate cuff pressure, or inflation of the cuff until end-inspiratory leaks are extinguished during positive-pressure ventilation, are not recommended because of their inaccuracy.[29] Tracheal cuff inflation pressures should be measured and recorded on a regular basis for purposes of quality assurance.

ORAL NUTRITION

The presence of a tracheostomy provides opportunity for oral nutrition in the mechanically ventilated patient, with its attendant psychological benefits, but it also complicates alimentation because of the interference of the tracheostomy tube with mechanisms of normal swallowing and airway control.[29] The presence of a tracheostomy inhibits physiologic upward movement of the larynx during deglutition, hinders glottic closure, and produces dysphagia due to mechanical compression of the esophagus. Further, an inflated tracheostomy balloon does not protect from aspiration. Patients with tracheostomies who are candidates for oral nutrition should mentate normally, have adequate oxygenation with low inspired oxygen concentrations (e.g., 30% FIO_2), and possess sufficient ventilatory reserve such that they can physiologically tolerate an episode of aspiration during the introduction of oral feeding. Initial efforts at feeding should be carefully supervised.

DECANNULATION

Patients who remain stable for 24 to 48 hours following discontinuation of mechanical ventilation may be evaluated for decannulation. The patient's ability to protect their airway should be assessed for 24 hours by deflating the tracheostomy tube balloon and observing for signs of aspiration. If aspiration is present, formal assessment of swallowing function should be undertaken prior to decannulation. In the absence of aspiration, the native airway can be assessed by deflating the tracheostomy tube balloon and occluding the tracheostomy tube. Patients who are able to breathe around a capped and deflated 8.0 tracheostomy tube most likely have adequate respiratory reserve and a sufficiently preserved native airway to tolerate decannulation. Patients who have difficulty breathing around a capped 8.0 tube should be reassessed with a capped 7.0 tracheostomy tube. Successful breathing with a capped and deflated 7.0 tube in place suggests that a patient will tolerate decannulation. Patients who fail breathing trials with capped tracheostomy tubes should undergo laryngoscopic evaluation to exclude the presence of tracheal stenosis. Many patients recovering from long-term mechanical ventilatory support may have normal airways but fail breathing around a capped 7.0 or 8.0 tracheostomy tube because of limited ventilatory reserve (e.g., due to generalized deconditioning or the presence of intrinsic lung disease). These patients may benefit from "downsizing" of the tracheostomy stoma using progressively smaller cuffless tracheostomy tubes, with intermittent capping using stomal obturators. Tracheostomy tubes with foam cuffs should not be used for decannulation trials because these cuffs spontaneously reinflate when exposed to ambient pressure, making assessment of airway stenosis difficult.

◼ Complications

A variety of complications resulting from tracheostomy placement have been described. A brief discussion of the more common complications occurring in the critical care setting and their management follows.

CUFF LEAKS

Cuff leak is a commonly encountered problem in patients with tracheostomies and may be manifest by either an audible leak around the tracheostomy tube or loss of returned volume in mechanically ventilated breaths. A mechanical problem with the tracheostomy tube should first be excluded by determining that the pneumatic cuff is functional (i.e., when the cuff is inflated, it does not leak air). A malfunctioning tracheostomy tube requires exchange (see earlier discussion). Once tracheostomy tube malfunction is excluded, the most common cause of cuff leak is tracheomalacia with resulting dilation adjacent to the tracheostomy tube cuff. This is particularly common in patients who have been maintained on mechanical ventilation for extended periods. It should *not* be treated by hyperinflating the tracheostomy tube cuff in an effort to achieve total occlusion, in that this will result in further dilation of the trachea and may lead to mucosal ischemia. If the cuff leak is well tolerated and the ability to ventilate the patient is not compromised, the author recommends maintaining the tracheostomy tube in place at the appropriate inflation pressure (e.g., 20 to 25 mm Hg). Conversely, if the cuff leak is sufficient so as to impair gas exchange, consideration should be given to exchanging the tracheostomy tube for a tracheostomy tube design that incorporates a large-volume, low-pressure cuff (such as a foam cuff tracheostomy tube).

TUBE OCCLUSION

A frequently encountered problem in patients with tracheostomies is tracheostomy tube occlusion. This is typically manifest by either high airway pressures or inability to pass a suctioning catheter. Tracheostomy tube occlusion is frequently the result of inspissated secretions. Many commonly used tube designs have a removable inner cannula to facilitate cleaning of the inner portion of the tracheostomy tube. A second common cause of tracheostomy tube occlusion is tube malpositioning such that the end of the tracheostomy tube abuts the tracheal wall, or the tube has migrated such that its tip resides in the pretracheal tissues. If tracheostomy malpositioning is suspected, the operating surgeon should assist in assessing it for either reinsertion or use of another tube design.

TUBE DISLODGEMENT

Although dislodgement of the tracheostomy tube may occur at any time following tracheostomy placement, this complication is most problematic in the immediate postoperative period, before the tracheostomy tract has matured. Factors predisposing to tracheostomy tube dislodgment include an inadequately secured tube, excessive coughing, and patient agitation. Tracheostomy tube dislodgement should be suspected when a patient is able to speak immediately following tracheostomy placement, the airway becomes obstructed, or respiratory distress develops. Because it may be technically difficult to reinsert the tracheostomy tube in this situation, the author recommends that the airway be reestablished via translaryngeal intubation. The tracheostomy should then be reinserted in the operating room with appropriate anesthetic assistance, lighting, and instrumentation. If tracheostomy tube dislodgement occurs once the tracheostomy track is sufficiently mature (that is, the tracheostomy track is at least 1 week old), it is generally technically feasible to reinsert the tracheostomy tube at the patient's bedside as noted earlier (see Exchanging Tracheostomy Tubes).

TRACHEOESOPHAGEAL FISTULA

The development of a tracheoesophageal fistula following tracheostomy is rare, occurring in fewer than 1% of patients, and is typically the result of pressure necrosis of the tracheal and esophageal mucosa from the tracheostomy tube cuff. A number of potential risk factors have been reported (e.g., high airway pressures, excessive cuff inflation pressures, use of nasogastric tubes, excessive tracheostomy tube movement). Clinical manifestations are nonspecific and include excessive tracheal secretions, coughing, and gastric distension. The presence of a tracheoesophageal fistula can be demonstrated on fiberoptic exam following removal or retraction of the tracheostomy tube. Because the use of fiberoptic exam alone is insensitive, it should be combined with an enterally contrasted esophageal evaluation if clinical suspicion exists (e.g., water-soluble contrast swallow, computed tomography [CT] scan).

Tracheoesophageal fistula requires surgical repair. Temporizing measures include positioning of an ETT cuff below the level of the fistula to limit aspiration, removal of nasogastric tubes, and placement of feeding gastrostomy tubes.[30]

TRACHEOINNOMINATE ARTERY FISTULA

Tracheoinnominate artery fistula (TIF) is a rare complication following tracheostomy formation and theoretically results from pressure necrosis or injury to the trachea adjacent to the course of innominate artery.[31] A number of risk factors have been postulated, including excessive tube movement, aberrant innominate artery anatomy, use of an excessively long or curved tracheostomy tube that erodes through the tracheal wall, inferior positioning of the tracheostomy tube, tracheal infection, and corticosteroid therapy.[31] A TIF may become apparent as quickly as a few days or as late as several months following tracheostomy placement. The classic presentation is of a "sentinel bleed," in which a large volume of blood emanates from the tracheostomy tube. Fiberoptic examination to evaluate for the presence of TIF should be performed in the operating room in the event airway manipulation results in massive hemorrhage. Temporizing measures in patients who develop massive bleeding include hyperinflation of the tracheostomy cuff, insertion of an ETT through the tracheostomy stoma in an effort to tamponade bleeding, or translaryngeal intubation and digital compression of the bleeding site through the tracheostomy stoma. Definitive repair entails median sternotomy, ligation of the innominate artery, and drainage of the mediastinum.

ANNOTATED REFERENCES

Ciaglia P, Firsching R, Syniec C. Elective percutaneous dilational tracheostomy. Chest 1985;87(6):715-9.
 The first article to describe percutaneous tracheostomy using a modified Seldinger technique. This approach has substantially changed tracheostomy practice.
Consensus conference on artificial airways in patients receiving mechanical ventilation. Chest 1989;96(1):178-80.
 The consensus recommendations regarding timing of tracheostomy continue to form the basis of practice for many intensivists.
Freeman BD, Borecki IB, Coopersmith CM, Buchman TB. Relationship between tracheostomy timing and duration of mechanical ventilation in critically ill patients. Crit Care Med 2005;33:2513-20.

 A detailed analysis of a large critical care database that provides insight into both the resource intensity of tracheostomy patients and the current variability in tracheostomy practice.
Freeman B, Kennedy C, Robertson TE, et al. Tracheostomy protocol: experience with development and potential utility. Crit Care Med 2008;36(6):1742-8.
 Describes a novel protocol-based approach to patient selection and timing of tracheostomy.
Heffner JE, Hess D. Tracheostomy management in the chronically ventilated patient. Clin Chest Med 2001;22(1):55-69.
 An excellent review of virtually all facets of tracheostomy care.

REFERENCES

Access the complete reference list online at http://www.expertconsult.com.

56

Hyperbaric Oxygen in Critical Care

STEPHEN R. THOM

Hyperbaric oxygen (HBO_2) treatment involves intermittent breathing of pure oxygen at greater than ambient pressure. Over the past 20 years, HBO_2 has undergone refinement, with increased understanding of mechanisms of action and clinical applications. Along with an expansion of the knowledge base, formalized education now exists for emergency, critical care/anesthesia, and surgically trained physicians, who may obtain special competency board certification through the American Board of Medical Specialists. This chapter will summarize existing literature on uses for hyperbaric oxygen therapy and some special issues related to care of critically ill patients.

Applications

HBO_2 treatment is carried out in either a monoplace (single person) or multiplace (typically 2 to 14 patients) chamber. Pressures applied while in the chamber are usually 2 to 3 atmospheres absolute (ATA), representing the sum of the atmospheric pressure plus additional hydrostatic pressure equivalent to 1 or 2 atmospheres. Treatments usually are for 2 to 8 hours, depending on the indication, and may be performed from 1 to 3 times daily. Monoplace chambers are usually compressed with pure oxygen. Multiplace chambers are pressurized with air, and patients breathe pure oxygen through a tight-fitting facemask, hood, or endotracheal tube. During treatment, the Pao_2 typically exceeds 2000 mm Hg, and levels of 200 to 400 mm Hg occur in tissues.[1]

HBO_2 should be viewed as a drug and the hyperbaric chamber as a dosing device. Elevating tissue oxygen tension is a primary effect. Although this may alleviate physiologic stress to hypoxic tissues, lasting benefits of HBO_2 must relate to abatement of underlying pathophysiologic processes. The accepted indications comprise a heterogeneous group of disorders (Box 56-1), thus implying that there are several mechanisms of action for HBO_2 (Box 56-2).[1-3]

ARTERIAL GAS EMBOLISM AND DECOMPRESSION SICKNESS

Among the earliest application of hyperbaric therapy was to treat disorders related to gas bubbles in the body. Compressed air construction work required exposure to elevated ambient pressure within compartments (caissons) for many hours to excavate tunnels or bridge foundations in muddy soil that otherwise would flood. In the 19th century, workers were noted to frequently experience joint pains, limb paralysis, or pulmonary compromise when they returned to ambient pressure. This condition—decompression sickness (DCS), caisson disease, or bends—was later attributed to nitrogen bubbles in the body, and recompression was found to relieve symptoms. The mechanism, based purely on Boyle's law, with reduction of gas bubble volume due to pressure, was later improved by adding supplemental oxygen to hasten inert gas diffusion out of the body. Similar observations were made at later times for scuba divers, who are also prone to develop arterial gas embolism (AGE) due to pulmonary overpressurization on decompression.

Iatrogenic AGE has been reported in association with cardiovascular, obstetric/gynecologic, neurosurgical, and orthopedic procedures and generally whenever disruption of a vascular wall occurs. Nonsurgical processes reported to cause AGE include overexpansion during mechanical ventilation, hemodialysis, and after accidental opening of central venous catheters.[4]

Treatment of gas bubble disorders includes standard support of airway, breathing, and circulation plus prompt application of HBO_2. Gas bubbles have been reported to persist for several days, and although delays should be avoided, HBO_2 may be beneficial even when begun after long delays.[5-9] Controlled animal trials support efficacy of HBO_2, but randomized clinical trials have not been done.[10] In their review of 27 case series, Moon and Gorman described substantial benefit with HBO_2 treatment—78% of 441 cases receiving HBO_2 fully recovered and 4.5 % died, whereas only 26% of 74 cases not undergoing HBO_2 treatment fully recovered and 52% died.[4]

Mechanisms of action of HBO_2 in AGE and DCS treatment include reduction of gas according to Boyle's law, hyperoxygenation to hasten inert gas diffusion, and an additional effect related to inhibition of leukocyte adherence to injured endothelium. Endothelial dysfunction occurs in association with mechanical interactions of bubbles at vessel walls and lumen occlusion.[11-15] Neutrophil activation and perivascular adherence occur and are associated with functional deficits post decompression.[16,4,17] Animals depleted of leukocytes before experimental cerebral air embolism suffer less severe reduction of cerebral blood flow and better neurologic outcome.[18] HBO_2 has been shown to temporarily inhibit human β_2-integrin adhesion function.[19] Inhibition of neutrophil β_2-integrin adhesion by HBO_2 has been described in a number of animal models including skeletal muscle ischemia-reperfusion, cerebral ischemia-reperfusion, pulmonary smoke inhalation injury, and brain injury after carbon monoxide (CO) poisoning.[20-23] The mechanism for this effect involves S-nitrosylation of cytoskeletal β-actin, which impedes the coordinated cell-surface β_2-integrin migration required for firm adherence.[24]

CARBON MONOXIDE POISONING

Carbon monoxide is the leading cause of injury and death by poisoning in the world.[25] The affinity of CO for hemoglobin, to form carboxyhemoglobin (COHb), is more than 200-fold greater than that of O_2. CO-mediated hypoxic stress is a primary insult, but COHb values correlate poorly with clinical outcome.* Pathologic mechanisms, in addition to elevations of COHb, include intravascular platelet-leukocyte aggregation, leukocyte-mediated oxidative injury to brain, excessive release of excitatory amino acids such as glutamate, impaired mitochondrial oxidative phosphorylation, and possible myocardial calcium overload.†

Survivors of acute CO poisoning are at risk for developing delayed neurologic sequelae (DNS) that include cognitive deficits, memory loss, dementia, parkinsonism, paralysis, chorea, cortical blindness, psychosis, personality changes, and peripheral neuropathy. DNS typically occurs from 2 to 40 days after poisoning, and the incidence is from 25% to 50% after severe poisoning.

Administration of supplemental oxygen is the cornerstone of treatment for CO poisoning. Oxygen inhalation will hasten dissociation of CO from hemoglobin as well as provide enhanced tissue oxygenation. HBO_2 causes carboxyhemoglobin dissociation to occur at a rate greater than that achievable by breathing pure oxygen at sea level. Additionally, HBO_2, but not ambient pressure oxygen treatment, has several actions that have been demonstrated in animal models to be beneficial in ameliorating pathophysiologic events associated with central nervous

---

*References 26-32.
†References 33-39.

system (CNS) injuries mediated by CO. These include an improvement in mitochondrial oxidative processes,[40] inhibition of lipid peroxidation,[41] and impairment of leukocyte adhesion to injured microvasculature.[22] Animals poisoned with CO and treated with HBO_2 have been found to have more rapid improvement in cardiovascular status,[42] lower mortality,[43] and lower incidence of neurologic sequelae.[44]

Despite online criticisms of their analysis, a meta-analysis by the Cochrane Library concluded that it is unclear whether HBO_2 reduces the incidence of adverse CO-mediated neurologic outcomes.[45] There are five prospective, randomized trials that have assessed clinical efficacy of HBO_2 for acute CO poisoning.[30,31,32,46,47] Several failed to find benefit,[30,47] but methodological weaknesses discussed by several authors[39,48] diminish their clinical impact. Only one clinical trial satisfies all items deemed to be necessary for the highest quality of randomized controlled trials.[49] HBO_2 treatment also appears to diminish acute mortality, based on a retrospective analysis.[48]

BLOOD LOSS ANEMIA

In rare instances when transfusion is not possible due to cross-matching incompatibilities or religious beliefs, intermittent use of HBO_2 has been applied to temporarily relieve physiologic stress from severe acute anemia. Anecdotal reports describe using 2.5 to 3.0 ATA O_2 to raise Pao_2 in plasma to meet metabolic needs.[50-53] Treatments are often administered for only brief times when physiologic decompensation occurs, because O_2 toxicity can be a problem (see later discussion). Short-term treatments, applied many times over several days, have

been used to support life until red cells become available or until adequate red cell mass is generated endogenously.

CLOSTRIDIAL MYONECROSIS (GAS GANGRENE)

Successful treatment of gas gangrene depends on prompt recognition and aggressive intervention. Mortality rates from 11% to 52% have been reported. There are five retrospective comparisons and 13 case series in the literature. These have been discussed in several reviews.[1,54,55] Because of difficulties with comparison among patient groups, impartial assessment of HBO_2 efficacy based on mortality or "tissue salvage" rates is difficult. Most authors comment on clinical benefits associated with treatment. Temporal improvement of vital signs in patients with gangrene can be among the most dramatic observations in day-to-day practice.

CRUSH INJURY

There is limited experience with HBO_2 for acute traumatic peripheral ischemia and suturing of severed limbs. A single randomized controlled trial (involving 36 patients) on this type of injury has been performed, which found HBO_2 to improve healing and reduce infection and wound dehiscence.[56] In a case series of 23 patients, HBO_2 was deemed to improve limb preservation, and it was also observed that the change in transcutaneous tissue oxygen level from ambient to hyperbaric conditions may predict outcome.[57] The rationale for considering HBO_2 is to temporarily improve oxygenation to hypoperfused tissues and because arterial hyperoxia will cause vasoconstriction that can diminish edema formation.[58,59] This latter mechanism has been demonstrated most convincingly in the context of experimental compartment syndrome.[60] Broad comparative evaluation of HBO_2 treatment for traumatic injuries is described as showing considerable benefit.[61]

PROGRESSIVE NECROTIZING INFECTIONS

The use of HBO_2 for treatment of necrotizing fasciitis and Fournier's gangrene, which are mixed aerobic-anaerobic infections, has been reported in six nonrandomized comparisons and four case series.* As with gas gangrene, variations in time of diagnosis and clinical status on admission compromise assessment of the existing literature. Most studies have reported that when HBO_2 is added to surgery and antibiotic therapy, mortality is reduced versus surgery and antibiotics alone. Animal trials have been difficult to assess because synergistic bacterial processes are difficult to establish. One report has found HBO_2 to potentiate antibiotics in streptococcal myositis),[72] and several animal models of polymicrobial bacteremia and sepsis have reported increased survival with HBO_2.[73-75] Mechanisms of action may include suppressed growth of anaerobic microorganisms and improved bactericidal action of leukocytes (that function poorly in hypoxic conditions).[11,76-78]

THERMAL BURNS

Some burn centers employ adjunctive HBO_2 for severe burns. This is not a universal practice, and controversy persists. Animal models have documented benefits with HBO_2 in reducing partial to full-thickness skin loss, hastening epithelialization, and lowering mortality.[1] Randomized clinical trials, albeit with small patient numbers, have reported improved rates of healing with shorter hospitalization stays and therefore reduced costs.[79-82] Uncontrolled series have also reported efficacy, but some studies have failed to find benefit.[83-85] The rationale for treatment has been based on reducing tissue edema and increasing neovascularization. The latter mechanism has not been directly shown with thermal injuries but is a well-documented effect in applications of HBO_2 for wounds.[3]

*References 62-71.

WOUND HEALING

Refractory cutaneous wounds are a frequent occurrence in the intensive care unit (ICU) setting, and HBO_2 may play a role if safe patient transport and monitoring are available. HBO_2 is used to treat refractory diabetic wounds and delayed radiation injuries. According to the most recent meta-analysis based on results from controlled clinical trials, employing HBO_2 as a component to refractory diabetic wound management decreases risk of a major amputation, with an odds ratio of 0.236 [95% confidence interval (CI) 0.133–0.418] and improves healing with an odds ratio of 11.64 [95% CI 3.457–39.196].[86] Another meta-analysis concluded that only four patients needed to be treated with HBO_2 to prevent one amputation.[87] The benefit of HBO_2 for radiation injury also has been shown in randomized trials and its utilization supported by independent evidence-based reviews.[88-90]

Critical Care in Hyperbaric Medicine

Hyperbaric treatment centers typically have the ability to manage patients who require critical care support. This is accomplished by close cooperation among the treating physicians, nurses, and respiratory therapists and the presence of specialized equipment to manage and monitor the patients.

Plans for treatment begin while the patient is still in the ICU, before transport to the hyperbaric chamber is initiated. Issues to be addressed include informed consent, determination that all intravenous/arterial lines and nasogastric tubes/Foley catheters are secured, capping all unnecessary intravenous catheters, placing chest tubes to one-way Heimlich valves, and adequately sedating or paralyzing the patient as clinically indicated. During transport, emergency drugs for advanced life support resuscitation should be available.

The environment of the hyperbaric chamber imposes limitations on equipment, including space restrictions, fire codes, and the effect of pressure on equipment function. Electrical components of equipment are located outside the hyperbaric chamber. Cables penetrate the chamber bulkhead to make connection to the pneumatic portion of ventilators, internal cardiac pacer wires, electrocardiogram attachments, and arterial line transducers. The patient is attached to equipment at ambient pressure before treatment, and once the treatment pressure is achieved, all settings are checked and transducers recalibrated. It is especially important to remember to check the cuff pressure of endotracheal tubes. Many centers make it a practice to replace the air in these cuffs with an equivalent volume of sterile saline before treatment to avoid volume changes related to pressurization.

There are several intravenous infusion pumps that operate normally in the multiplace chamber environment. If glass bottles, pressure bags, or any other gas-filled equipment are used inside a hyperbaric chamber, they must be adequately vented and closely monitored during a treatment.

Adverse Effects

Most HBO_2 chamber facilities have equipment and treatment protocols analogous to an ICU. The inherent toxicity of O_2 and potential for injury due to elevations of ambient pressure must be addressed whenever HBO_2 is used therapeutically.

BAROTRAUMA

Middle ear barotrauma is the most common adverse effect of HBO_2 treatment.[91] As the ambient pressure within the hyperbaric chamber is increased, a patient must be able to equalize the pressure within the middle ear by auto-insufflation, or else pain followed by hemorrhage, serous effusion, or rupture will develop. Standard protocols include instruction of patients on auto-insufflation techniques and adding oral or topical decongestants when needed. When these interventions fail,

tympanostomy tubes must be placed. The incidence of tube placement has been reported to be approximately 4% in one series.[92] Others report an overall incidence of aural barotrauma to be between 1.2% and 7%.[93,94]

Pulmonary barotrauma during HBO_2 treatment is extremely rare but should be suspected when any significant chest or hemodynamic symptoms occur during or shortly after decompression. Because the offending gas in virtually all cases will be pure O_2, absorption within the body may occur. If symptoms do develop, however, decompression should be stopped and the patient evaluated. If pneumothorax is suspected, placement of a chest tube is appropriate. Preexisting pneumothorax should be treated with chest tube drainage before initiating therapy.

OXYGEN TOXICITY

Biochemical toxicity due to O_2 can be manifested by injuries to lungs, CNS, and eyes. Pulmonary insults can impair mechanics (elasticity), vital capacity, and gas exchange.[94] These changes are typically observed only when treatment duration and pressures exceed typical therapeutic protocols. There is one report of reversible small-airway changes in 4 of 21 patients treated daily for 90 minutes at 2.4 ATA for 21 days.[95] Most studies have failed to identify any adverse pulmonary effect from standard protocols.[96,97,98]

CNS O_2 toxicity is manifested as a grand mal seizure. This occurs at an incidence of approximately 1 to 4 in 10,000 patient treatments.[93,99,100] The risk is higher in hypercapnic patients and possibly those who are acidotic or with compromise due to sepsis, because an incidence of 7% (23 in 322 patients) was reported in case series of HBO_2 treatment of gas gangrene.[54] Seizures are managed by reducing the inspired O_2 tension while leaving the patient at the same ambient pressure (to avoid pulmonary overexpansion injury when a patient is in tonic convulsion phase). Pathologic changes in association with isolated O_2-mediated seizures have not been found in studies with guinea pigs, rabbits, and humans.[101]

Progressive myopia has been reported in patients who undergo prolonged daily therapy, but this typically reverses within 6 weeks after termination of treatments.[102] There is a risk for nuclear cataract development, most typically when treatments exceed a total of 150 to 200 hours, but they may arise with less provocative exposures.[103,104] Although there is a theoretical risk for retrolental fibroplasia in neonates,[105] there are no reports of this having occurred. Currently, experimental and clinical evidence does not indicate that typical HBO_2 therapy protocols have detrimental effects on neonates or the unborn fetus.[106] This is likely due to the relatively short duration of hyperoxia.

OTHER RISKS

Confinement anxiety may occur and is typically managed with use of sedating agents. Any environment with an elevated concentration of O_2 presents a risk for fire. Scrupulous attention to avoiding an ignition source is standard in HBO_2 therapy programs.[107]

KEY POINTS

1. Several therapeutic mechanisms of action for hyperbaric oxygen therapy stem from two fundamental effects: hyperoxygenation of perfused tissues and reduction of gas bubble volume.

2. Safe treatment of critically ill patients can be accomplished in either one-man "monoplace" or larger multiple-person hyperbaric chambers.

3. Efficacy of hyperbaric oxygen therapy has been documented by randomized clinical trials for a heterogeneous group of disorders.

ANNOTATED REFERENCES

Bouachour G, Cronier P, Gouello JP, et al. Hyperbaric oxygen therapy in the management of crush injuries: a randomized double-blind placebo-controlled clinical trial. J Trauma 1996;41(2):333-9.

This blinded, randomized trial of 36 crush injury patients documented efficacy of hyperbaric oxygen therapy in improving wound healing and reducing repetitive surgery, particularly in those older than 40 years and with severe (grade III) injuries.

Goldman RJ. Hyperbaric oxygen therapy for wound healing and limb salvage: a systematic review. PM R 2009;1(5):471-89.

This recent meta-analysis provides a useful overview on the benefits of HBO₂ for refractory diabetic wound healing.

Marx RE, Johnson RP, Kline SN. Prevention of osteoradionecrosis: a randomized prospective clinical trial of hyperbaric oxygen versus penicillin. J Am Dent Assoc 1985;111(1):49-54.

This prospective randomized trial of 74 patients who required dental extractions after receiving in excess of 6800 cGy external beam radiotherapy demonstrated efficacy of prophylactic hyperbaric oxygen therapy in reducing the incidence and severity of postoperative osteoradionecrosis.

Weaver LK, Hopkins RO, Chan KJ, et al. Hyperbaric oxygen for acute carbon monoxide poisoning. N Engl J Med 2002;347(14):1057-67.

This prospective, randomized, placebo-controlled trial of 152 patients with carbon monoxide poisoning describes the efficacy of hyperbaric oxygen therapy in reducing neurologic morbidity among those with a history of unconsciousness, or with cerebellar dysfunction, or those with a carboxyhemoglobin level greater than 25%.

57

Imaging of the Chest

AMY E. MORRIS | JEFFREY P. KANNE | ERIC J. STERN

Chest imaging plays a central role in the management of critically ill patients. Bedside chest radiography and computed tomography (CT) are essential aids to both diagnosis and evaluating responses to therapy. In this chapter, we review chest imaging in the intensive care unit (ICU) setting, focusing on radiography and CT. Radiographic techniques used at the bedside and appropriate positioning of various monitoring and life support devices will be discussed. In addition, imaging findings of common pathologic processes encountered in critically ill patients are described.

Principles of Imaging in the Intensive Care Unit

Portable chest radiography plays a major role in patient care, especially in critically ill patients. Bedside chest radiographs are frequently obtained in ICU patients, and an understanding of how to interpret these films is important for ICU physicians. The American College of Radiology's current guidelines call for daily chest radiographs of all mechanically ventilated patients in the ICU,[1] but this approach is controversial. Some earlier studies supported this recommendation, arguing that early detection of unexpected findings on routine films may save money and decrease length of stay.[2-4] However, several recent and larger studies have refuted this, demonstrating that a small minority of routine chest radiographs have any significant impact on patient management. Further, these studies suggest that transition to on-demand imaging saves money and radiation exposure without prolonging length of stay or negatively impacting other safety parameters.[5-10]

Regardless of the frequency with which they are obtained, interpretation of bedside chest radiographs can be quite challenging because of variation in quality due to both technical and patient factors. The ill health of the patient and multiple cumbersome life support devices limit proper upright patient positioning, while difficulty controlling respiratory and body motion can blur the radiographic images, all potentially leading to low-quality radiographs. The importance of dedicated and competent radiology technologists and an effective quality assurance program cannot be overemphasized.

Conventional and Digital Radiography

With conventional portable radiography units, the maximum tube current and voltage are limited, so exposure times are relatively long, and image contrast may be excessive. Digital (or computed) radiography uses a phosphor plate in lieu of a film-screen combination to capture and store the radiographic image, which reduces the patient's radiation dose. When digital images are processed, the portion of the dynamic range containing the diagnostic information is identified, and the final output for display is adjusted to a consistent and optimized contrast and density. This obviates the need for repeated examinations because of errors in exposure and may improve diagnostic yield.[11] For these reasons, as well as the ease with which digital processing allows placement of images on a digital network, digital radiography has largely replaced conventional techniques.

Conventional and digital radiography share some disadvantages, however. The overall time required for obtaining the radiograph remains the same, and both portable techniques capture images in the anteroposterior projection. When combined with a shorter source image receptor distance, this leads to geometric magnification of anterior chest structures such as the heart. In addition, severe patient illness in the ICU often requires supine and semi-upright positioning, which may complicate interpretation of radiographs, particularly in cases of pneumothorax or pleural effusion.[12]

Computed Tomography

Computed tomography provides better anatomic detail and a higher degree of diagnostic accuracy than chest radiography, but for critically ill patients, transportation and cumbersome monitoring devices limit access to CT. Mobile CT scanners have been developed to image critically ill patients in the ICU and avoid the need for transportation. They are not yet in widespread use, in part due to image quality concerns, but have demonstrated utility in neurosurgical[13-16] and other intensive care applications,[17] including infectious disease outbreak situations.[18]

Picture Archiving and Communications System

Immediate access to bedside chest images is particularly useful in the ICU, where information is desired without delay. A picture archiving and communications system (PACS) permits transmission of medical images over a digital network for simultaneous display within minutes of their acquisition at multiple locations. In addition, PACS allows for rapid retrieval of previous examinations for comparison, and workstation tools enable accurate measuring and adjustment of digital image parameters such as window and level settings.

Interpreting the ICU Chest Radiograph

MONITORING AND SUPPORT DEVICES

Endotracheal Tubes

On the chest radiograph, the position of an endotracheal tube (ETT) is determined by the location of the tube's tip in relation to the carina with respect to the position of the patient's chin. With the chin in the neutral position, the tip of the ETT should be 3 to 7 cm above the carina (Figure 57-1). Alternatively, the tip of the ETT should project over the T3 or T4 vertebral body, because the carina is located between T5 and T7 on anteroposterior radiographs in most individuals. Neck flexion and extension can result in 2 cm of downward or upward displacement, respectively, of the ETT.[19] Projection of the anterior portion of the mandible over the lower cervical spine indicates neck flexion, whereas an unobscured cervical spine indicates neck extension.

The most common complication of ETT placement is inadvertent intubation of the right main bronchus (Figure 57-2) because of its shallower angle of departure from the trachea compared to the left main bronchus. Esophageal placement of the ETT can occur, although this is usually detected on physical examination. Radiographic findings of esophageal intubation include direct visualization of the ETT lateral to the tracheal wall, gaseous distention of the stomach, and displacement of the trachea by an overdistended balloon cuff.

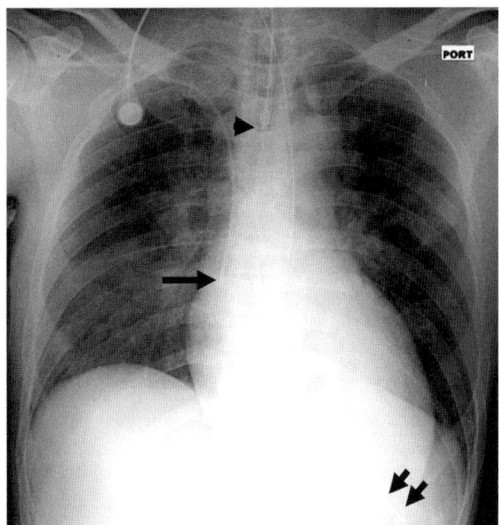

Figure 57-1 Typical normal line and tube positions. Note expected positions of endotracheal tube (superimposed over T3 vertebral body *[arrowhead]*), central venous catheter (in the origin of superior vena cava *[arrow]*), and nasogastric tube (in stomach *[double arrows]*).

Tracheostomy Tubes

The tip of a tracheostomy tube should be several centimeters above the carina, and the tube's diameter should be approximately two-thirds that of the trachea.[20] Unlike ETTs, chin position does not affect tracheostomy tube position. Air is commonly seen in the subcutaneous tissue of the neck and upper mediastinum immediately after tracheostomy tube placement and should resolve over time. Pneumothorax and mediastinal hematoma, the latter manifesting as a dense mediastinum with full, convex margins, are more worrisome complications of tracheostomy tube placement that should not be overlooked.

Central Venous Catheters

Central venous catheters are inserted from an internal jugular (IJ), subclavian (SC), or femoral approach. The optimal location of an IJ or SC catheter tip is within the superior vena cava downstream of the central venous valves. On the anteroposterior chest radiograph, the origin of the superior vena cava usually lies to the right of midline at the level of the first intercostal space (see Figure 57-1).[21] The catheter tip should remain proximal to the right atrium to reduce the risk of arrhythmias, myocardial perforation, or cardiac tamponade. Portable chest radiographs should be obtained immediately after central venous catheter placement to determine catheter position and identify any complications such as pneumothorax, vessel perforation (Figure 57-3),

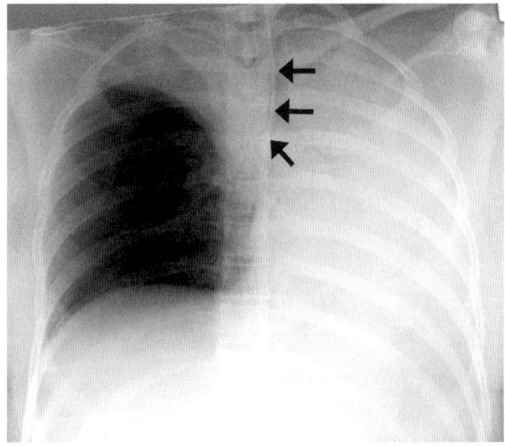

Figure 57-2 Anteroposterior chest radiograph shows endotracheal tube *(arrows)* extending into bronchus intermedius, with resulting collapse of left lung and right upper lobe from hypoventilation.

cardiac perforation, retained or fragmented catheter, or a knotted catheter.

Peripherally Inserted Central Catheters

Peripherally inserted central catheters (PICCs) are relatively new devices gaining widespread acceptance for long-term central venous access. The catheters are small, 2 to 5 French, and are placed into the superior vena cava through a large upper-extremity vein. PICCs may be difficult to identify on bedside chest radiographs because of their small size and faint opacity. They are also more susceptible to displacement than other intravenous catheters, owing to increased flexibility of the material (see Figure 57-3).

Pulmonary Artery Catheters

Pulmonary artery catheters measure intracardiac and intrapulmonary pressures reflecting volume status, cardiac function, and vascular tone. Their use is declining in many ICUs because recent studies demonstrate limited utility in affecting patient outcomes in a variety of clinical settings.[22,23] Nevertheless, when they are used, accurate placement is critical for proper interpretation. The catheters are usually introduced via an internal jugular or subclavian approach; less commonly they may be inserted through the femoral vein. They then traverse the central venous system into the right ventricle, through the pulmonic valve into the main, then right (less commonly left) pulmonary artery, then "wedge" in a proximal interlobar artery. If the tip extends beyond these larger arteries (Figure 57-4), pulmonary infarction from occlusion of the pulmonary vessel or development of a pseudoaneurysm

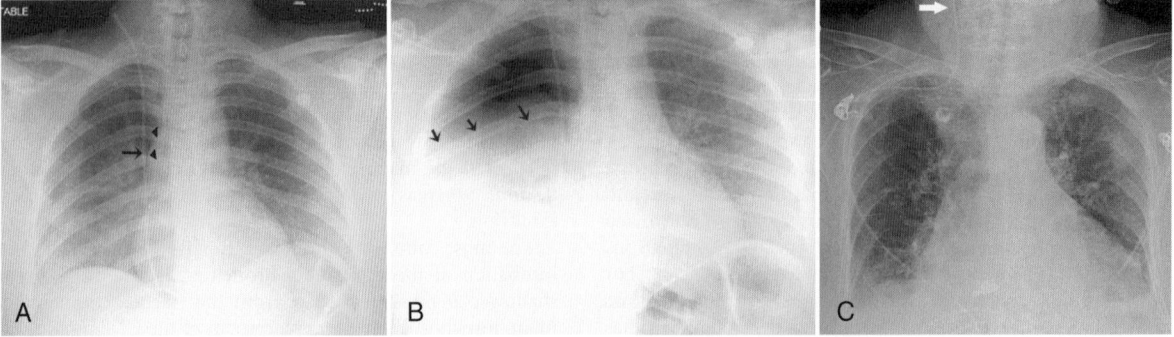

Figure 57-3 Complications of intravenous catheter placement. **A,** Right internal jugular (IJ) catheter *(arrow)* is lateral to right mediastinal margin *(arrowheads)*, indicating catheter is extravascular. **B,** Twelve hours later, a pleural fluid collection has developed from inadvertent infusion of saline into right pleural space *(arrows)*. **C,** In another patient, a peripherally inserted central catheter (PICC) line is malpositioned, with tip in internal jugular vein *(arrow)*.

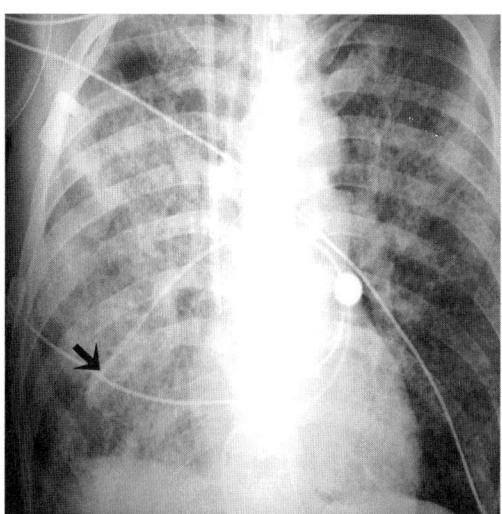

Figure 57-4 Tip of Swan-Ganz catheter extends into right lower lobe pulmonary artery. In this location, risk of vessel injury increases.

can ensue. The balloon at the catheter tip should be inflated only during placement or when obtaining pressure measurements, so an inflated balloon should never be present on a portable chest radiograph. Complications are similar to those that occur with other central venous catheters but also include pulmonary vascular perforation and pulmonary hemorrhage.

Intraaortic Balloon Pumps

Intraaortic balloon pumps (IABPs) assist left ventricular function in patients with severe left ventricular dysfunction, usually after myocardial infarction. They are essentially balloons approximately 16 cm in length that are inflated during systole to reduce afterload and augment coronary artery perfusion. IABPs are inserted into the common femoral artery and advanced into the descending thoracic aorta. On the frontal chest radiograph, the tip of the balloon should be visible within the descending thoracic aorta just distal to the origin of the left subclavian artery, typically at the level of aortic arch. A more upstream location of the balloon can result in occlusion of the subclavian and vertebral arteries, whereas a more downstream location can lead to occlusion of the mesenteric and renal arteries. IABPs can migrate, so position should be reassessed on subsequent chest radiographs.

Thoracostomy Tubes

Thoracostomy tubes are placed in the pleural space to drain fluid or air. On a chest radiograph, the side port of a thoracostomy tube is marked by a disruption in the radiographically opaque line and should be located medial to the inner margin of the ribs. A malpositioned

thoracostomy tube is often suspected when the tube does not drain as expected. It may not be inserted into the pleural space at all but instead tunnel through the subcutaneous soft tissues. Alternatively, the tip may lie within a pulmonary fissure, or rarely within the lung parenchyma. Subcutaneous placement can be very difficult to ascertain on chest radiograph, and an intrafissural location can only be suspected when the tube follows the course of one of the pulmonary fissures. The cross-sectional nature of CT scans provides an advantage to accurately identify the course of a thoracostomy tube and its relationship to abnormal air or fluid collections (Figure 57-5).

Enteric Tubes

Enteric tubes are placed into the stomach or proximal small bowel via a transoral or transnasal approach and come in a variety of sizes and configurations (see Figure 57-1). These tubes are frequently placed in ICU patients, especially those who are endotracheally intubated. Although the best position for feeding tubes is controversial, placement distal to the pylorus may decrease the risk of aspiration.[24] Usually, enteric tube position is easily determined by a chest or abdominal radiograph, although they may occasionally be obscured by excess soft tissue in obese patients. These tubes can coil in the pharynx or esophagus, putting the patient at risk for aspiration if tube feeds are initiated. Inadvertent insertion into the tracheobronchial tree (Figure 57-6) and esophageal perforation are rare but have more serious consequences.

Approach to ICU Chest Imaging

In many large hospitals, "the ICU" is not a single entity but a group of system- or illness-specific units. Certain diagnoses are more common in specific settings, and patient context must be considered when interpreting a chest radiograph. However, the general approach to interpreting a chest radiograph should be uniform across disciplines to avoid missing an unexpected finding. We have organized the rest of the chapter by anatomic location in the chest: lungs, pleura, mediastinum, and vasculature. Within each section we will address key findings specific to cardiac, trauma, neurologic, and neurosurgical patients, as well as those that may be found in any critically ill patient.

Lung Abnormalities

DIFFUSE LUNG OPACITIES

Cardiogenic Pulmonary Edema

Several conditions can cause the pattern of homogenous lung opacity that represents, or mimics, pulmonary edema. The classic appearance of cardiogenic pulmonary edema is that of bilateral perihilar fluffy opacities, sometimes called a *butterfly* or *bat-wing pattern*, in association with an enlarged heart, engorgement of central pulmonary veins, interstitial edema, and vascular redistribution or cephalization of vessels (Figure 57-7). Pleural effusions may also be present. The

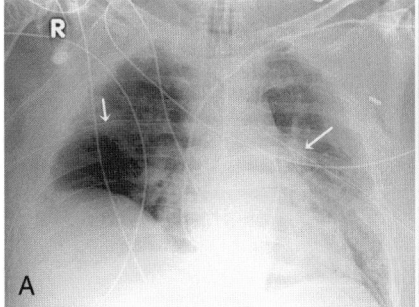
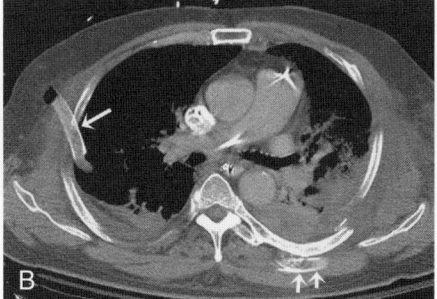
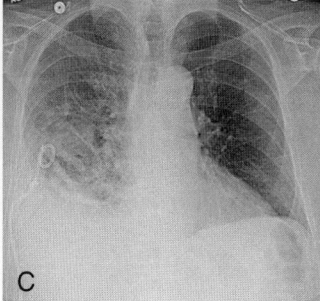

Figure 57-5 Malpositioned thoracostomy tube after bedside placement. **A,** Anteroposterior chest radiograph shows bilateral thoracostomy tubes (*arrows*) with tips and side ports projecting over lungs. **B,** Computed tomography shows left thoracostomy tube (*double arrows*) is in posterior chest wall. Right thoracostomy tube (*single arrow*) is in satisfactory position. **C,** In a different patient, a small-bore, curved "pigtail" catheter is appropriately placed for drainage of a right pleural effusion.

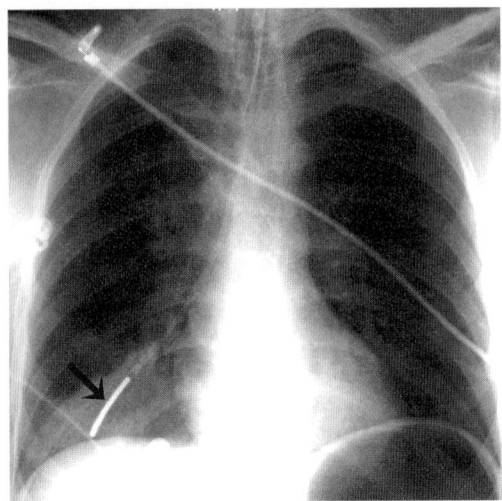

Figure 57-6 Distal-weighted enteric feeding tube *(arrow)* extending into right lower lobe bronchus.

opacities associated with cardiogenic pulmonary edema can fluctuate rapidly, a clue to its diagnosis. However, this classic appearance is rare in the ICU. The bat-wing pattern is seen in few patients with pulmonary edema; opacities may be asymmetrical due to variations in patient position and underlying cardiopulmonary disease, such as emphysema or mitral valve insufficiency. In addition, cephalization of the vasculature is not a very useful marker of edema in supine ICU patients. Finally, some patients, particularly those with milder disease or chronically elevated left ventricular pressures, may only have more subtle radiographic findings, such as peribronchial cuffing and indistinct vessels.[25,26] Serial measurements of vascular pedicle width may be a useful adjunct indication of intravascular volume status in these patients.[27]

Neurogenic Pulmonary Edema

Neurogenic pulmonary edema can occur in the setting of any cerebral insult, including intracranial hemorrhage or mass, head trauma, stroke, seizures, or infection. Elevated microvascular pressure and increased vascular permeability in the lung both appear to play a role in its development.[28] Neurogenic pulmonary edema can develop within hours after the neurologic insult or several days later. On the

chest radiograph, neurogenic edema usually manifests as a diffuse, homogeneous pulmonary opacity similar to that of cardiogenic edema, but without an enlarged cardiac silhouette and often without the indistinct vessels that suggest engorgement. (Figure 57-8). Occasionally, opacities may have a focal distribution reflecting gravity, patient position, and heterogeneity in pulmonary venous pressure. Rapid clearing of the lungs within days of resolution of the neurologic insult is characteristic, in contrast to other forms of noncardiogenic pulmonary edema in which opacity can persist.[28] It is important to note that some patients with neurologic injury are treated with large volumes of intravenous fluid, which may complicate the interpretation of pulmonary edema opacities on the chest radiograph.

Acute Lung Injury and Acute Respiratory Distress Syndrome

Acute lung injury (ALI) and acute respiratory distress syndrome (ARDS) are common in medical and surgical ICU patients and have a high mortality.[29-31] They are clinical syndromes defined by hypoxemia and diffuse bilateral lung opacities in the absence of left atrial hypertension.[32] Both result from a massive inflammatory reaction in the lungs incited by a variety of causes, and they are radiographically indistinguishable. The severity of hypoxemia alone differentiates the two, with ARDS the more severe manifestation. In the acute phase of ARDS, diffuse ill-defined opacities often predominate in the periphery of the lungs. As the disease progresses, the entire hemithorax can become opacified on chest radiographs (Figure 57-9), although CT typically demonstrates heterogeneity in lung aeration. This finding has led to much discussion regarding appropriate ventilator management of ARDS to balance alveolar recruitment while avoiding hyperinflation of spared lung tissue (see Chapter 58). During the subacute phase (5 to 10 days later), proliferation of endothelial cells and fibroblasts leads to a pattern of progressive lung destruction. Some patients recover from ARDS without any residual deficit in pulmonary function, but others progress to a chronic phase several weeks after the initial lung injury and have permanent respiratory sequelae. Fibrosis and focal emphysema are usually evident on these patients' radiographs or CT scans.

Fat Embolism Syndrome

This syndrome is a rare but serious complication of recent severe fracture, usually of a long bone, and is characterized by pulmonary, cerebral, and cutaneous manifestations 12 to 72 hours after the injury. In mild cases, the chest radiograph often shows no abnormality. In more severe cases, the initial chest radiograph may be normal, but within 12 to 72 hours, airspace and interstitial opacities develop that

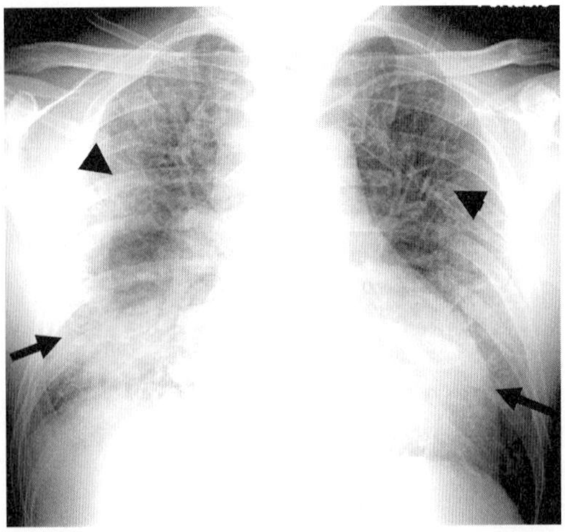

Figure 57-7 Cardiogenic pulmonary edema in a 54-year-old man with acute myocardial infarction. Chest radiograph shows an enlarged cardiac silhouette with bibasilar opacities and diffuse septal thickening in both lungs. Note Kerley's A *(arrowheads)* and Kerley's B lines *(arrows)*.

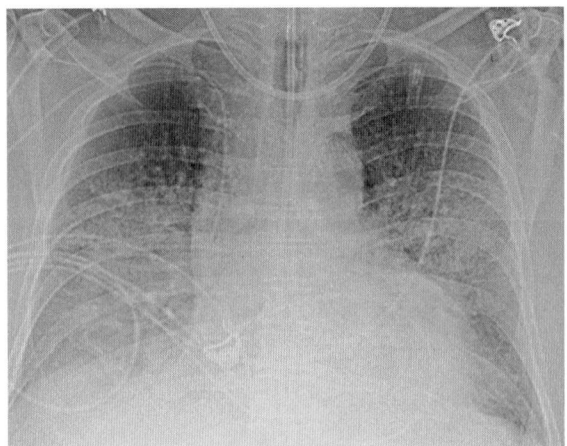

Figure 57-8 Neurogenic pulmonary edema in patient with large left middle cerebral artery stroke. Chest radiograph shows diffuse opacities similar to cardiogenic pulmonary edema, predominantly in the bases. Note normal cardiac silhouette. Echocardiogram confirmed absence of impaired cardiac function.

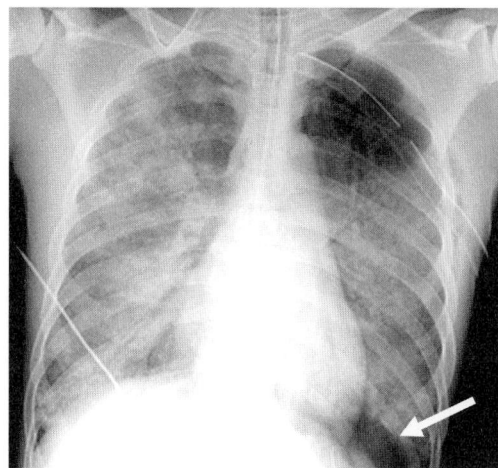

Figure 57-9 A 22-year-old man with clinical sepsis developed hypoxia 2 days after admission. Anteroposterior chest radiograph shows diffuse lung opacity with normal heart size, consistent with noncardiogenic pulmonary edema or acute lung injury/acute respiratory distress syndrome (ALI/ARDS). Also note pneumothorax in left costophrenic sulcus *(arrow)*.

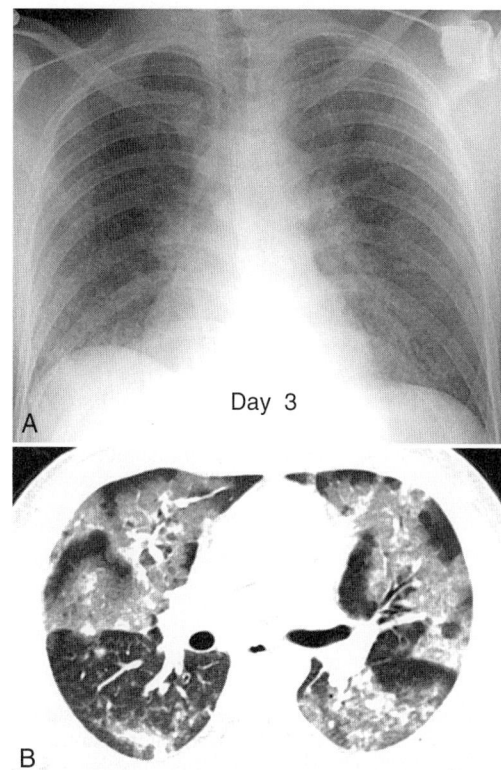

Day 3

Figure 57-10 A 33-year-old man presented with a left femur fracture and clinical fat embolism syndrome. Initial chest radiograph was normal. **A,** Seventy-two hours later, diffuse pulmonary opacity developed without an enlarged cardiac silhouette, coinciding with dyspnea, altered level of consciousness, and diffuse petechiae. **B,** Computed tomography image (same day) shows geographic appearance of ground-glass opacity in both lungs, consistent with noncardiogenic pulmonary edema.

resemble other causes of pulmonary edema (Figure 57-10), then resolve 10 to 14 days later in the absence of superimposed disease.[33] CT scans are often not performed in these patients, but when available, variable findings including focal or diffuse areas of consolidation or "ground-glass" appearance and small nodules have all been described.[34,35] Rarely, filling defects from fat emboli in pulmonary arteries are reported.[36] The history of fracture, associated nonpulmonary symptoms such as a petechial rash, and delay in onset of radiographic opacities are all clues to distinguish fat embolism syndrome from other causes of a pulmonary edema pattern on chest radiographs.

Unilateral Pulmonary Edema Pattern

Postpneumonectomy pulmonary edema is described later. Reexpansion pulmonary edema (RPE) rarely follows treatment of pneumothorax or pleural effusion. It is more likely to occur if the lung has been chronically collapsed, if large volumes of air or pleural fluid (greater than 1 L) are removed rapidly, or pleural pressure drops below −20 cm H_2O.[37] Recent studies call these absolute numbers into question, however.[38] Usually within a few hours after evacuation of air or fluid, patients develop symptoms such as cough, dyspnea, and tachypnea; hypotension due to third-spacing of edema fluid in the affected lung has been described. Chest imaging reveals diffuse homogeneous opacity on the affected side, and in rare cases, the contralateral lung may also demonstrate opacities.

FOCAL LUNG OPACITIES

In this section we will describe the most common etiologies of lung opacities of a more heterogeneous nature. This is a diverse group that includes lobar or multilobar opacities, nodular or multinodular abnormalities, or other scattered patches of density that do not resemble the bilateral, more diffuse pattern of pulmonary edema.

Aspiration

Patients with a decreased level of consciousness are at risk for aspiration. These include neurologic or neurosurgical patients who have suffered a stroke, head injury, or seizure, as well as medical or surgical patients who have esophageal disorders, altered mental status, or who have been pharmacologically sedated. The clinical severity and radiographic appearance of aspiration depend on both the amount and composition of aspirated fluid. Radiographically, aspiration can result

in unilateral or bilateral lobar or multilobar opacities. Opacities tend to be in the dependent portions of the lungs, including the posterior segments of the upper lobes and the superior and posterior basilar segments of the lower lobes (Figure 57-11). Occasionally, aspirated particulate matter or foreign bodies can obstruct the airways and cause volume loss.

Pneumonia

The radiographic hallmark of community-acquired bacterial pneumonia (CAP) is lung consolidation with air bronchograms in a segmental, lobar, or (less commonly) diffuse distribution (Figure 57-12). In comparison, the majority of patients with healthcare-associated or nosocomial pneumonia (HCAP), including ventilator-associated pneumonia, are more likely to have bilateral multilobar disease.[39] Radiographs typically demonstrate bronchopneumonia characterized by patchy peribronchial opacities, bronchial wall thickening, and sometimes volume loss.

CT scanning is unnecessary in most patients with community-acquired pneumonia and a typical chest radiograph as described; in such patients, a given radiographic pattern is poorly predictive of a specific causative organism.[40] CT scans may be helpful for patients whose chest radiographs are atypical or have nonresolving opacities, patients who are immunosuppressed, or patients who may require invasive procedures such as bronchoscopy. In these cases, CT can provide additional anatomic detail that may assist in identifying a pathogen or noninfectious etiology, or in guiding interventions. Ground-glass opacities are nonspecific, but airspace disease including consolidation and air bronchograms suggests bacterial, mycoplasma, or fungal pneumonia. Centrilobular nodules are infrequently found in

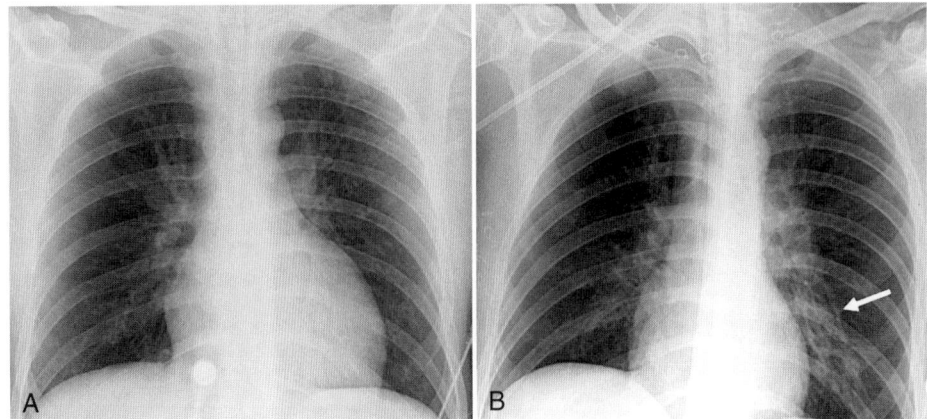

Figure 57-11 A 49-year-old man presented with seizure and witnessed aspiration. **A,** Initial anteroposterior chest radiograph is normal. **B,** Twenty-four hours later, patchy left lower lobe opacity *(arrow)* has developed, consistent with aspiration pneumonia. Note increased opacity behind heart.

bacterial pneumonia and instead suggest mycoplasma, fungal, or viral infection (Figure 57-13).

Chest radiography and CT may also show complications of pneumonia. Cavitation can occur in some bacterial infections, particularly in nosocomial pneumonia or immunocompromised patients, and may progress to larger abscess or pneumatocele formation. Pleural effusions are also more common in nosocomial pneumonia; a minority will become complicated and may develop into empyema (see later discussion).[39]

Septic Emboli

Septic emboli to the lungs come from a variety of sources, including infected right heart valves, peripheral and pelvic thrombophlebitis, and infected intravenous catheters. The usual radiographic findings of septic emboli are bilateral ill-defined nodules, predominantly in the lung periphery. These opacities classically develop at different times and show features of different stages of evolution; they often cavitate and may develop into larger abscesses. On CT, multiple lung cavitary and noncavitary nodules and wedge-shaped subpleural areas of consolidation are the usual findings (Figure 57-14).

PARENCHYMAL ABNORMALITIES SPECIFIC TO THORACIC SURGERY PATIENTS

Thoracoscopy or thoracotomy with lobectomy or pneumonectomy can alter the expected appearance of the intrathoracic structures, and knowledge of the normal expected findings after surgery allows for better identification of complications.

Pneumonectomy

Radiographs obtained immediately after pneumonectomy normally show midline position of the mediastinum and gas filling the pneumonectomy space. Over the first few days, the ipsilateral hemidiaphragm elevates, and fluid begins to accumulate within the pneumonectomy space as the gas is resorbed. In most cases, one-half to two-thirds of the hemithorax fills within the first week, and the remainder over the next several weeks to months.[41] The mediastinum shifts toward the operative side as the remaining lung hyperinflates and herniates across the midline, anterior to the heart. The degree of mediastinal displacement depends primarily on the compliance and the degree of hyperinflation of the remaining lung. Appropriate mediastinal displacement is the

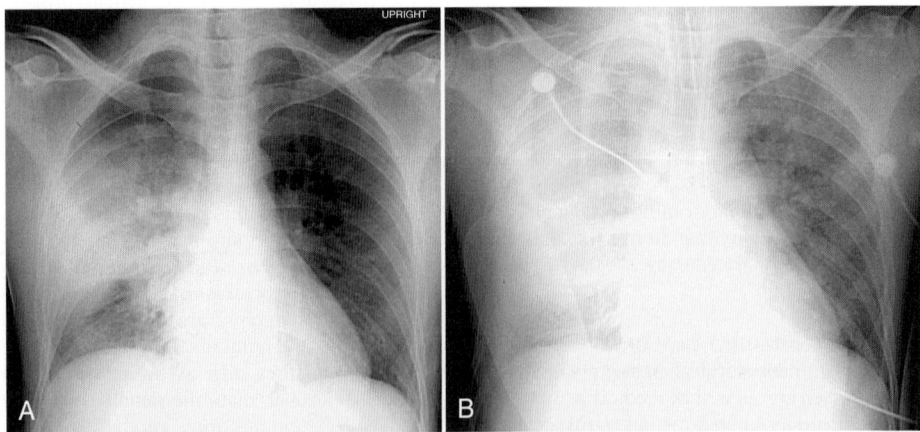

Figure 57-12 A 30-year-old man presented with *Klebsiella pneumoniae* infection. **A,** Initial chest radiograph shows right upper lobe opacity consistent with lobar pneumonia. **B,** Two days later, right lung is nearly completely consolidated, showing rapid spread of infection. Tube and line are in expected location. Pacing pad is superimposing on right chest.

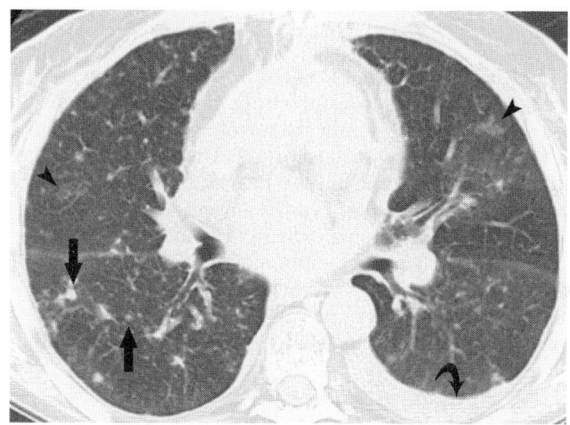

Figure 57-13 A 45-year-old woman with heart transplant and varicella pneumonia. Computed tomography shows multiple small lung nodules *(arrows)* and patchy foci of ground-glass opacity *(arrowheads)*. A small left pleural effusion is present *(curved arrow)*.

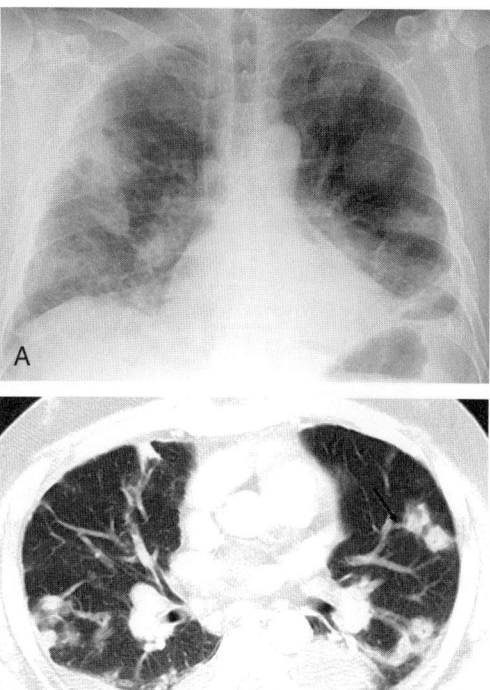

Figure 57-14 A 46-year-old intravenous drug abuser presented with septic emboli. **A,** Bedside chest radiograph shows multiple bilateral peripheral opacities, some of which are cavitary. **B,** Computed tomography shows multiple peripheral well-defined pulmonary nodules.

most reliable indicator of a normal course after pneumonectomy. Failure of the mediastinum to shift to the operative side indicates an abnormality in the pneumonectomy cavity such as bronchopleural fistula, hemothorax, or empyema. Postoperative complications of pneumonectomy can occur early (within a few days of surgery) or late; in this review, we will focus on the early complications.

Postpneumonectomy pulmonary edema is an uncommon condition with a high mortality rate, due at least in part to an increase in pulmonary capillary permeability. Radiographic features can be mild, with peribronchial cuffing and ill-defined vascular structures. In more severe cases, the pattern is identical to that of ARDS. Bronchopleural fistula is another infrequent but life-threatening complication of pneumonectomy, which manifests with dyspnea and sometimes hemoptysis. Both pulmonary edema and bronchopleural fistula are more common after right pneumonectomy; in the latter case, the shorter length of the bronchial stump predisposes to leakage. Radiographic findings of bronchopleural fistula include persistent pneumothorax or subcutaneous and mediastinal emphysema after surgery, a decrease in height of more than 1.5 cm of the gas-fluid level in the pneumonectomy cavity, and mediastinal shift away from the operative side rather than toward it (Figure 57-15).

Lobectomy

After uncomplicated lobectomy, the chest radiograph can show rotation and hyperinflation of the remaining lobe(s), change in the orientation of the remaining bronchovascular structures, linear atelectasis, and/or development of pleural effusion. Reorientation of the remaining bronchovascular anatomy should not be confused with atelectasis. Complications of lobectomy occur with less frequency than with pneumonectomy but are similar. In addition, lung torsion, which has a high mortality rate, occurs rarely and manifests as rapid opacification of a lobe or lung associated with unusual configuration of the hilum. Anastomotic suture lines are evident when the fissure incompletely divides the lung into lobes.

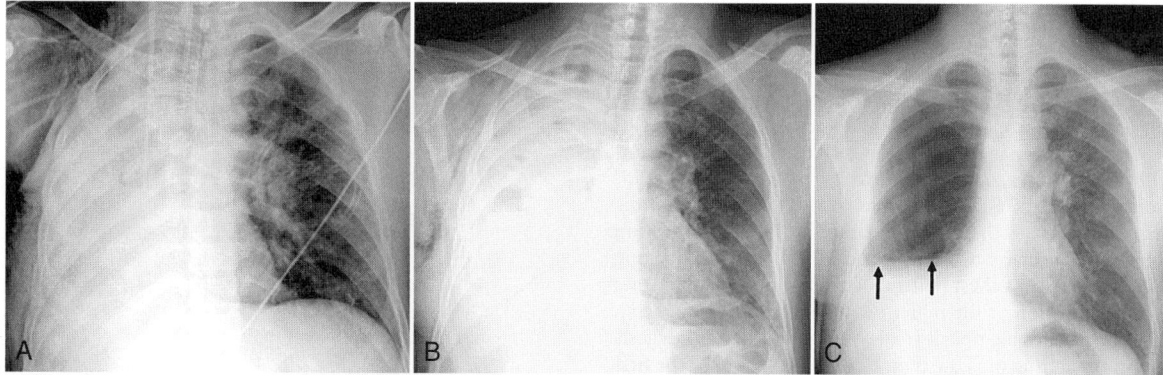

Figure 57-15 Serial chest radiographs after right pneumonectomy show development of a bronchopleural fistula. **A,** Supine view obtained the day after surgery shows fluid in right hemithorax and rightward deviation of mediastinum, as expected. Tube and line are in expected positions. **B,** Four days later, mediastinum is now shifted to the left, and several lucencies have developed in right hemithorax. **C,** Two weeks after pneumectomy, upright posteroanterior radiograph shows gas-fluid level *(arrows)* and leftward mediastinal deviation, opposite of what is expected, consistent with bronchopleural fistula from a stump leak.

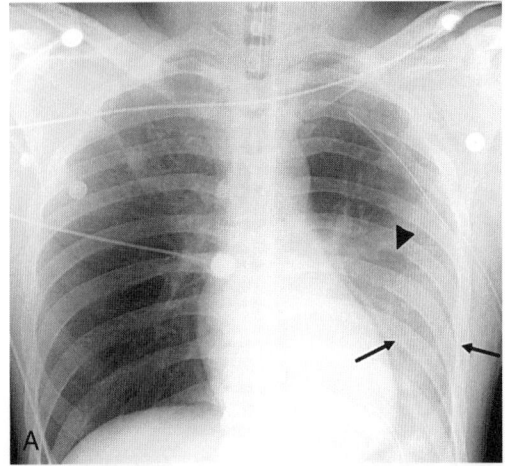

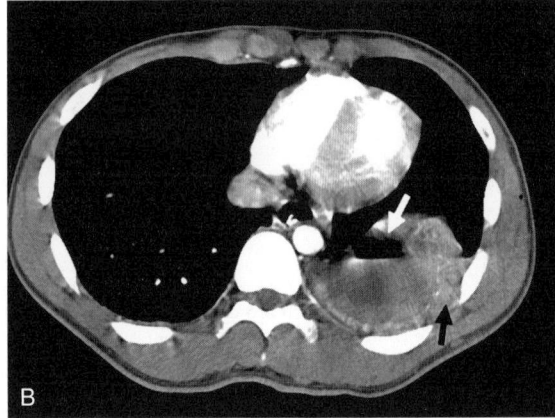

Figure 57-16 A 30-year-old man involved in motor vehicle crash. **A,** Chest radiograph shows a small lucent area *(arrowhead)* within an area of left lower lobe opacity *(arrows).* **B,** Computed tomography image of chest shows a "cavity" with an air-fluid level *(white arrow)* in left lower lobe, representing a pulmonary laceration surrounded by pulmonary contusion and hemorrhage *(black arrow).*

PARENCHYMAL ABNORMALITIES SPECIFIC TO TRAUMA PATIENTS

Imaging of trauma patients focuses on identifying acute complications from the trauma as well as recognizing additional injuries that may have been obscured or overlooked on initial evaluation.

Pulmonary Contusion

Contusion is the most common lung injury after blunt chest trauma, occurring in up to 70% of patients.[42] It is characterized by leakage of blood into the pulmonary interstitium and alveolar spaces and clinically presents with dyspnea, tachycardia, and hypoxia. On chest radiographs, the contusion manifests as pulmonary opacity in a nonanatomic distribution, in contrast to the usual segmental or lobar distribution of pneumonia or atelectasis. Contusion usually occurs in the lung periphery deep to the site of chest wall impact, although it is sometimes seen opposite the location of the injury owing to a contrecoup effect. The timing of the developing opacity on the chest radiograph suggests the diagnosis in the setting of acute trauma, presenting within the first several hours after injury and resolving within 14 days. CT is more sensitive than chest radiography for detecting pulmonary contusion as well as associated chest wall injuries.[43,44] The appearance on CT of lung contusion ranges from patchy, ground-glass opacity to dense consolidation in a nonsegmental distribution, often sparing 1 to 2 mm of subpleural lung (Figure 57-16).

Pulmonary Laceration

Pulmonary laceration is characterized by frank disruption of the lung parenchyma. Radiographic features of pulmonary laceration are often masked on chest radiography by the surrounding contusion during the first few days and are better seen on CT. The appearance will change over time. In the acute phase, the hematoma within the laceration appears as a well-circumscribed, homogeneous area of soft-tissue attenuation. As the hematoma evolves, a round or elliptical gas collection called a *pneumatocele* becomes more obvious (see Figure 57-16). Most pneumatoceles appear within a few days, but some may develop over several weeks. They can be single or multiple and can be several centimeters in diameter. Resolution occurs over several months.

PLEURAL DISEASE

Parapneumonic Effusion and Empyema

The nature of fluid within the pleural space can be difficult to determine on the chest radiograph. Pleural effusions can be transudative, exudative, purulent (empyema), bloody, or chylous. On the chest radiograph, pleural effusion causes increased opacity in the affected hemithorax, a crescentic opacity interposed between the inner margin of ribs and the lung, and an apical cap. In the setting of pneumonia, lateral decubitus films can often differentiate mobile from loculated fluid collections, with the latter suggesting active infection of the pleural space (empyema). However, loculations and gas within the pleural space, which also suggests frank empyema, are best detected on CT (Figure 57-17). Empyema can also complicate thoracic surgery, usually at least several days after the operation.

HEMOTHORAX AND CHYLOTHORAX

Hemothorax and chylothorax are most often seen in surgical patients following thoracic surgical procedures or penetrating (more common) or blunt chest trauma. Chylothorax is rare, but hemothorax occurs in up to 50% of blunt thoracic trauma.[45] Either process can also complicate pneumonectomy, causing opacification of the operative hemithorax with contralateral shift of the mediastinum, in contrast to the ipsilateral shift seen with normal filling of the pneumonectomy space. Hemothorax and chylothorax are less common in the medical ICU;

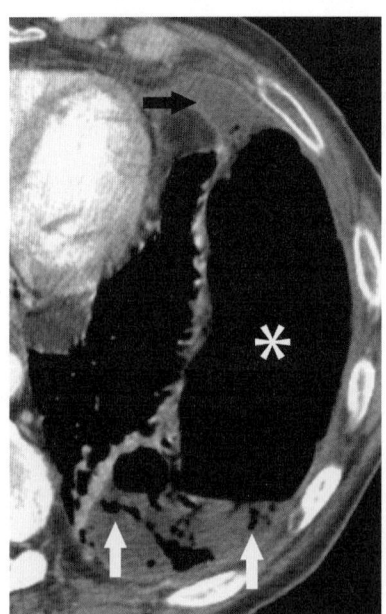

Figure 57-17 Coned-down contrast-enhanced computed tomography image of a 74-year-old man with left empyema from ruptured splenic abscess shows a complex pleural collection containing a large amount of gas *(asterisk)*, smaller gas loculations *(white arrows)*, and a loculated liquid component anteriorly *(black arrow)*.

the former is most often an iatrogenic complication of a procedure or anticoagulation, and chylothorax usually affects oncology patients or others with thoracic duct obstruction.

Regardless of the setting, rapid opacification of the pleural space following an acute inciting event likely indicates hemorrhage, whereas chylothorax accumulates more slowly over a period of several days. CT scanning with attenuation measurement will also help differentiate hemothorax from other causes of pleural effusion: liquid blood usually measures 30 to 45 Hounsfield units (HU), and clotted blood 50 to 90 HU. The two may mix in a hemothorax, giving an inhomogeneous or layered appearance that suggests the diagnosis.[43]

PNEUMOTHORAX

Pneumothorax can occur spontaneously, in association with malignancy or other destructive lung process, iatrogenically, or as a result of trauma. In the latter category, it is more common with blunt chest trauma than with penetrating injuries to the chest. The clinical significance of pneumothorax depends more on the patient's underlying cardiopulmonary function than the physical size of the pneumothorax, but all pneumothoraces can rapidly become life threatening if positive-pressure mechanical ventilation is instituted.

In the supine position, free gas will localize in the nondependent caudal and anteromedial aspects of the pleural space. Therefore, evidence of pneumothorax on the supine chest radiograph is often indirect and includes a low, sharp costophrenic sulcus (deep sulcus sign), relative basilar hyperlucency, increased sharpness of the ipsilateral hemidiaphragm, increased sharpness of cardiac border, presence of gas in the minor fissure, and caudal displacement of the ipsilateral hemidiaphragm (Figure 57-18). CT is more sensitive than chest radiography for detecting pneumothorax and is especially helpful in critically ill patients who cannot tolerate upright or lateral decubitus positioning. In tension pneumothorax, air enters the pleural cavity via a "ball-valve" mechanism by which it cannot escape. Chest radiographs demonstrate mediastinal shift away from the involved hemithorax, but this is infrequently captured on film owing to the clinical urgency of associated hypotension and hypoxia, mandating immediate bedside treatment.

DIAPHRAGMATIC RUPTURE

Rupture of the diaphragm is a rare complication in patients admitted with trauma; it is more common in penetrating trauma.[46] Delay in diagnosis is common, especially in patients receiving positive-pressure ventilation, because the injury is masked by the positive-pressure gradient between the thoracic and abdominal cavities. Radiographic findings of diaphragmatic rupture include a gas-filled viscus or the tip of a properly placed enteric tube above the diaphragm, irregularity of diaphragmatic contour, elevation of the affected hemidiaphragm without atelectasis, and contralateral shift of the mediastinum without

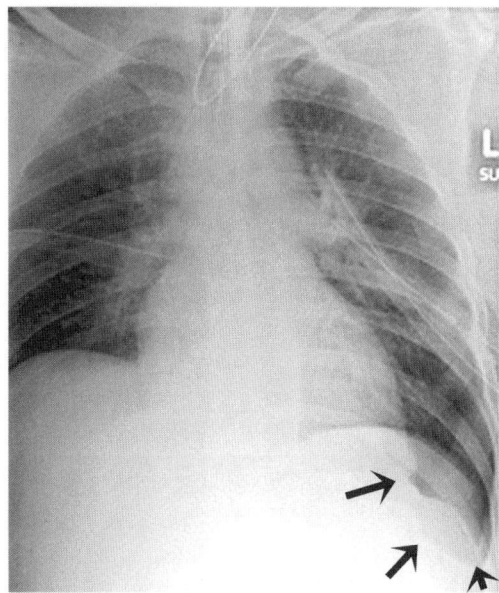

Figure 57-18 Bedside anteroposterior chest radiograph shows lucency without pulmonary vessels in lower left lateral hemithorax, expanding costophrenic sulcus *(arrows)* despite two left thoracostomy tubes, consistent with pneumothorax and reflecting "deep sulcus sign."

pleural effusion or pneumothorax. Diaphragmatic rupture is much more easily seen on CT, where findings include discontinuity of the diaphragm, visceral herniation, waist-like constriction of the bowel (collar sign), and layering of the herniated viscus against the posterior ribs (dependent viscera sign) (Figure 57-19).

MEDIASTINAL DISEASE

In this section we will focus on radiographic findings in several diagnoses that are relevant to the trauma population, with a particular emphasis on blunt trauma.

Acute Traumatic Aortic Injury

Tears of the thoracic aorta (Figure 57-20) are caused by acute deceleration injury such as occurs in a high-speed motor vehicle crash or a fall, or as a result of crush injury to the chest. A tear of the thoracic aorta almost always occurs in a transverse orientation, typically at the aortic isthmus. Tears of the ascending aorta or complete transection are nearly universally fatal, but if the adventitia remains intact, a pseudoaneurysm may form, usually with some amount of surrounding

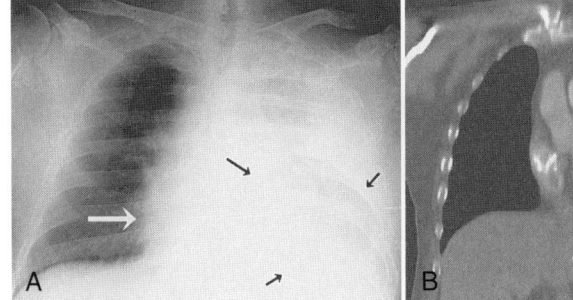
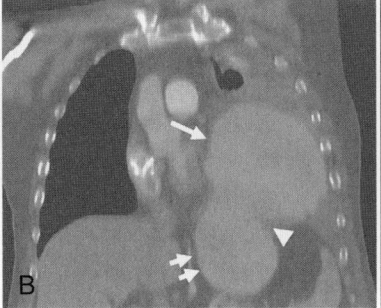
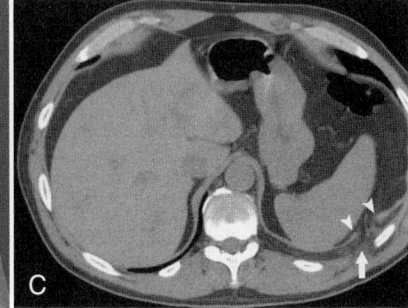

Figure 57-19 A 48-year-old man involved in a motor vehicle crash sustained a diaphragmatic injury. **A,** Bedside chest radiograph shows diffuse opacity in left hemithorax and rightward mediastinal displacement *(white arrow)*. A round lucency representing the gastric bubble is present within opacified left hemithorax *(black arrows)*. **B,** Coronal computed tomography re-formation shows partial herniation of stomach (gastric fundus *[single arrow]* and gastric body *[double arrows]*) into chest through a large defect in diaphragm *(arrowhead)*. **C,** More subtle diaphragmatic injury in a different patient subjected to blunt thoracic trauma. Diaphragm is ruptured *(arrowheads)*, leaving a small defect through which abdominal contents can herniate into thoracic cavity. Edema and hemorrhage surround area of injury *(arrow)*.

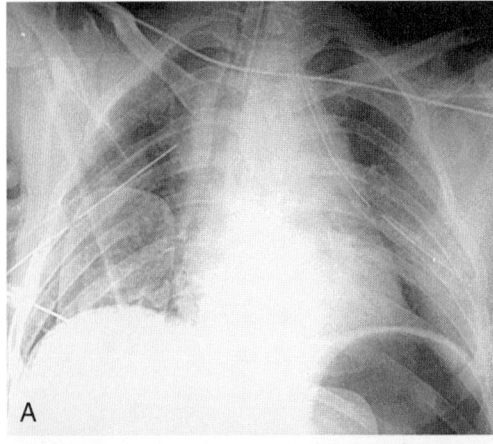

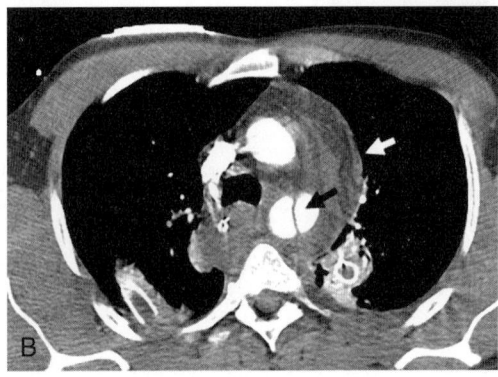

Figure 57-20 A 35-year-old man was involved in a high-speed motor vehicle crash. **A,** Anteroposterior chest radiograph shows abnormal contour of mediastinum, obscuration of aortic knob, and rightward displacement of trachea, consistent with mediastinal injury. Note tubes are in satisfactory position. **B,** Computed tomography shows intimal flap within aortic lumen *(black arrow),* representing aortic dissection surrounded by mediastinal hematoma *(white arrow).*

hemomediastinum. These may rupture at any time and require immediate surgical intervention.

Radiographic abnormalities that suggest aortic injury include a dense mediastinum with convex margins to the lungs, indistinct aortic contours, rightward deviation of the trachea, downward displacement of the left main bronchus, and thickening of the right paratracheal stripe Mediastinal widening is often mentioned as a sign of mediastinal hematoma, but this is an imprecise finding and not specific for aortic injury.[47,48] In patients whose chest radiographs are equivocal or highly suspicious for aortic injury, contrast medium–enhanced CT is indicated. CT findings of acute aortic injury include irregularity of the aortic wall, pseudoaneurysm, abrupt change in aortic caliber, intimal flap, extravasation of contrast material, and periaortic hematoma. Evidence of hemothorax may also be seen, usually on the left, on the chest radiograph or CT.

Tracheobronchial Tree Rupture

Rupture of the tracheobronchial tree is an uncommon consequence of blunt trauma, with bronchial rupture occurring more often than rupture of the trachea.[49] In bronchial rupture, the injury is usually located in the main bronchus near the carina. Disruption of the trachea typically involves the membranous portion just proximal to the carina.

Tracheobronchial disruption often causes pneumomediastinum or pneumothorax visible on chest radiographs and/or CT. The "fallen lung" sign (Figure 57-21), indicating complete bronchial disruption, describes the severed and collapsed lung lying against the

posterolateral aspect of the chest wall or the diaphragm. Other findings that suggest tracheobronchial injury include a large pneumothorax not responding to percutaneous drainage, or pneumothorax and pneumomediastinum in the absence of pleural effusion. However, it should be noted that pneumomediastinum is not specific for tracheobronchial or esophageal injury after blunt trauma.[50] Bronchoscopy is usually performed to confirm tracheobronchial injury, although CT with two-dimensional multiplanar reconstruction may prove a useful noninvasive alternative.[51]

Esophageal Rupture

Acute rupture of the esophagus can occur by iatrogenic means, from blunt chest trauma, or in the setting of severe retching or vomiting (Boerhaave syndrome). Trauma patients are more likely to have an injury in the upper thoracic esophagus, whereas Boerhaave syndrome usually involves the lower third of the esophagus.[52] Mediastinitis and septic shock rapidly follow esophageal rupture, accounting for the relatively high mortality rate. The radiographic findings of esophageal rupture include a dense mediastinum with convex margins to the lungs, pneumomediastinum, pleural effusion, pneumothorax, and hydropneumothorax. On CT, the area of greatest esophageal thickening often represents the perforation site. CT also provides more detailed information than radiography on developing complications. Contrast esophagography is the standard approach to confirm the diagnosis.

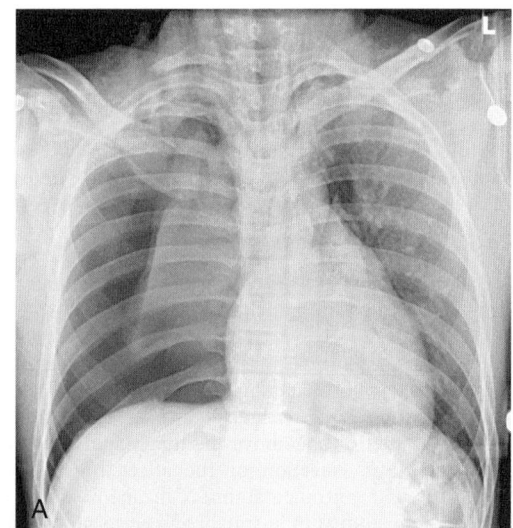

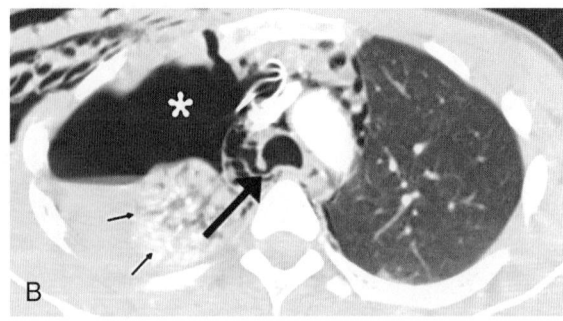

Figure 57-21 A 22-year-old man was involved in a high-speed motor vehicle crash. **A,** Anteroposterior chest radiograph shows right pneumothorax, pneumomediastinum, right lung collapse, and subcutaneous emphysema. **B,** Computed tomography shows tracheal laceration *(large arrow),* right pneumothorax *(asterisk),* and collapsed right lung *(small arrows)* in dependent portion of chest ("fallen lung sign").

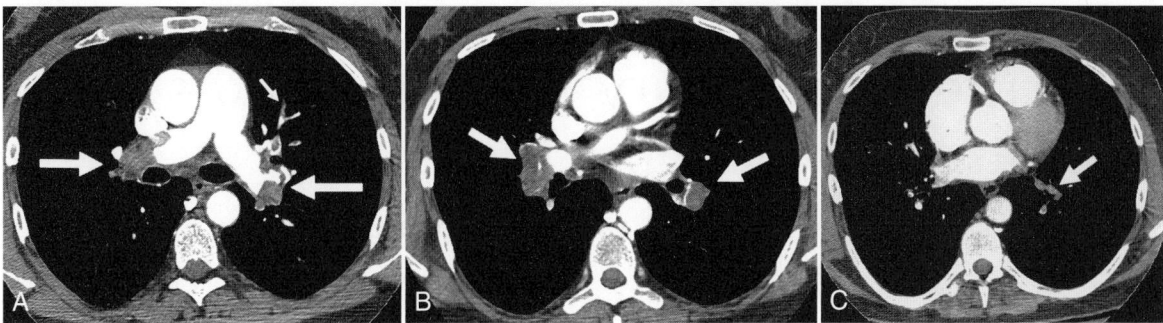

Figure 57-22 A 46-year-old woman presented with acute shortness of breath and hypoxia. Chest radiograph is normal. **A,** Chest computed tomography shows a low-attenuation filling defect in left and right main pulmonary arteries (*large arrows*) and left upper lobe segmental artery (*small arrow*), representing massive pulmonary embolism. Emboli extend to left and right interlobar arteries (*arrows*) as well as a left lower lobe segmental artery (*arrow*), seen in **B** and **C,** respectively.

Thoracic Duct Rupture

The most common cause of thoracic duct disruption is iatrogenic injury.[53] Thoracic duct injury from blunt chest injury is very rare and is thought to occur with hyperextension of the thoracic spine. Chylothorax, which usually develops several days to weeks after the trauma, is the typical radiographic finding. The delay in development of chylothorax is a clue to the diagnosis, particularly in differentiating it from traumatic hemothorax (see earlier discussion). The injury site is best identified with lymphangiography.

VASCULAR DISEASE

Pulmonary Thromboembolic Disease

Acute pulmonary embolism (PE) is a potentially lethal condition that can be difficult to diagnose clinically because of the nonspecific clinical presentation. Hospitalized patients are at increased risk of developing a PE. Although many imaging tests, including ventilation-perfusion scintigraphy and conventional pulmonary angiography, have been used to diagnose pulmonary embolism, CT pulmonary angiography (CTPA) has emerged as the initial imaging study of choice, given its high sensitivity and specificity and generally good interobserver agreement.[54-57] CTPA has the additional advantage of evaluating the entire thorax for other explanations for cardiopulmonary signs and symptoms. Specifically in ICU patients, CTPA appears to be an accurate diagnostic technique; indirect CT venography (CTV) compares favorably with ultrasound in evaluating venous thrombosis and improves the diagnostic yield of CTPA alone.[57-59] The addition of CTV to PE evaluation protocols is a controversial topic because it requires additional radiation and has not been conclusively demonstrated to improve patient outcomes compared to CTPA alone.[59] However, this has not yet been well studied in hospitalized or critically ill patients.

Many findings on conventional chest radiographs have been described in patients with pulmonary embolism, but they are inconsistently present and are nonspecific. Features diagnostic of acute pulmonary embolism on CTPA include a partial or complete filling defect in the pulmonary arteries (Figure 57-22). Associated lung abnormalities such as regional oligemia, volume loss, and a wedge-shaped subpleural opacity may also be present.

Conclusion

Chest imaging is an important component in diagnostic evaluation of critically ill patients. Although bedside chest radiography is limited by both technical and patient factors, knowledge of complications of various diseases and therapies as well as their respective radiographic appearances can lead to improvement in patient care. CT is an important adjunct modality when radiographic findings are equivocal, do not explain the patient's clinical picture, or provide inadequate anatomic detail for diagnosis.

KEY POINTS

1. Although portable chest radiographs are limited by both technical and patient factors, knowledge of complications of various diseases and therapies as well as their respective radiographic appearances can enhance patient care. Computed tomography scans provide additional anatomic detail that can also improve diagnosis and management of critical illness.

2. Knowledge of the normal positions of life-support devices on the chest radiograph is important so that malposition can be corrected and potential complications averted.

3. Many chest radiographs in the ICU setting have a similar appearance, particularly with respect to lung opacification. Understanding the diverse pathologies encountered in critical care and the specific clinical settings in which certain diagnoses are found provides a context for interpretation and may improve the diagnostic yield.

ANNOTATED REFERENCES

Hejblum G, Chalumeau-Lemoine L, Ioos V, et al. Comparison of routine and on-demand prescription of chest radiographs in mechanically ventilated adults: a multicentre, cluster-randomised, two-period crossover study. Lancet 2009;374(9702):1687-93.
This paper reports the results of a multicenter randomized study involving 849 patients, comparing the safety and utility of daily chest radiographs versus an on-demand strategy for mechanically ventilated patients. The results indicate that on-demand chest radiographs result in fewer x-rays for patients, without reduction in quality of care or safety. A brief review of the relevant literature is performed.
Hill JR, Horner PE, Primack SL. ICU imaging. Clin Chest Med 2008;29(1):59-76, vi.
Rubinowitz AN, Siegel MD, Tocino I. Thoracic imaging in the ICU. Crit Care Clin 2007;23(3):539-73.
These are concise, well-written, and well-illustrated reviews of thoracic radiology in the ICU. Both articles focus on the medical ICU population; findings specific to surgical and trauma patients are not discussed in depth.

Miller LA. Chest wall, lung, and pleural space trauma. Radiol Clin North Am. 2006;44(2):213-24, viii.
Sangster GP, González-Beicos A, Carbo AI, et al. Blunt traumatic injuries of the lung parenchyma, pleura, thoracic wall, and intrathoracic airways: multidetector computer tomography imaging findings. Emerg Radiol 2007;14(5):297-310.
These are excellent overviews of radiologic findings in the thoracic trauma patient population. Sangster et al. focuses on CT and is beautifully illustrated; Miller et al. provides a more general radiographic overview.
Moores LK, Holley AB. Computed tomography pulmonary angiography and venography: diagnostic and prognostic properties. Semin Respir Crit Care Med 2008;29(1):3-14.
This review summarizes landmark and recent studies evaluating the accuracy of CT pulmonary angiography in the diagnosis of pulmonary embolism. Issues specific to ICU patients are discussed, as are the data regarding the controversial topics of isolated subsegmental pulmonary emboli, indeterminate CT scans, and lower-extremity imaging by CT venography.

REFERENCES

Access the complete reference list online at http://www.expertconsult.com.

Acute Lung Injury and Acute Respiratory Distress Syndrome

JULIE A. BASTARACHE | LORRAINE B. WARE | GORDON R. BERNARD

Acute lung injury (ALI) and acute respiratory distress syndrome (ARDS) are common problems in the intensive care unit (ICU) and can complicate a wide spectrum of critical illnesses. First described by Ashbaugh in 1967,[1] the syndrome was initially termed *adult respiratory distress syndrome* to distinguish it from the respiratory distress syndrome of neonates. However, with the recognition that ALI/ARDS can occur in children, the term *acute* has replaced *adult* in the nomenclature in recognition of the typical acute onset that defines the syndrome. Although specific treatments for ALI/ARDS have been slow to emerge, the recent development of new strategies for mechanical ventilation that improve mortality, and fluid management strategies that reduce the length of mechanical ventilation, emphasizes the importance of identifying and appropriately treating all patients with ALI/ARDS. Although this point would seem to be straightforward, in practice, ALI/ARDS remains largely underdiagnosed,[2,3] and often expert practitioners disagree on the diagnosis,[4] which perpetuates inappropriate or inadequate treatment.

Epidemiology

The exact incidence of ALI/ARDS has been difficult to estimate for a variety of reasons. In the past, variable definitions of the syndrome were used.[5] The wide variety of causes and coexisting disease processes has also made identification of cases difficult, both at the clinical and administrative coding level.[6] The National Institutes of Health first estimated the incidence at 75 per 100,000 population in 1977,[7] but a number of studies since then have reported lower incidences.[6] Two prospective studies confirmed the higher original National Institutes of Health Estimate. The first utilized enrollment logs from the National Heart, Lung and Blood Institute–sponsored ARDS Network of 20 hospitals and estimated that the incidence could be as high as 64 cases per 100,000 population. This dataset has the advantage of being prospectively collected from a large number of academic medical centers. The second was a large prospective study of residents of King County, Washington. In that study, the crude incidence of ALI/ARDS in adults was 78.9 per 100,000 patient years.[8] A large prospective European study of the incidence of ARDS found that ALI occurred in 7.1% of all hospital admissions.[9] A third of these patients presented with only mild ALI, but of these, half progressed rapidly to ARDS. Some studies suggest a decline in the incidence of ARDS over time. A large prospective cohort of trauma patients at risk for ARDS and multisystem organ failure collected over time showed that the incidence of ARDS decreased from 43% in 1997 to 12% in 2004, a finding that may reflect advances in posttrauma critical care.[10] Regardless of the exact incidence, it is clear that ALI/ARDS is a major public health problem that will be encountered frequently by all physicians who care for critically ill patients.

Risk Factors

ALI/ARDS can occur as a result of either direct or indirect injury to the lungs (Table 58-1) in patients with a predisposing risk factor. The commonly associated clinical disorders can be separated into those that directly injure the lung and those that indirectly injure the lung. Although it is not always feasible to determine the exact cause of ALI/ARDS in a given patient, direct causes appear to account for

approximately half of all cases of ALI/ARDS.[11] It is not clear whether the distinction between direct and indirect lung injury is clinically useful.[12] Some investigators have demonstrated reduced respiratory system compliance in patients with ARDS due to direct pulmonary injury compared to indirect causes,[13] although total respiratory system compliance (including the chest wall) is similar.[14] Patients with direct lung injury may be more likely to have improved lung mechanics with the application of PEEP. However, in the largest cohort of patients studied to date, there was no difference in mortality between those with direct (pulmonary) and indirect (extrapulmonary) causes of lung injury.[11] Regardless of the underlying cause of ALI/ARDS, most patients with ALI/ARDS appear to have a systemic illness with inflammation and organ dysfunction not confined to the lung.[15]

Sepsis is the most common cause of indirect lung injury, with an overall risk of progression to ALI or ARDS of approximately 30% to 40%.[16-19] In a more recent prospective study of hospitalized patients with a risk factor for acute lung injury (e.g., sepsis, pneumonia) 6.5% of patients developed ALI, and 4% met criteria for ARDS; the risk was higher with multiple risk factors.[20] In addition to sepsis itself being a risk factor for development of ARDS, the site of infection may also influence the risk of lung injury. In patients with sepsis admitted to an ICU, patients who had pneumonia as the source of sepsis had an increased risk of ARDS compared to those with infections at other sites such as the abdomen, skin, or soft tissue.[21] Severe trauma with shock and multiple transfusions also can cause indirect lung injury. Although the other causes of indirect lung injury are less common, many, such as blood transfusions, are commonplace events in the ICU setting. The most common cause of direct lung injury is pneumonia, which may be of bacterial, viral, or fungal origin. The risk of developing ALI/ARDS increases substantially in the presence of multiple predisposing disorders.[19] Secondary factors may also increase the risk. Such factors include chronic lung disease,[18] chronic or acute alcohol abuse,[22,23] increasing age,[24] transfusion of blood products,[25-27] lung resection,[28] and obesity.[24] Emerging evidence has suggested that some at-risk patients may actually be protected from the development of ARDS. Several studies have shown that patients with diabetes are less likely to develop ARDS.[29-31] To some extent, every patient in the ICU is at risk for developing ALI/ARDS, and vigilance is required to recognize the diagnosis and treat appropriately.

Pathophysiology

The pathophysiology of ALI/ARDS is complex and remains incompletely understood. Microscopically, lungs from afflicted individuals in the early stages show diffuse alveolar damage with alveolar flooding by proteinaceous fluid, neutrophil influx into the alveolar space, loss of alveolar epithelial cells, deposition of hyaline membranes on the denuded basement membrane, and formation of microthrombi (Figure 58-1).[32] Alveolar flooding occurs as a result of injury to the alveolar-capillary barrier and is a major determinant of the hypoxemia and altered lung mechanics that characterize early ALI/ARDS.

The alveolar-capillary barrier is formed of two separate cell layers, the microvascular endothelium and the alveolar epithelium. Injury to the alveolar epithelium is a prominent histologic feature, with loss of alveolar epithelial barrier integrity and sloughing of alveolar epithelial

TABLE 58-1	Risk Factors Associated with Development of Acute Lung Injury and Acute Respiratory Distress Syndrome	
Direct Lung Injury		*Indirect Lung Injury*
Pneumonia		Sepsis
Aspiration of gastric contents		Multiple trauma
Pulmonary contusion		Cardiopulmonary bypass
Fat, amniotic fluid, or air emboli		Drug overdose
Near-drowning		Acute pancreatitis
Inhalational injury		Transfusion of blood products
Reperfusion pulmonary edema		

type I cells. Alveolar epithelial apoptosis is widespread and likely contributes to the loss of epithelium seen ultrastructurally.[33,34] Although endothelial injury is less obvious at the microscopic level, ultrastructural studies reveal that it is widespread.[35,36] Endothelial injury allows leakage of plasma from the capillaries into the interstitium and airspaces. Alveolar flooding in ALI/ARDS is characteristically with a protein-rich edema fluid, owing to the increased permeability of the alveolar capillary barrier, in contrast to the low-protein pulmonary edema that results from hydrostatic causes such as congestive heart failure or acute myocardial infarction.[37-40]

Neutrophils play an important role[41] in the initial inflammatory response in ARDS. Early ALI/ARDS is characterized by migration of neutrophils into the alveolar compartment.[35,36] Neutrophils can release a variety of injurious substances, including proteases such as neutrophil elastase, collagenase, and gelatinases A and B, as well as reactive

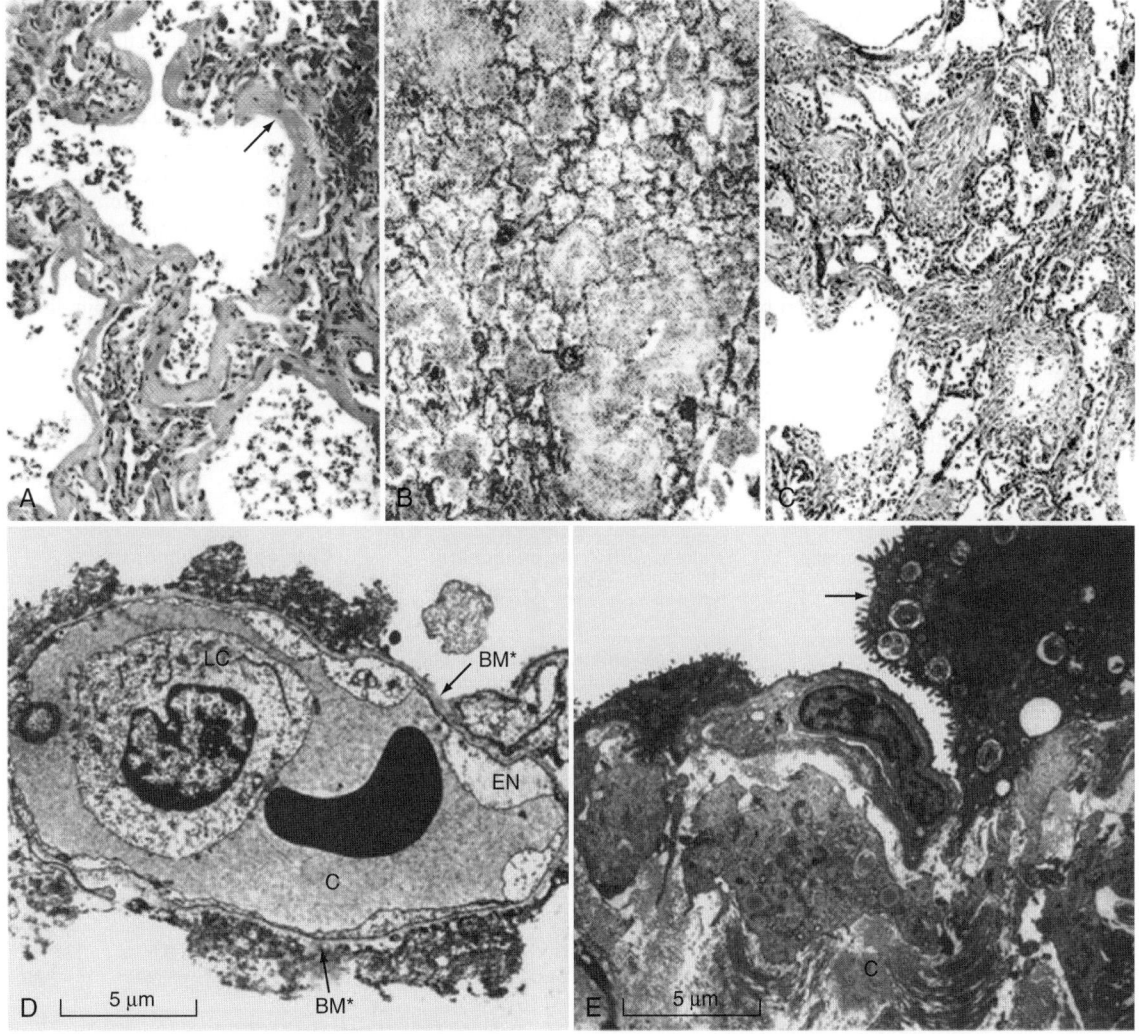

Figure 58-1 Histology. **A,** Lung biopsy specimen obtained from a patient 2 days after onset of acute respiratory distress syndrome (ARDS) as a result of aspiration of gastric contents. Characteristic hyaline membranes are evident *(arrow)*, with associated intraalveolar red cells and neutrophils, findings consistent with pathologic diagnosis of diffuse alveolar damage (hematoxylin and eosin, ×90). **B** and **C,** Lung biopsy specimens obtained 14 days after onset of sepsis-associated acute lung injury (ALI) and ARDS; **B** shows granulation tissue in distal air spaces, with chronic inflammatory-cell infiltrate (hematoxylin and eosin, ×60). Trichrome staining in **C** reveals collagen deposition (dark blue areas) in granulation tissue, a finding consistent with deposition of extracellular matrix in the alveolar compartment (×60). **D,** Specimen of lung tissue from a patient who died 4 days after onset of ALI/ARDS. There is injury to both capillary endothelium and alveolar epithelium. Note intravascular neutrophil (LC) in the capillary (C). Vacuolization and swelling of endothelium (EN) are apparent. Loss of alveolar epithelial cells is also apparent, with formation of hyaline membranes on epithelial side of basement membrane (BM*). **E,** Specimen of lung tissue obtained from a patient during fibrosing alveolitis phase; there is evidence of reepithelialization of epithelial barrier with alveolar epithelial type II cells. Arrow indicates a typical type II cell with microvilli and lamellar bodies containing surfactant. Epithelial cell immediately adjacent to this cell is in the process of changing to a type I cell, with flattening, loss of lamellar bodies, and microvilli. Interstitium is thickened, with deposition of collagen (C). *(With permission from Ware LB, Matthay MA. The acute respiratory distress syndrome. N Engl J Med. 2000;342[18]:1334-1349.)*

nitrogen and oxygen species. In addition, they can elaborate proinflammatory cytokines and chemokines which amplify the inflammatory response in the lung. Resident alveolar macrophages are also involved in initiating and sustaining a proinflammatory cytokine cascade that leads to recruitment of neutrophils into the lung.

In addition to acute neutrophilic inflammation and elaboration of a proinflammatory cytokine cascade, a variety of other abnormalities contribute to the pathogenesis of ALI/ARDS. Surfactant dysfunction is characteristic, with abnormalities in both the protein and lipid components.[42-45] This likely results from disruption of normal surfactant activity secondary to the influx of plasma proteins into the airspaces, intraalveolar proteolysis, and injury to the alveolar epithelial type II cells. Surfactant dysfunction may have important implications both for lung mechanics and host defense.[46] Activation of the coagulation cascade and impaired fibrinolysis are also apparent in patients with ALI/ARDS,[47,48] both in the lung[49-51] and systemically.[52,53] Alteration in the balance of endogenous oxidants and antioxidants, with a decrease in endogenous antioxidants[54] despite the increased oxidant production, has also been observed.[55]

The contribution of ventilator-associated lung injury to the pathogenesis of ALI/ARDS has been recognized. There are several mechanisms by which mechanical ventilation can injure the lung. Ventilation at very high volumes and pressures can injure even the normal lung, leading to increased permeability pulmonary edema due to capillary stress failure[56] and sustained elevations of circulating plasma cytokines.[57] In the injured lung, even tidal volumes that are well tolerated in the normal lung can lead to alveolar overdistension in relatively uninjured areas because the lung available for distribution of the administered tidal volume is greatly reduced and because of uneven distribution of inspired gas.[58,59] In addition to alveolar overdistension, cyclic opening and closing of atelectatic alveoli can cause lung injury even in the absence of alveolar overdistension. The combination of alveolar overdistension with cyclic opening and closing of alveoli is particularly harmful and can initiate a proinflammatory cascade.[60]

A ventilatory strategy that was designed to minimize alveolar overdistension and maximize alveolar recruitment ameliorated proinflammatory cytokine release.[61] This fundamental insight into the pathogenesis of clinical ALI/ARDS has led to multiple clinical trials of novel ventilatory strategies for patients with ALI/ARDS, including the landmark ARDS Network trial of 6 mL/kg versus 12 mL/kg tidal volume ventilation[62] (see Treatment section).

Diagnosis

In 1994, the American-European Consensus Conference published new clinical definitions for ALI and ARDS.[5] Prior to this time, a variety of definitions were used clinically, including the Murray Lung Injury Score.[63] To meet the Consensus diagnostic criteria for either ALI/ARDS, the acute onset of bilateral radiographic infiltrates is required. There should be no clinical evidence of left atrial hypertension, with a pulmonary artery occlusion pressure (PAOP) $\leq$ 18 mm Hg if measured. Although not strictly part of these definitions, an underlying cause of lung injury should be sought. In the absence of an identifiable underlying cause (see Table 58-1), particular attention should be given to the possibility of other causes of pulmonary infiltrates and hypoxemia, such as hydrostatic pulmonary edema. One potential limitation of the consensus definition is the need for arterial blood gas sampling to calculate a Pao_2/Fio_2 ratio. Recent work has shown good correlation between the Spo_2/Fio_2 ratio (measured by pulse oximetry) and the Pao_2/Fio_2 ratio,[64,65] with an Spo_2/Fio_2 ratio of 235 corresponding to a Pao_2/Fio_2 ratio of 200, and an Spo_2/Fio_2 ratio of 315 correlating to a Pao_2/Fio_2 ratio of 300. These calculations are valid only when the Spo_2 is less than 98%, because the oxyhemoglobin dissociation curve is flat above this level. Oxygen saturation is a noninvasive, continuously available measurement; use of the Spo_2/Fio_2 ratio may improve the ability of clinicians to diagnose ARDS.

Differentiating ARDS from hydrostatic edema can be difficult, and there may be significant overlap in the syndromes (Figure 58-2).[66] A

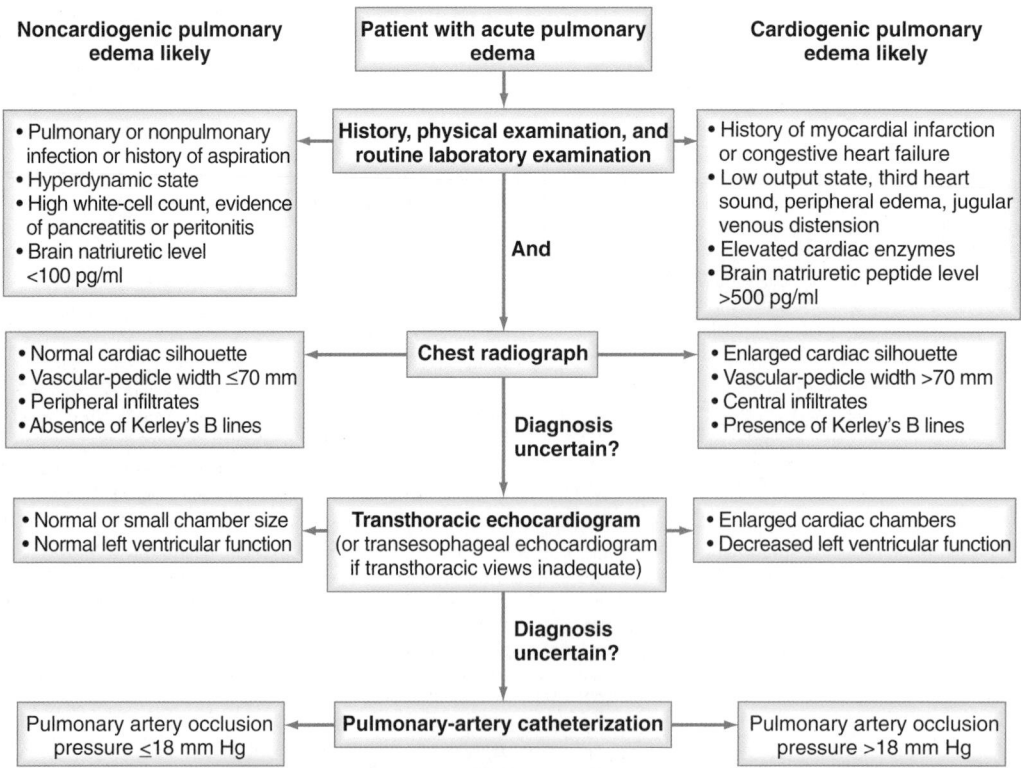

Figure 58-2 Algorithm for differentiating between cardiogenic and noncardiogenic pulmonary edema. *(With permission from Ware LB, Matthay MA. Clinical practice. Acute pulmonary edema. N Engl J Med. 2005;353[26]:2788-2796.)*

recent multicenter trial on intravenous catheter directed fluid management strategies in patients with ARDS showed that 29% of patients with clinically defined ARDS had a PAOP greater than 18 mm Hg at the time of pulmonary artery catheter insertion, but that 97% of patients had a normal or elevated cardiac index, suggesting they did not have clinical heart failure.[67] Other studies have shown similar rates of elevated PAOP in patients with ARDS.[68]

There are no specific clinical or laboratory studies that can reliably distinguish between ARDS and hydrostatic edema. A study examining the diagnostic utility of serum levels of B-type natriuretic peptide (BNP) showed that BNP measured at admission could not reliably differentiate between hydrostatic edema and ARDS. Furthermore, BNP levels in these patients did not correlate with invasive hemodynamic measurements.[69]

The standardization of definitions for ALI and ARDS has been helpful from several perspectives. For clinical research, it has been valuable in allowing the comparison of different studies and the rapid identification of patients for enrollment in clinical trials. Clinically, the new definitions are easy to apply and facilitate rapid identification and appropriate treatment of patients with ALI/ARDS. However, it should be noted the nature of ALI/ARDS is such that any definition will have significant shortcomings. First, the definitions must be based solely on clinical criteria, because currently there is no laboratory test that allows clinical assessment of the presence or absence of ALI/ARDS. Second, there is no reference to pathogenesis or underlying cause. This is because the list of potential causes of ALI/ARDS is so long, diverse, and common in the critically ill. Third, the presence or absence of multiorgan dysfunction, an important determinant of outcome, is not specified. Finally, though the presence of bilateral infiltrates has major prognostic significance and is clearly a hallmark of the syndrome, the radiographic findings are not specific for ALI/ARDS.[4,70] Diagnostic uncertainty in ALI/ARDS is a major barrier to initiation of appropriate therapy and one of the main reasons why clinicians fail to initiate lung-protective ventilation in clinically appropriate patients.[71]

Recent work has focused on alternative methods to increase sensitivity and specificity of the clinical definitions for ALI/ARDS. The pulmonary edema fluid–to–plasma protein ratio can reliably distinguish between low-permeability (hydrostatic edema) and high-permeability (ARDS) pulmonary edema if measured early after endotracheal intubation,[72] but prospective validation is still needed. Alternatively, circulating biomarkers may prove useful for the diagnosis of ALI/ARDS.[73] Despite its shortcomings, the current clinical definition of ALI/ARDS based on consensus criteria should be used to rapidly identify patients with ALI/ARDS so appropriate therapy can be initiated promptly.

In the majority of patients, the initial diagnosis of ALI/ARDS is made clinically. Invasive techniques for diagnosis are of limited clinical utility, and the benefits rarely outweigh the risks. Bronchoscopy may be indicated in the early phases of ALI/ARDS in patients in whom there is no identifiable predisposing risk factor. Rarely, an alternate treatable diagnosis is found, such as acute eosinophilic pneumonia, pulmonary alveolar proteinosis, diffuse alveolar hemorrhage, or unsuspected infection. Bronchoalveolar lavage for cultures and cytologic examination can identify the cause of pneumonia, and is particularly useful in the diagnosis of opportunistic infections. Lavage fluid usually has a predominance of neutrophils, and there may be evidence of diffuse alveolar hemorrhage. Cytologic examination can be used to confirm the presence of diffuse alveolar damage.[74]

In the past, open lung biopsy was obtained more frequently for diagnosis in patients with suspected ARDS. Interestingly, the degree of histologic abnormality on lung biopsy does not correlate with ultimate outcome as measured by pulmonary function.[75] Open or thoracoscopic lung biopsy may still be useful in some cases where the diagnosis is uncertain and the underlying cause is not apparent. Although open lung biopsy can provide findings that lead to a change in treatment, postoperative complications can occur in 20% of patients.[76] Several pathologic studies have shown that biopsy or autopsy can identify unsuspected diagnoses requiring specific therapy (e.g., miliary tuberculosis, pulmonary blastomycosis, aspergillosis, bronchiolitis

obliterans organizing pneumonia) in 40% to 60% of cases,[76-78] although the general applicability of these studies may be limited by the fact that they were retrospective case series.

In addition to familiarity with the Consensus definitions of ALI and ARDS, the critical care clinician should be aware that ALI and ARDS also have been called by a variety of other terms, some of which are seen mainly in older literature, but some that remain in clinical use. Some of the more common of these terms include *adult hyaline membrane disease*, *postperfusion lung* or *pump lung*, *shock lung*, *ventilator-associated lung injury*, and *adult respiratory insufficiency syndrome*. The terms *primary graft dysfunction*, *primary graft failure*, or *transplant lung* have been used to describe ALI/ARDS from reperfusion pulmonary edema occurring immediately after lung transplantation.

Regardless of the name applied, ALI/ARDS is a clinical syndrome that has prognostic and therapeutic implications above and apart from the underlying cause (i.e., infections, aspiration, trauma, etc.). This fact should not take away the imperative to identify these underlying causes if present and treat them aggressively.

Clinical Course

EARLY ALI/ARDS

The Consensus definitions are designed to identify ALI/ARDS patients early in their course, in the acute or exudative phase. Clinically, the acute phase is manifested by the acute onset of radiographic infiltrates consistent with pulmonary edema, hypoxemia, and increased work of breathing. Radiographic infiltrates are bilateral (by definition), but may be patchy or diffuse, fluffy or dense (Figure 58-3), and pleural effusions may occur.[79] Chest computed tomographic (CT) imaging, though rarely of use clinically, has been employed extensively as an investigative tool to better define the nature of the infiltrates in patients with ALI/ARDS. The distribution of infiltrates by CT is surprisingly patchy; areas of alveolar filling and consolidation occur predominantly in dependent zones, while non-dependent regions can appear relatively spared.[80-82] Even areas that appear spared in conventional radiographic images may have substantial inflammation when sampled using bronchoalveolar lavage[83] or using FDG-PET scanning.[84]

The hypoxemia that characterizes early ALI/ARDS is usually relatively refractory to supplemental oxygen. The increased work of breathing in the acute phase of ALI/ARDS is due to decreased lung compliance as a result of alveolar and interstitial edema combined with increased airflow resistance[85] and increased respiratory drive.[86] The combination of hypoxemia and increased work of breathing usually necessitates endotracheal intubation and mechanical ventilation, although occasionally patients can be managed with noninvasive ventilation (see Treatment section).

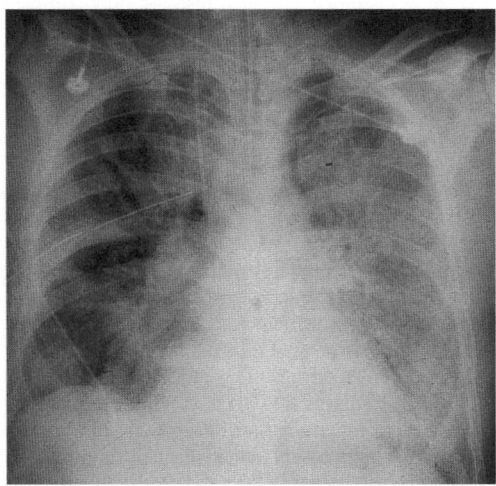

Figure 58-3   Chest radiograph.

In addition to hypoxemia and increased work of breathing, many patients with ARDS also develop evidence of increased pulmonary vascular resistance leading to pulmonary hypertension and RV failure. The prevalence of pulmonary hypertension in patients presenting to the hospital with ARDS may be as high as 92%,[87] and as many as 10% of patients with ARDS may have right ventricular (RV) failure defined by hemodynamic measurements.[88] Nevertheless, the presence of RV failure does not impact mortality. Attempts to reverse pulmonary hypertension and RV failure with pulmonary vasodilators such as sildenafil have led to decreased pulmonary artery pressure with treatment, as well as concomitant increases in shunt fraction and decreases in oxygenation.[89] These findings suggest that although patients with ARDS have evidence of pulmonary hypertension, it may in some cases be a beneficial physiologic response to reduce blood flow to areas of severely compromised lung.

LATE FIBROPROLIFERATIVE ALI/ARDS

In most patients, ALI/ARDS will substantially resolve after the acute phase. However, in others, the syndrome progresses to a fibrosing alveolitis. Fibrosing alveolitis usually becomes clinically apparent after 7 to 10 days, although evidence of deposition of extracellular matrix has been identified in alveolar lining fluid from patients as early as the first day after intubation.[90] Radiographically, linear opacities develop, consistent with the evolving fibrosis. Histologically, pulmonary edema and neutrophilic inflammation are less prominent. A severe fibroproliferative process fills the airspaces with granulation tissue that contains extracellular matrix rich in collagen and fibrin, as well as new blood vessels and proliferating mesenchymal cells.[91,92]

Clinically, the late fibroproliferative phase of ALI/ARDS is characterized by continued need for mechanical ventilation, often with persistently high levels of PEEP and FIO_2. Lung compliance may fall even further, and pulmonary dead space is elevated. If it has not developed in the acute phase, pulmonary hypertension may occur now owing to obliteration of the pulmonary capillary bed, and right ventricular failure may appear.[93] This phase of the illness can be prolonged, lasting weeks, and can be very frustrating for the clinician, patient, and family; small gains in pulmonary function are frequently offset by new problems such as hospital-acquired infections, organ failures, or barotrauma. Progressive deconditioning can make eventual weaning from mechanical ventilation difficult if the fibrosing alveolitis stage is prolonged. Based on improvement in number of ventilator-free days through use of lower tidal volumes, it seems likely the incidence of fibrosing alveolitis will fall.

RESOLUTION OF ALI/ARDS

Lung biopsies from ALI/ARDS survivors typically show normal or near-normal lung histology. For such histologically complete resolution of ALI/ARDS to occur, a variety of processes must be reversed. Alveolar edema is actively reabsorbed by the vectorial transport of sodium and chloride from the distal airway and alveolar spaces into the lung interstitium.[94] Water is passively absorbed along the osmotic gradient, probably through water channels, the aquaporins.[95] The majority of patients with early ALI/ARDS have impaired alveolar fluid transport, but in those with intact alveolar fluid transport, faster rates of alveolar epithelial fluid transport are associated with better outcomes.[37] Soluble and insoluble protein must also be cleared from the airspaces. Soluble protein probably diffuses by a paracellular route into the interstitium, where it is cleared by lymphatics. Insoluble protein probably is cleared by macrophage phagocytosis or alveolar epithelial cell endocytosis and transcytosis.[96]

The denuded alveolar epithelium in ALI/ARDS must be repaired. The alveolar epithelial type II cell serves as the progenitor cell for repopulating the alveolar epithelium. Type II cells proliferate, migrate, and differentiate to reconstitute a tight alveolar epithelial type I cell barrier. The inflammatory cell infiltrate must also resolve, but here the mechanisms are less clear. Resolution of neutrophilic inflammation may be predominantly via neutrophil apoptosis and phagocytosis by macrophages. However, one report suggests that neutrophil apoptosis is impaired in the lungs of patients with ALI/ARDS.[97] The resolution of fibrotic changes is also not well understood. Clearly, however, substantial remodeling is necessary to restore a normal or near-normal alveolar architecture. In patients with advanced fibrosis, this process likely takes place over many months; pulmonary function abnormalities continue to improve, sometimes remarkably so, out to the first year in survivors of ALI/ARDS (see later discussion).[98]

Treatment

STANDARD SUPPORTIVE THERAPY

The gradual decline in mortality attributable to ALI/ARDS over time likely reflects improvements in standard supportive therapy. Although it is beyond the scope of this chapter to discuss all aspects of supportive therapy in detail, a few aspects will be considered.

Treatment of Predisposing Factors

First and foremost, a search for the underlying cause of ALI/ARDS should be undertaken. Appropriate treatment for any precipitating infection such as pneumonia is critical to enhance the chance of survival. In the immunocompromised host or patients without predisposing risk factors, invasive diagnostic evaluation including bronchoscopy may be warranted to look for evidence of opportunistic infections or alternative specific causes of ARDS. In a patient with sepsis and ALI/ARDS of unknown source, an intraabdominal process should be considered. Timely surgical management of intraabdominal sepsis is associated with better outcomes.[99] In some patients, the cause of lung injury will not be specifically treatable (such as aspiration of gastric contents) or will not be readily identifiable.

Fluid and Hemodynamic Management

There are data supporting the use of early goal-directed therapy to support cardiac output and oxygen delivery within a set range with fluids, inotropes, and blood transfusions using central venous oxygen saturation as a therapeutic driver in patients who have severe sepsis and septic shock,[100] many of whom develop ALI/ARDS. But this approach has not been specifically studied in ALI/ARDS. Historically, patients with critical illness and ALI/ARDS received a pulmonary artery catheter (PAC) to manage fluid and hemodynamic status. A large, randomized European trial of PAC use versus no PAC use in all patients admitted with ARDS[101] showed no difference in clinical outcomes in either group, suggesting that routine PAC use in ARDS is not beneficial. The ARDS Clinical Trials Network tested the value of pulmonary artery catheterization in the context of specific fluid-management protocols and was unable to demonstrate improved outcomes through use of the PAC.[67] Some investigators have proposed that clinical outcomes in ALI/ARDS can be improved by delivery of supranormal levels of oxygen to the tissues using vigorous volume resuscitation and positive inotropes. However, no benefit to supranormal levels of oxygen delivery has been demonstrated in patients with ALI/ARDS.[102,103]

For decades there was disagreement as to the best fluid-management strategy in patients with ARDS. Proponents of a liberal fluid strategy reasoned that increased circulating volume would preserve end-organ perfusion and protect patients from the development of nonpulmonary organ failures. Reductions in intravascular volume can have adverse effects on cardiac output and tissue perfusion, factors that could contribute to multisystem organ failure. This is a legitimate concern, since mortality in ALI/ARDS is usually from non-pulmonary causes including other organ failures. Others supported a conservative fluid strategy in an attempt to reduce circulating volume, thereby reducing the driving force for pulmonary edema formation. In experimental lung injury, lower left atrial pressures are associated with less formation of pulmonary edema.[93,104] There is some clinical evidence to support this approach.[105-108] Given the equipoise with the approach to fluids in ALI/ARDS, the ARDS Network conducted a large, multicenter, randomized controlled trial of catheter-driven (central venous catheter versus PAC) fluid management in patients with ALI.[109] Once patients were out of shock, they were randomized to a liberal fluid treatment strategy that resulted in an average of 1 liter of fluid accumulation per day or to a conservative fluid treatment strategy with aggressive use of diuretics to achieve a goal central venous pressure (CVP) below 4 or a goal PAOP below 8, an approach that resulted in an average of zero net fluid accumulation by day 7. Although there was no difference in mortality at 60 days (the primary outcome of the study), patients in the conservative group had improved oxygenation and significantly more ventilator-free days without the development of additional organ failures. In this study, it did not matter whether treatment was guided by CVP measurements (derived from a central venous line) or from PAOP measurements (derived from a PAC).[110]

Despite the findings in support of conservative fluid management strategy in patients with ARDS, there continues to be a great deal of uncertainty about appropriate goals for hemodynamic therapy in ALI/ARDS. Currently, the recommended strategy is to aim to achieve the lowest intravascular volume that maintains adequate tissue perfusion as measured by urine output, other organ perfusion, and metabolic acid-base status, using CVP monitoring to direct therapy. If organ perfusion cannot be maintained in the setting of adequate intravascular volume, administration of vasopressors and/or inotropes should be used to restore end-organ perfusion.[93] Available evidence does not support the use of one particular vasopressor or combination of vasopressors. Once shock has resolved, patients should be managed with a conservative fluid strategy, with the goal of driving the CVP below 4 to keep each patient's fluid balance net zero over their ICU stay.

Nutrition

Standard supportive care for the patient with ALI/ARDS includes providing adequate nutrition. The NIH NHLBI ARDS Network is currently conducting a randomized trial of trophic (10 mL/h, well below caloric requirements) versus full-calorie enteral feeds in patients with ALI/ARDS. The enteral route is preferred to the parenteral route and is associated with fewer infectious complications.[111] Enteral feeding may also have other beneficial effects. Experimentally, lack of enteral feeding promoted translocation of bacteria from the intestine.[112] In normal volunteers, administration of parenteral nutrition with bowel rest increased circulating levels of tumor necrosis factor alpha (TNF-α), glucagon, and epinephrine, and increased febrile responses compared to volunteers who received enteral nutrition.[113]

Until the results of the ARDS Network study become available, the goals of nutritional support in any critically ill patient include providing adequate nutrients for the patient's level of metabolism and treating and preventing any deficiencies in micro- or macronutrients.[114] Whether a particular dietary composition is beneficial in patients with ALI/ARDS is unclear. Immunomodulation via dietary manipulation has been attempted in critically ill patients, using various combinations of omega-3 fatty acids, ribonucleotides, arginine, and glutamine. A meta-analysis of these trials suggested a beneficial effect on infection rate but not on overall mortality.[115] The ARDS Network recently conducted a large, multicenter, randomized placebo-controlled study of omega-3 fatty acid and antioxidant supplementation in patients with ALI/ARDS. This study was stopped early by the data safety monitoring board for a trend towards excess mortality in patients receiving the omega-3 fatty acid supplement (personal communication from Dr. Art Wheeler and Dr. Todd Rice). One other randomized controlled trial in ALI/ARDS studied the effects of an immunomodulatory nutritional formula.[116] In that trial, a diet rich in fish oil, γ-linoleic acid, and antioxidants was associated with a shorter duration of mechanical ventilation and fewer organ failures, but no difference in mortality. Using a different approach, a high-fat, low-carbohydrate diet reduced the duration of mechanical ventilation in patients with acute respiratory failure.[117] Although the mechanism of this beneficial effect was postulated to be due to reduction of the respiratory quotient and a resultant fall in carbon dioxide production, the most common cause of a high

respiratory quotient in critically ill patients is not dietary composition but simply overfeeding.[114] Overall, there is still no compelling evidence to support the use of anything other than standard enteral nutritional support, with avoidance of overfeeding, in patients with ALI/ARDS. There is evidence from one large study to suggest that omega-3 fatty acid and antioxidant supplementation may be deleterious, so this regimen is not recommended at present. How early to attempt institution of feeding remains an unanswered question.

MECHANICAL VENTILATION

Lung-Protective Ventilation

Although historically a tidal volume of 12 to 15 mL/kg was recommended in patients with ALI/ARDS, it is now clear that a low-tidal-volume, protective ventilatory strategy reduces mortality. In 2000, the NIH ARDS Network published the findings of their first randomized, controlled, multicenter clinical trial in 861 patients.[62] The trial was designed to compare a lower-tidal-volume ventilatory strategy (6 mL/kg predicted body weight, plateau pressure < 30 cm H_2O) with a higher tidal volume (12 mL/kg predicted body weight, plateau pressure < 50 cm H_2O). The rationale for the clinical trial was the growing body of clinical and experimental evidence suggesting that ventilation with high tidal volumes and high plateau pressures might be harmful to the injured lung (see earlier Pathophysiology section). In this trial, the in-hospital mortality rate was 40% in the 12 mL/kg group and 31% in the 6 mL/kg—a 22% reduction. Ventilator-free days and organ failure–free days were also significantly improved in the low-tidal-volume group. These findings were truly remarkable, since no prior large randomized clinical trial of any specific therapy for ALI/ARDS has ever demonstrated a mortality benefit.

The current recommended treatment strategy for patients with ARDS is summarized in Table 58-2. Predicted body weight is calculated based on measured height, using the equations provided. This is a key point often overlooked by clinicians; use of actual rather than predicted body weight can result in the use of erroneously high and potentially injurious tidal volumes. The tidal volume should initially be set at 6 mL/kg predicted body weight. Interestingly, a tidal volume of 6 mL/kg predicted body weight is similar to normal tidal volumes in spontaneously breathing adults at rest. So, although this size tidal volume is often referred to as low tidal volume, it is really *normal* tidal volume ventilation. *However*, if end-inspiratory plateau pressure (measured during a 0.5-second pause) is still above 30 cm H_2O, then tidal volume must be reduced in a stepwise fashion by 1 mL/kg to a minimum of 4 mL/kg. Ventilation with this size tidal volume is generally well tolerated. Some patients may have breath stacking or significant dyssynchrony with the ventilator. Increasing the inspiratory flow rate and, if necessary, the level of sedation is usually sufficient to manage these problems. Several studies have shown that on average, patients receiving lower-tidal-volume ventilation do not require increases in dose or duration of sedatives compared to patients receiving higher-tidal-volume ventilation.[118,119] As with any mode of ventilation in ALI/ARDS, occasionally patients will require neuromuscular blockade, but this should be used only as a last resort in patients with refractory hypoxemia, since use of paralytics may increase the risk of critical illness, polyneuropathy, and myopathy. Respiratory acidosis may develop but is usually not symptomatic. Increasing the respiratory rate is usually sufficient to compensate for the decreased tidal volume; a rate as high as 35 was used in the ARDSNet clinical trial.

In the ARDS Network protocol, the level of PEEP and F_{IO_2} was titrated according to a set of predetermined values (see Table 58-2). The optimal level of PEEP in ALI/ARDS has been controversial and is not yet established. Higher levels of PEEP may be beneficial in preventing alveolar collapse and minimizing injurious repeated opening and closing of alveoli. On the other hand, higher PEEP may overdistend and injure more complaint areas of the lung. Several studies have investigated the effects of different levels of PEEP in patients with ALI/ARDS.[120] One large multicenter trial conducted by the ARDS Network randomized patients with ARDS ventilated with low-tidal-volume

TABLE 58-2	Management of Patients with ARDS
Calculate Predicted Body Weight (PBW)	• Males: PBW (kg) = 50 + 2.3[(height in inches) − 60] or 50 + 0.91[(height in cm) − 152.4]. • Females: IBW (kg) = 45.5 + 2.3[(height in inches) − 60] or 45.5 + 0.91[(height in cm) − 152.4].
Ventilator Mode	Volume assist/control until weaning.

Tidal Volume (VT)	• Initial VT: 6 mL/kg predicted body weight.
	• Measure inspiratory plateau pressure (Pplat, 0.5 sec inspiratory pause) every 4 hours AND after each change in PEEP or VT.
	  ◦ If Pplat > 30 cm H_2O, decrease VT to 5 or to 4 mL/kg.
	  ◦ If Pplat < 25 cm H_2O and VT < 6 mL/kg PBW, increase VT by 1 ml/kg PBW.

Respiratory Rate (RR)	• With initial change in VT, adjust RR to maintain minute ventilation. • Make subsequent adjustments to RR to maintain pH 7.30-7.45, but do not exceed RR = 35/min, and do not increase set rate if $Paco_2$ < 25 mm Hg.
I : E Ratio	Acceptable range = 1 : 1 to 1 : 3 (no inverse ratio).
FIO₂ , Positive End-Expiratory Pressure (PEEP), and Arterial Oxygenation	Maintain Pao_2 = 55-80 mm Hg or Spo_2 = 88%-95% using the following PEEP/Fio_2 combinations:

FIO_2	0.3-0.4	0.4	0.5	0.6	0.7	0.8	0.9	1
PEEP	5-8	8-14	8-16	10-20	10-20	14-22	16-22	18-25

Acidosis Management	• If pH < 7.30, increase RR until pH ≥ 7.30 or RR = 35/min. • If pH remains < 7.30 with RR = 35, consider bicarbonate infusion. • If pH < 7.15, VT may be increased (Pplat may exceed 30 cm H_2O).
Alkalosis Management	If pH > 7.45 and patient not triggering ventilator, decrease set RR but not below 6/min.
Fluid Management	• Once patients are out of shock, adopt a conservative fluid management strategy. • Use diuretics or fluids to target a central venous pressure (CVP) of < 4 or a pulmonary artery occlusion pressure (PAOP) of < 8.

Liberation from Mechanical Ventilation	• Daily interruption of sedation.
	• Daily screen for spontaneous breathing trial (SBT).
	• SBT when all of the following criteria are present:
	  (a) Fio_2 < 0.40 and PEEP < 8 cm H_2O.
	  (b) Not receiving neuromuscular blocking agents.
	  (c) Patient awake and following commands.
	  (d) Systolic arterial pressure > 90 mm Hg without vasopressor support.
	  (e) Tracheal secretions are minimal, and the patient has a good cough and gag reflex.

Spontaneous Breathing Trial	• Place patient on 5 mm Hg pressure support with 5 mm Hg PEEP *or* T-piece. • Monitor HR, RR, oxygen saturation for 30-90 minutes. • Extubate if there are no signs of distress (tachycardia, tachypnea, agitation, hypoxia, diaphoresis).

ventilation to receive lower (mean PEEP levels on days 1 to 4 were 8.3 ± 3.2) versus higher levels of PEEP (mean PEEP levels on days 1 to 4 were 13.2 ± 3.5).[121] In this study, there were no differences between the groups in clinical outcomes, including ventilator-free days and mortality. Two other studies of the effects of PEEP in ARDS had similar results,[122,123] although one of the studies did show an increase in the number of ventilator-free days and organ failure–free days with application of higher PEEP.[123] None of these trials have shown significant increases in barotrauma related to higher PEEP levels. Although these three large studies have not shown beneficial effects of higher PEEP in all patients with ALI/ARDS, there may be a subset of patients who would benefit from higher PEEP. In a small trial, one investigator reported that a ventilator strategy that incorporated low tidal volume and titration of the PEEP level to above the lower inflection point on each individual patient's pressure volume curve improved mortality in ARDS.[124] However, measurement of the pressure-volume curve in any given patient is not practical clinically. Given the lack of compelling data favoring either a high PEEP or low PEEP strategy, current recommendations are to adjust the level of PEEP within an acceptable range (see Table 58-2) to achieve adequate oxygenation at a given Fio_2.

Noninvasive Ventilation

Noninvasive positive-pressure ventilation (NIV) delivered by nasal or full face mask has been highly successful in avoidance of intubation in patients with acute exacerbation of COPD.[125] NIV is commonly used in pediatric patients with ALI/ARDS,[126] but there is only one small randomized trial of 50 patients which showed that NIV improved oxygenation and prevented the need for endotracheal intubation in children admitted with acute respiratory failure. The role for NIV in adults with ALI/ARDS is still unclear. A growing number of small studies suggest that bilevel NIV with pressure-support ventilation and PEEP may reduce the need for intubation and improve outcomes in selected patients with ALI/ARDS.[127,128] However, data from large randomized controlled trials is still lacking. Furthermore, it seems likely that the majority of patients with ALI/ARDS will still require invasive

mechanical ventilation. In one large multicenter study of 354 of 2770 patients with acute hypoxemic respiratory failure *who were not already intubated*, NIV failed in 30% of patients but failed in 51% of patients with ARDS.[129]

One group of patients in whom NIV is particularly appealing is those patients who are immunosuppressed for various reasons and are at highest risk for nosocomial infections. Encouraging results have now been reported in a variety of patients with acute respiratory failure and immunosuppression.[130-132] Pending data from larger randomized clinical trials, a trial of noninvasive mechanical ventilation can be considered in a patient with ALI/ARDS who does not have a severe oxygenation defect, hemodynamic instability, or altered mental status, so long as the patient can be closely observed and readily intubated if NIV fails.

PHARMACOLOGIC THERAPY

There is no specific pharmacologic therapy for ALI/ARDS. A variety of treatment strategies have been investigated in large randomized trials, with a predominant focus on antiinflammatory strategies. Agents that appeared promising in experimental and early clinical studies but failed in large randomized trials include early glucocorticoids,[133,134] alprostadil,[135-137] surfactant,[138-140] ketoconazole,[141] N-acetylcysteine,[142] procysteine,[142] lisofylline,[143] and site-inactivated recombinant factor VIIa.[144] Some investigators have suggested that glucocorticoid therapy, although not helpful for the acute phase of ALI/ARDS, might hasten the resolution of late fibroproliferative ALI/ARDS. In one very small randomized study (plagued by crossovers such that only four patients remained in the placebo arm) there was a suggestion that glucocorticoid therapy might be beneficial in late ARDS.[145] This question was addressed in a randomized multicenter study conducted by the ARDS Network of 14 days of methylprednisolone in patients who had persistent ARDS for at least 7 days.[146] Compared to patients treated with placebo, those treated with methylprednisolone had an increase in the number of shock-free days and ventilator-free days by day 28, as well as improvements in oxygenation; but they did not have improved survival and had higher rates of reintubation, perhaps due to neuromuscular weakness. Given the serious concern about safety of high-dose glucocorticoids in critically ill patients, including the possibility of increasing the risk of nosocomial infections or critical illness polyneuropathy/myopathy, as well as the lack of improvement in mortality, routine use of glucocorticoids in ARDS cannot be recommended.

Despite the dismal findings in the numerous studies of pharmacologic therapy for ALI/ARDS to date, new therapeutic strategies are under investigation and may yet be beneficial. One area that has been largely ignored in the therapeutic realm is modulation of coagulation. There is mounting evidence that like sepsis, ALI/ARDS is a procoagulant, antifibrinolytic state[47,48] and that coagulation is activated and modulated locally in the airspace.[49,51] Modulation of coagulation by administration of recombinant human activated protein C (rhAPC; drotrecogin alfa) significantly reduces mortality in patients with severe sepsis, many of whom also had ALI/ARDS,[147] but the same therapy in patients with nonseptic ALI/ARDS did not show a mortality difference.[148] Likewise, a randomized trial of site-inactivated recombinant factor VIIa did not show benefit in patients with ALI/ARDS.[144] Another ongoing area of research involves the use of HMG-CoA reductase inhibitors (statins) in patients with ALI/ARDS. Some studies have shown that patients admitted to the hospital on statins have a lower mortality if they develop ALI/ARDS,[149] although other studies have not found the same association.[150] Another promising area of research is in modulating peroxisome proliferator–activated receptors using the glitazone class of diabetes medications in patients at risk for ALI/ARDS.[151] Clinical studies have shown a decreased incidence of ALI/ARDS in patients with diabetes,[29-31] but it is unclear whether this protection is a result of the diabetes itself or an effect of treatment. Another area that is actively under investigation involves strategies to hasten or facilitate the resolution of ALI/ARDS. Such therapies might be targeted at enhancing the rate of alveolar fluid clearance or modulating alveolar repair.

RESCUE THERAPIES

Despite appropriate treatment, some patients with ARDS will have profound and refractory hypoxemia. Initial management of these patients includes increased sedation and occasionally neuromuscular paralysis to maintain adequate oxygenation. In patients who do not respond to conventional treatment with low-tidal-volume ventilation and remain persistently hypoxemic, there are several unproven rescue therapies that may be tried to improve oxygenation in the acute setting (summarized in Table 58-3). Extracorporeal membrane oxygenation

(ECMO) has been used in patients with ARDS and severe hypoxemia. In specialized centers, ECMO has been used successfully to treat patients with severe ARDS,[152-154] but it has not proven effective at reducing mortality in small randomized trials.[155,156] One large trial randomized 180 patients with severe ARDS to ECMO versus conventional management and showed reduced mortality in patients treated with ECMO.[157] In this study, patients randomized to ECMO were transferred to a specialty center to receive therapy. Upon arrival, only 75% of patients in the ECMO group were actually treated with ECMO. Because of the study design, it is difficult to determine whether it was transfer to a specialty center for care or ECMO itself that conferred benefit. Although the results of this study are encouraging, the need for transfer to a specialty center and the dropout rate of 25% upon transfer limit the widespread use of ECMO in severe ARDS.

High-frequency oscillatory ventilation (HFVO) has been studied in several small randomized trials in patients with ARDS[158-162] and did improve oxygenation but not mortality in these studies. Likewise, prone positioning has been studied in several small[163-165] and three large trials[166-168] and has been associated with improvements in oxygenation but no reduction in mortality. Other rescue therapies include the use of a pulmonary vasodilator, such as inhaled nitric oxide (iNO) or inhaled prostacyclin. One clinical study showed that higher urinary NO excretion, a surrogate for endogenous NO activity, was associated with improved clinical outcomes in patients with ALI.[169] There have been several small, randomized clinical trials of iNO in ARDS, and although none have shown improved mortality, its use has been associated with improvements in oxygenation.[170] Inhaled prostacyclin is another pulmonary vasodilator that may be used as rescue therapy in severe refractory ARDS, although there are no randomized trials showing a mortality benefit.[171-173]

▣ Complications

Complications are common in any critically ill patient population. Supportive care for all critically ill patients must include vigilance in both preventing and diagnosing common complications such as pulmonary embolus, acute myocardial infarction, gastrointestinal bleeding, and nosocomial infection. Certain complications are more common in ALI/ARDS patients and deserve special mention.

BAROTRAUMA

Barotrauma occurs when air dissects out of the airways or alveolar space into surrounding tissues, leading to pneumothorax, pneumomediastinum, pneumatocele, or subcutaneous emphysema (Figure 58-4).

TABLE 58-3	Summary of Rescue Therapies for Acute Lung Injury and Acute Respiratory Distress Syndrome				
Rescue Therapy	*Year*	*How Studied*	*Number of Patients*	*Comments*	*References*
ECMO	1979	Phase II	90	In this relatively large, multicenter trial there was no benefit with the use of ECMO.	(156)
	2009	Phase III	180	This large randomized trial showed benefit to treatment with ECMO; however, 25% of patients assigned to ECMO did not receive this therapy, and the need for urgent transfer to specialized treatment centers limit general applicability of this trial.	(157)
ECCOR	1994	Phase III	40	This newer form of extracorporeal therapy did not improve mortality in ALI/ARDS.	(155)
Prone positioning	2001	Phase III	304	Although prone positioning improved oxygenation, there was no mortality benefit in this large multicenter trial.	(167)
	2009	Phase III	342	Patients were randomized according to severity of hypoxemia to receive 20 hours of prone positioning vs. usual care and had no reduction in mortality at 28 days or 6 months.	(168)
High-frequency oscillatory ventilation (HFOV)	2002	Phase III	148	HFOV group had improved oxygenation but no difference in mortality.	(160)
	2005	Phase III	61	No significant differences in any outcome between the groups.	(162)
Inhaled nitric oxide (iNO)	1998	Phase II	177	Although some patients will have improvement in oxygenation with inhaled nitric oxide, there was no mortality benefit in any of these large studies.	(214)
	1999	Phase III	203		(215)
	2004	Phase III	385		(216)

ECCOR, extracorporeal CO$_2$ removal; *ECMO*, extracorporeal membrane oxygenation; *PEEP*, positive end-expiratory pressure.

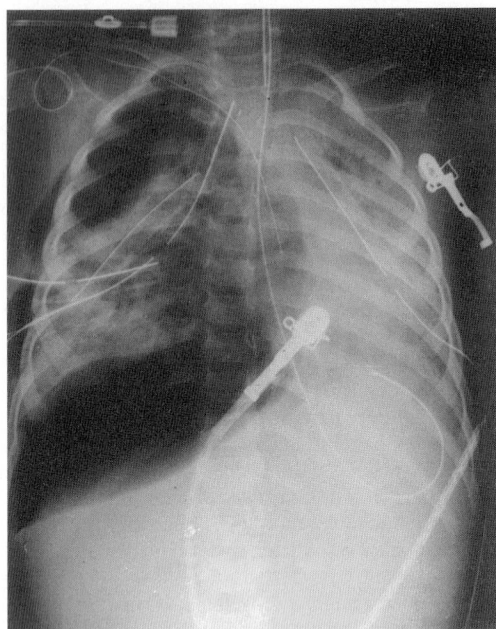

Figure 58-4 Barotrauma chest radiograph.

The exact incidence of pulmonary barotrauma in ALI/ARDS is unclear but appears to be declining. Data from two recent large randomized trials of protective ventilatory strategies suggest an incidence of early pneumothorax of 12% to 13%.[62,174] Higher incidences have been reported in the past, a finding that may have been the result of the use of mechanical ventilation with high tidal volumes and very high inspiratory plateau pressures.[175] In 861 patients enrolled in the NIH ARDS Network trial, approximately 10% of patients developed some form of barotrauma regardless of whether they were in the 6 or 12 mL/kg tidal volume arm. Further, PEEP level was the only factor that predicted the development of barotrauma in a multivariate analysis.[176]

Treatment of barotrauma depends on the location of the extravasated air. Pneumothorax can be life threatening, particularly if it is under tension; immediate diagnosis and tube thoracostomy are essential. Pneumothorax should be considered in any mechanically ventilated patient with ALI/ARDS who develops sudden unexplained worsening of hypoxemia, respiratory distress, or hemodynamic instability. A chest radiograph (preferably upright) is usually sufficient to make the diagnosis, but in many cases there may not be time to obtain one. Pneumomediastinum and subcutaneous emphysema can be painful, but other than analgesia, they do not require specific therapy. Air embolus is a potentially fatal complication of positive-pressure mechanical ventilation that has been reported occasionally in patients with ALI/ARDS[155,177,178] and usually occurs in conjunction with other evidence of pulmonary barotraumas, many times simultaneously.

NOSOCOMIAL PNEUMONIA

The incidence of nosocomial pneumonia in patients with ALI/ARDS is difficult to quantify. Depending on the diagnostic definition and/or strategy employed, estimates range from 15% to 60% of patients.[179,180] There is yet no consensus regarding the appropriate way to diagnose nosocomial pneumonia in the mechanically ventilated patient. Since patients with ALI/ARDS frequently die from uncontrolled infection, recognition (though notably difficult) and treatment of nosocomial pneumonia is an important part of caring for the ALI/ARDS patient. Clinical criteria commonly used in the diagnosis include fever, elevated white blood cell count, purulent secretions, and pulmonary infiltrates. However, these signs are often present in patients with ALI/ARDS even in the absence of nosocomial pneumonia.[181] Autopsy studies of patients dying with ALI/ARDS show a high incidence of unsuspected pneumonia.[182-184] Regardless of the methods used for diagnosis, early, appropriate, empirical therapy is the mainstay of treatment for nosocomial pneumonia. The adequacy and timeliness of initial empirical therapy are important determinants of outcome. Knowledge of local bacterial resistance patterns is crucial, and a high index of suspicion is required.

MULTISYSTEM ORGAN DYSFUNCTION

Although ALI/ARDS is often thought of as a primary pulmonary disorder, evidence is accumulating to suggest that ALI/ARDS is a systemic disorder with many similarities to sepsis or SIRS. Multisystem organ dysfunction is a common complication in ALI/ARDS. Organ dysfunction may result from the underlying cause of ALI/ARDS, such as sepsis, or occur independently. The exact incidence of multisystem organ dysfunction in ALI/ARDS is difficult to quantify. In the recent ARDS Network trial of low-tidal-volume ventilation, the mean number of non-pulmonary organ system failures per patient was 1.8.[62] Given the simultaneous occurrence of multiple organ failures, it is often difficult to determine the exact cause of death in ALI/ARDS patients, and survival ultimately depends on the successful support of the failing organs.

NEUROMUSCULAR WEAKNESS

Patients with ALI/ARDS are at high risk for developing prolonged muscle weakness that persists after resolution of pulmonary infiltrates and can complicate weaning from mechanical ventilation and rehabilitation. This clinical syndrome is commonly called *critical illness polyneuropathy*, but it actually has components of neuropathy and myopathy which can coexist or occur separately.[185] Although little prospective data are available, one study suggests that neuromuscular abnormalities are persistent in many survivors of critical illness, even when studied up to 5 years after ICU discharge.[186] Prolonged muscle weakness is most common in critically ill patients who are treated with glucocorticoids. In one study, use of corticosteroids was shown to be the best independent predictor of ICU-acquired paresis (odds ratio 14.9, 95% CI 3.2-69.8).[187] Neuromuscular blockade has also been implicated, and for this reason, the use of neuromuscular blockade should be reserved for those patients who are unable to be adequately oxygenated or who have problematic dyssynchrony with the mechanical ventilator despite deep sedation. In the absence of a compelling clinical indication, such as underlying connective tissue disease, the use of glucocorticoids should not be routine unless new clinical evidence in support of their clinical utility in ALI/ARDS becomes available.

Clinical Outcomes and Prognosis

Once a patient develops ALI/ARDS, there are several prognostic factors that can help clinicians predict outcome. Elevated pulmonary dead space fraction in ALI/ARDS is a reflection of extensive injury to the lung microcirculation, lung microvascular thrombi, and regional differences in pulmonary blood flow and is a predictor of death in patients with ARDS.[188,189] Although dead space fraction may predict mortality, it is not routinely measured in the ICU. For this reason, predictive models that use readily available clinical variables have been developed.[190] In addition to dead space fraction, a positive cumulative fluid balance at day 4 in patients with ARDS predicted increased mortality,[191] further supporting the use of a conservative fluid strategy.[109]

Mortality from ALI/ARDS appears to be gradually declining,[192] although this finding has not been consistent among retrospective studies.[193] Prior to the 1990s, mortality in clinical trials was approximately 40% to 60%.[194] Several recent single-center studies suggest that mortality rates measured in the same centers had declined over time.[195-198] In the ARDS Network study of 861 patients with ALI/ARDS, aggregate mortality to hospital discharge was 31% in the 6 mL/kg tidal volume arm and 40% in the 12 mL/kg tidal volume arm. However, mortality data from this study may significantly underestimate overall ALI/ARDS mortality, since many severely ill patients were excluded, including those with advanced liver disease, bone marrow transplantation, severe chronic respiratory disease, burns greater than 30% body surface area, or any other underlying condition with a likelihood of death greater than 50% within 6 months. As has previously been observed in other studies, in this study risk of in hospital mortality was highest in patients with sepsis (43%), intermediate in those with pneumonia (36%) or aspiration (37%), and lowest in those with multiple trauma (11%).[11] The low-tidal-volume strategy was effective at reducing mortality across all causes of ALI/ARDS.[11] Another study has shown that implementation of the ARDSNet low-tidal-volume ventilator strategy was associated with reducing hospital mortality compared to historical controls.[199]

Several recent multicenter studies in France,[200] Sweden,[201] Australia,[202] and Argentina[203] attempted to define mortality and prognostic variables in observational population-based studies rather than from clinical trial participants. In these studies, mortality was variable, ranging from 32% for ALI to 58% to 60% for ARDS. The highest mortality observed in patients who met Consensus definitions of ARDS was reported from the French study (60%). Factors that were independently associated with mortality from ALI/ARDS varied from study to study and included age, Acute Physiology Score, Pao_2/Fio_2 ratio, organ failures or septic shock, immunosuppression, cardiovascular failure, and chronic liver disease.[200-204] Two other U.S. studies of patients with ALI/ARDS predominantly from medical ICUs reported high overall mortality rates (58%).[205,206] Mortality was associated with chronic liver disease and other underlying diseases, including HIV infection or cancer. In summary, these studies suggest that while some improvements in ALI/ARDS mortality have been made, mortality remains quite high in population-based studies.

ALI/ARDS survivors frequently have long-term functional disability, cognitive dysfunction, and psychosocial problems.[207] Interestingly, pulmonary function frequently returns to normal or near normal in survivors. In a report of 1-year follow-up in 109 survivors from ARDS,[98] lung volumes and spirometry had returned to normal by 6 months. However, carbon monoxide diffusing capacity was persistently low at 12 months. Six-minute walk distances were persistently low at 12 months, largely due to muscle wasting and weakness rather than pulmonary function abnormalities.[98] Treatment with any systemic corticosteroid, the presence of illness acquired during the ICU stay, and the rate of resolution of the lung injury and multiorgan dysfunction during the ICU stay were the most important determinants of the 6-minute walk distance during the first year of follow-up. In other studies, patients who survive ALI/ARDS have been reported to have reduced health-related quality of life[208] and pulmonary disease–specific health-related quality of life,[209-211] as well as functional impairment that persist 2 years after ICU discharge.[212] In addition to physical and social difficulties after ARDS, survivors have high rates of depression and anxiety.[213]

ANNOTATED REFERENCES

Bernard GR, Artigas A, Brigham KL, et al. The American-European Consensus Conference on ARDS: definitions, mechanisms, relevant outcomes, and clinical trial coordination. Am J Respir Crit Care Med 1994;149(3 Pt 1):818-24.
This paper presents the findings of the American-European Consensus Conference on ARDS, including the new definitions for ALI and ARDS that are now widely used both clinically and in research studies.

Herridge MS, Cheung AM, Tansey CM, et al. One-year outcomes in survivors of the acute respiratory distress syndrome. N Engl J Med 2003;348(8):683-93.
In this multicenter study, the authors evaluated 109 survivors of ARDS at 3, 6, and 12 months after discharge from the hospital. Notably, functional disability was very common even at 12 months and was largely caused by muscle wasting and weakness. By contrast, pulmonary function was normalized, other than persistent decrements in the diffusing capacity for carbon monoxide.

Rubenfeld GD. Epidemiology of acute lung injury. Crit Care Med 2003;31(4 Suppl):S276-84.
This is a scholarly review of all the pertinent issues that hamper an accurate estimate of the incidence of ALI/ARDS.

The Acute Respiratory Distress Syndrome Network. Ventilation with lower tidal volumes as compared with traditional tidal volumes for acute lung injury and the acute respiratory distress syndrome. N Engl J Med 2000;342(18):1301-8.
This was a multicenter trial of 6 mL/kg compared with 12 mL/kg tidal volume in 861 mechanically ventilated patients with ALI or ARDS. The major finding was a reduction in hospital mortality in the 6 mL/kg group from 40% to 31%.

Ware LB, Matthay MA. Medical progress: the acute respiratory distress syndrome. N Engl J Med 2000;342(18):1334-49.
This review article presents a comprehensive overview of the pathogenesis, clinical features, and treatment of ALI and ARDS.

Ware LB, Matthay MA. Clinical practice. Acute pulmonary edema. N Engl J Med 2005;353(26):2788-96.
This case-based review article highlights the pathophysiologic and clinical differences between hydrostatic pulmonary edema and ARDS and provides a clinical algorithm for differentiating between the two.

The National Heart, Lung, and Blood Institute Acute Respiratory Distress Syndrome (ARDS) Clinical Trials Network. Pulmonary-artery versus central venous catheter to guide treatment of acute lung injury. N Engl J Med 2006;354(21):2213-24.

The National Heart, Lung, and Blood Institute Acute Respiratory Distress Syndrome (ARDS) Clinical Trials Network. Comparison of two fluid-management strategies in acute lung injury. N Engl J Med 2006;354(24):2564-75.
These companion papers present the main findings from the ARDS Network Fluid and Catheter Treatment Trial (FACTT). The major findings from these two manuscripts are that patients with ARDS who are not in shock should have central venous pressure–directed management of a conservative fluid strategy, with a goal CVP of below 4; such patients had more ventilator-free days compared to patients treated with a liberal fluid strategy.

Rice TW, Wheeler AP, Bernard GR, Hayden DL, Schoenfeld DA, Ware LB. Comparison of the Spo_2/Fio_2 ratio and the Pao_2/Fio_2 ratio in patients with acute lung injury or ARDS. Chest 2007 Aug;132(2):410-7.
This study compares the use of the Spo_2/Fio_2 ratio to the more invasive Pao_2/Fio_2 ratio, which requires blood gas analysis for the diagnosis of ARDS and should improve the rate of ALI/ARDS diagnosis among clinicians. In this study, an S/F ratio of 235 corresponded with a P/F ratio of 200, while an S/F ratio of 315 corresponded with a P/F ratio of 300.

REFERENCES

Access the complete reference list online at http://www.expertconsult.com.

59

Aspiration Pneumonitis and Pneumonia

PAUL E. MARIK

Aspiration is defined as the misdirection of oropharyngeal or gastric contents into the larynx and lower respiratory tract.[1] The pulmonary syndromes that commonly follow depend on the quantity and nature of the aspirated material, frequency of aspiration, and the nature of the host's defense mechanisms and response. The most important syndromes include *aspiration pneumonitis*, or Mendelson syndrome, a chemical pneumonitis caused by the aspiration of gastric contents; and *aspiration pneumonia*, an infectious process caused by the aspiration of oropharyngeal secretions colonized by pathogenic bacteria.[1] There is some overlap between these two syndromes, but they are distinct clinical entities (Table 59-1). Other aspiration syndromes include airway obstruction, lung abscess, exogenous lipoid pneumonia, chronic interstitial fibrosis, and *Mycobacterium fortuitum* pneumonia.

Aspiration Pneumonitis

Aspiration pneumonitis is best defined as acute lung injury (ALI) following the aspiration of regurgitated gastric contents.[1] This syndrome occurs in patients with a marked disturbance of consciousness such as drug overdose, seizures, massive cerebrovascular accident, following head trauma, and after or during anesthesia. Drug overdose is the most common cause of aspiration pneumonitis, occurring in approximately 10% of patients hospitalized following a drug overdosage. Adnet and Baut demonstrated that the risk of aspiration increases with the degree of unconscious (as measured by the Glasgow Coma Scale).[2] Historically, the syndrome most commonly associated with aspiration pneumonitis is Mendelson syndrome, reported in 1946 in obstetric patients who aspirated while receiving general anesthesia.[3] Mendelson's original report consisted of 44,016 non-fasted obstetric patients he studied between 1932 and 1945. Of these, more than half received an "operative intervention" with ether by mask without endotracheal intubation. He described aspiration in 66 patients (1:667). Although several became critically ill from their aspiration, "recovery was usually complete" within 24 to 36 hours, and only 2 patients died (1:22,008).

EPIDEMIOLOGY AND RISK FACTORS

Although aspiration is a widely feared complication of general anesthesia, clinically apparent aspiration in modern anesthesia practice is exceptionally rare, and in healthy patients the overall morbidity and mortality are low. The risk of aspiration with modern anesthesia is about 1 in 3000 anesthetics, with a mortality of approximately 1:125,000 and accounting for between 10% and 30% of all anesthetic deaths.[4,5] The risk of aspiration is greatly increased in patients intubated emergently in the field, emergency room, or intensive care unit (ICU). The risk factors for aspiration are listed in Table 59-2. In these patients, every effort should be made to reduce the risk of aspiration; this includes removing dentures, clearing the airway, and (in certain circumstances) placing a nasogastric tube to empty the stomach prior to intubation. If there is an immediate risk of airway compromise, endotracheal intubation should be performed prior to placement of a nasogastric tube. However, if the patient is likely to have a full stomach (upper-gastrointestinal bleed, small-bowel obstruction, ileus, etc.), it may be prudent to place a nasogastric tube prior to endotracheal intubation. When intubating emergently, suction equipment must be immediately available and rapid-sequence induction using cricoid pressure should be performed.

PATHOPHYSIOLOGY

Mendelson emphasized the importance of acid when he showed that unneutralized gastric contents introduced into the lungs of rabbits caused severe pneumonitis indistinguishable from that caused by an equal amount of 0.1 N hydrochloric acid.[3] However, if the pH of the vomitus was neutralized before aspiration, pulmonary injury was minimal. Experimental studies have demonstrated that the severity of lung injury increases significantly with the volume of aspirate and indirectly with its pH, with a pH of less than 2.5 being required to cause aspiration pneumonitis. However, the stomach contains a variety of other substances in addition to acid. Several experimental studies have revealed that aspiration of small particulate food matter from the stomach may cause severe pulmonary damage, even if the pH of the aspirate is above 2.5.

Aspiration of gastric contents results in a chemical burn of the tracheobronchial tree and pulmonary parenchyma, with an intense parenchymal inflammatory reaction. Proinflammatory cytokines, including tumor necrosis factor α (TNF-α) and CXC chemokines such as interleukin 8 (IL-8), are crucial to the development of aspiration pneumonitis by mediating neutrophil recruitment. Once localized to the lung, neutrophils play a key role in the development of lung injury through release of oxygen radicals and proteases. Gastric acid prevents the growth of bacteria, so stomach contents are normally sterile. Bacterial infection, therefore, does not play a significant role in the early stages of acute lung injury following aspiration of gastric contents. However, acid aspiration pneumonitis reduces host defenses against infection, increasing the risk of superinfection.[6] The incidence of this complication has not been well studied, but experimental models suggest that acid-aspiration pneumonitis "primes the lung," making secondary infection more severe.[6,7] Colonization of gastric contents by potentially pathogenic organisms may occur when the gastric pH is increased by the use of antacids, H₂ blockers, or proton pump inhibitors. In addition, gastric colonization by gram-negative bacteria occurs in patients receiving gastric enteral feedings, as well as in patients with gastroparesis and small-bowel obstruction. In these circumstances, the pulmonary inflammatory response is likely to result from both bacterial infection and the inflammatory response of the gastric particulate matter. It is also important to note that atrophic gastritis and gastric colonization is common in elderly patients; aspiration of vomitus by these patients is likely to result in an inflammatory response due to bacteria and particulate matter.

CLINICAL PRESENTATION

Aspiration of gastric contents can present dramatically with a full-blown picture that includes gastric contents in the oropharynx, wheezing, coughing, shortness of breath, cyanosis, pulmonary edema, hypotension, and hypoxemia, which may progress rapidly to severe acute respiratory distress syndrome (ARDS) and death. Many patients may not develop signs or symptoms associated with aspiration, whereas others may develop a cough or wheeze. In some patients, aspiration may be clinically silent, manifesting only as arterial desaturation, with radiologic evidence of aspiration. Warner and colleagues studied 67 patients who aspirated while undergoing anesthesia.[4] Forty-two (64%) of these patients were totally asymptomatic, 13 required mechanical ventilatory support for more than 6 hours, and 4 died.

TABLE 59-1	Contrasting Features of Aspiration Pneumonitis and Aspiration Pneumonia	
Feature	**Aspiration Pneumonitis**	**Aspiration Pneumonia**
Mechanism	Aspiration of sterile gastric contents	Aspiration of colonized oropharyngeal material
Pathophysiologic process	Acute lung injury from acidic and particulate matter	Acute pulmonary inflammatory response to bacteria and bacterial products
Bacteriologic findings	Initially sterile, with subsequent bacterial infection possible	Gram-negative rods, gram-positive cocci, and (rarely) anaerobic bacteria
Major predisposing factors	Depressed level of consciousness	Dysphagia and gastric dysmotility
Age group affected	Any age group, but usually young persons	Usually elderly persons
Aspiration event	May be witnessed	Usually not witnessed
Typical presentation	Patient with a history of depressed level of consciousness in whom a pulmonary infiltrate and respiratory symptoms develop	Institutionalized patient who presents with features of a "community-acquired pneumonia" with an infiltrate in a dependent bronchopulmonary segment
Clinical features	No symptoms; or symptoms ranging from a nonproductive cough to tachypnea, bronchospasm, bloody or frothy sputum, and respiratory distress 2 to 5 hours after aspiration	Tachypnea, cough, fever, and signs of pneumonia

Reproduced with permission from Marik PE. Aspiration pneumonitis and pneumonia: a clinical review. *N Engl J Med.* 2001;344(9):665-672.

MANAGEMENT

The upper airway should be suctioned following a witnessed aspiration. Endotracheal intubation should be considered in patients who are unable to protect their airway. While common practice, the prophylactic use of antibiotics in patients with suspected or witnessed aspiration is not recommended. Similarly, the use of antibiotics shortly after an aspiration episode in a patient who develops fever, leukocytosis, and a pulmonary infiltrate is discouraged, because it may select for more resistant organisms in a patient with an uncomplicated chemical pneumonitis. However, empirical antimicrobial therapy is appropriate in patients who aspirate gastric contents in the setting of small-bowel obstruction or in other circumstances associated with colonization of the stomach. Antimicrobial therapy should be considered in patients with an aspiration pneumonitis that fails to resolve within 48 hours. Empirical therapy with broad-spectrum agents is recommended. Antimicrobials with anaerobic activity are not routinely required. Lower respiratory tract sampling (protected specimen brush/bronchoalveolar lavage) and quantitative culture in intubated patients may allow targeted antimicrobial therapy and discontinuation of antibiotics in culture-negative patients.[8]

Immunomodulating Agents

Corticosteroids have been used in the management of aspiration pneumonitis since 1955.[9] However, limited data exist for evaluating the role of these agents, with only a single prospective placebo-controlled study having been performed. In that study, Sukumaran et al. randomized 60 patients with "aspiration pneumonitis" to methylprednisolone (15 mg/kg/day for 3 days) or placebo.[10] The patients were subdivided into two groups: a younger group with drug overdose as the predominant diagnosis and an older group with neurologic disorders. In the overdose group, 87% had an initial gastric pH below 2.5, compared to

12.8% in the neurologic group; 77.6 patients in the overdose group were admitted from the community, compared to 12.8% of patients in the neurologic group. Radiographic changes improved more rapidly in the steroid group, as did oxygenation. The number of ventilator and ICU days was significantly shorter in the overdose patients who received corticosteroids; however, these variables were longer in the neurologic group. There was no significant difference in the incidence of complications or outcome. The results of this study are somewhat difficult to interpret, as it is likely that the patients in the overdose group had true aspiration pneumonitis, whereas many patients in the neurologic group probably developed aspiration pneumonia. In addition, patients received a short course of high-dose corticosteroids. Current evidence suggests that patients with ARDS may benefit from a prolonged course of low-dose corticosteroids, but a short course of high-dose corticosteroids may be harmful.[11,12] Wolfe and colleagues performed a case-controlled study of 43 patients with aspiration pneumonitis, of whom 25 received high-dose corticosteroids (approximately 600 mg prednisolone/day for 4 days).[13] There was no difference in mortality, but secondary gram-negative pneumonia was reported to be more frequent in the steroid group (7/20 versus 0/13); however, ventilator days tended to be fewer in this group (4.3 versus 9.8 days). Based on these limited data, it is not possible to make evidence-based recommendations on the use of corticosteroids in patients with acid-aspiration pneumonia. However, more recent literature suggests that patients with ARDS may benefit from a prolonged course of low dose corticosteroids, so this approach should be considered.[11,12]

In animal models, a number of pharmacologic interventions (e.g., inhaled β_2-agonists, pentoxifylline, antiplatelet drugs, omega-3 fatty acids) have been shown to attenuate acute lung injury following acid aspiration,[14-19] but the role of these interventions in humans remains to be tested. Because of their inherent safety, these agents should at least be considered in patients with severe acid-aspiration pneumonitis.

Aspiration Pneumonia

Aspiration pneumonia develops after the aspiration of colonized oropharyngeal contents. Aspiration of pathogens from a previously colonized oropharynx is the primary pathway by which bacteria gain entrance to the lungs. Indeed, *Hemophilus influenzae* and *Streptococcus pneumoniae* first colonize the naso/oropharynx before being aspirated and causing community-acquired pneumonia (CAP).[20] However, when the term *aspiration pneumonia* is used, it refers to the development of a radiographic infiltrate in the setting of patients with risk factors for increased oropharyngeal aspiration. Approximately half of all healthy adults aspirate small amounts of oropharyngeal secretions

TABLE 59-2	Factors That Increase Risk of Aspiration During Endotracheal Intubation

Emergent situations
Upper gastrointestinal bleed
Difficult intubation/multiple intubation attempts
Advanced age (>70 years)
Seizures
Conditions predisposing to gastroesophageal reflux:
    Bowel obstruction
    Ileus
    Hiatal hernia
    Peptic ulcer disease
    Gastritis

during sleep. Presumably, the low virulent bacterial burden of normal pharyngeal secretions together with forceful coughing, active ciliary transport, and normal humoral and cellular immune mechanisms result in clearance of the inoculum without sequelae. If mechanical, humoral, or cellular mechanisms are impaired or if the aspirated inoculum is large enough, pneumonia may follow. Any condition that increases the volume and/or bacterial burden of oropharyngeal secretions in the setting of impaired host defense mechanisms may lead to aspiration pneumonia. Indeed, in stroke patients undergoing swallow evaluation, there is a strong correlation between the volume of aspirate and the development of pneumonia.[21] Factors that increase oropharyngeal colonization with potentially pathogenic organisms and that increase the bacterial load may augment the risk of aspiration pneumonia. The clinical setting in which pneumonia develops largely distinguishes aspiration pneumonia from other forms of pneumonia, but there is much overlap. For example, otherwise healthy elderly patients with CAP have been demonstrated to have a significantly higher incidence of silent aspiration when compared with age-matched controls.[22]

EPIDEMIOLOGY

Two principal factors make the epidemiologic study of aspiration syndromes difficult: (1) lack of specific and sensitive markers of aspiration and (2) the failure of most studies to make the distinction between aspiration pneumonitis and aspiration pneumonia. Nevertheless, several studies list "aspiration pneumonia" as the cause of CAP in 5% to 15% of cases.[23,24] CAP is a major cause of morbidity and mortality in the elderly, and it is likely aspiration is the major cause of pneumonia in these cases. Epidemiological studies have demonstrated that the incidence of pneumonia increases with aging, with the risk being almost six times higher in those older than 75 compared to those younger than 60 years of age.[25,26] The attack rate for pneumonia is highest among those in nursing homes, where pneumonia is the most common cause of death.[27]

DYSPHAGIA AND THE COUGH REFLEX

Swallowing is a complex and coordinated neuromuscular process that consists of both volitional and involuntary activity. Oropharyngeal aspiration due to abnormalities in swallowing and upper-airway protective reflexes is an important pathogenic mechanism leading to CAP. It has been estimated that in the United States, approximately 300,000 to 600,000 people each year are affected by dysphagia resulting from neurologic disorders.[28] These include patients with cerebrovascular accidents, Parkinson's disease, and dementia. Aspiration pneumonia is the major cause of death in these patients. In addition, the efficiency of the swallow mechanism decreases with aging, thereby increasing the risk of aspiration in the elderly. Kikuchi et al. evaluated the occurrence of silent aspiration in otherwise "healthy elderly patients" with CAP and age-matched control subjects using indium-111 chloride scanning.[22] Silent aspiration was demonstrated in 71% of patients with CAP, compared to 10% in control subjects.

An intact cough reflex is an important respiratory defense mechanism. Sekizawa and coworkers demonstrated a marked depression of the cough reflex in elderly patients with pneumonia.[29] Furthermore, the greater the derangement of the cough reflex, the greater the risk of pneumonia.[30] Nakazawa and colleagues demonstrated impairment of the swallow and the cough reflex in elderly patients with aspiration pneumonia but not in patients with dementia who had no prior history of aspiration pneumonia.[31]

Risk Factors for Dysphagia

The major risk factors for dysphagia are listed in Table 59-3. In patients with an acute stroke, the incidence of dysphagia ranges from 40% to 70%.[32] Dysphagic patients who aspirate are at an increased risk of developing pneumonia. Although dysphagia improves in most patients following a stroke, in many the swallowing difficulties follow a

TABLE 59-3	Risk Factors for Dysphagia and Aspiration Pneumonia
Cerebrovascular Disease	
Ischemic stroke	
Hemorrhagic stroke	
Subarachnoid hemorrhage	
Degenerative Neurologic Disease	
Alzheimer's dementia	
Multi-infarct dementia	
Parkinson's disease	
Amyotrophic lateral sclerosis (motor neuron disease)	
Multiple sclerosis	
Head and Neck Cancer	
Oropharyngeal malignancy	
Oral cavity malignancy	
Esophageal malignancy	

fluctuating course, with 10% to 30% continuing to have dysphagia with aspiration.[33,34]

RISK FACTORS FOR PNEUMONIA IN PATIENTS WHO ASPIRATE

Although the presence of dysphagia and the volume of aspirate are key factors that predispose patients to aspiration pneumonia, a number of other factors also play an important role.[21] As noted earlier, colonization of the oropharynx is an important step in the pathogenesis of aspiration pneumonia. The elderly have increased oropharyngeal colonization with pathogens such as *Staphylococcus aureus* and aerobic gram-negative bacilli (e.g., *Klebsiella pneumoniae* and *Escherichia coli*). Although the increased colonization may be transient, it underlies the increased risk in the elderly of pneumonia with these pathogens. The defects in host defenses that predispose to enhanced colonization with these organisms are uncertain, but dysphagia with a decrease in salivary clearance and poor oral hygiene may be major risk factors.[35] Edentulous patients appear to have a lower risk of aspiration pneumonia than dentate patients.[36]

DIAGNOSIS AND MANAGEMENT OF ASPIRATION PNEUMONIA

There is no gold standard test to diagnose aspiration pneumonia, and unlike the case with aspiration pneumonitis, aspiration that leads to pneumonia is generally not witnessed. The diagnosis is therefore inferred when a patient with known risk factors for aspiration has a radiographic infiltrate in a characteristic bronchopulmonary segment. In patients who aspirate in the recumbent position, the most common sites of involvement are the posterior segments of the upper lobes and the apical segments of the lower lobes. In patients who aspirate in the upright or semirecumbent position, the basal segments of the lower lobes are favored. The usual picture is that of an acute pneumonic process, which runs a course similar to that of a typical CAP. Untreated, however, these patients appear to have a higher incidence of cavitation and lung abscess formation.[37] Gram-negative pathogens and *S. aureus* are the likely pathogens in patients with CAP due to aspiration pneumonia.[38,39] El-Sohl and colleagues performed quantitative bronchial sampling in 95 institutionalized elderly with severe aspiration pneumonia.[40] Out of the 67 pathogens identified, gram-negative enteric bacilli were the predominant organisms isolated (49%), followed by anaerobic bacteria (16%) and *S. aureus*. Anaerobic isolates were recovered in conjunction with aerobic gram-negatives; in these patients clinical response was not related to the use of antibiotics with anaerobic activity.

Antimicrobial therapy is indicated in patients with aspiration pneumonia. The choice of antibiotics depends on the setting in which the aspiration occurs as well as the patient's premorbid condition.

However, antimicrobial agents with gram-negative activity, such as third-generation cephalosporins, fluoroquinolones, piperacillin, and carbapenems, are usually required.[38-41] Antibiotics with activity against methicillin-resistant *S. aureus* (MRSA) may also be required. Antimicrobials with specific anaerobic activity are not routinely warranted and may only be indicated in patients with severe periodontal disease, patients expectorating putrid sputum, and patients with a necrotizing pneumonia or lung abscess on chest radiograph.[1,38-41]

ASSESSMENT AND MANAGEMENT OF DYSPHAGIA

All elderly patients with CAP, patients with a recent cerebrovascular accident, and patients with degenerative neurologic diseases should be referred to a speech and language pathologist (SLP) for a formal swallow evaluation and for the development and implementation of a management program; this may include dietary modifications as well as various swallow maneuvers.[42,43] A clinician's bedside assessment of the cough and gag reflex is unreliable in screening for patients at risk of aspiration.

The management of patients with dysphagia requires the coordinated expertise of a number of healthcare professionals, including the patient's primary care physician, pulmonologist, SLP, clinical dietician, occupational therapist, physiotherapist, nurse, oral hygienist, and dentist, as well as the patient's primary caregivers. Goals are to optimize the safety, efficiency, and effectiveness of the oropharyngeal swallow, maintain adequate nutrition and hydration, and improve oral hygiene. Enhanced quality of life, wherever possible, should direct management. The emphasis should be to safely maximize oral nutritional intake and hydration.

Tube Feeding

Nutritional supplementation, as determined by the clinical dietitian, may be required. Tube feeding is not essential in all patients who aspirate. The practice of tube feeding in the end stages of degenerative illnesses in the elderly should be carefully considered. Finucane et al. found no data to suggest that tube feeding of patients with advanced dementia prevented aspiration pneumonia, prolonged survival, reduced the risk of pressure sores or infections, improved function, or provided palliation.[44] Short-term tube feeding, however, may be indicated in elderly patients with severe dysphagia and aspiration in whom improvement of swallowing is likely to occur. Nakajoh and colleagues demonstrated that the incidence of pneumonia was significantly higher in stroke patients with dysphagia who were fed orally, compared to those who received tube feeding (54.3% versus 13.2%, *P* <0.001), despite the fact that the orally fed patients had a higher functional status (higher Barthel index).[30] The FOOD trials consisted of two large randomized studies that enrolled dysphagic stroke patients.[45] In the first trial, patients enrolled within 7 days of admission were randomly allocated to early tube feeding or no tube feeding for more than 7 days. Early tube feeding was associated with an absolute reduction in risk of death of 5.8%. The second trial allocated patients to early nasogastric feeding or early feeding via a percutaneous endoscopic gastrostomy (PEG) tube. PEG feeding was associated with an absolute increase in the risk of death of 1% and an increased risk of death or poor outcome of 7.8%. Patients with a PEG were less likely to be transitioned to oral feeding than the NG group and were more likely to be living in an institution, perhaps explaining the higher mortality of the PEG fed patients. It was interesting to note that PEG-fed patients were more likely to develop pressure sores, suggesting that these patients may have been cared for differently. The results of the FOOD trials suggest that dysphagic stroke patients should be fed early via nasogastric or feeding tube and transitioned to oral feeding as their dysphagia resolves. Those patients whose dysphagia does not resolve may be candidates for placement of a PEG tube.

Colonized oral secretions are a serious threat to dysphagic patients, and feeding tubes offer no clear protection. There are no data to suggest that patients fed with gastrostomy tubes have a lower incidence of pneumonia than patients fed with nasogastric tubes.[46] The incidence of aspiration pneumonia has been shown to be similar in stroke patients with postpyloric as compared to intragastric feeding tubes.[47] Over the long term, aspiration pneumonia is the most common cause of death in gastrostomy tube–fed patients.[48]

Oral Hygiene

Institutionalized patients have been shown to have poor oral hygiene and rarely receive treatment from dentists and oral hygienists.[49] An aggressive protocol of oral care will reduce colonization with potentially pathogenic organisms and decrease the bacterial load—measures likely to reduce the risk of pneumonia.[50]

Pharmacologic Management

The neurotransmitter, substance P, is believed to play a major role in both the cough and swallow sensory pathways. Angiotensin-converting enzyme (ACE) inhibitors prevent the breakdown of substance P and may theoretically be useful in the management of patients with aspiration pneumonia. A number of studies have demonstrated a lower risk of aspiration pneumonia in stroke patients treated with an ACE inhibitor compared to other antihypertensive agents.[51,52]

Sedative medication has been demonstrated to increase the risk of pneumonia in residents of long-term care facilities and should therefore be avoided.[53] The prescription of phenothiazines and haloperidol should be very carefully considered, because they reduce oropharyngeal swallow coordination, causing dysphagia.[54,55] Medications that dry secretions, including antihistamines and drugs with anticholinergic activity, make it more difficult for patients to swallow and should therefore also be avoided.[54,56]

◼ Conclusions

Aspiration syndromes are common in hospitalized patients. Aspiration pneumonitis follows the aspiration of gastric contents, usually in patients with a marked decreased level of consciousness. Treatment of aspiration pneumonitis is essentially supportive; however, corticosteroids and other immunomodulating agents may have a role in these patients. Aspiration pneumonia occurs in patients with dysphagia and usually presents as a "CAP" with a focal infiltrate in a dependent bronchopulmonary segment. Patients with aspiration pneumonia require treatment with broad-spectrum antibiotics and management of the underlying dysphagia.

KEY POINTS

1. *Aspiration pneumonitis* is defined as acute lung injury following aspiration of regurgitated gastric contents; it results in a chemical burn of the tracheobronchial tree and pulmonary parenchyma, with an intense parenchymal inflammatory reaction.

2. The severity of lung injury after aspiration of gastric contents increases significantly with the volume of the aspirate and indirectly with its pH, with a pH less than 2.5 and a volume of 20 mL being required to cause aspiration pneumonitis.

3. The treatment of aspiration pneumonitis is essentially supportive; the role of corticosteroids is uncertain.

4. Aspiration pneumonia develops after the aspiration of colonized oropharyngeal contents in patients with dysphagia.

5. The most common causes of dysphagia leading to aspiration pneumonia include cerebrovascular and degenerative central nervous system disease.

6. Treatment of aspiration pneumonia includes antibiotics directed against the most likely pathogens (including aerobic gram-negative organisms) and evaluation and management by a speech and language pathologist.

ANNOTATED REFERENCES

Marik PE. Aspiration pneumonitis and pneumonia: a clinical review. N Engl J Med 2001;344(9):665-72.
  Classic review paper on aspiration syndrome.
Mendelson CL. The aspiration of stomach contents into the lungs during obstetric anesthesia. Am J Obstet Gynecol 1946;52(27):191-205.
  Classic paper on aspiration pneumonitis.
El-Sohl AA, Pietrantoni C, Bhat A, et al. Microbiology of severe aspiration pneumonia in institutionalized elderly. Am J Respir Crit Care Med 2003;167(12):1650-4.
  This study used quantitative bacterial cultures to determine the microbiology of aspiration pneumonia in institutionalized patients.
American Thoracic Society; Infectious Diseases Society of America. Guidelines for the management of adults with hospital-acquired, ventilator-associated, and healthcare-associated pneumonia. Am J Respir Crit Care Med 2005;171(4):388-416.

The American Thoracic Society (ATS) guidelines for the management of pneumonia in institutionalized patients.
Dennis MS, Lewis SC, Warlow C. FOOD Trial Collaboration. Effect of timing and method of enteral tube feeding for dysphagic stroke patients (FOOD): a multicentre randomised controlled trial. Lancet 2005;365(9461):764-72.
  This is an important study that evaluated the role of tube feeding and PEG tubes in patients with dysphagic stroke.
Finucane TE, Christmas C, Travis K. Tube feeding in patients with advanced dementia: a review of the evidence. JAMA 1999;282(14):1365-70.
  This paper evaluates the role of PEG tubes in patients with dementia

REFERENCES

Access the complete reference list online at http://www.expertconsult.com.

60

Severe Asthma Exacerbation

THOMAS C. CORBRIDGE | SUSAN J. CORBRIDGE

Magnitude of the Problem

Each year in the United States, acute asthma accounts for approximately 1.8 million emergency department visits, 497,000 hospitalizations, and 3800 deaths.[1] All too commonly, failure to achieve adequate outpatient control lies at the crux of the problem. Asthma control is achieved in a minority of patients, largely due to the underuse of antiinflammatory agents, and poor control is a risk factor for asthma exacerbation.[2] More than half of current asthmatics had one or more attacks during the preceding year, and there appears to be a subset of patients who are prone to exacerbations. Factors underlying the exacerbation-prone phenotype include cigarette smoking, medication nonadherence, psychosocial factors, poverty, obesity, and alterations in host cytokine response to viral infections.[3] The rate of asthma death is higher in blacks than whites and in patients aged 65 and older. Patients who require mechanical ventilation for asthma have a mortality rate of less than 10% and are most likely to die of tension pneumothorax or nosocomial infection.[4] Fortunately, the rate of asthma death (which had increased from 1980 to 1995) has decreased each year since 2000. Risk factors for fatal or near-fatal asthma are listed in Table 60-1.

Pathophysiology of Acute Airflow Obstruction

Less than 15% of asthmatics have rapid-onset exacerbations. These are predominantly bronchospastic events resulting in significant airflow obstruction within minutes to a few hours. They occur from exposure to an allergen or irritant, stress, inhalation of illicit drugs, or the use of a nonsteroidal antiinflammatory agent or beta-blocker in susceptible patients. The trigger is generally not infectious and may remain unidentified.

Asthma attacks most commonly evolve over 24 hours and are associated with increasing airway wall inflammation and mucus plugs. These exacerbations are commonly triggered by viral infections (e.g., rhinovirus, influenza virus, respiratory syncytial virus) or mycoplasma and take longer to resolve.

Regardless of the tempo of the attack, acutely ill asthmatics develop critical airflow obstruction. The time available for expiration (less than 2 seconds in a patient breathing 30/min) is insufficient for full exhalation, resulting in gas trapping and dynamic lung hyperinflation (DHI). Trapped gas elevates alveolar volume and pressure relative to mouth pressure at end-expiration, a state referred to as *auto-PEEP*.[5] Auto-PEEP must be overcome by forcefully lowering pleural pressure during spontaneous inspiration, which increases the inspiratory work of breathing. At the same time, dynamic hyperinflation increases elastic work of breathing. Dynamic hyperinflation also decreases diaphragm force generation by placing the diaphragm in a mechanically disadvantageous position. Dynamic hyperinflation may be self-limiting because increases in lung volume increase lung elastic recoil pressure and airway diameter to augment expiratory flow. In the end, an imbalance between increased respiratory system load (both resistive and elastic) and decreased respiratory muscle strength may result in respiratory failure.[6]

Hypoxemia results from decreased ventilation ($\dot{V}$) to perfused ($\dot{Q}$) alveolar-capillary units. The severity of hypoxemia roughly tracks the severity of obstruction, but in recovering patients, airflow rates may improve faster than Pao$_2$ and $\dot{V}/\dot{Q}$ inequality, indicating that larger airways recover faster than smaller airways. Multiple inert gas

elimination technique (MIGET) analysis also demonstrates small areas of high $\dot{V}$ relative to $\dot{Q}$ and slightly increased physiologic dead space in acute asthma. This may result from decreased blood flow to hyperinflated lung units. Elevated dead space and decreased minute ventilation in the critically hyperinflated and fatiguing patient underlie the development of hypercapnia in severe exacerbations.

Large swings in intrathoracic pressure accentuate the normal inspiratory fall in systolic blood pressure, a phenomenon referred to as *pulsus paradoxus*. During vigorous inspiration, intrathoracic pressure falls, lowering right atrial and right ventricular pressures and thereby augmenting right ventricular (RV) filling. Enhanced right-sided filling shifts the intraventricular septum leftward, causing a conformational change in the left ventricle (LV), LV noncompliance, and incomplete LV filling. Furthermore, LV filling may be impeded by dynamic hyperinflation, causing tamponade-like physiology; LV emptying is impaired by large negative pleural pressures and increased LV afterload.

During forced expiration, high intrathoracic pressures impede right-sided filling during asthma exacerbations. The net result of cyclical changes in pleural pressure is pulsus paradoxus. Importantly, however, an increase in pulsus paradoxus does not occur when decreased respiratory muscle strength limits the magnitude of pleural pressure change.

Clinical Features

Dyspnea, cough, wheeze, and increased work of breathing are the hallmarks of acute asthma. Patients with moderate to moderately severe attacks are tachypneic and in mild to moderate respiratory distress. They have expiratory phase prolongation, difficulty speaking in long sentences, and audible wheezes. Arterial blood gases commonly reveal hypoxemia and acute respiratory alkalosis. A more severe attack leads to upright positioning, diaphoresis, monosyllabic speech, respiratory rate above 30/min, accessory muscle use, pulse above 120/min, pulsus paradoxus greater than 25 mm Hg, hypoxemia, and normo- or hypercapnia. Depressed mental status, paradoxical respiration, bradycardia, absence of pulsus paradoxus from respiratory muscle fatigue, and a quiet chest signal an impending arrest. The emergence of wheezes in these patients is generally a good marker that airflow has improved. Thus posture, speech, and mental status allow for a quick appraisal of severity, response to therapy, and need for intubation.

The common cardiac response to acute asthma is sinus tachycardia. Supraventricular and ventricular arrhythmias occur rarely. Severe exacerbations may also cause right heart strain and myocardial ischemia.

Differential Diagnosis

"All that wheezes is not asthma" is an adage worth remembering. In heavy smokers over the age of 40, consider an acute exacerbation of chronic obstructive pulmonary disease. In patients with congestive heart failure, bear in mind that elevated left atrial pressure can cause wheezing. Pulmonary embolism rarely causes wheeze, but this possibility should be considered when dyspnea is out of proportion to signs and measures of expiratory flow. Vocal cord dysfunction (and other causes of upper airway obstruction) should be considered when there is stridor, normal oxygenation, or resolution of airflow obstruction after intubation. Tracheal stenosis (e.g., subglottic stenosis from prior intubation or bronchogenic cancer) may also present with breathlessness and wheezing. Finally, foreign-body aspiration should be considered in the very young and old, in individuals with altered mental status or

TABLE 60-1	Risk Factors for Fatal or Near-Fatal Asthma

Frequent ED visits and hospitalizations
Intensive care unit admission
Intubation (prior or current)
Hypercapnia
Barotrauma
Psychiatric illness
Medical noncompliance
Illicit drug use
Poverty
Inadequate access to medical care
Use of >two canisters/month of an inhaled β_2-agonist
Poor perception of airflow obstruction
Comorbidities (e.g., coronary artery disease)
Sensitivity to *Alternaria* species

neuromuscular disease, and if symptoms developed after eating or dental work. Pneumonia should be considered in the febrile patient with cough and phlegm when there are localizing signs on physical examination, and hypoxemia does not correct with low-flow oxygen.

Peak Flow Measurements

To avoid underestimating the severity of an asthma exacerbation, it is important to objectively measure the degree of airflow obstruction. Clinicians often underestimate the degree of obstruction and may alter therapy after peak expiratory flow rate (PEFR) determination. Patients perform slightly better than clinicians at estimating severity, but there is still variability in perception. Peak flow measurements should be deferred in patients with severe exacerbations; the maneuver can worsen bronchospasm even to the point of arrest.

The change in PEFR or FEV_1 (forced expiratory volume in the first second of expiration) predicts the need for hospitalization. Several studies have demonstrated that failure of initial therapy to improve expiratory flow significantly after 30 to 60 minutes predicts a refractory course requiring continued treatment in the emergency department (ED) or hospitalization.

Acid-Base Status

Arterial blood gas determination is recommended in patients with severe attacks (e.g., when FEV_1 is less than 1 L or PEFR is less than 200 L/min). However, serial blood gases are generally not necessary unless the patient is mechanically ventilated. Hypoxemia and respiratory alkalosis are common in mild to moderate exacerbations. Eucapnia and hypercapnia indicate a severe exacerbation, but they are in and of themselves not sufficient reasons for intubation, because these patients may still respond adequately to pharmacotherapy. Conversely, the absence of hypercapnia does not preclude a life-threatening attack.

In response to acute respiratory alkalosis of sufficient duration, there may be renal wasting of bicarbonate and development of a post-hypocapnic metabolic acidosis. Lactic acidosis occurs, particularly in patients with labored breathing who receive parenteral β-agonists.

Chest Radiography

In classic cases of acute asthma, the chest x-ray rarely affects management. A chest x-ray should be obtained when there are localizing signs on examination, concerns regarding barotrauma, or questions regarding diagnosis. Chest x-rays are also indicated in intubated patients to confirm proper endotracheal tube position.

Emergency Department Disposition

Asthmatic patients with inadequate response to albuterol in the ED invariably require hospital admission or prolonged treatment in an ED holding area (see later).[8] Approximately one-third of patients are non-responders to albuterol (Figure 60-1), which is not necessarily explained

by prior heavy use of this medication. Rather, nonresponsiveness suggests a significant component of airway wall inflammation and the presence of intraluminal mucus. Albuterol nonresponders have negligible (i.e., <10%) changes in their PEFR after 30 to 60 minutes of therapy. These patients should be admitted to the hospital, as should patients with other markers of a severe attack such as a PEFR less than 40% of predicted or personal best PEFR, or deterioration despite ED treatment. Patients with respiratory failure, need for frequent albuterol treatments, fatigue, altered mental status, and cardiac arrhythmias require intensive care unit admission. Patients with an incomplete response to treatment in the ED, defined by improved but persistent symptoms and a PEFR or FEV_1 between 40% and 69% of predicted, should be considered for admission, although selected patients safely return home with appropriate treatment and follow-up. Patients with a good response to treatment may be discharged home with appropriate instructions for anti-inflammatory therapy. These patients have a PEFR $\geq$ 70% an hour after their last treatment, a clear chest, and are in no distress.

Oxygen

Supplemental oxygen should be provided to maintain arterial oxygen saturations greater than 90% (>95% in pregnancy). This improves oxygen delivery to tissue beds including the respiratory muscles and reverses hypoxic pulmonary vasoconstriction. Oxygen further protects against β-agonist-induced pulmonary vasodilation and increased

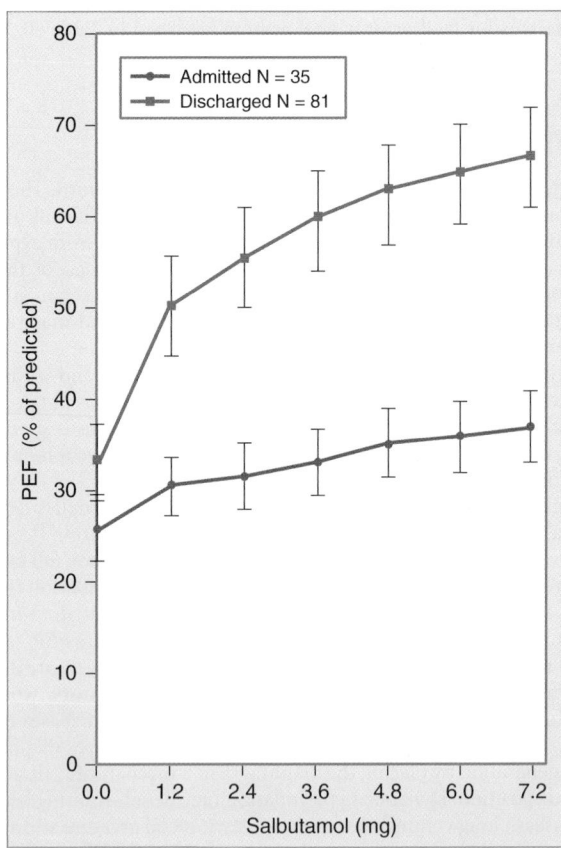

Figure 60-1 Dose-response relationship to albuterol 4 puffs (400 μg) every 10 minutes in 116 acute asthmatics. Sixty-seven percent of patients obtained discharge criteria after administration of 2.4 mg albuterol within 1 hour; half of responders met discharge criteria after 12 puffs. Patients with a blunted cumulative dose-response relationship were hospitalized. (*Reproduced with permission from Rodrigo C, Rodrigo G. Therapeutic response patterns to high and cumulative doses of salbutamol in acute severe asthma. Chest. 1998;113:593.*)

TABLE 60-2	Selected Drugs Used in the Treatment of Acute Asthma
Albuterol	2.5 mg in 2.5 mL normal saline by nebulization every 15-20 min × 3 in the first hour or 4-8 puffs by MDI with spacer every 10-20 min for 1 hour, then as required; for intubated patients, titrate to physiologic effect and side effects.
Levalbuterol	1.25 mg by nebulization every 15-20 min × 3 in the first hour, then as required.
Epinephrine	0.3 mL of a 1:1000 solution subcutaneously every 20 min × 3. Terbutaline is favored in pregnancy when parenteral therapy is indicated. Use with caution in patients older than age 40 and in patients with coronary artery disease.
Corticosteroids	Methylprednisolone IV or prednisone PO 40-80 mg/d in 1 or 2 divided doses until PEFR reaches 70% of predicted or personal best.
Anticholinergics	Ipratropium bromide 0.5 mg (with albuterol) by nebulization every 20 min, or 8 puffs by MDI with spacer (with albuterol) every 20 min.
Magnesium sulfate	2 g IV over 20 minutes, repeat once as required (total dose 4 g, unless hypomagnesemic).

IV, intravenous; *MDI,* metered-dose inhaler; *PEFR,* peak expiratory flow rate; *PO,* per os (oral).

blood flow to low $\dot{V}/\dot{Q}$ units. Oxygen saturation should be monitored until there is clear clinical progress, remembering that improved oxygenation may lag behind improved airflow rates.

Pharmacologic Management

Selected drugs used in the treatment of acute asthma are presented in Table 60-2. Brief discussions of a few of the more common therapeutic agents employed to treat severe asthma exacerbation follow.

β_2-AGONISTS

Inhaled short-acting β_2-agonists (SABAs) are the preferred drugs to treat the bronchospastic component of acute asthma. They should be delivered in a repetitive or continuous fashion depending on clinical response and side effects. A commonly recommended strategy is albuterol, 2.5 mg by nebulization, every 20 minutes during the first hour of ED management. In severe asthma exacerbations, continuous administration (same total dose) may be slightly superior to repetitive dosing, although there is little difference between the two strategies in most cases. Albuterol can be delivered effectively by metered dose inhaler (MDI); 4 to 8 puffs of albuterol by MDI with a spacer is equivalent to a 2.5-mg nebulizer treatment. MDIs with spacers are cheaper and faster; hand-held nebulizers require less supervision and coordination. Treatment frequency after the first hour depends on clinical response and side effects.

Although albuterol is the most widely used SABA, other SABAs are available, including levalbuterol, bitolterol, and pirbuterol. Levalbuterol in one-half the milligram dose of albuterol provides comparable efficacy and safety but has not been studied by continuous administration. Bitolterol and pirbuterol have not been studied in severe asthma exacerbations.

There is no advantage to subcutaneous epinephrine or terbutaline in the initial management of acute asthma unless the patient is unable to comply with inhaled therapy. In refractory cases, however, subcutaneous treatment in the absence of contraindications may confer additional benefit. β-Agonists are generally well tolerated in younger patients; tremor and tachycardia are common, but serious toxicity is rare. Subcutaneous injections are riskier and should be used with caution in older patients at risk for coronary artery disease. Long-acting β_2-agonists (LABAs) are not recommended for treatment of acute asthma, although limited data demonstrate formoterol (which has acute onset of action) is effective and safe in this setting. Combination therapy with a LABA and an inhaled corticosteroid (ICS) may be initiated or continued in hospitalized patients receiving rescue therapy.

LABA/ICS combination therapy may be required to achieve adequate outpatient asthma control and decrease the risk of future attacks.

IPRATROPIUM BROMIDE

The modest bronchodilator properties of ipratropium bromide preclude its use as a single agent in acute asthma. However, ipratropium bromide added to albuterol appears to be more effective than albuterol alone. The expert panel of the National Institutes of Health recommends adding ipratropium bromide to albuterol, particularly in patients with severe exacerbations, to improve flow rates and decrease hospitalizations. For nebulization in adults, 0.5 mg of ipratropium bromide is added to 2.5 mg of albuterol; by MDI, 8 puffs of ipratropium bromide are added to 4 to 8 puffs of albuterol by MDI. If a combination albuterol/ipratropium bromide inhaler is used, the recommended dose is 8 puffs every 20 minutes for the first 1 to 3 hours as guided by clinical response and toxicity.

CORTICOSTEROIDS

Most acutely ill asthmatics are not taking corticosteroids (either inhaled or oral) prior to ED arrival. In the ED, systemic corticosteroids are recommended for all patients save the rare patient who has a marked immediate and durable response to initial SABA therapy (who should invariably be started on an ICS before ED discharge).

Corticosteroids treat the inflammatory component of asthma by promoting new protein synthesis. Their effects are typically delayed, underlining the importance of early initiation. If initiated early in the ED, systemic corticosteroids decrease hospitalization rates. They also decrease the chance of relapse after discharge. In hospitalized patients, systemic corticosteroids improve the rate of recovery.

Oral steroids are as effective as parenteral steroids. Single-dose formulations of an intramuscular preparation should be considered in an ED patient who is deemed unlikely to take oral corticosteroids after discharge.

Various dosing regimens have been studied, and debate continues regarding the optimal dosing strategy. For hospitalized adults, the Expert Panel Report 3 recommends 40 to 80 mg/d of prednisone, methylprednisolone, or prednisolone in 1 or 2 divided doses until PEFR reaches 70% of predicted or the patient's personal best. For outpatients, a common strategy is to use prednisone, 40 mg/d for 5 to 10 days, with early follow-up to judge clinical response and optimize the outpatient regimen.

There is no established role for high-dose ICSs in acute asthma. However, ICSs play a pivotal role in achieving outpatient asthma control. Patients discharged from the ED or hospital after an asthma attack should be started on an ICS-based treatment program combined with adequate education regarding ICS use.

OTHER THERAPIES

Aminophylline does not confer additional bronchodilation in adults compared to standard care with β_2-agonists. It increases the frequency of adverse effects such as tachyarrhythmias, and therefore should only be used by seasoned clinicians facing refractory cases.

Prospective trials have yielded conflicting results regarding the use of magnesium sulfate ($MgSO_4$) in acute asthma. The general consensus is that intravenous (IV) $MgSO_4$ is not effective in mild to moderate exacerbations. In patients with severe exacerbations, however, $MgSO_4$ is safe and may improve airflow rates. The dose in adults is 2 gm by vein over 20 minutes. Additional, albeit limited, data support the use of inhaled $MgSO_4$ in acute asthma.

There are insufficient data to recommend leukotriene modifiers in acute asthma. The most compelling data come from randomized trials of IV montelukast in adults, but the IV formulation is not available in the United States.

Studies of heliox have been plagued by methodological differences, small patient numbers, and failure to control for concurrent upper airway obstruction (e.g., vocal cord dysfunction). Taken in sum, the available data do not support its routine use in acute asthma. However, heliox can be conditionally recommended in patients with severe asthma attacks as a way to potentially decrease work of breathing. The gas is easily administered by tight-fitting face mask, and its effects (or lack thereof) can be determined within seconds to minutes after administration. Limited data further support the use of heliox as a driving gas during albuterol nebulization to improve bronchodilator delivery.

Noninvasive Ventilation

Noninvasive ventilation (NIV) has not been studied extensively in acute asthma. There are no large, well-designed randomized trials to inform its use in this setting, but a recent systematic review of the available literature suggests it may be beneficial in selected patients with respiratory failure, perhaps by decreasing work of breathing. Data also suggest that the coupling of albuterol nebulization with noninvasive positive-pressure ventilation (NPPV) may be superior to nebulization alone in acute asthma.

Noninvasive ventilation includes the use of low levels of nasal continuous positive airway pressure (CPAP) of 5 to 7.5 cm H_2O or, more commonly, bilevel positive airway pressure (BiPAP). One approach to BiPAP use is to start with 8 cm H_2O inspiratory pressure support and 3 cm H_2O of expiratory positive airway pressure. These pressures can be adjusted as required to 15 cm H_2O for inspiration and 5 cm H_2O during expiration to achieve common endpoints of improved patient comfort, RR below 25 and tidal volume above 7 mL/kg.[9] Noninvasive ventilation should only be used in alert, cooperative, and hemodynamically stable patients who do not need an endotracheal tube for airway protection or secretion clearance.

Intubation and Mechanical Ventilation

Respiratory arrest or impending respiratory arrest (e.g., extreme exhaustion, a quiet chest, progressive hypercapnia, and altered mental status) are indications for intubation. Oral intubation is preferred because it allows for a larger endotracheal tube, which lowers airway

resistance and helps remove mucus plugs. Nasal intubation is not recommended because it necessitates a smaller tube and may be complicated by nasal polyps and sinusitis.

POSTINTUBATION HYPOTENSION

The time immediately after intubation can be difficult for patients with severe airflow obstruction, and care must be taken to stabilize the patient by the thoughtful use of sedatives, paralytics, bronchodilators, intravenous fluids, and positive-pressure ventilation. A common problem in the immediate postintubation period is hypotension which stems from loss of vascular tone with sedation or paralysis, hypovolemia, tension pneumothorax, and—importantly—overzealous mechanical ventilation.

Inappropriately fast respiratory rates during mechanical ventilation result in inadequate exhalation time and dangerous levels of dynamic hyperinflation. Clues to this condition include (1) excessive efforts required to deliver manual breathes during Ambu bag ventilation and high airway pressures and (2) hypotension and tachycardia. When critical dynamic hyperinflation is suspected, a trial of hypopnea (2-3 breaths/min) or apnea in a well-oxygenated patient for 30 to 60 seconds is both diagnostic and therapeutic. This maneuver lowers lung volumes and airway pressures and increases cardiac preload to help regain cardiopulmonary stability. However, close inspection of the chest radiograph is mandatory in all hypotensive patients to rule out pneumothorax, which invariably requires tube thoracostomy (unilateral or bilateral as required).

INITIAL VENTILATOR SETTINGS

Expiratory time (Te), tidal volume (VT), and the severity of airway obstruction determine the level of dynamic hyperinflation during mechanical ventilation (Figure 60-2).[10,11] Expiratory time is determined by minute ventilation (RR × VT) and the inspiratory flow rate. To illustrate this point, consider the following hypothetical ventilator settings: RR 15/min; VT 1000 mL, and an inspiratory flow rate of 60 LPM (or 1 LPS). In this example, the respiratory cycle time (the total amount of time allowed for one complete breath) is 4 seconds

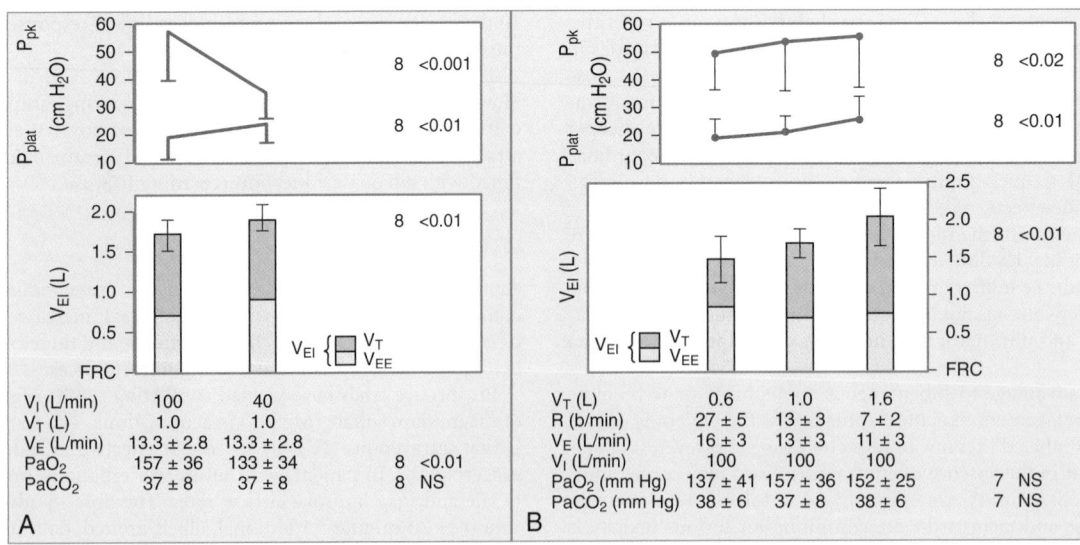

Figure 60-2 Effects of ventilator settings on airway pressures and lung volumes during normocapnic ventilation of eight paralyzed asthmatic patients. V_{EE}, lung volume at end-expiration; V_{EI}, lung volume at end-inspiration; P_{pk}, peak airway pressure; P_{plat}, end-inspiratory plateau pressure, V_E, minute ventilation, Vi, inspiratory flow. The numerals 7 and 8 are patient numbers. The numerals < 0.001, < 0.01, and < 0.02 are P values. **A,** As inspiratory flow is decreased from 100 L/min to 40 L/min at the same V_E, P_{pk} falls, but hyperinflation increases due to dynamic gas trapping. **B,** Dynamic hyperinflation is reduced by low respiratory rates and high tidal volumes (as long as V_E is decreased), but high tidal volumes result in high P_{plat}. *(Reproduced with permission from Tuxen DV, Lane S. The effects of ventilatory pattern on hyperinflation, airway pressures and circulation in mechanical ventilation of patients with severe air-flow obstruction. Am Rev Resp Dis. 1987;136:872.)*

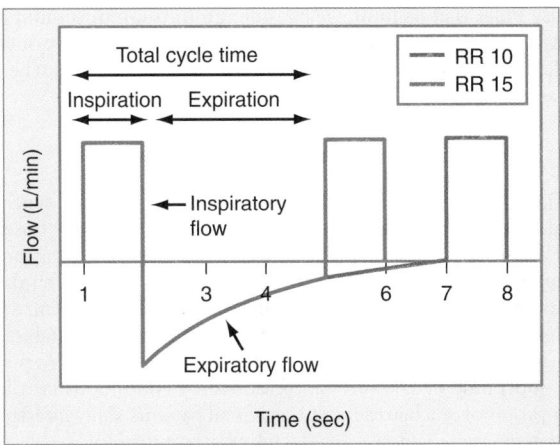

Figure 60-3 Effects of changing respiratory rate (RR) on expiratory time (Te) with a VT of 1000 mL and a constant inspiratory flow rate of 60 LPM (1 LPS). Note that with RR of 15/min (*solid line*), total cycle time (amount of time allowed for one complete breath) is 4 seconds. Inspiratory time (Ti) is 1 second, and Te is 3 seconds, resulting in an I:E of 1:3. By lowering RR to 10/min (*dotted line*) total cycle time increases to 6 seconds, and Te is 5 seconds, resulting in an I:E of 1:5. Lower RR allows for greater exhalation of the delivered breath and lower end-expiratory plateau pressure (not shown), although effects are modest because of low end-expiratory flow rates.

(Figure 60-3). Inspiratory time (Ti) is 1 second, and Te is 3 seconds, resulting in an I:E of 1:3. If these settings caused critical dynamic hyperinflation, lowering RR to 10/min would prolong respiratory cycle time to 6 seconds and Te to 5 seconds (I:E of 1:5), thus providing additional exhalation time. Granted, the additional volume of gas emptied by this strategy may be small because of low expiratory flow rates, but even small changes in lung volume may be clinically relevant. Now consider the effect of increasing inspiratory flow. If inspiratory flow is increased from 60 LPM to 120 LPM, then Ti would decrease to 0.5 seconds, and with a RR of 15/min, Te would increase from 3 seconds to 3.5 seconds. High inspiratory flow rates, however, increase peak airway pressures, and though high peak airway pressures themselves do not correlate with outcome, they might worsen patient-machine synchrony. Furthermore, high inspiratory flow rates may have the untoward effect of increasing respiratory rate in spontaneously breathing patients, thereby decreasing Te. On the other hand, if too low an inspiratory flow is used, Te falls and dynamic hyperinflation increases.

A reasonable compromise is to choose an inspiratory flow rate of 60 LPM and an initial minute ventilation of 7 to 8 L/min in a 70-kg patient to avoid dangerous levels of dynamic hyperinflation.[12] This can be achieved by setting the RR between 12 and 14/min and VT between 7 and 8 mL/kg. In spontaneously breathing patients, low levels of machine-set PEEP (e.g., 5 cm H_2O) decrease inspiratory work of breathing by decreasing the pressure gradient required to overcome auto-PEEP, without aggravating lung inflation. There are no randomized trials of ventilator mode in acute asthma. In paralyzed patients and other patients not breathing above the set respiratory rate, synchronized intermittent mandatory ventilation (SIMV) and assist-controlled ventilation (AC) are identical. In patients triggering the ventilator, AC may increase Ve more than SIMV, but SIMV may increase work of breathing. Depending on the institution, volume-controlled ventilation (VC) may be recommended over pressure-controlled ventilation (PC) because of greater staff familiarity with its use. Pressure control offers the advantage of limiting peak airway pressure to a predetermined set value (e.g., 30 cm H_2O) and has been used successfully in children with severe asthma exacerbation. During PC, VT is inversely related to auto-PEEP, and Ve is not guaranteed, requiring appropriate use of minute ventilation/tidal volume alarms.

ASSESSING LUNG INFLATION

In concept, the degree of dynamic hyperinflation is central to ventilator adjustments, but there are inherent problems with measuring the degree of hyperinflation in clinical practice. The only validated method is to measure the volume gas at end-inspiration, termed *Vei*, by collecting expired gas from total lung capacity (TLC) to functional residual capacity (FRC) during 40 to 60 seconds of apnea. Although Vei may underestimate air trapping in the presence of slowly emptying lung units, a Vei greater than 20 mL/kg correlates with barotrauma. The utility of this measure is limited by the need for paralysis and staff expertise with expiratory gas collection. Alternate measures of lung inflation include the single-breath plateau pressure (Pplat) and auto-PEEP. Accurate measurements of Pplat and auto-PEEP require patient-ventilator synchrony and the absence of patient interference. Paralysis is generally not required. However, neither pressure has been validated as a predictor of outcome. Pplat (or lung distension pressure) is an estimate of average end-inspiratory alveolar pressure that is determined by briefly stopping flow at end-inspiration (Figure 60-4), but Pplat is also affected by properties of the chest wall and abdomen. For example, Pplat will be higher in a patient with abdominal distension or obesity for the same degree of hyperinflation. Nevertheless, experience suggests that a Pplat less than 30 cm H_2O generally correlates with favorable outcomes.

Auto-PEEP is the lowest average alveolar pressure achieved during the respiratory cycle. It is obtained by measuring airway opening pressure during an end-expiratory hold maneuver (Figure 4) and does not estimate end-inhalation volume or pressure. Persistence of expiratory gas flow at the beginning of inspiration (which can be detected by auscultation or flow tracings) also suggests auto-PEEP (Figure 60-5). As with Vei, auto-PEEP may underestimate the severity of dynamic hyperinflation when there is poor communication between the alveoli and airway opening. In general, however, auto-PEEP less than 15 cm H_2O is likely acceptable.

VENTILATOR ADJUSTMENTS

We offer the following approach to ventilator adjustments in severe asthma (Figure 60-6). This approach relies on Pplat as the measure of dynamic hyperinflation and arterial pH as a surrogate marker of ventilation. If initial ventilator settings result in Pplat above 30 cm H_2O, RR

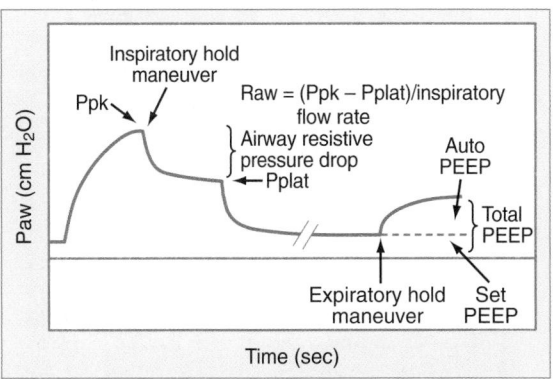

Figure 60-4 Pressure-time tracing during mechanical ventilation demonstrating measurement of peak inspiratory pressure (Ppk), plateau pressure (Pplat), and auto-PEEP. While delivering a constant inspiratory flow (not shown), airway pressure (Paw) increases to Ppk, the sum of airway resistive pressure and Pplat. Airway resistive pressure and Pplat are determined by an end-inspiratory hold maneuver during which inspiratory flow is temporarily stopped during one breath to eliminate airway resistive pressure, allowing Paw to fall from Ppk to Pplat. If inspiratory flow is set at 60 L/min, the resistance pressure drop equals airway resistance (Raw) in units of cm H_2O/L/sec. An end-expiratory hold maneuver is performed to measure auto-PEEP. During this maneuver, Paw increases by the amount of auto-PEEP present. Note that end-inspiratory and end-expiratory hold maneuvers are performed on different breaths.

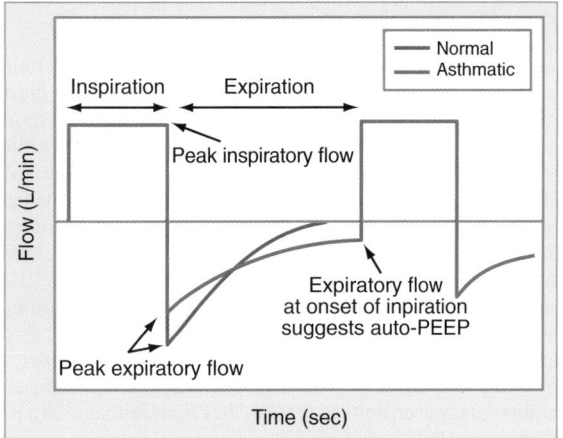

Figure 60-5 Flow-time tracings in a normal subject and a patient with asthma during mechanical ventilation. Note that peak expiratory flow rates are diminished in asthma because of increased airway resistance and that increased expiratory time is required to exhale the tidal breath. In the asthmatic patient, expiratory flow persists at the time of the next delivered breath (as demonstrated by failure of the exhalation flow tracing to return to baseline or zero flow), suggesting the presence of auto-PEEP.

should be reduced to decrease Pplat below 30 cm H_2O. Decreasing RR may cause hypercapnia. Fortunately, hypercapnia is generally well tolerated in this patient population. Anoxic brain injury and myocardial dysfunction are contraindications to permissive hypercapnia because of the potential for hypercapnia to dilate cerebral vessels, decrease myocardial contractility, and constrict pulmonary vasculature. Lowering RR may not increase Paco$_2$ as much as expected if it decreases the degree of hyperinflation and thereby lowers dead space. If hypercapnia results in a blood pH of less than 7.20, and RR cannot be increased

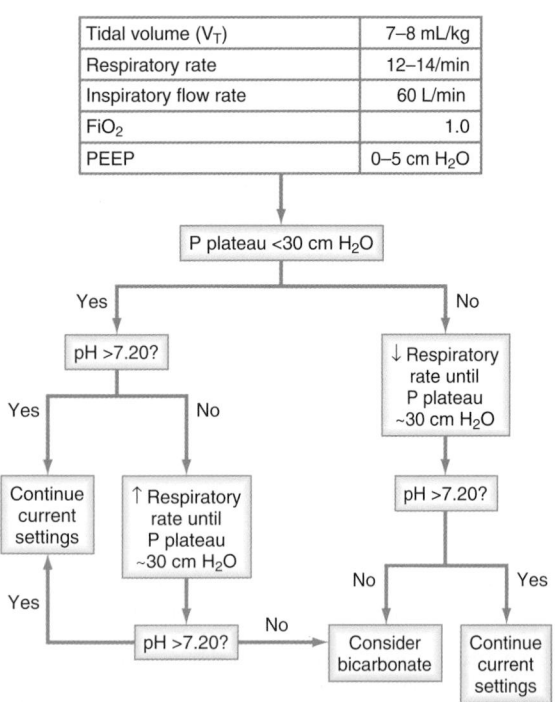

INITIAL SETTINGS

Tidal volume (V$_T$)	7–8 mL/kg
Respiratory rate	12–14/min
Inspiratory flow rate	60 L/min
FiO$_2$	1.0
PEEP	0–5 cm H$_2$O

Figure 60-6 Recommendations for initial ventilator settings and subsequent ventilator adjustments based on Pplat (end-inspiratory plateau pressure) and arterial pH in patients with severe asthma exacerbation.

because Pplat is at its limit, we consider an infusion of sodium bicarbonate, although bicarbonate has not been shown to improve outcome. If Pplat is less than 30 cm H_2O and pH is less than 7.20, RR can be safely increased until Pplat nears the 30 cm H_2O limit.

SEDATION AND PARALYSIS

Sedation improves comfort, safety, and patient-ventilator synchrony. In patients who may be extubated within hours (such as those with rapid onset asthma), propofol is recommended because it can achieve a deep level of sedation while allowing for rapid reversal after discontinuation. Benzodiazepines such as lorazepam and midazolam are less expensive alternatives, but time to awakening is less predictable.

To provide amnesia, sedation, analgesia, and suppress respiratory drive, morphine or fentanyl can be added by continuous infusion to either propofol or a benzodiazepine. For all patients, daily interruption of sedatives and analgesics avoids undue accumulation.

Ketamine is an IV anesthetic with sedative, analgesic, and bronchodilating properties. In most cases it is reserved for intubated patients with refractory and critical obstruction. Ketamine should be used with caution because of its sympathomimetic effects and ability to cause delirium.

When safe and effective mechanical ventilation cannot be achieved by sedation alone, consider short-term muscle paralysis. Cisatracurium is essentially free of cardiovascular effects, does not release histamine, and does not rely on hepatic and renal function for clearance. Pancuronium is a less expensive alternative, but it lasts longer and may increase heart rate. Pancuronium and atracurium both release histamine, but this is of unclear clinical significance in the setting of severe asthma exacerbations.

Paralytics may be given intermittently by bolus or continuous IV infusion. Continuous infusions mandate the use of a nerve stimulator (or interruption of drug every 4-6 hours) to avoid drug accumulation and prolonged paralysis. The use of paralytics has been associated with additional complications including myopathy, venous thromboembolism, and ventilator-associated pneumonia. Paralytics should be discontinued as soon as possible to minimize risk.

USE OF BRONCHODILATORS DURING MECHANICAL VENTILATION

Additional controlled trials are needed to inform the optimal use of bronchodilators in intubated patients and to provide additional evidence for or against current recommendations. One consistent observation is that intubated patients require higher drug dosages to achieve a clinical effect. This may reflect the refractory nature of these patients or inadequate dose or delivery. Whether bronchodilators are delivered by MDI or nebulizer, there is little doubt that good patient-ventilator synchrony helps delivery. When MDIs are used during mechanical ventilation, a spacing device on the inspiratory limb of the ventilator is mandatory. When nebulizers are used, they should be placed close to the ventilator, and in-line humidifiers should be stopped during treatments. Dropping the inspiratory flow rate to approximately 40 L/min during nebulization helps minimize turbulence, but this strategy may worsen the extent of hyperinflation and should be time-limited.

Regardless of whether an MDI with spacer or nebulizer is used, higher drug dosages are required, and the dosage should be titrated to achieve a fall in the peak-to-pause airway pressure gradient (Figure 60-7). When no measurable drop in airway resistance occurs, other causes of elevated airway resistance such as a kinked or plugged endotracheal tube should be excluded. Moreover, it may be reasonable to consider a drug holiday in patients who do not demonstrate a physiologic response to appropriately delivered medications.

OTHER CONSIDERATIONS

Rarely, the management strategies discussed are unable to stabilize the patient on the ventilator. In these situations, general anesthetic

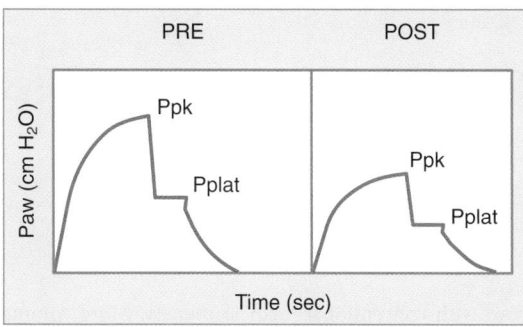

Figure 60-7 Pressure-time tracings before and after successful administration of a bronchodilator. Note the drop in both airway resistive pressure and end-expiratory plateau pressure (Pplat), reflecting increased airway diameter and decreased lung inflation, respectively.

bronchodilators such has halothane, isoflurane, and enflurane may reduce peak pressures and Paco$_2$. These agents are associated with hypotension and arrhythmias, and their benefits are short lived. Heliox delivered through the ventilator circuit may also decrease peak pressure and Paco$_2$. However, safe use of heliox requires significant institutional expertise and planning, which includes recalibration of gas density–dependent flow meters to low-density gas and the use of a spirometer to measure tidal volume.

EXTUBATION

Weaning and extubation criteria have not been validated for patients with acute asthma. One approach is to perform a spontaneous breathing trial once (1) Paco$_2$ normalizes without significant hyperinflation, (2) airway resistance is less than 20 cm H$_2$O/L/sec, (3) the patient is awake or easily arousable, (4) oxygen requirements are not excessive, (5) PEEP is ≤ 5 cm H$_2$O, (6) the patient is hemodynamically stable, and (7) secretions are not excessive. Patients with labile asthma may meet these criteria quickly after intubation; more commonly, 24 to 48 hours of treatment are required. After extubation, observation in an ICU is recommended for an additional 12 to 24 hours. During this time, the focus can switch to safe transfer to the ward and outpatient management.

Postexacerbation Management

The importance of patient education, adherence to daily antiinflammatory controller medications, environmental control, and close follow-up cannot be overstated. Patients who have experienced severe asthma exacerbations are at risk for subsequent attacks and asthma-related death. In this regard, a recent tri-society task force report provides recommendations for antiinflammatory treatment after discharge and follow-up after acute asthma episodes.[13,14]

KEY POINTS

1. Failure to achieve adequate control in the outpatient arena underlies many asthma exacerbations.

2. Severe exacerbations are characterized by diaphoresis, upright positioning, inability to speak in long sentences, use of accessory muscles, a widened pulsus paradoxus, and normo- or hypercapnia. Altered mental status, paradoxical breathing, bradycardia, and a quiet chest warn of imminent respiratory arrest.

3. Acutely ill asthmatics respond variably to inhaled β-agonists. Frequent (or continuous) administration of albuterol is recommended in refractory patients. Addition of ipratropium bromide to albuterol may confer additional benefit.

4. Systemic steroids are indicated for severe asthma exacerbations.

5. Limited data support the use of noninvasive ventilation (NIV) to decrease inspiratory work of breathing in selected patients.

6. Postintubation hypotension suggests inadequate expiratory time causing lung hyperinflation and decreased cardiac preload. A trial of apnea or hypopnea is both diagnostic and therapeutic in this setting. Tension pneumothorax is a competing concern in this clinical setting.

7. During mechanical ventilation, prolong the expiratory phase by setting low minute ventilation and an adequate inspiratory flow rate. Assess lung hyperinflation by measuring plateau pressure; if necessary, accept moderate hypercapnia to decrease lung hyperinflation.

8. Avoid prolonged paralysis and sedation during mechanical ventilation.

9. Establish a program to assess and achieve asthma control at the time of discharge to help prevent future exacerbations.

ANNOTATED REFERENCES

1. Moorman JE, Rudd RA, Johnson CA, et al. National surveillance for asthma—United States, 1980-2004. MMWR Surveill Sum 2007;56(8):1-54.
   This publication contains detailed national asthma data including information on ED visits, hospitalizations, and deaths stratified by age, gender, race, ethnicity, and income.
2. Bateman ED, Reddel HK, Eriksson G, et al. Overall asthma control: the relationship between current control and future risk. J Allergy Clin Immunol 2010;125(3):600-8.
   This study demonstrates that current asthma control predicts future exacerbations and that achieving adequate control with daily controller therapy reduces exacerbations.
3. Dougherty RH, Fahy JV. Acute exacerbations of asthma: epidemiology, biology and the exacerbation-prone phenotype. Clin Exp Allergy 2009;39(2):193-202.
   This study reviews asthma exacerbation risk factors, including features of the exacerbation-prone phenotype.
4. Afessa B, Morales I, Cury JD. Clinical course and outcome of patients admitted to an ICU for status asthmaticus. Chest 2001;120(5):1616-21.
   The authors report outcome data on 132 ICU admissions in 89 patients, reporting an in-hospital mortality of 8.3%. The most common causes of death were tension pneumothorax and nosocomial infection.
5. Pepe PE, Marini JJ. Occult positive end-expiratory pressure in mechanically ventilated patients with airflow obstruction: the auto-PEEP effect. Am Rev Respir Dis 1982;126(1):166-70.
   This landmark article is the first to describe the clinical implications and measurement of auto-PEEP during mechanical ventilation.
6. Corbridge T, Hall JB. The assessment and management of status asthmaticus in adults. State-of-the-art. Am Rev Respir Dis 1995;151:1296-316.
   This comprehensive review of the evaluation and management of acute asthma provides detailed information about pharmacotherapy and mechanical ventilation of patients with respiratory failure.
7. U.S. Department of Health and Human Services, National Institutes of Health, National Heart, Lung and Blood Institute, Expert Panel Report 3. Guidelines for the diagnosis and management of asthma. Available at: http://www.nhlbi.nih.gov/guidelines/asthma/asthgdln.pdf, 2007.
   The gold standard document for the evaluation and management of asthma. These guidelines are divided into sections that cover definition, pathophysiology, diagnosis, assessment, education, environmental control, and management of acute exacerbations.
8. McFadden ER Jr. Acute severe asthma: state of the art. Am J Resp Crit Care Med 2003;168(7):740-59.

   This state-of-the-art review covers assessment and management of acutely ill asthmatics and offers useful information about patient assessment and pharmacotherapy.
9. Nowak R, Corbridge T, Brenner B. Noninvasive ventilation. Proc Am Thorac Soc 2009;6(4):367-70.
   This systematic review was a part of the recent tri-society task force report on the management and follow-up of asthma exacerbations. The authors support the use of noninvasive ventilation in selected asthmatic patients and provide recommendations for its use.
10. Tuxen DV, Lane S. The effects of ventilatory pattern on hyperinflation, airway pressures, and circulation in mechanical ventilation of patients with severe air-flow obstruction. Am Rev Respir Dis 1987;136(4):872-9.
    This classic study demonstrated the relationship between inspiratory flow rate and minute ventilation and lung volumes in a small number of mechanically ventilated patients with obstructive lung disease.
11. Brenner B, Corbridge T, Kazzi A. Intubation and mechanical ventilation in the asthmatic patient in respiratory failure. Proc Am Thorac Soc 2009;6:371-9.
    This systematic review was included in the recent tri-society task force report on the management and follow-up of asthma exacerbations. The authors cover indications for intubation, intubation technique, and appropriate ventilator settings.
12. Williams TJ, Tuxen DV, Scheinkestel CD, Czarny D, Bowes G. Risk factors for morbidity in mechanically ventilated patients with acute severe asthma. Am Rev Respir Dis 1992;146(3):607-15.
    This is another landmark study looking at the relationship between minute ventilation, dynamic lung hyperinflation, and outcomes. The article provides recommendations for initial ventilator settings.
13. Krishnan JA, Nowak R, Davis SQ, Schatz M. Anti-inflammatory treatment after discharge home from the emergency department in adults with acute asthma. Proc Am Thorac Soc 2009;6:380-5.
    This is one of the papers contained in the recent tri-society task force report on the management and follow-up of asthma exacerbations. The authors provide recommendations for use of oral, intramuscular, and inhaled steroids in patients discharged from the ED.
14. Schatz M, Rachelefsky G, Krishnan JA. Follow up-after acute asthma episodes: what improves outcomes. J Allergy Clin Immunol 2009;124(2 Suppl):S35-42.
    This article was included in the recent tri-society task force report on the management and follow-up of asthma exacerbations. Recommendations include the use of the Expert Panel Report 3 by the National Institutes of Health to guide outpatient management, appropriate patient education, use of controller agents, the need to arrange follow-up visits, and referral to an asthma specialist.

Chronic Obstructive Pulmonary Disease

PETER M.A. CALVERLEY

Chronic obstructive pulmonary disease (COPD) is a major cause of death and disability worldwide and is one of the most common reasons for intensive care unit (ICU) admission. Several monographs review this complex disorder in some detail.[1,2] The intensivist's view of COPD is predominantly physiologic, focusing on the impact of disrupted function on the individual's normal homeostatic mechanisms. Although many important insights that have shaped our understanding of COPD have come from ICU studies, other aspects of this disorder must be considered if a rational approach to COPD management is to be developed.

Access to ICU care for sick COPD patients remains relatively inequitable among different healthcare systems. In North America and parts of Western Europe, most patients are offered ICU care, but in other relatively developed healthcare systems, such as in the United Kingdom, this is not the case. Even physicians in the same healthcare system differ significantly in their selection of patients for ICU referral.[3] These choices may be influenced by local resource availability, but they are also conditioned by the generally pessimistic view of the outcome achievable with this treatment intervention. However, poor response to treatment in the ICU is not universal, and extended periods of mechanical ventilation are not invariably required to successfully manage patients with COPD.[4] Nevertheless, intensivists often take a particularly bleak view of the prognosis of COPD patients compared with others entering their units. In one prospective study, intensivists estimated the survival of the sickest COPD patients to be 10% at 180 days post admission, when in fact it was 40%.[5] In a survivor population after mechanical ventilation, 96% were happy to have received ventilator support, despite their continuing physical problems.[6] Clearly, decisions about ventilator support should not be made in the emergency department without sufficient medical information or a proper discussion with the family. Supportive therapy should be offered until it is clear what the patient's wishes are and what the likely outcome of treatment will be.

Definition and Natural History

Although the most appropriate definition of COPD has been debated, it has less of an impact in the context of ICU care, where acute hospitalization is usual only in cases of severe and well-established disease. The currently favored definition, developed by the Global Initiative for Chronic Obstructive Lung Disease (GOLD), is:

"Chronic obstructive pulmonary disease (COPD) is a preventable and treatable disease with some extrapulmonary effects that may contribute to severity in individual patients. Its pulmonary component is characterized by airflow limitation that is not fully reversible. The airflow limitation is usually both progressive and associated with an abnormal inflammatory response of the lungs to noxious particles or gasses."[7]

The emphasis here is on incompletely reversible airflow obstruction that is persistent and progressive. Symptoms and disability usually parallel these processes, although some individuals can apparently cope with a severe degree of airflow limitation without seeking medical help. Such patients finally present to the emergency room when they develop a severe exacerbation of COPD. In this situation, it is wisest to offer ventilatory support until the patient has at least had a chance

to improve with conventional medical therapy. More common is a patient whose progressive illness is accompanied by repeated exacerbations, events that identify an accelerated decline in both lung function and health status.[8,9] Such patients have often been hospitalized previously, and their response to treatment is usually clearly established.

The usual inhaled particles or gases that produce COPD are a complex mixture of hydrocarbons and particulates derived from tobacco smoke. These are the principal causes of COPD in the United States and western Europe,[10] although other factors such as poor lung function during childhood, bronchial hyperresponsiveness, and low birth weight may also be important. The associated inflammatory changes, which persist when smoking stops,[11,12] are thought to explain the airway and parenchymal destruction and fibrosis within the lung, although this has not been conclusively established as the only mechanism.

The natural history of COPD explains why the number of patients presenting for ICU care has not diminished in the last 3 decades as might be expected, given the overall reduction in tobacco consumption in Western countries. This is illustrated by the classic study of Fletcher and Peto, which has now been confirmed by longitudinal data from the Framingham study[13,14] (Figure 61-1). Although the rate of decline of lung function is reduced in individuals who stop smoking, the lung function already lost is never regained, and even if the rate of decline of lung function returns to normal, these patients are still more likely to experience disability as they age. Thus, in an aging population that contains many former smokers, a significant number will still develop complications of COPD that require ICU care. The situation is complicated by the steadily rising number of women who smoke.[15] Women are at least as susceptible as male smokers and more likely to be symptomatic. Thus an early fall in the number of COPD cases is being offset by the changing demographics of the current and ex-smoking population.

The important role of comorbidities in COPD has now been recognized.[16] Most patients with significant symptoms due to COPD have at least one if not many comorbid diseases, especially cardiovascular problems.[17] Whether the association is causal or an epiphenomenon is of little relevance in the ICU, where a high index of suspicion for undiagnosed comorbid disorders is a useful aid to effective management.

Pathology

The pathologic features of COPD depend on the stage of the illness and the part of the lung examined.[18] Central airways show mucous gland hypertrophy and goblet cell metaplasia, whereas more peripheral airways show variable combinations of smooth muscle hypertrophy, peribronchial fibrosis, luminal occlusion by mucus, and enlarged lymphoid follicles. Alveoli are often but not invariably enlarged by the loss of alveolar walls, with an attendant loss of support for the small noncartilaginous airways in this region of the lung. There is evidence of persistent inflammation, with neutrophils in the airway lumen and macrophages in the airway wall. CD8+ T lymphocytes are more prominent in this response than in bronchial inflammation of an asthmatic type, although intermediate states appear to exist.[19] Inflammatory cells are also present adjacent to breaks in the alveolar wall.[20] Overall, as the clinical and spirometric severity of the disease increases, so do the numbers of each cell population involved in the inflammatory

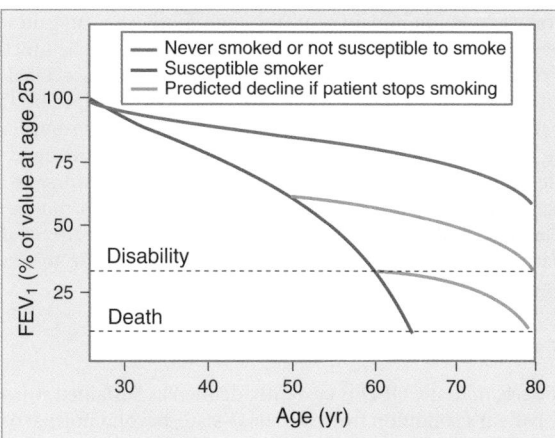

Figure 61-1 Natural history of chronic obstructive pulmonary disease and the effect of smoking cessation. Compared with lung function standardized to age 25, smokers show an accelerated rate of decline in forced expiratory volume (FEV$_1$), which returns to more normal values when they stop smoking. However, they are operating at a lower FEV$_1$ than predicted for their age, and physiologic decline continues. This explains why older ex-smokers can present to the ICU with severe disease despite years of abstinence. *(Adapted from Fletcher C, Peto R: The natural history of chronic airway obstruction. BMJ. 1977;1(6077): 1645-1648.)*

process.[21] In addition, extraluminal lymphoid follicles develop containing CD4$^+$ lymphocytes, possibly reflecting a response to repeated infective exacerbations.[21] Data obtained during exacerbations, though limited, support an increased role for neutrophils and, surprisingly, eosinophils.[22]

Physiology

The pathologic changes just described combine to produce the characteristic diagnostic finding of reduced forced expiratory flow (FEV$_1$) at a given lung volume, which is usually assessed on a time base as an FEV$_1$/forced vital capacity (FVC) ratio of less than 0.7. Technically, this should be 70% of the age-adjusted normal value for this ratio, because lung elastic recoil declines with age, even in healthy individuals. Use of the uncorrected ratio tends to overdiagnose COPD among the very elderly.[23] In practice, however, this does not cause problems for COPD patients admitted for ICU care, because they are invariably more severely affected.

COPD affects all aspects of lung function, but its primary impact is a change in lung mechanics. This is traditionally analyzed in terms of the static (no flow) and dynamic (flow) properties of the respiratory system.[24] Because chest wall mechanics are believed to be normal in COPD (although they are seldom measured directly), changes in the pressure-volume characteristics of the respiratory system are determined by alterations in lung compliance, often attributed to the loss of elastic recoil due to emphysema. How large a role this plays in changes in tissue compliance is not known. The resulting steeper slope, early-onset inspiratory plateau, and increase in end-expiratory lung volume are typical of the pressure-volume relationships in patients with COPD. Changes in end-expiratory lung volume and increases in residual volume change chest wall geometry favor a lower, flatter diaphragm and a more horizontal rib cage; these changes, in turn, impair the inspiratory muscles' ability to develop pressure, and increase the overall work of breathing.[25] Expiratory muscle activation is common in more severe COPD[26,27] even at rest, and provides a useful clinical marker of respiratory distress. Flattening of the diaphragm redirects the axis of shortening of the skeletal muscle and often produces paradoxical in-drawing of the lower thoracic rib cage (so-called Hoover's sign), which becomes more evident as pulmonary hyperinflation and respiratory drive to breathe rise. Patients with Hoover's sign are more

breathless and have more hyperinflation of their chest wall during exercise.[28]

The dynamics of the respiratory system are influenced by static properties but also differ significantly between inspiration and expiration. Maximum inspiratory flow is affected by inspiratory resistance as well as by the inspiratory muscles' ability to develop pressure (and thus indirectly by chest wall geometry). Maximum expiratory flow is influenced by expiratory pressure generation and, more importantly, by the onset of volume-related airflow limitation, best described by the maximum expiratory flow-volume loop. As lung volume falls during expiration, airways close or become flow limited; hence, the flow at a specific lung volume is reduced. Although an assessment of flow (FEV$_1$) relative to total volume change during expiration (FVC) is useful in defining COPD, an assessment of tidal flow limitation is more helpful in determining the degree of dyspnea experienced by the patient.[29] More attention is now being paid to the determination of expiratory flow limitation under tidal conditions. In the past, detection was difficult, involving invasive measurements or reliance on body plethysmography, which tended to overestimate the incidence of tidal expiratory flow limitation. The development of the negative expiratory pressure test and, more recently, within-breath variation in respiratory system reactance has changed this.[30] The within-breath method assesses more breaths, is less prone to observer error, and is likely to be automated in future for ICU application.[31]

In general, the lower the FEV$_1$, the greater the likelihood that expiratory flow limitation is present. However, some COPD patients are not flow-limited on every breath and regulate their end-expiratory lung volume to try to minimize this. When respiratory drive rises (e.g., during exercise), during disease exacerbations, or when minute ventilation has to increase to maintain gas exchange during ventilator weaning, this resting variation in expiratory lung volume is likely to decrease. If expiratory flow and hence tidal volume are to increase, end-expiratory lung volume must rise; this further increases the work of breathing and the sensation of respiratory distress. This process, described as *dynamic hyperinflation*, has been clearly demonstrated during exercise and can be lessened by bronchodilator treatment which aids lung emptying.[32]

In the ICU, patients have a high respiratory drive during weaning and adopt a rapid, shallow breathing pattern. Total respiratory muscle work increases, in part because of the increased operating lung volumes, but also because of the presence of intrinsic positive end-expiratory pressure (PEEPi). This represents the pressure that must be developed to overcome residual expiratory driving pressure before inspiratory flow can begin.[33] Calculating the size of this variable is fraught with technical difficulties beyond the problems of accurate placement of the balloon catheter system in intubated patients. Several methods have been proposed that correct for the effects of coexisting abdominal muscle activation, with recent work favoring a correction based on the total decay of gastric pressure.[34] However, the need to compute this variable in clinical practice has been questioned.[35]

What is clear is that the overall impairment of mechanical function in COPD is substantial and that both static and dynamic properties interact—a concept best captured by the time constant of the respiratory system, which is the product of the total respiratory system resistance in compliance. This is greatly lengthened in COPD and helps explain why lung emptying is delayed and dynamic hyperinflation occurs. There is substantial evidence of regional inhomogeneity in more severe COPD. Differences in the regional time constants explain why COPD patients are prone to barotrauma during mechanical ventilation, despite seemingly acceptable peak inspiratory pressures, as well as why gas exchange can be quite disordered in this population.

GAS EXCHANGE

Arterial hypoxemia is common in COPD but becomes clinically significant only when the partial pressure of oxygen in arterial blood (PaO$_2$) falls below 60 mm Hg, a problem largely confined to patients with an FEV$_1$ below 35% of their predicted value. It arises predominantly due to ventilation-perfusion mismatching, often worsens during exercise, and is readily corrected by a small increase in the inspired oxygen concentration, unless the situation is made worse by secretion retention or severe pneumonia.[36] Arterial hypercapnia is seen in some but not all hypoxemic patients who are clinically stable, but it is more frequent, at least temporarily, in hospitalized individuals.[37] A combination of ventilation-perfusion mismatching due to an increase in physiologic dead space and a degree of effective alveolar hypoventilation explains this phenomenon. Acute rises in the partial pressure of arterial carbon dioxide ($Paco_2$) precipitate respiratory acidosis, a more reliable guide to prognosis and the need for ventilation than the $Paco_2$ itself.[38,39]

CONTROL OF BREATHING

Despite years of study, there is no conclusive evidence that ventilatory control is abnormal in COPD patients. However, the response to sustained mechanical loading appears to be variable in healthy subjects[40] and may explain why some individuals adopt the breathing patterns they do. Traditional techniques of studying respiratory control, which involve stimulation with exogenous CO_2 or nitrogen, suggested that respiratory drive was reduced. However, studies using mouth occlusion pressure techniques or recording the electrical activation of inspiratory muscles suggest that respiratory drive is generally high, even in those COPD patients who tolerate relatively high levels of CO_2.[41-43] Studies of breathing pattern have been more instructive. In general, the lower the tidal volume, the higher the $Paco_2$.[44] This is because the ratio of dead space (its fixed, predominantly anatomically determined volume) to tidal volume increases as the latter is reduced. Small tidal volumes are accompanied by an increased respiratory frequency to maintain the somewhat higher-than-normal level of minute ventilation. The resulting shortening of inspiratory time is also associated with hypercapnia.[44] The system appears to be regulated to minimize peak inspiratory pressure generation, even at the cost of impaired gas exchange. There are theoretical reasons for believing that this is both energy efficient and likely to minimize the occurrence of inspiratory muscle fatigue.[45] This also explains the usefulness of rapid, shallow breathing as an index of weaning failure when neuromechanical coupling in the respiratory system is under considerable stress.[46]

PULMONARY CIRCULATION

In the past, considerable attention was paid to the determination of pulmonary artery pressure in COPD patients, but this is now thought to be less important. Undoubtedly, pulmonary artery pressure increases by day and at night[47] in hypoxemic COPD patients, reflecting a combination of hypoxic vasoconstriction and pulmonary vascular remodeling. How important this is in the daily limitation of exercise reported by these patients is not clear, but it is known that treatment with domiciliary oxygen prevents disease progression[48] and may even reduce pulmonary artery pressure. More specific attempts at therapy, including treatment with vasodilators, phosphodiesterase enzyme type V (PDEV) inhibitors, and nitric oxide—studied inside and outside the ICU—have been unsuccessful, usually resulting in unacceptable worsening of ventilation-perfusion mismatching.[49] In general, assessment of pulmonary hypertension has fallen out of favor as part of a routine evaluation in COPD patients, but its occurrence is important to note when interpreting changes in central venous pressure in instrumented patients. Acute rises in pulmonary arterial pressure can follow a pulmonary embolism. Although this can lead to rather atypical COPD exacerbations with persistent hypoxemia,[50] this is uncommon in routine practice.[51]

Systemic Effects

There is good evidence that systemic (extrapulmonary) factors are important in COPD. Patients with a reduced body mass index die sooner than better-nourished individuals with a similar degree of pulmonary function impairment, although those who can gain weight fare better.[52] There are data to show that peripheral muscle function is impaired,[53] fiber type is altered,[54] and exercise is associated with increased oxidative stress.[55] The earlier concept of a specific COPD myopathy has now largely been abandoned, as the major burden falls on the lower limb muscles, with preserved function in the upper limb muscle groups. This likely reflects inactivity, which is worse in those with exacerbated COPD.[56] Weakness of the quadriceps muscle is an independent guide to a poor prognosis.[57] In contrast, the wealth of circulating biomarkers in COPD have contributed little to practical management so far.[58]

Exacerbations

An *exacerbation* of COPD is currently defined as sustained worsening of the patient's condition from the stable state, beyond normal day-to-day variation, that is acute in onset and necessitates a change in regular medication.[7] The key feature is the sustained change from usual daily symptoms. The operational requirement for a change in treatment is more arbitrary but is almost always present in patients referred for ICU care. Disease exacerbation is the principal cause of ICU admission with COPD, and patients commonly have or are at risk of developing significant *respiratory failure*, defined as a Pao_2 below 60 mm Hg with or without an increase in $Paco_2$.[59] The most common causes of exacerbation are listed in Table 61-1. Viral and bacterial infections are both relevant,[54] with rhinoviruses commonly reported in most series; *Haemophilus influenzae* and *Streptococcus pneumoniae* are the principal microbial pathogens.[60,61] Some patients, particularly those with a regular cough and green sputum production, develop persistent lower respiratory tract colonization, making the interpretation of qualitative microbiology difficult.[62] Usually there is an increase in the absolute number of colony-forming units of microorganisms in these patients during exacerbations, reflecting an increased burden of infection, although more subtle changes have been reported involving the introduction of a different serotype of *H. influenzae*[63] without substantial changes in the total bacterial load.[64]

Not all exacerbations of COPD have an infectious precipitant, and changes in the degree of atmospheric pollution can precipitate events in some patients.[65] How frequently individuals develop exacerbations after exposure to a specific precipitating event is not clear, although the likelihood of meeting the consensus definition rises as spirometric impairment worsens.[66]

The physiologic consequences of increased airflow obstruction secondary to increased inflammation within the bronchial tree are summarized in Figure 61-2. Whatever the precipitant, the key event appears to be a change in lung mechanics. Previously, attention focused on alterations in respiratory system resistance, but more recent data emphasize that airway narrowing and closure may be more important, particularly by producing changes in operating lung volumes (see earlier discussion). Observations in patients recovering from hospitalized exacerbations have shown progressive improvements in

TABLE 61-1	Causes of Chronic Obstructive Pulmonary Disease Exacerbation

New infection:
    Bacterial (*Haemophilus influenzae, Streptococcus pneumoniae, Moraxella hemophilus*)
    Change in an existing strain (e.g., *H. influenzae*)
    Viral (influenza, rhinovirus, respiratory syncytial virus)
Atmospheric pollution:
    Sulfur dioxide, oxides of nitrogen
Temperature change:
    Often related to pollution episodes
Intercurrent illness*:
    Pneumonia, pulmonary embolus, pneumothorax
Postoperative:
    Especially after upper abdominal surgery

*Clinical presentation is dominated by the primary illness, but respiratory failure can occur.

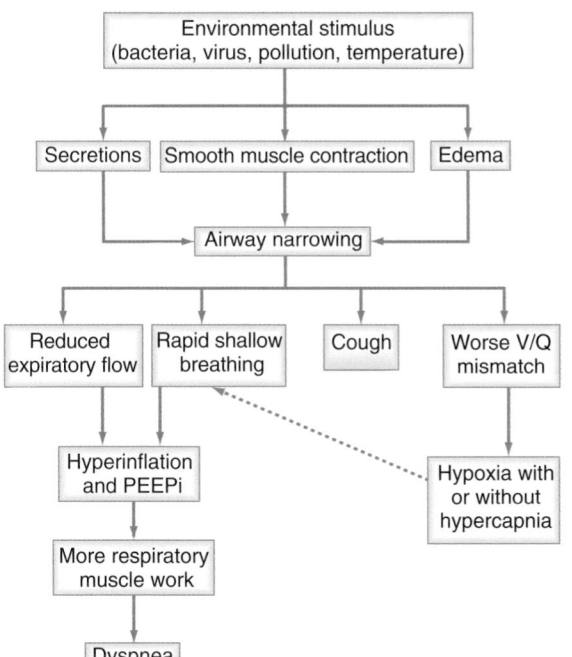

Figure 61-2 Schematic of principal physiologic changes that accompany an exacerbation of chronic obstructive pulmonary disease. Note that deterioration in one area tends to produce worsening in other areas and leads to a downward spiral in functional abnormality. PEEPi, intrinsic positive end-expiratory pressure; V/Q, ventilation-perfusion.

respiratory system reactance (a measure of inspiratory resistance and flow limitation) together with reductions in end-expiratory lung volume that are most evident in patients reporting less dyspnoea.[67] These changes are larger than those in spirometry and help explain why the small changes in FEV_1 associated with exacerbations can be associated with substantial deterioration in gas exchange and clinical well-being, leading to hospitalization.

Pneumonia is an important reason for hospitalization in COPD, is more frequently seen in these patients than in others, and is associated with worse outcomes.[68] Pneumonia is diagnosed more frequently in patients taking the inhaled corticosteroid, fluticasone propionate,[69] especially older patients with worse airflow obstruction.[70] These pneumonias are not necessarily associated with poor outcome in terms of mortality or health status[69] and are not seen with all types of inhaled corticosteroids.[71,72] At present the benefit of inhaled corticosteroid treatment, especially combined with a long-acting inhaled bronchodilator, outweigh the apparent risk of increased pneumonia events.

Clinical Features

Key clinical features of the acute presentation of COPD are summarized in Table 61-2. In addition to obtaining an appropriate history and performing a physical examination, with particular attention to the respiratory rate, it is necessary to assess the degree of abnormal gas exchange and the presence of acidosis by measuring arterial blood gases. In the context of an exacerbation, more direct measurements of lung mechanics are usually impractical, and the severity of the mechanical problem is evaluated indirectly by its effect on gas exchange. An urgent chest radiograph is useful for identifying specific precipitating factors, particularly alveolar shadowing due to infection, the presence of a pneumothorax, or radiographic features of pulmonary edema. The last is especially important, because it is commonly associated with hypercapnic respiratory failure, with the combination of an increased ventilatory drive and poor perfusion of respiratory muscles, together with further impairment of ventilation-perfusion matching favoring CO_2 retention. In this context, an electrocardiogram is invaluable to

TABLE 61-2	Clinical Features of Chronic Obstructive Pulmonary Disease Exacerbation

Sustained increase in dyspnea*
Increased cough (with or without sputum)*
Increased sputum volume or purulence*
Symptoms of upper respiratory tract infection (variable and should be accompanied by a major symptom)
Fever (infrequent in the absence of pneumonia)
Cyanosis (with advanced disease)
Tachypnea
Pursed-lip breathing
Accessory muscle use (including abdominals)
Pulmonary overinflation (reduced cricoid distance, Hoover's sign, resonant percussion over the heart)
Tachycardia
Boundary pulse
Hypotension†
Flapping tremor†
Impaired level of consciousness†

*Major symptom.
†Severe illness.

screen for both underlying ischemic heart disease and rhythm disturbances. If a major thromboembolic event is suspected on clinical grounds, quantitative D-dimer and urgent computed tomographic pulmonary angiography is the best way to establish this diagnosis. Simple laboratory tests, such as the hemoglobin and white cell count, can be valuable guides to the need for oxygenation and the likelihood of coexisting sepsis.

Exacerbation of airway inflammation is not the only reason for the deterioration of postoperative COPD patients, who are at significant risk after any type of surgery. This may reflect the consequences of anesthesia and impaired secretion clearance, the risks of lower respiratory tract infection after intubation, or the effects of surgery itself. Both pain and the drugs administered to relieve it are likely to depress ventilation in these patients. Thoracic and upper abdominal surgery impairs the function of the inspiratory and expiratory muscles, respectively. In patients with severe COPD, abdominal muscle activation is an important involuntary technique to "share" the work of breathing between the inspiratory and expiratory muscles; impairment of abdominal muscle activation commonly increases the degree of breathlessness and may precipitate respiratory muscle fatigue. Persistent smoking before elective procedures should be discouraged, because this further compromises the already reduced compensatory mechanisms in COPD patients. In this setting, it is not surprising that respiratory failure develops in a significant number of individuals with severe disease, necessitating ICU care.

Intensive Care Unit Referral

The need for ventilatory support is the primary reason for ICU referral among COPD patients. Although the various indications for mechanical ventilation (Table 61-3) vary in frequency from institution to institution, they represent the most common causes for ICU admission.

Before referring a patient for ICU care, and especially for any form of ventilatory support, it is important to determine what degree of

TABLE 61-3	Indications for Invasive Mechanical Ventilation

Severe dyspnea, with use of accessory muscles and paradoxical abdominal motion
Respiratory frequency >35 breaths/min
Life-threatening hypoxemia (Pao_2 <40 mm Hg or Pao_2/ Fio_2 <200 mm Hg)
Severe acidosis (pH <7.25) and hypercapnia ($Paco_2$ >60 mm Hg)
Respiratory arrest
Somnolence, impaired mental status
Cardiovascular complications (hypotension, shock, heart failure)
Other complications: metabolic abnormalities, sepsis, pneumonia, pulmonary embolism, barotrauma, massive pleural effusion
Noninvasive positive-pressure ventilation failure (or exclusion criteria)

Fio_2, inspired oxygen fraction; $Paco_2$, partial pressure of carbon dioxide in arterial blood; Pao_2, partial pressure of oxygen in arterial blood.

intervention is appropriate. Advance directives are becoming increasingly common among COPD patients, particularly in the United States. These are specific orders about the level of intervention desired by the patient, informed by discussions with his or her physician. These difficult and potentially upsetting discussions are necessary when patients are approaching the terminal phase of an illness, and they should be encouraged as a routine practice, particularly those who have already been admitted to an ICU and have a clear idea of what therapy involves. However, it is important to ensure that such interviews are conducted when the patient is clinically stable and capable of making rational judgments about what the future holds. We still have some way to go before this important aspect of care becomes a routine part of our clinical practice.

Principles of Treatment

Four general principles guide the management of COPD patients presenting acutely to the ICU, and each should contribute to shortening the duration of illness and stabilizing the patient physiologically until either the natural course of the disease or the effects of therapy lead to its resolution.

TREAT PRECIPITATING FACTORS

Bacterial infection is the most common reason for ICU admission in COPD patients. There is now good evidence that antibiotics shorten the symptomatic period, even when patients are treated with corticosteroids[73]; when given early, antibiotics are associated with lower mortality, fewer episodes of intubation, and shorter hospital stays.[74] Intravenous therapy with antimicrobials is generally required in patients sick enough to merit ICU admission. Radiographic evidence of pneumonia likely requires a broadening of the antibiotic spectrum, but whether the infection is confined to the airways or involves the alveoli, antibiotic therapy should follow locally established guidelines designed to minimize the development of resistance within the ICU and to address known patterns of drug resistance in the community and the hospital. Broad-spectrum penicillins or, more commonly, cephalosporins are usually recommended, often with an intravenous macrolide. Some advocate the prophylactic use of a quinolone in COPD patients in the ICU,[75] but this practice requires confirmation before being accepted as universally effective. Colonization with methicillin-resistant *Staphylococcus aureus* is a frequent problem and requires particular vigilance in the selection of antibiotics. Likewise, excessive use of broad-spectrum agents can produce superinfection, such as *Clostridium difficile* diarrhea. This can be particularly distressing in a patient with severe COPD and low body mass index and requires early identification and appropriate therapy.

The role of antiviral drugs, such as the neuraminidase inhibitors, in the management of acutely ill COPD patients remains to be determined. Surprisingly, H1N1 influenza infection has not been a major problem for COPD patients, possibly reflecting prior partial immunity.[76] If this virus is diagnosed, the use of antivirals such as oseltamivir is prudent but not likely to have a major effect on the natural history of the episode. Similar considerations apply to other viral pneumonias.

For those COPD patients with postoperative pain, epidural anesthesia is frequently helpful insofar as it permits adequate analgesia without unwanted ventilatory depressant effects. Prophylaxis for pulmonary embolism should follow established guidelines in other high-risk groups managed in the ICU setting.

REDUCE LUNG VOLUME AND INCREASE EXPIRATORY FLOW

Agents that improve lung emptying, commonly by increasing airway caliber or preventing airway closure, interfere with the vicious circle of pulmonary hyperinflation described in Figure 61-2. This has been demonstrated in stable patients using exercise as a model of hyperinflation,[32] but the data in spontaneously breathing COPD patients during exacerbations are much less satisfactory. Nonetheless, treatment with regular but high doses of short-acting nebulized β-agonists such as albuterol or ipratropium (2.5-5 mg or 250-500 μg, respectively), is usually recommended. There is no clear evidence that one drug is better than the other,[77] and combination therapy is commonly used. The outcomes of the few studies conducted in this setting were based on FEV_1 rather than symptoms or lung volume change. Intravenous theophylline, or one of its derivatives, is often added to these regimens but is no more effective than a placebo infusion.[78,79]

REDUCE PULMONARY INFLAMMATION

Several randomized, controlled trials have shown that oral corticosteroids shorten the duration of hospitalization and accelerate improvement of post-bronchodilator FEV_1 during an exacerbation of COPD.[80,81] Patients randomized to treatment with oral corticosteroids were less likely to relapse during the subsequent month and showed a number of other benefits, although these did not always reach statistical significance.[82] There does not appear to be any additional benefit from using particularly high doses of corticosteroids or prolonging treatment beyond 10 days to 2 weeks. In the ICU, corticosteroid treatment is often given peremptorily to patients on mechanical ventilation; caution should be exercised, however, because these individuals are often at risk for relatively acute-onset corticosteroid myopathy.[83] If corticosteroid therapy has been maintained for a longer-than-normal period, or if courses of oral corticosteroids to treat less serious exacerbations have been given frequently, a tapered dose-reduction plan should be introduced. Otherwise, treatment can be discontinued at the end of the normal 10 to 14 days. Patients given this therapy may benefit from subsequent treatment with inhaled corticosteroids, but they should be evaluated for significant side effects.[69] Osteoporosis is particularly common in COPD patients, whether they receive corticosteroid treatment or not, and it is probably worth identifying in any individual who requires ICU care.[84]

MANAGE GAS EXCHANGE

It is relatively easy to improve oxygenation in an uncomplicated exacerbation of COPD.[85] Raising the inspired oxygen concentration to 28% to 35% is usually sufficient to achieve a Pao_2 greater than 90 mm Hg. However, this can be accompanied by an undesirable increase in $Paco_2$, with its accompanying respiratory acidosis. Such an increase in $Paco_2$ impairs respiratory muscle function, at least during loaded breathing,[86] and often precedes more serious clinical deterioration, including impairment of consciousness. The reasons for this effect have been debated for many years, with some advocating a reduction in respiratory drive from the carotid chemoreceptors, and others citing a worsening ventilation-perfusion match as the cause.[85] Each view has evidence to support it, but the actual cause is likely a combination of both problems, with ventilation-perfusion mismatching being particularly important in severely ill patients, and hypoventilation playing a larger role in those not yet sick enough to require intubation.[87]

Although the phenomenon of oxygen-induced hypercapnia has been recognized for decades, it remains a real problem. In one large center in the United Kingdom, 34% of individuals showed evidence of oxygen-induced hypercapnia.[39] The use of high-flow oxygen in the emergency room is widespread, as is the false sense of security provided by a high oxygen saturation. Many intensivists have legitimate concerns about the failure to adequately oxygenate COPD patients with compromised circulation, along with the attendant risk of unanticipated mortality. However, the solution is to carefully consider the risks of excessive or insufficient oxygen in a given individual, rather than to slavishly adhere to one view or the other. Patients whose problems are predominantly due to COPD and who have a normal hemoglobin and preserved cardiac output can maintain adequate tissue oxygen delivery with an oxygen saturation as low as 85%, and they will do quite well if an arterial oxygen saturation (Sao_2) of 90% to 93% is maintained. The modest increase in inspired oxygen needed to achieve this (often 24%-28%) is accompanied by less hypercapnia and may avoid the need for ventilatory support. However, if cardiac output is impaired (reduced blood pressure, poor peripheral circulation) or tissue metabolic demands are increased (e.g., in sepsis secondary to pneumonia), a higher Sao_2 will be required to ensure sufficient oxygen delivery; in this case, the consequences of any resultant hypercapnia, including the need for ventilatory support, must be accepted.

Oxygen can be delivered accurately by facemask, using the Venturi principle of entraining room air into the mask. This is a precise method of giving a known inspired oxygen concentration to COPD patients,[88] but many patients dislodge facemasks and are unlikely to keep nasal prongs in place.[89] Nasal prongs allow the patients to speak and drink, but the inspired oxygen fraction (Fio_2) is more variable, and it may be necessary to monitor arterial blood gases more frequently. Institutions where nebulizers are used to deliver bronchodilator drugs should be cautious about nebulizing these drugs using wall oxygen, because this can produce severe hypercapnia. A better policy is to nebulize in air, with the patients keeping their nasal cannulas in place.

For many years, respiratory stimulants were used to waken semiconscious patients and permit physiotherapy and other forms of suction, but this approach was never tested scientifically and must be viewed with some skepticism. Although respiratory stimulants were recommended as a way of deferring the need for positive-pressure ventilation, the advent of nasal positive-pressure ventilation has changed this approach, and the only study that directly compared the effects of doxapram and this modality in COPD concluded that patients did better with noninvasive ventilation and were less likely to deteriorate.[90] If chemical ventilatory stimulants are used, they should be considered a short-term means of sustaining the patient until a more appropriate method of ventilation can be instituted. Ultimately, some kind of mechanical ventilatory support is the best way to address the problems of hypercapnia.

Noninvasive Ventilation

This topic is reviewed in detail in Chapter 51, but some key issues relevant to COPD are worth emphasizing. Many of the data supporting the use of noninvasive ventilation (NIV) were obtained in patients with hypercapnic respiratory failure due to COPD exacerbation, and several excellent reviews have analyzed these data.[91,92]

Noninvasive ventilation has a number of potentially beneficial effects in COPD. Intuitively, it seems reasonable to expect that it would increase tidal volume, improve CO_2 elimination, and hence reduce respiratory drive. Studies of gas exchange using a multiple inert gas elimination methodology confirmed that CO_2 elimination is increased, but overall ventilation-perfusion mismatch is not changed during NIV.[93] A more important effect is the unloading of the respiratory muscles, which are often close to fatigue conditions in severe episodes of respiratory failure. By assuming some of the additional work required to overcome intrinsic PEEP, NIV directly reduces the drive to breathe, and the respiratory rate falls, a good prognostic feature.[94] Data from randomized, controlled trials suggest that there is a mean fall of 3.1 breaths per minute (95% confidence interval 4.3 to 1.9) with the institution of NIV in COPD patients.[91] This allows more effective emptying of the lungs and less dynamic hyperinflation. The resulting improvement in the intensity of breathlessness is usually a much earlier sign of successful NIV treatment in COPD than are changes in blood gas tensions, which often lag behind evidence of clinical improvement.

Evidence-based reviews provide a reasonable series of recommendations based on the relative effectiveness of NIV. Key points, including the number of patients needed to be treated to prevent one significant event or complication, are shown in Table 61-4. Noninvasive ventilation is associated with less treatment failure, lower mortality, fewer complications, and a lower intubation rate compared with conventional medical treatment. It reduces ICU or hospital stay by approximately 3 days and favorably influences gas exchange. With NIV, pH

TABLE 61-4	Efficacy of Noninvasive Ventilation Compared with Usual Care		
Outcome	*Number of Patients Studied*	*Relative Risk (95% Confidence Interval)*	*NNT*
Treatment failure	529	0.51 (0.38-0.67)	5
Death	523	0.41 (0.26-0.64)	8
Intubation	546	0.42 (0.31-0.59)	5
Complications	143	0.32 (0.18-0.56)	3

NNT, number needed to treat—the number of patients who must be treated to prevent this outcome in one individual.

increases by a mean value of 0.03 (0.02-0.04), $Paco_2$ falls by 3 mm Hg (5.9-0.23 mm Hg), and Pao_2 rises by 2 mm Hg (−2 to +6 mm Hg). The lower rate of nosocomial pneumonia associated with NIV is a particular advantage.

Data support the use of NIV as a first-line treatment in patients with exacerbations of COPD and moderate respiratory acidosis (pH < 7.35) despite medical treatment. In general, most patients with pH in the range of 7.3 to 7.35 survive without NIV, although the number patients needed to prevent one intubation is still only 10.[95] As acidosis becomes more severe, the benefits of NIV become greater; this treatment should be encouraged in anyone with a pH less than 7.3. In patients with more severe acidosis (pH < 7.25), the benefit is less clear, and results in different trials suggest that such patients have a better outcome if they are managed in the ICU with mechanical ventilation and intubation; however, these trials are influenced by selection bias. In clinical practice, it is reasonable to offer a trial of NIV unless the patient has some of the established contraindications to this treatment (Table 61-5). Even then, there are occasions when NIV is appropriate first-line therapy—for example, if a patient does not wish to be intubated (as indicated in an advance directive) or has a "ceiling of treatment" determined by his or her prior health status.

Treatment failure, which occurs in approximately 30% of cases,[96] reflects an inability to adapt to NIV or progression of the underlying disease. Recent data suggest that patients likely to subsequently fail with NIV can be prospectively identified by a high blood sugar on admission (irrespective of having diabetes), a raised respiratory rate, or a high APACHE 2 score. All these variables are relatively effective predictors of risk, but combining them increases their discriminant power.[94] In COPD patients, failure to trigger the noninvasive ventilator or excess trigger sensitivity can lead to problems of coordination between patient and machine. Air leakage can be a problem when facemasks are used, the usual approach in patients with COPD. Reducing rather than increasing inspiratory positive airway pressure often lessens this complication and allows better patient-ventilator coordination. Some patients develop hypercapnia, occasionally due to rebreathing in the mask, but more often due to ineffective cough and retained secretions. Conversion to a nasal mask and chinstrap allows more effective cough without loss of ventilator support. Late failure (after 48 hours or more of NIV), suggested by worsening acidosis, is a poor prognostic sign; it usually reflects deterioration caused by the underlying lung disease. If this occurs, the institution of invasive mechanical ventilation needs to be considered.[97] Patients treated in this way may have a better prognosis, although the interpretation of data is difficult, given the nonrandomized design of the relevant study. What is clear is that extending the period of NIV in a patient with physiologic evidence of deterioration is not likely to produce a successful result.

TABLE 61-5	Contraindications to Noninvasive Ventilation

Impaired consciousness (unless oxygen induced)
Confusion, agitation
Significant risk of vomiting
Profound hypoxemia
Excessive secretions
Facial or upper airway trauma or surgery

In addition to its role in the acute phase of respiratory failure, NIV can be valuable as a "bridge" in helping patients wean from intermittent positive-pressure ventilation. In an important multicenter prospective trial, Nava and colleagues randomized people who had failed a T-piece weaning trial to either NIV or further mechanical ventilation.[98] Noninvasive ventilation was associated with fewer days of ventilatory support (10.2 versus 16.6, respectively), shorter ICU stay (15.1 versus 24 days), less nosocomial pneumonia, and better 60-day survival (92% versus 72%). These results were achieved in a unit with experience in NIV. The generic use of weaning by NIV has proven less successful, particularly if patients have significant cardiac disease or established acute respiratory distress syndrome (ARDS).[99] However, further data from Spain have confirmed the value of this approach in hypercapnic patients limited primarily by COPD.[100,101]

Mechanical Ventilation

Mechanical ventilation should be considered when NIV is not appropriate (see Table 61-5) or has failed. Patients with a pH below 7.25 are more likely to require this therapy, although most physicians now offer a trial of NIV unless the patient is hemodynamically unstable or the treatment is contraindicated. Persistent significant hypoxemia despite treatment, hypotension, and impaired mental state are all predictors of imminent respiratory arrest and the need for intubation and institution of mechanical ventilation.

The major risk during intubation is hypotension. This reflects a combination of problems, including reduced venous return secondary to positive intrathoracic pressures, direct vasodilatation, and reduced sympathetic tone produced by the anesthetic agents. Reoxygenation of the patient with rapid-sequence induction of anesthesia is recommended, and this is normally accompanied by cricoid pressure during intubation to reduce the risk of aspiration, although the benefits of this technique remain unclear.[102] Short-acting muscle relaxants are usually used. Because of concerns about the risk of hyperkalemia, nondepolarizing drugs are often preferred in this circumstance. Hypotension is normally combated with fluid replacement, and if it is persistent, it is sensible to disconnect the endotracheal tube from the ventilator and allow the patient to return to a true end-expiratory lung volume before resuming ventilation.

VENTILATION STRATEGIES

A wide range of ventilation strategies have been advocated for use in COPD, each with its own proponents; none has shown a clear advantage over its competitors, however. Familiarity with the equipment in the context of COPD patients is probably more important than the relatively minor differences between ventilator modes. The most commonly used approaches, together with their proposed advantages, are summarized in Table 61-6.

VENTILATOR SETTINGS

In general, a combination of a relatively low respiratory rate, prolongation of the expiratory time, and limited tidal volume minimizes the risks of barotrauma, reduces the degree of dynamic hyperinflation, and allows better synchronization between machine-delivered breaths and the patient's own lengthened respiratory time constants. In the United Kingdom, patients are commonly paralyzed for the first 12 to 24 hours of intermittent positive-pressure ventilation to heighten ventilator synchrony and stabilize gas exchange. Although a degree of permissive hypercapnia is usual with this regimen, it is generally well tolerated. Typical ventilator settings are a tidal volume of 8 to 12 mL/kg, a frequency of 10 to 14 breaths per minute, and an inspiratory-expiratory ratio of 1:2.5 or 1:3. Increasingly, pressure control ventilation is used; with this method, the respiratory flow more closely resembles the patient's own spontaneous breathing pattern, and there is more equal ventilation of all lung units rather than preferential ventilation of those with the highest compliance, as occurs during volume cycle ventilation.

TABLE 61-6	Modes of Ventilation	
Mode	**Method**	**Comment**
Assist-control	Preset tidal volume, patient triggered with backup rate	Patient still performs substantial work of breathing; dynamic hyperinflation worsens this
Spontaneous intermittent mandatory ventilation	Preset number of breaths of a preset volume—patient does the rest	Patient still makes an effort during part of machine breath—involves more patient work, especially at low respiratory rates
Pressure support ventilation	Pressure set to augment each inspiration—tidal volume depends on patient effort, pulmonary mechanics, and pressure applied	Basis of noninvasive ventilation therapy; pressure titrated to a respiratory rate below 27 breaths/min; asynchrony with machine breaths a problem at high pressures
Proportional assist ventilation	Flow and volume generated proportional to patient effort	Experimental technique; requires accurate measurement of elastance and resistance + an intact drive to breathe; proven effective in COPD patients

The optimal extrinsic PEEP remains contentious in this setting, as there is a risk of inducing hyperinflation if too much pressure is added. In general, 5 cm H_2O of PEEP is probably sufficient to overcome intrinsic load without risking passive hyperinflation.

ASSISTED VENTILATION AND WEANING

As acidosis resolves and oxygen requirements fall, it is possible to reduce the degree of sedation and allow the patient to make some contribution to ventilation before weaning. Several modes of ventilatory support are available in these circumstances, and again, there is no specific advantage of one over another.[103,104] There is an impression, however, that reliance on spontaneous intermittent mandatory ventilation prolongs subsequent weaning. Although not universally accepted, there are good data supporting the use of spontaneous breathing trials in clinically stable COPD patients to determine when they are ready to wean.[104-106] The ability to sustain ventilation in the absence of increasing CO_2, worsening acidosis, or clinical distress (reflected by an increase in blood pressure, heart rate, or restlessness) is generally agreed to be a predictor of future weaning success. Although COPD patients are less likely to achieve these goals as early as other ICU patients, the reintubation rate in those who do meet these criteria is low.[105,106] Unfortunately, breathing through the ventilator on a continuous positive airway pressure (CPAP) circuit may be associated with significant increases in inspiratory resistance,[107] and it is sensible to use pressure support to offset some of this additional respiratory work. This reflects the necessity of identifying patients who can be weaned using the ventilator alone and those who need more prolonged support. In the latter circumstance, weaning supported by NIV is particularly helpful.

A variety of predictors of weaning success have been developed to try to identify when successful weaning will occur. Unfortunately, none has proved entirely reliable, and relatively few have been assessed prospectively. An empirical approach based on the criteria listed in Table 61-7 is widely used. An aggressive policy toward weaning is justified in COPD patients, because an inability to wean is invariably associated with a worse prognosis and prolonged ventilation.

Nonventilatory Issues

Therapy employed in spontaneously breathing patients is still required in those undergoing mechanical ventilation. High-dose nebulized bronchodilators are commonly used, singly and in combination,[108,109] although it is important to pay attention to the details of drug delivery. Drug deposition within the ventilator circuit and endotracheal tube can

TABLE 61-7	Criteria for Weaning Failure

Increasing hypercapnia or worsening hypoxemia (<55 mm Hg)
pH < 7.32
Increased respiratory rate > 35 breaths/min
Increase in heart rate or blood pressure by 20% of baseline
Agitation, sweating, or impaired consciousness

lead to a significant loss of effective drug.[93] When using a nebulized drug, the nebulizer should be placed in the inspiratory line at least 30 cm from the endotracheal tube; this allows the tubing to act as a spacer device and increases the respirable fraction.[110] If a metered dose inhaler is used instead, it should always be given with some form of spacer device for the same reason. Parenteral corticosteroids are commonly administered. This is not without hazard, particularly because of the real risk of myopathy (see earlier). As noted previously, there does not seem to be any advantage in giving high doses of corticosteroids.

Clearance of secretions is important in ventilated patients, and it is essential that the patient's hydration state be maintained. Whether specific mucolytic drugs such as *N*-acetylcysteine are helpful is unclear, and no good scientific studies to support or reject their use are available. Introduction of a mini-tracheostomy often facilitates secretion clearance without compromising subsequent weaning. For patients requiring longer periods of ventilation, a formal tracheostomy is needed; the introduction of a speaking valve or fenestrated tube permits speech and improves patient communication and morale.

The benefits of nutritional support are unclear, although it is obviously needed in patients who are catabolic and poorly nourished. However, concerns about providing an excessive metabolic CO_2 load are unfounded. Simple nursing measures are often surprisingly effective; in particular, keeping the patient's head elevated prevents nosocomial pneumonia and is more effective than other approaches such as gut sterilization in patients with COPD.

Prognosis

The prognosis following an exacerbation of COPD is better than the gloomy outlook proposed by some physicians. Nonetheless, patients who experience exacerbations appear to have a more severe clinical course than those who do not, and they report a worse overall quality of life.[111] Mortality after an ICU admission is significant, at least in North American series[112]; 10% to 15% of such subjects die as inpatients, and over the next 2 years, 30% to 60% die. Patients with a low FEV_1, significant comorbidity, and a particularly poor performance status at home have the worst outlook.[113] These factors should be considered when decisions about the requirement for ventilatory support are made. However, as noted already, the physician's view of the very sick COPD patient can be unduly pessimistic. Exacerbations leave patients relatively immobile, and this has now been confirmed

objectively.[56] There are encouraging data suggesting that early rehabilitation can reduce subsequent hospital admissions, although the optimal place to organize such a program for patients post exacerbation has still to be determined.[114]

Changes in clinical practice continue to improve the outlook for COPD patients. The impact of NIV on their acute care has been enormous, as has closer adherence to evidence-based recommendations across the field of intensive care,[115] something about which both practitioners and their patients can feel proud.

KEY POINTS

1. The prognosis of patients with chronic obstructive pulmonary disease (COPD) admitted to the ICU is better than commonly believed.

2. The burden of symptomatic COPD is likely to rise for several decades more, despite effective smoking cessation programs in many countries.

3. Small changes in forced expiratory flow are associated with significant impairment in lung mechanics, particularly airway closure and dynamic hyperinflation, and worse gas exchange.

4. Common upper respiratory tract pathogens and respiratory viruses precipitate most exacerbations of COPD. Treatment aimed at these agents is useful, but it is not as important as improving lung emptying and maintaining gas exchange until the acute insult resolves.

5. Oral and intravenous corticosteroids shorten the duration of an exacerbation and reduce the risk of relapse. However, high-dose treatment beyond 2 weeks provides no advantage and actually poses a risk, especially in ventilated patients.

6. Maintaining oxygenation is relatively easy, but there are risks of carbon dioxide retention and acidosis if high-flow oxygen is administered. An oxygen saturation between 91% and 93% ensures adequate tissue oxygen delivery if the cardiac output is stable.

7. Respiratory acidosis is a poor prognostic marker in COPD exacerbations and a strong indicator of the need for assisted ventilation.

8. Unless contraindicated, noninvasive ventilation (NIV) is the safest and most effective way of managing acute respiratory failure. More acidotic patients should be managed in an ICU with the option of endotracheal intubation and mechanical ventilation if NIV fails.

9. COPD patients meet conventional weaning criteria less frequently than other ICU patients do, but they are more likely to wean successfully when they do meet the criteria.

10. Seriously ill COPD patients should be encouraged to make advance directives, particularly after an ICU admission involving any form of ventilatory support.

ANNOTATED REFERENCES

Aaron SD, Vandemheen KL, Hebert P, et al. Outpatient oral prednisone after emergency treatment of chronic obstructive pulmonary disease. N Engl J Med 2003;348(26):2618-25.

Davies L, Angus RM, Calverley PMA. Oral corticosteroids in patients admitted to hospital with exacerbations of chronic obstructive pulmonary disease: a prospective randomised controlled trial. Lancet 1999;354(9177):456-60.

Niewoehner DE, Erbland ML, Deupree RH, et al. Effect of systemic glucocorticoids on exacerbations of chronic obstructive pulmonary disease. N Engl J Med 1999;340(25):1941-7.
These three papers defined the evidence base for the use of oral and intravenous corticosteroids in COPD exacerbations.

Calverley PMA, MacNee W, Pride NB, Rennard SI, editors. Chronic Obstructive Pulmonary Disease. 2nd ed. London: Arnold; 2003.
Comprehensive and up-to-date overview of all aspects of COPD by a team of internationally respected authors.

Connors AFJ, Dawson NV, Thomas C, et al. Outcomes following acute exacerbation of severe chronic obstructive lung disease: The SUPPORT investigators (Study to Understand Prognoses and Preferences for Outcomes and Risks of Treatments). Am J Respir Crit Care Med 1996;154(1):959-67; erratum, Am J Respir Crit Care Med 1997;155(4 Pt 1):386.
Still the major study of outcomes in COPD patients managed in the ICU.

Lightowler JV, Wedzicha JA, Elliott MW, et al. Non-invasive positive pressure ventilation to treat respiratory failure resulting from exacerbations of chronic obstructive pulmonary disease: Cochrane systematic review and meta-analysis. BMJ 2003;326(7382):185.
Valuable overview of the relative benefits of noninvasive ventilation in the management of acute respiratory failure in COPD.

Soler N, Torres A, Ewig S, et al. Bronchial microbial patterns in severe exacerbations of chronic obstructive pulmonary disease (COPD) requiring mechanical ventilation. Am J Respir Crit Care Med 1998;157(5 Pt 1):1498-505.
Important paper describing the role of lower respiratory tract colonization in the genesis of COPD exacerbations in an ICU population.

Younes M. Dynamic intrinsic PEEP (PEEP(i), dyn): Is it worth saving? Am J Respir Crit Care Med 2000;162(5):1608-9.
Thoughtful overview of a physiologically important but technically difficult measurement.

Ferrer M, Sellares J, Valencia M, et al. Non-invasive ventilation after extubation in hypercapnic patients with chronic respiratory disorders: randomised controlled trial. Lancet 2009;374(9695):1082-8.
A prospective trial of the role of weaning with NIV in hypercapnic COPD patients; see also editorial by Calverley in the same issue.

REFERENCES

Access the complete reference list online at http://www.expertconsult.com.

62

Pulmonary Embolism

RUSSELL D. HULL | GRAHAM F. PINEO

Venous thromboembolism (VTE), deep venous thrombosis (DVT), pulmonary embolism (PE), or all three can complicate the course of sick hospitalized patients but may also affect ambulant and otherwise apparently healthy individuals.[1-3] Pulmonary embolism remains the most common preventable cause of hospital death and is responsible for approximately 150,000 to 200,000 deaths per year in the United States. Most patients who die from PE succumb suddenly or within 2 hours of the acute event before therapy can be initiated or can take effect.[4] Effective prophylaxis against VTE is now available for most high-risk patients.[5,6] Prophylaxis is more effective in preventing death and morbidity from VTE than is treatment of the established disease.

Pathophysiology

Venous thrombi are composed predominantly of fibrin and red cells and have a variable platelet and leukocyte component. The formation, growth, and dissolution of venous thromboemboli represent a balance between thrombogenic stimuli and protective mechanisms. The factors that predispose to the development of DVT are venous stasis, activation of blood coagulation, and vascular damage. The protective mechanisms that counteract these thrombogenic stimuli include (1) the inactivation of activated coagulation factors by circulating inhibitors (e.g., antithrombin III, α_2-macroglobulin, α_1-antitrypsin, and activated protein C); (2) clearance of activated coagulation factors and soluble fibrin/polymer complexes by the reticuloendothelial system and liver; and (3) dissolution of fibrin by fibrinolytic enzymes derived from plasma and endothelial cells, and digestion of fibrin by leukocytes.

Acquired and inherited risk factors for VTE have been identified and are shown in Table 62-1. The risk of VTE increases when more than one predisposing factor is present.[7,8]

Activated protein C resistance is the most common hereditary abnormality predisposing to VTE. The defect results from substitution of glutamine for arginine at residue 506 in the factor V molecule, making factor V resistant to proteolysis by activated protein C. The gene mutation is commonly designated *factor V Leiden* and follows autosomal dominant inheritance. Patients who are homozygous for the factor V Leiden mutation have a markedly increased risk of thromboembolism and present with clinical thromboembolism at a younger age (median 31 years) than those who are heterozygous (median age 46 years).[7,9] Factor V Leiden is present in approximately 5% of the normal Caucasian population, 16% of patients with a first episode of DVT, and up to 35% of patients with idiopathic DVT.[7,9,10]

Prothrombin G20210A is another gene mutation that predisposes to VTE. It is present in approximately 2% to 3% of apparently healthy individuals and in 7% of those with DVT.[9] An inherited abnormality cannot be detected in up to 40% to 60% of patients with idiopathic DVT, suggesting that other gene mutations are present and have an etiologic role.

Historically, VTE usually occurred in sick hospitalized patients. The burden of illness from VTE has shifted to the community setting such that most patients now present as outpatients to their primary care physician or to the emergency room. The main reason for this shift is the greatly reduced length of hospital stay for most surgical procedures or medical conditions and the discharge of patients from the hospital either before the period of risk of VTE has ended or where there is already the presence of subclinical venous thrombi that subsequently

evolve and lead to symptomatic DVT or PE. The shift in burden of illness from the hospital to the community setting has led to an emphasis on effective and safe methods for outpatient diagnosis and management.

Pulmonary embolism originates from thrombi in the deep veins of the leg in 90% or more of patients.[11-13] Other less common sources of PE include the deep pelvic veins, renal veins, inferior vena cava, right ventricle, and axillary veins. Most clinically important PE arise from thrombi in the popliteal or more proximal deep veins of the leg. Pulmonary embolism occurs in 50% of patients with objectively documented proximal vein thrombosis; many of these emboli are asymptomatic.[11] Usually only part of the thrombus embolizes, and 50% to 70% of patients with angiographically documented PE have detectable DVT of the legs at the time of presentation.[12] The clinical significance of PE depends on the size of the embolus and the cardiorespiratory reserve of the patient.

Clinical Features

The clinical features of DVT include leg pain, tenderness and swelling, a palpable cord, discoloration, venous distention, prominence of the superficial veins, and cyanosis. The clinical diagnosis of DVT is highly nonspecific because none of the symptoms or signs is unique, and each may be caused by nonthrombotic disorders. Patients with relatively minor symptoms and signs may have extensive DVT, whereas those with florid leg pain and swelling, suggesting extensive DVT, may have negative results on objective testing. Thus, objective testing is mandatory to confirm or exclude a diagnosis of DVT.[14-16]

The location of the initial DVT has an impact on the incidence of recurrence; thus the presence of an ilial femoral vein thrombosis was shown to have a higher rate of recurrent VTE compared with popliteal vein thrombosis.[17] Also, there is a high correlation between venographic results as measured by the Marder Score and recurrence of VTE.[18]

The clinical presentation of PE depends on the size, location, and number of emboli, and on the patient's underlying cardiorespiratory reserve. The clinical manifestations of acute PE generally can be divided into several syndromes that overlap considerably: (1) transient dyspnea and tachypnea in the absence of other associated clinical manifestations; (2) pulmonary infarction or congestive atelectasis (also known as *ischemic pneumonitis* or *incomplete infarction*), which includes pleuritic chest pain, cough, hemoptysis, pleural effusion, and pulmonary infiltrates on the chest x-ray; (3) right ventricular failure associated with severe dyspnea and tachypnea; (4) cardiovascular collapse with hypotension, syncope, and coma (usually associated with massive PE); and (5) less common and highly nonspecific clinical features including confusion and coma, pyrexia, wheezing, resistant cardiac failure, and unexplained arrhythmia.

The prognosis for long-term survival and recurrent VTE may be worse for patients presenting with PE as opposed to DVT. This may be a reason to treat patients presenting with PE more aggressively in the future, but at the present time, anticoagulant management for each entity is identical. Various studies have attempted to identify risk factors for recurrent VTE, including fatal PE, in patients presenting initially with PE. Factors contributing to recurrent VTE include length of initial hospitalization, presence of cancer, older age, hospitalization for multiple injuries, and surgery within 3 months.[19,20] Risk factors for

TABLE 62-1	Factors Predisposing to Development of Venous Thromboembolism

Clinical Risk Factors

Surgical and nonsurgical trauma
Previous venous thromboembolism
Immobilization
Malignant disease
Heart disease
Leg paralysis
Age (>40 years)
Obesity
Estrogens
Parturition

Inherited or Acquired Abnormalities

Factor V Leiden
Prothrombin 20210A
Protein C deficiency
Protein S deficiency
Antithrombin deficiency
Antiphospholipid antibody syndrome
Dysfibrinogenemia
Heparin-induced thrombocytopenia
Myeloproliferative syndromes

an adverse outcome include factors such as older than age 70, hypotension, congestive heart failure, chronic obstructive pulmonary disease (COPD), cancer, presence of a DVT, and right ventricular hypokinesis on echocardiography. Using a standardized Pulmonary Embolism Severity Index[21] and measurement of troponin and beta-type natriuretic peptides are useful in the initial diagnosis and in estimating prognosis in patients presenting with PE.[22-27]

Etiology and Pathogenesis

Pulmonary embolism occurs in at least 50% of patients with objectively documented proximal vein thrombosis.[1] Many of these emboli are asymptomatic. The clinical importance of PE depends on the size of the embolus and the patient's cardiorespiratory reserve. Usually only part of the thrombus embolizes, and 30% to 70% of patients with PE detected by angiography also have identifiable DVT of the legs.[11,12] Deep vein thrombosis and PE are not separate disorders but a continuous syndrome of VTE in which the initial clinical presentation may be symptoms of either DVT or PE. Therefore, strategies for diagnosis of VTE include both tests for detection of PE (lung scanning, computed tomography [CT], or pulmonary angiography)[8-10] and tests for DVT of the legs (ultrasound or venography)[11-13]

Prevention of Venous Thromboembolism

Over the years, numerous clinical trials have been carried out for the prevention of VTE, particularly in patients undergoing orthopedic surgery and in hospitalized medical patients. Agents tested include heparin, low-molecular-weight heparin, fondaparinux, warfarin, and more recently, specific inhibitors of activated factor X or thrombin. In addition, medical devices and, in particular, intermittent pneumatic compression alone or in addition to pharmacologic agents have been studied. Effective prophylaxis against VTE is now available for most high-risk patients; prophylaxis is more effective for preventing death and morbidity and more cost-effective than treatment of the established disease. Evidence-based recommendations for the prevention of VTE are available.[5,6]

Assessment of Clinical Probability

Management studies over the past 2 decades have demonstrated that patients can be assigned categories of pretest probability using decision rules such as the Geneva Score or the approach of Wells.[28-34] With the shift of the burden of thromboembolic disease to the out-of-hospital population, these clinical probability guidelines have proven to be extremely useful in stratifying patients into low, moderate, or high risk

for the diagnosis of PE. However, the prevalence of PE in these categories is not sufficiently low or high to withhold further investigations altogether based on the clinical probability assessment. The measurement of a D-dimer or performance of an objective diagnostic test is mandatory to exclude or confirm the presence of PE in many patients. The assessment of pretest probability and measurement of the D-dimer have now been integrated into diagnostic algorithms for PE (using either CT angiography [CTA] or ventilation/perfusion [V/Q] scanning) and for DVT (using ultrasonography to objectively confirm the diagnosis[28-34] (Figures 62-1, 62-2, and 62-3).

D-DIMER ASSAY

Measurement of the plasma D-dimer has been extensively studied for the exclusion of patients with suspected PE.[35-39] Numerous assays for the D-dimer exist, but the most extensively studied have been enzyme-linked immunosorbent assay (ELISA) and quantitative rapid ELISA, which have high sensitivity and negative likelihood ratios equal to a normal perfusion lung scan. A positive D-dimer result is not useful for the exclusion of PE. Numerous management studies have demonstrated that PE can be excluded without performing imaging studies in patients with a low clinical probability[35-39] (see Figures 62-2 and 62-3). Patients with a high clinical probability (i.e., PE likely) should not undergo D-dimer testing but go directly to objective diagnostic tests.

Differential Diagnosis

The differential diagnosis in patients with suspected PE includes cardiopulmonary disorders for each of the modes of presentation (see Clinical Features). For the presentation of dyspnea and tachypnea, they include atelectasis, pneumonia, pneumothorax, acute pulmonary edema, bronchitis, bronchiolitis, and acute bronchial obstruction. For pulmonary infarction exhibited by pleuritic chest pain or hemoptysis, they include pneumonia, pneumothorax, pericarditis, pulmonary or bronchial neoplasm, bronchiectasis, acute bronchitis, tuberculosis, diaphragmatic inflammation, myositis, muscle strain, and rib fracture. For the clinical presentation of right-sided heart failure, they include myocardial infarction, myocarditis, and cardiac tamponade. For cardiovascular collapse, they include myocardial infarction, acute massive hemorrhage, gram-negative septicemia, cardiac tamponade, and spontaneous pneumothorax.

Diagnostic Imaging

COMPUTED TOMOGRAPHY AND COMPUTED TOMOGRAPHY ANGIOGRAPHY

Spiral CT imaging has gained an increasingly important role in the diagnosis of PE in recent years and is now the primary imaging test in most centers. Single-detector spiral CT is highly sensitive for large emboli (segmental or larger arteries) but much less sensitive for emboli in subsegmental pulmonary arteries[40]; such emboli may be clinically important in patients with severely impaired cardiorespiratory reserve. Therefore, a negative result by single-detector spiral CT should not be used alone to exclude the diagnosis of PE. A filling defect of a segmental or larger artery on single-detector spiral CT is associated with a high probability (>90%) of PE.[40]

The development of multidetector row CT, together with the use of contrast enhancement, has further improved the utility of CT for the diagnosis of PE.[41-44] Contrast-enhanced CTA has the advantage of providing clear results (positive or negative) with a relatively low rate of non-diagnostic test results, good characterization of nonvascular structures for alternate or associated diagnoses, and the ability to simultaneously evaluate the deep venous system of the legs (CT venography [CTV]).

The accuracy and clinical utility of multidetector CTA and combined CTA-CTV was evaluated in the PIOPED II Study.[42] Among 824

SUSPECTED DVT

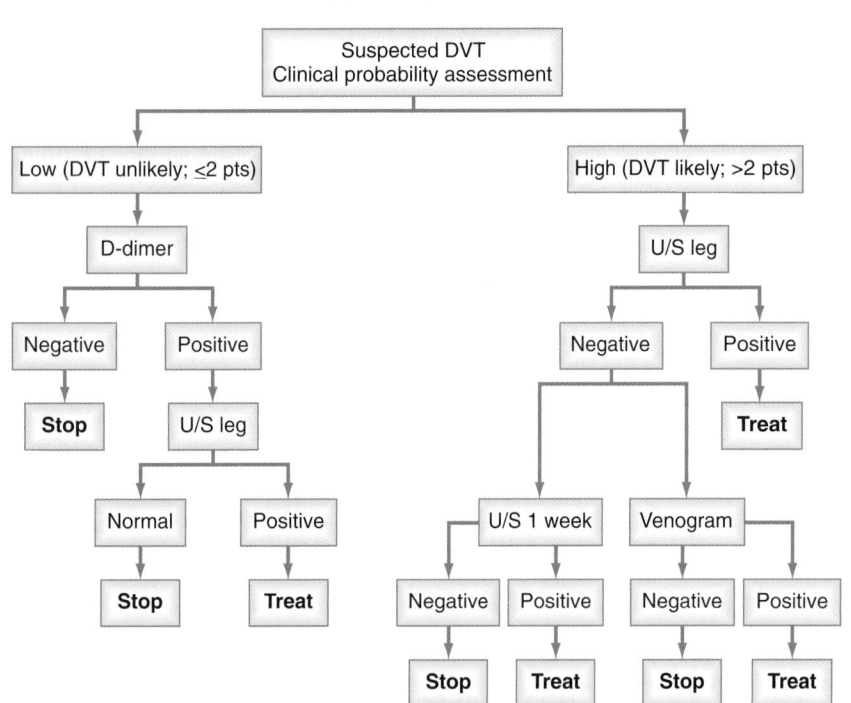

Figure 62-1 **Integrated strategy for diagnosis of deep venous thrombosis (DVT) using clinical probability assessment, measurement of D-dimer, and ultrasonography of legs as primary diagnostic tests.** If clinical probability is low (i.e., DVT unlikely and D-dimer negative), no further investigations are required. If D-dimer is positive, proceed to ultrasonography of legs; then either treat or stop investigations. If clinical probability is high (i.e., DVT likely) D-dimer measurement need not be carried out; proceed directly to ultrasonography of legs. If negative, options are to repeat ultrasound in 1 week or in some cases to perform an ascending venogram.

SUSPECTED PE (USING V/Q SCAN)

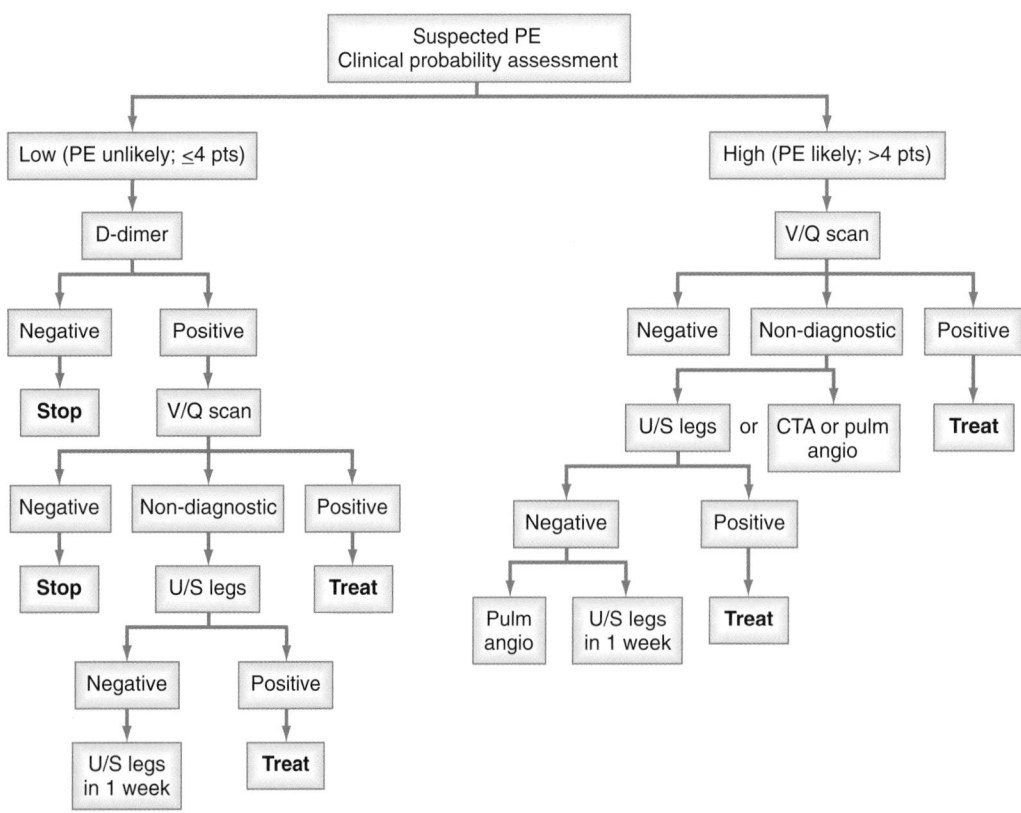

Figure 62-2 **Integrated strategy for diagnosis of suspected pulmonary embolism (PE) using clinical probability assessment, measurement of D-dimer, and ventilation/perfusion (V/Q) scan as primary imaging test.** Patients with low clinical probability (i.e., PE unlikely, negative D-dimer) need no further investigation. If D-dimer is positive, V/Q scan performed; if not diagnostic, proceed to ultrasound. Then either treat or repeat ultrasound in 1 week. Patients with high probability (i.e., PE likely) need not have D-dimer measured but should proceed directly to V/Q scan. If V/Q scan not diagnostic, options are to perform CTA, pulmonary angiography, or ultrasonography of legs. If ultrasonography is negative, either repeat in 1 week or perform pulmonary angiogram.

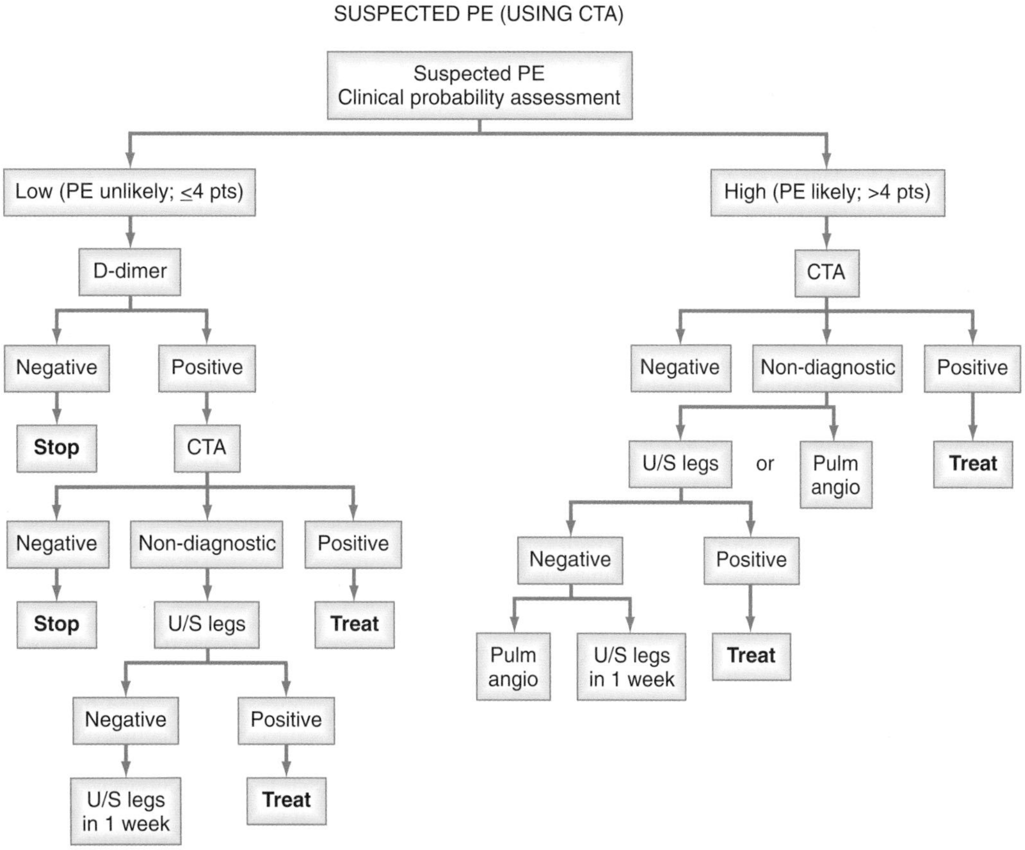

SUSPECTED PE (USING CTA)

Figure 62-3 **Integrated strategy for diagnosis of pulmonary embolism (PE) using clinical probability assessment, measurement of D-dimer, and computed tomography angiography (CTA) as primary imaging test.** Patients with low clinical probability (i.e., PE unlikely, negative D-dimer) need no further testing, but if D-dimer is positive, they should proceed to CTA, and if this is nondiagnostic, to ultrasonography of legs. Then either treat or repeat ultrasound in 1 week. Patients with high clinical probability (i.e., PE likely) need not have D-dimer measured but should proceed directly to CTA. If CTA is not diagnostic, options are to perform ultrasonography of legs or proceed to pulmonary angiogram. If ultrasound of legs is negative, options are to repeat in 1 week or proceed to pulmonary angiography.

patients with a reference diagnosis and a completed CT study, CTA was inconclusive in 51 (6%) because of poor image quality. Sensitivity of CTA was 83%, and specificity was 96%. CTA and CTV were inconclusive in 87 (11%) of 824 patients because the image quality of either CTA or CTV was poor. Multidetector CTA-CTV had a higher sensitivity (90%) than CTA alone (83%), with similar specificity (about 95%) for both testing techniques. Positive results on CTA in combination with a high or intermediate probability of PE by the clinical assessment, or normal findings on CTA with a low clinical probability, had a predictive value (positive or negative) of 92% to 96%.[32] Such values are consistent with those generally considered adequate to confirm or rule out the diagnosis of PE. Additional testing is necessary when clinical probability is discordant with CTA or CTA-CTV imaging results.[42]

RADIONUCLIDE LUNG SCANNING

Radionuclide V/Q scanning continues to have a role in the diagnosis of suspected PE. A normal perfusion lung scan excludes the diagnosis of clinically important PE.[45,46] A normal perfusion lung scan is found in approximately 10% of patients with suspected PE seen at academic health centers or tertiary referral centers. A high-probability V/Q scan result (i.e., large perfusion defects with ventilation mismatch) has a positive predictive value for PE of 85% and provides a diagnostic endpoint to give antithrombotic treatment in most patients.[45-47] A high-probability V/Q scan is found in approximately 10% to 15% of symptomatic patients. For patients with a history of PE, careful comparison of the lung scan results to the most recent lung scan is required to ensure the perfusion defects are new. Further diagnostic testing is indicated for patients with a high-probability V/Q scan who have a

"low" pretest clinical suspicion, and in those who are at high risk for major bleeding, to reduce the likelihood of a false-positive diagnosis.

The major limitation of V/Q scanning is that the results are inconclusive in most patients, even when considered together with the pretest clinical probability.[45] The nondiagnostic V/Q scan patterns are found in about 70% of patients with suspected PE.[12,45,47] These lung scan results have historically been called "low-probability" (matching ventilation/perfusion abnormalities or small perfusion defects), "intermediate probability," or indeterminate (because the perfusion defects correspond to an area of abnormality on chest x-ray film). Further diagnostic testing is required in most of these patients because regardless of the pretest clinical suspicion, the posttest probabilities of PE associated with these lung scan results are neither sufficiently high to give antithrombotic treatment nor sufficiently low to withhold therapy. The uncommon exception is the patient with a low clinical suspicion and a so-called low-probability V/Q scan result. However, even in these patients, objective testing for DVT with ultrasound may provide added diagnostic value. A randomized trial has established that CTA is not inferior to using V/Q scanning for excluding the diagnosis of PE when either test is used in an algorithm together with venous ultrasonography of the legs.[43]

MAGNETIC RESONANCE IMAGING

Magnetic resonance imaging (MRI) appears to be a promising diagnostic approach for PE. However, clinically important interobserver variation exists in the sensitivity for PE, ranging from 70% to 100%.[48,49] Further studies are required to determine the clinical role of MRI in the diagnosis of patients with suspected PE.

PULMONARY ANGIOGRAPHY

Pulmonary angiography using selective catheterization of the pulmonary arteries is a relatively safe technique for patients who do not have pulmonary hypertension or cardiac failure.[45,46] If the expertise is available, pulmonary angiography should be used when other approaches are inconclusive and when definitive knowledge about the presence or absence of PE is required.[12]

OBJECTIVE TESTING FOR DEEP VEIN THROMBOSIS

Objective testing for DVT is useful in patients with suspected PE, particularly those with nondiagnostic lung scan results[47] or inconclusive CT results.[42] Detection of proximal vein thrombosis by objective testing provides an indication for anticoagulant treatment regardless of the presence or absence of PE and prevents the need for further testing. However, a negative result by objective testing for DVT does not exclude the presence of PE.[12]

Currently, the primary role for using ultrasound testing of the legs is for those centers that do not have the capability for combined CTA-CTV, or if the results of such imaging are inconclusive. If the patient has adequate cardiorespiratory reserve, serial ultrasound testing for proximal vein thrombosis can be used as an alternative to pulmonary angiography in patients with non-diagnostic lung scan or CT results, and withholding anticoagulant therapy is safe if repeated ultrasound testing of the legs is negative.[50-53] The rationale is that the clinical objective in such patients is to prevent recurrent PE, which is unlikely in the absence of proximal vein thrombosis. Selective pulmonary angiography should be done among patients with features suggesting a possible source of embolism other than proximal DVT of the leg (e.g., upper-extremity thrombosis, renal vein thrombosis, pelvic vein thrombosis, or right-heart thrombus).

Integrated Strategies for Diagnosis of Pulmonary Embolism

Figure 62-3 summarizes the approach to diagnosis of suspected PE using CTA or CTA-CTV as the primary imaging test. Figure 62-2 summarizes the approach to diagnosis using V/Q scanning for settings in which CTA capabilities are not available. Figure 62-3 summarizes the approach to the diagnosis of DVT using ultrasonography. The specific approach used will depend on the local availability of technology, expertise with the different diagnostic techniques, and individual patient circumstances.

An appropriately validated assay for plasma D-dimer, if available, provides a simple and rapid first-line exclusion test in patients with low, intermediate, or unlikely clinical probability. The appropriate use of D-dimer can reduce the need for more expensive imaging tests without compromising patient safety. If a validated D-dimer test is not available or the patient has high clinical probability for PE, diagnostic imaging should be employed. If capability for combined CTA-CTV exists, that is the preferred approach for most patients because it provides a definitive basis to give or withhold antithrombotic therapy in about 90% of patients. Lung scanning may be indicated as the first-line imaging test in women of reproductive age, because the radiation exposure to the breast is significantly less than with CTA.[53]

When other approaches are inconclusive, selective pulmonary arteriography should be done unless contraindications exist, because the risk of arteriography in properly selected patients is less than the risk of unnecessary anticoagulant therapy.

ECHOCARDIOGRAPHY

Echocardiography provides a number of independent parameters related to pulmonary hemodynamics and, in addition to measurement of troponin and beta-type natriuretic peptide levels, can identify patients with non-massive PE who are at risk of dying or are candidates for thrombolytic therapy.[22-27] Transthoracic echocardiography is particularly useful for patients in the intensive care unit (ICU) and can further identify patients who are candidates for thrombolysis or catheter fragmentation or who may progress to chronic thromboembolic pulmonary hypertension.[23,24]

Clinical Course of Venous Thromboembolism

Proximal DVT is a serious and potentially lethal condition. Untreated proximal vein thrombosis is associated with a 10% rate of fatal PE. Inadequately treated proximal vein thrombosis results in a 20% to 50% risk of recurrent VTE events.[54,47,55] Prospective studies of patients with clinically suspected DVT or PE indicate that new venous thromboembolic events on follow-up are rare (≤2%) among patients in whom proximal vein thrombosis is absent by objective testing.[50-52] The aggregate data from diagnostic and treatment studies indicate that the presence of proximal DVT is the key prognostic marker for recurrent VTE.

Thrombosis that remains confined to the calf veins is associated with low risk (≤1%) of clinically important PE. Extension of thrombosis into the popliteal vein or more proximally occurs in 15% to 25% of patients with untreated calf vein thrombosis.[11] Patients with documented calf vein thrombosis should receive either anticoagulant treatment to prevent extension or undergo monitoring for proximal extension using serial noninvasive tests.

The postthrombotic syndrome is a frequent complication of DVT.[56,57] Patients with postthrombotic syndrome complain of pain, heaviness, swelling, cramps, and itching or tingling of the affected leg. Ulceration may occur. The symptoms usually are aggravated by standing or walking and improve with rest and elevation of the leg. A prospective study documented a 25% incidence of moderate to severe postthrombotic symptoms 2 years after the initial diagnosis of proximal DVT in patients who were treated with initial heparin and oral anticoagulants for 3 months.[56] The study also demonstrated that ipsilateral recurrent DVT is strongly associated with subsequent development of moderate or severe postthrombotic symptoms. Thus prevention of ipsilateral recurrent DVT likely reduces the incidence of the postthrombotic syndrome. Application of a properly fitted graded compression stocking, as soon after diagnosis as the patient's symptoms will allow and continued for at least 2 years, is effective in reducing the incidence of postthrombotic symptoms, including moderate to severe symptoms.[58]

Chronic thromboembolic pulmonary hypertension is a serious complication of PE. Historically, thromboembolic pulmonary hypertension was believed to be relatively rare and occur only several years after the diagnosis of PE. A prospective cohort study provides important information on the incidence and timing of thromboembolic pulmonary hypertension.[59-61] The results indicate that thromboembolic pulmonary hypertension is more common and occurs earlier than previously thought. On prospective follow-up of 223 patients with documented PE, the cumulative incidence of chronic thromboembolic pulmonary hypertension was 3.8% at 2 years after diagnosis despite state-of-the-art treatment for PE. The strongest independent risk factors were a history of PE (odds ratio 19) and idiopathic PE at presentation (odds ratio 5.7).[59] Further clinical studies on identification and prevention of chronic thromboembolic pulmonary hypertension are needed.

Objectives and Principles of Antithrombotic Treatment

The objectives of treatment in patients with established VTE are to (1) prevent death from PE, (2) prevent morbidity from recurrent DVT or PE, and (3) prevent or minimize the postthrombotic syndrome.

Recommendations for treatment of established VTE are linked to the strength of the evidence from clinical trials using the approach for grading evidence of the American College of Chest Physicians (ACCP) guideline committee.[55] Recommendations classified as 1A are supported by evidence from scientifically valid randomized clinical trials (grade A evidence), and the results provide a clear risk-to-benefit conclusion (grade 1). Such recommendations should be implemented for most patients. Grade 2A recommendations also are supported by definitive clinical trial evidence (grade A), but the results indicate a less clear risk-to-benefit conclusion (grade 2); therefore, such recommendations may or may not be appropriate for the individual patient. The remaining grades of recommendation are based on nondefinitive evidence (grade B or C) and are less strong.

Anticoagulant Therapy

Anticoagulant therapy is the treatment of choice for most patients with proximal DVT or PE (grade 1A). Absolute contraindications to anticoagulant treatment include intracranial bleeding; severe active bleeding; malignant hypertension; or recent brain, eye, or spinal cord surgery. Relative contraindications include recent major surgery, recent cerebrovascular accident, active gastrointestinal tract bleeding, severe hypertension, severe renal or hepatic failure, and severe thrombocytopenia (platelets < 50,000/μL).

HEPARIN THERAPY

Unfractionated Heparin Therapy

Unfractionated heparin (UFH) has been used extensively to prevent and treat VTE, but more recently, low-molecular-weight heparin (LMWH) has replaced UFH for the treatment of VTE in most cases, either entirely or predominantly in the out-of-hospital setting. However, there are patients in whom UFH by continuous infusion continues to be used primarily because the anticoagulant effect can be reversed by stopping the intravenous (IV) infusion and/or administering protamine sulphate.[62] Such patients include critically ill patients in the ICU or cardiovascular unit, patients who may be candidates for interventions requiring interruption of anticoagulant therapy (e.g., surgical procedures, thrombolysis), or patients with severe renal failure.[62] In some countries, UFH is the anticoagulant of choice for patients suffering PE who are hemodynamically unstable.

The anticoagulant activity of UFH depends upon a unique pentasaccharide that binds to antithrombin (AT) and potentiates the inhibition of thrombin and activated factor X (Xa) by ATIII.[62-64] About one-third of all heparin molecules contain the unique pentasaccharide sequence.[62-64] It is the pentasaccharide sequence that confers the molecular high affinity for AT.[62-64] In addition, heparin catalyses the inactivation of thrombin by another plasma cofactor, cofactor II, which acts independently of AT.[62]

Heparin has a number of effects other than inhibition of thrombin and activated factor X.[63] These include the release of tissue factor pathway inhibitor; suppression of platelet function; increase in vascular permeability, and binding to numerous plasma and platelet proteins, endothelial cells, and leucocytes. The anticoagulant response to a standard dose of UFH varies widely between patients. This makes it necessary to monitor the anticoagulant effects of UFH, using either the activated partial thromboplastin time (APTT) or heparin levels, and to titrate the dose to the individual patient.[62]

The simultaneous use of initial UFH and warfarin has become clinical practice for all patients with VTE who are medically stable.[62,65] Exceptions include patients who require immediate medical or surgical intervention, such as in thrombolysis or insertion of a vena cava filter, or patients at very high risk of bleeding. Heparin is continued until the International Normalized Ratio (INR) has been within the therapeutic range (2 to 3) for 2 consecutive days.[62]

It has been established from experimental studies and clinical trials that the efficacy of UFH therapy depends upon achieving a critical therapeutic level of UFH within the first 24 hours of treatment.[66-68] Data from double blind clinical trials indicate that failure to achieve the therapeutic APTT threshold by 24 hours was associated with a

23.3% subsequent recurrent VTE rate, compared with a rate of 4% to 6% for the patient group who were therapeutic at 24 hours.[67,68] Recurrences occurred throughout the 3-month follow-up period and could not be attributed to inadequate oral anticoagulant therapy.[67] The critical therapeutic level of UFH, as measured by the APTT, is 1.5 times the mean of the control value or the upper limit of the normal APTT range.[66-68] This corresponds to a UFH blood level of 0.2 to 0.4 U/mL by the protamine sulphate titration assay, and 0.35 to 0.70 by the antifactor Xa assay. It is vital for each laboratory to establish the minimal therapeutic level of UFH, as measured by the APTT, that will provide a UFH blood level of at least 0.35 U/mL by the antifactor Xa assay for each batch of thromboplastin reagent being used, particularly if a new batch of reagent is provided by a different manufacturer.[62]

Numerous audits of UFH therapy indicate that administration of IV UFH is fraught with difficulty, and that the clinical practice of using an ad hoc approach to UFH dose titration frequently results in inadequate therapy. Use of a prescriptive approach or protocol for administering IV UFH therapy has been evaluated in two prospective studies in patients with VTE.[66,68] Both protocols were shown to achieve therapeutic UFH levels in the vast majority of patients. Using the weight-based nomogram, there were fewer episodes of recurrent VTE as compared to standard care. Continued use of the weight-based nomogram has been shown to be similarly effective.[69]

Adjusted-dose subcutaneous UFH has been used in initial treatment of VTE.[70] Four randomized clinical trials compared the efficacy of subcutaneous UFH with subcutaneous LMWH in patients with proven VTE.[71-74] Nomograms have been developed for subcutaneous UFH. The importance of achieving the therapeutic range by 24 hours was reaffirmed.[75] The largest of these trials compared subcutaneous UFH dose adjusted with the use of APTT by means of a weight-adjusted algorithm with fixed-dose LMWH for the initial treatment of patients with VTE, 16% of who presented with PE.[74] Subcutaneous UFH was shown to be similar to fixed-dose LMWH in terms of efficacy and safety.[74]

Complications of Unfractionated Heparin Therapy. The main adverse effects of UFH therapy include bleeding, thrombocytopenia, and osteoporosis. Patients at particular risk of bleeding are those who have had recent surgery or trauma or who have other clinical factors that predispose to bleeding on heparin, such as peptic ulcer, occult malignancy, liver disease, hemostatic defects, weight, age older than 65 years, and female gender.

Management of bleeding on heparin will depend on the location and severity of bleeding, risk of recurrent VTE, and APTT; in these instances, heparin should be discontinued temporarily or permanently. Patients with recent VTE may be candidates for insertion of an inferior vena cava filter. If urgent reversal of heparin effect is required, protamine sulphate can be administered.[62]

Heparin-induced thrombocytopenia is a well-recognized complication of UFH therapy, usually occurring within 5 to 10 days after heparin treatment has started.[76,77] Approximately 1% to 2% of patients receiving UFH will experience a fall in platelet count to less than the normal range or a 50% fall in the platelet count within the normal range. In the majority of cases, this mild to moderate thrombocytopenia appears to be a direct effect of heparin on platelets and is of no consequence. However, patients receiving UFH may develop an immune thrombocytopenia mediated by immunoglobulin G (IgG) antibody directed against a complex of PF4 and heparin.[29] In some cases, neutrophil acting peptide 2 (NAP-2) and interleukin 8 (IL-8) also play a role in pathogenesis.

The incidence of heparin-induced thrombocytopenia (HIT) is lower with the use of LMWH[76,78-82]; however, the clinical manifestations may be as or more severe than those seen with UFH. Furthermore, the nadir of the platelet count, onset, and duration of thrombocytopenia have been shown to be somewhat different.[80] Recently, delayed onset of HIT has been described, with the onset being as long as several weeks after the end of exposure to heparin, thus making this syndrome sometimes more difficult to diagnose. Furthermore, the incidence and severity of

HIT varies among different patient populations, being more prevalent in patients having cardiac or orthopedic procedures than for medical patients.[83] The development of thrombocytopenia may be accompanied by arterial or DVT which may lead to serious consequences such as death or limb amputation.[76,83]

When a clinical diagnosis of HIT is made, heparin in all forms must be stopped immediately.[77,84] In most centers, the confirmatory laboratory test is an ELISA for the PF4-heparin complex but where possible, this should be confirmed with a functional assay such as the serotonin release assay.[83] In those patients requiring ongoing anticoagulation, an alternative form of anticoagulation must be undertaken immediately because of the high incidence of thrombosis when heparin is stopped.[85] Some authorities recommend the use of alternative anticoagulants in all patients once a diagnosis is made. The most common alternative agents are the specific antithrombin, argatroban,[77,86,87] or the direct thrombin inhibitor, lepirudin.[88-91] Both agents are given by IV infusion. Lepirudin, which is renally excreted, has the advantage that it can be given to patients with hepatic insufficiency,[77,85] but it has the disadvantage that with prolonged use, antibodies develop, and some of these can have series deleterious effects, including anaphylaxis.[92] Argatroban is only partially excreted by the kidney, so it can be used in persons with renal failure, but it cannot be used in patients with significant hepatic insufficiency.[77,85] Both agents can be used in conjunction with vitamin K antagonists, but it should be noted that argatroban by itself increases the INR beyond that observed with warfarin alone, and this must be taken into account in controlling the vitamin K antagonist.[87] The alternative antithrombotic agents should be continued until the platelet count is at least back to 100×10^9/L and/or the INR is therapeutic for 2 consecutive days.[77] The pentasaccharide, fondaparinux, has been used as an alternative antithrombotic agent in HIT patients, and it has the advantage that it is given by a once-daily subcutaneous injection.[93,94] Insertion of an inferior vena cava filter is seldom indicated.

Osteoporosis has been reported in patients receiving UFH in dosages of 20,000 U/day (or more) for more than 6 months.[62] Demineralization can progress to the fracture of vertebral bodies or long bones, and the defect may not be entirely reversible.[62] Laboratory and clinical studies indicate that the incidence of osteoporosis with use of long-term LMWH is low.[62]

Low-Molecular-Weight Heparin for Initial Treatment of VTE

Heparin currently in use clinically is polydispersed unmodified heparin with a mean molecular weight ranging from 10 to 16 kD. Low-molecular-weight derivatives of commercial heparin have been prepared that have a mean molecular weight of 4 to 5 kD.[62,95,96]

The LMWHs commercially available are made by different processes (e.g., nitrous acid, alkaline, or enzymatic depolymerization) and they differ chemically and pharmacokinetically.[95,96] The clinical significance of these differences, however, is unclear, and there have been very few studies comparing different LMWHs with respect to clinical outcomes.[96] The doses of the different LMWHs have been established empirically and are not necessarily interchangeable. Therefore, at this time, effectiveness and safety of each of the LMWHs must be tested separately.[96]

The LMWHs differ from UFH in numerous ways. Of particular importance are increased bioavailability (>90% after subcutaneous injection); prolonged half-life and predictable clearance, enabling once- or twice-daily injection; and predictable antithrombotic response based on body weight, permitting treatment without laboratory monitoring.[62,95,96] Other possible advantages are their ability to inactivate platelet-bound factor Xa, resistance to inhibition by platelet factor 4, and their decreased effect on platelet function and vascular permeability (possibly accounting for fewer hemorrhagic effects at comparable antithrombotic doses).

Subcutaneous unmonitored LMWH has been compared with continuous IV heparin in a number of clinical trials for the treatment of proximal DVT or PE using long-term follow-up as an outcome measure.[97-105] These studies have shown that LMWH is at least as effective and safe as unfractionated heparin in the treatment of proximal venous thrombosis. Pooling of the most methodologically sound studies indicates a significant advantage for LMWH in the reduction of major bleeding and mortality.[106] LMWH used predominantly out of hospital was as effective and safe as IV UFH given in hospital.[101-103] Economic analysis of treatment with LMWH versus IV UFH demonstrated that LMWH was cost-effective for treatment in hospital as well as out of hospital.[101,102] As these agents become more widely available for treatment, they have replaced IV UFH in the initial management of most patients with VTE. LMWH is now the recommended agent for initial treatment of VTE.[55]

There has been a hope that the LMWHs will have fewer serious complications such as bleeding,[69] heparin-induced thrombocytopenia,[80,81,107] and osteoporosis[108] when compared with unfractionated heparin. Evidence is accumulating that these complications are indeed less serious and less frequent with the use of LMWH.

Recent reviews suggest the absolute risk for heparin-induced thrombocytopenia with LMWH was 0.2%, compared with 2.6% with UFH. Accordingly, there is an advantage in this regard to using LMWH.[108]

In obese patients, the clinician should review the pharmacopeia recommendations for the particular LMWH agent being used concerning dosage guidelines.[62] For patients with significant renal impairment, the clinician should also review the pharmacopeia guidelines for dosage modifications for the individual LMWH agent. In patients with severe renal failure, it may be preferable to use UFH.[55,62]

Long-Term Low-Molecular-Weight Heparin

The use of LMWH for the long-term treatment of acute VTE has been evaluated in randomized clinical trials.[109-111] Taken together, these studies[110-111] indicate that long-term treatment with subcutaneous LMWH for 3 to 6 months is more effective in cancer patients with VTE than adjusted doses of oral vitamin K antagonist therapy (INR 2.0–3.0) for preventing recurrent VTE. The ACCP recommendation states: "For most patients with DVT and cancer, we recommend treatment with LMWH for at least the first 3 to 6 months of long-term treatment."[55]

ORAL VITAMIN K–ANTAGONIST THERAPY (WARFARIN)

The anticoagulant effect of warfarin is mediated by inhibition of the vitamin K–dependent γ-carboxylation of coagulation factors II, VII, IX, and X.[112,113] This results in the synthesis of immunologically detectable but biologically inactive forms of these coagulation proteins. Warfarin also inhibits the vitamin K–dependent γ-carboxylation of proteins C and S. Protein C circulates as a proenzyme that is activated on endothelial cells by the thrombin-thrombomodulin complex to form activated protein C. Activated protein C in the presence of protein S inhibits activated factor VIII and activated factor V activity.[112,113] Therefore, vitamin K antagonists such as warfarin create a biochemical paradox by producing an anticoagulant effect due to the inhibition of procoagulants (factors II, VII, IX, and X) and a potentially thrombogenic effect by impairing the synthesis of naturally occurring inhibitors of coagulation (proteins C and S). Heparin and warfarin treatment should overlap by 4 or 5 days when warfarin treatment is initiated in patients with thrombotic disease.

The anticoagulant effect of warfarin is delayed until the normal clotting factors are cleared from the circulation, and the peak effect does not occur until 36 to 72 hours after drug administration.[114,115] During the first few days of warfarin therapy, the prothrombin time (PT) reflects mainly the depression of factor VII, which has a half-life of 5 to 7 hours.[114] Equilibrium levels of factors II, IX, and X are not reached until about 1 week after the initiation of therapy. The use of small initial daily doses (e.g., 5-10 mg) is the preferred approach for initiating warfarin treatment.[116,119]

The dose-response relationship to warfarin therapy varies widely between individuals, so dosage must be carefully monitored to prevent overdosing or underdosing. A number of drugs interact with warfarin.[113] Critical appraisal of the literature reporting such interactions indicates that the evidence substantiating many of the claims is limited.[118] Nonetheless, patients must be warned against taking any new drugs without the knowledge of their attending physician.

Laboratory Monitoring and Therapeutic Range

The laboratory test most commonly used to measure the effects of warfarin is the one-stage PT test. The PT is sensitive to reduced activity of factors II, VII, and X but is insensitive to reduced activity of factor IX. Confusion about the appropriate therapeutic range has occurred because the different tissue thromboplastins used for measuring the PT vary considerably in sensitivity to the vitamin K–dependent clotting factors and in response to warfarin.[119,120]

To promote standardization of the PT for monitoring oral anticoagulant therapy, the World Health Organization (WHO) developed an international reference thromboplastin from human brain tissue and recommended that the PT ratio be expressed as the International Normalized Ratio, or INR.[62] The INR is the PT ratio obtained by testing a given sample using the WHO reference thromboplastin. For practical clinical purposes, the INR for a given plasma sample is equivalent to the PT ratio obtained using a standardized human brain thromboplastin known as the *Manchester Comparative Reagent*, which has been widely used in the United Kingdom.[55]

Warfarin is administered in an initial dose of 5 to 10 mg per day for the first 2 days.[116,117] The daily dose is then adjusted according to the INR. UFH or LMWH therapy is discontinued on the fourth or fifth day following initiation of warfarin therapy, provided the INR is prolonged into the recommended therapeutic range (INR 2 to 3).[55] Because some individuals are either fast or slow metabolizers of the drug, selection of the correct dosage of warfarin must be individualized. Therefore, frequent INR determinations are required initially to establish therapeutic anticoagulation.

Once the anticoagulant effect and patient's warfarin dose requirements are stable, the INR should be monitored at regular intervals throughout the course of warfarin therapy for VTE. However, if there are factors that may produce an unpredictable response to warfarin (e.g., concomitant drug therapy), the INR should be monitored frequently to minimize the risk of complications due to poor anticoagulant control.[55] Several warfarin nomograms and computer software programs are now available to assist healthcare givers in the control of warfarin therapy. Also, there is increasing interest in the use of self-testing with portable INR monitors and, in selected cases, self-management of oral anticoagulant therapy.

Adverse Effects of Oral Anticoagulants

Bleeding. The major side effect of warfarin therapy is bleeding.[113,119,120] A number of risk factors have been identified that predispose to bleeding on oral anticoagulants.[113,121,122] The most important factor influencing bleeding risk is the intensity of the INR.[121,122] Other factors include a history of bleeding, previous history of stroke or myocardial infarction, hypertension, renal failure, diabetes, and decreased hematocrit.[121] Efforts have been made to quantify the bleeding risk according to these underlying clinical factors.[121,122] Introduction of a multicomponent intervention combining patient education and alternative approaches to the maintenance of INR resulted in a reduced frequency of major bleeding in the patients in this group.[121] Furthermore, patients in the intervention group were within the therapeutic INR a significantly greater amount of time than were patients in the standard care group. In a retrospective cohort study of patients with an INR greater than 6.0, it was shown that a prolonged delay in the return of the INR to the therapeutic range was seen in patients who had an INR over 4.0 after two doses of warfarin were withheld, patients with an extreme elevation of the INR, and older age patients, particularly those with decompensated congestive heart failure or active cancer.[122,123] Numerous randomized clinical trials have demonstrated that clinically important bleeding is lower when the targeted INR is 2.0 to 3.0, and that bleeding increases exponentially when the INR increases above 4.5 or 5.0.[121,122] There is a strong negative relationship between the percentage of time patients are within the targeted range for INR and both bleeding and recurrent thrombosis.

Warfarin therapy in elderly patients can present problems.[124,125] Many of these patients require long-term anticoagulants because of underlying clinical conditions that increase with age, while they are more likely to have underlying causes for bleeding, including the development of cancer, intestinal polyps, renal failure, and stroke; and they are more prone to having frequent falls. The daily requirements for warfarin to maintain the therapeutic INR also decrease with age, presumably due to decreased clearance of the drug. Therefore, before initiating oral anticoagulant treatment in elderly patients, the risk/benefit ratio of treatment must be considered. If they are placed on oral anticoagulant therapy, careful attention to the INR is required.

Patients with cancer are more likely to bleed on warfarin treatment.[126] Compared with patients on oral anticoagulants who do not have cancer, patients with cancer have a higher incidence of both major and minor bleeding, and anticoagulant withdrawal is more frequently due to bleeding. Patients with cancer have a higher thrombotic complication rate and a higher bleeding rate regardless of the INR, whereas bleeding in non-cancer patients was seen only when the INR was greater than 4.5. Safer and more effective anticoagulant therapy is required for the treatment of VTE in patients with cancer.[126]

Management of Over-Anticoagulation. The approach to the patient with an elevated INR depends on the degree of elevation of the INR and the clinical circumstances.[113,127,128] Options available to the physician include temporary discontinuation of warfarin treatment, administration of vitamin K, administration of blood products such as fresh frozen plasma or prothrombin concentrate to replace the vitamin K–dependent clotting factors, or administration of activated factor VII. If the increase is mild and the patient is not bleeding, no specific treatment is necessary other than reduction in the warfarin dose. The INR can be expected to decrease during the next 24 hours with this approach. With more marked increase of the INR in patients who are not bleeding, treatment with small doses of vitamin K (e.g., 1 mg) given either orally or by subcutaneous injection should be considered.[127,128] With very marked increase of the INR, particularly in a patient who is either actively bleeding or at risk for bleeding, the coagulation defect should be corrected. Vitamin K can be given IV slowly or by the subcutaneous or oral routes.[113,127] Where possible, the oral route is preferred. If ongoing anticoagulation with warfarin is planned, repeated small doses of vitamin K should be given so there is no problem with warfarin resistance.[113,127]

Reported side effects of vitamin K include flushing, dizziness, tachycardia, hypotension, dyspnea, and sweating.[113] Intravenous administration of vitamin K_1 should be performed with caution to avoid inducing an anaphylactoid reaction; risk of anaphylactoid reaction can be reduced by slow administration. In most patients, IV administration of vitamin K produces a demonstrable effect on the INR within 6 to 8 hours and corrects the increased INR within 12 to 24 hours. Because the half-life of vitamin K is less than that of warfarin sodium, a repeat course of vitamin K may be necessary. If bleeding is very severe and life threatening, vitamin K therapy can be supplemented with concentrates of factors II, VII, IX, and X.

When bleeding occurs in a patient on warfarin, it is important to consider the site of bleeding. Bleeding from the upper gastrointestinal tract commonly is seen in patients on oral anticoagulants, and the concomitant use of other medications is often an association. Once bleeding is controlled, it is important to carry out the necessary investigations to identify bleeding lesions in the gastrointestinal or genitourinary tract, which are often unsuspected.

Temporary Interruption of Oral Anticoagulant Therapy. Bridging therapy should be considered if oral anticoagulant therapy needs to be temporarily placed on hold for surgery or a procedure.[129-135]

Long-Term Treatment of Venous Thromboembolism Using Vitamin K Antagonists

Patients with established DVT or PE require long-term anticoagulant therapy to prevent recurrent disease.[55,113] Warfarin therapy is highly effective[54,55] and is preferred in most but not all patients. Adjusted-dose subcutaneous heparin or unmonitored LMWHs have been used for the long-term treatment of patients in whom oral anticoagulant therapy proves to be very difficult to control,[109] and LMWH is the preferred treatment in patients with DVT and cancer.[109-111]

The preferred intensity of the anticoagulant effect of treatment with warfarin has been confirmed by the results of randomized trials.[55,113,136,137] The results of two recent randomized trials[136,137] indicate that although low-intensity warfarin therapy is more effective than placebo, it is less effective than standard-intensity therapy (INR 2-3), and does not reduce the incidence of bleeding complications. Additional important evidence regarding the intensity of anticoagulant therapy with warfarin is provided by a recent randomized trial[138] that compared standard-intensity warfarin therapy (INR 2-3) with high-intensity warfarin therapy (INR 3.1-4.0) for the prevention of recurrent thromboembolism in patients with persistently positive antiphospholipid antibodies and a history of thromboembolism (venous or arterial). High-intensity warfarin therapy (INR 3.1-4.0) did not provide improved antithrombotic protection. The high-intensity regimen has been previously shown to be associated with a high risk (20%) of clinically important bleeding in a series of randomized trials[138-141] in patients with DVT. The evidence outlined above provides the basis for recommending an INR of 2.0 to 3.0 as the preferred intensity of anticoagulant treatment with warfarin.

The safety of warfarin treatment depends heavily on the maintenance of a narrow therapeutic INR range. The importance of maintaining careful control of warfarin therapy is evident and may be enhanced with the use of anticoagulant management clinics if warfarin is going to be used for extended periods of time.

Duration of Anticoagulant Therapy and Recurrent Venous Thromboembolism

The appropriate duration of warfarin treatment for VTE has been evaluated by multiple randomized clinical trials.[55,142-148] Treatment should be continued for at least 3 months in patients with a first episode of proximal DVT or PE secondary to a transient (reversible) risk factor (grade 1A). Stopping treatment at 4 to 6 weeks resulted in an increased incidence of recurrent VTE during the following 6 to 12 months (absolute risk increase 8%). In contrast, treatment for 3 to 6 months resulted in a low rate of recurrent VTE during the following 1 to 2 years (annual incidence 3%).

Patients with a first episode of idiopathic VTE should be treated for 3 to 6 months[55] (grade 1A) and considered for indefinite anticoagulant therapy. This decision should be individualized, taking into consideration the estimated risk of recurrent VTE, risk of bleeding, and patient compliance and preference. Indefinite therapy is recommended for patients in whom risk factors for bleeding are absent and in whom good anticoagulant control can be achieved (grade 1A).[55] If indefinite anticoagulant treatment is given, the risk-benefit of continuing such treatment should be reassessed at periodic intervals.

Numerous attempts have been made to identify patients who are at particularly high risk for recurrent VTE when anticoagulant therapy is discontinued.[149-155] Measurement of the D-dimer either before anticoagulants are stopped or 1 month after discontinuation can help predict patients at risk of recurrent VTE if the D-dimer is elevated.[152,153,155] In a recent study, measurement of the D-dimer assay prior to discontinuing anticoagulants, combined with assessment of signs of postthrombotic syndrome, in consideration of age or those who are obese, can help identify patients at high or low risk for recurrent VTE. Similarly, assessment of residual proximal venous thrombosis based on non-compressibility of the previously involved segment of the vein can predict patients who are at higher risk for recurrent VTE.[149-151]

For patients with a first episode of VTE and documented antiphospholipid antibodies or two or more thrombophilic conditions (e.g., combined factor V Leiden and prothrombin 20210A gene mutations), indefinite anticoagulant treatment should be considered. For patients with a first episode of VTE who have documented deficiency of protein C or protein S, or the factor V Leiden or prothrombin 20210A gene mutation, or high factor VIII levels (>90th percentile), the duration of treatment should be individualized after the patients have completed at least 3 months of anticoagulant therapy. Some of these patients also may be candidates for indefinite therapy.

Warfarin treatment should be given indefinitely for most patients with a second episode of unprovoked VTE[55,113] (grade 1A), because stopping treatment at 3 to 6 months in these patients results in a high incidence (21%) of recurrent VTE during the following 4 years. The risk of recurrent VTE during 4-year follow up was reduced by 87% (from 21% to 3%) by continuing anticoagulant treatment; this benefit is partially offset by an increase in the cumulative incidence of major bleeding (from 3% to 9%).[55]

Use of LMWH for long-term treatment of VTE has been evaluated in clinical trials.[109-111] The studies indicate that long-term treatment with subcutaneous LMWH for 3 to 6 months is at least as effective as (and in cancer patients more effective than) warfarin adjusted to maintain the INR between 2.0 and 3.0. Therefore, patients with VTE and cancer should be treated with LMWH for the first 3 to 6 months of long-term treatment (grade 1A).[55] The patient then should receive anticoagulation indefinitely or until the cancer resolves. The regimens of LMWH that are established as effective for long-term treatment are dalteparin, 200 U/kg once daily for 1 month, followed by 150 U/kg daily thereafter; or tinzaparin, 175 U/kg once daily.

Fondaparinux and Related Compounds

Fondaparinux, a synthetic indirect inhibitor of factor Xa has been studied in a wide variety of patients for the prevention and treatment of VTE. Based on the results of such clinical trials, fondaparinux has been approved as a substitute for UFH or LMWH for the initial treatment of VTE.[156,157] Idraparinux, a derivative of fondaparinux, has a high affinity for antithrombin, and this high affinity prolongs the plasma half-life to 80 hours. Because of this long half-life, idraparinux can be given subcutaneously on a once-weekly basis. In a clinical trial in a treatment of DVT, idraparinux was given in a once-weekly subcutaneous injection and compared with either LMWH or UFH followed by warfarin for a 3-month period.[158] Idraparinux was similar in efficacy in terms of recurrent VTE, but clinically relevant bleeding was less common with idraparinux than with conventional therapy. However, in patients presenting with PE, idraparinux given by weekly subcutaneous injection for 3 months was less effective than conventional therapy with similar bleeding rates.[113] In a long-term study, idraparinux was compared with placebo in patients with DVT or PE who had had an initial 6-month treatment with standard therapy.[159] There was a significant reduction in the risk of recurrent VTE with idraparinux, but there was an increase in major bleeding, including three fatal intracranial hemorrhages. Given these results and the fact that the anticoagulant effect of idraparinux could not be blocked, this agent has not been further developed. However, a biotinylated form of idraparinux has been developed that provides the opportunity of removing the long-acting compound by administering an antibody to the biotin molecule. This agent is under investigation for the treatment of DVT and PE.

New Oral Anticoagulants

There has been much interest in developing new oral antithrombotic agents that may be able to replace warfarin. The most advanced agents are specific inhibitors of factor Xa or thrombin (factor 2). Advantages of these agents are that they can be given by the oral route once or twice daily, they require no laboratory monitoring, and in most cases, the same dose is taken by all patients. In clinical trials, all these agents are compared with enoxaparin, either 40 mg once daily beginning 12 hours prior to surgery, or 30 mg twice daily beginning 12 to 24 hours postoperatively in patients undergoing total hip or total knee replacement surgery.[160-165] These procedures carry a high risk for VTE, and because of the nature of the procedure, there is a significant risk of bleeding. Therefore, agents which can be shown to be effective and safe in this clinical situation show promise for prevention and treatment of VTE in other settings. To date, there has been publication of clinical trials in patients undergoing total hip or total knee replacement with the factor Xa inhibitors, rivaroxaban (Bayer Health Care) and apixaban (BMS-Pfizer), and the antithrombin agent, dabigatran (Boehringer-Ingelheim). Results have varied somewhat depending on the dosage of the comparative agent, enoxaparin, and the dose and timing of the investigative agent. Rivaroxaban and dabigatran have been approved by a number of agencies for thromboprophylaxis in hip and knee arthroplasty patients and are used in a number of countries, but neither has been approved by the U.S. Food and Drug Administration (FDA) at this time.

All three agents are being investigated for initial and/or extended treatment of VTE. In the RECOVER study, dabigatran etexilate, 150 mg twice daily, was compared with standard warfarin therapy, with an INR target of 2 to 3 in patients presenting with VTE who had an initial course of parenteral therapy, usually with LMWH for 8 to 11 days.[166] Treatment continued for 6 months, and there was a follow-up of 30 days. Dabigatran was shown to be non-inferior to standard therapy in the prevention of recurrent VTE or VTE-related death, and the incidence of major bleeding was comparable. However, the incidence of combined major and non-major clinically relevant bleeding was significantly less with dabigatran.

Thrombolytic Therapy

Thrombolytic therapy is indicated for patients with PE who present with evidence of vascular collapse (hypotension and/or syncope) and for selected patients with PE who have clinical findings of right ventricular failure or echocardiographic evidence of right ventricular hypokinesia.[55,167-169] Thrombolytic therapy provides more rapid lysis of PE and more rapid restoration of right ventricular function and pulmonary perfusion than anticoagulant treatment.[167-170]

Inferior Vena Cava Filter

Insertion of an inferior vena cava filter is indicated for patients with acute VTE and an absolute contraindication to anticoagulant therapy and for those rare patients who have objectively documented recurrent VTE during adequate anticoagulant therapy.[55,100,170]

Insertion of a vena cava filter is effective for preventing important PE. However, use of a permanent filter results in an increased incidence of recurrent DVT 1 to 2 years after insertion (increase in cumulative incidence at 2 years increases from 12% to 21%).[100] Therefore, if the indication for filter placement is transient, such as a contraindication to anticoagulation due to a temporary high risk of bleeding, a retrievable vena cava filter should be used.[171,172] A retrievable filter can then be removed after several weeks to months, once the filter is no longer required. If a permanent filter is placed, long-term anticoagulant treatment should be given as soon as safely possible to prevent morbidity from recurrent DVT.

Conclusions

Based on a large number of clinical trials, the accepted medical treatment for acute PE has been established. Historically this consisted of UFH given by continuous IV infusion, with warfarin starting on days 1 or 2 and continued for 3 months, with a targeted INR of 2.0 to 3.0. A number of LMWHs have been shown to be at least as effective as UFH in decreasing recurrent VTE and in fact are associated with less major bleeding. Low-molecular-weight heparin has become the treatment of choice for both in-hospital and out-of-hospital treatment of DVT and, more recently, submassive PE as well. Long-term LMWH is the therapy of choice in patients with VTE and cancer. Although warfarin has been used for years for the long-term treatment of patients suffering VTE, the optimal duration of treatment after a first episode or recurrent episodes of venous thrombosis remains uncertain. Patients with a first episode of idiopathic DVT require at least 3 to 6 months of anticoagulant treatment, and patients who have a first recurrence require at least 1 to 2 years of anticoagulant treatment. In all cases, the duration of therapy should be reviewed periodically. Because the risk of recurrent VTE continues even after these extended periods of treatment, recommendations have been made for longer periods of treatment, particularly if additional risk factors are present.[55] Indeed, current guidelines suggest considering indefinite anticoagulation in appropriate patients.[55] The advent of new oral anticoagulants which do not require laboratory monitoring will simplify long-term therapy.

ANNOTATED REFERENCES

Geerts WH, Bergqvist D, Pineo GF, et al. Prevention of venous thromboembolism: American College of Chest Physicians Evidence-Based Clinical Practice Guidelines. 8th ed. Chest 2008;133(6 Suppl):381S-453S.
The most recent guidelines from the ACCP for prevention of venous thromboembolism.
Mookadam F, Jiamsripong P, Goel R, Warsame TA, Emani UR, Khandheria BK. Critical appraisal on the utility of echocardiography in the management of acute pulmonary embolism. Cardiol Rev 2010;18(1):29-37.
A critical review of the utility of echocardiography in the management of acute pulmonary embolism.
Ceriani E, Combescure C, Le Gal G, et al. Clinical prediction rules for pulmonary embolism: a systematic review and meta-analysis. J Thromb Haemost 2010, Feb 9. [Epub ahead of print].
Clinical prediction rules have become a standard component for the diagnosis of VTE. This is a systematic review of the various prediction rules for the diagnosis of PE.
Stein P, Hull RD, Patel K, et al. D-dimer for the exclusion of acute venous thrombosis and pulmonary embolism. A systematic review. Ann Intern Med 2004;140(8):589-602.
This paper presents an exhaustive review of the D-dimer test for the exclusion of VTE, indicating that the ELISA D-dimer assay is the preferable test.
Stein PD, Woodard PK, Weg JG, et al. Diagnostic pathways in acute pulmonary embolism: recommendations of the PIOPED II Investigators. Am J Med 2006;119(12):1048-55.
Recommended diagnostic pathways for acute PE from the PIOPED II Investigators.
Kearon C, Kahn SR, Agnelli G, Goldhaber S, Raskob GE, Comerota AJ. Antithrombotic therapy for venous thromboembolic disease. American College of Chest Physicians Evidence-Based Clinical Practice Guidelines. 8th ed. Chest 2008;133(6 Suppl):454S-545S.
The most recent ACCP Guidelines for the treatment of VTE.
Hirsh J, Bauer KA, Donati MB, Gould M, Samama MM, Weitz JI. Parenteral anticoagulants: American College of Chest Physicians Evidence-Based Clinical Practice Guidelines. 8th ed. Chest 2008;133(6 Suppl):141S-59S.
This paper, part of the ACCP Supplement on Anti-thrombotic and Thrombolytic Therapy, reviews parenteral anticoagulants including heparin, low-molecular-weight heparin, fondaparinux, and the direct thrombin inhibitors.

Warkentin TE, Greinacher A, Koster A, et al. Treatment and prevention of heparin-induced thrombocytopenia: American College of Chest Physicians Evidence-Based Clinical Practice Guidelines. 8th ed. Chest 2008;133(6 Suppl):340S-80S.
A review of the prevention and treatment of heparin-induced thrombocytopenia by two of the leading investigators in the area.
Gould MK, Dembitzer AD, Doyle RL, Hastie TJ, Garber AM. Low-molecular-weight heparins compared with unfractionated heparin for treatment of acute deep venous thrombosis. A meta-analysis of randomized, controlled trials. Ann Intern Med 1999;130(10):800-9.
One of the best meta-analyses comparing LMWH and UFH for treatment of acute DVT; indicates a significant advantage for LMWH in reduction of major bleeding and mortality.
Ansell J, Hirsh J, Hylek E, Jacobson A, Crowther M, Palareti G. Pharmacology and management of the vitamin K antagonists: American College of Chest Physicians Evidence-Based Clinical Practice Guidelines. 8th ed. Chest 2008;133(6 Suppl):160S-98S.
A comprehensive review of the pharmacology and management of warfarin as part of the ACCP Supplement on Antithrombotic and Thrombolytic Therapy.
Douketis JD, Berger PB, Dunn AS, et al. The perioperative management of antithrombotic therapy: American College of Chest Physicians Evidence-Based Clinical Practice Guidelines. 8th ed. Chest 2008;133(6 Suppl):299S-339S.
A review of bridging therapy for the interruption of warfarin therapy in patients requiring surgical procedures, with guidelines from the ACCP Panel.
Young T, Tang H, Aukes J, et al. Vena caval filters for the prevention of pulmonary embolism. Cochrane Database Syst Rev 2007;(4):CD006212.
A Cochrane review of the role of vena caval filters for the prevention of PE.

REFERENCES

Access the complete reference list online at http://www.expertconsult.com.

63

Other Embolic Syndromes

CLAUS-MARTIN MUTH | ERIK S. SHANK

The presentation, pathophysiology, and treatment of embolic disease other than thromboembolic processes are discussed in this chapter. Included are emboli associated with iatrogenic complications of medical diagnostic and therapeutic manipulations as well as sequelae from skeletal trauma and pregnancy.

Air Embolism

Air embolism, the entry of gas into the vasculature, is a largely iatrogenic clinical entity that can result in serious morbidity and even mortality (Table 63-1).[1] This is one of the most serious problems in diving medicine.[2] The medical use of a variety of gases has created numerous types of gas embolisms, including carbon dioxide, nitrous oxide, and nitrogen emboli. There are two broad categories of gas embolism, venous and arterial, depending on the mechanism of gas entry and where the emboli ultimately lodge.

VENOUS GAS EMBOLISM

A venous gas embolism occurs as a result of the entry of gas into the systemic venous system.[3] The gas is then transported to the lungs via the pulmonary arteries, causing interference in gas exchange, arrhythmias, pulmonary hypertension, right ventricular strain, and cardiac failure. Predispositions that allow entry of gas into the venous system include incision of noncollapsed veins and the presence of subatmospheric pressure in these vessels. These conditions occur when the surgical field is above the level of the heart (for instance, during neurosurgical operations performed in the sitting position).[4] Other potential pathways include entry of air into central venous and hemodialysis catheters[1] and entry of air into the veins of the myometrium in the peripartum period.[1,5]

Pathophysiology

The most common scenario for venous gas embolism is insidious, where there is continuous entry of small gas bubbles into the venous system. With rapid entry or larger volumes of gas, increasing strain on the right ventricle follows because of the migration of the emboli to the pulmonary circulation. Pulmonary arterial pressure increases, while increased resistance to right ventricle outflow causes diminished pulmonary venous return. This is reflected in decreased left ventricular preload, resulting in diminished cardiac output and, ultimately, systemic cardiovascular collapse.[6] Quite often, tachyarrhythmias develop, but bradycardias are possible as well. When large quantities of gas/air (over 50 mL) are injected abruptly, acute cor pulmonale and/or asystole can occur.[3] These alterations of lung vessel resistance and ventilation/perfusion mismatch in the lung cause intrapulmonary right-to-left shunt with increased alveolar dead space, leading to arterial hypoxia and hypercapnia.

Diagnosis

The so-called mill-wheel cardiac murmur, a continuous churning murmur, is relatively typical of venous gas embolism and can be auscultated by a precordial or esophageal stethoscope. A capnometric decrease of end-tidal carbon dioxide suggests ventilation/perfusion mismatching resulting from obstruction of the pulmonary arteries.[7] Precordial Doppler ultrasonography is a sensitive and practical monitor to detect intracardiac air,[1,8] but an even more sensitive and specific monitor in procedures with a high risk for gas embolism is transesophageal echocardiography (TEE). TEE is the current gold standard for detecting intracardiac gas; however, this technique requires significant training in application and interpretation to be effective.[1,9]

Treatment

When a diagnosis of venous gas embolism is considered (Table 63-2), further entry of gas into the venous circulation must be avoided. Catecholamine therapy and cardiopulmonary resuscitation should be initiated for cardiovascular collapse. Adequate oxygenation is often only possible with a significant increase in the oxygen concentration of the inspired gas (i.e., 100% oxygen); 100% oxygen also reduces the size of the gas embolism by increasing the gradient for nitrogen egress from the bubble.[10] Rapid-volume resuscitation is recommended to elevate venous pressure, thus decreasing the continued entry of gas into the venous circulation. Some authors recommend attempting to evacuate air from the right ventricle by a central venous catheter (multi-orifice catheters may be more effective than a single lumen) or a pulmonary arterial catheter.[11] A left-lateral decubitus position had been recommended in the past but has largely been abandoned because recent hemodynamic studies showed no benefit. Hyperbaric oxygen therapy is not a first-line treatment but may be a useful adjunct in severe cases and should certainly be considered if there are neurologic findings. If central nervous system symptoms are present, a paradoxical embolism should be presumed.

PARADOXICAL EMBOLISM

A paradoxical embolism arises when air/gas entrained in the venous circulation enters the systemic arterial circulation, causing symptoms of end-artery obstruction. There are a number of mechanisms by which this can occur, such as the passage of gas across a patent foramen ovale to the systemic circulation. A patent foramen ovale is detectable in about 30% of the population and makes right-to-left shunting of gas bubbles possible.[12] Elevated pulmonary arterial pressure due to a venous gas embolism may be reflected in elevated right atrial pressures predisposing to bubble transport across a patent foramen ovale. In addition, the decrease in left atrial pressure caused by mechanical ventilation and use of positive end-expiratory pressure may create a pressure gradient across the patent foramen ovale favoring passage of gas into the systemic circulation.[1]

Venous gas may enter the arterial circulation by overwhelming the filtering capacity of the lungs that normally prevents arterial gas emboli. Clinical cases are documented in which a fatal cerebral arterial gas embolism developed as the result of a large venous gas embolism, but no intracardiac defects or shunt mechanisms could be demonstrated.[13] The filtration threshold of the pulmonary circulation for gas emboli can be affected by various anesthetic agents. In particular, in experimental studies, volatile anesthetics have been shown to reduce the threshold for spillover of venous bubbles into systemic arteries.[14]

Treatment

Therapy of paradoxical embolism is identical to that of a primary arterial gas embolism (see Table 63-2). It should be stressed that every venous gas embolism has the potential to evolve into an arterial gas embolism.

TABLE 63-1	Medical Specialties with Documented Cases of Gas Embolism
Specialty	*Mechanism of Gas Embolism*
All medical specialties	Inadvertent entry of air through peripheral intravenous circuits
All surgical specialties	Intraoperative use of hydrogen peroxide, generating arterial and venous oxygen emboli
Anesthesiology	Entry of air through disconnected intravascular catheters, inadvertent infusion of air through intravascular catheters
Cardiac surgery	Entry of air into extracorporeal bypass pump circuit, incomplete removal of air from the heart after cardioplegic arrest, carbon dioxide–assisted harvesting of peripheral veins
Cardiology	Entry of air through intravascular catheters during angiographic studies and procedures
Critical care/pulmonology	Entry of air through disconnected intravascular catheters, pulmonary barotrauma, rupture of intraaortic balloon pumps, entry of air in extracorporeal membrane oxygenator (ECMO) circuit
Diving medicine and hyperbaric medicine	Pulmonary barotrauma, paradoxical embolism after decompression injury, entry of gas through disconnected intravascular catheters
Endoscopic/laparoscopic surgery	Entry of gas into veins or arteries during insufflation of body cavities
Gastroenterology	Entry of gas into veins during upper and lower endoscopies and endoscopic retrograde pancreatography (ERCP)
Neonatology/pediatrics	Pulmonary barotrauma in treatment of infants with premature lungs
Nephrology	Inadvertent entry of air through hemodialysis catheters and circuits on hemodialysis machine
Neurosurgery	Entry of air through incised veins and calvarial bone, especially during sitting craniotomies
Obstetrics/gynecology	Cesarean sections, gas insufflation into veins during endoscopic surgery, intravaginal/intrauterine gas insufflation during pregnancy
Otolaryngology	Laser (Nd:YAG) surgery on the larynx and trachea/bronchi
Orthopedics	Gas insufflation into veins during arthroscopy, total hip arthroplasty, prone spine surgery
Radiology	Injected air/gas as contrast agent, inadvertent injection of air during angiographic studies
Thoracic surgery	Entry of air into pulmonary vasculature during lung biopsies and video-assisted thoracoscopy (VATS), chest trauma (penetrating and blunt), lung transplants
Urology	Transurethral prostatectomy (TURP), radical prostatectomy
Vascular surgery	Entry of air during carotid endarterectomies

ARTERIAL GAS EMBOLISM

Arterial gas embolism occurs though the entry of gas into the pulmonary veins or directly into the arteries of the systemic circulation. Mechanisms include overexpansion of the lung through decompression barotrauma in diving, pulmonary barotrauma from positive-pressure ventilation in critical care patients, and paradoxical embolism. Additionally, cardiac surgical procedures with extracorporeal bypass are a potential mechanism for these events.[1] The entry of even small amounts of gas into the arterial system leads to a flow of gas bubbles into functional end arteries and occlusion of these vessels. Although possible in all arteries, the embolic obstruction of the coronary arteries or the nutritive arteries of the brain, termed *cerebral arterial gas embolism*, is especially critical and can be fatal owing to the vulnerability of these organs to short periods of hypoxia.

Pathophysiology

Entry of gas into the aorta causes distribution of gas bubbles into nearly all organs. Small emboli in the vessels of the skeletal muscles or viscera are well tolerated, although organ dysfunction such as rhabdomyolysis and/or renal insufficiency may occur.[15] Embolization to the cerebral or coronary circulation may result in severe morbidity or death. Embolization into the coronary arteries can induce electrocardiographic changes typical of ischemia and infarction, with arrhythmias, myocardial depression, cardiac failure, and cardiac arrest. Circulatory responses may also be seen with embolization to the cerebral vessels.[16] Cerebral arterial gas embolization typically involves migration of gas to small arteries of the brain. The emboli generate pathology by two broad mechanisms: reduced perfusion distal to the obstruction and an inflammatory response to the bubble.[1]

Clinical Features

The signs and symptoms associated with cerebral arterial gas embolism can develop suddenly. The clinical presentation is determined by the absolute quantity of gas and the areas of the brain affected. Thus, the clinical picture can vary from minor motor weakness, headache, or moderate confusion to complete disorientation, hemiparesis, convulsions, loss of consciousness, and coma. Additionally, asymmetry of pupils, hemianopia, and impairment of respiratory and circulatory centers (bradypnea, Cheyne-Stokes breathing, cardiac arrhythmias, and circulatory failure) are all well-known complications. After surgical procedures with risks for the development of gas embolism, a delayed recovery from general anesthesia or a transitional stage of impaired consciousness can be a clue to a cerebral arterial gas embolism. The diagnosis in these cases is not easy because anesthesia

TABLE 63-2	Treatment of Gas Embolism	
	Venous Gas Embolism	*Arterial Gas Embolism*
Prevent further gas entry	Increase venous pressure (e.g., Valsalva, IV fluids) Identify and disable entryway for gas	Identify and disable the entryway for gas
Definitive therapy	Supportive	Hyperbaric oxygen therapy as soon as the patient is stable for transfer to a hyperbaric oxygen facility
Supportive therapy	Oxygen, intravascular volume expansion, catecholamines	Oxygen, intravascular volume expansion, catecholamines
Positioning	Supine	Supine
Evacuation of embolized gas	Aspiration of multilumen central venous catheter; patient in left lateral decubitus position	Hyperbaric oxygen
Adjunctive therapy	Hyperbaric oxygen	Lidocaine, antiepileptics

complications, such as central anticholinergic syndrome or residual anesthetic effects, can mimic a mild cerebral arterial gas embolism.

Diagnosis

The most important criterion is the patient's history, because the clinical suspicion of embolism is based on the initial neurologic symptoms and the direct temporal relation with an invasive procedure. The greatest risks for venous or arterial gas embolism are present in craniotomies performed in the sitting position, cesarean sections, hip replacements, and cardiac surgery using cardiopulmonary bypass. All of these procedures have in common an open vascular bed and a hydrostatic gradient favoring the intravascular entry of gas.

Differentiating a cerebral arterial gas embolism from cerebral infarct or intracerebral hemorrhage can sometimes be made using computed tomography (CT). However, pathologic changes are sometimes very subtle and not well visualized on CT, and the diagnosis of cerebral arterial gas embolism must be entertained early. Magnetic resonance imaging (MRI) can sometimes show local increase of water density concentrated in the injured tissue. But this method is not completely reliable and may fail when only mild symptoms are present. Another nonspecific finding is hemoconcentration with increased hematocrit, possibly the consequence of extravascular shift of fluid into the injured tissues.[17]

Treatment

Protection and maintenance of vital functions is the primary goal. For somnolent or comatose patients, endotracheal intubation should be performed to maintain adequate oxygenation and ventilation. Additionally, oxygen should be administered in as high a concentration as possible, ideally 100%.[1,18] This is important not only to treat hypoxia and hypoxemia but also to create a steeper diffusion gradient favoring egress of gas from the bubble. Current therapeutic recommendations include maintenance of a flat supine position for these patients, because neither a head-down nor an elevated head position provides any cardiovascular benefit and may aggravate the cerebral insult.

Cerebral gas embolism may be associated with the development of generalized seizures that resist management by benzodiazepines. In such cases, it is advised to suppress the seizure activity with barbiturates. It must be stressed, however, that with sufficient doses of barbiturates, respiratory drive is depressed, and the patient's ventilation must be supported.

Definitive treatment of arterial gas embolism is with hyperbaric oxygen therapy (HBOT),[19,20] with best results reported when HBOT is initiated as early as possible. HBOT involves placing the patient in an environment pressurized above sea level pressure while breathing 100% oxygen. This therapy causes a mechanical diminution of the gas bubble by both raising the ambient pressure and creating systemic hyperoxia. Hyperoxia produces a diffusion gradient for oxygen into the gas bubble, as well as for egress of nitrogen (or other gas) from the bubble. Hyperoxia also enables significantly larger quantities of oxygen to be dissolved in the plasma and increases the diffusion distance of oxygen in tissues. Improved oxygen-carrying capacity and delivery are important to offsetting the embolic insult to the microvasculature.

Hyperbaric oxygen has other postulated benefits after arterial air embolism. These include anti-edema effects and reducing blood vessel permeability while supporting the integrity of the blood-brain barrier.[21] In addition, there are experimental studies indicating that hyperbaric oxygen diminishes the adherent properties of leukocytes to the damaged endothelium.[22]

The aforementioned benefits suggest that all patients with the clinical symptoms of arterial gas embolism should receive treatment with hyperbaric oxygen. Although immediate institution of such therapy results in the best response, treatment in a hyperbaric chamber is still indicated after a longer period of time and may result in amelioration of the patient's condition. Thus, once the patient is stabilized from a cardiopulmonary standpoint, transfer to a hyperbaric oxygen facility should be accomplished without delay.

Further Therapeutic Measures

As a consequence of a gas embolism, hemoconcentration may occur, resulting in increased blood viscosity and further impairing the already compromised microcirculation. One important maneuver to optimize the microcirculation is therefore to achieve euvolemia. In animal studies, moderate hemodilution to a hematocrit of 30% leads to a reduction of the neurologic damage.[23] It is therefore acceptable to decrease the hematocrit within certain limits. Placement of a central venous catheter is strongly recommended to properly assess central venous pressure (CVP). CVP should be kept around 12 mm Hg. As a further monitor of normovolemia, urine output should be maintained and monitored by Foley catheter.

Anticoagulants may be useful in the treatment of arterial gas embolism, although no randomized studies in humans have been published. In an animal model of cerebral arterial gas embolism, the clinical course was less severe if the animals had been pretreated with heparin[24]; however, increased hemorrhage in infarcted areas of the spine and the brain may preclude the use of heparin. Low-dose or low-molecular-weight heparin may be given to patients when clinically indicated.

The use of corticosteroids has been controversial for arterial gas embolism. Because corticosteroids appear to be without benefit in cytotoxic edema and potentially may aggravate neuronal ischemic injury, they are not indicated in arterial gas embolism.[25] Although still experimental and an off-label use, there are suggestions that lidocaine may be beneficial.[26,27] In animals receiving prophylactic doses of lidocaine, the depressant effects of gas embolism on somatosensory evoked potentials and elevations in intracranial pressure could both be attenuated. In a clinical trial, cerebral protection during cardiac operations was demonstrated.[27] Therefore, a strong argument can be made for the administration of lidocaine in therapeutic concentrations after severe arterial gas embolism.

Fat Embolism Syndrome

Fat embolism syndrome (FES) is a clinical entity first described over 150 years ago by Bergmann.[28] It is very important to differentiate FES, a complex with potentially catastrophic cardiopulmonary and cerebral dysfunction, from fat embolization, a far more common and often subclinical entity.[29]

FES is most frequently seen after lower extremity and pelvic trauma, intramedullary nailing of long-bone fractures, hip arthroplasty, and knee arthroplasty.[30] However, FES has also been described in association with a diverse group of other medical conditions, including sickle cell disease, acute pancreatitis, and diabetes mellitus, with liposuction procedures, burns, decompression sickness, and total parenteral nutrition infusion.[31-33] In a retrospective review of patients with fractures of the long bones from trauma, the incidence of FES was 0.9%.[34]

FES always involves pulmonary compromise. The presentation may range from subclinical shunting to fulminant pulmonary failure. In response to the lodging of fat particles in the pulmonary vasculature, the patient may present with right-sided heart failure, cardiovascular collapse, or severe hypoxia. Frequently there is cerebral involvement. Cerebral symptoms may be due to paradoxical fat embolization to the central nervous system and/or a response to the severe hypoxia associated with this condition.

Intramedullary orthopedic surgery is the most common iatrogenic cause of FES. In hip and knee arthroplasties, manipulation of the femoral components can generate intramedullary pressures exceeding 800 mm Hg. Cementing the prosthesis can raise the intramedullary pressure even further.[35] However, one study suggested there is no additional risk of FES associated with cementing the prosthesis.[36]

The pathophysiology of FES is complex and probably has both a mechanical component and a secondary biochemical process. In the initial phase, fat and marrow are displaced from the bones, enter the venous system, and travel through the heart to enter the lungs. There the emboli may cause shunting, severe hypoxemia, and right ventricular dysfunction. Analogous to gas emboli, the fat may travel paradoxically to other organs via the systemic circulation, either by transpulmonary passage or through an intracardiac shunt, most commonly through a patent foramen ovale. The secondary phase may involve inflammatory mediators responsible for interstitial edema or acute respiratory distress syndrome. Additionally, bone marrow contains thromboplastin that may activate the coagulation cascade. These mechanisms may be responsible for the delayed petechial rash seen 24 to 48 hours after the initial event in approximately 50% of patients with FES.

The diagnosis of FES remains one of exclusion. A number of authors have suggested clinical criteria for diagnosing FES; most notable are Gurd,[37] Schonfeld,[38] and Lindeque.[39] All include acute respiratory collapse as a major criterion. Schonfeld and Gurd both highlight the presence of petechiae in their criteria for FES. Petechiae, as mentioned earlier, are not a consistent sign of FES and present relatively late in the process. Laboratory tests that may help in making the diagnosis of FES include arterial blood gases (hypoxia), electrocardiogram (right-sided heart strain), chest radiograph (diffuse bilateral infiltrates and opacities), MRI (for signs of cerebral FES), and CT.[40] Bronchoalveolar lavage (BAL) may help confirm the diagnosis by demonstrating fat droplets in alveolar macrophages, although the sensitivity and specificity of this test are unclear.[41,42] Intraoperative transesophageal echocardiography (TEE) will demonstrate multiple echogenicities in the right heart chambers in the presence of fat embolization. It may also show paradoxical echogenic particles in the left heart chambers, should a patent foramen ovale or other means for right-to-left intracardiac shunting be present.[43] A pulmonary arterial catheter may show elevations in right-sided heart pressures.[44]

Treatment of FES remains supportive; no specific drug regimens are recommended. Therapy should include maintaining an adequate cardiac preload and cardiac output with the use of inotropic agents if necessary. Some authors have suggested that volume expansion with albumin may be beneficial owing to albumin binding oleic acid, thereby decreasing its "edemogenic potential."[45] The severe hypoxemia associated with FES must be aggressively treated, usually with 100% oxygen via an endotracheal tube. Even with ideal pulmonary care, lung function may further deteriorate, with a clinical picture resembling acute respiratory distress syndrome. Prophylactic corticosteroid therapy may minimize the incidence of FES,[46] though this remains controversial. Other therapeutic regimens used after the development of FES, including heparinization, dextran, and parenteral ethanol, cannot be recommended.

◼ Amniotic Fluid Embolism

Amniotic fluid embolism was first described by Meyer[47] in 1926 and involves the introduction of amniotic fluid into the maternal circulation. In 1941, it was further characterized by two pathologists, Steiner and Lushbaugh, who reported the histologic findings in 42 women who died during the third trimester of pregnancy.[48] Nine of the women were found to have squamous cells and eosinophilic material possibly of fetal origin in their lungs. The pathologists suggested that this was a syndrome associated with tumultuous labor in multiparous older women. This description became the basis for the "classic" amniotic fluid embolism (AFE).

Estimates for the incidence of amniotic fluid embolism vary from 1 in 8000 to 1 in 80,000 pregnancies. It is currently the most common cause of peripartum deaths.[49] Clark and colleagues, reviewing the national registry of AFE, suggested the descriptive terminology "syndrome of acute peripartum cardiovascular collapse and coagulopathy" to describe AFE. They determined, in contrast to previously accepted notions, that no demographic variables, including maternal age, parity, race, or route of delivery of the infant, predicted elevated risk of AFE.[49] Fetal elements were present in the pulmonary vasculature of 73% of the patients with AFE. Interestingly, the syndrome was not associated more frequently with vasopressin-induced labor, nor was cesarean section an apparent risk factor. The authors did note a strong temporal association to placement of intrauterine monitoring devices or

artificial rupture of membranes and presentation of AFE symptoms. A significant association was made between AFE and male sex of the fetus.

Amniotic fluid embolism may present initially as seizures or seizure-like states or with cardiopulmonary symptoms including acute dyspnea, hypotension, pulmonary edema, or cardiac arrest.[50] Cardiac events are relatively evenly distributed between pulseless electrical activity, severe bradycardias, ventricular tachycardias, and asystole.

Patients with AFE who survive the initial insult usually proceed to a consumption coagulopathy. This is associated with fibrinogen depletion, increased fibrin split products, elevation of prothrombin and activated partial thromboplastin times, as well as decreased platelet levels.[51]

Unlike other embolic diseases discussed in this chapter, exposure to fetal products usually does not generate the AFE syndrome. In fact, it has been demonstrated that amniotic fluid infusion into the maternal circulation is generally innocuous.[52] This is fortunate because the outcome, over 50 years since the syndrome was described, remains dismal. Fewer than 15% of women who are stricken with AFE survive neurologically intact.[53]

Even with ideal care, AFE remains a disease with an extremely poor outcome. In spite of rapid and aggressive resuscitation, neurologic sequelae are common in the survivors. That AFE should present often as seizures or a seizure-like state is relatively surprising, but such presentations may be due to profound hypoxia as well as hypotensive insults to the central nervous system.

Clark and colleagues[49] have suggested that AFE may share similar mechanisms to septic shock and other anaphylactoid responses. The premise is that fetal components in the amniotic fluid initiate a complex inflammatory cascade with resultant cardiopulmonary collapse. The coagulopathy may be due to the activation of clotting cascades by amniotic fluid containing platelet factor III, factor X-like properties, as well as functionally active tissue factor.[53,54] Tissue factor when combined with maternal factor VII will activate the extrinsic coagulation pathway.[53]

The diagnosis of AFE is primarily one of exclusion. It should be entertained in any pregnant woman who experiences acute cardiovascular collapse or coagulopathy. It has been described in women undergoing first-trimester therapeutic abortions as well as during the peripartum period. There is no definitive diagnostic test for AFE. Demonstrating fetal matter in the pulmonary vasculature on autopsy supports the diagnosis but is nonspecific.[55] Aspirating from a wedged pulmonary artery catheter or sampling mixed venous blood for fetal elements may also help support the diagnosis,[56] although in one study only 50% of patients being resuscitated for presumed AFE had fetal elements aspirated by a wedged pulmonary artery catheter.

Treatment of AFE is largely supportive. Initial cardiopulmonary resuscitation should be performed, with left lateral displacement to maintain uterine perfusion and venous return. Management should be directed toward maintaining oxygenation, usually with 100% oxygen through an endotracheal tube. Additional cardiovascular support should be initiated rapidly with volume and pressors if necessary. If the fetus has not yet been delivered, this should be accomplished by emergent cesarean section.[57] An arterial line and pulmonary catheter may help guide therapy.[55] Epinephrine may be a first-line agent of choice, as it is in other anaphylactoid reactions. Corticosteroids may be helpful, but therapeutic heparinization to minimize consumption coagulopathy remains controversial.[55]

It is vital to aggressively follow the coagulation profile and treat the disseminated intravascular coagulation (DIC) that frequently ensues once the initial cardiovascular collapse has been managed. The mortality from DIC may be as great as 75% in spite of optimal therapy.[53] Treatment is usually with blood components, including red blood cells followed by platelets, fresh frozen plasma, and cryoprecipitate.[58] Use of recombinant factor VIIa[59] and aprotinin[60] have been reported in the literature, but studies are lacking. Recently, aprotinin has been withdrawn from the market based on increased adverse events compared to other antifibrinolytics.

KEY POINTS

Gas Embolism

1. Venous gas embolism may become an arterial embolism through intracardiac or extracardiac right-to-left shunting. Arterial gas embolus must be diagnosed early so hyperbaric therapy can be rapidly initiated.

2. Treatment of venous gas embolism is prevention of further air entry into the venous circulation and cardiopulmonary support with emphasis on reestablishing stable hemodynamics. For arterial gas embolism, the definitive therapy is hyperbaric oxygen therapy.

Fat Embolism Syndrome

3. Fat embolism syndrome presents as acute respiratory collapse. It is a diagnosis that should be entertained early after orthopedic surgeries and trauma to the long bones. It remains a diagnosis of exclusion.

Amniotic Fluid Embolism

4. Amniotic fluid embolism is managed initially with aggressive cardiopulmonary support. In the post-resuscitation period, the coagulation profile should be closely followed for the appearance of disseminated intravascular coagulation (DIC).

5. Amniotic fluid embolism may strike any woman in the peripartum period. Risk factors often cited for amniotic fluid embolus, such as tumultuous labor or multiparity in an older woman, have not been demonstrated in recent reviews. It is a syndrome of peripartum cardiovascular collapse and coagulopathy.

ANNOTATED REFERENCES

Conde-Agudelo A, Romero R. Amniotic fluid embolism: an evidence-based review. Am J Obstet Gynecol 2009;201(5):445.e1-445.e13.
An evidence-based review of the literature on amniotic fluid embolism cases. This review discusses the presentation, outcome, and possible pathophysiology while underscoring the difficulties in studying a rare event with much conflicting literature.
Georgopoulos D, Bouros D. Fat embolism syndrome: clinical examination is still the preferable diagnostic method (editorial). Chest 2003;123(4):982-3.
A well-written and compelling discussion of the new diagnostic modalities to aid in the diagnosis of fat embolism syndrome and the reasons why clinical criteria remain the preferred method for diagnosing FES.

Kim YH, Oh SW, Kim JS. Prevalence of fat embolism following bilateral simultaneous and unilateral total hip arthroplasty performed with or without cement. J Bone Joint Surg Am 2002;84-A(8):1372-9.
A randomized prospective study comparing the incidence of fat emboli in femoral necks that were cemented versus those that were not cemented during hip arthroplasties.
Muth CM, Shank ES. Gas embolism. N Engl J Med 2000;342(7):476-82.
This review article discusses the variety of iatrogenic mechanisms able to generate gas emboli and presents current recommendations for treatment.

REFERENCES

Access the complete reference list online at http://www.expertconsult.com.

64

Pulmonary Hypertension

LEWIS J. RUBIN

Pulmonary hypertension (PH) is defined as a pulmonary artery mean pressure (PAPm) of 25 mm Hg or greater and may be precapillary or postcapillary in etiology. Postcapillary causes include processes affecting the left side of the heart (e.g., left ventricular systolic or diastolic dysfunction, mitral stenosis or regurgitation, aortic valvular disease) or, more rarely, the pulmonary veins (pulmonary veno-occlusive disease). Management of postcapillary PH typically involves treating the underlying left-sided cardiac process. Medications used to treat precapillary PH are often not only ineffective for postcapillary PH but may in fact be harmful, potentially leading to the development of pulmonary edema.

Precapillary PH, or pulmonary arterial hypertension (PAH), can be idiopathic (IPAH—previously known as *primary pulmonary hypertension* [PPH]) or may occur in association with a variety of underlying disease processes such as collagen vascular disease, portal hypertension, congenital systemic-to-pulmonary shunts, drug or toxin exposure, or HIV infection.[1] IPAH is principally a disease of young women, but it can affect all age groups and both sexes. A genetic predisposition may underlie a substantial proportion of these cases.[2-8]

Initial therapy may be directed at an underlying cause or contributing factor, such as using continuous positive airway pressure (CPAP) and supplemental oxygen for PH associated with obstructive sleep apnea. Following identification and treatment of underlying associated disorders and contributing factors, specific therapy for PAH should be considered. IPAH carried a very poor prognosis (median survival approximately 2.8 years from the date of diagnosis) through the mid-1980s. Subsequently, a number of therapeutic options have been developed, and seven have been approved by the U.S. Food and Drug Administration (FDA), falling into three classes of drugs: (1) prostacyclins, including intravenous epoprostenol, treprostinil (subcutaneously, intravenously, and by inhalation), and inhaled iloprost; (2) endothelin receptor antagonists (bosentan, ambrisentan); and (3) phosphodiesterase type-5 inhibitors, including sildenafil and tadalafil. Other agents being studied for PAH include guanylate cyclase activators, tyrosine kinase inhibitors, and vasoactive intestinal peptide (VIP).

Diagnosis

SYMPTOMS, SIGNS, AND CLINICAL HISTORY

Because of the insidious onset of symptoms, PAH is often advanced at the time of diagnosis. Dyspnea on exertion is a common presenting symptom, but it is sometimes attributed to deconditioning or other cardiorespiratory ailment. Chest pain, mimicking angina pectoris, may occur. Patients with advanced disease may present with syncope or signs and symptoms of right-sided heart failure, including lower extremity edema, jugular venous distention, and ascites.

The clinical history should focus initially on exclusion of underlying causes of PH. Important clues to an underlying condition might include previous history of a heart murmur, deep venous thrombosis or pulmonary embolism, Raynaud's phenomenon, arthritis, arthralgias, rash, heavy alcohol consumption, hepatitis, heavy snoring, daytime hypersomnolence, morning headache, and morbid obesity. A careful family history should be obtained. Medication exposures, particularly to appetite suppressants and amphetamines, should be noted.

Cocaine is a powerful vasoconstrictor and may contribute to the development of PH. Intravenous drug abuse has been associated with the development of PAH.

PHYSICAL EXAMINATION

Signs of PAH may not become apparent until late in the disease. Findings such as an accentuated second heart sound, a systolic murmur over the left sternal border, jugular venous distention, peripheral edema, and/or ascites might suggest the presence of PH and right ventricular dysfunction. Associated systemic diseases such as collagen vascular disease or liver disease may also become apparent during routine examination.

LABORATORY EVALUATION

Laboratory evaluation can provide important information in detecting associated disorders and contributing factors. A collagen vascular screen including antinuclear antibodies, rheumatoid factor, and erythrocyte sedimentation rate is often helpful in detecting autoimmune disease, although some patients with IPAH will have a low-titer positive antinuclear antibody test.[9] The scleroderma spectrum of disease, particularly limited scleroderma, or the CREST syndrome (calcinosis, Raynaud's phenomenon, esophageal dysfunction, sclerodactyly, telangiectasias), has been associated with an increased risk for the development of PAH.[10,11] Liver function tests (aspartate aminotransferase, alanine aminotransferase, alkaline phosphatase) may be elevated in patients with right ventricular failure and passive hepatic congestion but may also be associated with underlying liver disease. Liver disease with portal hypertension has been associated with the development of PH. Thyroid disease may occur with increased frequency in patients with IPAH and should be excluded with thyroid function testing.[12] Human immunodeficiency virus (HIV) testing and hepatitis serologic studies should be considered in patients at risk. Routine laboratory studies such as complete blood cell count, complete metabolic panel, prothrombin time, and partial thromboplastin time are recommended during the initial evaluation and as indicated to monitor the patient's long-term clinical status.

ECHOCARDIOGRAPHY

Doppler echocardiography is useful in estimating the severity of PH and detecting left-sided heart disease. Findings may include enlargement of the right ventricle, flattening of the interventricular septum, and compression of the left ventricle. Bubble contrast echocardiography may detect a right-to-left shunt, but exclusion of a left-to-right intracardiac shunt may require cardiac catheterization with an oximetry series. Echocardiography may be a useful noninvasive means of long-term follow-up,[13,14] although not all patients have suitable echocardiographic windows.

RADIOGRAPHIC EVALUATION AND EXCLUSION OF THROMBOEMBOLIC DISEASE

Chest radiography may reveal enlargement of the central pulmonary vessels and evidence of right ventricular enlargement. Evidence of parenchymal lung disease may be apparent. When parenchymal lung disease is suspected, pulmonary function testing and high-resolution computed tomography (CT) of the chest may be indicated. Ventilation/perfusion (V/Q) lung scanning should be performed in an attempt to exclude chronic recurrent pulmonary thromboembolic disease, which is among the most preventable and treatable causes of PH. Diffuse mottled perfusion can be seen in IPAH, whereas larger segmental and subsegmental mismatched defects are suggestive of chronic recurrent pulmonary thromboembolic disease. Intermediate results on V/Q lung scanning may require pulmonary arteriography to obtain a definitive diagnosis. Although contrast medium–enhanced CT has been popularized recently for the diagnosis of acute pulmonary thromboembolic disease, there is limited experience with this technique in chronic thromboembolic disease. Accordingly, we recommend caution at present in using contrast-enhanced CT to exclude chronic recurrent thromboembolic disease.

PULMONARY FUNCTION TESTING

Pulmonary function testing is indicated to detect underlying parenchymal lung disease. The diffusing capacity is often reduced in pulmonary vascular disease, consistent with impaired gas exchange.

RIGHT-SIDED HEART CATHETERIZATION AND VASOREACTIVITY TESTING

Right-sided heart catheterization remains an important part of the evaluation. Left-sided heart dysfunction and intracardiac shunts can be excluded, the degree of PH can be accurately quantified, and cardiac output can be measured. Pulmonary vascular resistance can then be calculated. Acute pulmonary vasoreactivity can be assessed using a short-acting agent such as prostacyclin (epoprostenol), inhaled nitric oxide, or intravenous adenosine.[1] The consensus definition of a positive acute vasodilator response in a PAH patient is a fall of PAPm of at least 10 mm Hg to ≤40 mm Hg, with an increased or unchanged cardiac output. The primary objective of acute vasodilator testing in patients with PAH is to identify patients who might be effectively treated with oral calcium channel blockers. The acute response to a short-acting agent such as prostacyclin has been shown to be predictive of the response to a calcium channel blocker.[14] Unstable patients or those in severe right-sided heart failure who would not be candidates for treatment with calcium channel blockers need not undergo vasodilator testing.

Treatment

GENERAL CARE

Warfarin, Oxygen, Diuretics, Digoxin, and Vaccination

Improved survival has been reported with oral anticoagulation in IPAH.[15,16] The target International Normalized Ratio (INR) in these patients is 1.5 to 2.5. Anticoagulation of patients with PAH due to other underlying processes such as scleroderma or congenital heart disease is controversial. Generally, patients with PAH treated with chronic intravenous epoprostenol are anticoagulated in the absence of contraindications, owing in part to the additional risk of catheter-associated thrombosis.

Hypoxemia is a pulmonary vasoconstrictor and can contribute to the development or progression of PAH. It is generally considered important to maintain oxygen saturations at greater than 90% at all times. Supplemental oxygen use is more controversial in patients with Eisenmenger physiology but may decrease the need for phlebotomy and potentially reduce the occurrence of neurologic dysfunction and complications.

Diuretics are indicated in patients with evidence of right ventricular failure and volume overload (i.e., peripheral edema and/or ascites). Careful dietary restriction of sodium and fluid intake is important in the management of patients with PAH with right-sided heart failure. Rapid and excessive diuresis may produce systemic hypotension, renal

insufficiency, and syncope. Serum electrolytes and measures of renal function should be followed closely in patients receiving diuretic therapy.

Although not extensively studied in PAH, digitalis is sometimes utilized in refractory right ventricular failure or atrial dysrhythmias. Drug levels should be followed closely, particularly in patients with impaired renal function.

Because of the potentially devastating effects of respiratory infections in PAH, immunization against influenza and pneumococcal pneumonia is recommended.

Calcium Channel Blockers

Patients with IPAH who respond to vasodilators and calcium channel blockers[15] generally have improved survival. Unfortunately, this tends to represent a relatively small proportion of patients, comprising fewer than 20% of IPAH patients and even fewer patients with other causes of PAH.

Prostanoids

Prostacyclin, a metabolite of arachidonic acid produced primarily in vascular endothelium, is a potent systemic and pulmonary vasodilator that also has antiplatelet aggregatory effects. A relative deficiency of endogenous prostacyclin may contribute to the pathogenesis of PAH.[17]

Epoprostenol. Epoprostenol therapy is complicated by the need for continuous intravenous infusion. The drug is unstable at room temperature and is generally best kept cold before and during infusion. It has a very short half-life in the bloodstream (<6 minutes), is unstable at acidic pH, and cannot be taken orally. Because of the short half-life, the risk of rebound worsening with abrupt/inadvertent interruption of the infusion, and its effects on peripheral veins, it should be administered through an indwelling central venous catheter. Common side effects of epoprostenol therapy include headache, flushing, jaw pain with initial mastication, diarrhea, nausea, a blotchy erythematous rash, and musculoskeletal aches and pain (predominantly involving the legs and feet). These tend to be dose dependent and often respond to a cautious reduction in dose. Severe side effects can occur with overdosage of the drug. Acutely, overdosage can lead to systemic hypotension. Chronic overdosage can lead to the development of a hyperdynamic state and high-output cardiac failure.[18] Abrupt or inadvertent interruption of the epoprostenol infusion should be avoided because this may lead to a rebound worsening of PH, with symptomatic deterioration and even death. Other complications of chronic intravenous therapy with epoprostenol include line-related infections (which can range from small exit-site reactions to tunnel infections and cellulitis to bacteremic infections with sepsis), catheter-associated venous thrombosis, systemic hypotension, thrombocytopenia, and ascites.

Treprostinil. Treprostinil, a prostacyclin analog with a half-life of 3 hours, is stable at room temperature. An international placebo-controlled, randomized trial demonstrated that treprostinil improved exercise tolerance, although the 16-meter median difference between treatment groups in 6-minute walk distance was relatively modest.[19] Treprostinil also improved hemodynamic parameters. Common side effects included headache, diarrhea, nausea, rash, and jaw pain. Side effects related to the infusion site were common (85% of patients complained of infusion-site pain, and 83% had erythema or induration at the infusion site). Treprostinil is also approved for intravenous delivery based on bioequivalence with the subcutaneous route and is also approved as an inhaled preparation administered in doses of 6 to 54 μg, 4 times daily.[20]

Inhaled Iloprost. Iloprost is a chemically stable prostacyclin analog with a serum half-life of 20 to 25 minutes.[21] In IPAH, acute inhalation of iloprost resulted in a more potent pulmonary vasodilator effect than acute nitric oxide inhalation.[21,22] In uncontrolled and controlled studies of iloprost for various forms of PAH,[23,24] inhaled iloprost at a total daily dose of 30 to 200 μg divided in 6 to 12 inhalations improved functional class, exercise capacity, and pulmonary hemodynamics for periods up to 1 year of follow-up. The treatment was generally well tolerated except for mild coughing, minor headache, and jaw pain in some patients. The most important drawback of inhaled iloprost is the relatively short duration of action, requiring the use of 6 to 9 inhalations a day.

Beraprost. Beraprost sodium is an orally active prostacyclin analog[25] that is absorbed rapidly in fasting conditions. It has been evaluated in peripheral vascular disorders such as intermittent claudication,[26] Raynaud's phenomenon, and digital necrosis in systemic sclerosis,[27] with variable results. Although several small, open, uncontrolled studies reported beneficial hemodynamic effects with beraprost in patients with IPAH, two randomized double-blind, placebo-controlled trials have shown only modest improvement and suggest that beneficial effects of beraprost may diminish with time.[28,29]

Endothelin Receptor Antagonists

Endothelin-1 is a vasoconstrictor and a smooth muscle mitogen that may contribute to the pathogenesis of PAH. Endothelin-1 expression, production, and concentration in plasma[30,31] and lung tissue[32] are elevated in patients with PAH, and these levels are correlated with disease severity.

Bosentan. Bosentan is a dual endothelin receptor blocker that has been shown to improve pulmonary hemodynamics and exercise tolerance and delay the time to clinical worsening in PAH patients falling into NYHA Classes III and IV.[33,34] The most frequent and potentially serious side effect with bosentan is dose-dependent abnormal hepatic function (as indicated by elevated levels of alanine aminotransferase and/or aspartate aminotransferase). Because of the risk of potential hepatoxicity, the FDA requires that liver function tests be performed at least monthly in patients receiving this drug. Bosentan may also be associated with the development of anemia, which is typically mild; hemoglobin/hematocrit should be checked regularly.

Ambrisentan. Ambrisentan is a selective endothelin-A receptor antagonist that has been shown to be effective in PAH.[35] The usual doses are 5 to 10 mg daily.

Phosphodiesterase Inhibitors

Phosphodiesterases (PDEs) are enzymes that hydrolyze the cyclic nucleotides, cyclic adenosine monophosphate (cAMP) and cyclic guanosine monophosphate (cGMP), and limit their intracellular signaling. Drugs that selectively inhibit cGMP-specific PDEs (or type 5 PDE5 inhibitors) augment the pulmonary vascular response to endogenous or inhaled nitric oxide in models of PH.[36-37] PDE5 is strongly expressed in the lung, and PDE5 gene expression and activity are increased in chronic PH.[38]

Sildenafil. Sildenafil is a potent specific PDE5 inhibitor that is approved for erectile dysfunction. Recent reports have shown that sildenafil blocks acute hypoxic pulmonary vasoconstriction in healthy adult volunteers and acutely reduces PAPm in patients with PAH.[39] In comparison with inhaled nitric oxide, sildenafil produced similar reductions in PAPm; but unlike nitric oxide, sildenafil also had apparent systemic hemodynamic effects. When combined with inhaled nitric oxide, sildenafil appears to augment and prolong the effects of inhaled nitric oxide,[40] and it appears to prevent rebound pulmonary vasoconstriction after acute withdrawal of inhaled nitric oxide.[41] Several randomized studies have demonstrated sildenafil's efficacy in PAH, both as monotherapy and in combination with epoprostenol.[42,43] Sildenafil treatment in animal models with experimental lung injury reduced

PAP, but gas exchange worsened owing to impaired V/Q mismatch.[44,45] Accordingly, caution is advised when using sildenafil to treat PH in patients with severe lung disease.

Tadalafil. The FDA recently approved tadalafil, another PDE5 inhibitor previously approved for erectile dysfunction, for the treatment of PAH based on a randomized clinical trial.[46] Side effects appear similar to sildenafil. The recommended dosage is 40 mg daily.

Nitric Oxide

Nitric oxide contributes to maintenance of normal vascular function and structure. It is particularly important in normal adaptation of the lung circulation at birth, and impaired nitric oxide production may contribute to the development of neonatal PH. L-Arginine is the sole substrate for nitric oxide synthase and thus is essential for nitric oxide production.

Inhaled Nitric Oxide. Inhaled nitric oxide has been shown to have potent and selective pulmonary vasodilator effects during brief treatment of adults with IPAH.[47] It is a potent pulmonary vasodilator in newborns with PH (persistent pulmonary hypertension of the newborn [PPHN]), children with congenital heart disease, and patients with postoperative PH, acute respiratory distress syndrome, or undergoing lung transplantation.[48] It is of substantial benefit in PPHN, decreasing the need for support with extracorporeal membrane oxygenation (ECMO).[49] Although inhaled nitric oxide has been used in diverse clinical settings, especially in intensive care medicine, FDA approval for this therapy is limited to newborns with hypoxemic respiratory failure at this time.

In chronic PAH, the use of inhaled nitric oxide has been primarily for acute testing of pulmonary vasoreactivity during cardiac catheterization[1] (see earlier) or for acute stabilization of patients during deterioration.

LUNG TRANSPLANTATION

Lung transplantation for PAH is generally reserved for patients whose condition is failing despite the best available medical therapy. Whereas lung transplantation is challenging in general, it is even more so in the group of patients with PAH.[50] Worldwide, overall survival is approximately 77% at 1 year and 44% at 5 years.[51] Survival in PAH patients undergoing lung transplantation is 66% to 75% at 1 year (one center has reported 1- and 5-year actuarial survival of 75% and 57%, respectively).[52] The higher early mortality in PAH patients may be related to higher anesthetic and operative risks, the need for cardiopulmonary bypass,[53] and the increased occurrence of postoperative reperfusion pulmonary edema in patients with PAH undergoing single lung transplantation. In this situation, reperfusion pulmonary edema may be aggravated by the increased blood flow to the newly engrafted lung. In addition, V/Q mismatching can be particularly severe.[54] Most centers therefore seem to prefer bilateral lung transplantation for patients with PAH.[55] The timing of transplantation in PAH is challenging. It is probably most useful in patients showing clear evidence of deterioration such as decline in functional capacity and the development of right-sided heart failure despite maximal medical therapy.

▣ Special Situations in the Intensive Care Unit

DEEP VENOUS THROMBOSIS PROPHYLAXIS

Patients with PAH are likely at increased risk for the occurrence of deep venous thrombosis (DVT) and are certainly at increased risk for poor outcomes as a consequence of the development of DVT. Patients with PAH are prone to a more sedentary lifestyle and to chronic venous congestion of the lower extremities owing to increased right-sided cardiac filing pressures. Hospitalization in the ICU, often with discontinuation of anticoagulation in anticipation of invasive procedures, likely places these patients at even higher risk for DVT. For these reasons, meticulous attention must be paid to DVT prophylaxis.

PROCEDURES AND SURGERY

Procedures and surgery in patients with PAH can be associated with substantially increased operative and perioperative risks, and appropriate precautions should be undertaken to optimize outcomes. As always, careful consideration should be given to whether an invasive procedure is absolutely necessary.

Vasovagal Events

Patients with severe PAH are particularly prone to vasovagal events, which can lead to severe consequences including syncope, cardiopulmonary arrest, and death. Pain, nausea, vomiting, or even a bowel movement can lead to a vasovagal event in patients with severe PAH. Cardiac output may be particularly dependent on heart rate in this situation, and the bradycardia and systemic vasodilatation that accompany a vasovagal event can therefore result in an abrupt decrease in systemic arterial pressure. Patients should therefore have close monitoring of their heart rate during invasive procedures, with ready availability of atropine or a similar agent.

Avoidance of Hypoxemia and Hypercarbia

Hypoxemia and hypercarbia are both pulmonary vasoconstrictors and can contribute to the worsening of PH. Oversedation can lead to ventilatory insufficiency and precipitate clinical deterioration. Caution should be utilized in laparoscopic procedures in which carbon dioxide is used for abdominal insufflation, because absorption can lead to hypercarbia. The induction of anesthesia and intubation for surgical procedures can be a particularly high-risk time for patients with PAH, because they are at risk for vagal events, hypoxemia, hypercarbia, and shifts in intrathoracic pressure with associated changes in cardiac filling pressures.

PREGNANCY

The hemodynamic changes in pregnancy are substantial, and volume shifts occur immediately postpartum, with cardiac filling pressures increasing as a result of decompression of the vena cava and the return of uterine blood into the systemic circulation. The changes induced by pregnancy impose a significant hemodynamic stress in women with IPAH, leading to an estimated 30% to 50% mortality rate.[56,57] A meta-analysis of the outcome of pulmonary vascular disease and pregnancy reported a maternal mortality rate of 36% in Eisenmenger's syndrome, 30% in IPAH, and 56% in secondary PH.[58] Because of high maternal and fetal morbidity and mortality rates, most experts recommend effective contraception and early fetal termination in the event of pregnancy.[59] There have been case reports of successful treatment of pregnant IPAH patients with chronic intravenous epoprostenol,[60-62] inhaled nitric oxide,[63-65] and oral calcium channel blockers.[66] Endothelin receptor antagonists are classified as teratogenic and should be avoided in this setting. In general, management includes early hospitalization for monitoring, supportive therapy with cautious fluid management, supplemental oxygen, diuretics, and dobutamine, as needed. The use of a pulmonary artery catheter for close hemodynamic monitoring and titration of vasodilator and cardiotonic therapy has been recommended. Recommendations regarding mode of delivery remain controversial.

PORTOPULMONARY HYPERTENSION

Patients with chronic liver disease have an increased prevalence of pulmonary vascular disease.[67,68] Two forms of pulmonary vascular disease can complicate chronic liver disease: the hepatopulmonary syndrome and portopulmonary hypertension. Both tend to occur in patients with chronic, late-stage liver disease, and each may increase the risk associated with liver transplantation.

Hypoxemia and intrapulmonary shunting characterize the hepatopulmonary syndrome. Shunting may be manifest echocardiographically by the late appearance (after three to five cardiac cycles) of bubble contrast in the left side of the heart. Treatment is generally supportive, with supplemental oxygen. The syndrome may improve in some patients after liver transplantation. Severe hepatopulmonary syndrome may increase the risk associated with undergoing liver transplantation.

Portopulmonary hypertension occurs in patients with chronic, late-stage liver disease and/or portal hypertension.[69] Portopulmonary hypertension often differs hemodynamically from IPAH, and these differences may affect the approach to therapy. Patients with portopulmonary hypertension have lower pulmonary arterial diastolic and mean pressures, higher cardiac outputs, and lower pulmonary and systemic resistances.[70] Later-stage patients may develop hemodynamic findings more similar to those of patients with IPAH, and this group may have a poorer prognosis and be at higher risk with attempted liver transplantation. It is occasionally possible to make a borderline candidate for liver transplantation an acceptable one through aggressive treatment of the PAH. Supplemental oxygen should be used as needed to maintain saturations ≥ 91% at times. Diuretic therapy should be utilized to control volume overload, edema, and ascites. Anticoagulant therapy has not been carefully studied in this population and should probably be avoided in patients with significant coagulopathy due to impaired hepatic synthetic capability and in patients at increased risk of bleeding due to gastroesophageal varices. There have been a number of case reports and small case series describing the use of intravenous epoprostenol for treatment of portopulmonary hypertension.[71-75] Interestingly, some patients may demonstrate improvement in their PH after liver transplantation.[76] Other patients may develop worsening of their PH well after transplantation. It may be possible to wean an occasional patient off epoprostenol after liver transplantation. This should probably be done very gradually under close observation. The development of increasing dyspnea, fluid retention, or fatigue should prompt reevaluation and reinstitution of epoprostenol if necessary. Because of its potential for hepatoxicity, caution is advised in using the oral endothelin antagonists in this population.

KEY POINTS

1. The evaluation of patients with pulmonary hypertension (PH) is directed at the detection of underlying contributing factors and associated conditions such as left-sided cardiac dysfunction, underlying congenital heart disease, pulmonary thromboembolic disease, collagen vascular disease, parenchymal lung disease, obstructive sleep apnea, liver disease, amphetamine or appetite suppressant use, intravenous drug abuse, or human immunodeficiency virus (HIV) infection.

2. Patients with severe PH are particularly prone to vasovagal events, and when these occur they can lead to severe consequences, including syncope, cardiopulmonary arrest, and death.

3. Hypoxemia and hypercarbia are both pulmonary vasoconstrictors and can contribute to the worsening of pulmonary hypertension.

4. The induction of anesthesia and intubation for surgical procedures can be a particularly high-risk time for patients with PAH, as they are at risk for vagal events, hypoxemia, hypercarbia, and shifts in intrathoracic pressure with associated changes in cardiac filling pressures.

ANNOTATED REFERENCES

Barst RJ, Rubin LJ, Long, WA, et al. A comparison of continuous intravenous epoprostenol (prostacyclin) with conventional therapy for primary pulmonary hypertension. The Primary Pulmonary Hypertension Study Group. N Engl J Med 1996;334(5):296-302.
This prospective, multicenter, randomized, and controlled trial showed that chronic therapy with intravenous epoprostenol improved exercise capacity, cardiopulmonary hemodynamics, and survival in patients with IPAH.
Fuster V, Steele PM, Edwards WD, Gersh BJ, McGoon MD, Frye RL. Primary pulmonary hypertension: natural history and the importance of thrombosis. Circulation 1984;70(4):580-7.
This early study suggested that anticoagulation with warfarin improved survival in patients with IPAH.
International PPH Consortium, Lane KB, Machado RD, Pauciulo MW, et al. Heterozygous germline mutations in BMPR2, encoding a TGF-beta receptor, cause familial primary pulmonary hypertension. Nat Genet 2000;26(1):81-4.
Deng Z, Morse JH, Slager SL, et al. Familial primary pulmonary hypertension (gene PPH1) is caused by mutations in the bone morphogenetic protein receptor-II gene. Am J Hum Genet 2000;67(3):737-44.

These seminal papers report that mutations in the BMPR2 gene, encoding a TGF-beta receptor, cause familial PAH. This important discovery may provide critical insight into the mechanisms underlying the development of IPAH and ultimately lead to better-targeted and more effective therapy.
Rich S, Kaufmann E, Levy PS. The effect of high doses of calcium-channel blockers on survival in primary pulmonary hypertension. N Engl J Med 1992;327(2):76-81.
This study showed that a subset of patients with IPAH demonstrate vasoreactivity and will respond to chronic therapy with oral calcium channel blockers. It also supported the concept that anticoagulation with warfarin may improve survival in IPAH.
Rubin LJ, Badesch DB, Barst RJ, et al. Bosentan therapy for pulmonary arterial hypertension. N Engl J Med 2002;346(12):896-903.
This international, prospective, multicenter, randomized, placebo-controlled, double-blind trial showed that endothelin receptor blockade with bosentan improved exercise capacity in patients with IPAH and PAH occurring in association with collagen vascular disease.

REFERENCES

Access the complete reference list online at http://www.expertconsult.com.

65

Pleural Disease and Pneumothorax

J. TERRILL HUGGINS | PETER DOELKEN | STEVEN A. SAHN

Pleural disease is an unusual cause for admission to the intensive care unit (ICU). Exceptions are a large hemothorax for monitoring bleeding rate and hemodynamic status and an unstable secondary spontaneous pneumothorax or large unilateral or bilateral pleural effusions that have caused acute respiratory failure.

Pleural disease can be overlooked in the critically ill patient because it may be overshadowed by the presenting illness that has resulted in ICU admission. Furthermore, pleural disease is often a subtle finding on the clinical examination and supine chest radiograph. A pleural effusion may not be seen on the supine chest radiograph because a diffuse alveolar filling process can mask the posterior layering of fluid or because bilateral effusions without parenchymal infiltrates are misinterpreted as an underexposed film or objects outside the chest. Pneumothorax may remain undetected in the supine patient because pleural air tends to be situated anteriorly and does not produce the diagnostic visceral pleural line seen on an upright radiograph. When the patient on mechanical ventilation support is at increased risk for barotrauma because airway pressures are high, the index of suspicion for pneumothorax should be heightened; if there is evidence of pulmonary interstitial gas (see following discussion) or subcutaneous emphysema, appropriate radiologic studies should be obtained.

Radiologic Signs of Pleural Disease in the Intensive Care Unit

Because the distribution of fluid and air in the normal pleural space tends to follow gravitational influences, and because the lung has a tendency to maintain its normal shape as it becomes smaller, fluid initially accumulates between the bottom of the lung and the diaphragm, and air accumulates between the top of the lung and the apex of the thorax in the upright position. When chest radiographs are obtained in other than the erect position, free pleural fluid and air change position and result in a different radiographic appearance.

PLEURAL FLUID

Standard Chest Radiograph

In healthy humans in the supine position, the radiolucency of the lung base is equal to or greater than that in the lung apex.[1] Furthermore, when in the supine position, breast and pectoral tissue tend to fall laterally away from the lung base, so an effusion should be suspected if there is increased homogeneous density over the lower lung fields compared to the upper lung fields. As the pleural effusion increases, the increased radiodensity involves the upper hemithorax as well. However, failure of chest wall tissue to move laterally, cardiomegaly, prominent epicardial fat pad, and lung collapse or consolidation may obscure a pleural effusion on a supine radiograph. Patient rotation or an off-center x-ray beam can mimic a unilateral homogeneous density. An absent pectoral muscle, prior mastectomy, unilateral hyperlucent lung, scoliosis, previous lobectomy, hypoplastic pulmonary artery, or pleural or chest wall mass may lead to unilateral homogeneous increased density and mimic an effusion.

Approximately 175 to 525 mL of pleural fluid results in blunting of the costophrenic angle on an erect radiograph.[2] This quantity of effusion can be detected on a supine radiograph as an increased density over the lower lung zone. Failure to visualize the hemidiaphragm, absence of the costophrenic angle meniscus, and apical capping are less likely to be seen with effusions of less than 500 mL.[1] The major radiographic finding of a pleural effusion in a supine position is increased homogeneous density over the lower lung field that does not obliterate normal bronchovascular markings, does not show air bronchograms, and does not show hilar or mediastinal displacement until the effusion is massive. If a pleural effusion is suspected in the supine patient, ultrasonography should be performed.

Other Radiographic Imaging

Sonography. Ultrasonography (US) provides good characterization for pleural diseases and is a useful diagnostic modality for critically ill patients who cannot be transported for computed tomography (CT). US takes less time and is less expensive than CT, can be done at the bedside, and can be repeated serially. Disadvantages include hindrance of the ultrasonic wave by air, either in the lung or pleural space, a restricted field of view, inferior evaluation of the lung parenchyma compared to CT, and operator dependence. US was helpful in diagnosis in 27 (66%) of 41 patients and treatment in 37 (90%) of 41 patients, and had an important influence on treatment planning in 17 (41%) of 41 critically ill patients.[3]

US has also been demonstrated to be a useful modality to guide bedside thoracentesis in the mechanically ventilated patient, resulting in high success rate and excellent safety of the procedure.[4]

Computed Tomography. CT is recognized as providing increased resolution compared with conventional imaging. Although moving a critically ill patient for CT has potential risks, the diagnostic advantage is justified in the stable patient when the clinical course is incongruent with the proposed diagnosis suggested by the portable chest radiograph. In selected patients with multisystem trauma, chest CT often provides additional diagnostic information and positively affects patient management and outcome.

PNEUMOTHORAX

When supine, pneumothorax gas migrates along the anterior surface of the lung, making detection on the anteroposterior radiograph problematic. The base, lateral chest wall, and juxtacardiac area should be carefully visualized for evidence of pneumothorax. Accumulation of air along the mediastinal parietal pleura may simulate pneumomediastinum.[5] An erect or decubitus (suspected hemithorax up) radiograph should be obtained to assess for the presence of a pneumothorax. US is sensitive for the detection of pneumothorax by determining the presence or absence of "lung sliding."[6] In individuals without pneumothorax, the lung–chest wall interface, which represents a to-and-fro movement synchronized with respiration, can be identified. US visualization of lung sliding is correlated with the absence of pneumothorax, and from this sign alone, at least anterior pneumothorax can be excluded rapidly at the bedside of a mechanically ventilated patient. However, absence of lung sliding may be caused by the presence of large bullae or pleural symphysis caused by previous pleurodesis or pleural adhesions due to previous pleural disease. Hence, the absence of lung sliding is not specific for pneumothorax, but detection of lung sliding reliably excludes the presence of pleural air in the examined area.

The most common radiographic signs of tension pneumothorax are contralateral mediastinal shift, ipsilateral diaphragmatic depression, and ipsilateral chest wall expansion. Underlying lung disease may prevent total lung collapse even if tension is present; in patients on mechanical ventilation, little or no midline mediastinal shift may result from the tension.[7] In the latter, a depressed ipsilateral diaphragm is a more reliable sign of tension than mediastinal shift.

In patients with acute respiratory distress syndrome (ARDS), barotrauma can result in a localized tension pneumothorax with a subtle contralateral mediastinal shift, flattening of the cardiac contour, and depression of the ipsilateral hemidiaphragm.[8] Pleural adhesions and relative compressibility and mobility of surrounding structures, in addition to the supine position, probably account for these loculated tension pneumothoraces.

In a study of 88 critically ill patients with 112 pneumothoraces, the anteromedial and subpulmonic recesses were involved in 64% of patients in the supine and semierect position.[9] Furthermore, in 30% of the pneumothoraces in this study that were not initially detected by the clinician or radiologist, half the patients progressed to tension pneumothorax. Therefore, a high index of suspicion is necessary to avoid catastrophic situations.

Factors that may contribute to an improved ability to diagnose this potentially lethal problem include familiarity with atypical locations of pneumothoraces in critically ill patients, usually due to the supine or semierect position; the consequence of underlying cardiopulmonary disease; and knowledge of other risk factors contributing to misdiagnosis (e.g., mechanical ventilation, altered mental status, prolonged ICU stay, and development of pneumothorax after peak physician staffing hours).[10]

Evaluation of Pleural Effusion in the Intensive Care Unit

DIAGNOSTIC THORACENTESIS

Indications

Patients with a pleural effusion provide the opportunity to diagnose, at least presumptively, the underlying process responsible for pleural fluid accumulation. Pleural effusions are most commonly due to primary lung disease but may also result from disease in the gastrointestinal tract, liver, kidney, heart, or reticuloendothelial system.

Although disease of any organ system can cause a pleural effusion in critically ill patients, the diagnoses listed in Table 65-1 represent the majority of the causes seen in ICUs. The types of pleural effusions seen in medical and surgical ICUs are similar, but some causes related to surgical (coronary artery bypass grafting, chylothorax, abdominal surgery) and nonsurgical trauma (hemothorax) represent a substantial percentage of surgical ICU effusions.

When a pleural effusion is suspected on physical examination and confirmed radiologically, a diagnostic thoracentesis under ultrasonographic guidance should be performed in an attempt to establish the cause. Exceptions are patients with a secure clinical diagnosis and a small amount of pleural fluid, as in atelectasis, or patients with uncomplicated congestive heart failure (CHF).[13] Observation may be warranted in these situations, but thoracentesis should be performed if there are adverse changes.[11]

The indications for diagnostic thoracentesis do not change simply because the patient is in the ICU or on mechanical ventilation. In fact, establishing the diagnosis quickly in these critically ill patients may be more important and life saving than in non–critically ill patients. It has been well documented that even in patients on mechanical ventilation, diagnostic thoracentesis is safe if there is strict adherence to the general principles of the procedure and ultrasonography is used.[4,12] Pneumothorax, the most clinically important complication of thoracentesis,[13] is no more likely to occur in the patient on mechanical ventilation than in the patient who is not; however, if a pneumothorax does develop, the patient on mechanical ventilation is likely to develop a tension pneumothorax.

Contraindications

There are no absolute contraindications to diagnostic thoracentesis. If clinical judgment dictates that the information gained from the pleural fluid analysis may help in diagnosis and therapy, thoracentesis should be performed. Diagnostic thoracentesis with a small-bore needle can be performed safely in virtually any patient if meticulous technique is used. The major relative contraindications to thoracentesis are a bleeding diathesis or anticoagulation. A patient with a small amount of pleural fluid and a low benefit-to-risk ratio also represents a relative contraindication. Thoracentesis should not be attempted through an area of active skin infection.

Complications

Complications of diagnostic thoracentesis include pain at the needle insertion site, bleeding (local, intrapleural, or intraabdominal), pneumothorax, empyema, and spleen or liver puncture. Pneumothorax has been reported in prospective studies to occur in 4% to 30% of patients.[13,14-16] However, when ultrasound-guided thoracentesis is performed by experienced physician sonographers, pneumothorax or other injuries due to organ puncture appear to be rare events.[4] Liver or spleen puncture tends to occur when the patient is not sitting absolutely upright because movement toward recumbency causes cephalad migration of the abdominal viscera. The upward displacement of abdominal organs is readily detected by ultrasonography. However, even if the liver or spleen is punctured with a small-bore needle, generally the outcome is favorable if the patient is not receiving anticoagulants and does not have a bleeding diathesis.

THERAPEUTIC THORACENTESIS

Indications and Contraindications

The primary indication for therapeutic thoracentesis is relief of dyspnea. Contraindications to therapeutic thoracentesis are similar to those for diagnostic thoracentesis. However, there appears to be an increased risk of pneumothorax,[13] making a therapeutic thoracentesis in patients on mechanical ventilation potentially hazardous.

The technique for therapeutic thoracentesis is essentially the same as for diagnostic thoracentesis, except that a blunt-tip needle or plastic catheter, rather than a sharp-tip needle, should be used. This reduces the risk of pneumothorax, which may occur as fluid is removed and the lung expands toward the chest wall. Again, the use of sonographic guidance is recommended.[17]

The amount of fluid that can be removed safely from the pleural space at one session is controversial. Ideally, monitoring pleural pressure should dictate the amount of fluid that can be removed. As long as intrapleural pressure does not fall to less than −20 cm H_2O, fluid removal can continue.[18] However, intrapleural pressure monitoring is not done routinely. In the patient with contralateral mediastinal shift on chest radiograph who tolerates thoracentesis without chest tightness, cough, or light-headedness, probably several liters of pleural fluid can be removed safely, but neither the patient nor the operator

TABLE 65-1	Causes of Pleural Effusions	
In the Medical ICU	*In the Surgical ICU*
Atelectasis	Atelectasis
Congestive heart failure	Congestive heart failure
Pneumonia	Pneumonia
Hypoalbuminemia	Pancreatitis
Pancreatitis	Hypoalbuminemia
ARDS	Coronary artery bypass surgery
Pulmonary embolism	ARDS
Hepatic hydrothorax	Pulmonary embolism
Esophageal sclerotherapy	Esophageal rupture
Postmyocardial infarction	Hemothorax
Iatrogenic	Chylothorax
	Abdominal surgery
	Iatrogenic

ARDS, Acute respiratory distress syndrome; *ICU*, intensive care unit.

may be aware of a precipitous drop in pleural pressure. In patients without a contralateral mediastinal shift or with ipsilateral shift (suggesting an endobronchial obstruction), the likelihood of a precipitous drop in intrapleural pressure is increased, and pleural pressure should be monitored during thoracentesis. Alternatively, a small-bore catheter connected to a standard thoracostomy pleural drainage system may be temporarily inserted, thus avoiding excessively negative pleural pressure development during drainage. Simple gravity drainage or drainage using any system incorporating a non-return valve do not reliably guard against the development of excessively negative pressure.

Physiologic Effects and Complications

Improvement in lung volumes up to 24 hours after therapeutic thoracentesis does not correlate with the amount of fluid removed, despite relief of dyspnea in those patients.[19-21] In some patients, however, maximum spirometric improvement may not occur for several days. Patients with initial negative pleural pressures and those with more precipitous falls in pleural pressure with thoracentesis tend to have the least improvement in pulmonary function after therapeutic thoracentesis because many have a trapped lung or endobronchial obstruction.[18] The mechanism of dyspnea from a large pleural effusion probably is related to the increase in chest wall resting volume, resulting in shortening of the respiratory muscles' resting length and consequent decrease in contractile efficiency.[20] Drainage of moderately sized pleural effusions (1495 mL) does not appear to result in predictable changes in respiratory system compliance or resistances, although a systematic decrease in work performed by the ventilator as a consequence of thoracentesis has been reported.[22]

Complications of therapeutic thoracentesis are the same as those seen with diagnostic thoracentesis. Three complications unique to therapeutic thoracentesis are hypoxemia, unilateral pulmonary edema, and hypovolemia. After therapeutic thoracentesis, hypoxemia may occur despite relief of dyspnea[23,24] from worsening ventilation/perfusion relationships in the ipsilateral lung or clinically occult unilateral pulmonary edema.

Some investigators have concluded that the change in partial pressure of arterial oxygen (Pao_2) after therapeutic thoracentesis is unpredictable[24]; some have observed a characteristic increase in Pao_2 within minutes to hours,[19] and others suggest a systematic decrease in Pao_2 that returns to prethoracentesis values by 24 hours.[23] In the largest study including 33 patients with various causes of unilateral pleural effusions, a significant increase in Pao_2 was found at 20 minutes, 2 hours, and 24 hours after therapeutic thoracentesis.[25] This was in conjunction with a decrease in the alveolar-arterial oxygen gradient [$P(A-a)o_2$] and was accompanied by a small but significant decrease in shunt, without a change in the ratio of dead space to tidal volume (V_D/V_T). Data suggest an improved ventilation/perfusion relationship after therapeutic thoracentesis, with an increase in ventilation of parts of the lung that were previously poorly ventilated but well perfused. The relief of dyspnea in these patients cannot be explained by improved arterial oxygen tension.

Improvement in lung volumes is a constant finding after therapeutic thoracentesis but may take days or even weeks to maximize; immediate changes are usually modest and highly variable. Therefore, the relief of dyspnea cannot be adequately explained by changes in lung volume or in the mechanics of breathing but may be the result of decreased stimulation of lung or chest wall receptors, or both.[20]

The differential diagnosis of pleural effusions in critically ill patients is outlined in Table 65-2. Brief discussions of the more common etiologies follow.

ATELECTASIS

Atelectasis is a common cause of small pleural effusions in comatose, immobile, pain-ridden patients in ICUs[26] and after upper abdominal surgery.[27,28] Other causes include major bronchial obstruction from lung cancer or a mucous plug. Atelectasis causes pleural fluid because of decreased pleural pressure. With alveolar collapse, the lung and chest wall separate further, creating local areas of increased negative pressure. This decrease in pleural pressure favors the movement of fluid into the pleural space, presumably from the parietal pleural surface. The fluid accumulates until the pleural or parietal-pleural interstitial pressure gradient reaches a steady state.

Pleural fluid from atelectasis is a serous transudate with a low number of mononuclear cells, a glucose concentration equivalent to serum, and pH in the range of 7.45 to 7.55. When atelectasis resolves, pleural fluid dissipates during several days.

CONGESTIVE HEART FAILURE

CHF is the most common cause of transudative pleural effusions and a common cause of pleural effusions in ICUs. Pleural effusions due to CHF are associated with increases in pulmonary venous pressure.[29] Most patients with subacute or chronic elevation in pulmonary venous pressure (pulmonary capillary wedge pressure of at least 24 mm Hg) have evidence of pleural effusion on US or lateral decubitus radiograph. Isolated increases in systemic venous pressure tend not to produce pleural effusions. Thus, patients with chronic obstructive pulmonary disease (COPD) and cor pulmonale rarely have pleural effusions, and the presence of pleural fluid implies another cause.

Most patients with pleural effusions secondary to CHF have the classic signs and symptoms. The chest radiograph shows cardiomegaly and bilateral small to moderate pleural effusions of similar size (right slightly greater than left). There is usually radiographic evidence of pulmonary congestion, with the severity of pulmonary edema correlating with the presence of pleural effusion.[29]

The effusion associated with CHF is a transudate, with mesothelial cells and lymphocytes accounting for the majority of the less than 1,000 cells per μL.[12] Acute diuresis can raise the pleural fluid protein and lactate dehydrogenase into the range of an exudate.[30,31] In the patient with secure clinical diagnosis of CHF, observation is appropriate. Thoracentesis should be performed if the patient is febrile, has pleural effusions of disparate size, has a unilateral pleural effusion, does not have cardiomegaly, has pleuritic chest pain, or has a Pao_2 inappropriate for the degree of pulmonary edema.

Treatment consists of decreasing venous hypertension and improving cardiac output with diuretics, digitalis, and afterload reduction. In successfully managed heart failure, the effusions resolve during days to weeks after the pulmonary edema has cleared.

HEPATIC HYDROTHORAX

Pleural effusions occur in approximately 6% of patients with cirrhosis of the liver and clinical ascites. The effusions result from movement of ascitic fluid through congenital or acquired diaphragmatic defects.[32-34]

The patient usually has the classic stigmata of cirrhosis and clinically apparent ascites. The usual chest radiograph shows a normal cardiac silhouette and a right-sided pleural effusion, which can vary from small to massive; effusions are less likely isolated to the left pleural space or are bilateral.[32-35] Rarely, a massive pleural effusion may be found without clinical ascites (demonstrated only by US), implying the presence of a large diaphragmatic defect. The pleural fluid is a serous transudate with a low nucleated cell count and a predominance of mononuclear cells, pH greater than 7.40, and a glucose level similar to that of serum.[12] The fluid can be hemorrhagic due to an underlying coagulopathy or rupture of a diaphragmatic bleb. Demonstrating that pleural and ascitic fluids have similar protein and lactate dehydrogenase concentrations substantiates the diagnosis.[32] If the diagnosis is problematic, injection of a radionuclide into the ascitic fluid, with detection on chest imaging within 1 to 2 hours, supports a pleuroperitoneal communication through a diaphragmatic defect[36]; delayed demonstration of the tracer suggests that the pathogenesis of the effusion is via convection through the mesothelium.

Hepatic hydrothorax may be complicated by spontaneous bacterial empyema (SBE), which is analogous to spontaneous bacterial

TABLE 65-2	Differential Diagnosis of Pleural Effusions in Critically Ill Patients				
	Clinical Presentation	*Chest Radiograph*	*Pleural Fluid Analysis*	*Diagnosis*	*Comments*
Transudates					
Congestive heart failure	Usual signs and symptoms plus I > O, weight gain, worsening $(P_A\text{-}a)o_2$, ↓ C_{ST}	Bilateral effusions, right > left, cardiomegaly, extravascular lung water	Serous, nucleated cells <1000/μL, lymphocytes, mesothelial cells, pH 7.45-7.55	Presumptive	Associated with ↑ pulmonary capillary wedge pressure; acute diuresis may result in ↑ protein and LDH
Atelectasis	Asymptomatic or dyspnea, worsening $P(_A\text{-}a)o_2$	Small unilateral or bilateral effusions, volume loss	Serous, nucleated cells <1000/μL, lymphocytes, mesothelial cells, pH 7.45-7.55	Presumptive	Common after upper abdominal surgery, also with pulmonary embolism, mucous plug
Hepatic hydrothorax	Stigmata of liver disease, clinical ascites; asymptomatic or dyspnea, worsening $P(_A\text{-}a)o_2$, poor response to low-flow o_2	Unilateral right or bilateral effusions, small to massive, normal heart size, no other CXR abnormalities	Serous-serosanguineous, nucleated cells <1000/μL, lymphocytes, mesothelial cells, pH 7.40-7.55	Presumptive, PF protein and LDH similar to ascitic fluid	6% of patients with clinical ascites, fluid movement from abdomen to chest via diaphragm defect
Hypoalbuminemia	Asymptomatic or dyspnea, anasarca	Small to moderate bilateral effusions, normal heart size, no other CXR abnormalities	Serous, nucleated cells <1000/μL, lymphocytes, mesothelial cells, pH 7.45-7.55	Presumptive	Serum albumin <1.5 g/dL, never have isolated pleural effusion
Iatrogenic: extravascular migration of central venous catheter	Chest pain, dyspnea	Abnormal position of catheter, widening of mediastinum, small to large unilateral effusion	Serous-hemorrhagic or white, may contain PMNs, chemistries similar to infusate, PF/S glucose > 1.0	Presumptive	Highest incidence with left external jugular vein placement; aspiration or retrograde flow of blood confirms intravascular placement
Exudates					
Parapneumonic effusions: uncomplicated	Fever, chest pain, ↑ WBC, purulent sputum	New alveolar infiltrate, minimal to moderate ipsilateral free-flowing effusion	Turbid, PMNs, glucose >60 mg/dL, LDH <700 IU/L, pH ≥ 7.30	Presumptive	Effusion resolves without sequelae on antibiotics only
Parapneumonic effusions: complicated	Fever, chest pain, ↑ WBC, purulent sputum	New alveolar infiltrate, moderate to large ipsilateral effusion with or without loculation	Pus, positive bacteriology, pH <7.10, glucose <40 mg/dL, LDH >1000 IU/L	Based on PF acidosis, positive bacteriology, aspiration of pus, loculation	Putrid odor defines anaerobic empyema, requires pleural space drainage for resolution
Pancreatitis	Acute abdominal pain, nausea, vomiting, fever	Small, unilateral, left effusion (60%), atelectasis	Turbid, nucleated cells 10,000-50,000/μL, PMNs, pH 7.30-7.35, PF/S amylase >1.0	PF/S amylase >1.0 or > upper limits of normal for serum	Effusion resolves as pancreatitis resolves, without need for pleural space drainage
Pulmonary embolism	Acute dyspnea, tachypnea, chest pain, ↑ $P(_A\text{-}a)o_2$	Unilateral, small to moderate effusion, peripheral infiltrate, atelectasis	Serous-bloody nucleated cells 100-50,000/μL, PMNs or lymphocytes	Presumptive	20% transudates, effusion present on admission, ⅓ of hemithorax, reaches maximum volume by 72 h
Post–cardiac injury syndrome	Chest pain, pericardial rub, fever, dyspnea 3 d to 3 wk after cardiac injury, ↑ WBC, ↑ erythrocyte sedimentation rate	Left or bilateral small to moderate effusion, left lower lobe infiltrates	Serosanguineous-bloody, nucleated cells 500-39,000/μL, PMNs or lymphocytes, pH >7.30	Presumptive	Effusion resolves in 1-3 wk, may require steroids
Esophageal sclerotherapy	Chest pain following sclerotherapy with large sclerosant volume, effusion appears by 48-72 h	Small, unilateral or bilateral effusion	Serosanguineous, nucleated cells 100-38,000/μL, PMNs or mononuclear, pH >7.30	Presumptive	Requires no specific therapy, resolves in days to weeks
ARDS	Depends on cause	Bilateral alveolar infiltrates tend to mask small bilateral effusions	Serous-serosanguineous, PMNs	Presumptive	Requires no specific therapy, effusions resolve as ARDS resolves
Spontaneous esophageal rupture	Severe retching or vomiting followed by thoracoabdominal pain, fever, subcutaneous air	Subcutaneous/mediastinal air; left pneumothorax, followed by left effusion	Early: serous, pH >7.30; later: turbid-purulent effusion, PMNs, pH approaches 6.00, ↑ amylase	Pleural fluid pH < 7.00, with ↑ salivary amylase and positive bacteriology	With early diagnosis, prognosis good with primary closure and drainage
Hemothorax	Following blunt and penetrating chest trauma, invasive procedures, malignancy, anticoagulation	Small to massive unilateral effusion, other abnormalities depending on cause of hemothorax	Gross blood, PF/blood Hct >50%	PF/blood Hct > 50%	Often not appreciated on initial radiograph in setting of trauma; should be drained with chest tube
Coronary artery bypass graft	Asymptomatic, dyspnea	Small to moderate left effusion without parenchymal infiltrates, left lower lobe atelectasis, elevation of left hemidiaphragm	Hemorrhagic PF/blood Hct <5%, nucleated cells <10,000/μL, lymph predominant, pH >7.40	Presumptive	May require weeks for resolution, rarely results in trapped lung

TABLE 65-2	Differential Diagnosis of Pleural Effusions in Critically Ill Patients (Continued)				
	Clinical Presentation	*Chest Radiograph*	*Pleural Fluid Analysis*	*Diagnosis*	*Comments*
Abdominal surgery	Asymptomatic 48-72 h after upper abdominal surgery	Small bilateral effusions, atelectasis	Serous nucleated cells <10,000/μL (75%), pH usually >7.40	Presumptive	Larger left effusions following splenectomy, most commonly found with atelectasis and diaphragmatic irritation, resolves spontaneously
Chylothorax (traumatic)	Asymptomatic or dyspnea following intrathoracic surgery, especially coarctation repair and esophagectomy	Small to massive left, right, or bilateral effusion	Milky fluid, nucleated cells <7000/μL almost all lymphocytes, pH 7.40-7.80, ↑ triglycerides	Triglycerides >110 mg/dL, chylomicrons on lipoprotein electrophoresis	Defect in thoracic duct frequently closes spontaneously with tube drainage and minimizing chyle formation

ARDS, Acute respiratory distress syndrome; *CXR,* chest radiograph; ↓, decreased; Hct, hematocrit; ↑, increased; *I,* input; *LDH,* lactate dehydrogenase; *O,* output; *PF,* pleural fluid; *PF/S,* pleural fluid/serum; *PMN,* polymorphonuclear leukocyte; *WBC,* white blood cell.

peritonitis. The criteria for diagnosis of SBE are similar to those for the diagnosis of spontaneous bacterial peritonitis. SBE must be considered in the differential diagnosis of the infected cirrhotic patient, even in the absence of clinical ascites.[37,38] The pleural fluid culture and analysis may reveal positive culture, a total neutrophil count of more than 500 cells per μL, and a serum to pleural fluid albumin gradient greater than 1.1. The chest radiograph should not show a pneumonic process. Treatment of SBE is conservative with antibiotics unless purulence is present, in which case tube thoracostomy must be considered.

Treatment of hepatic hydrothorax is directed at resolution of the ascites, using sodium restriction and diuresis. The effusion frequently persists unchanged until all ascites is mobilized. If the patient is acutely dyspneic or in respiratory failure, therapeutic thoracentesis should be done as a temporizing measure. Care should be exercised with paracentesis or thoracentesis, because hypovolemia can occur with rapid evacuation of fluid. Chest tube insertion should be avoided, as it can cause infection of the fluid, and prolonged drainage can lead to protein and lymphocyte depletion and renal failure. Chemical pleurodesis via a chest tube is often unsuccessful owing to rapid movement of ascitic fluid into the pleural space. Treatment options in hepatic hydrothorax refractory to medical management include transjugular intrahepatic portal systemic shunt and video-assisted thoracoscopy to patch the diaphragmatic defect, followed by pleural abrasion or talc poudrage in the properly selected patient.[39,40]

HYPOALBUMINEMIA

Many patients admitted to a medical ICU have a chronic illness and associated hypoalbuminemia. When the serum albumin level falls below 1.8 g/dL, pleural effusions may be observed.[41] Because the normal pleural space has an effective lymphatic drainage system, pleural fluid tends to be the last collection of extravascular fluid that occurs in patients with low oncotic pressure. Therefore, it is unusual to find a pleural effusion solely due to hypoalbuminemia in the absence of anasarca. Patients with hypoalbuminemic pleural effusions tend not to have pulmonary symptoms unless there is underlying lung disease, since the effusions are rarely large. Chest radiograph shows small to moderate bilateral effusions and a normal heart size. The pleural fluid is a serous transudate with less than 1000 nucleated cells per μL, predominantly lymphocytes and mesothelial cells. The pleural fluid glucose level is similar to that of serum, and the pH is in the range of 7.45 to 7.55. Diagnosis is presumptive if other causes of transudative effusions can be excluded. The effusions resolve when hypoalbuminemia is corrected.

IATROGENIC CAUSES

Extravascular migration of a central venous catheter can cause pneumothorax, hemothorax, chylothorax, or a transudative pleural effusion.[42-44] Its incidence is estimated at less than 1% but may be considerably higher. Malposition of the catheter on placement should be suspected if there is absence of blood return or questionable central venous pressure measurements. The immediate postprocedure chest radiograph should be assessed for proper catheter placement; a catheter placed from the right side should not cross the midline. If the catheter is not in the appropriate vessel, phlebitis, perforation of a vein or the heart, or instillation of fluid into the mediastinum or pleural space can occur. In the alert patient, acute infusion of intravenous fluid into the mediastinum usually results in new-onset chest discomfort and dyspnea. Depending on the volume and the rate at which it is introduced into the mediastinum, tachypnea, worsening respiratory status, and cardiac tamponade may ensue. The chest radiograph shows the catheter tip in an abnormal position,[45,46] a widened mediastinum, and evidence of unilateral or bilateral pleural effusions. The effusion can have characteristics similar to those of the infusate (milky if lipid is being given) and may be hemorrhagic and neutrophil-predominant due to trauma and inflammation. The pleural fluid to serum glucose ratio is greater than 1.0 if glucose is being infused.[43] The pleural fluid glucose concentration can fall rapidly after glucose infusion into the pleural space, probably explaining the relatively low glucose concentrations in pleural fluid compared to the infusate.[47] Extravascular migration of a central venous catheter appears to be more common with placement in the external jugular vein, particularly on the left side. Left-sided catheters appear to put the patient at increased risk of perforation because of the horizontal orientation of the left compared to the right brachiocephalic vein. When catheters are introduced from the left side, they should be of adequate length for the tip to rest in the superior vena cava.

Free flow of fluid and proper fluctuation in central venous pressure during the respiratory cycle may not be reliable indicators of intravascular placement. This is probably because intrathoracic pressure changes are transmitted to the mediastinum and thus the venous pressure catheter. Aspiration of blood or retrograde flow of blood when the catheter is lowered below the patient's heart level should confirm intravascular catheter placement. If blood cannot be aspirated and the effusate is aspirated instead, extravascular migration is assured. The central venous catheter should be removed immediately. If there is a small effusion, observation is warranted. If the effusion is large, causing respiratory distress, or a hemothorax is discovered, thoracentesis or tube thoracostomy should be performed.

PARAPNEUMONIC EFFUSIONS

Community-acquired or nosocomial pneumonia is common in critically ill patients. The classic presentation is fever, chest pain, leukocytosis, purulent sputum, and a new alveolar infiltrate on chest radiograph. In the elderly debilitated patient, however, many of these findings may not be present. The chest radiograph commonly shows a small to large ipsilateral pleural effusion.[4,8,48-50] When the effusion is free flowing and anechoic on ultrasound, and thoracentesis shows a nonpurulent, polymorphonuclear (PMN) predominant exudate with a pH of 7.30 or greater, it is highly likely that the effusion will resolve during 7 to 14 days without sequelae with antibiotics alone (uncomplicated effusion). If the chest radiograph or CT demonstrates loculation and pus is aspirated, the diagnosis of empyema is established and immediate drainage is needed. In the free-flowing nonpurulent fluid, if Gram stain or culture is positive or pH is less than 7.30, the likelihood of a poor outcome increases, and the pleural space should be drained.

Although a meta-analysis found that low-risk patients with fluid pH between 7.20 and 7.30 may be managed without tube drainage, the patient admitted to the ICU typically cannot be considered low risk, and pH values of less than 7.30 should prompt drainage in most cases.[51-53] Drainage can be accomplished by standard chest tube or small-bore catheter. When loculations occur, pleural space drainage should be accomplished by placement of image-guided tubes or catheters with fibrinolytics or empyectomy and decortication.[54,55] Most thoracic surgeons routinely begin with thoracoscopy and, if not successful, proceed directly to a standard thoracotomy for empyectomy and decortication.[56-59]

PANCREATITIS

Pleuropulmonary abnormalities are commonly associated with pancreatitis, largely owing to the close proximity of the pancreas to the diaphragm. Approximately half of patients with pancreatitis have an abnormal chest radiograph, with pleural effusions in 3% to 17%.[60,61] Mechanisms that may be involved in the pathogenesis of pancreatic pleural effusion include direct contact of pancreatic enzymes with the diaphragm (sympathetic effusion), transfer of ascitic fluid via diaphragmatic defects, communication of a fistulous tract between a pseudocyst and the pleural space, and retroperitoneal movement of fluid into the mediastinum with mediastinitis or rupture into the pleural space.[60,62] Ascitic amylase moves into the pleural space via the previously mentioned mechanisms. The pleural fluid/serum amylase ratio is greater than one in pancreatitis because of slower lymphatic clearance from the pleural space compared with more rapid renal clearance.

The effusion associated with acute pancreatitis is usually small and left-sided (60%) but may be isolated to the right side (30%) or be bilateral (10%).[60] The patient usually presents with abdominal symptoms of acute pancreatitis. Diagnosis is confirmed by an elevated pleural fluid amylase concentration greater than that in serum. A normal pleural fluid amylase may be found early in acute pancreatitis but increases on serial measurements. The fluid is a polymorphonuclear (PMN)-predominant exudate with glucose values approximating those of serum. Leukocyte counts may reach 50,000 cells per µL. The pleural fluid pH is usually 7.30 to 7.35.

No specific treatment is necessary for the pleural effusion of acute pancreatitis; the effusion resolves as the pancreatic inflammation subsides. Drainage of the pleural space does not appear to affect residual pleural damage. If the pleural effusion does not resolve in 2 to 3 weeks, pancreatic abscess or pseudocyst should be excluded.

PULMONARY EMBOLISM

The presence of a unilateral pleural effusion may suggest pulmonary embolism or obscure the diagnosis by directing attention to a primary lung or cardiac process. Pleural effusions occur in approximately 40% of patients with pulmonary embolism.[63] These effusions result from several different mechanisms including increased pleural capillary permeability, imbalance in microvascular and pleural space hydrostatic pressures, and pleuropulmonary hemorrhage.[63,64] Ischemia from pulmonary vascular obstruction, in addition to release of inflammatory mediators from platelet-rich thrombi, can cause capillary leak into the lung and, subsequently, the pleural space, explaining the usual finding of an exudative effusion. Transudates, described in approximately 20% of patients with pulmonary embolism, result from atelectasis.[64]

With pulmonary infarction, necrosis and hemorrhage into the lung and pleural space may result. More than 80% of patients with infarction have bloody pleural effusions, but more than 35% of patients with pulmonary embolism without radiographic infarction also have hemorrhagic fluid.[63] The presence of a pleural effusion does not alter the signs or symptoms in patients with pulmonary embolism. Chest pain, usually pleuritic, occurs in most patients with pleural effusions complicating pulmonary embolism and is invariably ipsilateral.[63] The chest radiograph virtually always shows a unilateral effusion that occupies less than one-third of the hemithorax.[63] An associated pulmonary infiltrate (infarction) is seen in approximately half of patients with pulmonary embolism and effusion.

Pleural fluid analysis is variable and nondiagnostic.[64] The pleural fluid is hemorrhagic in two-thirds of patients, but the number of red blood cells exceeds 100,000 per µL in less than 20%.[64] The nucleated cell count ranges from less than 100 (atelectatic transudates) to greater than 50,000 per µL (pulmonary infarction).[64] There is a predominance of PMNs when a thoracentesis is performed near the time of the acute injury and of lymphocytes with later thoracentesis. The effusion due to pulmonary embolism is usually (92%) apparent on the initial chest radiograph and reaches a maximum volume during the first 72 hours.[63] Patients with pleural effusions that progress with therapy should be evaluated for recurrent embolism, hemothorax secondary to anticoagulation, an infected infarction, or an alternate diagnosis. When consolidation is absent on chest radiograph, effusions usually resolve in 7 to 10 days; with consolidation, the resolution time is 2 to 3 weeks.[64]

The association of pleural effusion with pulmonary embolism does not alter therapy. Furthermore, the presence of a bloody effusion is not a contraindication to full-dose anticoagulation because hemothorax is a rare complication of heparin therapy.[65] An enlarging pleural effusion on therapy necessitates thoracentesis to exclude hemothorax, empyema, or another cause. Active pleural space hemorrhage necessitates discontinuation of anticoagulation, tube thoracostomy, and placement of a vena cava filter.

POST–CARDIAC INJURY SYNDROME

Post–cardiac injury syndrome (PCIS) is characterized by fever, pleuropericarditis, and parenchymal infiltrates 3 weeks (2 to 86 days) after injury to the myocardium or pericardium.[66-68] PCIS has been described after myocardial infarction, cardiac surgery, blunt chest trauma, percutaneous left ventricular puncture, and pacemaker implantation. The incidence after myocardial infarction has been estimated at up to 4% of cases,[66] but with more extensive myocardial and pericardial involvement, it may be higher. It occurs with greater frequency (up to 30%) after cardiac surgery.[69] The pathogenesis of PCIS remains obscure; an autoimmune response in patients with myocardial or pericardial injury and possibly concomitant viral illness has been speculated.[70]

The diagnosis of PCIS remains one of exclusion, for no specific criteria exist. It is important to diagnose or exclude PCIS presumptively. Failure to diagnose accurately could lead to iatrogenic complications from inappropriate therapy, such as cardiac tamponade from anticoagulation for presumed pulmonary embolism and adverse effects related to antimicrobial therapy for presumed pneumonia.

Pleuropulmonary manifestations are the hallmark of PCIS. The most common presenting symptoms are pleuritic chest pain, found in virtually all patients, and fever, pericardial rub, dyspnea, and rales, which occur in half of patients.[68] Rarely, hemoptysis occurs, an important differential point when pulmonary embolism with infarction is in the differential diagnosis. Fifty percent of patients have leukocytosis, and almost all have an elevated erythrocyte sedimentation rate (average, 62 mm per hour).[68]

The chest radiograph is abnormal in virtually all patients, with the most common abnormality being left-sided and bilateral pleural effusions; a unilateral right effusion is unusual.[68] Pulmonary infiltrates are present in 75% of patients and are most commonly seen in the left lower lobe.[66] The pleural fluid is a serosanguineous or bloody exudate with a glucose level above 60 mg per dL and pleural fluid pH above 7.30. Nucleated cell counts range from 500 to 39,000 per μL, with a predominance of PMNs early in the course.[68] Pericardial fluid on echocardiogram is an important finding suggesting PCIS. The pleural fluid characteristics should help differentiate PCIS from a parapneumonic effusion and CHF, but do not exclude pulmonary embolism.

PCIS is usually self-limited and may not require therapy if symptoms are trivial. It usually responds to aspirin or nonsteroidal antiinflammatory agents, but some patients require corticosteroid therapy for resolution. In those who respond, the pleural effusion resolves within 1 to 3 weeks.

ESOPHAGEAL SCLEROTHERAPY

Pleural effusions are found in approximately 50% of patients 48 to 72 hours after esophageal sclerotherapy with sodium morrhuate and in 19% of patients after absolute alcohol sclerotherapy.[71-73] Effusions may be unilateral or bilateral, with no predilection for side. Effusion appears more likely with larger total volumes of sclerosant injected and larger volume injected per site.[71-72] The effusions tend to be small, serous exudates with variable nucleated (90 to 38,000 per μL) and red cell counts (126 to 160,000 per μL) and glucose concentration similar to that of serum.[71] These effusions probably result from an intensive inflammatory reaction after extravasation of the sclerosant into the esophageal mucosa, resulting in mediastinal and pleural inflammation. The effusion not associated with fever, chest pain, or evidence of perforation is of little consequence, requires no specific therapy, and resolves during several days to weeks.[71,72] However, late perforation may evolve in patients with apparent innocuous effusions. In patients with symptomatic effusions for 24 to 48 hours, diagnostic thoracentesis should be done and an esophagram considered.

ACUTE RESPIRATORY DISTRESS SYNDROME

The presence of pleural effusions in ARDS has not been well appreciated. In a retrospective study of 25 patients with ARDS, a 36% incidence of pleural effusions was found, a percentage similar to that found with hydrostatic pulmonary edema.[74] All patients had extensive alveolar pulmonary edema and endotracheal tube fluid that was compatible with increased permeability edema. Several experimental models of increased permeability pulmonary edema, including α-naphthyl thiourea, oleic acid, and ethchlorvynol, have been shown to produce pleural effusions. In the oleic acid and ethchlorvynol models, the development of pleural effusions lagged behind interstitial and alveolar edema by several hours. In the oleic acid model, 35% of the excess lung water collected in the pleural spaces. It appears that the pleura act as a reservoir for excess lung water in increased permeability and hydrostatic pulmonary edema. These effusions tend to be underdiagnosed clinically because the patient has bilateral alveolar infiltrates and the radiograph is taken with the patient in a supine position. Experimentally, the effusion is serous to serosanguineous, with a predominance of PMNs. These effusions usually require no specific therapy and resolve as ARDS resolves. However, in a series of positive end-expiratory pressure (PEEP)-unresponsive patients with ARDS, drainage of pleural effusion via tube thoracostomy has been shown to result in improved oxygenation.[75] The decision to proceed to pleural space drainage in ARDS should be approached on a case-by-case basis and is not generally recommended.

SPONTANEOUS ESOPHAGEAL RUPTURE

Esophageal rupture, a potentially life-threatening event, requires immediate diagnosis and therapy. The history in spontaneous esophageal rupture is usually severe retching or vomiting or a conscious effort to resist vomiting. In some patients, the perforation may be silent. Early recognition of spontaneous rupture depends on interpretation of the chest radiograph. Several factors influence chest radiograph findings:

the time between perforation and chest radiograph examination, site of perforation, and mediastinal pleural integrity.[76] A chest radiograph taken within minutes of the acute injury is usually unremarkable. Mediastinal emphysema probably requires at least 1 to 2 hours to be demonstrated radiographically and is present in less than half of patients; mediastinal widening may take several hours.[77] Pneumothorax, present in 75% of patients with spontaneous rupture, indicates violation of the mediastinal pleura; 70% of pneumothoraces are on the left, 20% are on the right, and 10% are bilateral.[77] Mediastinal air is seen early if pleural integrity is maintained, whereas pleural effusion secondary to mediastinitis tends to occur later. Pleural fluid, with or without associated pneumothorax, occurs in 75% of patients. A presumptive diagnosis should immediately be confirmed radiographically. Esophagrams are positive in approximately 90% of patients.[78] In the upright patient, rapid passage of the contrast material may not demonstrate a small rent; therefore, the study should be done with the patient in the appropriate lateral decubitus position.[79]

Pleural fluid findings depend on the degree of perforation and the timing of thoracentesis from injury. Early thoracentesis without mediastinal perforation shows a sterile, serous exudate with a predominance of PMNs, a pleural fluid amylase less than serum, and pH greater than 7.30.[80] Once the mediastinal pleura tears, amylase of salivary origin appears in the fluid in high concentration.[81] As the pleural space is seeded with anaerobic organisms from the mouth, the pH falls rapidly and progressively to approach 6.0.[80,82] Other pleural fluid findings suggestive of esophageal rupture include the presence of squamous epithelial cells and food particles. The diagnosis of spontaneous esophageal rupture dictates immediate operative intervention. If diagnosed and treated appropriately within the first 24 hours with primary closure and drainage, survival is greater than 90%.[77] Delay from the time of initial symptoms to diagnosis results in a reduced survival with any form of therapy.

HEMOTHORAX

Hemothorax (blood in the pleural space) should be differentiated from a hemorrhagic pleural effusion, because the latter can be the result of only a few drops of blood in pleural fluid. An arbitrary but practical definition of a hemothorax with regard to therapy is a pleural fluid/blood hematocrit ratio greater than 30%. The majority of hemothoraces result from penetrating or blunt chest trauma.[83] Hemothorax can also result from invasive procedures such as placement of central venous catheters, thoracentesis, and pleural biopsy, as well as from pulmonary infarction, malignancy, or ruptured aortic aneurysm. Bleeding can occur from vessels of the chest wall, lung, diaphragm, or mediastinum. Blood that enters the pleural space clots, rapidly undergoes fibrinolysis, and becomes defibrinogenated; thus, it rarely causes significant pleural fibrosis.

Hemothorax should be suspected in any patient with blunt or penetrating chest trauma. If a pleural effusion is found on the admitting chest radiograph, thoracentesis should be performed immediately and the hematocrit measured on the fluid. The hemothorax may not be apparent on the initial chest radiograph, which may be due to the supine position of the patient. Because bleeding may be slow and not appear for several hours, it is imperative that serial radiographs be obtained in these patients. The incidence of concomitant pneumothorax is high (approximately 60%).[83] Patients with traumatic hemothorax should be treated with immediate tube thoracostomy.[83-85] Large-diameter chest tube drainage evacuates the pleural space, may tamponade the bleeding (especially if the origin is from a pleural laceration), allows monitoring of the bleeding, and decreases the likelihood of subsequent fibrothorax.[85,86] If bleeding continues without signs of slowing, thoracotomy should be performed, depending on the individual circumstance.[85] Pleural effusions occasionally occur after removal of the chest tube from traumatic hemothoraces.[87] A diagnostic thoracentesis is indicated to exclude empyema. If empyema is excluded, the pleural effusion usually resolves without specific treatment and without residual pleural fibrosis.

Hemothorax is a rare complication of anticoagulation and has been reported in patients receiving heparin and warfarin. Coagulation studies are usually within the therapeutic range. The hemothorax tends to occur on the side of the pulmonary embolism. Anticoagulation should be discontinued immediately, a chest tube inserted to evacuate the blood, and a vena cava filter considered.

CORONARY ARTERY BYPASS SURGERY

A small, left pleural effusion is virtually always present after coronary artery bypass surgery. This is associated with left lower lobe atelectasis and elevation of the left hemidiaphragm on chest radiograph. Left diaphragm dysfunction is secondary to intraoperative phrenic nerve injury from cold cardioplegia, stretch injury, or surgical trauma.[88-90] The larger and grossly bloody effusions tend to be associated with internal mammary artery grafting, which causes marked exudation from the bed where the internal mammary artery was harvested.[91]

The pleural fluid is a hemorrhagic exudate with a low nucleated cell count, a glucose level similar to that of serum, and a pH greater than 7.40. Rarely, a loculated hemothorax may develop with trapped lung, resulting in clinically significant restriction.[92] If there is a large effusion that qualifies as a hemothorax (see previous section), the fluid should be drained by tube thoracostomy. It is also prudent to drain moderately large, bloody effusions to avoid later necessity for decortication.

ABDOMINAL SURGERY

Approximately half of the patients who undergo abdominal surgery develop small unilateral or bilateral pleural effusions within 48 to 72 hours of surgery.[27,28] The incidence is higher after upper abdominal surgery, in patients with postoperative atelectasis, and in patients who have free ascitic fluid at the time of surgery.[27] Larger left-sided pleural effusions are common after splenectomy.[27] The effusion is usually an exudate with less than 10,000 nucleated cells per µL. The glucose level is similar to that of serum, and pH is usually greater than 7.40.[27] The effusion usually is related to diaphragmatic irritation or atelectasis. Small effusions generally do not require diagnostic thoracentesis, are of no clinical significance, and resolve spontaneously. Pleural effusion from subphrenic abscess or pulmonary embolism is unlikely to occur within 2 to 3 days of surgery. The only indication for diagnostic thoracentesis would be to exclude infection if the effusion is relatively large or loculated.

CHYLOTHORAX

Trauma from surgery accounts for approximately 25% of cases of chylothorax, second only to lymphoma. Most series estimate an incidence of chylothorax of less than 1% after thoracic surgery,[93] but a 3% incidence has been reported after esophagectomy.[94] Virtually all intrathoracic procedures, including lobectomy, pneumonectomy, and coronary artery bypass grafting, have been reported to cause chylothorax. Other iatrogenic chylothoraces can be caused by complications of prolonged central vein catheterization. Nonsurgical trauma, such as penetrating and nonpenetrating neck, thoracic, and upper abdominal injuries, also has been associated with chylothorax.

When the thoracic duct is torn by stretching during surgery, chyle leaks into the mediastinum and subsequently ruptures through the mediastinal pleura. In the nonsurgical setting, penetrating injuries and fractures may directly tear the thoracic duct. Chylothorax from a central venous catheter usually involves venous thrombosis. Other rare causes of chylothorax include sclerotherapy of esophageal varices and translumbar aortography.[95-97]

The patient may be asymptomatic if the effusion is small and unilateral, or may present with dyspnea with a large unilateral effusion or bilateral effusions. The pleural fluid is usually milky, but 12% can be serous or serosanguineous,[98] with less than 7000 nucleated cells per µL, virtually all lymphocytes. The pleural fluid pH is alkaline

(7.40-7.80), and triglyceride levels are greater than plasma levels. Finding a pleural fluid triglyceride concentration of greater than 110 mg/dL makes the diagnosis of chylothorax highly likely.[98] If the triglyceride level is less than 50 mg/dL, chylothorax is highly unlikely. Triglyceride levels of 50 to 110 mg/dL indicate the need for lipoprotein electrophoresis[98]; the presence of chylomicrons confirms a chylothorax. The thoracic duct defect after trauma usually closes spontaneously within 10 to 14 days, with chest tube drainage as well as bed rest and total parenteral nutrition to minimize chyle formation. A pleuroperitoneal shunt relieves dyspnea, recirculates chyle, and prevents malnutrition and immunocompromise.

DUROPLEURAL FISTULA

Disruption of the dura and parietal pleura by surgical and nonsurgical trauma may result in a duropleural fistula with subsequent development of a pleural effusion.[99-102] The pleural fluid characteristics depend on the severity of the trauma and the delay between the trauma and the pleural fluid analysis. Pleural fluid due to a chronic duropleural fistula is usually a colorless transudate with low mononuclear cell count; a duropleural fistula associated with recent trauma may be a transudate or an exudate.[101,102] The diagnosis may even be delayed because of a coexisting process such as hemothorax. The diagnosis of duropleural fistula is established by the detection of β_2-transferrin in the pleural fluid.[103] Confirmation of the fistula by conventional or radionuclide myelography is recommended if surgical management is contemplated.

Pneumothorax

DEFINITION AND CLASSIFICATION

Pneumothorax refers to air in the pleural space. Free air may also be found in the adventitial planes of the lung or the mediastinum (pneumomediastinum). Spontaneous pneumothorax occurs without an obvious cause as a consequence of the natural course of a disease process. Primary spontaneous pneumothorax occurs without clinical findings of lung disease. Secondary spontaneous pneumothorax occurs as a consequence of clinically manifest lung disease, the most common being COPD. Traumatic pneumothorax results from penetrating or blunt chest injury. Iatrogenic pneumothorax occurs as an inadvertent consequence of diagnostic or therapeutic procedures.

PATHOPHYSIOLOGY

Pressure in the pleural space is subatmospheric throughout the normal respiratory cycle, averaging approximately −9 mm Hg during inspiration and −5 mm Hg during expiration. Owing to airway resistance, pressure in the airways is positive during expiration (+3 mm Hg) and negative (−2 mm Hg) during inspiration. In normal breathing, airway pressure is greater than pleural pressure throughout the respiratory cycle. Airway pressure may be increased markedly with coughing or strenuous exercise; however, pleural pressure rises concomitantly so that the transpulmonary pressure gradient is usually not substantially changed.

When there are rapid fluctuations in intrathoracic pressure, however, a large transpulmonary pressure gradient occurs transiently. Bronchial and bronchiolar obstruction, resulting in air trapping, can significantly increase the transpulmonary pressure gradient. The alveolar walls and visceral pleura maintain the pressure gradient between the airways and pleural space. When the pressure gradient is transiently increased, alveolar rupture may occur; air enters the interstitial tissues of the lung and may enter the pleural space, resulting in a pneumothorax. If the visceral pleura remain intact, the interstitial air moves toward the hilum, resulting in pneumomediastinum.[104-105] Because mean pressure within the mediastinum is always less than in the periphery of the lung, air moves proximally along the bronchovascular sheaths to the hilum and mediastinal soft tissues.

The development of pneumomediastinum after alveolar rupture requires continual cyclic respiratory efforts, which result in slow movement of air from the ruptured alveolus along a pressure gradient to the mediastinum.[105] Mediastinal air may decompress into the cervical and subcutaneous tissues or the retroperitoneum. With abrupt rise in mediastinal pressure or insufficient decompression to subcutaneous tissue, the mediastinal pleura may rupture, causing pneumothorax. Inadequate decompression of the mediastinum, rather than direct rupture of subpleural blebs into the pleural space, may be the major cause of pneumothorax.[104]

When pneumothorax occurs, the elasticity of the lung causes it to collapse. Lung collapse continues until the pleural defect seals or pleural and alveolar pressures equalize. When a ball-valve effect occurs at the site of communication between the pleural space and the alveolus, permitting only egress of air from the lung, there is a progressive accumulation of air within the pleural space, which can result in markedly increased positive pleural pressure, producing a tension pneumothorax. Tension pneumothorax compresses mediastinal structures, resulting in impaired venous return to the heart, decreased cardiac output, and at times, fatal cardiovascular collapse.[106-107] Rarely, tension along the bronchovascular sheaths and in the mediastinum can cause collapse of the pulmonary arteries and veins, resulting in cardiovascular collapse.[104]

Patients with primary spontaneous pneumothorax have a decrease in vital capacity and an increase in the $P(A-a)O_2$ gradient; they usually present with hypoxemia due predominantly to the development of an intrapulmonary shunt and areas of low ventilation/perfusion in the atelectatic lung.[108,109] Hypercapnia does not occur because there is adequate function in the uninvolved lung to maintain necessary alveolar ventilation. Patients with secondary spontaneous pneumothorax, in contrast, commonly develop hypercapnia because the gas exchange abnormality caused by the pneumothorax is superimposed on lungs with preexisting abnormal pulmonary gas exchange.

PNEUMOTHORAX IN THE INTENSIVE CARE UNIT

Patients with secondary spontaneous pneumothorax may be admitted to an ICU because they develop severe hypoxemic and, at times, hypercapnic respiratory failure. Patients with primary spontaneous pneumothorax rarely require ICU admission because the contralateral lung can maintain necessary alveolar ventilation, and the hypoxemia can be managed with supplemental oxygen. The most common causes of pneumothoraces in ICU patients are invasive procedures and barotrauma.

Iatrogenic Pneumothorax

Central Venous Catheters. Central venous catheters are used routinely in critically ill patients for volume resuscitation, parenteral nutrition, and drug administration. Approximately 3 million central venous catheters are placed annually in the United States, and this procedure continues to be associated with clinically relevant morbidity and some mortality. The morbidity and mortality associated with central venous catheter use are most commonly physician related.[42] Pleural complications of acquisition of venous access and the indwelling phase of central venous catheters include pneumothorax, hydrothorax, hemothorax, and chylothorax. In a recent study of mechanical complications of central venous catheters, 1.1% of 534 patients had pneumothorax.[110] This translates into approximately 33,000 pneumothoraces per year from central venous catheter insertions in critically ill patients in the United States. In the same study, none of the 405 patients developed pneumothorax when the central venous catheter was replaced over a guidewire.

The subclavian and internal jugular routes have been associated with pneumothorax, hemothorax, chylothorax, and catheter placement into the pleural space. Cannulation of the subclavian vein is associated with a higher risk of pneumothorax (less than 5%)[111] than cannulation of the internal jugular vein (less than 0.2%)[112]; with the external jugular venous approach, pneumothorax is avoided. There is a greater risk of pneumothorax with the infraclavicular compared to the supraclavicular approach to the subclavian vein. All complications of insertion, regardless of approach, can be reduced by appropriate physician training and experience. Operator inexperience appears to increase the number of complications with the internal jugular approach. It probably does not have as much impact on the incidence of pneumothorax with the subclavian vein approach, which accounts for 25% to 50% of all complications.[113]

Most pneumothoraces occur at the time of the procedure from direct lung puncture, but delayed pneumothoraces have been noted; therefore, it is prudent to view a chest radiograph 12 to 24 hours after the procedure. Up to half of patients with needle-puncture pneumothorax may be managed expectantly without the need for tube drainage. Bilateral pneumothoraces have been reported to occur from unilateral attempts,[113] and death can occur when there is a delay in the diagnosis of pneumothorax. As stated previously, a pneumothorax may be more difficult to detect while the patient is supine. Additional views should be taken, especially if the venous cannulation does not proceed as anticipated. With any newly placed central venous catheter, a postprocedure chest radiograph should be obtained, regardless of the site cannulated, to assure that the catheter tip is properly positioned. If a small pneumothorax is diagnosed by chest radiograph and the patient is asymptomatic and not on mechanical ventilation, the patient can be followed expectantly with repeat chest radiographs to assure that the leak has ceased. If the patient is on mechanical ventilation or the pneumothorax is large or has caused significant symptoms or gas exchange abnormalities, then tube thoracostomy should be performed as soon as possible.

Barotrauma. Pulmonary barotrauma is an important clinical problem because of the widespread use of mechanical ventilation. Barotrauma occurs in approximately 3% to 10% of patients on mechanical ventilation and includes parenchymal interstitial gas, pneumomediastinum, subcutaneous emphysema, pneumoperitoneum, and pneumothorax.[7,114-118] The most clinically important form is pneumothorax, occurring in 1% to 15% of all patients on mechanical ventilation. In patients with ARDS, rates of 6.5% to 87% have been reported.[117,118] The number of ventilation days, underlying disease (ARDS, COPD, necrotizing pneumonia), and use of PEEP have an impact on the incidence of pneumothorax.[114-116,119,120] When a pneumothorax develops in the setting of mechanical ventilation, 30% to 97% of patients develop tension pneumothorax.[7,115,119,120] The reported incidence of barotrauma varies widely between the studies, with the lowest incidences reported in the most recent large series.[118] This may be partly explained by the adoption of less aggressive ventilation strategies over time.

The initial radiographic sign of barotrauma is often pulmonary interstitial gas or emphysema.[117,121] In the early stages, however, interstitial gas may be difficult to detect radiographically. This harbinger of pneumothorax may be detected as distinct subpleural air cysts, linear air streaks emanating from the hilum, and perivascular air halos. Subpleural air cysts, most commonly seen in ARDS, tend to appear abruptly on the chest radiograph as single or multiple thin-walled, round lucencies, and are most often visualized at the lung bases, medially or diaphragmatically.[122] The cysts, which may expand rapidly, are usually 3 to 5 cm in diameter. Differentiating between peripheral subpleural air cysts and a localized basilar pneumothorax may be problematic. Pleural air cysts appear to be more common in younger patients, possibly because connective tissue planes of the lung are looser in younger patients than in older patients.[123] The risk of tension pneumothorax is substantial in patients who have developed subpleural lung cysts with continued mechanical ventilation. When mechanical ventilation is discontinued, the cyst may resolve spontaneously or become secondarily infected.

Ultrasonography has emerged as a bedside modality for the detection of pneumothorax. The absence of lung sliding is the finding associated with pneumothorax.[6] False-positive results may occur and are due to bullous lung disease or preexisting pleural symphysis.[6,124,125]

The disappearance of lung sliding that was present previously may be more specific for the development of pneumothorax—for example, after line placement. However, this subject awaits further study.

When evidence of barotrauma without pneumothorax is observed in any patient requiring continued mechanical ventilation, immediate attempts should be made to lower the plateau airway pressure. In ARDS, tidal volumes[126,127] and inspiratory flow rates should be lowered, an attempt should be made to reduce or remove PEEP, and neuromuscular blockers and sedation should be considered.[128] In status asthmaticus, in addition to the aforementioned maneuvers, controlled hypoventilation should be accomplished.[129,130] There is no evidence supporting the use of prophylactic chest tubes. However, the patient should be monitored closely for tension pneumothorax and provisions made for emergency bedside tube thoracostomy.

Tension Pneumothorax. Pneumothorax in the mechanically ventilated patient usually presents as an acute cardiopulmonary emergency, beginning with respiratory distress and, if unrecognized and untreated, progressing to cardiovascular collapse. In one report of 74 patients, the diagnosis of pneumothorax was made clinically in 45 (61%) patients based on hypotension, hyperresonance, diminished breath sounds, and tachycardia.[120] The mortality rate was 7% in these patients diagnosed clinically. In the remaining 29 patients, diagnosis was delayed between 30 minutes and 8 hours, and 31% of these patients died of pneumothorax. Other series of barotrauma in the setting of mechanical ventilation have reported mortality rates from 58% to 77%.[7,116]

Tension pneumothorax is lethal if diagnosis and treatment are delayed. The diagnosis should be made clinically at the bedside for the patient on mechanical ventilation who develops a sudden deterioration characterized by apprehension, tachypnea, cyanosis, decreased ipsilateral breath sounds, subcutaneous emphysema, tachycardia, and hypotension. The diagnosis may be problematic in the unconscious patient, the elderly, and the patient with bilateral tension, which may be more protective of the mediastinal structures and lessen the impact on cardiac output.

In the unconscious or critically ill patient, hypoxemia may be one of the earlier signs of tension pneumothorax. In the patient on mechanical ventilation, increasing peak and plateau airway pressure, decreasing compliance, and auto-PEEP should raise the possibility of tension pneumothorax. Difficulty in bagging the patient and delivering adequate tidal volumes may be noted.

When the clinical signs and symptoms are noted in mechanically ventilated patients, treatment should not be delayed to obtain radiographic confirmation. If a chest tube is not immediately available, placement of a large-bore needle into the anterior second intercostal space on the suspected side is life saving and confirms the diagnosis, as a rush of air is noted on entering the pleural space. An appropriately large chest tube can then be placed and connected to an adequate drainage system that can accommodate the large air leak that may develop in mechanically ventilated patients.[130]

On relief of the tension, there is a rapid improvement in oxygenation, increase in blood pressure, decrease in heart rate, and fall in airway pressures. In experimental tension pneumothorax, it has been observed that the inability to raise cardiac output in response to hypoxemia leads to a reduction in systemic oxygen transport and a decrease in mixed venous partial pressure of oxygen (Po_2), partially explaining the cardiovascular collapse seen in these patients.[107] In mechanically ventilated patients, a decrease in cardiac output is an inevitable consequence of tension pneumothorax.

Bronchopleural Fistula

DEFINITION AND CAUSES

Communication between the bronchial tree and the pleural space is a dreaded complication of mechanical ventilation.[131,132] There are three presentations of bronchopleural fistula (BPF): (1) failure to reinflate the lung despite chest tube drainage, or continued air leak

TABLE 65-3	Consequences of a Large Bronchopleural Fistula

Failure of lung reexpansion
Loss of delivered tidal volume
Inability to apply positive end-expiratory pressure
Inappropriate cycling of ventilator
Inability to maintain alveolar ventilation

after evacuation of pneumothorax in the setting of chest trauma; (2) complication of a diagnostic or therapeutic procedure such as thoracic surgery; and (3) complication of mechanical ventilation, usually for ARDS.[106] In ARDS, often a pneumothorax occurs under tension and is later associated with empyema, multiple sites of leakage, and a poor prognosis. A large air leak through a BPF can result in failure of lung reexpansion, loss of a significant amount of each delivered tidal volume, loss of the ability to apply PEEP, inappropriate cycling of the ventilator,[133] and inability to maintain alveolar ventilation (Table 65-3).

If there is a continued air leak for longer than 24 hours after the development of pneumothorax, then a BPF exists. The main factors that perpetuate BPF are high airway pressures that increase the leak during inspiration, increased mean intrathoracic pressures throughout the respiratory cycle (PEEP, inflation hold, high inspiratory/expiratory ratio) that increase the leak throughout the breath, and high negative suction. In severe ARDS, all these factors are present because they usually are necessary to support gas exchange and lung inflation.

MANAGEMENT

Given the frequency of barotrauma in BPF in mechanically ventilated patients, intensivists are called to give advice on the management of these difficult patients. Definitive therapy of BPF frequently involves invasive surgical approaches that include thoracoplasty, mobilization of the pectoralis or intercostal muscles, bronchial stump stapling, and decortication.[134-139] Although some of these techniques are still used today, there is a trend toward more conservative management of acute and chronic BPF, using innovations of standard techniques and new modalities that include chest tube management, drainage systems, ventilatory support, and definitive nonoperative therapy (Table 65-4). Even insertion of an endobronchial valve designed for the treatment of emphysema may be considered in selected patients.[140] Nonoperative therapy provides an alternative to the surgical approaches in patients who are poor operative candidates. Each patient with a BPF is unique and requires individual management based on the specific clinical setting. Attention to the basics of medical care of patients with BPF should not be neglected in the face of the potentially dramatic events related to the BPF. Nutritional status must be maintained, appropriate antibiotics used for the infected pleural space, and the space adequately drained.

TABLE 65-4	Management of Bronchopleural Fistula in Patients Requiring Mechanical Ventilation

Conservative

Adequate-size chest tube
Use of drainage system with adequate capabilities
Mechanical ventilation:
   Conventional (controlled, assist control, intermittent mandatory ventilation)
   High frequency
   Independent lung
Flexible bronchoscopy
Direct application of sealant

Invasive

Mobilization of intercostal or pectoralis muscles
Thoracoplasty
Bronchial stump stapling
Pleural abrasion and decortication

Chest Tubes

The initial therapy for pneumothorax in a patient on mechanical ventilation is placement of a chest tube in an attempt to reexpand the lung. The chest tube is initially necessary, can be detrimental later, and may play a role more important than that of a passive conduit. Air leaks in the setting of BPF range from less than 1 to 16 L per minute[141]; therefore, a chest tube that permits prompt and efficient drainage of this level of airflow is required. Gas moves through a tube in a laminar fashion and is governed by Poiseuille's law (v = [π r^4 P/8lV] t). In the clinical setting, the gas moving through a chest tube is moist; therefore, it is subject to turbulent flow and governed by the Fanning equation (v = [π r^2 r^5 P/fl]).[141-143] Therefore, both the length (l) and, even more so, the radius (r) are important when choosing a chest tube and connecting tubing to evacuate a BPF adequately (as flow varies exponentially to the fifth power of the radius of the tube). The smallest internal diameter that allows a maximum flow of 15.1 L per minute at −10 cm H_2O suction is 6 mm[141,142] (a 32 French chest tube has an internal diameter of 9 mm). A chest tube with a diameter adequate to convey the potentially large airflow of the BPF must be considered. A chest tube with too small a diameter can lead to lung collapse and tension pneumothorax in the setting of a mobile mediastinum.

Not only can the chest tube be used to drain pleural air, it can also be used to limit the air leak in certain situations. One modality is the application of intrapleural pressure equivalent to the level of PEEP during the expiratory phase of ventilation.[144-146] With positive intrapleural pressure applied through the chest tube, the air leak persists during the inspiratory phase of ventilation but decreases during expiration, allowing maintenance of PEEP in patients in whom it is necessary for adequate oxygenation. Synchronized closure of the chest tube during the inspiratory phase has also been used to control the air leak.[147,148] A combination of these techniques has been suggested for patients with significant BPF air leaks during both the inspiratory and expiratory phases of mechanical ventilation.[131,148] These techniques pose potential hazards, including increased pneumothorax and tension pneumothorax,[131,147] necessitating extremely close patient monitoring when such manipulations are used.

Instillation of chemical agents through the chest tube may potentially help close the BPF if the anatomic defect is small and single, but it is unlikely to be successful if the fistula is large or if there are multiple fistulas. Various agents have been successful in preventing recurrent pneumothoraces in patients who are not on mechanical ventilation,[149-152] but BPF in the setting of mechanical ventilation is a different situation. One study compared the recurrence of pneumothorax in 39 patients with BPF randomized to intrapleural tetracycline or placebo groups.[153] There was no evidence that intrapleural tetracycline facilitated closure of the BPF. No adverse effects were encountered from the instillation of tetracycline in patients with persistent air leaks.

The chest tube may be associated with adverse effects in patients with BPF. The gas escaping through the chest tube represents part of the minute ventilation delivered to the patient and makes maintenance of an effective tidal volume problematic.[154,155] Maintenance of a specific level of ventilation is not only affected by the amount of gas escaping through the fistula. The escaping gas does not passively flow from the airways into the BPF but is involved in physiologic gas exchange.[154,155] Approximately 25% of the minute ventilation has been found to escape via the BPF in patients with ARDS, with more than 20% of CO_2 excretion occurring by this route in half of the patients.[155] The role of the BPF in active CO_2 exchange is complex; proposed mechanisms include drainage of gas from alveoli in the area of the BPF and removal of gas from remote alveolar areas by pressure gradients created by the BPF.[156]

Carbon dioxide excretion and a reduction in minute ventilation occur to a lesser extent in BPF trauma victims.[154] In these patients, variable CO_2 excretion and loss of minute ventilation were dynamic and dependent on the level of chest tube suction. The difference between trauma and ARDS patients may have been due to the variability of lung compliance and the use of different ventilators.[155] Also, BPF may affect oxygen use, which generally decreases the use of inspired oxygen before it escapes through the fistula.[154] This relationship is variable but requires consideration in patients with oxygenation problems.

Negative pressure applied to the chest tube may be transmitted beyond the pleural space and into the airways, creating inappropriate cycling of the ventilator.[133,156] The increased flow through a BPF can occur with increased negative pleural pressure and may interfere with closure and healing of the fistulous site.[131] Therefore, the least amount of chest tube suction that keeps the lung inflated should be maintained in patients with BPF. The chest tube is a potential source of infection, both at the insertion site and within the pleural space.

Drainage Systems

As with the chest tube, the resistance of flow of gases is a consideration in the choice of the drainage system for the patient with a BPF.[141] The size of the air leak and the flow the drainage system can accommodate are necessary considerations. In an experimental model of BPF that simulated the type of air leak seen clinically (mean maximal flow, 5 L per minute), four pleural drainage units (PDU)—Emerson Post-Operative Pump (Emerson), Pleur-Evac (Teleflex Medical), Sentinel Seal (Tyco), and Thora-Klex (Avilor)—were tested at water seal, −20 cm H_2O, and −40 cm H_2O suction.[141] Compared to the water seal, −20 cm H_2O suction significantly increased the ability of all four PDUs to evacuate air via the chest tube, but an increase in suction to −40 cm H_2O did not significantly alter flow. When the air leak reached 4 to 5 L per minute, use of the Thora-Klex or Sentinel Seal became clinically impractical. The Pleur-Evac can handle flow rates up to 34 L per minute, but its use with rates over 28 L per minute is impractical owing to intense bubbling in the suction control chamber.[112] Air leaks of this magnitude are infrequent clinically in BPF and are likely to be seen only with major airway disruption or diffuse parenchymal leak secondary to ARDS with severe barotraumas.[156] In the latter situations, the low-pressure, high-volume Emerson suction pump remains the only PDU capable of handling the air leak.[141] The choice of PDU should be influenced by its physiologic capabilities and the type of BPF air leak encountered.

Mechanical Ventilation

Conventional Ventilation. The dilemma with a BPF in a mechanically ventilated patient is achieving adequate ventilation and oxygenation while allowing repair of the BPF to occur. Because air flow escaping through a BPF theoretically delays healing of the fistulous site, reducing flow through the fistula has been a major goal in promoting repair. The BPF provides an area of low resistance to flow and acts as a conduit for the escape of a variable percentage of delivered tidal volume during conventional positive-pressure mechanical ventilation. Thus the goal of management is to maintain adequate ventilation and oxygenation while reducing the fistula flow.[131] Using the lowest possible tidal volume, fewest mechanical breaths per minute, lowest level of PEEP, and shortest inspiratory time can do this. Avoidance of expiratory retard also reduces airway pressures. Using the greatest number of spontaneous breaths per minute, thereby reducing use of positive pressure, may also be advantageous. Intermittent mandatory ventilation may have an advantage over assist-control ventilation in BPF.

In a retrospective study of 39 patients with BPF who were maintained on conventional ventilation, only two patients developed a pH less than 7.30, despite air leaks of up to 900 mL per breath.[156] Overall, mortality was higher when the BPF developed late in the illness and was higher with larger leaks (more than 500 mL per breath).

High-Frequency Ventilation. Despite anecdotal reports, experimental data, and clinical studies involving high-frequency ventilation (HFV) in the setting of BPF, controversy exists. However, there appear to be subgroups of patients with BPF in whom HFV may be beneficial. Both animal[157] and human[158] studies suggest that HFV is superior to conventional ventilation in controlling P_{O_2} and partial pressure of carbon dioxide (P_{CO_2}) when there is a proximal (tracheal or bronchial) unilateral or bilateral fistula in the presence of normal lung parenchyma.

The use of HFV in BPF in patients with parenchymal lung disease such as ARDS is more controversial. Although some studies have shown that HFV improves or stabilizes gas exchange in patients with extensive parenchymal lung disease others have not shown a beneficial effect on gas exchange or a reduction in fistula outflow.[159,160] A trial of HFV appears reasonable in the patient with a proximal BPF and normal lung parenchyma; however, it is unclear whether HFV should be considered the primary mode of ventilation in this setting. Despite discrepancies in clinical results, a trial of HFV in a critically ill patient with a BPF and diffuse parenchymal disease who fails conventional ventilation appears justified. Caution must be exercised, however, with close monitoring of gas exchange parameters and fistula flow whenever HFV is used.

Other Modes of Ventilation. Other maneuvers during both conventional ventilation and HFV can be potentially helpful in patients with BPF. Selective intubation and conventional ventilation of the unaffected lung in patients with unilateral BPF may be useful but predisposes to the collapse of the nonintubated lung.[161-163] The use of differential lung ventilation with conventional ventilation may be of benefit in some patients.[159] Positioning of the patient such that the BPF is dependent has been shown to decrease fistula flow.[163]

Case reports and animal studies suggest other potential applications of HFV in BPF, including the use of independent lung ventilation with HFV applied to the BPF lung and conventional ventilation to the normal lung.[164] Another mode of HFV, ultra high-frequency jet ventilation, is being explored and has been used with some success in reducing BPF in humans[165] and animal models.[166] Independent lung ventilation with ultra high-frequency lung ventilation applied to the BPF lung and conventional ventilation to the normal lung led to rapid BPF closure in two of three patients.[165]

Flexible Bronchoscopy

The flexible bronchoscope can be valuable in the diagnosis of BPF.[167-169] Bronchoscopic therapy of BPF has several potential advantages, including low cost, shortened hospital stay, and relative noninvasiveness, particularly in poor operative candidates[167-169] (see Chapter 9). Proximal fistulas, such as those associated with lobectomy or pneumonectomy or stump breakdown, can be directly visualized through the bronchoscope. Distal fistulas cannot be visualized directly and require bronchoscopic passage of an occluding balloon to localize the bronchial segment leading to the fistula.[170-172] A balloon is systematically passed through the working channel of the bronchoscope and into each bronchial segment in question and then inflated; a reduction in air leak indicates localization of a bronchial segment communicating with the BPF. Once the fistula has been localized, various materials can be passed through a catheter in the working channel of the bronchoscope and into the area of the fistula.[167-176] Direct application of a sealant through the working-channel catheter onto the fistula site is the method generally used for directly visualized proximal fistulas. For distal fistulas, a multiple-lumen Swan-Ganz catheter has been used to localize the BPF and pass the occluding material of choice.[170]

Several agents have been used through the bronchoscope in an attempt to occlude BPF. These include fibrin agents,[169-170] cyanoacrylate-based agents,[167] absorbable gelatin sponge (Gelfoam [Pfizer]), blood-tetracycline,[171] and lead shot.[172] The reports on all of these agents are limited to only a few patients. The cyanoacrylate-based and fibrin agents have received the most attention but still have had less than 20 total cases reported. These patients have had at least a 50% reduction of fistula flow, and most had closure of the fistula subsequent to sealant application, although multiple applications were necessary in some patients. These agents appear to work in two phases, with the agent initially sealing the leak by acting as a plug and subsequently inducing an inflammatory process with fibrosis and mucosal proliferation permanently sealing the area.[167] They are not useful with large proximal tracheal or bronchial ruptures or multiple distal parenchymal defects.[170]

ANNOTATED REFERENCES

Anzueto A, Frutos-Vivar F, Esteban A, et al. Incidence, risk factors and outcome of barotrauma in mechanically ventilated patients. Intensive Care Med 2004;30(4):612-9.
  Barotrauma in mechanically ventilated patients. The incidence of barotraumas has decreased significantly when compared with historical data.
Doelken P, Abreu R, Sahn SA, Mayo PH. Effect of thoracentesis on respiratory mechanics and gas exchange in the patient receiving mechanical ventilation. Chest 2006;130(5):1354-61.
  A physiologic study of the effects of large-volume thoracentesis in mechanically ventilated patients. The effects on respiratory mechanics are small and unpredictable.

Heidecker J, Huggins JT, Sahn SA, Doelken P. Pathophysiology of pneumothorax following ultrasound-guided thoracentesis. Chest 2006;130(4):1173-84.
  An investigation into the causes of pneumothorax after thoracentesis. Postprocedure pneumothorax is most often due to unexpandable lung when ultrasound is used.
Lichtenstein DA, Menu Y. A bedside ultrasound sign ruling out pneumothorax in the critically ill. Lung sliding. Chest 1995;108(5):1345-8.
  Pneumothorax in the ICU. Lung sliding reliably rules out pneumothorax.

REFERENCES

Access the complete reference list online at http://www.expertconsult.com.

Community-Acquired Pneumonia

MICHAEL S. NIEDERMAN

Pneumonia is an infection of the gas-exchanging units of the lung that is most commonly caused by bacteria but occasionally due to viruses, fungi, parasites, and other infectious agents. It is the eighth leading cause of death in the United States and the number one cause of death from infectious diseases.[1] When this infection arises in patients who are residing out of the hospital, it is termed *community-acquired pneumonia* (CAP), although the population included in this definition is expanding. Currently the "community" includes complex patients such as those who have recently been hospitalized, those in nursing homes, and those with chronic diseases who are commonly managed in such facilities as dialysis centers or nursing homes. These patients are now referred to as having "healthcare-associated pneumonia" (HCAP), and it remains controversial whether their treatment should be similar to that for CAP or nosocomial pneumonia.[2]

Incidence

In 1994, over 5.6 million people were diagnosed with CAP in the United States. The majority, 4.5 million, were treated out of the hospital, and only a minority of hospitalized patients were cared for in the intensive care unit (ICU).[1,3] Although the majority of patients with CAP are managed in the outpatient setting, morbidity, mortality, and the major portion of the cost of treatment is focused on hospitalized patients, particularly those admitted to critical care units. In addition, those patients with comorbid illness and those of advanced age make up a large proportion of the hospitalized critically ill population. In particular, the elderly have a higher mortality from CAP than younger patients, generally as a reflection of the fact that they more commonly have comorbid illness.[3]

Although CAP can vary from being a mild to a severe illness, very few hospitalized patients are severely ill enough to require ICU admission.[4-5] Torres, et al. specifically examined all ICU admissions over a 4-year period and found that 10% were related to CAP.[4] In that study, CAP patients who required ICU care were admitted directly to the ICU 42% of the time, after admission to another ward 37% of the time, and after transfer from another hospital in 21% of patients.[4] In another study of 395 patients admitted to the hospital with CAP, only a total of 64 (approximately 15%) were admitted to the ICU.[6] Recently, Woodhead et al. found that CAP accounted for 5.9% of all ICU admissions, but that early admission (within 2 days of hospitalization) was associated with a lower mortality (46.3%) than late admission (>7 days in the hospital, 50.4% mortality).[7]

Kaplan and colleagues evaluated the cost of care for elderly patients with CAP in the United States.[5] Using Medicare data, they evaluated all individuals aged 65 or older admitted to nonfederal hospitals in 1997. A total of 623,718 patients were evaluated, with 86% being aged 70 or older, and the mean age was 77 years. Underlying illness was present in two-thirds, with congestive heart failure, the most common comorbidity, present in 32%. In this population, the use of ICU, mechanical ventilation, or both was common, with 140,226 patients having complex courses of illness. The overall mortality rate was 10.6% but rose higher with advancing age, nursing home residence, and comorbid illness. The mean length of stay was 7.6 days, with a mean cost of $6949, but costs were greater for patients with complex illness and mechanical ventilation and less for those with simple pneumonia. Costs generally paralleled length of stay but were disproportionately high for those needing mechanical ventilation, where the mean length of stay was 15.7 days and the cost $23,961. Interestingly, there was little

extra cost for nonsurvivors compared with survivors, except in the group with complex pneumonia as a whole but not in those requiring mechanical ventilation. The findings not only emphasize the high impact of CAP on costs and outcomes in the United States but also demonstrate the disproportionate increase in costs when patients are treated with mechanical ventilation, thereby raising for discussion the ethics and appropriateness of such care in the very elderly. Other studies of CAP have reported that costs are higher for patients with comorbid illness than those without, but in those without comorbid illness, the cost for those who died was less than for those who survived, while the opposite was true when the entire CAP population was considered.[8]

Risk Factors for Developing Severe CAP

In all studies of CAP, patients who are admitted to the hospital or ICU commonly have a number of coexisting illnesses, suggesting that individuals who are chronically ill have an increased risk of developing severe illness (Box 66-1). In one study, the mean age of all CAP patients was 59 years, coexisting illness was present in 46%, whereas 74% had a history of prior cigarette smoking.[6] Patients often have a history of coexisting illness, and the most common chronic illnesses in these patients are respiratory disease, cardiovascular disease, and diabetes mellitus, findings that have been echoed in a number of studies.[1,4,9] In studies of severe CAP, serious coexisting illness is present in 46% to 66% of all patients.[4,5,9] The most common respiratory illness in CAP patients is chronic obstructive pulmonary disease (COPD), a finding that applies to those with either mild or severe forms of CAP.[4] Among those with severe CAP, cigarette smoking and alcohol abuse are also quite common, and cigarette smoking has been identified as a risk factor for bacteremic pneumococcal infection.[4,10] Other common illnesses associated with CAP include malignancy, neurologic illness (including seizures), as well as AIDS.[1,9,11] One study identified alcohol abuse as a risk factor, along with the failure to receive antibiotic therapy before hospital admission, a finding suggesting that a delay in therapy may convert milder forms of pneumonia into a more severe illness.[9,11] In addition, genetic differences in the immune response may predispose certain individuals to more severe forms of infection and adverse outcomes, and may be reflected by a family history of severe pneumonia or adverse outcomes from infection.

Prognostic Factors

In a meta-analysis of 33,148 patients with CAP, the overall mortality rate (OR) was 13.7%, but those admitted to the ICU had a mortality rate of 36.5%.[12] Eleven prognostic factors were significantly associated with mortality:

1. Male sex (OR = 1.3)
2. Pleuritic chest pain (OR = 0.5)
3. Hypothermia (OR = 5.0)
4. Systolic hypotension (OR = 4.8)
5. Tachypnea (OR = 2.9)
6. Diabetes mellitus (OR = 1.3)
7. Neoplastic disease (OR = 2.8)
8. Neurologic disease (OR = 4.6)
9. Bacteremia (OR = 2.8)
10. Leukopenia (OR = 2.5)
11. Multilobar infiltrates (OR = 3.1)

Box 66-1

RISK FACTORS FOR DEVELOPING SEVERE COMMUNITY-ACQUIRED PNEUMONIA

Advanced age
Comorbid illness (e.g., chronic respiratory illness, cardiovascular disease, diabetes mellitus, neurologic illness, renal insufficiency, malignancy)
Cigarette smoking
Alcohol abuse
Absence of antibiotic therapy before hospitalization
Failure to contain infection to its initial site of entry
Immune suppression
Genetic polymorphisms in the immune response

In other studies, the clinical features that predict a poor outcome (Box 66-2)[1] include advanced age (>65 years), preexisting chronic illness of any type, absence of fever on admission, respiratory rate greater than 30 breaths/min, diastolic or systolic hypotension, elevated blood urea nitrogen (>19.6 mg/dL), profound leukopenia or leukocytosis, inadequate antibiotic therapy, need for mechanical ventilation, hypoalbuminemia, and the presence of certain "high-risk" organisms (type III pneumococcus, *Staphylococcus aureus*, gram-negative bacilli,

Box 66-2

RISK FACTORS FOR A POOR OUTCOME FROM COMMUNITY-ACQUIRED PNEUMONIA

Patient-Related Factors
Male sex
Absence of pleuritic chest pain
Nonclassic clinical presentation
Neoplastic illness
Neurologic illness
Age >65 years
Family history of severe pneumonia or death from sepsis

Abnormal Physical Findings
Respiratory rate >30 breaths/min on admission
Systolic (<90 mm Hg) or diastolic (<60 mm Hg) hypotension
Tachycardia (>125 beats/min)
High fever (>40°C) or afebrile
Confusion

Laboratory Abnormalities
Blood urea nitrogen >19.6 mg/dL
Leukocytosis or leucopenia (<4000/mm³)
Multilobar radiographic abnormalities
Rapidly progressive radiographic abnormalities during therapy
Bacteremia
Hyponatremia (<130 mmol/L)
Multiple organ failure
Respiratory failure
Hypoalbuminemia
Thrombocytopenia (<100,000/mm³)
Arterial pH <7.35
Pleural effusion

Pathogen-Related Factors
High-risk organisms:
    Type III pneumococcus, *Staphylococcus aureus*, gram-negative bacilli (including *Pseudomonas aeruginosa*), aspiration organisms, severe acute respiratory syndrome (SARS)
Possibly high levels of penicillin resistance (minimal inhibitory concentration of at least 4 mg/L) in pneumococcus

Therapy-Related Factors
Delay in initial antibiotic therapy (more than 4-6 hours)
Initial therapy with inappropriate antibiotic therapy
Failure to have a clinical response to empirical therapy within 72 hours

aspiration organisms, or postobstructive pneumonia). Other studies have found that when CAP patients have a delay in the initiation of appropriate antibiotic therapy, mortality is increased.[1,4,11,13]

One study of 3233 patients in Spain found that risk factors for all-cause mortality were a higher severity of illness on admission, need for ICU care, and the presence of multilobar infiltrates. However, late mortality (after at least 3 days) was reduced if blood cultures were negative, antibiotic therapy was consistent with guidelines, and if an etiologic agent was identified.[14] Thus severity of illness on admission most affects early mortality, while therapy-related, modifiable risk factors impact late mortality.

When these findings are viewed together, they suggest some general principles. Mortality is more likely in CAP patients who have severe physiologic derangements, serious underlying illnesses, delay in the initiation of appropriate antimicrobial therapy, and the presence of atypical clinical features. This last factor suggests that an unusual clinical presentation (low fever, nondistinct respiratory symptoms) is associated with mortality, which may be the result of its reflecting an inadequate inflammatory response to infection and because it can also lead to a delay in the recognition of pneumonia and the institution of appropriate therapy.

One approach to evaluating CAP patients is to use a scoring system to define prognosis and predict the risk of death. The investigators in the Pneumonia Outcomes Research Team (PORT) study have developed a mortality prediction rule that classifies all patients into one of five groups (Pneumonia Severity Index [PSI] classes I to V), each with a different risk for death.[15] Patients in classes IV and V have a predicted mortality risk of 8.2% to 9.3% and 27% to 31.1%, respectively, whereas those in classes I and II have a mortality risk of 0.1% to 0.4% and 0.6% to 0.7%, respectively, and those in class III have a risk of death of 0.9% to 2.8%. To use this scoring system, patients have points calculated based on such factors as age, sex, presence of comorbid medical disease, certain physical findings, and certain laboratory data.[15]

Although the PORT scoring system has been shown to be accurate for predicting mortality and prognosis, it is important to realize that it does not directly measure severity of illness, since many points in the scoring system are for comorbid conditions rather than features of illness. The investigators from the PORT study evaluated the use of ICU by patients with CAP and the ability of the scoring system to predict need for ICU care. From their original database, 170 patients were admitted to the ICU and compared to 1169 who were managed out of the ICU. While the PORT rule was useful for predicting mortality, there was a poor correlation between the need for ICU admission and the risk of death. In fact, 27% of the ICU patients were in PSI risk classes I to III, and this group, although needing intensive care, had a significantly lower mortality than patients in risk classes IV and V.[16] In another study, patients in PORT class V were evaluated, and only about 20% needed ICU admission; they had a 37% mortality compared to the 20% mortality of the PSI V patients who did not need the ICU.[17] In general, the PSI V patients who needed the ICU tended to get more of their points from acute illness, while those not needing the ICU tended to score points because of chronic disease factors. The findings are quite important for demonstrating that the need for ICU care does not always equate with a high risk of death. In the Infectious Diseases Society (IDSA)/American Thoracic Society (ATS) CAP guidelines, these limitations were discussed, including the fact that age and comorbidity are heavily weighted variables for defining mortality risk, tending to move all older patients into high PORT score classes.[1,18] On the other hand, in a young patient without comorbid illness, the pneumonia must be particularly severe to place the patient in a high-mortality risk group, and certain vital sign thresholds must be exceeded to accumulate points toward a poor prognosis. These thresholds are heart rate greater than 125 beats/min, respiratory rate greater than 30 breaths/min, and systolic blood pressure less than 90 mm Hg.

Although prognostic scoring systems can be complex and difficult to apply in clinical practice, the PORT prediction rule has been promoted as a way to avoid overestimating severity of illness, and calculation of the score has been advocated as a way of keeping some patients out of the hospital who have a low risk of death. For the critical care physician, the opposite problem—underestimating severity of illness—is a more serious concern, and the use of the CURB-65 approach, modified from the British Thoracic Society (BTS) rule, is a simple and accurate way to address this issue. *CURB-65*, an acronym for the clinical features used to assess pneumonia severity and prognosis,[18] assigns 1 point, on a 5-point scale, to confusion, blood urea >7 mmol/L (19.6 mg/dL), respiratory rate ≥30 breaths/min, blood pressure <90 mm Hg systolic or ≤60 mm Hg diastolic, and age ≥ 65 years. In one study, when the score was 0 to 1, the mortality rate was 0%, whereas mortality was more than 20% for a score of 3 or higher, and those with a score of 2 had a mortality of 8.3%.

Use of the CURB-65 rules may be a problem in the elderly, reflecting the altered clinical presentations of pneumonia in this population. In one study, a rule similar to CURB-65 had a 66% sensitivity and a 73% specificity for predicting mortality in a population that included 48% of patients who were at least 75 years of age.[19,20] Interestingly, although the rule was not optimal in an elderly population and did not work as well as it did in other populations, it had a higher sensitivity for predicting mortality than the Prognostic Scoring Index (PSI) derived from the PORT study.[15,20] Some studies have compared the PSI and CURB-65 and found them to be similar for identifying low-risk populations, but the CURB-65 may be more discriminating for identifying poor prognosis in those with severe illness, compared to the PSI.[21]

Other prognostic scoring systems have been developed to define the presence of severe pneumonia. One called the *CUR-XO* is based on defining the need for ICU admission by the presence of one of two major criteria: arterial pH < 7.30 or systolic BP < 90 mm Hg.[22] In the absence of these criteria, severe CAP can also be identified by the presence of two of six minor criteria including: confusion, BUN > 30 mg/dL, respiratory rate > 30/minute, Pao_2/Fio_2 ratio < 250, multilobar infiltrates, and age of at least 80. When these criteria were met, the tool was 92% sensitive for identifying those with severe CAP and was more accurate than the PSI or CURB-65 criteria, although not quite as specific as the CURB-65 rule.[22] Using this approach, some criteria (acidosis and systolic hypotension) are weighted more heavily than others, which contrasts with the approach of some of the other approaches to define severe CAP.

A different approach than assessing risk for death is to use scoring systems to define the need for ICU interventions such as intensive respiratory and vasopressor support (IRVS). The SMART-COP tool was developed to predict the need for IRVS.[23] Using a multi-variate model, there were eight clinical features associated with the need for IRVS: **s**ystolic blood pressure <90 mm Hg, **m**ultilobar infiltrates, **a**lbumin < 3.5 g/dL, **r**espiratory rate elevation (≥25 for those ≤age 50, and ≥30 for those >age 50), **t**achycardia (>125/min), **c**onfusion, low **o**xygen (<70 mm Hg if ≤age 50 or <60 mm Hg if >age 50), and arterial **p**H <7.35. The abnormalities in systolic blood pressure, oxygenation, and arterial pH each received 2 points, while the 5 other criteria received 1 point each, and with this system, the need for IRVS was predicted by a SMART-COP score of at least 3 points. Using this cutoff, the sensitivity for need for IRVS was 92.3% and the specificity 62.3%, with a positive and negative predictive value of 22% and 98.6%, respectively. The PSI and CURB-65 did not perform as well overall for predicting the need for IRVS.

Pathogenesis

Pneumonia results when host defenses are overwhelmed by an infectious pathogen. This may occur because the patient has an inadequate immune response, often as the result of underlying comorbid illness (congestive heart failure, diabetes, renal failure, COPD, malnutrition), because of anatomic abnormalities (endobronchial obstruction, bronchiectasis), as a result of acute illness-associated immune dysfunction (as can occur with certain viral infections), or because of therapy-induced dysfunction of the immune system (cor-

ticosteroids). Pneumonia can also occur in patients who have an adequate immune system if the host defense system is overwhelmed by a large inoculum of microorganisms (massive aspiration) or if the patient encounters a particularly virulent organism to which he or she has no preexisting immunity or to which the patient has an inability to form an adequate acute immune response.[24,25]

Most pneumonias result from microaspiration, but patients can also aspirate large volumes of bacteria if they have impaired neurologic protection of the upper airway (stroke, seizure) or if they have intestinal illnesses that predispose to vomiting. Other routes of entry include inhalation, which applies primarily to viruses, *Legionella pneumophila*, and *Mycobacterium tuberculosis*; hematogenous dissemination from extrapulmonary sites of infection (right-sided endocarditis); and direct extension from contiguous sites of infection (such as liver abscess). With this paradigm in mind, it is easy to understand why previously healthy individuals develop infection with virulent pathogens such as viruses, *L. pneumophila*, *Mycoplasma pneumoniae*, *Chlamydophila pneumoniae*, and *Streptococcus pneumoniae*. On the other hand, chronically ill patients can be infected by these organisms as well as by organisms that commonly colonize patients but only cause infection when immune responses are inadequate. These organisms include enteric gram-negative bacteria (e.g., *Escherichia coli*, *Klebsiella pneumoniae*, *P. aeruginosa*, *Acinetobacter* spp.) and fungi.

Recent studies have evaluated the normal lung immune response to infection and have shown that in most patients with unilateral CAP, the inflammatory response is limited to the site of infection, not spilling over to the uninvolved lung or the systemic circulation.[26,27] In patients with localized pneumonia, tumor necrosis factor alpha (TNF-α), interleukin (IL)-6, and IL-8 levels were increased in the pneumonic lung and generally not increased in the uninvolved lung or in the serum.[26,27] In patients with severe pneumonia, the immune response is characterized by a "spillover" of the immune response into the systemic circulation, reflected by increases in serum levels of TNF-α and IL-6.[28] It remains uncertain why localization does not occur in all individuals and why some patients develop diffuse lung injury (e.g., acute respiratory distress syndrome [ARDS]) or systemic sepsis as a consequence of pneumonia. These complications may result from an inability to develop a brisk lung immune response, as a consequence of either specific bacterial virulence factors, inadequate or delayed therapy, or genetic polymorphisms that affect the immune response. In fact, one study suggested that if bacteria persisted in the lung in spite of therapy, then inflammation in the form of IL-1β was persistent and at a high level, presumably being driven by the ongoing presence of the organisms.[29] Although there are a large number of genes that have been identified as being able to affect the severity and outcome of CAP by affecting the inflammatory response, the ability to use this information to impact patient management has not emerged.

Pneumonia-associated inflammation may also impact the long-term mortality of CAP. While the in-hospital mortality implications of CAP are well-known, there is also a high incidence of late mortality among hospitalized CAP patients. In one study of elderly patients hospitalized with CAP, the 1-year mortality rate exceeded 40%.[30] The explanation for this finding is unclear, but other studies have shown that patients with high levels of systemic inflammation (defined by serum levels of IL-6 and IL-10) on admission and on discharge have an increased mortality at 6 months to 1 year.[31] In addition, patients with evidence of cardiac dysfunction complicating CAP, as reflected by high serum levels of B-natriuretic peptide (BNP) are also likely to have increased disease-related mortality.[32]

Clinical Features

SYMPTOMS AND PHYSICAL FINDINGS

Patients with CAP and an intact immune system have a normal pulmonary response to infection and generally have respiratory symptoms such as cough, sputum production, and dyspnea, along with fever and other complaints. Cough is the most common finding and present in up to 80% of all patients but is less common in the elderly, those with serious comorbidity, or patients coming from nursing homes.[33] The elderly generally have fewer respiratory symptoms than younger individuals; as mentioned, the absence of clear-cut respiratory symptoms and an afebrile status have themselves been predictors of an increased risk of death.[1,18] Pleuritic chest pain is also common in patients with CAP, and in one study its absence was also identified as a poor prognostic finding.[34]

In the elderly patient, pneumonia can have a nonrespiratory presentation with symptoms of confusion, falling, failure to thrive, altered functional capacity, or deterioration in a preexisting medical illness such as congestive heart failure.[33,35] In one study, delirium or acute confusion were significantly more frequent in the elderly patients with pneumonia than in age-matched controls who did not have pneumonia.[35] In that study, there was no association between the type of isolated microorganisms and the clinical presentation of CAP, except for pleuritic chest pain, which was more common in pneumonia caused by bacterial pathogens such as *S. pneumoniae*. Approximately 16% of elderly patients with pneumonia were considered well nourished, compared with 47% of controls, with kwashiorkor-like malnutrition being the predominant type of nutritional defect and the one associated with delirium on initial presentation. Several other studies have examined the clinical presentation of pneumonia in the elderly and found that a nursing-home elderly population had a substantially higher mortality rate than other individuals with CAP. These findings may be a reflection of the fact that patients residing in a nursing home had a higher frequency of comorbid illness and dementia. Metlay and coworkers studied 1812 patients of all ages and found that with advancing age, patients tended to have a longer duration of symptoms such as cough, sputum production, dyspnea, fatigue, anorexia, myalgia, and abdominal pain.[33] In general, overall symptoms were less prominent in patients older than age 65 than in those who were younger.

Another study evaluated 1474 patients with CAP, of whom 305 were older than 80 years of age.[36] The population excluded individuals in nursing homes and severe immune suppression (neutropenia, AIDS, and transplant). Clinically, the very elderly had less pleuritic chest pain, headache, and myalgias and were more likely to be afebrile and to have altered mental status on admission. Overall mortality was higher in the older patients (15% versus 6%), as were in-hospital complications and early mortality (within 48 hours). The PSI values, as expected, were higher in the older population, in part because comorbid illness and age itself add to the PSI score; but still, the mortality rate for patients in PSI class V was 24% in the younger population versus 32% in the elderly.

Physical findings of pneumonia include tachypnea, crackles, rhonchi, and signs of consolidation (egophony, bronchial breath sounds, dullness to percussion). Patients should also be evaluated for signs of pleural effusion. In addition, extrapulmonary findings should be sought to rule out metastatic infection (arthritis, endocarditis, meningitis) or to add to the suspicion of an "atypical" pathogen such as *M. pneumoniae* or *C. pneumoniae*, which can lead to complications as bullous myringitis, rash, pericarditis, hepatitis, hemolytic anemia, or meningoencephalitis. One of the most important ways to recognize severe CAP early in the course of illness is to carefully count the respiratory rate. In the elderly, an elevation of respiratory rate can be the initial presenting sign of pneumonia, preceding other clinical findings by as much as 1 to 2 days.[37] In fact, in one study, tachypnea was the most common finding in elderly patients with pneumonia, being present in over 60% of all patients and occurring more often in the elderly than in younger patients with pneumonia.[33]

RADIOGRAPHIC FEATURES

For most patients, CAP is defined by a combination of clinical symptoms and the presence of a new radiographic infiltrate, but not all patients with this illness will have this finding when first evaluated.

Even when the radiograph is negative, if the patient has appropriate symptoms and focal physical findings, pneumonia may still be present. In one study, 47 patients with clinical signs and symptoms of CAP were evaluated with both chest radiography and high-resolution computed tomography (CT) of the chest.[38] Eight patients with a negative chest radiograph were identified by CT to have pneumonia and, in general, more extensive disease was found on CT than on chest radiography.[38] The findings of this study confirm the need to repeat the chest film after 24 to 48 hours in certain symptomatic patients with an initially negative chest film. Although some studies have suggested that febrile and dehydrated patients can have a normal chest radiograph when first admitted with pneumonia, the idea of hydrating pneumonia is in the realm of "conventional wisdom" and anecdotal reports.

The presence of alveolar densities (lobar or bronchopneumonic) has been associated with a high likelihood of a bacterial etiology, but it is extremely difficult to distinguish among specific pathogens by using patterns of radiographic abnormalities.[39] The chest radiograph may have prognostic value in patients with severe pneumonia, with multilobar infiltrates or rapid progression of infiltrates serving as poor prognostic signs, helping to identify patients who require intensive care.[1,4] Chest CT can also have value in the critically ill patient in situations when a noninfectious process is being considered, or when complications such as pneumothorax, empyema, or abscess are suspected. CT can suggest certain alternative noninfectious diagnoses such as granulomatous vasculitis, acute eosinophilic pneumonia, and bronchiolitis obliterans with organizing pneumonia.

When a pleural effusion appears on the initial chest radiograph, it is necessary to distinguish an empyema from a simple parapneumonic effusion, which is best done by sampling the pleural fluid. The presence of bilateral pleural effusions may be an independent predictor of short-term mortality in CAP. Pneumococcal pneumonia is the infection most commonly complicated by effusion (36% to 57% of patients), but other pathogens causing effusion include *H. influenzae*, *M. pneumoniae*, *Legionella* species, and tuberculosis.

TYPICAL VERSUS ATYPICAL PNEUMONIA SYNDROMES

In the past, the clinical and radiographic features of CAP have been organized into patterns of either "typical" or "atypical" pneumonia syndromes, with the idea being that specific patterns could suggest certain etiologic agents. The typical pneumonia syndrome is characterized by sudden onset of high fever, shaking chills, pleuritic chest pain, lobar consolidation, a toxic-appearing patient, and the production of purulent sputum. Although this pattern has been attributed to pneumococcus and other bacterial pathogens, these organisms do not always lead to such classic symptoms, particularly in the elderly. The atypical pneumonia syndrome, which is characterized by a subacute illness, nonproductive cough, headache, diarrhea, or other systemic complaints, is usually due to infection with *M. pneumoniae*, *C. pneumoniae*, *Legionella* species, or viruses. However, patients with impaired immune responses may present in this fashion, even with bacterial pneumonia. Thus, the ability to use the features on clinical presentation to predict the likely etiologic agents is limited and often misleading.[1,39-41]

In one study examining the microbial etiology and clinical presentation of CAP, clinical features were no more than 42% accurate in differentiating pneumococcus, *M. pneumoniae*, and other pathogens from one another.[40] In another study of 359 patients with CAP, a comparison of patients with *S. pneumoniae*, *H. influenzae*, *L. pneumophila*, and *C. pneumoniae* revealed no significant differences in their clinical presentations.[41] The limitations of clinical features in defining microbial etiology also apply to evaluations of radiographic patterns.[39]

USING CLINICAL FEATURES TO DEFINE SEVERE COMMUNITY-ACQUIRED PNEUMONIA

Although there is no uniformly accepted definition for severe CAP, this term generally refers to any patient who is admitted to the ICU because of CAP. Most of these patients have "respiratory failure" which is defined by the presence of hypoxemia or hypercarbia, and not all such patients require mechanical ventilation. Some patients with CAP are treated in the ICU because the pneumonia has led to clinical instability of an underlying disease, but the pneumonia itself may not be severe. Bacteremia does not always correlate with more severe illness, and its presence alone is not always a predictor of a poor outcome, with most episodes of bacteremia being due to pneumococcus. However, in the elderly with pneumococcal pneumonia, bacteremia is present in one fourth of patients with CAP and is often associated with azotemia and multilobe involvement.[42] When an infection such as pneumonia is complicated by severe sepsis or septic shock (not just bacteremia), outcome is adversely affected, with increases in mortality, length of stay, and costs for survivors.

For nearly 20 years, guidelines have attempted to define when patients should be admitted to the ICU, but the decision is still best made by careful clinical assessment. The 1993 ATS guidelines used the presence of any one of 10 criteria to define the patients who needed ICU admission.[1,6] However, subsequent studies showed that 65% of all admitted CAP patients (not needing ICU care) had one of these criteria present, and thus a more specific definition of the need for ICU admission was required.[6] Ewig and colleagues evaluated all 10 criteria in a patient cohort and suggested that ICU admission be considered if patients had two of three "minor criteria" present on admission or one of two "major criteria" present on admission or later in the hospital course.[6] The minor criteria were systolic blood pressure less than 90 mm Hg, Pao_2/Fio_2 ratio less than 250, or multilobar infiltrates, while the major criteria were need for mechanical ventilation or septic shock. This definition of need for ICU care had a sensitivity of 78%, a specificity of 94%, a positive predictive value of 75%, and a negative predictive value of 95%. As discussed earlier, another way to identify patients with more severe illness is to apply the BTS rule in its original or modified version. One study found that the use of the revised ATS criteria had a sensitivity of 70.7% and a specificity of 72.4% for predicting need for ICU admission.[16] The BTS criteria were much less sensitive with similar specificity, whereas the PORT rule (class IV or V) had similar sensitivity but lower specificity (although this latter rule was very effective at predicting risk of death).

The most recent IDSA/ATS guidelines for CAP suggested that ICU care be considered if the patient had one of two major criteria (need for mechanical ventilation or septic shock with the need for vasopressors), or 3 of 9 minor criteria.[1] The minor criteria include: respiratory rate ≥30 breaths/min, Pao_2/Fio_2 ratio ≤250, multilobar infiltrates, confusion/disorientation, uremia (BUN level >20 mg/dL), leukopenia (WBC count <4000 cells/mm³), thrombocytopenia (platelet count <100,000 cells/mm³), hypothermia (core temperature <36°C), and hypotension requiring aggressive fluid resuscitation. Other factors to consider in the decision making process are hypoglycemia (in a nondiabetic patient), hyponatremia, acute alcohol intoxication, cirrhosis, asplenia, and unexplained metabolic acidosis. The use of these minor criteria to define need for ICU admission requires validation. However, in one study, patients who met only minor criteria for ICU admission did not have an increase in mortality, whereas in another study, presence of four minor criteria was very accurate for defining the need for ICU care.[43,44]

There is some debate about the benefit of ICU care for patients with CAP, but the benefit seems most certain if patients are admitted early in the course of severe illness, thus emphasizing the need for sensitive criteria to define severe illness. In one recent study, patients with an obvious need for ICU care who were directly admitted to the ICU had a mortality rate of 10.9%, which was significantly lower than the 19.6% mortality rate of those without obvious need for ICU care who had delayed admission.[45] The measurement of admission respiratory rate is a simple and reliable assessment, and investigators have observed a linear relationship between admission respiratory rate (once it rose > 30 breaths/min) and mortality.[46] If patients are put in the ICU when they meet several "minor" criteria or when they have an elevated respiratory rate, this type of expectant management may have benefits and

may keep mortality rates in the 25% to 50% range. This is in marked contrast to the experience in older studies that reported mortality rates above 70% for pneumococcal bacteremia patients admitted to an ICU late in the course of illness, when nearly all admitted patients were mechanically ventilated on arrival to the ICU. In studies of severe CAP with good outcomes, approximately 60% of ICU admitted patients were intubated.[4,6]

Etiologic Pathogens

LIKELY PATHOGENS

Even with extensive diagnostic testing, an etiologic agent is defined in only about half of all patients with CAP, pointing out the limited value of diagnostic testing and the possibility that we do not know all the organisms that can cause CAP.[1,41] In the past 4 decades, a variety of new pathogens for this illness have been identified, including *L. pneumophila*, *C. pneumoniae*, severe acute respiratory syndrome coronavirus, novel H1N1 influenza, and hantavirus. In addition, antibiotic-resistant variants of common pathogens such as *S. pneumoniae* have become increasingly common. One of the ways CAP leads to respiratory failure is when it is complicated by ARDS. All of the bacteria and viruses listed here, as well as pneumonia due to aspiration, have been reported to cause ARDS.

The likely pathogens for infection vary depending on patient risk factors for specific microorganisms and the presence of certain comorbid illnesses, but for all patient groups, including those with severe CAP, pneumococcus is the most common pathogen.[1] In fact, in one study of lung puncture cultures, this organism was even identified as being common in patients who had no diagnosis established by routine diagnostic testing.[47] The incidence of antibiotic-resistant pneumococci has increased in recent years, and up to 40% of these organisms can have reduced sensitivity to penicillin or other antibiotics, although the clinical relevance of in vitro resistance is still uncertain.[1,48,49] Identified risk factors for drug-resistant *S. pneumoniae* (DRSP) include β-lactam therapy in the past 3 months, alcoholism, age older than 65 years, immune suppression, multiple medical comorbidities, and contact with a child in day care.[1,50,51] Other common infecting organisms in those with severe CAP include viruses (e.g., influenza, respiratory syncytial virus, and the coronavirus illness of severe acute respiratory syndrome [SARS]), *L. pneumophila*, *M. pneumoniae*, *M. tuberculosis*, and *H. influenzae* (especially in smokers). In the setting of severe pneumonia, patients can be infected with *S. aureus* (including methicillin-resistant forms, or MRSA) or enteric gram-negatives and (rarely) anaerobes. In the elderly, including those with aspiration pneumonia, healthcare-associated pneumonia, and in those with underlying cardiopulmonary disease, enteric gram-negative organisms are often seen.

The frequency of gram-negative CAP is difficult to define, but in one study of 559 hospitalized patients with CAP, 60 patients had gram-negative enteric infections, including 39 with *P. aeruginosa*.[1,52] Risk factors for gram-negative organisms were probable aspiration (OR=2.3), previous hospital admission within 30 days of admission (OR=3.5), previous antibiotics within 30 days of admission (OR=1.9), and presence of pulmonary comorbidity (OR=2.8). Risk factors for *P. aeruginosa* were pulmonary comorbidity (OR=5.8) and previous hospitalization (OR=3.8). Infection with a gram-negative pathogen led to ICU admission and mechanical ventilation more often than infection with other organisms. The mortality rate of CAP due to *P. aeruginosa* was 28%. In a more recent study from Korea, 10% of 912 CAP patients had gram-negatives, with *Klebsiella* spp. being twice as common as *P. aeruginosa*.[53] Patients with gram-negatives had a higher mortality than those without, and risk factors for gram-negative infection included septic shock, cardiac disease, smoking, hyponatremia, and dyspnea. Nursing home patients (HCAP) were included in the population of patients studied, again emphasizing the overlap between CAP and HCAP. Another recent study of 3272 episodes of CAP found that 2% were caused by enteric gram-negatives (most commonly *P.*

aeruginosa), and the risk factors for these organisms were COPD, current use of corticosteroids, prior antibiotic therapy, tachypnea ≥ 30/minute, and septic shock on admission.[54] Patients with these organisms needed ICU care more often and had a higher mortality and length of stay than those without these pathogens present.

Although aspiration has often been considered a risk factor for anaerobic infection, studies of severe CAP in elderly patients with aspiration risk factors suggested that this population is very likely to have gram-negative infection.[55,56] One study evaluated 95 residents of long-term care facilities who had pneumonia requiring ICU admission and risk factors for oropharyngeal aspiration such as swallowing disorders due to neurologic illness, disruption of the gastroesophageal junction, dysphagia, or anatomic abnormalities. Using protected bronchoalveolar lavage (BAL) sampling within 4 hours of admission, a total of 67 pathogens were identified, with enteric gram-negatives in 49%, anaerobes in 16%, and *S. aureus* in 12%.[55] Fifty-five percent of the anaerobes were recovered along with aerobic gram-negative co-infection. The presence of anaerobes did not correlate with oral hygiene but did correlate with functional status, being more common in patients who were totally dependent. Of the seven patients who received inadequate therapy for anaerobes, six recovered, raising a question about whether these organisms really need to be treated. These findings suggest that anaerobes may not really be pathogens but could simply be colonizers in the institutionalized elderly, including those with aspiration risks.[55]

Primary pulmonary infection with atypical pathogens has been reported for patients with severe CAP for many years. In fact, in one ICU in Spain, atypical pathogens were present in almost 25% of all patients, but the responsible organism varied over time. *Legionella* was the most common atypical pathogen leading to severe CAP in 14% of patients during one time period, but in the same hospital a decade later, it was seen in only 2%, having been replaced by *Mycoplasma* and *Chlamydophila* infection, which were found in 17% of patients compared with only 6% a decade earlier.[9,11] Several studies have shown that even if bacterial pathogens lead to CAP, they can be accompanied by atypical pathogens in the form of mixed infection.[57,58] Atypical pathogens can include *C. pneumoniae*, *M. pneumoniae*, and *L. pneumophila*, and some recent studies have shown that these infections are common in patients of all ages, not just young and healthy individuals; these organisms have even been reported among the elderly in nursing homes.[1,57,59] When mixed infection is present, it may lead to a more complex course and a longer length of stay than if a single pathogen is present, which may explain the increasing number of studies that show a reduction in CAP mortality, including those in the ICU, when initial therapy provides coverage for these organisms, compared with regimens that do not provide coverage.[60,61] Interestingly, multiple retrospective studies of pneumococcal bacteremia have shown a reduced mortality when dual therapy (usually involving a macrolide) rather than monotherapy is used, raising the possibility that even these patients have mixed infection with atypical pathogens.[62,63] The frequency of atypical pathogens can be as high as 60%, with as many as 40% of all CAP patients having mixed infection.[58] These high incidence numbers have been derived with serologic testing, which is of uncertain accuracy.

Atypical organism pneumonia may not be a constant phenomenon, and the frequency of infection may vary over the course of time and with geography. In fact, one study showed that the benefit of providing empirical therapy directed at atypical pathogens was variable, being more important in some calendar years than in others.[61] The incidence of *Legionella* infection among admitted patients has varied from 1% to 15% or more and is also a reflection of geographic and seasonal variability in infection rates, as well as a reflection of the extent of diagnostic testing.

In the past, *S. aureus* was an uncommon cause of CAP, but it was capable of leading to severe pneumonia. In the past several years, a community-acquired strain of MRSA (CA-MRSA) has emerged as a cause of severe CAP, particularly in patients without a history of previous hospitalization or chronic illness, often as a complication of

TABLE 66-1	Common Pathogens Causing Community-Acquired Pneumonia
Inpatient with no cardiopulmonary disease or modifying factors	*Streptococcus pneumoniae, Haemophilus influenzae, Mycoplasma pneumoniae, Chlamydophila pneumoniae,* mixed infection (bacteria plus atypical pathogen), viruses (including influenza), *Legionella* species, and others (*M. tuberculosis,* endemic fungi, *Pneumocystis jirovecii*)
Inpatient with cardiopulmonary disease and/or modifying factors	All of the above. but drug-resistant *S. pneumoniae* (DRSP) and enteric gram-negative organisms are more of a concern.
Severe community-acquired pneumonia (CAP) with no risks for *P. aeruginosa*	*S. pneumoniae* (including DRSP), *Legionella* species, *H. influenzae,* enteric gram-negative bacilli, *S. aureus* (including MRSA), *M. pneumoniae,* respiratory viruses (including influenza), others (*C. pneumoniae, M. tuberculosis,* endemic fungi)
Severe CAP with risks for *P. aeruginosa*	All of the pathogens above plus *P. aeruginosa*

influenza infection.[1,64,65] The organism can lead to a severe bilateral necrotizing pneumonia, often related to toxin production by the organism. This organism is distinct from the nosocomial strain of MRSA and is clonal in origin, usually due to the USA-300 strain.

RISK FACTORS FOR SPECIFIC PATHOGENS

Table 66-1 summarizes the common pathogens causing CAP in hospitalized patients, including those admitted to the ICU. The classification is based on the presence of clinical risk factors for specific pathogens, referred to as *modifying factors*. The modifying factors for DRSP are age older than 65 years, β-lactam therapy within the past 3 months, alcoholism, immune suppressive illness (including therapy with corticosteroids), multiple medical comorbidities, and exposure to a child in day care.[1,50] The modifying factors for enteric gram-negatives include residence in a nursing home (now defining the patient as having HCAP), underlying cardiopulmonary disease, multiple medical comorbidities, and recent antibiotic therapy. For the patient with HCAP, resistant gram-negatives and MRSA can occur, particularly if the patient has multiple risk factors in addition to nursing home residence. These risk factors include severe illness, poor functional status, immune suppression, recent antibiotic therapy, and recent hospitalization in the past 3 months.[2] In predicting the likely etiologic pathogens for those admitted to the ICU, patients are divided into a population at risk for pseudomonal infection and a population without this organism being likely. The risk factors for *P. aeruginosa* infection are structural lung disease (bronchiectasis), corticosteroid therapy (>10 mg prednisone/day), broad-spectrum antibiotic therapy for more than 7 days in the past month, and malnutrition.[1]

Table 66-2 shows that certain clinical conditions are associated with specific pathogens, and these associations should be considered in all patients when obtaining a history.[1] For example, if the presentation is subacute following contact with birds, rats, or rabbits, the possibility of psittacosis, leptospirosis, tularemia, or plague should be considered. Certain exposures should also raise concern about specific organisms. Thus, *Coxiella burnetii* (Q fever) is a concern with exposure to parturient cats, cattle, sheep, or goats; *Francisella tularensis* is a concern with rabbit exposure; hantavirus with exposure to mice droppings; *Chlamydophila psittaci* with exposure to turkeys or infected birds; and *Legionella* with exposure to contaminated water sources (saunas). Following influenza, superinfection with pneumococcus, *S. aureus* (including community-acquired MRSA), and *H. influenzae* should be considered. With travel to endemic areas in Asia, the onset of respiratory failure after a preceding viral illness should lead to suspicion of SARS or influenza. Endemic fungi (coccidioidomycosis, histoplasmosis, and blastomycosis) occur in well-defined geographic areas and may present acutely as symptoms that overlap with acute bacterial pneumonia.

TABLE 66-2	Clinical Associations with Specific Pathogens
Condition	*Commonly Encountered Pathogens*
Alcoholism	*Streptococcus pneumoniae* (including penicillin-resistant), anaerobes, gram-negative bacilli (possibly *Klebsiella pneumoniae*), tuberculosis
Chronic obstructive pulmonary disease/current or former smoker	*S. pneumoniae, Haemophilus influenzae, Moraxella catarrhalis*
Residence in nursing home	*S. pneumoniae*, gram-negative bacilli, *H. influenzae, Staphylococcus aureus, Chlamydia pneumoniae*; consider *Mycobacterium tuberculosis*. Consider anaerobes, but less common.
Poor dental hygiene	Anaerobes
Bat exposure	*Histoplasma capsulatum*
Bird exposure	*Chlamydia psittaci, Cryptococcus neoformans, H. capsulatum*
Rabbit exposure	*Francisella tularensis*
Travel to southwestern USA	*Coccidioidomycosis*; hantavirus in selected areas
Exposure to farm animals or parturient cats	*Coxiella burnetii* (Q fever)
Postinfluenza pneumonia	*S. pneumoniae, S. aureus* (including CA-MRSA), *H. influenzae*
Structural disease of lung (e.g., bronchiectasis, cystic fibrosis)	*P. aeruginosa, P. cepacia,* or *S. aureus*
Sickle cell disease, asplenia	Pneumococcus, *H. influenzae*
Suspected bioterrorism	Anthrax, tularemia, plague
Travel to Asia	Severe acute respiratory syndrome (SARS), tuberculosis, melioidosis

Although a variety of radiographic patterns can be seen in pneumonia, specific findings cannot generally be used to predict the microbial etiology in CAP, but there are certain patterns to keep in mind. Focal consolidation can be seen with infections caused by pneumococcus, *Klebsiella* species, aspiration (especially if in the lower lobes or other dependent segments), *S. aureus, H. influenzae, M. pneumoniae,* and *C. pneumoniae.* Interstitial infiltrates should suggest viral pneumonia as well as infection due to *M. pneumoniae, C. pneumoniae, C. psittaci,* and *P. jirovecii.* Lymphadenopathy with an interstitial pattern should raise concerns about anthrax, *F. tularensis,* and *C. psittaci,* whereas adenopathy can be seen with focal infiltrates in tuberculosis, fungal pneumonia, anthrax, and bacterial pneumonia. Cavitation can be the result of an aspiration lung abscess, infection with *S. aureus* or aerobic gram-negatives (including *P. aeruginosa)*, tuberculosis, fungal infection (aspergillus), nocardiosis, and actinomycosis.

FEATURES OF SPECIFIC PATHOGENS

Streptococcus Pneumoniae

The most common pathogen for CAP, *S. pneumoniae* (synonymous with *pneumococcus*) is a gram-positive, lancet-shaped diplococcus, of which there are 84 different serotypes, each with a distinct antigenic polysaccharide capsule. Eighty-five percent of all infections are caused by one of 23 serotypes, which are now included in a polysaccharide vaccine. Infection is most common in the winter and early spring, which may relate to the finding that up to 70% of patients have a preceding viral illness. The organism spreads from person to person and commonly colonizes the oropharynx before it leads to pneumonia. Pneumonia develops when colonizing organisms are aspirated into a lung that is unable to contain the aspirated inoculum. The classic radiographic pattern is a lobar consolidation, but bronchopneumonia can also occur, and in some series this is the most common pattern.[66] Bacteremia is present in up to 20% of hospitalized patients, and extrapulmonary complications include meningitis, empyema, arthritis, endocarditis, and brain abscess.

Since the mid-1990s, antibiotic resistance among pneumococci has become increasingly common, and penicillin resistance, along with

resistance to other common antibiotics (macrolides, trimethoprim/sulfamethoxazole, selected cephalosporins), is present in over 40% of these organisms.[1,48-51] Fortunately, most penicillin resistance is of the "intermediate" type (penicillin minimal inhibitory concentration [MIC] of 0.1 to 1.0 mg/L) and not of the high level type (penicillin MIC of 2.0 or more). Although the clinical impact of in vitro resistance is uncertain, one large database has data showing that only organisms with a penicillin MIC of more than 4 mg/L can lead to an increased risk of death.[1,48] Recently the definitions of resistance have been changed for non-meningeal infection, with sensitivity being defined by a penicillin MIC ≤ 2 mg/L, intermediate as a MIC of 4 mg/L, and resistant as a MIC ≥ 8 mg/L.[67] While the clinical impact of resistance on outcomes such as mortality was hard to show using older definitions, with the new definitions of resistance, very few pathogens will be defined as resistant, but those that are may affect outcome.

Although some studies did not show an increased mortality rate in patients infected with resistant strains of pneumococcus after adjusting for disease severity, more recent studies have not been so clear.[1,48,68,69] Turrett and colleagues studied a population of 462 patients with pneumococcal bacteremia, of which more than half were HIV positive, and high-level resistance was a predictor of mortality.[68] Other investigators did not find an increased risk of death from infection with resistant organisms but did find an enhanced likelihood of suppurative complications (empyema) and a more prolonged hospital length of stay.[69] The conflicting data in earlier reports may have been the result of studying relatively few patients. Feikin and colleagues studied the impact of pneumococcal resistance in 5837 patients with bacteremic CAP.[48] They found an increased mortality for patients with a penicillin MIC of at least 4 mg/L or greater or with a cefotaxime MIC of 2.0 mg/L or more. However, this increased mortality was only present if patients who died in the first 4 days of therapy were excluded from analysis. One limitation of these data was the failure to account for severity of illness or therapy choices. However, Moroney and associates used both cohort study and matched control methods and found that severity of illness, not resistance or accuracy of therapy, was the most important predictor of mortality.[70] Interestingly, in the case-control part of the study, severity of illness was greater in patients without resistant organisms, implying a loss of virulence among organisms that become resistant, a finding echoed in another study that found absence of invasive illness to be a risk factor for pneumococcal resistance.[50]

The relationship of prior antibiotic use to subsequent pneumococcal resistance has been known, and prior therapy with macrolides, β-lactams, and quinolones has been identified as a predisposing factor for subsequent resistance to the same class of antibiotic.[50,71-73] One study related the recent usage of certain specific antibiotic classes to the development of penicillin resistance.[73] In this study, 303 patients with pneumococcal bacteremia were evaluated, and 98 had penicillin-nonsusceptible strains. The use of penicillins, sulfonamides, and macrolides within either 1 or 6 months before infection was associated with an increased risk of bacteremia with penicillin-nonsusceptible *S. pneumoniae* (PNSP). The odds ratio of increased risk was from threefold to sixfold for β-lactams and pneumococci. Interestingly, the risk was no lower for therapy in the past 6 months compared with therapy in the past 1 month. Although quinolones were associated with a slightly increased risk of infection with PNSP, this increase was not statistically significant, but other studies have shown that quinolone therapy can predispose to subsequent pneumococcal resistance to this class of antibiotics.[71,72] Prolonged and repeated courses of therapy may be particular risk factors for promoting pneumococcal resistance to β-lactams, sulfonamides, and macrolides.[73] In another study of patients with pneumococcal bacteremia, pneumococcal resistance to β-lactams (penicillins and cephalosporins), macrolides, and quinolones was more likely if the patient had received the same agent in the past 3 months.[71] Although some studies have shown that discordant therapy of drug-resistant pneumococcus can be a risk factor for mortality, in one study discordant therapy was less likely if patients were treated with ceftriaxone or cefotaxime compared to other therapies.[74] Thus in clinical practice, resistance is not likely to affect outcome, since current guidelines for severe CAP recommend the use of these effective agents as empirical therapy. Macrolide-resistant pneumococci have also been described and can be either low- or high-level resistant, depending on whether the mechanism of resistance is efflux or ribosomal alteration, respectively. Although high-level resistance may be clinically relevant, this is generally not an issue in the management of ICU CAP, since all patients who receive macrolide therapy do so in combination with a highly active β-lactam which is effective against pneumococcus even if macrolide resistance is present.

Legionella Pneumophila

This small, weakly staining, gram-negative bacillus was first characterized after an epidemic in 1976 and can occur either sporadically or in epidemic form. Although multiple serogroups of the species *L. pneumophila* have been described, and these account for 90% of all cases of legionnaires' disease, serogroup 1 is responsible for the most cases. The other species that commonly causes human illness is *L. micdadei*. The organism is waterborne and can emanate from air-conditioning equipment, drinking water, lakes and river banks, water faucets, and shower heads.[75] Infection is generally caused by inhalation of an infected aerosol generated by a contaminated water source. When a water system becomes infected in an institution, endemic outbreaks may occur. In its sporadic form, *Legionella* may account for 7% to 15% of all cases of CAP, being a particular concern in patients with severe forms of illness.[1,11,75]

The classic *Legionella* syndrome is characterized by high fever, chills, headache, myalgias, and leukocytosis.[75] The diagnosis is also suggested by the presence of a pneumonia with preceding diarrhea, along with mental confusion, hyponatremia, relative bradycardia, and liver function abnormalities, but this syndrome is usually not present. Symptoms are rapidly progressive, and the patient may appear to be quite toxic. This classic syndrome is not always present, so this diagnosis should always be considered in patients admitted to the ICU with CAP and in those with rapidly progressive radiographic abnormalities.

To establish this diagnosis serologically, it is necessary to collect both acute and convalescent titers. The urinary antigen test is the single most accurate acute diagnostic test for *Legionella* but is specific only for serogroup 1 infection. In recent years, most cases have been diagnosed with urinary antigen, and there has been less reliance on serology and culture.[76] With this increased reliance on urinary antigen testing, the case fatality rate of legionellosis has fallen, possibly reflecting diagnosis of less severe illness than in the past.[76]

Staphylococcus Aureus

This organism can lead to severe forms of CAP which can be necrotizing, with a cavitary pneumonia and hematogenous dissemination to multiple sites in the body. The organism can also seed the lung hematogenously from a valvular vegetation in patients with right-sided endocarditis or from septic venous thrombophlebitis (from central venous catheter or jugular vein infection). When a patient develops postinfluenza pneumonia, *S. aureus* can lead to secondary bacterial infection and, in the United States, community-acquired strains of methicillin-resistant *S. aureus* (CA-MRSA) have emerged, primarily in skin and soft-tissue infections, but also as a cause of severe CAP. CA-MRSA is a clonal disease, emanating from the USA-300 clone of *S. aureus*, and is clinically and bacteriologically different from the strains of MRSA that cause nosocomial pneumonia.[64] In addition, it can infect previously healthy individuals, and the classic clinical presentation of this pathogen causing CAP is as a complication of a preceding viral or influenza infection. The illness is characterized by a severe bilateral necrotizing pneumonia, which may be related to staphylococcal virulence factors such as the Panton-Valentine leukocidin (PVL). Since the pathogenesis of pneumonia due to this organism may be related to toxin production by the bacteria, therapy may need to involve both an antibacterial agent and an antitoxin-producing agent.[65] The frequency of this illness is still relatively low, but it does occur sporadically, with certain geographic areas having a high frequency, especially during influenza season.

Other Organisms, Including Influenza

The incidence of viral pneumonia is difficult to define, but one careful study of over 300 non–immune compromised CAP patients looked for viral pneumonia by paired serologies and found that 18% had viral pneumonia, with about half being pure viral infection and the others being mixed with bacterial pneumonia.[77] Influenza (A more than B), parainfluenza, and adenovirus were the most commonly identified viral agents. Influenza should always be considered during epidemic times and can lead to a primary viral pneumonia or to secondary bacterial infection with pneumococcus, *S. aureus*, or *H. influenzae*. Viral illnesses that can lead to respiratory failure in addition to influenza include respiratory syncytial virus (which can affect the elderly), varicella (a particular concern in pregnant females with chickenpox), and hantavirus (endemic in the Four Corners area of New Mexico).[78]

Beginning in April 2009, an outbreak of H1N1 influenza infected approximately 61 million people worldwide, with as many as 13,000 deaths. H1N1 influenza, in contrast to seasonal flu, affected younger people more than the elderly, and high-risk populations included pregnant women and those with obesity. The CDC estimated that 90% of hospitalizations and 87% of deaths occurred in people younger than 65, whereas with seasonal influenza, about 60 percent of flu-related hospitalizations and 90 percent of flu-related deaths occur in people 65 years and older.[79] Over 90% of patients with this illness present with cough and fever, but patients may also have chills, muscle aches, and headache. The incubation period is 3 to 7 days, and spread is person to person and via aerosol droplets if the infected person is within 5 to 6 feet. In one series, 12% of all hospitalized patients with H1N1 infection were mechanically ventilated, and 6% of hospitalized patients died.[80] When H1N1 infection led to ICU admission, most patients had lung infiltrates which could have been due to viral pneumonia (usually in the first 3-5 days) or secondary bacterial infection (usually after 5-10 days). The frequency of documented bacterial pneumonia complicating this illness varied from less than 5% to more than 25% of patients with radiographic pneumonia. Antiviral therapy with zanamivir and oseltamivir may reduce the severity of illness, particularly if given early. The role of corticosteroids for patients with severe illness is uncertain.[81,82]

It important to always consider the diagnosis of tuberculosis in patients with severe CAP and, in endemic areas, fungal infection with coccidioidomycosis and histoplasmosis, especially in HIV-infected persons. Several rickettsiae can also cause CAP, including Q fever (*Coxiella burnetii*), which occurs worldwide, Rocky Mountain spotted fever (RMSF), and scrub typhus (*Rickettsia tsutsuga-mushi*) in Asia and Australia. Transmission typically involves an intermediate vector, often ticks (Q fever, RMSF) or mites (scrub typhus), but also sheep, cows, and contaminated milk (Q fever). These infections have a variable incubation period ranging from days to a few weeks, and are characterized by a febrile syndrome that may have a pneumonic component and a maculopapular rash (Q fever and RMSF).

Severe Acute Respiratory Syndrome

In late 2003, a respiratory viral infection caused by a coronavirus emerged in parts of Asia and was termed *severe acute respiratory syndrome* (SARS). The illness affected people from a variety of endemic areas in Asia, but was seen in North America when an outbreak occurred in Toronto, Canada. Importantly, worldwide as many as 20% of affected patients were healthcare workers, particularly those caring for patients admitted to the ICU. Transmission risk was greatest during emergent intubation and was also possible during noninvasive ventilation, making this latter modality of therapy contraindicated if SARS is suspected.[83] Infection control may be quite effective in preventing the spread of SARS to healthcare workers and includes careful handling of respiratory secretions, ventilator circuits, the use of N-95 respirator masks, and careful gowning and gloving.[84] Even more elaborate infection control measures, including personal air exchange units, are needed for healthcare workers involved in high-risk procedures such as intubation.

Clinically, SARS patients present after a 2- to 11-day incubation period with fever, rigors, chills, dry cough, dyspnea, malaise, headache, and frequently pneumonia and ARDS. Laboratory data show not only hypoxemia but also elevated liver function tests. In the Toronto experience, about 20% of hospitalized patients were admitted to the ICU, and 15% were mechanically ventilated. Respiratory involvement typically began on day 3 of the hospital stay, but respiratory failure was not until day 8.[84] The mortality rate for ICU-admitted SARS patients was over 30%; when patients died, it was generally from multiple-system organ failure and sepsis. There is no specific therapy, but anecdotal reports have suggested a benefit to the use of pulse doses of corticosteroids and ribavirin.

Bioterrorism Considerations

Certain airborne pathogens can cause pneumonia as the result of deliberate dissemination by the aerosol route in the form of a biological weapon, and they present a clinical syndrome of CAP. The pathogens most likely to be used in this fashion and that can lead to severe pulmonary infection are *Bacillus anthracis* (anthrax), *Yersinia pestis* (plague), and *F. tularensis* (tularemia).[85-89] The Centers for Disease Control and Prevention (CDC) has classified these agents as category A pathogens because of their high mortality rate and their potential impact on public health.[85] Other pneumonic pathogens could also serve as agents of biological warfare and are potentially less serious and are categorized as category B; these include *C. burnetii* and *Brucella* species. Certain emerging pathogens are categorized as category C agents and are not widely available as weapons but have the potential for high morbidity and mortality and include hantavirus and multidrug-resistant tuberculosis.[84] Some agents of bioterrorism can be spread via the aerosol route but do not generally present as pneumonia; they include smallpox and viral hemorrhagic fevers (Ebola, Marburg).

In the fall of 2001 in the United States, a series of intentional attacks with anthrax led to 11 confirmed cases of inhalational illness.[87,88] Anthrax is an aerobic gram-positive, spore-forming bacillus that had rarely led to disease before 2001. Particle size is essential in determining the infectiousness of the spores, and a size of 1 to 5 μm is required for inhalation into the alveolar space, but generally infection requires an inoculum size of 8000 to 40,000 spores. The organisms initially enter alveolar macrophages and are transported to mediastinal lymph nodes, where they can persist and germinate and produce two toxins (lethal toxin and edema toxin). Illness follows rapidly after germination.[87,88] Although respiratory symptoms are often present, anthrax is not a typical pneumonic illness but rather a disease characterized by hemorrhagic thoracic lymphadenitis, hemorrhagic mediastinitis, and pleural effusion. Whereas the incubation period of anthrax has varied from 2 to 43 days in prior outbreaks, in the October 2001 series the incubation period was from 4 to 6 days.[87] In the U.S. experience, all patients had chills, fever, and sweats and most had nonproductive cough, dyspnea, nausea, vomiting, and chest pain. Chest radiographs were abnormal in all of the first 10 patients, 7 had mediastinal widening, 8 had pleural effusions (generally bloody), and 7 had pulmonary infiltrates.[87,88] Blood cultures were positive in all 8 patients in whom they were obtained before therapy, but sputum culture and Gram stain are unlikely to be positive. Five of the 11 patients died.

Therapy for anthrax includes supportive management and antibiotics, with possibly some role for corticosteroids if meningeal involvement or mediastinal edema is present. Recommended therapy is ciprofloxacin (400 mg intravenously (IV) twice daily) or doxycycline (100 mg IV twice daily). Until the patient is clinically stable, one to two additional agents should be added, including clindamycin, vancomycin, imipenem, meropenem, chloramphenicol, penicillin, ampicillin, rifampin, and clarithromycin.[87] After an initial response, therapy should be continued with either ciprofloxacin or doxycycline for at least 60 days.[87] Postexposure prophylaxis can be done with ciprofloxacin or, alternatively, doxycycline or amoxicillin for a total of 60 days.

🔲 Diagnostic Evaluation

In the patient with severe CAP, diagnostic testing is done to define the presence of pneumonia, the severity of illness and its complications, and the etiologic pathogen. Most studies of severe CAP have not found that establishing an etiologic diagnosis can lead to improved outcome, and mortality is lowest when patients are given empirical therapy that is likely to be effective and leads to a good clinical response within 48 to 72 hours.[13] As discussed, the diagnosis of CAP is suggested by the history and physical examination and confirmed by chest radiograph. The history may suggest certain pathogens on the basis of epidemiologic considerations (see Table 66-2), but the clinical features and chest radiograph cannot give an exact etiologic diagnosis. An etiologic diagnosis is best established if blood or pleural fluid cultures identify a pathogen, if bronchoscopic techniques demonstrate an organism in high concentrations, or if serologic testing confirms a fourfold rise in titers to specific pathogens (comparing acute and convalescent samples collected weeks apart).

Although defining a specific etiologic diagnosis of CAP allows for focused antibiotic therapy, most patients do not have a specific pathogen identified. Many who do are diagnosed days or weeks later when the results of cultures or serologic testing become available. In addition, recent studies have emphasized the mortality benefit of prompt administration of effective antibiotic therapy, with a goal of administering IV antibiotics within 4 to 6 hours of admission to the hospital for those with moderate to severe illness.[90] Thus therapy should never be delayed for the purpose of diagnostic testing, and the diagnostic workup should be streamlined, with all patients receiving empirical therapy based on algorithms as soon as possible. With such empirical regimens, as many as 90% of admitted patients will have a prompt response to therapy.[91]

For ICU-admitted patients, after a chest radiograph defines the presence of pneumonia, testing should include an assessment of oxygenation (pulse oximetry or blood gas, the latter if retention of carbon dioxide is suspected), routine admission blood work, and two sets of blood cultures (Table 66-3).[1] Although blood cultures are positive in only 10% to 20% of CAP patients, they can be used to define a specific diagnosis and to define the presence of drug-resistant pneumococci.[1,48] Blood cultures are not routine for all admitted patients but should be done in those with severe illness, especially if the patient has not received antibiotics prior to admission, since the incidence of a true positive result is high in this population.[92] If the patient has a pleural effusion, this should be tapped and the fluid sent for culture and biochemical analysis. Sputum culture can help to identify the presence of a drug-resistant or unusual pathogen and should be obtained from all critically ill patients who are intubated.[1] Urinary antigen testing for pneumococcus or *Legionella* has some potential value for providing a rapid diagnosis. *Legionella* urinary antigen is specific to serogroup 1 infection and is positive in a little more than half of all infected patients, but it is the test most likely to be positive in the setting of acute illness.[93] Pneumococcal urinary antigen has a high sensitivity and specificity for diagnosing pneumococcal pneumonia, especially if concentrated urine is examined; it can be positive even in the presence of antibiotic therapy, but false-positive tests can occur in patients who have had recent pneumococcal infection.[94]

The role of Gram stain of sputum to guide initial antibiotic therapy is controversial, but this test has its greatest value in guiding the interpretation of sputum culture and can be used to define the predominant organism present in the sample. The role of Gram stain in focusing initial antibiotic therapy is uncertain because the accuracy of the test to predict the culture recovery of an organism such as pneumococcus depends on the criteria used. If the finding of any gram-positive diplococcus is used to define a positive test, the test will be sensitive but not very specific. On the other hand, the finding of a predominance of gram-positive diplococci will be specific but not sensitive for predicting the culture recovery of pneumococcus.[1] In one study, the practical limitations of the test were clear: of 116 patients with CAP, only 42

TABLE 66-3	**Diagnostic Testing for Community-Acquired Pneumonia**		
Test	*Sensitivity*	*Specificity*	*Comment*
Chest radiograph	65%-85%	85%-95%	CT is more sensitive to infiltrates. Recommended for all patients.
Computed tomography (CT)	Gold standard	Not infection specific	Should not be done routinely but helpful to identify cavitation and loculated pleural fluid. Recommended in the evaluation of nonresponding patients.
Blood cultures	10%-20%	High when positive	Usually shows pneumococcus (in 50%–80% of positive samples) and defines antibiotic susceptibility. Recommended in patients with severe community-acquired pneumonia (CAP), particularly if not on antibiotic therapy at the time of testing.
Sputum Gram stain	40%-100% depending on criteria	0%-100% depending on criteria	Can correlate with sputum culture to define predominant organism and can use to identify unsuspected pathogens. Recommended if sputum culture obtained. May not be able to narrow empirical therapy choices.
Sputum culture			Use if suspect drug-resistant or unusual pathogen, but positive result cannot separate colonization from infection. Obtain via tracheal aspirate in all intubated patients
Oximetry or arterial blood gas			Both define severity of infection, need for oxygen; if hypercarbia is suspected, a blood gas sample is needed. Recommended in severe CAP.
Serologic testing for *Legionella*, *Chlamydia pneumoniae*, *Mycobacterium pneumoniae*, viruses			Accurate, but usually requires acute and convalescent titers collected 4 to 6 weeks apart. Not routinely recommended.
Legionella urinary antigen	50%-80%		Specific to serogroup 1, but the best acute diagnostic test for *Legionella*
Pneumococcal urinary antigen	70%-100%	80%	False positives if recent pneumococcal infection. Can increase sensitivity with concentrated urine
Serum procalcitonin			Not a routine test, but if done, should be measured with the highly sensitive Kryptor assay. May help guide duration of therapy and need for ICU admission.

could produce a sputum sample, of which 23 were valid and only 10 samples were diagnostic, with antibiotics directed to the diagnostic result in only 1 patient.[95] Even if Gram stain findings were used to focus antibiotic therapy, this would not allow for empirical coverage of atypical pathogens that might be present with pneumococcus as part of a mixed infection. In spite of these limitations, Gram stain can be used to broaden initial empirical therapy by enhancing the suspicion for organisms not covered in routine empirical therapy (such as *S. aureus*, being suggested by the presence of clusters of gram-positive cocci, especially during a time of epidemic influenza).[1]

Routine serologic testing is not recommended.[1] However, in patients with severe illness, the diagnosis of legionellosis can be made by urinary antigen testing, the test most likely to be positive at the time of admission but specific only for serogroup 1 infection.[87] Bronchoscopy is not indicated as a routine diagnostic test and should be restricted to immune-compromised patients and to selected individuals with severe forms of CAP. In the patient admitted to the ICU with CAP, bronchoscopy with quantitative cultures is often done to be sure all efforts are being made to define the etiologic agent, but the benefit of this approach is unclear. As mentioned, several studies[13,91] have not shown any improvement in outcome when a specific etiologic diagnosis is made for patients with severe CAP. Rather, outcome is improved if the initial empirical therapy is accurate and the patient has a prompt clinical improvement.[13] However, patients who have rapidly progressive lung infection despite therapy may benefit from invasive diagnostic testing, but again a favorable impact of this testing on patient outcome has not been demonstrated. One population that should be considered for invasive testing is the corticosteroid-treated COPD patient who has a slowly responding or nonresponding pneumonia, because these individuals are at risk for infection with *Aspergillus*, and this organism can be recovered from a bronchoscopic sample. In addition, bronchoscopy may have value for the nonresponding patient or other immune-suppressed individuals; in one study, it provided diagnostically useful information for such patients.[96]

One study compared the management of CAP with empirical therapy versus a pathogen-directed approach.[97] In that study, even with extensive testing, nearly 40% of 262 patients had no etiology established. Although pathogen-directed therapy had no overall impact on mortality or length of stay, it did lead to less adverse events than empirical therapy and also was accompanied by lower mortality for patients admitted to the ICU.[97] In patients with severe CAP, diagnostic testing may be valuable for guiding modifications of antibiotic therapy rather than impacting the choice of initial therapy.[98] In one study, 214 patients with severe CAP were evaluated, and a microbiologic diagnosis was established in 57.3%. When the yield of specific tests was examined, the investigators found that sputum or tracheal aspirate cultures had the highest yield of any microbiologic investigation, being positive in 44.4% of all patients in which a sample was collected. Blood cultures were positive in 21.1% of the 189 patients sampled, whereas bronchoscopic protected specimen brush was positive in 25% of the 62 patients who were sampled, and bronchoalveolar lavage was positive in 34% of the 41 patients who were sampled. When diagnostic testing identified a cause, antibiotics were changed in 74.3% of patients, compared with 32.7% of patients without an etiologic diagnosis ($P < 0.05$). In most instances, the change in therapy was a simplification of the initial empirical antibiotic regimen that occurred in 65 patients.[98]

Although not part of routine management, measurement of serum levels of biomarkers such as C-reactive protein or procalcitonin (PCT) may be valuable in guiding management of antibiotics for CAP. PCT is an acute-phase reactant synthesized in the liver in response to bacterial but not viral infection. Studies in CAP have documented that serial measurement of levels of PCT, using the sensitive Kryptor assay, can guide the duration of antibiotic therapy, allowing cessation of therapy once levels fall and leading to a marked reduction in the duration of therapy, compared to clinical judgment.[99,100] In patients with severe CAP, measurement of initial and serial levels can help define those with a poor prognosis, and a low PCT value may distinguish which patients in PSI classes IV and V might be safely managed out of the ICU. In one study, patients with a higher PSI score or with complications or death had significantly higher procalcitonin levels than those with an uncomplicated clinical course.[101] In another study, Kruger et al.[102] reported that nonsurvivors had significantly higher median PCT levels than survivors (0.88 versus 0.13 ng/mL; P=0.0001). Low PCT accurately predicted patients at very low risk of death, even in patients falling in a high prognostic scoring category by the CURB-65 evaluation. Given its high negative predictive potential (98.9% with PCT level of <0.228 ng/mL), patients with low PCT might be safely treated out of the ICU.[102] Huang et al. found that 23.1% (126/546) of high-risk patients defined by PSI had low procalcitonin levels, and this subgroup had very low mortality, similar to low-risk patients.[103]

Therapy

Initial antibiotic therapy for severe CAP is necessarily empirical, with the goal of targeting the likely etiologic pathogens, based on the considerations in Tables 66-1 and 66-2, which categorize patients on the basis of severity of illness and risk factors for specific pathogens. The likelihood of organisms such as DRSP, enteric gram-negative organisms, and P. aeruginosa is determined by the presence of cardiopulmonary disease or "modifying factors."[1] Although a set of likely pathogens can be predicted for each patient (see Table 66-1), and this information can be used to guide initial empirical therapy, if diagnostic testing shows the presence of a specific pathogen, then therapy can be focused.

In choosing empirical therapy of CAP, certain principles and therapeutic approaches should be followed (Box 66-3). If these principles are followed and patients receive guideline-concordant therapy, outcomes such as duration of mechanical ventilation can be improved.[1,104] All individuals should be treated for DRSP and atypical pathogens, but only those with appropriate risk factors (see earlier discussion) should have coverage for P. aeruginosa, and patients with bilateral necrotizing pneumonia after influenza need coverage for CA-MRSA.[1] Although macrolide monotherapy (azithromycin) has been documented as effective for some non-ICU admitted patients, all patients admitted to the ICU require combination therapy using a β-lactam with either a macrolide or quinolone, plus the addition of other agents, depending on the clinical setting.[1,105] In one study of 529 patients with ICU-admitted CAP, combination therapy with a β-lactam plus either a macrolide or quinolone led to improved survival for the population with shock needing pressors (279 patients), compared to the use of monotherapy.[106] This recommendation to

avoid monotherapy is based not only on data such as these but also on the fact that the efficacy (especially for meningitis complicating pneumonia), effective dosing and safety of any single agent, including quinolone monotherapy, has not been established for ICU-admitted CAP patients. In one study comparing high-dose levofloxacin to a β-lactam/quinolone combination, the single-agent regimen was overall effective. However, patients in septic shock were excluded, and there was a trend to a worse outcome with monotherapy for individuals receiving mechanical ventilation.[105] In another study of severe CAP, use of a β-lactam/macrolide combination had a survival advantage compared to quinolone monotherapy.[107] From the available data, it appears that adding either a macrolide or a quinolone leads to similar results, although some data in patients with bacteremic CAP, especially with pneumococcus, suggest that a macrolide may have particular advantages, possibly because of its antiinflammatory effects.[62,63] One recent study looking at severe CAP (not all pneumococcal) also confirmed the benefit of adding a macrolide as part of initial empirical therapy, but not a quinolone, for reducing mortality.[108] In that study, 165 of the 218 pneumonia patients had sepsis or septic shock, and for these severely ill patients who received a macrolide in a combination regimen, the ICU mortality was 25% compared to a 46% mortality in those getting a quinolone as part of a combination regimen. If Legionella is suspected, the use of a quinolone may be preferable, since these agents have been highly successful in treating pneumonia caused by this organism, possibly more effective than macrolides.[109] In addition, the choice between a quinolone and macrolide may best be determined by using a regimen that is different from what the patient has recently received.

For patients with pseudomonal risk factors, therapy can be with a two-drug regimen using an antipseudomonal β-lactam (cefepime, imipenem, meropenem, piperacillin/tazobactam) plus ciprofloxacin (the most active antipseudomonal quinolone) or levofloxacin. Alternatively, a three-drug regimen can be used, combining an antipseudomonal β-lactam plus an aminoglycoside plus either an IV antipneumococcal quinolone (moxifloxacin or levofloxacin) or a macrolide.[1] If CA-MRSA is suspected, therapy can be with either vancomycin or linezolid, although other agents might be effective, since this pathogen is not as antibiotic resistant as nosocomial MRSA. However, since CA-MRSA is in part a toxin-mediated illness, the use of an agent that inhibits toxin production along with an antibacterial effect is recommended by some.[65] To do this, linezolid can be used alone (since it acts to inhibit protein synthesis), or clindamycin can be added to vancomycin.

Some patients with severe CAP can now be reclassified as having HCAP, because they come to the hospital from a nursing home or have had recent contact with a healthcare environment because of treatment with dialysis or hospitalization in the past 3 months. Some of these patients can be treated the same as other severe CAP patients, but some will need coverage for nosocomial pneumonia pathogens, including multidrug-resistant (MDR) gram-negatives and nosocomial MRSA.[2] Those who need coverage for MDR organisms are individuals with severe HCAP who have an additional risk factor (besides just residence in a nursing home), whereas those without such risk factors can receive the severe CAP regimens listed earlier. The risk factors for MDR pathogen infection include poor functional status, immune suppression, recent antibiotic therapy, or recent hospitalization.[2] Those at risk for MDR pathogens should receive dual antipseudomonal therapy (β-lactam plus an aminoglycoside) plus MRSA coverage (linezolid or vancomycin).

Although they should not be used as monotherapy for ICU-admitted CAP patients, the antipneumococcal quinolones have assumed great importance because they can cover pneumococcus (including DRSP), nonpseudomonal gram-negative organisms, and atypical pathogens.[1] Quinolones penetrate well into respiratory secretions and are highly bioavailable, achieving the same serum levels with oral or IV therapy and thereby allowing rapid switch to oral therapy in responding patients. The available IV agents active against pneumococcus are moxifloxacin and levofloxacin.[1] Based on in vitro activity,

---

Box 66-3

EMPIRICAL THERAPY REGIMENS FOR SEVERE COMMUNITY-ACQUIRED PNEUMONIA

No Pseudomonal Risk Factors
Selected β-lactam (cefotaxime, ceftriaxone)
plus
Intravenously administered macrolide *or* quinolone (moxifloxacin or levofloxacin*)

Pseudomonal Risk Factors Present
Selected antipseudomonal β-lactam (cefepime, piperacillin/ tazobactam, imipenem, meropenem)
plus
Ciprofloxacin or levofloxacin*
or
Selected antipseudomonal β-lactam
plus
Aminoglycoside
plus
Intravenously administered macrolide or antipneumococcal quinolone (moxifloxacin or levofloxacin*)

*For patients with normal renal function, the recommended dose of levofloxacin is 750 mg daily. Note: Although routine MRSA coverage is NOT recommended for all severe CAP, consider CA-MRSA, especially after influenza and with bilateral necrotizing pneumonia, and if suspected, treat by adding either linezolid or the combination of vancomycin and clindamycin.

the recommended doses for moxifloxacin are 400 mg daily and for levofloxacin 750 mg daily, with the need to adjust dosing of levofloxacin (but not moxifloxacin) in patients with renal insufficiency. The higher dose of levofloxacin is recommended because of reports of failures in pneumococcal pneumonia with levofloxacin, which have occurred in patients who were infected with levofloxacin-resistant organisms, particularly after a recent course of quinolone therapy or with the acquisition of resistance during therapy with the 500-mg dose.[1,71,72]

TIMELINESS OF INITIAL THERAPY OF HOSPITALIZED PATIENTS

For inpatients with CAP, the use of timely and accurate therapy is essential to reduce mortality. In patients with severe CAP, improved survival has been shown to occur if initial empirical therapy is accurate and if it leads to a rapid clinical response.[13,60,90] In one study, if initial therapy led to a clinical response within 72 hours, mortality of severe CAP was approximately 10%, compared with a mortality rate of 60% in patients who had initially ineffective therapy.[13] For CAP in general, early therapy within 4 to 6 hours of arrival to the hospital is associated with reduced mortality compared with therapy given later; but if the patient has pneumonia with sepsis and hypotension, the earlier the therapy is started, the greater the benefit, with mortality rising by nearly 8% for every hour of delay in starting therapy.[110]

THE NEED TO TREAT ALL POPULATIONS FOR ATYPICAL PATHOGEN INFECTION

Although the term *atypical* does not accurately describe a specific clinical pneumonia syndrome, it can be used to refer to a group of pathogens that includes *M. pneumoniae, C. pneumoniae,* and *Legionella.* This group of organisms cannot be reliably eradicated by β-lactam therapy (penicillins and cephalosporins) but must be treated with a macrolide, tetracycline, or a quinolone. In North American CAP guidelines, initial empirical therapy for all patients requires therapy for the possibility of atypical pathogen infection, either as primary infection or as part of a mixed infection, but such therapy is always necessary for ICU patients.[1] This recommendation is based on a number of studies, as mentioned earlier, that show a high frequency of these pathogens when using serologic diagnosis, often in the form of mixed infection coexisting with a bacterial pathogen.[57,58] In one study of inpatients in the United States, infection with atypical pathogens was more common in older individuals (65-79 years) than in those younger than 35, and other studies have shown these pathogens to be common in patients with severe CAP.[11,57]

A number of studies of large populations of inpatients, including those with severe CAP, have shown that when therapy includes a macrolide or a quinolone, outcomes including mortality are improved, compared with when a β-lactam is used by itself.[60,61,106] Although these findings are not definitive, they do suggest the need for routine therapy of atypical pathogens, a strategy that may even be needed in patients with bacteremic pneumococcal pneumonia. As mentioned, several studies have suggested that when patients with this infection receive a β-lactam alone, the mortality is higher than if they receive a β-lactam combined with a macrolide, and the mortality benefit is particularly high for those in the ICU.[62,63]

Legionella is a potentially important pathogen in patients with severe CAP, and there are many drugs available with in vitro activity against *L. pneumophila,* but there are limited prospective comparative data on the role of therapy in the outcome of this infection.[75] Retrospective data and clinical experience support the use of erythromycin at a dose of 4 g/day in the hospitalized patient with *L. pneumophila.* Rifampin should be added in patients with multilobar disease, organ failure, or severe immunosuppression and should be administered for the first 3 to 5 days.[1] Other macrolides (clarithromycin and azithromycin) are also effective, and azithromycin is available in an IV form. However, more recent data suggest that quinolones

(moxifloxacin, levofloxacin) may be an even more effective alternative, since they have been highly effective in animal models and in treating patients with *Legionella,* including those in the ICU.[109] If the patient has severe CAP following influenza, it may also be necessary to add an antiviral agent such as zanamivir or oseltamivir, which are both effective but not clearly proven to reduce the development of respiratory complications. In patients with documented influenza, including H1N1, early therapy provides the best chance for improved outcome.[81,82,111]

There is little information on the proper duration of therapy in patients with CAP, especially those with severe illness. Even in the presence of pneumococcal bacteremia, short durations of therapy may be possible, with a rapid switch from IV to oral therapy in responding patients.[112] Generally, *S. pneumoniae* can be treated for 5 to 7 days if the patient is responding rapidly and has received the correct dose of an accurate therapy. The presence of extrapulmonary infection (e.g., meningitis) and identification of certain pathogens (e.g., bacteremic *S. aureus* and *P. aeruginosa*) may require longer duration of therapy. Identification of *L. pneumophila* pneumonia may require at least 14 days of therapy, depending on severity of illness and host defense impairments, but shorter durations with quinolone therapy have been effective. Most therapy in the ICU will be given IV; however, recent studies using a variety of antibiotics have suggested that oral therapy may be instituted after as early as 2 to 3 days of parenteral therapy, assuming the patient's condition has stabilized and the patient is afebrile.[1] The switch to oral therapy, even in severely ill patients, may be facilitated by the use of quinolones that are highly bioavailable and achieve the same serum levels with oral therapy as with IV therapy.

ADJUNCTIVE THERAPY MEASURES

In addition to antibiotic therapy, the patient with severe CAP may require chest physiotherapy, especially if either an excessive volume of purulent sputum (>30 mL/day) or severe respiratory muscle weakness resulting in ineffective cough are present.[113] Aerosolized humidification has been used to reduce sputum viscosity, thereby enhancing clearance in patients who have generally ineffective cough. However, it is likely that much of the generated water vapor is deposited in the upper airway where it is likely to stimulate cough but unlikely to influence the rheologic properties of sputum. Bronchodilator therapy, which also enhances mucociliary clearance and ciliary beat frequency, is most likely to be of benefit in patients with pneumonia complicating COPD.

Activated protein C (drotrecogin alfa [activated]) infusion has been shown to reduce 28-day mortality in patients with severe sepsis and an APACHE II score of more than 25, but in the original trial, over half of the treated patients had pneumonia as the cause of sepsis, suggesting a role for this therapy in patients with severe CAP.[114] However, in a subsequent analysis of these data, although activated protein C had benefit in CAP, this benefit was most evident in patients who received inappropriate empirical antibiotic therapy, questioning the incremental benefit for patients being treated with the correct antibiotics.[114]

Several studies have looked at the use of adjunctive corticosteroids in patients with severe CAP and have shown possible benefit with no proven harm. However, a recent prospective randomized trial in 213 patients found no difference in clinical cure rates with corticosteroid treatment compared to placebo, although steroid-treated patients had faster defervescence but a higher rate of late failure.[115,116] Adjunctive immune therapy with granulocyte colony-stimulating factor (G-CSF) has also been used in severe CAP, with no benefit in mortality or in the course of illness resolution.[117] Although the role of corticosteroids as routine therapy of CAP is not established, steroids may be beneficial in patients with sepsis and relative adrenal insufficiency that occurs in a high proportion of patients with severe CAP.[118] Salluh et al. have shown that in patients with severe CAP, median cortisol levels were 15.5 μg per dL, and that 65% of patients met the criteria for adrenal insufficiency (cortisol levels less than 20 μg per dL).[118] Another setting in which corticosteroids may have benefit is in pneumococcal pneumonia that is complicated by meningitis, where pretreatment with corticosteroids prior to antibiotic therapy may lead to more favorable neurologic outcomes.[119]

EVALUATION OF RESPONSE TO THERAPY

The majority of patients will respond rapidly to accurate empirical therapy within 24 to 72 hours. Clinical response is defined as improvement in symptoms of cough, sputum production, and dyspnea, along with ability to take medications by mouth, declining white blood cell count, and an afebrile status on at least two occasions 8 hours apart.[1,112] In the critically ill patient, improvement in oxygenation may be one of the earliest signs of response to therapy, although few studies have examined mechanically ventilated patients. When a patient has met criteria for clinical response, it is appropriate to consider a switch to an oral therapy regimen if the patient is otherwise medically and socially stable.[1,112] Radiographic improvement lags behind clinical improvement, and in a responding patient, a chest radiograph is not necessary until 2 to 4 weeks after starting therapy. In general, 50% of patients with pneumococcal pneumonia have radiographic clearing at 5 weeks, whereas the majority clear in 2 to 3 months. With bacteremic disease, 50% of patients have a clear chest radiograph at 9 weeks, and most are clear by 18 weeks.[120] Radiographic resolution is most influenced by the number of lobes involved and the age of the patient. Radiographic clearance of CAP decreases by 20% per decade after age 20, and patients with multilobar infiltrates take longer to clear than those with unilobar disease.[120]

If the patient fails to respond to appropriate therapy in the expected time interval, it is necessary to consider infection with a drug-resistant or unusual pathogen (tuberculosis, *C. burnetii*, *Burkholderia pseudomallei*, *C. psittaci*, endemic fungi, or hantavirus); a pneumonic complication (lung abscess, endocarditis, empyema); or a noninfectious process that mimics pneumonia (bronchiolitis obliterans with organizing pneumonia, hypersensitivity pneumonitis, pulmonary vasculitis, bronchoalveolar cell carcinoma, lymphoma, pulmonary embolus).[1] The evaluation of the nonresponding patient should be individualized but may include CT of the chest, pulmonary angiography, bronchoscopy, and occasionally open lung biopsy.

▇ Prevention

Prevention of CAP is important for all groups of the population but especially the elderly patient, who is at risk for both a higher frequency of infection and a more severe course of illness. Appropriate patients should be vaccinated with both pneumococcal and influenza vaccines, and cigarette smoking should be stopped in all at-risk patients. Even for the patient who is recovering from CAP, immunization while in the hospital is appropriate to prevent future episodes of infection. Evaluation of all patients for vaccination need and provision of information about smoking cessation are now performance standards used to evaluate the hospital care of CAP patients.[1]

PNEUMOCOCCAL VACCINE

Pneumococcal capsular polysaccharide vaccine can prevent pneumonia in otherwise healthy populations, as was initially demonstrated in South African gold miners and American military recruits.[1,121] The benefits in individuals of advanced age or with underlying conditions in nonepidemic environments are less clearly defined. The vaccine efficacy has ranged from 65% to 84% in patients with diabetes mellitus, coronary artery disease, congestive heart failure, chronic pulmonary disease, and anatomic asplenia.[1,121] In immunocompetent patients over the age of 65, effectiveness has been documented to be 75%. In the immunocompromised patient, effectiveness has not been proven, and this includes patients with sickle cell disease, chronic renal failure, immunoglobulin deficiency, Hodgkin's disease, lymphoma, leukemia,

and multiple myeloma. One retrospective cohort study evaluated 47,365 patients older than 65 years to determine the impact of pneumococcal vaccination on three different clinical events: hospitalization for CA, outpatient therapy for CAP, and documented pneumococcal bacteremia.[122] The use of vaccination was associated with a significant reduction in the incidence of pneumococcal bacteremia (OR = 0.56) but no change in the frequency of pneumonia treated in or out of the hospital.

A single revaccination is indicated in a person who is older than age 65 years who initially received the vaccine more than 5 years earlier and was younger than age 65 on first vaccination.[1] If the initial vaccination was given at age 65 or older, repeat is not indicated unless the patient has anatomic or functional asplenia or has one of the immune-compromising conditions listed earlier. In these patients, revaccination is indicated, and the second dose is given at least 5 years after the original dose.

The available pneumococcal vaccine is widely underutilized, especially as the 23-valent pneumococcal vaccine contains 23 pneumococcal serotypes that cause 85% of all infections due to pneumococcus. Two protein-conjugated pneumococcal vaccines have been licensed and are more immunogenic than the older vaccine, but they contain only 7 and 13 serotypes, and are approved for use in children but not yet in adults.[1] However, the conjugate vaccine has had benefit for adults, even when given to only children, demonstrating a "herd immunity" effect. In one study of the heptavalent conjugated pneumococcal vaccine, benefit in reducing invasive illness occurred not only in the population immunized but in adults, particularly those over age 65, who were not the target of the immunization efforts, possibly by lowering the community incidence and pathogen reservoir and reducing the spread of invasive disease.[123] However, more recently, children who have received the 7-valent pneumococcal polysaccharide vaccine have developed infection with strains not included in the vaccine, leading to a higher frequency of severe necrotizing pneumonia, especially with serotype 3 pneumococcus.[124]

Hospital-based immunization could be highly effective because over 60% of all patients with CAP have been admitted to the hospital for some indication in the preceding 4 years, and hospitalization could be defined as an appropriate time for vaccination. Pneumococcal vaccine can be given simultaneously with other vaccines such as influenza vaccine, but each should be given at a separate site, and the vaccine can, and often should, be given before discharge in the patient admitted for CAP.

INFLUENZA VACCINATION

Influenza epidemics contribute to morbidity and mortality both by causing direct infection and by leading to postinfluenza complications. The influenza vaccine preparations are revised annually to account for changes in the antigenic nature of the virus (antigenic drift) that is present each season. Three strains are represented in each vaccine preparation: an influenza A strain (H3N2); an influenza A strain (H1N1); and one influenza B strain. Vaccination should be given to all patients older than age 65, to those with chronic medical illness (including nursing home residents), and to those who provide health care to patients at risk for complicated influenza.[1] It is given yearly, usually between September and mid-November. While the traditional influenza vaccine contains an inactivated virus, there is now an intranasal vaccine containing a live attenuated influenza virus. It is currently approved for individuals aged 5 to 49 years who are not immune suppressed or chronically ill and who do not have asthma.

When the vaccine matches the circulating strain, it can prevent illness in 70% to 90% of healthy persons younger than age 65.[1,125] For older persons with chronic illness, the efficacy is less, but the vaccine can still attenuate the influenza infection and lead to fewer lower respiratory tract infections and the associated morbidity and mortality that follow influenza. In many studies, the vaccine has been shown to be cost-effective and able to prevent severe illness and death and reduce the occurrence of secondary pneumonia and hospitalization.[125]

KEY POINTS

1. Community-acquired pneumonia (CAP) is a common illness, but only about 20% of all affected patients are admitted to the hospital, and only 10% to 20% of admitted patients require ICU care.

2. Risk factors for CAP becoming severe include smoking, alcohol abuse, serious comorbid medical illnesses, and advanced age. Risk factors for CAP mortality include severe physiologic abnormalities, delays in the initiation of appropriate antibiotic therapy, advanced age, genetic abnormalities in the immune response, rapid radiographic progression, development of respiratory failure, and the presence of certain high-risk pathogens.

3. Prognostic scoring systems are useful for predicting CAP mortality but are less accurate for identifying patients who require ICU care. ICU care is needed for patients with respiratory failure, multilobar infiltrates, severe hypoxemia (PaO$_2$/FIO$_2$ ratio < 250), and systolic blood pressure less than 90 mm Hg. Early recognition of severe CAP may allow the ICU to be used in a fashion that can reduce the mortality of this illness.

4. The failure to localize infection to a single site in the lung, with excessive systemic and pulmonary inflammation, is a common feature in patients with severe forms of CAP.

5. Clinical features of pneumonia cannot help predict the microbial etiology, especially in older patients with impaired immune response who commonly have less dramatic clinical findings than younger patients with a similar severity of illness.

6. The most common pathogens causing severe CAP include pneumococcus, atypical pathogens (*Legionella* species, *Mycoplasma pneumoniae*, and *Chlamydophila pneumoniae*), enteric gram-negatives (including *Pseudomonas aeruginosa*), *Staphylococcus aureus* (including community-acquired methicillin-resistant strains), and *Hemophilus influenzae*, but infection can also be the result of viral illness (influenza, SARS), bioterrorism (anthrax), and other miscellaneous organisms.

7. Antibiotic-resistant pneumococci are increasingly common and must be considered in the choice of initial antibiotic therapy for severe CAP, but the impact of resistance on the outcomes of patients is uncertain.

8. It may be difficult to establish an exact etiologic diagnosis in patients with severe CAP, but diagnostic testing should always include a chest radiograph, oxygenation assessment, and blood cultures. In selected patients, sputum Gram stain and culture, bronchoscopic culture, and urinary antigen testing for *Legionella* and pneumococcus should also be added.

9. Therapy for severe CAP must be done promptly and empirically, using multiple antibiotics directed against pneumococcus, atypical pathogens, enteric gram-negative organisms, and in some patients, *P. aeruginosa* and community-acquired methicillin-resistant *S. aureus*. This usually requires the combination of a specific β-lactam with either a macrolide or a quinolone and sometimes the addition of other agents. Quinolone monotherapy is not recommended for the empirical management of severe CAP. In patients with severe CAP after influenza, community-acquired methicillin-resistant *S. aureus* (CA-MRSA) should be considered.

10. Adjunctive therapies for severe CAP include chest physiotherapy, inhaled bronchodilators, and activated protein C, all used in carefully selected populations. Use of systemic corticosteroids has not been established as routine adjunctive therapy but may have value if the patient has adrenal insufficiency or pneumococcal pneumonia with meningitis.

11. Nonresponse in severe CAP can be recognized as early as 24 to 48 hours and requires consideration of unusual or drug-resistant pathogens, noninfectious diseases that mimic pneumonia, and pneumonia complications.

12. Prevention of pneumonia can be accomplished by focusing on smoking cessation and immunization for pneumococcus and influenza, with consideration of a hospital-based immunization program.

ANNOTATED REFERENCES

Baddour LM, Yu VL, Klugman KP, et al. Combination antibiotic therapy lowers mortality among severely ill patients with pneumococcal bacteremia. Am J Respir Crit Care Med 2004;170:440-4.

In a study of patients with documented pneumococcal bacteremia, the use of dual therapy was associated with a reduced mortality, compared to monotherapy, with the greatest impact being in those with critical illness. The findings corroborate other retrospective analyses, although the mechanism of benefit is unclear, but may relate to the antiinflammatory benefit of macrolides when they are used as the second agent.

Charles PG, Wolfe R, Whitby M, Fine MJ, Fuller AJ, Stirling R, et al. SMART-COP: a tool for predicting the need for intensive respiratory or vasopressor support in community-acquired pneumonia. Clin Infect Dis 2008;47:375-84.

No prognostic scoring tool is ideal for determining the need for ICU care, but this study focused on defining a tool that predicted the need for invasive or noninvasive ventilation or the need for pressors to support blood pressure. The scoring tool incorporated eight simple clinical assessments and weighted some abnormalities more than others. The predictive value of this tool for the need for advanced supportive care was superior to older prognostic scoring tools.

Christ-Crain, M, Stolz, D, Bingisser R, et al. Procalcitonin guidance of antibiotic therapy in community-acquired pneumonia: a randomized trial. Am J Respir Crit Care Med 2006;174:84-93.

A landmark prospective randomized trial of 302 patients with radiographic community-acquired pneumonia, showing that serial measurements of procalcitonin, using the sensitive Kryptor assay, could be used to guide duration of antibiotic therapy. Patients managed by procalcitonin data had a 55% shorter duration of therapy than those managed by clinical assessment, with no adverse consequences of shorter duration therapy.

El-Solh AA, Pietrantoni C, Bhat A, et al. Microbiology of severe aspiration pneumonia in institutionalized elderly. Am J Respir Crit Care Med 2003;167:1650-4.

Prospective microbiological evaluation of elderly patients admitted to the ICU from a nursing home; patients had severe CAP in the setting of risk factors for aspiration. The predominant organisms were gram negative and not anaerobic; even when anaerobes were identified, specific antibiotic therapy did not appear to be necessary.

Kumar A, Roberts D, Wood KE, et al. Duration of hypotension before initiation of effective antimicrobial therapy is the critical determinant of survival in human septic shock. Crit Care Med 2006;34:1589-96.

In a study of 2154 patients with septic shock, the investigators documented that the sooner patients received appropriate therapy, the lower the mortality. If therapy was started within the first hour of hypotension, survival was nearly 80%, but over the first 6 hours, dropped by 7.6% for each hour of delay after the onset of hypotension to the initiation of appropriate therapy.

Leroy O, Saux P, Bedos JP, Caulin E. Comparison of levofloxacin and cefotaxime combined with ofloxacin for ICU patients with community-acquired pneumonia who do not require vasopressors. Chest 2005;128:172-83.

A prospective randomized, open-label trial of 398 patients with severe CAP treated with either quinolone monotherapy (high-dose levofloxacin) or the combination of a β-lactam with a quinolone. Although both regimens were equivalent, there was a trend to for worse outcome (cure) with monotherapy in mechanically ventilated patients, and by design, patients with septic shock were excluded. Thus this study did not provide definitive evidence of the safety and efficacy of quinolone monotherapy for patients with severe CAP.

Mandell LA, Wunderink RG, Anzueto A, Bartlett JG, Campbell GD, Dean NC, et al. Infectious Diseases Society of America; American Thoracic Society. Infectious Diseases Society of America/American Thoracic Society consensus guidelines on the management of community-acquired pneumonia in adults. Clin Infect Dis 2007;44:S27-72.

Evidence-based guideline for CAP, focusing on epidemiology, bacteriology, and management. A definition of severe CAP is provided, relying on the presence of either one of two major risk factors or the presence of three minor risk factors. For patients with severe CAP, the likely etiologic pathogens are identified and accompanied by suggestions for initial empirical therapy that never includes monotherapy for any ICU-admitted patient.

Valencia M, Badia JR, Cavalcanti M, Ferrer M, Agusti C, Angrill J, et al. Pneumonia severity index class V patients with community-acquired pneumonia. Characteristics, outcomes, and value of severity. Chest 2007;132:515-22.

In a study of 457 patients with CAP falling into PSI class V, only 92 required ICU admission. Those needing ICU care received more of their PSI points from acute illness factors rather than from chronic disease factors. The findings point out that PSI class is not a direct measurement of pneumonia severity, even if it can predict mortality well, since patients can accumulate points for reasons other than the severity of the acute infection.

REFERENCES

Access the complete reference list online at http://www.expertconsult.com.

67

Nosocomial Pneumonia

GIANLUIGI LI BASSI | MIGUEL FERRER | ANTONI TORRES

Definitions

Nosocomial pneumonia is an infection of the pulmonary parenchyma caused by pathogens predominantly present in hospital settings.[1] Nosocomial pneumonia develops in patients admitted to the hospital for more than 48 hours, and usually the incubation period of this infection is no longer than 2 days. Nosocomial pneumonias include ventilator-associated pneumonia (VAP), which commonly develops in intensive care unit (ICU) patients who have been tracheally intubated and mechanically ventilated for at least 48 hours. Ventilator-associated tracheobronchitis (VAT) has not been as extensively studied as VAP in patients undergoing mechanical ventilation, but this disorder is characterized by signs of respiratory infection such as an increase in the volume and purulence of respiratory secretions, fever, and leukocytosis. However, in contrast to VAP, radiologic infiltrates suggestive of consolidation on chest x-ray are not observed.[1] Healthcare-associated pneumonia (HCAP) is a new clinical entity that has recently been defined in the latest guidelines of the American Thoracic Society[1] for the diagnosis and treatment of nosocomial pneumonia. Patients who develop HCAP are not hospitalized, but they present several risks for being colonized by pathogens present in hospital settings, including multiresistant microorganisms. Risk factors for developing HCAP are hospitalization for 2 days or more within the preceding 90 days, residence in a nursing home or extended care facility, home infusion therapy (including antibiotics), chronic dialysis within 30 days, home wound care, and a family member with multidrug-resistant (MDR) pathogen colonization or infection. Interestingly, there is still controversy about the etiology and definition of HCAP. Indeed, several North American studies have reported that HCAP is mostly caused by multiresistant microorganisms; conversely, European data show larger similarities between etiology of HCAP and community-acquired pneumonia.

Nosocomial pneumonia can also be classified based on the presence of microorganisms isolated through respiratory surveillance cultures and includes the following categories[2]:

1. Primary endogenous pneumonia: causative microorganisms are isolated in surveillance cultures on admission.
2. Secondary endogenous pneumonia: causative microorganisms are nosocomial pathogens not present in patients on admission; they colonize the oropharynx and gastrointestinal (GI) tract during the course of the patient's hospital stay and thereafter translocate into the lower respiratory tract.
3. Exogenous pneumonia: caused by microorganisms not originally isolated through surveillance cultures; hence the patient is not a previous carrier. Colonization of artificial airways (ventilatory tubes, humidifiers), bronchoscopes, and nebulizers plays an important role in this category.

The time of onset for nosocomial pneumonia also has important implications for possible etiology, empirical antimicrobial treatment, and outcomes. Langer et al.[3] first differentiated between nosocomial pneumonia at early onset (developing within the first 4 days after hospital admission) and late onset (5 days or more). However, there are no well-designed trials supporting these time cutoffs. An interesting trial performed by Trouillet et al.[4] found that three variables were significant for predicting infection with MDR VAP: duration of mechanical ventilation (MV) $\geq$ 7 days (odds ratio [OR] = 6.0), prior antibiotic use (OR = 13.5), and prior use of broad-spectrum drugs (third-generation cephalosporin, fluoroquinolone, and/or imipenem) (OR = 4.1).

Epidemiology

INCIDENCE

Nosocomial pneumonia is the second most common nosocomial infection and the leading cause of death from nosocomial infections for critically ill patients. The incidence of nosocomial pneumonia is age dependent, with 5 of every 1000 cases affecting hospitalized patients younger than 35 years of age and up to 15 of 1000 in hospitalized patients older than 65.[5] In earlier reports, nosocomial pneumonia increased hospital stay by 7 to 9 days per patient, accounting for up to 25% of all ICU infections and for more than 50% of the antibiotics prescribed.[6] A Spanish report by Sopena et al.[7] in 2005 studied the epidemiology of nosocomial pneumonia in 186 non-ICU patients from 12 hospitals and found that nosocomial pneumonia was observed mostly in elderly patients with underlying diseases and was primarily caused by *S. pneumoniae*, *Legionella pneumophila*, *Aspergillus* spp., and *P. aeruginosa*. The mortality rate was 26%, with an attributable mortality of 13%. Cook et al.[8] estimated that the risk of VAP is 1% per day on mechanical ventilation[8]; they also demonstrated that the risk changes over time, being 3% the first 5 days on mechanical ventilation, 2% from the 5th to 10th day, and 1% for the remaining days. Considering that most invasively ventilated patients are intubated for less than a week, nearly half of VAP cases occur during the first days of mechanical ventilation.

MORTALITY

The crude mortality from nosocomial pneumonia may be as high as 30% to 70%, although several cofactors influence mortality during critical illness and make it extremely difficult to determine attributable mortality.[9] Mortality caused by VAP has been defined as the percentage of deaths that would not have occurred in the absence of the infection. Several case-matching studies have estimated that one third to one half of all VAP-related deaths are the direct result of the infection, with a higher mortality rate in cases caused by *P. aeruginosa* or *Acinetobacter* spp. and associated with bacteremia.[10] The development of VAP is accompanied by a 1.8- to 4-fold increase in the risk of death. A multicenter French study[9] evaluated the attributable mortality and risk factors for death for late-onset pneumonia. They evaluated 764 patients admitted to the ICU for more than 96 hours and found a 47% mortality in patients with VAP versus 22% in the total population. Moreover, mortality was inversely related to adequacy of the initial empirical therapy. Similarly, Luna et al.[11] assessed the appropriateness and delay of antibiotic therapy in 76 mechanically ventilated patients with bacteriologically confirmed VAP and found an overall mortality of 52.6%. Based on current evidence, nosocomial pneumonia is associated with a high mortality rate, but precise estimates of mortality attributable to this condition are not possible, owing to heterogeneity between patient populations, microbial patterns, antibiotic treatment, and diagnostic methods.[12]

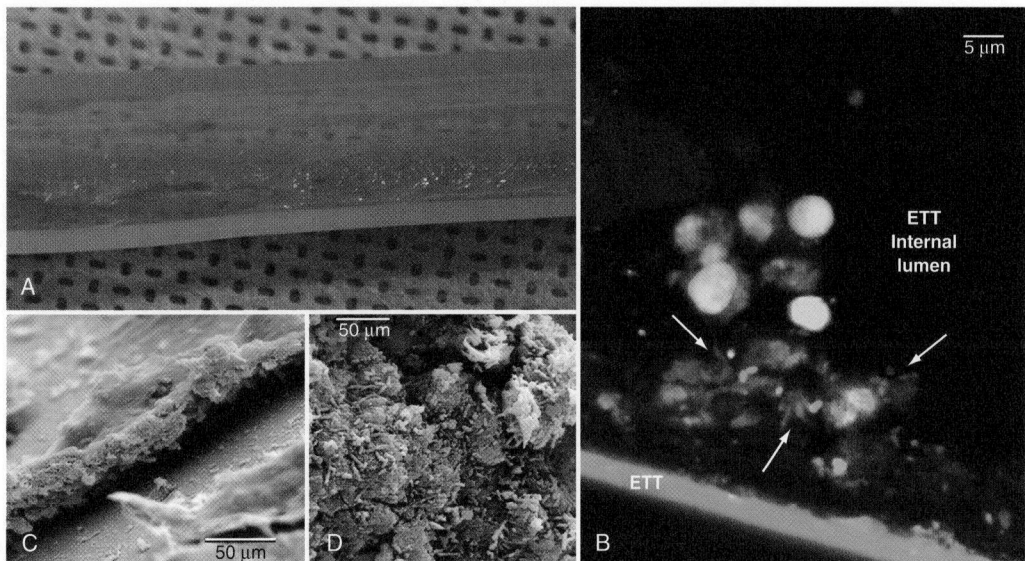

Figure 67-1 Laboratory studies to assess biofilm formation on internal surface of tracheal tube, following oropharyngeal challenge in pigs of *Pseudomonas aeruginosa* (strain PAO1) and 72 hours of mechanical ventilation. **A,** Internal surface of tracheal tube at extubation, largely covered by respiratory secretions. **B,** Cross-section of tracheal tube stained with LIVE/DEAD BacLight bacterial viability kit and imaged with confocal scanning laser microscopy. Bacterial biofilm adheres to internal ETT surface. *White arrows* indicate bacteria embedded into biofilm matrix. ETT, endotracheal tube. **C,** Scanning electron microscopy of tracheal tube lumen. Note presence of amorphous deposits on most of surface. **D,** Higher magnification of tracheal tube lumen through scanning electron microscopy. *P. aeruginosa* sessile cells are clearly visible within biofilm extracellular polymeric substance.

Pathogenesis

Extensive laboratory and clinical work has determined the key pathogenetic mechanisms of VAP. Pathogens must first gain access into the airways to cause pneumonia, and intubated patients are at high risk for aspiration of colonized oropharyngeal secretions. Patients can be colonized exogenously from the hands, apparel, or equipment of healthcare personnel, the hospital environment, and the use of invasive devices. Likewise, patients may be colonized from endogenous sources, including pathogens colonizing the GI tract, oropharynx, tracheal tube, and proximal trachea. In healthy, nonintubated patients, when bacteria gain access into the respiratory tract, colonization is prevented through defense mechanisms such as cough, mucus clearance, and cellular and humoral immune responses. Intubated patients are already at high risk for infection because of the underlying critical illness, comorbidities, malnutrition, and invasive devices/procedures; however, tracheal intubation is the "*conditio sine qua non*" for the development of pneumonia, because it facilitates aspiration of pathogens and hinders intrinsic respiratory defenses.

ROLE OF TRACHEAL TUBE IN THE PATHOGENESIS OF VENTILATOR-ASSOCIATED PNEUMONIA

Pulmonary aspiration of colonized oropharyngeal secretions across the tracheal tube cuff is the main pathogenic mechanism for development of VAP. The endotracheal tube (ETT), commonly used in the ICU for long-term mechanically ventilated patients, includes a high-volume, low-pressure (HVLP) cuff. HVLP cuffs were originally designed to control pressure exerted against the tracheal wall and prevent tracheal injury.[13-15] However, the potential diameter of the HVLP cuff is two to three times larger than the tracheal diameter, so when the tracheal cuff is inflated within the trachea, folds invariably form along the cuff surface, causing consistent micro- and macroaspiration of oropharyngeal secretions.[16]

Pathogens may also grow on the internal surface of the ETT and ultimately translocate into the lungs. The ETT is commonly made of polyvinyl chloride (PVC), and bacteria easily adhere to its internal surface to form a complex structure called *biofilm*[17,18] (Figure 67-1).

Biofilm is composed of sessile bacteria embedded within a self-produced exopolysaccharide matrix.[19] Biofilm on the internal surface of an ETT can be identified early following tracheal intubation.[20,21] Sessile bacteria undergo phenotypic differentiation from their planktonic counterparts, and most of such differentiation constitutes a survival advantage. Indeed, bacteria within the biofilm are difficult to eradicate, and antibacterial efficacy of the host's immune response and antibiotics are largely reduced. During mechanical ventilation, biofilm particles may dislodge into the airways as a result of inspiratory airflow[17] and invasive medical interventions such as tracheal aspiration[22] and bronchoscopy. Several studies have assessed the role of bacterial biofilm on pathogenesis of VAP and confirmed that the ETT biofilm is difficult to eradicate and constitutes a persistent source of colonization. Adair et al.[23] studied 40 tracheal tubes obtained from critically ill patients with and without VAP and compared the genotype of bacteria retrieved from the lower airways and the ETT. In 70% of the samples obtained from patients with VAP, the authors found the same genotype in bacteria from ETT biofilm and the patients' airways. Moreover, they confirmed that antibiotic susceptibility was lower in pathogens isolated from within the biofilm.

SOURCES OF COLONIZATION

Tracheally intubated patients in the ICU can be colonized either exogenously or endogenously. Patients are colonized exogenously by contaminated respiratory equipment, the ICU environment, and the hands of the ICU staff. Several reports have described ICU outbreaks due to colonized bronchoscopes,[24,25] water supply,[26,27] respiratory equipment,[28,29] humidifiers,[30] ventilator temperature sensors,[31,32] respiratory nebulizers,[33,34] and contaminated environment.[35] Several factors play a significant role in reducing risks for cross-transmission of pathogens. Indeed, in every ICU an adequate ratio of single rooms to open beds should be provided; healthcare personnel should be adequately trained on infection control and preventive strategies; strict sterilization protocols and hand washing with alcohol-based solutions should be implemented, and finally, lower patient-to-nurse ratios are advantageous.

Endogenous colonization is believed to be the primary pathogenic mechanism for VAP development. In the critically ill patient, the oral flora shifts early to a predominance of aerobic gram-negative pathogens,[36,37] *Pseudomonas aeruginosa*, and methicillin-resistant *Staphylococcus aureus* (MRSA). Therefore, pulmonary aspiration of oropharyngeal contents increases the risk for airway colonization and infection. Following aspiration and colonization of the airways, the occurrence of VAP primarily depends on the size of the inoculum, functional status, and the competency of host defenses. There is still controversy regarding the exact sequence of colonization and sources of infection in the pathogenesis of VAP. Early studies by Feldman et al.[38] found that in patients undergoing mechanical ventilation, the oropharynx is the first site to be colonized by pathogens (36 hours), followed by the stomach (36-60 hours), the lower respiratory tract (60-84 hours), and thereafter the tracheal tube (60-96 hours).

Dental Plaque

In the healthy human, oral colonization with pathogens is prevented by the physical-chemical properties of the oral mucosa surface, the salivary enzymatic content, and specific proteases and immunoglobulins. ICU patients are at higher risk for dental plaque colonization due to difficulties in oral hygiene, changes in salivary properties during critical illness, and change of oral flora by antibiotic therapy. An early study by Scannapieco et al.[39] showed that ICU patients are often colonized by aerobic pathogens on admission. More recently, Fourrier and collaborators[40] found that prolonged ICU stay increases risks for colonization of dental plaque by aerobic pathogens. Moreover, the authors found that colonization of dental plaque was highly predictive of concurrent or subsequent nosocomial infection. Azarpazhooh et al.[41] found evidence of an association of pneumonia with oral health (OR = 1.2 to 9.6, depending on oral health indicators). The authors reported that improved oral hygiene and frequent professional oral health care reduces the progression or occurrence of respiratory infection among high-risk elderly adults living in nursing homes and especially those in ICUs (number needed to treat [NNT] = 2-16; relative risk reduction [RRR] = 34%-83%). During critical illness and extensive antibiotic therapy, the oral flora may rapidly change; unfortunately, standard culture-based microbiological assays determine neither the dominant bacterial species nor the range of bacterial diversity within the community. In a study by Heo,[42] 18 ICU patients who developed VAP were studied, comparing genetic features of strains obtained from oral, tracheal, and bronchoalveolar lavage (BAL) samples. The authors found that oral respiratory pathogens were often genetically identical to pathogens recovered from the lower airways, and rapid changes of bacterial species in both oral and pulmonary sites appeared to occur.

Sinuses

The association between sinusitis and VAP has long been debated. Several studies have confirmed that orotracheal as compared to nasotracheal intubation is associated with a decreased incidence of sinusitis,[43-45] and that incidence of VAP is lower in patients who do not develop sinusitis.[46] A study by Holzapfel et al.[47] evaluated the incidence of nosocomial maxillary sinusitis and pneumonia in patients who underwent either nasotracheal or orotracheal intubation. The authors found that sinusitis increased the risk of nosocomial pneumonia by a factor of 3.8.

Stomach

According to the gastropulmonary hypothesis of colonization, the stomach of ICU patients is often colonized by pathogens as a consequence of alkalinization of gastric contents by enteral nutrition and drugs. Continuous gastroesophageal reflux facilitates translocation of microbes into the oropharynx, which are then aspirated across the ETT cuff. Several trials have investigated the benefits of selective gut decontamination and stress ulcer prophylaxis and confirmed that preventing gastric alkalinization and reducing the bacterial burden of the stomach is associated with a lower incidence of nosocomial respiratory infections.[48] Early studies have shown that in tracheally intubated patients,

gastric pH higher than 4 is consistently associated with gastric colonization with pathogens.[49,50] However, the association between gastric colonization and VAP found in early studies[51-53] has been challenged by more recent studies.[54-57] Overall, this area remains highly controversial, and several studies[38,54,58-63] have not found a relationship with bacteria causing VAP as first originating in the stomach.

IMPAIRMENT OF RESPIRATORY DEFENSE DURING CRITICAL ILLNESS AND TRACHEAL INTUBATION

In healthy subjects, the physiologic adduction of the true and false vocal folds provides full closure of the airways, and efficiently prevents aspiration of pathogen-laden oropharyngeal contents. The airways are additionally protected by the epiglottis, which moves over the top of the larynx to divert any fluid or solids from passing into the airways. Following intubation, the tracheal tube completely bypasses these anatomic barriers and creates a direct conduit for bacteria to be aspirated and reach lower airways. Cough is one of the most efficient mechanisms to prevent further translocation of pathogens that may have gained access into airways. In the healthy human, cough begins with an inspiratory effort followed by a forced expiratory effort against a closed glottis and ultimately, opening of the glottis to generate rapid expiratory airflow. Tracheal intubation prevents closure of the glottis, hence it fully hinders cough; moreover, intubated patients are often sedated and unable to generate high expiratory flows. Mucociliary clearance is the primary innate airway defense mechanism to clear pathogens. In young, healthy nonsmokers, the mucociliary velocity ranges between 10 and 15 mm/min. Studies in animals have consistently shown that inflation of the tracheal tube cuff within the trachea lowers mucociliary velocity by 37% within an hour, and 52% after 2 hours.[64] Clinical studies[65] in critically ill, tracheally intubated patients have confirmed those results and found that mucociliary velocity is very low (0.8-1.4 mm/min); lower mucociliary clearance has been associated with higher risks for pulmonary complications.

Although many ICU patients develop tracheal bacterial colonization during the course of mechanical ventilation, only a small proportion subsequently develop VAP. As previously mentioned, the daily hazard rate for developing VAP is higher during the first days of mechanical ventilation.[8] Investigators have found that a temporary immunoparalysis can be found early in the course of the critical illness and admission to the ICU.[66] In particular, researchers have focused on assessing human leukocyte antigen DR (HLA-DR) expression on peripheral monocytes as a marker of immune function.[67-69] According to the rationale that impaired immune function may predispose to the development of VAP, low levels of HLA-DR expression have been found in patients who subsequently developed nosocomial pneumonia.[70]

ETIOLOGIC AGENTS

Nosocomial pneumonia may be caused by a variety of pathogens and, in many patients, more than one pathogen may be isolated. Microorganisms responsible for nosocomial pneumonia differ according to the ICU population, the duration of hospital and ICU stays, and the specific diagnostic method(s) used. VAP is commonly caused by aerobic gram-negative bacilli such as *P. aeruginosa*, *Escherichia coli*, *Klebsiella pneumoniae*, or *Acinetobacter* species, while *S. aureus* is the predominant isolated gram-positive pathogen.[1,71-74] Data from 7087 infected patients (63.5% with respiratory tract infection) from the Extended Prevalence of Infection in Intensive Care (EPIC II) study[75] have confirmed that *Pseudomonas* spp. and *S. aureus* are the most common isolated pathogens in intensive care units.

Few studies have assessed whether the pathogens that cause pneumonia in ventilated patients differ from those in patients who are not mechanically ventilated. Weber et al.[76] evaluated 158,519 patients admitted to a single center over a 4-year period and identified 327 episodes of VAP and 261 episodes of nosocomial pneumonia. The infecting flora in ventilated patients mostly included MRSA (17.75%)

and gram-negative bacilli such as *P. aeruginosa* (59.0%), *Stenotrophomonas maltophilia* (17.50%), and *Acinetobacter* species (6.75%). Similarly, in 20.37% of the patients not requiring mechanical ventilation, MRSA was identified, while a lower incidence of nosocomial pneumonia due to *P. aeruginosa*, *Acinetobacter* spp., and *S. maltophilia* was found. Nevertheless, the overall frequency of infection with these gram-negative pathogens was sufficiently high to warrant the use of empirical therapy likely to be active against them.

The high rate of polymicrobial infection in VAP has been shown repeatedly. Combes and colleagues[77] studied 124 ICU patients, of whom 65 (52%) had monomicrobial VAP and 59 had (48%) polymicrobial VAP. In most patients, two different bacteria were isolated (42 patients, 34%); however, up to four different bacteria coexisted in 7 patients (6%). Interestingly, no differences were detected in mortality rate at 30 days between patients with polymicrobial or monomicrobial infection. A study by Teixeira et al.[78] investigated risk factors for inadequate empirical antimicrobial therapy in 151 ICU patients and found that 69 (45.7%) patients with a clinical diagnosis of VAP received inadequate empirical antimicrobial treatment. Multiple logistic regression analysis revealed that inadequate antimicrobial treatment was associated with polymicrobial VAP (OR, 3.67; 95% confidence interval [CI], 1.21-11.12; $P = 0.02$), and importantly, inadequate antimicrobial treatment was associated with higher mortality for patients with VAP.

Underlying diseases may predispose patients to infection with specific organisms, Patients with chronic obstructive pulmonary disease (COPD), for example, are at increased risk for *Haemophilus influenzae*, *Moraxella catarrhalis*, *P. aeruginosa*, or *Streptococcus pneumoniae* infections.[79,80] Patients with acute respiratory distress syndrome (ARDS) are at higher risk for developing VAP caused by *S. aureus*, *P. aeruginosa*, and *Acinetobacter baumannii*, and often in these patients, VAP is caused by multiple pathogens.[81,82] Finally, trauma and neurologic patients are at increased risk for *S. aureus*, *Haemophilus*, and *S. pneumoniae* infections.[83-85]

It is important to identify MDR pathogens in order to guide appropriate antibiotic treatment. Causative pathogens of VAP that are potentially multiresistant are *P. aeruginosa*, MRSA, *Acinetobacter* spp., *S. maltophilia*, *Burkholderia cepacia*, and extended-spectrum β-lactamase (ESBL+) *Klebsiella pneumonia*. Conversely, *S. pneumoniae*, *H. influenzae*, methicillin-sensitive *S. aureus* (MSSA), and antibiotic-sensitive *Enterobacteriaceae* are not considered MDR pathogens. Patients at risk of being colonized by MDR pathogens are extremely heterogeneous, often present several comorbidities, and many receive antibiotics prior to and during the course of their hospitalization. Therefore, it is extremely challenging to accurately define risk factors for carrying MDR pathogens. Langer et al.[3] tried to better classify patients who develop VAP, in order to provide data for guiding empirical antibiotic treatment. They compared early-onset and late-onset pneumonia and found that early-onset pneumonia is rarely caused by MDR pathogens, is less severe, and is associated with better outcome. However, recent reports are challenging such conclusions and demonstrate no association between MDR pathogens and time of onset of pneumonia.[86,87] Those data suggest the need for additional studies to accurately identify risk factors for harboring MDR pathogens, rather than risk stratification based on nonspecific factors such as severity of pneumonia and time of onset. The incidence of MDR pathogens is also closely linked to local factors and varies widely from one institution to another. Consequently, each ICU has to continuously collect accurate epidemiologic data. Rello et al.[88] analyzed variations of VAP etiology among three Spanish ICUs and compared them with data collected in Paris. The authors concluded that VAP pathogens varied widely among the four clinical centers, with marked differences in the microorganisms isolated from VAP episodes in Spanish centers as compared with the French site. Therefore, clinicians must be aware of the common microorganisms associated with both early-onset and late-onset VAP in their own hospitals to avoid the administration of inadequate initial antimicrobial therapy.

Legionella pneumophila as a cause of nosocomial pneumonia should be considered, particularly in immunocompromised patients.[89] Often the source of legionellosis outbreaks within the hospital is a water system that has become colonized by the microorganism.[90]

The role of anaerobes in the pathogenesis of VAP requires further assessment, since the primary mechanism for VAP development is through aspiration of oropharyngeal contents, and the oropharynx is highly colonized by anaerobes. Robert et al.[91] studied 26 mechanically ventilated patients and found that 15 patients became colonized with 28 different anaerobic strains. Similarly Dore et al.[92] found anaerobic bacteria in 30 (23%) of 130 patients diagnosed with VAP, but always in association with aerobic pathogens. Importantly, empirical antibiotic therapy active against anaerobic bacteria appears to improve short-term outcomes in patients with VAP.[93] Nevertheless, several authors[94,95] were unable to reproduce those data, and the role of anaerobes in VAP is still considered controversial. In particular, Marik et al.[95] studied microbiology of 185 episodes of suspected VAP through blind protected specimen brush sampling and mini-BAL and were unable to identify anaerobes as the causative pathogens of VAP.

Rarely, the causative organism of VAP is a fungus. *Candida* spp. and *Aspergillus fumigatus* are the most common isolated fungi, predominately in immunocompromised patients. In mechanically ventilated patients, the clinical significance of respiratory tract colonization by *Candida* is controversial. In a retrospective analysis of 639 patients from a Canadian study or VAP, 114 patients had *Candida* colonization of the respiratory tract.[96] Interestingly, patients with *Candida* colonization had a significant increase in hospital mortality (34% versus 21% in patients without *Candida* colonization, $P = 0.003$). However, it is still unclear whether *Candida* colonization is associated with or responsible for worse outcomes. Moreover, a recent report showed that in ICU patients, isolation of *Candida* species in respiratory samples demonstrates only colonization rather than *Candida* pneumonia.[97]

It is commonly reported that VAP is infrequently due to viruses; however, it should also be acknowledged that patients with clinical suspicion of VAP are rarely screened for viruses. Daubin et al.[98] studied 139 patients mechanically ventilated for more than 48 hours, of which 39 (28%) developed VAP. Although *P. aeruginosa* and MRSA still accounted for most of the VAP cases, herpes simplex virus type 1 was found in 12 cases of VAP and cytomegalovirus (CMV) in 1 case. Several studies have reported a high incidence of active CMV infection in mechanically ventilated patients.[99-101] Recently, Chiche et al.[102] studied 242 immunocompetent ICU patients and found active CMV infection in 39 (16%). At 28 days, only 15% of the patients with active CMV infection were weaned and alive, in comparison to 52% of patients free of CMV infection ($P < 0.001$).

Prevention

Nosocomial pneumonia is associated with high morbidity and mortality and constitutes an important burden for the healthcare system[1,103]; therefore, preventive strategies should be implemented to reduce overall incidence of the disease (Box 67-1). Strategies have focused on reducing cross-transmission, the likelihood of aspiration across the ETT cuff, and the bacterial load in the oropharynx. The Institute for Healthcare Improvement recommends that approaches with proven efficacy for reduction of morbidity and mortality related to infection control should be grouped and implemented together as a bundle, because together they are expected to result in a better outcome than when implemented individually. Designing a preventive bundle is just the first step and must be followed by continuous assessment of healthcare personnel compliance and improvements to implement interventions. Several reports[104-106] have found drastic reductions in the incidence of VAP following implementation of VAP preventive bundles.

GENERAL PROPHYLACTIC MEASURES

Maintaining high levels of education among ICU personnel relating to VAP pathophysiology and preventive strategies can be effective in

PREVENTIVE STRATEGIES FOR NOSOCOMIAL PNEUMONIA

- Implementation, as a bundle, of nosocomial pneumonia preventive strategies that have proven efficacy in reducing morbidity and mortality
- Implementation of educational programs for caregivers and frequent performance feedbacks and compliance assessment
- Strict alcohol-based hand hygiene
- Avoidance of tracheal intubation and use of NIV when indicated
- Daily sedation vacation and implementation of weaning protocols
- No ventilatory circuit tube changes unless the circuit is soiled or damaged
- Use of tracheal tube with cuff made of novel materials and shapes
- Use of silver-coated tracheal tube
- Application of low-level PEEP during tracheal intubation
- Aspiration of subglottic secretions
- Internal cuff pressure maintained within the recommended range and carefully controlled during transport of patients outside ICU
- Oral care with chlorhexidine
- Avoid stress ulcer prophylaxis in very low-risk patients for gastrointestinal bleed, and consider use of sucralfate when indicated.
- Semirecumbent patient positioning
- Continuous lateral rotation therapy
- Postpyloric feeding in patients who have impaired gastric emptying
- SDD for patients requiring >48 hours of mechanical ventilation

ICU, Intensive care unit; *NIV,* noninvasive ventilation; *PEEP,* positive end-expiratory pressure; *SDD,* selective digestive decontamination.

reducing incidence of this problem.[107-110] Respiratory care practitioners and nurses should be the primary recipients of education programs, and frequent performance feedback and compliance assessment should be undertaken.[111] Interestingly, Needleman et al.[112] studied administrative data from 799 hospitals in 11 states (covering 5,075,969 discharges of medical patients and 1,104,659 discharges of surgical patients) and found that a higher proportion of hours of care per day provided by registered nurses, compared to licensed practical nurses and nurses' aides, were associated with lower incidence of pneumonia.

Adherence to simple infection-control measures such as alcohol-based hand disinfection effectively reduces cross-transmission of pathogens and incidence of VAP.[113] The World Health Organization has endorsed hand hygiene as the single most important element of strategies to prevent healthcare-associated infections.[114] Overall, most studies conducted in ICUs have shown consistent results and temporal association between implementation of alcohol-based hand hygiene and reduction of nosocomial infections.[115-117]

Kollef et al.[118] demonstrated that patient transport outside the ICU was associated with increased risks for VAP. Clinicians and nursing staff should carefully carry out transport of intubated patients. In particular, the internal pressure of the ETT cuff should be always kept within the recommended range, particularly when the patient is expected to be maintained supine during diagnostic or therapeutic procedures; ventilator circuits should be carefully manipulated in order to prevent aspiration of colonized fluids from within the circuit.

Daily interruption or lightening of sedation to avoid constant impairment of respiratory defenses, as well as avoidance of paralytic agents, is highly recommended. It is well acknowledged that prolonged tracheal intubation is associated with VAP.[8] A report by Kress et al.[119] was recently confirmed by Schweickert et al.,[120] who studied 128 mechanically ventilated patients randomized to continuous infusions of sedation with or without daily interruption. The authors demonstrated reduction of duration of mechanical ventilation and length of

stay in the ICU when patients were allowed to wake up daily. Moreover, a trial by Schweickert et al.[121] has shown that early physical and occupational therapy during critical illness is associated with more ventilator-free days. In a study by Strøm et al.,[122] 140 critically ill adult patients expected to be intubated for more than 24 hours were randomized to receive no sedation or sedation with daily interruption until awake. Both groups were treated with bolus doses of morphine. In that study, patients receiving no sedation had significantly more days without ventilation and shorter stay in the ICU. Results from these clinical trials are challenging standard sedation protocols for intubated patients and hold promise for reducing length of stay on mechanical ventilation and, ultimately, risks for VAP.

There is evidence of shorter length of mechanical ventilation, reduced rate of failed extubation, and decreased incidence of VAP when protocol-driven weaning from the ventilator is implemented.[123,124] Marelich et al.[123] randomized 385 patients to receive either a protocol-driven weaning procedure or standard care and found that duration of mechanical ventilation was decreased from a median of 124 hours for the control group to 68 hours in the protocol-driven weaning group ($P = 0.0001$). Moreover, a trend toward less VAP was found in the treatment group ($P = 0.061$).

NONINVASIVE VENTILATION

Tracheal intubation and mechanical ventilation account for the main risk for nosocomial pneumonia and therefore should be avoided whenever possible. Noninvasive ventilation (NIV) is an attractive alternative for patients with acute exacerbations of COPD or acute hypoxemic respiratory failure and for some immunocompromised patients with pulmonary infiltrates and respiratory failure.[125-128] NIV can also be safely used to facilitate early extubation and avoid continued invasive weaning. A meta-analysis[129] evaluated 12 trials enrolling 530 participants, mostly with chronic obstructive pulmonary disease, and confirmed that noninvasive weaning is significantly associated with reduced mortality, VAP, and length of stay in the ICU and hospital. Another report[130] emphasized the role of NIV in preventing reintubation in recently extubated patients at risk for relapse and respiratory failure. Kohlenberg et al.[131] pooled data of 400 ICUs in Germany and found mean pneumonia incidence of 1.58 and 5.44 cases per 1000 ventilator days for NIV and invasive mechanical ventilation, respectively. Therefore, when indicated, NIV should be attempted to avoid tracheal intubation and reduce overall duration of tracheal intubation.

TRACHEAL TUBE CUFF

Several strategies have been applied to improve the design of tracheal tubes and reduce the likelihood of aspiration of pathogen-laden secretions across the cuff. Novel ETT cuffs made of new materials such as polyurethane,[16] silicone,[132] and latex[133,134] have been developed and tested in laboratory and clinical trials. Particularly, the polyurethane cuff has a thickness of 5 to 10 μm in comparison to 50 μm of PVC cuffs; hence, upon inflation, smaller folds form, and aspiration of secretions above the cuff can be prevented or reduced. Lorente et al.[135] compared a standard ETT to an ETT incorporating an ultrathin polyurethane cuff and intermittent aspiration of subglottic secretions and found a reduction of incidence of VAP from 22.1% to 7.9% between the standard and new tubes, respectively ($P = 0.001$). A single-center study by Miller et al.[136] tested the use of a polyurethane-cuff ETT versus a standard PVC cuff ETT, with a before and after design, and found that VAP rates decreased from 5.3 per 1000 ventilator days before the use of the polyurethane-cuffed ETT to 2.8 per 1000 ventilator days during the intervention year ($P = 0.0138$). The polyurethane-cuffed ETT has also shown benefits in reducing early postoperative pneumonia in cardiac surgical patients. Poelaert et al.[137] studied 134 cardiothoracic surgery patients and demonstrated that the incidence of early postoperative pneumonia was significantly lower in the polyurethane group than in the polyvinyl chloride group (23% versus 42%,

$P < 0.03$). Silicone[132,138] and latex[133,134,139] cuffs are low-volume, low-pressure cuffs and are promising alternatives to PVC cuffs. Upon inflation, folds are never formed, yet compliance of those materials is extremely high; thus they allow reliable control of the pressure exerted against the trachea. In a clinical trial on patients undergoing anesthesia or admitted to the ICU, Young et al.[132] demonstrated high effectiveness of a silicone cuff in reducing pulmonary aspiration.

The shape of the cuff plays an important role in prevention of aspiration.[133,140] In comparison to standard cuffs with cylindrical shapes, cuffs designed with a smooth, tapering shape allow elimination of folds for a full circumference of the trachea/cuff contact zone, irrespective of the cuff material.

It is important to maintain the internal pressure of ETT cuff pressure between 25 and 30 cm H_2O, particularly when no positive end-expiratory pressure (PEEP) is applied; this serves to prevent either macroleakage of contaminated secretions into the lower airways or tracheal injury. A recent study[141] demonstrated that frequently the ETT cuff was deflated or hyperinflated using standard management.

Ventilatory settings may play a role in pathogenesis of VAP. In particular, PEEP may decrease the incidence of VAP by counteracting hydrostatic pressure exerted by oropharyngeal secretions above the ETT cuff, hence reducing pulmonary aspiration.[142] A recent report[143] assessed effects of 5 to 8 cm H_2O in normoxemic ventilated patients and showed reduction of the rate of VAP (PEEP group 9.4%, control patients 25.4%, relative risk, 0.37; 95% CI = 0.15-0.84; $P = 0.017$).

TRACHEAL TUBES COATED WITH ANTIMICROBIAL AGENTS

Coating the ETT with antimicrobial agents such as silver is a promising strategy to prevent biofilm formation within its internal surface and VAP. Olson et al.[144] examined a silver-coated tracheal tube in comparison to standard tube in intubated dogs. The dogs were challenged with *P. aeruginosa* into the oropharynx. Using the new tube, the investigators were able to postpone colonization of the ETT inner surface (3.2 ± 0.8 versus 1.8 ± 0.4 days; $P = 0.02$) and reduce bacterial burden in the lung parenchyma (4.8 ± 0.8 versus 5.4 ± 9 log colony-forming unit [CFU]/g lung tissue; $P = 0.01$). Similarly, Berra et al.[20] randomized 16 sheep to be intubated with a standard ETT or a silver sulfadiazine/chlorhexidine–coated ETT. After 24 hours of mechanical ventilation, all eight ETTs and ventilatory circuits in the control group were heavily colonized, and biofilm was found within the ETT. Pathogenic bacteria colonized the trachea and the lungs in five of eight sheep (up to 10^9 CFU/g). In the study group, seven of eight ETTs and ventilator circuits showed no growth and no biofilm; moreover, there was no bacterial growth in the lungs and bronchi, except for one bronchus in one sheep. Interestingly, the efficacy of silver-based coatings seems to decrease over time. Indeed, animal studies consistently reported no colonization and biofilm formation after 24 hours of mechanical ventilation. However, heavy ETT colonization was reported when studies were prolonged after 72 hours. To date, only one laboratory study[145] has reported the absence of ETT colonization and biofilm formation following up to 168 hours of mechanical ventilation. In that study, the authors used ETTs internally coated with silver-sulfadiazine that were regularly cleaned with a novel concentric inflatable silicone device, the Mucus Shaver,[146] devised to keep the ETT lumen free of mucus. The North American Silver-Coated Endotracheal Tube (NASCENT) randomized trial[72] studied 1509 patients expected to require mechanical ventilation for more than 24 hours and randomized to be intubated with either a silver-coated or a conventional tube. The silver-coated ETT was associated with a lower incidence of microbiologically confirmed VAP (37/766 [4.8%] versus 56/743 [7.5%]; $P = 0.03$), for a relative risk reduction of 35.9%. More importantly, the silver-coated tube had its greatest impact during the first 10 days of tracheal intubation. A retrospective cohort analysis by Afessa et al.,[147] based on the NASCENT study, showed that the silver-coated ETT was associated with reduced mortality in patients with VAP (silver ETT versus control, 5/37 [14%] versus 20/56 [36%], $P = 0.03$), but mortality was higher in those without VAP (silver versus control, 228/729 [31%] versus 178/687 [26%], $P = 0.03$). In conclusion, there is promising evidence that ETTs coated with antimicrobial agents could reduce incidence of VAP. Nevertheless, clinicians should carefully consider benefits and limitations of these new ETTs and properly direct the use of silver-coated tubes to patients expected to be ventilated for longer periods of time and with higher associated risks for nosocomial pneumonia.

Shorr et al.[148] analyzed cost-effectiveness of the silver-coated ETT as a preventive tool for VAP. Based on the NASCENT trial, the authors assumed a reduction in the relative risk of VAP from 35.9% to 24%. Assuming marginal VAP costs of $16,620 and costs of $90.00 for coated and $2.00 for uncoated ETTs, the authors found that savings per case of VAP prevented were $12,840.

ASPIRATION OF SUBGLOTTIC SECRETIONS

Aspiration of colonized subglottic secretions through dedicated ETTs reduces hydrostatic pressure exerted above the cuff and potentially prevents macroleakage across the cuff. A meta-analysis[149] comprising data from five studies and 896 patients has shown that subglottic secretion drainage reduced the incidence of VAP by nearly half (risk ratio [RR] = 0.51; 95% CI, 0.37-0.71), primarily by reducing early-onset pneumonia. Likewise, in the trial by Bouza et al.[150] of 690 patients undergoing major cardiac surgery and on mechanical ventilation for more than 48 hours, the use of ETT tubes with aspiration of subglottic secretions was able to reduce incidence of VAP, median length of ICU stay, and antibiotic use and led to overall cost savings. In the multicenter trial by Lacherade et al.,[151] 333 patients were randomized to be intubated with either an ETT that allowed drainage of subglottic secretions or a standard ETT. Microbiologically confirmed VAP occurred in 14.8% of the patients in the treatment group, compared to 25.6% of the patients intubated with standard tube ($P = 0.02$). Importantly, this was the first trial reporting efficacy of subglottic secretions aspiration in reducing both early- and late-onset VAP in comparison to earlier studies (late onset VAP in 18.6% of patients in treatment group versus 33.0% of the patients in control group, $P = 0.01$). In more recent studies, aspiration of subglottic secretions was performed intermittently.[135,151] The benefits of intermittent subglottic suction were similar to studies in which continuous aspiration of subglottic secretions was used. Hence, based on current evidence, intermittent aspiration (every 4-6 hours) is advisable to avoid potential risks for tracheal injury using continuous aspiration.[152]

TRACHEOSTOMY

Tracheostomized patients present the same risks for aspiration of pathogen-laden secretions pooled above the cuff[153,154] as do orotracheally intubated patients. An observational study by Ibrahim et al.[155] on 880 mechanically ventilated patients demonstrated an association between tracheostomy and higher incidence of VAP (adjusted OR, 6.71; 95% CI, 3.91-11.50; $P < 0.001$). Conversely, a case-control study by Nseir et al.[156] on 354 patients mechanically ventilated for more than 7 days showed a lower rate of nosocomial pneumonia associated with tracheostomy (4.8 versus 9.2 episodes per 1000 ventilator days in patients with or without tracheostomy, respectively). Meta-analyses have assessed outcomes of early versus late tracheostomy.[157-159] Unfortunately, all included studies were highly heterogeneous owing to differences in studied populations and no clear classification of "early" versus "late" tracheostomy. Nevertheless, the meta-analyses failed to demonstrate benefits of early tracheostomy on reduction of VAP incidence. To date, the latest multicenter randomized trial[160] enrolled 419 mechanically ventilated patients to undergo either early or late tracheostomy. Patients in the early tracheostomy group underwent tracheostomy after a mean of 7 days, whereas patients in the late tracheostomy group underwent tracheostomy after a mean of 14 days. Although the authors found shorter length of mechanical ventilation and ICU stay with early tracheostomy, they were able to demonstrate only a trend toward a lower incidence of pneumonia and no difference in survival.

Clinicians should consider that early tracheostomy may offer several benefits for mechanically ventilated patients: improved patient comfort, ability to communicate, capability for oral feeding, less need for sedation and analgesia, and reduced airway resistance in comparison to standard ETTs, which could be extremely important during the weaning period to shorten the duration of tracheal intubation.

VENTILATOR CIRCUIT MANAGEMENT

Decreased frequency of ventilator circuit changes, replacement of heated humidifiers by heat and moisture exchangers, decreased frequency of heat and moisture exchanger changes, and closed suctioning systems have been tested as measures for preventing VAP. Results from clinical trials in adults[161-167] and meta-analyses[168,169] yield consistent evidence that routine change of the ventilator circuit does not decrease risks for VAP and costs. Therefore, circuits should not be changed unless the circuit is soiled or damaged. Importantly, inadvertent flushing of the contaminated condensate into the lower airways or nebulizers should be always avoided by careful emptying of ventilator circuits and water traps.[170-172]

Two meta-analyses assessed the effects of heated humidifiers (HH) and heat and moisture exchangers (HME) on prevention of nosocomial pneumonia. Kola et al.[173] pooled data from nine clinical trials on 1378 patients and found that the use of HME decreased the rate of VAP (relative risk = 0.7; 95% CI = 0.50-0.94). Conversely, a meta-analysis by Siempos et al.[174] including 13 studies on 2580 patients found no difference between HME and HH patients in the prevention of VAP and secondary outcomes such as ICU mortality, length ICU stay, duration of mechanical ventilation, or episodes of airway occlusion. Hence, to date there are no consistent data showing reduction in the incidence of VAP and better outcome using either HME or HH. Based on the ongoing controversy, neither humidification strategy can be recommended as a pneumonia prevention tool. However, it is rational to deliver inspiratory gases at body temperature or slightly below and at the highest relative humidity in order to prevent loss of heat and moisture from the airways and, more importantly, change in rheologic properties of secretions and impairment of mucociliary clearance.[175] Therefore, the use of HH is indicated particularly in patients with hypothermia, prolonged mechanical ventilation, thick secretions, and chronic respiratory disorders. Finally, studies that have evaluated the effect of less frequent changes of heat and moisture exchangers on the development of VAP have found no increased risks.[176-180] However, it is important to emphasize that when HMEs are used for prolonged periods of time, the technical performance of the devices should be periodically checked.

Closed tracheal suctioning systems have been introduced in clinical settings to avoid adverse events associated with ventilator disconnection during open tracheal suctioning and exogenous contamination of suction catheters entering the ETT. Three meta-analyses[181-183] have compared the closed tracheal suction system to the open tracheal suction system in mechanically ventilated patients and found no benefits on VAP prevention. One meta-analysis[182] evaluated nine randomized trials comprising 1292 patients and found no difference in the incidence of VAP between patients suctioned with closed or open systems (OR = 0.96, 95% CI 0.72-1.28). Moreover, data pooled from four of these nine studies showed a higher incidence of respiratory tract colonization in the group managed with a closed system (OR = 2.88, 95% CI 1.50-5.52).

The use of a saline solution instilled into the tracheal tube before tracheal suctioning remains controversial. Caruso et al.[184] published a report on 262 patients randomized to receive either isotonic saline instillation before tracheal suctioning or no treatment. The authors found a lower incidence of microbiologically proven VAP (saline instillation versus no treatment: 23.5% versus 10.8%; $P = 0.008$), and no significant differences were found in secondary outcomes such as the incidence of ETT obstruction, pulmonary and lobar atelectasis, mortality, and duration of mechanical ventilation and ICU stay. Theoretically, in sedated patients in the semirecumbent position and with the internal surface of the ETT highly colonized, saline instillation may increase risks for translocation of pathogens into the airways, so current limited evidence suggests that routine saline instillation should not be recommended.

BODY POSITION

Early studies clearly demonstrated that intubated patients are at higher risk for gastropulmonary aspiration when placed in the supine position (0 degrees) as compared with a semirecumbent position (45 degrees).[185,186] One randomized trial[187] demonstrated a reduction in the incidence of VAP in patients positioned in the semirecumbent position compared with patients treated completely supine. Moreover, the trial confirmed increased risk for VAP in patients enterally fed. A later randomized trial[188] studied the feasibility of maintaining the head of the bed oriented 45 degrees during mechanical ventilation. This study found that patients were positioned on average only 28 degrees above horizontal, and no difference on VAP incidence was found. Thus, as strongly suggested by the American[1] and European[189] guidelines, intubated patients should be preferentially kept in the semirecumbent position (30-45 degrees) rather than supine (0 degrees) to prevent aspiration, especially when receiving enteral feeding.

Laboratory reports[190,191] challenge the role of the semirecumbent position in patients with oropharyngeal colonization due to tracheal intubation or during the course of mechanical ventilation. Theoretically, in such patients a tracheal orientation above horizontal, as in the semirecumbent position, might facilitate aspiration across the tracheal tube cuff. Laboratory studies in animals[190,191] consistently found that tracheal orientation and body position to avoid aspiration across the ETT cuff enhance mucus drainage and decrease risks for VAP; however, such results need to be confirmed in humans.

ROTATING BED

Normal healthy people change body position, even during sleep, every few minutes. Conversely, when critically ill patients are tracheally intubated and on mechanical ventilation, they are maintained in the supine, semirecumbent position for days with few or no changes in body position. Several ICU beds allow rotation of patients in the longitudinal axis from one lateral position to the other and seem to reduce extravascular lung water, improve ventilation-perfusion ratio, and enhance mobilization of airway secretions.[192] Several studies have evaluated the effects of rotational therapy on VAP; however, most of these studies present limitations. For example, most studies used a clinical diagnosis of pneumonia, lack of standardization of VAP preventive measures, and included heterogeneity on the duration and type of rotation therapy. Three meta-analyses[193-195] showed significant reduction in the incidence of VAP in patients undergoing rotation therapy, but they consistently failed to show beneficial effects on secondary outcomes such as duration of mechanical ventilation, length of stay, and mortality. An article by Staudinger et al.[196] studied the effects of continuous lateral rotation therapy on the incidence of microbiologically confirmed VAP in 3 medical ICUs and found an incidence of 11% in the rotation group and 23% in the control group ($P = 0.048$), respectively. The authors also found that the duration of ventilation (8 ± 5 versus 14 ± 23 days, $P = 0.02$) and length of stay (25 ± 22 days versus 39 ± 45 days, $P = 0.01$) were significantly shorter in the rotation group. In conclusion, in patients at higher risk for prolonged immobilization and respiratory infection, continuous lateral rotation therapy should be considered as a feasible method exerting additive effects to other preventive measures for VAP.

STRESS ULCER PROPHYLAXIS AND ENTERAL FEEDING

There is clear evidence that in intubated and mechanically ventilated patients, the stomach is often colonized by pathogens. Early studies showed that in tracheally intubated patients, gastric pH higher than 4 was consistently associated with gastric colonization.[49,50] Alkalinization of gastric contents due to drugs for stress ulcer prophylaxis and continuous enteral nutrition were the main risk factors for gastric colonization.

In the ICU, stress ulcer prophylaxis is usually achieved with either sucralfate, histamine type 2 blockers (H_2 blockers), or proton pump inhibitors (PPI). Sucralfate is the only treatment that potentially prevents stress GI ulceration without raising gastric pH. Several randomized studies have compared the effects of drugs that alkalinize gastric contents to sucralfate.[52-57,197,198] Two studies compared either H_2 blockers[51] or sucralfate[199] to placebo. Nine studies assessed gastric pH and colonization and consistently found lower pH and gastric colonization with regular use of sucralfate. Conversely, studies conducted by Bonten et al.[54] and Thomason et al.[56] found gastric luminal alkalinization and colonization, irrespective of the use of sucralfate. Finally, Eddleston et al.[199] found no differences in gastric colonization when sucralfate was compared to placebo.

Randomized trials reported inconsistent results regarding stress ulcer prophylaxis and the incidence of VAP. In particular, early studies found a higher incidence of pneumonia in patients with alkalinized gastric contents,[51-53] while more recent studies have not found such an association.[54,55,124] Cook et al.[55] studied 1200 patients randomized to receive either H_2 blockers or sucralfate for stress ulcer prophylaxis. The authors found a higher risk for GI bleeding using sucralfate and no significant difference in VAP incidence, 19.1% and 16.2% in patients treated with H_2 blockers or sucralfate, respectively. A recent meta-analysis[200] on the efficacy and safety of PPIs in comparison with H_2 blockers pooled data by seven randomized controlled trials on 936 patients and found no difference between PPI and H_2-blocker therapy on the risk for pneumonia and ICU mortality. In conclusion, GI bleeding is a serious complication in critically ill patients at high risk for stress ulcers (i.e., patients with coagulopathy, need for prolonged mechanical ventilation, and history of GI ulceration or bleeding). The actual risk for VAP is unknown when accurate methods of enteral feeding (i.e., avoiding large gastric residual volumes) or other preventive measures are used in combination with stress ulcer prophylaxis. Therefore, clinicians must weigh the potential benefit of sucralfate (with potentially less VAP and more GI bleeding) versus H_2 blockers/PPI (with potentially more VAP and less GI bleeding) and probably limit stress ulcer prophylaxis to high-risk patients.

Enteral nutrition has been considered a risk factor for the development of nosocomial pneumonia, mainly because of increased risks for alkalinization of gastric contents, gastro-esophageal reflux, and gastropulmonary aspiration. However, its alternative, parenteral nutrition, is associated with higher risks for catheter-related infections, complications of line insertions, higher costs, and loss of intestinal villous architecture, which may facilitate enteral microbial translocation. A large meta-analysis[201] of 15 studies comprising 753 patients admitted to the ICU for trauma, head injury, burns, and abdominal surgery found a significantly lower incidence of infections and a reduced length of hospital stay associated with early enteral feeding. Conversely, studies in medical ICU patients have proven higher risk for VAP with early enteral feeding.[202,203] Nonetheless, in a study by Artinian et al.[202] the increased risk of VAP associated with early enteral feeding did not translate into an increased risk of death. Therefore, in medical ICU patients, the benefits of early nutrition should be balanced with associated increased risks for VAP.

A large number of studies have evaluated the risks for ICU-acquired pneumonia in patients randomized to either gastric or postpyloric feeding. Theoretically, many ICU patients present impaired gastric emptying; hence placement of the feeding tube beyond the pylorus has the potential to achieve nutrition goals without increased risks for gastropulmonary aspiration. A meta-analysis by Heyland et al.[204] found that small-bowel feedings were associated with a lower incidence of pneumonia (RR, 0.77; 95% CI, 0.60-1.0); conversely, a meta-analysis by Ho et al.[205] found no significant benefit on the risk of diarrhea, length of ICU stay, mortality, or risk of pneumonia. Therefore, ICU physicians should preferentially indicate postpyloric feeding in critically ill patients who have impaired gastric emptying.

MODULATION OF OROPHARYNGEAL AND GASTROINTESTINAL COLONIZATION

One of the most important factors in the pathogenesis of nosocomial pneumonia is the early shift of oral flora following tracheal intubation into a predominance of aerobic gram-negative pathogens. Therefore, extensive efforts have been devoted to modulating oropharyngeal flora of ICU patients and reducing the risks for aspiration of pathogens. Several antiseptics for oropharyngeal decontamination have been evaluated: chlorhexidine gluconate, iseganan, or povidone iodine; chlorhexidine has been the focus of most research. Chlorhexidine is a cationic chlorophenyl *bis*-biguanide antiseptic that has long been used as an inhibitor of dental plaque formation and gingivitis. Meta-analyses[206-208] of studies assessing the benefits of chlorhexidine on reduction of VAP have shown good results, particularly in cardiothoracic ICU patients. Results in noncardiac ICU populations are more uncertain. Most of the aforementioned studies used chlorhexidine concentrations of 0.12% and 0.2%. However, recent studies in general ICU patients have demonstrated significant reductions in VAP rates when chlorhexidine concentration was increased to 2%.[209,210] Therefore, oral decontamination with chlorhexidine should be routinely used, particularly in cardiothoracic patients. The usefulness of chlorhexidine as VAP preventive strategy in other ICU populations still requires more evidence before being put into general practice, but the use of higher chlorhexidine concentrations has showed promising results.

Since the original studies published by Stoutenbeek and coworkers,[211,212] selective decontamination of the digestive tract (SDD) has been used as a preventive strategy for nosocomial pneumonia for almost 3 decades. SDD comprises a combination of nonabsorbable antibiotics against gram-negative pathogens (i.e., tobramycin, polymyxin E) plus either amphotericin B or nystatin administered into the GI tract in order to prevent oropharyngeal and gastric colonization with aerobic gram-negative bacilli and *Candida* spp., while preserving the anaerobic flora. Some regimens include a short course of systemic antibiotics (most commonly cefotaxime) in addition to nonabsorbable GI antibiotics. Randomized clinical trials[213-215] and meta-analyses[216-218] confirm results of earlier studies and suggest that SDD confers protection against pneumonia. Interestingly, SDD is the only preventive strategy for VAP that has shown reduction of mortality rates. A clinical trial by de Smet et al.[214] evaluated the effectiveness of SDD and selective oropharyngeal decontamination in a crossover study using cluster randomization in 13 ICUs and applied SDD, oropharyngeal decontamination, or standard care in random order for 6 months. SDD consisted of 4 days of intravenous cefotaxime and topical application of tobramycin, colistin, and amphotericin B in the oropharynx and stomach. Oropharyngeal decontamination consisted of oropharyngeal application only of the same antibiotics. The authors enrolled a total of 5939 patients. Post hoc analysis in a random-effects logistic-regression model found that the odds ratio for death at day 28 in the oropharyngeal decontamination and SDD groups, as compared with the standard-care group, were 0.86 (95% CI, 0.74-0.99, P = 0.045) and 0.83 (95% CI, 0.72-0.97, P = 0.02), respectively.

It is important to acknowledge that prophylactic use of antibiotics to modulate GI flora may potentially increase risks for antibiotic resistance, and results from randomized clinical trials still remain controversial; moreover, standard SDD is aimed at preventing overgrowth of aerobic gram-negative bacteria, yet it could increase colonization by gram-positive bacteria such as MRSA and *Enterococcus* spp. A large Dutch randomized controlled trial[213] demonstrated that carriage of multiresistant gram-negative bacteria was actually reduced in patients who had SDD, compared with controls (RR, 0.61; 95% CI, 0.46-0.81). Overall, emergence of resistance of gram-negative bacteria was consistently a rare event with SDD. Recently, Bonten's group reported data[219] on bacterial ecology in 13 ICUs that participated in their previous study of SDD.[214] Rectal and respiratory samples were analyzed once monthly in all ICU patients and showed that during SDD, average proportions of patients with intestinal colonization with GNB resistant to either ceftazidime, tobramycin, or ciprofloxacin increased from 5%, 7%, and 7%, respectively to 15%, 13%, and 13% post intervention (*P* <0.05). During SDD/SOD, resistance levels in the respiratory tract were not more than 6% for all three antibiotics but increased gradually (for ceftazidime, *P* <0.05 for trend) during intervention and to levels of 10% or more for all three antibiotics post intervention (*P* <0.05).

Conclusions on the effect of SDD on VAP, based on the results of several meta-analyses and clinical trials, may be summarized as follows:

1. SDD reduces the incidence of VAP and is the only VAP preventive strategy that has shown survival benefits in ICU patients.

2. The long-term effects of SDD on emergence of bacterial resistance and risk of superinfections are still controversial. The antibiotics used in SDD achieve very high concentrations in the GI tract, hence improving bactericidal activity and reducing risks for development of antibiotic resistance. However, few studies have assessed the risks for development of new antimicrobial resistance upon recolonization of the GI tract. Therefore, during the course of SDD, it is highly recommended to conduct appropriate surveillance of antibiotic resistance patterns within the ICU and hospital.

3. The parenteral and enteral antimicrobials used in standard SDD regimens are only effective against aerobic gram-negative pathogens and may promote gut overgrowth of MRSA and *Enterococcus* spp. (including vancomycin-resistant *Enterococcus*). Some researchers recommend the use of enteral vancomycin in ICU settings with endemic MRSA. Several studies have evaluated the effects and safety of prophylactic vancomycin on MRSA carriage and infection.[220] Pooling data from those studies, neither vancomycin-intermediate *S. aureus* (VISA) nor vancomycin-resistant *S. aureus* (VRSA) were identified. Only one study[221] reported a time-limited outbreak of vancomycin-resistant *Enterococcus* controlled through implementation of infection control procedures. However, the use of vancomycin as prophylaxis raises concerns, because vancomycin is still a first-line agent against MRSA, a different situation from the antimicrobials against gram-negative pathogens and fungi used in standard SDD.

Early attempts at VAP prophylaxis using parenteral antibiotics were unsuccessful.[222] Only one study[223] showed that a short course of cefuroxime upon emergent intubation and during 48 hours following intubation in patients with structural coma or severe burns was an effective prophylactic strategy to decrease the VAP rate. However, routine use of parenteral antibiotics is not recommended until more data become available.

Several clinical trials have attempted to modify GI and oropharyngeal growth of pathogens through the use of probiotics. Probiotics are microorganisms that can be administered either as individual strains or in various combinations. These microorganisms are often administered with nondigestible food ingredients that facilitate bacterial growth and/or activity (prebiotics); products containing both probiotics and prebiotics are called *synbiotics*. A meta-analysis[224] on the effects of probiotics, pooling data from five randomized controlled trials in 689 patients, showed a lower incidence of VAP. The use of probiotics is a promising strategy for VAP; however, additional evidence is required before recommending its use in all mechanically ventilated patients, particularly owing to the heterogeneity of previous studies.

Diagnosis

The diagnosis of VAP is a controversial issue.[225,226] Clinical signs suggestive of pneumonia in non-ICU patients, such as fever, tachycardia, and leukocytosis, are too nonspecific to be of diagnostic value for ventilated patients.[103,227,228] Moreover, the chest radiograph is often difficult to interpret in intubated, critically ill patients. Indeed, when the chest radiograph is normal, pneumonia may not be completely ruled out because of the limited technical quality. Also, chest radiographs may not reveal subtle lung infiltrates that may be detected with computed tomography (CT) scans, particularly in patients with COPD.[229]

When infiltrates are evident, it is often difficult to differentiate among cardiogenic and noncardiogenic pulmonary edema, pulmonary contusion, atelectasis, and pneumonia.

Few studies have examined the accuracy of portable chest radiographs in the diagnosis of pneumonia in the ICU.[228,230-232] In mechanically ventilated patients with autopsy-proven pneumonia, no single radiographic sign had a diagnostic accuracy greater than 68%.[231] The presence of air bronchograms or alveolar opacities in patients without ARDS correlated with pneumonia; however, no such correlation was found for patients with ARDS. Many causes other than pneumonia can explain asymmetrical consolidation in patients with ARDS, and marked heterogeneity of radiographic abnormalities has also been reported in patients with uncomplicated ARDS.[233] A clinical study showed the presence of lung infection in only 42% of the patients with clinically suspected VAP, with frequent occurrence of multiple infectious and noninfectious processes,[234] indicating a poor correlation between clinical signs and bacteriologic demonstration of VAP.

The Clinical Pulmonary Infection Score (CPIS) is based on six clinical assessments—temperature, blood leukocyte count, volume and purulence of tracheal secretions, oxygenation, pulmonary radiographic findings, and semiquantitative culture of tracheal aspirate—each worth between 0 and 2 points (Table 67-1).[235] The CPIS showed a good correlation ($r = 0.84$, $P < 0.0001$) with quantitative bacteriology of BAL samples. Moreover, a value ≥ 6 was the threshold to accurately identify patients with pneumonia. Yet the value of CPIS remains to be validated in a large prospective study, especially in patients with bilateral pulmonary infiltrates.

The presence of bacteria in the lower airways of intubated patients is not sufficient to diagnose true lung infection. The tracheobronchial tree and the oropharynx of mechanically ventilated patients are frequently colonized by enteric gram-negative bacilli.[1,37,61] Cultures of endotracheal aspirate from patients with respiratory failure and histologically documented pneumonia, simultaneously obtained from the trachea and lung tissue, agreed in only 40% of cases, with a 82% sensitivity and 27% specificity.[236] Similarly, another study demonstrated that only 23% of colonized patients subsequently developed nosocomial pneumonia.[37]

Many sampling procedures of respiratory secretions, such as sputum collection, endotracheal aspirates, BAL, and protected specimen brush (PSB) are available. In addition, there are several microbiological techniques including Gram staining and intracellular organism count from specimens obtained via BAL. Each diagnostic technique has advantages as well as limitations and provides different diagnostic specificity/sensitivity.

Qualitative cultures of endotracheal aspirates have a high percentage of false-positive results due to frequent bacterial colonization of the proximal airways in ICU patients. Conversely, quantitative culture techniques of endotracheal aspirates may have an acceptable overall diagnostic accuracy. When patients develop pneumonia, pathogens are

TABLE 67-1	The Clinical Pulmonary Infection Score (CPIS)		
Criterion	*0*	*1*	*2*
Tracheal secretions	Absent	Not purulent	Abundant and purulent
Chest x-ray infiltrates	No	Diffuse	Localized
Temperature, °C	≥36.5 and ≤38.4	≥38.5 or ≤38.9	≥39 or ≤36
Leukocytes	≥4000 and ≤11000	<4000 or >11000	<4000 or >11000 + immature neutrophils >50% or >500
Pao₂/Fio₂	>240 or ARDS		≤240, no ARDS
Microbiology	Negative		Positive

Adapted from Pugin J, Auckenthaler R, Mili N, et al. Diagnosis of ventilator associated pneumonia by bacteriologic analysis of bronchoscopic and non-bronchoscopic "blind" bronchoalveolar lavage fluid. Am Rev Respir Dis 1991;143:1121-9.
CPIS is considered positive with a score greater than or equal to 6.
ARDS, acute respiratory distress syndrome.

present in the lower respiratory tract secretions at concentrations of at least 10^5 to 10^6 CFU/mL,[237-240] and contaminants are generally present at less than 10^4 CFU/mL. The current diagnostic threshold proposed for tracheal aspirates is 10^6 CFU/mL. Similarly, PSB collects between 0.001 and 0.01 mL of secretions; therefore the presence of more than 10^3 bacteria in the originally diluted sample (1 mL) actually represents 10^5 to 10^6 CFU/mL in pulmonary secretions. Finally, 10^4 CFU/mL is considered the cutoff for BAL, which collects 1 mL of secretions in 10 to 100 mL of effluent.

Results of quantitative endotracheal aspirate cultures cannot always be used to accurately predict which microorganisms found in the proximal trachea are actually present in the lungs. In one study,[240] only 40% of the microorganisms cultured in endotracheal aspirate samples coincided with those obtained from PSB specimens. Also, when quantitative cultures of different lower respiratory tract specimens were compared with postmortem quantitative lung biopsy cultures, all techniques for detecting VAP were of limited value.[241]

A major problem in the management of patients with suspicion of VAP is the use of antibiotics. The indiscriminate administration of antimicrobial agents for patients in the ICU may contribute to the emergence of multiresistant pathogens and increase the risk of severe superinfections with increased morbidity and mortality, as well as expose the patient to antibiotic-related adverse effects and higher costs.[242,243] On the other hand, correct and prompt treatment of pneumonia results in better patient survival.[103,244,245] Inappropriate therapy is strongly associated with worse survival.[56,246] Inadequate empirical antibiotic treatment initiated before obtaining the results of cultures from respiratory secretions was associated with greater hospital mortality rate compared with an antibiotic regimen that provided adequate antimicrobial coverage based on microbiologic culture results.[247-251] However, the choice of the initial antibiotic treatment is often difficult due to several factors: (1) high frequency of resistant organisms in ICU patients previously treated with antibiotics,[252] (2) high risks for MDR pathogens in late-onset pneumonia occurring more than 7 days after initiation of mechanical ventilation,[4] and (3) frequent isolation of multiple organisms from pulmonary secretions when the sampling technique is not specific enough to differentiate colonizing from infecting pathogens.[253-255]

The importance of a microbiological diagnosis of VAP is aimed not only at determining whether a patient has pneumonia but also in optimizing antimicrobial treatment.[189] To allow narrowing or de-escalation of the initial empirical treatment, antimicrobial susceptibility data should be available as soon as possible. Recently, several alternative techniques to microbial cultures have been developed to achieve a more rapid and accurate diagnosis of nosocomial pneumonia. Among the most recent improvements, the direct antibiogram using E-test strips applied directly to respiratory tract samples have proved to be both reliable and effective and can anticipate the availability of antimicrobial susceptibility data by more than 48 hours.[256,257] Other advances include clinical application of quantitative polymerase chain reaction (qPCR) for direct measurement of microbial genetic material in patient specimens.[258] The mecA gene that confers resistance to methicillin in *S. aureus* can be detected using qPCR; qPCR of mecA in mini-BAL samples was able to rapidly and accurately diagnose MRSA pneumonia.[259]

Diagnostic Strategies for Hospital-Acquired Pneumonia

An ideal diagnostic strategy for patients with clinically suspicion of hospital-acquired pneumonia should reach the following objectives:

1. Accurately identify patients with true pulmonary infection and isolate the causative microorganisms in order to promptly initiate appropriate antimicrobial treatment and then to optimize therapy based on susceptibility of the pathogens.
2. Identify patients with extrapulmonary sites of infection.
3. Withhold and/or withdraw antibiotics in patients without infection.

A diagnostic strategy should be sensitive enough to identify the greatest number of patients infected so as to initiate early adequate empirical antibiotic treatment and provide improvement in outcomes. On the other hand, the strategy must be able to discriminate patients without a true infection and avoid overtreatment with antimicrobial drugs, which may be associated with worse outcome due to selection of MDR microorganisms.

The diagnosis of nosocomial pneumonia begins with clinical suspicion. The presence of a new or progressive radiographic infiltrate plus at least two of three clinical criteria (fever greater than 38°C, leukocytosis or leucopenia, and purulent secretions) represents the beginning of diagnostic procedures.

Two diagnostic algorithms can be used following clinical suspicion of nosocomial pneumonia. The clinical approach recommends treating every patient with suspicion of having a pulmonary infection with new antibiotics even when the likelihood of infection is low (Figure 67-2). However, samples of respiratory secretions such as endotracheal

Figure 67-2 Clinical noninvasive strategy for diagnosis and management of VAP. ATB, antibiotic; LRT, lower respiratory tract; VAP, ventilator-associated pneumonia. *(Adapted from American Thoracic Society. Guidelines for the management of adults with hospital-acquired, ventilator-associated, and healthcare-associated pneumonia. Am J Respir Crit Care Med 2005;171:388-416.)*

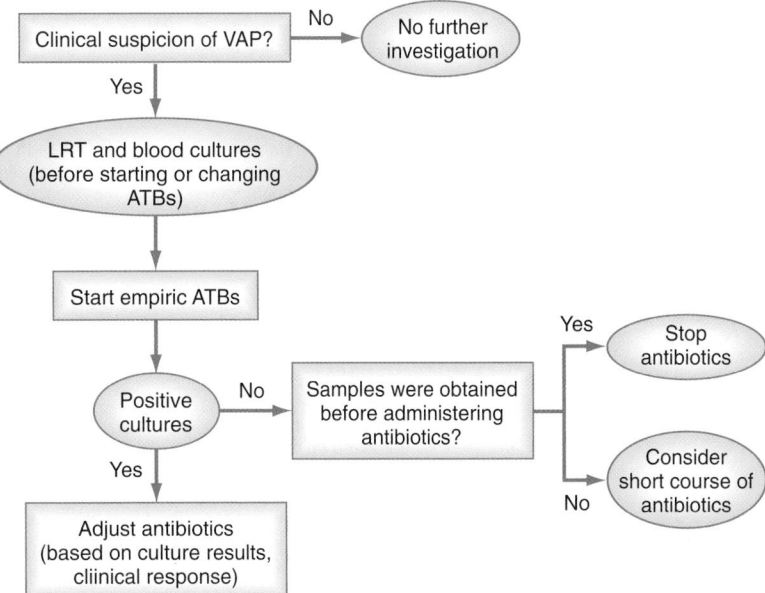

aspirate or sputum should be obtained before the initiation of antibiotic treatment. In this strategy, the selection of appropriate empirical therapy is based on risk factors and local resistance patterns. The etiology of pneumonia is defined by semiquantitative cultures of endotracheal aspirates or sputum, with initial microscopic examination of the Gram stain. Antimicrobial therapy is adjusted according to culture results or clinical response. Semiquantitative culture of tracheal aspirates has the advantage that no specialized microbiologic techniques are required, and the sensitivity is high. This clinical strategy provides antimicrobial treatment to the majority of the patients with suspicion of HAP and yields a low rate of false negatives. Still, if the tracheal aspirate culture does not demonstrate pathogens, and the patient has not received new antibiotics within the previous 72 hours, the diagnosis of pneumonia is unlikely.[251] This strategy is useful in centers where bronchoscopic methods are not always available for sampling the lower respiratory tract. The main drawback of this strategy is that the high sensitivity of semiquantitative cultures of tracheal aspirates leads to overestimation of the incidence of nosocomial pneumonia, hence antibiotic treatments can be administered to patients without pneumonia.

The bacteriologic strategy is based on the results of quantitative cultures of lower respiratory secretions (Figure 67-3). The procedure used to collect the samples (endotracheal aspirate, BAL, or PSB) may be invasive (bronchoscopic) or noninvasive (blind procedures). Specific threshold cutoffs for each test to discriminate between colonizing microorganisms and those producing infection are used in this strategy. The cutoff point used for BAL is 10^6 CFU/mL, 10^4 CFU/mL for BAL, and 10^3 CFU/mL for PSB. The bacteriologic strategy attempts to accurately identify patients with true nosocomial pneumonia so that only infected patients are treated and clinical outcomes are improved.[84,250,255,260] Such a strategy reduces risks for overuse of antibiotics, since quantitative cultures yield fewer microorganisms above the threshold in comparison to semiquantitative cultures. Among the disadvantages of the bacteriologic strategy is the possibility of obtaining false-negative results that lead to delayed antibiotic treatment in a patient with pneumonia. Moreover, results using the microbiology strategy may lack of reproducibility, and often no microbiological information is available at the time of initiation of empirical antibiotic therapy.

EVALUATION OF DIAGNOSTIC STRATEGIES

Four randomized controlled trials[250,261-263] have assessed the impact of diagnostic strategies on antibiotic use and outcome in patients with clinical suspicion of nosocomial pneumonia. In three small studies,[250,261,262] invasive diagnostic techniques resulted in a greater number of antibiotic changes than noninvasive techniques; however, no differences in mortality and morbidity were found when either invasive (PSB and/or BAL) or noninvasive (quantitative endotracheal aspirate cultures) techniques were used. By contrast, a larger trial[263] showed a reduction in mortality, better Sequential Organ Failure Assessment (SOFA) score at follow-up, reduced use of antibiotics, and increased number of antibiotic-free days using invasive diagnostic techniques. This study was limited, however, by the use of qualitative cultures of tracheal aspirates, thereby limiting comparison with other clinical trials. A meta-analysis by Shorr et al.[264] pooled data from these randomized studies on 628 patients and found that overall, an invasive approach did not alter mortality (OR, 0.89; 95% CI, 0.56-1.41). Invasive testing, though, affected antibiotic utilization (OR for change in antibiotic management after invasive sampling, 2.85; 95% CI, 1.45-5.59). Importantly, it should be realized that diagnostic cultures of pulmonary secretions after initiation of new antibiotic therapy in patients with suspicion of HAP can lead to a high number of false-negative results, irrespective of the sampling technique. In this clinical setting, a lower threshold should be used to define a positive quantitative result.[265,266] Nevertheless, it is strongly recommended that diagnostic sampling of the respiratory tract be obtained before starting any new antibiotic or changing previous antimicrobial therapy.

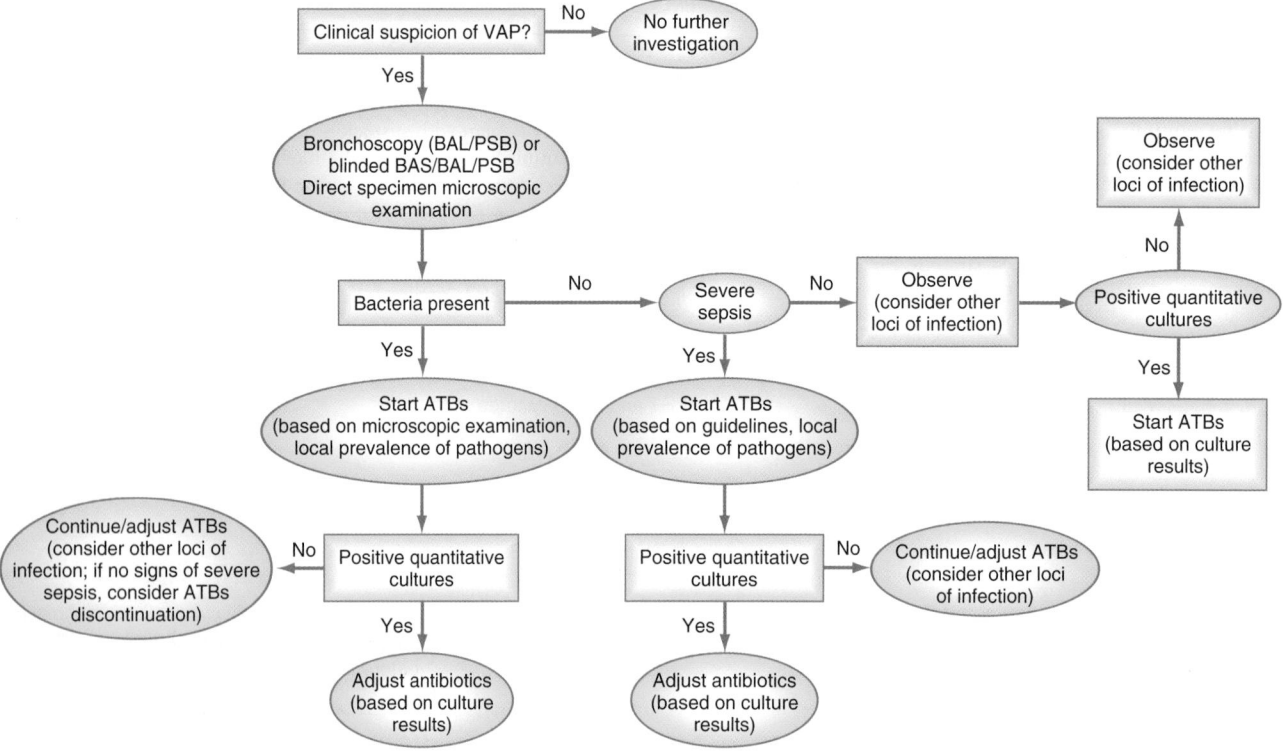

Figure 67-3 Invasive and quantitative culturing strategy for diagnosis and management of VAP. ATB, antibiotic; BAL, bronchoalveolar lavage; BAS, bronchial aspirate; PSB, protected specimen brush; VAP, ventilator-associated pneumonia. (*Adapted from American Thoracic Society. Guidelines for the management of adults with hospital-acquired, ventilator-associated, and healthcare-associated pneumonia. Am J Respir Crit Care Med 2005;171:388-416.*)

A clinical trial[267] compared quantitative culture of BAL fluid and culture of endotracheal aspirate in critically ill patients with suspected VAP. This study was part of a larger 2-by-2 factorial design also comparing empirical antimicrobial monotherapy (a carbapenem) and combination therapy (a carbapenem plus a fluoroquinolone). A total of 740 patients in 28 ICUs in Canada and the United States were enrolled, and the authors found no difference in the 28-day mortality rate between the BAL group and the endotracheal aspiration group (18.9% and 18.4%, respectively; $P = 0.94$). The BAL group and the endotracheal aspiration group also had similar rates of targeted therapy (74.2% and 74.6%, respectively; $P = 0.90$), days alive without antibiotics (10.4 ± 7.5 and 10.6 ± 7.9; $P = 0.86$), and maximum organ-dysfunction scores (mean [±SD], 8.3 ± 3.6 and 8.6 ± 4.0; $P = 0.26$). The two groups did not differ significantly in the length of stay in the ICU or hospital. Unfortunately, at least 40% of the screened patients were excluded because they were at risk for colonization with *Pseudomonas* spp. or MRSA or were immunosuppressed. Therefore, translation of these findings into clinical practice is a major concern, because many ICU patients evaluated for suspected VAP fall into these categories.

PRACTICAL IMPLEMENTATION OF A DIAGNOSTIC STRATEGY IN SUSPECTED VENTILATOR-ASSOCIATED PNEUMONIA

In practice, the development of local clinical guidelines can combine both clinical and bacteriologic strategies (Table 67-2). The diagnostic protocol begins with clinical suspicion of nosocomial respiratory infection (Figure 67-4). In mechanically ventilated patients, the presence of an infiltrate on chest radiograph differentiates between the possible presence of pneumonia and tracheobronchitis. The next step is to sample the lower respiratory tract (see Table 67-2) to identify the causative microorganism. Sampling should be performed before initiation or change of antibiotic treatment, even though it should not delay the administration of antibiotic therapy, particularly for septic patients. Respiratory tract specimens can be obtained through expectoration, bronchial aspirate, BAL, or PSB. The latter two techniques can be performed with bronchoscopy or blindly. Several other samples should also be collected, as noted in Table 67-2. With clinical suspicion of pneumonia, CPIS[235] should be calculated to improve objective assessment of the clinical parameters (see Table 67-1).

■ Treatment

Once the clinical decision to initiate antimicrobial therapy has been made, the following issues should be considered to achieve the best antimicrobial efficacy and reduce overuse of antibiotics:
- The most likely etiologic microorganisms
- Choice of the empirical antimicrobials likely to be active against these microorganisms

TABLE 67-2	Diagnostic Protocol to Combine Clinical and Bacteriologic Strategies for the Diagnosis of Ventilator-Associated Pneumonia

1. As soon as pneumonia or infection associated with mechanical ventilation is suspected and before initiating new empirical antibiotic treatment, collect samples as follows*:
   - Expectoration
   - Tracheobronchial aspirate (BAS)**
   - Bronchoalveolar lavage (BAL) or mini-BAL**
   - Protected brush specimen (PBS)**
2. Two blood cultures
3. In cases of evidence for parapneumonic effusion, obtain pleural fluid sample
4. Obtain *Legionella pneumophila* and *Streptococcus pneumoniae* antigens in urine
5. Other lab tests: complete blood cell count, serum electrolytes, liver and renal function tests, C-reactive protein, procalcitonin, arterial blood gases

*Samples should be sent to the microbiology department, or if not available, maintained in refrigerator at 4°C (only respiratory samples) for a maximum of 1 hour for Gram staining, intracellular organism counting (only in BAL and mini-BAL), and quantitative cultures. The collection of lower respiratory secretion samples should not delay the initiation of empirical treatment in patients with severe sepsis.

**These techniques may be performed by bronchoscopy or blind procedures. Quantitative cultures are performed with the respiratory secretions obtained by BAS, BAL, or PBS. The cutoff count to diagnose pneumonia is the following: BAS 10^6 CFU/mL; BAL 10^4 CFU/mL, and PSB 10^3 CFU/mL.

- Adjustment of therapy following microbiologic results and duration of treatment

LIKELY ETIOLOGIC MICROORGANISMS

The microorganisms most frequently isolated from the bronchial secretions of patients with VAP are *S. aureus* and *P. aeruginosa*, comprising around 50% of the isolates. These are followed, in order of frequency, by *Enterobacteriaceae* (*E. coli*, *Klebsiella* spp., *Enterobacter* spp., *Citrobacter* spp., *Serratia* spp., and *Proteus* spp.) representing 15%, nonfermentative gram-negative bacilli other than *P. aeruginosa* (*Acinetobacter* spp., *Stenotrophomonas* spp., and *Burkholderia* spp.) in 10%, and *H. influenzae* and *S. pneumoniae* (among others) in the remaining cases.[103]

The microorganisms causing VAP generally come from the oropharyngeal flora of the patient. Underlying chronic diseases,[268] specific risk factors, acute inflammatory processes, and factors specific to each hospital or ICU can facilitate abnormal bacterial colonization of the oropharynx and may predispose patients to infection with specific organisms.[1,269] Therefore, the selection of initial antimicrobial therapy must be tailored to the local prevalence of pathogens and antimicrobial patterns of resistance of each institution.[88,270] Healthy subjects rarely have significant colonization with gram-negative bacilli in the oropharynx, even after prolonged exposure to the hospital or ICU environment. Conversely, elderly individuals and patients with comorbidities and/or previous exposure to antibiotics may be at increased risk for abnormal oropharyngeal colonization.[271] The dynamics of change of oropharyngeal flora during hospital stay can be described as follows (Figure 67-5):

Figure 67-4 Clinical suspicion of nosocomial respiratory infection.

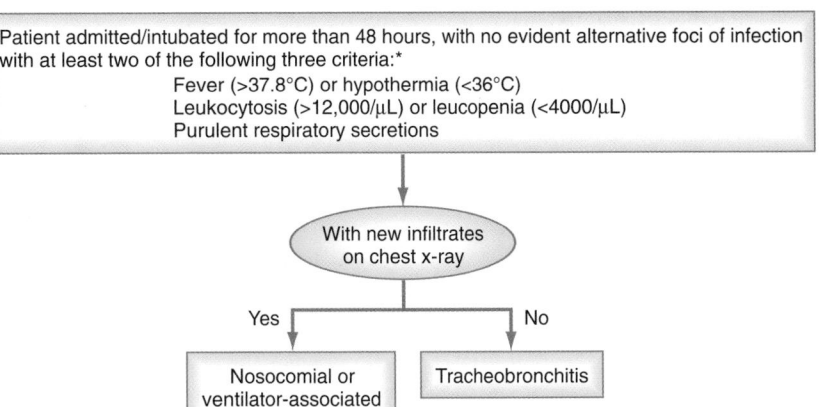

Patient admitted/intubated for more than 48 hours, with no evident alternative foci of infection with at least two of the following three criteria:*

Fever (>37.8°C) or hypothermia (<36°C)
Leukocytosis (>12,000/μL) or leucopenia (<4000/μL)
Purulent respiratory secretions

With new infiltrates on chest x-ray

Yes — Nosocomial or ventilator-associated pneumonia

No — Tracheobronchitis

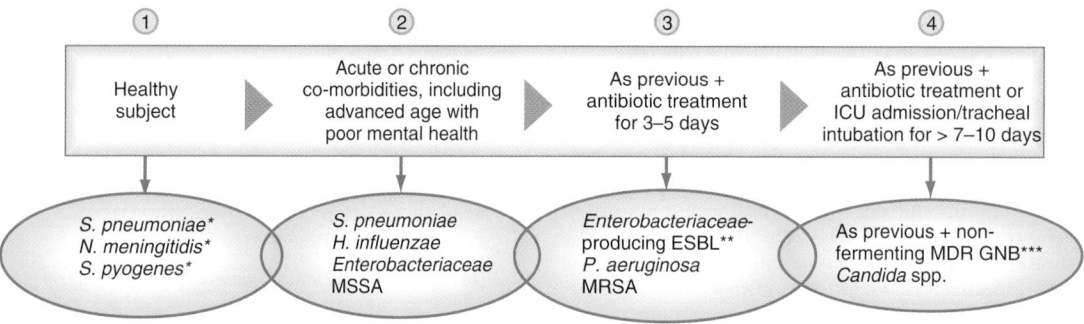

Figure 67-5 Evolution of potentially pathogenic microorganisms present in oropharyngeal flora, related to comorbidity, antibiotic treatment, and colonization pressure.
*Transitorily present in healthy carriers.
**Producers of ESBL or with type ampC chromosomal β-lactamases.
***_Pseudomonas aeruginosa_, _Stenotrophomonas_ spp., _Acinetobacter_ spp., _Burkholderia_ spp.
ESBL, extended-spectrum β-lactamase; GNB, gram-negative bacilli; MDR, multidrug-resistant; MRSA, methicillin-resistant _Staphylococcus aureus_; MSSA, methicillin-sensitive _S. aureus_.

1. Healthy subjects are colonized with normal oropharyngeal flora in which pathogenic microorganisms such as _S. pneumoniae_, group A streptococci, or meningococci may be transiently found.
2. Patients with chronic comorbidities or an acute inflammatory process have impairment of normal immune responses. As a result, _S. aureus_ and _Enterobacteriaceae_ can colonize the oropharynx.
3. Patients who have received antibiotic treatment become colonized with resistant pathogens, including ESBL+ _Enterobacteriaceae_, _Enterobacter_ spp., _P. aeruginosa_, or MRSA.
4. Patients who have received broad-spectrum antibiotics for more than 7 days are often colonized by multiresistant microorganisms. This leads to emergence of highly resistant gram-negative bacilli (_Acinetobacter baumannii_, _S. maltophilia_, _B. cepacia_) and gram-positive microorganisms (coagulase-negative _Staphylococcus_ and _Enterococcus_ spp.)

Changes in oropharyngeal flora tend to occur progressively such that the presence of microorganisms during one stage often overlaps with the next stage.

CHOICE OF EMPIRICAL ANTIMICROBIALS LIKELY TO BE ACTIVE AGAINST CAUSATIVE MICROORGANISMS

The latest guidelines of the American Thoracic Society and Infectious Diseases Society of America (ATS/IDSA) for the management of adult patients with nosocomial pneumonia[1] recommend that the selection of empirical antibiotic therapy for each patient should be based on the

timing of onset and presence of risk factors for MDR pathogens. Risk factors for MDR pathogens defined by the ATS/IDSA guidelines are summarized in Box 67-2. An algorithm for the initial management of patients with nosocomial respiratory infection and selection of appropriate antimicrobials is shown in Figure 67-6. The antibiotics recommended by the current ATS/IDSA guidelines are shown in Tables 67-3 and 67-4. Adequate dosing of antibiotics for empirical therapy is summarized in Table 67-5. Broad-spectrum empirical antibiotic therapy should be rapidly deescalated as soon as microbiological data become available in order to limit the emergence of resistance in the hospital. In brief, initial empiric therapy should be based on patient's risk of colonization by MDR organisms and managed as follows:

- Patients with early-onset pneumonia, no risk factors for MDR bacteria and who have not undergone antibiotic treatment within the previous month may be treated with monotherapy (see Figure 67-6 and Table 67-3). A β-lactam without antipseudomonal activity (e.g., third-generation cephalosporin such as ceftriaxone or cefotaxime, ertapenem, amoxicillin-clavulanate, or a fluoroquinolone with antipneumococcal activity (e.g., levofloxacin or moxifloxacin). Fluoroquinolones are not recommended as monotherapy in ICUs with high rate of _Enterobacteriaceae_ resistant to quinolones.
- Patients with late-onset pneumonia or early onset with risk factors for MDR bacteria are at increased risk of infection with resistant gram-negative bacilli. An antipseudomonal antibiotic is indicated if the infection is severe or the patient fulfills the risk factors of colonization by MDR microorganisms (antibiotic treatment or intubation for more than 7-10 days). Priority should be given to treatment with a β-lactam. The choice of the β-lactam should take into account the following: (1) in vitro susceptibility of _P. aeruginosa_ in the ICU, (2) the prevalence of _Enterobacteriaceae_

Box 67-2

RISK FACTORS FOR MULTIDRUG-RESISTANT PATHOGENS CAUSING NOSOCOMIAL PNEUMONIA

- Antimicrobial therapy in preceding 90 days
- Current hospitalization of 5 days or more
- High frequency of antibiotic resistance in the community or in the specific hospital unit
- Presence of risk factors for healthcare-associated pneumonia:
  - Hospitalization for 2 days or more in the preceding 90 days
  - Residence in a nursing home or extended care facility
  - Home infusion therapy (including antibiotics)
  - Chronic dialysis within 30 days
  - Home wound care
  - Family member with multidrug-resistant pathogen
- Immunosuppressive disease and/or therapy

Adapted from American Thoracic Society. Guidelines for the management of adults with hospital-acquired, ventilator-associated, and healthcare-associated pneumonia. Am J Respir Crit Care Med 2005;171:388-416.

TABLE 67-3	Initial Empirical Antibiotic Treatment in Nosocomial and Ventilator-Associated Pneumonia of Early Onset in Patients Without Risk Factors for Infection by Multidrug-Resistant Pathogens	
Probable Microorganism	**Recommended Antibiotic**	
Streptococcus pneumoniae	Ceftriaxone	
Haemophilus influenzae	_or_	
Methicillin-sensitive _Staphylococcus aureus_	Levofloxacin, moxifloxacin	
Enteric gram-negative bacilli	_or_	
Escherichia coli	Ampicillin/sulbactam	
Klebsiella pneumoniae	_or_	
Enterobacter spp.	Ertapenem	
Proteus spp.		
Serratia marcescens		

Adapted from American Thoracic Society. Guidelines for the management of adults with hospital-acquired, ventilator-associated, and healthcare-associated pneumonia. Am J Respir Crit Care Med 2005;171:388-416.

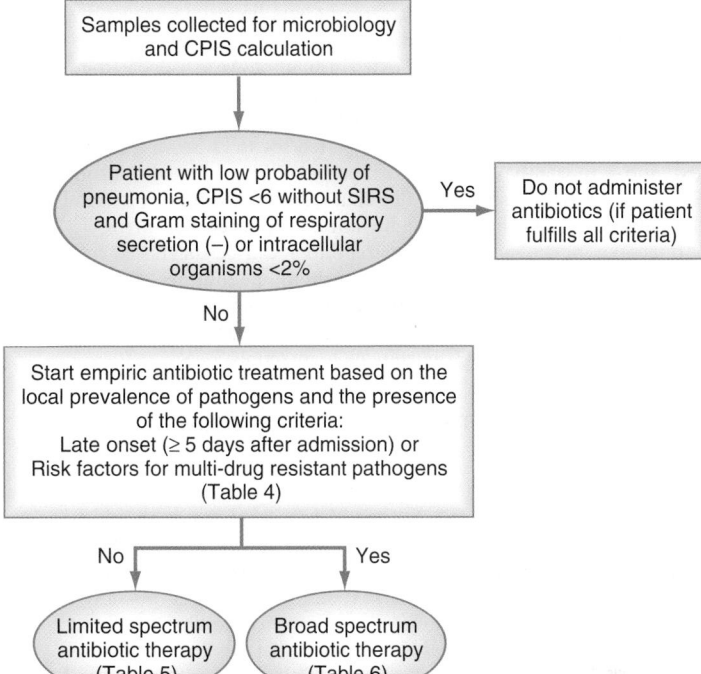

Figure 67-6 Algorithm for treatment of patients with suspicion of nosocomial respiratory infection. Systemic inflammatory response syndrome (SIRS) comprises at least two of the following: temperature >38°C or <36°C; heart rate > 90 beats/min; respiratory rate >20 breaths/min or $PaCO_2$ <32 mm Hg; and leukocytes > 12,000/mm³, <4000/mm³, or the preference of >10% immature neutrophils.

producing ESBL, (3) the results of previous cultures, and (4) antibiotics received by the patient. An antipseudomonal β-lactam would include a third-generation or four-generation cephalosporins (ceftazidime or cefepime), piperacillin-tazobactam, or a carbapenem (imipenem or meropenem; see Table 67-4).

ANTIMICROBIAL THERAPY IN SPECIAL SITUATIONS

The addition of antibiotics with activity against MRSA depends on the local prevalence of MRSA, the presence of risk factors for MRSA, and the severity of infection. In geographic areas with documented presence of community-acquired MRSA, severe pneumonia with radiologic images of cavitation and presence of gram-positive cocci in

TABLE 67-4	Initial Empirical Antibiotic Treatment for Nosocomial and Ventilator-Associated Pneumonia of Late Onset or in Patients with Risk Factors for Infection by Multidrug-Resistant Pathogens and Any Degree of Severity
Probable Microorganism	**Combined Antibiotic Treatment**
Microorganisms from Table 67-3 plus: *Pseudomonas aeruginosa* *Klebsiella pneumoniae* (ESBL+)[†] *Acinetobacter* spp.[†] Other nonfermenting gram-negative bacilli Methicillin-resistant *Staphylococcus aureus* (MRSA) *Legionella pneumophila*[‡]	Antipseudomonal cephalosporin (ceftazidime or cefepime)* *or* Carbapenem (imipenem, meropenem)* *or* β-lactam/β-lactamase inhibitor (piperacillin-tazobactam)* + Antipseudomonal fluoroquinolone (ciprofloxacin, levofloxacin)** *or* Aminoglycoside** (amikacin) ± Linezolid or vancomycin***

*The choice of β-lactam is made as follows: patients who have not received any antipseudomonal β-lactam within the last 30 days should be administered piperacillin-tazobactam or an antipseudomonal cephalosporin. Patients who have received these drugs should be given empirical therapy with a carbapenem. Patients with infection by ESBL-producing microorganisms should be treated with carbapenem regardless of the results of the antibiogram.

**For combined empirical therapy for multidrug-resistant GNB, an antipseudomonal fluoroquinolone should be used in cases of renal failure or concomitant use of vancomycin. In other settings, combined empirical therapy is initiated with amikacin and maintained for a 5-day period.

***Empirical therapy aimed against MRSA is initiated in patients with proven colonization (ψ), previous infection by this microorganism, or implementation of MV for more than 6 days. The antibiotic of choice is either vancomycin (except in patients allergic to this medication, with creatinine values ≥ 1.6 mg/dL, or in patients presenting signs of empirical treatment failure after 48 hours of antibiotic therapy) or linezolid. (Ψ) For epidemiologic surveillance, nasal and perineal cultures should be performed on admission and at 1-week intervals thereafter while remaining in the ICU.

[†]If an ESBL+ strain such as *K. pneumoniae* or *Acinetobacter* spp. is suspected, a carbapenem is the first choice.

[‡]If *L. pneumophila* is suspected, the combination antibiotic regimen should include a macrolide (e.g., azithromycin), or a fluoroquinolone (e.g., ciprofloxacin, levofloxacin) should be used rather than an aminoglycoside.

ESBL, extended-spectrum β-lactamase; GNB, gram-negative bacilli.

TABLE 67-5	Recommended Initial Intravenous Antibiotic Dosage for Empirical Treatment of Patients with Nosocomial and Ventilator-Associated Pneumonia		
Antibiotic	**Doses**	**Interval of Administration**	**Perfusion Time**
Non-antipseudomonal cephalosporin:			
Ceftriaxone	2 g	24 hours	1/2-1 hour
Cefotaxime	2 g	6 hours	1/2-1 hour
Antipseudomonal cephalosporin:			
Ceftazidime	2 g	8 hours	2-3 hours
Cefepime	1-2 g	8 hours	2-3 hours
Carbapenems:			
Imipenem	0.5 or 1 g	6 or 8 hours	1 hour
Meropenem	1 g	8 hours	2-3 hours
Piperacillin-tazobactam	4 g-0.5 g	6 hours	2-3 hours
Fluoroquinolones:			
Levofloxacin	500 mg	12 hours*	1/2 hour
Ciprofloxacin	400 mg	8 hours	1/2 hour
Amikacin	15-20 mg/kg	24 hours**	1/2-1 hour
Vancomycin	1 g	8-12 hours***	1-3 hours
Linezolid	600 mg	12 hours	1 hour

*Administer this dose for 3 days and after continue with 500 mg/24 h.

**Adjust the dosage according to PK/PD parameters.

***Initiate this dose with 24 hours, measure trough blood levels prior to the following dosage, and adjust the levels according to values.

Dosages are based on normal renal and hepatic function.

respiratory secretions, empirical treatment with linezolid or vancomycin may be appropriate. Recently an outbreak of MRSA and linezolid-resistant *S. aureus* (LRSA) was reported in an intensive care department of a 1000-bed tertiary care university teaching hospital in Madrid, Spain, and was associated with nosocomial transmission and extensive usage of linezolid.[272] In that report, 12 patients with LRSA were identified, and a mortality of 50% was reported. CFR-mediated linezolid resistance was demonstrated in all isolates. Tigecycline may be a useful alternative in this setting, although clinical experience is scanty.

Infections by *L. pneumophila* serogroup 1 can be diagnosed by a *Legionella* urinary antigen test. This test should be routinely obtained if the hospital water supply is known to be colonized with *L. pneumophila* serogroup 1. A fluoroquinolone or a macrolide would be appropriate treatment for *L. pneumophila* infection.

MODIFICATIONS OF THERAPY AND DURATION OF TREATMENT

A suggested flowchart for follow-up of patients with nosocomial pneumonia is shown in Figure 67-7. After 72 hours, treatment should be adjusted based on microbiological results. The initial β-lactam should be continued if the microorganism is susceptible to the empirical β-lactam originally prescribed. If not, another β-lactam, possibly a carbapenem, may be introduced. The empirical antibiotic against MRSA should be discontinued if the presence of this pathogen is not confirmed by cultures. Discontinuation of the fluoroquinolone and especially the aminoglycoside should be considered after 3 to 5 days of treatment. The bactericidal activity of aminoglycosides and fluoroquinolones leads to a rapid reduction in the bacterial load during the first days of treatment. After this time, monotherapy may be sufficient. This approach would decrease emergence of resistant mutants and minimize nephrotoxicity caused by aminoglycosides.

The majority of infections can be effectively treated with regimens lasting up to 8 days. Four situations may justify prolonged treatment: (1) infection by microorganisms that may multiply in the cellular cytoplasm, such as *Legionella* spp.; (2) the presence of biofilms or prosthetic devices; (3) the development of tissue necrosis, the formation of abscesses, or infection within a closed cavity, such as empyema; and (4) persistence of the original infection (such as perforation or endocarditis). If the clinical course from the pneumonia is favorable—as defined by defervescence, improvement in Pao$_2$/Fio$_2$, and reduction in C-reactive protein (CRP) levels within the first 3 to 5 days of antimicrobial therapy—treatment may be withdrawn after the completion of 7 days. If the causative microorganism is a nonfermenting gram-negative bacillus, the treatment can be extended beyond 14 days. A large prospective, multicenter, randomized trial study comparing the efficacy of 8-day and 15-day antibiotic regimens for treating VAP suggested that an 8-day regimen reduces antibiotic use and decreases the emergence of multiresistant bacteria in the lung, without modification of the prognosis.[273] However, this study observed that in cases of pneumonia produced by nonfermenting gram-negative bacilli, eradication of these microorganisms from bronchial secretions was lower with the shorter regimen.[273] On the other hand, the 14-day treatment regimen was associated with a greater trend to colonization by multiresistant flora and a greater frequency of reinfection.[274]

In patients with clinical suspicion of ICU-acquired pneumonia who have a CPIS lower than 6 on the third day of treatment, the treatment may be withdrawn. In this setting, the patient probably does not have pneumonia, or the pneumonia is sufficiently mild such that prolonged antibiotic treatment is not required.[235]

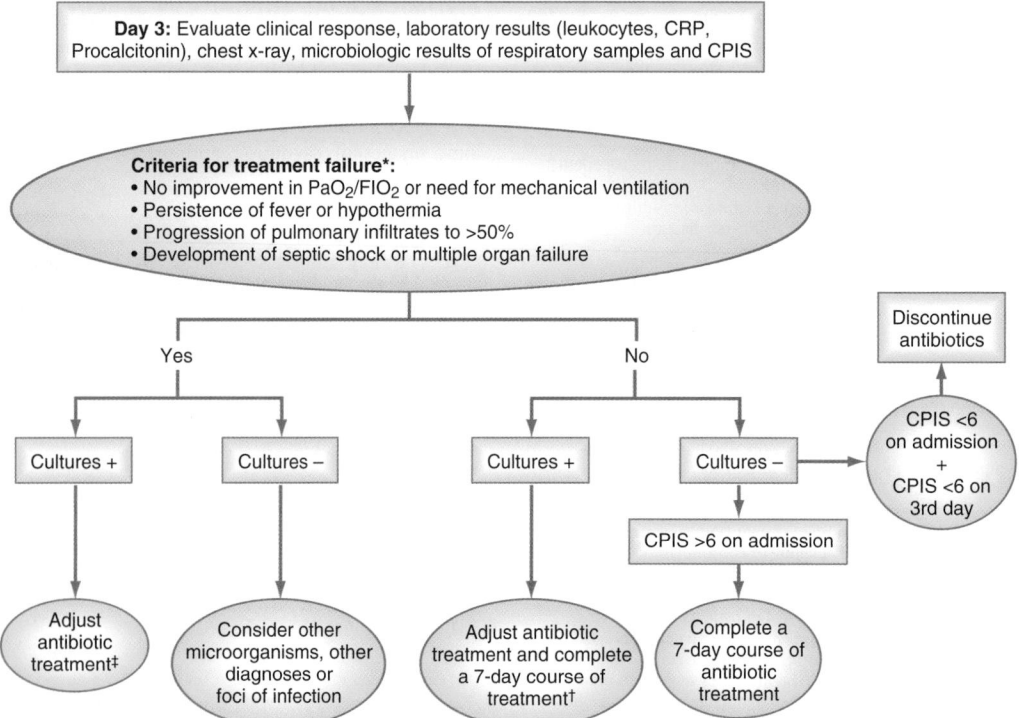

Figure 67-7   Suggested flowchart for follow-up of patients with nosocomial pneumonia and VAP.
*Criteria of treatment failure taken from Ioanas M, Ferrer M, Cavalcanti M et al. Causes and predictors of non-response to treatment of the ICU-acquired pneumonia. Crit Care Med 2004;32:938-45.
†In cases in which the etiologic agent is *Pseudomonas aeruginosa* or *Acinetobacter* spp., treatment should be maintained for 14 days.
‡Patients with criteria of treatment failure and in whom MRSA is isolated should be administered linezolid. If a GNB is isolated, consultation is recommended.

Implementation of Guidelines

There is evidence that appropriate and timely antibiotic treatment can improve outcome in patients with VAP. Guidelines can play a significant role in accomplishing this aim. However, to significantly reduce morbidity and mortality, guidelines should (1) be implemented in specific clinical settings and (2) guide appropriate antibiotic treatment, tailored on specific risk factors for acquiring MDR pathogens. Although guideline implementation is difficult to achieve and requires effort, there is evidence demonstrating that management and outcome of patients is improved. Our report[275] on the validation of the current 2005 ATS/IDSA guidelines demonstrates worse microbial prediction, in comparison to previous guidelines, in patients considered to be at low risk for acquiring MDR pathogens, and similar low prediction for fungi. Those data suggest the need for further research to improve the accuracy of future guidelines and, ultimately, the outcome of patients with VAP.

Although guideline-recommended strategies may provide significant benefits for patients, implementation is often hard to achieve.[276,277] Guidelines can be translated into clinical practice via education and behavioral changes of healthcare personnel, design and distribution of dedicated protocols, and frequent audit and feedback. Few studies have assessed the effects of the implementation of guidelines on outcomes. Soo-Hoo et al.[277] developed hospital guidelines to manage patients with severe hospital-acquired pneumonia based on the 1996 ATS guidelines.[269] Recommendations designed by a multidisciplinary taskforce focused particularly on empirical antibiotic treatment and specimen collection. A strict campaign to educate healthcare personnel was undertaken, and progress in guidelines implementation was frequently reviewed. After the guidelines were introduced into clinical settings, the authors found that adequate antibiotic therapy was administered in more than 81% of the patients with pneumonia, compared with 46% before implementation ($P < 0.01$). Moreover, a lower mortality at 14 days was found after guidelines implementation ($P = 0.03$). Similarly, Ibrahim and co-workers developed a protocol to provide appropriate initial antibiotic treatment for patients with VAP and encouraged a 7-day course of treatment.[270] The authors adapted the 1996 guidelines to the microbial patterns of their institution. Patients more often received adequate antimicrobial treatment after guidelines implementation (94%, in comparison to 48% before implementation; $P < 0.001$). Length of treatment was reduced by 6 days, and a second episode of VAP was less likely to occur after implementation.

FOCUS OF GUIDELINES ON PREVENTION AND MANAGEMENT OF VAP TO IMPROVE OUTCOME

Preventive approaches to VAP have focused on reducing cross-transmission, pulmonary aspiration across the ETT cuff, and reducing bacterial load in the oropharynx. Several strategies with proven efficacy in reducing morbidity and mortality related to mechanical ventilation have been grouped by the Institute for Healthcare Improvement as the "Ventilator Bundle." Although the bundle was not designed to specifically prevent VAP, interventions such as semirecumbent position[187] and sedation vacation[119,124] have proven to significantly reduce VAP rates.

The bundle was later modified to specifically address VAP by adding two strategies: daily oral use of chlorhexidine and subglottic secretion drainage. A 2-year multifaceted program to prevent VAP with eight targeted measures based on well-recognized published guidelines showed that increasing compliance with these measures was followed by an important reduction in the incidence of VAP.[111]

In conclusion, in an effort to improve survival of patients with nosocomial pneumonia and considering the impact of antibiotic therapy on outcome, clinicians should consider the following points:

1. The microbial prediction of guidelines should be highly accurate and the presence of MDR pathogens promptly identified. To achieve this goal, the guidelines should be adapted to the local microbiology, and the prevalence of specific bacteria and risk factors for harboring MDR pathogens assessed.
2. Viruses and fungi as causative pathogens of VAP should be considered and appropriate therapy administered.
3. Following clinical diagnosis of VAP, antimicrobial therapy should never be delayed.
4. Antimicrobial therapy should be adequate and, in particular, cover MDR pathogens when risk factors are present. The importance of designing guidelines and protocols and adapting them to local microbiology is essential to achieve this goal.
5. The dosage and duration of antibiotic treatment should be adequate.
6. A multitask educational approach for healthcare personnel should be initiated to implement guidelines into clinical settings.

KEY POINTS

1. Nosocomial pneumonia is a common complication occurring in critically ill patients and is the leading cause of nosocomial infection–related death. Tracheal intubation is the main risk factor for the development of nosocomial pneumonia.

2. Etiologic agents for nosocomial pneumonia differ according to the population of ICU patients, duration of hospital stay, and prior antimicrobial therapy. Nosocomial pneumonia due to multidrug-resistant pathogens is associated with the highest morbidity and mortality.

3. Preventive strategies, grouped as bundles, should be implemented in hospital settings. Several preventive strategies have shown efficacy in decreasing the incidence of pneumonia. In particular, the most effective strategies focus on reduction of cross-transmission, diminishing the likelihood of aspiration across the tracheal tube cuff, and decreasing bacterial load in the oropharynx.

4. In the presence of clinical suspicion of nosocomial pneumonia, diagnostic strategies should include early collection of respiratory samples *before* starting/changing antibiotics.

5. The choice of empirical treatment should be based on the most likely etiologic microorganisms and the antimicrobials likely to be active against these microorganisms. Therapy should be adjusted/de-escalated following microbiologic culture results.

ANNOTATED REFERENCES

American Thoracic Society. Guidelines for the management of adults with hospital-acquired, ventilator-associated, and healthcare-associated pneumonia. Am J Respir Crit Care Med 2005;171:388-416.
Latest guidelines published by a joint committee of the American Thoracic Society and the Infectious Disease Society of America. Prior antibiotic treatments and recent stay in hospital and healthcare-associated facility were identified as major risk factors for acquiring MDR pathogens. Moreover, the importance of choosing specific antimicrobials based on local prevalence of pathogens and antibiotic susceptibility is also emphasized.

Valles J, Pobo A, Garcia-Esquirol O, Mariscal D, Real J, Fernandez R. Excess ICU mortality attributable to ventilator-associated pneumonia: the role of early vs. late onset. Intensive Care Med 2007;33:1363-8.
Prospective case-control study that shows risks for increased mortality associated with VAP, particularly late-onset. In patients with late-onset VAP, observed mortality was higher than expected mortality (51.7 versus 26.7%, respectively, P < 0.01) with attributable mortality of 25% and an RR 1.9 (95% CI, 1.26-2.63).

Kollef MH, Afessa B, Anzueto A, et al. Silver-coated endotracheal tubes and incidence of ventilator-associated pneumonia: the NASCENT randomized trial. JAMA 2008;300:805-13.

First randomized multicenter clinical trial testing efficacy of a silver-coated tracheal tube versus standard tube on incidence of ventilator-associated pneumonia. A total of 2003 patients expected to require mechanical ventilation for 24 hours or longer were randomized. Rates of microbiologically confirmed VAP were 4.8% (silver-coated tube group) compared to 7.5% (control group, P = 0.03), with a relative risk reduction of 35.9%.

Giantsou E, Liratzopoulos N, Efraimidou E, et al. Both early-onset and late-onset ventilator-associated pneumonia are caused mainly by potentially multiresistant bacteria. Intensive Care Med 2005;31:1488-94.
Study challenges previous definitions of VAP based on onset. Among 408 patients with early- and late-onset VAP (cutoff 7 days), potentially multiresistant bacteria, mainly Pseudomonas aeruginosa and MRSA, were the most commonly isolated pathogens in both types of VAP.

Schweickert WD, Gehlbach BK, Pohlman AS, Hall JB, Kress JP. Daily interruption of sedative infusions and complications of critical illness in mechanically ventilated patients. Crit Care Med 2004;32:1272-6.
Study confirming previous results that in critically ill patients receiving mechanical ventilation, daily interruption of sedative infusions decreases duration of mechanical ventilation and ICU length of stay.

Importantly, the study clearly elucidates that shortening the length of mechanical ventilation reduces associated complications, including VAP.

Lorente L, Lecuona M, Alejandro J, Maria M, Antonio S. Influence of an endotracheal tube with polyurethane cuff and subglottic drainage on pneumonia. Am J Respir Crit Care Med 2007;176:1979-83.
Single-center study that proves that the use of a tracheal tube with an ultrathin polyurethane cuff, in addition to aspiration of subglottic secretions, can reduce the incidence of early- and late-onset VAP.

Lacherade JC, De JB, Guezennec P, et al. Intermittent subglottic secretion drainage and ventilator-associated pneumonia: a multicenter trial. Am J Respir Crit Care Med 2010;182:910-7.
The first study that demonstrates efficacy of intermittent aspiration of subglottic secretions on reduction of both early- and late-onset VAP.

Liberati A, D'Amico R, Pifferi S, Torri V, Brazzi L. Antibiotic prophylaxis to reduce respiratory tract infections and mortality in adults receiving intensive care. Cochrane Database Syst Rev 2009;4:CD000022.
The first study clearly identifying duration of mechanical ventilation and previous antibiotic usage as risk factors for multidrug-resistant pathogens in VAP.

Canadian Critical Care Trials Group. A randomized trial of diagnostic techniques for ventilator-associated pneumonia. N Engl J Med 2006;355:2619-30.
Latest meta-analysis including 36 studies involving 6914 patients treated in ICUs to investigate whether the use of antibiotics administered as preventive intervention reduce lower respiratory tract infections. The results show that fewer infections and deaths were associated with administration of a combination of topical plus systemic antibiotics.

Ferrer M, Liapikou A, Valencia M, et al. Validation of the American Thoracic Society–Infectious Diseases Society of America Guidelines for hospital-acquired pneumonia in the intensive care unit. Clin Infect Dis 2010;50:945-52.
The first study that validates 2005 guidelines for the management of patients with hospital-acquired pneumonia. The study demonstrates worse microbial prediction of 2005 guidelines, in comparison to previous guidelines, in patients considered at low risk for acquiring MDR pathogens, and similar low prediction for fungi.

REFERENCES

Access the complete reference list online at http://www.expertconsult.com.

68

Pulmonary Infections in the Immunocompromised Patient

CARLOS AGUSTÍ | CARMEN LUCENA | ANTONI TORRES

Improvements in solid-organ and hematopoietic stem cell transplantation (SOT and HSCT) techniques, expanded use of chemotherapeutic treatments and glucocorticoids, and the appearance of new immunomodulatory therapies contribute to the increasing numbers of immunocompromised patients.[1] Recognizing and managing pulmonary complications, particularly infections that result from immunosuppression, are challenging tasks for clinicians. Despite the introduction of potent broad-spectrum antimicrobial agents, complex supportive care modalities, and the use of preventive measures, pulmonary infections continue to be the most frequent complications in these patients and have a high associated mortality, especially when intubation and mechanical ventilation are required.[2] In a prospective study of 200 immunocompromised patients with lung infiltrates, infectious agents were isolated from more than three-fourths of patients.[3] Early diagnosis and intervention are essential to improving outcomes.

Evaluating the Net State of Immunosuppression

Proper assessment of factors involving the patient's net state of immunosuppression is of paramount importance (Table 68-1). Most important among them are the specific type of underlying immune deficiency, the immunosuppressive therapy received, and the epidemiologic exposures the patient has encountered in both the community and hospital. A timetable with intervals during which each type of infection and noninfectious pulmonary complication tend to be most prevalent have also been adapted for SOT and HSCT patients (Table 68-2). Knowledge of these time-related complications, as well as the individual characteristics of each patient, will help guide diagnostic tests and allow implementation of appropriate empirical therapy.

Etiology of Pneumonia in Intensive Care Patients

BACTERIAL INFECTIONS

Bacteria are the most frequent cause of pulmonary infections in immunocompromised patients. Jain et al., in a study evaluating 104 intensive care unit (ICU) patients with lung infiltrates, found that 49% of episodes were bacterial infections.[4] The specific bacterial etiology of pulmonary infections in immunocompromised patients differs in frequency depending on underlying immune defects. Encapsulated organisms such as *Streptococcus pneumoniae* and *Haemophilus influenzae* are particularly common in patients with immunoglobulin defects, such as those suffering from multiple myeloma or in patients with chronic lymphocytic leukemia. Infections caused by penicillin-resistant *S. pneumoniae* are on the rise,[5] and prophylactic use of antibiotics against gram-negative bacteria in patients with neutropenia has favored the emergence of *Staphylococcus aureus* infections (including methicillin-resistant [MRSA]) and multi-resistant gram-negative bacilli (*Pseudomonas aeruginosa*, *Acinetobacter* spp., and *Stenotrophomonas maltophilia*.)[6] Epidemiologic studies have shown that *Legionella* pneumonia is more prevalent in the ICU host, particularly in

renal transplant recipients and patients with lymphoma. It is important to consider that 15% to 30% of cases of bacterial pneumonia are mixed bacterial/opportunistic infections,[1] a finding of particular therapeutic importance in patients who do not respond to what was initially considered to be appropriate specific antibiotic treatment.

FUNGAL INFECTIONS

Aspergillus spp. are some of the most common microorganisms causing pneumonia in the ICU patient. Since neutrophils are the key cells in defense against *Aspergillus*, neutropenic patients, particularly HSCT recipients, are at special risk for this infection. Among recipients of solid-organ transplants, the incidence of invasive pulmonary aspergillosis (IPA) is highest after lung transplantation. A steady increase in documented cases of IPA after organ transplantation has been reported.[7] It is estimated that aspergillosis is found in 30% of patients with protracted severe neutropenia.[8]

Although mortality associated with IPA in IC patients has historically been as high as 80%, during the past 2 decades, the outcome of this infection seems to be changing. Early detection of infection using antigen-specific diagnostic techniques based on serum detection of either galactomannan or beta-D-glucan, two constituents of fungal cell walls, may improve diagnosis, particularly in patients with leukemia and HSCT recipients. Recent reports suggest that detection of galactomannan in bronchoalveolar lavage fluid might be more sensitive than detection in serum.[9] Diagnosis of invasive fungal diseases with the use of polymerase chain reaction (PCR) assay, although promising, is currently investigational.[10] Implementation of thoracic computed tomography (CT) scan in patients at high risk for invasive pulmonary aspergillosis may improve outcome.[11] Prompt institution of azoles appears to have resulted in improved survival.[12]

Candida species colonize the respiratory tract and are often recovered from pulmonary specimens in ICU patients, but are only considered truly pathogenic if fungemia occurs or lung tissue invasion can be demonstrated. With expanded use of new antifungal therapies, an increased incidence of infections due to *Candida krusei* and *Candida glabrata* has been reported. Other fungi that can infect immunocompromised patients as a result of environmental exposures (e.g., *Penicillium purpurogenum*,[13] *Scedosporium prolificans*[14]) can cause lethal infections.

A marked decrease in the incidence of *Pneumocystis jiroveci* pneumonia has been found recently, primarily owing to use of specific prophylaxis in patients at risk and the use of highly active antiretroviral therapy (HAART) in human immunodeficiency virus (HIV)-infected patients. In a recent report, *P. jiroveci* infection was documented in 2.5% of patients undergoing allogeneic HSCT. The majority of cases occurred late in the course following HSCT (median 14.5 months)[15] and with a CD4+ count less than 200 cells/mm[3].

MYCOBACTERIUM INFECTIONS

There has been a marked decrease in pulmonary tuberculosis in HIV-infected patients with the introduction of HAART.[16] However, remarkable geographic differences in the incidence of pulmonary tuberculosis in such patients have been reported.[17] A high level of suspicion

TABLE 68-1	Variables to Be Considered in Evaluating the Net State of Immunosuppression

Specific type of underlying immune deficiency:
  Neutrophil defect: aplasia, neutropenia, leukemia
  Immunoglobulin defect: multiple myeloma
  T-cell defect: acquired immunodeficiency syndrome (AIDS), solid organ transplant, lymphoma
Type, dose, and duration of immunosuppressive therapy
Type of organ transplanted
Presence or absence of leukopenia
Integrity of the mucocutaneous barriers
Timing between transplantation and development of pulmonary infiltrates
Disturbances secondary to transplant: graft-versus-host disease
Environmental exposures
Infection with immunomodulating viruses: cytomegalovirus, Epstein-Barr virus
Other metabolic conditions: uremia, diabetes

TABLE 68-2	Timetable of the Most Likely Pulmonary Complications in Immunocompromised Transplant Patients

First 30 Days After Transplant

Bacterial and fungal infections
Herpesvirus, respiratory viruses
Noninfectious complications: pulmonary edema, diffuse alveolar hemorrhage

2 to 6 Months After Transplant

Bacterial and fungal infections
Immunomodulatory viruses: cytomegalovirus, Epstein-Barr virus
Opportunistic infections: *Pneumocystis jiroveci*, *Listeria monocytogenes*

More Than 6 Months After Transplant

Community-acquired respiratory viruses and bacteria
In patients with poor allograft function, consider opportunistic infections.

is necessary to diagnose pulmonary tuberculosis in ICU patients; tuberculosis should be particularly considered in patients with T-cell defects (see Table 68-1). The typical radiologic pattern is often replaced by diffuse, basal, or miliary infiltrates as well as mediastinal lymph nodes. Although sputum analysis is a good noninvasive test for mycobacterium staining, most patients will undergo bronchoscopy, with a diagnostic yield of more than 90%.

Different PCR techniques have been developed to try to circumvent the problem of diagnostic delay in tuberculosis; however, false-positive results in patients shedding nonviable microorganisms limit the clinical use of these techniques. Atypical mycobacterial infections, particularly *Mycobacterium avium* complex, were previously common in HIV patients with less than 50 CD4$^+$ cells/mm^3. However, since the introduction of HAART, the incidence of these infections has dropped significantly. With the exception of lung transplant patients, atypical mycobacterial infections are rare in SOT recipients.

VIRUSES

Cytomegalovirus (CMV) is the most prevalent and lethal virus causing pneumonia in ICU patients. The incidence of CMV infection will depend on several factors: the type of transplant (highest in allogeneic HSCT recipients), degree of immunosuppression (highest when graft rejection is present and/or additional immunosuppressive treatment is required), and serologic status. The risk for CMV pneumonia without prophylaxis is greater in allogenic (20%-35%) than autologous transplantation (1%-6%). Patients receiving heart/lung or lung transplants are at high risk for CMV infections, probably because the lung harbors latent CMV, and therefore CMV can be transmitted into the allograft. The introduction of HAART has resulted in a drastic decrease in the number of cases of CMV disease in HIV-infected patients. CMV infection is extremely rare in patients with cancer.[18]

Since a third of patients with serologic evidence of previous CMV infection will develop CMV pneumonia, emphasis must be placed on the prevention of CMV disease in high-risk patients. In addition, reactivation of CMV probably contributes to the net state of immunosuppression, resulting in increased susceptibility to other infectious agents. CMV antigenemia based on the detection of the pp65CMV antigen in peripheral blood leukocytes, and quantitative PCR for early detection of viral DNA/RNA in serum, are used for early detection of active infection. Both assays have a sensitivity and specificity for the diagnosis of active infection of greater than 80% and diagnose active infection 1 to 3 weeks before conventional methodologies.[19] As a rule, symptomatic CMV infection will not develop before 2 to 3 weeks after transplantation. However, widespread use of anti-CMV prophylactic therapy has resulted in significantly delayed appearance of CMV among transplant recipients.[20]

The clinical and radiologic findings of CMV pneumonia are nonspecific. Occasionally, involvement of other organ systems with hepatitis, ulcerative gastroenteritis, hemorrhagic colitis, or retinitis may be a clue to the etiology of the pulmonary disease. Over the past decade, most centers have adopted preemptive antiviral treatment or prophylaxis strategies to prevent CMV disease. Both strategies are effective but also have shortcomings with presently available drugs. New treatment options for CMV are urgently needed and may be critical for the management of drug-resistant CMV disease, which will probably become more prevalent with increased use of antiviral drugs in ICU patients.[21] Before the development of surveillance and prophylactic measures, CMV pneumonia had a high mortality that reached 85%. Currently, mortality is between 30% and 50%.

Recent developments in molecular-based diagnostic tools have shown that conventional respiratory viruses (influenza, parainfluenza, RSV, adenoviruses, enteroviruses, rhinoviruses) are frequent causes of respiratory illnesses and are associated with high rates of morbidity and mortality among ICU patients.[22]

Diagnostic Approaches

Evaluation of pulmonary infiltrates in the ICU host remains a diagnostic challenge (Table 68-3). A confident diagnosis can seldom be made based on clinical and conventional radiology. Sputum cultures have a low sensitivity but are indicated because organisms isolated in the upper respiratory tract are likely to be the cause of the pneumonia. Since ICU patients with pulmonary infection are at risk for rapid dissemination of the disease with accompanying acute respiratory failure, fiberoptic bronchoscopy (FOB) should be considered early after the appearance of pulmonary infiltrates. Early use of FOB may add to prompt identification of the specific etiologic agent, facilitating an etiology-guided treatment and avoiding unnecessary and potentially harmful additional treatment. It has been shown that early diagnosis of both viral and fungal infections decreases mortality.[23] Fiberoptic bronchoscopy is a low-risk procedure that can be safely performed in most patients, including those with hypoxemia who are treated with supplemental oxygen or during noninvasive ventilation. In ICU patients, it provides a specific diagnosis in 50% to 80% of cases.[3,24,25]

Bronchoalveolar lavage (BAL) is a reliable technique for detecting opportunistic infections such as *P. jiroveci*, CMV, and fungi but also bacteria, mycobacteria, and other pathogens. It can still recover resistant pathogens even after several days of empirical treatment, thereby allowing modifications of the primary regimen. This bronchoscopic technique also provides useful information in diagnosing noninfectious etiologies such as diffuse alveolar hemorrhage or alveolar proteinosis that can occur in ICU patients.[26] The protected specimen

TABLE 68-3	Variables Related to Mortality in Different Groups of Immunocompromised Patients

APACHE II score > 20
Bilateral infiltrates in chest radiography
Mechanical ventilation requirement
Inadequate empirical treatment
Delay in diagnosis

brush (PSB) does not seem to add diagnostic information to BAL. By contrast, a simple, safe, and cost-effective technique such as tracheobronchial aspirate may complement BAL in diagnosing pneumonia in ICU patients.[32]

Rarely, an open lung biopsy will be needed for diagnostic purposes. Although its diagnostic yield is high and often leads to changes in therapy,[27] the indications and proper moment must be selected carefully, owing to potential morbidity and mortality.

Thoracic CT scan is an important diagnostic tool in invasive pulmonary aspergillosis (IPA). The halo sign (hemorrhagic pulmonary nodule) and air-crescent sign (cavitation) are early radiologic signs typical of IPA. This technique is also valuable in detecting pneumonic infiltrates in febrile neutropenic patients, particularly in transplant recipients,[28] since it can detect pulmonary infiltrates when the chest x-ray is normal and may provide a time gain of several days in diagnosis. On the other hand, neutropenic patients with fever and a normal HRCT scan have a very low risk of pneumonia. A potential drawback of the CT scan in evaluating pulmonary infiltrates in ICU patients is its incapacity to detect polymicrobial infections. The possibility of more than one etiologic agent can be as high as 15% in some groups of ICU patients.

Prognostic Factors for Pneumonia in Intensive Care Patients

Pneumonia in ICU patients carries a high mortality irrespective of the factors leading to the altered immune status. Those patients with the highest mortality rate are recipients of an HSCT. A number of additional prognostic factors have been identified that portend a poor prognosis.[29] Some of these factors are common to the different groups of ICU patients, whereas others relate to specific groups. Particularly relevant is the requirement for mechanical ventilation, which is associated with a grim prognosis, particularly in HSCT recipients, where the mortality rate is higher than 90%; very few survive 6 months after the onset of this pulmonary complication. Another prognostic factor that has a decisive influence on outcome is inadequacy of empirical antimicrobial treatment. The difficulty of making an appropriate antibiotic selection in light of growing resistance and the wide spectrum of potential etiologic factors emphasizes the importance of designing strategies aimed at obtaining an early diagnosis. The impact of diagnostic delay on mortality is an important theme in the care of seriously ill patients, particularly as it affects the adequacy of initial therapy.[29,30]

Therapeutic Strategies

NONINVASIVE VENTILATION

Patients requiring mechanical ventilation may have a worse prognosis than similar patients matched for general severity-of-illness scoring systems, such as APACHE II, because mechanical ventilation may be directly injurious to the lungs through increasing the risk

for nosocomial pneumonia.[30] Early implementation of noninvasive ventilation (NIV) is indicated in the early stage of hypoxemic acute respiratory failure in ICU patients, since it decreases the requirement for intubation and the incidence of nosocomial pneumonia.[31] However, there are concerns with the nonselective use of NIV in immunocompromised patients, especially insofar as it may have a deleterious impact on clinical course by delaying the institution of conventional mechanical ventilation in patients who have acute lung injury.[32]

EMPIRICAL TREATMENT OF SUSPECTED PNEUMONIA

Empirical treatment of pneumonia in ICU patients will vary depending on factors influencing the net state of immunosuppression (see Tables 68-1 and 68-2) and local patterns of microbial resistance.[33] For neutropenic patients with fever, administration of empirically chosen intravenous antibiotics is a widely accepted clinical practice.[34] However, there is considerable controversy regarding this topic. Often there is an unwise combination of potent broad-spectrum antimicrobial drugs for long periods of time. Clearly this approach is highly cost-ineffective and can cause harm due to toxicity and potential interactions of the drugs administered.[35]

Novel antifungal and antiviral (mainly CMV) diagnostic tests not only provide earlier diagnosis and need for treatment, but negative tests may support withholding specific therapy, thereby avoiding the risk of severe side effects.[35] Recently, considerable attention has been directed towards stratification of patients with febrile neutropenia according to their risk. Studies have shown that by using demographic and clinical data, as well as the evaluation of different inflammatory markers such as procalcitonin,[36] interleukin (IL)-6, and IL-8,[37] it is possible to identify patients at low risk for complication who might be safely managed with a more simplified antibiotic regime, even on an outpatient-monitored basis. These findings represent an important step forward in the rational use of antibiotic treatment, offering the potential for cost savings, reduction in adverse drug events, and decreases in antibiotic resistance and hospitalization.[35]

Conclusions

Pneumonia represents a serious challenge for clinicians caring for ICU patients. Mortality in these patients is high, particularly in those undergoing HSCT and those requiring mechanical ventilation. In the past several years, important advances in prophylactic, preemptive, and therapeutic measures have taken place. A number of diagnostic and laboratory procedures is currently available, and the clinician must define an appropriate evaluation strategy based on the net state of immunosuppression. Early diagnosis is advantageous, and fiberoptic bronchoscopy substantially increases diagnostic yield and changes empirical treatment in many patients. Neutropenic patients with fever of unknown origin and normal chest roentgenograms should undergo HRCT scan. Early application of NIV is warranted to avoid intubation and improve prognosis in patients with hypoxemia but no evidence of acute lung injury.

REFERENCES

Access the complete reference list online at http://www.expertconsult.com.

69

Lung Transplantation

DAVID WEILL

Historical Perspective

Lung transplantation evolved from heart-lung transplantation as a method by which donor organs could be used more efficiently. Heart-lung transplantation was first performed in 1981[1] and was initially the procedure of choice for diseases that are now more commonly treated by transplant using either bilateral sequential lung transplantation or single-lung transplantation. The appeal of developing the isolated lung transplant technique was improvement in donor organ utilization. Specifically, by using each of the three thoracic organs available from a single donor (i.e., two lungs and a heart), donor organ utilization can be maximized while achieving acceptable outcomes.

The double-lung transplant procedure, originally accomplished by en bloc replacement using a tracheal anastomosis, was first performed in 1983 in Toronto. The bilateral procedure is now performed as a sequential transplant using bilateral bronchial anastomoses. The bilateral sequential technique, as compared with the en bloc tracheal anastomotic technique, has been associated with fewer airway anastomotic complications, likely as a result of the superior blood supply from retrograde pulmonary artery flow.

Single-lung transplantation was first described in 1986.[2] The advantage of the procedure is that it has allowed maximal donor utilization while being associated with good patient outcomes. The single-lung procedure has historically been accepted as the procedure of choice for common transplant indications such as emphysema and idiopathic pulmonary fibrosis and is currently performed as commonly as the bilateral procedure.[3]

Survival and Demographics

Worldwide, 1200 to 1400 patients receive a lung transplant each year. Despite the yearly increase in patients on the transplant waiting list (recently nearly 4000 patients), the number of transplant procedures performed each year has been relatively stable over the past several years (Figure 69-1).[3] Significant discussion and research regarding methods to expand the donor pool are ongoing,[4] but until strategies to increase lung donor procurement are actually employed, the number of transplants performed each year will likely remain stable.

Long-term survival after lung transplantation is limited by the development of the bronchiolitis obliterans syndrome (BOS), which is commonly referred to as *chronic rejection*. BOS, defined by declining spirometry below the best postoperative level achieved, is variable in time to onset but increases in frequency as duration post transplant lengthens. Unfortunately, the etiology of BOS remains elusive, but it likely involves both immune and nonimmune mechanisms, including frequent early acute rejection episodes, infection with cytomegalovirus (CMV), severe early postoperative lung injury, and donor factors. Largely because the mechanism of BOS is unknown, satisfactory treatment is currently unavailable.

Indications and Procedure Choice

Indications for lung transplant are listed in Table 69-1 according to the generally accepted procedure choice. Although there are many end-stage lung diseases that can potentially be amenable to lung transplantation, four diseases account for the vast majority of lung transplant recipients: emphysema (both cigarette-induced and due to

alpha$_1$-antitrypsin deficiency), cystic fibrosis, primary pulmonary hypertension, and idiopathic pulmonary fibrosis.[3] Contraindications to transplant include evidence of extrapulmonary disease such as significant kidney, liver, or cardiac disease; poor nutritional or rehabilitation status; recent or current malignancy; and a poor psychosocial profile.

Generally the procedure of choice is the one that can be performed safely while utilizing the available donor organs most efficiently. Emphysema is the most common lung transplant indication and has consistently been associated with the best survival post transplant.[3] While some controversy exists regarding the optimal procedure choice (single versus double) in this group of patients,[5] most patients with emphysema who have undergone a lung transplant have received a single-lung transplant. Bilateral lung transplant has traditionally been reserved for suppurative lung diseases, such as cystic fibrosis, and other bronchiectatic disease where replacing as much infected lung tissue as possible is the primary goal. Patients with primary pulmonary hypertension generally receive a bilateral lung transplant because this prevents the potentially life-threatening situation that occurs when, in performing a unilateral transplant, nearly all cardiac output flows to the allograft, given its relatively lower vascular resistance compared to the native primary pulmonary hypertension lung. In the early transplant period when single lungs were transplanted for this indication, the result in most centers was profound unilateral pulmonary edema in the allograft.

Candidate Selection

Because of the rigors of a major thoracic surgery such as lung replacement, an extensive evaluation process occurs in all potential lung transplant recipients. The majority of the preoperative testing is directed toward excluding significant extrapulmonary disease, particularly those diseases that would lessen the chances of survival in the immediate postoperative period or make tolerance of the commonly used postoperative immunosuppression difficult. Occult coronary artery disease or malignancies are commonly uncovered as the evaluation proceeds, particularly in those patients who have significant cigarette-smoking histories. Other important goals of the evaluation process are to determine the likelihood of compliance with the complicated postoperative medical regimen and the existence of a solid support system to help with medical care once the patient leaves the hospital.

Waiting List Considerations

TIME ON WAITING LIST

Waiting times for lung transplant recipients are highly unpredictable and vary considerably geographically. Waiting list priority is strictly according to time, or "seniority," on the list. Currently there is no waiting list status system, although there likely will continue to be significant efforts to give priority to those on the waiting list who are more ill and who are most likely to do well post transplant. Unfortunately, devising such a system for lung allocation is problematic, primarily owing to the lack of compelling data correlating likelihood of waiting list mortality among the various disease groups with the highest probability of survival after transplantation. At most centers, as the numbers of patients referred for transplant increase and the

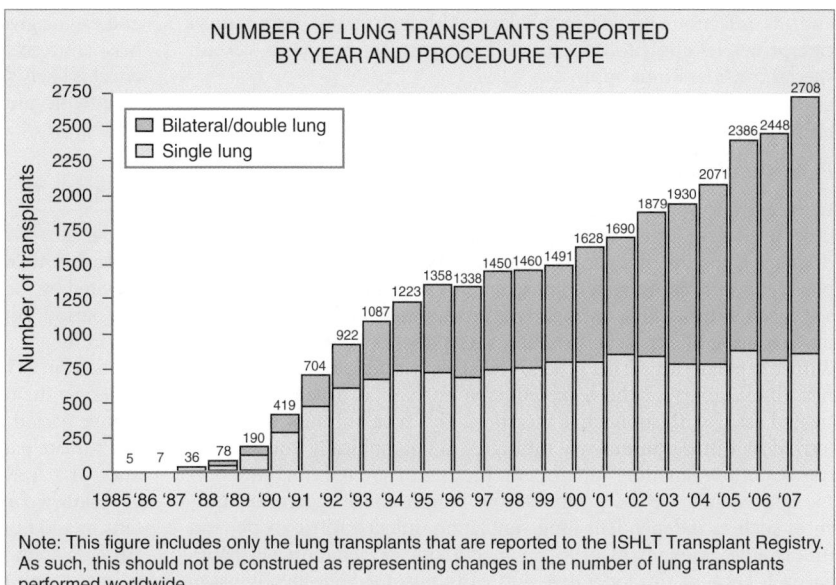

Figure 69-1 Number of lung transplants reported by year. (*Adapted from the International Society for Heart and Lung Transplantation [http://ishlt.org/].*)

length of the waiting list increases, waiting times continue to lengthen, and the mortality rate for patients on the waiting list will increase as well.

CARE OF PATIENTS ON WAITING LIST

Management of patients on the lung transplant waiting list involves close interaction with the referring physician. Treatment is directed toward the underlying disease process and is not generally affected by the patient's waiting list status. However, clinical activities that may affect transplant outcome should form prominent aspects of the medical care plan. For instance, enrollment and participation in a cardiopulmonary rehabilitation program is of paramount importance so waiting patients can develop or maintain the best cardiovascular fitness possible. Furthermore, weight management is often an important issue, and regular exercise can help avoid excessive weight gain, which is associated with poor outcomes after transplantation. Conversely, in patients with cystic fibrosis, weight maintenance can be achieved by regular consultation with nutritional support personnel familiar with patients in whom specific dietary needs exist. Other considerations requiring the attention of the transplant team include substantial increases in corticosteroid use, which although never definitively linked to poor outcomes post transplant, remain a theoretical concern in terms of bronchial anastomotic and wound healing. As lung transplant waiting lists grow at most centers, regular outpatient clinic visits to monitor patients on the waiting list will likely become more important so that clinical issues that may affect transplant success can be detected and addressed.

An important development in donor lung allocation occurred in 2005 with the institution of the Lung Allocation Score (LAS). Traditionally, lungs had been allocated using a time-based system governed by how long a patient had been on the lung transplant waiting list.

However, the new LAS system is based on two factors: (1) expected mortality on the waiting list for a given patient and (2) expected survival following lung transplant. These two factors are influenced by a number of clinical parameters that are measured by individual transplant centers and used to assign a score. The highest scores are assigned to patients with relatively high waiting list mortality (due to severity of illness) and an adequate or better chance of survival following lung transplantation. Familiarity with this system is particularly important for the ICU physician, who may encounter a patient with a high urgency score.

Donor Criteria

The expansion of lung transplantation as a therapy for end-stage lung disease is not limited by the number of potential recipients but rather by the availability of suitable donor organs. The standard, or "classic," lung donor criteria are well known, if not closely followed, among lung transplant practitioners. Although some of these criteria certainly make good sense (i.e., a clear chest radiograph, no bronchoscopic evidence of aspiration), nearly all the others are controversial, often ignored, and not based on convincing research data.[4] The standard or classic lung donor criteria are listed in Table 69-2. Whereas certain geographic regions in the United States, some countries in Europe, and Australia have adopted more aggressive donor management strategies that have resulted in more donor lungs, many areas with lung transplant programs have fewer than expected lung donors.

Postoperative Care

Early postoperative care of lung transplant recipients can be divided into four general categories: (1) hemodynamic management, (2) respiratory management, (3) initiation of an immunosuppression regimen,

TABLE 69-1	Lung Transplant by Procedure Type (in Order of Frequency)	
Single-Lung Transplant	***Double-Lung Transplant***	
Emphysema/chronic obstructive pulmonary disease (COPD)	Cystic fibrosis	
Idiopathic pulmonary fibrosis	Emphysema/COPD	
Alpha$_1$-antitrypsin deficiency	Alpha$_1$-antitrypsin deficiency	
Re-transplant	Idiopathic pulmonary fibrosis	
	Primary pulmonary hypertension	
	Bronchiectasis	

TABLE 69-2	Standard Lung Transplant Donor Criteria
Age <55 years	
ABO blood group compatibility	
Clear chest radiograph	
Pao$_2$ > 300 mm Hg on fractional inspired oxygen of 1.0 and positive end-expiratory pressure = 5 cm H$_2$O	
Less than 20-pack-year smoking history	
Absence of chest trauma	
No aspiration or sepsis	
Gram stain shows sputum sample free of bacteria, fungus, and significant number of white blood cells	

and (4) infectious disease prophylaxis. Although many basic critical care principles apply to the care of lung transplant recipients, certain special considerations apply.

HEMODYNAMIC MANAGEMENT

Fluid Administration

In the early postoperative period, proper fluid management may be the most important aspect of lung transplant care. Because the lymphatic drainage is disrupted during surgery, the transplanted lung has a propensity toward pulmonary edema, and this tendency is exacerbated by several conditions. First, owing to the procurement and reimplantation process, lung allografts suffer lung injury that is characterized by a diffuse capillary leak. This process, commonly referred to as *ischemia-reperfusion injury* or the *reimplantation response*, is usually mild and treated easily with supportive measures. This type of injury is characterized by diffuse pulmonary infiltrates radiographically and varying degrees of oxygenation impairment. In cases of severe injury, the pulmonary edema may be profound and require more aggressive measures such as independent lung ventilation, inhaled nitric oxide, and in extreme cases, extracorporeal membrane oxygenation (ECMO). Second, because intraoperative and early postoperative hypotension occurs commonly, overexuberant resuscitation with crystalloid solutions sometimes occurs and worsens the pulmonary edema. In some circumstances, hypotension or decreased urine output has been treated with starch solutions that, because of the large molecules they contain, results in passage of even greater amounts of fluid through the dilated capillary channels.

Especially in the first 72 hours after surgery, judicious use of intravenous fluids should be exercised, and efforts should be made to minimize fluid administration while maintaining adequate urine output. Use of pulmonary artery catheters is standard in the early postoperative care of transplant recipients and helps guide fluid management. Low central venous pressures (0–5 mm Hg) are the objective. Also, careful attention to input and output measurements provides additional information regarding volume status and is a reminder to administer only essential fluids. Generally, if renal function allows, an appropriate goal is to keep the patient 1 L negative for the first 3 postoperative days. This is best achieved with liberal use of loop diuretics and limiting extra fluid infusions.

Hypotension is common after lung transplantation. Not only is the patient (by design) intravascularly volume depleted but he or she is also receiving medications that cause hypotension: paralytics, sedatives, and analgesics. As a result, during the early postoperative period, patients typically will have episodes of hypotension that need to be addressed. Another important consideration is the effect of positive-pressure ventilation on the hemodynamics of a recent lung transplant recipient, particularly in those receiving a single-lung transplant for emphysema, owing to discrepancies in native lung and allograft compliance characteristics. These discrepancies, coupled with many recipients who not only have preoperative right ventricular dysfunction but also in whom postoperative intravascular volume depletion is intentionally achieved, can result in overinflation of the native lung. The concept of native lung hyperinflation is covered in more detail later in Ventilator and Respiratory Management, but one must consider whether early postoperative hypotension is best treated with ventilator management strategies that address overdistention of the native lung.

During periods where hypotension is found to be the result of profound intravascular volume depletion, fluid resuscitation should ideally include solutions that have the greatest tendency to remain in the vascular space and not simply migrate through the dilated pulmonary capillary channels. Colloid solutions such as albumin and packed red blood cells (RBCs) are ideal in this setting, as is replacement with clotting factors, particularly in the patient who has postsurgical consumption of these factors. Generally, in hypotensive patients with hemoglobin less than 10 g, use of packed RBCs is the treatment of choice. If a patient has very little postoperative bleeding, albumin infusions provide a temporary solution to intravascular volume depletion

and can be given in conjunction with a loop diuretic to achieve a more brisk diuresis by transiently increasing effective renal blood flow. This effect is likely short lived but nonetheless provides a temporary increase in oncotic pressure that may lessen the development of pulmonary edema.

VENTILATOR AND RESPIRATORY MANAGEMENT

Initial care of early postoperative lung transplant recipients is directed toward ventilatory stability. Selection of a ventilator mode is generally dictated by the patient's level of consciousness in the early postoperative period. For example, patients who are deeply sedated and/or under the influence of paralytic agents will obviously require full control of ventilation. The assist-control mode meets this requirement and is generally the preferred ventilatory modality in the immediate postoperative period. However, because an effort is made at many programs to extubate patients soon after surgery, use of less sedation and avoidance of paralytic agents are being employed. In such patients, less ventilatory control is required; patients usually do well with intermittent mandatory ventilation until early extubation is achieved. In patients with poor early graft function—for example, those with primary graft failure—ventilatory strategies that limit barotrauma are most efficacious and usually include pressure-control modalities. Certainly, with pressure-control ventilation, the use of sedation and paralytics is warranted, recognizing the potential deleterious neuromuscular effects of the latter when used in combination with high doses of corticosteroids and, in some instances, aminoglycoside antibiotics.

Use of Positive End-Expiratory Pressure

Positive end-expiratory pressure (PEEP) can be safely used in lung transplant recipients, especially those who have received a bilateral lung transplant. In double-lung recipients, the compliance characteristics of the two allografts will be similar; therefore, the positive pressure exerted on each lung will be nearly evenly distributed. PEEP of +5 to +15 is safe in this patient population. In fact, some believe that PEEP has a beneficial effect by decreasing postoperative bleeding by increasing intrathoracic pressure, which would lead to tamponade of the small blood vessels in the chest. This point, however, is not widely accepted and has not been supported by conclusive data.

In single-lung recipients, the use of PEEP can be more problematic. The differing compliance characteristics of the remaining native lung and the allograft lead to the potential for a majority of the positive pressure being directed at only one lung. This is particularly true in emphysema recipients who have a highly compliant native lung and a less compliant transplanted lung. In this situation, nearly all the positive pressure is exerted on the native lung, which leads to a situation known as *acute native lung hyperinflation*. The hyperinflated native lung can cause both cardiac tamponade, manifested as acute hypotension associated with a reduction in cardiac index, and allograft compression, manifested by hypoxemia and hypercarbia. Because of these potential problems, avoidance of PEEP in patients with emphysema undergoing single-lung transplantation is generally recommended. The use of PEEP in single-lung recipients with other disease processes is usually not problematic.

Chest Physiotherapy and Patient Positioning

Chest physiotherapy (CPT) is an essential part of postoperative respiratory management. Because the allograft is denervated, the cough reflex in lung transplant recipients is impaired; CPT therefore is imperative to clear retained mucus and blood in the airway. As postoperative recovery ensues, CPT is less important because patients learn to cough periodically, regardless of the impetus to do so. Before patients are trained to do this, aggressive CPT is used (i.e., usually every hour in the first few postoperative days while the patient is awake and every 2 hours during sleep) and includes vibratory percussion, intermittent positive-pressure ventilation, and patient-directed incentive spirometry. Whereas CPT devices that deliver excessive airway pressure are to be avoided owing to concerns of potential anastomotic disruption, positive-pressure devices using less than 20 cm Hg airway pressure are generally safe.

Patient positioning in the bed can help minimize development of pulmonary edema. The lung that is positioned toward the bed when the patient is in the lateral decubitus position receives relatively less blood flow than the upward positioned lung, primarily owing to the effects of gravity. This is especially important in single-lung transplant recipients because vascular compliance characteristics differ between the native lung and the allograft, with the newly transplanted lung receiving relatively more blood flow as a result of less vascular resistance. Of course, if the new lung experiences significant reperfusion injury after transplant, then the vascular resistance would likely be higher in the allograft. Regardless of the initial condition of the transplanted lung, the allograft side should be placed upward for the first 6 hours postoperatively while the patient is in the lateral decubitus position to diminish its blood flow and ideally its tendency to develop pulmonary edema. The single-lung recipient should then be positioned with the new lung down for 1 to 2 hours before being again placed with the allograft upward. Also of note, one can determine how well the allograft is functioning by comparing oxygenation when the native lung and allograft are receiving the majority of the blood flow. For instance, when the patient oxygenates better with the native lung downward (and therefore receiving the majority of the blood flow) than when the allograft is receiving most of the pulmonary blood flow, this indicates that the new lung is not yet functioning well. In double-lung recipients, which side is positioned downward is less important, and patients are simply turned from side to side periodically (e.g., every 2 hours).

Single-Lung Versus Double-Lung Issues

Management of the mechanical ventilator after lung transplant surgery is heavily influenced by the type of lung transplant procedure performed (i.e., a single- or double-lung transplant). In recipients who receive a bilateral transplant, ventilator management is very similar to that for nontransplant patients. However, in single-lung recipients, the compliance differences between the native lung and the allograft mandate different ventilator strategies. Different strategies are particularly important in single-lung recipients with emphysema, rather than in single-lung recipients with fibrotic lung, owing to the tendency of the native emphysematous lung to hyperinflate under the influence of positive pressure. This tendency is the reason some programs have advocated double-lung transplants routinely for patients with emphysema because of their potential for increased mortality with single-lung transplant.[6] Fortunately, proper ventilator management in single-lung recipients can prevent most of the problems with native lung hyperinflation, and concerns about this phenomenon should not influence procedure choice.[7]

Ventilator management in patients with emphysema who receive a single-lung transplant should be directed toward limiting airway pressure and allowing maximal expiratory time. Avoidance of PEEP and the use of excessively large tidal volumes limit the degree of native lung hyperinflation, because any degree of positive pressure will have a tendency to be directed to the highly compliant native emphysematous lung. Because some degree of native lung hyperinflation is unavoidable, strategies to allow maximal emptying of the native lung should be employed and include reducing the set respiratory rate and increasing inspiratory flow rate to allow a longer expiratory time. If the problems associated with acute native lung hyperinflation cannot be resolved with simple ventilator maneuvers, and if the patient has not experienced significant ischemia-reperfusion injury, extubation should be strongly considered because the removal of all positive pressure will resolve the problem. By using these management strategies and clearly understanding the physiology involved with single-lung transplant recipients, one can usually avoid the untoward effects of native lung hyperinflation and its associated morbidity and mortality.

Native lung hyperinflation is more common when acute lung injury is present in the allograft, because the compliance discrepancy between the native lung and the allograft is even more pronounced. In this rare circumstance, independent lung ventilation using a double-lumen endotracheal tube can be initiated and can provide a means to ventilate the native lung and allograft according to the compliance characteristics of each.[8] Independent lung ventilation outside of the operating room setting is associated with difficulties, particularly relating to endotracheal tube malpositioning and subsequent acute lobar or total lung collapse. Prevention and recognition of tube dislodgment requires constant surveillance, generally endoscopically, and is difficult unless personnel skilled with endoscopic endotracheal tube management skills are available on a continuous basis. Under these circumstances, diligent nursing care is required, including the administration of appropriate sedation and/or paralytic agents as well as the avoidance of routine repositioning of the patient.

Extubation

The extubation criteria in a lung transplant recipient are similar to those for other types of ventilated patients, particularly postsurgical patients. The patient should certainly be free of any lingering effects of the anesthetic and able to meet standard extubation criteria.[9] As more experience with lung transplant management has developed, the decision to extubate is being made sooner, and some centers are even trying to extubate patients in the operating suite soon after surgery.[10] Other programs, however, are reluctant to extubate this quickly because of concerns about delayed ischemia-reperfusion injury that would compromise allograft function or uncertainty about whether anesthetic medications have been completely cleared. Regardless, the dogma about leaving patients ventilated for a predetermined amount of time is now being challenged.

Chest Tube Management

Lung transplant recipients generally have two chest tubes per transplanted lung after surgery. A posterior tube is positioned to drain surgical bleeding, while the anterior tube evacuates air from the pleural space. The anterior tube is usually the first tube to be removed, given that in the absence of a bronchial anastomosis dehiscence, prolonged air leaks into the chest tube are uncommon. In fact, much of what is often mistakenly regarded as an air leak coming from the thorax is often air being introduced via the skin incision at the chest tube site. The posterior tube is removed when total 24-hour drainage from it is less than 150 mL. In a bilateral lung transplant, one should be cognizant that there is communication between the two hemithoraces because the pleural space has been opened. Because of this, chest tubes in bilateral transplants should be removed one tube per side at a time, with the anterior tubes being removed first followed by the posterior tubes.

Bronchoscopy After Lung Transplantation

The initial bronchoscopy after lung transplantation typically occurs in the operating room. The goal of the procedure is to assess the bronchial anastomoses and clear retained blood and sputum from the airway. Once the patient returns to the ICU, there is generally no need to bronchoscope the patient again in the first 24 postoperative hours unless complications develop. For instance, acute ventilatory insufficiency should prompt a bronchoscopic examination of the transplanted lung or lungs to make certain that acute mucus plugging of the airways is not accounting for the ventilatory insufficiency. Because of blood in the airway from the operation and caused by retained secretions from the native lung in single-lung recipients, mucus plugging is not rare. Serious complications from bronchoscopy early after surgery are rare. Transient oxygen desaturation during bronchoscopy is common but not generally harmful to the patient.

IMMUNOSUPPRESSIVE REGIMENS

Commonly Used Agents

Different transplant centers use different immunosuppressive regimens. However, general comments can be made about the more commonly used medications. Some programs use an induction strategy that involves the early administration of antibody, either directed directly at the lymphocyte ("lymphocyte-depleting") or against interleukin receptor sites.[11] Most antibodies delivered are monoclonal and are better tolerated than the polyclonal antibodies used in the earlier transplant era. Regardless of which induction agent is preferred, a primary advantage of this strategy involves the early avoidance of nephrotoxic immunosuppressive agents (such as calcineurin inhibitors like cyclosporine or tacrolimus), while still providing adequate immunosuppression. This benefit is particularly important during the immediate postoperative period when renal insufficiency is common owing to purposeful intravascular volume depletion, use of nephrotoxic antibiotics and antiviral agents, and the effects of cardiopulmonary bypass (if used).

Most lung transplant programs use a three-drug immunosuppressive regimen. Corticosteroids are a central part of the early strategy, particularly during the period when adequate blood levels of the other immunosuppressive agents are not yet achieved. Because of the large corticosteroid doses used immediately after surgery, a variety of side effects can be expected. For example, fluid retention, systemic hypertension, and poor glucose control should be anticipated. Acute changes in mental status can also occur and clinically present as delirium or psychosis. Many of these effects can be eliminated by administrating the corticosteroids in a tapering fashion that aims to reduce the dosage as quickly as it is safe to do so.

Calcineurin inhibitors, such as tacrolimus and cyclosporine-based medications, comprise the second part of the three-drug strategy. These medications are typically administered intravenously early in the postoperative period for a number of reasons. First, lung transplant recipients are generally unable to take oral medications in the first 24 hours after surgery. Second, intravenous absorption is more predictable and avoids the rapid absorption seen early after oral administration, which is highly desirable in lung recipients in whom one would like to avoid nephrotoxic effects that could impede good urine output. Finally, because intravenous delivery is highly amenable to dose titration, turning off the intravenous drip in response to reduced urine output can quickly reestablish adequate urine output and helps achieve the goal of relative intravascular volume depletion that is critical in the early postoperative period. In the first 48 hours after surgery, a cyclosporine level equal to or less than 100 ng/mL and a tacrolimus level no greater than 5 is desirable. Once urine output is adequate and renal function is stable, drug dosage can be increased to achieve more therapeutic medication blood levels.

The third part of the immunosuppressive regimen involves the use of either azathioprine or mycophenolate mofetil. Azathioprine is generally well tolerated and is usually associated with mild, reversible side effects such as leukopenia, anemia, thrombocytopenia, and liver function test abnormalities. Mycophenolate mofetil, a newer agent, can also cause leukopenia and anemia. In some circumstances, the drug can lead to nausea, vomiting, and abdominal pain, all of which can be ameliorated by reducing the dose or temporarily stopping the drug. Monitoring of mycophenolic acid blood levels is being performed in some solid organ recipients,[12,13] but the precise target levels in lung transplantation are unknown.

INFECTIOUS DISEASE PROPHYLAXIS

Infections after lung transplant are common and occur because of baseline immunosuppression, transmission from the donor, and ICU-related instrumentation (e.g., chest tubes, central venous catheters, endotracheal tubes). The antibiotic prophylactic regimen is directed toward preventing pneumonia, surgical site infections, and central line–related infections. Usually this goal is achieved through prophylactic use of late-generation cephalosporins and vancomycin. Because of their colonization with *Pseudomonas* species, patients with cystic fibrosis receive a third prophylactic antibiotic with good gram-negative coverage, such as an aminoglycoside.

Infection with CMV after transplant can lead to deleterious acute and chronic effects. Acutely, patients are at risk to develop CMV

TABLE 69-3	CMV Prophylaxis Protocol	
	Recipient Positive	*Recipient Negative*
Donor Positive	6 wk GCV* (2 wk IV and 4 wk PO)	12 wk GCV* (6 wk IV, PO)
	CMV-IG 3 doses (1 dose every 2 wk)	CMV-IG† 7 doses in 6 wk
Donor Negative	No prophylaxis used	

*Intravenous dose 5 mg/kg q 12 h adjusted for creatinine clearance.
†150 mg/kg within 72 h post transplant, then every 2 weeks for 4 doses, then 100 mg/kg every 4 weeks for 2 additional doses
CMV IG, cytomegalovirus hyperimmune globulin; *GCV*, ganciclovir; *IV*, intravenous; *PO*, per os (oral).

pneumonia which, in many instances, leads to severe morbidity and mortality. CMV syndrome, caused by CMV replication in the bloodstream, is heralded by the onset of malaise, fever, nausea, and vomiting. Furthermore, many believe that CMV infection (even asymptomatic) can lead to more long-term sequelae such as chronic allograft dysfunction (BOS).[14]

To prevent both the acute and chronic consequences of CMV infection, many programs have adopted an aggressive CMV prophylactic protocol. The more aggressive protocols include combination therapy using both ganciclovir and CMV hyperimmune globulin.[15] The duration of therapy is dependent on CMV serology status of the donor and the recipient and is outlined in Table 69-3. Other less aggressive strategies are also used and, although less expensive and associated with less treatment-associated toxicity, likely lead to an increased incidence of CMV-related diseases.

Prophylactic use of antifungal agents is controversial and varies among centers.[16] There are single-center studies that have demonstrated a reduction in invasive fungal disease after instituting a fungal prophylactic regimen.[17] Programs that do use antifungal prophylaxis generally use medications in the azole class or aerosolized amphotericin.[18,19] While there have been no conclusive studies in lung transplant to support an antifungal prophylactic strategy, some lung transplant physicians use these agents primarily for their ability to raise blood levels of the calcineurin inhibitors, which ultimately results in significant cost savings because the calcineurin inhibitor dose can be reduced.[20] One concern with this strategy, however, is the potential to select for resistant fungal infections, particularly candidal species.

Intensive Care Unit Issues

In the early postoperative period while the patient is mechanically ventilated, the use of sedative medications and paralytics is common. However, in most cases, when early allograft function is adequate, the routine use of paralytic medications can be avoided. Avoidance of these drugs is desirable given that paralyzing agents have been associated with prolonged paralysis, which in lung transplant recipients can impair ability to wean from mechanical ventilation and to participate fully in the postoperative physical therapy regimen. The deleterious effects of paralytic agents can be exacerbated by concomitant use of high-dose corticosteroids and aminoglycoside antibiotics,[21] both of which are commonly used in the early postoperative period in lung transplant recipients.

Strategies involving gastrointestinal prophylaxis and prophylaxis against deep vein thrombosis are similar to those employed in other thoracic surgical patients. Generally, gastrointestinal prophylaxis is achieved using H_2 blockers or a proton-pump inhibitor and is particularly important early postoperatively when the patient is exposed to high doses of corticosteroids. Most programs continue the gastrointestinal prophylactic measures indefinitely. Because of the risk of surgical bleeding, prophylaxis is initially achieved using antistasis devices to the lower extremities. As the risk of postoperative bleeding diminishes, standard prophylactic regimens for deep venous thrombosis using heparin-based drugs can be safely used until the patient is fully ambulatory.

EARLY POSTOPERATIVE COMPLICATIONS

Hemodynamic Instability

As discussed earlier, the immediate hemodynamic goal in the lung transplant recipient is intravascular volume depletion. Although achieving the goal of reducing the tendency toward pulmonary edema, this strategy often results in hypotension. Furthermore, the combination of intravascular volume depletion, a poorly compliant right ventricle requiring higher filling pressures, the use of sedative and paralytic medications that cause hypotension, and positive pressure provided by the mechanical ventilator can result in exacerbation of blood pressure difficulties. Fortunately, the hypotension that occurs commonly under these circumstances can be readily reversed by a few different measures. For example, gentle volume resuscitation with colloids, such as albumin or red blood cell transfusion, can reestablish an adequate blood pressure, while not contributing significantly to pulmonary edema development. In some patients with known preoperative right ventricular dysfunction, such as that seen in primary or secondary pulmonary hypertensives, maintaining adequate right ventricular filling pressures using volume expansion is important in ensuring adequate cardiac performance even in the presence of normal systemic blood pressures. The hemodynamic effect of positive-pressure ventilation has been discussed previously. If the lung transplant recipient experiences problems with positive-pressure-related hypotension, removal from the mechanical ventilator is the treatment of choice. Not only does this remove the hemodynamic effects of positive-pressure ventilation but it also obviates the need for administration of sedative and paralytic medications, all of which have hypotensive side effects. Rarely is there a need for inotropic or cardiopressor support, except in instances of early postoperative hypothermia or profound hemorrhage.

Ventilatory Instability

Ventilatory instability in the early postoperative period requires similar evaluation as any postsurgical patient. Initial efforts to determine the etiology of ventilatory problems should be directed at diagnosing mechanical problems related to the mechanical ventilator and the endotracheal tube. For instance, acute onset of hypercarbia in the early postoperative setting should lead to investigation of the patency of the endotracheal tube specifically and the bronchial tree generally. Plugging of the airways, either with retained mucus or blood, is very common in this setting and can cause rapid ventilatory insufficiency. Development of this problem is suggested by acute increases in ventilatory pressure, but it is definitively diagnosed by bronchoscopic examination of the airways. Treatment involves removal of mucus or blood blocking the airway. Of course, improper patient-ventilator synchrony can cause a similar clinical scenario and may result from inadequate patient sedation.

Problems with early allograft function lead to inadequate ventilation and oxygenation. These problems are usually temporary and are best managed through supportive measures. However, in the case of primary graft failure, oxygenation and ventilatory problems are more profound and require more complex management strategies. In the setting of a double-lung transplant, management should include the application of increased levels of PEEP and, if necessary, alterations of inspiratory-to-expiratory ratios. In single-lung recipients, one can selectively ventilate the native lung while other measures are taken to improve allograft performance. This strategy can be accomplished through the use of double-lumen endotracheal tubes, which allow independent lung ventilation.[22] In cases of significant allograft dysfunction, positioning the patient on the side with the native lung "down" can lead to increased perfusion to that side (i.e., the side with less pulmonary edema) and can lead to improvements in oxygenation.

Extracorporeal Membrane Oxygenation

In instances in which none of the measures described results in hemodynamic and ventilatory stability, ECMO is an alternative treatment strategy.[23-25] Although associated with significant morbidity, ECMO can rapidly restore hemodynamic and ventilatory stability. Important morbidity as a result of this therapy includes bleeding complications secondary to the anticoagulation necessary to maintain the ECMO circuit. Bleeding can occur anywhere and is particularly evident at the cannula insertion site. However, intracranial hemorrhage is the most catastrophic complication and the most common cause of death associated with ECMO.[26] The preferred ECMO method in lung transplant recipients is generally the venoarterial route, although the venovenous route has been used as well.[27] Insertion of the ECMO cannulas is best performed at the femoral site, because local control of bleeding can be achieved. Although associated with good hemodynamic stability, central cannulization often results in poorly controlled bleeding.

OPERATIVE COMPLICATIONS

Postoperative bleeding issues are similar to those present in other thoracic surgical patients and are best handled by correction of coagulopathies and replacement of red blood cells. As in other thoracic patients, careful chest tube output monitoring is essential in detecting and ultimately treating excessive bleeding. Return to the operating room for exploration in the presence of excessive bleeding is not uncommon after lung transplantation. Bleeding complications are generally more common in patients in whom dissection to free the native lung is difficult, such as in cystic fibrosis patients or in patients with fibrotic lung diseases. There is also a tendency toward more bleeding in patients who have required cardiopulmonary bypass.[28]

As improvements in surgical technique have developed, a decrease in airway, venous, and pulmonary artery anastomotic complications has occurred.[29] Although uncommon, anastomotic complications in the immediate postoperative period generally involve the vascular connections rather than the bronchial anastomosis. Complications with the bronchial anastomosis, such as dehiscence or stricture, usually occur later in the postoperative period. Conversely, problems with venous[30,31] or pulmonary artery anastomoses[32] manifest immediately postoperatively and are life threatening, particularly if not detected promptly.

Pulmonary artery stricture, or narrowing, is fortunately very uncommon. When it does occur, problems with oxygenation are seen and usually occur in the absence of radiographic abnormalities. The diagnosis is initially one of exclusion, where more common causes of poor oxygenation are investigated first. Once no evidence of other causes of poor allograft function can be found, evaluation of the pulmonary artery anastomosis should occur and usually is best accomplished via pulmonary angiography. Pulmonary perfusion scanning can, in some instances, be helpful and is noninvasive. However, nonspecific alterations in allograft blood flow do not distinguish among the usual causes of postoperative allograft dysfunction. Pulmonary angiography, on the other hand, can anatomically demonstrate pulmonary artery narrowing and provides the means to measure pressure gradients across the pulmonary artery anastomosis.[33] If a significant gradient across the pulmonary artery anastomosis were to exist, the suspicion of a pulmonary artery stricture would be high enough to warrant surgical re-exploration.

Of the complications associated with vascular anastomoses, problems with the venous anastomosis are most common. Because of the technical challenges associated with establishing the venous anastomosis and the low-flow state of the venous system, the venous anastomosis is susceptible to kinking or clot formation. Both of these complications cause impedance of venous return and backflow of blood into the pulmonary vasculature. This results in immediate and profound pulmonary edema that is refractory to all supportive measures. A clinical scenario of this kind should prompt immediate investigation, ideally via visualization and Doppler measurement of the venous anastomosis using transesophageal echocardiography.[34,35]

Transfer from the ICU

In uncomplicated cases, lung transplant recipients can generally be discharged from the ICU within 24 to 48 hours. Once the respiratory status is stable, plans can be made to transfer patients to less intensive care settings. Aside from reducing the potential for ICU-related infections, discharge from an ICU setting allows more freedom of movement so more effective pulmonary rehabilitation can occur. Additionally, from a psychosocial standpoint, patients feel less isolated and are able to visit more frequently with friends and family members in less acute care settings.

ANNOTATED REFERENCES

Garrity Jr ER, Villanueva J, Bhorade SM, Husain AN, Vigneswaran WT. Low rate of acute lung allograft rejection after the use of daclizumab, an interleukin 2 receptor antibody. Transplantation 2001;71(6):773-7.

Garrity and colleagues evaluated the impact of induction therapy using daclizumab on acute rejection incidence. They found that induction therapy with daclizumab significantly reduced the incidence of acute rejection and was not associated with a significantly increased incidence of infections.

Liu V, Zamora MR, Dhillon GS, Weill D. Increasing lung allocation scores predict worsened survival among lung transplant recipients. Am J Transplant 2010;10(4):915-20.

Liu and colleagues examined the United Network Organ Sharing (UNOS) database in order to determine whether increasing LAS scores negatively impacted outcomes following lung transplantation. The authors found that as LAS increased, specifically above a score of 60, outcomes worsened.

Meyers BF, Sundt 3rd TM, Henry S, et al. Selective use of extracorporeal membrane oxygenation is warranted after lung transplantation. J Thorac Cardiovasc Surg 2000;120(1):20-6.

The authors reviewed their experience using ECMO in post–lung transplant recipients. Although ECMO is associated with increased morbidity, it is a viable therapeutic option in patients with profound respiratory and hemodynamic embarrassment. The authors further explain the technical approach to ECMO therapy.

Weill D, Lock BJ, Wewers DL, et al. Combination prophylaxis with ganciclovir and cytomegalovirus (CMV) immune globulin after lung transplantation: effective CMV prevention following daclizumab induction. Am J Transplant 2003;3(4):492-6.

The authors compared monotherapy using intravenous ganciclovir to combination therapy using intravenous ganciclovir and hyperimmune CMV globulin. Weill and colleagues found that a significant reduction in CMV disease and infection was observed in the combination therapy, as compared with using ganciclovir alone.

Weill D, Torres F, Hodges TN, Olmos JJ, Zamora MR. Acute native lung hyperinflation is not associated with poor outcomes after single lung transplant for emphysema. J Heart Lung Transplant 1999;18(11):1080-7.

The authors report on the incidence and effect of acute native lung hyperinflation in the University of Colorado Lung Transplant Program. Acute native lung hyperinflation, while radiographically common, was not associated with increased morbidity or mortality. Consequently, aggressive measures to prevent acute native lung hyperinflation, such as dual lung ventilation, contralateral lung volume reduction surgery, or routine use of double-lung transplant for emphysema patients, are not warranted.

Yonan NA, el-Gamel A, Egan J, Kakadellis J, Rahman A, Deiraniya AK. Single lung transplantation for emphysema: predictors for native lung hyperinflation. J Heart Lung Transplant 1998;17(2):192-201.

Yonan and colleagues discuss factors that predict the development of acute native lung hyperinflation. The authors conclude that acute native lung hyperinflation was common and led to increased morbidity and mortality. Yonan suggested that acute native lung hyperinflation could be avoided by the routine use of contralateral lung volume reduction surgery, double-lung transplant, or dual lung ventilation.

REFERENCES

Access the complete reference list online at http://www.expertconsult.com.

70

Burns and Inhalation Injury

ANTHONY BALDEA | RICHARD L. GAMELLI

Inhalation injury often occurs in combination with thermal injury and leads to serious complications that manifest at different points in the disease process. Inhalation injury alone carries a 5% to 8% risk of mortality; when combined with burn injury, mortality from inhalational injury can increase to 20% or more.[1] These factors, combined with a complicated pathologic course, make inhalation injury a potentially difficult and dangerous disease process.

Classification of Injury

Classifications of inhalation injury have been developed according to several different schemes. One of the first schemes was developed as a result of observations made at the Cocoanut Grove fire of 1942 and grouped patients according to outcomes and their initial symptoms. Early signs of hypoxia that were directly attributable to respiratory tract injury had the highest and most immediate mortality. Signs of cyanosis and dyspnea that occurred within a few hours of the insult could be due to development of pulmonary edema. At 24 hours, upper airway edema was found to be increased and necessitated establishment of an airway (via intubation through a tracheostomy). After 48 hours, patients developed worsening respiratory symptoms due to atelectasis and subsequent pneumonia.[2]

Additional classification symptoms for inhalation injury were based on the anatomic location of injury. Upper airway injury involves the nasopharyngeal and oropharyngeal regions to the larynx. This damage results in massive edema and compromise of airway patency, often necessitating intubation or tracheostomy. Injury to distal parts of the tracheobronchial tree manifests at a later time after the inhalational injury. Tracheal and major bronchi injuries result in direct mucosal damage and desquamation of the epithelial lining. Injury to the distal alveoli results in atelectasis and predisposes to pneumonia.[3]

Initial Inhalation Insult

The initial manifestations of inhalation injury are due to direct damage to airway surfaces that result in inflammation and edema.[4] Clinically, patients initially present with symptoms of stridor, hypoxia, and respiratory distress.[5] Management of the initial insult incorporates a thorough physical examination as well as a careful and specific history that provides details about the extent of exposure to the inhaled substance and the nature of the substance itself. Physical examination should include inspection of the oropharynx for direct damage and documentation of stridor, cyanosis, and confusion; it is not unusual for there to be no obvious physical symptoms of inhalation injury at the time of original assessment. Initial management includes providing adequate oxygenation as well reevaluation and maintenance of airway patency.[6]

Environmental Variables That Determine Severity

The extent of inhalation injury is related to the duration of exposure and severity of trauma to the tracheobronchial tree. A major component of the degree of the initial inhalation energy is the amount of heat-carrying capacity of the inhaled substance. For example, dry heat has a low heat-carrying capacity and thus usually injures upper airway and supraglottic structures; steam has 4000 times the heat-carrying capacity of dry heat and tends to cause more extensive tracheobronchial damage.[7] Thermal injury produces direct injury to the mucosa of upper airway structures, manifesting clinically as upper airway edema within the first 24 hours.[3]

The level of injury produced by inhalation of particulate matter also depends on the diameter of the inhaled matter. Large-diameter particles (>100 µm) enter the airway but usually do not travel beyond the upper respiratory tract. Smaller particles (<10 µm) can reach the lower tracheobronchial tree, while even smaller particles (<5 µm) can reach the terminal bronchus and alveolus. Particulate matter can cause direct mechanical damage and can also transport toxins beyond the level of the initial inhalation.[3]

Pathology

UPPER AIRWAY INJURY

Upper airway structures that are in direct danger from inhalation injury include the mucous membranes of the nasopharynx, hypopharynx, epiglottis, glottis, and larynx, which can demonstrate a significant amount of inflammation due to direct injury. In addition, the cartilage of the glottis is intolerant of edema, and damage to this structure can produce life-threatening compromise of airway patency.[7]

Injury to the upper airway from direct thermal injury occurs very early and quickly manifests symptoms. Mucous membranes are damaged when the temperature of inhaled gases reaches 150°C. The resulting damage initiates an inflammatory cascade that leads to increased capillary permeability, histamine release, and inflow of transudative fluid, all of which result in edema. This process starts over the course of the first 24 hours post exposure, and the resultant edema typically resolves in 4 to 5 days. Airway compromise occurs when edema causes the airway diameter to fall below 8 mm and thus mandates the need for a mechanical airway.[7]

LOWER AIRWAY INJURY

Thermal Injury

Direct thermal injury to lower airway structures is an uncommon occurrence (5%). The low incidence of lower airway injury is due to the dissipation of heat during travel through the airway and to reflexive closing of the glottis at high temperatures (150°C). Small particulate matter (<5 µm) can travel to terminal bronchi and alveoli and cause damage to cell populations such as epithelial cells and alveolar macrophages.[8]

Tracheobronchial Injury

Cytoplasmic vacuolization and cytoplasmic blebbing are seen in epithelial cells of the bronchial tree 48 hours after severe smoke inhalation.[9] This is followed by epithelial necrosis, hemorrhage, and perivascular congestion. Such damage initiates an inflammatory cascade that recruits activated neutrophils and macrophages to the injured area, causing further damage.[10] Airway congestion and increased lymphatic flow lead to obstruction of bronchial segments and impaired gas exchange.

Parenchymal Damage

Direct damage to the lung epithelium causes the recruitment of inflammatory mediators that produce increased parenchymal damage; neutrophils are among the first mediators recruited. In addition to growth factors and cytokines, neutrophils release reactive oxygen species and proteases that cause direct cellular damage. Such damage triggers further inflammation and leads to pulmonary dysfunction.[11] This dysfunction includes evidence of increased apoptosis of lung epithelial cells, leading to decrease in surfactant release and defective surfactant mechanisms, resulting in obstruction and collapse of lung segments.[12] In addition, alveolar macrophages release free radicals that cause further damage to the pulmonary parenchyma.[13] With extensive destruction and inflammation, pulmonary compliance is reduced and gas exchange is impaired, leading to altered pulmonary blood flow patterns and ventilation/perfusion mismatches.[14]

▣ Damage From Asphyxiants

Smoke generates two compounds—carbon monoxide (CO) and cyanide—that are absorbed systemically and impair oxygen utilization and delivery. These compounds directly interfere with oxygen uptake and delivery mechanisms resulting in cellular and local tissue hypoxia and eventually organ failure and death.

CARBON MONOXIDE TOXICITY

CO is an odorless, nonirritating gas that is responsible for up to 600 accidental deaths per year. The pathology of CO poisoning is attributable to its ability to rapidly diffuse into the bloodstream and bind to the iron moiety of heme that is normally bound by oxygen. Because of higher affinity (240 times) for the heme-binding site, CO easily displaces oxygen and impairs the ability of hemoglobin to deliver oxygen. The stoichiometry of hemoglobin is also altered, further impairing oxygen delivery by the other sites of hemoglobin. CO also binds to enzymes within mitochondria involved in the utilization of oxygen by cells and tissues. By binding to these enzymes, myoglobin, cytochromes, and NAPDH reductase, cellular and local tissue acidosis increases, further impairing oxygen delivery. This results in progressive cellular dysfunction and ultimately organ failure.[15]

Neurologic symptoms are often the first manifestation of CO poisoning. Mild carboxyhemoglobin levels (5%–10%) are usually well tolerated. When concentrations reach 10% to 30%, symptoms usually begin to manifest. Headaches, nausea, and dizziness are the most common initial symptoms in mild to moderate CO poisoning. With severe poisoning (50% carboxyhemoglobin levels), more significant neurologic symptoms occur, such as syncope, seizures, and coma. The diagnosis of CO poisoning is made based on the combination of physical symptoms and elevated levels of systemic carboxyhemoglobin. Pulse oximetry values do not differentiate between carboxyhemoglobin and oxyhemoglobin and thus remain paradoxically elevated. Blood Po_2 level remains normal because it reflects oxygen dissolved in plasma that is not affected by CO.[16] Neurologic symptoms may persist in the form of delayed neuropsychiatric sequelae with symptoms that include a persistent vegetative state, parkinsonism, short-term memory loss, behavioral changes, hearing loss, and psychosis. These symptoms may manifest anytime from 3 to 240 days after recovery. Approximately 50% to 75% of patients with delayed neuropsychiatric sequelae recover fully in 1 year.[17]

The hallmark of treatment of CO poisoning involves maintaining adequate oxygenation. The CO half-life decreases from 6 to 8 hours to 40 to 80 minutes within 1 hour of treatment with 100% oxygen. Administration of 100% oxygen can be done via facemask or by mechanical ventilation. Hyperbaric oxygen treatment has been shown to have an advantage over normobaric oxygen treatment for CO poisoning; when administered in a hyperbaric chamber, the half-life of CO decreases to 15 to 30 minutes.[18] However, given the limited number of hyperbaric chambers available, the widespread use of hyperbaric therapy is limited.[17,19]

CYANIDE TOXICITY

Cyanide inhalation is a potentially life-threatening occurrence that requires immediate intervention. Once inhaled, cyanide rapidly crosses into the blood and disrupts normal cellular utilization of oxygen by binding to cytochrome oxidase, thus interfering with cellular respiration. As in CO toxicity, cellular lactic acid production is increased, and cellular dysfunction soon follows.[20]

Diagnosis of cyanide toxicity is made by careful review of the history of inhalation, duration of exposure, and clinical symptoms. Physical manifestations of cyanide poisoning include headache and confusion followed by fixed pupils, bradycardia, hypotension, seizures, arrhythmias, heart block, cardiac failure, and coma. Diagnosis is aided by measurement of blood concentrations of cyanide, which are considered toxic at levels greater than 0.5 mg/L.[20]

The treatment of cyanide toxicity includes administration of oxygen as well as decontamination agents. When cyanide toxicity is suggested, 100% oxygen should be administered immediately. This can be done under normobaric or hyperbaric conditions, but the use of hyperbaric chambers is yet to be proven to provide a benefit.[21] Amyl and sodium nitrates are often used as decontamination agents; these compounds induce the formation of methemoglobin, to which cyanide has high affinity. Methemoglobin thus acts as a scavenger for cyanide. Another utilized compound for treatment of cyanide toxicity is sodium thiosulfate, which acts by transferring a sulfur group to cyanide and converting it to renally excreted thiocyanate. Hydroxycobalamin (not approved by the U.S. Food and Drug Administration [FDA]) detoxifies cyanide by binding to it and forming cyanocobalamin, an inert vitamer of the vitamin B_{12} family.[22,23]

▣ Features of Specific Irritants

Smoke produces a variety of compounds that have been shown to cause or initiate damage to the lung. The mechanism of damage for many of these compounds is unknown, but the location of damage within the respiratory tract is related to the ability of the compound to reach that location (Table 70-1). The ability of gases and toxins to exert damage on the tracheobronchial tree depends on the capacity of the toxin to reach different areas of the airway.[5] Water solubility affects the location of deposit of gases and toxins. Mucous membranes line much of the upper respiratory tract, which allows gases that are highly water soluble to be absorbed in the upper respiratory tract and cause irritation to these structures. Because less-soluble gases are not absorbed in the upper airway, they travel to the lower airway and cause irritation and damage to those structures.[3]

ACROLEIN

Acrolein, a lipophilic aldehyde carbonyl with an attached vinyl group, is a toxic compound found in the inhalation of several materials,

TABLE 70-1	Specific Lung Irritants	
Chemical Irritants	**Properties**	**Mechanism of Toxicity**
Smoke		
Acrolein	Lipophilic	Direct epithelial damage
Industrial		
Chlorine	Water soluble	Forms free radicals
Phosgene	Low solubility	Causes the release of arachidonic acid metabolites
Nitric oxide	Lipid soluble	Causes lipid peroxidation
Sulfur dioxide	Water soluble	Causes lipid peroxidation
Ammonia	Water soluble	Forms hydroxyl ions and causes liquefactive necrosis

including tobacco smoke, vehicle exhaust, and wood smoke. Its lipophilic nature allows it to pass through the upper airway and penetrate lower airway structures, where it is eventually absorbed. Systemic acrolein is metabolized by the liver through reaction with glutathione, resulting in the generation of mercapturic acids that are renally excreted.[24] This transformation, however, does not occur as readily in the lung, and thus acrolein levels remain elevated in lung tissue and cause direct epithelial damage.[25,26]

HYDROGEN CHLORIDE

The toxicity of chlorine is related to its water solubility as well as duration of exposure. Chlorine is a moderately water-soluble gas that can penetrate deep into the lower lung structures. Within the upper airway, chlorine has a direct irritant effect that causes inflammation and edema. Within the lower airway, hydrogen chloride forms reactive ions that create free radicals that react with various compounds and ultimately lead to mucosal destruction, pulmonary edema, and parenchymal damage.[27,28]

PHOSGENE

Phosgene is an acylating agent found in plastics and aniline dyes. It is a low-soluble gas that when inhaled produces severe pathology within the bronchoalveolar spaces. Phosgene reacts with glutathionine and causes the release of arachidonic acid metabolites.[29-31]

AMMONIA

The inhaled form of ammonia, anhydrous ammonia, is highly water soluble and is mostly absorbed in the upper airway. However, owing to its toxic nature, lower airway structures can also be affected. Ammonia exerts its effects by reacting with tissues, creating hydroxyl ions, which results in liquefactive necrosis.[32]

NITROGEN OXIDE

Nitric oxides are highly lipid-soluble compounds that are absorbed in the lower lung regions. Nitric oxides exert their toxic effects by the production of free radicals through lipid peroxidation, leading to parenchymal damage and pulmonary edema.[33,34]

SULFUR DIOXIDE

Sulfur dioxide is a highly water-soluble gas that is mainly absorbed in the upper airways. Sulfur dioxide, like nitric dioxide, reacts with tissues to produce free radicals via lipid peroxidation.[35]

Role of a Cutaneous Thermal Injury

The combined effect of thermal injury and inhalation injury is synergistic on morbidity and mortality, creating increased pulmonary vascular changes and inflammation that lead to decreased pulmonary compliance and pulmonary function. Burn injury alone increases vascular permeability and can result in pulmonary edema. When associated with inhalation injury, this increase in pulmonary edema is exacerbated and results in a massive influx of inflammatory mediators, which increases damage to the lung parenchyma.[36] With increasing damage to lung parenchyma, pulmonary compliance decreases and ventilation/perfusion mismatch occurs. With the resulting edema, atelectasis and consolidation of the lung (from the increased vascular permeability and increased lymphatic flow) set the stage for secondary bacterial infections.[37-39] In addition, pulmonary edema and decreased pulmonary compliance result in increased intrathoracic pressure, which causes a left side–dominant myocardial depression and contributes to the altered hemodynamic profile observed in combined thermal and inhalation injury.[40]

Postinhalation Pulmonary Complications

Inhalation injury directly injures upper and lower airway structures through thermal energy, toxic irritants, and particulate matter deposition. Lung parenchymal damage caused by alveolar macrophages and toxin exposure contributes to pulmonary dysfunction, increased infectious complications, and the development of acute respiratory distress syndrome (ARDS). Concomitant burn injury also increases vascular permeability and causes a release of inflammatory mediators.

LOCAL FACTORS

Ciliary Dysfunction

Inhalation injury causes direct damage to mucosal and ciliary elements, leading to ciliary dysmotility. Such damage is caused by several agents, including acrolein and other aldehydes.[26] In addition, the release of inflammatory mediators (such as thromboxane) has been shown to decrease mucociliary activity.[41] This allows particles and toxins to exert their effects on local defense mechanisms as well as initiate a cascade that leads to parenchymal damage and bacterial infection.[42]

Pulmonary Alveolar Macrophage

Alveolar macrophage numbers increase in smoke inhalation injury, with resultant increases in circulating tumor necrosis factor alpha (TNF-α) and interleukin (IL)-8 within 24 hours of injury, leading to extensive subsequent tissue damage.[43] In addition, the phagocytic function of macrophages is diminished, which precipitates increased lung parenchymal exposure to various toxins and bacteria.[13,44]

Proteasomes

Analysis of bronchoalveolar lavage fluid obtained on admission following inhalation injury demonstrates decreased circulating levels of proteasome 26S, with reduced specific proteasome activity. Furthermore, decreased proteasome 26S concentrations are associated with increased rates of developing ventilator-associated pneumonia, suggesting that insufficient proteasome function may contribute to increased susceptibility for pulmonary complications following inhalation injury.[45]

Surfactant

Severe inhalation injury and subsequent increased capillary permeability alter surfactant production and function. In lung injury models, surface tension generated by surfactant is reduced, leading to a loss of the normal force that maintains alveolar patency; this ultimately results in alveolar collapse.[12] In addition, reduction in surfactant protein levels (SP-A, SP-B) may lead to reduced lung defense mechanisms, further enhancing evolving lung pathology following inhalation injury.[46]

Infections

Infectious complications are a common occurrence with burn injury. Pneumonia in particular can occur in up to 50% of severely burned patients, with the majority (65%) of these patients requiring mechanical ventilation.[47,48] The mortality rate doubles in patients with concomitant inhalation injury and nosocomial pneumonia, reaching rates as high as 86%.[49] The root cause of this synergistic effect has to do with both direct lung injury from inhalation and immune dysfunction and systemic inflammation, creating an environment susceptible to opportunistic infections such as *Pseudomonas aeruginosa* and *Acinetobacter* species and leading to fulminant nosocomial pneumonias.[50,51]

Pathogens. The organisms that cause infections in inhalation injury can be organized into groups according to the pathogens' exogenous/endogenous state or to the time from injury to infection. Organisms that are endogenous and cause infections are those present in the oral and respiratory tract or those in the gut at the time of admission. These include *Staphylococcus aureus*, *Streptococcus pneumoniae*, *Haemophilus influenzae*, *Proteus mirabilis*, and *Escherichia coli*. Exogenous organisms are those that are acquired during the hospital course and were not present in either the gastrointestinal or respiratory tract. These include methicillin-resistant *S. aureus*, *Acinetobacter*, *Pseudomonas aeruginosa*, and other opportunistic organisms (e.g., *Candida*). Within these groupings, early infections tend to be from endogenous organisms, whereas infections at a later time tend be from exogenous organisms.[47] *P. aeruginosa* infection has been shown to significantly increase mortality rates in burn-injured patients. The emergence of *Acinetobacter* species has increased in burn injury and is difficult to treat owing to its easy transmissibility and multidrug resistance.[52] Like *P. aeruginosa*, infections by *Acinetobacter* tend to occur later in the time course of treatment and carry a high mortality rate.[53] A thorough understanding of the pathogens involved in inhalation injury and the time course for the onset of these infections is important to tailor effective empirical antimicrobial therapy in order to avert serious complications.

Acute Respiratory Distress Syndrome

ARDS is characterized by pulmonary edema not of cardiac origin and pulmonary inflammation leading to alterations in ventilation and perfusion.[54] During thermal injury, inflammatory mediators are released systemically and travel to the highly vascular lung tissue, leading to increased vascular permeability, recruitment of activated immune cells, and reduced surfactant function.[10,55] This leads to alveolar collapse and ventilation/perfusion mismatches. Such effects are further exacerbated by inhalation injury, which causes direct lung damage and inflammation. Thus, burn and inhalation injury carry a significant risk for the development of ARDS, which results in a high mortality rate in this population (50%–60%).[56]

Endogenous Mediators of Lung Injury

Neutrophil. During inhalation injury, there is sequestration of activated neutrophils in the lungs, mediated by direct lung damage. Neutrophils release oxygen radicals, proinflammatory cytokines, and proteases, which result in further damage to lung parenchyma and epithelia. This causes further release of inflammatory mediators that increase pulmonary vascular permeability, resulting in pulmonary edema.[11] Mucosal damage and pulmonary edema lead to collapse of bronchial segments, changes in pulmonary blood flow, and decreased gas exchange. The importance of neutrophil-mediated lung injury in the pathology of ARDS during inhalation injury is further corroborated by studies showing that the inhibition of neutrophil rolling reduces epithelial injury and decreases vascular permeability, and may lead to improved outcomes.[57]

Endothelium. Lung injury induces changes in endothelial function that increase vascular permeability and polymorphonuclear leukocyte recruitment, leading to increased inflammation and lung damage. These changes include a reduction of vascular endothelial growth factor (VEGF) that occurs during inflammation and sepsis, which may impair repair mechanisms and lead to further inflammation. In addition, endothelial damage causes release of thromboxanes that cause further endothelial damage.[58]

Complement. In the lung, complement activation causes endothelial expression of P-selectin, a chemoattractant for neutrophils.[59] In addition, complement activation also causes the formation of cell-lysing complexes that are then activated by macrophages. Once activated, these lysing complexes further contribute to lung damage.[60]

Eicosanoids. Thromboxanes and leukotrienes, potent mediators of inflammation produced by the arachidonic acid pathway, amplify the inflammatory process initiated by injury. Thromboxane A_2 increases permeability in the lung and results in interstitial as well as pulmonary edema. Leukotriene B_4 functions as a potent chemoattractant for neutrophils, further exacerbating the damage caused by these cells.[61-63]

Activation of the eicosanoid pathway is mediated by phospholipase A_2. Phospholipase A_2 causes the release of arachidonic acid from phospholipids of cell membranes. Once released, arachidonic acid is metabolized by cyclooxygenases and lipoxygenases in the lung, generating a large amount of eicosanoids. Phospholipase A_2 levels have been shown to be elevated after inhalation injury.[64] This activation pathway has been investigated as a target for potential therapies in inhalation injury, and evidence shows that inhibition of phospholipase A_2 can attenuate lung injury in animal models.[65,66]

Ongoing Pulmonary Damage After Inhalation Injury

OXYGEN TOXICITY

Oxygen toxicity can complicate the treatment of inhalation injury. After 48 to 72 hours of exposure to elevated oxygen levels ($FIO_2 > 60\%$), there is evidence of damage and apoptosis of endothelial cells, with resultant interstitial edema and cellular necrosis.[67] After 72 hours of exposure, type I epithelial cells show evidence of damage. The mechanism by which this occurs is the generation of highly reactive oxygen radicals that cause direct DNA damage and induce cells to undergo apoptosis, leading to necrosis of epithelial structures.[68,69]

FLUID MANAGEMENT

A key to the initial management of inhalation injury and burns is adequate fluid resuscitation.[6] The parameters used to determine fluid management in this clinical setting include urine output, blood pressure, and other hemodynamic parameters. Because inhalation injury causes destruction of mucosal barriers that results in tissue damage and increases in pulmonary vascular permeability, increased fluid requirements can cause worsening of pulmonary edema. Studies have shown that combined burn and inhalation injuries have increased fluid requirements compared with burn injuries alone.[70] Patients presenting with concomitant burn and inhalation injuries with an initial $PaO_2:FIO_2$ ratio less than 350 have a statistically significant increase in fluid requirements to maintain organ perfusion in comparison with those with $PaO_2:FIO_2$ above 350. Interestingly, the degree of inhalation injury as assessed bronchoscopically did *not* correlate in an incremental manner with the degree of required fluid administration.[71]

LONG-TERM SEQUELAE

Inhalation injury produces changes in pulmonary architecture that have complex long-term consequences. Long-term studies of survivors of inhalation injury may have symptoms similar to asthma: cough, dyspnea, and symptoms of obstruction. The extent of obstruction is related to the extent of inhalation injury and the amount of smoke inhaled. Residual inhaled toxins and irritants are thought to underlie continued long-term bronchial obstruction.

Studies have shown persistence of inflammation in both bronchial lavage fluid and serum after inhalation injury. Increased levels of cytokines and lymphocytic inflammation continue to persist up to 6 months after the initial injury. In addition, carbonaceous material has been found in alveolar macrophages months after smoke inhalation and may provide the irritants necessary to create increased levels of inflammatory mediators and bronchial hyper-responsiveness.[72,73]

Long-term structural abnormalities from inhalation injury affect about 10% of patients. These include tracheal stenosis, found only in patients who required intubation or tracheostomy. Bronchiectasis and bronchiolitis obliterans are both rare occurrences that lead to pulmonary dysfunction and symptoms of obstruction. Bronchiolitis obliterans has been found after inhalation with toxic chemicals such as chlorine, phosgene, and ammonia and is thought to occur from residual toxins remaining in the lungs.[74]

Treatment

MEDICAL MANAGEMENT

Burn injury with inhalation injury initially necessitates stabilization and resuscitation of the patient. The cornerstones of management include adequate fluid resuscitation, maintenance of airway patency, effective mechanical ventilation when required, and vigilant surveillance for infectious complications. However, it is often noted that fluid needs may exceed calculated resuscitation in burn injury complicated by inhalation injury by over 50%.

PULMONARY TOILET

Endoscopic intervention has several roles in the evaluation and treatment of inhalation injury. In the initial injury period, airway edema and mucosal sloughing can present in the first 12 to 24 hours. Laryngoscopy and bronchoscopy are used in this period to evaluate the extent of injury to tracheobronchial mucosa and provide predictive indicators for airway patency and collapse. During the course of treatment, bronchoscopy is used for removal of debris and airway casts as well as for surveillance of infectious events.[75] Pulmonary toilet, such as frequent endotracheal suctioning and chest physiotherapy, are useful adjuncts in preventing pneumonia during treatment of inhalation injury.[76]

ANTIBIOTICS

Inhalation injury, especially with concomitant burn injury, predisposes the patient to nosocomial infections by opportunistic organisms. In an effort to reduce the rate of these infections, prophylactic antibiotic coverage has been studied and has been shown to be of no benefit. It may in fact lead to increased antimicrobial resistance by these organisms. Currently, broad-spectrum antibiotics are used when infections or sepsis is suspected; they are not initiated prophylactically.[42] Once an infectious agent is identified by culture or Gram stain, antibiotic therapy is appropriately directed at that source.[77]

STEROID THERAPY

In burn injury complicated by inhalation injury, systemic corticosteroid therapy is detrimental except for the treatment of severe bronchospasm. However, with isolated inhalation injury, corticosteroid therapy may be useful.[12] The use of corticosteroids early in the course of lung injury has shown confounding results and often results in deleterious outcomes. These studies have demonstrated no improvement in mortality rates compared with control groups, and in some cases, corticosteroid treatment leads to worse outcomes and complications.[78,79] One meta-analysis of corticosteroid therapy for lung injury has shown that use of systemic corticosteroids should be considered only in patients with persistent ARDS who have no septic or infectious complications.[80]

NEBULIZED SOLUTIONS

The use of nebulized albuterol, a β_2-agonist and bronchodilator, has been described as a potential therapy for acute inhalational lung injury.[81] In addition, nebulized unfractionated heparin has also been proposed to be of therapeutic benefit in patients with inhalation injury, owing to its effects on preventing airway cast formation. In one retrospective study, addition of nebulized heparin and N-acetylcysteine to nebulized albuterol showed a statistically significant improvement in lung injury scores, less hypoxia, improved lung compliance, and better overall survival when compared to nebulized albuterol alone.[82]

VENTILATOR MANAGEMENT

The hallmark of ventilator management during the treatment of inhalation injury is to minimize further damage and inflammation to lung tissue and provide adequate ventilation and oxygenation.[83] This management strategy has led to several schemes of mechanical ventilation aimed at reduced barotrauma and improved pulmonary gas exchange.[56]

Positive End-Expiratory Pressure

During inhalation injury, injury to the lung increases capillary permeability and results in influx of inflammatory mediators and edema. This causes an increase in the hydrostatic pressure across the alveolar regions of the lung, resulting in collapse. This, coupled with changes in surfactant due to lung injury, results in increased opening alveolar pressures and extensive atelectasis. Studies have shown that increasing positive end-expiratory pressure (PEEP) above that of hydrostatic pressures can prevent collapse of pulmonary subsegments.[84] However, because hydrostatic pressures are not evenly distributed, and atelectasis tends to occur in dependent lung regions, increasing PEEP to overcome the collapse in these regions could lead to overdistention of other regions, resulting in barotrauma.[85]

Inverse-Ratio Ventilation

With severe lung injury, mechanical ventilation leads to increase in shear forces and changes in pulmonary blood flow. This, coupled with reduction in elasticity (which results in decreased lung compliance), leads to further injury to the lung and ventilation/perfusion mismatches.[86,87] One way of counteracting the mechanical ventilation-induced damage to lung parenchyma and reducing shearing forces is to change the inspiratory-to-expiratory ratio.[88] By reversing the ratio from increased expiratory time to an increased inspiratory time, the peak inspiratory pressure of the lung is reduced and oxygenation is improved.[89] This is possibly a result of the prolonged inspiratory phase of ventilation that dissipates the shearing forces on the lung, increases distal alveolar pressure as well as delivered tidal volume, and results in less damage from mechanical ventilation. In addition, shortened expiratory time increases intrinsic PEEP, preventing alveolar collapse and increasing lung reruitment.[90] Despite the theoretical advantages of inverse-ratio ventilation, studies have yet to show an advantage for this approach over conventional ventilation.[91]

High-Frequency Ventilation

The high-frequency mode of ventilation uses rapid respiratory rates and small tidal volumes to achieve adequate oxygenation and ventilation while minimizing barotrauma.[92] There are three major types: high-frequency positive-pressure ventilation (HFPPV), high-frequency jet ventilation (HFJV), and high-frequency oscillation (HFOV). HFPPV and HFJV are the oldest forms of high-frequency ventilation and incorporate passive expiration dependent on chest wall elastic recoil. HFPPV delivers small tidal volumes (4 mL/kg) at high flow rates (250 L/min) and frequency (100 breaths/min). Because expiration with this mode is passive, there is an increased risk of air trapping and overdistention. HFJV also delivers small tidal volumes and high respiratory rates. The volume is determined by jet velocity and duration of flow. Like HFPPV, tidal volumes are difficult to measure and manipulate with HFJV and thus ventilation is adjusted empirically.[93] Also like HFPPV, expiration is passive and can result in air trapping. HFOV maintains open lung volumes by applying a constant airway pressure but does not allow for patient-triggered inspiratory flow. Thus, inspiration and expiration are active processes, and air trapping is reduced. Oxygenation is maintained by increasing the mean airway pressure until an adequate oxygen level is reached. Ventilation is achieved by oscillating the airway pressure through electromagnetically driven pistons that deliver cyclic tidal volumes and facilitate ventilation. The oscillatory frequency determines the piston displacement, and thus reduced frequency increases tidal volume delivery and improves ventilation.[94] The therapeutic advantage of HFOV is due to the maintenance of mean airway pressure that reduces the opening and closing of alveolar spaces at low lung volumes and thus reduces trauma due to shearing forces created by the decreased compliance. In addition, reduced tidal volumes and high frequency of ventilation result in increased end-expiratory volumes, increasing recruitment of atelectatic segments and reducing lung injury due to overdistention and shear forces.

Many recent studies investigating the usefulness of high-frequency ventilation have focused on HFOV because of this mode's theoretical protective advantage.[95] Several trials of HFOV in patients with acute lung injury and ARDS have shown improvements in oxygenation and ventilation. However, sample sizes for these studies have not been large enough to show a significant survival benefit.[96,97] In addition, more information is needed to refine algorithms for the use of HFOV.

Airway Pressure–Release Ventilation

Airway pressure–release ventilation (APRV) utilizes continuous positive airway pressure administered at a high level, with intermittent time-cycle releases of airway pressure. Since the diaphragm is relaxed in conventional forms of mechanical ventilation, gas preferentially distributes to the anterior nondependent regions of the lung. During spontaneous breathing, the posterior portions of the diaphragm move more than the anterior regions, so the dependent lung regions are better ventilated. The physiologic rationale behind APRV is that by more closely mimicking the gas distribution pattern of spontaneous breathing, the dependent lung regions are better ventilated by decreasing any ventilation/perfusion (V/Q) mismatch. APRV has been successfully employed in the setting of postinhalation injury ARDS, during which V/Q mismatch often occurs.[98-100]

EXTRACORPOREAL MEMBRANE OXYGENATION

Extracorporeal membrane oxygenation (ECMO) is used in situations in which mechanical ventilation fails to provide adequate oxygenation or elimination of carbon dioxide. Use of ECMO has shown variable results, but a few small studies have shown some improvement of survival.[101] However, large trials on the use of ECMO are lacking.[102,103] As ECMO technology improves, this alternative to mechanical ventilation in patients in pulmonary failure who do not respond to conventional interventions may become more widespread.

NONINVASIVE VENTILATION

Along the spectrum of pulmonary support for the burned patient lies noninvasive ventilation (NIV), which is positive-pressure ventilation of a spontaneously breathing patient without the use of an endotracheal tube. This is primarily accomplished via a face mask (or helmet) attached to a standard ventilator. NIV should be considered as an adjunct in the pulmonary support of awake, cooperative, spontaneously breathing patients, in an effort to avoid endotracheal intubation. Contraindications to its use include hemodynamic instability, presence of gross facial injuries, compromised cough/secretion clearance, and uncooperative patients.

The rationale for utilizing NIV is to avoid the complications associated with endotracheal intubation, including ventilator-associated pneumonia, trauma secondary to insertion, mucosal ulceration, aspiration, and impaired swallowing mechanisms. NIV may also be a way to improve patient comfort. Physiologically, NIV improves hypoxemic or hypercapnic respiratory failure by maintaining functional residual capacity (FRC) and vital capacity (VC). NIV in adult and pediatric case series has been shown to successfully avoid intubation[104] and is associated with a lower incidence of nosocomial infection, less antibiotic use,

reduced length of stay in intensive care units, and reduced mortality.[105]

The primary complication of NIV is prolonged pressure from the mask leading to focal skin necrosis; facial soft-tissue ulcers occur in 7% to 10% of patients receiving full-mask NIV.[106] Another complication is gastric distention in 1% to 2% of patients, with potential complications of emesis, aspiration, and pneumonia. However, studies designed to look at avoidance of gastric distention while using NIV have not shown any benefit in decreasing pneumonia rates by prophylactic nasogastric tube insertion.[107]

▣ Future Directions

Burn and inhalation injuries pose difficult challenges for clinicians. In particular, interventions such as mechanical ventilation aimed at treating pulmonary failure from lung injury often cause further injury. Future avenues of investigation should include a larger assessment of different ventilation modes (inverse-ratio ventilation, high-frequency ventilation) that reduce the damage inflicted on the lungs by mechanical ventilation. In addition, therapeutic interventions (surfactant replacement, antithrombolytic therapy) designed to attenuate the inflammatory response, which is responsible for much of the damage, also need further investigation.

KEY POINTS

1. Careful and focused history and physical examination, including the extent of exposure and the nature of inhaled substances, aid in the diagnosis and treatment of inhalation injury.

2. The nature of the inhaled substance, including physical properties and heat-carrying capacity, can give an indication of the level and extent of damage to the tracheobronchial tree.

3. Pathologic changes of inhalation injury include upper airway edema necessitating mechanical ventilation, and damage to the epithelial lining of the tracheobronchial tree resulting in increased generation of inflammatory mediators and further damage. Mortality from burn injury with inhalation injury is greater than either alone.

4. Pulmonary complications from inhalation injury are related to direct damage from thermal energy and toxins, infection from opportunistic organisms, damage caused by inflammatory mediators released by alveolar macrophages and neutrophils, reduction in surfactant production, and mucociliary dysfunctions.

5. Long-term complications from inhalation injury include persistence of symptoms such as cough, dyspnea, and symptoms of obstruction. Structural changes may include tracheal stenosis, bronchiectasis, and bronchiolitis obliterans.

6. Initial medical management includes adequate fluid resuscitation, maintenance of airway patency, and when needed, effective mechanical ventilation. Regular pulmonary toilet and appropriate antibiotic therapy are important after the initial injury period.

7. Mechanical ventilation during inhalation injury involves both providing adequate oxygenation and ventilation and minimizing further damage to lung tissue. The use of high-frequency ventilation and airway pressure–release ventilation may provide some benefit in patients with acute lung injury. Increasing use of noninvasive ventilation has led to fewer complications from endotracheal intubation.

ANNOTATED REFERENCES

Dries DJ. Key questions in ventilator management of the burn-injured patient (first of two parts). J Burn Care Res 2009;30(1):128-38.

Dries DJ. Key questions in ventilator management of the burn-injured patient (second of two parts). J Burn Care Res 2009;30(2):211-20.
Outlines the various ventilatory management strategies employed in the care of patients with inhalation injury.

Hollingsed TC, Saffle JR, Barton RG, Craft WB, Morris SE. Etiology and consequence of respiratory failure in thermally injured patients. Am J Surg 1993;166(6):592-6; discussion 596-597.

Provides information on pathologic consequences of inhalation injury and also gives information on the possible causes of respiratory failure.

Monafo WW. Initial management of burns. N Engl J Med 1996;335(21):1581-6.
Describes the initial evaluation and management of burn patients, as well as important clinical signs and symptoms.

Pruit Jr BA, Cioffi WG, Shimazu T, Ikeuchi H, Mason Jr AD. Evaluation and management of patients with inhalation injury. J Trauma 1990;30(12 Suppl):S63-8.

Outlines evaluation and initial management issues of patients with severe inhalation injuries and also provides valuable criteria for triage of inhalation injury.

Soejima K, Schmalstieg FC, Sakurai H, Traber LD, Traber DL. Pathophysiological analysis of combined burn and smoke inhalation injuries in sheep. Am J Physiol Lung Cell Mol Physiol 2001;280(6):L1233-41.

In a sheep model, provides information on the early physiologic and cellular dysfunctions that occur with inhalation injury.

Tasaki O, Goodwin CW, Saitoh D, et al. Effects of burns on inhalation injury. J Trauma 1997;43(4):603-7.

Evaluates the effect of burn injury on the pathology of inhalation injury as well as correlates outcomes of combined burn and inhalation injuries.

REFERENCES

Access the complete reference list online at http://www.expertconsult.com.

Drowning

DAVID SZPILMAN | JAMES P. ORLOWSKI | JOOST BIERENS

Drowning is usually related to a leisure situation that turned into a dramatic, life-threatening event. Parents, friends, relatives, babysitters, or guardians may feel not only profound loss and grief but also either guilt for failure to fulfill protection responsibilities or intense anger at others who did not provide adequate supervision or medical care. Nevertheless, drowning is a neglected public health problem.[1] Each year, drowning is responsible for an estimated 500,000 deaths around the world. The exact number is unknown because many deaths go unreported.[2]

Age, gender, alcohol use, socioeconomic status (as measured by income and/or education), and lack of supervision are key risk factors for drowning. Considering all ages, males die five times more often from drowning than females. An estimated 40% to 45% of deaths occur during swimming.[3] Young children, teenagers, and older adults are at highest risk of drowning.[4] In the age group of 5 to 14 years, drowning is the leading cause of death worldwide among males and the fifth leading cause of death for females.[4] The patterns of drowning are highly dependent on geographic factors. In the United States, drowning is the third most common cause of unintentional injury death for all ages and ranks second for people aged 5 to 44 years.[5] Considering all deaths by drowning in United States (3443 in 2007), 53% occurred in swimming pools.[3]

Drowning is the second leading cause of death for children aged 1 to 14 years and third cause of injury death for all ages in Brazil. With a population of 190 million inhabitants in 2007, a total of 7009 deaths by drowning in 2007 (3.7 per 100,000 inhabitants) were reported.[6] Ironically, 90% of all drowning deaths occur within 10 m of safety.[2] On Rio de Janeiro beaches, precipitant causes are discernable in 13% of all cases, with the most frequent being alcohol (37%), seizures (18%), trauma (including boating accidents; 16.3%), cardiopulmonary diseases (14.1%), snorkeling and SCUBA diving (3.7%), diving resulting in head or spinal cord injuries, and others (e.g., homicide, suicide, syncope, cramps, immersion syndrome (11.6%). It is important to recognize a precipitant cause to drowning, as this may guide specific approaches to rescue and resuscitation. In Brazil, freshwater drowning occurs more commonly in rivers and lakes, contributing to half of deaths by drowning.[7]

As a demonstration of geographic and cultural differences, in the Netherlands, there are more deaths by drowning that are secondary to suicide than occur from accidents, a situation markedly different from that found in the United States and Brazil. In the Netherlands, children are most at risk, but less than 6% of all drownings occur at beaches. Each year in the Netherlands, some 300 persons die from drowning, and 450 persons are admitted to hospitals. The average hospital stay is 11 days; 33% are dismissed within 48 hours, and 10% die.

A New Definition

Sound epidemiologic data on drowning are lacking. Data collection for such purposes has been hampered by the absence of a uniform and internationally accepted definition. A lack of consensus is present with respect to definitions and terminology used by different water safety and health organizations, experts in the field, papers in the scientific medical literature, and laypersons.[8] Within the framework of the first World Congress on Drowning (WCOD), a definition was developed to provide a common basis for future epidemiologic studies in all parts of the world. The following definition was adopted in June 2002:

"Drowning is the process of experiencing respiratory impairment from submersion or immersion in liquid."

The drowning process is a continuum beginning when the patient's airway is below the surface of the liquid, usually water, which—if this process continues—may or may not lead to death. A patient can be rescued at any time during the process and be given appropriate resuscitative measures, in which case the process is interrupted. Furthermore, any submersion or immersion incident without evidence of liquid aspiration should be considered a water rescue (i.e., events where no respiratory impairment is evident, whether with or without other injury or hypothermia). The term *near-drowning* was abandoned. Confusing terms like *dry drowning* and *secondary drowning* (delayed onset of respiratory distress) are now eliminated.[9]

Pathophysiology

Despite pathophysiologic differences between drowning in fresh or salt water in experimental models, from a clinical and therapeutic view, there are no important differences in humans. The most significant pathophysiologic alteration in drowning relates to hypoxia.[10] When there is no way to keep the airways out of water, breath holding is the first automatic response when there is no hypoxia and consciousness is still preserved. Water in the mouth is spit out or swallowed actively. When the first involuntary aspiration of water occurs, it produces coughing or rarely laryngospasm (less than 2%), leading to hypoxia. If laryngospasm occurs, hypoxia will lead to its rapid termination. More water is gradually aspirated into the lungs, leading to further hypoxia, loss of consciousness, irreversible apnea, and then asystole.

The respiratory disturbances depend less on the composition of the water and more on the amount of water aspirated. The aspiration of either fresh or salt water produces surfactant destruction, alveolitis, and a noncardiogenic pulmonary edema resulting in increased intrapulmonary shunt and hypoxia.[11] In animal research, the aspiration of 2.2 mL of water per kilogram of body weight decreases the arterial oxygen pressure (Pao_2) to approximately 60 mm Hg within 3 minutes.[12] In humans, it seems that as little as 1 to 3 mL/kg of water aspiration produces profound alterations in pulmonary gas exchange and decreases pulmonary compliance by 10% to 40%.[11] Humans rarely aspirate sufficient amounts of water to provoke significant electrolyte disturbances, and victims need no initial electrolyte correction.[13]

Ventricular fibrillation in humans, when it occurs, is related to hypoxia and acidosis, not to hemolysis and hyperkalemia. Hypoxia produces a well-established sequence of cardiac deterioration, with tachycardia, then bradycardia, then a pulseless phase of ineffective cardiac contractions (PEA phase) followed by complete loss of cardiac rhythm and electrical activity (asystole). Decreased cardiac output, arterial hypotension, increased pulmonary arterial pressure, and pulmonary vascular resistance are the results of hypoxia.[11] Intense peripheral vasoconstriction can also be caused by hypoxia, catecholamine release, and hypothermia.

A drowning victim can be rescued at any time during the process and may not require any intervention at all or may receive appropriate resuscitative measures, in which case the drowning process is interrupted. The victim may recover from the initial resuscitation efforts with or without subsequent therapy aimed at eliminating hypoxia, hypercarbia, and acidosis. In drowning, apnea is one of the first events, and if the victim is not ventilated soon enough, circulatory arrest will

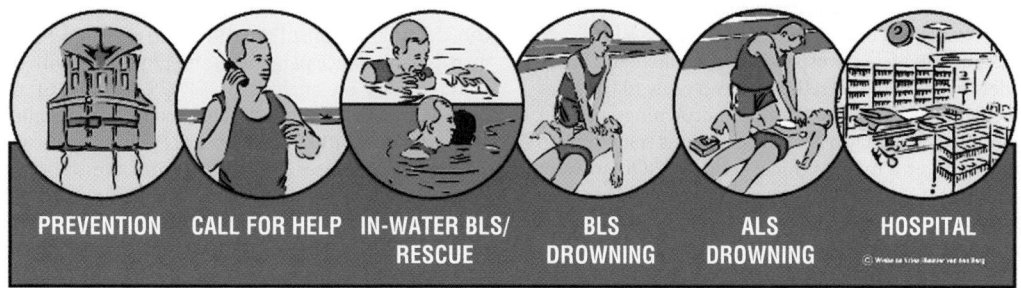

Figure 71-1 Drowning chain of survival. *(Adapted from Szpilman D, Morizot-Leite L, Vries W, et al. First aid courses for the aquatic environment. In: Bierens J, ed. Handbook on Drowning: Prevention, Rescue, and Treatment. Berlin: Springer-Verlag, 2006:342-7.)*

ensue and, in the absence of effective resuscitative efforts, death will result. It should be noted that the heart and brain are the two organs at greatest risk for permanent damage from relatively brief periods of hypoxia. The development of posthypoxic encephalopathy with or without cerebral edema is the most common cause of death and morbidity in hospitalized drowning victims.

Chain of Survival, Prevention to Hospital

In 2007, the United States Lifesaving Association reported 74,463 rescues on the shores of U.S. beaches, with estimates of 683 cases of rescues for each reported death (www.usla.org/Statistics/public.asp). On Rio de Janeiro beaches, approximately 290 rescues for each reported death (0.34%) occurred, and there was one death for each 10 victims admitted for medical care in the Drowning Resuscitation Center (DRC). In the past 31 years of work, the Rescue Service of Rio de Janeiro made approximately 166,000 rescues by lifeguards on the beaches, and 8500 victims needed medical attention in the DRC.[14] For drowning, rescue is an essential component to keep the patient alive, and the initial evaluation is made in a hostile environment (water). Therefore, it is essential for physicians to be aware of the drowning chain of survival,[15] from prehospital care to hospital admission (Figure 71-1).[15]

PREVENTION

Despite the emphasis on immediate treatment, the definitive therapy for drowning is prevention (Table 71-1). Prevention remains the most powerful therapeutic intervention and can be effective in more than 85% of drownings.

RECOGNITION OF THE INCIDENT

Initiation of help to a drowning victim must be preceded by a recognition that someone is drowning. Contrary to popular opinion, the victim (especially males) does not wave or call for help.[16] The victim is typically in an upright posture, with arms extended laterally, thrashing and slapping the water. Individuals close by may not recognize that the victim is struggling and may assume that the victim is playing and splashing in the water. The victim may submerge and resurface several times during this phase. Children can struggle for only 10 to 20 seconds before final submersion, and adults may be able to struggle for up to 60 seconds.[16] Because breathing instinctively takes precedence, the drowning victim is usually unable to cry for help.

IN-WATER BASIC LIFE SUPPORT AND RESCUE

For nonlifeguards, an attempt to help without becoming a second victim is the priority. If possible, potential rescuers can use techniques like "throw before you go and reach (with long objects) before you assist" or can advise the victim on how to get out of this situation (e.g., choosing a better way to escape, swim, float, reassuring the victim that assistance is coming). The decision when to do basic water life support

(BWLS)[15] is based on the victim's consciousness level. If conscious, rescue to land without any further medical care is the protocol.[17] The panicked and struggling victim can be dangerous to a would-be rescuer. A victim attempting to cling to life and breathe can drown a potential rescuer. For this reason, it is always best to approach a struggling victim with an intermediary object. Lifeguards use rescue or torpedo buoys for this purpose that also can double as a thorax and face flotation device to keep the head out of the water and the airways free.[16]

For an unconscious victim, the most important step is the immediate institution of resuscitative measures. Hypoxia caused by submersion results first in cessation of breathing, leading to cardiac arrest within a variable but short time interval if not corrected. In-water resuscitation (ventilation only) provides the victim a 3.15 times better chance of survival without sequelae. Rescuers should check ventilation and, whenever possible and if indicated, attempt to provide mouth-to-mouth resuscitation while still in the water. Unfortunately, external cardiac compressions cannot be performed effectively in the water, so assessment for pulse and compression must be delayed until the victim

TABLE 71-1	Preventive Measures

Watch children carefully; 84% of drownings occur because of inadequate adult supervision. Begin swimming lessons from 2 years of age.
Avoid inflatable swimming aids such as "floaties." They can give a false sense of security. Use lifejackets!
Never try to help rescue someone without being able to do so.
Avoid drinking alcohol before swimming.
Don't dive in shallow water—cervical spine injury could happen.

Beaches	*Pools and Similar*
Always swim in a lifeguard-supervised area.	Over 65% of deaths occur in fresh water, even on the coast.
Ask the lifeguard for safe places to swim or play.	Fence off your pool and include a gate. Appropriate fencing can decrease drowning by 50% to 70%.
Read and follow warning signs posted on the beach.	Avoid toys around the pool which are very attractive to children.
Do not overestimate your swimming capability—46.6% of drowning victims thought they knew how to swim.	Whenever infants or toddlers are in or around water, be within arm's length, providing "touch supervision."
Swim away from piers, rocks, and stakes.	Turn off motor filters when using the pool.
Take lost children to the nearest lifeguard tower.	Always use portable phones in pool areas so you are not called away to answer.
Over 80% of drowning occurs in rip currents (the rip is usually the most falsely calm place between two sand bars). If caught in a rip, swim transversally to the sand bar, or let it take you away without fighting and wave for help.	Use a pool sign to warn of shallow water.
If you are fishing on rocks, be cautious about waves that may sweep you into the ocean.	Learn CPR. Over 42% of pool owners are untrained in first aid techniques.
Keep away from marine animals.	Be careful!

is out of the water.[17] Very few studies have examined how often in-water cervical spine injury (CSI) occurs. In one study concerning sand beaches, 46,060 water rescues were retrospectively evaluated; this study found that the incidence of CSI in this setting was very low (0.009%).[18] In another retrospective survey of more than 2400 drownings, only 11 (<0.5%) had CSI, and all of these had a history of obvious trauma from diving, falling from height, or a motor vehicle accident.[19] Other water locations may have different rates of CSI depending on a wide variety of elements. Furthermore, any time spent on immobilizing the cervical spine in unconscious victims with no signs of trauma could lead to cardiopulmonary deterioration and even death.

Considering the low incidence of CSI and the high risk of wasted time in ventilation when needed, routine cervical spine immobilization of water rescues without reference to whether a traumatic injury was sustained is not recommended.[18,19] Rescuers who suspect a spinal cord injury should float the victim supine in a horizontal position, allowing the airways to be out of the water, and check to see if there is spontaneous breathing. If the victim is not breathing, protocols should be started for in-water resuscitation (mouth-to-mouth) while maintaining the head in a neutral position as much as possible. The rescuer should then use a jaw thrust without head tilt or chin lift to open the airway, without risking him- or herself or the victim. If there is spontaneous breathing, the rescuer's hands should be used to stabilize the victim's neck in a neutral position. If possible, a back-support device should be applied before moving the individual from the water. The victim should be rescued to a dry place, maintaining the neck in a neutral position as much as possible. The head, neck, chest, and body should be kept in alignment if the victim must be moved or turned.[10]

ON-LAND BASIC DROWNING LIFE SUPPORT

Removal of the victim from the water should be performed according to their level of consciousness, but preferably a vertical position should be adopted to avoid vomiting and further complications to the airways.[20] If the victim is exhausted, confused, or unconscious, transport should be in as near a horizontal position as possible but with the head still maintained above body level[20] (keep horizontal if prolonged immersion or a history of immersion in cold water). The airways must be kept open at all times. The first procedure in on-land basic drowning life support (BDLS) should be placing the victim in a position parallel to the waterline,[20] as horizontal as possible, lying supine, far enough away from the water to avoid incoming waves. If conscious, reposition the victim supine with head up. If breathing, place in recovery position (lateral decubitus position).[20] In a 10-year study in Australia, vomiting occurred in more than 65% of victims who needed rescue breathing and in 86% of those who required both rescue breathing and chest compressions.[21] Even in victims who required no interventions after water rescue, vomiting occurred in 50% once they reached shore. The presence of vomitus in the airway can result in further aspiration and impairment of oxygenation by airway obstruction; it can also discourage rescuers from attempting mouth-to-mouth resuscitation.[21] The abdominal thrust (Heimlich) maneuver should never be used as a means of expelling water from the lungs; it is ineffective and carries significant risks. During resuscitation, attempts at active drainage by placing the victim head down increases the risk of vomiting more than fivefold and leads to a small but significant increase in mortality (19%) when compared with keeping the victim in a horizontal position.[20] If vomiting occurs, turn the victim's mouth to the side, and remove the vomitus with a finger sweep, a cloth, or use of suction.

One of the most difficult medical decisions a lifeguard or an emergency medical technician (EMT) must make is how to treat a drowning victim appropriately. A cardiopulmonary or an isolated respiratory arrest occurs in approximately 0.5% of all rescues. The questions that arise are should the rescuer administer oxygen, call an ambulance, transport the person to a hospital, or observe for a time at the site? Even emergency physicians may be in doubt as to the most appropriate immediate support measures; drowning victims vary in the severity of injury. Based on these needs, a classification system was developed in Rio de Janeiro (Brazil) in 1972 and updated in 1997[22] to assist lifeguards, ambulance personnel, and physicians with treatment priorities. It was based on analysis of 41,279 rescues, of which 2304 (5.5%) needed medical attention. The system was revalidated in 2001 by a 10-year study with 46,080 rescues.[23] This classification (see Algorithm 71-1)[22] encompasses all support from the site of the accident to the hospital, recommends treatment, and shows the likelihood of death based on the severity of injury. Severity is easily assessed by an on-scene rescuer, EMT or physician using only clinical variables.[22]

ADVANCED DROWNING LIFE SUPPORT ON SITE

Advanced drowning life support (ADLS) on site is outlined in Algorithm 71-1, available in the online version of this chapter. To save precious time, medical equipment should be brought to the victim instead of the victim to the ambulance. Advanced medical treatment is given according to drowning classification.

Non-resuscitatable Condition

A victim with submersion time over 1 hour or with obvious physical evidence of death (rigor mortis, putrefaction, or dependent lividity will be in this category. Do *not* start resuscitation; follow to the morgue.

Grade 6: Cardiopulmonary Arrest

Resuscitation started by layperson or lifeguard at the scene must be continued by advanced life support (ALS) personnel until successful, or if there is no way to warm the victim appropriately at the scene. In this case, the victim should be transported while receiving resuscitation to a hospital where advanced warming measures can be accomplished. The first priority is adequate oxygenation and ventilation. The medical staff must keep doing cardiac compression while starting artificial ventilation using bag and facemask with 15 liters of oxygen until an orotracheal tube can be inserted. Once intubated, victims can be oxygenated and ventilated effectively even through copious pulmonary edema fluid. The Sellick maneuver should be used if possible during intubation to prevent regurgitation and aspiration. Aspirate the orotracheal tube only when fluid interferes with effective ventilation. Semiautomatic external defibrillation may have a role in cardiac rhythm monitoring. If the drowning victim is pulseless and hypothermic (<34°C), CPR must be continued. Although ventricular fibrillation (VF) is uncommon, especially in pediatric victims, some adults may develop VF as a consequence of coronary artery disease or from ALS therapies such as epinephrine. Peripheral venous access is the preferred route for drugs. Although some drugs can be administered endotracheally despite copious noncardiogenic pulmonary edema fluid, whether the drugs are absorbed and what doses to use are unresolved issues.[16] The epinephrine dose for resuscitation is still a controversial issue in the setting of a drowning, where the time elapsed to start resuscitation can be much longer and outcome much different from other causes. Both beneficial and toxic physiologic effects of epinephrine administration during CPR have been shown in animal and human studies. Initial or escalating high-dose epinephrine has occasionally resulted in return of spontaneous circulation and improved early survival. Higher doses of epinephrine have not improved long-term survival and neurologic outcome when used as initial therapy, but higher doses have not definitively been shown to cause harm either. Therefore, high-dose epinephrine is not recommended for routine use but can be considered if 1-mg doses fail.[24] Our recommendation is to use a first dose of 0.01 mg/kg IV after 3 minutes of CPR[26] and if no response is achieved, increase to 0.1 mg/kg each 3 minutes of CPR.[10]

Grade 5: Respiratory Arrest

Respiratory arrest is usually reversed when ADLS arrives at the scene. Oxygenation and ventilation protocols, as for grade 6, should be followed until spontaneous breathing is restored, then protocols for grade 4 followed.

Grade 4: Acute Pulmonary Edema With Hypotension

Oxygen with mechanical ventilatory support is the first-line therapy. Initially, oxygen should be administered by facemask at 15 L/min until an orotracheal tube can be inserted. Grade 4 needs early intubation in all cases, which is an optimal provision of positive airway pressure. Mechanical ventilation is indicated for SaO_2 of less than 90% with the use of 15 liters of oxygen by facemask, a $PaCO_2$ of more than 45 mm Hg, an abnormally high respiratory rate, or excessive patient effort to maintain adequate arterial blood gases (ABG), such that the patient is consuming large amounts of energy breathing and is likely to tire.[16] Patients should be sedated to tolerate intubation and artificial mechanical ventilation providing tidal volume of at least 5 mL/kg of body weight. FIO_2 can start at 1.0, but as soon as possible (usually less than 20 minutes) should be reduced to 0.45 or less to avoid oxygen toxicity. Positive end-expiratory pressure (PEEP) should be added initially at a level of 5 cm H_2O and then increased by 2 to 3 cm H_2O increments until the desired intrapulmonary shunt (QS:QT) of 20% or less, or PaO_2:FIO_2 of 250 or more is achieved. If low blood pressure is not corrected by oxygen, a rapid crystalloid infusion (independent of drowning water type) should be used before trying to reduce PEEP.[11,27]

Grade 3: Acute Pulmonary Edema Without Hypotension

Victims with SaO_2 > 90% with the use of 15 liters of oxygen by facemask can tolerate noninvasive ventilatory support in only 27.6% of cases and 72.4% of patients need intubation and mechanical ventilation, which follow the same protocols as grade 4.

Grade 2: Abnormal Auscultation with Rales in Some Pulmonary Fields

Victims only require oxygen by nasal cannula in 93.2% of cases or no oxygen assistance in fewer than 10% of cases.

Grade 1: Coughing with Normal Lung Auscultation

Victims do not need any oxygen or respiratory assistance.

Rescue: No Coughing or Difficulty Breathing, Normal Lung Auscultation

Evaluate and release from the accident site without further medical care.

HOSPITAL

Hospital admission in severe cases (grades 4 to 6) is only possible if adequate and prompt BDLS and ADLS prehospital care was accomplished. If this is not the case, the appropriate approach is to follow ADLS on-site protocols. Hospital care is recommended for grades 2 to 6. Decision making in the emergency department about admission to an intensive care unit (ICU) or hospital bed versus observation in an emergency department or discharge home should include a thorough history of the accident and previous illness, physical examination, and diagnostic studies including chest radiography and ABG measurement. Electrolytes, blood urea nitrogen, creatinine, and hemoglobin also should be assessed serially, although perturbations in these laboratory tests are unusual. In some cases, a toxicologic screen for suspected alcohol or drug ingestion might be warranted. Patients grade 3 to 6 should be admitted to an ICU for close observation and therapy. Patients grade 2 can be observed in the emergency room for 6 to 24 hours, but grade 1 and rescue cases with no complaints or associated illness or trauma should be released home. Table 71-2 shows general mortality rates for each grade of severity, hospitalization need, and prehospital and in-hospital mortality rates.

Patients grade 4 to 6 usually will arrive from prehospital ACLS care on mechanical ventilation with acceptable oxygenation. If not, the emergency department physician should follow grade 4 ventilation protocols. Grade 3 depends on clinical evaluation in the field. In any case, once the desired oxygenation is achieved at a given level of positive airway pressure, that level of PEEP should be maintained

TABLE 71-2	Classification, Mortality, and Hospital Needs (N = 1831*)			
Grade	No.	Overall Mortality (%)	Admission to Hospital (%)	Hospital Mortality (%)
Rescue	38,976	0 (0.0%)	0 (0.0%)	0 (0.0%)
1	1189	0 (0.0%)	35 (2.9%)	0 (0.0%)
2	338	2 (0.6%)	50 (14.8%)	2 (4.0%)
3	58	3 (5.2%)	26 (44.8%)	3 (11.5%)
4	36	7 (19.4%)	32 (88.9%)	7 (19.4%)
5	25	11 (44%)	21 (84%)§	7 (33.3%)
6	185	172 (93%)	23 (12.4%)§	10 (43.5%)
Total	1831†	195 (10.6%)	187 (10.2%)‡	29 (15.5%)
		P < 0.0001		

*Overall mortality was 10.6%.[22]
†The rescue cases were excluded.
‡Need of overall hospitalization (10.2%) in ND/D cases in association with the grade and mortality. Mortality in the hospital was 15.5%.
§Four patients grade 5 and 162 grade 6 out of this table were pronounced dead and taken directly to the morgue.[22]

unchanged for 48 hours before attempting to decrease it to permit adequate surfactant regeneration. During that time, if consciousness level allows the patient to breathe without fighting, continuous positive airway pressure (CPAP) plus ventilatory pressure support mode (PSV) can be a good choice. In selected cases, CPAP may be provided only by mask (e.g., in cooperative adolescents) or nasal cannula (in infants who are obligate nasal breathers), but usually this is tolerated by the patient. Pulmonary edema usually necessitates intubation. A clinical picture very similar to acute respiratory distress syndrome (ARDS) is common after significant drowning episodes (grade 3 to 6). Management is similar to that of other patients with ARDS, including efforts to minimize volutrauma and barotrauma. Lung-protective ventilation involving permissive hypercapnia probably is not suitable for drowning victims grade 6 with significant hypoxic-ischemic brain injury. Instead, a normocapnia is indicated together with other therapeutic measures to control cerebral edema.

Despite aggressive management, neurologic injury and sequelae, including persistent vegetative state, can occur in grade 6 drowning victims. In patients who are hemodynamically unstable or have severe pulmonary dysfunction (grade 4 to 6), pulmonary artery catheterization may provide useful information concerning Starling forces in the lungs and may help in managing pulmonary edema. Vasopressors should only be used in refractory hypovolemia when replacement with crystalloid was not enough to restore blood pressure. No evidence exists to support routine administration of hypertonic solutions and transfusions for fresh water drowning; similarly, there are no data to recommend use of hypotonic solutions in salt-water cases.[11,27] Echocardiography to assess cardiac function and ejection fractions can help to guide the clinician in titrating inotropic agents, vasopressors, or both if volume crystalloid replacement had failed. Some studies have shown that cardiac dysfunction with low cardiac output is common immediately after severe drowning cases (grades 4 to 6).[11] Important supportive measures include Foley catheter placement to monitor urine output. Low cardiac output is associated with high pulmonary capillary occlusion pressure, high central venous pressure, and high pulmonary vascular resistance and can persist for days after correction of oxygenation and perfusion abnormalities in drowning victims. Despite depressed cardiac output, furosemide therapy is not generally indicated. One study even has suggested that volume infusion benefits drowning victims. Studies suggest that dobutamine infusion to improve cardiac output is the most logical and potentially beneficial therapy in such cases.

Metabolic acidosis occurs in 70% of patients arriving at the hospital after a drowning episode.[13] It should be corrected when pH is lower than 7.2 or the bicarbonate is less than 12 mEq/L if the victim has adequate ventilatory support.[27] Significant depletion of bicarbonate is rarely present in the first 10 to 15 minutes of CPR, and its use is not indicated in the initial resuscitation period.[26]

Pools and beaches generally have insufficient bacteria to promote pneumonia in the immediate postdrowning period.[28] If the victim needs mechanical respiratory assistance, the incidence of secondary pneumonia increases from 34% to 52% in the third or fourth day of hospitalization when pulmonary edema is resolving.[29] Vigilance not only for pulmonary but also other infectious complications is important. Prophylactic antibiotics are of doubtful value in the intensive care management and tend to select out only more resistant and more aggressive organisms. An altered chest x-ray should not be interpreted as pneumonia, because it is usually the result of pulmonary edema and aspirated water in the alveoli and bronchi. It is preferable to monitor tracheal aspirates daily with Gram stain, culture, and sensitivity. At the first sign of pulmonary infection, usually after the first 48 to 72 hours (as gauged by prolonged fever, sustained leukocytosis, persistent or new pulmonary infiltrates, and leukocyte response in the tracheal aspirate), antibiotic therapy can be initiated on the basis of predominant organism and sensitivities. Fiberoptic bronchoscopy may be useful for evaluation of infection by obtaining quantitative cultures, determining the extent and severity of airway injury in cases of aspiration of solids, and for the rare occasions where therapeutic clearing of sand, gravel, and other solids is indicated. Corticosteroids for pulmonary injury are at best of doubtful value and should not be used except for bronchospasm.

The clinician must be aware of and constantly vigilant for potential complications associated with beta-adrenergic bronchodilators and underlying pulmonary injury in the drowning victim, especially volutrauma and barotrauma.[28] Spontaneous pneumothoraces are common (10%) secondary to positive-pressure ventilation and local areas of hyperinflation. Any sudden change in hemodynamic stability after mechanical ventilation should be considered to be due to pneumothorax or other barotrauma until proved otherwise. After a secure airway is established, nasogastric tube placement reduces gastric distention and prevents further aspiration. Rarely, drowning victims who seem healthy on assessment in the emergency department, including having normal chest radiography, develop fulminant pulmonary edema as long as 12 hours after the incident. Whether this late-onset pulmonary edema is delayed ARDS or neurogenic pulmonary edema secondary to hypoxia is unclear. Renal insufficiency or renal failure is rare in drowning victims but can occur secondary to anoxia, shock, or hemoglobinuria.

The most important complication after a drowning episode, beyond reversible pulmonary injury, is anoxic-ischemic cerebral insult. Most late deaths and long-term sequelae of drowning are neurologic in origin.[28] Although the highest priority in resuscitation after drowning is restoration of spontaneous circulation, every effort in the early stages after rescue should be directed at resuscitating the brain and preventing further neurologic damage. These steps include providing adequate oxygenation (Sat O_2 > 92% but not 100%) and cerebral perfusion (mean arterial pressure around 100 mm Hg). Any victim who remains comatose and unresponsive after successful CPR or deteriorates neurologically should undergo careful and frequent neurologic function assessment for the development of cerebral edema and should be treated with the following measures:

- Raise the head of the bed by 30 degrees (if there is no hypotension).
- Maintain adequate mechanical ventilation.
- Ensure appropriate respiratory toilet without provoking hypoxia.
- Treat for seizure activity.
- Avoid metabolic sudden corrections.
- Prevent interventions that increase intracranial pressure (ICP)—including urinary retention, pain, hypotension, or hypoxia—by using sedation or muscular relaxants as necessary.
- Frequently monitor blood glucose concentration, and maintain normoglycemic values.[7,27]

Continuous monitoring of core and/or brain (tympanic) temperature is mandatory in the emergency department and intensive care unit

(and in the prehospital setting if possible). Drowning victims with restoration of adequate spontaneous circulation who remain comatose should not be actively rewarmed to temperature values above 32°C to 34°C. If core temperature exceeds 34°C, hypothermia (32°C–34°C) should be achieved as soon as possible and sustained for 12 to 24 hours. Hyperthermia should be prevented at all times in the acute recovery period. Although there is insufficient evidence to support a specific target Paco₂ or oxygen saturation during and after resuscitation, hypoxemia should be avoided. Unfortunately, studies that have evaluated the results of cerebral resuscitation measures in drowning victims have failed to demonstrate that therapies directed at controlling intracranial hypertension and maintaining cerebral perfusion pressure (CPP) improve outcome. These studies have shown poor outcomes (i.e., death or moderate to profound neurologic sequelae) when the intracranial pressure was 20 mm Hg or more and the CPP was 60 mm Hg or less, even when therapies are directed at controlling and improving these pressures. More research is needed to evaluate specific efficacy of neuroresuscitative therapies in drowning victims.

New therapeutic interventions for drowning victims such as extracorporeal membrane oxygenation, artificial surfactant, nitric oxide, and liquid lung ventilation are still in the investigational stage.[30]

Outcome and Scoring Systems

Drowning victims with severities of grade 3 to 6 have the potential to develop multisystem organ failure.[16] Despite this, the prognosis for such patients is primarily based on neurologic outcome.[2] Drowning grade 1 to 5 patients return home safely without sequelae in 95% of cases.[22] Of major concern among researchers are grade 6 victims. Both at the rescue site and in the hospital, no one indicator for grade 6 appears to be absolutely reliable in terms of defining outcome.[31] Based on the longest submersion time registered in cold water (66 minutes) with complete recovery,[16] resuscitation should be started without delay in each victim without carotid palpable pulse who has been submerged for less than 1 hour or does not present obvious physical evidence of death (rigor mortis, putrefaction or dependent lividity).

Contrary to some research that affirms that prolonged submersion and successful resuscitation is only possible after exposure to cold or icy water, some anecdotal cases in warm water were described to survive without sequelae.[22,32,33] Multiple studies have established that outcome is almost solely determined by a single factor: duration of submersion (Table 71-3).[17,21,22,28,32-36] Basic and advanced life support enable victims to achieve their best outcome possible when the time of duration cardiopulmonary arrest (submersion time included) is minimized. Based on a report of a drowning victim successfully resuscitated after 2 hours of CPR,[28] efforts should stop only if asystole persists after rewarming the victim above 34°C.

Prognostic scoring systems have been developed to predict which patients will do well with standard therapy and which are likely to have a significant cerebral anoxic encephalopathy and will require aggressive measures to protect the brain. One of the best characterized prognostic factors is consciousness level related to the Glasgow Coma Scale at the period immediately after resuscitation (first hour; Conn & Modell Neurological Classification).[28,37] Because of the typical delay of 2 to 6

TABLE 71-3	Probability of Neurologically Intact Survival to Hospital Discharge*	
Duration of Submersion	**Death or Severe Neurologic Impairment**
0 to <5 minutes	10%
5 to <10 minutes	56%
10 to <25 minutes	88%
>25 minutes	100%

*Based on duration of submersion.[35] Note in these data how 5 more minutes of submersion in the 5 to <10-minute group increases mortality almost 6 times compared to the 0 to <5-minute group.

hours between rescue and transfer from an outlying emergency facility to a pediatric ICU, many patients with severe anoxic-ischemic cerebral insults and coma have had multiple determinations of neurologic status and level of consciousness before definitive therapy is begun. Data suggest that patients who remain profoundly comatose (i.e., decorticate, decerebrate, or flaccid) 2 to 6 hours after the drowning accident are brain dead or have moderate to severe neurologic impairment. Patients who are improving but remain unresponsive have a 50% likelihood of a good outcome. Most patients who are clearly improving and are alert, or are stuporous or obtunded but respond to stimuli 2 to 6 hours after the incident, have normal or near-normal neurologic outcomes. These prognostic variables are important in counseling family members of drowning victims in the early stages after the accident and in deciding which patients are likely to have a good outcome with standard supportive therapy and which victims should be candidates for more agressive attempt to cerebral resuscitation therapies[33,35] (Table 71-4).

TABLE 71-4	Clinical Prognostic Score for the Immediate Period Post Successful CPR*	
Neurologic Prognostic Score		
(Post Successful CPR on Drowning)		
A—First Hour	**B—After 5 to 8 Hours**	
Alert—10	Alert—9.5	
Confused—9	Confused—8	
Torpor—7	Torpor—6	
Coma with normal brainstem—5	Coma with normal brainstem—3	
Coma with abnormal brainstem—2	Coma with abnormal brainstem—1	
A + B		
Recovery Without Sequelae		
Excellent (≥13)	≥95%	
Very good (10-12)	75% to 85%	
Good (8)	40% to 60%	
Regular (5)	10% to 30%	
Poor (3)	≤5%	

*Based on Glasgow Coma Score.[22,28,36]

ANNOTATED REFERENCES

Szpilman D, Handley AJ, Bierens J, Quan L, Vasconcellos R. Drowning. In: Field JM, editor. The Textbook of Emergency Cardiovascular Care and CPR. Philadelphia: Lippincott Williams & Wilkins; 2009. p. 477-89. Co-sponsored by AHA & ACEP.
A very good review on drowning, with information on epidemiology, prevention, rescue, and treatment and special attention on the drowning chain of survival.

Field JM, editor. Drowning. In ACLS Resource Text for Instructors and Experienced Providers. Dallas: American Heart Association Inc.; 2008. p. 301-17.
Presents information on advanced cardiac life support and excellent flow charts to be followed as protocols.

Bierens J, editor. Handbook on Drowning: Prevention, Rescue and Treatment. Heidelberg, Germany: Springer-Verlag; 2006.
This is a unique book for those involved in aquatic incidents and more specifically, for those involved with drowning incidents. The most complete edition of drowning content, based on World Drowning Congress 2002—The Netherlands, contributed by world experts.

Orlowski JP, Szpilman D. Drowning. Rescue, resuscitation, and reanimation. Pediatr Clin North Am 2001;48(3):627-46.
A good review article highlighting issues such as prevention, physiopathology, basic life support for drowning, and treatment.

Szpilman D. Near-drowning and drowning classification: a proposal to stratify mortality based on the analysis of 1831 cases. Chest 1997;112(3):660-5.
This retrospective study reviewed 41,279 cases of water rescues to establish classifications for drowning according to severity, based on mortality rate of the subgroups.

Bierens JJ, van der Velde EA, van Berkel M, van Zanten JJ. Submersion in The Netherlands: prognostic indicators and results of resuscitation. Ann Emerg Med 1990;19(12):1390-5.
This retrospective study revealed important prognostic indicators, highlighting submersion time as the primary prognostic factor.

Cummins RO, Szpilman D. Submersion. In: Cummins RO, Field JM, Hazinski MF, editors. ACLS—The Reference Textbook. Vol 1. *ACLS for Experienced Providers.* Dallas: American Heart Association Inc.; 2003:97-107.
An excellent review article which highlights important issues such as in-water resuscitation, cervical trauma, and prognostic indicators in the prehospital setting.

REFERENCES

Access the complete reference list online at http://www.expertconsult.com.

72

Acute Parenchymal Disease in Pediatric Patients

KATHLEEN M. VENTRE | JOHN H. ARNOLD

Pulmonary parenchymal processes in children that the intensive care clinician may encounter include common and uncommon diseases of the lower airways, alveoli, and pulmonary interstitium. Among the more challenging conditions to manage in the intensive care unit (ICU) are those which include disease or dysfunction of all three of these components, such as bronchopulmonary dysplasia and congenital diaphragmatic hernia. This chapter will discuss the pathophysiology and management principles pertinent to each disease category, with emphasis given to common examples and conditions that are unique to the pediatric patient.

Diseases of the Airways

STATUS ASTHMATICUS

Although unusual anatomic conditions of the lower airways can occur in pediatric patients (Table 72-1), status asthmaticus and bronchiolitis are probably the most common causes of lower-airway disease encountered in the pediatric ICU. Asthma is common in the industrialized world, and the overall mortality rate attributable to asthma in the United States is estimated at 2.6 deaths per million children per year.[1] Recurrent hospitalizations, previous ICU admissions, and the need for mechanical ventilatory support have been identified as risk factors for death from asthma.[2] Status asthmaticus is characterized by acute, severe airway obstruction due to bronchoconstriction that is refractory to initial management with supplemental oxygen, inhaled bronchodilators, and corticosteroids. The pathophysiology of this condition begins with a precipitant that triggers contraction of hyperresponsive bronchial smooth muscle, mucus secretion, and mucosal edema, all of which lead to the obstruction of large and small airways (Figure 72-1). Hyperinflation from airflow limitation and premature closure of lower airways in expiration leads to increased end-expiratory lung volume[3] and an increased respiratory workload, which ultimately set the stage for alveolar hypoventilation and hypoxemia. An abrupt and profound acidosis can develop when respiratory compensation for accumulated inorganic acids ceases to occur.[3] On physical examination, the child with status asthmaticus can appear anxious or lethargic, will often demonstrate accessory muscle use, and depending on the quality of air entry, can demonstrate either cough with profound inspiratory and/or expiratory wheezing and prolongation of audible expiration, or a silent chest. An exaggerated pulsus paradoxus can often be demonstrated, a finding that reflects the profoundly negative intrapleural pressures generated by these patients during spontaneous respiration.

Therapy

Supportive therapy for status asthmaticus begins with maintaining the airway, monitoring the quality of respirations, and ensuring euvolemia. Standard medical therapies for these patients include bronchodilators and corticosteroids, and several adjunct therapies have been investigated as possible rescue agents in difficult cases (Table 72-2). Short-acting β-agonist agents, which mediate airway smooth muscle relaxation via local β₂ receptors,[3] are the most commonly used bronchodilators for status asthmaticus. Among these agents, albuterol is the most widely used. Unlike epinephrine and isoproterenol, albuterol is relatively β₂ selective,[3] and it is most commonly administered by nebulization. It is typically given at a dose of 0.15 mg/kg (up to 2.5 mg/dose) on a frequent intermittent basis, but only a small fraction of the nebulized dose may actually be delivered to the lung, particularly in critically ill infants and children who are intubated with small tracheal tubes.[4-6] Several studies have demonstrated that small doses of nebulized β-agonist given in rapid sequential fashion produce sustained improvements in forced expiratory volume more often than when larger doses are given less frequently,[7,8] and there is also evidence to suggest that continuous nebulization of the drug may actually lead to more rapid and sustained clinical improvement.[9]

In recent years, a preparation of the therapeutically active isomer of albuterol (levalbuterol) has become available. Levalbuterol appears to be effective when administered to children with stable asthma.[10] There are no controlled trials presently available to evaluate its use in children with acute exacerbations of the disease. Inhaled anticholinergic agents such as ipratropium also have a role in the management of severe bronchospasm in children with asthma. Addition of inhaled ipratropium to inhaled β-agonists has been associated with favorable changes in pulmonary function, especially in children with severe asthma.[11,12] For patients who do not respond to inhaled bronchodilators, it is possible to administer β-agonist therapy intravenously (IV). In some countries, the IV preparation of albuterol is available, which allows for an alternative administration route for this β₂-selective agent. In the United States where IV albuterol is not available, terbutaline, which has some β₂ selectivity, is a reasonable alternative. Although terbutaline has not been associated with clinically significant cardiac toxicity in most pediatric patients,[3,13] many clinicians advise monitoring the electrocardiogram (ECG) and serum troponin level during its administration.

For as long as the inflammatory basis for asthma has been recognized, corticosteroids have had an important role in the management of status asthmaticus. The use of corticosteroids has been demonstrated to significantly improve airways obstruction in patients with severe acute asthma.[14] The parenteral route is the method of choice for administering these agents to the critically ill child, and it is important to understand that fatal anaphylaxis to these drugs has been reported.[15,16] Methylprednisolone is one of the most commonly used agents for acute severe asthma. Because of its half-life, steady-state levels can be achieved relatively quickly, and although dosing regimens vary, it is probably most appropriate to dose the drug every 6 hours. There does not seem to be any advantage to administering massive doses of glucocorticoids in status asthmaticus.[17] If methylprednisolone is not available, equipotent doses of another glucocorticoid may be used.

Magnesium has been investigated for use in status asthmaticus because of its potential to augment the effects of bronchodilators by causing relaxation of airway smooth muscle. A recent randomized controlled trial in adults demonstrated that 2 g IV magnesium sulfate improves pulmonary function when administered as an adjunct to nebulized β-agonists and IV corticosteroids in patients with especially low forced expiratory volume in the first second of expiration (FEV₁) (<20% of predicted).[18] Although magnesium is occasionally added to standard therapy in pediatric status asthmaticus, the evidence supporting its use in this population is limited.[19]

Enthusiasm for the use of methylxanthines (theophylline, aminophylline) in pediatric asthma has fluctuated over time. These drugs act primarily as phosphodiesterase inhibitors, but the mechanism of their

TABLE 72-1	Anatomic Causes of Lower-Airway Dysfunction

Tracheomalacia, bronchomalacia:
   Vascular anomaly
   Tracheoesophageal fistula
   Idiopathic
Bronchiectasis
Congenital lobar emphysema
Cystic adenomatoid malformation
Pulmonary sequestration
Bronchogenic cyst

setting of acute respiratory illness. The primary cause of bronchiolitis is respiratory syncytial virus (RSV), which is responsible for 45% to 75% of cases, although parainfluenza viruses, rhinoviruses, adenoviruses, influenza viruses, enteroviruses, and *Mycoplasma pneumoniae* can produce the syndrome as well. RSV dependably produces yearly epidemics occurring during the winter and spring months. Infection with RSV is nearly universal among infants and children by 2 years of age. Although hospitalization rates vary seasonally and regionally, a recent study cited an average hospitalization rate between 3 per 1000 among children younger than 5 years of age, and 17 per 1000 among children younger than 6 months.[21] Among all hospitalized children, the percentage requiring intensive care has been reported as 7% to 9%

effects in asthma is not well understood. A recent randomized controlled trial investigated the effects of aminophylline in 163 children with status asthmaticus. Aminophylline was administered to these children as an adjunct to nebulized β-agonists, nebulized anticholinergics, and parenteral corticosteroids.[20] The results of this trial suggested that aminophylline improved pulmonary function and may have averted intubation in a portion of those patients who received it.[20] Although aminophylline may have a role in the treatment of severe status asthmaticus that is not responding to standard therapies, the potential for its widespread use is limited by its narrow therapeutic index.[3]

BRONCHIOLITIS

Bronchiolitis is a clinical term implying an invasion of the large and small airway respiratory epithelium by inflammatory cells in the

TABLE 72-2	Selected Pharmacotherapies for Status Asthmaticus
Nebulized Therapies	Albuterol (0.5%), 0.15 mg/kg/dose (0.03 mL/kg/dose) inhaled q 1-6 h as needed (PRN) Continuous inhalation 0.5 mg/kg/h Ipratropium, 0.25-0.5 mg inhaled q 4-6 h Racemic epinephrine (2.25%), 0.25-0.5 mL inhaled q 1 h PRN
Subcutaneous (SQ) Therapies	Epinephrine (1:1000), 0.01 mg/kg/dose (0.01 mL/kg/dose) SQ (max 0.5 mL/dose)
Intravenous (IV) Therapies	Terbutaline, 10 μg/kg IV × 1, followed by 0.4-6.0 μg/kg/min IV infusion Magnesium sulfate, 25-50 mg/kg IV over 20 minutes (max 2 g/dose) Methylprednisolone, 1 mg/kg/dose IV q 6 h

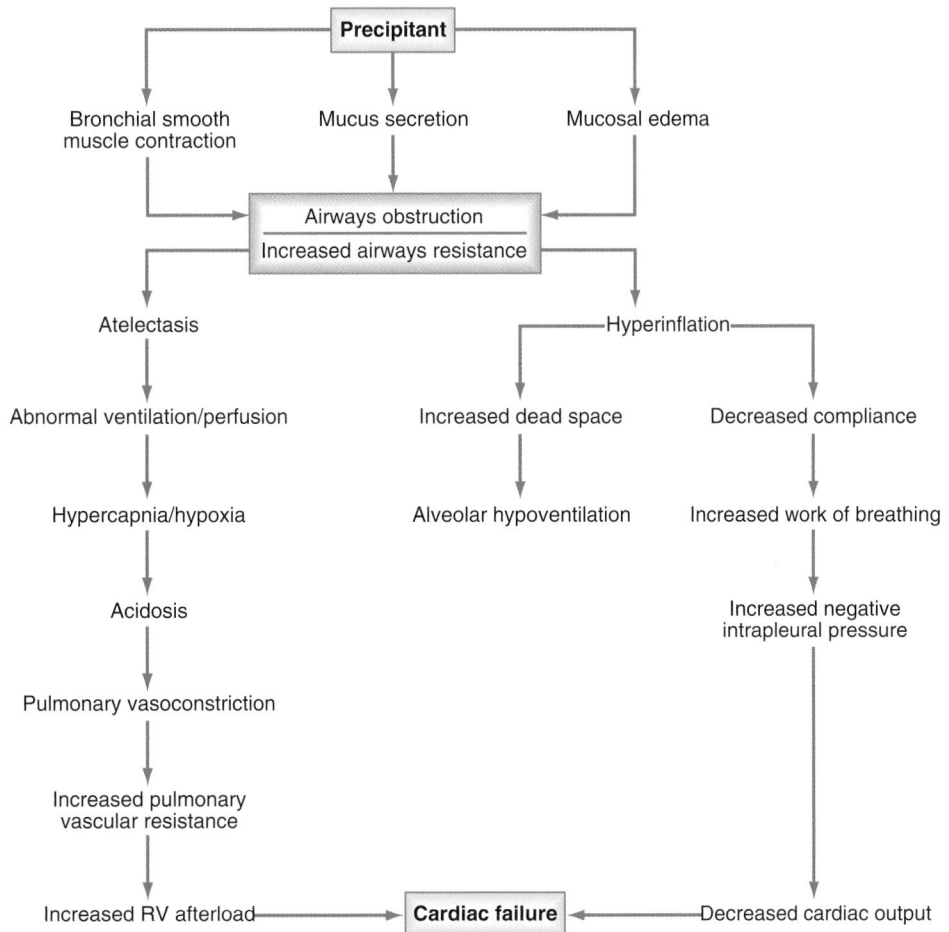

Figure 72-1 **Pathophysiology of status asthmaticus.** *(Modified from Helfaer M, Nichols D, Rogers M. Lower airway disease: bronchiolitis and asthma. In: Rogers M, editor. Textbook of Pediatric Intensive Care. 3rd ed. Baltimore: Williams and Wilkins; 1996, p. 141.)*

among patients without comorbidity and as high as 20% to 37% in those with preceding cardiac disease, chronic lung disease, prematurity, immunocompromise, and age younger than 6 weeks.[22] Patients with these coexisting conditions are also at increased risk of mortality from RSV[23] and have been identified as candidates to receive monthly prophylaxis with an RSV antigen–specific monoclonal antibody (Palivizumab [MedImmune Inc., Gaithersburg, Maryland]) during RSV season. However, recent epidemiologic data indicate that most RSV-infected children have no significant comorbidities, suggesting that prevention strategies targeting only medically complex patients may have minimal impact on the overall disease burden.[21]

RSV transmission can occur either by direct contact with contagious secretions or by exposure to aerosolized particles from the respiratory mucosa.[24] The incubation period varies from 2 to 8 days,[24] symptoms tend to escalate over 3 to 5 days, and convalescence can be prolonged up to several weeks in the most vulnerable small infants. On histologic examination, reappearance of ciliated respiratory epithelium commonly takes more than 2 weeks.[24] Viral shedding from the respiratory tract typically occurs over 3 to 8 days but may also continue for up to 4 to 6 weeks in small infants. Symptoms typically begin with signs of upper respiratory illness, including fever, coryza, and possibly otitis media. Small infants commonly present with lethargy and central apnea[25] early in the course of illness. Cough and tachypnea soon develop as the illness progresses to the lower airways, usually 1 to 3 days following incubation.[24] Wheezing produced by flow limitation in peripheral airways is a nearly universal finding and may be due in large part to intermittent obstruction of large and small airways with necrotic epithelial debris, edema, and mucus[24] rather than to the bronchospasm more commonly seen in asthma. Radiographic findings are often nonspecific but commonly include hyperinflation, peribronchial thickening, subsegmental consolidation, and multiple areas of atelectasis or infiltration involving most frequently the right middle and right upper lobes. A large prospective study of RSV-infected hospitalized children found that secondary bacterial infection occurred in only 1.2% of the study cohort, establishing that risk of bacterial disease is low in RSV bronchiolitis, despite potentially suggestive radiographic findings and the widespread empirical use of broad-spectrum antimicrobial agents in these patients.[26]

Therapy

Treatment of the infant or child with bronchiolitis is primarily supportive. Many years of clinical experience with empirical use of symptomatic medical therapies have failed to determine a clear role for any of these agents in the management of this disease. Data on the use of medical therapies in critically ill children with bronchiolitis is especially scant. Aerosolized ribavirin, a synthetic guanosine analog with broad-spectrum antiviral activity, is currently the only specific therapy approved for hospitalized infants with RSV bronchiolitis.[24] In general, it has been shown to improve oxygenation and clinical status scores and reduce inflammatory mediators associated with ongoing wheezing in patients with RSV.[24] A meta-analysis of three studies on the use of ribavirin in ventilated patients showed a small but significant decrease in ventilator days associated with the use of this agent.[27] Nonetheless, prospects for widespread administration of this agent or even additional large-scale trials to further evaluate its role are limited by the technical challenges, cost, and occupational hazards associated with its use.[28-30]

Widespread use of bronchodilators and corticosteroids for the management of bronchiolitis is common despite the absence of evidence for improved clinical outcomes in critically ill children.[27] There are presently no randomized controlled trials that have evaluated the efficacy of bronchodilators in critically ill children with bronchiolitis.[31] Moreover, a recent large randomized controlled trial,[32] as well as a systematic review,[33] have failed to establish that any bronchodilator produces a significant improvement in relevant outcome measures in less severely ill hospitalized children with bronchiolitis. A few small studies have associated some short-term physiologic benefit with the use of corticosteroids and immune globulin in critically ill infants and

children with bronchiolitis, but the efficacy of these therapies in altering outcomes in this population remains unproven.[27] Following from the observation that critically ill children with severe bronchiolitis demonstrate surfactant deficiency and dysfunction, a great deal of interest surrounds the use of exogenous surfactant to modify the course of bronchiolitis in intubated patients. A number of small underpowered trials have been conducted on this topic,[34-36] but the available data are not sufficient to provide a reliable estimate of surfactant's effects in this setting.[37] Moreover, the interpretation of this literature is complicated by the fact that the choice of surfactant preparation, the dosing regimen, and the mechanical ventilation strategy vary across studies, and each of these could have an important effect on outcome.[37] An ongoing multicenter randomized controlled trial evaluating the impact of the synthetic surfactant, lucinactant (Discovery Laboratories, Warrington, Pennsylvania), on duration of mechanical ventilation among children younger than 2 years of age with acute hypoxemic respiratory failure[38] may provide additional insight into surfactant's therapeutic role in critically ill patients with bronchiolitis. Because future prospects for providing lasting immunity to RSV remain doubtful,[24] there is an ongoing need for large multicenter studies to identify therapies which may benefit critically ill children with this disease.

Meanwhile, supportive care of the patient with bronchiolitis consists of an ongoing assessment of airway patency, the adequacy of respirations, and maintenance of adequate circulating volume. Supplemental oxygen is often required to reverse hypoxemia, and the clinician should be attentive to changes in mental status that could signal impending respiratory failure.

MECHANICAL VENTILATION

The need for mechanical ventilation in the patient with lower airways disease commonly arises from failure of ventilation and resulting hypercapnia. Hypoxemia and recurrent apnea, which are common in young infants with bronchiolitis, also frequently precipitate the institution of ventilatory support. Assuming adequate airway protection, oxygenation, and respiratory drive, it is probably best to avoid intubation in the patient with lower airways disease unless the overall clinical status of the child warrants the risk of augmenting airway hyperreactivity through airway instrumentation.[39] To this end, there are several adjunct therapies that may obviate the need for intubation when added to aggressively applied conventional therapies. An inspired mixture of helium and oxygen (heliox) has been used to alleviate airflow limitation in pediatric patients. Owing to its low density and reduced Reynolds number, helium is able to convert turbulent gas flow to laminar flow in airways, and its clinical effect is generally immediate. Because it is an inert gas, it can potentially lower airway resistance without toxicity. When given as 60% to 80% of the total inspired gas mixture, helium can produce more efficient delivery of oxygen as well as nebulized drugs.[40]

The use of heliox in patients with lower-airway disease has generally produced inconsistent results. A small randomized controlled trial in spontaneously breathing children with status asthmaticus demonstrated that administration of heliox improves respiratory mechanics by lowering the pulsus paradoxus, increasing peak flow, and decreasing the dyspnea index, which may decrease the need for mechanical ventilation.[41] In another small series, a 60:40 heliox mixture administered to 7 intubated patients resulted in a 15% to 50% reduction in peak inspiratory pressure and a 30% to 60% reduction in $Paco_2$.[42] A recent literature review on the use of heliox in patients of all ages with acute asthma concluded that it may be useful in the short-term management of these patients, but any clinical advantage attributable to its use seems to diminish over time.[43] There is little evidence available on the use of heliox in critically ill patients with bronchiolitis. This issue was prospectively investigated in a nonrandomized study of 38 nonintubated infants with RSV bronchiolitis admitted to an ICU.[44] The investigators were able to demonstrate favorable changes in respiratory status through the first 4 hours of heliox administration and a significant decrease in ICU length of stay among infants who received heliox therapy.[44] In a small randomized crossover study of RSV-positive, nonintubated patients, clinical indicators of respiratory status improved during heliox administration, particularly among children with more severe disease.[45] However, many of the patients required another form of respiratory support, and the study was not designed to evaluate longer-term outcomes such as ICU length of stay.[45]

The application of noninvasive forms of mechanical support such as continuous positive airway pressure (CPAP) or bilevel positive airway pressure (BiPAP) using either a nasal interface or full face mask has potential advantage in the patient with adequate respiratory drive. Careful titration of applied CPAP (or positive end-expiratory pressure [PEEP]) noninvasively may prevent premature airway closure during expiration and decrease gas trapping (see later discussion). The patient who develops high levels of intrinsic PEEP due to hyperinflation manifests an increased work of breathing and, ultimately, respiratory muscle fatigue, which may precipitate dramatic and rapid clinical deterioration. Noninvasive respiratory support may allow unloading of the muscles of respiration without adding to airway reactivity and has been used with success in managing asthma as well as bronchiolitis.[46-48]

In the patient with respiratory failure for whom noninvasive mechanical support is not feasible, intubation and mechanical ventilation is warranted. As tracheal intubation is performed in the patient with airways disease, the clinician should be watchful for complications arising from the transition to positive-pressure ventilation. In the spontaneously breathing child with severe airway obstruction, profoundly negative intrathoracic pressures develop in order to generate lung inflation. These conditions produce maximal venous return as right atrial pressure remains subatmospheric.[49] The transition to positive-pressure ventilation in this setting increases juxtacardiac pressures and right ventricular afterload, resulting in decreased venous return, decreased left ventricular compliance, and decreased left ventricular end diastolic volume,[49] with risk of hypotension and cardiac arrest.[3]

In intubated patients with status asthmaticus or bronchiolitis, low elastic recoil and increased airway resistance due to bronchoconstriction, airway edema, and mucus plugging contribute to regional gas trapping and dynamic hyperinflation (Figure 72-2, A). Gas trapping can also be exacerbated by the patient's forced expiratory efforts, during which increased abdominal pressure is transmitted to the pleural space, potentiating premature airway closure and the development of excess or intrinsic PEEP ("auto-PEEP"). The magnitude of the auto-PEEP reflects the degree of dynamic hyperinflation in patients with severe asthma.[50] Dynamic hyperinflation and auto-PEEP have an adaptive purpose in increasing the elastic recoil pressure of the lung to a level that would eventually allow complete evacuation of inhaled volume.[50] However, this increase in lung volume takes place at the expense of an unfavorable change in pulmonary compliance. Other potential consequences of dynamic hyperinflation and auto-PEEP include air leak, hemodynamic compromise from sustained elevations in pulmonary vascular resistance, and increased inspiratory workload from the patient's attempts to drop the ventilator circuit pressure below the total PEEP level (applied or set PEEP plus auto-PEEP) to trigger a breath (see Figure 72-2, B). The development of gas trapping and auto-PEEP can be inferred if the flow-versus-time waveform on the ventilator console shows initiation of inspiratory flow before the expiratory flow from the preceding breath reaches zero. Alternatively, the ventilator can quantify auto-PEEP by allowing the alveolar pressure to equilibrate with pressure at the airway opening during an end-expiratory hold maneuver. The accuracy and reliability of each of these techniques rest on the premise that all lung units communicate with the airway opening, which may not be true if bronchial obstruction is severe.[51]

Excessive gas trapping and auto-PEEP are managed though adherence to the basic principles of mechanical ventilatory support of patients with lower airways disease: (1) limitation of tidal volume, plateau pressure, and respiratory rate; (2) reducing inspiratory time, and (3) judiciously titrating applied PEEP. In the spontaneously

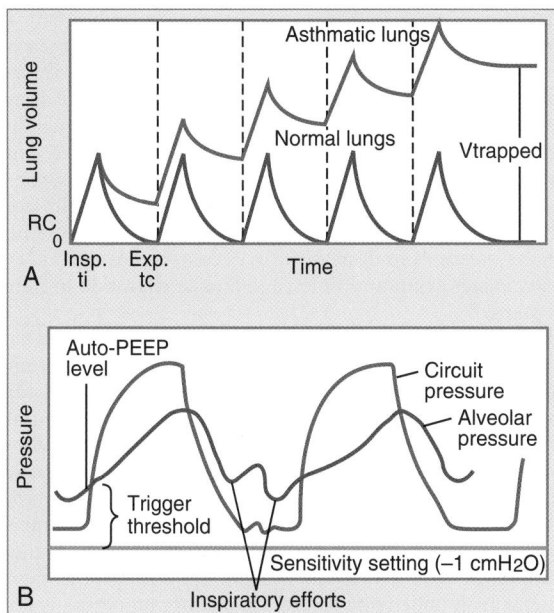

Figure 72-2 A, Dynamic hyperinflation. Expiratory flow limitation in the asthmatic lung *(upper tracing)* causes incomplete evacuation of lung volume at end exhalation. Repetitive cycles of gas trapping lead to excess pressure accumulation at end exhalation ("auto-PEEP"), with a progressive shift toward ventilation on the less compliant *(upper and outer)* portion of the pressure-volume curve (see also Figure 35-3). *(Adapted from Stather DR, Stewart TE. Clinical review: mechanical ventilation in severe asthma. Crit Care 2005;9:581-7.)* **B, Effect of auto-PEEP on inspiratory threshold load.** Ventilator circuit pressure, alveolar pressure, and trigger sensitivity setting are indicated. The difference between peak inspiratory circuit pressure and peak inspiratory alveolar pressure reflects increased airway resistance. Difference between end-expiratory circuit pressure and end-expiratory alveolar pressure reflects expiratory flow limitation and auto-PEEP. Pressure drop required to generate inspiratory flow ("trigger threshold") is the difference between end-expiratory pressure and sensitivity setting. Auto-PEEP will require the patient to generate a larger inspiratory pressure drop to generate inspiratory flow.

breathing mechanically ventilated patient, increases in applied PEEP can reduce auto-PEEP by reducing the tendency to premature airway closure during exhalation and restoring a pressure gradient between the alveoli and airway opening that favors a return toward normal end-expiratory lung volume. Reduction of auto-PEEP through this kind of maneuver can facilitate the triggering of ventilator breaths and decrease the inspiratory workload. However sound this concept may appear in theory, it can be difficult to optimize in practice. If increases in applied PEEP fail to improve respiratory mechanics or worsen gas trapping, the clinician may consider a trial of neuromuscular blockade in an effort to facilitate enforcement of permissive hypercapnia and further reductions in minute ventilation.

In summary, initial ventilator settings in patients with lower-airway disease should be guided by observation, auscultation, careful ventilator waveform analysis, and attention to inspiratory plateau pressure. Ultimately, the choice of ventilator mode is not as important as a thorough understanding of how any mode might be strategically manipulated to alleviate the pathophysiology of gas trapping and auto-PEEP. It is generally preferable to allow the patient to breathe in a spontaneous ventilator mode, using a strategy of permissive hypercapnia. In spontaneously breathing mechanically ventilated patients, applied PEEP can be titrated cautiously upward as needed to improve respiratory mechanics to a level not exceeding 80% of the auto-PEEP, or until the plateau pressure begins to exceed a tolerable limit, which is usually around 30 cm H_2O.[51,52] If controlled ventilation is necessary, it is preferable to apply the lowest minute ventilation that provides adequate gas exchange.[53] The use of neuromuscular blocking agents should be limited to the shortest feasible course because of their potentially detrimental effect on the relationship between ventilation and perfusion, and because of the risk of myopathy when these agents are administered together with corticosteroids.[54] High-frequency oscillatory ventilation (see later discussion) has been used to rescue a limited number of pediatric patients with asthma and bronchiolitis who demonstrate respiratory failure refractory to management with conventional ventilation.[55] One recent report recommends the use of high distending pressures to decrease airway resistance, as well as low frequencies, longer expiratory times, and muscle relaxation to minimize gas trapping.[56]

Sedation is an important component of managing intubated patients with lower-airway disease. Besides alleviating distress and promoting synchrony with the ventilator, sedative agents can be helpful adjuncts in limiting carbon dioxide production and reducing mechanical ventilatory requirements.[51] Ketamine, a dissociative anesthetic with sympathomimetic and bronchodilatory properties, is often used for sedation in the intubated asthmatic child.[57] Because of its favorable effects on airway reactivity, the inhalational anesthetic, isoflurane, may be a useful adjunct to managing severe status asthmaticus in the intubated child who is difficult to sedate or unresponsive to other therapies. The mechanism underlying its bronchodilatory properties is not well understood.[58] Although isoflurane has a better safety profile than halothane when used for this purpose, periodic monitoring of renal function may be advisable in the child who requires prolonged therapy with this agent.[58]

Diseases of the Alveoli

VIRAL PNEUMONIA

Defined as acute respiratory symptoms accompanied by parenchymal infiltrates on chest x-ray, pneumonia is a common syndrome in children and is most commonly caused by viral or bacterial pathogens.[59] Important viral pathogens responsible for pneumonia in infants and children include RSV, influenza, parainfluenza, and adenovirus. As previously discussed, each of these is agents is also capable of producing the clinical syndrome of bronchiolitis in infants and children. The precise infectious etiology for pediatric viral pneumonias may be suggested by the physical examination, the age of the patient, and seasonal incidence patterns. Confirmatory testing through microbiologic analysis is generally sought to facilitate therapeutic decision making and cohorting of similarly affected patients. RSV is the most common viral cause of lower respiratory infection in infancy[60] and primarily infects the small airways. Influenza is another very important cause of pediatric pneumonia. Infection rates in healthy children are estimated at 10% to 40% each year, and approximately 1% of these children require hospitalization.[60] The course of up to 25% of infected children is complicated by lower respiratory tract disease.[60] Neonates and children up to 5 years of age, especially those with underlying lung disease, congenital heart disease, immunocompromise, and other chronic conditions, seem to be at special risk for influenza pneumonia.[60] Neonates are at risk for especially severe influenza syndromes which may also include apnea and sepsis.[60] Infants and children older than 6 months of age, especially those in high-risk categories, are candidates for annual vaccination against influenza.[61] Antiviral therapy for A and B strains of influenza are now available and can be considered for patients of appropriate age who are at high risk of complicated or severe disease.[60] When administered within 48 hours of disease onset, amantadine, which is approved for use in children older than 1 year of age, may decrease the severity of influenza A disease, but data in young patients are limited.[60] Oseltamivir, a neuraminidase inhibitor active against both A and B strains of influenza, has been demonstrated to decrease symptom duration when administered early in disease. When originally licensed for pediatric administration, oseltamivir was not approved for use in infants younger than 1 year.[62] However, increased experience using oseltamivir in smaller infants during the 2009 H1N1

influenza pandemic produced some consensus on appropriate dosing guidelines in this age group.[63] Unlike RSV, influenza is commonly associated with secondary bacterial pneumonia that is typically caused by *Streptococcus pneumoniae* or *Staphylococcus aureus*, making it especially important to consider appropriate empirical antimicrobial therapy when clinically appropriate.[64,65] Parainfluenza viruses are also responsible for causing pneumonia in children, and seasonal epidemics commonly occur in autumn.[60] Primary infection tends to occur in young children 2 to 6 years of age, and recurrent infection is generally less severe, except perhaps in the immunocompromised host.[60] Finally, adenoviruses have been reported to cause up to 20% of pneumonias in children younger than 5 years of age, and the mortality rate attributable to the disease in this population has been reported as high as 20%.[66] In neonates, adenovirus can produce an especially severe syndrome of disseminated disease and sepsis, which can present in the first 10 days of life.[66] The incubation period is generally 2 to 14 days,[60] and the virus can produce a profound and destructive lower-respiratory process. Necrotizing bronchitis, purulent exudative alveolitis, and hyaline membrane formation have been identified on autopsy specimens of affected patients.[66] Survivors of severe adenoviral infections commonly demonstrate chronic sequelae such as recurrent wheezing and bronchiolitis obliterans.[66]

BACTERIAL PNEUMONIA

Most commonly, bacterial presence is established in the lower respiratory tract as a result of oropharyngeal overgrowth of environmentally acquired pathogens and subsequent introduction of these secretions into the lower airways. Children with aspiration syndromes, immunodeficiencies, and malformations of the respiratory tract are at increased risk of bacterial lower respiratory infection.[67] Bacterial pathogens remain an important cause of potentially lethal pediatric pneumonias in the developing world, and they are the most important cause of severe pneumonia in Europe and North America, especially when complicated by parenchymal necrosis and/or parapneumonic effusion.[59] It is challenging to establish a causal role for specific bacteria when these agents are normally found in the upper airway secretions, the specimen most commonly sampled for microbiologic diagnosis in children. The best data regarding the etiology of community acquired pneumonia come from lung-puncture studies revealing that *S. pneumoniae*, *Hemophilus influenzae*, and *S. aureus* are among the most important causes.[59] Since the introduction of a conjugate vaccine against *H. influenzae* type B (Hib) in 1988, the incidence of invasive disease in infants and young children attributable to this organism has declined by 99%.[60] Other serotypes of the organism, including nonencapsulated strains, may also cause pneumonia in children.[60]

A comprehensive review of necrotizing pneumonia cases occurring in predominantly immunocompetent children admitted to Children's Hospital Boston between 1990 and 2005 indicates that parenchymal necrosis appears to be an increasingly common complication of pediatric bacterial pneumonia.[68] In this series, *S. pneumoniae* was the predominant inciting organism, accounting for 22% of cases. Since 2002, many more organisms, including methicillin-sensitive *S. aureus*, methicillin-resistant *S. aureus*, *Fusobacterium* species, *Pseudomonas* species, and other *Streptococcus* species, have emerged as important causes of necrotizing pneumonia as well. Despite the short-term morbidity in these children, conservative management (consisting mainly of antibiotics and chest drainage) appeared sufficient to produce resolution of clinical symptoms within 2 months of hospital discharge, and marked improvement of imaging findings within 6 months.

Recent studies on the epidemiology of pediatric pneumonia complicated by parapneumonic effusion indicate that the incidence of empyema appears to have risen during the 1990s.[69-71] During that period, *S. pneumoniae* was isolated most commonly from patients with empyema, followed by *Streptococcus pyogenes* and *S. aureus*.[70,71] As in the case of necrotizing pneumonia, temporal trends in the epidemiology of pediatric empyema in the United States show a shift in causative organisms after the year 2000, when the heptavalent pneumococcal conjugate vaccine (PCV) was licensed for widespread use. A large case series reported from Texas Children's Hospital indicates that since 2000, S. aureus has overtaken S. pneumoniae as the most common bacterial pathogen isolated from children with empyema, and the majority of S. aureus isolates in this cohort were methicillin resistant.[69] In addition, nonvaccine serotypes (particularly serotypes 1, 3, and 19A) predominate among causes of pneumococcal empyema in the post-PCV era.[70,72] The overall impact of widespread vaccination with PCV on the incidence of pediatric empyema across the United States is less clear. In Utah, where pneumococcal serotype 1 has always been prevalent, the incidence of pediatric empyema is still rising, while data from Texas Children's Hospital show a decrease in the incidence of empyema since the vaccine became available.[69,70]

In neonates and young infants up to about 3 months of age, group B Streptococcus (GBS), Listeria monocytogenes, and gram-negative enteric organisms are the major causes of pneumonia and sepsis.[60,67] Widespread maternal intrapartum antibiotic prophylaxis has influenced the incidence of perinatal GBS infection as well as its antimicrobial resistance patterns.[73] The incidence of GBS sepsis has declined among very low-birth-weight infants in the era of ampicillin prophylaxis, while the incidence of Escherichia coli sepsis (largely resistant to ampicillin) has increased in the same time period.[73] Perinatally acquired Chlamydia trachomatis is another important cause of lower respiratory tract infection in infants up to 12 weeks of age.[67] Although uncommon, periodic epidemics of infection with Bordetella pertussis occur among incompletely immunized infants and children.[67] Apnea and intermittent cyanosis progressing to respiratory failure and shock can develop in young infants infected with B. pertussis, and clinicians should have a relatively low threshold for admitting these patients to the ICU.

Therapy

In the clinical setting, one is often faced with having to select empirical antimicrobial therapy before arriving at a definitive viral or bacterial diagnosis. The presence of a focal alveolar process on chest radiographs, especially if accompanied by significant parapneumonic effusion, evidence of parenchymal necrosis, and/or abnormal peripheral blood counts and C-reactive protein, all add considerably to the predictive value for the presence of bacterial disease.[59] Before demonstrating evidence of localized infection, neonates and young infants may demonstrate nonspecific but potentially ominous signs of lethargy, hypothermia, and apnea. Infants younger than 3 months of age should be treated with both ampicillin and gentamicin, and consideration should be given to adding a third-generation cephalosporin in severe cases.[59] Investigation and empirical coverage for infection with B. pertussis should also be considered in infants with severe respiratory disease that features profound peripheral lymphocytosis, paroxysmal cough, and/or apnea.

For the critically ill child with community-acquired bacterial pneumonia, reasonable coverage may be assured with a third-generation cephalosporin,[59,67] although some centers advocate the use of clindamycin as a second empirical agent. A macrolide antibiotic can be added in cases where infection with atypical agents such as Mycoplasma pneumoniae and Chlamydia pneumoniae is possible, particularly in patients with sickle cell disease.[59,74] Although emerging resistance to penicillins in S. pneumoniae is widely recognized, high doses of cephalosporins are still appropriate in the majority of penicillin-nonsusceptible strains, so long as concurrent meningitis is not suspected, but the addition of vancomycin may be warranted in some cases.[59,75] If infection with S. aureus is possible, an antistaphylococcal penicillin such as oxacillin should be added unless local resistance patterns warrant the use of vancomycin.[59] In patients at risk for aspiration pneumonia and in immunocompromised children, special consideration should be given to administration of two antibiotics effective against gram-negative organisms (such as Pseudomonas) and to optimizing coverage for anaerobic organisms.

Management of pleural effusion is another important consideration in the care of the patient with bacterial pneumonia. Although drainage of parapneumonic effusions is indicated under certain circumstances, satisfactory recovery may occur in many cases without intervention.[76] Recently an evidence-based clinical practice guideline was developed for the medical and surgical treatment of parapneumonic effusions in adults.[77] The panel issued management suggestions according to the underlying risk of poor clinical outcome, based on effusion size and loculation as well as chemical and microbiologic analysis of the pleural fluid.[77] Pleural fluid drainage was recommended for large effusions occupying more than 50% of the hemithorax, whether or not loculation or pleural thickening is present. Drainage was also recommended for purulent effusions, those with positive culture or Gram stain, or those with pH less than 7.20 as measured by a blood gas analyzer.[77] In situations where drainage is indicated, more complex or invasive options such as thoracoscopic or "open" procedures are likely to be necessary for sufficient control of the effusion.[77] It must be emphasized that the consensus panel's recommendations are based primarily on case series, historical controls, and expert opinion.[77]

The literature on parapneumonic effusion in children also does not presently provide robust evidence on which to base clinical intervention. The effect of image-guided needle aspiration versus percutaneous pigtail catheter drainage was examined in a 5-year retrospective study of pediatric parapneumonic effusions.[78] When comparing outcomes in the two groups, the authors found no difference in length of stay but did report a significant decrease in the need for second intervention in patients who received a chest drain.[78] Other independent predictors for second intervention in their study population included loculation of pleural fluid and pH less than 7.2. A combination of low glucose and low pH in the pleural fluid specimen was especially predictive of the need for reintervention.[78] The decision to perform thoracostomy drainage in pediatric patients with parapneumonic effusion may depend on the clinical context in which it occurs. In cases where significant pleural fluid organization has taken place, some favor the administration of intrapleural thrombolytics to facilitate evacuation of fluid through the chest drain.[79] Studies assessing the efficacy of this practice have produced conflicting results. In one uncontrolled case series, 54 of 58 children (93%) with pneumonia complicated by empyema who received intrapleural tissue plasminogen activator (tPA) did not require additional surgical drainage.[80] However a randomized controlled trial that enrolled 454 adults with empyema showed no outcome benefit attributable to the administration of intrapleural thrombolytics, compared to chest drainage and routine supportive care alone.[81] In recent years, video assisted thoracoscopic surgery (VATS) has gained popularity as a way to facilitate chest drainage through inspection of the pleural space, disruption of adhesions, and placement of chest drains in strategic locations.[79] To date, at least two prospective pediatric trials have failed to identify an outcome advantage attributable to VATS when compared to thrombolytic-enhanced chest drainage and routine supportive therapy for empyema.[82,83]

In summary, it is certainly important to drain large parapneumonic effusions when they are suspected of causing hemodynamic instability in the critically ill child. Pleural drainage may also be useful to relieve respiratory embarrassment that may contribute to respiratory failure or ongoing ventilator dependence. The best opportunity to achieve sufficient drainage is probably in the first 48 to 72 hours of disease, before organization of the effusion begins to take place. A randomized controlled trial will be necessary to resolve the issue of which pediatric patients with parapneumonic effusion would benefit from aggressive pleural drainage.

ACUTE LUNG INJURY AND ACUTE RESPIRATORY DISTRESS SYNDROME

What was once known as *adult respiratory distress syndrome* is now called *acute respiratory distress syndrome* (ARDS) in an effort to acknowledge its prevalence in the pediatric population. A syndrome of lung injury featuring permeability edema leading to hypoxic respiratory failure had been described in adults for many years, but consensus criteria for the diagnosis of the syndrome did not enter the scientific

TABLE 72-3	American-European Consensus Criteria for Acute Lung Injury and Acute Respiratory Distress Syndrome
Acute Lung Injury	**Acute Respiratory Distress Syndrome**
Acute onset	Acute onset
Bilateral pulmonary infiltrates on chest radiography	Bilateral pulmonary infiltrates on chest radiography
PAOP ≤ 18 mm Hg or no clinical evidence LA hypertension	PAOP ≤ 18 mm Hg or no clinical evidence LA hypertension
Pao_2/Fio_2 ratio ≤300	PaO_2/FIO_2 ratio ≤200

Adapted from Bernard GR, Artigas A, Brigham KL et al. The American-European Consensus Conference on ARDS. Definitions, mechanisms, relevant outcomes, and clinical trial coordination. Am J Respir Crit Care Med 1994;149:818-24.

literature until 1994.[84] Once clear diagnostic criteria were established for ARDS and acute lung injury (ALI), the less severe form of the disease, large-scale randomized controlled trials began and have added considerably to our understanding of the epidemiology and outcomes of both conditions (Table 72-3). Both ALI and ARDS may arise as a consequence of primary pulmonary disease or as a feature of systemic pathophysiology that is nonpulmonary in origin. Using contemporary diagnostic criteria, ARDS is estimated to account for 1% to 4% of all PICU admissions, or approximately 10% of all children requiring mechanical ventilatory support.[85,86] Pneumonia, which was responsible for 35% of cases in a recent epidemiologic study, appears to have overtaken sepsis as the most common cause of pediatric ARDS.[85] Reported mortality rates for pediatric ARDS have fluctuated over time, depending on the criteria used to identify cases, the presence of important comorbidities such as immunocompromise and nonpulmonary organ failures among patients in the cohort, and the quality and consistency of supportive care provided in the ICU. Recent reported mortality rates for pediatric ARDS range from 8% in a prone-positioning trial[87] in which the investigators protocolized nearly every conceivable aspect of supportive therapy, to 22% in a recent large prospective cohort study, a figure more comparable to the mortality rates reported from contemporary adult ARDS trials.[52,85] The last decade has seen the completion of many multicenter trials designed to investigate the effects of various adjuvant therapies in pediatric and adult ALI and ARDS (Table 72-4). So far, tidal volume reduction during mechanical ventilation stands as the only intervention proven to offer a significant mortality benefit to patients with ALI and ARDS.

MECHANICAL VENTILATION

Mechanical ventilatory support of the patient with ALI and ARDS is often necessary to provide adequate oxygenation. In relatively stable patients, noninvasive ventilation may be effective when instituted early in the disease process. This method has been used successfully in the management of acute hypoxic respiratory failure in a heterogenous population of adult patients[88] and in a more selected population of immunocompromised adult patients.[89] Each of these randomized controlled trials showed that early use of noninvasive ventilation decreased the need for intubation and reduced the risk of death in the ICU and in the hospital. Data on the use of noninvasive positive-pressure ventilation (NIPPV) in pediatric patients are limited, but several case series report success with the application of this technique in children with alveolar disease.[90,91] In one study, noninvasive BiPAP was used to support pediatric patients with pneumonia, acute chest syndrome and sickle-cell disease, underlying chronic hypoventilation syndromes, and postoperative hypoventilation with atelectasis.[90] The authors reported favorable changes in respiratory rate, heart rate, and oxygenation among all patients receiving noninvasive support, and 91% of respiratory failure episodes in their study were reversed without the need for intubation.[90]

When noninvasive techniques are not appropriate or have failed, tracheal intubation is warranted. It has been well established in a number of animal and human studies that the mechanical ventilation

strategy can have a profound influence on the course of disease and overall clinical outcome.[52,92-95] Chief among these is the landmark multicenter study conducted by the ARDS Network (ARDSnet) investigators, which established that ALI and ARDS patients randomized to receive tidal volumes of 6 cc/kg ideal body weight had a mortality reduction of 22% relative to those who received ventilation using "traditional" tidal volumes of 12 cc/kg ideal body weight.[52] Remarkably, this trial also demonstrated a greater reduction in plasma levels of the proinflammatory cytokine, interleukin 6 (IL-6), among those patients randomized to receive lower tidal volumes, suggesting that reducing the magnitude of phasic stretch during mechanical ventilation can actually attenuate the systemic inflammatory response. Over the last decade, much attention has been given to the provision of "lung-protective" mechanical ventilation in patients with acute lung injury and ARDS. Lung-protective ventilation involves (1) preservation of end-expiratory lung volume by judicious use of PEEP to minimize atelectrauma; (2) minimization of cyclic stretch; and (3) avoidance of parenchymal overdistension at end-inspiration by limiting tidal volume and transpulmonary pressure.[52,92-95]

When oxygenation failure is refractory to conventional ventilation, high-frequency oscillatory ventilation (HFOV) is an alternative modality that is well established in the pediatric population. During HFOV, lung recruitment is maintained by application of a relatively high mean airway pressure with superimposed pressure oscillations at a frequency of 3 to 15 Hz.[95] Because maximal recruitment is maintained throughout the respiratory cycle, and ventilation is achieved using very small phasic changes in pressure and volume, this technique allows the lung to be ventilated above the critical opening pressure of injured lung units while avoiding end-inspiratory overdistension of more compliant lung units (Figure 72-3).[96-98] This "open-lung" strategy of mechanical ventilation can capitalize on pulmonary hysteresis to achieve satisfactory gas exchange at lower alveolar pressures (see Figure 72-3). In 1994, a prospective multicenter randomized clinical study compared HFOV and conventional mechanical ventilation in pediatric patients with diffuse alveolar disease or air leak syndromes.[99] Patients in the HFOV arm showed rapid and sustained improvements in oxygenation without suffering adverse effects on ventilation.[99] Ultimately these patients showed a decreased incidence of ventilator-associated lung injury, as evidenced by a decreased need for supplemental oxygen at 30 days, and demonstrated improved outcomes compared to their cohorts in the conventional arm, particularly when HFOV was instituted within 72 hours of intubation.[99] The *oxygenation index* (OI), defined as $(MAP \times FIO_2 \times 100)/PaO_2$, used often in the pediatric literature to quantify oxygenation failure, was shown to discriminate between survivors and nonsurvivors in the first 72 hours of therapy.[99] Furthermore, the time at which changes in the OI were found to occur seemed to influence the likelihood of survival: an OI ≥42 at 24 hours predicted mortality with an odds ratio of 20.8, a sensitivity of 62%, and a specificity of 93%.[99] In the time since this study was published, other investigators have helped establish that the OI seems to be a time-sensitive predictor of survival in patients with hypoxic respiratory failure, and OI trends can be used to facilitate decisions about the need for extracorporeal support in patients with acute hypoxic respiratory failure.[100]

Diseases of the Interstitium

The interstitial lung diseases (ILD) in children are a diverse group of rare conditions that involve alteration of the alveolar wall, infiltration and fibrosis of the pulmonary interstitium, and loss of functional alveolar-capillary units.[101] The major clinical findings include abnormal gas exchange, tachypnea, and crackles, as well as the potential for both restrictive and obstructive pulmonary physiology.[102] There are numerous potential etiologies, ranging from primary congenital abnormalities of the alveolar-capillary unit which present in early infancy, to acquired syndromes of chronic interstitial disease referable to infection, recurrent aspiration, or symptomatic cardiovascular disease (Table 72-5).[101] In children, as in adults, the morbidity and

TABLE 72-4	Results of Selected Clinical Trials Evaluating Ventilation Strategies or Pharmacologic Therapies for Acute Lung Injury and Acute Respiratory Distress Syndrome				
Intervention	**Year**	**Number of Patients**	**Findings**	**Study**	
Low-tidal-volume mechanical ventilation	2000	861	*22% relative mortality benefit*	National Institutes of Health (NIH) Acute Respiratory Distress Syndrome Network. N Engl J Med 2000;342:1301-8.	
Prone positioning	2001	304	No mortality benefit	Gattinoni et al. N Engl J Med 2001;345:568-73.	
	2005[a]	102	No mortality benefit	Curley et al. JAMA 2005;294:229-37.	
	2006	136	No mortality benefit[b]	Mancebo et al. Am J Respir Crit Care Med 2006;173:1233-9.	
	2009	342	No mortality benefit	Taccone et al. JAMA 2009;302:1977-84.	
Conservative vs. liberal fluid administration strategy	2006	1000	No mortality benefit	NIH Acute Respiratory Distress Syndrome Network. N Engl J Med 2006;354:2564-5.	
Surfactant	1996	725	No mortality benefit	Anzueto et al. N Engl J Med 1996;334:1417-21.	
	2004	448	No mortality benefit	Spragg et al. N Engl J Med 2004;351:884-92.	
	2005[a]	152	Mortality benefit seen in surfactant group[c]	Willson et al. JAMA 2005;293:470-6.	
Corticosteroids	1998	24	Mortality benefit[d]	Meduri et al. JAMA 1998;280:159-65.	
	2006	180	No mortality benefit	NIH Acute Respiratory Distress Syndrome Network N Engl J Med 2006;354:1671-84.	
Inhaled nitric oxide	1998	177	No mortality benefit	Dellinger et al. Crit Care Med 1998;26:15-23.	
	1999[a]	108	No mortality benefit[e]	Dobyns et al. J Pediatr 1999;134:406-12.	
	2004	385	No mortality benefit	Taylor et al. JAMA 2004;291:1603-9.	
Increased recruitment vs. minimal alveolar overdistension in ALI and ARDS (PEEP titrated to Pplat 28-30 cm H_2O vs PEEP 5-9 cm H_2O)	2008	767	No mortality benefit	Mercat A et al. JAMA 2008;299:646-55.	
Activated protein C	2008	75	No mortality benefit	Liu et al. Am J Respir Crit Care Med 2008;178:618-23.	
Drug study of albuterol to treat acute lung injury	Terminated by DSMB (futile)	282 (of 1000)	No mortality benefit	Matthay M et al. Am. J Respir Crit Care Med 2009;179:A2166.	
Awaiting Results[k]					
Early vs. delayed enteral feeding and Ω-3 fatty acid (FA) and antioxidant supplementation for ALI/ARDS	Ω-3 FA and antioxidant arm terminated (futile)	272		NIH Acute Respiratory Distress Syndrome Network[e]	
Early vs. delayed enteral feeding	Recruiting	Est 1000		NIH Acute Respiratory Distress Syndrome Network[f]	
High-frequency oscillatory ventilation (HFOV) using high airway pressure (Paw)/low F_{IO_2} vs. HFOV using low Paw/high F_{IO_2}	Completed June 2009	100		Brower RG, principal investigator[g]	
Airway pressure-release ventilation vs. volume-cycled low-tidal-volume ventilation	Recruiting	Est 368		Tumlin JA, principal investigator[h]	
HFOV vs. conventional ventilation	Pilot phase completed	94		Ferguson ND and Meade MO, principal investigators[i]	
Surfactant (lucinactant)	Recruiting[a] (children up to 2 years of age)	Est. 172		Thomas N and Randolph AG, principal investigators[j]	

Adapted from Ventre KM, Arnold JH. Acute lung injury and the acute respiratory distress syndrome. In: Rogers M, editor. Textbook of Pediatric Intensive Care. 4th ed. Baltimore: Lippincott Williams and Wilkins; 2008.

[a]Pediatric study; [b]58% ICU mortality in control arm—study ultimately underpowered; [c]study ultimately underpowered; [d]small study; [e]crossover design, ClinicalTrials.gov identifier NCT0079301; [f]ClinicalTrials.gov identifier NCT00883948; [g]ClinicalTrials.gov identifier NCT00609180; [h]ClinicalTrials.gov identifier NCT00793013; [i]ClinicalTrials.gov identifier NCT00474656; [j]ClinicalTrials.gov identifier NCT00578734; [k]information available at www.ClinicalTrials.gov; accessed Jan 31, 2010.

mortality of these diseases are high,[103,104] but the frequency distribution of specific etiologies may be very different in the two populations. The prevalence of specific ILD subtypes in the pediatric population has shifted in recent years, following publication of an international consensus statement on ILD classification.[105] In the past, usual interstitial pneumonitis (UIP) and respiratory bronchiolitis had occasionally been described in children, but recent revisions to the classification and essential diagnostic criteria for each ILD subtype now cast doubt on whether either of these conditions actually exist in the pediatric population.[105] On the other hand, several varieties of ILD are uniquely found in infancy, such as disorders of lung growth and development, neuroendocrine cell hyperplasia, follicular bronchitis/bronchiolitis, cellular interstitial pneumonitis, idiopathic pulmonary hemorrhage of infancy, and chronic pneumonitis of infancy due to congenital abnormalities of surfactant dysfunction.[102] Overall, infectious etiologies may be relatively common in the pediatric population, accounting for perhaps 20% of pediatric ILD in some series.[101,103] Given the wide variety of potential etiologies in ILD, a systematic approach to the

diagnostic workup has been suggested.[103] While history and physical exam have a role in the initial evaluation of a child with suspected ILD, noninvasive tests such as serologies, cultures, chest radiographs, high-resolution chest computed tomography (CT) scans, pulmonary function testing, barium swallow, pH studies, and echocardiograms will more often allow the clinician to arrive at a specific diagnosis.[102,103] In those children in whom an etiology still cannot be determined, more invasive studies such as bronchoalveolar lavage, cardiac catheterization, and lung biopsy should be considered.[103] Results of biopsy specimens may be particularly important to guide decision making in critically ill children who are not responding to therapy.

THERAPY

As many of the etiologies for pediatric ILD may begin with an inflammatory response to lung injury, treatment of children with this condition commonly involves the use of antiinflammatory agents such as corticosteroids. A favorable response to corticosteroids among children

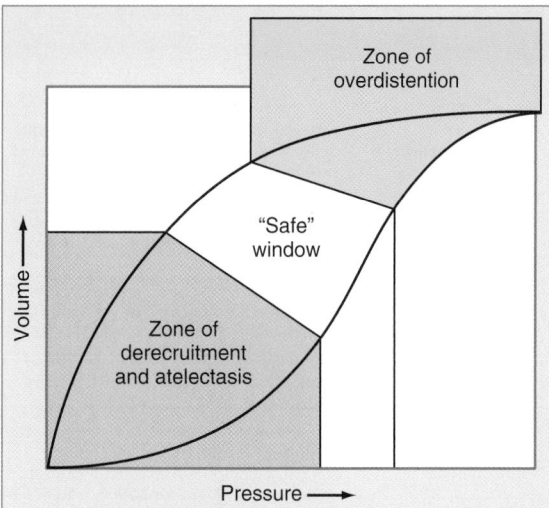

Figure 72-3 Pressure-volume relationships in acute lung injury. Lower curve shows pressure-volume relationships during inspiration. Upper curve shows pressure-volume relationships during exhalation. Note that during exhalation (compared to inspiration), larger lung volumes can be maintained at lower transpulmonary pressures. Combining moderate to high end-expiratory pressures with small tidal volumes minimizes potential for cyclic derecruitment (*lower left*) and overdistension (*upper right*). (*From Froese AB. High-frequency oscillatory ventilation for adult respiratory distress syndrome: let's get it right this time! Crit Care Med 1997;25:906-8.*)

with ILD may be evident in only 40% of cases,[106] and this variability may reflect the diverse potential causes of the disease. In cases where concerns about long-term administration of corticosteroids arise, steroid-sparing antiinflammatory agents such as azathioprine, cyclophosphamide, methotrexate, cyclosporine, and IV gammaglobulin have been used.[102] There is also a great deal of experience with the use of hydroxychloroquine in the management of pediatric ILD, although its use has been associated with the development of hepatic toxicity and retinopathy in children.[106] Ultimately, identifying and controlling underlying causes and contributing issues are very important when this is possible.

Complex Parenchymal Diseases

BRONCHOPULMONARY DYSPLASIA

Bronchopulmonary dysplasia (BPD) is a term used to describe histopathologic changes in the lungs of neonates exposed to mechanical ventilation who go on to demonstrate radiologic abnormalities and supplemental oxygen dependence at 36 weeks postmenstrual age.[107] Heterogeneous alveolar consolidation, squamous metaplasia of airway epithelium, hyperplasia of mucus glands, peribronchial fibrosis, airway smooth muscle hypertrophy, and vascular lesions of pulmonary hypertension once typified BPD-related histopathologic changes when the disease was first described by Northway and colleagues in 1967.[108,109] The past 2 decades have witnessed a shift in the histopathologic features of BPD away from cystic, metaplastic, and fibroproliferative changes toward a more uniform distribution of lung aeration across fewer, larger, and more simplified alveoli.[110,111] This progression likely documents the effects from more than 20 years of widespread intratracheal surfactant administration to preterm infants, as well as a trend toward the use of lung-protective ventilatory strategies and other improvements in the supportive care of these patients. Ten years ago, a consensus conference convened by the National Institutes of Health refined the diagnostic criteria for BPD in order to acknowledge its evolution into a disease with mild, moderate, or severe manifestations,

TABLE 72-5	Consensus Classification of Interstitial Lung Diseases
Histologic Patterns	***Clinical/Radiologic/Pathologic Diagnosis***
Usual interstitial pneumonia[1]	Idiopathic pulmonary fibrosis/ cryptogenic fibrosis alveolitis
Nonspecific interstitial pneumonia	Nonspecific interstitial pneumonia
Organizing pneumonia	Cryptogenic organizing pneumonia[2]
Diffuse alveolar damage	Acute interstitial pneumonia
Respiratory bronchiolitis[1]	Respiratory bronchiolitis interstitial lung disease
Desquamative interstitial pneumonia	Desquamative interstitial pneumonia
Lymphoid interstitial pneumonia	Lymphoid interstitial pneumonia
Other Forms of Interstitial Lung Disease	
Primary pulmonary disorders	Alveolar hemorrhage syndromes Aspiration syndromes Radiation or drug-induced lung disease Hypersensitivity pneumonitis Infectious or postinfectious chronic lung disease Pulmonary alveolar proteinosis Pulmonary infiltrates with eosinophilia Pulmonary lymphatic disorders Pulmonary microlithiasis Pulmonary vascular disorders
Systemic disorders with pulmonary involvement	Connective tissue disease Histiocytosis Lipid storage disease Neurocutaneous syndromes Malignancies Sarcoidosis Inborn errors of metabolism

Adapted from Fan LL, Deterding RR, Langston C. Pediatric interstitial lung disease revisited. Pediatr Pulmonol 2004;38:369–78.
[1]Not described in children; [2]Previously known as *bronchiolitis obliterans organizing pneumonia.*

depending on the intensity of respiratory support an infant requires at the point of assessment (Table 72-6).[112] The revised criteria better represent the array of clinical manifestations seen in contemporary BPD and should facilitate the execution of clinical trials to identify subpopulations of infants who are likely to benefit from specific therapies.

In the current era, BPD is most likely to develop in premature infants who are born at a gestational age when alveolar development is not yet complete, and whose birthweight is less than 1000 to

TABLE 72-6	Consensus Diagnostic Criteria for Bronchopulmonary Dysplasia (BPD)	
	Gestational Age	
	<32 Weeks	*≥32 Weeks*
Time point of assessment	36 weeks postmenstrual age or discharge to home*	>28 days but <56 days postnatal age or discharge to home*
Supplemental oxygen requirement	>21% for ≥28 days	>21% for ≥28 days
Disease severity — Mild	Breathing room air at 36 weeks postmenstrual age or at discharge*	Breathing room air by 56 days postnatal age or at discharge*
Moderate	Requires <30% oxygen at 36 weeks postmenstrual age or at discharge*	Requires <30% oxygen at 56 days postnatal age or at discharge*
Severe	Requires >30% oxygen, with or without mechanical ventilation or CPAP at 36 weeks postmenstrual age or at discharge*	Requires >30% oxygen with our without mechanical ventilation or CPAP at 56 days postnatal age or at discharge*

Adapted from Kinsella JP, Greenough A, Abman SH. Bronchopulmonary dysplasia. Lancet 2006;367(9520):1421-31.
*Whichever comes first.

1200 g.[108,113] Clinically, the BPD syndrome is associated with airway hyperreactivity and intermittent airway obstruction, leading to increased work of breathing, recurrent wheezing, chronic abnormalities of gas exchange, and potentially significant pulmonary hypertension.[108] Focal airway collapse consistent with tracheomalacia and/or bronchomalacia has also been documented in these infants,[114] but their pathogenesis in this context is unknown. The spectrum of pathology observed in BPD patients is believed to derive from an inflammatory response to lung injury; numerous investigations have identified mediators of inflammation in the bronchoalveolar lavage (BAL) fluid of infants with chronic lung disease.[115] Our present understanding of the pathogenesis of chronic lung injury in the neonate mirrors what has been learned from laboratory and clinical investigations of this process in older children and adults, but it is also important to recognize that in preterm infants, perinatally or postnatally acquired inflammatory lung injury takes place against a background of disrupted alveolar development. This is a key distinction between BPD and ARDS or ALI that develops in mature infants and older children, and likely accounts for the persistence of pulmonary morbidity in the BPD population into early adolescence.[111] In any event, preterm neonates with respiratory failure may be especially susceptible to ventilator-associated lung injury because surfactant deficiency, high chest wall compliance, and a dynamic functional residual capacity (FRC) that is near closing capacity in this age group may potentiate cycles of derecruitment and reinflation that have been shown to promote the development of lung injury in humans and animal models, including surfactant-deficient preterm animals.[92-94,116,117] Mechanical ventilatory techniques targeted to promote alveolar recruitment and maintain lung volume have in fact decreased the incidence of ventilator-associated lung injury in neonates. Numerous large prospective, randomized, controlled trials have found a lower incidence of chronic lung disease among high-risk infants supported with HFOV compared to cohorts who are supported with conventional phasic ventilation, with no apparent increase in the development of intracranial hemorrhage or other significant morbidities.[118-120]

Pulmonary edema from cardiogenic and noncardiogenic causes, infectious issues, and exposure to high concentrations of supplemental oxygen are other factors important in the pathogenesis of BPD. Premature infants may be at special risk from exposure to high concentrations of supplemental oxygen because they are deficient in the antiproteases and antioxidant enzymes that have a role in modulating the injurious effects from the proliferation of reactive oxygen species.[107]

Therapy

In the past 5 years, methylxanthines have emerged as having a potentially important role in the prevention of BPD. A large multicenter, randomized, controlled trial found that 36% of 963 very-low-birth-weight infants who received caffeine in the first 10 days of life remained dependent on supplemental oxygen at 36 weeks postmenstrual age, compared to 47% in the placebo group ($P < 0.001$).[121] Positive-pressure respiratory support was also discontinued 1 week earlier in the intervention group ($P > 0.001$). For those infants in whom BPD cannot be prevented, medications that may be useful in producing short-term improvements in their pulmonary mechanics include bronchodilators, corticosteroids, and diuretics (Table 72-7).[107,108,122] Aerosolized β-agonists may be useful in the management of smooth muscle–mediated bronchospasm in the infant with chronic lung disease, but the consequent decrease in airway smooth muscle tone may aggravate airway collapse in the infant with tracheomalacia or bronchomalacia.[114] Diuretics may be especially helpful in the management of these infants because many demonstrate a tendency to accumulate fluid in the pulmonary interstitium on the basis of alterations in pulmonary vascular resistance, plasma oncotic pressure, capillary permeability, and impaired lymphatic drainage.[115] Judicious use of diuretics can also facilitate the delivery of adequate nutrition to the infant with chronic lung disease.[115] Inhaled nitric oxide (iNO) has also been studied for its potential role in treating refractory hypoxemia in infants with chronic lung disease. Case series have documented improvements in oxygen-

TABLE 72-7	Pharmacotherapies Commonly Used in the Management of Infants with Bronchopulmonary Dysplasia
Inhaled Therapies	Albuterol (0.5%) 0.15 mg/kg/dose inhaled q 1-6 h PRN Continuous nebulization 0.5 mg/kg/h Ipratropium 0.25-0.5 mg/dose inhaled q 4-6 h Fluticasone 44 mcg BID (*maintenance therapy*) (Max 440 µg/d)
Diuretic Therapies	Furosemide 1-2 mg/kg/dose IV/po q 6 h Chlorothiazide 10-20 mg/kg/d IV divided q 12 h <6 months: 20-40 mg/kg/d PO divided q 12 h ≥6 months: 20 mg/kg/d PO divided q 12 h Spironolactone 1.5-3.3 mg/kg/d PO divided q 6-24 h
GI Therapies	Metoclopramide 0.1-0.2 mg/kg/dose IV/PO q 6 h (Max 10 mg/dose) Ranitidine 1 mg/kg/dose IV q 8 h 2-3 mg/kg/dose PO q 12 h
Other Therapies	Caffeine citrate 20 mg/kg IV × 1 (*load*) followed by 5 mg/kg/d

ation with the use of iNO, including in infants with intercurrent infection, with a sustained response reported in some cases.[123,124]

Lower respiratory tract infection is one of the most common reasons for hospital readmission in the first year of life for infants with BPD, and accounts for a significant fraction of these pulmonary exacerbations.[113] Other potential causes for BPD exacerbations include aspiration syndromes, worsening pulmonary hypertension, and the evolution of clinically important systemic-to-pulmonary collateral vessels.[108] Therefore, the diagnostic approach to the infant with BPD who demonstrates unexplained deterioration may include dynamic airway studies as well as echocardiography and in certain cases, cardiac catheterization.[108] Treatment of these episodes is supportive and often includes empirical antibiotic coverage for potential infectious causes.

CONGENITAL DIAPHRAGMATIC HERNIA

Management of the infant with congenital diaphragmatic hernia (CDH) is one of the greatest clinical challenges the intensive care clinician encounters. The Bochdalek hernia is the most common form and occurs when abdominal contents herniate into the thoracic cavity through a posterolateral diaphragmatic defect, usually at around the 10th week of gestation. This phase of gestation concurrently includes the branching of bronchi and pulmonary arteries, and this crucial process may be interrupted by the growing mass of herniated viscera.[125] On the other hand, the discovery that administering the teratogen nitrofen to mid-gestation rats results in diaphragmatic defects in the developing fetus as well as a spectrum of anomalies in other organ systems similar to what is seen in humans with CDH suggests that the pathogenesis of this syndrome may originate from fetal exposure to an agent that causes generalized maldevelopment from that point forward.[126-129] The complex pathology associated with congenital diaphragmatic hernia in humans includes a hypoplastic and abnormally muscularized pulmonary arterial tree.[125] Other congenital anomalies are associated with CDH in up to 39% of cases. Congenital cardiac disease is the most commonly associated feature and most frequently involves some degree of cardiac hypoplasia, although a wide variety of structural cardiac anomalies may be associated with CDH.[130] Genitourinary, gastrointestinal, neurologic, and skeletal defects are also commonly described.[125] Adjunct medical therapies have not managed to improve the discouraging survival statistics of these infants, whose mortality rate is traditionally reported in the range of 50%. Nonetheless, there are experienced centers that have reported more encouraging results in recent years by adopting strategic forms of mechanical support of these patients that incorporate much of what has been learned about modulating the pulmonary and hemodynamic consequences of mechanical ventilation.

Therapy

In infants with CDH, as in those with BPD, intensive care management is directed at managing their lower airways disease, alveolar disease, and abnormal pulmonary vascular reactivity. Initial medical stabilization of the infant with CDH includes endotracheal intubation and nasogastric decompression. It is preferable to obtain preductal (i.e., right radial) arterial access when possible. Information from preductal blood gases should guide clinical intervention, because it reflects the status of the cerebral circulation. Initially, echocardiography is suggested to rule out structural cardiac disease, and it may be repeated as necessary throughout the clinical course to determine evidence of ongoing right-to-left shunting as well as estimates of right ventricular pressure and function in response to therapy.[125] Inhaled nitric oxide has been used in infants with CDH with varying results, and a role for the drug in reducing the need for extracorporeal membrane oxygenation (ECMO) or in improving survival among these patients was not established by a large, randomized controlled trial on the use of iNO in neonates with pulmonary hypertension.[131] In general, evidence supporting the use of iNO in the management of infants with CDH is limited to small case series and individual case studies.[132-134] In CDH, as in BPD, deficient alveolar development may explain the limited potential benefit from iNO.[124] A limited number of reports have addressed the possibility of targeting an array of potential mechanisms behind pulmonary hypertension in CDH, including interference with calcium-mediated platelet activation and vasoconstriction (prostaglandin analogues), inhibition of endothelin-mediated vasoconstriction (bosentan), and inhibition of phosphodiesterase metabolism (sildenafil, milrinone), but none have been able to establish a clear outcome benefit for any of these agents in infants with this disease.[135] At least one source has raised concern about the potential for hepatotoxicity when bosentan is used in infants.[136]

Recommendations for the optimal timing of surgical repair in infants with CDH have evolved over time. It was once considered appropriate to refer these infants for immediate repair. Growing experience with the mechanical support of CDH patients, along with the observation that pulmonary vascular resistance and reactivity as well as pulmonary compliance could become more favorable within days after birth, have since created a trend toward delaying surgical repair until a satisfactory level of physiologic stability can be achieved.[125,137]

MECHANICAL VENTILATION

Given what is presently known about ventilator-associated lung injury, it is logical to apply lung-protective ventilation strategies to infants with chronic lung disease as well as to infants with CDH. Although the technique has not been traditionally applied to neonates, permissive hypercapnia is in fact well tolerated by most infants with these conditions.[138-140] Because of the heterogeneity of airspace involvement in BPD and CDH, regional hyperinflation can easily occur. Therefore it makes sense to maintain end-expiratory lung volume with a careful titration of PEEP, and limit tidal volume to 4 to 6 cc/kg in order to ventilate at the area of maximal compliance on the pressure-volume curve.[141] While managing these patients, monitoring tidal volume at the endotracheal tube is important because compressible volume losses in the ventilator circuit can be significant. Judicious use of sedation and the use of spontaneous ventilation (such as flow-triggered pressure support) may improve matching of ventilation to perfusion and may allow optimal patient-ventilator synchrony.

A review of all infants with CDH managed at Children's Hospital Boston revealed a significant increase in survival from 44% to 69% during the period in which permissive hypercapnia was used to manage these infants, with even higher survival rates noted in infants without coexisting heart disease (Table 72-8).[142] Of note, neither the introduction of ECMO nor delaying surgical repair was associated with significant increases in survival in this single-center historical experience.[142] Other case series have also reported favorable results using kinder and gentler ventilatory strategies rather than more aggressive techniques that attempt to control pulmonary vascular resistance.[137,143,144] These observations suggest that ventilator-associated lung injury greatly contributes to excess mortality in infants with CDH,[137,142] and it is possible that a survival benefit attributable to ECMO may emerge as lung-sparing mechanical ventilation is more widely applied.[142] At least one single-center experience suggests that epidural analgesia in the postoperative period facilitates spontaneous ventilation and may further improve pulmonary outcomes in these infants.[142]

Over the past decade, experience with the use of HFOV in infants with CDH has grown. For those clinicians who opt to use HFOV in this population, it is essential to understand that infants with CDH do not have inherently recruitable lungs, and attempts to improve gas exchange by applying high levels of mean airway pressure can actually increase the dead-space fraction and may result in both lung injury and potentially dangerous elevations in pulmonary vascular resistance.[145] Therefore, centers experienced in the use of HFOV in infants with CDH generally recommend trying to limit the mean airway pressure to 16 cm H_2O or less.[145] The Hospital for Sick Children in Toronto has developed an HFOV protocol for infants with CDH that emphasizes maintaining a preductal Sao$_2$ above 85%, tolerating hypercarbia with a compensated pH, and initiation of HFOV when the peak inspiratory pressure on conventional ventilation exceeds 25 cm H_2O. This group has reported a significant improvement in the survival of CDH infants since implementing this set of guidelines in 1995.[145]

Weaning the Pediatric Patient from Mechanical Ventilation

Although it is clear that it is best to discontinue mechanical ventilatory support as soon as feasible, a great deal of controversy surrounds ventilator mode selection, the pace of weaning, and timing of separation from mechanical support in children. In the largest pediatric study presently available in the literature, the use of specific weaning modes and ventilator weaning protocols was evaluated against standard care (no defined protocol) for mechanically ventilated infants and children.[146] Patients with alveolar disease as well as lower-airway disease were included, but those older than 2 years of age with status

TABLE 72-8	Therapeutic History and Outcomes for Congenital Diaphragmatic Hernia, Children's Hospital, Boston								
							Survival, Isolated CDH		
Year	*ECMO*	*Surgery*	*Ventilation*	*Paralysis*	*Analgesia*	*Monitoring*	*ECMO*	*CMV**	*Overall*
1981-84	N/A	Immediate	Hyper	Yes	High-dose fentanyl	Postductal	N/A	73%	73%
1984-87	Postop	Immediate	Hyper	Yes	High-dose fentanyl	Postductal	50%	67%	61%
1987-91	Preop	Delayed	Hyper	Yes	High-dose fentanyl	Postductal	48%	80%	57%
1991-94	Preop	Delayed	Permissive hypercapnia	No	Epidural	Preductal	71%	100%	84%
P value							NS	0.02	0.02

From Wilson JM, Lund DP, Lillehei CW, Vacanti JP. Congenital diaphragmatic hernia—a tale of two cities: the Boston experience. J Pediatr Surg 1997;32:401-5.
*Conventional mechanical ventilation.

asthmaticus and those with congenital diaphragmatic hernia were excluded. In this study, 182 intubated spontaneously breathing children who met standardized bedside criteria for extubation readiness were randomized to the protocolized application of pressure-support ventilation (PSV), volume-support ventilation (VSV), or no protocol.[146] There were no significant differences among the three treatment groups in extubation failure rates, and most children were weaned from the ventilator in 2 days or less.[146] In children who were successfully extubated, the median duration of ventilator weaning did not significantly differ according to mode of ventilation.[146]

Separating the infant or child with complex and/or chronic pulmonary disease from mechanical ventilation is challenging and requires an appreciation of the components of pulmonary dysfunction and timely recognition of acceptable mechanics and gas exchange in the spontaneously breathing patient. For example, the patient with a syndrome of alveolar hypoplasia is expected to be tachypneic at baseline, and this feature precludes the use of commonly applied criteria for extubation readiness. In these cases, weaning from mechanical ventilation can be guided by an ongoing assessment of tidal volume (measured at the tracheal tube), work of breathing, serum pH, and evidence of appropriate daily weight gain as pressure support is decreased.

Summary

A fundamental understanding of age-specific diagnostic and treatment considerations is required when caring for the pediatric patient with pulmonary disease. Although the capacity for physiologic compensation in infants and children is remarkably efficient, they are also prone to sudden and profound clinical deterioration, warranting the application of sophisticated supportive measures in the ICU. In recent years, work in the laboratory as well as the clinical arena has brought about an appreciation that in airway disease, alveolar disease, and complex conditions such as BPD and CDH, gentler strategies of mechanical ventilation may have a central role in improving functional outcomes. Thoughtful application of therapies proven to reverse pulmonary pathophysiology while promoting spontaneous ventilation as much as possible is likely to enhance already favorable survival statistics for even the most critically ill pediatric patients.

ANNOTATED REFERENCES

Ventilation with lower tidal volumes as compared with traditional tidal volumes for acute lung injury and the acute respiratory distress syndrome. The Acute Respiratory Distress Syndrome Network. N Engl J Med 2000;342:1301–8.

Landmark multicenter trial showing that in adult patients with ALI and ARDS ($Pao_2/Fio_2 \leq 300$), mechanical ventilation limiting tidal volumes to 6 cc/kg ideal body weight and plateau pressure ≤ 30 cm H_2O results in decreased mortality and more ventilator-free days when compared with tidal volumes of 12 cc/kg ideal body weight and plateau pressure ≤ 50 cm H_2O.

Flori HR, Glidden DV, Rutherford GW et al. Pediatric acute lung injury: prospective evaluation of risk factors associated with mortality. Am J Respir Crit Care Med 2005;171:995–1001.

Multicenter prospective cohort study describing the epidemiology of pediatric ALI and ARDS in the era of consensus diagnostic criteria.

Courtney SE, Durand DJ, Asselin JM, Hudak ML, Aschner JL, Shoemaker CT. High-frequency oscillatory ventilation versus conventional mechanical ventilation for very-low-birth-weight infants. N Engl J Med 2002;347:643–52.

Large multicenter, well-controlled trial demonstrating significant benefit of high-frequency oscillatory ventilation compared to conventional ventilation in very-low-birth-weight infants. Infants who received high-frequency oscillatory ventilation were successfully extubated earlier and were more likely to survive without need for supplemental oxygen at 36 weeks postmenstrual age. No increase was observed in the occurrence of intracranial hemorrhage or other complications referable to prematurity.

Inhaled nitric oxide and hypoxic respiratory failure in infants with congenital diaphragmatic hernia. The Neonatal Inhaled Nitric Oxide Study Group (NINOS). Pediatrics 1997;99:838–45.

Multicenter trial in which infants with isolated congenital diaphragmatic hernia and hypoxic respiratory failure were randomized to receive inhaled nitric oxide or 100% oxygen. The study was unable to show a survival benefit or reduction in need for extracorporeal membrane oxygenation among those infants who received nitric oxide.

Randolph AG, Wypij D, Venkataraman ST et al. Effect of mechanical ventilator weaning protocols on respiratory outcomes in infants and children: a randomized controlled trial. JAMA 2002;288:2561–8.

Large multicenter trial that evaluated standardized ventilator weaning protocols versus no defined protocol in pediatric patients mechanically ventilated for acute illness. Most of the study population was successfully weaned from the ventilator in 48 hours or less. Use of protocols for the gradual weaning of mechanical ventilatory support had no impact on the duration of mechanical ventilation.

REFERENCES

Access the complete reference list online at http://www.expertconsult.com.

73

Pulmonary Edema

ZVI VERED | SAAR MINHA | EDO KALUSKI | NIR URIEL

Definition

Pulmonary edema is a potentially life-threatening syndrome caused by excess fluid transition into the alveoli due to alternations in Starling's forces. This results in the disruption of gas exchange, tissue hypoxemia, respiratory acidosis, organ hypoxemia, and ultimately organ failure. Left untreated, this syndrome can rapidly progress to death.

Pulmonary Fluid Homeostasis

Pulmonary fluid homeostasis is dependent upon the equilibrium between forces that drive fluid into the alveolar space and counterforces responsible for its clearance—primarily lymphatics. One of the main regulatory forces for this fluid balance is the microvascular pressure in the alveolar capillaries, as presented by modification of the Starling's equation (Figure 73-1, *A*), which describes the balance between the hydrostatic pressure gradient and the oncotic pressure gradient. While the oncotic or osmolarity gradient is dependent mainly on protein concentrations, the pulmonary capillary hydrostatic pressure is dependent on pulmonary flow and resistance (see Figure 73-1, *B*). Pulmonary capillary pressure is regulated at the precapillary level by the arteriolar vasomotor tone, which determines the transmission of flow and pressures from the pulmonary artery to the capillary bed. By contrast, venous capillaries lack this protective mechanism, allowing unprotected transmission of elevated left ventricular pressure to the pulmonary capillary bed and excessive fluid accumulation.[1]

Protective mechanisms against fluid accumulation in the alveolar and interstitial space include both passive elements, such as the tight junctions between the alveolar epithelium, and active reabsorption of fluid from the airspace using Na^+ and Cl^- channels.[2] The primary sites of sodium and chloride reabsorption are the epithelial ion channels located on the apical membrane of alveolar epithelial cells (both type I and II) and the distal airway epithelial cells. Water will follow the osmotic gradient created by the reabsorption of Na^+ and Cl^-, preventing edema formation. Pulmonary edema will occur when this delicate balance is overwhelmed by one of three pathologic processes: impaired clearance mechanisms, increased hydrostatic pressures resulting in excessive pressure gradients, or increased permeability of the capillary alveolar barrier. When the main cause is related to increased pulmonary venous pressure, pulmonary edema is said to be *cardiogenic* in origin. In contrast, when other factors such as increased permeability prevail, the term *noncardiogenic pulmonary edema* is used. The interstitial fluid content in each etiology is different, owing to the underlying pathophysiology. Increased pulmonary venous pressures causing cardiogenic pulmonary edema will yield fluid with low protein content. Increased permeability of microvascular epithelium in noncardiogenic pulmonary edema will result in fluid with relatively high protein content.

Diagnosis and Assessment

HISTORY AND PRESENTING SYMPTOMS

The presenting signs and symptoms of pulmonary edema are dyspnea, tachypnea, and respiratory distress. Alveolar flooding can lead to cough and expectoration of frothy edema fluid. The history should focus on cardiogenic and noncardiogenic mechanisms contributing to pulmonary edema and elicit precipitating factors that might have led to edema formation. Common causes for cardiogenic pulmonary edema include ischemia, exacerbation of systolic or diastolic dysfunction (ischemia, infarct, or myopathic processes), severe valvular disease, or arrhythmias. A history of paroxysmal nocturnal dyspnea or progressive orthopnea usually indicates cardiogenic origin for pulmonary edema. However, silent ischemia may also present as pulmonary edema, with a paucity of clues provided by the history.[2] Noncardiogenic pulmonary edema is usually preceded by specific predisposing clinical situations such as pneumonia, sepsis, multiple blood transfusions, or intravenous (IV) illicit drug usage.

PHYSICAL EXAMINATION

Physical findings on lung examination are quite similar for cardiogenic and noncardiogenic pulmonary edema. The patient is usually tachypneic, pale, and diaphoretic with wet inspiratory rales/crackles heard over both lung fields, and most notably the bases. Patients with cardiogenic causes may present with an S_3 "gallop" on cardiac auscultation, indicating elevated left-ventricular diastolic pressures—a sign with high specificity (90%-97%) but low sensitivity (9%-51%).[2] Stenotic or regurgitant valvular murmurs on auscultation may indicate a cardiac cause but are not always related to the primary cause of the edema. Peripheral edema, which may be a sign for coexisting right heart failure, is neither sensitive nor specific for a cardiogenic origin of pulmonary edema. Most patients with cardiogenic causes for pulmonary edema will have cold, clammy skin, but some patients with noncardiogenic causes will present with warm skin, indicating decreased peripheral resistance.

AUXILIARY TESTS

Plain chest radiography has been reported to be more sensitive than clinical examination[3] for pulmonary edema, which makes it one of the cornerstones for this diagnosis. The first finding that indicates interstitial edema are "Kerley B" lines. These are 3- to 6-mm-long lines perpendicular to the pleural surface, usually at the bases (Figure 73-2). Another sign of interstitial edema is peribronchial cuffing resulting from edematous thickening of the bronchial wall. Redistribution of blood to the upper fields of the lungs results in upper-lobe blood vessel distension. When fluid eventually leaks to the alveoli, bilateral and diffuse opacities are seen, usually sparing the apices and extreme lung bases, causing a central "butterfly" distribution. As the process progresses, opacities may coalesce to produce a general "white-out" of the lungs.[4] Chest radiographs may aid in distinguishing between cardiogenic and noncardiogenic etiologies for pulmonary edema. In one study, it was demonstrated that in 50% of patients with cardiogenic edema there was upper-lobe blood diversion, whereas in patients with increased permeability edema due to acute respiratory distress syndrome (ARDS), only 10% showed this inverted pattern. Normal or "balanced" patterns were more commonly seen in ARDS. A peripheral distribution of edema was absent in patients with cardiogenic edema but was the most common pattern seen in patients with ARDS[5] (Figure 73-3). Unfortunately, about one out of five patients admitted for acute decompensated heart failure had no signs of congestion on chest radiograph[6]—a fact that emphasizes the importance of a holistic, integrative approach to the diagnosis of pulmonary edema.

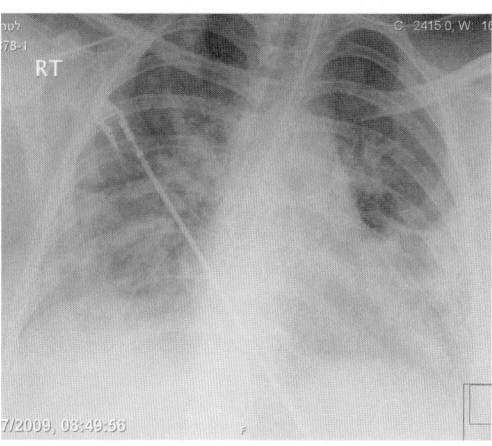

Figure 73-3 Chest x-ray images in ARDS. Diffuse bilateral opacities with involvement of peripheral lung fields.

$Q = K * (Pmv - Ppmv) - (\pi mv - \pi pmv)]$
Q = net transvascular flow of fluid
K = membrane (capillary) permeability
Pmv = hydrostatic pressure in the microvessels
Ppmv = hydrostatic pressure in the perimicrovascular interstitium
πmv = plasma protein oncotic pressure in the circulation
A πpmv = protein oncotic pressure in the perimicrovascular interstitium

$Pcap = LAP + (pulmRR * CO)$
Pcap = pulmonary capillary pressure
L_{ap} = left atrial pressure
pulmRR = pulmonary vascular resistance
B CO = cardiac output

Figure 73-1 A, Starling equation. **B,** Capillary pressure equation.

A novel approach utilizes ultrasound as a bedside tool to for the diagnosis of dyspnea and differentiation between pulmonary edema and other major dyspnea-causing diseases such as chronic obstructive pulmonary disease (COPD). Pulmonary edema induces abundant sonographic artifacts caused by interactions of water and air called *B-lines* or *comet tails* by some authors (Figure 73-4); these findings are usually not seen in other pulmonary diseases.[7] Electrocardiograms are useful in diagnosing active myocardial ischemia or to provide other clues regarding organic cardiac disease leading the pulmonary congestion.

BIOMARKERS

In recent years, a variety of biomarkers have been used to enhance the diagnostic accuracy of cardiogenic pulmonary edema. Brain natriuretic peptide (BNP) and N-terminal proBNP (NT-proBNP) are both secreted from the ventricles and correlate with the left ventricular (LV) end-diastolic pressure; however, heart failure with preserved LV function usually results in much lower BNP levels than heart failure with impaired LV systolic function. These biomarkers can be used for several indications in the intensive care unit (ICU). Among others, it may aid in differentiating between cardiogenic pulmonary edema and acute lung injury (ALI), monitor volume load in septic patients, and differentiate between septic and cardiogenic shock. Several conflicting reports have addressed the use of BNP/NT-proBNP for the differentiation between ALI and cardiogenic pulmonary edema.[8] Different cutoffs were used in the different trials, yielding various ranges of specificities and sensitivities for each diagnosis. It should be emphasized that these conflicting results arise in part from the fact that BNP increases with elevated right ventricular end-diastolic pressures and hypoxia, which are common properties of any severe lung disease. Based on currently available data, low levels of natriuretic peptide (BNP <100 pg/mL or NT-proBNP <250 pg/mL) may be used to exclude elevated cardiac filling pressures in patients presenting with respiratory failure with

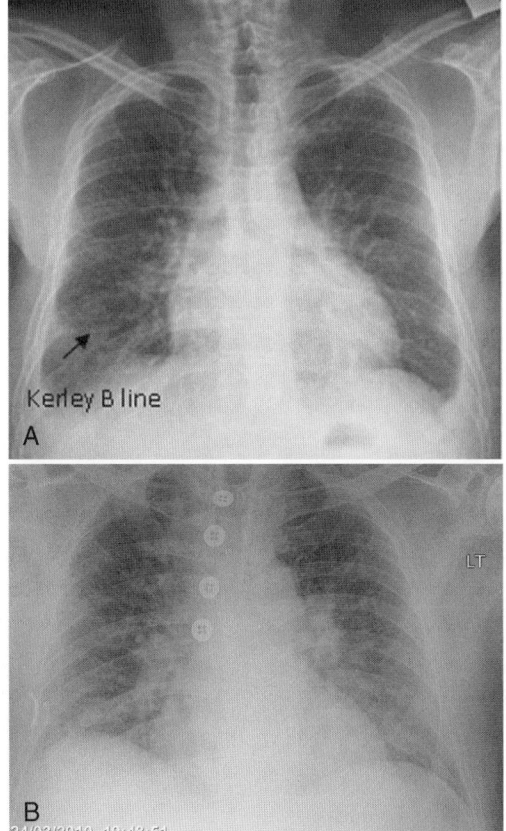

Figure 73-2   Chest x-ray images in pulmonary edema. A, Early stage of pulmonary edema/pulmonary congestion. Pulmonary congestion with redistribution of blood to upper lung fields, perihilar haze, and Kerley B lines. **B,** Pulmonary edema with perihilar diffuse densities and apical sparing ("butterfly" or "bat-wings".)

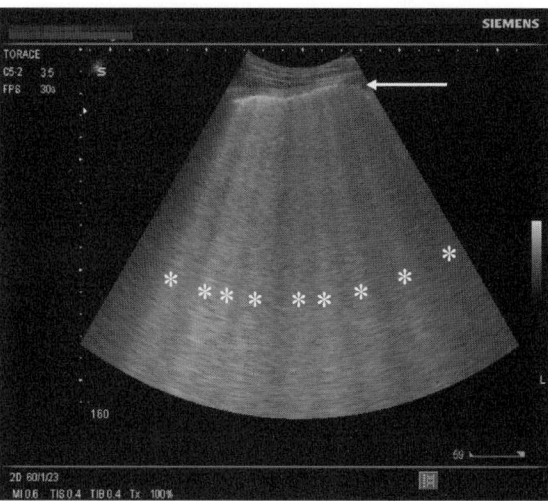

Figure 73-4 Ultrasound image demonstrating "B-lines" ("comet trails") in a dyspneic patient, indicating interstitial edema. *(Courtesy Giovanni Volpicelli, MD, FCCP, Department of Emergency Medicine, San Luigi Gonzaga University Hospital, Torino, Italy.)*

signs of pulmonary edema, whereas extremely elevated levels of these markers (BNP > 500 pg/mL and NT-proBNP > 1000 pg/mL) in the absence of signs and symptoms of septic shock will support a cardiogenic origin for pulmonary edema. The "gray zone" values between these extremes will necessitate further workup.[8] Cardiac troponin (cTn) I or T measurement are highly sensitive for myocardial injury, which can aid in the diagnosis of cardiac origin of pulmonary edema, but in the setting of critical illness, various nonischemic conditions (sepsis, stroke, pulmonary embolism, acute renal failure, etc.) can also induce elevation of cTn and should be excluded before concluding that the cTn elevation is "ischemic."

ECHOCARDIOGRAPHY

Transthoracic echocardiography (TTE) is used to assist with the diagnosis of myocardial, valvular, and structural pathologies that contribute to pulmonary edema and thus should be performed in any patient presenting with pulmonary edema. While severe valvular stenosis or regurgitation is readily visible on echocardiographic exam, evaluation of cardiac function is more challenging. Decreased myocardial function in patients presenting with pulmonary edema can be due either to past myocardial ischemia/infarction or a current, ongoing ischemic event complicated by pulmonary edema. Furthermore, depressed myocardial function is often seen in other conditions associated with critical illness, such as sepsis. On the other hand, preserved systolic LV function cannot exclude a cardiac origin of pulmonary edema, since patients can present with heart failure and preserved LV systolic function (formerly diastolic dysfunction), thus necessitating further evaluation. Echo-Doppler can also provide semiquantitative measurements of ventricular filling pressures, cardiac output, stroke volume, and pulmonary artery pressures. TEE is used to enhance and refine evaluation of structural and valvular pathologies such as native or prosthetic valve dysfunction, cardiac origins of embolism, infective endocarditis, and congenital diseases.[9] In one study performed in the ICU, TEE led to a significant change in management in 32% of cases,[10] emphasizing its diagnostic value.

HEMODYNAMIC ASSESSMENT

Pulmonary edema is a medical emergency and requires immediate medical therapy to alleviate symptoms. Dyspnea is the cardinal symptom of pulmonary edema and can be assessed subjectively (by analog scales of dyspnea severity) and objectively (by oxygen saturation, respiratory rate, alveolar-arterial difference, and acidemia). In most cases, the diagnosis, treatment, and monitoring of the patient with pulmonary edema is self-evident, but hemodynamic monitoring, either invasive or noninvasive, should be considered in selected patients. Since there are several techniques for hemodynamic assessment, the benefits and limitations of each technique should be considered prior to usage (Table 73-1).

Echo-Doppler

Echo-Doppler is part of the routine assessment of patients with pulmonary edema and can assess, in a semiquantitative manner, some of the hemodynamic parameters used for diagnosis and monitoring of response to therapy. However, echo-Doppler has shortcomings:

1. It is difficult to obtain reliable measurements of right heart pressures and estimate the left atrial pressure in a significant proportion of patients.
2. Although echo-Doppler can provide assessment of cardiac output (and hence cardiac index and cardiac power),[11] these measurements are time consuming, require an adequate ultrasound window, demand expertise, and are subject to considerable variability.
3. Echocardiography cannot provide the on-line continuous real-time monitoring or recording that is offered by right heart catheterization and impedance cardiography (ICG).

TABLE 73-1	Hemodynamic Monitoring Tools			
	Echo-Doppler	*Impedance Cardiography*	*Pulmonary Artery Catheter*	*Left Heart Catheterization*
Cardiac output, cardiac index, and cardiac power	+++	+++	+++	+
Right atrial pressure	++	−	+++	−
Right ventricular pressures	++	−	+++	−
Pulmonary artery pressures	++	−	+++	−
Left atrial pressures	+	−	++	+
Left ventricular pressures	+	−	−	+++
Systemic vascular resistance (SVR)	+	+++	+++	+
Pulmonary vascular resistance (PVR)	+	−	+++	−
Valvular disease	+++	−	TS, PS	AS, AI, MR
Diastolic dysfunction	+++	−	−	+
Systolic dyssynchrony	+++	−	−	+
Global and regional systolic function	+++	−	−	++
Thoracic fluid content	−	+++	−	−
Continuous on-line data monitoring and recording	−	+++	++	−
Shunt calculation	++	−	++ (Fluoroscopy guided)	−
Right heart saturations	−	−	+++ (Fluoroscopy guided)	−

AI, aortic insufficiency; *AS,* aortic stenosis; *MR,* mitral regurgitation; *PS,* pulmonic regurgitation; *TS,* tricuspid regurgitation.

4. Cardiac output (CO)/cardiac index (CI)/cardiac power (CP) obtained by echo-Doppler in its lower ranges are not reliable enough to discriminate between low cardiac output, such as in acute heart failure, and a cardiac output that is inconsistent with life ("cardiogenic shock").
5. Standard echocardiographic measurements of right atrial pressure and other derived right-sided pressures are often inaccurate in patients receiving mechanical ventilation.

Pulmonary Artery Catheterization and Other Invasive Modalities

Insertion of a pulmonary artery catheter permits measurement of the pulmonary capillary wedge pressure (PCWP), a method first described in 1970 by Swan and Ganz[12] and still considered to be the "gold standard" for diagnosis of pulmonary edema resulting from elevated LV diastolic filling pressures. Current monitoring systems that include cardiac output and systemic vascular resistance (SVR) calculators add further information and help distinguish cardiogenic pulmonary edema (high PCWP and high SVR) from noncardiac (low PCWP ± low/normal SVR). A wedge pressure of more than 18 mm Hg is indicative of elevated filling pressures of the left ventricle and usually indicates a cardiogenic origin of pulmonary edema. In addition to its utility in diagnosis, PCWP allows continuous monitoring of the LV filling pressure during treatment, facilitating the administration of appropriate therapy to alleviate pulmonary edema. It is recommended that pulmonary artery catheterization (PAC) be used in patients in whom a diagnostic dilemma exists, when echo-Doppler measurements are difficult to obtain, or in hemodynamically unstable patients not responding to conventional therapy.[13]

The clinical value and safety of PAC as a tool for hemodynamic assessment has been a subject of considerable debate. Gore[14] and Connors[15] demonstrated a neutral to negative effect of PAC on patient outcome. Meta-analyses assessing the effects of PAC on morbidity[16] and mortality[17] in clinical trials showed that mortality was unaffected, but morbidity was increased with the use of a PAC. There may be methodological issues in some of these studies; nevertheless, these publications resulted in a call for a moratorium[18] on PAC. In 1997, a consensus conference[19] attempted to reassess indications for PAC. Conditions that could be considered to benefit from PAC included myocardial infarction complicated by hypotension, shock, or mechanical complications, assessing and managing acute and chronic heart failure, and pulmonary hypertension. The ESCAPE study[20] enrolled patients with established heart failure who did not require PAC for their diagnosis or management. The results of the study have demonstrated no benefit of right heart catheterization in the study's primary endpoint (i.e., days alive out of hospital during the 6 months after randomization). Although the PAC is an invaluable tool for diagnostic, therapeutic, and prognostic assessment of PE, it should be used selectively by well-trained teams to address pertinent diagnostic and management issues.

Impedance Cardiography. Both thoracic impedance[21] and total body impedance[22,23] can accurately measure continuous CO and CI. ICG-derived COs appear to be less variable and more reproducible than CO measured by other techniques.[24] Some bioimpedance systems, however, do not provide accurate CO values[25] when compared to the gold standard of thermodilution.[26] However, bioimpedance devices that can measure CO reliably can serve as tools for assessing pump performance by providing noninvasive measurements of CP and cardiac power index (CPI). None of these systems provide assessment of right side pressures or pulmonary vascular resistance (PVR).

Beat-to-Beat Pulse Contour. Semi-invasive techniques utilizing beat-to-beat pulse-contour analysis are becoming available for continuous cardiac output monitoring. At present, there are conflicting reports regarding the usefulness of these techniques compared to invasively measured PCWP in assessing the presence of pulmonary edema in different ICU populations,[27-30] and no report has addressed the utility of pulse-contour analysis in differentiating between cardiac and noncardiac etiologies of pulmonary edema.

Noncardiogenic Pulmonary Edema

A variety of etiologies may lead to noncardiogenic pulmonary edema (Table 73-2), with a final common pathway of fluid accumulation in the lung interstitium due to either increased permeability of capillaries or decreased fluid clearance mechanisms without evidence of elevation of LV end-diastolic pressure.

ACUTE RESPIRATORY DISTRESS SYNDROME

ARDS is a severe form of ALI. This heterogeneous syndrome results from diffuse alveolar damage caused by excessive release of inflammatory mediators. These mediators activate neutrophils, macrophages,

TABLE 73-2	Etiology of Noncardiogenic Pulmonary Edema
Increased Capillary Permeability and Reduced Fluid Clearance	
Acute respiratory distress syndrome	
Neurogenic pulmonary edema	
Preeclampsia	
Transfusion related	
Toxins and Drugs	
Opiates	
Anticancer drugs	
Salicylate	
Thiazolidinedione	
Tricyclic antidepressants	
Alveolar-Capillary Pressure Imbalance	
Perioperative pulmonary edema	
Elevated Capillary Pressure (Fluid Shift/Excessive Fluid Transfusion)	
Peripartum pulmonary edema	
Ovarian hyperstimulation	
Exertional pulmonary edema	
Hypoxia Related	
High-altitude pulmonary edema	
Rapid Change in Intrathoracic Pressure	
Post upper airway obstruction	
Post pneumonectomy	
Post evacuation of pleural/pericardial effusion	

and other pulmonary cell populations which, in turn, release other mediators such as proteases that result in capillary endothelial damage, causing protein-rich fluid to leak into the interstitium and, at advanced stages, into the alveolar space. ARDS is manifested as acute-onset respiratory failure, hypoxemia (with $Pao_2/Fio_2 < 200$), and bilateral pulmonary infiltrates without evidence of elevated left atrial pressure. A wide variety of etiologies can lead to ARDS (e.g., sepsis, pneumonia, and multiple blood transfusions). ARDS may be confused with diffuse alveolar hemorrhage or malignancy (mainly lymphoma) involving both lungs; a thorough investigation must exclude such diagnoses.

PERIOPERATIVE PULMONARY EDEMA

Perioperative pulmonary edema can result from a wide variety of etiologies including volume overload, negative pressure pulmonary edema (resulting from exaggerated negative intrathoracic pressure generated by an inspiratory effort against a closed glottis), and transfusions. In one large trial including 8159 patients undergoing major outpatient surgical procedures, an incidence of 7.6% of postoperative pulmonary edema was noted with approximately 12% mortality; of note, prior reports had reported lower rates of pulmonary edema and mortality.[31,32] Excessive fluid administration during the postoperative period was associated with increased mortality, especially in patients without other comorbidities. Fluid overload during and after surgery can be attributed to exaggerated treatment for hypotension related to anesthesia, excessive blood loss, fluid shifts during surgery ("third spacing"), and postoperative fever. The relatively common incidence of pulmonary edema after surgery leads to a recommendation for close monitoring of fluid balance in the perioperative period, with special emphasis on monitoring patients at risk for developing pulmonary edema because of preexistent medical problems, including cardiac disease.

HIGH-ALTITUDE PULMONARY EDEMA

High-altitude pulmonary edema (HAPE) is the abnormal accumulation of edema involving the interstitial and alveolar spaces; it is due to a breakdown in the pulmonary blood-gas barrier. This is triggered by hypobaric hypoxia and rapid ascent to altitudes above 2500 m. Such hypoxia triggers a maladaptive mechanism including poor ventilatory response, increased sympathetic tone, exaggerated and uneven pulmonary vasoconstriction (pulmonary hypertension), and inadequate production of hormonal mediators (e.g., nitric oxide [NO]) that then lead to capillary leak and pulmonary edema.[33] The risk for developing HAPE depends on individual susceptibility, altitude ascent rate, and time spent at the altitude. The incidence of HAPE increases at different heights, ranging from 0.2% to 6% at 4500 m to 2% to 15% at 5500 m.[34] Clinical symptoms that precede presentation of pulmonary edema include shortness of breath, nonproductive cough, and difficulty in continuing to ascend to greater heights. such symptoms can easily be mistaken for exhaustion. The symptoms usually appear 2 to 4 days after arriving at a new altitude. It is unusual for HAPE to develop after more than 1 week at the same altitude. When symptoms progress, the patient becomes easily exhausted and may have productive pink sputum. In the later stages, the patient becomes severely hypoxemic, a situation that may be fatal without medical treatment. A favorable outcome depends on early recognition of the patient's signs and symptoms, using supplementary oxygen, rapid descent to lower altitude, or the use of a hyperbaric chamber. No pharmacologic intervention beyond oxygen has been proven to be beneficial for HAPE, but several pharmacologic agents have been examined. Nifedipine (calcium channel blocker) may aid in both lowering the elevated pulmonary pressure and the systemic resistance. Tadalafil and sildenafil are phosphodiesterase-5 inhibitors acting on the pulmonary vasculature by increasing the amount of available nitric oxide. These agents have been shown to be beneficial for prophylactic treatment of HAPE but have not been examined in the treatment of this condition. Salmeterol, an inhaled β-agonist, has been proposed as a prophylactic drug for HAPE that may also be useful for treatment.

PREGNANCY-RELATED PULMONARY EDEMA

Pregnancy causes significant hemodynamic changes in the cardiovascular system, including increase in plasma volume, cardiac output, heart rate, and capillary permeability, as well as decreased colloid osmotic pressure. In light of these and other factors, pulmonary edema may occur in pregnant women with preexisting cardiac conditions or abnormalities (cardiomyopathies and valvular disease) or with pregnancy-related abnormalities such as preeclampsia. The incidence of pulmonary edema ranges from 0.08% in normal pregnancies to 3.4% in preeclampsia and up to 5% in preterm labor.[35] In a large survey including 62,917 women, the overall incidence of pulmonary edema was 0.08%. Among the pregnant women who developed pulmonary edema, the most common attributable causes or associated conditions were tocolytic use (13 patients [25.5%]), cardiac disease (13 patients [25.5%]), fluid overload (11 patients [21.5%]), and preeclampsia (9 patients [18%]).[36] The diagnosis of pulmonary edema was made during the antepartum period in 24 patients (47%), the intrapartum period in 7 (14%), and the postpartum period in 20 (39%). The increased incidence of pulmonary edema in the intra- and postpartum period can be attributed to changes in the plasma colloid pressure. Plasma colloid pressure decreases from about 22 to 16 mm Hg at term after delivery in normal pregnancy, and from 18 to 14 mm Hg postpartum in preeclampsia complicated pregnancies. This reduction is attributed to blood loss and fluid shift due to increased vascular permeability, especially in pregnancies with preeclampsia, and leads to pulmonary edema occurring after delivery.[37] Women with preeclampsia are at increased risk for the development of pulmonary edema due to underlying endothelial damage and decreased colloid osmotic pressure, which cause leakage into the pulmonary interstitium or alveolar space.

The development of pulmonary edema associated with pregnancy appears to be influenced by maternal age, parity, and preexisting essential hypertension. In a small study examining the role of echocardiography in the diagnosis of pulmonary edema in the setting of preeclampsia, 25% of the patients had decreased systolic function, and a significant number of the remaining patients had elevated diastolic pressures when compared to other pregnant hypertensive/normotensive women without preeclampsia, thereby indicating that elevated filling pressure may be a part of the pathologic process in preeclampsia.[38]

Tocolytics are also a major cause for pulmonary edema during pregnancy. Therapy using β-agonists can cause increased hydrostatic pressure and lead to pulmonary edema.[39] Pulmonary edema has also been reported after usage of calcium channel blockers as tocolytics.[40] As in most patients with pulmonary edema, the mainstay of treatment includes fluid restriction, diuretics, and cessation of tocolytics.

There are a wide array of etiologies that may cause dyspnea in pregnant women, ranging from positional (supine) dyspnea to more severe conditions such as pulmonary embolism. Careful consideration of the differential diagnosis and risk factors in pregnancy will influence the intensity of the clinical workup while taking into account both maternal and fetal risks.

POSTOBSTRUCTIVE PULMONARY EDEMA

Postobstructive pulmonary edema (POPE) was first described in 1973 as sudden onset of pulmonary edema following relief of upper airway obstruction. The incidence may be up to 10% of cases after the relief of acute obstruction and up to 40% after relief of chronic obstruction.[41] Two types are described: type I POPE follows a sudden, severe episode of upper airway obstruction such as postextubation laryngospasm, epiglottitis, or croup and is seen in strangulation and hanging; type II POPE develops after surgical relief of chronic upper airway obstruction.[42] Type I POPE usually develops within 1 hour after the event, but it can be delayed up to 6 hours. In contrast, there is close proximity between the relief of the obstruction and the development of POPE in type II.

The etiology for type I POPE is multifactorial. Negative intrathoracic pressure is caused by inhaling against closed obstruction. This causes increased venous return, decreased cardiac output, and fluid transudation into the alveolar space.[43] Risk factors for type I POPE are young age (owing to increased ability to generate increased negative pressure), direct suctioning of the endotracheal tube during thoracotomy, narcotics, short neck, oral or pharyngeal surgery or pathology, vocal cord paralysis, conditions leading to increased capillary-alveolar pressure gradients, endotracheal tube obstruction, and premature extubation. The etiology for type II POPE, which is less frequent than type I, is less clear. It is suggested that the obstructive lesion causes constant positive end-expiratory pressure (PEEP) with increased end-expiratory lung volume. Relief of the obstruction causes immediate reduction of the lung volume that is postulated to result in increased pulmonary permeability and transudation of fluid. The diagnosis usually is suggested by physical findings after surgery of tachypnea, tachycardia, agitation, and frothy pulmonary secretions. The diagnosis is confirmed by x-ray. Most patients will respond quickly to standard therapy with adjunct support of PEEP (5 mm H_2O).

REEXPANSION PULMONARY EDEMA

Reexpansion pulmonary edema (REPE) after spontaneous pneumothorax is a rare complication of tube thoracostomy, with reported mortality ranging from 0 to 20%.[30,31,44,45] Most patients will present with symptoms as early as 1 hour after thoracostomy, but delayed presentation of up to 24 hours after thoracostomy has also been described. Tachypnea, tachycardia, and hypoxia are the main presenting signs and symptoms. The chest radiograph demonstrates unilateral pulmonary edema, although bilateral pulmonary edema has rarely been reported. In a recent study, many REPE cases were mild and asymptomatic and only diagnosed by computed tomography (CT) of the chest. Most cases will resolve within 24 to 72 hours.

The pathophysiology of REPE is unclear. The main hypothesis is that capillary leak is induced by a postexpansion inflammatory process. During reexpansion, mechanical injury to the alveolar-capillary membrane, together with reperfusion injury from the reinstitution of blood flow, initiates an acute inflammatory process. Predictive factors for REPE are age (20-39 years) and prolonged duration of pneumothorax prior to relief.[46] It was also suggested that REPE may be related to the application of negative pressure to the chest tube. No human study has been performed prospectively to determine whether the incidence of REPE would be less if the chest tube is put to water seal only. Unfortunately, REPE can also occur in patients whose lungs are reexpanded without suction. REPE therefore appears to be related to three factors: longer duration of pneumothorax, greater size of the pneumothorax, and a rapid rate of expansion after tube thoracostomy. Controlling for one factor may not prevent the process if one or two of the other factors are present. In lieu of a randomized controlled trial, the American College of Chest Physicians (ACCP) recommends that in the presence of a spontaneous pneumothorax in clinically stable patients with a large (≥30% of the lung field) primary pneumothorax, either a small-bore (14F or smaller) catheter or 16 to 22F chest tube with the tube connected to Heimlich valve or a water-seal device be placed. However, if the lung fails to reexpand, application of negative pressure to the chest tube is deemed appropriate.[47]

Therapy for REPE is supportive. Mechanical ventilation with PEEP and hemodynamic support may be appropriate. Some authors recommend nonsteroidal antiinflammatory drugs (NSAIDs), but there are no studies to support their use. Patient positioning also may be therapeutic when pulmonary edema is unilateral. In these cases, the lateral decubitus position with the affected side up will reduce intrapulmonary shunting and improve oxygenation.

TRANSFUSION-RELATED PULMONARY EDEMA

Acute onset of dyspnea shortly after blood transfusion can be attributed to two main etiologies: transfusion-associated cardiac overload (TACO) and immune-mediated ALI resulting from transfusion of plasma-containing products (transfusion-related ALI, or TRALI).[48] TRALI was defined by the National Heart, Lung, and Blood Institute Working Group as an ALI that develops within 6 hours after blood transfusion.[49] TRALI is considered to be the leading cause for transfusion-related mortality. Virtually all blood products can lead to TRALI, but infusions of whole blood, platelets, packed red blood cells, and fresh frozen plasma are the most commonly identified precipitating causes. Owing to nonuniformity of definitions, the true incidence of TRALI is uncertain, but when uniform definitions are used, the incidence is reported to be 1 case for every 1000 to 2400 units transfused, with equal incidence between men and women and wide age variability.[50] Risk factors for TRALI are prolonged storage of blood products, fresh frozen plasma infusion, and underlying conditions such as recent surgery, thrombocytopenia, and massive transfusions. The pathogenesis of TACO is similar to other causes of acute congestive heart failure: volume overload leading to increased central and pulmonary pressures resulting in increased hydrostatic pressure and extravasation of fluid into the alveolar space. The pathogenesis of TRALI is less obvious. Three hypotheses are proposed: (1) antigranulocyte antibodies in the donor's plasma (or less commonly, in the recipient's plasma) react with antigens on the recipient's (or less commonly, donor's) granulocytes to initiate an inflammatory response within the pulmonary microvasculature; (2) biologically active substances such as lipids and cytokines contained within the transfusions prime granulocytes in the pulmonary vasculature, contributing to increased vascular permeability; or (3) a "two-hit" hypothesis wherein the primary stimulus causes granulocyte sequestration in the pulmonary capillaries, and a secondary stimulus causes the granulocytes to "activate," damaging the endothelial layer such that fluid and protein leak into the alveolar space. Surgery, infections, and other situations can serve as the initial primer for this process.[51]

The clinical presentation of TACO is indistinguishable from other forms of cardiogenic and noncardiogenic PE, with tachypnea, tachycardia, and respiratory distress developing within several hours of blood-product infusion. Although TRALI can also present with some of these symptoms, specific clues can aid in the differentiation between these two entities: TRALI often presents with hypotension, fever, and transient leukopenia (leading to a clinical presentation similar to ARDS), whereas the absence of fever and the presence of hypertension usually suggests TACO. Pulmonary capillary wedge pressure is elevated in TACO and usually normal in TRALI. BNP levels may be higher than 1200 pg/mL in TACO, with transudative features in the pleural fluid analysis, as opposed to BNP less than 200 pg/mL and exudative features in TRALI.

The mainstay of TACO treatment is discontinuation of blood-product transfusion, respiratory support as needed, and diuretics. It has been suggested that subsequent blood products should be infused at a slower rate after the appearance of TACO, but no solid evidence supports this suggestion. TRALI treatment is mainly supportive: mechanical positive-pressure invasive ventilation and high concentrations of oxygen and PEEP. Although some authors have advocated the use of steroids for TRALI, this approach is still considered anecdotal.[52] The mortality rate for TRALI varies between 5% and 8%, but rates of up to 47% in critically ill patients have also been reported.[48] Most survivors recover completely with appropriate treatment. It is recommended that patients who recover from TRALI should not receive any other blood products from the same donor, but it seems they are not at increased risk for TRALI when receiving blood products from other donors.

DRUG TOXICITIES

Development of pulmonary edema has been linked to a number of drugs and substances.

Opiates

Opiate overdose can induce pulmonary edema due to increased capillary permeability. Interstitial protein content in this setting is similar to the plasma protein content. The pulmonary capillary wedge pressure is generally within the normal range. Direct toxic and hypoxic etiologies have also been suggested as contributing mechanisms in this clinical setting. The incidence of pulmonary edema in patients with heroin overdose is 0.8% to 2.4%,[53] with most of the symptoms developing over the first 2 hours of admission. The entire opiate family shares the ability to induce pulmonary edema, and even overdose of codeine has been linked to this condition.[54] Most patients require mechanical ventilation to correct severe hypoxia and respond within 24 to 36 hours to supportive care.

Salicylates

Salicylate intoxication can induce pulmonary edema. The mainstay of treatment for aspirin intoxication is volume resuscitation and bicarbonate, which can lead to volume overload and pulmonary edema that cannot be easily differentiated from ALI. Development of pulmonary edema in the setting of aspirin intoxication is an indication for immediate hemodialysis.[55]

Other Drugs

Other drugs, including thiazides, rituximab, propofol, and cytarabine, have been associated with noncardiogenic pulmonary edema.

NEUROGENIC PULMONARY EDEMA

Acute central nervous system (CNS) injury may lead to a clinical presentation similar to ARDS.[56] Symptoms develop within minutes to several hours after the offending injury. Classic signs and symptoms of pulmonary edema include tachycardia, tachypnea, basilar rales on auscultation, and bilateral infiltrates on chest radiograph. Both cardiac output and pulmonary capillary wedge pressure are normal in this situation. These signs and symptoms together with evidence of acute CNS injury establish the diagnosis. The most common causes for neurogenic pulmonary edema (NPE) are epileptic seizures, head injury, and cerebral hemorrhage, but any intracranial or spinal injury can be associated with this condition.[56]

There are several theories describing the precipitating factors leading to NPE. Excessive stimulation of the autonomic nervous system can result in pulmonary venous vasoconstriction, causing elevations in hydrostatic pressure and extravasation of fluid into the pulmonary interstitium. This mechanism is supported by data showing the ability of α-adrenergic agonists to alleviate pulmonary edema caused by cerebral stimulation in rats.[57] Furthermore, rapid elevation of pulmonary venous pressure may cause microvascular injury and excessive capillary permeability, leading to ALI. Two etiologies must be differentiated from NPE in the setting of an intubated head injured patient: aspiration pneumonia and ventilator-associated pneumonia (VAP). The treatment of NPE must first focus on treatment of the offending head/spinal injury. It is essential that hematomas are evacuated, intracranial pressure (ICP) decreased, and convulsions controlled. Other supportive therapies include ventilation that meets the oxygenation needs of the patient, with permissive hypercapnia allowed only in patients with ICP monitoring, and avoidance of high PEEP that may reduce cerebral perfusion. Hemodynamic support should aim to maintain low cardiac filling pressures without compromising cerebral perfusion. Invasive hemodynamic monitoring may be required. The exact place of α- and β-adrenergic agents in the therapy of NPE is not established. Most NPE episodes will resolve within 48 to 72 hours.

OTHER NONCARDIOGENIC ETIOLOGIES OF ACUTE PULMONARY EDEMA

Massive pulmonary embolism (PE) can cause pulmonary edema due to elevated hydrostatic pressure and injury to adjacent pleural and pulmonary vasculature. Viral infections can also induce pulmonary edema, as demonstrated in severe cases of Hanta virus infection.[58] Other viruses, including enteroviruses and coronavirus, can also lead to pulmonary edema.

There are reports of pulmonary edema in trained athletes after strenuous exercise such as marathon running or swimming. The theories that explain this phenomenon point to preexisting ventilation/perfusion mismatch in combination with increased cardiac output, causing elevated hydrostatic pressure that leads to pulmonary edema.[59,60] Cold water immersion can induce pulmonary edema by both increasing cardiac output and elevating pulmonary vascular resistance and pressures.

Cardiogenic Pulmonary Edema

DEFINITION AND PATHOPHYSIOLOGY

Pulmonary edema is a life-threatening presentation of acute heart failure (AHF). AHF is defined as rapid onset or change in the signs or symptoms of heart failure, resulting in the need for urgent therapy. It may be new or worsening of a preexisting condition.[13] During 2006 there were over 1 million admissions in the United States alone with AHF as the primary diagnosis and more than 3 million admissions with heart failure as a secondary diagnosis, with a direct and indirect cost of 25 million and 37.2 million U.S. dollars, respectively.

AHF is predominantly a disease of the elderly. The primary cardiac pathologies that predispose the patient to develop AHF can be related to ischemic, myocardial, valvular, pericardial, or rhythm disorders. Noncardiac factors may also contribute to the development of AHF by increasing pressure (hypertension) and volume overload (Table 73-3). The precipitating insult leading to the appearance of signs and symptoms of AHF are diverse and include (among others) active ischemia, increased afterload (hypertensive emergencies), increased preload (volume overload), circulatory failure due to high output state (sepsis, thyrotoxicosis, anemia), and drugs (NSAIDs or discontinuation of prescribed drugs).

Cardiogenic pulmonary edema results from transudation of protein-poor fluid from the alveolar interstitium into the alveolar space as a result of rapid increase in pulmonary capillary pressure overwhelming alveolar fluid reabsorption mechanisms. Mild elevations in LV and left atrial pressures (18-25 mm Hg) cause edema in the perimicrovascular and peribronchovascular interstitial spaces. As left atrial pressure rises further (>25 mm Hg), edema fluid floods the alveoli with protein-poor fluid, leading to the full-blown presentation of pulmonary

TABLE 73-3	Common Precipitating Factors for Acute Heart Failure	
Noncompliance with medical regimen, sodium and/or fluid restriction	Atrial fibrillation and other arrhythmias
Acute myocardial ischemia or ischemia	Recent addition of negative inotropic drugs (e.g., verapamil, nifedipine, diltiazem, beta-blockers)
Uncorrected high blood pressure	Pulmonary embolism
Nonsteroidal antiinflammatory drugs	Excessive alcohol or illicit drug use
Stress related cardiomyopathy	Concurrent infections (pneumonia, viral illnesses)
Cardiac toxicity: chemotherapy	Worsening lung disease (respiratory insufficiency or failure)
Anemia	Acute renal failure

Adapted from Hunt et al. 2009 focused update incorporated into the ACC/AHA 2005 Guidelines for the Diagnosis and Management of Heart Failure in Adults: a report of the American College of Cardiology Foundation/American Heart Association Task Force on Practice Guidelines. Circulation 2009;119:e391-479.

edema.[2] Cardiovascular failure leading to pulmonary edema may be the result of reduced LV contractility and increased systemic vascular resistance, or from impaired LV filling due to abnormal relaxation or excessive stiffness.

Traditionally it is thought that volume overload, nonadherence to medical therapy, ischemia, and arrhythmia can all induce decrease in cardiac contractility and progressive volume overload. It seems that all these factors may serve as triggers for cardiogenic pulmonary edema, but other factors are also crucial for the initiation of an acute episode of decompensated heart failure.[61] Vascular resistance and afterload mismatch are probably the predominant mechanisms in a substantial proportion of these events. Invasive monitoring of patients in AHF episodes often reveals decreased cardiac contractility compared to baseline and increased systemic vascular resistance (SVR)—a mismatch between rapidly increasing afterload (or SVR) and impaired systolic performance resulting in an acute elevation of LV end-diastolic pressures and decrease in cardiac output.

The exact mechanism responsible for the acute elevation of SVR in cardiogenic pulmonary edema is unknown, but it is likely that patients with chronic heart failure have increased arterial stiffness. Diastolic dysfunction is associated with elevated filling pressures and pulmonary congestion and has a role in triggering AHF. Systolic function (or reduced LVEF) was reported to correlate weakly with hemodynamic measures of contractility as well as outcome.

The association between AHF and decreased renal function (cardiorenal syndrome) is well established, and renal dysfunction is a powerful predictor of all-cause mortality in AHF patients. Regardless of the cause for renal function deterioration, the failing kidney leads to increased sodium retention and decreased water clearance. Another potential trigger for AHF is neurohormonal and inflammatory activation. Experimental models have demonstrated that inflammatory cytokines may induce diastolic dysfunction, reduce contractility, and increase capillary permeability.

As in chronic heart failure, the neurohormonal system in AHF shows increased activation, with release of norepinephrine, endothelins, angiotensin-2, aldosterone, antidiuretic hormone, and BNP; these mediators enhance arterial stiffness and elevated SVR. Other triggers for AHF include ventricular dyssynchrony, valvular disease, rhythm disorders, and noncardiac precipitators.

Cardiogenic pulmonary edema due to AHF can be considered a two-step process: induction and amplification (Figure 73-5). The initiation phase, or "cardiac pathway," is caused by low cardiac reserve in the cardiac pathway due to factors such as prior myocardial infarction or nonadherence to medications; such factors can be amplified by an acute decrease in contractility. This decrease is then exacerbated by an acute decrease in contractility due to arrhythmia, ischemia, or inflammatory activation. In contrast, the "vascular pathway" is activated in individuals with mild to moderate impairment in contractile reserve,

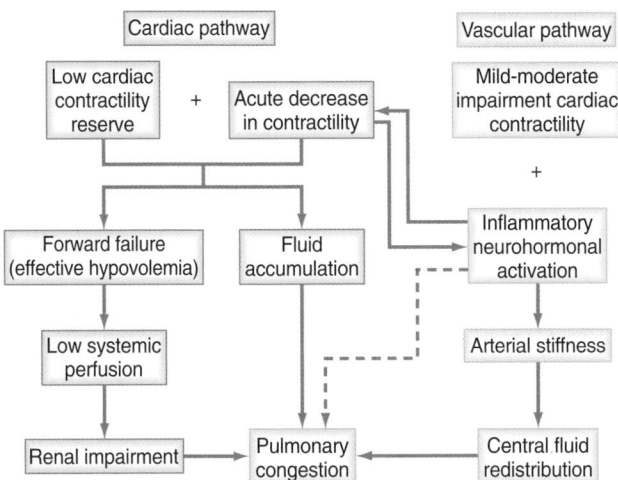

Figure 73-5 Early phases of acute heart failure. *(Adapted from Cotter G, Felker GM, Adams KF, Milo-Cotter O, O'Connor CM. The pathophysiology of acute heart failure—is it all about fluid accumulation? Am Heart J 2008;155:9-18.)*

but it rarely leads to AHF by itself. Here, a variety of offenders (neurohormonal activation, inflammation, aging processes) will abruptly lead to afterload mismatch, resulting in forward heart failure without a significant change in the LV systolic function (as assessed by LVEF). In most patients, both pathways coexist, and their combination may lead to the combination of excessive pulmonary venous pressure and pulmonary edema, along with reduced cardiac output, resulting in reduction of perfusion of vital organs. AHF can then be further exacerbated through additional mechanisms, including:

1. AHF induces hypoxia, acidosis, and hypoperfusion that then may provoke myocardial ischemia even if the offending trigger was not ischemic. These changes, along with platelet activation and resultant inflammatory processes, may cause further deterioration of myocardial contractility and exacerbation of heart failure.
2. Right ventricular failure caused by increased pulmonary venous and pulmonary arterial pressures due to fluid extravasation, hypoxia, and vasoconstriction will lead to disturbed interventricular interaction, further compromising LV performance.
3. Respiratory failure with decreased arterial oxygen saturation (yielding suboptimal tissue oxygenation) and ventilatory failure may be accompanied by respiratory acidosis, which may lead to decreased cardiac output, eventually resulting in respiratory failure superimposed on cardiovascular failure.
4. Leakage of the alveolar-capillary membrane and decreased alveolar fluid clearance as a result of initiation of pulmonary inflammatory processes. Although debated, it seems that inflammatory processes activated during pulmonary edema may interfere with fluid-clearance mechanisms, further enhancing pulmonary edema.
5. Most patients with cardiogenic pulmonary edema or AHF have renal function impairment at baseline. During pulmonary edema, they may develop the cardiorenal syndrome described earlier. Acute tubular necrosis can be induced by hypoperfusion, with resultant activation of neurohormonal protective mechanisms involving the renin-angiotensin system, sympathetic nervous system, vasopressin, and endothelin. Renal dysfunction, accompanied by renal hypoperfusion, may cause intravascular and extravascular fluid overload and exacerbation of symptoms.
6. Arrhythmias, especially atrial tachyarrhythmias, are common in AHF patients and can lead to decreased LV filling, with further augmentation of heart failure.

CLASSIFICATION

AHF leading to pulmonary edema reflects a wide spectrum of conditions. The European Society of Cardiology (ESC) has defined 6 possible clinical categories that may be complicated by pulmonary edema:

1. Worsening/decompensated heart failure: progression of known chronic heart failure presents as peripheral edema and/or pulmonary edema.
2. Pulmonary edema: severe respiratory distress, tachypnea, rales, and arterial oxygen saturation less than 90% on room air
3. Hypertensive heart failure: signs and symptoms of AHF in the setting of significantly elevated blood pressure and preserved LV systolic function. Patients usually present with signs of increased sympathetic tone and pulmonary edema, but without signs of peripheral edema.
4. Cardiogenic shock: tissue hypoperfusion due to heart failure after correction of preload and arrhythmia. The clinical signs and symptoms include signs of poor perfusion (low urine output), low blood pressure (<90 mm Hg systolic or a drop of >30 mm Hg in mean blood pressure).
5. Isolated right heart failure: low-output failure presenting with increased jugular venous pressure in the absence of pulmonary congestion and low LV filling pressures
6. Acute coronary syndrome (ACS) accompanied by heart failure: about 15% of patients with ACS present with signs of heart failure that are often associated with arrhythmia.

One of the most clinically applicable classifications of AHF is the modified Forrester classification[62] (Table 73-4). This classification utilizes a 4-square table to define the clinical status of the patient and establish treatment strategy. Most patients will present in category B (warm and wet) and will respond favorably to medical therapy (composed predominantly of loop diuretics and vasodilators). Patients in category C (cold and wet) will require inotropic agents and vasodilators to improve tissue perfusion and promote diuresis. Category A (warm and dry) is found in heart failure patients who present with dyspnea or edema that appears to be unrelated to the heart failure. In this setting, other causes such as respiratory disease or sepsis should be sought. Category L stands for "light," representing either a rare situation of overdiuresis of category-B patients or patients who are free of symptoms at rest but develop symptoms with exercise.

DIAGNOSIS

The etiology of cardiogenic pulmonary edema presenting as acute decompensated heart failure includes decreased contractility, increased systemic vascular resistance, or a combination of the two. Along with providing the immediate treatment needed for stabilization, initial assessment should focus on volume status, adequacy of vital organ perfusion, delineation of the cardiac pathology, and determination of the role of precipitating factors (see Table 73-3).

The history should include preexisting chronic diseases, such as diabetes mellitus and hypertension, and acute conditions that may have triggered the exacerbation, such as recent infection or a recent change in drug therapy. The diagnosis in a patient with known chronic heart failure is usually straightforward, but cases of new-onset AHF

TABLE 73-4	Modified Forrester Classification		
Congestion at rest (wet)? (Congestion – orthopnea, jugular venous pressure, edema)			
Yes	No		
B – Warm and wet	A –Warm and dry	No	Low perfusion at rest (cold)? (Low perfusion – narrow pulse pressure, cool extremities)
C – Cold and wet	L – cold and dry	Yes	

Modified from Stevenson LW. Tailored therapy to hemodynamic goals for advanced heart failure. Eur J Heart Fail 1999;1:251-7.

are more challenging, demanding exclusion of life-threatening situations including myocardial ischemia. The physical exam should focus on the signs and symptoms of heart failure mentioned earlier in this chapter. S_3 gallop, S_4, and new murmurs (especially new regurgitant or an altered mitral regurgitation murmur) must be sought, along with rales on lung auscultation. All patients must be evaluated for active unstable coronary disease by utilizing electrocardiography (ECG) and cardiac markers. ST-segment elevation or depression and new or dynamic T-wave changes may indicate acute coronary syndrome. Arrhythmias on ECG may serve as triggers for AHF and should be excluded. Elevated cardiac markers may establish the diagnosis of myocardial infarction, but mild elevations of cardiac troponin may also be caused by AHF; thus increases in cardiac troponin should be interpreted cautiously. A chest radiograph is mandatory for the diagnosis of pulmonary edema. Other laboratory tests include complete blood count for the exclusion of anemia and severe leukocytosis (indicating infection), blood chemistry for the evaluation of electrolytes and renal function, and other tests such as NT-proBNP that can aid in establishing the diagnosis when the etiology of dyspnea is equivocal. The roles of BNP/NT-proBNP level and Doppler-echocardiography have been discussed earlier. Other noninvasive imaging tests can aid in the diagnostic workup. Cardiac magnetic resonance (CMR) imaging is useful for the detection of myocardial alterations, including inflammatory or infiltrative processes, thus aiding in the diagnosis of myocarditis, cardiomyopathies, and storage and infiltrative diseases. CT coronary angiography, a new rapidly developing technique, may replace invasive coronary angiography in patients with low/moderate pretest probability for coronary artery disease.

Heart Failure with Preserved Ejection Fraction

Close to 50% of patients admitted with AHF have relatively preserved LV systolic ejection fraction (LVEF > 45%). Increasing age, female gender, hypertension, small size heart on chest radiograph, and an ischemia- or infarction-free ECG may suggest the diagnosis of heart failure with preserved ejection fraction (HFPEF; formally known as *diastolic dysfunction*). Pulmonary edema in this setting is related to complex pathophysiologic processes that are only partially elucidated. Stressors lead to increased venous vasoconstriction, which in turn increases the blood flow to the right ventricle, lung, and eventually the left ventricle. Owing to limitations in LV compliance, this excessive flow can not be accommodated by the left ventricle without considerable rise in left ventricular, left atrial, and pulmonary venous pressures. The elevated pulmonary venous and arterial pressures lead to

neurohormonal activation that increases the systemic vascular resistance, which further increases venous return and systemic blood pressure and amplifies the development of pulmonary edema.[63]

Various echo-Doppler indices are used for assessing the severity of diastolic function (Figure 73-6). Doppler measurements made in diastole across the mitral valve are useful in characterizing and quantifying diastolic dysfunction. However, these measurements may be affected by heart rate, afterload, and preload. E wave represents the early filling and the active relaxation of the LV, after which comes a plateau with absence of flow. The second wave, called the *A wave*, represents flow produced by atrial contraction. Measurements of isovolumic relaxation time (IVRT), E-wave deceleration time, the E wave, and the A wave peak velocity and ratio, as well as the pulmonary venous flow patterns, allow the clinician to define the nature and severity of "diastolic dysfunction." Tissue Doppler (TD) measures tissue velocity relative to the transducer, with high spatial (1 mm) and temporal resolution (>100 s⁻¹). The most frequently used modality of TD is measurement of LV basal ("annular"), longitudinal myocardial shortening. The early diastolic (E′) lengthening velocities are considered sensitive for diastolic dysfunction and E/E′ ratios correlate closely with LV filling pressures.[64]

Exclusion of Active Myocardial Etiologies as Causative or Aggravating Factors for AHF

Myocarditis or other cardiomyopathies, ischemic heart disease, valvular disease, and acquired heart disease must be excluded as part of the evaluation of pulmonary edema.

Myocarditis usually results from various viral infections, including those caused by adenovirus, coxsackievirus, and enterovirus. The clinical presentation can vary from asymptomatic with normal echocardiographic and electrocardiographic features to cardiogenic shock. Occasionally the patient will report nonspecific complaints (fever, malaise, and weakness sometimes progressing to dyspnea on exertion and palpitation) preceding the onset of heart failure and pulmonary edema. The diagnosis relies on ECG, echocardiographic, and laboratory tests indicating an active inflammatory process together with elevated cardiac troponin levels. The main differential diagnosis is acute coronary syndrome. Since establishing the diagnosis is crucial, invasive diagnostic procedures such as coronary angiography and endomyocardial biopsy are sometimes needed for this task. A small number of patients with severe LV dysfunction will require assist devices as a bridge to resolution and sometimes to transplantation.

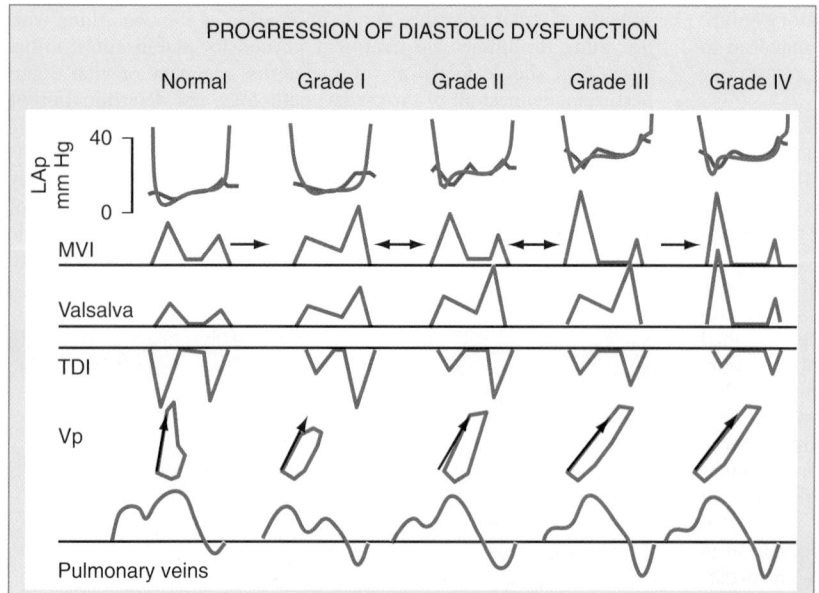

Figure 73-6 The progression of left ventricular diastolic dysfunction is assessed using various Doppler echocardiographic variables. Left panel: Normal LA pressure, mitral E/A >1.2, no significant change following Valsava; normal TDI velocities, Vp > 50 degrees; pulmonary diastolic wave > systolic. Each successive grade represents a worsening state of diastolic dysfunction. Furthermore, E/E′ values can provide further assessment of filling pressures: <8 = normal; >15 = elevated filling pressure. LAp, left atrial pressure; MVI, mitral valure inflow; TDI, tissure Doppler imaging; Valsava, response of mitral valve inflow to Valsava manoeuvre; Vp, mitral inflow propagation velocity. (*Adapted from:* S R Ommen, SR and Nishimure, RA. A clinical approach to the assessment of left ventricular diastolic function by Doppler echocardiography: update 2003. In: Heart 2003;89:iii18-iii23 doi:10.1136/heart.89.suppl_3.iii18.)

TABLE 73-5	Common Mechanical/Valvular Abnormalities Causing Heart Failure Decompensation

Severe aortic stenosis/regurgitation
Severe mitral stenosis/regurgitation (papillary or chordal tear)
Left ventricular outflow obstruction (sub-/supraaortic stenosis)
Hypertrophic/dilated cardiomyopathy
Mechanical valve dysfunction (pannus, thrombus, endocarditis, chordal/papillary tear)
Acquired ventricular septal defect (VSD); usually as a result of ischemia

Active ischemic heart disease can present as pulmonary edema both in patients with a prior history of ischemic disease and in those with first episode of a myocardial infarction, often involving occlusion of the proximal left anterior descending artery. In most patients, the diagnosis is straightforward, with typical complaints, echo and ECG features, along with elevated cardiac biomarkers. Most patients will undergo coronary angiography to revascularize the ischemic myocardium. Thrombolytic therapy may also be administered if primary percutaneous angioplasty is unavailable or to be performed at a later time.

Valvular and structural heart disease must be excluded as causative factors for pulmonary edema, using echocardiography. Echo-Doppler provides definitive diagnosis of abnormal flow velocities and pressure gradients over stenotic lesions as well as accurate assessment of LV function, the presence and degree of hypertrophy or ventricular dilatation, hypertrophic obstructive cardiomyopathy, sub-/supravalvular LV outflow obstruction, and prosthetic valves (Table 73-5). Some of these pathologies will necessitate prompt surgical intervention.

Determining Prognostic Factors and Assessing Severity

Although there is no established risk stratification score for patients with pulmonary edema and AHF, several factors should be noted and will influence the therapeutic strategy:

1. Baseline characteristics: older age (>65 years), male sex, low weight (<78 kg), hyponatremia (Na < 135 mEq/L), low hemoglobin (<11 g/dL) and impaired renal function (BUN > 45 mg/dL) have been correlated with worse outcome.
2. Findings on admission: oxygen desaturation and high respiratory and heart rates are associated with poor outcome. Blood pressure on admission correlates with outcome in a U-shaped pattern, where high values indicate high SVR, and low values indicate low contractility.
3. Cardiac contractility: cardiac power output (CPO) is the product of the simultaneous measurement of cardiac output and mean arterial pressure (MAP) and is calculated as CPO = CO × MAP × 0.022 (watts). This factor was reported to be a predictor of outcome in patients with chronic heart failure, cardiogenic shock, and AHF. CPO less than 0.5 W on admission is associated with recurrence of HF events, but since it requires right-heart catheterization, it is not used frequently.

TREATMENT

Pulmonary edema is one of the most common presentations of acute decompensated heart failure. The treatment goals for patients with pulmonary edema are described in Table 73-6.

Since pulmonary edema is a potentially life-threatening event, every effort must be undertaken to halt the vicious cycles responsible for further deterioration of cardiac contractility and elevation of systemic resistance. This is achieved by alleviating volume overload and pulmonary venous pressures, eliminating precipitating factors, improving oxygenation, and inducing both arterial and venous vasodilatation, thus decreasing vascular resistance and alleviating afterload mismatch.

Initial Stabilization

Stabilization measures include establishment/maintenance of the airway, oxygenation, and ventilation. Vital signs should be continuously monitored, with emphasis on oxygen saturation and blood pressure while following heart rate and watching for arrhythmias. When arrhythmias or conduction abnormalities are diagnosed, they should be treated promptly, especially atrial fibrillation and other hemodynamically significant arrhythmias. Ischemia and major severe valvular diseases should be sought and treated. Fluid-balance monitoring is best achieved by daily weight and closely following input and output. Hypoxemic patients should be treated with supplemental oxygen therapy to achieve the goal of oxygen saturation above 95% (>90% in COPD patients). Patients with respiratory distress, respiratory acidosis, or persisting hypoxemia should receive assisted ventilation using noninvasive positive-pressure ventilation (NIPPV). NIPPV should be considered as early as possible, since it improves LV function by reducing afterload (by decreasing systolic wall stress) and preload (by decreasing venous return). NIPPV should not be used in patients with cardiogenic shock or right ventricular involvement. Three meta-analyses reported short-term mortality benefit and decrease in need for intubation in patients who were treated early with NIPPV, but the benefit on mortality was equivocal.[13] Patients who fail NIPPV or do not tolerate it should undergo endotracheal intubation and conventional mechanical ventilation using PEEP.

Loop Diuretics

Loop diuretics have been the mainstay of AHF therapy for more than 200 years despite lack of adequate knowledge regarding their efficacy, safety, and dosing. Loop diuretics initially produce a rapid fall in both left and right heart pressures via venodilatation, resulting in improved cardiac function and symptom relief. However, diuretics activate the renin-angiotensin-aldosterone system. In later stages, by promoting fluid removal, loop diuretics serve as the mainstay of treatment in patients with volume overload. In most patients presenting with volume overload, diuretic therapy should be initiated in the emergency department (ED) without delay.[65] These agents should not be used in hypotensive patients and should be used cautiously in patients with hyponatremia and aortic stenosis. Diuretic dosing should be sufficient to cause a rate of diuresis that will cause relief of volume overload and signs of congestion without inducing complications. An initial dose of 20-40 mg of IV furosemide should be given in the ED, and further treatment should be guided according to renal function and prior usage of oral diuretics. The total furosemide dose should be less than 100 mg in the first 6 hours and 240 mg during the first 24 hours.[13] Further treatment should include multiple doses or continuous infusion of loop diuretics, with the goal of relieving signs of congestion. A

TABLE 73-6	Goals of Treatment in Acute Heart Failure*

Immediate (ED/ICU/CCU)

Improve symptoms.
Restore oxygenation.
Improve organ perfusion and hemodynamics.
Limit cardiac/renal damage.
Minimize ICU length of stay.

Intermediate (in Hospital)

Stabilize patient and optimize treatment strategy.
Initiate appropriate (life-saving) pharmacologic therapy.
Consider device therapy in appropriate patients.
Minimize hospital length of stay.

Long-Term and Predischarge Management

Plan follow-up strategy.
Educate and initiate appropriate lifestyle adjustments.
Provide adequate secondary prophylaxis.
Prevent early readmission.
Improve quality of life and survival.

*Adapted from Dickstein K, Cohen-Solal A, Filippatos G et al. ESC Guidelines for the diagnosis and treatment of acute and chronic heart failure 2008: the Task Force for the Diagnosis and Treatment of Acute and Chronic Heart Failure 2008 of the European Society of Cardiology. Developed in collaboration with the Heart Failure Association of the ESC (HFA) and endorsed by the European Society of Intensive Care Medicine (ESICM. European heart journal. Eur Heart J 2008;29(19):2388-442.

CCU, cardiac care unit; *ED*, emergency department; *ICU*, intensive care unit.

debate exists regarding the best approach for diuresis: continuous versus boluses. A recent trial showed no superiority for continuous diuresis.[66] Response to diuretic treatment may be optimized by a strict limitation of sodium intake. Urinary output, body weight, volume status, and laboratory indices should be monitored continuously both for signs and symptoms of resolution of heart failure and for complications of treatment such as deterioration of renal function and electrolyte imbalance. If a patient's status remains unchanged with this strategy, a second type of diuretic should be added, usually a thiazide (oral metolazone/IV chlorothiazide) or spironolactone. When these fail and the patient is still symptomatic, ultrafiltration should be considered.

Morphine

Morphine reduces patient anxiety and decreases the work of breathing, causing decreased sympathetic tone and leading to both arterial and venous dilatation and reduced filling pressures. Although this drug is used frequently in patients with pulmonary edema, its long-term benefits are controversial, and some authors have reported high rates of adverse effects, including the necessity of mechanical ventilation and increased mortality, highlighting the need to use this drug cautiously.[67,68]

Vasopressin Antagonists

Vasopressin (antidiuretic hormone [ADH]) is a peptide hormone secreted from the posterior pituitary gland that promotes vasoconstriction through interaction with V1 receptors and water retention through V2 receptors. Blockage of these receptors has the potential for augmenting the effect of diuretics through the increase in free water clearance. Tolvaptan is the most studied vasopressin antagonist. It is an oral V2-selective receptor antagonist. In the EVEREST trial, tolvaptan promoted weight loss and relieved symptoms of pulmonary edema, but without decrease in morbidity and mortality after 1 year.[69] Use of this and other vasopressin antagonists is still under investigation.

Ultrafiltration

Ultrafiltration is a mode of continuous renal replacement therapy that prompts fluid loss with minimal solute loss. Since the benefits of this method over diuretic therapy are not well established, it should be considered for patients resistant to medical therapy and those with severe renal insufficiency.[13,65]

Vasodilators

These agents should be considered in patients with volume overload without sufficient response to diuretics when the blood pressure is adequate to enable their use. Frequent monitoring should be employed during vasodilator treatment, owing to the hemodynamic effects of these agents. These drugs should be used when a rapid resolution of symptoms is needed, angina relief is necessary while waiting for coronary intervention, when control of hypertension is needed, and as bridging therapy prior to oral medication. Several agents can be used in these settings:

Nitrates. Nitrates are the vasodilators most frequently used for the treatment of pulmonary edema and result in preload reduction. Intravenous nitroglycerin added to diuretic therapy can contribute to rapid improvement of symptoms of pulmonary congestion.

Nitroglycerin: acts mainly as a venodilator, thus decreasing LV filling pressures. In high doses, it has the ability to decrease afterload and enhance cardiac output. Heart failure patients with hypertension, active ischemia, and significant mitral regurgitation are candidates for this therapy. High rates of tachyphylaxis require nitrate-free intervals during treatment. An initial dose of 10-20 μg/min IV titrated up every 3 to 5 min in 5 to 10 μg/min increments (range 10–200 μg/min) should be employed. Similar effects can be achieved with isosorbide dinitrate, but it should be used cautiously because of its long half-life. In view of nitrate tolerance

and tachyphylaxis, long-term continuous nitrate administration is discouraged, and if prescribed requires nitrate-free or nitrate-poor intervals to reduce the extent of tolerance.

Sodium nitroprusside: a balanced arterial and venodilator leading to preload and afterload reduction. The effect on afterload reduction makes this agent useful in the setting of hypertensive crisis, acute aortic/mitral insufficiency, or acute ventricular septal rupture. Its usage should usually include invasive monitoring because of the potential for marked hypotension and reflex tachycardia. The initial dose is 0.3 μg/kg/min titrated upward by 0.3 μg/kg/min every 5 minutes. A concern with the use of this drug is the potential for cyanide and thiocyanate toxicity, mainly in patients with renal failure and long-term infusion. This can be prevented by limiting the rate to less than 400 μg/min. Owing to the safety issues mentioned, sodium nitroprusside is usually used for durations of less than 48 hours.

Nesiritide: a recombinant human B-natriuretic peptide, has the ability to exert venous and arterial dilatation along with a modest diuretic effect. Like the nitrates, it should be considered as an adjunctive therapy, especially in hypertensive patients (increased SVR). Retrospective analyses of pooled data for nesiritide suggested the possibility of worsening renal function and increased mortality, leading to substantial controversy about the safety of this agent.[70,71] Nesiritide's relatively long half-life compared to nitrates also makes it a less favorable vasodilator. Drug administration starts with 2 μg/kg followed by infusion of 0.015–0.03 μg/kg/min.

Inotropic Agents

These agents should be employed in patients with signs of elevated filling pressures and hypoperfusion (cold skin, impaired liver/kidney function, impaired mentation) as well as blood pressure less than 90 mm Hg. Therapy should be initiated as soon as possible and tapered or withheld as soon as the perfusion is restored, since these drugs have the ability to increase myocardial oxygen demand and promote myocardial injury. Inotropes can also be used as bridging therapy in patients with cardiogenic shock until more definitive treatment, such as coronary revascularization or mechanical support, is instituted and in an inappropriately bradycardic patient with low cardiac output. In view of data suggesting that inotropes are associated with increased complication rates and higher long-term mortality, these agents should be used only after careful selection of appropriate patients. Routine invasive monitoring is usually not indicated, but right-heart catheterization should be considered in patients with low cardiac output whose filling pressures are unclear. These agents increase heart rate and myocardial oxygen consumption. They also share a tendency for arrhythmogenicity, necessitating close monitoring as mentioned. Several agents are available:

Dobutamine: acts mainly on β_1-adrenoreceptors (with minimal effect on β_2 and α_1) to activate adenylate cyclase, which in turn enhances the production of the secondary messenger cyclic-AMP, creating a dose dependant positive inotropic and chronotropic effect. The initial dose is 2-3 μg/kg/min titrated to the desired clinical effect with a maximal dose of 20 μg/kg/min. Patients pretreated with β_1-blockers will have a diminished response to dobutamine (as opposed to milrinone). Dobutamine may increase heart rate, myocardial oxygen consumption, arrhythmogenesis, and even myocardial necrosis.[72] Several studies have demonstrated increase in adverse events[73] and mortality in heart failure patients treated with dobutamine.

Dopamine: acts on both dopaminergic receptors and adrenoreceptors. At low doses (<2 μg/kg/min), it exerts its main effect on dopaminergic receptors, resulting in renal and mesenteric vasodilatation but with minor effects on diuresis. Higher doses (3–5 μg/kg/min) will cause β_1-activation, producing positive inotropic effect. Even higher doses (>5 μg/kg/min) will have an effect on the β_1-receptors, causing vasoconstriction with increased risk of tachyarrhythmia. Low doses of dopamine can be used with high doses of dobutamine to avoid the adverse effects noted. Both dobutamine and dopamine should be used cautiously in patients with heart rates above 100 beats/minute and in those with frequent arrhythmias. As with dobutamine, dopamine—especially in higher doses—may be associated with excessive morbidity.[74]

Milrinone: a phosphodiesterase inhibitor produces inotropic effects by increasing the intracellular concentration of cyclic adenosine monophosphate (cAMP) through prevention of cAMP degradation. Other effects of milrinone include decrease in the systemic and pulmonary vascular resistance and improvement of diastolic compliance. As opposed to sympathomimetics, its activity can be achieved even with the concomitant usage of a beta-blocker, but caution should be employed in patients with coronary artery disease, as the use of milrinone may increase medium-term mortality. Initiation of therapy includes a bolus of 25 to 75 µg/kg followed by continuous infusion of 0.375 to 0.75 µg/kg/min, with dose adjustments for renal failure.

Levosimendan: a calcium-sensitizing agent with three mechanisms of action: (1) enhanced cardiac troponin C sensitivity to intracellular calcium, (2) peripheral vasodilatation through opening smooth muscle adenosine triphosphate (ATP)-dependent potassium channels, and (3) PDE3-I activity. Similar to milrinone, it can be given to patients on beta-blocker therapy. It should first be given as a bolus of 3 to 12 µg/kg followed by infusion of a rate of 0.05 to 0.2 µg/kg/min. The bolus is skipped in patients with initial blood pressure less than 100 mm Hg. In one study of patients with heart failure, levosimendan use was associated with higher rates of cardiac adverse events and no mortality benefits at 90 and 180 days, respectively.[75]

Coronary Angiography and Intervention

The updated 2009 European and American guidelines suggest that coronary angiography should be considered in heart failure patients with high likelihood of clinically significant coronary artery disease including high cardiac risk profile, noninvasive tests suggesting ischemia or LV dysfunction due to ischemia, symptoms of angina, cardiac arrest, and acute coronary syndromes. Coronary angiography is indicated in patients with refractory heart failure or cardiogenic shock, especially following acute coronary syndromes or in the presence of severe valvular or structural heart disease prior to percutaneous or surgical correction, device therapy, or cardiac transplant.

Assist Devices

Some patients in cardiogenic shock are candidates for mechanical assistance for their failing heart. This may be a temporary measure used to overcome an acute episode of decompensation, while in other patients, it is used for longer periods of time.

Intraaortic Balloon Pump. The intraaortic balloon pump (IABP) is one of the most commonly used mechanical assistance devices. Between 1996 and 2001, more than 22,000 IABPs were used in 250 centers worldwide for various indications.[76] Apart from cardiogenic shock, the use of this device is supported by evidence in postinfarct angina, refractory ventricular arrhythmia, ventricular septal rupture, acute mitral insufficiency, and post acute myocardial infarction. Use of IABP in the setting of acute myocardial infarction complicated by hypotension unresponsive to other interventions is listed as a class I indication in both the American Heart Association (AHA)[77] and the European Society of Cardiology (ESC) guidelines. The IABP is a polyethylene balloon mounted on a catheter, which is inserted into the aorta through the femoral artery. The pump is available in a wide range of sizes (2.5 cc to 50 cc) that will fit patients of any age and size. The balloon is guided into the descending aorta and positioned approximately 2 cm from the left subclavian artery. Inflation of the IABP occurs at the beginning of diastole, on the dicrotic notch on the arterial waveform, causing augmentation of blood perfusion to the coronary

arteries. Deflation of the balloon should occur at the beginning of systole, immediately prior to the arterial upstroke, augmenting coronary perfusion. As the balloon deflates, blood is ejected from the left ventricle against a decreased afterload, causing an increase of cardiac output by as much as 40% and decrease in the LV stroke work and myocardial oxygen requirements.

Despite the guideline recommendations, the efficacy of routine IABP use adjunctive to primary percutaneous coronary intervention in cardiogenic shock was questioned in a meta-analysis.[78] The principal findings of the meta-analysis of randomized clinical trials of IABP therapy in myocardial infarction with ST-T wave abnormalities showed no efficacy benefit of adjunctive IABP therapy, including lack of 30-day survival benefit or improved LVEF. Instead, IABP therapy was associated with a significant increase in the rates of stroke and bleeding. These clinically relevant higher complication rates are not outweighed by any clinical benefit. Currently, only one prospective randomized study has been performed,[79] but it was underpowered to demonstrate any benefit of adding IABP to optimal medical therapy in reducing short-term morbidity in acute myocardial infarction patients with cardiogenic shock.

Contraindications to the use of IABP include severe aortic insufficiency (absolute), aortic dissection, severe peripheral vascular disease, and hypertrophic obstructive cardiomyopathy (HOCM) (relative).

Complications of IABP are vascular injury, peripheral embolization, bleeding, hemolysis, thrombocytopenia, infection, and limb ischemia.

Ventricular Assist Devices

Ventricular assist devices (VAD) are mechanical devices that, in contrast to IABP, reduce myocardial work by diminishing preload while maintaining systemic circulation. They can be used for support of the right ventricle (RVAD), left ventricle (LVAD) or both ventricles (BiVAD). Their use in support can be short term for helping recovery, long term while waiting for heart transplant, or permanent as a destination therapy.

Impella. The Impella LP 2.5 (Abiomed Europe GmbH, Aachen, Germany) is a catheter-based, axial-flow pump with a maximal flow of 2.5 L/min. The pump is inserted via a 13F sheath in the femoral artery and placed in retrograde fashion through the aortic valve. The microaxial pump continuously aspirates blood from the left ventricle and expels it to the ascending aorta, with a maximal flow of 2.5 L/min (Figure 73-7). The ISAR-SHOCK study prospectively followed 26

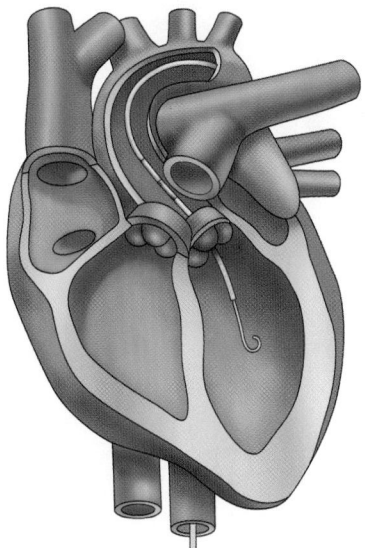

Figure 73-7 Impella Device. The ventricular pump withdraws blood from the left ventricle and then reinjects it into the ascending aorta.

patients with cardiogenic shock treated with either IABP or Impella 2.5. Though cardiac index significantly increased in patients with the Impella LP2.5 as compared with patients with IABP, mortality at 30 days was similar.[80] Impella 5, which can generate flows of up to 5 L/min is also available. The device is implanted via a cutdown (femoral or subclavian) and is used for the same indications as the Impella 2.5. Contraindications to use of the Impella devices include mechanical aortic valve, aortic valve stenosis/calcification, moderate to severe aortic insufficiency, and severe peripheral arterial obstructive disease. Complications of Impella device use include aortic valve injury, arrhythmia, bleeding, hemolysis, thrombocytopenia, infection, limb ischemia, and vascular injury.

Tandem Heart. The Tandem Heart system (Cardiac Assist Technologies Inc., Pittsburgh, Pennsylvania) is a percutaneous ventricular assist device (pVAD) indicated for the hemodynamic stabilization of patients with cardiogenic shock. The Tandem Heart largely serves to unload the left ventricle by providing a bypass circuit drawing blood from the left atrium and then perfusing the withdrawn blood into the descending aorta (Figure 73-8). A transseptally introduced left atrial cannula with multiple side holes withdraws blood to a centrifugal pump placed outside the patient's body. Using adjustable rotation, it then injects blood through an arterial cannula to the iliac artery or descending aorta. The size of the left atrial cannula is 21F, whereas the size of the arterial cannula ranges from 15- to 17F, capable of delivering up to 5 L/min of blood flow. As with the Impella device, the hemodynamic and metabolic parameters in cardiogenic shock can be reversed more effectively by Tandem Heart support as compared to standard IABP treatment.[81,82] However, there were more complications encountered by the Tandem system. Complications of the Tandem Heart support include puncture of the aortic root, coronary sinus, or posterior free wall of the right atrium, and thromboembolism, systemic hypothermia, canula dislodgment, bleeding, and infection.

Venous-Arterial Extracorporeal Membrane Oxygenation. The extracorporeal membrane oxygenation (ECMO) device is an easily applicable and widely accepted option for temporary mechanical circulatory support, allowing cardiac and pulmonary recovery or bridging until further therapeutic alternatives can be considered. There are two cannulation types: VA cannulation (femoral artery/axillary artery to femoral vein), which is used in patients who require cardiac support

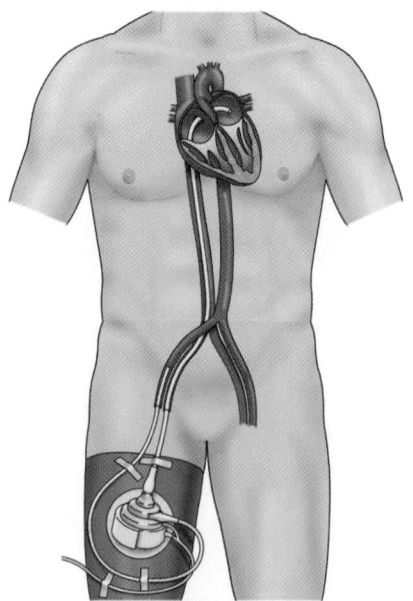

Figure 73-8 Tandem Heart. The left atrial cannula withdrawing blood is connected to the centrifugal pump outside the body and then reintroduced via the femoral artery to descending aorta.

in addition to respiratory support (Figure 73-9). In patients with pure respiratory failure, VV cannulation (usually via the femoral vein and internal jugular vein) is preferred.

Historically, ECMO has been used most frequently for support of respiratory failure,[83,84] but recently the use of ECMO has been evaluated in other patient populations. In a series of 517 patients with refractory postcardiotomy shock treated with ECMO, the overall hospital survival was 24.8%.[85] Given the poor prognosis of patients who have undergone ECMO for the treatment of postcardiotomy shock, ECMO may at best only function as salvage therapy in this setting. In pediatric patients undergoing CPR, ECMO has recently been demonstrated to be associated with survival rates to hospital discharge of 34% to 38%.[86]

ECMO usage is linked to a relatively high complication rate, mainly due to coagulation abnormalities, cerebrovascular events, limb ischemia, and bleeding.

CentriMag. The CentriMag Blood Pumping System (Levitronix LLC, Waltham, Massachusetts) is one of a new generation of magnetically levitated centrifugal pumps that produce unidirectional flow. The device is unique in that the absence of rotating seals or bearings allows for minimal friction and shear stress, resulting in lower levels of complement activation. This device also has the potential to produce higher flows (up to 10 L/min) at lower rotations per minute (rpm). The CentriMag system can be inserted in the operating room[87] or via a percutaneous approach.[88] Beside cardiocirculatory support of up to 10 L/min, the device provides the possibility to function as an ECMO. CentriMag has been used for postcardiotomy shock with encouraging results, achieving a survival rate of around 50%.[89] Complications with this system include vascular injury as well as peripheral embolization and infection.

In summary, although percutaneous VAD provides superior hemodynamic support in patients with cardiogenic shock compared with IABP, there is no evidence of improved early survival with the use of these more powerful devices (Table 73-7). The results of studies therefore do not yet support percutaneous VAD as a first-choice approach in the mechanical management of cardiogenic shock.

Treatment of Heart Failure with Normal Systolic Function

Although this is a common clinical entity, established evidence-based therapies are lacking. The goals of therapy are similar to those in other patients with heart failure: relieving signs of pulmonary congestion and improving hypoxemia. These patients respond favorably to the combination of diuretics and vasodilators, primarily nitrates, thus alleviating the vasoconstriction responsible for the initiation of the pathophysiologic cascade leading to heart failure.

1. The dose of diuretic should be tailored to the patient's symptoms and signs of heart failure. When symptoms cannot be controlled with moderate doses of loop diuretics, combination therapy should be implemented.
2. Beta-blockers: patients treated with beta-blockers prior to admission should be discharged on these agents, preferably at the preadmission dose. Recent studies suggested that beta-blocker continuation during AHF therapy is not harmful and may be linked with improved outcome.[90] Careful titration of dosage is often required, especially in subjects with hypotension, hypoperfusion, reduced heart rate, or conduction system disease.
3. Angiotensin-converting enzyme (ACE) inhibitors and angiotensin-receptor blockers (ARBs) should be initiated as soon as feasible, given their favorable hemodynamic effects. However, these medications should be held temporarily in hypotensive patients or patients with acute renal failure.
4. Aldosterone antagonists: both the ACC/AHA[65] and ESC[13] guidelines recommend using aldosterone antagonists in symptomatic patients with EF less than 35% in the absence of hyperkalemia and severe renal dysfunction.
5. Other medications: hydralazine and nitrates are endorsed by the American guidelines for both African Americans and other

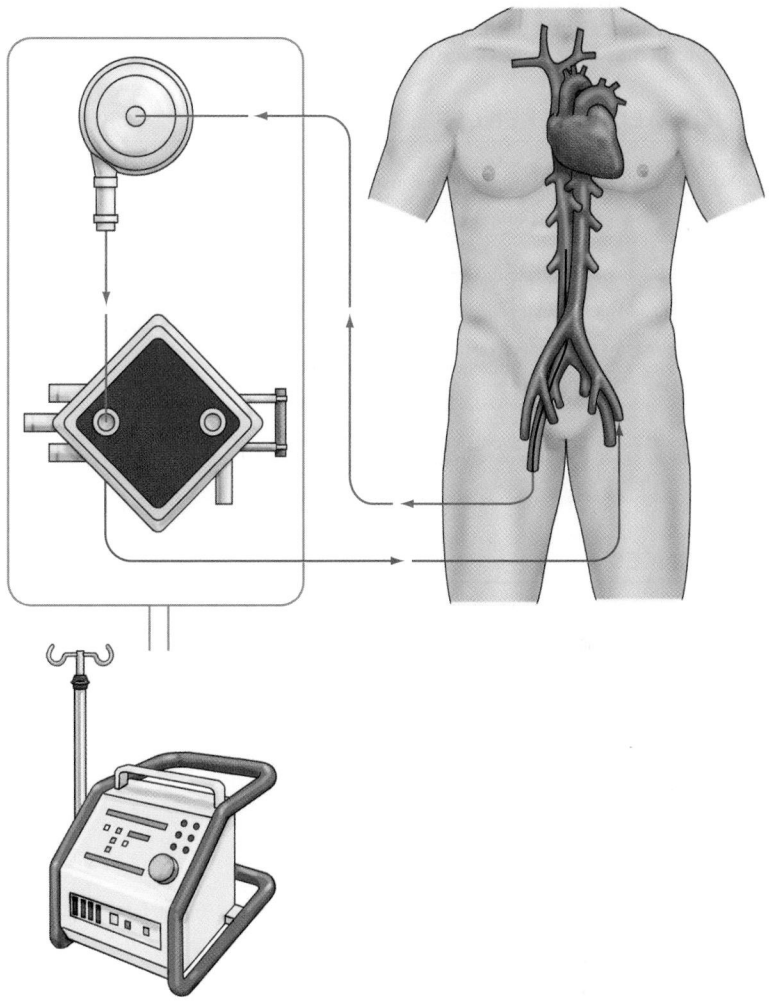

Figure 73-9 **VA ECMO.** Venous-arterial extracorporeal membrane oxygenation device. Femoral vein to femoral artery.

ethnic groups who are symptomatic after adequate doses of beta-blockers, ACE inhibitors or ARBs, and diuretics. Digoxin is indicated for symptomatic heart failure patients on baseline therapy. Routine use of aspirin, statins, warfarin, calcium channel blockers, nutritional supplements, antiarrhythmic therapy, and hormonal therapy should be discouraged in patients with acute or chronic heart failure.

Maintenance Therapy

After initial hemodynamic stabilization and symptom control, the medical team should initiate or reinstate chronic oral therapy for heart failure. Discharge of the patient should be considered when the patient's intravascular volume status has been optimized and the patient is tolerating oral therapy. Oral therapies should be chosen using similar guidelines as with chronic heart failure.

Upon discharge, it is important that the patient is familiar with the medical regimen, precipitating factors of pulmonary edema that are to be avoided, and the required follow-up plan. Emphasis should be given to behavior modification that should include modified physical activity, attention to weight control, dietary restrictions, and smoking or substance abuse cessation.

OUTCOME

Pulmonary edema is a severe presentation of AHF, with short-term mortality reported between 12% and 45%.[91] As stated earlier, several prognostic factors can be identified at presentation, such as advanced age, altered renal function, and diminished level of oxygenation. Reported rates of short-term mortality in patients with cardiogenic

TABLE 73-7	Mechanical Assist Devices Available for Treatment of Cardiogenic Shock					
	CentriMag	*ECMO*	*Tandem Heart*	*Impella 5*	*Impella 2.5*	*IABP*
Insertion	Percutaneous	Percutaneous	Surgical	Surgical/percutaneous	Surgical/percutaneous	Surgical/percutaneous
CO	Improved by 40%	2.5 liter	5 liter	5 liter/8 liter		10 liter
Ventricular support	Left	Left	Left	Left/right	Left/right	Left/Right
Pulmonary effects	No effect	No effect	No effect	No effect	Yes	Optional (oxygenator chamber)
Support time (off-label use)	Days	Days	Days	Weeks	Days	Weeks

CO, cardiac output; *ECMO,* extracorporeal membrane oxygenation; *IABP,* intraaortic balloon pump.

pulmonary edema and myocardial infarction ranged between 46% and 80%, while patients without infarction had a significantly lower rate of short-term mortality. Only a few studies in specific populations have addressed the long-term prognosis of patients treated for pulmonary edema.[92,93] These trials documented mortality rates as high as 40% at 1 year.

ANNOTATED REFERENCES

Noveanu M, Mebazaa A, Mueller C. Cardiovascular biomarkers in the ICU. Curr Opin Crit Care 2009;15:377-83. Available at: http://www.ncbi.nlm.nih.gov/pubmed/19606027.
A most important manuscript explaining in detail the value of biomarkers in the ICU.

Swan HJ, Ganz W, Forrester J et al. Catheterization of the heart in man with use of a flow-directed balloon-tipped catheter. N Engl J Med 1970;283:447-51. Available at: http://www.ncbi.nlm.nih.gov/pubmed/5434111.
A classic manuscript by Ganz and Swan describing the indications and method of use of the pulmonary artery catheter.

Dickstein K, Cohen-Solal A, Filippatos G, et al. ESC Guidelines for the diagnosis and treatment of acute and chronic heart failure 2008: the Task Force for the Diagnosis and Treatment of Acute and Chronic Heart Failure 2008 of the European Society of Cardiology. Developed in collaboration with the Heart Failure Association of the ESC (HFA) and endorsed by the European Society of Intensive Care Medicine (ESICM). Eur Heart J 2008;29:2388-442.
A summary of the most recent European Society of Cardiology Guidelines on AHF and its diagnosis and therapy.

Stream JO, Grissom CK. Update on high-altitude pulmonary edema: pathogenesis, prevention, and treatment. Wilderness Environ Med 2008;19:293-303. Available at: http://www.ncbi.nlm.nih.gov/pubmed/19099331.
The most up-to-date and complete manuscript describing high-altitude pulmonary edema.

Sciscione AC, Ivester T, Largoza M et al. Acute pulmonary edema in pregnancy. Obstet Gynecol 2003;101:511-5. Available at: http://www.ncbi.nlm.nih.gov/pubmed/12636955.
Important manuscript summarizing the most common reasons for pulmonary edema associated with pregnancy.

Paulus WJ, Tschöpe C, Sanderson JE et al. How to diagnose diastolic heart failure: a consensus statement on the diagnosis of heart failure with normal left ventricular ejection fraction by the Heart Failure and Echocardiography Associations of the European Society of Cardiology. Eur Heart J 2007;28:2539-50. Available at: http://www.ncbi.nlm.nih.gov/pubmed/17428822.

Hunt SA, Abraham WT, Chin MH et al. 2009 focused update incorporated into the ACC/AHA 2005 Guidelines for the Diagnosis and Management of Heart Failure in Adults: a report of the American College of Cardiology Foundation/American Heart Association Task Force on Practice Guidelines developed in collaboration with the International Society for Heart and Lung Transplantation. Circulation 2009;119:e391-479. Available at: http://www.ncbi.nlm.nih.gov/pubmed/19324966.

REFERENCES

Access the complete reference list online at http://www.expertconsult.com.

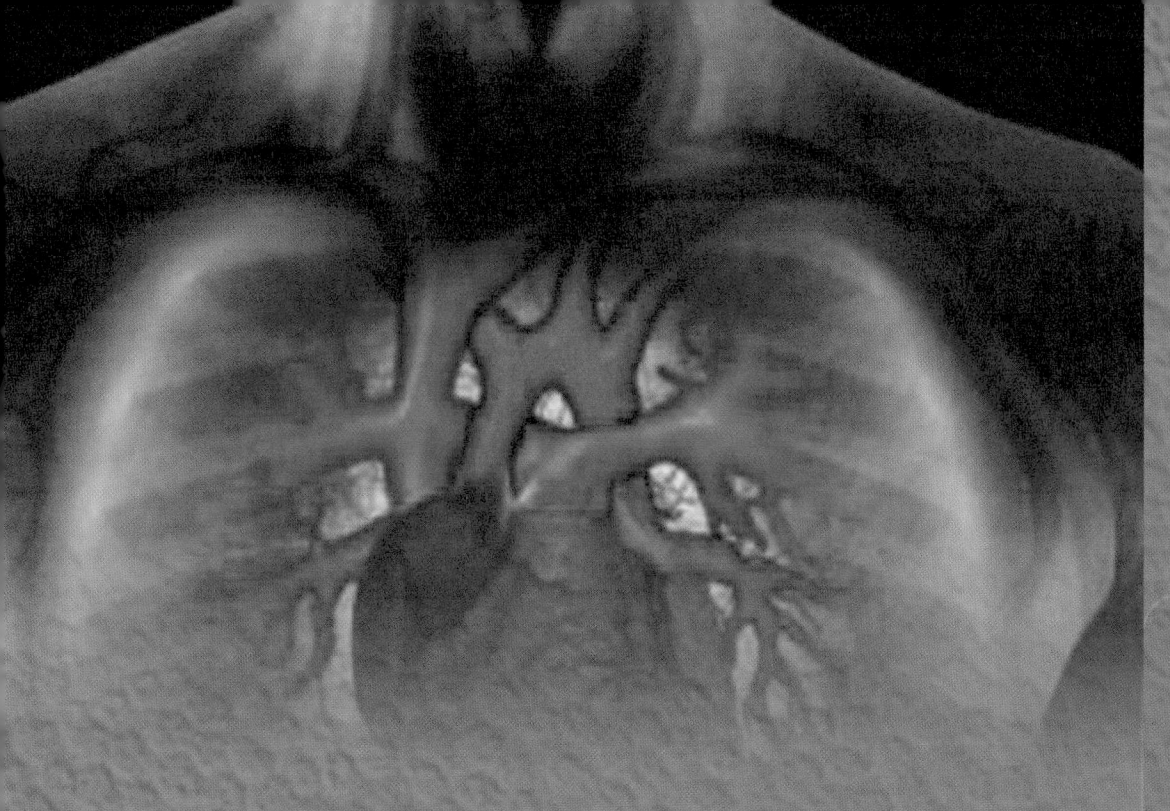

PART
4

Cardiovascular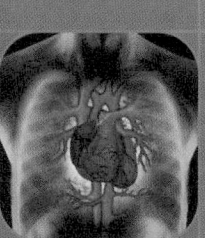

74

Hemodynamic Monitoring

ANDREW RHODES | R. MICHAEL GROUNDS | E. DAVID BENNETT

Hemodynamic monitoring is the intermittent or continuous observation of normal or altered physiologic parameters pertaining to the circulatory system, with a view to the early detection of need for therapeutic intervention. It also consists in observing how the cardiovascular system responds to illness, injury, and therapeutic intervention. Invasive hemodynamic monitoring has traditionally been within the realm of the intensive care unit (ICU) or operating theater, but attempts are now being made to improve noninvasive techniques and validate their use in other clinical settings. The main function of the hemodynamic forces that are measured is to transport substrates to, and clear metabolites from, the cells in order to allow adequate cellular function. Assessment of hemodynamics must therefore also take into account the metabolic status of the cells in particular relation to the supply of oxygen.

Techniques for hemodynamic monitoring have continued to evolve, and some of the technologies have markedly improved over the last decade. There are a number of different types of equipment utilizing a variety of different physical principles available for use in the ICU. Use of a particular method of monitoring should be adapted to the type of patient and is largely dependent on available technical expertise, cost effectiveness, and individual preference in each unit.

The primary objective of hemodynamic monitoring is to ensure that the patient is achieving an optimal tissue perfusion and oxygen delivery while maintaining adequate mean arterial pressure. Identification and correction of tissue hypoxia remains one of the central tenets of every protocol that aims to resuscitate patients from shock conditions. When monitoring circulation, it is imperative therefore that an estimate is made of the adequacy of circulation with respect to the likelihood of there being underlying tissue hypoxia. The monitors that are currently available in routine clinical practice are unable to assess tissue hypoxia at either a local or a cellular level. An extrapolation is therefore made from a number of globally measured variables that provides an estimate of the likelihood of underlying disturbance. This information can then be used to direct therapeutic decisions to benefit patients.[1-11] Ideally, targeting such goals should lead to significant reductions in morbidity and mortality. There is now evidence to show that such interventions can lead to reduced morbidity and mortality in some groups of patients.[1-3,11]

The key concepts of invasive monitoring revolve around two main principles: (1) the measurement of the physiologic variable can be achieved accurately and reproducibly, and the information obtained cannot be obtained by a less invasive method of measurement; and (2) the knowledge of this variable when used correctly can improve the outcome for that patient.[12,13]

It must be remembered that no monitoring therapy will improve patient outcome on its own. It must be linked to a clinical protocol or therapeutic target that has been proven to improve outcome. The type of monitoring is governed by the environment in which it is likely to be used. Above all, it is incumbent on us as clinicians to ensure the monitoring systems used do not harm the patient and should not add to the burden of complications or even death that may befall him or her.

Arterial Pressure Monitoring

Noninvasive measurement of blood pressure is one of the most widely undertaken procedures in clinical medicine. Invasive techniques are more commonly employed in intensive care patients for several reasons. Most importantly, the accuracy provided by intraarterial lines is vital to assess the mean arterial pressure in critically ill patients when they are hemodynamically unstable. In addition, continuous surveillance of arterial pressure is of paramount importance when vasoactive agents are used. Furthermore, frequent noninvasive arterial pressure monitoring adds to the discomfort of the patient. Finally, an arterial line also permits frequent arterial blood gas estimations. Historically it has been relatively easy to measure pressure in the major peripheral arteries. Reliance has therefore been put on the maintenance of systemic pressure under the assumption that adequate pressure will also provide adequate flow and thus adequate tissue perfusion.

Studies in intensive care patients where the focus has been the maintenance of blood pressure have not been particularly fruitful.[4] *Hypotension* is defined as a systolic pressure less than 90 mm Hg or a mean pressure less than 65 mm Hg. Most intensivists accept that pressure needs to be kept at a level that allows adequate tissue perfusion, particularly of the major organs, but that maintenance of blood flow through these organs is paramount.

Interpretation of the changes seen in the arterial waveform in relation to changes in intrathoracic pressure can now also give information about whether the patient is likely to respond to a fluid challenge (Box 74-1).[6,14] A greater than 10% or 12% variability of systolic pressure, pulse pressure, and/or stroke volume caused by the regular and consistent positive pressure associated with positive-pressure inspiration indicates that the patient is probably hypovolemic and is likely to respond to fluid resuscitation. It should be stressed, however, that this technique can only be used in sedated and ventilated patients in whom there is no spontaneous breathing. This is an important technological development because occult hypovolemia is probably not uncommon in critically ill patients and if unrecognized is likely to contribute to an increase in both morbidity and mortality.

Central Venous Pressure

Central venous pressure (CVP) is the intravascular pressure in the great thoracic veins, measured relative to atmospheric pressure. It is conventionally measured at the junction of the superior vena cava and the right atrium and provides an estimate of the right atrial pressure. The CVP is often used as a marker of volemic status or preload, although the ability of this measurement to provide this information is limited.

The CVP is influenced by the volume of blood in the central venous compartment and also the compliance of that compartment (Box 74-2). Starling[15] demonstrated the relationships between CVP and ventricular contraction and Guyton the relationship between venous return and CVP. By plotting the two relationships on the same set of axes, it can be seen that the "ventricular function curve" and the "venous return curve" intersect at only one point, demonstrating that if all other factors remain constant in an individual patient, a given CVP can, at equilibrium, be associated with only one possible cardiac output (Figure 74-1). Both curves can of course be affected by a number of factors: total blood volume and distribution of that blood volume between the different vascular compartments (determined by vascular tone). The inotropic state of the right ventricle will affect the shape of the ventricular function curve. When any one of these factors is altered, there will be an imbalance between cardiac output and venous return that will persist for a short time until a new equilibrium is reached at a new central venous blood volume and/or an altered central venous vascular tone.

Box 74-1

CHANGES IN DOPPLER WAVEFORM SHAPE ASSOCIATED WITH CHANGES IN PATIENT PHYSIOLOGY

Preload reduction
Preload increase
Afterload increase
Afterload reduction
Myocardial depression
Positive inotropes
Decrease flow time
Increase flow time
Decrease peak velocity and decrease flow time
Increase peak velocity and increase flow time
Decrease peak velocity and reduce mean acceleration
Increase peak velocity and increase mean acceleration

Box 74-2

FACTORS AFFECTING THE MEASURED CENTRAL VENOUS PRESSURE

Central Venous Blood Volume
Venous return/cardiac output
Total blood volume
Regional vascular tone

Compliance of Central Compartment
Vascular tone
Right ventricular compliance:
    Myocardial disease
    Pericardial disease
    Tamponade

Tricuspid Valve Disease
Stenosis
Regurgitation

Cardiac Rhythm
Junctional rhythm
Atrial fibrillation
Atrioventricular dissociation

Reference Level of Transducer
Positioning of patient

Intrathoracic Pressure
Respiration
Intermittent positive-pressure ventilation
Positive end-expiratory pressure
Tension pneumothorax

Normal CVP exhibits a complex waveform, illustrated in Figure 74-2. The a wave corresponds to atrial contraction and the x descent to atrial relaxation. The c wave that punctuates the x descent is caused by the closure of the tricuspid valve at the start of ventricular systole and the bulging of its leaflets back into the atrium. The v wave is due to continued venous return in the presence of a closed tricuspid valve. The y descent occurs at the end of ventricular systole when the tricuspid valve opens and blood once again flows from the atrium into the ventricle. This normal CVP waveform may be modified by a number of pathologic processes (Box 74-3).

If the CVP is to be used as an index of cardiac preload, the end-diastolic pressure at end expiration must be identified. The c wave marks the closure of the tricuspid valve at the beginning of ventricular systole, and immediately before its onset, the measured pressure should be equivalent to the right ventricular end-diastolic pressure (except in the case of tricuspid stenosis, in which a pressure gradient will always exist between the two chambers). Where no c wave is clearly visible, it is conventional to take the average pressure during the a wave. Where no a wave is visible (e.g., in atrial fibrillation), the pressure at the Z point (that point on the CVP waveform that corresponds with the end of the QRS complex on the electrocardiogram) should be used.

Taking all these factors into account, it is perhaps not surprising that the CVP will not provide a reliable estimate of preload in critically ill patients. The CVP correlates poorly with overall volemic status, right ventricular end-diastolic volume, stroke index, or an individual patient's response to a fluid challenge.[16] It is perhaps best used in non–critically ill patients when it can provide an estimate of the components to right ventricular filling and venous return because their vasculature is behaving in a normal physiologic manner.

Pulmonary Artery Catheter

Continuous, reliable, and accurate pressure and flow monitoring of cardiac performance helps in the early initiation of appropriate therapy toward precise hemodynamic goals. The pulmonary artery catheter with its measured and derived parameters (Boxes 74-4 and 74-5) helps direct therapy in the critically ill who balance their physiology precariously. The first double-lumen, balloon-tipped, flow-directed catheter was designed by Swan and Ganz in 1970.[17] Thereafter, there have been several modifications to the pulmonary artery catheter, which now enables continuous monitoring of cardiac output from a thermodilution technique, of intravascular pressures, and of mixed venous oxygen saturation (Svo_2).

The pulmonary artery catheter is used to gain a comprehensive overview of the circulation. Information can be obtained about the preload, contractility, and afterload of the heart. Modern pulmonary artery catheters also measure the mixed venous oxygen saturation,

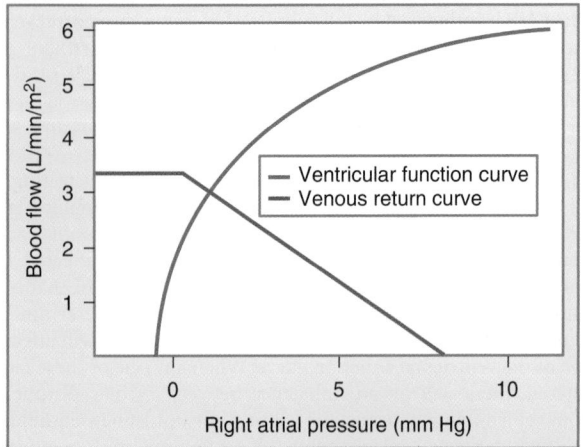

Figure 74-1   Ventricular function and venous return curves.

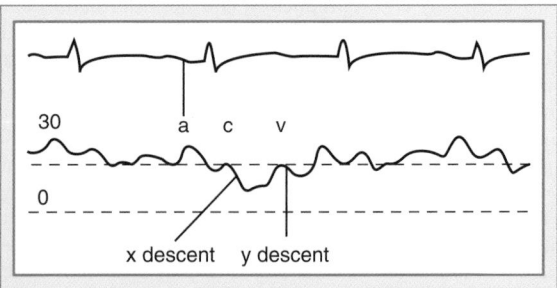

Figure 74-2   Central venous pressure waveform from a ventilated patient *(bottom)*, with time-synchronized electrocardiogram (ECG) trace *(top)*. The a wave represents atrial contraction and occurs immediately after atrial depolarization, as represented by the p wave on the ECG. The c wave represents bulging of the tricuspid valve in early ventricular systole and is followed by the v wave, caused by atrial filling during ventricular systole.

Box 74-3

DISEASE STATES THAT MODIFY THE CENTRAL VENOUS PRESSURE WAVEFORM

In atrial fibrillation, the a wave is lost and the c wave may become more prominent.

In the presence of atrioventricular dissociation or junctional rhythm, when atrial contraction may occur during ventricular systole, extremely tall cannon a waves occur due to atrial contraction against a closed tricuspid valve.

In tricuspid regurgitation, blood is ejected backward during ventricular systole from the right ventricle into the right atrium. This produces a large fused c-v wave on the central venous pressure trace.

In tricuspid stenosis, forward movement of blood from the right atrium into the ventricle occurs against a greater than normal resistance, leading to an accentuated a wave and an attenuated y descent.

Similarly, if right ventricular compliance is decreased by either myocardial or pericardial disease, the a wave will be accentuated.

With pericardial constriction, a short steep y descent will also be seen that allows differentiation from cardiac tamponade, where the central venous pressure will be monophasic with a single x descent.

Box 74-5

PARAMETERS CALCULATED USING THE PULMONARY ARTERY CATHETER

Systemic vascular resistance
Stroke volume
Oxygen delivery
Oxygen consumption
Pulmonary vascular resistance
Left ventricular stroke work index
Right ventricular stroke work index

---

enabling the clinician to make a judgment about the balance between the oxygen supply and demand. With this information, therapy can be tailored to the individual patient's requirements. Once correctly positioned, the balloon tip is inflated, temporarily occluding the pulmonary artery. Transducing the catheter port just distal to the balloon provides the pulmonary capillary occlusion pressure. The pressure in the left atrium becomes the main determinant of pressure distal to the inflated balloon because a static column of blood links the two points across the pulmonary capillary bed. This occlusion pressure therefore can provide an estimate of left ventricular preload. Accurate recognition of the waveform indicating the occlusion pressure is vital; however, the ability of clinicians to recognize this waveform is poor.[18-20] The catheter must be in the correct position and the point at the end of expiration must be identified to exclude interference from extravascular intrathoracic pressures.

For the pulmonary capillary occlusion pressure to give an accurate estimation of left ventricular preload, a number of criteria must be met:

- No impedance to flow across the pulmonary capillary beds
- No disease of the mitral valve
- A linear relationship between pressure and volume (compliance) in the left ventricle

Many of these criteria are not valid in the critically ill, and thus much like with the CVP, pulmonary capillary occlusion pressure represents only a poor marker of systemic preload.

Appropriate use of the pulmonary artery catheter relies on the user achieving an adequate level of cardiac output for any given situation. Cardiac output can be increased by increasing the preload of the heart (Table 74-1) and then by manipulation of either the right ventricular or left ventricular afterload. The adequacy of the cardiac output can

be assessed in relationship to the body's overall energy balance by a coordinated assessment of cardiac output and Svo2.

The Svo2 is the venous saturation of oxygen in the pulmonary artery. It enables a quantification to be made of the overall oxygen extraction of the blood. The normal value for this is in the region of 70% to 75%. Any decrease in this variable is due to either a decrease in oxygen delivery or an increase in oxygen utilization. A thorough understanding of the factors that derive these variables therefore enables a complete understanding of the circulatory dysfunction for any given patient. In recent years, use of the pulmonary artery catheter has been surrounded by controversy (Table 74-2) after the publication of a large observational study linking it with a poor outcome.[21] There have been suggestions[22-24] that use of the pulmonary artery catheter may not improve outcome, and there have been studies where use of the pulmonary artery catheter led to a worse outcome despite the fact that its use was restricted to sicker patients.[25,26] A further study started to resolve this confusion was stopped early.[27] Larger prospective randomized controlled trials have now been performed and have refuted earlier suggestions of harm with this tool.[28,29] What is clear from most of these studies is that if the pulmonary artery catheter is used without a clear protocol for treatment, then benefit is never demonstrated. With an appropriate protocol in the correct group of patients, however, improved outcomes can be shown.[1,2,30,31]

Pulse Contour Analysis

Analysis of the arterial pulse pressure wave obtained from an intraarterial line can provide a great deal of information over and above just the value of arterial pressure. This has led to development of technologies for continuous monitoring of cardiac output obtained by analyzing the pulse wave contour obtained from intraarterial catheters placed in either the radial or femoral arteries. Arterial pulse pressure analysis is a technique of measuring and monitoring stroke volume on a beat-to-beat basis from the arterial pulse pressure waveform. The concept is not new. Otto Frank developed the Windkessel model to simulate the heart-vessels interaction in 1899.[32] By 1904 Elanger and Hooker had proposed a correlation between stroke volume and change in arterial pressure and suggested there was a correlation between cardiac output and the arterial pulse contour.[33] This eventually led to the

---

Box 74-4

PARAMETERS MEASURED USING THE PULMONARY ARTERY CATHETER

Pulmonary artery pressure
Central venous pressure
Cardiac output
Pulmonary artery saturation
Mixed venous oxygen saturation
Core temperature

TABLE 74-1	Normal Values of Cardiac Pressures Obtained from a Pulmonary Artery Catheter in a Spontaneously Breathing Patient		
		Mean (mm Hg)	Range (mm Hg)
Right atrium		4	3-6
Right ventricle			
Systolic		25	20-30
Diastolic		4	2-8
Pulmonary artery			
Systolic		25	20-30
Diastolic		10	5-15
Mean		15	10-20
Pulmonary artery occlusion pressure		10	5-14

TABLE 74-2	Complications Associated with the Pulmonary Artery Catheter	
Complications Associated with Catheter Insertion		
Minor arrhythmias		48%
Sustained arrhythmias		Uncommon
Arterial puncture		1%
Pneumothorax		1%
Complications When Catheter Is in Place		
Infection of insertion site		0%-22%
Catheter-related sepsis		2%
Mural thrombus		28%-61%
Pulmonary infarction		0.1%-7%
Rupture of pulmonary artery		<0.1%
Death		<0.1%

development of algorithms relating the arterial pressure contour and cardiac output, and with recent advances in computer technology, this has led to the development of the principle to the point where it can be used in clinical practice. These technologies offer the ability to monitor stroke volume (and therefore cardiac output) on a near real-time basis. This has several advantages over existing technologies, because the majority of critically ill patients already have arterial pressure lines in situ, thus allowing the technology to be deemed relatively noninvasive. Fluctuations of blood pressure around a mean value are caused by the volume of blood (the stroke volume) forced into the arterial conduit by each systole. The magnitude of this change in pressure—known as the *pulse pressure*—is a function of the magnitude of the stroke volume.

A number of factors exist that have made the transition of this concept into clinical reality technically challenging:

- Compliance of the aorta is not a linear relationship between pressure and volume. This nonlinearity prevents any simple approach for estimating volumes from the pressure change. There needs to be correction for this nonlinearity for any individual patient.[34]
- Wave reflection. The pulse pressure measured from an arterial trace is actually the combination of an incident pressure wave ejected from the heart and a reflected pressure wave from the periphery. To calculate stroke volume, these two waves have to be recognized and separated. This is further complicated by the fact that the reflected waves change in size, depending on the proximity of the sampling site to the heart and also the patient's age.
- Damping. As the change in pressure around a mean value describes the stroke volume, accurate pressure measurements are imperative. Unfortunately, pressure transducer systems used in routine clinical practice often suffer from being either underdamped or overdamped, leading to imperfect waveforms and measurements.
- Aortic flow during systole. Although the filling of the aorta is on an intermittent pulsatile basis, outflow tends to be more continuous.

The systems require constant reappraisal during use, and the need for recalibration is paramount.[35-37] Taking all these problems into consideration, the ideal algorithm for arterial pulse contour analysis should contain the following features:

- The algorithm must work independently of whichever artery the blood pressure is being measured from—despite the known fact that the pressure waveform shape and pressure itself are changed by transmission through the arterial tree to the various peripheries.
- It must correct for known aortic nonlinearity and would need to be calibrated to take account of any individual's variation in aortic characteristics and therefore be able to measure individual stroke volume.
- It should not be affected by changes in systemic vascular resistance causing changes in reflected wave augmentation of the peripheral arterial pressure.
- It must not rely on identifying details of wave morphology.
- It must not be affected by any form of damping or distortion of the arterial cannulae and lines.

In recent years, a number of companies have developed systems to measure stroke volume from pulse pressure analysis techniques. Many of the companies developed methods for calibrating the pulse contour changes for individual patients. This compensated for the inability to determine arterial compliance. This has been achieved with either transpulmonary thermodilution (PiCCO),[34] lithium dilution (LiDCO),[38] or an internal "autocalibration" by the Vigileo system. With an accurate and precise calibration, the data obtained by these devices are as reliable as the pulmonary artery catheter. Many questions remain unanswered, however. For instance, when are the devices likely not to provide robust information, how are the algorithms affected by significant changes in vasomotor tone, and how frequently should the recalibration be performed? Recent data have shown that the devices can be used to titrate therapy in surgical patients, with resulting improvements in outcome.[39]

Esophageal Doppler

The 19th-century physicist Christian Doppler described the effect that bears his name, demonstrating that the shift in frequency emitted by, or reflected off, a moving object is proportional to the relative velocity between object and observer. Doppler derived a formula that related frequency shift to velocity, which included the variables that might distort this observation (such as the angulation of the point of observation to the path of the moving object and the speed sound). This observation has been widely used for measuring the speed of moving objects, ranging from stars to cars to red blood cells. Transcutaneous Doppler ultrasound has been in general clinical use for measuring blood velocity in both peripheral and central veins and arteries for a considerable time. In 1969, Light[40] demonstrated that it could be used to measure the velocity of blood in the human aorta. This has since been further developed and improved such that blood velocity can now be measured in the descending aorta, from which cardiac output can be calculated. The two most commonly used commercially systems both use a flexible probe which is inserted down into the esophagus to a length of approximately 40 cm from the mouth. One system (Deltex CardioQ[41]) has a piezoelectric crystal mounted at 45 degrees on the tip of the disposable probe which produces ultrasound at a continuous frequency of 4 MHz. The probe tip is adjusted to lie in the esophagus at a point alongside the descending aorta. The ultrasonic beam is transmitted into the lumen of the aorta, insonating the moving red cells. Some of the ultrasound is reflected back to the crystal at a frequency proportional to the velocity of the moving red cells. This shifted frequency is converted to a velocity using the Doppler equation:

$$V = f \times C / (2 \times Fo \times \cos Q)$$

where V = velocity of blood in cm/sec, f = Doppler shifted frequency, Fo = transmitted frequency, C = acoustic velocity in blood, and Q = angle of Doppler beam to blood vessel. The velocity of the red blood cells thus obtained is converted to flow using a propriety algorithm which assumes the cross-sectional diameter of the descending aorta based on a number of factors including age, gender, height, and weight. Because this measurement is made on the descending aorta, it does not take into account flow to head and arms, which is assumed to be a constant 30% of the total cardiac output. Beat-by-beat values for cardiac output and stroke volume are calculated, and these values have been shown to correlate well with cardiac output measured by thermodilution.[25] In contrast, the other commercially available product (Arrow Hemosonics[42]) uses a nondisposable probe over which is placed a disposable sheath; the whole device is then inserted into the esophagus. The pulsed Doppler transducer measures descending aortic red blood cell velocity. This is converted to flow by the continuous measurement of descending aortic diameter, which is obtained from an M-mode echo signal provided by a separate transducer incorporated in the probe. Good correlation with independent measurements of cardiac output have also been obtained with this device. This technique allows cardiac output and stroke volume to be measured rapidly and relatively noninvasively and requires less training than required for use of the pulmonary artery catheter. Most studies find a similar agreement with the values for cardiac output measured with this technique as compared to the pulmonary artery thermodilution catheter.[42-46] Operator experience is frequently cited as the cause of any inaccuracy. It can be difficult to ensure that the Doppler probe is correctly positioned in the esophagus to ensure that the probe tip is accurately measuring the maximal blood flow at the center of the aorta.[45] This technique has been used to improve the outcome of surgical patients by titrating fluid challenges to achieve a maximal stroke volume in the intraoperative setting.

Electrical Impedance Cardiography Technology

Electrical impedance cardiography technology measures the basal chest electrical impedance or resistance to flow in ohms.[47] The change of impedance across the chest wall is related to the change of flow of blood throughout the chest cavity. The impedance dz/dt (dz = change in impedance, dt = change in time) is produced by change in blood flow and volumes in the ascending aorta. In devices using baseline impedance, large amounts of thoracic fluid such as severe pulmonary edema may interfere with the impedance signal and dampen the waveform. The latest methods are baseline impedance independent. They provide continuous trends of heart rate and stroke volume and give derived cardiac output and index using stroke waveform morphology. Recent models of electrical impedance cardiography use advanced waveform morphology analysis to measure a filling index, the trend of which may be useful in monitoring response to therapy. Unfortunately, in view of its major limitations, its reliability in critically ill patients is very limited. Recent advancements in this technology use the concept of frequency amplification as opposed to amplitude modification (FM rather than AM), which leads to a much more robust signal-to-noise ratio. This is now known as *bioreactance*. Early data from this technique appear promising, although further validation is required.

Conclusion

There are a number of different technologies for measuring cardiac performance. The simplest and most reliable of these are measurements of pressure. Measurements of flow and other variables of cardiac performance are more complex and often more difficult to obtain. Individual clinicians must choose the appropriate parameters to measure and be aware of the various limitations of the measuring techniques. Whichever technique is chosen, it is important to remember that simply monitoring will derive no benefit to the patient unless the data obtained are linked to a therapeutic decision and/or protocol.

KEY POINTS

1. Hemodynamic monitoring plays a major role in assessing and managing critically ill patients.

2. Arterial lines provide not only a continuous systemic pressure display but also easy access for blood gas analysis and other laboratory tests.

3. Central venous lines provide useful information from careful interpretation of waveforms. Unfortunately there is no threshold value of central venous pressure that can differentiate patients who will respond to a fluid challenge from those who will not.

4. The pulmonary artery flotation catheter is able to measure the cardiac output, pressures in the right atrium and pulmonary arteries, and the mixed venous oxygen saturation. Modern catheters perform all of these functions on a semicontinuous basis and can also provide information about right ventricular volumes and ejection fraction. Recent studies have not shown that they increase the risks of complications to patients. Some studies have shown that when used to specifically target therapy to specific outcomes goals, their use will be associated with an outcome benefit for patients.

5. Transesophageal Doppler is a relatively noninvasive technique for the rapid beat-to-beat estimation of stroke volume and cardiac output. This can generally only be used in sedated and ventilated patients.

6. Pulse contour analysis of arterial waveforms provides beat-by-beat measurement and variability of stroke volume and cardiac output. There are a variety of proprietary monitors utilizing this technology.

7. All these techniques can be used to measure cardiac output and thus estimate global tissue oxygenation. Their therapeutic utility depends on correct training in their use and appropriate interpretation of the data they provide. Therapeutic decisions based on data obtained from hemodynamic monitors must also take into account information obtained from physical examination and laboratory results.

8. Use of a particular method of monitoring should be adapted to the type of patient and is largely dependent on available technical expertise, cost effectiveness, and individual preference in each unit.

9. Despite widespread use of these technologies, there are limited data showing clinical benefit, and thus their use should be weighed against their potential disadvantages and cost.

ANNOTATED REFERENCES

Iberti TJ, Fischer EP, Leibowitz AB, et al. Multicenter study of physicians' knowledge of the pulmonary artery catheter. Pulmonary Artery Catheter Study Group. JAMA 1990;264:2928-32.
This study showed that physician understanding and ability to interpret the information provided by the pulmonary artery catheter was poor.
Connors Jr AF, Speroff T, Dawson NV, et al. The effectiveness of right heart catheterization in the initial care of critically ill patients. SUPPORT Investigators. JAMA 1996;276:889-97.
This controversial study used propensity scoring to compare outcomes in patients who did and did not receive pulmonary artery catheters during the course of their treatment. It concluded that patients who received a pulmonary artery catheter had a worse outcome than those who did not.
Wilson J, Woods I, Fawcett J, et al. Reducing the risk of major elective surgery: randomised controlled trial of preoperative optimisation of oxygen delivery. BMJ 1999;318:1099-103.
This study clearly demonstrated that the insertion of a pulmonary artery catheter into high-risk surgical patients and the attainment in the perioperative period of an oxygen delivery of 600 mL/min/m² was associated with a significantly improved outcome.
Harvey S, Harrison DA, Singer M, Ashcroft J, et al. Assessment of the clinical effectiveness of pulmonary artery catheters in management of patients in intensive care (PAC-Man): a randomised controlled trial. Lancet 2005;366:472-7.
This multicenter study compared outcome in critically ill patients who did and did not receive pulmonary artery catheters and concluded there was no difference.

Perel A. Assessing fluid responsiveness by the systolic pressure variation in mechanically ventilated patients: systolic pressure variation as a guide to fluid therapy in patients with sepsis-induced hypotension. Anesthesiology 1998;89:1309-10.
This was one of the first papers to demonstrate that analyzing the reduction in systolic blood pressure resulting from an increase in intrathoracic pressure in ventilated patients would predict which patients would respond appropriately to fluid resuscitation. It led to this methodology becoming a widely accepted way of identifying patients who are clinically hypovolemic and their response to treatment.
Pearse R, Dawson D, Fawcet JT, Rhodes A, Grounds RM, Bennett ED. Early goal-directed therapy after major surgery reduces complications and duration of hospital stay. A randomised controlled trial. Crit Care 2005;9:687-93.
This paper was the first to demonstrate that targeting an oxygen delivery of 600 mL/min/m² in the immediate postoperative period in high-risk surgical patients, using calibrated pulse power technology, led to significant reduction in morbidity and length of hospital stay.
Cecconi M, Rhodes A, Poloniecki J, Della Rocca G, Grounds RM. Bench-to-bedside review: the importance of the precision of the reference technique—with specific reference to the measurement of cardiac output. Crit Care 2009;35:201-6.
This study demonstrated the importance of defining the precision of the reference technology used for measuring cardiac output to which newer technologies are being compared.

REFERENCES

Access the complete reference list online at http://www.expertconsult.com.

75

Acute Myocardial Infarction

JOHN RIORDAN | WILLIAM J. BRADY

Angina pectoris was recognized in the 18th century; myocardial infarction (MI), however, was described approximately 200 years later. Simultaneous to the identification of MI was the initial introduction and subsequent application of the electrocardiogram (ECG)—the first objective method of assessing the coronary origin of the presentation. In fact, early clinician investigators described the evolving "electrographic" changes during angina in 1918.[1] Over the next 50 years, angina pectoris and MI were further characterized and diagnosed; unfortunately, however, the management of ischemic heart disease did not progress as significantly. From this point in medical history until the 1960s, management consisted primarily of pain relief coupled with strict bed rest for prolonged periods and management of resultant congestive heart failure (CHF); acute complications such as cardiogenic shock and sudden cardiac death were invariably fatal events. Subsequently, the introduction and widespread use of cardiopulmonary resuscitation, external defibrillation, and antidysrhythmic agents gave the clinician powerful new tools in the management of sudden cardiac death and other malignant dysrhythmias. Overall management, however, was still aimed at the complications of ischemic heart disease rather than the syndrome itself.

With recognition of the thrombotic nature of the acute coronary syndrome within the last several decades, the stage was set for the next most significant advance in the management of more acute forms of ischemic heart disease, namely acute myocardial infarction (AMI). Early coronary angiography coupled with intraarterial administration of streptokinase ushered in the era of acute reperfusion therapies, certainly the most significant advancement in the recent past. Clinicians were now able not only to treat the acute complications of the illness but also to interrupt, if not halt, the primary process, thereby markedly reducing morbidity and mortality. Furthermore, aggressive antiplatelet and anticoagulant therapies as well as intracoronary stenting have increased rates of patency and reduced coronary reocclusion and reinfarction.

The most recent efforts in this important area of acute cardiac care focus on rapid recognition of acute coronary syndrome (ACS), use of various adjunctive therapies, and restoration of coronary perfusion. When applied to the patient with ST-segment elevation myocardial infarction (STEMI), this process can be described as a STEMI "system of care." In this system of care, STEMI is rapidly recognized; emergent reperfusion therapy, whether it be accomplished via medical fibrinolysis or catheter-based percutaneous coronary intervention (PCI), is quickly initiated while adjunctive antiplatelet and anticoagulant therapies are administered. This system of care spans from the ambulance with prehospital 12-lead ECG through the emergency department (ED) to the cardiac catheterization laboratory and coronary care unit (CCU).

Epidemiology

Globally, cardiovascular disease now ranks as the leading cause of death. It now causes one third of all deaths worldwide. The World Health Organization (WHO) in conjunction with the Centers for Disease Control and Prevention (CDC) published the *Atlas of Heart Disease and Stroke*; in this report, the WHO/CDC note a combined death toll of 17 million persons per year, with a potential increase to 24 million people per year by 2030.[2] In the United States, ischemic heart disease, particularly acute forms of the illness, is the leading cause

of death for adults. Unfortunately, half of these deaths result from sudden cardiac death unrelated to ACS, usually within the first 2 hours of symptom onset, either out of hospital or soon after arrival in the ED. Fifteen percent of the fatalities occur prior to age 65 years, with the majority in women. The "burden" placed on medical centers and other acute care facilities is tremendous, with an approximate 8 million people having been admitted to hospital in the past 20 years; 20% of these admissions involve AMI. Furthermore, while death from coronary heart disease has decreased in North America and many western European countries, there is an increased mortality in developing countries.[3,4]

According to the American Heart Association,[5] coronary heart disease caused approximately 1 of every 6 deaths in the United States in 2006. In 2010, an estimated 785,000 Americans will have a new coronary event, and approximately 470,000 will have a recurrent attack. It is estimated that an additional 195,000 "silent" first MIs occur each year. These events usually occur in patients over the age of 40 years, with an increasing occurrence as one ages. Approximately every 25 seconds, someone in the United States will have a coronary event, and approximately every minute someone will die of one such event.[5]

Pathophysiology

Ischemic heart disease describes an entire spectrum of illness, ranging from acute to chronic entities related to coronary artery disease, including angina pectoris, AMI, cardiomyopathy and malignant dysrhythmia. Acute coronary syndromes have been defined as unstable angina pectoris (USAP) and AMI. In the past, AMI was separated into Q-wave (transmural) and non–Q wave (nontransmural) events. This terminology was replaced by myocardial infarction with associated ST elevation (*STEMI*) and infarction without elevation of the ST segment (non-STEMI or *NSTEMI*). In STEMI, the patient's symptoms and ECG are relied upon to drive treatment. When diagnostically abnormal ST-segment elevation is not present, a rise in serum markers over time can indicate an NSTEMI, assuming the appropriate clinical conditions exist. While this terminology is still used, MI has been further defined and categorized to reflect the many possible clinical situations (please refer to the following discussions for further delineation of AMI).

Historically, the two primary intracoronary pathophysiologic events underlying the development of ACS include thrombus formation and vasospasm. In the setting of either a structurally normal artery or preexisting coronary artery disease, initial endothelial damage produces platelet aggregation and resultant thrombus formation. In most cases, disruption of an atherosclerotic plaque provides the endothelial injury. Occlusion of the coronary artery then results, ranging from minimal, transient, asymptomatic obstruction to complete occlusion usually associated with prominent symptomatology, namely AMI. Coronary artery obstruction can lead to myocardial ischemia, hypoxia, acidosis, and ultimately AMI. Vasospasm results when locally active substances are coupled with systemic mediators to produce a cascade of events resulting in worsened myocardial perfusion. Isolated vasospasm followed by thrombus is involved in approximately 10% of AMIs. Refer to Figure 75-1 for a depiction of the acute pathophysiology of AMI.

In the last decade, the definition of MI has evolved. The European Society of Cardiology and the American College of Cardiology published consensus criteria for "redefinition" of MI in 2000.[6] These

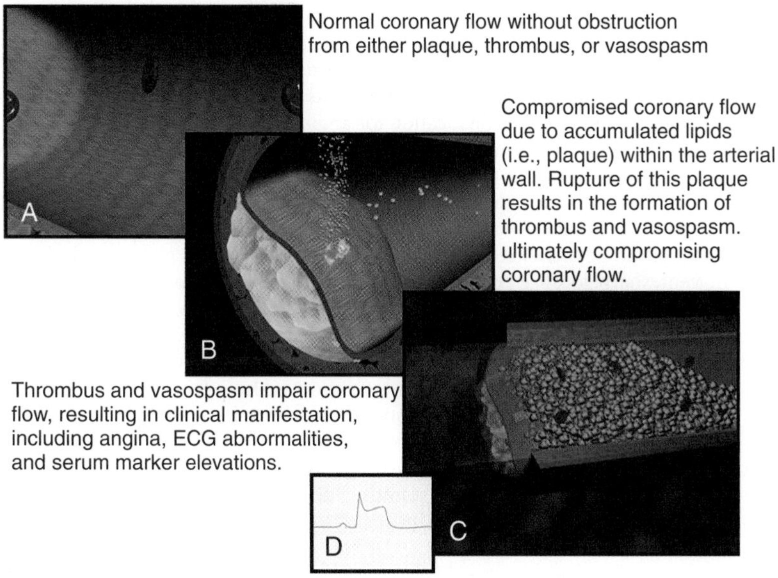

Normal coronary flow without obstruction from either plaque, thrombus, or vasospasm

Compromised coronary flow due to accumulated lipids (i.e., plaque) within the arterial wall. Rupture of this plaque results in the formation of thrombus and vasospasm. ultimately compromising coronary flow.

Thrombus and vasospasm impair coronary flow, resulting in clinical manifestation, including angina, ECG abnormalities, and serum marker elevations.

Figure 75-1 Pathophysiology of acute myocardial infarction. A, Normal coronary flow without obstructive lesions. **B,** Lipid accumulation with plaque formation and ultimate rupture, leading to thrombus formation and vasospasm. **C,** Significant compromised flow within the coronary artery, resulting in clinical manifestation, as noted in **D,** with ST-segment elevation, likely accompanied by chest discomfort or other symptoms. *(Figures courtesy Ashok Subramanian, MD.)*

criteria reflected the improvements in biomarker testing. Then in 2007, working groups from these organizations along with the World Heart Federation and American Heart Association published the "Universal Definition of Myocardial Infarction."[6] This expanded definition classifies infarction based on clinical situations resulting in myocardial necrosis/cell death.[6]

The term *myocardial infarction* should be used when there is evidence of myocardial necrosis in a clinical setting consistent with myocardial ischemia. Under these conditions, any one of the following criteria meets the diagnosis for myocardial infarction; the various subcategories of *acute* myocardial infarction are referred to as types 1 to 5[6]:

Type 1. Spontaneous myocardial infarction related to ischemia due to a primary coronary event such as plaque erosion. The type 1 AMI demonstrates a typical rise and/or fall of cardiac biomarkers (preferably troponin), with at least one value above the 99th percentile of the upper reference limit (URL) together with evidence of myocardial ischemia manifested by at least one of the following:
- Symptoms of ischemia
- ECG changes indicative of new ischaemia (new ST-segment and/ or T-wave changes or a new left bundle branch block [LBBB])
- Development of pathologic Q waves on the ECG
- Imaging evidence of new loss of viable myocardium or new regional wall motion abnormality

Type 2. Myocardial infarction secondary to ischemia due to either increased oxygen demand or decreased supply (e.g., coronary artery spasm, coronary embolism, anemia, arrhythmias, severe hypertension, or significant hypotension)

Type 3. Sudden, unexpected cardiac death involving cardiac arrest, often with symptoms suggestive of myocardial ischemia, and accompanied by presumably new ST elevation, or new LBBB, and/ or evidence of fresh thrombus by coronary angiography and/or at autopsy, but death occurring before blood samples could be obtained or at a time before the appearance of cardiac biomarkers in the blood

Type 4. Myocardial infarction associated with PCI, without or without intracoronary stent. For percutaneous coronary interventions (PCI) in patients with normal baseline troponin values, elevations of cardiac biomarkers above the 99th percentile URL are indicative of periprocedural myocardial necrosis. By convention, increases of biomarkers greater than 3×99th percentile URL have been designated as defining PCI-related myocardial

infarction. A subtype related to a documented stent thrombosis is recognized.

Type 5. Myocardial infarction associated with CABG. For coronary artery bypass grafting (CABG) in patients with normal baseline troponin values, elevations of cardiac biomarkers above the 99th percentile URL are indicative of periprocedural myocardial necrosis. By convention, increases of biomarkers greater than $5 \times$ 99th percentile URL plus either new pathologic Q waves, or new LLLB, or angiographically documented new graft or native coronary artery occlusion, or imaging evidence of new loss of viable myocardium have been designated as defining CABG-related myocardial infarction. Also, pathologic findings of an acute myocardial infarction define the type 5 AMI.[6]

Criteria for *prior* MI includes the following[6]:
- Development of new pathologic Q waves with or without symptoms
- Imaging evidence of a region of loss of viable myocardium that is thinned and fails to contract, in the absence of a nonischemic cause
- Pathologic findings of a healed or healing MI

Additional issues to consider in the pathophysiology of AMI focus on initial primary illness or concurrent medical events. Such considerations obviously have significant potential for impact on additional diagnostic and therapeutic issues; these presentations are reasonably likely in the undifferentiated, ill critical care patient. In the type 2 AMI presentation, the patient with shock of varying causes may experience AMI secondary to the physiologic insult placed on the heart. For instance, the patient with distributive shock resulting from urosepsis or the patient with hypovolemic shock due to gastrointestinal hemorrhage may experience either NSTEMI or STEMI. Furthermore, metabolic poisons such as cyanide, carbon monoxide, and hydrogen sulfide can disrupt myocardial cellular function, resulting in ACS.

Clinical Features

The history—and the clinician's interpretation of the available history—is vital. In the critical care unit, however, the patient may be unable to offer a thorough history because of either active illness or instrumentation such as endotracheal intubation. If available, an appropriate history will enable the clinician to focus the evaluation, provide adequate therapies, secure a safe disposition, and minimize the need for additional investigations.

Angina pectoris, the chest pain associated with ACS, by definition includes a sense of choking, strangulation, or constriction. Common descriptions of the discomfort include not only pain but also pressure, squeezing, fullness, or heaviness. In some patients, the symptoms are perceived as gastrointestinal. The location for angina is substernal and left chest with radiation to the shoulders, arms, neck, or jaw. Patients with AMI, however, may also present with pain in the right chest. The duration of chest pain is valuable in determining its cause. Angina pectoris generally is short-lived, lasting less than 15 minutes. Patients with AMI usually experience more than 30 minutes of chest pain. Intermittent, sharp, localized chest discomfort lasting less than several seconds usually is not due to ACS. The symptoms of angina pectoris improve dramatically within 2 to 5 minutes after rest or nitroglycerin. If the pain persists for more than 10 minutes, the diagnosis of ACS or a noncardiac origin should be considered. Caution is also advised in the chest pain patient who appears to respond to an antacid; overreliance on this response as a major decision point in "ruling out" ACS is not encouraged. Many AMI patients experience associated symptoms such as dyspnea, diaphoresis, nausea, vomiting, dizziness, and anxiety; these various symptoms may be the primary complaint in patients presenting with AMI.

Risk factors that increase the likelihood for atherosclerosis and AMI—male gender, family history, cigarette smoking, hypertension, hypercholesterolemia, and diabetes mellitus—should be sought. Personal habits such as cigarette smoking and use of illicit drugs, particularly sympathomimetic substances such as cocaine, should be reviewed. Artificial or early menopause and the use of contraceptive pills may increase the likelihood of ischemic heart disease in women. If a patient has a history of coronary artery disease, a risk-factor analysis is unwarranted, because the risk of coronary artery disease is 100%.

There has been disagreement over whether these coronary risk factors should be considered in the clinician's medical decision making. An early report[5] suggested that such factors, which were initially derived because of their ability to predict the development of coronary atherosclerosis and its complications over decades in association with other clinical variables such as ECG interpretation, have minimal predictive value acutely as to whether a patient is currently experiencing an AMI. More contemporary investigation in possible ACS patients suggests that the coronary risk factors do in fact have significant predictive value.[7,8,9] This important issue is still debated by the epidemiologists; for the clinician, a consideration of the risk-factor burden is one feature of the overall diagnostic analysis.

Because angina is a visceral sensation that is often diffuse, some patients may have an anginal equivalent syndrome. Such anginal equivalent presentations describe patients who are experiencing ACS yet do not complain of typical chest pain; rather, these patients note atypical pain, dyspnea, weakness, diaphoresis, or emesis—these complaints, in fact, are the manifestation of the ACS event. Patients with altered cardiac pain perception (e.g., the elderly or patients with long-standing diabetes mellitus) are potentially at risk to present with anginal equivalent syndromes. A recent large survey of 434,877 confirmed AMI patients reported that a significant minority of these individuals—approximately 30%—lacked chest pain on presentation, noting only the anginal equivalent complaints.[10] The most frequently encountered anginal equivalent chief complaint is dyspnea, which is found in 10% to 30% of patients with AMI, often due to pulmonary edema.[10,11,12] Isolated emesis and diaphoresis are quite rare.[11,12]

The geriatric patient may also present atypically with acute weakness (3%–8%) and syncope (3%–5%).[13] Unexplained sinus tachycardia, bronchospasm resulting from cardiogenic asthma, and new-onset lower extremity edema have all been reported as anginal equivalent presentations for AMI in this age group. Among the very elderly, anginal equivalent syndromes typically involve neurologic presentations with acute mental status abnormalities and stroke. From the perspective of acute delirium, less than 1% of such patients in an ED population with altered mentation will be found to have AMI. AMI associated with acute stroke is noted in approximately 5% to 9% of patients.[13]

PHYSICAL EXAMINATION

The physical examination in the patient with AMI rarely provides diagnostic confirmation of the illness; the examination can certainly suggest MI yet not confirm its presence. The ECG, serum markers, and other investigations interpreted in the context of the clinical event confirm the diagnosis. Specific examination findings resulting directly from ACS include anxiety, pale appearance, and diaphoresis. In fact, the presence of significant diaphoresis as a physical examination finding is strongly suggestive of AMI.[14] Significant physical examination findings encountered in the AMI patient most often result indirectly from the coronary event and result directly from complications of the AMI. These findings include hypotension, altered mentation, various other signs of poor perfusion, rales and low oxygen saturations related to pulmonary congestion, and heart sounds related to myocardial and/or valvular dysfunction.[15] Both brady- and tachydysrhythmias are seen as well. And, of course, the combination of poor peripheral perfusion—manifested by hypotension unresponsive to hemodynamic support—and pulmonary edema is considered cardiogenic shock.

The physical examination, although crucial to many life-threatening disease processes, is often unhelpful in diagnosing AMI; AMI may be suggested, however, in the patient with obvious cardiac dysfunction manifested by acute pulmonary edema or cardiogenic shock, or both. A change in mental status, poor peripheral perfusion, pronounced tachycardia, hypotension, diaphoresis, rales, jugular venous distension, and S_3 and S_4 heart sounds often provide evidence of significant myocardial dysfunction in patients with AMI. Patients with evidence of myocardial dysfunction, including S_3 heart sound, S_4 heart sound, or rales, on initial presentation are at much greater risk for adverse cardiovascular events, including nonfatal AMI, death, stroke, life-threatening dysrhythmia, and the requirement for cardiac surgery.

Caution should be exercised when attributing a chest wall source for pain based on palpation or movement. To safely relate the chest discomfort to a chest wall origin, the pain must be described as sharp or stabbing (i.e., pleuritic in nature) and be completely reproducible by palpation.[16] Up to 15% of patients with AMI may have some form of tenderness on chest wall palpation.[17]

Diagnostic Strategies

ELECTROCARDIOGRAM

In the chest pain patient (or patient with acute cardiorespiratory decompensation suspected of AMI), the ECG can be used to establish the diagnosis of AMI or other noncoronary ailment, select appropriate therapy, determine the response to treatments, determine the correct inpatient disposition location, and predict risk of both cardiovascular complication and death. The ECG is an extremely powerful diagnostic study, which, if used in appropriate fashion, can guide the clinician in the evaluation of the chest pain patient suspected of AMI. In fact, the ECG provides pivotal information in the patient with STEMI, allowing its diagnosis and guiding acute resuscitative therapies. In other coronary-related ailments, the ECG can provide useful information regarding diagnosis and management. An understanding of its shortcomings, however, in this application will only improve its use. From the perspective of the ECG diagnosis of AMI, the ECG has numerous shortcomings, including the "normal" and "nondiagnostic" interpretations, evolving AMI patterns, the NSTEMI ECG presentation, confounding and mimicking patterns, and the isolated acute posterior wall AMI.

The ECG may manifest a range of ECG abnormalities (Figure 75-2) in the patient with potential AMI, including the prominent T wave, T-wave inversion, ST-segment depression, ST-segment elevation, and QA waves, among other findings. The earliest ECG finding resulting from STEMI is the hyperacute T wave, which may appear minutes after the interruption of blood flow; the R wave also increases in amplitude at this stage. The hyperacute T wave, a short-lived structure that evolves rapidly on to ST-segment elevation over a 5- to 30-minute

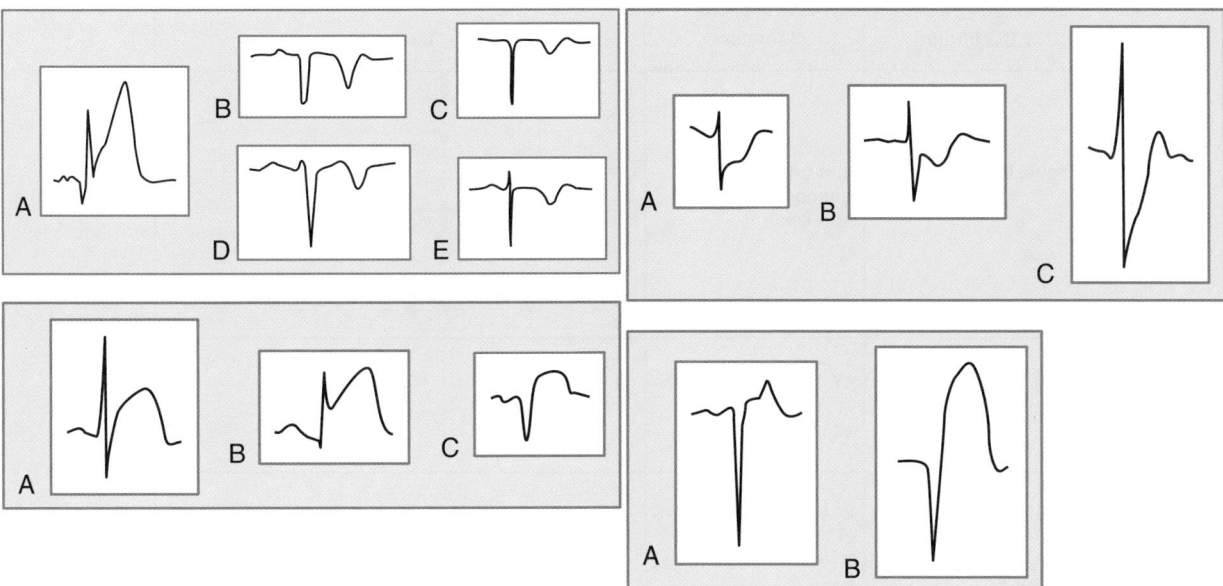

Figure 75-2 Electrocardiographic findings of acute myocardial infarction (AMI): **(1)** T-wave abnormalities of AMI. **A,** Prominent "hyperacute" T wave. **B-E,** T-wave inversions of non–ST-segment elevation MI (NSTEMI). **(2)** ST-segment depression. **A,** Flat. **B,** Downsloping. **C,** Upsloping. **(3)** ST-segment elevation. **A,** Convex ST-segment elevation. **B,** Obliquely straight ST-segment elevation. **C,** Convex ST-segment elevation. **(4)** Pathologic Q waves. **A,** Pathologic Q wave of completed myocardial infarction. **B,** Simultaneous ST-segment elevation with pathologic Q wave 2 hours into the course of ST-segment elevation MI (STEMI).

period, is often asymmetric with a broad base; these T waves are also associated not infrequently with reciprocal ST-segment depression in other ECG leads. Such a finding on the ECG is transient in the AMI patient; either apparent or progressive ST-segment elevation is usually encountered at this stage. As the infarction progresses, the hyperacute T wave evolves into the giant R wave, particularly in the anterior wall AMI. The giant R wave is a transition structure from the hyperacute T wave to typical ST-segment elevation; it essentially is a large monophasic R wave with pronounced ST-segment elevation. Prominent T waves may be seen in patients with AMI as well as hyperkalemia, acute myopericarditis, benign early repolarization, left ventricular hypertrophy, and bundle branch block.

Within moments, the ST segment assumes a more easily recognized morphology. In approximately 85% of STEMI patients, the initial upsloping portion of the ST segment is either convex or flat; if the ST segment is flat, it may be either horizontally or obliquely so. An analysis of the ST-segment waveform can be particularly helpful in distinguishing among the various causes of ST-segment elevation and identifying the AMI case. This technique uses the morphology of the initial portion of the ST segment/T wave—defined as beginning at the J point and ending at the apex of the T wave. Patients with noninfarctional ST-segment elevation (i.e., early repolarization or left ventricular hypertrophy-related change) tend to have a concave morphology of the waveform. Conversely, patients with ST-segment elevation due to AMI have either obliquely flat or convex waveforms. The use of this ST-segment elevation waveform analysis in emergency room chest pain patients increases specificity for the AMI diagnosis.[18] This morphologic observation should be used only as a guideline. As with most guidelines, it is not infallible.

Significant ST-segment elevation occurring in at least two anatomically oriented leads is the primary ECG indication for fibrinolysis or urgent PCI. In that ST-segment elevation represents a significant finding, a brief review of the various causes of ST-segment elevation in the chest pain patient is warranted. Unfortunately, ST-segment elevation in the chest pain patient less often results from AMI; in fact, only 20% to 30% of chest pain patients will have STEMI—the remainder of these patients will have noninfarctional causes of the ST-segment elevation.[18,19] Patients with chest pain may present electrocardiographically with ST-segment elevation due to AMI, confounding patterns,

or masquerading syndromes. In most instances, ST-segment elevation resulting from AMI is easily noted. Confounding patterns such as LBBB, ventricular paced rhythms, and left ventricular hypertrophy may obscure the typical ECG findings of AMI as well as produce noninfarctional ST-segment elevation, which may lead the uninformed clinician astray. Other ST-segment elevation patterns, including benign early repolarization and acute pericarditis, occur in the individual with chest discomfort and may suggest the incorrect diagnosis of AMI, exposing the patient to unnecessary and potentially dangerous therapies.

ST-segment depression is generally considered to represent subendocardial, noninfarctional ischemia, although it may be the presenting ECG finding in the NSTEMI patient. The morphology of subendocardial ischemic ST-segment depression is classically horizontal or downsloping; upsloping ST-segment depression is also seen, yet is less often associated with acute ischemia. With subendocardial ischemia, the ST-segment depression is often diffuse and can be located in both the anterior and the inferior leads. ST-segment depression also occurs as the primary ECG finding in NSTEMI as well as a secondary, though important, manifestation in STEMI, namely reciprocal ST-segment depression. Also, ST-segment depression in the right precordial leads may represent posterior wall AMI. Nonischemic causes of ST-segment depression include digoxin effect and repolarization changes seen in left ventricular hypertrophy, bundle branch block, and ventricular paced rhythm presentations.

Reciprocal ST-segment depression, also known as *reciprocal change*, is defined as ST-segment depression in leads separate and distinct from leads reflecting ST-segment elevation. Importantly, this form of ST-segment depression is not associated with situations in which altered intraventricular conduction produces deviation—such as bundle branch block, left ventricular hypertrophy, and ventricular paced rhythms. Reciprocal change in the setting of a STEMI identifies a patient with an increased chance of poor outcome and, therefore, an individual who may benefit from a more aggressive approach. Furthermore, its presence on the ECG supports the diagnosis of AMI with very high sensitivity and positive predictive values greater than 90%. The use of reciprocal change in both prehospital and emergency room chest pain patients increases the diagnostic accuracy in the ECG recognition of AMI.[20,21] Reciprocal change is seen in approximately 75% of cases

ECG finding	Comment	Example
New LBBB	New onset and with appropriate clinical correlation	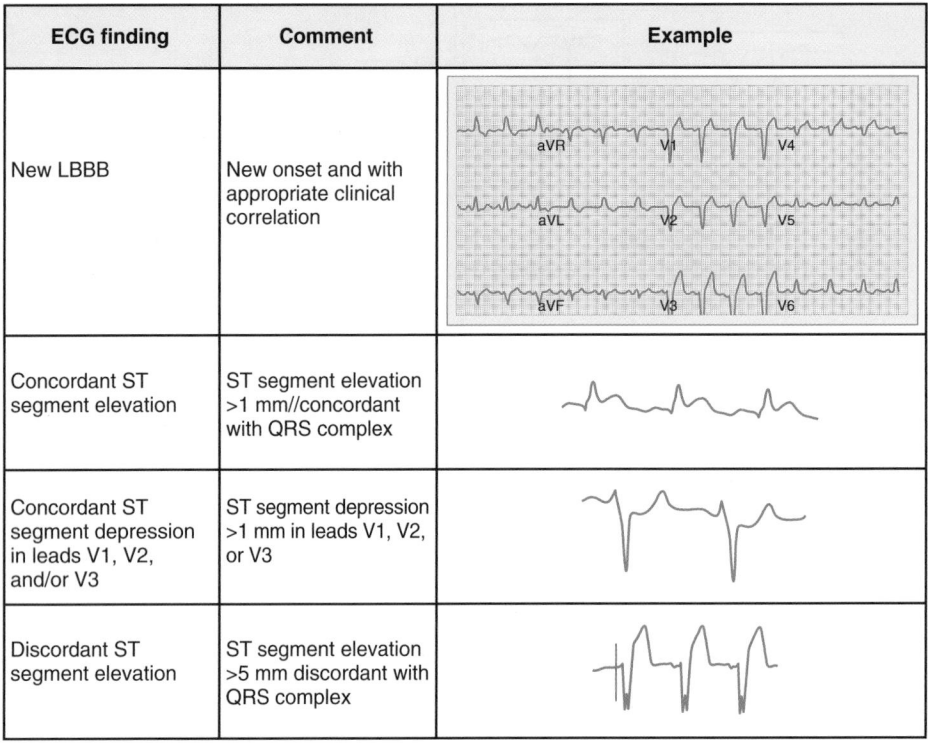
Concordant ST segment elevation	ST segment elevation >1 mm//concordant with QRS complex	
Concordant ST segment depression in leads V1, V2, and/or V3	ST segment depression >1 mm in leads V1, V2, or V3	
Discordant ST segment elevation	ST segment elevation >5 mm discordant with QRS complex	

Figure 75-3 Electrocardiographic indications for reperfusion therapy in the left bundle branch block presentation.

of inferior wall AMI and much less often in cases of anterior wall MI (30%).[20,21]

Inverted T waves produced by ACS are classically narrow and symmetric; they are morphologically characterized by an isoelectric ST segment that is usually bowed upward (i.e., concave) and followed by a sharp symmetric downstroke. The terms *coronary T wave* and *coved T wave* have been used to describe these T-wave inversions. Prominent, deeply inverted, and widely splayed T waves are more characteristic of the noninfarctional, nonischemic conditions such as cerebrovascular accident. An important subgroup of patients with noninfarctional angina often have deep T-wave inversions in the precordial leads (V$_1$ through V$_4$); the T wave may also be biphasic in this same distribution. The syndrome, termed the *left anterior descending T wave* or *Wellen syndrome*, is important to recognize because it is highly specific for stenosis of the left anterior descending coronary artery with anterior wall AMI as the natural history. T-wave inversion can also be caused by NSTEMI and evolving states of STEMI.

In general, Q waves represent established myocardial necrosis and rarely are the primary finding in the AMI patient. Pathologic Q waves may be caused by a previously unrecognized prior infarction, or conversely, a prior MI may mask ischemic extension in the same anatomic location. Q waves usually develop within 8 to 12 hours after a transmural AMI, yet they can be noted as early as 1 to 2 hours after the onset of complete coronary occlusion. As such, the simultaneous presence of Q waves and ST-segment elevation does not preclude consideration of fibrinolytic therapy.

The ECG changes discussed previously may all be encountered in the AMI patient. Two basic ECG presentations of AMI, the STEMI and NSTEMI, warrant further comment. The STEMI presents with ST-segment elevation in at least two anatomically contiguous leads—a reasonably straightforward principle. On the contrary, the NSTEMI can manifest with a range of ECG abnormalities, representing a diagnostic challenge and a potential failing of the ECG. Patients with NSTEMI may present with obvious abnormality such as ST-segment depression or T-wave abnormalities; these findings can be transient. In these cases, symmetric convex downward ST-segment depression or inverted or biphasic T waves are characteristically seen. Alternatively, the ECG may only reveal nonspecific findings or appear initially normal. Lastly, the NSTEMI patient may demonstrate only a confounding pattern such as LBBB. Regardless of the non–ST-segment elevation presentation, the NSTEMI patient is diagnosed with AMI only after the return of a positive serum marker.

Several ECG patterns confound the diagnosis of AMI, including LBBB, ventricular paced rhythms, and left ventricular hypertrophy. In the patient with LBBB, the anticipated or expected ST-segment/T-wave configurations are discordant, directed on the opposite side of the isoelectric baseline from the terminal portion of the QRS complex. This relationship is called *QRS complex–T wave axes discordance* (Figure 75-3).[22,23] Loss of this discordance in patients with LBBB may imply AMI. The clinician must realize, however, that the ECG is markedly compromised as a diagnostic tool in this setting. As with the LBBB pattern, the right ventricular paced rhythm and left ventricular hypertrophy patterns can both mimic and mask the manifestations of AMI. In ventricular paced rhythms, the principle of appropriate discordance should also be followed. An inspection of the ECG in patients with ventricular paced rhythms must be performed, looking for a loss of this QRS complex–T wave axes discordance. Loss of this normal discordance in patients with ventricular paced rhythms can suggest AMI.[24] Left ventricular hypertrophy is not uncommonly encountered on the ECG of chest pain patients. Its presence on the ECG, particularly the repolarization changes that alter the morphology of the ST segment and/or the T wave, can confound the early evaluation. These repolarization changes are seen in approximately 70% of cases and represent the new norm for the patient with electrocardiographic left ventricular hypertrophy.[25] Left ventricular hypertrophy is associated with poor R wave progression, producing a QS pattern in the right to mid-precordial leads. In most instances, the ST-segment elevation is seen here along with prominent T waves. ST-segment depression with inverted T wave is also seen in the lateral leads.

Several additional ECG tools can be employed by the clinician to further evaluate the chest pain patient suspected of AMI. These tools include additional ECG leads and ST-segment surveillance. The additional-lead ECG improves the diagnostic power of the standard 12-lead ECG; with the addition of three leads, the 15-lead ECG is produced. In the 15-lead ECG, the posterior leads V_8 and V_9 image the posterior wall of the left ventricle (posterior AMI) and lead V_4R evaluates the right ventricle (right ventricular infarction). The use of the additional leads can not only confirm the presence of AMI but also alter treatment decisions in ACS patients. In a study of all emergency room chest pain patients initially evaluated with a 12-lead ECG, Brady el al.[26] reported that the 15-lead ECG provided a more accurate description of myocardial injury in those patients with AMI yet failed to alter rates of diagnoses or the use of reperfusion therapies or change disposition locations. Looking at a more select population of chest pain patients, Zalenski and colleagues[27] investigated the use of the 15-lead ECG in chest pain patients with a moderate to high pretest probability of AMI who were already identified as candidates for critical care admission. In this study, the authors reported an approximate 12% increase in sensitivity for the diagnosis of AMI. Potential clinical indications for obtaining the 15-lead ECG in chest pain patients include: (1) ST-segment depression in leads V_1 through V_3; (2) STEMI of the lateral or inferior wall; (3) isolated ST-segment elevation in lead V_1 or ST-segment elevation in leads V_1 and V_2; and (4) the inferior or lateral AMI complicated by hypotension on presentation or after preload reducing medication administration. Figure 75-4, *A* is an example of a 15-lead ECG with inferoposterior AMI with right ventricular infarction. Note the ST-segment elevation in leads II, III, and aVf (inferior AMI), RV_4 (right ventricular infarction), and leads V_8 and V_9 (posterior AMI); the ST-segment depression with prominent R wave is also seen in leads V_1 to V_3.

ECG body mapping, an extrapolation of the additional-lead concept, more completely images the heart in an electrical sense. Contemporary body mapping systems rely on a more widely distributed lead distribution, focusing on areas of the myocardium which are not imaged appropriately by the traditional 12-lead ECG, including the electrocardiographically "near-silent" and "silent" areas. The "near-silent" areas include the far inferior and lateral walls as well as the septal region of the left ventricle; the "silent" areas include the posterior wall of the left ventricle and the entire right ventricle. Various systems are available in today's market, and most rely on a combination of torso mapping with ECG determination. An example of a body map is depicted in Figure 75-4, *B*; note the torso imaging with colorimetric depictions (green indicating normal ST segments, blue indicating ST-segment depression, and red indicating ST-segment elevation). The various ECG waveforms are also displayed for the entire body map, much more completely describing the heart when compared to the somewhat limited imaging of the 12-lead electrocardiogram. While body mapping has demonstrated increased rates of STEMI diagnosis, at this time, conclusive data noting improved patient outcomes is lacking.[28]

Serial monitoring of the ST segment can also aid the clinician in the diagnosis of AMI as well as monitor the response to therapy. This can be accomplished using two different approaches: serial 12-lead ECG acquisition or ST-segment trend monitoring. Either technique can demonstrate the evolution of ST-segment/T-wave changes in a number of different clinical scenarios, including the initially nondiagnostic ECG, the continuous chest pain patient with an initially nondiagnostic ECG, and the individual with a confounding or masquerading ECG pattern. This increased level of monitoring may provide earlier evidence of coronary occlusion in patients with non-AMI ACS presentations. Potentially, serial ECGs can furnish an increased level of ECG monitoring in patients presenting with chest pain and a nondiagnostic ECG on presentation.[29-33] In the coronary care unit setting, serial ST-segment surveillance initiated at admission offers additional clinical data, with approximately 20% of patients revealing dynamic ECG change in the early stages of the hospital course.[34] ST-segment monitoring has proved to be an effective method for noninvasive evaluation of reperfusion after delivery of fibrinolytic therapy in multiple investigations. In one series, Krucoff and colleagues[33] noted that angiographically proven reperfusion was detected with a sensitivity of 89% using serial ST-segment trend monitoring, with a corresponding specificity of 82%.

SERUM MARKERS

The elevation of serum cardiac markers over several days of hospitalization has traditionally been the standard method for diagnosing AMI. Whereas creatine phosphokinase (CK)-MB fraction once was the typical marker used by most clinical laboratories to indicate myocardial necrosis, now the troponins are the most commonly used serologic tests in the regions with established acute cardiac care. Previously, detection of AMI by enzyme elevations over 48 to 72 hours was sufficient to establish the diagnosis of AMI. Because of the evolution of acute interventional modalities, however, significant time-sensitive pressure now exists to identify patients with AMI earlier after onset of the ailment. Particularly in patients with a nondiagnostic ECG, early serum markers of myocardial necrosis have the potential to alter the diagnostic course and treatment plans. Further, there are now clear data that indicate that elevations in serum markers, even in those not meeting traditional criteria for AMI, independently identify those patients at risk for poor outcome.[35-37]

In the last decade, the ability to measure serum markers has improved greatly. This improved sensitivity has been mirrored by improved specificity. The current "gold standard" is the troponin molecule (specifically I and T). This intracellular peptide controls the interaction of actin and myosin in the cardiac myocyte. When injury occurs, these markers are released from the cell. Changes in the absolute value of these markers can be detected as soon as 2 to 3 hours in 80% of patients following MI, thus "ruling in" for MI. "Ruling out" MI can take longer. While most patients display positive markers in 6 hours, and a few more patients become positive after 8 hours, a full 12-hour rule out should be performed in highly suspicious clinical situations.

Once released into the blood, these markers are then cleared by the kidneys. A baseline elevation of these markers in the absence of MI has been termed a *troponin leak* and has been noted to occur under multiple clinical conditions (Box 75-1). In fact, previous studies have demonstrated elevated troponin levels in up to half of critical care patients, many of whom do not have evidence of clinically significant coronary artery disease or ACS. However, regardless of etiology, patients with elevated troponin values have a higher incidence of adverse outcome, including mortality. It is the rise or fall of theses values, with one above the 99th percentile of the upper reference limit (URL), coupled with evidence of myocardial ischemia that differentiates MI from other causes of high troponin. Troponin elevations can persist for 1 to 2 weeks following injury. However, they are usually not rising or falling rapidly at his time. A greater than or equal to 20% increase in the value of the sample during this period can indicate re-injury.

Box 75-1

CAUSES OF SERUM TROPONIN T AND I ELEVATIONS, INCLUDING BOTH ACUTE CORONARY SYNDROMES, NONCORONARY CARDIAC EVENTS, AND NONCARDIAC AILMENTS

Acute coronary syndrome/acute myocardial infarction
Shock of any form (cardiogenic, obstructive, distributive)
Myocarditis and myopericarditis
Cardiomyopathies
Acute congestive heart failure (pulmonary edema)
Sepsis
Pulmonary embolism
Renal failure
Sympathomimetic ingestions
Polytrauma
Burns
Acute CNS event
Rhabdomyolysis
Cardiac neoplasm, inflammatory syndromes, and infiltrative
 diseases
Congenital coronary anomalies
Extreme physical exertion

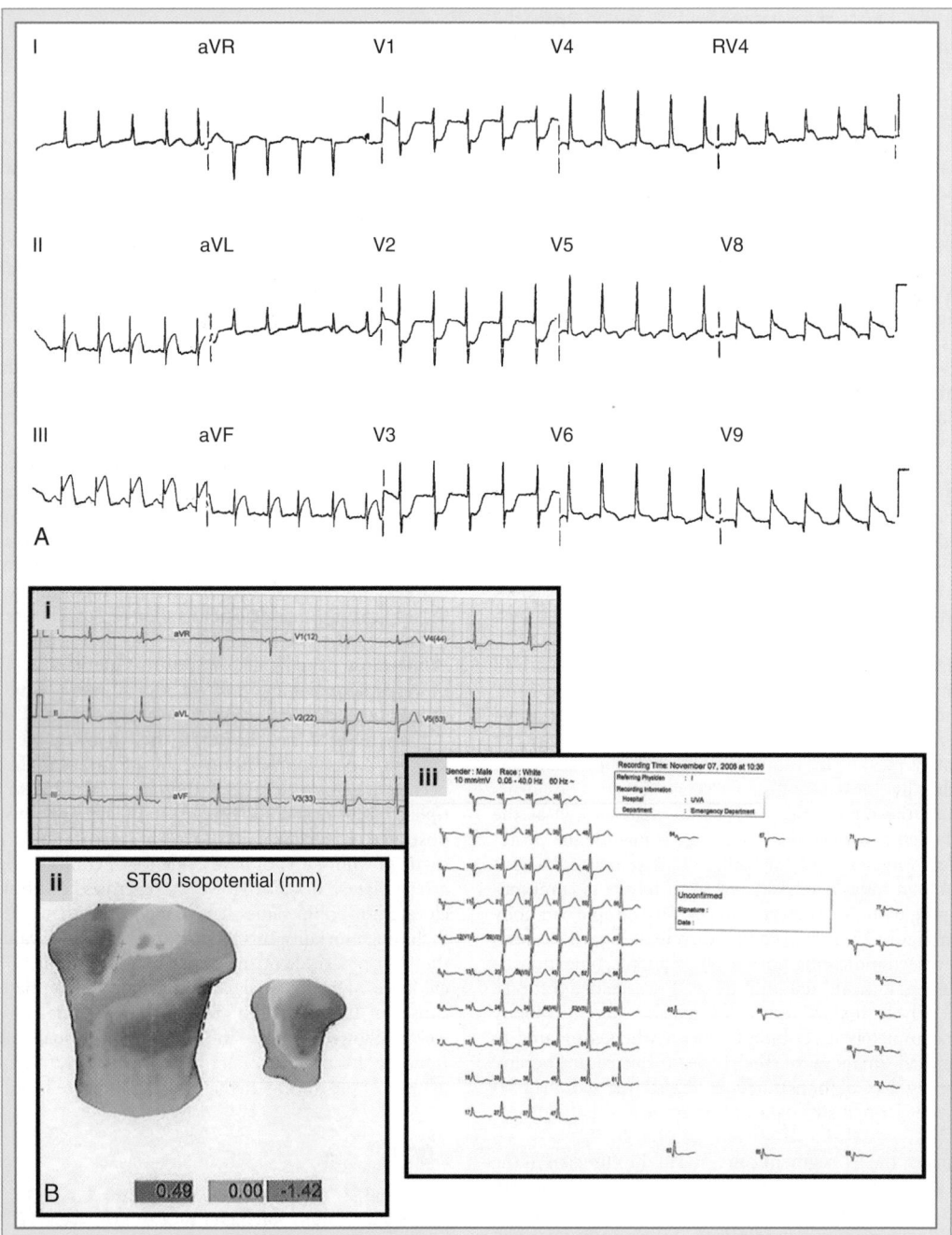

Figure 75-4 **A,** A 15-lead electrocardiogram showing inferoposterior acute myocardial infarction (AMI) with right ventricular (RV) infarction. Note the ST-segment elevation in leads II, III, and aVf (inferior AMI), RV$_4$ (RV infarction), and leads V$_8$ and V$_9$ (posterior AMI). The ST-segment depression with prominent R wave is also seen in leads V$_1$ to V$_3$. **B,** ECG body mapping. **i.** Non-diagnostic 12-lead ECG in an acutely ill patient with pulmonary edema. **ii.** Torso map demonstrating acute posterior and RV infarctions signified by the red coloration in the appropriate anatomic regions. **iii.** An 80-lead ECG with ST-segment elevation in the RV and posterior left ventricular leads, consistent with acute posterior AMI with RV infarction.

As already noted, two myocardial-specific proteins—myocardial troponin T and troponin I—are extremely important in the evaluation of patients suspected of having AMI and have largely replaced CK for biochemical determination of infarction. The cardiac troponins I and T are genetically distinct from those forms found in skeletal muscle, making them highly cardiac-specific markers. The biokinetics of troponin release are related to the location of the protein within the cell. Normally, small quantities of troponins are free in the cytosol, whereas the majority is entwined in the muscle fiber. Following injury, a biphasic rise in serum troponins is seen. This two-component pattern corresponds to the early release of the free cytoplasmic proteins followed by a prolonged rise with disruption of the actual muscle fiber, resulting in a sustained release of the troponins for approximately 7 days. Serum troponin concentrations begin to rise measurably in the serum at about the same time as CK-MB elevations become detectable—as early as 3 hours after onset—and therefore offer no particular benefit over the CK-MB regarding early detection of the event. The troponins, however, remain elevated for prolonged periods of time, ranging from 7 to 10 days. The cardiac-specific troponins are highly sensitive for the early detection of myocardial injury in patients with AMI. A positive test result is associated with significant risk, whereas negative study (i.e., serial troponins) findings predict low risk.[38]

The sensitivity of the troponins approaches 50% within 3 to 4 hours of the event. The test finding is positive for AMI in about 75% at 6 hours after onset of symptoms; at 12 hours, the test is almost 100% sensitive for AMI.[39] Moreover, the presence of a positive troponin, even in the face of a nondiagnostic ECG and negative CK-MB assay, independently confers a prognosis on the patient that is similar to those suffering STEMIs.[40,41] Thus, elevated troponin values appear to be excellent indicators of risk of subsequent death, AMI, and acute cardiovascular complications in all ACS patients, even those who do not meet traditional criteria for AMI. A negative test result, however, does not necessarily imply a favorable prognosis. One caveat for the troponins is that a number of systemic diseases can cause elevations in the serum levels of troponins without ACS.

If unable to measure troponin, then CK-MB should be measured by mass assay. It too should be scrutinized to the same URL as noted above. Unfortunately, CK-MB is less sensitive than the troponins in this determination and less frequently used by many health systems and medical centers. It typically rises in 2 to 4 hours and falls in 1 to 2 days.

Another widely employed serum marker is myoglobin. Myoglobin is a theoretically attractive indicator for myocardial injury, because levels are elevated in the serum within 1 to 2 hours after symptom onset and peak 4 to 5 hours after AMI. The sensitivity of myoglobin for AMI approaches 100% at 3 hours. Yet, its considerable lack of specificity markedly reduces the power of this test. Currently, myocardial myoglobin is not biochemically distinguishable from skeletal muscle myoglobin, reducing its specificity to approximately 80% compared with 94% for immunochemical CK-MB determination 3 hours after emergency room presentation. As with the troponins, myoglobin level is elevated in patients with renal failure because of reduced clearance, making this marker less useful in a patient population that tends to be at an elevated risk for ACS. Additionally, it also will be elevated in any clinical situation involving the skeletal muscle, such as trauma, exercise, and significant systemic illness.

Medical decision making regarding serum marker use in the suspected AMI patient is complex. Serum markers are most often used in a serial fashion. Relying solely on the result of a single negative assay can result in a missed diagnosis in up to 74% of patients.[42] Single testing strategies, however, may be of value when the clinician is evaluating a nonspecific presentation with illness course lasting greater than 72 to 96 hours. Trending results over time significantly reduces the chance of a missed diagnosis, particularly in acute presentations of short course. A number of studies support the assertion that the troponins approach 100% sensitivity and specificity for cardiac ischemia at 12 hours following an event.[39] These studies all caution, however, that such elevations will occur only with cell injury; hence, they are not appropriate markers for non-AMI ACS presentations. In the setting of an appropriate clinical history or diagnostic ECG changes, a strategy of serial cardiac marker testing is relatively straightforward. Depending on the particular investigation employed, the clinician looks for the characteristic rise and fall of serial markers over a time course for the diagnosis of AMI.[6] Most literature supports such serial testing in the acute setting for a period of 8 to 12 hours to adequately rule out MI.[6,43,44]

The more challenging diagnostic situation is found in the critically ill patient with minimal rise in the serum marker and absence of a distinct cardiac event. It is clear, for instance, that troponin levels can be elevated in patients with renal failure or skeletal muscle diseases in the absence of ischemic coronary artery disease. In the renal failure patient, clinical suspicion of ACS must guide evaluation and management decisions; furthermore, the trending of values over time, seeking the characteristic rise and fall of serial markers as well as comparisons to "baseline" values, will also improve the clinician's ability to use these diagnostic tests in appropriate fashion, thereby optimizing care. Patients with significant physiologic injury (e.g., sepsis, acute respiratory failure, multiple trauma, shock) have also been found to have elevated troponin values. In these populations, the elevated levels correlate with left ventricular function and the presence of organ dysfunction, yet the data addressing hospital survival and length of stay are conflicting.

CHEST RADIOGRAPHY

In the setting of AMI, the chest radiograph does not assist in arriving at the diagnosis; other ancillary studies such as the ECG, serum markers, and echocardiography are the primary investigations. Rather, its use provides important information concerning the appropriate application of therapies (i.e., an evaluation of mediastinal width in the consideration of fibrinolytic agent use, determination of pulmonary congestion in the consideration of acute parenteral β-adrenergic blocking therapy). Further, the presence of CHF on the chest radiograph places the patient in a higher-risk group of AMI patients who may benefit from an aggressive therapeutic approach.

The chest radiograph is obtained in the vast majority of patients who present with AMI. Evidence of pulmonary congestion is noted radiographically in approximately one third of such patients. Radiographic findings often parallel the clinical examination findings. AMI patients who develop CHF based on physical examination have an increased mortality risk, as reported by the Killip classification; the chest radiograph provides prognostic data. The chronicity of the CHF syndrome may also be suggested by the heart size. Patients who present with AMI complicated by pulmonary edema and who have a normal heart size most often have no past history of CHF. In fact, AMI is the most frequent cause of pulmonary edema with a normal cardiac size. In other instances, patients with AMI who manifest an enlarged cardiac silhouette on the chest radiograph frequently have a preexisting history of CHF, anterior wall infarct, and multiple-vessel coronary artery disease (Figure 75-5).[45]

ECHOCARDIOGRAPHY

Echocardiography is a very useful diagnostic tool in the cardiac evaluation of the critically ill patient. An adequate echocardiogram is an excellent way to assess cardiac function at the bedside. Basic two-dimensional images, with adequate windows, allow visualization of cardiac anatomy and function. Addition of color Doppler facilitates the assessment of valvular function and ejection fraction (EF). Addition of microbubble contrast agents helps delineate the endocardial border and can be useful in assessing myocardial perfusion and blood flow. In the MI patient, an echo can detect complications of acute infarction including rupture of the free wall or papillary muscle, valvular dysfunction, or regional wall motion abnormalities. While the latter can occur with both ischemia and infarction, a normal echo has a high negative predictive value for excluding infarction.

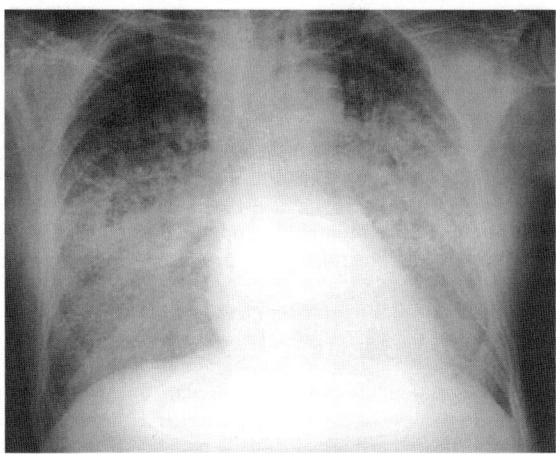

Figure 75-5 Chest radiograph showing cardiomegaly and pulmonary edema in an acute myocardial infarction patient with cardiogenic shock and multivessel coronary artery disease.

Transthoracic ECHO (TTE) can be performed at the bedside with very little preparation. However, this operator-dependent study can be technically difficult to perform in certain patients. Often, body habitus, clinical acuity, or limited cooperation can decrease the ability to perform a complete study.

Although technically more difficult, a transesophageal echo (TEE) is another valuable bedside test. Since it has significant risk of complication, careful patient selection is mandatory. The awake patient should be fully cooperative and NPO prior to the procedure. Conscious sedation is often required, and some patients may also require "prophylactic" endotracheal intubation. Complications from the procedure are usually due to mechanical injury. Therefore, patients at high risk (coagulopathy, esophageal disease) should be carefully screened and appropriately consented. The images from this test are often superior with regard to valvular and perivalvular pathology.

INVASIVE HEMODYNAMIC MONITORING

Invasive hemodynamic monitoring in the AMI patient includes intra-arterial line placement and right heart catheterization. The need for an arterial line for continuous systemic blood pressure monitoring in the AMI patient is unusual. In most instances, noninvasive blood pressure monitoring coupled with serial focused examinations of the patient suffice. Indications for intraarterial line placement for continuous systemic blood pressure monitoring include the continuous infusion vasoactive medications, cardiogenic shock, recurrent or persistent hypotension unresponsive to appropriate therapy, and severe pulmonary edema.

Right heart catheterization, the placement of a pulmonary artery (PA) catheter, allows for precise determination of the patient's hemodynamic status. Such information allows for determination of the cardiac output pulmonary artery balloon-occluded pressure and mixed venous oxygen saturation (Svo_2). Although the array of clinical data provided by right heart catheterization is impressive, the vast majority of AMI patients do not require such extensive and invasive hemodynamic monitoring; in fact, many intensivists have questioned the utility of right heart catheterization.[46] More useful monitoring techniques include continuous ECG monitoring (for dysrhythmia), ST-segment trend monitoring (for evolution of ACS), and noninvasive blood pressure determinations. Additionally, serial focused physical examinations provide important clinical data: repeat assessments of the patient's general appearance, mental status, jugular venous pressure, lung fields, and peripheral perfusion provide (in most instances) appropriate and adequate information regarding the patient's hemodynamic status.

In general, a PA catheter should be considered in patients with unexplained shock, with or without acute pulmonary edema. Such monitoring allows for precise and immediate titration of vasoactive medications. Diagnosis of the various functional and mechanical complications of AMI is best made using the examination and selected noninvasive investigations (ECG, chest radiograph, and echocardiogram). Potential indications for placement of a PA catheter in the AMI patient include cardiogenic shock, recurrent or persistent hypotension unresponsive to appropriate therapy, severe pulmonary edema, the combination of persistent hypotension with pulmonary congestion, concurrent use of intraaortic balloon counterpulsation, and various complications of AMI (left ventricular rupture, pericardial tamponade, papillary muscle dysfunction, and profound right ventricular infarction).

CARDIAC CATHETERIZATION

Cardiac catheterization, also known as *coronary angiography*, is used to evaluate the anatomy of the coronary arteries; left ventricular function can also be assessed. Access is usually obtained through the right femoral artery; the left femoral artery and both brachial and radial arteries, however, can be used as well. Once the coronary anatomy has been evaluated, coronary lesions (Figure 75-6) that are appropriate for

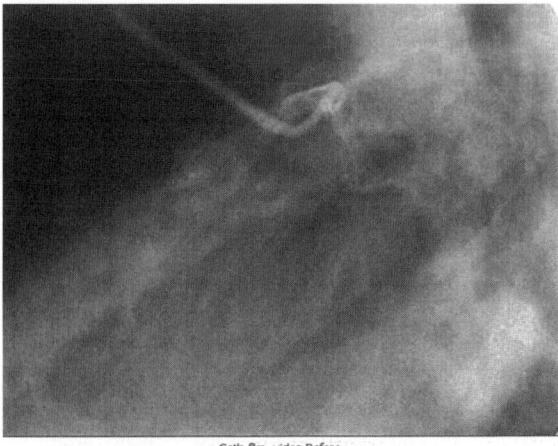

Cath film_video Before

Figure 75-6 Coronary angiography with obstructive coronary lesion and thrombus *(arrow)*. This figure corresponds to the pathophysiology depicted in Figures 75-1, *B* and *C*.

intervention can be treated with balloon angioplasty or coronary stent placement, or both. Fractional flow reserve is a technique that can be used to evaluate the significance of a lesion by measuring the pressures proximally and distally to the lesion.

In the critically ill patient, many clinical issues and scenarios exist that can be evaluated and addressed via coronary angiography, including diagnostic and therapeutic considerations. The diagnosis of AMI can be established via coronary angiography, although such information is usually obtained via other noninvasive means such as the ECG, serum markers, and echocardiogram. In situations in which the diagnosis is in question, however, coronary angiography provides information regarding the status of the coronary arteries and left ventricular function in the AMI setting. Furthermore, the patient who has suffered AMI and experiences recurrent ischemia or continued infarction despite adequate revascularization therapy can be studied in the catheterization laboratory. Current information suggests that rescue angioplasty may be advantageous in patients whose infarct-related arteries fail to reperfuse after fibrinolytic therapy. Some centers routinely catheterize patients after fibrinolytic therapy to determine whether successful reperfusion has occurred and to perform angioplasty if necessary and anatomically feasible. Other centers catheterize patients after fibrinolytic therapy only if there is clinical evidence that the infarct-related artery has failed to open, such as continued chest pain or persistent ST-segment elevation. Routine performance of coronary angiography after fibrinolysis for risk stratification prior to discharge represents an additional, though controversial, indication for cardiac catheterization.

The structure and function of both native and prosthetic valves can be assessed at the time of coronary angiography. Additional information obtained in the catheterization laboratory includes right heart catheterization and myocardial biopsy findings. The diagnosis of aortic dissection or aortic aneurysm can also be made in the catheterization laboratory via aortography. If aortic dissection or aneurysm is suspected, however, it should be investigated via CT angiography or conventional aortography prior to cardiac catheterization.

When preparing a patient for the cardiac catheterization laboratory, several important issues must be considered and addressed, *assuming the clinical situation permits*, including contrast dye allergy, renal function, intravascular volume status, and platelet count and coagulation ability. The physician should obtain a detailed allergy history from the patient. Patients who are allergic to contrast dye or shellfish need to be premedicated with prednisone and diphenhydramine. Also, contrast dye is nephrotoxic; patients who have a history of renal insufficiency may be candidates for *N*-acetylcysteine therapy prior to the study. These patients should also be adequately hydrated prior to receiving dye. Patients should have adequate platelet counts and normal to minimally abnormal coagulation times. Careful consideration must be made prior to sending a patient with thrombocytopenia or coagulopathy for a catheterization procedure. Complications of cardiac catheterization include hemorrhage (both local at the puncture site and regional to the retroperitoneum), pseudoaneurysm, arteriovenous fistula, AMI, stroke, cholesterol embolism, cardiac dysrhythmia, cardiac valve damage, and death.

KEY POINTS

1. The definition of myocardial infarction (MI) has evolved. Now, the patient's clinical presentation is considered in conjunction with highly sensitive and specific serum markers, the electrocardiogram (ECG), advanced imaging techniques and pathologic samples.

2. Atypical presentations of acute myocardial infarction (AMI) are seen in up to 30% of infarct patients. The rate of atypical presentation is highest among the very elderly in whom mental status change, syncope, and other nonspecific symptom/sign complexes are seen. Atypical presentations are more likely to be encountered in the ill critical care patient.

3. The ECG is diagnostic (i.e., ST-segment elevation or new left bundle branch block [LBBB]) for AMI in only 50% of patients ultimately diagnosed with acute infarction. The remainder of these AMI patients demonstrate normal, nonspecifically abnormal, abnormal but not diagnostic, and confounding patterns.

4. Cardiac troponin is the diagnostic marker of choice. While highly specific, serial measurements should be obtained to properly identify MI.

5. Echocardiography (ECHO) is a valuable noninvasive tool. It can be utilized under many clinical circumstances to help identify MI and its complications.

ANNOTATED REFERENCES

Thygesen K, Alpert JS, White HD, on behalf of the Joint ESC/ACCF/AHA/WHF Task Force for the Redefinition of Myocardial Infarction. Universal definition of myocardial infarction. Circulation 2007;116:2634-53.
This article is vital to the understanding of MI. Not only is myocardial infarction defined, the subtypes of AMI encountered in the critical care environment are also delineated. The "typical rise and fall" description of the serum marker pattern encountered in AMI is discussed; this portion of the paper is vital to understanding AMI and differentiating MI-related troponin elevations from noninfarction serum marker abnormalities.

Hoekstra JW, O'Neill BJ, Pride YB, et al. Acute detection of ST-elevation myocardial infarction missed on standard 12-lead ECG with a novel 80-lead real-time digital body surface map: primary results from the multicenter OCCULT MI trial. Ann Emerg Med 2009;54:779-88.
This paper investigates the use of the additional ECG lead concept taken to extreme—the use of ECG body mapping. In the discussion, the authors note that the traditional 12-lead ECG can and does "miss" a number of ACS events, including STEMI. They found that the ECG body map provided an incremental increase in STEMI detection as compared to the 12-lead; in fact, an increase in STEMI diagnosis by 28% was reported. Importantly, patients with ECG body map–only STEMI have adverse outcomes similar to those of 12-lead STEMI patients, yet these patients are managed much less aggressively in the early phase of presentation.

Lim W, Whitlock R, Khera V, et al. Etiology of troponin elevation in critically ill patients. J Crit Care 2010;25:322-8.
A small but interesting study exploring the etiology of elevated troponin values in the ICU patient. Interestingly, these investigators found that approximately half of the ICU patients with elevated troponin values experienced AMI; sepsis and renal failure accounted for the next most frequently encountered cause of elevated troponin.

Body R. Emergent diagnosis of acute coronary syndromes: today's challenges and tomorrow's possibilities. Resuscitation 2008;78:13-20.
This article nicely summarizes the pros and cons of the various diagnostic studies and diagnostic strategies in the evaluation of the patient suspected of AMI.

Goodacre S, Pett P, Arnold J, et al. Clinical diagnosis of acute coronary syndrome in patients with chest pain and a normal or non-diagnostic electrocardiogram. Emerg Med J 2009;26:866-70.
This paper investigates the patient with a nondiagnostic ECG who is ultimately diagnosed with ACS. It importantly makes the point that the ECG is a fallible study, and when the clinical situation suggests the diagnosis, ACS cannot be excluded based upon a normal or nondiagnostic ECG.

REFERENCES

Access the complete reference list online at http://www.expertconsult.com.

Acute Coronary Syndromes: Therapy

JOANNE MAZZARELLI | STEVEN M. HOLLENBERG

Definition and Clinical Manifestations

Acute coronary syndromes (ACS) account for nearly 2 million hospitalizations annually in the United States, and if patients who die before reaching the hospital are included, mortality may be as high as 25%. Acute coronary syndromes are a family of disorders that share similar pathogenic mechanisms and represent different points along a common continuum. They include ST-segment elevation myocardial infarction (STEMI), non–ST-segment elevation myocardial infarction (NSTEMI), and unstable angina pectoris. The common link between the various ACSs is the rupture of a vulnerable but previously quiescent coronary atherosclerotic plaque. Exposure of plaque contents to the circulating blood pool triggers the release of vasoactive substances and activation of platelets and the coagulation cascade. The extent of resultant platelet aggregation, thrombosis, vasoconstriction, and microembolization dictates the clinical manifestations of the syndrome.

Acute coronary syndromes have traditionally been classified into Q-wave myocardial infarction, non–Q wave myocardial infarction (NQMI), and unstable angina (UA). More recently, classification has shifted and is now based on the initial electrocardiogram (ECG). Patients are divided into three groups: those with STEMI, those without ST-segment elevation but with enzyme evidence of myocardial damage (NSTEMI), and those with UA. Classification according to presenting ECG coincides with current treatment strategies, since patients presenting with ST elevation benefit from immediate reperfusion and should be treated with fibrinolytic therapy or urgent revascularization, whereas fibrinolytic agents are not effective in other patients with ACS.

Pathophysiology of Acute Coronary Syndromes

Myocardial ischemia results from an imbalance between oxygen supply and demand, and usually develops in the setting of obstructive atherosclerotic coronary artery disease which limits blood supply. The pathophysiology of unstable coronary syndromes and myocardial infarction (MI) usually involves dynamic partial or complete occlusion of an epicardial coronary artery due to acute intracoronary thrombus formation.

The inciting event underlying the development of an ACS is rupture of an atherosclerotic plaque.[1] Possible sequelae of plaque rupture include thrombus formation with total occlusion, with likely development of STEMI; dissolution of thrombus and healing of the fissure, with clinical stabilization; and subtotal occlusion, which can lead to either NSTEMI or UA.

Atherosclerotic plaques are composed of a lipid core that includes cholesterol, oxidized low-density lipoproteins (LDL), macrophages, and smooth muscle cells, covered by a fibrous cap. Plaque rupture occurs when external mechanical forces exceed the tensile strength of the fibrous cap. After plaque rupture, the clinical consequences depend largely on the balance between prothrombotic and antithrombotic forces.[2] The lipid core contains tissue factor and other thrombogenic materials that lead to platelet activation and aggregation. Fibrinolytic factors such as tissue plasminogen activator, prostacyclin, and nitric oxide act to counteract the potential for thrombosis. A major factor in the outcome of plaque rupture is blood flow. With subtotal occlusion, high-grade stenosis, or vasospasm, thrombus begins to propagate

downstream in the arterial lumen. In contrast to the initial thrombi, which are platelet rich, these thrombi contain large numbers of red cells enmeshed in a web of fibrin. The former would be expected to respond best to antiplatelet therapy, the latter to antithrombotic and fibrinolytic therapy.

ST-Segment Elevation Myocardial Infarction

Symptoms suggestive of MI may be similar to those of ordinary angina but are usually greater in intensity and duration. Nausea, vomiting, and diaphoresis may be prominent features, and malaise and even stupor attributable to low cardiac output can occur. Compromised left ventricular (LV) function may result in pulmonary edema with development of pulmonary bibasilar crackles and jugular venous distention; a fourth heart sound can be present with small infarcts or even mild ischemia, but a third heart sound is usually indicative of more extensive damage.

Patients presenting with suspected myocardial ischemia should undergo a rapid evaluation and should be treated with oxygen, sublingual nitroglycerin (unless systolic pressure is <90 mm Hg), and aspirin, 160 to 325 mg orally.[3,4] Opiates relieve pain and also reduce anxiety, the salutary effects of which have been known for decades and should not be underestimated. A 12-lead ECG should be performed and interpreted expeditiously. Figure 76-1 shows a possible treatment algorithm for patients with STEMI.

ST-segment elevation of at least 1 mV in two or more contiguous leads provides strong evidence of thrombotic coronary occlusion, and the patient should be considered for immediate reperfusion therapy. The diagnosis of STEMI can be limited in the presence of preexisting left bundle branch block (LBBB) or permanent pacemaker. Nonetheless, new LBBB with a compatible clinical presentation should be treated as acute myocardial infarction (AMI) and treated accordingly. Indeed, recent data suggest that patients with STEMI and new LBBB may stand to gain greater benefit from reperfusion strategies than those with ST elevation.[5]

FIBRINOLYTIC THERAPY

Early reperfusion of an occluded coronary artery is indicated for all eligible candidates. Overwhelming evidence from multiple clinical trials demonstrates the ability of fibrinolytic agents administered early in the course of an acute MI to reduce infarct size, preserve LV function, and reduce short-term and long-term mortality.[6-8] Patients treated early derive the most benefit.[9] Multiple studies conclude that greatest mortality benefit is seen if fibrinolytics are administered within the first 12 hours of symptom onset,[8,10,11] but it is reasonable to administer fibrinolytics to patients whose onset of symptoms exceeds 12 hours but who have continued clinical or ECG evidence of ischemia.

Indications for and contraindications to fibrinolytic therapy are listed in Box 76-1. Because of the small but nonetheless significant risk of a bleeding complication, most notably intracranial hemorrhage, selection of patients with AMI for administration of a fibrinolytic agent should be undertaken with prudence and caution. That is of special importance in ICU patients who may have a predisposition to bleeding complications because of multiple factors. Contraindications can be regarded as absolute or relative. In the surgical patient, thrombolysis may pose a prohibitive risk, and emergent coronary

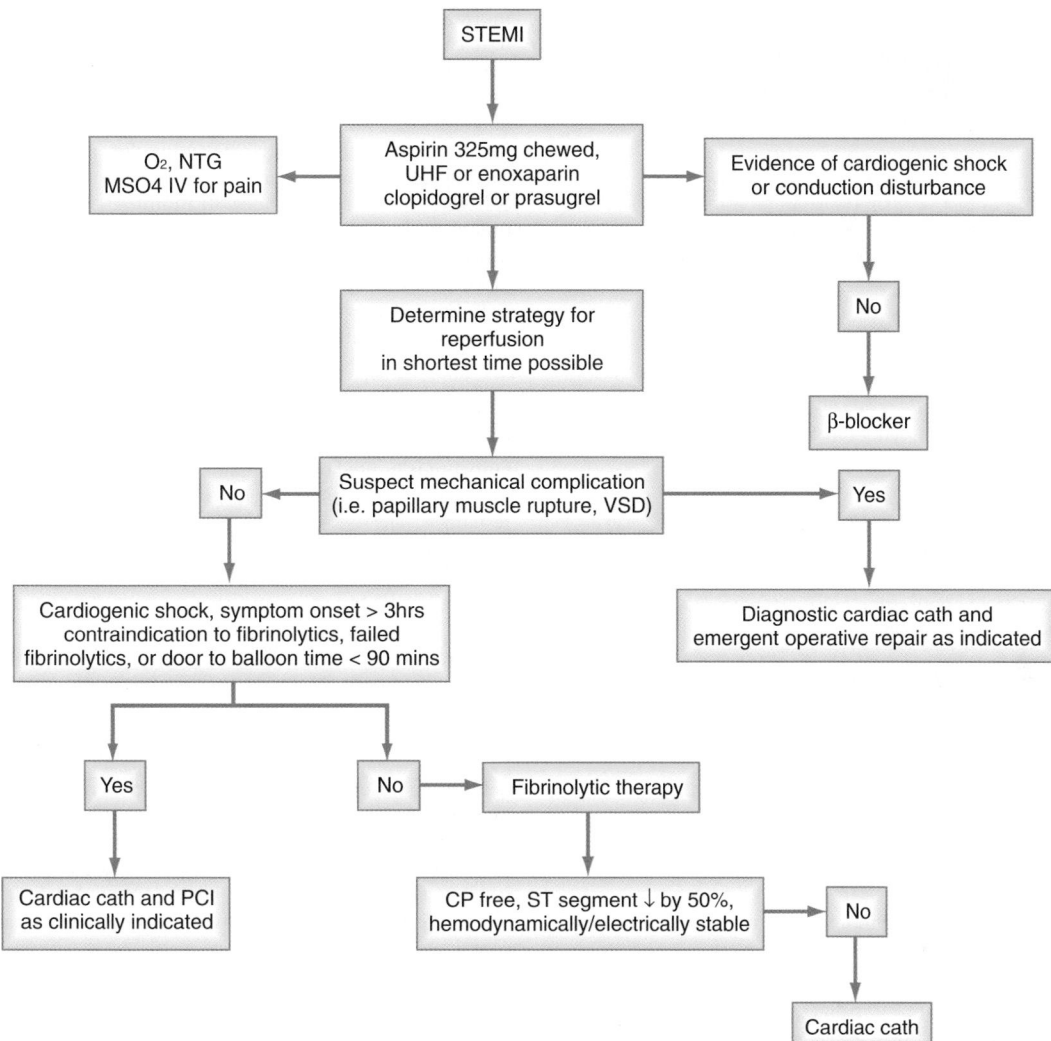

Figure 76-1 Treatment algorithm for ST-segment elevation myocardial infarction (STEMI). *CP*, chest pain; *MSO₄*, morphine; *NTG*, nitroglycerin; *O₂*, oxygen; *UFH*, unfractionated heparin; *VSD*, ventricular septal defect.

angiography (with percutaneous coronary intervention [PCI] as clinically indicated) may be preferable.

After administration of fibrinolytics for STEMI, the patient should be monitored for signs and symptoms of adequate reperfusion within 90 minutes, as indicated by relief of symptoms and/or hemodynamic/electrical instability coupled with at least a 50% resolution of the highest initial ST elevation.[12,13] If signs of adequate reperfusion are not evident within 90 minutes, patients should be taken to the cardiac catheterization lab and considered for PCI. More recent data support the notion that all patients who receive fibrinolytics for STEMI and have at least one high-risk feature should have cardiac catheterization for risk stratification and potential percutaneous revascularization,[14,15] even if this involves immediate transfer from the presenting hospital to a PCI-capable facility. Patients not considered high-risk may be observed in the initial facility where fibrinolytics were administered. High-risk features include extensive ST-segment elevation (>2 mm ST elevation in two anterior leads), new-onset LBBB, previous MI, Killip class 2 or 3 or left ventricular ejection fraction (LVEF) ≤ 35%, systolic blood pressure ≤ 100 mm Hg, heart rate ≥ 100 bpm, or right ventricular involvement.

In contrast to the treatment of STEMI, fibrinolytics have shown no benefit and an increased risk of adverse events when used for the treatment of UA/NSTEMI.[16] Based on these findings, there is currently no role for fibrinolytic agents in these latter syndromes.

Fibrinolytic Agents

Streptokinase was the original lytic agent used in MI, but it has now been superseded by tissue plasminogen activator (tPA),[6] which is more fibrin selective than streptokinase and produces a higher early coronary patency rate (70%-80%).[17,18] Administration of tPA usually follows an accelerated regimen consisting of a 15-mg bolus, 0.75 mg/kg (up to 50 mg) IV over the initial 30 minutes, and 0.5 mg/kg (up to 35 mg) over the next 60 minutes. Reteplase (rPA) is a deletion mutant of tPA with an extended half-life, and is given as two 10-U boluses 30 minutes apart. Reteplase was originally evaluated in angiographic trials that demonstrated improved coronary flow at 90 minutes compared to tPA, but subsequent trials showed similar 30-day mortality rates.[19] Tenecteplase (TNK-tPA) is a genetically engineered tPA mutant with amino acid substitutions that result in prolonged half-life, resistance to plasminogen activator inhibitor 1, and increased fibrin specificity. TNK-tPA is given as a single bolus adjusted for weight. A single bolus of TNK-tPA has been shown to produced coronary flow rates identical to those seen with accelerated tPA, with equivalent 30-day mortality and bleeding rates.[20]

Because these newer agents in general have equivalent efficacy and side-effect profiles, at no current additional cost compared to tPA, and because they are simpler to administer, they have gained popularity. An ideal fibrinolytic agent would have greater fibrin specificity, slower

INDICATIONS FOR AND CONTRAINDICATIONS TO FIBRINOLYTIC THERAPY IN ACUTE MYOCARDIAL INFARCTION

Indications
- Symptoms consistent with acute myocardial infarction
- ECG showing 1-mm (0.1 mV) ST elevation in at least two contiguous leads, or new left bundle-branch block
- Presentation within 12 hours of symptom onset
- Absence of contraindications

Contraindications
Absolute
- Active internal bleeding
- Intracranial neoplasm, aneurysm, or AV malformation
- Stroke or neurosurgery within 6 weeks
- Trauma or major surgery within 2 weeks which could be a potential source of serious rebleeding
- Aortic dissection

Relative
- Prolonged (>10 minutes) or clearly traumatic cardiopulmonary resuscitation*
- Noncompressible vascular punctures
- Severe uncontrolled hypertension (>200/110 mm Hg)*
- Trauma or major surgery within 6 weeks (but more than 2 weeks)
- Preexisting coagulopathy or current use of anticoagulants with INR > 2-3
- Active peptic ulcer
- Infective endocarditis
- Pregnancy
- Chronic severe hypertension

*Could be an absolute contraindication in low-risk patients with myocardial infarction.

clearance from the circulation, and more resistance to plasma protease inhibitors, but has not yet been developed.

PRIMARY PERCUTANEOUS CORONARY INTERVENTION IN ACUTE MYOCARDIAL INFARCTION

The major advantages of primary PCI over fibrinolytic therapy include a higher rate of normal flow (TIMI grade 3),[7] lower risk of intracranial hemorrhage, and the ability to stratify risk based on the severity and distribution of coronary artery disease. Patients ineligible for fibrinolytic therapy should obviously be considered for primary PCI. In addition, data from several randomized trials have suggested that PCI is preferable to fibrinolytic therapy for several subsets of AMI patients at higher risk.[21,22] The largest of these trials is the GUSTO-IIb Angioplasty Substudy, which randomized 1138 patients. At 30 days, there was a clinical benefit in the combined primary endpoint of death, nonfatal reinfarction, and nonfatal disabling stroke in the patients treated with percutaneous transluminal coronary angioplasty (PTCA) compared to tPA, but no difference in the "hard" endpoints of death and MI at 30 days.[22]

Recent meta-analyses comparing direct PTCA with fibrinolytic therapy have suggested lower rates of mortality and reinfarction among those receiving direct PTCA.[23,24] Thus direct angioplasty, if performed in a timely manner (ideally within 60 minutes) by highly experienced personnel, may be the preferred method of revascularization, since it offers more complete revascularization with improved restoration of normal coronary blood flow and detailed information about coronary anatomy.[3] There are certain subpopulations in which primary PCI is clearly preferred, and other populations in which the data are suggestive of benefit. These subsets are listed in Box 76-2. More important than the method of revascularization is the time to revascularization, and that this should be achieved in the most efficient and expeditious manner possible.[25] It is important to keep in mind that early, complete, and sustained reperfusion after MI is known to decrease 30-day

mortality. The preferred method for reperfusion in STEMI is PCI only if it can be done within a timely manner. Practical considerations regarding transport to a PCI-capable facility should be carefully reviewed before forgoing thrombolytics for PCI. Early recognition and diagnosis of STEMI are key to achieving the desired door-to-needle (or medical contact–to-needle) time for initiation of fibrinolytic therapy of 30 minutes or door-to-balloon (or medical contact–to-balloon) time for PCI under 90 minutes.[3] Achieving reperfusion in timely matter correlates with improvement in ultimate infarct size, LV function, and survival.[12,13] The ultimate goal is to restore adequate blood flow through the infarct-related artery to the infarct zone, as well as to limit microvascular damage and reperfusion injury. The latter is accomplished with adjunctive and ancillary treatments that will be discussed in the following sections.

Coronary Stenting

Primary angioplasty for AMI results in a significant reduction in mortality but is limited by the possibility of abrupt vessel closure, recurrent in-hospital ischemia, reocclusion of the infarct related artery, and restenosis. The use of coronary stents has been shown to reduce restenosis and adverse cardiac outcomes in both routine and high-risk PCI.[26] The PAMI Stent Trial was designed to test the hypothesis that routine implantation of an intracoronary stent in the setting of MI would reduce angiographic restenosis and improve clinical outcomes compared to primary balloon angioplasty alone. This large, randomized, multicenter trial involving 900 patients did not show a difference in mortality at 6 months but did show improvement in ischemia-driven target vessel revascularization and less angina in the stented patients compared to balloon angioplasty alone.[27] Despite the lack of definite data demonstrating mortality benefit, virtually all the trials investigating adjunctive therapy for STEMI have employed a strategy of primary stenting, and stenting has becoming the default strategy. Whether to use a bare metal stent or a drug-eluting stent in acute MI is a question that has not yet been addressed definitively by clinical trials; selection is currently based on both patient and angiographic characteristics.

Adjunctive Therapy to Primary PCI

Aspirin. Aspirin is the best known and the most widely used of all the antiplatelet agents because of low cost and relatively low toxicity. Aspirin inhibits the production of thromboxane A2 by irreversibly acetylating the serine residue of the enzyme prostaglandin H2 synthetase. Aspirin has been shown to reduce mortality in acute infarction to the same degree as fibrinolytic therapy, and its effects are additive to fibrinolytics.[28] In addition, aspirin reduces the risk of reinfarction.[29,30] Unless contraindicated, all patients with a suspected ACS (STEMI, NSTEMI, UA) should be given aspirin as soon as possible.

Thienopyridines. Thienopyridines are a class of oral antiplatelet agents that block the P2Y12 component of the adenosine diphosphate

SITUATIONS IN WHICH PRIMARY ANGIOPLASTY IS PREFERRED IN ACUTE MYOCARDIAL INFARCTION

Situations in which PTCA is clearly Preferable to Fibrinolytics:
- Contraindications to fibrinolytic therapy
- Cardiogenic shock
- Patients in whom uncertain diagnosis prompted cardiac catheterization which revealed coronary occlusion

Situations in which PTCA may be Preferable to Fibrinolytics:
- Elderly patients (>75 years)
- Hemodynamic instability
- Patients with prior coronary artery bypass grafting
- Large anterior infarction
- Patients with a prior myocardial infarction

PTCA, percutaneous transluminal coronary angioplasty.

receptor and thus inhibit the activation and aggregation of platelets. Currently used thienopyridines include clopidogrel and prasugrel.[32] Clopidogrel is a prodrug that is converted in the liver to the active thiol metabolite via the cytochrome P450 (CYP) 3A, 1A, 2B, and 2C subfamilies. The active metabolite irreversibly binds to the P2Y12 component of the ADP receptor on the platelet surface, which prevents activation of the GPIIb/IIIa receptor complex and reduces platelet aggregation for the remainder of the platelet's lifespan, approximately 7 to 10 days. Onset of inhibition of platelet aggregation (IPA) is dose dependent, with a 300- to 600-mg loading dose achieving inhibition of platelet within 2 hours, whereas a dose of 50 to 100 mg achieves inhibition of platelets in about 24 to 48 hours. Peak effect (time to maximal IPA) occurs at 6 hours with a loading dose of 300 to 600 mg[31] and 5 to 7 days with a dose of 50 to 100 mg.[32]

The efficacy of clopidogrel in combination with aspirin administered to patients with STEMI prior to PCI was tested in the COMMIT-CCS 2 and CLARITY TIMI-28 studies. CLARITY TIMI-28[33] randomized 3491 STEMI patients to clopidogrel (300-mg load followed by 75 mg daily) or placebo. All patients also received a fibrinolytic, aspirin, and when appropriate, heparin. Use of clopidogrel decreased the incidence of the primary composite efficacy endpoint (infarct artery patency or death or recurrent MI before angiography, 15.0 % versus 21.7%, $P < 0.001$), largely due to a difference in occlusion of the infarct-related artery (12% versus 18%), with no difference in mortality or major bleeding. In the 1863 patients in CLARITY TIMI-28 who underwent PCI (reported as CLARITY-PCI), retreatment with clopidogrel prior to PCI for STEMI resulted in a significant reduction in cardiovascular death, MI, or stroke at 30 days (7.5% versus 12.0%; $P = 0.001$) without causing excess bleeding.[34] It is therefore routine practice to administer a loading dose of clopidogrel, 300 mg or 600 mg, prior to PCI regardless of the physician's concern that the patient might need coronary artery bypass graft (CABG) in the near future.

Some patients are considered clopidogrel nonresponders, usually defined as a recurrence of cardiovascular events while on the recommended dose. Ex vivo assays measuring the degree of inhibition of platelet aggregation while on clopidogrel have demonstrated that 4% to 30% of patients do not have an adequate platelet response while on clopidogrel.[37-39] Despite these findings, testing for clopidogrel resistance has not become routine.

Prasugrel is a recently approved thienopyridine that irreversibly binds to the P2Y12 component of the ADP receptor with a more rapid onset of action.[40] Like clopidogrel, prasugrel is a prodrug metabolized to both an active and inactive metabolite, but a higher proportion is metabolized to an active metabolite, resulting in a higher level of inhibition of platelet aggregation than clopidogrel. The onset of inhibition of platelet aggregation is dose dependent and can be achieved in less than 30 minutes at a dose of 60 mg, but peak effect of IPA occurs in approximately 4 hours.[35] The randomized double-blind TRITON-TIMI 38 trial compared prasugrel (loading dose of 60 mg followed by maintenance dose of 10 mg) with clopidogrel (300-mg load followed by 75-mg maintenance) in 13,608 patients with UA/NSTEMI (n = 10,074) or STEMI (n = 3534) who underwent PCI.[36] All patients also received aspirin, and treatment with prasugrel or clopidogrel was continued for a median of 14.5 months. The primary endpoint, a composite of cardiovascular death, nonfatal MI, and nonfatal stroke, was less frequent among patients who received prasugrel (9.9% versus 12.1 %, $P < 0.001$). The rate of major bleeding was higher in the prasugrel group (2.4% versus 1.8 %, $P = 0.03$), as was the rate of life-threatening bleeding. A post hoc analysis of the TRITON TIMI-38 trial identified three ACS subgroups in which prasugrel was found to be harmful or showed no net benefit: patients with a history of transient ischemic attack (TIA) or stroke (net harm), age older than 75 (no net benefit), and body weight less than 60 kg (no net benefit). The FDA has labeled history of TIA and/or stroke as a contraindication to prasugrel use.[36]

Dual antiplatelet therapy with aspirin and thienopyridines is given to all patients undergoing PCI, as described above. However, data suggest that even patients not undergoing PCI benefit from the addition of clopidogrel to aspirin. COMMIT-CCS-2 randomized over 45,000 patients with suspected MI to 75 mg of clopidogrel daily (no loading dose).[37] The majority of patients had STEMI, but only 54% were treated with fibrinolytics. Clopidogrel was continued after hospital discharge for a mean duration of 14.9 days. The co-primary endpoint of all-cause mortality was reduced from 8.1% in the placebo group to 7.5% in the clopidogrel group (OR, 0.93 [95% CI, 0.87-0.99]; $P = 0.03$; NNT = 167), without increased bleeding in the clopidogrel group. On the basis of these data, patients presenting with MI should be considered for a thienopyridine regardless of whether or not they underwent reperfusion therapy. The duration of thienopyridine use in this population has yet to be defined.

Glycoprotein IIb/IIIa Receptor Antagonists

Glycoprotein IIb/IIIa receptor antagonists inhibit the final common pathway of platelet aggregation, blocking cross-linking of activated platelets, and are often-used percutaneous interventions.[38-42] In the era of dual antiplatelet therapy using a thienopyridine and aspirin, the role of addition of a glycoprotein IIb/IIIa inhibitor in primary angioplasty for STEMI is uncertain. Studies such as the ADMIRAL and CADILLAC trials conducted prior to the use of dual antiplatelet therapy established the efficacy of abciximab in primary PCI (with or without stenting) in patients with STEMI.[41] The results of recent clinical trials have raised questions about whether glycoprotein IIb/IIIa antagonists have additional utility when added to dual antiplatelet therapy in patients with STEMI.[43-45] The BRAVE-3 trial randomized 800 patients undergoing primary stenting to 600 mg of clopidogrel plus either placebo or abciximab prior to PCI and showed no difference at 30 days in either the primary endpoint of infarct size or the secondary composite endpoint of death, recurrent MI, stroke, or urgent revascularization of the infarct-related artery.[43] Similar findings were seen in ON-TIME2, in which 984 patients with STEMI were randomized to either high-dose tirofiban or placebo in addition to dual antiplatelet therapy prior to transport for PCI. Although patients who received high-dose tirofiban had improved resolution of ST-segment elevation before and after PCI, there was no significant difference in TIMI flow or the 30-day composite endpoint of death, recurrent MI, or urgent target-vessel revascularization between the two groups.[44] Given the present data, current guidelines suggest that when a STEMI patient is treated with a thienopyridine and aspirin plus an anticoagulant such as UFH or bivalirudin, the use of a glycoprotein IIb/IIIa inhibitor at the time of PCI may be beneficial but cannot be recommended as routine.[3]

Anticoagulants

Administration of full-dose heparin after fibrinolytic therapy with tPA is essential to diminish reocclusion after successful reperfusion.[6,28] Dosing should be adjusted to weight, with a bolus of 60 U/kg up to a maximum of 4000 U and an initial infusion rate of 12 U/kg/h up to a maximum of 1000 U/h, with adjustment to keep the partial thromboplastin time (PTT) between 50 and 70 seconds.[4] Heparin should be continued for 24 to 48 hours. For patients undergoing PCI who have already been treated with aspirin and a thienopyridine, both unfractionated heparin or bivalirudin (with or without prior heparin administration) are acceptable anticoagulant regimens.[3] Bivalirudin is a direct thrombin inhibitor that inhibits both clot-bound and circulating thrombin. It is administered as an initial bolus of 0.75 mg/kg, followed by a continuous infusion at 1.75 mg/kg/h for the duration of PCI, with adjustments for patients with renal dysfunction. Bivalirudin is an excellent alternative to unfractionated or low-molecular-weight heparin (LMWH) in patients with a history of heparin-induced thrombocytopenia. It is at least equivalent to heparin plus a glycoprotein IIb/IIIa inhibitor in reducing ischemic events associated with UA and/or NSTEMI, with the added benefit of a reduction in bleeding.[46] Up until recently, the role of bivalirudin in STEMI was uncertain. The HORIZONS-AMI trial randomized 3602 patients with STEMI undergoing primary PCI to UFH plus a glycoprotein IIb/IIIa inhibitor or to bivalirudin alone (with provisional glycoprotein IIb/IIIa in the cardiac catheterization lab).[47] Major adverse cardiac event (MACE) rates were equivalent, but use of bivalirudin alone was associated with a 40%

reduction in bleeding (4.9% versus 8.3%, $P < 0.001$;). However, at 1 year, MACE rates were similar in the two groups (11.9% versus 11.9%, HR 1.00, 0.82-1.21, $P = 0.98$), but there was a decrease in all-cause mortality with bivalirudin (3.4% versus 4.8%, $P = 0.03$).[48]

Enoxaparin is an LMWH with established efficacy as an anticoagulant in patients with STEMI who have received fibrinolytics or are undergoing PCI.[49,50] The standard dose of enoxaparin is a 30-mg intravenous (IV) bolus, followed 15 minutes later by subcutaneous injections of 1 mg/kg every 12 hours. Patients with decreased creatinine clearance or older than 75 are at higher risk of bleeding with standard-dose enoxaparin and should not receive a bolus, but can receive a reduced dose of 0.75 mg/kg every 12 hours. Patients undergoing PCI should have an additional bolus if the last dose was given 8 to 12 hours prior. Maintenance dosing of enoxaparin should be given during the hospitalization (up to 8 days).

Fondaparinux, also an LMWH, can be dosed daily in patients receiving fibrinolytics for STEMI (initial dose of 2.5 mg IV followed by subcutaneous injections of 2.5 mg once daily). The OASIS-6 trial randomized over 12,000 patients with STEMI to 2.5 mg of fondaparinux or placebo. Death or reinfarction at 30 days was significantly reduced in the fondaparinux group (9.7% versus 11.2%, $P = 0.008$) and were maintained at 6 months.[51] Severe bleeds were reduced with fondaparinux (61 versus 79, $P = 0.13$), and significant benefit was seen in patients who received fibrinolytics, as well those who were not reperfused. However, in patients undergoing PCI for STEMI, fondaparinux should not be administered alone, owing to an increased rate of catheter-related thrombosis observed in clinical trials.[51,52] If fondaparinux has been chosen, unfractionated heparin should be administered with fondaparinux in the catheterization laboratory. Table 76-1 summarizes typical antiplatelet and anticoagulant therapy for ACSs.

Nitrates

Nitrates have a number of beneficial effects in AMI. They reduce myocardial oxygen demand by decreasing preload and afterload, and they may also improve myocardial oxygen supply by increasing subendocardial perfusion and collateral blood flow to the ischemic region.[53] Occasional patients with ST elevation due to occlusive coronary artery spasm may have dramatic resolution of ischemia with nitrates. In addition to their hemodynamic effects, nitrates also reduce platelet aggregation. Despite these benefits, the GISSI-3 and ISIS-4 trials failed to show a significant reduction in mortality from routine acute and chronic nitrate therapy.[54,55] Nonetheless, nitrates are still first-line agents for the symptomatic relief of angina pectoris and when MI is complicated by congestive heart failure.

Beta-Blockers

Beta-blockers are beneficial both in the early management of MI and as long-term therapy. In the prefibrinolytic era, early IV atenolol was shown to significantly reduce reinfarction, cardiac arrest, cardiac rupture, and death.[56] In conjunction with fibrinolytic therapy with tPA, immediate β-blockade with metoprolol resulted in a significant reduction in recurrent ischemia and reinfarction, although mortality was not decreased.[57]

The COMMIT-CCS 2 trial of 45,852 patients with acute MI had a factorial arm (the clopidogrel arm was discussed earlier) and randomized patients—93% of whom had STEMI and 54% of whom were treated with lytics—to treatment with metoprolol (3 IV injections of 5 mg each followed by oral 200 mg/day for up to 4 weeks) or placebo.[58] Surprisingly, there was no difference in the primary endpoint of death, reinfarction, or cardiac arrest by treatment group (9.4% for metoprolol versus 9.9% for placebo, $P = NS$) or in the co-primary endpoint of all-cause mortality by hospital discharge (7.7% versus 7.8%, $P = NS$). Although reinfarction was lower in the metoprolol group (2.0% versus 2.5%, $P = 0.001$). there was an increase in the risk of developing heart failure and cardiogenic shock (5.0% versus 3.9%, $P < 0.0001$).[58] Death due to shock occurred more frequently in the metoprolol group (2.2%, versus 1.7%), while death due to arrhythmia occurred less frequently in the metoprolol group (1.7%, n = 388 versus 2.2%, n = 498). Based on these findings, routine use of *intravenous* beta-blockers in the absence of systemic hypertension is no longer recommended.[59]

In contrast to the use of early aggressive beta-blocker therapy, the long-term use of beta-blockers post MI has favorable outcomes on mortality.[60,61] The CARvedilol Post-infaRct survIval COntRolled evaluatioN (CAPRICORN) trial was a randomized placebo-controlled trial designed to test the long-term efficacy of carvedilol on morbidity and mortality in patients with LV dysfunction 3 to 21 days after MI who were already treated with angiotensin-converting enzyme (ACE) inhibitors.[62] After an average follow-up period of 1.3 years, cardiovascular mortality was lower in the carvedilol arm (11% versus 14% for placebo, $P = 0.024$), as was all-cause mortality or nonfatal MI (14% versus 20%, $P = 0.002$).[62] This study supports the claim that beta-blocker therapy after acute MI reduces mortality irrespective of reperfusion therapy or ACE inhibitor use. Relative contraindications to oral beta-blockers include heart rate less than 60 bpm, systolic arterial pressure less than 100 mm Hg, moderate or severe LV failure, signs of peripheral hypoperfusion, shock, PR interval greater than 0.24 second, second- or third-degree AV block, active asthma, or reactive airway disease.[59]

Angiotensin-Converting Enzyme Inhibitors

Angiotensin-converting enzyme generates angiotensin II from angiotensin I and also catalyzes the breakdown of bradykinin. Thus ACE inhibitors can decrease circulating angiotensin II levels and increase levels of bradykinin, which in turn stimulates production of nitric oxide by endothelial nitric oxide synthase. In the vasculature, ACE inhibition promotes vasodilation and tends to inhibit smooth muscle proliferation, platelet aggregation, and thrombosis.

ACE inhibitors have been shown unequivocally to improve hemodynamics, functional capacity and symptoms, and survival in patients with chronic congestive heart failure.[63,64] Moreover, ACE inhibitors prevent the development of congestive heart failure in patients with asymptomatic LV dysfunction.[65] This information was the spur for trials evaluating the benefit the prophylactic administration of ACE inhibitors in the post-MI period. The SAVE trial showed that patients with LV dysfunction (LVEF < 40%) after MI had a 21% improvement

TABLE 76-1	Antiplatelet/Anticoagulant Therapy in Acute Coronary Syndromes	
Drug	**Initial Medical Treatment**
Antiplatelet Drugs	
Aspirin	162 to 325 mg nonenteric formulation, orally or chewed
Clopidogrel	LD of 300 to 600 mg orally, MD of 75 mg orally per day
Prasugrel	LD of 60 mg orally, MD of 10 mg orally per day
Ticlopidine	LD of 500 mg orally, MD of 250 mg orally twice daily
Anticoagulants	
Unfractionated heparin	LD of 60 U per kg (max 4,000 U) as IV bolus MD of IV infusion of 12 U/kg/h (max 1000 U/h) to maintain APTT at 1.5 to 2.0 times control (approximately 50-70 sec)
Enoxaparin	LD of 30 mg IV bolus may be given MD of 1 mg/kg subcutaneously every 12 h; extend dosing interval to 1 mg/kg every 24 h if estimated creatinine clearance <30 mL/min
Fondaparinux	2.5 mg subcutaneously once daily. Avoid for creatinine clearance <30 mL/min
Eptifibatide	LD of IV bolus of 180 μg/kg MD of IV infusion of 2 μg/kg/min; reduce infusion by 50% in patients with estimated creatinine clearance <50 mL/min
Tirofiban	LD of IV infusion of 0.4 μg/g/min for 30 min MD of IV infusion of 0.1 μg/kg/min; reduce rate of infusion by 50% in patients with estimated creatinine clearance <30 mL/min
Bivalirudin	0.1 mg per kg bolus, 0.25 mg/kg/h infusion

Adapted from Anderson JL, Adams CD, Antam EM et al. ACC/AHA 2007 guidelines for the management of patients with unstable angina/non–ST-elevation myocardial infarction: a report of the American College of Cardiology/American Heart Association Task Force on Practice Guidelines. J Am Coll Cardiol 2007;50:e1-157.

LD, loading dose; *MD*, maintenance dose.

in survival after treatment with the ACE inhibitor, captopril.[66] A smaller but still significant reduction in mortality was seen when all patients were treated with captopril in the ISIS-4 study.[55] The HOPE trial randomized 9297 patients with documented vascular disease or those at high risk for atherosclerosis (diabetes plus at least one other risk factor) in the absence of heart failure to treatment with the tissue-selective ACE inhibitor, ramipril (target dose 10 mg/day), or placebo.[67] An impressive 22% reduction in the combined endpoint of cardiovascular death, MI, and stroke was observed, and the improved survival was additive to the benefits of aspirin and beta-blockers.[67] The mechanisms responsible for the benefits of ACE inhibitors probably include limitation in the progressive LV dysfunction and enlargement (remodeling) that often occur after infarction, but a reduction in ischemic events was seen as well.

Immediate IV ACE inhibition with enalaprilat has not been shown to be beneficial,[68] but oral ACE inhibition should be started early in the hospital course. Patients should be started on low doses of oral agents (captopril, 6.25 mg three times daily) and rapidly increased to the range demonstrated beneficial in clinical trials (captopril, 50 mg three times daily; enalapril, 10-20 mg twice daily; lisinopril, 10-20 mg once daily; or ramipril, 10 mg once daily).

Lipid-Lowering Agents

There is extensive epidemiologic, laboratory, and clinical evidence linking cholesterol and coronary artery disease (CAD). Total cholesterol level has been linked to the development of CAD events with a continuous and graded relation.[69] Most of this risk is due to LDL cholesterol. A number of large primary and secondary prevention trials have shown that LDL cholesterol lowering is associated with a reduced risk of coronary disease events. Earlier lipid-lowering trials used bile acid sequestrants (cholestyramine), fibric acid derivatives (gemfibrozil and clofibrate), or niacin in addition to diet. The reduction in total cholesterol in these early trials was 6% to 15% and was accompanied by a consistent trend toward a reduction in fatal and nonfatal coronary events.[70]

More impressive results have been achieved using HMG-CoA reductase inhibitors (statins). Statins have been demonstrated to decrease the rate of adverse ischemic events in patients with documented CAD in the 4S trial,[71] as well as in the CARE study[72] and the LIPID trial.[73]

The goal of treatment is an LDL cholesterol level less than 100 mg/dL.[74] Maximum benefit may require management of other lipid abnormalities (elevated triglycerides, low HDL cholesterol) and treatment of other atherogenic risk factors.

The use and efficacy of high-dose statin loading prior to PCI for STEMI was addressed in the STATIN STEMI trial; 171 patients were randomized to either 80 mg or 10 mg of atorvastatin in addition to 600 mg of clopidogrel prior to PCI for STEMI.[75] The 30-day incidence of death, MI, or target vessel revascularization was 5.8% in the high-dose statin group versus 10.6 % in the low-dose statin group ($P = 0.26$).[75] Although high-dose statin administration prior to PCI is not requisite, all patients with ACS should be started on a statin prior to discharge unless there is a contraindication.

Calcium Channel Blockers

Randomized clinical trials have not demonstrated that routine use of calcium channel blockers improves survival after MI.[76] In fact, meta-analyses suggest that high doses of the short-acting dihydropyridine, nifedipine, increase mortality in MI.[77] Adverse effects of calcium channel blockers include bradycardia, atrioventricular block, and exacerbation of heart failure. The relative vasodilating, negative inotropic effects, and conduction system effects of the various agents must be considered when they are employed in this setting. Diltiazem is the only calcium channel blocker that has been proven to have tangible benefits, reducing reinfarction and recurrent ischemia in patients with non–Q wave infarctions who do not have evidence of congestive heart failure.[78]

Calcium channel blockers may be useful for patients whose postinfarction course is complicated by recurrent angina, because these agents not only reduce myocardial oxygen demand but also inhibit coronary vasoconstriction. For hemodynamically stable patients, diltiazem can be given, starting at 60 to 90 mg orally every 6 to 8 hours. In patients with severe LV dysfunction, long-acting dihydropyridines without prominent negative inotropic effects, such as amlodipine, nicardipine, or the long-acting preparation of nifedipine, may be preferable; increased mortality with these agents has not been demonstrated.

Non–ST-Segment Elevation Myocardial Infarction

The key to initial management of ACS patients who present without ST elevation is risk stratification. The overall risk of a patient is related to both the severity of preexisting heart disease and the degree of plaque instability. Risk stratification is an ongoing process that begins with hospital admission and continues through discharge.

Braunwald has proposed a classification for UA based on severity of symptoms and clinical circumstances for risk stratification.[79] The risk of progression to acute MI or death due to ACS increases with age. ST-segment depression on the ECG identifies patients at higher risk for clinical events.[79] Conversely, a normal ECG confers an excellent short-term prognosis. Biochemical markers of cardiac injury are also predictive of outcome. Elevated levels of troponin T are associated with an increased risk of cardiac events and a higher 30-day mortality, and in fact, were more strongly correlated with 30-day survival than ECG category or CPK-MB level in an analysis of data from the GUSTO-2 trial.[80] Conversely, low levels are associated with low event rates, although the absence of troponin elevation does not guarantee a good prognosis and is not a substitute for good clinical judgment.

ANTIPLATELET THERAPY

As previously noted, aspirin is a mainstay of ACS therapy. Both the VA Cooperative Study Group[29] and the Canadian Multicenter Trial[81] showed that aspirin reduces the risk of death or MI by approximately 50% in patients with UA or NQMI. Aspirin also reduces events after resolution of an ACS and should be continued indefinitely.

In addition to patients with STEMI, patients with NSTEMI and suspected UA benefit from the use of a thienopyridine in addition to aspirin. This benefit, a decrease in cardiovascular death, MI, or stroke, is seen not only in patients who undergo PCI but also in patients who are managed medically. In the CURE trial, 12,562 patients were randomized to receive clopidogrel or placebo in addition to standard therapy with aspirin within 24 hours of UA symptoms.[82] Clopidogrel significantly reduced the risk of MI, stroke, or cardiovascular death from 11.4% to 9.3% ($P<0.001$).[82] It should be noted that this benefit came with a 1% absolute increase in major non-life-threatening bleeds ($P = 0.001$) as well as a 2.8% absolute increase in major/life-threatening bleeds associated with CABG within 5 days ($P=0.07$).[82] Because percutaneous revascularization was performed on only 23% of patients in the CURE trial during the initial hospitalization, the study provides convincing evidence that clopidogrel is beneficial in patients who are managed medically, in addition to those undergoing PCI. The optimal duration of therapy in this patient population, however, is unknown.

The PCI-CURE report examined the subset of patients (n = 2658) with UA/NSTEMI who underwent PCI.[83] Overall, including events before and after PCI, there was a 31% reduction in cardiovascular death or MI ($P<0.002$). There was no difference between the groups in major bleeding.[83] PCI-CURE suggests that patients with UA/NSTEMI who undergo PCI, pretreatment with clopidogrel followed by up to 1 year of clopidogrel therapy is beneficial in reducing major cardiovascular events. However, PCI-CURE did not adequately address the question of dose or timing of clopidogrel in relationship to PCI. The CREDO trial randomized 2116 patients to a 300-mg loading dose of clopidogrel or placebo (3-24 hours before PCI). Both groups received 325 mg of aspirin and were treated with 75 mg of clopidogrel daily for 1 year. Although there was no difference between groups in the 28-day composite endpoint of death, MI, or urgent target vessel revascularization, treatment with clopidogrel was associated with a 26.9% relative risk reduction in the 1-year composite endpoint of death, MI, or stroke.[84]

Clopidogrel has also been tested for secondary prevention of events. The CAPRIE trial, a multicenter trial of 19,185 patients with known vascular disease (prior stroke, MI, or peripheral vascular disease), randomized patients to either 75 mg/d of clopidogrel or 325 mg aspirin.[85] After an average follow-up of 1.6 years, patients treated with clopidogrel had significantly fewer cardiovascular events than patients treated with aspirin (5.8% versus 5.3%, a relative risk reduction of 8.7%).[85]

The TRITON TIMI-38 trial, as mentioned previously, included both STEMI (n = 3534) and UA/NSTEMI (n = 10,074) patients.[36] The primary endpoint, cardiovascular death, nonfatal MI, and nonfatal stroke, was significantly lower in the prasugrel group at the expensive of increased bleeding in the prasugrel-treated patients.[36] Although prasugrel is a reasonable choice of thienopyridine in patients with ACS, it should not be used in patients with a history of stroke or TIA, and it should be used with caution in patients older than 75 or weighing less than 60 kg.[3] The dosing regimen of prasugrel for patients with UA/NSTEMI is identical to the dose used in STEMI patients (60-mg loading and 10-mg maintenance).

Ticagrelor, which reversibly binds to the P2Y12 platelet receptor, exhibited greater efficacy than clopidogrel in the PLATO trial.[86] Major bleeding events did not differ between the groups, although bleeding unrelated to CABG occurred more often with ticagrelor. Both prasugrel and ticagrelor may have a quicker onset of action than clopidogrel and may prove to be very useful in patients who are clopidogrel resistant or have recurrent cardiovascular events while on clopidogrel.

The current guidelines recommend a loading dose of 300 to 600 mg of clopidogrel in patients with UA/NSTEMI, followed by 75 mg daily.[3] Prasugrel should be administered as a 60-mg loading dose followed by a 10 mg/d maintenance dose.[3] The duration of clopidogrel may depend on whether or not the patient has received a stent. Typically, patients who received bare metal stents (BMS) for at least 4 weeks and those with drug-eluting stents (DES) should remain on clopidogrel for at least 12 months.[3,87] For DES, however, adequate long-term data have not been sufficient to formulate a definite recommendation on the duration of therapy.

ANTICOAGULANT THERAPY

Heparin is an important component of primary therapy for patients with unstable coronary syndromes without ST elevation. When added to aspirin, heparin has been shown to reduce refractory angina and the development of MI,[30] and a meta-analysis of the available data indicates that addition of heparin reduces the composite endpoint of death or MI.[88]

Unfractionated heparin, however, can be difficult to administer because the anticoagulant effect is unpredictable in individual patients; this is due to binding of heparin to heparin-binding proteins and heparin inhibition by several factors released by activated platelets, most notably platelet factor 4. Therefore, the APTT (activated partial thromboplastin time) must be monitored closely. The potential for heparin-associated thrombocytopenia is also a safety concern.

Low-molecular-weight heparins, which are obtained by depolymerization of standard heparin and selection of fractions with lower molecular weight, have several advantages. Because they bind less avidly to heparin binding proteins, there is less variability in the anticoagulant response and a more predictable dose-response curve, obviating the need to monitor APTT. The incidence of thrombocytopenia is lower (but not absent, and patients with heparin-induced thrombocytopenia with anti-heparin antibodies cannot be switched to LMWH). LMWH is less susceptible to inactivation by platelet factor 4. Finally, LMWHs have longer half-lives and can be given by subcutaneous injection. These properties make treatment with LMWH at home after hospital discharge feasible. Since evidence suggests that patients with unstable coronary syndromes may remain in a hypercoagulable state for weeks or months, the longer duration of anticoagulation possible with LMWH may be desirable.

Several trials have documented beneficial effects of LMWH therapy in unstable coronary syndromes. The ESSENCE trial showed that the LMWH, enoxaparin, reduced the combined endpoint of death, MI, or recurrent ischemia at both 14 and 30 days when compared to heparin.[89] Similar results were found in the TIMI 11B trial comparing enoxaparin to heparin.[90] A meta-analysis of these two very similar trials demonstrated a 23% 7-day and an 18% 42-day reduction in the harder endpoint of death or MI.[90] Dalteparin, another LMWH, is also available, but the evidence for its efficacy is not nearly as compelling as that for enoxaparin.[91]

Although LMWHs are substantially easier to administer than standard heparin, and long-term administration can be contemplated, they are also more expensive. Specific considerations with the use of LMWHs include decreased clearance in renal insufficiency and the lack of a commercially available test to measure the anticoagulant effect. LMWH should be given strong consideration in high-risk patients, but whether substitution of LMWH for heparin in all patients is cost-effective is uncertain.

Direct Thrombin Inhibitors

Recombinant hirudin, argatroban, and bivalirudin are examples of direct thrombin inhibitors (DTIs). As opposed to heparin, they directly bind to both circulating and clot-bound thrombin and inhibit the conversion of fibrinogen to fibrin in the final step of the clotting cascade. Direct thrombin inhibitors have several theoretical advantages over heparin. Heparin binds to a number of tissue and plasma proteins, which alters its bioavailability and clearance. Heparin may also have a platelet-activating effect in ACS. Lastly, DTIs do not bind to platelet factor 4 and therefore avoid the problem of heparin-induced thrombocytopenia.

Bivalirudin is a 20–amino acid peptide based on the structure of hirudin, a natural anticoagulant isolated from the saliva of the medicinal leech, *Hirudo medicinalis*. Bivalirudin is the only DTI indicated for use in ACS. The REPLACE 2 trial compared bivalirudin plus provisional glycoprotein IIb/IIIa inhibitor to unfractionated heparin plus planned glycoprotein IIb/IIIa inhibitor in 6010 patients undergoing planned or urgent PCI.[46] Although 6-month event rates with bivalirudin were slightly higher (7.6 % versus 7.1%), bleeding with bivalirudin was lower, and the prespecified composite endpoint met statistical criteria for non-inferiority. Similar findings were seen in the ACUITY trial, which compared heparin with glycoprotein IIb/IIIa inhibitor to bivalirudin with glycoprotein IIb/IIIa inhibitor to bivalirudin alone with provisional glycoprotein IIb/IIIa inhibitor.[92] Bivalirudin alone, compared with heparin plus glycoprotein IIb/IIIa inhibitors, resulted in non-inferior rates of composite ischemia (7.8% versus 7.3%, $P = 0.32$). Major bleeding was again significantly reduced with bivalirudin alone. However, patients who got bivalirudin alone without a thienopyridine prior to angiography or PCI had a higher rate of composite ischemic events than patients who received heparin plus a glycoprotein IIb/IIIa inhibitor (9.1% versus 7.1%). Therefore, it is not recommended that bivalirudin be administered alone, particularly if there is a going to be a delay to angiography.

Glycoprotein IIb/IIIa Antagonists

Given the central role of platelet activation and aggregation in the pathophysiology of unstable coronary syndromes, attention has focused on platelet glycoprotein IIb/IIIa antagonists, which inhibit the final common pathway of platelet aggregation. Three agents are currently available. Abciximab, a monoclonal antibody Fab fragment; tirofiban, a small-molecule, synthetic nonpeptide agent; and eptifibatide, a small-molecule cyclic heptapeptide. The benefits of glycoprotein IIb/IIIa inhibitors as adjunctive treatment in patients with ACS have shown in several trials.[93-94] Meta-analyses have found a relative risk reduction of 11% in NSTEMI.[38] Additional analysis suggests that glycoprotein IIb/IIIa inhibition is most effective in high-risk patients, those with either ECG changes or elevated troponin.[38] The benefits appear to be restricted to patients undergoing PCI, which may not be entirely surprising.

The above mentioned studies were conducted prior to the era of dual antiplatelet therapy. As mentioned previously, it is common practice to administer a thienopyridine and aspirin in conjunction with an anticoagulant in patients with ACS. For patients with UA/NSTEMI undergoing an initial invasive approach, the most recent data suggest that either a glycoprotein IIb/IIIa inhibitor _or_ a thienopyridine can be given in addition to aspirin and an anticoagulant if the patient is considered low risk (troponin negative). However, _if_ the patient is considered high risk (troponin positive, recurrent ischemic features), both a glycoprotein IIb/IIIa inhibitor and clopidogrel can be given in addition to aspirin and an anticoagulant.[3,87]

INTERVENTIONAL MANAGEMENT

Cardiac catheterization may be undertaken in patients presenting with symptoms suggestive of unstable coronary syndromes for one of several reasons: to assist with risk stratification, as a prelude to revascularization, and to exclude significant epicardial coronary stenosis as a cause of symptoms when the diagnosis is uncertain.

An early invasive approach has now been compared to a conservative approach in several prospective studies. Two earlier trials, the VANQWISH trial[95] and the TIMI IIIb[16] study, were negative, but the difference in the number of patients who had been revascularized by the end of these trials was small. In addition, they were performed before widespread use of coronary stenting and platelet glycoprotein IIb/IIIa inhibitors, both of which have now been shown to improve outcomes after angioplasty.

The FRISC II,[96] TACTICS-TIMI 18,[97] and RITA III[98] trials each demonstrated that the composite endpoint of death, MI, or refractory angina was less frequent among patients who were randomized to the early invasive strategy, with the greatest benefit observed in high-risk patients, those with elevated cardiac biomarkers, extensive ST-segment depression, and hemodynamic features suggestive of large infarctions.[87]

The ICTUS trial enrolled 1200 patients with UA/NSTEMI who were initially treated with aspirin and enoxaparin before randomized assignment to one of two strategies: an early invasive strategy within 48 hours that included abciximab for PCI or a selective invasive strategy.[99] Patients who were assigned the latter strategy were selected for coronary angiography only if they had refractory angina despite medical treatment, hemodynamic or rhythm instability, or predischarge exercise testing demonstrated clinically significant ischemia. The trial showed no reduction in the composite endpoints of death, nonfatal MI, or rehospitalization for angina at 1 year among patients who were assigned to the early invasive strategy. After 4 years of follow-up, the rates of death and MI among the two groups of patients remained similar.[99] It is not clear why the results of ICTUS differ from previous trials. The more recent Timing of Intervention in Acute Coronary Syndromes (TIMACS) study randomized 3031 patients with UA/NSTEMI to undergo cardiac catheterization either within 24 hours of symptom onset or more than 36 hours later.[100] The median time to angiography was 14 hours for the early intervention group and 50 hours for the delayed-intervention group. There was no difference between the groups in the composite endpoint of death, MI, or stroke at 6 months.

Risk stratification is the key to managing patients with NSTEMI ACS. One possible algorithm for managing patients with NSTEMI is shown in Figure 76-2. An initial strategy of medical management with attempts at stabilization is warranted in patients with lower risk, but patients at higher risk should be considered for cardiac catheterization. Pharmacologic and mechanical strategies are intertwined in the sense that selection of patients for early revascularization will influence the choice of antiplatelet and anticoagulant medication. When good clinical judgment is employed, early coronary angiography in selected ACS patients can lead to better management and lower morbidity and mortality.

▓ Complications of Acute Myocardial Infarction

POSTINFARCTION ISCHEMIA

Causes of ischemia after infarction include decreased myocardial oxygen supply due to coronary reocclusion or spasm, mechanical

problems which increase myocardial oxygen demand, and extracardiac factors such as hypertension, anemia, hypotension, or hypermetabolic states. Nonischemic causes of chest pain such as postinfarction pericarditis and acute pulmonary embolism should also be considered.

Immediate management includes aspirin, β-blockade, IV nitroglycerin, heparin, consideration of calcium channel blockers, and diagnostic coronary angiography. Postinfarction angina is an indication for revascularization. PTCA can be performed if the culprit lesion is suitable. CABG should be considered for patients with left main disease, three-vessel disease, and those unsuitable for PTCA. If the angina cannot be controlled medically or is accompanied by hemodynamic instability, an intraaortic balloon pump should be inserted.

VENTRICULAR FREE WALL RUPTURE

Ventricular free wall rupture typically occurs during the first week after infarction. The classic patient is elderly, female, and hypertensive. Early use of fibrinolytic therapy reduces the incidence of cardiac rupture, but late use may actually increase the risk. Pseudoaneurysm with leakage may be heralded by chest pain, nausea, and restlessness, but frank free wall rupture presents as a catastrophic event with shock and electromechanical dissociation. Pericardiocentesis may be necessary to relieve acute tamponade, ideally in the operating room, since the pericardial effusion my be tamponading the bleeding. Salvage is possible with expeditious thoracotomy and repair, either with a patch or by direct suturing.[101] A pericardial effusion may be seen by echocardiography; contrast ventriculography is not a sensitive way to detect a small rupture.

VENTRICULAR SEPTAL RUPTURE

Septal rupture presents as severe heart failure or cardiogenic shock, with a pansystolic murmur and parasternal thrill. The hallmark finding is a left-to-right intracardiac shunt ("step-up" in oxygen saturation from right atrium to right ventricle), but the diagnosis is most easily made with echocardiography.

Rapid institution of intraaortic balloon pumping and supportive pharmacologic measures are necessary. Operative repair is the only viable option for long-term survival. The timing of surgery has been controversial, but most authorities now suggest that repair should be undertaken early, within 48 hours of the rupture.[102]

ACUTE MITRAL REGURGITATION

Ischemic mitral regurgitation is usually associated with inferior MI and ischemia or infarction of the posterior papillary muscle, although anterior papillary muscle rupture can also occur. Papillary muscle rupture has a bimodal incidence, either within 24 hours or 3 to 7 days after AMI. It presents dramatically with pulmonary edema, hypotension, and cardiogenic shock. When a papillary muscle ruptures, the murmur of acute mitral regurgitation may be limited to early systole because of rapid equalization of pressures in the left atrium and left ventricle. More importantly, the murmur may be soft or inaudible, especially when cardiac output is low.[103]

Echocardiography is extremely useful in the differential diagnosis, which includes free wall rupture, ventricular septal rupture, and infarct extension with pump failure. Hemodynamic monitoring with pulmonary artery catheterization may also be helpful. Management includes afterload reduction with nitroprusside and intraaortic balloon pumping as temporizing measures. Inotropic or vasopressor therapy may also be needed to support cardiac output and blood pressure. Definitive therapy, however, is surgical valve repair or replacement, which should be undertaken as soon as possible, since clinical deterioration can be sudden.[103,104]

RIGHT VENTRICULAR INFARCTION

Right ventricular infarction occurs in up to 30% of patients with inferior infarction and is clinically significant in 10%.[105] The combination

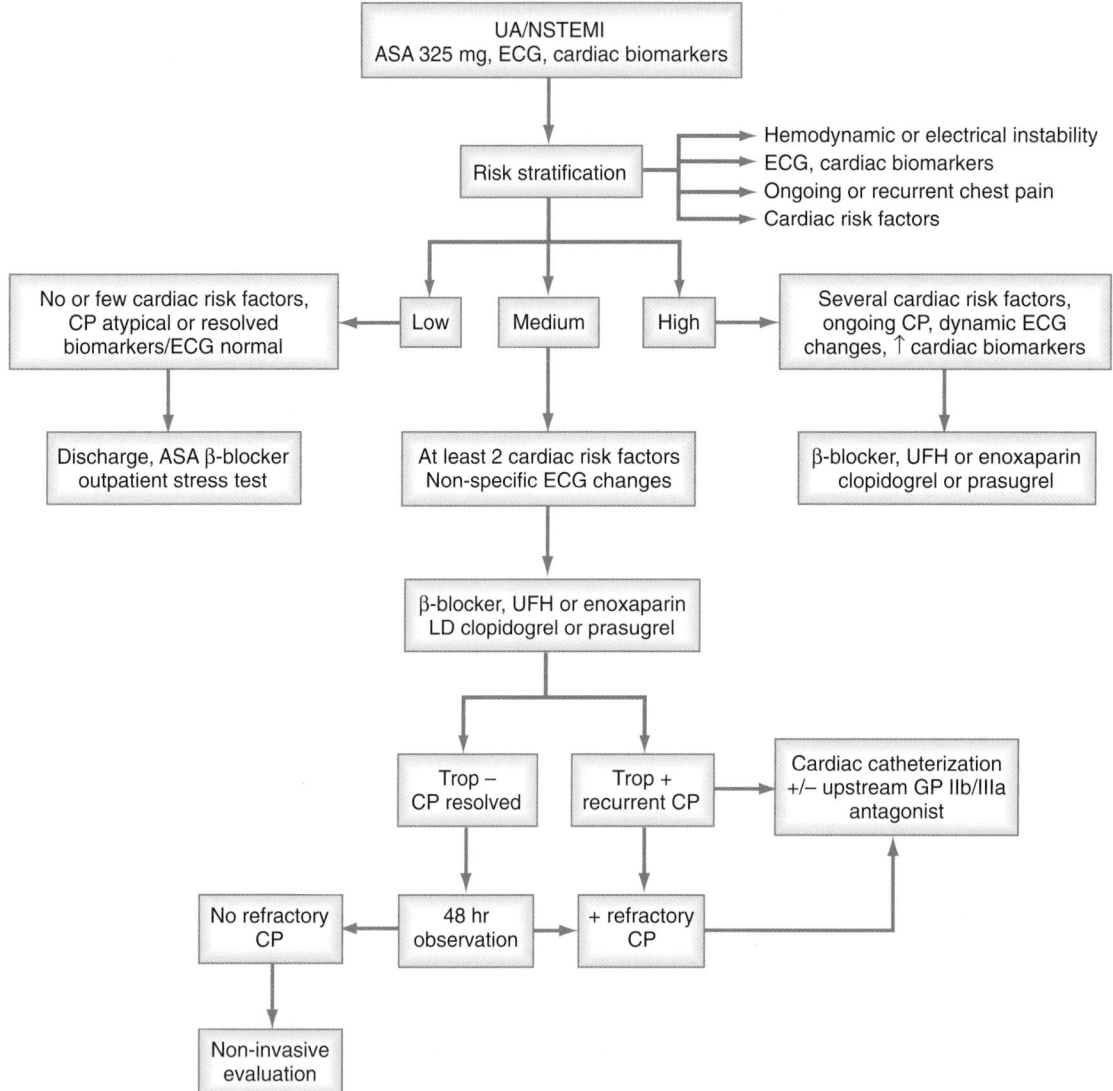

Figure 76-2 Possible treatment algorithm for patients with non–ST-segment elevation acute coronary syndromes. *ASA,* aspirin; *CP,* chest pain; *ECG,* electrocardiogram; *GPIIb/IIIa,* glycoprotein IIb/IIIa antagonist; *Trop,* troponin; *UFH,* unfractionated heparin.

of a clear chest x-ray with jugular venous distention in a patient with an inferior wall MI should lead to the suspicion of a coexisting right ventricular infarct. The diagnosis is substantiated by demonstration of ST-segment elevation in the right precordial leads (V_3R to V_5R) or by characteristic hemodynamic findings on right heart catheterization (elevated right atrial and right ventricular end-diastolic pressures, with normal to low pulmonary artery occlusion pressure and low cardiac output). Echocardiography can demonstrate depressed right ventricular contractility.[106] Patients with cardiogenic shock on the basis of right ventricular infarction have a better prognosis than those with left-sided pump failure.[105] This may be due in part to the fact that right ventricular function tends to return to normal over time with supportive therapy,[107] although such therapy may need to be prolonged.

In patients with right ventricular infarction, right ventricular preload should be maintained with fluid administration. In some cases, however, fluid resuscitation may increase pulmonary capillary occlusion pressure but may not increase cardiac output, and overdilation of the right ventricle can compromise LV filling and cardiac output.[107] Inotropic therapy with dobutamine may be more effective in increasing cardiac output in some patients, and monitoring with serial echocardiograms may also be useful to detect right ventricular overdistention.[107] Maintenance of atrioventricular synchrony is also

important in these patients to optimize right ventricular filling.[106] For patients with continued hemodynamic instability, intraaortic balloon pumping may be useful, particularly because elevated right ventricular pressures and volumes increase wall stress and oxygen consumption and decrease right coronary perfusion pressure, exacerbating right ventricular ischemia.

Reperfusion of the occluded coronary artery is also crucial. A study using direct angioplasty demonstrated that restoration of normal flow resulted in dramatic recovery of right ventricular function and a mortality rate of only 2%, whereas unsuccessful reperfusion was associated with persistent hemodynamic compromise and a mortality of 58%.[108]

CARDIOGENIC SHOCK

Epidemiology and Pathophysiology

Cardiogenic shock, resulting either from LV pump failure or mechanical complications, represents the leading cause of in-hospital death after MI.[109] Despite advances in management of heart failure and AMI, until very recently, clinical outcomes in patients with cardiogenic shock have been poor, with reported mortality rates ranging from 50% to 80%.[110] Patients may have cardiogenic shock at initial presentation, but shock often evolves over several hours.[111,112]

Cardiac dysfunction in patients with cardiogenic shock is usually initiated by MI or ischemia. The myocardial dysfunction resulting from ischemia worsens that ischemia, creating a downward spiral (Figure 76-3). Compensatory mechanisms that retain fluid in an attempt to maintain cardiac output may add to the vicious cycle and further increase diastolic filling pressures. The interruption of this cycle of myocardial dysfunction and ischemia forms the basis for the therapeutic regimens for cardiogenic shock.

Initial Management

Maintenance of adequate oxygenation and ventilation are critical. Many patients require intubation and mechanical ventilation, if only to reduce the work of breathing and facilitate sedation and stabilization before cardiac catheterization. Electrolyte abnormalities should be corrected, and morphine (or fentanyl if systolic pressure is compromised) used to relieve pain and anxiety, thus reducing excessive sympathetic activity and decreasing oxygen demand, preload, and afterload. Arrhythmias and heart block may have major effects on cardiac output and should be corrected promptly with antiarrhythmic drugs, cardioversion, or pacing.

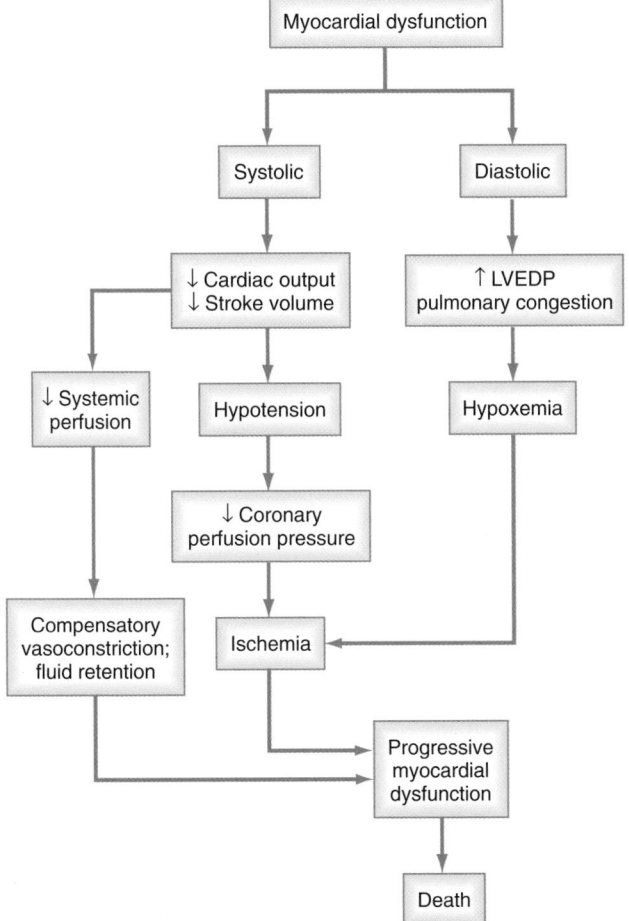

Figure 76-3 The "downward spiral" in cardiogenic shock. Stroke volume and cardiac output fall with left ventricular (LV) dysfunction, producing hypotension and tachycardia that reduce coronary blood flow. Increasing ventricular diastolic pressure reduces coronary blood flow, and increased wall stress elevates myocardial oxygen requirements. All of these factors combine to worsen ischemia. The falling cardiac output also compromises systemic perfusion. Compensatory mechanisms include sympathetic stimulation and fluid retention to increase preload. These mechanisms can actually worsen cardiogenic shock by increasing myocardial oxygen demand and afterload. Thus, a vicious circle can be established. *LVEDP*, left ventricular end-diastolic pressure. *(Adapted with permission from Hollenberg et al. Cardiogenic shock. Ann Intern Med 1999;131:47-59.)*

The initial approach to the hypotensive patient should include fluid resuscitation, unless frank pulmonary edema is present. Patients are commonly diaphoretic, and relative hypovolemia may be present in as many as 20% of patients with cardiogenic shock. Fluid infusion is best initiated with predetermined boluses titrated to clinical endpoints of heart rate, urine output, and blood pressure. Ischemia produces diastolic as well as systolic dysfunction, and thus elevated filling pressures may be necessary to maintain stroke volume in patients with cardiogenic shock. Patients who do not respond rapidly to initial fluid boluses or those with poor physiologic reserve should be considered for invasive hemodynamic monitoring. Optimal filling pressures vary from patient to patient; hemodynamic monitoring can be used to construct a Starling curve at the bedside, identifying the filling pressure at which cardiac output is maximized. Maintenance of adequate preload is particularly important in patients with right ventricular infarction.

When arterial pressure remains inadequate, therapy with vasopressor agents may be required to maintain coronary perfusion pressure. Maintenance of adequate blood pressure is essential to break the vicious cycle of progressive hypotension with further myocardial ischemia. Dopamine increases both blood pressure and cardiac output, but recent data suggest that norepinephrine may be a superior agent in patients with cardiogenic shock.[113] Phenylephrine, a selective α_1-adrenergic agonist, may be added when tachyarrhythmias limit therapy with other vasopressors. Vasopressor infusions must be titrated carefully in patients with cardiogenic shock to maximize coronary perfusion pressure, with the least possible increase in myocardial oxygen demand. Hemodynamic monitoring with serial measurements of cardiac output, filling pressures, (and other parameters such as mixed venous oxygen saturation) allows for titration of the dosage of vasoactive agents to the minimum dosage required to achieve the chosen therapeutic goals.[114]

Following initial stabilization and restoration of adequate blood pressure, tissue perfusion should be assessed. If tissue perfusion remains inadequate, inotropic support or intraaortic balloon pumping should be initiated. If tissue perfusion is adequate but significant pulmonary congestion remains, diuretics may be employed. Vasodilators can be considered as well, depending on the blood pressure.

In patients with inadequate tissue perfusion and adequate intravascular volume, cardiovascular support with inotropic agents should be initiated. Dobutamine, a selective β_1-adrenergic receptor agonist, can improve myocardial contractility and increase cardiac output; it is the initial agent of choice in patients with systolic pressures above 80 mm Hg. Dobutamine may exacerbate hypotension in some patients and can precipitate tachyarrhythmias. Use of dopamine may be preferable if systolic pressure is less than 80 mm Hg, although tachycardia and increased peripheral resistance may worsen myocardial ischemia. In some situations, a combination of dopamine and dobutamine can be more effective than either agent used alone. Phosphodiesterase inhibitors such as milrinone are less arrhythmogenic than catecholamines, but they have the potential to cause hypotension and should be used with caution in patients with tenuous clinical status. Levosimendan, a calcium sensitizer, has both inotropic and vasodilator properties and does not increase myocardial oxygen consumption. Several relatively small studies have shown hemodynamic benefits with levosimendan in cardiogenic shock after MI,[115,116] but survival benefits have not been shown either in cardiogenic shock or acute heart failure.[117]

Intraaortic balloon pump (IABP) counterpulsation reduces systolic afterload and augments diastolic perfusion pressure, increasing cardiac output and improving coronary blood flow.[118] These beneficial effects, in contrast to those of inotropic or vasopressor agents, occur without an increase in oxygen demand. IABP does not, however, produce a significant improvement in blood flow distal to a critical coronary stenosis and has not been shown to improve mortality when used alone without reperfusion therapy or revascularization. In patients with cardiogenic shock and compromised tissue perfusion, IABP can be an essential support mechanism to stabilize patients and allow time for definitive therapeutic measures to be undertaken.[118,119] In appropriate settings, more intensive support with mechanical assist devices may also be implemented.

Reperfusion Therapy

Although fibrinolytic therapy reduces the likelihood of subsequent development of shock after initial presentation,[112] its role in the management of patients who have already developed shock is less certain. The available randomized trials.[6,18,28,120] have not demonstrated that fibrinolytic therapy reduces mortality in patients with established cardiogenic shock. On the other hand, in the SHOCK Registry,[121] patients treated with fibrinolytic therapy had a lower in-hospital mortality rate than those who were not (54% versus 64%, $P = 0.005$), even after adjustment for age and revascularization status (OR 0.70, $P = 0.027$).

Fibrinolytic therapy is clearly less effective in patients with cardiogenic shock than in those without. The explanation for this lack of efficacy appears to be the low reperfusion rate achieved in this subset of patients. The reasons for decreased fibrinolytic efficacy in patients with cardiogenic shock probably include hemodynamic, mechanical, and metabolic factors that prevent achievement and maintenance of infarct-related artery patency.[122] Attempts to increase reperfusion rates by increasing blood pressure with aggressive inotropic and pressor therapy and IABP counterpulsation make theoretic sense, and two small studies support the notion that vasopressor therapy to increase aortic pressure improves fibrinolytic efficacy.[122,123] The use of intraaortic balloon pumping to augment aortic diastolic pressure may increase the effectiveness of fibrinolytics as well.

To date, emergency percutaneous revascularization is the only intervention that has been shown to consistently reduce mortality rates in patients with cardiogenic shock. An extensive body of observational and registry studies has shown consistent benefits from revascularization. Notable among these is the GUSTO-1 trial, in which patients treated with an "aggressive" strategy (coronary angiography performed within 24 hours of shock onset with revascularization by PTCA or bypass surgery) had significantly lower mortality (38% compared with 62%).[124] The National Registry of Myocardial Infarction–2 (NRMI-2) collected 26,280 shock patients with cardiogenic shock in the setting of MI between 1994 and 1997 and similarly supported the association between revascularization and survival.[125] Improved short-term mortality was noted in those who then underwent revascularization during

the reference hospitalization, either via PTCA (12.8% mortality versus 43.9%) or CABG (6.5% versus 23.9%).[125] These data complement the GUSTO-1 substudy data and are important not only because of the sheer number of patients from whom these values are derived but also because NRMI-2 was a national cross-sectional study which more closely represents general clinical practice than carefully selected trial populations. These studies cannot be regarded as definitive because of their retrospective design, but two randomized controlled trials have now evaluated revascularization for patients with MI.

The SHOCK study was a randomized, multicenter international trial that assigned patients with cardiogenic shock to receive optimal medical management—including IABP and fibrinolytic therapy—or to cardiac catheterization with revascularization using PTCA or CABG The primary endpoint, all-cause mortality at 30 days, was 46.7% in the revascularization group and 56% in the medical therapy group, a difference that did not reach statistical significance ($P = 0.11$).[126] Planned follow-up, however, revealed a significant benefit from early revascularization at 6 months and 1 year ($P < 0.03$).[127] Subgroup analyses also revealed benefit in patients younger than 75, those with prior MI, and those randomized less than 6 hours from onset of infarction.[126,127]

The SMASH trial was similarly designed but enrolled sicker patients.[128] The trial was terminated early owing to difficulties in patient recruitment and enrolled only 55 patients, but it showed a reduction in 30-day absolute mortality similar to that in the SHOCK trial (69% mortality in the invasive group versus 78% in the medically managed group, $P = NS$), and this benefit was also maintained at 1 year.[128]

When the results of both the SHOCK and SMASH trials are put into perspective with results from other randomized controlled trials of patients with AMI, an important point emerges: despite the moderate relative risk reduction (for the SHOCK trial 0.72, CI 0.54-0.95; for the SMASH trial, 0.88, CI 0.60-1.20) the absolute benefit is important, with 9 lives saved for 100 patients treated at 30 days in both trials, and 13.2 lives saved for 100 patients treated at 1 year in the SHOCK trial. This latter figure corresponds to a number needed to treat (NNT) of 7.6, one of the lowest figures ever observed in a randomized controlled trial of cardiovascular disease.

On the basis of these randomized trials, the presence of cardiogenic shock in the setting of acute MI is a class I indication for emergency revascularization, either by percutaneous intervention or CABG.[4]

ANNOTATED REFERENCES

Ambrose JA, Martinez EE. A new paradigm for plaque stabilization. Circulation 2002;105:2000-4.
A concise but thorough overview of the pathophysiology of plaque formation and stabilization in relation to the prevention and treatment of acute coronary syndromes.

Anderson JL, Adams CD, Antman EM, et al. ACC/AHA 2007 guidelines for the management of patients with unstable angina/non ST-elevation myocardial infarction: a report of the American College of Cardiology/American Heart Association Task Force on Practice Guidelines. Circulation 2007;106:803-77.
The most recent guidelines on the management of non-ST elevation myocardial infarction (NSTEMI). These guidelines incorporate the most recent data and recommendations on the use of glycoprotein IIb/IIIa receptor antagonists. Thienopyridines, and parenteral anticoagulants, as well as the role of coronary angiography, in patients with NSTEMI.

Kushner FG, HM, Smith SC, et al. 2009 Focused Updates: ACC/AHA Guidelines for the Management of Patients With ST-Elevation Myocardial Infarction (Updating the 2004 Guideline and 2007 Focused Update) and ACC/AHA/SCAI Guidelines on Percutaneous Coronary Intervention (Updating the 2005 Guideline and 2007 Focused Update): A Report of the American College of Cardiology Foundation/American Heart Association Task Force on Practice Guidelines. Circulation 2009;120:2271-306.
The most recent guidelines on the management Of ST elevation myocardial infarction (STEMI), incorporating the most recent data and recommendations on revascularization as well as fibrinolytic, antiplatelet, antithrombotic and antianginal therapy in patients with STEMI.

Mehta SR, GC, Boden WE, et al. Early versus delayed invasive intervention in acute coronary syndromes. N Engl J Med 2009;362:2165-75.
In patients presenting with NSTEMI or unstable angina, early intervention did not significantly reduce the primary composite endpoint of death, MI or stroke at 6 months. However, there was a relative reduction of 28% in the secondary outcome of death, myocardial infarction, or refractory ischemia in the early-intervention group. In addition, early intervention was superior to delayed intervention in high-risk patients.

De Backer D, BP, Devriendt J, et al on behalf of the SOAP II investigators. Comparison of Dopamine and Norepinephrine in the Treatment of Shock. N Engl J Med 2010;362:779-89.
1679 patients with shock (septic, cardiogenic, hypovolemic) were randomized to either dopamine or norepinephrine as first-line vasopressor agents. There was no significant difference in the rate of death

between the two groups; however, the use of dopamine was associated with a greater number of adverse events.

Cantor WJ, FD, Borgundvaag B, et al. Routine early angioplasty after fibrinolysis for acute myocardial infarction. N Engl J Med 2009;360:2705-18.
High risk patients with ST elevation myocardial infarction treated with fibrinolytics followed by early (<6 hours) rather than delayed percutaneous cornary intervention had significantly fewer rates of death, reinfarction, recurrent ischemia, new or worsening congestive heart failure, or cardiogenic shock at 30 days.

Wiviott SD, BE, McCabe CH, et al. Prasugrel versus clopidogrel in patients with acute coronary syndromes. N Engl J Med 2007;357:2001-15.
In patients with moderate-to-high-risk acute coronary syndromes undergoing planned percutaneous coronary intervention, prasugrel was associated with a decrease in ischemic events when compared to clopidogrel at the cost of higher bleeding rates, including fatal bleed. There was no difference in mortality.

Keeley EC, Boura JA, Grines CL. Primary angioplasty versus intravenous thrombolytic therapy for acute myocardial infarction: a quantitative review of 23 randomised trials. Lancet 2003;361:13-20.

Stone GW, MB, Cox DA, et al. Bivalirudin for patients with acute coronary syndromes. N Engl J Med 2006;355:2203-16.

Wiviott SD, AE, Gibson CM, et al. Evaluation of prasugrel compared with clopidogrel in patients with acute coronary syndromes: design and rationale for the TRial to assess Improvement in Therapeutic Outcomes by optimizing platelet Inhibition with prasugrel Thrombolysis In Myocardial Infarction 38 (TRITON-TIMI 38). Am Heart J 2006;152.

Chen ZM, JL, Chen YP, et al. Addition of clopidogrel to aspirin in 45,852 patients with acute myocardial infarction: randomised placebo-controlled trial. Lancet 2005;366:1607-21.

Chen ZM, PH, Chen YP, et al. COMMIT (ClOpidogrel and Metoprolol in Myocardial Infarction Trial) collaborative group. Early intravenous then oral metoprolol in 45,852 patients with acute myocardial infarction: randomised placebo-controlled trial. Lancet 2005;366:1622-32.

Kim JS, KJ, Choi D, et al. Efficacy of High-Dose Atorvastatin Loading Before Primary Percutaneous Coronary Intervention for ST-Segment Elevation Myocardial Infarction. J Am Coll Caridiol Intv 2010;3:332-9.

REFERENCES

Access the complete reference list online at http://www.expertconsult.com.

Invasive Cardiac Procedures

STÉPHANE MANZO-SILBERMAN | OLIVIER VARENNE

🖿 Percutaneous Transluminal Coronary Angioplasty

Chronic ischemic heart disease is usually due to obstruction of the coronary arteries by atherosclerosis. It is the leading cause of mortality and morbidity in economically developed countries. Percutaneous transluminal coronary angioplasty (PTCA) has emerged as a major therapeutic option in patients with coronary artery atherosclerosis. The first PTCA in a patient was performed by Andreas Grüntzig in Zurich in September 1977.[1] PTCA was initially limited to the treatment of discrete stenoses in proximal segments of a coronary artery. Improvements in equipment and technique have increased the success rate and have led to its use in patients with complex stenoses or in high-risk clinical situations such as acute coronary syndromes (ACS)[2,3] or cardiac arrest.[4] PTCA is currently the most widely used coronary revascularization technique.

PROCEDURE

Vascular access is obtained either through the femoral or radial artery, where a sheath is introduced with the use of local anesthesia. A 5F to 8F guiding catheter is advanced through the sheath to the ostium of the coronary artery to be dilated. Once the guiding catheter is positioned in the coronary ostium, angiography of the diseased artery is performed to visualize the stenosis and the arterial segments proximal and distal to it; intracoronary infusion of nitrates is mandatory for the diagnosis and accurate sizing of the lesions and the choice of stent (Figure 77-1, A). A flexible guidewire is advanced through the guiding catheter, navigated across the stenosis by rotating and advancing its angulated tip, and positioned in the distal arterial segment. The deflated balloon angioplasty catheter is advanced over the wire and positioned at the stenosis. The positions of the guidewire and balloon catheter are confirmed periodically by injecting contrast medium into the coronary artery through the guiding catheter. Once it is positioned, the balloon is usually inflated with a mixture of saline and contrast medium so the inflation can be visualized (see Figure 77-1, B and C). Most often, a stent is implanted after balloon angioplasty (Figure 77-2). Balloon-expandable stents are most commonly used. The stent-balloon device is positioned on the predilated site (see Figure 77-1, D), and the stent is implanted in the coronary artery wall by a short balloon inflation (see Figure 77-1, E). The balloon catheter is deflated and pulled out. The result is evaluated by injecting contrast medium (see Figure 77-1, F). If the result is satisfactory, the guidewire is removed. If the angiographic result is unsatisfactory, the guidewire remains in place. The balloon catheter can be replaced by a larger one, or another stent can be implanted. At the end of the procedure, a final angiogram is obtained to confirm that the result is satisfactory.

In noncalcified lesions, direct stent implantation without prior balloon dilation is often performed. Direct stenting shortens the duration of the procedure and reduces costs and is used in approximately 30% to 50% of cases.[5]

PREPROCEDURE AND POSTPROCEDURE MANAGEMENT AND MEDICATIONS

The combination of low-dose aspirin (75-325 mg) and clopidogrel has been shown to reduce the incidence of acute stent occlusion after PTCA and is considered essential therapy before coronary interventions.[6,7] If patients are not treated chronically or if there is doubt about medication compliance, a dose of aspirin (500 mg orally) should be given more than 3 hours prior, or at least 300 mg intravenously (IV) directly prior to the procedure. For chronic use, there is no need for doses higher than 100 mg daily.[8] Current guidelines recommend a loading dose of clopidogrel, 300 mg, administered at least 6 hours before the procedure. Higher loading doses (600 mg) lead to more rapid (around 2 hours) and long-lasting inhibition of platelet aggregation. The CURRENT-OASIS 7 trial compared 300-mg and 600-mg clopidogrel loading doses and demonstrated fewer adverse events with a loading dose of 600 mg of clopidogrel, followed by 150 mg daily for a week, and 75 mg daily for at least 3 weeks.[9]

Despite administration of dual antiplatelet therapy combining aspirin and clopidogrel, a small percentage (0.4-1.1%) still suffer subacute stent thrombosis. Variability in response to clopidogrel may account for some of these events,[10-12] and more potent antiplatelet agents have been investigated. Prasugrel, a novel oral thienopyridine, has a more rapid onset and predictable and potent antiplatelet effects.[13,14] In the TRITON-TIMI 38 trial,[15] 13,608 moderate to high-risk ACS patients were randomized to prasugrel (60-mg loading dose followed by 10 mg daily) or clopidogrel (300-mg loading dose followed by 75 mg daily). Follow-up was up to 15 months. Prasugrel was associated with a 19% reduction in the primary efficacy endpoint of cardiovascular death, nonfatal myocardial infarction (MI), and nonfatal stroke. This was accompanied by a 32% increase of major bleeding, especially in subgroups of patients with cerebrovascular accident, weight less than 60 kg, and older than 75 years of age. Ticagrelor, a reversible and direct-acting oral antagonist of the adenosine diphosphate receptor P2Y12, provides faster, greater, and more consistent platelet inhibition than clopidogrel. PLATO,[16] a multicenter double-blind, randomized trial compared ticagrelor (180-mg loading dose, 90 mg twice daily thereafter) and clopidogrel (300-mg to 600-mg loading dose, 75 mg daily thereafter) for the prevention of cardiovascular events in 18,624 patients with an ACS. At 12 months, ticagrelor significantly reduced the occurrence of the primary endpoint, a composite of death from vascular causes, MI, or stroke—9.8% of patients receiving ticagrelor as compared with 11.7% of those receiving clopidogrel (hazard ratio, 0.84; 95% confidence interval [CI], 0.77 to 0.92; $P < 0.001$). No significant difference in the rates of major bleeding was found between the ticagrelor and clopidogrel groups (11.6% and 11.2%, respectively; $P = 0.43$), but ticagrelor was associated with a higher rate of major bleeding unrelated to coronary artery bypass grafting (CABG) (4.5% versus 3.8%, $P = 0.03$), including more instances of fatal intracranial bleeding and fewer fatal bleeding of other types.

Intracoronary nitrates are given at the beginning of and during the procedure to prevent vasospasm. Unfractionated heparin (typically 5000 to 10,000 units) is administered IV during PTCA to decrease the incidence of coronary artery thrombosis,[17] but it is usually not continued after the procedure. Low-molecular-weight heparin has been suggested as an accepted alternative to unfractionated heparin.[18]

Although the mainstay of antiplatelet and anticoagulation therapy for PTCA is the combination of clopidogrel and aspirin before and after the procedure and heparin during it, the use of platelet glycoprotein IIb/IIIa inhibitors or the direct thrombin inhibitor, bivalirudin, have emerged as powerful adjunctive therapies. The platelet glycoprotein IIb/IIIa receptor binds fibrinogen to cross-link platelets and can

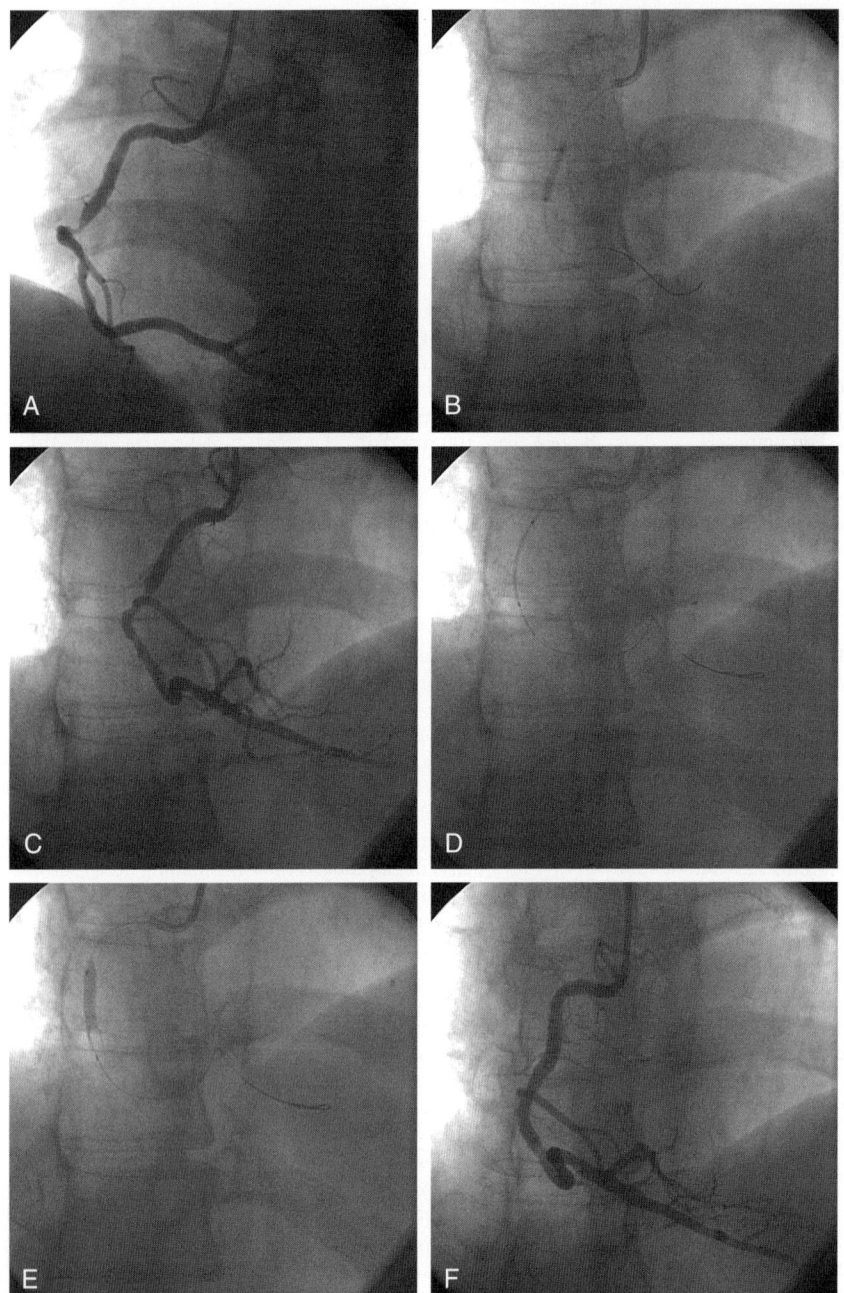

Figure 77-1 **Coronary angioplasty procedure. A,** Critical stenosis in midsegment of a right coronary artery. **B,** Inflation of a 3.5-mm-diameter angioplasty balloon. **C,** Angiographic control after balloon inflation. **D,** Placement of a 3.5-mm-diameter, 18-mm-long metal stent. **E,** Inflation of the balloon. **F,** Final result.

be blocked irreversibly by inhibitors such as abciximab, eptifibatide, and tirofiban. Several multicenter randomized studies have compared heparin and aspirin to an additional treatment with platelet glycoprotein IIb/IIIa receptor inhibitors in patients undergoing PTCA and showed a significant reduction in major clinical events.[19-21] The greatest treatment benefit of platelet glycoprotein IIb/IIIa inhibitors appears to be in procedures on high-risk lesions or in patients with severe clinical patterns, such as ACS with ST-segment changes or elevation of biological markers of myocardial necrosis.[22-24] Bivalirudin, when used instead of heparin plus glycoprotein IIb/IIIa inhibitors, has been shown in large-scale randomized trials to reduce major and minor bleeding and thrombocytopenia while resulting in similar rates of ischemia after percuteanous intervention (PCI) in patients with stable angina or ACS.[25]

The femoral arterial sheath is usually removed immediately after PTCA. Hemostasis is obtained by either manual compression or use of closure devices. Patients with stable angina and an uncomplicated procedure are usually discharged the day after removal of the sheath. Medications prescribed at the time of discharge depend on the underlying condition. Most often, the post-PTCA regimen includes low-dose aspirin, clopidogrel, a beta-blocker or a calcium antagonist, and a statin.

Although the femoral artery remains the most widely used approach in the United States for diagnostic and therapeutic procedures, the radial artery is used increasingly to reduce the local complication rate and increase the patient's comfort. The sheath is pulled out immediately after the procedure, and hemostasis is obtained by applying a pressure dressing for several hours.[26] Immediate ambulation is feasible, and hospital discharge on the same day is possible in selected cases.[27]

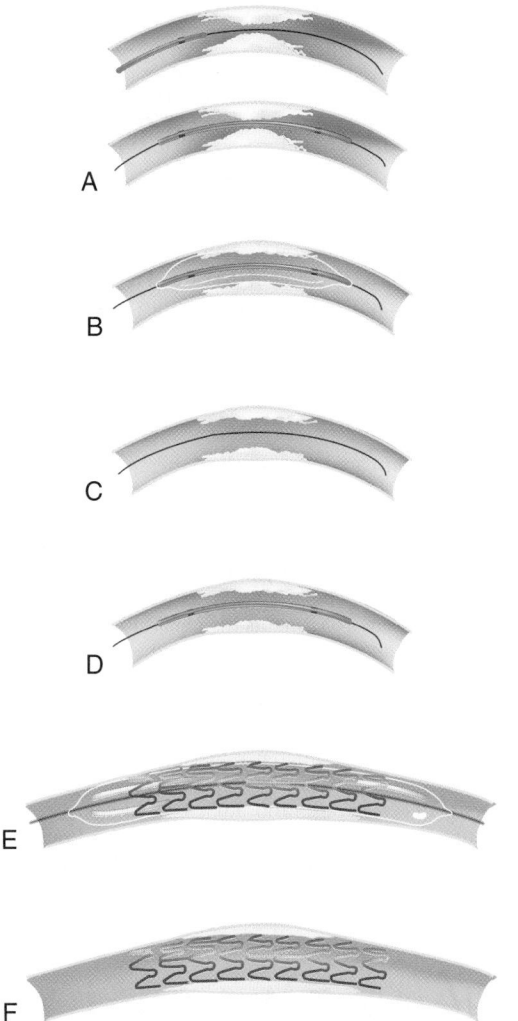

Figure 77-2 Implantation of a coronary stent. A, Placement of balloon catheter. **B,** Predilation with balloon catheter. **C,** Balloon is withdrawn. **D,** Placement of coronary stent, which has been crimped on a balloon catheter. **E,** Inflation of balloon and expansion of stent. **F,** Withdrawal of balloon catheter and final result.

EFFICACY OF THE PROCEDURE

PTCA of a nonoccluded coronary artery is successful in more than 97% of patients. In the remaining patients, PTCA is unsuccessful because the stenosis cannot be crossed with either the guidewire or the balloon catheter, or because the stenosis is not adequately dilated despite the use of an appropriately sized balloon and stents. In 2% to 3% of cases, the vessel abruptly occludes (abrupt closure) during or immediately after the procedure. Reopening of the artery is attempted with repeat balloon inflations and multiple stent implantations. Stenting for abrupt closure (bailout stenting) has virtually eliminated the need for urgent coronary bypass surgery after failed PTCA. The most challenging lesions (long, angulated, calcified, or associated with intraluminal thrombus) carry a lower success rate.[28] PTCA also has a lower initial success rate (50%-70%) in patients with chronically occluded arteries, because it may be difficult to manipulate the guidewire through a chronically occluded region.[29,30] In patients with recurrent angina after bypass surgery, the success rate of PTCA performed for properly selected stenosis of saphenous and arterial bypass grafts is close to that of native arteries, but the incidence of late events (MI, repeat PTCA, or other surgery) is higher.[31,32]

MECHANISMS OF CORONARY ARTERY DILATATION

The mechanisms by which PTCA increases the size of the arterial lumen have been studied in animals and cadavers.[33-36] Balloon-induced barotrauma causes endothelial denudation, cracking and disruption of the atherosclerotic plaque, and stretching or tearing of the media and adventitia (Figure 77-3). These brutal and profound changes account for the postballoon inflation angiographic features of intraluminal haziness, intimal flap, or dissection (Figure 77-4). Intracoronary ultrasound imaging, which provides a cross-sectional view of the artery within the lumen, detects dissection of the arterial wall—sometimes extensive—in 50% to 80% of patients who have undergone successful PTCA.[37,38] These morphologic alterations open up new pathways for blood flow, leading to an increased luminal size. Balloon inflation may be deleterious, however, causing plaque hemorrhage, extensive dissection resulting in luminal compromise, platelet deposition, and thrombus formation.

In the weeks after successful PTCA, favorable remodeling of the disrupted plaque and endothelialization at the sites of intimal injury result in an increased luminal size. Angiographic studies indicate that intimal disruption usually resolves within 1 month after successful PTCA.[39]

RESTENOSIS

In patients who have undergone successful PTCA, recurrence of the stenosis, or restenosis, was the main limitation to long-term, event-free survival. Restenosis occurs in about 30% to 50% of patients in whom a coronary artery stenosis has been dilated by balloon alone.[40-42] Restenosis typically occurs 1 to 6 months after PTCA.[40]

The process of restenosis is multifactorial. Injury of the vessel initiates release of thrombogenic, vasoactive, and mitogenic factors.[43] Endothelial and deep-vessel injury leads to platelet aggregation, thrombus formation, inflammation, and activation of macrophages. These events induce the production and release of growth factors and cytokines, which in turn may promote their own synthesis and release from target cells.[44] A self-perpetuating process is initiated that results

Figure 77-3 Pathologic specimen after coronary angioplasty. Balloon inflation has created plaque rupture with hemorrhage.

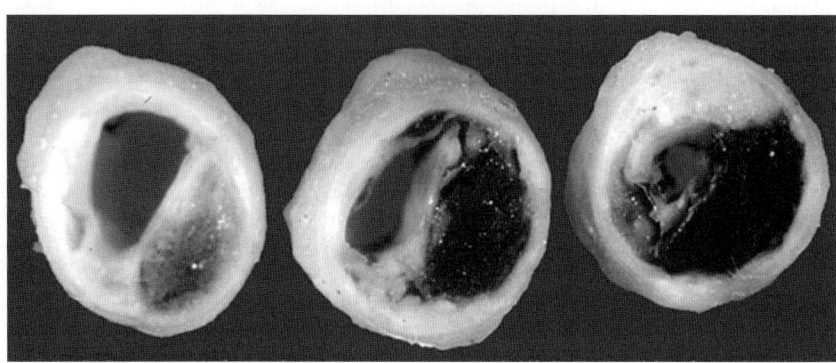

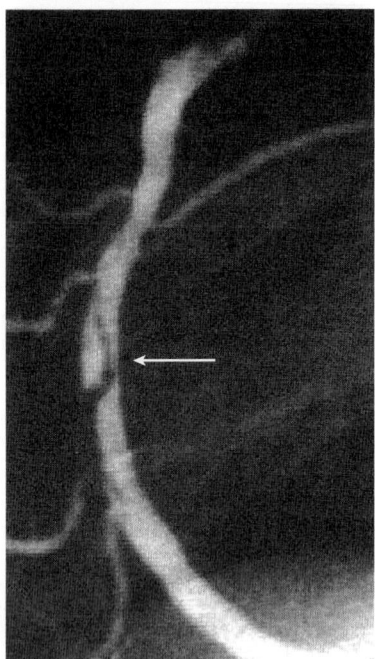

Figure 77-4 Arterial dissection *(arrow)* after balloon inflation in mid-segment of a right coronary artery.

in the migration of smooth muscle cells from their usual location in the arterial media to the intima, where they change to a synthetic phenotype, produce extracellular matrix, and proliferate, thereby resulting in a stenosis within the vessel lumen. Intimal thickening accounts for about 30% of the loss in lumen diameter 6 months after coronary interventions. In addition, arterial remodeling occurs in the weeks after PTCA and can be evaluated using serial intravascular ultrasound imaging to measure the reduction in the cross-sectional area of the vessel.[45,46]

Coronary stenting with bare metal stents significantly reduces the incidence of restenosis, because it produces large lumens and staves off pathologic remodeling.[47,48] Several multicenter randomized trials showed that the incidence of restenosis is 25% to 50% lower after coronary stenting than after balloon angioplasty. Drug-eluting stents have been developed to further reduce the restenosis rate. Stents are covered with a polymer that allows progressive delivery of antiproliferative drugs such as sirolimus, paclitaxel, or everolimus that inhibit smooth muscle cell proliferation. The restenosis rate has been virtually abolished with drug-eluting stents, with no increase in the acute complication rate.[49] Currently, drug-eluting stents are used in the majority of procedures.

An annual rate of 0.4 to 0.6% of late stent thrombosis has been noted after implantation of sirolimus- or paclitaxel-eluting stents, with no increase of death or MI.[50] Incomplete endothelial coverage of the stent and a prolonged inflammatory reaction to the polymer have been suggested as causal factors. Current guidelines recommend dual antiplatelet therapy for 12 months after implantation of drug-eluting stents, although no randomized trial has proved the efficacy of this strategy to prevent late stent thrombosis.[8,51] Interruption of clopidogrel administration after implantation of a drug-eluting stent is associated with acute stent thrombosis, especially during the first 6 months.[52] Management of dual antiplatelet therapy in patients with drug-eluting stents in the setting of surgical procedures requires a clear consensus between surgeons, anesthesiologists, and cardiologists.[53] Future developments to reduce the rate of late stent thrombosis include drug-eluting stents with bioabsorbable polymers (Figure 77-5) and nonmetallic stents which are completely bioabsorbed.[54]

Other Coronary Interventions

ROTATIONAL ATHERECTOMY

Rotational atherectomy uses a diamond-studded burr spinning at about 180,000 revolutions per minute to excavate calcified or fibrotic plaque.[55,56] This device is used for very calcified lesions.

Comparison of Clinical Applications

Whether to recommend medical therapy, angioplasty, or surgical treatment remains a tailored decision in the care of individual patients with coronary artery disease. Nonetheless, the results of several clinical trials allow general guidelines to be developed.

PERCUTANEOUS TRANSLUMINAL CORONARY ANGIOPLASTY VERSUS MEDICAL THERAPY

PTCA has been compared with medical therapy for stable angina in several studies. In the COURAGE trial,[57] 2287 patients who had stable angina with objective evidence of myocardial ischemia and significant coronary artery disease were randomized to PCI with optimal therapy or optimal medical therapy. The primary outcome was death from any cause and nonfatal MI. There was a statistically significant difference in the rates of freedom from angina throughout most of the follow-up period in favor of the PCI group. However, there was no difference at 4.6 years in the primary outcome, all-cause death, and nonfatal MI (19.0% in the PCI group and 18.5% in the medical therapy group; hazard ratio for the PCI group, 1.05; 95% CI, 0.87-1.27; $P = 0.62$). There were no significant differences between the PCI group and the medical therapy group in the composite of death, MI, and stroke (20.0% versus 19.5%; hazard ratio, 1.05; 95% CI, 0.87-1.27; $P = 0.62$); hospitalization for ACS (12.4% versus 11.8%; hazard ratio, 1.07; 95% CI, 0.84-1.37; $P = 0.56$); or MI (13.2% versus 12.3%; hazard ratio, 1.13; 95% CI, 0.89-1.43; $P = 0.33$). Therefore, in patients with stable angina,

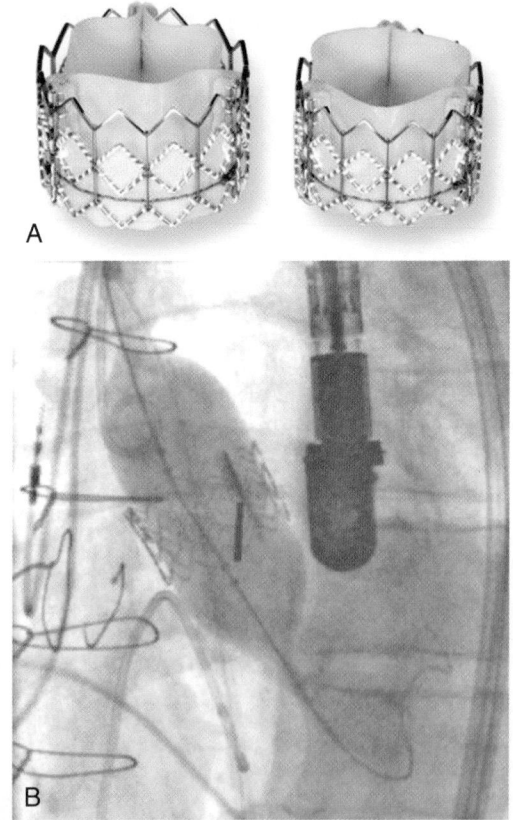

Figure 77-5 Sapiens aortic valve **(A)**. After implantation **(B)**.

even though PCI provides more optimal relief of symptoms, optimal medical therapy can be administered safely and angioplasty performed only in patients with persistent symptoms.

The TIMI IIIB study addressed the benefit of PTCA for patients with unstable angina or non–Q wave MI.[58] This study enrolled 2220 patients with unstable angina and MI without ST-segment elevation who had electrocardiographic (ECG) evidence of changes in the ST segment or T wave, elevated levels of cardiac markers, a history of coronary artery disease, or all three findings. Patients were randomly assigned to an early invasive strategy that included routine catheterization within 4 to 48 hours and revascularization as appropriate, or to a more conservative (selectively invasive) strategy, in which catheterization was performed only if the patient had objective evidence of recurrent ischemia or an abnormal stress test. At 6 months, the rate of the primary endpoint (a composite of death, nonfatal MI, and rehospitalization for ACS) was 15.9% with the early invasive strategy and 19.4% with the conservative strategy (odds ratio, 0.78; 95% CI, 0.62-0.97; $P = 0.025$). In the FRISC II trial,[59,60] 2457 patients were randomly assigned to invasive or noninvasive treatment and 3 months of dalteparin or placebo. After 1 year, in 100 patients, an invasive strategy saved 1.7 lives, prevented 2.0 nonfatal MIs and 20 readmissions, and provided earlier and better symptom relief at the cost of 15 more patients with CABG and 21 more with PTCA.[59] An invasive approach with early (<48 hours) angiography is therefore the preferred strategy in patients with unstable coronary artery disease and signs of ischemia on ECG or raised levels of biochemical markers of myocardial damage.

In patients with acute myocardial infarction (AMI), PTCA performed without prior thrombolytic therapy (primary PTCA) by an experienced team results in a lower risk of death or reinfarction than thrombolytic therapy.[2,3,61] In patients with AMI complicated by cardiogenic shock, emergency revascularization improves survival.[62,63] PTCA performed after failed thrombolytic therapy reduces adverse cardiac events and improves left ventricular function at 1 month.[64] In patients with right ventricular infarction, complete reperfusion of the right coronary artery by angioplasty results in dramatic recovery of right ventricular performance, as assessed by echocardiography, and an excellent clinical outcome.[65] In cardiac arrest, a strategy of immediate coronary angiography followed by angioplasty if necessary may increase survival.[4]

Thus, the results of clinical trials comparing PTCA with medical therapy suggest that the benefit of angioplasty depends on the severity and acuity of the clinical presentation. A gradient of risk extends across the spectrum of patients with coronary artery disease. At one end of the spectrum, patients with stable angina and one- or two-vessel disease treated medically are at low risk of nonfatal MI. PTCA reduces angina more effectively, with a low risk of complications, but it does not lower the risk of death, MI, or future revascularization procedures. In practice, initial revascularization by PTCA is proposed in this setting if the amount of myocardium at risk is high, and if the lesions seem at low risk for procedure-related complications. At the other end of the spectrum, ACS patients have a high risk of major complications and death that is significantly improved by PTCA and potent antithrombotic regimens.

PERCUTANEOUS TRANSLUMINAL CORONARY ANGIOPLASTY VERSUS BYPASS SURGERY

Several studies have compared PTCA with bypass surgery for patients with multivessel coronary artery disease. The SYNTAX trial randomly assigned 1800 patients with three-vessel or left main coronary artery disease to undergo CABG or PCI (in a 1:1 ratio).[66] For all these patients, the local cardiac surgeon and interventional cardiologist determined that equivalent anatomic revascularization could be achieved with either treatment. A non-inferiority comparison of the two groups was performed for the primary endpoint—a major adverse cardiac or cerebrovascular event (death from any cause, stroke, MI, or repeat revascularization) during the 12-month period after randomization. Rates of major adverse cardiac or cerebrovascular events at 12

months were significantly higher in the PCI group (17.8%, versus 12.4% for CABG; $P = 0.002$), in large part because of an increased rate of repeat revascularization (13.5% versus 5.9%, $P < 0.001$); as a result, the criterion for non-inferiority was not met. At 12 months, the rates of death and MI were similar between the two groups; stroke was significantly more likely to occur with CABG (2.2%, versus 0.6% with PCI; $P = 0.003$) The SYNTAX score was designed in this study to predict outcomes related to anatomic characteristics. In the group of patients with high SYNTAX scores, the composite rate of death, nonfatal MI, and stroke was raised in the PCI group.

In daily practice, in patients with the more diffuse and complex lesions leading to a high SYNTAX score, bypass surgery remains the preferred therapeutic option. Patients with multivessel coronary disease and less complex lesions (low or intermediate SYNTAX score) who are good candidates for either PTCA or bypass surgery can be reassured that both revascularization approaches are followed by equivalent rates of major complications. However, the invasive nature of bypass surgery must be weighed against the likelihood of repeated procedures after PTCA. Finally, PCI can be an alternative therapy in patients with highly complex lesions but with severe comorbidities that increase the risk of surgery (high Euroscore or high Parsonnet Score).

Mitral Valvuloplasty

In patients with severe mitral stenosis, surgical mitral commissurotomy alleviates symptoms and improves mid- and long-term prognosis. Percutaneous mitral valvuloplasty was first applied in 1984 to young patients with rheumatic mitral stenosis, using a transseptal approach.[67] The technique is widely accepted as a first-choice treatment in cases of severe but noncalcified mitral stenosis. Selection of patients is based on the echocardiographic features of the mitral valve.[68]

The transseptal approach is the most commonly used technique. After puncture of the intraarterial septum with a needle and a long sheath, a large (23- to 25-mm diameter) valvuloplasty balloon is advanced through the atrial opening and positioned across the mitral valve. Stepwise inflation of this balloon results in separation of the fused commissures, similar to the surgical technique of mitral commissurotomy.

Overall procedure mortality is 1% to 2%. Long-term follow-up studies demonstrate preservation of the improved mitral orifice.[69]

Aortic Valvuloplasty

Calcific aortic stenosis in an adult is the most common indication for the more than 25,000 aortic valve replacements performed in the Unites States each year. Percutaneous aortic balloon valvuloplasty was proposed as an alternative to surgery. The balloon catheter is advanced retrogradely through the aortic stenosis using a femoral approach in most cases. Mid- and long-term results are disappointing; improvement in the orifice area is less than that obtained with a valve replacement, and echocardiographic follow-up shows recurrence of aortic stenosis in most cases.[70] More recently, percutaneous transcatheter implantation of a heart valve prosthesis for aortic stenosis has been assessed in patients with contraindications to surgery[71] (Figure 77-6). Outcomes are encouraging despite a high rate of local femoral complications due to the size of the sheaths used to introduce the system. New systems are currently being developed with smaller insertion sheaths. Future trials will determine whether the percutaneous approach is equivalent to surgical replacement in patients with aortic stenosis and no contraindication to surgery.

Conclusion

The past 30 years have seen the explosive growth of interventional techniques. PTCA has become the most widely used method of

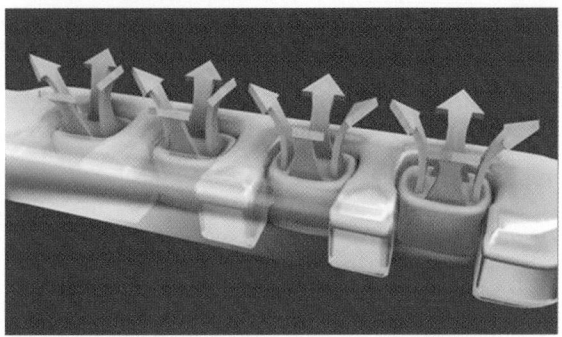

Figure 77-6 The NEVO stent (Cordis, Johnson and Johnson, Bridgewater, New Jersey). Reservoirs in the stent platform are filled with a blend of polymer and sirolimus which are eluted into the vessel wall to inhibit neointimal proliferation after stent implantation.

coronary revascularization. Coronary stenting has revolutionized the practice of interventional cardiology by partially overcoming the limitations of coronary balloon angioplasty, such as abrupt vessel closure and restenosis. Drug-eluting stents have virtually eliminated restenosis. In patients with stable angina, PTCA reduces symptoms effectively, with a low risk of complications. Patients with ACS have a high risk of major complications and death that can be significantly reduced by PTCA. Percutaneous aortic valve replacement can be used effectively in patients with contraindications to surgical replacement. New developments include drug-eluting metal stents with a bioabsorbable polymer and nonmetal entirely bioabsorbable stents to reduce polymer-induced inflammation and potentially very late stent thrombosis. As with all new techniques, careful validation of their utility will be necessary to ensure their optimal use in patient care.

KEY POINTS

1. Percutaneous transluminal coronary angioplasty (PTCA) is safe and effective and is currently the most widely used coronary revascularization technique.

2. Restenosis occurs in 10% to 30% of cases after angioplasty with bare metal stents 3 to 6 months after the procedure. Drug-eluting stents have virtually eliminated restenosis and are implanted in most lesions. Dual antiplatelet therapy must be prescribed before and after the procedure.

3. In patients with unstable coronary artery disease and signs of ischemia on electrocardiography or raised levels of biochemical markers of myocardial damage, an invasive approach with early (<48 hours) angiography is the preferred strategy.

4. Primary PTCA is the most effective therapy for acute myocardial infarction, especially in high-risk situations (cardiogenic shock, right ventricular infarction).

5. Transcatheter aortic valve replacement is an alternative to surgery in high-risk patients. Percutaneous mitral valvuloplasty is an accepted alternative to surgery in selected patients.

ANNOTATED REFERENCES

Andersen HR, Nielsen TT, Rasmussen K, et al. A comparison of coronary angioplasty with fibrinolytic therapy in acute myocardial infarction. N Engl J Med 2003;349:733-42.

In this study, 1572 patients with acute myocardial infarction were randomized to treatment with angioplasty or accelerated treatment with IV alteplase; 1129 patients were enrolled at 24 referral hospitals, and 443 patients were enrolled at 5 invasive treatment centers. The primary endpoint (a composite of death, reinfarction, or disabling stroke) was reached in 8.5% of the patients in the angioplasty group, compared with 14.2% of those in the fibrinolysis group (P = 0.002). A reperfusion strategy involving the transfer of patients to an invasive treatment center for primary angioplasty is superior to on-site fibrinolysis, provided the transfer takes 2 hours or less.

Bowers TR, O'Neill WW, Grines C. Effect of reperfusion on biventricular function and survival after right ventricular infarction. N Engl J Med 1998;338:933-40.

Echocardiographic studies were performed before and after angioplasty in 53 patients with acute right ventricular infarction. Complete reperfusion of the right coronary artery by angioplasty resulted in the dramatic recovery of right ventricular performance and an excellent clinical outcome. In contrast, unsuccessful reperfusion was associated with impaired recovery of right ventricular function, persistent hemodynamic compromise, and a high mortality rate.

Hochman JS, Sleeper LA, Webb JG, Dzavik V, Buller CE, Aylward P, et al. SHOCK Investigators. Early revascularization and long-term survival in cardiogenic shock complicating acute myocardial infarction. JAMA 2006;295:2511-5.

Patients with shock due to left ventricular failure complicating MI were randomly assigned to emergency revascularization (152 patients) or initial medical stabilization (150 patients). Revascularization was accomplished by either CABG or angioplasty. Intraaortic balloon counterpulsation was performed in 86% of the patients in both groups. Six-month mortality was lower in the revascularization group than in the medical therapy group (50.3% versus 63.1%; P = 0.027). The 6-year survival rates for the hospital survivors were 62.4% versus 44.4% for the early revascularization and initial medical stabilization groups, respectively, with annualized death rates of 8.3% versus 14.3% and, for the 1-year survivors, 8.0% versus 10.7%. Early revascularization should be strongly considered for patients with acute myocardial infarction complicated by cardiogenic shock.

Serruys PW, Morice MC, Kappetein AP, Colombo A, Holmes DR, Mack MJ, et al. SYNTAX Investigators. Percutaneous coronary intervention versus coronary-artery bypass grafting for severe coronary artery disease. N Engl J Med 2009;360:961-72.

Patients with multivessel disease were randomized to PCI with drug-eluting stents or surgical revascularization. Rates of major adverse cardiac or cerebrovascular events at 12 months were significantly higher in the PCI group because of an increased rate of repeat revascularization; as a result, the prespecified criterion for non-inferiority was not met. However, in the subgroups of patients with less complex lesions, PCI remains an acceptable alternative to surgery, with comparable rates of adverse events.

Wallentin L, Lagerqvist B, Husted S, et al. Outcome at 1 year after an invasive compared with a non-invasive strategy in unstable coronary-artery disease: the FRISC II invasive randomised trial. Lancet 2000;356:9-16.

In this study, 2457 patients were randomly assigned to invasive or noninvasive treatment. After 1 year, in 100 patients, an invasive strategy saved 1.7 lives, prevented 2.0 nonfatal myocardial infarctions and 20 readmissions, and provided earlier and better symptom relief. An invasive approach with early angiography is therefore the preferred strategy in patients with unstable coronary artery disease and signs of ischemia on ECG or raised levels of biochemical markers of myocardial damage.

REFERENCES

Access the complete reference list online at http://www.expertconsult.com.

78

Supraventricular Arrhythmias

JOHN CAMM | IRINA SAVELIEVA

Classification and Epidemiology

Supraventricular arrhythmias include rhythms arising from the sinus node and the adjacent atrial tissue (inappropriate sinus tachycardia, sinoatrial reentry tachycardia), both the right and left atria (atrial tachycardia, flutter, and fibrillation), the atrioventricular (AV) node (AV nodal reentry tachycardia, accelerated ectopic junctional rhythm), and the AV node, with involvement of an accessory pathway or multiple pathways (AV reentry tachycardia) (Figure 78-1).

ATRIOVENTRICULAR NODAL REENTRY TACHYCARDIA AND ATRIOVENTRICULAR REENTRY TACHYCARDIA

AV nodal reentry tachycardia and AV reentry tachycardia are usually referred to as *paroxysmal supraventricular tachycardias* and are often seen in young patients with little or no structural heart disease, although a congenital heart abnormality giving rise to increased atrial pressure and dilatation (e.g., Ebstein's anomaly, atrial septal defect, Fallot's tetralogy) can coexist in a small percentage of patients with these arrhythmias.[1] The first presentation is common between age 12 and 30 years, and the prevalence is approximately 2.5 per 1000. Women are twice as likely as men to present with AV nodal reentry tachycardia.

ATRIAL FLUTTER AND FIBRILLATION

Atrial fibrillation is the most common supraventricular arrhythmia, affecting 1% to 2% of the general population, especially the elderly. It is usually associated with cardiovascular pathologies, among which hypertension and congestive heart failure prevail.[2] About a third of patients, however, present with no underlying heart disease and are considered to have "lone" atrial fibrillation. The epidemiology of isolated atrial flutter is largely unknown and is believed to be in the range of 0.037% to 0.88% per 1000 person-years, but at least half these patients also have atrial fibrillation as a coexistent arrhythmia.

ATRIAL TACHYCARDIA

Atrial tachycardia affects 0.34% to 0.46% of patients with arrhythmias and is common in younger individuals following surgical correction of congenital heart disease and in the elderly, in whom it often occurs in association with atrial fibrillation.

OTHER SUPRAVENTRICULAR TACHYCARDIAS

Inappropriate sinus tachycardia and sinoatrial reentry tachycardia are less well-defined clinical and electrocardiographic entities, and their prevalence and associated conditions are not well appreciated. Sinoatrial reentry tachycardia is found incidentally in 1.8% to 16.9% of patients undergoing electrophysiologic study for other supraventricular tachyarrhythmias.

Clinical Presentation

The leading symptom of most supraventricular tachyarrhythmias, particularly AV nodal reentry tachycardia and AV reentry tachycardia, is rapid, regular palpitations, usually with an abrupt onset; they can occur spontaneously or be precipitated by simple movements. A common feature of tachycardias that involve circulation through the AV node is termination by the Valsalva maneuver. In younger individuals with no structural heart disease, the rapid heart rate can be the main pathologic finding. Other symptoms may include anxiety, dizziness, dyspnea, neck pulsation, central chest pain, weakness, and occasionally polyuria due to the release of atrial natriuretic peptide in response to increased atrial pressures (more common in atrial tachycardia and AV nodal reentry tachycardia). Prominent jugular venous pulsations due to atrial contractions against closed AV valves may be observed during AV nodal reentry or AV reentry tachycardia.

True syncope is relatively uncommon unless uncontrolled tachycardia over 200 beats per minute is sustained for a long period, especially in patients who remain standing. Syncope has been reported in 10% to 15% of patients, usually just after onset of the arrhythmia or in association with a prolonged pause following its termination. However, in older patients with concomitant heart disease such as aortic stenosis, hypertrophic cardiomyopathy, and cerebrovascular disease, significant hypotension and syncope may result from profound hemodynamic collapse associated with only moderately fast ventricular rates.

It is essential to recognize that patients presenting with AV reentry tachycardia may also present with atrial fibrillation. If an accessory pathway has a short antegrade effective refractory period (<250 msec), it may conduct to the ventricles at an extremely high rate and cause ventricular fibrillation. The incidence of sudden death is 0.15% to 0.39% per patient-year, and it may be the first manifestation of the disease in younger individuals.

Irregular palpitations may be due to atrial premature beats, atrial flutter with varying AV conduction block, atrial fibrillation, or multifocal atrial tachycardia. Although highly symptomatic, these arrhythmias usually have a benign hemodynamic prognosis. However, in patients with depressed ventricular function, uncontrolled atrial fibrillation can reduce cardiac output and precipitate hypotension and congestive heart failure. Atrial fibrillation in association with slow AV conduction or complete block (Frederick's syndrome) may result in hemodynamic collapse. Inappropriate sinus tachycardia and nonparoxysmal accelerated junctional rhythm are characterized by relatively slow heart rates and gradual onset and termination.

Electrocardiography

Whenever possible, a 12-lead electrocardiogram (ECG) should be taken during tachycardia. If a patient with an arrhythmia is hemodynamically unstable, a monitor strip should be obtained from the defibrillator before electrical discharge.

NARROW-COMPLEX TACHYCARDIAS

The typical ECG feature is narrow QRS complexes less than 120 msec. In this case, the tachycardia is almost always supraventricular, and the differential diagnosis relates to its mechanism (Figure 78-2).

WIDE-COMPLEX TACHYCARDIAS

The differential diagnostic features of wide-complex tachycardias favoring a supraventricular origin of the arrhythmia include, but are not limited to, preexistent bundle branch block; rate-dependent aberrancy; antidromic AV reentry tachycardia, when an accessory pathway conducts and excites the ventricles antegradely; and prominent

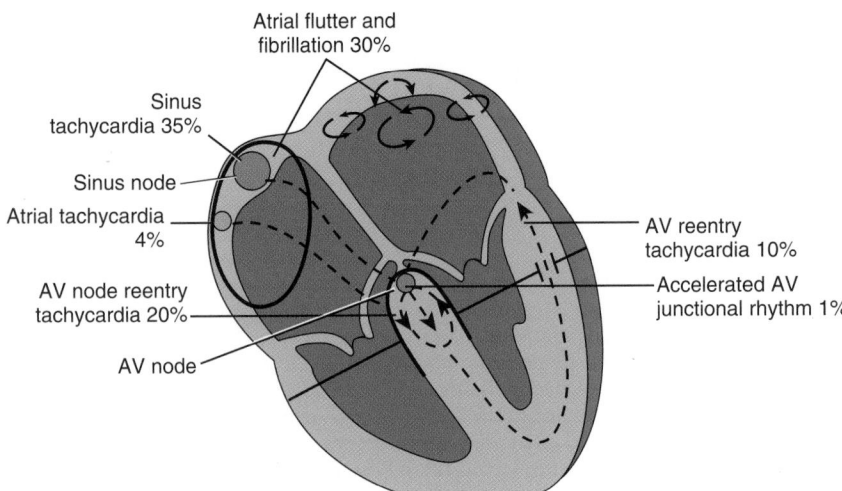

Figure 78-1 Supraventricular tachyarrhythmias encountered in the emergency setting. AV, atrioventricular.

electrolyte abnormalities (e.g., hypokalemia) or heart muscle disease (cardiomyopathy), all of which may result in QRS widening (Figure 78-3). If the diagnosis of supraventricular tachycardia cannot be proved, the patient should be treated as if ventricular tachycardia is present. Immediate direct-current (DC) cardioversion is the treatment for any hemodynamically unstable tachycardia.

Atrioventricular Nodal Reentry Tachycardia

MECHANISM

In AV nodal reentry tachycardia, there are two functionally and anatomically different pathways within the AV node: one is characterized by a short effective refractory period and slow conduction, and the other has a longer effective refractory period and faster conduction. In sinus rhythm, the atrial impulse that depolarizes the ventricles usually conducts through the fast pathway. If the atrial impulse (e.g., an atrial premature beat) occurs early, when the fast pathway is still refractory, the slow pathway takes over in propagating the atrial impulse to the ventricles; it then travels back through the fast pathway, which by then has recovered its excitability, thus initiating the most common "slow-fast," or typical, AV nodal reentry tachycardia.

ELECTROCARDIOGRAPHIC PRESENTATION

In sinus rhythm, the ECG is usually normal unless other unrelated abnormalities are present. During AV nodal reentry tachycardia, the

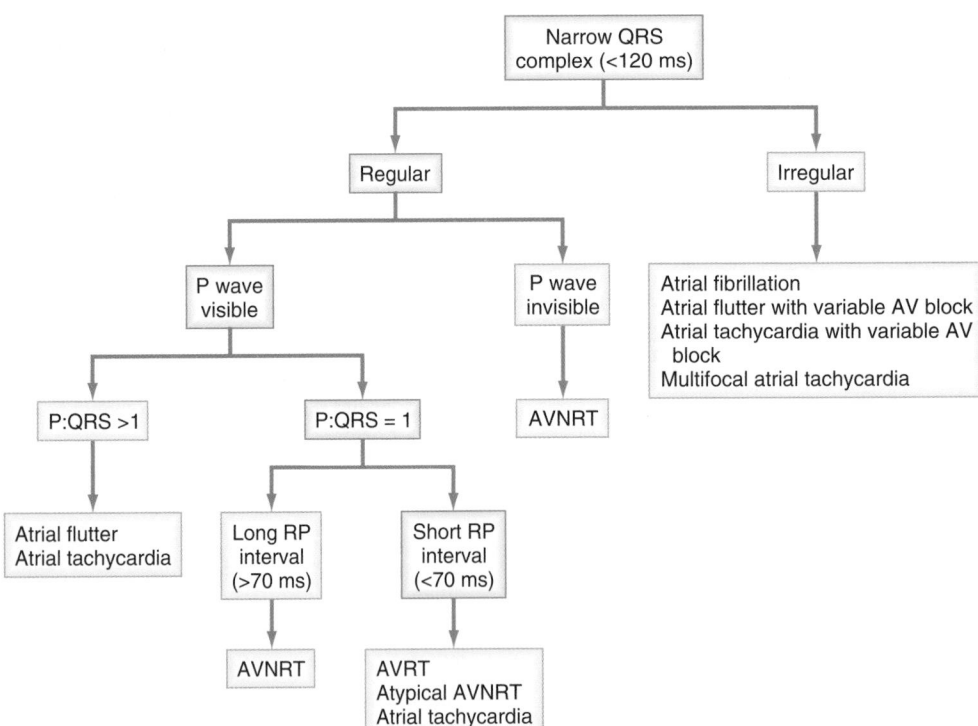

Figure 78-2 Differential diagnosis for narrow QRS complex (presumably supraventricular) tachycardias. Note that ventricular tachycardia may present with narrow QRS complexes (e.g., fascicular tachycardia). AV, atrioventricular; AVNRT, atrioventricular nodal reentry tachycardia; AVRT, atrioventricular reentry tachycardia.

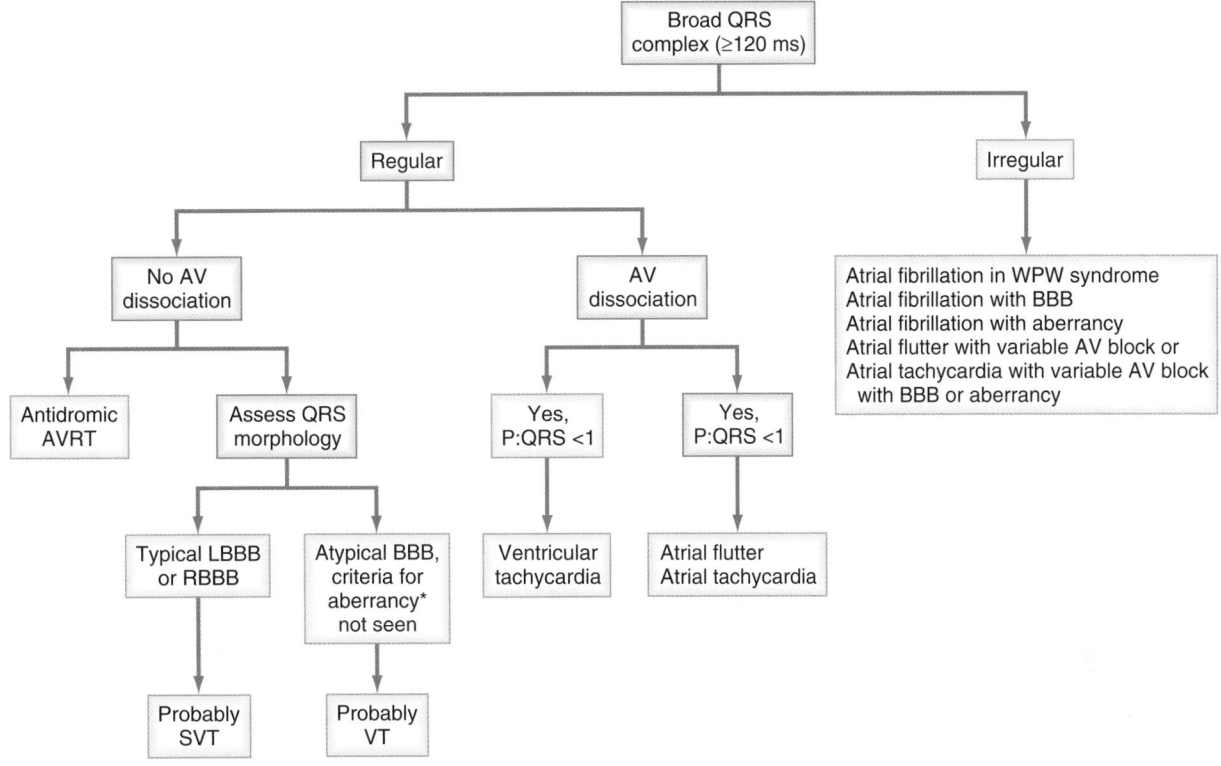

Figure 78-3   Differential diagnosis for wide QRS complex tachycardias. AV, atrioventricular; AVRT, atrioventricular reentry tachycardia; BBB, bundle branch block; LBBB, left bundle branch block; RBBB, right bundle branch block; SVT, supraventricular tachycardia; WPW, Wolff-Parkinson-White; VT, ventricular tachycardia. *Criteria for aberrancy: rate dependency, triphasic QRS complexes, rSR in V₁, with R >, QRS width < 140 msec, QRS deflections are discordant in precordial leads, absence of fusion and capture beats.

rhythm is regular, with narrow QRS complexes and a rate of 140 to 250 beats per minute. The atria are activated retrogradely, producing the inverted P waves in leads II, III, and aVF. Because atrial and ventricular depolarization occurs simultaneously, the P waves are often obscured by the QRS complexes and cannot be detected on the surface ECG (Figure 78-4, *A*). However, in about a third of cases of slow-fast AV nodal reentry tachycardia, a terminal positive deflection in lead aVR or V₁ (or both), imitating right bundle branch block or pseudo-S waves in the inferiorly oriented leads, may be present, reflecting retrograde activation of the atria. Tachycardia using these pathways in

reverse ("fast-slow," or long RP, tachycardia) is less common (5%-10% of cases).

Atrioventricular Reentry Tachycardia

ACCESSORY PATHWAYS

AV reentry tachycardia occurs as a result of an anatomically distinct AV connection termed an *accessory pathway*, produced by incomplete separation of the atria and ventricles during fetal development. The

Figure 78-4   A, Atrioventricular nodal reentry tachycardia, slow-fast type. Note narrow QRS complexes and absence of P waves. **B,** Atrioventricular reentry orthodromic tachycardia. Retrograde inverted P waves follow QRS complexes in leads II, III, and aVF. **C,** Atrioventricular reentry antidromic tachycardia with wide QRS complexes. Electrocardiogram during sinus rhythm with a QRS complex morphology identical to that seen during tachycardia may be helpful in the diagnosis. **D,** Atrial fibrillation in preexcitation syndrome with a fast ventricular rate response.

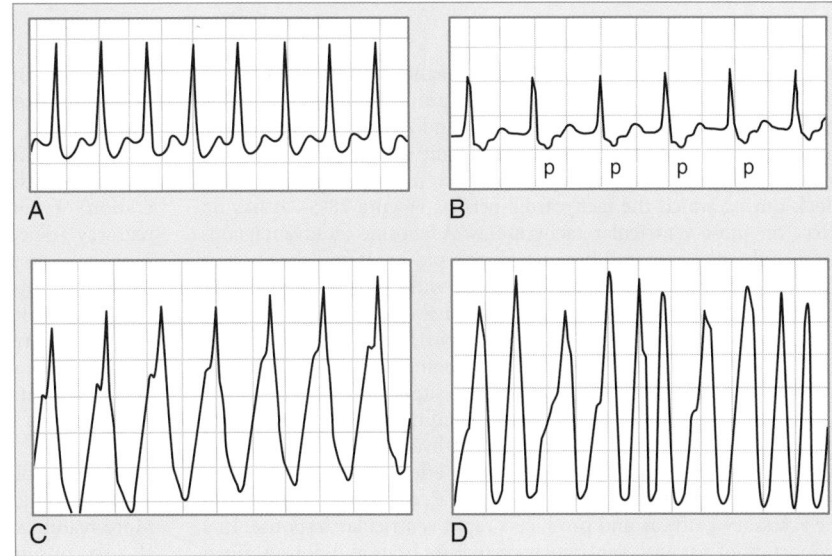

most common AV accessory pathways (often called a *Kent bundle*) is located around the mitral or tricuspid annulus. In about 10% of cases, there are multiple pathways.

Accessory pathways are capable of conduction in either or both directions. Accessory pathways that are capable of antegrade conduction are referred to as *manifest*, demonstrating a delta wave during sinus rhythm when the atrial impulses conduct over the accessory pathway without encountering AV delay. The PR interval is short (<120 msec), and the QRS complex is wide; this occurs because the atrial impulse enters a nonspecialized ventricular myocardium, and depolarization progresses slowly at first, giving rise to the delta wave before it is overtaken by a depolarization wavefront propagating via the normal conduction tissue. An accessory pathway that is capable of only retrograde conduction is termed *concealed* and does not produce a short PR interval or a delta wave during sinus rhythm.

MECHANISM AND ELECTROCARDIOGRAPHIC PRESENTATION

The reentry circuit of orthodromic AV reentry tachycardia involves the AV node and an accessory pathway, with the impulses conducting from the atria to the ventricles over the AV node and traveling in the reverse direction through the accessory pathway (see Figure 78-4, *B*). In antidromic AV reentry tachycardia, the reentrant impulses conduct antegradely from the atria to the ventricles via an accessory pathway and retrogradely via the AV node or a second accessory pathway (see Figure 78-4, *C*). Antidromic AV reentry tachycardia is uncommon (<10% of cases). Atrial fibrillation is usually encountered in patients with antegradely conducting pathways (see Figure 78-4, *D*).

ACUTE MANAGEMENT

In an emergency, distinguishing between AV nodal reentry tachycardia and AV reentry tachycardia may be difficult, but it is usually not critical, because both tachycardias respond to the same treatment. If the patient is hemodynamically stable, vagal maneuvers including carotid sinus massage, Valsalva maneuver, and facial immersion in cold water (diving reflex) can terminate tachycardia in about 50% of patients (Box 78-1).[3,4] Commercially available gel packs can be used as cold compresses instead of facial immersion, but the most important element is wet nostrils and breath-holding.

PHARMACOLOGIC TERMINATION

AV blocking agents such as adenosine, verapamil, diltiazem, and beta-blockers are effective in terminating both AV nodal reentry and AV reentry tachycardia (Table 78-1).[1]

Adenosine

Intravenous (IV) adenosine is effective in diagnosing, rate slowing, and often terminating narrow-complex tachycardias.[5] Adenosine usually terminates AV nodal reentry tachycardia and AV reentry tachycardia but rarely interrupts the atrial flutter circuit and does not suppress automatic atrial tachycardia; it can, however, produce high-degree AV block during which the tachycardia persists (Figure 78-5). It has no effect on most ventricular tachycardias. Adenosine is advantageous compared with verapamil because of its rapid onset and the absence of a negative inotropic effect in patients with poor left ventricular function and those with significant hypotension.

Adenosine is administered as a very rapid 3- to 6-mg IV bolus; if this is ineffective, another 6- to 12-mg bolus can be given 2 to 5 minutes later. Adenosine is metabolized very quickly, with an effective half-life of 10 seconds. Adverse effects including dyspnea, facial flushing, and chest tightness are therefore short-lived, but in about 12% of patients, adenosine may shorten the atrial effective refractory period and provoke atrial flutter or fibrillation or accelerate conduction over the accessory pathway and produce a rapid ventricular response. In a proportion of patients, ventricular premature beats and nonsustained

---

Box 78-1

VAGAL MANEUVERS TO TERMINATE TACHYCARDIA

Carotid Sinus Massage
Ensure that there is no significant carotid artery disease (carotid bruits).
Monitor the electrocardiogram continuously.
Place the patient in the supine position with the head slightly extended.
Start with right carotid sinus massage.
Apply firm rotatory or steady pressure to the carotid artery at the level of the third cervical vertebra for 5 sec.
If no response, massage the left carotid sinus.
Generally, right carotid sinus massage decreases sinus node discharge, and left carotid sinus massage slows atrioventricular conduction.
Do not massage both carotids at the same time.
A single application of carotid sinus pressure is effective in about 20% to 30% of patients with paroxysmal supraventricular tachycardias; multiple applications terminate tachycardia in about 50% of patients.
Asystole is a potential but rare complication.

Valsalva Maneuver
Valsalva maneuver involves an abrupt voluntary increase in intrathoracic and intraabdominal pressures by straining.
Monitor the electrocardiogram continuously.
Place the patient in the supine position.
The patient should not take a deep inspiration before straining.
Ideally, the patient blows into a mouthpiece of a manometer against the pressure of 30-40 mm Hg for 15 sec.
Alternatively, the patient strains for 15 sec while breath-holding.
Transient acceleration of tachycardia usually occurs during the strain phase as a result of sympathetic excess.
On release of strain, the rate of tachycardia slows because of the compensatory increase in vagal tone (baroreceptor reflex); it may terminate in about 50% of patients.
Termination of tachycardia may be followed by pauses and ventricular ectopics.

---

ventricular tachycardia may occur after the successful termination of supraventricular tachycardia.[6] Some individuals, particularly heart transplant recipients, are unusually sensitive to adenosine and require a lower dose (1 mg).

Verapamil and Diltiazem

Verapamil is administered IV as a 5- to 10-mg bolus over 2 minutes, and the effect on tachycardia is expected in 5 to 10 minutes. If necessary, a second bolus of 10 mg can be given 30 minutes after the initial dose. Vagal maneuvers can be effective at this stage. Verapamil should not be used for wide-complex tachycardias. IV verapamil is contraindicated in patients with poor left ventricular function or heart failure, and it should not be administered after pretreatment with oral and especially IV beta-blockers. It should not be used for atrial fibrillation associated with preexcitation syndrome, because it may result in acceleration of conduction over an antegradely conducting accessory pathway (especially with a short effective refractory period) a rapid ventricular response, and ventricular fibrillation. Diltiazem is an alternative to verapamil, but lower effective rates have been reported with this drug.[7] Diltiazem has the same contraindications as verapamil.

DC cardioversion or pharmacologic conversion with IV ibutilide, propafenone, or flecainide is appropriate for termination of atrial fibrillation with preexcitation.

Beta-Blockers

Among beta-blockers, esmolol, administered as an IV infusion at a rate of 50 to 200 μg/kg/min, is the agent of choice because of its rapid onset. More readily available IV metoprolol, atenolol, and propranolol can also be considered (see Table 78-1). Excessive bradycardia caused by

TABLE 78-1	**Acute Pharmacologic Rate Control in Atrial Tachyarrhythmias**				
Drug	*Route of Administration*	*Dose*		*Onset*	*Potential Adverse Effects*
Verapamil	Intravenous	5-10 mg (0.075-0.15 mg/kg) over 2 min; if no response, additional 5-10 mg after 15-30 min; 3-10 mg every 4-6 h for rate control		3-5 min	Hypotension, bradycardia, heart block, possible deterioration of ventricular function in the presence of organic heart disease
Diltiazem	Intravenous	0.25 mg/kg over 2 min; if no response, additional 0.35 mg/kg after 15-30 min; followed by 5-15 mg/h infusion for rate control		2-7 min	
Esmolol	Intravenous	0.5 mg/kg over 1 min, followed by 0.05-0.2 mg/kg/min for 4 min; if no response after 5 min, 0.5 mg/kg for 1 min, followed by 0.1 mg/kg for 4 min; infusion 0.05-0.2 mg/kg/min for rate control		2-3 min	Hypotension, bradycardia, heart block, possible deterioration of ventricular function in the presence of organic heart disease
Metoprolol	Intravenous	2.5-5 mg over 2 min followed by repeat doses if necessary (total 10-15 mg)		5 min	
Atenolol	Intravenous	2.5 mg over 2 min, followed by repeat doses if necessary (total 10 mg) or infusion 0.15 mg/kg for 20 min		5-10 min	
Propranolol	Intravenous	1 mg over 1 min (total 10-12 mg; 0.15 mg/kg)		5 min	
Digoxin	Intravenous	0.5-1 mg, followed by 0.25 mg every 2-4 h (maximum, 1.5 mg)		30-60 min	Bradycardia, atrioventricular block, atrial arrhythmias, ventricular tachycardia

Intravenous amiodarone can also be effective in rate control, especially in patients with poor left ventricular function, but there is insufficient evidence to support this recommendation. The rate-slowing effect of amiodarone is usually delayed by 1-2 hours.

AV node blocking agents can be countered with IV injection of atropine, 0.6 to 2.4 mg in divided doses of 0.6 mg.

Other Antiarrhythmic Agents

Because adenosine, verapamil, diltiazem, and beta-blockers are so highly effective in terminating AV nodal reentry tachycardia and AV reentry tachycardia, specific antiarrhythmic drugs such as propafenone, flecainide, sotalol, ibutilide, and amiodarone are seldom needed in the acute setting. Digoxin is not useful because it is often ineffective and may facilitate conduction over the accessory pathway, shorten the atrial effective refractory period, and promote atrial fibrillation.

ATRIAL PACING

In patients with implantable devices, antitachycardia pacing facilities can be used to terminate the arrhythmia. However, there is also a risk of inducing atrial fibrillation with a rapid ventricular response in a patient with an antegradely conducting accessory pathway.

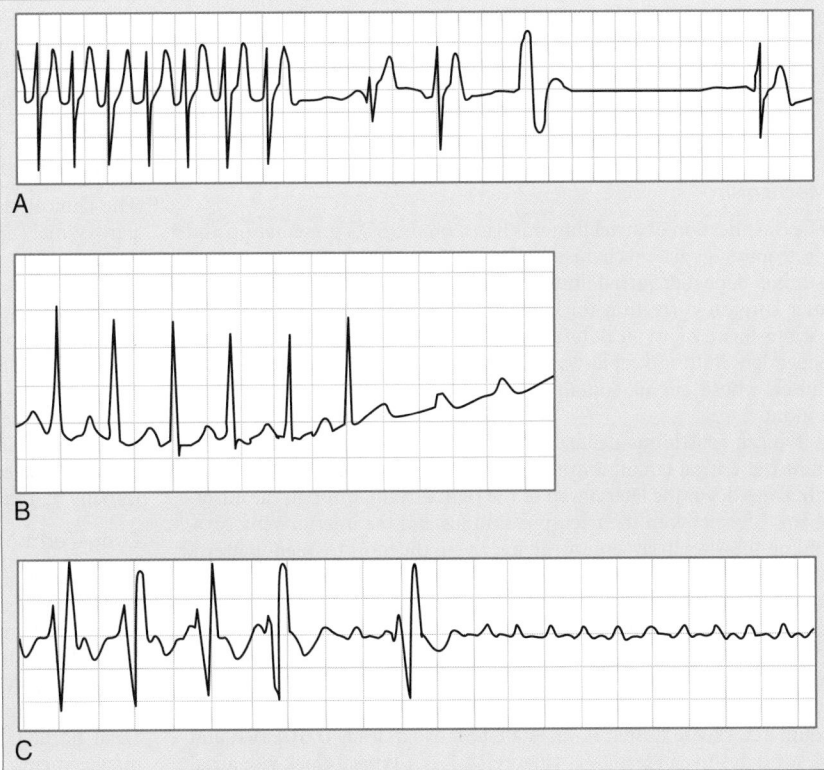

Figure 78-5 **A,** Adenosine usually terminates atrioventricular reentry tachycardias. **B** and **C,** It rarely interrupts the atrial flutter circuit or suppresses automatic focal atrial tachycardia but produces high-degree atrioventricular block during which the tachycardia persists.

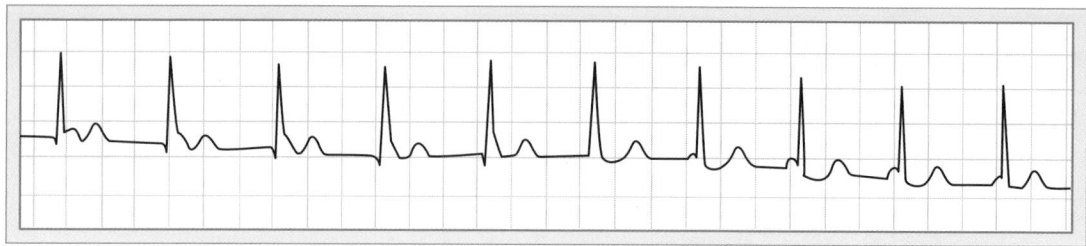

Figure 78-6   Accelerated junctional rhythm with independent sinus node activity.

LONG-TERM MANAGEMENT

Patients with AV nodal reentry tachycardia and AV reentry tachycardia should be referred to a cardiologist for electrophysiologic evaluation and long-term management. Both pharmacologic and nonpharmacologic alternatives, including ablation of an accessory pathway, are widely available.

Accelerated Atrioventricular Rhythm

Accelerated AV rhythm is produced by abnormal automaticity in the AV node. It is a narrow QRS complex tachycardia (unless bundle branch block is present), with the ventricular rate ranging from 70 to 250 beats per minute. AV dissociation is also present, because the atria are activated normally by the sinus node impulse while the ventricles are depolarized from an accelerated junctional site (Figure 78-6). This arrhythmia is commonly due to digitalis toxicity, and drug withdrawal is the usual therapy. If the rate of the AV node pacemaker is not fast, atropine can be given to increase the sinus node discharge until it resumes its dominance.

Atrial Fibrillation and Atrial Flutter

Atrial fibrillation with a fast ventricular response is the most common supraventricular arrhythmia encountered in the emergency department in both younger adults with first-onset arrhythmia and older patients presenting with decompensation. Atrial flutter shares these clinical presentations and requires similar initial therapy. The acute management of both arrhythmias is therefore considered together.

ATRIAL FLUTTER

Mechanism

The classification of atrial flutter is based on the ECG presentation and electrophysiologic mechanisms. The most common type is typical isthmus-dependent atrial flutter. Incisional reentry atrial flutter occurs after surgical correction for congenital heart disease. There are also various forms of atypical flutters, such as atypical right atrial isthmus-dependent flutter (double-wave and lower loop reentry) and left atrial flutter, whose circuit contains the pulmonary vein or mitral valve annulus.[8]

Typical, or isthmus-dependent, atrial flutter involves a macroreentrant right atrial circuit around the tricuspid annulus. The wavefront circulates down the lateral wall of the right atrium, through the eustachian ridge between the tricuspid annulus and the inferior vena cava, and up the interatrial septum, giving rise to the most frequent pattern, referred to as *counterclockwise flutter*. Reentry can also occur in the opposite direction (clockwise or reverse flutter).

Electrocardiographic Presentation

Atrial flutter is usually an organized atrial rhythm with an atrial rate typically between 250 and 350 beats per minute. In the more common counterclockwise flutter, F waves are negative in leads II, III, aVF, and V_{5-6} and positive in leads V_{1-2} (Figure 78-7, *A*). Typical clockwise atrial

flutter is characterized by positive F waves in leads II, III, and aVF and negative waves in leads V_{1-2}.

Treatment with propafenone, flecainide, and amiodarone to prevent recurrent atrial fibrillation without adding an AV blocking agent (beta-blocker or nondihydropyridine calcium antagonist) can organize the arrhythmia into typical atrial flutter with AV conduction of 1:1 or 2:1, producing a ventricular rate response of 150 beats per minute or higher (see Figure 78-7, *B*). The probability of 1:1 conduction is increased in the presence of an accessory pathway with a short effective refractory period.

Long-Term Management

The precise mechanism of atrial flutter is important for long-term management (e.g., catheter ablation) but has little influence on the initial approach. Patients with all types of atrial flutter should be referred for electrophysiologic evaluation with a view to ablation. Atrial fibrillation may develop even after successful ablation, and the patient should be followed up carefully.

ATRIAL FIBRILLATION

Electrocardiographic Presentation

Atrial fibrillation is defined as rapid oscillations or fibrillatory f waves that vary in size, shape, and timing (see Figure 78-7, *C*). The ventricular response rate is variable and depends on the rate and regularity of atrial activity, the refractory properties of the AV node itself, and the balance between sympathetic and parasympathetic tone. The RR intervals are irregular unless the patient has complete AV block or a paced rhythm.

Classification

The clinical classification of atrial fibrillation includes first detected, paroxysmal (up to 7 days), persistent (more than 7 days, long-standing persistent (>1 year), and permanent (accepted) forms of the arrhythmia and is essential for deciding between rhythm restoration and rate control. First-onset atrial fibrillation, if the duration of the episode is less than 48 hours, is a clear indication to restore sinus rhythm by either electrical or pharmacologic means. Because atrial fibrillation may be asymptomatic, the "first detected episode" should not be regarded as necessarily the true onset of the arrhythmia, in which case formal anticoagulation (see later discussion) and rate control may be preferential. Persistent or permanent atrial fibrillation should be treated initially by rate control and anticoagulation when appropriate.

Long-Term Management

Recognition of the pulmonary veins as the source of atrial premature beats or rapid atrial tachycardia that triggers atrial fibrillation or drives the atria prompted the development of ablation techniques that may "cure" the arrhythmia. In symptomatic permanent or persistent atrial fibrillation, AV node ablation and permanent pacing are effective in rate and symptom control. Any patient with first-onset or recurrent atrial fibrillation should be referred to a cardiologist for long-term management.

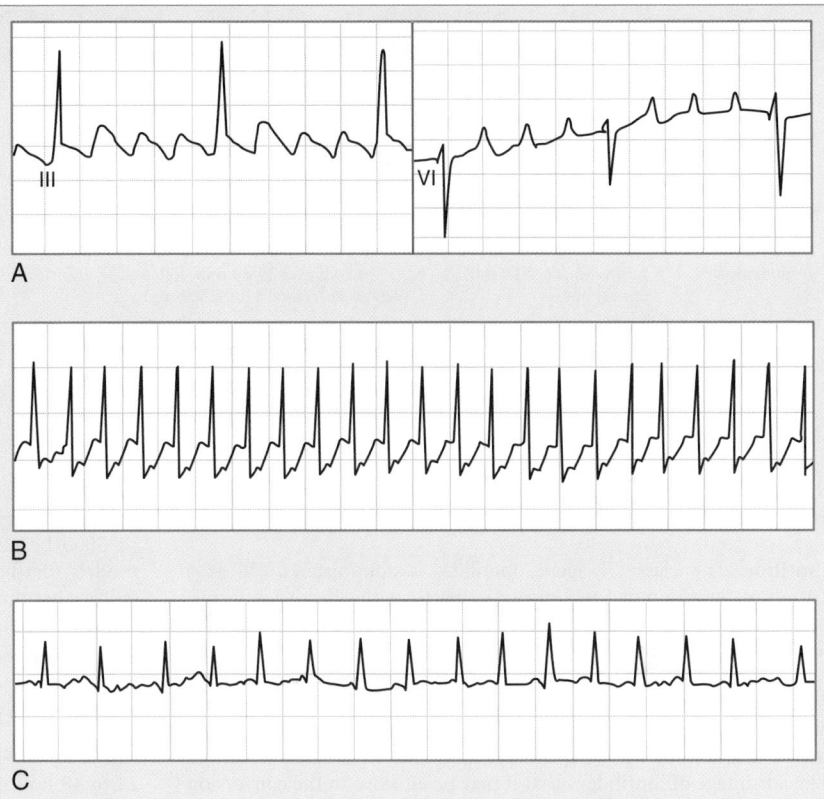

Figure 78-7 A, Typical counterclockwise atrial flutter. F waves are negative in leads II, III, aVF, and V$_{5-6}$ and positive in leads V$_{1-2}$. **B,** Atrial flutter with 1:1 atrioventricular conduction and a ventricular rate of 270 beats per minute in a patient treated with flecainide. **C,** Atrial fibrillation with fast, uncontrolled ventricular rates.

ACUTE MANAGEMENT

Acute therapy for atrial flutter and atrial fibrillation depends on the clinical presentation. Emergency electrical cardioversion is indicated for patients with hemodynamic collapse and progressively deteriorating left ventricular systolic function.

Direct-Current Cardioversion

Atrial flutter can be converted with DC shock energy as low as 25 to 50 J, but because a 100-J shock is virtually always successful, it should be considered as the initial shock strength. In recent-onset atrial fibrillation, sinus rhythm can be restored by a shock of 100 J, but it is recommended that cardioversion be started with an initial shock energy level of 200 J or greater. In patients with an arrhythmia of unknown duration, in heavier individuals, and in those with chronic obstructive lung disease and pulmonary emphysema, an initial setting of 300 to 360 J is appropriate. Success may occur on the third or subsequent attempt at an intensity that initially proved ineffective.

Rate Control

Rate control is pertinent to all atrial tachyarrhythmias, particularly if restoration of sinus rhythm is deferred. IV verapamil, diltiazem, and beta-blockers can rapidly control the ventricular response rate in atrial fibrillation[2] (see Table 78-1), but the efficacy may be less in atrial flutter. The decrease in the ventricular rate (approximately 20%-30%), time to maximal effect (20-30 minutes), conversion rate (12%-25%), and adverse reactions (usually hypotension and bradycardia, although left ventricular dysfunction and high-degree heart block may occur) are reportedly similar with both classes of drugs. Beta-blockers are preferable if thyrotoxicosis is suspected as a cause of the arrhythmia.

IV digoxin is no longer the treatment of choice when rapid rate control is essential because of the delayed onset of its therapeutic effect (>60 minutes). However, because of its positive inotropic action, digoxin may be safer to use in patients with poor ventricular function

and moderately fast ventricular rates. Digoxin may convert flutter to fibrillation, in which rate control is easier to accomplish.

There is evidence that IV amiodarone may be effective in rate control when other AV node blocking agents have no effect on ventricular response or are contraindicated.

Pharmacologic Cardioversion

If the arrhythmia is hemodynamically stable and is of recent onset, pharmacologic cardioversion can be effective.

Flecainide and Propafenone. Pharmacologic cardioversion of atrial fibrillation can be accomplished with the IC class of antiarrhythmic drugs—flecainide and propafenone administered orally as a single dose of 300 and 600 mg, respectively (Table 78-2).[2] Placebo-controlled randomized studies show an efficacy rate of 60% to 80% between the third and eighth hour after drug ingestion.[9,10] Both oral and IV routes of administration are equally effective, although with IV injection, restoration of sinus rhythm can be achieved more quickly.

Flecainide is given as a slow IV injection of 2 mg/kg over 10 to 30 minutes, up to the maximum dose of 150 mg. Propafenone is administered as a slow IV injection of 1.5 to 3 mg/kg, up to 300 to 600 mg. Because these drugs can significantly slow the atrial rate (from 300-350 beats/min to 200 beats/min), which may result in 1:1 AV conduction, beta-blockers or calcium antagonists with negative dromotropic effects on AV node conduction (verapamil, diltiazem) should be used concomitantly Other cardiovascular effects include reversible QRS widening and (rarely) left ventricular decompensation. Because of the negative inotropic effect, they are contraindicated in patients with severe structural heart disease and a poor ejection fraction.

Class IC drugs are usually ineffective for the conversion of atrial flutter, because they slow conduction within the reentrant circuit and prolong the flutter cycle length but rarely interrupt the circuit. These drugs pose the risk of increased (e.g., 2:1 or 1:1) AV conduction.

TABLE 78-2	Antiarrhythmic Drugs for Pharmacologic Conversion of Atrial Tachyarrhythmias		
Drug	*Route of Administration*	*Dose*	*Potential Adverse Effects*
Flecainide	Oral or intravenous	Loading oral dose 200-300 mg or slow injection 1.5-2 mg/kg over 10-20 min; if no response, infusion 1.5 mg/kg for 1 h, then 0.1-0.25 mg/kg over 24 h	Rapidly conducted atrial flutter, possible deterioration of ventricular function in the presence of organic heart disease, monomorphic ventricular tachycardia
Propafenone	Oral or intravenous	Loading oral dose 450-600 mg or 1.5-2 mg/kg over 10-20 min, followed by infusion 5-10 mg/kg if needed	
Ibutilide	Intravenous	1 mg over 10 min; if no response, additional 1 mg	QT prolongation, torsades de pointes, hypotension
Amiodarone	Intravenous (preferably central line)	5-7 mg/kg over 30-60 min, followed by infusion 20 mg/kg for 24 h (total 1200-1800 mg)	Hypotension, bradycardia, QT prolongation, torsades de pointes (?), gastrointestinal upset, constipation, phlebitis
Procainamide	Intravenous	1000 mg over 30 min, followed by 2 mg/min infusion	QRS widening, torsades de pointes, rapid atrial flutter
Vernakalant	Intravenous	3 mg/kg over 10 min; after 15 minute break 2 mg/kg unless arrhythmia terminated	Hypotension, postfibrillation bradycardia

Reported efficacy rates are as low as 13% to 40% with IV flecainide and propafenone.

Ibutilide. The class III agent, ibutilide, is administered IV as a 10-minute injection of 1 to 2 mg and is particularly effective in terminating atrial flutter, with a success rate of about 60%. Its administration may be associated with excessive QT interval prolongation, however, because of the rapid delayed rectifier potassium current (I_{Kr}) blockade and the risk of torsades de pointes.[11,12] It is less effective in atrial fibrillation. Higher doses of ibutilide administered as two successive infusions of 1 mg are usually required to terminate fibrillation. The advantage of ibutilide is that it may be effective in the conversion of arrhythmias of up to 30 days' duration, but the success rate drops significantly to 20% to 30%. The safety of ibutilide in patients with poor left ventricular function is unknown.

Amiodarone. Amiodarone administered IV at a dose of 5 mg/kg for 1 hour, followed by an infusion of 20 mg/kg over 24 hours, is effective in converting both atrial fibrillation and flutter, but the effect is significantly delayed.[13,14] However, because of its ability to control the ventricular rate, a low likelihood of torsades de pointes, and the absence of a negative inotropic effect, amiodarone can be used safely in patients with significant structural heart disease and those who are critically ill.

Procainamide and Sotalol. Procainamide administered as a slow IV injection of 1000 mg over 20 to 30 minutes, followed if necessary by an infusion of 2 mg/min over 1 hour, converts atrial flutter or fibrillation of less than 48 hours' duration, but its efficacy is limited in longer-lasting arrhythmias.[15] It is less effective than propafenone, flecainide, and ibutilide.

Sotalol is not indicated for the pharmacologic cardioversion of atrial flutter or fibrillation because its efficacy does not exceed 11% to 13%; however, it may satisfactorily control the ventricular rate.

Vernakalant. This drug is given by a short IV infusion (3 mg/kg over 10 minutes). If after a 15-minute waiting period the arrhythmia persists, a second infusion of 2 mg/kg may be given over 10 minutes. In recent-onset atrial fibrillation (<72 hours), about 50% of cases will terminate on average 12 minutes from the start of the first infusion. Vernakalant may be given to patients with underlying structural heart disease but not to patients with grade II/IV congestive heart failure. Proarrhythmia is uncommon, but hypotension and posttermination bradycardia may occur.[16]

The choice of an antiarrhythmic agent for cardioversion is illustrated in Figure 78-8.

Atrial Pacing

Burst overdrive atrial pacing can terminate atrial flutter in about 80% of cases and is feasible after cardiac surgery, when patients frequently have epicardial atrial pacing wires, or in patients with implantable dual-chamber pacemakers and defibrillators. High-frequency (50 Hz or 3000 beats/min) atrial pacing is available in some of the latest models for the termination of early-onset atrial fibrillation, but its efficacy has not yet been established. Atrial burst overdrive pacing may induce sustained atrial fibrillation, although short periods of fibrillation often precede conversion to sinus rhythm.

ANTICOAGULATION

Anticoagulation is imperative if the arrhythmia persists for more than 24 to 48 hours or if its duration is unknown. Atrial flutter and atrial fibrillation pose similar risks of thromboembolism, and the same criteria for anticoagulation should be applied in patients with either arrhythmia. In hemodynamically stable arrhythmias of more than 48 hours' or of unknown duration, rate control and 3 weeks' anticoagulation with warfarin (International Normalized Ratio 2.0 to 3.0) should be considered before any intervention (electrical or pharmacologic cardioversion, catheter ablation).[17]

TRANSESOPHAGEAL ECHOCARDIOGRAPHY–GUIDED CARDIOVERSION

If, for any reason, deferral of cardioversion is not indicated, the transesophageal echocardiography–guided approach, with short-term anticoagulation with low-molecular-weight heparin, is a safe and effective

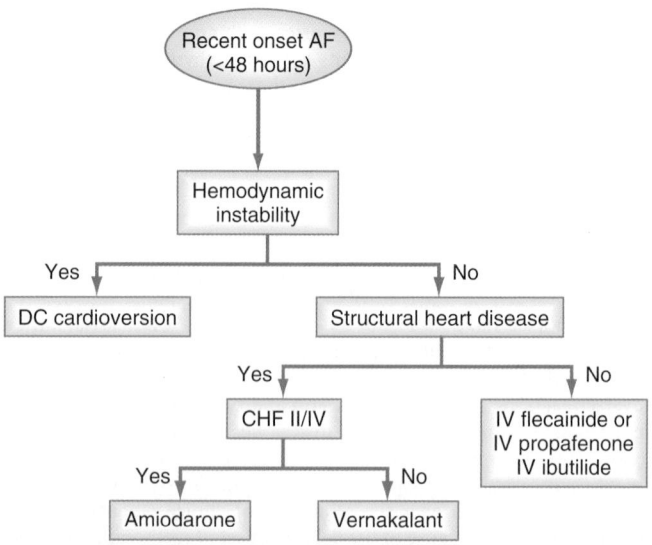

Figure 78-8 Choice of antiarrhythmic for pharmacologic cardioversion of atrial fibrillation.

Modified from Straus SE, Majumdar SR, McAlister FA. New evidence for stroke prevention: scientific review. JAMA 2002;288:1388-95.

INR, International Normalized Ratio.

TABLE 78-3	Risk Stratification and Indications for Anticoagulation in Atrial Fibrillation and Flutter	
Risk of Stroke	*Definition*	*Therapy*
Low (1%/yr)	Age < 65 yr; ejection fraction ≥ 0.50; no stroke or transient ischemic attack, hypertension, heart failure, or valvular heart disease	Aspirin 325 mg
Low to moderate (1.5%/yr)	Age 65-75 yr; no risk factors	Aspirin 325 mg
Moderate to high (2.5%/yr)	Age 65-75 yr and either diabetes or coronary heart disease	Warfarin (INR 2.0-3.0)
High (6%/yr)	Age < 75 yr and hypertension, heart failure, or ejection fraction < 0.50 Age > 75 yr, particularly women, even in the absence of risk factors	Warfarin (INR 2.0-3.0)
Very high (10%/yr)	Age > 75 yr and hypertension, heart failure, or ejection fraction < 0.50 Any age with a history of stroke or transient ischemic attack or valvular heart disease	Warfarin (INR 2.0-3.0)

alternative.[18] It may be clinically beneficial in patients with recent-onset arrhythmias or in individuals at high risk of bleeding complications during prolonged anticoagulation therapy.[19] Compared with unfractionated heparin, low-molecular-weight heparin therapy does not involve prolonged IV administration or laboratory monitoring and therefore has the potential to greatly simplify cardioversion-related anticoagulation therapy in low-risk individuals. Postcardioversion anticoagulation should be considered if atrial fibrillation has been present for 48 hours or more, or if thromboembolic risk factors are present (Table 78-3).[17,20]

Atrial Tachycardia

MECHANISM

The mechanism of atrial tachycardia is attributed to enhanced automaticity, triggered activity, or intraatrial reentry. Macroreentrant atrial tachycardia often occurs after surgery for congenital heart disease. Focal atrial tachycardia typically originates along the crista terminalis in the right atrium, in the pulmonary veins in the left atrium, or around one of the atrial appendages.

ELECTROCARDIOGRAPHIC PRESENTATION

The heart rate varies from 120 to 250 beats per minute, P waves precede the QRS complex, and PP intervals are regular (see Figure 78-5, *B*). The PR interval is linked to the rate of tachycardia and is longer than in sinus rhythm at the same rate. P wave morphology is usually different from that during sinus rhythm and depends on the site of origin. Left atrial tachycardia presents with the negative P waves in leads I,

aVL, V_5, and V_6. Automatic atrial tachycardia may present as an incessant variety, leading to tachycardia-induced cardiomyopathy

ATRIAL TACHYCARDIA WITH ATRIOVENTRICULAR BLOCK

Tachycardia with AV block occurs commonly in patients with organic heart disease, and in 50% to 75% of cases, it is due to digitalis toxicity (Figure 78-9). Digoxin-specific antibody fragments are available for the reversal of life-threatening overdosage.

MULTIFOCAL ATRIAL TACHYCARDIA

This tachycardia presents as rapid, irregular atrial activity with discrete P waves of varying morphology and is considered a transitional rhythm between atrial tachycardia and fibrillation. However, it may occur in patients with chronic severe pulmonary disease as a result of theophylline or β-agonist overdose. Elimination of the causative factor may reduce the need for antiarrhythmic therapy. IV verapamil can accomplish rate control.

ACUTE MANAGEMENT

DC cardioversion converts atrial tachycardia based on the reentry mechanism or triggered activity, but it may not terminate automatic tachycardia. Similarly, atrial overdrive pacing may slow the tachycardia rate but seldom suppresses the automatic focus.

It is generally accepted that beta-blockers and calcium antagonists, particularly verapamil, can either terminate the tachycardia or produce rate control. Adenosine can terminate atrial tachycardia, but the most common response to adenosine is to create AV block and thereby reveal the unaffected tachycardia (see Figure 78-5, *B* and *C*).

Flecainide, propafenone, sotalol, and amiodarone are effective in converting the arrhythmia. If tachycardia occurs as a result of digitalis intoxication, therapy includes the cessation of digoxin and IV administration of potassium.

LONG-TERM MANAGEMENT

Patients with atrial tachycardia should be referred to a cardiologist because the arrhythmogenic focus can be found and ablated in up to 86% cases.

Inappropriate Sinus Tachycardia

Inappropriate sinus tachycardia is a persistent increase in resting heart rate unrelated to or out of proportion with the level of physical or emotional stress. It is found predominantly in women and is not uncommon in health professionals. Sinus tachycardia due to intrinsic sinus node abnormalities such as enhanced automaticity or abnormal autonomic regulation of the heart, with excess sympathetic and reduced parasympathetic input, is not unusual. The main therapy is beta-blockers, although ivabradine, a drug which blocks the main current responsible for diastolic depolarization in the sinus node, is being increasingly used in Europe.[21] In general, sinus tachycardia is a secondary phenomenon, and the underlying causes should be actively

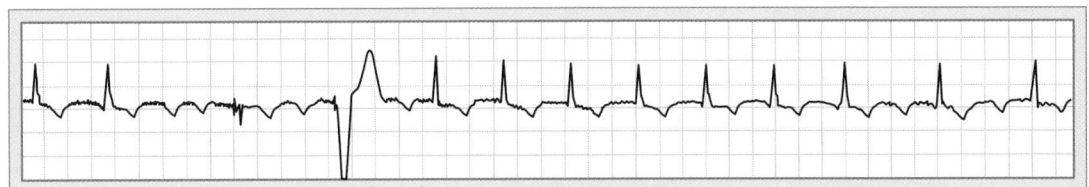

Figure 78-9 Atrial tachycardia with varying atrioventricular block due to digitalis toxicity.

investigated. Depending on the clinical setting, acute causes include fever, hypotension, infection, anemia, thyrotoxicosis, hypovolemia, acute heart failure, acute pulmonary embolism, and shock. Sinus tachycardia may be associated with the abuse of drugs such as amphetamines.

KEY POINTS

1. Supraventricular tachycardia (SVT) is characterized by narrow QRS complexes, but differentiating SVT from ventricular tachycardia may be necessary when bundle branch block, rate-dependent aberrancy, and antidromic atrioventricular (AV) reentry tachycardia are present.

2. If the diagnosis of SVT cannot be proved, the arrhythmia should be treated as ventricular tachycardia.

3. Immediate direct-current (DC) cardioversion is the treatment for any hemodynamically unstable tachycardia.

4. In hemodynamically stable paroxysmal junctional tachycardias (AV nodal reentry tachycardia and AV reentry tachycardia), vagotonic maneuvers should be tried first, because they may terminate tachycardia in about 50% of patients without the need to resort to pharmacologic therapy.

5. Intravenous (IV) adenosine, verapamil, and esmolol are first-line drug therapies for paroxysmal junctional tachycardias, but adenosine and verapamil should not be used for wide complex tachycardias and atrial fibrillation with preexcitation.

6. DC cardioversion or pharmacologic conversion with IV ibutilide or flecainide is appropriate for the termination of atrial fibrillation associated with preexcitation syndrome.

7. IV verapamil, diltiazem, esmolol, metoprolol, and propranolol can rapidly accomplish rate control in atrial fibrillation but may be less effective in atrial flutter.

8. Beta-blockers are preferable in atrial fibrillation associated with thyrotoxicosis.

9. Pharmacologic cardioversion of atrial fibrillation in the absence of severe underlying heart disease can be attained using oral or IV flecainide or propafenone, vernakalant, and IV ibutilide, but the last is more effective in atrial flutter.

10. Propafenone, flecainide, and vernakalant may result in atrial flutter with slow atrial rates and 2:1 or 1:1 AV conduction; verapamil, diltiazem, or beta-blockers should be available to treat this complication. Ibutilide can significantly prolong the QT interval and cause polymorphic ventricular tachycardia that, if sustained, may require DC cardioversion.

11. IV amiodarone should be considered as first-line drug therapy in patients with severely impaired left ventricular function.

12. Accelerated AV rhythm and atrial tachycardia with AV block commonly occur as a result of digitalis toxicity; digitalis withdrawal is the usual therapy.

13. Anticoagulation is indicated if atrial fibrillation or flutter persists for more than 48 hours or if the duration is unknown; anticoagulation and rate control should be the initial therapy in these patients.

14. An alternative approach is transesophageal echocardiography, to exclude the presence of atrial thrombi or dense spontaneous echocontrast, and short-term anticoagulation with low-molecular-weight heparin, followed by DC or pharmacologic cardioversion.

15. Patients with paroxysmal junctional tachycardias, atrial tachycardia, atrial flutter, and first-onset or recurrent atrial fibrillation should be referred to a cardiac electrophysiologist/cardiologist for assessment and long-term management planning; effective nonpharmacologic therapies are available for these arrhythmias.

ANNOTATED REFERENCES

Albers GW, Dalen JE, Laupacis A, et al. Antithrombotic therapy in atrial fibrillation. Chest 2001;119:194S-206S.

This paper focuses on the prevention of stroke in nonrheumatic atrial fibrillation and flutter and provides expert recommendations regarding risk stratification, anticoagulation strategies, cardioversion (including transesophageal echocardiography-guided cardioversion), and long-term management of patients at risk of thromboembolism. It contains a complete review of the evidence base for anticoagulation in atrial fibrillation.

Blomström-Lundvist C, Scheiman MM, Aliot EM, et al. ACC/AHA/ESC guidelines for the management of patients with supraventricular arrhythmias—executive summary. A report of the American College of Cardiology/American Heart Association Task Force on Practice Guidelines and the European Society of Cardiology Committee for Practice Guidelines (Writing Committee to develop guidelines for the management of patients with supraventricular arrhythmias). J Am Coll Cardiol 2003;42:1493-531.

These practice guidelines describe a range of generally accepted approaches to the diagnosis and management of supraventricular tachyarrhythmias (excluding atrial fibrillation) and provide insight into the multiple mechanisms defined by electrophysiologic studies, with a focus on both acute and long-term therapies.

Camm AJ. Atrial fibrillation: is there a role for low-molecular-weight heparin? Clin Cardiol 2001;24:I15-19.

This review paper summarizes evidence emerging from clinical studies that clearly supports both the use of transesophageal echocardiography-based cardioversion protocols and the introduction of low-molecular-weight heparin for anticoagulation in atrial fibrillation. Clinical settings in which low-molecular-weight heparin may offer advantages over unfractionated heparin and warfarin are discussed.

Fuster V, Rydén LE, Asinger RV, et al. Task force report: ACC/AHA/ESC guidelines for the management of patients with atrial fibrillation. Eur Heart J 2001;22:1852-923.

These guidelines incorporate a comprehensive review of the latest information about the classification, epidemiology, mechanisms, and clinical presentations of atrial fibrillation. Practical approaches to acute and long-term management of this arrhythmia are discussed at length. An extensive list of references covers various aspects of atrial fibrillation.

Mehta D, Wafa S, Ward DE, Camm AJ. Relative efficacy of various physical manoeuvres in the termination of junctional tachycardia. Lancet 1988;1:1181-5.

This paper compares the ability of four vagotonic physical maneuvers to terminate paroxysmal supraventricular tachycardias that involve the AV node as part of their reentrant circuits. It shows that these tachycardias can be terminated without resorting to pharmacologic therapy in more than half of patients. The paper provides a detailed methodological description and explains the physiologic effects of vagotonic maneuvers.

REFERENCES

Access the complete reference list online at http://www.expertconsult.com.

79

Ventricular Arrhythmias

RAÚL J. GAZMURI | CRISTINA SANTONOCITO

Abnormalities in impulse generation and conduction may lead to arrhythmic events in critically ill patients, some of which could be life threatening. These abnormalities may originate from primary cardiac events or from a myriad of "extracardiac" acute or acute-on-chronic conditions. The presence of arrhythmias or—more commonly—the presence of conditions that increase the risk of arrhythmias is frequently a reason for hospital admission to areas with capability for continuous monitoring of the electrocardiogram (ECG) and availability of personnel training for the prompt recognition and management of these arrhythmias (i.e., ICUs and telemetry units).

Arrhythmias that originate in atrial tissue and pulmonary veins are considered supraventricular. They may compromise stroke volume, leading to reductions in cardiac output and therefore hemodynamic instability consequent to excessive heart rate and/or disruption of ventricular filling after removal of the atrial contribution. However, in the absence of accessory conduction pathways (i.e., that bypass the atrioventricular [AV] node), supraventricular arrhythmias are rarely life threatening and can often be managed by nonemergent pharmacologic means or by electrical means (e.g., cardioversion or, more infrequently, override pacing). In contrast, arrhythmias that originate in ventricular structures may pose substantial risk of becoming life threatening, such as ventricular tachycardia (VT) and ventricular fibrillation (VF), requiring immediate recognition and treatment.

In this chapter, ventricular arrhythmias are discussed, with primary focus on mechanisms, predisposing conditions, incidence, diagnosis, and acute clinical management.

Normal Electrophysiology

ANATOMIC SYNOPSIS

The cardiac electrical impulse originates in the sinoatrial (SA) node, located high on the right atrium near its junction with the superior vena cava (Figure 79-1). The impulse then propagates through muscle fibers and specialized internodal pathways (composed of Purkinje-type fibers) to converge on the AV node, located in the interatrial septum near the tricuspid valve and the opening of the coronary sinus. From the AV node, the impulse travels through the bundle of His, its left and right branches, and the Purkinje system to simultaneously activate the right and left ventricles. A ring of fibrous tissue interposed between the atria and the ventricles prevents spread of the electrical impulse through the muscle fibers, enabling the AV node to function as a relay and filter structure limiting the number of impulses that can be transmitted to the ventricles and thus maintaining the ventricular rate within a range that is physiologically permissible for stroke volume generation. Thus, the AV node prevents a $1:1$ conduction under conditions of very rapid atrial activation such as atrial flutter (rate $\approx 300\ s^{-1}$) and atrial fibrillation (rate $\approx 350\ s^{-1}$ to $600\ s^{-1}$), typically preventing increases in ventricular rate above $150\ s^{-1}$ or $180\ s^{-1}$ in instances of atrial flutter or atrial fibrillation, respectively.

ACTION POTENTIAL AND PACEMAKER ACTIVITY

Action potential results from rapid depolarization and repolarization of polarized cells driven by a coordinated sequence of opening and closing of channels that regulate ion currents across the cell membrane.

The main ion currents are carried by channels that regulate influx of sodium ions (Na^+) and calcium ions (Ca^{2+}) (inward currents) and by efflux of potassium ions (K^+) (outward currents).[1-3]

The action potential is essential to initiate and propagate the electrical impulse throughout the conduction system and ultimately reach cardiomyocytes where the action potential signals activating of contractile activity and therefore pump function through Ca^{2+}-induced Ca^{2+}-release from the sarcoplasmic reticulum. Accordingly, the electrical impulse typically precedes mechanical activity. However, cardiomyocytes can also react to mechanical forces through stretch-activated ion channels and other related mechanisms including mechanical modulation of Ca^{2+} handling and interaction with other mechanosensitive cells in the heart.[4,5] This mechanism is in part responsible for commotion cordis,[6,7] precordial thump,[8] and fist pacing.[9]

The functional characteristics of the action potential differ contingent on the cell type. Cells from the Purkinje system and from atrial and ventricular muscle are primarily responsible for propagation of the action potential. These cells have a stable resting potential at approximately -90 mV (inside negative), which is largely the result of a K^+ current known as the *inward rectifier* (I_{K1}). I_{K1} "anchors" the membrane potential to a voltage close to the equilibrium potential of K^+;[2] it is turned off during depolarization (inward rectification). Initiation of an action potential requires depolarization of the membrane potential between -70 and -80 mV. This voltage is the threshold at which fast voltage-gated Na^+ channels are activated, prompting Na^+ influx driving an inward current (I_{Na}).[3] Depolarization to the threshold potential typically occurs upon arrival of an action potential. The I_{Na} drives the membrane potential toward the equilibrium potential of Na^+, causing further depolarization and reversal of the membrane potential to approximately $+20$ mV (overshoot). This phase is known as *phase 0* of the action potential and ushers in a 4-phase repolarization (Figure 79-2). Phase 1 is the initial early repolarization (action potential notch) and results from rapid inactivation of Na^+ channels (inner gate) and the opening of K^+ channels carrying a rapidly activating and rapidly inactivating "transient" outward current (I_{To}). Based on recovery time, two distinct subpopulations of channels can be recognized carrying a rapidly "fast" recovering current (I_{Tof}) and a slowly recovering current (I_{Tos}). The difference in these currents rely on distinct pore-forming α-subunits with Kv4.2/Kv4.3 (*KCND2/KCND3*) genes encoding I_{Tof} and Kv1.4 encoding I_{Tos}.[10] It appears that I_{Tof} is the predominant contributor to I_{To} in ventricular myocardium.[11] Because the K+ channels carrying I_{To} are expressed in the subepicardial and midmyocardial regions but not in the subendocardial region, they contribute to the inhomogeneity of repolarization.[12]

Phase 2 is the plateau phase of the action potential and results mainly from a Ca^{2+} current carried by the slow and prolonged opening of L-type voltage-gated Ca^{2+} channels (I_{Ca-L}).[13,14] Opening of these channels begins during phase 0 at a membrane potential of -30 to -40 mV. These channels are inactivated in response to increases in cytosolic Ca^{2+} and are strongly regulated by neurotransmitters. Phase 3 corresponds to late repolarization and follows the closing of Ca^{2+} channels and opening of K^+ channels with slow activation kinetics carrying currents known as *delayed rectifiers* (I_K). The I_K are the main repolarizing currents and have two components carried by distinct gene products: a rapid component (I_{Kr}) and a slow component (I_{Ks}).[15,16] Both are implicated in the heritable forms of long QT syndrome (see later discussion).[17] In addition, opening of I_{K1} (main contributor to the

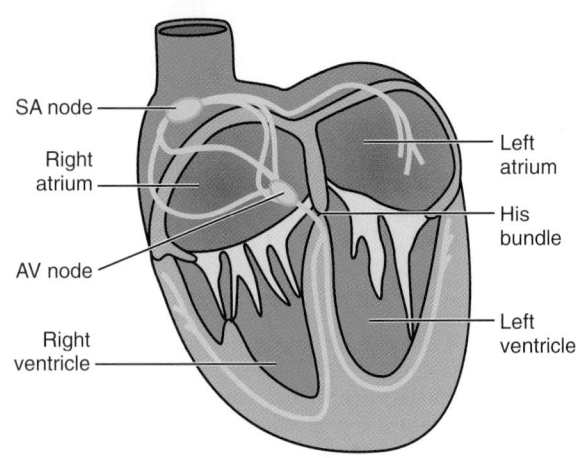

Figure 79-1 Conduction system of the heart. AV, atrioventricular; SA, sinoatrial.

resting membrane potential as described earlier) contributes to repolarization. Phase 4 represents return to the resting membrane potential and the interval during which ionic balance is restituted, largely through the action of the Na^+/K^+ pump.

Cells of the SA and AV nodes lack voltage-gated Na^+ channels, and phase 0 is carried by I_{Ca-L}.[18] Because of their slower opening kinetics (relative to Na^+ channels), they give rise to a slanted phase 0 and in

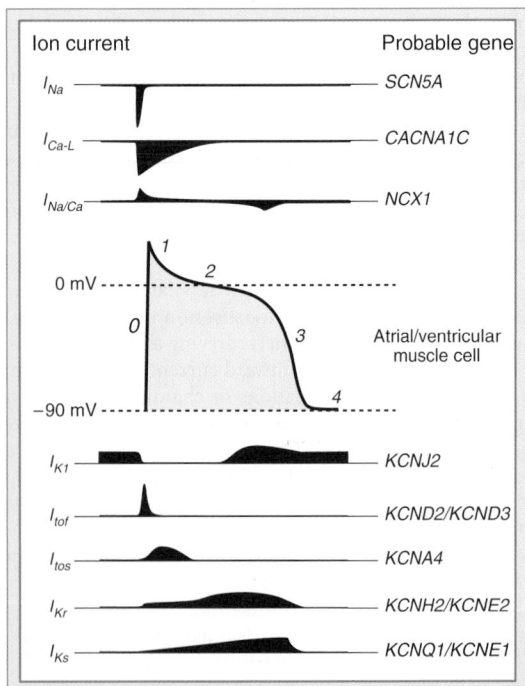

Figure 79-2 Action potential of a cardiac muscle cell, depicting the main underlying inward and outward currents and respective gene products. Distinctive phases of the action potential are numbered. *Voltage* (mV) refers to potential on intracellular side of plasma membrane relative to an outside reference. Notice that resting potential is negative inside at approximately −90 mV, indicating the cell at rest is polarized (phase 4). Beginning of action potential is signaled by rapid reduction in such potential, with inside voltage reaching 0 mV (depolarization) and then becoming transiently positive (overshoot) during phase 0, to be followed by phase 1, 2, and 3 as voltage returns to resting potential on phase 4.

part determine the lower conduction velocity of the SA and AV nodes (≈50 cm·s⁻¹) compared with the His-Purkinje system (≈400 cm·s⁻¹) and muscle cells (≈100 cm·s⁻¹). SA and AV node cells also have pacemaker activity and slowly depolarize during phase 4 to a threshold potential of approximately −40 mV. The slow depolarization is called *pre-potential* or *pacemaker potential* and involves a background Na^+ current (I_{Na-B}), a decay of K^+ currents, and the opening of T-type voltage-gated Ca^{2+} channels (I_{Ca-T}) at a potential between the thresholds for I_{Na} and IC_a-L, unleashing phase 0. Cells of the His-Purkinje system have latent pre-potential activity and can become active when SA or AV node activity is depressed or their impulse is blocked. Atrial and ventricular muscle cells exhibit pre-potential activity only under abnormal circumstances (see later discussion).

The preceding description is succinct and oversimplified. Various other ion channels, antiporters, pumps, and receptors play important roles in specific physiologic states and disease processes. For example, there is a nonselective cationic channel that is gated at resting potential by intracellular Ca^{2+} and produces an inward Na^+ current (I_{NS}).[19] This current may contribute to delayed afterdepolarizations following Ca^{2+} release by the sarcoplasmic reticulum. $I_{k(atp)}$ is a K^+ current carried through metabolically regulated channels that are inhibited by adenosine triphosphate (ATP) and opened under conditions of ischemia and hypoxia. $I_{k(atp)}$ is the main contributor to the shortening of the action potential duration and the characteristic ST-segment elevation observed in the surface electrocardiogram during myocardial ischemia.[20,21]

The sarcolemmal Na^+/Ca^{2+} exchanger is another important modulator of the action potential. Because it exchanges one Ca^{2+} for three Na^+, it is electrogenic and generates a current ($I_{Na/Ca}$) whose direction is determined by the Na^+ and Ca^{2+} gradients and the membrane potential.[21,22] In settings in which there is cytosolic Ca^{2+} overload (e.g., ischemia and reperfusion, digitalis toxicity), Ca^{2+} may trigger Ca^{2+} release from the sarcoplasmic reticulum during phase 4, which in turn prompts reverse-mode operation of the Na^+/Ca^{2+} exchanger, causing an inwardly directed $I_{Na/Ca}$ (Na^+ influx). This current contributes to the generation of delayed afterdepolarizations and triggered arrhythmias (see later discussion).

Adrenergic receptors also play important roles in modulating the action potential by modifying channel activity.[23-25] For example, stimulation of β-adrenergic receptors increases the activity of I_{Ca-L}, leading to increased Ca^{2+} influx, signaling increased contractile activity. β-Adrenergic receptor stimulation can also activate K^+ channels, shortening repolarization and the duration of the action potential.[26] $α_1$-Adrenergic receptors exert actions via G-protein on the Na^+/K^+ pump, K^+ channels, and phospholipase C and can alter impulse initiation and repolarization. $α_1$-Adrenergic stimulation has been linked to triggered rhythms via early and delayed afterdepolarizations and the development of abnormal automatic rhythms in the setting of ischemia and reperfusion.[27,28]

Alteration in the proteins forming these various channels—mostly genetic, but also acquired—may distort the normal action potential, yielding distinctive electrocardiographic patterns (e.g., long QT syndrome, Brugada syndrome) that are associated with increased risk of ventricular tachyarrhythmias.

Mechanisms of Ventricular Tachyarrhythmias

The mechanisms by which ventricular tachyarrhythmias develop encompass abnormalities in impulse generation and abnormalities in impulse conduction. Both mechanisms often coexist and orchestrate the initiation and maintenance of ventricular tachyarrhythmias. Identification of the arrhythmogenic mechanism is important because therapeutic strategies may be designed to target the vulnerable parameters responsible for the genesis and/or maintenance of the arrhythmia.

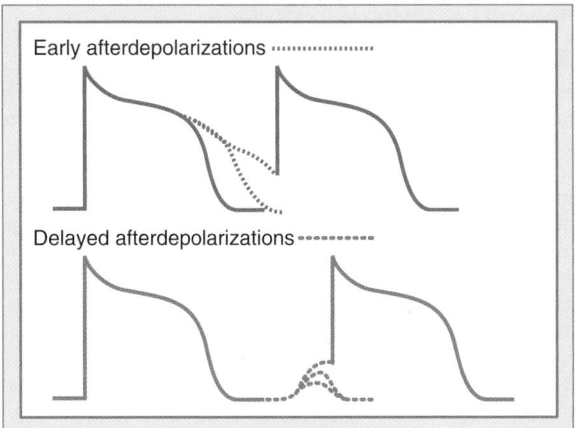

Figure 79-3 Afterdepolarizations *(dotted lines)*. Early afterdepolarizations are retardations in repolarization with prolongation in action potential duration *(upper figure)*. Delayed afterdepolarizations represent spontaneous depolarizations that occur after repolarization is over *(lower figure)*. Afterdepolarizations that reach threshold trigger an action potential.

ABNORMALITIES IN IMPULSE GENERATION

Abnormalities in impulse generation are generally the result of automaticity or triggered activity.

Automaticity

Automaticity refers to the emergence of ectopic pacemaker activity and may result from enhanced normal automaticity or from the development of abnormal automaticity.

Enhanced normal automaticity occurs when cells whose pacemaker potentials are normally under overdrive suppression (e.g., cells from the AV node or His-Purkinje system) fire at rates that escape the overdrive suppression of the SA node. This phenomenon may result from effects on phase 4 pre-potentials favoring earlier development of action potentials (i.e., less maximal polarization, faster depolarization, or lower threshold potential) or from shortening of the action potential duration, with an earlier return to phase 4. Enhanced normal automaticity is usually the result of adrenergic stimulation.

Abnormal automaticity refers to the generation of impulses in cells that normally do not exhibit pacemaker potential. This phenomenon can occur in cells that are partially depolarized as a result of a pathologic process (e.g., ischemia). Under these conditions, the reduction in the resting membrane potential (less negative; to −70 or even −50 mV) shifts the balance during phase 4 toward depolarizing currents.[29] Through this mechanism, automaticity can developed in atrial and ventricular muscle cells and in specialized tissues other than the SA in which the firing conditions can be altered. Examples of abnormal automaticity include accelerated idioventricular rhythms and some VTs that develop 24 to 72 hours after an acute myocardial infarction.[30,31]

Triggered Activity

Triggered activity refers to arrhythmias that arise from afterdepolarizations. Afterdepolarizations are alterations in membrane potential that occur during the repolarization phase without intervening external triggers or cell-to-cell interactions.[32] Afterdepolarizations can develop in different phases of the action potential. Those that develop during phase 2, phase 3, or early phase 4 and are called *early afterdepolarizations* and are characterized by transient retardations in repolarization with or without upturn of the membrane potential (Figure 79-3). An upturn of sufficient magnitude may trigger an "extra" action potential before the cycle is over. Early afterdepolarizations are typically associated with conditions that prolong the action potential duration, such as decreased inactivation of fast I_{Na} (e.g., long QT3 syndrome) or

decreased outward K$^+$ currents (e.g., I_{Ks} in long QT1 and I_{Kr} in long QT2 syndromes) prolonging Ca^{2+} entry through I_{Ca-L}.[33] The development of early afterdepolarizations in this setting is thought to trigger torsades de pointes. Early afterdepolarizations are also associated with increased sympathetic tone, use of catecholamines, hypoxia, acidosis, and bradycardia.

Afterdepolarizations that occur in late phase 4 are called *delayed afterdepolarizations* and are characterized by low-amplitude depolarizations that may reach threshold and trigger an action potential (see Figure 79-3). The main underlying abnormality in delayed afterdepolarizations is intracellular Ca^{2+} overload, promoting Ca^{2+} release from the sarcoplasmic reticulum[33] and depolarizing currents (i.e., inward $I_{Na/Ca}$ currents). Delayed afterdepolarizations are classically associated with digitalis toxicity; however, many other conditions favoring cytosolic Ca^{2+} overload can also produce delayed afterdepolarizations such as myocardial stretch, hypertrophy, catecholamines, ischemia, and reperfusion. In the setting of heart failure, increased expression of Na$^+$-Ca^{2+} exchanger along with abnormalities in the ryanodine receptor has been shown to predispose to delayed afterdepolarizations.

ABNORMALITIES IN IMPULSE CONDUCTION (REENTRY)

Abnormalities in impulse conduction account for the vast majority of sustained ventricular tachyarrhythmias consequent to a phenomenon known as *reentry*. Reentry occurs when a normally propagating impulse reenters a region of previously excited tissue after its refractory period is over and excites it again. Reentry can continue to repeat, originating a tachyarrhythmia. Several forms of reentry have been described, including circus movement, phase 2, and reflection.[34]

Circus Movement

Circus movement is the most widely studied mechanism and encompasses four distinct models: ring, leading circle, figure of eight, and spiral wave.

The *ring model* is the simplest of all[35] and can be used to illustrate the basic mechanism of reentry (Figure 79-4). The ring model requires two anatomically contiguous paths in specialized tissue or in muscle fibers separated by a central area of unexcitable tissue. One of these paths (*b* in Figure 79-4) must exhibit a zone of unidirectional block allowing the impulse to propagate in only one direction. The alternative path (*a* in Figure 79-4) allows the impulse to circumvent the unidirectional block. Conduction through this alternative path should be slow or refractoriness proximal to the path should be brief to allow recovery of excitability. Once the impulse reaches the distal end of the alternative path, it propagates in a retrograde manner through the path of unidirectional block to reenter the proximal end of the alternative path. For the cycle to repeat (and establish a reentry circuit causing tachyarrhythmia), the wavelength of the circling impulse must be shorter than or at least equal to the length of the reentry circuit (or path length), thus enabling the leading edge of the circling impulse to find the tissue in an excitable state. The *wavelength of the circling*

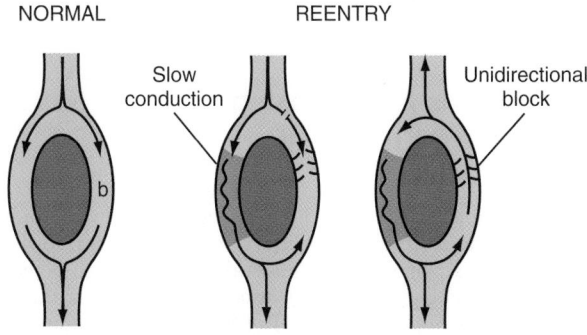

Figure 79-4 Ring model of reentry.

impulse is defined as the product of conduction velocity and duration of the refractory period.

Reentry is usually triggered by the arrival of a premature beat that finds the path of unidirectional block in a refractory period. Unidirectional block may result from increased refractoriness associated with either anatomic abnormalities (e.g., fibrosis, accessory pathway, bundle branch) or functional defects (e.g., ischemia, action of drugs). The ring model best applies to tachyarrhythmias that involve AV accessory pathways and the AV node.

The *leading circle model* is similar to the ring model but does not require anatomic obstacles and can develop in structurally uniform myocardium by a properly timed premature impulse.[36,37] The *figure-of-eight model* was first described in experimental myocardial infarction. It refers to two reentry circuits moving alongside a functional conduction block (ischemia or infarct) in opposite directions, forming a pretzel-like configuration.[38] The *spiral wave model* is considered a more complex version of the leading circle model. It involves a core and filaments and is usually described as reentry in two dimensions.[39,40] The spiral wave model has been used to explain the electrocardiographic patterns associated with monomorphic and polymorphic VTs and also VF. In monomorphic VTs, the spiral wave is thought to be anchored and unable to drift within the myocardium, whereas in polymorphic VTs, such as torsades de pointes, the spiral is thought to drift. In the case of VF, the spiral wave is believed to break up into multiple rotating spiral waves that are continuously extinguishing and recreating. However, some authors have proposed a single rapidly shifting spiral, and others have postulated a stationary rotor whose frequency of excitation is exceedingly high, resulting in multiple areas of intermittent block.[41]

Phase 2

Phase 2 reentry refers to the generation of local reexcitation as a result of increased heterogeneity of repolarization. This phenomenon occurs when repolarization is markedly shortened in certain regions of the myocardium—essentially obliterating phase 2 of the action potential (plateau phase)—but is maintained in others. This creates conditions conducive to local reexcitation, which may precipitate ventricular tachyarrhythmias during myocardial ischemia.[42] During ischemia, action potentials of normal duration alternate with ones of shorter duration, yielding beat-to-beat alternans (temporal dispersion) and site-to-site alternans (spatial dispersion) and promoting regions with conduction block and regions with injury current, leading to reentry and ventricular tachyarrhythmias. The degree of spatial and temporal dispersion progresses along with the duration of ischemia, suggesting that this mechanism may be an important trigger of VT and VF during acute myocardial ischemia.[43,44] In the surface ECG, dispersion of the action potential duration manifests as T-wave alternans, which is a predictor of VF.[45]

Reflection

Reflection refers to a back-and-forth propagation of the impulse over the same functionally unexcitable tissue, with recurrent activation of the proximal region as a result of electrotonic currents.[46,47] The area of unexcitable tissue could result from ischemia and lead to extrasystolic activity. Reflection differs from classic reentry in that the impulse travels along the same pathway in both directions.

▦ Conditions Predisposing to Ventricular Arrhythmias

CHANNELOPATHIES

The term "channelopathies" has been coined to identify a group of diseases characterized by abnormalities in the proteins that form ion channels.[48,49] These abnormalities distort the normal action potential, primarily accentuating the inherent instability of repolarization and increasing the risk of polymorphic VT of the torsades de pointes type. Channelopathies may be hereditary or acquired.

HEREDITARY CHANNELOPATHIES

Long QT Syndrome

The vast majority of hereditary channelopathies result from mutations in genes that encode for Na^+ and K^+ channels, with the most representative being the long QT syndrome.[50-52] The long QT syndrome was first described in 1957 by Jervell and Lange-Nielsen in a group of patients with long QT intervals, episodes of torsades de pointes, and deafness.[53] This syndrome is transmitted by autosomal recessive inheritance and is known as the *Jervell and Lange-Nielsen syndrome*. In 1963 and 1964, Romano and colleagues[54] and Ward[55] independently reported patients with an almost identical disorder but without deafness. This syndrome is transmitted by autosomal dominant inheritance and is known as the *Romano-Ward syndrome*.

It is now recognized that long QT syndrome results from mutations in at least 12 genes, leading to distinct types designated long QT1 through long QT12 (Table 79-1). Long QT1 is the principal genetic type responsible for both Jervell and Lange-Nielsen and Romano-Ward syndromes and accounts for nearly 50% of all genotyped families. Long QT2 accounts for nearly 40% and long QT3 for about 5%. The remaining types are much less frequent.[56]

Long QT1, QT2, QT5, QT6, QT7, and QT11 result from mutations in the genes *KCNQ1*, *HERG*, *KCNE1*, *KCNE2*, *KCNJ2*, and *AKAP9*, respectively, which encode various components of K^+ channels, leading to loss-of-function mutations and consequent decrease in the main repolarizing K^+ current, I_k, and thus prolongation of the QT interval.

Long QT3 stems from a mutation in *SCN5A*, the gene that encodes the α-subunit of the fast cardiac Na^+ channel. *SCN5A* mutation causes a gain of function leading to incomplete channel inactivation and persistence of I_{Na} during the plateau phase of the action potential.[57,58]

Long QT4 has been linked to a loss-of-function mutation in the *ANKB* gene.[59] This gene encodes ankyrin-B, which is a member of a family of versatile membrane adapters. Ankyrin-B, among other functions, coordinates the opening and closing of calcium, potassium, sodium, and chloride channels. The failure to properly coordinate the opening and closing of ion channels leading to long QT syndrome and arrhythmias illustrates a novel mechanism of arrhythmias.

Long QT8 stems from a mutation on the gene *CACNA1C*, which encodes the α_{1c}-subunit of I_{Ca-L}. The mutation causes a gain of function that leads to increased Ca^+ influx into cardiac cells. Long QT8 presents with an exaggerated QT interval prolongation and is associated with neurocognitive impairment, congenital structural heart disease, developmental abnormalities, and immunodeficiencies.

In long QT9, QT10, and QT12, the mutations affect the genes *CAV3*, *SCN4β*, and *SNTA1*, leading to a gain of function in I_{Na}, resulting in increased Na^+ influx within the cardiac cell.[60,61]

Accordingly, the common mechanistic thread among long QT syndromes is perturbation of the balance between I_{Na} and I_K during the plateau phase of the action potential, yielding prolongation of repolarization, a reduced rate of I_{Ca-L} inactivation, late Ca^{2+} influx, and early afterdepolarizations predisposing to torsades de pointes.[62]

The diagnosis is suspected in young individuals who present with syncope or episodes of sudden death typically during exercise, emotional distress, or exposure to factors that cause prolongation of the QT interval. A family history of unexplained syncope or sudden cardiac death, especially in young kindred, should raise suspicion. Sudden cardiac death occurs in approximately 4% of affected individuals. The diagnosis should be suspected when the corrected QT interval ($QTc = QT_{(ms)} \cdot \sqrt{R - R_{(s)}}$) exceeds 470 milliseconds in males (normal <422 milliseconds) and 480 milliseconds in females (normal <432 milliseconds) in the absence of other conditions that may lengthen the QT interval. In addition, there may be sinus bradycardia with sinus pauses in about one-third of individuals (especially in long QT3), QT dispersion, and various T-wave abnormalities (e.g., notched, bifid, biphasic). Factors predisposing to sudden cardiac death include recurrent syncope, survival from cardiac arrest, congenital deafness, female sex, relative bradycardia, corrected QT interval greater than 600

TABLE 79-1	Congenital Long QT syndromes						
Type	Frequency in LQT Patients (%)	Gene Chromosome	Protein	Mechanism, Mutation Effect	Genetic Transmission	Clinical Features	Syndrome Type
LQT1	40-55	KCNQ1 11p15.5	α-subunit, I_{Ks}	Loss-of-function↓ K efflux	Autosomal recessive or dominant	Broad-based and late-onset T wave, with (recessive) or without (dominant) bilateral sensory-neural deafness, ↑ risk of fatal arrhythmia	RWS, JLNS
LQT2	35-45	HERG 7q35-36	α-subunit, I_{Kr}	Loss-of-function↓ K efflux	Autosomal dominant	Widely split and low amplitude T wave; no associated defects	RWS
LQT3	2-8	SCN5A 3p21-24	α-subunit, I_{Na}	Gain-of-function↑ Na influx	Autosomal dominant	Late-onset, biphasic or peaked T wave; no associated defects	RWS
LQT4	<1	ANKB 4q25-27	Ankyrin-B	Loss-of-function↑ Na and ↓ Ca within cell	Autosomal dominant	Variable QT-interval prolongation; no associated defects	RWS
LQT5*	<1	KCNE1 21q22.1-2	β-subunit, I_{Ks}	Loss-of-function↓ K efflux	Autosomal recessive or dominant	With (recessive) or without (dominant) bilateral sensory-neural deafness, ↑ risk of fatal arrhythmia	RWS, JLNS
LQT6†	<1	KCNE2 21q22.1	Membrane protein, I_{Kr}	Loss-of-function↓ K efflux	Autosomal dominant	No associated defects	RWS
LQT7	<1	KCNJ2 17q23	α-subunit, I_{K1}	Loss-of-function↓ K efflux	Autosomal dominant	Mild prolongation of QT interval, prominent Q wave, bidirectional VT; periodic paralysis, dysmorphic features, and cardiac arrhythmias	AS
LQT8	<1	CACNA1C 12p13.3	α-subunit, I_{Ca}	Gain-of-function↑ Ca influx		Exaggerated QT-interval prolongation; neurocognitive impairment, congenital structural heart disease, developmental abnormalities, and immunodeficiencies	TS
LQT9	<1	CAV3 3p25	Caveolin-3 protein	Loss-of-function↑ Na influx	Autosomal dominant	No associated defects	RWS
LQT10	<0.1	SCN4β 11q23	β-subunit, I_{Na}	Loss-of-function↑ Na influx	Autosomal dominant	No associated defects	RWS
LQT11	<0.1	AKAP9 7q21-q22	Regulatory protein of α subunit, I_{Ks}	Loss-of-function↓ K efflux	Autosomal dominant	No associated defects	RWS
LQT12	<0.1	SNTA1 20q11.2	Scaffolding protein (I_{Na})	Loss-of-function↑ Na influx	Autosomal dominant	No associated defects	RWS

*KCNQ1 and KCNE1 gene products are assembled to form a complete I_{Ks} channel.

†HERG and KCNE2 gene products are assembled to form a complete I_{Kr} channel.

AS, Andersen syndrome; FREQ, relative frequency; JLNS, Jervell and Lange-Nielsen syndrome; RWS, Romano-Ward syndrome; TS, Timothy syndrome.

milliseconds, and kinship with a symptomatic patient.[50] Genetic testing for identifying the various long QT subtypes is becoming readily available, with its impact on risk stratification and guidance for placement of an implantable cardioverter-defibrillator (ICD) to be determined by future research.[56,60]

In addition to long QT syndromes, recent population studies[63] have shown that even milder prolongation of the QTc in adults (>450 milliseconds in men and > 470 milliseconds in women) increases the risk of sudden cardiac death by threefold after adjustment for age, gender, body mass index, hypertension, cholesterol/high-density lipoprotein ratio, diabetes mellitus, myocardial infarction, heart failure, and heart rate. In the same population, QTc prolongation was strongly associated with variant rs10494366 T>G and rs10918594 C>G of the nitric oxide synthase 1 adaptor protein (NOS1AP) gene.[64] More recent studies show that use of the calcium channel blocker, verapamil, in patients with these variants prompts a greater QTc prolongation than in patients with the wild genotype.[65]

Accordingly, this is an evolving concept showing the importance prolongation in repolarization has in the genesis of arrhythmias, not only in individuals with defined genetic abnormalities but also in individuals who appear to be phenotypically normal.

Short QT Syndrome

Short QT is a more recently described syndrome[66] characterized by tall and peaked T waves with QT interval ≤ 300 milliseconds, insensitive to changes in heart rate, and a structurally normal heart. Individuals are at risk of developing VF and also atrial fibrillation and may complain of palpitations and episodes of syncope. They may also have family members with a similar history or a history of unexplained or sudden death at a young age.

The underlying mechanism is increased outward potassium currents during phase 2 and phase 3 of the action potential, shortening its plateau phase. Mutations in the KCNH2, KCNJ2, and KCNQ1 gene products with an autosomal dominant pattern of inheritance have been associated with the short QT syndrome. A few affected families have been identified.

Current treatment is implantation of an ICD. A recent study suggests that quinidine could be beneficial by prolonging the action potential duration through action on I_K channels, which may benefit patients with ICDs and reduce the number of arrhythmic events, or become a useful treatment in affected individuals who are at risk of sudden cardiac death from birth.

Brugada Syndrome

Another important hereditary channelopathy is Brugada syndrome, described in 1992 by the Brugada brothers,[67-70] who noticed an association between sudden cardiac death and ST-segment elevation in V_1 to V_3, with a pattern resembling right bundle branch block in individuals with structurally normal hearts.

Brugada syndrome results in part from mutations in the SCN5A gene (encoding for the I_{Na} α-subunit). In contrast to long QT3—which also affects the SCN5A gene—the mutations in Brugada syndrome lead to a loss of function resulting in accelerated inactivation of I_{Na} during phase 1, leaving the repolarizing I_{To} current unopposed and consequently prompting rapid repolarization and shortening of the action potential duration (refer to Figure 79-2 for the I_{Na} and I_{To} contributions to the action potential). Because I_{To} is expressed predominantly in the epicardium, the normally depolarized endocardium can re-excite the prematurely repolarized epicardium, leading to phase 2 reentry and generation of a phase 2 reentrant premature beat that could capture a

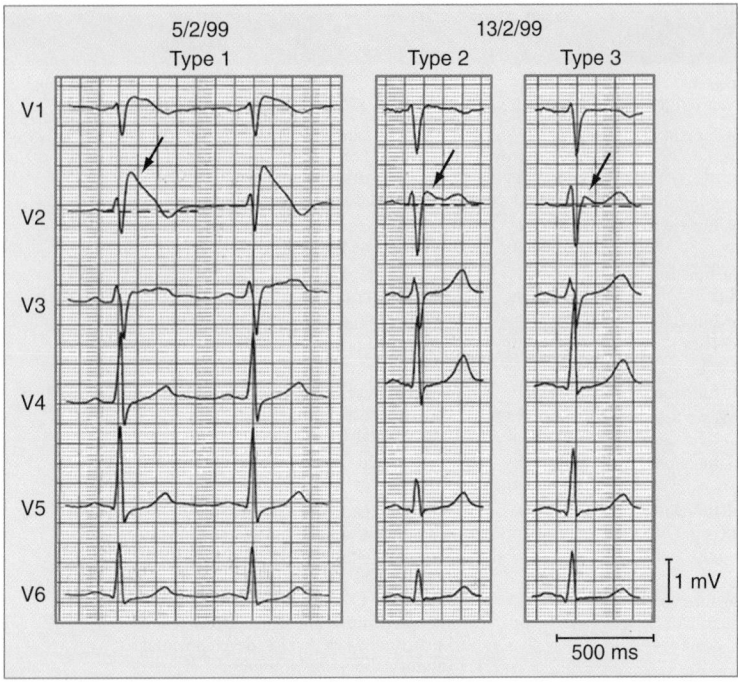

Figure 79-5 Representative tracings in a patient with Brugada syndrome, demonstrating dynamic changes in V_1 to V_2 after resuscitation from cardiac arrest. *Type 1* refers to the coved-type ST-T configuration, whereas *type 2* and *type 3* refer to the saddleback ST-T configuration. *(From Wilde AA, Antzelevitch C, Borggrefe M, Brugada J, Brugada R, Corrado D et al. Study Group on the Molecular Basis of Arrhythmias of the European Society of Cardiology. Proposed diagnostic criteria for the Brugada syndrome: consensus report. Circulation 2002;106:2514-9.)*

vulnerable window and precipitate VT (which is typically polymorphic) and/or VF.

Brugada syndrome exhibits predominantly an autosomal dominant pattern of inheritance, with an average worldwide prevalence of 5:10,000. More than 100 mutations in seven genes have been identified. Loss-of-function mutations in the *SCN5A* gene cause approximately 20% of cases. A few mutations have been described in the *GPD1L* gene, which encodes the glycerol-3-phosphate dehydrogenase-1 like protein; the *CACNA1C* gene, which encodes the α-subunit of the Ca(v)1.2 ion channel conducting the inward current (I_{Ca-L}); the *CACNB2* gene, which encodes the β2-subunit of the Ca(v)1.2 ion channel; the *SCN1B* and *SCN3B* genes, which in the heart encode the β-subunits of the Na(v)1.5 sodium ion channel; and the *KCNE3* gene, which encodes the ancillary inhibitory β-subunit of several potassium channels including the Kv4.3 ion channel conducting the repolarizing potassium current I_{Tos}.[71]

The ST-segment elevation can adopt various shapes that have been related to the severity of the I_{Na}/I_{To} imbalance, including—in order of increasing severity—saddleback, coved, and triangular shapes.[62] These changes are dynamic and can change in the same affected individual as shown in Figure 79-5.

Brugada syndrome is the major but not the only cause of sudden unexpected death syndrome (SUDS)[72,73] and is the most common cause of sudden death in young men without known underlying cardiac disease in Thailand and Laos.[74] However, Brugada syndrome exhibits variable expressivity, reduced penetrance, and "mixed phenotypes" where families may contain members with Brugada syndrome as well as members with short QT syndrome, long QT syndrome, atrial fibrillation, disease of the conduction system, and even structural heart disease.[71]

Patient with Brugada syndrome may have concealed or intermittent forms that can be unmasked (or precipitated) by febrile states, vagotonic agents, α-adrenergic agonists, β-adrenergic blockers, tricyclic or tetracyclic antidepressants, a combination of glucose and insulin and hypokalemia, and alcohol and cocaine toxicity.[75]

A useful clinical test to identify concealed Brugada syndrome is the administration of class IC antiarrhythmic drugs: Na+ channel blockers such as ajmaline (1 mg/kg intravenous (IV) in 5 minutes), flecainide (2 mg/kg IV in 10 minutes), or procainamide (10 mg/kg IV in 10 minutes). The test should be performed in an environment with

capability for immediate defibrillation, because there is a 0.5% risk of precipitating VF. Of the drugs listed above, ajmaline is the preferred drug because of its very short half-life.[76] The test is considered positive if an additional 1-mm ST-segment elevation (measured 0.08 seconds after the J point) occurs in leads V_1, V_2, and V_3. The test is highly specific and should be considered in patients who present with history of syncope of unknown origin or with idiopathic VF.

Patients with the Brugada syndrome must be treated with an ICD, because antiarrhythmic agents have not been found in general to be effective.[69] However, recent studies have shown that quinidine and hydroquinidine can prevent spontaneous ECG changes and reduce the risk of VT and VF, presumably through inhibition of I_{To}.[77,78] Although such a pharmacologic approach is currently regarded as an adjunct to ICD placement to reduce the number of shocks, it could be considered in high-risk patients when ICD placement is not possible.

ACQUIRED CHANNELOPATHIES

Acquired abnormalities in cardiac channels may result from a broad spectrum of conditions. One common mechanism is advanced heart failure affecting the expression of several ion channels regardless of the primary etiology.[79,80] For example, there is down-regulation of I_{To} and I_{K1}, leading to prolongation of the QT interval. Although such an effect could be considered adaptive, allowing more time for excitation-contraction coupling, it also predisposes to inhomogeneous repolarization and early afterdepolarizations. In addition, in heart failure there is up-regulation of the Na+/Ca2+ exchanger—consequent in part to down-regulation of the sarcoplasmic reticulum Ca2+-ATPase (SERCA2a)[81]—yielding larger $I_{Na/Ca}$, which predisposes to delayed afterdepolarizations and triggered arrhythmias, especially in the face of cytosolic Ca2+ overload.

Another increasingly important mechanism of acquired channelopathies is the use of medications that can interfere with channel function. By far the most common effect is prolongation of the QT interval leading to drug-induced long QT syndrome. Most of the drugs involved block the K+ repolarizing current carried by human ether-à-go-go (*HERG*) subunits corresponding to the I_{Kr} channel.[82] I_{Kr} carries the same K+ current that is affected in congenital long QT2. The list of medications is long and includes antiarrhythmic agents, in which the primary target is ion channels, and many other drugs in which

TABLE 79-2	Drugs Associated with QT Prolongation and Risk of Torsades de Pointes
Antiarrhythmic Agents	**Antipsychotic Agents**
Amiodarone	Chlorpromazine
Disopyramide	Haloperidol
Dofetilide	Mesoridazine
Ibutilide	Pimozide
Procainamide	Thioridazine
Quinidine	**Enterokinetic/Antinausea Agents**
Sotalol	Cisapride
Antibiotics	Domperidone
Clarithromycin	Droperidol
Erythromycin	Opiate Agonists
Chloroquine	Levomethadyl
Halofantrine	Methadone
Pentamidine	**Miscellaneous**
Sparfloxacin	Arsenic trioxide
Antihistaminic Agents	Probucol
Astemizole	
Terfenadine	

Data from www.QTdrugs.org (Torsades list: Drugs with a risk of torsades de pointes); revised on 03/25/2008.

prolongation of the QT interval is an unintended effect.[83] The intensivist should be familiar with this group of medications and capable of recognizing the arrhythmogenic risk of administering medications that could prolong the QT interval.

The University of Arizona, Health Sciences Center, maintains a list of drugs associated with risk of causing QT prolongation and promoting torsades de pointes (available at www.qtdrugs.org). Based on the risk level, drugs are classified by an advisory board as: (1) Torsades List, defined as drugs that are generally accepted to carry a risk of torsades de pointes; (2) Possible Torsades List, defined as drugs that prolong the QT interval and/or in some reports have been associated with torsades de pointes but lack substantial evidence for causing torsades de pointes; (3) Conditional Torsades List, defined as drugs that carry a risk of torsades de pointes and/or QT prolongation under certain conditions such as in patients with congenital long QT syndrome, drug overdose, or coadministration of interacting drugs; and (4) drugs to be avoided in patients with congenital long QT syndrome. Table 79-2 lists drugs from the Torsades List.

The importance of drug-induced long QT syndrome has mandated pharmaceutical companies to screen early in the process of drug selection to exclude compounds that can induce long QT syndrome, mostly screening for effects on the *HERG* gene products carrying the I_{Kr} current.[82]

OTHER CONDITIONS

The QT interval may also be prolonged by cocaine abuse, organ phosphorus compound poisoning, subarachnoid hemorrhage, stroke, myocardial ischemia, fasting using liquid-protein-modified diets, autonomic neuropathy, and human immunodeficiency virus disease.[84-88] Electrolyte abnormalities can not only prolong but also shorten the QT interval. Some of these conditions and others not associated with channelopathies are discussed next.

Electrolyte Abnormalities

Electrolyte abnormalities rarely precipitate but often contribute to the development of ventricular tachyarrhythmias, mostly in relation to abnormalities in serum K^+, Mg^{2+}, and Ca^{2+}.[89] Abnormalities in serum K^+ are among the most common electrolyte abnormalities in critically ill patients.

Hypokalemia (serum $K^+ < 3.5$ mM) decreases the resting membrane potential (making it more negative), rendering cells less excitable and lowering the firing rate of pacemaker cells. Hypokalemia also prolongs

the QT interval and flattens the T wave.[17] This effect is explained by the fact that conductivity of I_{kr} is proportional to the square root of external K^+. Thus, at lower K^+, I_{Kr} is reduced, prolonging repolarization. This effect is more pronounced in cells from the mid-myocardial region (which have a greater I_{Kr}/I_{ks} ratio). Hypokalemia can develop in various settings, including the use of thiazide and loop diuretics, diabetic keto-acidosis, gastrointestinal fluid losses, alcohol abuse, hypomagnesemia, administration of insulin, and use of β-receptor agonists.

Hyperkalemia (serum $K^+ > 5.5$ mM) exerts opposite effects. It lowers the resting membrane potential (making it less negative), rendering cells more excitable; however, with severe hyperkalemia, the rate of rise of phase 0 is reduced, slowing conduction velocity and leading—at very high potassium levels—to widespread blocks (widening of the P wave and the QRS interval). Rapidly rising serum K^+ can precipitate VF, probably as a result of reentry that follows areas of conduction block. Hyperkalemia, by increasing I_{Kr}, accelerates repolarization and shortens the action potential duration, yielding the characteristic peaked and tall T waves.

Magnesium plays an important electrophysiologic role. Mg^{2+} is a cofactor of the Na^+/K^+ pump and hence is important in maintaining the integrity of intracellular K^+ and the resting membrane potential. Mg^{2+} also modulates the effects of various K^+ and Ca^{2+} channels. Hypomagnesemia is associated with prolongation of the QT interval and increased risk of ventricular arrhythmias. This effect could be mediated in part through other electrolyte deficits, because hypomagnesemia is associated with hypokalemia and hypocalcemia.

Serum calcium is also important. Hypocalcemia increases the QT interval, predisposing to VTs. Hypercalcemia exerts the opposite effects, reducing the QT interval. Changes in intracellular calcium contribute to arrhythmias associated with acute ischemia and reperfusion and may be important in the genesis of VT induced by exercise and by digitalis.

Hypothermia

Moderate hypothermia (32°C to 35°C) and severe hypothermia (<32°C) can also predispose to ventricular tachyarrhythmias by causing prolongation of the QT interval and QT dispersion.[90] Typically, patients with hypothermia develop J waves (also known as *Osborn waves*) in the ECG, which reflects accentuation of the inhomogeneity of repolarization caused by the predominant distribution of I_{To} in subepicardial and mid-myocardial regions.[91] Hypothermia may be complicated by the ingestion of drugs and the presence of electrolyte abnormalities that further increase the risk of ventricular tachyarrhythmias.

Hypoglycemia

Recent studies have shown that acute hypoglycemia can trigger VT and VF in patients with diabetes mellitus.[92] The mechanism involves prolongation of the QT interval by direct suppression of repolarizing K^+ currents. In addition, episodes of hypoglycemia trigger a neuroendocrine stress response with release of catecholamines which favors intracellular Ca^{2+} entry and reduces serum K^+, further compounding the risk. Patient at particularly high risk are those with coronary artery disease or acute myocardial infarction, left ventricular hypertrophy, autonomic neuropathy, congestive heart failure, and on those taking medications that prolong the QT interval.

Arrhythmogenic Right Ventricular Cardiomyopathy

This disorder is characterized by progressive replacement of the normal right ventricular muscle cells by fibrous tissue and fat.[93] The condition may be familial with autosomal dominant inheritance.[94] Patients present with palpitations, syncope, and sometimes sudden death. It is considered an important cause of sudden death in subjects younger than 35 years, especially when related to exercise.[95,96] The ECG is abnormal in 90% of cases, showing T-wave inversions beyond lead V_1 and epsilon waves in leads V_1 to V_3. The QRS complex may be widened (>110 milliseconds), with complete or incomplete right bundle branch block morphology. There are ventricular premature beats with left bundle branch configuration.

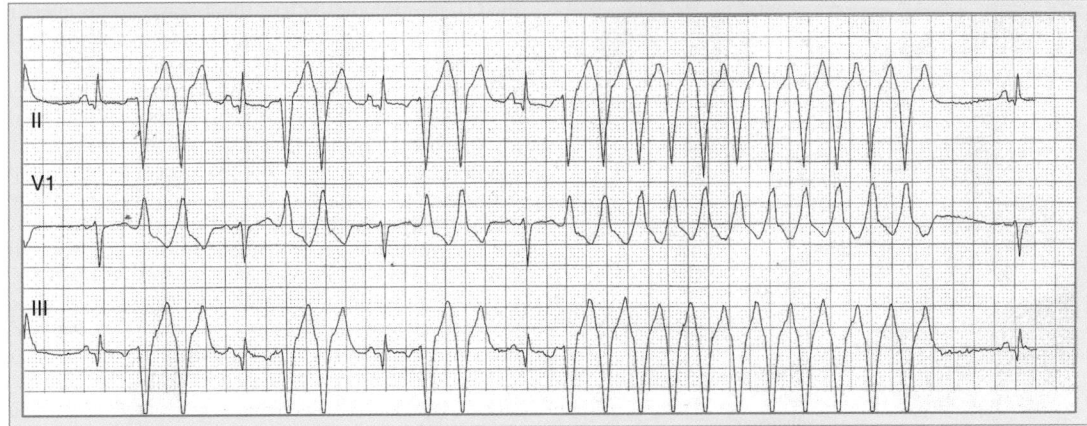

Figure 79-6 ECG tracing (lead II, III, and V₁) showing couplets followed by an 11-beat episode of nonsustained monomorphic ventricular tachycardia.

Clinical Diagnosis

Various types of ventricular arrhythmias can develop in critically ill patients, with different prognostic implication and management. The common element intensivists should first recognize is the presence of wide QRS complexes whose origin resides in ventricular tissue and defines ventricular ectopic activity. However, not all wide QRS complexes originate from ventricular tissue. Supraventricular activity originating from sinus node and atrial tissue (e.g., atrial fibrillation, atrial flutter, and multifocal atrial tachycardia) can produce a wide QRS because of preexistent or rate-dependent bundle branch blocks or intermittent aberrant pathways. The diagnostic clue for identifying ventricular ectopic activity is demonstration of dissociation from atrial activity, which is often difficult to establish having to rely on other features as discussed later. Ventricular ectopic activity may present clinically in many forms, as described next.

PREMATURE VENTRICULAR CONTRACTIONS

Premature ventricular contractions (PVCs) are isolated ventricular ectopic beats that may be found in normal, healthy individuals. However, they often accompany cardiac conditions (e.g., ischemia, cardiomyopathy, valvular heart disease), use of stimulants (e.g., caffeine, cocaine, alcohol, ephedrine, pseudoephedrine), electrolyte abnormalities (e.g., hypokalemia, hyperkalemia, hypomagnesemia), hypoxemia, catecholamine discharge, and medications (e.g., tricyclic antidepressants, antipsychotic medications, digoxin, flecainide, sotalol, quinidine). The ECG demonstrates a wide QRS complex with a bizarre axis, a T wave with polarity opposite to the QRS, and a full compensatory pause. PVCs usually do not produce symptoms. PVCs may present one after each normally conducted QRS in the form of bigemini and also as couplets (two consecutive PVCs).

VENTRICULAR TACHYCARDIA

VT is defined as three or more consecutive ventricular ectopic beats with a rate that typically exceeds 100 beats per minute and often ranges between 130 and 170 beats per minute. VT usually have QRS complexes of 120 msec or longer and is therefore classified as wide-complex tachycardia. However, wide-complex tachycardia, as described earlier, can also be supraventricular when the impulse originates above the bifurcation of the bundle of His but is conducted with aberrancy (see later).[97] VTs are classified as *monomorphic* if all QRS complexes have similar morphology and *polymorphic* if they have variable morphology. VTs are considered *sustained* if they last 30 seconds or longer and *nonsustained* if they last less than 30 seconds. Most sustained VTs present with palpitations, chest discomfort, and weakness or with more severe symptoms such as dizziness, angina, syncope, seizures, and even sudden cardiac death.[98]

Monomorphic Ventricular Tachycardia

Monomorphic VTs are the most common and are usually associated with structural heart disease, such as previous myocardial infarction and, less commonly, cardiomyopathy. The reentrant circuit can be small (microentry) or large (macroentry) and can be located in different regions of the myocardium. The mechanism is usually reentry operating within or around damaged myocardium. A representative tracing is shown in Figure 79-6.

Examination of the jugular veins may show cannon a-waves, indicative of AV dissociation. Variability in S₁ occurrence and intensity and variations in blood pressure are also findings consistent with AV dissociation.

In nonemergency settings, a standard 12-lead ECG should be obtained to determine whether a wide-complex tachycardia is present and whether it is monomorphic or polymorphic. If monomorphic, the possibility of supraventricular tachycardia (SVT) with aberrancy should be considered, although most wide-complex tachycardias are ventricular. The presence of shock, heart failure, or cardiac arrest favors VT. SVT with aberrancy (in a stable patient) should be suspected whenever there is a history of previous aberrant rhythms, accessory pathways, and baseline or rate-induced bundle branch block. The ECG should be carefully examined for evidence of AV dissociation, which is specific for VT.[99] If P waves are not visualized in V₁ or in any of the other standard leads, a Lewis lead (arm electrode positioned on the parasternal area) or an esophageal lead can be used.[100] AV dissociation is indicated by P waves and QRS complexes that present at different and uncoupled rates. Other manifestations of dissociation include captured beats (narrow QRS conducted beats) and fusion beats (merge of ectopic with conducted beats).

Other ECG clues include: (1) regularity of the R-R interval, which can be altered in SVT but usually not in monomorphic VT; (2) a QRS duration of 140 milliseconds or more with right bundle branch block pattern and 160 milliseconds or more with left bundle branch block (LBBB) pattern; however, the QRS duration can be shorter (110-114 milliseconds) in instances of fascicular tachycardia; (3) a QRS axis between −90 degrees and ±180 degrees; (4) a positive QRS concordance (positive QRS from V₁ to V₆); (5) combination of LBBB pattern and right axis; (6) monophasic or biphasic QRS complex with right bundle branch block pattern and slurred or prolonged S wave in V₁ with LBBB morphology.

ECG criteria and algorithms are available to help differentiate ventricular from SVT.[101-104] A widely accepted four-step algorithm developed by Brugada is shown in Figure 79-7.[102] A similar algorithm that incorporates pertinent clinical information can be found at http://www.anaesthetist.com/icu/organs/heart/ecg/wct.htm#step0.

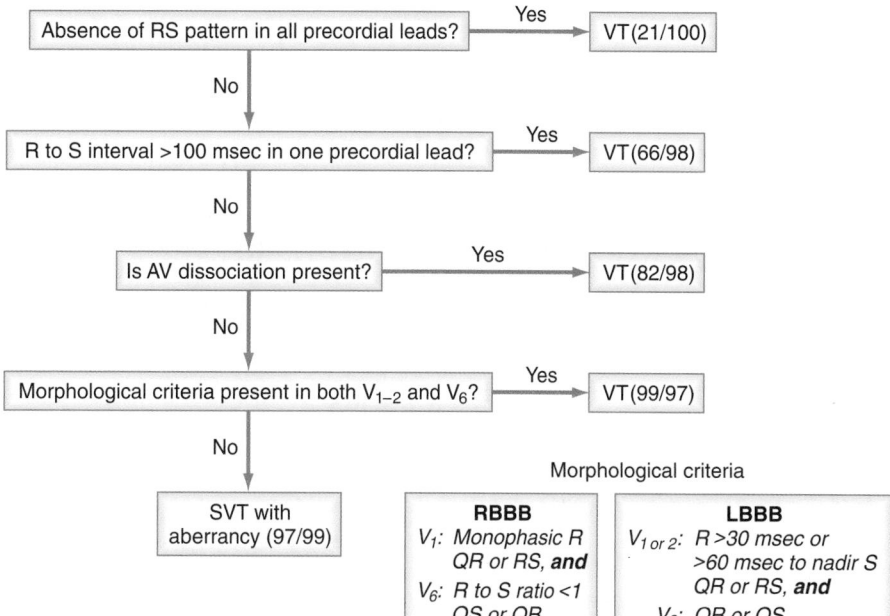

Figure 79-7 Four-step Brugada algorithm for diagnosis of wide-complex tachycardia. Ventricular tachycardia (VT) is diagnosed whenever an answer is positive within each successive step: in step 1, when an RS complex cannot be identified in any precordial lead; in step 2, when the longest RS complex (beginning of R to nadir of S) in a precordial lead exceeds 100 milliseconds; in step 3, when there is atrioventricular (AV) dissociation; and in step 4, when the morphologic criteria for tachycardia with right bundle branch block (RBBB) or left bundle branch block (LBBB) morphology are met. In parentheses are sensitivity and specificity reported in the original report based on 554 wide-complex tachycardias.[102] SVT, supraventricular tachycardia.

Some special forms of VT tend to be mistaken for SVT with aberrancy.[105] These include bundle branch reentrant tachycardia, in which the impulse travels down the right bundle branch, across the interventricular septum, and up the left bundle branch.[106,107] The morphology resembles SVT with LBBB and is common among patients with nonischemic dilated cardiomyopathy.[108] Right ventricular outflow tract tachycardia is another condition caused by triggered activity from delayed afterdepolarizations that most commonly originate in the right ventricular outflow tract.[109] The tachycardia usually presents with LBBB morphology and right axis deviation. Right ventricular outflow tract tachycardias occur in structurally normal hearts, typically in young individuals, and are responsive to verapamil or adenosine.[110] Finally, there are fascicular tachycardias that originate from either fascicle of the left bundle branch. They occur in structurally normal hearts, mimic SVT with aberrancy, and are responsive to beta-blockers and verapamil.[111]

Polymorphic Ventricular Tachycardia

Polymorphic VTs have irregular rhythms, usually compromise hemodynamic function, and may quickly degenerate into VF. Variation in QRS morphology represents changes in the electrical axis. One special form of polymorphic VT is *torsades de pointes*. This is a descriptive term denoting a rotating electrical axis in 180 degrees along an imaginary axis ("twisting points"); it is typically associated with long QT syndrome. Representative tracings are shown in Figure 79-8.

Accelerated Ideoventricular Rhythm

Accelerated idioventricular rhythm (AIVR) is a form of automatic ventricular arrhythmia and is characterized by the presence of regularly wide QRS complexes with a rate between 50 and 120 beats per minute. It is often, but not always, slightly faster than the underlying sinus rhythm. Accelerated idioventricular rhythm is an electrocardiographic diagnosis and does not produce symptoms. Identifying this rhythm is important because it usually indicates underlying myocardial ischemia, and the treatments for VT may not apply.[112]

Ventricular Fibrillation

VF is defined as the abrupt onset of irregular waveforms of varying contour, duration, and amplitude without identifiable QRS and T waves. VTs or SVTs that conduct through accessory pathways (e.g., Wolff-Parkinson-White syndrome) may be the initiating rhythm that

degenerates into VF. VF (and pulseless VT) causes immediate cessation of blood flow, precipitating unconsciousness within seconds. Generalized seizures and agonal breathing may follow, which should not distract from the primary diagnosis and the emergency treatment of cardiac arrest.

INCIDENCE IN THE CRITICAL CARE SETTING

The reported incidence of ventricular arrhythmias in critically ill patients is influenced by multiple factors including the underlying condition, predisposing factors, structural abnormalities, management in ICU, triggering events, and also the method for detection and the definition of the event.[113,114]

A recent multicenter study surveyed the incidence and prognostic implication of arrhythmias in critically ill patients in 26 ICUs over a period of 1 month.[115] The study included 1341 patients, of whom 163 (12%) had episodes of sustained arrhythmias, encompassing 8% with supraventricular arrhythmias (atrial fibrillation the most common), 2% with ventricular arrhythmias, and 2% with conduction abnormalities. The in-hospital mortality was 29% in patients with arrhythmias and 17% in those without. However, adjusting for prognosis factors—including older age, past medical history of cardiovascular disease, admission for acute medical illness, sepsis, central nervous system or cardiovascular disease, higher SAPS II score, and ventilator management or vasopressor agents—and propensity scores, only ventricular arrhythmias were associated with increased mortality (OR = 3.53; 95% CI, 1.19-10.42). Supraventricular arrhythmias and conduction abnormalities were instead markers of severity of illness without independent contribution to the risk of death.

In another study, Reinelt and colleagues[114] reported a higher incidence of ventricular tachyarrhythmias corresponding to 9% (65 of 756 patients), distributed among monomorphic VT in 83%, VF in 9%, and polymorphic VT in 8%. Factors present during the arrhythmic episodes included hypokalemia (10%), hypomagnesemia (12%), sedation (60%), mechanical ventilation (77%), and administration of catecholamines such as norepinephrine, epinephrine, or dobutamine (75%). In 23% of the episodes there was a history of previous myocardial infarction, and in 40% a history of recent myocardial infarction. Fifty-two percent of the episodes occurred during a postoperative period and 35% while a pulmonary artery catheter was in place. The presence of arrhythmias was associated with an increased length of stay and lower survival.

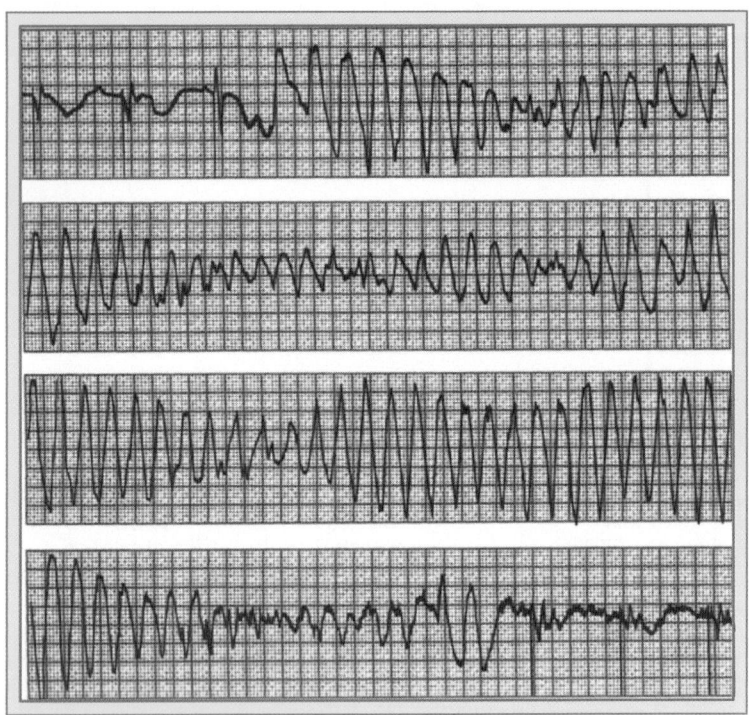

A

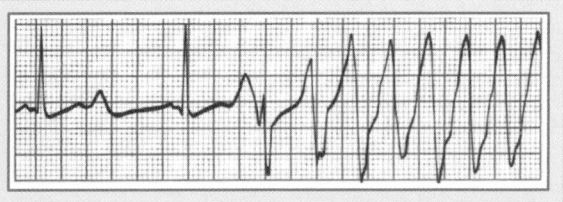

B

Figure 79-8   Torsades de pointes. **A,** Patient with a demand ventricular pacemaker developed QT prolongation (≈640 milliseconds, seen during paced rhythm) after treatment with amiodarone for recurrent ventricular tachycardia (VT). An episode of torsades de pointes developed that spontaneously terminated with resumption of a paced ventricular rhythm. **B,** Tracing from a young boy with congenital long QT syndrome and marked prolongation of the QTU interval (≈600 milliseconds). TU alternans is noted before a late premature complex, occurring on the downslope of the TU wave, initiates an episode of VT. *(From Braunwald E, Zipes D, Libby P, editors. Heart disease: a textbook of cardiovascular medicine, 6th ed. Philadelphia: Saunders; 2001, p. 868.)*

Special consideration should be given to patients admitted for evaluation of an acute coronary syndrome. Before the advent of thrombolysis in the 1980s, the incidence of VT ranged between 3% and 39%.[116] With the widespread use of thrombolysis, the incidence has decreased.[117] This is thought to reflect less ventricular dysfunction and dilatation as a result of successful reperfusion. For similar reasons, VT is less frequent in patients with non–ST-segment elevation (<1%) compared with those with ST-segment elevation (≈4%) myocardial infarction.[117]

Episodes of ventricular arrhythmias associated with acute myocardial infarction have different mechanisms contingent on whether they occur early or late and whether they are sustained or nonsustained. *Early* usually refers to the initial 48 hours after the onset of symptoms.[118] Early nonsustained VTs are relatively common, with an incidence between 9% and 12%,[119,120] and reflect electrical instability during the acute ischemic event but have little prognostic implication.[121] Early sustained VTs or VF occur less frequently[122] but identify a population at higher risk of death.[117]

In a recent study,[123] investigators analyzed the incidence and long-term prognosis of early VF or sustained VT (VF/VT) in 16,588 patients with acute myocardial infarction from the GUSTO V trial, and also examined the impact of baseline use of angiotensin-converting enzyme inhibitors (ACEI) and angiotensin receptor blockers (ARB). Early VF/VT occurred in 732 patients (4.4%). Compared to patients without VF/VT, the development of VF or VT was associated with significantly higher 30-day mortality (22% versus 5%, P < 0.001). Baseline use of an ACEI or ARB was associated with decreased incidence of VF/VT (OR 0.65, 0.47-0.89, P = 0.008). Moreover, of patients who developed VF/VT, those on baseline ACEI or ARB had a lower 30-day mortality compared with those not on an ACEI or ARB (17.7% versus 24.2%, P = 0.04). The association between baseline ACEI or ARB persisted after adjustment for multiple confounders.

Late VTs coincide with the phase of myocardial healing and may signal the presence of persistent ischemia, left ventricle dysfunction, or electrophysiologic instability.[118] Nonsustained VTs occur in approximately 6% of patients.[52,124] Sustained VTs occur in approximately 1% and convey a worse prognosis than do nonsustained episodes.[117,125]

One particularly arrhythmogenic period in patients with acute myocardial infarction is during reperfusion after thrombolysis.[52,119] There are frequent PVCs and episodes of nonsustained VT but rarely episodes of sustained VT or VF.[126] AIVR is also common, with an incidence as high as 50% to 75%. It occurs within 24 hours after the start of thrombolysis and then subsides.[112,126]

Efforts to predict life-threatening arrhythmias in the ICU have not been successful. In one study,[127] ECG markers of autonomic tone, ventricular irritability, and repolarization lability measured within 12 hours before an episode of monomorphic VT, polymorphic VT, or VF failed to predict the event.

■ Acute Management

PVCs and episodes of nonsustained VT have little immediate hemodynamic significance, and management should focus on identifying and removing contributing factors. The risk of degenerating into sustained ventricular tachyarrhythmias is low when PVCs occur with a frequency of less than 30 per hour but increases as PVCs occur with greater frequency, are multifocal, present in pairs or triplets, or exhibit the R-on-T phenomenon. Acute antiarrhythmic drugs are typically not required. Treatment of nonsustained VT that persists after the episode of critical illness should take into account the underlying cardiac substrate and triggers and include thorough assessment of mechanical and electrical function. In general, asymptomatic patients without structural heart disease require no specific therapy.

The management of sustained ventricular tachyarrhythmias requires a dynamic approach in which therapeutic interventions often parallel and occasionally precede diagnostic evaluation. This is particularly the case in instances of pulseless VT, polymorphic VT, and VF when delivery of unsynchronized electrical shocks and advanced cardiac life support may not be delayed. In less urgent situations (or after reestablishment of cardiac activity), treatment should focus on identifying and treating—if possible—the arrhythmogenic substrate as well as the triggering events and maintaining factors. Arrhythmogenic conditions commonly present in critically ill patients that should be sought include: (1) hemodynamic and respiratory abnormalities, (2) endogenous or exogenous adrenergic states, (3) acid-base and electrolyte imbalances, (4) presence of proarrhythmic drugs, (5) prolongation of the QT interval, (6) ongoing myocardial ischemia, and (7) mechanical stimulation of cardiac structures. Not infrequently, treatment of these factors alone terminates the arrhythmic episode (e.g., repositioning of a pulmonary artery catheter, reversal of myocardial ischemia, discontinuation of drugs that prolong the QT interval, correction of electrolyte imbalances, discontinuation of sympathomimetic agents, etc).

Specific antiarrhythmic interventions should take into consideration the type of rhythm and the degree of hemodynamic stability (discussed next).

VENTRICULAR ARRHYTHMIAS WITH PRESERVED BLOOD FLOW

Monomorphic Ventricular Tachycardia

Direct-current synchronized cardioversion and antiarrhythmic agents administered through the IV route are acceptable first-line options. Antiarrhythmic agents have the advantage that anesthesia is not needed and that the antiarrhythmic effect persists after termination of the event; however, patients may experience adverse effects including hypotension and (paradoxically) increased susceptibility to arrhythmia, given that most agents cause QT prolongation.

The American College of Cardiology/American Heart Association/European Society of Cardiology (ACC/AHA/ESC) 2006 Guidelines for management of patients with ventricular arrhythmias[128] recognize various drugs available in IV formulation that could be used for treating VT, including flecainide, propafenone, sotalol, procainamide, lidocaine, and amiodarone, with availability contingent on the specific country. The same 2006 Guidelines recommend IV procainamide (or ajmaline in some European countries) as a reasonable initial choice for patients with stable sustained monomorphic VT.[129,130] Close monitoring is recommended, as IV procainamide can cause transient hypotension,[131] especially in patients with severe left ventricular dysfunction. For patients with sustained monomorphic VT but who are hemodynamically unstable, are refractory to conversion after electrical shocks, or have recurrent episodes despite procainamide or other agents, IV amiodarone is considered a reasonable choice.[132-135] The initial effect of amiodarone is to slow down AV nodal conduction and block adrenergic stimulation. However, effects on ventricular conduction and refractoriness develop more gradually, achieving the maximal effect only after weeks or months of treatment.[136-138]

In patients in whom stable sustained monomorphic VT is specifically associated with an acute ischemic substrate (i.e., unstable angina or myocardial infarction), lidocaine is considered a reasonable initial choice.[139,140]

Calcium channel blockers such as verapamil and diltiazem should not be used in patients to terminate wide-QRS-complex tachycardia of unknown origin, especially in patients with a history of myocardial dysfunction.

Addition of a second antiarrhythmic agent is discouraged because proarrhythmic effects are compounded. Thus, a single agent should be used and proceed to direct-current synchronized electrical cardioversion if optimal dosing fails.

Direct-current synchronized cardioversion is a highly effective and accepted intervention and should be considered first-line treatment in patients who are unstable or in those who have borderline blood pressure that could be further decreased by the vasodilator and antiinotropic effects of antiarrhythmic agents. Monophasic waveform electric shocks at an initial energy of 100 J or higher have been shown to be effective. It likely that comparable or lower energy levels might be effective when using biphasic waveform electric shocks, but more data are needed before specific recommendations can be made for the equivalent energy level.

Transvenous pacing is also an option for terminating monomorphic VT and should be considered in instances of refractoriness to cardioversion or frequent recurrences despite antiarrhythmic medication.

VENTRICULAR ARRHYTHMIAS WITH CESSATION OF EFFECTIVE BLOOD FLOW

Ventricular arrhythmias that prompt cessation of effective blood flow include pulseless VT, VF, and polymorphic VT. The immediate priority is the reestablishment of an organized electrical activity with a mechanically competent pump function, which typically requires delivery of unsynchronized electric shocks and cardiopulmonary resuscitation contingent on the duration of the arrhythmia and response to electric shocks. If there is any doubt about the specific type of ventricular arrhythmia (i.e., whether it is monomorphic or polymorphic VT) and the patient lacks effective blood flow, shock delivery should not be delayed for detailed rhythm analysis.

Ventricular Fibrillation and Pulseless VT

Consistent with the AHA/ERC 2005 guidelines,[141] the energy levels of the initial electric shock depends on the waveform and specific device. For biphasic waveform defibrillators, the initial device-specific energy level typically ranges from 150 to 200 J. In the absence of a recommended dose, 200 J should be used. Equal or higher energy level dose is recommended for the second and subsequent shocks. If the available defibrillator uses monophasic waveforms, the energy level should be 360 J for all shocks. Following shock delivery, providers should be prepared to provide advanced cardiac life support according to the most recent guidelines for cardiopulmonary resuscitation and emergency cardiovascular care (i.e., 2010 Guidelines). A 1-shock strategy followed by immediate chest compression is now recommended to minimize interruptions on chest compression. The general goals of advanced cardiac life support are to reestablish and maintain a hemodynamically effective cardiac rhythm.

The time for appropriate intervention is critically important. The probability of survival after VF and pulseless VT is inversely related to the time elapsed between the onset of the arrhythmia and the delivery of electric shocks.[142,143] Recent studies have shown that immediate defibrillation is highly effective and is associated with high survival rates when the duration of untreated VF is short (<4 minutes).[144,145] With more protracted untreated VF, mounting evidence from animal and human studies indicates that a period of closed-chest resuscitation before attempting defibrillation could improve outcome.[144,146-148] For patients with shock-refractory VF or pulseless VT, use of amiodarone has been shown to facilitate the restoration of cardiac activity.[149,150]

Electrical storm is a rather uncommon but highly lethal phenomenon defined as recurrent episodes of VF, occurring mainly in the course of an acute myocardial infarction. Conventional antiarrhythmic drug therapy—including lidocaine and procainamide—often fails to secure a stable sinus rhythm. The underlying mechanism seems to be excessive (and probably unbalanced) sympathetic activity. Recent studies have shown that outcome can be dramatically improved by sympathetic blockade using IV beta-blockers or stellate ganglionic blockade.[151]

Polymorphic Ventricular Tachycardia

Polymorphic VT with cessation of effective blood flow is treated as VF using high-energy unsynchronized shocks at the same energy level for defibrillation. Delivery of synchronized electric shocks is not recommended because of unreliable synchronization to QRS complexes. As with all ventricular arrhythmias, substantial effort must be directed at identifying and correcting associated precipitating and maintaining factors. It is useful to distinguish polymorphic VT associated with normal or prolonged QT-interval, determined during periods of intervening sinus rhythm. Both VTs may present with similar irregularity of rate and QRS morphology, with phasic increase and decrease of QRS amplitude.

Polymorphic VT with a normal QT interval is most frequently seen when acute myocardial ischemia is present but is also associated with cardiomyopathies, idiopathic polymorphic VT, and catecholaminergic VT.[152,153] In this setting, use of IV beta-blockers[153] or IV amiodarone[154] has been shown to be effective. Coronary angiography should be considered in the setting of recurrent polymorphic VT when ischemia is suspected.[155]

Polymorphic VT with prolonged QT interval usually occurs associated with bradycardia. The mainstay in management includes discontinuation of drugs that prolong the QT interval, correction of electrolyte abnormalities, and avoidance of catecholamines. In the setting of congenital long QT syndrome, beta-blockers (or sympathetic interruption), pacing, and implantation of an internal cardioverter defibrillator device should be considered. In the acquired forms of long QT syndrome, IV magnesium, overdrive pacing, and beta-blockers after pacing are recommended interventions. Isoproterenol is contraindicated in congenital long QT syndrome because it can precipitate torsades de pointes.

Conclusion

Ventricular tachyarrhythmias are important and prevalent manifestations of cardiac and extracardiac abnormalities in critically ill patients. In addition to the traditional assessment based on ECGs and hemodynamic manifestations, understanding and recognition of the processes that affect ion channels, pumps, exchangers, and signaling mechanisms are important for proper management. There is also increased awareness that mutations affecting cardiac channels are prevalent and clinically relevant. The intensivist should be alert and prepared to identify them and provide the necessary initial treatment and an appropriate referral. Initial enthusiasm for antiarrhythmic agents has diminished as the pro-arrhythmic effects of various compounds have become evident. Some drugs are no longer recommended as first-line agents, whereas others have become components of accepted algorithms. More emphasis is currently being placed on understanding arrhythmogenic mechanisms and on correcting the precipitating and maintaining factors.

REFERENCES

Access the complete reference list online at http://www.expertconsult.com.

KEY POINTS

1. Hereditary and acquired abnormalities in cardiac ion channels can alter the action potential, mostly by prolonging repolarization, and predispose to ventricular tachyarrhythmias, especially torsades de pointes.

2. Ventricular arrhythmias are the result of abnormalities in impulse generation (automaticity and triggered activity) and impulse conduction (reentry).

3. Proper management of ventricular tachyarrhythmias requires assessment of precipitating and maintaining conditions; often, the removal of these conditions is all that is needed.

4. A long QT interval in the baseline electrocardiogram should prompt a diligent search for possible drugs and metabolic conditions involved.

5. Ventricular tachyarrhythmias in critically ill patients are often precipitated by cardiac, metabolic, and respiratory processes.

6. Atrioventricular dissociation is a reliable sign that a wide-complex tachycardia is ventricular; this may be evident on the surface 12-lead electrocardiogram or after analyzing an esophageal lead.

7. Direct-current synchronized cardioversion should be considered first-line treatment in patients with ventricular tachycardia who are hemodynamically unstable or have heart failure.

80

Conduction Disturbances and Cardiac Pacemakers

JASON KNIGHT | JOHN SARKO

Conduction Disturbances

Bradyarrhythmias and conduction blocks are common in the ICU. A broad range of clinical presentations and pathologic findings occurs in this group of arrhythmias. Some bradyarrhythmias are benign and asymptomatic and do not require treatment. Other atrioventricular (AV) blocks and arrhythmias are life threatening and warrant immediate intervention.

NORMAL CARDIAC CONDUCTION

Normal depolarization and impulse conduction are central to maintaining cardiac output. Two types of cells are found in the heart: (1) cells responsible for impulse generation and conduction, and (2) cells responsible for contraction. Depolarization of the myocardium begins in the sinoatrial (SA) node. The SA node is located in the posterior and superior portion of the right atrium and is innervated by the sympathetic and parasympathetic nervous systems.

The impulse is generated by a specialized group of cells with the ability to depolarize spontaneously. Initial depolarization of the SA node is not seen on the electrocardiogram (ECG). The P wave is generated when the impulse spreads throughout the atria. There is no specific conduction system in the atria to convey the SA node impulse to the AV node.[1] The impulse is transmitted by depolarization of adjacent atrial myofibrils. Approximately halfway through the P wave, the impulse reaches the AV node. The second half of the P wave is due to left atrial depolarization.

In a normal heart, the atria and ventricles are electrically isolated from each other except at the AV node. The AV node is located in the atrial septum near the apex of the triangle of Koch. The AV node is innervated by the sympathetic and parasympathetic nervous systems. Conduction through the AV node accounts for the majority of the PR interval. After emerging from the AV node, the impulse is conducted through the bundle of His. From there, the impulse travels down the right and left bundle branches and their fascicles to the Purkinje network, which causes ventricular contraction.

FAILURE OF IMPULSE CONDUCTION

Failure of conduction can occur anywhere along the conduction pathway. AV node block is most often caused by medications, increased parasympathetic tone, or ischemia. AV node blocks are usually reversible, except when infarction permanently damages a portion of the conduction pathway. Infranodal blocks are rarely caused by physiologic abnormalities. Structural heart disease and anatomic disruption of the conduction system are the main causes of infranodal heart block. Rare causes of infranodal block include disruption of the bundle of His from aortic valve calcification, Lenègre's disease (idiopathic degeneration of Purkinje fibers), and Chagas' disease.[2]

Once AV block is identified, it is helpful to determine the site of conduction pathology. The anatomic site can be identified in most cases by synthesizing the type of AV block, the width of the QRS complex, and the QRS morphology. When the QRS complex is narrow (<0.12 seconds), the site of pathology is most likely supraventricular.

When the QRS complex is wide, the most likely site of AV block is infranodal. Bundle branch and fascicular blocks produce various QRS morphologies that may aid in determining the specific anatomic location of pathology.

Clinical Presentation

Syncope and presyncope are the most dramatic symptoms of conduction disturbances; palpitations, dyspnea, angina, and fatigue are seen as well. Many patients are asymptomatic. A significant number of patients develop bradydysrhythmias after an acute myocardial infarction (AMI) (Table 80-1).[3]

Diagnostic Evaluation

A high-quality ECG is paramount for the appropriate evaluation of P waves and various intervals. Routine monitoring in the ICU is usually accomplished with a single or three-lead display at the bedside. The lead chosen should clearly delineate the P waves and QRS complexes. Complex arrhythmias may require Lewis leads, intraatrial leads, or esophageal ECG monitoring. Calipers significantly aid in the diagnosis of AV blocks and are helpful to "march out" P waves and intervals. Holter or continuous loop monitoring can also be an important tool in the evaluation of AV block.[4] These monitors allow one to evaluate the cardiac conduction system during a patient's activities of daily living. A monitoring period of at least 24 hours is recommended so that both daytime and nighttime activities are included.

SINUS NODE ABNORMALITIES

Sinus Bradycardia

Sinus bradycardia is defined as a sinus rhythm with a heart rate less than 60 beats per minute. Sinus bradycardia is divided into two categories: appropriate and inappropriate. Appropriate bradycardia is seen in young, healthy individuals and endurance athletes; the heart rate increases appropriately with exercise. Pathologic sinus bradycardia does not increase appropriately with exercise. Medications are the most common cause of inappropriate sinus bradycardia; autonomic influences, electrolyte abnormalities, and intrinsic structural disorders are others. In older individuals, sinus bradycardia can result from a decrease in the sinus node firing rate, which is a normal part of the aging process. Ischemia may also increase vagal tone and result in a slower heart rate.

Sinus Arrest

Sinus arrest occurs when the pacemaker cells in the SA node fail to depolarize. Pauses of less than 3 seconds may be seen in up to 11% of normal individuals and should not cause concern.[5] There is a higher incidence of sinus pause in athletes. Pauses longer than 3 seconds are usually considered pathologic and should be evaluated.

SA exit block and sinus arrest appear similar on ECGs, but they should be distinguished if possible. The duration of the pause in exit block is a multiple of the P-P interval. High-grade exit block cannot be distinguished from sinus arrest. The treatment is the same for both conditions.[6]

TABLE 80-1	Incidence of Bradydysrhythmias in Acute Myocardial Infarction	
Rhythm		*Incidence (%)*
Any bradydysrhythmia		25-30
Sinus bradycardia		25
Junctional escape rhythm		20
Idioventricular escape rhythm		15
First-degree atrioventricular (AV) node block		15
Second-degree AV block type I		12
Second-degree AV block type II		4
Third-degree block		15
Right bundle branch block		7
Left bundle branch block		5
Left anterior fascicular block		8
Left posterior fascicular block		0.5

Noninvasive testing includes ECG, carotid sinus massage, and a tilt table test. Carotid sinus massage is useful to diagnose carotid sinus hypersensitivity. Risks of carotid sinus massage include transient ischemic attack and stroke, and the test should not be performed on patients with carotid bruits. The tilt table test is helpful to determine whether syncopal episodes are due to autonomic dysfunction. Invasive diagnostic testing of the SA node can also be performed, although this is rarely necessary.

The treatment of sinus node dysfunction can be temporary or permanent. Atropine or an isoproterenol drip can be used in the ICU as a bridge to permanent pacemaker placement. Temporary pacing is indicated for patients who fail to respond to medical therapy.

Carotid Sinus Hypersensitivity

Carotid sinus hypersensitivity is diagnosed when ventricular asystole greater than 3 seconds' duration (usually due to a sinus pause or arrest) or a drop in systolic blood pressure greater than 50 mm Hg occurs in response to carotid massage. If symptoms occur, a 30 mm Hg drop in systolic blood pressure defines a positive response. Treatment is permanent pacing in symptomatic patients only.[7]

Postsurgical Bradydysrhythmias

Bradyarrhythmias are common after cardiac surgery. Valve surgery and septal myectomy can cause significant damage to the conduction system. Prolonged ischemia during heart transplantation may also result in sinus node or conduction system damage. The decision to place a permanent pacer should not be made until 5 to 7 days postoperatively, however, because the bradyarrhythmia may be temporary. Medication administered during surgery or reversible ischemia is often implicated. Pacing is required in 3.2% to 8.5% of patients with valve surgery and approximately 10% of patients with transplants.[8]

ATRIOVENTRICULAR NODE DYSFUNCTION

There are many causes and several manifestations of AV node dysfunction. Box 80-1 lists the causes of AV node abnormalities.

First-Degree Atrioventricular Block

First-degree AV block is characterized by a prolonged PR interval greater than 0.20 second in adults and 0.18 second in children who are not taking medications that can prolong the PR interval (Figure 80-1). All the P waves are conducted to the ventricles, and the PR interval is typically fixed. Potential causes of first-degree AV block include delayed conduction through the atria from the SA node to the AV node, a delay in AV node conduction, or prolonged infranodal conduction.

Conduction delays from the SA node to the AV node are typically due to structural causes such as right atrial enlargement or an ostium primum atrial septal defect. A delay in AV node impulse conduction is the most common cause of first-degree AV block. Patients with delayed conduction in the AV node often have a PR interval greater

---

Box 80-1

CAUSES OF ATRIOVENTRICULAR NODE DYSFUNCTION

Drugs:
  Digoxin
  Beta-blockers
  Certain calcium channel blockers
  Membrane-active antidysrhythmic drugs
Primary cardiac disease:
  Ischemic heart disease
  Idiopathic fibrosis of the conduction system
  Congenital heart disease
  Calcific valvular disease
  Cardiomyopathy
Metabolic:
  Hyperkalemia
  Hypermagnesemia
Infiltrative disease
Infectious/inflammatory disease
Collagen vascular disease
Endocrine:
  Addison's disease
Trauma
Radiation
Tumors
Neurally mediated:
  Carotid sinus syndrome
  Vasovagal syndrome
  Neuromyopathic disorders

Adapted from Wolbrette DL, Naccarelli GV. Bradycardias: sinus nodal dysfunction and atrioventricular conduction disturbances. In: Topol EJ, editor. Textbook of Cardiovascular Medicine. Philadelphia: Lippincott-Raven; 1998, p. 1655.

---

than 0.30 second. Infranodal causes of first-degree AV block are rare and are typically associated with a wide QRS complex due to disease in the fascicles or the bundle of His. First-degree AV block can also occur when each of these conduction times is at the upper limit of normal and summate to produce an overall prolongation of the PR interval.[7]

First-degree AV block is typically benign and asymptomatic. It can be seen in 0.5% of young adults without heart disease. In older people, first-degree block is most often the result of idiopathic degenerative disease. A prolonged PR interval is often an incidental finding when an ECG is ordered for other reasons. It rarely warrants further workup or treatment.

Second-Degree Atrioventricular Block Type I

Second-degree AV block type I, or a Wenckebach (or Mobitz type I) rhythm, is defined by a progressive prolongation of the PR interval with each successive beat, with eventual failure of a P wave to conduct to the ventricles (Figure 80-2). This results in a dropped beat and failure of the ventricles to depolarize. The P waves occur at regular intervals. As the PR interval lengthens, the RR interval becomes shorter, which eventually results in decremental conduction. There is a reciprocal relationship between the RP interval and the PR interval.

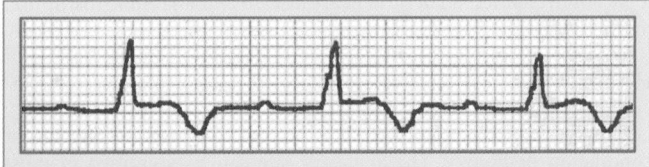

Figure 80-1   Electrocardiogram from patient with first-degree atrioventricular block. PR interval is approximately 0.29 second. All P waves are being conducted to ventricles. PR interval is constant.

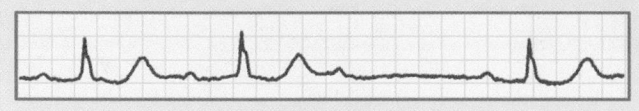

Figure 80-2 Electrocardiogram rhythm strip from patient with second-degree atrioventricular block type I. Note progressive prolongation of PR interval until a failure of conduction occurs. Also note reciprocal RP shortening. Pattern of conduction is 3:2.

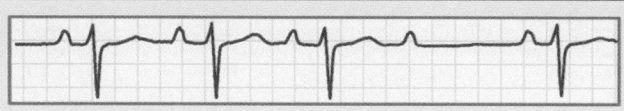

Figure 80-3 Electrocardiogram demonstrating second-degree atrioventricular block type II. PR interval is constant before and after blocked P waves. QRS complex is widened.

The pathophysiology of second-degree AV block type I is similar to that of first-degree AV block, except that intraatrial block is usually not a cause. For all practical purposes, second-degree AV block type I is caused by a block in AV node conduction. The QRS complex is generally narrow.

QRS complexes are typically grouped in twos, threes, fours, and so on. Group beating is characteristic of Wenckebach rhythms. The rhythm is described by recording the number of P waves and QRS complexes involved in the pattern of block (e.g., 4:3 or 3:2). During a dropped beat, a P wave is observed with no corresponding QRS complex. Second-degree AV block type I is a stable rhythm and has a much better prognosis than does a Mobitz type II rhythm. If the Wenckebach rhythm is due to medication, resolution of the block can be monitored with an ECG. Once the medication is discontinued, a shortening of the PR interval and a lengthening of the RP interval, with a corresponding improvement in AV node conduction, may be observed.

Second-Degree Atrioventricular Block Type II

Second-degree AV block type II (or Mobitz type II block) is characterized by a sudden nonconducted P wave without a change in the PR interval. A P wave with no corresponding QRS complex is observed on the ECG (Figure 80-3). This is an inherently unstable rhythm, and serious pathology may be present. In contrast to the Mobitz type I rhythm, type II is described as a high degree of AV block, with P wave–to–QRS ratios of 3:1 and 4:1. A Mobitz type II rhythm is almost always due to an infranodal conduction disturbance. The conducted QRS complexes are often wide, and a bundle branch block pattern is often observed. Second-degree AV block can result from anterior wall MI. Type II second-degree AV block can progress to complete heart block.

2:1 Atrioventricular Block

When conduction of every other P wave is blocked, 2:1 AV block is present. The PR interval of the conducted beat remains fixed. QRS complexes are regular and occur at half the atrial rate. 2:1 AV block can be caused by a Mobitz I (usually with a narrow QRS complex) or Mobitz II (with a wide QRS complex) rhythm, and the two entities are difficult to distinguish.

Third-Degree Atrioventricular Block

Third-degree AV block is characterized by complete AV dissociation. There is no conduction of the atrial signal through to the ventricle, so the atrial and ventricular systems operate independently. On ECGs, the P waves "march through" and are not associated with ventricular contraction. The PR intervals are irregular. The ventricular complexes may be junctional (narrow QRS complex; rate 40-60) or ventricular (wide QRS complex, rate <40). Depending on the escape heart rate, patients may present with tachypnea, dyspnea on exertion, fatigue, cyanosis, or syncope (Figure 80-4).

Third-degree block can be divided into congenital and acquired causes. Sixty percent of patients with congenital heart block are female. Patients with congenital third-degree block often have an escape rhythm with an adequate rate.[9] Acquired third-degree block occurs most frequently in the seventh decade of life and usually requires permanent pacing; these patients are often male. Specific causes include medications, ischemia, progression from Mobitz type II rhythm, and infarction. Acute MI results in third-degree heart block

in 14% of patients with inferior wall infarcts and 2% of patients with anterior infarcts. Third-degree block is usually observed within 24 hours after an MI. Third-degree block as a complication of inferior MI is usually temporary and may require only temporary pacing. Complete heart block as a result of anterior MI usually requires a permanent pacer.

Treatment involves correction of underlying disorders and immediate transcutaneous or transvenous pacing in unstable patients. If the primary cause cannot be medically managed, permanent pacing is required.

Diagnostic Pitfalls

Determining the degree of AV node block is usually straightforward if an adequate ECG has been obtained. There are circumstances, however, in which one may be misled to an incorrect diagnosis.

Third-degree block is occasionally misdiagnosed as second-degree block type II if there appears to be a constant PR interval. This may occur for short periods on an isolated rhythm strip. The clinician must therefore examine a strip for an appropriate length of time to make the correct diagnosis. Vagal maneuvers can also be attempted and may identify a second-degree AV block that is really a third-degree AV block.

With isorhythmic AV dissociation, the P waves and QRS complexes occur at a similar rate. The P waves may never "march out" long enough to determine whether they are all conducting. Interventions such as vagal maneuvers to change the PQRS relationship may aid in diagnosis.

When second-degree AV block is fixed (2:1, 3:1, 4:1), some P waves may be concealed during the repolarization phase of the ECG. This may occur in acute MI or with ischemia. Vagal maneuvers and examination of multiple leads may be necessary to correctly identify the AV block.

When complete AV dissociation occurs with accelerated junctional or ventricular rhythms, it is possible that some of the atrial impulses would be conducted if the heart rate were slower. It is best to designate these rhythms as complex AV dissociation.

Therapy

Medical therapy for AV block consists of atropine, adrenergic agents, Digibind (if appropriate), and pacing. Atropine decreases vagal tone and is useful for hypervagotonia but not AV node ischemia. It is more useful in inferior wall MI than anterior wall MI. Atropine will not improve third-degree AV block or a Mobitz type II block if the pathology is below the AV node, and it is ineffective in heart transplant patients. Atropine should be used with caution in patients with Mobitz type II rhythms, because a paradoxical decrease in heart rate can occur.

Digibind should be used in symptomatic patients with digoxin-induced AV block. The number of vials of Digibind required is approximately equal to the patient's weight (in kilograms) times the digoxin serum level (in ng/mL) divided by 100.

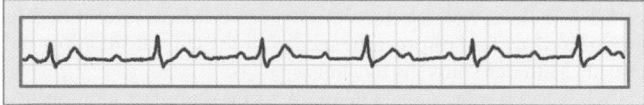

Figure 80-4 Complete heart block. PR intervals are irregular because ventricles and atria represent two independent sources of depolarization.

TABLE 80-2	NBG Pacemaker Code				
Position	I	II	III	IV	V
Category	Chamber paced	Chamber sensed	Response to sensing	Rate modulation or programmability	Antitachycardia functions
Letters used	A = atria V = ventricular D = dual (A+V)	A = atria V = ventricular D = dual (A+V)	T = triggered I = inhibited D = dual (T+I)	R = rate modulation P = simple programmable (rate or output) M = multiprogrammable O = none	P = pacing S = shock D = dual (P+S)

Data from Bernstein AD, Camm AJ, Fletcher AD. The NASPE/BPEG generic pacemaker code for antibradyarrhythmia and adaptive rate pacing and antitachycardia devices. Pacing Clin Electrophysiol 1987;10:794-8.

Pacemakers

Although pacemakers are reliable, patients occasionally present with abnormalities in one or more pacemaker functions that may impact their current illnesses. Intensivists can expect to encounter patients with pacemakers routinely, and it is helpful to be familiar with the basics of their functions and malfunctions.

The North American Society of Pacing and Electrophysiology and the British Pacing and Electrophysiology Group created a code consisting of five letters to describe pacemaker functions, known as the NBG pacemaker code (Table 80-2).[10] The first three letters describe the antibradycardia functions, the fourth describes the programmability of rate responsiveness, and the fifth describes any antitachycardia functions. A pacemaker may carry one classification (e.g., DDD) but be capable of several modes of function, depending on how it is programmed. Indications for permanent pacing were updated by the American College of Cardiology in 2002.[11]

The pacemaker itself consists of two components: a pulse generator and wire leads connecting the generator to the heart. The pulse generator consists of a lithium-based battery and the circuitry to detect and analyze the cardiac rhythm and produce the output. The battery can last more than 10 years, depending on the type of programming; at the end of its life, it shows a gradual rate decrease, not an abrupt drop-off.[12]

Pacemakers also contain a reed switch that can be used to assess the pacemaker's pacing ability. When an external magnet is placed over the pulse generator, the reed switch closes, disabling the sensing mechanism. The unit then fires asynchronously without regard for the patient's underlying rhythm. The pacing rate is unique to each model and manufacturer, and the magnet-programmed rate can vary depending on whether the battery is at the beginning or end of its life or at a time of elective replacement.

Each patient is given a card when a pacemaker is implanted that describes the manufacturer, model, and pacing parameters. The pacemaker itself also contains a radiopaque code, visible on x-ray, that identifies the unit. Pacemakers can be interrogated with a manufacturer-specific program that retrieves ECG information about the unit that can help assess its functioning. An electrophysiologist should be consulted when a malfunction is suspected.

Two types of lead systems exist: unipolar and bipolar. Bipolar leads are considered standard unless patient-specific factors warrant the use of a unipolar lead. Unipolar programming uses the lead in the endocardium as the cathode and the pacemaker unit itself as the anode. Because voltage in a unipolar lead is detected over a greater distance, the pacing spike is larger than with bipolar lead programming. Leads can be attached to the endocardium by active fixation (screwed into the myocardium) or passive fixation (held in place by fins). Passive fixation is associated with a greater incidence of dislodgment and perforation.[13]

Assessment of pacemaker function requires knowledge of its parameters. A pacing spike must be present on the ECG to properly evaluate the unit. If one is not present, a magnet can be placed over it and an ECG recorded. This can then be used with the clinical situation and prior ECG to determine its function.

Every pacer is programmed to fire after a maximum period in which no activity has been detected. This is called the *lower rate-limiting interval*, and it is the time between two consecutive paced beats. The *escape interval* is the time between a native complex and the following pacemaker spike. A slight delay beyond the lower rate-limiting interval can be programmed into the pacemaker when it senses a native QRS complex. This is an attempt to permit the heart to generate its own output and thus function in a more physiologic manner; this is called *rate hysteresis*, and it is found most often in ventricular demand pacemakers.[14] Dual-chamber pacers have an interval programmed between atrial and ventricular spikes called the *AV interval*, which functions basically as the PR interval. The interval between a ventricular spike and the next atrial pacing spike is the *ventriculoatrial interval*. The AV and ventriculoatrial intervals sum to equal the lower rate-limiting interval.

COMPLICATIONS

Failure to Sense (Undersensing)

Undersensing occurs when the pacemaker generates output regardless of the patient's underlying rhythm (Figure 80-5). A spike is seen at an interval earlier than the lower rate-limiting interval. Pacemaker output then competes with the patient's own intrinsic rhythm. Although ventricular pacing can present a problem when the threshold for ventricular capture has been altered (e.g., by ischemia), and atrial pacing can produce atrial fibrillation, these are rarely urgent problems.[15]

Specific causes of failure to sense are listed in Table 80-3. Blanking is not a true cause; rather, it is an instance of functional undersensing in dual-chamber pacemakers. To prevent a pacemaker-induced tachycardia, a 12- to 125-millisecond period of inactivity is programmed into the ventricular component after an atrial complex. If an intrinsic QRS complex occurs during this period, it will not be sensed. Scar tissue does not conduct impulses as easily as normal myocardium does, so sensing may not occur. Most pulse generators begin asynchronous pacing at a critical point at the end of their life and will not sense intrinsic activity. Defibrillation can damage the unit; placing the defibrillator pad in an anteroposterior position may help. The unit should be observed closely after shocks are delivered.

Failure to Pace (Generate Output)

This complication is noted when a pacemaker spike is not seen after the lower rate-limiting interval has been exceeded (except when hysteresis has been programmed; Figure 80-6). Oversensing occurs when stimuli are erroneously sensed as pacemaker output. As a result, the expected proper output is inhibited; this can be continuous or intermittent. Failure to pace can be a devastating complication for a pacemaker-dependent patient. It is important to determine whether output is truly occurring or not. A 12-lead ECG should be done, because spikes may be too small to be seen in a specific lead. Several causes are possible (Table 80-4).

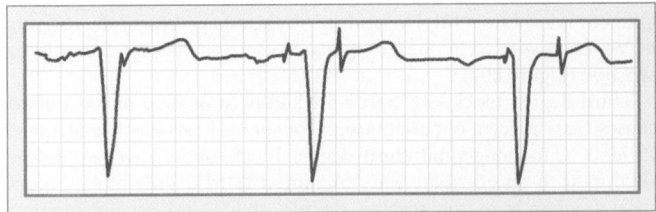

Figure 80-5 Failure to sense. Atrial and ventricular pacing spikes are seen around the intrinsic QRS complexes. Pacemaker activity does not lead to capture.

TABLE 80-3	Causes of Undersensing	
Cause	**Treatment**
Lead fracture	Replace lead
Lead dislodgment	Reposition lead or increase sensitivity
Insulation defect in pacing lead	Replace lead
Magnet interrogation	Remove magnet
Blanking	Decrease ventricular refractory period
Amplitude of P wave or QRS complex too low to be sensed	Increase sensitivity
Myocardial fibrosis	Increase sensitivity or reposition lead
Myocardial perforation	Increase sensitivity or reposition lead
End of battery life	Replace battery
Acute myocardial infarction	Treat myocardial infarction
Electrolyte disturbance	Correct electrolytes
Antidysrhythmic drugs	Increase sensitivity, change drug
Magnetic resonance imaging	Reprogram to VOO, AOO, or DOO mode
Defibrillation	Place defibrillator pads as far from pacemaker unit as possible, place in anteroposterior position
Complexes occurring in pacemaker's refractory period	None, or use new generator with shorter refractory period

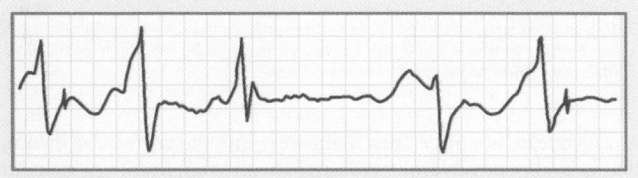

Figure 80-6 Failure to pace. An unduly long interval passes after the third QRS complex before another beat occurs. Pacemaker should have fired before this intrinsic beat.

Cross-talk is not a true malfunction of the pacemaker, but it can lead to an inhibition of activity. In a dual-chamber system, the output of one chamber is sensed as the output of the other, and no pacemaker spike is generated; this occurs more often in unipolar leads. This problem is corrected by programming a blanking period. For a brief period after the atrial output (12 to 25 milliseconds), the ventricular component is inhibited from firing. A second protection against cross-talk is to program the unit to fire depending on when in the AV interval the stimulus is detected. If it occurs immediately after the blanking period, a "safety" spike is generated because it is assumed that it is impossible to differentiate cross-talk from a native QRS complex.

TABLE 80-4	Causes of Failure to Pace	
Cause	**Treatment**
Lead fracture, loose connection, or insulation defect	Adjust or replace leads
Battery depletion	Replace battery
Pulse generator failure	Replace pulse generator
Cross-talk	Program a blanking period or safety pacing
Electromagnetic oversensing: Sensing P or T or U waves	Decrease sensitivity, or advance tip deeper into right ventricle
Myopotential sensing	Decrease sensitivity, or use bipolar sensing
Electrocautery	Decrease sensitivity, or electrically isolate patient
Extracorporeal shock wave lithotripsy	Decrease sensitivity, or use minimal equipment necessary
Transcutaneous electrical nerve stimulator (TENS)	Decrease sensitivity, stop TENS unit
Magnetic resonance imaging	Program to DOO, VOO, or AOO mode

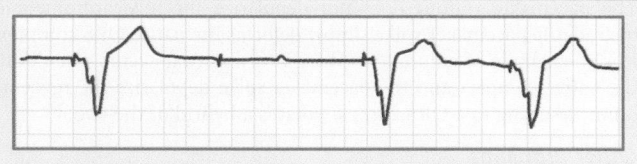

Figure 80-7 Failure to capture. After first QRS complex, a small pacemaker spike occurs that does not result in depolarization of ventricle. A nonconducted P wave follows, and then a pacemaker spike with capture occurs.

Failure to Capture

This complication occurs when a pacemaker fires as expected but fails to depolarize the myocardium. A pacer spike is seen on the ECG, but no QRS complex immediately follows it (Figure 80-7). This can be dangerous for a pacemaker-dependent patient and may require temporary pacing until the problem is fixed. Most cases are due to problems with the lead/tissue interface, although isolated problems in the leads or the myocardium can also occur (Table 80-5).[13,16]

When a lead is placed into the myocardium, tissue fibrosis occurs over the first 4 to 6 weeks. Because scar tissue does not conduct as well as normal myocardium, the output voltage may need to be increased. Twiddler's syndrome is seen when a patient fidgets with the generator and ends up pulling the leads from their attachments to the myocardium. It is confirmed by chest x-ray. The pacemaker is replaced and fixed tightly to the underlying fascia. Perforation of the ventricle typically occurs shortly after the leads are placed and is confirmed by a chest x-ray showing the tip of the lead outside the heart. It is suggested by a change in pacing to a right bundle branch pattern, failure to capture, contraction of the diaphragm or intercostal muscles with pacing, or development of a pericardial friction rub. Provided the patient is not anticoagulated, the perforation is usually well tolerated.[14] Echocardiography can assess for the presence of pericardial effusion or tamponade. Repositioning of the lead is typically performed in the operating room after any coagulopathy has been reversed.

An increased threshold for capture can also be caused by myocardial ischemia, metabolic abnormalities, or certain drugs. Definitive treatment involves correcting the underlying disorder.

When assessing for failure to capture, a distinction must be made between pseudofusion and fusion beats. A pseudofusion beat occurs when the pacemaker fires at the same time that an intrinsic beat occurs.

TABLE 80-5	Causes of Failure to Capture	
Cause	**Treatment**
Lead dislodgment from endocardial surface	Repair lead
Twiddler's syndrome	Fix unit to chest wall
Lead fracture or break in insulation	Replace lead
Improperly or inadequately programmed voltage	Reprogram voltage
Battery failure	Replace battery
Cardiac perforation	Reposition lead (in operating room) or increase voltage
Increased threshold for capture: Fibrosis or scar tissue at contact site	Increase voltage or reposition lead
Myocardial ischemia	Treat ischemia
Metabolic: Hyperkalemia Hypercarbia Hypoxemia Hypothyroidism	Treat abnormality
Drugs: Beta-blockers Class Ia antidysrhythmics Verapamil Flecainide	Remove drug and replace with another

The pacemaker output does not depolarize the myocardium, and instead, the pacemaker spike simply deforms the native QRS complex. It is an example of failure to capture. A fusion beat occurs when both the native complex and the pacemaker spike depolarize the myocardium, resulting in a QRS complex that is a hybrid of the two.

Other Problems

Pacemaker-mediated tachycardia, also called *endless loop* or *pacemaker reentrant tachycardia*, is a complication of dual-chamber units. A premature atrial contraction or premature ventricular contraction that travels in a retrograde manner into the atria is sensed by the atrial component of the pacemaker, which induces the ventricular component to fire. The resulting ventricular depolarization reenters the atria, and the cycle continues. An upper rate limit is programmed into the pacemaker, so the tachycardia will not exceed this rate. A tachycardia paced by atrial and ventricular spikes is seen. Application of a magnet terminates the dysrhythmia; adenosine may not reliably block it.[17] A blanking period must be programmed.

Pacemaker syndrome is seen when only the ventricle is paced. Patients present with lethargy, syncope, dizziness, weakness, fatigue, palpitations, or congestive heart failure. It occurs because of an inability to raise the heart rate with exercise and because of the loss of AV synchrony. Dual chamber pacing is required to correct this.

The diagnosis of MI in a patient with a functioning pacemaker is difficult. Criteria similar to those in patients with left bundle branch block have been proposed, but sensitivity and specificity are lower.[15]

Advanced Cardiac Life Support protocols are not contraindicated by the presence of a pacemaker. Defibrillator pads should be kept as far away from the pulse generator as possible to minimize any damage to the unit.

Examination by magnetic resonance imaging has been considered contraindicated because of the interaction between the strong magnetic field and the pulse generator. Increased pacing rates, decreased rates, and pacing at the magnet rate have all been seen. However, programming the pacemaker to an asynchronous mode (AOO, VOO, or DOO) and close monitoring of the patient, along with the use of lower magnetic fields, may allow safe imaging.[18]

Temporary Pacing

Temporary cardiac pacing may be required for emergent or elective reasons. In general, any patient with bradycardia causing symptoms or hemodynamic instability that is unresponsive to atropine ought to be considered for temporary pacing (Box 80-2).[19] In most cases, this occurs after acute MI,[19] but certain drug poisonings may benefit from pacing,[20,21] and some interventions may, because of underlying disease, predispose a patient to significant bradycardia.

MODES OF PACING

Several modes of temporary pacing are available. Transcutaneous pacing involves placing the pacing pads on either the chest wall and back (the usual locations) or in an anterolateral position (especially if external defibrillation may be required). The negative electrode is placed over the apex of the heart. This is the easiest mode to use, but it is uncomfortable for a conscious patient and may require analgesia or sedation.

Transvenous pacing is usually well tolerated by patients but requires a high degree of skill to correctly place the pacing electrode in the right ventricle. Therefore, the American College of Physicians and the American College of Cardiology recommend that only physicians formally trained in their use place these electrodes.[22] The right internal jugular vein approach is best because of its more direct route to the heart; the left subclavian vein approach can also be used but should be avoided, if possible, because it is a preferred site for placement of a permanent pacemaker.[19]

Transesophageal pacing allows pacing of either the atria or the ventricles, but it is not a commonly used modality. Transthoracic pacing,

---

Box 80-2

INDICATIONS FOR TEMPORARY CARDIAC PACING

Drug toxicity:
   Beta-blocker
   Calcium channel blocker
   Digitalis-induced dysrhythmia (when direct-current cardioversion is contraindicated)
Hyperkalemia with bradycardia or asystole
Hypothermia (transcutaneous pacing only)
Symptomatic bradycardia (including hemodynamic compromise, syncope, or ventricular ectopy in response to bradycardia) not responsive to atropine
Pacemaker malfunction with symptoms
Alternating BBB (after MI)
RBBB with alternating LAFB or LPFB (after MI not known to be old)
RBBB with LAFB or LPFB, or LBBB with first-degree heart block, not known to be old
Mobitz type II heart block
Asystole
LBBB not known to be old
Recurrent sinus pauses > 3 seconds not responsive to atropine
RBBB with first-degree heart block
Possibly helpful: bifascicular block or RBBB of unknown age

BBB, bundle branch block; *LAFB,* left anterior fascicular block; *LBBB,* left bundle branch block; *LPFB,* left posterior fascicular block; *MI,* myocardial infarction; *RBBB,* right bundle branch block.

in which leads are placed percutaneously into the ventricular myocardium, is also possible but is fraught with complications, including pericardial tamponade, pneumothorax, visceral injury, and coronary artery laceration. Pacing leads placed during open heart surgery can also be used.

Pacing threshold should be determined, and the pacing energy should then be set at two to three times this minimum output. Thresholds should be checked daily.

KEY POINTS

Conduction Disturbances

1. Atrioventricular (AV) node block is most often caused by medications, increased parasympathetic tone, or ischemia. Except when infarction permanently damages a portion of the conduction pathway, such blocks are usually reversible. Infranodal blocks, however, are rarely caused by physiologic abnormalities.

2. First-degree AV node block and Wenckebach block typically do not require treatment. Type II second-degree heart block and complete heart block usually do require treatment.

3. Therapy for AV block consists of atropine, adrenergic agents, Digibind (if appropriate), and pacing.

4. Bradyarrhythmias are common after cardiac surgery and may require temporary pacing, but a decision to place a permanent pacemaker should not be made until 5 to 7 days after surgery.

Pacemakers

1. A cardiologist or electrophysiologist should be consulted when a pacemaker or cardioverter-defibrillator malfunction is suspected.

2. Placing a magnet over the pacemaker disables the sensing mechanism, causing the pacemaker to fire at its preprogrammed rate regardless of the underlying intrinsic rhythm.

3. Magnetic resonance imaging may be safe in a pacemaker patient if the unit is programmed to an asynchronous mode and the patient is watched carefully.

4. Failure to sense occurs when the pacemaker generates output regardless of the patient's underlying rhythm; this is rarely an urgent problem.

5. Failure to pace is noted when a pacemaker spike is not seen when expected (after the lower rate-limiting interval has been exceeded); this can be devastating for a pacemaker-dependent patient, and temporary pacing may be required.

6. Failure to capture occurs when a pacemaker fires as expected but fails to depolarize the myocardium. This complication may require temporary pacing.

ANNOTATED REFERENCES

Epstein AE, DiMarco JP, Ellenbogen KA, et al. ACC/AHA/HRS 2008 guidelines for device-based therapy of cardiac rhythm abnormalities: executive summary: a report of the American College of Cardiology/American Heart Association Task Force on Practice Guidelines. J Am Coll Cardiol 2008;51:2085-105.
This guideline revises the indications for implantable pacemakers and cardioverter-defibrillators.
Bernstein AD, Camm AJ, Fletcher AD. The NASPE/BPEG generic pacemaker code for antibradyarrhythmia and adaptive rate pacing and anti-tachycardia devices. Pacing Clin Electrophysiol 1987;10:794-8.
The system for describing pacemakers is introduced and discussed in this article.

Roguin A, Schwiter J, Valhous C, et al. Magnetic resonance imaging in individuals with cardiovascular implantable electronic devices. Europace 2008;10:336-46.
This study reviews the evidence behind the traditional contraindication of performing MRI in patients with pacemakers and suggests that on a case-by-case basis, MRI may be performed safely. A strategy for the safe performance of an MRI in patients with pacemakers is proposed.

REFERENCES

Access the complete reference list online at http://www.expertconsult.com.

81

Sudden Cardiac Death: Implantable Cardioverter-Defibrillators

FRÉDÉRIC L. PAULIN | DEREK V. EXNER

Since its initial development in the 1970s[1] and its introduction to clinical practice in the 1980s,[2] the implantable cardioverter-defibrillator (ICD) has revolutionized the management of patients with or at risk for life-threatening ventricular arrhythmias. Large randomized controlled trials[3-13] have shown that these devices prevent death from ventricular tachycardia (VT) or ventricular fibrillation (VF). Device-based treatment of recurrent VT or VF is the initial treatment of choice for many patients who have experienced or are at high risk for experiencing these rhythm disturbances.[14] Device complexity makes a detailed understanding of ICD technology challenging for practitioners, but a general understanding of these devices and associated clinical problems is increasingly important because of their widespread use.

Epidemiology of Sudden Cardiac Death

Sudden cardiac death, arbitrarily defined as death from a cardiac cause occurring within 1 hour of cardiovascular symptom onset or without preceding symptoms,[15] is a major public health problem responsible for approximately 450,000 deaths annually in North America alone.[16] Out-of-hospital cardiac arrest carries a dismal prognosis, with reported rates of survival to hospital admission of 5% to 10% and minimal improvement in survival rates over the past several decades.[17] This poor outcome occurs despite public health efforts to improve public recognition of cardiac symptoms and shorten the time to therapy by means of bystander cardiopulmonary resuscitation (CPR) and better access to emergency medical services.[18] Among patients who survive to hospital admission, mortality and morbidity remain exceedingly high,[19,20] highlighting the need for preventive efforts.

A significant proportion of sudden cardiac deaths are due to a treatable arrhythmia such as VT or VF,[18,21] with the remainder being due to asystole or pulseless electrical activity (PEA). In autopsy studies, a majority of sudden cardiac death victims have pathologically apparent structural heart disease, particularly coronary atherosclerosis.[22] In many cases, recent unstable coronary disease can be demonstrated by pathologic evidence of recent plaque rupture, with or without thrombosis.[23] In cases in which cardiac monitoring was in place at the time of death, arrhythmia is commonly present.[24]

A significant proportion of sudden cardiac death occurs in patients without previously identified cardiac disease.[19,25] Currently there is no feasible means of screening the population at large to identify all individuals who are at risk for this catastrophic event. Prediction and prevention strategies have therefore focused on identifying patients with clinical characteristics that place them at particularly high risk for sudden cardiac death.[26,27] From the public health perspective, the most important conditions that predispose to a high risk of sudden cardiac death include cardiovascular risk factors, coronary artery disease, and left ventricular (LV) dysfunction of ischemic etiology and a variety of hereditary conditions that are listed in Box 81-1.

Approximately 50% of deaths in patients with heart failure are sudden.[27,28] The majority of these are due to ventricular tachyarrhythmias.[24] However, asystole and PEA are more common modes of sudden unexpected death in patients with end-stage heart failure.[29] Among the factors that predict sudden cardiac death, severity of LV systolic dysfunction and age are by far the strongest predictors.[30-32] Trials of ICD therapy have largely focused on patients with LV dysfunction, coronary disease, and spontaneous or inducible ventricular arrhythmias.[33]

Prevention of Tachyarrhythmic Sudden Cardiac Death: Non-Device Therapy

Previously, antiarrhythmic drugs were the cornerstone of treatment and prevention of recurrent VT and VF. However, it is recognized that these drugs are intrinsically hazardous, given their arrhythmogenicity and other adverse effects.[34-39] Currently, antiarrhythmic drugs retain a primary role in patients with other conditions for which these agents are indicated (e.g., concurrent atrial fibrillation) or to decrease the frequency of ICD shocks. In this instance, D-L sotalol, dofetilide, or amiodarone are most often utilized.

Although class IC antiarrhythmic drugs, including encainide, flecainide, and moricizine, are effective at suppressing ventricular ectopy, they have been shown to significantly increase mortality in the landmark Cardiac Arrhythmia Suppression Trials.[34,36] D-Sotalol, a pure class III antiarrhythmic agent, was evaluated in a randomized controlled trial and, similar to class IC agents, was found to increase mortality.[40] The L-isomer that confers the beta-blocking effect may attenuate this hazard.[41] Dofetilide, a class III agent, has been shown to be safe in patients with symptomatic heart failure and LV dysfunction when initiated in the hospital.[42] In contrast, dronedarone, a newer antiarrhythmic agent, was found to increase mortality in patients with advanced heart failure.[43] Thus, its role in the management of arrhythmias in patients with heart failure is unclear. Newer antiarrhythmic agents including azimilide, celivarone, and vernakalant are under investigation.

Amiodarone is the only available empirical choice for arrhythmia prevention in patients with heart failure or LV dysfunction. Several trials have shown decreased risk of death among patients treated with amiodarone after myocardial infarction (MI).[35,44] Among patients at risk for arrhythmic death, a meta-analysis of controlled trials showed a reduction in total, cardiac, and sudden cardiac deaths with amiodarone therapy.[45] In patients with heart failure, emperic amiodarone does not increase the risk of death (in contrast to class IC agents).[10,37]

Guided approaches to antiarrhythmic drug choice have also been evaluated.[46] This can be done noninvasively using serial ambulatory cardiac monitoring to assess the response to specific drug choices, or invasively using serial programmed electrical stimulation to evaluate the drug effect on inducibility of VT or VF. Both approaches have been evaluated and can predict response to medical treatment reasonably well.[47-49]

The high recurrence rates of VT/VF and medication-related adverse events limit both empirical and guided therapies.[38,50,51] For example, although amiodarone is the most effective antiarrhythmic drug for preventing the recurrence of VT and VF, a substantial proportion of patients (up to 20%) treated with amiodarone are unable to continue therapy in the long term owing to cumulative side effects, recurrent arrhythmia prompting a change in therapy, or death.[38,52]

Medications other than antiarrhythmic drugs have also been evaluated. Beta-blockers clearly reduce the risk of death among patients with

COMMON CAUSES OF SERIOUS VENTRICULAR ARRHYTHMIAS

Structural Disease
Left ventricular dysfunction
Coronary artery disease and acute myocardial infarction
Coronary artery anomalies
Hypertrophic cardiomyopathy
Arrhythmogenic right ventricular cardiomyopathy
Left ventricular noncompaction cardiomyopathy
Cardiac sarcoidosis

Primary Electrophysiologic Defects
Wolff-Parkinson-White syndrome
"Idiopathic" ventricular tachycardia or fibrillation
Catecholaminergic polymorphic ventricular tachycardia
Long QT syndrome (congenital or acquired)
Brugada syndrome
Early repolarization syndrome
Short QT syndrome

recent MI[53,54] and LV dysfunction,[55-57] and it appears that approximately 50% of this decreased risk is due to reductions in sudden death.[53] Beta-blockers have been shown to suppress ventricular arrhythmias among patients at elevated risk[58,59] and may reduce death when used as primary antiarrhythmic therapy.[60] Use of HMG-CoA reductase inhibitors ("statins") has been associated with a lower risk of sudden death compared with nonuse in several studies.[61-63] However, there are no large randomized controlled trials to confirm this finding. Trials of angiotensin-converting enzyme inhibitors and angiotensin receptor blockers in patients with heart failure and coronary disease have shown reductions in the risk of sudden cardiac death in these populations.[64] Omega-3 fatty acids ("fish oils") appear to reduce the risk of sudden cardiac death in epidemiologic studies[41,65] and in prospective randomized trials.[66,67] A report[68] has raised methodological concerns on one of these prospective trials.[67] A recent randomized trial designed to look at the effect of highly purified omega-3 fatty acids on secondary prevention of sudden cardiac death after MI showed no benefit,[69] possibly related to a low event rate in both groups. Aldosterone inhibition (spironolactone, eplerenone) has also been shown to be useful in preventing sudden death in patients with heart failure and after MI. While more widespread use of automated external defibrillator (AED) therapy was hoped to have a significant benefit in the prevention of sudden death, the Home AED Trial (HAT) failed to show a survival benefit of an AED in addition to CPR versus CPR alone among a large group of patients with a history of prior MI.[70]

Catheter ablation and surgery are often effective in preventing recurrent VT in patients who are difficult to treat by other means. Both techniques attempt to destroy or "ablate" involved myocardial tissue to interrupt reentrant VT circuits, thus preventing the development of sustained arrhythmias. In the past, VT surgery was considered a primary form of therapy in experienced centers, as it could offer a cure to patients with few other therapeutic options.[71-74] Currently, VT surgery has a limited role owing to very high operative morbidity and mortality and improved nonsurgical approaches. Catheter ablation is a technique using intracardiac catheters to induce VT, map the pathologic circuits or substrate, and ablate small areas of involved myocardial tissue with radiofrequency energy.[75,76] Ablation may carry a lower procedural risk than open surgical approaches, but a substantial number of patients have recurrent ventricular arrhythmias.[74,77] Thus, it is presently not a replacement for ICD therapy. VT related to ischemic heart disease may be difficult to manage with catheter ablative procedures,[77,78] owing to multiple pathologic intracardiac circuits. Like antiarrhythmic drugs, VT ablation is used as an adjunct to decrease the frequency of ICD therapy rather than a means to prevent sudden death.[79]

Revascularization is of primary importance in patients with coronary artery disease and malignant ventricular arrhythmias. One study evaluated the role of ICD in patients undergoing coronary artery bypass grafting (CABG) and showed no benefit in this population.[80] Other studies have demonstrated an association between CABG and decreased risk of sudden death.[11,81,82] Two randomized trials of ICD therapy early following MI found no difference in mortality with usual medical care versus an ICD[9,11] (see Clinical Trials).

Lifestyle factors have been associated with lower risks of sudden death. Tobacco avoidance, exercise, moderate alcohol consumption,[83] and a diet rich in fish[65] have all been shown to be protective, and lifestyle modification programs may prevent sudden death.[84,85]

Implantable Cardioverter-Defibrillator Therapy

DEVICE BASICS

The ICD is composed of two parts: the pulse generator and the leads. The generator consists of batteries; a capacitor for charging and discharging ("shocking"); electronic circuits that monitor, analyze, and guide treatment of arrhythmias; and information storage capabilities. Additional capabilities are available in current devices.

The pulse generators of early devices were large (approximately 250 cm³) and required surgical implantation in the abdomen. Leads were large (150 to 180 cm²) epicardial pads placed via a thoracotomy. Separate epicardial screw-in sensing leads were also required. Implantation was associated with significant perioperative morbidity and mortality. Rhythm analysis was rudimentary and relatively insensitive. Only medium- or high-energy shock therapy was available, and data storage capacity was limited to information regarding the number of shocks. When intracardiac electrogram storage and analysis became available, it was apparent that inappropriate shocks, predominantly for atrial fibrillation, were common.[86,87]

The initial primary purpose of the ICD was to detect VT and VF and terminate these arrhythmias with effective defibrillation. Reports of early experiences suggested a substantially lower annual mortality among ICD recipients versus similar historical comparative groups.[88] Recent refinements in ICD technology have improved the safety and tolerability of the devices substantially, but effective defibrillation remains the crucial lifesaving feature.

Current devices are much smaller, allowing subpectoral or subcutaneous implantation. Using nonthoracotomy lead systems, implantation methods are identical to permanent pacemaker implantation. Local anesthetic with mild sedation is used for implantation; heavy sedation or a brief general anesthetic is needed to test defibrillation thresholds. Operative mortality for nonthoracotomy systems is less than 0.5%.[89] The risk of defibrillator-threshold or safety-margin testing is estimated to be less than 0.05% for death or stroke and less than 0.2% for necessitating prolonged resuscitation, based on a large series of registry data.[90] This risk is higher in patients with severe LV dysfunction where even a brief induction of VF can have persistent and detrimental efffects.[90,91] Obesity, cachexia, limited vascular access, pulmonary hypertension, anticoagulation, bleeding disorders, and vascular or cardiac anomalies may increase the technical challenge of implantation. Tricuspid valve prosthesis or significant tricuspid valvular disease may preclude use of endocardial lead systems. Features of contemporary ICD systems are listed in Table 81-1.

COMPLICATIONS RELATED TO TRANSVENOUS ICD PLACEMENT

Although placement of a transvenous ICD system is routine in many centers, complications related to system placement do occur. Common procedural complications are summarized in Box 81-2.

THERAPEUTIC FUNCTIONS

Bradycardia and Pacing

Patients with significant heart failure commonly have symptomatic bradycardia due to conduction disturbances, inadequate chronotropic

TABLE 81-1	Features of Current Implantable Cardioverter-Defibrillators
Size	30-45 cm³
Weight	70-100 g
Batteries	Low-resistance lithium or silver vanadium for charging defibrillation capacitor; separate battery for pacing functions
Leads	Steroid-eluting, silicone- or polyurethane-coated, 4-9F (1.3–3 mm) caliber, depending on type; ports for ventricular, atrial, left ventricular (coronary sinus), and superior vena cava leads
Output, charge	30-39 J (delivered), 750-800 V
Battery life	3-8 yr, depending on manufacturer, device, and use
Arrhythmia detection	Rate-based; enhanced ventricular tachycardia detection features vary by device and manufacturer
Arrhythmia management	Defibrillation with biphasic waveform, low-energy cardioversion, antitachycardia pacing (ATP) features; atrial therapies, including ATP and cardioversion; bradycardic ventricular and dual chamber pacing; biventricular pacing
Storage capabilities	Device and lead identification, implantation date, physician contact; arrhythmia event data, including date and time, onset, heart rate, therapies delivered, shock counters, rate histograms, electrograms, marker channel; pacemaker functions, including pacing thresholds, lead impedances, R-wave and P-wave amplitude, percent pacing, heart failure diagnostic information
Programmable functions	Pacing parameters, tachyarrhythmic therapies, tiered therapy algorithms; many other refined programmed functions vary by manufacturer

responses, and medications that induce bradycardia.[29] Moreover, post-cardioversion and postshock bradycardia is common among ICD patients. To meet these needs, all current ICDs have pacing capabilities. ICD systems are available with ventricular, dual-chamber, or biventricular pacing modalities.

Although patients who receive an ICD may have an indication for single or dual-chamber pacing, there are concerns about the potential adverse effects of right ventricular pacing. One major trial showed that atrioventricular sequential pacing at a rate of 70 beats per minute was associated with higher rates of heart failure, hospitalization, or death when compared with backup ventricular pacing at 40 beats per minute.[92] This effect was ascribed to the untoward hemodynamic effects of right ventricular pacing. Other studies have supported this finding.[93] Furthermore, pacing can precipitate ventricular tachyarrhythmias in some patients.[94] Thus, the pacemaker backup rate should be turned down to the lowest acceptable rate in patients with LV dysfunction.

Biventricular pacing, or resynchronization therapy, is a pacing modality incorporated in some devices. The intent of biventricular pacing is not to treat bradycardia per se. Instead, it coordinates synchronous left and right ventricular contraction.[95] In the presence of left bundle branch block or right ventricular pacing, the interventricular septum moves rightward during systole. This decreases the

contribution of septal contraction to LV output, leading to less efficient LV systolic function. Biventricular pacing coordinates left and right ventricular contraction to minimize this effect. The left ventricle is approached through the venous system (coronary sinus) using specially designed leads to allow epicardial LV pacing.

Several studies evaluated biventricular pacing in patients with advanced symptomatic heart failure (NYHA III-IV) and significant intraventricular conduction delay (QRS duration ≥ 120 milliseconds).[13,96-98] Results show improvements in symptoms, exercise tolerance, and quality of life[99] among a significant proportion of these selected patients. A survival benefit has also been demonstrated (Table 81-2).[13,98,100] More recent studies looking at less severe heart failure (NYHA I-II) have demonstrated a decrease in symptomatic heart failure episodes and favorable LV remodeling without a survival benefit.[101,102] Another trial in less symptomatic patients (RAFT) will be reported later this year.[103] Heart failure patients with QRS durations less than 120 milliseconds have not been shown to benefit from cardiac resynchronization therapy (CRT),[104] but studies addressing methods other than QRS duration are ongoing (EchoCRT).

Tachyarrhythmia Detection

The primary method of detecting sustained VT is assessment of ventricular rate and duration of the tachycardia. Therapy is delivered for persistent heart rates exceeding a cutoff that is manually programmed. Different algorithms can be programmed for different rates (Figure 81-1). The major limitation of an exclusively rate-based rhythm analysis is that tachycardias other than VT (e.g., supraventricular tachycardia [SVT]) cannot be distinguished by rate alone.

Enhanced arrhythmia detection features in current dual-chamber systems enable sensitive and specific detection of VT and VF, decreasing the occurrence of inappropriate therapies.[105-110] Onset criteria allow the distinction between sinus tachycardia, which generally has a gradual onset, and VT, which is abrupt. Rate stability criteria distinguish irregular atrial fibrillation from VT. Devices also use the intracardiac electrogram to identify VT. Analysis of QRS morphology during tachycardia compared with a sinus rhythm template is a feature found in many single and dual-chamber devices. Dual-chamber devices use atrial lead sensing to evaluate the relationship between ventricular and atrial activity to distinguish supraventricular tachycardia from VT.[109] Judicious use of these features is highly sensitive for VT and specific for discrimination of SVT. Another method used to limit ICD shocks is to increase the number of intervals to detect before the device treats the arrhythmia. This prevents unnecessary therapies for arrhythmias that would otherwise have self-terminated, but with the tradeoff of an increased likelihood of syncope from the delay in administration of therapy.[111,112] Trials assessing the utility of delayed detection are ongoing.[113] Combining multiple algorithms to withhold unnecessary ICD shocks (SVT, noise, and more frequent use of antitachycardia pacing [ATP]) also holds promise.

Tachyarrhythmic Therapies: Tiered Therapy Algorithms

Using the methods outlined previously, the ICD detects arrhythmias and administers therapies as programmed. In contrast to early devices, current ICDs can deliver therapies other than defibrillation, including lower-energy cardioversion and ATP. Some devices also have atrial antitachycardia and cardioversion features, whose clinical benefit remains to be proven.[114,115] A tiered therapy algorithm (see Figure 81-1) uses different "zones" of detection to preferentially administer ATP or shocks depending on the rapidity of the detected rhythm.

High-energy defibrillation is the primary and most important function of the ICD. It is highly effective for VF or very rapid VT. Other therapies are intended to abort hemodynamically tolerated VT to obviate a painful high-energy shock. Typically, tachycardias above 200 beats per minute are promptly treated with high-voltage shocks. If the ICD detects a ventricular rhythm in the "VF zone," the battery charges the capacitor, which then discharges, or "shocks," if a second rhythm analysis confirms ongoing VF. Current is transmitted between the right ventricular lead and either the device itself ("active" or "hot" can) or

Box 81-2

COMPLICATIONS OF CARDIOVERTER-DEFIBRILLATOR IMPLANTATION

Direct anesthetic risks
Risk of inducing ventricular fibrillation/defibrillation
Atrial and ventricular arrhythmias
Bleeding/hematoma
Embolism (thrombus, air)
Vessel or organ injury (nerve, plexus)
Pneumothorax/hemothorax
Subclavian/axillary venous thrombosis or stenosis
Lead dislodgement
Extracardiac stimulation (e.g., phrenic nerve stimulation)
Cardiac valve injury
Cardiac perforation or pericardial tamponade
Infection

TABLE 81-2	Randomized Implantable Cardioverter-Defibrillator

Trials

Trial and Year of Publication	Sample Size (N)	Treatment Arms	Patient Characteristics	Mortality Benefit (Annualized Absolute Risk Reduction)	Comments
Cardiac Arrest Survivors (Secondary Prevention)					
AVID[3] 1997	1016	ICD vs amiodarone	Mixed etiologies (81% CAD) LVEF ≤ 0.40	4%	Largest secondary prevention trial Quality-of-life assessment showed neutral effects of ICD
CIDS[5] 2000	659	ICD vs amiodarone	Mixed causes (80%-90% CAD)	2%	Trends similar to AVID Possible benefit of ICD on quality of life
CASH[6] 2000	288	ICD vs amiodarone vs metoprolol	Mixed etiologies (75% CAD)	2%	Propafenone arm discontinued owing to increased mortality Metoprolol and amiodarone performed similarly
Patients at Risk of Sudden Death (Primary Prevention)					
MADIT[7] 1996	196	ICD vs no ICD	100% CAD LVEF ≤ 0.35 Inducible, nonsuppressible VT	5%	Demonstrated a benefit of primary prevention ICD therapy Small sample size
MADIT II[8] 2002	1232	ICD vs no ICD	100% CAD LVEF ≤ 0.30	3%	Survival benefit with ICD Largest primary prevention trial in patients with CAD
CABG-Patch[80] 1997	900	ICD vs no ICD	100% CAD undergoing CABG LVEF ≤ 0.35 Abnormal signal-averaged ECG	None	No survival benefit with ICD Revascularization in both groups may have attenuated benefits of ICD therapy
COMPANION[13] (2004)	1520	CRT-ICD vs CRT-pacer vs no device	Mixed etiologies (54%-59% CAD) LVEF ≤ 0.35 Symptomatic heart failure	7% CRT-ICD 4% CRT-pacer	CRT lowers risk of death Combination of an ICD + CRT had lowest risk of death CRT improved quality of life
DEFINITE[12] (2004)	458	ICD vs no ICD	Heart failure not related to CAD LVEF ≤ 0.35 Highly symptomatic heart failure	3%	Trend toward a survival benefit with ICD Non-CAD patients only
SCD-HeFT[10] (2005)	2521	ICD vs amiodarone vs placebo	Mixed etiologies (52% CAD) LVEF ≤ 0.35 Symptomatic heart failure	2%	Survival benefit with ICD Largest primary prevention trial Amiodarone did not alter survival
DINAMIT[11] (2004)	674	ICD vs no ICD	6-40 days post MI LVEF ≤ 0.35 Abnormal heart rate variability	None	No survival benefit with ICD Reduced rate of arrhythmic (4.9%) but increased rate of nonarrhythmic death (6.6%) with ICD over 2.5 years
IRIS[9] (2009)	898	ICD vs no ICD	5-31 days post MI EF ≤ 0.40 HR ≥ 90 BPM or NSVT ≥ 150 BPM	None	Similar to DINAMIT; no survival benefit with ICD Reduced rate of arrhythmic (5.9%) but increased rate of nonarrhythmic death (6.7%) with ICD over 3 years

AVID, Antiarrhythmics Versus Implantable Defibrillators; *CABG-Patch,* Coronary Artery Bypass Graft–Patch Trial; *CAD,* coronary artery disease; *CASH,* Cardiac Arrest Study Hamburg; *CIDS,* Canadian Implantable Defibrillator Study; *COMPANION,* Comparison of Medical Therapy, Pacing, and Defibrillation in Heart Failure; CRT, cardiac resynchronization therapy; *DEFINITE,* Defibrillators in Non-Ischemic Cardiomyopathy Treatment Evaluation; *DINAMIT,* Defibrillator in Acute Myocardial Infarction; *ICD,* implantable cordioverter-defibrillation; *LVEF,* left ventricular ejection fraction; *MADIT,* Multicenter Automatic Defibrillator Trial; SCD-HeFT, Sudden Cardiac Death Heart Failure Trial; *IRIS,* Immediate Risk-Stratification Improves Survival.

other electrodes or coils.[116] The current passes through ventricular myocardium and depolarizes a proportion of myocytes with 27 to 35 J of energy, depending on the manufacturer and configuration. This depolarized mass of myocardium interrupts the fibrillating electrical wavefronts and terminates VF. After each therapy, the device reinstates a diagnostic algorithm to detect ongoing VT/VF. If the arrhythmia persists, the capacitor recharges, discharges, and continues this cycle of behavior until another rhythm is detected or the therapies are exhausted (e.g., 4–6 consecutive high-energy shocks for a single episode).

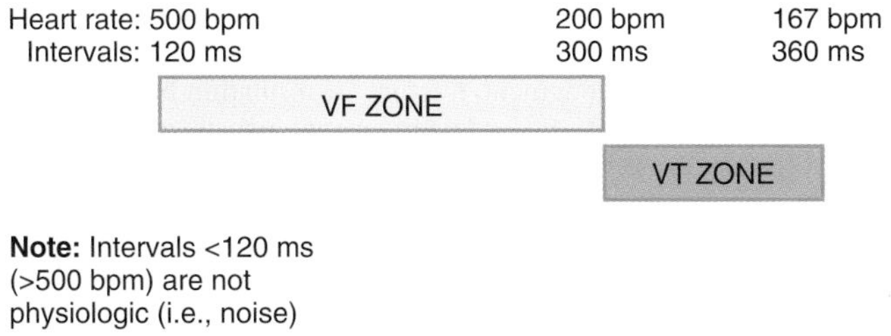

Heart rate: 500 bpm / 200 bpm / 167 bpm
Intervals: 120 ms / 300 ms / 360 ms

VF ZONE

VT ZONE

Note: Intervals <120 ms (>500 bpm) are not physiologic (i.e., noise)

Figure 81-1 Tiered ICD therapy zones. Contemporary ICD systems can be programmed with ventricular fibrillation (VF) and ventricular tachycardia (VT) detection zones to increase the use of antitachycardia pacing (ATP) therapies for slower rhythms (167-200 bpm) and shocks for fast arrhythmias over 200 bpm, as shown in this example.

The major limitation of high-energy shocks is the associated discomfort experienced if the patient remains conscious during the arrhythmia. Many patients report that shocks are painful and are associated with fear, embarrassment, or other unpleasant emotions.[117] Quality of life is significantly impaired in patients who receive ICD ≥ 5 shocks, from either the shock itself or the health condition necessitating the shock.[118,119] It is important to prevent ICD shocks, given that both appropriate and inappropriate shocks have been associated with an increased risk of death.[120] However, it is unclear whether the shock itself is responsible for the increased risk of death, or changes in the underlying condition both increase the occurrence of arrhythmias and the risk of death.

Low-energy cardioversion is an established method of terminating hemodynamically tolerated VT, with a success rate greater than 80%.[121,122] When the device detects a rhythm in the VT zone, it charges the capacitor and delivers a lower-energy shock synchronized to the R wave (see Figure 81-1). Energy outputs of 0.1 to 5 J can terminate some VT events. Patient discomfort increases substantially with increased output, particularly above 0.5 to 1 J. Above 5 to 10 J, no benefit is gained with low-energy cardioversion versus defibrillation in terms of patient comfort, although avoidance of high-energy output may prevent long-term device dysfunction[123,124] and prolong battery life. The other major risks of low-energy cardioversion are acceleration of the tachycardia rate, which occurs in up to 10% of cases, and delay of definitive therapy.[122] Less commonly, cardioversion can cause the rhythm to degenerate to polymorphic VT or VF, necessitating defibrillation. ATP is generally favored over shocks to limit the problem.

ATP, when effective, is ideal therapy for terminating hemodynamically tolerated VT. ATP is painless, although awareness of palpitations can occur. ATP is usually the initial therapy attempted for episodes of VT, because success rates are similar to those obtained with low-energy cardioversion; up to 90% of VTs can be terminated with pacing.[125-127]

ATP is more complex than defibrillation or cardioversion. The principle is to deliver pacing stimulation to the ventricle to gain control over the reentrant circuit that is perpetuating the tachycardia (overdrive suppression). If pacing is effective in entering the VT circuit, when pacing is terminated, the patient's native or paced control over ventricular depolarization is restored. In order to enter the circuit, pacing must occur in the excitatory gap when the ventricle is not refractory to stimulation, and the device must pace at a rate faster than the VT rate. Rates with a cycle length between 70% and 90% of the VT cycle length (i.e., approximately 10% to 40% faster) are most effective in terminating the tachycardia.[125,127] ATP techniques intended to improve entry into the circuit and termination of the tachycardia have been developed. Manufacturers do not share a standard nomenclature to describe ATP algorithms, but each method employs several comparatively simple principles. Burst pacing delivers a series of several beats at a fixed cycle length. Ramp pacing progressively shortens cycle length (i.e., accelerates). Adaptive therapy modes allow pacing at differing rates, depending on the VT rate. Scanning allows the device to introduce pacing at varying points in the VT cycle. In the setting of VT, the device delivers several different ATP protocols in an attempt to terminate the tachycardia.

Atrial therapies incorporated in some devices include ATP and cardioversion. Their effectiveness in preventing and terminating atrial arrhythmias has been demonstrated,[114,128,129] but the clinical value of this approach remains controversial. It is very uncommon to implant a device to treat atrial arrhythmias solely, but this is occasionally done in highly symptomatic patients who are intolerant of medical therapy.

Clinical Trials

As discussed earlier, prevention of sudden cardiac death has focused on a population of patients with LV dysfunction and heart failure, a group shown to be at high risk for arrhythmic death.

Many large (N > 100) randomized controlled trials assessing the efficacy of ICD therapy have been completed (see Table 81-2).[3-13,80] Three large trials assessed the role of ICD therapy as secondary prevention of sudden cardiac death among patients with ischemic LV dysfunction and sustained, hemodynamically significant ventricular arrhythmias.[3,5,6] The largest of these trials (Antiarrhythmics versus Implantable Defibrillators [AVID]) randomized 1016 patients with symptomatic VT or VF and LV dysfunction (LV ejection fraction < 0.40) to therapy with ICD versus antiarrhythmic drugs (82.4% amiodarone).[3] This study was stopped before completion of enrollment because of a statistically significant survival benefit (11.3% absolute risk reduction at 3 years) of the ICD. The Canadian Implantable Defibrillator Study (CIDS)[5] and the Cardiac Arrest Study Hamburg (CASH)[6] demonstrated trends toward decreased mortality, but these findings were not statistically significant. Meta-analysis of these three randomized trials supported data consistency, with a significant relative reduction in mortality risk of 28% (95% confidence interval [CI] 13%–40%).[130]

Several primary prevention trials assessed the role of ICD therapy among patients at risk for but without clinically sustained VT or VF.[4,7,8,80] Although inclusion criteria varied, enrollment in these trials focused on patients with LV dysfunction. Similar to the secondary prevention trials, results of the primary prevention trials were consistent. Mortality reductions in the primary and secondary prevention trials have demonstrated similar results (see Table 81-2). From these studies it is clear ICD therapy reduces annual mortality by 2% to 7% in most patient groups. These studies also indicate that patients with both ischemic and nonischemic etiologies of LV dysfunction benefit

from ICD therapy and that amiodarone has a limited role in the prevention of sudden death in patients with heart failure.

All but three of the primary prevention trials demonstrated a mortality benefit from ICD therapy. As previously discussed, routine aggressive coronary artery revascularization was likely responsible for the lack of benefit from routine ICD therapy in the CABG-Patch Trial.[80] This inference is supported by a lower than anticipated mortality rate in that trial and the fact that the ICD resulted in a significantly lower rate of arrhythmic death.[82] ICD therapy also did not reduce the risk of death in DINAMIT or IRIS (see Table 81-2). Similar to CABG-Patch, the proportion of arrhythmic deaths to the total deaths in these trials was also lower than anticipated.[9,11] The lack of benefit from ICD therapy in these three studies illustrates that when considering a patient for an ICD, careful thought must be given to the long-term risk of arrhythmic death and the competing modes of death. ICDs have less impact with reduced rates of arrhythmic death.

A marked increase in the number of ICDs is occurring because of these trials. It is worth emphasizing that ICD therapy is costly,[131,132] and the magnitude of benefit is sensitive to baseline risk.[133] Studies to date have assessed ICD therapy in relatively high-risk populations, but even within these populations, risk appears to vary substantially. For example, in AVID, no benefit was observed among the subgroup of patients with an LV ejection fraction greater than 0.35.[30] Whether ICD therapy is appropriate in lower-risk high-risk patients, particularly those with relatively preserved LV ejection fraction, remains to be determined. Further studies will aid in determining whether ICD therapy in such patients provides no benefit, small but costly benefit, small but clinically important benefit, or harm.

Device-Related Issues Among Patients in Intensive Care

DEVICE INTERROGATION

To perform device interrogation, an analyzer header must be placed directly over the generator or, in newer devices, the wireless connection must be initiated. Devices from different manufacturers require brand-specific programmers. ICD patients are provided with device information and contact telephone numbers so that device type can be determined in the event of an emergency. If this information is unavailable, an overpenetrated chest x-ray will reveal identifying markers on the pulse generator. Interrogation of the device determines the manufacturer, model, settings, recorded events, and battery and lead parameters. Implanting centers generally provide around-the-clock interrogation and reprogramming. In smaller and more remote facilities, if emergent device interrogation or reprogramming is required, the device manufacturer can generally provide guidance on how to get the device interrogated in that region and advise about the use of magnets for suspending therapies. It is worth reemphasizing that the application of a magnet will suspend detection of VT and VF by the ICD. In contrast, a magnet turns off sensing, resulting in asynchronous pacing (e.g., AOO, VOO or DOO pacing modes) when applied to a pacemaker.

LEAD FAILURE

Lead failure due to dislodgment, fracture, or insulation breach occurs in 5% to 10% of patients, and lead replacement is usually required.[134-136] Risk of lead failure is higher with a subclavian route compared with a cephalic vein approach, owing to the compressive effects of the clavicle and first rib on the subclavian vein.[135] Lead failure is also more likely in younger patients, as well as certain specific leads that have been subject to manufacture advisory.[137] Presenting complaints include inappropriate shocks, syncope or presyncope from device failure to deliver therapy, or proarrhythmia. Increased defibrillation thresholds can occur in the absence of lead defects, dislodgment, or change in physiologic conditions from ischemia, electrolyte abnormalities, or antiarrhythmic medications. This is thought to be due to myocardial fibrosis at the point of contact of the defibrillation lead. Frequent shocks appear to exacerbate this response. Steroid-eluting leads attenuate the inflammatory-fibrotic myocardial response and the associated increase in thresholds.

PACING FUNCTION PROBLEMS

Oversensing occurs when the pacemaker detects electrical activity that is not due to chamber depolarization. It is suspected when the heart rate falls below the programmed lower pacing rate limit or when surface lead channels or intracardiac electrograms appear "noisy." This activity may be due to electrical activity in another cardiac chamber (far-field sensing), T-wave sensing, diaphragmatic or pectoral myopotentials, or electromagnetic interference. In this situation, the device fails to pace appropriately. Solutions to oversensing include increasing the sensing thresholds, switching from unipolar to bipolar pacing mode, avoiding electromagnetic interference, or repositioning/replacing the lead.

Undersensing occurs when the device fails to detect chamber depolarizations. This is usually detected as extra pacing spikes, with or without associated capture, depending on the timing. Undersensing may be due to poor lead contact with the myocardium, defects of the lead insulation or coil, inadequate device programming, device malfunction, or changes in physiologic conditions such as myocardial ischemia or electrolyte abnormalities. Chest x-ray to assess lead position and integrity, as well as device interrogation to assess lead impedance, are required.

Failure to capture occurs when pacemaker spikes do not trigger ventricular depolarization. This may occur because the ventricle is refractory, insufficient energy is delivered, or the lead contact is inadequate. Chest x-ray and pacemaker interrogation are required to assess lead position and pacing thresholds.

Paced tachycardias can occur. This is due to either inappropriate tracking of atrial tachyarrhythmias or pacemaker-mediated (endless loop) tachycardia by a dual-chamber device. Dual-chamber pacemakers may sense atrial tachycardias such as atrial fibrillation or atrial flutter and pace the ventricle at inappropriately rapid rates. Pharmacologic management of the atrial arrhythmia, decreasing the upper pacing rate of the ventricle, or enabling mode-switching function to avoid tracking the atrial rhythm will correct this problem. Pacemaker-mediated tachycardia occurs with dual-chamber devices but is less common than in the past because of automatic recognition and prevention algorithms. When ventricular pacing is associated with ventricle-to-atrium conduction, an endless loop of ventricular pacing, ventricle-to-atrium conduction, atrial sensing, and ventricular pacing can develop. Reprogramming to extend the postventricular atrial refractory period (PVARP) resolves pacemaker-mediated tachycardia.

INFECTION

Infections involving ICDs have been reported to occur in 1% to 16% of patients.[138-140] This is a devastating complication carrying substantial morbidity and reported mortality as high as 10%.[141,142] *Staphylococcus epidermidis* and *Staphylococcus aureus* cause the majority of infections, although any pathogenic bacteria or fungus can theoretically seed the device. Infection in the first several months following implantation usually results from bacterial contamination with skin colonizers introduced during or immediately after the implantation procedure.[143] Late device infections (>1 year after implantation) are equally common[144] and usually implicate primary sources of bacteremia other than the ICD.[145-147]

Diagnosis of device infection is often challenging. Clinical suspicion must be high in patients with an implanted device who present with fever, weight loss, fatigue, systemic inflammation, or pulmonary embolism.[141,148] All ICD or pacemaker patients with fever of uncertain cause should undergo careful examination of the generator pocket site for signs of inflammation, and blood cultures should be performed. In patients with proven bacteremia or fungemia, transthoracic and transesophageal echocardiography may be helpful.[149] The presence of *S. aureus* bacteremia—given its association with device endocarditis (54%-72%)—should be approached with the presumption that the device is infected and warrants transesophageal echocardiography (TEE) to help guide duration of antibiotic therapy.[150]

Treatment of confirmed ICD system infection requires extraction of all device components, a prolonged (e.g., 2-6 weeks) intensive antibiotic course, and reimplantation.[144] The optimal duration of antibiotic therapy is uncertain, and individualized timing of reimplantation is important in patients at high risk for life-threatening arrhythmias or those who are pacemaker dependent. When infection is suspected but unconfirmed, a trial of prolonged antibiotic therapy and close clinical vigilance for relapse may obviate system extraction. The risk of occult lead infection among patients with staphylococcal bacteremia is high,[149,151] and consideration should be given to extraction,[151] especially if relapse of infection occurs.

Peri-implantation antistaphylococcal antibiotic prophylaxis for pacemakers and ICDs is recommended.[143,152,153] Endocarditis prophylaxis for subsequent invasive procedures, especially in the first 6 months post implant in patients with ICDs or pacemakers who have no other indications, remains controversial and is not universally recommended.[14]

ARRHYTHMIAS AND ANTIARRHYTHMIC DRUGS

Patients with ICDs are at high risk for atrial and ventricular tachyarrhythmias. Management of these arrhythmias generally does not differ from the usual therapy for patients without ICDs. In fact, more liberal use of rate-slowing and proarrhythmic medications is permissible owing to the protective effects of backup pacing and defibrillation. Observing device behavior during arrhythmias is important because it may influence management decisions. For example, if a short burst of rapid ventricular pacing is observed during a patient's tachycardia, it is likely that the device is undertaking an ATP algorithm for termination of VT. If the mechanism of the tachycardia is atrial fibrillation with rapid ventricular response, this will inevitably lead to the device escalating to shock therapy to treat the rhythm. Urgent slowing of the ventricular rate may prevent the impending inappropriate shocks. In patients with atrial or ventricular tachyarrhythmias, device-based termination with ATP should not be overlooked as a therapeutic option. Simple reprogramming of the device may be all that is required to resolve a failure of the device to detect and treat ventricular and regular atrial arrhythmia.

ICD patients often receive additional antiarrhythmic therapy to prevent device-provided therapies.[154] These antiarrhythmics may decrease the frequency of VT and VF and thus decrease the need for defibrillation therapies, avoiding patient discomfort. Moreover, most antiarrhythmics will increase the tachycardia cycle length and make the arrhythmia more hemodynamically stable. A handful of drugs have been studied in the prevention of ICD shocks:

- Sotalol has been shown to be effective at preventing shocks but carries an early drug discontinuation rate of approximately 25% over 1 year, mostly related to its beta-blocking side effects.[155-157]
- Beta-blockers are also effective at preventing shocks and, when compared to sotalol, are either equivalent,[158] superior,[159] or tend to be inferior.[157] Regardless of the exact magnitude of effect compared to sotalol, given the low risk associated with beta-blockers, this drug class should be used and maximized in every patient.
- Azimilide, a class III antiarrhythmic drug that blocks rapid and slow delayed rectifier potassium current appears to be a promising drug for ICD shock prevention. Trials show that this drug is highly effective at reducing ICD shocks,[160,161] as well as VT storm,[161] while being tolerated as well as placebo. Adverse effects under review for U.S. Food and Drug Administration (FDA) approval include a small risk of torsades de pointes and neutropenia.
- Amiodarone[154] is highly effective in treating VT and SVT. In the OPTIC trial,[157] amiodarone plus beta-blockers was superior to beta-blockers alone or sotalol in preventing ICD shocks. Early

drug discontinuation in this trial was similar for amiodarone and sotalol.

- Dofetilide may decrease time to first ICD shock but does not appear to decrease the frequency of ventricular arrhythmias and may cause torsades de pointes.[162]
- Dronedarone, although effective at suppressing ventricular arrhythmias, needs further large trial data before advocating its widespread use.
- Class I antiarrhythmic drugs, though avoided in general, are occasionally used in ICD patients to decrease occurrences of VT.

Using antiarrhythmic drugs is a double-edged sword. Despite their effectiveness, they each have their own known side-effect profile. Most will decrease the tachycardia cycle length. This makes the VT more hemodynamically stable and more amenable to termination with antitachycardia pacing. However, one has to consider the programmed tachycardia detection interval of the ICD to ensure that the VT is within its treatment range. This may also mean that a tachycardia that once caused syncope will now be treated while the patient is fully aware and conscious. Although it seems somewhat intuitive to consider reprogramming the ICD when managing VT/VF with antiarrhythmics, this process can easily be overlooked when the reason for initiating these drugs is to treat SVT, such as atrial fibrillation. Another important point to consider is the effects of these drugs on pacing and defibrillation threshold. Class I drugs, except propafenone,[163] and chronic amiodarone use[164] have this effect, which may be clinically important in patients whose defibrillation threshold is close to the maximum output of the device. In a substudy of OPTIC,[165] defibrillation threshold was increased by 1.29 J with amiodarone and beta-blocker, compared to a decrease of 0.89 J with sotalol and a decrease of 1.67 J with beta-blockers alone. In most patients, this variation is well within their defibrillator safety margin. However, if amiodarone therapy is initiated, consideration should be given to follow-up testing of device function in patients with high thresholds at baseline.[166] Another unintended effect of these drugs is that they may increase pacemaker dependence and result in increased right ventricular pacing which may have detrimental effects concerning LV function. In a monitored hospital setting, these issues are less important, but consultation with an electrophysiologist or a cardiologist familiar with the patient's device and its programming should be obtained with regard to introduction of antiarrhythmic drugs for long-term use.

CATHETER ABLATION TO REDUCE ICD THERAPIES

Aside from the issues with antiarrhythmics already discussed, these drugs are limited by their efficacy, patient compliance, and side-effect profiles. VT catheter ablation is an attractive option in some patients as a means to decrease ICD therapies. The efficacy of this approach has been demonstrated in two single-center trials.[76,167] Multicenter trials dealing predominantly with an ischemic heart disease population demonstrated a success rate of 41% for all inducible VTs, with a recurrence of sustained VT at 1 year of 56% in one trial,[168] compared to an another reporting a success rate of 49% for elimination of all inducible VTs with a recurrence of 47% at 6 months.[169] Although the absolute success rate is not fantastic, in both trials there was a substantial reduction in the frequency of VT documented in patients who had an ICD. There was, however, an increase in the frequency of VT in 20% of patients with an ICD in one of the studies.[169] Procedure-related deaths were 2.7% and 3% in these studies. There are no large multicenter trials for ICD patients with nonischemic VT, but this may be effective in some.

CARDIAC ARREST AND DIRECT-CURRENT CARDIOVERSION

Cardiopulmonary resuscitation and external direct-current cardioversion involve particular issues for patients with ICDs.[170,171] In principle, given the dire circumstances surrounding cardiac arrest, the presence of an ICD should not be a distraction to the resuscitation process.

Potential for device-related problems should be recognized. Cardiac compressions theoretically increase the risk of lead dislodgment, leading to asystole in pacemaker-dependent patients. Elective external cardioversion or emergent defibrillation exposes the device to potentially damaging high voltage.[172] Contemporary devices have incorporated elements that shunt energy away from the pulse generator. As a result, a circuit can develop, causing thermal damage at the lead/tissue interface and raise pacing and defibrillation thresholds.[173] Inadvertent reprogramming has been reported as well. Transient elevations in thresholds are common; however, failure to capture following cardiac arrest or cardioversion should prompt immediate assessment for lead dislodgment or potentially permanent lead failure. Direct-current cardioversion-defibrillation paddles should be placed as far from the pulse generator as possible in an anteroposterior position, and the lowest effective energy should be used.[170,171] Potential for electromagnetic interference from external defibrillation should be recognized, and applying a magnet over the ICD should be undertaken to disable the device.

For elective cardioversion, there are several special considerations.[170] Thought should be given to attempting programmed cardioversion through the device rather than externally. If external cardioversion is necessary, a device programmer should be available in the room for immediate assessment of abnormal device function. Given the potential for a transient increase in capture threshold, the practitioner should be prepared to externally pace if necessary. Pacing and sensing thresholds should be checked immediately after a successful cardioversion and then again in 24 hours if feasible. The local device clinic should be contacted before attempting elective cardioversion, if possible, to ensure that immediate assistance is available and to identify any device peculiarities in advance.

EVALUATION OF THE ICD RECIPIENT AFTER A SHOCK

Many ICD patients experience a shock within 2 years of implantation,[174] and most isolated appropriate device therapies do not require a change in treatment, although addition or increase of a beta-blocker, amiodarone, or sotalol may be considered. Symptoms and patient-perceived device behavior before the shock should be assessed. The presence of presyncope, syncope, or palpitations suggests that the shock was due to arrhythmia. It is important to identify precipitants of arrhythmia such as exercise, angina, noncompliance with medications, or symptoms of worsening heart failure. Unstable myocardial ischemia and electrolyte disturbances should be excluded and treated. Diagnosis of ischemic events after a shock is challenging, because pacing, antitachycardia pacing, and shocks can cause nonspecific abnormalities of the ST segments,[175] and cardiac markers are often transiently elevated.[176]

In addition to baseline clinical parameters, the initial assessment of a patient after a shock includes device interrogation. Patients' memory of the sequence of events can be inaccurate, and interrogation provides information about the heart rate and rhythm before therapy initiation, therapy attempts, rhythm response to therapy, and definitive therapy, including number of shocks. Such information is crucial for evaluating the appropriateness of the shock and possible precipitating events to allow tailored programming of the device. An approach to the management of a patient who has received ICD therapies is provided in Figure 81-2.

MULTIPLE SHOCKS AND ELECTRICAL STORM

Multiple repetitive shocks can occur in 10% to 20% of ICD patients.[174,177,178] When these occur, it is crucial to rapidly determine whether such therapies are appropriate. Frequent shocks are often highly psychologically distressing[179] and can result in a syndrome similar to posttraumatic stress disorder.[180] Sedation with benzodiazepines improves patient comfort and may decrease catecholamine-dependent arrhythmias.[181] If the shocks are inappropriate, tachyarrhythmia detection should be disabled by magnet application.

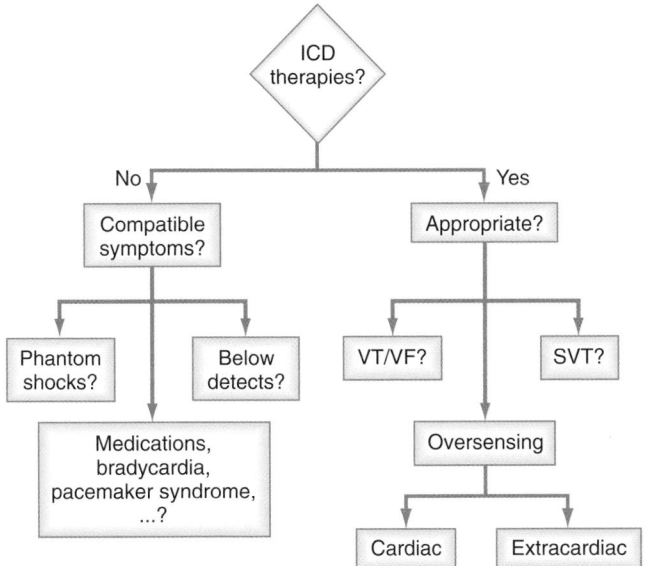

Figure 81-2 Approach to management of a patient with ICD therapies.

stepwise approach recommended for management of this condition is provided in Figure 81-3. After initial therapeutic maneuvers are performed, there may be a role in suppressing or limiting premature beats that may be triggering the arrhythmia. Transient overdrive pacing in this circumstance may be of some benefit. If AV conduction is intact, overdrive pacing from the atria might be less proarrhythmic than ventricular pacing. If amiodarone is ineffective, other antiarrhythmics may be used, depending on LV function. A recent single-center case series demonstrated the usefulness of VT ablation, where electrical storm was suppressed in 89% of patients after 1 to 3 procedures.[183]

ELECTROMAGNETIC INTERFERENCE

Several environmental and medical sources of electromagnetic interference can affect device functioning (Table 81-5).[170,184] Noise (electromagnetic interference) can be interpreted as rapid cardiac activity. Noise reversion algorithms on pacemakers prevent prolonged inhibition of pacing by activating an asynchronous pacing mode when prolonged noise is detected; however, asynchronous pacing can have adverse hemodynamic effects and can initiate ventricular arrhythmias. In ICDs, noise will be treated as VT/VF and if prolonged enough will result in therapies being delivered. In a pacemaker-dependent patient with an ICD, noise will result in inhibition of pacing until therapies are delivered, resulting in syncope which will mimic an appropriate shock.

MAGNETIC RESONANCE IMAGING

The functioning of ICDs can be adversely affected by magnetic resonance imaging (MRI) techniques and can create artifacts that limit image quality (see Table 81-5). There are several major potential risks of exposure to clinically relevant magnetic field strengths (0.2-3 T).[170,185] Magnetic force induces significant device torque, which can cause motion of the pulse generator, resulting in local pain, tissue damage, or device dislodgment.[186,187] Electromagnetic interference can precipitate rapid pacing or inadvertent therapies or interfere with sensing functions, leading to therapy inhibition. ICDs are more sensitive to inhibition of pacing than pacemakers are. Diathermy of the lead (heating) is well described, but its clinical significance is not known. Theoretically, heating of the lead tip can cause local tissue damage, myocardial perforation, or scar and increase sensing and pacing thresholds.[185] In addition to the risk to the patient, the presence of any foreign body with ferromagnetic properties can create imaging artifacts, limiting the diagnostic value of MRI scanning in the area of the pulse generator or leads.

The absolute risk of adverse events in routine clinical situations is unknown, because there are no large-scale studies. With current technology, the presence of an ICD or implanted pacemaker is considered a contraindication to MRI. In the rare case in which a patient is foreseen to require an implantable device but also requires an MRI, implantation may be deferred if the potential diagnostic benefit of MRI in the near future outweighs the risk of delaying device implantation. In situations in which the diagnostic value of MRI is considered essential to the care of an ICD patient, scanning should be considered

Urgent device reprogramming and therapy directed at the underlying condition (e.g., atrial tachyarrhythmias) is required. More than three episodes of VT/VF occurring within 24 hours is labeled an *electrical storm*. This ominous entity has been shown to predict an increased risk of non-sudden death in the next several months.[177] The incidence of electrical storm is approximately 1% to 2% per month in non-CRT recipients and less than 0.5% per month in CRT recipients (Table 81-3). The mean time to development of electrical storm is quite variable but is usually in the initial 6 months after ICD implantation.

Recurrent VT or VF is most appropriately treated with beta-blockade alone[182] or in combination with intravenous amiodarone.[174] Sedation with benzodiazepines may be beneficial. It is essential that potential precipitants for the electrical storm be sought. These include myocardial ischemia, electrolyte abnormalities, and a worsening in LV function/decompensated heart failure. Despite careful evaluation for such precipitants, a clear cause for the electrical storm event is not found in over half of patients (Table 81-4). Nonetheless, a careful search for these precipitants is necessary, since they are often amenable to intervention and will reduce the likelihood of recurrent VT/VF.[174] A

TABLE 81-3	Electrical Storm Triggers	
Myocardial ischemia/infarction		4-14%
Electrolyte/metabolic abnormality		4-10%
Worsening heart failure		9-19%
No clear cause		57-87%

TABLE 81-4	Electrical Storm Incidence							
	Year	N	Follow-Up (Months)	Storm		Time to Storm (Months)	Therapies	Higher Risk of Death
Villacastin[178]	1996	80	21	20%		—	Shocks	Yes
Credner[174]	1998	103	14	10%		4	Shocks/antitachycardia pacing (ATP)	Yes
Exner[177]	2001	457	31	20%	1%-2%	9	Shocks/ATP	Yes
Verma[189]	2004	2028	14	10%	per month	27	Shocks/ATP	Yes
Brigadeau[190]	2006	307	27	40%		<6	Shocks/ATP	No
Hohnloser[191]	2006	633	12	23%		3	Shocks/ATP	Yes
Sesselberg[192]	2007	719	21	4%	0.2%-0.4%	4	Shocks/ATP	Yes
Gasparini[193]	2008	631	19	7%	per month	6	Shocks/ATP	Yes

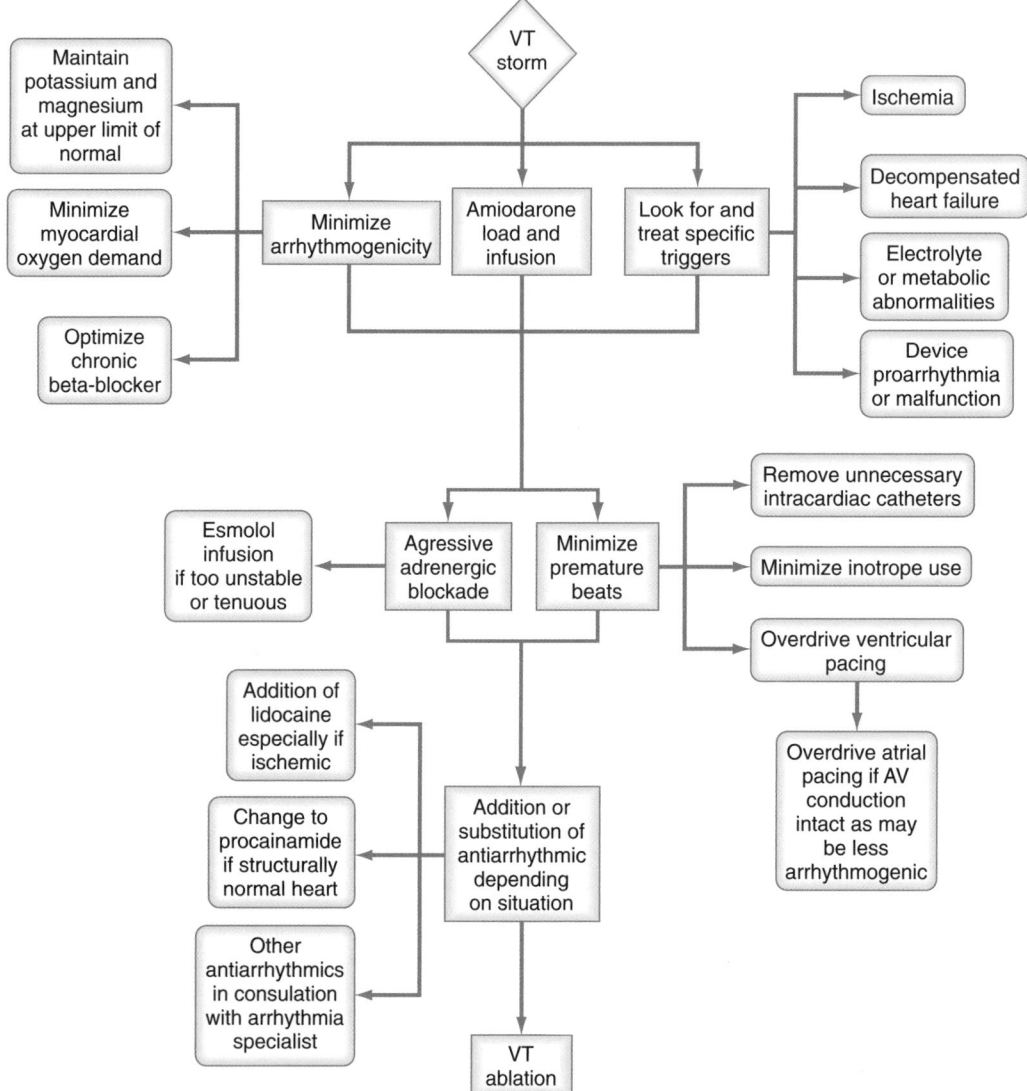

Figure 81-3   Stepwise approach to management of a patient with frequent, repetitive ICD therapies (electrical storm).

only after appropriately planning for the risks; a team prepared to address potentially life-threatening complications must be present to attend to the patient. Based on a few case series, MRI of extrathoracic regions can be undertaken with minimal risk as long as the proper precautions are taken.[188] "MRI-safe" ICDs and pacemakers represent a potential solution to this dilemma in some patients, and much progress has been made in their development over the last 5 years.

SURGERY

With careful planning, most if not all surgical procedures can be safely performed in ICD patients. ICD patients have a high burden of cardiovascular morbidity, and perioperative cardiac events (ischemia, heart failure, arrhythmias) are relatively common. Adherence to established guidelines for perioperative assessment,[171] appropriate consultation, and anticipation of potential complications may reduce complications. The greatest risks related to the device itself are malfunction due to electromagnetic interference, arrhythmia precipitation, and changes in defibrillation, pacing, and sensing thresholds due to anesthetic agents or metabolic changes.[171] Strategies to prevent complications from electromagnetic interference are listed in Table 81-5.

DISEASE PROGRESSION AND END-OF-LIFE ISSUES

Many ICD patients inevitably develop end-stage heart failure due to underlying disease progression. Upgrading an existing ICD system to include resynchronization should be considered. When standard therapies are exhausted, heart transplantation may be an option. In patients who are not transplant candidates, a symptom-directed palliative approach is undertaken. When patients indicate a desire for permanent disabling of the ICD VT/VF therapies, possible reversible transient precipitants such as depression or other mood disturbances should be sensitively explored. In many cases, deterioration in health such as an exacerbation of heart failure causes frustration, and patients may feel that treatments are futile.

Psychosocial support and discussion of the goals of therapy often clarify patients' motivations and desires. In truly terminal patients or in those who are clear and firm about their desire to discontinue ICD therapy, deactivation or disabling of VT/VF therapies, which is reversible, should be undertaken after full discussion of the medical, ethical, and legal ramifications. Disabling pacing functions is more challenging, particularly in those who are pacemaker dependent. This should be undertaken only after extensive discussion with the patient and family and should be performed in accordance with local policies.

TABLE 81-5	Sources of Electromagnetic Interference	
Source	*Potential Problems*	*Preventive Measures*
Imaging techniques (MRI)[170]	Device motion Diathermy (lead heating) Oversensing Reprogramming	MRI generally contraindicated. If unavoidable, program to asynchronous pacing mode and disable tachyarrhythmia therapies; resuscitation team must be available during imaging.
Surgical procedures involving electrosurgical (electrocautery) techniques[170,171,194]	Oversensing Spurious tachyarrhythmia therapies	Use alternative cutting and hemostatic techniques. Use bipolar electrocautery if working within 15 cm of the device and/or leads. Preoperative reprogramming (decrease sensitivity, asynchronous pacing, or noise reversion mode). Provide internal or external alternative pacing system for pacemaker-dependent patients. Peripheral monitoring (e.g., pulse oximeter). Place ground pad on leg to direct current away from pulse generator. Use brief bursts with pauses of at least 10 sec; use lowest power output possible and do not use near pulse generator. Assess and reprogram device immediately after procedure.
Muscle and nerve stimulators (including spinal, peripheral, and transcutaneous)	Oversensing	Test stimulator functioning, and interrogate device's sensed activity and response before use.
Radiotherapy	Cumulative dose-dependent pulse generator damage Prolonged charge time Battery depletion	Minimize dose. Shield device. Check device functioning after sessions.
Temporary intracardiac foreign bodies (including pulmonary artery catheters, temporary pacemakers, and instruments used in percutaneous coronary interventions)	Lead dislodgment	Avoid these manipulations with recently implanted devices. Use fluoroscopy or echocardiographic guidance if necessary.
Environmental (including cellular telephones, security systems [retail and airport], electrical equipment [including household appliances])[195]	Usually not problematic in an inpatient setting Possible interference with device sensing functions	Observe for unusual device behavior (rapid pacing, pacing inhibition, shocks) during use of electrical equipment near patient. Awareness of potential for interaction.
Other medical procedures (e.g., radiofrequency ablation, percutaneous coronary interventions, extracorporeal shock wave lithotripsy)[170]	Several case reports of interaction with devices	Device interrogation following exposure.

ATP, antitachycardia pacing; MRI, magnetic resonance imaging.

KEY POINTS

1. The implantable cardioverter-defibrillator (ICD) is the gold standard for treating patients with or at high risk of serious ventricular tachyarrhythmias. Familiarity with its function, malfunction, and associated clinical problems is required of all acute care practitioners.

2. Antiarrhythmic drugs and ablation methods may be used to treat concomitant arrhythmias or refractory life-threatening arrhythmias in ICD recipients.

3. Current ICDs have pacemaker (ventricular, dual chamber, or biventricular) functions and advanced anti-tachyarrhythmia therapies, including low-energy cardioversion, antitachycardia pacing (ATP), and defibrillation.

4. Device malfunction may include oversensing, undersensing, failure to capture, and paced tachycardias. Chest radiographs to assess lead position and device interrogation can help define the cause of abnormal device behavior.

5. ICD system infection is associated with high morbidity and mortality. Patients with unexplained fever, systemic inflammation, proven bacteremia, or pulmonary embolism should undergo careful examination of the pulse generator pocket, appropriate laboratory evaluation, and echocardiography to assess for lead vegetations.

6. Single ICD shocks are relatively common, and multiple repetitive shocks can occur. It is important to distinguish appropriate from inappropriate shocks and identify possible precipitants of ventricular arrhythmias such as exercise, myocardial ischemia, medication noncompliance, or electrolyte disturbance. If necessary, magnet application can suspend the tachyarrhythmia therapies to prevent repetitive non-lifesaving shocks.

7. Important medical interventions that may affect ICD function in the ICU include surgical electrocautery, magnetic resonance imaging, external cardioversion-defibrillation, cardiopulmonary resuscitation, insertion of pulmonary artery catheters, and the use of some antiarrhythmic drugs.

8. Disabling ICD functions should be performed only after considering and thoroughly discussing the medical, ethical, and legal implications.

ANNOTATED REFERENCES

Epstein AE, DiMarco JP, Ellenbogen KA, et al. ACC/AHA/HRS 2008 Guidelines for device-based therapy of cardiac rhythm abnormalities: a report of the American College of Cardiology/American Heart Association Task Force on Practice Guidelines. J Am Coll Cardiol 2008;51:e1-62. Available at http://content.onlinejacc.org/cgi/content/full/51/21/2085.
Summarizes expert opinion and evidence relevant to cardiac device utilization and provides guidelines for implantation and management of device therapy.
Poole JE, Johnson GW, Hellkamp AS, Anderson J, et al. Prognostic importance of defibrillator shocks in patients with heart failure. N Engl J Med 2008;359:1009-17.
Recent analysis of ICD shocks from a large clinical trial of patients with heart failure (SCD-HeFT). This work highlights the importance of ICD shocks, the need for careful patient evaluation, and for shock prevention where possible.

Mirowski M, Reid PR, Mower MM, et al. Termination of malignant ventricular arrhythmias with an implanted automatic defibrillator in human beings. N Engl J Med 1980;303:322-4.
Of historical interest, this original report of the effectiveness of the ICD to terminate recurrent life-threatening ventricular arrhythmias heralded the era of "device-based" therapy.
Pinski SL, Trohman RG. Interference in implanted cardiac devices. Pacing Clin Electrophysiol 2002;25:1367-81 (Part I) and 25:1496-1509 (Part II).
Two-part review of electromagnetic interference and ICD function; comprehensive summary of case reports and clinical studies. Recommendations for dealing with electromagnetic interference related to device therapy are included.

REFERENCES

Access the complete reference list online at http://www.expertconsult.com.

Severe Heart Failure

EDUARD SHANTSILA | BENJAMIN WRIGLEY | MICHAEL D. SOSIN | GREGORY Y.H. LIP

Heart failure is a very common condition with high mortality and morbidity rates. Data from the Framingham heart study suggest that at 40 years of age, the lifetime risk for congestive heart failure is 21.0% (95% confidence interval [CI], 18.7%-23.2%) for men and 20.3% (95% CI, 18.2%-22.5%) for women.[1] The prevalence of heart failure is between 2% and 3% and reaches 10% and 20% in those older than 70 years.[2] In the United States, approximately 5 million patients have heart failure, with over 550,000 new cases diagnosed each year.[3] Despite improvements in treatment, the overall prevalence of heart failure is increasing because of the aging of the population and better survival following myocardial infarction (MI).[3,4] Total heart failure–related costs were about $28 billion in 2005 and consume approximately 2% of national expenditure on health in Europe.[5] Patients with severe heart failure often present in extremis, and their condition may deteriorate rapidly, so a sound knowledge of immediate treatment is vital for critical care and emergency physicians. Such patients often respond rapidly to appropriate treatment, making this a very satisfying condition to treat. However, it is important to note that outlook remains poor despite initial clinical improvement.

In this chapter, we will discuss causes, presentation, investigation, treatment, and prognosis of severe heart failure, including new developments in the investigation and management of this common, serious condition.

Etiology

Ischemic heart disease is the most common cause of heart failure, commonly related to previous MI. Although epidemiologic surveys such as the Framingham study suggest a high prevalence of hypertension as the "cause" of heart failure, it is likely that associated ischemic heart disease or arrhythmias also contribute. Other studies have demonstrated similar findings (Table-82-1).

It should be pointed out that epidemiologic studies such as the Framingham study have been almost exclusively carried out in white populations, and etiologic factors may have different relative importance in other ethnic groups. For example, in Afro-Caribbeans, hypertension is the predominant etiologic factor, whereas in Indo-Asians, coronary artery disease and diabetes are common. It is important to note that different causes may coexist in the same patient.

ISCHEMIC HEART DISEASE

Ischemic heart disease is the most common cause of heart failure in the Western world. Many patients presenting with severe heart failure will give a history of previous MI. However, an episode of severe heart failure may also be the first manifestation of ischemic heart disease, either due to massive MI causing cardiogenic shock[6] or as a result of previous silent (or unreported) episodes of ischemia/infarction. It is therefore important to exclude MI in all patients presenting with severe heart failure. Additionally, once the patient is stabilized, adequate secondary preventive strategies are vital to prevent further ischemia or infarction. Some patients with ischemic cardiomyopathy may show evidence of "hibernation" of segments of myocardium,[7] and cardiac function in these patients may improve with revascularization (see later discussion).

HYPERTENSIVE HEART DISEASE

Hypertension causes a significant proportion of cases of heart failure. An episode of severe heart failure may be the first presentation of hypertension—such patients have had unrecognized severe hypertension for many years. The onset of heart failure may result in a previously raised blood pressure becoming normal or even low, which can make the diagnosis difficult in a patient with previously undiagnosed hypertension. Electrocardiography and echocardiography may show evidence of left ventricular hypertrophy. Patients with hypertension also commonly have diastolic dysfunction as a cause for heart failure. In this situation, systolic contraction is normal or minimally impaired, but the main abnormality is in diastolic relaxation and ventricular compliance. The incidence of diastolic abnormalities increases with age, and while the mortality rate associated with diastolic heart failure appears to be lower than that of systolic heart failure, it is still significant. To date, the ideal method of defining abnormal diastolic function has not been clearly ascertained.

DILATED CARDIOMYOPATHY

Dilated cardiomyopathy is defined as left ventricular dysfunction of unknown cause. It is therefore a diagnosis of exclusion, and a firm diagnosis of dilated cardiomyopathy can only be made in the presence of a normal coronary angiogram. Intensive investigation of patients with a label of dilated cardiomyopathy may yield a definite cause in at least 50% of cases (Table 82-2). As many as 30% of patients with dilated cardiomyopathy may have a genetic cause of the disease.[8]

Dilated cardiomyopathy can manifest at any age, and because heart failure may be perceived as a disease of the elderly, this can often result in misdiagnosis in younger patients.

VALVULAR HEART DISEASE

Structural Valve Disease

Valvular heart disease was once a leading cause of heart failure in the Western world. Owing to the rise in ischemic heart disease and the decrease in rheumatic fever, it is now less often the primary cause of an episode of severe heart failure. However, it is important not to discount significant valve disease in patients presenting with severe heart failure and to remember that signs may be difficult to elucidate in the acutely ill patient. Because all patients with severe heart failure should undergo echocardiography soon after admission, most if not all cases of significant valve disease should be detected. As noted earlier, after extensive MI, acute mitral regurgitation can develop, causing sudden-onset severe heart failure days after a patient's initial presentation with chest pain.

Functional Valve Disease

Patients with heart failure of any cause with dilation of the left ventricle and mitral valve ring can develop functional mitral regurgitation. This further reduces left ventricular performance; in selected patients, mitral valve repair or replacement may be indicated.

DIABETES

In addition to the role of diabetes as a risk factor for the development of ischemic heart disease and resultant heart failure, there is evidence

TABLE 82-1	Epidemiologic Studies of Etiology of Heart Failure			
Etiology	Teerlink et al. (31 Studies 1989-90) (%)	Framingham Heart Study* (%)		Hillingdon Study (%)
		Men	Women	
Ischemic	50	59	48	36
Nonischemic:	50	41	52	64
Hypertension	4	70	78	14
Idiopathic	18	0	0	0
Valvular	4	22	31	7
Other	10	7	7	10
Unknown	13	0	0	34

Data from Lip GYH, Beevers DG. ABC of heart failure: aetiology. BMJ 2000;320:104-7. Because of rounding, totals may not equal 100%.

*Total exceeds 100%, as coronary artery disease and hypertension were not considered as mutually exclusive causes.

for a distinct diabetic cardiomyopathy.[8] Current guidelines recognize diabetes as a risk factor for heart failure.[8] Hemoglobin A_{1c} levels have been shown to be an independent progressive risk factor for cardiovascular and total mortality and rehospitalization rate in heart failure patients.[9,10] All patients presenting with heart failure should be screened for diabetes, both for this reason and so that appropriate secondary prevention can be instituted.

OTHER POSSIBLE CAUSES OR EXACERBATING FACTORS

Rare causes of heart failure must always be considered, especially in younger patients, and these include amyloidosis and hemochromatosis. Another important cause is human immunodeficiency virus (HIV) infection, and HIV-associated cardiomyopathy has been well described. Given that HIV infection is considered pandemic by the World Health Organization, many more patients may present in this way in the future.

Patients with a long history of stable heart failure may decompensate as the result of a number of different factors. Intercurrent infection is a common cause of decompensation, and prompt recognition and treatment are important. Arrhythmias are also a common cause for decompensation of a previously stable heart failure patient, and a recent meta-analyses of 16 randomized clinical trials (53,969 patients) revealed that the presence of AF is associated with an adverse effect on total mortality, with an odds ratio of 1.40 (95% CI, 1.32-1.48).[11] Another common cause of decompensation is anemia, which is often poorly tolerated in patients with heart failure. A meta-analysis of 34

TABLE 82-2	Final Diagnoses in 1230 Patients with Initially Unexplained Cardiomyopathy	
Diagnosis	Number	Percentage
Idiopathic dilated cardiomyopathy	616	50
Myocarditis	111	9
Ischemic heart disease	91	7
Infiltrative cardiomyopathy	59	5
Peripartum cardiomyopathy	51	4
Hypertension	49	4
Human immunodeficiency virus infection	45	4
Connective tissue disease	39	3
Substance abuse	37	3
Familial	25	2
Valvular disease	19	1.5
Doxorubicin therapy	15	1
Endocrine disorder	11	1
Others	62	5.5

Data from Felker GM et al. Underlying causes and long term survival in patients with initially unexplained cardiomyopathy. N Engl J Med 2000;342:1077-84.

studies comprising 153,180 patients, of whom 37.2% were anemic, showed that adjusted mortality risk of anemia had a hazard ratio of 1.46 (95% CI, 1.26-1.69).[12] Poor prognosis associated with presence of atrial fibrillation or anemia was irrespective of left ventricular systolic function, either preserved or impaired.[11,12] It is vital to consider and treat such exacerbating conditions where appropriate.

Presentations of Severe Heart Failure

Severe heart failure can manifest in several ways. The patient may or may not have a previous history of heart failure or precipitating conditions such as angina or hypertension. It is important to note that gradual-onset heart failure can easily be mistaken for asthma, and patients presenting to an emergency department may well have been given a diagnosis of asthma in the weeks or months preceding their admission.

ACUTE PRESENTATION: PULMONARY EDEMA

The classic presentation of heart failure is with acute pulmonary edema. Such patients present with extreme shortness of breath, often unable to speak because of their rapid respiratory rate. Symptoms may come on very suddenly. Even patients with ischemic heart failure may not report chest pain, either because the ischemia is silent or because the pain is being masked by the profound shortness of breath. Many patients will be unable to give a history owing to their shortness of breath, and therefore examination findings and basic investigations are vital to make the diagnosis.

General Examination

Examination may often reveal pallor, sweating, and dyspnea. The patient will have a high respiratory rate and increased work of breathing, using accessory muscles of respiration. Peripheral edema is not always present, particularly in patients presenting with a first episode of heart failure. Equally, the jugular venous pulse may not be elevated.

Respiratory Examination

Percussion is unlikely to be of value, owing to difficulty in examining the patient. A pleural effusion large enough to cause such dyspnea as to simulate severe heart failure will usually be obvious on auscultation. Percussion can be performed afterward if needed to confirm such a diagnosis. Patients with heart failure may well have pleural effusions, but they are usually relatively small and unlikely to benefit from drainage. Auscultation usually reveals extensive fine crepitations, usually equal bilaterally and greatest at the lung bases. However, some patients have predominant wheeze due to edema of the bronchial walls, and this may cause diagnostic confusion. In such patients, the preferred option may be to treat both bronchospasm and pulmonary edema. Similarly, in the most severely affected and exhausted patients, the chest may be surprisingly silent because of reduced tidal volumes. A single dose of an intravenous (IV) diuretic agent is unlikely to cause harm to patients with breathlessness of other causes, and in situations of diagnostic difficulty, a rapid response to diuretics may be helpful.

Cardiovascular Examination

Examination of the pulse may reveal atrial fibrillation. Patients in sinus rhythm are usually tachycardic, although patients with a history of ischemic heart disease may well be taking beta-blockers, which mask tachycardia. Heart rate appears to be an independent and powerful factor of prognosis in heart failure. In the BEAUTIFUL study, heart failure patients with heart rates of 70 bpm or greater had 34% higher risk for cardiovascular death and 53% higher risk admission to hospital than those with heart rate blow 70 bpm. The study has shown 8% and 15% increments of cardiovascular death and hospital admission for every increase of 5 bpm.[13]

The blood pressure is preserved in approximately 80% of patients presenting with decompensated heart failure overall, but a significant number are hypotensive at presentation. This is the single most important factor affecting treatment (see later discussion) and is also likely to be altered by treatment, and so must be measured frequently. Palpation may or may not reveal a displaced apex beat, depending on the length of the history. There may be palpable heaves or thrills, but these are likely to be difficult to appreciate in the acutely breathless patient. Auscultation of the heart sounds may well be difficult. There may be a third or fourth heart sound, or there may be murmurs representing chronic stenotic or regurgitant valves, or an acute mitral valve prolapse or ventricular septal defect following MI. (These latter two conditions can even occur several days after admission in a patient with extensive MI.) It is important to reexamine the patient regularly; once initial treatment has commenced, the patient may become less breathless, and previously inaudible signs may become clear.

Abdominal Examination

Examination of the abdomen can also be difficult in the acutely breathless patient. Where possible, such examination may reveal ascites, edema of the abdominal wall or genitalia, and enlargement of the liver. Pulsation of the liver can indicate tricuspid regurgitation.

SUBACUTE PRESENTATION: SHORTNESS OF BREATH/PERIPHERAL EDEMA

Many patients with severe heart failure present less acutely with varying combinations of breathlessness and edema. This is often the case in patients with a previous diagnosis of heart failure and can be precipitated by intercurrent infection or withdrawal of diuretic or other medication (by the patient or a physician). In the early stages, edema may be more prominent unilaterally, and this may result in diagnostic difficulty. Such patients may be referred for exclusion of deep venous thrombosis (and it is important to be aware that the two conditions can coexist). These patients often report gradually increasing breathlessness with symptoms of orthopnea (shortness of breath occurring when lying supine) and paroxysmal nocturnal dyspnea (sudden shortness of breath waking the patient from sleep). Patients may resort to sleeping in a chair, leading to additional gravitational edema. Edema of the bowel can lead to reduced appetite, so called "cardiac cachexia," and further edema from hypoproteinemia. Peripheral edema is therefore often multifactorial in patients with heart failure. Differential diagnoses of peripheral edema are listed in Table 82-3.

Examination findings are similar to those for the acute presentation, although the patient is not in extremis and is able to speak sufficiently to give a full history. A full examination is possible more often in this situation, including auscultation of the heart sounds and abdominal examination. Peripheral edema may well be extensive, up to the abdominal wall and sacral areas. The jugular venous pulse may be elevated. Patients with extensive peripheral edema but a low jugular venous pulse may have hypoproteinemia rather than heart failure.

CHEST PAIN

As noted earlier, ischemic heart disease is an extremely common cause of heart failure. Patients presenting with chest pain thought to be ischemic in nature must be examined closely for subtle signs of heart failure. Patients presenting with extensive MI may develop symptoms and signs of heart failure hours or days after admission. This may be

TABLE 82-3	Causes of Peripheral Edema

Heart failure
Hypoproteinemia
Liver cirrhosis
Nephrotic syndrome
Lymphedema
Malnutrition
Gravitational edema

precipitated by treatment (such as acute use of beta-blockers or calcium channel blockers) or by a complication of the MI, such as ventricular septal defect or mitral valve prolapse due to chordal rupture.

COLLAPSE/CARDIAC ARREST

Patients with severe heart failure of any cause are at high risk for malignant arrhythmias and thromboembolic disease such as pulmonary embolism. It is therefore not unusual for patients with severe heart failure to present with collapse or cardiac arrest. In such patients, the outlook is extremely poor. Even for patients presenting with ventricular tachycardia or ventricular fibrillation who are successfully cardioverted, the chance of surviving to discharge from hospital is low. Such patients can be considered for implantable cardioverter-defibrillators (see later and Chapter 81). Pulmonary embolism and ventricular arrhythmias are covered in Chapters 62 and 79, respectively, so will not be discussed in detail here.

Investigations

ELECTROCARDIOGRAPHY

All patients presenting with severe heart failure require at least one electrocardiogram (ECG). In cases of diagnostic difficulty, an entirely normal ECG virtually excludes systolic heart failure as the cause of symptoms.[14] In heart failure, an ECG is essential to diagnose arrhythmias such as atrial fibrillation, which may complicate management, as well as to look for evidence of myocardial ischemia or infarction and conduction abnormalities such as left bundle branch block or bradycardia due to high-degree atrioventricular block, which may respond to pacing. In patients in whom ischemia is suspected, serial ECGs are recommended, as changes may evolve during the course of the patient's treatment. Patients with acute severe heart failure should have continuous ECG monitoring during the acute phase, as they are at high risk for malignant ventricular arrhythmias. Patients with biventricular pacemakers (discussed later) in situ may have paced QRS complexes that are narrower than in those with single-chamber right ventricular leads.

CARDIAC ENZYMES AND OTHER BIOMARKERS

All patients presenting with severe heart failure, either as a first presentation or an exacerbation, should raise the question of MI. As noted earlier, patients with ischemia often do not report chest pain in the setting of acute heart failure symptoms. Therefore, the use of biomarkers of cardiac muscle necrosis—ideally troponin I or T, assayed at presentation and repeated after 12 hours—is important for most patients presenting with heart failure, in conjunction with ECG findings, as noted earlier.

CHEST RADIOGRAPHY

Acutely, the chest radiograph is useful mainly in cases of diagnostic difficulty. In cases in which the diagnosis is reasonably clear from clinical information, treatment should not be delayed while waiting for a radiograph. However, most patients should have a chest radiograph early in the course of the admission.

The chest radiograph may show cardiomegaly, although this is poorly sensitive or specific for a diagnosis of heart failure (NB: portable films using anteroposterior projection may exaggerate the cardiac outline). A globular heart suggests the presence of pericardial fluid, which can be determined definitively by early echocardiography. Signs of pulmonary edema range from mild blunting of the costophrenic angles, perhaps with evidence of fluid in the horizontal fissure of the right lung, to upper lobe blood diversion (due to hypoxic vasoconstriction in the edematous dependent lung and opposite changes in the relatively edema-free upper lobes), to frank pulmonary edema. The chest radiograph may reveal signs of coexistent consolidation requiring antibiotic therapy. Pacemakers are also visible on chest radiographs, and it is important to examine and count the number of pacing leads to establish whether a patient has an implantable cardioverter-defibrillator (ICD) or biventricular pacemaker present. This is particularly important if the patient is unable to give an adequate history because of their acute clinical condition.

ECHOCARDIOGRAPHY

Echocardiography should be carried out early in all cases of suspected heart failure. In recent years, bedside echocardiography devices have been developed that can be useful in the emergency department to assess the left ventricle and valves initially. In all cases, a full echocardiogram should be carried out when the patient is sufficiently stabilized.

Echocardiography is useful both to determine the extent of left ventricular dysfunction and to identify the cause. In cases of ischemic cardiomyopathy, regional wall motion abnormalities are commonly seen (although these can occasionally occur in cases of cardiomyopathy of other causes). Valve disease is readily identified by echocardiography. Echocardiography can be used to calculate the left ventricular ejection fraction, but in experienced hands, a qualitative assessment of left ventricular function can be equally useful. Some patients presenting with severe heart failure have preserved systolic function, and echocardiography can also be used to assess diastolic function. In the patient presenting with shortness of breath, in whom the cause is unclear, echocardiography can readily determine the presence or absence of systolic heart failure. Although a number of diagnostic criteria have been developed for assessment of the diastolic left ventricular function, their reliability in predicting intracardiac filling pressures is not always satisfactory and needs further development.[15] A clear distinction can sometimes be made only by measurements of gas exchange or blood oxygen saturation or by invasive hemodynamic measurements during graded levels of exercise following the clinical stabilization.

It is important to emphasize that heart failure is not directly equivalent to the impairment of left ventricular contractility, and there is a poor correlation between parameters of myocardial function and the symptoms. About half of heart failure patients have preserved contractility. However, prognosis for patients presenting with symptomatic heart failure is equally poor for those with normal or decreased ejection fraction.

BRAIN NATRIURETIC PEPTIDE

Natriuretic peptides are currently emerging as a novel test in cases of heart failure. The group includes three structurally related peptides, with variable activity at three distinct natriuretic peptide receptor subtypes, of which two are of potential use in patients with heart failure. Atrial natriuretic peptide is released from the atria in response to wall stretch. Brain natriuretic peptide (BNP), so called because it was first identified in brain tissue, is mainly released by the cardiac ventricles in response to wall stretch.[16] All the natriuretic peptides are elevated in acute coronary syndromes and MI, owing to release from myocytes. In addition, decompensated heart failure is associated with elevations of natriuretic peptide levels. Many possible applications for assays of these peptides have been proposed, but at present the most widely accepted indications for use of BNP (which appears to have the best sensitivity/specificity of all the natriuretic peptides) are as follows:

1. In the acutely dyspneic patient in whom there is diagnostic difficulty, a high BNP level is very suggestive of underlying cardiac failure.
2. In the dyspneic patient with no clinical signs of heart failure, a normal BNP level has a high negative predictive value—that is, it is useful in *excluding* heart failure as a cause.

The use of BNP for monitoring progress in heart failure is controversial; some studies have suggested that BNP may be useful to guide treatment. Indeed, many studies have found that BNP levels may have prognostic implications. It is also important to note that BNP levels must be used in conjunction with clinical assessment of the patient, as unexpected values may occur in some patients, such as a high BNP level in a stable patient. Recent findings do not support routine use of the peptides in all dyspneic patients admitted to the emergency department.[17] Of particular note is the fact that patients with severe heart failure due to cardiogenic shock may exhibit a paradoxically normal or even low BNP level. It has been suggested that myocytes in such a situation are unable to produce BNP. This theory is supported by studies of serial BNP levels in patients recovering from an episode of cardiogenic shock. An initially low BNP level is followed by a high level as recovery of myocardial function begins, and as recovery continues, the level returns to normal.

However, the measurement of BNP during admission with acute decompensated heart failure may help to assess prognosis and guide therapy following stabilization.[18,19] A soluble form of ST2, an interleukin 1 (IL-1) receptor family member, has also been found to be potentially useful for identifying heart failure patients at risk of sudden cardiac death and may provide additional information to BNP.[20]

INVASIVE INVESTIGATIONS

Central Venous Catheter

Placement of a central venous catheter may be necessary for certain drugs such as inotropic agents or amiodarone, which cannot be given into a peripheral vein. The central venous pressure measurement may give some idea as to right-sided filling pressure but does not give reliable information about the status of the left ventricle. In situations in which detailed information regarding filling pressures would affect management of a seriously ill patient, the Swan-Ganz catheter should be considered instead.

Swan-Ganz Catheter

Insertion of a pulmonary artery (Swan-Ganz) catheter may provide additional hemodynamic information. The procedure has been associated with increased mortality and therefore should be used only in severely ill patients in whom the results are likely to influence management. It is important to note that echocardiography can provide much of the information obtainable by Swan-Ganz catheterization when adequate images can be obtained.

Treatment

ACUTE TREATMENT

Simple Measures

The patient should be in erect sitting position. High-flow oxygen therapy should be administered to hypoxic patients with pulmonary edema. A single small dose of opiate (such as morphine, 2.5 mg) may alleviate distress and also temporarily reduce cardiac preload; it is also clearly indicated for patients presenting with ischemic chest pain in addition to pulmonary edema.

Urinary catheterization is essential in the severely compromised patient to monitor urine output but may also be therapeutic to reduce the need for exertion, particularly if large doses of diuretics are to be used.

Diuretics

Although not supported by randomized trials, it is clear that IV diuretic therapy can cause rapid relief of pulmonary edema and symptoms of acute decompensated heart failure. Care is needed in patients with compromised renal function or hypotension, as diuretic therapy may exacerbate such problems. It is usual to give an initial bolus IV dose of diuretic, which should be tailored to the patient's previous use of diuretics. A diuretic-naïve patient will usually respond to a single 50-mg IV dose of furosemide, whereas patients already taking diuretics long term may need much larger doses. Subsequent therapy is often given as further boluses of IV diuretic at intervals, although there is some evidence that a continuous infusion of diuretic may be more efficacious and cause less renal dysfunction.

Some patients with significant fluid overload may require combination diuretic therapy—for example, with the addition of a thiazide diuretic such as metolazone. Metolazone is a weak diuretic when used alone, but increased sodium delivery to, and reabsorption in, the distal renal tubule resulting from the use of a loop diuretic is blocked by metolazone, resulting in a profound diuresis. Care is needed to avoid dehydration and hyponatremia with this strategy. An alternative may be to combine furosemide with an aldosterone blocker in the acute phase.

Thromboprophylaxis

Patients with severe heart failure are often poorly mobile due to breathlessness, peripheral edema, and the presence of monitoring and treatment equipment. They are at high risk for the development of deep venous thrombosis and pulmonary embolism. The MEDENOX (prophylaxis in MEDical patients with ENOXaparin) trial, which included 1102 hospitalized patients, including 376 with NYHA class III/IV heart failure, found that 14.9% of placebo-treated patients suffered venous thromboembolism. Importantly, in the group treated with enoxaparin, only 5.5% suffered venous thromboembolism.[21] This trial also included patients with other serious medical illnesses including cancer, so this may be an overestimate of the risk of thromboembolism in heart failure. In cases of moderate to severe heart failure, particularly in hospitalized patients, some of this increased risk may be related to immobility, which is a well-known risk factor for deep venous thrombosis. Indeed, in previous years when bed rest was standard treatment for patients with heart failure, the rate of pulmonary embolism was very high. All patients with severe heart failure who are not anticoagulated and in whom there are no contraindications (such as active bleeding) should receive thromboprophylaxis with unfractionated or low-molecular-weight heparin, with the dose adjusted according to the patient's body weight.

Vasodilators: Glyceryl Trinitrate/Sodium Nitroprusside

Infusion of glyceryl trinitrate has been a standard part of therapy for pulmonary edema with preserved blood pressure for many years. It is a direct-acting vasodilator that reduces left ventricular preload and afterload by release of the potent vasodilator, nitric oxide. Glyceryl trinitrate has a very short half-life and is given by continuous IV infusion, with dose titrated according to response and the patient's blood pressure. The most frequent adverse effect is hypotension, which is readily reversible on stopping or reducing the rate of infusion. Glyceryl trinitrate is additionally antianginal and therefore of particular benefit in the patient with ischemic chest pain and pulmonary edema. Patients receiving glyceryl trinitrate rapidly develop tolerance to the drug, which can limit its effectiveness if given for long periods.

Sodium nitroprusside is an alternative vasodilator that is also effective in patients with heart failure and preserved blood pressure. The drug is given by continuous infusion and must be protected from sunlight. However, its use is limited by concerns over the toxic effects of the metabolites of sodium nitroprusside: cyanide and thiocyanide.

Nesiritide

The natriuretic peptides have a variety of beneficial effects on the heart and circulation, causing diuresis, increasing sodium excretion, and reducing pre- and afterload by causing venous and arterial dilatation. They may also reduce left ventricular remodeling and fibrosis. These attributes have recently led to the therapeutic use of natriuretic peptides in heart failure, and short-term studies have shown that nesiritide infusion is at least as efficacious as standard therapy (dobutamine, milrinone, or glyceryl trinitrate) and is associated with reduced diuretic use in patients with acutely decompensated heart failure.[22] Nesiritide (recombinant human BNP) has been approved by the U.S. Food

and Drug Administration (FDA) for use in patients with acutely decompensated heart failure in whom systolic blood pressure is above 90 mm Hg. It is given by IV bolus (2 μg/kg) followed by continuous infusion (0.01 μg/kg/min) as an alternative to glyceryl trinitrate. Treatment is usually continued for 24 to 48 hours.

Inotropes

Approximately 80% of patients presenting with acute decompensated congestive heart failure have preserved blood pressure and can therefore receive cardiac load–reducing therapy such as glyceryl trinitrate or nesiritide. However, these treatments are contraindicated in hypotensive patients with heart failure. If such patients do not respond to initial diuretic therapy favorably or show evidence of deterioration, inotropic therapy may be considered. Long-term use of inotropic therapy is likely to be harmful in patients with heart failure,[23] but potentially appropriate uses of inotropes include use as temporary treatment of diuretic-refractory acute heart failure decompensations or as a bridge to definitive treatment such as revascularization or cardiac transplantation.

Experimental Agents

A number of novel and promising treatments for acute decompensated heart failure are currently under clinical development. Infusion of cinaciguat (BAY 58-2667), the first of a new class of soluble guanylate cyclase activators, has potent preload- and afterload-reducing effects, thereby increasing cardiac output.[24] Administration of relaxin, a natural human peptide that affects multiple vascular control pathways, improved symptoms and reduced cardiovascular death or readmission due to heart or renal failure at day 60 compared with placebo (2.6% [95% CI, 0.4-16.8] versus 17.2% [9.6-29.6]; $P = 0.053$). Both agents were safe and well tolerated, and further clinical development is warranted.[25]

Intraaortic Balloon Counterpulsation

Intraaortic balloon counterpulsation is an invasive strategy to preserve coronary flow in the presence of very poor cardiac output. A percutaneous approach is used to position a balloon in the descending aorta. The balloon is inflated during diastole, diverting blood into the coronary arteries. This technique may be used to maintain circulation to the heart and brain at the expense of other tissues as a bridge to transplantation or other surgical intervention. Use of intraaortic balloon counterpulsation is associated with a significant adverse event rate— up to 60% in one study of patients with cardiogenic shock.[26] There is no definite evidence that use of intraaortic balloon counterpulsation improves the mortality rate among patients in heart failure; however, a comparison of patients from the Global Utilization of Streptokinase and Tissue Plasminogen Activator for Occluded Coronary Arteries (GUSTO-I) study showed a significantly lower rate of mortality in those undergoing intraaortic balloon counterpulsation up to 1 day after admission as compared with all other patients (57% versus 67%).[27] It has been recently shown that continuous aortic flow augmentation improved cardiac performance and pulmonary capillary wedge pressure, but not clinical outcomes.[28]

Assisted Ventilation

Noninvasive Ventilation. Noninvasive ventilation is a form of ventilatory support that does not require paralysis and intubation. Positive pressure is provided via a tight-fitting mask that may lie over the nose only or over the full face. Some patients are unable to tolerate the mask or the sensation of assisted ventilation.

Continuous positive airway pressure (CPAP) has an accepted role in the treatment of sleep apnea syndromes. It is now recognized that sleep apnea is prevalent in patients with heart failure and may play a role in the development and progression of heart failure. In addition, noninvasive ventilation has favorable effects on intrathoracic and left ventricular transmural pressures in patients with congestive heart failure. Noninvasive ventilation has been used to treat acute heart failure. Several randomized trials have suggested that use of CPAP results in more rapid increase in Pao_2, decrease in Pco_2, and lower rates of intubation compared with standard treatment.[29] Noninvasive ventilation may be considered in patients with rising Pco_2 levels despite adequate medical therapy. Its use results in decreased blood pressure, so it may have a deleterious effect in patients who are already hypotensive. To be used successfully, noninvasive ventilation requires careful attention to mask fitting and close patient observation. It should be used only in a high-dependency setting with appropriately trained staff.

Intermittent Positive-Pressure Ventilation. Patients with evidence of exhaustion or worsening arterial blood gases despite adequate treatment may require invasive ventilation. The prognosis of patients with such refractory pulmonary edema is poor, but some patients show dramatic improvement after only a short period of intermittent positive-pressure ventilation. Intermittent positive-pressure ventilation results in decreased venous return due to increased intrathoracic pressure and therefore can have a deleterious effect on blood pressure. Blood pressure must be maintained (with inotropic agents if necessary) before intubation.

Surgery

Valve Replacement. Patients with severe heart failure due to valvular heart disease or functional mitral regurgitation may benefit from valve replacement or repair. Ideally, surgery should be delayed until the patient is stable, but selected patients not improving on initial therapy may benefit from emergency valve replacement, although such patients are inherently at high risk for such major surgery. A multidisciplinary team consisting of cardiologist, cardiovascular surgeon, and intensivist/anesthetist is needed to select suitable patients for intervention. A full discussion of indications for surgery is beyond the scope of this chapter.

Left Ventricular Assist Device. Left ventricular assist devices (LVADs) are surgically implanted devices developed to allow short- or long-term support to the failing left ventricle. Commonly, an inflow cannula receives blood from the left ventricle, which is then pumped out through a cannula in the ascending aorta. Although initially used as a bridge to transplantation, some studies have demonstrated recovery of function, allowing explantation of the device after a period of left ventricular support in certain subgroups of patients together with appropriate pharmacologic therapy.[30] LVAD therapy for patients with terminal heart failure but who are not eligible for heart transplantation has been shown in the Randomized Evaluation of Mechanical Assistance for the Treatment of Congestive Heart Failure (REMATCH) trial[31] to be superior to medical therapy in ameliorating symptoms and to produce a 48% mortality reduction at 2 years' follow-up. However, the frequency of serious adverse events in the LVAD group was more than twice that in the medical therapy group, mainly due to infection, bleeding, and malfunction of the device. A number of devices are available. Choice depends on availability and local expertise.

New continuous-flow devices are smaller and may be more durable than the pulsatile-flow devices. In one randomized trial, ,the continuous-flow device improved 2-year survival of patients with severe heart failure by 24% to 58%.[32]

The main complications of LVADs include thromboembolism, right ventricular failure, and device failure (equivalent to severe aortic regurgitation, as the devices do not have valves). Careful patient selection is necessary to gain most benefit from such devices.

Revascularization. In recent years, the phenomena of "stunned" and "hibernating" myocardium have been recognized and widely investigated. *Hibernating myocardium* is defined as poorly functioning myocardium caused by reduced perfusion, which may recover function if perfusion is restored. *Stunned myocardium* results from an episode of ischemia. The segment of myocardium regains normal blood flow after the episode, but recovery of function is delayed (although recovery

occurs spontaneously). In patients with chronic ischemic cardiomyopathy, revascularization may therefore result in improvement in left ventricular function. Patients with cardiogenic shock due to acute MI have a very poor prognosis (see later discussion), and in recent years several studies have addressed the possible benefits of acute revascularization in such patients. Retrospective analysis of the patients from the GUSTO-I study with cardiogenic shock (7.2%) showed that revascularization was associated with decreased mortality rate (overall 30-day mortality, 55%; patients undergoing coronary artery bypass grafting, 29%; patients undergoing percutaneous transluminal coronary angioplasty, 22%).[33]

The treatments were not allocated randomly, however. The two randomized controlled trials of medical therapy versus revascularization (Should We Emergently Revascularize Occluded Coronaries for Cardiogenic Shock [SHOCK][34] and Swiss Multicenter Angioplasty for SHOCK [SMASH][35]) had difficulties in recruitment, and both reported no significant difference in early mortality, although the SHOCK trial did show decreased mortality rate at 6 months in the intervention group. It is important to note that results from the SHOCK trial registry, which showed that patients selected to undergo angiography had better outcomes whether or not they went on to be revascularized, suggest that bias may be involved in the results of these studies. Furthermore, adding surgical ventricular reconstruction to coronary revascularization reduced the left ventricular volume, as compared with revascularization alone, but not the rate of death or hospitalization for cardiac causes.[36] Current evidence certainly does not support aggressive revascularization of all patients with cardiogenic shock, but revascularization may be appropriate in selected patients.

Stabilization and Chronic Treatment

A full discussion of long-term treatment for patients with heart failure is beyond the scope of this book. However, patients presenting with acute heart failure may need to be established on a variety of medications during their index admission, and so a brief summary of the main drugs used in heart failure treatment maintenance is presented here.

Loop Diuretics. As noted earlier, loop diuretic therapy may provide rapid symptom relief in patients with fluid overload. However, loop diuretics may be associated with a number of adverse effects such as volume depletion, and no mortality benefit has been demonstrated in cases of heart failure. Although some patients with chronic heart failure may be able to have diuretic therapy withdrawn once they are appropriately stabilized, most require at least a small dose of maintenance diuretic, tailored to clinical evidence of fluid overload. Regular weighing is a simple method of monitoring the fluid status of heart failure patients. Care must be taken to monitor renal function in patients on high doses of diuretics. Diuretics may cause hypokalemia, although combining them with angiotensin-converting enzyme (ACE) inhibitors and potassium-sparing diuretics such as spironolactone (see later discussion) may reduce this problem.

Angiotensin-Converting Enzyme Inhibitors/Angiotensin II Receptor Blockers. Multiple large randomized trials have shown that ACE inhibitors (e.g., ramipril, perindopril, lisinopril) are of unequivocal benefit in patients with heart failure and asymptomatic left ventricular dysfunction.[37] All patients should be started on an ACE inhibitor as soon as possible after a diagnosis of heart failure has been made—this is almost always during the index admission. Most patients will require gradual introduction of the drug, with monitoring of blood pressure and renal function. Effort should be made to achieve the highest tolerated dose of the chosen ACE inhibitor.

Some patients are unable to tolerate ACE inhibitors as a consequence of cough due to elevated levels of bradykinin, which is usually degraded by ACE. An alternative in such patients are angiotensin II receptor blockers, which directly block the angiotensin II receptor and do not cause bradykinin buildup. There is not yet sufficient evidence on angiotensin II receptor blockers to recommend them over ACE inhibitors as first-line therapy in heart failure patients. However, the recent Candesartan in Heart Failure—Assessment of Reduction in Mortality (CHARM) study demonstrated that in patients unable to tolerate ACE inhibitors, the angiotensin II receptor blocker, candesartan, provided similar mortality benefit.[38] Another arm of the CHARM study (CHARM-ADDED) showed additional benefit (reduction in the primary endpoint of cardiovascular death or hospital admission for congestive heart failure) when candesartan was added to ACE inhibitors.

Recently the Heart Failure End Point Evaluation of Angiotensin II Antagonist Losartan (HEAAL) trial showed that triple increase of losartan dose (150 mg daily compared with traditional 50 mg) is required to achieve maximal reduction of rate of death or admission in patients with heart failure.[39]

Beta-Blockers. For many years, beta-blockers were thought to be harmful in patients with heart failure because of their negative inotropic effect. More recently, however, several large randomized trials have demonstrated consistent benefit of beta-blockers such as carvedilol,[40] bisoprolol,[41] and metoprolol.[42] Beta-blockers are indicated in patients with stabilized heart failure and are rarely started during the index admission. Their use involves careful dose titration, best supervised in a specialist heart failure clinic. The degree of heart rate reduction is more important than the maximal dose of beta-blocker achieved, and for every heart rate reduction of 5 bpm, there is an 18% reduction in the risk for death (but no significant relationship between all-cause mortality and beta-blocker dosing).[39]

Aldosterone Inhibitors. The landmark Randomised Aldactone Evaluation Study (RALES) showed that in patients with severe heart failure, spironolactone reduced mortality by 30%.[43] More recently, a more selective aldosterone inhibitor, eplerenone, has been developed, which (because of its lack of action at sex hormone and glucocorticoid receptor sites) lacks the unpleasant side effects of spironolactone, such as painful gynecomastia. The recent EPHESUS study, which recruited 6642 post-MI patients with left ventricular ejection fraction less than 40% and clinical heart failure and randomized them to receive eplerenone or placebo (in addition to otherwise optimized medical therapy), demonstrated a 15% reduction in all-cause mortality among the eplerenone group after a mean follow-up period of 16 months.[44] It is likely that aldosterone antagonists will be used increasingly in the management of patients with chronic heart failure.

Aldosterone blockers may cause hyperkalemia, particularly in combination with ACE inhibitors; patients on this combination should have regular renal function testing. In the EPHESUS study, the eplerenone added to standard therapy significantly improved outcomes, without an excess risk of hyperkalemia when periodic monitoring of serum potassium was performed.[45]

Antithrombotic Therapy. Patients with heart failure and atrial fibrillation have clear indications for anticoagulation with adjusted-dose warfarin. There is no clear evidence for the use of antithrombotic therapy in patients with heart failure in sinus rhythm, although such patients fulfill Virchow's triad (abnormal flow, abnormal vessel wall, abnormal blood constituents) for a prothrombotic state. Recently completed trials also failed to demonstrate benefits of warfarin over antiplatelet agents in heart failure patients.[46]

Direct thrombin inhibitors (such as dabigatran etexilate) and factor Xa inhibitors (such as rivaroxaban) may become an alternative to warfarin and are currently being investigated for a number of indications. They have advantages over warfarin in that dose adjustment and INR monitoring are not required.

Digoxin. Digoxin therapy in patients with heart failure in sinus rhythm (i.e., for inotropic effect) is common practice in North America but is less frequently used in Europe. Evidence of benefit is somewhat limited. Withdrawal of digoxin from patients with symptomatic heart failure resulted in increased risk of heart failure decompensation.[47] The Digitalis Investigation Group (DIG) trial[48] demonstrated no difference in survival associated with the use of digoxin. A reduction in the risk of death from progressive heart failure in the DIG trial was balanced by an increase in the risk of sudden cardiac death. Digoxin may therefore be considered as additional therapy for patients on ACE inhibitors and beta-blockers but is not an alternative to these drugs.

Cardiac Resynchronization Therapy

Patients with heart failure may exhibit dyssynchronous contraction of the left ventricle resulting from abnormal electrical conduction pathways. Typically this results in septal contraction occurring some time before contraction of the free wall of the left ventricle. Such dyssynchronous contraction results in significant circulation of blood in the left ventricular cavity, rather than forward flow of blood. The use of biventricular pacing to restore synchronous contraction of the left ventricle (cardiac resynchronization therapy) has increased in popularity in recent years. However, the optimal method for selecting patients for cardiac resynchronization therapy is unclear. Current guidelines use duration of the ECG QRS complex, but recent studies have shown that some patients with narrow QRS complexes or even less advanced heart failure (i.e., with NYHA I-II functional class) may benefit from cardiac resynchronization therapy, and equally, not all patients with wide QRS complexes benefit.[49] Echocardiographic evidence of dyssynchronous contraction in combination with the ECG might prove to be a better method of selecting candidates for cardiac resynchronization therapy. More recent findings indicate that the benefit of cardiac resynchronization therapy can be maximized by simultaneous implantation of a defibrillator.[50,51]

Arrhythmia Therapy

Atrial Fibrillation. Atrial fibrillation can result in significant impairment of left ventricular function due to loss of atrial contraction and abnormal left ventricular filling. Atrial fibrillation in the presence of reduced left ventricular function results in a very high risk of thromboembolic stroke, so all patients with atrial fibrillation and reduced left ventricular function should be anticoagulated in the absence of contraindications. In the presence of poor left ventricular function or dilated left ventricle or left atrium on echocardiography, DC cardioversion is unlikely to cause sustained conversion to sinus rhythm but could be considered in situations in which palpitations due to atrial fibrillations cause significant distress to the patient. Pharmacologic rate control is likely to be more successful. Digoxin is commonly used for this purpose, although in the presence of renal impairment or diuretic-induced hypokalemia, toxicity is common. If tolerated, beta-blockers may achieve rate control, although the need to introduce such drugs gradually makes them less suitable for initial rate control. It may be possible to control the rate initially with careful digoxin therapy, then consider withdrawing digoxin once the patient is established on a sufficiently high dose of beta-blocker. Amiodarone is an alternative antiarrhythmic safe for use in heart failure patients, which can be used to control atrial fibrillation, although side-effects are problematic.

Ventricular Arrhythmias. Patients with heart failure frequently suffer from sudden death. Although it is now recognized that some episodes of sudden death are caused by thrombosis such as pulmonary embolism, it is clear that malignant arrhythmias are a common cause of death in heart failure. Surprisingly, therefore, multiple trials of a variety of antiarrhythmic drugs in patients with heart failure have failed to show a mortality benefit (amiodarone)[52] or have even shown a worsening of mortality (e.g., flecainide).[53] Routine use of antiarrhythmic drugs in patients with heart failure is therefore not recommended. In contrast, recent studies involving the use of ICD devices in patients with reduced ejection fraction following MI have shown reduced

TABLE 82-4	Indications for Implantable Cardioverter-Defibrillator Therapy in Patients with Heart Failure

Cardiac arrest due to ventricular fibrillation or ventricular tachycardia
Spontaneous sustained ventricular tachycardia
Syncope of unknown origin with inducible ventricular tachycardia or
ventricular fibrillation at electrophysiologic study
Nonsustained ventricular tachycardia with inducible ventricular fibrillation/
ventricular tachycardia at electrophysiologic study
Left ventricular ejection fraction < 30% at least 1 month after myocardial
infarction or 3 months after coronary artery bypass grafting

mortality. The recent COMPANION study,[54] which compared optimal medical treatment alone to optimal medical treatment plus cardiac resynchronization therapy plus or minus ICD therapy, found that combined cardiac resynchronization therapy/ICD reduced mortality but not hospitalization as compared with cardiac resynchronization therapy alone. At present, routine use of implantable cardioverter defibrillators (which in any case would be prohibitively expensive in most countries) in all heart failure patients cannot be recommended. Current indications for ICD therapy in heart failure are listed in Table 82-4.

Other Therapies

Anemia is common in heart failure and associated with a worse prognosis, but interventions directed at increasing hemoglobin levels (e.g., using erythropoietin) have shown inconsistent results. However a meta-analysis of randomized clinical trials suggests that administration of erythropoiesis-stimulating proteins is associated with a significantly lower risk of heart failure–linked hospitalizations.[55] Similar benefits were seen with IV ferric carboxymaltose.[56]

Although uniform conclusions cannot be drawn at present, statin use in patients with heart failure may be indicated. Some data are suggestive of potential benefits of administration of atorvastatin and possible simvastatin in terms of the prognosis, while rosuvastatin only appears to be of use in patients with heart failure due to ischemic heart disease who have relatively low levels of BNP.[57] However, treatment with statins is probably useful in those with hypercholesterolemia.

Of interest, long-acting testosterone administration has been shown to improve exercise capacity, muscle strength, and glucose metabolism in men with moderately severe heart failure, providing the basis for further development in this direction.[58]

Further Management: Specialist Heart Failure Clinic

Patients with heart failure are at high risk of further admissions and sudden death. Careful follow-up and adequate secondary prevention using the drugs and devices detailed here is essential to reduce the risk of readmission and other complications of heart failure. Ideally, such patients should be followed in a specialist heart failure clinic, with access to a cardiologist specializing in heart failure, specialist heart failure nursing, and access to investigations such as echocardiography, cardiac catheterization, and BNP. Nurse-led clinics are ideal for dose titration of beta-blockers and ACE inhibitors and also provide opportunities for monitoring of fluid status and symptoms. A recent meta-analysis has shown that remote patient monitoring may facilitate reduction of deaths and hospitalizations.[59] This can take place via different methods, including regular structured telephone contact between patients and healthcare providers and electronic transfer of physiologic data using remote-access technology via remote external, wearable, or implantable electronic devices. Intriguingly, patient self-monitoring of atrial pressures with implanted investigational left atrial pressure monitoring, followed by appropriate individualized adjustments of the therapy guided by these pressures, was associated

with highly significant improvement of event-free survival over a median follow-up of 25 months (hazard ratio, 0.16 [95% CI, 0.04-0.68], $P = 0.012$).[60]

Prognosis

Heart failure has a poor prognosis—diagnosis of chronic heart failure is associated with a mortality rate worse than that of many cancers.[61] As noted earlier, patients with severe heart failure often present in extremis but may respond rapidly to prompt effective management. However, their inpatient course is associated with a high risk of complications such as thromboembolism (particularly in the presence of atrial fibrillation) and sudden death, even in patients who show signs of recovery from their initial event. Close follow-up and secondary preventive measures are essential to improve prognosis in this high-risk group.

Summary

Severe heart failure is a common disorder, with high rates of mortality and morbidity. Patients often present in extremis, so good knowledge of initial treatment is essential for all physicians and emergency department staff. Patients often respond rapidly to effective initial treatment, making this a satisfying condition to treat. However, patients may also deteriorate rapidly and may require involvement of intensivists, cardiologists, and cardiac surgeons. Once stabilized, there are a number of evidence-based treatments that improve prognosis in these patients. Careful follow-up, ideally in a specialist heart failure clinic, is recommended after discharge.

KEY POINTS

1. Severe heart failure is a common emergency presentation associated with a high rate of mortality and a high rate of morbidity among survivors.

2. Ischemic heart disease is the most common underlying cause in the Western world, although the cause may differ between ethnic groups. Severe heart failure may be the first presentation of ischemic heart disease. Other common causes are hypertensive heart disease and dilated cardiomyopathy.

3. The diagnosis of heart failure is not always straightforward—it may be confused with asthma or chronic airway disease. Classic examination findings of heart failure are not sensitive or specific and require confirmation by the early use of investigations such as echocardiography.

4. Assessment for B-type natriuretic peptide may be a useful method of ruling out heart failure in the acutely breathless patient but is not sufficiently sensitive to diagnose heart failure without additional investigations.

5. Initial therapy for an episode of severe heart failure should involve diuretic therapy, and a single dose of IV morphine can be considered. In patients with preserved systolic blood pressure, an infusion of vasodilator or recombinant BNP (nesiritide) may be considered. In patients with hypotension, inotropic agents can be considered, although studies suggest increased risk of mortality with such agents.

6. Patients who do not show evidence of improvement, or whose condition deteriorates, should be considered for additional support such as intraaortic balloon counterpulsation or assisted ventilation early. Patients with cardiogenic shock due to ischemic heart disease should be considered for revascularization.

7. Once stabilized, patients must be established on appropriate secondary preventive therapy, including angiotensin-converting enzyme inhibitors and beta-blockers. Long-term follow-up is best provided by a specialist heart failure clinic.

ANNOTATED REFERENCES

ESC Committee for Practice Guidelines (CPG), Dickstein K, Cohen-Solal A, Filippatos G, McMurray JJ, Ponikowski P, Poole-Wilson Pa, et al. ESC Guidelines for the diagnosis and treatment of acute and chronic heart failure 2008: the Task Force for the diagnosis and treatment of acute and chronic heart failure 2008 of the European Society of Cardiology. Eur Heart J 2008;29:2388-442.

The last update of the recommendation of the diagnostics and management of heart failure issued by the European Society of Cardiology.

Hunt SA, Abraham WT, Chin MH, et al. 2009 Focused update incorporated into the ACC/AHA 2005 Guidelines for the diagnosis and management of heart failure in adults: a report of the American College of Cardiology Foundation/American Heart Association Task Force on Practice Guidelines. Developed in collaboration with the International Society for Heart and Lung Transplantation. J Am Coll Cardiol 2009;53:e1-90.

Current recommendation on the assessment and management of heart failure approved by the American College of Cardiology and the American Heart Association.

Halperin JL, for the Executive Steering Committee, SPORTIF III and V Study Investigators. Ximelagatran compared with warfarin for prevention of thromboembolism in patients with nonvalvular atrial fibrillation: rationale, objectives, and design of a pair of clinical studies and baseline patient characteristics (SPORTIF III and V). Am Heart J 2003;146:431-8.

The ongoing SPORTIF III (open label, 23 countries) and V (double blind, 409 U.S. centers) trials are comparing ximelagatran with adjusted-dose warfarin in patients with atrial fibrillation and at least one other risk factor (including heart failure).

MERIT-HF Investigators. Effect of metoprolol CR/XL in chronic heart failure: Metoprolol CR/XL Randomised Intervention Trial in Congestive Heart Failure (MERIT-HF). Lancet 1999;353:2001-7.

The benefit of beta-blockers in heart failure was proved in these randomized controlled studies (MERIT-HF, CIBIS-II, and U.S. Carvedilol Heart Failure Study), bringing to an end the idea that beta-blockade could be harmful in patients with heart failure.

Rich MW, Beckham V, Wittenberg C, et al. A multidisciplinary intervention to prevent the readmission of elderly patients with congestive heart failure. N Engl J Med 1995;333:1190-5.

This trial demonstrated that a multidisciplinary intervention involving nutritional advice, counseling, patient education, and exercise training could significantly reduce readmission rates and length of hospital stay in elderly patients with heart failure.

REFERENCES

Access the complete reference list online at http://www.expertconsult.com.

83 Myocarditis and Acute Myopathies

FREDRIC GINSBERG | JOSEPH E. PARRILLO

Myocarditis in the Intensive Care Unit

Myocarditis is defined as inflammation of heart muscle.[1] Many different etiologic agents have been implicated in this disease, but viral infections are the most common cause. Myocarditis is also associated with autoimmune and other systemic diseases.[2] The clinical picture of myocarditis varies widely, from asymptomatic patients who recover without specific therapy and suffer no long-term sequelae to critically ill patients with heart failure and cardiogenic shock. There are no standardized, specific, and widely agreed-upon criteria for making the diagnosis of myocarditis or for determining a cause in many patients.[3] Lastly, there has been controversy regarding the most appropriate medical therapy for this condition.

On pathologic examination of myocardial biopsy specimens or on autopsy series, myocarditis is usually apparent as infiltration of myocardium with lymphocytes and fibroblasts, accompanied by myocyte necrosis (myocytolysis).[3] It is this type of myocarditis, often termed *lymphocytic myocarditis*, that will be referred to in this chapter unless otherwise specified. Other types of inflammatory reactions can be seen less frequently in myocarditis, involving giant cells, eosinophils, or granulomas, which can be associated with specific clinical conditions.

In most patients with myocarditis, a specific cause is not found.[4] It is presumed that in North America and Europe, the most common etiologic agent is viral.[1] Coxsackie B enterovirus was felt to be the most common cause up to the 1990s, but adenoviruses and parvovirus 19 have been implicated as causative agents more frequently over the past 20 years. Other viral causes include hepatitis C, cytomegalovirus, and human herpesvirus 6.[2] Myocarditis is a common finding in patients infected with human immunodeficiency virus (HIV). However, the causative agent responsible in these cases may be a secondary viral infection such as cytomegalovirus or other opportunistic infection such as mycobacteria, fungi, or parasites, rather than HIV itself.[1,5,6] Infectious illnesses such as Lyme disease, acute rheumatic fever, and diphtheria often have myocarditis as a prominent feature. In Central and South America, the most common cause of myocarditis is the protozoan, *Trypanosoma cruzi*, the cause of Chagas' disease (Table 83-1). Systemic and autoimmune diseases such as systemic lupus erythematosus, polymyositis, scleroderma, sprue, Whipple's disease, and sarcoidosis can be complicated by myocarditis, and myocarditis can be a feature of the infiltrative cardiomyopathies seen in hemochromatosis or amyloidosis. Idiopathic specific forms of myocarditis include hypersensitivity or eosinophilic myocarditis, which has also been reported after smallpox vaccination,[7] and giant cell myocarditis.[8] Lastly, myocarditis can be associated with doxorubicin cardiomyopathy or with peripartum cardiomyopathy, or it can be a manifestation of a hypersensitivity reaction to medications[9,10] (Table 83-2).

Unfortunately, it is difficult to make a clinical diagnosis of a specific viral cause of myocarditis. This usually requires measurement of antiviral antibody titers in acute and convalescent-phase sera. Viral cultures of tissue specimens are unreliable.[4] Identification of viral genomes incorporated in myocyte DNA suggests but does not specifically prove that the virus is the cause.

Pathogenesis

Based on observations of human myocarditis, as well as murine models of the disease caused by coxsackie B3, the pathogenesis of viral myocarditis can be described in three stages.[2,11] The first stage is initiated by viral infection and replication within myocytes. Viral proteases and activation of cytokines may produce myocyte damage and apoptosis.[12] The presence of this viral replication phase is difficult to detect clinically because patients may be asymptomatic during this phase or only have nonspecific viremic symptoms. In addition, there is no rapid screening test to confirm viral infection.

The second stage involves host immune activation. Stimulation of cellular immunity and humoral responses attenuates viral proliferation and can result in recovery from the illness. However, unabated immune activation can result in activated T cells targeting myocardial antigens that cross-react with viral peptides. This leads to release of cytokines such as tumor necrosis factor (TNF), interleukin (IL)-1, and IL-6, resulting in further myocyte damage.[1,12] Activation of CD4 cells and antibody production plays a less important pathogenetic role. It is believed that this secondary immune response to viral infection plays a greater role in disease pathogenesis than the primary infection.[12]

Evidence supporting these mechanisms includes several key observations. Myocardial biopsy with recombinant DNA techniques can detect viral genomes in 20% to 35% of patients. Tissue-specific autoantibodies have been detected in 25% to 73% of patients with evidence of myocarditis on biopsy, with antibodies directed against contractile, structural, and mitochondrial myocyte proteins. Inappropriate expression of the major histocompatibility complex can frequently be demonstrated on biopsy specimens.[1] Elevated levels of inflammatory cytokines are detected in patients with active myocarditis.

Either persistent overactivation of cellular immune activity or incomplete clearing with persistent or recurrent viral replication can lead to the third stage, during which significant myocardial damage occurs. This leads to left ventricular (LV) dilatation and remodeling, LV systolic dysfunction, and manifestations of heart failure.[12] These processes can then abate, with reduction in LV size and improvement of LV function, or can continue to progress with development of dilated cardiomyopathy, worsening ventricular function, and chronic heart failure. Chronic dilated cardiomyopathy is the major long-term sequela of acute myocarditis (Figure 83-1).

Clinical Presentation and Diagnosis

The incidence of myocarditis is difficult to determine; many cases are mild with subclinical disease. Myocarditis is diagnosed on clinical grounds, as there are no specific clinical diagnostic criteria. The presentation of myocarditis varies widely. Patients can be asymptomatic insofar as myocarditis has been found in 1% to 10% of autopsy specimens of young adults who had no history of cardiac illness. Myocarditis can be found at autopsy in up to 20% of cases of young, apparently healthy adults who die suddenly and unexpectedly.[1,4,10]

Patients ill with myocarditis present with nonspecific symptoms of dyspnea (72%), chest pain (32%), and symptoms of arrhythmia (18%).[13] The presentation may be indistinguishable from acute coronary syndromes due to coronary artery disease. There may have been a preceding viral prodrome with fever, malaise, and arthralgias. Physical examination can show fever, tachycardia, S_3 and S_4 gallop sounds, and a pericardial rub if myopericarditis is present. Signs of heart failure can be present, including pulmonary rales and wheezes, elevated jugular venous pulse, and peripheral edema. Murmurs of mitral regurgitation and tricuspid regurgitation may be heard. Infrequently, the presentation is fulminant and severe, with acute heart failure, pulmonary edema, and cardiogenic shock.[4]

TABLE 83-1	Causes of Myocarditis*		
Infectious	**Immune-Mediated**	**Toxic Myocarditis**

Infectious	**Immune-Mediated**	**Toxic Myocarditis**
Bacterial: *Brucella, Corynebacterium diphtheriae,* gonococcus, *Haemophilus influenzae,* meningococcus, *Mycobacterium, Mycoplasma pneumoniae,* pneumococcus, salmonella, *Serratia marcescens,* staphylococcus, *Streptococcus pneumoniae, Streptococcus pyogenes, Treponema pallidum, Tropheryma whippelii,* and *Vibrio cholerae* Spirochetal: *Borrelia* and *Leptospira* Fungal: actinomyces, aspergillus, blastomyces, *Candida, Coccidioides, Cryptococcus, Histoplasma,* mucormycoses, *Nocardia,* and *Sporothrix* Protozoal: *Toxoplasma gondii* and *Trypanosoma cruzi* Parasitic: ascaris, *Echinococcus granulosus, Paragonimus westermani, Schistosoma, Taenia solium, Trichinella spiralis,* visceral larva migrans, and *Wuchereria bancrofti* Rickettsial: *Coxiella burnetii, Rickettsia rickettsii,* and *Rickettsia tsutsugamushi* Viral: **coxsackievirus,** cytomegalovirus, dengue virus, echovirus, encephalomyocarditis, Epstein-Barr virus, hepatitis A virus, hepatitis C virus, herpes simplex virus, herpes zoster, **human immunodeficiency virus,** influenza A virus, influenza B virus, Junin virus, lymphocytic choriomeningitis, measles virus, mumps virus, parvovirus, poliovirus, rabies virus, respiratory syncytial virus, rubella virus, rubeola, vaccinia virus, varicella-zoster virus, variola virus, and yellow fever virus	Allergens: acetazolamide, amitriptyline, cefaclor, colchicine, furosemide, isoniazid, lidocaine, methyldopa, penicillin, phenylbutazone, phenytoin, reserpine, streptomycin, tetanus toxoid, tetracycline, and thiazides Alloantigens: heart transplant rejection Autoantigens: **Chagas' disease,** *Chlamydia pneumoniae,* Churg-Strauss syndrome, inflammatory bowel disease, giant cell myocarditis, insulin-dependent diabetes mellitus, Kawasaki's disease, myasthenia gravis, polymyositis, **sarcoidosis, scleroderma, systemic lupus erythematosus,** thyrotoxicosis, and Wegener's granulomatosis	Drugs: amphetamines, **anthracyclines,** catecholamines, cocaine, cyclophosphamide, **ethanol,** fluorouracil, hematin, interleukin-2, lithium, and trastuzumab Heavy metals: copper, iron, and lead Physical agents: electric shock, hyperpyrexia, and radiation Miscellaneous: arsenic, azides, bee and wasp stings, carbon monoxide, inhalants, phosphorus, scorpion bites, snake bites, and spider bites

From Feldman A, McNamara D. Myocarditis. N Engl J Med 2000;343:1388-98.
*The most common causes are shown in **boldface** type.

TABLE 83-2	Distinct Forms of Myocarditis

Active viral
Postviral (lymphocytic): common form of acute myocarditis
Hypersensitivity
Autoimmune
Infectious
Giant-cell myocarditis

From Haas G. Etiology, evaluation, and management of acute myocarditis. Cardiol Rev 2001;9:88-95.

The differential diagnosis includes acute myocardial infarction (AMI), pericarditis, or chest pain from pulmonary causes including pulmonary embolism or pneumonia. Generalized sepsis is also a consideration.

Laboratory findings can include leukocytosis, eosinophilia, and an elevated erythrocyte sedimentation rate. Cardiac biomarkers such as creatine kinase, troponin T, and troponin I may be elevated, with sensitivity of troponin I reported at 34% and specificity of 89%.[14] Rheumatologic serologic markers and HIV status should be evaluated.

The 12-lead electrocardiogram (ECG) is an insensitive test for the diagnosis of myocarditis. It shows sinus tachycardia and nonspecific ST-segment depression and T-wave inversion most often. Patients may

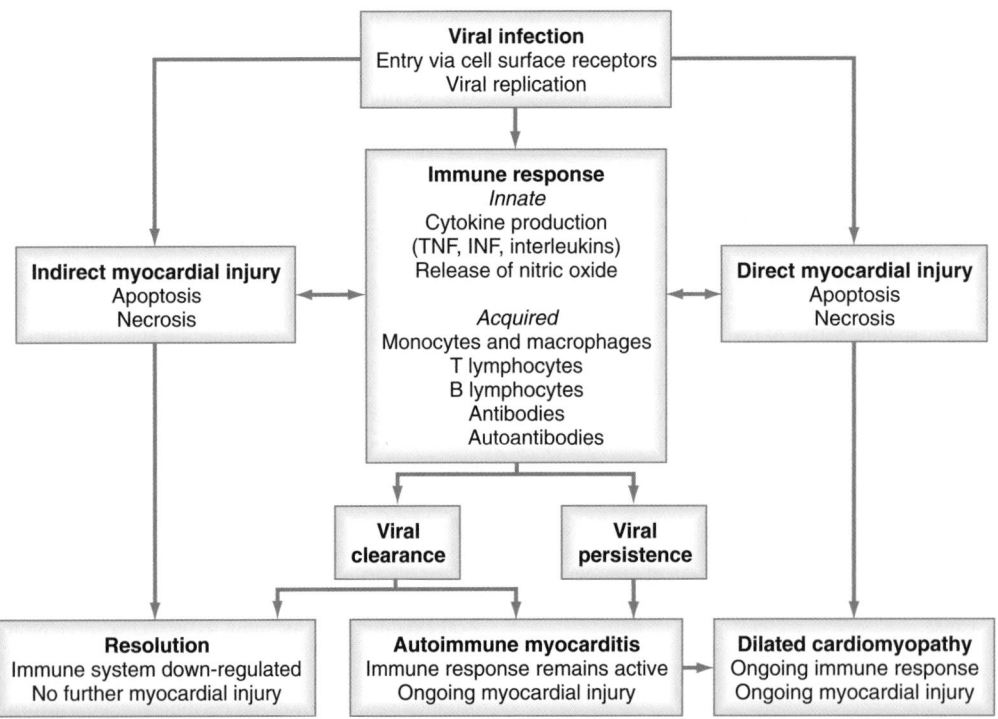

Figure 83-1   Pathogenesis of viral myocarditis involves direct myocardial injury from viral infection as well as immune-mediated myocyte damage from cytokines, proteases, and autoantibodies. The outcome of these processes can be healing of inflammation and resolution, ongoing active myocarditis, or chronic dilated cardiomyopathy. (*Adapted from Blauwer LA, Cooper LT. Myocarditis. Prog Cardiovasc Dis 2010;52:274-88.*)

present with chest pain and ST-segment elevation, with a picture mimicking AMI. More severe cases can be associated with supraventricular or ventricular arrhythmias, conduction disturbances, and heart block.[1]

Echocardiography is essential to diagnose and quantitate regional or global LV wall-motion abnormalities, left ventricular and right ventricular size and function, the presence of pericardial effusion, and valvular regurgitation. Fulminant myocarditis is characterized by a nondilated left ventricle, with severe systolic dysfunction and increased wall thickness reflecting myocardial edema.[15] Findings on myocardial nuclear scintigraphy are frequently abnormal, but this test is not useful in the diagnosis of myocarditis. Cardiac catheterization and coronary angiography are often necessary to exclude acute ischemia as the cause of chest pain or acute heart failure.

There is increasing use of cardiac magnetic resonance imaging (CMR) in the diagnosis of myocarditis.[16,17,18] This technique has the potential to offer a noninvasive means to make this diagnosis. CMR should be considered in symptomatic patients with a high clinical suspicion of disease when the results are likely to affect management decisions. Diagnostic criteria include: (1) focal or diffuse myocardial edema in T2-weighted images, (2) early gadolinium enhancement indicating inflammation, and (3) late gadolinium enhancement in subepicardial or mid-myocardial areas indicating necrosis and fibrosis. Abnormalities may be diffuse or patchy, often confined to the lateral free wall of the left ventricle or the base of the interventricular septum (Figure 83-2). Diagnostic accuracy of CMR is reported at 78% when 2 or 3 criteria are present and 68% when only late gadolinium enhancement is present. CMR is more likely to be abnormal when performed more than 7 days after onset of symptoms. CMR may also detect pericardial effusion (seen in 32%-57% of patients) and gives information regarding LV function. CMR can also be used to direct myocardial biopsy in patients with patchy uptake. The value of CMR for assessing prognosis is unknown, and this presently represents a major limitation of this diagnostic technique.[19,20,21]

Endomyocardial Biopsy

Percutaneous endomyocardial biopsy (EMB) is currently used to aid in the diagnosis of myocarditis and is considered the definitive diagnostic technique. The Dallas criteria have been accepted as the standard for histopathologic diagnosis. These criteria define *active myocarditis* as the presence of an inflammatory myocardial infiltrate (more than five lymphocytes per high-power field) accompanied by myocyte necrosis. *Borderline myocarditis* is defined as inflammation without myocyte necrosis. However, there is no difference in prognosis in patients with either of these biopsy results.[9] Thus, lymphocyte infiltration (with or without myocyte necrosis) is the most important diagnostic criterion.

Although EMB is useful for diagnostic purposes, there are a number of significant limitations. A high frequency of interobserver variation has been noted among pathologists in applying the Dallas criteria. Biopsies are not sensitive in diagnosing myocarditis; various series have reported positive right ventricular biopsy results in only 10% to 67% of patients with myocarditis suspected on clinical grounds or with recent-onset idiopathic dilated cardiomyopathy. This variability may relate to the timing of biopsies in respect to the stage or chronicity of the patient's illness. In addition, the myocardial inflammation may not be diffuse and may be patchy, or may predominantly involve the left ventricle, so random right ventricular biopsies may miss affected myocardium.[22] Thus, performing a biopsy earlier in a patient's clinical course, taking multiple biopsy specimens, and performing LV biopsies are ways of improving diagnostic yield. In addition, immunohistochemical staining for human leukocyte antigens can improve diagnostic sensitivity.[11,23] EMB should be performed in centers with a high-volume experience, with proven safety and availability of appropriate pathologic techniques.[24] However, it is important to emphasize that a negative biopsy finding does not preclude the diagnosis of myocarditis.

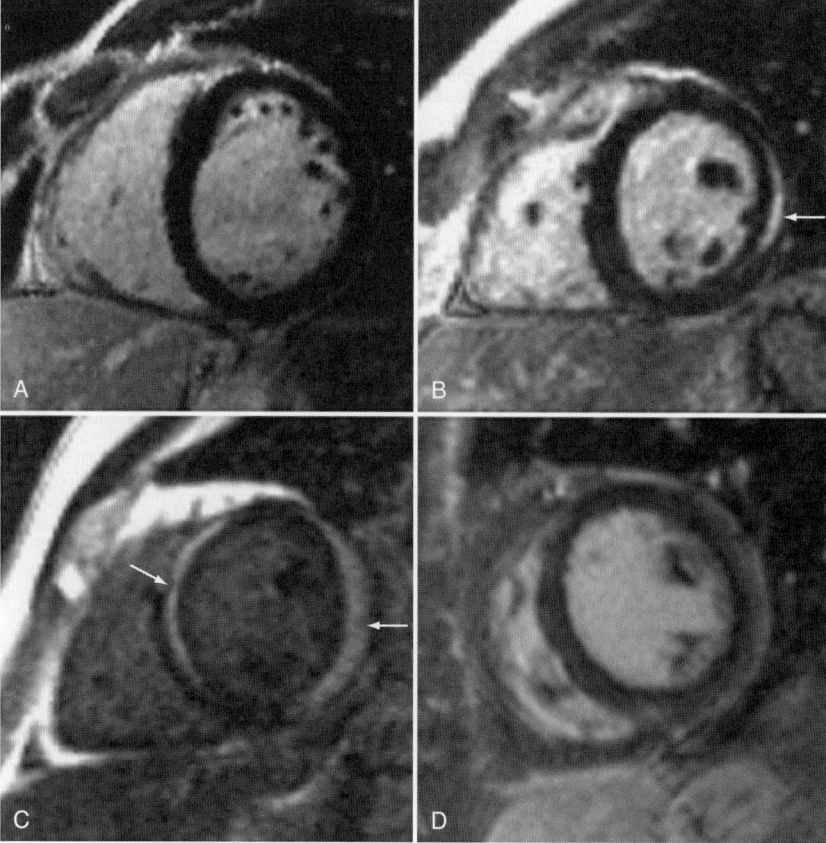

Figure 83-2 Cardiovascular magnetic resonance (CMR) with late gadolinium enhancement—normal and abnormal findings in myocarditis. **A,** Normal myocardium with no evidence of irreversible myocyte injury. **B,** Regional subepicardial enhancement of the lateral wall *(arrow)*. **C,** Subepicardial enhancement of lateral and midwall enhancement of the septal wall *(arrows)*. **D,** Diffuse subepicardial enhancement. *(From Friedrich MG, Sechtem U, Schulz-Menger J, Holmvang G, Alakija P, Cooper LT et al. Cardiovascular magnetic resonance in myocarditis: a JACC White Paper. J Am Coll Cardiol 2009;53(17):1475-87.)*

Although EMB is an insensitive test with a number of problems, a positive biopsy finding has a high positive predictive value.[9] Some authors question the benefits of performing biopsy with standard staining techniques as a routine in suspected myocarditis cases, but this remains the best diagnostic test currently available. Other analyses such as examining specimens for viral genomes utilizing polymerase chain reaction (PCR) or using immunohistochemistry technology to identify up-regulated HLA proteins may offer improved diagnostic yield.[22]

Endomyocardial biopsy should be strongly considered in cases of suspected myocarditis when pathology results will affect management decisions. A recent American Heart Association/American College of Cardiology/European Society of Cardiology (AHA/ACC/ESC) scientific statement offered recommendations concerning the appropriate use of EMB based on patients' clinical presentations.[25] EMB was deemed useful, beneficial. and effective (class I indication) in patients with acute heart failure with hemodynamic compromise, after causes such as coronary artery disease are excluded. EMB is this setting is necessary to differentiate giant cell myocarditis and eosinophilic myocarditis from lymphocytic myocarditis, since immunosuppressive therapy is mandated in the first two conditions (see later). A class I indication for EMB was also recommended for patients with new-onset subacute heart failure, with duration of illness of 2 weeks to 3 months, who fail to improve with medical therapy for heart failure or who demonstrate severe ventricular arrhythmia or advanced heart block. EMB should be considered if causes such as sarcoidosis or collagen vascular disease are suspected and should be performed to diagnose giant cell myocarditis or eosinophilic myocarditis.[26] Endomyocardial biopsy should always be performed prior to initiating immunosuppressive therapy (Table 83-3).

TABLE 83-3	Indications for Endomyocardial Biopsy

Exclusion of potential common etiologies of dilated cardiomyopathy (familial, ischemic, alcohol, postpartum, cardiotoxic exposures) and the following:

Subacute or acute symptoms of heart failure refractory to standard management

Substantial worsening of ejection fraction despite optimized pharmacologic therapy

Development of hemodynamically significant arrhythmias, particularly progressive heart block and ventricular tachycardia

Heart failure with concurrent rash, fever, or peripheral eosinophilia

History of collagen vascular disease such as systemic lupus erythematosus, scleroderma, or polyarteritis nodosa

New-onset cardiomyopathy in the presence of known amyloidosis, sarcoidosis, or hemachromatosis

Suspicion for giant cell myocarditis (young age, new subacute heart failure, or progressive arrhythmia without apparent etiology)

Adapted with permission from Wu L, Lapeyre A, Cooper L. Current role of endomyocardial biopsy in the management of dilated cardiomyopathy and myocarditis. Mayo Clin Proc 2001;76:1030-8.

An algorithm has been proposed outlining the steps in evaluating patients suspected of having acute myocarditis (Figure 83-3).

Clinical Course and Prognosis

The clinical course and prognosis of acute myocarditis is variable. The majority of patients diagnosed with myocarditis will improve. Patients with mild symptoms most often recover without complications. Eight to 12% of young, apparently healthy adults who die suddenly from a cardiac cause are found to have myocarditis at autopsy, suggesting that

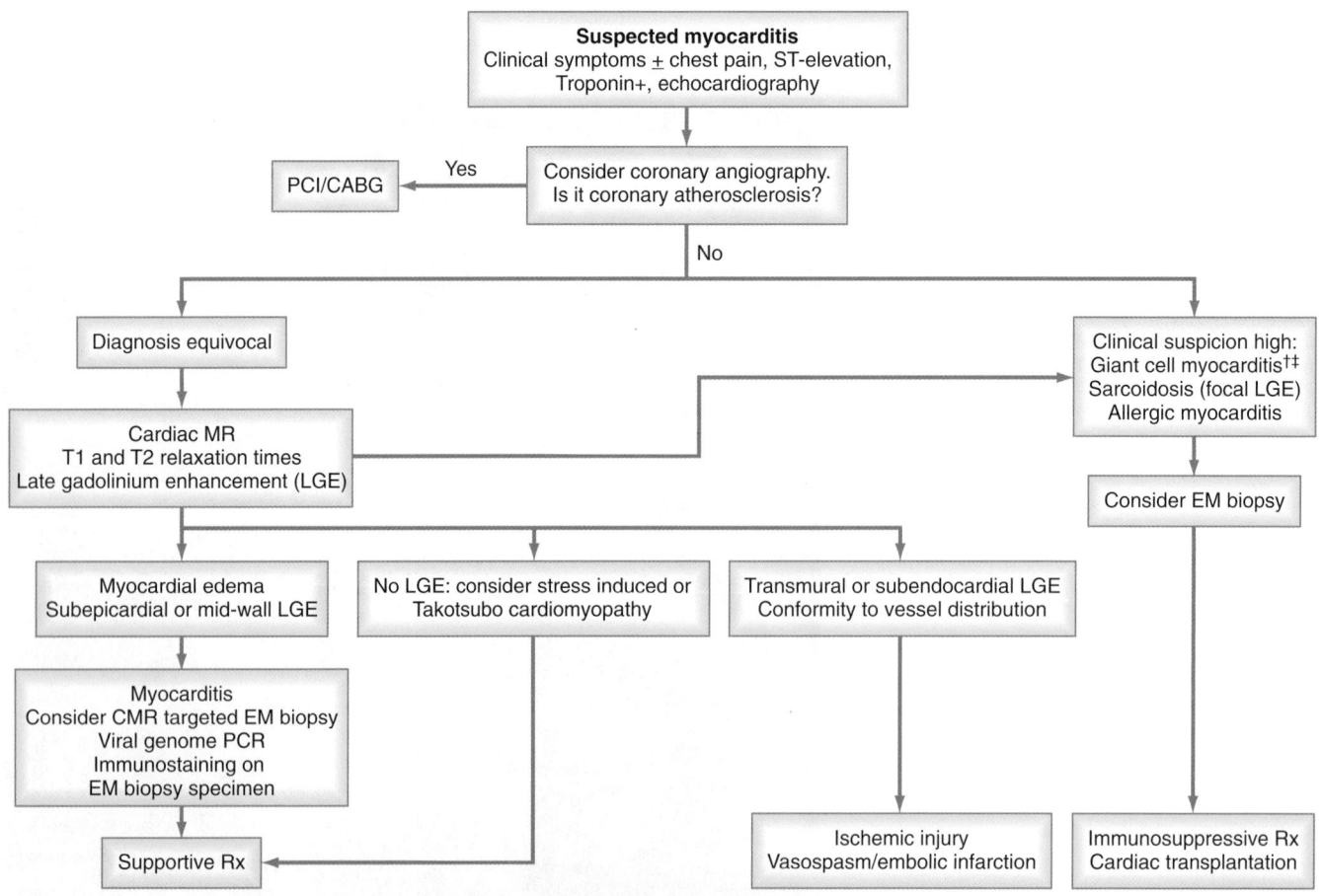

Figure 83-3 Diagnostic algorithm for suspected acute myocarditis. *(Adapted from Nelson KH, Li T, Afonso L. Diagnostic approach and role of MRI in the assessment of acute myocarditis. Cardiol Rev 2009;17:24-30.)*

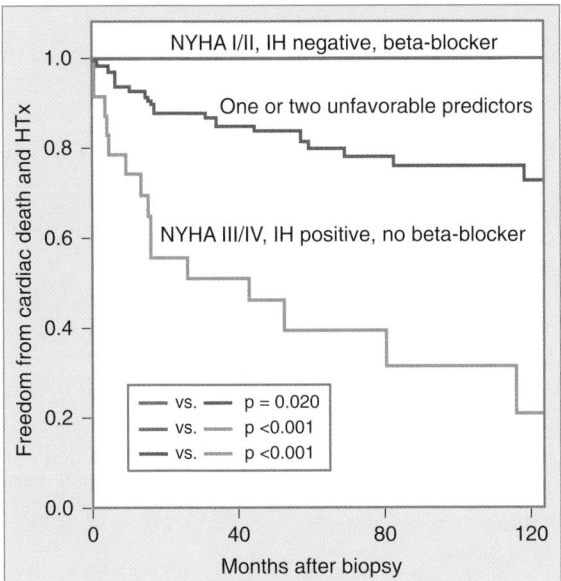

Figure 83-4 Prognosis for patients with acute myocarditis was predicted by three factors: New York Heart Association functional class, positive immunohistology for myocarditis at endomyocardial biopsy, and therapy with beta-blockers. *(Adapted from Kindermann I, Kindermann M, Kandolf R et al. Predictors of outcome in patients with suspected myocarditis. Circulation 2008;118:639-48.)*

patients even with apparently mild illness can suffer fatal arrhythmias.[11] Some patients with myocarditis will progress to chronic dilated cardiomyopathy with manifestations of systolic heart failure,[3] although a precise incidence is not known. Fifteen to 25% of patients who present with new-onset dilated cardiomyopathy have evidence for antecedent myocarditis.[3] Patients with heart failure and LV dysfunction will experience spontaneous resolution of their illness within 12 months in up to 40% of cases, without long-term sequelae. Roughly one-quarter of patients with acute myocarditis and ejection fraction less than 35% will improve, half will develop chronic cardiomyopathy and heart failure, and one-quarter will deteriorate and may be candidates for cardiac transplantation.[27]

It is important to examine the patient population under study and the criteria used for diagnosing myocarditis in any series assessing prognosis and mortality. No clinical markers reliably predict which patients with myocarditis will recover or worsen.[9] In the Myocarditis Treatment Trial, 1-year mortality rate was 20% and 5-year mortality was 56% in patients with biopsy-confirmed lymphocytic myocarditis.[28] A series of 21 patients with active myocarditis on biopsy was analyzed for predictors of disease course. Variables assessed included baseline hemodynamics, use of ventilatory and circulatory support, and serum cardiac biomarkers. Overall, there was a 37% mortality rate (8 of 21), with death occurring at 27.6 ± 6.9 days. Factors predicting a worse prognosis included hypotension (mean 84/49 mm Hg), higher pulmonary capillary wedge pressure (mean of 24 mm Hg), and use of mechanical ventilation. Factors that were not predictive of mortality included sex, age, heart rate, cardiac index, peak creatine kinase, or the use of intraaortic balloon counterpulsation for circulatory support.[29] Another trial reported 181 patients with myocarditis confirmed by EMB utilizing the Dallas criteria, immunohistochemical staining and PCR, which assesses for viral genome. LV biopsy was performed in 90% of patients. Patients were followed for an average of 59 months, and 22% died or received cardiac transplantation. Multivariate analysis concluded that functional class III and IV heart failure and a positive immunohistochemical result were the only predictors of poor outcome, and treatment with beta-blockers was associated with better outcomes[23] (Figure 83-4). Other series have reported that LV ejection

fraction (LVEF) less than 40% and right ventricular dysfunction also predict a poorer prognosis.[11]

FULMINANT MYOCARDITIS

A small percentage of patients with acute myocarditis present critically ill with acute severe heart failure and cardiogenic shock. This presentation is termed *fulminant myocarditis*. Most often these patients give a history of recent fever and symptoms of a viral illness, with a distinct time of onset of heart failure symptoms. This presentation can be contrasted with that of patients with myocarditis who have acute heart failure but not cardiogenic shock, who demonstrate a less distinct time of onset of heart failure symptoms and less severe hypotension.

In a study of 147 patients presenting with heart failure due to biopsy-positive active myocarditis with ejection fraction less than 40%, 10% of patients were diagnosed with fulminant myocarditis and 90% with acute lymphocytic myocarditis.[8] The patients with fulminant myocarditis needed hemodynamic support with high-dose vasopressors or left ventricular assist devices (LVADs). The acute myocarditis patients had more stable hemodynamics and did not require vasopressors or received them at low doses. Patients with fulminant myocarditis tended to be younger and had higher heart rates and lower systemic blood pressure. There was no difference between the groups in mean pulmonary capillary wedge pressure or cardiac index.

With aggressive treatment, patients with fulminant myocarditis actually had better survival rates: 93% at 1 year and 93% at 11 years. Patients with acute myocarditis had an 85% 1-year survival rate and a 45% survival rate at 11 years. Patients with lower pulmonary capillary wedge pressure or higher cardiac index at presentation also had better survival.

In summary, fulminant myocarditis has a distinct clinical course, with critical illness at presentation but with excellent long-term survival once patients recover from the acute phase of their illness. Healing of myocardial injury and significant improvement of LV systolic function can be expected. Therefore, an aggressive approach to therapy, including the use of ventricular assist devices or other mechanical assist devices, without resorting to early cardiac transplantation, is warranted (Figure 83-5).[9]

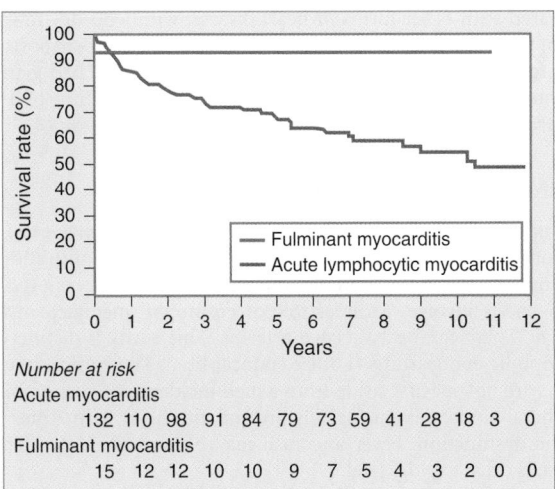

Figure 83-5 Unadjusted transplantation-free survival according to clinicopathologic classification. Patients with fulminant myocarditis were significantly less likely to die or require heart transplantation during follow-up than were patients with acute myocarditis (*P* = 0.05 by the log-rank test). *(From McCarthy RE III, Boehmer JP, Hruban RH, Hutchins GM, Kasper EK, Hare JM et al. Long-term outcome of fulminant myocarditis as compared with acute (nonfulminant) myocarditis. N Engl J Med 2000;342:690-5.)*

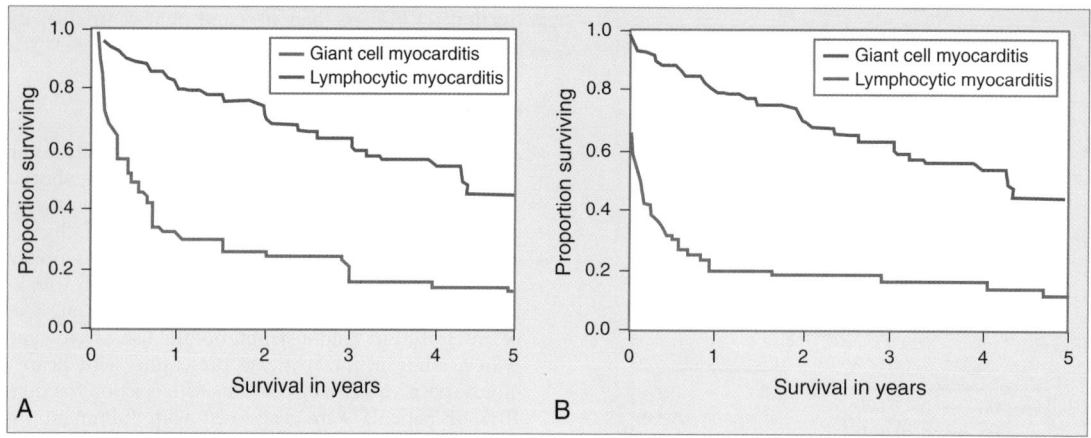

Figure 83-6 Line graphs showing the Kaplan-Meier survival curves for patients with giant cell myocarditis and lymphocytic myocarditis from the onset of symptoms **(A)** and from time of presentation to the referring center **(B)**. In each case, survival was significantly shorter among those with giant-cell myocarditis. *(From Cooper LT Jr, Berry GJ, Shabetai R. Idiopathic giant cell myocarditis—natural history and treatment. Multicenter Giant Cell Myocarditis Study Group Investigators. N Engl J Med 1997;336:1862.)*

GIANT CELL MYOCARDITIS

Giant cell myocarditis is a distinct form of myocarditis, generally with a rapidly progressive course without significant likelihood of spontaneous resolution. On endomyocardial biopsy, infiltration with inflammatory giant cells is seen. Although the pathogenesis is not clear, it is believed to be an autoimmune disorder, and CD4 T lymphocytes are thought to play an important role. A total of 63 patients with biopsy-confirmed giant cell myocarditis were studied retrospectively.[30] Heart failure was the presentation in 75% of cases; 14% presented with ventricular arrhythmias, and 11% presented with chest pain, an abnormal ECG, or heart block. There was an association with inflammatory bowel disease in 8% of cases. Survival was poor, with a median time of 5.5 months to death or cardiac transplantation (Figure 83-6). In this uncontrolled series, immunosuppressive therapy was associated with prolonged survival from 3 months in 30 patients not given immunosuppressive drugs and 3.8 months in patients treated with prednisone, to 11.5 months in patients given prednisone plus azathioprine and 12.6 months in patients who were given cyclosporine as part of their regimen. Prognosis after cardiac transplantation was also worse when compared with other forms of heart disease, with a 30-day mortality rate of 15% and a 26% mortality rate during the 3.7-year posttransplant follow-up period. Twenty-six percent of patients had giant cell infiltrates seen in their transplanted heart at an average time of 3 years after transplant.

EOSINOPHILIC MYOCARDITIS

Eosinophilic myocarditis, also termed *hypersensitivity myocarditis*, is a rare form of myocarditis characterized by eosinophilic infiltration and degranulation seen on endomyocardial biopsy. It is believed that pathogenesis involves a direct role of eosinophil-mediated myocyte damage. There can be associated arteritis. This entity is distinct from eosinophilic endocarditis (Löffler endocarditis). The clinical manifestations are not specific, aside from a high incidence of eosinophilia in peripheral blood. Patients usually present with heart failure due to LV systolic dysfunction. Fever and rash may be present. Untreated, the disease is often rapidly fatal.[7]

The cause is believed to be a hypersensitivity reaction, usually to medication or rarely in association with parasitic infections. Drugs most often implicated are sulfonamides, diuretics, angiotensin-converting enzyme (ACE) inhibitors, cephalosporins, digoxin, or dobutamine. Eosinophilic myocarditis has been reported to occur weeks after smallpox vaccination, with an incidence of 1 in 16,000 vaccinated.[31] The clinical course is unfavorable, often with rapidly worsening heart failure and sudden death due to ventricular arrhythmia. Treatment involves the discontinuation of all potentially offending medication and the use of high-dose corticosteroids. Excellent responses to corticosteroids, as well as some spontaneously resolving illness, have been reported.[32,33]

Eosinophilic myocardial infiltration has been reported in 2% to 7% of myocardial biopsy specimens of patients awaiting cardiac transplantation, or in the explanted heart after transplant. The cause is unclear, but dobutamine therapy, sodium bisulfite used as a preservative in dobutamine solutions, and use of LVADs have been implicated. The presence of eosinophilic myocarditis in this setting did not have an adverse affect on posttransplant survival and did not recur in the transplanted heart.[34,35]

Therapy

GENERAL MANAGEMENT OF HEART FAILURE

Treatment of myocarditis is based on the clinical presentation. Patients with mild disease can be treated expectantly, with dietary sodium restriction and avoidance of strenuous exercise for several weeks or months.[3] Animal models indicate that strenuous exercise can worsen myocarditis. Elimination of unnecessary medications is important in patients with eosinophilia.

Nonsteroidal antiinflammatory drugs should be avoided because they may worsen myocarditis.[4] The routine use of anticoagulants for prophylaxis of systemic emboli is not recommended. Patients who present with symptoms of arrhythmia or heart failure should be hospitalized, with continuous cardiac rhythm monitoring performed for evaluation of potential life-threatening arrhythmias or conduction abnormalities. If these are diagnosed, they are treated in a similar matter as in patients with other causes of heart disease, utilizing antiarrhythmic drugs or pacemakers. However, a period of observation is recommended to assess for improvement of cardiac function prior to implantation of an implantable cardioverter-defibrillator (ICD).

There are data in murine models of myocarditis supporting the use of ACE inhibitors, angiotensin blockers, and beta-blockers. These drugs reduce inflammation and lessen necrosis and fibrosis.[2,3,11,19] There are convincing data in humans supporting the use of these medications, as well as aldosterone antagonists in patients with dilated cardiomyopathy. Therefore, in patients with myocarditis and heart failure, the use of standard multidrug medical therapy for heart failure and LV systolic dysfunction is indicated.[3,10] These medications have been shown to improve symptoms, prolong life, and regress the adverse LV remodeling in patients with dilated cardiomyopathy of various causes.[36,37,38]

Treatment with ACE inhibitors should be initiated at low doses, with upward titration to maximally tolerated doses. Patients should be closely monitored for potential side effects including renal insufficiency, hyperkalemia, and angioedema. Relative contraindications to the use of ACE inhibitors include renal failure, hyperkalemia, bilateral renal artery stenosis, and hepatic failure. Patients with hypotension should be treated with parenteral vasopressors or circulatory assist devices prior to initiation of low-dose ACE inhibitor therapy.

As described earlier, β-adrenergic blockade was associated with improved survival in a multivariate analysis of patients with acute myocarditis.[23] Large randomized controlled clinical trials, which included patients with idiopathic dilated cardiomyopathy, have unequivocally shown benefit from beta-blockers in patients with LV systolic dysfunction,[39-43] and these agents should also be used in patients with heart failure due to myocarditis. Beta-blockers should be initiated after patients are on a stable dose of ACE inhibitors and when signs of fluid overload have resolved. Contraindications to beta-blocker therapy include bronchospastic disease or severe chronic obstructive lung disease, heart block, or significant underlying bradycardia. Hypotension should be corrected prior to initiating beta-blocker therapy.

Digoxin has been shown in animal models to decrease levels of cytokines, but digoxin was associated with adverse outcomes in one murine model of myocarditis. Digoxin can be useful in helping to control ventricular rates in patients with atrial fibrillation. After ACE inhibitors and beta-blockers have been initiated, the use of digoxin should be considered in patients with significant LV systolic dysfunction. However, no survival benefit for digoxin has ever been shown in patients with heart failure due to dilated cardiomyopathy.[44] Contraindications to the use of digoxin include renal failure or heart block.

Use of the aldosterone antagonist, spironolactone, has been shown to have symptomatic and survival benefit in patients with class III-IV chronic systolic heart failure.[45] In experimental models, these agents can reverse the progressive myocardial fibrosis that occurs in the remodeling process of dilated cardiomyopathy. These agents have not been studied in patients with myocarditis, but their use should be strongly considered in patients with severe LV dysfunction (ejection fraction less than 35%) and symptomatic heart failure.[2] Contraindications to the use of aldosterone antagonists include renal insufficiency, serum creatinine levels above 2.0 mg%, or hyperkalemia. Serum potassium levels must be carefully monitored during initiation and dose titration.

In critically ill patients with severe heart failure and low cardiac index, parenteral vasodilators should be used. Intravenous (IV) nitroprusside is a powerful venous and arterial dilator which significantly reduces systemic vascular resistance, mean systemic arterial pressure, and pulmonary capillary wedge pressure, raising cardiac index. It must be administered in the intensive care unit (ICU), with invasive hemodynamic monitoring with a pulmonary artery catheter, to best gauge the appropriate dose of medication and accurately assess response to therapy. Prolonged use of nitroprusside is associated with accumulation of the toxic metabolites thiocyanate and cyanide, and serum levels of these compounds must be monitored. Intravenous nitroglycerin is also an effective venodilator and coronary vasodilator, with less arterial dilating property than nitroprusside. The use of nitroglycerin in cases of myocarditis has not been studied. Patients often develop tolerance to this drug.[46-48]

Patients with severe myocarditis may develop cardiogenic shock, with hypotension, respiratory failure, and signs of end-organ hypoperfusion. In these instances, initial treatment with inotropic agents or vasopressors is indicated. Dobutamine is a potent β₁-agonist with less β₂- and α-agonist properties. Dobutamine has favorable short-term hemodynamic effects with increasing myocardial contractility, reducing systemic vascular resistance and reducing pulmonary capillary wedge pressure. However, dobutamine can be proarrhythmic, and patients can develop tolerance to the drug. Routine use of dobutamine in patients with exacerbations of chronic systolic heart failure was associated with increased mortality rates when compared with placebo.[49]

Milrinone is another parenteral inotropic agent that works by inhibiting phosphodiesterase. This drug leads to increased inotropy and decreased systemic vascular resistance and pulmonary capillary wedge pressure, with resultant increased stroke volume and cardiac index. Milrinone may cause hypotension. It is less proarrhythmic than dobutamine, and it does not induce tolerance.[50,51]

Arterial vasoconstrictors such as norepinephrine and dopamine can be used in patients with refractory hypotension for short-term urgent blood pressure support. However, these agents cause increased myocardial oxygen consumption and can have deleterious effects on myocardial function.

In patients with fulminant myocarditis or cardiogenic shock not responding to pharmacologic therapy, intraaortic balloon counterpulsation should be utilized. Mechanical ventricular assist devices (VADs) are used for patients requiring greater hemodynamic support. These devices are mechanical pumps which provide physiologic cardiac output and LV afterload reduction and may provide time for spontaneous improvement or recovery of normal LV function. VADs are usually univentricular but can be biventricular, supporting both right and LV function. With improved technology, these devices are smaller and can be implanted through smaller incisions or percutaneously. VADs are connected to an external power pack via a driveline through the skin. The power pack is now small and portable, so patients have freedom of movement and can participate in rehabilitation efforts during VAD use. Routine anticoagulation therapy is not required. Complications of VADs include local site infection, sepsis, thromboemboli, and device failure.[52,53]

In patients with myocarditis, VADs can be used to provide circulatory needs and improve coronary flow during the time necessary for spontaneous resolution of myocarditis to occur. Beneficial reverse remodeling may occur while patients are on VAD support, resulting in improved myocyte structure and function. VADs can provide support for months or even years. Some authors believe that patients with fulminant myocarditis should be given every opportunity to recover ventricular function with VAD use, and that cardiac transplantation should be used only as a last resort when severe heart damage is irreversible.[54]

There are several unresolved issues regarding VAD usage in patients with myocarditis. These include appropriate patient selection, timing of VAD placement, best medical therapy during VAD support, and optimal duration of VAD support. A 50-day course of VAD support in the study described earlier allowed identification of 50% of those patients who ultimately recovered, and a 90-day course identified 80% of patients who recovered. The optimal means of serial assessment of native heart function while on VAD support needs to be delineated, and the best weaning protocol also needs definition.

Cardiac transplantation is the final option for treating critically ill patients with myocarditis. However, these patients have a higher rate of transplant rejection and a lower survival rate when compared with patients transplanted for ischemic or other causes of cardiomyopathy. Myocarditis has been reported to recur in the transplanted heart (Figure 83-7).[10]

IMMUNOSUPPRESSIVE THERAPY

Because autoimmune mechanisms are responsible for myocardial injury and the clinical manifestations of myocarditis, therapy with immunosuppressive drugs has been studied. However, given the high rate of spontaneous recovery of LV function, placebo-controlled trials are essential to properly evaluate the effects of therapy. In addition, heterogeneous patient populations consisting of patients with acute myocarditis and chronic dilated cardiomyopathy have been included in immunosuppressive trials, confounding the interpretation of results.

High-dose daily prednisone therapy was used for a 3-month course in 102 patients with dilated cardiomyopathy, 59% of whom were classified as having "reactive" myocarditis on endomyocardial biopsy.[55] The authors found a significant improvement in LVEF at 3 months in treated patients with reactive myocarditis (Figure 83-8), but this

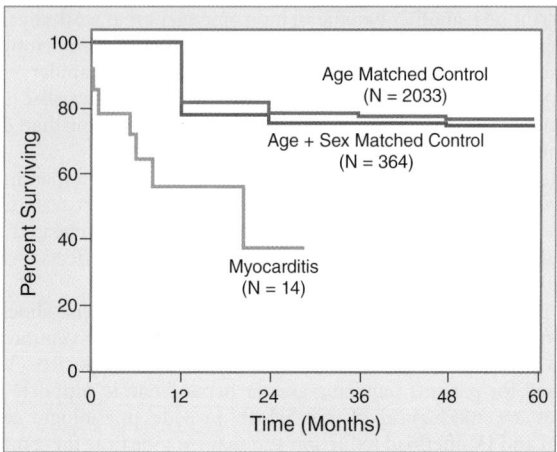

Figure 83-7 Graph showing actuarial survival duration of heart transplant recipients with active lymphocytic myocarditis (green) compared with that of age-matched (red) and age- plus sex-matched (purple) control patients. (*From Haas G. Etiology, evaluation, and management of acute myocarditis. Cardiol Rev 2001;9:88-95.*)

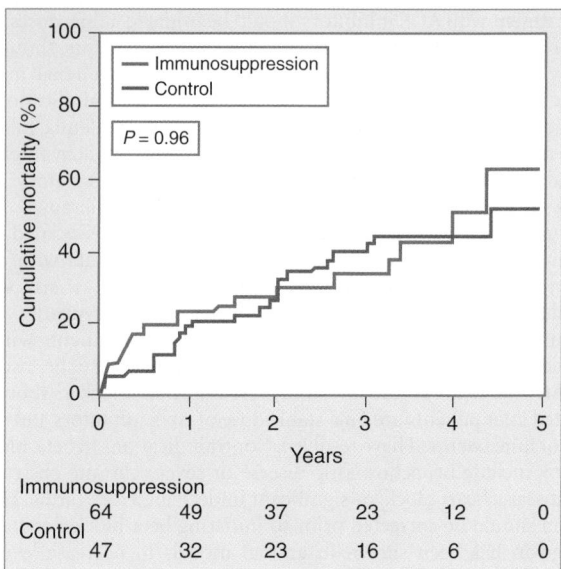

Figure 83-9 Actuarial mortality (defined as deaths and cardiac transplantations) in immunosuppression and control groups. Numbers of patients at risk are shown at the bottom. There was no significant difference in mortality between the two groups. (*From Mason JW, O'Connell JB, Herskowitz A, Rose NR, McManus BM, Billingham ME et al. A clinical trial of immunosuppressive therapy for myocarditis. The Myocarditis Treatment Trial Investigators. N Engl J Med 1995;333:269-75.*)

improvement was not sustained at 9 months. Improvement did not occur in patients with nonreactive biopsies treated with prednisone. No significant mortality benefit from immunosuppressive treatment was noted, although this was not a prespecified primary endpoint.

The Myocarditis Treatment Trial enrolled 111 patients with a positive endomyocardial biopsy finding and LVEF less than 45%, with a duration of illness of less than 2 years.[28] Three treatment groups were compared: daily prednisone plus azathioprine, prednisone plus cyclosporine, and placebo. Mortality was 20% at 1 year and 56% at 3 years. These investigators found no difference in ejection fraction at week 28 or week 52, no change in LV size at week 28, and no difference in 1-year mortality between treated and untreated groups. Their conclusion was that these immunosuppressive strategies were not beneficial. Significant limitations of this study include a 30% dropout rate and significant interobserver variability among pathologists' diagnoses of biopsy specimens, despite utilizing the Dallas criteria (Figure 83-9).

In view of the limitations of histopathologic diagnosis using the Dallas criteria, another group of investigators used immunohistologic markers of inflammation, up-regulation of HLA, to diagnose active myocarditis as an indication for immunosuppressive therapy.[56] This criterion has the advantage of indicating that autoimmunity is playing a role in pathogenesis. Also, since HLA is distributed throughout the entire myocardium, biopsy sampling error is eliminated as a confounding variable in assessing response to therapy. In this study, 84 of 202 patients with chronic (>6 months) idiopathic dilated cardiomyopathy (ejection fraction < 40%) were found to have strong expression of HLA in biopsy specimens and were randomized to receive placebo or prednisone plus azathioprine for 3 months. At 3 months' follow-up, a significant improvement in the prespecified secondary endpoints of LVEF, LV volumes, and functional capacity was seen in the treated

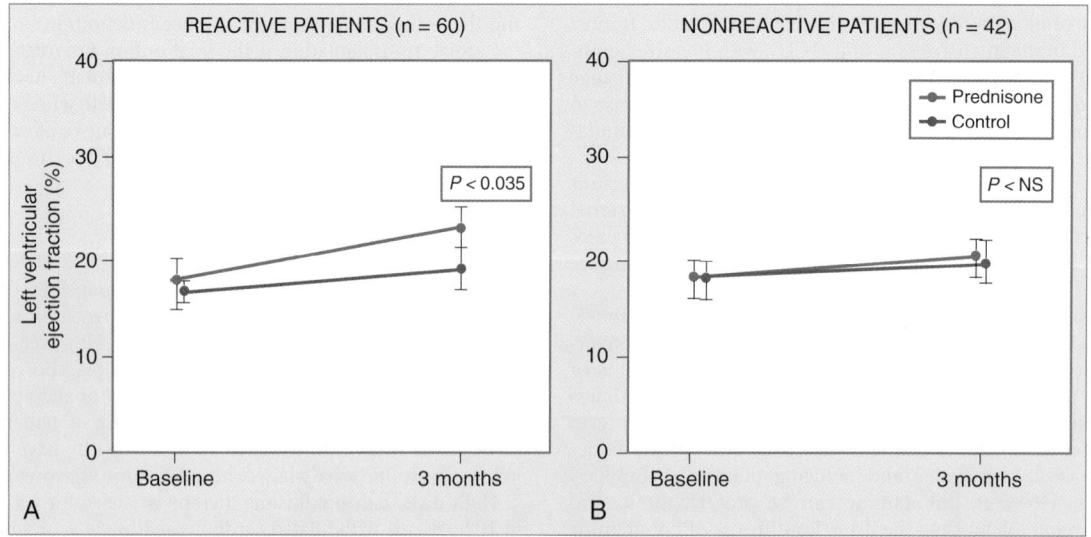

Figure 83-8 **A,** Ejection fraction in reactive dilated cardiomyopathy patients at 3 months. **B,** Prednisone does not change ejection fraction in nonreactive patients in 3 months. (*From Parrillo JE, Cunnion RE, Epstein SE, Parker MM, Suffredini AF, Brenner M et al. A prospective, randomized, controlled trial of prednisone for dilated cardiomyopathy. N Engl J Med 1989;321:1061-8.*)

group, and this improvement was maintained at 2 years (71.8% improvement in the treated group versus 30.8% in the untreated group). However, there was no improvement in the prespecified composite primary endpoint of death, cardiac transplant, or hospital readmission. This study was limited by a 31% dropout rate.

In another study, patients with positive endomyocardial biopsy specimens and progressive heart failure who responded to 6 months of therapy with prednisone and azathioprine were more likely to have circulating cardiac autoantibodies and no viral genome in their myocardium as compared with nonresponders.[57]

Studies have suggested that in patients with heart failure and low ejection fraction, IV immunoglobulin has a pronounced antiinflammatory effect, as measured by circulating levels of inflammatory markers.[58] Uncontrolled studies suggested benefit in patients with myocarditis from treatment with IV immunoglobulin.[59,60] However, a placebo-controlled double-blind trial of IV immunoglobulin in patients with myocarditis or idiopathic dilated cardiomyopathy of less than 6 months' duration showed no significant improvement with therapy, as assessed by ejection fraction or functional capacity at 6 and 12 months.[50] In this study, average LVEF improved from 25% ± 8% at baseline to 41% ± 17% at 6 months in both treated and untreated groups. One-year event-free survival rate was 91.9% in both groups, indicating a favorable prognosis.

In summary, there is no evidence that patients with lymphocytic myocarditis or idiopathic dilated cardiomyopathy benefit from routine use of immunosuppressive therapy. However, this treatment approach should be considered in patients with myocarditis and positive endomyocardial biopsy findings, those who develop early signs of severe heart failure, and those who are shown to experience progressive worsening of LV function. Lastly, immunosuppressive therapy should be used in patients with myocarditis associated with connective tissue diseases such as systemic lupus erythematosus (SLE), eosinophilic or granulomatous forms of the disease, and in giant cell myocarditis (Figure 83-10).

Current investigations are evaluating antiviral therapies in the acute stage of myocarditis as well as the use of antiviral vaccine in the prevention of disease. Appropriately powered, controlled, prospective studies of homogeneous patient groups utilizing immunosuppressive therapy

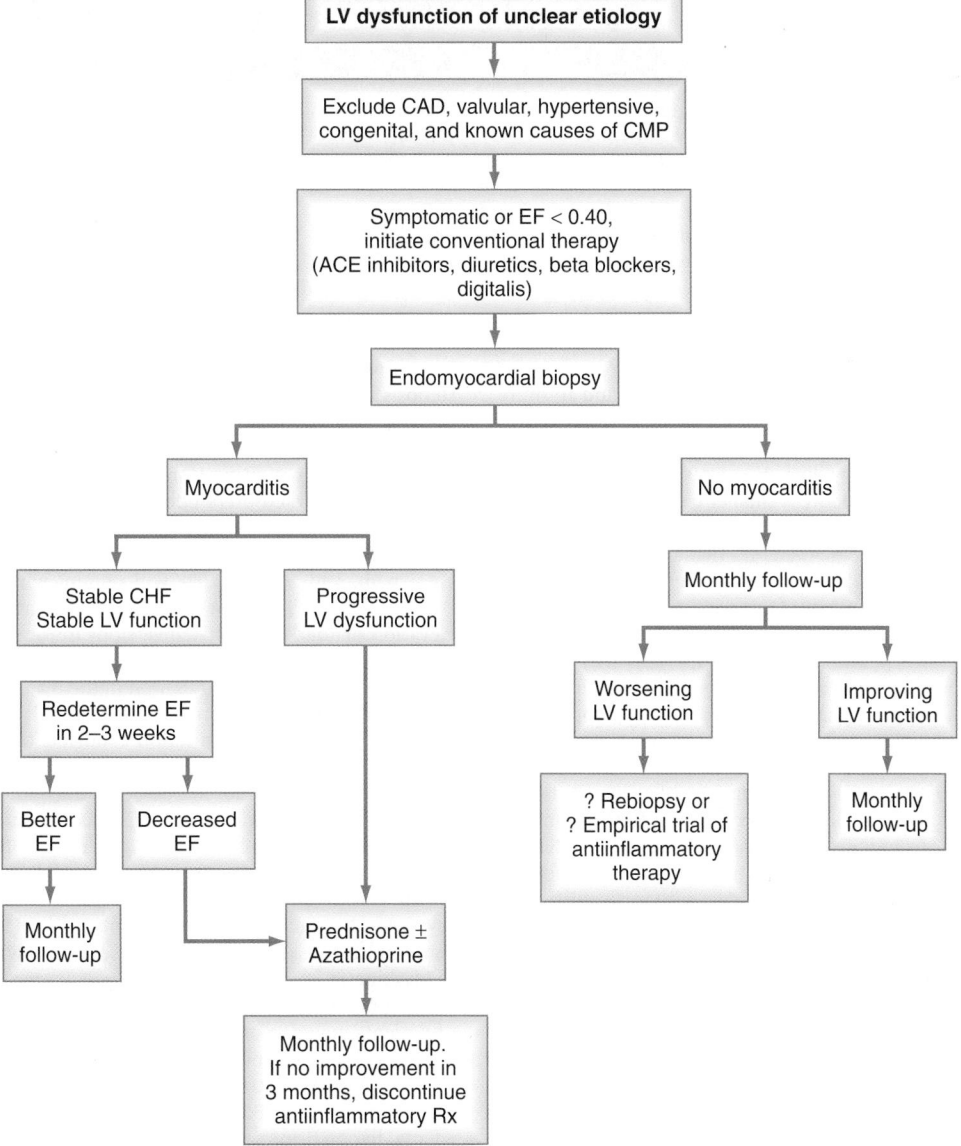

Figure 83-10 Algorithm describing a reasonable approach to myocarditis management based on currently available data. ACE, angiotensin-converting enzyme; CAD, coronary artery disease; CHF, congestive heart failure; CMP, cardiomyopathy; EF, ejection fraction; LV, left ventricular. *(From Parrillo J. Myocarditis: how should we treat in 1998? J Heart Lung Transplant 1998;17:941-4.)*

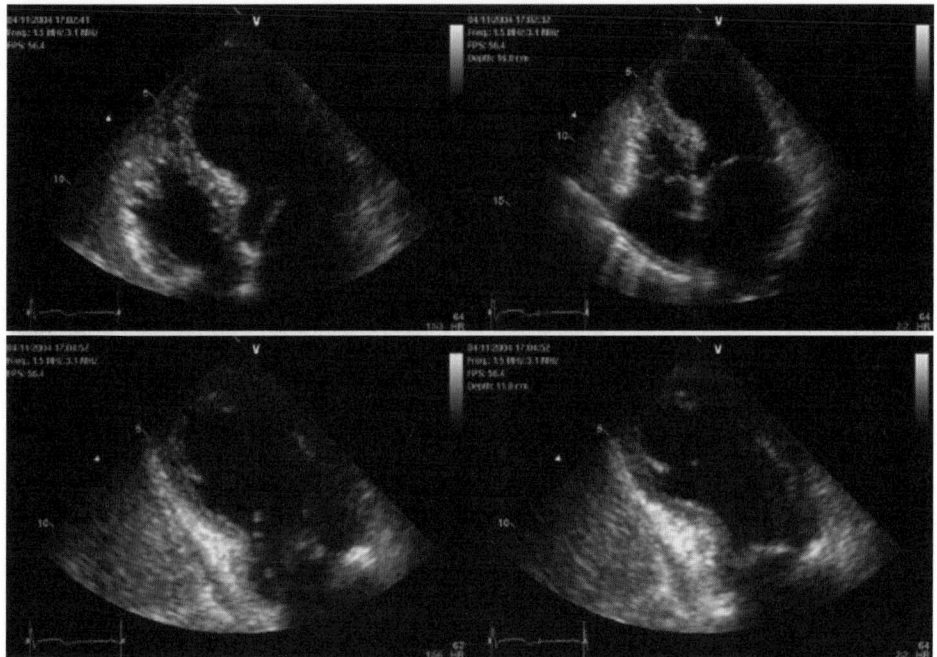

Figure 83-11   End-diastolic and end-systolic apical four-and-two-chamber echocardiographic views demonstrating typical apical and mid-ventricular LV wall-motion abnormalities of a patient with transient apical ballooning syndrome. *(From Gianni M, Dentali F, Grandi AM, Sumner G, Hiralal R, Lonn E. Apical ballooning syndrome or takotsubo cardiomyopathy: a systematic review. Eur Heart J 2006;27:1523-9.)*

are still needed. Evaluating the mechanisms of myocardial recovery during VAD support may also help direct research toward novel approaches to the treatment of myocarditis.

SUMMARY

The most common cause of myocarditis is viral infection, and autoimmune mechanisms are involved in pathogenesis. Patients with myocarditis can present with acute chest pain, mimicking acute ischemic heart disease or other cardiopulmonary illnesses, or can present with heart failure due to dilated cardiomyopathy. A smaller percentage of patients present with acute heart failure due to severe LV systolic dysfunction. Oral and parenteral pharmacologic therapies that are used in patients with heart failure of the more common causes are also used in these patients. Patients can also present with fulminant myocarditis, characterized by severe heart failure and cardiogenic shock. These patients need intensive, aggressive pharmacologic therapy and may require support with VADs, because they very often show significant improvement in LV function such that pharmacologic and VAD support can be weaned and discontinued without having to resort to cardiac transplantation.

Endomyocardial biopsy is used in the diagnosis of myocarditis and for directing therapy, although it is limited by sampling error and current histopathologic techniques for assessing disease activity. Newer immunohistologic methods may better define those patients who will respond to immunosuppressive therapy. Patients with myocarditis and progressive myocardial failure despite conventional heart failure therapy should be considered for immunosuppressive therapy on a case-by-case basis. Such patients should be followed with serial measures of LV performance and endomyocardial biopsies.

Transient Apical Ballooning Syndrome

A distinctive cardiomyopathy with acute onset, frequently precipitated by emotional or physical stress, is termed *transient apical ballooning syndrome* (TABS) owing to a distinctive LV wall-motion abnormality. This cardiomyopathy was first described in patients in Japan in 1991,[61] and the syndrome has subsequently been described in the United States

and Europe.[62,63] It is characterized by the sudden onset of chest pain and/or dyspnea, ECG changes mimicking AMI, and mild elevation of serum myocardial biomarkers. The syndrome is precipitated by extreme emotional or physical stress in over 70% of cases.[64] The characteristic LV wall-motion abnormality is akinesis or dyskinesis of a large area of the LV apex (Figure 83-11 and 83-12). Coronary artery stenosis is not present. TABS is also known as *stress cardiomyopathy* or *takotsubo cardiomyopathy*, so named because the takotsubo pot used by Japanese fishermen to trap octopus has a shape similar to the left ventricle in this condition ("short neck, round flask").[63-66]

There is a marked preponderance for elderly females to be affected by this condition—86% to 100% in reported series, with a mean age of 63 to 67 years. Between 66% and 90% of patients will present with chest pain, and 15% to 20% will present with dyspnea, pulmonary edema, or shock. The most common ECG changes seen are ST-segment elevation or marked T-wave inversions in the precordial leads. These findings are indistinguishable from AMI. Elevation of creatine kinase MB (CK-MB) and troponin is seen in the majority of patients, but the enzyme rise is typically milder than would be expected, given the marked ECG and LV wall-motion abnormalities.

Precipitators of TABS have included arguments with family members, the death of loved ones, or sudden financial setbacks. Physical stresses have included medical procedures such as thoracentesis or biopsy, institution of cancer chemotherapy or hemodialysis, and hip fracture and noncardiac surgeries.

Echocardiography and left ventriculography show moderate to severe LV dysfunction in these patients, with characteristic hyperkinesis of inferior-basal and basal-septal segments, with severe hypokinesis or dyskinesis involving mid-anteroseptal, apical, and inferior-apical wall segments. Acutely, LVEF is reduced to 20% to 40%.[64,65] Up to 20% of patients may demonstrate a LV outflow tract gradient due to basal septal hyperkinesis and transient systolic anterior motion of the anterior leaflet of the mitral valve.[61,62,66]

Patients with TABS often present critically ill, with pulmonary edema, hypotension, and shock. Cardiogenic shock develops secondary to marked LV systolic dysfunction and decreased stroke volume. Shock can also be exacerbated by the development of an LV outflow tract gradient.[68] Cardiogenic shock has been reported in 5% of patients

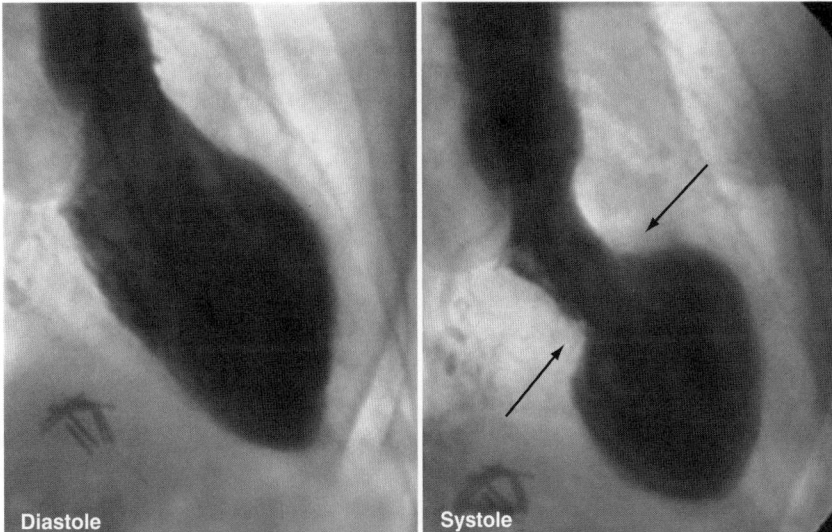

Figure 83-12 Left ventriculogram showing typical left ventricular wall-motion abnormalities in transient apical ballooning syndrome. Arrows in systole indicate hyperkineses of basal inferior and anterior segments, with severe hypokinesis of remaining wall segments. *(From Sharkey SW, Lesser JR, Zenovich AG, Maron MS, Lindberg J, Longe TF et al. Acute and reversible cardiomyopathy provoked by stress in women from the United States. Circulation 2005; 111:472-9.)*

at presentation and has occurred during the course of the illness in 6% to 46% of patients in different series.[63-66,69]

Suspicion of TABS and urgent diagnosis are important, since therapy and prognosis differ substantially from AMI. TABS should not be treated with thrombolytic therapy, as coronary occlusion is not involved in the pathogenesis. If cardiogenic shock develops, treatment with intraaortic balloon pump (IABP) counterpulsation is indicated. Inotropic therapy should be used judiciously or not at all. Dobutamine and other β-agonists may worsen cardiogenic shock by increasing hyperkinesis of the basal portion of the heart and causing or aggravating an LV outflow tract gradient. There have been several case reports of patients with TABS with hypotension who develop frank cardiogenic shock after initiation of inotropic therapy. Since a hyperadrenergic state has been proposed to be a major pathogenic mechanism, empirical use of beta-blockers while patients are being supported with IABP counterpulsation has been used successfully. Echocardiography can be useful to guide therapy. For those with extensive wall-motion abnormalities but no outflow obstruction, IABP support without beta-blockers is recommended. Administration of the α-agonist, phenylephrine, can also be considered in cases with a high LV outflow tract gradient, because this drug increases afterload, causing LV dilatation and a decrease in mitral valve systolic anterior motion and lowering of intraventricular gradients.[67]

TABS is associated with a good prognosis; therefore aggressive therapy of hemodynamic compromise and cardiogenic shock is indicated. In almost all patients, the marked apical wall-motion abnormalities begin to improve within days, and LV function can be expected to recover to normal during the ensuing weeks or months. Follow-up in various series has shown recovery of LVEF to normal in most instances. In-hospital mortality in larger series has been reported at 0% to 4%.[62,64-66,69,70] The large majority of survivors will recover completely, with normal functional status. The long-term prognosis is good. In one series, only 2 out of 72 patients had recurrence of TABS within 13 months.[63] In another series, the recurrence of TABS was calculated at 2.9% per year. Over a 4-year follow-up, long-term survival of patients who recovered from TABS was equivalent to sex- and age-matched control groups without a history of TABS.[70]

The pathogenesis of TABS is unknown. Transient multivessel coronary spasm has been proposed, but this has not been demonstrated at the time of acute coronary angiography in the vast majority of patients. In most patients, the extent of LV wall-motion abnormality is larger than the distribution of a single coronary artery.[62,63] Cardiac MRI has not shown evidence of infarction or myocarditis.[71] In our judgment, a hyperadrenergic state precipitated by acute stress and causing myocardial stunning is the most attractive hypothesis. One study documented

supraphysiologic levels of serum catecholamines and stress neuropeptides in patients during the acute phase of TABS, likely due to adrenal and sympathoneuronal hyperactivity. The apex of the left ventricle may be more sensitive than other LV wall segments to the deleterious effects of adrenergic hyperstimulation.[65]

TABS has been reported to occur in approximately 1.7% to 2.2% of admissions for acute coronary syndrome in Japan and 2% of cases of acute heart failure due to acute coronary syndrome.[69,71] TABS may be more common than currently recognized. Correct diagnosis is more likely to be made in centers where emergency coronary angiography and primary percutaneous coronary intervention are used in the treatment of acute coronary syndrome and ST-segment elevation myocardial infarction (STEMI).

In summary, TABS should be suspected in patients who present with symptoms and ECG findings consistent with AMI, who have a large apical wall-motion abnormality seen on echocardiography or left ventriculography, and whose symptoms were precipitated by severe emotional or physical stress. Diagnosis is confirmed when urgent cardiac catheterization and coronary angiography demonstrate no significant coronary artery occlusion or stenosis.

Tachycardia-Induced Cardiomyopathy

A sustained rapid heart rate can lead to the acute development of LV dilation and dysfunction with symptoms of heart failure. This is termed *tachycardia-induced cardiomyopathy* (TICMP) and can occur in otherwise normal hearts or can exacerbate heart failure in patients with preexisting cardiomyopathy. Supraventricular or ventricular arrhythmias of any type can lead to this syndrome. Arrhythmias which may be responsible for TICMP include atrial fibrillation, atrial flutter, automatic atrial tachycardia, AV node reentry tachycardia, supraventricular tachycardia involving accessory pathways, accelerated junctional tachycardia, ventricular tachycardia (from RV and LV sites) and even prolonged, sustained ventricular bigeminy.[72] It is not known how long the tachycardia needs to be present in order to cause LV dysfunction, but sustained arrhythmia for days to weeks is likely necessary. The presence of an underlying predisposing substrate has been postulated, as not all patients with sustained tachycardia will develop cardiomyopathy.[73]

Animal models of TICMP have been established and studied to elucidate pathophysiologic mechanisms and clinical correlates. In these models, sustained, rapid atrial or ventricular pacing leads to severe biventricular systolic and diastolic dysfunction with four-chamber dilation. Within 24 hours of initiating rapid pacing, there is a fall in cardiac output and an increase in ventricular filling pressures.

Neurohormonal activation occurs, typical for dilated cardiomyopathy. Cardiac output, ejection fraction, and ventricular volume continue to deteriorate over 3 to 5 weeks. When pacing is discontinued, cardiac output improves to near normal in 48 hours, and hemodynamics are normal within 4 weeks. Ejection fraction recovers to normal in 1 to 2 weeks, although end-diastolic volume remains high at 12 weeks, suggesting persistent remodeling. Structural cardiac changes seen include myocyte hypertrophy and apoptosis and altered extracellular matrix. Proposed pathophysiologic mechanisms include myocardial energy depletion, ischemia, and altered myocyte handling of calcium.[73-75]

There currently are no data in humans regarding the time course, mechanisms, or cellular biochemical alterations. TICMP can occur at any age, from infants to the elderly. TICMP has been reported to occur in fetuses with sustained supraventricular tachycardia, which resolved with correction of the arrhythmia.[74] It is not known if there is a minimal heart rate necessary to induce cardiomyopathy. The longer the duration of arrhythmia, the more likely cardiomyopathy is to occur and the more severe it will tend to be. The incidence and prevalence of TICMP are not known.

The diagnosis of TICMP should be suspected in any patient with impaired ventricular function in the setting of sustained supraventricular tachycardia or ventricular tachycardia. The diagnosis is clear when LV function prior to the onset of tachycardia was demonstrated to be normal, and no intercurrent illness other than the arrhythmia has occurred. The diagnosis is confirmed when LV function rapidly improves with correction of the arrhythmia.

Treatment of TICMP is to rapidly restore normal heart rate. This can be done with parenteral rate-slowing medication, including beta-blockers such as esmolol or metoprolol or calcium channel blockers such as diltiazem. Verapamil may aggravate hypotension and LV dysfunction and should be avoided. Adenosine can rapidly convert atrioventricular nodal reentry tachycardia to sinus rhythm. Intravenous digoxin can also be considered, although its onset of action is delayed. Type I drugs such as procainamide can be prescribed for supraventricular tachycardia associated with accessory pathways. Electrical cardioversion can rapidly terminate supraventricular and ventricular tachycardia and restore sinus rhythm. In patients with atrial flutter or atrial fibrillation, reliable control of the heart rate to a range of 60 to 90 bpm is a reasonable alternative to conversion of the arrhythmia to sinus rhythm.

In patients with TICMP who have received appropriate arrhythmia therapy, heart failure symptoms improve rapidly. LV systolic function will generally recover to normal within 4 weeks if there is no other underlying heart disease. Cardiac rhythm monitoring for 24 to 48 hours is often necessary to ensure that heart rate is controlled during activity as well as at rest.[74] In a report of 11 patients with atrial flutter and abnormal systolic function who underwent atrial flutter ablation, ejection fraction improved from an average of 31% at baseline to 41% within 7 months of ablation. Lack of resolution of cardiomyopathy was predicted by a lower baseline ejection fraction.[76] A series of 24 patients with TICMP was reported whose cardiomyopathy initially resolved with arrhythmia control, but who experienced repeated rapid decline in LV function and recurrent heart failure when their arrhythmias reoccurred. These patients again had improvement or normalization of ejection fraction following repeated arrhythmia control within 6 months. However, three of the patients died suddenly and unexpectedly, emphasizing that structural and electrical abnormalities may persist on a chronic basis.[77]

KEY POINTS

1. Myocarditis is most often caused by a viral infection. Myocardial damage is mediated through activation of cellular immune mechanisms.

2. The clinical course of myocarditis can be benign, with complete resolution, or the illness can be more severe, with the development of dilated cardiomyopathy and congestive heart failure. Fatal arrhythmia can occur.

3. The pharmacologic therapy of heart failure associated with myocarditis is similar to therapy used in other forms of dilated cardiomyopathy. Severe cases may require the use of a ventricular assist device.

4. Fulminant myocarditis is an unusual complication, with a rapidly progressive course resulting in cardiogenic shock. These cases should be aggressively managed with pharmacologic therapy and ventricular assist devices, because significant improvement in left ventricular function will often occur.

5. Endomyocardial biopsy is frequently used to make the diagnosis of myocarditis and to direct therapy, although there are limitations in the interpretation of biopsy results.

6. Immunosuppressive therapy should not be used routinely in the treatment of myocarditis but should be strongly considered in patients who have severe heart failure early in the course of the illness or whose condition deteriorates despite the use of conventional heart failure treatment.

7. Transient apical ballooning syndrome, or stress cardiomyopathy, is an acute severe cardiomyopathy often precipitated by emotional or physical stress, with a presentation similar to acute myocardial infarction and a generally good prognosis after a period of aggressive supportive care.

ANNOTATED REFERENCES

Cooper LT, Baughman K, Feldman AM, et al. The role of endomyocardial biopsy in the management of cardiovascular disease: a scientific statement from the American Heart Association, the American College of Cardiology and the European Society of Cardiology. Circulation 2007;116:2216-33.
This paper presents the ACC/AHA/ESC recommendations for the indications for and utility of endomyocardial biopsy.
Cooper L, Berry G, Shabetai R. Idiopathic giant cell myocarditis—natural history and treatment. N Engl J Med 1997;336:1860-6.
The Multicenter Giant Cell Myocarditis Study Group investigators describe the clinical course, prognosis, and treatment of patients with this disease.
Gianni M, Dentali F, Grandi AM, Sumner G, Hiralal R, Lonn E. Apical ballooning syndrome or takotsubo cardiomyopathy: a systematic review. Eur Heart J 2006;27:1523-9.
A comprehensive review of the reported series of patients with this condition.
Magnani JW, Dec GW. Myocarditis. Current trends in diagnosis and treatment. Circulation 2006;113:876-90.
An excellent overview of the etiology, pathogenesis, diagnosis, and treatment of myocarditis.

Mason J, O'Connell J, Herskowitz A, et al. A clinical trial of immunosuppressive therapy for myocarditis. N Engl J Med 1995;333:269-75.
Despite limitations in patient follow-up and biopsy interpretation, this controlled trial showed no difference in survival between patients treated with an immunosuppressive regimen and control patients.
McCarthy R, Boehmer J, Hruban R, et al. Long-term outcome of fulminant myocarditis as compared with acute (nonfulminant) myocarditis. N Engl J Med 2000;342:690-5.
These authors describe and compare the clinical course of patients with fulminant myocarditis with acute myocarditis, defining fulminant myocarditis as a distinct clinical illness.
Parrillo JE, Cunnion RE, Epstein SE, Parker MM, Suffredini AF, Brenner M, et al. A prospective randomized controlled trial of prednisone for dilated cardiomyopathy. N Engl J Med 1989;321:1061-8.
This study by members of the National Heart, Lung, and Blood Institute concluded that prednisone treatment delivered "only marginal clinical benefit, and should not be administered as standard therapy for dilated cardiomyopathy."

REFERENCES

Access the complete reference list online at http://www.expertconsult.com.

84

Acquired and Congenital Heart Disease in Children

DUNCAN MACRAE

Physiology

CIRCULATORY CHANGES AT BIRTH

During the transition from intrauterine to extrauterine life, major circulatory changes occur which have important implications for the clinical care of the newborn.[1,2] At birth in the normal newborn, the low-resistance placenta is eliminated from the circulation, resulting in an immediate increase in systemic vascular resistance (SVR). The pulmonary vascular resistance (PVR) falls when the lungs become responsible for gas exchange, and the fetal channels, foramen ovale, and arterial duct become redundant and close. In addition to altered hemodynamics in babies born with congenital heart disease, some babies with structurally normal hearts have a persistent right-to-left shunt after birth due to failure of the transition from fetal to postnatal circulation. Babies with this circulatory pattern, which is characterized by failure of the PVR to fall, have persistent pulmonary hypertension of the newborn (PPHN).[3] PPHN is one of the two principal causes of nonpulmonary cyanosis in the neonate, the other being cyanotic congenital heart disease.

The right ventricle (RV) and left ventricle (LV) contribute equally to fetal cardiac output. At birth, the LV becomes responsible for the systemic circulation, characterized by its high vascular resistance. The PVR falls suddenly at birth to approximately 50% of fetal levels to facilitate the required increase in pulmonary blood flow. It continues to fall to adult values during the first 6 to 8 weeks of life as the smooth muscle layer in the media of the pulmonary arterioles progressively thins out. The LV progressively adapts to its high-pressure role by rapid myocardial growth, in contrast to the RV, which regresses to its low-pressure subpulmonary role. The presence of congenital heart defects can profoundly alter these adaptive processes (see later).

PHYSIOLOGY OF THE NEONATAL MYOCARDIUM

The neonatal myocardium is functionally immature.[4] Age-dependent changes in intrinsic function and integration with a maturing circulation determines its response to insults such as hypoxia and ischemia.[5]

The myocardium matures in the postnatal period by increasing the number, volume, and conformation of its myocytes. The cell membrane (sarcolemma) develops the T-tubular system, which facilitates rapid conduction of the action potential to the center of the cell, and the arrangement of myofibrils gradually becomes more uniform, improving its contractile function. In parallel with these structural changes, myocellular metabolism matures. Proper contractile function of the cardiac myocyte depends on an efficient excitation-contraction process, which is activated by the binding of calcium to troponin C. In the adult heart, calcium release from the sarcoplasmic reticulum (SR) is the predominant source of calcium for troponin C activation. In contrast in the neonate, activation relies substantially on calcium influx through the L-type calcium channels. Optimal function of the neonatal myocardium is therefore exquisitely dependent on maintenance of normal extracellular calcium concentrations. Other elements of myocyte function are age dependent, such as the sarcoplasmic reticulum calcium-ATPase (SERCA) which is present in reduced quantities in the immature heart. This results in relatively inefficient calcium re-uptake and therefore slower diastolic relaxation of the neonatal compared to the adult

myocyte and is at least in part responsible for the prominence of diastolic dysfunction in the failing neonatal myocardium.

Healthy infants have higher plasma concentrations of catecholamines and higher-density cardiac sympathetic innervation than older children and adults. This may partly explain the reduced ability of neonates to increase cardiac output in response to endogenous or exogenous catecholamines. Children in heart failure also have higher plasma catecholamine concentrations[6] but reduced densities of β-adrenergic receptors compared to age-matched controls.[7] The effects of this are similar to those seen with exogenous agonist-induced desensitization. Children with severe heart failure show evidence of uncoupling of β₁-adrenergic receptors from the enzyme adenylcyclase[7] and other maladaptive responses that result in reduced response to receptor agonists. In addition to heart failure, chronic hypoxia, such as is seen in cyanotic congenital heart disease, induces activation of the sympathetic nervous system, with resultant adrenergic receptor desensitization. Developmental aspects of myocardial support have recently been reviewed.[8] The characteristics of the neonatal ventricle are listed in Table 84-1.

CONGESTIVE HEART FAILURE

Although the basic pathophysiologic mechanisms of heart failure have age-independent common mechanisms, the presentation and management of heart failure changes with age. The overwhelming cause of heart failure in the first year of life is congenital heart disease, usually with an intracardiac left-to-right shunt or a ventricular obstructive lesion (Table 84-2). By contrast, the primary abnormality in adult heart failure is usually left ventricular dysfunction. Heart failure in adults is often gradual in onset; the neonate has little functional reserve, resulting in rapid decompensation and an emergent presentation.

The clinical features[9] of heart failure in infants are listed in Table 84-3. A prominent sign of cardiac failure in infancy is difficulty in feeding secondary to increased respiratory rate and effort. This equates to exertional dyspnea in the older child or adult. Failure to thrive results and leads to the classic "wizened" appearance. Although hepatomegaly is a common sign of heart failure in infants (resulting from an increase in total circulating volume and hepatic venous congestion), peripheral edema, ascites, and pericardial or pleural effusions are much less commonly seen than in adults. One relatively common feature of severe heart failure in infancy is the occurrence of compression of the bronchial tree—particularly the left mainstem or lower lobe bronchus—secondary to extrinsic compression by an enlarged left atrium or pulmonary artery. This can cause airway obstruction and associated lobar collapse, or localized hyperinflation due to distal air-trapping. Long-standing extrinsic compression may rarely cause tracheobronchomalacia, resulting in long-term respiratory difficulties even after resolution of heart failure.

CYANOSIS

Cyanosis is the visible manifestation of greater than 5 g/dL of reduced deoxygenated hemoglobin in cutaneous blood vessels, and is a prominent feature in many types of congenital heart disease. *Peripheral cyanosis* results from high oxygen extraction ratios across the tissue vascular

TABLE 84-1	Characteristics of the Neonatal Ventricle
	Comparison to Mature Ventricle
Contractility	Contractility of the neonatal ventricle is reduced compared to the mature ventricle.
Compliance	Neonatal ventricle inherently noncompliant compared to mature ventricle
Augmentation cardiac output	Little stoke volume reserve due to low compliance. Therefore cardiac output is highly heart-rate dependent in neonates.
Afterload	Neonatal ventricle tolerates increased afterload poorly.
Energy substrate	Lactate is primary substrate of neonatal ventricle under aerobic conditions. Glucose metabolized under anaerobic conditions. By 1-2 years, changes over to primary adult substrate, free fatty acids.

TABLE 84-3	Clinical Features of Heart Failure in Infants

Respiratory Signs
- Initially tachypnea
- Dyspnea manifesting as poor feeding
- Later signs: retractions, intercostal recession, nasal flaring
- Pulmonary wheeze/rales

Other Signs
- Tachycardia; little variability even at rest
- Gallop rhythm
- Hepatomegaly
- Cardiomegaly
- Poor peripheral perfusion; in severe failure, ashen appearance

bed, reflecting low tissue blood flow or high tissue oxygen demand. *Central cyanosis* results from desaturation of arterial blood, which may be due to pulmonary disease or right-to-left shunting of deoxygenated systemic venous blood in association with a congenital heart defect. Pulmonary and cardiac causes of central cyanosis can usually be differentiated by allowing the child to breathe 100% oxygen (a "hyperoxic test"), which will result in a substantial improvement in oxygen saturation the case of cyanosis of pulmonary origin but have little effect on the child with cyanosis due to right-to-left shunt.[10] During administration of 100% oxygen, arterial oxygen tensions (Pao_2) above 160 mm Hg are highly suggestive of a noncardiac diagnosis, and a Pao_2 over 250 mm Hg excludes it. Occasionally, *differential cyanosis* is seen where one or both of the upper limbs are normally saturated and the lower limbs cyanosed. The cause is deoxygenated blood traversing the arterial duct to enter the aorta distal to the origin of one or both subclavian arteries and supplying the lower limbs, while oxygenated blood from the left ventricle predominantly supplies the upper limbs.

Chronic hypoxemia induces the twin physiologic responses of erythropoiesis, resulting in polycythemia and an increase in blood volume in a compensatory attempt to maintain oxygen-carrying capacity. However, as hemoglobin concentrations rise, blood viscosity increases and ultimately leads to sluggish flow in the peripheral circulation, cellular aggregation, and the occurrence of thrombotic lesions. Polycythemic patients are at high risk of thrombotic complications in situations of increased fluid loss (e.g., intercurrent diarrheal illness) or

inadequate fluid intake (e.g., preoperative fasting). In addition to polycythemia, most children with chronic cyanosis develop finger clubbing, the result of an increased number of capillaries laid down in the vascular beds of the fingers and toes. Rare but important complications of severe cyanosis arise primarily from hypoxemia and polycythemia and include cerebral and pulmonary thrombosis and cerebral abscess.

PULMONARY VASCULATURE AND PULMONARY HYPERTENSION

The pulmonary vascular bed is of central importance to the manifestations of congenital heart disease from the first hours of life. Pulmonary vascular resistance usually falls dramatically in response to aeration of the lungs with the first breaths. Thereafter, the smooth muscle of the pulmonary vascular bed thins gradually during the first months of life, with associated fall in PVR to adult values by approximately 2 months of age. In infants with congenital heart lesions where an intracardiac communication between the systemic and pulmonary circulations is present, such as a ventricular septal defect (VSD), the fall in PVR encourages flow into the low-resistance pulmonary vascular bed, and a left-to-right shunt develops. In response to the increased flow and subsequent shear stress this induces, progressive structural changes occur in the pulmonary arteries and arterioles. Initially these changes consist of accelerated extension of muscle to the distal "non-muscular" pulmonary arteries and medial muscular hypertrophy in the proximal muscular arteries. Later changes involve gradual hypertrophy of the arterial intima, with deposition of collagen and elastin leading to gradual luminal obstruction and eventual occlusion. Associated with this is the development of plexiform lesions, the histologic hallmark of pulmonary vascular disease. Mild pulmonary vascular changes are of little significance to the cardiac intensivist; however, children with more extensive medial muscular hypertrophy of the pulmonary arteries are at risk of labile pulmonary hypertension (PHT) in the postoperative period (see later). The extent of pulmonary hypertensive changes frequently determine the feasibility of surgical options. Children with established fixed high PVR are unsuitable for corrective surgery, as surgical separation of the two circulations in the face of fixed high PVR will result in immediate right ventricular failure. Smaller elevations in PVR determine operability in the single-ventricle Fontan circulation (discussed later). Calculation of PVR and the response to varying vasodilators can be achieved following a pulmonary reversibility study in the cardiac catheter laboratory.[11-13]

Circulatory Support in Children

Children presenting with circulatory failure[14] must initially be assessed and managed according to standard resuscitation algorithms. These require that adequate oxygenation and circulating volume be achieved. If cardiac output remains low, cardiovascular drug therapy is usually indicated. The developmental differences previously noted serve to emphasize the need to adopt age-appropriate pharmacologic strategies when supporting the failing myocardium of the neonate and infant.[15-17] If cardiac output remains low despite application of such measures, mechanical circulatory support should be considered (Figure 84-1).

TABLE 84-2	Common Causes of Heart Failure in Childhood		
Neonate < 2 Weeks Age	**Neonate > 2 Weeks Age, Infant**	**Older Child**	
Congenital Heart Disease			
LEFT-SIDED OBSTRUCTIVE LESIONS	LEFT-TO-RIGHT SHUNT LESIONS	ANY LESION	
• Critical aortic stenosis • Aortic coarctation • Hypoplastic left heart syndrome	• Ventriculoseptal defect • Atrioventriculoseptal defect • Truncus arteriosus • Total anomalous pulmonary venous drainage	• Following surgery • Late deterioration of ventricle in palliated circulations	
Other Causes		ACQUIRED HEART DISEASE	
ARRHYTHMIAS		• Cardiomyopathies (idiopathic or specific)	
• Incessant supraventricular tachycardia		• Myocarditis • Rheumatic fever	
CONGENITAL MYOCARDITIS		• Infective endocarditis • Arrhythmias	
SEVERE VENTRICULAR DYSFUNCTION		• Severe anemia • Nutritional deficiencies	
• Due to birth asphyxia, sepsis, or severe metabolic disorders			

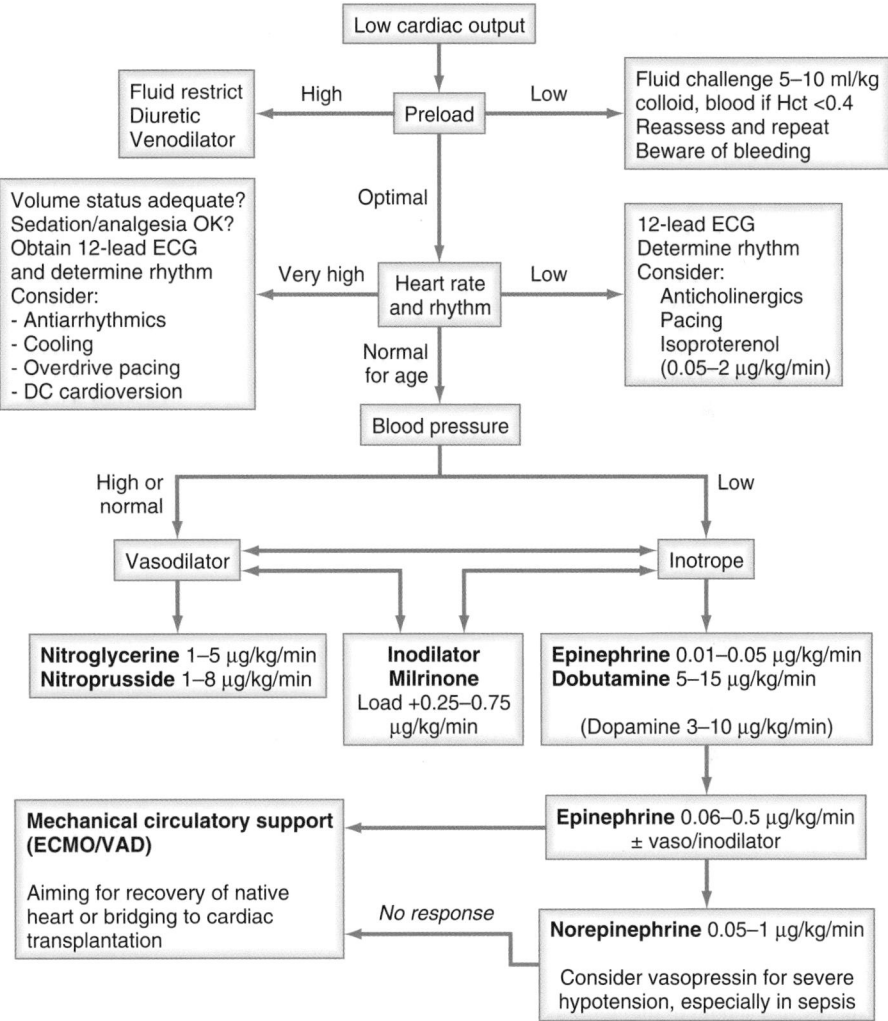

Figure 84-1 Management of low cardiac output in children.

PHARMACOLOGIC SUPPORT

β-Adrenergic Agonists

Clinical and experimental studies have demonstrated marked age-related differences in the hemodynamic response to inotropic therapy. Although some of the observed differences may be accounted for by differences in drug pharmacokinetics, the variable maturation of the sympathetic nervous system, its receptors, and the cardiac myocytes mitigate against the recommendation of narrow specific dose ranges for the use of catecholamines in neonates and children.[8]

In clinical pediatric practice, adrenergic agonists are titrated to hemodynamic effect much as they are in adults (Table 84-4). When systolic ventricular function is impaired, low-dose epinephrine is commonly used as the first-line inotrope, although dobutamine and dopamine still have their advocates. Dopamine was formerly preeminent but is now less favored because of its noncardiac adverse effects.[18] Additional agents should be administered according to assessment of response, judged clinically and from available hemodynamic monitoring. Higher-dose epinephrine, norepinephrine, or vasopressin can be used in refractory circulatory failure, particularly if vasodilation is present, such as occurs occasionally after cardiopulmonary bypass in children.[19,20] Isoproterenol is a nonspecific β-adrenergic agonist whose principal cardiovascular effects are vasodilation and increasing heart rate. The drug is rarely used in intensive care except as a chronotropic agent where heart rate is critically low and cardiac pacing not yet established. Caution is needed when higher-dose catecholamine support is used in the neonate, as these can induce a rise in ventricular end-diastolic pressure (EDP) in a ventricle already developmentally noncompliant. Catecholamine-induced myocardial necrosis has been identified in neonatal animal models.[21,22]

Phosphodiesterase Inhibitors

Phosphodiesterase (PDE) inhibitors have emerged as important agents in the management of neonates and children with cardiac failure. The

TABLE 84-4	Vasoactive Agents in Children

Adrenergic Agonists

	Intravenous Dose Range	Alpha 1	Beta 1	Beta 2	Dopa	Comments
Dopamine	1-5 µg/kg/min 5-15 µg/kg/min	0 0/++	+/++++		++++	Beta-mediated inotropic effects at lower doses; alpha-mediated vasoconstriction at higher doses
Dobutamine	2-15 µg/kg/min	0	+/+++	0/++	0	
Epinephrine	0.02-0.1 µg/kg/min 0.2-0.4 µg/kg/min	0/++++/+++	++/+++++++	++/++++++	0 0	β_2 Effect prominent at lower doses; alpha constrictor effects at higher doses
Norepinephrine	0.2-0.5 µg/kg/min	++/++++	+	0	0	Increases SVR. Reserved for treatment of severe hypotension associated with vasodilatation
Isoproterenol	0.02-0.4 µg/kg/min	0	++++	++++	0	Prominent chronotropic activity. Vascular β_2 effects cause vasodilatation

Other Cardiovascular Drugs

	Dosage	Effects
PDE3 Inhibitors		
Amrinone	Neonates: 4 mg/kg over 15 minutes, then 3-5 µg/kg/min IV >4 weeks age: 1-3 mg/kg over 30 minutes, then 5-15 µg/kg/min IV	Cardiac: mild nonadrenergic inotropic and lusitropic effects Vascular: systemic and pulmonary vasodilator
Milrinone	All ages: 50-75 µg/kg over 20 minutes Maintenance: 0.5-0.75 µg/kg/min IV	Amrinone may cause thrombocytopenia Reduce amrinone dose in slow acetylators Reduce milrinone dose in renal failure
Levosimendan	0.05-0.2 µg/kg/min IV for 24 hours	Duration of effect 3-7 days
Digoxin	Initial dose 15 µg/kg, then 5 µg/kg after 6 hours. Thereafter, 5 µg/kg 12 hourly. Slow IV or oral.	Delays AV conduction Used in management of supraventricular tachycardia Mild inotropic properties; may provide symptomatic relief in congestive heart failure Bradycardia, supraventricular or ventricular dysrhythmias in overdose Aim for plasma level 0.8-2.0 ng/mL Dose adjustment required in renal failure
Esmolol	Short-term management of SVT and perioperative hypertension 5-200 µg/kg/min IV	Bradycardia Hypotension Bronchospasm
Nitroprusside	0.5-5 µg/kg/min IV Direct blood pressure monitoring required	Systemic and pulmonary vasodilation Systemic hypotension prominent Cyanide toxicity: • Metabolic acidosis earliest sign • Monitor thiocyanate levels when used > 48 hours or in renal failure
Captopril	Oral administration; 0.05 mg/kg as a test dose, then incremental increases to 0.4 mg/kg (occasionally up to 1 mg/kg), titrated to effect (systemic blood pressure); 8 hourly dosing	Systemic vasodilatation/hypotension Small increase in plasma potassium levels
Nitroglycerin	0.5-8 µg/kg/min IV Direct blood pressure monitoring required	Systemic and pulmonary vasodilation
Propranolol	Relief of spasmodic RV outflow obstruction in emergency management of hypercyanosis in tetralogy of Fallot: 0.05-0.1 mg/kg IV stat Systemic hypertension: 2-6 mg/kg in 4-6 divided doses	Bradycardia Hypotension Bronchospasm Lethargy

cardiovascular actions of the clinically available PDE3 inhibitors, amrinone,[23] milrinone,[24] and enoximone, are similar (Table 84-5). By inhibiting breakdown of cyclic adenosine monophosphate (cAMP), intracellular calcium accumulation is promoted and augments the contractile state of the myocyte. In addition, reuptake of calcium—a cAMP-dependent process—is also augmented, and these agents may therefore enhance diastolic relaxation, a particularly important aspect of neonatal cardiac function. In a recent multicenter randomized controlled study of neonates and young children following cardiac surgery, prophylactic administration of milrinone reduced the incidence of low cardiac output.[25] Clinical studies in infants and children have demonstrated a synergistic effect when β_1-agonists and PDE inhibitors such as amrinone, milrinone, or enoximone are coadministered, and this effect may be greater in neonates than in adults. In clinical use, the vasodilating action of the PDE3 inhibitors is prominent, a useful property given the usual well-documented pattern of low cardiac output associated with rising SVR and PVR in young patients following cardiac surgery.[26]

Systemic Vasodilators

Systemic vasodilators are indicated in situations where lowering SVR will reduce LV afterload and improve cardiac output. This is especially so in the neonatal setting, where elevation of the SVR is poorly tolerated by the myocardium. Vasodilators are also employed in the management of systemic hypertension as occurs in children following repair of aortic coarctation or other left-sided obstructive lesions. Vasodilators have variable effects on preload through concomitant venodilatation, the manifestations of which are dependent on the position the resultant end-diastolic pressure occupies on the ventricular function curve (VFC). If preload reduction brings the EDP to the pre-plateau sloping portion of the VFC, stroke volume can only be maintained or augmented if preload is optimized by appropriate fluid administration. Directly placed systemic left atrial pressure monitoring lines are commonly used to determine systemic ventricular loading conditions in neonates. Systemic vasodilators should be used with extreme caution in patients with systemic hypotension and those with left ventricular outflow obstruction, since they are at risk of uncompensated severe systemic hypotension and myocardial ischemia.

In children, sodium nitroprusside is frequently the systemic vasodilator of choice because of its powerful arteriolar dilating properties and short half-life which render it both effective and highly titratable. Nitroglycerin is an alternative short-acting drug which acts as an arteriolar dilator at higher doses but is an effective venodilator at lower

TABLE 84-5	Strategies to Prevent and Treat Pulmonary Hypertension
Strategy	**Comment**
Anatomic investigation	Rule out residual or undiagnosed anatomic abnormalities
Permit right-to-left decompression	Deliberate residual ASD acts as "pop-off" in at-risk situations
Analgesia/sedation	Facilitate ventilation; minimize sympathetic influences
Avoid acidosis	Respiratory and metabolic acidosis raise PVR
Maintain oxygenation	Normal/high alveolar and mixed venous Po_2 lower PVR
Optimize hematocrit	Ensures optimal oxygen delivery and higher mixed venous Po_2
Optimize cardiac output	Ensures optimal oxygen delivery and higher mixed venous Po_2
Pulmonary vasodilators	Selectively reduce PVR

doses. Phentolamine, a long-acting α-adrenergic blocker, is used in some centers for children undergoing surgery for congenital heart disease.[27,28]

For longer-term vasodilator therapy in children able to absorb enterally administered drugs, angiotensin-converting enzyme (ACE) inhibitors such as captopril and enalapril are used.[29] They have peripheral vascular and neurohormonal effects, as well as direct effects on the myocardium through activation of intracellular signaling pathways involved in growth and apoptosis of cardiac myocytes and fibroblasts. Studies in adults have established that ACE inhibitors improve survival and symptoms in heart failure, in part because of their favorable effects on cardiac remodeling. Evidence for the use of ACE inhibitors in children is much less clear. Acute hemodynamic benefits have been demonstrated in children with heart failure due to left-to-right shunts and systolic dysfunction of the systemic ventricle. Prolonged treatment with ACE inhibitors has been shown to be effective in reducing not only LV volume overload but also LV hypertrophy in the hearts of growing children with chronic LV volume overload.[30,31] The results of a randomized controlled trial of the use of ACE inhibitors in infants with single-ventricle circulations is awaited.[32]

Digoxin

Digoxin may have weak inotropic actions through its inhibitory effect on Na^+/K^+-ATPase and may also have peripheral effects that attenuate the actions of the neurohormonal system. Several adult studies have shown that digoxin improves symptoms in heart failure.[33] Although no studies have shown survival improvement,[33,34] there is a resurgence of interest in defining the role of digoxin in the management of heart failure. Digoxin is widely used to treat heart failure in children, although as in adults there are few data supporting or refuting its use.[17]

Diuretics

Standard practice is to use diuretics in virtually all children with heart failure.[17] There are no pediatric studies showing that diuretic therapy reduces morbidity or mortality, but a recent adult study has shown that the diuretic, spironolactone, improves survival in adults with heart failure.[35]

Potent diuretics such as furosemide are widely used in heart failure treatment in childhood[36]; in the perioperative period, controlling fluid balance is crucial, and renal function may be impaired. The intravenous (IV) route is preferred in these situations. Studies have shown that continuous infusion leads to smoother control of fluid and electrolyte shifts than intermittent IV bolus administration.[36]

Beta-Blockers

Although there is increasing evidence of survival benefits accruing from beta-blocker therapy in adults with moderate and severe heart failure,[37,38] evidence of similar benefits in children with heart failure is limited.[29,39,40] A recent publication suggests that the benefit of adding beta blockade to ACE inhibition is minimal.[41] While it might be reasonable to extrapolate adult survival advantages to older children with heart failure, extreme caution should be exercised in seeking to apply such therapy in the neonatal period.

Beta-blockers have established roles in children in managing both hypertension and ventricular outflow tract obstruction such as that which occurs in tetralogy of Fallot.

Levosimendan

Levosimendan offers new therapeutic possibilities in the management of patients with severe ventricular dysfunction by improving cardiac contractility and vasodilatation without affecting intracellular free calcium.[46] This drug enhances the sensitivity of cardiac myofilaments to calcium. The myocardial effects of levosimendan show improvement not only in systolic function but also in improved diastolic function, which is significantly impaired in severe heart failure. Anecdotes about the efficacy of levosimendan continue to be reported[47] to add to the small previously published studies such as that of Namachivayam et al.[48] It is, however, disappointing not to be able to report the results of more substantive pediatric trials. One of the problems with understanding the clinical utility of levosimendan has been to quantify the magnitude of its lusitropic effects, separating this from inotropic and chronotropic effects. Recently Jorgensen et al.[49] published an elegant study of the use of levosimendan in a carefully monitored group of adult patients with aortic valve disease. This study demonstrated unequivocally that levosimendan exerts a direct positive lusitropic effect, shortening isovolumic relaxation time and improving LV filling.

The potential for tight control of blood glucose to improve cardiac outcomes in children has recently been highlighted.[50] Further evidence from clinical trials such as the CHiP trial[51] are required before tight control is routinely adopted in pediatric critical care.

Other Inotropic Agents

Triiodothyronine (T_3) plays an important role in the regulation of heart metabolism,[42] up-regulating β-adrenoceptors and increasing cardiac myocyte contractility.[43] Clinical studies have shown that T_3 supplementation can produce elevation in heart rate without concomitant decrease in systemic blood pressure[44] and may enhance cardiac function reserve in infants after cardiopulmonary bypass. A recent double-blind placebo-controlled trial investigated the use of triiodothyronine supplementation in children younger than 2 years of age undergoing cardiopulmonary bypass. Although some indices of cardiac function assessed by echocardiography were judged better in the T_3 group, no significant differences were found in clinical endpoints including time to extubation or intensive care unit (ICU) discharge.[45]

PULMONARY VASODILATORS AND OTHER STRATEGIES TO PREVENT AND TREAT PULMONARY HYPERTENSION[11]

Oxygen alone is a potent dilator of the pulmonary vascular bed, with both alveolar oxygen concentration and systemic oxygen saturation having a favorable influence. Pulmonary vascular resistance is also influenced by lung volume, being raised at both low and very high lung volumes. Avoiding atelectasis, alveolar hypoxia, and pulmonary arteriolar hypoxia are simple strategies to minimize PVR and pulmonary artery pressure. Historically, most IV drugs used to treat PHT had nonselective effects, dilating both the pulmonary and systemic vascular beds. Tolazoline, prostaglandin E1, and prostacyclin are among many agents which have been used as pulmonary vasodilators. Prostacyclin is a short-acting vasodilator which acts via increasing levels of the intracellular messenger, cAMP, which has been widely used in the treatment of primary PHT in children.[52] The pulmonary effects of such nonselective agents are frequently limited by their nonspecific action leading to clinically important systemic hypotension. In contrast, nitrates, sodium nitroprusside, and indeed nitric oxide act via the activation of guanylate cyclase and hence increase cellular levels of cyclic guanosine monophosphate (cGMP) which is then inactivated by PDE5.

Elevation of PVR is seen in all children following cardiopulmonary bypass (CPB),[26] with reactive postoperative pulmonary hypertensive episodes typically occurring in children following correction of left-to-right shunt lesions or in those with preoperative pulmonary venous hypertension.[53] These crises are particularly associated with long CPB durations and late presentation for surgery. In the current era, early corrective surgery has dramatically reduced the numbers of infants in whom PHT is a major perioperative issue. Postoperative PHT is still seen in neonates and infants in association with lesions such as obstructed total anomalous pulmonary venous drainage, truncus arteriosus, and mitral valve replacement for congenital mitral stenosis. Children with lesser elevations in PVR may also benefit from pulmonary vasodilatation, including children with predominant RV dysfunction, for instance following cardiac transplantation[54] and in Fontan circulations and relatively high PVR.[55] General measures associated with the prevention and treatment of PHT should be considered before deploying specific pulmonary vasodilators (see Table 84-5). In patients at high risk of PHT following cardiac surgery, left ventricular filling can be maintained by right-to-left shunting through a small, surgically created atrial septal defect (ASD). Right-to-left shunt acts as a safety valve, and while some systemic desaturation occurs, LV filling and hence cardiac output are maintained.

Nitric oxide is an endogenous endothelial-derived vasodilator and a gas at room temperature. If added to inhaled gas mixtures in children with reactive PHT, it induces selective pulmonary vasodilation.[56] It is distributed to ventilated alveoli, from where it diffuses into the adjacent pulmonary arteriolar smooth muscle. Inhaled nitric oxide (iNO) has been shown in randomized controlled trials to be effective and safe therapy in neonates with PPHN. Although the evidence for outcome benefit is limited to one randomized controlled study,[57] there is a substantial body of evidence to show that iNO is effective in pediatric cardiac patients, including those with acute postoperative PHT following congenital heart surgery[58,59] and following pediatric heart transplantation. Inhaled nitric oxide can also be used in preoperative assessment of patients with PHT.[13,60]

Other candidate selective pulmonary vasodilators undergoing investigation in children include inhaled prostacyclin[61]; the PDE5 inhibitor, sildenafil[62-64]; and bosentan, an endothelin-1 receptor blocker.[65-67]

MECHANICAL CIRCULATORY SUPPORT

Extracorporeal membrane oxygenation (ECMO) is a mature technology which has been used to support over 27,000 neonates with respiratory failure, in whom survival rates of 70% to 80% are expected. Its use in this indication is supported by randomized controlled trials that demonstrate good short- and medium-term outcomes.[68] ECMO and ventricular assist devices (VADs) have subsequently been used to provide temporary circulatory support in children with intractable circulatory failure (see Chapter 93). Indications for mechanical circulatory support include selected children with problems including severe ventricular failure, refractory arrhythmias, and cardiac arrest.[69,70] The aim of mechanical circulatory support in such circumstances is to provide optimal cardiac output while resting the heart, awaiting its recovery, or to achieve survival by successful support of the child to cardiac transplantation. Single-center series[71] and collaborative registry figures of ECMO[72] or VAD for acute postoperative indications report similar figures for survival to hospital discharge (~40%) in children who (it is assumed) would not have survived without mechanical support. Rapid-deployment ECMO has recently been reported as an effective intervention for the management of cardiac arrest in the pediatric cardiac ICU and cardiac catheter laboratory.[73] Hospital survival figures for CPR-ECMO seem encouraging,[74] but long-term neurodevelopmental follow-up studies are urgently needed before such strategies can be recommended unequivocally.[75,76]

Cardiomyopathies

The two most common causes of heart failure in children are congenital heart disease and cardiomyopathy. Cardiomyopathies are primary myocardial diseases of either known or unknown cause, characterized by left or biventricular dilatation and impaired contractility; they occur in children and adults of all ages. Additional information on cardiomyopathy in adults is provided in Chapter 83. Key aspects germane to pediatrics are provided in the following discussions.

Nugent et al. reported the incidence of pediatric cardiomyopathy in a 10-year population-based study in Australian children as 1.24 cases per 100,000 children younger than 10 years of age,[77] a remarkably similar finding to a recently reported U.S. study.[78] Of 314 cases of cardiomyopathy reported by Nugent et al., 184/314 (59%) were dilated cardiomyopathy, 80 (25%) hypertrophic cardiomyopathy, 8 (2.5%) restrictive cardiomyopathy, and 42 (13%) unclassified, of which 29 (69%) exhibited LV non-compaction. In this study, 20% of cardiomyopathies were classified as familial, and in 8.9%, specific mitochondrial or metabolic disease etiologically linked to cardiomyopathy were identified. Of the children in Nugent's study who underwent myocardial biopsy, 40.3% had histologic evidence of lymphocytic myocarditis according to the Dallas criteria,[79] which contrasts with an incidence of lymphocytic myocarditis in adult studies of only 10%.[80]

PRESENTATION

Most children present with signs and symptoms of heart failure including dyspnea, upper abdominal discomfort, nausea, and vomiting. Abdominal symptoms are often misdiagnosed as indicative of gastroenteritis, although the astute clinician will note the absence of diarrhea. It is presumed that these abdominal symptoms result from hepatic congestion and gut edema as a result of right heart failure or ischemia (from splanchnic vasoconstriction). A history of an antecedent flulike illness is strongly suggestive of a diagnosis of myocarditis. Some children with myocarditis follow a fulminant course typified by rapid onset of cardiogenic shock.[81,82]

The chest x-ray in acutely presenting cardiomyopathies typically shows cardiomegaly and pulmonary venous congestion. An echocardiogram will reveal left atrial and ventricular dilatation and impaired systolic and diastolic function and often mitral or tricuspid regurgitation. Electrocardiographic (ECG) features are mostly nonspecific and include ST and T-wave changes and arrhythmias. The presence of Q waves may indicate anomalous origin of the left coronary artery from pulmonary artery (ALCAPA). If ALCAPA cannot be unequivocally excluded by echocardiography, coronary angiography must be undertaken.

As cardiomyopathies result from a variety of acquired or inherited disorders, the differentiation of secondary (and possibly treatable) causes of dilated cardiomyopathy from the idiopathic form of the disease is of the greatest importance. Endomyocardial biopsies can be obtained to assist in the diagnosis of myocarditis and other specific myocardial diseases.

PROGNOSIS

Recent studies have reported 5-year survival rates in childhood cardiomyopathy of between 64% and 84%, although the impact of cardiac transplantation on survival rates is not clear in all studies. In contrast to myocarditis, sudden death is uncommon in children with other forms of dilated cardiomyopathy. Children with cardiomyopathies who fail to respond to conservative treatment, and especially those with ongoing requirement for IV inotropic support, ventilatory support, or mechanical circulatory support and children with recurrent arrhythmias are candidates for early cardiac transplantation.[83] Late recovery of ventricular function is, however, possible.[84] The prognosis for cardiomyopathy due to myocarditis in children appears to differ from adults, with survival of up to 80% among children who reach the hospital alive.[85,86] Many children who survive the acute phase go on to recover normal cardiac function—in marked contrast to adults, in whom mortality rates of 20% at 1 year increased to 56% at 5 years.[80]

ICU MANAGEMENT OF DILATED CARDIOMYOPATHY AND MYOCARDITIS

In children presenting with acute heart failure, hypotension, or cardiogenic shock, β-adrenergic agonists may improve systolic ventricular function. PDE3 inhibitors such as milrinone are of hemodynamic benefit in acute heart failure, although large trials in adult heart failure have failed to show clear benefit from chronic administration.[87] While metoprolol and carvedilol may be of benefit in chronic heart failure,[29,39,40] they should be avoided in hemodynamically unstable children. Nasal or mask continuous positive airway pressure (CPAP) has been shown to result in symptomatic improvement both by unloading of respiratory muscles and lowering of LV afterload as a consequence of raising intrathoracic pressure.[88] Children in severe heart failure have high SVRs and no ventricular reserve. Great care is therefore needed if sedative agents are administered to facilitate tracheal intubation or ICU procedures. Agents with the least effects on the cardiovascular system should be chosen and allowance made for slow circulatory times when titrating sedative doses.

The use of mechanical circulatory support with ECMO or ventricular-assist systems can be life saving in children with myocarditis or cardiomyopathy who develop cardiogenic shock.[89,90] A high proportion of children who receive mechanical support for fulminant myocarditis will recover ventricular function. Those who do not may be bridged to cardiac transplantation. Clearly, survival with a recovered native ventricle is a better outcome for a child than survival via cardiac transplantation. A multicenter series[86] documented a median time to return of ventricular function of 9 days in those who survived without transplantation. The absolute time limits for recovery of native ventricular function have not been established, although pragmatic decisions on whether or not to proceed to cardiac transplantation should probably be made if cardiac recovery has not occurred after 10 to 14 days of support.[91]

▓ Congenital Heart Disease

Congenital heart disease (CHD) classified as moderate or severe is detected in approximately 6/1000 live births, of whom between 2.5 and 3 will require expert cardiologic care soon after birth. The presence of extracardiac anomalies in children with CHD is associated with poorer outcomes. Syndromes associated with cardiovascular involvement are of particular significance to the pediatric intensivist who must coordinate care of the cardiac and extracardiac aspects of care.[92] Trisomy 21 (Down's syndrome) is associated with a high incidence of congenital heart disease, in particular atrioventricular septal defects. Deletion of the q11 region of chromosome 22 is associated with a spectrum of cardiac conotruncal defects (e.g., truncus arteriosus, tetralogy of Fallot) and extracardiac abnormalities.[93] Of the later, thymic aplasia places infants at risk from hypocalcemia secondary to hypoparathyroidism and impaired cellular immunity.

Many classifications of congenital heart lesions have been proposed. A sequential approach to the description of cardiac anatomy is most frequently employed by pediatric cardiologists, but a broader physiologic approach is more useful to the non-specialist. It is beyond the scope of this chapter to present a detailed overview of all aspects of CHD. A brief overview is presented, focusing on common lesions and information of particular importance to intensivists. Readers are directed elsewhere for more detailed coverage of pediatric cardiology,[94] pediatric cardiac surgery,[95] and pediatric cardiac intensive care.[96]

LESIONS WITH PREDOMINANT LEFT-TO-RIGHT SHUNT

Ventricular septal defect is the archetypal lesion associated with left-to-right shunting of blood. VSDs may occur in isolation or in

association with other cardiac anomalies. Ventricular output will follow the path of least resistance, resulting in blood shunting across the defect and into the lungs, as the PVR is lower than the SVR. The magnitude of the shunt, usually expressed as the ratio of pulmonary blood flow to systemic blood flow (Qp : Qs), depends on the size of the VSD and the level of the PVR. Small-diameter defects offer resistance at the level of the ventricular septum, limiting flow from the left to right ventricle and maintaining a pressure gradient between the two chambers. Larger-diameter defects are unrestrictive, with no pressure gradient between the two ventricles, and in this situation, flow is solely dependent on the ratio of PVR to SVR. Small, restrictive VSDs rarely result in symptoms in infancy, typically presenting when a cardiac murmur is detected as an incidental finding. Infants with larger unrestrictive VSDs gradually develop congestive cardiac failure due to the increase in pulmonary blood flow which occurs as the developmental fall in PVR falls in the first weeks of life.[97] Thus the consequences of a moderate or large unrestrictive VSD are increased pulmonary blood flow (high Qp : Qs) and extra volume work demanded of the left ventricle. The volume overload of the LV results in LV enlargement and failure. If large left-to-right shunts are left untreated, PVR gradually rises. Although the initial rise is the result of pulmonary arteriolar muscular hypertrophy which is reversible, irreversible pulmonary vascular obstructive disease[98] eventually ensues and may result in the onset of right-to-left shunt (Eisenmenger syndrome). For this reason, steps must be taken in all children with congenital heart lesions and raised pulmonary blood flow to correct the lesion or protect the lungs by either a corrective procedure or a palliative procedure such as pulmonary artery banding before severe pulmonary vascular changes develop. With the exception of isolated atrial septal defects, most left-to-right shunt lesions which require surgical intervention present in the first year of life, with heart failure and associated development of PHT. The principal lesions are described next.

Ventricular Septal Defect

Anatomy. Ventricular septal defects occur in any part of the interventricular septum and are classified by location.[99,100]

Pathophysiology. Left-to-right shunting at the ventricular level leads to left atrial dilatation, left ventricular volume overload, and increased pulmonary blood flow. The degree of left-right shunt is determined by the size of the defect and the PVR. If a defect is small, shunt flow is determined mainly by the size of the defect. Left-to-right flow across larger unrestrictive defects is determined principally by PVR—the lower the PVR, the greater will be the shunt and pulmonary blood flow.

Many small VSDs close spontaneously,[101] but if closure does not occur, infants with unrestrictive defects will fail to thrive and develop congestive heart failure as the PVR falls in early infancy. Untreated VSD leads to PHT and eventual progression to fixed pulmonary vascular obstructive disease. Eventually, pulmonary artery pressure and vascular resistance exceeds that of the systemic circulation, leading to shunt reversal and cyanosis (Eisenmenger syndrome). Patients with a fixed high PVR are not suitable for VSD closure, since the right ventricle will not tolerate the excessive afterload of the hypertensive pulmonary vascular bed.

VSD Closure. Most VSDs are repaired as a primary surgical procedure.[102] Occasionally, pulmonary artery banding is undertaken to reduce pulmonary blood flow and protect the pulmonary vascular bed in neonates in whom primary repair is high risk. This may be the case with complex defects such as multiple defects or in very small premature infants. These conservative strategies are questioned by some surgeons.[103,104] Although most VSDs are closed surgically with a sutured patch during CPB, some defects can be closed at cardiac catheterization with an occlusion device.[105]

Postoperative Management. Most children undergoing elective VSD closure progress rapidly to extubation. Patients with severe cardiac failure or high pulmonary artery pressures preoperatively benefit from a more cautious approach in the early postoperative period, as do those with complex associated lesions. Low cardiac output or pulmonary edema may be noted in the early postoperative period as a consequence of generalized myocardial hypocontractility or due to the presence of a residual VSD. Pulmonary hypertension is relatively rare in the current era of early primary repair of VSD. Late-presenting cases may have PHT, and life-threatening pulmonary hypertensive crises can occur in the postoperative period. Surgically placed pulmonary artery catheters greatly assist in the early detection and management of such episodes.[106] Junctional ectopic tachycardia (JET)[107,108] and complete heart block are generic risks of surgery in the vicinity of the ventricular septum. Compete heart block may be transient, but if AV synchrony has not returned by 7 to 10 days, a permanent pacing system is required.[109]

Atrial Septal Defect

Anatomy. Anatomically, interatrial communications[99,110] are of four types. *Ostium secundum* defects are the most common form of ASD and are centrally located in the atrial septum. *Ostium primum* defects are part of the atrioventriculoseptal defect spectrum (see later). *Sinus venosus* defects occur close to the RA-SVC or RA-IVC junction and are commonly associated with partial anomalous pulmonary venous drainage. Coronary sinus defects describe a type of ASD associated with absence of the wall between the left atrium and coronary sinus, which allows left atrial blood to reach the right atrium via the coronary sinus.

Pathophysiology. Left-to-right shunting of blood at the atrial level leads to right atrial and ventricular dilatation with increased pulmonary blood flow. Congestive heart failure occurs in up to 5% of children with ASD in the first year of life. Pulmonary hypertension in association with ASD is relatively rare in childhood, with an incidence of 13% in unoperated children younger than 10 years of age, although if defects are not closed, patients may progress to irreversible PHT.[111] Occasionally infants or young children with primary PHT, pulmonary hypoplasia, or similar conditions present with apparently symptomatic ASD with right-to-left shunting. In these situations, the ASD is beneficial, decompressing the right heart, and symptoms being a consequence of PHT rather than simply the presence of an ASD.

ASD Closure. Centrally located secundum ASDs are frequently closed by placement of an ASD closure device at cardiac catheterization.[112,113] Occasionally, surgery is required in association with immediate or long-term complications of ASD device closure.[114] Large defects and nonsecundum defects are closed surgically using CPB. Defects are typically closed if a child becomes symptomatic or electively at between 3 and 5 years of age. There is essentially no mortality risk associated with closure of an isolated ASD, and good long-term morbidity-free survival is expected.[115]

Postprocedure Management. The vast majority of elective ASD closures progress rapidly to extubation post procedure (hours). Specific postoperative problems seen following ASD closure include *sinoatrial node dysfunction*, which manifests as an inappropriate chronotropic response or as atrial or junctional arrhythmias. The problem is caused either by direct trauma to the sinoatrial node or interruption to its blood supply during surgery. *Post-pericardotomy syndrome* manifests as fever, malaise, lymphocytosis, nausea, vomiting, or abdominal pain in the weeks following surgery. The symptoms are due to a sterile inflammatory process which can cause pericardial fluid to accumulate to the point at which pericardial tamponade is manifest. A history of recent cardiac surgery with symptoms as described should raise suspicion of the syndrome and of potential tamponade, particularly if cardiomegaly is present on chest x-ray. *Pulmonary hypertension* is relatively rare in children after ASD repair. A previously undiagnosed ASD presenting in adulthood is more likely to be associated with PHT. *Venous obstruction* of pulmonary veins or vena cava may occur in association with repair of sinus venosus defects. *LV dysfunction* manifesting as

transiently elevated LA pressure and pulmonary edema is occasionally seen after ASD closure in older patients, owing to chronic RV overload and decreased LV compliance.

Atrioventriculoseptal Defect

Anatomy. Atrioventriculoseptal defects (AVSDs)[116] result from failure of the lower part of the atrial septum to fuse with the upper part of the ventricular septum. The hallmark of all atrioventricular septal defects is the presence of a common atrioventricular (AV) junction and valve (AVV) with two bridging and three smaller leaflets. The common AVV has varying degrees of competence. There are three potential components of this defect, an ostium primum atrial septal defect, a ventriculoseptal defect, and abnormal formation of the AVVs. The condition presents as partial AVSDs (sometimes referred to as *primum ASDs*), where an ASD and cleft AV valve are present, and complete AVSDs, which in addition have a VSD. AVSD spectrum lesions commonly occur in children with Down's syndrome.

Pathophysiology. Partial defects behave like a secundum ASD, with left-to-right shunt at atrial level causing RA and RV volume overload. Associated incompetence of the left AVV may lead to significant regurgitation and worsening symptoms. In complete defects, left-to-right shunting of blood at ventricular level leads to congestive heart failure by about 2 months of age. Pulmonary hypertension and pulmonary vascular obliterative disease occur if repair is not undertaken by 6 to 9 months of age.

Surgery. Partial or complete AVSDs are repaired under cardiopulmonary bypass. Partial defects are usually repaired electively at between 1 and 5 years, whereas complete defects are usually repaired between 3 and 6 months to avoid severe pulmonary hypertensive complications.[116]

Postoperative Management. Afterload reduction with sodium nitroprusside or milrinone is useful if mild AV valve regurgitation is present following repair. If residual valve incompetence persists or increases, the operation should be revised. Problems seen after AVSD surgery include PHT,[117] which is, however, uncommon in the current era of early surgical repair. Residual lesions such as residual left AVV regurgitation or residual VSD will slow postoperative recovery and require prompt diagnosis and aggressive management including re-operation if necessary. Elevated LAP following AVSD repair can occur for reasons including the presence of residual left AVV regurgitation, left AVV stenosis, left ventricular outflow tract obstruction, residual VSD, and left ventricular myocardial dysfunction. The precise cause of elevated LAP must be diagnosed and appropriate management instituted.

Patent Ductus Arteriosus

Anatomy. A ductus arteriosus is a vascular communication necessary in the fetal circulation. It is located between the junction of the main and left pulmonary arteries and the lesser curvature of the aorta and normally closes within 2 weeks of birth. Persistent patency occurs as an isolated defect, in premature neonates, and in association with other congenital heart lesions.

Pathophysiology. The key pathophysiologic abnormality in patent ductus arteriosus (PDA), as in VSD, is left-to-right shunting leading to increased pulmonary blood flow, PHT, and left ventricular volume overload.[118] Neonates with this condition usually present with congestive heart failure, apneas, or respiratory problems. In term infants and older children, isolated PDA may present incidentally or with the onset of cardiac failure or problems with recurrent pulmonary infections. Pulmonary hypertension progressing to pulmonary vascular obstructive disease can occur within the first year of life, the rate of onset of symptoms depending on the size of the duct.

Management. Indomethacin or ibuprofen are used to induce closure of patent ductus in premature neonates, acting through inhibition of the vasodilatory prostaglandin production, with success in approximately 70% of cases.[119] Transcutaneous catheter occlusion can be effective in suitable cases, with a low incidence of associated complications.[120] Surgical ligation or division are required in very small subjects and in older children with large ducts in whom occlusion devices cannot be safely deployed. Surgical closure is carried out via a lateral thoracotomy or as a video-assisted thoracoscopic procedure.[121]

Postprocedural Issues. The principal complications of conservative treatment of PDA with indomethacin or ibuprofen in preterm neonates are failure to induce closure and renal failure.[119] Surgical approaches may be complicated by occlusion failure and complications of thoracotomy, including infection and hemorrhage. Adjacent structures including the thoracic duct, phrenic nerve, and the recurrent laryngeal nerve may be damaged during surgery. Complications following transcatheter closure include residual shunt, embolization of closure device, and hemolysis.

Truncus Arteriosus

Truncus arteriosus is caused by the failure of the common arterial trunk to divide into the aorta and pulmonary artery.

Anatomy. A single arterial vessel originates from both ventricles, overriding the ventricular septum and supplying the coronary, pulmonary, and systemic circulations. Anatomic variations depend on the respective origins of the right and left branch pulmonary arteries from the common arterial trunk, main pulmonary artery or aorta. A VSD lies immediately below a single ventriculoarterial truncal valve, which is commonly dysplastic, leading to stenosis or regurgitation. Coronary artery abnormalities are common and may lead to difficulties when conducting surgical repair. Ten percent to 15% of cases have associated hypoplasia, coarctation, or interruption of the aortic arch, and a small proportion have stenosis or hypoplasia of the pulmonary arteries.

Aorto-pulmonary window is a rare lesion in which an abnormal vascular communication exists between the ascending aorta and the main pulmonary artery. Like truncus arteriosus, this lesion is associated with 22q11 chromosomal deletion.[122,123]

Pathophysiology. The RV and LV are pressure and volume overloaded, particularly if truncal valve stenosis or regurgitation are present. Runoff into the pulmonary circulation, due to low PVR, and into the ventricles, due to truncal valve regurgitation, leads to a low diastolic pressure, which in the presence of high ventricular end-diastolic pressures may exacerbate myocardial ischemia. Pulmonary blood flow depends on the PVR and the presence or absence of stenoses in the proximal pulmonary arteries. Most commonly, therefore, pulmonary overcirculation and congestive heart failure result as PVR falls in the first weeks of life. The defect is commonly associated with 22q11 chromosomal deletion (DiGeorge syndrome, Sphrintzen's syndrome). The important clinical manifestations associated with these include scanty or absent T cells and the consequent risk of graft-versus-host reactions if transfused with viable leucocytes. Irradiation of all blood products is recommended unless normal T-cell status is confirmed. There is some evidence that children with 22q11 microdeletions have more postoperative complications than children undergoing identical surgery without deletions.

Surgery.[124,125] The pulmonary arteries are removed from the arterial trunk, leaving a vessel which becomes the "neo-aorta." A valved conduit is then placed from the right ventricle to the pulmonary arteries, and the VSD is closed. Mortality risk is less than 10% if the truncal valve is functionally normal, no other lesions are present, and the child is of an acceptable weight. Long-term results are encouraging, although the valved conduit will require upsizing during childhood.[126]

Postoperative Management. Specific postoperative problems associated with repair of truncus include PHT and low cardiac output. Inotropic support is required routinely, and delayed sternal closure

may be employed to prevent tissue tamponade in the early postoperative period. Intensivists must be aware of the possibility of right-to-left shunting, as surgeons may leave a smaller interatrial communication to decompress the RV (see Pulmonary Hypertension). Failure to appreciate this mechanism may lead to an inappropriate focus on pulmonary causes of cyanosis. Right bundle branch block is common after truncus repair, owing to the surgical right ventriculotomy. Heart block and atrial or junctional arrhythmias are also seen.

LEFT HEART OBSTRUCTION

Obstruction to the exit of blood from the LV can occur at subvalvar, valvar, or supravalvar levels or more distally in the aortic arch. Babies with severe obstruction of the aortic valve or arch present in the neonatal period with either heart failure or cardiogenic shock. Aortic coarctation, aortic interruption, and critical aortic stenosis are associated with a duct-dependent systemic circulation and typically present in the first few days of life as the arterial duct closes. Less severe obstruction may be detected later as an incidental finding (murmur) or with the gradual onset of signs and symptoms including those of LV failure. Chronic obstruction to LV outflow causes LV hypertrophy, and while systolic function may initially be well preserved, reduced diastolic compliance may occur early in the clinical course. If the obstruction is unrelieved, the subendocardial region becomes ischemic, and endocardial fibrosis occurs. Papillary muscle ischemia may also occur and results in acquired mitral valve regurgitation.

Valvar Aortic Stenosis

Anatomy. Aortic stenosis (AS) at valve level is the most common form of aortic stenosis and may be associated with other left heart abnormalities (e.g., supravalvular AS, mitral valve anomalies, aortic coarctation), aortic insufficiency (AI), and endocardial fibroelastosis. In neonatal AS,[127] the LV and other left-sided structures may be hypoplastic.

Pathophysiology. Neonates with clinically apparent valvar aortic stenosis present with acute left ventricular failure or shock. Systemic perfusion may be maintained by right-to-left shunting of blood across a patent ductus, with consequent systemic desaturation and the risk of reduced systemic perfusion if the ductus closes spontaneously. The LV exhibits poor performance in both diastole and systole, and as a consequence there are high left atrial pressures. Pulmonary edema is a prominent clinical feature. End-organ ischemic damage including renal failure and necrotizing enterocolitis are frequently seen as a consequence of poor systemic perfusion. Less severe aortic stenosis typically presents later in infancy or childhood with exercise-induced syncope, chest pain, or sudden death. In these patients, concentric LV hypertrophy induced by chronic pressure overload is usually seen.

Surgery. A number of treatment options are available, with the choice of procedure dependent on age, clinical status of the child at presentation, associated anomalies, and anatomic complexity. The simplest procedure, percutaneous balloon valvotomy, is appropriate in patients with mild to moderate stenosis and favorable aortic valve anatomy.[128] Open aortic valve surgery is an alternative to balloon valvoplasty and may be favored if additional procedures such as duct ligation are required. If the native aortic valve cannot be salvaged or reconstructed, surgical choices include replacement of the aortic valve with a homograft or valved conduit, or placement of the patient's own pulmonary valve into the aortic position with associated pulmonary homograft autograft (the Ross procedure).[129-131] A variant of the Ross procedure, the Ross-Konno procedure, is indicated for complex LV outflow tract obstruction; in addition to the Ross operation, annular enlargement or aortoventriculoplasty are undertaken.[132]

Postoperative Management. Most neonates presenting in heart failure or shock who undergo urgent procedures remain critically ill postoperatively and require ongoing multiorgan support.[133] If low cardiac output persists following repair, residual aortic stenosis or regurgitation must be excluded. Inotropic and vasodilator support of the failing myocardium should be guided by serial hemodynamic and echocardiographic evaluations. Relief of aortic stenosis in older children may be associated with systemic hypertension secondary to the unrestrained force of contraction of the hypertrophied LV. Children undergoing prosthetic valve replacement require long-term anticoagulation therapy.[129,134]

Subvalvar Aortic Stenosis

Subaortic stenosis[135] is seen in various forms including a fibrous diaphragm-like ring with a central orifice, a fibromuscular tunnel (frequently associated with hypoplasia of ascending aorta and LV anomalies), or simply as dynamic obstruction due to hypertrophy of LV outflow.

Sub-AS presents in neonates in association with other lesions including malalignment-type VSD, double-outlet right ventricle, and aortic or aortic valvar lesions or as an isolated lesion in childhood.

Pathophysiology. Similar to valvar AS, pressure overload in the LV leads to hypertrophy with resultant raised pressure overload.

Surgery. The choice of surgical procedure depends on the anatomic substrate. Membranous sub-AS requires simple resection. The tunnel form may be suitable for resection or require a more extensive Konno or Ross-Konno procedure. Finally, the hypertrophic form of sub-AS requires a Ross-Konno operation with resection of LV myocardium.[129,132] Some children with a small-diameter aortic valve and endocardial fibroelastosis of the LV with poor function may not be suitable for biventricular repair and are palliated by creation of cavopulmonary circulations.

The perioperative course is usually uneventful after resection of membranous sub-AS, although later recurrence is common. Following surgery for tunnel and hypertrophic forms of sub-AS, the recovery pathway is determined by the age of the child, the nature and complexity of surgery performed, and most critical of all, the size and function of the LV. Specific postoperative problems include residual LV outflow tract stenosis, mitral regurgitation, VSD with left-right shunt, and left bundle branch block or complete heart block secondary to resection of left ventricular myocardium.

Supravalvular Aortic Stenosis

Supravalvular aortic stenosis occurs in isolation and in association with Williams syndrome (supravalvar AS, RV outflow tract obstruction, peripheral pulmonary stenoses, renal artery stenoses).[136,137] It may be a localized or diffuse narrowing above the sinotubular junction. The stenosis is occasionally associated with a hypoplastic ascending aorta, and there may be compromise to coronary filling.

Pathophysiology. Similar to valvular AS, pressure overload in the LV leads to hypertrophy, with resultant raised pressure overload. In addition, coronary arteries fill under high pressure and may become tortuous and dysplastic.

Surgery. Patch angioplasty is performed in most cases. There is a significant risk of postprocedural coronary ischemia, as coronary perfusion pressure is acutely lowered when the supraaortic obstruction is released.

Postoperative Management. Postoperative course is usually uneventful. Specific postoperative problems include residual aortic or LV outflow tract stenosis leading to cardiac failure and coronary ischemia, which occurs if the repair has disturbed the coronary arteries or if LV hypertension and LV subendocardial ischemia persist.

Aortic Coarctation

Anatomy. Aortic coarctation is a constriction of the thoracic aorta in the region of the left subclavian artery where the ligamentum arteriosum originates. The complexity of the lesion varies from a discrete narrowing to more extensive aortic-arch hypoplasia extending back to the proximal aortic arch.[138] Coarctation commonly coexists with VSD[139] and can also be associated with other left-sided lesions including aortic and mitral valve stenosis.

Pathophysiology. In the neonatal presentation of aortic coarctation, a normal circulation is maintained until ductal tissue contracts, at which point distal aortic flow is severely reduced, leading to a clinical presentation of heart failure or shock and characteristic loss of lower limb pulses.[140] Prostaglandin E1 or E2 infusion should be started as soon as the diagnosis of a duct-dependent lesion is suspected in order to reopen or maintain patency of the ductus arteriosus. Following initial resuscitation, urinary output and resolution of metabolic acidosis are early indicators of successful reperfusion of the distal aorta. Early surgical repair is indicated.

Beyond the early neonatal period, aortic coarctation presents as progressive onset of cardiac failure or as an incidental finding (murmur, upper limb hypertension, absent weak femoral pulses) later in childhood. Thoracic aortic collaterals develop and may be noted as rib notching on a plain chest x-ray.

Surgery. In the newborn period, surgical resection of the narrowed aortic segment and associated ductal tissue and either direct anastomosis or repair with a subclavian flap or similar angioplasty without CPB are performed.[141] If aortic arch hypoplasia is more extensive, a homograft or prosthetic tube graft may be incorporated in the repair and CPB may be required.[142] Neonatal coarctation associated with VSD can be palliated by resection of the coarctation and banding of the pulmonary artery to restrict pulmonary blood flow, with delayed VSD repair. Alternatively, both lesions can be corrected in the neonatal period.[139] The mortality rate for repair of neonatal coarctation is low. Kanter et al. reported 91% survival in a series which included both isolated and complex coarctation.[143] In older children it is less than 1%, although paraplegia secondary to interruption of spinal cord perfusion remains a concern.

Balloon angioplasty with or without endovascular stent placement is frequently used to alleviate recurrent aortic coarctation and is increasingly being used, with apparent success, to address native coarctation, particularly in older patients. Balloon angioplasty is not favored in symptomatic neonates.[141,144]

Postoperative Management. Specific postoperative problems include systemic hypertension, which is thought to be due to multiple factors including altered baroceptor and adrenal catecholamine and renin-angiotensin axes.[145,146] Persistent hypertension is less common following neonatal repair, and when present it usually responds to short-term vasodilator therapy.[147,145] Additional β-adrenergic blockade (esmolol,[148] propranolol, or labetalol) may be required, particularly with late-presenting coarctation, but should be used with caution if ventricular function is impaired. Some children have persistent hypertension following repair[149] and require long-term antihypertensive therapy. Post-coarctectomy syndrome[150] occurs in older patients and is thought to be the result of restoration of higher-pressure pulsatile flow to the mesenteric arterial tree; this condition presents as abdominal distension, abdominal pain, ascites, or occasionally enteric infarction. The condition is best managed by avoiding enteral feeding for 24 hours following repair and aggressive treatment of systemic hypertension. The necessity of aortic clamping during surgical repair interrupts distal aortic flow and may result in spinal cord ischemia (rare in neonates, 0.4% incidence in older patients) or renal ischemia. The intensivist must seek positive confirmation of lower limb movement and adequate renal function in the early postoperative period. In neonates, low cardiac output due to preexisting ventricular dysfunction may persist, although residual coarctation should be excluded. Structures near the aortic arch prone to surgical injury include the thoracic duct, recurrent laryngeal nerve, and phrenic nerve, leading to postoperative chylothorax, stridor, or hemidiaphragm paralysis.

Interrupted Aortic Arch

Anatomy. In interrupted aortic arch (IAA), the aortic arch is either atretic or interrupted, creating either complete disruption or luminal obstruction (without external interruption). A patent arterial duct is necessary to maintain perfusion of the distal aortic arch, closure of which leads to emergent presentation. A VSD and obstruction of the left ventricular outflow tract commonly coexist. The more common form of IAA (type B) is associated with 22q11 chromosomal deletion[122,123] (see earlier).

Pathophysiology. IAA can be regarded as a severe form of aortic coarctation with duct-dependent distal aortic perfusion and requires similar initial management.[140]

Surgery. Surgical reconstruction of the aortic arch and closure of the associated VSD are usually undertaken under cardiopulmonary bypass in the neonatal period.

Specific postoperative problems seen after repair of IAA include PHT, residual aortic arch obstruction, and residual VSD. There is a risk of transfusion-associated graft-versus-host disease and hypocalcaemia in children with type B IAA with 22q11 deletion and DiGeorge phenotype.[151]

Anomalous Pulmonary Venous Connection

Anatomy. Pulmonary veins drain anomalously into systemic venous structures and subsequently to the right atrium rather than directly into the left atrium. The condition may affect all pulmonary veins (total anomalous pulmonary venous connection [TAPVC]) or fewer, typically one vein (partial anomalous pulmonary venous connection). In *supracardiac TAPVC* (45% of cases) the pulmonary veins drain via a vertical vein to the innominate vein or connect directly into the SVC. In *intracardiac TAPVC* (25% of cases), the venous confluence drains via the coronary sinus into the RA; and in *infracardiac TAPVC* (25% of cases), the veins drain into the IVC or portal veins. Mixed forms also exist (5% of cases).[152] TAPVC is associated with an obligate ASD to allow mixing of systemic and pulmonary venous return to access the left ventricle and systemic circulation.

Pathophysiology. In the case of TAPVC, two patterns emerge depending on presence of obstruction to the PV return. Obstruction of the pulmonary venous pathway is common and causes pulmonary venous hypertension, pulmonary venous edema, reflex pulmonary artery vasoconstriction, and subsequent right heart failure. If obstruction is not present, the main pathophysiologic effects result from complete mixing of systemic and pulmonary venous blood in the right heart, with RV volume overload and failure.

Surgery. The pulmonary veins are anastomosed or baffled into the left atrium. In the current era, the expected operative mortality is less than 5%, although higher risks are reported in complex cases with associated lesions.[153]

Specific Postoperative Problems. Pulmonary hypertension, which may on occasion be severe or even life threatening, is common in infants following surgery for obstructed anomalous pulmonary veins.[117] If high pulmonary artery pressure occurs postoperatively, it is essential to rule out residual pulmonary venous obstruction. Late restenosis is seen in up to 10% of cases and carries a poor prognosis, often related to a progressive fibrotic process occluding the lumen of the pulmonary veins.[154]

CYANOTIC LESIONS

Tetralogy of Fallot

Anatomy. Tetralogy of Fallot (TOF)[155] was initially described in the 19th century as an association of four anatomical findings: VSD, sub-pulmonary stenosis, aortic override of the ventricular septum, and right ventricular hypertrophy. The four lesions are actually the result of just one central problem, anterior and superior malalignment of the infundibular septum with respect to the muscular septum, which creates an obstruction in the right ventricular outflow tract and leads to the four features seen. Children presenting with TOF should be investigated for a 22q11 microdeletion (see earlier).

Pathophysiology. Preoperative physiology depends mainly on the degree of right ventricular outflow tract obstruction (RVOTO). Patients with minimal RVOTO have unrestricted pulmonary blood flow with left-to-right shunt through the VSD. Conversely, patients with severe obstruction will be cyanosed, with saturations in the 70% to 80% range preoperatively as a result of right-to-left shunting across the VSD. Right ventricular outflow tract obstruction is often dynamic and may cause profound cyanosis ("hypercyanotic spells") which require treatment aimed at alleviating the dynamic right ventricular outflow tract obstruction and maintaining right heart output. Treatment of such episodes requires oxygen, sedation, and volume expansion. The knee-chest or over-shoulder positions compress the liver and increase RV filling. If such maneuvers fail, beta blockade (propranolol, 0.1 mg/kg) or vasoconstriction (e.g., phenyl-ephrine, 5-20 μg/kg IV) may be required, or as a last resort, preoperative ECMO support.

Surgery. The timing and type of surgical intervention in TOF is controversial.[156,157] Complete repair is usually undertaken in the first year of life, although some centers adopt a two-stage approach with initial placement of a modified Blalock-Taussig shunt in cyanotic infants. Complete repair is then undertaken when the child is bigger.

Specific Postoperative Problems. Residual VSD is poorly tolerated after TOF repair and requires early surgical closure. Moderate degrees of residual right ventricular outflow tract obstruction may be well tolerated in the early postoperative period, but severe residual obstruction demands early reinvestigation and reoperation, with placement of a larger RV outflow tract patch or valved RV-PA conduit. All patients with a right ventricular incision develop right bundle branch block. Junctional ectopic tachycardia is poorly tolerated after Fallot repair.[107] Low cardiac output due to RV dysfunction is relatively common and should be suspected if the child is hypotensive, tachycardic, and has a raised CVP and hepatomegaly. The problem is predominantly one of poor RV compliance, often referred to as *RV restriction*,[158] and typically resolves in 3 to 5 days. Until recovery occurs, the heart should be supported by optimizing RV filling and ensuring atrioventricular synchrony. Negative pressure ventilation has been shown to improve cardiac output where RV restriction exists.[14,159]

Pulmonary Atresia with Intact Ventricular Septum[160]

Anatomy. In pulmonary atresia with intact ventricular septum (PA/IVS), there is complete obstruction to the outflow of the right ventricle, along with a variable degree of hypoplasia of the RV and tricuspid valve (TV). The TV may also be incompetent. Pulmonary blood flow occurs via a PDA. Coronary artery sinusoids or fistulae are often found in severe PA/IVS with a small right ventricle. Some 10% of cases will have an RV-dependent coronary circulation, where coronary sinusoids/fistulae are associated with proximal stenosis, and perfusion of areas of myocardium is dependent on flow via the right ventricle. In some patients, the pulmonary arterial supply is abnormal, with segments of the lungs being supplied solely or partially (dual supply) from systemic collateral vessels termed *major aortopulmonary collateral arteries* (MAPCA).[161] Children presenting with this condition should be investigated for a 22q11 microdeletion (see earlier).

Pathophysiology. Preoperatively there is complete mixing of systemic and pulmonary venous return in a duct-dependent circulation. The RV may be very hypertensive, since there is no path for egress of blood. Some blood may pass via coronary sinusoids, if present, or back through a regurgitant tricuspid valve.

Surgery. The goal of treatment is to provide a secure source of pulmonary blood flow balanced to systemic flow, and to permit the right ventricle to develop to its maximal potential, always aiming for a two-ventricle repair where possible.[161,162] Interventional procedures are needed in all cases in the fetal[163] or neonatal period[164,165] because of duct dependency. Subsequent strategies are chosen according to individual anatomic findings.

In severe forms of the condition (severe RV hypoplasia ± coronary fistulae) a two-ventricle repair will never be possible, and a palliative approach is adopted. Initial palliation secures pulmonary blood flow with systemic pulmonary artery shunts (30%-40% PA/IVS), with the ultimate aim being a single-ventricle Fontan circulation (see later). In contrast, babies with a normal-sized RV may be suitable for RV outflow tract reconstruction in the neonatal period, therefore avoiding a shunt and ending up with early anatomic correction (10% of cases). An intermediate group of patients—the majority of cases of PA/IVS—need initial palliation with decompression of the RV by radiofrequency perforation of the atretic pulmonary valve or outflow tract patch, and often require a systemic–pulmonary artery shunt. Progression to either a single, "one-and-a-half,"[166] or biventricular repair depends on subsequent development of the RV and pulmonary arteries. Fetal cardiac valvoplasty may have a role in the management of this condition in the future.[163]

Specific postoperative problems include low cardiac output due to excessive runoff through the shunt, myocardial ischemia due to decompressed coronary fistulae, or low systemic diastolic pressure due to excessive shunt runoff.[167]

D-Transposition of the Great Arteries

Anatomy. In D-transposition of the great arteries (TGA),[168,169] which accounts for 5% to 7% of all congenital heart lesions, the great vessels are transposed so that the aorta arises from the anatomic right ventricle and the pulmonary artery from the left ventricle, so-called ventriculo-arterial discordance. The condition occurs with a VSD in approximately 40% of cases. Other commonly associated lesions include coarctation (10%), left ventricular outflow tract obstruction (5%), and coronary abnormalities (33%).

Pathophysiology. The predominant finding in TGA is cyanosis due to parallel rather than serial function of the pulmonary and systemic circulations, with the greatest proportion of the output of a ventricle being recirculated to that ventricle. Survival is therefore dependent on the presence of mixing between the two circulations (Figure 84-2). The presence of either a PDA or VSD (alone or in combination) without an atrial communication does not ensure adequate mixing of the two circulations. If the diagnosis is suspected in a neonate, an infusion of prostaglandin E1 or E2 should be established to maintain ductal patency, and following echocardiographic confirmation of the diagnosis, a balloon atrial septostomy is sometimes necessary to enlarge the foramen ovale and secure mixing at atrial level, particularly if the foramen ovale is restrictive, leading to high pulmonary venous pressures. Saturations typically increase from very low levels (<50%) to 65% to 85% following these interventions, and it is then usually possible to discontinue the prostaglandin infusion.

Surgery. The preferred surgical option in the current era is the arterial switch (Jatene) operation,[168-170] although long-term results following Senning operations also appear to be acceptable.[171] The switch operation is usually performed within the first 2 weeks of life, beyond which the left ventricle (functioning as a low-pressure subpulmonary or right ventricle since birth) is less able to cope with systemic pressures.[172] Babies with a large VSD have equal ventricular pressures, and repair can be delayed a little longer, although in practice most surgeons repair TGA with VSD within the first month of life. The operation consists of transection of the aorta and pulmonary artery, with reconstruction of the vessels in their anatomic position, which necessitates transfer of the coronary arteries from the PA to the neo-aorta.

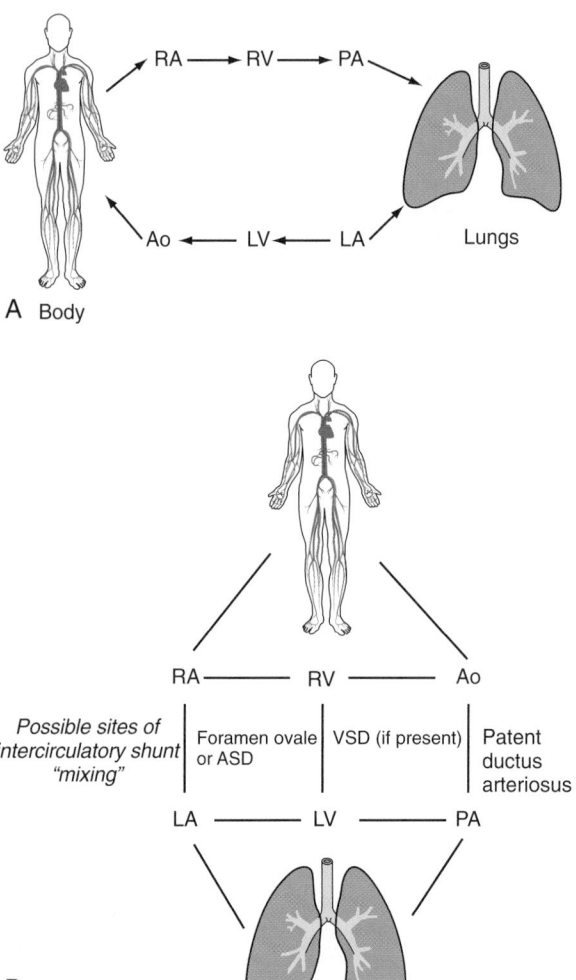

Figure 84-2   A, Normal series circulatory arrangement. **B,** Parallel circulation of transposition of the great vessels.

Specific Postoperative Problems. Left ventricular dysfunction is common in babies during the first 12 hours following the arterial switch operation.[26] It may be a sign of coronary insufficiency,[173] acute dysfunction secondary to an unprepared/involuted LV, or simply nonspecific post-CPB low cardiac output. In the absence of ECG or echocardiographic evidence of regional coronary ischemia, low cardiac output is managed conservatively. The postoperative LV of the neonate is poorly compliant. Rapid volume infusion should be avoided, as LV distension and ischemia may result. Preload should be augmented gradually, titrating volume infused against measured left atrial pressure.

Alternative Surgical Techniques. Atrial switch operations (Senning and Mustard procedures) are alternatives to the arterial switch and may be chosen in infants presenting beyond the early neonatal period in whom a one-stage arterial switch is not possible owing to deconditioning of the left ventricle. In atrial switch operations, blood is diverted by an atrial baffle to establish a series circulation, leaving the RV as the systemic ventricle. It is believed that the burden of late complications such as RV failure is greater after atrial switch procedures. An alternative strategy for late-presenting transposition is a two-stage repair, with initial banding of the pulmonary artery to condition the LV, with switch once the ventricle is conditioned.[174]

Postoperative Care. Atrial switch procedures are usually performed outside the neonatal age group and compared to arterial switch patients, have a relatively uneventful postoperative course. Atrial volumes and compliance are reduced by the procedure such that post-operatively, left and right atrial pressures must be maintained at higher-than-normal levels to maintain ventricular filling. Slow heart rates and arrhythmias are poorly tolerated.

Complex Single-Ventricle Circulations

Some defects are such that they can never be corrected to provide two functioning ventricles.[175,176] These complex arrangements include any heart in which one ventricle is hypoplastic such that it would be incapable of supporting either the pulmonary or systemic circulation independently. Examples of such situations include tricuspid atresia or double-inlet left ventricle. In these examples, the right ventricle has failed to develop adequately and is connected to a dominant left ventricle via a VSD. Flow to the circulation supplied by the rudimentary ventricle originates from the dominant chamber and is dependent on an adequate VSD. Children with this type of anatomy will always have two ventricles, even if one is hypoplastic, but physiologically they behave as if the heart consists of only a single ventricle.

Complex single-ventricle hearts can be palliated with a series of interventions leading to creation of a Fontan circulation in which the systemic and pulmonary circulations are completely separated.[177] Initially, adequate intracardiac communications are established to ensure both systemic and pulmonary venous return have unobstructed access to the dominant ventricle to supply both systemic and pulmonary blood flow. If necessary, pulmonary flow is augmented by the use of a systemic-to–pulmonary artery shunt or right ventricle–to–pulmonary artery conduit. Systemic and pulmonary blood flow are assured at the expense of mixing of pulmonary and systemic venous returns, with consequent cyanosis and volume loading of the single ventricle.

Subsequently, if hemodynamic conditions are favorable, the Fontan circulation is established, usually in two staged procedures. Initially a bidirectional cavopulmonary or a hemi-Fontan anastomosis is created in which the SVC is connected to the proximal right pulmonary artery. This has the benefit of reducing the volume load placed on the systemic ventricle by previously placed systemic/pulmonary shunt. Finally, venous return form the IVC is also directed to the pulmonary circulation. This is achieved by forming a lateral tunnel[178] or using a synthetic extracardiac conduit[179] to channel blood from the IVC to the inferior aspect of the right pulmonary artery, completing the total cavopulmonary connection or Fontan circulation.

In the Fontan circulation, there is no subpulmonary ventricle, all ventricular tissue having been incorporated into the single ventricle, which receives pulmonary venous return and ejects into the systemic circulation. This establishes a form of series circulation and results in normal systemic oxygenation and equality of pulmonary and systemic blood flow. Pulmonary blood flow in the Fontan circulation is driven by the transpulmonary hydrostatic gradient and is only viable if the PVR and systemic ventricular end-diastolic pressures (pulmonary venous pressures) are low. The presence of good systemic ventricular function and low PVR are crucial determinants of operability. Patients with a Fontan circulation tolerate factors which impede systemic venous return such as dehydration, pneumothorax, pericardial effusion, positive pressure ventilation,[88] raised PVR, or compromised ventricular or respiratory[180] function very poorly. Perioperative use of ACE inhibitors[181] has been shown to reduce the severity and duration of pleural drainage,[182] a common problem caused by high postoperative systemic venous pressures. A communication or fenestration between the systemic venous pathway and pulmonary venous atrium may be created in patients thought to be at higher risk of complications such as effusions or perioperative low cardiac output as a result of relatively high PVR.

Long-term follow-up studies have demonstrated that systemic ventricular function remains abnormal after Fontan procedures.[183] Ultimately the Fontan circulation may fail, and cardiac transplantation must be considered.

Hypoplastic Left Heart Syndrome

Hypoplastic left heart syndrome (HLHS) is a term encompassing a range of hypoplastic abnormalities of the left-sided cardiac structures and connections including the ascending aorta.[184] The condition is usually palliated in three stages, although some authorities prefer to offer cardiac transplantation without prior palliative surgery.[185] The first-stage procedure secures systemic and pulmonary blood flow with either a Norwood procedure or similar or a hybrid procedure.[186,187] The Norwood approach consists of reconstruction of the aortic arch, with the establishment of pulmonary blood flow via a central systemic/pulmonary artery shunt. Some advocate replacing the systemic/pulmonary artery shunt of the classical Norwood with an RV-PA conduit, which may be easier to manage postoperatively because there is potentially less diastolic runoff, with less risk of coronary ischemia than occurs across the central shunt of the classical Norwood operation.[184,188] Balancing the pulmonary and systemic circulations in the immediate postoperative period can be challenging. Interventions such as sudden hyperventilation or increases in oxygen concentration which lower PVR should be avoided. Strategies to manage the postoperative Norwood patient include the use of long-acting vasodilators such as phenoxybenzamine[27,28] and close monitoring of cerebral oxygenation, venous oxygen saturation, and plasma lactate. ACE inhibitors are subsequently introduced and very close inter-stage monitoring may be undertaken in an attempt to minimize inter-stage morbidity and mortality.

Following the first-stage procedure, a bidirectional cavopulmonary anastomosis is undertaken, typically between 2 and 6 months of age, and finally a completion to a Fontan circulation follows at 18 to 24 months of age. Fetal diagnosis facilitates early and appropriate management and may contribute to improved outcomes in HLHS,[189] although there is known to be significant risk of poor neurodevelopmental status in survivors of neonatal HLHS interventions.[190]

Surgical Control of Pulmonary Blood Flow.

Pulmonary Artery Banding. Pulmonary artery banding is a surgical procedure in which a constriction is created in the main pulmonary artery, with the aim of limiting pulmonary blood flow to protect the lungs from overcirculation, usually as a primary palliative procedure ahead of a later definitive repair. It is performed without CPB through either a left thoracotomy or median sternotomy. The procedure is undertaken to restrict pulmonary blood flow, aiming to maintain a balance between the systemic and pulmonary circulations and to prevent the onset of PHT in some complex anomalies unsuitable for early anatomic repair.[191] PA banding is a palliative procedure and is usually a stepping stone to a more complex repair.

Physiology. A PA band reduces pulmonary blood flow and therefore volume loading of the systemic or single ventricle. The intracardiac shunt is predominantly right to left following banding, and systemic arterial saturations are typically 75% to 85% following effective banding. The pressure gradient across an effective PA band in a neonate is typically in the range of 40 to 60 mm Hg.

Specific Management Issues. Oxygen saturations may be an issue. Very low Sao_2 postoperatively (<70%) may indicate that the band is too tight—that is, the pulmonary blood flow is too restricted. Urgent echo evaluation of the band gradient[192] and exclusion of other causes of hypoxemia should be undertaken. If hypoxemia persists, and particularly if significant metabolic acidosis develops, urgent removal of the band may be indicated. PA bands may occasionally be too loose to adequately reduce pulmonary blood flow, resulting in arterial oxygen saturations in excess of 90%. Signs of congestive cardiac failure may be noted and require medical treatment (diuretics) or further surgical intervention (re-banding or correct lesion.)

OTHER LESIONS

Vascular Rings and Slings

Vascular rings and slings[193] result from abnormal branching or positioning of the great vessels, which result in encirclement or compression of the trachea and/or esophagus. They are seen in isolation or in association with intracardiac defects.

Anatomy. Three common types occur either in isolation or in association with other cardiac lesions including right aortic arch, tetralogy of Fallot, and AVSD:

1. Double aortic arch. This results from failure of the embryonic regression of one of the arches. The right arch, which is commonly dominant and usually larger, passes posterior to the esophagus and trachea to connect to the left-sided descending thoracic aorta, forming a vascular ring. The left arch is commonly smaller and may exhibit varying degrees of hypoplasia, coarctation, or true atresia. The carotid and subclavian arteries originate from both arches. Sometimes a persistent ductus or ligamentum arteriosum forms a true ring around the trachea.

2. Right aortic arch with aberrant left subclavian artery. In this condition, the left subclavian has its origin from the ascending aorta and courses to the left behind the esophagus, with the vascular ring completed by the ligamentum arteriosum.

3. Pulmonary artery sling. The left pulmonary artery (LPA) arises from the right pulmonary artery and passes to the left by passing behind the trachea. The trachea is squeezed between the aorta and LPA, and a true ring may be formed by a persistent ductus or ligamentum arteriosum.

Pathophysiology. Vascular rings have the potential to compress both trachea and esophagus. PA slings usually cause chronic tracheal compression which eventually results in destruction of the tracheal skeleton, with resultant tracheal stenosis in 50% of cases.

Surgery.[194,195] Vascular rings are usually approached via a lateral thoracotomy (usually left). The left arch or ligamentum are divided to release the ring, and the descending aorta is dissected away from the esophagus. To correct PA sling, the anomalous LPA is transected and rerouted anteriorly and reanastomosed to the central PA.

Postoperative Care. This is usually uneventful. Extubation at the end of anesthesia or early in the ICU course is expected. Tracheomalacia may persist or present postoperatively, especially after PA sling surgery, and may require long periods of respiratory support postoperatively via a tracheostomy.

Anomalous Left Coronary Artery from the Pulmonary Artery

Anatomy. Anomalous left coronary artery from the pulmonary artery (ALCAPA) usually occurs as an isolated lesion in which the left coronary artery arises from the pulmonary artery rather than the aorta.

Pathophysiology. Symptoms develop gradually as PVR falls during early infancy. There is progressive onset of myocardial ischemia as left coronary flow falls in parallel with the fall in PA pressure. The myocardium is initially well perfused by desaturated PA blood, but as coronary flow falls, severe left ventricular ischemia and dysfunction occur.

Surgery. Surgical intervention is necessary to reconnect the left coronary with the aorta, and this can be achieved either by creating a tunnel from the left coronary orifice to the aorta[196] (the Takeuchi operation) or by directly reimplanting the coronary artery.[197]

Postoperative Care. The principal perioperative problem in infants with symptomatic ALCAPA is management of low cardiac output. β-Adrenergic agonists, PDE3 inhibitors such as milrinone,[25] and occasionally mechanical circulatory support may be required.

Specific Issues for the Intensivist

DELAYED STERNAL CLOSURE

Complex cardiac surgery involving cardiopulmonary bypass results in edema of the myocardium and other mediastinal tissues. Under these circumstances, sternal closure at the end of the surgical procedure may cause cardiac compression ("tissue tamponade") which decreases ventricular compliance and leads to reduced cardiac output and elevated pulmonary venous pressures.[198,199] The child may therefore be returned to the ICU, where the sternum may be closed once the hemodynamic situation has improved. Transient deteriorations at delayed closure are usually self-limiting and can be tolerated, but hypotension, oliguria, rising plasma lactate, or falling venous saturations suggest closure will not be tolerated.[200]

INFECTIVE ENDOCARDITIS

Infective endocarditis is a condition characterized by microbial infection of the heart valves or other structures and is associated with substantial morbidity and mortality in both children and adults. The subject has recently been extensively reviewed.[201] While prophylactic antibiotic treatment prior to non-cardiac procedures is no longer recommended in children and young people,[202] intensivists should aim to minimize the risk of line-related bloodstream infection complications by employing best-practice guidelines in the care and surveillance of central venous lines.[203]

KEY POINTS

1. The immature myocardium has little functional reserve, poorly tolerating both increased preload and afterload.

2. Cardiac output in the neonate is critically heart rate dependent.

3. A hyperoxic test will usually differentiate cyanosis resulting from intracardiac shunting of deoxygenated blood and that due to intrapulmonary ventilation/perfusion mismatch.

4. Manipulation of the pulmonary circulation, especially pulmonary vascular resistance and the function of the subpulmonary (right) ventricle, are critical to understanding and managing many congenital heart lesions.

5. Systemic vasodilators play a prominent role in balancing shunted circulations and in the management of heart failure in children.

6. Mechanical circulatory support is effective in bridging many children with severe heart failure to recovery or cardiac transplantation.

7. In the era of mechanical circulatory support, acute fulminant myocarditis in children should be regarded as a recoverable condition.

8. Appropriate intensive care management of the congenital heart patient must be based on a sound understanding of the anatomy and pathophysiology of the child's circulation.

9. Issues relating to the management of intracardiac shunts, cyanosis, and the management of the pulmonary circulation and right ventricle are of great importance in managing children with congenital heart disease.

10. Specialist advice should be sought early if children with known or suspected heart disease are admitted to non-specialist pediatric or adult facilities.

REFERENCES

Access the complete reference list online at http://www.expertconsult.com.

85

Pericardial Diseases

BERNHARD MAISCH | ARSEN D. RISTIC

Etiology and Classification of Pericardial Disease

The spectrum of pericardial diseases consists of congenital defects, pericarditis (dry, effusive, effusive-constrictive, constrictive), neoplasm, and cysts. The etiologic classification comprises infectious pericarditis, pericarditis in systemic autoimmune diseases, type 2 (auto) immune process, post-myocardial infarction syndrome, and autoreactive (chronic) pericarditis.[1-3]

Pericardial Syndromes

CONGENITAL DEFECTS OF THE PERICARDIUM

Congenital defects of the pericardium occur in 1 in 10,000 autopsies. Pericardial absence can be partial left (70%), right (17%), or total bilateral (rare). Additional congenital abnormalities occur in approximately 30% of patients.[4] Most patients with a total pericardial absence are asymptomatic. Homolateral cardiac displacement and augmented heart mobility impose an increased risk for traumatic aortic dissection.[5] Partial left-side defects can be complicated by herniation and strangulation of the heart through the defect (chest pain, shortness of breath, syncope, or sudden death). Surgical pericardioplasty (Dacron, Gore-Tex, or bovine pericardium) is indicated for imminent strangulation.[6]

ACUTE PERICARDITIS

Acute pericarditis is dry, fibrinous, or effusive, independent of its etiology. Major symptoms are retrosternal or left pre-cordial chest pain (which radiates to the trapezius ridge, can be pleuritic or simulate ischemia, and varies with posture) and shortness of breath. A prodrome of fever, malaise, and myalgia is common, but elderly patients may not be febrile. The pericardial friction rub can be transient and monophasic, biphasic, or triphasic. Pleural effusion may be present. Heart rate is usually rapid and regular. Echocardiography is essential to detect effusion and concomitant heart or paracardial disease (Table 85-1).[7-19]

Hospitalization and symptomatic treatment is warranted. Nonsteroidal anti-inflammatory drugs (NSAIDs) are the mainstay. Indomethacin should be avoided in elderly patients, owing to its effect on reducing flow in the coronaries. Ibuprofen (300 to 800 mg tid) is preferred for its rare side effects, favorable impact on coronary flow, and large dose range.[7] Colchicine 0.5 mg at least twice daily for 3 months added to an NSAID or to aspirin reduced the recurrence rate impressively in the COPE trial[20] even at the first episode of pericarditis or even as monotherapy in "idiopathic" effusions. It is well tolerated with fewer side effects than NSAIDs. Systemic corticosteroids should be restricted to connective tissue diseases and autoreactive or uremic pericarditis. Intrapericardial steroid application as long-acting crystalloid triamcinolone is effective for autoreactive effusions and avoids systemic side effects.[2]

CHRONIC PERICARDITIS

Chronic (>3 months) pericarditis includes effusive (inflammatory or hydropericardium in heart failure), adhesive, and constrictive forms.[7]

Symptoms are usually mild (chest pain, palpitations, fatigue), related to the degree of cardiac compression and pericardial inflammation. The detection of the curable causes (e.g., tuberculosis, toxoplasmosis, myxedema, viral, autoimmune, and systemic diseases) allows successful specific therapy. Symptomatic treatment and pericardiocentesis should be applied if indicated. For recurrences the etiology should be investigated intensely and if no specific therapy is effective, balloon pericardiotomy or pericardiectomy may be considered.[22,23]

RECURRENT PERICARDITIS

The term *recurrent pericarditis* encompasses (1) the intermittent type (symptom-free intervals without therapy) and (2) the incessant type (discontinuation of anti-inflammatory therapy ensures a relapse). Massive pericardial effusion, overt tamponade, or constriction is rare. Symptomatic management relies on exercise restriction and the regimen used in acute pericarditis. Colchicine may be effective when NSAIDs and corticosteroids failed to prevent relapses.[20,21,24,25] It should be considered first-choice treatment for recurrent pericarditis according to the CORE trial.[21] Corticosteroids should be used only in patients with poor general condition or in frequent crises.[7] A common mistake could be to use a dose too low to be effective or to taper the dose too rapidly. The recommended regimen is prednisone, 1 to 1.5 mg/kg, for at least 1 month. If patients do not respond adequately, azathioprine (75 to 100 mg/day) or cyclophosphamide can be added.[26]

Corticosteroids should be tapered over a 3-month period. Toward the end of the taper, introduce antiinflammatory treatment with colchicine (0.5 mg bid or tid) or an NSAID. Renewed treatment should continue for 3 to 6 months. Recently it was demonstrated in "idiopathic" pericarditis that previous corticoid treatment was even a risk factor for recurrence or chronicity. Therefore corticoids should be administered after definite exclusion of viral or bacterial infection of the pericardium. Pericardiectomy is indicated only in frequent and highly symptomatic recurrences resistant to medical treatment.[27]

PERICARDIAL EFFUSION AND CARDIAC TAMPONADE

Pericardial effusion may appear as transudate (hydropericardium), exudate, pyopericardium, or hemopericardium. Large effusions are common with neoplastic, tuberculous, cholesterol, uremic, myxedema, and parasitoses pericarditis.[28] Loculated effusions are more common when scarring has supervened (e.g., postsurgical, post trauma, purulent pericarditis). Effusions that develop slowly can be remarkably symptomatic, whereas rapidly accumulating smaller effusions can present as tamponade. Cardiac tamponade is the decompensated phase of cardiac compression caused by effusion accumulation and the increased intrapericardial pressure. Heart sounds are distant. Orthopnea, cough, and dysphagia, occasionally with episodes of unconsciousness, can be observed. Insidiously developing tamponade may present as the signs of its complications (renal failure, abdominal plethora, shock liver, worsening of glaucoma,[29] and mesenteric ischemia). Tamponade without two or more inflammatory signs (typical pain, pericardial friction rub, fever, diffuse ST-segment elevation) is usually associated with a malignant effusion (likelihood ratio 2.9).[30]

Electrocardiography demonstrates low QRS and T-wave voltages, PR-segment depression (Figure 85-1), ST-segment/T-wave changes, bundle branch block, and electrical alternans (rarely seen in the

TABLE 85-1	Diagnostic Pathway and Sequence of Performance in Acute Pericarditis	
Diagnostic Measure	*Characteristic Findings*	
Obligatory		
Auscultation	Pericardial rub (monophasic, biphasic, or triphasic)	
ECG*	*Stage I:* anterior and inferior concave ST segment elevation. PR segment deviations opposite to P wave polarity	
	Early stage II: all ST junctions return to the baseline. PR segments deviated.	
	Late stage II: T waves progressively flatten and invert	
	Stage III: generalized T wave inversions in most or all leads	
	Stage IV: ECG returns to prepericarditis state	
Echocardiography	Effusion types B to D (Horowitz)	
	Signs of tamponade	
Blood analyses	Erythrocyte sedimentation rate, C-reactive protein, lactate dehydrogenase, leukocytes (inflammation markers)	
	Troponin I†, CK-MB (markers of myocardial involvement)	
Chest radiograph	Ranging from normal to "water bottle" shape of the heart shadow	
	Performed primarily to reveal pulmonary or mediastinal pathology	
Mandatory in Tamponade, Optional in Large/Recurrent Effusions or if Previous Tests Inconclusive in Small Effusions		
Pericardiocentesis/drainage	Polymerase chain reaction and histochemistry for etiopathogenetic classification of infection or neoplasia	
Optional or if Previous Tests Inconclusive		
CT	Effusions, pericardium, and epicardium	
MRI	Effusions, pericardium, and epicardium	
Pericardioscopy, pericardial/epicardial biopsy	Establishing the specific etiology	

*Typical lead involvement: I, II, aVL, aVF, and V3-V6. The ST segment is always depressed in aVR frequently in V1, and occasionally in V2. Stage IV may not occur, and there are permanent T wave inversions and flattenings. If ECG is first recorded in stage III, pericarditis cannot be differentiated by ECG from diffuse myocardial injury, "biventricular strain," or myocarditis. ECG in early repolarization is very similar to stage I. Unlike stage I, this ECG does not acutely evolve and J-point elevations are usually accompanied by a slur, oscillation, or notch at the end of the QRS just before and including the J point (best seen with tall R and T waves—large in early repolarization pattern). Pericarditis is likely if in lead V6 the J point is greater than 25% of the height of the T wave apex (using the PR segment as a baseline).

†A cTnI rise was detectable in 38/118 patients (32.2%), more frequently in younger, male patients, with ST-segment elevation and pericardial effusion at presentation. An increase beyond 1.5 ng/mL was rare (7.6%), and associated with CK-MB elevation. cTnI increase was not a negative prognostic marker regarding the incidence of recurrences, constrictive pericarditis, cardiac tamponade, or residual left ventricular dysfunction (Imazio). Data from references 2, 3, and 7 to 19.

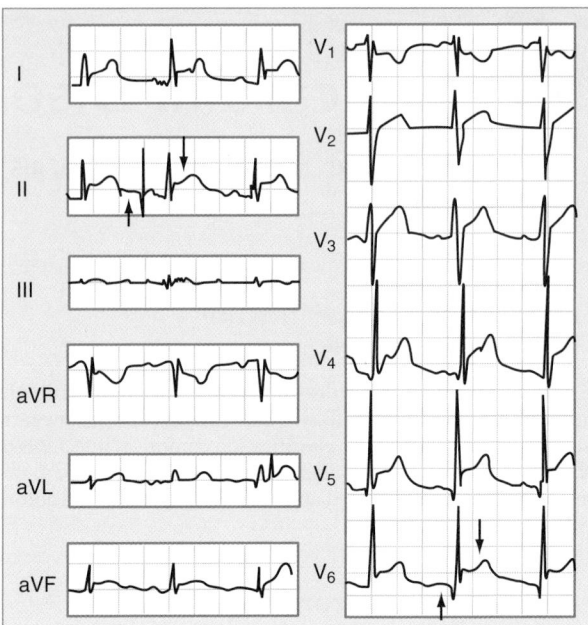

Figure 85-1 Typical electrocardiographic changes in acute pericarditis: PR depression *(small arrow)* and concave ST segment elevation *(large arrow).*

CONSTRICTIVE PERICARDITIS

Constrictive pericarditis is a rare but severely disabling consequence of the chronic inflammation of the pericardium, leading to an impaired filling of the ventricles and reduced ventricular function. Until recently, increased pericardial thickness has been considered an essential diagnostic feature of constrictive pericarditis. However, in the large surgical series from the Mayo Clinic constriction was present in 18% of the patients with normal pericardial thickness.[42] Tuberculosis, mediastinal irradiation, and previous surgical procedures are frequent.[43] Constrictive pericarditis may rarely develop only in the epicardial layer in patients with previously removed parietal pericardium.[44] Transient constrictive pericarditis is an uncommon but important entity, because pericardiectomy is not indicated in these patients.[45]

Patients complain about fatigue, peripheral edema, breathlessness, and abdominal swelling, which may be aggravated by a protein-losing enteropathy. In decompensated patients venous congestion, hepatomegaly, pleural effusions, and ascites may occur. Hemodynamic impairment can be additionally aggravated by a systolic dysfunction due to myocardial fibrosis or atrophy. Differential diagnosis has to include acute dilatation of the heart, pulmonary embolism, right ventricular infarction, pleural effusion, chronic obstructive lung diseases,[46] and restrictive cardiomyopathy. The best way to distinguish constrictive pericarditis from restrictive cardiomyopathy is the analysis of respiratory changes with or without changes of preload by Doppler and/or tissue Doppler echocardiography,[47] but physical findings, electrocardiogram (ECG), chest radiography (see Figure 85-2, *Right*), computed tomography (CT) (Figure 85-4, *Left*), magnetic resonance imaging (MRI) (see Figure 85-4, *Right*), hemodynamics, and endomyocardial biopsy may be helpful as well.[7]

Pericardiectomy is the only treatment for permanent constriction. The indications are based on clinical symptoms, echocardiography findings, CT/MRI, and heart catheterization. A primary installation of cardiopulmonary bypass (CPB) is not recommended (diffuse bleeding following systemic heparinization). Pericardiectomy for constrictive pericarditis has a mortality rate of 6% to 12%.[48-51] The complete normalization of cardiac hemodynamics is reported in only 60% of patients.[48,50] Major complications include acute perioperative cardiac insufficiency and ventricular wall rupture.[52] Cardiac mortality and

absence of tamponade).[7] Microvoltage and electrical alternans are reversible after effusion drainage and resolution of the inflammatory process.[19] In chest radiography large effusions are depicted as globular cardiomegaly with sharp margins ("water bottle" silhouette) (Figure 85-2).[12] The size of effusions can be graded in echocardiography as (1) small (echo-free space in diastole < 10 mm), (2) moderate (10 to 20 mm) (Figure 85-3), (3) large (≥20 mm), or (4) very large (≥20 mm and compression of the heart). In large pericardial effusions, the heart may move freely within the pericardial cavity ("swinging heart") inducing pseudoprolapse and pseudosystolic anterior motion of the mitral valve, paradoxical motion of the inter-ventricular septum, and midsystolic aortic valve closure (Table 85-2).[31-41] Up to one third of patients with an asymptomatic large pericardial chronic effusion develop unexpected cardiac tamponade.[22] Triggers for tamponade include hypovolemia, paroxysmal tachyarrhythmia, and intercurrent acute pericarditis.

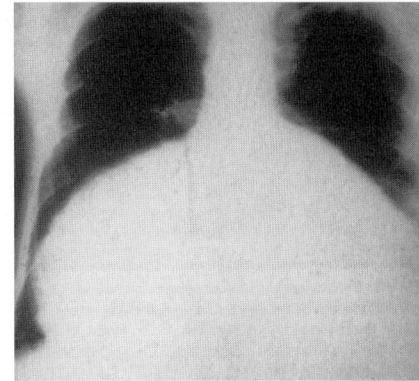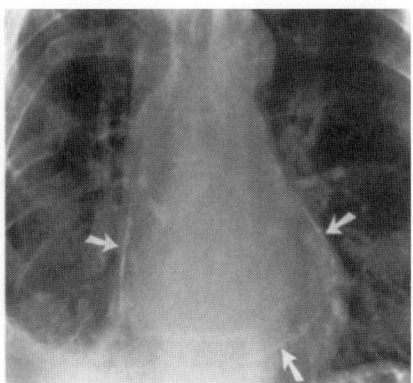

Figure 85-2 Chest radiographs in a patient with very large pericardial effusion—"water bottle" sign *(left)*—and in a patient with constrictive pericarditis and pericardial calcifications *(white arrows, right)*.

morbidity at pericardiectomy are mainly caused by the presurgically unrecognized presence of myocardial atrophy or myocardial fibrosis.[43] Exclusion of patients with extensive myocardial fibrosis and/or atrophy reduced the mortality rate for pericardiectomy to 5%. Postoperative low cardiac output[52] should be treated by fluid substitution and catecholamines, high doses of digitalis, and intra-aortic balloon pump in most severe cases. If the indication for surgery is established early, long-term survival after pericardiectomy corresponds to that of the general population.[49,50] However, if severe clinical symptoms were present for a longer period before surgery, even a complete pericardiectomy may not achieve a total restitution.

PERICARDIAL CYSTS

Congenital pericardial cysts are uncommon; they may be unilocular or multilocular, with the diameter ranging from 1 to 5 cm.[53] Inflammatory cysts comprise pseudocysts as well as encapsulated and loculated pericardial effusions, caused by rheumatic pericarditis, bacterial infection, particularly tuberculosis, trauma, and cardiac surgery. Most patients are asymptomatic and cysts are detected incidentally on chest radiographs as an oval, homogeneous radiodense lesion, usually at the right cardiophrenic angle.[54] However, the patients can also present as chest discomfort, dyspnea, cough, or palpitations, owing to the compression of the heart. Echocardiography is useful, but additional imaging by CT (density readings) or MRI is often needed.[55] The treatment of congenital and inflammatory cysts is percutaneous aspiration and ethanol sclerosis.[56,57] If this is not feasible, video-assisted thoracotomy or surgical resection may be necessary. Echinococcal *cysts*

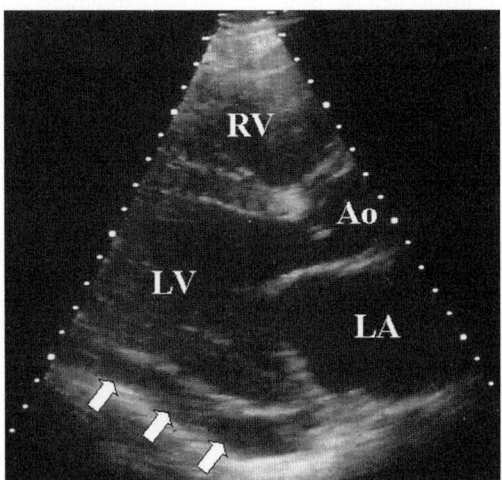

Figure 85-3 Echocardiographic findings in a small-moderate pericardial effusion *(white arrows)*. Long-axis parasternal view. LV, left ventricle; LA, left atrium; RV, right ventricle; Ao, aortic root.

usually originate from ruptured hydatid cysts in the liver and lungs. Their surgical excision is not recommended, instead percutaneous aspiration and instillation of ethanol or silver nitrate after pretreatment with albendazole (800 mg/day 4 weeks) is recommended.[57]

Specific Forms of Pericarditis

VIRAL PERICARDITIS

Viral pericarditis is the most common infection of the pericardium. Inflammatory abnormalities are due to direct viral attack, the immune response (antiviral or anticardiac), or both.[3,58] Early viral replication in pericardial and epimyocardial tissue elicits cellular and humoral immune responses against the virus and/or cardiac tissue. Deposits of IgM, IgG, and occasionally IgA can be found in the pericardium and myocardium for years.[58] Various viruses can cause pericarditis (e.g., enteroviruses, echoviruses, adenoviruses, cytomegaloviruses, Epstein-Barr virus, herpes simplex, herpes humanus 6(HHV6), influenzaviruses, parvovirus B19(PVB19), hepatitis C, human immunodeficiency virus [HIV]), whereby in the last few years PVB19 and HHV6 have been increasing and entero-, echo- and adenoviruses have been decreasing as has also been observed in myocarditis. Attacks of enteroviral pericarditis follow the seasonal epidemics of coxsackievirus A+B and echovirus infections.[59] Cytomegalovirus (CMV) pericarditis has an increased incidence in immunocompromised and HIV-infected hosts.[60] Infectious mononucleosis may also present as pericarditis.

The diagnosis of viral pericarditis is not possible without the evaluation of pericardial effusion and/or pericardial/epicardial tissue, preferably by polymerase chain reaction (PCR) or in-situ hybridization. A fourfold rise in serum antibody levels is suggestive but not diagnostic for viral pericarditis.

Treatment of viral pericarditis is directed to resolve symptoms (see acute pericarditis), prevent complications, and eradicate the virus. In patients with chronic or recurrent symptomatic pericardial effusion and confirmed viral infection the following specific treatment is under investigation[61]:

1. CMV pericarditis: hyperimmune globulin—once per day 4 ml/kg on days 0, 4, and 8; 2 ml/kg on days 12 and 16.
2. Coxsackievirus B pericarditis: interferon alfa or beta 2.5×10^6 IU/m² subcutaneously three times per week.
3. Adenovirus, parvovirus B19 and HHV6 perimyocarditis: immunoglobulin treatment with 20 g or even more intravenously on days 1 and 3 for 6 to 8 hours, which may be repeated and combined with gancyclovir to become effective for virus elimination.

Pericardial manifestations of HIV infection can be due to infective, noninfective, and neoplastic diseases (Kaposi's sarcoma and/or lymphoma). Infective (myo) pericarditis results from the local HIV infection and/or from other viral, bacterial (*Staphylococcus aureus, Klebsiella pneumoniae, Mycobacterium avium,* and *M. tuberculosis*), and fungal co-infections (*Cryptococcus neoformans*).[62] In progressive disease the

TABLE 85-2	Diagnosis of Cardiac Tamponade
Clinical presentation	Elevated systemic venous pressure,* hypotension,[†] pulsus paradoxus,[‡] tachycardia,[§] dyspnea, or tachypnea with clear lungs
Precipitating factors	Drugs (cyclosporine, anticoagulants, thrombolytics), recent cardiac surgery, indwelling instrumentation, blunt chest trauma, malignancies, connective tissue disease, renal failure, septicemia[∥]
ECG	Can be normal or nonspecifically changed (ST-T wave), electrical alternans (QRS, rarely T), bradycardia (end stage), electromechanical dissociation (agonal phase)
Chest radiograph	Enlarged cardiac silhouette with clear lungs
M-mode/two-dimensional echocardiogram	Diastolic collapse of the anterior RV free wall,[¶] RA collapse, LA and rarely LV collapse, increased LV diastolic wall thickness "pseudohypertrophy," IVC dilatation (no collapse in inspiration), "swinging heart"
Doppler	Tricuspid flow increases and mitral flow decreases during inspiration (reverse in expiration)
	Systolic and diastolic flows are reduced in systemic veins in expiration and reverse flow with atrial contraction is increased
M-mode color Doppler	Large respiratory fluctuations in mitral/tricuspid flows
Cardiac catheterization	Confirmation of the diagnosis and quantification of the hemodynamic compromise
	RA pressure is elevated (preserved systolic × descent and absent or diminished diastolic y descent)
	Intrapericardial pressure is also elevated and virtually identical to RA pressure (both pressures fall in inspiration)
	RV mid-diastolic pressure is elevated and equal to the RA and pericardial pressures (no dip-and-plateau configuration)
	Pulmonary artery diastolic pressure is slightly elevated and may correspond to the RV pressure
	Pulmonary capillary wedge pressure is also elevated and nearly equal to intrapericardial and right atrial pressure
	LV systolic and aortic pressures may be normal or reduced
	Documenting that pericardial aspiration is followed by hemodynamic improvement**
	Detection of coexisting hemodynamic abnormalities (LV failure, constriction, pulmonary hypertension)
	Detection of associated cardiovascular diseases (cardiomyopathy, coronary artery disease)
RV/LV angiography	Atrial collapse and small hyperactive ventricular chambers
Coronary angiography	Coronary compression in diastole

*Jugular venous distention is less notable in hypovolemic patients or in "surgical tamponade." An inspiratory increase or lack of fall of the pressure in the neck veins (Kussmaul sign), when verified with tamponade or after pericardial drainage, indicates effusive-constrictive disease.

[†]Heart rate is usually greater than 100 beats/min but may be lower in hypothyroidism and in uremic patients.

[‡]Pulsus paradoxus is defined as a drop in systolic blood pressure greater than 10 mm Hg during inspiration, whereas diastolic blood pressure remains unchanged. It is easily detected by simply feeling the pulse, which diminishes significantly during inspiration. Clinically significant pulsus paradoxus is apparent when the patient is breathing normally. When this sign is present only in deep inspiration it should be interpreted with caution. The magnitude of pulsus paradoxus is evaluated by sphygmomanometry. If the pulsus paradoxus is present, the first Korotkoff sound is not heard equally well throughout the respiratory cycle, but only during expiration at a given blood pressure. The blood pressure cuff is therefore inflated above the patient's systolic pressure. Then it is slowly deflated while the clinician observes the phase of respiration. During deflation, the first Korotkoff sound is intermittent. Correlation with the patient's respiratory cycle identifies a point at which the sound is audible during expiration but disappears when the patient breathes in. As the cuff pressure drops farther, another point is reached when the first blood pressure sound is audible throughout the respiratory cycle. The difference in systolic pressure between these two points is the clinical measure of pulsus paradoxus. Pulsus paradoxus is absent in tamponade, complicating atrial septal defect, and in patients with significant aortic regurgitation.

[§]Occasional patients are hypertensive, especially if they have preexisting hypertension.

[∥]Febrile tamponade may be misdiagnosed as septic shock.

[¶]Right ventricular collapse can be absent in elevated right ventricular pressure and right ventricular hypertrophy or in right ventricular infarction.

**If after drainage of pericardial effusion intrapericardial pressure does not fall below atrial pressure, the effusive-constrictive disease should be considered.

LA, left atrium; LV, left ventricle; RA, right atrium; RV, right ventricle; IVC, inferior vena cava.

Data from References 31 to 41.

incidence of echocardiographically detected pericardial effusion may be up to 40%.[63] Cardiac tamponade is rare.[64] During treatment with retroviral compounds, lipodystrophy can develop (best demonstrated by MRI) with intense paracardial fat deposition leading to heart failure. Treatment is symptomatic, whereas in large effusions and cardiac tamponade pericardiocentesis is necessary. The use of corticosteroid therapy is contraindicated except in patients with secondary tuberculous pericarditis, as an adjunct to tuberculostatic treatment.[65]

BACTERIAL PERICARDITIS

Purulent pericarditis in adults is rare but always fatal if not treated.[66-69] The mortality rate in treated patients is 40%, mostly due to cardiac tamponade, toxicity, and constriction. It is usually a complication of an infection originating elsewhere in the body, arising by contiguous spread or hematogenous dissemination.[70] Predisposing conditions are pericardial effusion, immunosuppression, chronic diseases (e.g., alcohol abuse, rheumatoid arthritis), cardiac surgery, and chest trauma. The disease appears as an acute, fulminant infectious illness with short

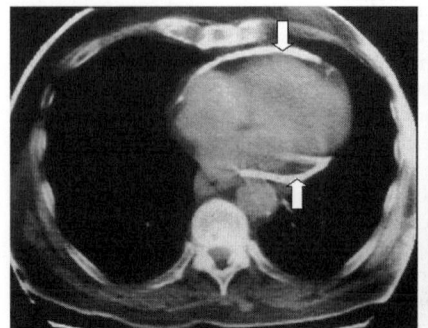 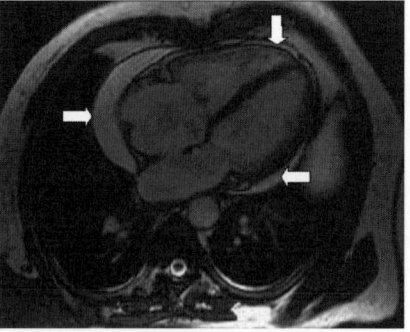

Figure 85-4 Computed tomography (CT) findings in constrictive pericarditis *(left)*. White vertical arrows are depicting thickened pericardium and pericardial calcification. Magnetic resonance image (MRI) of a patient with effusive-constrictive pericarditis is shown on the right-sided image. *Horizontal arrows* show loculated pericardial effusion, and the *vertical arrow* shows thickened pericardium.

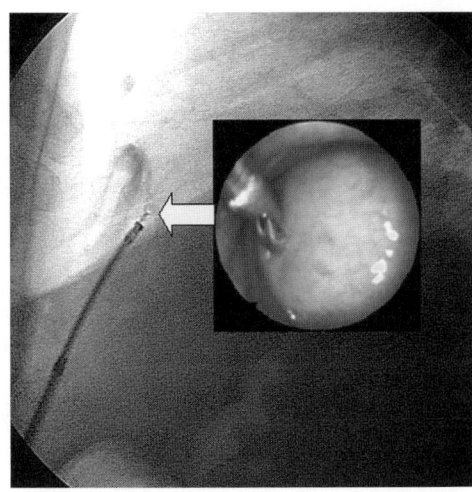

Figure 85-5 Flexible percutaneous pericardioscopy and epicardial biopsy (*arrow*).

duration. Percutaneous pericardiocentesis must be promptly performed, and obtained pericardial fluid should undergo Gram, acid-fast, and fungal staining, followed by cultures of the pericardial and body fluids. Rinsing of the pericardial cavity, combined with effective systemic antibiotic therapy is mandatory (antistaphylococcal antibiotic plus aminoglycoside, followed by tailored antibiotic therapy according to pericardial fluid and blood cultures).[67] Intrapericardial instillation of antibiotics (e.g., gentamicin) is useful but not sufficient. Frequent irrigation of the pericardial cavity with urokinase or streptokinase, using large catheters, may liquefy the purulent exudate,[68,69] but open surgical drainage through subxiphoid pericardiotomy is preferable.[66] Pericardiectomy is required in patients with dense adhesions, loculated and thick purulent effusion, recurrence of tamponade, persistent infection, and progression to constriction.[67] Surgical mortality is up to 8%.

TUBERCULOUS PERICARDITIS

In the past decade, tuberculous pericarditis in developed countries has been primarily seen in immunocompromised patients (acquired immunodeficiency syndrome [AIDS]).[71] The mortality rate in untreated effusive tuberculous pericarditis approaches 85%. Pericardial constriction occurs in 30% to 50%.[72,73]

The clinical presentation is variable: acute pericarditis with or without effusion; cardiac tamponade; silent, often large pericardial effusion with a relapsing course; toxic symptoms with persistent fever; acute constrictive pericarditis; subacute constriction; effusive-constrictive or chronic constrictive pericarditis; and pericardial calcifications.[3,74] The diagnosis is made by the identification of *M. tuberculosis* in the pericardial fluid or tissue and/or the presence of caseous granulomas in the pericardium.[71] Importantly, PCR can identify DNA of *M. tuberculosis* rapidly from only 1 µl of pericardial fluid.[75,76] Increased adenosine deaminase activity and interferon gamma concentration in pericardial effusion are also diagnostic, with a high sensitivity and specificity. Both pericardioscopy and pericardial biopsy have also improved the diagnostic accuracy for tuberculous pericarditis (Figure 85-5).[15] Pericardial biopsy enables rapid diagnosis with better sensitivity than pericardiocentesis (100% vs. 33%).

Pericarditis in a patient with proven extracardiac tuberculosis is strongly suggestive of tuberculous etiology (several sputum cultures should be taken).[77] The tuberculin skin test may be false negative in 25% to 33% of tests[72] and false positive in 30% to 40% of patients.[71] The more accurate enzyme-linked immunospot (ELISPOT) test detects T cells specific for *M. tuberculosis* antigen.[78] Perimyocardial tuberculous involvement is also associated with high serum titers of antimyolemmal and antimyosin antibodies.[79] The diagnostic yield of pericardiocentesis in tuberculous pericarditis ranges from 30% to 76% according to the

methods applied for the analyses of pericardial effusion.[72,75] Pericardial fluid demonstrates high specific gravity, high protein levels, and high white blood cell count (from 0.7 to 54×10^9/L).[71]

Various antituberculous drug combinations of different durations (6, 9, 12 months) have been applied.[71,72,77,80-83] Prevention of constriction in chronic pericardial effusion of undetermined etiology by "ex iuvantibus" antitubercular treatment was not successful.[80] The use of corticosteroids remains controversial.[77,81-84] A meta-analysis of patients with effusive and constrictive tuberculous pericarditis[82,83] suggested that tuberculostatic treatment combined with corticosteroids might be associated with fewer deaths and less frequent need for pericardiocentesis or pericardiectomy.[77,85] If given, prednisone should be administered in relatively high doses (1 to 2 mg/kg/day) because rifampicin induces its liver metabolism.[7] This dose is maintained for 5 to 7 days and progressively reduced in 6 to 8 weeks. If, in spite of combination therapy, constriction develops, pericardiectomy is indicated.

PERICARDITIS IN RENAL FAILURE

Renal failure is a common cause of pericardial disease producing large pericardial effusions in up to 20% of patients.[86] Two forms have been described:

1. Uremic pericarditis—in 6% to 10% of patients with advanced renal failure (acute or chronic) before dialysis has been instituted or shortly thereafter.[87] It results from inflammation of the visceral and parietal pericardium and correlates with the degree of azotemia (blood urea nitrogen > 60 mg/dL).

2. Dialysis-associated pericarditis—in up to 13% of patients on maintenance hemodialysis[88] and occasionally with chronic peritoneal dialysis due to inadequate dialysis and/or fluid overload.[89] Pathologic examination of the pericardium shows adhesions between the thickened pericardial membranes ("bread and butter" appearance). The clinical features may include transient pericardial rubs, fever and pleuritic chest pain, but many patients are asymptomatic. Because of autonomic impairment in uremic patients, heart rate may remain slow (60 to 80 beats/min) during tamponade, despite fever and hypotension. Anemia, due to induced resistance to erythropoietin, may worsen the clinical picture.[90] The ECG may not show the typical diffuse ST-segment/T-wave elevations observed with other causes of acute pericarditis, owing to the lack of the myocardial inflammation.[91] If the ECG is typical of acute pericarditis, intercurrent infection must be suspected.

Most patients with uremic pericarditis respond rapidly to hemodialysis or peritoneal dialysis with resolution of chest pain and pericardial effusion. To avoid hemopericardium heparin-free hemodialysis should be used. Hypokalemia and hypophosphatemia should be prevented by supplementing the dialysis solution when appropriate.[92] Intensified dialysis usually leads to resolution of the pericarditis within 1 to 2 weeks.[93] Peritoneal dialysis, which does not require heparinization, may be therapeutic in pericarditis resistant to hemodialysis or if heparin-free hemodialysis cannot be performed. NSAIDs and systemic corticosteroids have limited success when intensive dialysis is ineffective.[94] Cardiac tamponade and large chronic effusions resistant to dialysis must be treated with pericardiocentesis. Large, nonresolving symptomatic effusions should be treated with intrapericardial instillation of corticosteroids after pericardiocentesis or subxiphoid pericardiotomy (triamcinolone hexacetonide, 50 mg every 6 hours for 2 to 3 days).[88,94] Pericardiectomy is indicated only in refractory, severely symptomatic patients owing to its potential morbidity and mortality. After renal transplantation, pericarditis has also been reported in 2.4% of patients.[95] Uremia or infection (CMV) may be the causes.

AUTOREACTIVE PERICARDITIS AND PERICARDITIS IN SYSTEMIC AUTOIMMUNE DISEASES

The diagnosis of autoreactive pericarditis is established using the following criteria[2]:

1. Increased number of lymphocytes and mononuclear cells greater than 5000/mm^3 (autoreactive lymphocytic) or the presence of antibodies against heart muscle tissue (e.g. antisarcolemmal) in the pericardial fluid (autoreactive antibody-mediated)
2. Inflammation in epicardial/endomyocardial biopsies by more than 14 cells/mm^2
3. Exclusion of active viral infection both in pericardial effusion and endomyocardial/epimyocardial biopsies (no virus isolation, no IgM-titer against cardiotropic viruses in pericardial effusion, and negative PCR for major cardiotropic viruses)
4. Tuberculosis, *Borrelia burgdorferi*, *Chlamydia pneumoniae*, and other bacterial infection excluded by PCR and/or cultures
5. Neoplastic infiltration absent in pericardial effusion and biopsy samples
6. Exclusion of systemic metabolic disorders and uremia. Intrapericardial treatment with triamcinolone is effective with rare side effects

Pericarditis occurs in systemic autoimmune diseases: rheumatoid arthritis, systemic lupus erythematosus, progressive systemic sclerosis, polymyositis/dermatomyositis, mixed connective tissue disease, seronegative spondyloarthropathies, systemic and hypersensitivity vasculitides, Behçet's syndrome, Wegener's granulomatosis, and sarcoidosis.[7] Intensified treatment of the underlying disease and symptomatic management is indicated.

THE POST–CARDIAC INJURY SYNDROME: POSTPERICARDIOTOMY SYNDROME

Post–cardiac injury syndrome develops within days to months after cardiac or pericardial injury or both.[7,96,97] It resembles the post–myocardial infarction syndrome, both appearing to be variants of a common immunopathologic process. Pericardial effusion also occurs after orthotopic heart transplantation (21%). It is more frequent in patients receiving aminocaproic acid during the operation.[98] Cardiac tamponade after open heart surgery is more common after valve surgery than coronary artery bypass grafting and may be related to the preoperative use of anticoagulants.[99]

Warfarin administration in patients with early postoperative pericardial effusion imposes the greatest risk, particularly in those who did not undergo pericardiocentesis and drainage of the effusion.[100] Symptomatic treatment is as in acute pericarditis (NSAIDs or colchicine for several weeks or months,[101] but has been questioned recently.[102] If symptomatic treatment with NSAIDs or colchicines also reduces the effusion and not only symptoms is tested in the COPPS trial.[103] Long-term (3 to 6 months) oral corticosteroids or preferably pericardiocentesis and intrapericardial instillation of triamcinolone (300 mg/m^2) are therapeutic options in refractory forms. Redo surgery is rarely needed.

POSTINFARCTION PERICARDITIS

Two forms of postinfarction pericarditis can be distinguished: an "early" form (pericarditis epistenocardiaca) and a "delayed" form (Dressler's syndrome).[104] Epistenocardiac pericarditis, caused by direct exudation, occurs in 5% to 20% of transmural myocardial infarctions but is clinically discovered rarely. Dressler's syndrome occurs from 1 week to several months after clinical onset of myocardial infarction with symptoms and manifestations similar to the post-cardiac injury syndrome. It does not require transmural infarction[105] and can also appear as an extension of epistenocardiaca pericarditis. Its incidence is 0.5% to 5%[106] and is lower still in patients treated with thrombolytics (<0.5%)[107] but more frequent in cases of pericardial bleeding after antithrombotic treatment.[104,108] Of note, ECG changes are often overshadowed by myocardial infarction changes. Stage one ECG changes are uncommon and suggest "early" post-myocardial infarction syndrome, whereas failure to evolve or "resurrection" of previously inverted T waves strongly suggests myocardial infarction pericarditis.[109,110] Postinfarction pericardial effusion greater than 10 mm is most frequently associated with hemopericardium, and two thirds of these patients may develop tamponade/free wall rupture.[111] Urgent surgical treatment is lifesaving. If the immediate surgery is not available or contraindicated, pericardiocentesis and intrapericardial fibrin-glue instillation could be an alternative in subacute tamponade.[111,112] Ibuprofen, which increases coronary flow, is the agent of choice.[113] Aspirin, up to 650 mg every 4 hours for 2 to 5 days, has also been successfully applied. Corticosteroids can be used for refractory symptoms but may delay the healing after infarction.[7]

TRAUMATIC PERICARDIAL EFFUSION AND HEMOPERICARDIUM IN AORTIC DISSECTION

Direct pericardial injury can be induced by accidents or iatrogenic wounds.[114-117] Iatrogenic tamponade occurs most frequently in percutaneous mitral valvuloplasty, during or after transseptal puncture, particularly if no biplane catheterization laboratory is available and a small left atrium is present. Whereas the puncture of the interatrial septum is asymptomatic, the passage of the free wall induces chest pain immediately. If high-pressure-containing structures are punctured, rapid deterioration occurs. However, if only the atrial wall is passed, the tamponade may be delayed for 4 to 6 hours. Rescue pericardiocentesis is successful in 95% to 100%, with a less than 1% mortality.[118]

Transection of the coronary artery and acute or subacute cardiac tamponade occur very rarely during percutaneous coronary interventions.[119,120] A breakthrough in the treatment of coronary perforation has been the development of membrane-covered graft stents.[121,122]

During right ventricular endomyocardial biopsy the catheter may pass the myocardium, particularly when the bioptome has not been opened before reaching the endocardial border or it is directed to the right ventricular free wall instead of to the septum. Frank cardiac perforations are accompanied by sudden bradycardia and hypotension.[123] A perforation rate of 0.3% to 5% was reported, leading to tamponade and circulatory collapse in less than half of the cases.[123-125] The incidence of pericardial hemorrhage in left ventricular endomyocardial biopsy is lower (0.1% to 3.3%). Severe complications, leading to procedure-related mortality, were reported in only 0.05% in a worldwide survey of more than 6000 cases[124] and in none of the 2537 patients in our center.[125]

Pacemaker leads penetrating the right ventricle or epicardial electrodes may cause pericarditis with tamponade, adhesions, or constriction.[126-129] A right bundle branch block instead of a usually induced left bundle branch block is a clue.

Blunt chest trauma is the major risk of car accidents. The deceleration force can lead to myocardial contusion with intrapericardial hemorrhage, cardiac rupture, pericardial rupture, or herniation. Transesophageal echocardiography or immediate CT should be performed.[130,132] Pericardial laceration and partial extrusion of the heart into the mediastinum and pleural space may also occur after injury.[115]

In dissection of the ascending aorta, pericardial effusion can be found in 17% to 45% of the patients and in 48% of the autopsy cases.[130] In a clinical series of aortic dissection, pericardial tamponade was found by CT,[132] MRI,[133] or echocardiography[134] in 17% to 33% of patients with type I dissection, 18% to 45% in type II dissection, and 6% in type III dissection.[132] Pericardiocentesis is contraindicated, owing to the risk of intensified bleeding and extension of the dissection.[135,136] Surgery should be performed immediately.

NEOPLASTIC PERICARDITIS

Primary tumors of the pericardium are 40 times less common than metastatic ones.[7] Mesothelioma, the most common of the primary tumors, is almost always incurable. The most common secondary malignant tumors are lung cancer, breast cancer, malignant melanoma, lymphomas, and leukemia. Effusions may be small or large with an imminent tamponade (frequent recurrences) or constriction. Tamponade may even be the initial sign of malignant disease.[137] With small effusions most patients are asymptomatic. The onset of dyspnea, cough, chest pain, tachycardia, and jugular venous distention is observed when the volume of fluid exceeds 500 mL. Pulsus paradoxus, hypotension, cardiogenic shock, and paradoxical movement of the jugular venous pulse are important signs of cardiac tamponade. The diagnosis is based on the confirmation of the malignant infiltration within the pericardium by cytology or biopsy. Of note, in almost two thirds of the patients with documented malignancy pericardial effusion is caused by nonmalignant diseases (e.g., radiation pericarditis or opportunistic infections).[138,139] The chest radiograph, CT, and MRI may reveal mediastinal widening, hilar masses, and pleural effusion.[7] The analysis of pericardial fluid and pericardial or epicardial biopsy are essential for the confirmation of malignant pericardial disease.

Cardiac tamponade is an absolute indication for pericardiocentesis. In suspected neoplastic pericardial effusion without tamponade, systemic antineoplastic treatment as baseline therapy can prevent recurrences in up to 67% of cases.[137] However, pericardial drainage is recommended in all patients with large effusions because of the high recurrence rate (40% to 70%).[110-146] Prevention of recurrences may be achieved by intrapericardial instillation of sclerosing, cytotoxic agents, or immunomodulators. Intrapericardial treatment tailored to the type of the tumor indicates that administration of cisplatin is effective in secondary lung cancer, and intrapericardial instillation of thiotepa appears to be highly effective in breast cancer pericardial metastases.[147-152] No patient showed signs of constrictive pericarditis. Tetracyclines as sclerosing agents also control the malignant pericardial effusion in around 85% of cases, but side effects and complications are quite frequent: fever (19%), chest pain (20%), and atrial arrhythmias (10%).[137,145,146] Although intrapericardial administration of radionuclides has yielded very good results, it is not widely accepted because of the logistic problems connected with their radioactivity.[153] Radiation therapy is very effective (93%) in controlling malignant pericardial effusion in patients with radiosensitive tumors such as lymphoma and leukemia. However, radiotherapy of the heart can cause myocarditis and pericarditis by itself.[137]

Rare Forms of Pericardial Disease

Fungal pericarditis occurs mainly in immunocompromised patients or in the course of endemic, acquired fungal infections.[154] It is due to endemic (Histoplasma, Coccidioides) or opportunistic fungi (Candida, Aspergillus, Blastomyces) and semifungi (Nocardia, Actinomyces).[155-157] Diagnosis is obtained by staining and culturing pericardial fluid or tissue. Antifungal antibodies in serum are also helpful in establishing the diagnosis.[3] Treatment with fluconazole, ketoconazole, itraconazole, amphotericin B, liposomal amphotericin B, or amphotericin B lipid complex is indicated. NSAIDs can support the treatment with antifungal drugs. Patients with histoplasmosis pericarditis do not need antifungal therapy but respond to NSAIDs given for 2 to 12 weeks. Sulfonamides are the drugs of choice for nocardiosis. Combination of three antibiotics including penicillin should be given for actinomycosis. Pericardiocentesis or surgical treatment is indicated for hemodynamic impairment. Pericardiectomy is indicated in fungal constrictive pericarditis.

Radiation pericarditis may begin already during exposure (very rare) or months and years later—with latency of up to 15 to 20 years. Its occurrence is influenced by the applied source, dose, fractionation, duration, radiation exposed volume, form of mantel field therapy, and the age of the patient.[158] The effusion may be serous or hemorrhagic, later on with fibrinous adhesions or constriction, typically without tissue calcification. The symptoms may be masked by the underlying disease or the applied chemotherapy. Imaging should start with echocardiography, followed by cardiac CT or MRI if necessary. Pericarditis without tamponade may be treated conservatively but effusions respond favorably to intrapericardial triamcinolone instillation. Pericardiocentesis and fluid analysis can rule out neoplastic progression to the pericardium.[159] Pericardial constriction occurs in up to 20% of patients, requiring pericardiectomy. The operative mortality is high (21%) and the postoperative 5-year survival is poor (1%), mostly owing to myocardial fibrosis.[160]

Chylopericardium refers to a communication between the pericardium and the thoracic duct, as a result of trauma or congenital anomalies, or as a complication of open-heart surgery,[161] mediastinal lymphangiomas, lymphangiomatous hamartomas, lymphangiectasis, and obstruction or anomalies of the thoracic duct.[162] Infection, tamponade, or constriction may aggravate the prognosis.[163] The pericardial fluid is sterile, odorless, and opalescent with a milky white appearance and the microscopic finding of fat droplets. The chylous nature of the fluid is confirmed by its alkaline reaction, specific gravity between 1010 and 1021, Sudan III stain for fat, and the high concentrations of triglycerides (5 to 50 g/L) and protein (22 to 60 g/L).[164,165] Enhanced CT, alone or combined with lymphography, can identify not only the location of the thoracic duct but also its lymphatic connection to the pericardium.[166,167]

Treatment depends on the etiology and the amount of chylous accumulation.[168] Chylopericardium after thoracic or cardiac operation is preferably treated by pericardiocentesis and diet (medium-chain triglycerides).[169,170] If further production of chylous effusion continues, surgical treatment is mandatory. When conservative treatment and pericardiocentesis fail, a pericardioperitoneal window is a reasonable option.[171,172] Alternatively, when the course of the thoracic duct is precisely identified, its ligation and resection just above the diaphragm is the most effective treatment.[173]

Drug- and toxin-related pericarditis, tamponade, adhesions, fibrosis, or constriction may be induced by several drugs.[7,174] Mechanisms include drug-induced lupus reactions, idiosyncrasy, "serum sickness," foreign substance reactions, and immunopathy. Management is based on the discontinuation of the causative agent and symptomatic treatment.

Pericardial effusion in hypothyroidism occurs in 5% to 30% of patients.[7] Fluid accumulates slowly and tamponade occurs rarely. In some cases, cholesterol pericarditis may be observed. The diagnosis is based on serum levels of thyroxine and thyroid-stimulating hormone. Bradycardia, low voltage of the QRS and T wave inversion or flattening in the ECG, cardiomegaly on the radiograph, and pericardial effusion on echocardiography, as well as a history of radiation-induced thyroid dysfunction, myopathy, ascites, pleural effusion, and uveal edema may be observed.[175-179] Therapy with thyroid hormone decreases pericardial effusion.

Pericardial effusion and constriction in pregnancy may manifest as a minimal to moderate clinically silent hydropericardium by the third trimester. Cardiac compression is rare.[180] ECG changes of acute pericarditis in pregnancy should be distinguished from the slight ST-segment depressions and T-wave changes seen in normal pregnancy.[180,181] Occult constriction becomes manifest in pregnancy owing to the increased blood volume.[181] Most pericardial disorders are managed as in nonpregnant women.[182,183] Caution is necessary because high-dose aspirin may prematurely close the ductus arteriosus, and colchicine is contraindicated in pregnancy. Pericardiotomy and pericardiectomy can be safely performed if necessary and do not impose a risk for subsequent pregnancies.[183,184]

Fetal pericardial fluid can be detected by echocardiography after 20 weeks' gestation and is normally 2 mm or less in depth. More fluid should raise questions of hydrops fetalis, Rh disease, neoplasia, hypoalbuminemia, immunopathy, or maternally transmitted mycoplasmal or other infections.[185]

KEY POINTS

1. The diagnosis of acute pericarditis is based on clinical presentation (chest pain, pericardial friction rub) and typical four-stage ECG changes. For etiologic diagnosis, pericardiocentesis, pericardioscopy, and pericardial/epicardial biopsy may be necessary.

2. Echocardiography is essential in all patients with pericarditis to detect pericardial effusion and determine its physiologic significance, as well as to check for signs of constriction, concomitant heart disease, or paracardial pathology.

3. A large proportion of patients usually classified as having "idiopathic" pericarditis actually have viral and autoreactive pericarditis. The diagnosis of viral pericarditis is not possible without the evaluation of pericardial effusion and/or pericardial/epicardial tissue, preferably by polymerase chain reaction (PCR) or in-situ hybridization.

4. PCR identification of *Mycobacterium tuberculosis*, high adenosine deaminase activity, and interferon gamma concentration in pericardial effusion are diagnostic with a high sensitivity and specificity for tuberculous pericarditis.

5. Pericardiocentesis is indicated for cardiac tamponade, for a high suspicion of purulent, tuberculous, or neoplastic pericarditis, or in patients with very large effusions without signs of tamponade (>20 mm in echocardiography in diastole). Electrical alternans and pulsus paradoxus are clinically important signs of advanced stage of cardiac tamponade and indicate the need for prompt pericardial drainage.

6. Aortic dissection is a major contraindication to pericardiocentesis. Relative contraindications include uncorrected coagulopathy; anticoagulant therapy; thrombocytopenia less than 50,000/mm^3; and small, posterior, and loculated effusions.

7. In cardiac wounds, postinfarction myocardial rupture, or dissecting aortic hematoma emergency cardiac surgery is lifesaving. Loculated effusions may require open surgery or thoracoscopic drainage.

8. Postinfarction pericardial effusions larger than 10 mm in diastole are frequently associated with cardiac rupture. Urgent surgical treatment is indicated.

9. Intrapericardial instillation of antineoplastic (e.g., cisplatin, thiotepa) and/or sclerosing agents (e.g., gentamycin) can prevent recurrences of neoplastic pericardial effusions. Intrapericardial instillation of triamcinolone is highly efficient in preventing recurrences in patients with autoreactive pericardial effusion, mainly avoiding adverse effects of systemic corticosteroid therapy.

10. Pericardiectomy is the only treatment for permanent constrictive pericarditis. However, surgery should not be indicated too early to avoid operating on patients with transient constriction. Even more important is not to perform surgery too late or in patients with myocardial fibrosis and/or atrophy. If the indication for surgery is established early enough, long-term survival after pericardiectomy corresponds to that of the general population.

ANNOTATED REFERENCES

Maisch B, Seferovic PM, Ristic AD, et al. Guidelines on the diagnosis and management of pericardial diseases executive summary; the Task Force on the Diagnosis and Management of Pericardial Diseases of the European Society of Cardiology. Eur Heart J 2004;25:587-610.
  First ESC guidelines for the diagnosis and treatment of pericardial diseases.
Maisch B, Ristic AD, Pankuweit S. Intrapericardial treatment of auto reactive pericardial effusion with triamcinolone: The way to avoid side effects of systemic corticosteroid therapy. Eur Heart J 2002;23:1503-8.
  First clinical study on autoreactive pericarditis and intrapericardial treatment with triamcinolone, showing high efficacy and low incidence of side effects during follow-up.
Maisch B, Ristic AD, Pankuweit S, et al. Neoplastic pericardial effusion: Efficacy and safety of intrapericardial treatment with cisplatin. Eur Heart J 2002;23:1625-31.

Study on intrapericardial treatment of neoplastic pericardial effusion revealing higher efficacy of cisplatin in lung cancer than in breast cancer patients.
Maisch B, Ristic A, Seferovic PM, Tsang TS. Interventional pericardiology. 2011 Springer.
  Most recent book on pericardial diseases focusing on recent advances in diagnosis and interventional treatment including original data on pericardioscopy, pericardial and epicardial biopsy as well as pericardiocentesis, percutaneous balloon pericardiotomy, and surgical procedures for pericardial diseases.
Seferovic PM, Ristic AD, Maksimovic R, et al. Diagnostic value of pericardial biopsy: Improvement with extensive sampling enabled by pericardioscopy. Circulation 2003;107:978-83.
  Recent study on pericardial biopsy revealing contribution of endoscopic guidance to the diagnostic value of the procedure.

REFERENCES

Access the complete reference list online at http://www.expertconsult.com.

86

Emergent Valvular Disorders

CATHERINE M. OTTO

In the critical care setting, there are two distinct presentations of valvular heart disease: acute valve dysfunction resulting in acute heart failure and chronic valve disease with decompensation due to increased metabolic demands (Table 86-1).[1] Valve regurgitation is the most common type of acute valve dysfunction. Valve stenosis, with rare exceptions, is a chronic slowly progressive disease. However, in patients with asymptomatic chronic valve stenosis, acute deterioration can occur if there is a superimposed hemodynamic burden. For example, patients with previously asymptomatic mitral stenosis may present with pulmonary edema in the setting of a systemic infection. Another example is the elderly adult with asymptomatic aortic stenosis who presents with cardiogenic shock in the setting of an acute gastrointestinal bleed. Prosthetic valve dysfunction also can present emergently, particularly mechanical valve thrombosis.

The key concepts in management of the critically ill patient with valvular heart disease are the use of echocardiography to provide an accurate diagnosis of disease severity and the appropriate use of invasive hemodynamic monitoring to optimize loading conditions. Handheld echocardiography may provide clues to the presence of valve disease but does not replace the need for a complete diagnostic study when this diagnosis is suspected. With acute valve regurgitation or prosthetic valve thrombosis, urgent surgical intervention can be life saving.

Mitral Regurgitation

ETIOLOGY

Mitral regurgitation may be caused by disease or distortion of any component of the mitral valve apparatus—the mitral annulus, leaflets, chordae, and papillary muscles—as well as by alterations in left ventricular (LV) geometry or systolic function (Figure 86-1).[2] Primary causes of chronic mitral regurgitation include myxomatous valve leaflets (mitral valve prolapse) and rheumatic disease. Chronic secondary mitral regurgitation may be due to dilated cardiomyopathy or to coronary artery disease with regional or global LV dysfunction.

Acute mitral regurgitation also may be due to involvement of the valve leaflets or the left ventricle. Patients with myxomatous mitral valve disease may develop acute regurgitation due to spontaneous chordal rupture.[3] Bacterial endocarditis results in acute mitral regurgitation due to destruction of valve tissue, often with leaflet perforation. Moderate to severe mitral regurgitation due to papillary muscle involvement or regional myocardial dysfunction complicates 12% of acute myocardial infarctions and is associated with an increased risk of heart failure or death.[4]

CLINICAL PRESENTATION

Although patients with chronic mitral regurgitation may be asymptomatic for many years, the regurgitant lesions impose a volume load on the left ventricle, because an increased total stroke volume is needed to maintain a normal forward cardiac output. Left ventricular volume overload results in progressive LV dilation and may lead to an irreversible decline in ventricular contractility, even in the absence of clinical symptoms. Evaluation of ventricular contractility is problematic in patients with mitral regurgitation, given that measures of ventricular performance are affected by preload and afterload.[5] However, based on

outcomes after mitral valve surgery, the empirical parameters of ventricular end-systolic dimension and ejection fraction can be used to optimize the timing of surgical intervention. Thus, patients with moderate to severe chronic regurgitation undergo periodic echocardiography, with valve repair or replacement recommended when the end-systolic dimension is ≥ 40 mm and the ejection fraction is ≤ 60%.[6]

Chronic mitral regurgitation usually is well tolerated even when there is a superimposed hemodynamic load such as systemic infection, pregnancy, or trauma. However, mitral regurgitant severity may acutely worsen by at least two mechanisms. An increase in afterload, for example with a hypertensive crisis, may increase regurgitant severity due to an increased driving pressure from the left ventricle to the left atrium. Alteration in LV geometry, for example with ventricular dilation due to decompensated heart failure, may change the orientation of the papillary muscles such that leaflet closure is impaired, resulting in a larger regurgitant orifice area.[7] In this situation, a vicious cycle may ensue where LV dilation worsens mitral regurgitant severity, which increases LV dilation, and so forth.

Acute mitral regurgitation presents with acute pulmonary edema and is a surgical emergency (Figures 86-2 and 86-3). Mitral chordal rupture results in the acute presentation of heart failure, often in patients who were unaware of a diagnosis of mitral valve prolapse. Patients with mitral valve perforation due to endocarditis present with pulmonary edema superimposed on signs and symptoms of endocarditis. Papillary muscle rupture or dysfunction after MI usually presents several days after acute MI; in some cases, the initial presentation is acute pulmonary edema, with the MI being clinically silent.

DIAGNOSIS

A high level of clinical suspicion is needed to make the diagnosis of acute mitral regurgitation (Table 86-2). Acute pulmonary edema often obscures the signs and symptoms of the underlying disease process. The classical finding is a holosystolic murmur at the apex, radiating to the axilla. Although there is some correlation between the loudness of the murmur and regurgitant severity with chronic regurgitation, the murmur may be soft with acute severe mitral regurgitation. In patients with severe mitral regurgitation after MI, a murmur cannot be appreciated at all in up to 50% of patients.

Thus, in patients presenting with acute pulmonary edema or cardiogenic shock, prompt echocardiography is essential. Transthoracic images often are diagnostic, allowing identification of the etiology of valve dysfunction, quantitation of regurgitant severity, estimation of pulmonary pressures, and measurement of ventricular size and systolic function. If transthoracic images are nondiagnostic, transesophageal echocardiography (TEE) can be performed at the bedside in the intensive care unit (ICU). TEE provides excellent images of valve anatomy and Doppler evaluation of valve function.

Other diagnostic tests are based on the clinical presentation. Multiple blood cultures should be obtained in febrile patients with systemic or pulmonary edema to exclude the possibility of endocarditis. In patients with an abnormal electrocardiogram (ECG), chest pain, or a history of coronary artery disease, coronary angiography may be needed.

In the patient with acute pulmonary edema or cardiogenic shock after MI, the differential diagnosis includes acute mitral regurgitation, a ventricular septal defect, or a contained rupture of the ventricular

TABLE 86-1	Causes of Acute Valve Dysfunction
Mitral regurgitation	Myxomatous disease with flail leaflet
	Spontaneous chordal rupture
	Endocarditis
	Acute myocardial infarction:
	Papillary muscle rupture
	Regional wall motion abnormality
	LV dilation and systolic dysfunction
Aortic regurgitation	Endocarditis
	Spontaneous rupture of a congenital fenestration
	Aortic dissection
Tricuspid regurgitation	Endocarditis
	Penetrating chest trauma
	Blunt chest wall trauma
Prosthetic valves	Endocarditis
	Valve thrombosis
	Paravalvular dehiscence
	Leaflet tear

TABLE 86-2	Diagnostic Approach to Acute Valve Dysfunction
Physical examination	Unreliable
	Consider valve dysfunction in all patients with pulmonary edema
Echocardiography (transthoracic)	Accurate diagnosis of etiology of disease
	Quantitation of severity of stenosis or regurgitation
	Measurement of ventricular ejection fraction
	Estimation of pulmonary pressures
Transesophageal echocardiography	Sensitive for detection of valvular vegetations
	Detection of paravalvular abscess
	Essential for prosthetic mitral valve dysfunction
	Useful for prosthetic aortic valve dysfunction
Right heart catheterization	Not reliable for diagnosis of valve disease
	May be helpful for optimizing loading conditions
Chest computed tomography	Sensitive and specific for diagnosis of aortic dissection
Angiography	Used when coronary angiography is needed

free wall. All these possibilities can be diagnosed by echocardiography in an experienced center.

Invasive hemodynamic monitoring with a Swan-Ganz catheter for measurement of pulmonary pressures and cardiac output is needed in the patient with suspected acute mitral regurgitation. At the time of placement, oxygen saturations in the right atrium, right ventricle, and pulmonary artery should be measured. A ventricular septal defect results in a "step-up" in oxygen saturation between the right atrium and ventricle secondary to oxygenated blood from the left ventricle entering the right ventricle. The pulmonary artery balloon-occluded (wedge) pressure tracing should be examined for the presence of a "v-wave," which supports the diagnosis of acute mitral regurgitation but is not always present.

MANAGEMENT

In patients with chronic mitral regurgitation and heart failure, management is directed at treating the process leading to decompensation and optimizing loading conditions (Table 86-3). For example, in a

patient with a systemic infection, treatment of the infection, control of fever and tachycardia, and invasive monitoring to optimize preload and afterload are utilized. Medical therapy typically includes afterload reduction with nitroprusside or other vasodilators and preload reduction with diuretics.[8,9] The goal is to support the patient through the

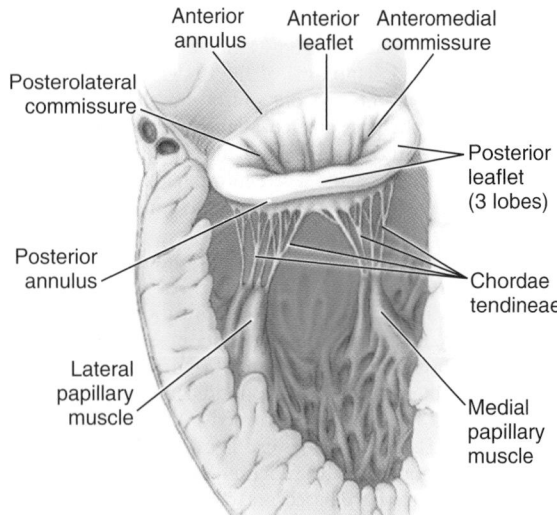

Figure 86-1 Mitral valve anatomy: mitral annulus, anterior and posterior leaflets, chordae tendineae, and papillary muscles. Mitral regurgitation may be due to a disease that primarily affects the valve leaflets (e.g., mitral valve prolapse, rheumatic mitral valve disease) or may result from alterations in function or structure of the left ventricle, such as those induced by ischemic disease or dilated cardiomyopathy. *(From Otto CM. Clinical practice. Evaluation and management of chronic mitral regurgitation. New Engl J Med 2001;345:740-6.)*

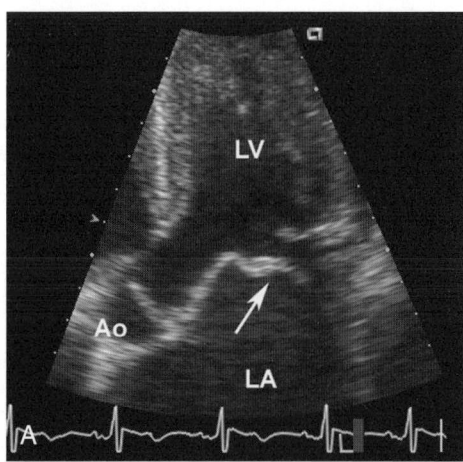

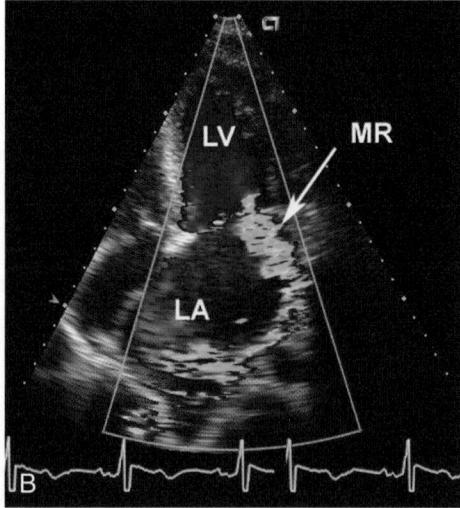

Figure 86-2 In this 24-year-old man with chronic mitral prolapse, chordal rupture resulted in a flail anterior leaflet, seen in apical four-chamber view *(panel **A**, arrow).* Severe mitral regurgitation (MR) was seen with a posterior and laterally directed jet on Doppler color-flow imaging *(panel **B**, arrow).* Ao, aorta; LA, left atrium; LV, left ventricle.

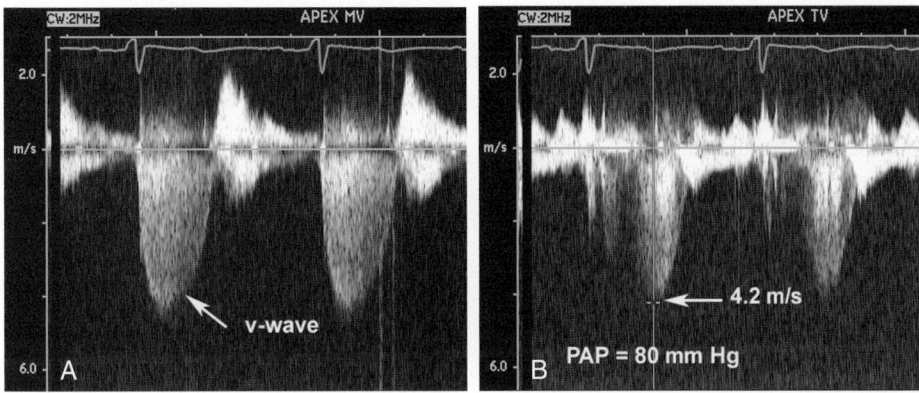

Figure 86-3 In the same patient as Figure 86-2, severe mitral regurgitation was recorded with continuous wave Doppler ultrasound **(A)**. The rapid rise in left atrial pressure due to the regurgitant jet entering the left atrium results in a rapid decline in Doppler velocity in late systole—the Doppler equivalent of the v-wave seen on a pulmonary wedge pressure tracing. The continuous-wave Doppler recording of maximum tricuspid regurgitant jet velocity **(B)** of 4.2 m/sec indicates a right ventricular–to–right atrial pressure difference of 70 mm Hg. The patient's right atrial pressure was estimated to be 10 mm Hg, based on size and respiratory variation in the inferior vena cava, so the estimated pulmonary systolic pressure is 80 mm Hg.

period of decompensation. Typically, hemodynamics return to the baseline compensated state after the acute illness.

In contrast, acute severe mitral regurgitation is a surgical emergency. Mortality is extremely high without restoration of valve competence; even with prompt valve surgery, 30-day mortality is 23%.[10] Medical stabilization should occur concurrently with consultation by a cardiac surgeon. Acutely, placement of an intraaortic balloon pump (IABP) provides optimal afterload reduction while improving diastolic coronary blood flow.

The timing and risk of surgical intervention depend on the etiology of acute mitral regurgitation. Spontaneous chordal rupture usually can be treated early with mitral valve repair. Compared to valve replacement, mitral valve repair is associated with a lower operative mortality, improved preservation of LV function, and better long-term survival. In addition, the risks of a prosthetic valve and anticoagulation are avoided.

The timing of surgery for endocarditis depends on the disease course in that individual, but most centers now advocate early surgical intervention in the patient with heart failure or severe valve regurgitation to prevent progressive valve damage and paravalvular abscess formation.[11,12] In a large prospective multicenter study, early surgery was associated with a lower mortality than medical therapy (12% versus 21%).[13] Valve repair is preferred but may not be possible, depending on the extent of tissue destruction. Early surgery is particularly beneficial in patients with paravalvular complications or systemic embolization.[14]

In patients with acute ischemic mitral regurgitation, treatment depends on the exact etiology of valve dysfunction.[15] In patients with acute mitral regurgitation due to a regional wall-motion abnormality, myocardial function may improve after percutaneous revascularization.[16] In these patients, use of an IABP and medical therapy may be

advantageous during the acute episode, with weaning of therapy as myocardial function improves.

Mitral regurgitation due to partial or complete papillary muscle rupture requires surgical intervention. Although the risk of surgery is high, with an operative mortality rate of about 50%, outcome is even worse with medical therapy, with a mortality of 75% at 24 hours and 95% within 2 weeks after complete papillary muscle rupture.[17] With the use of echocardiography, partial papillary muscle rupture can be recognized; prognosis in these patients depends on the extent of myocardial damage and severity of mitral regurgitation.[18] With partial papillary muscle rupture, some surgeons prefer to stabilize the patient and delay surgery for 6 to 8 weeks after MI to avoid operating on the necrotic myocardial tissue. However, many patients cannot be stabilized, so acute intervention must be considered. Again, valve repair is preferred, but myocardial necrosis may necessitate valve replacement. Risk factors for surgery include older age, female gender, and poor LV systolic function. In some patients, the risk of surgical intervention may be so high as to be futile.

Aortic Regurgitation

ETIOLOGY

Chronic aortic regurgitation most often is due to a congenital bicuspid valve, rheumatic valve disease, or aortic root dilation. There are numerous causes of aortic root dilation, including hypertension, cystic medial necrosis, Marfan syndrome, and a bicuspid aortic valve.[19] The most common causes of acute aortic regurgitation are endocarditis, rupture of a congenital fenestration, and acute aortic dissection.[1] Endocarditis results in aortic regurgitation by destruction of the valve leaflet tissue, with a high percentage of cases also having paravalvular abscess formation. Aortic dissection results in acute aortic regurgitation either due to enlargement of the aortic annulus or to extension of the dissection into the valve region, resulting in a flail aortic valve leaflet.

CLINICAL PRESENTATION

The acute backflow of blood from the aorta into the left ventricle in diastole results in an acute elevation in LV end-diastolic pressure, with consequent pulmonary edema. Because there has been no time for compensatory LV dilation, forward cardiac output falls abruptly owing to the regurgitant flow across the valve in diastole, so patients with acute aortic regurgitation also may be in cardiogenic shock. Decreased

TABLE 86-3	Therapeutic Approach to Acute Valve Dysfunction

1. Accurate diagnosis with echocardiography; differentiate acute valve dysfunction from acute decompensation with chronic valve disease.
2. Treat the underlying disease process associated with decompensation (endocarditis, acute myocardial infarction, anemia, etc.).
3. Optimize loading conditions using diuretics, vasodilators, and other agents, with invasive hemodynamic monitoring.
4. Consult the cardiac surgery team as soon as the diagnosis is made.
5. Intraaortic balloon pump for acute mitral regurgitation.
6. Consider surgical or percutaneous intervention.

coronary perfusion pressure results in diffuse subendocardial ischemia, further impairing ventricular function.

DIAGNOSIS

The clinical diagnosis of acute aortic regurgitation differs markedly from chronic aortic regurgitation (Figure 86-4). In contrast to the high-pitched diastolic decrescendo murmur of chronic aortic regurgitation, there is a "to-and-fro" murmur across the aortic valve which many clinicians fail to recognize as indicating aortic regurgitation. The pulse pressure is narrow due to the low forward stroke volume, and peripheral signs of aortic regurgitation are not seen. As with acute mitral regurgitation, the physical examination findings often are subtle, so a high index of suspicion and prompt echocardiography are needed to make this diagnosis.

Acute aortic regurgitation should be considered in the patient with signs or symptoms of endocarditis, in patients with a personal or family history of aortic root disease, and in those with a presentation consistent with acute aortic dissection.[20]

Echocardiography allows imaging of the aortic valve and root and determination of the severity of aortic regurgitation based on a combination of two-dimensional (2D) imaging and pulsed, continuous-wave, and color Doppler modalities[21] (Figures 86-5, 86-6, and 86-7). The continuous-wave Doppler curve shows a steep diastolic slope corresponding to the rapid equalization of diastolic pressure in the aorta

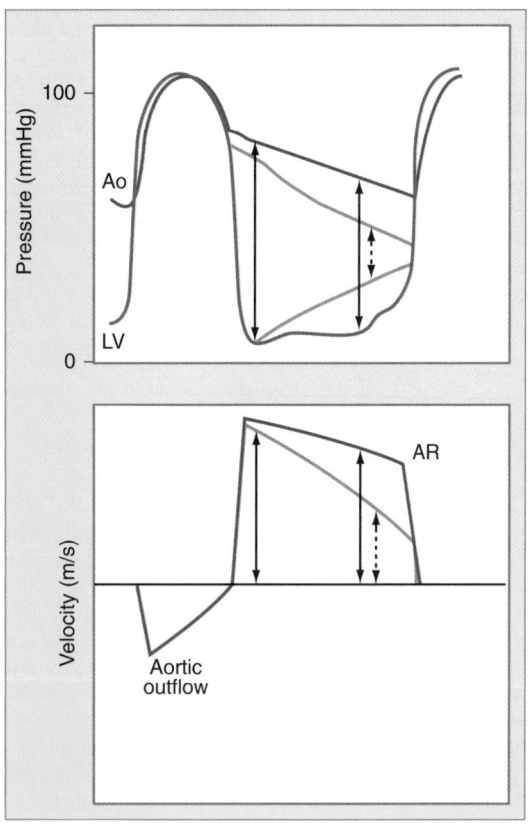

Figure 86-4 Left ventricular (LV) and central aortic (Ao) pressures and corresponding Doppler velocity curves are shown for chronic *(purple lines)* and acute *(green lines)* aortic regurgitation. The shape of velocity curve is related to the instantaneous pressure differences across the valve, as stated in the Bernoulli equation. With acute aortic regurgitation (AR), aortic pressures fall more rapidly, and ventricular diastolic pressure rises more rapidly, resulting in a steeper deceleration slope on Doppler curve. *(From Otto CM. Textbook of clinical echocardiography. 4th ed. Philadelphia: Saunders; 2009, p. 303.)*

and left ventricle. With severe acute regurgitation, there is no pressure gradient at end-diastole, so cuff diastolic blood pressure is equal to LV end-diastolic pressure. Echocardiography also allows accurate assessment of LV size and systolic function. When the differential diagnosis includes aortic dissection, transthoracic echocardiography is inadequate to exclude this possibility. Instead, TEE or computed tomography (CT) images should be obtained.

MANAGEMENT

Acute aortic regurgitation is a surgical emergency.[1] Preoperative management is supportive, with ventilatory support and invasive hemodynamic monitoring. While the diagnosis is being made, therapy may include the use of diuretics, inotropic agents, and nitroprusside or other vasodilators in an attempt to stabilize hemodynamics.[1,9] However, an IABP is contraindicated, as inflation of the balloon in the descending thoracic aorta in diastole will increase the amount of backflow across the aortic valve.

If acute aortic regurgitation is due to aortic dissection, acute surgical intervention is needed. The surgical approach may be replacement of the ascending aorta and valve with a combined prosthetic valve and fabric tube. When the valve leaflets are normal, some centers will preserve the native valve by resuspension of the leaflets in the prosthetic conduit (called *the David procedure*).

When acute aortic regurgitation is due to endocarditis, surgical options include a mechanical valve, a heterograft tissue valve such as a porcine aortic valve or bovine pericardial valve, or a cryopreserved homograft aorta valve. Rarely, the patient may undergo valve repair if there is a simple perforation with adjacent normal leaflet tissue.

Mitral Stenosis

ETIOLOGY AND CLINICAL PRESENTATION

Mitral stenosis is nearly always due to rheumatic disease, with only rare cases of calcific mitral stenosis seen in the elderly. Rheumatic mitral stenosis is a slowly progressive disease with an insidious decline in exercise tolerance and symptom onset over many years.[22] However, in the asymptomatic patient with compensated moderate or severe mitral stenosis, acute decompensation can occur in the setting of increased systemic hemodynamic demands. Because mitral stenosis is more common in women (80% of cases) and occurs during the reproductive years, the most common emergency presentation of mitral stenosis is a pregnant woman with heart failure. Many of these patients are unaware of underlying valve disease and are initially diagnosed during pregnancy. The clinical presentation may also be due to or exacerbated by the onset of atrial fibrillation.

A large atrial myxoma may mimic the clinical presentation of mitral stenosis, presenting with acute hemodynamic compromise due to obstruction of the mitral valve orifice by the tumor mass.

DIAGNOSIS

The apical diastolic rumble and opening snap of mitral stenosis is challenging to appreciate even in a quiet room with optimal patient positioning and frequently is inaudible in the ICU setting. However, the diagnosis is easily made by transthoracic echocardiography, with the mitral leaflet showing the characteristic findings of rheumatic disease: commissural fusion, chordal shortening and fusion, and restriction of the diastolic opening of the leaflets (Figure 86-8).[23] Mitral stenosis severity can be quantitated by calculation of valve area by 2D planimetry or by the Doppler pressure half-time method, with moderate to severe stenosis defined as a valve area less than 1.5 cm^2 (Figure 86-9). Transthoracic echocardiography also provides information on LV size and systolic function, left atrial size, pulmonary pressures, and any associated valve lesions. If evaluation for left atrial thrombus is needed, TEE has a sensitivity of only 60% compared to a sensitivity of nearly 100% from the transthoracic approach.

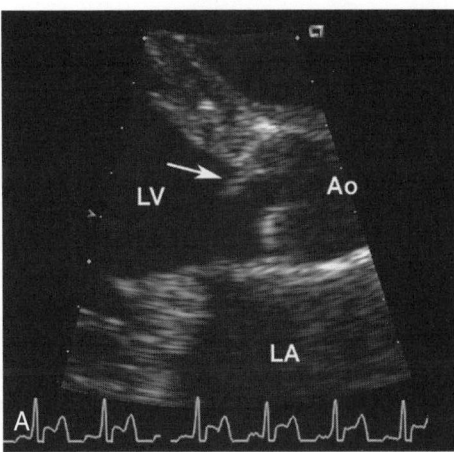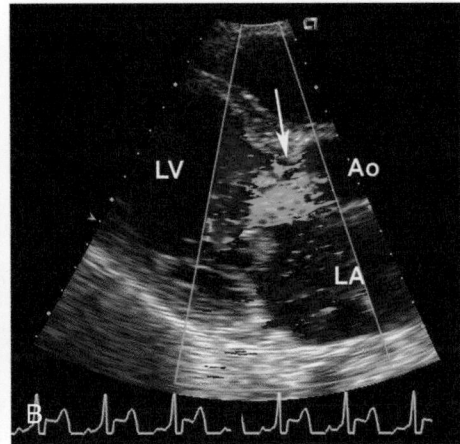

Figure 86-5 Endocarditis resulting in acute severe aortic regurgitation. In a long-axis view of the aortic valve **(A),** a flail aortic valve leaflet is seen (*arrow*), with the leaflet (*arrow*) prolapsing into the left ventricular (LV) outflow tract in diastole. Color-flow Doppler imaging **(B)** in the same view shows a broad jet of diastolic flow filling the outflow tract, consistent with severe regurgitation. Ao, aorta; LA, left atrium; LV, left ventricle.

MANAGEMENT

Most patients with mitral stenosis and acute decompensation can be managed conservatively with treatment of the superimposed illness.[9] Efforts should be directed towards decreasing overall metabolic demand and increasing oxygen delivery by controlling fever, maintaining a normal hemoglobin level, and providing supplemental oxygen. If atrial fibrillation is present, rate control is essential, preferably with conversion back to sinus rhythm. Even when sinus rhythm is present, beta-blockers may improve ventricular diastolic filling by prolonging the duration of diastole as heart rate is decreased.[24] Invasive hemodynamic monitoring and ventilatory support may be needed when severe heart failure is present.

In patients who do not respond to conservative therapy, emergency intervention should be considered. The optimal intervention is percutaneous balloon mitral valvotomy (PBMV), which typically results in an increase in mitral valve area to more than 1.5 cm^2.[25-27] PBMV can be safely performed even during pregnancy.[28-30] Patients with a left

atrial thrombus, coexisting moderate to severe mitral regurgitation, or heavily calcified and deformed mitral valves are not candidates for PBMV; in theses patients, surgical mitral valve replacement may be needed.

Aortic Stenosis

ETIOLOGY AND CLINICAL PRESENTATION

Valvular aortic stenosis in adults is most often due to calcification of a normal trileaflet or congenital bicuspid valve (Figure 86-10). Rheumatic aortic stenosis is less common and is invariably accompanied by mitral valve involvement. In younger adults, congenital aortic stenosis may be encountered; some of these patients have restenosis after prior commissurotomy in childhood.

Like mitral stenosis, aortic valve stenosis is a chronic, slowly progressive disease that presents acutely only in patients who have not been receiving regular medical care.[31-33] As in mitral stenosis, acute

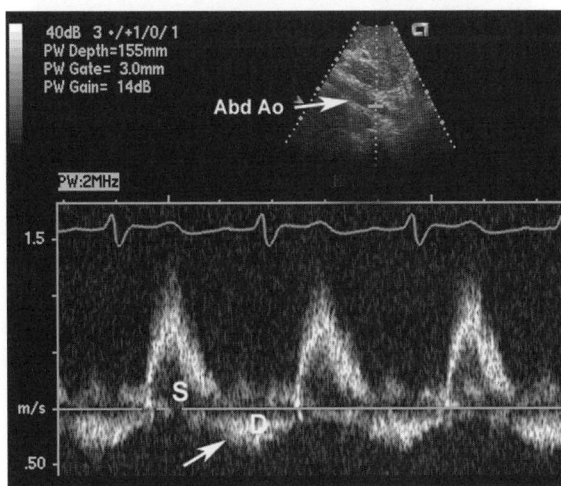

Figure 86-6 Same patient as Figure 86-5. Pulsed Doppler flow in the proximal abdominal aorta (Ao) shows normal forward flow in systole (S), with abnormal reversed flow in diastole (D) that extends throughout diastole. This finding is highly specific for severe aortic regurgitation and can be helpful in the acute setting.

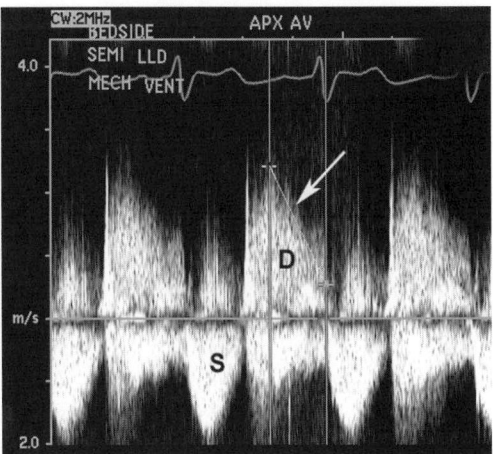

Figure 86-7 Same patient as Figure 86-5. Continuous-wave Doppler recording of flow across the aortic valve shows an increased antegrade velocity in systole (S) consistent with a high transaortic stroke volume. In diastole (D), a dense signal of retrograde flow is seen, with a steep deceleration slope (*arrow*) consistent with equalization of pressures between the aorta and left ventricle in diastole.

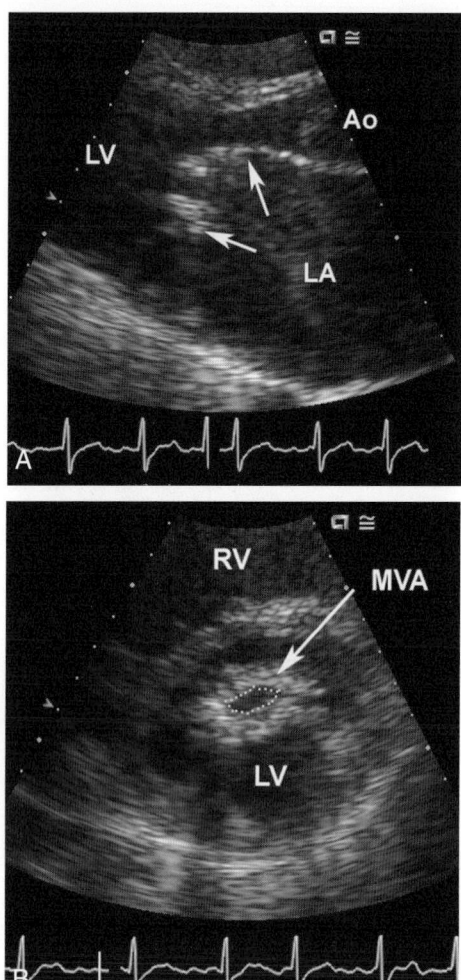

Figure 86-8 In a patient with mitral stenosis the long axis view **(A)** demonstrates the classic findings of diastolic doming of leaflets *(arrows)* due to commissural fusion, with thickening predominantly at the leaflet tips. In the short-axis view **(B)**, the restricted mitral orifice with fusion of the commissures is visualized, providing accurate measurement of valve area by direct planimetry. In this case, the valve area of 0.7 cm^2 indicates severe valve obstruction. Ao, aorta; LA, left atrium; LV, left ventricle; RV, right ventricle.

decompensation may occur with a superimposed systemic condition. Young women with congenital aortic stenosis may present with angina or heart failure during pregnancy. In older adults, asymptomatic patients with moderate to severe valve obstruction may present with heart failure in the setting of pneumonia, anemia, or other condition with increased metabolic demands.

DIAGNOSIS

The classic physical examination findings for aortic stenosis include a delayed and decreased carotid upstroke, a narrow pulse pressure, a single second heart sound (S$_2$), and a systolic ejection murmur at the aortic region that radiates to the carotids. However, while a grade 4 murmur (palpable thrill) with a single S$_2$ and diminished carotids is specific for severe stenosis, these findings are very insensitive for the diagnosis.[34] Particularly when the patient is decompensated, the murmur may be soft, and carotid upstrokes may be altered by coexisting vascular disease or loading conditions.

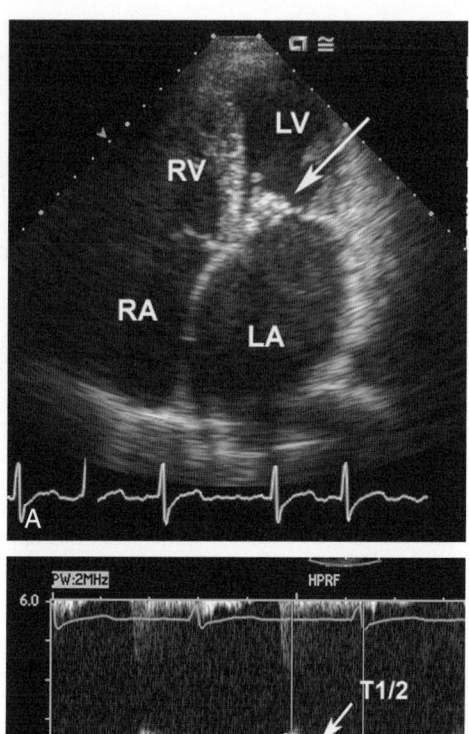

Figure 86-9 Same patient as Figure 86-10. Apical four-chamber view **(A)** shows severe left atrial enlargement due to mitral obstruction, with thickened valve leaflets *(arrow)*. Haziness in left atrium is due to stasis of blood flow, with spontaneous contrast on echocardiography. Continuous-wave Doppler recording of flow across mitral valve shows increased velocity corresponding to transvalvular pressure gradient. Pressure half-time (T1/2) can be used to accurately calculate mitral valve area (0.7 cm^2).

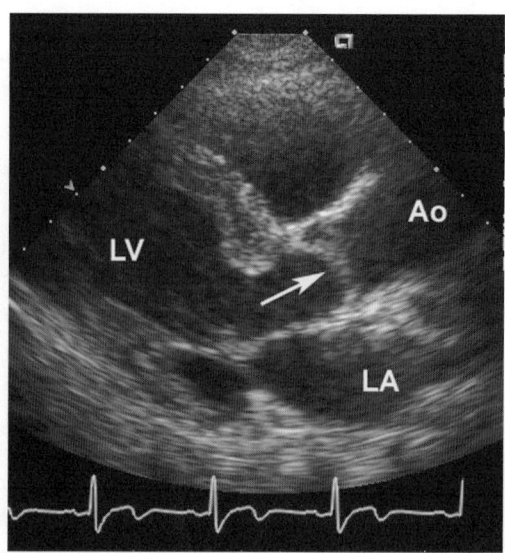

Figure 86-10 In this 26-year-old pregnant woman with a loud systolic murmur, the long-axis view shows doming of the aortic valve in systole *(arrow)*. Short axis images confirmed a unicuspid aortic valve. Ao, aorta; LA, left atrium; LV, left ventricle.

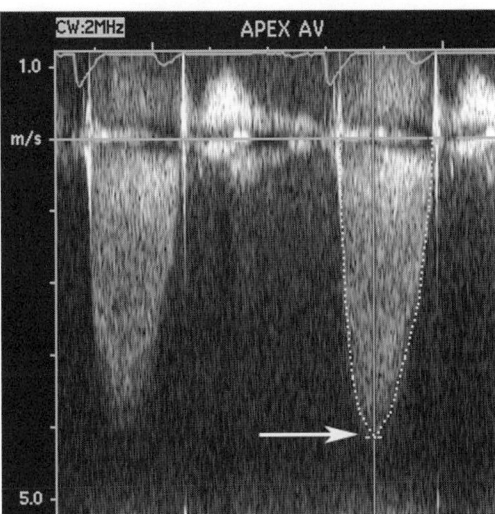

Figure 86-11 Continuous-wave Doppler examination of the aortic valve (same patient as Figure 86-8) demonstrates a high-velocity signal consistent with severe aortic stenosis. The maximum velocity of 4.2 m/sec corresponds to a maximum transaortic pressure gradient of 69 mm Hg and a mean gradient of 41 mm Hg. Valve area, calculated by the continuity equation, was 0.8 cm^2.

Echocardiography provides reliable evaluation of aortic stenosis severity based on the maximum velocity through the narrowed orifice and valve area, calculated with the continuity equation (Figure 86-11). Disease severity is a continuum, and velocities may be relatively low despite severe stenosis when cardiac output in reduced. In general, stenosis can be graded as severe (valve area <1.0 cm^2 or jet velocity >4 m/sec), moderate (valve area 1.0-1.5 cm^2 or jet velocity 3-4 m/sec) or mild (valve area >1.5 cm^2 or jet velocity <3 m/sec). Echocardiography also allows evaluation of ventricular systolic and diastolic function and any associated valve disease.[23]

MANAGEMENT

As with mitral stenosis, most patients with decompensated aortic stenosis can be managed conservatively by (1) treating the underlying disease process that led to decompensation and (2) restoring the patient's normal loading conditions. However, in the patient who has denied symptoms or has not been receiving medical care, the first presentation of aortic stenosis may be syncope or pulmonary edema. In these patients, aortic stenosis is the cause of decompensation, as evidenced by very severe valve obstruction, often with a low ejection fraction. Treatment is urgent aortic valve replacement. Some centers advocate the use of balloon aortic valvuloplasty in these patients, but the magnitude and duration of benefit is limited. Cautious use of nitroprusside may improve hemodynamics prior to valve replacement in severe decompensated aortic stenosis if mean arterial pressure is above 60 mm Hg,[35,36] and some patients can be managed with careful diuresis. However, in unstable patients who are surgical candidates, it is more prudent to proceed promptly to valve replacement. Transcatheter aortic valve implantation is currently in clinical trials for high-risk patients with severe aortic stenosis and may become an option for acutely ill patients in the future.[37]

Right-Sided Valve Disease

Pulmonic valve disease is nearly always congenital in origin, with a chronic disease course. Tricuspid valve stenosis is rare and usually accompanies rheumatic mitral valve disease. Tricuspid valve endocarditis often results in acute severe regurgitation; pulmonic valve endocarditis is rare. Cases of acute traumatic disruption of the tricuspid

valve with blunt chest trauma have been described, although myocardial contusion or thoracic aorta disruption is more common.[38,39] Acute severe tricuspid regurgitation results in a low forward cardiac output and signs of an elevated right atrial pressure.

Prosthetic Valves

MECHANICAL VALVES

Prosthetic mechanical heart valves are very durable, with complications most often due to valve thrombosis or paravalvular regurgitation.[40] Valve thrombosis occurs in the setting of inadequate anticoagulation and may result in functional valve stenosis if movement of the valve occluder is restricted, or valve regurgitation if the clot prevents full closure of the valve. The clinical presentation of valve thrombosis is similar to that of native valve stenosis or regurgitation. Again, echocardiography provides key information on the presence and severity of valve dysfunction (Figure 86-12).[41] TEE is especially

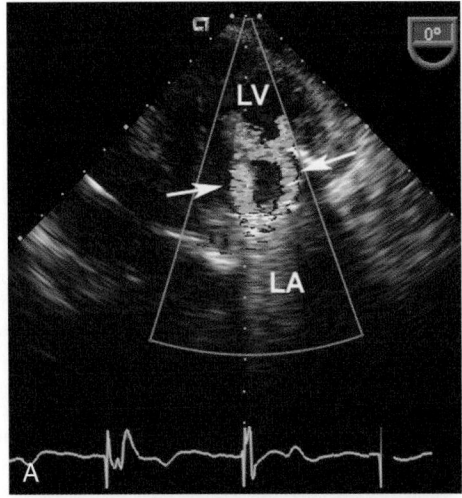

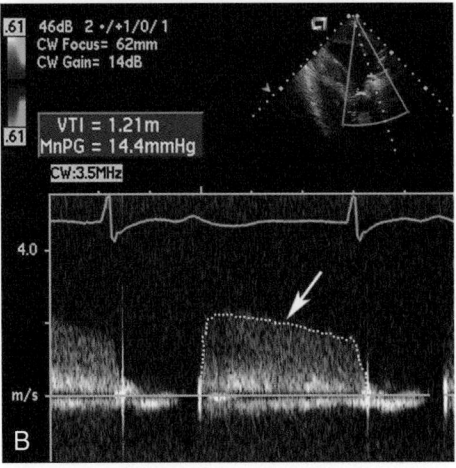

Figure 86-12 Acute prosthetic mitral valve thrombosis in an 82-year-old man 29 years after valve replacement. Patient presented acutely with pulmonary edema and a right upper extremity thrombotic occlusion after anticoagulation was temporarily discontinued owing to a gastrointestinal bleed. Color Doppler imaging **(A)** shows only narrow jets *(arrows)* of flow antegrade across the mitral valve replacement (MVR), and continuous-wave Doppler signal **(B)** shows a high gradient and very prolonged deceleration slope, consistent with severe obstruction to flow. After careful discussion, given his high risk for surgery, he was treated with thrombolytic therapy, which resulted in normalization of his mitral valve Doppler flows and resolution of pulmonary edema.

important with mitral prosthetic valves; the valve itself blocks ultrasound penetration from a transthoracic approach.

Treatment of prosthetic valve thrombosis is controversial. When only a small thrombus and mild hemodynamic compromise are present, conservative therapy with full-dose intravenous anticoagulation for several days may be adequate. With severe hemodynamic compromise, surgical intervention with repeat valve replacement may be necessary, although operative mortality is reported to be high, ranging from 17% to 40%.[6] Systemic thrombolytic therapy can restore valve function in about 80% of patients but is associated with death in 20%, systemic embolism due to fragmentation of the valve thrombosis in 16%, and the need for emergency surgery in 20%.[6] The duration of thrombolytic therapy is based on the resolution of Doppler echocardiographic evidence of resolution of thrombus and valve dysfunction (see Figure 86-12). Current guidelines recommend emergency operation for left-sided valve thrombosis and severe symptoms or a large clot burden, except in patients with excessively high surgical risk. Fibrinolytic therapy is reasonable for right-sided valve thrombosis, for left-sided thrombosis with mild obstruction or a small clot burden, and for patients who are not surgical candidates.[6,42,43]

Paravalvular regurgitation early after valve replacement may be related to suture dehiscence at a site of annular calcification. Paravalvular regurgitation may be associated with hemolytic anemia, which can be treated conservatively if mild but may require reoperation if severe recurrent anemia is present. The new onset of paravalvular regurgitation should prompt careful evaluation for endocarditis (see Chapter 87).

TISSUE VALVES

Tissue valves are subject to degeneration of the leaflets, with superimposed calcification that may result in stenosis or regurgitation. Usually this is a slowly progressive process with presentation 10 to 15 years after valve implantation.[44] As with native valve disease, acute decompensation may occur in patients with chronic prosthetic valve dysfunction if there is a superimposed hemodynamic stress.

Acute regurgitation of a tissue valve can result from endocarditis or from a leaflet tear due to tissue degeneration. Tears in the valve leaflet typically occur adjacent to an area of calcification secondary to the increased stress on the normal leaflet tissue. As with mechanical valves, both transthoracic and transesophageal imaging are needed for full evaluation of suspected prosthetic tissue valve dysfunction. Treatment is similar to that for native valves, with medical stabilization followed by surgery for repeat valve replacement.

KEY POINTS

Acute Mitral Regurgitation

1. Causes include endocarditis, mitral prolapse, and acute myocardial infarction.
2. Presents with pulmonary edema.
3. Murmur may be soft or absent.
4. Prompt echocardiography is essential.
5. Pulmonary wedge v-wave is not always seen.
6. Intraaortic balloon pump improves hemodynamics.
7. Definitive treatment is mitral valve surgery.

Acute Aortic Regurgitation

1. Causes include endocarditis and aortic dissection.
2. Diastolic murmur may be soft.
3. Prompt echocardiography is essential.
4. Treatment is emergency surgery.

Mitral Stenosis

1. Rheumatic mitral stenosis typically occurs in young women.
2. May present during pregnancy.
3. Echocardiography is diagnostic.
4. Acute decompensation can be treated conservatively.
5. Percutaneous balloon mitral valvuloplasty is the optimal intervention.

Aortic Stenosis

1. Aortic stenosis is common in the elderly.
2. Decompensation occurs with increased hemodynamic demand.
3. Physical examination shows a systolic murmur.
4. Echocardiography is diagnostic.
5. Conservative management for decompensation is appropriate.
6. Severe symptomatic disease requires aortic valve replacement.

Prosthetic Valves

1. Mechanical valves are at risk of valve thrombosis.
2. Management of prosthetic valve thrombosis is controversial.
3. Tissue valves undergo degeneration 10 to 15 years after implantation.
4. Acute regurgitation is similar to native valve disease.

ANNOTATED REFERENCES

Stout KK, Verrier ED. Acute valvular regurgitation. Circulation 2009;119:3232-41.
   Detailed summary of the literature on acute valve regurgitation, clinical presentation, diagnostic approach, and management. Surgical considerations in the decision for valve repair versus replacement are reviewed. References to earlier publications can be found here.
Prendergast BD, Tornos P. Surgery for infective endocarditis: who and when? Circulation 2010;121:1141-52.
   Review paper that summarizes the literature on timing of surgery for infective endocarditis and provides a practical approach for patient management.
Lalani T, Cabell CH, Benjamin DK, et al. Analysis of the impact of early surgery on in-hospital mortality of native valve endocarditis: use of propensity score and instrumental variable methods to adjust for treatment-selection bias. Circulation 2010;121:1005-13.
   In this prospective study of 1552 patients with native valve endocarditis, the 46% who underwent early surgery were compared to the 54% treated medically. Overall survival was significantly better with early surgery, with an estimated absolute risk reduction of 11%. Propensity score subgroup analysis identified

patients most likely to benefit from early surgery as those with paravalvular complications, systemic embolization, infection with Staph aureus, and stroke.
Chandrashekhar Y, Westaby S, Narula J. Mitral stenosis. Lancet 2009;374:1271-83.
   Review of mitral stenosis including epidemiology and pathology, diagnosis, clinical course, and management. The management of mitral stenosis during pregnancy and the role of percutaneous mitral valvotomy are emphasized.
Sun JC, Davidson MJ, Lamy A, Eikelboom JW. Antithrombotic management of patients with prosthetic heart valves: current evidence and future trends. Lancet 2009;374:565-76.
   This review of antithrombotic therapy for prosthetic valves covers preventive anticoagulation and management of thrombotic complications. For obstructive valve thrombosis, the authors recommend thrombolytic therapy and echocardiographic monitoring, with surgery reserved for patients with contraindications to thrombolysis or those who do not respond to thrombolytic therapy. Smaller (<5 mm) nonobstructive thrombi usually can be managed with standard anticoagulation alone.

REFERENCES

Access the complete reference list online at http://www.expertconsult.com.

87

Infectious Endocarditis

MICHEL WOLFF | JEAN-FRANÇOIS TIMSIT | BRUNO MOURVILLIER

Infectious endocarditis is associated with a myriad of complications, both cardiac and extracardiac, that may require intensive care unit (ICU) admission. Local progression of the infection causes destruction of valve cusps or leaflets and chordae and may extend to peri- and paravalvular structures. Hemodynamic deterioration leads to secondary organ failure. Finally, embolization of infected tissues may damage vital organs and cause peripheral abscesses. Intensivists are often confronted with complex treatment decisions, such as the indication and timing of cardiac surgery and the management of hemodynamic and neurologic complications. Therefore, treatment of patients with complicated infectious endocarditis requires close cooperation between intensivists, infectious disease specialists, cardiologists, and cardiac surgeons. This chapter focuses on the changing epidemiology and progress made during the past 2 decades in the diagnosis and management of complicated infectious endocarditis.

Pathophysiology

Infectious endocarditis is a microbial infection of the endocardial surface of the heart. The process is initiated by bloodborne microorganisms that adhere directly to the endothelium or by nonbacterial thrombotic endocarditis. The most important factors facilitating nonbacterial thrombotic endocarditis are organic valvular lesions, with associated perturbation of blood flow, and prosthetic valves. Circulating microorganisms can adhere to microscopic lesions, which explains why some patients with infectious endocarditis have no previously known valvular abnormality.[1]

In simple infectious endocarditis, infection is limited to the valve cusps or leaflets and chordae and consists of vegetations (Figure 87-1) which are formed by pathogens, platelets, fibrin, and inflammatory cells. In advanced infectious endocarditis, deep tissue invasion results in the destruction or invasion of valvular and perivalvular structures. The infection may spread as cellulitis, with the formation of an abscess or pseudoaneurysm that can rupture to another heart chamber or even the pericardium.

In prosthetic valve endocarditis (PVE), lesions may differ according to the type of prosthesis. With biological prostheses or homografts, the infection may be limited to cusps, whereas with mechanical prostheses, involvement of the sewing ring and the valve annulus is the rule. Bacterial adherence to the prosthesis results from a complex relationship among the biomaterial, plasma proteins (e.g., fibronectin, laminin, thrombospondin, fibrinogen), and bacterial adhesion proteins. Staphylococci express numerous surface factors: clumping factors A and B, which promote their adhesion to fibrinogen and fibrin, and fibronectin-binding proteins A and B, which permit adhesion to fibronectin.[2] In addition, once staphylococci have escaped the microbicidal effects of platelet peptides, they can bind to the platelet surface by a series of pathogenetic steps including direct binding to the platelet surface, up-regulation of platelet surface receptors for fibrinogen, and interaction between specific bacterial proteins and platelet surface receptors. Surface charge modifications are associated with increased in vitro resistance profiles of *Staphylococcus aureus* to a number of endogenous cationic antimicrobial peptides such as α-defensins.[3,4]

Incidence and Classification

The incidence of infective endocarditis ranges from one country to another within 3 to 10 episodes/100,000 person-years. This may reflect methodological differences between surveys rather than true variations.[5] The overall annual incidence of infectious endocarditis in Europe and the United States is between 15 and 60 cases per million. In a study conducted in France, the crude annual incidence of infectious endocarditis was 30 (95% confidence interval [CI], 27 to 33) per million inhabitants.[1] Infectious endocarditis can be classified into three groups that differ markedly in terms of incidence, clinical presentation, microbiological features, and outcome: left-sided native valve, right-sided native valve, and PVE.

Left-sided native valve infectious endocarditis traditionally occurs in patients with underlying heart disease but may affect patients with no known valvular disease, especially when endocarditis is caused by highly virulent bacteria such as *S. aureus* or *Streptococcus pneumoniae*. Most infections are community acquired, but nosocomial cases are becoming more common.

Right-sided native valve infectious endocarditis is usually associated with intravenous (IV) drug use and still accounts for 10% of all infectious endocarditis episodes.[6] Nosocomial cases are frequently a consequence of catheter-related infections. In most cases of pacemaker and implantable cardioverter-defibrillator infectious endocarditis, vegetations are located only on leads, but tricuspid valve involvement may also occur.[7]

Prosthetic valve endocarditis occurs in 1% to 6% of patients with valve prosthesis, with an incidence of 0.3% to 1.2% per patient year.[4] It accounted for 21% of 2781 patients with definite infective endocarditis in the ICE Prospective Cohort Study[6] (ICE-PCS). Early PVE is classically defined as occurring within 1 year of surgery, and late PVE beyond 1 year, because of significant differences between the microbiological profiles observed before (usually nosocomial origin) and after this time point (predominance of community-acquired pathogens).[8] However, a recent large prospective multicenter international registry found that 37% of all PVE was associated with nosocomial infection or non-nosocomial healthcare-associated infections in outpatients with extensive healthcare contact.[9]

Demographics and Etiologic Profiles

CLASSIC AND CHANGING PATIENT CHARACTERISTICS

The demographic characteristics of patients who develop infectious endocarditis have changed over the last few decades. Today, patients tend to be older, and their underlying diseases have changed.[10,11] In ICE-PCS, 38% of all definite infectious endocarditis occurred in patients older than 65 years.[11] In developing countries, rheumatic heart disease remains the most frequent underlying cardiac condition predisposing patients to infectious endocarditis. In contrast, in the United States and Western Europe, nonrheumatic heart abnormalities, including mitral valve prolapse, aortic valve calcification, aortic bicuspid valve, and hypertrophic obstructive cardiomyopathy, are the main risk factors. For patients with mitral valve prolapse, risk factors include mitral regurgitation and thickened mitral leaflet. However, results of a 1-year survey of infectious endocarditis in France showed a significantly lower incidence of known underlying heart disease between 1991 and 1999. Nowadays, congenital heart diseases are rarely involved, except bicuspid aortic valve. Other conditions including diabetes mellitus, long-term hemodialysis, and immunosuppression are associated with a higher incidence of infectious endocarditis. At Duke University Medical Center, rates of hemodialysis dependence and

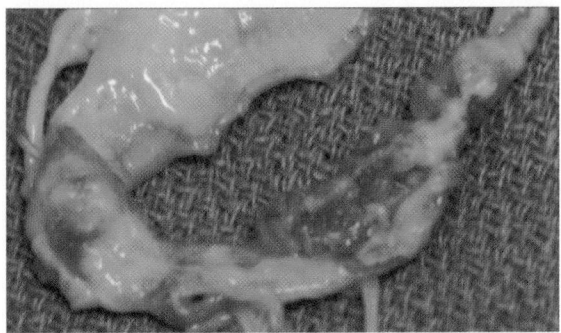

Figure 87-1 Vegetations on native mitral valve in a patient with streptococcal endocarditis.

immunosuppression among 329 patients with infectious endocarditis rose significantly between 1993 and 1999.[12] Moreover, a recent study showed that more than one third of cases of native valve endocarditis in non–injection drug users involve contact with health care. Such episodes of endocarditis maybe nosocomial if they occur in a patient hospitalized for more than 48 hours before the onset of signs or symptoms consistent with infective endocarditis. A higher proportion of non-nosocomial healthcare-associated endocarditis is now observed in patients with extensive out-of-hospital contact with healthcare interventions or systems (wound care, receipt of hemodialysis or IV chemotherapy, residence in a nursing home or long-term care facility).[13]

CAUSATIVE ORGANISMS

Overall Distribution

Most Frequently Isolated Pathogens. Streptococci are traditionally the most common causative agent of infectious endocarditis, but the results of the ICE-PCS show that streptococci had fallen into second place to staphylococci as the leading cause.[6] However, this apparent temporal shift from predominantly streptococcal to predominantly staphylococcal infective endocarditis may be partly due to recruitment/referral bias in specialized centers, since this trend is not evident in population-based epidemiologic surveys of infective endocarditis.[14] *Streptococcus* species (mainly *Streptococcus mitis, Streptococcus sanguis, Streptococcus mutans*), which abound in the mouth and nasopharynx, are associated with dental procedures and diseases. Poor dental hygiene and minor or unrecognized periodontal disease may be the source of *Streptococcus viridans* infectious endocarditis. *Streptococcus gallolyticus* (previously *S. bovis*) may be involved in valve infection of dental or buccal origin. In addition, the association of *S. gallolyticus* with carcinoma or other lesions of the colon (e.g., diverticulitis, polyps) is well known. Beta-hemolytic streptococci (groups A, B, C, and G) and *Streptococcus milleri* are isolated from 6% of patients with infectious endocarditis,[1] with the predominant species being group B. The majority of nonpregnant patients with group B streptococcal infectious endocarditis have an underlying condition such as diabetes mellitus, breast cancer, decubitus ulcer, or cirrhosis.[15]

Enterococci, mainly *Enterococcus faecalis* and *Enterococcus faecium*, account for only 10% of cases of infectious endocarditis.[6] These pathogens affect older patients, as demonstrated by a description of 93 episodes of enterococcal infectious endocarditis occurring in patients with a mean age of 74 years.[16] The portals of entry are the gastrointestinal and urogenital tracts through a lesion or a procedure (e.g., injection sclerosis of esophageal varices, transurethral prostate resection, urethral dilatation) resulting in transient bacteremia, in which case the infection is healthcare associated.

Staphylococcus aureus is now implicated in approximately 30% of all cases of left-sided native valve infectious endocarditis,[6] in 23% of PVE,[9] and is the most common cause of healthcare-associated infections.[15] *S. aureus* is also the causative agent in most acute infections, with about half of patients having no previously known heart disease.

A clinically identifiable focus of infection (e.g., carbuncle, cellulitis, bursitis, ulcer, burn, osteomyelitis) may be present. However, in 50% to 60% of cases, no obvious portal of entry is detected, although the skin is probably the source in many of them. The relationship between *S. aureus* nasal carriage and infection has been established in specific subsets of patients, especially in IV drug users and patients with diabetes mellitus or on hemodialysis.[12] Methicillin-resistant strains are isolated in healthcare-associated endocarditis, although rare cases of community-acquired methicillin-resistant endocarditis have been reported.

Coagulase-negative staphylococci (CoNS), in a recent international study, were found to cause 16% of 537 cases of definite noninjecting drug use–associated PVE. Nearly 50% of patients with CoNS PVE presented between 60 days and 365 days of valve implantation. Methicillin resistance was present in 68% of CoNS strains.[17] CoNS are also a well-documented, albeit rather rare, cause of native valve infectious endocarditis. Most patients have documented valvular abnormalities, especially mitral valve prolapse. A substantial subset of CoNS infective endocarditis has been identified as being due to *Staphylococcus lugdunensis*, which causes destructive cardiac lesions; its differentiation from other CoNS species in the laboratory may be difficult.

Overall, staphylococci, streptococci, and enterococci account for more than 80% of microorganisms responsible for infective endocarditis.

Infrequent Pathogens. Enterobacteriaceae and HACEK Group. Despite the high frequency of Enterobacteriaceae bacteremia leading to severe sepsis or septic shock, infectious endocarditis caused by these pathogens is extremely uncommon, probably because gram-negative bacilli adhere less avidly to the endothelium than gram-positive cocci do. Most cases of native valve infectious endocarditis develop in patients with severe comorbidities, including cirrhosis or immunosuppression.[18] Gram-negative bacilli are usually encountered in early and late PVE, but they account only for 2% of the cases. Bacteria of the HACEK group (fastidious organisms) originate from the oropharyngeal or urogenital flora and include *Haemophilus aphrophilus* or *paraphrophilus* (H), *Actinobacillus actinomycetemcomitans* (A), *Cardiobacterium hominis* (C), *Eikenella corrodens* (E), and *Kingella* species (K). These HACEK pathogens are implicated in 2% of cases of infectious endocarditis on either native or prosthetic valves.[6]

Streptococcus pneumoniae infectious endocarditis occurs more commonly in alcoholics, but other patients, such as those with diabetes, malignancy, or chronic obstructive pulmonary disease, may be affected. Approximately 65% to 80% of patients have no known predisposing cardiopathy. The primary infection focus is the lungs, and meningitis is present in 40% to 60% of cases.[19]

Fungi are a rare cause of infective endocarditis, being isolated in 2% of cases but in 4% of those patients with prosthetic valve infection. Although injection drug use was traditionally an important risk factor, a recent study showed that patients with *Candida* infective endocarditis were more likely to have a prosthetic valve, short-term indwelling catheters, and healthcare-associated infections.[20] Other fungi such as *Aspergillus* spp. are even less frequently encountered. Fungi are frequently responsible for mural endocarditis.

Patients with Negative Blood Cultures. Five main points should be emphasized: (1) *Abiotrophia* spp. (previously classified as nutritionally variant streptococci) are the main cause of culture-negative infectious endocarditis in patients who have recently received antibiotics. (2) Only 5% to 7% of patients who have not recently taken antibiotics have negative blood cultures. Polymerase chain reaction (in blood, excised vegetation, or systemic emboli) can be used to identify the causative organism, such as *Bartonella* spp., *Tropheryma whippelii*, or *Coxiella burnetii*, but also streptococci or other pathogens not isolated from blood cultures.[21] (3) Serologic tests are useful to diagnose infectious endocarditis caused by those organisms or by *Brucella* and *Legionella* species. (4) HACEK organisms may require prolonged incubation and subculturing. (5) *Candida* (but not *Aspergillus)* spp. are usually isolated

TABLE 87-1	Causative Agents of Left-Sided Native Valve Infectious Endocarditis	
Microorganisms	ICE-PCE (2781 patients)[6] Number (%)	Bichat-Claude Bernard ICUs (120 patients): Number* (%)[22]
Streptococci	810 (29)	42 (35)
Staphylococcus aureus	869 (31)	48 (40)
Enterococci	283 (10)	4 (3)
CoNS	304 (11)	2 (1)
Streptococcus pneumoniae	NR	5 (4)
HACEK	44 (2)	NR
Fungi	45 (2)	4 (3)
Other	121 (4)	9 (7)
Negative blood cultures	277 (10)	10 (8)

*The number of microorganisms exceeds the number of patients because some cases were polymicrobial.

CoNS, coagulase-negative staphylococci; HACEK, *Haemophilus aphrophilus* or *paraphrophilus, Actinobacillus actinomycetemcomitans, Cardiobacterium hominis, Eikenella corrodens,* and *Kingella* species; NR, not reported.

from routine blood cultures, but in some cases, fungi are recovered only from excised vegetations or peripheral emboli.

Specific Microbiologic Characteristics of Infectious Endocarditis in ICU Patients

The microbiological characteristics of infectious endocarditis in patients who require ICU admission differ from those in the overall population. Analysis of a large series of infectious endocarditis patients hospitalized in two medical ICUs in a Parisian teaching hospital between 1994 and 2001 showed that *S. aureus* was the leading pathogen responsible for left-sided native valve and PVE[22] (Tables 87-1 and 87-2). Those figures were confirmed by an Austrian study of 33 ICU patients with infectious endocarditis: *S. aureus* was isolated from 36% of them, versus 15% *S. viridans* and 12% enterococci.[23] In a French multicenter study, *S. aureus* accounted for 46% of 198 critically ill patients with definite endocarditis according to Duke criteria (see later discussion).[24] Clearly these findings are largely explained by *S. aureus* causing valve destruction, septic shock, and emboli to vital organs such as brain.

Clinical Characteristics and Diagnosis

In 1994, a new set of diagnostic criteria for the diagnosis of infectious endocarditis, including two major and six minor criteria—known as the *Duke criteria*—was proposed. Modifications of these criteria were proposed in 2000 to take into account transesophageal echocardiography and to consider all *S. aureus* bacteremias and positive Q fever serology as major criteria.[25]

CLINICAL CHARACTERISTICS

In ICU patients, the clinical presentation of infectious endocarditis often includes extracardiac manifestations or findings associated with cardiac complications. Patients are generally referred to the ICU for cardiogenic or septic shock, pulmonary edema caused by valvular or prosthetic dysfunction, neurologic events, acute renal failure, or respiratory failure in the setting of pulmonary emboli complicating right-sided infectious endocarditis. Two salient features, usually associated with high-grade fever, strongly suggest the diagnosis of infectious endocarditis: (1) a heart murmur (most commonly preexisting) or a prosthetic valve and (2) petechiae on the skin (especially the extremities; Figure 87-2) and conjunctivae. A typical ICU candidate has an acute febrile and toxic illness with heart murmur, petechiae, and meningeal signs. Cerebrospinal fluid examination finds pleocytosis and gram-positive cocci. Blood cultures yield *S. aureus*, and echocardiography confirms left-sided infectious endocarditis. In patients with catheter-related bacteremia, the diagnosis of infective endocarditis may be suggested by persistent positive blood cultures 3 to 5 days after the onset of antimicrobial treatment and removal of the catheter.

ECHOCARDIOGRAPHY

Echocardiography has the following objectives: (1) to detect vegetations and determine their size, (2) to diagnose paravalvular extension of the infection, (3) to evaluate myocardial function, (4) to detect pericardial effusion, and (5) if cardiac surgery is being considered, to measure the valve ring to choose the appropriate prosthetic valve for replacement. Transthoracic echocardiography is rapidly obtained and noninvasive, but its overall sensitivity is only 40% to 65%. False-negative results are obtained when the examination is inadequate (especially in those with obesity or chronic obstructive pulmonary disease) or when vegetations are less than 5 mm. Transesophageal echocardiography associated with color Doppler techniques is more

TABLE 87-2	Causative Agents of Prosthetic Valve Endocarditis (PVE)	
Microorganisms	Early PVE (n = 51) Number (%)	Late PVE (n = 331) Number (%)
Staphylococcus aureus	19 (37)	61 (18)
Coagulase-negative staphylococci	9 (17.5)	66 (20)
Streptococcus viridans	1 (2)	34 (10)
Streptococcus bovis	1 (2)	22 (7)
Other streptococci	0	11 (3)
Enterococci	4 (8)	42 (13)
Streptococcus pneumoniae	0	3 (1)
Propionibacterium	0	5 (1.5)
HACEK	0	7 (2)
Enterobacteriaceae	2 (4)	3 (1)
Pseudomonas aeruginosa	1 (2)	1 (0.3)
Fungi	5 (10)	11 (3)
Other	0	5 (1.5)*
Culture negative	9 (17.5)	41 (12)

Adapted from Wang A, Athan E, Pappas PA, et al. Contemporary clinical profile and outcome of prosthetic valve endocarditis. JAMA 2007;297:1354-61.

*Other: *Listeria monocytogenes*, 2; *Micromonas*, 2; *Mycobacterium* spp., 1.

HACEK, *Haemophilus aphrophilus* or *H. paraphrophilus, Actinobacillus actinomycetemcomitans, Cardiobacterium hominis, Eikenella corrodens,* and *Kingella* species.

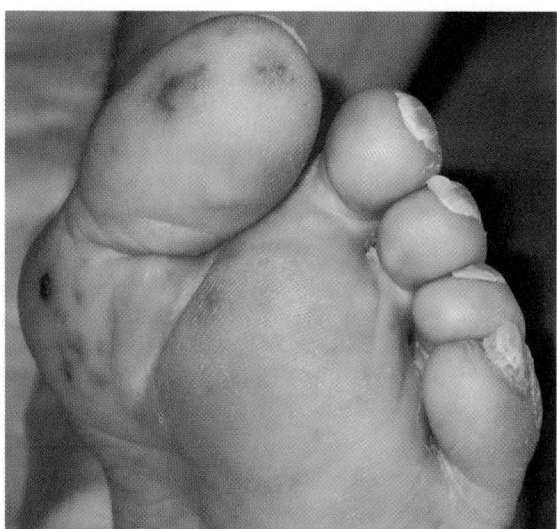

Figure 87-2 Typical purpuric lesions in a patient with *Staphylococcus aureus* mitral valve endocarditis.

invasive, but its sensitivity for detecting vegetations is 90% to 100%.[5] Transesophageal echocardiography is particularly useful in patients with suspected valve perforation or extension of perivalvular infectious endocarditis and in those with PVE. Its sensitivity and specificity for the detection of cardiac abscess are 80% and 95%, respectively. This technique is necessary for all patients undergoing valve surgery and may be repeated at close intervals to help the physician decide when to operate. However, transesophageal echocardiography should be used cautiously in nonintubated critically ill patients with respiratory failure. Follow-up echocardiography to monitor complications and response to treatment is mandatory.[5]

Complications

Cardiac complications and hemodynamic failure, central nervous system (CNS) complications, and acute renal failure are the leading causes of ICU admission for patients with infectious endocarditis. Other complications are not addressed in detail.

CARDIAC COMPLICATIONS AND HEMODYNAMIC FAILURE

Congestive heart failure (CHF) is usually caused by infection-induced valvular damage or prosthesis dysfunction. CHF is observed in 50% to 60% of cases overall and is more frequently associated with aortic than mitral disease. CHF caused by aortic failure may require urgent valve replacement. Perivalvular extension of infectious endocarditis is frequently associated with CHF, and spread into the septum may lead to heart block. Erosion of a mycotic aneurysm of the sinus of Valsalva can cause hemopericardium and tamponade or can create fistulas to the right or left ventricle. Myocardial infarction due to coronary artery embolization is a rare event. Hemodynamic failure can also be caused by septic shock, especially during the bacteremic phase of *S. aureus* infectious endocarditis.[22] All these complications may require the administration of positive inotropes or vasoconstrictors and the use of mechanical ventilation before valve replacement.

NEUROLOGIC COMPLICATIONS

CNS complications of infectious endocarditis occur frequently. They may be the first or predominant manifestation of the disease and can arise through several mechanisms. CNS complications are a leading cause of death due to infectious endocarditis, and their specific management may be complex.

Frequency, Microbiology, and Timing

In most series, CNS involvement during the course of infectious endocarditis occurs in 20% to 40% of cases. Among 1329 episodes of infectious endocarditis from seven series described between 1985 and 1993, 437 (33%) were accompanied by CNS manifestations.[26] In a Finnish teaching hospital, 55 of 218 infectious endocarditis (25%) were associated with neurologic complications.[27] However, two other studies reported lower rates: in France, strokes occurred in 17% of 264 infectious endocarditis cases caused by staphylococci or streptococci[1]; in the United States, among 513 episodes of complicated, left-sided, native valve infectious endocarditis, focal neurologic signs or altered mental status were observed in 18% and 16% of cases, respectively.[10] Experience from the large, contemporary, and multinational ICE-PCS study reported a similar (17%) incidence of strokes.[6] The use of sensitive methods of detection such as magnetic resonance imaging (MRI) indicates that silent cerebral complications are frequent. Among 60 patients who experienced episodes of left-sided infective endocarditis, 35% had a symptomatic neurologic event, while silent cerebral complications were detected in another 30%.[28] In a recently published study involving 127 patients with definite endocarditis who underwent systematic MRI, cerebral lesions were detected in 106, most being asymptomatic.[29] Not surprisingly, the incidence of symptomatic neurologic complications is much higher in the subset of patients with infective

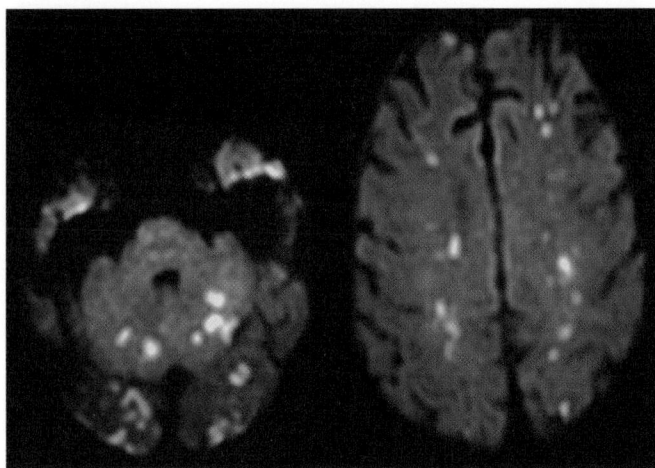

Figure 87-3   T2-weighted magnetic resonance imaging sequence performed at the acute phase of aortic valve *Staphylococcus aureus* endocarditis, showing multiple ischemic cerebral lesions.

endocarditis requiring admission to the ICU. A multicenter study showed a 55% incidence of symptomatic neurologic events among 198 critically ill patients with left-sided endocarditis.[24] Neurologic complications are a hallmark of left-sided abnormalities of either native or prosthetic valves. When neurologic complication rates were assessed as a function of the causative agent, the frequency of CNS involvement was two to three times higher with *S. aureus* than with other pathogens.[27]

Most neurologic complications are already evident at the time of hospitalization or develop within a few days. The probability of developing these complications decreases rapidly once antimicrobial therapy has been started. In the ICE-PCS study, the crude incidence of stroke in patients receiving appropriate antimicrobial therapy was 4.82/1000 patient days in the first week of therapy and fell to 1.71/1000 patient days in the second week. This rate continued to decline with further therapy.[30] Moreover, recurrent neurologic events, although possible even late, are uncommon.

Pathogenesis and Distribution

Neurologic complications of infectious endocarditis can arise through various mechanisms, but the major mechanism is cerebral embolization. Cerebral emboli (Figure 87-3) result from dislodgment or fragmentation of cardiac vegetations, followed by vessel occlusion; this results in various degrees of ischemia and infarction, depending on the vessels and the collateral blood flow. Occlusion of cerebral arteries, with either stroke or transient ischemic attack, accounts for 40% to 50% of the CNS complications of infectious endocarditis.[26-27] Cerebral hemorrhage may be the consequence of different mechanisms, each of which accounts for one-third of bleeding complications: rupture of an intracranial aneurysm; septic erosion of the arterial wall, without a well-delineated aneurysm (acute necrotizing arteritis); or hemorrhagic transformation of ischemic brain infarcts, especially in anticoagulated patients. Overall, intracranial hemorrhage represents 10% of CNS complications. Brain hemorrhage is more frequent during the bacteremic phase of *S. aureus* infectious endocarditis and is made more likely by severe thrombopenia and anticoagulant therapy.[22] A case-control study using diffusion-weighted MRI (Figure 87-4) has revealed that cerebral microbleeds were observed in 57% of patients with in infective endocarditis compared to 15% of control subjects.[31] Meningitis, occurring in 5% to 40% of patients with CNS manifestations of infectious endocarditis, can be the consequence of a wide variety of mechanisms; the cerebrospinal fluid may be purulent with positive cultures, clear with moderate pleocytosis, or hemorrhagic. Brain abscesses associated with infectious endocarditis are uncommon; they account for less than 5% of CNS events, but the rate depends on the

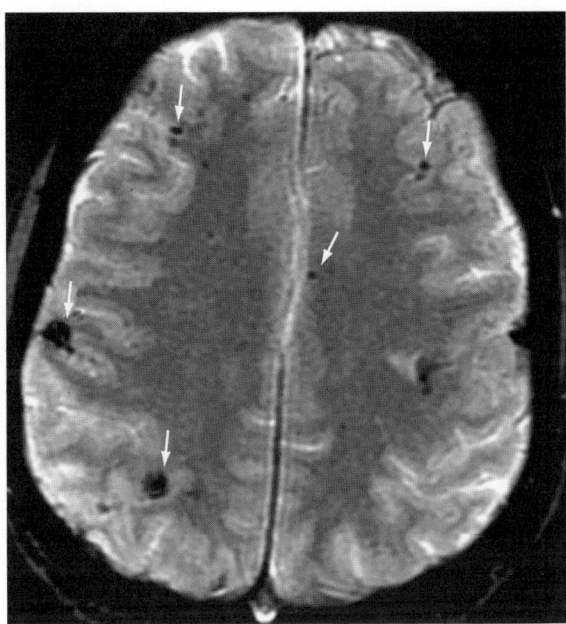

Figure 87-4 T2-weighted magnetic resonance imaging sequence performed at the acute phase of definite mitral valve *Staphylococcus aureus* endocarditis, showing multiple cerebral microbleeds *(arrows)*.

imaging technique used. In addition, many small abscesses or areas of cerebritis resolve with antibiotics alone. Finally, *toxic encephalopathy*, defined as mental changes or stupor without focal neurologic manifestations and without computed tomographic (CT) abnormalities, is often included among the CNS complications of infectious endocarditis. Obviously this manifestation can have different causes, such as subtle cerebral lesions, or may be present in the setting of severe sepsis.[24]

Specific Management

Infectious endocarditis occurring in patients receiving anticoagulant therapy poses a difficult problem. In the absence of CNS complications or in patients with nonhemorrhagic neurologic lesions, warfarin should be discontinued and replaced by heparin. However, in the presence of brain hemorrhage, anticoagulant therapy should be temporarily discontinued. CT scanning is essential for the diagnosis and management of CNS events associated with infectious endocarditis. In addition, it may be the only technique available for unstable ICU patients, especially those on mechanical ventilation. CT may show intracranial bleeding, ischemic lesions, or a pattern consistent with cerebral abscess. MRI is more sensitive for most lesions and should be performed in hemodynamically stable patients, because it can modify clinical management.[29] Although conventional four-vessel angiography remains the gold standard for the evaluation of mycotic aneurysms, magnetic resonance angiography is a promising technique. In the absence of randomized trials, which are difficult (if not impossible) to organize, the respective roles of medical, endovascular, and neurosurgical treatment of intracranial aneurysms are not easily assessable. Endovascular treatment (coil embolization) seems to be a reliable and safe technique that should be considered when cerebral mycotic aneurysms are diagnosed.[32]

ACUTE RENAL FAILURE

Acute renal failure occurs in up to 40% of complicated infectious endocarditis cases necessitating ICU admission[2,23] and may result from several mechanisms. It is often the consequence of cardiogenic or septic shock (with or without multiorgan failure) leading to acute tubular necrosis. Drugs, such as the combination of a glycopeptide and an aminoglycoside, and the use of iodine contrast medium for radiologic investigations may further deteriorate renal function. In some patients with streptococcal or staphylococcal infectious endocarditis, acute renal failure is caused by severe glomerulonephritis. Acute renal failure may require the initiation of dialysis.

OTHER COMPLICATIONS

Systemic embolism can involve many organs such as the spleen and kidneys; rarely, the liver or the iliac, mesenteric, or peripheral arteries are involved. Splenic abscesses are caused mainly by *S. aureus* or *S. viridans*. Abdominal CT is the best procedure to detect splenic abscesses, which may require percutaneous drainage or splenectomy. Pulmonary emboli, the hallmark of right-sided endocarditis, may be responsible for respiratory failure or even acute respiratory distress syndrome, especially in IV drug users with *S. aureus* infectious endocarditis.

Medical and Surgical Treatment

In the absence of large prospective randomized studies, which present a considerable challenge, the overall strategy for infectious endocarditis treatment is derived mainly from retrospective series, clinical judgment, and expert recommendations.

ANTIBIOTIC TREATMENT

Certain general principles underlie the current guidelines[5,33] for infectious endocarditis treatment. In cases of streptococcal infectious endocarditis, determination of the minimal inhibitory concentration of penicillin is necessary to choose the best regimen. Parenteral antibiotics are recommended over oral drugs because of the importance of sustained antibacterial activity, which requires high dosages (e.g., 150 to 200 mg/kg of amoxicillin for streptococcal infectious endocarditis). However, oral antibiotics may be considered for right-sided *S. aureus* infectious endocarditis after a few days of parenteral antibiotics when IV administration is not possible because of poor venous access. In that case, a combination of a fluoroquinolone and rifampin is an acceptable regimen. Many experts recommend using a combination of agents with activities against the cell wall (β-lactams or glycopeptides) plus an aminoglycoside (gentamicin) for most cases of infectious endocarditis, especially complicated cases such as those in ICU patients. Gentamicin can be administered in one or two daily doses, except for infective endocarditis due to enterococci, for which two doses are recommended. The use and duration of aminoglycosides depend on the pathogen and, for streptococci, their susceptibility to penicillin G and the presence of a prosthesis (Table 87-3). Although a shorter course of aminoglycosides has been proposed for enterococcal infectious endocarditis,[16] no controlled study has confirmed the safety of this strategy. For staphylococcal infectious endocarditis, a triple regimen including rifampin is recommended,[34] especially for patients with PVE. Short-term therapy (15 days) was shown to be effective in selected cases of uncomplicated *S. aureus* right-sided infectious endocarditis or left-sided native valve infectious endocarditis due to highly susceptible streptococci. However, most current recommendations emphasize prolonged antibiotic administration (4-6 weeks or even 8 weeks) for *S. aureus* PVE. Valve cultures, but not positive Gram staining or positive PCR, should be taken into account to decide how long to continue antimicrobial therapy after valve replacement.[5]

The role of new molecules in the treatment of infective endocarditis remains to be evaluated. Daptomycin is a bactericidal lipopeptide which can be used in methicillin-resistant *S. aureus*[35] and vancomycin-resistant enterococci infective endocarditis[36]

SURGICAL MANAGEMENT

In recent series,[6,9] 48% to 50% of patients (up to 75% in specialized medical-surgical centers) undergo valve replacement during the acute

TABLE 87-3	Antibiotic Treatment of Complicated Infectious Endocarditis as a Function of Valve Type, Pathogen, and Susceptibility	
Microorganism	*Native Valve Infectious Endocarditis*	*Prosthetic Valve Endocarditis*
Penicillin-susceptible streptococci (MIC < 0.125 mg/L)	Penicillin G, amoxicillin, or ceftriaxone for 4 wk*	Penicillin G or amoxicillin for 6 wk + gentamicin for 2 wk*
Relatively penicillin-resistant streptococci (MIC ≥ 0.125-2 mg/L)	Penicillin G or amoxicillin for 4 wk + gentamicin for 2 wk*	Penicillin G or amoxicillin for 4-6 wk + gentamicin for 4 wk*
Streptococci with penicillin G MIC > 2 mg/L, enterococci, and *Abiotrophia* spp.	Penicillin G or amoxicillin for 4-6 wk + gentamicin for 4 wk*	Penicillin G or amoxicillin for 6 wk + gentamicin for 6 wk*
MSSA	Nafcillin or oxacillin for 4-6 wk + gentamicin for 3-5 days[†]	Nafcillin or oxacillin + rifampin for ≥ 6 wk + gentamicin for 2 wk[†]
MRSA	Vancomycin + rifampin for 4-6 wk + gentamicin for 3-5 days	Vancomycin + rifampin for ≥ 6 wk + gentamicin for 2 wk
HACEK organisms	Ceftriaxone or cefotaxime for 4 wk	Ceftriaxone or cefotaxime for 6 wk
Enterobacteriaceae	Ceftriaxone or cefotaxime for 4 wk + gentamicin or amikacin for 1 wk[‡]	Ceftriaxone or cefotaxime for 6 wk + gentamicin or amikacin for 2 wk[‡]
Bartonella spp.	Ceftriaxone or doxycycline for 6 wk + gentamicin for 2-3 wk	Ceftriaxone or doxycycline for 6 wk + gentamicin for 2-3 wk
Coxiella burnetii	Doxycycline or ofloxacin + hydroxychloroquine for ≥ 18mo	Doxycycline or ofloxacin + hydroxychloroquine for ≥ 18mo
Candida spp.	LF AmB[§] with or without 5-FC[§§] or AmB with or without 5-FC or an echinocandin for 2 wk, then fluconazole for susceptible organism in stable patient with negative blood culture results for 4 wk	LF AmB[§] with or without 5-FC[§§] or AmB with or without 5-FC or an echinocandin for 2 wk, then fluconazole for susceptible organism in stable patient with negative blood culture results for 4 wk Lifelong suppressive therapy for prosthetic valve endocarditis if valve cannot be replaced is recommended.

*Vancomycin or teicoplanin therapy is indicated for patients who are allergic to β-lactam antibiotics. Optimal antimicrobial therapy is not available for high-level aminoglycoside-resistant and vancomycin-resistant enterococci. Eradicating these pathogens requires consultation with an infectious disease specialist or a microbiologist.

[†]A first-generation cephalosporin is indicated for patients who are allergic to penicillin, except for those with immediate-type hypersensitivity reactions to β-lactam antibiotics, who should be treated with a glycopeptide.

[‡]The results of susceptibility tests might indicate the need to adapt the initial regimen.

[§]Lipid formulation of amphotericin B.

[§§]5-Fluorocytosine.

HACEK, *Haemophilus aphrophilus* or *paraphrophilus*, *Actinobacillus actinomycetemcomitans*, *Cardiobacterium hominis*, *Eikenella corrodens*, and *Kingella* species; MIC, minimal inhibitory concentration; MRSA, methicillin-resistant *Staphylococcus aureus*; MSSA, methicillin-susceptible *S. aureus*.

phase of infectious endocarditis before the completion of antibiotic treatment.

Indications for and Timing of Cardiac Surgery

Absolute indications are CHF caused by valvular insufficiency, prosthesis obstruction or dehiscence, periannular abscess, or *S. aureus* or fungal PVE. These microorganisms cannot be eradicated without removal of the prosthesis. Development of CHF in the setting of infectious endocarditis generally requires cardiac valve replacement regardless of the number of days on antibiotics. Emergency cardiac surgery is recommended for the following situations: (1) aortic or mitral infective endocarditis with severe acute regurgitation or valve obstruction, causing refractory pulmonary edema or cardiogenic shock and (2) aortic or mitral infective endocarditis with fistula into a cardiac chamber or pericardium, causing pulmonary edema or shock.[5]

Relative indications requiring case-by-case evaluation are persistent bacteremia beyond 7 days despite appropriate antibiotic therapy, non–*S. aureus* PVE, and difficult-to-treat organisms such as *C. burnetii*, *Bartonella* spp., multiresistant enterococci, or *P. aeruginosa*, especially in patients with PVE.

With regard to other potential indications, contraindications, and timing of valve replacement, the following factors should be emphasized: (1) Although the risk of systemic embolization is higher in patients with large vegetations on the mitral valve, vegetation characteristics alone rarely justify valve surgery. The decreasing risk of emboli with time, especially after the first week of effective antibiotic therapy, should be considered when deciding whether to operate.[30] (2) In patients with neurologic complications, a conservative approach is to delay cardiac surgery for 2 or 3 weeks after an embolic event and for at least a month after cerebral bleeding. However, in the case of CHF, the valve can be replaced within 7 days or less after an embolic infarct, especially when it is of limited size and the patient's good mental status prevails.[5] (3) In that case, there is a high probability of complete neurologic recovery.[37] True contraindications of valve surgery are rare and

include uncontrolled septic shock, unhealed sternal wound infection, and severe coagulation disorders.

Coronary angiography is recommended for patients older than 40 years and those with at least one risk factor, except when emergency surgery is needed.[5]

Surgical Technique

Surgery includes complete removal of all infected and necrotic tissue, followed by valve reconstruction. In selected cases, good results have been achieved with conservative mitral valve valvuloplasty. In most patients, valve replacement with a mechanical or biological prosthesis or a homograft is necessary. The use of cryopreserved homografts has been suggested to reduce the risk of persistent or recurrent infection. However, mechanical prostheses and xenografts compare favorably, with improved durability.[38]

Outcome and Prognostic Factors

The overall in-hospital mortality was 18% in the large, contemporary, and multinational ICE-PCE study.[6] This figure includes all types of infectious endocarditis, however, and warrants refinement according to different categories of disease. Another recent cohort of 513 patients with complicated left-sided native valve infectious endocarditis had a 6-month mortality rate of 26%.[10] Two studies found mortality rates for PVE of 33% and 22%, respectively.[9,36] In the international ICE collaborative study, healthcare-associated native valve endocarditis was associated with higher in-hospital mortality (25%) compared to community-acquired endocarditis (13%).[13] Survival of ICU patients with infective endocarditis is lower. Among 228 patients with infectious endocarditis referred to the two ICUs in our hospital, the in-hospital mortality rate was 45%.[22] It was 42% in a multicenter study involving 198 critically ill patients with infective endocarditis.[24]

Prognostic factors of survival have been studied by several authors. In most cases, these reflect the site of infectious endocarditis (see earlier discussion), comorbidities, causative agent, and type of complications. CHF, septic shock, neurologic events, *S. aureus* PVE, increasing age, and paravalvular complications are associated with in-hospital mortality in most studies.[6,10,13,23,24] The hemodynamic status of the patient at the time of valve replacement is the main determinant of perioperative mortality, with a poorer prognosis for patients with pulmonary edema or impaired left ventricular function.[3,7] Neurologic events markedly increase the risk of death, which can reach 50% in patients with altered mental status.[10] Among microorganisms, *S. aureus* is associated with higher mortality rates than streptococci for left-sided native valve and PVE.[13,25,26] Finally, mounting evidence shows that for both complicated left-sided native valve infectious endocarditis and *S. aureus* PVE, valve replacement during active endocarditis combined with medical therapy is associated with a better outcome than medical treatment alone.[6,12,13,39,40] The reoperation rate, mainly for prosthesis dehiscence or new infectious endocarditis, is 2% to 3% per year, and the 5-year survival rate is approximately 80% to 90% for native valve infectious endocarditis and 60% for PVE. A scoring system taking into account mental status, comorbidity, CHF, microbiology, and the use of surgical treatment in left-sided native valve infectious endocarditis was recently published.[41]

Conclusion

Despite advances in both diagnosis and treatment, infectious endocarditis still carries high morbidity and mortality rates, especially for patients requiring ICU admission. Improvement of outcome requires a multidisciplinary approach to optimize medical treatment and decision making concerning valve surgery.

ANNOTATED REFERENCES

Heiro M, Nikoskelainen J, Engblom E, et al. Neurologic manifestations of infective endocarditis: a 17-year experience in a teaching hospital in Finland. Arch Intern Med 2000;160:2781-7.
Neurologic complications are evident before antimicrobial treatment is started in the vast majority of patients and are significantly associated with Staphylococcus aureus.
Murdoch DR, Corey R, Hoen B, et al. Clinical presentation, etiology, and outcome of infective endocarditis in the 21st century: the International Collaboration on Endocarditis–Prospective Cohort Study. Arch Intern Med 2009;169:463-73.
The results of the largest series of patients (more than 2700) with infective endocarditis included in the ICE-PCS (International Collaboration on Endocarditis–Prospective Cohort Study).
Wang A, Athan E, Pappas PA, et al. Contemporary clinical profile and outcome of prosthetic valve endocarditis. JAMA 2007;297:1354-61.
A detailed description of prosthetic valve endocarditis from the same ICE-PCS. Complications of PVE strongly predict in-hospital mortality, which remains high (23%) despite prompt diagnosis and the frequent use of cardiac surgery.
Duval X, Iung B, Klein I, et al. Effect of early cerebral magnetic resonance imaging on clinical decisions in infective endocarditis. A prospective study. Ann Intern Med 2010;152:497-504.
Cerebral lesions were identified by MRI in most patients with endocarditis, including those without neurologic symptoms. The MRI findings affected both diagnostic classifications and clinical management plans.
The Task Force on the Prevention, Diagnosis, and Treatment of Infective Endocarditis of the European Society of Cardiology (ESC). Guidelines on the prevention, diagnosis, and treatment of infective endocarditis (new version 2009). Eur Heart J 2009;30:2369-413.
The most recently available guidelines for prevention, diagnosis, and treatment of infective endocarditis.

REFERENCES

Access the complete reference list online at http://www.expertconsult.com.

Hypertensive Crisis: Emergency and Urgency

STUART L. LINAS

Hypertension is a common problem, and its incidence may be increasing in adults.[1] Population data also suggest hypertension is increasing globally; 972 million individuals worldwide now have hypertension,[1] and 30% of hypertensive individuals are unaware of their diagnosis.[2] Of the 59% of hypertensive individuals being treated for hypertension, only 34% have a blood pressure less than 140/90 mm Hg.[2] The exact risk of hypertensive crisis is not clear, but most authors estimate the risk to be less than 1%; it may be increasing.[3,4]

Hypertensive emergency is defined as an elevated blood pressure associated with evidence of acute end-organ damage. With acute damage to vital organs such as the kidney, heart, and brain, there is a significant risk of morbidity in hours without therapeutic intervention. Both the absolute level of blood pressure as well as the time course of blood pressure elevation determines the development of crisis. In general, with hypertensive crisis, the diastolic blood pressure is above 120 mm Hg. However, in children, gravid females, and previously normotensive individuals, hypertensive crises may occur with relatively minor increases in blood pressure. It is very important to identify this syndrome early to prevent end-organ damage and institute appropriate therapy as soon as the diagnosis is realized. Malignant hypertension is a specific syndrome in which a markedly elevated blood pressure is associated with hypertensive neuroretinopathy.

Individuals with *hypertensive urgency* have an elevated blood pressure (systolic blood pressure often >180 and diastolic pressure often >115 mm Hg) without evidence of acute end-organ damage. Hypertensive urgency may be associated with chronic, stable complications such as stable angina, previous myocardial infarction, chronic congestive heart failure, chronic renal failure, previous transient ischemic attacks, or previous cerebrovascular accident with no threat of an acute insult. Hypertensive urgency may also be associated with inadequately treated blood pressure or noncompliance. Complications from hypertensive urgency are not immediate. In contrast to hypertensive crisis, a more gradual blood pressure reduction over hours is recommended.

An increased blood pressure can occur in the absence of acute or chronic target organ dysfunction. When the etiology of hypertension is not identified, the blood pressure is lowered over days to weeks. However, occasionally an elevated blood pressure may result from drug use, including over-the-counter medications such pseudoephedrine and elicit substance abuse, as for example with cocaine. In these situations, the blood pressure is lowered rapidly. The focus of this chapter is hypertensive emergencies including hypertensive crisis and hypertensive urgency.

Pathophysiology of Hypertensive Crisis

The precise pathophysiology of hypertensive crisis is unknown. An abrupt increase in blood pressure is one of the initiating events in the transition from simple hypertension or normotension to hypertensive crisis. The product of cardiac output and peripheral vascular resistance determines blood pressure. The initial blood pressure increase is likely secondary to an increase in vascular resistance. Considerable evidence suggests that mechanical stress in the arteriolar wall leads to disruption of endothelial integrity.[5] With disruption of vascular integrity, diffuse

microvascular lesions develop.[6,7] Fibrinoid necrosis of the arterioles is seen in vulnerable organs and is considered the histologic hallmark of hypertensive crisis.[6,7] It is unclear whether hypertension alone causes the development to hypertensive crisis or whether other factors are necessary. For example, increases in peripheral vascular resistance result in part from activation of the renin-angiotensin-aldosterone system. Evidence suggests angiotensin II may directly injure the vascular wall by activation of genes for proinflammatory cytokines (interleukin 6) and also of nuclear factor κB.[8,9] Other vascular-toxic influences may contribute to increased peripheral vascular resistance, including hyperviscosity, immunologic factors, and other hormones including catecholamines, vasopressin, and endothelin.[10-12] The end result of these changes is a significant increase in peripheral vascular resistance, with ischemia of heart, brain, and kidneys.

In considering hypertensive crisis and treatment, the impact of blood pressure on cerebrovascular physiology is important. For example, hypertensive encephalopathy is a distinct clinical syndrome that occurs when rapidly rising central perfusion pressures exceed the ability of the central nervous system (CNS) to autoregulate. *Autoregulation* of cerebral blood flow refers to the ability of the brain to maintain a constant cerebral blood flow as the cerebral perfusion pressure varies between 60 to 150 mm Hg. In the setting of chronic hypertension, the range of autoregulation is increased from 60 to 150 mm Hg to 80 to 160 mm Hg. Autoregulation of cerebral blood flow (CBF) is a function of cerebral perfusion pressure (CPP, derived from the mean arterial pressure [MAP] minus the venous pressure) and cerebral vascular resistance, according to the following equation:

$$CBF = CPP \div CVR$$

Under normal physiologic conditions, the backflow in the cerebral venous system or venous pressure is near zero, and the arterial pressure determines the CPP. With acute brain jury, as seen with subarachnoid hemorrhage, stroke, and intracranial hemorrhage, the ability of the brain to autoregulate and maintain cerebral blood flow is impaired. Inability to autoregulate cerebral blood flow is also seen in hypertensive crisis when the MAP is greater than 140 mm Hg.

Diagnosis of Hypertensive Emergencies

MEDICAL HISTORY, PHYSICAL EXAMINATION, AND LABORATORY EVALUATION

Hypertension from any cause may enter an "emergent" phase. Although hypertensive emergency usually occurs in individuals with a history of essential hypertension, it is also is seen in individuals with secondary hypertension and in individuals with no hypertensive history, as in preeclampsia, pheochromocytoma, drug withdrawal, and acute glomerulonephritis. A medication history, including over-the-counter medications and illegal drug use, should be ascertained from every patient. Malignant hypertension is a unique clinical/pathologic syndrome that is associated with hypertensive crisis. Increases in blood pressure and target-organ damage are caused by changes in the vasculature characterized by fibrinoid necrosis and a proliferative endarteritis. Risk factors associated with the development of malignant hypertension include age between 30 and 50 years,[13] male gender,[5] African American background,[14] and smoking (increases the risk by 2.5- to 5-fold).[15]

Patients with hypertensive crisis present with a variety of symptoms. The most common is headache. It is either sudden in onset or represents a change from a usual headache pattern and is often worst in the morning. The location is generally occipital or anterior, with a steady quality. Other symptoms include visual complaints (scotoma, diplopia, hemianopsia, blindness), neurologic symptoms (focal deficits, stroke, transient ischemic attacks, confusion, somnolence), ischemic chest pain, renal symptoms (nocturia, polyuria, hematuria), back pain (aortic aneurysm), and gastrointestinal complaints (nausea, vomiting). Weight loss occurs as the high levels of circulating renin and angiotensin induce a diuresis.[16] These patients often present with intravascular volume depletion, which has strong implications for treatment.

The blood pressure is measured in both arms and also with the patient lying and standing. In hypertensive emergency, diastolic blood pressures are usually above 120 mm Hg. Pathologic processes that cause stiffening of the vascular wall can prevent vessel compression by external compression with a blood pressure cuff. This results in an artificial increase (at times extreme) in the systolic and diastolic blood pressure, or "pseudohypertension." Pseudohypertension can occur in atherosclerosis, Monckeberg's medial calcification, and metastatic calcification, as experienced in end-stage renal disease. Clues to pseudohypertension include a markedly elevated blood pressure in an individual without evidence of end-organ damage. The diagnosis is suggested by a palpable radial artery after proximal compression (Osler's maneuver).[17]

A dilated funduscopic examination should be performed on all individuals. Arteriolar thickening reflects chronic hypertension and is manifested by increased light reflex, vascular tortuosity, and arteriovenous nicking where the arterioles cross the venules. These funduscopic findings reflect chronic hypertension and have no prognostic significance with regard to hypertensive crisis. As hypertension increases in severity, there are additional findings caused by the breakdown of the blood-retina barrier, leading to retinal hemorrhage and leakage of lipids, causing hard exudates. Additional findings as the blood pressure continues to increase may include cotton-wool spots as a result of nerve ischemia and swelling of the optic nerve with papilledema.[18]

A complete cardiovascular examination should include a careful cardiac evaluation for evidence of left ventricular hypertrophy, which can occur with long-standing hypertension. Examination of the abdomen should include evaluation for a enlarged kidneys, as seen with polycystic kidney disease, as well as for evidence of aortic aneurysm. Lastly, a careful neurologic examination should be done to rule out any evidence of a cerebral vascular accident. Alterations in mental status may indicate a stroke or hypertensive encephalopathy. Symptoms of hypertensive encephalopathy include headache, visual changes, and seizures. Focal neurologic symptoms are unusual without an associated cerebral bleed. Hypertensive neuroretinopathy is usually present but may be absent in patients in whom the pressure increase has been very abrupt, such as in cases of acute glomerulonephritis or catecholamine excess states.

The initial laboratory evaluation should include a serum sodium, chloride, potassium, bicarbonate, creatinine and blood urea nitrogen, complete blood count (with a peripheral smear to identify schistocytes), prothrombin time, activated partial thromboplastin time, serum and urine toxicology screen, pregnancy test when appropriate, an electrocardiogram, and a urinalysis. Evidence of intravascular hemolysis is common and may make it difficult to differentiate hypertensive crisis from primary vasculitis with secondary hypertension.[19,20] The renin-angiotensin-aldosterone axis is markedly activated, as evidenced by hypokalemia and metabolic alkalosis.[3,21] The blood urea nitrogen and creatinine are often elevated. The urinalysis may show small amounts of proteinuria as well as hematuria with occasional erythrocyte casts.[5] Marked increases in proteinuria suggest a primary glomerular process such as glomerulonephritis as the etiology of the elevated blood pressure.

Box 88-1

DIFFERENTIAL DIAGNOSIS OF HYPERTENSIVE ENCEPHALOPATHY

Cerebral infarction
Subarachnoid hemorrhage
Intracerebral hemorrhage
Subdural or epidural hematoma
Brain tumor or other mass lesion
Seizure disorder
Central nervous system vasculitis
Encephalitis/meningitis
Drug ingestion
Drug withdrawal

If hypertensive encephalopathy is suspected, magnetic resonance imaging (MRI) should be performed. With hypertensive encephalopathy, edema may occur in the posterior regions of the cerebral hemispheres, particularly in the parieto-occipital regions, a finding called *posterior leukoencephalopathy* on MRI. However, brainstem involvement on MRI has also been reported.[22,23] It is important to consider and eliminate other conditions with a similar clinical presentation (Box 88-1). Several important diagnostic considerations help exclude other causes of altered mental status: (1) symptoms of generalized brain dysfunction tend to develop over time (12-24 hours) with hypertensive encephalopathy, as compared to acutely with ischemic stroke or cerebral hemorrhage; (2) focal neurologic findings are unusual with hypertensive encephalopathy unless there is an associated bleed; (3) papilledema is almost always noted with hypertensive encephalopathy and if absent should raise suspicion of another etiology; (4) in comparison to an acute CNS bleed, mental status with hypertensive encephalopathy improves within 24 to 48 hours of treatment.

Treatment of Hypertensive Emergency

Patients with hypertensive crisis are best treated parenterally with intensive care monitoring by arterial cannulation or automated blood pressure cuff measurement. In general, the need to lower the blood pressure and the rate at which this should occur is dictated by the clinical setting. Excessive falls in pressure should be avoided, given the potential negative impact on renal, cerebral, and coronary ischemia.

In most but not all settings, blood pressure can be reduced acutely by 20% to 25% within minutes to hours.[3] After the patient is stabilized at this pressure, the blood pressure may be further decreased to 160/100-110 mm Hg over the next 2 to 6 hours.[3] If the patient is clinically stable, the blood pressure may then be decreased toward a normal blood pressure over the next 24 to 48 hours.[3] With these decreases in blood pressure, CNS blood flow autoregulation is usually maintained. Clinical settings where additional considerations and alternative approaches to reducing blood pressure should be considered include (1) ischemic stroke where immediate reduction of blood pressure is usually not indicated except when the blood pressure is over 220/120 or the patient requires thrombolytic therapy, (2) acute aortic dissection where a rapid blood pressure reduction in 15 to 30 minutes to a systolic blood pressure under 100 mm Hg is clinically warranted if the patient tolerates, and (3) in previously normotensive subjects with abrupt increases in BP.

More rapid reduction in blood pressure is also recommended in patients with active unstable angina or congestive heart failure with pulmonary edema. Exceptions to rapid blood pressure reduction may include older patients with carotid stenosis. Older adults are particularly susceptible to CNS hypoperfusion. In addition, recent data (discussed later) suggest that significant reduction of blood pressure in older adults in the setting of ischemic stroke may not be beneficial.

Blood pressure management in patients with stroke or intracranial bleeding is controversial, since the loss of CNS blood flow autoregulation and the presence of brain edema require high systemic pressures to provide adequate cerebral perfusion.

From 40% to 50% of hypertensive crises arise in patients with pre-existing hypertension without identifiable secondary causes.[24,25] Essential hypertension is the underlying disorder in the majority of African American individuals.[26-28] In contrast, from 50% to 60% of white patients with malignant hypertension have an identifiable cause (Box 88-2). Renovascular hypertension secondary to either fibromuscular dysplasia or atherosclerosis is not uncommon. Up to 20% of cases of malignant hypertension occur in patients with underlying chronic glomerulonephritis. Other renal causes include reflex nephropathy (particularly in children) and analgesic nephropathy.[3]

Box 88-2

SYNDROMES OF HYPERTENSIVE CRISIS

Malignant hypertension
Non-malignant hypertension with target-organ disorders:
   Patient requiring emergency surgery with poorly controlled hypertension
   Hyperviscosity syndrome
   Postoperative patient
   Renal transplant patient: acute rejection, transplant renal artery stenosis
   Quadriplegic patient with autonomic hyperreflexia
   Severe burns
   Acute aortic dissection
   Intracranial hemorrhage, ischemic stroke, or subarachnoid hemorrhage
   Hypertensive encephalopathy
   Myocardial ischemia/acute left-ventricular failure
   Preeclampsia/eclampsia
   Antiphospholipid antibody syndrome
   Acute renal failure:
      Scleroderma renal crisis
      Chronic glomerulonephritis
      Reflux nephropathy
      Analgesic nephropathy
      Acute glomerulonephritis
      Radiation nephritis
      Ask-Upmark kidney
      Chronic lead intoxication
   Renovascular hypertension:
      Fibromuscular dysplasia
      Atherosclerosis
   Endocrine hypertension:
      Congenital adrenal hyperplasia
      Pheochromocytoma
      Oral contraceptives
      Aldosteronism
      Cushing's disease/syndrome
   Systemic vasculitis
   Atheroembolic renal crisis
   Drugs:
      Oral contraceptives
      Nonsteroidal antiinflammatory agents
      Atropine
      Corticosteroids
      Sympathomimetics
      Erythropoietin
      Lead intoxication
      Cyclosporine
   Catecholamine excess states:
      Pheochromocytoma
      MAO/tyramine interaction
      Antihypertensive withdrawal
      Cocaine intoxication, sympathomimetic overdose

Specific Treatment Recommendations for Hypertensive Crisis Based on Etiology

GENERAL COMMENT ON MEDICATION USED TO TREAT HYPERTENSIVE CRISIS

The classes of parenteral antihypertensive agents available to treat hypertensive crisis include direct vasodilators (sodium nitroprusside, nitroglycerin), α- and β-adrenergic blockers (labetalol), α-adrenergic blockade (phentolamine), angiotensin-converting enzyme (ACE) inhibitors (enalaprilat), calcium channel blockers (nicardipine), and dopamine agonists (fenoldopam). Some of the advantages and disadvantages of these medications are detailed in Table 88-1. There is no consensus on the most effective antihypertensive medications in the setting of a CNS insult and no large randomized trials demonstrating the superiority of a given agent. Rather, the choice of antihypertensive therapy should be individualized to the patient and clinical setting. However, most authors now caution the use of nitroprusside in the setting of increase in intracranial pressure. Vasodilators increase blood volume and therefore have the potential to increase the intracranial pressure (ICP). Animal and human studies in the setting of a normal ICP show no effect of nitroprusside on ICP.[19-21] However, in studies on animals and humans with preexisting increased ICP, nitroprusside increased the ICP, likely reflecting vasodilatation on the background of decreased cranial compliance.[29-33] When sodium nitroprusside is contraindicated, other treatment options include labetalol and nicardipine. Fenoldopam, which is an agonist of the vasodilator dopamine-1 receptor, shares with nitroprusside a rapid onset and short duration of action. In addition, fenoldopam, in contrast to nitroprusside, increases renal blood flow, induces natruresis, and produces no toxic metabolites.[34-38]

MALIGNANT HYPERTENSION

Malignant hypertension is specific syndrome characterized by markedly elevated pressures in conjunction with hypertensive neuroretinopathy. Funduscopic examination often reveals flame-shaped hemorrhages, cotton-wool spots, or papilledema. Malignant hypertension is also associated with nephropathy, encephalopathy, microangiopathic hemolytic anemia, and cardiac ischemia. Untreated malignant hypertension is a rapidly fatal disorder, with a mortality of more than 90 % within 1 year, as reported in a classic series by Kincaid-Smith.[6] In this series, deaths were due to renal failure (19%), congestive heart failure (13%), renal failure plus congestive heart failure (48%), stroke (20%), and myocardial infarction (1%).

Aggressive therapy to prevent progressive ischemic injury in malignant hypertension is critical. Although the autoregulatory range of CNS blood flow is reset upwards in chronic hypertension, the lower limit of the autoregulation remains approximately 25% below the resting mean blood pressure in patients with both normotension and chronic hypertension.[39] When the arterial blood pressure falls below this lower limit, cerebral blood flow decreases progressively, and symptoms of low CNS flow including nausea, yawning, hyperventilation, clamminess, and syncope develop. To protect cerebral function, after initial reduction of blood pressure by 20% within the first hour, blood pressure is further reduced over the next 2 to 6 hours to the 160/110 range as long as the patients remains stable. Nitroprusside is one of the most useful intravenous agents for hypertensive emergency. Some patients are highly sensitive to treatment owing to coexisting hypovolemia; therefore, low-dose nitroprusside (0.3 μg/kg/min or less, with titration every 3-5 minutes) is used to reach goal blood pressure. A number of parenteral agents have been used as successful alternatives to nitroprusside, including labetalol, fenoldopam, and nicardipine. Premature discontinuation of parenteral therapy may cause rebound hypertension. Oral therapy is usually started after the pressure has been stabilized on parenteral therapy. Parenteral therapy is then slowly weaned.

Renal failure is common with malignant hypertension. For patients with worsening renal failure due to malignant hypertension, renal

TABLE 88-1	Treatment of Hypertensive Crisis: Intravenous Medication	
Drug Name and Mechanism of Action	*Indications/Advantages/Dose*	*Disadvantages/Adverse Effects/Metabolism Cautions*
Sodium nitroprusside: Nitric oxide compound; vasodilation of arteriolar and venous smooth muscle. Increases cardiac output by decreasing afterload	Useful in most hypertensive crisis. Onset of action immediate, duration of action 1-2 min. Dose: 0.25 μg/kg/min. Maximum dose: 8-10 μg/kg/min	Contraindicated in high-output cardiac failure, congenital optic atrophy. Anemia and liver disease at risk of cyanide toxicity: acidosis, tachycardia, change in mental status, almond smell on breath. Renal disease at risk of thiocyanate toxicity: psychosis, hyperreflexia, seizure, tinnitus. Cautious use with increased intracranial pressure. Do not use maximum dose for more than 10 minutes. Crosses the placenta.
Nitroglycerin: Directly interacts with nitrate receptors on vascular smooth muscle. Primarily dilates venous bed. Decreases preload	Use with symptoms of cardiac ischemia, perioperative hypertension in cardiac surgery. Initial dose: 5 μg/min. Maximum dose: 100 μg/min	Contraindicated in angle-closure glaucoma, increased intracranial pressure. Blood pressure decreased secondary to decreased preload, cardiac output—avoid when cerebral or renal perfusion compromised. Caution with right ventricular infarct.
Labetalol: β-Adrenergic blockade and α-adrenergic blockade IV. α:β-Blocking ratio is 1:7	Onset of action 2-5 min. Duration 3-6 hours. Bolus 20 mg, then 20-80 mg every 10 min for maximum dose 300 mg. Infuse at 0.5-2 mg/min	Avoid in bronchospasm, bradycardia, congestive heart failure, greater than first-degree heart block, second/third trimester pregnancy. Use caution with hepatic dysfunction, inhalational anesthetics (myocardial depression). Enters breast milk.
Esmolol: Cardioselective β$_1$-adrenergic blocking agent	Use with aortic dissection. Use during intubation, intraoperative, and postoperative hypertension. Onset 60 seconds, duration 10-20 min. 200-500 μg/kg/min for 4 min, then infuse 50-300 μg/kg/min	See labetalol. Not dependent on renal or hepatic function for metabolism (metabolized by hydrolysis in RBC).
Fenoldopam: Postsynaptic dopamine-1 agonist; decreases peripheral vascular resistance; 10 times more potent than dopamine as vasodilator	May be advantageous in kidney disease, increases renal blood flow, increases sodium excretion, no toxic metabolites. Initial dose: 0.1 μg/kg/min, with titration every 15 min. No bolus	Contraindicated in glaucoma (may increase intraocular pressure) or allergy to sulfites; hypotension, especially with concurrent beta-blocker. Check serum potassium every 6 hours. Concurrent acetaminophen may significantly increase blood levels. Dose-related tachycardia.
Hydralazine: Primarily dilates arteriolar vasculature	Primarily used in pregnancy/eclampsia. Dose: 10 mg every 20-130 min; maximum dose 20 mg. Decreases blood pressure in 10-20 min. Duration of action 2-4 h	Reflex tachycardia; give beta-blocker concurrently. May exacerbate angina. Half-life 3 hours, affects blood pressure for 100 hours. Depends on hepatic acetylation for inactivation.
Phentolamine: α-Adrenergic blockade	Used primarily to treat hypertension from excessive catecholamine excess (e.g., pheochromocytoma). Dose: 5-15 mg. Onset of action 1-2 min, duration 3-10 min	β-blockade is generally added to control tachycardia or arrhythmias. As in all catecholamine excess states, beta-blockers should never be given first, as the loss of β-adrenergically mediated vasodilatation will leave α-adrenergically mediated vasoconstriction unopposed and result in increased pressure.
Nicardipine: Dihydropyridine calcium channel blocker; inhibits transmembrane influx of calcium ions into cardiac and smooth muscle	Onset of action 10-20 min, duration 1-4 h. Initial dose: 5 mg/h to maximum of 15 mg/h	Avoid with congestive heart failure, cardiac ischemia. Adverse effects include tachycardia, flushing, HA.
Clevidipine: Short-acting dihydropyridine calcium channel hypertension[99]	Initial dose: 1 mg/h; can be increased to 21 mg/h	Reduces blood pressure without affecting cardiac filling pressures or causing reflex tachycardia
Enalaprilat: Angiotensin-converting enzyme inhibitor	Onset of action 15-20 min, duration 12-24 h. Dose: 1.25-5 mg every 6 h	Response not predictable, with high renin states may see acute hypotension. Hyperkalemia in setting of reduced glomerular filtration rate. Avoid in pregnancy.
Trimethaphan: Nondepolarizing ganglionic blocking agent; competes with acetylcholine for postsynaptic receptors	Used in aortic dissection. Dose: 0.5-5 mg/min	Does not increase cardiac output. No inotropic cardiac effect. Disadvantages include parasympathetic blockade, resulting in paralytic ileus and bladder atony, and development of tachyphylaxis after 24-96 hours of use.

failure exacerbates the hypertension. Aggressive treatment can arrest and reverse renal damage. Since the arteriolopathy of malignant hypertension includes fixed anatomic lesions, initial lowering of blood pressure may worsen renal function. Dialysis may be required in patients with a presenting creatinine greater than 4.5 mg/dL.[40] In the majority of patients, renal function begins to improve after 2 weeks of therapy. Of the patients who require dialysis, 50% will regain sufficient function to discontinue dialysis.[41] Recovery of renal function is predicted when the combined length of both kidneys is 20.2 cm or more, but is felt to be unlikely when the length is 14.2 or less.[42] The mean time to recovery is approximately 2 to 3 months, but recovery after up to 26 months has been reported.[43] In patients with malignant hypertension secondary to glomerulonephritis, eventual deterioration to end-stage renal disease (ESRD) may occur despite blood pressure control.[44] In contrast, renal function tends to remain well preserved in patients without underlying glomerulonephritis if blood pressure is well controlled.

Nitroprusside has been one of the preferred agents to treat hypertension and renal failure. The metabolism of nitroprusside results in the production of cyanide, which is taken up by red blood cells and conjugated to thiocyanate in the liver. Cyanide toxicity occurs in patients with anemia or liver disease, whereas thiocyanate toxicity is seen in the setting of renal disease (see Table 88-1). Thiocyanate levels should be monitored and the duration of therapy kept to less than 72 hours whenever possible. Fenoldopam has no toxic metabolites and may protect renal function.[34-38]

Controversy exists as to the management of the relatively asymptomatic malignant hypertensive patient (i.e., with neuroretinopathy alone).[45,46] Although oral medication under close observation has been used successfully,[47] we prefer initial parenteral therapy. The progressive breakdown of CNS autoregulation in these patients enhances the sensitivity to ischemia, with abrupt decreases in blood pressure. Of the oral agents, calcium antagonists and minoxidil are effective and safe.

ACE inhibitors may cause hyperkalemia in undialyzed patients with significant renal insufficiency.

HYPERTENSIVE ENCEPHALOPATHY

In hypertensive encephalopathy, the MAP exceeds the limits of autoregulation, and brain edema develops from extravasation of plasma proteins. If hypertensive encephalopathy is untreated, coma and death may follow.[48] The challenge of hypertensive encephalopathy is appropriate lowering of blood pressure in the setting of CNS ischemia and edema. The hallmark of hypertensive encephalopathy is improvement within 12 to 24 hours of adequate blood pressure reduction. The MAP should be cautiously reduced by no more than 15% over 2 to 3 hours. Neurologic complications have been reported from reductions in MAP of 40% or more.[49]

Hypertensive encephalopathy is one of the medical conditions believed to cause reversible posterior leukoencephalopathy, a condition that results from reversible vasogenic subcortical edema without infarction.[22,23] This syndrome is characterized by headache, decreased alertness, changes in behavior including confusion and diminished speech, seizures, and alterations in visual perceptions and is rapidly reversible with lowering of the blood pressure.[22,23] An MRI examination shows characteristic findings including white matter edema in the posterior cerebral hemispheres.[22]

There is a growing literature supporting a shared pathologic process between hypertensive encephalopathy and eclampsia. Both clinical syndromes share the same clinical features and imaging findings. Eclampsia during pregnancy, as well as postpartum eclampsia, has also been associated with reversible posterior leukoencephalopathy.[22,23]

In previously normotensive patients, including those with eclampsia, blood pressure should be normalized. If the mental status worsens with treatment, the pressure should be allowed to increase until neurologic symptoms resolve and then be reduced to within the normal range over several days to allow restoration of autoregulation.

ISCHEMIC CEREBRAL INFARCTION

When the CPP decreases below the level of autoregulation, ischemia develops. In response, there may be a marked elevation in arterial blood pressure, which tends to spontaneously return to baseline 24 to 48 hours after the acute event. Following ischemic cerebrovascular accident (CVA), it is also important to consider other causes that may contribute to an increase in blood pressure, including a full bladder, nausea, pain, preexisting hypertension, hypoxia, or increased ICP. The role of blood pressure treatment in this setting is controversial. Oftentimes, simply calming the patient, treating pain, and relieving a full bladder may reduce the blood pressure.

Data from animal studies show that in the area surrounding the ischemic infarct, there are "neurons at risk" that rely on collateral circulation to maintain perfusion.[55] These neurons are nonfunctional—not dead—and potentially can be "rescued" by reperfusion, a phenomenon referred to as *ischemic penumbra*.[50] The degree to which this occurs in humans is not known. In addition, in acute stroke, autoregulation is impaired, and cerebral blood flow is therefore not preserved in a predictable manner. As a result of these changes, acute reductions in blood pressure could potentially increase the area of infarct, resulting in severe clinical consequences.

Comprehensive guidelines for the treatment of stroke were recently updated by the American Heart Association/American Stroke Association Stroke Council, Clinical Cardiology Council, Cardiovascular Radiology and Intervention Council, and the Atherosclerotic Peripheral Vascular Disease and Quality of Care Outcomes in Research Interdisciplinary Working Groups and affirmed by the American Academy of Neurology.[51] In patients determined to be candidates for administration of intravenous recombinant tissue plasminogen activator (tPA), the blood pressure must be reduced if the systolic blood pressure is > 185 mm Hg or the diastolic blood pressure is > 110 mm Hg, and the patient must be carefully monitored before, during, and after administration of this compound. Recombinant tissue plasminogen activator is contraindicated if the systolic blood pressure is >185 mm Hg or diastolic blood pressure is >110 mm Hg.[51]

Questions remain as to how to manage individuals with ischemic stroke who are not candidates for intravenous recombinant tissue plasminogen activator. There are no large randomized trials to guide this therapy. If there is no indication for acute lowering of the blood pressure (acute ischemic damage to vital organs such as cardiac ischemia, aortic dissection), the current recommendation is that a systolic blood pressure over 220 mm Hg or a diastolic blood pressure over 120 mm Hg be treated to lower the blood pressure 15% to 25% over the first 24 hours.[51]

However, a recent prospective observational study analyzed the impact of blood pressure lowering in the setting of ischemic stroke in 1092 patients.[52] The data suggest an improved outcome at 3 months with modest reductions in blood pressure between 10 and 27 mm Hg. Interestingly, the authors noted that the benefit of blood pressure reduction waned with age. In patients with more than 27 mm Hg blood pressure reduction, a poorer outcome was multiplied by 6 in patients aged 70 to 76 years, by 10 in patients 76 to 80 years, and by 15 in patients older than 80 years.[52] The authors recommend that the treatment regime for patients eligible to receive thrombolytic therapy be applied to all patients suffering from ischemic stroke but that sudden decreases in blood pressure to above 10% from baseline be avoided.[52]

SUBARACHNOID HEMORRHAGE

Approximately 10% of cerebrovascular accidents are due to subarachnoid hemorrhage; ruptured congenital berry aneurysms are the most common cause. Aneurysmal subarachnoid hemorrhage remains a devastating entity, with a mortality rate of 50% to 60% at 30 days despite improvement in care and early surgical intervention. Of those who do survive, 50% remain dependent.[53] The level of consciousness when the patient presents, global cerebral edema, the size of the subarachnoid blood collection on computed tomography (CT), and a recurrent hemorrhage have been associated with outcome.[53] Worse outcomes have also been associated with age, hyperglycemia, and medical complications.[53] Subarachnoid hemorrhage increases ICP and decreases cerebral perfusion, causing global ischemia. Complications include an intracerebral hemorrhage or the development of hydrocephalus. Management of these patients is significantly different from those with ischemic stroke. In contrast to ischemia, intracranial bleed induces intense vasospasm in neighboring vessels 4 to 12 days after the initial bleed, increasing the risk for significant cerebral ischemia. The mental status evaluation may be used to guide therapy, with an intact mental status supporting adequate cerebral perfusion.

Markedly elevated pressures increase the risk of rebleeding. The goal is a 20% to 25% reduction in blood pressure over 6 to 12 hours, but to not less than 160 to 180/100 mm Hg.[54] Labetalol is the preferred agent, as there are no significant adverse effects on ICP or CPP.[3] Given the potential increase in cerebral blood volume and ICP associated with vasodilators, sodium nitroprusside and nitroglycerin are not usually first-line treatments. There are clinical data to show that treatment with oral nimodipine within 4 days of the acute event decreases vasospasm and cerebral ischemia.[55] Nimodipine may also directly protect against ischemic damage to nerve cells by blocking calcium uptake into cells.

INTRACEREBRAL HEMORRHAGE

Intracerebral hemorrhage accounts for 10% to 20 % of all strokes.[56] Hypertension is a major risk factor; 75% of affected individuals have preexisting hypertension.[57] Although patients with intracerebral hemorrhage may present with nausea, vomiting, change in mental status, hypertension, headache, and a focal neurologic examination, the definitive diagnosis must be made by neuroimaging. Unlike ischemic stroke, where blood pressure generally returns to normal within 24 to 48 hours, in intracerebral hemorrhage, the most rapid decline in blood pressure occurs in the first 24 hours, but the blood pressure may remain elevated for 7 to 10 days.[50] The hematoma compresses normal tissue, creating an area of ischemia, increasing ICP and further decreasing CPP. Autoregulation is altered, making cerebral perfusion critically dependent on systemic blood pressure.[58] The prognosis overall is not encouraging. A retrospective analysis of 411 patients with intracerebral hemorrhage showed that 30% died before reaching the hospital and an additional 50% died within 28 days.[59] Independent risk factors associated with this early death included unconsciousness, lateral shift of midline structures, MAP ≥ 134 mm Hg, hyperglycemia, anticoagulant therapy, and ventricular extrasystoles.[59]

There is no clear consensus on the appropriate treatment of hypertension in the setting of acute intracranial hemorrhage. The decision to treat or not treat blood pressure should be made based on individual considerations including baseline blood pressure, etiology of hemorrhage, age, and elevated ICP, as well as a careful literature review. The central issue is whether aggressive lowering of blood pressure reduces the risk of intracerebral bleeding without disrupting blood flow to collateral areas. Some argue that decreasing blood pressure decreases risk of hemorrhage extension, edema, and associated systemic complications, particularly when systolic blood pressure exceeds 200 mm Hg, a level associated with hematoma growth in some studies.[56-58] A retrospective analysis of 76 patients with intracerebral hemorrhage and hypertension showed that maximum systolic blood pressure was significantly associated with hematoma enlargement.[60] Furthermore, this analysis suggested that systolic blood pressure ≥160 mm Hg is associated with enlargement of hematoma when compared to a systolic blood pressure ≤150 mm Hg.[60] Others argue that not treating hypertension allows continued perfusion of areas at risk from low blood flow.[58] It was previously thought rebleeding was rare in the first 24 hours. More recent data suggest that it is more common than thought, occurring in up to a third of affected individuals.[57,61] The greatest risk is in the first few hours after the initial insult.[61,62] An increased risk of bleed is associated with an initial large irregular bleed,[63] coagulopathy, liver disease,[64] and a low platelet count.[64] No studies have demonstrated a clear relationship between acute hypertension after an intracerebral bleed and the risk of rebleed.[58]

A recent[65] consensus was that (1) aggressive lowering of blood pressure using intravenous medication and blood pressure monitoring every 5 minutes should be considered when the systolic blood pressure is over 200 mm Hg or the mean arterial blood pressure is over 150 mm Hg; (2) in the setting of suspected intracranial hypertension, in addition to ICP monitoring, aggressive lowering of blood pressure with continuous or intermittent intravenous medication should be considered when the systolic blood pressure is over 180 mm Hg or the MAP is over 130 mm Hg, keeping the CPP above 60 to 80 mm Hg; and (3) if there is no suspected elevation of the ICP and the systolic blood pressure is over 180 or the MAP is over 130, consider lowering the target blood pressure to 160/90 mm Hg or to a MAP of 110 mm Hg.

There is no consensus on the agent of choice. Concern revolves around the impact of different antihypertensives on ICP. Common to all agents is a decrease in MAP and a decrease in CPP. Vasodilating agents may increase cerebral blood flow, and in the setting of decreased cranial compliance may potentially increase ICP, further decreasing CPP.[32,58] The combination of decreased cerebral compliance, decreased cerebral blood flow, and altered autoregulation—as occurs in chronic hypertension—makes the administration of any antihypertensive agent potentially dangerous. No large randomized studies are available to guide therapy. Combination α- and β-blockers are recommended when antihypertensive treatment is indicated in intracerebral hemorrhage. Risks of this therapy include worsening of bradycardia associated with the Cushing response. However, in the setting of normal cranial compliance and an increased ICP, vasodilators are probably safe. Because of the very high levels of circulating catecholamines with an intracerebral bleed, β-blockade is added when vasodilator therapy alone is ineffective.

HEAD TRAUMA

Head trauma complications include skull fractures, epidural hematomas, subdural hematomas, intracerebral hematomas, and diffuse axonal damage. With trauma, there is often edema. Acute increases in ICP are initially prevented by flow of blood and CSF from the cranial vault. However, with increasing edema, ICP eventually increases. In most trauma centers, ICP monitoring has become the standard of care.[66] Anywhere from 31% to 61% of patients with a closed head injury may have defective autoregulation.[67] If autoregulation is intact, increasing the MAP will cause vasoconstriction and produce no change in ICP. With altered autoregulation, increasing the MAP may cause vasodilatation, increasing blood volume and causing edema and increased ICP. The goal is to maintain a minimum CPP of 70 mm Hg and a MAP above 90 mm Hg. If an antihypertensive agent is needed, a major consideration is its impact on ICP. A combination alpha- and beta-blocker or nicardipine may be preferred when there is decreased intracranial compliance and increased ICP.[68,69] In the absence of intracranial hypertension, vasodilators may be preferred.

AORTIC DISSECTION

Aortic dissection begins with a tear in the intima of the aorta that is propagated by the aortic pulse wave (dP/dt). Myocardial contractility, heart rate, and blood pressure contribute to the aortic pulse wave. There are two types of aortic dissection, type A and type B. Type A dissections are often associated with a tear in the intima of the proximal aorta next to a coronary artery and may extend to the aortic arch.[70] Type B dissections occur in the descending aortic arch and usually begin with an intimal tear next to the subclavian artery.[71] Risk factors for dissection include advanced atherosclerosis, Marfan syndrome, Ehlers-Danlos syndrome, and coarctation of the aorta.[72] Symptoms occur as the expanding hematoma causes pressure on the vasculature. This may cause myocardial infarction, stroke, spinal cord/bowel infarction, and acute renal failure. Ischemic kidney may develop, leading to refractory hypertension.[73] Dissection to the aortic root can precipitate acute aortic insufficiency.[74] Rupture of the ascending aorta leads to hemopericardium and tamponade.[74]

Both types of dissection may present with severe, often tearing pain in the chest, back, or abdomen, accompanied by diaphoresis, nausea, or vomiting. They are often but not always associated with hypertension.[75] Discrepancies in peripheral pulses may be observed. The chest was present in only one half of individuals with type B dissection.[76] The diagnosis may be confirmed with CT or MRI. Multiplane transesophageal echocardiography is also used. Type A dissections usually require surgery to prevent the catastrophic consequences of great-vessel occlusion, aortic insufficiency, or tamponade. Type B dissections may usually be treated medically[77,78] unless there is rupture, in which case open repair or endovascular repair is indicated. A recent meta-analysis suggested that endovascular repair may be preferred.[77]

Treatment for both type A and type B dissections is initiated based on clinical suspicion alone, given the high mortality associated with this entity. The goal of treatment is to first decrease myocardial contractility and heart rate with β-blockade. β-Blocking agents are preferred. Next, the blood pressure is reduced to the lowest tolerable level until pain is relieved. Relief of pain suggests arrest of ongoing aortic dissection. The most widely used agent is nitroprusside. Nitroprusside is titrated to a systolic pressure of 100 to 120 mm Hg or to as low as 70 to 80 mm Hg. Prior treatment with β-blockade prevents reflex cardiac stimulation and a potential increase in the aortic pulse wave seen with nitroprusside.

An alternative regimen, preferred by some because of a more potent reduction in the steepness of the pulse wave contour, involves use of the ganglionic blocking agent, trimethaphan.[76] This agent prevents increases in cardiac output and left ventricular ejection rate.[73,76] The rapid onset (1-2 minutes) and short duration (10 minutes) of action of this drug allows precise pressure control. Any mild reflex increase in heart rate may be treated with subsequent β-blockade. Hydralazine is avoided because it causes unwanted reflex cardiac stimulation.

Even normotensive individuals should be treated with antihypertensive medications to keep the heart rate and shear forces low.

PULMONARY EDEMA

Many patients who present with pulmonary edema have long-standing antecedent hypertension with concentric left ventricular hypertrophy and well-preserved systolic contraction.[79,80] They develop acute diastolic dysfunction in response to abrupt increases in cardiac afterload due to increased systemic blood pressure.[81] With poor diastolic relaxation, the left ventricle requires markedly elevated filling pressures, leading to pulmonary venous hypertension and edema. The therapeutic goal is to decrease afterload, improve diastolic relaxation, and decrease pulmonary pressure. Vasodilators are the agents of choice, as they improve diastolic relaxation and lower pulmonary venous pressure.[82] A beta-blocker may also be used. Nitroprusside is often used because it reduces preload and afterload, improving left ventricular function and reducing myocardial oxygen demand. Modest decreases in pressure improve symptoms markedly. In less emergent settings, ACE inhibitors or calcium channel antagonists have been shown to improve diastolic function and cause regression of concentric ventricular hypertrophy.[83]

In patients with left ventricular failure secondary to poor systolic function, vasodilators are the agents of choice. Nitroglycerin is preferred with cardiac ischemia. Nitroprusside may be used in patients refractory to nitrites. Whereas nitroglycerin dilates intercoronary collateral vessels more than small resistance arterioles and improves perfusion of ischemic myocardium, nitroprusside dilates resistance arterioles predominantly, thereby resulting in a potential steal of blood flow away from ischemic areas. Diuretics are used to reduce left ventricular end-diastolic volume.

In the setting of acute myocardial infarction, acute catecholamine release and sympathetic outflow contribute to hypertension. The hypertension usually resolves in a few hours with sedation and pain control alone. Diastolic blood pressures over 100 mm Hg, should be treated with nitroglycerin. The pressure is rapidly, but cautiously, reduced to near-normotensive levels; overshoot hypotension can worsen coronary perfusion. Therapy can usually be stopped within 24 hours. There is considerable evidence that the early use of β-blocking agents may reduce ultimate infarct size independent of blood pressure control.[84]

PERIOPERATIVE HYPERTENSION

Perioperative hypertension is a major risk factor for the development of postoperative hypertension.[85] Whenever possible, it is preferred to postpone elective surgery until the blood pressure has been well controlled over days to weeks. However, when waiting is not an option, lowering the blood pressure to below 180/110 prior to noncardiac surgery is recommended.[85] In patients with chronic hypertension on adequate treatment, oral medications should be taken the morning of surgery.

Induction of anesthesia increases sympathetic activity, causing elevated blood pressure, a response that may be exaggerated in uncontrolled hypertension. As anesthesia continues, there is generally a fall in blood pressure. Rapid and wide fluctuations in blood pressure leading to intraoperative hypotension, stroke, myocardial ischemia, or acute renal failure are more common in individuals with a hypertensive history.

Patients taking hypertensive therapy prior to surgery should continue treatment after surgery, changing to an equivalent intravenous medication if they are unable to take oral medications. If patients have been on a beta-blocker or clonidine, this medication should be continued postoperatively to prevent "rebound" hypertension. If intravenous medication is necessary, propranolol or methyldopa may be used. The high incidence of increased blood pressure results from the decreased use of "deep" anesthesia and absence of prolonged sedation following surgery. As a result, there is increased sympathetic response to surgical stimuli such as pain, hypoxia, and the anesthetic agents themselves. Effective pain control and avoidance of hypoxia may be sufficient to treat the hypertension. Adequate blood pressure control reduces the risk of bleeding from suture lines, premature graft closure, and ischemic damage to organs at risk. Nitroprusside is widely used. Nitroglycerin is preferred for the post–coronary bypass patient. Fenoldopam, with its impact on increasing renal blood flow, is also recommended, especially in clinical settings where renal ischemia is a risk.

CATECHOLAMINE-ASSOCIATED HYPERTENSION

Hypertensive crisis related to excess catecholamine secretion can result from the ingestion of sympathomimetic agents such as cocaine, amphetamines, phencyclidine, phenylpropanolamine (diet pills), decongestants such as ephedrine and pseudoephedrine, and other agents including atropine, ergot alkaloids, and tricyclic antidepressants. It may also be caused by tyramine ingestion in conjunction with monoamine oxidase (MAO) inhibitor therapy, autonomic dysfunction, withdrawal from certain antihypertensive medications, and pheochromocytoma. Critically elevated pressures can result and cause myocardial infarction, aortic dissection, and stroke.

Pheochromocytoma is a very rare cause of hypertension.[86] Excess catecholamine secretion by the tumor results in a sustained elevation of blood pressure in the majority of cases, while peripheral catecholamine uptake and storage leads to paroxysmal symptoms when the catecholamines are released in response to stimuli. Symptoms of pheochromocytoma include headache, palpitations, hypertension, anxiety, abdominal pain, and diaphoresis. Patients may present with orthostatic changes in blood pressure, a clue to the diagnosis.[87] For the patient with hypertensive emergency, the treatment of choice is the short-acting parenteral α-antagonist, phentolamine. Following blood pressure reduction, β-blockade is generally added to control tachycardia or arrhythmias. As in all catecholamine excess states, beta-blockers should not be used as initial therapy. Loss of β-adrenergically mediated vasodilatation leaves α-adrenergically mediated vasoconstriction unopposed and results in increased pressure. An oral regimen of the nonselective α-antagonist, phenoxybenzamine, can be used in less critical situations. Labetalol has been effective in treating hypotension related to pheochromocytoma in selected patients. However, as its β-blockade exceeds its α-blocking effect, severe hypertension has been reported.[88]

Significant rebound hypertension may develop 12 to 72 hours after abrupt discontinuation of chronic beta-blocker therapy or centrally acting α-agonist antihypertensives, such as clonidine or methyldopa, from increased sympathetic outflow. With severe hypertension, headache, diaphoresis, anxiety, nausea, tachycardia, and abdominal pain are reported. In cases of moderate hypertension, simply restarting the antihypertensive agent may control the blood pressure. With more severe blood pressure elevations, intravenous therapy should be started.

In patients on MAO-inhibitor therapy, ingestion of foods containing tyramine or sympathomimetic amines can result in hypertension (Table 88-2). Tyramine is metabolized by an alternative pathway to octopamine, which releases catecholamines from peripheral sites by

TABLE 88-2	Tyramine-Containing Foods	
Chianti wine		Chicken liver
Soy sauce		Yeast
Avocados		Fermented sausage
Bananas		Canned figs
Coffee		Certain beers
Chocolate		Unpasteurized cheese
Pickled herring		

acting as a false neurotransmitter. Nitroprusside or phentolamine is used, with the addition of β-blockade as needed for tachycardia. The episodes are self-limited and last 6 hours or less.

GESTATIONAL HYPERTENSION/ PREECLAMPSIA/ECLAMPSIA

Gestational hypertension is defined as a systolic blood pressure of at least 140 mm Hg and a diastolic blood pressure of at least 90 mm Hg on two separate blood pressure measurements done 6 hours apart. It occurs after 20 weeks of pregnancy in patients known to previously be normotensive.[89] Up to 50% of these women develop preeclampsia if gestational hypertension develops before 30 weeks of gestation. *Preeclampsia* is defined as gestational hypertension with 300 mg of protein on a 24-hour urine (urine dipstick 1+). A 24-hour urine is necessary because dipstick urine protein correlates poorly with 24-hour urine protein in gestational hypertension.[90] Preeclampsia should also be suspected in patients with hypertension developing after 20 weeks' gestation and associated with nausea, vomiting, cerebral symptoms, abnormal liver function tests, and thrombocytopenia, even in the absence of proteinuria. Preeclampsia develops in 5% of all pregnancies and occurs twice as often in primigravid versus multigravid women.[91] In women with a history of multiple pregnancies but with a new partner,[91] preeclampsia also appears. In the setting of molar pregnancy, it is seen in up to 70% of individuals.[92] During normal pregnancy, blood pressure is initially decreased and then slowly rises toward the normal range during the third trimester. In preeclampsia, intravascular volume is low despite peripheral edema, and the renin-angiotensin system is activated. Progression to seizures defines eclampsia and may occur with diastolic pressures of as low as 100 mm Hg. Clinical treatment includes bed rest and parenteral magnesium.

With regard to hypertensive treatment in pregnancy, the optimal blood pressure has not been defined. The goal is to prolong the pregnancy until the fetus can be delivered. In the case of mild preeclampsia, there are no large studies to guide therapy.[91] With more severe preeclampsia, treatment is initiated to prevent cerebral hemorrhage. The recommendation is to initiate antihypertensive therapy when the systolic blood pressure is above 160 mm Hg or the diastolic blood pressure is above 110 mm Hg. Usually, preferred medications include hydralazine and labetalol administered to keep the systolic blood pressure 140 to 155 mm Hg and the diastolic blood pressure 90 to 105 mm Hg.[91] Nitroprusside should be avoided owing to the risk of cyanide toxicity in the fetus. ACE inhibitors should also be avoided because of their potential impact on the fetus's kidney.

OTHER HYPERTENSIVE SITUATIONS

The renal crisis of scleroderma is an aggressive form of malignant hypertension in which proliferative endarteritis precedes hypertension. Ischemic-induced activation of the renin-angiotensin system causes the hypertension. The incidence of this condition among patients with scleroderma ranges from 8% to 13%, and it is more common among blacks.[93] Progression to ESRD occurs in 1 to 2 months without treatment. Aggressive pressure control with ACE inhibitors leads to a long-term survival of about 50% to 70%.[94]

Hypertension is a feature of both primary and secondary antiphospholipid antibody syndromes, occurring in up to 93% of patients.[95] Malignant hypertension occurs in this syndrome secondary to both microvasculopathy and emboli to the renal artery. Antihypertensive treatment is similar to malignant hypertension. Successful treatment outcomes have been reported with anticoagulation.[95]

One-fourth of patients with extensive second- or third-degree burns develop severe hypertension in the first few days, likely due to high

---

> **Box 88-3**
>
> **SEVERE UNCOMPLICATED HYPERTENSION**
>
> Severe hypertension (diastolic >115 mm Hg) in association with one or more of the following:
> Chronic renal failure
> Chronic congestive heart failure
> Stable angina
> Previous myocardial infarction
> Transient ischemic attacks
> Previous cerebrovascular accident

levels of circulating catecholamines and renin. Nitroprusside or phentolamine (in countries where it is still available) are other treatments.

Patients with transverse spinal cord lesions at the T6 level or higher, including patients with Guillain-Barré syndrome, have dysreflexia in which noxious stimulus in dermatomes below the level of lesion trigger a massive sympathetic discharge. This leads to severe hypertension, bradycardia, diaphoresis, and headache. In 90% of patients, distention of the bladder or bowel causes the dysreflexia, and prompt decompression leads to resolution of hypertension.[96] Drugs that have been used successfully in treating this condition include nitroprusside, phentolamine, and labetalol.

Hypertension in the renal transplant recipient may be caused by acute rejection, vascular anastomotic stenosis, obstructive uropathy, corticosteroid use, cyclosporine, and native-kidney renin release.[97] Oral calcium channel antagonists are effective and well tolerated in these patients. Other rare causes of hypertension include erythropoietin-associated hypertension. This is treated with phlebotomy and dose reduction in conjunction with antihypertensive drugs.[98] Diabetics on beta-blockers can experience severe hypertension with hypoglycemic episodes, presumably due to catecholamine release.

Hypertensive Urgency

Hypertensive urgency refers to patients in whom blood pressure is severely elevated, but based on detailed history, physical examination, and laboratory evaluation, there is no evidence of acute end-organ damage. This clinical situation is quite different from that of patients with severe hypertension and chronic stable complications such as those with stable chronic renal failure or stable angina. The decision to treat the latter group in the inpatient or outpatient setting often depends on the associated end-organ involvement (Box 88-3) and reliability of patient follow-up.

The third (and most common) treatment category, termed *severe uncomplicated hypertension* (see Box 88-3), is used to describe patients with severe blood pressure elevation but no end-organ involvement. Despite markedly elevated pressures (e.g., diastolic of pressures 140 mm Hg at times), these patients are at low risk of immediate complications. Hypertension-related morbidity tends to occur over months to years. The treatment of choice is gradual pressure reduction over a few days in the outpatient setting. The major risk of therapy is rapid pressure reduction. The choice of antihypertensive agent is based on ease of administration and side-effect profile rather than on rapid blood pressure reductions. Frequently, restarting a previously effective regimen is all that is necessary. It is critically important to follow these patients over the next 24 to 48 hours to ensure the blood pressure is appropriately reduced. While medicolegal issues may pressure physicians into loading these patients with medication to observe on-the-spot control of their blood pressure, this practice has recently been questioned as having no clear rational scientific basis.

ANNOTATED REFERENCES

Adams Jr HP, del Zoppo G, Alberts MJ, et al. Guidelines for the early management of adults with ischemic stroke: a guideline from the American Heart Association/American Stroke Association Stroke Council, Clinical Cardiology Council, Cardiovascular Radiology and Intervention Council, and the Atherosclerotic Peripheral Vascular Disease and Quality of Care Outcomes in Research Interdisciplinary Working Groups. Stroke 2007;5:1655-711.
Recent guidelines on total management (including BP) after ischemic CVA.

Freedman BI, Sedor JR. Hypertension-associated kidney disease: perhaps no more. J Am Soc Nephrol 2008;19:2047-51.
Editorial review of the role of BP in the pathogenesis of ESRD. Raises the interesting suggestion that excess risk of ESRD in African Americans is related to a genetic variant of motor protein non-muscular myosin 2 a (MYH9).

Fleisher LA, Beckman JA, Brown KA, Calkins H, Chaikof E, Fleischmann KE, et al. ACC/AHA 2007 guidelines on perioperative cardiovascular evaluation and care for noncardiac surgery: executive summary. A report of the American College of Cardiology/American Heart Association Task Force on Practice Guidelines (Writing Committee to Revise the 2002 Guidelines on Perioperative Cardiovascular Evaluation for Noncardiac Surgery). Circulation 2007;116;1971-96.
Consensus statement on management of hypertension (and other CV issues) in the perioperative period.

Wadei HM, Textor SC. Hypertension in the kidney transplant recipient. Transplant Rev 2010;24:105-20.
Careful recent review of diagnosis and management of hypertension after kidney transplantation.

Kincaid-Smith P, McMichael J, Murphy EA. The clinical course and pathology of hypertension with papilledema (malignant hypertension). Q J Med 1958;27:117.
Classical description of clinical events in malignant hypertension.

Lee VH, Wijdicks EF, Manno EM, Rabinstein AA. Clinical spectrum of a reversible posterior leukoencephalopathy syndrome. Arch Neurol 2008;2:205-10.
Retrospective review of a single-center experience with RPLS. Largest series to document neuroimaging improvement in association with clinical improvement.

Ohwaki K, Yano EM, Nagashima H, Hirata M, Nakagomi T, Tamura A. Blood pressure management in acute intracerebral hemorrhage: relationship between elevated blood pressure and hematoma enlargement. Stroke 2004;35:1364-7.
Retrospective assessment of 170 consecutive patients with acute intracerebral hemorrhage and relationship between blood pressure and hematoma enlargement. BP less than 150 mm Hg may prevent risk.

Trivedi M, Coles JP. Blood pressure management in acute head injury. J Intensive Care Med 2009;24:96-107.
Review of physiology of cerebral autoregulation and options for managing cerebral hemodynamics and systemic BP after head injury.

REFERENCES

Access the complete reference list online at http://www.expertconsult.com.

89

Cardiac Surgery: Indications and Complications

FRÉDÉRIC VANDEN EYNDEN | JACQUES P. GOLDSTEIN

Since the first clinical use of the heart-lung machine developed by Gibbon in 1953, cardiac surgery has become a standard technique worldwide for the treatment of congenital and acquired cardiac diseases. Sixty years of trial and error since then have seen much progress: the development of mechanical assist devices, percutaneous valve therapies, and robotic surgery to name just a handful. This chapter reviews the specific indications for cardiac surgery and discusses some of the most frequent postoperative complications.

Surgical Indications for Coronary Artery Diseases

In the early 1990s, three large multicenter randomized trials were undertaken in Europe and the United States. The Veterans Administration Cooperative Study, the European Coronary Surgery Study, and the Coronary Artery Surgery Study indicated that patients who underwent coronary artery bypass grafting (CABG) always had extended survival compared with medically treated patients.[1] Since then, medical treatment has evolved, with the advent of plaque stabilizers and percutaneous coronary angioplasty (PTCA). Nowadays, referring a patient to medical treatment or PTCA or surgery is an expert decision based on appropriateness criteria[2] and often discussed on multidisciplinary rounds. In patients with myocardial ischemia, indications for surgery will be based on symptoms (Canadian Cardiovascular Society classification [CCS]), medical history (left ventricular [LV] function, diabetes), and sets of lesions defined by the anatomic localization of the coronary artery stenosis on a coronarography and best defined by the Syntax score.[3]

In acute coronary syndromes, most clinical scenarios are amenable to revascularization, except for ST-segment elevation myocardial infarction (STEMI) with onset of symptoms later than 12 hours. Even patients in shock will benefit from revascularization compared with medical treatment.[4,5] In less acute ischemia, the indication for revascularization will depend on symptoms classified according to the CCS. Most asymptomatic patients will benefit from medical treatment, whereas most symptomatic patients will benefit from invasive treatment. Surgery is preferred over PTCA in three situations:

- Left main stenosis of more than 50% or a left main equivalent disease (>70% stenosis in the proximal left anterior descending and proximal circumflex arteries)
- Triple-vessel disease, defined as significant lesions (>70%) in all three coronary territories (right, anterior, and lateral)
- Significant proximal left anterior descending stenosis with two-vessel disease

The improvement of long-term survival is even more striking in the presence of LV dysfunction and diabetes.

Use of a saphenous graft has been supplanted by total arterial revascularization.[6,7,8] Although surgery is certainly the best method to restore coronary flow, it is also the most invasive one, with attendant complications. Less invasive CABG procedures may broaden surgical indications by reducing morbidity and mortality. Efforts have been made to reduce handling of the heart to cannulate, avoid cardiopulmonary bypass (CPB), and avoid sternal splitting. Current efforts are made in various directions.

While initially very promising, off-pump CABG performed via sternotomy on a beating heart—avoiding CPB and heart handling—has somehow failed to show real advantages, mainly because it is more technically demanding, and studies may have suffered from performance biases.[9] Minimally invasive direct coronary artery bypass (MIDCAB) performed via a small left thoracotomy without CPB is widely accepted but limited to bypass of one artery: the left anterior descending (LAD) artery. CABG with femorofemoral CPB or off-pump techniques using thoracoscopic instruments and the support of a robot (da Vinci system) are under investigation worldwide and need large-scale validation but are certainly part of the armamentarium of tomorrow.[10] These newer techniques are also combined with PTCA in hybrid procedures, narrowing the gap between cardiology and cardiac surgery.[11]

Surgical Indications for Aortic Valve Surgery

AORTIC STENOSIS

Echocardiography is the most efficient technique to evaluate the degree of stenosis, LV hypertrophy, and LV function in patients with aortic valve stenosis.[12] The American College of Cardiology/American Heart Association Task Force on Practice Guidelines has graded the degree of aortic stenosis as mild (effective valve area >1.5 cm^2), moderate (area >1 to 1.5 cm^2), or severe (area ≤1 cm^2).[13] When stenosis is severe and cardiac output is normal, the mean transvalvular pressure gradient is generally greater than 50 mm Hg. Symptomatic patients (dyspnea, angina, or palpitations) with severe stenosis are candidates for surgery (class 1 recommendation), as are asymptomatic patients with reduced ventricular function (left ventricular ejection fraction [LVEF] <50%) or patients undergoing any other cardiac surgery (CABG, mitral valve, or thoracic aorta). When cardiac output is reduced, transvalvular gradient is reduced (low flow/low output), and estimation of the severity of the stenosis may require advanced diagnostic tools such as stress test, echocardiography, or pressure measurement in the cath lab. An accurate estimation of the degree of stenosis is essential in those patients with low cardiac output who, despite being at high risk for surgery, do better than with medical treatment if correctly diagnosed.[14]

Management of patients with coronary artery disease who will have CABG and are incidentally diagnosed with mild to moderate aortic stenosis during workup is controversial. For asymptomatic patients with mild aortic stenosis (mean gradient between 30 and 50 mm Hg) who require CABG, it may be reasonable to replace the valve (class IIa recommendation). For patients with lower mean gradient, leaving the native valve is advised unless there is a risk of rapid progression, such as important calcification (class IIb).[15] In very high risk patients, transcatheter aortic valve implantation (TAVI) is presently in its evaluation phase.[16]

AORTIC REGURGITATION

Chronic aortic regurgitation is usually well tolerated, and pure regurgitation is not considered for surgery unless severe (i.e., regurgitant volume >60 mL per beat or regurgitant orifice >0.3 cm^2) in a symptomatic patient at rest (class I) or on exercise testing (class I) or in an asymptomatic patient with LV dysfunction (LVEF <50%) (class I) or with LV enlargement (end-systolic diameter >55 mm or end-diastolic diameter >75 mm) (class IIa).[13] Symptomatic patients with mild aortic regurgitation should be investigated for other causes (ischemic cardiomyopathy). Regurgitation due to cusp lesions such as calcifications or destruction due to endocarditis are indications for valve replacement, except perhaps in very experienced hands in which repair is sometimes performed. Regurgitation due to annular enlargement with none or very little cusp lesion is now usually repaired with good results.[17,18] In the latter, annular enlargement is often concomitant with ascending aortic enlargement, and the aorta is replaced by a valve conduit if repair is not feasible or by a straight Dacron tube, with the native valve resuspended.[19]

Surgical Indications for Mitral Valve Surgery

Indications for mitral valve surgery have changed with the extension of mitral valve repair. With a better understanding of the specific anatomic lesions of the mitral valve associated with improvements in the surgical techniques, successful mitral repair can be achieved in specific ischemic and nonischemic mitral regurgitation.[13]

MITRAL STENOSIS

Moderate or severe mitral stenosis (mitral valve area ≤1.5 cm^2) in symptomatic patients is usually treated with percutaneous mitral balloon valvuloplasty, except when there is concomitant moderate to severe mitral regurgitation, left atrial thrombus, or the valve is not suitable for a percutaneous approach (echo score > 8); in the latter case, mitral valve replacement is performed.

MITRAL REGURGITATION

Mitral regurgitation is responsible for pulmonary hypertension, left atrial enlargement with atrial fibrillation, and excessive workload on the heart, leading to dyspnea. Much work has been done on the mechanisms and causes of mitral regurgitation, pioneered by Carpentier and colleagues in the early 1980s; advances include the development of repair techniques other than systematic valve replacement. In experienced hands, more than 90% of regurgitant valves are repaired, avoiding problems associated with prosthetic valves (degeneration, need for anticoagulation, prosthetic valve infection). The lower morbidity related to valve repair has broadened the indication for mitral valve surgery to asymptomatic patients with no ventricular dysfunction and no pulmonary hypertension or atrial fibrillation, if the regurgitant surface is more than 40 mm. In those patients, repair is mandatory, whereas in patients with any of the aforementioned complications of regurgitation, replacement is an option.[20,21] Recently, minimally invasive approaches through a 5-cm thoracotomy have been successfully applied to mitral repair and are gaining wide acceptance.[22,23]

Most mitral valves successfully repaired suffer from structural abnormalities and are identified as *organic mitral regurgitation*. *Functional mitral regurgitation* is the term used when the valve has no anatomic defect but is incompetent secondary to LV dysfunction, annulus dilation, or papillary muscle dysfunction. In some cases, CABG alone may improve LV function and reduce mitral regurgitation. Some advocate the use of ring annuloplasty or ventricular reduction surgery, but results are less convincing than in structural disorders.[24]

In long-standing mitral regurgitation, chronic right ventricular overload causes tricuspid regurgitation and atrial enlargement, promoting atrial fibrillation. Tricuspid regurgitation and atrial fibrillation also have to be assessed during the intervention, with a tricuspid annuloplasty and lesions made to the atria to stop reentrant circuits causing the arrhythmia.[25,26]

ASCENDING AORTA

Dilation of the ascending aorta is associated with hypertension, atherosclerotic disease, and structural (bicuspid aortic diseases)[27] and genetic factors that arise with entities such as Marfan or Ehlers-Danlos syndromes. When reaching threshold values[28] or when rapidly enlarging, dilated ascending aortas present a risk of rupture and dissection, prompt surgery is indicated.[29] In patients with structural arterial wall abnormalities, surgery is warranted when the largest diameter is 45 mm, while in general population 55 mm is the cutoff value for surgery.[30]

Dissection of the ascending aorta presents in almost every patient with pain, cardiac tamponade, or acute or poorly tolerated aortic regurgitation requiring urgent surgical correction.

Axillary cannulation and selective cerebral perfusion have permitted more thorough repair of aneurysm and dissection of the ascending aorta, prolonging in the aortic arch. Actual development is directed towards one-step treatment of the entire thoracic aorta.[31]

MISCELLANEOUS

Besides the indications discussed, some less frequent conditions can be encountered, which are usually referred to centers with specific expertise. Surgery for terminal heart failure, long dominated by heart transplantation, is nowadays (mainly because of organ shortage) a field of active research for the ideal mechanical substitute to be used as a bridge to transplantation or as a definitive organ substitute (destination therapy).

Large pulmonary emboli unresponsive to thrombolysis can be surgically removed from the pulmonary arteries, as can the organized fibrotic material found in chronic thromboembolic disease. Isolated tricuspid disease, rhythm restoring surgery, and adult congenital surgery are other indications.

Complications After Cardiac Surgery

Patients after cardiac surgery under CPB require close observation and prompt intervention if required.

BLEEDING AND CARDIAC TAMPONADE

Hemostasis is deeply altered after cardiac surgery under CPB.[32] Problems include decreased platelet numbers and function and activation of the coagulation and fibrinolytic cascade. All these factors, associated with cytokine activation and kallikrein stimulation of neutrophils, lead to a propensity for patients to bleed after the procedure.

Besides careful surgical techniques, diffuse bleeding can be prevented.[33] Patients should be rapidly rewarmed at 37°C, since hypothermia inhibits coagulation and alters platelet function. Arterial hypertension should be aggressively treated in the first 24 hours with short-acting drugs. Even if transfusion affects long-term outcome,[34-36] one should not be afraid to transfuse blood components: packed red blood cells, platelets, and plasma are to be given in a bleeding patient even before coagulation results are available. Correction of fluid deficits with crystalloid or colloid infusion induces some degree of hemodilution, contributing to altered hemostasis. If the patient is bleeding, correcting hemostasis according to lab results actually corrects a past situation, so blood components must be given on an empirical basis. When the coagulation tests are available, specific measures are taken; prolonged partial thromboplastin time (PTT) should be treated with a protamine supplement first, before fresh frozen plasma (FFP) is considered. Whereas prolonged prothrombin time is treated with FFP and cryoprecipitate, low platelet count should be corrected by platelet transfusion. A normal platelet count does not exclude platelet dysfunction, so a platelet transfusion may be indicated even in the presence of a normal platelet count if the patient had been treated by antiplatelet agents, is uremic, or is suspected of von Willebrand disease. In the latter patients, the use of desmopressin is warranted. The use of aprotinin, once commonly given to reduce bleeding in cardiac surgery, has been abandoned in view of its serious side effects.

Blood losses must be monitored as long as drains are in place. Reoperation must be considered if the bleeding rate exceeds 300 mL/h for 3 consecutive hours or 1000 mL/h during the first 4 to 5 hours after the procedure in adult patients. Early reexploration for bleeding is indicated in 0.5% to 5% of cardiac surgery patients, depending on institutional criteria. Early reoperation generally stops the bleeding even if no bleeding origin is found.

Cardiac tamponade may occur if excessive bleeding persists. To prevent it, chest drainage must be placed properly in the operating room, and aspiration must be applied early to avoid blood accumulation in the pericardium and pleural space. Hypotension and pulsus paradoxus are early signs of tamponade; suspicion should be high if the bleeding abruptly decreases, and transesophageal echo is mandatory to diagnose it. Tamponade can result from circumferential effusion or from a local hematoma compressing the left or right atrium. Delayed cardiac tamponade may also occur within days after cardiac surgery. If required, drainage is performed via a reopening of the incision below the xiphoid process.

MYOCARDIAL DYSFUNCTION AFTER CARDIAC SURGERY

Most cardiac interventions are done under cardiac arrest; the heart is isolated from the circulation and hence not perfused for some time, causing ischemia-reperfusion injury. Schematically, there is an overload of intracellular calcium during ischemia and generation of reactive oxygen species during reperfusion. This cellular environment is responsible for various protein activation, leading to depressed cellular contractility (myocardial stunning), apoptosis, or cell necrosis. Various forms of myocardial protection have been developed to prevent myocardial injury, including intermittent cross-clamping, cold crystalloid, or cold or warm blood cardioplegia. While cold blood cardioplegia is the most used technique worldwide, it should be emphasized that there is no definitive evidence favoring one strategy over another.[37,38] Failing to protect the myocardium during surgery leads to 2% to 7% of diffuse ventricular failure. Although most patients will respond to inotropic support and recover global function after a few hours or a few days—depending on the extent of injury—patients with extensive apoptosis and necrosis evidenced as cardiac marker elevation will have a statistical survival impairment. Patients with preoperative cardiac dysfunction and diffuse coronary disease are more at risk for myocardial protection deficit. Segmental myocardial zones might be electively damaged in incomplete revascularization, technical failure to complete anastomoses, or distal disease impeding delivery of the cardioplegic solution. STEMI and NSTEMI may occur, requiring specific treatment, possibly including the need for coronary angiogram. Electrocardiographic (ECG) interpretation is difficult in the perioperative period, and biomarker assays are delayed.[39] Liberal use of echocardiography is advised to discern segmental ischemia from diffuse dysfunction; any other causes of low cardiac output will be diagnosed along.

Treatment involves preload, afterload, and rhythm optimization and administration of inotropic agents like dobutamine and levosimendan.[40] Should all these measures fail, the use of mechanical devices to support the circulation is indicated. All devices have advantages and risks. The first device generally considered is the intraaortic balloon pump (IABP). Contraindications include aortic regurgitation, dissecting thoracic aortic aneurysm, and synthetic thoracic aortic graft. At best, cardiac output may be increased by 20% by an IABP, depending on the extent of myocardial injury and preexisting myocardial function. If the IABP fails to increase cardiac output to a sufficient level, one should consider the insertion of an extracorporeal membrane oxygenation[41,42] and/or a ventricular assist device.[43,44] These supports generally require anticoagulation to avoid embolic complications and may induce severe hemorrhagic complications.

RIGHT VENTRICULAR FAILURE

In the absence of pulmonary hypertension, the right ventricle plays a marginal role at rest. This is illustrated by the Fontan operation (bypassing the right ventricle) as a successful operation in congenital surgery. Nevertheless, in adult cardiac surgery, pulmonary hypertension is common and can be due to intrinsic disease of the pulmonary vasculature (chronic obstructive pulmonary disease [COPD], etc.) or secondary to left-sided heart disease[45]; hence, patients with pulmonary hypertension, even mild forms, need acceptable right ventricular function to overcome this increased afterload. The right ventricle is more vulnerable to the aggressions of surgery because of less myocardial protection (anatomically less topical cooling, less retroplegic protection).[46,47] Isolated right ventricular failure is observed, and treatment must be tailored: preload optimization (fluids should be administered to bring the central venous pressure up to 15-20 mm Hg); AV conduction through dual-chamber pacing or cardioversion; and postcharge control through avoiding hypoxemia, hypercarbia, acidosis, excessive positive end-expiratory pressure, or inspiratory plateau pressures over 30 mm Hg. One should consider the administration of inhaled nitric oxide (iNO) or prostanoids and the administration of inotropes like dobutamine. Right ventricular failure might also benefit from right ventricular assist devices.

CARDIAC ARRHYTHMIAS

Postoperative cardiac arrhythmias are very frequent and have various causes ranging from even moderate electrolyte imbalances to structural irreversible heart lesions.

Ventricular epicardial pacing wires and often atrial wires are placed during the operation and left for up to 10 postoperative days to help in the treatment of arrhythmia through external pacing. Some patients with cardiac asynchrony and poor ventricles (LVEF < 30%) may benefit from biventricular pacing.[48]

Atrial Arrhythmias

Atrial fibrillation: after open heart procedures, up to 40% of patients may develop atrial fibrillation. Flutter is generally more difficult to treat than fibrillation. Age, previous history of atrial fibrillation, mitral valvular disease, increased left atrial size, right coronary disease, and previous cardiac surgery are risk factors for postoperative atrial fibrillation. Postoperative atrial fibrillation is related to an increase in in-hospital stroke (3.3% versus 1.4% with sinus rhythm) and an increase in long-term mortality in the CABG population, but these observations could be related to underlying comorbidities.[49] Nevertheless, such observations have led to recommendations for prophylactic therapy before surgery or as soon as possible after surgery with beta-blockers in most patients. If beta-blockers are contraindicated, amiodarone can be used in high-risk patients (especially after mitral valve surgery and in those with a history of atrial fibrillation).[50] Although prophylactic therapy decreases the incidence of atrial fibrillation by up to 60%, about one patient out of five will still develop atrial arrhythmias.[51] If hemodynamic instability occurs, aggressive treatment is warranted and mostly achieved through electrical cardioversion with or without pharmacologic support (with ibutilide or amiodarone). If this therapy is ineffective, intravenous esmolol can be given to control heart rate.

In stable patients, spontaneous reversion to sinus rhythm is observed in 80% of patients and 90% by 8 weeks. One treatment option is rate control with beta-blockers and anticoagulation; if atrial fibrillation persists after 48 hours,[52] rhythm control might be preferred when anticoagulation is to be avoided. Class Ia, (quinidine, procainamide) class Ic (propafenone, flecainide), and class III (ibutilide, dofetilide, amiodarone) are equivalent in reversing atrial fibrillation, but class Ia and Ic might increase the atrioventricular (AV) conduction rate transiently, inducing a badly tolerated rapid ventricular response before conversion to sinus rhythm occurs, hence class III should be preferred (except sotalol, considered less effective and not recommended).

A bolus of 5 mg/kg of amiodarone is given initially over 20 minutes, followed by 15 mg/kg during the first 24 hours. Oral therapy is continued for 3 months.[53]

Sinus bradycardia: many patients are appropriately treated perioperatively with beta-blockers, often inducing sinus bradycardia. In the immediate postoperative setting, low cardiac rhythms may be inappropriate; this is easily managed on demand with external pacing wires.

Ventricular Arrhythmias

Ventricular fibrillation (VF) and ventricular tachycardia (VT): ventricular electrical instability occurs after cardiac surgery in 1% to 3% of patients. Perioperative infarction or ischemia may trigger ventricular fibrillation or tachycardia, but reperfusion of a previously under- or unperfused area may be a cause as well. Besides technical difficulties during surgery, common risk factors are low ejection fraction (<40%), previous MI or unstable angina, and revascularization of an artery irrigating a myocardial area not previously collateralized, especially if it is the left anterior descending artery (such revascularization brings flow to a formerly poorly perfused territory and is prone to arrhythmic induction). Patients with sustained VT/VF, once classical measures of life support (cardiopulmonary resuscitation, defibrillation) have been successfully conducted, should be assessed for ongoing ischemia. Electrolyte imbalances should be promptly corrected, and amiodarone administration is beneficial in the perioperative setting. Electrophysiologic studies are warranted, especially in cases of low LVEF before patient discharge.

Torsades de pointes is a variant of VF/VT promoted through long QT intervals; it is triggered by hypokalemia and by various medication prolonging the QT interval such as haloperidol, droperidol, procainamide, or sotalol. Besides electrical cardioversion, rapid correction of hypokalemia and administration of magnesium sulfate are warranted.

Premature ventricular complexes (isolated bigeminy, trigeminy) are often observed and usually benign. They may result from multiple cardiac and extracardiac triggers (catheters, epicardial leads, inotropes, etc.) and could be promoted by poor myocardial protection. Treatment relies on correction of electrolyte imbalances and atrial overpacing or the administration of amiodarone (or lidocaine).

Conduction Disturbances

About 25% of patients develop conduction disturbances after cardiac surgery. Ischemic and cold injuries are usual suspects, and the block reverses after 1 to 2 days. When left bundle branch block persists, especially in the context of coronary disease, perioperative infarction should be suspected. Aortic valve surgery carries a higher risk for permanent atrioventricular conduction block; extensive decalcification into the annulus can irreversibly interrupt the His bundle, requiring definitive pacemaker placement. Mitral approach through a septal biatrial approach (Guiraudon incision) interrupts the sinus node artery and is also at risk for definitive conduction deficits.

Treatment of conduction disturbances is easily managed with external pacing through temporary epicardial leads.

MEDIASTINITIS AND STERNAL DEHISCENCE

Wound complications and infections are uncommon in cardiac surgery and generally include sternal dehiscence and mediastinitis.[54] Deep sternal wound infection occurs in 1% to 4% of patients after cardiac surgery and has an overall mortality of around 25%. Risk factors of mediastinitis are imperfect aseptic technique, prolonged operative time, harvesting both internal mammary arteries, undrained retrosternal hematoma, insecure sternal closure, obesity, diabetes mellitus, COPD, prolonged mechanical ventilation, long-term corticosteroid treatment, and male gender.[55] Early diagnosis is one of the cornerstones in the management of mediastinitis. The gold-standard treatment in early diagnosed mediastinitis includes early radical débridement to remove all the infected tissue, and closed drainage techniques. Severe mediastinitis necessitates complete sternal resection and associated techniques using omental or bilateral pectoralis major flap transposition to achieve chest stabilization and restore pulmonary function.

PHRENIC NERVE INJURY AND PARALYSIS

Phrenic nerve paralysis may enhance the risk of postoperative respiratory dysfunction (Figure 89-1). Consequences of postoperative phrenic nerve palsy range from asymptomatic radiographic abnormality, to severe respiratory failure requiring prolonged mechanical ventilation, to other associated morbidities and even mortality.

Several conditions may injure the phrenic nerve. The most common is a transient paralysis of the left phrenic nerve related to topical cooling of the heart.

Transient or definitive phrenic nerve injury may be the result of internal mammary artery pedicle mobilization, ductus arteriosus closure, and aortic coarctation surgery. Reoperations in cardiac surgery enhance the risk of phrenic nerve injury, leading even to double phrenic nerve injury.[56]

AORTIC DISSECTION AFTER CARDIAC SURGERY

Acute aortic dissection after cardiac surgery is a feared complication in which the blood leaves the normal aortic channel, the true lumen,

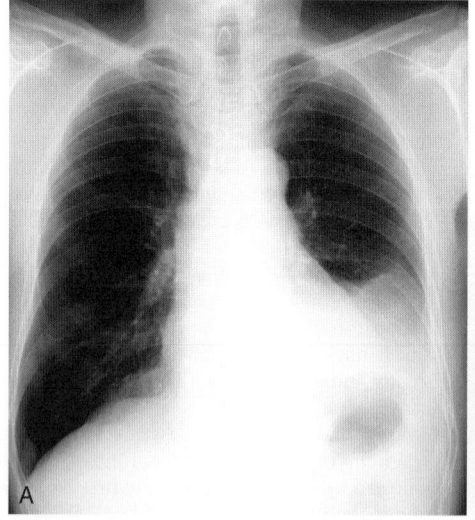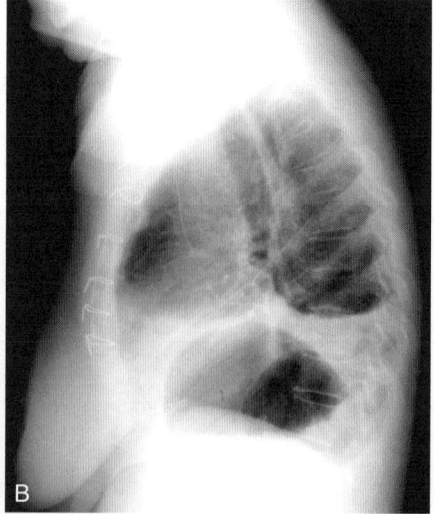

Figure 89-1 A, Posteroanterior chest x-ray of a left phrenic nerve injury after coronary bypass surgery. **B,** Lateral chest x-ray of a left phrenic nerve injury after coronary bypass surgery.

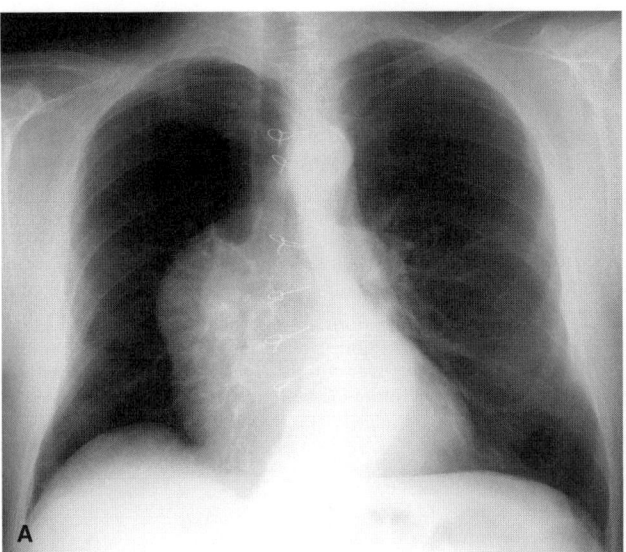
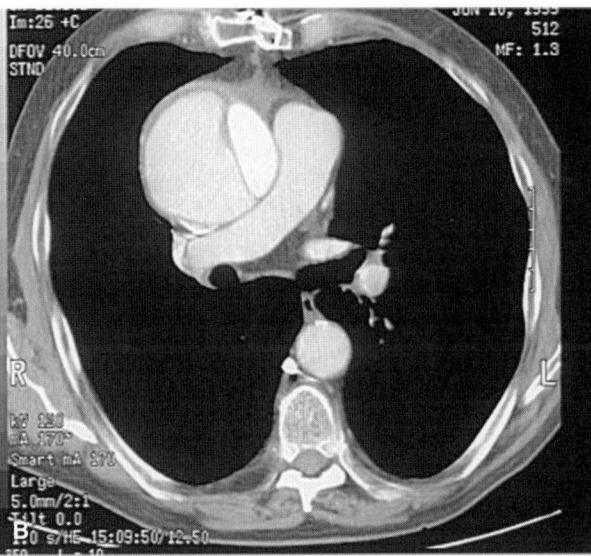

Figure 89-2 **A,** Chest x-ray of a patient with aortic dissection after aortic valve replacement. **B,** Computed tomography scan of a patient with aortic dissection after aortic valve replacement.

and dissects the media to produce a false lumen (Figure 89-2). Cardiac surgery also may lead to aortic dissection. Aorta cannulation or partial clamping in the presence of excessive aortic pressure may induce shear stress and subsequent intimal tears.[57]

Diagnosis

Symptoms are generally due to vessel occlusion. Cardiac ischemia and arrest may occur secondary to coronary arteries shearing off from their aortic origin after aortic dissection. Also, massive hemorrhage may occur after free rupture of the false lumen into the pericardium, pleura, or peritoneum. Aortic valvular incompetence may appear secondary to aortic valve involvement by the dissection. Oliguria or anuria also may appear. Neurologic complications, including stroke (secondary to aortic arch vessel occlusion) and paraplegia (secondary to medullar hypoperfusion), may be observed. During or immediately after cardiac surgery, signs induced by aortic dissection and surgeon visualization of a large adventitial hematoma are important. The gold-standard test to confirm aortic dissection is transesophageal echocardiography, which is easily applicable in the operating room as well as the ICU. The intimal flap is easily identified in the aortic lumen, and Doppler evaluation may help locate the entry point of the dissection. Echocardiography may help to identify aortic valve regurgitation, assess LV contractility, and possibly recognize a pericardial effusion. Computed tomography (CT) with contrast injection also has been used for the diagnosis of aortic dissection and evaluation of the extent of the dissection, including involvement of the abdominal aorta. Complications including stroke, renal hypoperfusion, or mesenteric ischemia also may be diagnosed by CT scan.

Treatment

After diagnosis of an acute postoperative dissection, an aggressive surgical approach is mandatory. Surgery is performed to prevent death from hemorrhage and to reestablish blood flow in nonperfused organs. Limited ascending aortic replacement, associated with intimal tear resection, if any, is the standard procedure for a Stanford A dissection.[29]

LEFT VENTRICULAR RUPTURE AFTER MITRAL VALVE REPLACEMENT

Left ventricular rupture may occur immediately after discontinuing CPB or shortly thereafter in mitral valve replacement. Risk factors are the presence of a small left ventricle, female gender, and advanced age. Excessive papillary muscle traction, decalcification of the mitral annulus, and ventricular mobilization (especially if the apex is tipped up) after valve replacement generally are involved in LV rupture near the posterior atrioventricular groove. This complication, if it occurs in the ICU, is generally fatal.

ORGAN DYSFUNCTION AFTER CARDIAC SURGERY

Pulmonary Dysfunction

Nearly all patients after cardiac surgery with CPB have an increased alveolar-arterial oxygen gradient resulting from right-to-left shunting. Hypoxemia is due to alterations in alveolar-capillary barrier permeability after CPB. Atelectasis also tends to develop, in part because of the absence of pulmonary ventilation during CPB. Left lower lobe atelectasis is the most common.

Risk factors for acute respiratory failure after cardiac surgery[58] include older age (>60 years), pulmonary hypertension, COPD, hemodynamic pulmonary edema due to elevated left atrial pressure, prolonged mechanical ventilation, and phrenic nerve paralysis.[59] Pulmonary dysfunction may lead to acute respiratory distress syndrome (ARDS). Mild pulmonary dysfunction generally resolves slowly after the patient is extubated and can be treated with ambulation and breathing exercises, but residual dysfunction may persist 10 days after operation. More severe cases are treated according to the underlying disease (infection, left heart failure, etc.).[60]

Neurologic Complications

After cardiac surgery under CPB, neurologic complications may be attributed to hypoxia, metabolic abnormalities, emboli, or hemorrhage. One may identify two types of complications, occurring with the same frequency[61]: a type 1 complication (3%) is a major focal deficit, stupor, or coma; and a type 2 complication (3%) is intellectual dysfunction. Cautious surgical technique to avoid microemboli shedding, avoidance of perioperative hypotension, placing a sterile ultrasound probe on the aorta to guide the cannulation site (epiaortic ultrasound), and preoperative carotid ultrasound (to screen for patients who could benefit from simultaneous carotid endarterectomy)[62] can be useful to reduce the incidence of neurologic complications.

Renal Dysfunction

Up to 10 % of patients who undergo cardiac surgery with CPB develop renal dysfunction in the postoperative period,[63] as defined by increases in serum creatinine levels above 2 mg/dL; 20% of these patients require dialysis. Overall mortality in those is 20%, and it may increase to 75% in patients who require dialysis. Predictive factors of renal dysfunction include advanced age, history of congestive heart failure, prior bypass surgery, type 1 diabetes, prior renal disease, and preoperative advanced renal dysfunction.[64] The association between preoperative renal dysfunction and adverse events after cardiac surgery has been reported to be stronger if renal dysfunction is defined using creatinine clearance rather than the plasma creatinine concentration, particularly in patients with normal plasma creatinine levels.[65]

KEY POINTS

1. With the progress of medical treatment, patients are referred later to cardiac surgery, they are older, and they present with multiple organ dysfunction. Along with good surgical technique, precise indications and careful postoperative care are essential to a successful cardiac surgery program. Teamwork is crucial.

2. Most procedures include the use of a bypass circuit, with continuous rather than pulsatile flow; the prolonged contact of the blood with extrinsic material and the use of oxygenators are physiologic insults that can induce dysfunction in virtually all organs.

3. Two major complications after cardiac surgery are bleeding and myocardial dysfunction; both require prompt recognition and prompt reaction, with therapeutic decision based on clinical judgment even before lab testing (i.e., transfusion before coagulation results).

ANNOTATED REFERENCES

Yusuf S, Zucker D, Peduzzi P, Fisher LD, Takaro T, Kennedy JW, et al. Effect of coronary artery bypass graft surgery on survival: overview of 10-year results from randomised trials by the Coronary Artery Bypass Graft Surgery Trialists Collaboration. Lancet 1994;344:563-70.

A systematic overview using data from the seven randomized trials that have compared a strategy of initial CABG surgery with one of initial medical therapy to assess the effects on mortality in patients with stable coronary heart disease at 10 years. A strategy of initial CABG surgery is associated with lower mortality than one of medical management with delayed surgery if necessary, especially in high-risk and medium-risk patients with stable coronary heart disease. In low-risk patients, the limited data show a non-significant trend towards greater mortality with CABG.

Enriquez-Sarano M, Avierinos JF, Messika-Zeitoun D, Detaint D, Capps M, Nkomo V, et al. Quantitative determinants of the outcome of asymptomatic mitral regurgitation. N Engl J Med 2005;352:875-83.

A prospective study showing a survival benefit at 5 years for patients with asymptomatic mitral regurgitation, based on quantitative grading of mitral regurgitation. Patients with an effective regurgitant orifice of at least 40 mm² should promptly be considered for cardiac surgery, providing they can be offered a mitral plasty.

David TE, Feindel CM, Bos J. Repair of the aortic valve in patients with aortic insufficiency and aortic root aneurysm. J Thorac Cardiovasc Surg 1995;109:345-51; discussion 351-2.

Since the early 1990s, Dr. David and Sir Yacoub practiced different techniques of aortic valve repair rather than replacement in cases of aortic insuficency, especially in annuloaortic ectasia. This article showed good results of aortic valvuloplasty, not only in terms of feasability and immediate result but also in midterm follow-up. Many surgeons started to follow the road paved by those two leaders, and more complex disease (bicuspid, etc.) were adressed with those techniques. Nowadays, David's operation is a standard of care in annulo-aortic disease.

Elefteriades JA. Natural history of thoracic aortic aneurysms: indications for surgery, and surgical versus nonsurgical risks. Ann Thorac Surg 2002;74:S1877-80.

A pivotal study about the natural history of thoracic aortic aneurysm, with 3000 patient-years of follow-up. The authors recommend intervention for the ascending aorta at 5.5 cm and for the descending aorta at 6.5 cm; those thresholds are still used.

Serruys PW, Morice MC, Kappetein AP, Colombo A, Holmes DR, Mack MJ, et al. Percutaneous coronary intervention versus coronary-artery bypass grafting for severe coronary artery disease. N Engl J Med 2009;360:961-72.

A prospective study comparing PCI and CABG in the modern era (optimal medical treatment and drug-eluting stents) and favoring CABG for patients with three-vessel or left main coronary artery disease. This study introduces a more accurate scoring of coronary lesions: the SYNTAX score.

REFERENCES

Access the complete reference list online at http://www.expertconsult.com.

90

Pathophysiology and Classification of Shock States

MARK E. ASTIZ

Pathophysiology of Shock

Circulatory shock represents a final common pathway of cardiovascular failure. The mortality rate remains high, particularly for patients in cardiogenic and septic shock, for whom the overall mortality rate approximates 50%.[1,2] From a physiologic perspective, *circulatory shock* can be defined as a syndrome in which tissue perfusion is reduced such that blood flow is inadequate to meet cellular metabolic requirements. Clinical manifestations of shock are those of organ hypoperfusion: altered mental status; cool, clammy extremities; decreased blood pressure; decreased pulses; and oliguria.

MECHANISMS UNDERLYING IMPAIRED CARDIOVASCULAR PERFORMANCE

The development of shock is related to alterations in one or more components of the circulatory system that regulate cardiovascular performance. The first component is intravascular volume, which regulates mean circulatory pressures and venous return to the heart. Decreases in intravascular volume limit venous return to the heart and cardiac output. The heart is the second component. Cardiac output is determined by heart rate, contractility, and loading conditions. Abnormalities in rhythm and heart rate may limit cardiac output. Impaired cardiac contractility decreases effective ventricular ejection and compromises stroke volume. Abnormalities in valvular function may also limit cardiac output. The third component is the resistance circuit and consists of the arteriolar bed, where the major decreases in vascular resistance occur. Arteriolar tone plays an important role in ventricular loading conditions, arterial pressure, and the distribution of systemic blood flow. Excessive decreases in arteriolar tone produce hypotension and limit effective organ perfusion, whereas excessive increases in arteriolar tone impede cardiac ejection by increasing ventricular afterload. Differences in arteriolar tone between organs can result in maldistribution of blood flow and mismatching of blood supply with tissue metabolic demands. The capillaries are the fourth component. They are the site of nutrient exchange and fluid flux between the intravascular and extravascular spaces. Increases in capillary permeability result in tissue edema and loss of intravascular volume. Decreases in capillary cross-sectional area, due to either obstruction or impairment in endothelial cell function, compromise nutrient blood flow. The opening of arteriovenous connections which bypass the capillary network may play a role in tissue hypoperfusion. The venules are the fifth component. They are the site of lowest shear stress in the circulatory system, and thus the site most prone to occlusion from alterations in cell rheology. Venular resistance contributes 10% to 15% of total vascular resistance. Increases in venular tone increase capillary hydrostatic pressures, thereby promoting the extravascular movement of fluid. The sixth component is the venous capacitance circuit. More than 80% of the total blood volume resides in the large-capacitance vessels. Increases in venous tone decrease venous capacitance, redistributing blood volume centrally and thereby increasing venous return to the heart. Decreases in venous tone increase venous capacitance and decrease effective arterial blood volume and venous return. The seventh component is mainstream patency. Obstruction of the systemic or pulmonary circuit impedes ventricular ejection, while venous obstruction limits venous return to the ventricles.

HEMODYNAMIC ASSESSMENT

Circulatory performance can be assessed from hemodynamic parameters. A low heart rate may limit cardiac output, whereas increased heart rates can compromise stroke volumes by limiting ventricular filling times. Bradyarrhythmias indicate structural abnormalities, the effects of drugs, hypoxia, or other metabolic stimuli. Severe bradyarrhythmias can also represent reflex-mediated responses, as occurs in cases of severe hemorrhagic shock, acute inferior wall myocardial infarction, and neurocardiogenic syncope (although not a true shock state). Tachyarrhythmias may be due to underlying cardiac disease and pharmacologic or environmental stimuli. Alternatively, increases in heart rate may reflect compensatory responses to maintain cardiac output.

In patients with circulatory shock, blood pressure should be monitored using intravascular measurements. Vasoconstriction due to compensatory mechanisms to maintain arterial pressure and the use of pharmacologic agents limits the accuracy of noninvasive measurements. This is particularly true in hypodynamic forms of circulatory failure.[3]

For most vital organs, autoregulatory and neuronal mechanisms maintain blood flow independent of blood pressure at a mean arterial pressure of 60 to 130 mm Hg.[4] At either higher or lower levels of pressure, blood flow becomes linearly dependent on blood pressure. Diseases such as hypertension can shift this relationship and increase the critical level of arterial pressure required for organ perfusion. Similarly, impaired autoregulatory mechanisms present in a variety of pathologic states expand the range of pressure-dependent blood flow.

The level of arterial pressure is not a reliable indicator of circulatory performance and tissue perfusion.[5,6] In states of hypodynamic circulatory shock, hypotension is a late marker of critical hypoperfusion. As cardiac output falls, blood pressure is initially maintained by increases in peripheral vascular resistance largely mediated by the sympathoadrenal system, and it is only after these mechanisms have been exhausted that hypotension develops. In this setting, tissue hypoperfusion may be present despite normal levels of blood pressure as blood flow is redirected toward more vital organs.[7,8] Conversely, hypotension may exist without evidence of organ hypoperfusion. In some vasodilated states, increases in cardiac output maintain vital organ blood flow despite decreased levels of arterial pressure.

Pulmonary artery wedge pressure and central venous pressure are indirect measures of ventricular preload. These measurements correlate poorly with blood volume, end-diastolic volumes, and fluid responsiveness.[9,10] Filling pressures are determined by ventricular compliance, venous return, and systolic function. Factors such as ventricular interactions, positive airway pressure, and intrinsic cardiac disease may decrease ventricular compliance and lead to an overestimation of ventricular preload.[9] Echocardiographic techniques can provide a more accurate assessment of ventricular loading conditions, while dynamic indicators such as pulse pressure variation or stroke volume variation may provide greater insight as to fluid responsiveness.[11,12]

Cardiac output can be measured by multiple techniques. Pulmonary artery thermodilution has been augmented by less invasive techniques including transpulmonary thermodilution and lithium dilution, echocardiography, esophageal Doppler, and arterial pulse contour analysis. End-systolic pressure-volume measurements are independent of

TABLE 90-1	**Circulatory Shock Hemodynamic Profiles**					
	MAP	PAWP	CO	SVR	SvO₂	Lactate
Hypodynamic						
Hypovolemic hemorrhage, dehydration	↓	↓	↓	↑	↓	↑
Cardiogenic myocardial infarction	↓	↑	↓	↑	↓	↑
Obstructive pulmonary embolism, pericardial tamponade, tension pneumothorax	↓	↔↑	↓	↑	↓	↑
Hyperdynamic						
Distributive sepsis, adrenal insufficiency, anaphylaxis	↓	↔↓	↔↑	↓	↔↑	↑

CO, cardiac output; *MAP*, mean arterial pressure; *PAWP*, pulmonary arterial wedge pressure; *SvO₂*, venous oxygen saturation; *SVR*, systemic vascular resistance.

loading conditions and are the most reliable measurement of cardiac contractility. Echocardiographic measurements and esophageal Doppler can be used to assess ventricular ejection. The response of stroke volume to changes in ventricular loading during fluid infusion is also useful to assess cardiac contractility. However, the adequacy of cardiac output in meeting tissue metabolic demands must be assessed independently by monitoring indices of tissue perfusion and oxygen metabolism. A low cardiac output may be adequate when metabolic requirements are decreased—for example, deep sedation or hypothermia. In contrast, an increased cardiac output may not be adequate when metabolic requirements are increased or maldistribution of blood flow exists, such as in septic shock.

Systemic vascular resistance is an indicator of arterial tone and is calculated from cardiac output and arterial pressure. Increases in systemic vascular resistance are due to vasoconstriction and represent compensatory mechanisms directed at maintaining blood pressure in the setting of decreased cardiac output. Excessive increases in vascular resistance increase ventricular afterload and the impedance to ejection. Decreases in vascular resistance are due to vasodilation, decreases in blood viscosity, or the presence of arteriovenous connections. Vasodilation may be pathologic, as occurs in septic shock and liver disease, or it may be adaptive, as occurs in hyperdynamic stress following major surgery and traumatic injury. Venous tone is much harder to assess clinically. In most cases, changes in venous tone will parallel changes in arterial tone. Modest increases in central venous pressures in the setting of large-volume infusion and the absence of intravascular volume loss suggest decreased venous tone.

▣ Classification of Shock

Hinshaw and Cox proposed a classification of circulatory shock involving four subsets: hypovolemic, cardiogenic, distributive, and obstructive shock.[13] This classification can be simplified into two categories with typical hemodynamic profiles (Table 90-1). The first category is hypodynamic shock, which includes the hypovolemic, cardiogenic, and obstructive shock subsets. The second category, hyperdynamic shock, includes distributive shock.

The central features of hypodynamic shock are a low cardiac index and a high-resistance vasoconstricted state. Increased oxygen extraction and lactic acidosis usually parallel the decrease in cardiac output. In cases of hypodynamic shock, the development of organ dysfunction is directly related to inadequate global blood flow. Common causes of hypovolemic shock are hemorrhage, dehydration, and massive capillary leak. Acute decreases in blood volume of 25% result in tachycardia and orthostatic hypotension, whereas decreases of 40% are associated with significant decreases in systolic blood pressure. Decreased filling pressures are the hallmark of hypovolemic shock, in contrast to

cardiogenic shock where they are elevated. Acute myocardial infarction involving 40% or more of the ventricular mass is the most common cause of cardiogenic shock.[14] Cardiomyopathies and severe valvular lesions are other important causes of cardiogenic shock. Finally, obstructive shock is most commonly due to pericardial tamponade, acute pulmonary embolism, and tension pneumothorax. Since filling pressures are usually increased in these settings (due to outflow obstruction, impaired ventricular filling, and decreased ventricular compliance), distinguishing between obstructive shock and cardiogenic shock can be difficult.

Hyperdynamic circulatory shock is characterized by a high cardiac output and a low-resistance vasodilated state. Filling pressures can be increased or normal depending on volume status and myocardial competence. Common causes of hyperdynamic shock include sepsis, anaphylaxis, some drug intoxications, spinal shock, and adrenal insufficiency. The underlying hemodynamic defect is maldistribution of blood flow and/or blood volume such that effective nutrient blood flow is compromised. In contrast to hypodynamic shock, oxygen extraction may be normal or decreased despite evidence of hypoperfusion.[15] Direct mediator-related effects coupled with tissue hypoperfusion produce cellular injury and organ dysfunction in patients with septic shock.

Considerable overlap may exist between these different syndromes. Early in septic and anaphylactic shock, prior to fluid infusion, a significant hypovolemic component usually exists.[16] Hypovolemia may be present in a small group of patients presenting with shock due to acute myocardial infarction.[17] In the presence of severe sepsis-related myocardial depression, patients with septic shock can develop a hypodynamic profile. Similarly, patients in cardiogenic shock after myocardial infarction and cardiac surgery may demonstrate significant vasodilation due to the activation of mediator cascades while on cardiopulmonary bypass.[1,18]

PROGRESSION OF SHOCK

Critical reductions in tissue perfusion elicit a complex set of reflexes that are directed at maintaining cardiac output and arterial pressure.[4] Activation of the sympathetic system increases heart rate and contractility. The release of catecholamines, angiotensin, vasopressin, and endothelins increases arteriolar and venous tone, thereby increasing arterial blood pressure and shifting blood volume from the capacitance vessels to the central circulation. In addition, blood flow is redirected from skeletal muscle, subcutaneous tissue, and the splanchnic circulation to the heart and brain. Vasopressin and activation of the renin-angiotensin system serve to enhance water and sodium retention, thereby protecting intravascular blood volume.

Progression of the shock state is marked by further declines in blood pressure that compromise coronary perfusion and cardiac performance. Increases in peripheral vascular resistance impede left ventricular ejection by increasing left ventricular afterload. Terminal phases of shock are marked by vasomotor dysfunction characterized by loss of arteriolar tone with paradoxical increased venular resistance. The resulting increase in capillary hydrostatic pressure coupled with increased microvascular permeability leads to a loss of intravascular volume and worsening of the shock state. Leukostasis and changes in erythrocyte rheology further impair microvascular blood flow. In animal models of hemorrhagic shock, a state of irreversible shock evolves from which the animals cannot be successfully resuscitated.[19]

This pathophysiology is altered in patients with hyperdynamic forms of circulatory failure such as septic shock, where inflammatory mediators play a prominent role.[20] These patients are characterized by arterial and venous dilation and increased cardiac output. The influence of vasodilatory substances such as nitric oxide predominates over the effects of endogenous and exogenous vasopressor substances. In some forms of vasodilatory shock, inappropriately low levels of vasopressin and cortisol may contribute to vasodilation and refractoriness

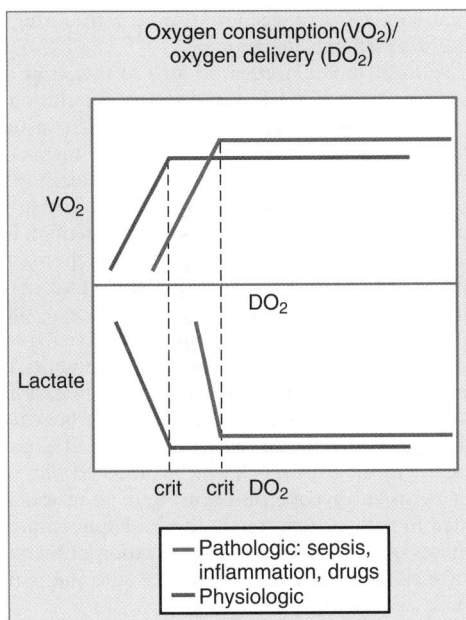

Figure 90-1 **Oxygen consumption/oxygen delivery relationships.** Oxygen consumption (VO_2) is independent of oxygen delivery (DO_2) until a critical level of DO_2 is reached at which oxygen extraction has been maximized. At that level of oxygen delivery (DO_2crit), VO_2 becomes linearly dependant on DO_2, and anaerobic metabolism manifested by lactic acidosis ensues. This relationship shifts upward and to the right when the ability of the tissues to extract oxygen is impaired due to alterations in the distribution of blood flow.

CELLULAR OXIDATIVE METABOLISM

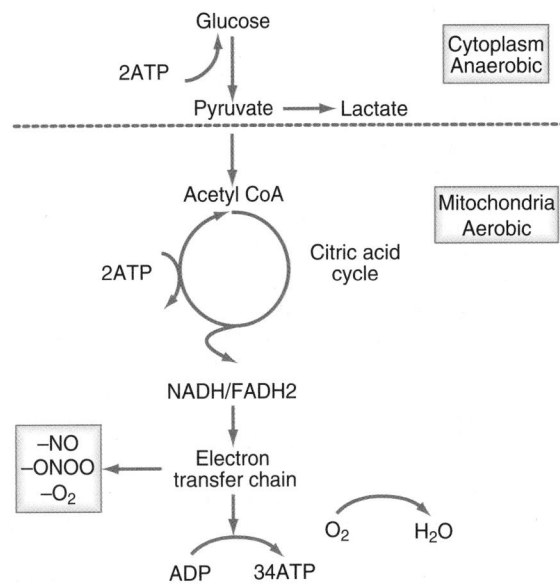

Figure 90-2 **Cellular oxidative metabolism.** Glucose is metabolized anaerobically in the cytoplasm and aerobically in the mitochondria under conditions of normal tissue perfusion. In conditions of shock, high-energy phosphate generation (ATP) is limited to anaerobic pathways. Nitric oxide (NO), peroxynitrite ($ONOO^-$), and superoxide (O_2^-) are potential inhibitors of the electron transfer chain.

to catecholamines.[21,22] Decreases in capillary cross-sectional area due to the interactions of activated leukocytes, platelets, endothelial cells, and the clotting cascade limit effective nutrient blood flow despite the increase in cardiac output.[23,24] Progressive hypotension refractory to fluid infusion and vasopressors results in worsening tissue hypoperfusion, acidosis, and organ failure. A hypodynamic circulation develops as a terminal event.

OXIDATIVE METABOLISM IN SHOCK

The primary metabolic defect in circulatory shock is impaired oxidative metabolism with resulting cellular and organ failure. This impairment is most commonly due to decreases in tissue oxygen supply caused by either global decreases in blood flow or maldistribution of blood flow on a regional or microcirculatory level. Systemic oxygen consumption may initially be increased yet inadequate to meet tissue metabolic requirements; however, the terminal phases of all forms of shock are characterized by decreases in oxygen consumption. In experimental studies, the risk of mortality is directly related to the total amount of accumulated oxygen debt.[25]

Oxygen delivery is determined by cardiac output, hemoglobin concentration, and the arterial oxygen saturation. Under normal circumstances, oxygen consumption is independent of oxygen delivery and cardiac output (Figure 90-1). Increases in cellular oxygen extraction from a normal level of 25% to a maximum of level of 80% maintain oxygen consumption as blood flow is reduced. When oxygen extraction is maximized, a critical level of oxygen delivery (DO_2crit) is reached below which oxygen consumption decreases and anaerobic metabolism ensues. Alterations in vasomotor reflexes due to sepsis or drugs limit maximal oxygen extraction, resulting in critical tissue hypoxia and anaerobic metabolism at higher levels of oxygen delivery.[26,27]

Aerobic adenosine triphosphate (ATP) generation is dependent on glycolysis occurring in the cytoplasm and oxidative phosphorylation

occurring in the mitochondria (Figure 90-2). Under anaerobic conditions, ATP generation is limited to the two ATP generated in the cytoplasm, as compared to the 38 ATP generated aerobically. The decreased entry of pyruvate into the citric acid cycle results in the accumulation of lactic acid and the generation of additional hydrogen ions from the hydrolysis of ATP. Accordingly, the presence of lactic acidosis serves as an indicator of critical cellular deficits in high-energy phosphate metabolism. The normal level of lactate is 0.4 mEq/L to 1.2 mEq/L; levels greater than 2 mEq/L are associated with an increased mortality rate.[28]

Oxidative metabolism may also be impaired by mechanisms independent of tissue hypoperfusion. A number of inflammatory mediators including nitric oxide, endotoxin, oxygen radicals, calcium, and tumor necrosis factor impair mitochondrial function. Mitochondrial abnormalities have been observed in animal models of septic shock and in cases of reperfusion injury.[29] Serum from patients with septic shock inhibits mitochondrial respiration and decreases cellular ATP concentration in vitro.[30] A potential pathway of direct mitochondrial impairment involves nitric oxide and its metabolite, peroxynitrite. Both of these substances can directly impair mitochondrial electron chain complexes.[31]

Accumulation of tissue carbon dioxide (CO_2) parallels the development of oxygen debt in circulatory shock.[32] Clinically, increases in tissue CO_2 levels are manifested by venous hypercapnia and decreases in venous pH. The result is a widening of the arterial-venous CO_2 gradient proportional to the degree of circulatory failure. The normal gradient is less than 5 mm Hg, and it can increase to 40 mm Hg during cardiac arrest.[33] Decreased clearance of CO_2 generated by oxidative processes is responsible for the initial increase in tissue CO_2 levels. With the onset of anaerobic metabolism, tissue CO_2 excess is largely generated from titration of anaerobically derived acids by bicarbonate. The increase in tissue CO_2 levels may have physiologic significance and has been associated with impaired myocardial performance in vitro.

MONITORING PERFUSION FAILURE

Controversy exists over the optimal manner in which to monitor tissue perfusion in patients with circulatory shock. Commonly utilized parameters such as heart rate, arterial pressure, and cardiac output correlate poorly with survival in critically ill patients.[5,6] This is particularly true in patients with septic shock and traumatic injury, in whom underlying deficits in tissue perfusion may exist despite initial resuscitative efforts.[5,34] These observations have led to the use of indices of tissue oxygen metabolism as markers of tissue perfusion and the adequacy of resuscitative efforts.

Mixed venous oxygen saturation (Svo_2) measured on blood taken from the pulmonary artery is used as an index of tissue oxygenation. Venous blood is in equilibrium with the tissues. Mixed venous blood, representing a weighted mean of all the venous effluents, reflects overall tissue oxygenation. Since increased oxygen extraction is the primary compensatory mechanism to maintain oxygen consumption, decreases in Svo_2 are an early marker of compromised tissue perfusion. In cardiogenic shock, Svo_2 tracks cardiac function and systemic perfusion.[35] The same is not true in septic shock and other settings where the relationship between venous blood and tissue oxygenation is altered by maldistribution of blood flow.[15] In these circumstances, the ability of the tissues to extract oxygen is limited by decreases in effective nutrient flow such that Svo_2 may be increased or normal despite the presence of tissue hypoxia and anaerobic metabolism. Accordingly, while mixed venous desaturation is indicative of tissue hypoxia, normal levels do not preclude tissue hypoperfusion.

Central venous oxygen saturation ($Scvo_2$) measured on samples taken from the superior vena cava and right atrium serves as an alternative to Svo_2.[36,37] In critically ill patients, the $Scvo_2$ is generally 5% higher than Svo_2; however, their correlation is inconsistent, depending in part on the location of the tip of the central venous catheter. In one study, patients with septic shock demonstrated improved survival when therapy was titrated to $Scvo_2 \geq 70\%$.[36]

Lactate concentration is a useful marker of critical hypoperfusion. Increases in lactate levels indicate the presence of anaerobic metabolism and tissue energy deficits.[28] Although the initial blood level of lactate has prognostic significance, the inability to clear lactate over time is more discriminating.[38,39] In patients with septic shock, factors other than hypoperfusion may contribute to lactate accumulation. These factors include increased muscle ATPase activity, increased hepatic flux of alanine from skeletal muscle, decreased pyruvate dehydrogenase activity, decreased hepatic clearance of lactate, and dysfunctional mitochondrial respiration. Despite these concerns, increases in lactate concentration are associated with decreases in the intracellular redox potential in patients with septic shock, suggesting that it is a useful marker of cellular energy metabolism.[40] When titration of therapy to $Scvo_2$ above 70% was compared to achieving a lactate clearance of 10% over 6 hours in patients with septic shock, the outcome was similar.[41]

Oxygen consumption and oxygen delivery are global markers of systemic oxygen metabolism. Oxygen consumption, a measure of overall metabolic requirements, is calculated from cardiac index, hemoglobin, and arterial and venous oxygen saturation. It can also be measured directly from expired gases. Oxygen delivery is calculated from cardiac output, hemoglobin, and arterial saturation and is a measure of the total amount of oxygen being delivered to the tissues. Although increased values of oxygen consumption and oxygen delivery have been observed in survivors compared with non-survivors, considerable overlap exists between the two groups. Efforts to titrate therapy to values associated with survival—"optimal goals"—have produced mixed results.[42,43] These differences may in part reflect the varying metabolic requirements of individual patients.

The decrease in CO_2 clearance in circulatory shock is the basis for end-tidal CO_2 and tissue CO_2 measurements. End-tidal CO_2 measurements are useful in monitoring perfusion during cardiopulmonary resuscitation.[44] Cardiac arrest results in marked decreases in pulmonary blood flow and accompanying decreases in CO_2 excretion. Con-sequently, end-tidal CO_2 values move toward zero during arrest and increase with successful resuscitation.

There have been multiple attempts to use measures of local or regional perfusion as indices of overall systemic perfusion. Toe temperature, subcutaneous oxygen tensions, transcutaneous oxygen tension, and laser Doppler are some examples of regional measures previously studied. Gastric tonometry, and more recently sublingual tonometry, have been used to assess those vascular beds for CO_2 excess as a marker of systemic hypoperfusion. Current attention has focused on two measures of microvascular blood flow. One approach is the use of near-infrared spectroscopy (NIRS) to assess the level of oxygenated hemoglobin in thenar skeletal muscle. Both the actual value and the response of tissue hemoglobin saturation to reactive hyperemia have been reported to predict survival.[45,46] The other techniques, orthogonal polarization spectral (OPS) imaging and sidestream dark-field (SDF) imaging, have been used to directly visualize microcirculatory flow. Decreases in capillary blood flow have been observed in patients with septic shock and cardiogenic shock which correlated with survival.[24,47] Evidence of persistent hypoperfusion using these measurements has been reported in patients with septic shock, despite improvement in systemic indices of perfusion.[48] Whether titration of therapy to these measures of local perfusion will impact on outcome remains to be determined.

ORGAN FAILURE

The primary causes of organ dysfunction in circulatory shock are ischemic injury, mediator-related organ dysfunction, and reperfusion injury. Ischemic injury occurs when anaerobic metabolism ensues and high-energy phosphate production falls below the level required for cellular function and membrane integrity. It is the major factor contributing to organ failure in patients with cardiogenic and hypovolemic shock. The direct effect of inflammatory mediators, coupled with an ischemic injury, plays a major role in organ dysfunction in septic shock. Tumor necrosis factor, nitric oxide, and superoxide radicals are examples of mediators directly affecting cellular and organ function. Reperfusion injury occurs upon restoration of tissue perfusion following an absence of blood flow (Figure 90-3). Activated neutrophils, oxygen radicals, endothelial cell dysfunction and apoptosis play important roles in this process.[49] Reperfusion injury may be important in hemorrhagic and traumatic shock; its role in cardiogenic shock and septic shock is less clear.

In cases of acute myocardial infarction shock, cardiac dysfunction is related to ischemia and myocardial necrosis. Reperfusion injury may also play a role in patients following acute coronary revascularization. Cardiac dysfunction is frequently observed in patients in shock. Myocardial depressant substances cause myocardial depression in patients in septic shock and may also play a role in cases of hemorrhagic shock.[50] Down-regulation of β-receptor density and affinity contribute to myocardial failure in sepsis and other syndromes. Increases in pulmonary vascular resistance are the cause of acute right ventricular failure in patients with pulmonary embolism and may also be important in septic shock, particularly when it is complicated by the acute respiratory distress syndrome.

Minute ventilation and respiratory rate increase in patients with shock. Overt respiratory failure may result from pulmonary edema or acute lung injury and leads to additional increases in the work of breathing. Decreased respiratory muscle perfusion coupled with hypoxia contributes to respiratory muscle failure. In patients with septic shock, inflammatory mediators may also directly impair respiratory muscle activity.[51]

Renal dysfunction in shock is related to ischemic and reperfusion injury. Initially, as cardiac output decreases, glomerular filtration is maintained by increases in efferent arteriolar tone. Release of atrial natriuretic peptide due to increased atrial pressures may help protect renal blood flow in patients with cardiogenic shock. However, as shock progresses, the increases in afferent arteriolar tone result in renal ischemia and acute tubular necrosis. Activation of neutrophils, dendritic

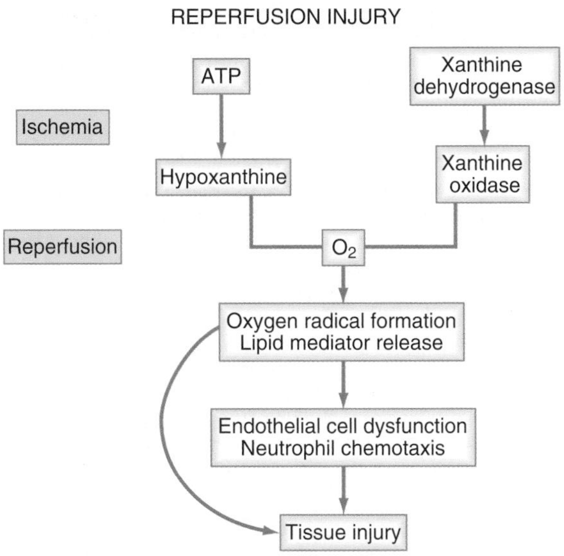

REPERFUSION INJURY

Figure 90-3 Reperfusion injury. Under ischemic conditions, ATP is metabolized to hypoxanthine and xanthine dehydrogenase is converted to xanthine oxidase. During reperfusion, superoxide is produced from hypoxanthine and oxygen by xanthine oxidase. Superoxide and its metabolites produce cellular injury and membrane disruption, resulting in the release of prostanoids and leukotrienes. The lipid mediators and oxygen radicals act as chemoattractants for neutrophils, which injure tissues through the release of elastases, proteases, and additional oxygen radicals.

cells, and lymphocytes during reperfusion all play an important role in renal injury associated with shock.[52] In septic shock, alterations in intrarenal blood flow may also impair effective glomerular filtration.

A characteristic pattern that involves centrilobar necrosis and marked transaminase elevation is observed in patients with ischemic hepatic injury associated with hypodynamic circulatory states.[53] Activation of Kupffer cells and the release of inflammatory mediators exacerbate ischemic injury in patients in septic shock and traumatic shock. In septic shock, canalicular cell function is impaired, resulting in intrahepatic cholestasis. Hepatic metabolic failure and impaired amino acid clearance are also features of septic shock.

Splanchnic mucosal blood flow is compromised early in shock. Intestinal injury may result from hypoperfusion and/or the release of oxygen radicals and activation of neutrophils during reperfusion. Loss of the integrity of the intestinal barrier can lead to translocation of bacteria and toxins, which in turn contributes to organ failure.[54] Splanchnic hypoperfusion related either to shock or to the use of vasopressors also contributes to the development of stress ulceration, acalculous cholecystitis, intestinal necrosis, and pancreatitis. Pancreatic hypoperfusion may also predispose to the release of myocardial depressant factors.

Thrombocytopenia is observed in a majority of patients with septic shock. The coagulation cascade is activated in septic and traumatic shock by the cytokines, tissue factors, and bacterial toxins. Disseminated intravascular coagulation is marked by impaired fibrinolysis and increased consumption of clotting factors. Clinical manifestations are bleeding and microvascular thrombosis. Large-volume asanguineous fluid resuscitation may exacerbate these tendencies by additional hemodilution of clotting factors and platelets. The development of hypothermia will exacerbate coagulopathies in patients with circulatory shock.

Disorientation and delirium are common in patients in shock. Hypotension, metabolic abnormalities, and hypoxia all contribute to neurologic dysfunction. Alterations in cerebral vascular reactivity and direct toxic effects of inflammatory mediators may also play a role in cerebral injury.[55] Severe hypotension, mean arterial pressure well below 60 mm Hg, can result in ischemic injury of the arterial border zones in the cortex and spinal cord.

Microvascular blood flow is impaired in all forms of circulatory failure.[24,47,56] The microcirculation is characterized by heterogeneous blood flow and decreased capillary perfusion. Rheologic abnormalities of neutrophils and erythrocytes impede microvascular blood flow. Increased expression of the neutrophil integrins, platelet P-selectin, and the endothelial cell adhesion molecules result in cellular aggregation and microvascular obstruction. Platelet-fibrin interactions mediated through platelet expression of glycoprotein IIB/IIIA receptors accentuate this process.[23] Decreased endothelial cell nitric oxide synthetase activity impairs normal vasodilatory reflexes and decreases the microvascular response to hypoxia. Increased microvascular permeability and tissue edema may also impede the diffusion of oxygen from the capillaries into the cells.

Shock is associated with down-regulation of immunologic function. Immunosuppressive substances including interleukin (IL)-10, prostaglandin E_2, and adenosine are released and decrease cellular and humoral immunity. Dendritic cell– and monocyte-mediated antigen processing is impaired, as is neutrophil function. Apoptosis of lymphocytes, dendritic cells, and monocytes is increased. An immunologic profile of decreased monocyte HLA-DR expression and impaired monocyte responsiveness to inflammatory stimuli has been associated with an increased risk of secondary infection and mortality.[57,58]

Clinical Aspects of Shock

INITIAL APPROACH TO CIRCULATORY SHOCK

The approach to patients with circulatory shock involves a rapid assessment of the underlying disease process and restoration of cardiopulmonary stability. The patient should be assessed for the cause of the shock syndrome and for evidence of end-organ hypoperfusion. A complete blood cell count, coagulation studies, blood gases, and electrolytes measurement should be performed. Blood lactate measurement is helpful to confirm the severity of perfusion failure. An electrocardiogram and chest radiograph should also be obtained. The need for additional studies such as cultures, cardiac enzymes, and other tests depends on the suspected cause of the shock state. Efforts to achieve cardiopulmonary stability should occur simultaneously. The VIP approach can be used to prioritize these efforts by focusing on *v*entilation, *i*nfusion, and *p*ump activity.[59] A systematic approach that incorporates physiologic endpoints for resuscitation with monitoring indices of systemic perfusion and an algorithm for therapeutic interventions based on the pathophysiology of the underlying shock state results in the best outcomes.[60]

Oxygenation and adequate ventilation must be ensured. High-flow oxygen systems can be employed initially; however, evidence of respiratory muscle fatigue, refractory hypoxia, or severe acidosis should prompt intubation and the initiation of mechanical ventilation. Reduction in the work of breathing may reduce physiologic stress and allow for redistribution of blood flow away from the respiratory muscles to other hypoperfused areas of the body.

Multiple studies have failed to demonstrate a benefit in mortality associated with the use of the pulmonary artery catheter. Less invasive techniques are being utilized to assess cardiac output and function, including transpulmonary thermodilution and lithium dilution, echocardiography, esophageal Doppler, and arterial pulse contour analysis. Nonetheless, information gained from a pulmonary artery catheter can be extremely helpful in guiding management in treating more complicated shock patients, particularly those with combined renal failure and respiratory failure.

Critical hypovolemia is present in the majority of patients presenting with circulatory shock in the medical-surgical setting and a significant portion of patients presenting with shock and acute myocardial infarction. Fluids should be infused in boluses and titrated to specific endpoints of heart rate, blood pressure, urine output, central venous or mixed venous saturation, and clearance of blood lactate. Determining the adequacy of fluid infusion based on intracavitary measurements such as central venous pressure may be difficult and should be guided by dynamic measurements when possible.[10-12] Attention should be given to the hemoglobin level, which will decrease with significant asanguineous fluid resuscitation. Although many patients tolerate a hemoglobin level of 7 g/dL to 10 g/dL, higher levels may be required in patients with cardiac dysfunction.

Disturbances of cardiac rhythm should be addressed rapidly. Bradycardia associated with hypotension may require a pacemaker or pharmacologic therapy to increase the heart rate. Tachyarrhythmias that are not compensatory may require cardioversion. In the appropriate clinical setting, consideration should always be given to possible cardiac tamponade and tension pneumothorax, since these are rapidly reversible causes of shock.

Continued evidence of hypoperfusion despite initial resuscitation efforts requires the initiation of vasoactive drugs. The choice of agents should be predicated on the goal of therapy. Persistent hypotension requires the use of a pressor agent such as norepinephrine to restore blood pressure to a level of mean arterial pressure associated with adequate end-organ perfusion. For many patients, this will be a mean arterial pressure from 60 to 70 mm Hg, which is within the autoregulatory range for most organs; however, this level may vary in individual patients. When hypotension is accompanied by impaired cardiac performance, an inotropic agent such as dobutamine should be added.

The treatment of lactic acidosis with alkali solutions is controversial. Sodium bicarbonate solutions increase serum osmolality and potentially worsen intracellular acidosis as bicarbonate is titrated to CO_2 and water. Prospective randomized trials have not demonstrated any benefit in either oxygen metabolism or circulatory function after alkali infusion for severe lactic acidosis.[61]

Definitive therapy depends on the cause of the shock state and may require additional diagnostic and therapeutic interventions. These efforts should be pursued in a timely manner. Endoscopic or surgical interventions may be required for patients in hemorrhagic and traumatic shock. Circulatory assist devices coupled with prompt efforts at revascularization enhance outcome in patients with cardiogenic shock.[1] Antibiotics and drainage procedures are required for septic shock. Steroids and activated protein C may also benefit patients with septic shock.[22,62] Acute pulmonary embolism and shock can be treated with thrombolysis, catheter embolectomy, or, in more extreme circumstances, surgical embolectomy.

NEWER THERAPIES

There is continuing interest in modulating the activity of inflammatory mediators in septic shock, hemorrhagic shock, and even cardiogenic shock.[1] Similarly there is an ongoing focus on attenuating reperfusion injury through interventions directed at neutrophils, reactive oxygen species, and reactive nitrogen species in multiple settings.[49] Efforts to avoid the adverse sequelae of resuscitation including the use of excessive fluids and the use of fluids that may exacerbate the inflammatory response are being examined. Newer fluids are being developed which, in addition to their volume-expanding capacity, have antiinflammatory activity. The role of the cholinergic antiinflammatory pathway and its manipulation is being elucidated. Hydrogen sulfide is being studied for its antiinflammatory and metabolic effects. Mitochondrial targeted therapies are being investigated in an effort to enhance mitochondrial function and recovery in shock. The role of apoptosis in the development of immune dysfunction and organ failure is being examined, with possible interventions directed at altering this process. Finally, the genetic underpinning of the immune response and its role in circulatory shock is another area of active interest.[63] Progress in this important area will ultimately allow for the development of more focused interventions that have the greatest likelihood of benefiting individual patients.

KEY POINTS

1. The development of shock is related to alterations in one or more components of the circulatory system that regulate cardiovascular performance. These are intravascular volume, cardiac function, arteriolar resistance, the capillary circulation, the venules, the venous capacitance circuit, and mainstream patency.

2. Circulatory performance can be assessed from the cardiac rate and rhythm, arterial blood pressure, cardiac filling pressures, cardiac output, and systemic vascular resistance. Although shock is frequently defined by low pressure, the level of arterial pressure is not a reliable indicator of circulatory performance and tissue perfusion.

3. Circulatory shock can be divided into four subsets: hypovolemic, cardiogenic, distributive, and obstructive shock. This classification can be simplified into two broad categories with typical hemodynamic profiles. The first category is hypodynamic shock, which includes the hypovolemic, cardiogenic, and obstructive shock subsets. The second category, hyperdynamic shock, includes distributive shock. The central features of hypodynamic shock are a low cardiac output and vasoconstriction manifested by a high vascular resistance. Hyperdynamic circulatory shock is characterized by a high cardiac output and vasodilation manifested by a low vascular resistance.

4. Critical reductions in tissue perfusion elicit a complex set of reflexes that are directed at maintaining cardiac output and arterial pressure. Progression of the shock state is marked by declines in blood pressure that compromise coronary perfusion, cardiac performance, and microcirculatory integrity.

5. The primary metabolic defect in circulatory shock is impaired oxidative metabolism. This impairment is most commonly caused by decreases in tissue oxygen supply due to either global decreases in blood flow or maldistribution of blood flow. Cellular oxidative metabolism may also be impaired by mechanisms independent of tissue hypoperfusion. Accumulation of tissue carbon dioxide (CO_2) parallels the development of tissue hypoxia in circulatory shock.

6. Controversy exists over the optimal manner in which to monitor tissue perfusion in patients with circulatory shock. Commonly utilized variables such as heart rate, arterial pressure, and cardiac output correlate poorly with survival in critically ill patients. These observations have led to the use of indices of systemic oxygen metabolism and CO_2 accumulation as markers of tissue perfusion and the adequacy of resuscitative efforts. More recent attention has focused on assessment of microcirculatory blood flow using measures of tissue oxygenation and direct visualization of capillary blood flow.

7. The primary causes of organ dysfunction in circulatory shock are ischemic injury related to tissue hypoperfusion, mediator-related organ dysfunction, and reperfusion injury. The relative importance of these mechanisms varies with the underlying cause of the shock state and the specific organ being examined.

8. The approach to patients with circulatory shock involves a rapid assessment of the underlying disease process and restoration of cardiopulmonary stability. The patient should be assessed for the etiology of the shock syndrome and for evidence of organ hypoperfusion. Simultaneous efforts to achieve cardiopulmonary stability should focus on ventilation, fluid infusion, and cardiac function. Definitive therapy depends on the etiology of the shock state.

9. There are several areas of active experimental interest. Therapies that modulate the activity of proinflammatory mediators and cellular apoptosis are being studied. The genetic underpinning of the immune response and its role in circulatory shock is another area of active interest. Mitochondrial-based interventions are also being examined.

ANNOTATED REFERENCES

Brealey D, Brand M, Hargreaves I, et al. Association between mitochondrial dysfunction and severity and outcome in septic shock. Lancet 2002;360:219-23.

This study was one of the first studies to correlate evidence of mitochondrial dysfunction in patients with septic shock with nitric oxide-mediated pathways.

Hinshaw LB, Cox BG. The fundamental mechanisms of shock. New York: Plenum Press; 1972.

The subsets of shock described in this text form the basis for all subsequent classifications of shock.

Rivers E, Nguyen B, Havstad S, et al. Early goal-directed therapy in the treatment of severe sepsis and septic shock. N Engl J Med 2001;345:1368-77.

This study involves septic hypotensive patients. The study illustrates the importance of an integrated approach to resuscitating patients with shock, which includes hemodynamic and perfusion-related endpoints.

Weil MH, Afifi AA. Experimental and clinical studies in lactate and pyruvate as indicators of the severity of acute circulatory failure (shock). Circulation 1970;41:989-1000.

This is a classic study defining the importance of monitoring lactate in assessing perfusion failure in critically ill patients. A relationship between increased lactate levels and mortality was demonstrated. No added discrimination was observed when lactate levels were compared to lactate/pyruvate ratios.

Weil MH, Rackow EC, Trevino R, et al. Differences in acid-base state between venous and arterial blood during cardiopulmonary resuscitation. N Engl J Med 1986;315:153-6.

This study was one of the first to reexamine the significance of CO_2 accumulation in patients with circulatory failure. Marked increases in mixed venous Pco_2 in patients during cardiac arrest were reported.

REFERENCES

Access the complete reference list online at http://www.expertconsult.com.

91

Resuscitation from Circulatory Shock

BENOÎT VALLET | EMMANUEL ROBIN | GILLES LEBUFFE

Circulatory failure results in a decrease in oxygen delivery (Do_2) associated with a decrease in cellular partial pressure of oxygen (Po_2). When a critical Po_2 value is reached, oxidative phosphorylation is limited and leads to a shift from aerobic to anaerobic metabolism. The result is a rise in cellular and blood lactate concentrations associated with a decrease in adenosine triphosphate (ATP) synthesis. Adenosine diphosphate (ADP) and hydrogen ions accumulate and together with the raised serum lactate level lead to metabolic lactic acidosis. This state is called *dysoxia* and can be accepted as a definition for "shock," a state in which inadequate tissue oxygenation produces cellular injury. Shock often, but not only, results from circulatory failure and decreased Do_2.

Resuscitation from "circulatory shock" requires an emergency and global approach that is based on limited clinical features for establishing diagnosis and probabilistic therapy. The efficacy of this initial therapeutic strategy then becomes part of the diagnostic approach: if the chosen therapy is successful, it confirms the diagnosis retrospectively. This initial diagnostic approach is essentially based on physician knowledge of global hemodynamics and oxygen-derived parameters. It can be helped by rapidly available oxygen-derived biological markers.

Understanding Underlying Pathophysiology of Global Flow and Oxygen Delivery

ADDRESSING GLOBAL ADEQUACY OF TISSUE OXYGENATION

Adequacy of tissue oxygenation is defined as an adapted oxygen supply (or Do_2) to oxygen demand.[1] Oxygen demand varies according to tissue type and according to time. Although oxygen demand cannot be measured or calculated, oxygen uptake or consumption ($\dot{V}o_2$) and Do_2 both can be quantified; they are linked by a simple relationship:

$$\dot{V}o_2 = Do_2 \times ERo_2$$

where ERo_2 represents oxygen extraction ratio (ERo_2 in %; $\dot{V}o_2$ and Do_2 in mL O_2/kg/min). Do_2 represents the total flow of oxygen in the arterial blood and is given as the product of cardiac output ($\dot{Q}$) by arterial oxygen content (Cao_2):

$$Do_2 = \dot{Q} \times Cao_2$$

with Cao_2 being the product of hemoglobin (Hb, g/100 mL) by arterial oxygen saturation (Sao_2, %) and Hb O_2 capacity (1.39 mL O_2/g Hb): $Cao_2 = Hb \times Sao_2 \times 1.39$.

Under physiologic control, oxygen demand equals $\dot{V}o_2$ ($\approx$2.4 mL O_2/kg/min for a 12 mL O_2/kg/min Do_2, which corresponds to a 20% ERo_2). The rate of oxygen delivered by blood is physiologically larger than the rate of $\dot{V}o_2$: Do_2 is adapted to oxygen demand. When oxygen demand increases (e.g., during exercise), Do_2 has to adapt and increase.

During circulatory shock and/or severe hypoxemia, as Do_2 declines secondary to a decrease in $\dot{Q}$ and/or a decrease in Cao_2, $\dot{V}o_2$ can be maintained by a compensatory increase in ERo_2, $\dot{V}o_2$ and Do_2 remaining therefore independent. But as Do_2 falls further, a critical point (DO_2 crit) is reached; ERo_2 can no longer compensate for this fall in Do_2, and at this critical level, $\dot{V}o_2$ becomes DO_2 dependent (Figure 91-1). At this DO_2 crit (4 mL/kg/min), for a $\dot{V}o_2$ of about 2.4 mL/kg/min, ERo_2 reaches its critical point (ERO_2 crit) of 60%. When $\dot{V}o_2$ is higher, DO_2 crit is higher as well. Increase in oxygen extraction occurs via two fundamental adaptive mechanisms[2]: (1) redistribution of blood flow among organs via an increase in sympathetic adrenergic tone and central vascular contraction (this is responsible for a decreased perfusion in organs with low ERo_2, such as the skin and splanchnic area, and a maintained perfusion in organs with high ERo_2, such as heart and brain); and (2) capillary recruitment within organs responsible for peripheral vasodilation (opposite to central vasoconstriction).

USING MIXED VENOUS OXYGEN SATURATION TO ASSESS ADEQUACY OF GLOBAL TISSUE OXYGENATION

In the clinical setting, mixed venous oxygen saturation (Svo_2) can be used for assessing whole-body $\dot{V}o_2$-to-Do_2 relationships. Indeed, according to the Fick equation, tissue $\dot{V}o_2$ is proportional to cardiac output:

$$\dot{V}o_2 = cardiac\ output \times (Cao_2 - Cvo_2)$$

where Cvo_2 is mixed venous blood oxygen content. To some extent, $\dot{V}o_2$ is approximately equal to cardiac output $\times$ ($Sao_2 - Svo_2$) $\times$ Hb $\times$ 1.39, and Svo_2 is approximately equal to $Sao_2 - \dot{V}o_2/(\dot{Q} \times Hb \times 1.39)$.

Four situations can be responsible for a decrease in Svo_2: a decrease in Sao_2 (hypoxemia), in Hb (anemia) or in cardiac output, or an increase in $\dot{V}o_2$ (like in exercise). At DO_2 crit, Svo_2 is about 40% (Svo_2 crit) with an ERo_2 of 60% and a Sao_2 of 100%. This Svo_2 crit has been identified in humans.[3] It is important to emphasize that for the same decrease in Cao_2 (induced by a decrease of Hb or Sao_2), the decrease in Svo_2 will be more pronounced if cardiac output cannot adapt. Hence, Svo_2 represents adequacy of global flow to Cao_2 decrease. A 40% Svo_2 can be taken as an imbalance between arterial blood oxygen supply and tissue oxygen demand with evident risk of dysoxia. In the clinical setting, a decrease of Svo_2 of 5% from its normal value (77%-65%) is representative of a significant fall in Do_2 and/or an increase in oxygen demand (Figure 91-2). If initial probabilistic treatment (fluid resuscitation and/or low-dose inotropes and/or red blood cell transfusion) does not allow Svo_2 to be restored to a minimal 65%, Hb, Sao_2, and cardiac output should then be individually measured to introduce the appropriate treatment.

ASSESSING GLOBAL FLOW

Global flow (i.e., cardiac output) is dependent on preload, myocardial contractility, afterload, and heart rate. Regional flow distribution is not homogeneous and is dependent on central and peripheral vascular tone, which ultimately results in the composite systemic vascular resistances (SVR). As an oversimplification, mean arterial pressure (MAP) can be estimated as the product of cardiac output by SVR. When flow decreases, MAP remains stable when SVR increases; this corresponds to increased sympathetic adrenergic tone and central vascular contraction in low ERo_2 organs, and preserved peripheral vasodilation in high ERo_2 organs. Overall, ERo_2 increases and Svo_2 decreases.

Minimal data exist to guide selection of the threshold for blood pressure maintenance. Arbitrary values of a systolic blood pressure of

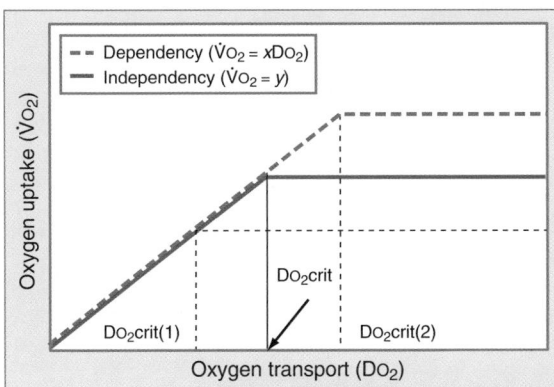

Figure 91-1 O₂ uptake (V̇O₂)-to-O₂ supply (DO₂) relationship. When V̇O₂ is supply independent ("independency") following the relation V̇O₂ = y, whole body O₂ needs are met. When V̇O₂ becomes DO₂ dependent ("dependency") according to the relation V̇O₂ = x DO₂, V̇O₂ starts to be linearly dependent on DO₂ at the critical DO₂ value (DO₂ crit), which corresponds to dysoxia (insufficient ATP synthesis as related to needs) and shock state. DO₂ crit is influenced by global organism O₂ needs: when V̇O₂ is decreased (e.g., by rest, sedation, hypothermia), the DO₂ crit is decreased as well *(lower dotted line; DO₂ crit[1])*; conversely, increased V̇O₂ (e.g., by increased muscle activity, awakening, hyperthermia, sepsis) is associated with increased DO₂ crit *(upper dotted line; DO₂ crit[2])*.

90 mm Hg or a MAP of 60 to 65 mm Hg have traditionally been chosen. Observation of an inappropriate tissue perfusion (e.g., raised blood lactate level, metabolic acidosis, Svo₂ lower than 65%, decreased urinary flow) and its persistence despite probabilistic therapy (fluid, low-dose inotropes, red blood cells) should lead to optimizing flow according to the Frank-Starling curve. This can be assessed by invasive and noninvasive investigative procedures (see later).

During circulatory shock, V̇o₂-to-Do₂ dependency with a rise in blood lactate levels implies oxygen debt. Several authors have reported that oxygen debt is related to the likelihood of multiple organ failure and mortality in postoperative or polytrauma patients.[4,5] Patients who survive multiple organ failure have been shown to have higher cardiac index, lower SVR, higher V̇o₂, and higher Svo₂ than nonsurvivors.[6,7] Rixen and Siegel[5] demonstrated that the degree of tissue oxygen debt is related to an enhanced inflammatory response, associated with an increased risk of acute respiratory distress syndrome and higher mortality rates.

Recent research has emphasized the potential interest of central venous oxygen saturation (Scvo₂) for detecting global oxygenation impairment.[7] Experimental studies reported that changes in Svo₂ and Scvo₂ closely reflect circulatory disturbances during periods of hypoxia, hemorrhage, and subsequent resuscitation (Scvo₂ being approximately 5% higher than Svo₂ in the critically ill). Fluctuations in these two parameters correlated relatively well, although absolute values differed.[8] Finally, observational data found Scvo₂ to be a useful parameter in detecting occult tissue hypoperfusion in both sepsis and cardiac failure.[9,10] An important feature with Scvo₂ monitoring is that Scvo₂ can be continuously provided by central venous catheters equipped with optic fibers (e.g., PreSep oximetry catheter [Edwards Lifesciences, Irvine, California]). In initial resuscitation of circulatory shock, insertion of a central venous catheter is a standard, rapid, and easy approach, much easier than any other invasive hemodynamic monitoring, especially in patients who are not yet sedated, intubated, and ventilated.

In a landmark trial by Rivers et al., patients with severe sepsis and septic shock admitted to the emergency department were randomized to standard therapy (n = 133) or to early goal-directed therapy (n = 130) targeted to achieve a central Scvo₂ of greater than 70%.[11] Standard therapy included antibiotics, fluid resuscitation, and vasoactive drugs to achieve a central venous pressure between 8 and 12 mm Hg, MAP greater than 65 mm Hg, and urine output greater than 0.5 mL/kg/h. Patients in the early goal-directed therapy group, in addition to the standard goals, had to reach an Scvo₂ of greater than 70% by optimizing fluid administration, hematocrit above 30%, and/or prescription of an inotrope (dobutamine < 20 μg/kg/min). Initial Scvo₂ in both groups was quite low (49 ± 12%), confirming that severe sepsis is hypodynamic before any fluid resuscitation has started. This study demonstrated a significant reduction in hospital mortality: 30.5% in the early goal-directed therapy group compared with 46.5% in the standard therapy group (P = .009). An important point in this study is that 99.2% of patients receiving early goal-directed therapy achieved their hemodynamic goals within the first 6 hours, compared with 86% of those receiving standard therapy. From the first to the 72nd hour, total fluid loading was not different between the two groups (approximately 13,400 mL); in contrast, from the first to the seventh hour, the amount of fluid received was significantly larger in the early goal-directed therapy patients (approximately 5000 mL versus 3500 mL). In the follow-up period between the seventh and the 72nd hour, in patients receiving early goal-directed therapy, mean Scvo₂ was higher (70.6 ± 10.7% versus 65.3 ± 11.4%; P = .02), mean arterial pH was higher (7.40 ± 0.12 versus 7.36 ± 0.12; P = .02), and lactate plasma levels were lower (3.0 ± 4.4 mmol/L versus 3.9 ± 4.4 mmol/L; P = .02), as was base excess (2.0 ± 6.6 mmol/L versus 5.1 ± 6.7 mmol/L; P = .02). The multiple organ failure score was significantly altered in patients receiving standard therapy when compared with early goal-directed therapy patients. This was the first study demonstrating that early identification of patients with sepsis, associated with early initiation of

Figure 91-2 Venous O₂ saturation (Svo₂)-to-cardiac index (CI) relationship. According to the modified Fick equation, the relationship Svo₂/CI is curvilinear. Subsequently, when O₂ uptake (V̇o₂) is constant, CI variations lead to large variations in Svo₂ when the initial CI value is low. In contrast, when initial CI values are already high, CI variations do not influence Svo₂ very much. These relationships are modified when CI variations are associated with large modifications in V̇o₂.

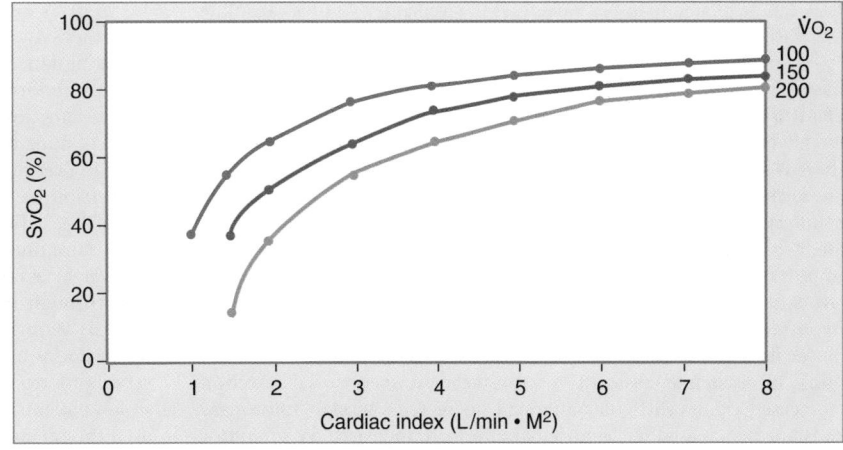

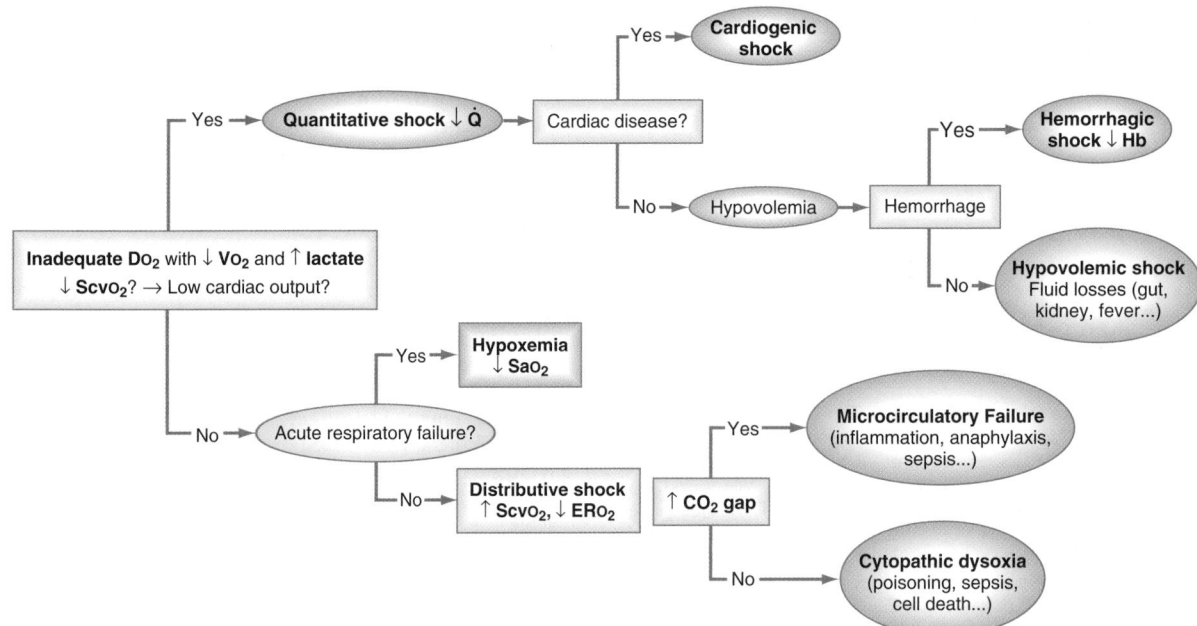

Figure 91-3 **Initial interpretation of a shock state.** CO_2 gap, central venous-to-arterial CO_2 difference; DO_2, O_2 supply; ERO_2, oxygen extraction ratio; *Hb*, hemoglobin; SaO_2, O_2 arterial saturation; $ScvO_2$, central venous O_2 saturation; $\dot{Q}$, cardiac output; $\dot{V}O_2$, O_2 uptake.

goal-directed therapy to achieve adequate tissue oxygenation by O_2 delivery ($ScvO_2$ monitoring), significantly improves mortality rates.[11] This study was then supported by more than 10 following trials,[12] and further multicentric prospective studies are under way.

Deciding Diagnostic and Treatment Strategy

Treatment strategy relies on shock definition (dysoxia) and starts with an early and rapid estimation of O_2 deficit, rapidly followed by an early probabilistic treatment (Figure 91-3). The response to this early probabilistic treatment (modification of lactate, arterial pH, $ScvO_2$ or SvO_2) then suggests which complementary investigation should be conducted (e.g., echocardiography, esophageal Doppler, computed tomography [CT] scan) and which type of monitoring should be installed (e.g., invasive systolic arterial blood pressure variations, noninvasive or invasive assessment of cardiac output), which will help refine the diagnosis and optimize treatment.

DIAGNOSING SHOCK TYPE

Quantitative Shock (Decreased DO_2)

Decreased Flow (Hypovolemic, Cardiogenic Shock). Decrease in flow can be related to either a decrease in circulatory volume (absolute or relative hypovolemia) or to a failure of the cardiac pump.

Hypovolemia is "absolute" after severe hydration defects, plasma, or blood losses; it can be "relative" when fluid administration is insufficient to compensate a loss in vascular tone in the context of sepsis or anaphylaxis (or use of large doses of sedative drugs). In that context, there is an inadequacy between the content (volume) and the vascular capacity, and abnormal sympathetic tone is associated with an altered capillary recruitment. Relative hypovolemia is therefore often associated with altered redistribution of flow among and within organs. It is important to notice that shock can result from a mixture of quantitative and distributive features and a mixture of absolute and relative hypovolemia.

Cardiac failure can result from either myogenic injury (infectious, viral, or ischemic disease) or "obstacle" to ventricular ejection (increased right ventricular afterload, increased vascular pulmonary resistance, increased left ventricular afterload, increased SVR) and/or a lack of ventricular filling (decreased right or left ventricular preload, valvulopathy, decrease in filling time by tachycardia).

Decreased CaO_2 (Hemorrhagic Shock, Acute Respiratory Failure, Poisoning). A decrease in Hb is not necessarily associated with hypovolemia (hemodilution in which decreased DO_2 remains modest). When associated with an acute hemorrhage (hypovolemia), the decrease in DO_2 is higher inasmuch as the decrease in flow is larger.

Hemoglobin capacity to carry O_2 can also be limited. During carbon monoxide poisoning, a decrease in DO_2 results from a loading competition on Hb between carbon monoxide and O_2 and is "maximized" by abnormal O_2 utilization (carbon monoxide interacts with oxidative phosphorylation) and a decrease in ERO_2 capabilities. In this particular case, shock is both quantitative and distributive.

In an acute respiratory disorder (altered gas exchange or abnormal central or peripheral respiratory control), decreased SaO_2 leads to a decreased CaO_2 and DO_2 as soon as cardiac output can no longer compensate.

Distributive Shock (Decreased ERO_2)

This type of shock is linked to:
- An altered flow redistribution among organs secondary to inflammation, anaphylaxis, or abusive use of sedative agents
- A decrease in capillary recruitment secondary to altered vascular reactivity, increased intravascular coagulation, increased blood cell adhesion, and/or endothelial edema
- An abnormal mitochondrial function (mitochondrial injury or dysfunction) described in "cytopathic hypoxia"[13] or more precisely as cytopathic dysoxia, a situation in which despite sufficient global DO_2, cells cannot synthesize ATP

Distributive shock may coexist with hypovolemic and/or cardiogenic shock. Because decreased ERO_2 is present, an elevated SvO_2 or $ScvO_2$ does not preclude that tissue hypoperfusion no longer exists. It is nevertheless possible to further detect abnormalities in tissue perfusion through bedside microcirculatory exploration or by using the central venous-to-arterial carbon dioxide difference $P(cv\text{-}a)CO_2$ (central venous PCO_2 as a surrogate for mixed venous PCO_2).[14] Central venous-to-arterial PCO_2 above 6 mm Hg can help in detecting septic shock patients who currently may remain inadequately resuscitated even though an $ScvO_2$ above 70% has been reached. In these patients, when compared to those who presented with a $P(cv\text{-}a)co_2$ below 6 mm Hg, cardiac index was much smaller (2.7 ± 0.6 L/min/m^2 versus 4.3 ± 1.6 L/min/m^2), lactate concentration remained higher (7.5 ± 3.7 versus 5.6 ± 3.6 mmol/L), and organ failure score was about to increase over a 24-hour time period. These results support the concept that hemodynamics required further optimization in these patients with impaired ERo_2, and that targeting a $P(cv\text{-}a)co_2$ less than 6 mm Hg could be used as a complementary tool to do so (see Figure 91-3).

DECIDING WHEN TO ADMIT PATIENT TO INTENSIVE CARE UNIT

Admission to the intensive care unit (ICU) is requested when hemodynamic instability is present and requires use of inotropes (inoconstrictors or inodilators). This occurs when shock does not readily respond to initial fluid therapy, requires ventilatory support (with a noninvasive interface or after intubation) or imposes hemofiltration (severe electrolyte disorder, fluid overflow, poisoning), and more generally when invasive procedures become necessary (invasive blood pressure monitoring). A patient becomes eligible for an ICU bed at the time failure of one or more organs develops.

CHOOSING APPROPRIATE MONITORING

The discussion on types of monitoring has no meaning until the cardiorespiratory emergency has been treated. The minimal monitoring device consists of electrocardiography, pulse oximetry, and rapid arterial pressure recordings (every 5 minutes and, at best, continuous and invasive). A central venous catheter allows measurement of central venous pressure, which often cannot help much in deciding fluid administration (except when it remains lower than 5-8 mm Hg), but which facilitates infusion of drugs, crystalloids, or colloids. The central venous line also allows for monitoring and/or sampling of $Scvo_2$ (surrogate for mixed Svo_2) if the catheter is not equipped with optic fibers. Central venous catheters are easier, should be cheaper, and carry less iatrogenic risk than Swan-Ganz catheters.

A Swan-Ganz catheter (with continuous cardiac output and Svo_2 monitoring) and/or any noninvasive flow assessment (transesophageal echography, esophageal Doppler echography) is recommended when optimized cardiac output is doubtful. This requires that some preliminary cardiorespiratory stability has been obtained. In that context, fluid administration should be continued (the heart is preload dependent) until cardiac output increases no further (becomes preload independent). When cardiac output is insufficient to maintain MAP or urine output, when Svo_2 remains low, or when lactate concentration remains elevated, an inotrope should be given. Cardiac echography must be performed in the context of congestive heart failure and/or myocardial ischemia to diagnose ventricular or valvular dysfunction. In the sedated, intubated, and ventilated patient, recordings of systolic pressure variation or pulse pressure variation can be helpful: the heart remains preload dependent until systolic pressure variation is smaller than 10 mm Hg or pulse pressure variation is less than 10%, or both.[15] Arrhythmia and tidal volume below 7 mL/kg limit this type of evaluation.

Iterative blood gas analysis (another approach justifying insertion of an arterial line), metabolic acidosis and lactate concentration evaluation, is a way to assess global tissue oxygenation and completes $Scvo_2$ or Svo_2 information.

▣ Therapeutic Principles: Symptomatic and Etiologic Treatments

SYMPTOMATIC TREATMENT

Emergency therapeutic principles of care need to be decided at the time the initial diagnostic strategy is considered. It is necessary to give supplemental O_2 and ventilatory support in response to acute respiratory failure (acute lung injury, mechanical failure, respiratory distress) either through a face mask or by endotracheal intubation and ventilation. Acute circulatory failure is treated by initial fluid loading in the absence of left ventricular failure (see later). If decreased global contractility is present, inotropic support is considered with either dobutamine or dopamine. In case of anaphylactic shock, emergency treatment is to give intravenous epinephrine to treat allergy-induced vasodilation.

Fluid loading is the first step in treatment, and its first goal is to optimize left ventricular preload to improve Do_2 by increasing cardiac output.[16] There is, however, an associated risk of interstitial edema, in particular pulmonary edema. Unless the patient has an acute lung injury, fluid loading aims at maximizing cardiac output[16] according to the Frank-Starling relationship, decreased lung gas exchange being detected by a decrease in Sao_2 (or by a decrease in its surrogate, pulse oximetry).

Swan-Ganz catheter–derived pulmonary artery occlusion pressure has long been the most used static clinical variable for guiding fluid infusion. In septic shock, it was accepted that maximal cardiac output was obtained for values between 12 and 15 mm Hg.[17] To better estimate left ventricular preload, left ventricular end-diastolic surface has now been proposed. In fact, in the sedated, intubated, and ventilated patient, ventilatory-induced systolic pressure variation predicts increased systolic ejection volume to fluid loading much better than pulmonary artery occlusion pressure.[18]

Synthetic colloids are first-line agents. They may induce less pulmonary edema than crystalloids, especially in patients in septic shock. Crystalloids are recommended as first-line agents during anaphylactic shock. Normalization of hemoglobin concentration, [Hb], by red blood cell transfusion is not required. However, a [Hb] between 8 and 10 g/dL[16] might be preferred in patients with severe sepsis and/or coronary disease and/or decreased cardiac contractility. In those latter cases, decreased [Hb] is not compensated by increased cardiac output, and Do_2 crit is reached more rapidly. In each case targeting a $Scvo_2$ larger than 70% may be a helpful guide for transfusion.[19]

Catecholamines help in restoring perfusion pressure and maintaining cardiac output, thus allowing sufficient Do_2; this should allow regional flow distribution and improved ERo_2. All catecholamines are inotropes; they can be divided into (1) inodilators when they combine inotropic and vasodilatory properties (low-dose dopamine, any dose of dobutamine or dopexamine); or (2) inoconstrictors when they combine inotropic and vasoconstricting properties (high-dose dopamine, any dose of epinephrine or norepinephrine). Inodilators increase flow; inoconstrictors increase perfusion pressure. Because of variable individual sensitivity to catecholamines, dose titration is strongly recommended.[17] More potent vasopressors such as vasopressin have been tested with conflicting results, in particular as regards regional circulation. More recently, in a large multicenter, randomized, double-blind trial, vasopressin showed no benefit as a first-line vasopressor in comparison to norepinephrine in septic shock.[20] It is important to emphasize that a rise in blood pressure may not be a surrogate of clinical benefit. Indeed, in a large placebo-controlled clinical trial, administration of the nonselective nitric oxide inhibitor, N^G-methyl-L-arginine, in septic shock produced both significant increases in blood pressure and significant increases in mortality.[21]

In septic shock, several studies demonstrated that increasing MAP from 65 to 85 mm Hg was associated with no difference in organ perfusion variables.[16] Because increasing blood pressure through vasoconstriction may be associated with a decrease in flow, a tradeoff may exist between raising blood pressure and decreasing cardiac index that will vary depending on the specific vasopressor or combined inotrope/vasopressor.[17] Applying such principles for symptomatic treatment in septic shock patients has resulted in decreasing unadjusted hospital mortality from 37% to 31% over 2 years ($P = .001$). The adjusted odds ratio for mortality improved the longer a site was involved in the Surviving Sepsis Campaign, resulting in an adjusted absolute drop of 0.8% per quarter and 5.4% over 2 years (95% CI, 2.5%-8.4%).[22]

OTHER THERAPEUTIC PRINCIPLES

The importance of correction of metabolic acidosis and the use of intravenous bicarbonate for shock-induced anion gap acidosis have been overemphasized in the past. Indeed, clinical studies, including one randomized, prospective trial, failed to show any hemodynamic benefit from bicarbonate therapy either to increase cardiac output or to decrease vasopressor requirements, regardless of the degree of acidemia. Cardiac function does not appear to be significantly decreased when the arterial pH remains higher than 7.00. Bicarbonate infusion, apart from renal or digestive losses, is therefore not recommended unless the patient has hyperkalemia.[23]

In patients with septic shock, stress-dose (low-dose) steroid therapy (hydrocortisone 200 mg/day) needs to be considered, especially if the decrease in blood pressure requires high or increasing concentrations of vasopressors, once appropriate antibiotics are being given or the infectious site is controlled.[16] Steroid therapy may be weaned once vasopressors are no longer required. Beyond 72 hours, absence of any hemodynamic improvement suggests the hydrocortisone treatment is futile.

Although not oriented toward better circulatory efficacy, a number of treatments are essential in septic shock.[16] Control of the infectious source is essential. Empirical or probabilistic antibiotics must be directed against gram-negative microorganisms but also against potentially resistant pathogens. This justifies double or sometimes triple antibiotherapy. It theoretically offers the following advantages: widening of the spectrum of activity, antibacterial synergy, increased bactericidal speed, and decreased risk for emergent resistant germs.

Prognosis

The main prognostic factors for circulatory shock are the number of organ failures present on admission, the delay to start of treatment, and the response to symptomatic treatment. In cases of septic shock, control of the infectious source and its sensitivity to medical and surgical treatment is essential. The early timing of goal-directed therapy certainly influences the severity of multiple organ failure and the prognosis. This point has been clearly demonstrated by the recent trial and earlier studies from Rivers and his colleagues.[9-12]

KEY POINTS

1. Circulatory shock occurs when a critical cellular partial pressure of oxygen (P_{O_2}) is reached, a state at which inadequate tissue P_{O_2} produces cell dysoxia (cell oxygen consumption and ATP production are oxygen-limited) and injury.

2. Shock often, but not always, results from circulatory failure and decreased oxygen delivery (D_{O_2}).

3. Initial resuscitation from circulatory shock consists of (1) addressing the global adequacy of tissue oxygenation, (2) assessing the global flow, (3) diagnosing the shock type, and (4) deciding the best probabilistic treatment.

4. Treatment aims at (1) reducing preload dependency, (2) restoring cardiac contractility, (3) improving perfusion pressure, (4) reaching oxygen supply-to-oxygen needs independency, and (5) eliminating disease sources (e.g., anaphylaxis, infection, myocardial ischemia).

ANNOTATED REFERENCES

Dellinger RP, Levy MM, Carlet JM, Bion J, Parker MM, Jaeschke R, et al. Surviving Sepsis Campaign: international guidelines for management of severe sepsis and septic shock: 2008. Intensive Care Med 2008;34:17-60.

The objective of the Surviving Sepsis Campaign, an international effort to increase awareness and improve outcome in patients with severe sepsis, was to develop management guidelines for severe sepsis and septic shock that would be of practical use for the bedside clinician. The process included a modified Delphi method, a consensus conference, several subsequent smaller meetings of subgroups and key individuals, teleconferences, and electronic-based discussion among subgroups and among the entire committee. Evidence-based recommendations, with their renewal in 2008, were made in 2004 regarding many aspects of the acute management of sepsis and septic shock that will hopefully translate into improved outcomes for the critically ill patient. The impact of these guidelines was formally tested and published in 2010 (see below).

Levy MM, Dellinger RP, Townsend SR, Linde-Zwirble WT, Marshall JC, Bion J, et al. The Surviving Sepsis Campaign: results of an international guideline-based performance improvement program targeting severe sepsis. Intensive Care Med 2010;36:222-31.

The Surviving Sepsis Campaign (SSC or "the Campaign") developed guidelines for management of severe sepsis and septic shock. A performance improvement initiative targeted changing clinical behavior (process improvement) via bundles based on key SSC guideline recommendations on process improvement and patient outcomes. A multifaceted intervention to facilitate compliance with selected guideline recommendations in the ICU, emergency departments, and wards of individual hospitals and regional hospital networks was implemented voluntarily in the United States, Europe, and South America. Elements of the guidelines were "bundled" into two sets of targets to be completed within 6 hours and within 24 hours. The Campaign was associated with sustained, continuous quality improvement in sepsis care. Although not necessarily cause and effect, a reduction in reported hospital mortality rates was associated with participation. Data from 15,022 subjects at 165 sites (included from January 2005 through March 2008) were analyzed to determine the compliance with bundle targets and association with hospital mortality. Compliance with the entire resuscitation bundle increased linearly from 10.9% in the first site quarter to 31.3% by the end of 2 years (P <.0001). Compliance with the entire management bundle started at 18.4% in the first quarter and increased to 36.1% by the end of 2 years (P = .008). Unadjusted hospital mortality decreased from 37 to 30.8% over 2 years (P = .001). The adjusted odds ratio for mortality improved the longer a site was in the Campaign, resulting in an adjusted absolute drop of 0.8% per quarter and 5.4% over 2 years (95% CI, 2.5%-8.4%).

Michard F, Boussat S, Chemla D, Anguel N, Mercat A, Lecarpentier Y, et al. Relation between respiratory changes in arterial pulse pressure and fluid responsiveness in septic patients with acute circulatory failure. Am J Respir Crit Care Med 2000;162:134-8.

In mechanically ventilated patients with acute circulatory failure related to sepsis, the authors investigated whether the respiratory changes in arterial pulse pressure (ΔPP) could be related to the effects of volume expansion (VE) on cardiac index. It was concluded that in that particular population of patients, analysis of ΔPP is a simple method for predicting and assessing the hemodynamic effects of VE.

Rivers E, Nguyen B, Havstad S, Ressler J, Muzzin A, Knoblich B, et al. Early goal-directed therapy in the treatment of severe sepsis and septic shock. N Engl J Med 2001;345:1368-77.

Goal-directed therapy involves adjustments of cardiac preload, afterload, and contractility to balance oxygen delivery with oxygen demand. The purpose of this study was to evaluate the efficacy of early goal-directed therapy before admission to the ICU. Early goal-directed therapy provided significant benefits with respect to outcome in patients with severe sepsis and septic shock.

Vallée F, Vallet B, Mathe O, Parraguette J, Mari A, Silva S, et al. Central venous-to-arterial carbon dioxide difference: an additional target for goal-directed therapy in septic shock? Intensive Care Med 2008;34:2218-25.

This study tested the hypothesis that, in resuscitated septic shock patients, central venous-to-arterial carbon dioxide difference [P(cv-a)CO₂] may serve as a global index of tissue perfusion when the central venous oxygen saturation (ScvO₂) goal value has already been reached. In a prospective observational study, 50 consecutive septic shock patients with ScvO₂ >70% were included immediately after their admission into the ICU (T0) following early resuscitation in the emergency unit. Patients were separated in Low P(cv-a) CO₂ group (Low gap; n = 26) and High P(cv-a)CO₂ group (High gap; n = 24) according to a threshold of 6 mmHg at T0. Measurements were performed every 6 hours over 12 hours (T0, T6, T12). At T0, there was a significant difference between Low-gap patients and High-gap patients for cardiac index (4.3 ± 1.6 versus 2.7 ± 0.8 L/min/m², P <.0001) but not for ScvO₂ values (78 ± 5 versus 75 ± 5%, P = .07). From T0 to T12, the clearance of lactate was significantly larger for the Low-gap group than for the High-gap group (P <.05), as well as the decrease of SOFA score after 24 hours (P <.01). At T0, T6, and T12, cardiac index and P(cv-a)CO₂ values were inversely correlated (P <.0001). Therefore, when the 70% ScvO₂ goal is reached, the presence of a P(cv-a)CO₂ > 6 mmHg might serve as a useful tool to identify patients who remain inadequately resuscitated.

REFERENCES

Access the complete reference list online at http://www.expertconsult.com.

92

Inotropic Therapy

JEAN-LOUIS TEBOUL | **XAVIER MONNET** | **CHRISTIAN RICHARD**

Rationale for Using Inotropic Therapy in the Critically Ill

On can consider two objectives for inotropic therapy in the critically ill: (1) to restore an adequate cardiac output through an improvement in cardiac function in patients with low blood flow related to reduced myocardial contractility and (2) to achieve supranormal cardiac output values to prevent or reduce complications in some high-risk situations; in this setting, inotropes could be given after volume resuscitation, even in patients with normal myocardial contractility.

USE OF INOTROPES FOR REVERSING IMPAIRED MYOCARDIAL CONTRACTILITY

The first category of situations where inotropic therapy is generally considered includes cardiogenic shock, acute heart failure, or acute exacerbation of chronic heart failure. However, although the use of such therapy in these clinical conditions seems logical on a purely pathophysiologic basis, no demonstration of a beneficial impact on morbidity and mortality can be found in the literature. Moreover, almost all the commercially available inotropes have been shown to be associated with increased mortality rates when given on a long-term basis to patients with chronic heart failure. It has been postulated that the long-term use of inotropes may lead to deterioration of left ventricular function through acceleration of myocardial cell apoptosis.[1] Additionally, the beneficial effects on mortality of agents known to have negative inotropic effects, such as β-blockers, is now well established in patients with chronic heart failure.[2,3] Therefore, inotropic therapy is generally reserved for patients with cardiogenic shock or for patients with advanced heart failure whose condition is refractory to standard therapy including diuretics, digoxin, β-blockers and angiotensin-converting enzyme (ACE) inhibitors. Under these conditions, clinicians can expect short-term positive effects of intravenous (IV) inotropic therapy, allowing cardiovascular stabilization. In patients with refractory heart failure who are candidates for cardiac transplantation, this therapy can be used as a bridge to transplantation. In those with potentially reversible causes of acute heart failure (such as myocardial infarction or acute myocarditis), short-term inotropic therapy must be considered as an appropriate bridge to coronary revascularization or recovery. The development of bedside echocardiography in the intensive care unit (ICU) should allow appropriate use of inotropic therapy, since this method provides a more accurate assessment of systolic cardiac function than traditional invasive methods like pulmonary artery catheterization.

USE OF INOTROPES FOR ACHIEVING SUPRANORMAL LEVELS OF OXYGEN DELIVERY

High-Risk Surgical Patients

The concept of attempting to achieve supranormal hemodynamic end-points emerged from studies in high-risk surgical patients. In a prospective study in high-risk patients undergoing surgery, Shoemaker et al. showed that the use of supranormal hemodynamic values as therapeutic endpoints was associated with a reduction in mortality from 33% to 4%.[4] In the protocol group, dobutamine and dopamine were given as inotropic drugs—even in the absence of evidence of reduced cardiac contractility—when volume resuscitation (and packed red blood cells if necessary) failed to achieve supranormal values of myocardial oxygen delivery (DO_2)[4] $(DO_2 > 600 \text{ mL/min/m}^2)$. In other randomized studies performed in high-risk patients undergoing surgery, the deliberate perioperative increase in DO_2 above supranormal values using fluid infusion and various inotropic drugs (dobutamine, dopamine, epinephrine, dopexamine) were associated with decreased mortality and postoperative complications.[5] It remains unclear, however, whether the benefits were related to the increased DO_2 per se or to other antiinflammatory effects of catecholamines.[6] The issue of drug dose is also essential. A recent meta-analysis has suggested that in the setting of major surgery, dopexamine at low doses but not at high doses could improve outcome.[7] From all these findings, it is reasonable to consider the increase of cardiac output and DO_2 towards supranormal values during the perioperative period in high-risk patients undergoing elective major surgery.

Critically Ill Patients

Whether this therapeutic approach could also be applied to patients admitted to the ICU for established acute illnesses has been a matter of debate. On the one hand, a pathologic myocardial oxygen consumption/oxygen delivery (VO_2/DO_2) dependency, presumably due to impaired oxygen extraction capabilities, has been reported in various categories of acute illnesses such as sepsis[8] and acute respiratory distress syndrome.[9] Such a phenomenon was reported to correlate with the presence of increased blood lactate, a marker of global tissue hypoxia,[8] and to be associated with a poor outcome.[10] This so-called pathologic oxygen consumption/supply dependency would incite the clinician to increase DO_2 towards supranormal values to overpass its critical level. However, such an aggressive therapeutic approach has been seriously questioned since the publication of randomized clinical trials performed in patients with acute illnesses that did not demonstrate any benefit from deliberate manipulation of hemodynamic variables toward values higher than physiologic values.[11,12] In one of these studies, the mortality rate was even higher in the group of patients assigned to receive an aggressive treatment aimed at achieving supranormal values of DO_2.[11] It was postulated that deleterious consequences of the use of high doses of dobutamine in patients of the protocol group were responsible for the increased mortality. It has to be noted that (1) the patients of the protocol group received high doses of the inotropic agent despite the absence of evidence for an altered contractility, and (2) in most of these patients, the aggressive inotropic support failed to achieve the target value of VO_2 (170 mL/min/m²). The analysis of the subgroup of septic patients of this study showed that the survivors were characterized by ability to increase both DO_2 and VO_2 regardless of their group of randomization.[13] The non-survivors were characterized by an inability to increase their VO_2 despite the increase in DO_2, suggesting a more marked impairment of peripheral oxygen extraction in non-survivors than in survivors.[13] In addition, the ability to increase cardiac output and DO_2 was also significantly reduced in non-survivors in comparison with survivors, suggesting a decrease in cardiac reserve in those patients who will die.[13] This is not a surprising finding, since the degree of myocardial dysfunction in septic shock correlates with increased risk of death. In this regard, it has been suggested that the response to a dobutamine challenge could have a prognostic value in septic patients. Indeed, in two prospective studies, survivors were able to increase both VO_2 and DO_2

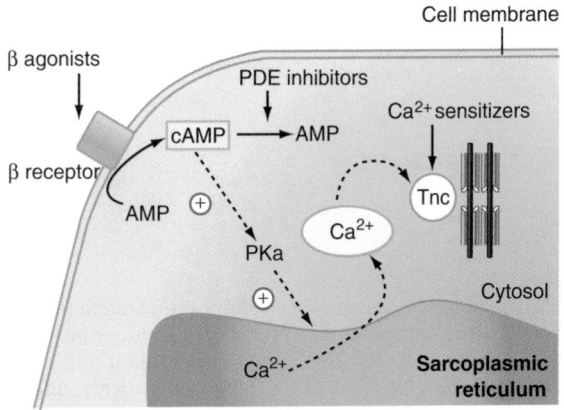

Figure 92-1 **Mechanisms of action of inotropic agents at the cellular level.** Schematic representation. β-Agonist agents fix the β receptor and stimulate formation of cyclic AMP (cAMP) from AMP through adenylate cyclase. Cyclic AMP activates protein kinase A (PKa), which provokes extrusion of Ca^{2+} from the sarcoplasmic reticulum into the cytosol through phosphorylated ryanodine receptors. Ca^{2+} fixes troponin C (Tnc) and finally activates fixation of actin on myosin filaments. Phosphodiesterase (PDE) inhibitors also increase cAMP concentration by inhibiting its degradation. The mechanism by which Ca^{2+} sensitizers increase inotropism is enhancement of troponin C sensitivity for Ca^{2+}. Cardiac myosin activators increase activity of the ATPase of myofibrils, increasing the contractile force of cardiomyocytes without increasing the amount of ATP molecules required for contraction. Istaroxime is a new drug that inhibits Na^+/K^+-ATPase, increasing activity of sarcoendoplasmic reticulum calcium ATPase pump and increasing reuptake of Ca^{2+} by the sarcoplasmic reticulum.

in response to dobutamine, while non-survivors were unable to increase either DO_2 or VO_2 or both.[14,15]

From all the results of randomized controlled studies, the deliberative attempt to achieve supranormal hemodynamic targets in the general population of critically ill patients is no longer recommended.[16,17] However, in the early phase of septic shock when blood flow and DO_2 are generally low, an aggressive hemodynamic therapy including inotropes, aimed at rapidly normalizing DO_2, was demonstrated to result in a better outcome in a randomized control trial.[18] Thus, in the early phase of septic shock and maybe in other acute illnesses, it could be essential to rapidly restore normal global blood flow to avoid further deleterious consequences of systemic hypoperfusion. In later stages of the disease, with inflammatory processes and organ dysfunction already developed, no evidence of benefit from a further increase in DO_2 has been shown. However, it seems likely that cardiac output should be kept in the normal range by using volume and/or inotropes to prevent worsening of the insult.

Pharmacologic Properties of Inotropic Agents

Different inotropic drugs are available. Some of them act on adrenergic receptors located at the surface of cardiomyocytes; others exert their effects within the myocardial cell.

ADRENERGIC SIGNALING

Natural as well as synthetic catecholamines enhance the Ca^{2+} cytosolic amount, which is directly related to the force of contraction (Figure 92-1). Ca^{2+} fixes on the troponin C Ca^{2+}-specific binding site, inducing a conformational change that leads to the fixation of the myosin head to the actin filament. Hydrolysis of the adenosine monophosphate (ATP) molecule located on the myosin head to adenosine diphosphate (ADP) simultaneously induces the flexion of the myosin neck and the shortening of the contractile apparatus.

A rapid overview of the physiologic response to adrenergic-receptor stimulation is essential to understand the pharmacologic properties of these drugs. Receptors of the adrenergic system are classed as α_1, α_2, β_1, β_2, and dopaminergic receptors. Activation of the β_1 receptors, and to a lesser degree the α_1 receptors, is responsible for the inotropic effect of adrenergic agents.

β_1-Adrenergic Receptors

β-Adrenergic receptors are transmembrane proteins located in the sarcolemma. The β_1 receptor subtype is mainly represented in the human heart. Its stimulation induces inotropic, lusitropic, chronotropic, and dromotropic effects, and all these effects result from the enhancement in Ca^{2+} cytosolic concentration. Binding of a β_1-agonist agent to its receptor stimulates the G_s protein. The guanosine diphosphate, normally fixed to the stimulatory α_s subunit of G_s protein, is replaced by guanosine triphosphate, and the α_s-guanosine triphosphate complex binds to adenylcyclase, which then becomes activated. Cyclic adenosine monophosphate (cAMP) is formed from ATP and activates protein kinase A. Protein kinase phosphorylates and activates several cellular structures as follows:

- The ryanodine receptors of the sarcoplasmic reticulum, leading to enhanced extrusion of Ca^{2+} out of the sarcoplasmic reticulum. Indeed, the main part of the Ca^{2+} cytosolic content needed for contraction is provided by the sarcoplasmic Ca^{2+} store. The entry of Ca^{2+} through the membrane L-type channels modifies the molecular conformation of the ryanodine receptor of the sarcoplasmic reticulum. Parts of these ryanodine receptors are Ca^{2+} channels that enable massive release of Ca^{2+} out of the sarcoplasmic reticulum (see Figure 92-1).
- The sarcolemmal L-type Ca^{2+} channels, increasing their opening time. This leads to an increased amount of cytosolic Ca^{2+} available for sarcoplasmic reticulum Ca^{2+} release and for contraction.

The increase in intracytosolic Ca^{2+} concentration also leads to the activation of calmodulin. This ubiquitous protein enables the phosphorylation of other proteins once it has fixed Ca^{2+}:

- The myosin light chain through the myosin light chain ATPase. This phosphorylation enhances the responsiveness of the cardiac contractile protein to Ca^{2+} and helps increase the affinity of myosin for actin, thus participating in the inotropic effect.
- The phospholamban and the sarcolemmal Na^+/Ca^{2+} exchanger, leading to a faster decrease in Ca^{2+} cytosolic concentration after contraction and accounting for the lusitropic effect.

Indeed, relaxation is dependent on Ca^{2+} reuptake by the sarcoplasmic reticulum through the sarcoendoplasmic reticulum calcium ATPase pump. The activity of sarcoendoplasmic reticulum calcium ATPase is normally inhibited by the phospholamban located in the sarcoplasmic reticulum membrane near the Ca^{2+} pump. Phosphorylation of phospholamban relieves this inhibition, and Ca^{2+} uptake by the sarcoplasmic reticulum is thus stimulated.

β_2-Adrenergic Receptors

The β_2 receptor subtype is mainly represented in noncardiac structures. β_2-Adrenergic stimulation induces arterial and venous relaxation. The effects of β_2 stimulation in vascular smooth muscle result from a different activation pathway: once Ca^{2+} intracytosolic amount increases, it fixes the calmodulin regulatory protein, and the Ca^{2+}-calmodulin complex activates the myosin light chain kinase, leading to inhibiting phosphorylation of the myosin light chain, and finally smooth muscle relaxation.

α-Adrenergic Receptors

When an agonist fixes the α_1-receptor, G_h, one of the G-protein family, stimulates phospholipase C, which splits phosphatidyl inositol in inositol triphosphate and 1,2-diacylglycerol. Inositol triphosphate-3 stimulates the release of Ca^{2+} from the sarcoplasmic reticulum. α_2-Adrenoreceptor stimulation inhibits adenylate cyclase and reduces the cAMP intracellular content. α-Adrenoreceptors are not prominent in the cardiac tissue but are in the vascular wall. The cardiac α_1

stimulation induces a positive inotropic effect; α_1 and α_2 stimulation induces a potent arterial and venous constriction.

PHARMACOLOGIC PROPERTIES OF THE INOTROPIC AGENTS USED IN CLINICAL PRACTICE

Epinephrine

Epinephrine is the main physiologic adrenergic hormone of the adrenal medullar gland. It is a potent stimulator of α, β_1, and β_2 receptors. The α-adrenergic effect is responsible for a marked arterial and venous vasoconstriction. Epinephrine increases systolic arterial pressure, but its effect on vasculature is partly counteracted by the β_2-mediated vasodilation. The diastolic blood pressure is thus only slightly affected by epinephrine, and the increase in mean arterial pressure (MAP) is less than with norepinephrine.

Through cardiac β_1 stimulation, epinephrine increases heart rate and inotropism. The combination of the latter effects and the α-mediated venous constriction promoting venous return and cardiac preload results in increase in cardiac output. Epinephrine also facilitates ventricular relaxation and enhanced coronary blood flow through the increase in myocardial VO_2.

Norepinephrine

Norepinephrine is the physiologic mediator released by the postganglionic adrenergic nerves. It is a potent α- and β_1-adrenergic agonist, but it has little activity on β_2 receptors. Through its α-adrenergic effect, norepinephrine induces potent arterial and venous constriction. It increases systolic as well as diastolic blood pressure, left ventricular afterload, venous return, and cardiac filling pressures. The β_1 stimulation results in a positive inotropic effect and an increase in stroke volume. However, the chronotropic effect is counteracted by baroreflex stimulation following vasoconstriction. Consequently, the heart rate is unchanged or reduced, and the cardiac output can be unchanged. Coronary blood flow is enhanced by norepinephrine because of coronary vasodilation secondary to enhanced cardiac metabolism and because of normalization of diastolic blood pressure when low.

Dopamine

Dopamine is the immediate physiologic precursor of norepinephrine and epinephrine. The cardiovascular effects of dopamine are mediated by several types of receptors that are activated at different levels of dopamine concentration and by norepinephrine produced by the transformation of dopamine.

At low rates of administration (<5 μg/kg/min), dopamine activates D_1 receptors located in renal, mesenteric, cerebral, and coronary vessels and induces vasodilation without affecting arterial blood pressure. At higher and intermediate rate of administration (5-10 μg/kg/min), dopamine predominantly stimulates the β_1-adrenergic receptor and thus enhances inotropism and increases heart rate. At such rates of infusion, dopamine increases systolic blood pressure without altering diastolic blood pressure, because stroke volume is enhanced and arterial vascular tone only slightly altered. Norepinephrine resulting from dopamine transformation contributes to these cardiovascular effects. At higher rates of administration (10-20 μg/kg/min), dopamine predominantly activates vascular α_1-adrenergic receptors and induces arterial and venous vasoconstriction, counteracting the D_1-receptor mediated vasodilation. This vasoconstriction increases arterial blood pressure, venous return, and cardiac filling pressures. At higher rates of administration, dopamine hemodynamic effects are similar to those of norepinephrine.

Dobutamine

Dobutamine is a synthetic adrenergic agonist derived from dopamine. Its effects on adrenergic receptors are complex but do not result from endogenous transformation to norepinephrine. Dobutamine simultaneously activates different adrenergic receptors with some opposite effects. In fact, the clinically used drug is a racemic mixture of a ($-$) enantiomer, activating α_1-adrenergic receptors, and a ($+$) enantiomer,

activating β_1 and β_2 receptors. The α_1- and β_1-adrenergic stimulation results in inotropic and chronotropic effects. Dobutamine exerts no intrinsic vascular effect, because the vasoconstriction induced by α_1 stimulation is counteracted by the β_2 vasodilating effect.

Dopexamine

Dopexamine is a synthetic catecholamine inducing β_2 and dopaminergic receptor activation, with no effect on α-adrenergic receptors and a weak direct effect on β_1-adrenergic receptors. It also exerts indirect effects through inhibition of neuronal reuptake of norepinephrine. Its administration induces vasodilation and inotropic effect with substantially increased stroke volume.

Isoproterenol (or Isoprenaline)

Isoproterenol (or isoprenaline) is a potent synthetic β-adrenergic agonist with a very low affinity for α-adrenergic receptors. Through its potent β_2 vasodilating effect it induces a fall in diastolic and mean blood pressure, whereas systolic blood pressure is increased owing to the increase in stroke volume related to its β_1-adrenergic activation. The combination of the latter effect and the marked increase in heart rate leads to enhanced cardiac output. The resulting increase in myocardial VO_2 is not compensated by coronary blood flow enhancement, so isoproterenol infusion may lead to myocardial ischemia, especially if there is preexisting coronary artery disease. Because of its proischemic and hypotensive effects, isoproterenol is no longer used as an inotropic agent in clinical practice in the absence of bradycardia.

Phosphodiesterase Inhibitors

Despite the major role of catecholamines in the management of critically ill patients with inadequate cardiac output, problems such as tachycardia, arrhythmias, increased myocardial VO_2, excessive vasoconstriction, or loss of effectiveness with prolonged exposure to β-agonists may occur. Thus, other inotropic drugs such as phosphodiesterase inhibitors (milrinone and enoximone) have been proposed for the management of myocardial dysfunction. These synthetic drugs inhibit the peak III isoform of phosphodiesterase, which catalyses cAMP (see Figure 92-1). By increasing intracellular cAMP concentration, they induce a potent vasodilation of arterial and venous systems through relaxation of vascular smooth muscle. The left ventricular preload is reduced to a greater extent than with dobutamine. At the cardiac level, phosphodiesterase inhibitors induce an inotropic effect similar to that induced by dobutamine. The heart rate is increased only at high rates of administration. The resulting effect is an increase in cardiac output. Because the enhancement of cAMP intracellular concentration also promotes the reuptake of Ca^{2+} by the sarcoplasmic reticulum, phosphodiesterase inhibitors facilitate ventricular relaxation. Finally, since β-agonists exert their action by increasing the production of cAMP, phosphodiesterase inhibition could enhance their adrenergic effects. This is the pharmacologic basis for the synergic association of β-agonists and phosphodiesterase inhibitors.

Calcium Sensitizers

Calcium sensitizers increase the sensitivity of troponin C for Ca^{2+} and hence the force and duration of the cardiomyocytes' contraction (see Figure 92-1). To date, levosimendan is the only calcium sensitizer approved for clinical use. The advantage of levosimendan over classical inotropes would be to increase the force of contraction without enhancing the influx of Ca^{2+} into the cytosol and thus without increasing the risk of arrhythmias related to this ionic alteration. Some degree of phosphodiesterase III inhibitory activity probably also contributes to the inotropic effect of these drugs. It also induces vasodilation by opening ATP-dependent K^+ channels.[19]

Cardiac Myosin Activators

Cardiac myosin activators belong to a new class of inotropes. They increase the activity of the ATPase of the myofibrils, increasing the contractile force of the cardiomyocytes without increasing the amount of ATP molecules required for contraction—that is, without increasing the myocardial VO_2.[20] Additionally, these substances increase the cardiac contractile force without the potentially deleterious increase in intracytoplasmic Ca^{2+} concentration. Cardiac myosin activators have been tested in animal studies in which their inotropic properties have been well demonstrated. Pharmacologic studies in humans are ongoing.

Istaroxime

Istaroxime is a new drug that inhibits the Na^+/K^+-ATPase, increasing the activity of the sarcoendoplasmic reticulum calcium ATPase pump. It induces some inotropic and lusitropic effects.[21] In animals, istaroxime was demonstrated to decrease the end-diastolic volume of the left ventricle and to increase the left ventricular ejection fraction. In patients with decompensated heart failure without hypotension, istaroxime decreased the pulmonary artery occlusion pressure and improved the diastolic function of the left ventricle.[22] This drug is still under clinical evaluation.

DECREASE IN β-ADRENERGIC RESPONSE

It is well recognized that response to β-adrenergic stimulation is decreased in chronic cardiac failure. This may be a response to increased activity of the sympathetic nervous system, which may itself be a response to reduced cardiac output. Therefore, this negative retrocontrol of the β-adrenergic response could act as a protection against excessive adrenergic stimulation. The cellular mechanisms involved are down-regulation of $β_1$-adrenergic receptors and stimulation of the G_i protein of the adenylcyclase system. The decrease in $β_1$-adrenergic receptors could result from a decrease in β-adrenergic receptor messenger RNA and to an increased internalization and degradation of these receptors. These latter mechanisms are mainly related to the phosphorylation of $β_1$-adrenergic receptors by the β-adrenoreceptor kinase, which is activated. The high level of nitric oxide (NO) production during heart failure also contributes to attenuation of β-adrenergic response. The effects of exogenous catecholamines during exacerbations of chronic heart failure can thus be reduced.

Similarly, there is evidence for a decreased responsiveness of the myocardium to β-adrenergic stimulation during septic shock.[23] This may be explained by the inhibition of adenylcyclase activation due to an overexpression of G_i protein[24] at the gene level.[25]

Hemodynamic Effects of Inotropic Agents in Critically Ill Patients

EFFECTS ON CARDIAC OUTPUT

Dobutamine and Dopamine

Dobutamine and dopamine are the β-adrenergic agents most widely used in critically ill patients when an increase in cardiac output through an increase in myocardial contractility is desired.

In patients with acute heart failure, the effects of these two agents were compared in a crossover trial.[26] Whereas dobutamine (2.5-10 µg/kg/min) increased cardiac output through an increase in stroke volume in a dose-response fashion, dopamine increased stroke volume and cardiac output at 4 µg/kg/min but not at higher doses, presumably because of an increase in left ventricular afterload. It was also reported that pulmonary artery occlusion pressure decreased with dobutamine while it increased with dopamine. Similar findings were observed in patients with respiratory failure in whom dopamine also increased the left ventricular end-diastolic volume measured using isotopes, while dobutamine did not.[27] This suggests an increase in left ventricular preload only with dopamine.

In patients with septic shock, in addition to hypovolemia, severe systemic vasodilation is associated with a variable degree of depressed myocardial contractility.[28] Dopamine at median or high doses has been proposed as one of the first-line catecholamines when arterial pressure remains low despite adequate volume resuscitation,[19] as it can exert

both an α-mediated increase in arterial tone and a β-mediated increase in myocardial contractility. However, it was reported that restoration of an adequate MAP with dopamine was mainly produced by the increase of cardiac output through an increase in stroke volume and, to a lesser extent, increase in heart rate; whereas minimal effects on systemic vascular resistance (SVR) were observed despite relatively high doses of this agent.[29] Dopamine was even demonstrated to increase cardiac output markedly while SVR fell in septic patients without shock.[30] Conversely, in another study in patients with severe septic shock, cardiac output did not increase significantly with dopamine at doses up to 25 µg/kg/min while SVR either did not change or significantly increased.[31] This emphasizes the great heterogeneity in the response to dopamine among septic patients and hence the difficulty to predict clinical hemodynamic effects from pharmacologic properties because of interindividual differences in terms of severity of the insult, underlying diseases, comorbidities, integrity of the neurovegetative status, drugs concomitantly prescribed, and other factors.

In patients with septic shock and depressed myocardial function, dobutamine is expected to increase stroke volume and heart rate owing to its $β_1$-adrenergic properties but a vasodilatory effect owing to its $β_2$-adrenergic properties. Accordingly, an increase in cardiac output and a decrease in SVR with dobutamine were reported in septic patients.[32,33] This emphasizes the need to give a potent vasopressive agent to septic shock patients when dobutamine is administered to support cardiac function in the presence of depressed myocardial contractility. One potential advantage of dobutamine is the decrease in cardiac filling pressures that could allow an additional volume infusion to improve further cardiac output when necessary. A change from dopamine to dobutamine was shown to result in lower right and left ventricular filling pressures and an increase in right ventricular ejection fraction for the same pulmonary artery pressure and right ventricular end-diastolic volume suggesting that dobutamine can exert a more favorable effect on cardiac contractility than dopamine.[34] This has justified the recommendation to give dobutamine rather than dopamine when use of an inotropic drug is judged necessary in patients with severe sepsis or septic shock.[17] However, because of the alteration of the β-adrenergic pathway in the septic heart, the effect on stroke volume and cardiac output of a β-agonist agent such as dobutamine may be attenuated in septic patients in comparison with nonseptic patients. In this regard, infusion of dobutamine at 5 µg/kg/min, a dose able to increase cardiac output substantially in patients with congestive heart failure,[35] has been reported to exert variable effects in the context of sepsis. For example, dobutamine at 5 µg/kg/min was reported to induce a substantial increase in cardiac output in some studies in patients with severe sepsis[32,36] and to have no significant effect on cardiac output in some studies investigating patients with septic shock.[37-41] It is likely that these differences in response to dobutamine were related to various individual factors, including differences in the vasopressor treatment coadministered, in the degree of myocardial depression and/or β-receptor down-regulation. In this regard, Silverman and associates showed that incremental doses of dobutamine (0, 5, 10 µg/kg/min) produced a dose-related increase in cardiac output in septic patients without shock but no positive effect on cardiac output in patients with septic shock, even for the highest dose.[23] Interestingly, they also found that post-β-adrenergic receptor signal transmission was impaired only in patients of the septic shock group and that impairment of β-adrenergic receptor responsiveness found in both groups was significantly more marked in the septic shock group.[23] These findings which allow the divergent results of numerous studies to be reconciled[32,36-43] emphasize the unpredictability of the effects of β-agonist agents in patients with sepsis. It must be stressed that the absence of positive cardiac response to dobutamine seems a marker of poor outcome in septic shock patients.[14,15,40] Because dobutamine also has potentially harmful effects (e.g., myocardial ischemia, cardiac arrhythmias), monitoring its effects on cardiac output to check its efficacy is the minimum required. However, no high-level recommendation on which method of cardiac output monitoring (e.g., pulmonary artery catheter, transesophageal Doppler, pulse contour method) is the more appropriate in this setting is currently available.

Epinephrine and Norepinephrine

Although these agents have β_1-adrenergic properties and thus are able to increase myocardial contractility, they are used as vasoconstrictive agents in cases of severe hypotension, since they also have potent α-adrenergic properties. Yet, significant increases in cardiac output with these drugs, consistent with potent inotropic effects, have been reported in septic patients.[29,44,45] In this regard, norepinephrine was shown to increase cardiac output to the same extent as dopamine for the same increase in MAP.[29] However, analysis of the existing literature indicates that the effects of norepinephrine on cardiac output are highly variable among septic patients.[46,47] By contrast, epinephrine appeared to be a potent inotropic agent in most studies in septic patients.[39,48-50]

Dopexamine

The pharmacologic properties of dopexamine should result in a combination of inotropic, afterload-reducing, and renal-vasodilating effects which could be useful for the management of acute exacerbation of congestive heart failure. In this regard, dopexamine was reported to substantially increase cardiac output in patients with heart failure without altering blood pressure: at doses up to 4 μg/kg/min, the majority of the effects resulted from increase in stroke volume. At higher doses, the increase in heart rate made a greater contribution.[51] In cases of human sepsis, dopexamine produced dose-dependent increases in stroke volume and heart rate but dose-dependent decrease in SVR.[52] This underlines the marked vasodilating effect of this drug, which should not be administered in severe sepsis in the absence of a potent vasopressor. Under these conditions, dopexamine at doses ranging drom 1 to 4 μg/kg/min could still enhance cardiac output without altering blood pressure.[53]

Phosphodiesterase Inhibitors

In patients with heart failure, phosphodiesterase inhibitors significantly increased cardiac output and stroke volume, whereas blood pressure slightly decreased due to decrease in SVR, confirming the combined inotropic and vasodilating effects of these agents.[54] Because of the ability of β-agonist agents to increase cAMP levels, thereby providing increased substrate for phosphodiesterase inhibitors, the combination of these two types of drugs would be attractive. Synergic effects on cardiac output of dobutamine and enoximone have been observed in patients with heart failure.[55]

Calcium Sensitizers

Levosimendan has stimulated many clinical studies during recent years. It is well demonstrated that it can induce some beneficial hemodynamic effects in patients with acute heart failure, enhancing cardiac output and decreasing pulmonary artery occlusion pressure.[56] In the LIDO study, levosimendan was even demonstrated to improve hemodynamic performance more effectively in patients with low-output heart failure.[56] Unlike dobutamine, levosimendan can keep its effects on cardiac performance in patients receiving β-blockers.[56]

EFFECTS ON ARTERIAL OXYGEN CONTENT

The aim of inotropic therapy in critically ill patients with reduced cardiac contractility is not only to increase cardiac output but ultimately to improve DO_2 to the tissues. Thus, attention should also be paid to the effects of these drugs on arterial oxygen content. Inotropes may affect arterial oxygen tension through several mechanisms. First, the reduction of lung filtration pressure resulting from improvement in cardiac function may decrease intrapulmonary shunt fraction and thus improve arterial oxygenation. Second, the increase in cardiac output may result in an increased venous admixture.[57] On the other hand, the increased mixed venous blood oxygen tension resulting from increased cardiac output may improve arterial oxygenation

in the presence of ventilation/perfusion mismatching and thus may compensate for the increased venous admixture. Accordingly, when looking at the published data, it appears that even if venous admixture increased with administration of an inotropic agent, no significant change in arterial oxygen tension was observed.[58,59] Therefore, when an inotropic agent increases cardiac output in critically ill patients, it generally increases DO_2 to the same extent.[29,32,60]

EFFECTS ON TISSUE OXYGEN UTILIZATION

Even though an inotropic agent produces a large increase in DO_2, its effectiveness in reducing oxygen deficit depends on its capacity to provide oxygen in the most hypoxic tissues. This concern is particularly crucial since first, redistribution of blood flow is a characteristic pattern of shock states, and second, inotropic drugs may also have vasoactive properties that interact with blood flow distribution.

Cardiogenic Shock

In this setting, redistribution of flow is recognized as a potent compensatory mechanism which, in response to reduced global DO_2, attempts to deviate blood flow from nonvital organs with low oxygen extraction ratio towards vital organs with oxygen high extraction ratio, such as the heart or brain. It must be kept in mind that administration of drugs with vasoactive properties may interfere with vasoregulation of regional blood flow. The extent to which this interference is beneficial in increasing oxygen supply and VO_2 in hypoxic areas remains speculative. This emphasizes the need to monitor as far as possible perfusion and/or function of critical organs.

Septic Shock

The maldistribution of flow at the macrocirculatory level as well as the microcirculatory level mainly contributes to defective tissue utilization and eventually to tissue oxygen debt in sepsis, even when systemic oxygen transport is greater than normal. Besides sepsis-induced microthrombosis, sepsis-induced alteration in vascular reactivity is a major cause of altered distribution of blood flow between and within organs. In addition, severe sepsis can modify the impact of endogenous catecholamines and adrenergic drugs on regional blood flows, since a depressed vascular responsiveness to vasoactive agents is likely to occur in this setting. This hypothesis may account for the absence of reduction of renal blood flow observed during norepinephrine administration in bacteremic animals in comparison with controls.[60]

In cases of human sepsis, numerous studies examined the effects of adrenergic agents on splanchnic perfusion. Their findings have sometimes varied, either because of differences in the methods used for assessing this regional circulation (e.g., gastric tonometry, laser-Doppler flowmetry, indocyanine green dilution) or because of the heterogeneity of the studied populations (e.g., differences in the severity of the septic insult, in the underlying diseases, in the therapy coadministered). However, from findings of the majority of these studies, some reasonable conclusions can be drawn. First, dobutamine is likely to exert a beneficial effect on the gut mucosal perfusion,[33,38,39,43,61] probably via a β_2-adrenergic effect.[62] Second, dopamine may have deleterious effects on gut mucosal perfusion[29] despite its potential vasodilating action through mesenteric dopaminergic receptors. Third, epinephrine is probably the adrenergic agent with the least desirable effects on the splanchnic vasculature. Most studies showed a lower splanchnic blood flow with epinephrine than norepinephrine alone[63] or in combination with dobutamine,[38,39,64] even for similar global hemodynamic effects. Fourth, dopamine can exert a favorable effect on splanchnic perfusion[65] comparable to that of dobutamine[37] and likely to be related to a β_2-adrenergic effect.

Regarding the effects of inotropic agents on the renal circulation in septic patients, two major points must be kept in mind. First, an α-adrenergic agent such as norepinephrine is able to increase renal blood flow and urine output[31,66-68] despite its potential vasoconstricting effect on the afferent glomerular arteries. This is probably due to the beneficial effect of increasing MAP when the renal blood flow is dependent on arterial pressure, as occurs in the presence of profound systemic hypotension. Otherwise, sepsis-induced depressed responsiveness of afferent glomerular arteries to the action of norepinephrine cannot be excluded. Accordingly, there is no evidence that norepinephrine decreases renal blood flow and urine output when given to septic patients to increase MAP toward normal values. Moreover, it has been demonstrated in patients with septic shock that elevating MAP up to 85 mm Hg with incremental doses of norepinephrine was not associated with a decrease in urine output.[66,69,70] Second, although dopamine at low doses (<5 μg/kg/min) is pharmacologically able to vasodilate renal arteries through its action on dopaminergic receptors, the systematic administration of low doses of dopamine in critically ill patients, including patients with sepsis, does not result in improved outcome[71] and must no longer be recommended.

Catecholamines can also exert proper effects on the microcirculation. Administration of 5 μg/kg/min of dobutamine was demonstrated to improve sublingual microvessel perfusion measured with orthogonal polarizing spectral imaging in patients with septic shock.[72] Interestingly, these changes were independent of changes in systemic hemodynamic variables.[72] Two studies showed no significant effect of increasing MAP with norepinephrine on sublingual microvessels in patients with septic shock who had already been resuscitated.[44,45] However, a possible favorable effect of norepinephrine on microcirculation cannot be excluded when norepinephrine is used to reverse life-threatening hypotension. Finally, inotropic drugs may also exert non-hemodynamic effects that could affect cellular metabolism and/or organ function.[6,73] For example, administration of epinephrine in patients with septic shock was demonstrated to increase blood lactate level independently of tissue hypoxia by stimulation of the skeletal muscle cell Na^+/K^+-ATPase, which accelerates aerobic glycolysis and thus the production of pyruvate and hence of lactate into the cell.[74] This metabolic effect is assumed to be related to activation of the β_2-adrenergic receptors located at the surface of the skeletal muscle cells.[75] In addition, catecholamines may modulate cytokine response to sepsis, trauma, or major surgery through β-adrenergic receptor activation.[6] Whether this effect (inhibition of proinflammatory cytokines and enhancement of proinflammatory cytokine production) plays a beneficial role in the reversal of tissue hypoxia and organ dysfunction remains to be evaluated.

Main Indications for Inotropic Therapy in Patients with Circulatory Failure

ACUTE HEART FAILURE AND CARDIOGENIC SHOCK

In the American College of Cardiology Federation/American Heart Association guidelines, inotropic agents are indicated to improve symptoms and end-organ function in patients with low output syndrome, left ventricular systolic dysfunction, and systolic blood pressure below 90 mm Hg despite adequate filling pressure.[76] In the European Society of Cardiology guidelines, inotropic agents are indicated in patients with values ≤ 100 mm Hg.[77] These indications clearly limit use of inotropic agents only for those patients with acute heart failure and low systolic blood pressure, who are most likely to have increased mortality rates with a strong inverse correlation between systolic blood pressure and survival.[78]

Dopamine is classically recommended as the inotropic agent of choice in the presence of severe hypotension, whereas dobutamine is considered first-line therapy in the presence of predominant pump failure and volume overload but normal or moderately reduced blood pressure.[79,80] Accordingly, the SHOCK trial registry (1190 patients) reported that dopamine and dobutamine were used in 89% and 70%, respectively, of patients with cardiogenic shock due to massive acute myocardial infarction.[81] The combination of dopamine and dobutamine at low doses has been considered a therapy of interest when dobutamine alone fails to restore an adequate MAP in cardiogenic shock. Nowadays, however, the use of dopamine is a matter of debate. In a recent study comparing dopamine and norepinephrine as the first-line vasopressor agent in the treatment of shock, dopamine was associated with a greater number of cardiac arrhythmias.[82] In addition, in a predefined subgroup analysis, the authors reported that dopamine was associated with increased risk of death in the subgroup of 280 patients with cardiogenic shock.[82]

It must be stressed, however, that IV administration of a catecholamine such as dobutamine is associated with an increased risk of death in acute heart failure patients.[83,84] This emphasizes their restrictive use for those patients with severe hypotension and peripheral hypoperfusion.[76,77]

Phosphodiesterase inhibitors have been proposed as an alternative to β-adrenergic agents. However, results of trials of long-term oral phosphodiesterase inhibitor therapy in chronic heart failure and of the OPTIME-CHF study in acute decompensation of congestive heart failure[85] have been disappointing. Thus, the use of these agents is limited to just a few categories of patients: (1) patients with advanced heart failure awaiting transplantation, in whom IV milrinone could be better tolerated than dobutamine, and its use may allow continuation of β-blocker therapy for controlling arrhythmias or myocardial ischemia[86]; (2) patients with acute decompensation of chronic heart failure unable to achieve stabilization with standard treatment; and (3) patients with long-term β-blocker use, in whom short-term IV milrinone may even be preferred to dobutamine.

There is now clear evidence that inotropic agents such as β-agonist agents and phosphodiesterase inhibitors can exert both short-term beneficial hemodynamic effects and serious adverse effects that make them even deleterious in terms of long-term outcome. It is likely their adverse effects (e.g., arrhythmias, increased risk of myocardial ischemia) are related to the increased cAMP concentration in the cytosol of the cardiomyocyte.[87]

The initial enthusiasm for calcium sensitizers in heart failure patients has also been attenuated in the recent years. In the LIDO study, compared to dobutamine, levosimendan significantly decreased mortality and improved the hemodynamic condition.[56] Nevertheless, these positive results have been contradicted by two large-scale studies. In the REVIVE study,[88] even though levosimendan improved a composite judgment criteria of clinical signs of heart failure at 5 days compared to placebo, the mortality rate was not significantly changed. In the SURVIVE study,[89] levosimendan was not better than dobutamine for increasing the survival rate in patients with acute heart failure requiring an inotropic support. A recent meta-analysis concluded that levosimendan improved hemodynamic parameters when compared with placebo but without showing evidence of survival benefit.[90] All these negative results have impeded the commercialization of levosimendan in many countries.

Nitric oxide synthase inhibitors have been proposed for use in patients with cardiogenic shock, in whom NO production is increased and may exert deleterious effects on cardiac function and vascular tone.[80] Tilarginine is a nonselective NO synthase inhibitor developed for treating acute heart failure. However, in the TRIUMPH study, tilarginine was unable to improve the survival rate of patients with cardiogenic shock at 3 months in comparison with placebo.[91] These negative results have interrupted clinical development of this new drug.

SEPTIC SHOCK

In cases of septic shock, dobutamine is generally considered the inotropic drug of choice when myocardial contractility is severely depressed.[19] Detection of a marked decrease in left ventricular ejection fraction using bidimensional echocardiography[92] can help diagnose a severe decrease in cardiac contractility and thus suggest the use of dobutamine when signs of peripheral hypoperfusion persist despite volume resuscitation and restoration of perfusion pressure with vasopressors. However, bedside bidimensional echocardiography is not yet available in all general ICUs, so the recommendation for using an inotrope such as dobutamine in septic shock is still based on the presence of a low cardiac output and high cardiac filling pressures after fluid resuscitation and an adequate MAP.[19] Since dobutamine can exert a vasodilatory effect, its use requires concomitant use of a vasopressor such as norepinephrine. Epinephrine is a potent inotrope with vasopressive properties that could be used as an alternative to the combination of dobutamine and norepinephrine. A randomized study in patients with septic shock and a presumed cardiac dysfunction found no significant difference in patient outcome between epinephrine alone and norepinephrine plus dobutamine.[93] However, this study has been criticized for a lack of statistical power. In the condition of depressed vascular tone and reduced myocardial function, epinephrine was shown to be inferior to the combination of dobutamine and norepinephrine in terms of splanchnic perfusion, despite similar effects on systemic blood flow and pressure.[38,39,64] For all these reasons, epinephrine is not recommended as the first-choice drug when treatment of impaired cardiac contractility is considered.[19]

Use of new inotropic drugs such as levosimendan has been proposed as an alternative to dobutamine in case of severe septic myocardial depression that no longer responds to dobutamine administration.[94] The rationale for using levosimendan is that the sensitivity of calcium to myofilament is reduced during sepsis, probably because of an abnormal phosphorylation of the troponin complex at the site where the calcium ion binds to troponin C.[95] Because levosimendan can improve not only left ventricular function but also right ventricular performance[96,97] through pulmonary vasodilation,[96] it might be useful in cases of septic myocardial depression with associated lung injury. However, more studies are needed to reach definitive conclusions about the utility of levosimendan in septic shock with myocardial depression.[98]

In summary, given all the available data, when inotropic therapy is used to reverse cardiac dysfunction in severe sepsis, the combination of norepinephrine and dobutamine is still recommended.[19]

KEY POINTS

1. Inotropic therapy is often considered in patients with cardiogenic shock or advanced heart failure whose condition is refractory to standard therapy. In these conditions, clinicians expect short-term positive effects of intravenous inotropic drugs, allowing cardiovascular stabilization.

2. Inotropic therapy may also be considered in high-risk surgical patients, even in the absence of reduced myocardial contractility, to achieve supranormal levels of oxygen delivery (DO_2) during the perioperative period to prevent tissue hypoxia and organ dysfunction. Such a therapeutic attitude is not recommended routinely for critically ill patients with established circulatory shock.

3. Most inotropic agents enhance myocardial contractility by increasing the Ca^{2+} concentration in the cytosol of cardiomyocytes after producing an increase in cytosolic cyclic adenosine monophosphate (cAMP). Synthetic and natural catecholamines enhance cAMP formation after fixing β_1-adrenergic receptors at the cellular surface. Phosphodiesterase inhibitors decrease cyclic AMP degradation.

4. The β_1-adrenergic agents, such as dobutamine, dopamine, and epinephrine, are the most potent inotropic agents.

5. Because of down-regulation of β_1-adrenergic receptors, the myocardial effects of exogenous catecholamines can be attenuated after a few days of administration.

6. Sepsis-induced decreased responsiveness of the myocardium to β-adrenergic stimulation also results in attenuation of cardiac effects of exogenous catecholamine administration in patients with septic shock.

7. The drugs given to increase cardiac contractility may also exert vasoactive effects that may interfere with the regulation of regional blood flow. The extent to which this interference is beneficial in increasing oxygen supply in hypoxic areas remains speculative. This emphasizes the need to monitor (as far as possible) perfusion and/or function of critical organs when such agents are given in patients in circulatory shock.

ANNOTATED REFERENCES

De Backer D, Biston P, Devriendt J, et al. Comparison of dopamine and norepinephrine in the treatment of shock. N Engl J Med 2010;362:779-89.
In this multicenter randomized trial, patients with shock (n = 1679) were assigned to receive either dopamine or norepinephrine as first-line vasopressor therapy to restore and maintain blood pressure. Although there was no significant difference in the rate of death between the two groups of patients, the use of dopamine was associated with a greater number of adverse events. A subgroup analysis showed that dopamine, as compared with norepinephrine, was associated with an increased rate of death at 28 days among the 280 patients with cardiogenic shock. This study will probably result in changes in international recommendations regarding the use of first-line vasopressor in the treatment of shock, at least in cases of cardiogenic shock.

Hayes MA, Timmins AC, Yau E, et al. Elevation of systemic oxygen delivery in the treatment of critically ill patients. N Engl J Med 1994;330:1717-22.
This randomized study showed that attempting to achieve supranormal values of oxygen delivery in patients with an established critical illness may worsen rather than improve outcome.

Mebazaa A, Nieminen MS, Packer M, et al. Levosimendan vs dobutamine for patients with acute decompensated heart failure: the SURVIVE Randomized Trial. JAMA 2007;297:1883-91.
In 1327 patients with acute decompensated heart failure requiring inotropic support, levosimendan was compared to dobutamine in a randomized double-blind design. Despite an initial reduction in plasma B-type natriuretic peptide level in patients receiving levosimendan, levosimendan did not significantly reduce all-cause mortality at 180 days or affect any secondary clinical outcomes. These disappointing results impeded the commercialization of levosimendan in many countries over the World.

Morelli A, De Castro S, Teboul JL, et al. Effects of levosimendan on systemic and regional hemodynamics in septic myocardial depression. Intensive Care Med 2005;31:638-44.
In 28 septic patients with persisting cardiac dysfunction after 48 hours of dobutamine administration, compared to dobutamine continuation, levosimendan improved systemic hemodynamics, improved gastric mucosal perfusion and renal function, and decreased lactate. This study suggests that levosimendan might be an alternative to dobutamine for treating sepsis-induced cardiac dysfunction.

Silverman HJ, Penaranda R, Orens JB, et al. Impaired beta-adrenergic receptor stimulation of cyclic adenosine monophosphate in human septic shock: association with myocardial hyporesponsiveness to catecholamines. Crit Care Med 1993;21:31-9.
This clinical study demonstrated that patients in septic shock exhibit a decreased hemodynamic response to dobutamine when compared to septic patients without shock. Moreover, the stimulation of circulating lymphocytes of the studied population showed that in patients with septic shock, the degree of impairment of β-adrenergic receptor responsiveness as well as that of post-β-adrenergic receptor signal transmission was higher than in septic patients without shock. This study provides strong evidence of a septic shock–related myocardial hyporesponsiveness to catecholamines that may contribute to the reduced myocardial performance observed in this critical illness.

The TRIUMPH Investigators. Effect of tilarginine acetate in patients with acute myocardial infarction and shock: the TRIUMPH randomized controlled trial. JAMA 2007;297:1657-66.
In this large-scale study, 658 patients with refractory shock due to myocardial infarction were randomized to receive either tilarginine, a nonselective inhibitor of NO synthase, or placebo. Tilarginine did not improve the mortality rates compared to placebo. This study has interrupted the development of tilarginine as a new drug for cardiogenic shock.

REFERENCES

Access the complete reference list online at http://www.expertconsult.com.

Mechanical Support in Cardiogenic Shock

JAY K. BHAMA | ROBERT L. KORMOS | THOMAS G. GLEASON

An estimated 61.8 million people in the United States have heart disease, among whom 950,000 die annually.[1] Of these, 540,000 people suffer myocardial infarctions each year; 193,000 succumb to complications directly related to the infarction. The leading cause of death among hospitalized patients with acute myocardial infarction (AMI) continues to be cardiogenic shock.[2] The incidence of cardiogenic shock complicating AMI (approximately 7%) has remained constant over the past 25 years. Accurate statistics on the worldwide utilization of all mechanical support for cardiogenic shock are not known. However, estimates on the use of intraaortic counterpulsation for patients in shock after AMI suggest a rate of use in only 22% of eligible patients.[3] The reasons for the apparent underutilization of this readily available modality are not clear. Accordingly, the indications, benefits, and limitations of mechanical cardiac support are outlined in this chapter.

Historical Background

The evolution of mechanical cardiac support dates to the early 1950s when Gibbon developed the prototype cardiopulmonary bypass (CPB) apparatus.[4] In the years following, Lillehei, Kirklin, and others applied the heart-lung machine to facilitate open-heart surgery; their pioneering work and early observations led directly to the development of modern mechanical cardiac support systems.[5-7] These surgeons recognized that some patients had improved outcomes after surgery if they were weaned slowly rather than abruptly from CPB support. Their initial publications introduced the concept that left ventricular (LV) decompression and myocardial rest could afford enhanced cardiac recovery after the insult of open-heart surgery. Clinical use of extracorporeal CPB for heart surgery became widespread in the early 1960s. Simultaneously, several groups of investigators were testing means of mechanical cardiac assistance for use outside the operating room for support of patients in cardiogenic shock. The current modes of mechanical support are derivations of those originally developed and include aortic counterpulsation, continuous flow pumps with or without an oxygenator, and pulsatile pumps.

HISTORY OF AORTIC COUNTERPULSATION

The concept of arterial counterpulsation was introduced in 1961 by Clauss and coworkers and involved use of an external "ventricular" chamber that filled with blood from a catheter in the iliac artery[8] and was subsequently compressed by a piston. Compression of the "ventricle" was synchronized to either the QRS complex of an electrocardiogram (ECG) or the impulse of a pacemaker, so that a counter pulse of blood was delivered into the arterial system during diastole. It was demonstrated in dogs that cardiac stroke work and LV end-systolic pressures could be substantially reduced with the use of a counterpulsation into the aorta. The following year, Moulopoulos and associates adapted the model to create an intraaortic balloon pump (IABP) that could provide a similar counterpulsation without the need for blood reservoirs.[9] The investigators used a balloon that was rapidly inflated and deflated with carbon dioxide during native diastole. The IABP was subsequently adapted and described for clinical use by Kantrowitz and colleagues in 1968.[10]

The original polyurethane balloon measured 1.8 cm in diameter by 14.8 cm in length when inflated (helium was used because its low density allows rapid delivery to and from the balloon) and displaced 32 mL of blood. There is little difference in the modern IABP and that originally described, other than the availability of different-sized balloons (30- to 50-mL balloons) and subtle differences in the materials used to make the catheters. The extracorporeal components of the IABP now include an electronically controlled pump with a solenoid valve in continuity with a pressurized helium source. The valve controls the flow of helium into and out of the balloon at intervals timed to either pressure changes on an arterial transducer, ECG signals (i.e., the QRS complex), or a ventricular pacer signal. This timing of balloon inflation and deflation is critical to attain optimal physiologic benefit of the cardiac support.

The physiologic rationale for the efficacy of the IABP is that balloon deflation provides a rapid, synchronized reduction in impedance (afterload) during isovolemic LV contraction. This is followed by a rapid, synchronized increase in aortic pressure during isovolemic LV relaxation (diastolic augmentation) caused by balloon inflation. In combination, these events achieve two important goals. First, LV systolic unloading directly reduces stroke work, which in turn reduces myocardial oxygen consumption during the cardiac cycle. Second, diastolic augmentation raises arterial blood pressure and provides better coronary arterial perfusion during diastole, yielding increased oxygen delivery to the myocardium. The IABP does not directly move or redistribute blood flow; however, peak diastolic coronary flow velocity can be increased as much as 87% with IABP augmentation and peak diastolic flow velocity by as much as 117%.[11] Since introduction into clinical use in 1968, the IABP has remained an important adjunct to supporting patients in cardiogenic shock. Myocardial recovery is promoted by the reduction of cardiac work and the simultaneous increase in myocardial oxygen supply. However, therapeutic success is dependent on the patient having a minimum degree of LV function that, in combination with IABP support, facilitates an adequate cardiac output to sustain end-organ function. When this minimal cardiac output is not met, alternative mechanical cardiac assistance must be considered.

HISTORY OF MECHANICAL ASSIST DEVICES

The need for effective mechanical cardiac assist devices became apparent in the 1950s during the development of CPB for open-heart surgery. Initial attempts with prolonged postoperative CPB demonstrated that the bypass circuit was damaging to both end-organ function and blood constituents after several hours of use.[12] The first attempt at isolated extracorporeal LV support was with a simple roller pump in 1962.[13] Subsequently, femoral venous–to–femoral arterial CPB was successfully used by Spencer and colleagues in four patients with postcardiotomy cardiac failure.[14]

Simultaneous to Spencer and colleagues' work with extracorporeal systems, DeBakey designed the first intracorporeal LV assist device (LVAD), the DeBakey blood pump.[15] This device consisted of a Dacron-reinforced silicone rubber tube with an inner chamber of blood from the left atrium that was connected to the descending thoracic aorta. Pressurized air was instilled into the outer chamber by an external pneumatic controller to compress the inner blood chamber, timed to the R wave of the QRS complex. Blood flow was directed from the left atrium to the descending aorta with the use of ball valves at both the inflow and outflow ends of the device. The DeBakey blood pump was first used in a patient who died 4 days postoperatively of neurologic complications. A remodeled extracorporeal version was subsequently used for postcardiotomy failure in a 37-year-old woman after aortic and mitral valve replacements. The device was needed for 10 days, but the patient survived.[16]

By 1972, investigators at the Texas Heart Institute had developed a pneumatically driven LVAD designed to be implanted in the abdomen.[17] This device had a blood chamber compressed by pulses of air delivered into the pump by a percutaneous driveline. Modern devices have chamber compression that is electrically powered via percutaneous drivelines. Paracorporeal, pneumatically driven devices were a parallel development. Paramount to the evolution of these devices was the sponsorship of the Artificial Heart Program of the National Heart, Lung, and Blood Institute, which was chartered in 1964.

By the 1960s, continuous flow, as compared to pulsatile, pumps were under development.[18,19] Over the subsequent 15 years, centrifugal pumps were perfected and introduced into clinical use. These pumps work on the principle of a forced, constrained vortex devised from three magnetic cones.[20-22] They have been shown to be useful in a variety of clinical settings where short-term mechanical support is needed and an IABP is inadequate. Several types of small, axial-flow or rotary pumps have also been developed, including some that allow for percutaneous deployment.[23-36] These are generally constructed of a magnetically suspended impeller that rotates at extremely fast rates (25,000 to 35,000 rpm). The axial rotary pump technology has some potential advantages over pulsatile devices; they are quite small with few moving parts and do not require a compliance chamber. The latest generation of rotary pump technology utilizes fully magnetically levitated rotors that completely eliminate the need for seals or bearings. This technology reduces the risk of damage to blood elements and may lead to lower rates of thromboembolism.

Current Mechanical Support Devices
COUNTERPULSATION/INTRAAORTIC BALLOON PUMP

Indications

The absolute indications for IABP placement include cardiogenic shock, uncontrolled angina pectoris, acute postinfarction ventricular septal defect or mitral regurgitation, and postcardiotomy left-sided heart failure with low cardiac output. In these settings, IABP should be considered a primary therapy that should not be delayed until noncardiac injury is clinically evident. It is important to recognize that blood pressure alone is not an adequate indication of hemodynamic or cardiac stability. Limb perfusion, renal function, mental status, and even gastrointestinal function need to be considered in the assessment of adequate resuscitation and homeostasis. Additional measurable indices include arterial (Sao_2) and mixed venous oxygen saturation (Svo_2), acid-base status, urine output, and body temperature. A multivariate analysis of data accrued from 391 postcardiotomy patients requiring IABP demonstrated that epinephrine requirements greater than 0.5 µg/kg/min, a left atrial pressure greater than 15 mm Hg, urine output less than 100 mL/h, and Svo_2 less than 60% correlated with mortality.[37] These criteria were used to help predict mortality and the need for subsequent mechanical support.

Other relative indications for IABP use include (1) high-risk, catheter-based interventional procedures such as left main coronary artery angioplasty, (2) after unsuccessful attempts at catheter-based intervention in patients with poorly controlled ventricular arrhythmias, and (3) concomitant poor LV function, and (4) in settings of persistent stunned, ischemic myocardium. These are all circumstances in which reduction of LV systolic wall tension and oxygen consumption by the IABP might enhance myocardial recovery after intervention. Conversely, the use of an IABP had no impact on mortality in a population of patients without hemodynamic instability undergoing high-risk angioplasty randomized in a prospective trial reported in 1997.[38] More recently, the Benchmark Counterpulsation Outcomes Registry of IABP use in 22,663 patients from 250 hospitals worldwide demonstrated that cardiogenic shock and high-risk angioplasty were the most common indications for utilization of the device.[39] Table 93-1 depicts a further characterization of the Benchmark report with respect to indications for use of the IABP and subsequent interventions.[40] Nevertheless, despite the widespread use of the IABP in over 150,000 patients worldwide each year,[41] no prospective randomized trial has ever demonstrated a survival benefit with IABP use in the patient population undergoing high-risk catheter intervention. In contrast, the SHOCK trial showed that early revascularization of patients with coronary artery disease and shock after an AMI, often facilitated by IABP use (86%), yielded a lower 6-month mortality rate (50%) than with medical therapy alone (63%).[2] Additional studies have shown that in patients undergoing urgent or emergent revascularization after an AMI, those supported preoperatively with an IABP had a lower operative mortality than those in whom an IABP was not used (5.3%-8.8% versus 11.8%-28.2%).[42,43] These data seem to justify a strategy of aggressive IABP use to facilitate early revascularization in the postinfarction patient.

TABLE 93-1	Indications for Use						
	Total Population (n = 16,909)	Diagnostic Catheterization (n = 1576)	Catheterization Only & PCI Only (n = 3882)	Surgery CABG (n = 9179)	Non-CABG (n = 1086)	No Intervention (n = 1186)
Support and stabilization (%)	20.6	21.4	54.4	9.7	5.0	7.8
Cardiogenic shock (%)	18.8	33.1	23.7	12.3	23.8	29.4
Weaning from cardiopulmonary bypass (%)	16.1	0.4	0.1	24.9	31.4	7.1
Preop: high risk CABG (%)	13.0	4.6	0.2	22.1	6.4	1.9
Refractory unstable angina (%)	12.3	15.3	8.3	15.8	2.2	3.0
Refractory ventricular failure (%)	6.5	9.1	2.5	5.9	15.7	12.7
Mechanical complication due to AMI (%)	5.5	9.8	7.0	4.2	5.2	5.1
Ischemia related to intractable VA (%)	1.7	1.6	1.5	1.9	1.7	1.6
Cardiac support for high-risk general surgery (%)	0.9	2.1	0.2	0.5	4.3	1.1
Other (%)	0.8	0.7	0.2	0.8	2.5	2.0
Intraoperative pulsatile flow (%)	0.4	0.1	0.1	0.7	0.5	0.2
Missing indication (%)	3.3	1.8	1.9	1.2	1.5	28.1

Modified from Ferguson JJ 3rd, Cohen M, Freedman RJ Jr et al. The current practice of intra-aortic balloon counterpulsation: results from the benchmark registry. J Am Coll Cardiol 2001;38:1456-62.

AMI, acute myocardial infarction; *CABG*, coronary artery bypass graft; *PCI*, percutaneous coronary intervention; *VA*, ventricular arrhythmias.

| TABLE 93-2 | IABP Outcomes and Complications |

| | Total Population (n = 16,909) | Diagnostic Catheterization (n = 1576) | Catheterization Only & PCI only (n = 3882) | Surgery | | No Intervention (n = 1186) |
				CABG (n = 9179)	Non-CABG (n = 1086)	
In-hospital mortality (%)	21.2	32.2	18.4	16.8	37.8	34.1
Mortality: balloon in place (%)	11.6	17.6	10.1	9.2	19.8	20.2
IABP-related mortality* (%)	0.05	0.1	0.1	0.0	0.0	0.1
Amputation†	0.1	0.0	0.1	0.1	0.1	0.0
Major limb ischemia‡ (%)	0.9	0.6	0.5	1.2	1.0	0.5
Any limb ischemia (%)	2.9	3.2	1.9	3.5	2.5	1.7
Severe access site bleeding (%)	0.8	0.8	1.2	0.7	0.7	0.3
Any access site bleeding (%)	2.4	2.7	4.4	1.7	1.3	1.4
Balloon leak (%)	1.0	0.9	0.8	1.1	0.5	1.6
Composite Outcomes						
Major IABP complication§ (%)	2.8	2.8	2.2	3.0	2.9	2.4
Any IABP complication‖ (%)	7.0	7.6	7.5	7.1	6.0	5.2
Any unsuccessful IABP¶ (%)	2.3	2.5	1.7	2.5	2.4	2.7

From Ferguson JJ 3rd, Cohen M, Freedman RJ Jr et al. The current practice of intra-aortic balloon counterpulsation: Results from the benchmark registry. J Am Coll Cardiol 2001;38:1456-62.

*Death as direct consequence of IABP therapy.
†All major limb ischemia.
‡Loss of pulse or sensation, abnormal limb temperature, or pallor, requiring surgical intervention.
§Balloon leak, severe bleeding, major limb ischemia, or death as a direct consequence of IABP therapy.
‖Any access site bleeding, any limb ischemia, balloon leak, poor inflation, poor augmentation, insertion difficulty, or death as direct result of IABP therapy.
¶Balloon leak, poor inflation, poor augmentation, or insertion difficulty.
CABG, coronary artery bypass graft; *IABP,* intra-aortic balloon pump; *PCI,* percutaneous coronary intervention.

Technical Considerations

The optimal site of insertion of an IABP is a common femoral artery that can be accessed either percutaneously with the use of a guidewire or by surgical cutdown. Modern intraaortic balloon catheters are available for adults and children according to the appropriate size and length for a given height and weight of the patient. Adult intraaortic balloons have a range in volume filled between 25 and 50 mL, with a standard balloon size holding 40 mL of helium. IABP catheters placed through the femoral artery are positioned so that the tip is just distal to the takeoff of the left subclavian artery in the proximal descending thoracic aorta. Optimally, the tip of the catheter should be positioned with transesophageal echocardiographic (TEE) or fluoroscopic guidance.[44] To reduce the diameter of femoral cannulation, a sheathless IABP technique can be utilized and is our preferred method.[45]

Inflation of the balloon should be timed with closure of the aortic valve (at the dicrotic notch of the aortic pressure tracing) and should be inflated to nearly occlude the descending thoracic aorta. Timing can be synchronized in one of three ways: (1) using an arterial (preferably aortic) pressure tracing in synchrony with the dicrotic notch, (2) using the descent of the R wave on a rhythm tracing, or (3) timed after a ventricular pacing spike when a pacemaker is in use.[46-50] The effectiveness of IABP is significantly improved by proper timing of inflation and deflation, which can be difficult when there is an accelerated heart rate, cardiac rhythm disturbances, atrioventricular dyssynchrony, or low mean arterial pressure. IABP timing should be adjusted to maximize diastolic augmentation; hence, deflation should be as late as possible but just before opening of the aortic valve. If this cannot be gauged by the pressure tracing, it can be timed to the onset of the R wave on the ECG tracing or with the use of M-mode echocardiography.[51]

IABP catheters should not be left in place after weaning because of the risk of thrombus formation and embolization. An IABP should be weaned stepwise from a rate that is equivalent to heart rate (1:1) down to a ratio of 1:3 just before removal. Balloon catheters placed via an open surgical technique should also be removed surgically. Percutaneous removal of catheters placed in the iliac artery above the inguinal ligament (often done in obese individuals) can result in significant retroperitoneal bleeding. Consideration of operative removal is warranted.

When femoral arterial cannulation is not desirable because of aortoiliac occlusive disease or extensive peripheral vascular disease, the subclavian artery or the ascending aorta can be utilized.[52-56] With either technique, the IABP catheters are advanced antegrade down the descending thoracic aorta so that the balloon tip sits above the level of the diaphragmatic hiatus, and the most proximal end of the balloon is distal to the takeoff of the left subclavian. These antegrade balloons should always be placed with either fluoroscopic or echocardiographic guidance. They should be removed with open arterial repair in all cases.

Relative contraindications to IABP use include severe atheromatous and atherosclerotic descending thoracic aorta, descending aortic dissection or aneurysm, recent descending thoracic aortic surgery, and mild to moderate aortic insufficiency. Severe aortic insufficiency is an absolute contraindication to use, because diastolic augmentation cannot be accomplished, and LV end-diastolic volume and pressure are actually increased rather than decreased.

Complications

The overall complication rate of IABP utilization is between 5% and 10%. Major complications occur at a rate of about 3% and include severe bleeding, major limb ischemia or amputation, infection, visceral or spinal cord ischemia, and attributable IABP mortality.[39,43] A summary of IABP complications as they occur in relation to subsequent percutaneous or operative coronary revascularization from the Benchmark Registry are listed in Table 93-2.[40] In this registry, rates of complications were quite low, the most common being access-site bleeding (4.3%) and limb ischemia (2.3%).[39] The rates of amputation, stroke, visceral or spinal cord ischemia and IABP-related mortality are all 0.1% or less.[39] Intraaortic balloon entrapment is a rare complication.[57-59] The incidence of major vascular complications according to the STS National Database (1996-1997) and the Benchmark Registry (1997-1999) is 5.4% and 1.4%, respectively.[40,43] Ipsilateral limb ischemia should be immediately addressed after its recognition. This usually requires removal of the IABP, with

	Hospital Mortality (Outcome Parameter) for Patients Undergoing Cardiac Surgery Who Either Received Preoperative IABP or Intra-/Postoperative IABP Support		
TABLE 93-3			
Type of Therapy	*Benchmark Registry 1997-1999 Mortality/Total Operations with IABP, n (%)*	*STS National Database 1996-1997 Mortality/Total Operations with IABP, n (%)*	*STS National Database 1996-1997 Mortality/Total Operations without IABP, n (%)*
Preoperative IABP	8.8 (329/3721)	9.5 (2487/26,077)	2.9 (10,919/378,810)
Intraoperative/ postoperative IABP	28.2 (954/3380)	23.6 (3528/14,933)	2.5 (9878/389,954)

Based on data from the Benchmark Counterpulsation Registry 1997-1999 and the STS National Database 1996-97 compared with hospital mortality for patients who had neither preoperative nor intraoperative/postoperative IABP support.

From Christenson JT, Cohen M, Ferguson JJ 3rd, et al: Trends in intraaortic balloon counterpulsation: complications and outcomes in cardiac surgery. Ann Thorac Surg 2002;74:1086-1090.

replacement at another location if it is still indicated. The ischemic limb may require thrombectomy with or without revascularization and fasciotomy.[60-66]

Outcomes

In the absence of prospective randomized data, it is difficult to ascribe outcome secondary to IABP placement. The Second Angioplasty in Myocardial Infarction (PAMI-II) Trial data examined high-risk patients with acute myocardial infarction revascularized by percutaneous intervention only and demonstrated a modest survival advantage at 6 months with the use of periprocedural IABP support.[38] When evaluating hospital mortality rates among patients undergoing coronary artery bypass graft (CABG) and/or valve surgery who received preoperative IABP or required intraoperative/postoperative IABP support, it is evident that mortality was significantly lower among patients supported preoperatively, as depicted in Table 93-3.[40,43] Hence, there appears to be a survival advantage to earlier IABP support for patients with AMI and cardiogenic shock who need revascularization. In the setting of an acute ventricular septal defect (VSD) or acute mitral regurgitation after an AMI, IABP support can offer a dramatic improvement in the hemodynamic response of the patient.[67-71] Figures

93-1 and 93-2 stratify hospital mortality rates associated with IABP use in patients with AMI by principal usage indication or by performance of percutaneous or surgical coronary revascularization. It is clear that the mortality rate of cardiogenic shock after AMI remains high at 39%. However, IABP support combined with revascularization portends a better prognosis than adjunctive IABP use with medical therapy alone.[39]

CONTINUOUS FLOW PUMPS

Both roller pumps and centrifugal pumps deliver continuous flow but have other distinct limitations. Roller pumps remain in widespread use for cardiopulmonary support during cardiac surgery; applications outside the operating room have been virtually abandoned for several reasons. Roller pumps are insensitive to changes in arterial line resistance that may cause disruption of the apparatus. They require unobstructed venous flow. The rollers eventually cause spallation of tubing, leading to particle emboli and weakening of the tubing.[72] Roller compression causes hemolysis after prolonged use.[73] Alternatively, centrifugal pumps are sensitive to both outflow resistance and filling pressure, offering a safer applicability outside the operating room. Centrifugal pumps like the BioMedicus Bio-Pump (Medtronic Corp., Minneapolis, Minnesota) generate a constrained vortex within an acrylic shell that houses concentric magnetic cones. The cones rotate as a magnetic rotary motor spins adjacent to the base of the cones[20-22] and can generate very high flows with less trauma to blood cells than roller pumps.[73-75]

The technology of centrifugal pumps, axial flow pumps, and membrane oxygenators has remarkably improved. Pump durability and reduced blood cell trauma have been demonstrated.[19,26,73-76] As a result, considerable experience has accumulated with the use of centrifugal pumps (cardiopulmonary support) for postcardiotomy LV failure, fulminant myocarditis, or cardiogenic shock after AMI.[32,77-93] Newer devices have incorporated design modifications that allow for improved pump performance as well as percutaneous application.

A novel centrifugal blood pump, the CentriMag system, utilizes fully magnetically levitated technology (Figure 93-3) to provide external mechanical circulatory support in a fashion similar to the BioMedicus Bio-Pump. The CentriMag system has many advantages that make it attractive for short-term mechanical support in the acute setting.[94] These advantages include ease of implantation, direct outflow cannulation of the ventricle for improved decompression, minimal need for

Figure 93-1 In-hospital mortality of 5495 patients with acute myocardial infarction (AMI) requiring intraaortic balloon pump counterpulsation, stratified by principal usage indication. AMI, acute myocardial infarction; PCI, percutaneous coronary intervention. *(From Stone GW, Ohman EM, Miller MF et al. Contemporary utilization and outcomes of intra-aortic balloon counterpulsation in acute myocardial infarction: the benchmark registry. J Am Coll Cardiol 2003;41:1940-5.)*

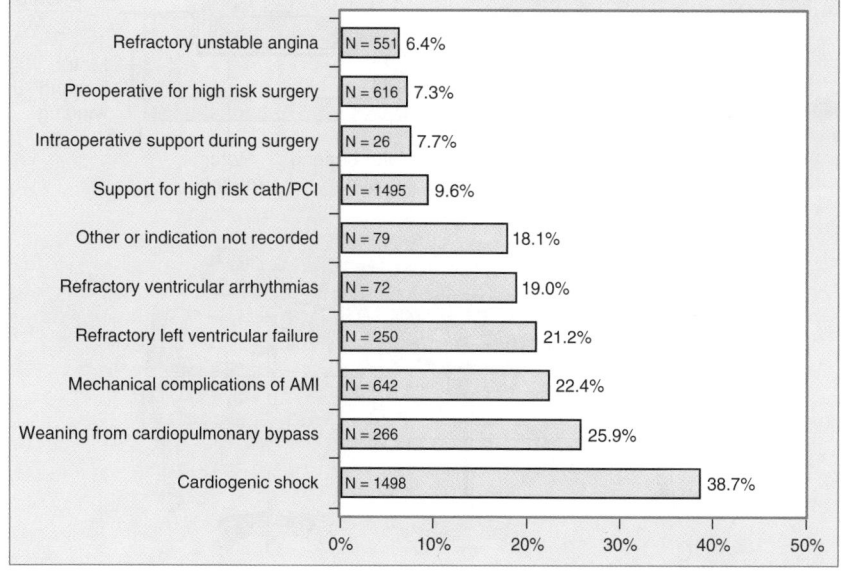

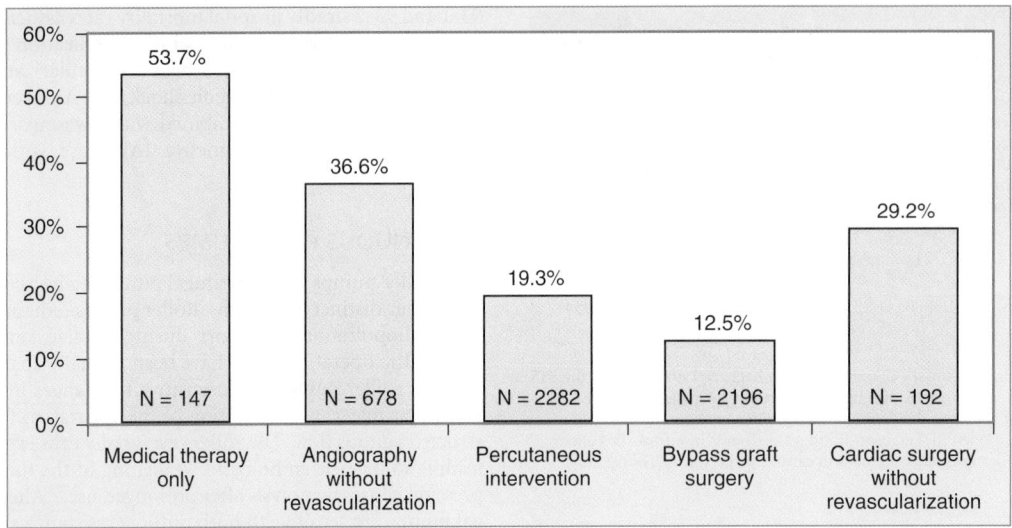

Figure 93-2 In-hospital mortality stratified by the performance of angiography and percutaneous or surgical coronary revascularization. *(From Stone GW, Ohman EM, Miller MF et al. Contemporary utilization and outcomes of intra-aortic balloon counterpulsation in acute myocardial infarction: the benchmark registry. J Am Coll Cardiol 2003;41:1940-5.)*

anticoagulation, and less damage to blood elements compared to traditional devices such as the BioMedicus pump. It has been used effectively for uni- or biventricular support in the setting of postcardiotomy cardiac failure as a bridge to decision, recovery, or long-term mechanical circulatory support device. For patients who also require pulmonary support, an oxygenator may be added to the circuit, effectively converting it to an ECMO system.

The Tandem Heart System (Cardiac Assist Inc., Pittsburgh, Pennsylvania) is an external centrifugal pump system that allows for percutaneous LV support (Figure 93-4).[95] Utilizing a percutaneous venous cannula that crosses the atrial septum, this pump can provide LV assistance without performing a sternotomy. This device has been

utilized both for short-term support in the catheterization suite or as a bridge to recovery, more definitive mechanical circulatory support (i.e., implantable device), or transplantation.

The most recent addition to the armamentarium for acute short-term mechanical circulatory support is the Impella Recover axial flow pump (Abiomed Inc., Danvers, Massachusetts). This device can be placed percutaneously or directly via the open chest during cardiac surgery (Figure 93-5). It has been used for partial support during percutaneous coronary interventions as well as for postcardiotomy cardiogenic shock as a bridge to recovery or a more definitive long-term device.[96] Important limitations for the use of this device include aortic stenosis that precludes proper positioning of the device as well

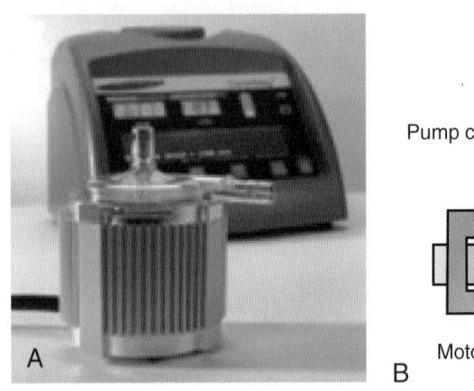

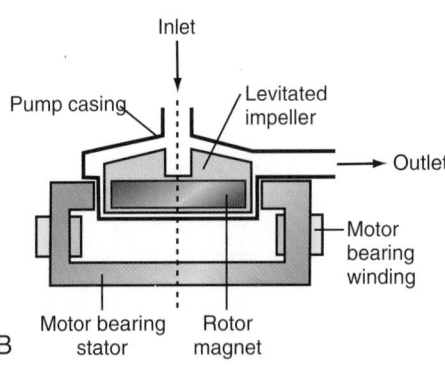

Figure 93-3 A, Levitronix CentriMag rotor and bearingless pump. **B,** Schematic representation of the pump. **C,** Console as seen in clinical use. *(From Bhama J, Kormos RL, Toyoda Y et al. Clinical experience utilizing the Levitronix CentriMag system for temporary right ventricular mechanical circulatory support. J Heart Lung Transplant 2008;28:971-6. Copyright 2009, International Society of Heart and Lung Transplantation.)*

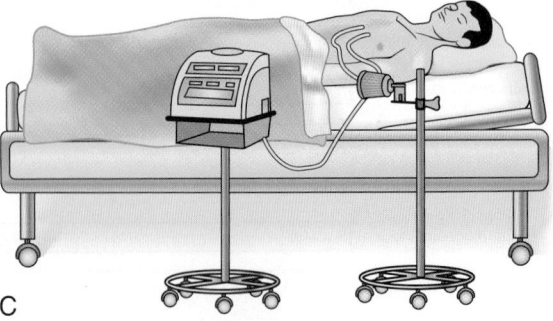

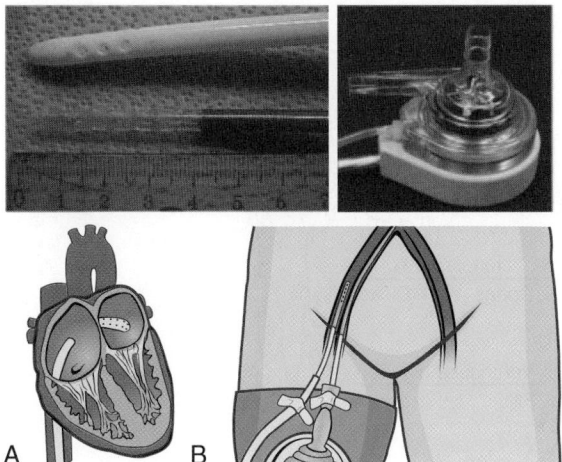

Figure 93-4 A, Components of the TandemHeart device: 21F left atrial drainage cannula and 15-17F femoral arterial cannula *(left)*; continuous flow centrifugal pump *(right)*. **B,** Schematic demonstrating transseptal left atrial drainage and femoral access points. *(From Windecker S. Percutaneous left ventricular assist devices for treatment of patients with cardiogenic shock. Curr Opin Crit Care 13:521-7. Copyright 2007, Lippincott Williams & Wilkins.)*

as peripheral vascular disease that may make percutaneous deployment impossible or mandate a surgical cutdown for placement. This device cannot be used in patients who have had a previous mechanical aortic valve replacement.

Indications

Short-term cardiopulmonary support for cardiogenic shock has emerged as an important adjunctive therapy. It is a relatively simple means of establishing immediate and complete circulatory support, requiring no additional equipment other than that needed for standard CPB support during cardiac surgery. Cardiopulmonary support can be initiated percutaneously via the common femoral artery and vein. Alternatively, when faced with postcardiotomy LV failure, cardiopulmonary support can facilitate patient stabilization for subsequent transport to a tertiary medical center for VAD placement. Cardiopulmonary support circuits can be converted to longer-term support (beyond 6-8 hours) by upgrading the oxygenator.[97,98] A standard

microporous hollow-fiber oxygenator (the type used in most CPB circuits) has a lifespan of 6 to 12 hours.[99] Changing to a solid-silicone membrane oxygenator (not microporous) will lengthen the lifespan of the cardiopulmonary support circuit up to 21 days; this conversion constitutes extracorporeal membrane oxygenation (ECMO) support. ECMO is generally used in the adult population for periods of 1 to 10 days when there is marked concomitant pulmonary insufficiency and cardiac failure. ECMO is also used for short-term (1-3 days) support when the neurologic status of a patient is unclear and longer-term support (i.e., VAD support) may not be appropriate until this status is clarified. Thus, ECMO can be used as a bridge to a longer-term, pulsatile flow assist device once the suitability of the patient is determined.

Technical Considerations and Complications

Disadvantages to the use of peripheral cardiopulmonary support or ECMO include the greater potential for ipsilateral limb complications, higher rates of hemolysis, the requirement for anticoagulation to prevent thrombosis of the oxygenator and circuit, and failure to adequately decompress the left ventricle.[100-106] Inadequate LV decompression with peripheral cardiopulmonary support/ECMO systems may be the mechanism responsible for some treatment failures. Regardless of the etiology of cardiogenic shock, a rested ventricle (i.e., decompressed) has a better chance of recovery than a distended ventricle.

Outcomes

The use of ECMO in the adult population for reasons other than primary cardiac failure with secondary pulmonary insufficiency has limited advantages over conventional therapies.[107,108] However, a substantial subset of patients who present with cardiogenic shock and are initially resuscitated with cardiopulmonary support/ECMO survive to revascularization, transplantation, or recovery, with survival rates as high as 75%.[77,78,81,82,109-116] ECMO used as a bridge to VAD placement for profound cardiogenic shock ("double bridge" mechanical assistance) can yield survival rates greater than 40%.[80] This strategy is pragmatic and offers immediate end-organ support while a subsequent definitive treatment plan can be designed.

VENTRICULAR ASSIST DEVICES

Pulsatile Pumps

There is a growing body of evidence suggesting that pulsatile assisted circulation, in the setting of acute cardiogenic shock, offers improved

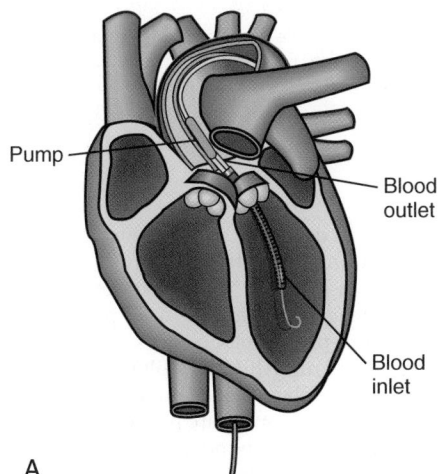

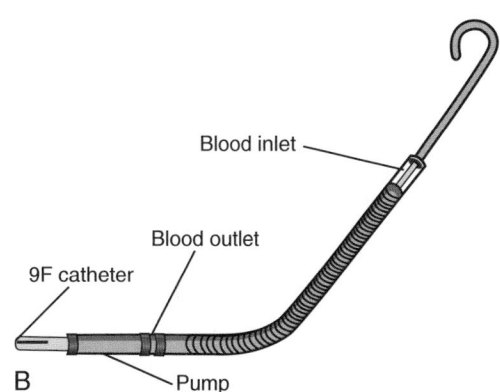

Figure 93-5 A, Schematic demonstrating retrograde placement of the Impella Recover LP 2.5 device across the aortic valve. **B,** Components of the device. Blood from the ventricle enters the inlet portion of the device and is propelled by a 12F microaxial pump to the outlet portion positioned in the ascending aorta, establishing left ventricular decompression. *(From Windecker S. Percutaneous left ventricular assist devices for treatment of patients with cardiogenic shock. Curr Opin Crit Care 13:521-7. Copyright 2007, Lippincott Williams & Wilkins.)*

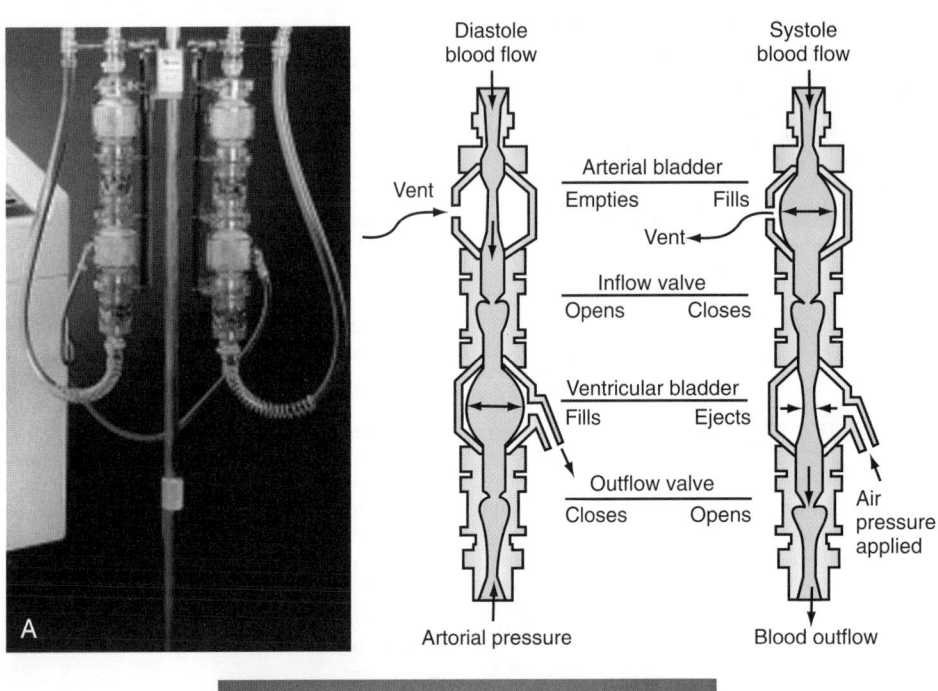

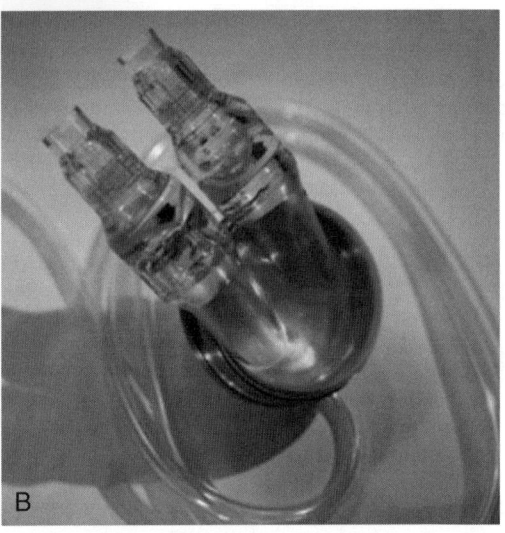

Figure 93-6 The ABIOMED BVS 5000 & AB 5000. **A,** In the BVS5000 model, the atrial chamber empties through a one-way valve into the ventricular chamber (diastole). The pneumatically driven pump compresses the ventricular chamber, and blood flows through a one-way valve into the patient (systole). The atrial chamber fills by gravity during pump systole. **B,** In the AB 5000 model, a single ventricular blood chamber fills by vacuum assistance, and blood is ejected by pneumatic inflation of a polyurethane bladder housed within the pump casing. (*From Couper GS, Dekkers RJ, Adams DH. The logistics and cost-effectiveness of circulatory support: advantages of the ABIOMED BVS 5000. Ann Thorac Surg 1999;68:646-9. Copyright 1999, The Society of Thoracic Surgeons; Moazami N, McCarthy PM. Temporary circulatory support. In: Cohn LH, Edmunds LH Jr, editors. Cardiac surgery in the adult. New York: McGraw-Hill; 2003.*)

end-organ perfusion and lymphatic flow and is thus beneficial.[117-119] VADs that utilize direct cardiac outflow cannulation (VAD inflow) provide better ventricular decompression and rest than peripheral bypass support systems. There are now several mechanical assist devices that achieve these goals, including the extracorporeal ABIOMED AB 5000 (Abiomed) and the paracorporeal Thoratec VAD system (Thoratec Corp., Pleasanton, California). Two other implantable intracorporeal pulsatile VADs that were designed for patients with chronic heart failure may have roles in certain subsets of patients with acute cardiogenic shock. These are the HeartMate LVAS XVE (Thoratec) and the intracorporeal Thoratec VAD system (Thoratec).

Extracorporeal Short-Term Support. The recently FDA-approved ABIOMED AB 5000 "ventricle" replaces the previously utilized BVS

5000 which was developed in the 1980s and was granted approval for use for postcardiotomy heart failure by the U.S. Food and Drug Administration in 1992.[116] Since that time, indications for the device have been broadened to include most patients with either postcardiotomy shock or precardiotomy shock who do not adequately respond to inotropes and an IABP. The ABIOMED system is a pneumatically driven, dual-chamber blood pump that delivers pulsatile flow. ABIOMED inflow cannulas are placed in the left and/or right atrium for univentricular or biventricular support. Outflow cannulas are housed with a Hemashield graft (Meadox Medicals Inc., Oakland California) and are sewn to the aorta and/or pulmonary artery for left-sided and/or right-sided heart support. The pumps, as depicted in Figure 93-6, are extracorporeal (BVS5000) or paracorporeal (AB5000). In the BVS5000, the upper (first) chamber fills passively by gravity, and the lower chamber serves as the pumping chamber. The two chambers are separated by a polyurethane trileaflet inflow valve; the lower chamber is separated from the arterial circulation by an outflow valve that prevents retrograde flow. As the pumping chamber is filled with blood, the surrounding air within the polycarbonate housing is displaced back into the drive console. This is sensed by the console; the console delivers compressed air back into the pumping chamber, which compresses the bladder and forces a pulse of blood into the arterial circulation.[120] The stroke volume that results is 70 to 80 mL, with VAD output dependent on the rate of upper-chamber filling. The AB5000 "ventricle" has a single ventricular blood chamber that fills by vacuum assistance from a portable console. Blood is ejected by pneumatic inflation of polyurethane bladder housed within the pump casing. Valves constructed of Angioflex, ABIOMED's proprietary polyether-based polyurethane plastic, insure unidirectional flow. Typically, flows of 5 L/min are achieved with either of the ABIOMED systems. Both of these devices require anticoagulation, particularly for LV assistance. The BVS5000 is generally useful for short-term (<7-10 days) support because of the increased risk of thromboembolic complications or device malfunction beyond this period. If longer support (2-3 months) is necessary, the ABIOMED pump can be exchanged with AB5000 or converted to a longer-term VAD system such as the Thoratec p-VAD or HeartMate.

ABIOMED cannulation can be achieved either on or off CPB and with or without aortic cross-clamping. However, the condition of the patient is typically unstable, and cannulation—particularly of the pulmonary artery and aorta—may be safer on bypass with a decompressed, supported heart. Access is obtained via median sternotomy, with all cuffed cannulas brought out of the chest through separate subcostal incisions. The cuffs allow soft tissue growth and adherence to reduce the incidence of infection of the cannulas and endocardium. Approximately 6000 ABIOMED VADs have been placed worldwide for precardiotomy or postcardiotomy cardiac failure.[118,120-123] Survival and hospital discharge rates have ranged from 20% to 45%, depending on the indication for the ABIOMED and the hemodynamic condition of the patient before surgery.[118,120-122] The most common complications directly attributed to this VAD include bleeding, stroke, and infection, with rates of 20% to 40%.[118,120,122] Hemolysis is not a common problem.

Paracorporeal Longer-Term Support. The Thoratec paracorporeal VAD (p-VAD) system is composed of a single chamber with a polyurethane seamless bladder housed in a rigid casing (Figure 93-7).[124] VAD inflow cannulas are either atrial or ventricular. Outflow cannulas have a polyester graft attached for direct connection to the aorta or pulmonary artery, similar to the ABIOMED cannulas. There are Bjork-Shiley tilting disc valves at both the inflow and outflow connections to the bladder to ensure unidirectional flow; they require anticoagulation. A pneumatic driveline is connected to the rigid casing and supplies alternating vacuum and pressure to facilitate bladder filling and emptying, respectively. The blood pump can be adjusted to accommodate changing preload and afterload. The pneumatically driven pulses (systole) can be controlled in three different modes: asynchronous, synchronous, and volume. The asynchronous mode maintains a fixed rate, but stroke volume may vary. The synchronous mode provides counterpulsation by timing ejection to the patient's R wave—this provides both a variable rate and variable stroke volume. The volume mode delivers a fixed stroke volume triggered by bladder filling, but the rate will vary. The volume mode is usually the most practical because the VAD output changes with the patient's physiologic condition.

The Thoratec p-VAD is similar to the ABIOMED but is more portable and has the potential for outpatient use in patients who are bridging to recovery or transplantation.[124-127] Two advantages to the Thoratec p-VAD system are the ability of secure ventricular inflow (VAD) cannulation and the applicability of long-term utilization. LV cannulation provides better ventricular decompression than atrial cannulation.[128-132] This is important because LV distention or inadequate decompression will limit ventricular recovery in some patients.

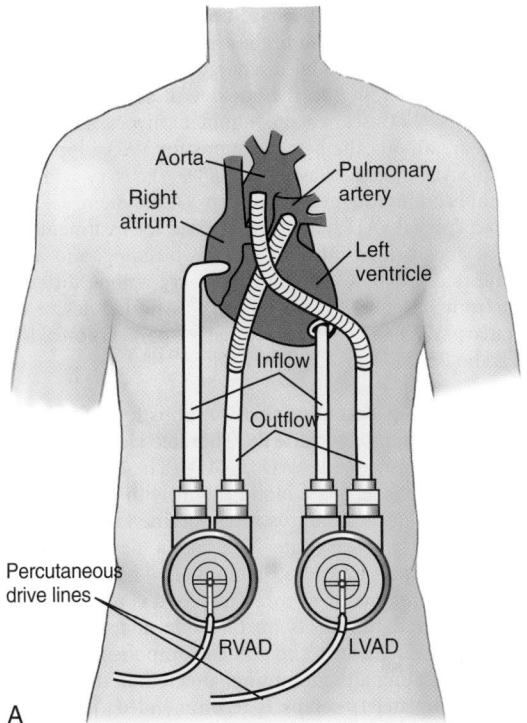

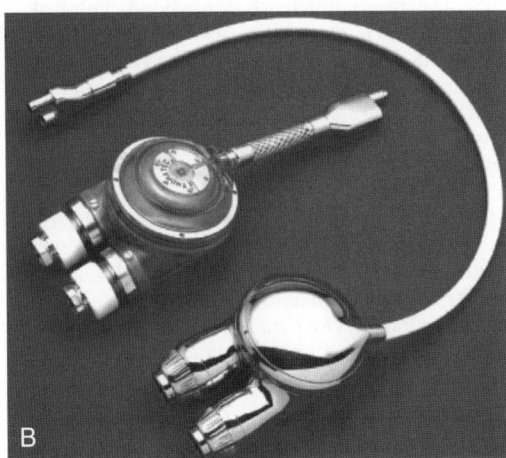

Figure 93-7 Thoratec ventricular assist system: a pneumatically powered system configured for uni- or biventricular support with paracorporeal (p-VAD) and intracorporeal (i-VAD) options. **A,** Schematic demonstrating configuration for right and left ventricular support. **B,** The i-VAD (*below*) shown next to a p-VAD (*above*). The smooth, contoured, polished titanium housing and the polyester velour-covered driveline allow for implantability with i-VAD. (*From Hunt SA, Frazier OH. Mechanical circulatory support and cardiac transplantation. Circulation 1998;97:2079-90. Copyright 1998, American Heart Association; Slaughter et al. Results of a multicenter clinical trial with the Thoratec implantable ventricular assist device. J Thorac Cardiovasc Surg 2007;133:1573-80. Copyright 2007, The American Association for Thoracic Surgery.*)

Ventricular cannulation also provides better VAD performance and reduces the risk of thrombotic complications, particularly in the setting of AMI.[111,128,130,132] Right ventricular cannulation provides similar advantages over right atrial cannulation. However, these advantages may not be manifest if the tricuspid valve is left intact, because the tricuspid leaflets are often in close proximity to the cannulation tip and can obstruct VAD inflow.[133] In this situation, the advantages and disadvantages of right atrial versus right ventricular cannulation must be weighed to direct the best approach.

Over 3700 Thoratec p-VADs have been placed worldwide in over 2400 patients[134]; more than half of these patients received biventricular support. Survival and hospital discharge rates vary widely between 20% and 80%, depending on the etiology of shock and the medical center.[77,80,124,131,135-137] Cases of acute fulminant myocarditis with cardiogenic shock are among the best situations for VAD support with the Thoratec p-VAD system, having an 88% recovery-with-discharge rate.[77] Complications of the Thoratec p-VAD system are similar to other extracorporeal VAD systems when used for treatment of cardiogenic shock and include infection, stroke, bleeding, and acute renal failure. The rates of these complications vary among different series but range from 10% to 60%.[122,124,131,135,137-142] Another device similar to the Thoratec p-VAD and commonly used for paracorporeal long-term support is the Berlin Heart EXCOR device.[143,144]

Intracorporeal Long-Term Support. Options for pulsatile intracorporeal long-term support include the Thoratec HeartMate LVAS XVE and the Thoratec implantable VAD (i-VAD). The Heartmate XVE has a fully implanted pusher-plate blood pump with externalized drivelines (Figure 93-8). It uses bioprosthetic porcine valves to ensure unidirectional flow. The HeartMate XVE has a flexible polyurethane diaphragm that pushes against a titanium alloy housing generating a maximum stroke volume of 83 mL. The blood contact surface is textured with polyurethane fibrils on one side and sintered titanium spheres on the housing. Fibrin and cellular components react and bond to the surface, creating a pseudointima, precluding the need for anticoagulation. Antiplatelet therapy is recommended. The i-VAD is an implantable version of the Thoratec p-VAD with identical internal components. The major difference is a smooth polished titanium housing that facilitates implantability (see Figure 93-7). A third device, the Novacor LVAS, is similar in design to the Heartmate XVE LVAS, with a fully implantable pusher plate blood pump and externalized drive lines. It was widely used as a bridge to transplantation in the early experience with LVAD support but is currently not in use and is largely of historic interest.

Both implantable pulsatile systems have variable modes that can generate fixed rates or demand-sensitive rates. Both are approved for use for the treatment of end-stage heart failure, but they may have a selective role for cardiogenic shock. These devices are practical alternatives for use in a "double-bridge" setting with initial resuscitation using a temporary device (i.e., ECMO/cardiopulmonary support or ABIOMED) for stabilization and pulmonary recovery.[80,112,113,145,146] Results with these devices have been favorable and, in certain subsets of patients, better than longer-term support with other systems.[77,142,147-152] Complications have been similar to other VADs and include bleeding, infection, stroke, thrombotic complications, and renal insufficiency.

NonPulsatile (Continuous Flow) Pumps

There are several miniaturized rotary continuous flow (nonpulsatile) pumps that have been designed for long-term (potentially permanent) mechanical assistance, including the MicroMed-DeBakey pump, the Jarvik 2000, the HeartMate II, and the HeartWare (Figure 93-9).[153-164] These devices are being studied in clinical trials for use as a bridge to transplantation, recovery, or permanent replacement therapy.[154,163] They are relatively costly, provide isolated LV support, and require specialized training to implant. Consequently, they have not yet received widespread use for acute cardiogenic shock.

◼ Treatment of Cardiogenic Shock: Algorithm for Mechanical Support

The hallmarks of cardiogenic shock are low cardiac output, hypotension, peripheral vasoconstriction, cold extremities, poor urine output, and altered mental status. As the pathophysiologic state progresses, pulmonary insufficiency and pulmonary edema ensue. Extrinsic causes of cardiogenic shock most commonly manifest as circulatory collapse secondary to pericardial tamponade. Acute tamponade is easily

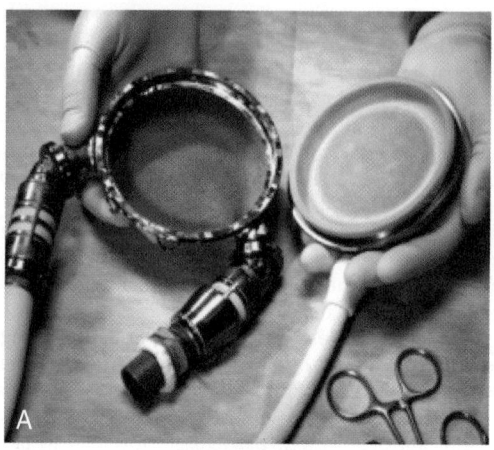

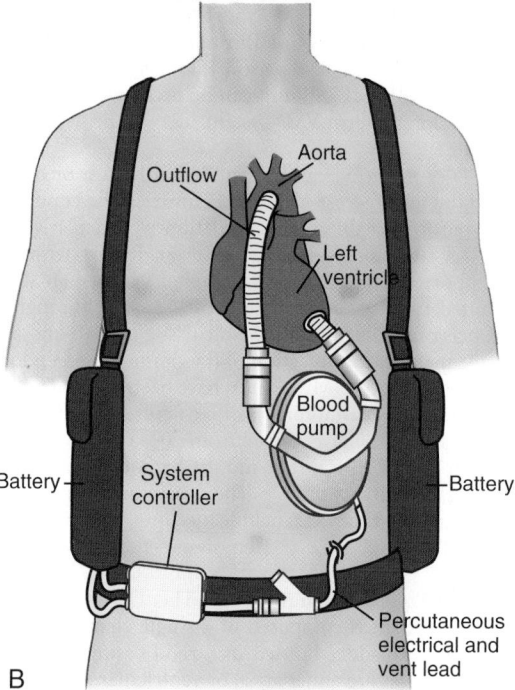

Figure 93-8 The HeartMate vented electric left ventricular assist device (HeartMate XVE): an intracorporeal electrically powered system. **A,** Textured surface designed to reduce thrombogenicity. **B,** Schematic demonstrating position of pump and related components. (From Loisance D. Mechanical circulatory support: a clinical reality. Asian Cardiovasc Thorac Ann 2008;16:419-31. Copyright 2008, Asia Publishing Exchange Ltd.; Hunt SA, Frazier OH, Mechanical circulatory support and cardiac transplantation. Circulation 1998;97:2079-90. Copyright 1998, American Heart Association.)

diagnosed by echocardiography and requires surgical or percutaneous evacuation and subsequent treatment of that which caused the tamponade (e.g., traumatic injury, aortic dissection, ruptured aneurysm). Extrinsic causes of cardiogenic shock usually require immediate surgical intervention but rarely necessitate mechanical assistance. However, intrinsic causes of acute cardiogenic shock can be refractory to both medical and surgical therapies and may require mechanical assistance. Intrinsic causes of cardiogenic shock can be divided into four pathophysiologic classifications: (1) acute valvular insufficiency, (2) AMI, (3) acute myocarditis, and (4) postcardiotomy cardiac failure.

Irrespective of the etiology of cardiogenic shock, the approach toward the initial management of patients should be fairly uniform, and a suggested management algorithm is outlined in Figure 93-10.

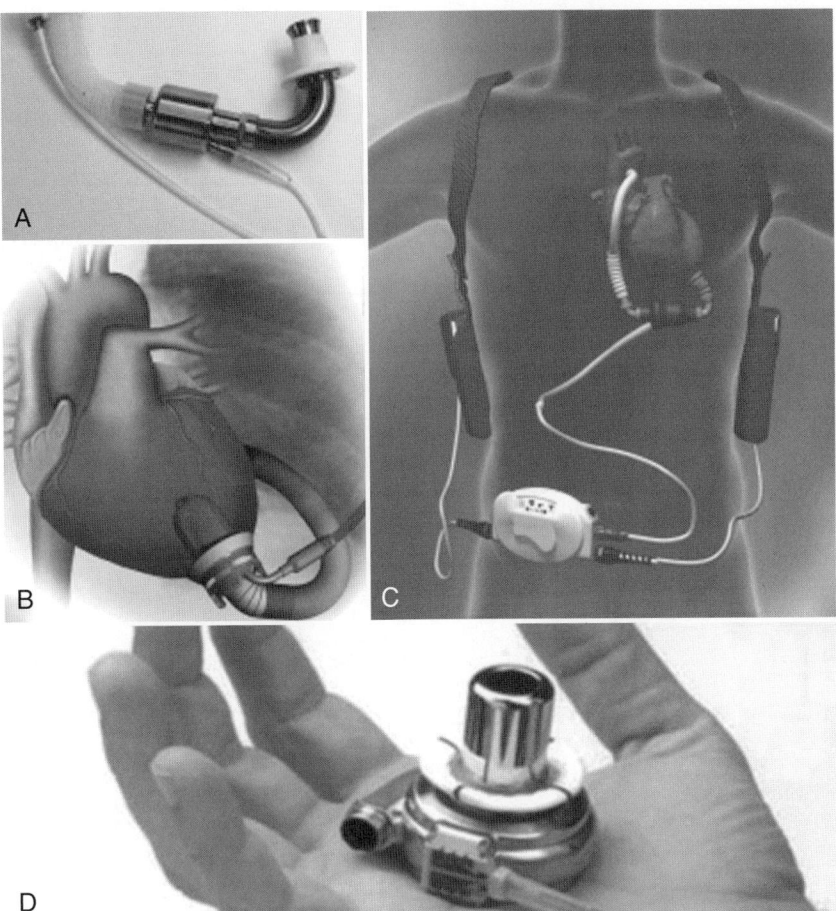

Figure 93-9 Implantable continuous flow ventricular assist devices currently in clinical use. **A,** MicroMed-DeBakey. **B,** Jarvik 2000. **C,** HeartMate II. **D,** HeartWare. *(From Mitter N, Sheinberg R. Update on ventricular assist devices. Curr Opin Anaesthesiol 23:57-66. Copyright 2010, Wolters Kluwer Health, Lippincott Williams & Wilkins.)*

First, insertion of a pulmonary arterial balloon catheter and echocardiography should be done to help formulate a differential diagnosis. Severe valvular insufficiency can usually be effectively excluded at this juncture. If severe aortic insufficiency is present, chronotropic control (heart rate 80-100 beats/min) and afterload reduction with inotropic support should be the initial maneuvers. An IABP is contraindicated because aortic regurgitation will worsen, and the patient should be prepared for immediate aortic valve replacement. Likewise, acute, severe mitral regurgitation can be readily identified with an echocardiogram and hemodynamic assessment. An IABP should be placed immediately in conjunction with inotropes and/or afterload reduction. Surgical intervention should proceed emergently and cardiac catheterization pursued preoperatively only if the patient can be adequately stabilized.

Acute fulminant myocarditis usually presents in a previously healthy individual with no history of cardiac disease. Patients with presumed myocarditis who do not stabilize after the insertion of an IABP and concomitant inotropic infusion should be diverted to VAD support expeditiously. A remarkable percentage of these patients will recover if adequately supported during the acute phase of this disease. Short-term to intermediate-term VADs are optimal in these patients because of the ease of their insertion and removal and the anticipation for relatively short-term recovery. Giant cell myocarditis is one exception to this rule, because most patients with this diagnosis will require transplantation.[165-168]

Cardiogenic shock after AMI requires immediate IABP placement, often with additional pharmacologic support. If a mechanical complication (i.e., severe mitral regurgitation or VSD) has occurred,

immediate surgical intervention is usually required. An expeditious cardiac catheterization is reasonable if the patient can be stabilized or placed on percutaneous bypass for the procedure. If no mechanical complication has occurred and the patient has been stabilized with IABP and medical therapy, cardiac catheterization may proceed. The number of diseased arteries usually determines subsequent allocation to percutaneous or surgical revascularization. Patients whose condition is unstable after an AMI, with continued cardiogenic shock despite IABP and inotropic support, should be considered for VAD support (see Figure 93-10).

Postcardiotomy cardiogenic shock should be managed intraoperatively with an initial trial of IABP and inotropic support. If there is persistent shock or an inability to be weaned from CPB, VAD implantation is the next therapeutic step, provided a meaningful recovery is predictable or a plan for transplantation or permanent therapy can be clarified.

The mode of mechanical support used for cardiogenic shock is determined by a number of factors. The first is the degree of pulmonary insufficiency. If there is pulmonary failure with a very large alveolar-to-arterial oxygen gradient on maximal ventilatory support, ECMO support is indicated. A small percentage of ECMO patients in this setting will recover, some will require VAD placement as a bridge to transplantation, fewer still will bridge to VAD and then to recovery. If the degree of pulmonary insufficiency is limited to pulmonary edema that is likely to recover with adequate cardiac output, patients should undergo VAD placement directly. The choice of VAD in this situation is also dependent on several factors including the predicted need for short- or longer-term support, the need for biventricular

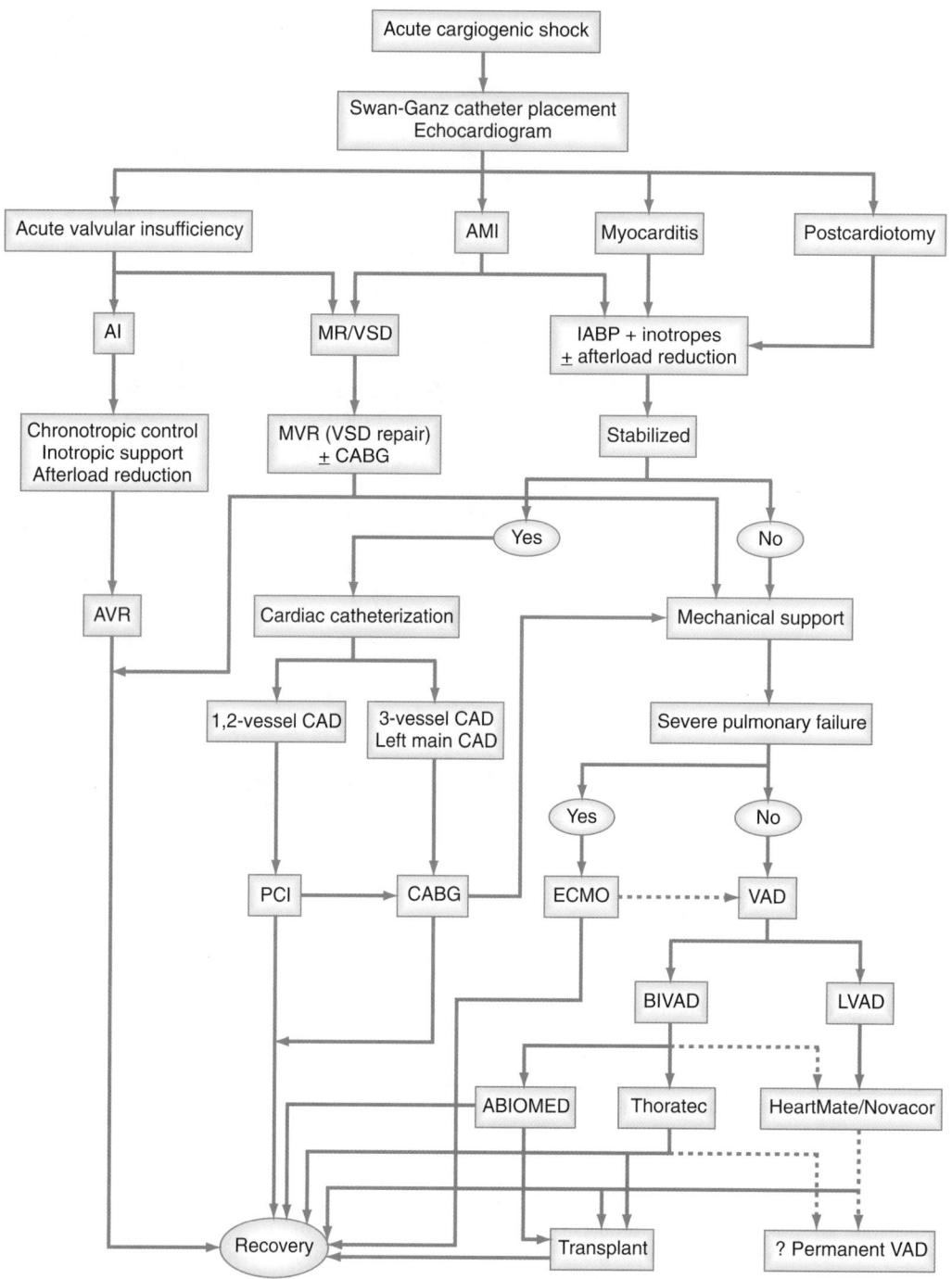

Figure 93-10 Algorithm for the management of acute cardiogenic shock.

versus univentricular support, the chance of ventricular recovery, the institutional experience with different devices, device availability, and the relative risks of anticoagulation.

The ABIOMED and Levitronix CentriMag systems are attractive options for postcardiotomy cardiac failure in those patients predicted to recover within days to a week of surgery, for cases when neurologic function is not known or is markedly compromised, and for patients who are not candidates for transplantation but may bridge to recovery or bridge to a longer-term and ambulatory device once stabilized with either device. Both are easy to insert, so in cases of profound

cardiogenic shock when operative brevity may be beneficial to patient recovery, these devices may be beneficial. Additionally, both allow for atrial cannulation, which may make conversion to other longer-term VAD systems technically easier.

The Thoratec p-VAD system is the most versatile VAD and remains the support used most frequently at our institution for the treatment of refractory cardiogenic shock. The device is relatively easy to install, may be used for short-term or long-term univentricular or biventricular support, and allows the potential for ambulation. VAD inflow cannulation can be either via the atria or ventricles. Ventricular cannulation is preferable even in the case of AMI because of its hemodynamic efficiency, reliability, and better ventricular decompression. Despite the friability of freshly infarcted myocardium, the Thoratec ventricular cannulas are safe to insert through infarcted tissue. Once a patient is stabilized with the Thoratec system, a management strategy can be mapped out as a bridge to recovery, transplantation, or permanent therapy with an intracorporeal device.

Initial placement of implantable pulsatile or continuous flow VADs (e.g., HeartMate XVE or Heartmate II) for mechanical support in patients with cardiogenic shock is generally not indicated. These devices may be used as a second bridge ("bridge-to-bridge") toward recovery, transplantation, or permanency. There may be a select group of patients in whom these intracorporeal VADs have a primary role in cardiogenic shock: (1) patients who require a larger cardiac output than other devices can generate (large individuals needing a cardiac output greater than 6 L/min to reverse the shock state); (2) patients who are more stable, can sustain longer operative times, and are unlikely to achieve myocardial recovery; and (3) patients in whom anticoagulation is contraindicated, making the HeartMate XVE device potentially safer.

■ Conclusion

Cardiogenic shock remains a lethal problem with a mortality rate as high as 75%.[2,169,170] Patients who cannot be stabilized with inotropic support and an IABP should be considered for mechanical assistance with a VAD. The ideal assist device that can be easily placed, is versatile and portable, has minimal risk of complication, offers a normal cardiac output with physiologically equivalent characteristics such as pulsatile flow, and is easily removed does not yet exist. Currently there are three modes of mechanical cardiac assistance that have received widespread use in the patient population with cardiogenic shock: ECMO/cardiopulmonary support, the ABIOMED AB 5000, and the Thoratec p-VAD system. Implantable devices such as the HeartMate LVAS XVE and Heartmate II have occasionally been used in this moribund population but have a more defined role in the subacute and chronic heart failure population.

The use of mechanical assistance for acute cardiogenic shock has facilitated impressive improvements in survival for certain disease cohorts such as those with acute myocarditis, with survival rates over 70%.[77] VADs have had a less remarkable impact on patients with postcardiotomy shock or AMI-induced shock,[111] but results in these patient populations are improving annually. Inherent to achieving better results is our understanding that patients who present with cardiogenic shock typically have significant underlying comorbidities with multiple-system organ dysfunction and marked derangements in both coagulation and inflammatory mediators that complicate management. They need to be approached by an integrated multidisciplinary team that includes cardiologists, cardiac surgeons, anesthesiologists, critical care specialists, and experienced nursing staff to implement efficient and decisive treatment plans. These integrated systems offer the greatest chance for success. Technologies expand and improve exponentially every year, and it is clear that mechanical assistance will continue to play a pivotal role in the management of these difficult patients.

KEY POINTS

1. The leading cause of death among hospitalized patients with acute myocardial infarction (AMI) continues to be cardiogenic shock.

2. Intraaortic counterpulsation for patients in shock after AMI is used in only 15% to 40% of eligible patients.

3. Pioneering surgeons recognized by the 1960s that left ventricular decompression and myocardial rest could afford enhanced cardiac recovery after the insult of open-heart surgery.

4. The physiologic rationale for the efficacy of the intraaortic balloon pump (IABP) includes (1) left ventricular systolic unloading directly reduces stroke work, which in turn reduces myocardial oxygen consumption during the cardiac cycle, and (2) diastolic augmentation which raises arterial blood pressure and provides better coronary arterial perfusion during diastole, yielding increased oxygen delivery to the myocardium.

5. The absolute indications for IABP placement include cardiogenic shock, uncontrolled angina pectoris, acute postinfarction ventricular septal defect or mitral regurgitation, and postcardiotomy left-sided heart failure with low cardiac output. IABP should be considered a primary therapy that should not be delayed until noncardiac injury is clinically evident.

6. Cardiogenic shock and high-risk angioplasty are the most common indications for use of the IABP.

7. The SHOCK trial showed that early revascularization of patients with coronary artery disease and shock after AMI, often facilitated by IABP use (86%), yielded a lower 6-month mortality rate (50%) than with medical therapy alone (63%).

8. Timing of IABP can be synchronized in one of three ways: using an arterial (preferably aortic) pressure tracing in synchrony with the dicrotic notch, using the descent of the R wave on a rhythm tracing, or timed after a ventricular pacing spike when a pacemaker is in use.

9. The effectiveness of IABP is significantly improved by proper timing of inflation and deflation.

10. Relative contraindications to IABP use include severe atheromatous and atherosclerotic descending thoracic aorta, descending aortic aneurysm, recent descending thoracic aortic surgery, and mild to moderate aortic insufficiency.

11. The incidence of major vascular complications according to the STS National Database (1996-1997) and the Benchmark Registry (1997-1999) is 5.4% and 1.4%, respectively.

12. It is clear that the mortality rate of cardiogenic shock after AMI remains high at around 40%.

13. IABP support combined with revascularization portends a better prognosis than adjunctive IABP use with medical therapy alone.

14. Short-term cardiopulmonary support for cardiogenic shock has emerged as an important adjunctive therapy. It is a relatively simple means of establishing immediate and complete circulatory support, requiring no additional equipment other than that needed for standard cardiopulmonary bypass support during cardiac surgery.

15. VADs that utilize direct cardiac outflow cannulation (VAD inflow) provide better ventricular decompression and rest than peripheral bypass support systems.

16. The hallmarks of cardiogenic shock are low cardiac output, hypotension, peripheral vasoconstriction, cold extremities, poor urine output, and altered mental status.

17. Intrinsic causes of cardiogenic shock can be divided into four pathophysiologic classifications: (1) acute valvular insufficiency, (2) acute myocardial infarction, (3) acute myocarditis, and (4) postcardiotomy cardiac failure.

18. Insertion of a pulmonary arterial balloon catheter and echocardiography should be done to help formulate a differential diagnosis.

19. Cardiogenic shock after AMI requires immediate IABP placement, often with additional pharmacologic support.

20. Initial placement of implantable VADs (e.g., HeartMate) for mechanical support in patients with cardiogenic shock is generally not indicated.

ANNOTATED REFERENCES

Farrar DJ. The Thoratec ventricular assist device: A paracorporeal pump for treating acute and chronic heart failure. Semin Thorac Cardiovasc Surg 2000;12:243-50.

The experience with use of the Thoratec system through May 2000 is reviewed. The results of over 1300 implants are discussed. Survival rates among patients transplanted and weaned from the Thoratec VAD support were 86% and 59%, respectively.

Hochman JS, Sleeper LA, Webb JG, et al. Early revascularization in acute myocardial infarction complicated by cardiogenic shock. SHOCK Investigators. Should We Emergently Revascularize Occluded Coronaries for Cardiogenic Shock. N Engl J Med 1999;341:625-34.

Results from the randomized SHOCK trial are reported. Emergency revascularization did not significantly reduce 30-day mortality, but it did reduce mortality at 6 months, and IABP placement helped facilitate early revascularization.

Pagani FD, Lynch W, Swaniker F, et al. Extracorporeal life support to left ventricular assist device bridge to heart transplant: a strategy to optimize survival and resource utilization. Circulation 1999;100:II206-10.

Experience using ECMO for initial resuscitation and as a bridge to left ventricular assist device placement and subsequent heart transplantation in patients with severe hemodynamic instability is presented. ECMO can be used to salvage some survivors from this very high-risk cohort before the utilization of LVAD resources.

Samuels LE, Holmes EC, Thomas MP, et al. Management of acute cardiac failure with mechanical assist: experience with the ABIOMED BVS 5000. Ann Thorac Surg 2001;71:S67-72; discussion S82-5.

Results of use of the ABIOMED ventricular assist device in pre- and postcardiotomy shock from one of the initial testing centers are outlined. An algorithm and standardized protocol for management of refractory cardiogenic shock with VAD insertion is presented.

Stone GW, Ohman EM, Miller MF, et al. Contemporary utilization and outcomes of intra-aortic balloon counterpulsation in acute myocardial infarction: the benchmark registry. J Am Coll Cardiol 2003;41:1940-5.

This study reviews the indications and outcomes for the usage of the intraaortic balloon pump (IABP) from 1996-2001. Data were collected prospectively in 250 medical centers with over 22,000 IABPs placed worldwide.

REFERENCES

Access the complete reference list online at http://www.expertconsult.com.

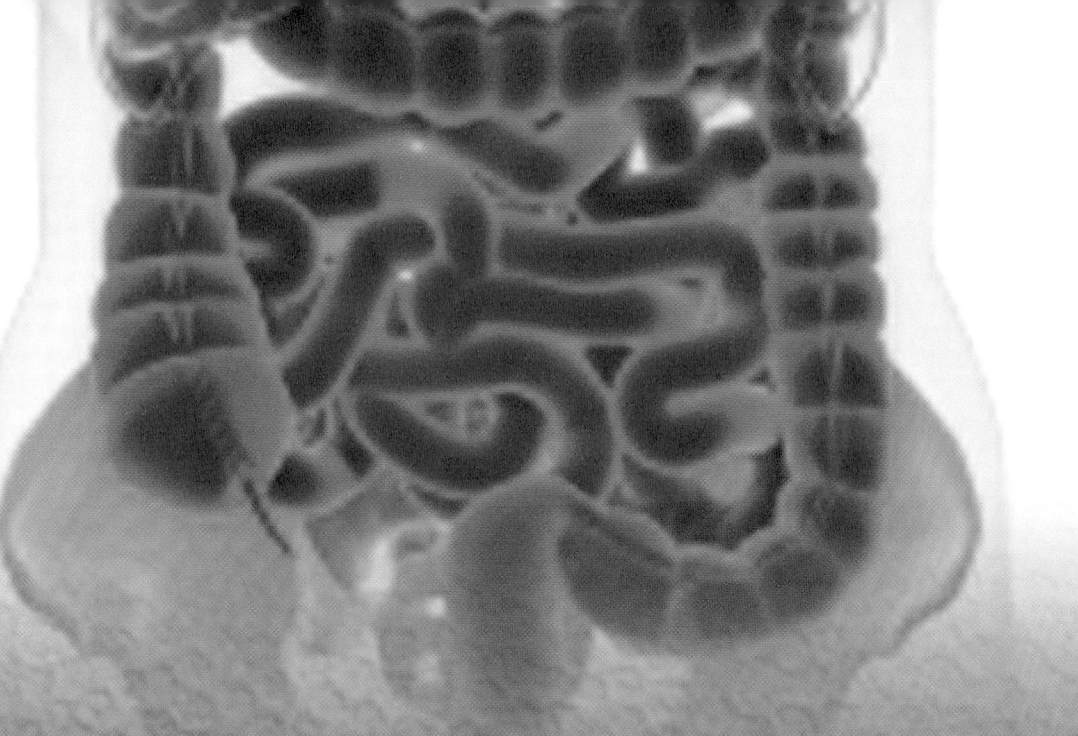

Gastrointestinal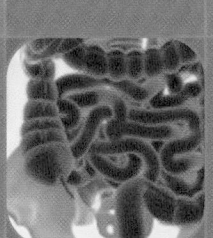

94

Critical Care Nutrition

JUAN B. OCHOA | DAREN K. HEYLAND | STEPHEN A. McCLAVE

The overall efficacy of nutritional support, the need to start nutritional therapy (NT) in the first place, and its likelihood to impact patient outcome are all determined by a number of clinical factors. All patients need a thorough and careful evaluation of their capacity to eat and the quantity and quality of their nutritional intake. When spontaneous oral intake is not possible or insufficient, or feeding patterns are disrupted, nutritional intervention is valuable. The quantity and quality of nutritional intake varies constantly to adjust to physiologic needs and thus is highly individualized. Individual evaluations and plans for NT in patients who cannot eat should also be highly individualized. The appropriate route or specific design of therapy for one disease process cannot necessarily be extrapolated (or expected to be effective) for a different disease process. Severity of illness within the patient population, level of physiologic stress, and baseline nutritional status before injury often determine a patient's need for and response to NT. Even when NT is indicated, factors related to overall amount, content, route, and timing may determine whether nutritional support influences outcome or is rendered ineffective.

Thinking about the true value of nutritional support in the intensive care unit (ICU) setting has undergone a paradigm shift. In the past, goals of nutritional support were to provide adjunctive therapy to support the stress response, provide exogenous nutrients to reduce the drain on endogenous stores and the depletion of lean body mass, and prevent the consequences of protein-calorie malnutrition. Today, providing early enteral feeding to critically ill patients is seen as a therapeutic tool or strategy to attenuate disease severity, modulate the immune response, restore or maintain gastrointestinal (GI) physiology, and through these effects, favorably impact patient outcome. Basic laboratory research and extensive clinical trials provide the basis for provision of NT to those patients who need it.

Less than ideal NT is unfortunately provided to a significant proportion of ICU patients. A recent evaluation of nutrition practices in 158 ICUs across 20 countries by Cahill et al.[1] reported significant deficits in meeting caloric and protein goals and adhering to the provision of specialized nutrition. For example, delivery of protein goals was only achieved 60.3% of the time.

One of the complex reasons for failing to prescribe and deliver NT as a standard of care is lack of awareness of its importance. Thus, this chapter emphasizes the importance of timely and adequate NT. Attaining access and initiating enteral feeding is considered part of the basic resuscitation of critically ill patients. Although any artificial nutritional support involves some risk, providing early enteral feeding is clearly an integral component of what should be considered optimal care.

Gut Use and Differential Response to Feeding and Starvation

Lack of adequate food intake is a frequent problem in the ICU. Diseases are frequently associated with significant anorexia and/or inability to eat. Surgical procedures and diagnostic tests often demand an empty stomach. A nil per os (NPO) order is too easily written even in the absence of a logical reason to do it. Despite physiologic differences between starvation in a healthy individual and lack of adequate intake during illness, it is essential to study starvation as an important aspect of nutritional care in the critically ill patient. The functional and structural integrity of the GI tract is affected by whether the gut is used and the patient receives enteral feeding. Animal and human studies suggest that enteral feeding maintains mucosal mass, stimulates cellular proliferation and production of brush-border enzymes, and maintains villus height.[2-4] Enteral nutrients maintain the integrity of tight junctions between intestinal epithelial cells, stimulate blood flow to the gut, and promote release of a variety of endogenous agents such as cholecystokinin, gastrin, bombesin, and bile salts—substances with trophic effects on intestinal epithelium. Bombesin, for example, can reverse all the histologic and functional deficits caused by parenteral feeding,[5] and gastrin and cholecystokinin can encourage partial recovery of gut-associated lymphoid tissue after the use of parenteral nutrition (PN).[6] Secretory immunoglobulin A (sIgA) and the production of bile salts help coat bacteria within the GI tract, preventing adherence. Along with the production of mucus and good GI contractility, this helps wash away bacteria in a caudad direction.[3] These mechanisms, together with antimicrobial secretions such as pancreatic enzymes, proteases, and lactoferrin help keep the total number of bacteria in check. The normal predominant anaerobic flora of the gut is maintained, preventing overgrowth of more pathogenic organisms such as Enterobacteriaceae, a process referred to as colonization resistance.[7]

Gut disuse, with or without PN, can lead to deterioration of the functional and structural integrity of the gut. In animals, gut disuse is associated with a marked reduction in villus height, cellular proliferation, mucosal mass, and brush-border enzymes. Intestinal changes caused by starvation in humans are less pronounced than in rodents, but whereas gut disuse may result in a 40% decrease of mucosal mass in rats, the decrease in humans still appears to be about 10% to 15%.[2] In humans, loss of villus height in response to pancreatitis is diminished by enteral feeding.[4] Villus atrophy is perpetuated in a time-dependent fashion with parenteral feeding.[3] Starvation alone may be insufficient to increase gut permeability, but injury followed by starvation increases mucosal permeability proportional to the severity of disease.[3,8] Increased permeability is prevented through early feeding, and in burns inversely correlates with the amount of enteral feeding delivered.[9] Increases in gut permeability are associated with systemic endotoxemia in humans.[8,10] Among burn patients, infection is associated with increased gut mucosal permeability.[9] Increases in gut permeability in critically ill patients correlate with the development of organ dysfunction.[11]

Lack of feeding in animals results in bacterial overgrowth and loss of mucosal defenses against bacterial invasion.[7,12] Reduced peristalsis (ileus) can contribute to bacterial overgrowth. Reduced secretions of bile salts and sIgA promote bacterial adherence to the mucosa. Bacterial translocation, a process whereby bacteria transgress the mucosal barrier, is associated with aerobic bacterial overgrowth and decreased intestinal sIgA levels.[3] Recent animal studies suggest that these gut-derived factors can reach the systemic circulation via the lymphatic system rather than via the portal bloodstream and thereby cause distant organ injury.[13] Thus, animal models suggest that bacterial overgrowth in the lumen leads to bacterial translocation, potentially being a portal for development of sepsis and organ failure.

The significance of bacterial translocation in humans as a cause of systemic illness is still unclear.[14,15] Translocation of bacterial products such as endotoxin may also occur. Endotoxin itself, when infused in even small doses in normal volunteers, increases gut mucosal permeability.[7] The intestinal secretion of sIgA is diminished within 5 days of gut disuse, with or without PN.[5,16] Respiratory tract secretion of IgA may be diminished even sooner. Reduction in the mucosal mass of gut-associated lymphoid tissue and decreased sIgA production increase susceptibility to infections normally controlled by IgA-mediated defenses in experimental animals.[17] In mice, as little as 5 days of gut disuse with PN results in loss of protection against respiratory viral infection and reduces clearance of the virus.[18] Refeeding with enteral nutrients restores antiviral defenses. Established antiviral mucosal immunity is lost when the GI tract is not stimulated by enteral feeding.[17]

Dendritic macrophages act as antigen-presenting cells that release cytokines and activate naive CD4$^+$ helper T cells (T$_H$0).[19] Secretion of interleukin (IL)-12 stimulates the naive cells to differentiate into T helper 1 (T$_H$1) lymphocytes, favoring a proinflammatory response and release of other proinflammatory cytokines such as IL-2, interferon gamma (IFN-γ), and tumor necrosis factor (TNF). T$_H$1 responses are associated with increased inflammation and are essential for host defenses against infection. Uncontrolled T$_H$1 responses, however, can result in self-injury. Production of IL-4 also stimulates differentiation of T$_H$0 into T$_H$2 lymphocytes,[19] leading to secretion of additional IL-4, IL-6, and IL-10. The T$_H$2 response tends to curb or check the T$_H$1 inflammatory response. T$_H$2 responses are essential to prevent self-injury caused by inflammation. However, excessive regulation of inflammatory responses by T$_H$2 cytokines can lead to immune suppression.[19]

Gut disuse, with or without PN, alters the balance of these lymphocyte populations and the profile of associated cytokines. In animals, gut disuse with PN for 5 days decreases IL-4 and IL-10 secretion and markedly reduces sIgA levels.[17] In human babies, use of PN reduces sIgA in intestinal immunocytes.[20] IFN-β, IL-5, and IL-6 production by T$_H$1 lymphocytes is not affected by gut disuse and PN.[21] Thus, the absence of enteral nutrition (EN) can unbalance the ratio of proinflammatory to antiinflammatory responses.

Gut disuse affects expression of adhesion molecules required for proper homing by naive B cells to the intestinal lamina propria and gut-associated lymphoid tissue. MADCAM-1 is the primary ligand required for the proper homing of B cells, and decreased expression of this molecule interferes with the normal migration of B cells from the vascular space into the lamina propria, leading to atrophy of Peyer's patches. In animals, there is a 60% decrease in MADCAM-1 expression within 4 days of initiating PN.[17] Within 3 days of starting PN, the number of T and B cells in the lamina propria and Peyer's patches decreases by about 50%.[3] In this model, secretion of the T$_H$1 cytokine, IFN-γ, is unchanged, but secretion of the T$_H$2 cytokines, IL-4 and IL-10, decreases. Decreased production of IL-4 and IL-10 leads to increased expression of the adhesion molecules, ICAM-1 and E-selectin, in both the intestinal and pulmonary microvasculature. Increased E-selectin expression on endothelial cells in the pulmonary microvasculature promotes sequestration and extravasation of polymorphonuclear neutrophils.[22-24] As a result, any subsequent injury (e.g., ischemia-reperfusion) can promote accumulation of polymorphonuclear neutrophils in the lungs, exacerbating organ injury and even increasing mortality.[25,26] Abundant data demonstrate that gut disuse through starvation, either caused by disease or through ill-advised physician orders or neglect, is a real problem that contributes to development of systemic infections, a systemic inflammatory response, and development of multiple organ failure.

EN, particularly if started early, prevents the ill effects of starvation. Normal enteral feeding stimulates proliferation of T$_H$2 CD4$^+$ helper T lymphocytes and the production and release of IgA-stimulating cytokines including IL-4, IL-5, IL-6, IL-10, and IL-13.[27] This process is normally counterbalanced by proliferation of T$_H$1 CD4$^+$ helper T lymphocytes and IgA-inhibitory cytokines including IFN-β, TNF, and IL-2. IL-4 stimulates naive CD4$^+$ helper T lymphocytes to convert to IgA-positive B cells in Peyer's patches. IL-10, IL-5, and IL-6 stimulate the differentiation of IgA-positive B cells into sIgA-secreting plasma cells in the lamina propria.[17]

Approximately 1 ton of food passes through the intestinal tract of an adult human every year.[20] About 1/100,000 of this intake represents intact immunologic gantigen.[20] *Oral tolerance* refers to the process whereby the immune response is down-regulated to prevent excessive

responses to common antigens found in food and in the commensal bacterial flora of the GI tract. During the induction of oral tolerance, an alternative pathway for CD4$^+$ helper T-cell activation leads to proliferation of special regulatory T cells (T$_H$3 and Tr1) which produce the counter-regulatory cytokines, IL-10 and transforming growth factor beta (TGF-β).[20] The stimulation and proliferation of T$_H$3 cells induced by enteral feeding therefore promotes expression of a balanced T$_H$2/T$_H$1 profile. The large dietary and indigenous microbial antigenic load is extremely important for maintaining normal mucosal immunity.[20] Antigenic constituents of food clearly exert a stimulatory effect on the intestinal B-cell system, helping to explain why enteral feeding supports a high density of IgA-secreting immunocytes within the intestinal lamina propria. Continued enteral feeding, as well as maintenance of the indigenous microbial flora in the gut, may help keep a balance between the T$_H$1 and T$_H$2 profile and prevent an exaggerated T$_H$1 inflammatory response.

The importance of EN for modulating the inflammatory response was illustrated by a classic study of human volunteers challenged with a small dose of *Escherichia coli* lipopolysaccharide (endotoxin).[28] One group of subjects was maintained for 1 week without feeding and received PN, whereas another group was fed enterally during the same period. After 7 days of either PN or EN, both groups were challenged with lipopolysaccharide. The subjects in the PN group had an exaggerated response to the proinflammatory stimulus, manifested by higher circulating levels of cortisol and TNF, among other findings. Similarly, following injury or an inflammatory disease process, early enteral feeding can blunt the hypermetabolic response.[29,30] Among patients with acute pancreatitis, those fed enterally rather than parenterally had significantly lower circulating levels of C-reactive protein, less evidence of oxidative stress, faster resolution of systemic inflammatory response syndrome (SIRS), and a greater decrease in their Acute Physiology and Chronic Health Evaluation (APACHE) II scores over a week of nutritional therapy.[14] In another study of patients with acute pancreatitis, there was faster resolution of the disease process among patients treated with enteral feeding compared with similar patients receiving PN.[31]

The traditional model of SIRS and the compensatory antiinflammatory response syndrome (CARS) described in trauma and sepsis may be influenced by the differential immunologic response between enteral feeding and starvation or gut disuse.[32] In SIRS, there appears to be an up-regulated, nonspecific activation of the innate immune system, with an increase in the expression of proinflammatory cytokines such as IL-1, TNF, IL-2, and IFN-γ. This profile is similar to that of the T$_H$1 subset response (in which IFN-γ, TNF, and IL-2 are produced). Intracellular bacteria and viruses absorbed through the intestinal epithelium may activate dendritic cells, macrophages, and natural killer cells to produce IL-2 and IFN-γ, which causes naive CD4 cells to proliferate into T$_H$1 cells. CARS, in contrast, appears to be a pattern of macrophage deactivation, reduced antigen presentation, and T-cell anergy, which results in a shift of the T–helper cell pattern to a T$_H$2 response.[32] Gut disuse following injury or illness may promote a SIRS response through stimulation of both the innate immune system (causing a hyperinflammatory response from macrophages and natural killer cells) and the acquired immune system (resulting in a shift from a T$_H$2 to a T$_H$1 profile).

Compared with the metabolic response to enteral feeding, this exaggerated stress response to gut disuse with or without PN has been shown to exacerbate disease severity, increase the rate of complications, and lead to prolongation of the disease process.[14,31] There is thus little justification to prolonging NPO status in critically ill patients beyond the period absolutely necessary during resuscitation, surgery, or other procedures. Process-improvement efforts aimed at minimizing starvation is an important goal of any modern ICU.

Impact of Enteral Nutrition on Outcome

Based on the theoretical rationale presented so far, EN should be associated with improved clinical outcomes in critically ill patients. To

Comparison: 01 EN vs PN
Outcome: 02 Mortality

Study	EN n/N	PN n/N	RR (95% CI random)	Weight %	RR (95% CI random)	Year
Adams	1/23	3/23		3.5	0.33 (0.04, 2.97)	1986
Borzotta	5/28	1/21		3.8	3.75 (0.47, 29.75)	1994
Cerra	7/31	8/35		14.1	0.99 (0.40, 2.41)	1998
Dunham	1/12	1/15		2.4	1.25 (0.09, 17.98)	1994
Hadfield	2/13	6/11		7.6	0.28 (0.07,1.13)	1995
Hadley	3/21	2/24		5.5	1.71 (0.32, 9.30)	1986
Kalfarentzos	1/18	2/20		3.1	0.56 (0.05, 5.62)	1997
Kudsk	1/51	1/45		2.3	0.88 (0.06, 13.70)	1992
Moore 1992	8/118	11/112		14.5	0.69 (0.29, 1.65)	1992
Rapp	9/18	3/20		10.2	3.33 (1.07, 10.43)	1983
Woodcock	9/17	5/21		14.2	2.22 (0.92, 5.40)	2001
Young	10/28	10/23		18.9	0.82 (0.42, 1.62)	1987
Total (95% CI)	57/378	53/370		100.0	1.08 (0.70,1.65)	

Test for heterogeneity chi-square = 14.70 df = 11 p = 0.2
Test for overall effect z = 0.34 p = 0.7

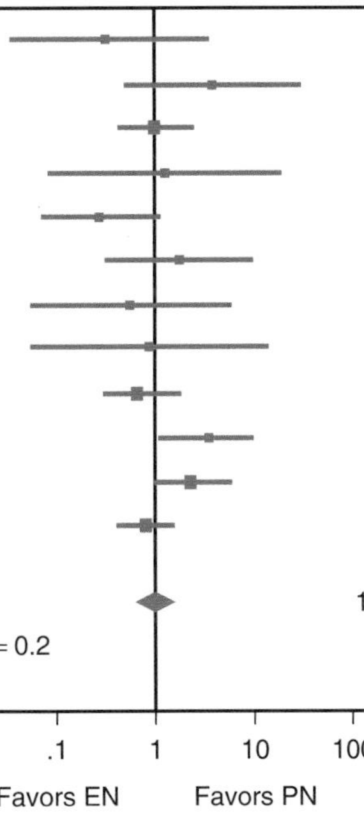

.01 .1 1 10 100
Favors EN   Favors PN

Figure 94-1 Studies comparing parenteral nutrition (PN) and enteral nutrition(EN) in terms of effect on mortality. CI, confidence interval; RR, relative risk.

evaluate the clinical evidence in support of using EN, we considered three groups of studies. The first are randomized trials that directly compared EN and PN. The second group includes studies that compared early EN (started within 24-48 hours of resuscitation) to more delayed forms of nutritional support (e.g., delayed EN, PN, or oral diet). The third group includes studies that evaluated various methods of delivering EN.

A recently published systematic analysis reviewed data from 13 randomized controlled studies comparing EN and PN in heterogeneous populations of ICU patients, including those with head trauma,

abdominal trauma, sepsis, and severe acute pancreatitis, among other conditions.[33] When a meta-analysis was carried out, there was no apparent difference in mortality rate between patients treated with EN and those treated with PN (relative risk [RR] 1.08; 95% confidence interval [CI], 0.70-1.65; Figure 94-1). However, compared with PN, EN was associated with a significant reduction in infectious complications (RR 0.61; 95% CI, 0.44-0.84; Figure 94-2).

Eight randomized controlled trials that compared early EN with more delayed forms of nutrition were recently reviewed and analyzed.[33] When these studies were aggregated, early EN was associated

Comparison: 01 EN vs PN
Outcome: 01 Infectious complications

Study	EN n/N	PN n/N	RR (95% CI random)	Weight %	RR (95% CI random)	Year
Adams	15/23	17/23		28.2	0.88 (0.60, 1.30)	1986
Kalfarentzos	6/18	15/20		14.6	0.44 (0.22, 0.90)	1997
Kudsk	9/51	18/45		14.8	0.44 (0.22, 0.88)	1992
Moore 1992	19/118	39/112		22.9	0.46 (0.29, 0.75)	1992
Woodcock	6/16	11/21		13.2	0.72 (0.34, 1.52)	2001
Young	5/28	4/23		6.3	1.03 (0.31, 3.39)	1987
Total (95% CI)	60/254	104/244		100.0	0.61 (0.44, 0.84)	

Test for heterogeneity chi-square = 7.94 df = 5 p = 0.16
Test for overall effect z = 3.00 p = 0.003

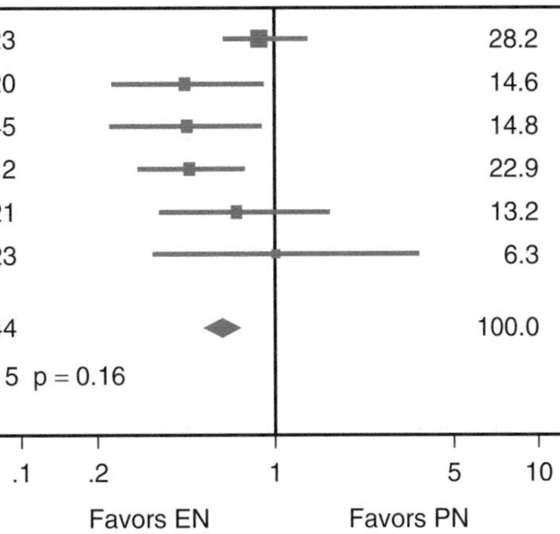

.1 .2 1 5 10
Favors EN   Favors PN

Figure 94-2 Studies comparing parenteral nutrition (PN) and enteral nutrition (EN) in terms of effect on infectious complications. CI, confidence interval; RR, relative risk.

Comparison: 01 early EN vs delayed nutrient intake
Outcome: 01 Mortality

Study	Early EN n/N	Delayed n/N	RR (95% CI random)	Weight %	RR (95% CI random)
Chiarelli	0/10	0/10		0.0	Not estimable
Chuntrasakul	1/21	3/17		11.1	0.27 (0.03, 2.37)
Eyer	2/19	2/19		15.3	1.00 (0.16, 6.39)
Kompan	0/14	1/14		5.4	0.33 (0.01, 7.55)
Minard	1/12	4/15		12.4	0.31 (0.04, 2.44)
Moore	1/32	2/31		9.5	0.48 (0.05, 5.07)
Pupelis	1/30	7/30		12.7	0.14 (0.02, 1.09)
Singh	4/21	4/22		33.6	1.05 (0.30, 3.66)
Total (95% CI)	10/159	23/158		100.0	0.52 (0.25, 1.08)

Test for heterogeneity chi-square = 4.05 df = 6 p = 0.67
Test for overall effect z = 1.76   p = 0.08

```
        .01    .1     1     10    100
       Favors early EN     Favors delayed
```

Figure 94-3   Studies comparing early versus delayed nutrient intake in terms of effect on mortality. CI, confidence interval; EN, enteral nutrition; RR, relative risk.

with treatment benefits that approached statistical significance. Early EN was associated with reduced mortality (RR 0.52; 95% CI, 0.25-1.08; Figure 94-3) and fewer infectious complications (RR 0.66; 95% CI, 0.36-1.22; Figure 94-4) compared with delayed nutrient intake. These differences approached but did not achieve statistical significance. No differences in length of hospital stay were observed between the groups. All seven studies that reported nutritional endpoints (e.g., nitrogen balance) showed a significant benefit for early EN. There were no differences in complications between the groups.

A number of strategies can be employed to maximize the delivery of EN while minimizing the risks of gastric colonization, gastroesophageal regurgitation, and pulmonary aspiration (Box 94-1). By delivering enteral feeds into the small bowel beyond the pylorus, the frequency of regurgitation and aspiration is decreased.[34] In a recent meta-analysis, there were seven randomized trials that evaluated the effect of route of feeding on rates of ventilator-associated pneumonia.[35] When these results were aggregated, there was a significant reduction in ventilator-associated pneumonia with feeding distal to the pylorus (RR 0.76; 95% CI, 0.59-0.99). These studies also demonstrated that small-bowel feeding is associated with an increase in protein and calories delivered and a shorter time to attain the target dose of nutrition.

Unless logistic problems represent an unacceptable hurdle, we recommend routine use of small-bowel feedings. If routine use of this strategy is not feasible, small-bowel feedings should be considered for patients at high risk for intolerance to EN (e.g., patients receiving inotropic or vasoactive drugs, continuous infusion of sedatives, or paralytic agents; or those with large volumes of nasogastric drainage) or at high risk for regurgitation and aspiration (e.g., patients kept supine). Finally, if obtaining small-bowel access is not feasible (e.g., because access to fluoroscopy or endoscopy is limited and blind techniques are not reliable), small-bowel feedings should be considered for selected patients who repeatedly have large gastric residual volumes

Comparison: 01 early EN vs delayed nutrient intake
Outcome: 02 Infectious complications

Study	Early EN n/N	Delayed n/N	RR (95% CI random)	Weight %	RR (95% CI random)	Year
Minard	6/12	7/15		37.7	1.07 (0.49, 2.34)	2000
Moore	3/32	9/31		20.3	0.32 (0.10, 1.08)	1986
Singh	7/21	12/22		42.0	0.61 (0.30, 1.25)	1998
Total (95% CI)	16/65	28/68		100.0	0.66 (0.36, 1.22)	

Test for heterogeneity chi-square = 3.00 df = 2 p = 0.22
Test for overall effect z = 1.32   p = 0.19

```
        .01    .1     1     10    100
       Favors early EN     Favors delayed
```

Figure 94-4   Studies comparing early versus delayed nutrient intake in terms of effect on infectious complications. CI, confidence interval; EN, enteral nutrition; RR, relative risk.

STRATEGIES TO OPTIMIZE BENEFITS AND MINIMIZE RISKS OF ENTERAL NUTRITION

Initiate early, within 24-48 h of admission.
Use small-bowel feedings.
Elevate head of the bed.
Use motility agents.
Reduce dose of narcotics prescribed.
Use feeding protocol that enables consistent evaluation of gastric residual volume and specifies when feeds should be interrupted.

and are not tolerating adequate amounts of EN intragastrically.[33] Additional strategies to maximize the benefits of EN while minimizing the risks (see Box 94-1) include caring for the patient with the head of the bed elevated 30 to 45 degrees,[36] using GI promotility agents, reducing doses of opioids,[37] and using nurse-directed feeding protocols that include frequent checking of gastric residual volumes.[38,39]

When data from all sources are considered, there is substantial clinical evidence, supported by a compelling theoretical rationale, that EN influences the clinical outcome of critically ill patients. EN is preferable to PN, and methods to maximize delivery and minimize risks should be considered in all critically ill patients receiving specialized nutritional support.

Assessment of the Critically Ill Patient

The clinician must first evaluate the level of stress in a critically ill patient to determine the likelihood of deterioration in nutritional status and to assess the overall need for aggressive nutritional support. Standardized scoring systems such as APACHE II or APACHE III, the Injury Severity Score (ISS), and the Abdominal Trauma Index (ATI) can be helpful for determining the level of stress and the likelihood of deterioration in nutritional status.[40,41] Scoring systems have also been used to assess the need for nutritional support in patients with acute pancreatitis.[42] Patients with an APACHE II score greater than 10 and having more than three Ranson's criteria require additional nutritional support.[42]

Assessment of the patient's nutritional status is difficult in the ICU. Classic chemical biomarkers, such as circulating levels of albumin and prealbumin, and immunologic parameters, such as lymphocyte counts, are all affected by the inflammatory response observed in critical illness. It is also the case for other parameters such as isokinetic dynamometry. Clinicians therefore have to be diligent at obtaining an excellent history and physical examination, identifying clinical signs of malnutrition. A history of poor nutrient intake and recent weight loss should alert the clinician that gut assimilation may be a problem, that more aggressive delivery of enteral or parenteral nutrients is appropriate, and that there is a greater need to meet calorie and protein requirements sooner in the hospital course (see Figure 94-2).

If the overall level of stress and severity of illness indicate the need for nutritional support, the clinician must next evaluate the status of the GI tract. Intravascular volume status should be optimized before initiating enteral feeds. It is not safe to infuse nutrients into the gut if there is ongoing ischemia or a high risk of mesenteric hypoperfusion. Feeding standard enteral formulas to patients with hypotension, hypovolemia, or septic shock, especially when vasopressors are being used to support blood pressure, may precipitate bowel ischemia.[43]

The concept of ileus and the clinical impression that the gut is "not working" can be misleading because intestinal motility is segmental in nature. The adequacy of gastric emptying can be evaluated by determining the presence or absence of nausea and vomiting, high residual volumes, or high output from the nasogastric tube. Colonic motility is evaluated by determining whether the patient is passing stool or gas. Small-bowel motility is evaluated by determining the presence or

absence of abdominal distention and bowel sounds. However, absorption of nutrients from the small bowel does not require intestinal motility. Infusing nutrients into the lumen of the small intestine (with or without simultaneous gastric decompression) actually can stimulate intestinal motility via the release of gastrin, bombesin, motilin, and other promotility hormones. Thus, the possible presence of ileus should not be used as an excuse to withhold oral or enteral intake; gut motility actually can improve with aggressive attempts to provide nutrition enterally.

When EN is started soon after the onset of critical illness (i.e., enteral nutrients have been lacking only a short time), one can presume that the integrity of the intestinal mucosa is well maintained, and a standard enteral formula can be used. If the period of gut disuse has been more prolonged, the clinician must consider the possibility that mucosal integrity is not normal. If there is evidence of malassimilation and diarrhea, enteral formulas containing oligopeptides may enhance absorption and assimilation of protein.[44] In a recent review of 19 prospective randomized trials in humans, 11 studies showed evidence of clinical benefit when oligopeptide-containing formulas were used instead of standard enteral (intact protein) formulas. Although there was no impact on patient outcome, the benefits of oligopeptide-based diets included significantly improved nitrogen absorption, higher visceral protein levels, more weight gain, less frequent stooling, and reduced stool volume.[44]

Once EN is started, the clinician must monitor tolerance. Overall assimilation of nutrients by the enteral route is assessed clinically by checking for the presence or absence of diarrhea. Additionally, it is important to monitor circulating concentrations of glucose, triglycerides, urea nitrogen, and creatinine ratio. Risk factors for aspiration include age older than 60 years, decreased level of consciousness, bolus feeding, and supine position.[45-47] Gastric residual volumes, output from the gastric port of an aspiration or feeding tube, and passage of stool and gas are valuable indices of intestinal motility.

Practical Considerations

All critically ill patients require a nutritional evaluation, and many benefit from receiving nutritional therapy. The complexity and degree of nutritional intervention necessary is proportional to the patient's severity of illness. In the ICU, nutritional intervention is subject to the same rules of any medical therapy demonstrating a mechanism of action, a benefit in clinical outcome, acceptable risks and side effects, and ideally a cost benefit. The form of nutritional intervention a given patient should get is not necessarily intuitive. In certain disease processes associated with high severity of illness—trauma, burns, acute pancreatitis, acute respiratory failure requiring mechanical ventilation, for example—the decision to use the parenteral rather than the enteral route for feeding can significantly affect outcome.[48,49]

The greater importance of EN among sicker patients was first shown by evaluating septic complications in trauma patients randomized at the time of surgery to receive either PN or EN.[50] Patients were ranked for severity of disease by their ATI scores. Among patients with ATI scores higher than 24, the incidence of septic complications was greater in the PN group than in the EN group (47.6% versus 11.1%; $P < 0.05$). Among patients with moderate illness and ATI scores lower than 24, there was no significant difference in the incidence of septic complications between the PN and EN groups (29.2% versus 20.8%; $P = NS$).[50]

Further evidence of the importance of maintaining gut integrity in patients with more severe disease was provided by a series of prospective randomized controlled trials of EN versus PN in patients with acute pancreatitis.[14,51,52] In the first trial published, feeding by the enteral route was shown to be safe, but only 19% of the patients had severe pancreatitis, and there were no differences in the rates of nosocomial infection, organ failure, or overall complications.[52] In a second study, 38% of the patients had severe pancreatitis, and a significantly greater percentage of those fed enterally rather than parenterally had resolution of SIRS over the first week of therapy (81% versus 17%;

$P<0.05$); nevertheless, there were no differences between the groups with respect to rates of nosocomial infection or complications.[14] In a third study, 100% of the patients had severe pancreatitis, and septic complications were reduced from 50% in the PN group to 28% in the EN group ($P<0.05$); the overall rate of complications was reduced from 75% in the PN group to 44% in the EN group ($P<0.05$).[51]

For EN support, clinicians must determine caloric requirements in order to set a goal or mandatory threshold for the volume, or "dose," of enteral feeding provided. Use of indirect calorimetry or simplistic equations (e.g., 25 kcal/kg/d) to estimate caloric requirements can help identify this threshold amount. Focusing on such a goal volume allows clinicians to determine a dose/response effect of enteral tube feeding; that is, the percentage of this goal volume required to achieve desired therapeutic endpoints (maintenance of gut integrity, containment of intestinal permeability, attenuation of the stress response, reduction of overall disease severity). In the early stages of critical illness, patients are in the throes of the hypermetabolic stress response and more prone to ileus owing to higher doses of narcotics, electrolyte abnormalities, and shifts in fluid volume. In this situation, it is difficult to provide full caloric requirements. The minimum amount or volume of feeds (as a percentage of total caloric requirements) sufficient to achieve the desired therapeutic effect is not known. Recent evidence suggests that "trophic" or "trickle" rates of feeding (usually meaning 10-30 mL/h of a nutritional formula containing ≈1 kcal/mL) are probably inadequate to provide demonstrable benefits. Data from clinical studies indicate that 50% to 65% of goal calories are needed to prevent increases in intestinal permeability in burn victims[9,53] and bone marrow transplant patients (M.T. Demeo, personal communication), promote better and faster return of cognitive function in head injury victims,[54] and reduce the duration of mechanical ventilation and ICU and hospital length of stay in critically ill patients.[55] When higher feeding rates are not feasible, trickle feeds may have limited value and should be provided, but efforts to infuse greater volumes should be continued.

Immunonutrition

An additional strategy to maximize the benefits of EN is to use formulas supplemented with specific nutrients thought to modulate the immune system, facilitate wound healing, and reduce oxidative stress. Enteral formulas have been developed that contain certain compounds such as L-glutamine, L-arginine, and omega-3 fatty acids, as well as selenium, vitamins E, C, and A, and beta carotene in supraphysiologic concentrations. Use of these products has been called *immunonutrition*, and these products have been called *immune-enhancing diets*. Although the overall effect of these individual nutrients in critically ill patients remains unknown, we have endeavored to review the efficacy and safety of products supplemented with arginine, glutamine, fish oils, and antioxidants.

L-ARGININE

The amino acid, L-arginine, plays fundamental roles in protein metabolism and polyamine synthesis and is a critical substrate for nitric oxide (NO) production.[56] L-Arginine stimulates the release of growth hormone, insulin growth factor, and insulin, all of which may stimulate protein synthesis and promote wound healing. The enzyme, L-arginase, metabolizes L-arginine to L-ornithine, an amino acid implicated in wound healing. NO is produced by a family of enzymes called *nitric oxide synthases* (NOSs) which exist in constitutive and inducible isoforms.[57] Under normal conditions and in some disease states, small quantities of NO are synthesized by the constitutive forms, which have a beneficial effect on tissue oxygenation, vasodilation, and immune function.[58]

In the absence of illness, L-arginine supplementation fails to demonstrate any significant effects on immune function. Upon immune activation, L-arginine transport is significantly increased in both myeloid and lymphoid cells, although the metabolic effects of L-arginine in these cell lineages is significantly different. L-Arginine is an essential compound for T-lymphocyte proliferation. In the absence of L-arginine, T lymphocytes lose membrane expression of the T-cell receptor complex and expression of the ζ chain, which is an intracellular peptide of the T-cell receptor. Production of some cytokines such as IFN-γ is quite sensitive to L-arginine. IL-2 production is also decreased, albeit more modestly than IFN-γ. The development of memory also appears to be compromised.

Myeloid cells can metabolize L-arginine through two different enzymes: inducible nitric oxide synthase (iNOS) or arginase-1 (ARG1). Classic inflammatory signals such as IL-1, TNF, IFN-γ, and endotoxin induce iNOS expression and the production of large amounts of NO. Classically, large amounts of NO are produced in septic patients, where excess NO production may be responsible for uncontrolled vasodilation and hemodynamic instability. Myeloid cells that produce NO are (in general) mature macrophages.

In contrast, signals that induce ARG1 expression include prostaglandin E$_2$, IL-4, IL-13, TGF-β, and IL-10, which are classically described as antiinflammatory. Up-regulation of ARG1 results in depletion of L-arginine, which can be observed in local tissues (e.g., spleen, possibly thymus) or systemically. Myeloid cells that express ARG1 are for the most part immature cells. Through L-arginine depletion, these cells regulate T-cell function and NO production; hence, these cells are called *myeloid-derived suppressor cells* (MDSC).

Yet a third state of myeloid activation can result in induction of both ARG1 and iNOS. Under these conditions, L-arginine myeloid cells paradoxically may generate reactive oxygen and nitrogen species such as hydrogen peroxide and peroxynitrite.

A growing number of illnesses exhibit a significant decrease in circulating L-arginine associated with the presence of MDSC expressing ARG1. T-lymphocyte dysfunction is characterized by loss of membrane expression of the T-cell receptor (TCR), loss of the ζ chain, and decreased production of IL-2 and IFN-γ. These disease states include certain cancers such as renal cell carcinoma, infections such as tuberculosis, and after physical injury (including trauma and elective surgery). Interestingly, L-arginine plasma levels in sepsis vary significantly, and low, normal, or elevated L-arginine plasma levels have been reported in the literature.

The dichotomy of L-arginine metabolism observed in myeloid cells (ARG1 versus iNOS) is thus best characterized by two disease processes: physical injury and sepsis, though obviously, a significant amount of overlap exists. Because L-arginine metabolism can take such significantly different routes, its supplementation in the diet can have significantly different biological consequences and affect clinical outcomes. Patient selection is thus an essential aspect of any clinical trial designed to evaluate the value of L-arginine supplementation.

L-Arginine is traditionally ordered at supraphysiologic doses along with omega-3 fatty acids, nucleotides, and other so-called immune nutrients and has been tested in patients recovering from elective surgery, trauma victims, and other critically ill patients, including those with sepsis.

Immunonutrition is the best studied aspect of NT in the ICU, and L-arginine remains the best studied compound in this context. Significant confusion regarding interpretation and results of these studies exists in the literature, in great part because a mechanistic hypothesis was poorly delineated. However, clear guidelines now have been reported by different organizations so that clinicians can safely incorporate the use of L-arginine into clinical practice. These guidelines are the result of improved understanding of L-arginine metabolism, the discovery of disease processes associated with severe L-arginine depletion, the negative biological consequences stemming from L-arginine deficiency, and a more careful analysis of the multiple clinical studies available. Guidelines for arginine supplementation can be summarized as follows:

1. Higher than normal (supraphysiologic) L-arginine supplementation is necessary. Normal L-arginine intake is 3 to 5 g/d. Diets available contain significant variation in the amount of L-arginine. In general, effectiveness of L-arginine as a dietary supplement is observed with diets containing higher concentrations of this compound.

2. Dietary supplementation with L-arginine alone should not be used, as only diets that contain a combination of L-arginine, omega-3 fatty acids, and nucleotides have been extensively tested and proven to provide a clear clinical benefit. Interactions among the different "immune nutrients" has not been systematically evaluated, although it is possible that omega-3 fatty acids modulate the appearance of MDSC and blunt ARG1 expression, hence increasing L-arginine availability.

3. Patients undergoing major elective surgery benefit from the use of immunonutrition formulas containing L-arginine. The risk of infections is reduced approximately 40% ($P < 0.0001$). In addition, there is significant reduction in the number and severity of other complications. All these benefits translate to a decrease in length of stay of approximately 2 to 3 days ($P < 0.0001$).[59,60] Cost benefits of these diets have been best studied in patients undergoing surgery for cancer, demonstrating savings of several thousand dollars per patient in a given surgical practice[61]; L-arginine-containing diets are now standard of care. There is no controversy regarding this point; it has been endorsed as a grade A recommendation by all major nutrition societies and the Society of Critical Care Medicine (SCCM).[62,63]

4. Immunonutrition incorporating supraphysiologic quantities of L-arginine ideally should be started preoperatively as an oral dietary supplement and continued in the postoperative period as early as possible, delivered in an enteral presentation if the patient cannot eat. In general, these diets should be started 5 days prior to surgery and continued 5 to 10 days postoperatively.

5. All elective surgical patient populations, including patients undergoing operations for head and neck cancer and patients undergoing cardiac or GI surgery, appear to benefit from the use of immunonutrition formulas containing L-arginine. A significant number of these patients will be considered critically ill and thus admitted to an ICU.

6. Trauma patients may benefit from the use of immunonutrition formulas containing L-arginine.[64] Immunonutrition containing glutamine (which is metabolized to arginine when given enterally) may be of particular benefit in trauma and burn patients.[65,66] Harm has not been reported. However, the number of patients studied is low, and further research is advisable. Benefits from these diets appear to be observed in those trauma patients who receive higher volumes and have lesser degrees of injury.[62,63]

7. A clear benefit of L-arginine-containing immunonutrition has not been observed in medical patients, particularly those with sepsis. Thus, for these patients, administration of L-arginine in pharmacologic doses remains controversial. Potential evidence of harm has been suggested in severely septic patients.[67] It remains theoretically possible that increased L-arginine availability results in increased NO production and worsening of the hemodynamic state. This possibility, however, has not been demonstrated in clinical practice. The lack of clarity both in understanding basic L-arginine metabolism during sepsis and confusing clinical results (showing both increased and decreased mortality) has led to highly divergent clinical recommendations.[68] For example, the SCCM suggests a grade B recommendation in the presence of sepsis,[62,63] while others recommend immunonutrition containing supraphysiologic quantities of L-arginine be withheld.[67] The authors of this chapter err on the safe side of clinical practice and urge caution with use of these diets during sepsis.

OMEGA-3 FATTY ACIDS

Dietary omega-3 and omega-6 fatty acids are incorporated into phospholipids and thereby influence the structure and function of cellular membranes. Omega-3 and omega-6 fatty acids also serve as substrates for the enzymes cyclooxygenase, lipoxygenase, and cytochrome P450 oxidase, leading to the formation of prostaglandins, thromboxanes, leukotrienes, and lipoxins. Metabolism of omega-6 fatty acids leads to the formation of arachidonic acid. Metabolism of arachidonate via the cyclooxygenase pathway results in the production of compounds containing two double bonds which are called *bisenoic prostanoids* and are designated by a subscript 2 (e.g., prostaglandin [PG]E$_2$). Metabolism of omega-3 fatty acids leads to the formation of eicosapentaenoic acid (EPA). Trienoic prostanoids (e.g., PGE$_3$) are derived from EPA. Products derived from arachidonic acid via the 5-LO pathway are designated by a subscript 4 (e.g., leukotriene [LT]B$_4$), whereas products resulting from the action of 5-lipoxygenase (5-LO) on EPA are designated by a subscript 5 (e.g., LTB$_5$). The 2-series prostanoids and the 4-series leukotrienes are potent biological mediators. In contrast, the 3-series prostanoids and the 5-series leukotrienes derived from EPA are much less active.

Experimentally increasing the quantity of omega-3 fatty acids (found in fish oils) in the diet reduces platelet aggregation, slows blood clotting, and limits the production of proinflammatory cytokines.[69] Data from studies using animal models suggest that a diet enriched with fish and borage oils can ameliorate inflammation-induced acute lung injury.[70,71] The only clinical study of fish oil (omega-3 fatty acid) supplementation pertinent to the care of critically ill patients was carried out by Gadek and colleagues.[72] In a randomized multicenter double-blind clinical trial, these investigators studied the effects of a diet (Oxepa7; Ross Products, Columbus, Ohio) supplemented with fish oils (containing EPA and docosahexaenoic acid), borage oil (rich in γ-linolenic acid), and antioxidants on markers of lung inflammation and survival. Patients (n=146) with acute respiratory distress syndrome (ARDS) were randomized within 24 hours of meeting entrance criteria to either a high-fat, low-carbohydrate control diet or the experimental diet. Only 98 of the 146 patients were deemed evaluable and included in the efficacy analysis. Among the evaluable patients, those who received the experimental diet had higher plasma phospholipid fatty acid levels (i.e., dihomo-γ-linolenic acid, EPA, and EPA/arachidonic acid ratio) and fewer total cells and neutrophils recovered from bronchoalveolar lavage fluid obtained on study days 4 and 7.

In addition, Pao$_2$/Fio$_2$ ratios on days 4 and 7 showed greater improvement in patients receiving the experimental diet compared with control patients. There was a non-significant improvement in survival in the experimental group compared with controls (16% versus 25%; P=0.17). Patients fed the experimental diet required fewer days on supplemental oxygen (13.6 versus 17.1; P=0.078), required significantly fewer days of ventilatory support (9.6 versus 13.2; P=0.027), spent less time in the ICU (11.0 versus 14.8 days; P=0.016), and had fewer new organ failures (10% versus 25%; P=0.018). Thus, the findings from this study support the view that administration of dietary lipids rich in omega-3 fatty acids can modify the lipid profile and favorably affect clinical outcome among critically ill patients with ARDS. However, a high-fat diet may be harmful, at least in critically ill burn victims,[73] so the results of the Gadek study may be confounded by use of a high-fat control formula.[72] Further, because of the addition of supplements other than fish oils (e.g., antioxidants), it is not possible to definitively attribute the beneficial effects of the experimental diet to its higher content of omega-3 fatty acids.

L-GLUTAMINE

The amino acid, L-glutamine, plays a central role in nitrogen transport within the body. It is used as a fuel by rapidly dividing cells, particularly lymphocytes and gut epithelial cells,[74-76] and is also a substrate for synthesis of the important endogenous antioxidant, glutathione. Although L-glutamine is not an essential amino acid under normal conditions, plasma L-glutamine concentration decreases during critical illness, and low circulating levels of L-glutamine have been associated with immune dysfunction[77] and increased mortality.[78] Thus, L-glutamine may be regarded as a "conditionally essential" amino acid.

The effects of L-glutamine supplementation on clinically important outcomes have been assessed in several randomized trials of surgical and critically ill patients,[79] and the results from these studies have been subjected to meta-analysis.[80] In the aggregate, L-glutamine supplementation is associated with a significant reduction in mortality (RR 0.78;

95% CI, 0.61-0.99; $P=0.04$), a trend toward a reduction in infectious complications (RR 0.89; 95% CI, 0.73-1.08; $P=0.2$), and no overall effect on length of stay (weighted mean difference in days, −1.30; 95% CI, −4.77 to 2.17). When route of administration (parenteral versus enteral) was assessed in a subgroup analysis, the majority of the treatment effect with respect to mortality and infectious complications was associated with parenteral administration of L-glutamine in patients receiving PN. Because the majority of L-glutamine provided enterally is metabolized in the gut and liver, it may not have a systemic effect. Only one small study in burn patients demonstrated a reduction in mortality with enteral L-glutamine.[81] In a study of trauma patients, administration of an enteral formula supplemented with L-glutamine was associated with a non-significant decrease in the number of infections compared with the number of infections observed with administration of the control formula (20 of 35 [57%] versus 26 of 37 [70%]).[82]

Therefore, for critically ill patients requiring PN, we recommend L-glutamine supplementation as long as the patient remains on PN. Enteral diets supplemented with L-glutamine can be considered for patients with major burns or trauma. Recommendations regarding L-glutamine supplementation (enteral or parenteral) in other critically ill patient populations are premature and warrant further study.

L-Glutamine unfortunately is unstable in aqueous solutions. To overcome this problem, L-glutamine is added to TPN solutions as a dipeptide (L-alanyl-L-glutamine). In patients receiving EN, L-glutamine powder can be dissolved into the nutrition formulation.

ANTIOXIDANTS, VITAMINS, AND TRACE MINERALS

For a variety of inflammatory, infectious, and ischemic diseases, reactive oxygen species (ROS) represent a final common pathway. These toxic mediators (e.g., superoxide anion, hydroxyl radical, hydrogen peroxide, hypochlorous acid) can cause cellular injury by numerous mechanisms including destruction of cell membranes through the peroxidation of fatty acids; disruption of organelle membranes, such as those bounding lysosomes and mitochondria; degradation of hyaluronic acid and collagen; and disruption of key proteins and enzymes such as Na^+/K^+-ATPase or alpha$_1$-proteinase inhibitor. To protect tissues from ROS-induced injury, the body maintains a complex endogenous defense system including enzymes such as superoxide dismutase, catalase, glutathione peroxidase, and glutathione reductase. These enzymes all have metals—notably, manganese, selenium, copper, or zinc—at their active sites. When these enzymatic antioxidants are overwhelmed, ROS are free to react with susceptible target molecules and cause cellular damage. Thus, cells have a secondary means of scavenging ROS using nonenzymatic antioxidants that are either water soluble, such as glutathione and vitamin C, or lipid soluble, such as vitamin E and beta carotene.[83]

In critical illness, oxidative stress arises as the result of an imbalance between protective antioxidant mechanisms and generation of ROS. This imbalance may be due to excess generation of ROS, low antioxidant capacity, or both. Plasma and intracellular concentrations of the various antioxidants are abnormally low in subpopulations of critically ill patients.[84-86] In critical illness, evidence of oxidative stress includes high circulating levels of byproducts of lipid per oxidation, markers of protein oxidation, nitration or nitrosylation, or increased activity of ROS-producing enzymatic systems.[87]

In a recent meta-analysis,[88] we aggregated results from 12 randomized trials that were designed to assess the value of administering exogenous antioxidants to critically ill patients.[87,89-99] Of the included studies, several examined the effects of a single nutrient with antioxidant properties.[90,92-94,96] In most cases, the nutrient evaluated was selenium,[90,92-94] but one study assessed the effect of zinc supplementation on outcome in ventilated patients with head trauma.[96] The effects of selenium combined with other antioxidants were assessed in four studies,[89-91,99] and four studies focused on the effects of vitamin A, vitamin C, vitamin E, N-acetylcysteine, and glutathione.[87,95,97,98] When the 12 trials were aggregated, antioxidants were associated with a

significant reduction in mortality (RR 0.66; 95% CI, 0.45-0.95; $P=0.03$). Only five of these studies reported on infectious complications.[87,90,91,95,97] When these results were aggregated, antioxidants had no effect on infectious complications (RR 0.94; 95% CI, 0.63-1.40; $P = 0.8$). In further subgroup analysis, the majority of the treatment effect seemed to be related to parenteral rather than enteral administration of antioxidants or antioxidant nutrients, especially selenium. Thus for critically ill patients, selenium supplementation in combination with other antioxidants (vitamin E or alpha tocopherol, vitamin C, N-acetylcysteine, zinc) may be beneficial.

Appropriate Use of Total Parenteral Nutrition in the Intensive Care Unit

The enteral route of feeding is always preferable to the parenteral route, but EN is not always available, reliable, or safe. PN may be effective in specific circumstances when used correctly; in other circumstances, no nutritional therapy may be the most appropriate management. In the critical care setting, EN is clearly the first choice. In most cases, no nutritional support (other than glucose-containing intravenous fluids) is the second best alternative when EN is unavailable, impractical, or unsafe. PN is usually the choice of last resort.

PATIENT SELECTION

In almost all critical care patient populations involving a wide range of disease processes (from surgery and pancreatitis to trauma, burns, and critically ill patients on mechanical ventilation), EN is first-line therapy and should be chosen before PN. Reduction of infections by the use of EN compared with PN is consistent regardless of whether patients have cancer or protein-energy malnutrition.[100] In the critical care of an average patient with an intact GI tract, PN should never be selected ahead of EN. When studies from diverse critical care patient populations are combined, "standard therapy" in which no artificial nutritional support is provided has a more favorable impact on patient outcome than PN does. In a recent meta-analysis, Braunschweig and colleagues showed a statistically significant reduction in infections with standard therapy compared with PN (RR 0.77; 95% CI, 0.65-0.91).[100] If the patients were clearly well nourished, an even greater reduction in the incidence of infections was seen with standard therapy compared with PN (RR 0.61; 95% CI, 0.50-0.76).[100] There was a trend toward reduced overall complications with standard therapy, which just missed statistical significance (RR 0.87; 95% CI, 0.74-1.03).[100] Hospital length of stay was reduced significantly in 8 of the 14 studies reviewed by Heyland and coworkers in which standard therapy was compared with PN.[101]

The presence of protein-calorie malnutrition (PCM) reverses the choice between standard therapy and PN. In general, PN has greater efficacy in patients with PCM, and the chance of a favorable impact on patient outcome is more likely with PN than with standard therapy. PCM is most commonly defined by a greater than 10% to 15% weight loss[101] or a low body mass index.[102] In patients with severe PCM, PN reduces infectious morbidity, overall major complications, and even mortality in comparison to standard therapy. In their meta-analysis, Heyland and coworkers showed a 48% reduction in risk of major complications with the use of total PN compared with standard therapy in malnourished surgery patients (RR 0.52; 95% CI, 0.30-0.91).[101] In a diverse population of malnourished patients, giving no nutritional support and providing standard therapy are associated with a trend toward increased infection (RR 1.17; 95% CI, 0.88-1.56) and a significant threefold increase in mortality (RR 3.0; 95% CI, 1.09-8.56).[100] Those patients with severe PCM, the ones most likely to benefit from PN, usually represent a very small minority of patients. The prevalence of severe PCM in some studies of ICU patients ranged from 8.3% to 12.6%.[103-105]

Critically ill patients with sepsis and multiple organ dysfunction respond poorly to PN. Heyland et al. showed a trend toward a 2.5-fold increase in complications (RR 2.40; 95% CI, 0.88-6.58) and a significant twofold increase in mortality (RR 0.178; 95% CI, 1.11-2.85) from the use of PN compared with standard therapy with no nutritional support.[101]

Thus, for critical care nutrition in general, the clinician should rarely choose PN over EN. Aggressive EN appears to be the first-line therapy for nutritional support in critical care and is associated with lower infectious morbidity compared with the parenteral route. EN appears to be superior to both PN and standard therapy with no nutritional support across diverse patient populations. When EN is not feasible, aggressive nutritional support may have to be held for 7 to 10 days following an injury or an acute event. These patients, despite critical illness, sepsis, and multiple organ dysfunction, are better managed by standard therapy with no PN support over this initial period. Only if there is evidence of PCM (and EN is not feasible) should PN be given preferentially over standard therapy in the first week.

LIPID CONTENT

Use of emulsified lipids (Intralipid) with PN is controversial because previous studies have shown that long-chain fats can cause immune suppression.[106] Intralipid can promote dysfunction of the reticuloendothelial system, enhance formation of prostanoids and leukotrienes, increase generation of ROS, and adversely affect the composition of cell membranes.[106]

Several reports demonstrate that intravenous lipids can adversely affect immune status and clinical outcome.[106-108] Results of a meta-analysis of PN suggest that the adverse effects of lipids may negate any beneficial effects of nonlipid PN supplementation.[101] Two studies compared the use of lipids to no lipids in PN.[106,109] Among trauma patients, the use of PN without lipids versus with lipids was associated with a significant reduction in pneumonia (48% versus 73%; P=0.05), catheter-related sepsis (19% versus 43%; P=0.04), length of ICU stay (18 versus 29 days; P=0.02), and length of hospital stay (27 versus 39 days; P=0.03).[110] In another study, the group that received no lipids (hypocaloric group) showed a trend toward a reduction in infections compared with the group that received lipids (29% versus 53%; P=0.2).[109] Combining these two studies, a meta-analysis showed a significant reduction in infections in the group that received no lipids (RR 0.63; 95% CI, 0.42-0.93) and no difference in mortality (RR 1.29; 95% CI, 0.16-10.7).[101]

The long-term effects of fat-free PN are unknown. However, some fat—at least 5% of total calories—has to be provided as lipid emulsion to prevent essential fatty acid deficiency, although this issue is usually not important until after the first 10 days of hospitalization.[102] Therefore, lipid-free PN is probably best given to those patients requiring only short-term PN (<10 days). This recommendation cannot be extrapolated to those who have an absolute contraindication to EN and need PN for a longer duration.

EFFECT OF HYPERGLYCEMIA

Hyperglycemia might be a key factor in the reduced efficacy and increased rate of complications associated with PN. Hyperglycemia impairs neutrophil chemotaxis and phagocytosis,[100] leads to glycosylation of immunoglobulins,[111] impairs wound healing,[112] alters function of the complement cascade,[113] and exacerbates inflammation.[110]

Compared with EN, PN more frequently leads to hyperglycemia. For a variety of reasons, patients receiving EN often receive fewer total calories than those receiving PN.[100] Whereas PN formulas typically contain 60% to 75% carbohydrate, EN formulas usually contain 40% to 55% carbohydrate.[100] The parenteral route of feeding has been shown to lead to an increased stress response compared with enteral feeding. This effect in turn may increase endogenous glucose production and decrease glucose oxidation.[100]

The results from a number of early studies highlight the relationship between hyperglycemia and incidence of nosocomial infection. In an early meta-analysis by Moore et al. comparing parenteral and enteral

routes of feeding in trauma patients, mean blood glucose concentration was greater than 200 mg/dL in the PN group on postoperative days 7 to 9, whereas it was only 132 mg/dL during the same period in patients receiving EN (P<0.05).[110] Incidence of infection was 44% in the PN group and 17% in the EN group (P<0.05).[110] In a different study, Kudsk and colleagues provided further evidence that hyperglycemia increases risk of infection.[111] Among trauma patients randomized to EN or PN, those with a blood glucose concentration greater than 220 mg/dL had a 53% incidence of infection, whereas those with a blood glucose concentration less than 220 mg/dL had 23% incidence of infection (P<0.03).

Van den Berghe et al. compared intensive insulin therapy (target range for blood glucose concentration, 4.4-6.1 mmol/L) and conventional treatment (target range for blood glucose concentration, 10.0-11.1 mmol/L) in critically ill patients receiving nutritional support.[114] This was a large study (n=1548) of surgical ICU patients (predominantly elective cardiovascular surgery) with relatively low APACHE II scores (median 9). Study patients were started on a glucose load (200-300 g/day) and then were advanced to PN, combined PN-EN, or EN after 24 hours of admission. Intensive insulin therapy was associated with a lower incidence of sepsis (P=0.003), a trend toward a reduction in ventilator days, reduced ICU length of stay (P<0.04), and decreased hospital mortality (P=0.01) compared with conventional insulin therapy.[114]

Initial enthusiasm with Van den Berghe's study led to widespread adoption of tight glycemic control even in the absence of additional trials. In 2009, results of the NICE-SUGAR trial became available. NICE-SUGAR (Normoglycemia in Intensive Care Evaluation–Survival Using Glucose Algorithm Regulation) was a prospective trial that randomized 6104 patients to tight glycemic control (80-108 mg/dL) or conventional glucose management (glucose < 180 mg/dL). A small but significant decrease in mortality was observed for the control group when compared to those receiving intensive insulin therapy (27.5% versus 24.9%, P=0.02). In addition, significantly more patients exhibited hypoglycemia (P < 0.0001). Differences in trial design between Van den Berghe's study and the NICE-SUGAR study may account for these disparate results. For one, high glucose infusions were used in Van den Berghe's trial. In addition, the studies used different techniques for glucose measurement.

From these studies, one can infer that hyperglycemia (defined as a circulating glucose concentration > 200 mg/dL) is associated with poor outcome in different critically ill patient populations including trauma, strokes, and acute coronary syndromes.[115-118] Using conventional glucose monitoring systems, glucose levels below 180 mg/dL should be maintained in critically ill patients.

CALORIC PROVISION—PERMISSIVE UNDERFEEDING

Several studies have shown a correlation between provision of excessive amounts of calories and increased rates of insulin resistance, infectious morbidity, and mortality. Hyperglycemia (blood glucose concentration > 220 mg/dL) has been shown to occur in greater than 50% of nondiabetic patients receiving PN in excess of 35 kcal/kg actual body weight per day.[119] In a retrospective study, patients who received a high dose of carbohydrates (77% of total calories and 42.4 kcal/kg/d on average) were compared with patients who received a lower dose of carbohydrates (60.6% of total calories and 34.3 kcal/kg/d on average).[120] The group that received more carbohydrates had significantly more episodes of sepsis (14 episodes in 26 patients versus 4 episodes in 17 patients; P < 0.05) and significantly higher mortality (28% versus 10%; P < 0.05).[120] Although the group on the higher-carbohydrate regimen received less protein than the group on the lower-carbohydrate regimen (82.5 versus 98.7 g/day), this difference did not reach statistical significance.[120]

In another study, children with greater than 60% total body surface area burns were randomized to either a control group that received a high-carbohydrate, normal-protein regimen of PN or a study group that received a reduced-carbohydrate, high-protein regimen.[121] The control group received 87% of goal calories, whereas the study group received only 77.7% of goal calories (*P*<0.002). The number of bacteremic days was 11% in the control group but only 8% in the experimental group (*P*<0.05). Mortality was 44% in the control group and 0% in the experimental group (*P*<0.03).[121]

Two additional studies evaluated the effect of hypocaloric feeding in critically ill patients. To achieve a hypocaloric dose of PN, Choban et al.[122] reduced both carbohydrates and lipids in morbidly obese critically ill patients, whereas McCowen et al.[109] withheld lipids in a heterogeneous group of patients including critically ill patients. In the study by McCowen's group, hypocaloric feeding was associated with a trend toward a reduction in infectious complications (*P*=0.2)[109]; infectious complications were not reported in the study by Choban's group.[122] There were no significant differences in mortality or length of stay between groups in either study.

Results of these studies suggest that insulin-resistant patients get hyperglycemic at lower rates of energy intake. Gain in body fat mass in response to excessive PN provision enhances the propensity to hyperglycemia and results in an increased incidence of sepsis. Isocaloric diets can have different effects depending on insulin resistance. Malnutrition and loss of body fat may increase insulin sensitivity. Patients with some degree of malnutrition seem to tolerate an infusion of carbohydrate and fat without hyperglycemia and hypertriglyceridemia and thus respond to nutritional support without added risk. Standard energy intake in patients with sepsis may actually exacerbate morbidity and mortality.

Thus, although increased protein intake is good, high nonprotein energy intake (from carbohydrates and fats) may reduce the benefits of nutritional support. "Permissive underfeeding," in which total caloric provision is set at 20 kcal/kg actual body weight (or even ideal body weight) per day may optimize the efficacy of PN in critically ill (especially septic) patients.

SUPPLEMENTAL TOTAL PARENTERAL NUTRITION

Few studies have looked at the impact of supplemental PN in patients receiving an insufficient volume of enteral feeding. In a study of 120 critically ill patients, Bauer and colleagues compared a control group receiving EN alone with a study group treated with EN supplemented with PN; both groups were fed for at least 4 to 7 days after starting nutritional support.[123] Overall, there was no difference in morbidity or mortality between the two groups. Duration of stay in the ICU, duration of mechanical ventilation, incidence of respiratory infection, and mortality were equal between the two groups. Hospital length of stay was shorter in the study group receiving supplemental PN than in the control group (31.2 versus 33.7 days; *P*=0.002), but this effect was easily explained by a statistically significant earlier date of entry into the study (1.1 versus 1.5 days; *P*=0.002). The cost of nutritional support was doubled by the addition of supplemental PN.

Of greater concern was a study by Herndon and colleagues of patients with greater than 50% total body surface area burns.[124] Mortality was significantly higher among the 16 study patients treated with EN and supplemental PN than it was in the 23 control patients treated with EN alone (63% versus 26%; *P*<0.05). Supplemental PN added to EN in the study group decreased the amount of enteral calories patients tolerated. Although both groups exhibited depressed natural killer cell activity from days 0 to 14, the group receiving supplemental PN experienced greater depression of T cell helper-suppressor ratios from days 7 to 14.

A recent meta-analysis evaluated five randomized trials that addressed the clinical benefits of supplemental PN in critically ill patients.[125] The aggregated results demonstrated a trend toward increased mortality associated with the use of combination EN and PN (RR 1.27; 95% CI, 0.82-1.94; *P*=0.3). Supplemental PN was not associated with a difference in the incidence of infection (RR 1.14; 95% CI, 0.66-1.96; *P*=0.6). Supplemental PN had no effect on hospital stay (standardized mean difference −0.12 days; 95% CI, −0.45 to 0.2 days; *P*=0.5) or ventilator days. Thus, there appears to be no clinical evidence

to support the practice of supplementing EN with PN when EN is initiated. Supplemental PN adds nothing and may actually worsen the outcome for patients already on EN.

DURATION AND TIMING OF PARENTERAL NUTRITION

When EN is not feasible, providing standard therapy with no artificial nutritional support may be better than PN in well-nourished patients, regardless of their disease process. The timing of PN initiation is based on the underlying nutritional status of the patient. In a previously well-nourished but otherwise critically ill patient who has not resumed oral intake, it is reasonable to wait 7 to 10 days before initiating PN.[100,126] Some experts recommend a longer waiting period (10 to 14 days) before initiating PN in a previously well-nourished patient who is not expected to resume oral intake soon.[92,93] However, after 14 days, increased mortality is seen in most patients who are not yet eating and remain on standard therapy with no nutritional support.[127] After 14 days, initiating PN is clearly associated with less mortality than providing no nutritional support.[127] PN is indicated over standard therapy for the first 7 to 10 days when the enteral route is not available in malnourished patients (usually characterized by >10%-15% weight loss). PN should not be initiated unless more than 7 to 10 days of therapy is anticipated. No studies of short-term PN (<7 days) have shown it to be efficacious or to impact favorably on patient outcome.

▣ Future Considerations

In the future, nutritional prescriptions will likely be complex recommendations that continue to consider protein and calorie requirements but, in addition, consider the key nutrients needed to modulate the stress response, maintain gut integrity, and ameliorate the pathophysiology of the underlying critical illness (Figure 94-5). It may turn out that prescription of key substrates will have a greater effect on outcome than provision of calories or protein per se. For example, consider a critically ill patient with clinical or biochemical evidence of hypoperfusion. Early in the course of the illness, current thinking would say that EN is contraindicated. However, providing L-glutamine or antioxidants enterally may be exactly what this patient needs to recover from the oxidative stress associated with critical illness. The need to meet protein and calorie requirements might occur much later in the course of the illness (see Figure 94-5). Although this example represents an extreme case, nutritional prescriptions in the future will have to be more cognizant of evolving pathophysiology and the ability of nutrients to modulate the integrity of the immune system, systemic inflammatory response, and the underlying disease in the early phases of the clinical course.

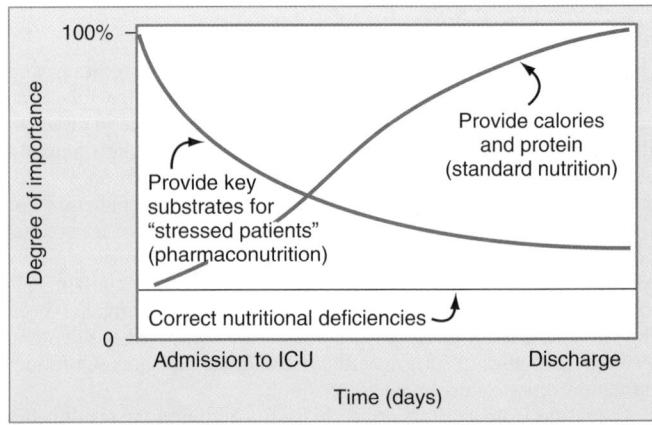

Figure 94-5 Pattern of prescriptions and goals of specialized nutritional support.

Greater understanding of the pathophysiologic mechanisms that underlie critical illness and the systemic inflammatory response may help forge new strategies for nutritional support in the future. Early on, clinicians may separate pharmaconutrition from provision of protein and calories, the latter of which may be limited by patient intolerance. Efforts to better delineate the dose/response effect of EN on gut integrity may help guide the "ramp-up" and degree of aggression with which feeding rates are advanced. Monitoring immune responses and alterations in the cytokine profile may help clinicians in the future decide whether to stimulate or up-regulate the immune response (through provision of arginine or nucleotides) or to down-regulate responses (through provision of omega-3 fatty acids and borage oil) as the patient proceeds through the hospital course.

KEY POINTS

1. Optimized nutrition therapy (NT) improves patient outcomes in critically ill patients and because of this is no longer considered adjunctive supportive care but rather a primary therapeutic strategy.

2. Spontaneous oral intake is not possible for many critically ill patients. For these patients, NT is necessary. NT maintains functional and anatomic integrity of the gut.

3. The therapeutic value of NT extends beyond meeting classic nutritional goals and includes modulating and restoring physiologic immune responses to critical illness.

4. A number of management strategies help reduce the risk of enteral nutrition: feeding distal to the stomach directly into the small bowel, elevating the head of the bed 30 to 45 degrees, using promotility agents, and using nurse-directed feeding protocols.

5. The greater the severity of critical illness, the more important the issues of gut integrity and permeability become, and the more likely it is that enteral nutrition will improve clinical outcome compared with parenteral nutrition.

6. Small-volume "trophic" or "trickle" feeds may not be sufficient to maintain gut integrity and normal mucosal permeability; 50% to 60% of goal calories (i.e., caloric requirements) may be needed to achieve the therapeutic endpoints of enteral nutrition.

7. Compared with standard enteral formulas, arginine-supplemented immune formulas improve outcome (lower incidence of infection and shorter hospital length of stay) in selected groups such as patients undergoing major elective surgery; however, arginine-supplemented formulas may worsen outcome (cause excess mortality) in other groups such as patients who are septic.

8. Glutamine supplementation (parenterally more so than enterally) may reduce mortality and infectious complications in certain critically ill populations.

9. Although the enteral route is always the first choice for nutritional support in critically ill patients, standard therapy (i.e., no artificial nutritional support) is associated with a better outcome than parenteral nutrition over the first 7 to 10 days when enteral nutrition is not feasible.

10. Parenteral nutrition should be started earlier in severely malnourished patients and is particularly important in patients with a nonfunctional gastrointestinal tract. In the few specific circumstances when parenteral nutrition is indicated, its efficacy may be maximized by strict control of blood glucose, permissive underfeeding, and withholding lipids for the first 7 to 10 days.

ANNOTATED REFERENCES

Brandtzaeg PE. Current understanding of gastrointestinal immunoregulation and its relation to food allergy. Ann N Y Acad Sci 2002;964:13-45.
This paper provides an excellent review of gut immunology and provides the reader with an understanding of how events at the level of the gut serve to shape the stress response and modulate systemic immunity.

Taylor SJ, Fettes SB, Jewkes C, Nelson RJ. Prospective, randomized, controlled trial to determine the effect of early enhanced enteral nutrition on clinical outcome in mechanically ventilated patients suffering head injury. Crit Care Med 1999;27:2525-31.
This study in trauma patients with head injury shows how modifying enteral feeding protocols to be more aggressive (faster ramp-ups in rate, higher gastric residual volumes) results in a greater percentage of goal calories being infused and better subsequent clinical outcome.

Van den Berghe G, Wouters P, Weekers F et al. Intensive insulin therapy in critically ill patients. N Engl J Med 2001;345:1359-67.
This landmark study clearly shows the tremendously favorable impact of tight glycemic control on patient outcome in critical illness.

Windsor AC, Kanwar S, Li AG et al. Compared with parenteral nutrition, enteral feeding attenuates the acute phase response and improves disease severity in acute pancreatitis. Gut 1998;42:431-5.
This prospective randomized trial of enteral versus parenteral feeding in patients with acute pancreatitis shows the degree to which enteral feeding can attenuate the stress response and thereby reduce overall disease severity (compared with parenteral feeding).

Young B, Ott L, Kasarskis E et al. Zinc supplementation is associated with improved neurologic recovery rate and visceral protein levels of patients with severe closed head injury. J Neurotrauma 1996;13:25-34.
This meta-analysis beautifully outlines which patient populations benefit most from enteral feedings, describes situations in which standard therapy (no artificial nutritional support) is most appropriate, and delineates those few circumstances in critical illness when parenteral nutrition is indicated.

REFERENCES

Access the complete reference list online at http://www.expertconsult.com.

95 Nutrition Issues in Critically Ill Children

DAVID M. STEINHORN | LAURA T. RUSSO

Nutritional support is a central therapy in the management of critically ill patients. Specific populations such as premature infants have unique requirements, which are beyond the scope of this chapter. In contrast, term infants and older children appear to have a graduated set of nutritional/metabolic requirements based upon age and body size which ultimately achieve those requirements typically administered to adult patients. In caring for critically ill children, it is useful to understand the fundamental differences seen in children of differing ages and conditions. It is perhaps somewhat ironic that our well-intended efforts to "increase" nutritional support may at times lead to greater harm than benefit through the provision of protein, carbohydrate, and fat beyond what the critically ill child can utilize. In addition, metabolic complications such as total parenteral nutrition (TPN)-associated cholestasis, hepatic steatosis, and increased catheter-related infections are new morbidities that have arisen with the advent of advanced nutritional methods.

Recent reviews of the literature on nutritional support for critically ill children details the lack of definitive or reliable studies to guide our practice based upon scientific evidence.[1,2] Therefore, many of the recommendations made rest upon "good practice" principles which rely upon expert consensus and avoidance of known harm whenever possible. The American Society of Parenteral and Enteral Nutrition (A.S.P.E.N.) has promulgated a set of expert guidelines for supporting critically ill children that represent a reasonable standard of care for children in the pediatric intensive care unit (PICU).[3]

The goal of this chapter is to provide the critical care clinician with a fundamental understanding of the issues necessary for providing effective and safe nutrition to acutely ill children in the PICU and those recovering from life-threatening illness. The material represents core concepts and approaches with wide acceptance by experts practicing in contemporary critical care where a range of enteral and parenteral nutrition aids are available.

Role of Nutritional Support for Critically Ill Children

Contemporary nutritional support depends upon a balanced approach that provides macronutrients (e.g., protein or amino acids, carbohydrate, and fat) as well as a corresponding amount of micronutrients (e.g., minerals, trace elements, vitamins). While clinicians tend to take each of these components for granted, one must consider that the macronutrients must be processed via intermediary metabolic pathways to produce adenosine triphosphate (ATP) when and where needed and to provide structural molecules for tissue repair, maintenance of organ integrity, and immunoglobulin synthesis. The metabolic processes associated with biotransformation of macronutrients for both kidney and liver may produce further demands on organs that often are already working at limited capacity owing to perfusion deficits and humoral factors such as lipopolysaccharides (LPS), proinflammatory cytokines that tend to limit reserve capacity. Excess calories can be stored, whereas excess protein beyond what the body can utilize is rapidly degraded to urea as the final byproduct.

The protein pools of the body are conceptualized as existing in two compartments. The first compartment, referred to as the *visceral protein pool*, represents those proteins that can easily be accessed and

degraded to provide amino acids when nutritional intake is inadequate. The visceral compartment includes plasma proteins, immunoglobulins, cytosolic enzymes, and so on that can be turned over readily. The second compartment, referred to as the *somatic protein pool*, represents primarily structural proteins in brain, heart, kidney, bone, and the like; this compartment is less accessible than the visceral pool. Protein is stored to a very limited extent when taken in beyond momentary need. Carbohydrate is generally stored to a limited extent as glycogen, beyond which it is converted into triglycerides under the influence of insulin. Fats must be taken up and cleared from the plasma through complex mechanisms involving lipoprotein lipase, which is impaired during stress states. Thus all three major macronutrients, when provided to patients by enteral or parenteral approach, depend upon a multitude of internal processes frequently altered by critical illness, leading to additional stress with no survival benefit. After decades of clinical research, the conclusion must be that excess nutritional support is to be avoided in favor of thoughtful moderation in providing nutrients.

Contemporary nutritional support has three primary goals: (1) preservation of lean body mass to minimize the catabolic consequence of critical illness, (2) provision of suitable substrates to permit restoration of immune function and repair of body tissues, and (3) prevention of nutrition-related complications including aspiration risks in patients receiving enteral nutrition and the avoidance of nutrient-induced organ overload, whether through excess carbohydrate (increased CO_2 production and hepatic steatosis) or excess protein/nitrogen load to the liver and kidney. Understanding the risks and realistic benefits of nutritional support are vital in current PICU care.

Impact of Physiologic Stress on Children

Alterations in protein and energy metabolism are hallmarks of critical illness and have been studied for many decades.[4] This work has demonstrated a great difference between short-term starvation states in otherwise healthy individuals and the dramatic "autocannibalism" seen in critically ill patients who are not receiving appropriate nutritional support as summarized in Table 95-1.

The events that lead to ICU admission are extremely varied, yet the body's response to acute physiologic stress tends to be similar whether the inciting event is sepsis, ischemia-reperfusion, trauma, burns, or other inflammatory conditions. Beyond low levels of stress, such as minor elective surgery, life-threatening illness, burns, organ transplantation, or major surgical procedures elicit dramatic systemic inflammatory responses due to activation of the immune system, clotting mechanisms, and the endothelium. The patient's ability to withstand the metabolic responses to such stresses and ultimately to reverse the process is central to recovery. A complete discussion of the metabolic response to stress is beyond the scope of this chapter; the reader is referred to other sources.[5,6]

The initial response to injury is to activate endothelial cells and to prime inflammatory cells such as neutrophils, macrophages, and lymphocytes through proinflammatory mediators including tumor necrosis factor, interleukin 2, histamine, eicosanoids, heat-shock proteins, free radicals, platelet-activating factor, and tryptases.[7] These same signals that produce activation of the endothelium lead to permeability changes, activation of clotting mechanisms, and changes in hepatic and

TABLE 95-1	Comparison of Nutrient Metabolism in Starvation Versus Sepsis/Trauma	
	Starvation	*Sepsis/Trauma*
Protein breakdown	++	+++
Hepatic protein synthesis	++	++++
Ureagenesis	++	++++
Gluconeogenesis	++	++++
Energy expenditure	Reduced	Increased
Mediator activity	Low	High
Hormone counterregulatory capacity	Preserved	Poor
Use of ketones	+++	+
Loss of body stores	Gradual	Rapid
Primary fuels	Fat	Amino acids, glucose, triglycerides

Adapted from Barton R, Cerra FB. The hypermetabolism-multiple organ failure syndrome. Chest 1989;96:1153-60.

peripheral protein metabolism.[8] If recovery is to occur, this process must be extinguished by a decrease in the inflammatory state and an increase in tissue repair.[9] Although it may seem that simply shutting off the proinflammatory signals should lead to resolution, the process of resolving inflammation appears more complex.[10] Studies show the importance of many of the proinflammatory stimuli in regeneration and repair, and the timing of interventions is important.[11] In response to injury, a wide range of neurohumoral reactions occur, forming the classic "stress response," which includes elevation of growth hormone, endogenous catecholamines, glucagon, and cortisol. Recognition of the role of insulin-like growth factor-1 along with growth hormone in promoting protein synthesis and counter-regulating inflammatory states suggests important potential treatment options that have been best studied in burns. Despite these studies showing benefit from growth hormone supplementation, evidence of increased mortality rate after growth hormone supplementation also has been reported.[12] Clinicians must balance the relative benefit of hormonal manipulation with potential risks.

In the inflammatory state, unremitting gluconeogenesis occurs through the release of glycerol and gluconeogenic amino acids from the periphery with their conversion to glucose in the liver and kidney. Hyperglycemia frequently is associated with this state and may induce glycosuria and an osmotic diuresis. Insulin activity becomes impaired at the tissue level, leading to so-called insulin resistance in the face of the powerful gluconeogenesis driven by the stress hormones. It seems that the impairment of insulin results from decreased phosphorylation of the insulin receptor and second messengers.[11] In the last decade, evidence from adult ICU experience has suggested a benefit from the use of insulin infusions to maintain tight control over serum glucose level.[13] Although much of the preceding information derives from adult studies, it has found its way into contemporary pediatric practice in many centers in children of various ages. This question is receiving intense scrutiny in critically ill children through multicenter trials which are currently underway. The use of insulin infusions to control hyperglycemia in premature infants continues to be standard practice; however, the potential to produce marked hepatic steatosis under the influence of insulin should be born in mind when choosing the amount of carbohydrate to provide.

The breakdown of protein is a central theme in the body's response to stress, which has wide-ranging significance beyond simple protein losses. The conversion of certain amino acids to glucose and the oxidation of others in peripheral tissues lead to the liberation of large quantities of amino-nitrogen, which would become toxic if not for the efficient conversion to urea. A dramatic increase in the rate of urea production is seen in critically ill patients. Concomitantly, other non-urea nitrogen is liberated in the form of uric acid and creatine and accounts for the dramatic increase in nitrogen wasting seen during stress states. Total urinary nitrogen losses in critically ill children may be 0.3 g/kg/d, which represents the loss of approximately 1.8 g/kg/d of whole protein catabolized. In parallel with the increased turnover of proteins, the metabolic rate for oxidation of energy substrates may increase following acute critical illness during the recovery phase (see subsequent section on energy expenditure).

The body's response to withholding feeding (i.e., starvation) in healthy individuals is qualitatively and quantitatively different than that seen when nutrient intake is absent during critical illness. These differences are fundamental to understanding nutritional support in the ICU and are summarized in Table 95-1. In simple starvation, the body's regulatory mechanisms for sparing lean tissue and using triglycerides as the primary energy source are intact, whereas under the influence of the stress response, rapid depletion of lean tissues occurs with oxidation of amino acids, carbohydrate, and fat as energy substrates.

One of the major consequences of life-threatening physiologic stress is the net depletion of body protein representing the somatic protein pool (e.g., skeletal muscle mass) and functional (e.g., plasma proteins, enzyme systems, antibodies) tissues contained in the visceral protein pool. With protein catabolism rates increased up to twofold, synthesis does not keep pace, and a state of negative nitrogen balance ensues when patients are not given adequate calories and protein.[14] These changes produce depressed function of T and B lymphocytes, monocytes, and neutrophils as cumulative protein loss increases. The synthesis of antibodies, chemotaxis, phagocytosis, and bacterial killing is impaired in the face of advanced protein-calorie malnutrition.[15] A decrease in total lymphocyte count may be seen in many patients, but a total lymphocyte count less than 1200/mm³ should raise concern for the presence of possible immune dysfunction. These alterations lead to impairment of host defense mechanisms. As noted earlier, for resolution of the inflammatory response, the patient's immune system plays a central role in recovery of wound healing and recovery of immune competence.[16] It is likely that the syndrome of multiple organ dysfunction seen in critically ill patients is due in part to the inability of the immune system to down-regulate the inflammatory response to injury in specific organs, as well as acquired mitochondrial dysfunction leading to ineffective cellular energy production.[17] Nutritional support of a critically ill patient is thought to be essential to achieving recovery and minimizing the subsequent period of convalescence.

Considerable attention currently is focused on the use of modified nutritional support regimens in critically ill adults to modify the inflammatory response and reduce secondary organ system dysfunction.[18] A wide range of substances have been studied in an attempt to improve outcome or minimize nitrogen loss during critical illness in specific populations of patients. Glutamine supplementation appears to benefit critically ill adults, particularly those with burns.[18] Omega-3 fatty acids appear to also be beneficial in patients with sepsis and systemic inflammatory response syndrome (SIRS). The results in adults suggest that formulas supplemented with these products improve oxygenation and reduce the alveolar inflammatory response during acute respiratory distress syndrome (ARDS). While trials of these agents are underway in critically ill children, there is still not a strong enough consensus among pediatric specialists to consider their use as standard therapy.[3]

Nutrition Assessment

The nutrition assessment of hospitalized children is a central and critical part of the initial examination and evaluation of all patients. The existence of chronic malnutrition as well as the development of acute malnutrition during critical illness has been recognized in pediatric critical care for many years[19-21] and appears to be an unmet need even today.[22] Therefore, clinicians must assess newly admitted patients for the presence of malnutrition that may complicate the response to therapies or impair recovery (Box 95-1). The presence of previous severe malnutrition may complicate critical care management through the presence of marasmic cardiomyopathy, severe intracellular energy deficiency, and the development of refeeding disequilibrium when nutrients are provided in the ICU.[23]

ASSESSMENT OF NUTRITION STATUS ON ADMISSION

1. Physical exam: Obvious wasting? Skin and hair normal?

2. Plot on growth chart: weight, height, head circumference (<24 months)[24]

3. Determine: percent height for age*[25] and BMI†

4. Measure: serum albumin and transferrin

Height for age <90 and BMI <5 percentiles
Serum albumin <2.5 g/dL or transferrin <180 mg/L

Yes — Malnutrition likely
No — Malnutrition unlikely

Consider:
Dietary/gastrointestinal consult
Nutritional support as soon as appropriate
Measure total protein, total lymphocyte count
Anthropometrics: measure triceps skin fold and midarm circumference

Ongoing assessment during hospitalization

From Statistics NCfH. CDC growth charts, United States, 2000. Available at: http://www.cdc.gov/growthcharts; and from Waterlow J. Classification and definition of protein-calorie malnutrition. Br J Med 1972;3:566-9.
*Actual height (cm) × 100/expected height at 50th percentile for age.
†BMI (kg/m^2) = body mass index: actual weight (kg)/[actual weight × height (m)]^2

The initial nutrition evaluation consists of assessing the patient's weight, height, historical evidence for recent weight loss, and anthropometric measurements including midarm circumference and skinfold determination (when edema is not present). Nutrition history must include the presence and duration of nausea, vomiting, diarrhea, fever, frequent infections, fatigue, food aversion, abdominal discomfort, or feeding intolerance. For growth standards, norms exist reflecting age and gender.[24] Ethnic background and considerations such as the presence of certain syndromes (e.g., Down syndrome) or the child's birth status (e.g., premature, growth restricted, etc.) may affect the child's growth status.

In particular, determination of body mass index (BMI, previously known as *weight-for-height*) for children older than 2 years of age provides important information regarding the previous nutritional status (see Box 95-1). In children younger than 2 years, the weight-for-age in light of the previous growth status is most useful. These straightforward measurements have withstood the test of time and were used by Pollack and coworkers to estimate the risk of malnutrition in critically ill children admitted to a multidisciplinary PICU.[19,20,25] Their findings demonstrated higher rates of preexisting malnutrition than had been previously thought. In addition, there was an unexpected deterioration in nutrition indices following admission, suggesting the powerful effects of life-threatening illness on nutritional stores and status even with excellent clinical care. Clinicians caring for children who will experience more than a few days of hospitalization must therefore be especially aware of the potential for acquired nutritional depletion. Potential sources of error exist in interpreting anthropometric measurements that are primarily related to changes in body water associated with many acute critical illnesses in children (i.e., conditions producing capillary leak syndrome or defects in renal water clearance).

Such conditions may invalidate the measurement of skinfold or midarm circumference; however, their longitudinal use in patients can be very useful in estimating the accretion of fat and lean tissue stores. It is standard practice to measure these parameters in patients at risk for malnutrition, such as those with cystic fibrosis, short bowel syndrome, and other conditions in which malabsorption or chronically elevated metabolic demands exist (e.g., congenital heart failure, bronchopulmonary dysplasia, and similar chronic conditions).

The triceps and scapular skin folds measure the subcutaneous tissue compartment (consisting primarily of adipose tissue) but also tissue edema in patients with anasarca from any cause. Triceps skin fold is measured by standardized skin caliper and is subject to considerable error if not performed in a consistent manner midway between the acromion and olecranon. The midarm circumference should be measured at the same point with a nonstretchable tape measure. The two indices taken together permit a reliable estimate of muscle mass. In general, good correlation exists between skinfold and arm circumference and weight-for-height percentile.[26] During critical illness, anasarca may obscure the loss of lean tissue, which may only be apparent following resolution of edema when successful diuresis has occurred. A very reliable indicator of global loss of lean body mass can be seen in the wasting of the interosseous and thenar muscles of the hand, which becomes apparent 2 or 3 weeks after hospitalization with resolution of edema.

In addition to anthropometric measurements, longitudinal determination of specific plasma proteins including albumin, transferrin, and prealbumin have demonstrated value in assessing the response of patients to nutritional support. Frequently serum proteins will be decreased during acute critical illness without reflecting preceding malnutrition. This phenomenon occurs with capillary leak syndrome, seen in the first hours following PICU admission in patients with sepsis, cardiopulmonary bypass operations, ischemia-reperfusion injury, and similar stresses. Loss of endothelial barrier function causes large molecules such as albumin, which are normally three to four times more concentrated in the vascular compartment than in the interstitial fluid, to move into the extravascular space, lowering their concentration without a concomitant decrease in the *total body pool* of albumin. This effect may be very pronounced in patients who have received large volumes of crystalloid fluid during their resuscitation. Clinicians must guard against the tendency to replace albumin during acute critical illness solely based upon a low albumin level. Measures to correct the underlying pathophysiology should be considered before administering albumin. Serum albumin in healthy children is generally above 3.0 g/dL, and edema is rarely seen in otherwise healthy children until the albumin falls below 2.0 g/dL, such as in nephrotic syndrome.

Shorter half-life serum proteins such as prealbumin [$T_{1/2}$ = 2 days] and transferrin [$T_{1/2}$ = 7 days] also reflect nutrition status and respond more quickly to changes in anabolic state.[27] As noted earlier, the pool of proteins in the plasma, interstitial space, and some intracellular proteins represent a relatively labile pool of protein referred to as the *visceral protein pool*. Visceral proteins are rapidly turned over relative to structural proteins that comprise the somatic protein pool. In critical illness, the synthesis of specific proteins such as C-reactive protein, ceruloplasmin, and α_2-macroglobulin is increased, whereas the synthesis of other proteins such as albumin [$T_{1/2}$ = ~20 days] is decreased.[28] These changes may be seen within 6 hours of the onset of severe physiologic stress. This response to physiologic stress is under the regulation of complex neurohumoral control and is referred to as the *acute phase response*. It is largely responsible for the increase in erythrocyte sedimentation rate associated with acute inflammatory conditions.[29] When followed longitudinally, the return of previously depressed levels of certain visceral proteins such as albumin, transferrin, retinol-binding protein, or prealbumin represents the abatement of physiologic stress or improvement in nutrition when levels are low due to protein-calorie malnutrition. Such positive changes herald the impending return to a state of growth and tissue accretion, barring reentry into a new inflammatory state.

Energy Expenditure

All cellular processes require energy, generally in the form of ATP which is produced through oxidation of metabolic fuels, with heat and water as byproducts. The production of ATP is closely coupled to cellular metabolism and must be maintained to prevent cell death. As ATP levels fall, ionic gradients cannot be maintained, excitatory cells cannot depolarize, the synthesis of new cells and repair of damaged cell constituents cannot occur, and mechanical work such as cardiac pump function and respiratory activity cease. Thus, the body has numerous mechanisms for efficiently producing energy from a wide variety of substrates including protein, fat, and carbohydrates. Following the adaptation to decreased nutrient intake, an otherwise healthy individual will rely upon ketone bodies derived from the breakdown of fat stores to provide critical intracellular energy. Protein stores are relatively spared as the decrease in insulin output allows the metabolism to shift to a ketone-based state. As indicated in Table 95-1, critical illness prevents the body's conservational mechanisms in response to decreased intake, leading to relatively rapid depletion of carbohydrate and available protein stores.

The close coupling between oxidative metabolism and substrate utilization is reflected in the amount of oxygen consumed (V_{O_2}) and carbon dioxide produced (V_{CO_2}) through the pathways of intermediary metabolism, which include the glycolytic pathway and the tricarboxylic acid cycle. Specific substrates such as fat, protein, and various carbohydrates have a characteristic relationship between V_{O_2} and V_{CO_2} based upon the stoichiometry of their unique oxidation. This relationship is referred to as the *respiratory quotient* ($RQ = V_{CO_2}/V_{O_2}$) and may be measured through the quantification of respiratory gas exchange through the patient's lung. The overall metabolic rate is most easily determined in the clinical setting through the process of *indirect calorimetry*, a process that estimates the resting energy expenditure (REE) based upon V_{O_2} and V_{CO_2}.[30] Indirect calorimetry is well established in clinical nutrition but has been elusively difficult to perform with consistent results and easily applied technology in children. The respiratory quotient for fats is around 0.707 and for proteins around 0.80 and, in conjunction with urinary nitrogen determination, forms the basis for determining the specific substrates being utilized.[30] This concept is demonstrated for the aerobic metabolism of glucose:

$$C_6H_{12}O_6 + 6O_2 \rightarrow 6CO_2 + 6H_2O \text{ (energy liberated} = 686 \text{ kcal/mole)}$$

$$RQ = 6CO_2/6O_2 = 1$$

The availability of equipment to reliably perform indirect calorimetry in children has been a major obstacle to its widespread application. Several factors limit the reliability with which indirect calorimetry can be performed in young children, including non–steady state due to patient movement and nursing interventions, use of uncuffed endotracheal tubes producing loss of respiratory gases, high bias flows on infant ventilators, use of elevated inspired oxygen in nonintubated infants, as well as the small tidal volumes seen in the smallest patients. When indirect calorimetry is not feasible, V_{O_2} can be calculated in many patients via the Fick equation ($A \times V_{dO_2} \times$ cardiac output) when a reliable measure of cardiac output is available. Based upon a conversion factor of approximately 5 kcal of energy per liter of oxygen consumed, one can closely estimate metabolic rate[30] if the oxygen consumption is known and the RQ is assumed to be in a normal range.

Through indirect calorimetry it has become clear that patients with similar clinical appearances may have widely differing metabolic rates when adjusted for age and weight.[3,31-34] The differences may be as great as 300%, suggesting the potential for severe over- or undernutrition depending upon the values assumed.[35] Thus, clinicians generally must rely upon information provided in controlled studies to guide the delivery of calories, since most will not have a means of easily determining the REE. A wide range of predictive equations have been devised which attempt to predict energy requirements of critically ill

children, but it is clear that no single method of estimating caloric expenditures will be successful for all critically ill children.[3,4,36]

In very young infants, the effects of environmental cold stress is recognized as a source of unnecessary morbidity.[37] The thermal neutral zone in infants up to 1 year of age tends to be several degrees higher than that for burned adults or older children. Heat lost to the environment produces rapid drops in core temperature in young children, with concomitant increase in metabolic demands. Maintaining the environment in a range of 30°C to 34°C with servo-controlled heaters or other means can significantly reduce energetic requirements in critically ill infants.

Nutritional Support for the Critically Ill Child

Nutritional support for critically ill children is fundamentally different than conventional nutrition of healthy children because of the alterations in metabolism outlined previously. During periods of critical illness, utilization of nutrients for growth is markedly inhibited by hormonal response to stress and circulating inflammatory mediators. Utilization of calories for activity is much lower than under normal conditions. In addition, diet-induced thermogenesis is also affected in hospitalized patients by the different routes and formulations of nutrients provided. Estimates of increased caloric and protein requirements during acute illness and recovery indicate that compared to critically ill adults, children have greater requirements for both on a body weight basis. Therefore, one of the most important points for clinicians prescribing nutritional support is to provide calories in a thoughtful manner based upon the guidelines that follow and to *avoid excess caloric intake* during the acute phase of illness. During acute critical illness in children, many investigators have found REE to be less elevated than previously expected, with significant risk for overfeeding.[33,35]

MAINTENANCE FLUIDS

Maintenance fluids for most patients can be estimated based upon body weight as indicated in Table 95-2. Children have generally increased requirements in relation to body weight for fluid, energy, protein, and many of the micronutrients. Water metabolism is closely coupled to metabolic activity because of the central role water plays in intermediary metabolism. For the term newborn, these amounts should be reduced during the first few days of life, owing to their increased intrinsic total body water. Premature infants have other considerations (e.g., high insensible losses), and consultation with a pediatrician or neonatologist is critical to provide appropriate and adequate fluid. Volumes must be increased for fever or persistent tachypnea to compensate for increased insensible fluid losses. Additional fluids must be provided to cover abnormal losses due to diarrhea, nasogastric drainage, or wound loss in burns or from other sites. Composition of the replacement fluid is based upon the content of sodium, potassium, bicarbonate, and chloride lost and conforms to conventional surgical and medical guidelines for fluid replacement. Typical maintenance fluids should provide sodium (3-5 mEq/kg/d) and potassium (2-3 mEq/kg/d) salts as well as a modest amount of glucose (5% or 10% if younger than 6 months of age). Recent trends in providing electrolytes has favored a balanced electrolyte solution that contains acetate salts of 1 to 2 mEq/kg/d to minimize development of critical

TABLE 95-2	Approximate Parenteral Maintenance Fluid Requirements
Body Weight	**Fluid Volume (Parenterally)**
First 10 kg	100 mL/kg/d
Second 10 kg	50 mL/kg/d
Additional kg	20 mL/kg/d

hyperchloremic metabolic academia in the young child. Provision of glucose in maintenance fluids is intended to spare lean tissue through the elicitation of insulin release, which exerts an anticatabolic effect in minimally stressed patients.

PRESCRIBING NUTRITIONAL SUPPORT

The decision to provide nutrition via a parenteral or enteral route takes many factors into consideration, including anticipated time to resumption of normal dietary intake, available routes of nutrient administration, underlying metabolic or endocrine conditions, and the existence of organ dysfunction. When patients will not receive conventional nutrition for a prolonged period of time, it is appropriate to consider support via the gut or intravenously (IV). There is general agreement that the enteral route is superior to TPN when a patient is able to tolerate it. Advantages of the enteral route include better maintenance of gut structure and function, reduced bacterial translocation, fewer metabolic complications, decreased intrahepatic cholestasis, greater ease and safety of administration, better outcomes, and reduced cost.[3]

Nutrition is frequently started as soon as the patient is metabolically stable; however, reliable data regarding the necessity or benefits of nutritional support in the first 5 days of critical illness have not be convincing.[3] For a critically ill patient, sufficient metabolic stability has been achieved when aggressive correction of electrolyte derangements has been achieved and the acid-base status no longer requires aggressive correction.

Once the decision has been made to start nutritional support, it is important to establish clear goals. During most acute critical illness, it is unreasonable to anticipate significant somatic growth, and the energy required for normal daily activities is markedly decreased. It is more realistic to employ nutritional support during this phase of illness to minimize the loss of lean body bass and support the synthesis of critical visceral proteins required for organ function, antibody production, and the mass of the immune system, as well as to provide substrate for wound healing. The requirements for nutrients can be divided into the macronutrients—consisting of carbohydrate, protein, and fat—and the micronutrients—consisting of minerals, vitamins, and trace elements. Vitamins and trace elements play key roles as essential cofactors in protein synthesis and intermediary metabolism.

Carbohydrate

Carbohydrate serves predominantly as an energy source. The carbon backbone of sugars also provides the basis for synthesis of many nonessential nutrients in the body. Carbohydrate is provided as sugars or starches in enteral formulas and as dextrose in parenteral nutrition. The caloric density of common dietary carbohydrate is generally 4 kcal/g, except for dextrose solutions, which provide 3.4 kcal/g because of energy lost through the process of hydration in solution. As the primary energy source, the rate of infusion should be adjusted to achieve the goals outlined in Table 95-3.

In general, the cellular energy requirements of most critically ill children and adults can be met and euglycemia can be maintained through the infusion of 5 to 8 mg/kg/min of dextrose. This range represents about 25 to 40 kcal/kg/d of carbohydrate calories and is a close first approximation of basal energy expenditure seen in many hospitalized children. In healthy nonstressed individuals, ketosis ensues when glucose entry into the circulation falls below 1.5 to 2 mg/kg/min. As an additional point of reference, infusion of over 10 to 12 mg/kg/min of glucose results in net lipogenesis and excess carbon dioxide production in most hospitalized patients. When hyperglycemia develops in the face of *appropriate* rates of glucose infusion, it has become routine to administer insulin as a continuous infusion. Recent reports suggest that maintaining serum glucose in a narrow euglycemic range in critically ill adults may be associated with greater morbidity due to hypoglycemia and offers limited actual benefit.[38] This practice has become commonplace in pediatric critical care, with several multicenter trials of this approach currently underway. Clinicians can expect the rate of insulin infusion required to control the serum glucose to be as much as 2 to 3 times higher than is routinely used in the treatment of diabetes as a result of the *insulin resistance* seen during critical illness.

Fat

Intravenous fat emulsions were originally developed to prevent essential fatty acid deficiency that can arise in a matter of days in critically ill children. A maximum of 20% to 30% of the caloric intake should be derived from fat. Intravenous fat should be infused as a 20% emulsion in infants to provide a concentrated calorie source (2 kcal/mL) as well as to supply essential fatty acids and lipid critical to central nervous system development and cell membrane repair. Intravenous fat emulsions are administered continuously unless rising plasma triglyceride levels suggest inadequate clearance. During periods of high physiologic stress, triglyceride levels are frequently elevated due to decreased peripheral clearance of triglycerides secondary to impaired lipoprotein lipase activity, increased generation of triglycerides from excess carbohydrate infusions, and elevation of lipolytic hormones in response to stress. To assess clearance, a minimum period of 4 hours without lipid infusion is needed to approximate the actual triglyceride level. A typical maximum for IV fat emulsion is 2.5 to 3.5 g/kg/d. Patients on enteral feedings may tolerate medium-chain triglycerides (MCT) better than long-chain fats following bowel injury or with right-sided heart failure. MCT are absorbed directly into the portal circulation, avoiding the complex absorptive process needed to digest long-chain fats. Formulas developed for patients with biliary disease typically contain a greater content of MCT, and many of the formulas developed for patients with absorption difficulties provide a significant portion of the triglyceride in the form of MCT.

Protein

Protein requirements are met through the provision of conventional enteral formulas or formulas containing hydrolysates of complex proteins that provide oligopeptides. Enteral formulas containing primary amino acids tend to be hypertonic with limited absorptive advantages, owing to the presence of mucosal transporter mechanisms that absorb di- and tripeptides more efficiently. The high rate of protein turnover during critical illness is associated with an increase in ureagenesis and urinary nitrogen losses that may amount to as much as 1 to 2 g/kg/d of protein equivalent. The supraphysiologic ureagenesis may represent additional metabolic stress on the liver and kidneys. To minimize nitrogen loss and assure that no amino acid falls to a level that would limit protein synthesis, high-quality nutritional protein must be given through the acute and convalescent phase of illness. Conceptually, proteins must be administered in amounts sufficient to replace losses, with additional protein to synthesize new tissue. Table 95-4 provides guidelines for the administration of protein to children in the ICU. It is important to recognize that nitrogen balance in response to nutritional support represents a continuum. In one recent study, the authors found that nitrogen balance was obtained at an intake of 2.8 g/kg/d.[39] Positive nitrogen balance was only achieved with amino acid infusion rates at the upper end of those typically used by clinicians. Furthermore, calories must be provided in sufficient quantity to ensure that protein can be used for synthesis rather than as an energy substrate.

TABLE 95-3	Target Goals for Nonprotein Calories When Resting Energy Expenditure Determination Not Available	
	Acute Phase (First 3-5 Days; kcal/kg/d)	Convalescent Phase (After 5 Days; kcal/kg/d)
Young children (<10 kg)	50-80	80-120
Children (1-7 years)	45-65	75-90
Children (>7 years)	30-50	30-75

TABLE 95-4	Protein Requirements	
	Acute Phase (First 3-5 Days; g/kg/d)	Convalescent Phase (After 5 Days; g/kg/d)
Infants/Children < 7 years	1.5-2.5	2.0-3.0
Children > 7 years	1.5-2.0	1.5-2.0

The concept of calorie-to-nitrogen ratio derives from the concept that protein should be used for synthesis of functional and structural molecules rather than used as energy. Thus, energy must be provided in adequate amounts. For a typical healthy individual, the ratio of enteral nonprotein calories to nitrogen ranges from 250-350:1. Because of the obligatory oxidation of amino acids during catabolic states, the ratio of nonprotein calories to nitrogen is generally much lower, in the range of 100-250:1. This ratio provides a convenient method for checking that protein infusion is in line with nonprotein calories. Very low ratios suggest either excess protein delivery or inadequate calories.

Special Considerations

Patients with hepatic failure require a restriction of protein intake. Typically, patients with elevated plasma ammonia levels due to hepatic insufficiency should be restricted to around 1 g/kg/d of protein regardless of age. This may be provided as a conventional enteral formula or as parenteral nutrition. One must remember that the blood products frequently administered in support of patients with liver failure contain significant amounts of protein that must be considered in the total nitrogen intake. Children with inborn errors of metabolism require care tailored to their specific metabolic problem. Their nutritional needs are best determined by a clinician or dietitian experienced in the management of children with metabolic disorders.

Patients with renal insufficiency should receive nutrition optimized to achieve wound healing, without excessive concern for the increase in blood urea seen. In general, the increased nitrogen load is handled through dialysis, so optimal nutrition can be provided to promote recovery. Patients receiving continuous renal replacement therapies are at risk for both amino acid and micronutrient loss across the dialysis membrane and should have their nutritional support adjusted correspondingly.[40]

Micronutrients

Multivitamin preparations are provided either as unit doses by the pharmacy in parenteral nutrition or as MVI in standard formulas. Occasionally, additional vitamins or trace elements will be required for specific deficiency states or diseases, but fine tuning of micronutrients other than minerals and electrolytes has been difficult to achieve clinically. Current recommendations are given in Table 95-5.[41]

ROUTE OF ADMINISTRATION

Nutrition should be provided via the gastrointestinal tract whenever possible, supplementing with peripheral or central parenteral nutrition when adequate enteral intake cannot be achieved.[3] In patients with significant burns, an enteral feeding tube should be placed within the first hours of hospitalization. Continuous drip feedings should begin

TABLE 95-5	Micronutrients			
Weight (Kg)	Copper	Zinc	Manganese	Chromium
<3	20*	300*	10*	0.2*
3-25	20*	100*	10*	0.2*
>25	1 mg/d	2.5-5 mg/d	0.25 mg/d	10 mg/d

From Energy and protein requirements. Report of a Joint FAO/WHO/UNU Expert Consultation. Geneva: World Health Organization; 1985.
*μg/kg/d.
Multivitamins as per hospital standard per age.

within hours to minimize bowel dysmotility and feeding intolerance often seen if feeding is delayed in such patients. In other patients, initiating feedings on the second hospital day is feasible in most cases and should be provided initially as a continuous infusion at a minimal rate of about 1 mL/kg/h and advanced as tolerated. The provision of *trophic* feedings is thought to provide a number of benefits even though significant nutritional intake cannot be achieved. These benefits include maintenance of gut motility, improved mesenteric blood flow, the release of trophic factors from the gut and pancreas, which maintain enterocyte mass and hepatocyte function.[42] In addition, enterocytes derive a significant portion of their nutrient and energetic requirements from the luminal contents during digestion, making enteral nutrition ideal when tolerated.

During acute critical illness, continuous drip feedings are often better tolerated than bolus feedings, especially in patients with respiratory distress. Transpyloric feeding when possible via weighted Silastic feeding tubes should be used to minimize the risk of gastroesophageal reflux and aspiration. It has been used with excellent results in critically ill children.[43] Placement of transpyloric feeding tubes can be done blindly by some experienced clinicians[44] or may be done by a radiologist under fluoroscopic guidance. Occasionally, metoclopramide or erythromycin may facilitate passage of a transpyloric tube. Even when a transpyloric feeding tube cannot be placed, continuous enteral feeding via a nasogastric tube may confer most of the benefits, although the risk of gastroesophageal reflux is somewhat greater. For young infants, the availability of breast milk is the optimal nutrient source and can be easily delivered by feeding tube when the infant cannot nurse. In older patients, the initial enteral nutrition formula for most critically ill children should be lactose free, have some of the fat provided as medium-chain triglycerides, and contain easily absorbed proteins such as di- and tripeptides (see earlier discussion). Most of the currently available formulas developed for children between the ages of 1 and 10 years of age conform to these recommendations. A wide variety of formulas exist; availability may vary from region to region. The hospital dietitian is best prepared to help select appropriate formulas and knows which products are available locally.

While beyond the scope of the current discussion, special considerations for premature infants and newborns include the use of formulas supplemented with docosahexaenoic acid (DHA) and arachidonic acid (ARA).[45] DHA and ARA are long-chain polyunsaturated fatty acids found in breast milk and recently added to infant formulas. Their importance in infant nutrition was recognized by the rapid accretion of these fatty acids in the brain during the first postnatal year. Subsequent reports of enhanced intellectual development in breastfed children and recognition of the physiologic importance of DHA in visual and neural systems from studies in animal models has led to formulas being developed that contain them.[46] It is becoming routine in the neonatal population to supplement DHA and ARA when providing enteral feedings.

Infants younger than 6 months of age should receive isotonic or hypotonic feedings initially until tolerance has been demonstrated. Young children between 1 and 5 years of age should receive an age-appropriate formula or an adult formula with appropriate supplements of protein, vitamins, and trace elements. Critically ill children older than 10 generally tolerate enteral formulas developed for adult patients, with supplementation of vitamins and micronutrients as needed for age. Enteral formulas should be initially iso- or hypotonic in order to minimize the possibility of diarrhea from excess osmotic load to the gut and to facilitate absorption. Infusion rates are begun conservatively at around 1 mL/kg/h, with a stepwise increase every 4 to 6 hours as tolerated up to the desired final rate. Once an acceptable rate is achieved, caloric density may be increased as tolerated. The clinician must maintain vigilance for evidence of feeding intolerance. In patients with poor tissue perfusion, enteral feedings are feasible; however, the risk of necrotizing enterocolitis is increased slightly when using the gut for nutrition. Thus, any signs of pronounced abdominal distension, profuse diarrhea, severe gastroesophageal reflux, or development of a new metabolic acidemia should lead to a hold on feedings

TABLE 95-6	Enteral Feeding Intolerance	
Problem	**Possible Reason**	**Possible Remedy**
Diarrhea, malabsorption	Delivery too fast	Decrease delivery rate
	High osmotic load	Reduce osmolarity or volume
	Mucosal injury	Start TPN, continuous slow enteral feeding to allow bowel recovery
	Substrate intolerance	Use elemental formula, especially disaccharide-free with MCT
Gastric retention/ gastroesophageal reflux	Hypertonic formula	Decrease osmolarity, dilute.
	High long-chain fat content	Change to MCT containing formula
	Hypodynamic gut	Positioning right-side down, consider prokinetic agent (e.g., Reglan, opiate antagonist)
Abdominal distension	Ileus, constipation	R/O surgical abdomen, R/O constipation
		Add bulking agent or stool softener

MCT, medium-chain triglycerides; *R/O*, rule out; *TPN*, total parenteral nutrition.

and assessment of the abdomen prior to reinstituting feedings. Common manifestations of enteral feeding intolerance are outlined in Table 95-6.

PARENTERAL NUTRITION

One of the great achievements of nutrition science has been the development of effective and safe nutrients to provide IV TPN over prolonged periods of time. For critically ill infants and children, TPN has been invaluable in the survival of premature infants, children with congenital or acquired bowel defects, and those who do not tolerate enteral nutrition due to malabsorption, surgery, or other causes of bowel dysfunction. However, we have learned that TPN may come with a significant cost in terms of iatrogenic electrolyte and acid-base disturbance, cholestasis, and hepatic fibrosis. Following prolonged TPN, especially in infants with short-bowel syndrome, excess carbon dioxide production and increased risk of bacterial and fungal infection are known problems. The goals of TPN support during critical illness should be clarified and kept realistic to avoid adding unnecessary metabolic stress to already compromised pulmonary, renal, and hepatic function. Excess TPN may contribute to organ dysfunction by increasing demands on those organs to regulate nutrients infused directly into the circulation, bypassing the first-pass counter-regulation that occurs with enteral nutrition.

Amino acid solutions developed for neonates (e.g., TrophAmine, which contains taurine, tyrosine, cysteine, and histidine) provide an advantage for select newborns and young infants with biliary disease, sepsis, or under high physiologic stress. This effect derives from increased branched-chain amino acids, the presence of amino acids which are conditionally "essential-for-age" in infants, and a reduction in nonessential amino acids. In premature infants or those on prolonged TPN, IV carnitine supplementation has been advocated to aid in triglyceride clearance through enhanced beta-oxidation of fatty acids.[47] In older children, conventional amino acid solutions provide adequate dietary nitrogen.

The provision of nutrients via TPN should be consistent with the guidelines set forth previously. Although an occasional patient may become acutely glucose intolerant or experience dramatic electrolyte changes following initiation of TPN, most patients will tolerate it well and can be advanced to full TPN within just a few days. Pediatricians have had a habit of starting with dilute solutions of TPN and increasing both protein and calorie intake slowly over many days as tolerance is demonstrated. This approach has little scientific basis so long as nurses and physicians observe for signs of intolerance such as hyperglycemia, glycosuria, acidemia, and hyperlipidemia.

A key point to getting patients quickly up to their desired goal is to order the TPN solution at the intended final concentration and begin at half the intended ultimate infusion rate. For example, if the goal for TPN will be a 20% dextrose solution with 2 g/kg/d of protein to run at 44 mL/hr, the pharmacy can compound that goal solution, but it should be started at 22 mL/h until tolerance is demonstrated by glucose monitoring. For comparison, this rate of infusion would be equivalent to a 10% solution with 1 g/kg/d of protein if it were running at the full 44 mL/h, a formulation most clinicians would be comfortable starting. If the patient tolerates the infusion (e.g., no acidemia, hyperglycemia, glycosuria) for 6 to 8 hours at the slower rate, the solution can be increased to 33 mL/h. After an additional period of demonstrated tolerance, the solution is increased to its intended final rate. This approach reduces the potential to waste TPN and reduces a source of possible error in compounding the subsequent days' TPN. Daily changes in electrolyte content must be made as indicated by serum levels. The essential issue when taking this approach is to supplement with conventional maintenance IV fluids while the TPN is being increased. Another useful approach to pediatric TPN is to plan for the entire day's nutrients to be placed in a volume of fluids equal to half to two-thirds of the total allowed daily fluid volume. The remaining maintenance volume of fluid is made up with proprietary crystalloid, maintenance solutions that can be increased or decreased as demanded by the patient's fluid status without affecting the amount of nutrients delivered. Taking this approach also lets the clinician reduce total fluid intake without sacrificing prescribed nutritional support. Using the two solutions allows one to titrate intake as required by changing clinical situations without abandoning TPN for day completely.

Assessment of Response to Nutritional Support

It is important to monitor the response to nutritional support. Intolerance of enteral support frequently manifests through abdominal distension, vomiting, or other physical signs. With TPN, intolerance manifests in iatrogenic derangements of minerals, electrolytes, and acid-base status. Hyperglycemia was discussed previously but may represent a complication of TPN administration. Standard nutrition assessment should be considered for each patient after the initial stress phase of critical illness. End-organ response to nutritional support is monitored by assessing whether serum transferrin or prealbumin is rising or falling and whether genuine weight gain is occurring in convalescing patients.

In some circumstances, a patient may not respond adequately to nutritional support and may benefit from a more detailed examination including the measurement of albumin, total protein, and transferrin, a 24-hour urine collection for nitrogen balance determination, and if possible, measurement of energy expenditure via indirect calorimetry. However, in general such a detailed and cumbersome approach has not consistently improved the status of the critically ill child. In circumstances in which clinicians believe the response to nutritional support could be improved, a consultation with a pediatric dietitian or gastroenterologist may be required. The use of total urinary nitrogen determination to assess nitrogen balance in critically ill children remains more useful in research studies than in practical patient care. Finally, indirect calorimetry can provide practical information regarding overall energy expenditure and substrate utilization when cardiopulmonary function is stable and lactic acidosis is not present; however, its utility in improving patient outcomes has not been confirmed.

Summary

Nutritional support of critically ill children is a central part of modern intensive care medicine. The complexity of pediatric disease and the wide range of nutrient options available necessitate close collaboration with dietary specialists who are familiar with children's nutrition requirements during critical illness. It has become almost axiomatic in critical care nutrition that giving ever more nutrition will only produce undesired complications while not improving outcomes. Enteral nutrition will continue to be the preferred route of nutrition when it is tolerated and provides the more efficient and cost-effective means of transitioning patients to conventional dietary intake when critical illness has resolved.

ANNOTATED REFERENCES

Pollack MM, Ruttiman UE, Wiley JS. Nutritional depletions in critically ill children: associations with physiologic instability and increased quantity of care. JPEN J Parenter Enteral Nutr 1985;9:309-13.
A classic work highlighting earlier observations of early nutritional depletion in critically ill children and the ramifications for physiologic stability and intensity of care. Brings together Pollack's earlier work on malnutrition in the PICU with his interest in physiologic stability, which set the stage for developing the PRISM scoring system.

Joffe A, Anton N, Lequier L, Vandermeer B, Tjosvold L, Larsen B et al. Nutritional support for critically ill children. Cochrane Database Syst Rev 2009;2:CD005144.
An up-to-date assessment of the evidence base for nutritional support in critically ill children, with a good review of the extant literature and its reliability in clinical management.

Mehta NM, Compher C; A.S.P.E.N. Board of Directors. Clinical Guidelines: nutrition support of the critically ill child. JPEN J Parenter Enteral Nutr 2009;33:260-76.
A comprehensive review and evaluation of the research behind current feeding guidelines for critically ill children. Contains excellent references and basic information for prescribing nutritional support. Discusses caloric, macro-, and micronutrient guidelines as well as aspects of immunomodulatory nutrition pertaining to children.

Le HD, Fallon EM, de Meijer VE, Malkan AD, Puder M, Gura KM. Innovative parenteral and enteral nutrition therapy for intestinal failure. Semin Pediatr Surg 2010;19:27-34.
A review of the unique nutritional considerations in caring for patients with short-bowel syndrome and intestinal failure. Discusses strategies for managing liver disease associated with intestinal failure and long-term parenteral nutrition.

Diamond IR, Pencharz PB, Wales PW. What is the current role for parenteral lipid emulsions containing omega-3 fatty acids in infants with short bowel syndrome? Minerva Pediatr 2009;61:263-72.
Contemporary discussion of omega-3 fatty acid supplementation in liver failure associated with long-term parenteral nutrition. Provides a good discussion of the theory behind the use of omega-3 supplements and provides a basis for clinicians to understand the increasing role omega-3 fatty acids may play in clinical medicine.

REFERENCES

Access the complete reference list online at http://www.expertconsult.com.

96

Portal Hypertension

JULIA WENDON | PABLO SOLIS-MUÑOZ

Anatomy and Physiology of the Portal System

The term *portal system* refers to a venous system that begins and ends in capillaries. The portal venous system commences in the capillaries of the intestine and ends in the hepatic sinusoids. The portal venous system drains blood from the gastrointestinal (GI) tract, pancreas, gallbladder, and spleen. The portal vein originates from the confluence of the splenic vein and the superior mesenteric vein. The inferior mesenteric vein and short gastric veins drain into the splenic vein. The superior mesenteric vein drains all the blood from the small bowel and the right colon, while the inferior mesenteric vein drains the blood from the remainder of the colon and most of the rectum. Flow in the portal vein is normally about 1 L/min (approximately 20% cardiac output) with a mean pressure of 7 mm Hg. Although the blood in the portal vein is the outflow from capillary beds and therefore has relatively low oxygen content, 70% of hepatic oxygenation is derived from portal flow. The blood flowing through the hepatic artery supplies the remainder of hepatic oxygen consumption and is the primary blood supply to the biliary tree. The portal vein carries a high concentration of nutrients and hormones, facilitating the liver's central role in fat, carbohydrate, drug, and protein metabolism. Toxic substances are removed by hepatocytes, and bacteria (and bacterial products) are removed by Kupffer cells. Portal venous blood and hepatic arterial blood mix at the sinusoidal level, and there exists an adenosine-mediated local hepatic arterial autoregulatory "buffer response" that increases arterial inflow in response to low portal flow; however, total hepatic flow is not preserved when hepatic arterial flow is decreased. This buffer response is also dysregulated in sepsis.[1]

Postsinusoidal blood drains through hepatic venules into hepatic veins and then into the inferior vena cava to return to the systemic circulation. A variety of pathologic processes can result in portal venous flow becoming "obstructed." Regardless of the cause (i.e., intra- or extrahepatic obstruction), this resistance to portal flow increases portal pressure and leads to the development of what is called the *portal hypertension syndrome*, which is characterized by the formation of portosystemic collaterals. Under these circumstances, only a portion of the blood flow that originates within the portal system reaches the liver; the remainder is diverted through collaterals and enters the systemic circulation directly.

The major sites of collateral remodeling are the gastroesophageal region, between the inferior mesenteric vein and the hemorrhoidal vein, the umbilical veins and cutaneus veins of the abdominal wall, and via retroperitoneal systems into the azygous system and the vena cava. Collateral vessels (varices) also may develop at the sites of previous surgery, trauma, or adhesions and may similarly be found at ileostomy or colostomy stomas (ectopic varices). In addition to the formation of discrete collateral vessels, there are also more generalized changes within the GI tract, leading to vascular ectasia or so-called portal hypertensive enteropathy. Bleeding may result from varices or portal hypertensive enteropathy.

Patients with portal hypertension exhibit characteristic splanchnic and systemic circulatory changes. Key to these manifestations is abnormal vasodilatation. Decreased arteriolar tone in the splanchnic vessels leads to splanchnic hyperemia and hypervolemia, but also a reduction in effective central blood volume, with the majority of the excess blood volume being within the splanchnic bed. These circulatory changes prompt homeostatic systemic responses, with activation of the vasoconstrictor and sodium-retaining mechanisms. Overall, these changes comprise a hyperdynamic circulation characterized by increased cardiac output and heart rate to maintain blood pressure in the face of decreased systemic vascular resistance, with an overall increase in total plasma volume.

Pathophysiology

According to Ohm's law (as applied to the cardiovascular system rather than an electrical circuit), the pressure within a vessel is determined by the flow of the blood in that vessel divided by the resistance. Apparent resistance depends upon a number of factors, including the length of the vessel, the radius of the vessel, and the viscosity of the blood. Since length and blood viscosity remain relatively constant, changes in radius are of paramount importance for determining changes in apparent resistance. An increase in blood flow in the portal vein and hepatic artery are important to the development of portal hypertension in some cases, but the increase in resistance seems to be the most important factor and is used to classify portal hypertension (PHT). The origin of PHT can be divided into cirrhotic and noncirrhotic and presinusoidal, sinusoidal, and postsinusoidal (Table 96-1). In response to PHT, vascular collaterals develop, and vascular resistance drops in the splanchnic bed, leading to the development of a hyperdynamic circulation. As a consequence, splanchnic and portal venous inflow increases, and PHT persists even with the development of vascular collaterals. As the pressure within the portal system continues to rise, portal blood flow decreases and hepatic perfusion deteriorates. The liver is deprived of portal blood, and this tends to accelerate the progression of liver disease. The hyperdynamic circulation and PHT also contribute to the development of portopulmonary syndrome (pulmonary hypertension and PHT), hepatopulmonary syndrome (hypoxia and intrapulmonary shunting in association with PHT), cirrhotic cardiomyopathy, ascites, and hepatorenal syndrome.

Increased vascular resistance in the portal system is the most important factor in the development of the PTH syndrome. Disorders as diverse as splenic vein or portal venous thrombosis, cirrhosis, or constrictive pericarditis can result in PHT even though their clinical manifestations differ. The site of increased resistance in cirrhosis was initially thought to be post-sinusoidal in nature, but increasingly it is recognized that sinusoidal and pre-sinusoidal factors contribute. The increased resistance to flow has both a static and a dynamic component. The static component in cirrhotic livers is due to distortion of liver architecture with reduced hepatic microcirculation. These vascular changes, together with compression of the portal vein branches by regenerative nodules, increase vascular resistance. Furthermore, fibrosis initially develops in the space of Disse, where hepatic stellate cells produce collagen and further compress the sinusoids. In clinical studies, measured portal pressure correlates with the extent of fibrosis in liver biopsy specimens. Also, the size of the hepatocytes is important. Treatments which are known to increase the size of hepatocytes increase portal pressure. This observation may explain, at least partially, why portal pressure frequently falls with abstinence from alcohol consumption. The dynamic component is mostly related to endothelins and nitric oxide. After activation, hepatic stellate cells, or Ito cells, become myofibroblasts and express endothelin (ETa and ETb) receptors and contract after exposure to endothelin-1, resulting in an

TABLE 96-1	Etiology of Portal Hypertension						
Condition	**Site of Increased Resistance**	**FHVP**	**WHVP**	**HVPG**	**SPP**	**Liver Disease**
Cirrhosis	Intrahepatic sinusoidal	Normal	Increased	Increased	Increased	Yes
Alcoholic hepatitis	Intrahepatic sinusoidal	Normal	Increased	Increased	Increased	Yes
Extrahepatic portal, splenic, or mesenteric vein thrombosis	Extrahepatic presinusoidal	Normal	Normal	Normal	Increased	No
Early primary biliary cirrhosis, PSC, sarcoid, schistosomiasis, congestive heart failure, noncirrhotic portal fibrosis, NRH	Intrahepatic presinusoidal	Normal	Normal/?raised	Normal/?raised	Increased	No
Hemochromatosis, peliosis, infiltrative disease, acute fatty liver of pregnancy	Intrahepatic sinusoidal hypertension	Normal	Increased	Increased	Increased	Yes
Veno-occlusive disease, posttransplant rejection	Intrahepatic postsinusoidal hypertension	Normal	?Increased	?Decreased	Increased	Yes
Budd-Chiari syndrome (noncirrhotic)	Extrahepatic postsinusoidal hypertension	Increased	Increased	Normal	Increased	Depends on severity
Constrictive pericarditis, inferior vena cava obstruction, congenital inferior vena cava web, right heart failure	Extrahepatic postsinusoidal hypertension	Increased	Increased	Normal	Increased	Depends on severity

FHVP, free hepatic venous pressure; *HVPG*, hepatic venous pressure gradient; *SPP*, systolic pulse pressure; *WHVP*, wedged hepatic venous pressure.

increase in portal pressure. The dynamic nature of portal pressure changes and Ito cell function are important, both in terms of the pathogenesis of acute bleeding and as a target for pharmacotherapy.

Diagnosis of Portal Hypertension

PHT is defined as a portal pressure that is 5 mm Hg greater than the pressure measured in the inferior vena cava or a pressure of more than 15 mm Hg in the splenic vein or portal pressure measured at surgery. If the gradient is greater than 10 mm Hg, then clinically significant PHT is present. The direct consequences of PHT are formation of portosystemic collaterals and splenomegaly. Portosystemic collaterals can become clinically apparent as gastric or esophageal varices, umbilical vein recanalization, retroperitoneal collaterals, and/or rectal or ileostomy varices. The complications of PHT are variceal bleeding, ascites, spontaneous bacterial peritonitis, hepatic encephalopathy, hyperdynamic circulation, and hypersplenism. Varices are rarely (maybe never) seen if the gradient is less than 10 mm Hg.[2] Variceal bleeding is not observed if the pressure gradient is less than 12 mm Hg, and protection from variceal bleeding is gained if the pressure gradient can be manipulated to less than 12 mm Hg or a 20% reduction in pressure is achieved.[3]

Direct measurement of the hepatic vein wedge pressure or the portal venous pressure requires invasive means, most often transjugular catheterization. The advantage of this approach is that caval and hepatic venous pressures can be measured during the same procedure. Less frequently, a transhepatic approach is adopted, and rarely, portal venous pressures are measured directly (by cannulating a branch of the superior mesenteric vein) at the time of a surgical procedure. Very rarely, splenic pulp pressure is measured.

Indirect measurements also can be used to assess the portal pressure gradient. This procedure involves measurement of the free and wedged hepatic venous pressure using catheterization of the right hepatic vein. Wedged hepatic venous pressure (measured using a balloon-tipped catheter) reflects the pressure in a static column of blood from the hepatic vein to the sinusoid. It is an assessment of sinusoidal pressure rather than portal venous pressure and therefore may underestimate the portal pressure gradient in disease states characterized by pre-sinusoidal hypertension (see Table 96-1). The free hepatic venous pressure is obtained with the catheter in the hepatic vein and gives an assessment of caval pressure. Free hepatic venous pressure is not elevated in patients with diseases characterized by pre-sinusoidal and sinusoidal PHT, but it is characteristically raised in post-hepatic (or extrahepatic postsinusoidal) etiologies. The gradient between the two measurements is called the *hepatic venous pressure gradient* and is the most commonly quoted parameter in the medical literature regarding management of PHT. Both the absolute value of

hepatic venous pressure gradient and the change in hepatic venous pressure gradient with pharmacotherapy have prognostic significance related to the risk of variceal bleeding.[4]

It can be appreciated that even indirect methods of measuring portal pressure are not readily available in most settings. Instead, most clinicians rely on the clinical manifestations of PHT: esophagogastric varices, splenomegaly, edema, and ascites.

Complications of Portal Hypertension

VARICES

Bleeding from varices is a major cause of morbidity and mortality in patients with significant PHT. Life expectancy after variceal bleeding is considerably curtailed, both as an immediate consequence of hemorrhage (and related complications, such as sepsis and renal failure) and in the longer term due to rebleeding.

Two main mechanisms have been implicated in the pathogenesis of variceal hemorrhage in patients with established varices and PHT: erosions secondary to acid reflux and spontaneous rupture. Effects related to ascites and changes in plasma volume also have been implicated in the genesis of bleeding. Ascites may be a factor in variceal hemorrhage, because ascites can transmit intraabdominal pressure and thereby increase the pressure inside the esophageal varices. Some studies have shown a decrease up to 10% in the hepatic vein pressure gradient (HVPG) and a decrease in portal flow with paracentesis. Drainage of large volume of ascites can decrease intraabdominal pressure, leading to splanchnic dilation and increased blood flow against a fixed resistance in the liver.[5] This circumstance would increase portal pressure and, hence, the risk of bleeding. The pressure inside the varices does seem to be affected by intraabdominal pressure, but whether this affects the risk of bleeding is not known. Erosions secondary to esophagitis also have been suggested as an important factor for the bleeding process.[6,7] However, there was no evidence of acid reflux in patients studied with a pH electrode, and treatment with cimetidine did not affect the rates of rebleeding from varices.[8]

The pressure inside the varices is directly dependent on the portal pressure and also on the radius of the varix. The pressure within the varix is inversely proportional to wall thickness. Therefore, varices are more likely to bleed when they are larger and have a thinner wall. Large, thin-walled varices are generally located near the gastroesophageal junction where the veins are more superficial and less surrounded by other tissues. There is a relationship between the risk of bleeding and portal pressure. If the HVPG is greater than 20 mm Hg after an initial bleed, it is a poor prognostic sign, and there is a substantial risk of rebleeding and mortality.[9] In a recent study, patients underwent portal pressure measurement after initial endoscopy and control of bleeding.

Those whose pressure was above 20 mm Hg were randomized to early transjugular intrahepatic portosystemic shunt (TIPS) or conventional treatment. The group who underwent TIPS shunt insertion had an improved outcome compared to the standard-of-care high-risk group and similar to that of the low-risk group. Recent work has also suggested that portal pressure may be equally predicted by Child-Pugh score, and thus in this group of patients, consideration should be given to early TIPS shunt insertion.

It may be equally possible to measure variceal pressure at the time of endoscopic band ligation. This appears to be feasible and safe, although it remains at present an experimental method, and more studies are required.[10]

The main risk factors for rebleeding and mortality according to the North Italian Group of Portal Hypertension are the Child-Pugh class, the size of the varix, and the presence or absence of red wale markings and/or cherry spot at endoscopy.

There is increasing evidence to suggest that an episode of infection is the precipitating event in most cases of variceal bleeding. Infection is thought to trigger the release of cytokines and other proinflammatory mediators, resulting in increased hepatic resistance and possibly increased portal venous flow, with a sudden rise in portal pressure. A postprandial increase in splanchnic blood flow also may contribute to an acute rise in portal pressure.

Gastroesophageal varices are present in approximately 50% of cirrhotic patients and are large in 20%. Approximately one-third of patients with varices have bleeding complications. The patients at greatest risk of bleeding are those with advanced liver disease and large varices and high-risk stigmata. It is important, therefore, to identify the population at risk and modify their risk of bleeding. In patients with cirrhosis, the incidence of varices is 5% per year.

Gastric varices can be classified into four different groups: GOV1 is the gastric varix that is a direct continuation of an esophageal varix; GOV2 are also a continuation of a esophageal varix, but are more extensive and reach the fundus of the stomach; IGV1 are fundal varices that are not in continuity with an esophageal varix; and IGV2 are gastric varices that do not originate from a esophageal varix and are located in the body of the stomach. GOV2 and particularly IGV1 bleed more commonly than other gastric varices.

Portal hypertensive gastropathy is a complication of PHT that causes flow and pressure changes in the gastric mucosa. Mild or chronic bleeding is observed in 35% of the patients with mild gastropathy and 90% of those with severe gastropathy. Overt bleeding happens in 30% of those with mild and in 60% of those with severe gastropathy.[11] The administration of propranolol decreases gastric mucosal blood flow and is effective in reducing bleeding in portal hypertensive gastropathy.[12,13] TIPS and transplant are effective modes of treatment.

Another form of gastropathy is gastric antral vascular ectasia (GAVE). This lesion is localized at the antrum, and is associated with poor hepatic function. GAVE carries a high risk of bleeding. It is best managed with endoscopic therapy, generally with sessions of argon plasma coagulation (APC) until hepatic transplantation can be performed.

Diagnosis of Variceal Bleeding

When a patient with a possible hepatic disorder presents with hematemesis or melena, the most common cause of bleeding is from varices.[14] Sometimes it is useful to insert a nasogastric tube followed by lavage of the stomach, both as a diagnostic tool and also to clear the gastric cavity before endoscopy. Since patients with PHT also can bleed from gastritis, esophagitis, Mallory-Weiss tears, and peptic ulcers, the most accurate method for the diagnosis of bleeding varices is upper endoscopy; accuracy exceeds 90%. Frequently one or two doses of 250 mg of erythromycin are administered before the procedure to help clear the stomach before the procedure.

Acute Variceal Hemorrhage

The patient should be placed in a suitable environment. Frequently a high-dependency area will provide optimal monitoring and level of intervention. Cultures should be taken from blood, urine, and ascites if possible, and therapy with antibiotics commenced.

Because of the high risk of infection in this population of patients, it is necessary to give prophylactic antibiotics. In a recent meta-analysis, treatment with antibiotics was associated with an increase in hospital survival and decrease in infection. The risk of rebleeding also was lower in patients receiving antibiotics.[14,15] Oral norfloxacin, 400 mg twice a day; intravenous (IV) ciprofloxacin, 400 mg twice a day; or levofloxacin, 500 mg twice a day are the recommended antibiotics in 5-day courses.

Resuscitation should follow standard guidelines, and steps should include securing the airway, ensuring adequate respiratory function, and obtaining IV access to enable circulatory resuscitation. In particular, early intubation should be considered in the face of the high risk of aspiration due to the combination of encephalopathy and a stomach full of blood and ongoing hemorrhage. Endotracheal intubation also increases the safety of esophagogastroduodenoscopy, which may often be prolonged with need for intervention.

The lack of tachycardia or hypotension in these patients is not indicative of stability, because up to 25% of blood volume may be lost without any hemodynamic changes.[16] Blood volume should be restored, and coagulation factor support in the form of fresh frozen plasma and platelets may be required.

After initial stabilization, standard liver function tests and liver imaging should be undertaken. Patency of the portal vein should be verified and screening tests for hepatocellular carcinoma undertaken.

▣ Treatment

PHARMACOTHERAPY

At the same time as resuscitation, first-line treatment of suspected variceal hemorrhage in patients classified as high risk should include pharmacotherapy with a vasoactive drug prior to endoscopy. Treatment in this way will decrease portal flow, pressure, and variceal bleeding and frequently increase systemic arterial blood pressure.

Terlipressin (Glypressin) is a prodrug of vasopressin that has some intrinsic activity. It acts on vasopressin-1 receptors within arteriolar smooth muscle and induces vasoconstriction via phospholipase C–dependent signaling.[17] Treatment with terlipressin results in splanchnic vasoconstriction and decreases splanchnic inflow, thereby reducing portal pressure. Terlipressin also reduces collateral blood flow and variceal pressure.[18]

Compared with vasopressin, terlipressin is associated with a lower incidence of systemic ischemic events, and unlike vasopressin, terlipressin can be used safely without coadministration of nitroglycerin or other organic nitrates. Terlipressin has a longer half-life than vasopressin and can be administered intermittently. A dose of 2 mg IV given four times daily is as effective as endoscopic sclerotherapy for achieving initial control of variceal bleeding and preventing early rebleeding.[19] Terlipressin has been shown to decrease mortality and length of stay when administered to a high-risk population of patients presenting with acute upper GI hemorrhage.[20]

Terlipressin is well tolerated and has few side effects and may represent first-line treatment in acute hemorrhage until endoscopy can be performed in a controlled environment. In a recent meta-analysis, terlipressin was more effective than placebo but less effective than octreotide for controlling bleeding.[21] Despite these findings, a recent study showed equivalence between terlipressin and octreotide.[22,23]

The duration of treatment should be governed by the clinical situation. After 48 hours of therapy, however, the dose should be tapered (initially halved), seeking to achieve a course of therapy lasting 6 to 7 days. A recent study compared endoscopic banding therapy and banding in addition to 5 days of terlipressin.[24] Outcome was improved in the cohort that received combined therapy.

Treatment with somatostatin also may be considered. The dose of somatostatin is 250 µg as a bolus followed by 250 µg every hour as an infusion. The efficacy of somatostatin in the control of bleeding is not totally clear. In a recent meta-analysis of studies of somatostatin compared to control or no treatment, the use of somatostatin was associated with initial hemostasis but not with a decrease in mortality or rebleeding.[25] The treatment effect of somatostatin amounted to lowering the transfusion requirement by 0.5 units of blood per patient. In view of these findings, somatostatin cannot be recommended as the first-line agent for the control of variceal bleeding.

The somatostatin analogue, octreotide, may act by blocking the acute rise in portal pressure associated with fluid resuscitation in the face of GI hemorrhage. Its use is associated with improved outcome after therapeutic endoscopy. Octreotide is a somatostatin analog that has much longer half-life and therefore can be given as a bolus or infusion. Octreotide acts by blocking the vasodilatory effects of glucagon and vasoactive intestinal peptide. The side-effect profile for octreotide is more favorable than the side-effect profiles for terlipressin or vasopressin. In a recent meta-analysis, octreotide was more effective than no treatment or vasopressin/terlipressin.[18]

In a recent study, vapreotide was given for 5 days to patients acutely bleeding from varices.[26,27] A decrease in the number of bleedings during the index endoscopy and in the next 5 days was observed.

THERAPEUTIC ENDOSCOPY

Endoscopy should be undertaken after the patient is resuscitated. With the advent of pharmacotherapy, endoscopy does not need to be performed immediately, but should be carried out at the earliest opportunity by an experienced operator in the appropriate environment. None of the endoscopic methods of therapy reduce portal pressure; instead, they act by interrupting the abnormal collateral flow either by occlusion (band ligation, glue techniques) or by the induction of thrombosis (sclerotherapy).

The timing of endoscopy has recently been addressed; one study suggested that the determinants of outcome following acute variceal hemorrhage were "door-to-needle time" (threshold value: 15 hours) and Model for End-stage Liver Disease (MELD) score.[28] A similar study from a Canadian group did not show any effect of door-to-needle time.[29] However, in this study, hemodynamically unstable patients were excluded and underwent endoscopy within 4 hours. Determinants of outcome were infection on admission, albumin level, and MELD score.

SCLEROTHERAPY

In the sclerotherapy approach, a sclerosant is injected directly into the varix. A variety of sclerosants are in use, but ethanolamine and sodium tetradecyl sulfate are the most common. The immediate effect of controlling bleeding is probably due to edema caused by the injection of the sclerosant; thrombosis occurs later. Injection sclerotherapy can be accompanied by complications (Table 96-2). The rate of mortality related to severe complications is approximately 15%. The most common long-term complication is esophageal stricture.

TABLE 96-2	Complications of Endoscopic Sclerosant Therapy	
Site	*Complication*
Local	Ulcers
	Bleeding
	Stricture
	Esophageal dysmotility
Regional	Perforation
	Mediastinitis
	Pleural effusion
Systemic	Sepsis
	Aspiration

BAND LIGATION THERAPY

In band ligation therapy, a rubber band is placed on a variceal column that has been aspirated into a cylinder attached to the endoscope. The initial hemostatic effect is caused by strangulation of the vessel that is the source of variceal hemorrhage; later, thrombosis and ischemia result, leaving a shallow mucosal ulcer. Endoscopic band ligation is associated with fewer complications than endoscopic sclerotherapy, and systemic complications are rare.[30]

Although superficial ulceration is a side effect of endoscopic band ligation, stricture formation is rare. The most hazardous complication is rebleeding associated with early shedding of the band. In a recent meta-analysis, band ligation was as effective as sclerotherapy in the control of bleeding.[31] But because it is associated with fewer side effects and better long-term control of the varices, band ligation is preferred. However, results from a recent study suggest that there is an increased risk of infections as the number of band ligations is greater.[32]

A recently published meta-analysis demonstrated that combined pharmacologic and endoscopic treatments is better than each of these treatments alone.[33,34]

GLUE (BUTYL CYANOACRYLATE)

Results from a recent study of a small number of patients with decompensated liver disease and severe esophageal variceal hemorrhage suggest that injection of tissue glue rather than a sclerosant may result in improved initial hemostasis, reduced rebleeding, and improved survival.[35,36] However, this approach requires further study and comparison with endoscopic band ligation and other therapies before it is universally adopted.

Esophageal Varices Versus Gastric Varices

First-line treatment of gastric varices includes the injection of cyanoacrylate. The GOV occasionally can be treated with banding but may also require treatment with cyanoacrylate. Other sclerosants should not be administered.

Gastric varices can be subclassified according to their anatomic position, relationship to esophageal varices, and whether they are primary in origin or whether they develop as a result of obliteration of esophageal varices. Endoscopic management of bleeding gastric varices can be technically demanding. Recent evidence shows that cyanoacrylate is the treatment of choice for most gastric varices.[37] Cyanoacrylate injection can cause complications such as embolic phenomena.

If treatment fails to control the bleeding, early TIPS should be considered. If the bleeding is not controlled acutely, temporary hemostasis may be achieved with placement of a tamponade-inducing device such as a Sengstaken-Blakemore tube or, more safely, a Minnesota balloon. Prior to placing this sort of device, the vast majority of patients should be endotracheally intubated and mechanically ventilated to protect the airway and prevent aspiration.[8]

▦ Failure of Therapy/Salvage

Therapy failure is defined as:
- Inability to achieve initial control of bleeding
- Need for alternative therapy
- Early rebleeding
- Death within 5 days of first bleeding event

In 10% to 20% of patients, initial methods fail to control variceal bleeding.[38] This group of patients is at high risk for having a poor outcome, as discussed later. Salvage therapy relies on other modalities for halting ongoing bleeding.

MECHANICAL SALVAGE METHODS

The use of balloon tamponade to control variceal hemorrhage has decreased dramatically with the widespread use of vasoactive agents and therapeutic endoscopy. Nonetheless, balloon tamponade still has a role in the emergency management of uncontrollable bleeding from varices. Inflation of the gastric balloon results in tamponade of the varices, reduces blood flow into the plexus, and controls bleeding. The use of balloon tamponade effectively controls bleeding in 90% of patients.[39]

In the vast majority of cases, adequate control is achieved by inflation of the gastric balloon plus adequate traction without inflation of the esophageal balloon.[40,41] It is rarely necessary to inflate the esophageal balloon, and it is important to appreciate that this maneuver contributes significantly to the incidence of potentially life-threatening complications. Constant pressure on the gastroesophageal junction is achieved with skin traction or fixed traction using a helmet.

In approximately 50% patients, bleeding recurs upon deflation of the gastric balloon.[42,43] Potential complications associated with the use of compression devices include pulmonary aspiration, esophageal mucosal ischemia and ulceration, and misplacement of the device with gastric balloon inflation in the esophagus, leading to esophageal perforation.

Ideally, the balloons should be filled with a mixture of water and radiocontrast material, allowing good delineation of position on chest radiograph. It is normally essential to endotracheally mechanically intubate and ventilate patients who require balloon tamponade, to minimize the risk of aspiration and provide control of the airway. Balloon tamponade should be viewed as a short-term solution only (ideally for not > 12 hours duration). It should be viewed as a temporizing measure until either endoscopic therapy or another definitive therapy (e.g., TIPS) can be undertaken. Regardless of other forms of salvage therapy, intermittent deflation of the gastric balloon is essential to avoid mucosal perfusion.

A recent study proposes an alternative in the form of a self-expandable metal stent to compress the esophageal varices. Placement of this device does not require endoscopy. Experience with this device is limited, and therefore more studies are needed on this topic.[44] In addition, it should be recognized that this option would not be effective if bleeding is originating from gastric varices.

SHUNT SURGERY/INTERVENTIONAL RADIOLOGY

Traditionally, two types of surgical interventions have been used in the management of PHT: operations aimed at decompressing the portal system and devascularization procedures. A third and more definitive alternative is liver transplantation.

Acute shunt surgery has been performed for more than 50 years. Although effective at lowering portal pressure (and thus decreasing the risk of further bleeding), shunting procedures can precipitate acute deterioration of hepatic function and encephalopathy by diverting portal blood flow away from the liver. The degree of these predictable events is somewhat dictated by whether the shunt is total, partial, or selective, as well as the ability of the hepatic arterial autoregulation buffer response to increase hepatic arterial flow.

Side-to-side portacaval shunt is an example of a total shunt that is achieved either by direct anastomosis of the portal vein to the inferior vena cava or anastomosis using a short interpositional graft. Traditionally, the graft diameter is greater than 12 mm, producing total portal decompression. This procedure controls variceal bleeding in 95% to 98% of patients and controls ascites in more than 90% of patients. The encephalopathy rate is 30% to 40%. If the diameter of the graft is reduced to 8 mm, this type of shunt is known as a *partial shunt*. It does not provide total portal decompression, thus the risk of rebleeding is higher, but rates of both encephalopathy and ascites/liver failure are lower.[45,46]

"Selective" shunts, such as the distal splenorenal shunt, aim to address the issue of portal flow diversion. The aim of this shunt is to decompress the gastroesophageal junction and the spleen through the splenic vein to the renal vein. PHT is thus maintained in the superior mesenteric and portal vein to maintain blood flow to the liver.[47,48]

TIPS achieves the same effect in terms of decompression of the portal system without the operative risk. Depending on the diameter of the intrahepatic shunt, TIPS can be viewed as either a total or a partial shunt. It can be used in the setting of refractory acute hemorrhage when both endoscopic and pharmacologic strategies have failed. Use of TIPS, however, is not clearly associated with a survival benefit. TIPS carries a higher risk of precipitating encephalopathy and is significantly more expensive than either endoscopic or pharmacologic strategies.[49,50] The exact subgroup of patients for whom salvage TIPS leads to a favorable outcome has not been characterized.[51,52]

New radiologic methods have been developed that can be performed with fluoroscopy or even at the bedside of the patient in an intensive care environment. One such method is percutaneous transhepatic variceal embolization (PTVE) with 2-octyl cyanoacrylate (2-OCA). The effectiveness of PTVE with 2-OCA for controlling bleeding from esophageal varices is dependent upon the site and range of embolization. If the lower-esophageal and periesophageal varices and/or the cardial submucosal and perforating vessels are sufficiently obliterated, PTVE with 2-OCA can preventing variceal recurrence and rebleeding.[53]

Devascularization procedures combine components of splenectomy and gastric and esophageal devascularization. The aim of these procedures is to reduce inflow to variceal beds and thereby reduce the risk of bleeding. Because portal flow is maintained, the risk of encephalopathy is low (10%-15%). In patients with extensive portomesenteric venous occlusion or previous splenectomy, devascularization may offer an alternative decompressive strategy in selected cases when anatomic considerations make surgical or radiologic shunting impossible. Generally, it is felt that Child-Pugh B and C patients are likely to do less well with a surgical operative procedure than a TIPS shunt, owing to the risks of hepatic decompensation. Recent studies compared surgical and medical shunts and showed that outcomes were similar, although proper selection of patients was important.[54,55]

LIVER TRANSPLANTATION

Liver transplantation provides the ultimate in decompressive therapy, but its role in the salvage management of refractory variceal hemorrhage remains minor due to the scarcity of donor organs. In selected circumstances, however, orthotopic liver transplantation can successfully arrest both ongoing bleeding and, in the longer term, remodeling of the splanchnic circulation.

Prognosis

The mortality rate following a variceal bleed is often quoted as in the range of 30% to 60%.[56] Several reports of improved outcome since the introduction of therapeutic endoscopy may alter this estimate.[57,58]

The overall improvement in survival over the last 20 years is attributed to decreased early mortality, largely due to effective control of bleeding and prevention of rebleeding (due to treatment of the initial bleed, use of antibiotics, and secondary prophylaxis), rather than modification of the natural history of the disease. Survival increased both at 30 days and 6 years after hemorrhage in historical cohorts compared to those treated contemporaneously.[59] A recent publication predicted 6-week outcome looking at the values of creatinine, Child-Pugh score, and number and type of infections.[60]

Poor prognostic indicators in the short term include:
- Failure to control bleeding (ongoing bleeding, early rebleeding)
- Sepsis
- Renal failure
- Severe liver disease (ascites, coagulopathy)
- Encephalopathy

Poor prognostic indicators in the long term include:
- Advanced age
- Presence of hepatocellular carcinoma
- Presence of complications
- Intolerance of secondary prophylaxis

Complications

SEPSIS, RENAL FAILURE, MULTIPLE ORGAN DYSFUNCTION SYNDROME

As mentioned earlier, failure to control initial bleeding is associated with high risk of death in the short term. The high risk of death is due to both the immediate consequences of massive blood loss and ongoing shock, as well as to the consequences of end-organ insults, leading to multiple organ dysfunction syndrome.

Significantly, bacterial infection is associated with both an increase in failure to control bleeding and early rebleeding. Bacterial infection is associated with poor short-term prognosis. The use of broad-spectrum antibiotics after variceal hemorrhage has been shown to reduce the infection rate, decrease the rebleeding rate, and more importantly, improve early survival.[61]

A large proportion of the deaths attributed to variceal bleeding are not directly caused by hemorrhage but a complication of variceal bleeding and decompensated liver disease. Importantly, renal failure in association with advanced liver disease (e.g., Child-Pugh score > 10) and variceal hemorrhage predicts a very poor short-term prognosis and correlates strongly with early death (<30 days). Development of renal failure is associated with severity of bleeding (reflected by hemodynamic parameters, transfusion requirement, and findings at endoscopic examination), severity of liver disease (determined by Child-Pugh score), and presence or absence of bacterial infection. The prognosis of renal failure developing in association with variceal bleeding is similar to that for patients developing renal failure in association with spontaneous bacterial peritonitis and type 1 hepatorenal syndrome.

Primary Prophylaxis

All cirrhotic patients should be screened for esophageal varices with endoscopy. If moderate to large varices are found, it is necessary to start prophylactic treatment with a nonselective β-adrenergic blocker such as propranolol or nadolol. The dose of the drug should be titrated to achieve a heart rate that is 25% lower than baseline, or 55 bpm. If the patient bleeds while on β-adrenergic blocker prophylaxis, band ligation should be performed while the patient continues to be on β-adrenergic blocker therapy to avoid bleeding from portal hypertensive gastropathy and to prolong the durability of the endoscopic treatment. If a patient is intolerant to β-adrenergic blocker therapy, band ligation should be performed as primary prophylaxis.[62] There is marked up-regulation of the hepatic and mesenteric expression of β_3-adrenergic receptors (ARs) in human cirrhosis and in two different animal models of cirrhosis. β_3-AR-agonists should be further evaluated for therapy of PHT.[63] A recent study has shown carvedilol to be as effective as propranolol in primary prophylaxis.[64,65]

Preprimary Prophylaxis

Based on two small studies, β-adrenergic blocker therapy cannot be recommended for preprimary prophylaxis—that is, to prevent the development or slow the growth of esophageal varices. The risk of bleeding of these patients is very small compared to the side effects they experience while on drug therapy. More studies on this area are needed.

Secondary Prophylaxis

After an initial variceal bleed, as many as 60% of untreated patients will bleed again. Rebleeding is most frequent in the 6 weeks following an index variceal bleed and is seen in up to 40% of patients.[66] Risk factors for early rebleeding include age older than 60 years, high severity of initial bleed, renal failure, ascites, active bleeding on endoscopy, red signs, clot on varix, hypoalbuminemia, and hepatic venous pressure gradient greater than 20 mm Hg. The risk of late rebleeding is related to the severity of liver disease, endoscopic findings indicative of high risk of rebleeding, and continued alcohol intake, along with the poor prognostic indicators mentioned earlier.

Cirrhotic patients who survive an episode of variceal hemorrhage remain at high risk for rebleeding. Different modalities of treatment are all effective at reducing this risk. With the exception of therapeutic endoscopy, all act to reduce portal pressure. Adverse prognostic indicators include age, presence of renal failure or encephalopathy, and advanced Child-Pugh severity score.

All patients who survive an episode of variceal bleeding should receive some form of effective treatment to prevent rebleeding. The available options include pharmacotherapy, endoscopic therapy, radiologic TIPS, surgical shunt, and liver transplantation. Currently, first-line secondary prophylaxis of variceal hemorrhage consists of treatment using a nonselective β-adrenergic antagonist. A combination of treatment with a β-adrenergic blocker and several sessions of band ligation is the treatment of choice.

ASCITES

Accumulation of fluid in the peritoneal cavity is called *ascites*. The most common cause is cirrhosis.[67] Ascites is present in 20% to 60% of cirrhotic patients at the time of presentation. Leakage of sinusoidal fluid in cirrhosis happens as a result of sinusoidal hypertension due to the regenerative nodules and surrounding fibrosis. The other factor related to the pathogenesis of ascites in cirrhosis is expansion of plasma volume as a consequence of excessive renal retention of salt and water. The symptoms are increased abdominal girth, weight gain, and frequently edema. Tense ascites can result in respiratory compromise due to diaphragmatic splinting and or hydrothorax. The best method for diagnosing ascites is abdominal ultrasound, which can detect as little as 100 mL of ascites. Ascites total protein and serum ascites albumin gradient (SAAG) are important in determining the etiology of the ascites. If total protein concentration in ascitic fluid is greater than 25 g/dL, the diagnosis is likely malignancy, tuberculosis, or a postsinusoidal form of PHT such as Budd-Chiari syndrome. In these cases, the SAAG will be less than 1:1. If the SAAG is more than 1:1 is and the total protein concentration in ascetic fluid is less than 2.5 g/dL, then the most likely diagnosis is cirrhosis.

Ascites should be treated with sodium restriction. Sodium restriction to 90 mEq day (i.e., 2 g of salt per day) is a realistic goal for outpatients. Diuretics should be used, knowing that they can promote deterioration of renal function. Spironolactone is the drug of choice, since these patients have secondary hyperaldosteronism. However, this drug can take from 1 to 3 days to achieve full effect, so a faster-acting drug such as furosemide is frequently needed. The goal is to achieve a loss of 0.3 to 0.5 kg/d in patients without edema or 0.5 to 1 kg/d in patients with edema. If that is not achieved in 3 days, the dose of spironolactone and furosemide should be increased. If ascites cannot be controlled and/or renal deterioration appears, then there is evidence of refractory ascites, a condition associated with a very poor prognosis. A short course of terlipressin can be considered. Refractory ascites should be treated with paracentesis for the comfort of the patient. TIPS should also be considered as a bridge to liver transplantation, if this is deemed appropriate.

ABDOMINAL COMPARTMENT SYNDROME

Abdominal compartment syndrome is relatively common in patients with massive ascites, but it can occur in other situations such as ileus or abdominal trauma with active bleeding. The intraabdominal pressure can be measured with a urinary catheter or nasogastric tube. Normal values are less than 10 cm H_2O. A value over 15 cm H_2O defines the abdominal compartment syndrome and may be associated with failure of other organs. Treatment with paracentesis, nasogastric and rectal tubes (even decompressive colonoscopy), or surgery may be considered. In the context of liver disease, decompression can be achieved easily with small-volume paracentesis.

Large-volume paracentesis puts patients at risk of further central volume depletion and, hence, cardiovascular and renal dysfunction. It is normal to administer 20% albumin IV to prevent these complications. Most papers suggest that removing less than 5 L of ascites will not put the patient at risk of a post paracentesis cardiovascular disfunction syndrome; however, most physicians administer a vial of 100 mL of 20% albumin for every 2 L evacuated.[68]

SPONTANEOUS BACTERIAL PERITONITIS

Spontaneous bacterial peritonitis (SBE) is the development of infection in ascites in the absence of an obvious source of infection (intestinal perforation or abdominal abscess) or another site of inflammation, such as cholecystitis or pancreatitis. The most common pathogens are *Escherichia coli*, *Streptococcus pneumonia*, and *Klebsiella* spp., although there has been an increase in other gram-positive organisms in the last decade, possibly related to the increased use of norfloxacin in the community setting as primary prophylaxis to decrease the incidence of bacterial peritonitis.[69] Recent data suggest that some genetic variants of NOD2 are related not only to the development of SBP but also with risk of death.[70]

SBE is the most common type of infection in cirrhotic patients and accounts for about 25% of all infections.[71] Patients may present with signs of generalized peritonitis (diffuse pain, abdominal tenderness, fever, decreased bowel sounds), however, the clinical picture may be very mild, and a high level of suspicion is needed in any patient with cirrhosis who presents unwell with ascites. A diagnostic paracentesis should be performed in all patients with suspected SBP and also in those admitted to the hospital for the first time with ascites and in those presenting with encephalopathy or renal failure.

Ascitic cultures are negative in up to 40% of patients with clinical suspicion of SBP. Accordingly, an increase in polymorphonuclear (PMN) count is diagnostic when it reaches 250 PMN/µL. In hemorrhagic ascites, 1 PMN should be subtracted from the count for every 250 red blood cells. Normally, antibiotic treatment consists of a third-generation cephalosporin, but drug choice should be guided by hospital and community bacterial resistance patterns.

Renal impairment is a major cause of death in SBP. In addition to antibiotic therapy, albumin therapy decreases renal dysfunction and in-hospital mortality. The albumin dose should be 1.5 g/kg during the first 6 hours and 1 g/kg on the third day.

Patients with recent previous SBP or total ascitic protein less than 1 g/dL should be considered for prophylaxis to prevent SBP, with norfloxacin, 400 mg once a day, or twice a day if the patient has had a variceal bleed.

Other Complications of Portal Hypertension Syndrome

HEPATORENAL SYNDROME

Hepatorenal syndrome (HRS) is a clinical condition that appears in patients with advanced chronic liver disease, impaired renal function, and abnormalities in the renal circulation. HRS is characterized by renal vasoconstriction and decreased glomerular filtration rate. At the same time, marked arterial vasodilatation is apparent in the systemic (extrarenal) circulation.[72]

HRS usually occurs in patients with advanced cirrhosis, although it can also be seen in other situations such as acute liver failure or severe alcoholic hepatitis. There are two types of HRS: type I, associated with a worse prognosis and generally rapidly progressive; and type II, defined as impairment in renal function that does not meet criteria for type I and probably involves several different types of renal injury. HRS is characterized by oliguria, a rapid and progressive rise in serum creatinine concentration in less than 2 weeks, and urinary sodium of less than 10 mEq/L. It is also necessary to differentiate HRS from the more common prerenal azotemia. Whereas prerenal kidney dysfunction responds to intravascular volume expansion, HRS does not respond to IV fluid administration or the removal of diuretics. In addition, renal causes of renal dysfunction should be excluded by urinalysis, imaging, blood tests, and if necessary, renal biopsy (usually via the transjugular route). Venovenous hemofiltration as well as terlipressin or noradrenaline are beneficial in some cases.[73] In a recent meta-analysis, administration of terlipressin and albumin increased short-term survival in HRS type I, but there is a lack of data to provide clear recommendations for HRS type 2.[74] Recently, a study has shown that a positive

response to midodrine, octreotide, and albumin can select a population of patients whose renal function can respond completely to TIPS as a second-line treatment.[75]

HEPATIC ENCEPHALOPATHY

Hepatic encephalopathy (HE) is a neuropsychiatric syndrome in patients with liver disease and/or major portosystemic shunting. The classic definition of Adams and Foley[76,77] led to several different definitions of HE. Currently, three different types of HE are recognized. Type A (*A* is for *acute*) refers to HE seen in acute liver failure. In Type A HE, cerebral edema is almost always present. Cerebral edema can lead to intracranial hypertension and its associated complications. Type B (*B* is for *bypass*) appears in patients with significant portosystemic shunts without intrinsic liver disease and is very rare. Finally, type C (*C* is for *chronic* or *cirrhosis*) is seen in patients with chronic liver disease and PHT. In these patients, many of the products that normally are filtered and eliminated by the liver are delivered to the systemic circulation and, hence, the brain. There are several hypotheses for the pathogenesis of HE, including excessive production of ammonia, systemic inflammation, high levels of the neurotransmitter, gamma-aminobutyric acid (GABA), false neurotransmitters, and endogenous benzodiazepines.[78,79] In patients presenting with HE, possible triggering factors should be identified and treated. These potential triggering factors include infection, bleeding, constipation, and electrolyte and acid-base abnormalities. There are five grades of HE. Grade 0, or subclinical, can only be detected with psychometric tests. In grade 1, the patient is euphoric or depressed and has sleep pattern alterations, frequently associated with vivid nightmares. In grade 2, the patient tends to sleep but is easily arousable, while in grade 3, calling vigorously or inflicting pain are needed to wake the patient. In grade 4, the patient is in a coma, and diagnosis is based on the previous medical history of the patient, physical examination that can show extrapyramidal signs such as rigidity of the limbs or clonus, and the electroencephalogram, which will show triphasic delta waves in the frontal lobe. Treatment is based on avoidance and prevention of precipitating factors and in improving protein intake by feeding dairy products and vegetable-based diets. Laxatives in the form of lactulose or other disaccharides may be used, aiming for two to three soft bowel movements per day. Antibiotics are reserved for patients who respond poorly to disaccharides. Rifaximin recently has been proposed in this context, and it appears to be an effective and safe treatment option for HE.[80] Artificial liver support devices, specifically the MARS device, have been shown to result in more rapid resolution of HE.[81] L-Ornithine L-aspartate (LOLA) also may ameliorate encephalopathy,[82] although further studies are required. A recent randomized controlled study in acute liver failure was not able to demonstrate any improvement in HE or survival in the LOLA-treated population.[83] The definitive treatment for HE is liver transplantation.[84,85]

Patients with grade III-IV HE require endotracheal intubation to protect the airway from aspiration. In acute liver failure, pathogenesis and treatment are different and centered in early detection and aggressive treatment of intracranial hypertension.

KEY POINTS

1. *Portal hypertension* is defined as the presence of a raised portocaval pressure gradient.

2. Cases with hepatic dysfunction (cirrhosis) have a worse prognosis than cases without hepatic dysfunction.

3. Portal hypertension results from both increased resistance to portal flow and an absolute increase in portal flow, despite portosystemic collateral remodeling.

4. Manifestations of portal hypertension are variceal hemorrhage, portosystemic shunting with risk of encephalopathy, ascites, and decreased renal blood flow with risk of hepatorenal failure.

ANNOTATED REFERENCES

Garcia-Tsao G, Groszmann RJ, Fisher RL, et al. Portal pressure, presence of gastroesophageal varices and variceal bleeding. Hepatology 1985;5:419-24.

This classic paper from the Yale University School of Medicine studied the relationship between the gradient of portal pressure measured invasively and the presence of esophageal varices, their size, and their risk of bleeding.

Gonzalez R, Zamora J, Gomez-Camarero J, Molinero LM, Bañares R, Albillos A. Meta-analysis: combination endoscopic and drug therapy to prevent variceal rebleeding in cirrhosis. Ann Intern Med 2008; 149:109-22.

Recent meta-analysis in which the combination of endoscopic and pharmacologic treatment was significantly better than each of these treatments alone.

Boyer TD, Haskal ZJ. American Association for the Study of Liver Diseases. The role of transjugular intrahepatic portosystemic shunt (TIPS) in the management of portal hypertension: update 2009. Hepatology 2010;51:306.

Recent update of the guidelines of the American Association for the Study of Liver Diseases dealing with the most important features of this interventional modality of treatment of portal hypertension.

Lee SW, Lee TY, Chang CS. Independent factors associated with recurrent bleeding in cirrhotic patients with esophageal variceal hemorrhage. Dig Dis Sci 2009;54:1128-34.

Recent paper showing the important relation between infection and rebleeding from esophageal varices as well as with repeated endoscopic band ligations.

Bernard B, Grangé JD, Khac EN, Amiot X, Opolon P, Poynard T. Antibiotic prophylaxis for the prevention of bacterial infection in cirrhotic patients with gastrointestinal bleeding: a meta-analysis. Hepatology 1999;29:1655-61.

First publication to show an increase in survival with antibiotic prophylaxis, not only a decreased number of spontaneous bacterial peritonitis and other infections.

Davenport A. Management of acute kidney injury in liver disease. Contrib Nephrol 2010;165:197-205.

Very complete paper from the nephrologic perspective on the causes and management of kidney disorders in patients with liver disease.

Blei AT, Córdoba J. Practice Parameters Committee of the American College of Gastroenterology. Hepatic encephalopathy. Am J Gastroenterol 2001;96:1968-76.

A review of the current recommendations for management of hepatic encephalopathy.

REFERENCES

Access the complete reference list online at http://www.expertconsult.com.

97

Ascites

LENA M. NAPOLITANO

Definition and Diagnosis

Ascites is the abnormal accumulation of fluid in the peritoneal cavity.[1] Patients with ascites generally present on clinical examination with abdominal distention and a fluid wave or shifting dullness on abdominal percussion, but the abdominal examination findings also may be normal if the amount of ascites is not massive.

Diagnostic imaging can confirm the diagnosis of ascites. Ultrasonography is the easiest and most sensitive technique for the detection of ascitic fluid, being capable of visualizing very small volumes (5-10 mL). Computed tomography (CT) is also very sensitive for detecting ascites (Figure 97-1). Small amounts of ascitic fluid localize in the perihepatic area and in Morrison's pouch (the hepatorenal space).

A diagnostic paracentesis (20 mL)[2] is performed to determine the etiology of the ascites as well as to exclude or establish a diagnosis of spontaneous bacterial peritonitis (SBP). A diagnostic paracentesis should be performed in any person with new-onset ascites. Paracentesis to evaluate for SBP is also indicated for cirrhotic patients with known ascites who require hospitalization or sustain clinical deterioration, such as worsening encephalopathy or unexplained fever. A missed or delayed diagnosis of SBP can lead to sepsis and significant morbidity and mortality.

Peritoneal fluid from patients with new-onset ascites of unknown origin should be assayed for cell count, albumin level, culture, total protein concentration, Gram stain, and cytologic analysis.[3] Serum albumin concentration should be measured as well.

The serum ascites albumin gradient (SAAG, serum albumin concentration—ascitic fluid albumin concentration) is the best diagnostic measure for classification of ascites (Table 97-1).[4] The SAAG is very specific and sensitive for distinguishing ascites due to portal hypertension (SAAG > 1.1 g/dL) from that occurring as a result of other pathogenetic mechanisms such as inflammation or peritoneal malignancy (SAAG ≤ 1.1 g/dL). Ideally, specimens should be obtained simultaneously. In the past, ascites was classified as being an exudate (protein concentration ≥ 2.5 g/dL) or a transudate (protein concentration < 2.5 g/dL), but this classification scheme is no longer used because of its poor sensitivity and specificity.[5] The total protein level may provide additional clues about diagnosis when used with the SAAG; that is, high SAAG and high protein concentration is seen in most cases of ascites due to hepatic congestion, whereas low serum ascites albumin gradient and high protein concentration characterizes malignant ascites. The terms *high albumin gradient* and *low albumin gradient* should replace the terms *transudate* and *exudate* in the description of ascites.

The ascitic fluid cell count and differential cell count are important in the evaluation of cases of possible SBP and other inflammatory peritoneal conditions. Normal peritoneal fluid contains less than 500 leukocytes/μL and less than 250 polymorphonuclear leukocytes/μL. A peritoneal fluid neutrophil count above 250 cells/μL is consistent with bacterial peritonitis. In tuberculous peritonitis and peritoneal carcinomatosis, most leukocytes in peritoneal fluid are lymphocytes. A sample of ascites should be inoculated into blood culture bottles for detection of SBP. Gram stain is not sensitive for the detection of SBP because of the low numbers of bacterial organisms present in the ascites.

The sensitivity of cytologic analysis for detecting malignancy is 58% to 75% if a large volume of fluid is analyzed. Laparoscopy is an additional invasive diagnostic study that also may be indicated if a diagnosis of malignant ascites is considered. Peritoneal or tumor implant biopsy samples can be obtained at the same time for histologic diagnosis.

Pathophysiology

Ascites is the most common complication related to liver disease and cirrhosis.[6] It is associated with profound changes in the splanchnic and systemic circulation and with renal abnormalities (Figure 97-2). However, the pathogenesis of renal sodium retention and ascites formation in cirrhosis remains a subject of much controversy.

One accepted theory of ascites formation is the *forward theory*, which states that the development of ascites is related to the existence of severe sinusoidal portal hypertension that causes marked splanchnic arterial vasodilation and a forward increase in the splanchnic production of lymph.[7] Splanchnic arterial vasodilation also produces arterial vascular underfilling, a significant reduction of the effective blood volume, and arterial hypotension. These pathophysiologic changes lead to compensatory activation of sodium- and water-retaining mechanisms (the renin-angiotensin-aldosterone system, sympathetic nervous system, and nonosmotic release of vasopressin) and promote ascites formation. Therefore, according to this theory, derangements in the splanchnic arterial circulation rather than the venous portal system are primary in the pathogenesis of ascites formation.[8]

This theory is supported by the observation that interventions that markedly decrease portal pressure, such as surgical portacaval shunts or transjugular intrahepatic portosystemic shunts (TIPS), reduce ascites. In the advanced stages of cirrhosis, the extreme underfilling of the arterial circulation leads to maximal stimulation of vasoconstrictor mechanisms which override the protective effects of renal vasodilator factors and cause renal vasoconstriction, further aggravating ascites formation and leading to functional renal insufficiency. Renal insufficiency is also one of the main causes of resistance to diuretic therapy.

Patients with advanced cirrhosis and portal hypertension often show an abnormal regulation of extracellular fluid volume, resulting in the accumulation of fluid as ascites, pleural effusion, or edema. The mechanisms responsible for ascites formation include alterations in the splanchnic circulation as well as renal functional abnormalities that favor sodium and water retention.[9] The renal functional abnormalities occur in the setting of a hyperdynamic circulatory state that is characterized by increased cardiac output, decreased systemic vascular resistance, and activation of neurohormonal vasoactive systems. This circulatory dysfunction, due mainly to intense arterial vasodilation in the splanchnic circulation, is considered to be a primary feature in the pathogenesis of ascites.

A major factor involved in the development of splanchnic arterial vasodilation is increased synthesis of nitric oxide (NO), a potent vasodilator that is elevated in the splanchnic circulation of patients with cirrhosis. Excessive production of NO decreases effective arterial blood volume and leads to fluid accumulation and renal function abnormalities, which are a consequence of the homeostatic activation of vasoconstrictor and antinatriuretic factors triggered to compensate for a relative arterial underfilling. The net effect is avid retention of sodium and water as well as renal vasoconstriction.

The *peripheral arterial vasodilation hypothesis* incriminates relative underfilling of the arterial vascular compartment as the primary problem. Relative arterial underfilling leads to the same neurohumoral

Ascites

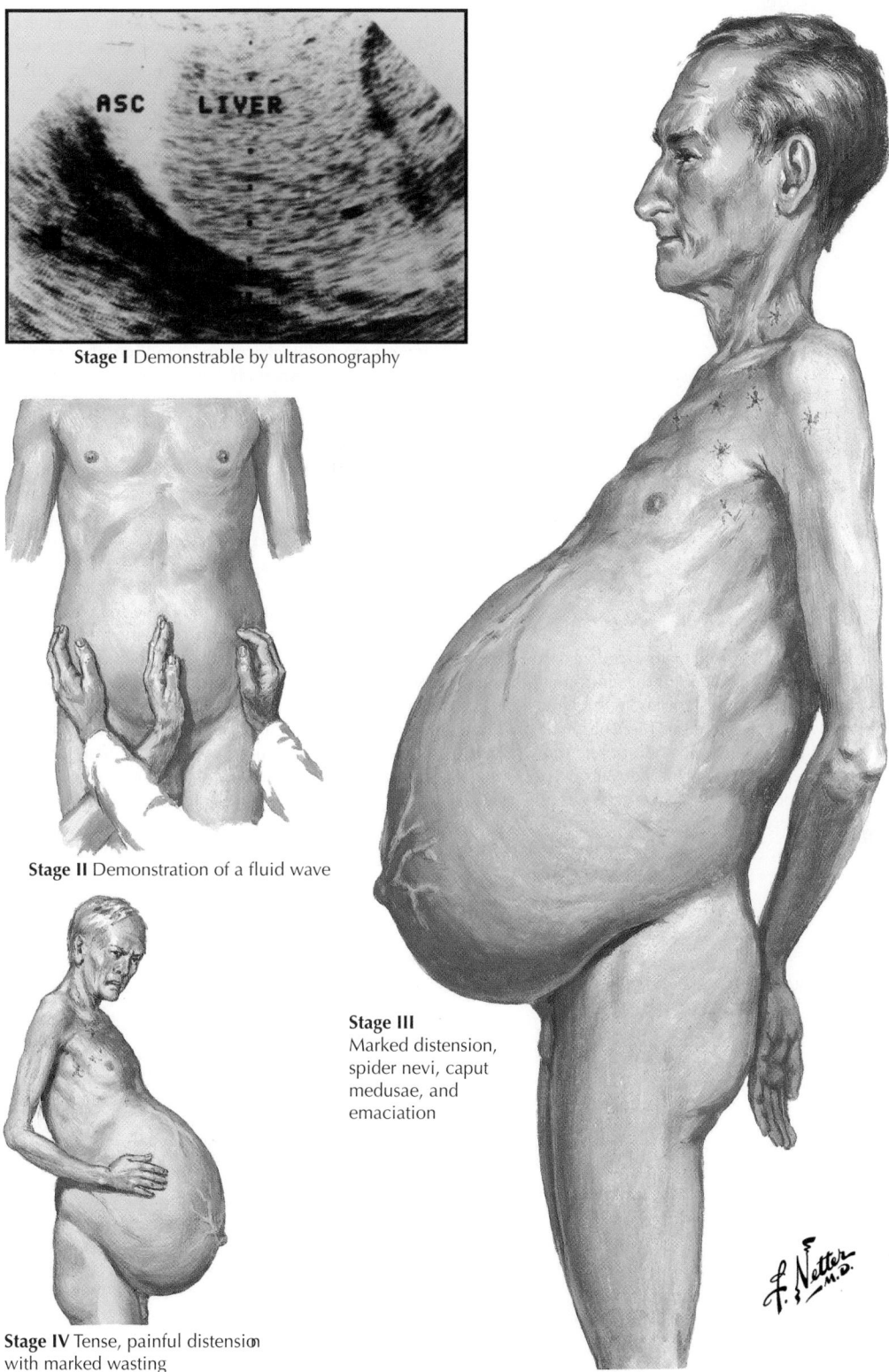

Stage I Demonstrable by ultrasonography

Stage II Demonstration of a fluid wave

Stage III
Marked distension, spider nevi, caput medusae, and emaciation

Stage IV Tense, painful distension with marked wasting

Figure 97-1 Ascites appearance on ultrasound (Netterimages.com) of abdomen and pelvis.

TABLE 97-1	Causes of Ascites Based on Normal or Diseased Peritoneum and Serum-to-Ascites Albumin Gradient (SAAG)

Normal Peritoneum

Portal Hypertension (SAAG > 1.1 g/dL)

Hepatic congestion
  Congestive heart failure
  Constrictive pericarditis
  Tricuspid insufficiency
  Budd-Chiari syndrome

Liver disease
  Cirrhosis
  Alcoholic hepatitis
  Fulminant hepatic failure
  Massive hepatic metastases

Hypoalbuminemia (SAAG < 1.1 g/dL)

Nephrotic syndrome
Protein-losing enteropathy
Severe malnutrition with anasarca

Miscellaneous Conditions (SAAG < 1.1 g/dL)

Chylous ascites
Pancreatic ascites
Bile ascites
Nephrogenic ascites
Urine ascites
Ovarian disease

Diseased Peritoneum (SAAG < 1.1 g/dL)

Infections
  Bacterial peritonitis
  Tuberculous peritonitis
  Fungal peritonitis
  HIV-associated peritonitis
Malignant Conditions
  Peritoneal carcinomatosis
  Primary mesothelioma
  Pseudomyxoma peritonei
  Hepatocellular carcinoma

Other Rare Conditions
  Familial Mediterranean fever
  Vasculitis
  Granulomatous peritonitis
  Eosinophilic peritonitis

The pathogenesis of peripheral arterial vasodilation in cirrhosis is not completely elucidated, but there is evidence for a major role of NO.[11] Increased vascular NO production has been demonstrated in cirrhosis. In patients with ascites, the hepatic artery produces more NO than it does in patients without ascites. In a rat model of cirrhosis, normalization of vascular NO production with administration of a NO synthase inhibitor corrects the hyperdynamic circulation, improves sodium and water excretion, and decreases neurohumoral activation. This insight into the mechanisms of the peripheral arterial vasodilation in cirrhosis should provide new tools in the treatment of edema and ascites, a major cause of morbidity and mortality in patients with cirrhosis.

The generally accepted peripheral arterial vasodilation hypothesis seems to best explain the mechanism of sodium retention and other clinical findings such as hyperdynamic circulation in patients with cirrhosis. However, recent data in patients with pre-ascites or early ascites do not seem to conform to the peripheral arterial vasodilation hypothesis.[12] Renal sodium handling abnormalities can be demonstrated in patients with cirrhosis prior to the development of ascites when these individuals are challenged with a sodium load. These changes are apparent even in the absence of systemic vasodilation or arterial underfilling. Therefore, an alternative hypothesis with a direct hepatorenal interaction, acting via sinusoidal portal hypertension and/ or hepatic dysfunction as the effector mechanism, is proposed to be the initiating event promoting renal sodium retention in patients with cirrhosis. The second and later process is the development of systemic arterial vasodilation, possibly due to the presence of excess systemic vasodilators and/or decreased responsiveness of the vasculature to endogenous vasoconstrictors. These changes in turn lead to a relatively underfilled circulation with consequent activation of neurohumoral systems, promoting further renal sodium retention as described by the peripheral arterial vasodilation hypothesis. When compensatory natriuretic mechanisms fail, refractory ascites develops and hepatorenal syndrome sets in. Thus renal sodium retention in patients with cirrhosis is the result of an interplay of many factors; direct hepatorenal interaction predominates in the earlier stages of the cirrhotic process, whereas systemic vasodilation becomes a more important pathogenetic mechanism as the disease progresses.

responses that occur in states characterized by low cardiac output (e.g., chronic congestive heart failure).[10] Activation of the renin-angiotensin-aldosterone axis and the sympathetic system, as well as nonosmotic release of vasopressin, are well documented in cases of cirrhosis. This sequence of events results in renal water and sodium retention, failure to escape from the sodium-retaining effect of aldosterone, and renal resistance to atrial natriuretic peptide. Dilutional hyponatremia is the strongest predictor of the occurrence of hepatorenal syndrome.

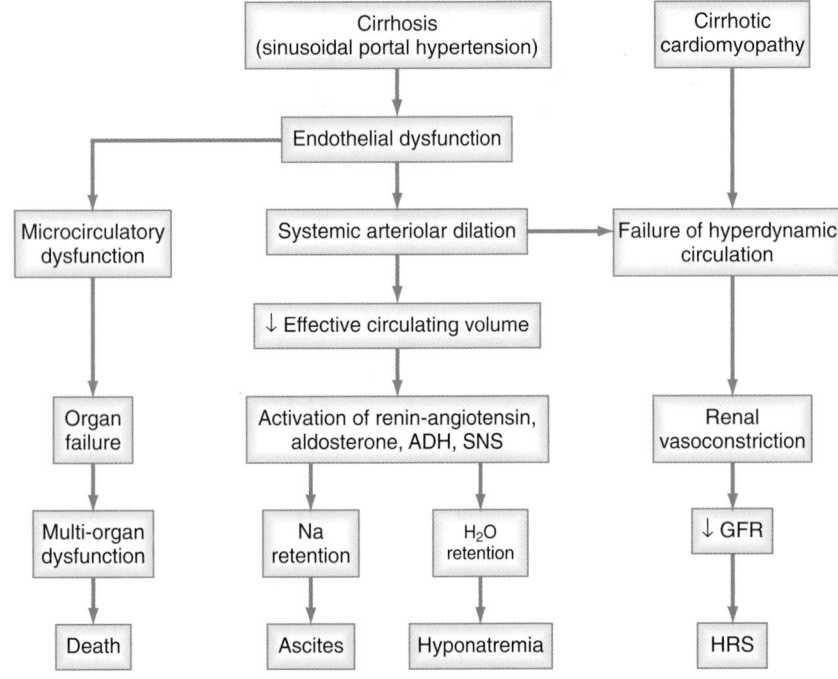

Figure 97-2 Pathophysiology of cirrhosis and ascites. Cirrhosis is associated with splanchnic arterial vasodilation, leading to a decrease in effective circulating volume and a hyperdynamic circulation. The decrease in effective circulating volume causes activation of renal sodium and water retentive pathways (e.g., RAAS, renal SNS, and ADH). Resulting sodium and water retention leads to ascites due to spillage of excess sodium and water from hepatic lymph into peritoneal cavity. As disease progresses, progressive decrease in effective circulating volume develops, causing severe renal vasoconstriction and decrease in glomerular filtration rate. Onset of cirrhotic cardiomyopathy accentuates this problem and tips patient into hepatorenal syndrome. Accompanying circulatory disturbance leads to organ failure and death. Sepsis is frequently associated with this process. (*From Salerno F, Camma C, Enea M, Rossle M, Wong F. Transjugular intrahepatic portosystemic shunt for refractory ascites: a meta-analysis of individual patient data. Gastroenterology 2007;133: 825-34.*)

TABLE 97-2	Grades of Ascites and Recommended Treatment	
Grade	*Definition*	*Treatment*
Grade 1	Mild ascites only detectable by ultrasonographic examination	No specific treatment Dietary sodium restriction Careful follow-up
Grade 2	Moderate ascites manifest by moderate symmetrical distention of the abdomen	Dietary sodium restriction Diuretics (spironolactone with or without furosemide, amiloride for patients with nonactivated renin-angiotensin-aldosterone system)
Grade 3	Large or gross ascites with marked abdominal distention	Paracentesis (total or large-volume, with colloid volume expansion) Dietary sodium restriction Diuretics

Adapted from Moore KP, Wong F, Gines P, et al. The management of ascites in cirrhosis: report on the Consensus Conference of the International Ascites Club. Hepatology 2003;38:258-66.

Etiology

Liver disease, particularly cirrhosis, is a common cause of ascites. In patients with liver disease, ascites develops as a result of portal hypertension, which can be prehepatic (e.g., due to portal vein thrombosis), intrahepatic (e.g., due to cirrhosis), or posthepatic (e.g., due to Budd-Chiari syndrome). Patients with chronic liver disease develop portal hypertension and subsequent ascites from increased resistance of blood flow through the hepatic parenchyma. Circulatory changes such as increased plasma volume and increased cardiac output develop in conjunction with decreased systemic vascular resistance and blood pressure.

Ascites is one of the most frequent complications of cirrhosis, accounting for approximately 85% of cases of ascites in the United States. Its appearance is considered a key marker of the transition from the compensated to the decompensated stage of the disease. In compensated cirrhotic patients, ascites develops at a 5-year cumulative rate of approximately 30%. The appearance of ascites also has prognostic significance, as it causes a sharp drop in the expected survival rate. Once ascites develops, the 1-year survival rate is 50% compared with the 1-year survival rate of over 90% in patients with compensated cirrhosis. Prognosis is particularly poor in patients who develop refractory ascites or hepatorenal syndrome.

Most cases of ascites are due to liver disease. However, a number of disorders may be associated with ascites, and these include portal vein thrombosis, cardiac disorders (constrictive pericarditis, congestive heart failure), liver cancer, nephrotic syndrome, protein-losing enteropathy, and pancreatitis (see Table 97-1). Nonhepatic causes include cardiac failure, malignancy, renal failure, and intraabdominal inflammation. It is important to diagnose nonhepatic causes of ascites such as malignancy, tuberculosis, and pancreatic ascites, since these occur with increased frequency in patients with liver disease.

Management

Ascites is the most common presentation of decompensated cirrhosis. It occurs in more than half of all patients with cirrhosis, and its development heralds a poor prognosis (50% 2-year survival rate). Ascites is characterized by three grades of severity, and treatment is based on grade (Table 97-2). Effective first-line medical therapy for ascites includes dietary sodium restriction (2 g/d) and use of diuretics.[13]

MEDICAL MANAGEMENT

Management of uncomplicated ascites includes salt restriction, diuretics, and large-volume paracentesis (LVP) (Table 97-3). Diuretics are the mainstay of medical therapy in the treatment of ascites. Initially, an aldosterone antagonist (spironolactone) is used. Spironolactone

TABLE 97-3	Management of Uncomplicated Ascites	
General Management	Treat ascites once complications have been treated. Avoid NSAIDs. Norfloxacin prophylaxis (400 mg PO once daily) in patients with an ascites protein level of <1.5 g/dL, impaired renal function (serum creatinine level ≥ 1.2 mg/dL, BUN ≥ 25 mg/dL, serum sodium level ≤ 130 mEq/L, or severe liver failure (CTP score ≥ 9 points with serum bilirubin level ≥ 3 mg/dL)	
Specific Management	Salt restriction	1-2 g/day Liberalize if restriction results in poor food intake.
	Diuretics	Spironolactone based: spironolactone alone (start at 50-100 mg once daily, single morning dose) *or:* Spironolactone (50-100 mg once daily) + furosemide (start 20-40 mg once daily, single morning dose)
	LVP	Use as initial therapy only in patients with tense ascites; administer intravenous albumin (6-8 g/L of ascites removed).
Follow-up and Goals	Adjustment of diuretic dosage should be performed every 4-7 days. Patient should be weighed at least weekly, and BUN, creatinine, and electrolytes measured every 1-2 weeks while adjusting dosage. Double dosage of diuretics if: Weight loss < 4 lb (2 kg) a week *and* BUN, creatinine, and electrolytes stable Halve the dosage of diuretics or discontinue if: Weight loss ≥ 1 lb (0.5 kg/day) *or* if there are abnormalities in BUN, creatinine, or electrolytes Maximum diuretic dosage is spironolactone, 400 mg once daily, and furosemide, 160 mg once daily.	

Data from Garcia-Tsao G, Lim JK; Members of the Veterans Affairs Hepatitis C Resource Center Program. Management and treatment of patients with cirrhosis and portal hypertension: recommendations from the Department of Veterans Affairs Hepatitis C Resource Center Program and the National Hepatitis C Program. Am J Gastroenterol 2009;104:1802-29.

BUN, blood urea nitrogen; *CTP,* Child-Turcotte-Pugh; *LVP,* large volume paracentesis; *NSAIDs,* nonsteroidal anti-inflammatory drugs; *PO,* orally.

competes with aldosterone for receptor sites in the distal renal tubules, increasing salt and water excretion and promoting retention of potassium and hydrogen ions. Spironolactone is usually initiated at a dose of 100 mg per day. The addition of a loop diuretic (e.g., furosemide) may be necessary in some cases to increase the natriuretic effect. The dosage of both the aldosterone antagonist and the loop diuretic should be increased sequentially until an adequate diuretic response is observed. Sodium restriction and diuretic therapy are initially effective in approximately 95% of patients. Water restriction is used only if persistent hyponatremia is present.

PARACENTESIS

In the treatment of ascites, paracentesis is reserved for patients refractory to medical management. As a therapeutic intervention, abdominal paracentesis is usually performed to drain a large volume of abdominal ascites.[14] When tense or refractory ascites is present, LVP (removal of more than 5 L of ascitic fluid) is safe and effective and has the advantage of producing immediate relief from ascites and its associated symptoms.[15] Total paracentesis—removal of all ascites (even >20 L)—usually can be performed safely. Recent studies demonstrate that intravenous (IV) infusion of 5 g of albumin for each liter of ascites removed (>5 L) decreases complications of paracentesis such as electrolyte imbalances and increased serum creatinine concentration secondary to large shifts of intravascular volume. LVP provides rapid resolution of symptoms with minimal complications and is well tolerated by most patients. Paracentesis-induced circulatory dysfunction (PICD) may

TABLE 97-4	Revised Diagnostic Criteria of Refractory Ascites

Treatment duration: Patients must be on intensive diuretic therapy (spironolactone 400 mg/d and furosemide 160 mg/d) for at least 1 week and on a salt-restricted diet of less than 90 mmol or 5.2 g of salt/day.

Lack of response: Mean weight loss of <0.8 kg over 4 days and urinary sodium output less than the sodium intake

Early ascites recurrence: Reappearance of grade 2 or 3 ascites within 4 weeks of initial mobilization

Diuretic-Induced Complications:

Diuretic-induced hepatic encephalopathy is the development of encephalopathy in the absence of any other precipitating factor.

Diuretic-induced renal impairment is an increase of serum creatinine by >100% to a value >2 mg/dL in patients with ascites responding to treatment.

Diuretic-induced hyponatremia is a decrease of serum sodium by >10 mmol/L to a serum sodium concentration of <125 mmol/L.

Diuretic-induced hypo- or hyperkalemia is a change in serum potassium to <3 mmol/L or >6 mmol/L despite appropriate measures.

Adapted from Moore KP, Wong F, Gines P et al. The management of ascites in cirrhosis: report on the Consensus Conference of the International Ascites Club. Hepatology 2003;38:258-66.

TABLE 97-5	Management of Refractory Ascites	
Definitions	Ascites that is not eliminated even with maximum diuretic therapy	
	Ascites that is not eliminated because maximum dosages of diuretics cannot be attained, given the development of diuretic-induced complications	
Recommended Therapy	Total paracentesis + IV albumin (6-8 g/L of ascites removed)	
	If <5 L of ascites is removed, a synthetic plasma volume expander may be used instead of albumin.	
	Continue with salt restriction and diuretic therapy as tolerated.	
Alternative Therapy	TIPS for patients who require frequent paracenteses (every 1-2 weeks) and whose CTP score is ≤11	
	Peritoneovenous shunt for patients who are not TIPS or transplant candidates	

Data from Garcia-Tsao G, Lim JK; Members of the Veterans Affairs Hepatitis C Resource Center Program. Management and treatment of patients with cirrhosis and portal hypertension: recommendations from the Department of Veterans Affairs Hepatitis C Resource Center Program and the National Hepatitis C Program. Am J Gastroenterol 2009;104:1802–29.

CTP, Child-Turcotte-Pugh; *IV,* intravenous; *TIPS,* transjugular intrahepatic portosystemic shunt.

occur after LVP and is characterized by hyponatremia, azotemia, and increased plasma renin activity. PICD is associated with increased mortality and may be prevented by administration of albumin IV (6–8 g/L of ascites removed).

The International Ascites Club, representing the spectrum of clinical practice from North America to Europe, has developed consensus guidelines for the management of cirrhotic ascites from the stage of early ascites to the stage of refractory ascites.[16] Mild to moderate ascites should be managed by modest salt restriction and diuretic therapy with spironolactone or an equivalent. Diuretics should be added in a stepwise fashion while maintaining sodium restriction. Gross ascites should be treated with therapeutic paracentesis followed by colloid volume expansion and diuretic therapy. Refractory ascites is managed by repeated LVP or insertion of a TIPS shunt. Successful placement of TIPS results in improved renal function, sodium excretion, and general well-being but has not been shown to improve survival. Clinicians caring for these patients should be aware of the potential complications of each treatment modality and be prepared to discontinue diuretics, or not proceed with TIPS placement, if complications or contraindications develop. Liver transplantation should be considered for all patients with ascites and cirrhosis. Ideally, liver transplantation should be performed prior to the development of renal dysfunction to minimize the risk of mortality.

REFRACTORY ASCITES

Refractory or recurrent ascites is a clinical challenge frequently encountered in patients with cirrhosis.[17,18] Ascites becomes refractory to medical treatment in 10% of cirrhotic patients. The diagnosis of refractory ascites recently has been revised (Table 97-4). Refractory ascites is a poor prognostic sign; as many as 50% of patients with this condition die within 6 months of its development.

The only definitive therapy for refractory ascites with cirrhosis is orthotopic liver transplantation. The other options that are available include LVP, peritoneovenous shunts, and TIPS (Table 97-5). TIPS is contraindicated in patients who have advanced liver failure, because it can hasten death in such individuals. Peritoneovenous shunts are associated with a high incidence of complications and frequent occlusion. They are therefore rarely used for management of refractory ascites. The initial treatment option for refractory ascites is repetitive LVP or total paracentesis.[19,20]

An early report describing experience with TIPS management of refractory ascites documented that ascites was markedly reduced after this procedure.[21] In responders, plasma aldosterone and renin activity decreased, serum creatinine concentration decreased, and urinary sodium excretion increased. However, new-onset hepatic encephalopathy was seen in 14 of 30 patients studied. Severe disabling chronic encephalopathy occurred in 5 patients but was successfully reversed by balloon occlusion of the shunt in 3 patients. Cumulative survival in this study was 41% and 34% at 1 and 2 years, respectively.

Clinicians would find it useful to have a way to predict a favorable clinical response to TIPS for refractory ascites. Accordingly, a prospective cohort study of 53 cirrhotic patients without organic renal disease and with refractory ascites was conducted.[22] Some of the patients were "responders" to TIPS. Responders included patients who survived for more than 6 months without severe chronic hepatic encephalopathy and with good control of ascites. The following parameters were examined for prognostic value: age, creatinine clearance, plasma renin activity, plasma aldosterone concentration, and Pugh score. Good control of ascites was obtained in 90% of patients, and 47% were responders to TIPS. The cumulative survival rate was 54% at 6 months, 48% at 1 year, and 39% at 2 years. The majority of patients died of complications of hepatic insufficiency. Severe chronic hepatic encephalopathy developed in 26% of patients. Creatinine clearance was the only factor that was a significant independent predictor of good clinical response to TIPS for refractory ascites. In patients with poor renal function, therefore, TIPS should not be considered.

A randomized prospective trial compared LVP and TIPS in 60 patients with cirrhosis and refractory ascites in Germany.[23] Multivariate analysis confirmed that TIPS was independently associated with survival without the need for transplantation ($P = .02$), with a mean follow-up of 45 months. At 3 months, 61% of the TIPS patients had no ascites, compared to 18% of the paracentesis group ($P = .006$).

A similar study performed in Spain randomized 70 patients with cirrhosis and refractory ascites to TIPS or repeated paracentesis plus IV albumin.[24] Recurrence of ascites and development of hepatorenal syndrome were lower in the TIPS group compared with the paracentesis group, whereas the frequency of severe hepatic encephalopathy was greater in the TIPS group. TIPS did not improve survival and was associated with higher costs.

The North American Study for the Treatment of Refractory Ascites multicenter clinical trial enrolled a larger sample size (n = 109) than prior studies.[25] Patients with refractory ascites were randomized to medical therapy (sodium restriction, diuretics, and total paracentesis, n = 57) or medical therapy plus TIPS (n = 52). The principal endpoints were recurrence of tense symptomatic ascites and mortality. A technically adequate shunt was created in 49 of 52 subjects. TIPS plus medical therapy was significantly superior to medical therapy alone in preventing recurrence of ascites ($P < .001$), but no difference in mortality was identified (21 deaths occurred in each group). There was a higher incidence of moderate to severe encephalopathy in the TIPS group (20 of 52 versus 12 of 57, $P = .058$), but no difference in the incidence of liver failure, variceal hemorrhage, or acute renal failure. No differences in frequency of emergency department visits, medically indicated hospitalizations, or quality of life were identified. Although TIPS plus medical therapy was superior to medical therapy alone for the control of ascites, TIPS did not improve survival, affect hospitalization rates, or improve quality of life.

The Cochrane Database Systematic Review of TIPS versus paracentesis for cirrhotic patients with refractory ascites included 5 randomized trials, which collectively enrolled 330 patients.[26] Mortality at 30 days (OR 1.00, 95% CI 0.10–10.06, $P = 1.0$) and 24 months (OR 1.29, 95% CI 0.65–2.56, $P = 0.5$) did not differ significantly between TIPS and paracentesis. Patients randomized to TIPS has significantly decreased reaccumulation of ascites at 3 months (OR 0.07, 95% CI 0.03–0.18, $P < .01$) and 12 months (OR 0.14, 95% CI 0.06–0.28, $P < .01$). Hepatic encephalopathy occurred significantly more often in the TIPS group (OR 2.24, 95% CI 1.39–3.6, $P < .01$), but gastrointestinal bleeding, infection, and acute renal failure did not differ significantly between the two groups. This meta-analysis supports that TIPS was more effective at removing ascites than paracentesis, without a significant difference in mortality, gastrointestinal bleeding, infection, and acute renal failure. However, TIPS patients developed hepatic encephalopathy significantly more often.

The unavailability of individual data, however, precluded the possibility of analyzing survival as a time-dependent variable and separating the confounding effect liver transplantation had on survival of patients with advanced cirrhosis. The proportion of patients who underwent liver transplantation in the five randomized trials ranged from 5% to 20%. A new meta-analysis used individual patient data of four randomized trials[27] but excluded one trial[28] because refractory ascites was not defined according to the International Ascites Club criteria, and mortality was not the primary endpoint of the study. This meta-analysis (305 patients: 149 TIPS, 156 paracentesis) documented that TIPS significantly reduced the recurrence of tense ascites (42% versus 89%, $P < .0001$) and significantly improved transplant-free survival of cirrhotic patients with refractory ascites (Figure 97-3). The average number of hepatic encephalopathy episodes was significantly higher in the TIPS group, although the cumulative probability of developing the first episodes of hepatic encephalopathy was similar between the groups.

Historically, the peritoneovenous shunt was an alternative for patients with medically intractable ascites. There is no evidence that these shunts improved survival, and with the advent of the TIPS procedure, this form of therapy has been abandoned.

MALIGNANT ASCITES

Malignant ascites is associated with intraabdominal and pelvic malignancies, and the pathophysiology includes lymphatic obstruction by tumor cells, excess vascular permeability, hormonal effects, and excess metalloproteinase production. Palliative therapies included fluid restriction, diuretics, paracentesis, implantation of drainage catheters (including the PleurX catheter approved by the U.S. Food and Drug Administration [FDA] in 2005), and surgical shunting techniques (peritoneovenous shunts.)[29] New approaches to the management of malignant ascites include administration of octreotide as an antisecretory agent, administration of metalloproteinase inhibitors such as batimastat, intraperitoneal immunotherapy (interferon, tumor necrosis factor alpha), and intraperitoneal administration of trifunctional antibodies (e.g., catumaxomab)[30,31] that attach to specific overexpressed surface markers on tumor cells and trigger an immune response leading to cytoreductive effects.

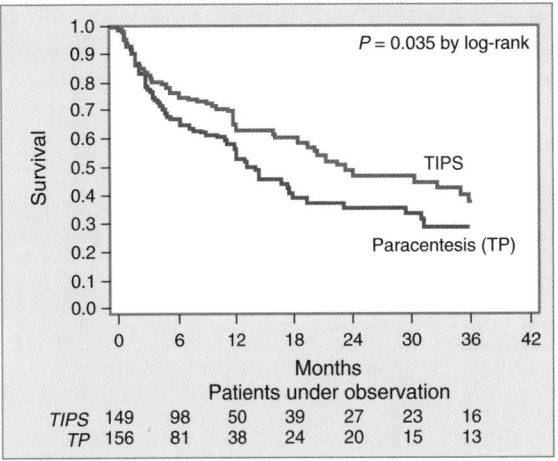

Figure 97-3 Cumulative probability of transplant-free survival according to treatment with TIPS or total paracentesis. *(From Salerno F, Camma C, Enea M, Rossle M, Wong F. Transjugular intrahepatic portosystemic shunt for refractory ascites: a meta-analysis of individual patient data. Gastroenterology 2007;133:825–34.)*

Complications

PARACENTESIS-INDUCED CIRCULATORY DYSFUNCTION

PICD, or postparacentesis effective hypovolemia, is a complication that may occur after LVP or total paracentesis. This complication is characterized by worsening hypotension and arterial vasodilation, hyponatremia, azotemia, and increased plasma renin activity. PICD is associated with an increased mortality rate and may be prevented with the administration of plasma expanders.

A study randomized 72 patients to receive albumin or saline after total paracentesis.[32] The incidence of PICD was significantly higher in the saline-treated group as compared with the albumin-treated group (33.3% versus 11.4%, $P = .03$). However, no significant differences were found when 6 L of ascitic fluid was evacuated (6.7% versus 5.6%, $P = .9$). Significant increases in plasma renin activity were found 24 hours and 6 days after paracentesis when saline was used, whereas no changes were observed when albumin was infused. Albumin was more effective than saline for the prevention of PICD but is not required when less than 6 L of ascitic fluid is evacuated. Therefore, administration of IV albumin (6 to 8 g/L of ascites removed) is recommended with LVP.

Nine randomized controlled trials (n = 806 procedures) have examined the use of plasma expanders for therapeutic paracentesis.[33-38] This systematic review identified no significant differences between therapeutic paracentesis with and without volume expansion with albumin, nor with nonalbumin plasma expanders compared with albumin for hyponatremia, renal impairment, encephalopathy, or death. However, these studies did not specifically examine prevention of PICD (defined by an increase in plasma renin activity or aldosterone concentration), and some studies determined that albumin prevented PICD more effectively than synthetic plasma expanders.[25]

SPONTANEOUS BACTERIAL PERITONITIS

SBP is a common complication of cirrhotic ascites.[39] It can precipitate hepatorenal syndrome. The overall mortality rate from an episode of SBP is approximately 20%, and following an episode, the 1-year mortality rate approaches 70%.

The prevalence of SBP in cirrhotic patients with ascites admitted to the hospital has been estimated at 10% to 30%. Any patient with ascites and fever or deterioration in renal or hepatic function should undergo diagnostic paracentesis. The fluid should be cultured and a cell count obtained. Empirical antibiotic therapy should be initiated until the results of these tests are available, and antibiotics should be adjusted

TABLE 97-6	Diagnosis and Management of Spontaneous Bacterial Peritonitis (SBP)
Diagnosis	Consider SBP and perform diagnostic paracentesis if: Symptoms/signs (abdominal pain, fever, chills) Patient is in emergency room or admitted Worsening renal function or encephalopathy SBP present if ascites PMN count > 250 cells/μL (if fluid bloody, subtract 1 PMN per 250 RBC/μL)
General Management	Avoid therapeutic paracenteses during active infection. IV albumin (1 g/kg of body weight) if BUN > 30 mg/dL, bilirubin > 4 mg/dL; repeat at day 3 if renal dysfunction persists. Avoid aminoglycosides.
Specific Management	Cefotaxime (2 g IV every 12 h) *or* Ceftriaxone (2 g every 24 h) *or* Ampicillin/sulbactam (2 g/L g IV every 6 h)
Follow-up	Continue therapy for 7 days. Repeat diagnostic paracentesis at day 2. If ascites PMN count decreases by at least 25% at day 2, IV therapy can be switched to oral therapy (quinolone such as ciprofloxacin or levofloxacin, 250 mg PO BID) to complete 7 days of therapy.

Data from: Garcia-Tsao G, Lim JK; Members of the Veterans Affairs Hepatitis C Resource Center Program. Management and treatment of patients with cirrhosis and portal hypertension: recommendations from the Department of Veterans Affairs Hepatitis C Resource Center Program and the National Hepatitis C Program. Am J Gastroenterol 2009;104:1802-29.

BID, twice a day; *BUN,* blood urea nitrogen; *IV,* intravenous; *PMN,* polymorphonuclear (neutrophil) cell count; *PO,* orally; *RBC,* red blood cell count.

TABLE 97-7	Management Strategy for the Prevention of Recurrent SBP
Recommended Therapy	Oral norfloxacin, 400 mg PO once daily (preferred) *or* Oral ciprofloxacin, 250-500 mg once daily* *or* Oral levofloxacin 250 mg once daily*
Alternative Therapy	TMP-SMX 1 double-strength tablet PO once daily (Patients who develop quinolone-resistant organisms may also have resistance to TMP-SMX.)
Duration	Prophylaxis should be continued until the disappearance of ascites or until liver transplantation.

Data from Garcia-Tsao G, Lim JK; Members of the Veterans Affairs Hepatitis C Resource Center Program. Management and treatment of patients with cirrhosis and portal hypertension: recommendations from the Department of Veterans Affairs Hepatitis C Resource Center Program and the National Hepatitis C Program. Am J Gastroenterol 2009;10:1802-29.

*Empirical doses.

PO, orally; *SBP,* spontaneous bacterial peritonitis; *TMP-SMX,* trimethoprim-sulfamethoxazole.

once culture results determine the pathogenic bacteria and antimicrobial susceptibilities are available for review.

To diagnose SBP, ascitic fluid should be examined by microscopy and inoculated directly into blood culture bottles. An ascitic fluid neutrophil count ≥ 250 polymorphonuclear cells/μL is diagnostic of SBP, but a Gram stain of the ascitic fluid is usually uninformative (Table 97-6).[40]

Gram-negative aerobic bacteria are the most common organisms isolated from ascites.[41] The three most common isolates are *Escherichia coli, Klebsiella pneumoniae,* and *Streptococcus pneumoniae.* Although the number of bacteria present in an episode of SBP is very low, they excite an intensive inflammatory response. Hospitalized patients should be treated with appropriate IV antibiotics.

Patients who have survived an episode of SBP have a 40% to 70% 1-year probability of a further episode. A randomized placebo-controlled trial examined the efficacy of antibiotic treatment purely for secondary prophylaxis of SBP.[42] Long-term treatment with norfloxacin reduced the recurrence of SBP at 1 year from 68% to 20%. The treatment effect was mostly due to a reduction of SBP secondary to gram-negative pathogens.

A meta-analysis of 8 prospective studies with a total of 647 patients randomized to oral antibiotic prophylaxis for SBP compared with placebo or no intervention documented an overall mortality benefit (RR = 0.65; 95% CI 0.48-0.88) for antibiotic treatment groups. The overall mortality rate was 16% for treated patients and 25% for the control cohort. Groups treated with prophylactic antibiotics also demonstrated a lower incidence of all infections (including SBP) of 6.2% compared with the control group rate of 22.2% (RR = 0.32; 95% CI 0.20-0.51).[43] A Cochrane meta-analysis of 9 trials concluded that antibiotic prophylaxis might be prudent among cirrhotic patients with ascites, but poor trial methodology, concern for systematic bias in publication and design, and concern regarding potential development of resistant pathogens for both the patient and society were articulated clearly.[44] On the basis of these results, long-term oral antibiotics are advised for patients recovering from an episode of SBP until resolution of ascites, transplantation, or death (International Ascites Club recommendations). Furthermore, specific patients at high risk of a first episode of SBP (patients with a protein level < 1 g/dL in ascitic fluid and those hospitalized with gastrointestinal hemorrhage) should also receive prophylaxis with orally administered antibiotics, usually a fluoroquinolone, as a management strategy for prevention of SBP (Table 97-7).[36,37]

HEPATORENAL SYNDROME

Hepatorenal syndrome (HRS) is a serious complication of end-stage liver disease, occurring mainly in patients with advanced cirrhosis and ascites who have marked circulatory dysfunction. In spite of its functional nature, HRS is associated with a poor prognosis[45] HRS can be precipitated by management of ascites with LVP, and therefore knowledge regarding pathophysiology and treatment of HRS is of paramount importance in treating the patient with ascites related to liver disease. For an in-depth discussion of hepatorenal syndrome, see Chapter 99.

Prognosis and Outcomes

The short-term prognosis of acutely ill patients with cirrhosis is influenced by the degree of hepatic insufficiency and by dysfunction of extrahepatic organ systems. The Child-Turcot-Pugh classification system (Table 97-8) was initially described for estimating outcome in cirrhotic patients undergoing surgery. One important component of this classification is the degree of ascites present, graded as absent, slight, or moderate.

TABLE 97-8	Child-Turcot-Pugh Scoring System*		
	Points Scored for Increasing Abnormality		
Clinical and Biochemical Measurements	*1*	*2*	*3*
Albumin (g/dL)	>3.5	2.8-3.5	<2.8
Bilirubin (mg/dL)	1-2	2-3	>3
For cholestatic disease: bilirubin (mg/dL)	<4	4-10	>10
Prothrombin time (seconds above normal)†	1-4	4-6	>6
or:			
International normalized ratio†	<1.7	1.7-2.3	>2.3
Ascites	Absent	Slight	Moderate
Encephalopathy (grade)	None	1 and 2	3 and 4

Data from Pugh RHW, Murray-Lyon IM, Dawson JL et al. Transection of the esophagus for bleeding esophageal varices. Br J Surg 1983;60:646.

*Scoring for Child class A = 5-6 points; B = 7-9 points; C = 10-15 points.

†Prothrombin time or international normalized ratio can be used for scoring.

A study[46] compared the Child-Pugh classification, the Acute Physiology and Chronic Health Evaluation (APACHE) II system, and the Sequential Organ Failure Assessment (SOFA) for predicting hospital mortality in patients (n = 143) with cirrhosis when used 24 hours after admission to a medical intensive care unit (ICU). Cumulative mortality rates were 36% in the ICU, 46% in the hospital, and 56% at 6-month follow-up. By using the area under receiver operating characteristic (ROC) curves, the SOFA score showed an excellent discriminative power (0.94) which was clearly superior to the APACHE II (0.79) and the Child-Pugh system (0.74). Hospital mortality rates below and above a cutoff of 8 SOFA points were 4% and 88%, respectively (P < .0005). The SOFA score also reflected resource use during the ICU treatment, as measured by daily workload and length of stay. The SOFA score is an easily applied tool with excellent prognostic abilities and can be used to enhance clinical judgment of prognosis as well as to provide patients and families with objective information. A similar study in 111 critically ill cirrhotic patients compared organ system failure scores obtained on the first day of ICU admission to the Child-Pugh classification in predicting hospital mortality.[47] The overall hospital mortality rate was 64.9%. Similarly, the organ system failure score (ROC 0.901) was superior to the Child-Pugh score (ROC 0.748) in prediction of hospital mortality in these ICU patients with cirrhosis.

In contrast, the prognostic accuracy of the Child-Pugh score was superior to either the APACHE II or III scores in prediction of short-term hospital mortality of patients with liver cirrhosis (n = 147) admitted to a medical ward and not the ICU.[48] Overall mortality in this study was 11.5%. Discrimination was excellent for Child-Pugh (ROC 0.859) and APACHE III (ROC 0.816) scores and acceptable for APACHE II score (ROC 0.759). Although the Hosmer-Lemeshow statistic revealed adequate goodness-of-fit for Child-Pugh score (P = .192), such was not the case for APACHE II and III scores (P = .004 and .003, respectively). This study documented that of the three models, the Child-Pugh score had the least statistically significant discrepancy between predicted and observed mortality.

KEY POINTS

1. The serum ascites albumin concentration gradient (serum albumin concentration—ascitic fluid albumin concentration) is the best diagnostic measure for the classification of ascites.

2. Diagnostic paracentesis must be performed in all patients with new-onset ascites.

3. Ascites is the most common complication related to liver disease and cirrhosis.

4. Ascites is characterized by three grades of severity, and treatment is based on grade.

5. The only definitive therapy for refractory ascites with cirrhosis is orthotopic liver transplantation. Other therapy includes large-volume paracentesis (LVP), transjugular intrahepatic portosystemic shunt (TIPS), and peritoneovenous shunts.

ANNOTATED REFERENCES

Garcia-Tsao G, Lim JK, Members of Veterans Affairs Hepatitis C Resource Center Program. Management and treatment of patients with cirrhosis and portal hypertension: recommendations from the Department of Veterans Affairs Hepatitis C Resource Center Program and the National Hepatitis C Program. Am J Gastroenterol 2009;104:1802-29.

This comprehensive review provides evidence-based recommendations for management of the cirrhotic patient with either compensated or decompensated cirrhosis, including management of ascites, refractory ascites, spontaneous bacterial peritonitis, and other complications including hepatorenal syndrome.

Salerno F, Camma C, Enea M, Rossle M, Wong F. Transjugular intrahepatic portosystemic shunt for refractory ascites: a meta-analysis of individual patient data. Gastroenterology 2007;133:825-34.

This meta-analysis of individual patient data from four prospective randomized clinical trials documented that TIPS significantly reduced the recurrence of tense ascites (42% versus 89%, P <.0001) and significantly improved transplant-free survival of cirrhotic patients with refractory ascites despite a significantly higher average number of hepatic encephalopathy episodes in the TIPS group.

Wong CL, Holroyd-Leduc J, Thorpe KE, Straus SE. Does this patient have bacterial peritonitis or portal hypertension? How do I perform a paracentesis and analyze the results? JAMA 2008;299:1166-78.

This publication includes a systematic review of nine randomized controlled trials (n = 806 procedures) that examined the use of plasma expanders for therapeutic paracentesis. No significant differences were identified between therapeutic paracentesis with and without volume expansion with albumin, nor with nonalbumin plasma expanders compared with albumin for hyponatremia, renal impairment, encephalopathy, or death. However, these studies did not specifically examine prevention of PICD (defined by an increase in plasma renin activity or aldosterone concentration), and some studies determined that albumin prevented PICD more effectively than synthetic plasma expanders.

Saab S, Hernandez JC, Chi AC, Tong MJ. Oral antibiotic prophylaxis reduces spontaneous bacterial peritonitis occurrence and improves short-term survival in cirrhosis: a meta-analysis. Am J Gastroenterol 2009;104:993-1001.

This meta-analysis of 8 prospective clinical trials with a total of 647 patients randomized to oral antibiotic prophylaxis for SBP compared with placebo or no intervention documented an overall mortality benefit (RR = 0.65; 95% CI 0.48-0.88) for antibiotic treatment groups. The overall mortality rate was 16% for treated patients and 25% for the control cohort. Groups treated with prophylactic antibiotics also demonstrated a lower incidence of all infections (including SBP) of 6.2% compared with the control group rate of 22.2% (RR = 0.32; 95% CI 0.20-0.51)

REFERENCES

Access the complete reference list online at http://www.expertconsult.com.

98 Gastrointestinal Hemorrhage

HORACIO HOJMAN | CHRISTINA J. WAI | STANLEY A. NASRAWAY

■ Definitions

Gastrointestinal (GI) bleeding can occur from anywhere throughout the GI tract. Classically, GI hemorrhage was classified into upper (source proximal to the ligament of Treitz) and lower (source distal to the ligament of Treitz) subgroups. However, new insights into the pathology of bleeding and therapeutic strategies have led to proposals for new categories. Bleeding that originates from the small bowel is now viewed as a separate entity,[1,2] and the term *lower GI hemorrhage* is reserved for bleeding that arises in the colon and/or rectum. This chapter follows this classification scheme.

■ Epidemiology

Upper GI bleeding occurs more frequently than lower GI bleeding.[3] In the United States, the annual incidence of hospitalization for upper GI bleeding is approximately 100 cases per 100,000 adults compared to about 20 cases per 100,000 patients for lower GI bleeding.[2,4] GI hemorrhage is most common among the elderly; in this population, the reported incidence is as high as 500 cases per 100,000 people per year. As demographic trends lead to increased numbers of elderly people in the general population, the incidence of GI hemorrhage is expected to steadily rise in the coming years.[5,6] Compared to patients with upper GI bleeding, patients with lower GI hemorrhage are less likely to experience shock and usually require fewer blood transfusions.[2] Despite improvements in the management of GI bleeding, mortality has remained relatively constant over the last 60 years.[7,8] Proposed reasons for the persistence of high mortality include an elderly patient population with many associated comorbidities.[9-11] This leads to a high death rate independent of the GI bleeding, with 80% of the mortality attributable to other causes.[12]

■ Initial Assessment and Management

Patients with GI bleeding need to be approached like any patient with potentially life-threatening hemorrhage. Although most bleeding episodes are of low magnitude and self-limited, the potential for significant bleeding warrants a thorough evaluation of the patient. Evaluation begins with assessing vital signs and looking for signs of hemodynamic instability. As with any actively bleeding patient, obtaining adequate vascular access is essential. Preferably a large-bore intravenous (IV) catheter (at least 16 gauge) should be inserted in the antecubital fossa of each arm. If quick and easy access is needed due to instability of the patient, a central venous catheter can be inserted. However, the most commonly used central venous catheters are those designed for multiple infusions; since these catheters have multiple lumens with relatively small diameter and the catheters are relatively long, resistance to flow is higher than for short, wide-bore peripheral IV catheters, and achievable fluid administration rates are correspondingly slower.[13]

Initial resuscitation begins with a crystalloid solution. With ongoing bleeding, packed red blood cell transfusions may become necessary.

The initial laboratory panel should include a complete blood count, serum electrolytes, and a coagulation profile. If coagulopathy is detected, every effort should be made to correct the problem. Extra attention should be paid to certain patient populations. Cirrhotic patients and those taking warfarin will have decreased levels of coagulation factors reflected by an elevated international normalized ratio

(INR). Consequently, fresh frozen plasma (FFP) should be administered to correct the coagulopathy. Platelets will be dysfunctional in patients taking aspirin or clopidogrel, and platelet transfusions may be indicated. Patients with renal failure and uremia or those with von Willebrand disease may respond to the administration of IV desmopressin (1-deamino-8-D-arginin vasopressin [DDAVP]; 0.3 µg/kg), a vasopressin analog that promotes von Willebrand factor release from endothelial cells.[14,15]

Routine endotracheal intubation is not recommended.[16-18] However, the threshold for intubation should be low for patients who may be at high risk for aspiration secondary to severe vomiting or mental status changes secondary to conditions like shock or hepatic encephalopathy.

Once stabilized, the source of bleeding should be identified to direct treatment. Active vomiting of blood is indicative of a source of bleeding located in the upper GI tract. For patients who are passing blood per rectum, the bleeding can originate from either the upper GI tract (due to brisk bleeding) or the lower GI tract. A nasogastric tube should be inserted first.[2] If the nasogastric aspirate contains bile without blood, it is safe to assume the source of bleeding is distal to the ligament of Treitz.[19] A rectal examination should always be performed to rule out anorectal pathology and evaluate the color of stool.[2]

Although frequently described as essential in aiding diagnosis, a complete history is generally not too useful and may be difficult to obtain from patients who are endotracheally intubated or in shock. The history also can obscure the diagnosis. For example, a history of cirrhosis secondary to alcohol abuse or hepatitis C may lead the clinician to suspect a variceal bleed when the actual bleeding source is a duodenal ulcer or gastric tumor. All potential etiologies for bleeding must be considered.

Whatever the type of GI bleeding, prompt endoscopy is of paramount importance, as this modality not only can help identify the source of bleeding but also offer therapeutic options.[20,21] For patients with lower GI bleeding, quick preparation of the colon is usually necessary to allow adequate visualization.[6,22] If the patient is hemodynamically unstable and cannot undergo timely colonic preparation, angiography is an alternative to identify and potentially treat the source of bleeding. Angiography can detect a bleeding vessel if the rate of hemorrhage is ≥0.5 mL/min.[3] Once an arterial source is identified, treatment with embolization is performed, with a success rate of greater than 90%. Ischemic complications are rare in the upper GI tract, owing to the abundance of collaterals as compared to the lower GI tract.

Although done infrequently out of concerns for uncontrolled bleeding, provocative mesenteric angiography can reveal the source of bleeding in up to 60% of patients when an initial angiogram failed to do so.[23] This procedure entails systemic heparinization followed by sequential angiographic injections of a vasodilator and tissue plasminogen activator.

Another useful diagnostic modality is computed tomography (CT) angiography. Its role in the management of GI bleeding is less clear. Although CT angiography appears to be as accurate as conventional angiography for identifying the source of massive GI bleeding,[24,25,26] this modality is not useful therapeutically. If a bleeding site is identified using CT angiography, an additional procedure (i.e., surgery or conventional angiography) will be required for treatment.[27] Therefore, CT angiography should be employed only when conventional angiography is unavailable. Another proposed use is for identifying bleeding sources originating from the pancreatic ducts or biliary system, as these are not accessible by endoscopy.[28]

Obtaining a gamma camera scan after injecting autologous technetium-99 (^{99m}Tc)-labeled ("tagged") red blood cells is another way to localize bleeding. This modality is more sensitive than angiography, since tagged red blood cell scans can detect bleeding at rates as low as 0.1 mL/min.[3] Studies have shown that scans which become positive within 2 hours are more accurate at identifying the source of bleeding (95%–100%) than scans that show extravasation after 2 hours.[2,29] Once the source of bleeding is identified, treatment is determined by the stability of the patient. If the patient is hemodynamically unstable, emergency surgery should be performed, whereas a second attempt at angiographic embolization is reasonable for more stable patients.

Unstable patients always should be admitted to an intensive care unit (ICU). For stable patients, the decision is based on clinical judgment. Criteria for ICU admission are hemodynamic instability, two or more comorbidities, age older than 60 years, and/or the need for hemodynamic monitoring or mechanical ventilation.

Upper GI Hemorrhage

Patients with upper GI bleeding tend to present with hematemesis. Upon evaluation, the nasogastric tube aspirate is often bloody. These patients commonly also have melena. If the bleeding is significant, it can be accompanied by hematochezia.[2] There are a multitude of potential etiologies for upper GI bleeding, including peptic ulcer disease, variceal hemorrhage, Dieulafoy's lesion, stress ulceration, Mallory-Weiss tear, esophagitis, and aortoenteric fistulas. Careful evaluation of the patient will help make the appropriate diagnosis.

COMMON CAUSES OF UPPER GI BLEEDING

Peptic Ulcer Disease

Peptic ulcer disease (PUD) is the most common cause of upper GI bleeding. Common underlying etiologies for PUD include the use of nonsteroidal antiinflammatory drugs (NSAIDs) and *Helicobacter pylori* infection. Many patients with PUD do not have *H. pylori* infection of the stomach.[30] Even when *H. pylori* infection is present, eradication of *H. pylori* is unnecessary in the acute setting but is important for long-term prevention of recurrence.[31]

Significant PUD bleeding is frequently due to a posterior penetrating ulcer in the first portion of the duodenum that erodes into the gastroduodenal artery. The bleeding stops spontaneously in approximately 80% of cases. However, the remaining 20% of patients have recurrent bleeding or do not stop bleeding spontaneously at all.[32,33] Historically, surgery was indicated to control the bleeding in a significant number of patients. It is rarely required these days because other less invasive therapies are available.

Early initiation of therapy with a proton pump inhibitor (PPI) is effective in reducing intragastric pH and the need for endoscopic treatment.[34] PPIs are more effective than histamine receptor 2 (H_2) blockers[35-37] or somatostatin.[38,39] Administration of large doses of omeprazole after endoscopy (80 mg bolus injection followed by 8 mg/h continuous infusion for 72 hours, and then 40 mg/d orally for 1 week) compared to standard doses has been found to decrease the incidence of recurrent bleeding,[32,38,40,41] decrease the need for surgery, and prevent development of shock that leads to death. Unless there is a contraindication, a PPI always should be administered.

Prompt endoscopy is essential, as it allows identification and treatment of the bleeding vessel.[20] Some groups report performing endoscopy within 3 hours of admission.[9] Endoscopy within 24 hours[10,42] has been associated with significant decreases in the incidence of recurrent bleeding, need for surgery, and length of stay. Administration of the prokinetic agent, erythromycin (3 mg/kg IV), before endoscopy can improve visibility during the procedure.[43,44]

Local injection of epinephrine, thermocoagulation, and application of endoscopic clips are approaches that can be used to stop bleeding. When used alone or in combination,[45] these methods are successful in over 90% of cases.[46] A detailed description of these endoscopic

procedures is beyond the scope of this chapter and will therefore only be discussed briefly to inform the intensivist about possible complications. Injection of diluted epinephrine (1:10,000 solution) is effective in stopping bleeding, especially when used in higher volumes.[47,48] Several proposed mechanisms include direct vasoconstriction, a tamponade effect related to the volume of injection, and induction of platelet aggregation. Although less frequent with high-volume injections,[49] rebleeding can occur in up to 20% of patients treated with epinephrine alone.[32] Thermal coagulation is more effective than epinephrine in preventing rebleeding and the need for surgery,[32] but it is associated with a 1% risk of perforation.[33] Hemoclips can also be applied endoscopically to control a bleeding vessel.[50,51] Although very safe, they are difficult to deploy and require expertise that is unavailable in many centers.

Even after initial endoscopic control, rebleeding occurs in as many as 20%[33] of patients, resulting in a significant increase in morbidity and mortality.[52] In a review of the literature, Elmunzer et al.[46] reported several predictive factors for rebleeding, including hemodynamic instability, multiple comorbidities, active bleeding, large ulcer size (>2 cm),[33] a posterior duodenal ulcer, and a lesser curvature ulcer.

Identification and treatment of those ulcers with potential for rebleeding is necessary to avoid complications. The Forrest classification is very useful at predicting recurrent bleeding.[53] There are three categories based on endoscopic findings. Forrest I lesions are those that are actively bleeding. Forrest II lesions have stigmata of recent bleeding. They are further classified into Forrest IIa lesions where a non-bleeding vessel is visible and Forrest IIb lesions defined by the presence of an adherent clot. Forrest III lesions are those that do not have signs of recent bleeding. Forrest I and II lesions have a high incidence of rebleeding. Nearly all Forrest I lesions rebleed.[54] In some series, Forrest IIa lesions have rebleeding rates as high as 81%,[55-57] although 40% is probably a more accurate number.[58] They also are associated with a high mortality rate of 11%. Endoscopic treatment is recommended for Forrest I and IIa lesions.[59] The role of endoscopic treatment for Forrest IIb lesions is less clear. Consensus is lacking on the definition of an adherent clot. Many clinicians are reluctant to mobilize a clot because of the potential to promote bleeding.[60] Nevertheless, administration of PPIs at high doses can help stabilize the clot and decrease the rebleeding rate.[32] Due to poor interobserver reliability in identifying a visible vessel,[61,62] Doppler ultrasound has been proposed as another diagnostic modality. Riemann and Rosenbaum[55] reported in a prospective randomized controlled trial that Doppler ultrasound is more effective than direct visualization for locating vessels. Patients treated after identification with Doppler ultrasound had a lower incidence of rebleeding and a significant decrease in mortality (0% versus 10%).

Angiography may be needed for patients who continue to bleed despite endoscopic treatment[63] or in whom endoscopy cannot be performed. Super-selective embolization controls the bleeding and decreases the complication rate.[64] Embolization of an actively bleeding vessel has a high success rate. If a bleeding site cannot be identified, blind embolization is not recommended. However, if the source of bleeding was previously identified endoscopically, blind embolization of the suspected vessels can be as effective as targeted embolization.[65-67] A metallic clip placed at the time of endoscopy may be helpful for identifying the area where bleeding occurred.[68] If rebleeding takes place, embolization can be attempted a second time for a combined success rate of 95%.[65] A potential complication of embolization is contrast-induced acute renal failure, particularly when infusion of a dye load occurs in combination with intravascular volume depletion secondary to hemorrhage.[63] Duodenal ischemia is rare and usually can be treated conservatively with PPIs. Mortality is in the range of 10% to 45%, and death is most often related to the presence of comorbid conditions.[69,70]

A minority of patients require surgical intervention to control the bleeding.[71,72] Because surgery is usually performed after failure of endoscopic and/or angiographic embolization, the patients are usually sicker and have a higher mortality rate. Although the reported mortality with surgery is similar to angiographic embolization, the mortality rate after failed embolization has been reported to be as high as 83%.[63] The procedure of choice is oversewing of the bleeding vessels with or without an acid-reducing procedure such as a vagotomy and pyloroplasty, a vagotomy and antrectomy, or a highly selective vagotomy. With the current availability of highly effective acid-suppressive medications and *H. pylori* treatment, extensive surgery is not indicated in these very sick patients.

Variceal Hemorrhage

The second most common cause of upper GI bleeding is variceal hemorrhage. Varices are present in approximately 50% of patients with cirrhosis and become more prominent with advanced liver disease.[73] They commonly develop in the lower esophagus and stomach secondary to portal hypertension. The hepatic vein pressure gradient is the main determinant of the propensity for variceal bleeding.[74,75] These thin-walled varicose veins, located in the weak lamina propria of the lower esophagus, are especially predisposed to rupture and bleeding.[76]

Despite recent improvements in medical management of these patients, mortality remains high at 20% in the first 6 weeks.[73,77] The rebleeding rate ranges between 30% and 40% in the first 6 weeks and is associated with a 30% mortality rate.[78] Because of the high mortality rate, prompt management is crucial. If the diagnosis of variceal hemorrhage is suspected, pharmacologic therapy should be instituted in transit to the hospital.[79] If not initiated during transport, vasopressin, the vasopressin analog, terlipressin, somatostatin, or the somatostatin analog, octreotide,[80] should be administered upon arrival at the hospital. These agents are effective at controlling hemorrhage from varices in up to 80% of cases. These medications also can facilitate endoscopic visualization by reducing the rate of active bleeding.[77,81]

Terlipressin is the only agent proven to reduce mortality.[82-84] Unfortunately, terlipressin is not available in the United States. It is administered at a dose of 2 mg every 4 to 6 hours for the first 48 hours, followed by half this dose for up to 5 days.[85-89] Somatostatin causes splanchnic arteriolar vasoconstriction and decreases the portal venous pressure by decreasing inflow into the portal circulation. It is administered as an initial bolus of 250 µg, which can be repeated up to three times, followed by an infusion of 250 µg/h for up to 5 days to prevent rebleeding.[85]

The role of octreotide is unclear. Although it has a longer half-life compared to somatostatin, its hemodynamic effects are not as pronounced. It is administered by continuous infusion at 25 or 50 µg/h preceded by a 50- or 100-µg bolus. Although somatostatin and octreotide are similarly successful for controlling variceal hemorrhage, use of these agents alone has not been shown to decrease mortality.[90-92] Accordingly, these agents should be used in combination with endoscopic therapy.

Historically, vasopressin has been used successfully to control acute variceal hemorrhage.[93] However, administration of vasopressin is associated with serious side effects (myocardial ischemia, mesenteric and limb ischemia, cerebrovascular accidents, and hyponatremia) in a significant number of patients, and it requires the concurrent administration of IV nitroglycerin (10 to 50 µg/minute). Vasopressin is administered as an infusion starting at 0.4 U/min, and the infusion rate can be increased incrementally to 1 U/minute as indicated by the clinical response. Although it controls bleeding in up to 80% of the cases, it does not decrease mortality, most likely because of its propensity to promote ischemia in other vital organs. Therefore, vasopressin should be reserved for those rare circumstances when other more effective drugs are unavailable.

Antibiotics should be started early in a prophylactic fashion, since as many as 20% of patients with cirrhosis and GI bleeding develop infections. Antibiotics have been shown to be effective in reducing the number of infections in these patients, and early administration of appropriate antibiotics has been shown to decrease the incidence of early rebleeding and improve survival.[94,95] Ceftriaxone (1 gm IV daily) is the recommended antibiotic. Studies show it to be superior to fluoroquinolones.[77] For patients with a history of penicillin allergy, fluoroquinolones can be used as an alternative.[73,77]

Patients should be admitted to an ICU for close monitoring and management. Endotracheal intubation is usually indicated,[77] as these patients are at risk for aspiration and/or hepatic encephalopathy. Resuscitation with crystalloids and packed red blood cells should be initiated promptly to avoid hypovolemia and subsequent complications like renal failure. However, hypervolemia should be avoided. Intravascular volume overload has the potential to exacerbate variceal bleeding.

Upper endoscopy should be performed next to determine the exact source of bleeding. Despite esophageal and gastric varices being a common source of bleeding in patients with cirrhosis, in as many as 25% of cases, acute GI bleeding arises from a non-variceal source.

Esophageal varices can be treated with sclerotherapy or band ligation. The type of endoscopic treatment depends on the experience and expertise of the endoscopist as well as the magnitude of bleeding. Band ligation appears to be superior for reducing the risk of recurrent bleeding after the acute event and has been associated with fewer complications. However, band ligation can be difficult to perform in patients with massive bleeding. In these cases, sclerotherapy is preferred.[77] The success of endoscopic treatment is similar to vasoactive drugs, with a rate of 80% to 85%.[77,96-99] However, despite similar success rates to vasoactive drugs for controlling bleeding, a recent Cochrane meta-analysis found that sclerotherapy could not be recommended as a first-line treatment, given its higher complication rate. Its use should be reserved for pharmacologic failures.[100] Conversely, the combination of pharmacologic and endoscopic treatment in selected patients appears to be superior to vasoactive drugs alone.[96,101]

Gastric varices bleed less frequently but more intensely than esophageal varices, leading to higher transfusion requirements and mortality.[102] The recommended treatment is sclerotherapy with histoacryl glue (*N*-butyl-2-cyanoacrylate).[103] Complications include ulceration of the mucosa and embolic events from the glue.[32,77]

With massive bleeding, a Sengstaken-Blakemore (S-B) tube or one of its variations can be inserted as a temporizing measure. The S-B tube has fallen out of favor as more effective therapies have become available. The risks of its use include aspiration, esophageal rupture, and an inability to control the bleeding.[104-107] However, for selected patients, it can be life saving. The S-B tube has a gastric and an esophageal balloon. The tube does not have to be cooled before insertion.[108] Tube placement should be preceded by endotracheal intubation. The tube should be introduced through the nose or, more frequently, through the mouth into the stomach. The position of the distal tube in the stomach should be confirmed by insufflation of air combined with auscultation. Radiographic confirmation has been advocated to avoid insufflation of the gastric balloon in the esophagus, resulting in esophageal rupture.[109] After confirming the position of the S-B tube, the gastric balloon is inflated with 500 mL of saline, and gentle traction is applied (approximately 1 kg or the weight of a 1-L IV bag). This maneuver stops bleeding from varices high in the fundus and occludes collaterals from the stomach to the submucosa of the esophagus. If the bleeding stops, the balloon is secured in place using a football helmet or a pulley system connected to an IV pole. If esophageal bleeding persists, the esophageal balloon is inflated next. The inflation port is connected to a manometer, and pressure is gradually increased until the bleeding stops or the pressure equals 45 mm Hg, whichever comes first. Once the bleeding is controlled, the S-B tube is kept in place, usually for 24 hours, before deflating the balloons. This allows preparation for other therapies such as endoscopy or a transjugular intrahepatic portosystemic shunt (TIPS). If bleeding recurs after deflation, the balloons can be reinflated. A method of inserting the S-B under direct vision by endoscopy has been described[110]; however, it is not clear that this approach reduces the incidence of complications.

If the previously described treatments are unsuccessful, TIPS should be attempted. TIPS placement reduces the hepatic vein pressure gradient and effectively controls bleeding in 90% to 100% of the cases.[78] However, emergency TIPS placement is associated with a high incidence of hepatic encephalopathy and a mortality rate as high as 50%.[111] In the event TIPS placement is unavailable, a surgical porto-systemic shunt should be considered. One surgical approach entails interposition of an 8-mm ringed polytetrafluoroethylene shunt between the portal vein and the inferior vena cava.[112] Because of the relatively small diameter of the graft, its placement creates only a "partial" portocaval shunt with preservation of hepatopetal flow, leading to a lower incidence of encephalopathy. In experienced hands, the graft has a 95% patency rate at 7 years. However, even its advocates advise against using this approach if the patient is a candidate for liver transplantation.[113] A splenorenal shunt (with or without splenectomy) is another surgical option. The operative mortality for distal sple-norenal shunt placement has been reported to be less than for porto-caval shunt placement; however, not all experts share this view.[113] Although some studies report a similar complication rate and mortal-ity compared to TIPS,[114] only a few specialized centers have surgeons who are experienced in performing these difficult procedures for very sick patients.

LESS COMMON CAUSES OF UPPER GI BLEEDING

Dieulafoy's Lesion

A Dieulafoy's lesion is a large anomalous artery located in the digestive tract; it is responsible for approximately 2% of upper GI bleeds.[115-117] These lesions usually are located along the lesser curvature of the stomach near the cardia but can be present anywhere along the GI tract from the mouth to the anal canal.[118,119] Dieulafoy's lesions are most often identified in elderly patients but can occur in younger patients.[120,121] Although these lesions may remain asymptomatic, erosion of the overlying mucosa and subsequently into the artery leads to intermittent brisk bleeding. The treatment used to be surgical, but most cases are now treated endoscopically with epinephrine injections, thermal probe coagulation, and/or clips.[32,122,123] Occasionally, angio-graphic embolization is needed to control the bleeding.[63,65] Mortality remains high, around 20%, because patients typically have many asso-ciated comorbidities.[115]

Stress Ulceration

Critically ill patients are susceptible to stress-related mucosal damage of the esophagus, stomach, and duodenum. These lesions initially were thought to arise from excessive acid production, but they are now thought to occur as a consequence of insufficient mucosal perfu-sion. When stress ulcers were first described in the 1960s, approxi-mately 10% to 20% of patients admitted to ICUs with multiple organ failure developed overt hemorrhage; 2% to 5% of them progressed to more extensive and even lethal bleeding. In the past, surgery was commonly needed to control the bleeding, although surgical inter-vention for stress ulceration is now exceedingly rare. Several surgical procedures were employed, including vagotomy and pyloroplasty, antrectomy, total gastric devascularization, and total or near-total gas-trectomy, but the mortality rate for these operations was exceedingly high (33% to 48%).[124] In recent years, the combination of stress ulcer prophylaxis, improvements in resuscitation, and other aspects of sup-portive care have led to a marked decrease in the incidence of hemor-rhage from stress erosions. In a landmark paper, Cook et al.[125] demonstrated that significant bleeding occurred only in patients who required mechanical ventilation for more than 48 hours or were coag-ulopathic. The group even suggested that prophylaxis could be with-held unless those risk factors were present. PPIs increase intragastric pH more effectively than H$_2$ blockers[126] and are more effective for preventing aspirin-related erosions.[127] However, data are insufficient to conclude that PPIs are superior to H$_2$ blockers for preventing stress ulcers.[128]

Mallory-Weiss Tear

Mallory-Weiss tears are longitudinal lacerations of the mucosa of the distal esophagus, cardia, or a combination of both, resulting in bleed-ing from submucosal vessels.[129] The incidence is variable in different series, but Mallory-Weiss tears account for 3% to 8% of cases of upper GI hemorrhage.[10,52,116,117] The laceration is thought to be caused by retching that accompanies vomiting. Mallory-Weiss tears are associ-ated with alcohol abuse, hiatal hernia, and possibly even *H. pylori* infections. The diagnosis is usually made by endoscopy. The bleeding stops spontaneously in approximately 90% of cases. If the bleeding persists, band ligation or hemoclips are usually effective in controlling it.[129,130] Hemoclips appear to be more effective than epinephrine injec-tions. The use of thermocoagulation has not been fully evaluated.[32]

Esophagitis

Esophagitis previously has been reported as a cause of 5% to 20% of upper GI bleeds.[7,116,117] However, recent series report an incidence of around 2%. A possible explanation for this discrepancy is that esopha-gitis is often observed at endoscopy and presumed to be the source of GI hemorrhage, without actual confirmation that the esophageal mucosa is the site of bleeding.[7] Serious bleeding requiring ICU admis-sion is rare and usually caused by an ulcer in the distal esophagus. Hemorrhage from esophagitis is more common in elderly patients,[131] and several medications such as potassium chloride and NSAIDs have been associated with this problem.[5] The diagnosis is usually made at endoscopy. Treatment, if needed, consists of removing offending medi-cations while adding acid-suppression treatment. Deep ulcers may need endoscopic treatment similar to those described for peptic ulcer disease.

Aortoenteric Fistulas

An aortoenteric fistula is a direct communication between the aorta, or occasionally an iliac artery, and the GI tract. It can happen at any level of the GI tract but is most common at the third portion of the duodenum. Aortoenteric fistula formation is usually the result of aortic reconstruction with a synthetic graft, although other causes have been described, including idiopathic,[132] trauma, radiation,[133] mycotic aneu-rysms,[134] diverticulitis, and foreign bodies.[135-137] Massive bleeding can occur suddenly and is usually fatal, although many patients present with a sentinel bleed days or even weeks prior to the onset of life-threatening hemorrhage. Endoscopy is frequently nondiagnostic, and the diagnosis is usually made by CT scan or angiogram. Endovascular repair has been reported,[138-140] but because of the high incidence of delayed bleeding and associated sepsis, it should be used only as a temporizing measure before definitive surgical treatment.[141,142] However, for selected patients with a short life expectancy, such as those with advanced cancer, endovascular repair may be an adequate option.[143] Definitive treatment involves surgical repair with removal of the graft and creation of an extra-anatomic bypass.

▣ Small-Bowel Bleeding

Bleeding originating in the small bowel has traditionally been classified as lower GI bleeding. However, new diagnostic and therapeutic impli-cations merit its description as a distinct entity. The reported incidence is between 1% and 7% of patients who present with blood per rectum.[1,144,145]

Prakash and Zuckerman[1] described a cohort of 29 patients whose source of bleeding was in the small bowel. In their series, patients bleeding from the small bowel had significantly worse outcomes com-pared to patients with colonic bleeding. The patients with small-bowel hemorrhage had also undergone more studies before diagnosis of the source was made. A normal upper endoscopy and colonoscopy should alert clinicians to the possibility that the source of bleeding is within the small bowel.

The most common cause of small-bowel bleeding is angiodysplasia, followed by small-bowel tumors.[146] Angiodysplasia is associated with advanced age and chronic renal failure.[147] Less frequently, the bleeding is caused by inflammation associated with Crohn's disease,[148,149] Meckel's diverticulum, NSAID or aspirin use,[144] Dieulafoy's lesions,[145,150] or small intestinal varices in patients with cirrhosis and portal hypertension.[151]

The diagnosis is difficult to make and usually is achieved only with the aid of a combination of studies.[150] Because of its wide availability, ^{99m}Tc-tagged RBC scan is the most commonly used test.[1,144] However, because of the high rate of false-positive and false-negative results, the use of this test cannot be recommended.[144,152] The intermittent nature of bleeding also results in angiography being positive in only about 50% of cases. Radiographic contrast studies of the small bowel are not advocated. Small-bowel follow-through has very poor sensitivity for identifying the source of bleeding. Enteroclysis, a procedure whereby contrast is instilled directly into the duodenum together with methylcellulose and air to improve visualization, is only marginally better.[5]

Some experts advocate "push enteroscopy," whereas others are proponents of capsule endoscopy. Push enteroscopy with a dedicated video enteroscope allows for visualization of the proximal 50 to 100 cm of the small bowel. The advantage of push enteroscopy is that it can be both diagnostic and therapeutic. Although capsule endoscopy appears to be more sensitive than push enteroscopy,[153] some patients undergoing this diagnostic approach may need additional procedures afterwards.[154,155] In cases of active bleeding, capsule endoscopy has a sensitivity as great as 92%,[156] but sensitivity is below 50% in cases characterized by intermittent bleeding.

Double-balloon enteroscopy is a relatively new technique that allows for complete visualization of the small bowel.[144,145,150] It uses a dedicated 200-cm enteroscope with two balloons. One of them is attached to the tip of an endoscope and the other to the tip of a flexible overtube. The balloons are sequentially inflated, allowing them to grip the mucosa of the small bowel and advance the endoscope without looping. The enteroscope can be inserted orally, transanally, or both to examine the entire small bowel. Like push endoscopy, double-balloon enteroscopy permits obtaining biopsies and offers the potential for control of the bleeding source. Unfortunately, double-balloon enteroscopy is not yet widely available.

Meckel's diverticulum is the most common congenital anomaly of the gut and is present in about 1% of the population. Complications due to the presence of a Meckel's diverticulum are rare. Occasionally, heterotopic gastric mucosa in the diverticulum can cause bleeding. Bleeding related to a Meckel's diverticulum occurs most frequently in children but should be considered in any patient younger than 40 years of age with evidence of bleeding from the small intestine. If the diagnosis is not established by the techniques discussed earlier, ^{99m}Tc-pertechnetate scintigraphy ("Meckel's scan") can be used to establish the diagnosis. Surgical resection is the treatment of choice.[144]

Finally, for patients who continue to bleed, exploratory laparotomy with or without intraoperative enteroscopy is an option to identify and treat the source of bleeding.[150]

▧ Lower GI Hemorrhage

Lower GI bleeding patients present with hematochezia or blood per rectum. Occasionally, bleeding from the right colon may present as melena because of longer transit time. Common causes of lower GI hemorrhage include colonic diverticula, angiodysplasia, inflammatory bowel diseases, and neoplasms. Rectal bleeding is a distinct entity.

COLONIC DIVERTICULA

Diverticulosis of the colon is an acquired condition that results in herniation of the mucosa through the muscular layer of the colon. Colonic diverticula are prevalent in the western hemisphere but rare in Africa and Asia. Diverticulosis develops with age, being rare before age 40, but with a prevalence of greater than 65% by age 80.[2,157] The cause of bleeding episodes is erosion of a vessel (vasa recta) into the diverticulum. Although diverticula are more common in the left colon, a significant number of bleeds originate from the right side. Bleeding stops spontaneously in 80% of cases.[2] Identification of the source is usually made with the aid of colonoscopy, which also can be therapeutic. Treatment includes thermocoagulation or epinephrine injection. The use of hemoclips also has been described.[158] If endoscopy cannot

be performed, angiography can be diagnostic and therapeutic.[159] The reported success rate with super-selective embolization exceeds 85%, and the incidence of clinically significant colonic ischemia is very low (<5%).[160]

Because bleeding tends to be intermittent, and an estimated bleeding rate of greater than 0.5 mL/min is necessary for angiographic visualization, the radiographic procedure sometimes is nondiagnostic. In such cases, provocative angiography can be helpful, leading to identification and successful embolization of the offending vessel in about 30% of cases.[23] Provocative angiography entails systemic heparinization plus selective transcatheter injection of a vasodilator and tissue plasminogen activator into the suspected arteries.

If angiography is not possible or available, localization using CT scan may be an option.[24,26,161] A limited surgical resection can be undertaken if the source of bleeding is identified. Surgery is indicated when bleeding does not stop. Mortality is high in these patients, approaching 20% even in tertiary centers.[160] It is critical to identify the site of bleeding before surgery.[162] In retrospective reviews, blind segmental resection is prone to failure and has been associated with a high mortality rate. A subtotal colectomy rather than segmental resection is therefore recommended in those cases where the source cannot be identified preoperatively.[157]

ANGIODYSPLASIA

Angiodysplasias are small, ectatic blood vessels found in the mucosa and submucosa of the GI tract. They are also known as *arteriovenous malformations* (AVM) or *vascular ectasias*. Angiodysplastic lesions are present in the GI tract in about 1% of the population.[29] They usually are asymptomatic. Angiodysplasia occurs more often in older individuals, and most lesions are located in the right colon, although they can be found in other regions of the GI tract.[3] Even though angiodysplasias are arguably the second most common cause of lower GI bleeding, the reported frequency as a cause for lower GI bleeding varies widely from 3% to 37%.[22,29,163]

Identification by colonoscopy is usually difficult, particularly after administration of opioids or cold water irrigation, as these decrease mucosal blood flow.[2] Avoidance of narcotics during colonoscopy or use of a narcotic antagonist have been proposed in small studies as means to facilitate endoscopic visualization of angiodysplasia. However, this approach has not been validated in larger studies.[29] Even when angiodysplasias are identified by colonoscopy, they should not be assumed to be the cause of lower GI bleeding unless stigmata of bleeding are visualized.[2] Endoscopic treatment entails thermal probe coagulation and injection of epinephrine. It is recommended that for actively bleeding angiodysplasias, treatment should start at the periphery of the lesions to address the feeding vessels before treating the area that is actively bleeding.

Angiography is reserved for patients who cannot undergo colonoscopy because of massive bleeding, or when colonoscopy fails to establish a diagnosis.[2] Angiographic diagnosis of angiodysplasia is made by identification of early filling of ectatic veins. Transcatheter embolization can be therapeutic but carries the risk of inducing significant ischemia.[3]

In selected cases, CT angiography can be as accurate as angiography for establishing the diagnosis and localizing the source of bleeding.[24,164,165] If the bleeding cannot be controlled by endoscopic means or angiographic embolization, surgery is indicated.

INFLAMMATORY BOWEL DISEASE

Severe inflammation of the colon accounts for 1%[148] to 5%[149,166,167] of cases of lower GI hemorrhage. Severe life-threatening bleeding is the primary indication for 10% of emergency colectomies performed for management of complications related to ulcerative colitis. About 1% of patients with Crohn's disease will also need emergency surgery.[29] Medical treatment should be initiated first. Endoscopy can be diagnostic and occasionally therapeutic. Angiography also may have a role in the diagnosis and treatment of these patients. Surgery should be reserved for patients who continue to bleed or experience recurrent bleeding. Colonic bleeding due to ulcerative colitis is usually associated with severe pancolitis[149] and should be treated with a subtotal colectomy and ileostomy.[168] Identification of the source of hemorrhage is very important in patients with Crohn's disease; bleeding originates in the small bowel in approximately two-thirds of cases. Limited resections are recommended for these patients.

NEOPLASMS

Although chronic bleeding from colonic adenocarcinoma or polyps is common,[2] massive hemorrhage requiring ICU admission is rare. Colonic polyps can bleed spontaneously or, more commonly, after colonoscopic resection. Nevertheless, in recent series, the incidence of significant post-polypectomy bleeding has been very low (less than 1%).[29,120] Major bleeding after polyp resection is usually arterial. It can be treated endoscopically with a combination of thermocoagulation and epinephrine injection.[22]

RECTAL BLEEDING

Massive rectal bleeding is uncommon, accounting for around only 2% of lower GI hemorrhage. Hemorrhoids are the most frequent cause, but substantial bleeding is rare except in patients with portal hypertension. If the bleeding does not stop spontaneously, band ligation is a safe option.

In the elderly population, solitary rectal ulcer must be considered as a possible etiology of lower GI bleeding.[169] Patients with this problem usually are bedridden and debilitated with multiple medical comorbidities.[170,171] Bleeding can be profuse and life threatening. Multiple therapeutic approaches have been described to control the bleeding, including endoscopic thermocoagulation, placement of vascular clips, and transanal sutures.[172]

Another cause of rectal bleeding is from radiation-induced proctitis after treatment for prostatic cancer. The mechanism is radiation-induced endarteritis obliterans, which results in neovascularization and the formation of telangiectasias that are prone to bleeding.[6] The presentation of bleeding usually occurs within months of radiation but can be delayed for several years.[4]

Ischemic proctitis,[4,173] Dieulafoy's lesions not associated with solitary rectal ulcers,[171,174-176] and stercoral ulcers are less common causes of rectal bleeding and usually can be treated with some variation of the methods described above.

Conclusion

GI hemorrhage encompasses a wide spectrum of disease processes. The first and most important goal is to stabilize the patient. Once hemodynamic stability is achieved, careful evaluation of the patient can lead to a correct diagnosis. Understanding the source of bleeding will then allow the clinician to appropriately manage and treat the patient.

KEY POINTS

1. Patient stabilization is the most important first step in treating gastrointestinal (GI) hemorrhage.

2. When patients are passing bright red blood per rectum, a nasogastric tube should be inserted to exclude an upper GI source.

3. Endoscopy or colonoscopy should be performed urgently as the first test to localize and potentially treat the source(s) of bleeding.

4. In selected cases, angiography is an alternative means to identify and control sources of bleeding.

5. When other methods of treatment are either unsuccessful or contraindicated for some reason, surgery is often the last resort for control of GI hemorrhage.

6. Peptic ulcer disease is the most common cause of upper GI hemorrhage; the second most common cause is rupture of esophageal and/or gastric varices.

7. Colonic diverticula and angiodysplasia are frequent causes of lower GI hemorrhage.

8. Small-bowel bleeding should be considered a separate entity from other forms of lower GI hemorrhage and is managed differently.

ANNOTATED REFERENCES

Lau J, Sung JJ. From endoscopic hemostasis to bleeding peptic ulcers: strategies to prevent and treat recurrent bleeding. Gastroenterology 2010;138:1252-4.
Although initial hemostasis can be achieved in 94% of bleeding peptic ulcers, there is a subgroup of patients who will experience recurrent bleeding. This is associated with a high mortality rate. This article describes the strategies to prevent and treat recurrent bleeding.
Bendtsen F, Krag A, Møller S. Treatment of acute variceal bleeding. Dig Liver Dis 2008;40:328-36.
This review article summarizes the current available data on the pathophysiology, diagnosis, and treatment of acute variceal bleeding.
Bai Y, Li ZS. Management of variceal hemorrhage: current status. Chin Med J 2009;122:763-5.
This editorial offers a concise summary of the current strategies to stop acute variceal bleeding.

Prakash C, Zuckerman GR. Acute small bowel bleeding: a distinct entity with significantly different economic implications compared with GI bleeding from other locations. Gastrointest Endosc 2003; 58:330-5.
Landmark study where the concept of small-bowel bleeding as a distinct entity, with significantly worse outcomes compared to colonic and upper gastrointestinal bleeding, was enunciated.
Barnert J, Messmann H, Medscape. Diagnosis and management of lower gastrointestinal bleeding. Nat Rev Gastroenterol Hepatol 2009;6:637-46.
A comprehensive review of the causes, diagnosis, and management of lower GI bleeding.

REFERENCES

Access the complete reference list online at http://www.expertconsult.com.

Hepatorenal Syndrome

ANAHAT DHILLON

An association between advanced liver disease, ascites, and renal failure was described as early as 1861. It is a form of renal failure occurring in the setting of severe liver disease. Helvig and Schutz gave this association its current name of *hepatorenal syndrome* in 1932.[1] Shortly thereafter, hepatorenal syndrome (HRS) was found to be a functional form of renal failure without renal histologic changes.[2] Significant advances in understanding the pathogenesis and treatment of the syndrome have been made in the past 2 decades. HRS is characterized by intense renal vasoconstriction, peripheral arterial vasodilation, impaired renal perfusion, and low glomerular filtration rate (GFR).[3] The annual incidence of HRS is variably reported at 8% to 40% in patients with cirrhosis.[4,5] The variability in incidence is related to the degree of liver dysfunction; the higher the Model for End-stage Liver Disease (MELD) score, the greater the incidence of HRS. HRS has a very high mortality, with nearly half the patients with type 1 HRS dying within 2 weeks of the diagnosis.[4,6]

Mechanisms of Renal Dysfunction in Cirrhosis

Sodium retention, impaired free-water excretion, and decreased renal perfusion and glomerular GFR are the main renal function abnormalities in cirrhosis. The onset of each of these abnormalities differs in time, and consequently, the course of cirrhosis can be divided in phases according to renal function. Renal dysfunction in cirrhosis usually follows a progressive course. Therefore, at the latest phase of the disease when HRS develops, all three abnormalities are invariably present.

IMPAIRMENT IN RENAL SODIUM METABOLISM WITHOUT ACTIVATION OF VASOACTIVE SYSTEMS

Chronologically, the first renal functional abnormality in cirrhosis is reduced ability to excrete sodium. When cirrhosis is still compensated (i.e., ascites is absent), subtle abnormalities in renal sodium metabolism already can be detected. Patients may not be capable of escaping from the effect of mineralocorticoids and develop continuous sodium retention. Arterial vasodilatation is already present in compensated cirrhosis with portal hypertension.[7]

With disease progression, the impairment in sodium handling increases. At a critical point, patients are unable to excrete the amount of sodium normally ingested in the diet. Sodium is retained and accumulates as ascites. Renal perfusion, GFR, the renal ability to excrete a free-water load, plasma renin activity, and the plasma concentrations of aldosterone and norepinephrine are normal.[8]

STIMULATION OF THE RENIN-ANGIOTENSIN AND SYMPATHETIC NERVOUS SYSTEMS AND ANTIDIURETIC HORMONE WITH PRESERVED RENAL PERFUSION AND GLOMERULAR FILTRATION RATE

In cases of alcoholic cirrhosis, hepatic, circulatory, and renal function may improve if alcohol consumption is discontinued. In all other forms of cirrhosis and alcoholic cirrhosis with ongoing ethanol abuse, the degree of sodium retention increases progressively with progression of disease. When renal sodium avidity is extremely high, the plasma renin activity and the plasma concentrations of aldosterone and norepinephrine are elevated.[7,9] Circulatory dysfunction is greater at this stage of the disease because increased activity of the sympathetic nervous system and the renin-angiotensin system is needed to maintain arterial pressure.

Renal perfusion and GFR are normal or moderately decreased, but renal perfusion is critically dependent on increased renal production of prostaglandins. These lipid mediators are vasodilators that antagonize the vasoconstricting actions of angiotensin II and norepinephrine. A syndrome indistinguishable from HRS can be produced in patients with cirrhosis, ascites, and increased plasma renin activity if prostaglandin synthesis is inhibited with nonsteroidal antiinflammatory drugs (NSAIDs).[9,10] In addition, prostacyclin and nitric oxide cooperate to maintain renal perfusion in cirrhosis.[11,12]

Pathogenesis

Development of HRS represents the terminal phase of the disease. HRS is characterized by low arterial blood pressure; marked increased plasma levels of renin, norepinephrine, and antidiuretic hormone; and very low GFR (<40 mL/min).[2] Impairment in GFR in HRS occurs because of decreased renal perfusion secondary to renal vasoconstriction, peripheral vasodilation, and impairment in cardiac function.[13] Renal histology is bland. Because renal vascular resistance correlates closely with activity of the renin-angiotensin and sympathetic nervous systems in cirrhosis,[14-18] HRS is thought to be related to extreme stimulation of these systems.

Urinary excretion of prostaglandin E$_2$, 6-keto-prostaglandin F$_{1\alpha}$ (a prostacyclin metabolite), and kallikrein is decreased in patients with HRS, indicating that renal production of these substances is reduced.[19,20] Renal failure in HRS, therefore, might be the consequence of an imbalance between the activity of vasoconstrictor systems and the renal production of vasodilators. The observation that HRS can be reproduced in nonazotemic, hyperreninemic, cirrhotic patients with ascites with NSAIDs is compatible with this hypothesis.[10] Another possibility, however, is that renal vasoconstriction caused by the renin-angiotensin and sympathetic nervous systems is the primary cause of HRS.

Peripheral arterial vasodilation has been implicated in HRS, but vasodilation is mainly present in the splanchnic arterial vascular bed. Doppler ultrasonography studies have consistently shown arterial vasoconstriction in renal, brachial, femoral, and cerebral beds.[21-22] Several endogenous vasodilators have been implicated as being responsible for splanchnic arteriolar vasodilation, including nitric oxide, carbon monoxide, glucagon, prostacyclin, and endogenous opiates.[23-25]

End-stage liver disease is associated with reduced systolic and diastolic response to stress, enlarged cardiac chambers, and repolarization changes, termed *cirrhotic cardiomyopathy*.[26] The development of HRS has been associated with a lower arterial pressure, a marked decrease in cardiac output, and increase in plasma renin activity and plasma norepinephrine.[20] The decrease in cardiac output is likely related to decreased effective circulating volume, as evidenced by low filling pressures and improvement with volume expansion; however, further studies are warranted (Figure 99-1).

Diagnosis

The first step in the diagnosis of HRS is demonstration of reduced GFR, and this is not easy in advanced cirrhosis.[2,27] Muscle mass and, therefore, the release of creatinine is considerably reduced in these

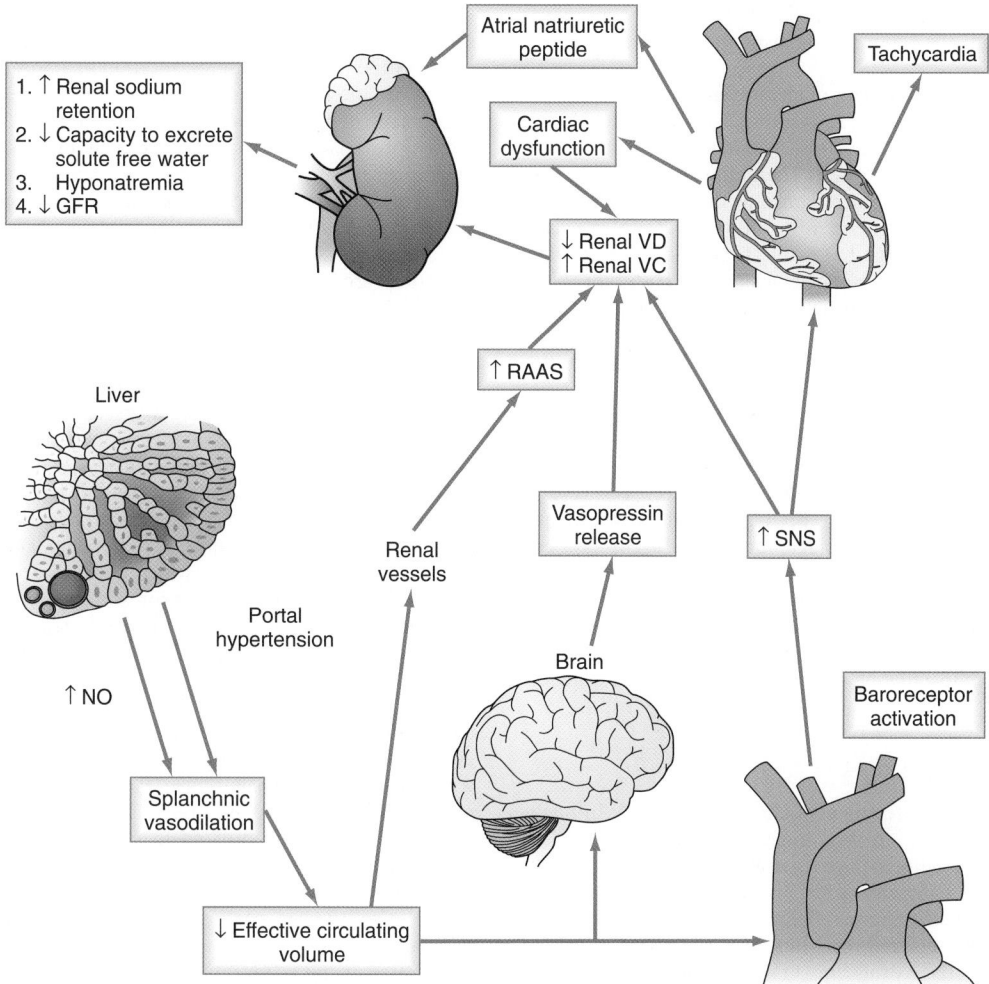

Figure 99-1 Pathophysiologic mechanisms of hepatorenal syndrome (HRS). *Renal VC,* renal vasoconstrictors; *Renal VD,* renal vasodilators; *SNS,* sympathetic nervous system. *(From Wadei HM, Mai ML, Ahsan N, Gonwa TA. Hepatorenal syndrome: pathophysiology and management. Clin J Am Soc Nephrol 2006;1:1066-79.)*

patients, and they can have a normal serum creatinine concentration despite having a very low GFR. Similarly, urea is synthesized by the liver, and urea synthesis may be reduced as a consequence of hepatic insufficiency, so failure to appropriately diagnosis HRS is relatively common.[28,29]

In 1996 and again in 2006, the International Ascites Club proposed different diagnostic criteria of HRS.[31,32] Serum creatinine concentration should be greater than 1.5 mg/dL in the absence of other potential causes of renal failure (Table 99-1).[30] The diagnosis of HRS requires exclusion of other causes of renal failure in cirrhotic patients. These other causes of renal dysfunction include prerenal failure related to

diuretics or lactulose, and acute kidney injury in the setting of shock. Additionally, the use of nephrotoxic medications such as aminoglycosides, NSAIDs, and vasodilators should be excluded as the cause of renal failure. When interpreting results, it is important to note that much of the research cited was performed prior to the revision in definition.

CLINICAL TYPES

HRS is classified into two types according to the severity and form of presentation of renal failure.[32] HRS type 1 is characterized by severe and rapidly progressive renal failure. It has been defined by doubling of the serum creatinine concentration to at least 2.5 mg/dL in less than 2 weeks. Although HRS type 1 may arise spontaneously, it frequently occurs in close relationship with a precipitating factor such as severe bacterial infection, gastrointestinal hemorrhage, major surgical procedure, or acute hepatitis superimposed on cirrhosis. The association of HRS and spontaneous bacterial peritonitis (SBP) has been carefully investigated.[33-35] HRS type 1 develops in approximately 30% of patients with SBP despite rapid and successful treatment of the infection with non-nephrotoxic antibiotics. Patients with an intense systemic inflammatory response and high cytokine levels in plasma and ascitic fluid are especially prone to develop HRS type 1 after infection. Patients with HRS type 1 after SBP show signs and symptoms of severe liver failure and circulatory dysfunction that worsen with the impairment in renal

TABLE 99-1	Major Diagnostic Criteria of Hepatorenal Syndrome (International Ascites Club)

Cirrhosis with ascites

Creatinine > 1.5 mg/dL

No improvement of serum creatinine (decrease to a level of 133 mmol/L) after at least 2 days with diuretic withdrawal and volume expansion with albumin. The recommended dose of albumin is 1 g/kg of body weight per day up to a maximum of 100 g/d

Absence of shock

No current or recent treatment with nephrotoxic medications

Absence of parenchymal kidney disease as evidenced by proteinuria, microhematuria and/or abnormal renal ultrasound

function, evolving to multiorgan failure.[36] HRS type 1 is the complication of cirrhosis with the poorest prognosis, with a 2-week median survival.

HRS type 2 is characterized by a moderate and steady decrease in renal function (serum creatinine < 2.5 mg/dL). Patients with HRS type 2 show signs of liver failure and arterial hypotension but to a lesser degree than patients with HRS type 1. The dominant clinical feature is severe ascites with poor or no response to diuretics, a condition known as *refractory ascites*. Patients with HRS type 2 are especially predisposed to develop HRS type 1 after infections or other precipitating events.[33-35] The median survival of patients with HRS type 2 is 6 months, and it is worse than for patients with nonazotemic cirrhosis with ascites.

Treatment

Treating the underlying etiology with liver or combined liver-kidney transplant is the goal of therapy. Given the pathophysiology of extreme renal vasoconstriction, splanchnic vasodilation, and decreased cardiac output, many vasoactive drugs have been evaluated as therapeutic agents to reverse HRS. To date, no single therapeutic agent has been found to permanently reverse HRS. As such, the current goals in treatment are as a bridge to hepatic transplantation and possibly improved long-term survival. Dopamine, fenoldopam, endothelin antagonists, natriuretic peptides, and angiotensin-converting enzyme (ACE) inhibitors have been shown to either have no benefit or worsen the outcome of HRS.[37]

LIVER TRANSPLANTATION

Liver transplantation is the treatment of choice for HRS.[38-42] Immediately after transplantation, further impairment in GFR may be observed, and many patients require renal replacement therapy; 35% of patients with HRS compared with 5% of patients without HRS require renal replacement therapy.[38] Because cyclosporine or tacrolimus can contribute to impaired renal function, it has been suggested that administration of these drugs should be delayed until renal function begins to recover, usually 48 to 72 hours after transplantation.[43] After the initial deterioration in renal function, GFR starts to improve and reaches an average of 30 to 40 mL/min by 1 to 2 months postoperatively. This level of moderate renal failure persists during follow-up and is more marked than is observed after hepatic transplantation in patients without HRS.[32] The hemodynamic and neurohormonal abnormalities associated with HRS disappear within the first month after the operation, and patients regain normal sodium and free-water clearance.

Patients with HRS who undergo transplantation have more complications, spend more days in the ICU, and have a higher in-hospital mortality rate than transplantation patients without HRS.[38-42] The long-term survival of patients with HRS after liver transplantation, however, is good. The 3-year probability of survival is 60%.[38-42] This survival rate is only slightly less than survival rates for liver transplant recipients without HRS (70% and 80%).[38,41]

VOLUME EXPANSION AND VASOCONSTRICTORS

Treatment with arterial vasoconstrictors and volume expansion is the most promising approach for medically treating patients with HRS. This therapeutic strategy is intended to increase renal perfusion by causing splanchnic vasoconstriction and reversal of the decreased effective circulating volume, leading to improved renal perfusion. Over the past decade, many small studies have been performed to evaluate various vasoconstrictors. The volume expander of choice has been albumin.

Monotherapy with either albumin or vasoconstrictor has not been as effective as combined therapy. Martin-Lalhi and colleagues[44] randomized 46 patients to terlipressin plus albumin or albumin alone. Improvement in renal function was better with combination therapy (43.5% versus 8.7% $P = .017$). Conversely, Ortega and colleagues[45] randomized 21 patients to terlipressin with or without albumin, with an improved response with the addition of albumin (77% versus 25% $P = .03$). One-month survival without transplantation was 87% in patients receiving terlipressin plus albumin and 13% in patients receiving terlipressin alone. Typical dosing of albumin, and as recommended by the consensus panel, is 1 g/kg on day 1 of therapy, using 25% albumin as the preferred formulation of the colloid.

Vasopressin is an endogenous hormone with three major identified receptors. The V1 receptor, found on vascular smooth muscle, promotes vasoconstriction. The V2 receptor is involved in osmoregulation in the kidney. The V3 receptor affects corticotropin secretion. The V1 receptor has been the target of interest for vasopressin analogs designed to increase splanchnic vasoconstriction.[37,46] The original studies were conducted with ornipressin, but the recent focus has been on terlipressin, which has a greater effect on the V1 receptor and fewer side effects.[47] Two meta-analyses have shown improved outcome with the use of terlipressin versus placebo.[47,48] Fabrizi and colleagues[47] analyzed 10 clinical trials and found reversal of HRS in 52% of cases, with a 29% incidence of side effects, most of which responded to reducing the dose of terlipressin. Dobre and colleagues[48] identified eight eligible trials which enrolled a total of 320 patients. Four of the studies compared terlipressin to placebo, with an improvement in the terlipressin group with regard to several outcomes, including reversal of HRS (OR of 7.47), improvement in mean arterial pressure, improvement in urine output, and reduction of serum creatinine. Sanyal and colleagues[49] conducted a multicenter randomized trial of 112 patients. The terlipressin group received 1 mg of the drug every 6 hours and was more likely to have reversal of HRS compared with placebo (34% versus 12.5%, $P = .008$). Importantly, a subgroup of patients who received terlipressin for more than 3 days had a greater response to therapy compared to placebo (52.8% versus 18%, $P = .002$). These data support the contention that length of therapy may contribute to some of the variability in efficacy of therapy. Sanyal et al.[50] also showed that earlier therapy increases probability of reversal.

Terlipressin and intravenous (IV) albumin seems to be a promising therapy for type 1 HRS. The dose ranges used vary from 1 to 2 mg every 4 to 6 hours. One algorithm used starts terlipressin at 1 mg every 6 hours until the serum creatinine decreases to less than 1.5 mg/dL on two measurements. If there is no improvement in creatinine concentration after 3 days of therapy, the dose is increased to 2 mg every 6 hours.[49] A maximal dose of 12 mg a day has been proposed. The proposed minimum duration of therapy is 3 to 5 days.[46] Early initiation of therapy and close monitoring are important. There are varying data on the rates of recurrence of HRS after discontinuation of therapy; estimates range from 5.3% recurrence rate to 50% recurrence rate.[36,37,46] However, recurrence with terlipressin is less frequent than with placebo; survival with terlipressin is improved. Further large multicenter studies to evaluate dosing and time for treatment are pending.

α-Adrenergic agonists also have been used in an effort to augment renal perfusion. Duvoux and coworkers[51] treated 12 patients with HRS type 1 with IV albumin (to maintain central venous pressure >7 mm Hg) and norepinephrine (0.5 to 3 mg/h) for a minimum of 5 days. A significant improvement in serum creatinine concentration in association with a marked suppression of plasma renin activity was observed in 10 patients. Transient myocardial ischemia was observed in one patient. Three patients underwent transplantation, and three were still alive after 8 months of follow-up. Two randomized control studies have compared norepinephrine to terlipressin.[52,53] In the first (n = 22), reversal of HRS occurred in 70% of the norepinephrine group versus 83% of the terlipressin group ($P = NS$). In the second (n = 20), norepinephrine was effective for increasing mean arterial pressure (MAP), increasing urine output, and decreasing serum creatinine concentration; the efficacy of norepinephrine was not significantly different from the efficacy of terlipressin. There were no differences in outcomes or the incidence of adverse events in either study. Treatment algorithms target an increase in MAP of 10 mm Hg.

Angeli and associates[54] used oral midodrine, an α-adrenergic agonist, IV albumin, and subcutaneous octreotide (a somatostatin analog to suppress glucagon) in five patients with HRS type 1. Midodrine dosage was adjusted to increase MAP by more than 15 mm Hg. Patients received treatment for at least 20 days in hospital and subsequently continued treatment at home. In all cases, there was a dramatic improvement in renal perfusion, GFR, blood urea nitrogen concentration, serum creatinine concentration, and serum sodium concentration. Plasma levels of renin, aldosterone, and antidiuretic hormone decreased to normal or near-normal levels. Two patients were transplanted 20 and 64 days after enrollment while on therapy. One patient who was not a candidate for liver transplantation was alive without treatment 472 days after being discharged from the hospital. The remaining two patients died 29 and 75 days after enrollment. The control group received dopamine therapy, with seven of the eight patients dying by day 12. Esralian and colleagues[55] retrospectively evaluated 60 patients, comparing midodrine plus octreotide to untreated controls. Forty percent of treated patients had an improvement in renal function as compared to 10% of controls ($P = .03$). In addition, treatment with midodrine plus octreotide was associated with an improvement in 30-day mortality (43% versus 71%, $P = .03$). Their data showed that patients who received the highest dose of 15 mg 3 times a day were more likely to respond to therapy. In a prospective observational study, Skagen[56] and colleagues studied midodrine and octreotide in both type 1 and type 2 HRS. The treatment group of 75 patients was compared to historical controls. The 1-month GFR was improved in the treatment group (48 versus 34 mL/min, $P = .03$). Median survival also was improved for type 1 HRS (40 versus 17 days, $P = .007$) and type 2 HRS (>12 months versus 22 days, $P = .0004$). Studies of monotherapy of octreotide have not shown benefit over placebo. The combination of midodrine plus octreotide is a promising regimen for HRS 2 patients and for patients who are treated as outpatients.

These studies show the following:

1. HRS type 1 is reversible after treatment with IV albumin and vasoconstrictors.
2. Both components of the treatment are important because HRS does not reverse when vasoconstrictors or plasma volume expanders are given alone.
3. The constant infusion of vasoconstrictors (ornipressin or norepinephrine) is associated with ischemic complications (a feature not observed when they are given intermittently).
4. There is a delay of several days between the improvement in circulatory function and the increase in GFR.
5. Reversal of HRS improves survival, and a significant number of patients live long enough to obtain liver transplantation.

TRANSJUGULAR INTRAHEPATIC PORTOSYSTEMIC SHUNT

Because portal hypertension is the initial abnormality with regard to circulatory dysfunction in cirrhosis, decreasing portal pressure by portosystemic anastomosis is a rational approach for the treatment of HRS. There are several case reports showing reversal of HRS after surgical portosystemic shunt.[57,58] However, major surgical procedures in patients with HRS are not likely to be tolerated well. The development of transjugular intrahepatic portosystemic shunt (TIPS) has reinvigorated the idea of treating HRS by reducing portal pressure.

Several studies assessing TIPS in the management of HRS type 1 have been reported.[59-61] The first study included 14 patients with type 1 HRS who were not candidates for transplantation. At 3, 6, and 12 months after TIPS, survival rates were 54%, 50%, and 20%, respectively.[59] In one study, which specifically investigated the effect of TIPS on neurohormonal systems, improvement in GFR and serum creatinine concentration was related to marked suppression of the plasma levels of renin and antidiuretic hormone.[60] The most recent study included 14 patients with type 1 HRS who were initially treated with midodrine and octreotide.[62] Ten of the 14 patients responded to vasoconstrictor therapy, and five subsequently underwent TIPS. These patients had an improvement in renal function, sodium excretion, and portosystemic gradient. These studies strongly suggest that TIPS is useful in the management of HRS type 1 and may be beneficial in combination with vasoconstrictor therapy.

OTHER THERAPEUTIC METHODS

Hemodialysis and arteriovenous or venovenous hemofiltration are frequently used in patients with HRS. Extracorporeal albumin dialysis uses an albumin-containing dialysate that is recirculated and perfused through charcoal and anion-exchanger columns. This modality has been shown to improve systemic hemodynamics and reduce plasma levels of renin in patients with HRS type 1.[63,64] In a small series of patients, improved survival was reported.[62] Newer modalities such as the Prometheus system and single-pass albumin dialysis have been used in a few patients with some success.[65,66] Further studies are needed to confirm these findings.

Prevention

Three randomized controlled studies enrolling large series of patients have shown that HRS can be prevented in specific clinical settings. In the first study,[67] albumin (1.5 g/kg IV at infection diagnosis and 1 g/kg IV 48 hours later) together with cefotaxime was compared to cefotaxime alone in patients with cirrhosis and SBP. Treatment with albumin markedly reduced the incidence of impaired circulatory function and the occurrence of HRS type 1. Moreover, the hospital mortality rate (10% versus 29%) and the 3-month mortality rate (22% versus 41%) were lower in patients receiving albumin plus antibiotics versus antibiotics alone. The second study showed that oral prophylaxis using norfloxacin decreased the 1-year probability of developing SBP and type 1 HRS and improved survival.[68] In a third study,[68] administration of the tumor necrosis factor synthesis inhibitor, pentoxifylline (400 mg TID), to patients with severe acute alcoholic hepatitis reduced the occurrence of HRS (8% in the pentoxifylline group versus 35% in the placebo group) and hospital mortality (24% versus 46%, respectively). Because bacterial infections and acute alcoholic hepatitis are two important precipitating factors of HRS type 1, these prophylactic measures may decrease the incidence of this complication.

Conclusion

HRS is a major clinical event during the course of decompensated cirrhosis. Although the most characteristic feature of the syndrome is functional renal failure caused by intense renal vasoconstriction, it is a more generalized process affecting the whole body. There are two types of HRS. Type 1 is characterized by rapid and progressive deterioration of circulatory and renal function. It usually develops in close chronologic relationship with a precipitating event, particularly severe bacterial infection; acute alcoholic, toxic, or viral hepatitis; or major surgical procedures. HRS type 1 carries a very poor prognosis (median survival rate < 2 weeks). HRS type 2 is characterized by steady deterioration of circulatory and renal function. Patients with HRS type 2 have a median survival of 6 months, and their main clinical problem is refractory ascites. The pathogenesis of HRS is decreased effective arterial blood volume due to splanchnic arterial vasodilatation and reduced venous return and cardiac output. The syndrome can be reversed by the simultaneous administration of IV albumin and arterial vasoconstrictors. Intrarenal mechanisms also are important and require a prolonged improvement in circulatory function to be deactivated. Systemic vasoconstriction, increased intrahepatic vascular resistance and portal pressure, and impaired hepatic function are other components of the syndrome. Long-term administration of IV albumin and vasoconstrictors and correction of portal hypertension with TIPS are effective treatments for HRS. These approaches improve survival and may serve as a bridge to liver transplantation, which is the ultimate treatment of choice in these patients.

KEY POINTS

1. Ascites is a common complication of liver cirrhosis, preceding the development of severe complications such as dilutional hyponatremia, refractory ascites, and hepatorenal syndrome (HRS) that carry an extremely poor prognosis.

2. Renal functional abnormalities in cirrhosis start with reduced ability to excrete sodium, sodium retention, and accumulation of ascites. As the disease progresses, circulatory dysfunction increases as a consequence of the activation of endogenous vasoactive systems (sympathetic nervous system and the renin-angiotensin system).

3. The final step leading to HRS is decreased renal perfusion due to an imbalance between extremely high vasoconstrictor tone and decreased production of renal vasodilators.

4. Diagnosis of HRS follows the criteria of the International Ascites Club (see Table 99-1) and mainly consists of the presence of serum creatinine level above 1.5 mg/dL in the absence of other potential causes of renal failure.

5. HRS is classified into two types:
   a. Type 1: severe and rapidly progressive renal failure, usually following a precipitating event, carrying an extremely poor prognosis (median survival: 2 weeks)
   b. Type 2: moderate and steady development of renal failure, clinically characterized by refractory ascites and associated with a slightly better prognosis (median survival: 6 months)

6. Liver transplantation is the treatment of choice for HRS. The recovery of renal function as well as the reversal of the hemodynamic and neurohumoral abnormalities associated with the syndrome may take 1 month after the operation.

7. The 3-year probability of survival in transplanted patients with HRS is 60%, slightly less than in recipients without HRS.

8. Recent studies have shown that HRS type 1 is reversible after treatment with intravenous albumin and vasoconstrictors.

9. Successful prevention of HRS has been achieved in specific clinical settings such as spontaneous bacterial peritonitis (by administration of albumin + antibiotics) and acute alcoholic hepatitis (by giving pentoxifylline).

ANNOTATED REFERENCES

Salerno F, Gerbes A, et al. Diagnosis, prevention and treatment of hepatorenal syndrome in cirrhosis. Gut 2007;56:1310-8.
  This paper resulted from a large consensus conference as a follow-up to the original conference in 1996. The authors clarified the definition of hepatorenal syndrome, providing a rationale for comparing different therapeutic approaches and performing meta-analysis.
Ginés A, Escorsell A, Ginés P, et al. Incidence, predictive factors, and prognosis of hepatorenal syndrome in cirrhosis. Gastroenterology 1993;105:229-36.
  This retrospective study established the natural history of type 1 hepatorenal syndrome and provided epidemiologic and prognostic data to compare with and to design future prospective studies.
Sanyal A, Boyer T, et al. A randomized, prospective, double-blind, placebo controlled trial of terlipressin for type 1 hepatorenal syndrome. Dig Dis Sci 2008;53:830-5.
  This recent prospective randomized trial established the benefit of terlipressin in the treatment of type 1 hepatorenal syndrome. They showed an improvement in renal function.

Sort P, Navasa M, Arroyo V, et al. Effect of plasma volume expansion on renal impairment and mortality in patients with cirrhosis and spontaneous bacterial peritonitis. N Engl J Med 1999;341:403-9.
  This important prospective, randomized, controlled trial showed that preventing renal impairment in spontaneous bacterial peritonitis resulted in an improvement in survival in those patients, and that this prevention was achieved by the administration of albumin to cause plasma volume expansion. The paper emphasizes the critical importance of improving renal perfusion in circumstances known to deteriorate it and to cause hepatorenal syndrome.
Alessandria C, Ottobrelli A, et al. Noradrenalin vs. terlipressin in patients with hepatorenal syndrome: a prospective, randomized, unblinded, pilot study. J Hepatol 2007;47:499-505.
  This prospective pilot study established the potential for equal efficacy of noradrenaline and terlipressin for the treatment of hepatorenal syndrome.

REFERENCES

Access the complete reference list online at http://www.expertconsult.com.

100

Hepatopulmonary Syndrome

DAVID KAUFMAN | ANNE MARIE MATTINGLY

Definition

Hepatopulmonary syndrome (HPS) is defined by abnormal oxygen exchange in association with intrapulmonary vascular dilatation (IPVD) in patients with liver disease.[1] The presence of other cardiopulmonary disease that alters gas exchange does not exclude this diagnosis.[2-5] HPS is most commonly associated with cirrhosis[1] and portal hypertension, but neither of these are required.[6] The correlation between the degree of liver dysfunction and the presence[7-8] and severity[3-4,7,9-10] of this syndrome is debated.

Clinical Features

HPS usually presents as dyspnea[6,11] in patients who are already known to have liver disease. HPS-induced shortness of breath often is relieved when the patient is lying down,[11-12] and therefore is referred to as *platypnea*. There are no consistently noted physical examination findings.[6,13] Hypoxia is often worse in the standing position (orthodeoxia),[12] and it generally can be corrected with sufficient supplemental oxygen.[1,3,4,10,14]

Pathophysiology

Dilated precapillary vessels and pleural-based arteriovenous connections are noted at autopsy in cases of HPS.[15] Current thinking suggests that these abnormal vessels develop due to a functional excess of pulmonary vasodilators[1]; they cause hypoxia through ventilation/perfusion (V/Q) mismatching, arteriovenous (AV) shunting, and limitation of oxygen diffusion to red blood cells (RBCs) in the center of the vessel.[15-17] The hyperdynamic circulation, which is characteristic of cirrhosis, likely exacerbates this problem by decreasing RBC transit time through the pulmonary capillaries, further limiting oxygen diffusion.[15,17] Orthodeoxia is due to a worsening of V/Q mismatch and AV shunting in the standing position.[18]

Nitric oxide (NO) has been implicated as a key vasodilator in HPS. Exhaled NO levels are increased in patients with cirrhosis compared to healthy controls and in HPS patients compared to cirrhotic patients without HPS; NO levels correlate with the severity of cirrhosis and gas exchange abnormalities.[19] In rat models of HPS induced by ligation of the common bile duct (CBDL), increased levels of endothelial[20] and inducible NO synthase (eNOS and iNOS, respectively) have been observed, and administration of a nitric oxide synthase inhibitor prevents the development of pulmonary vasodilation and HPS.[21]

Excess eNOS is located in the pulmonary arteries and capillaries and is associated with impaired vasoconstriction; levels of this enzyme correlate with the degree of gas exchange abnormalities.[20] CBDL rats demonstrate increased hepatic production of endothelin-1 (ET-1)[22] and increased vascular expression of the endothelin-B receptor (ET-B)[23] in proportion to the severity of gas exchange abnormalities[22,24]; interaction between ET-1 and the ET-B receptor, therefore, is believed to be the trigger for increased eNOS expression. This theory is further supported by data that show a reduction in eNOS expression and an improvement in HPS when CBDL animals are treated with endothelin-B receptor antagonists.[24]

iNOS is expressed in macrophages found in the lungs of CBDL rats,[21] while treatment of these rats with norfloxacin is associated with a reduction in the rate of gram-negative bacterial translocation, accumulation of pulmonary macrophages, production of iNOS, and

severity of HPS.[25] Pulmonary macrophages in CBDL rats also have been noted to express elevated levels of heme-oxygenase-1 (HO-1), an enzyme that catalyzes formation of the vasodilating gas, carbon monoxide (CO).[26] Increased levels of carboxyhemoglobin (COHb) have been observed in rat[26] as well as human[27] subjects with HPS, and treatment with an HO-1 inhibitor normalizes COHb levels and partially alleviates HPS in CBDL rats.[26] These data suggest that CO also contributes to pulmonary vasodilation in this syndrome. Finally, tumor necrosis factor alpha (TNF-α) rises in CBDL animals in association with ET-1 and endotoxin levels, and it has been proposed to influence accumulation of the iNOS- and HO-1-producing pulmonary macrophages.[28] Administration of pentoxifylline, a phosphodiesterase inhibitor that suppresses production of TNF-α, is associated with a reduction in TNF-α levels, pulmonary macrophage accumulation, ET-B receptor and eNOS expression, and severity of HPS.[29]

Diagnosis

HPS should be considered in any patient with liver disease and dyspnea or hypoxia. Evaluation begins with an arterial blood gas (ABG), with the patient resting in the seated position and breathing room air.[6,17] No specific gas exchange criteria for HPS have been universally accepted,[30] but a 2004 European Respiratory Society (ERS) task force advised further evaluation when the Pao$_2$ is less than 80 mm Hg or the alveolar-arterial oxygen gradient (A-a gradient) is 15 mm Hg or greater (≥20 mm Hg for patients over age 64).[17]

Accurate HPS diagnosis requires the presence of ABG changes that cannot be fully explained by comorbid cardiopulmonary disease. Conditions that frequently coexist with cirrhosis that may influence gas exchange include chronic obstructive pulmonary disease (COPD), congestive heart failure, restrictive lung disease due to ascites or hepatic hydrothorax, α$_1$-antitrypsin deficiency, and portopulmonary hypertension (distinguished from HPS by its increased pulmonary artery pressure and vascular resistance; in HPS, pulmonary artery pressure and vascular resistance are low).[31] Patients should have a chest x-ray (CXR) and pulmonary function tests[12] to assess for pulmonary disease; of note, increased markings at the lung bases on CXR[1,6,8] and/or a reduced diffusion capacity for carbon monoxide (DLCO)[3-4,7,13,18] are common findings in HPS and, in isolation, do not exclude the diagnosis. Cardiac function is evaluated by echocardiogram, often concurrently with IPVD assessment (see later discussion).

When a gas exchange abnormality is present and not fully explained by another cardiopulmonary disease, the patient should be evaluated for the presence of IPVDs. Contrast-enhanced echocardiography (CEE) is commonly used for this purpose; advantages include that it is widely available, it permits concurrent evaluation for cardiac causes of abnormal gas exchange, and it can distinguish intracardiac from intrapulmonary shunt based on the number of cardiac cycles required for agitated saline to pass from the right to left atrium.[12] CEE is highly sensitive for the presence IPVDs[30] and may document them in up to 82% of patients tested.[32] Compared with patients without IPVDs, those with a positive CEE have a greater incidence of dyspnea[33] and abnormal CXRs,[9,33] as well as more severe cirrhosis[9,32-33] and gas exchange abnormalities.[9,33] However, many patients with IPVDs demonstrated by CEE do not have gas exchange abnormalities,[5,8,13,32-33] and so this test is not very specific for HPS.[30]

Technetium-99m-labeled macroaggregated albumin (^{99m}Tc MAA) lung perfusion scanning is an alternative test for IPVDs. It is expensive, requires radiation exposure,[13] and cannot document the site of shunting, but it is able to provide a quantitative shunt fraction[13,17,30] that correlates directly with the A-a gradient[3,10,14] and inversely with the room air Pao$_2$[3,10,14,34] and oxygen saturation.[34] Perfusion scanning is less sensitive than CEE for the detection of IPVDs,[5] but positive results are rare in patients without HPS.[5,10,34] Because of these test characteristics, CEE has been advocated as the first-line modality for evaluating patients with liver disease and abnormal gas exchange.[5,10,17] If CEE is positive but the relative contributions of other cardiopulmonary disease and possible HPS are not clear, lung perfusion scanning can determine if HPS is present.[5,10,12,17]

Prevalence

The prevalence of HPS varies greatly depending on how it is diagnosed. When abnormal gas exchange is defined by widening of the A-a gradient, more patients meet HPS criteria than when a reduction of Pao$_2$ is used,[9] because hyperventilation can maintain a normal Pao$_2$ while the A-a gradient is still elevated due to decreased Paco$_2$.[15] HPS prevalence is also affected by the sensitivity of the IPVD evaluation method used; IPVDs are found more frequently with CEE compared to lung perfusion scanning[5] and with TEE compared to TTE,[35] thereby increasing HPS diagnosis rates.[5,35] For example, HPS was diagnosed in 3 of 40 (7.5%) cirrhotic patients when a Pao$_2$ of less than 70 mm Hg and a positive lung perfusion scan were required[5]; when criteria consisted of an A-a gradient more than 15 mm Hg and a positive CEE, the prevalence of HPS among patients with cirrhosis was reported as 32% (31 of 98 patients).[9]

Prognosis

In the absence of liver transplantation, patients with HPS have a poorer functional status, reduced self-reported quality of life,[8] and a worse survival[7-8,36] than non-HPS controls matched for severity of liver disease. HPS patients who die during follow-up have been noted to have greater room air Pao$_2$ reductions, A-a gradient elevations, and shunt fractions than those who survive,[3,7,36] but this is not a universal finding.[8] Without a transplant, HPS patients demonstrate progressive hypoxemia.[36] Despite this, death is usually due to complications of liver disease,[7,17,36] and mortality from primary respiratory failure is rare.[36]

Therapy

Multiple medical therapies have been tried for HPS without clear efficacy, including inhibitors of nitric oxide[37-39] and TNF-α production,[40] as well as antibiotics to reduce macrophage accumulation.[41] Case reports have documented improvement in HPS after transjugular intrahepatic portosystemic shunt (TIPS) placement, but this therapy is still considered experimental.[12,42] Pulmonary angiography with embolization of dilated capillaries[43] or arteriovenous communications[44] also has been effective in case reports. Some authors advise pursuing pulmonary angiography in HPS patients with a poor response to administration of 100% oxygen,[1,3,44] since these patients are more likely to have large shunts that may improve with embolization. Oxygen therapy also has been recommended.[1,6,11-12,17]

Liver transplantation is the only definitive therapy for HPS and should be considered when patients are symptomatic or have a Pao$_2$ less than 60 mm Hg.[6,17] Owing to the increased mortality associated with HPS and the lack of other effective therapies, the United Network for Organ Sharing (UNOS) has adjusted organ allocation algorithms to prioritize patients with HPS and a Pao$_2$ below 60 mm Hg.[45]

Patients with HPS who receive liver transplants have been observed to have a greater postoperative mortality than their non-HPS counterparts in two series (33% of 9 HPS patients versus 9.2% of 76 non-HPS patients at 6 months[46]; 29% of 24 HPS patients versus 8%–10% of historical controls at 1 year[14]), although data from the largest available HPS population (24 transplanted HPS and 30 transplanted non-HPS patients) showed no survival difference between HPS and non-HPS transplant recipients when followed for over 7 years.[36] A preoperative Pao$_2$ $\leq$ 50 mm or shunt fraction $\geq$ 20% was predictive of postoperative mortality in one report (mean Pao$_2$ 59 mm Hg versus 43 mm Hg, and shunt fraction 18% versus 41% in 17 survivors versus 7 nonsurvivors).[14] A subsequent series of 24 transplanted HPS patients also showed a trend toward increased mortality after transplant among HPS patients with preoperative Pao$_2$ $\leq$ 50, although this difference did not reach statistical significance ($P = .08$).[36] Another small series noted a non-significant correlation between mortality and shunt fraction, observing that 3 out of 6 patients with HPS and preoperative shunt fractions over 30% died during the first 60 days after liver transplant, while only 1 of 6 HPS patients with a shunt fraction $\leq$ 30% died (at day 71).[3] Among those patients who survive the perioperative period, improvement in or resolution of HPS is noted in the majority of cases,[4,14,36,46] although the amelioration of symptoms may require a year or more to occur.[4,14,36]

KEY POINTS

1. Hepatopulmonary syndrome (HPS) consists of a triad of liver disease, abnormal pulmonary gas exchange, and intrapulmonary vascular dilatation. It most commonly presents as dyspnea or hypoxia in patients already known to have liver disease.

2. HPS is believed to result from excessive pulmonary vasodilation, mediated primarily by nitric oxide. Pulmonary vasodilatation leads to hypoxia through ventilation/perfusion mismatching, arteriovenous shunting, and limitations to oxygen diffusion.

3. Diagnosis of HPS requires a seated, room air, arterial blood gas to document abnormal gas exchange, as well as confirmation of intrapulmonary shunt using echo or lung perfusion scanning. The reported prevalence of HPS varies widely because of different diagnostic criteria with variable sensitivity and specificity.

4. Patients with liver disease and HPS have an increased risk of death relative to patients with liver disease alone. Liver transplantation is the only effective therapy and improves or resolves HPS in most cases. Transplant evaluation should be pursued in patients with HPS who are symptomatic or have a seated room air Pao$_2$ less than 60 mm Hg.

ANNOTATED REFERENCES

Rodriguez-Roisin R, Krowka MJ. Hepatopulmonary syndrome: a liver-induced lung vascular disorder. N Engl J Med 2008;358:2378-87.
A general review of the clinical features, diagnostic criteria, and treatment options for HPS.

Rodriguez-Roisin R, Krowka MJ, Hervé P, Fallon MB; ERS Task Force Pulmonary-Hepatic Vascular Disorders (PHD) Scientific Committee. Pulmonary-hepatic vascular disorders (PHD). Eur Respir J 2004;24:861-80.
An international consensus statement that summarizes current opinion on the pathophysiology, diagnosis, and treatment of HPS.

Mandell MS. The diagnosis and treatment of hepatopulmonary syndrome. Clin Liver Dis 2006;10:387-405.
A discussion of the challenges inherent in characterizing HPS due to variable diagnostic criteria.

Schenk P, Fuhrmann V, Madl C, Funk G, Lehr S, Kandel O, et al. Hepatopulmonary syndrome: prevalence and predictive value of various cut offs for arterial oxygenation and their clinical consequences. Gut 2002;51:853-9.

An analysis of the how the prevalence of HPS varies when different criteria for abnormal oxygenation are applied.

Abrams GA, Jaffe CC, Hoffer PB, Binder HJ, Fallon MB. Diagnostic utility of contrast echocardiography and lung perfusion scan in patients with hepatopulmonary syndrome. Gastroenterology 1995;109:1283-8.
A comparison of the sensitivity and specificity of contrast-enhanced echo and lung perfusion scanning for the diagnosis of HPS.

Krowka MJ, Wiseman GA, Burnett OL, Spivey JR, Therneau T, Porayko MK, et al. Hepatopulmonary syndrome: a prospective study of relationships between severity of liver disease, Pao$_2$ response to 100% oxygen, and brain uptake after ^{99m}Tc MAA lung scanning. Chest 2000;118:615-24.
An analysis of the associations between severity of liver disease, degree of hypoxia, shunt fraction, and mortality in patients with HPS.

Swanson KL, Weisner RH, Krowka MJ. Natural history of hepatopulmonary syndrome: impact of liver transplantation. Hepatology 2005;41:1122-9.

A case-control study of outcomes in patients with and without HPS, examining the relationships between oxygenation, shunt fraction, severity of liver disease, transplantation status, and survival.

Taillé C, Cadranel J, Bellocq A, Thabut G, Soubrane O, Durand F, et al. Liver transplantation for hepatopulmonary syndrome: a ten-year experience in Paris, France. Transplantation 2003;79:1482-9; discussion 1446-7.

An observational study that describes the postoperative course of 23 adult patients with HPS who underwent liver transplantation.

Schiffer E, Majno P, Mentha G, Giostra E, Burri H, Klopfenstein CE, et al. Hepatopulmonary syndrome increases the postoperative mortality rate following liver transplantation: a prospective study in 90 patients. Am J Transplant 2006;6:1430-7.

A comparison of survival rates after liver transplantation in patients with and without HPS.

Arguedas MR, Abrams GA, Krowka MJ, Fallon MB. Prospective evaluation of outcomes and predictors of mortality in patients with hepatopulmonary syndrome undergoing liver transplantation. Hepatology 2003;37:192-7.

A prospective assessment of the association between preoperative oxygenation and shunt fraction and postoperative survival in HPS patients undergoing liver transplantation.

REFERENCES

Access the complete reference list online at http://www.expertconsult.com.

101

Hepatic Encephalopathy

ALVARO MARTINEZ-CAMACHO | BRETT E. FORTUNE | GREGORY T. EVERSON

Hepatic encephalopathy encompasses a spectrum of neuropsychiatric abnormalities that occur in patients with liver disease in the absence of other brain disease.[1-2] The spectrum includes personality changes, impaired mental function, motor abnormalities (asterixis, tremor, hyperventilation, hyperactive reflexes), and altered consciousness. A consensus panel of experts proposed classification of hepatic encephalopathy into type A, associated with acute liver failure; type B, associated with portal-systemic bypass without intrinsic liver disease; and type C, associated with chronic liver disease.[3]

The encephalopathy accompanying acute hepatic failure (type A) is commonly associated with cerebral edema and increased intracranial pressure (ICP), exhibits abrupt onset with a short prodrome and rapid progression, and often ends with the death of the patient.[4-6] Patients sequentially experience drowsiness, delirium, agitation or convulsions, decerebrate rigidity, unresponsiveness, and deep coma within a comparatively short period of time, usually hours to days. Irreversible neurologic damage may occur as a result of brain ischemia or herniation. Patients who develop coma in the setting of acute liver failure have a grave prognosis; fewer than 20% survive without hepatic transplantation.[7]

In patients with chronic liver disease, encephalopathy (type C) develops insidiously and often is heralded by a change in mental or behavioral status. Encephalopathy may be episodic, persistent, or minimal and subclinical.[3] Episodes are sporadic, characterized by exacerbations and remissions, and generally are precipitated by inciting events.[1-2] Although the initial manifestation of portosystemic encephalopathy (PSE) is usually a subtle change in mentation, neurologic dysfunction may progress and be classified according to confusion, lethargy, and even coma (Table 101-1).[8] Neurologic signs vary and fluctuate but usually include asterixis, hyperreflexia, clonus, and an extensor plantar response. Causes of PSE may not always be apparent, but azotemia, sepsis, gastrointestinal (GI) bleeding, dehydration, electrolyte imbalances, and sedatives are frequent precipitants (Box 101-1). In some patients, chronic encephalopathy may not be clinically obvious, but only detectable by psychometric testing. By these tests, about two-thirds of cirrhotic patients with portal hypertension have unsuspected subclinical hepatic encephalopathy.[9-12] Patients who undergo portal-systemic shunt or bypass, either surgical or transjugular intrahepatic portosystemic shunt (TIPS), often develop encephalopathy (type B) which is similar to the encephalopathy experienced by patients with chronic liver disease.

General Principals

No single abnormality of hepatic or neurologic metabolism adequately explains all of the clinical, biochemical, physiologic, or experimental findings of encephalopathy occurring in patients or animal models.[1-2,6] Abnormalities of multiple neurotransmitters including glutamate, γ-aminobutyric acid (GABA), dopamine, serotonin, and opioids have been described, and plasma levels of a wide array of potential neurotoxins (ammonia [NH_3], GABA, short-chain fatty acids, methanethiols) are increased (Box 101-2).[13-14] Despite this seeming confusion, several lines of investigation focus on NH_3 as a key factor in the pathogenesis of hepatic encephalopathy. Ammonia accumulation deranges glutamate and glutamine metabolism in the central nervous system (CNS) and alters the metabolism of GABA and its function as an inhibitory neurotransmitter. In addition, benzodiazepine receptors in the CNS are physically linked to GABA receptors. The latter finding provides an explanation for the increased sensitivity of patients with liver disease to the sedative and hypnotic effects of benzodiazepines and a rationale for use of benzodiazepine antagonists in the treatment of PSE. Hepatic encephalopathy occurring in the setting of either acute liver failure or chronic liver disease is also associated with marked changes in CNS glial cells on neuropathologic examination. Encephalopathy of acute liver failure is characterized by astrocytic swelling, but chronic encephalopathy is characterized by Alzheimer type II astrocytosis.[15]

CEREBRAL BLOOD FLOW

In acute liver failure, the brain is potentially subject to hypoxic injury due to complications such as systemic arterial hypotension, respiratory failure, and reduction in cerebral blood flow that accompanies cerebral edema and intracranial hypertension. Therapy is often directed at optimal oxygenation, maintenance of cerebral perfusion pressure (goal > 40 mm Hg), and reduction of ICP (goal < 20 mm Hg).[4,9] Paradoxically, increases in cerebral blood flow, however, may aggravate cerebral edema and worsen neurologic damage. In humans with acute liver failure, cerebral blood flow has been measured primarily by the xenon-133 washout technique.[16-20] These data suggest that cerebral blood flow is initially relatively low but then increases with increasing blood concentration of NH_3, which decreases cerebral arteriolar tone.

CEREBRAL GLUCOSE AND OXYGEN METABOLISM

Brain energy metabolism is unique in that glucose is the only substrate under normal physiologic conditions, and its uptake and utilization by the brain is independent of insulin.[21-25] Under stress, the brain can utilize β-hydroxybutyrate and acetoacetate. Ammonia accumulation during hepatic failure in humans or in experimental models of hyperammonemia is associated with altered cerebral glucose metabolism. In early acute liver failure, prior to onset of intracranial hypertension, cerebral glucose metabolism and cerebral oxygen consumption are proportionally diminished.[21] There is no evidence of cerebral hypoxia, implying that the reduced glucose and oxygen utilization reflect diminished metabolic demand by the brain at this early stage. Cerebral lactate uptake is increased despite sufficient glucose delivery and preserved oxidative metabolism. Acute short-term mechanical ventilation, resulting in moderate reduction in PCO_2 and cerebral blood flow, does not adversely affect oxidative brain metabolism. Thus, prior to the development of intracranial hypertension, cerebral glucose and oxygen metabolism are reduced, but these changes are consistent with normal aerobic metabolism and physiologic regulation. After development of intracranial hypertension, oxygen metabolism remains reduced, but measurements of cerebral glucose utilization vary from reduced rates to increased rates, and glycolysis may be accelerated.[22-23,25] These findings suggest that progression of acute liver failure and development of intracranial hypertension are associated with relative cerebral hypoxia and a switch to anaerobic metabolism.

AMMONIA HYPOTHESIS

The *ammonia hypothesis* states that the major mechanism of hepatic encephalopathy is excessive accumulation of NH_3, which induces neuronal metabolic derangements but also promotes astrocytic swelling.[26] In addition, NH_3 perturbs cerebral nitric oxide metabolism, which can

TABLE 101-1	Stages of Encephalopathy in Chronic Liver Disease
Stage	*Clinical Signs*
Stage I	Mental slowness, euphoria or anxiety, shortened attention span, impaired calculating ability
Stage II	Lethargy or apathy, inappropriate behavior, personality change, more obvious problems with calculations
Stage III	Lethargic, somnolent, marked confusion and disorientation, but responds to verbal stimuli
Stage IV	Coma, patient may or may not respond to noxious stimuli

Patients with chronic liver disease rarely, if ever, demonstrate cerebral edema, regardless of the stage of encephalopathy.

Box 101-2

BRAIN NEUROTOXINS OR NEUROINHIBITORS THAT ACCUMULATE IN HEPATIC FAILURE

Ammonia
Manganese
Glutamine
GABA
Taurine
Benzodiazepine receptor ligands
Monoamines
Opioids
Methanethiols

---

mediate some of the effects.[27] Studies using positron-emission tomography (PET) and magnetic resonance spectroscopy have demonstrated an increase in cerebral metabolic rate and increased permeability of the blood-brain barrier for NH_3.[28-34] Blood NH_3 originates mainly from four sources: intrahepatic deamination of amino acids, extrahepatic metabolism of nucleotides, gut metabolism of glutamine, and bacterial degradation of intestinal protein and urea.[35] More than 50% of blood NH_3 is derived from the latter source. NH_3 is normally metabolized by the liver to either urea or glutamine by the actions of carbamoyl-phosphate synthetase I (the initiating enzyme of the urea cycle) and glutamine synthetase, respectively. Patients with hepatic failure have impaired NH_3 metabolism related to a reduction in liver metabolism and an increase in portal-systemic shunting. As a result, an elevation in blood NH_3 concentration is a characteristic feature of severely impaired hepatic function.

Certain clinical and experimental observations link the increase in blood NH_3 concentration to hepatic encephalopathy.[13,15,36-37] Hyperammonemia and elevated concentrations of NH_3 within the cerebrospinal fluid (CSF) are features of acute and chronic hepatic encephalopathy, Reye syndrome, deficiencies of urea cycle enzymes, and sodium valproate toxicity. In cirrhotics or patients with portocaval shunts, ingestion of NH_3-generating substances (proteins, amino acids, urea, ammonium salts) may precipitate encephalopathy. In animal models, chronic administration of ammonium salts results in Alzheimer type II astrocytosis, a change indistinguishable from that observed in patients with chronic hepatic encephalopathy.[15]

GLUTAMINE-GLUTAMATERGIC NEUROTRANSMITTER SYSTEM

The glutamatergic excitatory neurotransmitter system in the CNS is markedly altered in patients with both acute and chronic liver disease and in animal models of hepatic encephalopathy.[6,26-27] CNS astrocytes

---

Box 101-1

CLINICAL EVENTS PRECIPITATING HEPATIC ENCEPHALOPATHY IN CIRRHOTIC PATIENTS

Gastrointestinal hemorrhage
Infection
Spontaneous bacterial peritonitis
Pneumonia
Sepsis
Dehydration
Imbalance of electrolytes or acid-base
Renal failure
Drugs, toxins, medications
Illicit substances
Alcohol
Sedatives, hypnotics
Narcotics
Dietary indiscretion (excessive protein intake)

---

are a major regulatory cell in the glutamatergic system.[15] Normally the astrocyte avidly takes up excess glutamate from the synaptic cleft (against a 3000-10,000 fold concentration gradient), an important function that terminates glutamate-induced neuroexcitation. Once glutamate is taken up by the astrocyte, it is metabolized to glutamine via the action of glutamine synthetase, which utilizes blood-derived NH_3 (Figure 101-1). The hyperammonemia of liver failure favors the formation of glutamine but also impairs the release of glutamine from the astrocyte. The accumulation of osmotically active glutamine in the astrocyte is associated with cell swelling. Normally, glutamine is actively extruded from the astrocyte and then taken up by presynaptic nerve terminals for conversion back to glutamate and subsequent utilization in neurotransmission. Under the conditions of liver failure and hyperammonemia, glutamate uptake into neurons and astrocytes is diminished, and glutamate accumulates in the extracellular fluid. Clinically, levels of glutamine and glutamate increase in CSF fluid during hyperammonemic states, and CSF concentrations of glutamine correlate loosely with the stage of encephalopathy. In animal models of acute encephalopathy, blockade of glutamine production by an inhibitor of glutamine synthetase, methionine sulfoximine, decreases cerebral edema and reduces astrocyte swelling.[14] Production of NH_3 from the intestine is reduced by orally administered nonabsorbable antibiotics such as rifaximin and neomycin, as well as nonabsorbable disaccharides including lactulose, lactitol, and lactose (in lactase-deficient patients). These treatments lower plasma NH_3 concentration and improve subjective and objective measures of encephalopathy.

Other clinical and experimental observations refute the link between NH_3 and hepatic encephalopathy. Blood levels of NH_3 are elevated in cirrhotic patients regardless of the presence or absence of encephalopathy. Some patients with hepatic encephalopathy have normal blood levels of NH_3. The grade of hepatic encephalopathy does not correlate with the blood concentration of NH_3. Seizures and hyperexcitability are commonly observed in animal models of NH_3 intoxication and in human congenital hyperammonemia but are rarely observed in patients with chronic hepatic encephalopathy. Administration of ammonium chloride to cirrhotic patients induces a mild hyperkinesis but fails to exacerbate typical chronic encephalopathy.[13]

γ-AMINOBUTYRIC ACID-BENZODIAZEPINE RECEPTOR HYPOTHESIS

GABA is an inhibitory neurotransmitter found throughout the CNS.[38] The *GABA hypothesis* states that an excess of GABA or increased sensitivity to GABA is responsible for hepatic encephalopathy.[14,38-39] Observations in rabbits with galactosamine-induced hepatic failure provided the initial support for this hypothesis. GABA originates from the intestine, and plasma levels increase in hepatic failure due to inadequate hepatic extraction. During acute liver failure, the blood-brain barrier becomes more permeable, and increased amounts of GABA enter the CNS. Once in the brain, GABA binds to its receptor to produce neuroinhibition and clinical encephalopathy. A key component to understanding the relationship of GABA and benzodiazepines was the recognition that the GABA receptor was tightly linked and

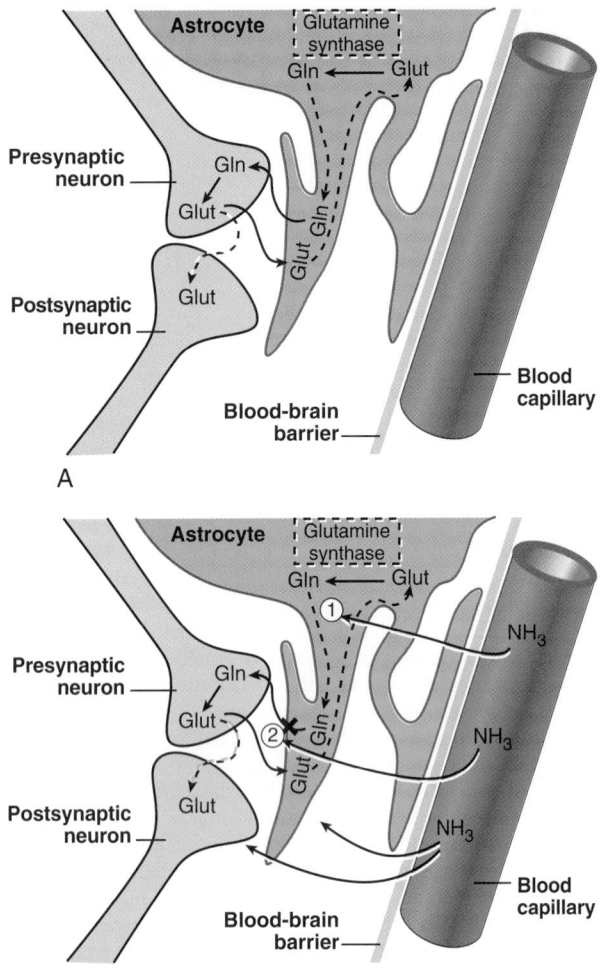

Figure 101-1 **A,** Glutamine forms predominantly in the astrocyte, is pumped out, and taken up by presynaptic neurons where it is converted to glutamate. Nerve stimulation releases glutamate from the presynaptic neuron to serve as an excitatory neurotransmitter. Astrocytes avidly take up glutamate from the synaptic cleft, to abolish neuronal stimulation. **B,** Ammonia freely diffuses across the blood-brain barrier and stimulates formation of glutamine by the astrocyte via the action of glutamine synthase (1). Ammonia also blocks the export of glutamine from the astrocyte at the synaptic cleft (2). The net effect of these two actions is increased concentration of glutamine within astrocytes, which promotes astrocyte swelling.

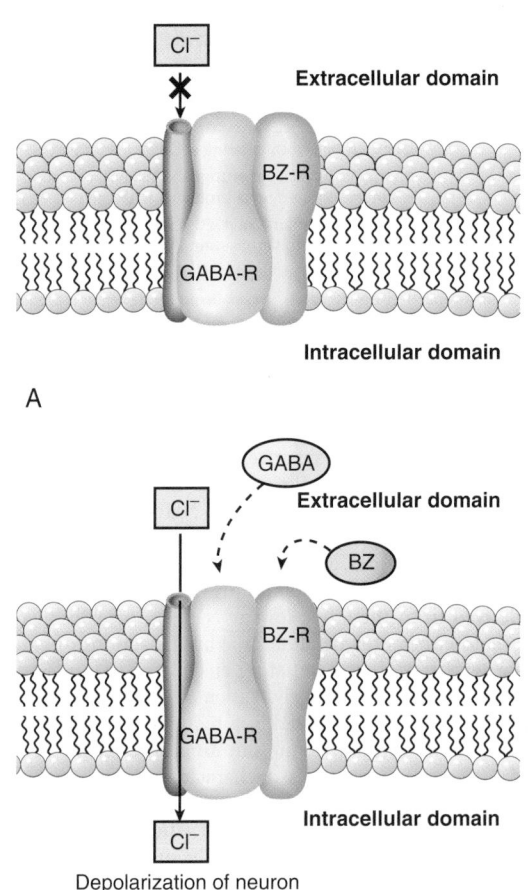

Figure 101-2 **A,** The GABA receptor complex is composed of the GABA receptor (GABA-R), central benzodiazepine receptor (BZ-R), and chloride channel (adjacent cylinder). **B,** Binding of GABA to GABA-R opens the chloride channel, depolarizes the neuronal membrane, and inhibits neurotransmission. Activation of the BZ-R by BZ or BZ-like compounds potentiates the binding of GABA to GABA-R.

modulated by the benzodiazepine receptor.[40-43] Binding of benzodiazepines to the benzodiazepine receptor induces a conformational change in the GABA receptor enhancing the binding of GABA and neuroinhibition. Activation of the GABA receptor opens a chloride channel, the third component of the GABA receptor complex (Figure 101-2). In summary, GABA-induced inhibition of neurotransmission is enhanced by binding of benzodiazepines or related compounds to the benzodiazepine receptor, increasing the number of GABA receptors, increasing the activity of the GABA receptor, or opening the GABA-associated chloride channel.

The GABA hypothesis predicts that benzodiazepines would increase the severity of hepatic encephalopathy, and benzodiazepine antagonists such as flumazenil might ameliorate hepatic encephalopathy. Clinical experience clearly suggests that cirrhotic patients, especially those with encephalopathy, are particularly sensitive to the amnesic and sedative effects of benzodiazepines. In our experience, use of benzodiazepines and other sedative/hypnotics is a common reason for exacerbations of hepatic encephalopathy. Recent studies have demonstrated that patients with hepatic encephalopathy have increased plasma levels of benzodiazepines or "natural" benzodiazepine-like compounds that then may act as "false neurotransmitters."[44-47] Some have suggested that patients with hepatic encephalopathy are particularly sensitive to GABA neuroinhibition, owing to an increase in background benzodiazepine stimulation of the GABA receptor.

DOPAMINERGIC SYSTEM

Patients with chronic hepatic encephalopathy often have abnormal motor function and can manifest signs such as tremor, slowness of gait, ataxia, and even rigidity. Although they typically lack other features of Parkinsonism (pill-rolling, resting tremor, mask-like facies, cogwheel rigidity), the motor abnormalities have prompted investigators to suggest that patients with hepatic encephalopathy may have impairment of the dopaminergic system. It is postulated that "false" neurotransmitters occupy dopaminergic binding sites within the CNS and inactivate and inhibit dopaminergic activity. However, clinical trials in humans have failed to provide much support for this hypothesis. Both levodopa (L-dopa) and bromocriptine, an L-dopa agonist, are ineffective therapies for PSE (see later discussion).

SEROTONERGIC SYSTEM

A number of alterations in CNS serotonin metabolism and/or signaling have been described in both humans and experimental animal models of hepatic encephalopathy. CNS levels of serotonin, serotonin receptors, and monoamine oxidases are increased. However, the exact role of serotonin in hepatic encephalopathy remains undefined.

TAURINE

Taurine is an inhibitory neurotransmitter which is increased in brains of animal models of experimental hepatic encephalopathy and in the CSF of primates with encephalopathy secondary to portocaval shunts. Plasma levels of taurine are greatest in patients with the greatest degrees of encephalopathy, suggesting that this inhibitory neurotransmitter may be involved in hepatic encephalopathy.[48] Additional neurotransmitters that may be altered in hepatic encephalopathy include endogenous opioids and melatonin.

METHANETHIOLS

Interest in methanethiol as a potential neurotoxin began with the finding of methanethiol in the urine of a patient with fetor hepaticus. Subsequently, levels of methanethiol, 4-methylthio-2-oxobutyrate, and methanethiol-mixed disulfides were found to be elevated in the plasma of cirrhotic patients.[49] It was suggested that these compounds may exacerbate the toxic effects of NH_3 and short-chain fatty acids. However, blood levels of methanethiols are similar in deeply comatose patients and those with only mild cerebral dysfunction, and there is little correlation between grade of encephalopathy blood levels of methanethiol.

FATTY ACIDS

Levels of short-chain fatty acids (SCFAs) are increased in the peripheral circulation of cirrhotic patients with hepatic encephalopathy. Normally the liver metabolizes these fatty acids after absorption from the gut, but this function is impaired in cirrhotics, and SCFA levels increase. The clinical severity of encephalopathy correlates poorly with plasma levels of acetic, propionic, butyric, valeric, and octanoic acids, and SCFAs have been administered to patients with cirrhosis without worsening of encephalopathy. SCFAs are not likely to cause hepatic encephalopathy.

MANGANESE, ZINC

The liver is responsible for manganese excretion, and liver disease is associated with manganese accumulation. Magnetic resonance imaging (MRI) studies of the brain in patients with cirrhosis reveal pallidal hyperintensity on T_1-weighted images (Figure 101-3), which correlates with the presence of extrapyramidal signs and symptoms and blood levels of manganese.[50] Manganese concentrations in the globus pallidus are markedly increased in autopsy studies of cirrhotics who died in hepatic coma. PET imaging reveals reduced cerebral glucose utilization in these areas. Such findings suggest a relationship between manganese, brain hypometabolism, and some of the neuropsychiatric and motor abnormalities of hepatic encephalopathy.

Zinc deficiency is common in long-standing cirrhosis. Its importance to the pathogenesis of hepatic encephalopathy is unknown, and three randomized controlled trials of zinc supplementation have yielded conflicting results as regards improvement in encephalopathy (one positive, two negative).[51-53]

Encephalopathy in the Setting of Acute Hepatic Failure

DEFINITION

Acute liver failure is defined by the development of coagulopathy (prothrombin time [PT] >20 sec prolonged with an international normalized ratio [INR] >1.5) in a patient with acute hepatitis who lacks underlying chronic liver disease (exception in Wilson's disease).[54-56]

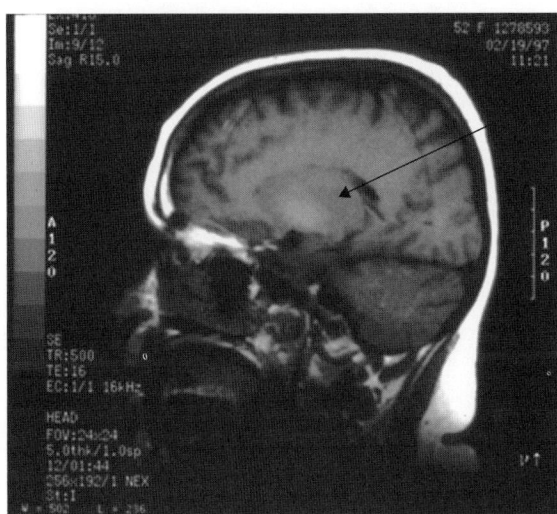

Figure 101-3 Magnetic resonance image (MRI) of a T_1-weighted sagittal view of the brain demonstrating hyperintensity of the globus pallidus (whitish area indicated by *arrow*) that may be related to manganese deposition.

Patients with acute liver failure usually have extreme elevations of aspartate aminotransferase (AST) and alanine aminotransferase (ALT) with the initial injury (1000 to 5000 IU/L), often are jaundiced, and exhibit constitutional symptoms. They are at risk for encephalopathy, although most recover uneventfully. Progressive hepatic encephalopathy is a poor prognostic sign and signals the need for hepatic transplantation.

ETIOLOGY

There are approximately 2000 cases of acute liver failure in the United States each year.[57,58] Among the most common causes are acetaminophen toxicity, other types of acute drug toxicity, and hepatitis A and B virus (HAV, HBV) infection. However, the second leading diagnostic category for fulminant hepatic failure (FHF) is cryptogenic, cause unknown (Table 101-2). Recent data obtained since 1998 indicate that over 50% of cases of FHF in the United States are due to acetaminophen overdosage (38%) or idiosyncratic drug reactions (~14%).[58] Many cases of acetaminophen-induced liver failure are due to "therapeutic misadventure" due to self-administration of as little as 4 grams/day over several days in the setting of fasting and alcohol use. Sporadic cases of FHF due to both cocaine and Ecstasy have recently been described. FHF from mushroom poisoning occasionally occurs with inexperienced amateur mushroom fanciers. Infiltration of the liver with rapid progression of tumor growth can lead to FHF and has been described for cases of metastatic breast carcinoma, lymphoma, and

TABLE 101-2	Causes of Acute Liver Failure	
Acetaminophen		20%
Cryptogenic		15%
Non-acetaminophen drug toxicity		12%
Hepatitis B		10%
Hepatitis A		7%
Autoimmune hepatitis		6%
Wilson's disease		6%
Miscellaneous*		24%

Adapted from Schiodt FV, Atillasoy E, Shakil O et al. Etiologic factors and outcome for 295 patients with acute liver failure in the United States. Liver Transplant Surg 1999;5: 29-34.

*Budd-Chiari syndrome, herpes simplex, paramyxovirus, Epstein-Barr virus, amanita poisoning, ischemia, malignant infiltration.

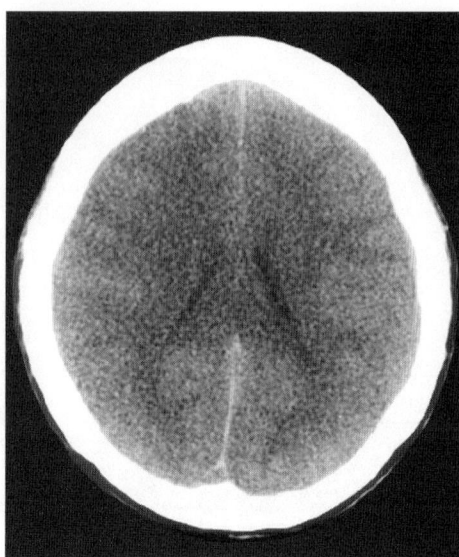

Figure 101-4 Computed tomographic (CT) scan of the brain of a patient with fulminant hepatic failure, stage IV hepatic coma, and cerebral edema. Note the diminished sulci and lack of distinction between white and grey matter. This patient resolved her cerebral edema with medical management and was subsequently transplanted. She achieved complete neurologic recovery post transplant.

Box 101-3

USE OF *N*-ACETYLCYSTEINE IN TREATMENT OF ACETAMINOPHEN OVERDOSE

Oral Dosing Schedule
1. Avoid use of activated charcoal, since it will bind *N*-acetylcysteine, reducing its efficacy.
2. Place nasogastric tube for administration of *N*-acetylcysteine. *N*-acetylcysteine is highly unpalatable; most patients cannot tolerate its oral administration. The NG tube is necessary to insure dosing of the medication.
3. Dosage: 140 mg/kg initially, followed by 70 mg/kg q 4 h, to a total of 17 doses of *N*-acetylcysteine.
4. Toxicity: nausea, vomiting.

Intravenous Dosing Schedule (Limited Availability in Research Centers)
1. Intravenous access for administration.
2. Obtain informed consent.
3. Dosage: Dilute in crystalloid solution to final concentration of 3%. Doses are infused over 1 hour through a 0.22-micron filter. Loading dose is 140 mg/kg initially, followed by 70 mg/kg q 4 h, to a total of 12 doses of *N*-acetylcysteine.
4. Adverse reactions occur in approximately 15%: flushing and transient skin rash (usually responds to diphenhydramine), wheezing, nausea, vomiting. Patient should be monitored for anaphylaxis (treat with epinephrine, H_1 and H_2 blockers, supportive care).

---

melanoma. Biopsy of the liver is required to establish the latter diagnoses. FHF also may occur in the third trimester of pregnancy, related to acute fatty liver of pregnancy, HELLP syndrome, or disseminated herpes infection.

PROGNOSIS

A major determinant of prognosis is the level of encephalopathy (see Table 101-1). Patients with acute liver failure who have progressed to higher stages of encephalopathy (stage III or IV) have the worst prognosis. Glasgow Coma Scale is useful in assessing need for transplantation.[59] Cerebral edema on computed tomography (CT) scan of the brain is a late feature of progressive encephalopathy (Figure 101-4). Additional clinical features that indicate a poor prognosis include metabolic acidosis, renal failure, severe jaundice, or markedly prolonged prothrombin time.[56,59-60] The likelihood of survival varies with the cause of acute liver injury. Patients with acetaminophen overdose have a relatively favorable outcome, and over 50% survive.[61] Patients with fulminant HAV and HBV infection have an intermediate prognosis, and 30% to 50%[62] survive. In contrast, patients with a fulminant presentation of Wilson's disease or severe sporadic non-A, non-B, non-C hepatitis have a survival of less than 10%.[63]

GENERAL CLINICAL MANAGEMENT

Once recognized, patients with acute liver failure with encephalopathy should be transferred to a center with expertise in managing hepatic failure where liver transplantation can be offered if indicated.

All patients should be placed on needle (HBV, NANBV) and stool (HAV) precautions but not in isolation. Gloves should be worn when handling biological specimens, and specimens should be clearly labeled (Hepatitis Patient). All used instruments should be autoclaved or appropriately disposed. FHF due to acute viral hepatitis is not reversible by antiviral therapy, although some advocate use of lamivudine or related drugs for severe acute HBV. Corticosteroids are contraindicated, as they may increase the risk of developing chronic hepatitis and are ineffective in treatment of encephalopathy or cerebral edema in this setting. Removal of the offending drug, toxin, or alcohol is the mainstay of therapy of drug-induced and alcoholic hepatitis,

respectively. *N*-acetylcysteine is an effective primary intervention for hepatic injury related to acetaminophen[64] and is currently under investigation in the treatment of FHF due to other etiologies (Box 101-3).

The coagulopathy of acute liver failure is due to depletion of clotting factors related to inadequate hepatic production. Some patients exhibit features of disseminated intravascular coagulation or primary fibrinolysis. Once the patient is diagnosed with severe acute liver failure or fulminant hepatic failure, we recommend administration of Mephyton (vitamin K) 10 mg/d subcutaneously (SQ) for 3 days. Prophylactic infusions of clotting factors are of unproven benefit. Use of clotting factors such as fresh frozen plasma, cryoprecipitate, activated factor VII, and platelets should be restricted to ongoing bleeding such as GI hemorrhage, or for invasive procedures such as placement of an intracranial monitor. Prophylaxis against peptic disease and GI bleeding with proton-pump inhibitors is recommended.

Infection is a leading comorbidity in patients with acute liver failure.[56-60] Blood, urine, and sputum should be cultured frequently (even in absence of fever or other signs of infection) and antibiotic therapy instituted only for positive cultures and directed against specific organisms. Fever is not a feature of most forms of acute liver injury and if present usually signifies concurrent infection. Febrile patients should be cultured immediately and treated empirically with antibiotics. The most common sources of infection are the respiratory tract, the urinary tract, and line sepsis. Currently, we use vancomycin with a broad-spectrum cephalosporin such as cefotaxime or a fluoroquinolone such as levofloxacin as initial treatment, and then tailor antibiotic use once results of cultures are known.

▣ Use of Intracranial Pressure Monitoring

ADVANTAGES

The use of ICP monitoring for managing high-grade encephalopathy in acute liver failure remains controversial. Several studies advocate ICP monitoring for its ability to provide important prognostic information about neurologic recovery after hepatic transplantation and in managing intracranial hypertension (ICH) while awaiting liver transplantation.[65-67] Therefore, ICP monitoring could be considered for patients with high-grade encephalopathy (stage III or IV) who are waiting on the transplant list. Also, centers could consider ICP monitoring in nontransplant candidates if there is a reasonable likelihood of spontaneous recovery, such as in acetaminophen-induced acute liver failure. In addition to helping with the management of ICH, ICP monitoring also assists with close monitoring during the crucial perioperative period of liver transplantation, since it has been found that there is a transient increase in ICP that can last for about 12 hours postoperatively, after the dissection of native liver and the reperfusion of the graft.[68]

DISADVANTAGES

However, the use of ICP monitoring may lead to severe complications such as intracranial hemorrhage in these already critically ill patients. In addition, several nonrandomized studies have failed to demonstrate an improvement in survival with the use of ICP monitoring.[65-67] One prospective study of 92 out of 332 patients with acute liver failure, high-grade encephalopathy, and ICP monitoring found a 10.3% rate of intracranial hemorrhage.[67] However, nearly half of the cases of intracranial bleeding were incidental radiographic findings without clinical consequence. Regardless of ICP use, 30-day survival post transplant was approximately 85%. Other reports confirm that bleeding complications from the placement of ICP monitoring devices in patients with acute liver failure are mostly mild and without clinical significance.[65-67,69] Use of ICP monitoring remains controversial, but experts agree that these devices should not be used in patients with mild hepatic encephalopathy (grades I or II) or in patients with evidence of cerebral herniation, hypotension, or imminent death.

Management of Encephalopathy and Intracranial Hypertension

Encephalopathy is a hallmark of acute liver failure. It is also observed in patients with underlying chronic liver disease who sustain superimposed acute liver injury. The encephalopathy of acute hepatic failure is related to both metabolic factors, such as progressive elevation in blood NH_3 concentration, and cerebral edema. Progressively worsening encephalopathy is an ominous clinical feature; development of grade III or IV encephalopathy may herald the death of the patient due to cerebral edema, increased ICP, and central herniation of the brain. Efforts to control the encephalopathy of acute liver failure are directed at preventing or resolving cerebral edema (Box 101-4).[16,67,70-73] Because emerging evidence suggests that NH_3 may play a role in the development of cerebral edema, we recommend that administration of protein should be limited to less than 40 grams/d in adults, and lactulose (20-40 g/d in divided doses) should be administered enterally to purge the bowel. However, one must exercise caution when using lactulose in the setting of FHF; dosing should be monitored carefully and adjusted to avoid excessive diarrhea and alterations in electrolytes and volume depletion. If oral (PO) lactulose is given simultaneously with intravenous (IV) mannitol, marked deficits of free water can develop, inducing severe hypernatremia. Although one recent study suggested that infusion of hypertonic (3%) saline to maintain serum sodium concentration between 145 and 155 mEq/L is beneficial,[74] rapid shifts in sodium concentration have been associated with central pontine myelinolysis. Further discussion of hypertonic saline is provided later in this chapter. Administration of terlipressin or vasopressin may worsen intracranial hypertension and should be avoided.[75]

Reversal of coagulopathy (PT/INR < 1.5, platelets > 60,000/μL) prior to placement of ICP transducers is recommended. However, reversal of coagulopathy may be difficult and require large volumes of fresh frozen plasma (FFP), potentially contributing to volume overload and worsening of cerebral edema. Recombinant human factor VIIa infusion (40 μg/kg bolus, repeated as needed every 4 hours to correct INR) may be preferred over FFP in this setting by limiting volume infusion and rapidly correcting the PT/INR.

Box 101-4

MEASURES USED TO MONITOR AND CONTROL CEREBRAL EDEMA DUE TO FULMINANT HEPATIC FAILURE

1. Correction of metabolic abnormalities.
   - Electrolytes (Na, K, Cl, HCO_3).
   - Acid-base (if patient is on mechanical ventilation, induce mild respiratory alkalosis).
   - Glucose (maintenance intravenous glucose infusion).
2. Avoid overtransfusion or overhydration.
   - Carefully match intake and output once patient is euvolemic.
   - Daily weight.
   - Avoid use of blood products unless indicated for ongoing bleeding and correction of coagulopathy or to maintain hemostasis when intracranial monitor has been placed. In the latter circumstance, the patient may require diuresis to avoid an excess intravascular volume, especially from plasma.
3. Institute dialysis in patients in renal failure.
   - Continuous arteriovenous or venovenous hemodialysis is preferred over standard hemodialysis.
   - Avoid severe volume shifts, stabilize blood pressure, maintain euvolemia, correct electrolyte and acid-base abnormalities.
4. Mechanical ventilation (worsening encephalopathy, >grade II).
   - Main indication in liver failure is airway protection to prevent aspiration pneumonia.
   - Induce mild respiratory alkalosis (pH 7.45-7.50, PCO_2 20-30 mm Hg).
   - Elevate head of bed 15-30 degrees.
   - Use sedation to avoid having the patient "fight the ET tube."
5. Consider placement of intracranial pressure (ICP) monitor in the epidural space.
   - Should be considered when patients evolve from stage II (agitated confusion) to stage III (stuporous) encephalopathy.
   - Maintain adequate platelet count (>60,000) with platelet transfusions and INR <1.5 with fresh frozen plasma if necessary.
   - Mannitol is used to control ICP in patients with intact renal function or in those on dialysis. Mannitol is given in 0.5-1 g/kg doses. Serum electrolytes, glucose, and osmolarity should be checked every 4-6 hours. If ICP elevated, osmolarity < 310, and Na < 145, then give mannitol. Mannitol should be held if the patient has excessive serum osmolarity or significant hypernatremia.

Hepatic glycogen, the main storage supply of glucose, is depleted early in the course of acute liver failure, predisposing to severe, potentially life-threatening hypoglycemia and worsening of cerebral energy metabolism. All patients with acute liver failure should be treated with glucose infusions, and blood glucose concentration must be monitored frequently.

SECOND-LINE THERAPIES FOR TREATMENT OF MANNITOL-REFRACTORY INTRACRANIAL HYPERTENSION

Hypothermia in ALF

Therapeutic hypothermia or intentional reduction of body core temperature has been increasingly used to treat hypoxic brain injury after cardiac arrest as well as in the traumatic setting. Animal models of acute liver failure suggest that hypothermia may be effective in the prevention of cerebral edema.[76-78] Several case reports suggest that hypothermia can be used as an effective form of supportive therapy while awaiting liver transplantation.

A series of cases reported by Jalan et al. demonstrated that use of hypothermia in 38 patients with acute liver failure and uncontrolled

ICH reduced cerebral edema and ICP.[24,79-83] In these studies, patients had high-grade hepatic encephalopathy (grades III or IV) and ICP above 25 mm Hg despite two doses of mannitol. Body temperature reduction to 32°C to 33°C for 8 to 14 hours decreased mean ICP from 45 to 16 mm Hg, and cerebral blood flow dropped from 103 to 44 mL/100 g/min. Cerebral perfusion pressure increased from 45 to 70 mm Hg. Unfortunately, those who were not deemed transplant candidates died after rewarming. Later cases showed similar findings and support the notion that hypothermia provides some neurologic benefits in transplant candidates. Although these studies show potential benefit, a randomized controlled trial to further validate the use of hypothermia is still needed to define its role.

Hypertonic Saline in ALF

Another possible method to treat refractory ICH during acute liver failure is hypertonic saline. There has been great concern for the use of hypertonic saline because of the potential consequence of osmotic shifts across the blood-brain barrier (BBB). However, a presumed advantage for hypertonic saline to treat ICH is a higher osmotic reflection coefficient across the BBB.[84-86] Thus, hypertonic saline could potentially lead to edema reduction, lower ICPs, and better perfusion by developing a higher osmotic gradient in the cerebral vascular compartment. In a randomized placebo-controlled study, Murphy et al. studied the effect of hypertonic saline infusion on ICP and clinical outcomes among ICU patients with acute liver failure.[74] Thirty patients were treated with hypertonic saline 30% (5-20 mL/hour) to maintain serum sodium levels at 145 to 155 mmol/L. After 24 to 72 hours, ICP was significantly lower in the treated group ($P = 0.04$) compared to the standard care group. However, high osmolar loads and continuous hemofiltration were required, and mortality was similar among the treated and standard care groups. The use of hypertonic saline in the management of ICH in acute liver failure warrants further investigation.

L-Ornithine-L-Aspartate (LOLA)

As already stated earlier in the chapter, NH_3 is thought to be a key neurotoxin in acute liver failure. Higher blood levels of NH_3 have been correlated with higher mortality, higher grades of hepatic encephalopathy, increased frequency of ICH, and severe complications. L-Ornithine-L-aspartate (LOLA) may be useful for both acute and chronic hepatic encephalopathy. This compound salt has been found to reduce NH_3 levels by increasing NH_3 disposal through enhanced peripheral metabolism.[87] LOLA increases the activity of hepatic urea cycle enzymes and also increases the rate of glutamine production within skeletal muscle.

The largest randomized controlled trial to test the efficacy of LOLA in high-grade encephalopathy on patients with acute liver failure was performed by Acharya et al.[87]; 201 patients with acute liver failure were randomized to either standard of care or LOLA (30 g daily infusion for 3 days). The primary endpoint, mortality, was not improved by LOLA (RR 1.27, $P = 0.204$). In a multivariate analysis, only blood NH_3 level was an independent predictor of survival, and this parameter also was not significantly affected by treatment with LOLA. Accordingly, LOLA is not currently recommended in the management of severe encephalopathy from acute liver failure.

OTHER OPTIONS FOR REFRACTORY ICH

Other potential therapies that can be considered in acute liver failure patients with refractory ICH include pentobarbital or thiopental and indomethacin. By inducing a comatose state and reducing cerebral edema, barbiturates such as pentobarbital (3-5 mg/kg IV load, then 1-3 mg/kg/h infusion) or thiopental (5-10 mg/kg load, then 3-5 mg/kg/h infusion) have been shown to have some benefit in refractory ICH.[65-67,88] However, severe side effects such as arterial hypotension, hypokalemia, and prolonged coma limit their use. These medications also often require coadministration of vasopressors in order to maintain cerebral perfusion pressure above 50 mm Hg, and require a

provider to have prior experience using these drugs. Indomethacin (dosed at 25 mg IV over 1 minute) also has the potential to cause an acute decrease in ICP and an acute increase in CPP by causing cerebral vasoconstriction. Therefore, these medications may also play a role as second- or third-line options for patients with persistent refractory ICH.[65,89-90]

EXPERIMENTAL THERAPIES

Several other methods have been tested in FHF: exchange blood transfusion, plasmapheresis, cross-circulation with human and baboon donors, hemoperfusion through isolated human or animal livers, hemodialysis (conventional and polyacrylonitrate), and column hemoperfusion (microencapsulated charcoal, albumin-covered Amberlite XAD-7 resin). Only exchange transfusion and charcoal hemoperfusion have been evaluated in controlled trials, and these studies found that mortality was either similar or greater in the treated groups. Since none of these techniques has been demonstrated to improve survival, their use in FHF is not currently recommended (unless under IRB-approved protocols in major liver centers).

Albumin Dialysis

Stange et al. recently reported use of an extracorporeal liver assist device based on albumin dialysis (MARS) in 26 patients with chronic liver disease who had either acute or chronic liver failure.[91] The treatments lowered plasma bilirubin and bile acid levels, but the effect on clinical outcome was unclear: nine patients with advanced liver disease died within an average of 15 days, but the remainder survived and were thought to have benefited. Further studies will be needed to define benefit and overall utility.

Bioartificial Liver

Bioartificial liver (BAL) machines recently have emerged as potential therapeutic interventions in the treatment of FHF. The major principal of BAL is the use of a "bioreactor" which contains liver cells external to the dialytic tubing in a dialysis cartridge through which blood or plasma flows. The liver cells used in these reactors vary from primary porcine hepatocytes to transformed human hepatocyte-like cells (HepG2-C3A). "Toxins" or metabolites diffuse across the capillary membrane, where the liver cells can remove, metabolize, or inactivate them. Experimental models suggest that removal of toxins and metabolites may reduce the neurotoxicity of FHF by inhibiting the formation of cerebral edema. In clinical terms, the goal is stabilization of neurologic function to allow for hepatic regeneration or to bridge the patient to liver transplantation. To date, there has been only one large randomized multicenter trial of the use of BAL in acute liver failure.

Demetriou et al. reported the results of multicenter randomized controlled trial of a porcine hepatocyte-based BAL in 171 patients with acute liver failure (n = 147) and primary nonfunction after liver transplantation (n = 24).[92] In both the group as a whole and the subgroup of acute liver failure, 30-day patient survival was slightly, but insignificantly, higher in the BAL group (entire cohort: 71% versus 62%, P = NS; acute liver failure: 73% versus 59%, P = NS). A major confounding variable in this study was the overwhelmingly positive effect of hepatic transplantation. Transplanted patients (55% of cohort) experienced a 70% reduction in relative risk (RR) of death ($P < .0001$). Additional analysis of survival in the subgroup of patients with acute liver failure, after controlling for impact of transplantation, suggested survival benefit for BAL-treated patients (RR death = 0.56, $P = 0.048$). Although this initial report is encouraging, additional studies will be needed to determine the efficacy and role of BAL in treatment of acute liver failure.

Hepatocyte Transplantation

The principals guiding use of hepatocyte transplantation are similar to those of the bioartificial liver: provide support during a period of critical need so the patient can be bridged to recovery or transplantation.[93-95] One potential advantage of hepatocyte transplantation is the ability of liver stem cells to regenerate, raising the potential for repopulation of a dying or dead liver by allogeneic donor hepatocytes. The latter theoretical consideration has not been proven in humans with acute liver failure. Experience with hepatocyte transplantation in FHF is limited. Our center reported the outcome of six patients who were not candidates for liver transplantation due to active substance abuse or prohibitive underlying medical illness, and one patient listed for transplantation who had disseminated herpes infection. Despite a suggestion of improvement in neurologic status after hepatocyte transplantation, all seven died. Currently, hepatocyte transplantation for acute liver failure should be viewed as unproven and experimental.

LIVER TRANSPLANTATION

Liver transplantation is the only treatment that has been proven to improve survival in patients with acute liver failure and grade III or IV encephalopathy.[7] Survival without transplantation is 10% to 20%. Survival increases to 60% to 80% with liver transplantation. In the study of BAL by Demetriou et al. noted above, the survival of patients with acute liver failure who underwent hepatic transplantation was 92%.[92]

Resolution of Cerebral Edema

At some stage, cerebral edema is irreversible and patients, despite transplantation, will experience brain death or massive irreversible brain injury.[96-97] Risk of irreversible neurologic injury is greatest in those with CPP less than 40 mm Hg for more than 4 hours. Lesser increases in ICP may be associated with neurologic injury, but usually the cerebral edema resolves in the posttransplant period, and complete or partial neurologic recovery may be expected. In most cases of acute liver failure, all the manifestations of the neurologic illness (cerebral edema, encephalopathy, coma) totally reverse without sequelae following successful hepatic transplantation. One complication, central pontine myelinolysis, may occur in the absence of cerebral edema and may be related to fluctuations in plasma sodium during resuscitative measures in the ICU, such as IV fluids, transfusions, antibiotics, sedatives, narcotics, invasive procedures, and ventilatory support. Central pontine myelinolysis may result in significant neurologic impairment, requiring prolonged support and rehabilitation (physical therapy, speech therapy). Despite the serious nature of central pontine myelinolysis , significant neurologic recovery can occur.[98]

Living Donor Liver Transplantation

Donor safety is a major concern in the performance of living donor liver transplantation (LDLT). Current statistics suggest that donor mortality is approximately 0.13% for adult-to-pediatric cases and 0.25% for adult-to-adult cases.[99] This procedure should be used with caution and only performed by centers with extensive experience and expertise in hepatic transplantation and liver resection.

Experience with LDLT for acute liver failure is limited worldwide. Japan has reported the largest number of LDLT cases for acute liver failure, largely because more than 99% of all liver transplants in Japan are from living donors.[100] In the largest series of LDLT for acute liver failure, Lee et al. report patient survival as 82.3% at 1 and 5 years after transplantation for 57 recipients.[101] These results are similar to those of cadaveric transplantation for acute liver failure and also demonstrate the durability of living donor allografts.

Encephalopathy in the Setting of Chronic Liver Disease

Patients with cirrhosis of any cause and chronic PSE may present with a host of neuropsychiatric symptoms, ranging from subtle changes in mental status to coma.[1-3] Fetor hepaticus is common but not invariable. Asterixis, the "flapping tremor," is due to involuntary intermittent relaxation of sustained motor activity, but is less specific than fetor hepaticus for hepatic encephalopathy and is usually only present during the late stages of encephalopathy. Asterixis is most easily elicited with the patient's arm outstretched, fingers separated, and wrists hyperextended. Although reported, cerebral edema rarely occurs in patients with encephalopathy in the setting of chronic liver disease. As the patient recovers from hepatic encephalopathy, asterixis and other manifestations of encephalopathy disappear.

RISK FACTORS AND PRECIPITATING EVENTS: IMPLICATIONS FOR DIAGNOSTIC TESTING AND TREATMENT

Flares of chronic encephalopathy may occur spontaneously, without an identifiable precipitant, in patients with very severe hepatic impairment and extensive portosystemic shunting. However, in the majority of cases, acute worsening of chronic encephalopathy is precipitated by one or more of a number of common events.

Gastrointestinal Hemorrhage

Hemodynamically significant GI hemorrhage is a major precipitant of hepatic encephalopathy. Delivery of a large protein load to the GI tract via hemorrhage stimulates bacterial metabolism of luminal blood and release of NH_3, GABA, and other chemicals or compounds that may inhibit neurotransmission. Poor hepatic function or shunting of portal blood via portosystemic collaterals impairs hepatic clearance and enhances delivery of these molecules to the brain. Rapid diagnosis and treatment of GI hemorrhage requires urgent esophagogastroduodenoscopy (EGD), initiation of endoscopic therapy, and administration of a somatostatin analog (octreotide) or other vasoactive treatments. TIPS may be used to control recalcitrant hemorrhage, but encephalopathy may worsen after this procedure.

Infection

Infection, in particular sepsis, may precipitate hepatic encephalopathy in patients with chronic liver disease. Spontaneous bacterial peritonitis (SBP) always should be considered in the differential diagnosis of patients with ascites and new onset of encephalopathy. Fever may be absent, and clinical signs (abdominal pain, ileus) may be lacking. SBP is presumptively diagnosed if the absolute neutrophil count in ascites fluid exceeds 250 cells/mL. Patients with cirrhosis and malnutrition are susceptible to infections due to reduced leukocyte migration, decreased serum bactericidal activity, depressed white cell mobilization, and impaired phagocytosis. Infection increases protein catabolism, releasing aromatic amino acids that may contribute to the encephalopathy. Primary therapy is directed against the infection.

Medications (Sedatives)

There are no safe sedatives for administration to cirrhotic patients who have hepatic encephalopathy. Because liver metabolism is usually severely impaired in these patients, the clearances of benzodiazepines, barbiturates, chlorpromazine, morphine, and opioid derivatives such as methadone, meperidine, and codeine are reduced. With repeated dosing, all these compounds tend to accumulate in cirrhotic patients, increasing the degree and prolonging the duration of sedation.

Renal Failure

A common precipitant of hepatic encephalopathy is excessive diuresis, resulting in relative depletion of intravascular volume and prerenal azotemia. Factors contributing to the encephalopathy include: electrolyte imbalances, disordered acid-base metabolism, reduced fluid volume, and impaired renal clearance of metabolites, drugs, and toxins. Acute decompensation of intrinsic or chronic renal disease may be another cause of encephalopathy. Certain renal disorders have a predilection to occur in the setting of liver disease: IgA nephropathy (Laënnec's), membranoproliferative glomerulonephritis (viral hepatitis), nephrolithiasis (primary sclerosing cholangitis with inflammatory bowel disease), medullary sponge kidney (congenital hepatic fibrosis), and autosomal dominant polycystic kidney (polycystic liver).

Fluid, Electrolyte, and Acid-Base Imbalance

Hepatic encephalopathy may be precipitated by dehydration, hypokalemia, and alkalosis. Metabolic alkalosis promotes an increase in levels of nonionic NH_3, which diffuses very rapidly into the CNS. Diffusion of NH_3 into the brain and enhanced glutamine production may precipitate encephalopathy due to either astrocyte swelling and dysfunction or impairment of glutamatergic neurotransmission. With hepatic impairment, the kidneys produce glucose from branched-chain amino acids (gluconeogenesis) in an attempt to maintain peripheral energy supply. This process results in decreased circulating levels of branched-chain amino acids and an increase in the circulating levels of the relatively more toxic aromatic amino acids, which may diffuse into the brain.

Hepatocellular Carcinoma

Hepatocellular carcinoma commonly occurs in cirrhotic patients (estimated risk of 1%-3% per year) and may be heralded by the onset of spontaneous encephalopathy, usually in association with portal vein thrombosis. When evaluating a patient with encephalopathy, the diagnosis of hepatocellular carcinoma should be entertained, and α-fetoprotein and imaging studies of liver (ultrasound, CT scan, MRI) performed.

Surgical Shunt Procedure or TIPS

Hepatic encephalopathy is a common complication of portal diversion following surgical portal-systemic shunts or TIPS (see Table 101-3).[102-103] Predictors of post-shunt encephalopathy include pre-shunt encephalopathy, severe liver disease (Child-Pugh score > 10 or Model-for-End-Stage-Liver-Disease [MELD] score > 15), poor clearance of indocyanine green and lidocaine, and elderly age. The mechanisms of hepatic encephalopathy after placement of a portal-systemic shunt include: lack of compensatory dilatation of the hepatic artery, lack of perfusion of the liver via the portal vein, and reduction in hepatocyte function. Clinically apparent encephalopathy after placement of a shunt usually responds to medical treatment (low-protein diet, lactulose, neomycin). In rare circumstances, narrowing of the shunt with a flow-reducing stent or occlusion of the shunt may be necessary to control encephalopathy.[104]

Noncompliance with Therapy

One of the most common factors precipitating encephalopathy is noncompliance to prescribed outpatient medical treatments (e.g., lactulose and neomycin). A careful history, focusing on adherence to medical therapy, is necessary in the evaluation of encephalopathic patients.

DIAGNOSIS

The diagnosis of PSE is based upon clinical suspicion in patients with chronic liver disease, and the impression is confirmed by resolution following medical therapy. Occasionally it may be necessary to employ additional testing to confirm the diagnosis of PSE. Additional testing is particularly useful when encephalopathy is the primary clinical manifestation of otherwise unsuspected liver disease, or if the manifestations of encephalopathy are predominantly a change in behavior or an unusual neurologic syndrome (seizures, focal neurologic deficits). Rarely, cerebral edema complicates chronic liver disease.[105]

Plasma Ammonia

Elevated blood NH_3 level is common in cirrhotic patients, especially those with encephalopathy. Some studies have demonstrated a correlation between blood NH_3 levels and the presence and grade of encephalopathy, while others have not. In general, blood NH_3 levels might be useful as a marker of liver disease but are of little diagnostic or clinical value in managing the cirrhotic patient with hepatic encephalopathy.

CSF Glutamine

Chronic elevation in NH_3 level leads to accumulation of glutamine in the CNS. CSF glutamine may be useful in confusing cases where the diagnosis of high-grade (III or IV) hepatic encephalopathy is uncertain or questionable. A normal CSF glutamine level would virtually exclude the diagnosis; increased CSF glutamine concentration could provide evidence in favor of the diagnosis.

Electroencephalography

Electroencephalographic (EEG) abnormalities are relatively nonspecific in hepatic encephalopathy, and are similar to changes observed in patients with other causes of metabolic encephalopathy. Two findings have some specificity as regards hepatic encephalopathy: reduced brainstem auditory-evoked potentials and diminished visual-evoked potentials. In various studies, the percentage of encephalopathic cirrhotics with EEG abnormalities is highly variable, ranging from 14% to 78% of patients. Despite this variation in sensitivity, EEG findings are objective and can be used as an endpoint of response to therapy or medical interventions.

Radiologic Imaging

Standard CT scans or nuclear brain scans exhibit little or no specific distinguishing features, although loss of cortical volume may be common in patients with Laënnec's cirrhosis and chronic encephalopathy. CT may be used to document cerebral edema or to exclude CNS complications such as tumor, infection, or hemorrhage. MRI imaging studies have revealed a few features relatively unique to hepatic encephalopathy. One feature, hyperintensity on T_1-weighted images of the globus pallidus (see Figure 101-3), correlates with (extrapyramidal) motor disorders and excess accumulation of manganese.

Neuropsychiatric Testing

In general, neuropsychiatric testing is used primarily to follow efficacy of treatment. A battery of tests is employed to distinguish hepatic encephalopathy and organic brain syndrome from other causes of encephalopathy and underlying psychiatric disease. These tests are itemized in Table 101-3. Poor performance on number connection tests correlates reasonably well with severity of encephalopathy and Child-Pugh and/or MELD classification.

THERAPEUTIC OPTIONS

Traditional treatment for hepatic encephalopathy has included a protein-restricted diet of 40 grams or less per day.[106-108] However, cirrhotic patients often develop severe muscle wasting; thus, in patients with advanced disease, unnecessary protein restriction might further worsen the poor nutritional state. Most hepatologists currently avoid

TABLE 101-3	Neuropsychiatric Tests Used to Evaluate Hepatic Encephalopathy
Cerebral Function	**Test**
Learning and delayed recall	Story Memory Test Figure Memory Test
Concentration	Digit Vigilance Test
Fine motor coordination	Grooved Pegboard
Sequential procedures	Trail Making Test
Problem solving	Wisconsin Card Sorting Test
Attention	WAIS-R* Digit Symbol Subtest
Vocabulary	WAIS-R Vocabulary Subtest
Verbal fluency skills	Controlled Oral Word Association Animal Naming
Auditory comprehension	Complex Material
Visual-spatial analysis	WAIS-R Block Design Subtest
Psychological function	MMPI-2†

*WAIS-R, Wechsler Adult Intelligence Scale–Revised
†MMPI-2, Minnesota Multiphasic Personality Inventory

use of protein restriction in management of chronic hepatic encephalopathy.

Branched-Chain Amino Acids

Early studies demonstrated that cirrhotic patients had an increase in aromatic amino acids and a decrease in branched-chain amino acids (BCAAs) in blood samples. Subsequent clinical work suggested that patients with the greatest imbalance in plasma amino acids were more likely to be encephalopathic and to experience early and higher mortality. For this reason, there have been at least 14 controlled trials of the use of BCAAs in the treatment of cirrhotic patients with chronic encephalopathy. A recent well-controlled trial suggested efficacy.[109-110] However, results of these trials have been inconsistent, and separate meta-analyses yielded opposite conclusions regarding efficacy.[108,111] In addition, BCAA preparations are much more expensive than standard amino acid supplements. A trial of BCAA might be considered in patients who develop encephalopathy on standard protein diets and manifest protein-calorie malnutrition. BCAA supplements may allow adequate protein intake in this select group of patients without increasing the frequency of attacks of encephalopathy.

Total Parenteral Nutrition

It is common for the wasted, cirrhotic patient to be considered for total parenteral nutrition (TPN). However, use of TPN is often inappropriate, expensive, and associated with other complications (electrolyte imbalances, fluid overload, and infection). In most cases, TPN should be avoided and enteral feedings used in its place, but care must be taken to avoid high enteral osmotic loads which may precipitate diarrhea as well as fluid and electrolyte imbalances. In addition, many enteral preparations are relatively high in protein for the amount of calories delivered. Occasionally, TPN is indicated when adequate calories cannot be delivered by the enteral route or when concurrent disease (infection, diarrhea, bowel obstruction, forced purgation) exists and complicates the use of the enteral route for nutritional support.

Lactulose

One of the most successful treatments for hepatic encephalopathy is lactulose, a nonabsorbable disaccharide which is fermented by bacteria in the intestine to yield acetic, butyric, propionic, and lactic acids.[112-116] The fermentation of lactulose produces an acidic milieu that alters the composition of the bacterial flora, lowers colonic pH, and produces an osmotic diarrhea. Each of these effects may be responsible for the ameliorative effects of lactulose on hepatic encephalopathy. Changing the composition of the bacterial flora may alter the metabolism of fecal contents and reduce the production of toxins, NH_3, and methanethiols that are responsible for the encephalopathy. The acidic luminal milieu creates an environment capable of trapping NH_3:

$$NH_3 + H^+ \Rightarrow NH_4^+$$

Ammonia is neutral and freely diffuses across the mucosal barrier of the colon, where it then can enter portal blood for delivery to the body. In contrast, the ammonium ion (NH_4^+) produced from the reaction of NH_3 with hydrogen ions is ionized, highly polar, and unable to diffuse readily across the lipid bilayer of mucosal cells. The ammonium ion is "trapped" in the fecal effluent and eliminated with passage of the bowel movement. In addition to these properties, the breakdown of each molecule of lactulose produces at least four osmotically active particles. Water diffuses into the lumen, down the osmotic gradient, increasing fecal water content, and if enough lactulose is given a dose-dependent osmotic diarrhea results. The purgative effect of lactulose also may be responsible for altering the composition of colonic bacteria and helps to eliminate toxins and wastes that might otherwise accumulate. The usual recommendation is that enough lactulose be given to produce two to three loose, semiformed stools each day. Excessive dosing with lactulose will produce severe diarrhea with large volume losses and electrolyte imbalances and should be avoided.

Neomycin

Neomycin is highly nephrotoxic and should never be given IV or parenterally. Orally administered neomycin, on the other hand, is poorly absorbed and has a limited entrance to the circulation and is therefore much less nephrotoxic. The goal of therapy with oral neomycin is to alter the bacterial composition of the colonic flora. The major advantage of neomycin over lactulose is that it does not cause diarrhea. The main disadvantage is that despite its poor absorption, some neomycin does gain entry to the body which can contribute to nephrotoxicity. We recommend use of neomycin in patients who are intolerant of lactulose (usually due to diarrhea). Also, we may add neomycin to a lactulose-based regimen to improve efficacy for controlling encephalopathy.[8,117-119] Some have recommended that neomycin be given in short courses lasting only 2 to 8 weeks.

Metronidazole

Studies have demonstrated that oral metronidazole (500 mg to 1.5 g/d given for 1 week) was well tolerated, safe (no obvious neurotoxicity), and as effective as neomycin or lactulose in controlling encephalopathy. Others have not observed similar efficacy and have measured little effect of metronidazole on blood NH_3 levels.[119] The advantages of metronidazole are that it does not cause diarrhea and it is not nephrotoxic. A disadvantage is that many patients complain of epigastric discomfort with its use (poor compliance with long-term treatment). Maintenance therapy can be expected to cause peripheral neuropathy (already a problem in patients with advanced liver disease), and metronidazole has been reported to cause the "disulfiram reaction" when alcohol is consumed. The physician prescribing metronidazole to cirrhotic patients also should be aware that this drug undergoes extensive hepatic metabolism. One study of cirrhotics with encephalopathy revealed a threefold reduction in hepatic elimination and maintenance of therapeutic levels with as little as 500 mg given every 24 to 48 hours.

Helicobacter pylori

Published reports have suggested that *Helicobacter pylori* infections might increase blood NH_3 levels and precipitate hepatic encephalopathy in patients with cirrhosis. Controlled trials of interventions to eradicate *H. pylori* have failed to confirm this initial observation.[120-122]

Dopaminergic Agents

One of the theories regarding the pathogenesis of encephalopathy is that cirrhotic patients may have a relative deficiency of dopaminergic activity within the CNS. There have been three trials using L-dopa and the dopaminergic compound, bromocriptine, to treat hepatic encephalopathy. These studies were conducted in patients with chronic PSE and indicated that L-dopa was ineffective in improving clinical encephalopathy, EEG, and encephalopathy scores. However, L-dopa was also associated with impaired bowel motility and caused obstipation, an effect which counteracted the potentially beneficial CNS effects of the drug. For this reason, bromocriptine, an L-dopa agonist that increases CNS L-dopa concentrations without causing obstipation, was studied. However, it too failed to demonstrate a benefit. For these reasons, dopaminergic agents have not been used in the treatment of encephalopathy in clinical practice.

Benzodiazepine Antagonists

There have been several randomized controlled trials of short-term administration of flumazenil in the treatment of hepatic encephalopathy.[123-131] In some studies, flumazenil was superior to placebo in improving the grade of encephalopathy; 30% to 60% of encephalopathic patients improved after administration of flumazenil, and EEG changes paralleled this improvement. In other studies, flumazenil was no better than placebo in ameliorating the symptoms of encephalopathy, and EEGs did not improve. A recent meta-analysis suggested benefit of flumazenil over placebo.[132] Flumazenil has a limited role in the treatment of hepatic encephalopathy, and additional trials of larger numbers of subjects with varying grades of encephalopathy are needed.

The mentioned studies are provocative. The striking reversal of encephalopathy in some patients suggests that the GABA-benzodiazepine receptor system is one factor that may contribute to hepatic encephalopathy. These studies further emphasize the need to screen patients for use of benzodiazepines, which can be a cause of hepatic encephalopathy.

LOLA

Although studies using LOLA in acute liver failure did not find significant changes in survival, other studies investigated its potential use in hepatic encephalopathy from chronic liver disease. One prospective study, which used eight Child-Pugh B or C patients without baseline hepatic encephalopathy and seven cirrhotic patients with TIPS, tested to see if LOLA dosing could prevent or reduce glutamine-induced hepatic encephalopathy. After each subject was given two doses of glutamine (20-gram challenges), each subject was randomly selected to receive either 5 g of IV LOLA once or placebo infusion. Blood NH_3 levels, psychometric tests, and electroencephalography were tested in both groups, and LOLA was found to provide significant benefit of reducing encephalopathy symptoms when compared to placebo in non-TIPS patients, as well as minimizing the negative psychometric measurements after glutamine challenge.[133] A meta-analysis was also performed to analyze the effects by LOLA on chronic hepatic encephalopathy. The meta-analysis included three randomized trials which pooled 212 patients. This analysis found an overall significant effect on improvement of chronic hepatic encephalopathy symptoms (RR 1.89; 95% CI: 1.32-2.71, $P = 0.0005$). However, most benefit was seen in the grade I or II patients (RR 1.87, 95% CI: 1.30-2.68, $P = 0.0007$).[134]

Rifaximin

Rifaximin is the newest agent developed for the treatment of hepatic encephalopathy. It is a nonabsorbable antibiotic derivative of rifamycin with broad antimicrobial activity.[135] In comparison studies of rifaximin with lactulose, patients treated with rifaximin showed greater improvement in the degree of hepatic encephalopathy, had lower NH_3 levels, and had lower PSE index scores.[136] A recent randomized controlled trial of 299 patients demonstrated reduction of recurrent hepatic encephalopathy episodes (HR 0.42, 95% CI: 0.28-0.64, $P < 0.001$) and number of hospitalizations due to hepatic encephalopathy (HR 0.5, 95% CI: 0.29-0.87, $P = 0.01$).[135,137-138] Rifaximin is likely to become a first-line agent for the treatment of chronic hepatic encephalopathy.

HEPATIC TRANSPLANTATION

The development of encephalopathy in a patient with chronic liver disease indicates severe portal-systemic shunting and hepatic dysfunction. The prognosis for patients who develop this complication is grim; one recent study indicated that the 1-year survival rate is 42% and the 3-year survival rate is 23%.[139] In addition, there are numerous comorbidities in encephalopathic patients, including inability to continue gainful employment, poor function at home, nursing strains on spouse or family, inability to drive a vehicle, and inability to handle personal finances. Although medical therapies can ameliorate the major symptoms of encephalopathy, they rarely are effective enough to return the patient to full function. Often the patient with encephalopathy is at risk for other life-threatening complications of liver disease such as variceal hemorrhage and spontaneous bacterial peritonitis. Posttransplant 1-year survival rates are 80% to 85%, doubling 1-year survival rates for patients with hepatic encephalopathy without a transplant. For all the above reasons, any patient with hepatic encephalopathy should be considered for hepatic transplantation.

Summary

This chapter has discussed several key issues regarding hepatic encephalopathy, including definitions, clinical syndromes, diagnostic tests, precipitants, prognosis, and outcomes with therapy including hepatic transplantation. The section on pathogenesis defines current knowledge regarding mechanisms of encephalopathy in both acute liver failure and chronic liver disease. The clinician faced with neuropsychiatric syndromes in patients with liver disease must differentiate the nature of the underlying liver disorder (acute liver failure versus chronic liver disease), evaluate diagnostic tests, and institute appropriate therapy. Generally, the intensivist will work in cooperation with a team composed of hepatologists, transplant surgeons, anesthesiologists, and nephrologists. Overall outcomes of patients with encephalopathy depend on the general condition of the patient, severity of underlying liver disease, comorbid conditions, and when in acute liver failure, the presence of cerebral edema and intracranial hypertension. Liver transplantation, including the option of living donor liver transplantation, may yield favorable outcomes without neurologic sequelae if instituted prior to excessive and prolonged intracranial hypertension in the case of acute liver failure, or prior to multiorgan failure in the case of chronic liver disease.

ANNOTATED REFERENCES

Vaquero J, Fontana RJ, Larson AM, et al. Complications and use of intracranial pressure monitoring in patients with acute liver failure and severe encephalopathy. Liver Transpl 2005;11:1581-9.
Largest study to evaluate the major complications of ICP monitors in patients with acute liver failure and severe encephalopathy.
Acharya SK, Bhatia V, Sreenivas V, Khanal S, Panda SK. Efficacy of L-ornithine L-aspartate in acute liver failure: a double-blind, randomized, placebo-controlled study. Gastroenterology 2009;136:2159-68.
Largest study to evaluate the efficacy of LOLA to treat hepatic encephalopathy in acute liver failure.
Bass NM, Mullen KD, Sanyal A, et al. Rifaximin treatment in hepatic encephalopathy. N Engl J Med 2010;362:1071-81.
Critical paper to demonstrate efficacy of rifaximin to treat hepatic encephalopathy.

Bustamante J, Rimola A, Ventura PJ, et al. Prognostic significance of hepatic encephalopathy in patients with cirrhosis. J Hepatol 1999;30:890-5.
Significant paper describing the survival of patients with hepatic encephalopathy without transplantation.
Ferenci P, Lockwood A, Mullen K, Tarter R, Weissenborn K, Blei AT. Hepatic encephalopathy—definition, nomenclature, diagnosis, and quantification: final report of the working party at the 11th World Congresses of Gastroenterology, Vienna, 1998. Hepatology 2002;35:716-21.
Most recent definition of the different grades of hepatic encephalopathy.

REFERENCES

Access the complete reference list online at http://www.expertconsult.com.

102

Fulminant Hepatic Failure

SU MIN CHO | RAGHAVAN MURUGAN | ALI AL-KHAFAJI

Acute liver failure (ALF), also known as *fulminant hepatic failure* (FHF), embraces a spectrum of clinical entities characterized by acute liver injury, severe hepatocellular dysfunction, and hepatic encephalopathy. This condition is uncommon but not rare; it affects approximately 2000 to 2800 people annually in the United States, with a mortality of 3.5 per million despite intensive support.[1] Loss of hepatocyte function sets in motion a vicious multiorgan dysfunction syndrome, with ensuing death even when the liver has begun to recover. Complications of FHF include encephalopathy, cerebral edema, sepsis, acute respiratory distress syndrome (ARDS), hypoglycemia, coagulopathy, gastrointestinal bleeding, pancreatitis, and acute renal failure (ARF). Acetaminophen toxicity, idiosyncratic drug reactions, and hepatotropic viruses remain the most common cause of FHF in the United States. FHF accounts for 5% to 6% of liver transplantation, which is currently the only proven and definitive treatment option for patients who are unlikely to recover spontaneously. Unfortunately, many patients die before a suitable organ can be identified. Thus, the dominant medical interventions for acute liver failure in the critical care setting are supportive. Alternative "liver replacement" therapeutic strategies are under clinical investigation.

Definitions

The terms *fulminant hepatic failure* and *acute liver failure* are often used interchangeably. FHF is defined as the presence of encephalopathy (regardless of grade) and coagulopathy (international normalized ratio [INR] > 1.5) within 26 weeks of the appearance of symptoms in patients with no previous history of underlying liver disease. Since the original definition of FHF proposed by Trey and Davidson in 1970, several other classifications have emerged (Box 102-1).[2-6] In different classifications, the interval between the onset of symptoms or jaundice and the appearance of encephalopathy allows grouping of patients with similar causes, clinical characteristics, and prognosis.

Etiology

Viral hepatitis remains the most common identifiable cause of FHF in the developing world, whereas acetaminophen toxicity and idiosyncratic drug reactions have replaced viral hepatitis as the most frequent apparent causes of FHF in the United States and Europe. Both prognosis and management are determined in part by the underlying etiology of FHF.

ACETAMINOPHEN TOXICITY

Acetaminophen overdose is now the leading cause of FHF in the United States and accounts for 40% to 50% of cases. This type of liver injury occurs both after attempted suicide by acetaminophen overdose and after unintentional "therapeutic misadventures" caused by use of the drug for pain relief in excess of the dose specified in the package labeling, typically over a period of several days.[7] A careful medical history clarifies the quantity ingested; blood levels can be confirmatory but may not be elevated in cases of unintentional overdose. Doses considered nontoxic (<4 g/day in adults, <8 mg/kg in infants) might cause hepatotoxicity if other concurrent factors exist, such as alcohol ingestion, fasting, or malnutrition. Hepatotoxicity usually develops 1 to 2 days after the overdose, and circulating alanine aminotransferase

(ALT) levels and INR values reach their peak around day 3. A continued increase of INR after day 3 is associated with a 90% mortality rate. Acetaminophen is also nephrotoxic, and renal failure may occur in the absence of liver necrosis.

Acetaminophen undergoes phase 1 metabolism by hepatic cytochrome P_{450} 2E1 (CYP2E1) enzymes to a toxic intermediate compound, *N*-acetyl-*p*-benzoquinone imine (NAPQI), which is rapidly detoxified by hepatic glutathione into a nontoxic metabolite. Under normal conditions, little NAPQI accumulates. However, in an overdose, owing to depletion of glutathione stores, unconjugated NAPQI accumulates and causes hepatocellular necrosis. The amount of liver injury is directly related to the amount of ingested acetaminophen and the amount of NAPQI produced. In a recent study, the dose of acetaminophen ingested did not correlate with the overall prognosis.[8] Enzyme inducers such as alcohol, antiepileptic drugs, and cigarette smoke can enhance acetaminophen-mediated hepatotoxicity. Chronic alcohol consumption induces synthesis of CYP2E1 enzymes and, to a lesser extent, depletes glutathione stores. Substrate competition for CYP2E1 occurs between ethanol and acetaminophen when the two drugs are taken simultaneously. During the metabolism of acetaminophen, NAPQI formation is diminished when alcohol is present. The rate at which CYP2E1 degrades is also slowed, and the half-life of the enzyme increases from 7 hours to 37 hours. As long as ethanol remains in the body, there is competition between acetaminophen and ethanol for CYP2E1; however, once ethanol is removed, NAPQI formation is enhanced, resulting in enhanced hepatic injury in the 24 hours after cessation of alcohol consumption. Genetic variability within the population affecting expression of the cytokine, tumor necrosis factor alpha (TNF-α), also has been implicated as a determining factor in the severity of drug reactions related to acetaminophen.[9]

IDIOSYNCRATIC DRUG REACTIONS

Drug-induced liver damage is a significant cause of death in patients with FHF in Western countries (Box 102-2). The most common implicated drugs are antibiotics, central nervous system (CNS) agents, herbal/dietary supplements, and immunomodulatory agents.[10] Hepatocellular injury is common in younger patients, whereas a cholestatic picture is more common in the elderly. Dose, duration, and the hepatic metabolism of the drug all may play a role in the development of drug-induced liver injury.

Most idiosyncratic drug reactions are due to single agent, but multiple medications are implicated in some patients. Women generally predominate among patients with idiosyncratic drug-induced liver injury. Other risk factors for drug-induced hepatotoxicity include extremes of age, abnormal renal function, obesity, preexisting liver disease, and concurrent use of other hepatotoxic drugs. Idiosyncratic drug toxicities are immunologically mediated by the drug itself or its metabolites. Most idiosyncratic reactions occur within 4 to 6 weeks after initiation of treatment, although rare cases have occurred months or years later.

Idiosyncratic hepatic injury is mediated by several mechanisms, including disruption of intracellular calcium homeostasis, injury to canalicular transport pumps, such as multidrug resistance–associated protein 3 (MRP3), T cell–mediated immunologic injury, triggering of apoptotic pathways by TNF-α, and inhibition of mitochondrial beta oxidation.[11] Isoniazid, pyrazinamide, antimicrobials

CLASSIFICATIONS OF ACUTE LIVER FAILURE

Trey and Davidson[2]
Fulminant hepatic failure: development of HE within 8 weeks of onset of symptoms

British Classification[6]
Acute liver failure (includes only patients with encephalopathy)
Subclassification depending on the interval between jaundice and HE:
- Hyperacute liver failure: 0 to 7 days
- Acute liver failure: 8 to 28 days
- Subacute liver failure: 29 to 72 days
- Late-onset acute liver failure: 56 to 182 days

French Classification[3]
Acute hepatic failure: a rapidly developing impairment of liver function
Severe acute hepatic failure: prothrombin time or factor V concentration below 50% of normal with or without HE
Subclassification:
- Fulminant hepatic failure: HE within 2 weeks of onset of jaundice
- Subfulminant hepatic failure: HE between 3 and 12 weeks of onset of jaundice

International Association for the Study of Acute Liver Failure[5]
Acute liver failure (occurrence of HE within 4 weeks after onset of symptoms)
Subclassification:
- Acute liver failure—hyperacute: within 10 days
- Acute liver failure—fulminant: 10 to 30 days
- Acute liver failure—not otherwise specified
- Subacute liver failure (development of ascites and/or HE from 5 to 24 weeks after onset of symptoms)

HE, hepatic encephalopathy.

(amoxicillin-clavulanate, tetracyclines, and macrolides), anticonvulsants, antidepressants, nonsteroidal antiinflammatory drugs (NSAIDs), and halothane are most frequently implicated in FHF. There is an association between certain HLA genotypes (e.g., B*5701) and the risk of flucloxacillin-induced liver injury.[12] Two histologic patterns are usually distinguished, one being characterized by confluent necrosis (isoniazid or halothane) and the other by hepatocyte microvesicular fatty change (valproic acid or tetracyclines). Reemergence of tuberculosis—a public health problem in the past decade—has increased the frequency of FHF caused by isoniazid. Concurrent treatment with rifampicin and pyrazinamide may increase the risk of isoniazid toxicity.

Hepatotoxic herbal medicines (kava kava, St. John's wort) and certain dietary supplements are emerging as potential causes in a high proportion of patients with FHF. Mushroom poisoning due to *Amanita phalloides* is relatively common in Europe, and more sporadic cases occur in the United States. Florid muscarinic effects such as sweating or watery diarrhea occur early, whereas FHF usually occurs 4 to 8 days after mushroom ingestion. Other toxins (e.g., carbon tetrachloride, yellow phosphorus, aflatoxins) are rare causes of FHF. Liver biopsy is seldom helpful for establishing the diagnosis. Treatment with *N*-acetylcysteine (NAC) has been shown to improve transplant-free survival compared to placebo and should be used in drug-induced liver injury, even if not related to acetaminophen.[13]

VIRAL HEPATITIDES

Whereas viral hepatitides remain the most common identifiable cause of FHF worldwide, considerable geographic variation exists in the subtype of hepatitides. Thus, hepatitis B virus (HBV) is a common cause of FHF in the Far East, and hepatitis E virus (HEV) is more prevalent in the Indian subcontinent.[14] In the United States,

approximately 12% of FHF referred for liver transplants are due to hepatitis A and B. Occurrence of FHF within the larger number of patients with viral hepatitis, however, is rare (0.2%-0.4% for hepatitis A, 1%-4% for hepatitis B).

Hepatitis A virus (HAV) is associated with a higher risk of developing FHF if infection is acquired in older adulthood. Thus, vaccination is recommended for adults traveling from developed countries to endemic areas. The relevance of HAV as a cause of FHF in patients with preexisting chronic liver disease has been recognized recently. HAV vaccination in this high-risk group has been suggested. Postexposure prophylaxis with immune serum globulin may reduce the incidence of hepatitis A, but only when administered within 14 days of exposure.

HBV can result in FHF through several mechanisms: acute primary HBV infections, reactivation of hepatitis B in patients with chronic HBV, or superinfection with hepatitis D virus. Acute HBV infection is diagnosed by the detection of immunoglobulin M (IgM) antibodies against hepatitis B core antigen (HbcAg), because a substantial number of patients have negative serum hepatitis B surface antigen (HBsAg) and serum HBV-DNA. Low or absent levels of HBsAg and HBV-DNA are associated with better prognosis and lower rate of recurrence after orthotopic liver transplantation (OLT). FHF after reactivation of chronic hepatitis B has been described mainly in immunosuppressed male patients; this form of the disease usually has a subfulminant course and a poor prognosis.

Most studies indicate that hepatitis C virus (HCV) infection alone does not result in FHF. However, isolated cases of HCV-RNA in serum or tissue of patients with FHF and negative markers for other viruses have been noted in Western countries.[15] Involvement of HCV in FHF is slightly more common in the Far East.[16] An increased risk of FHF in patients with chronic hepatitis B and superinfection by HCV has been suggested.

FHF is seen in 2.5% to 6% of hepatitis D virus cases. Coinfection with HBV and hepatitis D virus (HDV) or superinfection by HDV in patients with chronic hepatitis B also can cause FHF. The incidence of coinfection is higher when intravenous (IV) drug abuse is present. Diagnosis of acute infection by HDV is made by the presence of HDV antigen, anti-HDV IgM antibody, or HDV-RNA.

Infection by hepatitis E virus (HEV) is uncommon in Western countries but occurs in travelers to endemic areas. Pregnant women infected by HEV seem to have a special propensity for developing FHF. Diagnosis is made by detection of anti-HEV IgM antibodies.

Other viruses have been implicated in the pathogenesis of FHF of indeterminate etiology. These viruses include cytomegalovirus (CMV), human herpesvirus-6 (HHV-6),[17,18] Epstein-Barr virus (EBV), hepatitis G virus (HGV),[19] herpes simplex virus (HSV),[20,21] varicella-zoster virus (VZV), parvovirus B19 in children, and togavirus, adenovirus, paramyxovirus, yellow fever, Q fever, and most recently, SEN virus and TT virus.[22] Although these causes are rare, they must be excluded, because some patients may benefit from specific antiviral therapy.

Miscellaneous cardiovascular, metabolic, and other disorders account for 2% to 10% of cases of FHF. Acute liver ischemia secondary to shock states can result in hepatocellular necrosis; however, the prognosis remains good if the primary condition can be corrected. The prognosis is worse when FHF is due to other causes such as Budd-Chiari syndrome, veno-occlusive disease, or malignancies associated with impaired hepatic blood flow. Rarely, the first manifestation of Wilson's disease is FHF, which sometimes occurs in patients without evidence of chronic liver disease. Death is universal without OLT. Acute fatty liver of pregnancy is rare, occurring in the third trimester of pregnancy, and usually responds well to fetal delivery. Other causes of FHF are autoimmune hepatitis, non-Hodgkin's lymphoma, or Reye syndrome, the last being less common in the pediatric population since aspirin use has been curtailed.

Prognostic Scoring Systems

Survival in patients with FHF depends on many factors, including etiology, age, severity of liver dysfunction, degree of liver necrosis,

Box 102-2

ETIOLOGIC CLASSIFICATION OF ACUTE LIVER FAILURE

Acetaminophen Toxicity
Idiosyncratic Drug Injury
Infrequent agents:
Isoniazid
Valproate
Halothane
Phenytoin
Sulfonamides
Propylthiouracil
Amiodarone
Disulfiram
Dapsone
Bromfenac
Troglitazone
Zidovudine
Lamivudine
Lamotrigine
Gatifloxacin
Methotrexate
Miscellaneous agents:
Ecstasy
Cocaine
Phencyclidine
Rare agents:
Carbamazepine
Ofloxacin
Ketoconazole
Lisinopril
Nicotinic acid
Labetalol
Etoposide
Imipramine
Interferon alfa
Flutamide
Tolcapone
Nefazodone
Oral contraceptives

Combination agents with enhanced hepatotoxicity:
Alcohol-acetaminophen
Trimethoprim-sulfamethoxazole
Rifampicin-isoniazid
Amoxicillin-clavulanic acid

Viral Hepatitides
Hepatitis A, B, C, D, E, G
Human herpesvirus
Cytomegalovirus
Epstein-Barr virus
Herpes simplex virus
Varicella-zoster virus
Paramyxovirus
Parvovirus B19
Adenovirus
Togavirus
Parvovirus
SEN virus
TT virus
Yellow fever virus

Toxins
CCL_4
Amanita phalloides
Yellow phosphorus
Herbal products

Vascular
Ischemic
Veno-occlusive disease
Budd-Chiari syndrome
Malignant infiltration
Non-Hodgkin's lymphomas

Miscellaneous
Wilson's disease
Autoimmune hepatitis
Acute fatty liver of pregnancy
Reye syndrome

nature of complications, and duration of illness. Patients with grade IV encephalopathy have a higher than 80% mortality without OLT. The successful use of OLT in FHF has created a need for early prognostic indicators to select patients most likely to benefit from OLT. Various prognostic scoring systems exist (Box 102-3), However, many of these are subject to debate because of bias and equating death with liver transplant, which falsely elevates the positive predictive value of any prognostication method.[23]

For patients with acetaminophen overdose, HAV infection, shock liver, or pregnancy-related acute liver failure, the short-term survival without transplantation is over 50%. Short-term transplant-free survival is lower (<25%) for patients with FHF of indeterminate cause or FHF caused by these factors: drugs other than acetaminophen, HBV infection, autoimmune hepatitis, Wilson's disease, Budd-Chiari syndrome, or cancer. The King's College prognostic criteria are the most widely used. These criteria provide a reasonable prediction of the likelihood of death and the need for transplantation in FHF patients.[24] The criteria are different for acetaminophen and non–acetaminophen-induced FHF (see Box 102-3), and experts have criticized the King's College criteria on the basis of low sensitivity and negative predictive value, especially for causes of FHF other than acetaminophen poisoning.

The APACHE II system has been found to be equal to King's College criteria for accuracy in predicting death in acetaminophen-induced FHF.[25] Other approaches include the Cliché criteria,[26] which use factor V assay, factor VIII/V ratio, serial α-fetoprotein levels, and plasma group-specific component protein (Gc globulin) levels.[27,28] Liver volume decreases with progression of the disease, and its measurement

with computed tomography (CT) may help assess prognosis. Other proposed prognostic tools include the proportion of necrosis as assessed by histologic examination of specimens obtained by liver biopsy, amount of fresh frozen plasma (FFP) required to correct coagulopathy, or determination of somatosensory evoked potentials. Other proposed markers for poor prognosis include serum levels of phosphate above 1.2 mmol/L on day 2 or 3, blood lactate concentration over 3.0 mmol/L, or Model for End-stage Liver Disease (MELD) score higher than 32.[29-31]

Role of Liver Biopsy

Liver biopsy can confirm the suspected cause of FHF and determine the degree of hepatocyte necrosis. Greater than 70% necrosis in a liver biopsy specimen is associated with 90% mortality without transplantation.[31,32] Because severe coagulopathy precludes safe percutaneous liver biopsy, the transjugular approach is often preferred. Although a liver biopsy is not mandatory, it can be valuable for determining prognosis, ruling out the presence of cirrhosis, and making the decision for early transplantation. Liver biopsy can help exclude occult malignancy in enigmatic cases and also can be used to assess the liver for evidence of regeneration, as manifested by the presence of liver cell mitosis. In rare cases, the liver biopsy can provide etiologic information that enables specific therapy to be instituted, as in the cases of HSV, CMV, adenovirus, and paramyxovirus hepatitis infections. Because of the variable nature of liver biopsies in patients with FHF, a minimum of three, and ideally six, specimens of the hepatic parenchyma should be obtained for histologic evaluation. In addition, if Wilson's disease or hepatic iron

VARIOUS PROGNOSTIC CRITERIA USED FOR LIVER TRANSPLANTATION IN PATIENTS WITH FULMINANT HEPATIC FAILURE

King's College Criteria[24]
Acetaminophen overdose:
- Arterial pH < 7.3 (irrespective of grade of encephalopathy or
- PT > 100 sec (INR > 6.5)
- Serum creatinine > 3.4 mg/dL (>300 μmol/L)
- Patients with grade III and IV hepatic encephalopathy

Non-acetaminophen liver injury:
- PT > 100 sec (INR > 6.5) (irrespective of grade of encephalopathy) or any three of the following variables:
  - Age < 10 or > 40 years
  - Non-A, non-B hepatitis, halothane hepatitis, idiosyncratic drug reactions
  - Jaundice > 7 days before onset of encephalopathy
  - Serum bilirubin 17.4 mg/dL (300 μmol/L)
  - PT > 50 sec

Cliché Criteria[26]
- Factor V < 20% in person < 30 years or both of the following:
  - Factor V < 30% in patients > 30 years
  - Grade III or IV encephalopathy

Serum Gc Globulin Levels[27,28]
Decreasing Gc levels due to dying hepatocytes

Serum α-Fetoprotein Level
Serial increase from day 1 to day 3 has shown correlation with survival

Liver Biopsy[32]
70% necrosis is discriminant of 90% mortality

Gc, plasma group-specific component protein; *INR*, international normalized ratio; *PT*, prothrombin time.

toxicity is a possible diagnosis, a separate core of liver tissue should be obtained for quantitative hepatic iron and copper determinations.

Pathogenesis and Clinical Features of Acute Liver Failure

FHF has a particular constellation of clinical features that are distinct from those seen with chronic hepatic insufficiency, regardless of the etiology. Typically, nonspecific symptoms such as malaise or nausea develop in a previously healthy person, followed by jaundice, rapid onset of altered mental status, and coma. Altered mentation and a prolonged INR are the hallmarks of the diagnosis. Supportive laboratory findings include high levels of ALT, a variable elevation of serum total bilirubin concentration, low serum glucose levels, and arterial blood gas studies showing respiratory alkalosis and/or metabolic acidosis. Patients with subfulminant hepatic failure (SFHF) have a more gradual onset of hepatic insufficiency accompanied by ascites, renal failure, and a very poor prognosis. Cerebral edema is infrequent in such patients. The magnitude of elevation of aminotransferase levels and rate of decline does not affect the prognosis. When patients spontaneously recover, the serum bilirubin concentration and INR normalize, whereas when the disease progresses, bilirubin levels continue to increase (due to intrahepatic cholestasis), and INR remains prolonged despite declining ALT levels. The high mortality rates associated with FHF are caused by complications such as cerebral edema, renal failure, sepsis, pancreatitis, and cardiopulmonary collapse, which results in multisystem organ failure.

ENCEPHALOPATHY

The presence of encephalopathy is the essential clinical feature that differentiates FHF from acute severe hepatitis, and the time to onset after the appearance of jaundice distinguishes FHF from SFHF. The onset of encephalopathy is often abrupt and occasionally may precede the appearance of jaundice. Agitation, delusional ideas, and hyperkinesis are common but short-lived symptoms; coma rapidly ensues. The overall prognosis for those with stable grade I or II encephalopathy is good, whereas the prognosis for patients with grade III or IV encephalopathy is much poorer. In cases of acetaminophen overdose, encephalopathy usually occurs on the third or fourth day after ingestion and rapidly progresses to grade IV within 24 to 48 hours.

The pathophysiology of hepatic encephalopathy is poorly understood and is probably multifactorial. Ammonia buildup in the brain is believed to be the main offender.[33-35] Elevated serum ammonia concentration is exacerbated by decreased urea synthesis in the injured liver.[36] Endogenous substances, false neurotransmitters, short-chain fatty acids, benzodiazepines, and γ-aminobutyric acid are additional factors that lead to encephalopathy. The electroencephalogram (EEG) typically shows diffuse slowing of cortical activity and high-amplitude waveforms at 5 to 7 cycles per second. Subclinical seizure activity is often present in patients with grade III and IV encephalopathy, emphasizing the importance of EEG monitoring in these patients. Prophylactic therapy with phenytoin has been shown to reduce seizure activity and reduce cerebral edema.[37] Seizure activity in FHF has been linked to excessive CNS glutamine, the main excitatory neurotransmitter in the brain. Newly synthesized glutamine is transported from the cytoplasm into mitochondria and is metabolized by glutaminase, yielding glutamate and ammonia. The generation of ammonia in the small mitochondrial compartment may reach extremely high levels, leading to induction of the mitochondrial permeability transition (MPT), production of free radicals, and potentially to oxidative damage of mitochondrial constituents. Thus, glutamine acts like a "Trojan horse," serving as a carrier of ammonia into mitochondria.[38] The glutamine-derived ammonia within mitochondria leads to astrocyte dysfunction, including cell swelling.

CEREBRAL EDEMA

Cerebral edema is estimated to occur in 75% to 80% of patients who progress to grade IV encephalopathy, and it is the leading cause of death in these patients. The mechanism(s) responsible for cerebral edema are only partially understood. Possible contributing factors include cerebral hyperemia, vasogenic edema due to disruption of the blood-brain barrier with rapid accumulation of low-molecular-weight substances, cytotoxicity due to the osmotic effects of ammonia, glutamine, and other amino acids, as well as the deleterious effects of pro-inflammatory cytokines and dysfunction of the sodium-potassium ATPase pump with loss of autoregulation of cerebral blood flow.[39,40] Intracranial blood flow is markedly reduced in patients with chronic hepatic encephalopathy; the decrease in perfusion appropriately matches the reduction in cerebral metabolic rate (CMR). However, patients with FHF often develop either relative or absolute cerebral hyperemia; thus, perfusion is not well matched to the reduced CMR present in evolving or established hepatic coma. An early indicator of this pathologic process is either a decrease in the transcranial oxygen content difference (arterial oxygen content − jugular bulb oxygen content) to less than 4 mL/dL or an increase in middle cerebral artery systolic blood flow velocity. Serial transcranial Doppler ultrasonographic monitoring of cerebral blood flow velocity helps detect early cerebral hyperperfusion or hypoperfusion suggesting impaired cerebral autoregulation.[41,42] Cerebral ischemia and permanent neurologic sequelae may occur (even after OLT) if cerebral perfusion pressure (CPP), calculated as mean systemic arterial blood pressure minus intracranial pressure, is not maintained above 40 to 50 mm Hg. However, there have been some reports of full neurologic recovery after OLT, despite high ICP and low CPP. CT of the brain often fails to demonstrate cerebral edema in patients with elevated ICP. Late clinical stages of cerebral edema include systemic hypertension, decerebrate rigidity, hyperventilation, pupillary dilation, seizures, and brainstem herniation. An arterial ammonia level above 200 μg/dL in grade III and grade IV encephalopathy is a strong predictor of brain herniation.[43] Full recovery of cerebral function is the rule if normal liver function returns, but permanent brain damage has been observed in patients making an otherwise complete hepatic recovery.

COAGULOPATHY

Severe alterations in coagulation are typical of FHF and are due to impaired hepatic synthetic function, leading to inadequate production of coagulation factors. Decreased levels of factors II, V, VII, IX, and X account for the prolongation of INR and activated partial thromboplastin time (APTT). Failure to observe an increase in circulating levels of the vitamin K–dependent factor VII by 25% after IV administration of vitamin K suggests that hepatic synthetic reserve is inadequate.[44] Many anticoagulation factors, such as proteins C and S, are synthesized by the liver, and activated coagulation factors are removed by the liver. Disruption of the balance between procoagulant and anticoagulant factors may result in excessive thrombosis and disseminated intravascular coagulation (DIC), and the laboratory distinction between the two is often difficult. Platelet counts are below 100,000/µL in two-thirds of patients at some point in their clinical course, and platelet function is altered. Hemorrhage from the gastrointestinal tract or elsewhere is common in FHF and most often correlates with a low platelet count; platelet transfusion may be necessary for patients with counts less than 50,000/µL. FFP has not been shown to be of value in the absence of bleeding.

METABOLIC DERANGEMENTS

FHF results in myriad metabolic abnormalities. Hypoglycemia is seen in up to 45% of patients with FHF. This abnormality is caused by depletion of hepatic glycogen stores and impaired gluconeogenesis and may be refractory to infusion of IV dextrose solution. Hepatic insulin resistance and impaired peripheral insulin sensitivity are often present.[45] Metabolic acidosis is common in acetaminophen-induced FHF and carries a poor prognosis. Hyponatremia, alkalosis, hypokalemia, hypophosphatemia, and lactic acidosis are common. Ionized hypocalcemia may indicate concomitant pancreatitis. Acute renal failure is seen in 30% to 70% of patients with acute liver failure and results from a combination of several factors such as intravascular volume depletion, sepsis, DIC, or direct nephrotoxicity from drugs such as acetaminophen or NSAIDs. Adrenal insufficiency has been described in up to 62% of patients with FHF when assessed by the change in plasma cortisol concentration after injection of synthetic ACTH (cosyntropin stimulation testing).[46] Hemodynamically unstable patients with adrenal dysfunction may benefit from replacement stress doses of hydrocortisone.

CARDIOVASCULAR, HEMODYNAMIC, AND RESPIRATORY COMPLICATIONS

Circulatory dysfunction accompanying FHF often mimics sepsis. Typically, patients are hyperdynamic, and calculated systemic vascular resistance is low. Vasodilation is thought to be due to the proinflammatory effects of circulating endotoxin and cytokines. Relative hypovolemia secondary to reduced systemic vascular resistance can make it difficult to assess the adequacy of intravascular volume, prompting insertion of pulmonary artery catheters. Cardiac arrhythmias occur frequently, owing to either electrolyte imbalances or increased circulating levels of catecholamines (from endogenous release or deliberate infusion). Severe peripheral shunting has been observed in FHF and may result from the plugging of small vessels by platelets, interstitial edema, or abnormal vasomotor tone, although the exact mechanism is unclear. Severely diminished tissue oxygen extraction is more common in nonsurvivors. An abnormal pattern of oxygen supply dependency results in oxygen extraction over a wider than normal range of oxygen delivery, presumably as a compensatory mechanism. Prostacyclin, which has microcirculatory vasodilatory effects, has been shown to increase peripheral oxygen uptake.[47]

Hyperventilation, hypercapnia, and respiratory alkalosis occur during acute liver failure and may worsen encephalopathy. Arterial hypoxemia is universal and is caused by a combination of intrapulmonary shunting, ventilation/perfusion mismatching, sepsis, aspiration, and ARDS.

SEPSIS

FHF is associated with impaired host resistance to and enhanced risk for bacterial and fungal infections. Common infections are aspiration pneumonia and primary bloodstream infections, including those caused by *Candida* spp. The most common microbial causes are gram-positive bacteria (*Staphylococcus aureus*, enterococci), enteric gram-negative bacilli (*Escherichia coli*, *Klebsiella* spp.), and *Candida* spp. Diminished hepatic reticuloendothelial function and opsonic activity, defective polymorphonuclear leukocyte function, and impaired cell-mediated and humoral immunity are the major predisposing mechanisms. In one prospective study of 50 patients, 80% had culture-proven infection, and in half of the remaining patients, infection was suspected but cultures were negative.[48] Regular microbial surveillance and aggressive treatment of presumed infection are essential, because prophylactic antibiotic regimens have shown little benefit.

▣ Management

Optimal management of FHF begins with the recognition that any patient with acute liver disease can die suddenly and is best cared for in an intensive care unit (ICU), preferably in a transplant center. Because the transportation of patients with advanced levels of coma is hazardous and the disease often worsens rapidly, transfer to a liver transplantation center should be considered at the time of admission of any patient with FHF. Because the liver has a unique ability to regenerate after acute, self-limited injury, treatment is limited to general supportive measures until the liver recovers. Elucidation of the cause of hepatic failure allows some patients to benefit from specific therapies and may influence posttransplant management if a transplant is performed.

THERAPY DIRECTED AT THE SPECIFIC ETIOLOGY OF FHF

Depending on the suspected or confirmed FHF etiology, a number of therapies may exist that can ameliorate or reverse the degree of liver injury. NAC should be given to all patients with FHF, regardless of the cause. NAC is a specific antidote for acetaminophen overdose; if given within the first 8 to 10 hours after an acute overdose, it replenishes glutathione stores and prevents development of hepatotoxicity. The efficacy of NAC declines progressively thereafter, but NAC may be effective up to 72 hours after acetaminophen ingestion.[49]

IV NAC is preferred over the enteral route. The dose is 150 mg/kg over 15 minutes, followed by 50 mg/kg given over 4 hours, followed by 100 mg/kg administered over 16 hours. Some experts recommend continued treatment until the INR normalizes. However, prolonged NAC therapy has been shown to impair murine liver regeneration and may impair liver regeneration following acetaminophen poisoning.[50] Currently, the optimal duration of treatment with NAC remains unclear.

Benefits of NAC on survival, brain edema, hemodynamics, oxygen delivery, and oxygen consumption were found in patients with established FHF.[49] A randomized, controlled trial of NAC by the U.S. Acute Liver Failure Study Group in patients with non–acetaminophen-induced FHF documented improved transplant-free survival.[13]

In *Amanita* intoxication, beneficial effects have been reported with the use of penicillin G (250 mg/kg/d) or silibinin, 20 to 50 mg/kg/h for a total of 1400 mg/d for 3 to 4 days.[51,52] These drugs may be useful if they are given early after mushroom ingestion. In severe cases, OLT is often required.

Hepatitis secondary to HSV may be missed because of its nonspecific presentation and the absence of typical mucocutaneous lesions. Most patients with HSV hepatitis are immunoincompetent hosts. If

HSV hepatitis is suspected, treatment with parenteral acyclovir or ganciclovir should be started.

In patients with Wilson's disease, plasma exchange with FFP replacement is preferred, because this intervention can remove relatively large amounts of copper in a short period of time. Net copper removal is proportional to plasma concentration and can reach 12 mg per session. However, plasmapheresis only helps to bridge patients to transplant and carries no survival benefit.[53] Chelating agents like penicillamine are ineffective in the setting of Wilson's disease–induced FHF. Hemofiltration and albumin dialysis also have been described as temporizing measures before OLT.[54]

The role of corticosteroids such as methylprednisolone (40 to 60 mg every 6 hours) or immunosuppressive agents in the setting of autoimmune hepatitis has not been well established.[55] Patients who do not respond to treatment after 2 weeks (as evidenced by persistently elevated bilirubin and aminotransferase levels) often die without liver transplantation.[55] Acute fatty liver of pregnancy usually responds to fetal delivery, and maternal mortality is improved after aggressive maternal care and early delivery. Fetal mortality, on the other hand, is only minimally improved after early delivery. Urgent chemotherapy is indicated for FHF caused by massive infiltration of the liver by lymphoma. Acute Budd-Chiari syndrome may be amenable to thrombolytic therapy or to transjugular intrahepatic portosystemic shunt (TIPS) placement. Administration of L-ornithine-L-aspartate (LOLA) in patients with FHF was ineffective in reducing circulating ammonia levels or improving survival. Patients who were treated with LOLA had a trend towards increased seizure activity.[56] L-Ornithine phenylacetate is a promising agent that facilitates excretion of glutamine and ammonia and may serve as a temporizing measure until transplantation is done.

HEPATIC ENCEPHALOPATHY

The treatment of encephalopathy associated with FHF is directed at limiting gut ammonia production and the avoidance of aggravating factors such as infection, ileus, obstipation, gastrointestinal hemorrhage, and other CNS depressants. Endotracheal intubation for grade III and IV hepatic encephalopathy (see Chapter 101) is essential. Lactulose (30 g every 1-2 hours) may be useful in the treatment of patients with grade I or II encephalopathy; however, administration of lactulose does not improve survival in advanced encephalopathy. The efficacy of lactulose in FHF has not been tested in clinical trials. This agent should be used with caution because of the risk of hypernatremia, dehydration due to diarrhea, and ileus. Lactulose by enema (300 g in 700 mL saline every 4-6 hours) remains an option in FHF patients who are unable to tolerate oral or nasogastric administration.

Oral metronidazole (500 mg/d), neomycin (4-12 g/day), and rifaximin (800-1200 mg/d) directed against ammonia-producing gut flora have been employed. However, metronidazole may be neurotoxic in hepatic failure; and neomycin, although minimally absorbed, can still cause nephrotoxicity and ototoxicity. Rifaximin is very expensive, and comparative studies, especially studies of cost-effectiveness, should be conducted before it is recommend it for routine use.

Endogenous benzodiazepine-like substances have been identified in the cerebrospinal fluid of patients with hepatic encephalopathy. Flumazenil, a benzodiazepine receptor antagonist, has been used (0.2-20 mg) with some success to provide short-term improvement in patients with hepatic encephalopathy.[57] Various experimental therapies such as exchange transfusion, charcoal hemoperfusion, and plasmapheresis have been used to lower circulating ammonia levels; however, none of these treatment approaches has been shown to improve survival.

CEREBRAL EDEMA

The optimal management of cerebral edema requires maintaining the delicate balance between mean arterial pressure (MAP) and ICP to preserve adequate cerebral perfusion (Box 102-4). Combined cerebral

---

Box 102-4

PREVENTIVE AND THERAPEUTIC INTERVENTIONS FOR PATIENTS WITH CEREBRAL EDEMA AND INTRACRANIAL HYPERTENSION

General Measures
Head of bed elevation to 30-degree angle, and maintain patient's neck in neutral position.
Endotracheal intubation for grade III or IV hepatic encephalopathy
Minimize tactile and tracheal stimulation, including airway suctioning.
Avoid hypovolemia and hypervolemia.
Avoid hypertension.
Avoid hypercapnia and hypoxemia.
Monitor and maintain ICP < 15 mm Hg.
Maintain CPP > 50 mm Hg.
Monitor and maintain Svjo₂ between 55% and 85%.
Use serial transcranial Doppler monitoring to titrate therapy.

Management of Intracranial Hypertension
Mannitol boluses, 0.5-1.0 g/kg body weight
Hyperventilation titrated to a Pco₂ of 28-30 mm Hg
Induced moderate hypothermia to 32°C-33°C
Achieve serum sodium levels of 145-155 mEq/L.
Induced coma with propofol or pentobarbital titrated to burst suppression of 5-10 cycles/sec
CVVH for oliguria and hyperosmolarity (>310 mOsm/L)

Other Unproven Therapies
Prophylactic phenytoin
Indomethacin, 25 mg intravenous bolus
Plasmapheresis
Total hepatectomy as a bridge to transplant

CPP, cerebral perfusion pressure; *CVVH*, continuous venovenous hemofiltration; *ICP*, intracranial pressure; *Svjo₂*, jugular bulb oxygen saturation.

---

edema and intracranial hypertension is the most common cause of death in patients with FHF when ICP is above 30 mm Hg. An arterial ammonia level over 200 μg/dL predicts brain herniation.[58] ICP monitoring may help to diagnose intracranial hypertension and guide management, especially in grade III or IV encephalopathy, although its use has never been shown to decrease mortality.[59,60] ICP should be maintained below 20 mm Hg, and CPP should be maintained above 50 mm Hg, although transplant-free recovery has been reported in acetaminophen-induced FHF patients despite impaired cerebral perfusion for 2 to 72 hours.[61]

Most centers prefer epidural to subdural or intraparenchymal transducers for monitoring ICP because of the lower rate of hemorrhagic and infectious complications.[62] Monitoring jugular bulb oxygen saturation with a reversed jugular bulb venous catheter also can guide interventions to avoid or treat intracranial hypertension. Decreased venous oxygen saturation (<55%) indicate cerebral ischemia, and high venous oxygen saturation (>85%) indicates either decreased metabolic demands of the brain or cerebral hyperemia (more commonly the latter).

Current recommendations include maintaining the patient's head at midline and a 30-degree upright angle to improve jugular venous outflow. In episodes of intracranial hypertension, a bolus of 0.5 to 1 g/kg of mannitol can be administered IV and repeated until plasma osmolarity reaches 310 mOsm/L. Patients with oliguria and renal failure may require hemodialysis to avoid hyperosmolarity. The role of high-dose corticosteroids has not been confirmed, and these agents are not effective in the treatment of cerebral edema associated with FHF. Attempts also should be made to avoid prolonged coughing or tracheal stimulation during suctioning to prevent an acute rise in ICP.

Hyperventilation reduces cerebral blood flow by 2% to 3% for every millimeter of mercury reduction in Paco₂. Moderate hyperventilation (Paco₂ = 28-30 mm Hg) can be employed to reduce ICP, but not all patients respond to reductions in Paco₂, and the efficacy of hyperventilation can wane after 48 hours, owing to normal equilibration mechanisms. Excessive cerebral vasoconstriction can be detected as widening of the cerebral arteriovenous oxygen content difference. Serial transcranial Doppler studies help detect early changes in cerebral blood flow in response to therapy.[63] Induction of mild to moderate hypothermia (core temperature 32°C-33°C), which can be induced with cooling blankets or a special intravascular catheter, has been shown to reduce ICP and cerebral blood flow and improve CPP in patients with FHF.[64,65] Care must be taken to avoid both cardiac depression and shivering during induced hypothermia. Induction of a barbiturate coma by administering parenteral sodium pentobarbital, sodium pentothal, or propofol titrated to the appearance of 5 to 10 cycles per second of EEG burst suppression can further reduce both cerebral metabolic rate and cerebral blood flow in refractory patients. However, adverse effects such as myocardial depression or arterial hypotension may create the need for inotropic or vasopressor support to preserve CPP in the minimally adequate range. Limited evidence supports the use of hypertonic saline to induce hypernatremia (serum sodium concentration 145-155 mEq/L).[66]

Indomethacin (25 mg IV bolus) has been shown to reduce cerebral blood flow and prevent brain edema in experimental models of FHF and in isolated cases of FHF in humans, with encouraging results.[67] Prophylactic infusion of phenytoin has been studied in two controlled studies which gave different conclusions in regard to its efficiency in preventing seizures, cerebral edema, and survival.[37]

COAGULOPATHY

Despite severe coagulopathy, patients with FHF seldom have spontaneous hemorrhage. Routine use of FFP is not recommended unless spontaneous bleeding occurs or an invasive procedure is being contemplated. Platelets should be transfused before invasive procedures if the platelet count is less than 50,000 cells/μL. Administration of FFP does not increase survival and may cause intravascular volume overload and worsen cerebral edema in addition to the potential risk of developing transfusion-related acute lung injury (TRALI). Recombinant activated factor VII offers advantages of shorter half-life and avoidance of volume overload compared with FFP; however, more studies using this agent are needed.[69] When evaluation of mental state is not possible, monitoring coagulation parameters helps assess improvement or worsening of liver function.

ACUTE RENAL FAILURE

Renal failure develops in up to 70% of patients with FHF, and the presence of FHF and renal failure has a grave prognosis without renal support. Mechanisms leading to acute tubular necrosis (ATN) include renal hypoperfusion (due to intravascular volume depletion and reduced mean arterial pressure), systemic inflammatory response syndrome (SIRS), hepatorenal syndrome, and direct toxic effects of the etiologic agent responsible for liver injury (e.g., acetaminophen). The presence of SIRS predicts renal failure in non–acetaminophen-induced FHF.[70] Optimal fluid balance is paramount in patients with FHF to avoid prerenal azotemia and progression to ATN. Frequent monitoring of serum creatinine level, urinary output, and urinary sodium concentrations is required. Diuretics and "renal dose" dopamine (2-4 μg/kg/min) have no protective value in the therapy for acute renal failure and are potentially harmful. Nephrotoxic drugs such as aminoglycosides or radiographic contrast agents should be avoided. Continuous venovenous hemofiltration (CVVH) is preferred over intermittent hemodialysis, because this modality avoids the rapid fluid shifts and abrupt changes in ICP that are associated with intermittent dialysis.[71]

MISCELLANEOUS THERAPY

Glycemic control is vital in patients with deep encephalopathy. Constant infusion of 10% to 20% glucose is preferable to bolus administration for maintenance of euglycemia. FHF is a catabolic state, and protein-caloric malnutrition develops quickly. Thus, nutrition should be started soon and adjusted individually to maintain an adequate caloric intake. Enteral nutrition through a nasogastric or nasojejunal tube is preferred to parenteral nutrition. Although aromatic amino acid–free enteral formulas are commercially available, their clinical efficacy and cost-effectiveness are not established. Correction of hypomagnesemia, hypokalemia, or hypophosphatemia is accomplished by supplementation of these formulations. H_2-receptor antagonists, proton pump inhibitors, or sucralfate are used to reduce the incidence of gastrointestinal ulceration or erosive gastritis.

A high index of suspicion should be maintained for the presence of infection, because fever and leukocytosis are absent in up to 30% of infected patients. Infection must be suspected in the presence of any sudden clinical deterioration, such as worsening encephalopathy or hemodynamic instability, especially when liver function has started to recover.[72] Microbiological cultures should be obtained from appropriate sites, and empirical antibiotics covering both enteric gram-negative and gram-positive bacteria should be started. Antifungal coverage should be initiated, particularly in patients already on broad-spectrum antibacterial coverage who have new-onset clinical deterioration. There are no generally accepted guidelines regarding use of prophylactic antibiotics. Their use is supported by recent studies that suggest that infection and progression to deep encephalopathy are highly correlated.[73,74] Selective enteral decontamination may reduce the risk of infection due to gram-negative bacilli, but there are insufficient data to support its routine use.[75]

HEPATIC REPLACEMENT THERAPIES

Liver Transplantation

OLT is the only measure that can radically influence the course of FHF. FHF accounts for about 5% to 10% of liver transplants performed in the USA. Spontaneous survival has improved from 15% to 40% thanks to advances in critical care support. The survival rate is further improved to 60% after OLT. However, transplantation is an expensive and high-risk procedure with considerable morbidity. Moreover, OLT commits the patient to a lifetime of iatrogenic immunosuppression. In most series, patients transplanted for FHF have a lower 1-year survival than those transplanted for other causes, in part because of their poor clinical condition at the time of the procedure. Clinical liver transplantation continues to evolve, but availability of this therapy is hampered by continued shortages in donor organs. Contraindications to transplantation include irreversible brain damage, uncontrolled infection, severe pancreatitis, and malignancy. Early identification of patients who are likely to survive without OLT is a very important objective. Both the King's College and the Cliché criteria are used most often to identify such patients (see Box 102-3). Liver biopsy, although not mandatory, may help decide the need for early transplantation. In general, patients with ≤60% are likely to survive without the need for transplantation, whereas those with ≥90% necrosis are unlikely to survive without transplantation.[26,76] The prognosis without transplantation is less clear for patients in between these boundaries. These patients require the most aggressive care and attention.

Decisions regarding transplantation do not have to be made at the time of admission, but rather at the time a donor organ has been identified. This is because the typical waiting time for a donor organ for a United Network for Organ Sharing (UNOS) status 1 patient (those with FHF) is 2 to 3 days or more in the United States.[77] Various surgical options exist for liver transplantation in patients with FHF (Box 102-5). The most frequently utilized procedure is cadaveric whole organ transplantation, with the donor organ being placed in the orthotopic position. However, continued efforts are being made to assess ways of expanding the donor pool by using marginal donors, living donor liver transplantation, cadaveric split liver transplantation, and various hepatic support systems to prolong survival long enough for the patient to undergo liver transplantation. Therapeutic hepatectomy with temporary portocaval anastomosis in FHF has been reported to stabilize FHF patients until a suitable liver donor organ was

Box 102-5

HEPATIC REPLACEMENT THERAPEUTIC OPTIONS AVAILABLE TO PATIENTS WITH FULMINANT HEPATIC FAILURE

Liver Transplantation
Cadaveric transplantation
Whole liver
Reduced-size liver
Split liver
Auxiliary partial liver
Orthotopic position
Heterotopic position
Auxiliary whole liver
Heterotopic position
Living-related transplantation
Left lateral segment
Left lobe
Extended left lobe
Right lobe

Artificial Liver Assist Devices
Non–cell-based systems
Charcoal hemoperfusion
High-volume plasmapheresis
Continuous high-frequency hemodiafiltration
Molecular adsorbent recirculating system (MARS)
Cell-based systems (bioartificial liver assist devices)
Primary porcine hepatocytes
Human hepatoblastoma cells
(Extracorporeal liver assist device [ELAD])

Hepatocyte Transplantation

procured.[78-80] The anhepatic periods were 14 hours in two cases and 66 hours in a third report.

Artificial and Bioartificial Liver Assist Devices

The use of artificial and bioartificial liver support devices in FHF has been shown to improve biochemical and physiologic indices of liver function (e.g., serum bilirubin concentration, INR, ICP, and CPP). However, the use of these devices has never been shown to improve transplant-free or overall survival.[81-83] The MARS system utilizes a hollow-fiber, double-sized, albumin-impregnated dialysis membrane to extract protein-bound toxins into an albumin-containing dialysate. The Prometheus system utilizes fractionated plasma separation and adsorption. Bioartificial systems can use either porcine hepatocytes or human hepatoblastoma cells, and studies are underway to evaluate the role of these approaches in the management of FHF.[84]

Hepatocyte Transplantation

Hepatocyte transplantation has been attempted in patients with FHF to accomplish the same goals as with the hepatic liver assist systems. The rationale is to deliver a sufficient supply of hepatocytes to maintain liver function until regeneration of native liver occurs or a graft for organ transplantation becomes available. Human hepatocytes from livers not used for transplantation can be cryopreserved, making them readily available if needed. Experimental studies in models of FHF showed engraftment and function of transplanted hepatocytes and increased survival. In patients with grade III and IV encephalopathy and severe coagulopathy, intrasplenic or intrahepatic injection of human hepatocytes has been performed.[85,86] In two studies, improvements have been noted in several parameters, including encephalopathy score, hemodynamic parameters, and serum ammonia and bilirubin levels. Pulmonary embolism of hepatocytes occurred when the injection was intraportal but not when hepatocytes were injected into the splenic artery.[85] Other concerns about this technique include transplantation and acquisition of an adequate number of hepatocytes (only 0.15-80 g have been injected compared with 300 g [20% of

normal liver mass required] to replace liver function), use of immunosuppression in FHF, and the need for a 48-hour period for engraftment and function. New sources of hepatocytes (e.g., stem cells and/or progenitor cells) are needed to increase the number of patients who might be candidates for hepatocyte transplantation. Future trials using this concept are likely if results with hepatocyte liver assist systems prove disappointing.

Conclusion

FHF remains a rare but a devastating illness with high mortality. The treatment of FHF poses a great challenge to intensive care clinicians. Early transfer to a transplant center is preferable not only because of the availability of transplantation, but also because of the availability of experienced clinician as these specialized centers. A multidisciplinary approach to critical care management is clearly required to address the multitude of organ derangements that are sequelae of FHF. Currently, only liver transplantation can radically alter the course of the disease process. Although transplant surgery including immunosuppressive therapy has considerably advanced over the past decade, this intervention is expensive and associated with complications related both to the procedure and the need for lifelong immunosuppression. Therefore, liver replacement strategies that are less invasive and permanent are urgently required. The current experience with nonbiological and biological artificial devices are encouraging but clearly require validation of their safety and efficacy by randomized controlled trials.

KEY POINTS

1. Fulminant hepatic failure (FHF) is distinguished from severe acute hepatitis by the presence of hepatic encephalopathy. Without liver transplantation, the mortality rate for FHF is 50% to 80%.

2. Intentional or accidental acetaminophen overdose remains the dominant cause of FHF in the United States. The hepatotoxic effects of acetaminophen are potentiated by concurrent alcohol ingestion, glycogen depletion, and/or anticonvulsant medications.

3. The King's College Criteria remain the most widely used prognostic scoring system for FHF; however, failure to fulfill the criteria does not reliably predict survival.

4. Transjugular liver biopsy may be valuable for determining prognosis based on the amount of hepatic necrosis and/or the presence of hepatic regeneration and may help to determine the etiology in enigmatic cases.

5. The onset of grade III or IV hepatic encephalopathy prognosticates a higher risk for mortality. The onset of grade III or IV encephalopathy is an indication for endotracheal intubation and the performance of diagnostic and therapeutic modalities for intracranial hypertension.

6. Intracranial hypertension is the major cause for early mortality in FHF and is due to cerebral hyperemia, osmotic factors, and derangements of the blood-brain barrier.

7. Cerebral hyperemia can be detected by a decreased cerebral arteriovenous oxygen content difference or by transcranial Doppler showing elevated systolic blood flow velocity.

8. Continuous monitoring of intracranial pressure should be initiated when grade III encephalopathy is present and is most safely performed with an epidural pressure transducer.

9. Elevated ICP can be managed with hyperventilation, mannitol, mild hypothermia, therapeutic sedation, and other less proven interventions; however, the optimal management of this condition remains unknown.

10. Prophylactic administration of fresh frozen plasma does not improve survival and may aggravate volume overload and cerebral edema.

11. Continuous venovenous hemofiltration is the preferred method for artificial renal replacement to avoid hemodynamic fluctuations, which can aggravate cerebral hyperperfusion or hypoperfusion.

12. Liver transplantation is the only proven liver replacement therapy to reduce mortality. Both biological and nonbiological artificial liver replacement therapies remain unproven to reduce transplant-free mortality.

ANNOTATED REFERENCES

O'Grady JG, Alexander GJ, Hayllar KM, Williams R. Early indicators of prognosis in fulminant hepatic failure. Gastroenterology 1989;97:439-45.

The classic paper that established the most widely used criteria (Kings College Criteria) for predicting liver transplant-free mortality in a large cohort of patients with either acetaminophen- or non–acetaminophen-induced FHF.

Polson J, Lee WM. AASLD position paper: the management of acute liver failure. Hepatology 2005; 41:1179-97.

A comprehensive review with many references related to management of acute liver failure.

Tunon MJ, Alvarez M, Culebras JM, Gonzalez-Gallego J. An overview of animal models for investigating the pathogenesis and therapeutic strategies in acute hepatic failure. World J Gastroenterol 2009; 15:3086-98.

A comprehensive review of the treatment strategies currently available in animal models of acute liver failure.

Ding GK, Buckley NA. Evidence and consequences of spectrum bias in studies of criteria for liver transplant in paracetamol hepatotoxicity. QJM 2008;101:723-9.

A review of prognostic models for predicting poor outcome in acute liver failure and their limitations.

Heard KJ. Acetylcysteine for acetaminophen poisoning. N Engl J Med 2008;359:285-92.

Review of the role of acetaminophen in the management of acute liver failure.

Bjerring PN, Eefsen M, Hansen BA, Larsen FS. The brain in acute liver failure. A tortuous path from hyperammonemia to cerebral edema. Metab Brain Dis 2009;24:5-14.

Great review of the pathogenesis of cerebral edema in the setting of ALF.

Dmello D, Cruz-Flores S, Matuschak GM. Moderate hypothermia with intracranial pressure monitoring as a therapeutic paradigm for the management of acute liver failure: a systematic review. Intensive Care Med 2010;36:210-3.

A comprehensive review of hypothermia's role in treatment of acute liver failure–induced cerebral edema.

REFERENCES

Access the complete reference list online at http://www.expertconsult.com.

103

Calculous and Acalculous Cholecystitis

SAMUEL A. TISHERMAN

Evaluating the patient with a possible acute abdomen in the intensive care unit (ICU) can be challenging. Patients frequently have multiple potential sources of sepsis and are often unable to describe symptoms or localize tenderness on physical examination. In addition, many imaging studies require transporting the patient off the unit, which can be risky. These confounding factors can be important in the evaluation of any intraabdominal process, but may be especially troublesome in the case of acute cholecystitis.

Acute cholecystitis has long been recognized as a complication of surgery or acute critical illness. The first reported case of acute postoperative cholecystitis, described in 1844, was a lethal complication that occurred in a patient who had been treated for a strangulated femoral hernia.[1] In 1902, Kocher and Matti described successful operation for gangrenous cholecystitis complicating a ventral herniorrhaphy.[2] In 1962, Thompson et al. reported a series of 98 patients who developed acute cholecystitis in the postoperative period.[3] Seventy-six percent were men, and 47% did not have gallstones. Twelve percent of the patients developed perforation of the gallbladder. It is noteworthy that Glenn and Becker showed that the incidence of acalculous and postoperative cholecystitis increased between 1955 and 1979.[4]

The pathophysiology of cholecystitis in critically ill patients is different from that in the general population. At least half of the cases are acalculous.[5] Understanding this disease process can help increase the index of suspicion and lead to early diagnosis and treatment, which is necessary for good outcomes in the already critically ill patient.

Risk Factors and Pathophysiology

In general, acute cholecystitis is associated with the presence of gallstones, which develop as a result of decreased solubility of cholesterol and bile salts in bile. Normally, the concentrations of conjugated bile salts, cholesterol, and phospholipids in bile keep these components in solution. If the balance of these components is altered, stones may form. Risk factors for gallstones include age, female sex, recent pregnancy, positive family history for gallstones, and hemolysis. Patients with gallstones may develop acute cholecystitis at any time. Occasionally, acute calculous cholecystitis can occur during hospitalization for other reasons.

Acalculous cholecystitis also can spontaneously occur under certain circumstances. In outpatients, risk factors for acalculous cholecystitis include diabetes mellitus, vasculitis, older age, and male sex.[6] Acalculous cholecystitis also has been reported in cancer patients and patients with systemic infections and the acquired immunodeficiency syndrome (AIDS). Indeed, acute cholecystitis is the most common indication for exploratory laparotomy or laparoscopy in AIDS patients.[7] Most have acalculous disease. Not surprisingly, the mortality rate is high. In children, the majority of cases of acute cholecystitis are acalculous.[8] The etiology appears to be dehydration or lymphadenopathy secondary to viral infections. Congenital biliary tract anomalies also need to be considered.

Acute cholecystitis has been described in multiple reports as a complication of a variety of surgical procedures,[9-14] trauma,[15-20] burns,[21] sepsis,[22] cardiovascular diseases, and malignancy.[23,24] There also has been an association with total parenteral nutrition and biliary stasis.[25-28] The pathophysiology, however, remains unclear.

Theories regarding the pathogenesis of acalculous cholecystitis in critically ill and postoperative patients have evolved over the years.

Sparkman was the first to suggest that gastrointestinal hypomotility and biliary stasis were causative factors.[29] Glenn and Wantz added that the lack of enteral feeding in the postoperative period increased the concentration of bile salts and cholesterol in bile.[30] They further noted acute onset of cholecystitis with refeeding, suggesting impaction of stones or viscous bile in the cystic duct, with gallbladder contractions. Thompson et al., having noted gallbladder mucosal necrosis, arterial thrombosis, gangrene, and perforation, suggested that hypoperfusion may be the critical mechanism for acalculous cholecystitis.[3] A recent histopathologic study found that two-thirds of surgical and trauma patients who developed acute cholecystitis had ischemic cholecystitis histologically.[31] Hakala et al. performed ex vivo microangiography of gallbladders immediately after cholecystectomy.[32] Patients with stones had normal vasculature, whereas those with acalculous disease had poor and irregular capillary filling, suggesting that microvascular disturbances may play a role in the pathogenesis of this disease. Hypoperfusion, particularly of the splanchnic circulation, is common in critically ill patients. Etiologic factors include hemorrhage, dehydration, heart failure, and/or sepsis. The use of vasopressors can exacerbate the situation. Mechanical ventilation with positive end-expiratory pressure (PEEP) can increase hepatic venous pressure and thereby decrease portal perfusion.[34]

Orlando et al. suggested that in addition to hypoperfusion, increased intraluminal pressure may be a critical factor.[33] Biliary stasis secondary to fasting and narcotics may play a critical role in increasing intraluminal pressure in the gallbladder. The combination of hypoperfusion and increased luminal pressure leads to a decrease in gallbladder perfusion pressure. Bacterial invasion can subsequently occur in the ischemic tissue.

The use of parenteral nutrition has been implicated in the pathogenesis of acalculous cholecystitis. In addition to the effects of fasting, parenteral nutrition can decrease bile production, worsening biliary stasis. Biliary sludge can be found in almost all patients on long-term parenteral nutrition.[25-28] Many go on to form gallstones. Trauma patients also develop sludge over time, and this factor may play a role in the development of cholecystitis, as well as pancreatitis.[35]

Eosinophilic infiltration of the inflamed gallbladder has been seen in patients developing acute acalculous cholecystitis after administration of antibiotics for other reasons, suggesting the possibility that a hypersensitivity reaction to the antibiotic played an etiologic role.[36] This theory has not been substantiated.

It has been suggested that the pigment load from massive transfusions can lead to changes in the relative concentrations of bile pigments compared to cholesterol and lecithin in bile, increasing risk of acalculous cholecystitis. Long et al., however, found no relationship between transfusion requirements and risk of cholecystitis.[34]

Incidence

The incidence of acute cholecystitis in the ICU is difficult to determine given the great diversity of ICU patient populations and illness severity. Among cardiac surgical patients, acute cholecystitis is second only to upper gastrointestinal hemorrhage as an indication for abdominal operation.[37] About half the cases of acute cholecystitis in this population are due to acalculous disease. Visceral hypoperfusion related to left ventricular dysfunction has been implicated as an etiologic factor. Rady et al. found that early predictors of acute cholecystitis included arterial occlusive disease, low preoperative oxygen delivery, longer cardiopulmonary bypass times, need for surgical re-exploration, cardiac arrhythmias, mechanical ventilation for ≥ 3 days, bacteremia, and nosocomial infections.[13] The common threads of these factors are decreased tissue perfusion and oxygenation, significant surgical trauma (which would be expected to lead to production of inflammatory mediators), and perhaps bacterial translocation from the gut lumen. These authors went so far as to suggest that patients who have had a complicated postoperative course should be followed by serial ultrasonography of the gallbladder. Hagino et al. found that 6 of 7 patients who developed cholecystitis after aortic reconstruction had prolonged hypotension and developed multiple organ dysfunction; 5 died.[14]

In the general population of postoperative patients, acute cholecystitis appears to occur with or without gallstones. Mortality is about 30%. Among trauma patients, about 90% of cases of acute cholecystitis are acalculous.[15-20] The percentage of cases of acute cholecystitis that are acalculous has increased significantly over time.[4] Because the incidence of the disease is low, but the many risk factors for the disease are common, it is difficult to identify specific groups of ICU patients who might benefit from selective screening for acute cholecystitis.

Clinical Presentation

Given that the underlying pathophysiology of cholecystitis in the ICU often involves gallbladder wall ischemia, there is significant risk for rapid progression to gangrene and perforation. Consequently, even though other causes of sepsis in the ICU are more common, one needs to have a low threshold for considering cholecystitis in the differential diagnosis of patients who may have intraabdominal sepsis.

The signs and symptoms of acute cholecystitis do not generally differ between calculus and acalculous disease. Typically, patients with acute cholecystitis present with right upper quadrant or epigastric pain, often associated with a fatty meal. The pain may radiate to the back. Anorexia, nausea, and vomiting are common findings, as are fever and chills. If the patient is receiving enteral nutrition, the symptoms may be related to meals or tube feedings.

On examination, the most consistent finding is fever. Focal tenderness in the right upper quadrant or epigastrium is typically found, often with evidence of peritoneal irritation. Rarely, the gallbladder is palpable. There may be abdominal distention and loss of bowel sounds. Jaundice may be present if the patient develops choledocholithiasis, Mirizzi's syndrome (external compression of the common hepatic duct by a stone impacted in the cystic duct), or liver dysfunction from sepsis.

In critically ill patients, symptoms and physical findings are frequently difficult to assess because of alterations in the patient's mental status and concurrent disease. Typical physical findings are frequently absent.

The most consistent laboratory finding is a leukocytosis. Elevated circulating levels of liver enzymes and bilirubin are common, but not necessarily present. Clinical findings and laboratory studies are not very sensitive or specific for cholecystitis even in the general population[38,39] and are less so in critically ill patients. Consequently, radiologic studies are necessary.

Imaging Studies

Ultrasonography has proven to be an accurate radiologic test for acute cholecystitis in the general population. In the ICU, the presence or absence of gallstones does not help with the diagnosis. The most useful ultrasonographic findings indicative of acute cholecystitis are thickening of the gallbladder wall and pericholecystic fluid (Figure 103-1). Ultrasonographic findings correlate well with operative findings. False-positive findings may occur with sludge, non-shadowing stones, cholesterolosis, ascites, hypoalbuminemia, and portal hypertension. Other ultrasonographic findings indicative of acute cholecystitis include the "double wall sign," representing edema of the gallbladder wall; the "halo sign," representing sloughed gallbladder mucosa; intramural gas; distention of the gallbladder; and the "sonographic Murphy's sign,"

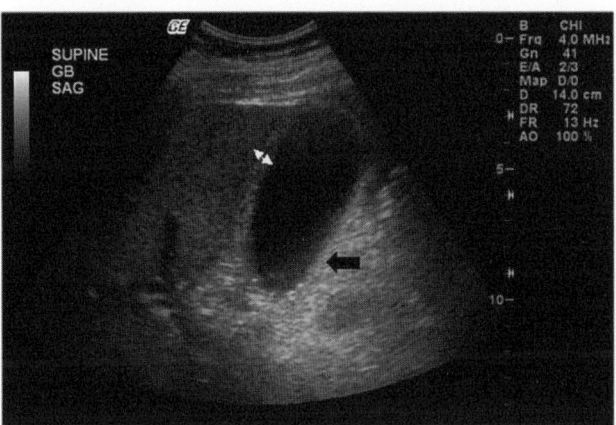

Figure 103-1 Ultrasound of gallbladder, demonstrating wall thickening (*double arrows*) and sludge (*black arrow*).

demonstrating point tenderness over the gallbladder. The sensitivity of ultrasound for detecting acalculous cholecystitis is 81% to 92%. The specificity is 60% to 96%.[38-42,47,48] One problem is that the typical ultrasonographic findings of cholecystitis can be seen in ICU patients without other evidence of cholecystitis. For example, Boland et al. performed ultrasound examinations of the gallbladder twice a week in a variety of ICU patients.[40] Half of the patients without calculi developed at least one ultrasonographic finding of acute cholecystitis. Helbich et al.[41] attempted to apply a scoring system to the ultrasonographic findings characteristic of acute cholecystitis, suggesting that patients with several findings should undergo more aggressive diagnostic evaluation and perhaps therapeutic interventions.[40] In equivocal cases, serial examinations may demonstrate increasing wall thickness which should increase the suspicion for cholecystitis.[42]

Scintigraphy of the gallbladder frequently has been used when acute cholecystitis is suspected, but the findings from other tests such as ultrasound are inconclusive or contradictory. Gallbladder scintigraphy is performed by administering technetium-labeled iminodiacetic acid (IDA). Cholecystitis is diagnosed if the radioactive tracer is visualized in the small bowel without visualization of the gallbladder within 4 hours, suggesting occlusion of the cystic duct (Figure 103-2). Delayed visualization of the gallbladder may represent chronic cholecystitis. The rate of false-positive tests is significant in fasting patients, particularly those receiving parenteral nutrition. The use of intravenous morphine to increase tone in the sphincter of Oddi and thereby increase pressure within the biliary system can decrease the risk of a falsely positive test.[43] The sensitivity of scintigraphy is 91% to 97%. The specificity is 38% to 99%.[43,44,48] Scintigraphy is a useful complement to ultrasonography when ultrasonography alone does not provide enough information to permit a sufficiently early decision regarding intervention.[44]

CT of the abdomen can be used to make the diagnosis of acute cholecystitis.[45,46] The criteria for a positive study include wall thickness greater than 4 mm, pericholecystic fluid, intramural gas, sloughed mucosa, or subserosal edema without ascites (Figure 103-3). If intravenous contrast is administered, enhancement of the gallbladder wall may be seen. Although CT may not be as sensitive as the other studies for determining the presence of gallstones or acute cholecystitis, it has the advantage of being able to detect or rule out other causes of an acute abdomen. A great disadvantage for critically ill patients, however, is the need to transport the patient to the scanner.

In critically ill patients, ultrasound is usually the first test requested because it can be performed at the bedside in the ICU and carries no risk. It also can be repeated readily. Because the study is operator-dependent, the reliability of the test, particularly its sensitivity, can be variable.[47] Specificity is good. Frequently, however, additional studies are necessary. Ultrasound and scintigraphy, in particular, complement each other well.[48] The results of any imaging studies need to be

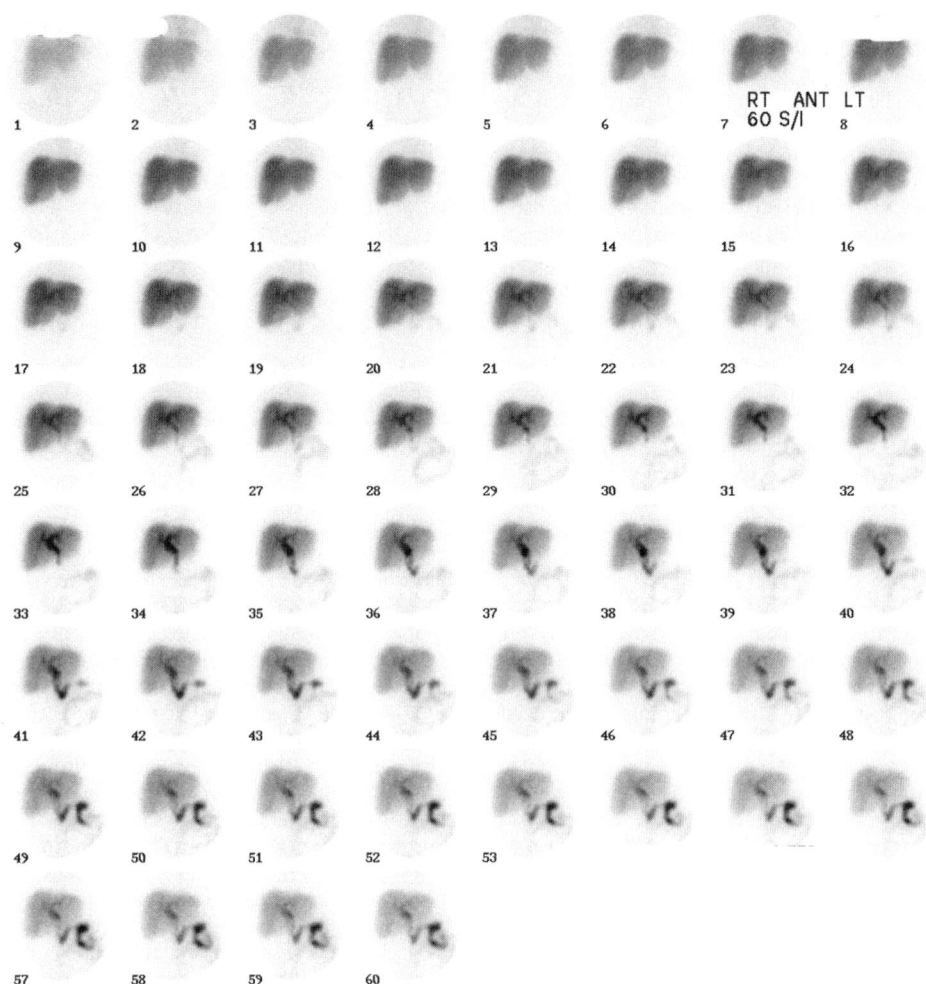

Figure 103-2 Scintigraphy of biliary tree, demonstrating concentration of tracer in liver, followed by flow into biliary tree and small bowel. Gall-bladder is not visualized, even after administration of morphine.

considered in the context of the patient's underlying disease(s), physical findings, and laboratory studies.

Management

The standard initial medical treatment for acute cholecystitis includes antibiotics, analgesia, and, at least during the early phase, bowel rest. Antibiotics for uncomplicated cholecystitis should cover enterococcal species and gram-negative rods, particularly *Escherichia coli* and *Klebsiella* spp.[49] Among patients who have previously received antibiotics, more resistant and unusual organisms are often cultured from gallbladder bile in patients with acute cholecystitis. These organisms can include *Staphylococcus* spp., resistant gram-negative bacilli, anaerobic bacteria, and fungi. Older patients are also more apt to have infected bile. In patients with empyema of the gallbladder, Tseng et al. found that bile cultures were positive in 83% of the cases.[50] Gram-negative bacteria (e.g., *E. coli*, *K. pneumoniae*, *Morganella morganii*, *Pseudomonas aeruginosa*, and *Salmonella* spp.) were found in 75%, gram-positive bacteria (e.g., *Enterococcus* spp.) in 30%, and obligate anaerobes in 7%. Broader coverage may be required for empirical coverage until cultures are obtained and coverage can be more tailored.

The next question, however, is whether to drain or remove the gallbladder acutely. There is a lack of any prospective randomized trials to help clarify this issue. Early surgical consultation is critical. The decision regarding radiographic or surgical intervention must be made with consideration of both the critical care and general surgical issues. If the patient can tolerate transport to the operating room and a

general anesthetic, cholecystectomy remains the most definitive therapy, particularly in light of the risk of the gallbladder gangrene and perforation. Frequently, however, critically ill patients with acute cholecystitis, particularly those with significant respiratory dysfunction or hemodynamic instability, are thought to be too ill for this approach. With advances in the ease of image-guided drainage, bedside cholecystostomy using ultrasonographic guidance has been utilized more commonly.

IMAGE-DIRECTED DRAINAGE

Image-directed cholecystostomy can readily be performed using either ultrasound or CT. This procedure was first used for palliation of obstructive jaundice in 1979.[51] In 1980, successful drainage of empyema of the gallbladder was reported.[52] The first large series of percutaneous cholecystostomy for acute cholecystitis was reported in 1985[53]; 113 of 114 patients were treated successfully.

Percutaneous cholecystostomy and bile culture have been performed occasionally in patients with unexplained sepsis in the ICU. In patients who have cholecystitis, cultures are often positive if performed 72 hours after the onset of symptoms. Culture of bile is sterile in approximately 50% of patients with acute cholecystitis.[49] Boland et al. tested the efficacy of percutaneous cholecystostomy as a diagnostic and therapeutic maneuver in 82 patients in the ICU with persistent unexplained sepsis[54]; 48 of 82 patients improved. Sonographic findings were not helpful in predicting response to percutaneous cholecystostomy. In a separate study of 24 such patients, 14 patients improved after

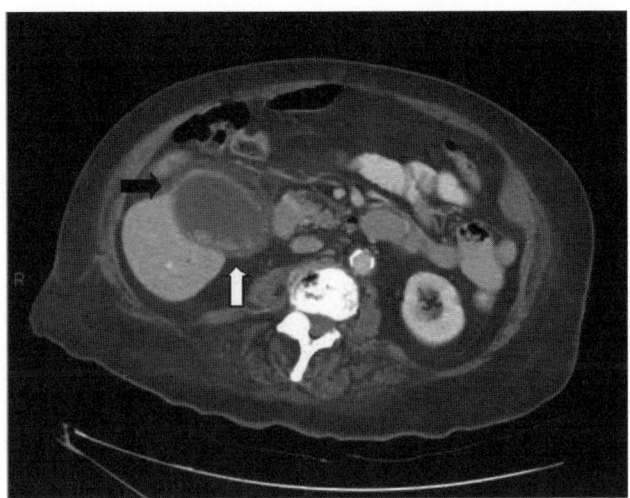

Figure 103-3 Computed tomographic study of abdomen, demonstrating thickening of gallbladder wall, with infiltration of pericholecystic fat *(black arrow)* and gallstones *(white arrow)*.

cholecystostomy.[55] Of the remaining patients, three had pneumonia and the others did not have a source of sepsis identified. Of the patients who improved, only four had positive bile cultures. Thus, in critically ill patients without a definitive diagnosis of acute cholecystitis, the role of percutaneous cholecystostomy and bile culture remains unclear. Since the risk of this procedure is low, percutaneous cholecystostomy should be considered when the index of suspicion for acute cholecystitis is high enough.

Percutaneous cholecystostomy is contraindicated if the patient has evidence of diffuse peritonitis suggesting gallbladder perforation. On the other hand, if imaging studies suggest a pericholecystic abscess, concomitant drainage of the abscess or surgical exploration is indicated.

Percutaneous cholecystostomy is most appropriate for patients with acute cholecystitis who are too unstable to tolerate a general anesthetic. The procedure is done under ultrasound or CT guidance. A needle is inserted into the gallbladder, usually via a transhepatic approach. The tract is dilated using a standard Seldinger technique. A pigtail catheter is advanced over the wire into the gallbladder. Some use a trocar technique instead. The catheter is then attached to a drainage bag.

Van Sonnenberg et al. reported a series of percutaneous cholecystostomies in 127 patients.[56] Indications included acute cholecystitis, obstructive jaundice, gallbladder perforation, need for percutaneous removal or dissolution of gallstones, need for diagnostic cholecystocholangiography, and gallbladder biopsy. The procedure was successful in 125 cases. Eleven patients (8.7%) had major complications, including bile peritonitis, bleeding, vagal reactions, hypotension, catheter dislodgement, and acute respiratory distress. Five (3.9%) had minor complications. No deaths were related to the procedure itself.

Overall mortality for percutaneous cholecystostomy is about 10%, similar to open cholecystostomy.[56-59] The limiting factor for success of percutaneous drainage is the viability of the gallbladder. Focal ischemia or necrosis is unlikely to improve without cholecystectomy and predisposes the patient to perforation. Cholecystectomy should be considered in patients who do not improve with cholecystostomy. Lo et al. found in their series that all six patients who failed to respond to cholecystostomy had transmural inflammation; five had a gangrenous gallbladder wall.[57]

Appropriate management following cholecystostomy is not completely clear. Once the patient has recovered, one can readily obtain a cholangiogram through the catheter. If gallstones are present, elective cholecystectomy at a later date is recommended. On the other hand, if no stones are present, cholecystostomy may obviate the need for cholecystectomy, as patients do well without cholecystectomy.[58,59]

A novel technique for drainage of the gallbladder involves a transpapillary endoscopic approach.[60] This approach may be helpful if other indications for endoscopic evaluation or intervention are present. It seems that the intervention is more successful if the ultrasound demonstrates that the gallbladder is not severely distended or thick.[61]

SURGICAL MANAGEMENT

Surgical options include cholecystostomy and cholecystectomy. Surgical cholecystostomy can be accomplished via a small right subcostal incision using local anesthesia or via laparoscopy. This procedure largely has been supplanted by image-guided percutaneous cholecystostomy, as described above.

Cholecystectomy may be advantageous compared to cholecystostomy, since it allows one to examine the entire right upper quadrant for other pathology and to completely drain any fluid collections around the gallbladder. It also alleviates the risk of gallbladder perforation. When cholecystectomy is performed, a laparoscopic approach can usually be attempted, recognizing that one may need to abandon the attempt and proceed with an open procedure because of difficulty with the dissection. The timing of cholecystectomy for acute cholecystitis remains controversial[62] but definitely should be considered if the patient is not responding to nonoperative management. If a patient undergoes cholecystostomy, it may be beneficial to delay the cholecystectomy for at least 2 weeks.

Bedside laparoscopy can be performed for evaluation of the acute abdomen in critically ill patients. If acute cholecystitis is identified, a cholecystostomy can be performed readily, or the patient can be taken to the operating room for a cholecystectomy.[63,64] If the diagnosis of cholecystitis is excluded, the patient may be spared an unnecessary trip to the operating room.

Complications and Outcome

Complications of acute cholecystitis are much more common in critically ill patients than in the general population. Elderly patients are particularly at risk. Among patients with acalculous cholecystitis, Kalliafas et al. found that 17 of 27 had gangrene, four had perforation, and one had an abscess.[38] Mortality was 41%.

Gangrene may be present in as many as 59% of cases.[9-22] Shapiro et al. found gangrene or frank necrosis in 13 of 22 patients undergoing cholecystectomy for acute cholecystitis that developed in the ICU.[22] Cornwell et al. found necrosis or gangrene in 6 of 14 trauma patients who developed acute acalculous cholecystitis.[65]

Compared to patients without gangrene, those with gangrene are at greater risk of perforation or failure of percutaneous drainage. Some of these patients have emphysematous cholecystitis (gas in the wall of the gallbladder), a diagnosis that carries an even greater risk of perforation. Emphysema can be identified by plain abdominal radiographs, CT, or ultrasound. Antibiotics should cover gas-forming anaerobic organisms. Although percutaneous drainage may be effective,[66] early cholecystectomy is indicated if the patient does not improve promptly.

Perforation of the gallbladder occurs in approximately 10% of cases.[9-22] Usually the resulting fluid collection is localized and amenable to percutaneous drainage. Free perforation also can occur, and when it does, the risk of mortality is markedly increased.[67] The clinical problem, however, is that preoperative imaging may not demonstrate evidence of perforation.[68] The risk of perforation increases with delay in drainage or operation. Cholecystectomy is indicated for free perforation or for patients failing to rapidly respond to percutaneous drainage.

Empyema of the gallbladder also greatly increases mortality.[69] This complication may be amenable to percutaneous drainage,[50,70] but the risks of failure or perforation are substantial.

The risk of mortality from cholecystitis in the ICU mainly reflects the underlying disease processes and comorbidities. Overall mortality is around 30%.[9-22] Hadas-Halpern et al. found that 10 of 80 patients undergoing percutaneous cholecystostomy for acute cholecystitis died of comorbid disease, whereas only two died of biliary peritonitis.[71]

Prevention

No intervention has been shown conclusively to prevent development of cholecystitis in ICU patients. If the theories regarding the pathophysiologic mechanisms are correct, the incidence of the disease should be reduced by aggressively resuscitating patients with shock, avoiding biliary stasis by implementing early enteral feeding, and minimizing the use of narcotics. Intermittent doses of cholecystokinin or deoxycholic acid have been shown to increase bile flow and, therefore, may decrease the risk of acalculous cholecystitis in patients receiving parenteral nutrition,[72-74] though studies in ICU patients are needed.

Summary

The diagnosis of acute cholecystitis in critically ill patients is difficult because patients frequently do not present with the usual symptoms and signs. Laboratory tests are nonspecific. The best initial radiographic study is ultrasound. Scintigraphy and CT also may be helpful.

Management includes antibiotics and bowel rest. Percutaneous cholecystostomy may be utilized in unstable patients, although cholecystectomy remains the most definitive treatment if this intervention can be accomplished safely.

KEY POINTS

1. Critically ill patients frequently do not present with the usual symptoms and signs of cholecystitis.

2. Laboratory tests for cholecystitis are not specific.

3. The best initial imaging study is ultrasound, but scintigraphy or computed tomography may be needed as well.

4. Management begins with antibiotics and bowel rest.

5. While cholecystectomy is the most definitive procedure, image-guided percutaneous cholecystostomy is indicated for patients too unstable to undergo cholecystectomy.

ANNOTATED REFERENCES

Boland G, Lee MJ, Mueller PR. Acute cholecystitis in the intensive care unit. New Horiz 1993;1:246-60.
  This paper is an extensive review of the pathophysiology, presentation, and management of acute cholecystitis in the ICU.
Thompson JW III, Ferris DO, Beggenstoss AH. Acute cholecystitis complicating operation for other diseases. Ann Surg 1962;155:489.
  This is one of the first papers to postulate that the critical pathophysiologic mechanism for acalculous cholecystitis is hypoperfusion.
Helbich TH, Mallek R, Madl C, Wunderbaldinger P, Breitenseher M, Tscholakoff D, et al. Sonomorphology of the gallbladder in critically ill patients. Value of a scoring system and follow-up examinations. Acta Radiol 1997;38:129-34.
  Ultrasound examinations of the gallbladder of patients in the ICU frequently reveal equivocal findings. This group tried to quantify these findings, coupled with serial examinations, to improve the diagnostic accuracy of ultrasonography in this setting.

Flancbaum L, Alden SM, Trooskin SZ. Use of cholescintigraphy with morphine in critically ill patients with suspected cholecystitis. Surgery 1989;106:668-73.
  The addition of morphine to cholescintigraphy can improve the diagnostic accuracy of this test for diagnosing cholecystitis in critically ill patients.
vanSonnenberg E, D'Agostino HB, Goodacre BW, Sanchez RB, Casola G. Percutaneous gallbladder puncture and cholecystostomy: results, complications, and caveats for safety. Radiology 1992;183:167-70.
  These authors describe a large series of patients who underwent percutaneous cholecystostomy with excellent results.

REFERENCES

Access the complete reference list online at http://www.expertconsult.com.

104

Acute Pancreatitis

PAMELA A. LIPSETT

The term *acute pancreatitis* describes a wide spectrum of disease ranging from a mild edematous form of acute pancreatitis to severe acute necrotizing pancreatitis. Acute pancreatitis is the third most common gastrointestinal disease requiring hospitalization in the United States and accounts for annual costs of more than $2 billion.[1,2] The mild form of acute pancreatitis is a self-limited disease associated with little or no distant organ dysfunction; it has a mortality rate of less than 1% and usually resolves in 3 to 4 days. Patients with this form of acute pancreatitis rarely need intensive care unit (ICU) therapy or pancreatic surgery. Although most (80%) patients with acute pancreatitis have mild disease, 10% to 15% develop the systemic inflammatory response syndrome (SIRS) and run a fulminant clinical course leading to pancreatic necrosis and multisystem organ injury.[3-5] The mortality rate for severe acute pancreatitis is 15% to 30%, whereas the overall mortality rate for all patients presenting with acute pancreatitis is less than 5%.[4,5] The natural course of severe acute pancreatitis occurs in two phases. The first 7 to 14 days of this disease process are characterized by SIRS and resulting end-organ dysfunction. Inflammatory mediators are released into the systemic circulation, and patients manifest signs and symptoms of cardiorespiratory and renal failure.[6] Pancreatic infection is uncommon during this early phase of acute pancreatitis and SIRS, but bacteremia and pneumonia have been identified at a median of 7 days.[7] Attempts to modify the course of the disease by instituting therapy with protease inhibitors, octreotide, or platelet-activating factor receptor antagonists have been unsuccessful.[8-10]

Since the 1980s, the morbidity and mortality associated with acute pancreatitis have decreased substantially.[11-14] The reasons for the decrease in mortality in severe acute pancreatitis are uncertain but may reflect improved critical care services and better strategies for surgical management. In general, mortality from severe acute pancreatitis is related to infection.[13,14] Infection of the necrotic pancreas (and associated tissues) typically develops in the second and third weeks of the disease and is reported to occur in 40% to 70% of patients with pancreatic necrosis.[7,13,14] Multiple organ system dysfunction syndrome is the main life-threatening complication, and mortality rates of 50% have been reported.[15] Infected necrosis is the most important risk factor for death secondary to necrotizing pancreatitis.[13-16] Prevention, diagnosis, and optimal treatment of infection in severe acute pancreatitis are crucial for improving outcome for patients with this disease.

This chapter discusses the etiology, pathophysiology, severity and staging, and management of patients with severe acute pancreatitis. Chronic pancreatitis is not discussed in this chapter. Several authors and/or societies have proposed guidelines and protocols for management of severe acute pancreatitis.[4,14,17-19]

Etiology and Epidemiology

In 2001 in California, the rate of hospital admission with an initial attack of acute pancreatitis was 44 per 100,000 per year, an increase of more than 32% over the decade of the study. Overall rates of hospitalization in the Unites States over the last 20 years has increased from 40 per 100,000 to 80 per 100,000 and included both sexes and all age groups.[20] The increasing incidence of acute pancreatitis is believed to be related to increases in alcohol consumption and gallstone disease in some societies. Acute pancreatitis is slightly more common in men than in women, with a male-to-female ratio of 1 : 1.2 to 1 : 1.5. Predisposing factors related to race have not been identified, but both

hospitalization rates and emergency department visits for patients diagnosed with acute pancreatitis are higher for blacks than for whites. Pancreatitis can occur in any age group, but cases in the very young (<3 years) are likely to be related to a systemic disease such as hemolytic uremic syndrome or cystic fibrosis. On the other hand, alcohol-related acute pancreatitis has a peak incidence between 45 and 55 years of age, with a gradual decline thereafter. Gallstone pancreatitis can occur in any age group, but its frequency increases with age. Biliary pancreatitis is more common in women, and alcohol-related acute pancreatitis is more common in men.

Understanding the etiology of a particular case of pancreatitis is important; evaluation and treatment depend to some extent on the predisposing disease process.[6,17] Gallstones are the leading cause of acute pancreatitis in developed countries and account for 45% of all cases. A biliary etiology should be suspected in female patients older than age 40 with a serum alanine aminotransferase level greater than three times the upper reference limit. Gallstone pancreatitis is the commonest form of pancreatitis in older patients. Since the frequency of gallstones increases with age, gallstones should be suspected in elderly patients.

Alcohol abuse typically accounts for about 35% of cases of acute pancreatitis; however, it is unclear whether acute alcoholic pancreatitis ever arises in the absence of chronic injury to the gland.[21] Infrequent, but not rare, causes of pancreatitis include drug reactions (usually idiosyncratic), pancreatic and ampullary tumors, hypertriglyceridemia, hypercalcemia (almost always secondary to hyperparathyroidism), hypothermia, congenital abnormalities of the biliary or pancreatic duct (e.g., choledochal cyst), trauma (including acute pancreatitis after endoscopic retrograde cholangiopancreatography), and infectious or parasitic organisms. Rare causes include bites of certain spiders, scorpions, and the Gila monster lizard. Unidentified causes are termed *idiopathic*. The roles of sphincter of Oddi dysfunction, pancreas divisum, and bile crystals or sludge in the development of acute pancreatitis are less clear.[20]

Pathogenesis and Genetic Susceptibility

Regardless of the actual underlying cause, pancreatitis is an inflammatory process that can initiate SIRS.[6] In spite of much investigation into the molecular pathogenesis of acute pancreatitis, the exact intracellular mechanisms initiating and accelerating pancreatitis are not completely understood. Three phenotypic responses occur in the acinar cell in the early phases of acute pancreatitis[22,23]: changes in secretions, intracellular activation of proteases, and generation of inflammatory mediators. Shortly after an appropriate stimulus, secretions are released from the apical cells into the pancreatic duct. This process entails exocytotic fusion of zymogen granules with the apical plasma membrane; the granules do not fuse with the basolateral membrane. However during acute pancreatitis, there is (1) markedly decreased apical secretion from the acinar cell, (2) disruption of the paracellular barrier in the pancreatic duct with leakage of contents into the paracellular space, and (3) redirection of secretion from zymogen granules from the apical pole to the basolateral regions of the acinar cell. Inappropriate activation of the proteolytic enzyme, trypsin, is thought to be the initial step in the development of acute pancreatitis. Trypsinogen activation is promotion by cationic trypsinogen mutations (PRSS1+), active trypsin, high calcium ion concentration, and low pH. Calcium levels

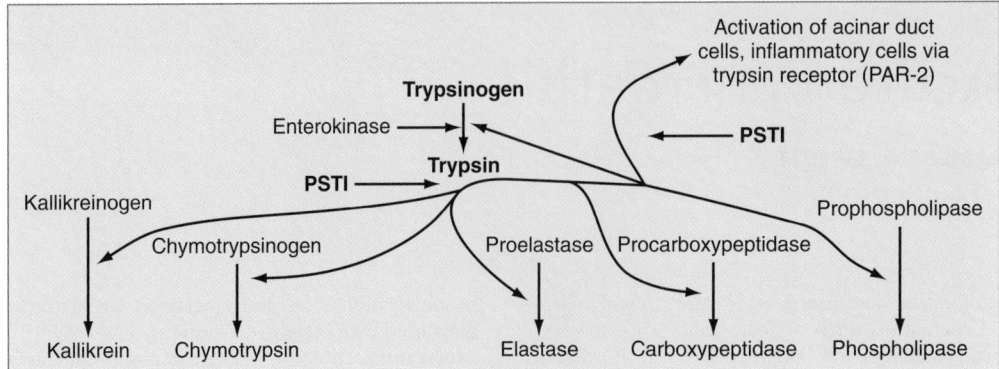

Figure 104-1 Activation pathways of proenzymes and protease-activated receptor (PAR)-2 by trypsin. When trypsin is activated, it is capable of activating many digestive proenzymes. Trypsin also activates inflammatory cells via PAR-2. Trypsin activity in the pancreas is mainly controlled by pancreatic secretory trypsin inhibitor (PSTI). When trypsinogen is activated into trypsin in the pancreas, PSTI immediately binds to trypsin to prevent further activation of pancreatic enzymes.

are regulated in part by calcium-sensing receptors (CASR) and dys-regulated by ethanol.[22,23] Degradation of active trypsin is blocked by high calcium ion concentration. If trypsin in active within the pancreas, inflammation results and this up-regulates serine protease inhibitor Kazak 1 (SPINK1), which further blocks activation of trypsinogen.[22] Trypsin also activates cells via the trypsin receptor, also known as *protease-activated receptor 2 (PAR-2)* (Figure 104-1).[22] Pancreatic acinar and duct cells abundantly express PAR-2. Trypsin activity in the pancreas is controlled mainly by the pancreatic secretory trypsin inhibitor (PSTI), also called *serine protease inhibitor Kazal type 1 (SPINK1)*.[22] PSTI is synthesized in pancreas acinar cells and acts as a potent natural inhibitor of trypsin. Normally when trypsinogen is cleaved to release trypsin in the pancreas, PSTI immediately binds to the enzyme to prevent further activation of additional pancreatic enzymes. PSTI also blocks further activation of pancreatic cells via the trypsin receptor, PAR-2.

Several additional protective systems prevent pancreatic autodigestion by trypsin, and the genetic expression of these systems may contribute to the risk of developing acute pancreatitis or modulate the severity of the disease when it occurs. Trypsin-activated trypsinlike enzymes such as mesotrypsin degrade trypsinogen. Bicarbonate-rich pancreatic secretions are affected by abnormal expression of the cystic fibrosis transmembrane conductance receptor. A mutation in SPINK1, N34S, has been reported in people with familial pancreatitis,[24] in children with idiopathic chronic pancreatitis,[25,26] and in 2% of the control population.[26] Because these mutations in SPINK1 are much more common than pancreatitis, this mutation probably is a disease modifier rather than a causative factor underlying the development of acute pancreatitis.

Genetic linkage and candidate gene studies have identified six pancreas-targeting factors that are associated with changes in susceptibility to acute and/or chronic pancreatitis, including cationic trypsinogen (PRSS1), anionic trypsinogen (PRSS2), serine protease inhibitor Kazal 1 (SPINK1), cy regulator (CFTR), chymotrypsinogen C (CTRC) and calcium-sensing receptor (CASR).[22]

Diagnosis

The diagnosis of acute pancreatitis is relatively straightforward when acute upper abdominal pain and tenderness, nausea, vomiting, and hyperamylasemia or hyperlipasemia are present.[27] These clinical and biochemical signs are nonspecific, however, and can be present in many other acute intraabdominal conditions such as acute perforation of a hollow organ or mesenteric infarction. Many cases of acute pancreatitis still are diagnosed at autopsy. The diagnosis of acute pancreatitis can be particularly difficult in postoperative patients. Acute pancreatitis also can be hard to diagnose in patients receiving drugs for sedation and patients who are hypothermic or unable to complain of abdominal pain. The Cullen sign and the Grey Turner sign (periumbilical and flank bruising, respectively) are rare and can be present with any disease associated with retroperitoneal hemorrhage. Although hyperamylasemia is common in patients with acute pancreatitis, normal circulating amylase levels are present in 10% to 20% of all cases of acute pancreatitis. Normal serum amylase concentrations are seen predominantly in acute pancreatitis secondary to hyperlipidemia, acute exacerbations of chronic pancreatitis, and late in the course of acute pancreatitis.[28] Advantages of serum amylase determination include its technical simplicity, wide availability, and sensitivity.[29] This diagnostic test is plagued by low specificity, however. Serum lipase concentration increases within 4 to 8 hours of the onset of acute pancreatitis, peaks at 24 hours, and returns to normal after 8 to 14 days.[29] The major advantage of serum lipase determination as a diagnostic test is its excellent sensitivity in acute alcoholic pancreatitis. Measurement of serum lipase activity also is valuable when patients present to an emergency department days after the onset of the disease, because serum lipase levels remain elevated longer than amylase levels.[29] Although serum lipase formerly was believed to be a specific marker for acute pancreatitis, increased circulating levels of serum lipase can occur in many other diseases. Simultaneous estimation of amylase and lipase levels does not improve accuracy.[29] Other pancreatic enzymes such as P-isoamylase, macroamylases, immunoreactive trypsinogen, and elastase generally are not considered useful for making the diagnosis of acute pancreatitis.

Serum triglyceride levels should be determined when an etiology of pancreatitis is uncertain and lipemic serum is suspected. Hydrolysis of triglycerides by pancreatic lipase and formation of free fatty acids that induce inflammatory changes are postulated to account for the pathophysiology of this form of pancreatitis. While it has never been proven, circulating triglyceride levels above 1000 mg/dL (11.3 mm/L) are believed to trigger pancreatitis.

Severity and Scoring

Prediction of the severity of the disease at the time of admission can be difficult, and patients can appear clinically well at admission but clinically deteriorate within 48 hours. Several different prognostic scoring systems with clinical, laboratory, and radiologic criteria have been proposed, yet none of the proposed scoring systems have a high sensitivity, specificity, positive predictive value, or negative likelihood ratio, and frequent clinical assessment is essential for identifying patients with severe disease.[30] Ranson's criteria (Table 104-1),[31] the Imrie[32] (Glasgow) score, the Acute Physiologic and Chronic Health Evaluation (APACHE) II and III scores,[33] the simplified acute physiology score, and Balthazar's computed tomography (CT) index (Table 104-2)[34-36] are the most popular scoring systems and often are used to determine the need for admission to an ICU. Ranson's criteria are

TABLE 104-1	Ranson's Criteria for Patients with Non–Gallstone-Associated Pancreatitis	
At Presentation		*During Initial 48 Hours*
Age > 55 years		Hematocrit fall > 10%
White blood cell count > 16,000/μL		Blood urea nitrogen > 5 mg/dL
Blood glucose > 200 mg/dL		Serum calcium < 8 mg/dL
Serum alanine transferase > 250 U/dL		Arterial Po_2 < 60 mm Hg
Serum lactate dehydrogenase > 350 IU		Base deficit > 4 mEq/L
		Estimated fluid sequestration > 6 L

Modified from Blamey SL, Imrie CW, O'Neill J, Gilmour WH, Carter DC. Prognostic factors in acute pancreatitis. Gut 1984;25:1340-6.

based on 11 prognostic signs present at presentation and 48 hours later.[31] A meta-analysis of studies using the Ranson criteria reported the following with regard to predicting severe acute pancreatitis (SAP): sensitivity, 74%: specificity, 77%; positive predictive value, 49%; and negative predictive value, 91%.[30] The Glasgow (Imrie) severity score system collects data on 9 variables at admission but is not complete until 48 hours after admission. Many institutions routinely utilize the APACHE scoring system for all patients admitted to the ICU.[33] Patients with SAP and an APACHE II score above 8 have severe disease and are likely to develop organ failure. Key statistical parameters related to APACHE II score of above 7 and the prediction of SAP are as follows: sensitivity, 65%; specificity, 76%; positive predictive value, 43%; and negative predictive value, 89%. Balthazar's CT index[34-36] uses both fluid collections and amount of pancreatic necrosis to predict outcome. A recent international group of experts concluded that an additional group of patients should be identified: those with moderately severe acute pancreatitis (MSAP).[37] This is a large group of patients who meet the Atlanta classification of severe disease but do not develop organ failure. Patients in the MSAP group often develop local complications and often have long hospitalizations with significant morbidity but without mortality. In a strategy to identify those patients who will not need ICU care, Lankish et al. proposed and validated a "harmless acute pancreatitis score (HAPS)." Using this scoring system, 98% of 204 patients were correctly identified as having non-severe disease within 30 minutes of presentation.[38] These simple measures included rebound or guarding on clinical examination, hematocrit greater than 43% in men and greater than 39.6 in women, and serum creatinine concentration above 2 mg/dL. Imamura and colleagues have recently proposed a simplified grading of early CT scans based on the presence or loss of enhancement of the renal rim fat. This simple assessment compared favorably with all the commonly used scoring systems.[39]

TABLE 104-2	Calculation of Balthazar's Computed Tomography Scoring System for Acute Pancreatitis			
Inflammatory Process		*Grade*	*Score*	*Subtotals*
Normal		A	0	
Focal or diffuse enlargement		B	1	
Contour irregularity				
Inhomogeneous attenuation				
Grade B *plus* peripancreatic haziness/mottled densities		C	2	
Grades B, C *plus* one ill-defined peripancreatic fluid collection		D	3	
Grades B, C *plus* two ill-defined fluid collections or gas		E	4	
Necrosis:				
None		0	0	
<30%			2	
50%			4	
>50%			6	
Total				

Modified from Balthazar EJ, Robinson DL, Megibow AJ, Ranson JH. Acute pancreatitis: value of CT in establishing prognosis. Radiology 1990;174:331-6.

Many investigators have studied and proposed a variety of serum biomarkers as predictors of the severity and prognosis of acute pancreatitis.[40-42] High circulating levels of C-reactive protein (CRP) (cutoff 150 mg/L) are associated with pancreatic necrosis, but there is a 48-hour latency before CRP increases, limiting its utility as an early predictor. This marker has a sensitivity and specificity of 80%. Although not ideal predictors of severity, serum concentrations of procalcitonin and interleukins (IL) 6 and 8 have some predictive value.[40-42] Certain urinary markers also have some predictive value. While not used extensively clinically at the current time, procalcitonin appears to offer the greatest promise. Serum procalcitonin levels higher than 3.8 ng/mL accurately predict later organ dysfunction (sensitivity, 79%; specificity, 93%).[42]

The scoring systems mentioned help quantify the degree of illness, but it is essential that clinicians identify patients with impending or actual organ failure. Patients with signs of SIRS are especially at risk for further organ dysfunction.[45] In a review of 259 patients with acute pancreatitis, mortality was significantly higher in patients who developed or had persistent SIRS at 48 hours (25.4%) than in patients who had transient SIRS (8%) or no SIRS in the first 48 hours (0.7%).[37]

An update of the Atlanta Classification system for severity of acute pancreatitis is expected soon; the system developed at the initial consensus meeting in 1992 has allowed comparisons among clinical trials and different treatment strategies.[36] It defined SAP by its association with organ failure, local complications such as necrosis, abscess, or pseudocyst, or both. By consensus, the Atlanta Classification also defined SAP based upon the presence of ≥3 of Ranson's criteria or an APACHE II score ≥ 8. Most often, SAP is a clinical expression of the development of pancreatic necrosis. Less commonly, patients with interstitial (edematous) pancreatitis can present with SAP. In addition to the previously proposed scoring systems, there is another very simple scoring system termed the *Panc 3 Score*.[46] Three findings—hematocrit over 44 mg/dL, body mass index above 30 kg/m², and a pleural effusion on chest x-ray—were the most sensitive predictors of overall severity. In the validation set of data, when all three of these findings were present and the pretest probability of pancreatitis was between 12% and 25%, the posttest likelihood of severe disease was 99%.[43]

Serum concentrations of CRP, neutrophil elastase, pancreatitis-associated peptide, IL-6, IL-8, IL-1, IL-10, and soluble tumor necrosis factor (TNF) receptors might be useful for the early prediction of severity of disease in acute pancreatitis.[40] Circulating CRP concentration is an independent predictor of outcome in acute pancreatitis, but it is not predictive of severity at presentation.[44] Laboratory tests also can be used for severity stratification; serum IL-6 concentration greater than 2.7 pg/mL within 48 hours from disease onset and a serum CRP level above 150 mg/L at 48 hours after pain onset can both be used. A recent meta-analysis of the role of procalcitonin in the identification of patients with SAP suggested that the test has a sensitivity of 0.72 for the diagnosis, a specificity of 0.86, and an area under the curve of 0.87, but the studies showed a fair amount of heterogeneity.[42] Trypsinogen-2 can be measured via a simple serum immunofluorometric assay or urine dipstick assay, using a threshold of 50 μg/L.[41]

Imaging

ULTRASONOGRAPHY AND ENDOSCOPIC ULTRASONOGRAPHY

Ultrasonography should be considered as an initial test in all patients with pancreatitis, especially if gallstones are suspected.[5,17,19] By aiding in the diagnosis of gallstones, common bile duct stones, common bile duct dilation, and free peritoneal fluid, ultrasonography can be useful for determining the cause of pancreatitis.[47] Ultrasonography currently has little role in the grading of severity of acute pancreatitis or determination of extent of pancreatic necrosis. However, this situation may change because of the evolution of contrast-enhanced ultrasonography. This technique employs microbubbles as a blood-pool contrast medium to allow visualization of tissue vascularization. Early in the course of pancreatitis, inflammation is associated with hyperemia. Later in the course of severe disease, contrast-enhanced ultrasonography can reveal confluent necrotic areas of devitalized pancreatic tissue.[48] The value of ultrasonography is compromised by overlying bowel gas in at least 25% to 30% of cases.

Endoscopic ultrasonography (EUS) combines ultrasonography and endoscopic evaluation. It is less invasive than endoscopic retrograde cholangiopancreatography (ERCP) and has been shown to be clinically useful in diagnosing acute pancreatitis and choledocholithiasis.[47] Endoscopic ultrasonography may be useful when CT and ultrasonography fail to show common bile duct stones. Endoscopic ultrasonography also may be useful for selecting patients who might benefit from endoscopic retrograde cholangiopancreatography and early stone extraction. Petrov et al. reviewed studies of patients randomized to EUS-guided ERCP (n = 213) versus ERCP alone (n = 210). These authors showed that ERCP could be avoided in 67.1% patients when EUS failed to identify gallstones.[47] The use of EUS significantly reduced the risk of overall complications [relative risk (RR) 0.35, 95% confidence interval (CI) 0.20-0.62] and post-ERCP pancreatitis (RR 0.21, 95% CI 0.06-0.83). One additional advantage of endoscopic ultrasonography is that it can be performed in pregnant women, patients with metallic implants, and patients who are too unstable to be transported out of the ICU.[47]

COMPUTED TOMOGRAPHY

Contrast-enhanced CT is considered the gold standard for diagnosing pancreatic necrosis and peripancreatic collections and for grading acute pancreatitis (see Table 104-2).[34-36] Necrosis is detected by CT as focal or diffuse areas of diminished pancreatic parenchymal contrast enhancement (<50 Hounsfield units). The accuracy of this test is greater than 90%. CT findings of acute pancreatitis include diffuse or segmental enlargement of the pancreas (interstitial edema), irregularity of the contour of the pancreas with obliteration of the peripancreatic fat planes, heterogeneous appearance with areas of decreased density within the pancreas, and variable ill-defined fluid collections (Figures 104-2 and 104-3).[34-36] The Balthazar index ranges from 0 to 10 and is obtained by adding the points attributed to the extent of the inflammatory process to the volume of pancreatic necrosis. Although CT findings correlate with clinical course and severity of patients with acute pancreatitis,[36] it is not necessary to obtain this study in patients with mild pancreatitis. In a recent Dutch observational study of 166 patients admitted with acute pancreatitis, early CT (within 4 days of admission) was performed in 47% of all patients. However, only 18 of the 166 patients had severe disease, and 11 eventually developed pancreatic necrosis. No changes in clinical management resulted from obtaining early CT scans. These data suggest that the use of early CT, especially in patients with mild disease, should be discouraged.[49] CT can be helpful when the diagnosis is in doubt or when complications of pancreatitis may be developing. In general, contrast-enhanced CT scans should not be performed during the first 72 hours of the disease, because necrosis may not be fully established until after 96 hours, and there have been isolated reports of intravenous (IV) contrast material causing derangements of the pancreatic microcirculation.[49] Contrast administration also can trigger or exacerbate renal insufficiency.

ENDOSCOPIC RETROGRADE CHOLANGIOPANCREATOGRAPHY

Endoscopic retrograde cholangiopancreatography is an effective means for treating common bile duct stones.[47] Endoscopic retrograde cholangiopancreatography is not indicated for the management of mild pancreatitis or nonbiliary pancreatitis, and its overall use in patients with acute pancreatitis continues to be debated.[50-58] Guidelines from England, Japan, and the United States indicate that ERCP is indicated in the management of patients with biliary pancreatitis and biliary obstruction or cholangitis.[17-19,52] There remains controversy regarding

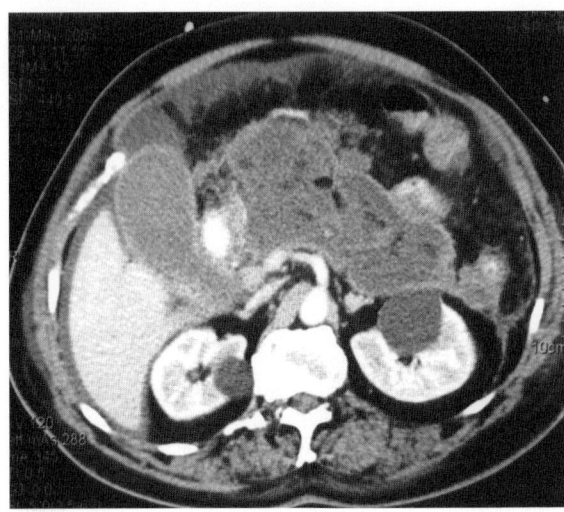

Figure 104-2 Computed tomography scan of a patient with severe necrotizing pancreatitis and Balthazar grade E scan; more than 50% necrosis of the gland was seen on previous scans of the gland, giving the patient a Balthazar index of 10. The patient developed pancreatic infection more than 4 weeks into his hospital course.

the role of ERCP for the management of patients with biliary pancreatitis but without bile duct obstruction. Five clinical trials have sought to determine whether ERCP plus sphincterotomy or conservative management is more appropriate for patients with acute pancreatitis.[53-57] In a study of 121 patients randomized to ERCP or conservative treatment within 72 hours of onset, there was a significant reduction in morbidity (17% versus 34%; P=.03) but no significant difference in mortality (2% versus 8%; P=.23).[53] The differences in morbidity seen in this trial cannot be explained by differences in the severity of pancreatitis between the two groups.[53]

In another study that enrolled 195 patients, ERCP performed within 24 hours was compared with conservative therapy. ERCP was associated with a significant reduction in morbidity (biliary sepsis; P = .001) without a significant reduction in mortality (five deaths with ERCP versus nine deaths with conservative treatment).[54] Included in this study were patients with nonbiliary pancreatitis such as alcohol-related and parasite-related disease. In another trial with a similar design, 280 patients were randomized to receive ERCP within 24 hours or conservative treatment[55]; 75 of the 178 patients in the ERCP arm had impacted

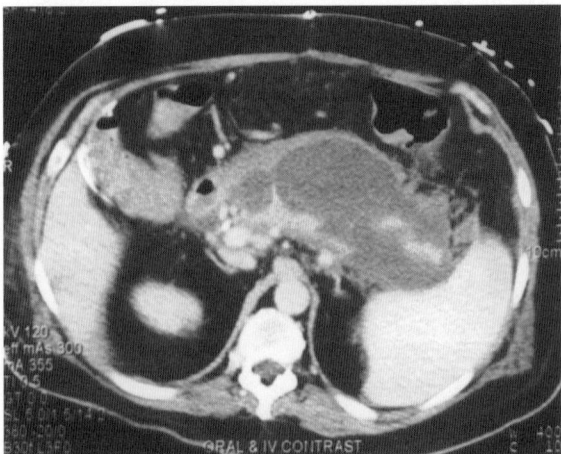

Figure 104-3 Computed tomography scan of a patient with severe acute pancreatitis, a large fluid collection, and significant (>50%) necrosis. Pancreatic infection occurred on hospital day 17.

biliary stones. This study is the only one that showed a significant reduction in morbidity and mortality.

The study by Folsch and colleagues[56] was a multicenter trial of ERCP versus conservative management. Patients with biliary sepsis and obstruction were excluded from study entry because efficacy in this group has been established. In contrast to the previous studies, this study showed a significant increase in complications in the ERCP group compared with the conservatively managed group (respiratory failure, 12% versus 4% [$P = .03$]; renal failure, 7% versus 4% [$P = .10$]). In addition, the mortality rate was higher in the ERCP group compared with the control group (11% versus 6%), requiring premature termination of the study.[56] The results of this large clinical trial suggest that in the absence of biliary obstruction or sepsis, ERCP may be harmful, and a conservative approach is preferred.

Oria and colleagues studied 102 patients with acute pancreatitis and an APACHE II score higher than 6; the subjects were randomized to receive ERCP within 72 hours or conservative management. Three patients in each group suffered local complications.[57] Petrov and colleagues performed a meta-analysis of these trials.[58] These authors concluded that the early use of ERCP did not significantly reduce the risk of local pancreatic complications in patients with either mild or severe pancreatitis.

In contrast, Dutch investigators reported their observational results of the use of ERCP as part of another clinical trial on the use of probiotics in SAP. Of the 153 patients enrolled, 81 underwent ERCP and 72 received conservative management. Of the 153 patients, 78 patients with cholestasis had fewer complications when ERCP was utilized [OR 0.35; 95% CI, 0.13-0.99], but there was no significant effect on mortality, and no reduction of complications or mortality if cholestasis was not present in patients with predicted SAP.[51] The role of ERCP in idiopathic pancreatitis also is unclear. Advances in ultrasonography and magnetic resonance cholangiopancreatography (MRCP) suggest that these modalities may have a preferred role when diagnostic considerations are the issue in acute pancreatitis, especially in view of the potential for complications with ERCP.[59] As noted previously, endoscopic ultrasound may have an increasing role in identifying patients with suspected choledocholithiasis who might benefit from ERCP.

MAGNETIC RESONANCE CHOLANGIOPANCREATOGRAPHY

Magnetic resonance imaging (MRI) and MRCP are noninvasive imaging modalities that are useful for depicting abnormalities of the pancreatic duct and parenchyma.[60-62] These imaging techniques can identify acute fluid collections and necrosis in SAP. MRI has several advantages over CT: there is no risk from radiation with MRI, it can detect pancreatic duct disruption, and it can help identify the etiology of acute pancreatitis. Without injection of gadolinium, MRI can discriminate between normal pancreatic parenchyma, the presence of edema, and the presence of necrosis as well as differentiate between solid and liquid fluid collections. In a study of 90 patients, 28 had gallstones, 9 had common bile duct stones, and 10 had pancreatic divisum.[60,62] MRCP can be performed when ERCP has failed or is not possible, although ERCP is not only a diagnostic modality but also a therapeutic one, because the endoscopic approach permits sphincterotomy and removal of common duct stones.[61]

Contrast-enhanced CT is the gold standard for documenting pancreatic necrosis and assessing the severity of acute pancreatitis. Nevertheless, results from a few studies suggest that MRCP compares favorably with contrast-enhanced CT for the diagnosis and grading of severe acute pancreatitis.[60,62] The major advantage of MRCP for SAP is that MRCP obviates the necessity for the infusion of iodinated contrast media and thereby may lower the risk for acute renal dysfunction in these critically ill patients.[60,62] Bowel peristalsis, vascular motion artifacts, gastrointestinal air, and the presence of metallic clips all can degrade the quality of the images obtained with MRCP. One disadvantage of MRI and MRCP is that acquisition of the image takes longer than with CT.

Management

GENERAL SUPPORT

Monitoring and Resuscitation

Several publications suggest that patients with SAP should be managed in an ICU, preferably by a specialist team.[17-19,52] Ongoing monitoring for signs of distant organ dysfunction is crucial. Resuscitation of intravascular volume is a key component of the initial management, regardless of the etiology and severity of acute pancreatitis. Sequestration of fluid into the so-called third space (i.e., the extravascular extracellular compartment) can lead to loss of as much as a third of plasma volume. Rapid restoration and maintenance of intravascular volume is essential because hypovolemia and shock probably are important factors contributing to the high incidence of acute renal failure among patients with severe acute pancreatitis.[30,63] It is common for patients with SAP to require administration of crystalloid fluid at rates as great as 500 mL/h, at least for a while.

Recently, 76 patients with SAP were randomly assigned to receive rapid infusion of IV fluid at either 10 to 15 mL/kg/h or 5 to 10 mL/kg/h, both groups receiving more than 10 L of fluid during their first 3 days of ICU care.[64] The investigators in this study suggested that several outcomes were better in the group that received more gradual fluid expansion. The results of this trial are interesting but require confirmation before there is widespread adoption of the authors' recommendations.

Single-organ or multiorgan dysfunction is common, and monitoring of respiratory status is essential. Respiratory and cardiovascular dysfunction are common and require prompt identification and supportive care. Adequate oxygen delivery to tissues and prevention of splanchnic ischemia are essential to prevent further organ injury. Vasoactive agents may be required, but they should be considered only after ensuring that intravascular volume has been repleted. In addition, because rapid administration of large volumes of IV fluid may be indicated, abdominal compartment syndrome should be considered and assessed.[65]

Even when systemic signs of adequate resuscitation are present, local inflammation in the pancreas can continue, leading to ongoing production of cytotoxic mediators. Accordingly, investigators have been interested in targeting this aspect of the disease process. Treatment with protease inhibitors has been successful in experimental models of acute pancreatitis and is used via continuous arterial infusion in Japan.[63,68] A trial was carried out that compared no infusion with continuous regional arterial infusion of the protease inhibitor, gabexate mesilate, plus antibiotics.[66] Treatment with gabexate mesilate shortened the duration of abdominal pain, duration of SIRS, and decreased the length of hospital stay. Circulating levels of several markers of inflammation also were decreased with the protease inhibitor.[66] A national survey of clinicians in Japan indicated the following: severe pain disappeared after a short period of time of infusion of a protease inhibitor; infected necrosis was less common when both a protease inhibitor and antibiotic infusion were infused; and mortality was lower when continuous arterial infusion was initiated within 2 days.[67]

Although there has been significant interest in decreasing cytokine production by administering an anti-TNF antibody, this approach has not been shown to be beneficial in clinical trials, perhaps owing to the early peak of TNF in the disease process. Similarly, although administration of an IL-1 receptor antagonist has been beneficial in animal models of SAP, this approach has not yet been applied successfully in clinical practice. One of the more interesting potential therapeutic approaches is directed at decreasing calcium ion–dependent cytokine release by using administering a calcium channel antagonist. In one animal study, treatment with a calcium channel blocker use was associated with a dramatic reduction in TNF release and an associated improvement in survival from 40% to 80%.[69] However, these data are experimental, and although of interest, both further experimental data and results from clinical trials would be needed before this strategy could be advocated for the care of patients with SAP.

Pulmonary Dysfunction

Respiratory dysfunction is a major component of multiple organ system dysfunction syndrome secondary to acute pancreatitis, and most patients with this syndrome require ventilatory support.[30,63] Acute respiratory distress syndrome (ARDS) is characterized by diffuse pulmonary infiltrates on the chest radiograph, arterial hypoxemia, pulmonary hypertension, and decreased pulmonary compliance.

Pulmonary Management

Patients with SAP must be monitored closely for hypoxic and/or hypercarbic respiratory failure. Supplemental oxygen is almost uniformly required, and mechanical ventilation is often required.[17-19,54,63] Noninvasive positive-pressure ventilation (NIPPV) may be used to avoid endotracheal intubation in carefully selected patients; however, NIPPV usually is not well tolerated. SAP often is associated with marked abdominal distention and diminished functional residual capacity on this basis. Management of acute lung injury and ARDS secondary to SAP is similar to the management of these conditions associated with other primary problems (e.g., sepsis).

Pain Relief

Provision of pain relief to patients with severe acute pancreatitis is not only humane but also may improve pulmonary dysfunction.[70-72] In studies outside the United States, buprenorphine was noted to have a superior effect to procaine and did not exacerbate acute pancreatitis by promoting contraction of the sphincter of Oddi.[70] Pentazocine was found to have a superior analgesic effect to procaine. In a single trial comparing metamizole and morphine, no difference in analgesia was seen.[72] Although IV narcotics are useful and effective, epidural analgesia with local anesthetics also should be considered.[73]

SPECIFIC SUPPORT

Nutrition

Traditionally, patients with acute pancreatitis have been managed by providing IV fluids and nutrition and avoiding enteral feeding to "rest" the inflamed pancreas and prevent stimulation of exocrine function and the release of proteolytic enzymes.[17-19,54] Nevertheless, most patients with mild acute pancreatitis can begin oral supplementation within a few days of their presentation with pain and do not require supplemental nutrition.[54]

In the past, the primary approach for providing nutritional support for patients with SAP was total parenteral nutrition (TPN). TPN is expensive, however, and may increase the risk of sepsis or metabolic derangements.[74] TPN also has been associated with alterations in gut barrier function.[74,75] Accumulating data support the view that enteral nutrition is safe and cost-effective in patients with SAP.[76-83] A meta-analysis of several trials of enteral versus parenteral nutrition for patients with SAP revealed that enteral nutrition reduced the frequency of infections, decreased the need for surgery, and shortened length of hospital stay.[76] One trial demonstrated that enteral nutrition instead of TPN markedly decreased medical costs per capita.[81] Similarly, the Cochrane Group reviewed 8 trials of enteral versus parenteral nutrition (total of 348 patients) and concluded that the relative risk of death with enteral nutrition was 0.50 (95% CI 0.28-0.91), RR for multiple organ failure was 0.55 (95% CI 0.37-0.81), RR for systemic infection was 0.39 (95% CI 0.23-0.65), RR for operative interventions was 0.44 (95% CI 0.29-0.67), RR for local septic complications was 0.74 (95% CI 0.40-1.35), and RR for other local complications was 0.70 (95% CI 0.43-1.13). Mean length of stay was reduced by 2.37 days (95% CI 7.18-2.44) in the enteral group. The main findings were also sustained in a subgroup of patients with severe AP.[80]

If a nasoduodenal or nasojejunal tube is placed, care should be taken if blind manipulation through the duodenum is attempted. Although blind placement is possible, the duodenum is often distorted in patients with acute pancreatitis, and the risk of perforation is increased.

Fluoroscopic or endoscopic guidance of the tube into a postpyloric, even jejunal, position may be preferable. Petrov et al. reviewed four studies totaling 92 patients with acute pancreatitis who received nasogastric rather than nasojejunal enteric feedings in randomized controlled trials.[84] Patients were moderately to severely ill with evidence of end organ failure, typically respiratory failure, but were found to tolerate gastric feedings as well as nasojejunal feedings. By the 7th day, 78.8% of patients were able to achieve their goal feeding, and 79.3% of patients were able to sustain full tolerance of gastric enteral feeds. The total number of patients in the comparator groups, especially those with SAP, does not support a uniform suggestion to use nasogastric feeds rather than nasojejunal feeds at this time. Supplemental TPN may be valuable when nutritional requirements cannot be achieved using enteral nutrition alone or enteral access cannot be established. Ileus is not an absolute contraindication to enteral feeding, and most patients tolerate continuous feeding at a slow rate.[85]

Resting energy expenditure varies widely among patients with SAP, depending on the magnitude of the regional inflammatory process and the presence of additional complications, especially infection. Infection can increase energy expenditure by 5% to 20%, but overfeeding should be avoided, nutritional guidelines should be considered, and glucose control should be employed.[85] Although triglyceride levels should be monitored and not be allowed to escalate to levels above normal, administration of lipids is safe and appropriate.[79] Pancreatic secretion is not stimulated by IV lipids, whereas the anatomic site of nutrient administration determines the degree and extent of pancreatic stimulation after enteral nutrition. There is no proven causal relationship between infusion of exogenous fat and the development of pancreatitis.

The timing of oral refeeding must be based on clinical judgment. Consideration for feeding is based on resolution of ileus, improvement in signs of retroperitoneal inflammation, improvement in distant organ dysfunction, and absence of an enterocutaneous fistula.

Pathogenesis of Pancreatic Infection and Antibiotic Prophylaxis

Microorganisms can gain access to necrotic pancreatic and peripancreatic tissue via several routes, bacterial translocation from the colon being the most likely. Failure of the intestinal barrier permits bacteria and yeast to translocate from the lumen of the gut into ascites, mesenteric lymph, the bloodstream, and the pancreatic phlegmon.[74,75] The notion that pancreatic infection in acute pancreatitis is due to infection by gut-derived organisms is supported by the observation that most pancreatic infections are monomicrobial and caused by gram-negative bacteria, at least when prophylactic antibiotics have not been administered (Figure 104-4).[74,75,86,87] Further support for the intestinal origin of pancreatic infection in acute pancreatitis derives from data obtained in a clinical trial of selective decontamination of the gut, wherein enteral administration of poorly absorbed antimicrobial agents was associated with a significant reduction in late mortality, principally owing to decreased incidence of pancreatic gram-negative infection.[85] Microorganisms also can gain access to pancreatic necrosis through hematogenous dissemination from infected central venous catheters,[88] via the biliary tree, or via the pancreatic duct from the lumen of the duodenum. Besselink and colleagues demonstrated clear links among intestinal barrier dysfunction, greater intestinal permeability, bacteremia, and infected necrosis.[74] However, these authors were unable to demonstrate a connection between measured enterocyte damage and intestinal permeability.

The wisdom of using prophylactic antibiotics for managing acute pancreatitis has been debated for more than 50 years. This question has been addressed by many small (relatively underpowered) randomized controlled clinical trials,[85-111] several meta-analyses of these same trials, and numerous observational or retrospective studies.[85-111] When more than 30% of the gland is necrotic, pancreatic infection occurs in over 30% of patients with acute pancreatitis. Approximately 80% of deaths due to acute pancreatitis are related to infectious complications.

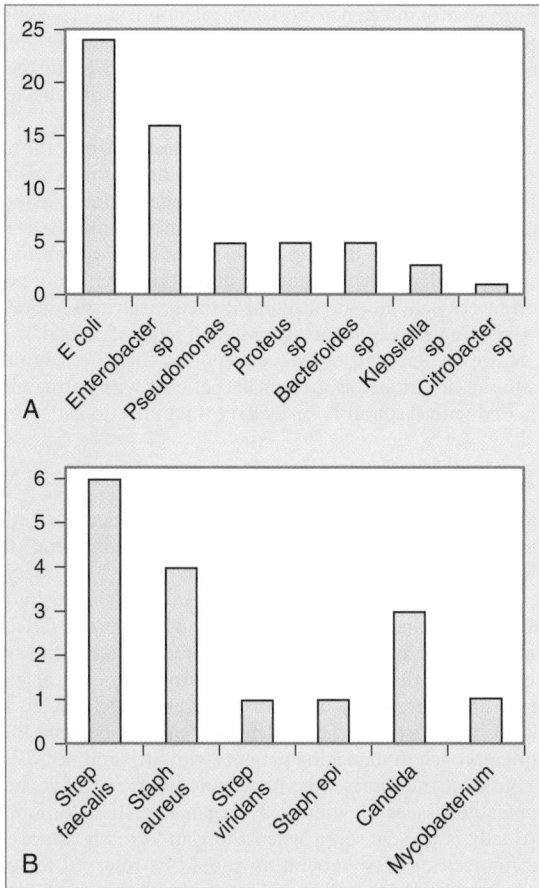

Figure 104-4 A, Gram-negative bacteria isolated from 45 patients with infected pancreatic necrosis in the preantibiotic era. **B,** Gram-positive organisms, yeasts, and mycobacteria isolated from 45 patients with infected pancreatic necrosis in the preantibiotic era. *(From Hartwig W, Werner J, Uhl W, Büchler MW. Management of infection in acute pancreatitis. J Hepatobiliary Pancreat Surg 2002;9:423-8.)*

Thus it is reasonable to consider whether administration of prophylactic antibiotics can decrease the incidence of either local or distant infections or the morbidity and mortality associated with pancreatic necrosis. Initial work in this area focused on the specific characteristics of antibiotics and whether or not the drugs penetrate into pancreatic tissue.[109] Trials in the 1970s used antibiotics that either do not penetrate well into pancreatic tissue[99] or did not have an adequate spectrum of antimicrobial activity. Aminoglycosides penetrate tissues poorly, whereas cephalosporins (e.g., cefotaxime), ureidopenicillins (e.g., piperacillin), fluoroquinolones (e.g., ciprofloxacin, ofloxacin, perfloxacin), metronidazole, and imipenem all penetrate well into pancreatic tissue.[109]

The most widely quoted trials in support of antibiotic prophylaxis for acute pancreatitis include the trial by Pederlozi et al.[89] of 74 patients randomized to receive either imipenem (0.5 g every 8 hours for 14 days) or placebo, the trial by Sainio et al.[90] of 60 patients randomized to receive either cefuroxime (1.5 g IV every 8 hours) or placebo, and the trial by Luiten et al.[85] of 102 patients randomized to receive selective digestive decontamination versus standard therapy. In the Pederlozi trial,[89] the secondary rate of pancreatic infection decreased from 30% in the control group to 12% in the imipenem group (P = .10). There were three deaths in each group, and there were no beneficial effects on organ failure, mortality, or avoidance of surgery. The trial by Saino and associates[90] enrolled mostly young patients with alcoholic pancreatitis and found that infectious complications were more common in the group not treated with antibiotic prophylaxis

compared with the group treated with cefuroxime (1.8 per patient versus 1 per patient; P=.10), as was mortality (7 versus 1; P=.03). Coagulase-negative *Staphylococcus* was cultured from unspecified sites in four of the eight patients who died. In the experimental arm of the selective digestive decontamination trial, colistin, amphotericin, and norfloxacin were administered via the oral and rectal routes. In addition, patients in this arm received a short course of therapy with cefotaxime. There were 18 deaths among the 52 patients in the control group (35%) and 11 deaths among the 50 patients in the selective digestive decontamination group (22%; P = .048).[85]

In a retrospective review of 180 patients with SAP, Ho and Frey[94] found a mortality rate of 18% and a pancreatic infection rate of 76% among patients who did not receive prophylactic antibiotics, whereas the mortality rate was only 5%, and the infection rate was 27% among patients who were treated with prophylactic imipenem.

Two well-designed randomized trials in the last 5 years have failed to show benefit from antibiotic prophylaxis. Intravenous ciprofloxacin (Cip) and metronidazole (Met) were compared with placebo in 114 patients with SAP; 12% of patients in the Cip/Met group developed pancreatic infection, whereas 9% of placebo patients (P = 0.585) developed pancreatic infection. Mortality was not different (5% versus 7%, respectively).[95] In a more recent trial of 100 randomized patients, meropenem (1 g/8 h) was compared with outcomes from a placebo group.[97] There were no differences between the groups for these parameters: incidence of infected necrosis, need for surgical intervention, or mortality. Imipenem prophylaxis was studied in 72 patients with SAP, and use of imipenem was associated with fewer complications (12/35 versus 22/35) and infections (5/35 versus 16/35).[97] However, the authors were unable to find a difference in the need for ICU care, overall hospital length of stay, need for surgical intervention, or 30-day mortality rate. Garcia-Barrasa et al. reported a randomized controlled trial of 21 patients randomized to either ciprofloxacin or placebo.[99] They were unable to demonstrate a difference between the groups for any outcome measure.

The literature is replete with papers attempting to summarize benefits and justify antibiotic prophylaxis for SAP. A systematic review and several recent meta-analyses have been conducted to try to answer the question of whether or not antibiotic prophylaxis is beneficial.[99-111] Using a fixed effects model, Hart et al. concluded that infected pancreatic necrosis (RR 0.72, 95% CI 0.46-1.16) and mortality (RR 0.71, 95% CI 0.41-1.23) were not dependent upon treatment group. However, these authors found that extrapancreatic infections were decreased when prophylaxis was used (RR 0.51, 95% CI 0.32-0.82).[106] Xu et al. also concluded that mortality was not different (RR 0.76, 95% CI 0.5-1.18), nor was the need for surgical intervention (RR 0.90, 95% CI 0.66-1.23) reduced when patients were treated with prophylactic antibiotics. However these authors concluded that peripancreatic infection (RR 0.69, 95% CI 0.48-0.91) and extrapancreatic infection (RR 0.66, 95% CI 0.48-0.91) were reduced by administration of antibiotics.[108]

Instead of using IV antibiotics, a recent trial considered whether administration of probiotics could be used to decrease pancreatic infection.[7] Infections occurred in 30% of patients in the probiotic group and 28% of patients in the placebo group. Death occurred in 16% of patients in the probiotic group and 6% of the patients in the placebo group. Importantly, nine patients in the probiotic group developed bowel ischemia, whereas none of the patients in the placebo group developed this complication. Based on this study, a probiotic strategy employing the multispecies product used in this study is not recommended. This same group of authors reported early nonpancreatic infection in 731 patients with pancreatitis over a 3-year period, with 173 patients developing a documented infection.[112] Pneumonia was identified in 84 (11.5%) patients at a median of 9 days (interquartile range [IQR] 4-17) and bacteremia in 107 (14.6%) on day 10 (IQR 3-23). Infected necrosis was identified later at a median of 26 days (IQR 17-37). These data suggest that patients with SAP, like all ICU patients, are at risk for nosocomial infections. However, whether prophylactic antibiotics should be broadly applied for these indications is a controversial topic. One of the most concerning issues with respect to the routine use of prophylactic antibiotics is the change in microbial species over the past decade, with resistant bacterial species and fungal pathogens being commonly identified.[5,87,112,113]

In addition, several reports of SAP have documented changes in the microbial spectrum of pancreatic infections characterized by an increased incidence of fungal species and more antibiotic-resistant bacterial species.[112,113] Fungal infection in SAP is a risk factor for morbidity and possibility mortality.[113] These studies raise the possibility that prophylaxis with any broad-spectrum antibiotic may be associated with increased risk of infection with fungal species or resistant bacteria. If broad-spectrum bacterial agents are used, prophylactic use of an antifungal agent may be warranted.[114] Although prophylactic antimicrobials administered IV or enterally are uniformly used in some institutions, I cannot recommend the widespread use of prophylactic antimicrobials without further data supporting the benefits of use over the apparent increase in antimicrobial resistance being reported in current series and seen in my own institution.

Management of Pancreatic Necrosis and Abscess

Pancreatic necrosis is defined by the presence of diffuse or focal areas of nonviable pancreatic parenchyma, often associated with peripancreatic fat necrosis.[36] Necrosis either can be sterile or infected; infection usually is confirmed by fine-needle aspiration.[115,116] Pancreatic infection occurs in about 10% of all cases of acute pancreatitis, but in 30% to 70% of cases with necrosis. Contrast-enhanced CT is currently the gold standard for documenting the presence of nonperfused pancreatic parenchyma, although as noted earlier, MRI also can show both fluid collections and nonperfused pancreatic parenchyma. A pancreatic abscess is a circumscribed intraabdominal collection of pus, usually in close proximity to pancreatic necrosis, which arises as a consequence of acute pancreatitis.[36]

Infected pancreatic necrosis should be suspected in patients with acute pancreatitis with clinical signs of sepsis. This diagnosis also should be suspected when patients fail to improve with supportive therapy or regress after an initial period of improvement.[47] Patients suspected of having infected pancreatic necrosis should undergo contrast-enhanced CT scan or ultrasound-guided fine-needle aspiration.[112,115,116] This approach is a safe and reliable way to differentiate between sterile and infected necrosis. Complication rates of this procedure are low. Rare serious complications include bleeding and aggravation of acute pancreatitis. With Gram staining and culture of aspirated material, fine-needle aspiration by ultrasonography has a diagnostic sensitivity of 88% and specificity of 90%.[115] Because there is a possibility of contamination of sterile necrosis, fine-needle aspiration is indicated only in these groups of patients: those with signs and symptoms of sepsis, those who fail to improve, and those who worsen after initial clinical improvement.[117] Outside of a clinical trial, fine-needle aspiration should not be performed as a matter of routine for patients with SAP who are doing well.[118,119] Studies have confirmed infection rates of 2.8% to 22% in the first week and 28.8% to 55% in the second to fourth weeks. The timing of fine-needle aspiration should be based on the probability of infection, based on time of onset from the disease and the current clinical condition of the patient. Some authors do not support the practice of needle aspiration of infection because they use prophylactic antibiotics and would not perform an "early" operation based on cultures obtained from a fine-needle aspirate. Rather, they wait 3 to 4 weeks and if the patient is unwell, operate at that time, whether or not presence of infection has been proven.[118]

LABORATORY MARKERS OF INFECTED NECROSIS

No reliable blood test has been developed to establish the diagnosis of infected necrosis.[114-117] Measurement of serum CRP concentration was the best available blood test for identification of pancreatic necrosis; CRP concentrations greater than 120 mg/L are associated with necrosis.[120] There is no correlation, however, between the serum CRP level

and the presence of infected necrosis. Procalcitonin is a 116–amino acid propeptide of calcitonin that has been shown to be a marker for severe bacterial and fungal infection. In the meta-analysis by Mofidi et al., the sensitivity and specificity of procalcitonin for predicting infected pancreatic necrosis were 0.80 and 0.91, respectively.[42]

Clinicians must pursue the possibility of infected pancreatic necrosis in order to tailor the use of antibiotics and other forms of therapy. While fine-needle aspirates are an invasive modality and can be subject to sampling error, procalcitonin can be obtained noninvasively and is not altered by antibiotic therapy. Importantly, the clinician must recognize that procalcitonin elevation is a nonspecific marker of potential infection in critically ill patients, and if the procalcitonin level is elevated, a systematic search for all potential sites of infection should follow. However, Rau and colleagues reported that the magnitude of procalcitonin elevation was greatest in patients with intraabdominal as compared with respiratory or urinary tract infections.[121]

INDICATION AND TIMING OF OPERATIVE INTERVENTION

Although there is no consensus about the timing of operative intervention for pancreatic necrosis, most experts now recommend delaying operation until infection has been identified.[86,112,122,123] An intervention may be delayed until the third or fourth week of ICU care. In the past there was some belief that early surgery might improve outcome by removing necrotic tissue and decreasing the stimulus for systemic inflammation, but this notion has been disproved by clinical trials and experience and now is only of historic interest.[124] Delaying as long as possible for any sort of invasive débridement has become the most common approach to managing patients with SAP and necrosis. Early in the course of the disease, the pancreatic tissue is friable, however, and nonviable tissues are not well demarcated. In addition, viable tissue usually is present, even when the gland grossly appears to be completely necrotic. Early operation should be reserved for patients with proven infected necrosis or patients with other surgical complications such as massive bleeding or bowel perforation.[118]

STERILE NECROSIS

Before 1990, the standard surgical practice was to débride necrotic pancreatic tissue operatively, even in the absence of infection.[123] Nonoperative management of sterile necrosis is now the standard of care according to several published guidelines. In selected cases, patients with extensive necrosis may not improve, and after a prolonged period of observation (6-8 weeks), operative débridement may be warranted.[86,125,126] Sterile pancreatic necrosis has a mortality rate of 0% to 10% when managed using a conservative nonoperative approach.[125-127]

OPERATIVE PROCEDURES

Although there is general agreement that infected necrosis requires operative débridement, there is no consensus about the best approach to achieve this goal, and there are increasing concerns about early open débridement.[122,123] When a patient is very ill with sepsis, the primary treatment goal is to achieve drainage of infected material. Open necrosectomy has been associated with high rates of complications (34%-95%)[122,123] and death (11%-39%).[122,123] Recently the results of the Step-up Approach versus Open Necrosectomy trial were reported. In this trial, the "step-up approach" consisted of percutaneous drainage followed by minimally invasive retroperitoneal necrosectomy, if needed, and this strategy was compared with open necrosectomy.[122] Thirty-five percent of patients were able to be treated with percutaneous drainage only. The trial's primary endpoint was a composite of the complications related to the aggressiveness and type of therapy, such as multiple organ failure, bleeding, perforation, and enterocutaneous fistula. Patients who received the step-up approach were less likely to develop complications (40% versus 69%, respectively). Additionally, with the step-up approach, there was less organ failure (12% versus 40%), lower rate of incisional hernia (7% versus 24%), and lower incidence of new-onset diabetes mellitus (16% versus 38%). This important trial is unique because it was a randomized study of the surgical care of infected necrosis rather than a case series reported from one or more institutions. Interestingly, 35% of patients were able to progress to a clinical cure with percutaneous drainage alone. This finding suggests that drainage of purulent material allowed the necrosis to "regress" to sterile necrosis. The findings from this study also suggest that the step-up approach may be beneficial because of a lower level of surgical trauma and therefore activation of inflammatory mediators. The results of this trial are consistent with results of minimally invasive necrosectomy and other less invasive procedures.[128-133] However, it is important to note that the trial did not compare open necrosectomy with minimally invasive retroperitoneal drainage.

As shown in older case series, percutaneous drainage of infected necrosis can be achieved in selected patients, especially when the infected material is not too viscous or too loaded with necrotic tissue. Drainage can be achieved via anterior or retroperitoneal approaches and is best achieved using a large-diameter catheter (12-14F).[129-133]

In recently reported studies, an endoscopic approach has been used to achieve drainage.[131-133] Pancreatic drainage can be achieved using natural orifice transluminal endoscopic surgery (NOTES). Endoscopic ultrasound is used to identify collections through the wall of the stomach. Using a Seldinger-type (guidewire-based) technique, the collection is accessed and dilated serially with 10- to 15-mm balloons. The goal is to create a channel large enough to permit the endoscope to enter the cavity. Once the endoscope is in the cavity, débridement is accomplished using typical endoscopic instruments, paying careful attention to hemostasis. Copious irrigation is carried out before placing a drain. A nasocystic drain is then placed over the wire and is used to retain access and allow irrigation of the collection. Although a few patients have been successfully managed with this approach, it should be noted that they have been highly selected.

Open treatment of infected pancreatic necrosis is still the most commonly employed modality for débridement, but fewer surgeons are using an open approach as the initial treatment modality.[122-124] However, even the open surgical treatment has been widely varied, and no study has systematically examined one open approach versus another. The surgeon may elect to perform open necrosectomy and either open or closed drainage, and may plan for selective or routine re-laparotomy. Irrigation and lavage may occur only in the operating room, or irrigation can be carried for intermittent periods postoperatively. Alternatively, irrigation can be performed continuously. Each of these techniques has been used successfully at different centers. Most experienced centers treating this disease now report mortality rates between 10% and 20% for infected pancreatic necrosis.

As previously noted in the step-up approach, the advent of minimally invasive techniques now allows several new approaches to drainage of infected pancreatic material.[122] Video-assisted retroperitoneal drainage (VARD) has been popular since 2000.[134] VARD drainage uses either a rigid nephroscope or a zero-degree laparoscope to access the retroperitoneum over a wire previously placed into the infected cavity, typically by CT scan. A 5-mm scope and instruments can be used in some patients. The lesser sac has also been approached via the base of the mesocolon with laparoscopic instruments, using hand access for débridement.[134-138] A recent report of 18 patients with infected necrosis who were treated using this less invasive strategy demonstrated a length of stay of 16 days and a reduction in major wound complications.[138] While VARD has the potential advantage of eliminating peritoneal contamination, commonly many procedures are needed, and the colon and other abdominal contents cannot be examined or treated if needed.

In the past, open surgical approaches have been based on institutional experience and not based on comparative trials. All methods aim to remove infected tissue while preserving most of the gland. Whether the step-up approach will fully replace open surgical débridement remains uncertain; the randomized trial studied only 88 patents, and in experienced hands, open techniques have lowered mortality rates for SAP to less than 15%.

Conventional Resection

In the past, formal pancreatic resections were performed for acute pancreatitis. These procedures have been abandoned in the treatment of SAP, however, because of excessively high rates for complications and mortality.[86,26] These procedures do not remove the surrounding necrotic tissue and needlessly remove healthy tissue.

Necrosectomy

Necrosectomy removes devitalized tissue from the pancreas and surrounding retroperitoneum and now can be performed by open or less invasive endoscopic or laparoscopic techniques.[125-138] The tissue generally is removed by gentle finger fracture technique when an open approach is employed, and by gentle separation when a less invasive approach is used. Necrosectomy is designed to remove most of the devitalized tissue without injuring major blood vessels; hemostasis must be carefully obtained before the procedure is completed. Repeated drainage procedures may be necessary.

While the general approach for the management of infected pancreatic necrosis is to delay drainage and perform drainage in a less invasive manner, some patients may require open procedures. The open packing technique originally was popularized by Bradley[87] et al. and was associated with a mortality of 15%, but morbidity was extensive and included external pancreatic fistulas in 46% of cases, hernias in 32% of cases, and massive venous hemorrhage in 7% of cases. Other centers have employed planned staged procedures or open drainage followed by the placement of drains. In case series using surgical management with drains, the overall mortality rate was only 6.2%. The authors noted a significantly better outcome when surgery was delayed beyond the fourth week. Alternatively, necrosectomy can be followed by closed-suction lavage of the retroperitoneum using 35 to 40 L/d of peritoneal lavage solution for each of the first 7 postoperative days. This approach was successfully used in 42 of 121 patients with pancreatic necrosis. Of the 121 patients, 12 (9.9%) died, including nine patients who were treated surgically and three patients who were treated conservatively.[138] Morbidity included pancreatic fistulas in 8 of 42 (19%) surgically treated patients. Pancreatic fistulas after pancreatitis usually close spontaneously eventually if pancreatic ductal obstruction is not present. In a few cases, enteric internal drainage or pancreatic resection may be required to achieve closure of pancreatic fistulas.

Aside from pancreatic infections, patients with SAP are at risk for the usual gamut of nosocomial infections, including catheter-related bloodstream infections, urinary tract infections, and ventilator-associated pneumonia.[7] Additional abdominal complications in patients with acute pancreatitis include concurrent biliary tract problems, stress gastritis and related bleeding, necrosis of the transverse colon, hemorrhage from gastric varices secondary to splenic vein thrombosis, and catastrophic bleeding from ruptured pseudoaneurysms involving the gastroduodenal artery or branches of the superior mesenteric artery. Should massive gastrointestinal bleeding occur, and a gastric or proximal duodenal source is excluded, arteriography should be considered. Necrosis of the transverse colon should be considered in a patient with abdominal tenderness and distention and sepsis. Patients with colonic necrosis are usually dramatically ill. Enterocutaneous fistulas are seen commonly when the open packing technique is used and less commonly when other methods of management are employed.

Outcome

With an increasing number of patients surviving SAP, attention has been focused on the quality of life and long-term outcome of surviving patients.[140-143] This patient population is subject to a wide range of medical problems, including diabetes mellitus, symptoms of polyneuropathy, recurrent pancreatitis, and continual abdominal pain, with endocrine or exocrine dysfunction occurring in the majority of patients.[141] Major social problems also can be an issue, especially among patients with alcohol-induced pancreatitis. Abdominal hernias may be present, especially in patients managed using open packing; future repairs may be needed. Chronic pancreatitis and related problems including pseudocysts, splenic vein thrombosis, and mesenteric pseudoaneurysms can occur but are not discussed here in further detail.

In one study, 35 patients after acute pancreatitis treated with open necrosectomy were evaluated for results on the Short-Form 36 assessment of health-related quality of life.[139] Among this cohort of 35 patients, 32 were employed at the time of their SAP, and 12 patients returned to work within 6 months of discharge. SF-36 scores were above 60% in all patients, and 20 of 32 patients has a good quality of life (>70%).[139] Patients with alcoholic pancreatitis had the worst outcomes. In 20 survivors of long-term (>30 days) hospital stay after an episode of SAP, 12 of 20 experienced morphologic or endocrine sequelae.[141] Problems noted more than 6 months after discharge from the hospital included pancreatic fistulae, stenosis of both the pancreatic and biliary tree, and chronic abdominal pain.[133]

▣ Summary

Acute pancreatitis is a widely variable disease that is usually mild in severity. SAP is a life-threatening disease, however, that can require intensive support, especially during the initial inflammatory period of SIRS, when massive fluid resuscitation and ventilatory, cardiovascular, renal, and nutritional support may be required. In patients with ongoing signs of SIRS beyond the second or third week of disease, progression from SAP with sterile necrosis to infected necrosis should be considered. Fine-needle aspiration should be employed to diagnose pancreatic infection. Débridement of infected pancreatic necrosis is required, but the exact method of surgical débridement is controversial, and a step-up approach to therapy may be best. Although SAP is a life-threatening disease, the overall survival of patients is about 90% at centers with expertise in the management of this complex syndrome.

KEY POINTS

1. Severe acute pancreatitis accounts for 10% to 15% of all patients presenting with pancreatitis and for virtually all the morbidity and mortality associated with the disease.

2. The early phase of severe acute pancreatitis is characterized by systemic inflammatory response syndrome and end-organ dysfunction, often requiring intensive support of the cardiopulmonary system. Respiratory dysfunction is a major component of multiple organ system dysfunction syndrome secondary to acute pancreatitis, and most patients with this syndrome require ventilatory support. Resuscitation of intravascular volume is an important component of initial management, regardless of the etiology and severity of acute pancreatitis. Sequestration of fluid can lead to loss of as much as one third of plasma volume.

3. Necrosis of more than 50% of the pancreas is associated with increased risk for complications, especially pancreatic infection. Infected pancreatic necrosis is the most important risk factor for death secondary to necrotizing pancreatitis. Prevention, diagnosis, and treatment of infection in severe acute pancreatitis are crucial.

4. Understanding the cause of severe acute pancreatitis may dictate therapeutic options. A biliary origin should be suspected in female patients older than 40 years of age with a serum alanine aminotransferase level more than three times the upper reference limit.

5. Contrast-enhanced computed tomography (CT) is considered the gold standard for diagnosing pancreatic necrosis and peripancreatic collections and for grading acute pancreatitis. The Balthazar index ranges from 0 to 10 and is calculated by adding the points attributed to the extent of the inflammatory process to the volume of pancreatic necrosis. Although CT findings correlate with clinical course and severity of acute pancreatitis, it is not necessary to obtain this study in patients with mild pancreatitis. Magnetic resonance imaging (MRI) may be useful in patients who are at high risk for complications related to infusion of iodinated contrast medium. MRI also can be useful when a pancreatic duct abnormality is suspected.

6. Approximately 80% of deaths due to acute pancreatitis are related to infectious complications. Although prophylactic administration of antibiotics is often employed, the quality of evidence supporting this practice is relatively weak. Moreover, problems associated with resistance to antibiotics have been observed in some recent clinical trials. Therefore, prophylactic antibiotics should not be used routinely unless new data from additional randomized controlled trials become available to support this practice.

7. Patients with severe necrotizing acute pancreatitis require nutritional supplementation. Enteral nutrition is safe and efficacious and may be delivered best distal to the pylorus. Some patients are so catabolic that enteral and parenteral nutrition may be required to support nutritional needs. Although triglyceride levels should be monitored, lipids can be used for supplementation in most patients.

8. Pancreatic infection should be suspected in three groups of patients: patients who fail to improve, patients who worsen, and patients with initial improvement who regress. A contrast-enhanced CT scan and fine-needle aspiration should be considered to rule out infection.

9. Pancreatic débridement and/or drainage should be performed in patients with infected pancreatic necrosis. The specific approach depends on local considerations, and no single method has been proven to be superior to another.

10. Increasingly, infected pancreatic necrosis is being managed using a more conservative staged or "step-up" approach and less invasive means of drainage in selected patients.

ANNOTATED REFERENCES

Bradley EL 3rd, Dexter ND. Management of severe acute pancreatitis: a surgical odyssey. Ann Surg 2010;251:6-17.
   This paper places the current interventional management of acute pancreatitis in context of prior surgical approaches.

Babu BI, Sheen AJ, Lee SH, et al. Open pancreatic necrosectomy in the multidisciplinary management of postinflammatory necrosis. Ann Surg 2010;251:783-6.
   This article reviews the care provided for 1535 patients with severe pancreatitis in the context of multidisciplinary care. Open necrosectomy was performed in 28 patients, but radiologic drainage was used both before and subsequent to surgery in the majority of patients.

Besselink MG, van Santvoort HC, Boermeester MA, et al. Timing and impact of infections in acute pancreatitis. Br J Surg 2009;96:267-73.
   The focus of this paper is on the large local national experience of a large cohort of patients and the timing and outcome of infectious complications in association with acute pancreatitis.

Gaisano HB, Gorelick. New insights into the mechanisms of pancreatitis. Gastroenterology 2009;136:2040-4.
   This article discusses mechanisms of pancreatitis and provides state-of-the-art thinking about pathophysiology and underlying molecular mechanisms of this disease.

Pezzelli R. Pharmacotherapy for acute pancreatitis. Expert Opin Pharmacother 2009;10:2999-3014.
   This article is an excellent current review of potential therapeutic options, with robust references for interventions suggested for care.

van Santvoort HC, Besselink MG, Bakker OJ, Hofker HS, Boermeester MA, Dejong CH, et al; Dutch Pancreatitis Study Group. A step-up approach or open necrosectomy for necrotizing pancreatitis. N Engl J Med 2010;362:1491-502.
   This article is an excellent randomized controlled trial of the aggressiveness of management for patients with infected pancreatic necrosis.

REFERENCES

Access the complete reference list online at http://www.expertconsult.com.

105

Peritonitis and Intraabdominal Infection

DAVID C. CHEN | PHILIP S. BARIE | JONATHAN R. HIATT

Critically ill patients with intraabdominal infection are at high risk for treatment failure and other serious complications. Failure can occur because of inadequate primary source control (percutaneous drainage or surgical therapy) or the development of secondary complications such as abdominal compartment syndrome or fistula formation. Since there are few controlled studies of the management of critically ill patients with peritonitis, recommendations often are based on expert opinion and extrapolation from animal models and sometimes on clinical data.

Basic management principles for patients with intraabdominal infection include adequate and timely resuscitation to optimize tissue perfusion and oxygenation. Effective resuscitation can mitigate or avoid certain manifestations of intraabdominal infection in critical illness such as ischemic colitis or acute acalculous cholecystitis. Source control also must be adequate and timely. Depending on the problem, source control can include draining intraabdominal abscesses, débriding devitalized tissue, closing perforations, reducing the burden imposed by bacteria and their toxins, and providing appropriate and timely broad-spectrum antimicrobial therapy. Optimal management of these patients also requires a basic understanding of peritoneal defense mechanisms, the limitations of these defenses, relevant microbiology, and factors that predict adverse outcomes in critical illness.

Pathogenesis

HOST DEFENSES

The peritoneal cavity is a complex space lined with mesothelial cells in visceral and parietal layers. The healthy peritoneal cavity is quiescent immunologically but responds rapidly to bacterial contamination. Normally, about 50 to 100 mL of peritoneal fluid circulates freely among several potential and actual spaces within the peritoneal cavity.[1] Net fluid movement is cephalad toward the diaphragm, facilitated by normal peristalsis, normal diaphragmatic excursions, splanchnic blood flow, and factors that maintain normal membrane permeability of the microcirculation. Conversely, ileus, mechanical ventilation, splanchnic hypoperfusion, and intraperitoneal inflammation can disrupt normal fluid movement and cause intraperitoneal fluid sequestration.

The three major intraperitoneal host defense mechanisms include clearance of bacteria by lymphatics, phagocytosis of bacteria by immune cells, and mechanical sequestration with abscess formation. A few phagocytic cells circulate as peritoneal macrophages, and opsonic proteins that facilitate phagocytosis are present. Experimentally, a small bacterial inoculum placed in the peritoneal cavity is cleared within a few minutes when the peritoneal fluid is absorbed by specialized lacunae on the undersurface of the diaphragm.[1] The bacteria then pass into the central venous system via diaphragmatic and mediastinal lymphatics for disposition by systemic host defenses. When an infectious inoculum is introduced, a brisk inflammatory response attempts to localize the infection, leading to abscess formation rather than generalized peritonitis. Intraabdominal abscess formation is a source-containment process; mortality is lower for patients with abscess(es) than for patients with generalized peritonitis.[2,3]

Intraabdominal infection stimulates both local and systemic inflammatory responses. Locally, influx and activation of phagocytic cells (neutrophils, monocytes, and macrophages) promotes bacterial killing but also impairs microvascular integrity and fosters interstitial edema and formation of exudative ascites. The surface area of the peritoneum is approximately the same as the skin, so edema of the submesothelial interstitial space to a thickness of 1 mm sequesters about 1.7 L of fluid in a 70-kg patient. Large volumes of interstitial and free peritoneal fluid can accumulate, requiring very large infusions of intravenous (IV) fluid to correct intravascular hypovolemia, a common occurrence in patients with generalized peritonitis. Intraperitoneal fluid accumulation is detrimental to intraabdominal host defenses, diluting opsonins and impairing neutrophil function, but there is no alternative to fluid administration for the hypovolemic patient.

With inflammatory injury, peritoneal mesothelial cells are denuded, exposing the underlying basement membrane. When platelets and fibrin come into contact with the basement membrane, fibrin polymerization occurs and produces a typical exudative rind on peritoneal surfaces. Fibrin and apoptotic neutrophils contribute to the formation of adhesions and the walls of abscesses. Normally the process is self-limited by up-regulation and/or activation of fibrinolytic factors such as plasminogen within the first week after mesothelial injury. If the insult is self-limited, peritoneal repair occurs within 3 to 5 days. Under local hypoxic conditions, the adhesions are invaded by fibroblasts, angiogenesis is up-regulated, and the adhesions become tenacious.[4]

MICROBIOLOGY

Most of the bacteria normally resident in the gut are commensal flora that play little if any role in the pathogenesis of intraabdominal infections. Currently it is estimated that more than 500 bacterial species are present within the lumen of the healthy human colon. Most of these species are obligate anaerobes. Under normal conditions, the intestinal microbiota supports enterocyte and colonocyte function and prevents overgrowth of more pathogenic species, including *Bacteroides fragilis*, *Escherichia coli*, *Klebsiella* spp., and *Enterobacter* spp. Overgrowth of these potentially pathogenic microbes can occur after patients are treated with broad-spectrum antibiotics.

Gastrointestinal perforation releases bacteria into the peritoneal cavity. Bacterial density within the gut lumen increases along the length of the gastrointestinal tract from the stomach to the colon. The bacteria must proliferate to cause infection, while local host defenses seek to prevent or contain the establishment of infection. In addition to the microbes present in peritoneal fluid, microbial colonization of peritoneal surfaces occurs rapidly after perforation or penetrating injury as a result of expression by the microorganisms of specific adherence factors. Enterobacteriaceae predominate within the first 4 hours but are superseded within 8 hours by members of the *B. fragilis* group. Adherent bacteria are difficult to eradicate by operative peritoneal lavage.[5]

Besides adherence factors, bacteria possess several other features that can enhance their virulence. Peptidoglycans and lipoteichoic acid in the cell walls of gram-positive bacteria, especially streptococci and staphylococci, stimulate a proinflammatory response. These organisms can elaborate exotoxins and proteases that cause tissue injury and promote the dissemination of the bacteria. Lipopolysaccharide (LPS) in the outer cell wall of gram-negative bacteria can interact with many cell types to stimulate an inflammatory response. As bacteria proliferate and the size of the inoculum increases, acidic bacterial metabolites can impair neutrophil function.[6] Larger inocula can render antibiotics, particularly β-lactams, ineffective via a process called the *inoculum effect.*[7] Additionally, bacteria demonstrate a quorum-sensing effect that maximizes survival and reproduction by altering their behavior based upon signaling pathways.[8]

Synergistic interactions, usually among members of the *B. fragilis* group and either facultative gram-negative bacilli or enterococci, can suppress local host defenses and promote bacterial survival and growth.[1] *B. fragilis* produces a capsular polysaccharide antigen that suppresses complement activation and inhibits leukocyte recruitment and function.[9] Anaerobic bacteria produce short-chain fatty acids that can impair the function of neutrophils. Facultative bacteria consume residual oxygen in the microenvironment, permitting the survival and proliferation of obligate anaerobes. Anaerobic bacteria lower the redox potential in the microenvironment, also favoring their growth. Aerobic and anaerobic bacteria can enhance the growth of other species by providing crucial nutrients or the producing enzymes that inactivate antibiotics.

In some respects, bacteria have evolved to take advantage of host defenses. As an example, bacterial adherence to colonocytes and bacterial growth is enhanced by physiologic concentrations of norepinephrine, which is secreted as part of the counter-regulatory response to stress, as well as being administered as an exogenous drug to promote arteriolar constriction and increase myocardial contractility.[10]

PERITONITIS

Peritonitis can be classified as primary, secondary, or tertiary. Most critically ill patients with intraabdominal infection have secondary or tertiary peritonitis. The bacteriology characteristic of these classes of peritonitis is shown in Table 105-1.

Primary, or spontaneous bacterial, peritonitis develops in the absence of gastrointestinal perforation and rarely causes critical illness. This type of peritonitis, which afflicts adults with hepatic cirrhosis or collagen vascular disease or children with certain glomerulopathies, is almost always monomicrobial. The typical pathogen is usually an enteric gram-negative bacillus such as *E. coli* or *Klebsiella* spp., although infection with streptococci is also known to occur. Definitive diagnosis is made by paracentesis and culture, and operative treatment is not indicated. Polymicrobial or anaerobic flora confirm the presence of an occult perforation that must be found and treated.

Device-associated peritonitis is a variant of primary peritonitis that also almost always is monomicrobial. The great majority of cases occur with chronic ambulatory peritoneal dialysis (CAPD) catheters, which become infected as often as once per year of dialysis.[11] The most common pathogens are *Staphylococcus aureus* and species of *Pseudomonas* and *Candida*. Catheter removal is usually necessary to eradicate these infections, especially when caused by *P. aeruginosa* or *Candida* spp. Although rare, recurrent CAPD-related peritonitis due to methicillin-resistant *S. aureus* (MRSA) has been associated with the emergence of vancomycin-resistant strains after treatment with multiple courses of vancomycin.[12]

Secondary peritonitis follows perforation of a hollow gastrointestinal viscus. The vast majority of cases are community acquired. Appendicitis is the most common cause, and the polymicrobial bacterial flora

typically are highly susceptible to antibiotics. Thorough microbiologic analysis of a carefully collected specimen of purulent peritoneal fluid from a patient with secondary peritonitis yields an average of five organisms. *B. fragilis* the most commonly isolated obligate anaerobe, and *E. coli* is the most commonly isolated facultative organism. Less common isolates include *Enterococcus* spp., *Candida* spp., *Clostridium* spp., and *P. aeruginosa*. These uncommon isolates do not need to be covered by the antibiotic regimen if the patient was previously healthy and does not have comorbid conditions that increase the risk for an adverse outcome. Early operative source control, combined with a short course of broad-spectrum antibiotics, are curative in more than 85% of all cases and more than 90% of appendicitis cases.[13] Most cases of community-acquired peritonitis do not result in severe illness, and these cases seldom require care in an intensive care unit (ICU).

Tertiary peritonitis describes recurrent or persistent intraabdominal infection after failure of more than one source control procedure to control the infection.[14-16] The flora usually include one or more strains of staphylococci (often methicillin-resistant *S. epidermidis* or MRSA) and *Enterococcus* spp., *Candida* spp., or *Pseudomonas* spp.[17-19] It is debated whether tertiary peritonitis represents invasive infection or permissive colonization of the peritoneal cavity in the face of devastated host defenses. The notion that host defenses are compromised is supported by the observation that fluid collections are often poorly localized and serosanguineous rather than purulent. Cases of tertiary peritonitis are fortunately uncommon, but class I data regarding management are lacking.

ADJUVANTS

Adjuvant substances act to decrease the bacterial inoculum necessary for infection. Adjuvants can increase virulence or interfere with host defenses and invariably are present to some degree in every patient with gastrointestinal perforation. Common adjuvants include ascites, blood, fibrin, bile, urine, chyle, pancreatic juice, and platelets.[20] The most important adjuvant is blood. Hemoglobin, fibrin, and platelets all impair host defenses, and iron, which is essential for bacterial growth, also depresses phagocyte function. Fibrin promotes bacterial trapping and abscess formation and can sequester bacteria from neutrophils. Bile salts impair host defenses and are toxic to neutrophils.[21] Pancreatic enzymes can be activated by bacterial infection, producing necrotic tissue that is an excellent culture medium.

Foreign materials also can act as adjuvants, serving as prime loci for bacterial adherence and sequestration from phagocytes. The foreign material also can elicit an inflammatory reaction, thereby reducing the size of the inoculum needed for infection. Adjuvant foreign materials include surgically placed drains, nonabsorbable suture material, fibers from gauze sponges, prostheses such as vascular grafts and mesh, topical hemostatic agents, talc, barium sulfate, necrotic tissue, and feces. Barium produces a marked chemical peritonitis and activates coagulation via the intrinsic pathway; the combination of barium and feces can be lethal.

🔲 At-Risk Patient

Fortunately, most patients with intraabdominal infection are not so sick as to require care in an ICU. In a population-based study of hospital discharges for peritonitis, severe sepsis developed in only 11% of cases (Table 105-2) but increased the mortality risk by 19-fold.[2] Similarly, only about 15% of patients enrolled in clinical trials of antimicrobial therapy for secondary peritonitis have an APACHE II score above 15 points.[22]

Some patients with community-acquired secondary peritonitis have critical illness as a result of delayed presentation, immunosuppression, or extremes of age. However, most patients with critical illness have hospital-acquired peritonitis (Table 105-3). The leading causes of hospital-acquired peritonitis are gastrointestinal anastomotic dehiscence and splanchnic ischemia due to various causes including hypovolemia, distributive shock, atheroembolism, and thromboembolism.

TABLE 105-1	Microbiology of Intraabdominal Infection	
Primary (Monomicrobial)	**Secondary (Polymicrobial)**	**Tertiary (Polymicrobial)**
Escherichia coli	*Bacteroides fragilis* group	*Acinetobacter* spp.
Enterococcus spp.	*Clostridium* spp.	*Enterobacter* spp.
Klebsiella spp.	*E. coli*	*Enterococcus* spp.
Streptococcus pneumoniae	*Klebsiella* spp. Other anaerobes	*Pseudomonas* spp. *Staphylococcus* spp. *Staphylococcus epidermidis* *Streptococcus* spp. *Candida* spp.

TABLE 105-2	Risk Factors for Severe Sepsis in Patients with Intraabdominal Infections	
Parameter	*Relative Risk*	*95% Confidence Intervals*
Age (Years)		
<20		1.0
20-39	1.4	0.8-2.5
40-59	3.2	1.8-5.6
60-79	4.6	2.6-8.0
>79	6.5	4.7-11.8
Site		
Appendix		1.0
Gallbladder	2.7	1.9-3.8
Colon	3.9	2.6-5.8
Stomach/duodenum	6.9	4.6-10.3
Small bowel	9.0	6.1-13.4
Extent		
Localized		1.0
Abscess	1.2	0.8-1.8
Diffuse	1.5	1.1-1.9
Comorbidities		
Congestive heart failure	1.2	1.0-1.6
Stroke	1.8	1.2-2.7
Liver dysfunction	2.0	1.4-2.8
Renal dysfunction	2.0	1.4-2.9

Data from Anaya and Nathens.[2]

Hospital-acquired peritonitis is usually polymicrobial, and commonly cultured organisms include *Enterococcus* spp., *Candida* spp., *Pseudomonas aeruginosa*, and other antibiotic-resistant organisms such as MRSA.[14,18,19]

The frequency of intraabdominal infection encountered in a particular ICU is variable. Surgical ICUs that care for patients with multiple trauma or following emergency surgery are likely to have more cases of intraabdominal infection than medical ICUs. Surgical patients that have required an operation for source control or have a postoperative secondary nosocomial infection account for 25% to 40% of patients with severe sepsis. However, units with a low prevalence must be equally vigilant in their surveillance and assessment, because a missed intraabdominal infection is almost always fatal.[23]

When patients with intraabdominal infection are critically ill, mortality exceeds 25%. The risk of failure increases with increasing severity of illness, inadequate empirical antibiotic therapy, delayed surgical therapy, and failure of source control.[14,18] Most clinical failures are not associated with multidrug-resistant pathogens, although some data

TABLE 105-3	Clinical Factors Predicting High-Risk Intraabdominal Infection

Shock
Advanced age
Acute Physiology and Chronic Health Evaluation (APACHE) II score >15
Isolation of enterococci
Impaired consciousness
Inadequate empirical antibiotics
Poor nutritional status
Cardiovascular disease
Inability to obtain source control
Immunosuppression
Hypoalbuminemia
Thrombocytopenia
Diffuse versus localized peritonitis
Symptoms more than 24 h before definitive intervention
Subsequent nosocomial infection
Protein C concentration below 66% of normal
Hospitalization >48 h
Malignancy
Postoperative infection
Recent antibiotic therapy
Residence in skilled nursing care or long-term care facility

Data from Pieracci et al.[13] and Solomkin et al.[18]

suggest that resistant pathogens cause clinical failure in cases of postoperative peritonitis.[24,25]

Spectrum of Disease Causing Critical Illness

ABSCESS OF SOLID ORGANS

Abscesses of solid organs are rare but must be recognized, as they can be lethal if untreated. Most cases arise as a complication of a community-acquired infection, but on occasion they can be a complication of medical care. The liver is affected most commonly, followed by the spleen and kidney.

Liver abscess is most often the result of ascending biliary infection (cholangitis) or portal bacteremia that complicates an enteric infection (typically colonic diverticulitis). The most common causative organisms, including *E. coli*, *Klebsiella* spp., and *Enterococcus* spp., reflect these pathogenic mechanisms. Systemic sources for bacteremia also can cause liver abscesses and include dental abscess (viridans streptococci) or vascular catheters (*S. aureus*, *Candida albicans*, and others). Devitalized liver, as can be present after trauma, angioembolization, or ablation of neoplasms, is at particular risk for infection. The lesions can be solitary or multiple. In rare instances, miliary liver abscesses develop.

Treatment of liver abscesses should be individualized. A source of origin should be sought and treated. Antibiotics are mandatory, and a prolonged course for more than 14 days may be necessary. If feasible, based upon the size and location of the abscess, percutaneous drainage always should be attempted.[26,27] Operative drainage may be required for abscesses that cannot be drained percutaneously. Overall mortality rate is approximately 25% but is higher for patients with multiple abscesses that are too small to drain.[28]

Splenic abscesses are uncommon and are the result of hematogenous or local contamination. Hematologic sources include endocarditis, urinary tract infections, pneumonia, osteomyelitis, otitis, mastoiditis, and pelvic infections. Splenic abscesses have been reported with other systemic infections including typhoid, paratyphoid, malaria, and candidiasis. Direct extension from adjacent infections of the pancreas, retroperitoneum, subdiaphragmatic spaces, and diverticulitis can involve the spleen. Systemic disorders such as hemoglobinopathies or sickle cell disease, can cause splenic infarction. Devitalized splenic tissue resulting from trauma, infarction, or embolization can become infected and evolve into splenic abscesses.[29]

S. aureus is the most common pathogen in splenic abscesses, while gram-negative organisms are relatively unusual. Anaerobic infections (e.g., due to *Clostridium perfringens*) have been described. Empirical antibiotic therapy should address all likely pathogens. Percutaneous drainage can be attempted if conditions are favorable, but splenectomy and drainage are usually definitive as therapy. Overall mortality rate is approximately 20%.

Despite the frequency of urosepsis, true abscesses of the kidney are uncommon compared to either hepatic or splenic abscesses. Ascending infection from the lower urinary tract is the usual source; therefore, any common urinary tract pathogen (*E. coli*, *Klebsiella* spp., *Enterococcus* spp., *S. aureus*) can be causative, and broad-spectrum antibiotic therapy is necessary until microbiologic data become available. Surgical drainage may be required for nonresponders or patients with recurrent sepsis.

ACUTE ACALCULOUS CHOLECYSTITIS

In contrast to cholecystitis due to gallstones, the etiology of acute acalculous cholecystitis is gallbladder ischemia; infection of the organ occurs secondarily.[30] Although acute acalculous cholecystitis can complicate many illnesses, splanchnic hypoperfusion is the common feature. Risk factors in medical patients include congestive heart failure, diabetes mellitus, abdominal vasculitis, and malignancy (including after bone marrow transplantation). Acalculous cholecystitis is more common in surgical patients and can occur following burns, trauma, cardiopulmonary bypass, biliary instrumentation, and emergency aortic surgery.[30]

The diagnosis of acute acalculous cholecystitis can be challenging, and a high index of suspicion is required. Prompt diagnosis and therapy are necessary, as the disease can be fulminant. Necrosis of the gallbladder occurs in 50% of patients, and perforation of the gallbladder occurs in 20%. Fever and hyperbilirubinemia are common associated findings.[29] Serum transaminase and alkaline phosphatase levels also may be elevated. When signs and symptoms can be localized to the right upper quadrant, the differential diagnosis includes gastroduodenal perforation, acute pancreatitis, right colonic ischemia, and acute hepatitis.

Bedside ultrasonography is favored for the diagnosis of acute acalculous cholecystitis; the most accurate diagnostic features are gallbladder wall thickness greater than 3.5 mm and presence of pericholecystic fluid. Computed tomography (CT) is equally accurate and can be utilized when there are no localizing findings and the patient is a candidate for intrahospital transport. Hepatobiliary scintigraphy is not useful to identify or exclude acute acalculous cholecystitis, owing to a high incidence of false-positive findings that result in part from a lack of dietary stimulus for gallbladder contraction. Coadministration of morphine sulfate, which increases biliary hydrostatic pressure, can promote filling of the gallbladder and increase diagnostic accuracy of hepatobiliary scintigraphy.[31]

Percutaneous cholecystostomy is the treatment of choice for acute acalculous cholecystitis in the critically ill patient. Success rates exceed 90% for control of acute acalculous cholecystitis, although the overall mortality rate remains about 30%. When percutaneous cholecystostomy fails to provide adequate control of acute acalculous cholecystitis, the diagnostic possibilities include malposition of the drainage catheter, uncontrolled gallbladder perforation, or another diagnosis. If a cholecystostomy tube study confirms the absence of gallstones once the patient has recovered, the drain can be removed. Interval cholecystectomy is unnecessary if the drain is removable.

ISCHEMIC COLITIS AND ENTERITIS

Intestinal ischemia is a dangerous and relatively common complication of critical illness that can progress within hours to gangrene, perforation, and generalized peritonitis.[32] The splanchnic circulation is especially vulnerable to low cardiac output, particularly when the cardiac index is less than 2 L/min/m². Most cases are caused by nonocclusive ischemia; the origin is often multifactorial, including hypovolemia, shock, and administration of vasopressors. A number of other causes have been identified. Acquired protein C/protein S deficiency induces a hypercoagulable state that has been associated with mesenteric arterial and venous thrombosis. Chronic atrial fibrillation or dilated cardiomyopathy can lead to mesenteric arterial thromboembolism. Arteriography can cause cholesterol embolization from dislodgement of an atherosclerotic plaque. Intestinal obstruction also must be considered, and this diagnosis may not be obvious with partial or proximal obstructions.

The pattern of injury with intestinal ischemia is variable depending on the mechanism, the presence of heart disease, and the status of the collateral circulation via the celiac and inferior mesenteric arteries. Large thrombi usually occlude the superior mesenteric artery where it narrows just distal to origin of the middle colic artery. The first 30 to 45 cm of small bowel and the left colon may be spared. Smaller emboli are more likely to infarct the small bowel and possibly the ascending colon (Figure 105-1); the distribution can be patchy. Nonocclusive ischemia classically occurs in watershed areas of the mesenteric circulation where collateral vessels bridge the two arterial distributions. A typical site is the splenic flexure of the colon at the watershed junction of the superior and the inferior mesenteric arteries. Although any segment of intestine can be affected by nonocclusive ischemia, the cecum (the point farthest from inferior mesenteric artery collaterals)

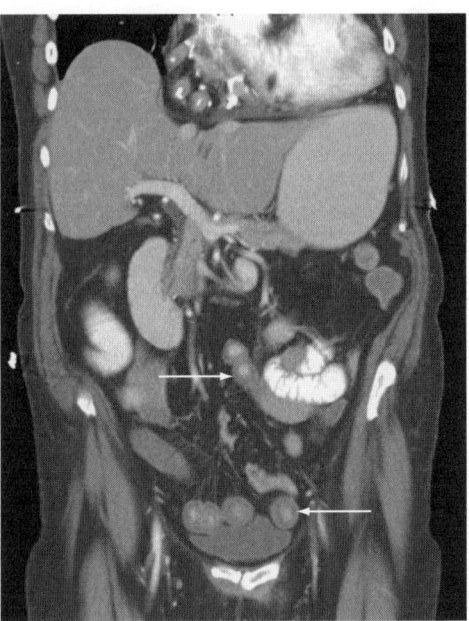

Figure 105-1 CT after administration of oral and intravenous contrast in a patient with embolic occlusion of superior mesenteric artery and patchy ischemia of small bowel and right colon. Bowel ischemia is evident by marked thickening of intestinal wall.

and the left colon are most likely to be affected (Figure 105-2). The left colon is particularly vulnerable after abdominal aortic operations, especially when the inferior mesenteric artery has been ligated during the procedure.

Patients with intestinal ischemia are profoundly ill and will die without prompt intervention. As the blood supply to the mucosa is more vulnerable than to seromuscular layers, transmural necrosis represents late-stage disease. Patients can develop severe sepsis or septic shock before transmural gangrene or perforation. The protean manifestations of the syndrome, including the potential for ischemia

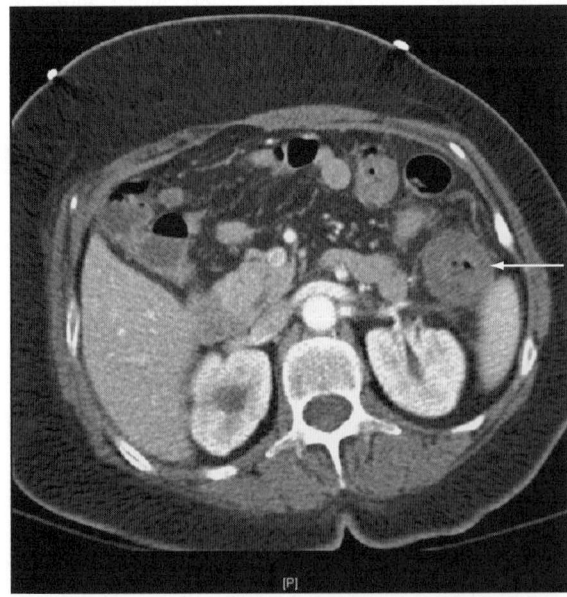

Figure 105-2 CT with oral and intravenous contrast in a patient with nonocclusive mesenteric ischemia of colon at splenic flexure. Ischemia of colon is evident by marked thickening of wall of colon.

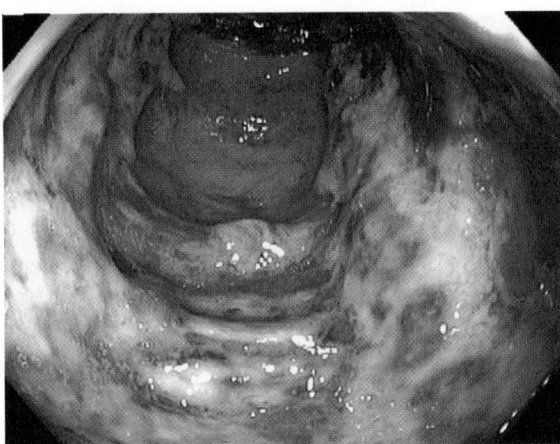

Figure 105-3 Colonoscopy is the preferred modality to assess for colonic ischemia but visualizes mucosa only and may underestimate extent of disease.

anywhere from the ligament of Treitz to the midrectum, make the diagnosis challenging.

Among communicative patients, pain that is disproportionately severe compared with tenderness and other objective findings is the diagnostic hallmark. Among intubated, sedated patients, the clinical features can be subtle. Abdominal distention, hypovolemia, hemoconcentration, unexplained and refractory metabolic acidosis, or occult rectal bleeding can be the only signs. Hematochezia following abdominal aortic surgery or resuscitation from shock is strongly suggestive of colon ischemia.

Given the propensity for left colonic involvement, lower endoscopy at the bedside is usually the first diagnostic modality to be employed, but a number of pitfalls should be recognized. Flexible sigmoidoscopy is simple and safe but may miss ischemia at or proximal to the splenic flexure; accordingly, colonoscopy is preferred (Figure 105-3). Endoscopy visualizes only the mucosa and can underestimate the extent of disease. CT and CT angiography are increasingly useful diagnostically and have largely supplanted use of formal arteriography (Figure 105-4).

Bedside diagnostic laparoscopy represents a new technique to identify intraabdominal pathology in an ICU setting, but reports to date are anecdotal. Laparoscopy should be considered when transfer of the patient to radiology or the operating room is considered unsafe or when routine radiologic examinations are inconclusive.[33,34] Diagnostic testing should be foregone entirely in favor of immediate laparotomy if signs of peritonitis are present.

Surgical therapy is individualized based on the location and extent of intestinal compromise and the physiologic state of the patient. Infarcted bowel is resected, but bowel of questionable viability can be left for reinspection at a "second-look laparotomy" in 12 to 24 hours, particularly if a massive resection would otherwise be needed. Anastomosis can be performed in the stable patient without peritonitis or deferred in unstable patients by leaving the occluded ends of bowel in temporary discontinuity until the second-look procedure. Creation of a temporary ostomy is a third option but is performed with decreasing frequency. If there is confidence that a second-look procedure is unnecessary, the abdominal fascia can be closed. If reoperation is planned, or if bowel edema and distention are such that definitive closure would risk the development of intraabdominal hypertension and abdominal compartment syndrome, damage-control principles are utilized, and a temporary abdominal wall closure is performed. Methods for temporary closure include closure of skin only or closure with absorbable mesh, biological material, or plastic sheeting, usually in conjunction with a negative pressure system.[35]

The wide spectrum of disease in patients with intestinal ischemia makes mortality estimates difficult, but the condition is highly morbid.

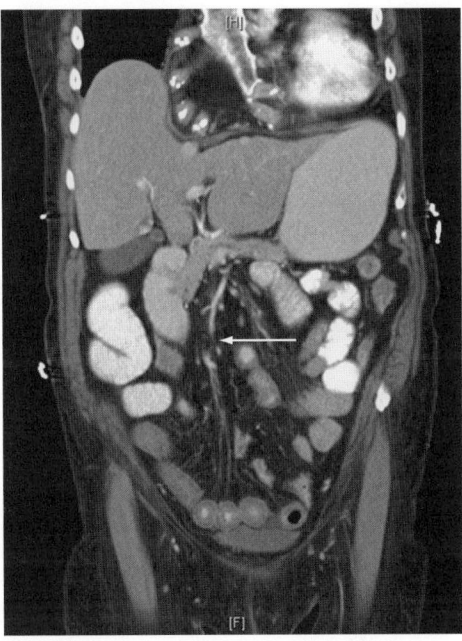

Figure 105-4 CT after administration of oral and intravenous contrast in patient with embolism to superior mesenteric artery and ischemia of small bowel and right colon. Arrow points to embolus in superior mesenteric artery.

Acute colonic ischemia following repair of a ruptured abdominal aortic aneurysm has a mortality risk as high as 80%.

CLOSTRIDIUM DIFFICILE COLITIS

The incidence and severity of *Clostridium difficile* infections (CDI) are increasing. CDI remains the most common nosocomial gastrointestinal infection, with significant morbidity and mortality. Early diagnosis and treatment are essential for a favorable outcome. A highly virulent and resistant strain, PCR ribotype 027, has been associated with recent outbreaks in North America and Europe characterized by increased incidence and a higher risk of death.[36] The ICU patient is at increased risk for CDI, and in these patients the disease is more frequent, more severe, more refractory to medical therapy, and subject to higher rates of relapse.[37] In one study, emergency colectomy was needed in 25% of patients with CDI requiring ICU admission. Other risk factors for CDI include preoperative antibiotic usage, uremia, burns, chronic obstructive pulmonary disease, cancer, abdominal surgery, cesarean section, antiperistaltic medications, proton pump inhibitors, ICU stay, prolonged hospital stay, chemotherapy, and postpyloric tube feeds.[36,37]

Clinical examination of patients with CDI may not demonstrate significant findings of peritonitis unless megacolon or perforation has developed. CT can demonstrate typical findings of colonic wall thickening, dilation, and the so-called accordion sign (thickened haustral fold and trapped contrast material, ascites, and/or pericolonic stranding; Figure 105-5). Measurement of stool toxin titers and endoscopy are useful diagnostic adjuncts, but definitive management in patients with evidence of refractory fulminant colitis should not be delayed as a consequence of waiting for the results of these tests. Routine cases of CDI are treated with oral or IV metronidazole. Severe disease is treated with oral vancomycin; administration of this antibiotic via the enteral route leads to high luminal concentrations of the drug owing to lack of absorption across the mucosa of the gut.

Fulminant CDI with perforation, toxic megacolon, severe ileus, hypotension, or refractory septicemia occurs in approximately 3% to 8% of patients. Patients who have a history of inflammatory bowel disease, recent surgery, prior treatment with IV immunoglobulin, vasopressor requirements, leukocytosis, or increased blood lactate

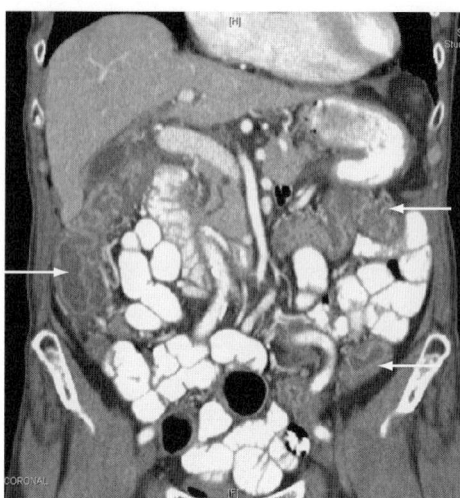

Figure 105-5   CT with oral and intravenous contrast in patient with *Clostridium difficile* colitis. Typical findings include colonic wall thickening, dilation, and accordion sign (thickened haustral fold and trapped contrast material, ascites, and pericolonic stranding).

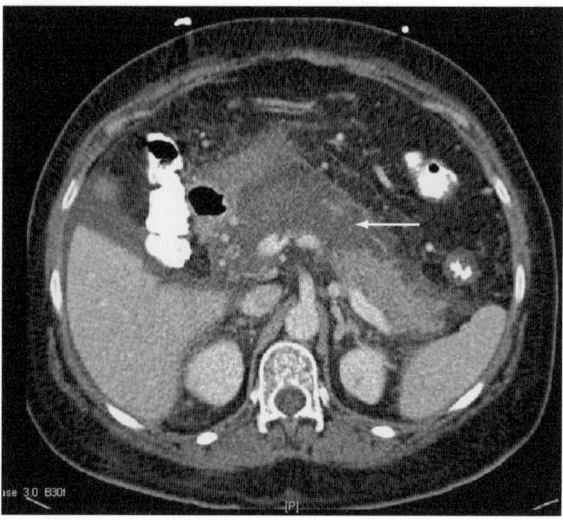

Figure 105-6   CT with oral and intravenous contrast in patient with severe acute pancreatitis. Borders of pancreas are indistinct from marked surrounding inflammation. Hypodense area in body of pancreas is an area of pancreatic necrosis. Study should be performed with contrast infusion and thin cuts through region of pancreas.

concentration should have early surgical consultation. Mortality was notably decreased in patients who had no more than 6 days of medical treatment prior to operation, supporting consideration of early subtotal colectomy.[36-39]

ACUTE PANCREATITIS

Gallstones and alcohol together account for about 80% of cases of pancreatitis, with the remainder due to trauma, upper abdominal surgery, or cardiopulmonary bypass. Approximately 85% of cases are self-limited and have a good prognosis. The remaining 15% of cases account for most of the morbidity and all of the mortality. Infection is the most common complication and can lead to multiple organ dysfunction syndrome and death. Mortality risk is associated with large IV fluid requirement, acidosis, and hypocalcemia.[40]

Pancreatic infections include infected pseudocysts, discrete pancreatic abscesses, or infected pancreatic necrosis. The last is a poorly localized process that affects the retroperitoneal fat as well as the pancreas itself. Infection can develop as early as 5 days after the onset of acute pancreatitis, with peak incidence at day 14. Almost any common organism can cause infection, including staphylococci, enteric gram-negative bacilli, obligate anaerobes, *P. aeruginosa*, and *Candida* spp. Assuming appropriate microbial susceptibility, imipenem, meropenem, doripenem, or a fluoroquinolone plus metronidazole are recommended empirical antimicrobial agents, based on kinetic studies of drug accumulation in normal pancreas or pancreatic juice. Fluconazole achieves adequate concentrations in pancreatic tissue, whereas aminoglycosides do not.[41]

Many aspects of the prevention and management of pancreatic infection are controversial, including the role of antibiotic prophylaxis, diagnostic methods, and techniques and timing of surgical drainage and débridement. Antibiotic prophylaxis of severe pancreatitis with imipenem is employed by many physicians and surgeons, but this practice is not supported by class I data and has been associated with an increased risk of fungal infection.[42] Regardless of the severity of illness, all patients with pancreatitis should undergo biliary ultrasonography in search of gallstones. Pancreatic protocol CT is the best study to define anatomic severity and infection. The study should be performed with contrast infusion and thin cuts through the region of the pancreas to assess for viability and presence of devitalized tissues (Figure 105-6). When peripancreatic infection is suspected, CT-guided fine-needle aspiration can be performed to obtain material for culture.

Source control is essential for patients with established pancreatic infection. Newer techniques with acceptable outcomes and lower morbidity have begun to replace traditional open drainage and surgical necrosectomy. These techniques include minimally invasive endoscopic, radiologic, and laparoscopic approaches. Endoscopic ultrasonography as a guide to drainage and laparoscopic pancreatic necrosectomy has demonstrated success in managing pancreatitis necrosis (Figure 105-7).[43,44] Recent results from the Dutch Pancreatitis Study Group demonstrated a significant reduction in major complications (new-onset multiple-organ failure, incisional hernias, and new-onset diabetes) following the step-up approach for managing infected pancreatic necrosis. This approach consists of percutaneous drainage followed (if necessary) by minimally invasive retroperitoneal necrosectomy.[45] Improvements in resuscitation and operative management of infectious complications have reduced the mortality rate to about 20%, half that of an earlier era.

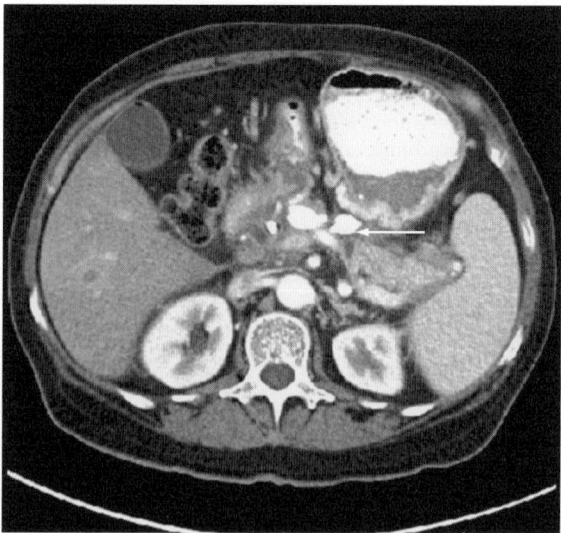

Figure 105-7   Interval CT in same patient as Figure 105-6, with pancreatic necrosis and pseudocyst formation. There has been significant resolution after internal endoscopic drainage, with two stents functioning as a cystogastrostomy.

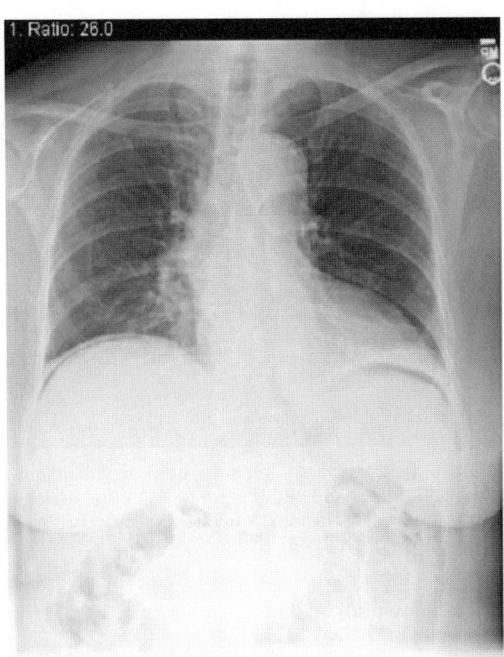

Figure 105-8 Pneumoperitoneum (crescent-shaped lucency) is evident under right hemidiaphragm on upright chest radiograph of patient with perforated sigmoid diverticulitis. Crescent-shaped lucency under left hemidiaphragm is stomach bubble.

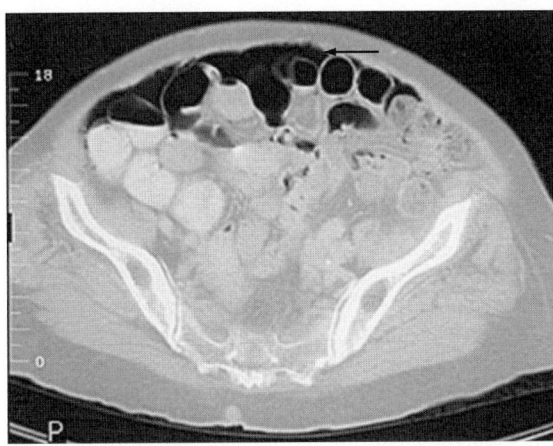

Figure 105-9 CT with oral and intravenous contrast in patient with pneumoperitoneum from perforated viscus. Multiple pockets of extraluminal gas are evident, particularly anterior to loops of small bowel.

Operation for patients with pancreatic necrosis and organ dysfunction without infection is a matter of debate. Current opinion favors a conservative approach with aggressive critical care support, reserving operation for confirmed infections. This strategy is meant to minimize the complications associated with difficult and potentially morbid procedures, including hemorrhage, intestinal fistulas, multiple reoperations, open abdomen, and abdominal wall hernias.

Diagnosis

Diagnosis of intraabdominal infection in critically ill patients can be challenging. Medical history is often unobtainable, and altered mental status can mask the physical findings. At times, the only clue may be unexplained signs of sepsis or organ dysfunction. Radiologic testing is utilized in most patients and can be diagnostic.

Although good-quality plain abdominal radiographs are difficult to obtain at the bedside, pneumoperitoneum (Figure 105-8), intestinal obstruction, or signs of intestinal ischemia may be found. Pneumoperitoneum can be an innocuous finding in mechanically ventilated patients and for as long as 7 days after abdominal operations.[46,47] Plain radiography can be augmented by water-soluble contrast injection of drains, fistulas, or sinuses to define the anatomy of complex infections or monitor resolution after drainage.

Ultrasonography can be performed at the bedside and provides excellent visualization of the biliary tree. Ultrasonography can detect abscesses, particularly in the pelvis when transvaginal or transrectal probes are used, and can be used to guide percutaneous drainage procedures. With the addition of color Doppler blood flow analysis, visceral blood flow can be assessed. Ultrasonography is operator dependent; visualization is limited in the presence of bowel gas, and dressings, stomas, and drains can impede positioning of the probe.

CT with oral and IV contrast is the primary radiologic imaging tool for the abdomen and pelvis.[48-50] CT signs of intraabdominal infection include extraluminal gas (Figure 105-9), free fluid, contrast extravasation, fat stranding, and presence of a contrast-enhancing rim that is characteristic of abscess (Figure 105-10). CT is now the test of choice for diagnosis of intestinal obstruction. Intramural gas may be

identified when mesenteric ischemia is present; occasionally, a thrombus is seen in a visceral vessel (see Figure 105-4). CT-guided percutaneous drainage of abscesses and intraabdominal fluid collections is the treatment of choice for source control in the absence of generalized peritonitis or disruption of visceral structures.[26,27,50]

Although CT is an excellent diagnostic modality, obtaining an adequate study in critically ill patients can be problematic. When patients are hemodynamically unstable or dependent on a high level of mechanical ventilatory support, transport out of the ICU can be risky.[51] Iodinated contrast agents can precipitate or aggravate renal dysfunction. If the need for CT can be anticipated 24 hours in advance, pretreatment with *N*-acetylcysteine and IV sodium bicarbonate can limit the risk of contrast-induced nephropathy.[52]

Other radiologic modalities used commonly in elective evaluations have limited value in critical illness. Radionuclide imaging and magnetic resonance are used rarely for ICU patients with intraabdominal infection.

Principles of Management

SOURCE CONTROL

Source control for complicated intraabdominal infections remains the most important component of successful treatment. Consensus

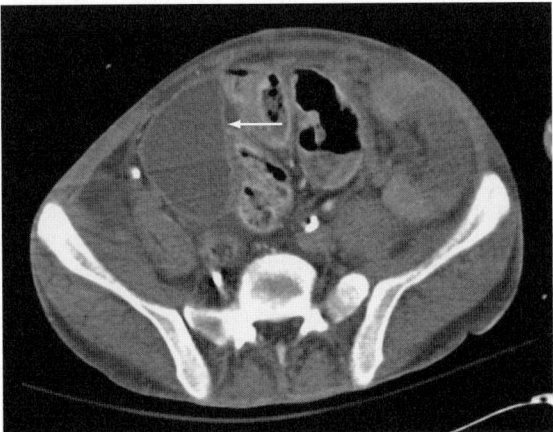

Figure 105-10 CT with oral and intravenous contrast material in patient with large pelvic abscess. Abscess cavity demonstrates classic rim enhancement of abscess wall. Percutaneous drainage should be performed under image guidance.

guidelines aim to implement source control interventions within the first 6 hours of management.[53,54]

The elements of definitive source control include removal of infected or nonviable material, closure or control of perforations, and reduction of peritoneal contamination by bacteria and toxins. Multiple staged operative procedures may be needed. Failure to obtain adequate source control reportedly occurs in 10% to 25% of cases of intraabdominal infection, depending on the severity and complexity of the infection.[14,54]

ABSCESS

Abscesses are characterized by low oxygen tension, poor antibiotic penetration, and impaired leukocyte function. Small abscesses may resolve with antibiotics alone. Source control with percutaneous drainage is the treatment of choice for most abscesses, provided adequate drainage is possible and no débridement or repair of anatomic structures is necessary.[12,53] Percutaneous decompression of abscesses is successful and produces rapid clinical improvement in 85% of cases.[26,27] Formal operative intervention should be performed without delay if clinical improvement does not occur promptly following drainage.

PERITONEAL TOILET

Once source control has been achieved, additional intraoperative measures to cleanse the peritoneal cavity of microscopic infection, including irrigation with fluid or antibiotic solutions and débridement of peritoneal surfaces, are ineffective and may be deleterious.[55-57] Bacteria adhere to mesothelial cells on the serosal surfaces in peritonitis, rendering them resistant to removal by passive irrigation.[57-59] Moreover, animal studies suggest that irrigation fluids disseminate infection by hindering the normal immunologic function of the peritoneum. Irrigation with antibiotic solutions is of no benefit if parenteral antibiotics are administered.[4] High-volume lavage and pulse irrigation used in fecal and purulent peritonitis may be of benefit but also can increase the risk of fistula formation.[57-59] Closed-suction drains do not prevent recurrent fluid collections and are ineffective at draining the peritoneal cavity.

OPEN ABDOMEN

Open abdomen techniques are used in selected patients with diffuse peritonitis, inadequate primary source control, intestinal ischemia and discontinuity, abdominal compartment syndrome, or necrotizing infections of the anterior abdominal wall.[60,61] Open abdomen is a component of the damage-control strategy used in unstable patients with massive trauma. In cases of peritonitis, goals of damage control include reassessment of intestinal viability, decompression of the abdomen, and access for peritoneal toilet. Open abdomen management has disadvantages including promotion of excessive losses of fluid and protein, ileus, fistula formation, and ventral hernias. Neither planned re-laparotomy nor open abdomen management offer a survival benefit as compared with on-demand re-laparotomy.[62]

Many variations in open abdomen techniques have been reported. Most often, a negative-pressure system is utilized with a fenestrated nonadherent material to cover the bowel, suction drains to aspirate fluid above this layer, and an airtight adherent outer drape to maintain a vacuum and prevent evisceration until adhesions form (Figures 105-11 and 105-12). Nasogastric and urinary catheter decompression are maintained, and parenteral nutritional support is provided to prevent bowel distention. At reexploration, the abdomen is lavaged, and loculated fluid collections are evacuated. After achieving resuscitation and adequate source control, aggressive diuresis should begin to reverse edema and facilitate closure of the abdomen. In a substantial percentage of patients, the fascia cannot be closed primarily; absorbable mesh or biological grafts, skin grafts, and enteral nutrition allow healing to occur, and ventral hernias are repaired electively when all

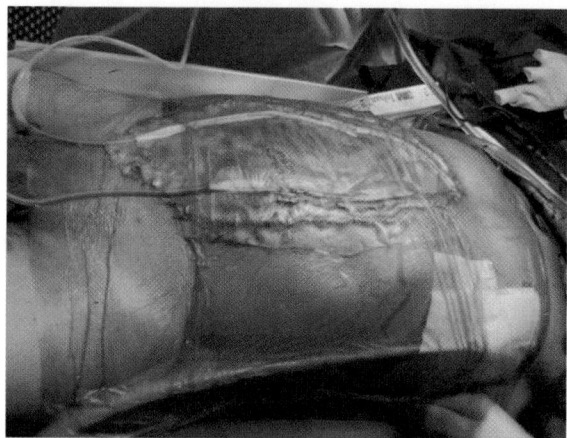

Figure 105-11 Open abdomen management of abdominal compartment syndrome. Sterile saline bag is sewn to skin edges. Closed suction drains are placed to limit fluid accumulation, and occlusive dressing is applied to cover abdominal wall. *(Courtesy Brian J. Kimbrell, MD.)*

acute problems have resolved, but no earlier than 3 to 6 months after the acute episode.

ANTIBIOTIC THERAPY

Optimal antibiotic therapy for intraabdominal infection requires an agent or combination of agents active against gut-derived facultative enteric gram-negative bacilli as well as obligate anaerobes.[12,13] Initial antibiotic therapy should be empirical, because the source is not always known.

A 2005 Cochrane review of 40 studies with 5094 patients comparing 16 different antibiotic regimens for empirical first-line therapy demonstrated equivalent efficacy and made no specific recommendations based on class I evidence.[21] Given this equivalence (Table 105-4), the selection of a regimen should be based on considerations of cost, availability, ease of administration, susceptibilities, and the risk of toxicity, including allergy to β-lactam agents.[12,63]

Evidence-based guidelines for selection of antimicrobial therapy for high-risk patients with intraabdominal infections have been formulated by both the Surgical Infection Society and the Infectious Diseases Society of America.[12] The most commonly accepted empirical treatment regimens for complicated intraabdominal infections include

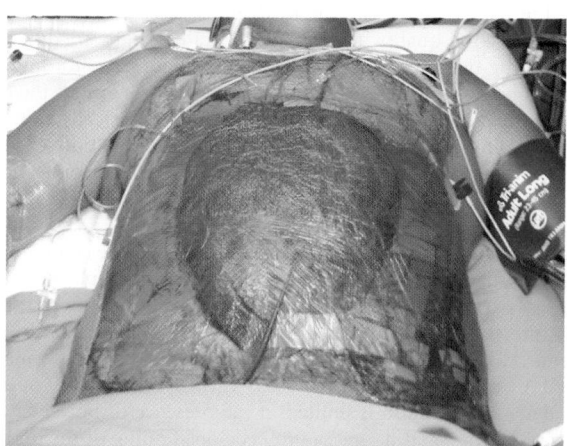

Figure 105-12 Open abdomen management of abdominal compartment syndrome using a VAC system closure. Bowel is covered with omentum if possible. Nonadherent dressing is layered under VAC sponge, or smaller pore sponge is used against viscera. Negative pressure is applied to wound closure to drain fluid, facilitate closure, and prevent evisceration. *(Courtesy Brian J. Kimbrell, MD.)*

TABLE 105-4	Antimicrobial Agent Regimens for Therapy of Serious Intraabdominal Infections

Single Agents

β-Lactam/-lactamase inhibitor combinations:
- Ampicillin/sulbactam
- Piperacillin/tazobactam
- Ticarcillin/clavulanic acid

Carbapenems:
- Imipenem-cilastatin
- Meropenem
- Ertapenem
- Doripenem

Cephalosporins:
- Cefotetan
- Cefoxitin

Fluoroquinolones:
- Moxifloxacin

Glycylcyclines:
- Tigecycline

Combination Agents

Aminoglycoside plus an antianaerobic agent:
- Amikacin, gentamicin, netilmicin, or tobramycin plus clindamycin or metronidazole

Aztreonam plus clindamycin:
- Combination of aztreonam plus metronidazole is devoid of coverage against gram-positive cocci

Fluoroquinolone plus metronidazole:
- Ciprofloxacin, levofloxacin, gatifloxacin, moxifloxacin

Third- or fourth-generation cephalosporin plus an antianaerobic agent

Data from Solomkin et al.[18] and Mazuski et al.[19]

extended-range β-lactam/β-lactamase agents such as piperacillin/tazobactam, carbapenems such as imipenem-cilastatin, meropenem, and ertapenem, or a third- or fourth-generation cephalosporin plus metronidazole.

In hospital-acquired peritonitis, local antimicrobial resistance patterns should be considered. Although mortality appears to be higher when an *Enterococcus* spp. is isolated from polymicrobial intraabdominal infections, there is no evidence that antienterococcal therapy improves outcome.[12,24,64] Combination therapy directed against a specific pathogen (e.g., double-drug coverage of *P. aeruginosa*) has no demonstrated benefit in sepsis and can worsen outcomes. Newer agents including the glycylcycline antibiotic, tigecycline; the carbapenems, ertapenem and doripenem; and the fluoroquinolone, moxifloxacin also have equivalency in the treatment of complicated intraabdominal infections and provide new options in dealing with the problems of emerging bacterial resistance.[65-70]

Fungal species are common components of the normal intestinal flora, and fungi are common isolates from peritoneal fluid during operations for perforated viscera. Treatment of fungal isolates in an otherwise immunocompetent patient has not been found to improve survival.[71] Because fungal colonization usually precedes invasive infection in surgical patients, some experts advocate systemic antifungal treatment when fungal species are recovered from peritoneal fluid.[12,72,73] Empirical antifungal therapy is warranted with isolation of fungi from two or more normally sterile sites, from the bloodstream of critically ill patients with fungal abscesses, and in immunosuppressed patients.[2,3,12,74] Fungal species cultured from an abscess or peritoneal fluid in a profoundly immunosuppressed patient also should be treated.[2,3,12] In the critically ill patient, initial antifungal therapy with an echinocandin (caspofungin, micafungin, anidulafungin) instead of a triazole is recommended.[12,71]

Shorter courses of antimicrobial therapy and modification of agents once susceptibilities are obtained are safe in patients with adequate source control and will limit intraabdominal infections caused by multidrug-resistant pathogens.[75-77] When source control is adequate, generalized peritonitis can be treated with antibiotics for as few as 3 to 5 days.[77] The duration of therapy should typically be limited to 7 to 10 days. In hospital-acquired peritonitis, the duration of therapy is less defined and is based upon clinical parameters such as fever, abdominal pain, leukocytosis, and return of gastrointestinal function. Persistent sepsis should raise the possibility of inadequate source control, other nosocomial infections, or tertiary peritonitis. Rather than broadening antibiotic coverage or continuing the current regimen, a complete diagnostic reevaluation with physical examination, cultures, and imaging is indicated to identify any source of ongoing infection.

The concept of deescalation, where empirical broad-spectrum antibiotics are replaced by targeted narrower-spectrum agents once susceptibilities are obtained, is safe and should help reduce the risk of emergence of antibiotic-resistant isolates. While evidence-based recommendations are unequivocal, compliance with deescalation is poor.[76] When intestinal function returns, oral antibiotics with good bioavailability can be administered to complete the course of therapy.[12,78]

The role of antibiotics for tertiary peritonitis is even less well defined. There is little proven benefit to empirical antibiotics, and most bacterial isolates tend to be resistant to standard regimens. Empirical coverage of isolated *Enterococcus* spp. and *Candida* spp. has been well studied and is without clearly defined benefit. Such coverage is recommended for complicated, nosocomial infections in immunosuppressed patients, critically ill patients, and patients with valvular heart disease or implanted prosthetic materials.[12] Antibiotics for tertiary peritonitis should be of narrow spectrum and administered briefly; anti-anaerobic therapy is probably unnecessary.

Complications

The complications of failed source control include abscess formation, anastomotic dehiscence, wound infections, recurrent or persistent peritonitis, fistula formation, sepsis, and multiple organ dysfunction syndrome, which is the leading cause of death. While abscess, anastomotic dehiscence, and fistula formation are most commonly attributable to failure of source control procedure, persistent peritonitis and sepsis are often attributable to failure of host defenses.

ENTEROCUTANEOUS FISTULA

Fistula formation is a dreaded complication of peritoneal inflammation and bowel injury. More than 80% of fistulas occur postoperatively, whereas fistulas that arise primarily from infection or irradiated bowel are rare.[79,80] A fistula can be an occult source of sepsis before drainage to the skin makes the diagnosis obvious. A fistula can contain an abscess cavity along its tract or exist internally as a connection between two intraabdominal structures.

When a fistula develops, initial care should be supportive. Therapy is directed at appropriate antibiotic therapy if signs of secondary infection are present, along with bowel rest, skin care, and parenteral nutritional support. Administration of octreotide may reduce fistula output, minimize losses of fluid, electrolytes, and proteins, and facilitate spontaneous closure.[81,82] Spontaneous closure with nonoperative therapy occurs in 30% to 50% of fistulas, usually within 3 to 4 weeks.[80]

Mortality

Significant progress in the management of peritonitis and intraabdominal infection has been made over the past century, but mortality remains about 25% for critically ill patients.[3] Age and severity of illness at the time of presentation are more important predictors of mortality than the site of infection within the abdomen.[3] Failure of the initial source control procedure is more likely to result in death than infection caused by a multidrug-resistant pathogen.

Organ dysfunction is present to some degree in every patient dying with intraabdominal infection. Early recognition of organ dysfunction as a sign of persistent intraabdominal infection offers an opportunity to intervene while the process is still reversible.[83-85] The key elements of management to minimize mortality include early recognition of the problem, rapid resuscitation, timely and correct performance of source control procedures, and administration of appropriate broad-spectrum antibiotics.

Administration of glucocorticoids in patients with septic shock has not demonstrated a survival benefit or clinical improvement of sepsis and increases the risk of superinfection.[86] Judicious transfusion of red blood cell concentrates may be of benefit as an adjunct in sepsis, but additional data are needed for confirmation.[87] The concept of very tight control of serum glucose concentration in the management of the critically ill patient with sepsis has been controversial, but recent results indicate that this practice increases complications and mortality and should be avoided.[88-91] One recent trial demonstrated that therapy with drotrecogin alfa (recombinant human activated protein C) improves survival among patients with severe sepsis and a high risk of death (APACHE II score ≥ 25 points or dysfunction of at least two organs), but follow-up studies failed to confirm this finding.[92-94] Surgical patients had more significant bleeding complications during the 96-hour infusion period, but most were treated successfully. At the time of this writing, a second multicentric pivotal trial of drotrecogin alfa (activated) is in progress, and results should be available soon. Based on currently available evidence, therapy with drotrecogin alfa (activated) should be considered for patients with severe abdominal sepsis associated with a high risk of death.[62,93,94]

KEY POINTS

1. Critically-ill patients with intraabdominal infection are at high risk for treatment failure.

2. Adequate and timely resuscitation ensure tissue perfusion and oxygenation and can prevent the life-threatening complications associated with splanchnic hypoperfusion.

3. Source control also must be adequate and timely and should include débridement of devitalized tissue, closure of perforations, drainage of infected collections, reduction of bacterial and toxin burden, and use of appropriate broad-spectrum antimicrobial therapy.

4. Acute acalculous cholecystitis is an ischemic process and only secondarily an infection. The diagnosis is challenging, and a high index of suspicion is required.

5. Intestinal ischemia is a dangerous and relatively common complication of critical illness, which can progress within hours to gangrene, perforation, and generalized peritonitis.

6. Early diagnosis and treatment, including operative intervention where appropriate, are essential to decrease the high mortality associated with fulminant colitis caused by *Clostridium difficile*.

7. Computed tomography is the primary radiologic modality for imaging the abdomen and pelvis in critically ill patients.

8. Percutaneous decompression of intraabdominal abscesses is successful in about 85% of cases and often can be definitive treatment. Patients who do not improve promptly following percutaneous drainage should undergo formal operative intervention without delay.

9. Optimal antibiotic therapy for secondary peritonitis requires an agent or combination therapy active against both aerobic gram-negative bacilli and anaerobes. High-risk patients with nosocomial intraabdominal infections should be treated with broader-spectrum empirical regimens, including selective use of agents effective against resistant gram-negative organisms, enterococcal species, and *Candida* species.

10. Shorter courses of antimicrobial therapy and modification of agents once susceptibilities are available are safe in patients with adequate source control and will decrease the risk of infections caused by multidrug resistant pathogens.

11. Complications associated with inadequate source control include abscess formation, anastomotic dehiscence, wound infection, recurrent or persistent (secondary or tertiary) peritonitis, fistula formation, abdominal compartment syndrome, sepsis, and multiple organ dysfunction syndrome.

12. Neither planned relaparotomy nor open abdomen techniques offer a survival benefit when compared with on-demand relaparotomy in achieving adequate source control.

13. Multiple organ dysfunction syndrome is present in virtually every patient who dies from intraabdominal infection.

14. Despite the risk of bleeding complications in surgical patients, recombinant human activated protein C should be considered for patients with severe abdominal sepsis.

ANNOTATED REFERENCES

Mazuski J, Solomkin J. Intraabdominal infections. Surg Clin N Am 2009;89:421-37.
Nonoperative management is safe and appropriate for highly selected patients with a well-controlled infectious source. Community-acquired intraabdominal infections should receive narrower-spectrum agents that provide coverage against the common gram-negative and gram-positive aerobic and obligate anaerobic microorganisms. Higher-risk nosocomial infections should be treated with broader-spectrum agents to treat resistant gram-negative organisms, Enterococcus spp., and Candida spp. Shorter durations of empirical antimicrobial therapy are both safe and effective with treatment generally limited to no more than 4 to 5 days in most patients who demonstrate satisfactory clinical response.

Bradley JS, et al. Diagnosis and management of complicated intra-abdominal infection in adults and children: guidelines by the Surgical Infection Society and the Infectious Diseases Society of America. Surg Infect 2010;11:79-109.
Evidence-based guidelines for intraabdominal infection were prepared by an expert panel of the Surgical Infection Society and the Infectious Diseases Society of America. These replace guidelines previously published in 2002 and 2003.

Wong PF, Gilliam AD, Kumar S, Shenfine J, O'Dair GN, Leaper DJ. Antibiotic regimens for secondary peritonitis of gastrointestinal origin in adults. Cochrane Database Syst Rev 2005;2:1-78.
This Cochrane review compares 40 studies of 16 different antibiotic regimens for peritonitis in 5094 patients. All regimens were comparable in terms of clinical success and mortality. Other factors such as local guidelines and preferences, ease of administration, costs, and availability must therefore be used for antibiotic selection.

Rivera-Sanfeliz G. Percutaneous abdominal abscess drainage: a historical perspective. AJR Am J Roentgenol 2008;191:642-3.
Since its first reported use 30 years ago, percutaneous abscess drainage has become a standard of care for treatment of abdominal and thoracic collections, replacing more invasive surgical procedures in all but the most difficult cases.

Sailhamer EA, Carson K, Chang Y et al. Fulminant Clostridium difficile colitis: patterns of care and predictors of mortality. Arch Surg 2009;144:433-9.
The incidence and severity of CDI are increasing. Fulminant CDI is a life-threatening disease, and early diagnosis and treatment are essential. Early surgical intervention with subtotal colectomy should be used in patients who are unresponsive to medical therapy. Mortality was notably decreased when patients had no more than 6 days of medical treatment.

van Santvoort HC, Besselink MG, Bakker OJ et al; Dutch Pancreatitis Study Group. A step-up approach or open necrosectomy for necrotizing pancreatitis. N Engl J Med 2010;362:1491-502.
A minimally invasive step-up approach to manage infected pancreatic necrosis may decrease the morbidity associated with open necrosectomy. This approach consists of percutaneous drainage followed, if necessary, by minimally invasive retroperitoneal necrosectomy; 35% were treated with percutaneous drainage only. New-onset multiple-organ failure, incisional hernias, and new-onset diabetes occurred less frequently in patients randomized to this less invasive study arm. The rate of death did not differ significantly between groups.

Dellinger RP, Levy MM, Carlet JM, et al. Surviving Sepsis Campaign: International guidelines for management of severe sepsis and septic shock: 2008. Intensive Care Med 2008;34:17-60.
This summary provides evidence-based guidelines for the management of severe sepsis, including specific recommendations regarding the management of peritonitis. The targets include early goal-directed resuscitation, prompt imaging studies, initiation of broad-spectrum antibiotics in the first hour of recognition, deescalation and shorter durations of antibiotic therapy, prompt identification of a specific anatomic site of infection, and expeditious implementation of source control measures as soon as possible following resuscitation. Consider rhAPC in patients with sepsis-induced organ dysfunction and high risk of death if there are no contraindications.

Blot SI, Vandewoude KH, De Waele JJ. Candida peritonitis. Curr Opin Crit Care 2007;13:195-9.
Systemic antifungal therapy for treatment of Candida spp. isolated from critically ill patients with intraabdominal infections is controversial. Treatment of Candida isolated from cases of CA-IAI in the immunocompetent host does not impact upon survival. However, Candida isolates from critically ill patients who are immunocompromised or have severe sepsis warrant initiation of empirical antifungal therapy.

De Waele JJ, Ravyts M, Depdt P, Blot SI, Decruyenaere J, Vogelaers D. De-escalation after empirical meropenem treatment in the intensive care unit: fiction or reality? J Crit Care 2010 Jan 13. [Epub ahead of print].
Deescalation of antimicrobial therapy is advocated to reduce the use of broad-spectrum antibiotics in critically ill patients, but application of this strategy in daily clinical practice is variable. In this study, deescalation after empirical treatment with meropenem occurred in fewer than half of the patients. Reasons included the absence of conclusive microbiology and colonization.

Finfer S, Chittock DR, Su SY, et al; NICE-SUGAR Study Investigators. Intensive versus conventional glucose control in critically ill patients. N Engl J Med 2009;360:1283-97. Epub 2009 Mar 24.

This study reports on the results of the 2009 NICE-SUGAR trial (Normoglycemia in Intensive Care Evaluation and Survival Using Glucose Algorithm Regulation), a large international RCT of 6100 patients including both surgical and medical ICU patients. The study found an increased absolute risk of death of 2.6% at 90 days as well as an increased risk of complications due to severe hypoglycemia. Based on this definitive study, tight glycemic control should be avoided.

Payen D, Sablotzki A, Barie PS, et al. International integrated database for the evaluation of severe sepsis and drotrecogin alfa (activated) therapy: analysis of efficacy and safety data in a large surgical cohort. Surgery 2006;140:726-39.

Persistent infections and the subsequent inflammatory responses are associated commonly with inadequate source control and unremitting coagulopathy. The use of drotrecogin alfa in surgical patients demonstrated a significant absolute reduction in risk of 28-day mortality, with this benefit most clearly defined in patients with severe sepsis and a high risk of death (APACHE II score = 25 points or dysfunction of at least two organs). Surgical patients did experience a greater proportion of serious bleeding events during the 96-hour infusion period, but most were managed without fatal consequences.

REFERENCES

Access the complete reference list online at http://www.expertconsult.com.

106 Ileus and Mechanical Bowel Obstruction

RAJEEV DHUPAR | JUAN B. OCHOA

Definition

Ileus is defined as the absence of physiologic motility of the bowel leading to a disturbance in the progression of bowel contents through the gastrointestinal (GI) tract. Ileus must be distinguished from *mechanical bowel obstruction*, which is defined as the presence of anatomic barriers, either extrinsic or intrinsic, that prevent the normal progression of bowel contents through the GI tract.

Pathophysiology

NORMAL GASTROINTESTINAL MOTILITY

Coordinated contraction of the GI tract can be measured by evaluating its electrical and motor activity. During fasting states, the coordinated contractions are called *migrating motor complexes* (MMC) and are divided into three phases: resting phase, intermittent contractions of moderate amplitude, and high-pressure waves.[1] When a food bolus is introduced into the intestine, the organized MMC disappear, and digested food (chyme) is propelled through the GI tract by spikes in the contraction of smooth muscle in the wall of the gut. Longitudinal progression of intestinal contents (made up by food and secretions) occurs through the coordinated response of several systems. These are:

1. Autonomic nervous system. Activation of the sympathetic nervous system decreases GI motility. Activation of the parasympathetic nervous system increases GI motility.[2]
2. Interstitial cells of Cajal (ICC). ICC are distributed throughout the tunica muscularis and are electrically coupled with one another. These cells, which are mesenchymal in origin, are responsible for the pacemaker activity of the GI tract.[1]
3. Myenteric and submucosal nerve plexi. These plexi integrate with the autonomic nervous system. Nitric oxide produced by neuronal nitric oxide synthase (nNOS) induces smooth muscle relaxation.
4. Endocrine system. Multiple endocrine substances affect GI motility. Some of these substances, including motilin, gastrin, and cholecystokinin, increase GI motility. Other hormones such as somatostatin and glucagon decrease GI motility.
5. Smooth muscle. Although there are differences in the muscular layers of the stomach, small bowel, and colon, intestinal motility depends on the coordinated contraction of an outer longitudinal layer and an inner circular layer.
6. Immune system. Activation of the innate immune system can produce profound alterations in GI motility. This appears to be especially evident after surgical manipulation of the small bowel and colon. Inflammatory mediators such as nitric oxide, cytokines, prostaglandins, and oxygen free radicals have direct inhibitory effects on normal contractile activity and may play an important role in the development of ileus due to sepsis and/or after abdominal operations.[3,4]

Integration of the aforementioned processes results in coordinated muscular contractions in the wall of the stomach and intestine that move fluids in the GI tract in an aboral direction. Additionally, this activity helps to ensure that food is adequately mixed with GI secretions and digested. When motility is normal, there is adequate contact time between the absorptive surfaces of the bowel and chyme to permit absorption. Normal motility ultimately leads to the evacuation of undigested food as fecal matter.

Clinical Consequences of Ileus

Ileus results in the inability to tolerate enteral feeding, nausea, vomiting, constipation, and obstipation. Accumulation of fluid and air in the bowel results in abdominal distention. Symptoms and consequences of ileus can range from minimal to life threatening. Serious consequences of ileus can include electrolyte abnormalities, intestinal ischemia, intestinal perforation, and abdominal compartment syndrome. Intolerance of enteral nutrition compromises the ability to provide adequate nutritional support to critically ill patients.

Diagnosis

Tools to aid clinicians in identifying and diagnosing GI dysfunction are poorly developed. Ileus is diagnosed by clinical evaluation of the following signs and symptoms:

1. Abdominal distention
2. Nausea, vomiting, or high output through a nasogastric (Salem sump) tube
3. Reflux of enteral tube feedings
4. Abdominal pain and discomfort (either spontaneous or elicited by palpation of the abdomen)
5. Decreased or absent bowel sounds
6. Constipation and obstipation
7. Suggestive radiologic patterns including increased air in the small intestine, bowel distention, and presence of air-fluid levels

There is no objective measure that defines abnormal abdominal distention or excessive nasogastric output. The true incidence of ileus in critical illness is therefore unknown.

Ileus is often diagnosed by challenging the patient with an enteral diet. Gastric ileus (i.e., absence of normal gastric emptying) is observed in as many as one third of all critically ill patients and is more common in hemodynamically unstable patients. Thus, clinicians often attempt to place feeding tubes into the small bowel, where success in achieving nutritional goals is more commonly achieved.

Three types of clinical ileus are observed: adynamic ileus, spastic ileus (observed rarely in diseases such as porphyria or lead poisoning), and ischemic ileus, identified in hemodynamically unstable patients with low-flow states and classified as nonocclusive mesenteric ischemia (NOMI).

Treatment

1. Adequate hemodynamic resuscitation. This helps to ensure adequate organ blood flow. It is especially important to minimize the infusion of exogenous catecholamines, since these agents can promote the development of ileus.
2. Judicious administration of intravenous fluids. Excessive fluid infusion can result in bowel edema, thereby decreasing intestinal blood flow and increasing intraabdominal pressure.
3. Maintaining electrolyte balance. The presence of hypokalemia prevents normal muscle contraction and nerve depolarization. It is also important to prevent or treat acidemia as well as maintain normal concentrations of other electrolytes (e.g., sodium ion, calcium ion, magnesium ion).
4. Avoid or minimize opioid use. Morphine and other opioids decrease coordinated contractions of the gut and

forward propulsion of chyme. These effects may be a particularly prominent cause of ileus and intolerance to oral or enteral nutrition in postoperative or trauma patients.

5. Avoid prolonged starvation. Starvation and parenteral nutrition are associated with GI mucosal atrophy.[5] Early use of the GI tract (within the first 24-48 hours of the onset of critical illness) is associated with better clinical outcomes.[6] Early enteral nutrition is associated with earlier achievement of caloric goals, earlier time to bowel movements, shorter lengths of stay, and a trend toward lower mortality. The initial goal of early enteral nutrition is to prevent intestinal atrophy, and thus low infusion rates (e.g., 10-20 mL/h) have been advocated. The benefits, risks, and indications of so-called "trickle tube feeds" are still unclear.

6. Do not assume that a patient has ileus and should not be fed enterally. It is unnecessary to wait for the passage of flatus and/or the presence of bowel sounds before attempting to feed enterally.[7] It also is untrue that the bowel "needs to rest" for adequate healing of intestinal anastomoses. On the contrary, provision of enteral nutrition is associated with more deposition of collagen and increased bursting strength in wounds.[8] Virtually all hemodynamically stable postoperative patients should be fed enterally as soon as hemodynamic stability and adequate resuscitation are achieved.

7. Total parenteral nutrition (TPN) is not an ideal substitute for enteral nutrition. TPN rarely achieves adequate nitrogen retention in critical illness and is associated with increased incidence of complications including infections. There are no data to support indiscriminate use of TPN in patients with ileus.[9]

8. Use nonsteroidal antiinflammatory agents (NSAIDs). In surgical patients, the use of systemic NSAIDs such as ketorolac is associated with earlier bowel movements and tolerance to oral diet. This is thought to be due to a quelling of the inflammatory response, as well as a resultant decrease in narcotic use.[10] In animals subjected to surgical manipulation of the GI tract, ketorolac is associated with faster gastric emptying and restoration of normal migrating motor complexes.[11]

9. Promotility agents. Although use of promotility agents has not been routinely implicated, recent protocols advocate starting these early with the objective of achieving caloric goals. There is a paucity of evidence, however, to support the view that systemic promotility agents such as metoclopramide, erythromycin, or cholecystokinin affect overall outcome.[12] Newer agents are being tested for clinical use to aid in the prevention of or hasten the resolution of ileus. These agents include mu-opioid antagonists, motilin analogs, and intestinal chloride channel modifiers.[13]

▓ Conclusions

Ileus can lead to significant adverse clinical consequences and mortality, especially if the problem is not recognized and adequately treated. The criteria and tools for the diagnosis of ileus are poorly developed, which hinders progress in this area. Inappropriately diagnosing ileus often leads to the unnecessary starvation of patients and/or inappropriate use of parenteral nutrition. Progress in understanding the mechanisms that lead to the development of ileus will permit the implementation of logical treatments.

ANNOTATED REFERENCES

Kalff JC, Schwarz NT, Walgenbach KJ, Schraut WH, Bauer AJ. Leukocytes of the intestinal muscularis: their phenotype and isolation. J Leukoc Biol 1998;63:683-91.
> *Provides a careful evaluation of infiltrating leukocytes to the intestine and their possible effect on intestinal motility.*

Moore EE, Jones TN. Benefits of immediate jejunostomy feeding after major abdominal trauma—a prospective, randomized study. J Trauma 1986;26:874-81.
> *A landmark article that demonstrates the feasibility of early enteral nutrition in severely traumatized patients. The authors also report a significant decrease in infectious complications associated with early enteral nutrition in severely traumatized patients.*

Moore FA, Feliciano DV, Andrassy RJ, et al. Early enteral feeding, compared with parenteral, reduces postoperative septic complications. The results of a meta-analysis. Ann Surg 1992;216:172-83.
> *A meta-analysis of 8 prospective randomized trials that compare the results of early enteral nutrition (EEN) over that of TPN. Overall, patients who received EEN had significantly fewer complications (18%) when compared to those receiving TPN (35%) (P = 0.01). This article provides strong evidence that EEN should be adopted as the standard of care if at all possible.*

Tadano S, Terashima H, Fukuzawa J, Matsuo R, Ikeda O, Ohkohchi N. Early postoperative oral intake accelerates upper gastrointestinal anastomotic healing in the rat model. J Surg Res 2010 Feb 4. Epub ahead of print.
> *This article provides a physiologic basis to challenge the belief that oral intake is associated with increased risk of anastomotic breakdown. While it is impossible to demonstrate increased anastomotic collagen deposition in humans in response to early oral intake, it is possible to demonstrate that early oral intake improves anastomotic strength.*

Traut U, Brügger L, Kunz R, Pauli-Magnus C, Haug K, Bucher H, et al. Systemic prokinetic pharmacologic treatment for postoperative adynamic ileus following abdominal surgery in adults. Cochrane Database Syst Rev 2008;1:CD004930.
> *A systematic analysis of 39 trials and 4615 patients studied to receive medications and/or dietary therapy to resolve postoperative ileus. Overall there are significant limitations to these studies.*

REFERENCES

Access the complete reference list online at http://www.expertconsult.com.

107

Toxic Megacolon and Ogilvie's Syndrome

H.M. OUDEMANS-VAN STRAATEN

Acute megacolon refers to a syndrome presenting as marked colonic distension in the absence of mechanical obstruction. It results from disturbed colonic motility[1,2] and may be a manifestation of Ogilvie's syndrome or toxic megacolon. Ogilvie's syndrome, or acute colonic pseudo-obstruction (or its precursor, critical illness–related colonic ileus [CIRCI]),[3] is a disease of seriously ill hospitalized patients and associated with myriad hemodynamic, metabolic, pharmacologic, inflammatory, and postoperative conditions. In toxic megacolon, distension is caused by severe colitis and is associated with systemic toxicity. Toxic megacolon is classically described as a complication of inflammatory bowel disease (IBD), usually ulcerative colitis, but in the critically ill, toxic megacolon mostly occurs as a complication of severe infectious colitis generally caused by *Clostridium difficile*. Whether secondary to IBD or *C. difficile* colitis, progressive colonic distension can lead to gut barrier failure, sepsis, ischemia, perforation, and multiple organ dysfunction. These potentially life-threatening complications must be prevented. This chapter focuses on toxic megacolon and Ogilvie's syndrome in critically ill patients admitted to the intensive care unit (ICU) and proposes prevention strategies.

Clinical Features

OGILVIE'S SYNDROME OR ACUTE COLONIC PSEUDO-OBSTRUCTION

The hallmark of Ogilvie's syndrome is abdominal distension with or without tenderness in hospitalized patients with serious comorbid disease.[4-6] Patients may present with constipation, but flatus or stools may pass as well. Bowel sounds are normal, diminished, or high, and percussion is hypertympanic. Tenderness is most pronounced over the cecum. Nausea and vomiting may occur, but gastric retention is often minimal, and enteral feeding may be tolerated. If diagnosis and treatment are delayed, progressive distension may cause peritoneal signs, respiratory compromise, nutritional depletion, sepsis, multiple organ failure, ischemia, and perforation. Perforation most commonly occurs in the cecum. The risk of perforation is unlikely when cecal diameter is less than 12 cm but increases sharply when cecal diameter is 12 cm or more. CIRCI is characterized by constipation for many days without marked colonic distension. This syndrome may herald development of Ogilvie's syndrome.[3]

TOXIC MEGACOLON

Toxic megacolon is a serious complication of colitis. Patients present with fever, abdominal tenderness, and distension or even with an acute abdomen. IBD or infectious colitis commonly present with diarrhea, but a decrease in stool frequency may herald the onset of megacolon and delay diagnosis.[2,7] Altered consciousness, dehydration, hypotension, tachycardia, leukocytosis, thrombocytopenia, low albumin, and electrolyte disturbances are common. In severe cases, systemic toxicity leads to septic shock and multiple organ failure.[8-10] Ascending pylephlebitis and septic emboli in the superior mesenteric vein and liver are rare complications. Patients with ulcerative colitis are at highest risk of developing toxic megacolon early in their disease.[11] Factors that may trigger toxic megacolon are early discontinuation or decrease in medications, use of antidiarrheal agents such as loperamide or opioids, severe hypokalemia, barium enema, and colonoscopy.

GASTROINTESTINAL MOTILITY

Intestinal motility is mainly under control of the enteric nervous system, an independently functioning complex network regulated by entero-enteric reflex pathways, the so-called enteric minibrain.[12]

Several types of motor activity are involved in intestinal propulsion; local reflex peristalsis after feeding and the migrating motor complex (MMC) during fasting are the most important.[13] Local reflex peristalsis is activated by intraluminal distension (food), which stimulates the release of the neurotransmitter, serotonin. Release of serotonin triggers afferent neurons that activate excitatory motor neurons proximal to the site of the stimulus to release acetylcholine and substance P, resulting in contraction. Distal to the site of distension, inhibitory neurons are activated to release nitric oxide (NO) and vasoactive intestinal peptide (VIP), leading to relaxation.[14] This nonadrenergic, noncholinergic, intrinsic inhibitory innervation (NANCI) is more pronounced in organs with a reservoir function, explaining why the stomach and proximal colon are more susceptible to distension than the small intestine.[15]

The MMC or interdigestive motility pattern is initiated by the hormone, motilin. The motilin receptor is expressed on enteric neurons of the human duodenum and colon.[16] Many peptides, autacoids, and hormones influence MMC activity, including insulin, cholecystokinin, serotonin, opioids, dopamine, norepinephrine, somatostatin, and NO.[17-19]

The enteric nervous system is modulated by the central autonomic nervous system; the parasympathetic nerves promote and the sympathetic nerves suppress motility.[20,21] Parasympathetic nerves to the right and transverse colon originate from the vagal nerve and those to the distal colon from the spinal cord (S2-4); they release acetylcholine. Sympathetic innervation of the colon runs through the spinal cord and the celiac and mesenteric ganglia. Sympathetic activations suppress contractions via the release of norepinephrine, causing a presynaptic inhibition of acetylcholine release from enteric neurons and also the release of other excitatory neurotransmitters such as serotonin from enteric nerve cells.[22,23] Apart from inhibiting motility, sympathetic activation contracts the sphincters by a direct effect of norepinephrine on the smooth muscle; norepinephrine released by sympathetic neurons also affects vascular tone.

Pathogenesis of Megacolon

COLONIC ILEUS AND OGILVIE'S SYNDROME

The pathophysiology of Ogilvie's syndrome is not fully understood. Increased sympathetic and suppressed or interrupted parasympathetic activity play a role. In addition, neurotransmitters, inflammatory mediators, metabolic derangement and pharmacologic interventions are directly or indirectly involved.[20,21]

Abdominal surgery induces hypomotility by a complex interaction of neurogenic and inflammatory mechanisms. Intestinal manipulation initiates norepinephrine release via sympathetic nerves from the spinal cord, as well as NO and VIP release via vagal nerve stimulation, causing inhibition of contractile activity and relaxation.[21] Prolonged postoperative ileus involves inflammation of the intestinal muscularis, initiated by activation of peritoneal mast cells and resident macrophages. Activated mast cells release histamine and proteases, which recruit leukocytes and temporarily increase intestinal permeability with translocation of bacteria and bacterial products. Activated mast cells also stimulate resident macrophages to release cytokines such as tumor necrosis factor (TNF) and up-regulate inducible nitric oxide synthetase (iNOS) and cyclooxygenase (COX-2) expression; collectively, all of these factors inhibit motility. Local inflammation by influx of leukocytes in the muscularis mucosa and circulating cytokines subsequently activate neurogenic inhibitory adrenergic pathways, causing generalized hypomotility.[21] In addition, activation of peripheral opioid receptors in the gastrointestinal (GI) tract inhibits acetylcholine release from motor neurons and promotes transmitter release from inhibitory neurons.[24] Opioid receptors are stimulated by endogenous opioids, which are locally secreted upon surgical stress. Exogenous opioids used for analgesia also act on peripheral opioid receptors in the GI tract, inhibiting motility. Peritonitis and pain cause a generalized inhibition of motility via spinal afferents that connect in the spinal cord to sympathetic efferents.[20]

Colonic hypomotility in critically ill patients may be related to circulating bacterial products and/or proinflammatory cytokines (e.g., lipopolysaccharide or TNF), leading to increased expression of iNOS and COX-2.[25,26] Colonic hypomotility also may be related to ischemia and reperfusion, causing an energy deficit, *functio laesa*, and oxidant-mediated tissue damage. Finally, distal colonic distension induces inhibition of proximal colonic motility, the so-called colo-colonic reflex, which passes by the paravertebral ganglia and activates inhibitory sympathetic nerves.[22] In this way, colonic dilation perpetuates itself.

Predisposing Factors

OGILVIE'S SYNDROME

Clinical factors predisposing to Ogilvie's syndrome are summarized in Box 107-1.[5,27,28] The syndrome was first described by Sir William Heneage Ogilvie (1887-1971) in two patients with malignant infiltration of the celiac plexus.[29] After surgery and trauma of spine, hip, and pelvis, dysfunction of the sacral parasympathetic nerves may impair motility of the distal colon, causing atony with functional obstruction.[30] In a series reporting 400 patients with Ogilvie's syndrome, the most common underlying conditions were trauma, cardiovascular disease, and infections.[5] In another series, the majority of patients had cardiovascular disease.[31] Both drugs and ischemia may play a role in cardiovascular disease. Exogenous catecholamines have dose-dependent effects on intestinal motility; low doses promote and high doses suppress motility.[18,32] α-Adrenergic agonists are stronger inhibitors of acetylcholine release than β-adrenergic agents. Dobutamine and dopexamine have little effect on intestinal peristalsis. Dopamine not only inhibits upper GI motility but also distal colonic motility.[17,19,33] The use of dopamine is associated with late defecation.[34] Clonidine and dexmedetomidine, central α2-adrenergic receptor agonists, decrease fasting colonic smooth muscle tone[35] and are associated with Ogilvie's syndrome.[36] Opioids suppress the phase III migrating motor contractions.[37] This inhibiting effect on gut motility is mediated by activation of mu-opioid receptors in the GI tract, reducing the release of acetylcholine from the myenteric plexus.[38] Ogilvie's syndrome with life-threatening complications is reported with the use of antipsychotic agents such as clozapine that cause generalized GI hypomotility by anticholinergic and antiserotonergic mechanisms.[39,40] In patients with sepsis, bacterial products (e.g., lipopolysaccharide), proinflammatory cytokines (e.g., TNF) and NO produced by the inducible enzyme, iNOS, suppress intestinal motility.[25,41,42]

TOXIC MEGACOLON

The incidence of toxic megacolon in IBD has substantially decreased with better management of severe colitis.[43] The most common cause of toxic megacolon in the critically ill is pseudomembranous colitis caused by overgrowth of *C. difficile*.[44] However, other pathogens such as enterotoxin-producing strains of *Clostridium perfringens*,

Staphylococcus aureus, and *Klebsiella oxytoca* can cause colitis after antibiotic use.[45] Sporadic cases of megacolon due to infections caused by *Salmonella* spp.,[46] *Shigella* spp., *Amoeba*, herpesvirus, or cytomegalovirus (CMV) have also been described.[11] In patients with human immunodeficiency virus (HIV), toxic megacolon may be a primary manifestation of the HIV infection or be related to infection with *C. difficile* or CMV.[47] Causes of toxic megacolon are summarized in Box 107-2.

Box 107-1

CLINICAL FACTORS PREDISPOSING TO OGILVIE'S SYNDROME OR ACUTE COLONIC PSEUDO-OBSTRUCTION

Cardiovascular
- Heart failure, stroke
- Gut ischemia

Critical illness
- Severe sepsis
- Acute pancreatitis
- Shock or hypoxemia

Postoperative state or trauma
- Intestinal manipulation
- Peritonitis
- Immobility and dehydration
- Vertebral, pelvic or hip fracture/surgery
- Retroperitoneal hematoma

Metabolic factors
- Hypokalemia and hyperglycemia
- Hypothyroidism, diabetes mellitus
- Liver or renal failure
- Amyloidosis

Drugs
- α-Adrenergic agonists, dopamine[18]
- Clonidine and dexmedetomidine[36]
- Opioids[88]
- Anticholinergics, calcium channel antagonists
- Antipsychotics[39,40]
- Antidepressants[92]
- High-dose phosphodiesterase inhibitors[93]

Gastrointestinal infections
- Cytomegalovirus, herpes zoster
- Tuberculosis

Neurologic
- Transsection of the spinal cord
- Low spinal cord disease
- Parkinson's disease

Obstetric
- Caesarian section
- Normal delivery

Box 107-2

DISORDERS ASSOCIATED WITH TOXIC MEGACOLON

Inflammatory bowel disease
- Ulcerative colitis
- Crohn's disease

Infectious colitis
- *Salmonella*, *Shigella*, amoebic colitis
- *Clostridium difficile*
- Cytomegalovirus colitis
- HIV infection

Cancer chemotherapy

Ischemia

HIV, human immunodeficiency virus.

The pathogenesis of toxic megacolon is not well understood.[2,11] In infectious colitis, inflammation extends into the deeper layers of the colonic wall, whereas the inflammation in ulcerative colitis is typically limited to the mucosa. Deep infiltration, microabscesses, edema, and necrosis may paralyze colonic smooth muscle and lead to dilatation. Bacterial toxins permeating through ulcerations activate the release of cytokines, with subsequent systemic toxicity. NO, locally generated in excessive amounts secondary to increased expression of iNOS in inflammatory and smooth muscle cells, is the key mediator of diminished smooth muscle function in toxic megacolon.[48,49]

CLOSTRIDIUM DIFFICILE INFECTION

Clostridium difficile is a gram-positive spore-forming rod. Pathogenic strains produce two major exotoxins: A and B. Both activate cell-signaling molecules including the transcription factor, nuclear factor-κB, and mitogen-activated protein kinases in monocytes, leading to the production and release of proinflammatory cytokines. Both toxins induce colitis in humans.[50] Colonic injury results from alterations of the enterocyte cytoskeleton, with disruption of tight junction function and marked inflammation in the lamina propria. Severe pseudomembranous colitis occurs in 3% to 5% of carriers. Recurrent sepsis or toxic megacolon are rare but severe complications.

Colonization with *C. difficile* results from alterations in the composition of the indigenous colonic microflora. Enemas containing normal human feces appear to be effective in the treatment of infected patients.[51,52] Mechanisms of suppression include the production of volatile acids, hydrogen sulfide, and secondary bile acids.[53] The most frequently identified clinical risk factor for *C. difficile*–associated diarrhea is the antecedent use of antibiotics affecting indigenous colonic microflora.[54] The opportunity to acquire the organism increases with prolonged hospital stay,[55] and it may spread by nosocomial transmission.[56] Whether a person remains an asymptomatic carrier or develops colitis depends on the size of the *C. difficile* population, toxigenicity of the strain, toxin-neutralizing effects of the indigenous gut flora, and underlying disease (Box 107-3).[53,57,58] Susceptibility is further increased by poor GI defense mechanisms resulting from the use of gastric acid–inhibiting drugs that facilitate intestinal transit of the bacteria,[54,55] total parenteral nutrition, postpyloric enteral feeding, or recent GI surgery.[59-61] A combination of factors increases the risk.

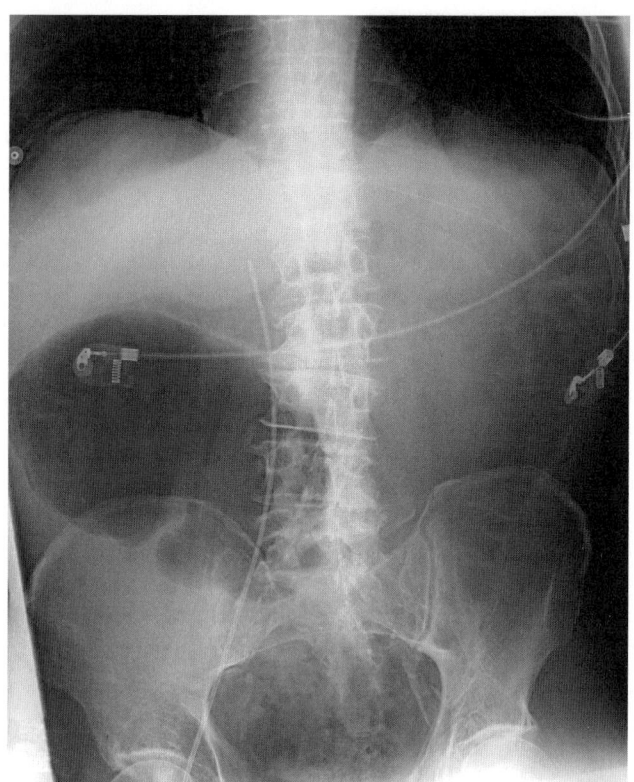

Figure 107-1   Plain abdominal radiograph of patient with respiratory insufficiency due to severe emphysema and Ogilvie's syndrome 10 days after dynamic hip screw implantation for femoral fracture. Dilatation is most pronounced in cecum and ascending colon. Gas and fecal pattern in distal colon are normal. Patient was successfully treated with intravenous neostigmine.

Box 107-3

FACTORS ASSOCIATED WITH COLONIZATION AND SUBSEQUENT INFECTION WITH *CLOSTRIDIUM DIFFICILE*

Disruption of indigenous microflora
- Antibiotics suppressing indigenous microflora
- Cancer chemotherapeutics with antimicrobial activity
- Preoperative bowel preparation

Opportunity of infection
- Prolonged hospital stay

Microbial factors
- Toxigenicity and adhesion

Diminished gastrointestinal defense
- Reduced or suppressed gastric acid secretion
- Parenteral nutrition
- Postpyloric enteral nutrition
- Gastrointestinal surgery

Antibody response of the host

Poor underlying condition
- High age
- Cancer
- Renal insufficiency
- Long-term use of corticosteroids
- Bedridden state

Diagnosis and Differential Diagnosis of Acute Megacolon

Besides history and clinical features, plain abdominal radiography is crucial for diagnosis and follow-up. Dilatation is most pronounced in the cecum, ascending, and right transverse colon. The size of the cecum may range from 6 to 20 cm. In Ogilvie's syndrome, colonic diameter typically decreases gradually to a collapsed bowel and a normal gas and fecal pattern in the rectum (Figure 107-1). Dilation of the left colon may occur as well (Figure 107-2). Mechanical obstruction is excluded if gas is visible in all colonic segments, including the rectosigmoid. If not, an enema should be administered. The osmotic effect of water-soluble contrast medium is diagnostic and may be therapeutic in decompressing the colon.[62] Some air/fluid levels and dilatation of the small bowel may be present. In Ogilvie's syndrome, the colonic haustral and mucosal pattern is maintained, whereas the pattern is disturbed or lost in toxic megacolon. Deep ulcerations may be visible between large pseudopolypoid projections into the lumen. Pneumatosis of the bowel wall is a sign of ischemic necrosis and free peritoneal air of perforation. A diagnosis of severe colitis can be made with computed tomographic (CT) scan, but findings are nonspecific for the underlying cause.[63] The scan shows a diffusely thickened or edematous colonic wall with pericolonic inflammation. CT scan may be helpful in patients presenting without diarrhea, with acute abdomen, for differential diagnosis, or to show or exclude complications.

The underlying cause of toxic megacolon, IBD, or infectious colitis must be identified (see Boxes 107-2 and 107-3). The history may reveal chronic abdominal complaints, diarrhea, bloody stools, familial occurrence of IBD, recent travel, intake of contaminated food, hospitalization,

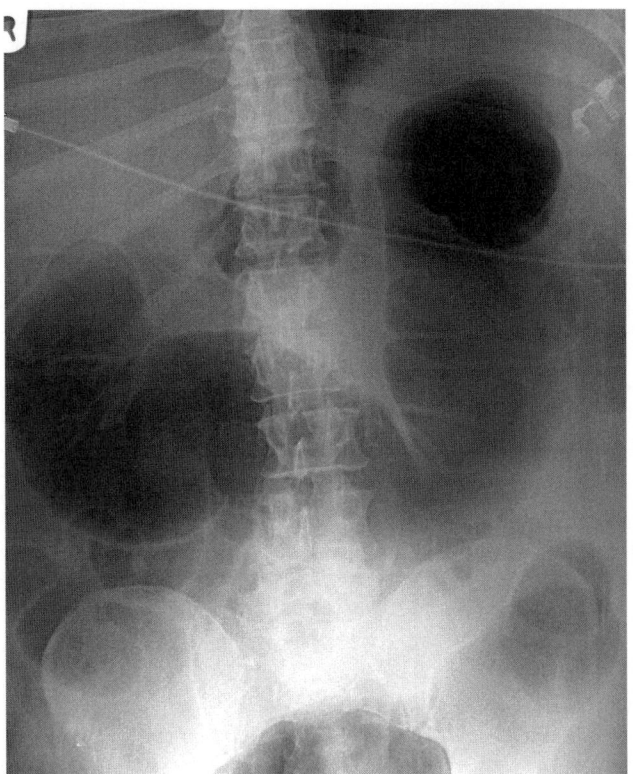

Figure 107-2 Plain abdominal radiograph of patient with Ogilvie's syndrome 11 days after surgery for ruptured aneurysm of abdominal aorta. Dilatation (probably due to ischemia) is present in both right and left colon. Syndrome resolved with vasodilators and intravenous neostigmine.

use of antibiotics, risk factors for HIV infection, or immunosuppression. Infection with CMV or *C. difficile* may precipitate toxic megacolon in ulcerative colitis.[64] If unresponsive to therapy, both Ogilvie's syndrome and ischemic colitis may be complicated by progressive distension with bacterial overgrowth and systemic toxicity, mimicking toxic megacolon.

For microbiological diagnosis of infectious colitis, a fresh fecal sample should immediately be submitted to the laboratory for culture on specific media. For screening of a *C. difficile* infection, stool can be tested for the presence of toxicogenic *C. difficile*. The screening assay is inexpensive, quick, and highly sensitive. Unfortunately, its specificity is low.[65] To improve diagnosis, a two-stage testing strategy is recommended with an initial highly sensitive rapid screening test capable of detecting both toxin A and B, followed by a confirmatory test capable of detecting neutralizable *C. difficile* toxin in cell culture.[65] Final results take 2 to 5 days. Although the test is positive in asymptomatic carriers, a positive test in a patient with antibiotic-associated megacolon makes infection with *C. difficile* highly probable. Surveillance cultures of feces are advocated to detect other pathogens such as enterotoxin-producing *C. perfringens*, *S. aureus*, and *K. oxytoca*. Blood cultures are warranted in all cases of toxic megacolon. They are generally positive in severe cases of typhoid fever. If stool and blood cultures remain negative, a bone marrow culture may still yield *Salmonella* spp. after 5 days despite antibiotic use.

Limited endoscopy with biopsy may provide useful information. Inflammatory bowel disease is characterized by diffusely abnormal crypt structure, whereas the architecture of the crypts is intact in bacterial colitis. In CMV colitis, inclusion bodies are present. Mild cases of *C. difficile* colitis are associated with nonspecific findings of colitis. In severe cases, focal ulcerations covered by purulent material,

presenting as yellow or white plaques 2 to 4 cm in diameter, are found with normal intervening mucosa. Pseudomembranous colitis may not be detected if flexible sigmoidoscopy is performed.[66] Full colonoscopy in patients with acute megacolon carries the risk of perforation, however.

Management

OGILVIE'S SYNDROME

An early proactive strategy for preventing Ogilvie's syndrome is advocated (Box 107-4). Awaiting resolution, the distended colon is at risk for life-threatening complications that need to be prevented. To exclude obstruction, a water-soluble contrast enema can be given unless the patient displays peritoneal irritation. Concomitantly, conditions that can impair colon motility must be corrected. All motility-inhibiting medications should be minimized or withdrawn. Alternatives are generally available; for example, opioids can be replaced by thoracic epidural anesthesia, an intervention that improves motility by inducing sympathetic blockade.[67,68] Efforts should be made to reduce infusion rates of norepinephrine and especially dopamine.

If these measures are not effective, neostigmine is the drug of choice. In a double-blind crossover trial in a non-ICU population, an intravenous (IV) bolus of 2 mg neostigmine led to rapid colonic decompression in the majority of the patients.[69] Since severe bradycardia is feared in the critically ill, a continuous infusion with neostigmine is safer. In a double-blind, placebo-controlled cross-over study in critically ill, ventilated patients with CIRCI, continuous IV administration of neostigmine at 0.4 to 0.8 mg/h resulted in defecation in 80% of the patients, whereas no defecation occurred during placebo infusion.[3] If defecation does not occur, the neostigmine dose should be increased at 4-hour intervals. With this regimen, neostigmine is tolerated well, adverse events present slowly, and if necessary, the dose can be reduced. Adverse events include bradycardia, increased salivation and bronchorrhea, bronchospasm, and abdominal cramps if motility recovers. Repeat radiographs are obtained for follow-up assessment of colonic diameter.

Several case reports showed effective colonic decompression with cisapride,[70] which enhances acetylcholine release in the mesenteric plexus. However, the drug was withdrawn from the U.S. market in 2000 because of its propensity to induce severe ventricular dysrhythmias. Erythromycin, a motilin agonist, also may improve colonic motility.[71] Recommended dose is low (200 mg twice daily IV), since higher doses can actually inhibit motility.[72]

Box 107-4

STRATEGIES TO PREVENT OGILVIE'S SYNDROME IN THE CRITICALLY ILL

- Early resuscitation of the circulation
- Minimizing prolonged infusion of high doses of α-adrenergic drugs
- Minimizing the use of dopamine
- Minimizing the prolonged use of opioids
- Use of thoracic epidural anesthesia
- Minimally invasive or laparoscopic surgery
- Selective decontamination of the digestive tract
- Avoiding antibiotics that disrupt growth of anaerobic fecal bacteria
- Early oral or enteral feeding
- Avoidance of proton pump inhibitors
- Early mobilization and ambulation
- Promoting timely defecation with
- Oral polyethylene glycol from day 3
- Intravenous neostigmine from day 5

Endoscopic decompression may be indicated if decompression with neostigmine fails.[73] In our experience, this intervention is seldom necessary. Colonoscopy in this setting is time consuming, difficult to perform, and not without hazards. The unprepared bowel contains copious amounts of stool. Inflation of air may increase colonic distension, impair ventilation, and lead to perforation. It is advocated to avoid the liberal use of air insufflation. Advancing the scope as far as the hepatic flexure may be sufficient to obtain adequate decompression.[74] Gas should be aspirated. Colonoscopy is successful in 70% to 80% of patients, but the recurrence rate is 15% to 40%. Recurrence may be reduced if a decompressive tube is left in place, but controlled trials with this intervention are not available. Mortality rate associated with colonoscopy is between 1% and 5% in experienced hands. If signs of ischemia are encountered, the procedure should be discontinued.

Indications for surgery are failure of conservative treatment, with clinical signs of impending or actual ischemia or perforation. For surgical management, the reader is referred to the specific literature.[6,28,75] The type of surgery depends on the state of the colon. If the colon is viable, some sort of venting stoma is placed. Tube cecostomy is a simple procedure and carries a lower mortality than resection.[5] A large Foley catheter is left in place for 2 to 3 weeks. Stomas have relatively low immediate morbidity but relatively high late morbidity. CT-guided transperitoneal percutaneous cecostomy may be considered for patients unresponsive to medical treatment and unfit for surgery.[28]

TOXIC MEGACOLON

The main initial goal of treatment is to reduce the severity of colitis and restore motility.[11] Medical treatment is successful in about 50% of cases, but the patient should be assessed daily by the intensivist and the surgeon. Conditions impairing colonic motility must be corrected as far as possible (see Box 107-1). Antiperistaltic agents for diarrhea are absolutely contraindicated. Patients need general support with IV fluids, electrolyte and vitamin replacement, early optimization of circulation and, if necessary, mechanical ventilation. They are additionally treated with IV antibiotics, corticosteroids, selective decontamination of the digestive tract (SDD), and enteral nutrition. Tolerance of nutrition is monitored by gastric retention and abdominal signs. TPN offers no proven benefit.[11]

Systemic antibiotics are necessary to reduce septic complications and peritonitis. Systemic antibiotics should have an anaerobic and gram-negative spectrum guided by local susceptibility patterns and adjusted to fecal surveillance cultures. It is important to select antibiotics that give the least disturbance of the indigenous anaerobic flora, and in case of C. difficile, the culprit antibiotic is discontinued. SDD with the correct antibiotics (polymyxin 100 mg, tobramycin 80 mg, and amphotericin B 500 mg 4 times daily)[76,77] attacks overgrowth of aerobic gram-negative bacteria and yeast species, reduces the fecal endotoxin pool, and leaves the protective flora intact.[78] Systemic toxicity and associated infections are thus limited.[77,79,80] In animal studies, decontamination of the bowel with oral nonabsorbable broad-spectrum antibiotics reduces iNOS expression and prevents dilatation.[48] A trial with neostigmine may be useful to promote motility and defecation, allowing the oral antibiotics to reach the entire GI tract, clear bacterial overgrowth, and mitigate associated systemic toxicity.

There are two effective drugs for the treatment of C. difficile–associated diarrhea: vancomycin and metronidazole. Oral vancomycin is not absorbed, and high fecal concentrations are achieved. IV vancomycin is not effective. IV metronidazole may be secreted through an inflamed mucosa. In patients with active disease receiving oral or IV metronidazole, bactericidal fecal concentrations were achieved, but concentrations fell as the diarrhea improved, and neither substance was detectable in the feces after recovery.[81] Although an older randomized controlled trial showed no difference between oral vancomycin 500 mg 4 times daily and oral metronidazole 250 mg 4 times daily,[82] a recent trial comparing oral vancomycin 125 mg 4 times daily to oral metronidazole 250 mg 4 times daily for 10 days showed that metronidazole and vancomycin are equally effective for the treatment of mild C. difficile associated diarrhea, while vancomycin was superior for patients with severe diarrhea.[83] Notably, treatment of asymptomatic carriers is not recommended.[84] For antibiotic treatment of toxic megacolon due to C. difficile colitis, IV metronidazole (500 mg 3 times daily) may be considered in addition to vancomycin (500 mg 4 times daily, administered via the nasogastric tube).[50,85] Vancomycin retention enemas might be administered as well (500 mg vancomycin in 100 mL normal saline). CMV colitis requires specific treatment with ganciclovir (5 mg/kg IV, with dose adjustment in patients with renal dysfunction).

All patients with severe colitis should be treated with corticosteroids.[86] Corticosteroids are potent inhibitors of inflammation and specifically inhibit iNOS expression, preventing further colonic dilatation.[48]

Patients with toxic megacolon need surgery without delay if they are unresponsive to medical treatment. Surgical intervention should be considered when the patient has progressive signs of organ failure despite medical treatment, a worsening CT scan, or signs of peritonitis. Subtotal colectomy with end-ileostomy is the treatment of choice for urgent surgery.[11,43,44]

Outcome

With appropriate management, pseudo-obstruction usually resolves within a couple of days. However, hospitalization may be prolonged[30] and mortality rate may be high because megacolon affects debilitated patients with other organ failure. Mortality is related to underlying disease, cecal diameter, delay in decompression, the kind of intervention, or the presence of an ischemic or perforated cecum.[5,11,75] In patients with pseudo-obstruction needing surgery, mortality was 30% compared to 14% after early conservative treatment.[5] In one series, all patients who died had coronary artery disease.[31] In the presence of perforation, mortality rate may increase to 50%.[75] Notably, none of these studies used neostigmine early after presentation. Colonic pseudo-obstruction reflects a failing organ, one that is not scored in the presently available organ failure scores.

In severe ulcerative colitis, the fatality of toxic megacolon is high, especially if surgery is delayed. The development of multiple organ failure predicts a fatal outcome.[9] Mortality of toxic megacolon due to C. difficile infection rises to 80%.[87] In a cohort of 59 intensive care patients with C. difficile colitis, one-fifth of the patients required surgery for progressive toxicity or peritonitis. In the surgical patients, APACHE scores at diagnosis were higher, and mortality rate was 42% compared to 15% in medical patients.[44]

Strategies to Prevent Megacolon in the Critically Ill

In contrast to the wide attention paid in the literature to gastric emptying, little notice is taken of defecation. Among critically ill patients, it is not unusual for the first stools to be passed after more than a week.[34] Defecation removes bacteria from the gut and reduces overgrowth of pathogenic bacteria and yeasts. With respect to the potentially lethal complications of Ogilvie's syndrome and toxic megacolon, clinical awareness and a strategy of care for the colon are crucial (see Box 107-4). This strategy includes early resuscitation of the circulation, tailored infusion therapy,[88] correction of hypokalemia and hypomagnesemia, minimizing prolonged infusion of high doses of α-adrenergic drugs and dopamine,[13] restrictive use of opioids, thoracic epidural anesthesia,[89] avoiding antibiotics, which disrupt the growth of anaerobic fecal bacteria, early enteral feeding, avoiding routine use of proton pump inhibitors, promoting defecation, and early mobilization and ambulation. Nutrients in the gut directly stimulate proliferation of enterocytes and motility by the production of GI messengers, acting via autocrine, paracrine, and endocrine pathways. The use of antibiotics that affect the growth of indigenous protective colonic microflora should be avoided whenever possible. SDD is advocated in patients with an expected stay of more than a few days. Proper SDD[76] prevents overgrowth of aerobic gram-negative bacteria and yeasts and reduces the fecal endotoxin pool and associated motility disorder, systemic toxicity,[78] gram-negative infections, and mortality.[77,80] With these measures, *C. difficile* colitis is virtually absent in the ICU. If defecation does not occur spontaneously, an enema and oral polyethylene glycol (PEG 13.125 g in 100 mL water 3 times daily) is advocated from day 3.[90,91] Compared to PEG, Ogilvie's syndrome was more often seen with lactulose. When stools do not pass and physical examination of the abdomen is without suspicion, neostigmine is started. By implementation of a protocol promoting defecation, deterioration of the patient's condition by dilatation of the colon can be prevented.

KEY POINTS

1. Acute megacolon is a nonobstructive motility disorder of the colon associated with many hemodynamic, metabolic, pharmacologic, inflammatory, and postoperative conditions. Main predisposing conditions are increased sympathetic or dopaminergic activity, ischemia, inducible nitric oxide synthase (iNOS) expression, and the use of opioids.

2. Clinical awareness and a strategy of care for the colon can prevent the development of acute megacolon and its potentially lethal complications.

3. A continuous infusion of neostigmine is a safe and generally effective treatment for nonobstructive megacolon in critically ill patients.

4. Toxic megacolon is a complication of severe colitis, which is most often caused by *Clostridium difficile* in critically ill patients.

ANNOTATED REFERENCES

Saunders MD, Kimmey MB. Colonic pseudo-obstruction: the dilated colon in the ICU. Semin Gastrointest Dis 2003;14:20-7.
Prognosis in acute colonic pseudo-obstruction is determined by the severity of underlying disease, the maximal cecal diameter, the delay in colonic decompression, and the status of the bowel.

Fruhwald S, Holzer P, Metzler H. Gastrointestinal motility in acute illness. Wien Klin Wochenschr 2008;120:6-17.
This review focuses on select motility disturbances such as gastroparesis, postoperative ileus, and Ogilvie's syndrome. Generally effective methods to treat these conditions are given. Finally, we focus on special management options to prevent such motility disturbances or to reduce their severity.

Boeckxstaens GE, de Jonge WJ. Neuroimmune mechanisms in postoperative ileus. Gut 2009;58:1300-11.
Ileus after abdominal surgery is caused by early neurogenic and late inflammatory mechanisms. Inflammation underlies long-lasting postoperative ileus.

Lomax AE, Sharkey KA, Furness JB. The participation of the sympathetic innervation of the gastrointestinal tract in disease states. Neurogastroenterol Motil 2010;22:7-18.
This study highlights the interaction between the sympathetic nervous system and inflammation, and the influence of sympathetic transmitters on gut flora.

Van der Spoel JI, Oudemans-van Straaten HM, Stoutenbeek CP, Bosman RJ, Zandstra DF. Neostigmine resolves critical illness-related colonic ileus in intensive care patients with multiple organ failure—a prospective, double-blind, placebo-controlled trial. Intensive Care Med 2001;27:822-7.
A continuous infusion of neostigmine is a safe and effective treatment for decompression of nonobstructive megacolon in the critically ill.

van der Spoel JI, Oudemans-van Straaten HM, Kuiper MA, van Roon EN, Zandstra DF, van der Voort PH. Laxation of critically ill patients with lactulose or polyethylene glycol: a two-center randomized, double-blind, placebo-controlled trial. Crit Care Med 2007;35:2726-31.
Both lactulose and polyethylene glycol are more effective in promoting defecation than placebo. Irrespective of study medication, early defecation was associated with a shorter length of stay.

Saunders MD, Cappell MS. Endoscopic management of acute colonic pseudo-obstruction. Endoscopy 2005;37:760-3.
Colonic decompression is the initial invasive procedure of choice for patients with marked cecal distension (>10 cm) of significant duration (>3 ± 4 days), who fail to respond to pharmacologic therapy with neostigmine. A tube for decompression should be placed in the right colon with the aid of a guide wire under fluoroscopic guidance to prevent recurrence.

Zar FA, Bakkanagari SR, Moorthi KM, Davis MB. A comparison of vancomycin and metronidazole for the treatment of *Clostridium difficile*-associated diarrhea, stratified by disease severity. Clin Infect Dis 2007;45:302-7.
The study suggests that metronidazole and vancomycin are equally effective for the treatment of mild C. difficile–associated diarrhea, but vancomycin is superior for severe cases.

REFERENCES

Access the complete reference list online at http://www.expertconsult.com.

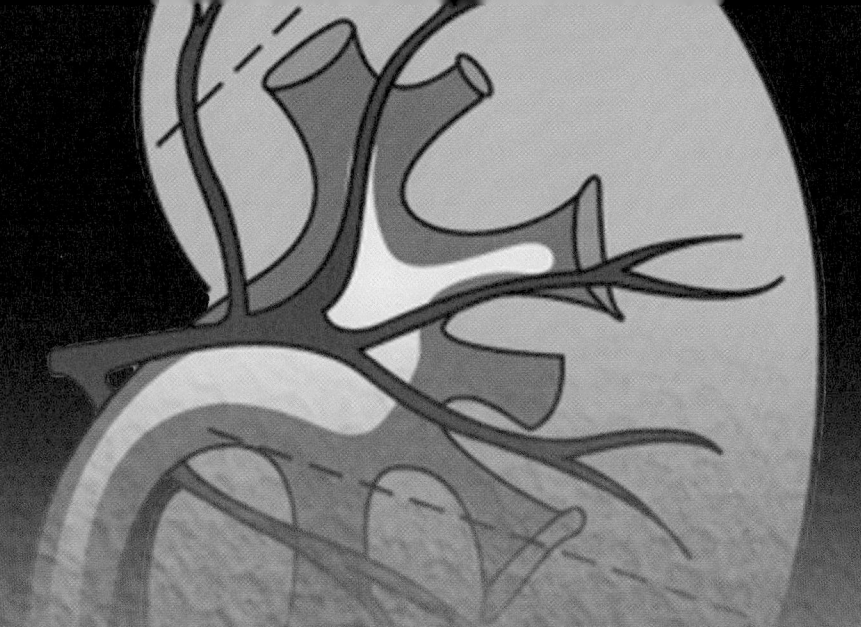

Renal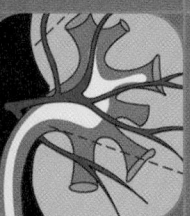

108

Clinical Assessment of Renal Function

TODD W.B. GEHR | ANTON C. SCHOOLWERTH

Five to 15 percent of patients in intensive care units (ICUs) experience acute deterioration in renal function.[1,2] Conversely, renal dysfunction adds substantially to the morbidity and mortality of these patients. Moreover, changes in renal function directly affect drug disposition. Thus, a means to assess renal function is essential for optimal management. The glomerular filtration rate (GFR) is the standard measure of renal function. It reflects overall renal functional capacity and, in renal failure, correlates with structural damage to the kidney. This chapter reviews selected aspects of renal physiology with an emphasis on measurement of renal function, consequences of altered function, and approaches to improving renal function. The focus is on measurement and optimization of glomerular filtration rate (GFR) and renal blood flow (RBF).

Renal Blood Flow

Under physiologic conditions, blood flow to the kidneys is 20% of cardiac output. This high rate of blood flow (1-1.2 L/min) is particularly remarkable in that the kidneys make up only 0.5% of total body weight. The high blood flow rate is due, at least in part, to the unique anatomic arrangement of the renal vasculature, with the interlobar and arcuate vessels offering little resistance to flow. This in turn is because the interlobular arteries originate from the arcuates in a parallel arrangement and because the afferent arterioles also arise in a parallel arrangement from the interlobular vessels. It is this parallel arrangement that accounts for the low resistance, because the total resistance of n equals parallel paths, each with a resistance R, is R/n^3. Major resistance vessels in the kidney are the afferent and efferent arterioles that bound the glomerular capillary network. Although total resistance is a function of resistance across each of these vessels, it is a unique feature of the kidney that variations in the individual resistances across the afferent and efferent arterioles, respectively, may lead to alterations in glomerular capillary pressure and, hence, in GFR.[3]

Despite a wide range of perfusion pressures, RBF and GFR are maintained relatively constant, a process described as *autoregulation*. The term *autoregulation* generally refers to the relative constancy of GFR over a range of perfusion pressures but also refers to the regulation of RBF. Emphasis has been placed on the preglomerular vasculature, mainly the afferent arterioles, as the major site at which renal perfusion is regulated. However, studies also suggest that the larger vessels, such as the interlobular vessels, may respond to a variety of vasoactive stimuli and participate in an autoregulatory phenomenon. A variety of hypotheses have been generated to explain the autoregulatory response of the kidney with respect to RBF. There is evidence to suggest mediation by neural, humoral, or intrarenal factors that regulate the renal circulation.[4]

The renin-angiotensin pathway has a significant effect on renal hemodynamics. Renin, elaborated in the juxtaglomerular cells, may be released in response to a decrease in renal perfusion pressure and to altered sodium chloride delivery to the ascending limb and macula densa cells. Increased renin secretion in turn leads to augmented angiotensin II (AII) formation at the local nephron level. AII, in turn, affects renal vascular resistance by an effect on both the afferent and efferent arterioles, with the effect predominating on the latter vessels.

Renal eicosanoids also affect renal hemodynamics. Eicosanoids are biologically active fatty acid products of arachidonic acid and are synthesized in the kidney in response to a variety of stimuli, with local release and effect on the renal vasculature. Stimulation of the cyclooxygenase pathway and prostaglandin synthetases leads to the formation of endoperoxides (PGG_2, PGH_2), prostaglandins (PGD_2, PGE_2, $PGF_{2\alpha}$, PGI_2), and thromboxane A_2, (TXA_2). Leukotrienes are synthesized by another major pathway involving the enzyme, lipoxygenase. In the kidney, the major products of arachidonic acid metabolism are PGE_2 and PGI_2 and, to a lesser extent, $PGI_{2\alpha}$. These compounds have a predominant effect of relaxing renal vascular smooth muscle and lead to vasodilatation, whereas TXA_2 is a vasoconstrictor prostanoid. It is believed that in disease states, endogenous vasodilator prostaglandins serve a protective function to maintain renal perfusion and GFR in response to vasoconstrictor stimuli, including AII and enhanced sympathetic nervous system activity. In contrast, release is inhibited by nonsteroidal antiinflammatory drugs.

Other vasoactive compounds that affect the renal circulation include the plasma and glandular kallikreins and kinins and endothelium-derived vasoactive factors such as nitric oxide and endothelin.[4] Among the catecholamines, α- and β-adrenergic agonists are known to affect renal vascular tone by causing vasoconstriction and vasodilatation, respectively. In addition, dopamine in low doses leads to renal vasodilatation. Emphasis has more recently been placed on atrial natriuretic peptide and purinergic agents such as adenosine. The effect is likely to be influenced by changes in salt intake and extracellular fluid volume as well as by hydration status. For example, the influence of AII on renal hemodynamics is greater in sodium depletion, which also activates the sympathetic nervous system. In response to mild nonhypotensive hemorrhage, renal hemodynamics are relatively well maintained. However, with further reductions in volume associated with a more severe hemorrhage, renal ischemia mediated by activation of the renin-angiotensin system, renal efferent adrenergic nerves, and circulating catecholamines may occur.[4]

Finally, modification of dietary protein and amino acid intake may affect renal hemodynamics. Dietary protein intake in excess of 1 g/kg/d has been associated with renal vasodilatation, as have infusions of casein hydrolysates and amino acids.[5,6] Conversely, chronic consumption of a low-protein diet may be associated with renal vasoconstriction.

MEASUREMENT OF RENAL BLOOD FLOW

Renal blood flow is measured conventionally by the clearance of infused para-aminohippurate (PAH), which is cleared almost totally from the arterial plasma by both filtration and secretion. Thus, its clearance approximates the rate of renal plasma flow (RPF):

$$RPF = U_{PAH} \cdot V/P_{PAH}$$

where U_{PAH} and P_{PAH} refer to urine and plasma PAH concentration, respectively, and V is urine flow rate in milliliters per minute.

RBF can be estimated by correction for the hematocrit (Hct):

$$RBF = RPF/[1 - Hct]$$

Although available, this test is rarely used in clinical practice. In fact, direct quantitation of RPF and RBF is rarely indicated outside research studies; however, sometimes it is necessary to document that the kidneys are being perfused. In this case, one of three additional methods may be utilized: (1) selective arteriography, including CT angiography and MR angiography, (2) Doppler ultrasonography, and (3) external radionuclide scanning.

Because the latter two methods are noninvasive, they are preferred. With respect to the nuclide study, until recently, scanning was usually performed utilizing ^{125}I-iodohippurate sodium; however, the poor radiologic characteristics of ^{131}I limit its use in renal imaging.[7] More recently, other agents such as ^{127}I-orthoiodohippurate and ^{99m}Tc-L, L-ethylenedicysteine may prove to be superior.[7,8]

CLINICAL CORRELATES

Although a significant body of data has been obtained to indicate a complex relationship between neurocirculatory factors and renal hemodynamics, several points can be made from a clinical perspective. Optimization of cardiac output and extracellular fluid (ECF) volume, including the intravascular space, is essential for the maintenance of renal perfusion. Particularly because the effects of vasoactive compounds such as AII and catecholamines are accentuated in the presence of renal hypoperfusion and volume contraction, attention should be directed to an assessment of ECF volume, with correction of any deficits, and to optimizing cardiac function. Frequently, pharmacologic agents have been employed to maintain renal perfusion in situations in which this may be compromised. Specifically, there has been widespread use of so-called low-dose or renal-dose dopamine infusions. This is based on the observation that in low doses (<3 µg/kg/min) dopamine leads to renal vasodilatation.[9] At higher doses, renal vasoconstriction may occur.

The beneficial effects of dopamine infusion have not been documented in patients who are depleted of sodium chloride and volume, and the use of dopamine has not been shown to be effective beyond a short period of infusion.[9-11] That is, infusions of renal-dose dopamine for 24 to 36 hours may be beneficial in the appropriate circumstance, but there is no evidence supporting the long-term use of this agent. Thus, justification for prolongation of its use beyond several days is not supported by available data. Furthermore, reports suggest that adverse outcomes may be associated with the use of dopamine.[11] Continuous infusions of fenoldopam mesylate, a potent dopamine A-1 receptor agonist, have been employed in an attempt to preserve renal function in a variety of clinical settings. A meta-analysis of 16 randomized trials in critically ill patients showed that fenoldopam significantly reduced the risk of acute kidney injury, need for renal replacement therapy, and in-hospital death.[12] Beyond anecdotal evidence, there are no compelling data to support the use of other potential vasodilator substances such as prostaglandins. Although high-protein feeding and amino acid infusions may increase RBF by an undefined mechanism, there is no justification for utilizing these therapies solely from a hemodynamic point of view.[5,6]

Glomerular Filtration Rate

Of the 500 to 700 mL of plasma delivered per minute to the kidneys (corresponding to a renal blood flow of 1-1.2 L/min), 20% to 25% is filtered. Glomerular filtration is a major function of the kidney and averages approximately 130 mL/min/1.73 m^2 in normal males and 120 mL/min/1.73 m^2 in females. Estimation or direct assessment of GFR remains one of the most important measurements of renal function and is widely utilized in clinical practice.

MEASUREMENT OF GLOMERULAR FILTRATION RATE

GFR is classically measured as the clearance of inulin (C_{In}), a fructose polymer with a mean molecular weight of approximately 5 kD. Because this substance is not present endogenously, it must be given by constant infusion after a loading dose. Inulin is available commercially but is expensive, often difficult to obtain, and cumbersome to utilize. As a result, C_{In} is rarely used in clinical practice except for research protocols. Although inulin is generally measured chemically, ^{3}H-labeled and ^{14}C-labeled inulin are also available but are expensive.

More recently, other radiolabeled nuclides have been found to be satisfactory substitutes for inulin and have advantages in the measurement of GFR.[7,8,13,14] Particularly ^{99m}Tc-labeled diethylenetriamine pentaacetic acid (DTPA) and ^{125}I- or ^{131}I-labeled iothalamate clearances closely approximate the C_{In}.[15,16] ^{99m}Tc-DTPA has been utilized and found to give measurements that correlate closely with C_{In} in ICU patients.[17,18] In addition, the clearance of gentamicin has been utilized in a limited fashion to measure GFR.[19,20] At the present time it is not common for GFR to be measured directly. Rather, GFR is estimated by the endogenous creatinine clearance or serum creatinine determination (see later).

The normal values for GFR given previously apply for individuals from the teenage years through approximately age 35. Thereafter, GFR declines in most individuals. Whereas this decline was formerly thought to occur at a relatively constant rate of approximately 10 mL/min per decade,[21-23] more recent data obtained in a longitudinal fashion indicate that this reduction is not so predictable.[24] In addition, a circadian rhythm for GFR has been described.[25,26] GFR is maximal in the daytime, whereas a minimal value during the night has been found in normal individuals. Whether this circadian pattern of GFR occurs in critically ill hospitalized patients is not known.

Creatinine Clearance and Serum Creatinine

CREATININE CLEARANCE

The endogenous creatinine clearance (C_{Cr}) enjoys widespread use as a reasonable gauge of GFR when great precision is not demanded, which it rarely is in clinical practice. The use of creatinine as a marker of GFR has the advantage that creatinine is endogenously produced and is easily measured by inexpensive methods. Creatinine, like inulin, is freely filtered and absorbed minimally if at all by the tubules. However, creatinine is secreted, and the contribution of secretion to total excretion is greater as the GFR decreases and serum creatinine rises. At GFRs below 40 mL/min, C_{Cr} exceeds C_{In} by 50% to 100%.[15,27] When GFR is significantly depressed and it is deemed important to get a more precise measurement of GFR, one of the previously mentioned methods to estimate GFR directly might be utilized. Additionally, because C_{Cr} overestimates GFR and the clearance of urea underestimates GFR, the mean value of simultaneously obtained creatinine and urea clearances has been shown to provide a close estimation of C_{In} when the latter is below 20 mL/min.[28]

Because cimetidine competes with creatinine for tubular secretion (see later), administration of cimetidine may increase the accuracy both of creatinine clearance in 24-hour collections (when given for several days beforehand) and of 4-hour, water-loaded clearances.[29-31] Taking advantage of this effect results in a more accurate estimate of GFR. Specifically, C_{Cr} obtained in the presence of cimetidine (400 mg as a priming dose followed by 200 mg every 3 hours) yielded values that closely approximated C_{In}.[29,30] Volume expansion in humans causes a small rise in GFR, whereas volume depletion, severe heart failure, hypotension, anesthesia, surgery, trauma, sepsis, and even mild intestinal bleeding without frank hypotension may depress GFR substantially.

Various methods are available to measure creatinine. Creatinine is frequently measured using the Jaffé alkaline picric acid reaction. Although this method is widely utilized, this reaction also measures other chromogens, which may lead to a false elevation in the estimated serum creatinine (S_{Cr}) measurement. Substances such as acetoacetate (in ketoacidosis), pyruvate, ascorbate, 5-flucytosine, certain (but not all) cephalosporin antibiotics, and very high urate artifactually raise S_{Cr} in normal subjects by 0.5 to 2 mg/dL.[32-38] These substances are excreted into the urine but contribute trivially compared with overall urine creatinine (U_{Cr}). Thus, noncreatinine chromogens affect the S_{Cr} but have little effect on the U_{Cr}.

In individuals with normal renal function, the contribution of serum noncreatinine chromogens to raising the S_{Cr} is approximately equal to the contribution of secretion to creatinine excretion, such that the C_{Cr} closely approximates GFR. As GFR decreases, the contribution of noncreatinine chromogens to the total measured S_{Cr} becomes less than the secreted moiety, and the C_{Cr} overestimates GFR to a greater extent. Direct enzymatic creatinine measurements are not affected by noncreatinine chromogens. Very high levels of serum glucose (>1000 mg/dL) and 5-flucytosine may interfere with the enzymatic reaction, whereas high levels of bilirubin (>5 mg/dL) affect the autoanalyzer method[36] and lead to falsely low S_{Cr} values. It is therefore important to know the method by which a given laboratory measures S_{Cr}. Competing for the same proximal tubular organic base secretory site as creatinine, certain pharmacologic agents may suppress this process and lead to a rise in S_{Cr}. Trimethoprim, probenecid, and cimetidine, but not ranitidine, are organic bases that inhibit creatinine secretion competitively and can result in a mild elevation in S_{Cr}, usually 0.5 mg/dL or less.[39-42]

As with all clearance methods, the C_{Cr} is subject to errors that may amount to as much as 10% to 15% or more. In addition to potential problems in estimating S_{Cr} and U_{Cr}, errors in timing of urine collection, incomplete collection, and inaccurate measurement of urine volume are other factors that contribute to errors.[43] Although 24-hour U_{Cr} clearances have been widely utilized, no specified time period is required for the clearance to be obtained. In fact, shorter collection periods of several hours may be more accurate in patients passing adequate amounts of urine (not oliguric), particularly if the patient is not in a steady state (see later). To reduce errors in volume measurement, one can induce a water diuresis in stable subjects before beginning the test,[44] although this is rarely practical in the ICU setting. Nevertheless, because many ICU patients have indwelling Foley catheters, it should be possible for accurately timed urine collections to be obtained and for C_{Cr} to be measured with reasonable accuracy.

SERUM CREATININE

Because of the practical and technical problems in obtaining estimates of GFR by clearance methods, renal function is most commonly estimated by following the S_{Cr} in hospitalized patients. Creatinine is formed nonenzymatically from creatine and phosphocreatine in muscle cells and is normally present in the serum at a concentration of 0.8 to 1.4 mg/dL in adults and 0.3 to 0.6 mg/dL in children and pregnant subjects. The measured S_{Cr} depends on the method of measurement, as discussed previously, GFR, rate of creatinine production, volume of distribution (e.g., S_{Cr} is lower in anasarca), and extent of its tubular secretion and intestinal degradation.[3] Because creatinine production is closely related to muscle mass, S_{Cr} is generally less in females than in males and decreases as muscle mass is lost with aging or with debilitating illnesses.

The relationship between S_{Cr} and C_{Cr} (and hence GFR) can be described by a rectangular hyperbola[43]; however, this relationship applies in the steady state and assumes a constant rate of creatinine production (Figure 108-1). Thus, a doubling of the S_{Cr}, reflects a 50% decrease in C_{Cr}, a fourfold increase in S_{Cr}, a 75% drop in GFR, and so on. Because creatinine production may not remain constant, S_{Cr} may underestimate the decrease in GFR in critically ill patients who have a decrease in muscle mass secondary to an ongoing catabolic state. Moreover, it should be appreciated that S_{Cr} is an insensitive marker of change early in the course of renal disease. Thus, a 33% fall in GFR may raise the S_{Cr} from 0.8 to 1.2 mg/dL, a value still within the normal range. If the prior value is not known, this fall in GFR may go unrecognized.

S_{Cr} provides a close estimate of GFR only in the steady state. With an abrupt decrease in GFR, as may occur in acute renal failure, creatinine production would be expected to continue unchanged, but because of the decrease in GFR, creatinine excretion will be impaired. As a result, the S_{Cr} increases until a new steady state is obtained, at which time the amount of creatinine produced equals the amount filtered (GFR – S_{Cr}) and excreted (U_{Cr} – V). Depending on the extent of damage and decrease in GFR, it may take several days for a new

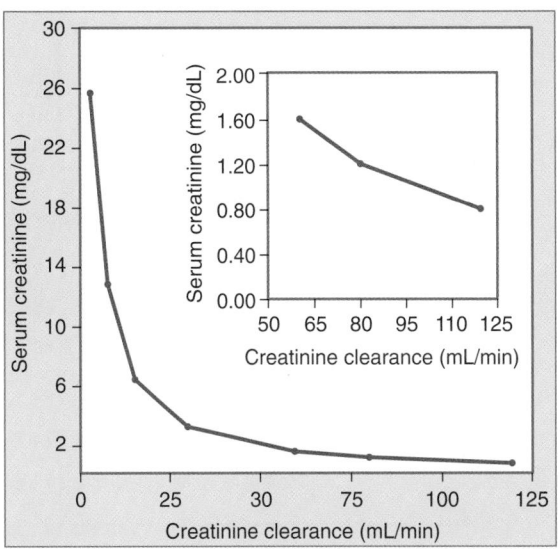

Figure 108-1 Relationship between creatinine clearance and serum creatinine. In steady state, serum creatinine should increase twofold for each 50% reduction in creatinine clearance. Inset represents enlarged view of changes in serum creatinine as creatinine clearance decreases from 120 to 60 mL/min. If serum creatinine is 0.8 mg/dL when creatinine clearance is 120 mL/min, creatinine clearance can decrease by 33% such that increased serum creatinine is still within normal range.

steady state to be achieved (Figure 108-2). Therefore, following an insult leading to an abrupt decrease in GFR, the S_{Cr} rises progressively over the next several days. This should not be interpreted as a new insult each day, but rather that a steady state has not yet been obtained. While the S_{Cr} is changing, its absolute value cannot be used as an accurate measure of the decrease in GFR. If an accurate measurement of GFR is needed during this time, a short C_{Cr} can be obtained.

A variety of equations have been developed to estimate C_{Cr} based on the S_{Cr} without collection of urine.[45,46] Table 108-1 is a compilation of the more commonly used equations.[47] These equations generally take into consideration muscle mass (estimated as body weight), sex (males having a higher GFR than females), and age. Aging, hepatic diseases, excessive muscle wasting, severe muscular atrophy or dystrophy, hyperthyroidism, paralysis, and chronic glucocorticoid therapy have been associated with reduced creatinine generation.[17] In addition, particularly at low levels of GFR, correction for nonrenal creatinine metabolism is also recommended.[48,49] One of the most commonly utilized equations is that developed by Cockcroft and Gault[50]:

$$C_{Cr} = \frac{(140 - age) \cdot lean\ wt\ in\ kg}{72 \cdot S_{Cr}}$$

where age is expressed in years. The preceding expression is used for men. The formula for women is the preceding formula multiplied by 0.85.

The reliability of this equation as a measure of GFR has been assessed in patients with diabetes, pregnant women with renal disease,[51] obese individuals,[52] elderly individuals,[53,54] and black Americans with hypertensive renal disease.[55] It has also been assessed in critically ill patients.[56] These studies have indicated that the accuracy of GFR estimates using the Cockcroft-Gault equation is similar to or greater than 24-hour C_{Cr}, and the precision is better. This equation seems to be most accurate for estimating GFR when the latter is in the range of 10 to 100 mL/min.[52,55,56] The advantage of this formula is that it is simple and underscores the essential determinants of C_{Cr}.

The MDRD (Modification of Diet in Renal Disease) study equation has gained widespread acceptance by most clinical laboratories, which

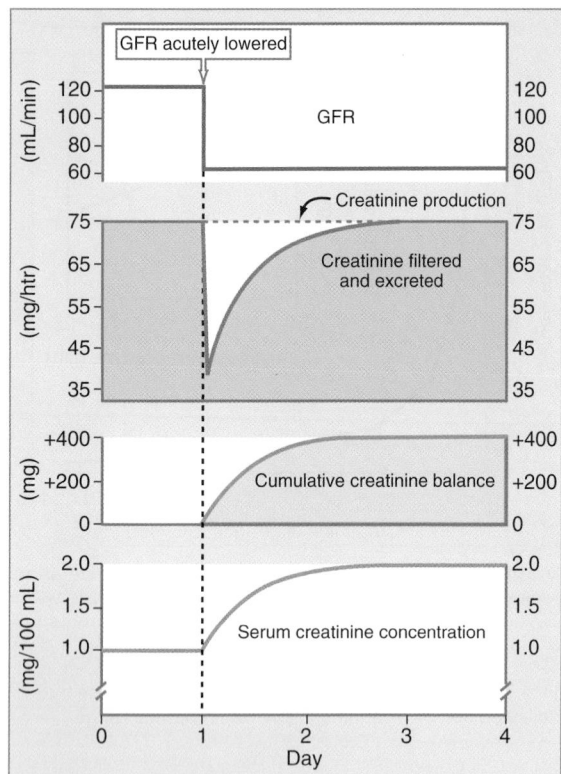

Figure 108-2 Expected changes in serum creatinine resulting from acute fall in glomerular filtration rate (GFR) and attainment of a new steady state. Between days 0 and 1, patient is excreting all creatinine produced, and serum creatinine is stable at 1 mg/dL. A 50% reduction in GFR on day 1 results in abrupt fall in filtered (and, therefore, excreted) creatinine. Release of creatinine from muscle remains constant; as a result, creatinine is retained and its serum concentration is increased. As creatinine concentration rises progressively, filtered (and excreted) creatinine also increases until excreted creatinine returns to control levels and matches creatinine production. New steady state (days 3 to 4) is achieved by doubling of serum creatinine concentrations, which maintains filtered creatinine load at control levels in the face of halving of GFR. Larger decrease in GFR would lead to greater increase in steady state (e.g., 90% reduction in GFR would lead to 10-fold rise in serum creatinine) and would take longer to achieve. *(From Kassirer JP. Clinical evaluation of kidney function-glomerular function. N Engl J Med 1971;285:385. Reprinted with permission from The New England Journal of Medicine.)*

	Common Equations for Estimating Glomerular Filtration Rate or Creatinine Clearance

TABLE 108-1

Cockcroft-Gault ($C_{Cr} \cdot BSA/1.73$ m^2)
For men: $C_{Cr} = [(140 - \text{age}) \cdot \text{weight (kg)}]/S_{Cr} \cdot 72$
For women: $C_{Cr} = ([(140 - \text{age}) \cdot \text{weight (kg)}]/S_{Cr} \cdot 72) \cdot 0.85$

MDRD (1)
GFR $= 170 \cdot [S_{Cr}]^{-0.999} \cdot [\text{age}]^{-0.176} \cdot [0.762$ if patient is female$] \cdot [1.18$ if patient is black$] \cdot [\text{BUN}]^{-0.170} \cdot [\text{Alb}]^{0.318}$

MDRD (2)
GFR $= 186 \cdot [S_{Cr}]^{-1.154} \cdot [\text{age}]^{-0.203} \cdot [0.742$ if patient is female$] \cdot [1.212$ if patient is black$]$

Jellife (1) ($C_{Cr} \cdot BSA/1.73$ m^2)
For men: $(98 - [0.8 \cdot (\text{age} - 20)])/S_{Cr}$
For women: $(98 - [0.8 \cdot (\text{age} - 20)])S_{Cr} \cdot 0.90$

Jellife (2)
For men: $(100/S_{Cr}) - 12$
For women: $(80/S_{Cr}) - 7$

Mawer
For men: weight $\cdot [29.3 - (0.203 \cdot \text{age})] \cdot [1 - (0.03 \cdot S_{Cr})]$
For women: weight $\cdot [25.3 - (0.175 \cdot \text{age})] \cdot [1 - (0.03 \cdot S_{Cr})]$

Bjornsson
For men: $[27 - (0.173 \cdot \text{age})] \cdot$ weight $\cdot 0/S_{Cr}$
For women: $[25 - (0.175 \cdot \text{age})] \cdot$ weight $\cdot 0.07/S_{Cr}$

Gates
For men: $(89.4 \cdot S_{Cr}^{-1.2}) + (55 - \text{age}) \cdot (0.447 \cdot S_{Cr}^{-1.1})$
For women: $(89.4 \cdot S_{Cr}^{-1.2}) + (55 - \text{age}) \cdot (0.447 \cdot S_{Cr}^{-1.1})$

Salazar-Corcoran
For men: $[137 - \text{age}] \cdot [(0.285 \cdot \text{weight}) + (12.1 \cdot \text{height}^2)]/(51 \cdot S_{Cr})$
For women: $[146 - \text{age}] \cdot [(0.287 \cdot \text{weight}) + (9.74 \cdot \text{height}^2)]/(60 \cdot S_{Cr})$

SERUM UREA NITROGEN

Less accurate as a marker of GFR than the S_{Cr}, serum urea nitrogen (SUN) (or blood urea nitrogen [BUN]) is still used extensively in clinical practice to estimate renal function. Although this was the earliest available indicator of renal function, several other factors should be appreciated regarding the use of this substance. Urea, like creatinine, is freely filtered and is retained in the blood as GFR falls. However, in contrast to creatinine, urea may be reabsorbed to a significant extent, its excretion tending to be increased with increasing urine flow rates, whereas its excretion is reduced when tubular fluid reabsorption is enhanced. Of greater importance, urea production is more variable than creatinine. Produced in the liver, urea increases with high protein intake, amino acid infusions, and hypercatabolic states. In addition, endogenous sources of protein such as absorbed hemoglobin from gastrointestinal bleeding may contribute to increased urea synthesis. Even at a constant GFR, SUN may rise in subjects on high protein intake and fall with protein restriction or on refeeding of previously starved, nonhypercatabolic subjects.

Several pharmacologic agents also may affect urea nitrogen formation. Tetracyclines may lead to an increase in SUN by an anti-anabolic effect without any detectable change in GFR, whereas glucocorticoids and severe illnesses or trauma do the same by inducing endogenous protein hypercatabolism. Because of the widespread use of hyperalimentation in ICU patients, an impairment in renal function is often associated with a marked disproportion in the elevation of SUN compared with S_{Cr}. For this reason, the issue is raised as to whether SUN elevation itself poses an important threat to the patient if the GFR is in a range that should not lead to enhanced morbidity by itself. In those circumstances, it is useful to measure the rate of urea appearance (or generation) to estimate whether other factors such as gastrointestinal bleeding, excessive amino acid infusions, and protein administration are contributing to the increase in SUN above that expected by the decrease in GFR.[47,48] Urea nitrogen (UN) appearance can be determined from urine urea nitrogen (UUN), SUN, and body weight as follows:

$$UN = UUN \cdot V + \Delta \text{ body pool UN}$$

where UUN $\cdot$ V is 24-hour UN excretion, and Δ body pool UN = 0.6 − nonedematous weight (kg) $\cdot \Delta$ SUN/day.

now routinely report estimated GFR values for blacks and nonblacks when a serum creatinine is ordered.[57-59] Its major limitations are imprecision and underestimation of measured GFR at high GFR values (GFR > 60 mL/min/1.73 m^2). The MDRD equation is generally more precise than the Cockroft-Gault equation.[60]

Limitations at higher GFR values prompted a recent modification by the Chronic Kidney Disease Epidemiology Collaboration Research Group.[61] This equation offers improved precision, especially with higher GFR values up to 90 mL/min/1.73 m^2.

CKD-EPI equation for estimated GFR (natural scale):

Blacks:
Female ($S_{Cr} \leq 0.7$) GFR $= 166 \cdot (S_{Cr}/0.7)^{-0.329} \cdot (0993)^{\text{Age}}$
Female ($S_{Cr} > 0.7$) GFR $= 166 \cdot (S_{Cr}/0.7)^{-1.209} \cdot (0993)^{\text{Age}}$
Male ($S_{Cr} \leq 0.9$) GFR $= 163 \cdot (S_{Cr}/0.9)^{-0.411} \cdot (0993)^{\text{Age}}$
Male ($S_{Cr} > 0.9$) GFR $= 163 \cdot (S_{Cr}/0.9)^{-1.209} \cdot (0993)^{\text{Age}}$

White or other:
Female ($S_{Cr} \leq 0.7$) GFR $= 144 \cdot (S_{Cr}/0.7)^{-0.329} \cdot (0993)^{\text{Age}}$
Female ($S_{Cr} > 0.7$) GFR $= 144 \cdot (S_{Cr}/0.7)^{-1.209} \cdot (0993)^{\text{Age}}$
Male ($S_{Cr} \leq 0.9$) GFR $= 141 \cdot (S_{Cr}/0.9)^{-0.411} \cdot (0993)^{\text{Age}}$
Male ($S_{Cr} > 0.9$) GFR $= 141 \cdot (S_{Cr}/0.9)^{-1.209} \cdot (0993)^{\text{Age}}$

If the weight is changing[47,48]:

$$\Delta \text{ body pool UN} = (0.6 \cdot \text{nonedematous weight} \cdot \Delta \text{ SUN}) + (\Delta \text{ weight} \cdot \text{final SUN})$$

Nitrogen balance (BN) is equal to:

$$BN = IN - UN - NUN$$

where IN is urea nitrogen intake, and NUN is nonurea nitrogen excretions.[48]

NUN, which includes fecal nitrogen, urinary creatinine, uric acid, and unmeasured nitrogen, averages 0.031 g nitrogen/kg/d.[48] The data obtained from the just-described measurements may be quite useful in evaluating the cause of disproportionate elevations in SUN. If the patient is in a steady state (with a stable weight and SUN), BN = 0, and IN can be estimated from UN + NUN.[48] Because catabolism, except for *severe* trauma and burns, is usually 2 to 4 g nitrogen per day, additional conclusions can be drawn if the patient is not in the steady state. For example, if it is known that IN is less than UN + NUN, gastrointestinal bleeding with or without excess catabolism would be suggested. Similarly, one can evaluate if the increase in SUN is a reflection of excessive exogenous protein and amino acid administration (usually >1.5 g/kg/d; g UN 0.16 = g protein or amino acids). If IN is above UN, such as in severe liver disease, the clinician might more carefully evaluate changes in weight and SUN as well as clearances, because the latter may be more severely depressed than initially suspected.

Sodium Balance and Extracellular Fluid Volume

Sodium is the primary cation of the ECF, present in a concentration of 140 to 142 mmol/L. The volume of the ECF is approximately 20% of total body weight and represents a third of total body water. Regulation of ECF volume is governed by factors regulating sodium balance and sodium excretion. The reader is referred to an excellent review on this topic.[62] For the purposes of this discussion, several factors are emphasized. Under physiologic conditions and in the steady state, sodium balance is maintained because the amount of sodium excreted equals that which enters the body by oral and intravenous routes. Sodium excretion and the fraction of filtered sodium that is excreted (FE_{Na}) can be readily determined. Absolute sodium excretion is measured as the product of the urine sodium concentration and the urine volume:

$$Na^+ \text{ excretion} = (U_{Na} \cdot V)$$

FE_{Na} can be determined as follows:

$$FE_{Na} = U_{Na} \cdot V/GFR \cdot S_{Na}$$

For practical reasons, the C_{Cr} ($= U_{Cr} \cdot V/S_{Cr}$) is used to estimate GFR, such that:

$$FE_{Na} = U_{Na} \cdot V/UC_r \cdot V/SCr \cdot S_{Na}$$

Because the V term in the numerator and denominator cancels out:

$$FE_{Na} = U_{Na}/S_{Na} \cdot S_{Cr}/U_{Cr}$$

Thus, FE_{Na} can be calculated from the sodium and creatinine determined in a random urine sample and serum (or plasma) simultaneously. The resulting calculation is expressed as a percentage by multiplying by 100. This test is of value in the setting of acute renal failure to aid in distinguishing a prerenal from a renal parenchymal etiology.[63] It is not usually helpful in aiding in the diagnosis of urinary tract obstruction or in the presence of underlying chronic renal insufficiency. The reason for the difficulty in interpretation in chronic renal insufficiency can be illustrated by the following considerations. At a GFR of 130 mL/min and a dietary sodium intake of 3 g of sodium (130 mmol), an individual in sodium balance will excrete 0.5% of the filtered load (FE_{Na} = 0.5%). For sodium balance to be maintained at lower levels of GFR with the same sodium intake, FE_{Na} must be

increased progressively. Successive decreases in GFR by 2 from 130 would result in an FE_{Na} of 1%, 2%, 4%, and 8%, respectively. Thus, interpretation of the FE_{Na} in a patient with acute renal failure superimposed on chronic renal insufficiency is problematic unless the prior steady-state FE_{Na} is known. This is rarely the case.

The fractional excretion of chloride (FE_{Cl}) has been suggested to be more accurate than that of sodium in helping to distinguish prerenal from parenchymal causes of acute renal failure.[64] This is particularly so in the situation in which acute renal failure occurs with simultaneous metabolic alkalosis. If the urine contains substantial amounts of bicarbonate urinary pH ($U_{pH} > 7$), sodium excretion increases to maintain electroneutrality. Under these circumstances, the FE_{Na} may give misleading information, but the FE_{Cl} can be used to obtain the same information.

Although urinary sodium excretion can be used to help make determinations with respect to ECF volume under certain circumstances, this may be fraught with potential errors. No laboratory test is available to provide this information. Rather, the astute clinician must rely on bedside evaluation complemented, where appropriate, with measurements of central venous pressure and pulmonary capillary wedge pressure to assist in making determinations with respect to ECF volume status. For example, a low FE_{Na} (<1%) in the setting of acute renal failure usually indicates a decrease in renal perfusion but does not provide information on the status of the patient's ECF volume. Because a low FE_{Na} can be seen with either ECF volume contraction or severe congestive heart failure, these conditions must be distinguished at the bedside. Moreover, sometimes a low FE_{Na} exists even in the presence of parenchymal renal disease, such as acute glomerulonephritis, severe burns, and radiocontrast nephropathy. Finally, administration of potent diuretic agents can alter the FE_{Na} and may result in misleading interpretations. For this reason, urine samples should be obtained before diuretics are administered. However, it may not be possible to obtain urinary sodium or chloride values while a patient is not receiving diuretics. In this setting the fractional excretion of urea nitrogen has been employed to distinguish prerenal from renal causes of acute kidney injury. In a well-hydrated individual, the Fe_{UN} is 50% to 65%,[65] whereas in oliguric prerenal azotemia, the Fe_{UN} is below 35%. The use of Fe_{UN} in the setting of acute kidney injury has not attained widespread acceptance owing to variable results on comparative trials.[65,66]

A few additional points are worthy of note with respect to diuretic use. There is now ample evidence that in a patient in positive sodium balance, diuretic therapy should not be utilized without simultaneously restricting sodium intake, including intravenous saline, if negative sodium balance and reduction in edema fluid are desired.[67] In general, this requires restriction of dietary sodium intake, usually to less than 2 g of sodium per day (0.88 mmol) if the patient is in an edema-forming state. Although a diuresis can be effected even with liberal sodium intake, this requires higher doses of diuretics and more frequent administration of these agents. The coexistence of hyponatremia should not deter clinicians from restricting sodium intake, but rather should cause them to address solute-free water intake as well. Of course, under certain circumstances, obligatory intakes make it difficult to achieve optimal restriction to assist diuresis. That is, with various pharmacologic drips, blood products, and feeding regimens necessary in acutely ill patients in the ICU, this may become a difficult problem. Under those circumstances, increasing doses of diuretics, including continuous infusions of loop diuretics, may be required.

KEY POINTS

1. Acute deterioration of renal function is common in the ICU and contributes significantly to overall morbidity and mortality.

2. The serum creatinine concentration often underestimates the decrease in GFR and may be abnormal only after marked reductions in GFR.

3. Utilizing equations to estimate renal function should be routine in the ICU.

ANNOTATED REFERENCES

Chertow GM, Sayegh MH, Allgren RL, Lazarus JM. Is the administration of dopamine associated with adverse or favorable outcome in acute renal failure? Am J Med 1996;101:49-53.

One of the first large, randomized trials exploring the use of low-dose dopamine (<3 μg/kg/min) and high-dose dopamine in ICU patients. The study revealed that there was no evidence that low-dose dopamine improved survival or obviated the need for dialysis, and its use should be discouraged.

Levey AS, Stevens LA, Schmid CH, Zhang Y, Castro III AF, Feldman HI, et al. A new equation to estimate glomerular filtration rate. Ann Intern Med 2009;150;604-12.

Comprehensive review of the use of equations used to predict GFR and the presentation of a newly derived equation using large clinical data sets. The CKD-EPI equation is probably the best equation to estimate GFR in the steady state.

Robert S, Zarowitz BJ, Peterson EL, Dumler F. Predictability of creatinine clearance estimates in critically ill patients. Crit Care Med 1993;21:1487-95.

Creatinine clearance, inulin clearance, and estimates of GFR based on the Cockcroft-Gault equation were compared in 20 ICU patients. This study emphasized the inaccuracies of obtaining creatinine clearances in

the ICU setting. The Cockcroft-Gault equation accurately predicted GFR as determined by inulin clearances.

Wilcox CS, Mitch WE, Kelly RA, Skorecki K, Meyer TW, Friedman PA, et al. Response of the kidney to furosemide: I. Effects of salt intake and renal compensation. J Lab Clin Med 1983;102:450-8.

Classic study on the pharmacodynamics of furosemide showing the importance of salt intake and homeostatic mechanisms activated by diuretic use.

Wharton 3rd WW, Sondeen JL, McBiles M, Gradwohl SE, Wade CE, Ciceri DP, et al. Measurement of glomerular filtration rate in ICU patients using ^{99m}Tc-DTPA and inulin. Kidney Int 1992;42:174-8.

This study in 18 ICU patients compared clearances of inulin, creatinine, and ^{99m}Tc-DTPA to estimated Cockcroft-Gault clearance. The clearance of DTPA correlated best to inulin clearance throughout the entire range of clearances studied. DTPA clearance was also simple and inexpensive to perform in the ICU setting.

REFERENCES

Access the complete reference list online at http://www.expertconsult.com.

109

Metabolic Acidosis and Alkalosis

THOMAS D. DUBOSE, JR. | PIROUZ DAEIHAGH

Acid-Base Disorders

The appropriate diagnosis and management of acid-base disorders in acutely ill patients necessitates accurate and timely interpretation of the specific acid-base disorder. Precise interpretation involves simultaneous measurement of plasma electrolytes and arterial blood gases as well as an appreciation by the clinician of the physiologic adaptations and compensatory responses that occur with specific acid-base disturbances. In most circumstances, these compensatory responses can be predicted through an analysis of the prevailing disorder. The severity of illness encountered in the intensive care unit (ICU), along with variety of therapeutic interventions in that setting, specifies that complicated acid-base disturbances are observed commonly and more regularly than on the typical internal medicine service. Hypotension, sepsis with multiorgan failure such as liver or kidneys, drug overdose, and diabetes all result in disturbances of acid-base homeostasis. In addition, therapeutic interventions in the ICU may extend and complicate acid-base equilibrium. Because disturbances of pH affect a wide variety of physiologic functions and have clinically significant consequences, timely and accurate characterization of these disturbances becomes an essential component of critical care medicine. Identification of an acid-base disturbance should prompt a search for the cause of the disturbance itself. A thoughtful evaluation of all acid-base disturbances is of primary importance, and efforts to normalize pH should be cause specific and based on proven therapeutic efficacy.

LABORATORY ASSESSMENT OF ACID-BASE STATUS

Evaluation of acid-base status requires analysis of both the arterial blood gas and an electrolyte panel. These collections should be obtained simultaneously or within a brief span. Use of a low-friction syringe allows ease of arterial puncture and collection. Excess heparin should be avoided to limit hemodilution and air bubbles removed from the syringe promptly to prevent gas exchange between blood and the air trapped in the syringe. Analysis should follow shortly. Mixed venous blood gas measurement is complicated by disassociation in arterial and venous $Paco_2$, especially in the presence of poor tissue perfusion. On-line continuous monitoring of blood gas values may offer advantages in the future but is not yet generally available. The anion gap (AG) should be calculated from the electrolyte panel in *every* instance because it may reveal a high-AG metabolic acidosis, even in the setting of a mixed disorder where arterial pH, bicarbonate, or $Paco_2$ may be in the normal range.

NORMAL ACID-BASE HOMEOSTASIS

Systemic arterial pH is maintained between 7.35 and 7.45 by extracellular and intracellular chemical buffering together with respiratory and renal regulatory mechanisms. The control of $Paco_2$ by the central nervous system (CNS) and respiratory systems and the control of the plasma bicarbonate by the kidneys stabilize the arterial pH by excretion or retention of acid or alkali. The metabolic and respiratory components that regulate systemic pH are described by the Henderson-Hasselbalch equation:

$$pH = pK_a + \log_{10} \frac{HCO_3}{P_{CO_2} \times 0.0301}$$

Under most circumstances, CO_2 production and excretion are matched, and the usual steady-state $Paco_2$ is maintained at 40 mm Hg. Primary changes in $Paco_2$ can cause acidosis or alkalosis, depending on whether $Paco_2$ is above or below the normal value (respiratory acidosis or alkalosis, respectively). Underexcretion of CO_2 produces hypercapnia, and overexcretion causes hypocapnia, both of which will affect the systemic pH. The $Paco_2$ is regulated primarily by neural respiratory factors and is not subject to regulation by the rate of CO_2 production; therefore, hypercapnia is usually the result of hypoventilation rather than of increased CO_2 production. Increases or decreases in $Paco_2$ may represent primary derangements of the ventilatory function of the lungs (under neural respiratory control) or may be due to compensatory changes in response to a primary alteration in the plasma $[HCO_3^-]$.[1]

A decrease in systemic pH is termed *acidemia*, whereas an increase in pH is called *alkalemia*. Conversely, such changes in pH can occur with changes in $Paco_2$ or serum bicarbonate, which are referred to as *alkalosis* or *acidosis*. An example of a simple disorder would be a patient with acute pancreatitis with profound vomiting (loss of acid) who will have alkalemia (pH 7.49) due to metabolic alkalosis, with bicarbonate of 35 mEq/L and a respiratory acidosis ($Paco_2$ 47.5 mm Hg) as compensatory response (see later discussion).

Primary alteration of $Paco_2$ evokes two metabolic mechanisms to limit change in systemic pH: the fast-acting cellular buffering and the renal-adaptive response, a slower process that becomes more efficient with time. This metabolic response would be secondary (or compensatory) to the primary respiratory disorder. A primary change in the plasma $[HCO_3^-]$ as a result of metabolic or renal factors results in compensatory changes in ventilation that blunt the changes in blood pH that would occur otherwise. Such respiratory alterations are referred to as *secondary* or *compensatory* changes because they occur in response to primary metabolic alterations.[1]

The kidneys regulate plasma $[HCO_3^-]$ through three main processes: (1) "reabsorption" of filtered HCO_3^-, (2) generation of "new" HCO_3^-, which is accomplished by formation of titratable acid, and (3) excretion of NH_4^+ in the urine. The kidney filters approximately 4000 mEq of HCO_3^- per day, and between 80% and 90% of HCO_3^- is reabsorbed in the proximal tubule. The distal nephron reabsorbs the remaining HCO_3^- and more importantly, secretes protons generated from dietary protein intake to defend systemic pH. Metabolism of the average diet rich in protein produces fixed acids that consume bicarbonate on entry into the extracellular fluid. Although the quantity of protons from dietary protein metabolism is small (40-60 mEq/day), it must be secreted to prevent chronic positive H^+ balance and metabolic acidosis. This quantity of secreted protons (net acid) is represented in the urine as titratable acid and NH_4^+. Metabolic acidosis in the presence of normal renal function augments net acid excretion by markedly increasing NH_4^+ production and excretion. It is important to note that this vital compensatory mechanism is impaired in chronic renal failure, hyperkalemia, and renal tubular acidosis.[1,2]

In sum, these regulatory responses—chemical buffering, regulation of $Paco_2$ by the respiratory system, and regulation of $[HCO_3^-]$ by the kidneys—act in concert to maintain a systemic arterial pH between 7.35 and 7.45.

Diagnosis of Types of Disturbances

Historically, two different conceptual frameworks have evolved among clinicians and physiologists for interpreting acid-base phenomena. The traditional or bicarbonate-centered framework relies quantitatively on the Henderson-Hasselbalch equation (see later), whereas the Stewart or strong-ion approach utilizes the original Stewart equation to calculate the H^+ concentration. The traditional approach has not only proven to be a mechanistic formulation that reflects the acid-base status at the tissue level but is also considerably easier to use in daily clinical practice, given the complexity of the Stewart theory and its associated fromulas.[3]

The most common clinical disturbances are simple acid-base disorders—that is, one of the metabolic disturbances (metabolic acidosis or alkalosis) or one of the respiratory disturbances (respiratory acidosis or alkalosis) occurring alone rather than in combination. Because *physiologic compensation is not complete* and cannot achieve a normal pH, the pH remains *abnormal* in simple disturbances. More complicated clinical situations can give rise to mixed acid-base disturbances through simultaneous expression of more than one simple disturbance, and in this setting the pH may be at a dangerous extreme or appear normal.[1,3]

SIMPLE ACID-BASE DISORDERS

Primary respiratory disturbances (primary changes in $Paco_2$) invoke compensatory metabolic responses (secondary changes in $[HCO_3^-]$), and primary metabolic disturbances elicit predictable compensatory respiratory responses by causing changes in $Paco_2$.

The degree of primary alteration and secondary compensation in either or both of these two variables (acidosis or alkalosis) determines the systemic pH (acidemia or alkalemia). For example, metabolic acidosis due to an increase in endogenous acids (e.g., ketoacidosis) lowers extracellular fluid $[HCO_3^-]$ and decreases systemic pH. This stimulates the medullary chemoreceptors to increase ventilation and to return the ratio of $[HCO_3^-]$ to $Paco_2$, and thus pH, toward normal, although not to normal. Table 109-1 contains the acid-base disturbances along with the appropriate compensatory response for simple disorders. The degree of respiratory compensation expected in a simple form of metabolic acidosis can be predicted from the relationship $Paco_2 = (1.5 \times [HCO_3^-]) + 8 \pm 2$; that is, the $Paco_2$ is expected to decrease 1.25 mm Hg for each mEq/L per liter decrease in $[HCO_3^-]$. Thus, a patient with metabolic acidosis and $[HCO_3^-]$ of 12 mEq/L would be expected to have a $Paco_2$ between 24 and 28 mm Hg. Values for $Paco_2$ below 24 or greater than 28 mm Hg define a mixed disturbance (metabolic acidosis plus respiratory alkalosis or metabolic acidosis plus respiratory acidosis, respectively). A readily available (though not as reliable) method of determining the nature and degree of compensatory response is the use of nomograms (Figure 109-1).[1,4] If the arterial acid-base value falls within one of the shaded bands in Figure 109-1, one may assume that a simple acid-base disorder is present, and a tentative diagnostic category can be assigned. Values that fall outside the shaded area suggest the presence of a mixed disorder. These nomograms, though helpful, are not substitutes for an appreciation of the limits of compensation as displayed in Table 109-1.[4]

MIXED ACID-BASE DISORDERS

Mixed acid-base disorders, defined as independently coexisting disorders, not merely compensatory responses, are more often seen in patients in ICUs and can lead to dangerous extremes of pH. A patient with diabetic ketoacidosis (DKA; high-AG metabolic acidosis) may develop an independent and superimposed respiratory problem leading to respiratory acidosis or alkalosis. Patients with underlying pulmonary disease may not respond to metabolic acidosis with an appropriate ventilatory response because of insufficient respiratory reserve. Such imposition of respiratory acidosis on metabolic acidosis can lead to severe acidemia and a poor outcome. When metabolic acidosis and metabolic alkalosis coexist in the same patient, the pH may be normal or near normal. When the pH is normal, an elevated AG (see later) denotes the presence of a metabolic acidosis. Patients who have ingested an overdose of drug combinations such as sedatives and salicylates may have mixed disturbances as a result of the acid-base response to the individual drugs (metabolic acidosis mixed with respiratory acidosis or respiratory alkalosis, respectively). Even more complex are triple acid-base disturbances. For example, patients with metabolic acidosis due to alcoholic ketoacidosis may develop metabolic alkalosis due to vomiting and superimposed respiratory alkalosis due to the hyperventilation of hepatic dysfunction or alcohol withdrawal.[1] In general, a normal arterial pH in face of abnormal bicarbonate level, $Paco_2$, or AG is highly suggestive of a complex and mixed acid base disorder.

PATHWAY TO DIAGNOSIS OF ACID-BASE DISORDERS

A stepwise approach to the diagnosis of acid-base disorders follows and is summarized in Table 109-2. In the determination of arterial blood gases by the clinical laboratory, both pH and $Paco_2$ are measured, and the $[HCO_3^-]$ is calculated from the Henderson-Hasselbalch equation. This calculated value should be compared with the measured $[HCO_3^-]$ (or total CO_2) on the electrolyte panel. These two values should agree within 2 mEq/L. If they do not, the values may not have been drawn simultaneously, a laboratory error may be present, or an error could have been made in calculating the $[HCO_3^-]$. After verifying the blood acid-base values, one can then identify the precise acid-base disorder.[1]

TABLE 109-1	Acid-Base Abnormalities and Appropriate Compensatory Responses for Simple Disorders				
Primary Acid-Base Disorders	**Primary Defect**	**Effect on pH**	**Compensatory Response**	**Expected Range of Compensation**	**Limits of Compensation**
Respiratory acidosis	Alveolar hypoventilation ($\uparrow Pco_2$)	↓	↑ Renal HCO_3^- reabsorption ($HCO_3^- \uparrow$)	Acute: $\Delta[HCO_3^-] = +1$ mEq/L for each ↑ ΔPco_2 of 10 mm Hg Chronic: $\Delta[HCO_3^-] = +4$ mEq/L for each ↑ ΔPco_2 of 10 mm Hg	$[HCO_3^-] = 38$ mEq/L $[HCO_3^-] = 45$ mEq/L
Respiratory alkalosis	Alveolar Hyperventilation ($\downarrow Pco_2$)	↑	↓ Renal HCO_3^- reabsorption ($HCO_3^- \downarrow$)	Acute: $\Delta[HCO_3^-] = -2$ mEq/L for each ↓ ΔPco_2 of 10 mm Hg Chronic: $\Delta[HCO_3^-] = -5$ mEq/L for each ↓ ΔPco_2 of 10 mm Hg	$[HCO_3^-] = 18$ mEq/L $[HCO_3^-] = 15$ mEq/L
Metabolic acidosis	Loss of HCO_3^- or gain of H^+ ($\downarrow HCO_3^-$)	↓	Alveolar hyperventilation to ↑ pulmonary CO_2 excretion ($\downarrow Pco_2$)	$Pco_2 = 1.5[HCO_3^-] + 8 \pm 2$ $Pco_2 =$ last 2 digits of pH $\times 100$ $Pco_2 = 15 + [HCO_3^-]$	$Pco_2 = 15$ mm Hg
Metabolic alkalosis	Gain of HCO_3^- or loss of H^+ ($\uparrow HCO_3^-$)	↑	Alveolar hypoventilation to ↓ pulmonary CO_2 excretion ($\uparrow Pco_2$)	$Pco_2 = +0.6$ mm Hg for $\Delta[HCO_3^-]$ of 1 mEq/L. $Pco_2 = 15 + [HCO_3^-]$	$Pco_2 = 55$ mm Hg

Adapted from Bidani A, Tauzon DM, Heming TA. Regulation of whole body acid-base balance. In: DuBose TD, Hamm LL, editors. Acid base and electrolytes disorders: a companion to Brenner and Rector's the kidney. Philadelphia: Saunders; 2002, p. 1-21.

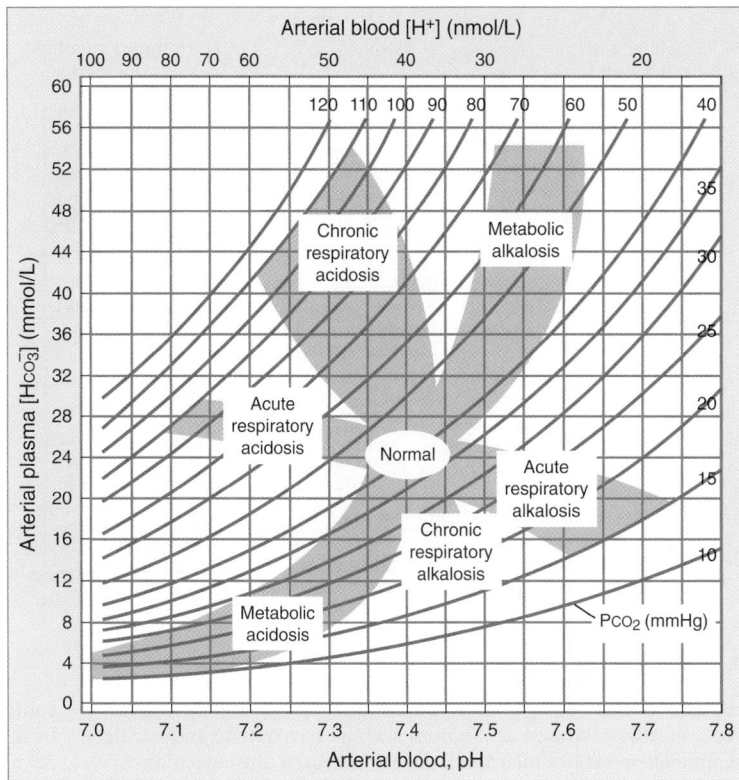

Figure 109-1 Acid base normogram. Shaded areas represent 95% confidence limits of normal respiratory and metabolic compensations for primary disturbances. Points outside shaded areas represent a mixed disorder, assuming absence of laboratory error.

The most common causes of acid-base disorders should be kept in mind while probing the history for clues about the etiology. For example, established chronic renal failure is expected to cause a metabolic acidosis, and chronic vomiting frequently causes metabolic alkalosis. Patients with pneumonia, sepsis, or cardiac failure frequently have respiratory alkalosis, and patients with chronic obstructive pulmonary disease or a sedative drug overdose often display a respiratory acidosis. The drug history is important because loop or thiazide diuretics may cause metabolic alkalosis, and the carbonic anhydrase inhibitor, acetazolamide, can result in metabolic acidosis.

Blood for electrolytes and arterial blood gases should be drawn simultaneously before therapy, because an increase in [HCO$_3^-$] occurs with metabolic alkalosis and respiratory acidosis. Conversely, a decrease in [HCO$_3^-$] occurs in metabolic acidosis and respiratory alkalosis.[1,2]

Metabolic acidosis often leads to hyperkalemia as a result of cellular shifts in which H$^+$ is exchanged for K$^+$ or Na$^+$. For each decrease in blood pH of 0.10, the plasma [K$^+$] should rise by 0.6 mEq/L. This

relationship is not invariable, however. DKA, lactic acidosis, diarrhea, and renal tubular acidosis are regularly associated with potassium depletion because of urinary K$^+$ wasting.[1]

By definition, a high-AG acidosis has two identifying features: a low [HCO$_3^-$] and an elevated AG. This means that the elevated AG will persist even if another disorder coincides to modify the [HCO$_3^-$] independently. In such a situation, one will be faced with an apparent normal bicarbonate level (and perhaps a normal pH) despite acid accumulation.

ANION GAP

Calculation of the anion gap is a key step in evaluation of acid-base disorders (see Table 109-2). Because normally the total unmeasured anions exceed the total unmeasured cations as indicated by the electrolyte panel, there exists an AG of 9 ± 3 mEq/L in plasma. The concentration of potassium in the blood usually is relatively small compared with that of sodium, chloride, and bicarbonate, so many clinicians omit this variable when calculating the AG.[5]

Simply put, AG represents unmeasured anions in plasma and is calculated as shown in the following equation. The various contributors to plasma AG in normal physiologic state and in metabolic acidosis are depicted in Figure 109-2. Patients with underlying pulmonary disease may not respond to metabolic acidosis with an appropriate ventilatory response because of insufficient respiratory reserve. Such imposition of respiratory acidosis on metabolic acidosis can lead to severe acidemia and a poor outcome. When metabolic acidosis and metabolic alkalosis coexist in the same patient, the pH may be normal or near normal. When the pH is normal, an elevated AG (see later) denotes the presence of a metabolic acidosis.

$$AG = Na^+ - (Cl^- + HCO_3^-)(Normal\ 9 \pm 3\ mEq/L)$$

The unmeasured anions include predominately anionic proteins such as albumin but also phosphate, sulfate, and organic anions. An increase in the AG is most often due to an increase in unmeasured anions and less commonly is caused by a decrease in unmeasured

TABLE 109-2	Steps in Acid-Base Diagnosis

1. Obtain arterial blood gases (ABG) and electrolytes simultaneously.
2. Compare [HCO$_3^-$] on ABG and electrolytes to rule out error due to specimen handling or measurements.
3. Calculate anion gap (AG). Correct for low albumin if indicated.
4. Screen for four common causes of high-AG acidosis:
   • Ketoacidosis
   • Lactic acid acidosis
   • Renal failure
   • Toxins
5. Know two causes of non-gap acidosis:
   • Bicarbonate loss from gastrointestinal tract
   • Renal bicarbonate wasting
6. Estimate compensatory response (see Table 109-1).
7. Compare ΔAG and ΔHCO$_3^-$.
8. Compare change in [Cl$^-$] with change in [Na$^+$].

Adapted in part from DuBose TD Jr. Acid-base disorders. In: Brenner BM, editor Brenner and Rector's the kidney 8th ed. Philadelphia: Saunders; 2008, p. 513.

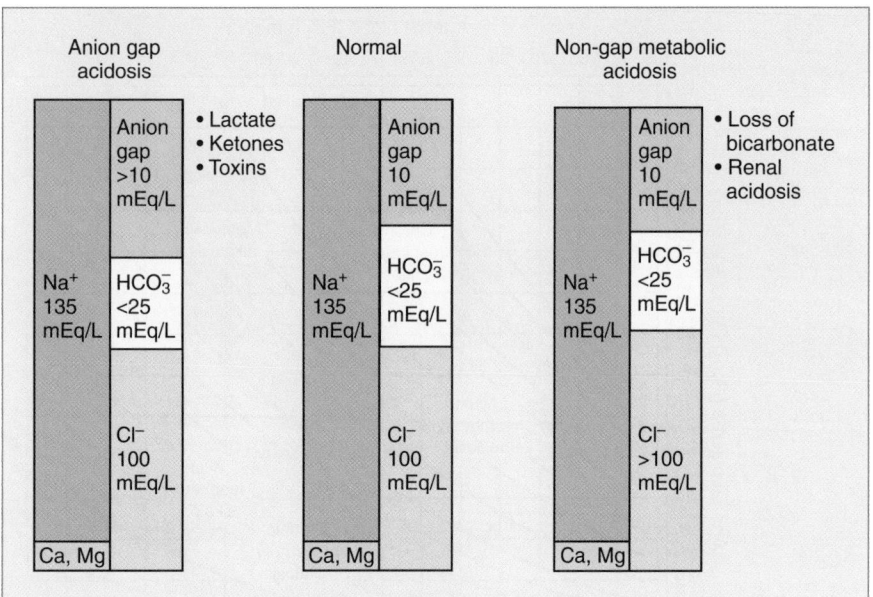

Figure 109-2 Contributors to plasma anion gap in normal physiologic state and in metabolic acidosis. (*Data from Gamble JL. Chemical anatomy, physiology, and pathology of extracellular fluid. 6th ed. Cambridge: Harvard University Press; 1954; and from Stewart PA. How to understand acid-base. New York: Elsevier; 1981.*)

cations (calcium, magnesium, potassium) (Table 109-3).[1] When endogenously produced acid anions such as acetoacetate and lactate accumulate in extracellular fluid, the AG increases, causing a high-AG acidosis. In addition, the AG may increase with an increase in anionic albumin, either because of increased albumin concentration due to profound volume depletion or alkalosis, which alters albumin charge (increased negative charge).[6]

A low serum AG is not an uncommon occurrence and most frequently is the result of severe hypoalbuminemia. Albumin is the major

contributor to serum AG, and a decline of 1 g/dL in serum albumin from the normal value of 4.5 g/dL will cause a reduction of 2.3 to 2.5 mEq/L in AG. Given the pivotal role of AG in formulating differential and treatment plans in acid-base disorders, it is extremely important to correct for low albumin when calculating AG in setting of hypoalbuminemia (see Table 109-3). Other causes of a low AG include:

1. Elevation of unmeasured serum cations such as magnesium and calcium
2. Addition of exogenous cations such as lithium (Li^-) intoxication
3. Elevation in plasma proteins, as in plasma cell disorders

Besides hypoalbuminemia, polyclonal gammopathy and monoclonal gammopathy with excessive accumulation of cationic immunoglobulin (Ig)G are the most common clinical disorders associated with a low serum AG. Therefore, once laboratory error and hypoalbuminemia have been excluded, a search for accumulation of IgG should be initiated. In patients with disturbed mentation or unexplained clinical findings, the possibility of lithium ingestion, bromism, or iodide intoxication should be considered. When the serum AG is negative in the absence of laboratory error, an extremely uncommon situation, bromide intoxication and iodide intoxication, should be excluded.[5]

In the face of a normal serum albumin, a high AG is usually due to non–chloride-containing acids that contain inorganic (phosphate, sulfate), organic (ketoacids, lactate, uremic organic anions), exogenous (salicylate or ingested toxins with organic acid production), or unidentified anions. As mentioned earlier, a high-AG acidosis has two identifying features: a low [HCO_3^-] and an elevated AG. The latter is present even if an additional acid-base disorder is superimposed to modify the [HCO_3^-] independently. Metabolic acidosis of the high-AG variety, concomitant with either chronic respiratory acidosis or metabolic alkalosis, represents a situation for which [HCO_3^-] may be normal or increased. Nevertheless, the AG is elevated, signaling the *presence of the acidosis* (see Table 109-3). In a typical simple AG metabolic acidosis, one would expect an equal but reciprocal change in serum bicarbonate and the AG, but this relationship does not hold when mixed disorders are present. Therefore, ΔAG versus ΔHCO_3^- is an important tool to search for a concealed acid-base disorder. For example, the combination of metabolic acidosis and metabolic alkalosis is expected to be present in a patient with advanced renal failure with several days' history of vomiting. This mixed disorder would be most easily recognized when the AG is elevated but the HCO_3^- concentration and pH

TABLE 109-3	Anion Gap in the Diagnosis of Metabolic Acidosis Anion Gap = $Na^+ - (Cl^- + HCO_3^-)$ = 9 + 3 mEq/L

Decreased Anion Gap	Increased Anion Gap

Increased cations (not Na^+):
↑ Ca^{++}, Mg^{++}
↑ Li^+
↑ IgG
Decreased anions:
(not Cl^- or HCO_3^-)
Hypoalbuminemia*
Acidosis
Laboratory error:
 	
Hyperviscosity
Bromism
	Increased anions (not Cl^- or HCO_3^-):
	↑ Albumin concentration
	Alkalosis
	↑ Inorganic anions:
	  Phosphate
	  Sulfate
	
	↑ Organic anions:
	  L-Lactate
	  D-Lactate`
	  Ketones
	  Uremic
	↑ Exogenously supplied anions:
	  Toxins:
	    Salicylate
	    Paraldehyde
	    Ethylene glycol
	    Methanol
	    Toluene
	    Pyroglutamic acid
	↑ Unidentified anions:
	  Uremic
	  Hyperosmolar, nonketotic states
	  Myoglobinuric acute renal failure
	Decreased cations (not Na^+):
	  ↓ Ca^{++}, Mg^{++}

Adapted from Emmett M, Narins RG. Clinical use of the anion gap. Medicine 1997;56:38-54; from Oh MS, Carroll HJ. The anion gap. N Engl J Med 1977;297:814-7; and from Kraut JA, Madisa NE. Serum anion gap: its uses and limitations in clinical medicine. Clin J Am Soc Nephrol 2007;2:162-74. Epub 2006 Dec 6.

*Albumin is the major unmeasured anion. A decline in serum albumin of 1.0 g/dL from the normal value of 4.5 g/dL decreases the anion gap by 2.3-2.5 mEq/L. Correction is very important to diagnose anion gap acidosis in setting of hypoalbuminemia.

are near normal ($\Delta AG > \Delta HCO_3^-$). In general, a $\Delta AG/\Delta HCO_3^-$ value of 1 is typical of pure high-AG acidosis such as lactic or DKA acidosis.[7] A ratio significantly greater than 1 suggests the presence of metabolic acidosis and metabolic alkalosis, whereas a ratio less than 1 suggests the presence of mixed gap and non-gap metabolic acidosis. However, studies have indicated variability in the $\Delta AG/\Delta HCO_3^-$.[5] This observation undercuts the ability to use this ratio alone to detect complex acid-base disorders, thus emphasizing the need to consider additional information to obtain the appropriate diagnosis.

To further illustrate the importance of anion gap as the only clue to the presence of an acid-base disorder in face of normal values in the ABG, consider the following case: A 49-year-old male with a history of heavy alcohol consumption and poor dietary intake is admitted for persistent vomiting of several days' duration. He is found to have metabolic alkalosis, with a pH of 7.55, $Paco_2$ of 48 mm Hg, $[HCO_3^-]$ of 40 mEq/L, $[Na^+]$ of 135 mEq/dL, $[Cl^-]$ of 80 mEq/dL, and $[K^+]$ of 2.8 mEq/L. If such a patient were then to develop a superimposed alcoholic ketoacidosis with a $[\beta\text{-hydroxybutyrate}]$ of 15 mM, arterial pH would fall to 7.40, $[HCO_3^-]$ to 25 mEq/L, and $Paco_2$ to 40 mm Hg. Although these blood gas findings are normal, the AG is elevated at 30 mEq/L, indicating a mixed metabolic alkalosis and metabolic acidosis.

▉ Metabolic Acidosis

Metabolic acidosis can occur because of an increase in endogenous acid production (such as lactate and ketoacids), loss of bicarbonate (as in diarrhea), or accumulation of endogenous acids (as in renal failure). Metabolic acidosis along with an elevated AG have profound effects on patient survival.[8]

EFFECTS OF ACIDOSIS

The effects of acidemia on the body are multiple (Table 109-4). The fall in blood pH is accompanied by a characteristic increase in ventilation, especially the tidal volume (Kussmaul respiration). Intrinsic cardiac contractility may be depressed, but inotropic function can be normal because of catecholamine release. Both peripheral arterial vasodilation and central venoconstriction can be present; the decrease in central and pulmonary vascular compliance predisposes to pulmonary edema with even minimal volume overload. CNS function is depressed, with headache, lethargy, stupor, and in some cases, even coma. Glucose intolerance may also occur.[1]

TABLE 109-4	Systemic Effects of Acidosis

Neurologic
- Obtundation and coma
- Hyperactivity of sympathetic nervous system
- Decreased cerebral metabolism
- Decreased response to catecholamines

Respiratory
- Increased minute ventilation
- Subjective dyspnea
- Respiratory muscle fatigue

Cardiovascular
- Decreased contractility of myocardium
- Core vasculature blood pooling (venoconstriction and arterial dilatation)
- Decreased cardiac response to catecholamines
- Tachyarrhythmias

Metabolic
- Hyperkalemia (inorganic acidemia)
- Hyperphosphatemia
- Increased protein catabolism

Adapted in part from Whitney GM, Szerlip HM. Acid-base disorder in critical care setting. In: DuBose TD, Hamm LL, editors. Acid-base and electrolytes disorders: a companion to Brenner and Rector's the kidney. Philadelphia: Saunders; 2002, p. 165-83.

GENERAL APPROACH IN TREATMENT OF METABOLIC ACIDOSIS

The treatment of metabolic acidosis with alkali should be reserved for severe acidemia, except when the patient has no "potential $[HCO_3^-]$" in plasma. Potential $[HCO_3^-]$ can be estimated from the increment (Δ) in the AG (ΔAG = patient's AG − 10).[1,9] It must be determined if the acid anion in plasma is metabolizable (i.e., β-hydroxybutyrate, aceto-acetate, and lactate) or non-metabolizable (anions that accumulate in chronic renal failure and after toxin ingestion with subsequent kidney injury). The latter requires return of renal function to replenish the $[HCO_3^-]$ deficit, a slow and often unpredictable process. Consequently, patients with a normal AG acidosis (hyperchloremic acidosis), a slightly elevated AG (mixed hyperchloremic and AG acidosis), or an AG attributable to a non-metabolizable anion in the presence of renal failure should receive alkali therapy, either orally ($NaHCO_3$ or Shohl's solution) or intravenously ($NaHCO_3$), in an amount necessary to slowly increase the plasma $[HCO_3^-]$ into the 20- to 22-mEq/L range. Controversy exists, however, in regard to the use of alkali in patients with a pure AG acidosis from accumulation of a metabolizable organic acid anion (ketoacidosis or lactic acidosis).[1] In general, severe acidosis (pH < 7.15) warrants the intravenous (IV) administration of 50 to 100 mEq of $NaHCO_3$ over 30 to 45 minutes during the initial 1 to 2 hours of therapy. Provision of such modest quantities of alkali in this situation seems to provide an added measure of safety, but it is essential to monitor plasma electrolytes during the course of therapy, because the $[K^+]$ may decline as pH rises. The goal is to increase the $[HCO_3^-]$ to no more than 15 mEq/L and the pH to 7.25. The goal is never to increase these values to the normal values of 25 mEq/L and 7.40, respectively. It is important to point out that studies in humans and animals have failed to conclusively show any significant and positive effect with bicarbonate therapy on hemodynamic parameters or patient outcome in the ICU setting.[1] However, the use of alkali remains a common practice in patients with profound acidosis or acidemia. There are two major clinical categories of metabolic acidosis: high AG and normal AG.

▉ High–Anion Gap Acidosis

High-AG acidosis is the most common form of metabolic acidosis encountered in the ICU. There are four principal causes of a high-AG acidosis (Figure 109-3; Tables 109-5 and 109-6)[1,4]:
1. Lactic acid acidosis
2. Ketoacidosis
3. Toxin induced
4. Acute and chronic renal failure

Initial screening to identify the cause of the high-AG acidosis should include (1) a search in the history for evidence of drug or toxin ingestion (ethylene glycol, methyl alcohol, salicylates); (2) determination of whether diabetes mellitus is present (DKA); (3) a search for evidence of alcoholism or increased levels of β-hydroxybutyrate (alcoholic keto-acidosis); (4) observation for clinical signs of uremia and determination of the blood urea nitrogen and creatinine (uremic acidosis); (5) inspection of the urine for oxalate crystals (ethylene glycol); and (6) recognition of the common clinical settings in which lactate levels may be increased (hypotension, septic or hemorrhagic shock, cardiac failure, leukemia, cancer, and drug or toxin ingestion).[1]

LACTIC ACIDOSIS

Lactic acidosis is one the most common causes of high-AG acidosis in the ICU. An increase in plasma L-lactate is most commonly due to increased production of lactate in setting of an imbalance in oxygen supply and demand at the tissue level (type A). Thus type A lactic acidosis is thought to be caused by tissue hypoperfusion and/or severe hypoxemia, although in recent years this view is thought to be an oversimplification. Non-hypoxic conditions can also generate significant lactic acidosis (type B) in a variety of clinical settings such as

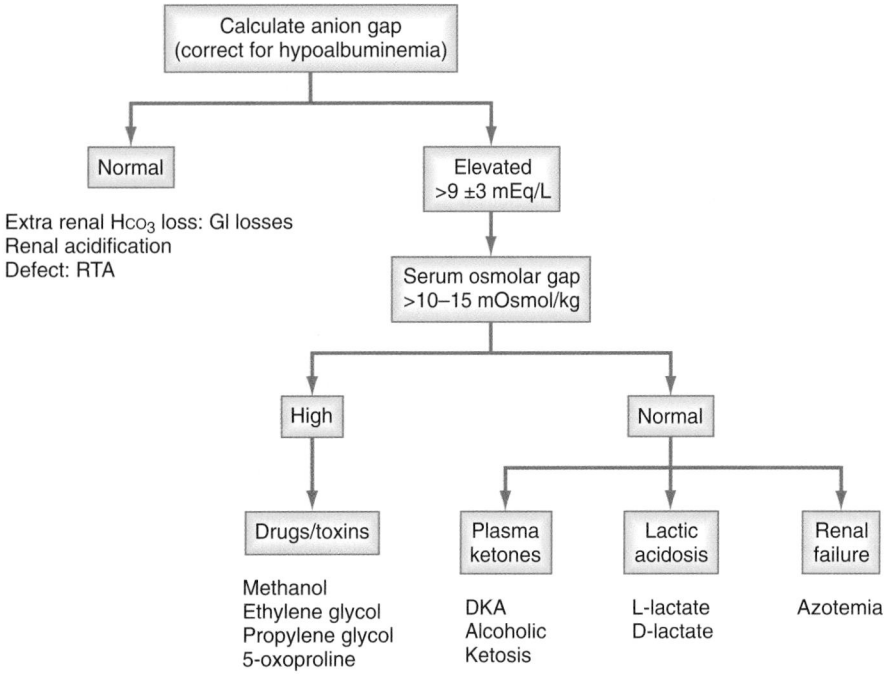

Figure 109-3 Anion gap acidosis workup. *(Data from Finkle KW, DuBose TD Jr. Metabolic acidosis. In: Dubose TD Jr, Hamm LL, editors. Acid-base and Electrolyte disorders: a companion to Brenner and Rector's the kidney. Philadelphia: Saunders; 2002, p. 55-66.)*

malignancies, hepatic failure, or ingestion of drugs/toxins. The following are some of the causes of lactic acidosis in clinical setting (also see Table 109-6):

- Poor tissue perfusion and/or hypoxia (type A)—imbalance in O_2 supply and demand
- Circulatory insufficiency (septic, cardiogenic, or hypovolemic shock)
- Severe hypoxia (hypoxemia, carbon monoxide poisoning, cyanide, severe anemia)

TABLE 109-5	Clinical Causes of High Anion Gap and Normal Anion Gap Acidosis

High Anion Gap

Ketoacidosis:
   Diabetic ketoacidosis (acetoacetate)
   Alcoholic (β-hydroxybutyrate)
   Starvation
Lactic acid acidosis (see table 109-6):
   L-Lactic acid acidosis (types A and B)
   D-Lactic acid acidosis
Renal failure: sulfate, phosphate, urate, hippurate
Ingestions (toxins and their metabolites):
   Ethylene glycol → glycolate, oxalate
   Methyl alcohol → formate
   Salicylate → ketones, lactate, salicylate
   Paraldehyde → organic anions
   Toluene → hippurate (commonly presents with normal AG)
   Propylene glycol → lactate
   Pyroglutamic acidosis (acetaminophen use) → 5-oxoproline

Normal Anion Gap

Gastrointestinal loss of HCO_3^- (negative urine anion gap):
   Diarrhea
   Fistula, external
Renal loss of HCO_3^- or failure to excrete NH_4^+ (positive urine anion gap):
   Proximal renal tubular acidosis (RTA type 2)
   Acetazolamide
   Classic distal renal tubular acidosis (low serum K^+) RTA type 1
   Generalized distal renal tubular defect (high serum K^+) RTA type 4
Miscellaneous:
   NH_4Cl ingestion
   Sulfur ingestion
   Dilutional acidosis
   Late stages in treatment of diabetic ketoacidosis.

Adapted in part from DuBose TD Jr. Acid-base disorders. In: Brenner BM, editor. Brenner and Rector's the kidney. 8th ed. Philadelphia: Saunders; 2008, p. 513-46.

TABLE 109-6	Etiologies of Lactic Acidosis

L-Lactic Acidosis

Conditions associated with type A lactic acidosis:
   Poor tissue perfusion
   Shock
   Cardiogenic
   Hemorrhagic
   Septic
   Profound hypoxemia:
     • Severe asthma
     • Severe anemia
   Carbon monoxide poisoning
Conditions associated with type B lactic acidosis:
   Liver disease
   Diabetes mellitus
   Catecholamine excess:
     • Endogenous
     • Exogenous
   Thiamine deficiency
   Ketoacidosis
   Seizure
   Malignancy
   Intracellular inorganic phosphate depletion
   Intravenous (IV) fructose
   IV xylose
   IV sorbitol
   Alcohols metabolized by alcohol dehydrogenase:
     • Ethanol
     • Methanol
     • Ethylene glycol
     • Propylene glycol
   Mitochondrial toxins:
     • Salicylate intoxication
     • Cyanide poisoning
     • 2,4-Dinitrophenol ingestion
     • Non-nucleoside antireverse transcriptase drugs
   Metformin
   Inborn errors of metabolism
   Pyroglutamic acidosis
   Kombucha tea

D-Lactic Acidosis

Short bowel syndrome
Ischemic bowel
Small bowel obstruction

Adapted in part from DuBose TD Jr. Acid-base disorders. In: Brenner BM, editor. Brenner and Rector's the kidney. 8th ed. Philadelphia: Saunders; 2008, p. 513-46.

- Normal tissue oxygenation (type B)
- Associated with systemic disorders: malignancies, diabetes mellitus, hepatic failure
- Drugs/toxins: metformin, ethanol, methanol, ethylene glycol, isoniazid, antiretroviral agents, and fructose
- Inborn errors of metabolism: impaired mitochondrial oxidation of pyruvate, G6PD deficiency

Among the most common causes of lactic acid acidosis in medical ICUs is unrecognized bowel ischemia or infarction in a patient with severe atherosclerosis or cardiac decomposition receiving vasopressors.[10] Moreover, independent of the cause of hemodynamic instability, use of catecholamines, especially epinephrine, also results in lactic acidosis, presumably by stimulating cellular metabolism such as hepatic glycolysis.[9]

D-Lactic acid acidosis is due to formation of D-lactate by gut bacteria and may cause both an increased AG and hyperchloremia (see Table 109-6).[9,10] This condition is caused by overgrowth of intestinal flora and may be associated with jejunoileal bypass or intestinal obstruction.

Lactic acidosis is among the most frequent and critical of all AG acidoses observed in the acute care setting. A study of 50 ICUs revealed an incidence of elevated lactate levels in over 60% of patients.[11] Whether lactic acidosis represents a unique entity or is a consequence of a variety of other conditions common to the ICU has been debated. Lactate concentrations are mildly elevated in nonpathologic states (such as exercise), but the magnitude of elevation is generally small. For purposes of definition, a serum L-lactate level greater than 4 mEq/L (normal being 1 mEq/L) is thought to represent a clinically significant lactic acidosis and is the initiating point for resuscitative protocols in many critical care units. Nevertheless, some patients in the ICU maintain serum lactate levels between 2 to 4 mEq/L, and it is uncertain whether such patients progress to frank lactic acidosis, but studies are suggestive of higher mortality for patients with even intermediate rises in serum lactate.[12]

L-Lactic acid is the product of the anaerobic metabolism of pyruvate, which is derived from glucose by means of the Embden-Meyerhof pathway. Under aerobic conditions, pyruvate is oxidized to acetyl CoA. In the absence of oxygen, however, pyruvate is reduced instead to lactate. Lactate is converted back to pyruvate by both the liver and the kidney via the Cori cycle, assuming normal liver function. Hepatic dysfunction, therefore, predisposes to the development of lactic acidemia in the presence of tissue hypoperfusion.

Whereas the lactic acid acidoses have been classified by Huckabee and Cohen into two types—type A (hypoxic) and type B (non-hypoxic) as noted earlier[13]—it has been recognized that lactic acidosis is often the result of the simultaneous existence of both hypoxic and non-hypoxic factors, and in many cases the precise etiology is difficult to establish. Decreased arterial perfusion to peripheral tissues in shock despite adequate arterial oxygen content, for example, results in L-lactic acid accumulation. Severe acidemia decreases portal blood flow and hepatic clearance of lactic acid.[1] Moreover, in sepsis there is both a decrease in tissue perfusion and a decrease in oxygen utilization. Technically, therefore, the classification of lactic acidosis is primarily of conceptual interest.

Numerous drugs have been implicated in the occurrence of lactic acidosis (see Table 109-6). Of particular note is biguanide (metformin) and antiretroviral therapy, specifically the nucleoside reverse transcriptase inhibitors (NRTIs) used in treatment of HIV infection. The biguanide family of hypoglycemic agents, which includes metformin, have been associated with mild elevation in serum lactate (usually <2 mEq/L) in patients with otherwise normal renal and hepatic function. Cases of severe lactic acidosis associated with use of metformin are typically accompanied by presence of sepsis and/or profound renal failure. The mechanism is largely unknown,[14] and the current recommendations are that the drug not be used in patients with congestive heart failure, liver disease, and significant renal insufficiency (creatinine >1.5 mg/dL in men, or >1.4 mg/dL in women).[9,15] Nucleoside analogs used in treatment of HIV infections inhibit mitochondrial polymerase and lead to lactic acid accumulation. Hyperlactemia is common with NRTI therapy, especially stavudine and zidovudine, but the serum lactate is mildly elevated and well compensated. Risk factors for NRTI therapy–associated lactic acidosis include a creatinine clearance less than 70 mL/min and a low CD4$^+$ T-lymphocyte count.[9,16]

Carbon monoxide poisoning produces lactic acidosis by reducing the oxygen-carrying capacity of the hemoglobin, resulting in tissue hypoxia. A newly recognized and not too uncommon cause of lactate accumulation is propylene glycol. This agent is used as carrier for a variety of IV medications used in ICU setting, most notably diazepam, lorazepam, nitroglycerin, and etomidate. Metabolism of propylene glycol by alcohol dehydrogenase in the liver results in lactate formation, which is then converted to pyruvate and shunted to glycolytic pathways. There have been numerous reports of high-AG acidosis and elevated serum osmolarity in patients receiving benzodiazepine infusions in the critical care setting.[17]

Critically ill patients with a significantly elevated AG or low serum bicarbonate should be suspected of having a lactic acidosis, particularly in the presence of hepatic insufficiency. A high index of suspicion must be maintained, however, because the AG is a relatively insensitive reflection of lactic acidosis. Iberti and coworkers reported a poor correlation between arterial pH, the AG, and serum lactate levels.[18] Fifty percent of patients with serum lactate levels above 5 and less than 9.9 mmol/L displayed a normal AG.

Several investigators have sought to characterize the prognostic value of serum lactic acid levels. Studies have found an inverse correlation between mortality and L-lactate levels above 2.0 to 2.5 mmol/L.[19-21] Prognosis is related to lactate concentration, as well as the ability to metabolize a lactic acid load after a resuscitative effort. Although lactic acidemia is associated with adverse outcome during critical illness, it does not appear to be a direct causative agent, rather a marker of poor prognosis. Therapeutic interventions that target the primary pathophysiology rather than the lactic acidosis per se have been shown to have outcome benefits.[22] Moreover, normalization of elevated lactic acid levels regardless of causative source is associated with better outcome in patients with sepsis, but this may be a surrogate for the acuity of the illness and index of organ dysfunction.[23] Falk and associates observed that the ability to lower serum lactate levels by 50% within 18 hours after resuscitation correlated with a significantly greater rate of survival.[24] Other studies have reinforced these findings, revealing both significantly lower lactate levels and increased ability to clear lactate in survivors as opposed to nonsurvivors.[25] To add to this argument, dichloroacetate, which indirectly decreases lactic acid level, has not been shown to improve survival, suggesting that elevated lactate level is an epiphenomenon with varying prognostic value in different clinical settings.[26]

Treatment of Lactic Acidosis

Therapy of lactic acidosis has two distinct goals. The first is to identify and remedy the defect in the oxidative metabolism (hypoperfusion and hypoxemia being the most common causes) in order to halt further production of lactate. The second is to raise the serum pH toward normal. If the underlying pathophysiologic state is effectively treated, the excess lactate production and acidemia often correct without specific interventions. As mentioned earlier, there is controversy as to whether lactic acidosis directly contributes to mortality or is simply a marker of the severity of the underlying illness,[9,10] and this has led to added debate on recommendations for use of buffers in the management of lactic acidosis. Nevertheless, *the basic principle and most effective therapy for L-lactic acidosis is that the underlying condition disrupting the normal lactate metabolism must first be corrected.*

To that end, optimizing cardiac output and tissue oxygenation through supportive therapies should be of primary consideration in management. Mechanical ventilation is instituted to reduce the metabolic work of breathing and optimize ventilation; fluids and inotropic agents are helpful in restoring adequate cardiac output. Septic shock requires control of the underlying infection, and volume resuscitation is the main goal in hypovolemic shock. Interruption in the cytokine cascade has theoretical advantages, but no widely applicable method is yet available. Vasoactive drugs should be used cautiously based on an understanding of the underlying hemodynamics and knowledge of the mechanisms of action of the drugs. Vasoconstrictors should be avoided if possible, because they may worsen tissue perfusion. Alkali therapy is generally advocated for acute, severe acidemia (pH < 7.15) to improve cardiac function. However, NaHCO₃ therapy may paradoxically depress cardiac performance and exacerbate acidosis by enhancing lactate production (higher intracellular pH stimulates phosphofructokinase activity, leading to increased pyruvate formation). While the use of alkali in moderate lactic acidosis is controversial, it is generally agreed that attempts to return the pH or [HCO₃⁻] to normal by administration of exogenous NaHCO₃ are deleterious.

Fluid overload occurs rapidly with NaHCO₃ administration because of the massive amounts required in some cases, along with high sodium content of the solution. In addition, central venoconstriction and decreased cardiac output are common, which lead to tissue hypoperfusion and further end-organ dysfunction—specifically, reduced glomerular filtration. As such, the volume overload and acidemia may precipitate the need for renal replacement therapy which can simultaneously deliver HCO₃⁻, remove lactate and excess extracellular fluid (ECF) volume, and correct electrolyte abnormalities. Although use of continuous hemofiltration (HF) in critically ill patients provides minimal additional lactate clearance, perhaps due to the high rate of its production,[27] the ultrafiltration accomplished with continuous renal replacement therapy may offer additional benefits in terms of volume and electrolyte management. The use of bicarbonate-based replacement fluid or dialysate is thought to convey better acid-base control when compared to lactate based solutions, though controlled studies have shown controversial results.[28,29] There are theoretical advantages of extracorporeal therapies such as HF or hemodiafiltration in treatment of sepsis with lactic acidosis. These include enhanced removal of inflammatory mediators and endotoxin while providing early and effective management of volume and acid-base disturbances. However, as yet, the evidence in humans is too limited to recommend HF as an adjunctive therapy for critically ill patients with sepsis or systemic inflammatory response syndrome (SIRS). Regarding the many uncertainties about optimal volume (high or very high) and type of membrane, clinical studies should first focus on endpoints as recovery from organ failure and length of treatment before survival studies are started.[30] Recently, smaller uncontrolled trials have shown promising effects of HF in refractory shock,[31] which raises the need for additional large-scale studies to further define the role of renal replacement therapy in treatment of sepsis and shock.

If the underlying cause of the L-lactic acidosis can be remedied, it is anticipated that the lactate will be reconverted to HCO₃⁻. HCO₃⁻ derived from lactate conversion, and any new HCO₃⁻ generated by renal mechanisms during acidosis and IV-administered bicarbonate are all additive and may result in overshoot alkalosis.[32]

Sodium Bicarbonate. Despite highly debated and somewhat discouraged practice of its use, bicarbonate therapy remains the most commonly administered agent in treatment of lactic acidosis. Two major factors contribute to this common practice: bicarbonate is readily available to physicians who feel obliged to react to a low pH; and bicarbonate use is often associated with some degree of rather immediate improvement in measured pH which may, often unrealistically, be interpreted as a sign of improvement in the metabolic derangements and patient condition. Although severe acidosis is classically thought to have a deleterious effect on cardiopulmonary performance, recent studies have actually shown an improvement in cardiac performance in the presence of a mild to moderate acidosis.[10] Accordingly, the pH below which most clinicians feel obligated to use NaHCO₃ has declined. Therefore, the recommendation for administration of NaHCO₃ in the treatment of severe acidosis when the pH is less than 7.15 seems reasonable. At this pH, as predicted by the Henderson-Hasselbalch equation, minor changes in bicarbonate or Pco₂ will result in a large

decrease in pH.[33] However, there are no data supporting a specific pH at which therapy must be instituted.

A prospective study evaluating NaHCO₃ in patients with lactic acidosis showed an increase in serum pH but no improvement in hemodynamics when compared with normal saline.[34] The use of NaHCO₃ also failed to increase hemodynamic responsiveness to circulating catecholamines concomitant with a decrease in serum ionized calcium.[35-38] It is important to note, however, the numerous deleterious effects of bicarbonate therapy in treatment of lactic acidosis. NaHCO₃ therapy can cause fluid overload and hypertension, because the amount required can be massive when accumulation of lactic acid is relentless. Fluid administration is poorly tolerated because of central venoconstriction, especially in the oliguric patient, and can worsen the state of volume overload. If the underlying cause of the lactic acidosis can be remedied, blood lactate will be converted to HCO₃⁻ and may result in an overshoot alkalosis. Sodium bicarbonate may also result in impaired utilization of oxygen and increase anaerobic metabolism through stimulation of phosphofructokinase (by raising cellular pH), which leads to further lactate accumulation. Finally, sodium bicarbonate IV administration generates CO₂ ($HCO_3^- + H^+ \rightarrow H_2O + CO_2$). With depressed cardiac output or ventilatory capacity of lungs, CO₂ can accumulate, causing intracellular acidosis and a further reduction in cardiac output. Other possible adverse effects of bicarbonate infusion include hypernatremia, hyperosmolarity, hypocalcaemia, and hypokalemia.

A reasonable approach in treatment of profound acidemia with bicarbonate is to raise the plasma bicarbonate to 15 mEq/L and the pH to 7.2. How much bicarbonate to administer is another unclear variable in the formula of alkali therapy for lactic acidosis. The volume of distribution of bicarbonate is roughly the same as the total body water, or about 50% of total body weight in kilograms. One approach, therefore, is to estimate the required bicarbonate therapy as:

$$\text{Bicarbonate deficit} = (\text{desired} - \text{actual HCO}_3^- \ [\text{mEq/L}]) \times 0.5 \ \text{L/kg} \times \text{body weight (kg)}$$

This must be viewed as a very rough estimate with considerable variability in the clinical setting. Constant infusion of hypertonic bicarbonate has many disadvantages and is discouraged to minimize the rapid development of fluid overload. The use of continuous renal replacement therapy is common in patients with overt shock and lactic acidosis, as frequently simultaneous acute kidney injury exists in such a setting. Though the extracorporeal removal of lactate is negligible and likely bears no effect on treatment of underlying cause,[27] effective alkali therapy can be provided with minimal volume overload using the newer bicarbonate-based dialysate or replacement fluid formulations.

Dichloroacetate. Dichloroacetate stimulates the activity of pyruvate dehydrogenase, thereby increasing the rate of oxidation of pyruvate and limiting the generation of lactate. Initial animal studies showed improved aerobic glucose utilization and an increase in intracellular adenosine triphosphate. A large multicenter trial showed a significant reduction in serum lactate, an increase in arterial pH, and an increase in the number of patients able to resolve hyperlactemia from 43% to 58%.[26] Nevertheless, although dichloroacetate was effective in improving lactic acidosis, there was no decrease in mortality. Chronic use of dichloroacetate has been associated with neurologic toxicity, including limb paralysis and neuropathies.[39] In summary, dichloroacetate is not recommended in the therapy for lactic acid acidosis.

Other Agents. Tromethamine (THAM) is a non–sodium containing buffer that accepts proton and generates bicarbonate. It does not raise the CO₂ content of the blood, thereby avoiding a fall in intracellular and cerebrospinal fluid pH. Despite this theoretical advantage, this agent has not proven to be any better than bicarbonate in managing lactic acidosis.[9] THAM is excreted in the urine and should be avoided in renal insufficiency. Severe hyperkalemia, hypoglycemia, ventilatory depression, and hepatic necrosis in neonates have been reported.[40] Given the risks of serious side effects, THAM should be used only after careful consideration or not at all. Other buffers such as Carbicarb (mixture of sodium bicarbonate and sodium carbonate) or Tribonat (a mixture of THAM, acetate, $NaHCO_3$, and phosphate) have not shown any survival advantage. Methylene blue was once advocated as a means of reversing the altered redox state to enhance lactate metabolism, but there is no evidence from controlled studies for its use.[1]

D-Lactic Acidosis

D-Lactic acidosis should be considered in patients with a history of intestinal disease who present with confusion and AG metabolic acidosis. Overproduction of D-lactate may occur when there is overgrowth of gut bacteria.[41] Patients present with an AG acidosis, normal L-lactate levels, and neurologic findings such as confusion, ataxia, and loss of memory (see Table 109-5). Symptoms are worsened after high-carbohydrate meals or oral hyperalimentation or tube feedings. In patients with short bowel syndrome or who have undergone jejunoileal bypass, there not only is an overgrowth of bacteria but also accumulation of carbohydrate in the colon. Sufficient D-lactate can be produced to overwhelm enzymatic clearance. Treatment is directed at decreasing the overgrowth of bacteria with antibiotics and the avoidance of high-carbohydrate feeding. D-Lactate is not measured on routine laboratory testing unless specifically ordered. Serum D-lactate levels of greater than 3 mmol/L confirm the diagnosis.[1]

KETOACIDOSIS

(See Table 109-5.)

Diabetic Ketoacidosis

DKA is caused by increased fatty acid metabolism and the accumulation of ketoacids (acetoacetate and β-hydroxybutyrate) due to insulin deficiency or resistance, along with elevated glucagon levels. DKA usually occurs in insulin-dependent diabetes mellitus in association with cessation of insulin or with an intercurrent illness such as pneumonia, gastroenteritis, pancreatitis, or myocardial infarction. Each of these conditions increases insulin requirements temporarily and acutely. The accumulation of ketoacids accounts for the increment in the AG and is accompanied most often by hyperglycemia glucose (300 mg/dL). It should be noted that insulin administration completely prevents production of ketones, with subsequent resolution of acidosis.

Treatment of Diabetic Ketoacidosis. The general principles of treatment of DKA include (1) frequent monitoring and recording of electrolyte values, (2) fluid replacement to correct the consequences of the preceding osmotic diuresis, (3) identification of the precipitating cause of the ketoacidosis (commonly an infectious process), and (4) anticipation of the consequences of therapy, especially if alkali therapy is included in the regimen. Most patients with DKA require correction of the volume depletion that almost invariably accompanies the osmotic diuresis and ketoacidosis. Extreme caution needs to be exercised in patients with history of end-stage renal disease (ESRD), as the hyperglycemia has limited to no diuretic effect in such patients, and aggressive fluid therapy may have a deleterious effect. The serum Na^+ concentration may be arithmetically corrected for the degree of hyperglycemia to determine the type of IV fluid needed (i.e., correct Na^+ by 1.6 to 1.8 mEq/L for each 100 mg/dL increment in plasma glucose). In general, it seems prudent to initiate therapy with isotonic saline at a rate of 1000 mL IV per hour. When the pulse and blood pressure have stabilized and the corrected serum Na^+ concentration is in the range 130 to 135 mEq/L, switch to 0.45% sodium chloride. Use of lactated Ringer's should be avoided. If the blood glucose level falls below 300 mg/dL, 0.45% sodium chloride with 5% dextrose should be administered.[42]

Low-dose IV insulin therapy (0.1 U/kg/h) smoothly corrects the biochemical abnormalities and minimizes hypoglycemia and hypokalemia.[42] Usually, in the first hour, a loading dose of the same amount is given initially as an IV bolus. Although regular insulin may also be administered intramuscularly (0.1 U/kg initially, then 0.1 U/kg/h), it should be noted that intramuscular insulin may not be effective in patients with volume depletion, which often occurs in ketoacidosis.

Total body K^+ depletion is usually present, although the K^+ level on admission may be elevated or normal. Because the plasma K^+ concentration should increase 0.6 mEq/L for each 0.1-unit decline in arterial blood pH, a normal or reduced K^+ value on admission indicates severe K^+ depletion and should be approached with caution. Administration of fluid, insulin, and alkali may cause the K^+ level to plummet. When the urine output has been established, 20 mEq of potassium chloride should be administered in each liter of fluid as long as the K^+ value is less than 4.0 mEq/L. Equal caution should be exercised in the presence of hyperkalemia, especially if the patient has renal insufficiency; additional measures including renal replacement therapy may be needed to correct the hyperkalemia. Never administer potassium chloride empirically.

The arguments for and against alkali therapy have been summarized previously. The young patient with a pure AG acidosis ($\Delta AG = \Delta HCO_3^-$) usually does not require exogenous alkali, because the metabolic acidosis should be entirely reversible. Elderly patients, patients with severe high-AG acidosis (pH < 7.15), or patients with a superimposed hyperchloremic component may receive small amounts of sodium bicarbonate by slow IV infusion (no more than 44-88 mEq in 60 minutes). Thirty minutes after this infusion is completed, arterial blood gas analysis should be repeated. Alkali administration can be repeated if the pH is 7.20 or less or if the patient exhibits a significant hyperchloremic component, but it is rarely necessary. The AG should be followed closely during therapy, because it is expected to decline as ketones are cleared from plasma and herald an increase in plasma HCO_3^- as the acidosis is repaired. Therefore, it is not necessary to monitor blood ketone levels continuously. Hypokalemia and other complications of alkali therapy dramatically increase when amounts of sodium bicarbonate exceeding 400 mEq are administered. However, the effect of alkali therapy on arterial blood pH needs to be reassessed regularly and the total administered kept at a minimum if necessary.[42]

Routine administration of PO_4^{-3} (usually as potassium phosphate) is not advised because of the potential for hyperphosphatemia and hypocalcemia.[42] A significant proportion of patients with DKA have significant hyperphosphatemia before initiation of therapy. In the volume-depleted, malnourished patient, however, a normal or elevated PO_4^{-3} concentration on admission may be followed by a rapid fall in plasma PO_4^{-3} levels within 2 to 6 hours after initiation of therapy.

Alcoholic Ketoacidosis

Chronic alcoholics who discontinue solid food intake while continuing alcohol use can develop ketoacidosis when alcohol consumption is abruptly curtailed. Usually, the onset of vomiting and abdominal pain leads to cessation of alcohol use prior to presentation to the hospital. The glucose concentration is low or normal, and acidosis may be severe because of elevated ketones, predominantly β-hydroxybutyrate. Mild lactic acidosis may coexist because of alteration in the redox state. The nitroprusside ketone reaction (Acetest) can detect acetoacetic acid but not β-hydroxybutyrate, so the degree of ketosis and ketonuria can be underestimated. Typically, insulin levels are low and concentrations of triglyceride, cortisol, glucagon, and growth hormone are increased. This disorder is not rare and is underdiagnosed. The clinical presentation of alcoholic ketoacidosis (AKA) is complex owing to the fact that mixed disorders frequently exist. The vomiting can lead to a metabolic alkalosis, respiratory alkalosis may be present in setting of chronic liver disease, hypoperfusion due to volume depletion can cause mild lactic acidosis, and hyperchloremic acidosis can be present due to renal excretion of ketoacids. Moreover, the osmolar gap may be elevated if blood alcohol level is elevated, though the differential in such settings should always include ethylene glycol, methanol, or other ingestions.[1,43]

Treatment of Alcoholic Ketoacidosis. Extracellular fluid deficits should be repleted by IV administration of saline and glucose (5% dextrose in 0.9% NaCl), and insulin should be avoided. Glucose in isotonic solution, not normal saline, is the mainstay of therapy. Hypophosphatemia, hypokalemia, and hypomagnesemia may coexist and should be corrected. Hypophosphatemia usually emerges 12 to 24 hours after admission, may be exacerbated by glucose infusion, and if severe may induce rhabdomyolysis, aspiration, and platelet dysfunction. Therefore, serum electrolytes—especially serum phosphorus, magnesium, and potassium—should be checked frequently. One such schedule may be blood draws at 4, 6, 12, and 18 hours post admission. Upper gastrointestinal (GI) hemorrhage, pancreatitis, and pneumonia may accompany this disorder.[42,44]

INGESTION-INDUCED ACIDOSIS

(See Tables 109-5 and 109-6.)

Salicylates

Salicylate intoxication in adults usually causes respiratory alkalosis (most common), mixed metabolic acidosis–respiratory alkalosis, or a pure high-AG metabolic acidosis. In the latter example, which is less common, only a portion of the AG is due to the salicylates. Lactic acid production is also often increased. Generally, the presentation is one of respiratory alkalosis with metabolic acidosis. The uncoupling of oxidative phosphorylation is thought to be the cause of the metabolic acidosis. Acidosis can lead to further movement of salicylate into the CNS. High ketone concentration is reported in as many as 40% of adult salicylate poisoning patients, which is thought to be as a result of salicylate-induced hypoglycemia.[45] Treatment should begin with vigorous gastric lavage with isotonic saline (not $NaHCO_3$) followed by administration of activated charcoal. In the acidotic patient, to facilitate removal of salicylate, IV $NaHCO_3$ is administered in amounts adequate to alkalinize the urine and maintain urine output (urine pH >7.5). While this form of therapy is straightforward in acidotic patients, a coexisting respiratory alkalosis may make this approach hazardous. Acetazolamide may be administered when an alkaline diuresis cannot be achieved, but this drug can cause systemic metabolic acidosis if HCO_3^- is not replaced. Hypokalemia may occur with an alkaline diuresis from $NaHCO_3$ and should be treated promptly and aggressively. Glucose-containing fluids should be administered because of the danger of hypoglycemia. Excessive insensible fluid losses may cause severe volume depletion and hypernatremia. Hemodialysis may be necessary for severe poisoning, especially if renal failure coexists, and is preferred with severe intoxication (level >100 mg/dL). Hemodialysis is superior to other dialytic modalities such as hemofiltration for simultaneous management of electrolyte abnormalities.[10,45]

Alcohols

Under most physiologic conditions, sodium, urea, and glucose generate the osmotic pressure of blood. Plasma osmolality is calculated according to the following expression using conventional laboratory values in which glucose and BUN are expressed in milligrams per deciliter (mg/dL):

$$P_{osm} = 2Na^+ + Glu/18 + BUN/2.8$$

The calculated and determined osmolality should agree within 15 mOsm/kg. When the measured osmolality exceeds the calculated osmolality by more than 10 to 15 mOsm/kg, one of two circumstances prevails. Either the serum sodium is spuriously low, as with hyperlipidemia or hyperproteinemia (pseudohyponatremia), or osmolytes other than sodium salts, glucose, or urea have accumulated in plasma. Examples include mannitol, radiocontrast media, isopropyl alcohol, ethylene glycol, ethanol, methanol, and acetone. In this situation, the difference between the calculated osmolality and the measured osmolality (osmolar gap) is proportional to the concentration of the unmeasured solute. With an appropriate clinical history and index of suspicion, identification of an osmolar gap is helpful in identifying the presence of poison-associated AG acidosis.

Ethylene Glycol

Ingestion of ethylene glycol (commonly used in antifreeze) leads to a metabolic acidosis and severe damage to the CNS, heart, lungs, and kidneys. Early on, the patient appears intoxicated and may develop seizures or frank coma. In the next 12 to 24 hours, signs of cardiopulmonary collapse ensue, along with development of renal failure due to intratubular obstruction by oxalate crystals. The increased AG and osmolar gap are due to ethylene glycol and its metabolites, oxalic acid, glycolic acid, and other organic acids. Lactic acid production increases secondary to inhibition of the tricarboxylic acid cycle and altered intracellular redox state.[10,46] Recognizing oxalate crystals in the urine, the presence of serum osmolar gap and high-AG acidosis facilitate diagnosis. Treatment should not be delayed while awaiting measurement of ethylene glycol levels in this setting. Treatment includes the prompt institution of a saline or osmotic diuresis, thiamine and pyridoxine supplements, fomepizole or ethanol, and hemodialysis.[10,47] The IV administration of the alcohol dehydrogenase inhibitor, fomepizole (4-methylpyrazole; 7 mg/kg as a loading dose), or IV ethanol to achieve a level of 22 mmol/L (100 mg/dL) serves to lessen toxicity, because both compete with ethylene glycol for metabolism by alcohol dehydrogenase. Fomepizole offers the advantages of a predictable decline in ethylene glycol levels without the adverse effects, such as excessive obtundation, associated with ethyl alcohol infusion. Once the above measures are undertaken, hemodialysis is performed to remove ethylene glycol and its metabolites from the blood.

Fomepizole is dialyzable, and the frequency of its dosing should be increased to every 4 hours during hemodialysis. An additional dose should be given at the beginning of hemodialysis if 6 or more hours have elapsed since the prior dose. If the patient is receiving IV ethanol, the rate of infusion needs to be adjusted to maintain a blood alcohol level of 100 to 150 mg/dL.

Methanol

Ingestion of methanol (wood alcohol) causes metabolic acidosis; its metabolites, formaldehyde and formic acid, cause severe optic nerve and CNS damage. Lactic acid, ketoacids, and other unidentified organic acids may contribute to the acidosis. Because of its low molecular weight (32 D), an osmolar gap is usually present. Treatment is similar to that for ethylene glycol intoxication, including general supportive measures, fomepizole or ethanol administration, and hemodialysis.

Ethanol

After absorption of ethanol from the GI tract, it is oxidized to acetaldehyde, acetyl coenzyme A, and CO_2. A blood ethanol level greater than 500 mg/dL is associated with high mortality. Acetaldehyde levels do not increase appreciably unless the load is exceptionally high or compounds such as disulfiram, insecticides, and sulfonylurea hypoglycemia agents that inhibit the acetaldehyde dehydrogenase step are also present in the patient's serum. Such agents in the presence of ethanol result in severe toxicity. Ethanol does not cause an increase in the AG or acidosis unless hypotension from profound intoxication ensues. The contribution of ethyl alcohol to serum osmolality can be estimated by dividing the blood alcohol level by 4.

Isopropyl Alcohol

Rubbing alcohol poisoning is usually the result of accidental oral ingestion or absorption through the skin. Although isopropyl alcohol is metabolized by the enzyme alcohol dehydrogenase, as is methanol and ethanol, isopropyl alcohol is not metabolized to a strong acid. Isopropyl alcohol is metabolized to acetone, and the osmolal gap increases as the result of accumulation of both acetone and isopropyl alcohol. Despite a positive nitroprusside reaction from acetone, the AG, as well as the blood glucose, is typically normal, not elevated, and the plasma HCO_3^- is not depressed. Thus, isopropyl alcohol intoxication does not typically cause metabolic acidosis. Treatment is supportive, with attention to removal of unabsorbed alcohol from the GI tract and IV fluids. Hemodialysis is effective but not usually necessary. Patients with severe isopropyl alcohol intoxication (blood levels >100 mg/dL) may develop cardiovascular collapse and lactic acidosis. Such severe intoxication may benefit from more aggressive therapy, including hemodialysis.[10]

Paraldehyde

Intoxication with paraldehyde is now very rare but is due partly to acetic acid, the metabolic product of the drug from acetaldehyde and other organic acids.[48]

Pyroglutamic Acidosis

Pyroglutamic acid, or 5-oxoproline, is an intermediate in the synthesis of glutathione. Acetaminophen ingestion rarely depletes glutathione stores, resulting in an imbalance in the precursors of this compound and excess formation of pyroglutamic acid.[49] Most of the cases of 5-oxoproline-induced acidosis has been in patients with sepsis who were receiving full doses of acetaminophen, with all showing an elevated plasma level of pyroglutamic acid and elevated AG. It is conceivable that heterozygosity for glutathione synthase deficiency could be the underlying risk factor for development of this newly appreciated form of metabolic acidosis. It is important to note that only a minority of critically ill patients on acetaminophen develop this condition.[1,49]

RENAL FAILURE

The hyperchloremic acidosis of moderate renal insufficiency is eventually converted to the high-AG acidosis of advanced renal failure. Poor filtration and reabsorption of organic anions contribute to the pathogenesis. As renal disease progresses, the number of functioning nephrons eventually becomes insufficient to keep pace with net acid production. Uremic acidosis is characterized, therefore, by a reduced rate of NH_4^+ production and excretion, primarily due to decreased renal mass. $[HCO_3^-]$ rarely falls below 15 mEq/L, and the AG rarely exceeds 20 mEq/L. The acid retained in chronic renal disease is buffered in part by alkaline salts from bone. Despite significant retention of acid (up to 20 mEq/day), the serum $[HCO_3^-]$ does not decrease further, indicating participation of buffers outside the extracellular compartment. Chronic metabolic acidosis results in significant loss of bone mass due to reduction in bone calcium carbonate. Chronic acidosis also increases urinary calcium excretion, proportional to cumulative acid retention.

Treatment of Renal Failure Acidosis

Both uremic acidosis and the hyperchloremic acidosis of renal failure require alkali replacement to maintain the $[HCO_3^-] \geq 20$ mEq/L. This can be accomplished most readily with relatively modest amounts of oral alkali (1-1.5 mEq/kg/day) on a chronic basis. It is assumed, but not proven, that alkali replacement prevents the harmful effects of H^+ balance on bone and prevents or retards muscle catabolism. For patients in the ICU, oral bicarbonate therapy may not be possible, and small amounts of daily IV bicarbonate supplement may be necessary. The development of acute renal failure with metabolic acidosis may necessitate the replacement of renal function by dialysis. Dialysis can provide sufficient replacement of bicarbonate through the use of bicarbonate-based dialysate. Bicarbonate is the preferred buffer for dialysis in the acute care setting, whether dialysis is provided intermittently or continuously. Occasionally, citrate may be used in continuous renal replacement therapy as a regional anticoagulant. Citrate anticoagulation, though effective, has the added risk of severe hypocalcemia and hypernatremia, requiring constant IV calcium infusion and frequent monitoring.

Non–Anion Gap (Hyperchloremic) Metabolic Acidoses

Alkali can be lost from the GI tract in diarrhea or from the kidneys (renal tubular acidosis [RTA]). Because a reduced plasma $[HCO_3^-]$ and elevated $[Cl^-]$ can also occur in chronic respiratory alkalosis as compensatory response, it is important to confirm the presence of acidemia by measuring the arterial pH. In hyperchloremic metabolic acidosis, reciprocal changes in $[Cl^-]$ and $[HCO_3^-]$ result in a normal AG

TABLE 109-7	Differential Diagnosis of Hyperchloremic Metabolic Acidosis

Gastrointestinal Bicarbonate Loss

Diarrhea
External pancreatic or small bowel drainage
Ureterosigmoidostomy, jejunal loop
Drugs:
    Calcium chloride (acidifying agent)
    Magnesium sulfate (diarrhea)
    Cholestyramine (bile acid diarrhea)

Renal Acidosis

Hypokalemic:
    Proximal RTA (type 2) (see table 109-8)
    Distal (classic) RTA (type 1)
    Drug-induced hypokalemia:
        Acetazolamide (proximal RTA)
        Amphotericin B (Distal RTA)
Hyperkalemic:
    Generalized distal nephron dysfunction (type 4 RTA) (see table 109-8)
    Mineralocorticoid deficiency or resistance (pseudohypoaldosteronism type 1) PHA-I, PHA-II
    ↓ Na^+ delivery to distal nephron
    Tubulointerstitial disease
    Ammonium excretion defect
    Drug-induced hyperkalemia:
        Potassium-sparing diuretics (amiloride, triamterene, spironolactone)
        Trimethoprim
        Pentamidine
        Angiotensin-converting enzyme inhibitors and angiotensin II receptor blockers
        Nonsteroidal antiinflammatory drugs
        Cyclosporine, tacrolimus
Normokalemic:
    Early renal insufficiency

Other

Acid loads (ammonium chloride, hyperalimentation)
Loss of potential bicarbonate: ketosis with ketone excretion
Dilution acidosis (rapid saline administration)
Hippurate
Cation-exchange resins

Adapted in part from DuBose TD Jr. Acid-base disorders. In: Brenner BM, editor. Brenner and Rector's the kidney. 8th ed. Philadelphia: Saunders; 2008, p. 513-46.

(Table 109-7). In pure hyperchloremic acidosis, therefore, the increase in $[Cl^-]$ above the normal value approximates the decrease in $[HCO_3^-]$. The absence of such a relationship suggests a mixed disturbance.

GASTROINTESTINAL TRACT LOSS

With diarrhea, stools contain a higher $[HCO_3^-]$ and decomposed HCO_3^- than plasma, so metabolic acidosis develops along with volume depletion. Instead of an acid urine pH (as anticipated with systemic acidosis), urine pH is usually around 6, because metabolic acidosis and hypokalemia increase renal synthesis and excretion of NH_4^+, thus providing a urinary buffer that increases urine pH despite increased net acid excretion. Metabolic acidosis due to GI losses with a high urine pH can be differentiated from RTA, because urinary NH_4^+ excretion is typically low in RTA and high with diarrhea.[50] Urinary NH_4^+ levels can be estimated by calculating the urine AG (UAG):

$$UAG = [Na^+ + K^+]_u - [Cl^-]_u$$

When $[Cl^-]_u$ is greater than $[Na^+ + K^+]$, and the UAG is negative, the urine ammonium level is appropriately increased, suggesting an extrarenal cause of the hyperchloremic acidosis. In such a setting, urinary fractional excretion of Na will also be less than 1% to 2% owing to volume loss from the GI tract. Conversely, when the UAG is positive, the urine ammonium level is low, suggesting a renal cause of the acidosis. Note that this qualitative test is useful in differential diagnosis of a hyperchloremic metabolic acidosis. Furthermore, it is not reliable in the presence of large amounts of other anions in the urine (ketonuria, penicillins, or aspirin).[51] Gastrointestinal HCO_3^- loss, as well as proximal RTA (type 2) and cDRTA (type 1), results in ECF contraction and stimulation of the renin-aldosterone system, leading typically to hypokalemia. The serum K^+ concentration, therefore, serves to distinguish these disorders with a low K^+ from either generalized distal nephron dysfunction (e.g., type 4 RTA) in which the renin-aldosterone–distal nephron axis is abnormal and hyperkalemia exists, and the acidosis of progressive chronic kidney disease in which normokalemia is common (see later discussion of different types of RTA).

In addition to GI tract HCO_3^- loss, external loss of pancreatic and biliary secretions can cause a hyperchloremic acidosis. Cholestyramine, calcium chloride, and magnesium sulfate ingestion can also result in a hyperchloremic metabolic acidosis (see Table 109-7), especially in patients with renal insufficiency. Coexistent L-lactic acid acidosis is common in severe diarrheal illnesses but will increase the AG.

Severe hyperchloremic metabolic acidosis with hypokalemia may occur in patients with ureteral diversion procedures. Because the ileum and colon are both endowed with Cl^-/HCO_3^- exchangers, when the Cl^- from the urine enters the gut or pouch, the HCO_3^- concentration in the urine increases as a result of the exchange process. Moreover, K^+ secretion is stimulated, which, together with HCO_3^- loss, can result in a hyperchloremic hypokalemic metabolic acidosis. This defect is particularly common in patients with ureterosigmoidostomies and is more common with this type of diversion because of the prolonged transit time of urine caused by stasis in the colonic segment.

RENAL TUBULAR ACIDOSIS

Loss of functioning renal parenchyma due to progressive renal disease leads to hyperchloremic acidosis when the glomerular filtration rate (GFR) is between 20 and 50 mL/min and typically changes into a high-AG acidosis when the GFR falls to less than 20 mL/min.[52] Such a progression occurs commonly with tubulointerstitial forms of renal disease, but hyperchloremic metabolic acidosis can persist with advanced glomerular disease. In advanced renal failure, ammoniagenesis is reduced in proportion to the loss of functional renal mass, and ammonium accumulation and trapping in the outer medullary collecting tubule may also be impaired. Because of adaptive increases in K^+ secretion by the collecting duct and colon, the acidosis of chronic renal insufficiency is typically normokalemic[52] (see Table 109-7).

Proximal RTA (type 2 RTA) is commonly due to generalized proximal tubular dysfunction manifested by glycosuria, generalized aminoaciduria, and phosphaturia (Fanconi's syndrome). With a low plasma $[HCO_3^-]$, the urine pH is acid (pH < 5.5); the serum HCO_3^- concentration usually reaches a nadir of 15 to 18 mEq/L, which limits further filtration and delivery of bicarbonate, so systemic acidosis is not progressive. The fractional excretion of $[HCO_3^-]$ may exceed 10% to 15% when the serum HCO_3^- is greater than 20 mEq/L. Because HCO_3^- is not reabsorbed normally in the proximal tubule, therapy with $NaHCO_3$ will enhance renal potassium wasting and hypokalemia. The two most common causes of acquired proximal RTA in adults are multiple myeloma, in which increased excretion of immunoglobulin light chains injures the proximal tubule epithelium, and chemotherapeutic drug injury of the proximal tubule (ifosfamide). Table 109-8 lists disorders associated with renal tubular acidosis.

Classic distal RTA (RTA type 1) is characterized by inability to acidify urine appropriately during spontaneous or chemically induced acidosis. The defect limits the ability of the collecting duct to excrete $NH4^+$ and other titratable acids, resulting in a net positive acid balance. The typical findings in classic distal RTA include hypokalemia, hyperchloremic acidosis, low urinary NH_4^+ excretion (positive UAG), and inappropriately high urine pH (urine pH > 5.5 despite systemic acidosis). Most patients have hypocitraturia and hypercalciuria, so nephrolithiasis, nephrocalcinosis, and bone disease are common. If bicarbonate administration has been high in an attempt to repair the acidosis, the bicarbonaturia will drive kaliuresis, and the hypokalemia may be severe.[2] Most studies suggest that the acquired or inherited forms of cDRTA are due to defects in the basolateral Cl^-/HCO_3 exchanger or subunits of the H^+-ATPase. Other examples include an abnormal leak pathway (e.g., amphotericin B)[2,53] or abnormalities of the H^+/K^+-ATPase (see Table 109-8). Correction of chronic metabolic acidosis can

---

TABLE 109-8 List of Select Disorders Associated with Renal Tubular Acidosis*

Renal Defect in Net Acid Excretion, Classic Distal Renal Tubular Acidosis (RTA 1)

Systemic or Tubulointerstitial Disease

Medullary sponge kidney
Cryoglobulinemia
Balkan nephropathy
Nephrocalcinosis
Chronic pyelonephritis
HIV nephropathy
Renal transplant
Sjögren syndrome
Thyroiditis
Hyperparathyroidism

Drug or Toxin Induced

Ifosfamide
Amphotericin B
Foscarnet
Toluene
Mercury
Classic analgesic nephropathy

Renal Defect in HCO_3^- Reclamation, Proximal Renal Tubular Acidosis (RTA 2)

Selective (Unassociated with Fanconi Syndrome)

Idiopathic:
 Carbonic anhydrase deficiency or inhibition
 Drugs such as acetazolamide
 Carbonic anhydrase II deficiency with osteopetrosis (Sly syndrome)

Generalized (Associated with Fanconi Syndrome)

Primary: inherited or sporadic
Genetically transmitted systemic diseases: cystinosis, Lowe syndrome, Wilson
 syndrome
Dysproteinemic states:
 Multiple myeloma
 Monoclonal gammopathy
Secondary hyperparathyroidism with chronic hypocalcemia:
 Vitamin D deficiency or resistance
 Vitamin D dependency
Drugs or toxins:
 Ifosfamide
 Lead
 Outdated tetracycline
 Streptozotocin
 Mercury
 Amphotericin B (historic)
Tubulointerstitial diseases:
 Sjögren syndrome
 Medullary cystic disease
 Renal transplantation

Generalized Defect of the Distal Nephron with Hyperkalemia (RTA 4)

Mineralocorticoid Deficiency

Primary aldosterone deficiency:
 Adrenal disease (hemorrhage, destruction, infarction)
 Heparin (Low MW or unfractionated)
 Persistent hypotension in critically ill patient
 Renin angiotensin system modulating agents (ACEI, ARB)
Secondary aldosterone deficiency (hyporeninemic hypoaldosteronism):
 Diabetic nephropathy
 HIV disease
 Tubulointerstitial nephropathy
 NSAID use

Renal Tubular Dysfunction (Voltage Defect)

Drugs that interfere with Na channel or Na^+/K^+-ATPase:
 Amiloride
 Pentamidine
 Triamterene
 Trimethoprim
 Cyclosporine
 Tacrolimus
Disorders associated with tubulointerstitial disease:
 Renal failure
 Lupus nephritis
 Obstructive uropathy
 Renal transplant rejection
 Sickle cell disease

*See following source for complete list of disorders.
Adapted in part from DuBose TD Jr. Acid-base disorders. In: Brenner BM, editor. Brenner and Rector's the kidney. 8th ed. Philadelphia: Saunders; 2008, p. 513-46.

usually be achieved readily in patients with cDRTA by administration of alkali in an amount sufficient to neutralize the production of metabolic acids derived from the diet.[2] In adult patients with distal RTA, this is may be equal to no more than 1 to 3 mEq/kg/d.[54]

In type 4 RTA, generalized distal nephron (collecting tubules) dysfunction is manifested by coexistence of hyperchloremic acidosis and hyperkalemia. In the differential diagnosis, it is important to evaluate the functional status of the renin-aldosterone system and ECF volume, which can effect renal perfusion and function. The specific disorders causing hyperkalemic hyperchloremic metabolic acidosis are outlined in detail in Table 109-8.[55]

Although metabolic acidosis and hyperkalemia occur with regularity in advanced renal insufficiency of any cause (e.g., diabetic nephropathy or tubulointerstitial disease), hyperkalemia with type 4 RTA is disproportionate to the reduction in glomerular filtration rate.

The regulation of potassium excretion is primarily the result of regulation of potassium *secretion*, which responds to hyperkalemia, aldosterone, sodium delivery, and nonreabsorbable anions in the CCD. A useful tool in determining appropriate renal response to hyperkalemia is transtubular potassium gradient (TTKG). This is a clinical estimate of K^+ transfer into the CCD and is helpful in recognizing hyperkalemia of renal origin. An abnormally low fractional excretion of potassium or TTKG in the face of hyperkalemia defines hyperkalemia of renal origin. The following formula is used to calculate the TTKG:

$$TTKG = (Urine\ K/Serum\ K)/(Urine\ osm/Serum\ osm)$$

When the TTKG is low in a hyperkalemic patient (<8), it reveals that the collecting tubule is not responding appropriately to the prevailing hyperkalemia and that potassium secretion is impaired. In contrast, in hyperkalemia of nonrenal origin, the kidney should respond by increasing K^+ secretion, as evidenced by a sharp increase in the TTKG. An important point to consider is that with high urine flow rates, the TTKG underestimates K^+ secretory capacity in the hyperkalemic patient.[1]

The underlying abnormalities that result in RTA type 4 are mineralocorticoid deficiency/resistance or renal tubular dysfunction (voltage defect). The former is most commonly present in older adults with diabetes mellitus or tubulointerstitial disease and renal insufficiency, although other conditions or medications can induce aldosterone deficiency or interfere with its effects (see Tables 109-8 and 109-9).[2] Independent of the tubular defect, hyperkalemia inhibits ammoniagenesis at the proximal tubule and contributes to development of metabolic acidosis. The importance of hyperkalemia as a cause of metabolic acidosis is underscored by the frequent observation that correction of it is associated with a marked increase in net acid excretion and a parallel correction in acidosis.[55]

A variety of clinical conditions and medications result in hyperkalemia with or without associated metabolic acidosis (Table 109-9). Commonly encountered disorders associated with type 4 RTA include diabetic kidney disease, obstructive uropathy, tubulointerstitial disease, and human immunodeficiency virus (HIV)-associated nephropathy (see Table 109-8).

DILUTIONAL AND TOTAL PARENTERAL NUTRITION–ASSOCIATED ACIDOSIS

A rapid increase in extracellular volume (ECV) or addition of exogenous acid (or acid equivalents) to blood can result in the development of hyperchloremic metabolic acidosis (see Table 109-7).[10] Examples of exogenous acid loads include infusion of arginine or lysine during parenteral hyperalimentation. This effect is thought to be secondary to an excess of cationic amino acids as compared with anionic amino acids present in these formulas. The severity of the acidosis associated with the use of protein solutions is less than that encountered with the older protein hydrolysate formulations.[10] Large amounts of normal saline infusion, especially in patients with limited renal function, can cause a decline in serum bicarbonate concentration and is referred to

TABLE 109-9	Causes of Drug-Induced Hyperkalemia

Impaired Renin-Aldosterone Elaboration/Function

Cyclooxygenase inhibitors (NSAIDs)
β-Adrenergic antagonists
Spironolactone
Angiotensin-converting enzyme inhibitors and angiotensin II receptor blockers
Heparin

Inhibitors of Renal Potassium Secretion

Potassium-sparing diuretics (amiloride, triamterene)
Trimethoprim
Pentamidine
Cyclosporine
Digitalis overdose
Lithium

Altered Potassium Distribution

Insulin antagonists (somatostatin, diazoxide)
β-Adrenergic antagonists
α-Adrenergic agonists
Hypertonic solutions
Digitalis
Succinylcholine
Arginine hydrochloride, lysine hydrochloride

Adapted in part from DuBose TD Jr. Acid-base disorders. In: Brenner BM, editor. Brenner and Rector's the kidney. 8th ed. Philadelphia: Saunders; 2008, p. 513-46.

as *dilutional acidosis*. This phenomenon is thought to occur as a result of a change in the volume of distribution of bicarbonate which leads to a decrease in its serum concentration, with reciprocal increase in serum chloride concentration.[53] Nevertheless, Garella and associates have demonstrated that the serum bicarbonate is only diluted modestly by large increases in ECV.[56] Thus, a clinically significant metabolic acidosis would occur only with massive fluid administration. Dilutional acidosis, however, is not uncommon in the ICU, and the intensivist should recognize this phenomenon and consider using solutions with lower chloride concentrations if large amounts of IV fluids are administered. A similar situation may arise from endogenous addition of ketoacids during recovery from ketoacidosis when the sodium salts of ketones may be excreted by the kidneys and lost as potential HCO_3^-.[42]

Metabolic Alkalosis

Metabolic alkalosis in its simplest from is revealed by an elevated arterial pH (alkalemia) and an increase in $Paco_2$ as a result of compensatory alveolar hypoventilation. It is often accompanied by hypochloremia and hypokalemia. The patient with a high $[HCO_3^-]$ and a low $[Cl^-]$ has either metabolic alkalosis or chronic respiratory acidosis. The arterial pH establishes the diagnosis, as it is increased in metabolic alkalosis but decreased or normal in respiratory acidosis. As shown in Table 109-1, the $Paco_2$ increases 6 mm Hg for each 10 mEq/L increase in the $[HCO_3^-]$ above normal. Stated differently, in the range of $[HCO_3^-]$ from 10 to 40 mEq/L, the predicted $Paco_2$ is approximately equal to the patient's $[HCO_3^-] \pm 15$ mEq/L. Metabolic alkalosis is one of the more common acid-base disorders in hospitalized patients and occurs as both a simple and a mixed disorder.[57] Metabolic alkalosis is also frequently observed not as a pure or simple acid-base disturbance, but in association with other disorders such as respiratory acidosis, respiratory alkalosis, and metabolic acidosis (mixed disorders). Mixed metabolic alkalosis–metabolic acidosis can be appreciated only if the accompanying metabolic acidosis is a high-AG acidosis. The mixed disorder can be appreciated by comparison of the increment in the AG above the normal value of 10 mEq/L (ΔAG = Patient's AG − 10), with the decrement in the $[HCO_3^-]$ below the normal value of 25 mEq/L (ΔHCO_3^- = 25 − Patient's HCO_3^-). A mixed metabolic alkalosis–high-AG metabolic acidosis is recognized because the delta values are not similar, and the delta/delta ratio is significantly greater than 1. Often, there is no bicarbonate deficit, yet the AG is significantly elevated. Thus, in a patient with an AG of 20 but near-normal bicarbonate, mixed metabolic alkalosis–metabolic acidosis should be considered.

Common examples include renal failure acidosis (uremic) with vomiting or DKA with vomiting.[1]

PATHOGENESIS AND DIFFERENTIAL DIAGNOSIS

Metabolic alkalosis occurs as a result of net gain of $[HCO_3^-]$ or loss of nonvolatile acid (usually HCl by vomiting) from the extracellular fluid. Because it is unusual for alkali to be added to the body, the disorder involves a generative stage in which the loss of acid usually causes alkalosis, and a maintenance stage in which the kidneys fail to compensate (by excreting HCO_3^-) because of limiting factors such as volume contraction, a low GFR, or depletion of Cl^- or K^+.[1,58]

Under normal circumstances, the kidneys have an impressive capacity to excrete HCO_3^-. Continuation of metabolic alkalosis represents a failure of the kidneys to eliminate HCO_3^- in the usual manner. For HCO_3^- to be added to the extracellular fluid (ECF), it must be administered exogenously or synthesized endogenously, in part or entirely by the kidneys. The kidneys will retain rather than excrete the excess alkali and maintain the alkalosis if one of the following mechanisms is operative:

1. Cl^- deficiency (ECF contraction) exists concurrently with K^+ deficiency, leading to a reduction in GFR and/or enhanced HCO_3^- reabsorption. This combination evokes secondary hyperreninemic hyperaldosteronism and stimulates H^+ secretion in the collecting duct and ammoniagenesis. Repair of the alkalosis may be accomplished by saline and K^+ administration.
2. Hypokalemia exists because of autonomous hyperaldosteronism unresponsive to increased ECF. Correction of alkalosis in such setting requires pharmacologic or surgical intervention, not saline administration.[58]

To establish the cause of metabolic alkalosis (Table 109-10), it is necessary to assess the status of the ECV (orthostatic vitals), the serum $[K^+]$, and the renin-aldosterone system.[1] For example, the presence of chronic hypertension and chronic hypokalemia in an alkalotic patient suggests either some type of primary mineralocorticoid excess or that the hypertensive patient is receiving diuretics. Low plasma renin activity and normal urine $[Na^+]$ and $[Cl^-]$ in a patient who is not taking diuretics indicate a primary mineralocorticoid excess syndrome. The combination of hypokalemia and alkalosis in a normotensive, nonedematous patient can be a challenging problem. The possible causes to consider include Bartter or Gitelman syndrome, Mg^{2+} deficiency, surreptitious vomiting, exogenous alkali, and diuretic ingestion. Determination of urine electrolytes (especially the urine $[Cl^-]$) and screening of the urine for diuretics may be helpful (Table 109-11). If the urine is alkaline with an elevated $[Na^+]$ and $[K^+]$ but low $[Cl^-]$, the diagnosis is usually either prolonged vomiting (overt or surreptitious) or alkali ingestion. If the urine is relatively acid and has low concentrations of Na^+, K^+, and Cl^-, the most likely possibilities are prior vomiting, the posthypercapnic state, or prior diuretic ingestion. If, on the other hand, urine sodium, potassium, or chloride concentrations are not depressed, magnesium deficiency, Bartter's or Gitelman's syndrome, or current diuretic ingestion should be considered. Bartter's syndrome is distinguished from Gitelman's syndrome by hypocalciuria and hypomagnesemia in the latter disorder. The genetic and molecular basis of these two disorders has been elucidated.[1,57]

ALKALI ADMINISTRATION

Chronic administration of alkali to individuals with normal renal function rarely causes alkalosis, because the kidney has a high capacity for bicarbonate excretion. However, in patients with coexistent hemodynamic disturbances, alkalosis can develop because the normal capacity to excrete HCO_3^- may be exceeded or there may be enhanced reabsorption of HCO_3^-. Such patients include those who receive oral or IV HCO_3^-, acetate loads (parenteral hyperalimentation solutions), citrate loads (transfusions or continuous renal replacement therapy), or antacids plus cation-exchange resins (aluminum hydroxide and sodium polystyrene sulfonate).

TABLE 109-10	Causes of Metabolic Alkalosis

Exogenous HCO_3^- Loads
Acute alkali administration
Milk-alkali syndrome

Effective Extracellular Volume Contraction, Normotension, Hypokalemia, and Secondary Hyperreninemic Hyperaldosteronism
Gastrointestinal origin:
  Vomiting
  Gastric aspiration
  Congenital chloridorrhea
  Villous adenoma
  Combined administration of sodium polystyrene sulfonate (Kayexalate and aluminum hydroxide)
Renal origin:
  Diuretics (especially thiazides and loop diuretics)
  Acute
  Chronic
  Edematous states
  Posthypercapnic state
  Hypercalcemia-hypoparathyroidism
  Recovery from lactic acidosis or ketoacidosis
  Nonreabsorbable anions such as penicillin, carbenicillin
  Mg^{++} deficiency
  K^+ depletion
  Bartter's syndrome (loss-of-function mutation of Cl^- transport in thick ascending limb of Henle's loop)
  Gitelman's syndrome (loss-of-function mutation in Na^+/Cl^- cotransporter)
  Carbohydrate refeeding after starvation

Extracellular Volume Expansion, Hypertension, K^+ Deficiency, and Hypermineralocorticoidism
Associated with high renin:
  Renal artery stenosis
  Accelerated hypertension
  Renin-secreting tumor
  Estrogen therapy
Associated with low renin:
  Primary aldosteronism
  Adenoma
  Hyperplasia
  Carcinoma
  Glucocorticoid suppressible
Adrenal enzymatic defects:
  11_β-Hydroxylase deficiency
  17_α-Hydroxylase deficiency
Cushing's syndrome or disease:
  Ectopic corticotropin
  Adrenal carcinoma
  Adrenal adenoma
  Primary pituitary
Other:
  Licorice
  Carbenoxolone
  Chewer's tobacco
  Lydia Pinkham tablets

Gain-of-Function Mutation of ENaC with Extracellular Fluid Volume Expansion, Hypertension, K^+ Deficiency, and Hyporeninemic Hypoaldosteronism
Liddle's syndrome

METABOLIC ALKALOSIS ASSOCIATED WITH EXTRACELLULAR FLUID VOLUME CONTRACTION, HYPOKALEMIA, AND HYPERRENINEMIC HYPERALDOSTERONISM

(See Table 109-10.)

Gastrointestinal Origin

Gastrointestinal loss of H^+ from vomiting or gastric aspiration results in retention of HCO_3^-. The loss of fluid and NaCl in vomitus or nasogastric suction results in contraction of the ECV and an increase in the secretion of renin and aldosterone. Volume contraction causes a reduction in GFR and an enhanced capacity of the renal tubule to reabsorb HCO_3^-. During active vomiting, there is continued addition of HCO_3^- to plasma in exchange for Cl^-, and the plasma $[HCO_3^-]$ exceeds the reabsorptive capacity of the proximal tubule. The excess $NaHCO_3$

TABLE 109-11	Diagnosis of Metabolic Alkalosis	
Saline-Responsive Alkalosis	**Saline-Unresponsive Alkalosis**
LOW URINARY [Cl⁻]	HIGH OR NORMAL URINARY [Cl⁻]
Normotensive	Hypertensive
Vomiting, nasogastric aspiration	Primary aldosteronism
Diuretics	Cushing's syndrome
Post hypercapnia	Renal artery stenosis
Bicarbonate therapy of organic acidosis	Renal failure plus alkali therapy
K⁺ deficiency	Normotensive
Hypertensive	Mg⁺⁺ deficiency
Liddle's syndrome	Severe K⁺ deficiency
	Bartter's syndrome
	Gitelman's syndrome
	Diuretics

reaches the distal tubule, where H⁺ secretion is enhanced by aldosterone and the delivery of the poorly reabsorbed anion HCO_3^-.[57] Because of contraction of the ECV and hypochloremia, Cl⁻ is avidly conserved by the kidney, as recognized by a low urinary chloride concentration (see Table 109-11). Correction of the contracted ECV with NaCl and repair of K⁺ deficits corrects the acid-base disorder. Metabolic alkalosis has been described in cases of villous adenoma and is ascribed to adenoma-derived high K⁺ secretion. The K⁺ and volume depletion likely causes the alkalosis, because colonic secretion is alkaline.

Renal Origin

Diuretics. Drugs that induce chloruresis without bicarbonaturia, such as thiazides and loop diuretics (furosemide, bumetanide, and torsemide), acutely diminish the ECV without altering the total-body bicarbonate content. The serum $[HCO_3^-]$ increases and "contraction" alkalosis ensues. The chronic administration of diuretics tends to generate an alkalosis by increasing distal salt delivery, so that K⁺ and H⁺ secretion are stimulated. The alkalosis is maintained by persistence of the contraction of the ECV, secondary hyperaldosteronism, K⁺ deficiency, and the direct effect of the diuretic (as long as diuretic administration continues). Repair of the alkalosis is achieved by providing isotonic saline to correct the ECV deficit.

Bartter's Syndrome. Three types of Bartter's syndrome have been described, and all are inherited as autosomal recessive disorders. Both classic Bartter's syndrome and the antenatal Bartter's involve impaired Cl⁻ absorption, which results in salt wasting, volume depletion, and activation of the renin-angiotensin system. Excessive prostaglandin elaboration commonly found with this disorder is in response to volume depletion, hypokalemia, and high angiotensin II levels.[59-64] These phenotypes are the result of loss-of-function mutations of one of the genes that encode three transporters involved in vectorial NaCl absorption in the thick ascending limb of Henle's loop.[65] The most prevalent disorder is a mutation of the gene that encodes the bumetanide-sensitive Na⁺ 2Cl⁻ K⁺ co-transporter (NKCC2 or BSC1) on the apical membrane. A second mutation has been discovered in the gene that encodes the apical K⁺ conductance channel (ROMK),[65] which operates in parallel with the Na⁺ 2Cl⁻ K⁺ transporter to recycle K⁺.[66] A third defect, in the basolateral Cl⁻ channel which transports Cl⁻ out of the cell, has been described. All three defects have the same net effect: loss of Cl⁻ transport in the thick ascending limb of Henle's loop.[67,68] Such defects would predictably lead to extracellular fluid contraction, hyperreninemic hyperaldosteronism, and increased delivery of Na⁺ to the distal nephron and thus alkalosis and renal K⁺ wasting and hypokalemia. Secondary overproduction of prostaglandins, juxtaglomerular apparatus hypertrophy, and vascular pressor unresponsiveness would then ensue.

Distinction from surreptitious vomiting, diuretic administration, and laxative abuse is necessary to make the diagnosis of Bartter's syndrome.[1] The finding of a low urinary Cl⁻ concentration is helpful in identifying the vomiting patient (see Table 109-11).[69,70] The urinary

Cl⁻ concentration in Bartter's syndrome would be expected to be normal or increased rather than depressed.

Treatment of Bartter's syndrome is generally focused on the repair of hypokalemia by inhibition of the renin-angiotensin-aldosterone or the prostaglandin-kinin system. K⁺ supplementation,[71] Mg⁺⁺ repletion,[72,73] propranolol,[74,75] spironolactone,[74,75] prostaglandin inhibitors,[74,75] and angiotensin-converting enzyme inhibitors[76,77] have all been advocated, but each has met with limited success.

Gitelman's Syndrome. Gitelman's syndrome resembles Bartter's syndrome in that an autosomal recessive Cl⁻-resistant metabolic alkalosis is associated with hypokalemia, a normal to low blood pressure, volume depletion with secondary hyperreninemic hyperaldosteronism, and juxtaglomerular hyperplasia.

Gitelman's syndrome, which occurs more often in adults, is distinguished from Bartter's syndrome, which occurs more commonly in children, by the presence of hypocalciuria, hypermagnesuria, and hypomagnesemia.[78-80] These unique features mimic the effect of chronic thiazide diuretic administration. Gitelman's syndrome is the result of missense mutations (several have been described) in the gene SLC12A3, which encodes the thiazide-sensitive distal convoluted tubule Na⁺/Cl⁻ co-transporter (NCCT).[80-82] Loss of activity of the NaCl co-transporter increases tubule Ca⁺⁺ absorption, leading to the classic finding of hypocalciuria. A large study of adults with proven Gitelman's syndrome and NCCT mutations showed that salt craving, nocturia, cramps, and fatigue were more common than in sex- and age-matched controls.[82] Women experienced exacerbation of symptoms during menses, and many had complicated pregnancies. Treatment of Gitelman's syndrome, as with Bartter's syndrome, consists of liberal dietary sodium and potassium salts, but with the addition of magnesium supplementation in most patients. Angiotensin-converting enzyme inhibitors have been suggested to be helpful in selected patients but can cause frank hypotension.

Nonreabsorbable Anions and Magnesium Deficiency. Administration of large quantities of nonreabsorbable anions such as penicillin or carbenicillin can enhance distal acidification and K⁺ secretion by increasing the transepithelial potential difference (lumen negative). Mg⁺⁺ deficiency results in hypokalemic alkalosis by enhancing distal acidification through stimulation of renin and hence aldosterone secretion.[83]

Potassium Depletion. Pure K⁺ depletion causes metabolic alkalosis, although generally of only modest severity. One reason the alkalosis is usually mild is that K⁺ depletion also causes positive sodium chloride balance with or without mineralocorticoid administration. The salt retention in turn antagonizes the degree of alkalemia. When access to salt as well as to K⁺ is restricted, more severe alkalosis develops. Activation of the renal H⁺/K⁺-ATPase in the collecting duct by chronic hypokalemia likely plays a major role in maintenance of the alkalosis. Specifically, chronic hypokalemia has been shown to markedly increase the abundance of the colonic H⁺/K⁺-ATPase mRNA and protein in the outer medullary collecting duct. In animals, the alkalosis is maintained in part by reduction in GFR without a change in tubule HCO_3^- transport. In humans, the pathophysiologic basis of the alkalosis has not been well defined. Alkalosis associated with severe K⁺ depletion, however, is resistant to salt administration. Repair of the K⁺ deficiency is necessary to correct the alkalosis.[83]

After Treatment of Lactic Acidosis or Ketoacidosis. When an underlying stimulus for the generation of lactic acid or ketoacid is removed rapidly, as with repair of circulatory insufficiency or with insulin therapy, the lactate or ketones are metabolized to yield an equivalent amount of HCO_3^-. Other sources of new HCO_3^- are additive with the original amount generated by organic anion metabolism to create an excess of HCO_3^-. The sources of the additional alkali include (1) new HCO_3^- added to the blood by the kidneys as a result of enhanced acid excretion during the preexisting period of acidosis and (2) alkali therapy during the treatment phase of the acidosis. Acidosis-induced contraction of the ECV and K^+ deficiency act to sustain the alkalosis.[57]

Post Hypercapnia. Prolonged CO_2 retention with chronic respiratory acidosis enhances renal HCO_3^- absorption and the generation of new HCO_3^- (increased net acid excretion). If $Paco_2$ is returned to normal, the metabolic alkalosis results from the persistently elevated $[HCO_3^-]$. Alkalosis develops if the elevated $Paco_2$ is abruptly returned toward normal by a change in mechanically controlled ventilation. Associated ECV contraction does not allow complete repair of the alkalosis by correction of the $Paco_2$ alone, and alkalosis persists until Cl^- supplementation is provided.

METABOLIC ALKALOSIS ASSOCIATED WITH HYPERVOLEMIA, HYPERTENSION, AND HYPERALDOSTERONISM

Mineralocorticoid administration or excess production (primary aldosteronism of Cushing's syndrome and adrenal cortical enzyme defects) increases net acid excretion and tends to result in metabolic alkalosis. The degree of alkalosis is augmented by the simultaneous increase in K^+ excretion leading to K^+ deficiency and hypokalemia. Salt intake for sufficient distal Na^+ delivery is also a prerequisite for the development of both the hypokalemia and the alkalosis. Hypertension develops partly as a result of ECF expansion from salt retention. The alkalosis is not progressive and is generally mild. Volume expansion tends to antagonize the decrease in GFR and/or increase in tubule acidification induced by hypermineralocorticoidism and K^+ deficiency. The kaliuresis persists and causes continued K^+ depletion with polydipsia, inability to concentrate the urine, and polyuria. Increased aldosterone levels may be the result of autonomous primary adrenal overproduction or of secondary aldosterone release due to renal overproduction of renin. In both situations, the normal feedback of ECV on net aldosterone production is disrupted, and hypertension from volume retention can result (see Table 109-10). States associated with inappropriately high renin levels include renovascular disease and accelerated and malignant hypertension. Estrogens increase renin substrate and, hence, angiotensin II formation. Primary tumor overproduction of renin is another rare cause of hyperreninemic hyperaldosterone–induced metabolic alkalosis.[83]

Primary adrenal overproduction of mineralocorticoid suppresses renin elaboration and can be seen in adrenal adenoma or hyperplasia. Abnormally high glucocorticoid production (Cushing's disease or syndrome) caused by adrenal adenoma or carcinoma or due to ectopic corticotropin production may also cause metabolic alkalosis. The alkalosis in this setting may be ascribed to coexisting mineralocorticoid (deoxycorticosterone and corticosterone) hypersecretion but also the fact that glucocorticoids have the capability of occupying and activating the mineralocorticoid receptors.

Ingestion of licorice, carbenoxolone, chewer's tobacco, or nasal spray can cause a typical pattern of hypermineralocorticoidism. These substances inhibit 11_β-hydroxysteroid dehydrogenase (which normally metabolizes cortisol to an inactive metabolite), and the cortisol buildup results in interaction and activation of type 1 renal mineralocorticoid receptors, mimicking aldosterone.[1]

Liddle's syndrome results from increased activity of the collecting duct Na^+ channel (ENaC). Liddle's syndrome is a rare inherited disorder associated with hypertension due to volume expansion, manifested as hypokalemic alkalosis and normal aldosterone levels.

Symptoms of Metabolic Alkalosis

With metabolic alkalosis, changes in central and peripheral nervous system function are similar to those of hypocalcemia; symptoms include mental confusion, obtundation, and a predisposition to seizures, paresthesia, muscular cramping, tetany, aggravation of arrhythmias, and hypoxemia in chronic obstructive pulmonary disease. Related electrolyte abnormalities include hypokalemia and hypophosphatemia.

Treatment of Metabolic Alkalosis

The maintenance of metabolic alkalosis represents a failure of the kidney to excrete bicarbonate efficiently because of chloride or potassium deficiency, or continuous mineralocorticoid elaboration, or both. Treatment is primarily directed at correcting the underlying stimulus for HCO_3^- generation and restoring the ability of the kidney to excrete the excess bicarbonate.[1,58] Assistance is gained in the diagnosis and treatment of metabolic alkalosis by paying attention to the urinary chloride concentration, the arterial blood pressure, and the volume status of the patient (particularly the presence or absence of orthostasis) (see Table 109-11 and Figure 109-4).[1] Particularly helpful in the history is the presence or absence of vomiting, diuretic use, or alkali therapy. A high urine chloride concentration and hypertension suggests that mineralocorticoid excess is present. If primary aldosteronism is present, correction of the underlying cause will reverse the alkalosis (adenoma, bilateral hyperplasia, Cushing's syndrome). Patients with bilateral adrenal hyperplasia may respond to spironolactone. Normotensive patients with a high urine chloride may have Bartter's or Gitelman's syndrome if diuretic use or vomiting can be excluded. A low urine chloride and relative hypotension suggests a chloride-responsive metabolic alkalosis such as vomiting or nasogastric suction. $[H^+]$ loss by the stomach or kidneys can be mitigated by the use of proton pump inhibitors or the discontinuation of diuretics. The second aspect of treatment is to remove the factors that sustain HCO_3^- reabsorption, such as ECV contraction or K^+ deficiency. Although K^+ deficits should be repaired, NaCl therapy is usually sufficient to reverse the alkalosis if ECV contraction is present, as indicated by low urine $[Cl^-]$.

Patients with congestive heart failure or unexplained volume overexpansion represent special challenges in the ICU. Patients with a low urine chloride concentration, which is usually indicative of a "chloride-responsive" form of metabolic alkalosis, may not tolerate normal saline infusion. Renal HCO_3^- loss can be accelerated by administration of acetazolamide (250-500 mg IV), a carbonic anhydrase inhibitor, if associated conditions preclude infusion of saline (elevated pulmonary capillary wedge pressure, or evidence of CHF.[1] Acetazolamide is usually very effective in patients with adequate renal function but can exacerbate urinary K^+ losses. Dilute hydrochloric acid (0.1 N HCl) is also effective but can cause hemolysis and may be difficult to titrate. If used, the goal should be to not restore the pH to normal but to a pH of approximately 7.50. Alternatively, acidification can also be achieved with oral NH_4Cl, which should be avoided in the presence of liver disease. Hemodialysis against a dialysate low in $[HCO_3^-]$ and high in $[Cl^-]$ can be effective when renal function is impaired. Patients receiving continuous renal replacement therapy in the ICU are prone to development of metabolic alkalosis due to bicarbonate-based replacement fluid/dialysate or when citrate regional anticoagulation is employed.

KEY POINTS

Diagnosis of types of disturbances

1. Simple and mixed disturbances can be differentiated through appreciation of the limits of compensation and calculation of the anion gap (AG).

2. Mixed disorders are more common in critically ill patients.

3. A pathway to correct diagnosis involves a stepwise approach.

Metabolic acidosis

1. Two broad types of acidosis can be defined by calculation of the AG, including high-AG and normal-AG acidosis.

2. $AG =$ unmeasured anions − unmeasured cations $= Na − (Cl + HCO_3) = AG$ (normal 9 ± 3 mEq/L)

3. AG must be corrected for hypoalbuminemia. Expected $AG = [\text{albumin}] \times 2.5$.

4. Compensation for metabolic acidosis: $\downarrow Paco_2 = (1.5 \times [HCO_3]) + 8$ or $1.25 \times \Delta HCO_3$.

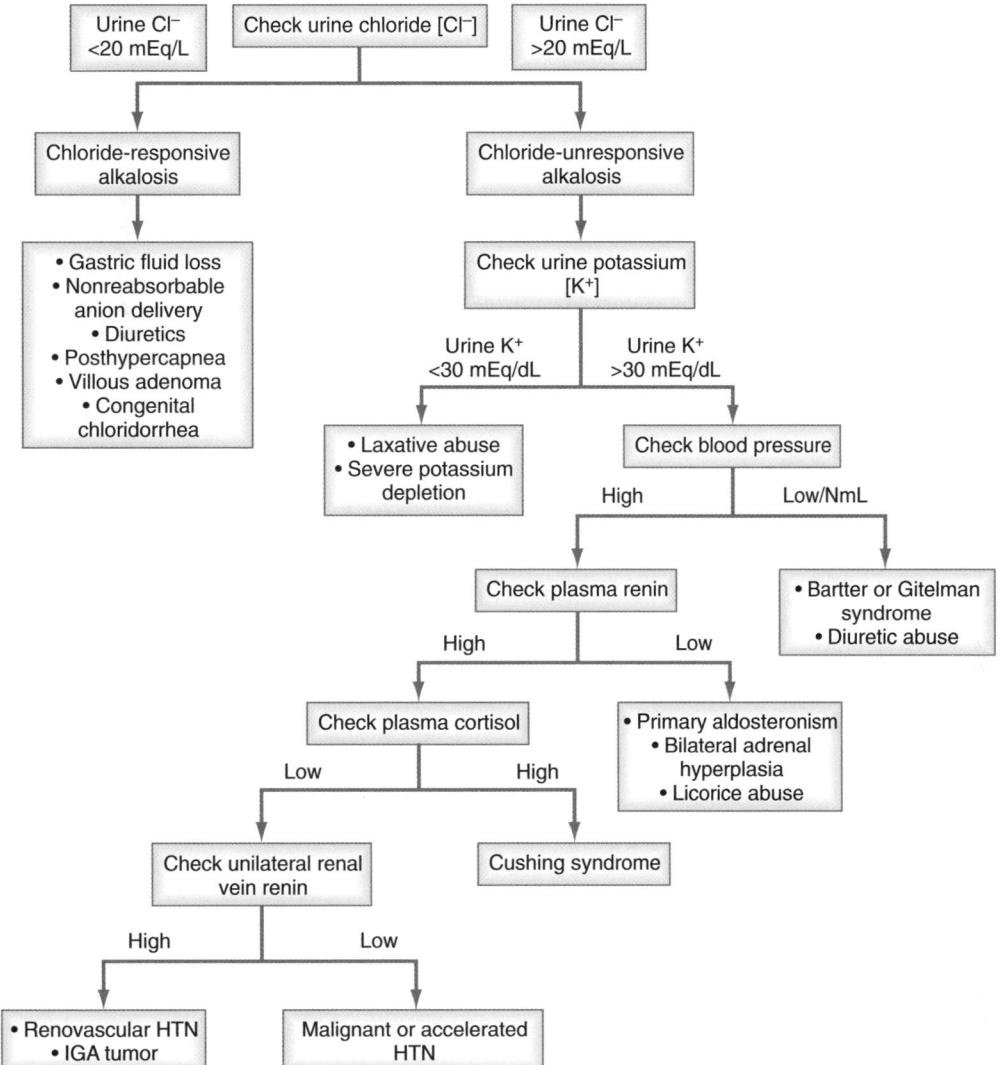

Figure 109-4 Workup of metabolic alkalosis. *(Data from DuBose TD Jr. Acid-base disorders. In: Brenner BM, editor. Brenner and Rector's the kidney. 8th ed. Philadelphia: Saunders; 2008, p. 513.)*

5. Treatment of acidosis requires consideration of the concept of "potential" bicarbonate.

High–anion gap acidoses

1. Four categories of high-AG acidosis can be identified readily through simple clinical laboratory tests. These include lactic acidosis, ketoacidosis, renal failure, and ingestions.

2. L-Lactic acid acidosis is the most common type of high-AG acidosis in the ICU.

L-Lactic acidosis

1. L-Lactic acid acidosis occurs with or without hemodynamic compromise in the ICU.

2. Type A results from impairment in tissue oxygenation (hypoperfusion or hypoxemia). However, there is no obvious impairment of either in type B lactic acidosis.

3. Bowel ischemia (type A) and therapy for HIV infection with nucleoside reverse-transcriptase inhibitors (type B) are frequent causes.

4. Therapy should first be directed to the underlying cause of lactate generation.

5. Alkali therapy has many disadvantages and should be administered with understanding of the pathophysiology of lactate generation.

Ketoacidosis

1. Diabetic ketoacidosis (DKA) is common, but alcoholic ketoacidosis is often missed. Distinguishing features include the degree of ketonemia and the relative level of β-hydroxybutyrate—the latter being a characteristic of alcoholic ketoacidosis, not DKA.

2. DKA responds to low doses of regular insulin and volume reexpansion with 0.9% NaCl.

3. Clearing of ketones in plasma is reflected by progressive correction of the anion gap.

Ingestion-induced acidosis

1. Toxins such as ethylene glycol and methyl alcohol increase the osmolar gap (OG). An OG greater than 10 to 15 mOsm/kg suggests ingestion.

2. OG = measured serum osmolarity − calculated serum osmolarity. Calculated osmolarity = (2 × Na) + (glucose/18) + (BUN/2.8)

3. Treatment should not be delayed and should include intravenous (IV) ethyl alcohol or fomepizole, IV fluids, NaHCO$_3$, thiamine, and hemodialysis.

Non-gap or hyperchloremic metabolic acidoses

1. Hyperchloremic acidosis is characterized by a normal anion gap, high chloride, and low bicarbonate.

2. Renal causes can be distinguished from gastrointestinal causes by calculation of the urine anion gap (UAG), which is an indirect assay for renal acid (NH_4^+) excretion.

3. $UAG = [Na^+ + K^+]_u - [Cl^-]_u$.
   Negative UAG = increased renal NH_4^+ excretion (appropriate renal response) = GI cause.
   Positive UAG = failure of kidneys to secrete NH_4^+ = renal cause.

4. UAG interpretation assumes patient is not hypovolemic and does not have a high-AG acidosis.

Metabolic alkalosis

1. Once generated by bicarbonate gain or acid loss, metabolic alkalosis is maintained by renal mechanisms that encourage bicarbonate retention rather than excretion.

2. Measurement of urine [Cl^-] and clinical estimation of extracellular fluid (ECF) volume status is helpful in evaluation of the causes of metabolic alkalosis.

3. Compensation for metabolic alkalosis: $\uparrow Pa_{CO_2} = 0.75 \times \Delta HCO_3$

4. Metabolic alkalosis in the ICU may occur in combination with other acid-base disorders (mixed acid-base disorders).

5. Combined metabolic and respiratory alkalosis can result in extreme elevation of the pH and is associated with high mortality.

6. Unique causes of alkalemia in the ICU include nasogastric suction, vomiting, diuretics, alkali administration, steroids, mechanical ventilation, hyperalimentation, magnesium deficiency, potassium deficiency, and third-space sequestration of ECF volume.

ANNOTATED REFERENCES

Bonnet F, Bonarek M, Morlat P, et al. Risk factors for lactic acidosis in HIV-infected patients treated with nucleoside reverse-transcriptase inhibitors: A case-control study. Clin Infect Dis 2003; 36:1324-8.
The problem of NRTI-induced lactic acid acidosis in patients with HIV is evaluated by a case-controlled study to determine risk factors. Two factors were identified to be associated with an increased risk of lactic acidosis: (1) creatinine clearance less than 70 mL/min and (2) a low CD4⁺ T-lymphocyte count before inception of therapy. Interestingly, the total cumulative exposure to NRTIs was not associated with an increased risk of lactic acid acidosis. Therefore, creatinine clearance and CD4⁺ T-lymphocyte count should be monitored in patients infected with HIV and could lead to modifications in antiretroviral therapy to diminish the risk of occurrence of lactic acidosis.

Bouman CS, Oudemans-van Straaten HM, Schultz MJ, Vroom MB. Hemofiltration in sepsis and systemic inflammatory response syndrome: the role of dosing and timing. J Crit Care 2007;22:1-12. Epub 2007 Jan 31.
The use of continuous forms of renal replacement therapy to control volume overload and correct electrolyte abnormalities in the ICU setting is common, and the potential role in treating sepsis with renal replacement therapy techniques may prove to be a milestone in critical care medicine.

Halperin ML, Hammeke M, Jose RG, et al. Metabolic acidosis in the alcoholic: a pathophysiologic approach. Metabolism 1983;32:308.
Alcoholic ketoacidosis is underdiagnosed clinically. This disorder cannot only result in life-threatening acidemia but, as a result of malnutrition, causes life-threatening hypophosphatemia. This scholarly review explains the pathophysiology and provides a basis for appreciation of the clinical syndrome.

Ogedegbe AE, Thomas DL, Diehl AM. Hyperlactatemia syndromes associated with HIV therapy. Lancet Infect Dis 2003;3:329-37.
The incidence of hyperlactatemia, as revealed in this study, is now approaching 20% in HIV-infected patients receiving NRTIs. The reported incidence probably underestimates the actual occurrence of lactic acidosis in such patients, especially because recognition may be difficult because many patients remain asymptomatic. However, studies show that life-threatening metabolic acidosis with hepatic steatosis occurs with NRTI therapy. This important public health problem is summarized thoroughly in this paper.

Mizock BA, Belyaev S, Mecher C. Unexplained metabolic acidosis in critically ill patients: the role of pyroglutamic acid. Intensive Care Med 2004;30:502-5.
This paper identifies an important and recently realized cause of high-AG acidosis in the critical care setting. This is an unsuspecting yet very common setting in which metabolic acidosis due to accumulation of this compound may develop, hence this information is critical to the clinician when formulating diagnostic and therapeutic plans for high-AG acidosis.

Stacpoole PW, Nagaraja NJ, Hutson AD. Efficacy of dichloroacetate as a lactate-lowering drug. J Clin Pharmacol 2003;43:683-91.
This paper by the same senior author who performed the first controlled clinical trial of dichloroacetate for treatment of lactic acidosis in adults demonstrates that the maximum lactate-lowering effect of dichloroacetate is dose dependent but independent of time after administration. The study suggests that dichloroacetate could be effective in reducing lactate levels in patients with mild hyperlactatemia. This may be an important observation for ongoing investigation in low-level hyperlactatemia as it applies to a number of clinical circumstances.

REFERENCES

Access the complete reference list online at http://www.expertconsult.com.

110

Disorders of Water Balance

S. ROB TODD

Water, the body's most abundant constituent, accounts for approximately 50% of lean body mass in females and 60% of lean body mass in males. As shown in Figure 110-1, total body water is distributed between the intracellular compartment (two-thirds of total body water) and the extracellular compartment (one-third of total body water). The extracellular compartment is subdivided into the interstitial compartment (three-fourths of extracellular body water) and the plasma compartment (one-fourth of extracellular body water).[1]

The concentration of solutes in body fluids, as reflected in extracellular fluid by the serum sodium ion concentration, is tightly regulated between 138 and 142 mmol/L. This precise control is achieved by the maintenance of water balance; intake and losses are matched in a steady-state situation, despite marked fluctuations in daily solute and water intake. Water intake is determined primarily by thirst. Water excretion is controlled by the hypothalamic secretion of vasopressin (antidiuretic hormone [ADH]) and its target tissue, the renal collecting tubule. This allows for enormous flexibility because the kidney is able to dilute or concentrate urine (osmolality as low as 50 mOsm/kg H_2O or as high as 1200 mOsm/kg H_2O), depending on the body's need to excrete or retain water, respectively. Under water-loading conditions, the kidney can excrete up to 20 to 25 L of urine a day. Likewise, the kidney has the ability to excrete as little as 0.5 L of urine per day (under conditions of water deprivation).[1]

Control of Serum Sodium Concentration

Sodium is the most abundant cation in the extracellular compartment and is therefore the major determinant of plasma osmolality (Posm):

$$Posm\,(mOsm/kg) = 2[Na\,(mEq/L)] + [Blood\ urea\ nitrogen\ (mg/dL)/2.8] + [Glucose\,(mg/dL)/18]$$

Under normal physiologic conditions, plasma osmolality is maintained between 280 and 290 mOsm/kg. Fluctuations in plasma osmolality outside this range are sensed by osmoreceptors in the hypothalamus, which is normally the primary determinant of the secretion of vasopressin, a cyclic octapeptide synthesized and secreted by supraoptic and paraventricular nuclei within the hypothalamus. The threshold for the osmotic release of vasopressin is 280 to 290 mOsm/kg, and the receptors are sensitive to changes in plasma osmolality of as little as 1% (Figure 110-2). The stimulus for vasopressin release is not limited to changes in osmolality. The primary nonosmotic stimulus for vasopressin secretion is decreased effective arterial blood volume, which can achieve a far greater rise in vasopressin levels than hyperosmolality can. Additional nonosmotic stimuli for vasopressin secretion include nausea, hypotension, and pain.

The primary site of action for vasopressin is within the principal cells of the renal collecting ducts. As illustrated in Figure 110-3, vasopressin binds to the V2 receptors on the basolateral membrane of these cells. Through a G protein–activated cascade, this results in increased insertion of a specific water (aquaporin 2) in the luminal membrane[2] and renders the collecting tubule permeable to water.

Thirst also plays an important role in water balance. The most potent stimulus for thirst is hypertonicity; a change of 2% to 3% in plasma osmolality produces a strong desire to consume water. The threshold that triggers the sensation of thirst is higher than that for the release of vasopressin and usually occurs at a plasma osmolality of 290 to 295 mOsm/kg (see Figure 110-2). A decrease in effective arterial blood volume also stimulates thirst.

Protection against states of water excess is provided by the normally functioning renal diluting system. The three essential components of the diluting mechanism are depicted in Figure 110-4. First, because the major site of urine dilution is the water-impermeable ascending limb of the loop of Henle and the distal convoluted tubule, it is necessary to have normal delivery of tubular fluid to the distal nephron. Therefore, either a decreased glomerular filtration rate or increased proximal tubule fluid reabsorption limits the volume of dilute urine available for excretion. Second, the diluting segment of the nephron must be functioning normally. Thiazide diuretics, for example, impair the distal convoluted tubule's ability to maximally dilute tubular fluid by blocking the thiazide-sensitive Na^+/Cl^- channel. Third, in order to excrete a dilute urine, vasopressin must be absent so that the collecting duct remains impermeable to water. With this diluting system intact, the kidney can handle a large load of free water (up to 1 L/h) without changes in serum sodium and thus serum osmolality.

An individual's average daily solute load is approximately 600 mOsm. In states of low water intake, the kidney can concentrate the urine to 1200 mOsm/kg, therefore allowing for the excretion of as little as 0.5 L of urine per day. For this to occur, the renal concentrating mechanism must operate normally. The determinants of the renal concentrating mechanism are depicted in Figure 110-5. The water-impermeable thick ascending loop of Henle actively reabsorbs sodium chloride into the medullary interstitium while leaving water behind in the tubular fluid. The reabsorbed sodium increases the osmolality of the interstitium, which reaches its maximum at the papillary tip of the medulla. In the presence of vasopressin, water in the collecting duct is able to travel down its osmotic gradient and is reabsorbed. Once vasopressin is secreted, the collecting duct must be able to respond to it. Any disorder or pharmacologic agent that impairs the ability of vasopressin to act on the collecting ducts will incapacitate the renal concentrating mechanism and lead to dilute urine excretion.

Figure 110-6 summarizes the mechanisms that maintain plasma tonicity and culminate in altered serum sodium values when impaired. These disorders arise whenever there is a disturbance in the body's regulation of the relative amount of water to sodium. Hypernatremia results from a decrease in water relative to sodium (a water deficit state), and hyponatremia is caused by an increase in water relative to sodium (a water excess state).

Hypernatremia

Hypernatremia is defined as a serum sodium concentration greater than 145 mEq/L. Its incidence in hospitalized patients ranges from 0.63% to 2.23%, with the elderly being more susceptible.[3] Hypernatremia results in significant morbidity and mortality, ranging from 42% to 70% in adult patients. Acute elevations of serum sodium above 160 mEq/L are associated with a mortality rate of 75%, whereas mortality in chronic hypernatremia is 10%.

Hypernatremia develops whenever intake is less than the sum of extrarenal and renal water losses or, less commonly, when too much salt is introduced without adequate water intake. The primary defense mechanism against water depletion and hyperosmolarity is the renal

TOTAL BODY WATER IN A 70-KG MAN = 42L

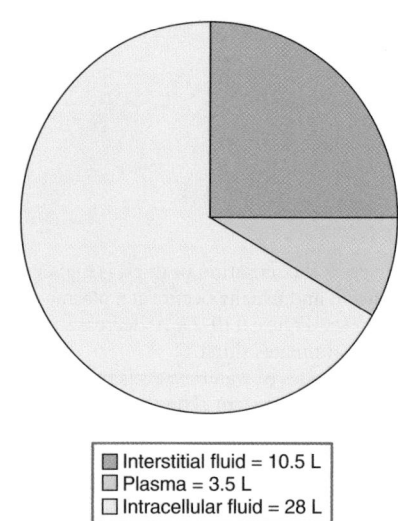

Interstitial fluid = 10.5 L
Plasma = 3.5 L
Intracellular fluid = 28 L

Figure 110-1 Body water distribution into different compartments. Extracellular fluid volume (14 L) is sum of interstitial fluid (10.5 L) and plasma fluid (3.5 L).

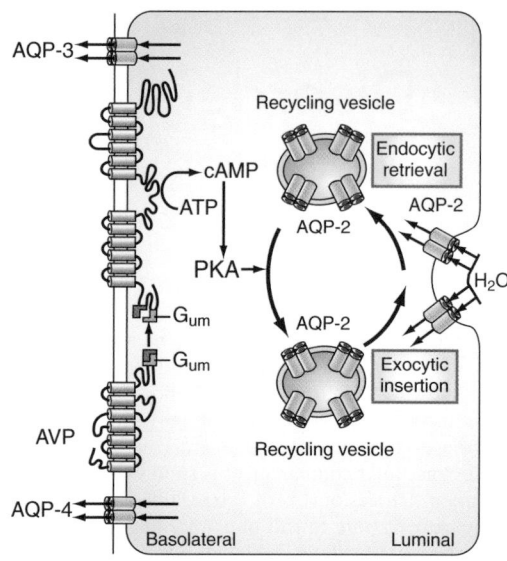

Figure 110-3 Intracellular action of vasopressin by its interaction with V2 receptor on basolateral membrane of collecting duct. This interaction leads to increased adenylate cyclase activity via the stimulatory G protein (Gs), which in turn causes vesicles in cytoplasm carrying water-channel protein, aquaporin (AQP)-2, to move throughout cell and fuse with luminal membrane, thus increasing water permeability of collecting duct cells. Water channels are then recycled by endocytosis when cell is no longer stimulated by vasopressin. ATP, adenosine triphosphate, AVP, arginine vasopressin; cAMP, cyclic adenosine monophosphate; PKA, protein kinase A. (*From Kumar S, Berl T. Disorders of water metabolism. In: Schrier RW, editor. Atlas of disease of the kidney. Philadelphia: Current Medicine; 1999, p. 1.9–.22.*)

concentrating capacity. However, even maximally concentrated urine does not prevent all water losses. Thirst also plays an important role in preventing water depletion. So long as water losses can be replaced, normal serum sodium concentration can be maintained. Most hypernatremic patients therefore have either an inability to obtain free water or an impaired thirst sensation. Both hypernatremia and hyponatremia can be assessed by the extracellular volume state: hypovolemic, isovolemic, or hypervolemic (see Figure 110-6).

HYPOVOLEMIC HYPERNATREMIA

Hypovolemic hypernatremia is the most common cause of hypernatremia. Patients who sustain losses of both sodium and water, but with comparatively greater water losses, are at risk of developing hypovolemic hypernatremia. Classically, these patients present with signs of volume depletion including orthostatic hypotension, decreased skin turgor, dry mucous membranes, flattened neck veins, and tachycardia. The urinary sodium concentration can aid in determining whether the water losses are primarily renal or extrarenal in nature, with a urinary sodium greater than 20 mmol/L indicating renal losses and less than 20 mmol/L indicating extrarenal losses.

ISOVOLEMIC HYPERNATREMIA

These patients have water losses without a change in total body sodium. Again, water losses alone do not always lead to hypernatremia; however, if water intake is also impaired, the serum sodium will increase. The water losses can be extrarenal (skin, respiratory tract), in which case urine osmolality will be elevated; or they can be renal, from impaired vasopressin production or collecting tubule response. The urine sodium in all cases varies depending on the individual's water intake.

Specific Isovolemic Hypernatremic Disorders

Central Diabetes Insipidus. Central diabetes insipidus results from impaired secretion of vasopressin from the supraoptic and paraventricular nuclei of the hypothalamus. Known causes include congenital defects and infection, tumor, or trauma affecting the central nervous system (CNS); however, approximately 50% of cases are idiopathic (Box 110-1). Differentiating central diabetes insipidus, nephrogenic diabetes insipidus, and primary polydipsia can be a diagnostic challenge because all three present with polyuria and polydipsia. Several clinical features may assist in this effort. Central diabetes insipidus is often abrupt in onset with patients experiencing a constant need for water, whereas a compulsive water drinker often provides a more vague history of onset. Similarly, nocturia is common in patients with central diabetes insipidus but is unusual in compulsive water drinkers. The plasma osmolality is also a helpful measurement, with values above 295 mOsm/kg suggestive of central diabetes insipidus and values below 270 mOsm/kg favoring a diagnosis of compulsive water drinking. Distinguishing among the three entities is best accomplished by measuring vasopressin levels and monitoring the response to a water deprivation test followed by vasopressin administration (Table 110-1). Pituitary magnetic resonance imaging (MRI) can also be used to make the diagnosis of central diabetes insipidus. The T_1-weighted images of a healthy posterior pituitary gland demonstrate a hyperintense signal, whereas this signal is absent in most patients with central diabetes

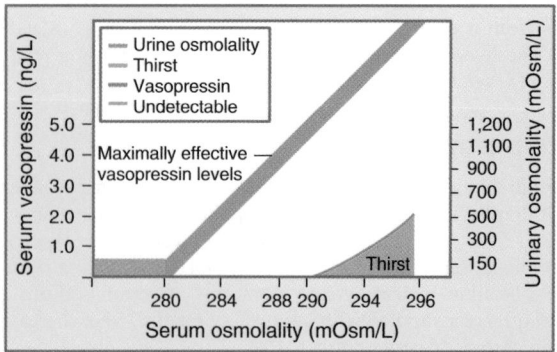

Figure 110-2 Mechanisms maintaining plasma osmolality. Response of thirst, vasopressin levels, and urinary osmolality to changes in serum osmolality. (*From Johnson R, Feehally J, editors. Comprehensive clinical nephrology. St Louis: Mosby; 2003, p. 83.*)

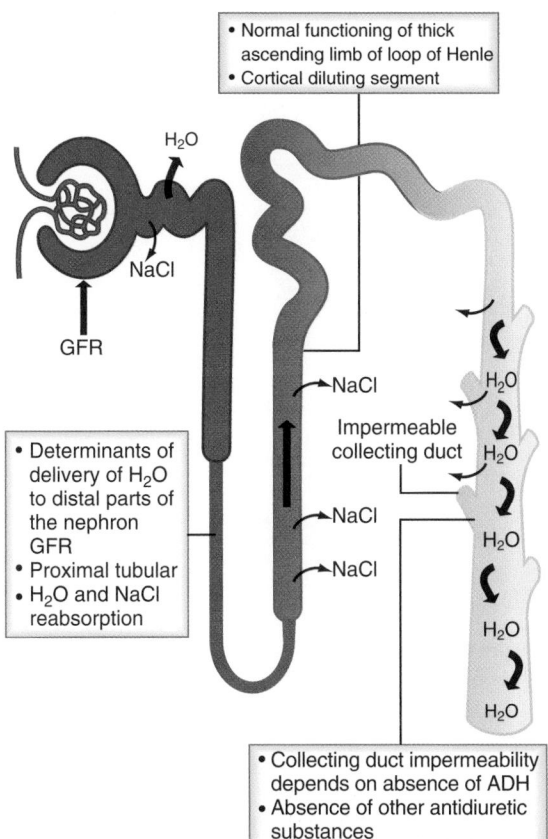

Figure 110-4 Determinants of urinary dilution mechanism include (1) delivery of water to thick ascending limb of loop of Henle, distal convoluted tubule, and collecting system of nephron; (2) generation of maximally hypotonic fluid in diluting segments (i.e., normal thick ascending limb of loop of Henle and cortical diluting segment); and (3) maintenance of water impermeability of collecting system, as determined by absence of antidiuretic hormone (ADH) or its action and other antidiuretic substances. GFR, glomerular filtration rate; H_2O, water; NaCl, sodium chloride. *(From Kumar S, Berl T. Disorders of water metabolism. In: Schrier RW, editor. Atlas of disease of the kidney. Philadelphia: Current Medicine; 1999, p. 1.9-.22.)*

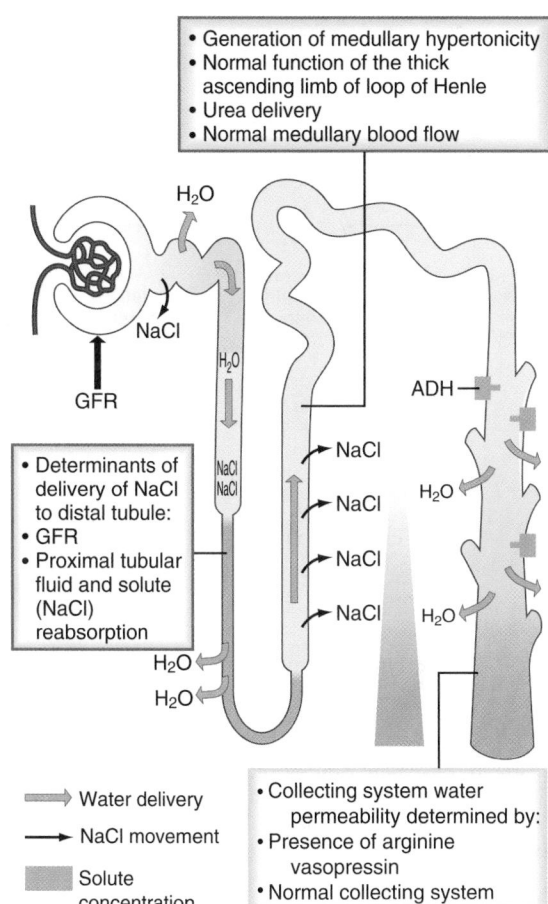

Figure 110-5 Determinants of renal concentrating mechanisms. Delivery of sodium chloride (NaCl) to diluting segments of nephron (thick ascending limb of loop of Henle and distal convoluted tubule) is determined by glomerular filtration rate (GFR) and proximal tubule function. Generation of medullary interstitial hypertonicity is determined by normal functioning of thick ascending limb of loop of Henle, urea delivery from medullary collecting duct, and medullary blood flow. Collecting duct permeability is determined by presence of antidiuretic hormone (ADH) and normal anatomy of collecting system, leading to formation of concentrated urine. *(From Kumar S, Berl T. Disorders of water metabolism. In: Schrier RW, editor. Atlas of disease of the kidney. Philadelphia: Current Medicine; 1999, p. 1.9-.22.)*

insipidus (although it may be present in rare inherited forms of the condition).[4]

The treatment of central diabetes insipidus relies primarily on pharmacologic agents (Table 110-2). In the acute setting, aqueous vasopressin (Pitressin) is advantageous; its short duration of action makes complications such as water intoxication less likely. For a patient with chronic central diabetes insipidus, desmopressin acetate (DDAVP) is the agent of choice; it has a long half-life and can be administered intranasally (10-20 μg) every 12 to 24 hours. DDAVP does not have the strong vasoconstrictive properties of aqueous vasopressin, which must be used with caution in patients with coronary and peripheral vascular disease. In patients with partial diabetes insipidus, additional agents that increase the release of vasopressin (e.g., carbamazepine, chlorpropamide, clofibrate) can be used.

Nephrogenic Diabetes Insipidus. Nephrogenic diabetes insipidus is either congenital or acquired. The diagnosis of congenital nephrogenic diabetes insipidus is made early in infancy with a presentation of hypoosmolar urine, severe dehydration, fever, vomiting, and hypernatremia. An intact thirst mechanism and access to free water are absolute necessities for survival, because pharmacologic therapies are ineffective. Rehydration therapy should consist of hypotonic glucose solutions,

because isotonic solutions promote further water losses via the excretion of solutes. Solute intake should also be limited by using low-sodium and low-protein diets.

One form of congenital nephrogenic diabetes insipidus follows an X-linked inheritance pattern, with only males exhibiting the complete disease phenotype. Females can have a subclinical form, which suggests the presence of variable penetrance. Affected males with X-linked congenital nephrogenic diabetes insipidus have an inability to concentrate urine in the presence of vasopressin. The defect has been located on the X chromosome where the V2 receptor protein is encoded. There appear to be multiple disease-causing mutations in this area of the X chromosome; 87 such mutations in the V2 receptor were found in 106 presumably unrelated affected families.[5] The autosomal recessive form of congenital nephrogenic diabetes insipidus is the result of mutations in the gene encoding for aquaporin-2 *(AQP2)*. This form is much less common than the X-linked variety, but multiple disease-causing mutations have been described.[6]

Acquired nephrogenic diabetes insipidus is more common but usually less severe, with partial preservation of urine-concentrating mechanisms. Urinary volumes are therefore much less (>3-4 L/day) in

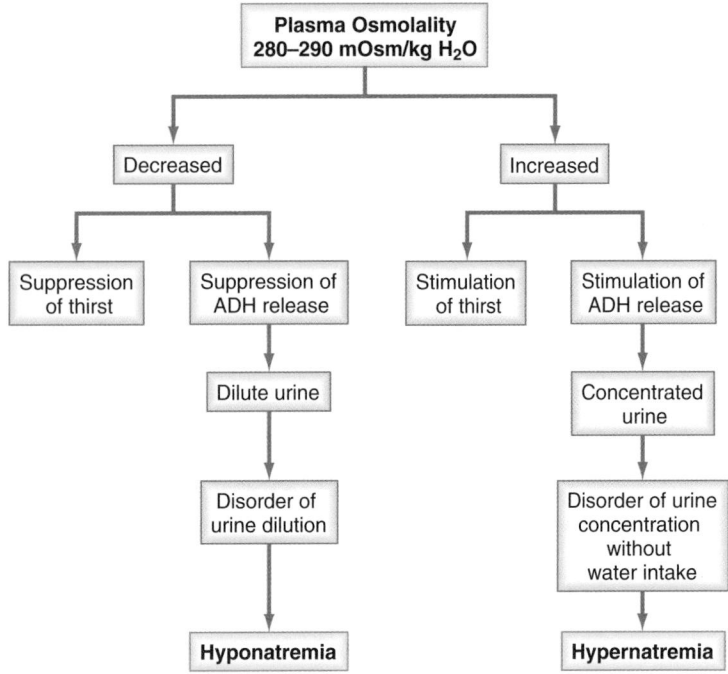

Figure 110-6   Plasma osmolality and pathogenesis of dysnatremias. *ADH*, antidiuretic hormone.

comparison to congenital nephrogenic diabetes insipidus, central diabetes insipidus, or compulsive water drinking. Common causes include hypercalcemia, hypokalemia, sickle cell anemia, demeclocycline therapy, lithium therapy, pregnancy, and chronic renal failure.

HYPERVOLEMIC HYPERNATREMIA

This is the least common form of hypernatremia (hypertonic fluid gain). Potential causes include hypertonic solution resuscitation, administration of sodium bicarbonate, or ingestion of excessive amounts of table salts. Congestive heart failure patients taking loop diuretics may also be prone to developing hypervolemic hypernatremia.

HYPERNATREMIA CLINICAL PRESENTATION

Hypernatremia always represents a hyperosmolar state, and as such, most of the signs and symptoms are reflections of CNS disturbances. These include altered mental status, lethargy, seizures, irritability, hyperreflexia, and spasticity. Patients can also exhibit nausea, vomiting,

fever, respiratory distress, and intense thirst. Certain patients are at increased risk for developing severe life-threatening hypernatremia. These include infants, elderly patients, certain hospitalized patients (those receiving hypertonic infusions, tube feedings, osmotic diuretics, lactulose, or mechanical ventilation), patients with altered mental status, and those with uncontrolled diabetes or an underlying polyuric disorder.

HYPERNATREMIA MANAGEMENT

Hypernatremia requires prompt treatment tailored to the patient's volume status, with the end goal being restoration of serum tonicity (Figure 110-7). The rate of correction of hypernatremia depends on its rate of development and on the presence or absence of neurologic symptoms. If corrected too rapidly, water moves into the brain cells, resulting in cerebral edema. If symptoms are present and the hypernatremia is thought to be acute in onset, rapid correction over the first several hours is appropriate, with the maximum correction rate not exceeding 2 mEq/L/h. An accepted goal is to correct half the water deficit over the first 24 hours, with the remaining deficit being

---

Box 110-1

CAUSES OF CENTRAL DIABETES INSIPIDUS

Congenital
Autosomal dominant
Autosomal recessive

Acquired
Posttraumatic
Iatrogenic (postsurgical)
Tumor (metastatic from breast, craniopharyngioma, pinealoma)
Histiocytosis
Granuloma (tuberculosis, sarcoid)
Aneurysm
Meningitis
Encephalitis
Guillain-Barré syndrome
Idiopathic

TABLE 110-1   Water Deprivation Test

Diagnosis	Urine Osmolality with Water Deprivation (mOsm/kg H$_2$O)	Plasma AVP After Dehydration	Increase in Urine Osmolality with Exogenous AVP
Normal	>800	>2 pg/mL	Little or none
Complete central diabetes insipidus	<300	Undetectable	Substantial
Partial central diabetes insipidus	300-800	<1.5 pg/mL	>10% of urine osmolality after water deprivation
Nephrogenic diabetes insipidus	<300-500	>5 pg/mL	Little or none
Primary polydipsia	>500	<5 pg/mL	Little or none

AVP, arginine vasopressin.

TABLE 110-2	Treatments for Diabetes Insipidus	
Type of Diabetes Insipidus	*Drug*	*Dose*
Complete central	DDAVP	10-20 g intranasally every 12-24 h
Partial central	Aqueous vasopressin	5-10 U subcutaneously every 4-6 h
	Chlorpropamide	250-500 mg/d
	Clofibrate	500 mg 3-4 times daily
	Carbamazepine	400-600 mg/d
Nephrogenic	Thiazide diuretics NSAIDs	
	Amiloride (for lithium-related disease)	5 mg/d
Gestational	DDAVP	As for complete central

Adapted from Lanese D, Teitelbaum I. Hypernatremia. In: Jacobson HR, Striker GE, Klahr S, editors. The principles and practice of nephrology. Philadelphia: CV Mosby; 1998.

DDAVP, desmopressin; *NSAIDs,* nonsteroidal antiinflammatory drugs.

The sum total of the water deficit and ongoing urinary water losses serves as a guide to the amount and duration of water replacement, with the understanding that these calculations are not static and may need frequent adjustments. In the case of acute severe central diabetes insipidus, in addition to the preceding water replacement therapy, it may be necessary to use short-acting aqueous vasopressin (Pitressin, 5 U subcutaneously every 6 hours), depending on the response to therapy. In the chronic setting, DDAVP should be used as previously described. In patients with chronic nephrogenic diabetes insipidus, the primary intervention is treatment or removal of the underlying cause. A rare form of diabetes insipidus can occur with pregnancy when the placenta produces vasopressinase. These patients respond to treatment with DDAVP, which is not degraded by this enzyme.[7]

The goal of hypervolemic hypernatremia therapy is to promote natriuresis with loop diuretics, along with the administration of 5% dextrose. Patients should be monitored closely to prevent overzealous sodium removal and volume depletion. If there is significant renal dysfunction, the volume overload and hypertonicity may require dialysis.

corrected over the next 48 hours. The serum sodium should be closely monitored during the course of treatment, with careful assessment of ongoing fluid losses.

In the setting of hypovolemic hypernatremia, initial management is fluid resuscitation using isotonic saline solutions or other plasma expanders. Once the intravascular volume has been restored, administration of hypotonic solutions can further restore normal serum tonicity.

For patients with isovolemic hypernatremia, the primary therapy is a 5% glucose solution. It is important to replace not only the water deficit but also any ongoing fluid losses. The water deficit can be calculated from the serum sodium concentration, using the assumption that 60% of the body weight is water:

$$\text{Water deficit} = 0.6 \times \text{Body weight (kg)} \times (P_{Na}/140 - 1)$$

To take into account any ongoing urinary water losses, it is necessary to calculate an electrolyte-free water clearance:

$$cH_2Oe = V[1 - (U_{Na} + U_K/P_{Na})]$$

Hyponatremia

Hyponatremia is defined as a serum sodium less than 135 mEq/L and is among the most common electrolyte disorders encountered in clinical practice.[8] It is generally associated with hypo-osmolality. There are, however, clinical settings in which plasma osmolality is normal or even high (Figure 110-8).

Translocational hyponatremia occurs when water moves from the intracellular space to the extracellular space in response to an osmotically active solute; as such, this does not reflect a change in total body water. In clinical practice, translocational hyponatremia is most frequently associated with hyperglycemia, which accounts for 15% of hyponatremia in hospitalized patients.[9] The decrease in plasma sodium can be approximated as 1.6 mEq/L for every 100 mg/dL increase in plasma glucose concentration. However, this correction factor has been challenged in that it leads to a serious underestimation of serum sodium values in association with serum glucose concentrations over 500 mg/dL. It has been recommended that a correction factor of 2.4 be used in patients with severe hyperglycemia.[10] This hyponatremia resolves with correction of the serum glucose.

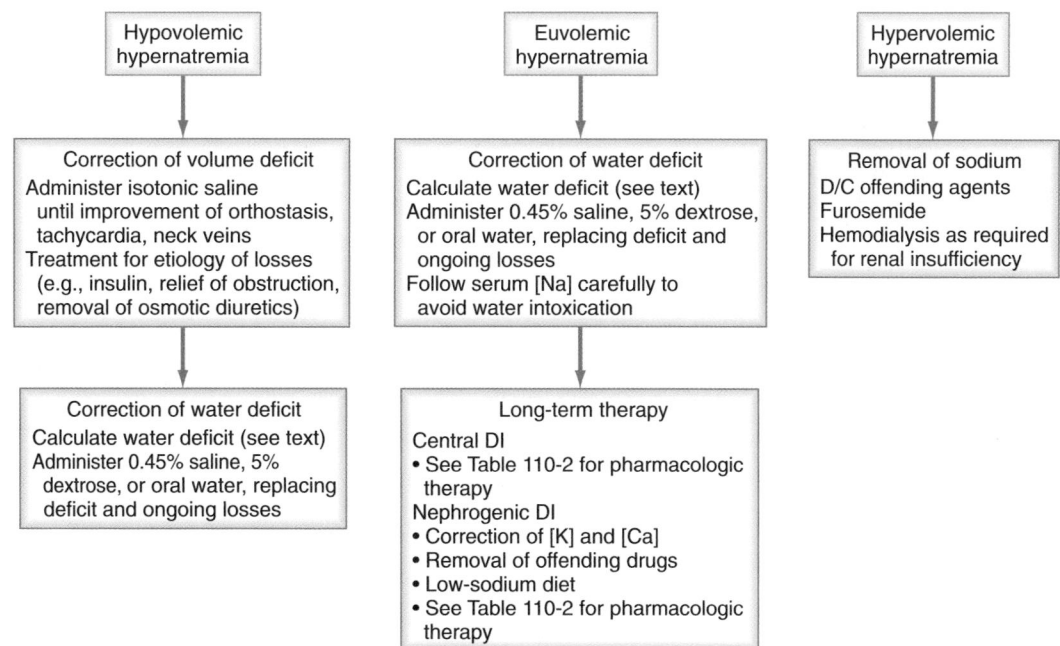

Figure 110-7 Therapeutic approach to hypernatremia. *D/C,* discontinue; *DI,* diabetes insipidus.

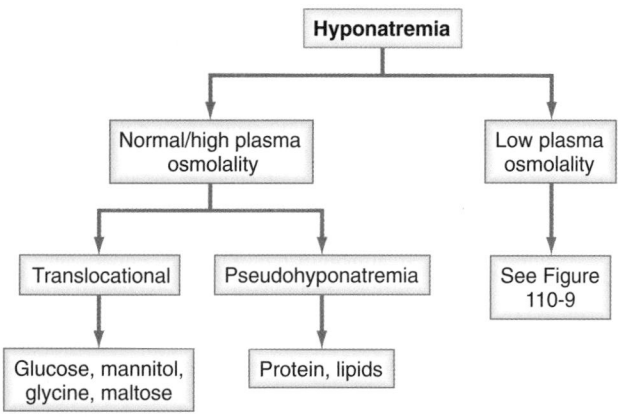

Figure 110-8 Diagnostic approach for patients with hyponatremia.

Pseudohyponatremia occurs when the solid phase of plasma is increased by large quantities of lipids or proteins. A rise in plasma lipids of 4.6 g/L or plasma protein concentrations greater than 10 g/dL will decrease the sodium concentration by approximately 1 mEq/L. This occurs because the flame photometry method of measuring sodium uses whole plasma rather than just the liquid phase. This is corrected by employing methods that use only the liquid phase to measure sodium concentration, such as direct potentiometry in an undiluted sample.

Once it is established that a patient has true hypotonic hyponatremia, it is helpful to determine the patient's volume status as previously stated. A thorough history and physical examination, supported by measurements of urinary sodium concentration, are essential in making this categorization (Figure 110-9).

HYPOVOLEMIC HYPONATREMIA

Hypovolemic hyponatremia occurs when a patient has both a total body sodium and water deficit, with the former exceeding the latter.

The underlying cause is the nonosmotic release of vasopressin in response to hypovolemia. Clinically this occurs in patients with high gastrointestinal or renal losses of solute and water in combination with the intake of hypotonic fluids. These patients exhibit signs of hypovolemia including tachycardia, orthostatic hypotension, flattened neck veins, dry mucous membranes, and decreased skin turgor.

Patients experiencing vomiting or diarrhea are volume contracted, and the kidney responds by avidly retaining sodium and chloride, thereby reducing the urinary sodium to less than 10 mmol/L. A similar response is seen in disorders such as pancreatitis, peritonitis, or burns, in which third-spacing of fluid leads to intravascular volume depletion and renal sodium conservation. An exception occurs in patients with vomiting and metabolic alkalosis. In this situation, bicarbonaturia results in increased urinary sodium excretion (>20 mmol/L) despite sometimes profound volume depletion. This results from the fact that bicarbonate is a non-reabsorbable anion, and its excretion requires the excretion of cations as well, most notably sodium.

Diuretic use is one of the more common causes of hypovolemic hyponatremia, particularly thiazide diuretics. Loop diuretics inhibit the sodium-potassium-chloride pump in the thick ascending loop of Henle, resulting in urine sodium levels above 20 mmol/L (see Figure 110-5). However, because this inhibition also interferes with generation of the hypertonic medullary interstitium, the responsiveness to vasopressin is decreased, and adequate urine dilution is still possible. In contrast, thiazide diuretics block the sodium-chloride co-transporter in the distal tubule, directly impairing the urinary diluting capacity (see Figure 110-4). Underweight women and elderly patients appear to be especially at risk for developing hyponatremia with thiazide use. Several proposed mechanisms for diuretic-induced hyponatremia, which usually occurs within 2 weeks after starting the drug, have been put forth. One is that hypovolemia causes increased vasopressin secretion, decreased delivery of fluid to the diluting segment of the nephron, and potassium depletion, resulting in increased thirst by alterations in osmoreceptor sensitivity.

Osmotically active, non-reabsorbable solutes also lead to renal sodium wasting (urine sodium >20 mmol/L) and hypovolemia. As long as water intake persists, a diabetic patient with glucosuria, a patient with urea diuresis after recovery from post-obstructive acute

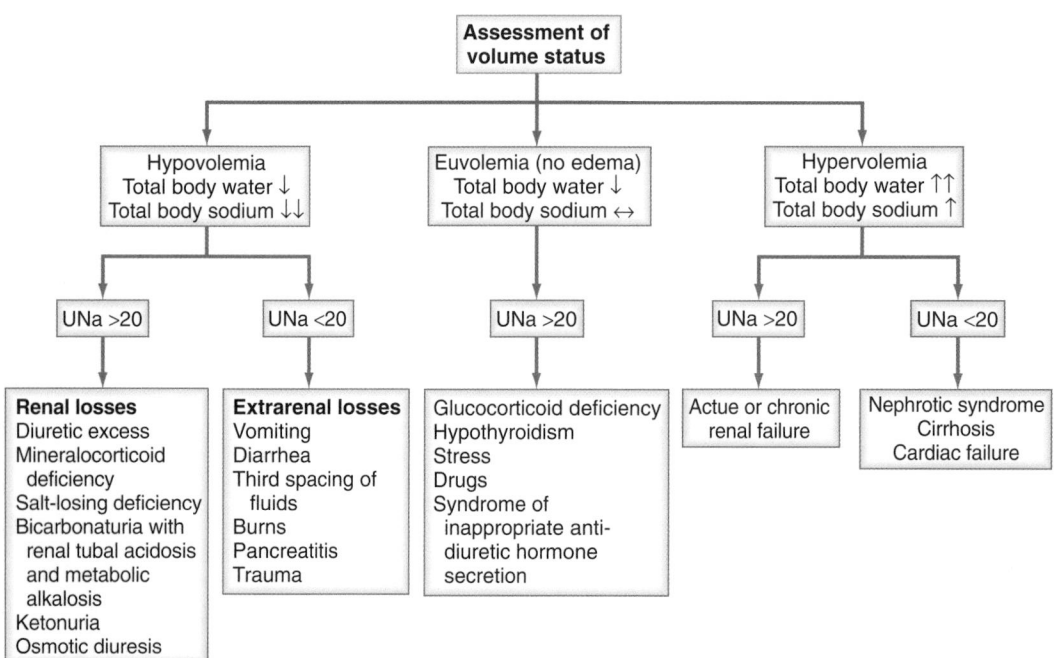

Figure 110-9 Diagnostic algorithm for hyponatremia. UNa, urinary sodium concentration. (*Adapted from Parix G, Kumar S, Beil T. Disorders of water metabolism. In: Johnson R, Feehally J, editors. Comprehensive clinical nephrology. St Louis: Mosby; 2003, p. 93.*)

DRUGS ASSOCIATED WITH HYPONATREMIA

Vasopressin Analogs
Desmopressin (DDAVP)
Oxytocin

Drugs That Enhance Vasopressin Release
Chlorpropamide
Clofibrate
Carbamazepine, oxcarbazepine
Vincristine
Nicotine
Narcotics
Antipsychotics, antidepressants
Ifosfamide

Drugs That Potentiate Renal Action of Vasopressin
Chlorpropamide
Cyclophosphamide
Nonsteroidal antiinflammatory drugs
Acetaminophen (paracetamol)

Drugs with Unknown Mechanism for Causing Hyponatremia
Haloperidol
Fluphenazine
Amitriptyline
Thioridazine
Fluoxetine
Sertraline

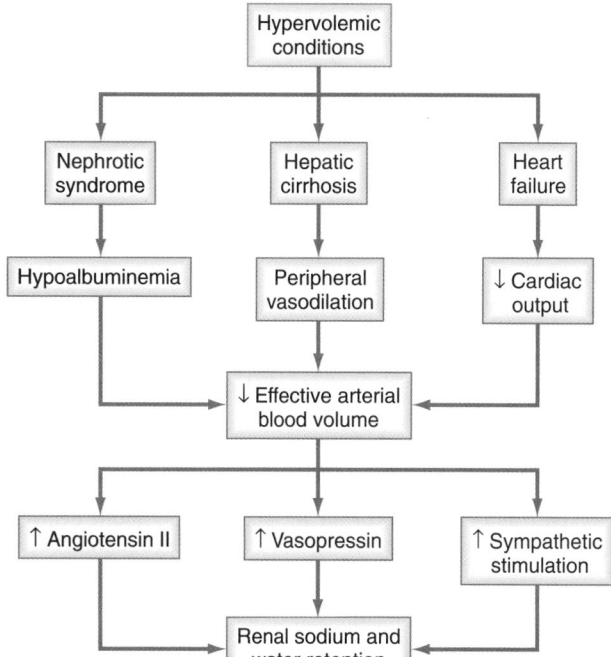

Figure 110-10 Pathophysiology of salt and water retention in hypervolemic disorders.

renal failure, and a patient with mannitol diuresis will all have urinary sodium losses in excess of water losses, leading to hyponatremia.

ISOVOLEMIC HYPONATREMIA

Isovolemic hyponatremia is the most commonly encountered dysnatremia in hospitalized patients. These patients have increased total body water but no clinical signs of increased total body sodium. There are many causes of isovolemic hyponatremia (see Figure 110-9), including many pharmacologic agents (Box 110-2), hypothyroidism, and glucocorticoid deficiencies. The most common cause, however, is the syndrome of inappropriate antidiuretic hormone (SIADH) secretion. This syndrome is characterized by an impaired suppression of vasopressin secretion relative to the degree of hypotonicity. CNS disturbances, certain solid organ tumors, and human immunodeficiency virus (HIV) are some of the more notable causes, although many others exist. SIADH remains a diagnosis of exclusion, and certain criteria need be met. Essential diagnostic criteria are a plasma osmolality less than 270 mOsm/kg H$_2$O, inappropriately concentrated urine osmolality greater than 100 mOsm/kg H$_2$O, clinical isovolemia, elevated urine sodium concentration under conditions of normal salt and water intake, and absence of adrenal, thyroid, pituitary, or renal insufficiency or diuretic use.[11]

HYPERVOLEMIC HYPONATREMIA

Congestive heart failure, cirrhosis, nephrotic syndrome, and renal failure can all result in hypervolemic states with increased total body sodium and water. Hyponatremia occurs when the increase in total body water exceeds that of sodium. All these conditions are associated with impaired water and salt excretion (Figure 110-10).

In congestive heart failure, the decrease in effective arterial blood volume leads to vasopressin release through the activation of aortic and carotid baroreceptors. Water excretion is further limited by stimulation of the renin-aldosterone-angiotensin and sympathetic nervous system pathways. This results in a reduction in glomerular filtration rate. The low cardiac output and increased production of angiotensin

II also potently stimulate thirst, leading to further hypotonicity. Patients with cirrhosis develop splanchnic arterial vasodilatation and arteriovenous fistulas, which also lead to a decreased effective arterial blood volume, increased vasopressin release, and in the end, impaired water excretion and hyponatremia.

In contrast to those with congestive heart failure and cirrhosis, most patients with nephrotic syndrome have intravascular volume contraction resulting from an alteration in Starling forces from hypoalbuminemia and lowered plasma oncotic pressure. Volume contraction has been shown to stimulate vasopressin release in nephrotic subjects.[12] In advanced renal failure, the water-excreting capacity of the kidney is greatly reduced. Just as edema occurs when sodium intake exceeds the excretory capacity of the diseased kidney, hyponatremia occurs when the free water intake is greater than the ability to excrete solute-free water. Even with maximum suppression of vasopressin, a patient with a glomerular filtration rate of 5 mL/min may be able to excrete only a little more than 2 liters of solute-free urine daily.[9]

HYPONATREMIA CLINICAL PRESENTATION

Patients with serum sodium concentrations above 125 mmol/L are usually asymptomatic, although some patients may have nausea and vomiting. Once serum sodium concentrations go below 125 mmol/L, neuropsychiatric symptoms predominate, mostly as a result of increasing cerebral edema. These include headaches, lethargy, ataxia, psychosis, seizures, coma, and death. Severe cerebral edema resulting in tentorial herniation can also occur, more commonly with the rapid development of hyponatremia. The mortality of severe hyponatremia approaches 50% if left untreated; therefore, the presence of any signs and symptoms warrants prompt intervention.[13,14]

HYPONATREMIA MANAGEMENT

Certain patient populations are at increased risk of developing cerebral edema during hyponatremia (Table 110-3). Postoperative premenopausal women with hyponatremia are more likely to develop neurologic complications than are either postmenopausal women or men;

TABLE 110-3	Hyponatremic Patients at Risk for Neurologic Complications	
Acute Cerebral Edema	*Osmotic Demyelination Syndrome*	
Postoperative menstruant females	Alcoholics	
Elderly women taking thiazides	Malnourished patients	
Children	Hypokalemic patients	
Psychiatric polydipsic patients	Burn patients	
Hypoxemic patients	Elderly women taking thiazides	

thus, hypotonic fluids should not be used perioperatively in these patients. Patients on thiazide diuretics, particularly elderly women, are more susceptible to severe hyponatremia and its complications. Children, psychiatric polydipsic patients, and patients with hypoxia also seem to be at higher risk.

Certain subpopulations of patients are at greater risk of developing osmotic demyelination syndromes during treatment for hyponatremia (see Table 110-3). Susceptibility to osmotic demyelination is related to the severity and chronicity of the hyponatremia. Osmotic demyelination is rarely seen with serum sodium greater than 120 mmol/L or if the duration of hyponatremia is less than 24 to 48 hours. Severely hyponatremic patients with alcoholism, malnutrition, hypokalemia, or severe burns, as well as elderly women prescribed thiazide diuretics, appear to be at increased risk.[15] Osmotic demyelination initially presents as a generalized encephalopathy associated with the rapid correction of serum sodium. The classic symptoms follow 2 to 3 days after the serum sodium is corrected; these include behavioral changes, cranial nerve palsies, and quadriplegia with a "locked-in" syndrome. MRI is diagnostic, but the typical lesions may not appear for up to 2 weeks after symptoms begin.[16]

The optimal treatment strategy for hyponatremia should focus on four factors: (1) presence or absence of symptoms, (2) duration of

hyponatremia if known, (3) patient's volume status, and (4) degree of hyponatremia (Figure 110-11).

Rapid correction is indicated for patients with acute (<48 hours) symptomatic hyponatremia. In these circumstances, the risk of cerebral edema far exceeds the risk of treatment-related complications such as osmotic demyelination. The goal should be a rise in serum sodium of 2 mmol/L/h until symptoms have resolved. Although it is not necessary to correct to normal serum sodium levels, doing so appears to be safe. Correction can usually be achieved using 3% hypertonic saline solutions at a rate of 1 to 2 mL/kg/h. If the patient is having severe symptoms (seizures, coma), higher rates of infusion can be used. The goal of this infusion is strictly to increase the serum tonicity rapidly. Administration of a loop diuretic will help normalize the serum sodium concentration more readily by enhancing free water excretion and will prevent volume expansion. Patients receiving hypertonic saline solutions need to be monitored very closely, with frequent assessments of volume status, output, and electrolytes.

Symptomatic hyponatremia for more than 48 hours must be approached with extreme caution; these patients have the greatest risk of complications. Partial correction of serum sodium in patients with chronic symptomatic hyponatremia should proceed without delay, because failure to correct is associated with poor outcome.[17] Cerebral water increases by about 10% during severe hyponatremia. With this in mind, it is safe to increase the serum sodium by 10%, followed by water restriction. This aggressive treatment should continue until either the symptoms resolve or this 10% increase is reached. Thereafter, the correction rate should be less than 0.5 mmol/L/h and should certainly not exceed 1 to 1.5 mmol/L/h or 12 mmol/L/d. To prevent overcorrection, it is important to monitor the rate and electrolyte content of infused fluids and urine output.

The approach to patients with chronic asymptomatic hyponatremia is different. For those with isovolemic hyponatremia, a search for underlying reversible causes should be undertaken. If SIADH is

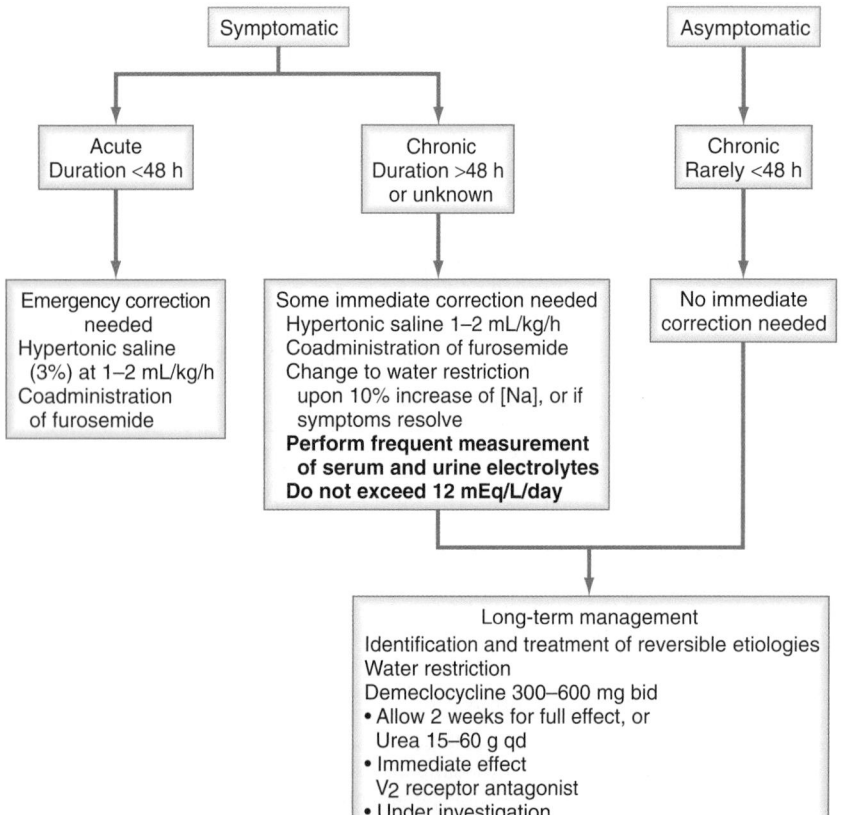

Figure 110-11 Treatment of severe (<125 mM/L) euvolemic hyponatremia. *(Adapted from Thurman JM, Halterman RK, Berl T. Theory of dysnatremic disorders. In: Brady H, Wilcox C, editors. Therapy in nephrology and hypertension. 2nd ed. Philadelphia: Saunders; 2003, p. 335-48.)*

determined to be the diagnosis, and if the cause is either unknown or untreatable, a conservative approach is appropriate. The hallmark of this treatment strategy is fluid restriction. Calculating a patient's electrolyte-free water excretion can help guide the degree of water restriction necessary:

$$cH_2Oe = V[1 - (UNa + UK)/PNa]$$

where cH_2Oe is electrolyte-free water clearance, V is urine volume, UNa is urinary sodium concentration, UK is urinary potassium concentration, and PNa is serum sodium concentration. To increase serum sodium, the amount of water intake has to be less than the sum of the insensible losses and the free water excretion. This formula can be used to guide therapy as follows[15]:

If $(UNa + UK)/PNa$ is greater than 1, water intake should be less than 500 mL/day.

If $(UNa + UK)/PNa$ is approximately 1, water intake should be 500 to 700 mL/day.

If $(UNa + UK)/PNa$ is less than 1, water intake should be up to 1 L/day.

Free water restriction is usually successful so long as the patient is compliant. This becomes difficult in an outpatient setting if intake is restricted to less than 1 L/day. In these circumstances, alternative treatments such as enhancing solute excretion or pharmacologic inhibition of vasopressin may be necessary.

Demeclocycline may be used to suppress vasopressin in patients with SIADH unresponsive to free water restriction. The usual oral dose is 600 to 1200 mg/d, and this should be adjusted to the lowest dose that keeps the serum sodium in the desired range with unrestricted water intake. Side effects of demeclocycline include skin photosensitivity and polyuria. Nephrotoxicity can also be seen, particularly in patients with liver disease who have impaired hepatic drug metabolism. However, the side-effect profile is far superior to that of lithium, which has been used in the past. Lithium, though effective in its antagonism of vasopressin, is limited by its neurotoxicity, nephrotoxicity, and narrow therapeutic window.

Secondary to its pivotal role in body water regulation, vasopressin has long been considered a potential target for the treatment of hyponatremia. Several oral nonpeptide vasopressin antagonists have been introduced in recent years.[18] A 2010 systematic review and meta-analysis evaluated the short-term efficacy and safety of vasopressin receptor antagonists.[19] The authors concluded that vasopressin antagonists are effective and safe for the treatment of isovolemic and hypervolemic hypernatremia. Further studies are needed to elucidate their exact role in this electrolyte disorder.

Another option for patients who remain unresponsive to or noncompliant with fluid restriction is to enhance solute excretion. One approach is to increase sodium intake (2-3 g of additional salt in the diet) in combination with a single dose of a loop diuretic (40 mg of furosemide is usually sufficient). The administration of urea (30-60 g/d) has a similar effect by promoting an osmotic diuresis. The major limitation to urea is the occurrence of gastrointestinal side effects.

Treatment of chronic hypovolemic hyponatremia requires repletion of volume. In this situation, neurologic symptoms are rare, because losses of both sodium and water limit osmotic shifts within the brain. Restoring effective arterial volume will inhibit further vasopressin release and help normalize serum sodium levels.

Hypervolemic hyponatremia can be very difficult to treat because it is often a sign of severe underlying cardiac, hepatic, or renal disease. Water restriction is important; however, these patients often experience extreme thirst, making compliance difficult. Loop diuretics increase free water excretion and can therefore be beneficial in raising serum sodium values as well as treating edema. Thiazide diuretics should generally be avoided because they impair urinary dilution and may worsen the hyponatremia. Vasopressin receptor antagonists are also under investigation in these disorders but are not yet available for clinical use.[20] A study by Wong and colleagues investigated the efficacy of the vasopressin V2 antagonist, VPA-985, in correcting hyponatremia in a group of patients including 33 with cirrhosis and 6 with congestive heart failure.[21] VPA-985 produced a significant aquaresis, with significant increases in free water clearance and serum sodium levels. Unless the underlying disease process can somehow be improved, treating hyponatremia in these cases represents a significant clinical challenge.

KEY POINTS

1. The concentration of sodium in extracellular fluid is a reflection of the tonicity of body fluids, not of total body sodium content.

2. The intake of water and the osmotic release of antidiuretic hormone maintain the concentration of sodium in a very narrow range (138-142 mEq/L), despite great variation in water intake.

3. Hyponatremia can occur with low, normal, or high total body sodium. A measurement of urinary sodium is helpful in differentiating extrarenal and renal sodium losses in hypovolemic hyponatremia.

4. Euvolemic hyponatremia is the most commonly encountered form, and the syndrome of inappropriate antidiuretic hormone (SIADH) secretion is most common in this setting.

5. The duration of hyponatremia and the presence or absence of neurologic symptoms determine the therapeutic approach.

6. Acute hyponatremia should be treated rapidly, but chronic hyponatremia requires careful monitoring to prevent an excessively rapid increase in serum sodium and demyelination.

7. Vasopressin antagonists are now under investigation for the treatment of hyponatremia.

8. Disorders in thirst and vasopressin release or action lead to hypernatremia.

9. Most patients admitted with hypernatremia are elderly; most hospital-acquired hypernatremia is caused by inadequate water intake in patients with water losses due to either loop diuretics or high (parenteral or oral) protein loads leading to an osmotic urea diuresis.

10. The treatment of hypernatremia requires administration (orally or parenterally) of electrolyte-free water; ongoing losses should not be ignored.

ANNOTATED REFERENCES

Rozen-Zvi B, Yahav D, Gheorghiade M, Korzets A, Leibovici L, Gafter U. Vasopressin receptor antagonists for the treatment of hyponatremia: systematic review and meta-analysis. Am J Kidney Dis 2010;56:325-37. Epub 2010 Jun 9.
This systematic review and meta-analysis provides an excellent review of the latest in the utilization of vasopressin antagonists in the management of hyponatremia.

Decaux G. Long-term treatment of patients with inappropriate secretion of antidiuretic hormone by the vasopressin receptor antagonist conivaptan, urea or furosemide. Am J Med 2002;110:582-4.
An excellent report on the use of a new V2 antagonist in the treatment of hyponatremia in SIADH. These drugs may soon be available for such purposes.

Furst H, Hallows KR, Post J, Chen S, Kotzker W, Goldfarb S, et al. The urine/plasma electrolyte ratio: a predictive guide to water restriction. Am J Med Sci 2000;319:240-4.

This physiologic analysis can serve as a guide to the degree of water restriction required to treat hyponatremia. An excellent review of the significance of urinary sodium and potassium concentrations.

Knepper MA. Molecular physiology of urinary concentrating mechanisms: regulation of aquaporin water channels by vasopressin. Am J Physiol 1997;272:F3-12.
This is an excellent review of the cellular biology of vasopressin action, with an emphasis on the regulation of AQP-2—the vasopressin-dependent water channel.

Palevsky PM, Bhagrath R, Greenberg A. Hypernatremia in hospitalized patients. Ann Intern Med 1996;124:197-203.
This study on the epidemiology of hypernatremia found that approximately 50% of patients admitted with this disorder are elderly.

REFERENCES

Access the complete reference list online at http://www.expertconsult.com.

111

Disorders of Plasma Potassium Concentration

KAMEL S. KAMEL | MITCHELL L. HALPERIN

Dyskalemias are common electrolyte disorders in the critical care setting that may predispose a patient to serious cardiac arrhythmias.[1] The pathophysiology of these electrolyte disturbances can be more easily understood if examined in the context of the major concept for the transport of potassium ions (K^+) across membranes. This process has two components, an open channel for K^+ in the cell membrane and a force to cause K^+ to move across cell membranes.

Potassium Channels

There are an insufficient number of K^+ channels in an open configuration in cell membranes to permit K^+ to diffuse to electrochemical equilibrium. When the number of open K^+ channels increases, K^+ move out of cells via open $[K]_{ATP}$ channels, and the voltage in the intracellular fluid (ICF) becomes more negative.

CLINICAL EXAMPLES

Sulfonylurea drugs stimulate the release of insulin.[2] They act by diminishing the open probability of the K_{ATP} channels. When fewer K^+ ions exit from pancreatic β cells, the ICF voltage becomes less negative. This causes voltage-gated calcium ion (Ca^{2+}) channels to open, and thereby the concentration of Ca^{2+} in the ICF rises, which provides a signal for the release of insulin from these cells. By virtue of a similar cascade of events, sulfonylurea drugs can cause vasoconstriction by raising the concentration of Ca^{2+} in the ICF in vascular smooth muscle and hence can be used to improve hemodynamics in patients with septic shock[3] (Figure 111-1).

Driving Forces

K^+ will move into a compartment that has a more negative voltage when K^+ channels are open. To create this negative voltage in cells, cations are exported at a faster rate than anions. The cations are usually sodium ions (Na^+) because of their abundance and the presence of a means to cause their movement out of cells, the activity of the electrogenic Na^+/K^+-ATPase. This ion pump is electrogenic because it exports 3 Na^+ while importing only 2 K^+ (Figure 111-2). Because Na^+ movement is not accompanied by movement of ICF anions (because macromolecular phosphates such as RNA, DNA, and phospholipids are impermeable), a negative intracellular voltage is generated. Open KCHJ10 K^+ ion channels in the immediate vicinity of the Na^+/K^+-ATPase in the plasma membrane serve the purpose of providing K^+ to the K^+ binding site of the Na^+/K^+-ATPase to permit continuing function of this critical electrogenic system (see Figure 111-2).

Regulation of Potassium Homeostasis

Regulation of K^+ homeostasis has two important aspects. First, the control of the transcellular distribution of K^+, which is vital for survival, as it acts to limit acute changes in the concentration of K^+ in plasma (P_K). Second, the regulation of K^+ excretion by the kidney, which maintains overall K^+ balance; this is however, a relatively slow process.

DISTRIBUTION OF POTASSIUM BETWEEN EXTRACELLULAR AND INTRACELLULAR FLUID COMPARTMENTS

K^+ are held inside the cell by an electrical force (cell interior negative voltage). To shift and maintain more K^+ inside cells, their interior voltage must become more negative. This can be achieved by activating the electrogenic Na^+/K^+-ATPase in cell membranes. β₂-Adrenergic agonists activate the Na^+/K^+-ATPase via a cyclic adenosine monophosphate (cAMP)-dependent mechanism that leads to phosphorylation of this ion pump. The quantity of Na^+ exported is also higher when the concentration of Na^+ rises in cells, but its impact on the net cell voltage depends on whether the entry process for Na^+ into cells was electroneutral or electrogenic.

Electroneutral Entry of Sodium into Cells

This occurs when Na^+ enters cells in exchange for hydrogen ions (H^+) via the Na^+/H^+ exchanger (NHE) (see Figure 111-2).[4] The NHE is normally inactive in cell membranes, as can be deduced from the fact that it catalyzes an electroneutral exchange and that the concentrations of its substrates (Na^+ in the ECF and H^+ in the ICF compartment) are considerably higher than that of its products (Na^+ in the ICF and H^+ in the ECF compartment) in steady state. The two major activators of NHE are insulin and a higher concentration of H^+ in the ICF compartment (Figure 111-2).

Electrogenic Entry of Sodium into Cells

The negative voltage in cells regulates the conductance of Na^+ channels in cell membranes. When open, one cationic charge enters per Na^+ transported. Since only one-third of a charge exits per Na^+ ion pumped via the Na^+/K^+-ATPase, this diminishes the net negative cell interior voltage; hence K^+ will exit from cells.

HORMONES THAT AFFECT THE DISTRIBUTION OF POTASSIUM

Catecholamines

β₂-Adrenergic agonists activate the Na^+/K^+-ATPase via a cAMP-dependent mechanism that leads to phosphorylation of this ion pump[5] and the export of preexisting intracellular Na^+. Therefore, hypokalemia may develop in conditions where there is a surge of catecholamines (e.g., patients with a subarachnoid hemorrhage, myocardial ischemia, and/or an extreme degree of anxiety). β₂-Agonists may be used to cause a shift of K^+ into cells in the emergency treatment of patients with hyperkalemia. On the other hand, non-selective β-blockers have been used in the treatment of patients with thyrotoxic hypokalemic periodic paralysis and are a potential therapy for other conditions of acute hypokalemia due to shift of K^+ into cells owing to a surge of catecholamines.

Insulin

The effect of insulin to shift K^+ into cells is due primarily to an augmentation of the electroneutral entry of Na^+ into cells via NHE.[4] This, in conjunction with stimulating the electrogenic Na^+/K^+-ATPase, causes the voltage in cells to become more negative (see Figure 111-2). This effect of insulin is utilized clinically in the emergency treatment of patients with hyperkalemia.[6,7]

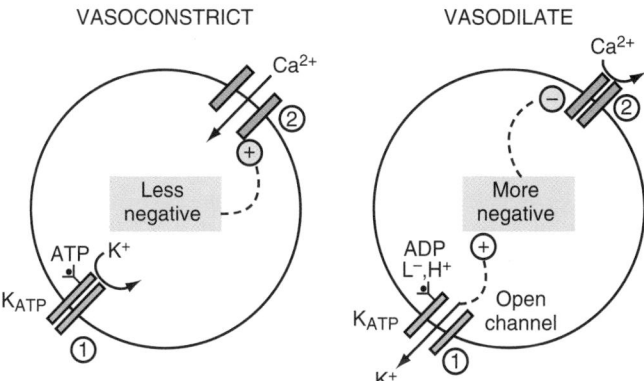

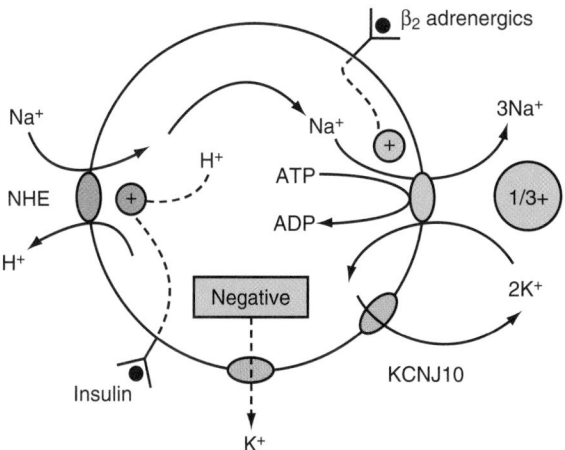

Figure 111-1 Vasoconstrictor tone in vascular smooth muscle cells. Circles represent a cell. *Left,* When K_{ATP} ion channels are largely closed, intracellular fluid (ICF) has a less negative voltage and voltage-gated calcium ion channels are in an open configuration, permitting a sustained rise in ICF calcium ion concentration. Hence vasoconstriction will be the dominant response in vascular smooth muscle cells, or release of insulin from pancreatic β cells. In contrast, when K_{ATP} channels are opened by adenosine diphosphate (ADP), for example, *(right)* ICF voltage will be more negative and voltage-gated Ca^{2+} channels will be closed. As a result, vascular cells will relax, whereas pancreatic β cells will not release insulin. *(From Halperin ML. The ACID truth and BASIC facts—with a sweet touch, an enLYTEnment. 5th ed. Toronto: RossMark Medical Publishers; 2003. Reproduced with permission. Ref 74)*

ACID-BASE INFLUENCES

Acids That May Cause a Shift of Potassium Into Cells

When an acid is added to the body, most of its H^+ are buffered in the ICF compartment.[8] Only monocarboxylic acids, however, can enter cells via a specific transporter, and this is an electroneutral process.[9] Once a monocarboxylic acid such as L-lactic acid enters cells on this transporter, its H^+ are released, and if this occurs in close approximation to NHE in the cell membrane, it becomes activated, and the net result is the electroneutral entry of Na^+ into these cells, which causes a rise in their intracellular concentration of Na^+. This in turn causes more Na^+ and positive voltage to exit from cells. The net result is the generation of a more negative voltage, which causes the retention of K^+ in these cells (Figure 111-3).[10]

Clinical Pearls. The hyperkalemia seen in patients with diabetic ketoacidosis (DKA) or hypoxic lactic acidosis likely reflects the lack of insulin in the former and diminished ion pumping by insufficient adenosine triphosphate (ATP) for the Na^+/K^+-ATPase in the latter.

Acids That May Cause a Shift of Potassium Out of Cells

A shift of K^+ out of cells may occur in patients with metabolic acidosis due to acids that are not substrates for the monocarboxylic acid transporter (e.g., HCl, citric acid). In this setting, the mechanism begins with the net exit of bicarbonate ions (HCO_3^-) from cells.[11] This exit is an electroneutral process because it occurs on the Cl^-/HCO_3^- anion exchanger (AE) (Figure 111-4). Nevertheless, the process becomes electrogenic because it results in a rise in the concentration of Cl^- in the ICF compartment. Since virtually all cells have Cl^- channels in their cell membranes,[12] the usual negative voltage forces some of these Cl^- to exit cells in an electrogenic fashion. As a result of the less negative voltage inside these cells, more K^+ will exit.[13]

Clinical Pearls. Although the addition of inorganic acids (e.g., HCl) causes a shift of K^+ out of cells, patients with chronic hyperchloremic metabolic acidosis (e.g., patients with chronic diarrhea or those with renal tubular acidosis [RTA]) usually have a low P_K because of excessive loss of K^+ in the diarrhea fluid[14] or in the urine.[15] Although

Figure 111-2 Na^+/K^+-ATPase activity and export of positive voltage. Na^+/K^+-ATPase *(yellow oval)* generates the electrical driving force for K^+ entry into cells, providing the source of Na^+ pumped out is Na^+ that existed in cells or Na^+ that entered cells via the electroneutral Na^+/H^+ exchanger (NHE) *(pink oval)*. K^+ channel conductance *(pale purple oval)* does not limit exit of K^+ to a major extent. Notwithstanding, the higher concentration of K^+ in the ICF compartment, which results from ion pumping by Na^+/K^+-ATPase, causes electrogenic exit of K^+ via the KCNJ10 K^+ channel *(darker purple oval)*, and this ensures an adequate concentration of K^+ outside cells for the Na^+/K^+-ATPase. *(From Halperin ML. The ACID truth and BASIC facts—with a sweet touch, an enLYTEnment. 5th ed. Toronto: RossMark Medical Publishers; 2003. Reproduced with permission. Ref 74)*

hypokalemia is a common finding in patients with metabolic alkalosis,[16] this usually reflects renal K^+ wasting for the most part due to the underlying disorder (e.g., vomiting, diuretic use, primary hyperaldosteronism) rather than the small effect of alkalemia to shift K^+ into cells. Respiratory acid-base disorders cause only small changes in the P_K, because there is little movement of Na^+ across cell membranes in these disorders.[17]

Tissue Anabolism/Catabolism

Hypokalemia may develop in conditions with rapid cell growth if insufficient K^+ is given. Examples include the use of total parenteral nutrition (TPN), rapidly growing malignancies, and during treatment of DKA or pernicious anemia. On the other hand, hyperkalemia may be seen in patients with crush injury or tumor lysis syndrome.[18] In these patients, factors that compromise the kidney's ability to excrete K^+ are usually present. In patients with DKA, there is total body K^+ depletion,[19] but hyperkalemia is present because there is a shift of K^+ from cells secondary to a lack of insulin. The corollary is that during therapy, complete replacement of the deficit of K^+ must await the provision of cellular constituents (phosphate, amino acids, Mg^{2+}, etc.) and the presence of anabolic signals.

Long-Term Regulation of Potassium Homeostasis

Control of the renal excretion of K^+ maintains overall daily K^+ balance. Although the usual intake of K^+ in adults eating a typical western diet is close to 1 mmol/kg body weight, K^+ excretion can decline to a nadir of 10 to 15 mmol/d when there is virtually no K^+ intake,[20] whereas the rate of excretion of K^+ can match an intake of more than 200 mmol/d with only a minor rise in the P_K.

Control of K^+ excretion occurs primarily in the late distal convoluted tubule up to the end of the cortical collecting duct (the abbreviation *CCD* will be used in this chapter to indicate all of these nephron segments).[19] There are two components that affect the rate of excretion of K^+: the flow rate in the CCD and the net secretion of K^+ by principal cells in the CCD. It is the latter which adjusts the luminal concentration of K^+ ($[K^+]_{CCD}$) and thereby regulates the rate of excretion of K^+:

$$K \text{ excretion} = \text{Flow rate}_{CCD} \times [K^+]_{CCD}$$

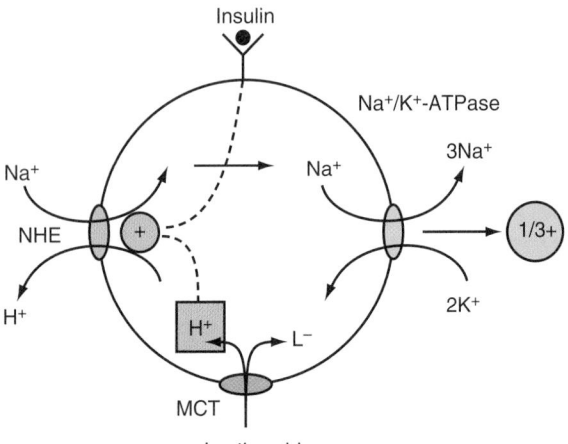

Figure 111-3 Interaction of monocarboxylic acid transporter and Na^+/ H^+ exchanger (NHE) to cause a shift of K^+ into cells. Circle represents the cell membrane of liver cells and the monocarboxylic acid transporter (M-CT; *red oval, bottom of cell*) and the NHE (*pink oval, left of cell*). When L-lactic acid enters, it dissociates, and this causes a local large increase in H^+ concentration at the inner surface of the cell membrane (*pink rectangle*), the location where NHE exists. This local high concentration of H^+ activates NHE by binding to its modifier site. This process requires the presence of insulin. As a result of activation of NHE, more Na^+ enters the cell in an electroneutral fashion. This Na^+ is subsequently pumped out of cells in an electrogenic fashion via the Na^+/K^+-ATPase (*orange oval*). Accordingly, the interior of the cell becomes more negative, and this causes more K^+ to be retained inside the cell.

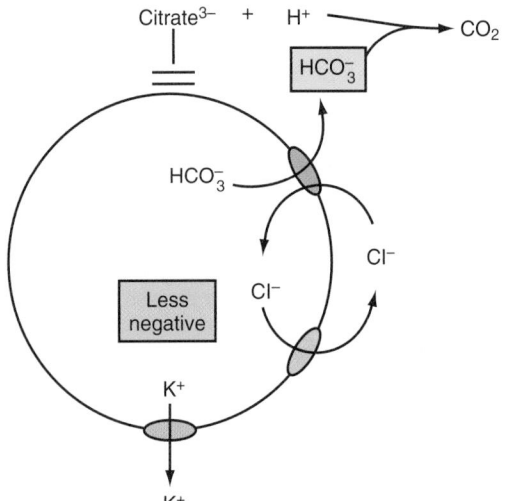

Figure 111-4 Role of Cl^-/HCO_3^- anion exchanger in the exit of K^+ from cells. Circle represents a cell membrane. Anion exchanger (AE; *blue oval*) is normally inactive in cell membranes but becomes active when pH in the ECF falls. When AE becomes active, HCO_3^- will be exported out of cell, and Cl^- will enter cell in a 1:1 electroneutral stoichiometry. Intracellular negative voltage will drive subsequent exit of Cl^- from the cell in an electrogenic fashion via Cl^- channels (*green oval*), which makes the interior of the cell less negative. As a result, K^+ will exit via K^+ channels (*purple oval*). (From Halperin ML. *The ACID truth and BASIC facts— with a sweet touch, an enLYTEnment.* 5th ed. Toronto: RossMark Medical Publishers; 2003. Reproduced with permission 74 ref.)

FLOW RATE IN THE LATE CORTICAL DISTAL NEPHRON

When vasopressin acts, the flow rate in the CCD is determined by the rate of delivery of osmoles, because the osmolality of fluid in the terminal CCD is fixed (equal to the plasma osmolality (P_{osm})[21]:

$$\text{Flow rate}_{CCD} = (\text{Number of osmoles delivered to the CCD})/P_{Osm}$$

The major osmoles in the lumen of CCD are Na^+, Cl^-, and urea. Owing to urea recycling within the nephron, almost 75% of osmoles delivered to the CCD are urea (see Reference 22 for more detailed information).

Clinical Example

A patient with HIV and pneumocystis carinii pneumonia is treated with trimethoprim and develops hyperkalemia.[23] Because his dietary intake is poor, the rate of delivery of osmoles (mainly urea) to the CCD is low, which means that the flow rate in his CCD is also diminished. This increases the concentration of trimethoprim in the lumen of the CCD (same quantity of trimethoprim is now contained in a smaller volume). Hence the ability of trimethoprim to block epithelial Na^+ channels (ENaC) in principal cells in the CCD will be enhanced.[24] Furthermore, in the presence of diminished ability to secrete K^+ in the CCD owing to a less negative TE luminal voltage, the low flow rate in CCD will further compromise the ability to excrete K^+. Increasing the rate of delivery of Na^+ and Cl^- with a loop diuretic can help augment the rate of excretion of K^+ by increasing the flow rate in the CCD. Of greater importance, it will lower the concentration of trimethoprim in the luminal fluid in the CCD, and hence trimethoprim becomes less effective in blocking ENaC.[25]

POTASSIUM CONCENTRATION IN THE LUMEN OF THE LATE CORTICAL DISTAL NEPHRON

The secretory process for K^+ in principal cells has two elements. First, a lumen negative voltage must be generated via electrogenic reabsorption of Na^+ via ENaC. Actions of aldosterone increase the number of open ENaC. The steps for aldosterone action include its binding to the cytoplasmic aldosterone receptor in principal cells, entry of this hormone-receptor complex into the nucleus, and then the synthesis of new proteins including the serum and glucocorticoid regulated kinase (SGK).[26] SGK phosphorylates and inactivates Nedd4-2 (Figure 111-5). As a result, this increases the number of open ENaC units in the luminal membrane of principal cells in the CCD. Second, open K^+ channels must be present in the luminal membranes of principal cells in the CCD. K^+ channels (ROMK) are abundant and have a high open probability in the absence of hypokalemia, and therefore they do not seem to be rate limiting for net secretion of K^+ in most patients.

The net activity of a complicated mixture of kinases and phosphatases lead to the phosphorylation or dephosphorylation of ROMK, which regulates how many of these K^+ channels remain in the luminal membrane of principal cells. For example, when the P_K falls to the lower end of its normal range, open ROMK are removed from the luminal membrane of principal cells. In contrast, when the P_K rises to the higher end of its normal range (e.g., after the intake of a K^+ load), more open ROMK are inserted into the luminal membranes of principal cells.

Glucocorticoids do not usually stimulate the secretion of K^+ in the CCD because principal cells have a pair of enzymes called 11β-hydroxysteroid dehydrogenase (11β-HSDH). These enzymes convert cortisol to a metabolite (cortisone) that does not bind to the mineralocorticoid receptor (see Figure 111-5). Cortisol, however, can exert a mineralocorticoid effect if the activity of 11β-HSDH is decreased or if it is overwhelmed by an abundance of cortisol.

Under most circumstances, variations in the concentration of Na^+ in the luminal fluid in the CCD does not regulate the secretion of K^+.[27] The reabsorption of Na^+ in the CCD can be electroneutral or electrogenic, depending on whether the same quantity of Cl^- (electroneutral) or a smaller quantity of Cl^- (electrogenic) is reabsorbed as compared to Na^+. The pathway(s) for the reabsorption of Cl^- in the CCD is (are)

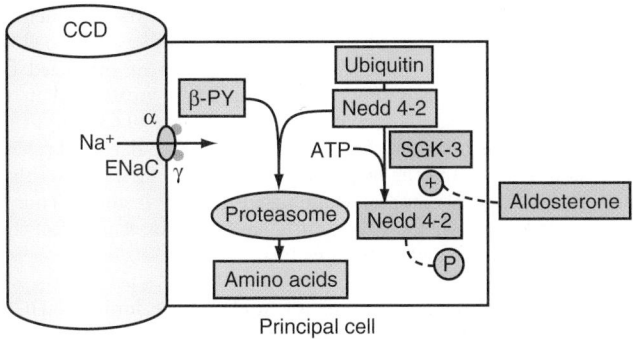

Figure 111-5 Model for control of epithelial Na$^+$ channel (ENaC) in principal cells in late cortical distal nephron (CCD). The barrel-shaped structure represents late cortical distal nephron, where secretion of K$^+$ occurs when more Na$^+$ than Cl$^-$ is reabsorbed (i.e., a lumen-negative voltage is created). The rectangle represents a principal cell, and the brown oval in its luminal membrane is the α subunit (channel pore) of ENaC. There are two ways to influence the number of open ENaC units in the luminal membrane of principal cells. First, ENaC can be removed as illustrated in purple. The β and γ subunits of ENaC have a PxYY motif which faces the interior of the cell. When Nedd4-2 binds to this motif, ENaC are removed from the luminal membrane into the cytoplasmic compartment, and ubiquitin is attached, which targets the complex to proteasomes and the ultimate degradation of ENaC. Second, more open ENaC units can be inserted in the luminal membrane of principal cells when aldosterone acts, as illustrated in brown shading. The major effect of aldosterone actions is activation of SGK-3, which regulates this process. SGK-3 phosphorylates and hence inactivates Nedd4-2, and thereby there are more open ENaC units in the luminal membrane of principal cells.

not well defined, but it is likely that paracellular pathways play an important role.[28,29]

Reabsorbing more Na$^+$ than Cl$^-$ in the CCD can occur if there is high mineralocorticoid activity (e.g., primary hyperaldosteronism, in conditions in which cortisol acts as a mineralocorticoid (e.g., apparent mineralocorticoid excess syndrome, ingestion of licorice, or large excess of cortisol, as in a patient with an ACTH-producing tumor) or if ENaC is constitutively active (e.g., Liddle's syndrome).

Reabsorbing less Cl$^-$ than Na$^+$ in the CCD can occur for three reasons, as depicted in Figure 111-6. First, Na$^+$ is delivered to the CCD with little Cl$^-$. A key finding in these patients is a Cl$^-$-poor urine.[30] Second, reabsorption of Cl$^-$ in the CCD may be inhibited; this mechanism is suspected when the urine is not Cl$^-$-poor. It appears that HCO$_3^-$ and/or an alkaline luminal pH in the CCD may inhibit

Cl$^-$ reabsorption[31] (see Figure 111-6, middle panel). Third, a greater lumen-negative voltage in the CCD could develop when the delivery of Na$^+$ and Cl$^-$ are very high and if the capacity for Cl$^-$ reabsorption is less than that for Na$^+$. This requires a stimulated reabsorption of Na$^+$ via ENaC in the CCD (see Figure 111-6, right panel).

If there are near-equal rates of absorption of Na$^+$ and Cl$^-$ in the CCD, an appreciably greater lumen-negative voltage cannot be generated, and hyperkalemia will develop if the intake of K$^+$ remains high.[28,32]

Tools to Assess Control of Renal Excretion of Potassium

EXAMINE RATE OF EXCRETION OF POTASSIUM

To assess the renal response in a patient with hypokalemia or hyperkalemia, we use the expected rate of K$^+$ excretion when these electrolyte abnormalities are due to nonrenal causes. With a K$^+$ deficit, the expected response is to excrete less than 15 mmol of K$^+$/d.[20,45] With a surfeit of K$^+$, the expected response is to excrete greater than 200 mmol/d, values observed in response to a K$^+$ load with a minor increase in P$_K$.[33]

To assess the rate of excretion of K$^+$, a 24-hour urine collection is not necessary. One can use the U$_K$/U$_{Creatinine}$ ratio in a spot urine sample even though there is a diurnal variation in K$^+$ excretion,[21] because creatinine is excreted at a near-constant rate throughout the day.[34] Moreover, the U$_K$/U$_{Creatinine}$ in spot urine samples provides more relevant information because it can be evaluated relative to the P$_K$ at that time. The expected U$_K$/U$_{Creatinine}$ ratio in a patient with hypokalemia is less than 1 mmol K$^+$/mmol creatinine (less than 10 mmol K$^+$/g creatinine), whereas in a patient with hyperkalemia, the expected U$_K$/U$_{Creatinine}$ ratio is greater than 15 mmol K$^+$/mmol creatinine (greater than 150 mmol K$^+$/g creatinine).

Establish Basis for Abnormal Rate of Excretion of Potassium

In a patient with hypokalemia, a higher than expected rate of excretion of K$^+$ implies that the lumen-negative voltage is abnormally more negative and that open luminal K$^+$ channels (likely ROMK) are present in the luminal membranes of the CCD.[39] The greater lumen negative voltage is due to reabsorbing more Na$^+$ than Cl$^-$ per unit time in the CCD. The converse is true in a patient with hyperkalemia where there is a lower than expected rate of excretion of K$^+$.

The clinical indices that help in the differential diagnosis of the pathophysiology of the abnormal rate of electrogenic reabsorption of Na$^+$ in CCD are an assessment of the ECF volume and the ability to conserve Na$^+$ and Cl$^-$ in response to a contracted effective arterial blood volume. The measurement of the activity of renin (P$_{Renin}$) and

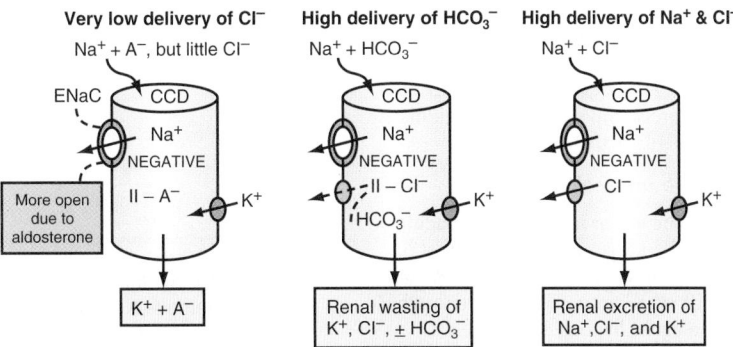

Figure 111-6 Less reabsorption of Cl$^-$ as the basis for a high [K$^+$]$_{CCD}$. The barrel-shaped structures represent the late cortical distal nephron (CCD). In all three settings, there is electrogenic reabsorption of Na$^+$ because of a lower rate of Cl$^-$ reabsorption in these nephron segments. Electrolyte excretions are shown in yellow shaded rectangles. *Far left,* Low distal delivery of Cl$^-$ is the reason for reabsorbing more Na$^+$ than Cl$^-$ in CCD (urine contains very little Cl$^-$). *Middle,* Urine contains abundant Cl$^-$. The reason for reabsorbing more Na$^+$ than Cl$^-$ in CCD is that HCO$_3^-$ and/or an alkaline luminal pH decreases permeability for Cl$^-$ in CCD. *Far right,* There is a large delivery of Na$^+$ and Cl$^-$ to the CCD, owing to inhibition of their reabsorption in an upstream nephron segment and presence of aldosterone to open epithelial Na$^+$ channel (ENaC) units, permitting reabsorption of more Na$^+$ than Cl$^-$ in the CCD. (*From Halperin ML. The ACID truth and BASIC facts—with a sweet touch, an enLYTEnment. 5th ed. Toronto: Ross-Mark Medical Publishers; 2003. Reproduced with permission 74 ref.*)

PLASMA RENIN AND ALDOSTERONE VALUES TO ASSESS THE BASIS OF HYPOKALEMIA OR HYPERKALEMIA

Lesions That Cause Hypokalemia		
Renin		Aldosterone
Adrenal Gland		
Primary hyperaldosteronism	Low	High
Glucocorticoid remediable hyperaldosteronism	Low	High
Kidney		
Renal artery stenosis	High	High
Malignant hypertension	High	High
Renin-secreting tumor	High	High
Liddle's syndrome	Low	Low
Disorders involving 11β-HSDH	Low	Low
Lesions That Cause Hyperkalemia		
Adrenal Gland		
Addison's disease	High	Low
Kidney		
Pseudohypoaldosteronism type 1	High	High
Hyporeninemic hypoaldosteronism	Low	Low

the level of aldosterone in plasma ($P_{Aldosterone}$) are also helpful in this setting (Box 111-1).[35]

HYPERKALEMIA

Therapy of Hyperkalemia

MEDICAL EMERGENCIES

The major danger of a severe degree of hyperkalemia is a cardiac arrhythmia. Because mild electrocardiographic (ECG) changes may progress rapidly to a dangerous arrhythmia, any patient with an ECG abnormality related to hyperkalemia should be considered as a medical emergency. We would aggressively treat patients with a P_K greater than 7.0 mmol/L, even in the absence of ECG changes—the exceptions include those who develop hyperkalemia after extreme exercise (the super-marathon[47]).

Antagonize the Cardiac Effects of Hyperkalemia

Ca^{2+} is the best agent, and its effects should be evident within minutes. It is usually given as 20 to 30 mL of a 10% calcium gluconate solution (2-3 ampules) or 10 mL of 10% $CaCl_2$ (one ampoule). Both solutions are equally effective, but the former is probably safer should the solution extravasate during the IV infusion. This dose can be repeated in 5 minutes if ECG changes persist. The effect usually lasts 30 to 60 minutes. Extreme caution should be exercised in patients on digitalis, because hypercalcemia may aggravate digitalis toxicity.

Induce a Shift of Potassium Into the Intracellular Fluid

Insulin. A number of studies support the use of insulin to treat acute hyperkalemia (reviewed in Reference 6). Large doses of insulin (20 units of regular insulin) are needed to have high enough levels of insulin in plasma for a maximal shift of K^+ into cells. Give enough glucose, and monitor $P_{Glucose}$ closely to avoid hypoglycemia.

β₂-Adrenergic Agonists. Although a number of studies suggest that β₂-agonists (e.g., 20 mg of nebulized albuterol) is effective treatment to lower P_K rapidly, we do not use these agents as a primary treatment of emergency hyperkalemia for two reasons. First, in a number of studies it was noted that 20% to 40% of patients with end-stage renal disease are resistant to this therapy, and it is not possible to predict who the non-responders will be. Second, we are concerned

about the safety of these drugs in the doses used for the treatment of hyperkalemia; these doses, which are 4 to 8 times those prescribed for the treatment of acute asthma. The combination of nebulized β₂-agonists and insulin was reported to produce a greater fall in P_K (1.2 mmol/L) compared with either drug alone (~0.65 mmol/L).[48] One should note, however, that only 10 units of regular insulin were given in this study, and the magnitude of the fall in P_K was lower than that observed in other studies using higher doses of insulin.[49] Thus, it remains uncertain whether β₂-agonists have a P_K-lowering effect that is additive to that of higher doses of insulin.

Sodium Bicarbonate. A number of studies have found $NaHCO_3$ therapy to be ineffective, as the sole treatment of hyperkalemia.[49-51] Notwithstanding, these studies were performed in stable hemodialysis patients who did not have significant acidemia. Studies that examined the combined use of $NaHCO_3$ with insulin also have yielded conflicting results.[52,53] Thus the question remains, *Would $NaHCO_3$ be effective in patients with a more significant degree of acidemia?* There are no data in the literature to answer this question definitively (for review, see Reference 6). Given this uncertainty, we only use $NaHCO_3$ in addition to other therapies to treat emergency hyperkalemia in patients with a significant degree of acidemia. Caution is warranted because an excessive administration of $NaHCO_3$ has the risk of inducing hypernatremia, ECF volume expansion, carbon dioxide retention, and acute hypocalcemia.

Clinical Approach

It is imperative to recognize when hyperkalemia represents a medical emergency because therapy must take precedence over diagnosis (Figure 111-7). A step-by-step approach to diagnosis of hyperkalemia is illustrated in Figures 111-8 and 111-9.

In Box 111-2, we provide a list of causes of hyperkalemia and of hypokalemia based on the presence or absence of hypertension.

1. Is hyperkalemia acute and/or was K^+ intake very low? If the answer is yes, consider factors that could cause a shift of K^+ from cells or the release of K^+ from cells due to cell destruction (e.g., crush injury). In their absence, rule out pseudohyperkalemia.
2. Are there laboratory or technical problems? Hemolysis, megakaryocytosis, fragile tumor cells, a K^+ channel disorder in red blood cells,[36] and excessive fist clenching during blood sampling[37] should be excluded. Pseudohyperkalemia can be present in cachectic patients, because the normal T-tubule architecture in skeletal muscle may be disturbed. This permits more K^+ to be released into venous blood, even without excessive fist clenching.

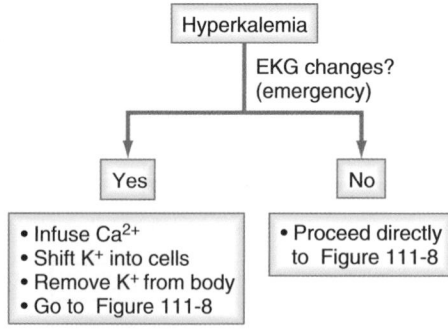

Figure 111-7 Initial clinical approach for the patient with hyperkalemia. If an emergency is present (usually cardiac), intravenous Ca^{2+} must be given immediately. Efforts are then made to shift K^+ into cells and remove K^+ from the body. If there is no emergency present, one can proceed to diagnosis of the cause of hyperkalemia. (*From Halperin ML. The ACID truth and BASIC facts—with a sweet touch, an enLYTEnment. 5th ed. Toronto: RossMark Medical Publishers; 2003. Reproduced with permission ref 74.*)

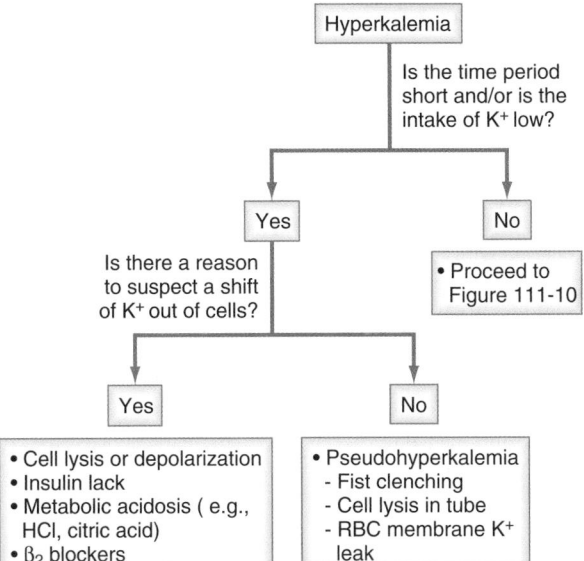

Figure 111-8 Initial steps in the clinical diagnosis of the cause of hyperkalemia. The most important issue is to determine if a shift of K^+ out of cells is likely; this is done by assessing the time course for the rise in the P_K and whether there was little intake of K^+. If that was the case and there is no reason to suspect a shift of K^+ out of cells, pseudohyperkalemia should be ruled out. In this latter setting, there should not be ECG changes related to hyperkalemia. If this is ruled out, proceed to Figure 111-9, and examine the rate of excretion of K^+. *(From Halperin ML. The ACID truth and BASIC facts—with a sweet touch, an enLYTEnment. 5th ed. Toronto: RossMark Medical Publishers; 2003. Reproduced with permission ref 74.)*

Since chronic hyperkalemia is usually associated with hyperchloremic metabolic acidosis because of inhibition of ammonium (NH_4^+) production by the associated rise in pH in proximal tubule cells, suspect that pseudohyperkalemia may be present if the concentration of HCO_3^- concentration in plasma (P_{HCO3}) is elevated.

3. What is the rate of K^+ excretion? If the rate of K^+ excretion is considerably less than 150 mmol/day (or <15 mmol K^+/mmol creatinine), this indicates a renal defect in excretion of K^+ due to a low $[K^+]_{CCD}$.
4. Why is $U_K/U_{Creatinine}$ abnormally low? Seek the basis for a diminished negative luminal voltage in the CCD—either a diminished

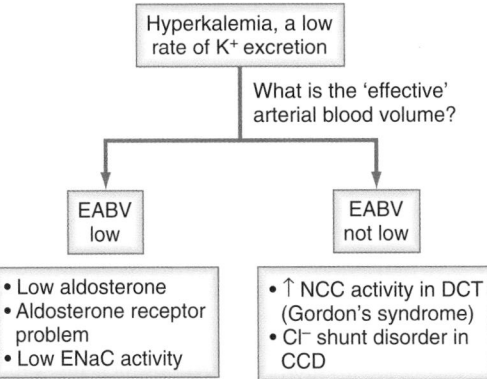

Figure 111-9 Basis for the low rate of excretion of K^+. Patients with chronic hyperkalemia can be divided into two groups based on their effective arterial blood volume (EABV). In this analysis, we have assumed an adequate distal delivery of Na^+. *(From Halperin ML. The ACID truth and BASIC facts—with a sweet touch, an enLYTEnment. 5th ed. Toronto: RossMark Medical Publishers; 2003. Reproduced with permission, ref 74.)*

Na^+ reabsorption via ENaC in the CCD or reabsorption of Na^+ and Cl^- at near-equal rates in the CCD.

DIMINISHED REABSORPTION OF SODIUM VIA ENaC IN CORTICAL COLLECTING DUCT

The first subgroup of patients with this type of disorder are those with marked decrease in their effective circulating volume and a sufficiently low distal delivery of Na^+ to CCD. The second subgroup of patients with this type of disorder includes those who have lesions that lead to a diminished number of open ENaC units in the luminal membrane of principal cells in CCD. These lesions include low aldosterone actions (e.g., adrenal insufficiency, drugs that block the aldosterone receptor in principal cells (e.g., spironolactone), molecular defects that lead to a lower number of open ENaC units in the luminal membrane of principal cells, and cationic compounds in the luminal fluid in the CCD that block ENaC (e.g., amiloride or triamterene or cationic antimicrobial agents such as trimethoprim). These patients often have a low effective arterial blood volume, a higher than expected rate of excretion of Na^+ and Cl^- in their urine considering the presence of a contracted effective arterial blood volume, and a high P_{Renin}. The measurement of $P_{Aldosterone}$ is helpful to determine the basis of diminished reabsorption of Na^+ via ENaC in CCD.

REABSORPTION OF SODIUM AND CHLORIDE AT NEAR-EQUAL RATES IN THE CORTICAL COLLECTING DUCT

One subgroup of patients with these types of disorder seems to have an increased permeability for Cl^- in CCD (a Cl^- shunt disorder). In another subgroup, the site of the lesion seems to be in the early distal convoluted tubule. The hyperkalemia in patients with type II pseudohypoaldosteronism (Gordon's syndrome) may be an example for this later pathophysiology. Two factors are important to achieve these near-equal rates of ion transport in the CCD in these patients. First, low delivery of Na^+ and Cl^- to the CCD due to a higher rate of reabsorption of Na^+ and Cl^- in the distal convoluted tubule occurs because of increased activity of Na^+ and Cl^- cotransporter (NCC). Second, effective arterial blood volume expansion, which suppresses the release of aldosterone and leads to less number of open ENaC units in luminal membrane of principal cells in CCD.

Regardless of the site of the lesion, these patients will tend to have an expanded effective arterial blood volume, hypertension, and a very low P_{Renin}. They are, however, able to excrete urine with little Na^+ and Cl^- when the effective arterial blood volume is contracted (e.g., after giving a diuretic plus a low salt diet).

▓ Specific Causes of Hyperkalemia

A list of the causes of hyperkalemia based on their possible underlying pathophysiology is provided in Box 111-3.

ADDISON'S DISEASE

The most common cause of this disorder used to be bilateral adrenal destruction with tuberculosis, but now autoimmune adrenalitis accounts for the majority of cases. Additional causes include other infectious diseases (disseminated fungal infection), adrenal replacement by metastatic carcinoma or lymphoma, adrenal hemorrhage or infarction, and drugs that impair the synthesis of aldosterone (e.g., ketoconazole and possibly fluconazole).

Patients with chronic primary adrenal insufficiency may present with chronic malaise, fatigue, anorexia, and weight loss. In most patients, the blood pressure is low, and postural symptoms of dizziness and syncope are common. The P_K is usually close to 5.5 mmol/L unless a significant degree of intravascular volume depletion diminishes the flow rate in CCD. Nevertheless, hyperkalemia is not seen on presentation in approximately a third of cases.[38] The diagnosis can be established by finding a low $P_{Aldosterone}$ and cortisol levels, high P_{Renin} (see Box 111-1), and a blunted cortisol response to the administration of ACTH. Both glucocorticoid and mineralocorticoid replacement are required.

Adrenal crisis is an emergency that requires immediate restoration of the intravascular volume with the administration of intravenous (IV) saline and correction of the cortisol deficiency (administer

dexamethasone or hydrocortisone). Beware of raising the P_{Na} too rapidly if hyponatremia is present because of the risk of osmotic demyelination in a catabolic patient.[39]

PSEUDOHYPOALDOSTERONISM TYPE I

The underlying pathophysiology is a fewer number of open ENaC units in the CCD. In the autosomal recessive form, most mutations are in the α subunit of ENaC.[40] These patients usually present in the neonatal period with renal salt wasting, hyperkalemia, metabolic acidosis, weight loss, and failure to thrive. ENaC activity is also impaired in the lung, leading to excessive airway fluid and recurrent lower respiratory tract infections. The autosomal dominant form this disorder is due to mutations involving the mineralocorticoid receptor.[41] The clinical disorder is usually milder and may remit with time.

Patients with this syndrome fail to respond to exogenous mineralocorticoids, and their $P_{Aldosterone}$ and P_{Renin} are markedly elevated. Treatment includes supplementation with NaCl and inducing the loss of K^+ through the gastrointestinal tract.

SYNDROME OF HYPORENINEMIC HYPOALDOSTERONISM

These patients represent a heterogeneous group with regard to the pathophysiology of their disorder.

Group 1: Patients with Low Capability of Producing Renin

This is a less common group in which there seems to be either destruction of or a biosynthetic defect in the juxtaglomerular apparatus that leads to a low P_{Renin} and thereby a low $P_{Aldosterone}$. Hyperkalemia is due to a diminished electrogenic reabsorption of Na^+ in the CCD. The effective arterial blood volume will tend to be low. These patients should have a significant rise in their rate of excretion of K^+ with the administration of mineralocorticoids.

Group 2: Patients with Low Stimulus to Produce Renin

Subgroup One. Patients in this category have Gordon syndrome, a disorder where there is a low delivery of Na^+ and Cl^- to the CCD due to their enhanced reabsorption in the early distal convoluted tubule. The activity of the thiazide-sensitive NCC is increased in this disorder.[32] Hypertension and hyperkalemia are common presenting features. The P_{Renin} is suppressed, and the $P_{Aldosterone}$ is inappropriately low considering that hyperkalemia is present (see Box 111-1). Thiazide diuretics are particularly helpful in these patients in treating both the hypertension and the hyperkalemia.[42]

The molecular basis involves mutations in the family of WNK (meaning *with no lysine*, where *K* is the single letter symbol for *lysine*) kinases (Figure 111-10). Major deletions in the genes encoding for WNK kinase 1 and WNK kinase 4 were reported in these patients. WNK kinase 4 normally causes a decrease in luminal NCC activity.[32] Therefore if WNK kinase 4 were deleted, reabsorption of Na^+ and Cl^- by NCC in the early distal convoluted tubule will be augmented. The molecular defect in WNK kinase 1 is the removal of intron bases that leads to a gain of function. WNK kinase 1 normally inactivates WNK kinase 4, hence a gain in WNK kinase 1 function leads to the presence of more open NCC units in the luminal membranes of the early distal convoluted tubule.

Subgroup Two. Hyperkalemia is due to less electrogenic reabsorption of Na^+ in the CCD. The underlying pathophysiology may involve augmented reabsorption of Na^+ and Cl^- in the early distal convoluted tubule, or some of these patients may have a Cl^- shunt disorder in CCD. There is no known molecular basis for the latter, and the most common setting is in patients with diabetic nephropathy. The P_{Renin} is suppressed, and the $P_{Aldosterone}$ is inappropriately low considering that hyperkalemia is present (see Box 111-1). In patients with a Cl^- shunt disorder, there is a significant increase in the rate of excretion of K^+ when bicarbonaturia is induced by the administration of acetazolamide.[25,43,44]

Box 111-3

CAUSES OF HYPERKALEMIA

High Potassium Intake
Only if combined with low excretion of K^+

Shift of Potassium Out of Cells
Cell necrosis
Lack of insulin
Use of nonselective beta-blockers
Metabolic acidosis where anions are largely restricted to the extracellular fluid compartment (e.g., HCl, citric acid)
Rare causes (e.g., hyperkalemic periodic paralysis, barium)

Diminished Potassium Loss in Urine
Advanced chronic renal insufficiency
Low $[K^+]_{CCD}$

Primary Decrease in Flux of Na^+ Through Epithelial Na^+ Channel (ENaC)
Very low delivery of Na^+ to the CCD
Low levels of aldosterone (e.g., Addison's disease)
Blockade of the aldosterone receptor (e.g., spironolactone)
Low ENaC activity (hereditary disease)
Blockade of ENaC (e.g., amiloride, triamterene, trimethoprim-like drugs)

Cl^- Reabsorbed at Similar Rate as Na^+ in CCD
Increased reabsorption of Na^+ and Cl^- in distal convoluted tubule (e.g., Gordon's syndrome [WNK kinase 4 and/or 1 mutations])
Cl^- shunt disorder in CCD (e.g., diabetic nephropathy, drugs such as cyclosporin)

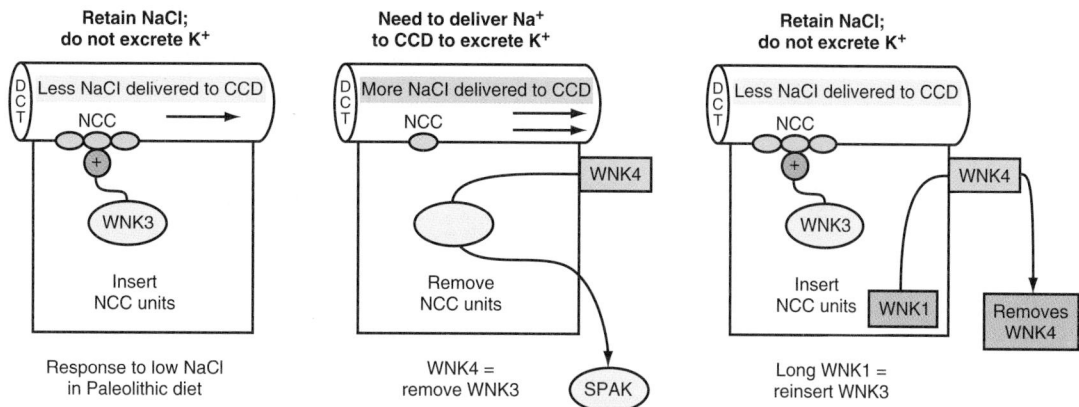

Figure 111-10 Effect of WNK kinases on reabsorption of Na$^+$ and Cl$^-$ and secretion of K$^+$. Horizontal cylinders represent lumen of early distal convoluted tubule (DCT); rectangle below these cylinders represents their cells. Effect of WNK kinases on NaCl and K$^+$ homeostasis can be understood from a Paleolithic perspective as diet contained little NaCl, while intake of K$^+$ was large but episodic. *Far left*, WNK-3 is present in their cytoplasm *(brown shading)*; this occurs when little NaCl is consumed (i.e., in a Paleolithic diet). As a result, more Na$^+$/Cl$^-$ co-transporters (NCC) reside in the luminal membrane of these cells. When there is a large intake of K$^+$ salts while little NaCl is consumed, SPAK is removed, owing to actions of WNK-4 *(green shading)*. Hence NCC is internalized, and there is a larger delivery of Na$^+$ and Cl$^-$ to cortical collecting duct (CCD) to facilitate secretion of K$^+$ *(middle portion of figure)*. *Far right, brown shading*, NaCl must be retained when there is no longer a need for K$^+$ secretion. Thus NCC must be reinserted into the early DCT. This is achieved when WNK-1 *(purple shading)* removes WNK-4 and hence reestablishes effects of SPAK. *(From Halperin ML. The ACID truth and BASIC facts—with a sweet touch, an enLYTEnment. 5th ed. Toronto: RossMark Medical Publishers; 2003. Reproduced with permission ref 74.)*

DRUGS ASSOCIATED WITH HYPERKALEMIA

1. **Drugs that affect cellular redistribution of K$^+$.** Nonselective β_2-adrenergic blockers may diminish the β_2-adrenergic mediated shift of K$^+$ into cells. In general, only a minor rise in P$_K$ is observed in patients taking this class of drugs. Digitalis overdose may be accompanied by hyperkalemia due to inhibition of Na$^+$/K$^+$-ATPase in cell membranes of skeletal muscles. The use of depolarizing agents such as succinylcholine during anesthesia may cause a shift of K$^+$ out of cells and hyperkalemia. Drugs that have an α-adrenergic agonist effect may cause hyperkalemia by inhibiting the release of insulin.

2. **Drugs that interfere with renal K$^+$ excretion.** With respect to many of these drugs, the mechanisms for the defect in K$^+$ excretion have not been studied in sufficient detail to draw unequivocal conclusions about how each drug may cause hyperkalemia.

Drugs that Inhibit Release of Renin

Nonsteroidal Antiinflammatory Drugs and Cyclo-oxygenase-2 Inhibitors. Secretion of renin by cells in the juxtaglomerular arterioles and by cells of the macula densa in the early distal tubule appears to be mediated in part by locally produced prostaglandins. As a result, inhibition of prostaglandin synthesis will cause both the P$_{Renin}$ and the P$_{Aldosterone}$ to be low. Nevertheless, the rise in the P$_K$ is very small in normal subjects, but a significant degree of hyperkalemia may develop in the presence of kidney diseases or with the intake of other drugs that may also impair the renal excretion of K$^+$.

Drugs that Interfere with the Renin-Angiotensin-Aldosterone Axis

The first class of drugs includes angiotensin-converting enzyme (ACE) inhibitors, angiotensin II receptor blockers, and renin inhibitors. In more detail, the two major stimuli for the release of aldosterone are angiotensin II and a high P$_K$. Although it is estimated that the overall incidence of hyperkalemia is approximately 10% in patients taking this class of drugs, nevertheless, the rise in the P$_K$ is less than 0.5 mEq/L in patients with relatively normal renal function. In contrast, a more severe degree of hyperkalemia may be seen in patients with renal insufficiency or the concurrent use of a drug that impairs renal K$^+$ excretion, such as a potassium-sparing diuretic or a nonsteroidal antiinflammatory drug (NSAID).

The second class of drugs that interfere with the renin-angiotensin-aldosterone axis are drugs that inhibit the synthesis of aldosterone. Aldosterone synthesis is selectively reduced in patients who are treated with heparin. Again, severe hyperkalemia occurs only if some other cause of impairment in K$^+$ excretion is present such as renal insufficiency or the intake of an ACE inhibitor or a potassium-sparing diuretic. Hyperkalemia has also been noted in patients receiving low-molecular-weight heparin.

The third class of drugs in this group are those that compete with aldosterone for binding to its receptor. Hyperkalemia is a potential problem in patients taking the nonspecific mineralocorticoid receptor antagonist, spironolactone, or the selective mineralocorticoid receptor antagonist, eplerenone. The incidence of hyperkalemia is dose dependent, with detectable effects even at doses of 25 mg spironolactone per day. At higher doses, the risk of severe hyperkalemia increases. Of special concern is the rise in use of these drugs after the demonstrated improved survival with the use of aldosterone antagonists in patients with congestive heart failure.

The fourth class of drugs that interfere with the renin-angiotensin-aldosterone axis block ENaC in the luminal membrane of principal cells in the CCD (e.g., amiloride, trimethoprim, and pentamidine). The cationic form of these drugs causes hyperkalemia and salt wasting. Patients with HIV and *Pneumocystis carinii* pneumonia treated with trimethoprim may develop hyperkalemia. Although this has been attributed to the use of high doses of trimethoprim in these patients, trimethoprim may cause a rise in the P$_K$ even when used in conventional doses. Another factor that may contribute to the development of hyperkalemia in patients taking these drugs is a low flow rate in the terminal CCD due to poor dietary intake and hence low rate of delivery of osmoles (urea and NaCl) to the CCD. This in turn increases the concentration of trimethoprim in the lumen of the CCD for a given rate of excretion of this drug (same quantity of trimethoprim is now in a smaller volume).

The fifth class of drugs in this group may cause a Cl$^-$ shunt–type disorder. Hyperkalemia develops in some patients receiving the calcineurin inhibitors, cyclosporin or FK506 following organ transplantation. The pathophysiology of hyperkalemia, the clinical signs in these patients (presence of hypertension, an ECF volume that is not low, suppressed P_{Renin}), and the finding that bicarbonaturia leads to an increase in the rate of excretion of K^+ resemble those of an increased permeability for Cl^- in the CCD (a Cl^- shunt disorder).

HYPERKALEMIC PERIODIC PARALYSIS

This syndrome has an autosomal dominant inheritance and is the result of a mutation in the α-subunit of the skeletal muscle Na^+ channel gene.[46] This leads to failure to completely close these voltage-gated Na^+ channels when the concentration of K^+ in the ECF is raised—hence there is a diminished electrical excitability of skeletal muscle cells. Symptoms of weakness and ultimately paralysis in association with hyperkalemia usually follow bouts of exercise. Acetazolamide seems to be effective in preventing these episodes, although its mechanism of action is not clear.

NO MEDICAL EMERGENCY

Removal of Potassium from the Body

It is important to appreciate that very much less K^+ loss is needed to lower the P_K from 7.0 to 6.0 mmol/L than to lower it from 6.0 to 5.0 mmol/L.[54] Hence creating a relatively small K^+ loss can be very important when there is a severe degree of hyperkalemia.

Enhancing Excretion of Potassium in Urine

If K^+ excretion is low because of a low urine volume, but with a high U_K, a loop diuretic may induce kaliuresis by increasing the flow rate in the CCD. One can avoid unwanted effective arterial blood volume contraction by replacing the Na^+ and Cl^- lost in the urine. This NaCl should be given at the same tonicity as the urine to avoid creating a dysnatremia. If the U_K is unduly low, depending on the possible pathophysiology of hyperkalemia, giving a mineralocorticoid (100 μg of Florinef) or inducing bicarbonaturia with a carbonic anhydrase inhibitor may cause a significant kaliuresis. To avoid the development of metabolic acidosis, the HCO_3^- lost in the urine may need to be replaced.

Cation Exchange Resins for Treatment of Hyperkalemia

A cation exchange resin can exchange bound Na^+ (Kayexalate) or Ca^{2+} (calcium resonium) for cations including K^+. Kayexalate contains 4 mEq of Na^+ per gram. The only favorable location for the exchange of Na^+ for K^+ is in the lumen of the colon. Based on data from patients with ileostomy, the amount of K^+ delivered to the colon that would be available for this exchange is close to 5 mmol/L. Furthermore, other cations such as NH_4^+, Ca^{2+}, and Mg^{2+} may exchange for resin-bound Na^+ apart from K^+. One possible theoretical benefit of using cation exchange resins is if they were to lower the concentration of K^+ in luminal water in the lower intestinal tract and thereby enhance the secretion of K^+ by the rectosigmoid colon. Even if more K^+ were secreted, the low stool volume would limit the total K^+ loss. For example, if the lumen-negative transepithelial voltage were −90 millivolts, and the P_K were 5 mmol/L, the concentration of K^+ in stool water would be 75 mmol/L. With a usual stool volume of 125 mL, of which 75% is water, only close to 7 mmol of K^+ would be lost by this route. Hence we feel that there is virtually no theoretical benefit to using resins for acute hyperkalemia and little benefit to adding resins to cathartics in the setting of chronic hyperkalemia.[6]

Dialysis

Hemodialysis is more effective than peritoneal dialysis for removing K^+. Removal rates of K^+ can approximate 35 mmol/h with a dialysate bath K^+ concentration of 1 to 2 mmol/L. A glucose-free dialysate is preferable to avoid the glucose-induced release of insulin and subsequent shift of K^+ into cells, lessening the rate of removal of K^+.

Box 111-4

CAUSES OF HYPOKALEMIA

Decreased Potassium Intake
Rarely a primary cause unless K^+ intake is very low and duration is prolonged
Can augment the degree of hypokalemia if there is ongoing K^+ loss

Shift of Potassium Into Cells
Hormones (insulin and β-adrenergics are most important)
Metabolic alkalosis (not a major mechanism for hypokalemia)
Anabolic state (e.g., recovery from diabetic ketoacidosis)
Rare (e.g., hypokalemic periodic paralysis)

Excessive Renal Potassium Loss
More reabsorption of Na^+ than Cl^- in CCD
High aldosterone levels
Cortisol acts as a mineralocorticoid
Low 11β-HSDH activity (apparent mineralocorticoid excess syndrome)
Inhibitors of 11β-HSDH (e.g., licorice)
Very high cortisol level (e.g., ACTH-producing tumor)
Constitutively active ENaC (e.g., Liddle's syndrome)
Artificial ENaC (e.g., amphotericin B)
Less reabsorption of Cl^- than Na^+ in the CCD
Delivery of Na^+ without Cl^- to the CCD and low extracellular fluid volume
Inhibition of Cl^- reabsorption in the CCD (e.g., bicarbonaturia)
High delivery of Na^+ and Cl^- to the CCD and a V_{max} for Na^+ reabsorption which exceeds that for Cl^- (inhibition of NaCl reabsorption an upstream nephron segment, plus effective arterial blood volume contraction)

Loss of Potassium via Gastrointestinal Tract
Diarrhea (infectious, some cases of laxative abuse, villous adenoma, short bowel syndrome)

Loss of Potassium via Skin
Conditions with increased loss of K^+ in sweat (e.g., fever in a patient with cystic fibrosis)

HYPOKALEMIA

Clinical Approach

A list of causes of hypokalemia is provided in Box 111-4.
1. **Deal with medical emergencies:** Emergencies that may be present on presentation must be addressed first , one must also, anticipate and prevent risks that may arise during therapy (Figure 111-11).
2. **Determine if the major basis for hypokalemia is an acute shift of K^+ into cells** (Figure 111-12).

The most important initial step is to establish whether the duration of illness is short. The following characteristics should be present if the basis of hypokalemia is a shift of K^+ into cells. The most important etiology is an adrenergic surge that lasts for many hours (e.g., post myocardial infarction, head trauma[55]) or the presence of hyperthyroidism in Asian patients with acute hypokalemia and extreme weakness.[56] There should be a minimum rate of excretion of K^+. A significant degree of metabolic acidosis or metabolic alkalosis should not be present.

Having established that there is an acute shift of K^+ into cells, the next step is to determine if an adrenergic surge may have caused this shift. In these settings, tachycardia, a wide pulse pressure, and systolic hypertension are often present. It is very important to recognize this group of patients, because administration of nonspecific beta-blockers can lead to very prompt recovery (i.e., within 2 hours) without the need for a large infusion of KCl, and hence avoids the development of rebound hyperkalemia when the stimulus for this shift of K^+ abates.

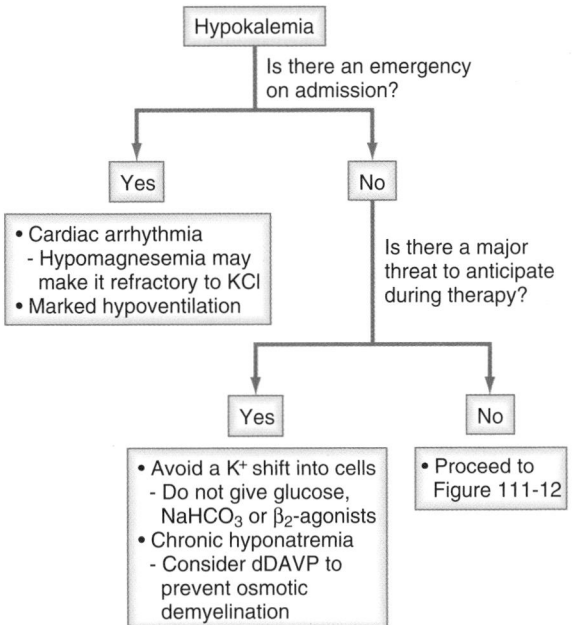

Figure 111-11 **Initial clinical approach for the patient with hypo-kalemia.** The steps are to deal with emergencies and anticipate and prevent dangers during therapy. *(From Halperin ML. The ACID truth and BASIC facts—with a sweet touch, an enLYTEnment. 5th ed. Toronto: RossMark Medical Publishers; 2003. Reproduced with permission ref 74.)*

PLASMA ACID-BASE STATUS AND HYPOKALEMIA

Patients with Hyperchloremic Metabolic Acidosis

Gastrointestinal loss of $NaHCO_3$ (e.g., diarrhea, laxative abuse, fistula, ileus, ureteral diversion)

Overproduction of an acid with a high rate of excretion of its conjugate anion in the urine (e.g., hippuric acid in patients with toluene abuse)

Reduced reabsorption of $NaHCO_3$ in the proximal convoluted tubule (e.g., proximal renal tubular acidosis treated with large amounts of $NaHCO_3$, use of acetazolamide)

Distal renal tubular acidosis:
- Low distal H^+ secretion subtype
- High distal secretion of HCO_3^- (e.g., Southeast Asian ovalocytosis with second mutation involving the Cl^-/HCO_3^- anion exchanger)

Patients with Metabolic Alkalosis

Vomiting, nasogastric suction, some types of diarrhea

Diuretic use or abuse

Other disorders—can be classified based on blood pressure and/or P_{Renin}:
- Patients with a low effective arterial blood volume, absence of hypertension, (e.g., Bartter's syndrome, Gitelman's syndrome, ligand binding to Ca-SR in thick ascending limb of the loop of Henle)
- Patients with a high effective arterial blood volume, hypertension, (e.g., primary hyperaldosteronism, renal artery stenosis, malignant hypertension, glucocorticoid remedial aldosteronism, Liddle's syndrome, apparent mineralocorticoid excess syndrome, Cushing's syndrome).

3-WHAT IS THE RATE OF EXCRETION OF POTASSIUM?

To assess the renal response to hypokalemia, we use the expected rate of K^+ excretion when hypokalemia was due to nonrenal causes—i.e., less than 10-15 mmol/d or close to 1 mmol K^+/mmol creatinine.[20] The rate of renal excretion of K^+ may be low in a patient with chronic hypokalemia due to extrarenal loss of K^+ or a renal loss of K^+ in the recent past.

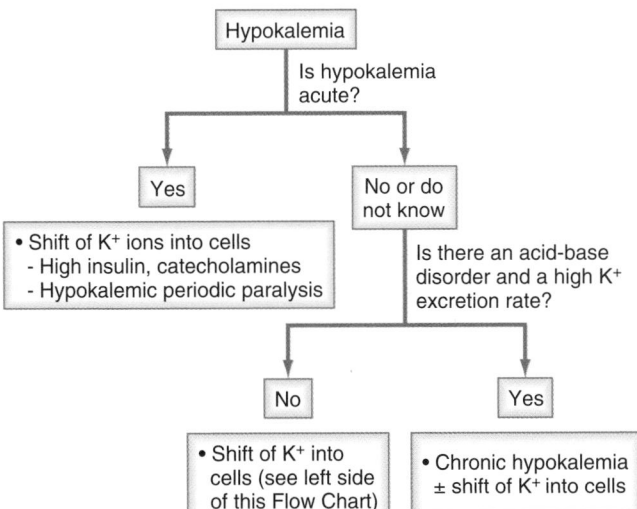

Figure 111-12 **Initial steps in the clinical diagnosis of hypokalemia.** If hypokalemia is known to be acute, its basis is a recent shift of K^+ into cells. In the absence of this evidence, the steps to follow are illustrated in brown shading, and the final diagnostic categories are in the boxes preceded by a bullet symbol. *(From Halperin ML. The ACID truth and BASIC facts—with a sweet touch, an enLYTEnment. 5th ed. Toronto: RossMark Medical Publishers; 2003. Reproduced with permission.)*

4-WHAT IS THE ACID-BASE STATUS?

Patients with chronic hypokalemia can then be divided into two groups based on their metabolic acid-base disorder (Box 111-5).

Patients with Chronic Hypokalemia and Metabolic Acidosis

These patients can be divided into two further categories based on their rate of excretion NH_4^+ (Figure 111-13). The rate of excretion of NH_4^+ can be estimated from the calculation of the urine osmolal gap.

Patients with Chronic Hypokalemia and Metabolic Alkalosis

These patients can be classified into two groups based on whether the loss of K^+ is nonrenal or renal with the use of the $U_K/U_{Creatinine}$ ratio in a spot urine sample (Figure 111-14).

Patients with Chronic Hypokalemia, Metabolic Alkalosis, and High Renal Excretion of Potassium. These patients have a high $[K^+]_{CCD}$ in

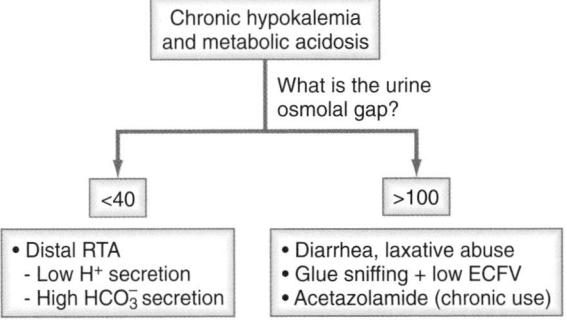

Figure 111-13 **Chronic hypokalemia and metabolic acidosis.** The first step in these patients is to estimate the concentration of NH_4^+ in the urine, using the osmolal gap. *(From Halperin ML. The ACID truth and BASIC facts—with a sweet touch, an enLYTEnment. 5th ed. Toronto: RossMark Medical Publishers; 2003. Reproduced with permission ref 74.)*

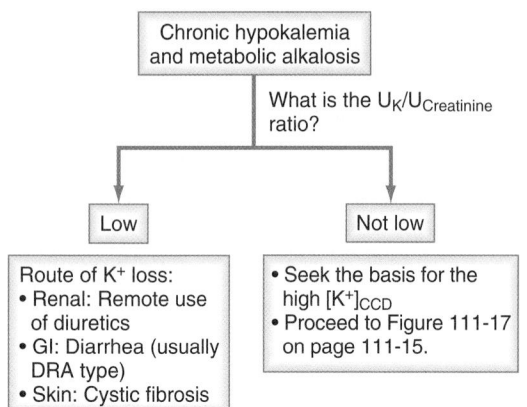

Figure 111-14 Chronic hypokalemia and metabolic alkalosis. In a patient with chronic hypokalemia and metabolic alkalosis, the first step is to determine the $U_K/U_{Creatinine}$. If this estimate of the rate of excretion of K^+ is definitely low, look for a nonrenal and/or a prior renal loss of K^+. On the other hand, if the $U_K/U_{Creatinine}$ is *not* low, determine why the $[K^+]_{CCD}$ is higher than expected. $[K^+]_{CCD}$ represents concentration of K^+ in the lumen of terminal CCD. DRA = down regulated in adenoma. *(From Halperin ML. The ACID truth and BASIC facts—with a sweet touch, an enLYTEnment. 5th ed. Toronto: RossMark Medical Publishers; 2003. Reproduced with permission.)*

the presence of hypokalemia. The most common cause of high $[K^+]_{CCD}$ is a more negative voltage in the lumen of the CCD. This higher lumen negative voltage may be due to disorders that cause more reabsorption of Na^+ than Cl^- in the CCD or disorders that may cause less reabsorption of Cl^- than Na^+ in the CCD. These two types of disorders can be differentiated with assessment of effective arterial blood volume and measurement of blood pressure (see Box 111-2 and Figure 111-15).

Disorders with More Reabsorption of Sodium than Chloride in the Cortical Distal Nephron. Patients with these types of disorders are expected to have hypertension and an effective arterial blood volume that is not contracted. Based on measurement of $P_{Aldosterone}$, these patients can be classified into two groups: those with conditions in

which the $P_{Aldosterone}$ is high and those with conditions in which the actions of aldosterone are mimicked and hence the $P_{Aldosterone}$ is low (see Figure 111-15 and Figure 111-16).

Disorders with Less Reabsorption of Chloride than Sodium in the Cortical Collecting Duct. These patients are expected to have a contracted effective arterial blood volume and the absence of hypertension (unless patients are given diuretics for treatment of hypertension; see Figure 111-15). The most common causes are protracted vomiting or the use of diuretics. The use of urine electrolytes in the differential diagnosis in patients with hypokalemia and a contracted effective arterial blood volume is illustrated in Box 111-6.

Specific Causes of Hypokalemia

HYPOKALEMIA AND A LOW EXTRACELLULAR FLUID VOLUME

Diuretic-Induced Hypokalemia

Two factors contribute to the development of hypokalemia in patients receiving diuretics: a high flow rate in the CCD and an increased secretion of K^+ in these nephron segments. The latter requires an enhanced electrogenic reabsorption of Na^+ via ENaC due to effects of aldosterone. Hypokalemia is usually modest in degree; a P_K less than 3 mmol/L is observed in less than 10% of patients and usually within the first 2 weeks of therapy.[57]

Diuretic abuse should be considered if little Na^+ and Cl^- are found in a single urine collection, as this reflects the normal renal response to a low effective arterial blood volume (see Box 111-6). The urine should be screened for diuretics, the assay should be performed on a urine sample that contains abundant Na^+ and Cl^- (i.e., a urine sample that reflects the action of a diuretic).

In the absence of diuretic use, Bartter's syndrome or Gitelman's syndrome should be suspected. Other diagnoses to rule out include hypercalcemia and other ligands that bind the calcium-sensing receptor in the loop of Henle (e.g., cationic drugs such as gentamicin, cationic proteins).

Four issues about hypokalemia and diuretic use are worth highlighting. First, since the risk of developing hypokalemia is dose dependent

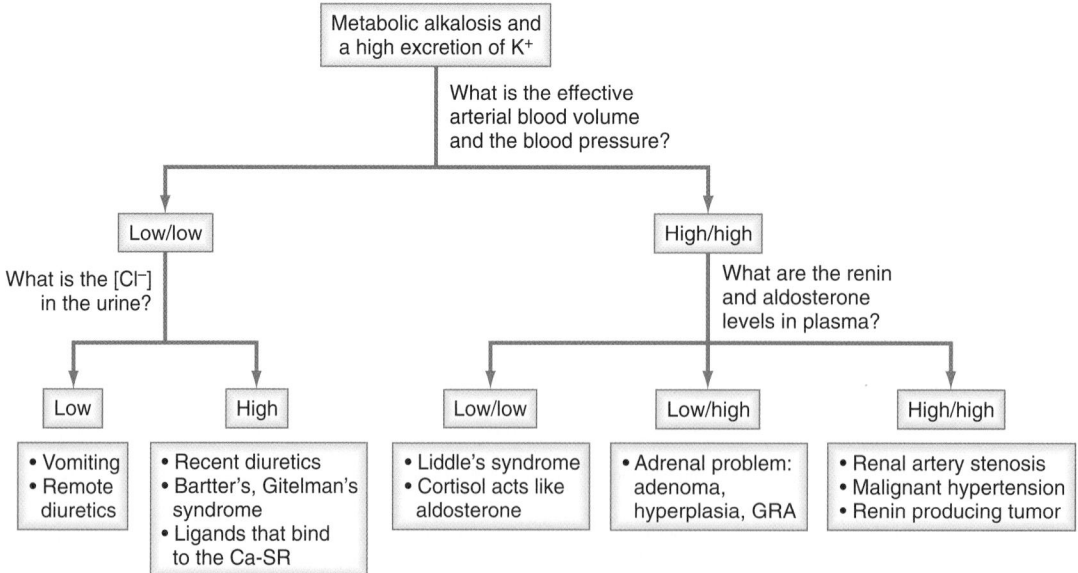

Figure 111-15 Chronic hypokalemia, metabolic alkalosis, and a high $K/U_{Creatinine}$. The goal is to determine why the $[K^+]_{CCD}$ is higher than expected in a patient with hypokalemia, metabolic alkalosis, and a $U_K/U_{Creatinine}$ that is definitely not low. Major clues are an estimate of the effective arterial blood volume and blood pressure. If both are low (*left side* of figure), the next step is to examine the concentration of Cl^- in the urine. On the other hand, if the effective arterial blood volume is not low and the blood pressure is high, the differential diagnosis is based primarily on the P_{Renin} and $P_{Aldosterone}$ (see Box 111-1). *(From Halperin ML. The ACID truth and BASIC facts—with a sweet touch, an enLYTEnment. 5th ed. Toronto: RossMark Medical Publishers; 2003. Reproduced with permission, ref 74.)*

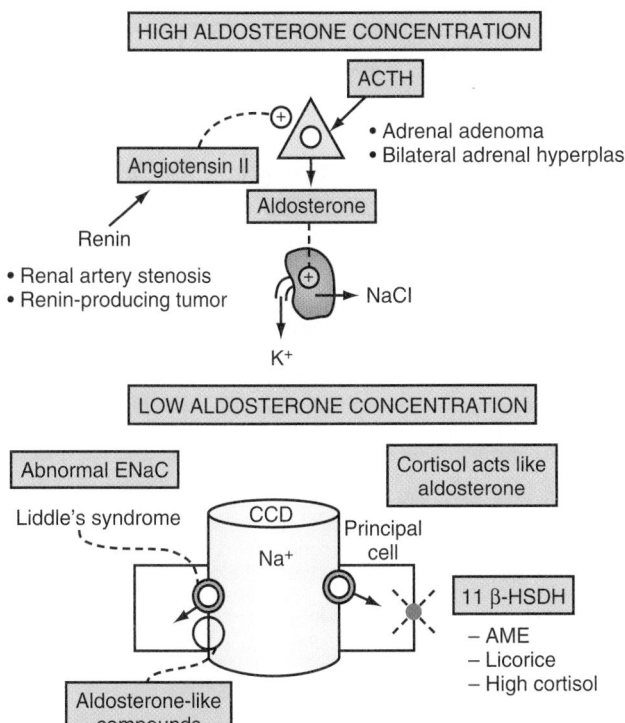

Figure 111-16 Conditions causing hypokalemia with more reabsorption of Na⁺ than Cl⁻. Conditions in which there is both hypokalemia and an abnormally high $P_{Aldosterone}$ are illustrated in upper portion of figure in brown shading. In contrast, conditions with hypokalemia but low $P_{Aldosterone}$ are illustrated in lower portion of figure in green shading. ACE, angiotensin-converting enzyme; ACTH, adrenocorticotropic hormone; AME, apparent mineralocorticoid excess syndrome; ENaC, epithelial Na⁺ channel; GRA, glucocorticoid remediable aldosteronism; 11β-HSDH, 11β-hydroxysteroid dehydrogenase. *(From Halperin ML. The ACID truth and BASIC facts—with a sweet touch, an enLYTEnment. 5th ed. Toronto: RossMark Medical Publishers; 2003. Reproduced with permission.)*

and increasing the thiazide dose does not usually result in further benefit in blood pressure control, the lowest effective dose of this drug should be used. Second, restricting the intake of NaCl to less than 100 mmol/d may minimize the degree of renal K⁺ wasting. Third, the use of a K⁺-sparing diuretic may reduce the renal loss of K⁺. Fourth, whether a mild degree of hypokalemia due to the use of diuretics should be treated is debatable. Because patients with ischemic heart disease, left ventricular hypertrophy, and/or those treated with digitalis may be at increased risk for arrhythmias, even a modest degree of hypokalemia should be prevented in these patients.

Vomiting-Induced Hypokalemia

Since the K⁺ concentration in gastric fluid is usually less than 15 mmol/L,[14] hypokalemia in patients with vomiting or nasogastric suction results primarily from the loss of K⁺ in the urine due to a higher rate of electrogenic reabsorption of Na⁺ in the CCD. This is due to actions of aldosterone released in response to decreased effective arterial blood volume, along with distal delivery of Na⁺ with nonabsorbable anions (SO_4^{2-} anions from metabolism of sulfur-containing amino acids in the early phase of vomiting, organic anions in the later phase of vomiting).[31] To a lesser extent, hypokalemia may be the result of a shift of K⁺ into the ICF compartment due to the alkalemia. Key diagnostic elements are a history of vomiting or a strong concern about body weight, a significant degree of hypokalemia, metabolic alkalosis, and especially a very low U_{Cl} (see Box 111-6). In a patient with recent vomiting, the urine may contain a considerable amount of Na⁺ despite ECF volume contraction, because the

---

Box 111-6

URINE ELECTROLYTES* IN THE DIFFERENTIAL DIAGNOSIS OF HYPOKALEMIA

Condition	Urine Electrolyte	
	Na⁺	Cl⁻
Vomiting		
Recent	High†	Low‡
Remote	Low	Low
Diuretics		
Recent	High	High
Remote	Low	Low
Diarrhea or Laxative Abuse	Low	High
Bartter's or Gitelman's Syndrome	High	High

*Do not use the urine electrolytes in this fashion during polyuric states.
†High = urine concentration > 15 mmol/L.
‡Low = urine concentration < 15 mmol/L.

excretion of HCO_3^- obligates the excretion of Na⁺. Other causes of hypokalemia with a low effective arterial blood volume must be considered (see Box 111-6).

Therapy must deal with the underlying cause of vomiting and the administration of KCl.[16,58] If the patient has a contracted effective arterial blood volume, NaCl should be administered as needed.

Hypokalemia in Patients with Hyperchloremic Metabolic Acidosis

Rare causes of excessive excretion of K⁺ and metabolic acidosis include distal RTA due to a low rate of secretion of H⁺ in the distal nephron[15] and inhibition of renal carbonic anhydrase (see Box 111-5). Hypokalemia is also seen in patients who sniff glue and overproduce hippuric acid.[59] Excessive excretion of K⁺ in this setting is due to an open ENaC in the CCD owing to the effect of aldosterone released in response to a contracted effective arterial blood volume and the distal delivery of Na⁺ with hippurate anions instead of Cl⁻.

In patients with a secretory type of diarrhea (e.g., cholera), much K⁺ can be lost in K⁺-rich colonic fluids.[14] Nevertheless, despite the large K⁺ deficit, hypokalemia is usually not present on presentation because the severe degree of intravascular volume depletion leads to an α-adrenergic surge, which inhibits the release of insulin. Hypokalemia becomes evident after therapy is initiated and the effective arterial blood volume is expanded. Patients with diarrhea due to a defect that leads to diminished reabsorption of Na⁺ and Cl⁻ in the colon usually have a low P_K but only a modest deficit of K⁺ unless there is also a reason for increased delivery of Na⁺ and Cl⁻ to the colon (intake of certain types of laxatives). The low P_K in these patients likely reflects a shift of K⁺ into cells due to a β₂-adrenergic response to the mild degree of contraction of effective arterial blood volume.

Abuse of laxatives may be denied, so measurement of urine electrolytes may provide helpful clues (see Box 111-6). The U_{Na} will be low if the effective arterial blood volume is contracted, but the U_{Cl} is characteristically high, reflecting the high rate of excretion of NH_4^+ in response to metabolic acidosis and/or hypokalemia. At times, one might have to rely on measurements of stool electrolytes and other evidence for laxatives in the stool to confirm the diagnosis.[60]

Bartter's Syndrome

Bartter's syndrome is a disease of children for the most part. Mutations that cause Bartter's syndrome have been identified in five separate genes that impact on NaCl transport in the thick ascending limb of the loop of Henle (the luminal Na⁺, K⁺, 2 Cl⁻ cotransporter, ROMK channel, the basolateral Cl⁻ channel, β subunit of Cl⁻ channel; Barttin, and also activating mutations in the calcium sensing receptor). There is often a positive family history and/or consanguinity. The clinical picture is dominated by effective arterial blood volume contraction, and the major laboratory features include hypokalemia, renal wasting of Na^+, Cl^-, and K^+, and metabolic alkalosis. The pathophysiology of Bartter's syndrome can be thought of as having a loop diuretic acting 24 hours a day, producing a higher than expected rate of excretion of Na^+ and Cl^- in the face of a contracted effective arterial blood volume, an inability to have a sufficiently high U_{osm} when vasopressin acts, and renal calcium wasting as evidenced by a high urine calcium/creatinine ratio. Renal K^+ wasting is due to both a high flow rate in the CCD and a high $[K^+]_{CCD}$. The high $[K^+]_{CCD}$ occurs because of an enhanced distal delivery of Na^+ and Cl^- to the CCD, together with more reabsorption of Na^+ than Cl^- in this nephron site. Although a considerable amount of magnesium is reabsorbed in the loop of Henle, hypomagnesemia is not a common finding in patients with Bartter's syndrome because downstream sites can reabsorb virtually all of this higher distal delivery of magnesium.

Gitelman's Syndrome

Gitelman's syndrome is a disease of young adults for the most part. The main clinical symptoms are tetany and weakness.[61] Mutations that cause Gitelman's syndrome have been identified in three separate genes that affect NaCl transport in distal convoluted tubule. Most patients have mutations in the gene encoding for the NaCl cotransporter in the early distal convoluted tubule. Other mutations involve the basolateral Cl^- channel or the γ subunit of Na^+/K^+-ATPase in the basolateral membrane. One can anticipate other molecular causes that enhance WNK 4 kinase or lower WNK 1 kinase activity. The clinical picture is dominated by effective arterial blood volume contraction, while hypokalemia, renal wasting of Na^+, Cl^-, and K^+, as well as metabolic alkalosis are the major laboratory findings. Because the thick ascending limb of the loop of Henle is not abnormal, patients can have a high U_{osm} when vasopressin acts. There is little calcium excretion in these patients (very low urine calcium/creatinine ratio). Hypomagnesemia is a common finding in patients with longer-standing Gitelman's syndrome.[62]

Gitelman's syndrome can be thought of as having a thiazide diuretic acting 24 hours a day. The combination of enhanced distal delivery of Na^+ and Cl^- to the CCD, together with a higher rate of reabsorption of Na^+ than Cl^- in this nephron site, leads to a higher luminal negative voltage in the CCD and an enhanced K^+ secretion 10.

Correction of hypokalemia is extremely difficult in patients with Bartter's and Gitelman's syndromes, even with large supplements of K^+. Correction of hypomagnesemia with oral magnesium is limited by gastrointestinal side effects. ACE inhibitors have been used with variable success, but hypotension is a potential problem with this therapy. We are concerned about the prolonged use of NSAIDs because of the potential for chronic renal dysfunction. K^+-sparing diuretics in large doses may help conserve K^+, but they may exacerbate renal salt wasting. A common clinical observation is that even high doses of amiloride may fail to curtail the excessive kaliuresis in patients with Bartter's and Gitelman's syndromes. Part of the explanation for this diminished effect is the high-volume delivery to the CCD.

Hypokalemia Due to Cationic Drugs Like Gentamicin and Tobramycin

Gentamicin and tobramycin are cationic antibiotics that bind to the calcium-sensing receptor on the basolateral aspect of cells of the loop of Henle.[63] This leads to inhibition of the luminal ROMK channel and thereby to "Lasix-like" effects.

HYPOKALEMIA AND A NORMAL OR HIGH EXTRACELLULAR FLUID VOLUME

Primary Hyperaldosteronism

Hypersecretion of aldosterone may be due to an adrenal adenoma or bilateral adrenal hyperplasia. This diagnosis should be suspected in patients with hypertension and unexplained hypokalemia with renal K^+ wasting. Nevertheless, a significant proportion of these patients do not have hypokalemia and/or hypertension.[64] An elevated $P_{Aldosterone}$ and a very low P_{Renin} are characteristic findings (see Box 111-2). A high

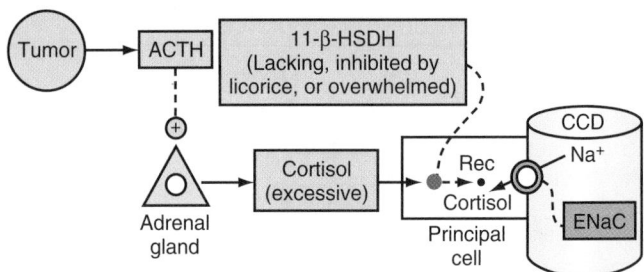

Figure 111-17 **Influence of 11β-HSDH on aldosterone-like actions of cortisol in principal cells the CCD.** Cortisol has a very high affinity to aldosterone receptor. When cortisol enters principal cells of the cortical collecting duct (CCD), 11β-HSDH *(larger solid dot in membrane)* inactivates it before it can bind to aldosterone receptor *(Rec; smaller dot in cell)*. There are three circumstances in which enough cortisol will bind to the aldosterone receptor, and more open epithelial Na^+ channel (ENaC) units will be present in principal cell luminal membranes *(brown shading)*. First, when a genetic disease causes a deficiency of 11β-HSDH (apparent mineralocorticoid excess syndrome); second, when an inhibitor of 11β-HSDH is present (e.g., licorice); third, when supply of cortisol exceeds ability of 11β-HSDH to inactivate it (e.g., ectopic production of ACTH by a tumor—*purple shading*). (From Halperin ML. *The ACID truth and BASIC facts—with a sweet touch, an enLYTEnment.* 5th ed. Toronto: RossMark Medical Publishers; 2003. Reproduced with permission ref 74.)

$P_{Aldosterone}$-to-P_{Renin} ratio in a random blood sample is usually a sufficient screening test. Primary hyperaldosteronism must be confirmed by finding of a non-suppressible high $P_{Aldosterone}$ or 24-hour urinary aldosterone excretion during salt loading. A computed tomography (CT) scan is the best imaging test to detect an adrenal adenoma. If surgery to remove the adenoma is an option, adrenal vein sampling should be done to confirm that the lesion detected on CT is a functioning adenoma.

The finding of very low P_{Renin} with high $P_{Aldosterone}$ separates patients with primary hyperaldosteronism from those with other causes of hypertension and hypokalemia (see Box 111-1). The differential diagnosis includes patients with glucocorticoid-remediable aldosteronism (GRA). These latter patients have elevated $P_{Aldosterone}$ and suppressed P_{Renin}, but they are unique because of suppression of aldosterone with the administration of dexamethasone.[65]

In patients with an adrenal adenoma, unilateral laparoscopic adrenalectomy is usually the preferred treatment. In patients with bilateral adrenal hyperplasia and those with adrenal adenomas who are not candidates for surgery, medical therapy is recommended. The goals of therapy, however, are not only to control the hypertension and correct the hypokalemia but also to reverse the unwanted effects of high aldosterone on the heart. Hence, the administration of a mineralocorticoid receptor antagonist (spironolactone or eplerenone) is recommended. Amiloride is an alternative in patients who are intolerant of these drugs. The effects of amiloride are more evident in patients who are salt restricted (lower flow rate in the CCD and thereby a higher concentration of amiloride for any given amount of the drug).

ACTH-Producing Tumor or Severe Cushing's Syndrome

The clinical picture is similar to primary hyperaldosteronism, but the level of aldosterone in plasma is low. Because of an overabundance of cortisol, the activity of 11β-HSDH is insufficient to inactivate all the cortisol that enters principal cells (Figure 111-17). As a result, cortisol binds to the mineralocorticoid receptor and exerts mineralocorticoid activity.

Plasma ACTH levels will be markedly suppressed in patients with Cushing's syndrome and high if there is an ACTH-producing tumor (e.g., oat cell carcinoma of the lung). In patients with ACTH-producing tumors, overt signs of glucocorticoid excess may not be evident at the time of diagnosis. The P_K is often below 2 mmol/L; $P_{Aldosterone}$ and P_{Renin}

are both suppressed. Therapy is directed at the primary disorder. Large supplements of KCl and drugs that inhibit ENaC are often necessary to treat the hypokalemia.

Syndrome of Apparent Mineralocorticoid Excess

The clinical picture is of hyperaldosteronism, but the level of aldosterone in plasma is low. Because of decreased activity of the enzyme 11β-HSDH, cortisol binds to the mineralocorticoid receptors and exerts mineralocorticoid activity (see Figure 111-17).[66] $P_{Aldosterone}$ and P_{Renin} are both suppressed (see Box 111-1). The diagnosis is confirmed by finding an elevated urinary cortisol-to-cortisone ratio. Blood pressure control and correction of hypokalemia are achieved with administration of aldosterone receptor blocker or an ENaC blocker (e.g., amiloride with the same caveat noted earlier for the need for salt restriction).

A similar clinical picture can be induced with chronic ingestion of licorice or other compounds that contain glycyrrhetinic acid.[67]

Liddle's Syndrome

The clinical picture is of hyperaldosteronism, but the level of aldosterone is low (see Box 111-2 and Figure 111-16). The pathophysiology of this disorder is one of a constitutively active ENaC in the CCD.[68] Several mutations in the genes encoding for the β or γ subunits of ENaC have been described in patients with this syndrome[69,70] (see Figure 111-5). One finds an autosomal dominant inherited disorder with early onset of severe hypertension and hypokalemia. Interestingly, a number of patients with this disorder, however, do not have hypokalemia. A positive family history of early-onset hypertension and hypokalemia and very low $P_{Aldosterone}$ and P_{Renin} are key elements in the diagnosis. There is no excess secretion of cortisol, and the urine cortisol-to-cortisone ratio is not elevated. Control of hypertension and correction of hypokalemia can be achieved by the administration of large doses of ENaC blockers (e.g., amiloride) but not with mineralocorticoid receptor antagonists (e.g., spironolactone).

HYPOKALEMIA DUE TO DRUGS LIKE AMPHOTERICIN B

Amphotericin B–induced hypokalemia can be thought of as a disorder in which there are artificial and unregulated cation (Na^+ and K^+) channels that are permanently in an open configuration in luminal membranes in the CCD. Treatment is to correct the electrolyte abnormalities, discontinue the drug if possible, and wait for its side effects to wear off. Try to avoid a large IV infusion of fluid when giving this drug, because this will minimize the risk of a very large flow rate in the CCD when amphotericin B acts.

HYPOKALEMIC PERIODIC PARALYSIS

This disorder is characterized by episodes of a transient shift of K^+ from the ECF to the ICF compartment of skeletal muscle. Thyrotoxic hypokalemic paralysis is more common in Asian and Hispanic males, and the first attack typically occurs between 20 and 50 years of age.[56] A familial nonthyrotoxic variety is more common in Caucasian males younger than 20 and is inherited as an autosomal dominant disorder. Genetic analyses have suggested that the abnormality in these patients is linked to the gene that encodes for the dihydropyridine-sensitive Ca^{2+} channel in skeletal muscles; it is not clear how this leads to hypokalemia. While it is stated that these attacks can be provoked by a large carbohydrate meal (release of insulin) or strenuous exercise (adrenergic surge), this association is not impressive when large groups of patients are studied.

Acute hypokalemia and paralysis can also occur in other conditions in which there is a prolonged adrenergic surge. These include exogenous causes (e.g., ingestion of amphetamines, excessive intake of caffeine, use of $β_2$-adrenergics to treat asthma) and endogenous causes (conditions associated with extreme stress (e.g., myocardial infarction, trauma, subarachnoid hemorrhage, insulin release from an insulinoma, pheochromocytoma).

Laboratory findings are very helpful to differentiate this acute hypokalemia from an acute shift of K^+ into cells in a patient with chronic hypokalemia.[56] First, there is an absence of acid-base disorders. Second, one should anticipate a low rate of excretion of K^+ as manifested by a low $U_K/U_{Creatinine}$. Patients with hypokalemic periodic paralysis usually need far less KCl to normalize their P_K than do patients who have a chronic K^+-wasting disease together with a reason to shift K^+ acutely into cells (~1 versus > 3 mmol KCl/kg body weight).

An acute attack is treated with the administration of KCl. There is, however, the risk of posttreatment hyperkalemia when K^+ moves back into the ECF compartment. Patients with the thyrotoxic variety of hypokalemic periodic paralysis can be treated with a nonselective beta-blocker and a much smaller administration of KCl.[71]

Therapy is largely symptomatic or empirical. Hyperthyroidism, if present, is treated in the usual fashion. Patients are advised to avoid carbohydrate-rich meals and vigorous exercise. Nonselective beta-blockers may reduce the number of attacks of paralysis, with little effect on the degree of fall in the P_K.[72] Acetazolamide, 250 to 750 mg per day, has been used successfully in patients with the familial form of hypokalemic periodic paralysis, although the basis of its beneficial effect is unclear.

Therapy of Hypokalemia

MEDICAL EMERGENCIES

These emergencies include cardiac arrhythmias, extreme weakness causing respiratory failure, and hepatic encephalopathy. When present, enough K^+ must be given to raise the P_K quickly. The total body K^+ deficit should be replaced much more slowly. Because large doses and high concentrations of K^+ might be needed, K^+ must be administered via a central vein, and the patient should be on a cardiac monitor. In general, the infusion should not contain glucose or HCO_3^-, because this might aggravate the degree of hypokalemia.

Clinical Example

A patient had an acute traumatic brain injury.[55] Within the first few hours, his P_K fell to a nadir of 1.3 mmol/L, and ventricular tachycardia developed. The basis for the fall in P_K was a sudden and marked shift of K^+ into cells secondary to the extreme adrenergic response and the administered adrenergic agents to maintain hemodynamics.

Therapy

The goal is to have a sustained rise in P_K by 1 mmol/L. To achieve this goal, 3 mmol of K^+ should be infused per minute in the first few minutes (cardiac output is 5 L/min, blood volume is 5 L, and the plasma volume is 3 L). Notwithstanding, the increase in the concentration of K^+ in the interstitial fluid bathing cardiac myocytes would be much smaller. Following this initial K^+ bolus, the rate of infusion of K^+ should be reduced, and the P_K should be measured (stopping the infusion for at least 60 seconds to avoid a spuriously high P_K). If the ECG changes did not improve and the P_K is appreciably lower than 3 mmol/L, this procedure would be repeated.

NO MEDICAL EMERGENCIES

Hypokalemia Due to an Acute Shift of Potassium Into Cells

In the absence of a cardiac or respiratory emergency, small doses of KCl should be given in patients with hypokalemic periodic paralysis to minimize the risk of severe rebound hyperkalemia, because they do not have a large deficit of K^+. If associated with hyperthyroidism or a condition in which there is a large adrenergic surge, a nonselective beta-blocker (propranolol 3 mg/kg) can provide effective therapy.[72]

Magnitude of the Potassium Deficit

There is no useful quantitative relationship between the P_K and the total body K^+ deficit, because there may also be a shift of K^+ into cells.[54] Hence, careful monitoring of P_K during replacement of the K^+ deficit is mandatory.

Route of Potassium Administration

The oral route is preferred if bowel sounds are present. When a peripheral IV route is used, the concentration of K^+ should not be greater than 40 mmol/L. The rate of administration of K^+ should not be greater than 60 mmol/h in all but emergency settings.

Potassium Preparations

Increasing the intake of K^+-rich foods (e.g., bananas, fruit juice) has the danger of inducing a large weight gain. Oral KCl (e.g., salt substitutes like co-salt, which provide 14 mmol of K^+ per gram) is generally well tolerated and inexpensive. Liquid K^+ supplements have an unpleasant taste and are often poorly tolerated. Most preparations used are "slow release," either microencapsulated or in a wax matrix. Although usually well tolerated, they may cause ulcerative or stenotic lesions in the gastrointestinal tract.

In patients with a deficit of KCl (e.g., chronic vomiting or diuretics), KCl is needed, whereas in patients with a $KHCO_3$ deficit (e.g., diarrhea), K^+ with HCO_3^- or a precursor of HCO_3^- (e.g., citrate) is needed. Because the administration of HCO_3^- may lead to a shift of K^+ into cells, KCl should be given initially, and alkali should be withheld until the P_K approaches a safe level (~3 mmol/L) unless there are ongoing and large losses of HCO_3^-. K^+ phosphate may be needed when there is rapid anabolism and little oral intake. We give K^+ as KCl to treat DKA and rely on the patient's diet to supply the phosphate needed to restore a normal ICF composition later in time. If given, limit phosphate infusion to less than 50 mmol/8 h to minimize the risk of hypocalcemia and metastatic calcification.

ADJUNCTS TO THERAPY

K^+-sparing diuretics will reduce the renal loss of K^+, but this is only useful on a chronic basis. Amiloride and triamterene are better tolerated than spironolactone, since they lack the gastrointestinal and hormonal (amenorrhea, gynecomastia, decreased libido) complications of spironolactone. Eplerenone is a highly selective mineralocorticoid receptor antagonist associated with a lower incidence of these endocrine side effects, but it is also significantly more expensive than spironolactone. Hyperkalemia may develop when K^+ is given with K^+-sparing diuretics, especially if other conditions that compromise K^+ excretion are present; note that these drugs have a long half-life.

RISKS OF THERAPY

With prolonged hypokalemia, the CCD may become temporarily hyporesponsive to the kaliuretic effect of aldosterone (reviewed in Reference 73). Hence, it is important to monitor the P_K frequently during the treatment of hypokalemia. Hyperkalemia has been observed in about 4% of patients taking K^+ supplements. The risk is highest in patients with renal failure and diabetes mellitus. The simultaneous use of ACE inhibitors, beta-blockers, or NSAIDs may also predispose to the development of hyperkalemia.

ANNOTATED REFERENCES

Kamel KS, Wei C. Controversial issues in treatment of hyperkalemia. Nephrol Dialysis Transplant 2003;18:2215-8.
This paper provides the most compelling arguments concerning the therapy for patients with hyperkalemia.

Juel C, Halestrap AP. Lactate transport in skeletal muscle—role and regulation of the monocarboxylate transporter. J Physiol 1999;517:633-42.
In this manuscript, the transport of lactate across cell membranes by the monocarboxylate transporter and its regulation are described. This provides the background to understand how HNE may be regulated in vivo, and thereby the driving force to shift K^+ into cells.

Halperin ML, Kamel KS, Oh MS. Mechanisms to concentrate the urine: an opinion. Curr Opin Nephrol Hypertens 2008;17:416-22.
In this paper, the authors provide a provocative interpretation of the factors that may control the reabsorption of Na^+ and Cl^- in the loop of Henle. The analysis of the recycling of urea has particular relevance to our understanding of the factors influencing the flow rate in the CCD, and thereby, how the examination of the urine should be used to deduce how much filtrate is delivered to the CCD in patients.

Carlisle EJF, Donnelly SM, Ethier J, Quaggin SE, Kaiser U, Vasuvattakul S, et al. Modulation of the secretion of potassium by accompanying anions in humans. Kidney Int 1991;39:1206-12.
In this study, the authors raise the possibility that the distal delivery of bicarbonate and/or the luminal fluid pH in the CCD helps to generate a higher concentration of K^+ owing to a greater lumen-negative voltage in these nephron segments.

Lin SH, Lin YF, Halperin ML. Hypokalemia and paralysis: clues on admission to help in the differential diagnosis. Quart J Med 2001;94:133-9.
This article describes the tools to suspect that the acute hypokalemia (and weakness) is due to a shift of K^+ into cells (e.g., thyrotoxic hypokalemic periodic paralysis).

Lin SH, Lin YF. Propranolol rapidly reverses paralysis, hypokalemia and hypophosphatemia in thyrotoxic periodic paralysis. Am J Kidney Dis 2001;37:620-4.
This article describes the optimal way to correct hypokalemia quickly when the cause is an adrenergic surge (e.g., thyrotoxic hypokalemic periodic paralysis).

REFERENCES

Access the complete reference list online at http://www.expertconsult.com.

112

Disorders of Calcium and Magnesium Metabolism

MICHELLE K. MCNUTT | ROSEMARY A. KOZAR

Serum Calcium Concentration

The calcium concentration is essential to many physiologic phenomena, including preservation of the integrity of cellular membranes, neuromuscular activity, regulation of endocrine and exocrine secretory activities, blood coagulation, activation of the complement system, and bone metabolism.

TOTAL SERUM CALCIUM CONCENTRATION

The normal range for total serum calcium must be established for each laboratory and varies according to the method used. Calcium exists in three forms: protein-bound calcium, ionized calcium, and nonionized calcium.[1]

Protein-Bound Calcium

Approximately 40% of total calcium is bound to serum proteins, and 80% to 90% of this calcium is bound to albumin. Variations in serum protein alter proportionately the concentration of the protein-bound and total serum calcium. An increase in serum albumin concentration of 1 g/dL increases protein-bound calcium by 0.8 mg/dL, whereas an increase of 1 g/dL of globulin increases protein-bound calcium by 0.16 mg/dL. However, the validity of this correction in critical illness has been questioned, with multiple authors emphasizing the importance of directly measuring serum ionized calcium concentration in this patient population.[2,3] Marked changes in serum sodium concentration also affect the protein binding of calcium. Hyponatremia increases, whereas hypernatremia decreases, protein-bound calcium. Changes in pH also affect protein-bound calcium, and an increase or decrease of 0.1 pH, respectively, increases or decreases protein-bound calcium by 0.12 mg/dL. In vitro, freezing and thawing serum samples may decrease the binding of calcium as well.

FREE (IONIZED) CALCIUM

Ionized calcium is the biologically active form of calcium responsible for most physiologic actions of calcium in the body. Serum ionized calcium concentration in normal subjects ranges from 4.0 to 4.9 mg/dL or 47% of total serum calcium. The ionized calcium level can be altered by environmental factors. Acidosis decreases protein binding, thereby increasing the ionized fraction of calcium. An increase in serum pH of 0.1 unit may cause a decrease in ionized calcium of 0.16 mg/dL. Freezing and thawing of serum may also alter the level of ionized calcium.

NONIONIZED CALCIUM

The nonionized form of calcium is also called *complexed calcium*. The calcium complexes are formed with bicarbonate, phosphate, and acetate and constitute approximately 13% of total serum calcium. Complexed calcium has been found to be increased twofold in patients with uremia.

CYTOSOLIC FREE CALCIUM

The normal concentration of cytosolic calcium is 100 nM/L, which is 10,000-fold lower than the concentration of extracellular calcium. This very steep gradient is maintained by an energy-driven calcium pump known as the *plasma membrane Ca^{++}-ATPase* (PMCA). In certain types of cells a Na$^+$/Ca^{++} exchanger energized by Na$^+$ gradient helps drive cytosolic calcium into the extracellular space. Part of cellular calcium is sequestered in intracellular organelles including endoplasmic reticulum, sarcoplasmic reticulum in muscle cells, and mitochondria. These organelles are endowed with their own calcium pumps that help preserve the very low free cytosolic calcium. The calcium-dependent intracellular signaling generally requires a 10-fold increase in free cytosolic calcium. With each heartbeat, the cytosolic calcium concentration in cardiac myocytes is elevated 10-fold, from a resting level of 100 nM to 1000 nM. Likewise, in other signaling events such as T-cell activation, which triggers the transcription of interleukin (IL)-2, a 10-fold increase in cytosolic calcium serves as the signal for the response. Elevation in cytosolic calcium is mediated by the activation of calcium channels, which allows passive calcium flux down its electrochemical gradient.[4]

VITAMIN D METABOLISM

Vitamin D (where D represents D$_2$ or D$_3$) is biologically inert and metabolized in the liver to 25-hydroxyvitamin D [25(OH)D], the major circulating form of vitamin D. 25(OH)D is activated in the kidneys to 1,25-dihydroxyvitamin D [1,25(OH)2D], which regulates calcium, phosphorous, and bone metabolism.[5]

CALCIUM HOMEOSTASIS

Calcium is regulated by a combination of bone exchange, renal excretion, and intestinal absorption. Decreased ionized calcium increases PTH (parathyroid hormone) and 1,25-dihydroxyvitamin D$_2$, both of which increase osteoclastic activity and thus stimulate bone resorption. Renal excretion of calcium is regulated by PTH and vitamin D, which increase distal tubular reabsorption of calcium, and by calcitonin, which inhibits calcium reabsorption. Intestinal absorption of calcium depends primarily on 1,25-dihydroxyvitamin D$_2$, which stimulates calcium absorption from all parts of the small intestine.[6]

Hypocalcemia

Disorders associated with hypocalcemia can be classified into disorders related to vitamin D and disorders related to parathyroid hormone.

DISORDERS RELATED TO VITAMIN D DEFICIENCY

Vitamin D Deficiency

Hypocalcemia is a common feature of vitamin D deficiency. The common causes of vitamin D deficiency are listed in Box 112-1. Lack of sunlight exposure impairs endogenous vitamin D synthesis. Because vitamin D is a fat-soluble vitamin, nutritional osteomalacia usually is associated with a deficient intake of food products containing fatty substances. Gastrectomy may lead either to dietary deficiency due to avoiding fatty products and/or due to malabsorption of vitamin D, as noted with Billroth type II surgery, in which a vitamin D–absorbing bowel segment is bypassed. Deficiency of bile salts impairs vitamin D

COMMON CAUSES OF VITAMIN D DEFICIENCY

Lack of exposure to sunshine
Nutritional
Malabsorption:
  Following gastrectomy
  Tropical and nontropical sprue
  Chronic pancreatitis
  Biliary cirrhosis
  Ingestion of cathartics
  Intestinal bypass
  Anticonvulsant therapy
Abnormal metabolism of vitamin D:
  Vitamin D–dependent rickets
  Ingestion of barbiturates and anticonvulsants
  Renal insufficiency
  Hepatic dysfunction
  Calcium deprivation
Renal losses of vitamin D:
  Nephrotic syndrome
  Fanconi's syndrome

absorption. Small-bowel diseases, laxative abuse, and certain anticonvulsants (phenytoin) interfere with absorption. Urinary losses of vitamin D were linked to Fanconi's syndrome and nephrotic syndrome.[7] Because hepatic formation of 25(OH) vitamin D from vitamin D is not tightly controlled and depends primarily on the availability of vitamin D, the serum level of 25(OH) vitamin D_3 is utilized as a measurement of body stores of vitamin D; low levels of 25(OH) vitamin D indicate vitamin D deficiency.[1]

Impaired Metabolism of Vitamin D

Hypocalcemia in patients ingesting phenobarbital is associated with low levels of circulating 25(OH) vitamin D. Half-life of vitamin D and 25(OH) vitamin D are shortened by barbiturates, owing to induction of microsomal enzymes in the liver. Low circulating levels of 25(OH) vitamin D also have been observed in patients with hepatic failure due to reduced transformation of vitamin D to 25(OH) vitamin D in the liver.[8]

Dietary calcium deprivation increases the clearance and inactivation of 25(OH) vitamin D and causes vitamin D deficiency. This variety of vitamin D deficiency may be caused by secondary hyperparathyroidism, which augments renal synthesis of 1,25(OH)$_2$ vitamin D and in turn enhances the degradation of 25(OH) vitamin D to inactive metabolites.

Hypothetically, this mechanism may account for vitamin D deficiency in clinical states of calcium malabsorption, including gastrointestinal (GI) diseases, anticonvulsant therapy (e.g., phenytoin), and certain drugs such as colchicine, fluoride, and theophylline. Likewise, increased intake of foods rich in phytate, oxalate, and citrate that chelate calcium in the GI tract and render it nonabsorbable may cause vitamin D deficiency.[1,9]

Vitamin D–dependent rickets type I (VDDR-1), also designated as *pseudovitamin D deficiency*, is inherited as an autosomal recessive disorder in which 25(OH) vitamin $D_{1\alpha}$-hydroxylase in the proximal tubules is deficient due to defects in the 1α-hydroxylase gene. It is manifested by early hypocalcemia, hypophosphatemia, severe secondary hyperparathyroidism, and severe rickets. The serum 1,25(OH)$_2$ vitamin D is undetectable or very low, whereas 25(OH) vitamin D levels are normal. The clinical abnormality can be reversed completely by the administration of pharmacologic doses of vitamin D or physiologic doses of 1,25(OH)$_2$ vitamin D. Linkage analysis in families with VDDR-1 mapped the disease locus to chromosome 12q13-14.[10]

End-Organ Resistance to 1,25(OH)$_2$ Vitamin D

Hypocalcemia refractory to 1,25(OH)$_2$ vitamin D_3 was described as type II vitamin D–dependent rickets, also known as *hereditary*

1,25(OH)$_2$ *vitamin D_3–resistant rickets*. This familial disorder is inherited by autosomal recessive transmission and is characterized by hypocalcemia, impaired intestinal absorption of calcium, rickets, and alopecia, which reflects a defect in the physiologic action of 1,25(OH)$_2$ vitamin D in the skin. In contrast to vitamin D–dependent rickets type I, in type II the serum 1,25(OH)$_2$ vitamin D level is elevated, and patients either respond to pharmacologic doses of 1,25(OH)$_2$ vitamin D_3 or do not respond at all. In some patients with this disorder, an abnormal nuclear uptake, abnormal cytosol receptor binding of 1,25(OH) vitamin D, or both are present. These findings suggest that the mechanism of the end-organ resistance is a defect in the receptor. Mutations of vitamin D receptor genes have been identified.

DISORDERS RELATED TO PARATHYROID HORMONE

Reduced Production of PTH

Hypoparathyroidism. Hypoparathyroidism is a disorder characterized by hypocalcemia and hyperphosphatemia due to a deficient or absent secretion of PTH.

Hypoparathyroidism is a common cause of hypocalcemia. It commonly presents as paresthesias, muscle spasms (i.e., tetany), and seizures. However, mild chronic hypoparathyroidism may cause hypocalcemia so gradually that the only symptoms may be visual impairment from cataracts after years of hypoparathyroidism.

Hypoparathyroidism may be either an acquired abnormality designated as *secondary hypoparathyroidism*, or primary hypoparathyroidism, also known as *idiopathic hypoparathyroidism*.

Secondary Hypoparathyroidism. Hypoparathyroidism may be caused by surgery. This variety of hypoparathyroidism may result from accidental removal of parathyroids or traumatic interruption of their blood supply. Hypocalcemia that appears after excision of parathyroid adenoma results from functional suppression and hypofunctioning of the remaining normal glands and is frequently transient. "Hungry bone syndrome" can develop following parathyroidectomy in patients with markedly elevated preoperative PTH levels. Decreased postoperative levels of PTH cause a "rebound" recalcification of bones secondary to unbalanced osteoblast and osteoclast activity. This results in profound hypocalcemia, hypophosphatemia, and elevated alkaline phosphatase. Similarly, hypocalcemia has been reported to occur in 15% of patients after thyroidectomy.[11]

Hypoparathyroidism may be a component of multiple endocrine dysfunctions, including adrenal insufficiency, pernicious anemia, thalassemia, and Wilson's disease. In the last two disorders, the deposition of iron and copper, respectively, in the parathyroid glands is the likely underlying mechanism.[12]

Hypocalcemia may occur in magnesium depletion.[13] It has been shown that the chronic state of low serum magnesium diminishes the release of PTH.[13] Hypomagnesemia has been reported to induce skeletal resistance to PTH.[14] Magnesium level should always be checked during the workup of profound refractory hypocalcemia. The mechanisms that underlie the effects of hypomagnesemia on serum calcium are poorly understood. It may be speculated, however, that magnesium depletion may impair the activity of the calcium pump and thus alter the distribution of calcium between the extracellular and intracellular spaces.

Hypocalcemia in association with hypomagnesemia has been reported in 60% of patients with severe acute respiratory syndrome.[15] Hypocalcemia may follow therapeutic use of magnesium sulfate (e.g., in preeclampsia) secondary to magnesium-induced suppression of PTH. Aminoglycosides and cytotoxic agents may exert a toxic effect on parathyroid glands, leading to hypocalcemia.[1,13] Symptomatic hypoparathyroidism has been observed in association with HIV infection.[1]

Primary (Idiopathic) Hypoparathyroidism. Primary hypoparathyroidism may occur in association with other endocrine disorders or as an isolated entity. The latter is termed *isolated hypoparathyroidism*, and it may occur as a sporadic or familial disorder, inherited as both an autosomal dominant and recessive form.[14]

Aplasia or hypoplasia of the parathyroids is most commonly caused by the DiGeorge velocardiofacial syndrome, associated with deletions of chromosome 22q11.2. Most cases are sporadic, but familial cases with autosomal dominant inheritance have been reported. Affected patients have abnormalities in organs derived from the third and fourth branchial arches including the parathyroid glands, thymus, and outflow tract of the heart. These patients typically present in the first week after birth with signs of hypocalcemia such as tetany and seizures. They have characteristic facial features, an upturned nose, and a widened distance between the inner canthi (telecanthus), with short palpebral fissures. Cardiac defects include truncus arteriosus, tetralogy of Fallot, or interrupted aortic arch. Thymic hypoplasia leads to immune deficiencies. *CATCH 22 syndrome* is an acronym for *c*ardiac defects, *a*bnormal facies, *t*hymic hypoplasia, *c*left palate and *h*ypocalcemia caused by chromosome *22*q11 deletions.[16]

Autoimmune hypoparathyroidism is commonly a part of polyglandular autoimmune syndrome type I, which is a familial syndrome. It occurs during childhood, is inherited as an autosomal recessive trait, and is associated with mucocutaneous candidiasis and adrenal insufficiency. It can present as hypoparathyroidism in the absence of the two other disorders. Adrenal insufficiency is a late phenomenon in this syndrome. The acronym *APECED* stands for *a*utoimmune *p*olyglandular *e*ndocrinopathy with *c*andidiasis and *e*ctodermal *d*ystrophy, including vitiligo, alopecia, nail dystrophy, enamel hypoplasia of teeth, and corneal opacities.[17]

Hypoparathyroidism was also reported in association with two mitochondrial cytopathies with mitochondrial DNA mutations: Kearns-Sayre syndrome and Kenny-Caffey syndrome.[18]

Impaired Action of PTH Due to Peripheral Resistance

Pseudohypoparathyroidism. Pseudohypoparathyroidism is a rare inheritable disorder characterized by mental retardation, moderate obesity, short stature, brachydactyly with short metacarpal and metatarsal bones, exostoses, radius curvus, and an expressionless face.[19] The biochemical abnormalities are hypocalcemia and hyperphosphatemia. Some patients exhibit only the biochemical abnormalities. Thus, the disorder may be subdivided into pseudohypoparathyroidism type IA, which is also known as *Albright's hereditary osteodystrophy*, and type IB. Pseudohypoparathyroidism type IA is associated with both the somatic and biochemical abnormalities, and type IB presents as the biochemical defect without the somatic abnormalities. Because of the hypocalcemic stimulus, secondary hyperparathyroidism may develop in some patients, leading to osteitis fibrosa cystica. Failure of the kidney to form $1,25(OH)_2$ vitamin D_3 in response to PTH results in a low circulating level of this metabolite.

Calcitonin. Calcitonin binds to specific cell membrane receptors on bone-resorbing osteoclasts and depresses their activity. In this regard, it antagonizes the effect of PTH on bone.

Medullary carcinoma of the thyroid is derived from parafollicular cells of ultimobranchial organ, which secrete calcitonin. It may present as a familial and autosomal dominant or sporadic disorder. Patients with this tumor have high circulating levels of calcitonin, and hypocalcemia has been reported in some patients.[20]

Hypocalcemia has been described in critically ill patients admitted to intensive care units (ICUs).[21] The degree of hypocalcemia correlated with the severity of the disease and was most commonly detected in patients who were septic. The mechanism of this abnormality is unknown. Circulating levels of calcitonin precursors (CTpr) increase up to several thousandfold in response to microbial infections, and this increase correlates with the severity of the infection and mortality. The relationship of elevated CTpr to the emergence of hypocalcemia needs to be investigated.[22]

Bisphosphonates. Hypocalcemia has been reported in patients with bone metastases of solid tumors who were treated with pamidronate[23]

Box 112-2

HYPERPHOSPHATEMIA AS A CAUSE OF HYPOCALCEMIA

Administration of phosphate:
 Oral phosphate
 Cow's milk in infants
 Laxatives containing phosphate
 Potassium phosphate tablets
 Phosphate-containing enemas
 Intravenous phosphate
Renal diseases:
 Acute renal failure
 Chronic renal failure
Neoplasms treated with cytotoxic agents:
 Lymphomas
 Leukemia
 Tumor lysis
 Rhabdomyolysis

---

and in a patient treated with alendronate for osteoporosis. In both cases, bisphosphonate induced skeletal resistance, and PTH was proposed as a possible mechanism. Hypomagnesemia may cause hypocalcemia by a similar mechanism.[24]

Rapid Removal of Calcium from the Circulation

Malignant Neoplasms. Hypocalcemia may develop in patients with malignant neoplasms in association with osteoblastic bone-forming metastases, most commonly cancer of the prostate and breast. These lesions may lead to rapid deposition of mineral in the newly formed matrix, thus causing hypocalcemia.

Hyperphosphatemia. The various causes of hyperphosphatemia that may lead to hypocalcemia are listed in Box 112-2. The oral or intravenous (IV) administration of phosphate lowers serum calcium concentration in normal animals and hypercalcemic human subjects, which formed the basis for the clinical use of phosphate administration in states of hypercalcemia. The association of hyperphosphatemia and hypocalcemia has been reported to occur in a variety of circumstances. Hyperphosphatemia has been observed in persons ingesting large quantities of phosphate-containing laxatives or receiving enemas with phosphate. Hyperphosphatemia and hypocalcemia with tetany may develop in infants fed cow's milk, which contains 1220 mg of calcium and 940 mg of phosphorus per liter (human milk contains 340 mg of calcium and 150 mg of phosphorus per liter).[25,26] The mechanism responsible for lowering serum calcium concentration by the administration of phosphate is not entirely understood. One possibility is that the decrease in serum calcium concentration is caused by deposition of calcium phosphate in the bone, soft tissues, or both.

In chronic renal failure, a constant increase in serum phosphorus concentration is observed when the glomerular filtration rate is 30 mL/min or less, and hyperphosphatemia is a common accompaniment of acute renal failure.

In patients undergoing chemotherapy for neoplastic diseases, particularly of lymphatic origin, large quantities of phosphates may be released into the circulation as a result of the cytolysis. Spontaneous tumor lysis may cause hyperphosphatemia and, consequently, hypocalcemia.

Acute Pancreatitis. The hypocalcemia associated with acute pancreatitis is not well understood. The precipitation of calcium soaps in the abdominal cavity, which results from the release of lipolytic enzymes and fat necrosis, has been suggested as the mechanism of hypocalcemia. Recently, endotoxemia has been implicated.[27]

Citrate, Lactate, Bicarbonate, Na-EDTA, Foscarnet, and Poisoning with Ethylene Glycol. Citrate is present in stored blood products (such as plasma and platelets) as an anticoagulant that exerts its action through the binding of ionized calcium. Patients receiving a massive transfusion frequently experience hypocalcemia; however, this is usually transient secondary to the rapid hepatic metabolism of citrate.[28] The ionized hypocalcemia (with a normal total calcium concentration) can lead to tetany, myocardial dysfunction, or hypotension. The same applies to IV lactate and Na-EDTA, which causes ionized hypocalcemia. Bicarbonate may directly complex calcium or may increase protein binding of calcium from the resulting alkalosis. Low serum ionized calcium may be a complication of ethylene glycol (antifreeze) poisoning because of calcium binding by oxalic acid, which is the metabolite of the poison. An analog of the pyrophosphate, foscarnet, used to treat cytomegalovirus infection in HIV-infected patients causes ionized hypocalcemia secondary to chelation of calcium by foscarnet.[1]

CLINICAL CONSEQUENCES OF HYPOCALCEMIA

The clinical presentation of hypocalcemia depends on its severity, rapidity of the fall in serum calcium concentration, age of the patient, chronicity of hypocalcemia, and comorbid conditions.

Most infants with hypocalcemia are asymptomatic. Among those who become symptomatic, the characteristic sign is increased neuromuscular irritability. Generalized or focal clonic seizures may be the first indication of hypocalcemia. Other manifestations may include stridor caused by laryngospasms and wheezing caused by bronchospasms. Vomiting may be caused by pylorospasm.

Neuromuscular manifestations in adults with hypocalcemia are variable (Table 112-1). The characteristic symptom is tetany, which includes perioral numbness and tingling, paresthesias in the extremities, carpopedal spasm, laryngospasm, and focal and generalized seizures. The spasms of the diaphragm and of intercostal muscles may cause respiratory arrest and asphyxia.

The characteristic physical findings in patients with hypocalcemia that are indicative of latent tetany are Trousseau's sign (carpal spasm) and Chvostek's sign (facial muscle contraction). Visual impairment may by caused acutely by papilledema, whereas usually chronic hypocalcemia, when due to hypoparathyroidism, causes cataracts. Myocardial functional and anatomic abnormalities have been associated with hypocalcemia. Acute hypocalcemia may be associated with hypotension. Very often the absence of the compensatory reflex tachycardia aggravates the condition. The typical ECG change consists of prolongation of the QT interval. Hypocalcemia prolongs phase 2 of the action potential and thus prolongs repolarization time, because inward calcium currents are one of the factors determining the plateau configuration of the action potential. QT prolongation is associated with a variety of ventricular arrhythmias, most characteristically torsades de pointes. These abnormalities can be reversed with calcium replacement.

TABLE 112-1	Clinical Manifestations of Abnormalities in Magnesium and Calcium	
Increased Serum Levels		
System	Magnesium	Calcium
Gastrointestinal	Nausea/vomiting	Anorexia, nausea/vomiting, abdominal pain, constipation
Neuromuscular	Weakness, lethargy, ↓ reflexes	Depression, confusion, coma, muscle weakness, back and extremity pain
Cardiovascular	Hypotension, cardiac arrest	Hypotension, arrhythmias
Renal	—	Polydipsia, polyuria
Decreased Serum Levels		
System	Magnesium	Calcium
Gastrointestinal		
Neuromuscular	Hyperactive reflexes, muscle tremors, tetany, delirium, seizures	Hyperactive reflexes, paresthesias, weakness, paralysis, tetany, seizures, carpopedal spasm, seizures
Cardiovascular	Arrhythmia	Heart failure

Calcium therapy significantly shortens the repolarization intervals and decreases the frequency of ventricular premature contractions.[29] Chronic hypocalcemia may infrequently cause hypocalcemic cardiomyopathy, which is a dilated cardiomyopathy. Partial recovery of cardiac function has been reported after restoration of normocalcemia.[30]

TREATMENT OF HYPOCALCEMIA

Symptomatic hypocalcemia generally responds promptly to IV administration of calcium. The commonly used preparations are 10% calcium gluconate (10-mL ampules containing 90 mg of elemental calcium) and 10% calcium chloride (10-mL ampules containing 360 mg of elemental calcium). The treatment should be instituted immediately, because delay may be associated with further aggravation of tetany and lead to generalized seizures and even cardiac arrest.

The IV administration of 100 to 200 mg elemental calcium (5-10 mEq) should be slow to avoid complications. Then the administration of calcium can be continued as a slow drip of 100 to 200 mg of elemental calcium, diluted in 250 to 500 mL of 0.45% NaCl or D_5W, given over several hours until oral calcium takes over. Calcium extravasation should be avoided because it causes local irritation and thrombophlebitis.

Chronic treatment with oral calcium should follow the IV therapy in patients with chronic hypocalcemia due to irreversible causes such as hypoparathyroidism. Oral calcium administration constitutes the best initial therapy in mild cases. The commonly used preparations are in tablet form: calcium lactate, 300 mg (60 mg of elemental calcium); chewable calcium gluconate, 1 g (90 mg of elemental calcium); calcium carbonate (Os-Cal), 250 mg of elemental calcium; calcium carbonate, 650 mg (250 mg of elemental calcium); and calcium citrate, 950 mg (200 mg of elemental calcium).

Oral calcium also may be used for patients for whom the diagnosis of irreversible hypoparathyroidism has not been established with absolute certainty. In patients who fail to respond to oral calcium, vitamin D in large doses is the only available treatment. The commonly used preparations are capsules containing 1.25 mg (50,000 units) of vitamin D_2 (ergocalciferol). The average dose ranges between 1.25 and 3.75 mg/d. DHT3 is three times as potent as vitamin D_2 in raising serum calcium concentration. Each capsule contains 0.125 mg of DHT3. The average daily dose ranges between 0.25 and 1 mg of DHT3. Both vitamins are available in liquid oil solutions as well. Both hypoparathyroidism and pseudohypoparathyroidism respond to physiologic doses of $1,25(OH)_2$ vitamin D_3 and $1\alpha(OH)$ vitamin D_3 with restoration of serum calcium concentration to normal. Calcitriol is marketed as Rocaltrol and is dispensed in capsules containing 0.25 and 1 μg. Chlorothiazides may enhance the calcemic action of vitamin D and its analogs, whereas furosemide may aggravate the hypocalcemia through its hypercalciuric action.

Patients in whom hypocalcemia is associated with hypomagnesemia respond poorly to IV calcium, but the serum calcium concentration is restored to normal levels with correction of the hypomagnesemia.

Symptoms rarely develop in patients with chronic renal failure and hypocalcemia. However, very often reduction of elevated serum phosphorus with phosphate-binding antacids causes an increase in serum calcium concentrations.

Hypocalcemia associated with osteomalacia resulting from vitamin D deficiency is rarely symptomatic. It usually responds to physiologic doses of vitamin D and increased oral calcium intake.

Hypercalcemia

Primary hyperparathyroidism and malignancy account for 80% to 90% of all cases of hypercalcemia.[31] Primary hyperparathyroidism is the leading cause of hypercalcemia in the outpatient setting. Its incidence is 1% in the normal population.[32] Hypercalcemia is most often detected in routinely tested blood specimens. Malignancy is the prevalent cause of hypercalcemia in hospitalized patients. The most common iatrogenic hypercalcemia is milk-alkali syndrome, which ranks third

DISORDERS ASSOCIATED WITH HYPERCALCEMIA

Primary hyperparathyroidism
Adenoma and carcinoma:
    Hyperplasia
    Multiple endocrine adenomatosis
    Ectopic secretion of parathyroid hormone by neoplasms (rare)
Secondary hyperparathyroidism:
    Malabsorption and vitamin D deficiency
    Chronic renal failure
    Following kidney transplantation
Familial hypocalciuric hypercalcemia
Hypercalcemia associated with malignancy:
    Lytic bone metastases
Circulating tumor-secreted factors:
    Parathyroid hormone–related protein
    1,25-Dihydroxyvitamin D_3–induced hypercalcemia
Locally acting, noncirculating, tumor-secreted cytokines:
    Interleukin (IL)-1 and IL-6
    Tumor necrosis factor beta (TNF-β)
    Granulocyte-macrophage colony-stimulating factor
    Transforming growth factor alpha (TGF-α)
    Prostaglandins
Hypercalcemia in patients with hyperabsorptive hypercalciuria
Hypervitaminosis D
Hypervitaminosis A
Granulomatous diseases:
    Sarcoidosis
    Tuberculosis
    Histoplasmosis
    Coccidioidomycosis
    Leprosy
Foreign body granuloma
Hyperthyroidism
Adrenocortical insufficiency
Infantile hypercalcemia
Immobilization
Milk-alkali syndrome
Hypophosphatasia
Parenteral nutrition
Hypercalcemia associated with acute renal failure
Medications:
    Thiazides
    Lithium
    Theophylline
    Calcium ion exchange resins

after malignancy and hyperparathyroidism and accounts for 10% to 15% of cases with hypercalcemia. The free over-the-counter access to the generic brands of calcium carbonate and their widespread use for heartburn, osteoporosis, and as an alleged prevention of colon cancer may be the underlying cause for the rise in the incidence of milk-alkali syndrome.[33]

Hypercalcemia presents a challenge to every clinician. In some instances, the cause of hypercalcemia is self-evident on the basis of the circumstantial clinical findings, whereas extensive efforts are required to establish the etiology in other situations. The important causes of hypercalcemia are listed in Box 112-3.

HYPERPARATHYROIDISM

Primary hyperparathyroidism is present in 10% to 20% of all patients with hypercalcemia.[1] Making the diagnosis of hyperparathyroidism is important because of its amenability of surgical cure. The disease is more common in females than in males; the incidence increases in women after menopause but is less frequent in older men. Primary hyperparathyroidism is caused by a solitary adenoma in 80% to 85% of patients, multigland hyperplasia in 15% to 20%, and parathyroid carcinoma in less than 1% of patients.[34]

The morphologic differentiation between adenomas and hyperplasia sometimes is very difficult. The presence of a capsule and a rim of compressed normal gland tissue around the periphery of an adenoma may be helpful in making a definitive diagnosis. The persistence or recurrence of hypercalcemia after surgery for a purported adenoma should raise the suspicion of parathyroid hyperplasia. If more than one gland shows histologic features of hyperplasia, a subtotal or total parathyroidectomy is recommended. Some patients with primary hyperparathyroidism have especially pronounced hypercalciuria despite a very mild degree of hypercalcemia and minimal or no bone disease. In patients with primary hyperparathyroidism, a very strong positive correlation was found between 1,25(OH)$_2$ vitamin D_3 in the serum and the urinary calcium excretion. Patients with nephrolithiasis and hypercalcemia had circulating levels of 1,25(OH)$_2$ vitamin D_3 higher than those present in hyperparathyroid patients without renal stones. The reason for this difference in the 1,25(OH)$_2$ vitamin D_3 levels is unknown, but it stresses the importance of vitamin D metabolism in the clinical presentation of primary hyperparathyroidism.[1]

Hyperparathyroidism is also associated with multiple endocrine neoplasia (MEN) type 1 and 2, both of which are inherited in an autosomal dominant fashion. MEN 1 syndrome is characterized by parathyroid hyperplasia, neuroendocrine tumors of the pancreas and duodenum, and pituitary adenomas. Hyperparathyroidism occurs in over 95% of patients with MEN 1. MEN 2 syndrome includes MEN 2A and MEN 2B. MEN 2A syndrome is characterized by pheochromocytoma, parathyroid hyperplasia, and medullary thyroid cancer. MEN 2B syndrome includes medullary thyroid cancer, pheochromocytoma, mucosal neuromas, and a distinct physical appearance but does not involve hyperparathyroidism. Establishing the diagnosis of hyperparathyroidism associated with MEN syndrome has important surgical implications.[35,36] The diagnosis of primary hyperparathyroidism requires the findings of elevated serum calcium and intact PTH (iPTH) levels, normal renal function, and normal or increased urinary calcium excretion. Patients presenting with bone, renal, GI, or neuromuscular symptoms are considered symptomatic and are best treated with surgical excision. Asymptomatic patients with primary hyperparathyroidism are surgical candidates if they meet the criteria established by the National Institutes of Health (NIH Criteria for Parathyroidectomy).[37,38] These criteria include markedly elevated serum calcium (>12 mg/dL), history of life-threatening hypercalcemia, creatinine clearance reduced by 30%, markedly elevated 24-hour urine calcium (>400 mg/d), nephrolithiasis, age younger than 50, osteitis fibrosa cystica, and substantially reduced bone mass (>2 SD below control).

Recent advances in technology have allowed the surgeon to localize the parathyroid adenoma preoperatively or intraoperatively, thus allowing a minimally invasive surgical approach. Options include the ^{99m}Tc-sestamibi scan with or without single photon emission computed tomography (SPECT), computed tomography (CT), ultrasonography, magnetic resonance imaging (MRI), and thallium-201/technetium pertechnetate scanning. The most promising perioperative adjunct, however, seems to be intraoperative PTH monitoring.[39]

Familial hypocalciuric hypercalcemia is an unusual form of parathyroid hyperplasia with autosomal dominant transmission. It is usually asymptomatic and incidentally diagnosed by an elevated serum calcium level and confirmed by a low urinary calcium level. The clinical course is relatively benign with an absence of nephrolithiasis and an infrequent occurrence of pancreatitis and chondrocalcinosis and usually requires no specific therapy.

MALIGNANCY ASSOCIATED WITH HYPERCALCEMIA

Hypercalcemia is most commonly produced by tumors of lung, breast, kidney, and ovary and by hematologic malignancies. Two main mechanisms are known to mediate the hypercalcemia of malignancy: local and humoral.[40] The local mechanism is manifested by the presence of osteolytic lesions in the skeleton. The malignant cells may act to destroy the bone directly; however, even local osteolysis is mediated by activated osteoclasts in most instances. The humoral factor most commonly associated with hypercalcemia of malignancy is parathyroid hormone–related protein (PTHrP).[41] PTHrP induces osteoclastic resorption of bone, increases tubular reabsorption of calcium in the kidneys, and inhibits osteoblast activity through the action of cytokines such as IL-6.[42] These factors explain why serum calcium rises rapidly in cancer patients in contrast to the gradual rise in hyperparathyroidism.

MULTIPLE MYELOMA AND HYPERCALCEMIA

Hypercalcemia occurs in about a third of patients with myeloma. Osteolytic bone lesions are the most common skeletal radiographic findings. The bone destruction in myeloma is mediated by osteoclasts that accumulate adjacent to the collections of myeloma cells. This association of myeloma cells with osteoclasts is most likely related to the osteoclast-activating effect of cytokines that are locally secreted by the malignant cells. Myeloma cells produce in vitro several osteoclast-activating factors, including TGF-β, IL-1, and IL-6. The increase in bone resorption in most cases is associated with a suppressed osteoblastic bone-forming activity. This explains the depressed skeletal uptake of bone-seeking radiolabeled elements in myeloma, resulting in negative bone scans in the majority of the affected patients. Myeloma cells exhibit a unique capability to grow rapidly in the bone. Myeloma cells secrete osteoclast-mobilizing and osteoclast-stimulating cytokines, whereas osteoclasts secrete IL-6, which is a major growth factor of the myeloma cells. This relationship between myeloma cells and osteoclasts explains the rapid destruction of bone in this malignancy.[43,44]

VITAMIN D INTOXICATION AND HYPERCALCEMIA

All patients receiving vitamin D, other than in small doses, for the treatment of hypoparathyroidism may develop hypercalcemia, with the attendant risk of renal failure. The appearance of hypercalcemia in hypoparathyroid patients receiving pharmacologic doses of either ergocalciferol (vitamin D_2) or DHT3 is almost unpredictable, because the margin between normocalcemic and hypercalcemic doses of the vitamin is very narrow. Some episodes of hypercalcemia may pass unnoticed and yet may be the underlying cause of reduced renal function in these patients. Hypercalcemia associated with vitamin D intoxication may be present from 1 to 6 weeks after discontinuation of the treatment, and normocalcemia may persist for an additional 4 months without any treatment. The toxic effect of vitamin D excess is associated with a high circulating level of 25(OH) vitamin D_3, which is continuously produced by the liver from the adipose tissue stores of vitamin D. The serum level of 1,25(OH)$_2$ vitamin D_3 generally is not elevated and even may be reduced; however, the free non-protein-bound 1,25(OH)$_2$ vitamin D_3 levels may be elevated. The hypercalcemia associated with 1,25(OH)$_2$ vitamin D_3 administration, however, is much more short lived (3-7 days).[45]

Various factors may alter the response to vitamin D. The inhibitory effect of estrogens on bone resorption may be absent after menopause, which allows more calcium to be released from the bone for any given dose of vitamin D. The administration of corticosteroids may reduce the effect of vitamin D; in fact, corticosteroids may be used to treat vitamin D intoxication. The most important precaution in preventing the complications of vitamin D intoxication is to measure serum calcium concentrations frequently in these patients. Likewise, the presence of excessive hypercalciuria, even in the absence of hypercalcemia, is a risk factor for nephrocalcinosis and renal failure. Thus, monitoring of urinary calcium excretion in these circumstances is recommended as well.

VITAMIN A INTOXICATION AND HYPERCALCEMIA

Hypercalcemia is also associated with excessive intake of vitamin A,[46] which is readily available in various pharmaceutical preparations. Isotretinoin, a derivative of vitamin A that is effective in the treatment of severe acne, has been reported as a cause of hypercalcemia. The main symptom of vitamin A intoxication is painful swelling over the extremities. Prolonged hypercalcemia in this condition also has been associated with nephrocalcinosis and impairment of renal function. In experimental animals, excessive amounts of vitamin A cause fractures, increased number of osteoclasts, and calcification of soft tissues. In human subjects, periosteal bone deposition constitutes the typical radiographic feature.

SARCOIDOSIS AND HYPERCALCEMIA

Sarcoidosis is a systemic granulomatous inflammatory disease characterized by noncaseating granulomas in multiple organ systems. Hypercalciuria is the most common defect in calcium metabolism; however, hypercalcemia occurs in approximately 5% of patients.[47] In a small proportion of patients, very high serum calcium concentration leads to metastatic calcifications and eventual death from uremia.

Seasonal incidence of hypercalcemia in sarcoidosis is directly related to the amount of sunlight exposure. Plasma levels of 1,25(OH)$_2$ vitamin D_3 have been found to be increased in patients with sarcoidosis and hypercalcemia, a finding that accounts for the abnormal calcium metabolism in this disease. In most of the patients, glucocorticoids can normalize the level of calcium and 1,25(OH)$_2$ vitamin D_3 in the serum. Serum immunoreactive PTH has been found to be low in patients with sarcoidosis, regardless of the presence or absence of hypercalcemia.[47]

HYPERTHYROIDISM, HYPOTHYROIDISM, AND HYPERCALCEMIA

Hyperthyroidism is associated with accelerated bone turnover, which is caused by direct stimulation of bone cells by the high thyroid hormone concentrations.[48] Biochemical markers of bone formation and resorption (osteocalcin, alkaline phosphatase, bone-specific alkaline phosphatase, and urinary collagen pyridinoline) are elevated in hyperthyroid patients, indicating increased bone turnover in favor of osteoclastic bone resorption.[49] The resultant hypercalcemia may be reversed by antithyroid therapy.[50]

Serum calcium and phosphate levels are normal and alkaline phosphatase is low in the vast majority of patients with hypothyroidism; however, some patients may manifest hypercalcemia. Calcium balance in patients with hypothyroidism tends to be positive as a result of increased intestinal absorption and reduced urinary excretion. Both changes predispose to the development of hypercalcemia. The bone turnover in hypothyroid patients is reduced.

ADRENAL INSUFFICIENCY AND HYPERCALCEMIA

Hypercalcemia is a common abnormality in adrenal insufficiency. The mechanism of hypercalcemia in this clinical setting is not well understood. One study indicates that the increase in serum calcium concentration is due to an increase in the protein-bound fraction of serum calcium that results from accompanying volume depletion. The volume depletion also may cause an increase in the renal tubular reabsorption of calcium, and vitamin D's enhancement of calcium absorption from the intestine may be greater in the absence of glucocorticoid hormone.[51]

IDIOPATHIC INFANTILE HYPERCALCEMIA

Idiopathic infantile hypercalcemia (IIH) is a rare cause of hypercalcemia in the first year of life and is a diagnosis of exclusion. It usually presents between the ages of 3 and 7 months, with clinical features including vomiting, irritability, constipation, increased thirst, and failure to thrive.[52] The pathophysiology of IIH remains unclear, but some authors attribute the hypercalcemia to intestinal vitamin D sensitivity that leads to increased calcium absorption and contributes to persistent hypercalciuria.[53] Treatment options for IIH include corticosteroids, low-calcium diet, calcitonin, and cellulose phosphate. The natural history of this disease remains elusive, but patients usually experience spontaneous resolution of hypercalcemia (usually before age 3), persistent hypercalciuria, and increased risk of nephrocalcinosis.

JANSEN'S METAPHYSEAL CHONDRODYSPLASIA

Jansen's metaphyseal chondrodysplasia is characterized by short limbs, mild hypercalcemia, and low serum PTH levels. It is caused by activating mutations of the PTH/PTHrP receptor and is inherited as an autosomal dominant trait. It is associated with increased proliferation and delayed maturation of chondrocytes.

IMMOBILIZATION AND HYPERCALCEMIA

Immobilization may be associated with excessive loss of bone minerals, hypercalcemia, and rapidly developing osteoporosis. The lack of postural mechanical stimuli to the skeleton disturbs the balance between bone formation and resorption, thus leading to loss of bone mass and its minerals. Usually the amount of calcium released from bone is excreted in the urine and does not increase serum calcium concentrations. Owing to reduced ability to excrete calcium in the urine, patients with preexisting renal impairment are prone to develop immobilization hypercalcemia.[54]

MILK-ALKALI SYNDROME

Milk-alkali syndrome (MAS) may occur in patients who ingest large amounts of milk and alkali as a therapy to relieve the symptoms of peptic ulcers. The syndrome is characterized by hypercalcemia, hyperphosphatemia, alkalosis, metastatic calcifications, and progressive renal failure. It has been shown that these abnormalities may be reversed by discontinuation of the therapy. Ingestion of large amounts of calcium carbonate (at least 4-5 grams daily) and absorbable alkali is a prerequisite for establishing the diagnosis.[33] For hypercalcemia to develop, calcium intake must be excessive, but inability to excrete this excessive calcium may also be important. Preexisting renal insufficiency has been implicated in the pathogenesis of MAS, as well as medications that affect renal calcium excretion, such as thiazide diuretics.

THIAZIDE DIURETICS AND HYPERCALCEMIA

Chronic administration of thiazide diuretics may lead to hypercalcemia in patients treated with large doses of vitamin D (hypoparathyroid patients and patients with osteoporosis) and in patients with hyperparathyroidism. The mechanism of action may involve: (1) reduced urinary excretion of calcium due to a direct tubular effect, or extracellular fluid depletion with secondary increase in tubular reabsorption of sodium and calcium, or both; and (2) increased bone responsiveness to the resorptive actions of vitamin D and PTH.

LITHIUM AND THEOPHYLLINE TOXICITY

Patients treated chronically with lithium may develop hypercalcemia with elevated PTH levels. The incidence of primary hyperparathyroidism in patients with bipolar affective disorders treated with lithium is 47-fold higher than in the general population. To date, 50 cases of parathyroid adenomas and hyperplasia that were associated with chronic lithium therapy have been reported.[55,56] Theophylline toxicity may be associated with hypercalcemia, probably due to stimulation of β-adrenergic receptors in bone.

CLINICAL MANIFESTATIONS OF HYPERCALCEMIA

The symptoms of hypercalcemia depend on its rate of onset, magnitude, duration, the underlying disorder, and comorbid conditions. Acute hypercalcemia may induce acute renal failure due to extracellular volume contraction and direct renal vasoconstriction. This abnormality is reversible, whereas chronic hypercalcemia may cause nephrolithiasis and nephrocalcinosis with tubulointerstitial scarring and chronic renal failure. Hypercalcemia may cause constipation, nausea and vomiting, and peptic ulcer disease. Polyuria is caused both by its natriuretic effect and impaired urinary concentration, with features of nephrogenic diabetes insipidus.

Hypercalcemia leads to membrane hyperpolarization with shortened QT interval on an ECG. Cardiac arrhythmias are rare. Neuromuscular effects include impaired concentration and memory, muscle weakness and fatigue, confusion, lethargy, stupor, and coma (see Box 112-3). Bone pain can occur in patients with hyperparathyroidism or malignancy. Osteoporosis of the cortical bone is associated with hyperparathyroidism. Compression fractures of the vertebral bodies, sometimes with sudden onset of paralysis, may be the first manifestation of multiple myeloma. Familial hypocalciuric hypercalcemia is rarely associated with the bone disease, but chondrocalcinosis and pseudogout have been reported to occur in high frequency. Hypercalcemic crisis is a life-threatening emergency that warrants aggressive treatment. It may be a complication of primary hyperparathyroidism, malignancy, and other hypercalcemic disorders. It is characterized by very high serum calcium levels exceeding 15 mg/dL. The treatment is aimed at restoring extracellular volume to normal and lowering serum calcium levels. Acute hemodialysis with calcium-free dialysate may become a necessity.

TREATMENT OF HYPERCALCEMIA

Lowering of serum calcium concentration can be produced by (1) inhibiting calcium release from the bone, increasing its deposition in the bone and other tissues, or both; (2) increasing removal of calcium from the extracellular fluid or inhibiting its absorption in the bowel; and (3) decreasing the ionized fraction by complex formation with chelating substances.

Hypercalcemia augments urinary losses of sodium and water, resulting in the contraction of extracellular volume and reduced glomerular filtration rate. The latter leads to diminished urinary excretion of calcium and further aggravation of hypercalcemia. Therefore, the first therapeutic goal is to restore the extracellular volume to normal by IV administration of normal saline. This usually requires 3 to 4 L of saline. This therapeutic action per se lowers the serum calcium concentration, partly by the dilutional effect and partly by increased urinary excretion of calcium. There is a risk of extracellular volume overload during rapid IV administration of saline, which is particularly hazardous in elderly patients. Therefore, monitoring of central venous pressure in this situation may be very helpful. Likewise, addition of loop diuretics as an adjunct therapy not only may minimize the risk of fluid overload but also may substantially increase the urinary excretion of calcium. The effect of loop diuretics as calciuretic agents requires prompt replacement of urinary losses of sodium and water. The use of loop diuretics may be particularly beneficial in patients who develop hypercalcemia as a result of excessive secretion and high serum levels of PTH, PTHrP, or both. Hormone-induced excessive tubular reabsorption of calcium plays a major role in the development and maintenance of hypercalcemia in these circumstances.

Bisphosphonates

Bisphosphonates (formerly diphosphonates) represent a group of drugs with a high therapeutic potential for the treatment of hypercalcemia in general and that associated with malignancy in particular. Bisphosphonates have a great affinity for bone and bind tightly to calcified bone matrix, impairing both the mineralization and resorption of bone. In addition, they interfere with the function of osteoclasts. They appear to have several direct effects on osteoclast function, including prevention of osteoclast attachment to bone matrix and prevention of osteoclast differentiation and recruitment. Bisphosphonates also inhibit the motility of isolated osteoclasts. Thus, they are very potent inhibitors of bone resorption.

The first of the bisphosphonates, ethane hydroxybisphosphonate (etidronate [Didronel]), is available for clinical use, but its potency as an antihypercalcemic agent is limited, at least when given orally.

Probably this is because its effect to reduce bone resorption is offset by its effect to inhibit bone mineralization. Reduction of serum calcium concentration has been achieved more successfully with the second generation of bisphosphonates, including dichloromethylene bisphosphonate (clodronate) and amino-hydroxypropylidene bisphosphonate (pamidronate; ADP), which causes a reduction in bone resorption with a dose that has a negligible effect on bone mineralization. Pamidronate and etidronate are approved for treatment of hypercalcemia of malignancy in the United States. In clinical trials, pamidronate and clodronate have been demonstrated to inhibit hypercalcemia, bone pain, and pathologic fractures in patients with malignancy-associated hypercalcemia. Pamidronate is most effective when given IV; a single infusion of 30 mg achieved normocalcemia in 90% of patients in one study. When compared, the effect of 30 mg of pamidronate is equal to 600 mg of clodronate and 1500 mg of etidronate in controlling hypercalcemia. The third generation of bisphosphonates, including alendronate, risedronate, and tiludronate, in preliminary studies is 500 times more efficient in inhibiting bone resorption than clodronate. Zoledronic acid is one of a new generation of nitrogen-containing bisphosphonates that in clinical studies was superior to pamidronate. This agent has been approved for clinical use.

Glucocorticoids

Glucocorticoids are effective in lowering serum calcium in states of vitamin D intoxication; possible mechanisms are suppression of bone resorption and decreased intestinal absorption. It has been pointed out that glucocorticoids are more effective in hypercalcemia associated with lymphoma, leukemia, and multiple myeloma than with other neoplasms. This effect of glucocorticoids might be related to a tumor lytic effect, interference with the production of osteoclast-activating cytokines, or both. The average dose is 3 to 4 mg/kg/d of hydrocortisone given IV or orally. The fall in serum calcium concentration occurs 1 to 2 days after starting the therapy.

Calcitonin

Calcitonin lowers serum calcium concentration by inhibiting bone resorption and increasing urinary calcium excretion. Administration of calcitonin is associated with negligible toxicity; however, its therapeutic action has a limited duration because of the osteoclast escape phenomenon, which is apparent several days after starting therapy. Addition of glucocorticoids may be helpful to maintain efficacy.

Mithramycin (Plicamycin)

Mithramycin is a cytotoxic substance derived from an actinomycete of the genus *Streptomyces* and is used mainly in the treatment of testicular tumors. Mithramycin lowers serum calcium concentration by suppressing bone resorption. The dose, which is lower than the antitumor dose and has fewer side effects, is 25 μg/kg, given IV. The drug is available commercially as Mithracin. The effect starts 24 to 48 hours after injection and lasts several days. Side effects are suppression of bone marrow activity and hepatocellular and renal toxicity, which usually occurs with repeated doses.

Phosphate

Oral and IV salts of phosphorus lower serum concentration and reduce urinary excretion of calcium. This effect has been variously attributed to (1) deposition of mineral in the bone; (2) increased deposition of calcium in soft tissues; and (3) suppression of bone resorption. The major untoward side effects of this therapy are extraskeletal calcifications, including nephrocalcinosis with resulting renal failure. Thus, the use of phosphates to treat hypercalcemia should be discouraged in patients with high serum phosphates and renal insufficiency. Phosphates may be given IV at a dose of 20 to 30 mg of elemental phosphorus per kilogram of body weight over 12 to 16 hours. Serum calcium concentration should be determined at close intervals. The commercially available preparation for IV use is InPhos; 40 mL of the solution contains 1000 mg of phosphorus, 65 mEq of sodium, and 8 mEq of potassium.

Other Therapies

Gallium nitrate has been approved by the Food and Drug Administration for treatment of hypercalcemia. It inhibits bone resorption by reducing the solubility of hydroxyapatite crystals. Nephrotoxicity is a major side effect of gallium nitrate. The use of a somatostatin congener (lanreotide) has been reported to successfully inhibit hypercalcemia in a patient with a PTHrP secreting pancreatic neoplasm. The calcium-lowering effect was associated with suppression of the serum levels of PTHrP.

The hypercalcemia associated with thyrotoxicosis and theophylline toxicity has been successfully treated with IV propranolol.

Intestinal absorption of calcium may be reduced by dietary restrictions and binding of calcium in the bowel with cellulose phosphate and sodium phytate to form nonabsorbable complexes.

Calcium also may be removed directly from the extracellular fluid with hemodialysis or peritoneal dialysis by employing calcium-free dialysate solution.

Reduction of serum ionized calcium may be accomplished with IV Na-EDTA, which is a chelating agent. The complexed calcium then is excreted in the urine. The main disadvantage of this therapy is the nephrotoxicity of EDTA.

Disorders of Magnesium Metabolism

Magnesium is the second most abundant intracellular cation. The intracellular concentration of magnesium ranges between 10 and 20 mEq/L; however, most of it is bound to organic compounds, including adenosine triphosphate (ATP). Of the fraction found in the extracellular space, one-third is bound to serum albumin. Therefore the plasma level of magnesium may be a poor indicator of total body stores in the presence of hypoalbuminemia. The exchange between the extracellular and intracellular compartments appears to be slow, and changes in intake and intestinal absorption are tightly balanced by parallel changes in urinary excretion.[57,58]

The renal tubular handling of magnesium displays a Tm (tubular maximum) with serum levels being close to the Tm threshold values. Thus, any rise in serum level and in the filtered load is counterbalanced by urinary spillover, and vice versa, a fall in filtered load leads to a sharp decline in urinary excretion almost down to zero. Therefore, in the presence of normal kidney function, serum levels are maintained at nearly constant values ranging form 1.4 to 1.7 mEq/L (1.7-2.1 mg/dL). Hypermagnesemia can be encountered primarily with impaired kidney function and excessive oral or parenteral load. Hypomagnesemia results from decreased dietary intake, intestinal malabsorption, or renal losses.[57]

Magnesium plays an important role in the function of many key enzymes including ATP, Na^+/K^+-ATPase, creatine kinase, and adenylate cyclase. Intracellular magnesium is key to protein synthesis, oxidative phosphorylation, nucleic acid stability, storing and utilization of energy, and enzymatic reactions. Extracellular magnesium is essential to nerve conduction, neuromuscular transmission, cardiac conduction and contractility, and vascular tone.

Though total serum magnesium concentration is commonly utilized to measure magnesium, it may not be the best test.[59] Changes in serum protein concentrations may affect total concentration but are not reflective of total body magnesium. A magnesium tolerance test can be used to determine magnesium status but requires calculating the amount of retained parenteral magnesium. Finally, ionized magnesium measurement devices are available but not yet readily available.

Hypomagnesemia and Magnesium Depletion

Hypomagnesaemia is a common problem in hospitalized patients, particularly in the ICU. The kidney is primarily responsible for magnesium homeostasis through regulation by calcium/magnesium receptors on renal tubular cells that sense serum magnesium levels.[60] Hypomagnesemia results from a variety of etiologies ranging from poor intake, increased renal excretion, GI losses, malabsorption, and a variety of endocrine dysfunctions. The causes of hypomagnesemia can be divided into two major categories: (1) extrarenal magnesium losses, including deficient intake, and (2) renal losses.

EXTRARENAL LOSSES

Dietary deprivation, prolonged malnutrition, tube feedings, and parenteral nutrition deficient in magnesium may induce cumulative magnesium depletion and hypomagnesemia. GI losses may be caused by steatorrhea, severe diarrhea, or acute pancreatitis. Hypomagnesemia may also follow surgery for morbid obesity with short bowel syndrome and diarrhea.[57]

Endocrine causes include hyperthyroidism, hypercalcemia associated with malignancy, and hyperaldosteronism.[61] Hungry bone syndrome after parathyroidectomy may lead to both hypocalcemia and hypomagnesemia owing to increased deposition of both divalent ions in the newly deposited bone mineral.

Chronic alcoholism is one of the leading causes of magnesium depletion. Poor nutrition, diarrhea, chronic pancreatitis, and possibly a renal tubular defect may contribute to hypomagnesemia.[62] Severe burns may lead to sequestration of magnesium in the necrotic tissue, including necrotic fat, leading to magnesium depletion. Finally, acute dialysis for severe refractory hypercalcemia without addition of magnesium to the dialysate may cause hypomagnesemia.

RENAL LOSSES

Osmotic diuresis induced by IV salt loads, diabetic ketoacidosis, and mannitol administration all increase urinary excretion of many electrolytes, including magnesium. During recovery from ketoacidosis, especially after phosphate replacement, a precipitous fall in serum magnesium may occur.

Hypercalcemia as seen with primary hyperparathyroidism, hyperthyroidism, and IV administration of calcium causes renal losses of magnesium as both divalent cations compete for the same reabsorption mechanism in Henle's loop. Similarly, loop diuretics cause renal magnesium and calcium wasting, whereas thiazides enhance urinary excretion of magnesium but cause tubular retention of calcium. Primary hyperaldosteronism and the syndrome of inappropriate antidiuretic hormone (SIADH) are associated with modest increases in urinary magnesium excretion.

Renal magnesium wasting has been observed in patients treated with aminoglycosides, amphotericin B, and cisplatin.[63-65] These agents may lead to potassium wasting and renal tubular acidosis. Cyclosporine and tacrolimus cause magnesium wasting with potassium retention. Loop diuretics can also lead to magnesium wasting. The diuretic phase of acute renal failure also may lead to magnesium loss.

Inherited Disorders of Renal Magnesium Losses

Isolated Dominant Hypomagnesemia. Patients with isolated dominant hypomagnesemia (IDH) present with generalized seizures in childhood, but their mothers may be asymptomatic with less pronounced hypomagnesemia. Many affected members of the family may be asymptomatic. Hypocalciuria but not hypocalcemia is present.

Isolated Recessive Hypomagnesemia. Individuals affected by isolated recessive hypomagnesemia (IRH) present with symptoms of hypomagnesemia early during infancy. Hypomagnesemia due to increased urinary magnesium excretion is the only biochemical abnormality. Linkage analysis has thus far excluded all established gene loci.[63]

Familial Hypomagnesemia with Hypercalciuria and Nephrocalcinosis (FHHNC). FHHNC is an autosomal recessive hypomagnesemia characterized by renal magnesium and calcium wasting, bilateral nephrocalcinosis, and nephrolithiasis with progressive renal failure. FHHNC patients present during early childhood with recurrent urinary tract infection, polyuria and polydipsia, failure to thrive, abdominal pain, vomiting, tetanic episodes, and generalized seizures. PTH levels are increased before renal failure.

Autosomal Dominant Hypocalcemia. Activating mutations of the calcium sensing receptor lead to hypocalcemia, hypocalciuria, and in about 50% of patients, hypomagnesemia. The diminished PTH secretion and decreased reabsorption of divalent cations in the cortical thick ascending limb of Henle's loop and distal convoluted tubule lead to urinary loss of calcium and magnesium. Inhibition of calcium and magnesium reabsorption in the loop of Henle is thought to be secondary to selective reduction in paracellular permeability and/or reduction in the lumen-positive transepithelial voltage.

Classic Bartter Syndrome. Classic Bartter syndrome is caused by mutations in the *CLCNKB* gene encoding the basolaterally located renal chloride channel ClC-KB, which mediates chloride efflux from the tubular epithelial cells to the interstitium. Hypomagnesemia is detected in up to 50% of patients with mutations in *CLCNKB* in chromosome 1p36.[63]

Gitelman's Syndrome. Gitelman's syndrome (GS) is an autosomal recessive disorder. Major symptoms include muscle weakness and tetanic episodes that are related to profound hypomagnesemia. Patients always present with hypocalciuria; the presence of both hypomagnesemia and hypocalciuria is diagnostic. Loss-of-function mutations in the gene coding for NaCl cotransporter (NCCT) of the distal convoluted tubule is the underlying abnormality. Hypocalciuria is explained by reduced entry of NaCl into distal convoluted tubule cells, leading to apical membrane hyperpolarization. This increases calcium absorption mediated by apical entry via the epithelial calcium channel and basolateral extrusion through the Na^+/Ca^{++} exchanger.

CLINICAL CONSEQUENCES OF MAGNESIUM DEPLETION

The clinical manifestations of hypomagnesemia depend on its severity, duration, and coexistent electrolyte abnormalities. Hypomagnesemia and depletion of intracellular stores, especially in cardiac muscle, have been considered to underlie cardiovascular and other functional abnormalities including cardiac arrhythmias such as atrial fibrillation and torsades de pointes, impairment of cardiac contractibility, and vasoconstriction. This may be especially important in patients undergoing coronary artery bypass graft surgery.[66] Depletion is also characterized by neuromuscular and central nervous system hyperactivity, and symptoms are similar to those of calcium deficiency, including hyperactive reflexes, muscle tremors, and tetany with a positive Chvostek's sign (see Table 112-1). Severe deficiencies can lead to delirium and seizures.

Hypomagnesemia is important not only for its direct effects on the nervous system but also because it can produce hypocalcemia and lead to persistent hypokalemia. When hypokalemia or hypocalcemia coexist with hypomagnesemia, magnesium should be aggressively replaced to assist in restoring potassium or calcium homeostasis. Prolonged insufficiency of magnesium supply[67] results in anorexia, nausea, vomiting, and weakness within weeks and in paresthesias and muscle weakness, cerebral seizures, and cardiac manifestations within months.

ECG changes in magnesium depletion include widening of QRS complex and peaking of T waves, followed by prolongation of PR interval and diminution of T waves. Ventricular arrhythmias are more common during myocardial ischemia after cardiopulmonary bypass. Magnesium prevents the increase in action potential duration and the prolongation in membrane repolarization, which normally occurs in ischemic myocardium.[66]

TREATMENT OF HYPOMAGNESEMIA

The amount and route of magnesium replacement depend on the degree of hypomagnesemia and severity of symptoms. In patients with asymptomatic hypomagnesemia, treatment of the underlying disorder (e.g., diarrhea) and dietary adjustments may solve the problem. Correction can be oral if asymptomatic and mild. Oral magnesium can lead to diarrhea, which may limit its utility. Magnesium oxide tablets have high magnesium content (550 mg of elemental magnesium per 1 g or 46 mEq/g) compared to other oral preparations such as magnesium chloride, magnesium sulfate, and magnesium acetate, which contain approximately 100 mg of elemental magnesium per 1 g (8-10 mEq/g). Oral replacement also can be made with antacids that contain both magnesium and aluminum in patients who develop diarrhea from magnesium oxide. If hypomagnesemia is associated with use of diuretics that need to be continued, addition of potassium-sparing diuretics such as amiloride may be helpful. Amiloride may also be considered in other states of magnesium wasting such as Bartter's or Gitelman's syndrome.

IV repletion depends on the severity and symptoms. For those with severe deficits (<1.0 mEq/L) or those who are symptomatic, administer 1 to 2 g of magnesium sulfate IV over 15 minutes. Caution should be exercised when giving large amounts of magnesium, as magnesium toxicity may develop. Administration of simultaneous calcium gluconate will counteract the adverse side effects of a rapidly rising magnesium level and correct hypocalcemia, which is frequently associated with hypomagnesemia.

In states of emergency such as torsades de pointes tachyarrhythmia, 2 g of magnesium sulfate over 2 minutes is recommended to suppress early depolarization. Magnesium is also a first-line drug for use in eclampsia.[68] Magnesium has a potentially deleterious effect on arteriovenous conduction; therefore, it is relatively contraindicated in greater than first-degree arteriovenous block and sinus bradycardia.

Hypermagnesemia

The normal kidney can dispose of large filtered loads of magnesium by attenuating tubular reabsorption to a minimum after the renal tubular Tm is exceeded. Thus, intact kidneys are the major regulating organ for maintaining magnesium balance. The most common cause of hypermagnesemia is concurrence of excessive magnesium load in the presence of impaired renal function. Very often a large magnesium load is the consequence of therapeutic employment of magnesium salts as laxatives or enemas. Hypermagnesemia may be more common in the elderly, who often consume magnesium salts as antacids and laxatives and display aging-related reduction in renal function.

Attempts to release bowel obstruction with magnesium salts may be detrimental. The magnesium salt is retained in the bowel and can generating local hypertonicity as it displaces large volumes of extracellular fluid into the distended bowel, leading to volume contraction with reduced renal function. The trapped magnesium diffuses into the circulation in massive amounts, and in the presence of impaired renal function raises the serum magnesium level.

Endogenous magnesium loads may be released in rhabdomyolysis from necrotic muscles and in tumor lysis from malignant cells destroyed by chemotherapy. Acute IV magnesium loads such as given in preeclampsia may cause transient hypermagnesemia occasionally accompanied by hypocalcemia as a result of acute suppression of PTH by high serum magnesium. Children born to mothers with preeclampsia may have hypermagnesemia as well.

Patients with chronic renal failure may present with mild elevation of serum magnesium; however, ingestion of magnesium salts should be avoided because they may induce life-threatening hypermagnesemia.

Adrenal insufficiency, primary hyperparathyroidism, milk-alkali syndrome, and familial hypocalciuric hypercalcemia may be associated with hypermagnesemia. Lithium and theophylline have also been reported to cause hypermagnesemia.

CLINICAL MANIFESTATIONS

Mild hypermagnesemia with serum magnesium levels less than 3 mEq/L (3.6 mg/dL, 1.5 Mm/L) is usually asymptomatic. Above these values, the severity of symptoms parallels the magnitude of serum magnesium. The major manifestations are neuromuscular, central nervous system, and cardiovascular abnormalities (see Table 112-1).

Neuromuscular manifestations relate to the curare-like action of hypermagnesemia, hindering the neuromuscular impulse transmission. It is first manifested as reduced deep tendon reflexes progressing to areflexia, muscle paralysis, and apnea. Central nervous system abnormalities consist of lethargy and coma.

The cardiovascular effects of hypermagnesemia may be related to its effects as ion channel blockers. These effects lead to bradycardia and hypotension and may progress to cardiac arrest. ECG abnormalities are similar to those seen with hyperkalemia and consist of increased PR interval, widened QRS, and peaked T waves. With a rise in serum magnesium above 10 mEq/L, complete heart block and cardiac arrest are the terminal events.

TREATMENT OF HYPERMAGNESEMIA

Treatment for hypermagnesemia consists of measures to withhold exogenous sources of magnesium, correct volume deficit, and correct acidosis if present. To manage acute symptoms, calcium chloride (5-10 mL) should be administered to antagonize the cardiovascular effects. If elevated levels or symptoms persist, dialysis is indicated.

KEY POINTS

Hypocalcemia

1. Serum levels of 25(OH) vitamin D serve as an estimate of body stores of vitamin D. Low serum concentrations of 25(OH) vitamin D indicate a state of vitamin D deficiency.

2. Hypoparathyroidism is a common cause of hypocalcemia. Magnesium depletion inhibits parathyroid hormone (PTH) secretion and peripheral responses to PTH and to vitamin D; it also blunts the calcemic effect of intravenous calcium. Thiazides enhance the calcemic effect of vitamin D, whereas furosemide aggravates the hypocalcemia.

3. Neuromuscular manifestations of hypocalcemia include confusion or coma, focal and generalized seizures, and respiratory arrest. Cardiovascular complications of acute hypocalcemia include hypotension, bradycardia, and ventricular arrhythmias such as torsades de pointes.

4. Hypoparathyroidism, and particularly the variant autosomal dominant hypocalcemia, should be treated cautiously. Raising serum calcium levels may cause hypercalciuria with increased risk of nephrocalcinosis and renal failure.

Hypercalcemia

1. Malignancy is the prevalent cause of hypercalcemia, accounting for 70% to 80% of all cases, and is most commonly seen in hospitalized patients. Primary hyperparathyroidism is common in the outpatient setting, accounting for 10% to 20% of all cases of hypercalcemia. Milk-alkali syndrome ranks third.

2. Hypercalcemia with undetectable PTH and high urinary cyclic adenosine monophosphate (cAMP) is consistent with humoral hypercalcemia of malignancy (HHM). Detection of parathyroid hormone-related protein (PTHrP) does not rule out parathyroid adenoma; rather, the absence of PTH and the presence of PTHrP rule out adenoma and support HHM.

3. Familial hypocalciuric hypercalcemia is a form of parathyroid hyperplasia with autosomal dominant transmission. It is caused by an inactivating mutation of a calcium-sensing receptor. The clinical course is benign, without nephrolithiasis, but hypermagnesemia, pancreatitis, and chondrocalcinosis may occur.

4. Hypercalcemic crisis is a life-threatening emergency. It may be a complication of primary hyperparathyroidism, malignancy, and other hypercalcemic disorders. It warrants aggressive treatment to lower the serum calcium concentration.

5. The first goal in treating hypercalcemia is to restore the extracellular volume to normal by intravenous administration of normal saline.

Hypomagnesemia

1. Hypomagnesemia is common in hospitalized patients (>10%) and even more so in the ICU setting (>50%). Concerns regarding hypomagnesemia are focused on its potential role in cardiac arrhythmias (e.g., torsades de pointes) and sudden death.

2. Hypomagnesemia leads to renal losses of potassium, and vice versa, hypokalemia augments urinary losses of magnesium. In the former, hypokalemia may be refractory to potassium replacement unless magnesium repletion is accomplished first.

Hypermagnesemia

1. The most common cause of hypermagnesemia is concurrence of excessive magnesium loads in the presence of impaired renal function. Very often a large magnesium load comes from therapeutic use of magnesium salts as laxatives or enemas.

2. Neuromuscular manifestations of hypermagnesemia relate to its curare-like effect, leading to loss of reflexes, muscle weakness and paralysis, and apnea. Central nervous system abnormalities are lethargy, drowsiness, dilated pupils, and coma.

3. The cardiovascular effects of hypermagnesemia consist of bradycardia and hypotension. The electrocardiogram (ECG) shows increased PR interval and QRS complex. Complete heart block and cardiac arrest is the terminal event.

ANNOTATED REFERENCES

Awad SS, Miskulin J, Thompson N. Hyperparathyroidism in patients with prolonged lithium therapy. World J Surg 2003;27:486-8.

This report calls attention to the association of chronic lithium therapy for bipolar disorders with the development of hypercalcemia with elevated PTH levels. The incidence of primary hyperparathyroidism in patients treated with lithium is 47-fold higher than in the general population. The most common cause of primary hyperparathyroidism is parathyroid adenoma.

Information from NIH conference. diagnosis and management of asymptomatic primary hyperparathyroidism: consensus development conference statement. Ann Intern Med 1991;114:593-7.

This landmark article summarizes the diagnosis and management of asymptomatic primary hyperparathyroidism, specifically the indications for surgical therapy, from the National Institutes of Health Consensus Development Conference Panel composed of endocrinologists, surgeons, radiologists, epidemiologists, and primary health providers.

Zivin JR, Gooley T, Zager RA, et al. Hypocalcemia: a pervasive metabolic abnormality in the critically ill. Am J Kidney Dis 2001;37:689-98.

This article presents an interesting finding that hypocalcemia was present in 88% of critically ill patients who were admitted to ICUs. The level of hypocalcemia correlated with the severity of the disease. The mechanism of this abnormality is unknown.

Konrad M, Weber S. Recent advances in molecular genetics of hereditary magnesium-losing disorders. J Am Soc Nephrol 2003;15:249-60.

This is a comprehensive, in-depth review of recently unfolding information on abnormalities associated both with intestinal and renal causes of magnesium wasting. The paper focuses on the molecular aspects of hereditary genetically transmitted defects in tubular epithelial and in intestinal magnesium transport causing hypomagnesemia.

Swaminathan S. Magnesium metabolism and its disorders. Clin Biochem Rev 2003;24:47-110.

This is a comprehensive review of magnesium balance with an in-depth classification of hypomagnesaemia and magnesium deficiency as well as hypermagnesemia.

REFERENCES

Access the complete reference list online at http://www.expertconsult.com.

Fluids and Electrolytes in Children

DESMOND BOHN

The fundamental principles that govern fluid and electrolyte physiology in pediatrics are in many instances similar to those in adults, particularly in older children. However, there are some important differences in factors that affect fluid management which apply mainly to infants and young children and have to be taken into account when prescribing fluids in critical care. In addition, many of the principles used to estimate fluid losses and the requirements for replacement of normal fluid losses (maintenance fluids) are based on limited studies published 50 years ago at a time when the complexity of illness was far less than is seen today. Also, these formulae were based on principles established for normal physiology and did not take into account the fact that the hormonal influences that govern fluid and electrolyte balance may be seriously perturbed in critical illness. The challenge now is to rethink some of these principles in the light of new knowledge of how acute illness may influence them.

Body Water Distribution in Children

Body water content changes significantly with age in children.[1,2] Total body water (TBW) is high in the fetus and preterm infant. During early fetal life, TBW represents 90% of total body weight, with 65% being in the extracellular fluid (ECF) compartment. By term, ECF and intracellular fluid (ICF) volume has fallen to 45% and 30% of TBW, respectively (Figure 113-1). The preterm infant has a relative expansion of both TBW and ECF volume expansion, and a diuresis in the first few days of postnatal life is a common finding. Fractional excretion of sodium is inversely correlated with age in the preterm, who is susceptible to both sodium loss and sodium and volume overload.[3] In addition, glomerular filtration rate is lower than in the term infant, and the large surface area–to–body weight ratio leads to considerable evaporative losses.[4-7] Further discussion of fluid and electrolyte physiology in the preterm infant is beyond the scope of this chapter.

Significant changes occur in TBW over the first year of life, from 75% of body weight at birth to 65% at 6 months and 60% at 1 year (Table 113-1). Some of this is accounted for by an increase in body fat. By puberty, TBW is approximately 60% of body weight in males, with a slightly lower percentage in females. Extracellular fluid volume decreases over the first year of life to 30% of TBW and decreases with age thereafter, reaching adult values early in childhood. The relatively high ECF volume in infancy is largely due to the larger interstitial lymph space. In contrast, the ICF volume remains relatively constant during childhood.

Fluid Homeostasis in Children

To achieve normal fluid homeostasis, fluid intake must balance losses. The latter consist of urine output plus insensible losses (evaporative from the skin surface and respiratory tract), with the addition of fluid loss in the stool, which in the absence of diarrhea should be minimal. Insensible losses are mainly in the form of electrolyte-free water (EFW) from the respiratory tract (15 mL/100 kcal/d). This loss is eliminated during positive-pressure ventilation. Sweat contains mainly water with a small amount of sodium, except in situations where sweat glands contain excessive amounts of sodium, such as in patients with cystic fibrosis. Evaporative losses also increase with elevations in body temperature; during thermal stress, water losses may increase to as much as 25 mL/100 kcal/d (Table 113-2).

Obligate water excretion in the urine is dependent upon solute load and the ability to concentrate and dilute urine. The average osmolar excretion in newborn infants receiving infant formula is 16 to 20 mOsm/kg/d.[2] Infants are somewhat disadvantaged compared to the older child and adult in that they cannot maximally dilute (infant 200 mOsm/L versus adult 80 mOsm/L) and concentrate urine (infant 800 mOsm/L versus adult 1200 mOsm/L). In addition, the infant's high metabolic rate and the solute load from enteral feeding formula means they require more water excretion per unit solute amount. High solute load and limited urine concentrating ability makes them prone to significant ECF contraction (dehydration) when there are excessive amounts of water loss. Typically this occurs in gastroenteritis, where reduced oral intake is combined with excessive water and electrolyte loss in the stool.

Urine is the major source of electrolyte loss in the body except when there are fluid losses from the gastrointestinal tract. The commonly used values for sodium (Na) and potassium (K) requirements in parenteral fluids in children are 2 to 3 mmol/kg/d and 1 to 2 mmol/kg/d. This assumes that these are the amounts of cations needed for normal homeostasis. However, in critically ill children, urinary Na and K concentration may be much higher.

In the normal healthy individual, water intake is regulated by thirst stimulated via osmoreceptors in the hypothalamus. Infants and small children are unable to regulate their intake because they do not have access to water for the same reasons that apply in older children or adults in coma or with reduced levels of consciousness. When oral intake is replaced by parenteral fluids in children, the amount of fluid (i.e., water) given depends on body weight and energy expenditure. In 1957, Holliday[8] published a formula that linked body weight to energy expenditure (Table 113-3). An allowance of 100 mL/100 kcal/d was made for insensible water loss, with 66.7 mL/100 kcal/d to replace urine output. Factoring in water of oxidation of 16.7 mL/100 kcal/d leaves a total of 100 mL/100 kcal/d for replacement of normal losses. The estimates for Na (3 mmol/100 kcal/d) and K (2 mmol/100 kcal/day) in maintenance fluids were calculated from the sodium and potassium concentration of cow's milk and breast milk.

This paper by Holliday became the standard reference text for parenteral fluid administration in pediatrics. Although convenient and simple to use, the assumptions made about daily requirements for sodium, potassium, and EFW mandate the use of hypotonic intravenous (IV) solutions, which has been almost universal practice in pediatric medicine for almost 50 years (Table 113-4). However, nonphysiologic stimuli for antidiuretic hormone (ADH) secretion, which inhibits excretion of EFW (e.g., pain, anxiety, narcotics, positive-pressure ventilation), are common in critically ill patients. It is therefore not surprising that mild degrees of hyponatremia are a common finding in pediatric patients receiving parenteral fluid therapy. In a study by Gerigk[9] of 103 children admitted to the hospital with acute medical illnesses, the median plasma Na value was 136 mmol/L, with plasma ADH levels that were higher than would be expected for that degree of hyponatremia. In 31 control patients (elective surgical admissions), median serum Na levels were 139 mmol/L, with lower ADH levels. We have made a similar observation in patients with hospital-acquired hyponatremia, who received twice as much EFW compared with a control group.[10] The nonphysiologic secretion of ADH has been reported in association with many acute medical illnesses including meningitis, bronchiolitis, encephalitis, traumatic

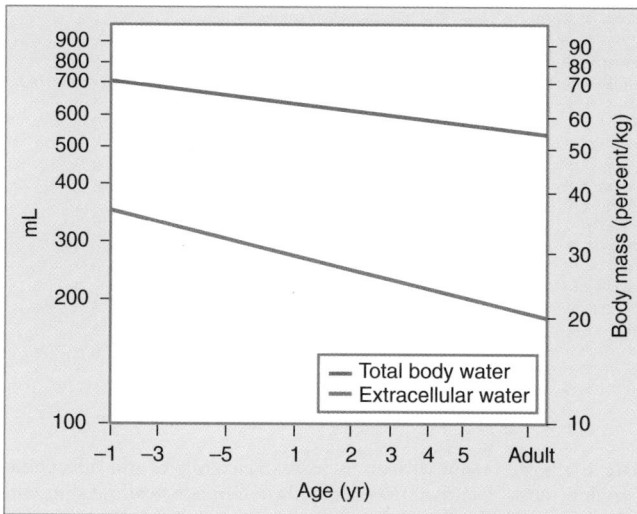

Figure 113-1 Changes in total body water (TBW) with age. Intracellular water is represented by the difference between the two diagonal lines. *(Adapted from Kooh SW Metcoff J. Physiologic considerations in fluid and electrolyte therapy with particular reference to diarrheal dehydration in children. J Pediatr 1963;62:107-31, with permission.)*

brain injury, and gastroenteritis.[11-22] An increasing number of publications are now recommending the use of isotonic or near-isotonic fluids for standard maintenance in pediatrics to avoid administration of EFW, which is potentially hazardous in situations where ADH secretion is not inhibited.[10,23-26] Hypotonic fluids should be reserved for patients with a demonstrated need for EFW (serum Na$^+$ > 145 mmol/L).

Perioperative Fluid Management

Standard practice in perioperative fluid management has been to replace intravascular volume loss with blood or colloid solutions and to use electrolyte solutions to provide for ongoing fluid requirements, replacement of losses from exposed serosal surfaces in open body cavities in thoracic and abdominal surgery, and losses from third-space fluid sequestration (Table 113-5). Extra fluid is also frequently administered to treat hypotension due to the vasodilating effects of anesthetic agents. The preferred electrolyte solution used by most anesthesiologists for intraoperative fluid administration is now Ringer's lactate or isotonic saline because of concerns about the development of postoperative fluid retention and hyponatremia associated with elevated ADH levels.[27-29] The potential for this is increased when hypotonic dextrose/saline solutions are used.[28,30-32] This inability to excrete a sodium-free water load is amply illustrated in scoliosis surgery, where patients seem to be particularly at risk for the development of hyponatremia postoperatively.[33] Two nonrandomized studies have shown

TABLE 113-2   Water Losses in Normal Children (mL/100 kcal/24 h)

Source	Newborn-6 Months	6 Months-5 Years	5-10 Years	Adolescence
Insensible	40	30	20	10
Urine	60	60	50	40
Fecal	20	10	—	—
Total	120	100	70	50

that the degree of hyponatremia is less when isotonic or near-isotonic solutions are used.[34,35] In a nonrandomized trial, Burrows[35] compared Ringer's lactate with 0.2% sodium chloride (NaCl) infusion in a group of children following scoliosis surgery. He found that the postoperative plasma Na level fell in both groups, but that the reduction was marked in those patients receiving the hypotonic fluid. Although at first glance, the explanation for this is EFW retention due to nonphysiologic stimulation of ADH secretion, it does not explain the reduction in plasma Na seen with Ringer's lactate.

Further insights to explain this observation come from the study by Steele,[36] where plasma and urine Na were measured in adult patients undergoing elective surgery, all of whom received Ringer's lactate as their perioperative fluid. They found that the urine Na concentration was consistently above 150 mmol/L and as high as 350 mmol/L in some instances. This was associated with a significant positive water balance and a fall in the plasma Na, a process they termed *postoperative desalination*. In a similar study of children undergoing elective surgery, all of whom received Ringer's lactate, we found similar levels of urinary Na loss (unpublished observations). We think that this desalination process is consistent with the kidney's attempts to deal with a volume overload situation after the vasodilating effects of anesthetic agents are no longer present, but ADH is still being actively secreted. In this situation, it would be unwise to prescribe hypotonic fluids in the postoperative period and impose an extra burden of more EFW to be excreted by the kidney.

Further evidence has now emerged that supports the use of isotonic rather than hypotonic fluid in the perioperative period. A prospective observational study in patients admitted to the intensive care unit (ICU) postoperatively documented an increased risk of development of hyponatremia associated with use of hypotonic saline; water retention and increased sodium excretion are to blame.[37] Two recent prospective randomized trials have compared the use of isotonic with hypotonic saline. Both have shown that the incidence of hyponatremia was significantly reduced with isotonic saline, and in neither study did the patients develop hypernatremia.[38,39]

Disorders of Sodium Homeostasis

Sodium is the principal cation of the ECF compartment. Movement of Na into the ICF compartment is reversed by activation of the Na$^+$/K$^+$-ATPase pump. Sodium is absorbed in the proximal tubule under the influence of aldosterone. The serum Na reflects the osmolality and the ECF water volume, which is tightly regulated by ADH secretion.

HYPONATREMIA

Hyponatremia (serum Na <136 mmol/L) is the commonest electrolyte disorder seen in a hospitalized population and implies an expansion

TABLE 113-1   Water Content of Body Compartments in Children

Age	Total Body Water (% Body Weight)	Extracellular Fluid (% Body Weight)	Intracellular Fluid (% Body Weight)
Premature	80	45	35
Full-term newborn	75	40	35
1 month to 1 year	65	30	35
1 to 12 years	60	20	40
Adolescents:			
Males	60	20	40-45
Females	55	18	40

TABLE 113-3   Requirements for Maintenance Parenteral Fluids*

Body Weight	0-10 kg	10-20 kg	>20 kg
Water requirements	100 mL/kg/d	1000 mL + 50 mL/kg/d for each kg >10 kg	1500 mL + 20 mL/kg for each kg >20 kg

*Based on the formula of Holliday in Holliday MA, Segar WE. The maintenance need for water in parenteral fluid therapy. Pediatrics 1957;19:823-32.

TABLE 113-4	Water and Electrolyte Content of Commonly Used Intravenous Fluids						
Fluid Type	Na+ mmol/L	Cl− mmol/L	Osmolality	Osmolality with 20 mmol KCl/L Added	pH	Electrolyte-Free Water/L
0.9% NaCl	154	154	308	348	5.5	0
0.45% NaCl	77	77	154	194	5.5	500
0.9% NaCl 5% dex	154	154	560	600	4	0
5% dex 0.45% NaCl	77	77	406	446	4	500
5% dex 0.2% NaCl	34	34	321	361	4	780
4% dex 0.18% NaCl	31	31	284	324	4	800
5% dex	0	0	252	292	4	1000
Ringer's lactate	130	109	272	312	6.5	114
Ringer's lactate 5%	130	109	525		6.5	114
3% NaCl	513	513	1027		5.5	0

Cl−, chloride ion; *dex*, dextrose; *KCl*, potassium chloride; *Na+*, sodium ion; *NaCl*, sodium chloride.

of the ICF compartment. It is caused by either water gain (e.g., use of hypotonic fluids) or salt loss (e.g., gastroenteritis) (Table 113-6).

Acute hyponatremia, defined as a fall in plasma Na to less than 130 mmol/L within 48 hrs, leads to rapid movement of water from the ECF to the ICF compartment and can cause cerebral edema, with catastrophic outcomes reported in children.[30,40,41] Clinical findings are those of raised intracranial pressure (nausea, vomiting, headache), frequently undiagnosed until the onset of seizures. This is usually followed by apnea, indicating that brainstem coning has occurred. Symptomatic hyponatremia rarely occurs below a serum Na level of 125 mmol/L, but when it does, it constitutes a medical emergency. The primary objective is to raise serum Na to above this level to prevent brainstem herniation. This can be most effectively achieved with the use of hypertonic saline.[42] Once this threshold has been reached, the serum Na can be allowed to correct by fluid restriction with or without the use of furosemide. IV mannitol has also been used successfully in the emergency treatment of acute symptomatic hyponatremia.[43]

Chronic hyponatremia is a common finding in patients with heart failure and renal failure and is associated with increased TBW and salt retention. It is not associated with cerebral edema, but correction of chronic hyponatremia with isotonic or hypertonic saline has been associated with central pontine demyelination.[44-46]

HYPERNATREMIA

Hypernatremia is defined as a serum Na greater than 145 mmol/L and is caused by either water deficit or salt gain (Table 113-7). The former is seen in infants with severe gastroenteritis with a loss of water in excess of sodium, sometimes compounded by increased solute intake from incorrect mixing of infant formula. The absence of ADH secretion causing diabetes insipidus is seen in patients with pituitary tumors, traumatic brain injury, and central nervous system (CNS) infections.[47-50] Water loss in critically ill children may also be associated with the use of loop diuretics or mannitol. Hypernatremia secondary to salt gain is seen with the excessive use of isotonic or hypertonic saline solutions or with the administration of IV bicarbonate.

A rise in serum Na is associated with movement of water from the ICF to the ECF compartment and development of a hyperosmolar state. Brain cells adapt with an increase in electrolytes and "ideogenic" osmoles (inositol, taurine), which tends to mitigate the fluid shift with partial restoration of intracellular osmolality and brain cell volume.[51-53] Levels of Na over 155 mmol/L are frequently associated with abnormal CNS findings, and there is an increased risk of subdural hemorrhage and infarction in infants with hypernatremic dehydration and serum Na levels higher than 160 mmol/L.[54-57] There is also the added danger of development of brain edema during the attempt to correct these hyperosmolar states rapidly, using solutions that are hypo-osmolar compared to the ICF compartment.[58-63] Published recommendations suggest that the rate of correction of serum Na should be less than 0.5 mmol/L/h using the following formula for correction, which estimates the effect of 1 L of any infusate on serum Na:

$$\text{Change in serum Na} = \frac{\text{Infusate Na} - \text{Serum Na}}{\text{TBW} + 1}$$

In severe hypernatremia (serum Na > 170 mmol/L), it is recommended that the maximum Na concentration not be corrected to below 150 mmol/L in the first 48 to 72 hrs.[64]

The epidemiology of hypernatremia in children has changed recently from gastroenteritis with dehydration as the principal cause to one of a hospital-acquired problem in association with either excess salt administration or a free-water deficit. In a study by Moritz of children with a serum Na above 150 mmol/L, the problem was hospital acquired in 60%, and the mortality was 11%.[65] In a similar series of adult patients, the ICU mortality rate for patients with plasma Na levels above 150 mmol/L was 30%.[66]

Management of Acute Water and Sodium Deficits in Children

Two major problems of acute water and electrolyte deficits are worthy of specific mention because of the potential for serious adverse outcomes associated with both.

TABLE 113-5	Electrolyte Composition of Body Fluids (mmol/L)			
	Na+	K+	Cl−	HCO3−
Sweat	50	5	55	0
Saliva	30	20	35	15
Gastric juice	60	10	90	0
Bile	145	5	110	40
Duodenum	140	5	80	50
Ileum	130	10	110	30
Colon	60	30	40	20

TABLE 113-6	Principal Causes of Hyponatremia
Water Gain	
Excessive water ingestion	
Hypotonic fluid administration	
Syndrome of inappropriate antidiuretic hormone (SIADH) secretion	
Congestive heart failure	
Chronic renal failure	
Salt Loss	
Gastroenteritis	
Cerebral salt wasting	

TABLE 113-7	Causes of Hypernatremia

Water Loss

Gastroenteritis
Central diabetes insipidus
Nephrogenic diabetes insipidus
Use of loop diuretics
Use of osmotic diuretics
Use of radiology contrast medium
Excessive insensible cutaneous loss (burns, sweating)
Diabetic ketoacidosis or hyperosmolar nonketotic diabetes

Salt Gain

Use of high–sodium content solutions (hypertonic saline, IV bicarbonate)
Hypertonic enteral feeding formulas
Cathartic agents

WATER AND ELECTROLYTE DEFICITS IN DIABETIC KETOACIDOSIS

Diabetic ketoacidosis (DKA) is characterized by losses of water and electrolytes due to hyperglycemia-induced osmotic diuresis. The high osmolality of the ECF results in shift of water from the ICF compartment. Studies performed in adult humans with type 1 diabetes where insulin therapy has been withheld have shown fluid deficits of 5 to 10 L together with up to 20% loss of total body sodium and potassium.[67] At the time of presentation, patients are ECF contracted, and clinical estimates of the deficit are usually in the range of 7% to 10%, although shock with hemodynamic compromise is a rare event in DKA in children. The hyperglycemia in DKA results in a hyperosmolar state, but serum Na concentration is an unreliable measure of the degree of ECF contraction, owing to the dilutional effect of fluid shift from the ICF to the ECF compartment. The *effective* osmolality (2 [Na + K] + glucose, all in mmol/L) at the time of presentation is frequently in the range of 300 to 350 mOsm/L. An elevated hematocrit may be a useful marker of severe ECF contraction. Urea is not an effective osmole because it moves freely across the cell membrane and is therefore not included in the calculation. An estimate of true ECF deficit can be made by "correcting" the measured serum Na for the increase in ECF water using the formula developed by Katz[68]:

$$\frac{Na + [Glucose\,(mmol/L) - 5.6]}{5.6} \times 1.6$$

The ECF contraction is associated with a reduction in GFR which results in reduced glucose and ketone clearance from the blood and worsening DKA. Studies in humans have shown that IV fluid administration alone results in substantial falls in blood glucose before insulin has been given; this is due to the increase in GFR.[69] Serum K is also frequently elevated at the time of presentation[70] but falls rapidly as GFR increases and insulin re-primes the Na^+/K^+-ATPase cell membrane pump.[71]

Cerebral edema as a complication of diabetic ketoacidosis (CE-DKA) was first described by Dillon in 1936.[72] Although originally reported in adults,[73-76] it is much more common in children and accounts for the majority of morbidity and mortality associated with DKA in this age group.[77] The reported occurrence rate in the pediatric literature varies between 0.2% and 1%.[78-81] However, this is likely to be an underestimate, as it is based on retrospective reviews relying on the clinical diagnosis of increased intracranial pressure. The incidence is also reported to be higher in new-onset diabetes and in younger children.[78,81,82] Series of brain imaging studies in children with DKA have shown decreased ventricular size either early (<12 hours) in the treatment course[83] or even before therapy has commenced.[84] The ultimate consequence of this, namely brainstem herniation, has been reported to be 5.8% (9/153) in one series of all children presenting with DKA.[85] The total adverse outcome rate (death or permanent neurologic injury) in CE-DKA is as high as 40% to 50% in some series, with few intact survivors where brainstem herniation has occurred.[78,86,87] For these

reasons, children with severe DKA (pH < 7.2) should be admitted to the ICU for close monitoring of CNS status during the first 24 hours of correction of the fluid deficit. Symptoms such as diminished level of consciousness, headache, or vomiting are signs of impending cerebral edema.

Many theories have been advanced to explain brain swelling in association with DKA, including overzealous rehydration with hypotonic IV fluids, rapid reduction of blood glucose with insulin, activation of the sodium/hydrogen ion (Na^+/H^+) transporter system, change in oncotic pressure, increased permeability of the blood-brain barrier, and changes in cerebral blood flow.[78,81,85,86,88] Most of these have been developed from individual case reports or small case series. Although the precise cause is not fully understood, there is general agreement that the pathogenesis of CE-DKA involves an osmolar shift that results in fluid accumulation in the ICF compartment and cell swelling.

Although the cause of cerebral edema in DKA is a subject of much controversy,[89] several case series have focused on fluid rehydration. The standard approach formerly was to give a bolus of between 10 and 30 mL/kg of fluid at the time of presentation, often with a bolus of insulin (0.1 units/kg). IV fluids were then administered depending on the clinical diagnosis of the degree of dehydration. This was done by calculating the fluid deficit and replacing this over 24 to 36 hours using a hypotonic fluid, generally 0.45% NaCl with added potassium. In the late 1980s and early 90s, a number of groups began to question the wisdom of this approach[86,90,91] based on experiences with CE-DKA. They noted that in many cases of CE-DKA, the measured serum Na failed to rise during fluid resuscitation as expected, indicating a failure to protect against a rapid fall in the effective osmolality. As a result, they advocated a more conservative therapeutic approach, limiting the total fluid to under 4 L/m²/d and increasing the tonicity of IV fluids. Using this approach, Harris et al. reported a decrease in the incidence of symptomatic cerebral edema but not its elimination.[90] In a second series by the same authors using the same approach, mannitol was administered for increasing obtundation in only 4/231 episodes, and there were no adverse outcomes in the total series.[91] However, the practice of aggressive fluid resuscitation still persists. Roberts[92] has recently reported a case series of 11 children who developed CE-DKA, most of whom received large amounts of IV fluid (>40 mL/kg in the first 4 hours). All received mannitol and, with one exception, recovered.

The issue of changes in serum osmolality as a risk factor has been identified in several series (Figure 113-2). A rapid reduction in effective osmolality is associated with either a fall in blood glucose or serum Na, or both, due to the rapid administration of IV fluid and possibly by bolus-dose insulin. Insulin administration is also known to activate the Na^+/H^+ ion exchanger, increasing the ICF Na concentration.[88] Water follows the osmotic gradient back into the ICF compartment. Hale,[93] in a retrospective series, found that CE-DKA developed in children when there was a progressive fall in serum Na and osmolality compared to patients without brain swelling, where effective osmolality did not change. In a large series that included age-matched controls, other identified risk factors for development of cerebral edema were a low $Paco_2$ and a high urea at the time of presentation.[81] These are probably reflective of the severity of the acidosis and ECF contraction. The only treatment variable that was associated with CE-DKA in this series was the use of bicarbonate therapy.

Although there is no clear consensus as to the most appropriate fluid resuscitation in DKA to prevent cerebral edema, most would agree that large amounts of hypotonic fluids are not appropriate.[86,91,93-96] The practice of using an IV bolus dose of insulin at the initiation of DKA treatment is now far less common and has largely been replaced by a more conservative rate of continuous infusion. Although the role of insulin in the development of CE-DKA remains speculative, bolus insulin at the start of therapy does not appear to provide a therapeutic benefit, and we believe its use should be avoided on sound theoretical grounds.

In the absence of a single unifying hypothesis as to the cause of cerebral edema in DKA, it is not possible to provide a definitive

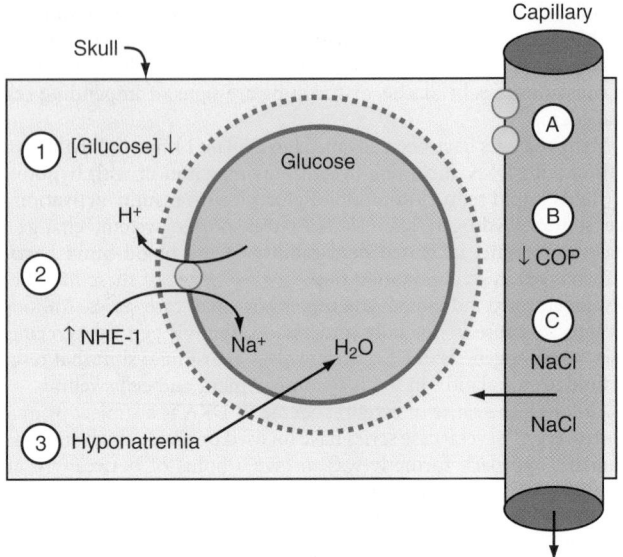

Figure 113-2 Risk factors for cerebral edema in DKA. Rectangle represents skull. Three risk factors for swelling of brain cells include higher concentration of glucose and/or its metabolites in the brain due to rapid lowering of P_{Glu} (site 1), activation of Na^+/H^+ exchanger (NHE) by insulin (site 2), and/or development of hyponatremia (site 3). Expansion of ECF volume could be the result of a less restrictive blood-brain barrier (site A), a fall in colloid osmotic pressure (COP) in plasma (site B), and/or excessive administration of saline (site C). *(From Carlotti AP, Bohn D, Halperin ML. Importance of timing of risk factors for cerebral oedema during therapy for diabetic ketoacidosis. Arch Dis Child 2003;88:170-3, with permission.)*

treatment approach that will predictably prevent CE-DKA. It remains likely that the pathogenesis of CE-DKA is multifactorial in nature and includes both patient and treatment-related factors. The objective of treatment should be gradual reduction in serum osmolality, which can be achieved by conservative fluid resuscitation and avoidance of hypotonic fluids in the initial resuscitation period.[97] A general rule is that failure of the serum Na to rise during IV fluid replacement indicates too rapid a rate of infusion. Our own approach is to use no more than 7.5 to 10 mL/kg over the first hour of treatment of normal saline (0.9% NaCl), with a reduction to 3.5 to 5 mL/kg/h thereafter.[95] In addition, insulin is given as a continuous infusion at the rate of 0.1 unit/kg/h, with the dose adjusted to avoid a drop in blood glucose concentration greater than about 5 mmol/h. It remains to be seen whether this approach will lower the risk of cerebral edema associated with the onset and management of DKA in children. This is consistent with the approach of Harris and others advocated more than 10 years ago.[90] A recent retrospective study from our center demonstrates that the use of isotonic saline, with the associated rise in serum sodium as the glucose falls, protects against the development of cerebral edema.[98]

Children presenting with DKA require close monitoring for alteration in level of consciousness and other signs of increased ICP such as headache and vomiting. This level of care is best provided in an ICU setting. In the event cerebral edema is suspected, serum osmolarity should immediately be raised by the administration of mannitol, 1 gm/kg IV,[92] or 2 to 3 mL/kg of 3% saline[99] and a decrease in the IV fluid and insulin infusion. This should be done without waiting for a computed tomography (CT) scan, which may fail to demonstrate cerebral edema.

FLUID AND ELECTROLYTE DEFICITS IN GASTROENTERITIS

Acute gastroenteritis is the commonest form of disturbance of fluid and electrolyte homeostasis seen in childhood. Infants with diarrhea are particularly vulnerable to significant losses of fluid, sodium, chloride, and bicarbonate from the small intestine and present with what is frequently classified as hypotonic, isotonic, or hypertonic dehydration based on the serum Na level. This terminology is technically incorrect; only in the hypertonic form is there loss of fluid from the ICF compartment, and these patients are truly dehydrated. Patients with diarrheal illnesses associated with fluid loss with normal or reduced serum Na have loss of TBW and ECF with normal or increased ICF volume.[100] Infants with hypernatremic dehydration are the ones at greatest risk of an adverse neurologic event (see earlier), but seizures from severe hyponatremia have been reported in infants presenting with acute gastroenteritis due to oral salt-free fluids being given as replacement.[11,101,102] Assessment of the degree of ECF deficit is usually made on clinical grounds using the time-honored clinical signs of capillary refill time, dry mucous membranes, skin turgor, and so on.[103] However, these are open to subjective interpretation, and there may be a tendency to overestimate the degree of ECF contraction in less severely ill children. In a study by Mackenzie,[104] the fluid deficit in children with gastroenteritis and mild to moderate "dehydration" was overestimated, which resulted in overuse of IV fluids. Skin turgor, increased capillary refill time, high urea, low pH, and increased base deficit all correlated with the degree of ECF contraction but not the presence of thirst or oliguria. Other studies have shown that a reduced bicarbonate is the most common electrolyte abnormality associated with significant ECF contraction in gastroenteritis.[105,106]

Patients with gastroenteritis whose serum is isotonic and hypotonic should be managed with isotonic saline, and those who are hypertonic should receive solutions that contain EFW. An observational study has found that ADH levels are frequently elevated in these patients.[107] A randomized controlled trial of IV fluid rehydration in children with gastroenteritis has shown that the use of isotonic saline protected against the development of hyponatremia without the development of hypernatremia when compared with hypotonic.[22] Infants with severe hypernatremia should have their free-water deficit corrected slowly because of the dangers of rapid fluid shift to the ICF compartment (see earlier). There is an increasing trend to rapidly rehydrate these patients with IV solutions in the emergency department prior to discharging them home,[108,109] but a more simple and effective technique is to use oral rehydration therapy (ORT), which has a proven efficacy in clinical trials of patients with acute gastroenteritis. These solutions contain Na concentrations of between 45 and 90 mmol/L.[109-112]

Chloride

Chloride is the principal anion of the ECF compartment. It is filtered at the glomerulus, and 80% is reabsorbed in conjunction with sodium in the proximal tubule. It is also re-absorbed in the ascending limb of the loop of Henle, a process that is blocked by furosemide. Chloride (Cl^-) is exchanged for bicarbonate (HCO_3^-) in the distal tubule. In ECF volume depletion, excess Cl along with Na is reabsorbed in the proximal tubule, resulting in lower distal delivery and less HCO_3 secretion. With chloride depletion, less Na^+ is reabsorbed in the proximal tubule. Increased distal delivery results increased exchange with K^+ and H^+. This contraction alkalosis is invariably associated with hypochloremia, most commonly due to overuse of loop diuretics. Hypochloremia is also caused by gastric suctioning and respiratory acidosis. In addition, many of the conditions that cause hyponatremia also result in hypochloremia.

Hyperchloremia is seen in association with respiratory alkalosis, hypernatremic dehydration, and administration of isotonic saline. Large amounts of isotonic saline used during fluid resuscitation can result in a hyperchloremic metabolic acidosis.[113] If the serum Cl is not measured, an increased base deficit could be wrongly interpreted as indicating inadequate volume resuscitation in shock.[114]

Plasma chloride measurements are an integral part of the calculation of the anion gap, which is important for the diagnosis of metabolic acidosis.[115] This is the difference between the measured cations

(Na^+) and anions ($Cl^- + HCO_3^-$), which is normally in the range of 12 to 16. The anion gap is increased when unmeasured anions are present, such as lactate and the accumulation of β-hydroxybutyrate in DKA. A normal or reduced anion-gap acidosis is seen in association with hyperchloremia from saline administration or other situations where there is an increase in serum Cl.[113,116,117]

Potassium

Potassium is the major cation of the ICF compartment. The intracellular concentration is 150 mmol/L. Measurement of serum K reflects the ECF concentration, which is only 2% of total body K. The gradient between the ICF and ECF compartments is maintained by activation of the Na^+/K^+-ATPase pump in the cell membrane. The movement of K from the ECF to ICF compartment is enhanced by insulin, hypothermia, alkalosis, catecholamines, and β-agonist therapy.

Potassium filtered at the glomerulus is reabsorbed in the proximal tubule and the thick ascending limb of the loop of Henle. It is secreted in the distal nephron under the influence of aldosterone, plasma K^+ concentration, and urine flow rate.

HYPOKALEMIA

Hypokalemia in children is commonly seen with gastroenteritis and diarrhea where ECF contraction leads to stimulation of aldosterone secretion. There is also total body potassium depletion in DKA, although the initial measured level is high due to the acidosis.[70] Adolescents with anorexia nervosa can present with profound degrees of hypokalemia, and it is a known cause of sudden death in this syndrome.[118] In the critical care setting, hypokalemia is most commonly associated with diuretic use, nasogastric suction, hypomagnesemia, and metabolic alkalosis. In acute metabolic alkalosis, each 0.1-unit rise in pH results in a fall of between 0.2 and 0.4 mmol/L in the serum K.[119] In chronic metabolic alkalosis, K is exchanged for hydrogen ion in the distal nephron. Increased K output in the urine is also associated with renal tubular defects (Bartter's syndrome, renal tubular acidosis) and the use of drugs such as amphotericin, ticarcillin, carbenicillin, and steroids.[120]

Potassium supplementation therapy in the critical care setting is usually in the form of KCl, as there is frequently an associated Cl deficiency. Acetate and phosphate can be used as alternative anions in the hyperchloremic state (e.g., DKA).

The clinical manifestations of hypokalemia include muscle weakness (which may prolong the effect of neuromuscular blockers), intestinal ileus, and cardiac arrhythmias. The latter are rarely a problem except in children with congenital heart disease, particularly in the post cardiopulmonary bypass setting. The potential for digoxin toxicity is enhanced with hypokalemia. In situations where hypokalemia needs to be treated in the setting of fluid restriction, high-concentration K infusions (up to 0.5 mmol/mL) can be infused through central lines, with frequent measurements of serum K levels. Hypokalemia may remain resistant to treatment when significant hypomagnesemia is present.

HYPERKALEMIA

Hyperkalemia is caused by either failure of potassium excretion (renal failure) or in the movement of K from the ICF to the ECF compartment. Common causes of the latter are seen in cellular breakdown or injury in tumor lysis syndrome, rhabdomyolysis, burns, and trauma.

The use of the depolarizing neuromuscular blocker, succinylcholine, in this setting or in patients with muscle dystrophy or spinal cord injury can lead to an abrupt rise in serum K and cardiac arrest. Severe hyperkalemia is also seen in malignant hyperthermia and is due to a combination of hemolysis and acidosis. Both captopril and propranolol can cause hyperkalemia by decreasing the amount of aldosterone synthesis. Propranolol also blocks β-adrenergic-mediated movement of K across the cell membrane. Acute metabolic acidosis also results in rapid movement of K from the ICF to ECF compartment, and severe hyperkalemia is frequently seen during cardiac arrest and CPR, without necessarily implying causality.

Acute hyperkalemia represents a medical emergency; serum levels in excess of 6 mmol/L can result in cardiac arrest and sudden death, particularly in the post cardiopulmonary bypass setting. Frequently the only clinical manifestation is the finding of tall, peaked T waves and widening of the QRS complex on the ECG tracing, but the absence of these findings does not exclude the diagnosis. Patients with borderline high levels of serum K can develop life-threatening hyperkalemia with the development of an acidosis. Because it is the extracellular K level which is harmful, emergency measures should be directed at increasing the transmembrane flux from ECF to the ICF compartment. These include the use of bicarbonate to correct acidemia, β-agonist therapy, and use of glucose/insulin.[119,121] IV calcium chloride will help protect the heart against the development of cardiac rhythm disturbances. These are temporizing measures while steps are taken to increase K removal from the body either by using sodium/potassium exchange resins (rectally or via NG tube) or acute dialysis.

Calcium

The ECF concentration is maintained under the control of vitamin D, parathyroid hormone, and calcitriol. The majority is in the bone, and in the absence of parathyroid hormone, there is reduced calcium reabsorption from bone and increased urinary secretion because of the decreased renal production of calcitriol. Forty percent of calcium is protein bound, and the most common cause of a low total calcium in critically ill children is hypoalbuminemia. In this situation, the ionized level is normal. Conversely, the ionized level is reduced when there is increased protein binding.

Hypocalcemia is seen in neonates with birth asphyxia, preterm infants, term newborns in the first week of life, and infants of diabetic mothers. It is an invariable finding in newborn infants with DiGeorge syndrome, where it is seen in association with conotruncal congenital heart defects, typically truncus arteriosus and interrupted aortic arch. The majority of these infants have microdeletions of the long arm of chromosome 22 (22q minus syndrome) and immunodeficiency. For this reason, all transfused blood products must be irradiated. Hypocalcemia is a common finding in critically ill older children, with a reported incidence of 49% in one study.[122] Causes include cardiopulmonary bypass, use of citrated blood and blood products, albumin transfusions, burns, sepsis, use of loop diuretics, and aminoglycosides. Hyperphosphatemia, seen in tumor lysis syndrome and renal failure, can also result in hypocalcemia.

Hypercalcemia in critically ill children is usually the result of excessive calcium administration, frequently in association with diuretic administration. The end result may be the development of nephrocalcinosis. Other less common causes include neonatal severe primary hyperthyroidism caused by mutations of the *CaSR* gene and Williams syndrome, where it is associated with supravalvular aortic stenosis and peripheral pulmonary artery stenosis.

ANNOTATED REFERENCES

Holliday MA, Segar WE. The maintenance need for water in parenteral fluid therapy. Pediatrics 1957;19:823-32.
   The original publication used as the basis for prescribing IV fluids in children, which has resulted in the use of hypotonic saline for the past 50 years. Assumptions about insensible losses and failure to recognize the problem of nonphysiologic ADH secretion frequently result in administration of excessive electrolyte-free water.

Hoorn EJ, Geary D, Robb M, Halperin ML, Bohn D. Acute hyponatremia related to intravenous fluid administration in hospitalized children: an observational study. Pediatrics 2004;113:1279-84.
   An observational case-control study of the incidence of hyponatremia in children admitted to the emergency department who received IV fluid. Patients who developed hyponatremia had twice the amount of electrolyte-free water administered compared to controls.

Duke T, Molyneux EM. Intravenous fluids for seriously ill children: time to reconsider. Lancet 2003;362:1320-3.

A review article which highlights the dangers of acute hyponatremia together with the groups of children at risk. The author recommends that the standard should become isotonic saline at amounts less than traditionally recommended in the formula for calculating maintenance fluids in children.

Neville KA, Verge CF, Rosenberg AR, O'Meara MW, Walker JL. Isotonic is better than hypotonic saline for intravenous rehydration of children with gastroenteritis: a prospective randomised study. Arch Dis Child 2006;91:226-32.

A randomized controlled trial of the use of hypotonic versus isotonic saline for fluid replacement in gastroenteritis. The use of isotonic saline resulted in a reduced incidence of hyponatremia without the development of hypernatremia.

Eulmesekian PG, Perez A, Minces PG, Bohn D. Hospital-acquired hyponatremia in postoperative pediatric patients: prospective observational study. Pediatr Crit Care Med 2010;11:479- 83.

A prospective observational study of the incidence of hyponatremia associated with the use of hypotonic saline in the postoperative period in children admitted to PICU. Of these children, 31% had a plasma sodium of less than 135 mmol/L at 24 hours postop. This was caused by a positive water and negative sodium balance.

Steele A, Gowrishankar M, Abrahamson S, Mazer CD, Feldman RD, Halperin ML. Postoperative hyponatremia despite near-isotonic saline infusion: a phenomenon of desalination. Ann Intern Med 1997;126:20-5.

A landmark study on causes of postoperative hyponatremia. Blood and urine levels of sodium were measured for 24 hours after elective surgery in patients receiving near-isotonic IV fluid. The serum sodium fell due to a combination of water retention (nonphysiologic ADH secretion) and high losses of sodium in the urine. The authors coined the term "desalination" to explain this.

Montanana PA, Modesto I, Alapont V, Ocon AP, Lopez PO, Lopez Prats JL, et al. The use of isotonic fluid as maintenance therapy prevents iatrogenic hyponatremia in pediatrics: a randomized, controlled open study. Pediatr Crit Care Med 2008;9:589-97.

A prospective randomized trial of isotonic versus hypotonic saline in a postsurgical pediatric population. The use of hypotonic saline was associated with an increased risk of the development of hyponatremia. Isotonic saline did not cause hypernatremia.

Neville KA, Sandeman DJ, Rubinstein A, Henry GM, McGlynn M, Walker JL. Prevention of hyponatremia during maintenance intravenous fluid administration: a prospective randomized study of fluid type versus fluid rate. J Pediatr 2010;156:313-9 e1-2.

A prospective randomized controlled trial comparing the sodium content versus administration rate of IV fluid in a postoperative patient population. This study was designed to address the question of whether the risk of hyponatremia could be reduced by using hypotonic fluids in lower amounts rather than isotonic fluids at recommended "maintenance" levels. Patients received IV hypotonic and isotonic fluids at either 100% maintenance amounts, based on the traditionally used formula, or 50% maintenance. The incidence of hyponatremia was decreased by the use of isotonic saline but not by the combination of hypotonic saline and fluid restriction.

Wolfsdorf J, Craig ME, Daneman D, Dunger D, Edge J, Lee W, et al. Diabetic ketoacidosis in children and adolescents with diabetes. Pediatr Diabetes 2009;10:118-33.

Consensus guidelines for the management of DKA in children, using up-to-date evidence. Recommends cautious IV rehydration to prevent the development of cerebral edema.

REFERENCES

Access the complete reference list online at http://www.expertconsult.com.

114

Acute Kidney Injury

ELWALEED A. ELHASSAN | ROBERT W. SCHRIER

Acute kidney injury (AKI) is characterized by an abrupt decrease in the glomerular filtration rate (GFR) that results in accumulation of nitrogenous waste products and an inability to maintain fluid and electrolyte homeostasis.[1] AKI can result from decreased renal perfusion not severe enough to cause cellular injury; an ischemic, toxic, or obstructive injury of the renal tubule; a tubulointerstitial process with inflammation and edema; or a primary reduction in the filtering capacity of the glomerulus. If renal tubular and glomerular function is intact, but solute clearance is limited by factors compromising renal perfusion, the injury is termed *prerenal azotemia*. If renal dysfunction is related to obstruction of the urinary outflow tract, it is termed *postrenal azotemia*. AKI due to a primary intrarenal cause is called *intrinsic renal injury* or *renal azotemia*. Prerenal azotemic and intrinsic renal injury due to ischemia and nephrotoxins are responsible for most episodes of AKI.[2,3]

Renal blood flow is approximately 1200 mL/min and constitutes 20% of cardiac output. Given this apparently generous perfusion, it may seem surprising that the kidneys are so susceptible to hemodynamic insults. The majority of this perfusion (80%-90%), however, is to the renal cortex, where glomerular filtration occurs. The medulla is designed to concentrate and dilute urine. During urine concentration, the high osmotic gradient required for reabsorption of water is associated with a low rate of blood flow. In fact, oxygen tension in the outer medulla in the region of the metabolically active thick ascending limb of Henle is only around 10 mm Hg.[4] This combination of low blood flow and oxygen tension in a metabolically active environment makes the kidneys very susceptible to ischemic injury.

Prerenal Causes

Prerenal azotemia is a consequence of reduction in renal perfusion without cellular injury. As such, this is a reversible process if the underlying cause is corrected. It may be secondary to decreased blood volume, as occurs with vomiting, dehydration, and hemorrhage, or it may be due to a reduction in the effective arterial blood volume, as in congestive heart failure and cirrhosis. Further, the administration of medications that interfere with the normal autoregulatory ability of the kidney can contribute to prerenal azotemia. In settings of diminished renal perfusion, administration of nonsteroidal antiinflammatory drugs (NSAIDs) or angiotensin-converting enzyme (ACE) inhibitors can precipitate overt prerenal azotemia.[3]

During prerenal azotemia, the renin-angiotensin-aldosterone system becomes activated secondary to a decrease in renal blood flow accompanied by increased activity of the adrenergic nervous system. Increased levels of angiotensin II and adrenergic activation serve to increase the proximal reabsorption of sodium, whereas aldosterone increases sodium reabsorption in the distal tubule. Together these actions decrease urine sodium concentration to less than 20 mmol/L and fractional excretion of sodium (FE_{Na}) to less than 1%.[5]

Prerenal azotemia accounts for approximately 70% of community-acquired cases of AKI[6] and 40% of hospital-acquired cases.[7] Therefore, prerenal causes should be excluded in all cases of AKI. Therapy of prerenal AKI involves reversing the underlying cause, such as volume replacement or discontinuation of offending agents.

Postrenal Causes

Postrenal AKI occurs when there is bilateral (or unilateral in the case of a single kidney) obstruction of urine flow. Intratubular pressure increases and in turn decreases net glomerular filtration pressure. Obstruction of urine flow is a relatively uncommon cause of AKI and is more common in the community than in the intensive care unit (ICU). Several series have placed the incidence of postrenal AKI at 3% to 25% of all cases of AKI.[8,9,10] Postrenal AKI can be divided into renal and extrarenal causes. Extrarenal causes include prostatic disease, pelvic malignancy, and retroperitoneal disorders. Intrarenal causes include crystal deposition, as occurs in ethylene glycol ingestion, or uric acid nephropathy in tumor lysis syndrome. Cast formation and tubular obstruction also occur in light-chain diseases such as multiple myeloma.

Postrenal causes of AKI should be evaluated with renal ultrasonography and measurement of postvoid residual urine in the bladder (>50 mL is abnormal). It is important to rule out these causes rapidly, because the potential for renal recovery is inversely related to the duration of obstruction.[11]

Intrarenal Causes

Intrarenal causes of AKI can be classified according to the anatomic location of the injury: glomerulus, tubule, vasculature, or interstitium. Suspicion of glomerulonephritis or vasculitis should be raised in a patient with renal failure who has an active urine sediment with red cells and red cell casts. In contrast, acute interstitial nephritis classically presents with pyuria and white cell casts in the urine; on occasion, hematuria is also present. Most cases of AKI from interstitial nephritis are drug related, commonly due to antibiotics or NSAIDs. Recovery usually occurs with removal of the offending agent and may be hastened by a short course of steroids, such as 60 to 80 mg of prednisone for 10 days. Tubular injury is most often either ischemic or toxic in nature and presents as acute tubular necrosis (ATN). This is the most common form of AKI encountered in the hospital and ICU[10,12,13] and is the focus of this chapter.

In ischemic AKI, there is both tubular and vascular injury. In the tubules, an increase in intracellular calcium after ischemic injury activates the cysteine proteases calpain and caspase. This leads to necrosis and apoptosis as well as relocation of Na^+/K^+-ATPase from the basolateral membrane to the cytosol. This relocation interferes with normal vectorial transport of sodium and increases distal delivery of sodium chloride (NaCl). An increase in delivery of NaCl to the macula densa in the distal tubule activates tubuloglomerular feedback and further decreases GFR. Further, ischemia increases production of nitric oxide, which also causes cellular damage and detachment of epithelial cells from the basement membrane. Much of the deleterious action of nitric oxide is mediated through the generation of peroxynitrite from the combination of reactive oxygen species and nitric oxide. Cellular detachment is responsible for cast formation and tubular obstruction. These mechanisms all independently contribute to the decrease in renal function seen in ATN.[14]

TABLE 114-1	Laboratory and Microscopic Findings in Prerenal Azotemia and Acute Tubular Necrosis	
Laboratory Test	*Prerenal Azotemia*	*Acute Tubular Necrosis*
Urine osmolality (mOsm/kg H₂O)	>500	<400
Urine sodium (mEq/L)	<20	>40
Urine plasma/creatinine ratio	>40	<20
Fractional excretion of sodium (%)	<1	>2
Urinary sediment	Normal, occasional hyaline cast	Renal tubular epithelial cells, granular and muddy brown casts

Data from Esson ML, Schrier RW. Diagnosis and treatment of acute tubular necrosis. Ann Intern Med 2002;137:744-52.

In ischemic injury, the vascular endothelium is damaged and displays an exaggerated response to vasoconstrictor stimuli such as angiotensin II and endothelin-1 and a decreased response to vasodilators such as acetylcholine and bradykinin. In addition, there is a loss of autoregulatory capability. This loss of autoregulation in the setting of otherwise minor hemodynamic changes is likely responsible for the fresh ischemic lesions often seen on biopsy when recovery from AKI is delayed.[15]

The kidney's susceptibility to toxic injury can be attributed to its functional properties. The kidneys receive 20% to 25% of the cardiac output, and there is extensive reabsorptive capacity as well as concentrating ability. All these factors contribute to the delivery of large amounts of toxin to the tubular epithelial cells. In addition, there is extensive biotransformation, generating toxic metabolites, and the high energy consumption with marginal oxygen delivery renders the tubules susceptible to toxic injury.[16]

An increasingly common form of AKI in the hospital is secondary to the use of contrast media. Nash and colleagues found contrast nephropathy to be the third most common form of AKI in the hospital.[7] The pathogenesis involves both hemodynamic and toxic effects. Contrast media cause renal vasoconstriction and medullary ischemia as well as direct tubular toxicity.[17] Patients with preexisting renal disease and diabetes are at high risk, as are patients who are volume depleted.

Differentiation of ATN from prerenal azotemia can be aided by evaluating urinary indices (Table 114-1).[18] In established ATN, tubular function is impaired, and tubular sodium reabsorption is hindered. This results in a urine sodium value greater than 40 mmol/L and an FE$_{Na}$ greater than 2%. Urine concentrating ability is also abnormal, resulting in isosthenuria with urine osmolality less than 350 mOsm/

kg H₂O.[19] However, a low FE$_{Na}$ may be seen in entities causing ATN, such as rhabdomyolysis and myoglobinuria,[20] as well as in contrast-mediated AKI[21] and sepsis.[22] In patients with prerenal azotemia who are treated with diuretics that may obscure the FE$_{Na}$, fractional excretion of urea (FE$_{Urea}$) or urine-to-plasma ratio of creatinine may be more discriminatory. An FE$_{Urea}$ less than 35% or a urine-to-plasma ratio of creatinine higher than 15 is indicative of prerenal azotemia.[23] However, a subsequent study indicates that in patients with AKI administered diuretics, the distinction between transient and persistent AKI cannot be made accurately by means of FE$_{Urea}$ because it lacks specificity.[24]

Epidemiology

When the RIFLE criteria (*r*isk, *i*njury, *f*ailure, *l*oss, *e*nd-stage renal failure) are employed, AKI is a common complication occurring in up to a third of ICU patients and is usually a manifestation of multiorgan failure syndrome.[25-27]

The most common cause of intrinsic renal failure is ATN.[3] Specific causes of ATN can be classified as hemodynamically mediated AKI, such as in prolonged prerenal azotemia, hypotension, and sepsis; toxic AKI, secondary to antibiotics, chemotherapeutic agents, and contrast media; or postsurgical AKI. In a large prospective analysis by Liano and coworkers, sepsis was the most common cause (35%); postsurgical (25%) and toxic (31%) causes were also common.[10] Many, if not most, patients have a multifactorial cause of AKI (Figure 114-1). Despite ever-improving supportive interventions in the ICU, the mortality rate for AKI has not changed in the last 3 decades, remaining at 40% to 80% depending on the study.[28] It has been hypothesized that this continued poor prognosis is due to the changing patient population cared for in the ICU. Today, patients are older with greater comorbidities, and their renal disease most often develops in the setting of multiorgan failure.[10,29] This high incidence of multiorgan failure has made it difficult to discern whether AKI itself causes increased mortality or whether it is a marker of severely ill patients. Several recent studies have found that AKI does in fact contribute to excess mortality in the setting of contrast nephropathy and cardiac surgery.[30,31] In those patients who do survive, there is significant morbidity, with about 33% requiring long-term renal replacement therapy (RRT) and 28% requiring long-term institutionalization.[32] As explained later, increasing RIFLE severity grades correspond with increasing mortality in patients. Hoste et al. reported that patients with a maximum score of RISK had a mortality rate of 8.8%, compared to 11.4% for INJURY and 26.3% for FAILURE. On the other hand, patients who had no evidence of AKI had a mortality rate of 5.5%.[33]

PATHOPHYSIOLOGY OF ISCHEMIC ACUTE KIDNEY INJURY

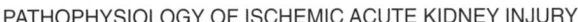
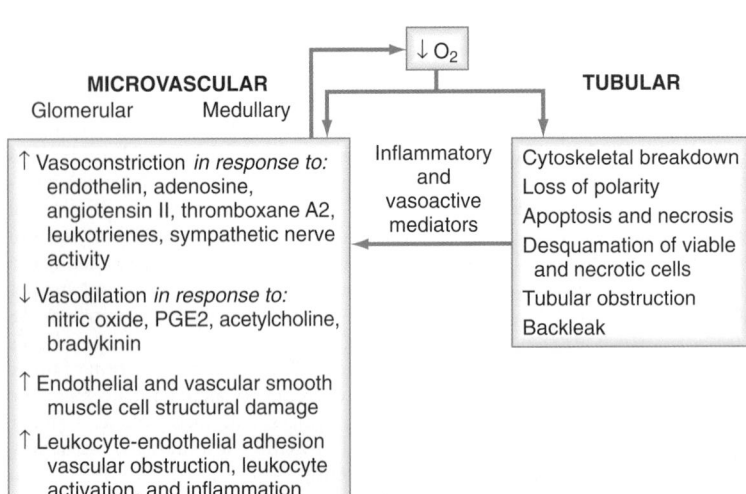

Figure 114-1 Pathophysiology of ischemic acute kidney injury (AKI). Interacting microvascular and tubular events contribute to the physiology of ischemic acute renal failure. PGE2, prostaglandin E2. (*Adapted from Bonventre JV, Weinberg JM. Recent advances in the pathophysiology of ischemic acute renal failure. J Am Soc Nephrol 2003;14:2199-210.*)

<table>
<tr><td>TABLE
114-2</td><td>Risk Factors for Developing Acute Kidney Injury</td></tr>
</table>

Age >65 years
Infection on admission
Cardiovascular failure
Cirrhosis
Respiratory failure
Chronic heart failure
Lymphoma or leukemia

Adapted from de Mendonca A et al. Acute renal failure in the ICU: risk factors and outcome evaluated by the SOFA score. Intensive Care Med 2000;26:915-21.

The risk of developing AKI in the ICU was evaluated by de Mendonca and associates, who found that seven characteristics, if present on admission, were associated with a high risk of developing AKI (Table 114-2).[29] Several other studies addressed risk factors for mortality in the setting of AKI.[7,10,12,34] As indicated in Table 114-3, the risk of death in those with AKI is increased by the presence of nonrenal organ failure; more severe renal dysfunction, as indicated by oliguria; sepsis; advanced age; and male gender. Liano and colleagues found that as the number of organ failures increased, mortality increased.[10] With two organ failures, mortality was 53%; this increased to 80% with three organ failures and 100% with five organ failures.

To further stratify the probability of death in critically ill patients, several severity-of-illness scoring systems have been developed. These indices help compare patients enrolled in clinical trials and better utilize finite resources to help those patients with the best chance of recovery. In large populations, these scoring indices have been successful in predicting outcome[35]; however, they do not discriminate well in patients with AKI.[36] The renal parameters used in these scores consist of blood urea nitrogen (BUN), serum creatinine, and total urine output per day. With the latest version of the Acute Physiology and Chronic Health Evaluation (APACHE III), oliguric AKI constitutes just 12.7% of the maximal score, thereby underestimating the effect of AKI on mortality.[37] Further, there is no correction for patients with AKI and a low serum creatinine, who also have a poor outcome, probably reflective of poor nutritional status.[37] An attempt has therefore been made to develop more disease-specific indices, such as Liano and colleagues' individual severity index, the Cleveland Clinic Foundation severity score, and the Project to Improve Care in Acute Renal Disease index. The majority of these indices were developed at single centers, and few have been validated outside the original institution. Also, the patient populations to which the indices were applied have differed, such as using all AKI patients or only dialyzed patients. Thus, there is no completely generalizable, validated bedside predictor for mortality in AKI patients.

▓ Definition

Acute renal failure (ARF) has traditionally been defined as an abrupt decrease in GFR with resultant retention of urea and other nitrogenous waste products along with dysregulation of body fluids and electrolytes. However, this is only a qualitative definition and not very helpful clinically, where a quantitative definition is required. Until recently, no agreement existed about how to best define, characterize, and study acute renal failure. This lack of a standard definition has been a major

<table>
<tr><td>TABLE
114-3</td><td>Risk Factors for Mortality in Acute Kidney Injury</td></tr>
</table>

Higher severity index score
Age > 65 years
Male gender
Oliguric acute renal failure
Sepsis
Nonrenal organ failure: (cardiovascular, hepatic or respiratory failure)
Thrombocytopenia
Mechanical ventilation
Prior compromised health status

hindrance to the progress of clinical and basic research in this field. The term *acute kidney injury* was proposed by the Acute Kidney Injury Network (AKIN) as an alternative to ARF in order to encompass the entire range of failure based on recent data showing that a small change in serum creatinine influences outcome. The Acute Dialysis Quality Initiative (ADQI) was created to develop consensus and evidence-based guidelines for treatment and prevention of acute renal failure, with the goal of comparing studies and advancing research.[38] The ADQI group proposed a consensus categorized definition—the RIFLE criteria[39]—which were validated and shown to correlate with hospital mortality and patient outcomes in several populations in large international databases. Subsequently, AKIN proposed a revision of the RIFLE criteria[40,41,42] to better account for small changes in serum creatinine not captured by RIFLE. The following modifications were made (Table 114-4):

1. The RIFLE severity grading system was reconfigured, with the *R* category becoming stage 1, *I* becoming stage 2, and *F* becoming stage 3, which also includes anyone who receives acute RRT, irrespective of their preceding serum creatinine increase or urine output.

2. The diagnosis of AKI could be made with a period of oliguria of at least 6 hours or a serum creatinine increase of ≥0.3 mg/dL from baseline. AKIN criteria caution that adequate volume resuscitation should be ascertained and urinary tract obstruction ruled out prior to using urine output to identify AKI. However, it should be noted that the change in urine flow is less helpful as a diagnostic criterion because of the high incidence of nonoliguric AKI.[43] Inclusion of the aforementioned absolute serum creatinine increase in the AKI definition was based on the repeated finding from several large studies that such serum creatinine increments are associated with increased mortality.[44,45]

3. Diagnostic increments of serum creatinine should occur during a period of no more than 48 hours, compared to 7 days for the RIFLE criteria.

Existing evidence supports the validity of both RIFLE and AKIN criteria to identify groups of hospitalized patients with increased risk of death and/or need for RRT.[39,40,46] Staging of AKI is relevant because with increased stage of AKI, the risk of death increases. Moreover, there is now mounting evidence of long-term risk of subsequent development of cardiovascular disease or chronic kidney disease and mortality even after resolution of AKI.[47] Lo et al. recently studied the long-term sequelae of AKI in a retrospective analysis of the large Kaiser Permanente database using the years 1996-2003.[48] This paper explored AKI and its correlation with long-term kidney disease and mortality in comparison with enrollees of the same healthcare organization who

<table>
<tr><td colspan="6">TABLE 114-4   Contrast Between Acute Kidney Injury Staging By *Rifle* and *Akin* Systems*</td></tr>
<tr><th>RIFLE Stages[†]</th><th>RIFLE Serum Creatinine Increase[‡]</th><th>RIFLE and AKIN Urine Output Criteria</th><th>AKIN Serum Creatinine Increase</th><th>AKIN Stages</th></tr>
<tr><td>Risk</td><td>≥150% to 200%</td><td><0.5 mL/kg/h for >6 h</td><td>≥0.3 mg/dL or ≥150% to 200%</td><td>1</td></tr>
<tr><td>Injury</td><td>>200% to 300%</td><td><0.5 mL/kg/h for >12 h</td><td>>200% to 300%</td><td>2</td></tr>
<tr><td>Failure</td><td>>300%, or serum creatinine >4 mg/dL, or GFR decrease by 75%</td><td><0.3 mL/kg/h for >24 h, or anuria ≥12 h</td><td>>300% or acute RRT</td><td>3</td></tr>
</table>

*Adapted from Bellomo R, Ronco C, Kellum JA, Mehta RL, Palevsky P. Acute renal failure—definition, outcome measures, animal models, fluid therapy and information technology needs: the Second International Consensus Conference of the Acute Dialysis Quality Initiative (ADQI) Group. Crit Care 2004;8:R204-12; and from Mehta RL, Kellum JA, Shah SV, Molitoris BA, Ronco C, Warnock DG, Levin A. Acute Kidney Injury Network: report of an initiative to improve outcomes in acute kidney injury. Crit Care 2007;1;11:R31.
†The remaining RIFLE stages are loss (persistent acute renal failure = complete loss of kidney function of >4 weeks) and end-stage renal disease (>3 months).
‡Serum creatinine increase from baseline.
GFR, glomerular filtration rate; *RRT,* renal replacement therapy.

did not develop AKI and served as controls. Compared with controls, patients who suffered dialysis-dependent AKI during their hospitalization had a 28-fold increased risk of developing stage 4 or 5 CKD. There was also a more than twofold long-term risk of death in this group.

Given the difficulties of measuring function as an index of injury, there has been a search for identifying kidney injury markers of critically ill patients. This approach would be optimal because it could identify patients early in the course of AKI who would benefit from intervention. Several biomarkers have been proposed and are currently being investigated.[49-51] These biomarkers include:

1. Serum cystatin C[52,53]
2. Urinary interleukin (IL)-18[54] and tubular enzymes such as the intestinal form of alkaline phosphatase, N-acetyl-α-glucosaminidase, and alanine aminopeptidase.[55]
3. Neutrophil gelatinase–associated lipocalin (NGAL)[56]
4. Kidney injury molecule 1 (KIM-1)[57]

Further studies are required to establish any of these or other potential biomarkers as practical diagnostic tools in the early clinical diagnosis of AKI. Such tools should facilitate timely and aggressive therapeutic interventions. Currently, urine sediment (i.e., epithelial cells) and urine indices (i.e., FE_{Na}) are early and sensitive harbingers of ATN.

▓ Treatment

In light of its dismal outcome, it is imperative that therapies to prevent or ameliorate AKI be developed. To that end, several trials for both prevention and treatment of AKI have been conducted with multiple agents.

With the increasing use of contrast agents in diagnostic and therapeutic procedures, prevention of contrast-mediated nephropathy has been studied extensively. Intravenous fluids have long been used to prevent contrast nephropathy, but in patients with chronic renal insufficiency, the incidence is still high. Therefore, multiple other agents have been studied. Solomon and coworkers found that both furosemide and mannitol when given with saline produced a worse outcome than saline alone in patients with chronic renal insufficiency.[58] Dopamine[59] and atrial natriuretic peptide[60] have also failed to reduce contrast nephropathy. Two agents, acetylcysteine[61] and fenoldopam,[62] were found to decrease the incidence of contrast nephropathy in high-risk patients, but these findings were not verified in a study by Allaqaband and associates.[63] In that trial, acetylcysteine and fenoldopam offered no additional benefit in patients with chronic renal insufficiency undergoing cardiovascular procedures. Landoni et al. recently performed a meta-analysis of 16 randomized trials of fenoldopam versus placebo or dopamine in 1290 patients who were in a variety of ICU or perioperative settings. They found that fenoldopam reduced the need for renal replacement and mortality in patients with AKI. However, because of the small size and heterogeneity of the studies included, a large multicenter appropriately powered trial will be needed to better define the role of fenoldopam in AKI.[64] Currently, our recommendation for preventing contrast nephropathy in high-risk patients (Table 114-5) is adequate hydration, preferably with isotonic sodium bicarbonate,[65,66,67] administration of 1200 mg acetylcysteine orally twice daily the day before and day of the procedure (given its tolerability and relative low cost), and the use of low-osmolar[68] or iso-osmolar[69] contrast media.

Dopamine has long been used to treat AKI. The renal effects of dopamine include an increase in GFR and an increase in sodium and water excretion. Clinically, the first response is an increase in diuresis.[70] These responses occur in patients with normal renal function, but it is unknown whether they are also seen in those with AKI. In patients with early renal dysfunction (serum creatinine > 1.8 mg/dL or urine output < 0.5 mL/kg/h), dopamine did not alter peak serum creatinine or the need for RRT.[71] This was confirmed in a meta-analysis to determine whether progression of AKI, need for RRT, or mortality were affected by dopamine.[72]

Aside from its lack of efficacy in AKI, dopamine has deleterious side effects. It hastened the onset of gut ischemia in an experimental model,[73] and clinically it worsened contrast nephropathy.[74] In cardiac surgery patients, dopamine was independently associated with an increased risk of postoperative atrial fibrillation.[75] Higher doses may increase mortality,[76] perhaps by worsening myocardial ischemia.[77] Therefore, low-dose dopamine currently has no role in the treatment or prevention of AKI.

Diuretics are also frequently used in patients with AKI, especially in an attempt to convert oliguric into nonoliguric AKI, given the improved prognosis of the latter.[78-80] Loop diuretics, most commonly furosemide, inhibit Na^+/K^+-ATPase in the thick ascending loop of Henle and therefore decrease the active reabsorption of sodium. Theoretically, this has some potential benefits, such as decreasing energy expenditure and increasing flow rate to flush out tubular casts. In the experimental setting, loop diuretics can be protective if administered before the insult. However, even when patients are successfully converted to nonoliguria, there is no reduction in the need for RRT or mortality.[81,82] Cantarovich and colleagues studied the role of high-dose loop diuretics in a placebo-controlled clinical trial of 388 dialysis-requiring AKI patients. Despite the increase in urine output, there were no differences between the two groups in terms of patient survival, renal recovery rates, number of dialysis sessions required, or time on dialysis. In addition, cardiac surgery patients and patients with contrast nephropathy who were treated with furosemide had a worse outcome.[83,84] A study by Mehta and coworkers found an increased mortality in AKI patients treated with diuretics.[85] It is unclear why this occurred, but the authors speculated about a possible nephrotoxic effect of diuretics or a delay in the initiation of RRT because of increased urine output. However, the increased mortality occurred in patients who were not diuretic responsive, likely because of more severe AKI. These patients already had a worse prognosis, and whether diuretics may have worsened the outcome is unknown. Ho et al. recently conducted a comprehensive systematic review of the use of furosemide in AKI.[86] They have shown that furosemide is not associated with any significant clinical benefits in the prevention or treatment of ARF in adults. High doses may be associated with an increased risk of ototoxicity. Although the use of loop diuretics in early or established AKI facilitates management of fluid balance, hyperkalemia, and hypercalcemia, and is indicated for these clinical purposes, any putative role in prevention or amelioration of AKI course is unproven. Therefore, if diuretics are temporarily employed for such indications, care must be taken to avoid delaying initiation of dialysis if clinically necessary.

Atrial natriuretic peptide is a hormone secreted by the cardiac atria that increases GFR and glomerular filtration pressure by dilating the afferent arteriole and constricting the efferent arteriole.[87] It also decreases tubular reabsorption of sodium and chloride,[88] redistributes medullary blood flow,[89] disrupts tubuloglomerular feedback,[90] and reverses endothelin-induced vasoconstriction.[91] Mentzer and colleagues studied the perioperative effects of nesiritide (BNP type) in 303 patients with left ventricular dysfunction who were undergoing coronary artery bypass graft.[92] They demonstrated short-term benefits of nesiritide on perioperative renal function as assessed by an attenuated increase in levels of serum creatinine, a reduction in calculated GFR loss, and a greater urine output 24 hours after surgery. This trial and other reports that have studied administration of natriuretic peptides during cardiac surgery were recently reviewed by Murray, who emphasized that in addition to such surrogate renal endpoints, future studies must demonstrate beneficial effects on overall survival and/or dialysis-free survival.[93] Pending further studies, atrial

TABLE 114-5	Risk Factors for Contrast Nephropathy

Preexisting renal impairment
Diabetes mellitus
Decrease in effective arterial volume (congestive heart failure, volume depletion, cirrhosis)
High dose of contrast media
Concurrent use of nephrotoxic agents (nonsteroidal antiinflammatory drugs, angiotensin-converting enzyme inhibitors)

natriuretic peptide cannot be recommended for prevention or therapy of ATN.

Hemodynamic Management

Intravascular volume is critical in maintaining hemodynamic stability, tissue oxygenation, and organ function.[94] In critically ill patients, it is increasingly being recognized that accurate assessment of volume status and appropriate use of fluid replacement may lead to better outcomes. In a study by Rivers and associates, it was shown that early goal-directed therapy (EGDT) based on optimizing the mixed control venous oxygen saturation in the first 6 hours resulted in decreased mortality in septic patients.[95] Subsequent studies have replicated those results,[96,97] and one of them showed a significantly improved prevention of AKI in patients randomized to EGDT compared to the standard care group.[98] However, supranormal levels of cardiac index or mixed venous oxygen saturation did not decrease mortality.[99] In addition, studies have shown increased mortality in patients with positive fluid balance and acute respiratory distress syndrome (ARDS).[100-102]

We have coined the term *pseudo-* or *pre-ARDS* to focus on a common and clinically important situation in ICUs. Just as prolonged prerenal azotemia may eventually lead to ischemic ATN, prolonged pseudo- or pre-ARDS may lead to ARDS in association with evidence of pulmonary capillary damage and stiff lungs, as diagnosed clinically by a decrease in pulmonary compliance. Thus, pseudo- or pre-ARDS describes a clinical syndrome of noncardiogenic pulmonary edema in the absence of evidence of decreased pulmonary compliance. Although many clinicians group these clinical entities together as ARDS—independent of pulmonary compliance—we believe that from a pathophysiologic, prognostic, and therapeutic viewpoint, these clinical entities may be substantially different.

Both pseudo-ARDS and ARDS are frequently associated with sepsis. Sepsis is a vasodilated state in which systemic vascular resistance decreases and cardiac output increases. Studies in renal experimental animals have shown that vasodilatation with an arterial vasodilator such as minoxidil is associated with an increased albumin distribution space and a failure of interstitial hydrostatic pressure to rise during saline administration.[103] These changes in interstitial Starling forces favor an increase in interstitial fluid volume during saline infusion. We frequently consult on ventilated ICU patients with AKI who have a 20-L positive fluid balance that has not been recognized in a quantitative sense because the pulmonary capillary wedge pressures are not considered elevated (<18 mm Hg). Excess saline fluid has been administered to resuscitate these vasodilated septic patients, leading to pulmonary edema, hypoxia, and ventilatory support. In the early stages, the majority of these patients do not have decreased pulmonary compliance (i.e., stiff lungs). However, these septic ICU patients with renal failure on prolonged respiratory support ultimately have a mortality as high as 80%. Patient mortality has been reported to begin increasing after 48 hours on a respirator. The potential barotrauma, oxygen toxicity, and pulmonary infections that may occur with prolonged ventilatory support frequently lead to stiff lungs and what virtually all authorities would term *bona fide ARDS*.

We believe that not distinguishing clinically between pseudo-ARDS and ARDS may be detrimental to ICU patients. Marked improvement in the pulmonary edema of pseudo-ARDS by diuresis or ultrafiltration may allow much earlier extubation and removal of ventilatory support before the development of pulmonary capillary damage and stiff lungs (i.e., ARDS). With ARDS and prolonged ventilatory support, a very high mortality occurs, particularly in the presence of renal failure and thus multiorgan failure. Recently, Bouchard and colleagues have reported results of a prospective multicenter observational study of 618 patients that aimed to determine whether fluid overload (>10% increase in body weight) in critically ill patients with AKI is associated with increased mortality. After adjustment for severity of illness, the study has shown that fluid overload was independently associated with mortality in those AKI patients who did and did not receive dialysis therapy.[104] A randomized study by the ARDS clinical trials network

demonstrated that pulmonary function in critically ill patients was worse in those treated with a liberal fluid management strategy (to achieve a mean central venous pressure [CVP] of ~12 mm Hg) than in those who were treated with a conservative strategy (to achieve a mean CVP ~8 mm Hg).[105] Moreover, fewer patients in the conservative strategy group required dialysis than in the liberal strategy group. Several pediatric studies comprising more than 400 children have demonstrated an association between worsening fluid overload (higher than 10% to 20%) and mortality.[106-108] Thus, there are reasons to believe that fluid overload is not just a marker but rather a pathologic factor in the high mortality of critically ill patients with AKI. Prospective randomized clinical trials will be needed to confirm this possibility. Until such studies are available, however, we recommend the avoidance of fluid overload in patients with AKI on the basis of knowledge of body weight changes and cumulative fluid balance for these patients.[109]

To aid in appropriate hemodynamic support, invasive monitoring has been used to guide therapy. Techniques such as the pulmonary artery catheter rely on measurement of filling pressures (e.g., CVP, pulmonary artery occlusion pressure) to estimate preload responsiveness. In critically ill patients, the relation between filling pressures and ventricular end-diastolic volume (preload) is often obscured by changes in ventricular compliance or changes in the pericardium or thorax.[110] In addition, the pulmonary artery catheter has been linked to a worse outcome in patients.[111,112] A positive response to fluid challenge can be predicted in mechanically ventilated patients by analyzing respiratory variations in pulse pressure. It has been shown that a change in pulse pressure greater than 15% during a single breath is more accurate in predicting an increase in cardiac output in response to volume loading than either right atrial pressure or wedge pressure.[113,114]

Fluid management in critical illness is aimed at improving organ perfusion. However, in inflammatory states such as sepsis, there may be major fluid shifts resulting in tissue edema despite intravascular depletion. Aside from the inflammatory cascade, vasodilatation itself can result in an increase in interstitial fluid volume, likely secondary to albumin escape from the vasculature.[115] There are currently no clinical methods to detect the presence of capillary leak, apart from fluid administration having no effect on intravascular volume.[110] Therefore, if only transient improvements in hemodynamics occur with fluid administration, or if there is a continuing need for fluid, it is likely the patient will best be served by a change to vasopressor agents.

When volume replacement is indicated, there is controversy over the optimal type of fluid. Crystalloids are the most common form of volume replacement, but their effect on plasma volume is limited. Each liter of fluid administered increases plasma volume 200 mL, but the intravascular half-life is only 20 to 30 minutes.[94]

Colloidal substances such as albumin, dextran, and hydroxyethyl starches, because they are macromolecules, are better retained within the intravascular space and have a greater effect on plasma volume. Albumin has been used for decades, but it is expensive and may cause an increase in mortality, according to the Cochrane Injuries Group.[116] Nevertheless, a randomized controlled trial was conducted to compare human albumin with crystalloid in ICU patients (Saline versus Albumin Fluid Evaluation [SAFE] study). It indicated that albumin is safe, albeit no more effective than saline for fluid resuscitation. SAFE demonstrated no difference in renal outcomes, at least based on duration of RRT.[117] Dextran cannot be recommended for plasma volume expansion because of serious side effects such as coagulation abnormalities[118] and AKI.[119]

Hydroxyethyl starches (HESs) are polymers of amylopectin that vary in molecular weight and number of substitutions of hydroxyethyl groups. As molecular weight and number of substitutions increase, side effects also increase. HES 200/0.5 is a compound with a middle molecular weight and low substitution number. It has been studied in a number of situations such as perioperative volume replacement, cardiac surgery, trauma, and sepsis.[120-122] A recent trial compared a "modern" HES preparation with a low-molecular-weight and low-molar substitution and a human albumin solution, given in cardiac surgery patients with preoperative compromised kidney function, showed that this type of HES solution had no negative influence on kidney integrity.[123] In another study (Efficacy of Volume Substitution and Insulin Therapy in Severe Sepsis [VISEP]), severely septic patients were randomly assigned to receive either 10% pentastarch, a low-molecular-weight hydroxyethyl starch (HES 200/0.5), or modified Ringer's lactate for fluid resuscitation. HES appeared to be harmful, leading to higher rate and longer duration of AKI, and its toxicity increased with accumulating doses.[124] Aside from coagulation disorders, all hyperoncotic colloids may induce a pathologic entity known as *osmotic nephrosis* with potential impairment of kidney function.[125] A systematic review of randomized controlled trials (RCTs) on the use of HES for fluid management in patients with sepsis (totaling 1062 patients) showed an almost twofold increased risk of AKI with HES compared with crystalloids.[126] Lastly, a recent comprehensive Cochrane review concluded there is no evidence from RCTs that resuscitation with colloids instead of crystalloids reduces the risk of death in patients with trauma, burns, or following surgery.[127] There is even evidence that colloids may be associated with a higher incidence of AKI. Given the relative efficacy and safety of crystalloids, it is prudent to utilize them in fluid resuscitation and limit colloid use to the framework of clinical trials.

In sepsis and septic shock, there is hypotension despite normal or increased cardiac output.[128] The hypotension in sepsis is often unresponsive to fluid and requires administration of vasopressor agents. Because these agents cause vasoconstriction, there has been concern about their use in AKI. Norepinephrine causes a reduction in renal blood flow in healthy animals and humans.[129] The ultimate effect of norepinephrine on renal blood flow, however, depends on the resulting increase in blood pressure and vascular resistance. Norepinephrine increases blood pressure via an α_1-mediated increase in systemic vascular resistance and a β_1-mediated increase in cardiac output. The increase in resistance can potentially decrease cardiac output by increasing afterload. In the kidney, the effect on renal vascular resistance depends on the increase in systemic pressure, with a decreased renal sympathetic tone causing vasodilatation as well as an autoregulatory vasoconstriction secondary to increased perfusion pressure and α_1-mediated renal vasoconstriction.[130] In a nonrandomized study, it was demonstrated that norepinephrine increased arterial blood pressure, urine output, and GFR.[131] A large randomized trial comparing dopamine to norepinephrine as initial vasopressor in patients with septic shock showed no significant differences between groups with regard to renal function or mortality, though norepinephrine was associated with less tachycardia in the first hours and was superior with regard to survival in cardiogenic shock patients (De Backer et al., in press).

Vasopressin is a hormone secreted by the posterior pituitary; it increases systemic vascular resistance by activating V_{1a} receptors on vascular smooth muscle. During septic shock, there is a biphasic response, with early high levels of endogenous vasopressin followed by a decrease.[132] The renal effects of vasopressin are complex and involve an interplay between V_1 and V_2 receptors that regulates the antidiuretic function of vasopressin.[132] Vasopressin is gaining attractiveness in the treatment of norepinephrine refractory shock patients.[133] It increases blood pressure and enhances diuresis in hypotensive oliguric patients but has not yet been proven to enhance survival nor been shown to prevent or ameliorate AKI in the critically ill.[134]

It has been proposed that tight glycemic control can reduce the incidence and severity of AKI in critical patients. Recently Schetz et al. combined the renal endpoints of patients in a secondary analysis of two large randomized clinical trials.[135] They demonstrated that tight glycemic control significantly reduced the incidence of severe AKI from 7.6% to 4.5%. The need for RRT was not decreased in the overall population, but it was significantly lower in surgical ICU patients than in medical ICU patients. However, further studies have highlighted significant concerns regarding the effectiveness and safety of using intensive insulin therapy with tight glycemic control to prevent or ameliorate morbidity and mortality of AKI and other forms of organ injury. The international Normoglycemia in Intensive Care Evaluation and Survival Using Glucose Algorithm Regulation (NICE-SUGAR) study was recently published.[136] This large trial enrolled over 6000 patients and set out to definitively determine the risk/benefit of tight glycemic control in critically ill patients. It showed that in contrast to conventional insulin therapy, intensive glucose control increased mortality among these patients. A blood glucose target of ≤180 mg/dL resulted in lower mortality than a target of 81 to 108 mg/dL. It may therefore be prudent to use conventional insulin therapy in ICU patients at risk of AKI to target plasma glucose of less than 150 mg/dL, using a protocol to avoid hypoglycemia.

Nutritional Support

Nutritional support in patients with AKI does not differ significantly from that of critically ill patients in general. The goals of nutritional support are preservation of lean body mass, stimulation of immune competence, repair, and wound healing. AKI affects water, electrolyte, and acid-base balance, but it also induces a change in protein, carbohydrate, and lipid metabolism.[137] In patients with uncomplicated renal failure, oxygen consumption is approximately that of normal subjects. In the presence of sepsis or multiorgan failure, however, oxygen consumption is increased 20% to 30%.[138] Therefore, energy expenditure is determined more by the underlying disease. Energy substrate should not exceed this requirement, and it is better to err on the side of slight underfeeding than overfeeding. Patients with AKI should be supplemented with 20 to 30 kcal/kg body weight per day. Even in hypermetabolic states such as sepsis, energy expenditure is rarely greater than 130% of calculated basic energy expenditure. In a randomized trial in AKI patients, comparing 30 and 40 kcal/kg/d energy provision, the higher energy prescription did not induce a more positive nitrogen balance but was associated with a higher incidence of hyperglycemia and hypertriglyceridemia and more positive fluid balance.[139] Therefore, supplementation should not exceed 30 kcal/kg body weight per day.

The hallmark of metabolic alterations in AKI is activation of protein catabolism and release of amino acids from skeletal muscle. This process is responsible for the negative nitrogen balance encountered in critically ill patients. An underlying mechanism of protein catabolism is insulin resistance, which may be associated with increased mortality in AKI patients.[140] Plasma insulin levels are elevated, but maximal insulin-stimulated glucose uptake is decreased by 50%. This insulin resistance leads to stimulated hepatic gluconeogenesis fueled by protein catabolism.[141] The elevated level of gluconeogenesis coupled with insulin resistance also frequently leads to hyperglycemia. Other factors such as inflammatory cytokines (namely, tumor necrosis factor) and catecholamines are also involved in the hypercatabolism.[142] To combat malnutrition in this setting, it is often necessary to use nutritional supplementation in the form of enteral or parenteral feeding.

Enteral nutrition has become the standard form of nutritional support in critically ill patients. Enteral feeding helps maintain gastrointestinal function, including acting as a barrier to microorganisms. Two clinical studies have suggested that enteral feeding is associated with improved outcome and survival in ICU patients.[143,144] A meta-analysis by Heyland and colleagues reviewed 26 randomized trials comparing total parenteral nutrition with standard care and found no survival benefit and possible harm in medical ICU patients fed parenterally.[145] Therefore, enteral support is recommended in critically ill patients with or without AKI.

Traditionally, nutrition has been delivered in the form of 50% to 80% carbohydrates. Recently, this has been the subject of study. In addition to providing calories, lipids also provide essential fatty acids. Essential fatty acids such as omega-3 polyunsaturated fatty acids and amino acids such as arginine have been found to stimulate the immune system. A prospective randomized trial of "immune-enhancing" enteral nutrition found that in patients who received adequate nutrition, those who received the immune-enhancing diet had a decrease in mortality and hospital stay.[146] This study did not address AKI patients, but it is likely they would also benefit.

In the past, protein restriction was employed in AKI patients to control uremia, but this is likely to be detrimental to the patient and results in a profoundly negative nitrogen balance.[147] With the advent of continuous modalities of RRT, it is possible to adequately supplement protein and control uremia. Therefore, some authors recommend aggressive protein replacement at 2.5 g/kg/d, as opposed to the standard 1 to 1.5 g/kg/d.[147] However, no compelling data are currently available concerning the efficacy and safety of such high protein intakes. Also, it is important to realize that hypercatabolism cannot be simply overcome by increasing protein or amino acid intake. We suggest administering 0.8 to 1.2 g/kg/d of protein in patients with AKI without the need for dialysis, and 1 to 1.5 g/kg/d in patients with AKI on RRT.

Indications for Nephrology Consultation

Currently there are wide variations in the timing of nephrology consultation in patients with AKI. Some physicians prefer to consult at the first rise in serum creatinine, whereas others wait until RRT is needed. In a study evaluating the effect of nephrology consultation on patient outcome, Mehta and associates found that a delay in nephrology consultation (>48 hours after ICU admission with AKI) led to higher mortality.[148] In this study, patients with delayed consultation had a lower serum creatinine concentration and higher urine output but more organ failure and higher total body water. In the multivariate analysis, delayed consultation was no longer significant, but the trend was there. Why would early consultation affect mortality? It could result from delayed recognition of renal failure. Higher total body water likely leads to tissue edema and organ dysfunction (i.e., pulmonary edema), so in ICU patients, early recognition of AKI and its appropriate management may lead to better outcomes.

Renal Replacement Therapy

INDICATIONS

As mentioned previously, up to a third of patients in the ICU develop AKI. Of those, 30% to 70% require RRT.[25,26,27] Many practitioners delay initiating RRT as long as possible because of concerns that dialysis may delay the recovery of renal function.[149,150] The optimal timing of initiation of dialysis is not defined. There is little disagreement in commencing dialysis in the presence of life-threatening conditions such as diuretic-resistant volume overload, severe hyperkalemia, acidosis, azotemia, or overt symptoms and signs of uremia such as encephalopathy and pericarditis. Medical treatment approaches for hyperkalemia accomplish intracellular shifts. When intermittent hemodialysis is used to correct hyperkalemia after such measures have been utilized, dialytic potassium removal will be reduced, and greater levels of post-dialysis potassium can occur.[151] Metabolic acidosis is common in severe AKI but can be corrected with bicarbonate and should rarely require urgent dialysis if not accompanied by volume overload or uremia.[152] Some poisons, drug overdose, and toxic compounds can contribute to acid-base disturbances and AKI. In such cases, dialysis can be supportive and facilitate removal of these substances and their metabolites. In acute salicylate poisoning, RRT is indicated when serum concentration is above 100 mg/dL and the patient exhibits altered mental status, pulmonary or cerebral edema, renal impairment, fluid overload that prevents administration of sodium bicarbonate, or clinical deterioration despite aggressive and appropriate supportive care.[153] Ethylene glycol and methanol poisoning are important causes of anion-gap metabolic acidosis. Dialysis treatment has been shown to reduce development of subsequent AKI and organ dysfunction.[154] Metformin-associated lactic acidosis may be an indication for dialysis, especially in critical patients who are more prone to death. According to a recent study, these are patients who show a low pH (<6.9) and high serum lactate and metformin concentrations.[155]

The level of azotemia at which RRT should begin is unknown. Several early retrospective studies that used blood urea or

BUN suggested that early initiation of RRT resulted in survival improvements.[156,157] More recent studies have continued to focus on BUN as the marker for starting dialysis. Single-center observational studies that were restricted to AKI after trauma[158] and coronary artery bypass surgery[159,160] suggested a benefit to dialysis initiation at lower BUN concentrations. A prospective multicenter observational study analyzed dialysis initiation, as inferred by BUN concentration, in 243 geographically and ethnically diverse patients.[161] Survival rates were slightly lower for patients who started dialysis at higher BUN concentrations, despite a lower burden of organ system failure. In a prospective multicenter observational trial study conducted at 54 ICUs in 23 countries, timing of RRT was stratified into "early" or "late" by median urea at the time RRT started and also categorized temporally from ICU admission into early (<2 days), delayed (2-5 days), or late (>5 days).[162] Timing by serum urea showed no significant difference in mortality. However, when timing was analyzed in relationship to ICU admission, late RRT (this may also be late AKI) was associated with greater crude mortality and covariate-adjusted mortality. Overall, late RRT was associated with a longer duration of RRT and stay in hospital and greater dialysis dependence.

Serum concentrations of BUN and creatinine are recognized to be inherently subject to a multitude of factors other than kidney function, such as catabolic rate, volume status, age, race, and muscle mass. It would therefore be prudent not to base dialysis initiation decision on a single BUN and creatinine threshold, but rather on the broader clinical context and trends of laboratory tests. Finally, it is important to consider the volume status when deciding the time for initiating RRT, because volume overload, as previously elaborated, emerged as an important factor associated with mortality in AKI. Table 114-6 depicts accepted indications for initiating RRT in the ICU.

ADEQUATE DOSING

In chronic hemodialysis patients, adequacy of dialysis is primarily determined by the level of small-solute (urea) clearance. This is determined by the Kt/V formula, where K is the dialysis membrane clearance of urea, t is the time on dialysis, and V is the volume of distribution of urea, which is equal to total body water. In chronic hemodialysis, a Kt/V of 1.2 per session is considered adequate.[163] As can be seen from the formula, to increase urea clearance, one can increase the time on dialysis or increase the dialyzer clearance. Dialyzer clearance depends on blood flow and dialysate flow rates, as well as the inherent properties of the membrane.

In the United States, intermittent hemodialysis and continuous RRT are the most commonly used modalities of RRT, with sustained low-efficiency dialysis and other "hybrid" treatments used in fewer than 10% of patients. Intermittent hemodialysis is most commonly provided on a thrice-weekly or every-other-day schedule.[164] Concerning intermittent modalities, there is no standard Kt/V for adequate dialysis in AKI currently, but it has been suggested that a higher target Kt/V

TABLE 114-6	Potential Indications for Renal Replacement Therapy in the ICU

Nonobstructive oliguria (urine output <200 mL/12 h) or anuria
Severe acidemia
Azotemia (blood urea nitrogen >80 mg/dL)
Hyperkalemia (K$^+$ >6.5 mmol/L)*
Uremia (encephalopathy, pericarditis, neuropathy, myopathy)
Severe dysnatremia (Na$^+$ >160 or <115 mmol/L)
Hyperthermia (temperature >39.5°C)
Clinically significant organ edema (especially lung)
Drug overdose with dialyzable toxin
Coagulopathy requiring large amounts of blood products in a patient at risk for adult respiratory distress syndrome

NOTE: Any one of these indications is sufficient to consider initiating renal replacement therapy. Two of these indications make renal replacement therapy desirable.

Adapted from Bellomo R, Ronco C. Continuous haemofiltration in the intensive care unit. Crit Care 2000;4:339-45.

*Intermittent hemodialysis removes K$^+$ more efficiently than continuous modalities.

confers better patient outcomes. Schiffl and colleagues studied 160 patients with AKI who were divided into two groups: one received daily hemodialysis, and the other alternate-day hemodialysis. It was found that daily hemodialysis resulted in less hypotension, sepsis, gastrointestinal bleeding, and respiratory failure, as well as a significant decrease in mortality.[165] This study has been criticized because the Kt/V delivered to the alternate-day group was only 0.94, which is significantly less than the prescribed dose of 1.2. Therefore, the results could be explained by the fact that the alternate-day group received inadequate dialysis. In contrast, the VA/NIH Acute Renal Failure Trial Network Study (ATN study) did not find a benefit for a more intensive dosing strategy for RRT.[166] This study compared intermittent hemodialysis (hemodynamically stable patients) or sustained low-efficiency dialysis (hemodynamically unstable patients) performed 3 (less intensive) versus 6 (more intensive) times a week in 563 critically ill patients with AKI and failure of at least one nonrenal organ or sepsis. The prescribed Kt/V per session was 1.2 to 1.4, and the actual delivered mean dose was 1.3 in the less intensive arm. The 60-day mortality rate and percentage of patients recovering renal function were similar in both groups. The Hannover Dialysis Outcomes study was a prospective randomized parallel group study that used intensified extended dialysis (dosed to maintain plasma urea levels <90 mg/dL) versus standard dialysis (dosed to maintain plasma urea levels between 120 and 150 mg/dL) on 14- and 28-day mortality and renal function.[167] Mortality and frequency of renal function recovery were similar between the two groups. Based on these two well designed and performed clinical trials, it appears that increasing urea target clearances does not improve mortality or rates of renal recovery. Therefore, at least the smaller dose used in these trials should be pursued, with monitoring of the delivered dose of therapy to ascertain a minimum delivered Kt/V of 1.2 per treatment, or maintenance of plasma urea around 110 mg/dL when using extended or intermittent RRT in AKI patients. The significant difference between prescribed and delivered dialysis dose was studied by Evanson and coworkers, who found that the prescribed dose was a Kt/V of 1.25, whereas the dose delivered was only 1.04.[168] These authors found that the most significant factor predicting actual delivered dose was the patient's predialysis weight. It follows that a higher weight in critically ill patients represents higher total body water and therefore a larger volume of distribution of urea. This would be expected to decrease the Kt/V if it were not accounted for in the prescription of dialysis.

CRRT has been advocated in patients with AKI because of its ability to more efficiently remove solute[169] and provide hemodynamic stability,[170] but the optimal dosing in CRRT is not known. This form of RRT depends on convection, not diffusion, for solute clearance, which means that there is no dialysate involved, and solute is removed with water during ultrafiltration. Ronco and colleagues randomized 425 patients with AKI to increasing doses of continuous venovenous hemofiltration (CVVH).[171] These investigators used three increasing doses of ultrafiltration—20, 35, and 45 mL/kg per hour—and found that mortality was 41%, 57%, and 58%, respectively. Survival was significantly lower in the 20 mL/kg group than in the other two groups. If the patient was septic, using the highest dose was beneficial.[170,171] A more recent study by Bouman et al. in severely ill, ventilated patients with high severity scores was unable to detect a difference in mortality between high ultrafiltration volume (48 mL/kg/h) and low ultrafiltration volume (20 mL/kg/h).[172] In the mentioned VA/ATN study, an approximate number of 201 patients received predilutional continuous venovenous hemodiafiltration (CVVHDF) in the less intensive arm (mean delivered effluent of 22 mL/kg/min) and 179 in the intensive therapy group (mean delivered effluent of 36 mL/kg/min).[166] A higher dose of CRRT did not influence either mortality or renal recovery. The recently reported Randomized Evaluation of Normal versus Augmented Level of RRT (RENAL) study was conducted in 35 centers in Australia and New Zealand.[173] It compared the effects of postdilutional CVVHDF doses of 25 and 40 mL/kg/h in 24-day and 90-day mortality rates of 1508 critically ill AKI patients. Treatment with higher-intensity regimen did not reduce mortality at 90 days. In conclusion, the results

of these two recent well-designed and executed large clinical trials (ATN and RENAL) did not show any benefit of higher CRRTs doses for critical AKI patients beyond a threshold dose necessary to optimize clinical outcome. Therefore, when using CRRT for treating such patients, a minimum dose to be targeted may be the minimal efficient one proved in those trials: 20 to 25 mL/kg/h. However, it is important to pay careful attention to ensure that interruptions of treatment in the ICU are minimized. Beyond small-solute clearance, other aspects of dialysis adequacy such as volume management should be well attended to.

MODALITY

When RRT is indicated in the ICU for severe AKI, physicians have to choose between intermittent techniques such as traditional intermittent hemodialysis (IHD; used in end-stage kidney disease), slow low-efficiency dialysis (SLED), or continuous therapies such as CVVH and peritoneal dialysis (PD) (Table 114-7). SLED is performed by utilizing dialysis machines to deliver a slow dialysate flow for periods ranging from 8 to 12 hours per day. Advantages with this technique include high hemodynamic tolerance, excellent solute-removal capability, and capacity to be instituted using regular hemodialysis machines without acquiring new equipment. Availability and expertise with the technique, as well as the hemodynamic status of the patient, are typical determining factors for modality choice for AKI.

RRT is required in severe AKI to remove uremic toxins and maintain fluid, electrolyte, and acid-base balance. CRRT and IHD are effective therapies that may be utilized and exchanged according to the hemodynamic status or coagulation problems of the patient. The effect of these modalities on patient outcomes has been evaluated. Lins et al. performed a multicenter randomized controlled trial to study the effect of intermittent versus continuous dialysis modalities for the treatment of 316 AKI patients who were admitted to the ICU.[174] They demonstrated that ICU stay, hospitalization, mortality, and renal recovery rates were not different between the groups. Moreover, two recent systematic reviews that collectively analyzed 45 studies found that outcomes were similar in critically ill AKI patients (stratified according to severity of illness) with CRRT and IHD for hemodynamically stable patients for relative risk of death, ICU mortality, in-hospital mortality, length of hospitalization, and requirement for chronic dialysis or renal recovery in survivors.[175,176]

Control of both uremia and volume is the major goal of RRT in AKI. A few studies have suggested that CRRT has advantages over intermittent therapies, including hemodynamic stability, improved survival, greater likelihood of renal recovery,[175,177,178] and better fluid balance.[179] IHD is complicated by hypotension in 20% to 30% of patients[180]; in hemodynamically unstable patients, this can significantly limit therapy and delay recovery of renal function. Therefore, some clinicians favor initiating CRRT for hemodynamically unstable patients with AKI, but this has not been supported by a prospective randomized trial[181] or the earlier-mentioned systematic reviews.[175,176] Moreover, Bagshaw et al. recently performed a systematic review and meta-analysis of nine randomized trials and concluded that it is impossible to make definitive recommendations about the initial RRT modality because of

TABLE 114-7	Practical Comparison of Acute Renal Replacement Therapy Modalities		
	Intermittent Hemodialysis	Sustained Low-Efficiency Dialysis	Continuous Renal Replacement Therapy
Session duration in hours	3-5	8-12	24
Blood flow, mL/min	300-400	200-300	100-200
Dialysate flow, mL/min	500-800	200-350	25-40
Anticoagulant requirement	Heparin or none	Heparin or none	Heparin or regional citrate

Data from Fieghen H, Wald R, Jaber BL. Renal replacement therapy for acute kidney injury. Nephron Clin Pract 2009;112:222-9.

numerous issues related to study design, conduct, and quality of these trials.[182] The main disadvantage of CRRT is the need for prolonged anticoagulation. SLED is gaining popularity as an intermittent modality in ICUs because of the aforementioned multiple advantages. Two RCTs that compared SLED with CVVH or CVVHD[183,184] found similar outcomes with regard to hemodynamic stability and uremic clearance; furthermore, a decreased anticoagulation requirement was reported for SLED.[184] Based on such evidence, all these modalities should be viewed as complementary. CRRT or SLED may be utilized for severe AKI with hemodynamic instability and transitioned to IHD once stability is attained. Peritoneal dialysis is an alternate modality for AKI where vascular access may be difficult, in conditions where anticoagulation may be problematic, in under-resourced regions, or following large disasters with mass casualties.[185] A prospective randomized study of daily IHD versus PD in 120 AKI patients showed no difference in survival or recovery of renal function.[186] These results contrast to a previous study that showed decreased survival associated with PD in comparison to CVVH[187] and suggest that PD remains an acceptable option to CRRT when dosed appropriately.

In certain situations, CRRT is preferable to IHD, including in patients with or at risk for increased intracranial pressure. Studies have shown that CRRT prevents the increase in intracranial pressure associated with intermittent RRT.[188,189] The use of CRRT in patients with severe sepsis or septic shock has also received much attention. Sepsis is associated with hemodynamic instability, making CRRT an attractive option. It has been shown that CRRT has beneficial effects on hemodynamics in animal models of sepsis.[190] This is thought to be secondary to the removal of inflammatory cytokines by both convective and adsorptive measures. Hemofiltration membranes allow the ultrafiltration of mid-molecular-weight molecules such as cytokines. Further, the continuous blood/membrane contact allows the membrane to adsorb more mediators. There is some evidence that hemofiltration may provide some benefit in those with sepsis and AKI.[191,192] Larger and adequately powered studies are needed to better define the role of this modality in AKI and sepsis.

Despite potential hemodynamic advantage over IHD, CRRT has some disadvantages as well. With CRRT, there is generally a need for continuous anticoagulation to prevent clotting of the filter. Although this is usually done with low-dose heparin, there is the risk of bleeding or heparin-induced thrombocytopenia. When a patient is a bleeding risk, a trial of no anticoagulation can be carried out, or regional anticoagulation with citrate is used in some centers. CRRT also requires more nursing support and is considerably more expensive than IHD.[193]

DIALYSIS MEMBRANE

Early dialysis membranes were made of cellulose or its derivatives, and it has been shown that the hydroxyl radicals on the cellulose membranes were able to activate the complement system.[194] These older membranes were thus not biocompatible. Newer synthetic polymers are less able to activate the complement cascade and also have the ability to bind activated complement, thereby decreasing systemic effects.[195] Because of this decrease in immune activation, these membranes are considered biocompatible. In CRRT, there is continuous contact between the blood and membrane, making this interaction quite important. Despite mechanistic advantages, a recent meta-analysis found no advantage to biocompatible versus bio-incompatible membranes in terms of adult patient mortality and kidney function recovery rates.[196]

Membranes may also play a role in blood purification beyond that of solute clearance. There is interest in the ability of membranes to adsorb and bind cytokines from the blood. This is particularly attractive in sepsis, when there is dysregulation of the immune system with both pro- and antiinflammatory effects. A recent prospective RCT evaluated the use of polymyxin B hemoperfusion in patients with abdominal sepsis to reduce circulating endotoxin levels and improve clinical outcomes. Patients were randomized to conventional therapy or conventional therapy plus two sessions of polymyxin B

hemoperfusion. The study showed that polymyxin B hemoperfusion added to conventional therapy significantly improved hemodynamics and organ dysfunction and reduced 28-day mortality.[197] Abundant clinical studies show an association between inflammation and mortality in patients with AKI. Some investigators have suggested a potential role for using CRRT[198,199] or IHD[200] to remove cytokines and/or diminish the inflammatory response in septic patients with AKI. Such an approach is still experimental, and inadvertent removal of other potentially desirable middle molecules may be undertaken.

BUFFER

In determining the adequacy of dialysis, factors other than solute clearance must be considered. One goal of RRT is to maintain normal acid-base balance in patients with AKI to prevent the complications of acidemia with regard to cardiovascular performance, hepatic metabolism, and hormonal response. To maintain normal pH, the dialysate must contain a buffer. Traditionally, the buffer choice was between bicarbonate and lactate, which metabolizes in the liver to bicarbonate on an equimolar basis under physiologic conditions. However, in critically ill patients with organ dysfunction and disordered tissue perfusion, it is possible that not all the anion will be converted to bicarbonate, resulting in increased serum lactate levels. Moreover, the increased lactate, without its redox partner pyruvate, can result in increased protein catabolism, myocardial depression,[201] and worsening acidosis in patients with preexisting lactic acidosis.[202,203]

Bicarbonate-based solutions are currently the buffer of choice and are available in separated solutions that are mixed just before use. In a study by Barenbrock and colleagues, bicarbonate-based versus lactate-based fluid replacement was studied in patients with AKI treated with CVVH.[204] They found that serum lactate concentration was significantly higher and bicarbonate lower in patients treated with lactate-based solution. In addition, they showed an increase in cardiovascular events and hypotension in patients treated with lactate solution.

MEDICATION DOSING

During AKI, drugs normally eliminated by the kidney exhibit a markedly decreased clearance. The physiochemical characteristics of drugs affect their removal by dialysis and hemofiltration. The amounts of drug removed during these procedures can be sufficient to require supplemental dosing. For patients on hemodialysis, a supplemental dose of drug is most commonly given at the completion of the dialysis session.[205] Drug clearance with CVVH is through convective transport, and it approximates the unbound drug concentration in plasma multiplied by the ultrafiltration rate.[206] Drugs with molecular weights of less than 500 D are readily removed by either conventional hemodialysis or CVVH, but those with higher weights of 1000 to 5000 D are eliminated more efficiently by CVVH because of the use of high-flux membranes that allow the passage of larger molecules.

The volume of distribution greatly impacts the clearance of a drug, in that those with large distributions are likely to be more bound in the tissues. Therefore, only a small amount has access to the vasculature at any time. For these drugs, clearance with CVVH is greater than with intermittent therapies because of the continuous nature of the clearance.[207] The extent of protein binding of a drug is important because the protein-drug complex is generally greater than 50,000 D. At this size, neither intermittent nor continuous therapies will efficiently remove the drug. However, the extent of protein binding is dependent on pH, uremia, concentration of free fatty acids, heparin therapy, and relative concentrations of drug and protein.[208] In critically ill patients, serum albumin is often decreased, thereby making more drug available for clearance during RRT. Because of the potential toxicities, as well as the need to maintain therapeutic levels of multiple medications, it is important to consider and adjust medication dose during AKI and its therapy with RRT. Dosages of medications must be adjusted for the type of RRT, as well as for the specific characteristics of the drug.

TABLE 114-8	Recommendations for Evaluation and Treatment of Acute Kidney Injury

Evaluate patient for AKI when serum creatinine increases by >0.5 mg/dL.

Exclude prerenal causes (volume depletion, CHF, cirrhosis, NSAIDs, ACE inhibitors).

Exclude postrenal causes with renal ultrasonography and postvoid residual.

Review urine sediment (muddy brown casts, ATN; RBC casts, glomerulonephritis or vasculitis; pyuria, acute interstitial nephritis; bland sediment, prerenal or postrenal azotemia).

Evaluate urine electrolytes in absence of diuretics.

After exclusion of pre- and postrenal azotemia and confirmation of ATN by urine sediment and electrolytes, notify a nephrologist when serum creatinine >2 mg/dL.

Note the projected need for dialysis: oliguric ATN (urine volume <400 mL/24 h), 60%-70% of patients; nonoliguric ATN (urine volume >400 mL/24 h), 30%-40% of patients.

Avoid excessive fluid resuscitation leading to pseudo-ARDS, ventilator support, and multiorgan complications.

Avoid hypotension (generally there is no need to treat hypertension aggressively in the absence of hypertensive crisis).

Maintain fluid balance and treat hyperkalemia; do not use "renal-dose" dopamine.

Review active medications for necessary dose adjustments.

When indicated, use enteral rather than parenteral alimentation.

Discuss timing for initiation and mode of renal replacement with nephrologist (intermittent versus continuous hemodialysis and use of biocompatible membrane).

ACE, angiotensin-converting enzyme; ARDS, acute respiratory distress syndrome; AKI, acute renal failure; ATN, acute tubular necrosis; CHF, congestive heart failure; NSAIDs, nonsteroidal antiinflammatory drugs; RBC, red blood cell.

From Esson ML, Schrier RW. Diagnosis and treatment of acute tubular necrosis. Ann Intern Med 2002;137:744-52.

Conclusion

Despite extensive clinical experience and improvements in supportive care, the mortality rate of critically ill patients with AKI has not changed over the last 3 decades. However, new information is emerging about the diagnosis and treatment of AKI. Table 114-8 summarizes current recommendations for the care of patients with AKI.[18] These recommendations are based on evidence from clinical trials as well as clinical judgment.

KEY POINTS

Prerenal Causes

1. Prerenal azotemia accounts for 70% of community-acquired acute kidney injury (AKI) and 40% of hospital-acquired AKI.

2. Because there is no cellular injury in prerenal azotemia, it is reversible with correction of causative factors such as volume depletion, use of nonsteroidal antiinflammatory drugs, or congestive heart failure.

3. It is characterized by bland urine sediment and a fractional excretion of sodium (FE$_{Na}$) less than 1%.

Postrenal Causes

1. Postrenal azotemia occurs when there is bilateral obstruction to urine flow.

2. It is an uncommon cause of AKI in the ICU.

3. Evaluation includes renal ultrasonography and postvoid residual, which should be less than 50 mL.

Intrarenal Causes

1. These causes are defined according to the anatomic location of injury—glomerulus, tubule, interstitium, or vasculature.

2. In the ICU, acute tubular necrosis is the most common form of AKI and includes both tubular and vascular injury.

3. Differentiation from prerenal azotemia is accomplished by examination of the urine sediment, which is characterized by muddy brown casts, as well as an FE$_{Na}$ greater than 1%. Novel biomarkers are promising to determine kidney injury early and allow timely interventions.

Epidemiology

1. AKI is a common complication, occurring in up to a third of ICU patients.

2. In the majority of patients, it is multifactorial in nature, with components of hypotension, sepsis, and drugs.

3. AKI mortality is high—up to 50% of patients—and generally part of multiorgan failure.

4. The risk of developing AKI increases with age and in the presence of baseline chronic kidney disease, oliguria, and sepsis.

Definition

1. Blood urea nitrogen (BUN) and creatinine are the most common parameters measured, but they are not sensitive indicators of renal dysfunction in the acute setting. Ongoing research is evaluating early diagnostic roles of injury biomarkers.

2. Recently the term *AKI* was introduced as an alternative to acute renal failure (ARF) in order to encompass the entire range of failure, based on recent data showing that even small changes in serum creatinine influence outcome.

3. The Acute Dialysis Quality Initiative (ADQI) has proposed a categorized definition of ARF called the *RIFLE criteria*, which were subsequently revised by the Acute Kidney Injury Network (AKIN) to better account for the small changes in serum creatinine not captured by RIFLE and shorten the necessary time to establish the diagnosis.

4. AKIN has defined AKI as an increase in serum creatinine (Scr) from baseline to 48 hours: stage 1, an increase in Scr of 0.3 mg/dL or 150% to 200%; stage 2, an increase in Scr of 200% to 300%; stage 3, an increase in Scr of greater than 300% or greater than 4 mg/dL, or acute renal replacement therapy (RRT) commencement (irrespective of the preceding Scr increase or urine output).

Treatment

1. To prevent contrast-induced AKI in patients at risk, hydration with isotonic sodium bicarbonate is most beneficial, with the possible addition of *N*-acetylcysteine before and after the procedure.

2. There is no role for dopamine in the treatment of AKI.

3. Diuretics have not been shown to prevent or ameliorate AKI. They can be used in the initial management of AKI to facilitate fluid balance and treat hyperkalemia or hypercalcemia, but their use should not delay commencing RRT when deemed clinically necessary.

Hemodynamic Management

1. Early goal-directed management may reverse adverse hemodynamics before tissue injury occurs and result in a better outcome.

2. Recognition of the clinical entity, pseudo–acute respiratory distress syndrome, and management with ultrafiltration may improve patient outcome.

3. Available evidence supports crystalloids use for resuscitating volume-depleted patients when the condition is not due to hemorrhage.

4. When vasopressors are indicated, the effect on systemic hemodynamics generally outweighs the direct renal vasoconstriction, but in cases of sepsis, vasopressin may be preferable because it may improve hemodynamics in refractory septic shock.

Nutritional Support

1. Patients with AKI have increased protein catabolism due to insulin resistance.

2. Enteral nutrition is recommended.

3. Caloric supplementation should be 20 to 30 kcal/kg/d.

4. Protein restriction has no role in the management of AKI.

Indications for Nephrology Consultation

1. Early nephrology consultation may lead to improved outcome due to earlier recognition of AKI.

Renal Replacement Therapy

1. It is likely that early initiation of renal replacement therapy is beneficial.

2. Dialysis initiation decision should not be based on a single BUN and creatinine threshold, but rather on the broader clinical context (e.g., volume status, pericarditis), trends of laboratory tests, and metabolic indicators (e.g., refractory hyperkalemia and acidosis).

3. When using extended or intermittent dialysis in AKI, monitoring the delivered dose of therapy is recommended to ascertain a minimum delivered Kt/V of 1.2 per treatment.

4. With continuous venovenous hemofiltration, ultrafiltration rates of at least 20 mL/kg/h should be attained.

Modality

1. Patients with delayed recovery from acute tubular necrosis often have fresh areas of necrosis on renal biopsy. This is likely exacerbated by dialysis-associated hypotension.

2. Current evidence does not support the superiority of CRRT over intermittent therapies in the treatment of AKI.

3. RRT modalities should be viewed as complementary; CRRT or hybrid therapies may be utilized for severe AKI with hemodynamic instability and transitioned to IHD once stability is attained.

4. Drawbacks to the use of CRRT include an increase in nursing care, higher expense, and the need for continuous anticoagulation.

Dialysis Membrane

1. The interaction between blood and the dialysis membrane can initiate an inflammatory response. This response has been shown to elicit vasoconstriction and may prolong the course of AKI.

2. Biocompatible membranes may decrease immune activation but have not been consistently shown to result in improved AKI outcomes.

Dialysis Buffer

1. Lactate buffer is associated with hyperlactatemia in patients with hypotension or liver dysfunction. Elevated serum lactate levels contribute to protein catabolism.

2. Lactate buffer is also associated with decreased hemodynamic stability.

3. Bicarbonate-based buffer is now the standard.

Medication Dosing

1. In critical illness, both the volume of distribution and the extent of protein binding of drugs change.

2. Owing to potential toxicities, it is important to consider the degree of renal function when determining medication dosing.

ANNOTATED REFERENCES

Bellomo R, Ronco C, Kellam JA, Mehta RL, Palevsky P. Acute Dialysis Quality Initiative workgroup. Acute renal failure—definition, outcome measures, animal models, fluid therapy and information technology needs: the Second International Consensus Conference of the Acute Dialysis Quality Initiative (ADQI) Group. Crit Care 2004;8:R204-12.

Mehta RL, Kellum JA, Shah SV, Molitoris BA, Ronco C, Warnock DG. Acute Kidney Injury Network. Acute Kidney Injury Network: report of an initiative to improve outcomes in acute kidney injury. Crit Care 2007;11:R31.
These two papers present the currently adopted classification systems for AKI, the RIFLE and AKIN criteria. Both criteria were shown to identify groups of hospitalized patients with increased risk of mortality and/or need for RRT.

Chertow GM, Burdick E, Honour M, Bonventre JV, Bates DW. Acute kidney injury, mortality, length of stay, and costs in hospitalized patients. J Am Soc Nephrol 2005;16:3365-70.
This is a large retrospective review which demonstrated that even small increases in serum creatinine are associated with significant increases in mortality, length of stay, and costs of hospitalized patients.

Bagshaw SM, Uchino S, Bellomo R, Morimatsu H, Morgera S, Shetz M, et al. Timing of renal replacement therapy and clinical outcomes in critically ill patients with severe acute kidney injury. J Crit Care 2009;24:129-40.
This prospective multicenter observational study showed that timing of RRT might exert an important influence on patient survival. Late RRT (days from admission) was associated with a longer duration of RRT, longer hospital stay, and higher dialysis dependence.

VA/NIH Acute Renal Failure Trial Network, Palevsky PM, et al. Intensity of renal support in critically ill patients with acute kidney injury. N Engl J Med 2008;3(359):7-20.

RENAL Replacement Therapy Study Investigators, Bellomo R, et al. Intensity of continuous renal-replacement therapy in critically ill patients. N Engl J Med 2009;22;361:1627-38.
These two prospective randomized clinical trials have shown that intensive RRT in critically ill patients with AKI did not decrease mortality, improve recovery of kidney function, or reduce the rate of nonrenal organ failure as compared with less intensive therapy.

REFERENCE

Access the complete reference list online at http://www.expertconsult.com.

115

Renal Replacement Therapy

CLAUDIO RONCO | ZACCARIA RICCI | RINALDO BELLOMO | VINCENZO D'INTINI

Severe acute kidney injury (AKI) causes dysregulation in the homeostasis of fluid, potassium, metabolic acids, and waste products, which can lead to life-threatening complications. Extracorporeal blood purification techniques can be applied to prevent these complications and improve homeostasis. Various techniques of renal replacement therapy include continuous venovenous hemodiafiltration, intermittent hemodialysis, and peritoneal dialysis, each with its technical variations but with a common fundamental principle of removing unwanted solutes and water through a semipermeable membrane. The membranes used are either biological (peritoneum) or artificial (hemodialysis or hemofiltration membranes) and have characteristics with advantages and disadvantages.

Principles of Renal Replacement Therapy

The principles of renal replacement therapy have been extensively studied and described.[1-3] The two fundamental principles of renal replacement therapy particularly relevant to critical care physicians are summarized here.

WATER REMOVAL

The removal of unwanted solvent (water) is therapeutically as important as the removal of unwanted solute (e.g., acid, uremic toxins, potassium). During renal replacement therapy, water is removed through a process called *ultrafiltration*. This process is essentially the same as that which occurs in the glomerulus. It requires a driving pressure greater than the oncotic pressure to drive fluid across a semipermeable membrane. This pressure is achieved by:

1. Generating a transmembrane pressure (as in hemofiltration or during intermittent hemodialysis) greater than the oncotic pressure
2. Increasing osmolality of the dialysate with osmotic agents (as in peritoneal dialysis)

SOLUTE REMOVAL

The removal of unwanted solutes can be achieved by creating an electrochemical gradient across the membrane by using a flow-past system with toxin-free dialysate (diffusion), intermittent hemodialysis, and peritoneal dialysis. This process is called *diffusion* and defines the movement of solute with a statistical tendency to reach the same concentration of solute in the available distribution space on each side of the membrane. Solute transport is governed by the following formula:

$$JD = DTA \, (dc/dx)$$

where J is solute flux, D is diffusion coefficient, T is temperature of the solution, A is membrane surface area, dc is concentration gradient between the two compartments, and dx is diffusion distance (thickness of the membrane). In dialysis, blood and dialysate are separated by a membrane. Bidirectional diffusive transport of molecules occurs in response to a concentration gradient.

Solutes also can be removed by creating a "solvent drag"—solutes moving together with solvent across a porous membrane—convection. In this process, the ultrafiltrate is discarded and replaced with toxin-free replacement fluid—hemofiltration. Solvent drag occurs when water is driven by a hydrostatic or an osmotic force across a

semipermeable membrane, carrying with it solutes that can pass through uninhibited. The solutes retain a similar concentration to the original solution, whereas larger molecules are retained. Filtration occurs in response to a transmembrane pressure gradient according to the formula:

$$Qf = Km \times TMP = Km \, (Pb - Puf - \pi)$$

where *Qf* is filtration, *Km* is coefficient of permeability of the membrane, *TMP* is transmembrane pressure, *Pb* is hydrostatic pressure of blood, *Puf* is hydrostatic pressure in the ultrafiltrate compartment, and π is oncotic pressure of blood. In convective treatments, the transport (*Jc*) of solute *x* is governed by the formula:

$$Jc = UF \, [x]_{UF}$$

where *UF* is volume of ultrafiltrate, and $[x]_{UF}$ is concentration of solute *x* in ultrafiltrate. From this, we may derive that clearance in convective treatments is as follows:

$$K = Qf \, [x]_{UF}/[x]_{PW}$$

where *Qf* is ultrafiltration rate, and $[x]_{UF}/[x]_{Pw}$ is the ratio of the solute concentrations in the ultrafiltrate and plasma water or the sieving coefficient *S*. From this formula, it may be observed that when the sieving coefficient is 1, clearance equals ultrafiltration rate.

Despite these distinctions, diffusion and convection often act simultaneously, and it is almost impossible to divide these transport mechanisms physically. The term *hemodialysis* may not aptly describe the mode of treatment in the case of highly permeable membranes. A more suitable term would be *hemodiafiltration* (if replacement solution is needed) or *high-flux dialysis* (if a filtration-back filtration mechanism is present and no replacement fluid is required). The various modalities are described in Figure 115-1.

The rate of diffusion of a given solute depends on its molecular weight, porosity of the membrane, blood flow rate, dialysate flow rate, protein binding, and concentration gradient across the membrane. If standard, low-flux, cellulose-based membranes are used, middle molecules of molecular weight of greater than 500 D are insufficiently removed. Synthetic high-flux membranes (cutoff at 20-40 kD) can remove larger molecules. When such membranes are used, convection is superior to diffusion in achieving the clearance of middle molecules. During peritoneal dialysis, larger molecules (albumin) also can be removed because of the porosity of the peritoneal membrane. Because blood flow rate across the peritoneal membrane is limited, however, clearances also are limited.

Indications for Renal Replacement Therapy

The treatment of AKI requires a different style and philosophy from renal replacement therapy for chronic renal failure. In a critically ill patient, renal replacement therapy should be initiated early. It is physiologically irrational and clinically dangerous to wait for complications to appear before intervening. Fear of early dialysis stems from the well-known adverse effects of conventional intermittent hemodialysis with cuprophane membranes, especially hemodynamic instability, and from the risks and limitations of continuous or intermittent peritoneal dialysis.[4-7] If extended dialysis techniques are used, they are minimized.[8] Accordingly, the time-honored criteria for initiation of renal replacement therapy in patients with chronic renal failure may be

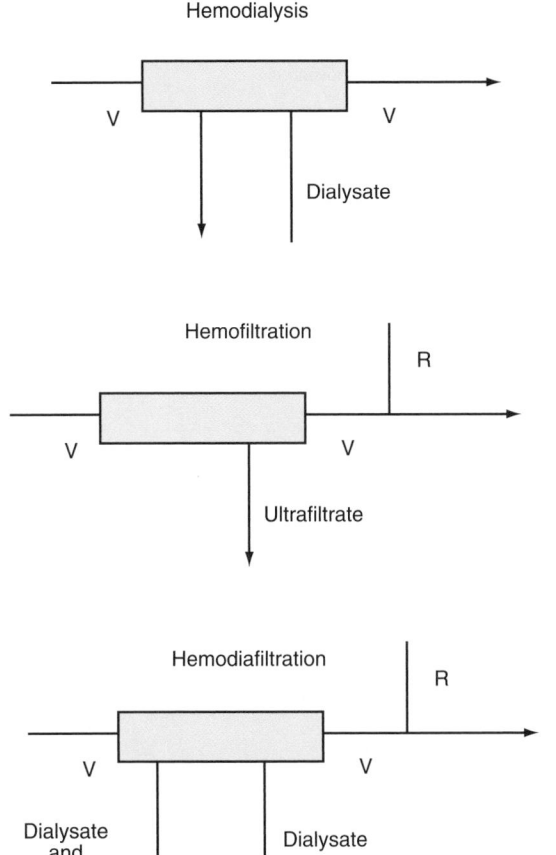

Figure 115-1 Solute removal methods: hemodialysis, hemofiltration, and hemodiafiltration. V, venous blood prefilter and postfilter; R, replacement fluid.

inappropriate in critically ill patients.[9] Modern criteria for initiation of renal replacement therapy in the intensive care unit (ICU) are presented in Table 115-1.

Once intermittent hemodialysis or continuous hemofiltration has been started, there are limited data on what is an "adequate" dose of dialysis. The concept of dialysis adequacy in AKI remains controversial and ill defined, and the current goal is maintenance of homeostasis at all levels.[10] Emerging data suggest that better uremic control may translate into better survival.[11-13] Patients at least should have urea levels maintained between 10 and 20 mmol/L throughout the treatment period. This level of uremic control should occur despite adequate nutrition support with a protein intake around 1.5 g/kg/d. If intermittent hemodialysis is used, daily treatment and/or extended treatment

TABLE 115-1	Modern Criteria for Initiation of Renal Replacement Therapy in the ICU*
Oliguria (urine output < 200 mL/12 h)	
Anuria (urine output 0-50 mL/12 h)	
[Urea] > 35 mmol/L	
[Creatinine] > 400 µmol/L	
[K⁺] > 6.5 mmol/L or rapidly rising	
Pulmonary edema unresponsive to diuretics	
Uncompensated metabolic acidosis (pH < 7.1)	
[Na⁺] < 110 mmol/L and >160 mmol/L	
Temperature > 40°C	
Uremic complications (encephalopathy, myopathy, neuropathy, pericarditis)	
Overdose with a dialyzable toxin (e.g., lithium)	

*If one criterion is present, renal replacement therapy should be considered. If two criteria are simultaneously present, renal replacement therapy is strongly recommended.

are more desirable,[8] with the goal of ensuring at least some adequacy for small-solute removal. This means intermittent hemodialysis must guarantee at least a daily urea clearance in liters greater than or equal to the patient's total body water. Total body water can be calculated from tables or simply as 60% of body weight. This relationship will be treated extensively in the following discussion.

Mode of Renal Replacement Therapy

There is a great deal of controversy as to which mode of renal replacement therapy is "best" in the ICU. This controversy arises from the lack of randomized controlled trials comparing different techniques. Trials of sufficient statistical power are difficult to conduct and may never be performed. In the absence of direct comparisons of suitable statistical power and design, techniques of renal replacement therapy may be judged on the basis of the following criteria:

1. Hemodynamic side effects
2. Ability to control fluid status
3. Biocompatibility
4. Risk of infection
5. Uremic control
6. Avoidance of cerebral edema
7. Ability to allow full nutritional support
8. Ability to control acidosis
9. Absence of specific side effects
10. Cost

In our opinion, the evidence available supports the view that peritoneal dialysis and conventional intermittent hemodialysis (3–4 h/d, 3–4 times/wk) are inferior to continuous renal replacement therapy and probably slow low-efficiency extended dialysis. Some salient aspects of continuous renal replacement therapy, intermittent hemodialysis, and peritoneal dialysis require discussion, however.

Continuous Renal Replacement Therapy

Continuous renal replacement therapy (CRRT) is now the most common form of renal replacement therapy in Australian and European ICUs. In the United States, however, CRRT reportedly is used in only 10% to 20% of ICU patients.[14] CRRT has undergone several technical modifications since it was first described in 1977. Initially it was performed as an arteriovenous therapy (continuous arteriovenous hemofiltration) in which blood flow through the hemofilter was driven by the patient's blood pressure. Clearances were low, however, and countercurrent dialysate flow soon was added to double or triple solute clearances (continuous arteriovenous hemodialysis/diafiltration) with or without spontaneous ultrafiltration. Double-lumen catheters and peristaltic blood pumps have come into use with or without control of ultrafiltration rate.

Whatever the technique of CRRT, the clearances achieved can be adjusted by adjusting ultrafiltration rate or dialysate flow rate or both, typically aiming to achieve a daily clearance at least equal to the patient's total body water. A standardized nomenclature is now available for CRRT techniques.[15] To make the reading easy and to make the reader familiar with the most accepted definitions and treatment schemes, we have summarized in Figure 115-2 the complete set of available techniques, including some hints on operational parameters. No matter what technique is used, the following outcomes are predictable, and the most important will be described:

1. Continuous control of fluid status
2. Hemodynamic stability
3. Control of acid-base status
4. Ability to provide protein-rich nutritional support while achieving excellent uremic control
5. Control of electrolyte balance
6. Control of phosphate and calcium balance
7. Prevention of swings in intracerebral water
8. Minimal risk of infection
9. High level of biocompatibility

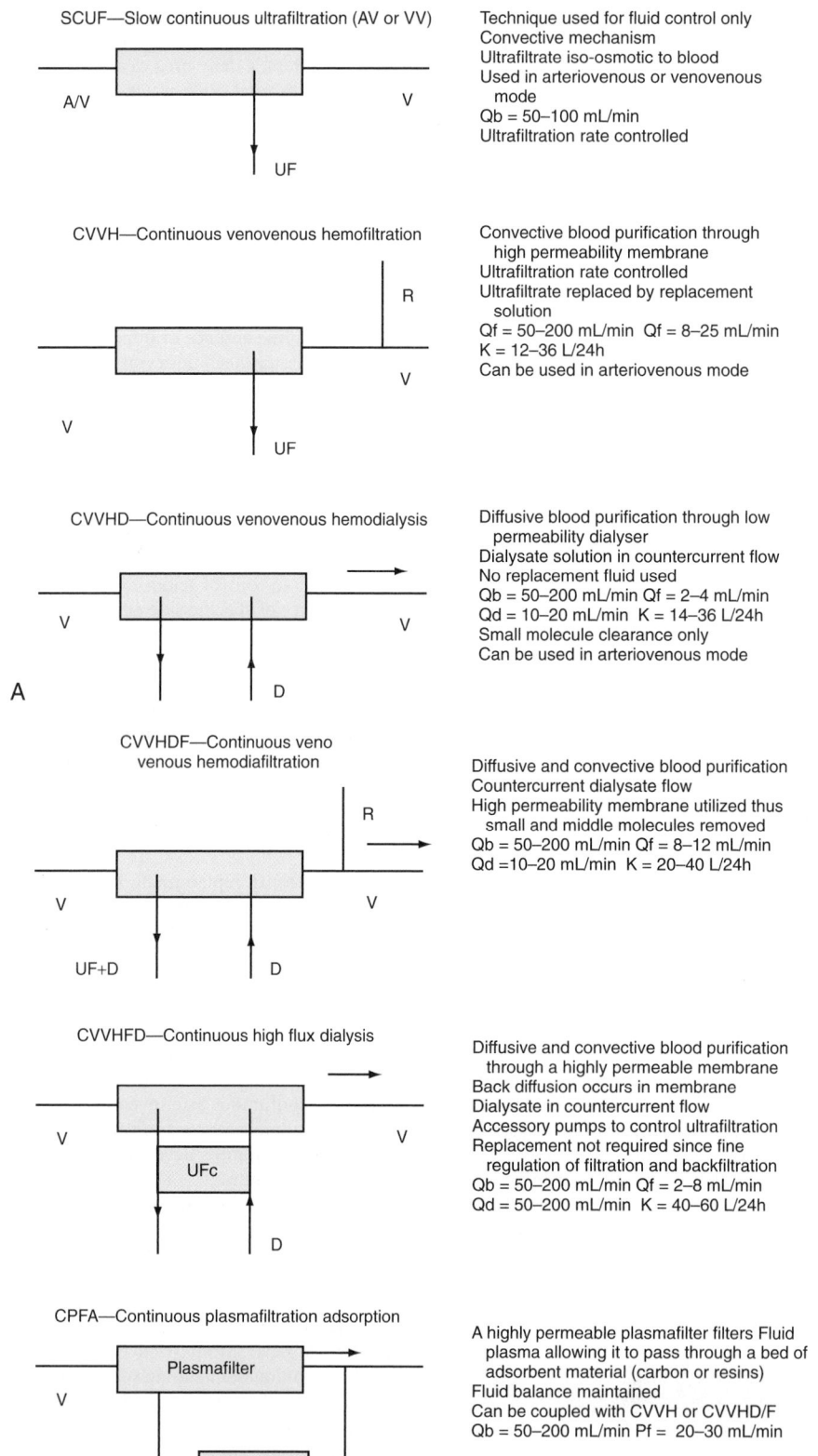

SCUF—Slow continuous ultrafiltration (AV or VV)

Technique used for fluid control only
Convective mechanism
Ultrafiltrate iso-osmotic to blood
Used in arteriovenous or venovenous
   mode
Qb = 50–100 mL/min
Ultrafiltration rate controlled

CVVH—Continuous venovenous hemofiltration

Convective blood purification through
   high permeability membrane
Ultrafiltration rate controlled
Ultrafiltrate replaced by replacement
   solution
Qf = 50–200 mL/min   Qf = 8–25 mL/min
K = 12–36 L/24h
Can be used in arteriovenous mode

CVVHD—Continuous venovenous hemodialysis

Diffusive blood purification through low
   permeability dialyser
Dialysate solution in countercurrent flow
No replacement fluid used
Qb = 50–200 mL/min   Qf = 2–4 mL/min
Qd = 10–20 mL/min   K = 14–36 L/24h
Small molecule clearance only
Can be used in arteriovenous mode

CVVHDF—Continuous veno venous hemodiafiltration

Diffusive and convective blood purification
Countercurrent dialysate flow
High permeability membrane utilized thus
   small and middle molecules removed
Qb = 50–200 mL/min   Qf = 8–12 mL/min
Qd =10–20 mL/min   K = 20–40 L/24h

CVVHFD—Continuous high flux dialysis

Diffusive and convective blood purification
   through a highly permeable membrane
Back diffusion occurs in membrane
Dialysate in countercurrent flow
Accessory pumps to control ultrafiltration
Replacement not required since fine
   regulation of filtration and backfiltration
Qb = 50–200 mL/min   Qf = 2–8 mL/min
Qd = 50–200 mL/min   K = 40–60 L/24h

CPFA—Continuous plasmafiltration adsorption

A highly permeable plasmafilter filters Fluid
   plasma allowing it to pass through a bed of
   adsorbent material (carbon or resins)
Fluid balance maintained
Can be coupled with CVVH or CVVHD/F
Qb = 50–200 mL/min   Pf = 20–30 mL/min

Figure 115-2   Schematic representation and definitions of the different continuous renal replacement therapies according to standard nomenclature. Functional capabilities are described. A, artery; D, dialysate; K, clearance; Pf, plasma filtration rate; Qb, arterial flow; Qd, dialysate flow; Qf, ultrafiltration rate; UF, ultrafiltrate; UFc, ultrafiltrate control pump; V, vein.

All critically ill patients need a high daily amount of volume infusions: blood and fresh frozen plasma, vasopressors and other continuous infusions, parenteral and enteral nutrition, which should be delivered without restriction or interruption. It is not uncommon for patients with AKI and associated septic shock to receive large amounts of fluid resuscitation, leading to fluid overload. The consequent positive fluid balance and tendency to interstitial edema causes the necessity for water removal and possibly the achievement of a negative daily fluid balance. Extracorporeal renal replacement therapies are typically utilized for ultrafiltration. Ultrafiltered water has a similar osmolarity to plasma water; for this reason, the process of "isolated ultrafiltration" substantially corresponds to blood dehydration, with possible increase of hematocrit values and smallest modification of solutes concentration.[16] CRRT slowly and continuously removes a patient's plasma water, mimicking urine output, whereas thrice-weekly intermittent hemodialysis must extract in few hours the equivalent of 2 days of administered fluids plus excess body water that may be present in the anuric patient. Intravascular volume depletion associated with excessive ultrafiltration rate is due to both the high rate of fluid removal required and the transcellular and interstitial fluid shifts caused by the rapid dialytic loss of solute. The major consequence of rapid fluid removal is hemodynamic instability. Consider the case of a septic patient with AKI who is receiving a high amount of vasopressors because of hemodynamic instability and needs appropriate fluid resuscitation, supplementation of nutrition, and blood product administration. The renal replacement modality of choice seems to be the one that warrants slow fluid removal, prolonged for many hours a day, to easily meet the highly variable required daily fluid balance. In particular, when volemic and uremic control is not a problem, an aggressive protein-rich nutritional policy (1.5-2.5 g/d) can be implemented in the care of AKI patients receiving CRRT, resulting in a marked improvement in daily nitrogen balance with possible favorable effects on immune function and overall outcome.[17] Safe prescription of fluid loss during renal replacement therapy requires intimate knowledge of the patient's underlying condition, understanding of the process of ultrafiltration, and close monitoring of the patient's cardiovascular response to fluid removal. To preserve tissue perfusion in patients with AKI, it is important to optimize fluid balance by removing the patient's excess water without compromising effective circulating fluid volume. It is still a matter of controversy which clinical parameter (actual patient weight/patient dry weight, mean arterial pressure, central venous pressure, wedge pressure, systemic saturation, mixed venous saturation, bioimpedance, etc.) or currently available monitoring (central venous catheter, Swan-Ganz catheter, transesophageal echocardiography, etc.) should be utilized to uniformly define the concept of "volume overload." In patients who are clinically fluid overloaded, however, it is extremely important to accurately evaluate the amount of fluid to remove[18]; one of the main features of slow and constant ultrafiltration is the possibility for interstitial fluid to slowly and constantly refill the "dehydrated" bloodstream. This phenomenon is driven by hydrostatic and osmotic forces and allows for elimination of high plasma water volumes per day, with a reduced risk of hypovolemia and hypotension. In critically ill children, correction of water overload is considered a priority; it has been shown and recently confirmed that restoring adequate water content in small children is the main independent variable for outcome prediction.[19] Similar results have been recently found in a large cohort of adult critically ill patients with AKI.[20]

Solute removal is a very broad concept generally described by the elimination of a marker solute. This marker solute should be reasonably representative of all solutes normally removed from blood by the kidney. Unfortunately, a reference solute that represents all the solutes accumulating during AKI is currently unavailable because kinetics and volume of distribution are different for each molecule. "Single-solute control" during RRT represents only a rough estimate of treatment efficiency. With these specifications, urea is generally utilized as an imperfect marker molecule because of its accumulation in all patients with AKI and the ease of serum level measurement. Furthermore, despite its moderate toxicity, urea is the final product of protein metabolism; its accumulation describes the need for dialysis, and its removal describes treatment efficiency. It is a small molecule, and its volume of distribution is similar to total body water. It is not bound to protein and freely passes through tissues and cell membranes. Creatinine has similar characteristics and is another commonly used marker solute.

One of the measures utilized to quantify urea/creatinine removal is dialysis dose. One of the main aspects of dose to be understood is the concept of clearance (K): K is the volume of blood cleared from a given solute over a given time. K does not reflect the overall solute removal rate (mass transfer) but rather its value normalized by the serum concentration. Even when K remains stable over time, the removal rate will vary if the blood levels of the reference molecule change. K depends on solute molecular size, intercompartmental transmittance (K_c), transport modality (diffusion or convection), and circuit operational characteristics (blood flow rate, dialysate flow rate, ultrafiltration rate, hemodialyzer type, and size). As originally conceived, K is utilized to evaluate renal function among disparate individuals whose kidneys are operating 24 hours a day and urea/creatinine blood levels are at steady state. For this reason, the concept of K is easily applicable to continuous treatments, and its use to describe intermittent therapy efficiency is a sort of adaptation. Because K represents only the instantaneous efficiency of the system, during treatments with different time schedules, information about the time span during which K is delivered is fundamental to compare the different RRT doses. For example, K is typically higher in IHD than in CRRT and sustained low-efficiency daily dialysis. However, daily mass removal may be greater during CRRT or sustained low-efficiency daily dialysis because the K is applied for 12/24 hours (Table 115-2). In any case, from a physiologic point of view, even if a continuous and an intermittent therapy were prescribed in order to provide exactly the same marker solute removal, still they could not be comparable: during continuous treatments, where a relatively low K is applied, a slow but prolonged removal of solutes approaches a pseudo-steady state slope (Figure 115-3). In highly intermittent therapies, the intensive K, limited to 4 to 6 hours per day, thrice a week, causes the sawtooth slope in solute removal and eventual rebound during the time span without treatment. These peaks and valleys of solutes, bicarbonate, electrolytes, plasma osmolarity, and volemia are not physiologic and might have a detrimental impact on a patient's hemodynamics and the balance of electrolytes, acid-base, and other "osmoles." Furthermore, in the case of intermittent hemodialysis, the K_c (i.e., the variable tendency of different tissues to "release" a solute into the bloodstream) is much more relevant than during low-efficiency treatments. As a matter of fact, solute control is optimized during CRRT.

It has been calculated that if the solute target in a 70-kg patient was, for example, a mean blood urea nitrogen level of 60 mg/dL, this would be easily obtainable with a "standard" continuous venovenous hemofiltration dose, but it might be very difficult to be reached by even intensive intermittent hemodialysis regimens.[16] Some authors have recently suggested expressing CRRT daily dose as K indexed to patient body weight. The current recommendation is to administer a CRRT

TABLE 115-2	Quantitative Blood Purification		
	Daily Short Hemodialysis	*SLEDD*	*CVVH*
Clearance (mL/min)	200	80	20
Urea [C]o (mg/dL)	110	110	70
Urea [C]t (mg/dL)	30	30	65
Treatment time (min)	180	480	1440
Kt/V	1.12	1.24	0.8
Total clearance (L)	36	38.4	28.8
Urea removed (g)	18	27	30.6

CVVH, continuous venovenous hemofiltration; SLEDD, slow low-efficiency extended daily dialysis; [C]o, concentration of urea at zero; [C]t, concentration of urea at end of treatment.

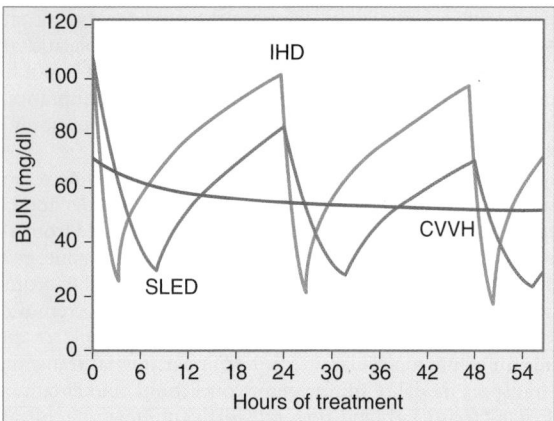

Figure 115-3 Patterns of solute removal during different renal replacement therapies. Slow and steady clearance of continuous treatments allows lower average serum urea levels than during intermittent therapies and avoids potentially dangerous peaks of solute increase. Importantly, since clearance does not reflect overall solute removal rate (mass transfer) but rather its value normalized by the solute serum concentration, when solute concentration rapidly decreases (intermittent dialysis), it ends up with a lower mass transfer than when solute levels are steady (continuous treatments). BUN, blood urea nitrogen; CVVH, continuous venovenous hemofiltration; IHD, intermittent hemodialysis; SLED, slow low-efficiency dialysis.

dose between 25 and 35 mL/h/kg per 24 hours.[21] Simplifying for low-molecular-weight solutes, K equals replacement solution and/or dialysate flow, and "standard" dose of a CRRT session may be expressed in a 70-kg patient as about 2500 mL/h (35 mL/h × 70 kg) per 24 hours or 60 L/day (2500 mL/h × 24 h) of replacement solution during continuous venovenous hemofiltration (CVVH) or of dialysate during continuous venovenous hemodialysis (CVVHD). It is expected this recommended dose will be modified in the next years, after the production of new evidence in this field (see later).

Oligoanuric patients often have mild acidemia secondary to increased unmeasured anions (strong ion gap [SIG] 12.3 mEq/L), hyperphosphatemia, and hyperlactatemia. This acidosis is attenuated by the alkalizing effect of hypoalbuminemia. Uchino and coworkers[22] compared the effect on acid-base balance of intermittent hemodialysis and continuous venovenous hemodiafiltration. Before treatment, metabolic acidosis was common in both groups (63.2% for intermittent hemodialysis and 54.3% for continuous venovenous hemodiafiltration). Both intermittent hemodialysis and continuous venovenous hemodiafiltration corrected metabolic acidosis, but the rate and degree of correction differed significantly. Continuous venovenous hemodiafiltration normalized metabolic acidosis more rapidly and more effectively during the first 24 hours than did intermittent hemodialysis ($P < 0.01$). Intermittent hemodialysis was also associated with a higher incidence of metabolic acidosis than was continuous venovenous hemodiafiltration during the subsequent 2-week treatment period. Accordingly, continuous venovenous hemodiafiltration can be considered physiologically superior to intermittent hemodialysis in the correction of metabolic acidosis.

In a comparison between CVVH and peritoneal dialysis, all patients randomized to CVVH achieved correction of acidosis by 50 hours of treatment, compared with only 15% of those treated by peritoneal dialysis ($P < 0.001$).[23]

Rocktaschel showed that once CVVH is commenced, acidemia is corrected within 24 hours. This change is associated with a decreased SIG and decreased phosphate and chloride concentrations. After 3 days of CVVH, patients develop alkalemia secondary to metabolic alkalosis due to a further decrease in SIG and a decrease in serum phosphate concentration in the setting of persistent hypoalbuminemia.[24]

ANTICOAGULATION DURING CONTINUOUS RENAL REPLACEMENT THERAPY

The flow of blood through an extracorporeal circuit causes activation of the coagulation cascade and promotes clotting of the filter and circuit itself. To delay such clotting and achieve acceptable operational life (≈24 hours) for the circuit, anticoagulation frequently is used.[25] Circuit anticoagulation increases the statistical risk of bleeding for the patient, however. The clinician must weigh the risks and benefits of more or less intense anticoagulation. In this regard, the intensivist has several strategies available (Table 115-3).

In most patients, low-dose heparin (<10 units/kg/h) is sufficient to achieve adequate filter life.[26] Heparin is easy and inexpensive to administer, easy to reverse, and at these doses has almost no effect on the patient's coagulation tests. In some patients, a higher dose is necessary. In others (pulmonary embolism, myocardial ischemia), full heparinization may be indicated concomitantly and should be pursued. Regional citrate anticoagulation is effective but requires that the hospital pharmacy or ICU use a special dialysate or replacement fluid. Citrate anticoagulation is expensive and more complex to organize. Nonetheless, it provides excellent and effective anticoagulation at minimal risk to the patient and has become a first choice of anticoagulation in many centers.[25] Regional heparin/protamine anticoagulation also is complex but may be useful if frequent filter clotting occurs and further anticoagulation of the patient is considered dangerous. Low-molecular-weight heparin also is efficacious but more expensive and hard to reverse because it accumulates in renal failure. It has not been shown to provide any advantages over unfractionated heparin. Heparinoids and prostacyclin may be useful if the patient has developed heparin-induced thrombocytopenia and thrombosis and citrate is not available. Serine proteinase inhibitors have been used but are not available outside Japan. Finally, in perhaps 10% to 20% of patients, anticoagulation is best avoided because of endogenous coagulopathy or recent surgery. In such patients, mean filter life of greater than 24 hours can be achieved provided that blood flow is kept at 200 mL/min and vascular access is reliable.[27]

Many circuits clot for mechanical reasons (inadequate access, unreliable blood flow from double-lumen catheter, depending on patient position, and kinking of catheter). Responding to frequent filter clotting by simply increasing anticoagulation without making the correct etiologic diagnosis (checking catheter flow and position, taking a history surrounding the episode of clotting, identifying the site of clotting) is often futile and exposes the patient to unnecessary risk of bleeding.

CONTINUOUS RENAL REPLACEMENT THERAPY TECHNOLOGY

The increasing use of venovenous CRRT has led to the development of a series of CRRT technologies that offer different kinds of machines to facilitate its performance.[28] Some understanding of these devices is important for the successful implementation of CRRT in any ICU. The simplest technical approach is to allow ultrafiltration to occur

TABLE 115-3	Strategies for Circuit Anticoagulation During Continuous Renal Replacement Therapy

No anticoagulation
Low-dose prefilter heparin (<500 units/h)
Medium-dose prefilter heparin (500-1000 units/h)
Full heparinization
Regional anticoagulation (prefilter heparin and postfilter protamine usually at a 100 units:1 mg ratio)
Regional citrate anticoagulation (prefilter citrate and postfilter calcium—special calcium-free dialysate needed)
Low-molecular-weight heparin
Prostacyclin
Heparinoids
Serine proteinase inhibitors (nafamostat mesilate)

spontaneously, measure it, and replace it as indicated. In such a system, hourly measurement of effluent is necessary, and the only requirement is that of a blood pump to deliver blood to the filter and a volumetric pump to administer replacement fluid at the appropriate rate. This approach is clearly inadequate in a modern ICU; such a system is inherently unsafe and labor intensive. A volumetric pump can regulate effluent flow easily, however. One can have a simple blood pump with safety features (air bubble trap and pressure alarms) and use widely available volumetric pumps to control replacement or dialysate flow and effluent flow. Such adaptive technology is inexpensive (approximately $10,000 U.S. dollars) but is not user-friendly. Also, volumetric pumps have an inherent inaccuracy of about 5%, which in a system exchanging 50 L/d can cause problems.[28] Various manufacturers have produced custom-made machines for hemofiltration. For a detailed discussion of such machines, the reader is referred to specialist textbooks.[28] These machines are safer and have much more sophisticated pump-control systems, alarms, and graphic displays. They are much more user-friendly, especially with the setup procedure. Most if not all ICUs in developed countries now conduct CRRT with third-generation devices characterized by advanced built-in technology and a high degree of automation.

Intermittent Hemodialysis

Intermittent hemodialysis remains dominant in the United States. Vascular access is typically by double-lumen catheter as in continuous hemofiltration. Intermittent hemodialysis machines use high dialysate flows (300-400 mL/min), however, and generate dialysate by using purified water and concentrate. Conventionally, intermittent hemodialysis is applied for short periods (3-4 hours), usually every second day. These features are summarized in Figure 115-4. The same applies to acid-base control. Limited fluid and uremic control imposes unnecessary limitations on nutritional support. Rapid solute shifts increase brain water content and intracranial pressure.[29] Finally, much controversy has surrounded the issue of membrane bioincompatibility. Standard low-flux dialyzing membranes made of cuprophane are known to trigger the activation of several inflammatory pathways, much more so than high-flux synthetic membranes (also used for continuous

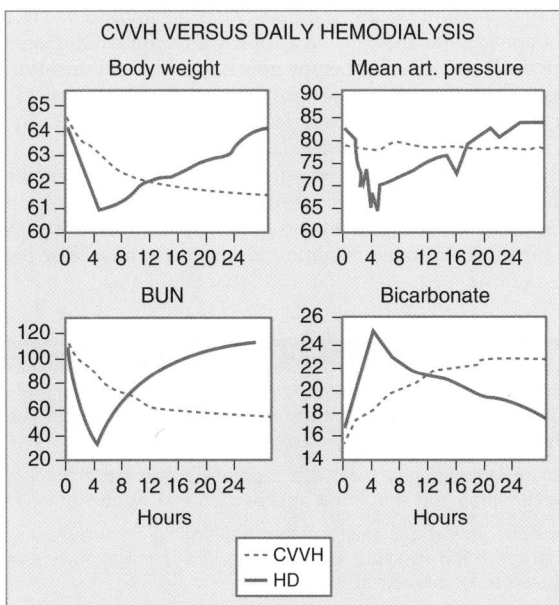

Figure 115-4 Comparisons of mean arterial pressure, body weight, blood urea nitrogen (BUN), and bicarbonate control with continuous and intermittent therapies, showing smoother and less varied control of all parameters with continuous treatment. CVVH, continuous venovenous hemofiltration; HD, hemodialysis.

hemofiltration). It is possible that such a proinflammatory effect contributes to further renal damage and delays recovery or even affects mortality.[30,31]

The serious limitations of applying "conventional" intermittent hemodialysis (3-4 h/d every second day) to the treatment of AKI have been highlighted,[8] and new approaches to intermittent therapies (so-called hybrid techniques) such as slow extended dialysis, slow low-efficiency daily dialysis, and intermittent extended hemofiltration are emerging. These techniques seek to adapt intermittent hemodialysis to the clinical circumstance and increase its tolerance and clearances. In our opinion, such hybrid approaches represent a welcome improvement in dialysis support and a clear recognition that AKI patients should not receive the dialysis offered to patients with end-stage renal failure.

Peritoneal Dialysis

Peritoneal dialysis is not commonly used in the treatment of adult AKI, either in the United States or elsewhere.[32] Typically, access is by the surgical insertion of an intraperitoneal catheter. Glucose-rich dialysate is inserted into the peritoneal cavity and acts as the "dialysate." After a given "dwell time," it is removed and discarded with the extra fluid and toxins that have moved from the blood vessels of the peritoneum to the dialysate fluid. Machines also are available that deliver and remove dialysate at higher flows through a double-lumen peritoneal catheter, providing intermittent treatment and higher solute clearances. Several major shortcomings make peritoneal dialysis relatively unsuited to the treatment of adult AKI:

1. Limited, sometimes inadequate solute clearance
2. High risk of peritonitis
3. Unpredictable hyperglycemia
4. Fluid leaks
5. Protein loss
6. Interference with diaphragm function

There have been no reports since the 1980s of the sole use of peritoneal dialysis for treatment of adult ICU patients with AKI. Despite this, the new technique called *continuous flow peritoneal dialysis* might offer something new in this field. No studies have been conducted so far. Peritoneal dialysis is a frequently used option in the case of pediatric AKI, and the typical patient is the post–cardiac surgery neonate; in these patients, peritoneal dialysis is a fundamental contributor in optimization of fluid balance.[33]

Drug Prescription During Dialysis Therapy

AKI and the need for renal replacement therapy profoundly affect drug clearance. A comprehensive description of changes in drug dosage according to the technique of renal replacement therapy, residual creatinine clearance, and other determinants of pharmacodynamics is beyond the scope of this chapter and can be found in specialist textbooks.[34] Table 115-4 provides general guidelines for the prescription of drugs that are commonly used in the ICU.

Controversies in Renal Replacement Therapy

Several controversies currently surround the use, timing, dose, and choice of renal replacement therapy. The most pressing question if continuous hemofiltration is used is the dose of treatment and whether it may be an important determinant of outcome. Furthermore, it is still not clear that CRRT, apart from theoretical discussions, offers an actual important survival advantage over intermittent hemodialysis in the management of AKI.

A single-center randomized controlled trial showed that increasing the ultrafiltration rate from 20 to 35 mL/kg/h significantly increased survival.[11] After this landmark study, up to 2007, the best evidence supported use of at least 35 mL/kg/h for CRRT. Lower doses of renal

TABLE 115-4	Drug Dosage During Dialytic Therapy*	
Drug	*CRRT*	*IHD*
Aminoglycosides	Normal dose q 36 h	Half normal dose q 48 h; two-thirds redose after IHD
Cefotaxime or ceftazidime	1 g q 8-12 h	1 g q 12-24 h after IHD
Imipenem	500 mg q 8 h	250 mg q 8 h and after IHD
Meropenem	500 mg q 8 h	250 mg q 8 h and after IHD
Metronidazole	500 mg q 8 h	250 mg q 8 h and after IHD
Co-trimoxazole	Normal dose q 18 h	Normal dose q 24 h after IHD
Amoxicillin	500 mg q 8 h	500 mg daily and after IHD
Vancomycin	1 g q 24 h	1 g q 96-120 h
Piperacillin	3-4 g q 6 h	3-4 g q 8 h and after IHD
Ticarcillin	1-2 g q 8 h	1-2 g q 12 h and after IHD
Ciprofloxacin	200 mg q 12 h	200 mg q 24 h and after IHD
Fluconazole	200 mg q 24 h	200 mg q 48 h and after IHD
Acyclovir	3.5 mg/kg q 24 h	2.5 mg/kg/d and after IHD
Ganciclovir	5 mg/kg/d	5 mg/kg/48 h and after IHD
Amphotericin B	Normal dose	Normal dose
Liposomal amphotericin B	Normal dose	Normal dose
Ceftriaxone	Normal dose	Normal dose
Erythromycin	Normal dose	Normal dose
Milrinone	Titrate to effect	Titrate to effect
Amrinone	Titrate to effect	Titrate to effect
Catecholamines	Titrate to effect	Titrate to effect
Ampicillin	500 mg q 8 h	500 mg daily and after IHD

*These values represent approximations and should be used as a general guide only. Critically ill patients have markedly abnormal volumes of distribution for these agents, which affects dosage. CRRT is conducted at variable levels of intensity in different units, also requiring adjustment. The values reported here relate to continuous venovenous hemofiltration at 2 L/h of ultrafiltration. Vancomycin is variably removed during continuous venovenous therapies, and constant evaluation of serum levels is recommended. IHD also may differ from unit to unit. The values reported here relate to standard IHD with low-flux membranes for 3 to 4 hours every second day.

CRRT, continuous renal replacement therapy; *IHD,* intermittent hemodialysis.

replacement therapy (RRT) were not recommended. More evidence finally came from two very recent trials. A small randomized controlled trial on 200 critically ill patients with AKI concluded that patient survival or renal recovery was not different between patients receiving high-dose (35 mL/kg/h) or standard-dose (20 mL/kg/h) continuous venovenous hemodiafiltration.[35] A second trial under the sponsorship of the Veterans Affairs/National Institutes of Health (VA/NIH) Acute Renal Failure Trial Network, randomly assigned 1124 critically ill patients with AKI and failure of at least one nonrenal organ or sepsis to receive intensive or less intensive RRT.[36] In both groups, only hemodynamically stable patients underwent intermittent hemodialysis, whereas hemodynamically unstable patients underwent continuous venovenous hemodiafiltration or sustained low-efficiency dialysis. Patients receiving the intensive treatment strategy underwent intermittent hemodialysis (Kt/V 1.2) and sustained low-efficiency dialysis 6 times per week and continuous venovenous hemodiafiltration at 35 mL/h/kg of body weight. For patients receiving the less intensive treatment strategy, corresponding treatments were provided thrice weekly and at 20 mL/h/kg. Sixty-day mortality was 53.6% with intensive therapy and 51.5% with less intensive therapy. There was no significant difference between the two groups in duration of renal replacement therapy or rate of recovery of kidney function or nonrenal organ failure. After this trial, operators might reasonably change their standard RRT dose prescriptions to a lower level than previously recommended; nonetheless, many concerns about the study have risen. On a time-averaged basis, greater urea removal occurred in patients receiving less intensive continuous renal replacement on a given day than in those receiving intensive intermittent hemodialysis. This uncertain separation of the dose during periods of unknown duration makes failure to observe a treatment effect unsurprising in the study.

Of note, despite being judged clinically hemodynamically stable, the relatively high rate of severe hypotensive events in patients treated with intermittent hemodialysis may argue the ATN approach to modality assignment and suggests that from a hemodynamic point of view, a greater number of patients may have benefited from more liberal use of continuous renal replacement than that chosen for the study. In any case, it is possible that strategies other than only increasing dialysis dose might help AKI patients. Current approaches to dialysis are probably inadequate to fully replace critical functions such as regulation of fluid balance, electrolyte and acid-base homeostasis, and efficient down-regulation of the inflammatory response, which might play a major role in the pathophysiology of AKI.

The Randomized Evaluation of Normal versus Augmented Level Replacement Therapy (RENAL) Trial was planned to test the hypothesis that higher-dose continuous venovenous hemodiafiltration at an effluent rate of 40 mL/kg/h would increase survival compared to continuous veno-venous hemodiafiltration at 25 mL/kg/h of effluent dose.[37] This trial randomized 1508 critically ill patients in 35 ICUs in Australia and New Zealand: 747 were randomly assigned to higher-intensity therapy and 761 to lower-intensity therapy. The two study groups received treatment for an average of 6.3 and 5.9 days, respectively. At 90 days after randomization, 322 deaths had occurred in the higher-intensity group and 332 deaths in the lower-intensity group, for a mortality of 44.7% in each group. Overall, the mortality rates were significantly lower, and recovery of kidney function in surviving patients was more common in the RENAL study than in the ATN study. It is possible that these differences are related to alternative strategies for the timing of initiation of RRT and to greater use of continuous therapy, as compared with intermittent therapy, as the initial mode of renal replacement in the RENAL Study. However, they may also be due to differences between the two study populations. Results of the ATN and RENAL studies imply that if a threshold dose of therapy must be achieved to optimize clinical outcomes, increasing the intensity of therapy beyond this dose seems not to provide further clinical benefit. Unfortunately, as recently shown by the DoReMi study group, such minimal dosing threshold is often not achieved.[38]

Summary

Renal replacement therapy has undergone remarkable changes and is continuing to evolve rapidly. Technology is being improved to facilitate clinical application, and new areas of research are developing. Continuous renal replacement therapy now is firmly established throughout the world as perhaps the most commonly used form of RRT. Conventional dialysis, which was slowly decreasing in use, is reappearing in the form of slow extended dialysis and slow low-efficiency daily dialysis, especially in the United States. Meanwhile, novel membranes, sorbents, and different intensities of treatment are being explored in the area of sepsis management and liver support. Intensivists need to keep abreast of this rapid evolution if they are to offer their patients the best of care.

KEY POINTS

1. Uremia is the accumulation of uremic toxins of different molecular weights associated with pathogenicity secondary to kidney dysfunction.

2. Acute kidney injury (AKI) is a separate syndrome from chronic renal failure and should be approached in a distinct manner.

3. Specific indications exist for the initiation of renal replacement therapy (RRT) in acute kidney injury. Early initiation has been shown to be beneficial.

4. Multiple therapeutic modalities of RRT exist to treat AKI. No modality is clearly superior to another. Treatments should be tailored depending on the clinical scenario.

5. Knowledge of prescribed drug pharmacokinetics is important when dosing patients on renal replacement therapy.

ANNOTATED REFERENCES

Bellomo R. Continuous hemofiltration as blood purification in sepsis. New Horiz 1995;3:732-7.

This article represents the beginning of the use of renal replacement therapy for the treatment of sepsis.

Bellomo R, Ronco C. Adequacy of dialysis in the acute renal failure of the critically ill: the case for continuous therapies. Int J Artif Organs 1996;19:129-42.

This is the first article to deal with adequacy of renal replacement therapy in critically ill patients.

Kellum JA, Mehta RL, Angus DC, et al. The first international consensus conference of CRRT. Kidney Int 2002;62:1855-63.

This is the first consensus publication on renal replacement therapy in the ICU provided by the Acute Dialysis Quality Initiative.

Ronco C, Bellomo R. Acute renal failure and multiple organ dysfunction in the ICU: from renal replacement therapy (RRT) to multiple organ support therapy (MOST). Int J Artif Organs 2002;25:733-47.

This article describes the first approach to multiple organ dysfunction with a complex and articulated extracorporeal system as a platform for therapy.

Ronco C, Bellomo R, Homel P, et al. Effects of different doses in continuous veno-venous haemofiltration on outcomes of acute renal failure: a prospective randomized trial. Lancet 2000;355:26-30.

This article reports on the largest randomized prospective trial on dose of renal replacement therapy in the ICU. This article has set the standard for dialysis dose in the ICU.

RENAL Replacement Therapy Study Investigators; Bellomo R, Cass A, Cole L, Finfer S, Gallagher M, Lo S, et al. Intensity of continuous renal-replacement therapy in critically ill patients. N Engl J Med 2009; 361:1627-38.

A landmark randomized clinical trial that shows the absence of beneficial effects from increasing continuous renal replacement dose from 25 to 40 mL/kg/h.

VA/NIH Acute Renal Failure Trial Network; Palevsky PM, Zhang JH, O'Connor TZ, Chertow GM, Crowley ST, Choudhury D, et al. Intensity of renal support in critically ill patients with acute kidney injury. N Engl J Med 2008;359:7-20.

The largest clinical trial on "routine" renal replacement therapy delivery in the United States (using both intermittent and continuous techniques). According to these authors, intensive renal replacement approach does not improve survival.

Kellum JA, Ronco C. Dialysis: results of RENAL—what is the optimal CRRT target dose? Nat Rev Nephrol 2010;6:191-2.

An interesting commentary that tries to synthesize the results of the recent randomized trials on the issue of dialysis dose.

REFERENCES

Access the complete reference list online at http://www.expertconsult.com.

Urinary Tract Obstruction

ISAAC TEITELBAUM | SCOTT LIEBMAN

A patent urinary tract is necessary for optimal kidney function. Under normal circumstances, urine passes unimpeded from the renal pelvises to the tip of the urethra. Obstruction can occur anywhere along this pathway and may lead to both acute and progressive kidney parenchymal damage.

Several definitions may be encountered when considering urinary tract obstruction:

- *Obstructive uropathy* refers to disorders that interfere with drainage of the urine. Obstructive uropathy can result from pathology within the urinary tract itself (intrinsic obstruction) or from pathology originating outside the urinary tract that causes external compression of the system (extrinsic obstruction). It may be acute or chronic and either partial or complete; the resulting symptom complex typically depends on both the acuity and severity.
- *Obstructive nephropathy* refers to cases in which obstructive uropathy causes a decline in renal function.
- *Hydronephrosis* refers to dilatation of the urinary collecting system, with renal parenchymal changes. Typically, however, the term is used to describe any dilatation of the urinary tract, regardless of renal parenchymal involvement. Hydronephrosis is usually, but not exclusively, seen in obstructive disorders. Nonobstructive pathogenesis of hydronephrosis includes vesicoureteral reflux or excessive flow through the collection system, such as with habitual water drinking or diabetes insipidus.

Epidemiology

Urinary tract obstruction is a common disorder. On autopsy, 3.1% of adults have hydronephrosis.[1] Data from the Healthcare Cost and Utilization Project's National Inpatient Sample (based on ICD-9 codes) indicate that 1.75% of all hospital discharges are complicated by either hydronephrosis or obstruction.[2] When hydronephrosis is excluded, urinary tract obstruction occurs in approximately 1% of hospital discharges.[2] Urinary tract obstruction accounts for approximately 10% of community-acquired acute kidney failure[3-5] and is a factor in 2.6% of acute kidney failure cases in the intensive care setting.[6]

Etiology

Many disorders may lead to urinary tract obstruction. A useful classification is to first divide causes by the level of obstruction: upper (from the renal pelvis to the ureterovesicular junction) or lower (from the bladder to the urethra) urinary tract. This approach may then be refined into intrinsic versus extrinsic causes.

CONGENITAL CAUSES

Congenital anomalies may result in obstruction at various levels of the urinary tract. This discussion will be limited to congenital ureteropelvic junction obstruction (UPJO), as this is the congenital disorder most likely to present in adulthood.

Congenital UPJO is usually due to disease intrinsic to the urinary tract. Often an adynamic segment of ureter results in failure of peristalsis at the ureteropelvic junction (UPJ).[7] Ureteral kinks or valves are another intrinsic cause of UPJO. Potential extrinsic causes of UPJO include abnormal rotation of the kidney during development, leading to ureteral compression and entrapment of the ureter by blood vessels, although significant controversy exists regarding the latter.[7,8]

Patients with UPJO often present with intermittent abdominal or flank pain, sometimes accompanied by nausea and vomiting. Alternatively, patients may present with hematuria or azotemia, or the condition may be uncovered after an imaging study done for an unrelated problem.

The widespread use of maternal prenatal ultrasound has lead to more antenatal diagnosis of UPJO. The diagnosis may be made by ultrasound, intravenous urography, or in equivocal cases, isotope renography (see later imaging section).

ACQUIRED CAUSES

There are many causes of acquired obstructive uropathy which may affect the urinary tract at any location from the renal tubules to the tip of the urethra. This discussion will consider upper and lower urinary tract obstruction separately, further dividing the causes into intrinsic versus extrinsic.

UPPER URINARY TRACT OBSTRUCTION

Intrinsic Causes

Intrinsic urinary tract obstruction may be due to pathology within the lumen (intraluminal) or within the walls of the collecting system (intramural).

Intraluminal Causes. Obstruction at the level of the renal tubules may be due to crystal-induced disease, uric acid nephropathy (as in the tumor lysis syndrome), or cast nephropathy due to multiple myeloma. Crystal-induced nephropathy has been classically described with sulfadiazine, acyclovir, indinavir, triamterene, and methotrexate.[9] Newer literature also implicates orlistat[10] and ciprofloxacin.[11]

Nephrolithiasis is a common cause of upper urinary tract obstruction at the level of the ureter, with the size of the stone determining the likelihood of obstruction. Stones ≤2 mm, 3 mm, 4 to 6 mm and larger than 6 mm will pass spontaneously 97%, 86%, 50%, and 1% of the time, respectively.[12] Typically the obstruction occurs at one of the three narrowest portions of the ureter: the UPJ, the ureterovesicular junction (UVJ), or at the point where the ureter crosses over the pelvic brim. The obstruction is usually, but not always, acute and symptomatic. Neoplasms, blood clots, and sloughed renal papillae are rarer causes of intrinsic obstruction at the level of the ureter.

The causes of intraluminal obstruction at the level of the bladder are similar to those affecting the ureter, with urolithiasis, blood clots, and neoplasms being most common. Worldwide, infection with *Schistosoma hematobium* with resulting fibrosis is a common cause of bladder obstruction.[13] Although rare in industrialized nations, it should be suspected in patients from endemic areas such as Africa and the Middle East.

Intramural Causes. Obstruction due to intramural causes is most often seen in the lower urinary tract. Disorders affecting the neuromuscular control of bladder emptying, such as cerebrovascular accidents,[14] spinal cord injury,[15] multiple sclerosis,[16] and diabetic neuropathy[17] may lead to bladder outlet obstruction. Multiple medications, including anticholinergics, opioid analgesics, nonsteroidal antiinflammatory agents, α-adrenoreceptor antagonists, benzodiazepines, and calcium channel blockers have also been associated with urinary retention.[18] Stricture of the urethra may also lead to obstruction.

One potential intramural cause affecting the upper tract is ureteral stricture due to genitourinary tuberculosis.

Extrinsic Compression

Pregnancy is typically associated with right-sided dilation of the renal pelvis, calyx, and ureter. Hormonal mechanisms and mechanical compression from an enlarging uterus and an enlarging ovarian vein plexus have been implicated in these changes.[19] Clinically meaningful obstruction from the gravid uterus is extremely rare.

Malignancies may cause obstruction by several different mechanisms. Local ureteric compression may be seen in metastatic cancers of the cervix, bladder and prostate, as well as with expanding retroperitoneal soft-tissue masses. Alternatively, the ureters may be compressed or encased by metastatic retroperitoneal lymphadenopathy from a distant primary.[20]

Retroperitoneal fibrosis may lead to obstruction of one or both ureters via inflammation. It is an uncommon disorder, with a reported incidence rate of 1.3 case per million population and a male/female ratio of 3.3:1.[21] Although the majority of these cases are idiopathic (>75%),[22] numerous conditions are suspected to cause retroperitoneal fibrosis, including malignancies, medications, infection, trauma, or radiation.[23] Treatment of idiopathic retroperitoneal fibrosis is initially with steroids, but recurrences are common. Case reports describe the use of cyclophosphamide, azathioprine, colchicine, mycophenolate, or tamoxifen for treatment relapses or steroid-resistant disease, although conclusive data are absent.[22] Abdominal aortic aneurysms (AAA) may also cause obstruction due to compression of the ureter or via inflammation. A recent series evaluated 999 cases of inflammatory AAA and found preoperative hydronephrosis in 7.4%.[24]

Extrinsic compression of the lower urinary tract is more common in males. The etiology is usually either benign prostatic hypertrophy or prostate cancer.

The clinician must always bear in mind that hydroureter and/or hydronephrosis may be absent in obstruction due to retroperitoneal processes. Thus, one must maintain a high degree of suspicion and use alternative imaging modalities when considering these disorders.

The etiology of urinary tract obstruction is summarized in Box 116-1.

Clinical Presentation

The clinical presentation of urinary tract obstruction depends on the location, duration, and severity of obstruction and may therefore be quite variable.

PAIN

Acute ureteral obstruction often presents with severe flank pain, otherwise known as *renal colic*. This is usually due to urolithiasis but may be due to other causes of ureteral obstruction (see earlier). Obstruction causes increased intraluminal pressure and spasm of the ureteral muscles, which are responsible for the colicky pain.[25] Partial ureteral obstruction may present with a chronic dull pain. Bladder outlet obstruction may lead to distention and subsequent abdominal discomfort.

CHANGES IN URINE OUTPUT

One pitfall in the diagnosis of obstruction is the expectation that patients will be anuric. While true of patients with obstruction of all functioning renal mass—complete bilateral ureteral obstruction, complete obstruction of a solitary functioning kidney, or complete obstruction distal to the bladder neck—this is not the case in patients with less severe disease. The degree of urine output does not reliably predict

---

Box 116-1

CAUSES OF URINARY TRACT OBSTRUCTION

Intrinsic Causes
Intraluminal
  Renal tubules:
    Crystal-induced disease
    Uric acid nephropathy
    Cast nephropathy (in multiple myeloma)
  Upper urinary tract:
    Nephrolithiasis
    Neoplasms
    Blood clots
    Sloughed renal papillae
  Lower urinary tract:
    Urolithiasis
    Blood clots
    Neoplasms
    Schistosomiasis
Intramural
  Upper urinary tract:
    Congenital ureteropelvic junction obstruction
    Genitourinary tuberculosis
  Lower urinary tract:
  Disorders affecting neuromuscular control:
    Cerebrovascular accident
    Spinal cord injury
    Multiple sclerosis
    Diabetic nephropathy
  Medications:
    Anticholinergic agents
    Opiates
    Nonsteroidal antiinflammatory agents
    α-Adrenoreceptor antagonists
    Benzodiazepines
    Calcium channel blockers
  Urethral structure

Extrinsic Causes
Upper urinary tract:
  Pregnancy
  Malignancy
  Retroperitoneal fibrosis
  Abdominal aortic aneurysms
Lower urinary tract:
  Benign prostatic hypertrophy
  Prostate cancer

---

the presence or absence of obstruction; patients may present with normal urine output or even polyuria due to the effects of obstruction on renal salt and water handling (reviewed later).

LOWER URINARY TRACT SYMPTOMS

Obstruction of the lower urinary tract often presents with some or all of a predictable constellation of symptoms known collectively as *lower urinary tract symptoms*, or *LUTS*. LUTS include voiding symptoms (difficulty urinating, incomplete emptying), postmicturition symptoms (post-void dribbling), and storage symptoms (urgency, frequency, hesitancy, incontinence).[26] Alternatively, patients with lower urinary tract obstruction may be asymptomatic.

KIDNEY DYSFUNCTION

If asymptomatic, the initial clue to underlying obstruction may be an elevated creatinine level on a blood sample drawn for an unrelated reason. The fact that urinary tract obstruction may be asymptomatic mandates its inclusion in the differential diagnosis of unexplained kidney failure. If blood work is not obtained during the course of the obstruction, the kidney function may deteriorate such that the first presentation is with uremic symptoms and need for dialysis.

INFECTION

The urinary retention associated with lower urinary tract obstruction provides an excellent culture medium for bacteria. Patients may present with cystitis, pyelonephritis, or sepsis. An obstructing renal stone may also be a nidus for infection. Recurrent infection should raise suspicion for possible anatomic abnormalities, especially in men. In one study, 25 out of 83 men (30%) with a febrile urinary tract infection (UTI) had anatomic lesions in the lower urinary tract, supporting imaging of the lower tract in men with this presentation.[27] More recent data refute this finding in men younger than 45 years old.[28]

LABORATORY VALUES

There are no laboratory values specific to obstruction. Blood tests may show no abnormalities or may show values consistent with kidney failure, such as elevated blood urea nitrogen, creatinine, potassium, and phosphorus levels and decreased calcium, bicarbonate, and hemoglobin values. The blood tests may also be indicative of a renal tubular acidosis (see later). The urinalysis may be bland or may include red blood cells (in the setting of a stone or malignancy) or white cells (in the setting of infection). An experienced observer may also be able to discern crystals in a freshly voided urine. The fractional excretion of sodium (FE_{Na}) may be less than 1% in acute obstruction, but it is generally greater than 1% when the obstruction is chronic, owing to renal tubular dysfunction.

◼ Imaging in Urinary Tract Obstruction

Various imaging modalities may be used to diagnose obstruction: plain abdominal radiography, ultrasound, CT, intravenous urography, retrograde pyelography, and nuclear scanning. It is important to understand the indications and limitations of each modality.

PLAIN ABDOMINAL RADIOGRAPHY

Abdominal radiography (kidney, ureter, and bladder [KUB]) is often the first imaging modality preformed in patients with acute flank pain. Although most stones are composed of calcium and should in theory be visible, only 59% of stones are detected on plain film.[29] Compared to CT scanning, the sensitivity and specificity of abdominal films were 45% to 59% and 77%, respectively.[29] Further, plain films may not always be able to differentiate phleboliths from calculi. This limits the utility of plain abdominal films to the diagnosis of recurrent disease in those with known radioopaque stones.

ULTRASOUND

Ultrasound (US) is inexpensive, does not expose the patient to radiation, and is typically readily available. Its accuracy in detecting hydronephrosis makes US a good screening tool for obstruction in the patient with unexplained kidney failure, or the patient with suspected lower urinary tract obstruction (Figure 116-1). US has been largely superseded by noncontrast CT in the detection of nephrolithiasis and stone-related obstruction. When CT is used as a reference, US has a sensitivity of 24% and a specificity of 90% for the detection of kidney stones and is likely to miss those less than 3 mm.[30] Another disadvantage of US compared to CT is that bowel gas may obscure visualization of the ureters.[31] Thus despite its ability to detect hydronephrosis, US may be limited in its ability to demonstrate the cause or site of an obstruction. Other conditions such as peripelvic cysts and renal artery aneurysms may mimic hydronephrosis on US.[31] These conditions are easily distinguished via CT scanning.

Features such as ureteral jets and resistive indices have been previously advocated as useful adjuncts in the diagnosis of obstruction, but evidence as to their utility is lacking. Despite its limitations, US may be the initial imaging modality of choice when radiation is contraindicated, such as in pregnant women and children.

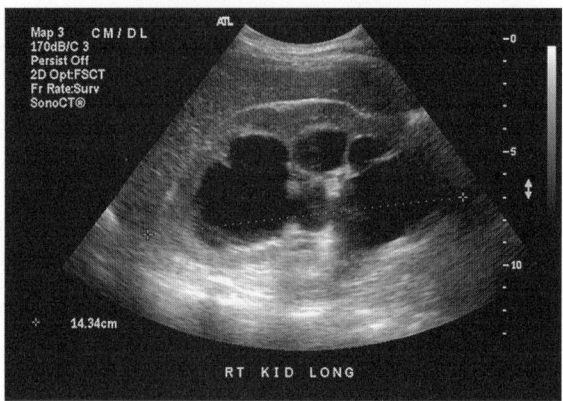

Figure 116-1 Typical appearance of a hydronephrotic kidney, showing renal pelvis and calyceal dilatation. Note the increase in kidney length (14.34 cm) compared with normal (~10-11 cm).

COMPUTED TOMOGRAPHY

The major utility of CT scanning as it relates to urinary tract obstruction is in the evaluation of acute flank pain and suspected nephrolithiasis (Figure 116-2). In this setting, CT offers a sensitivity of 96% and a specificity of 98% for detection of stones.[32] The retroperitoneum is also well visualized, making CT ideal to detect retroperitoneal fibrosis or obstruction due to retroperitoneal lymphadenopathy. In addition to defining the anatomy of the collecting system, CT has the added benefit of visualizing other organ systems, thereby providing information regarding other conditions in the differential diagnosis of acute flank pain.

One concern raised with CT scanning is the high radiation dose administered. Each CT scan is equivalent to approximately 10 KUBs.[33] Recent work has focused on lower-dose radiation protocols. One study found that lower-dose radiation CT scan (equivalent to that of a plain film) had a sensitivity of 97% and a specificity of 96% for the diagnosis of acute renal colic when compared with standard dose. The lower-dose CT was inferior at detecting stones less than 3 mm in size,[34] which may impair its ability to diagnose noncollecting system pathology.

ISOTOPE RENOGRAPHY

In conventional renography, radiographic tracers are injected into the patient's blood stream, and renal uptake and excretion are measured

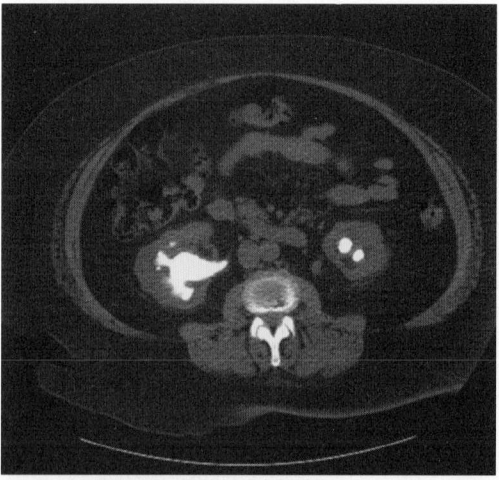

Figure 116-2 Bilateral nephrolithiasis on an unenhanced computed tomography (CT) scan. Note the staghorn appearance on the left.

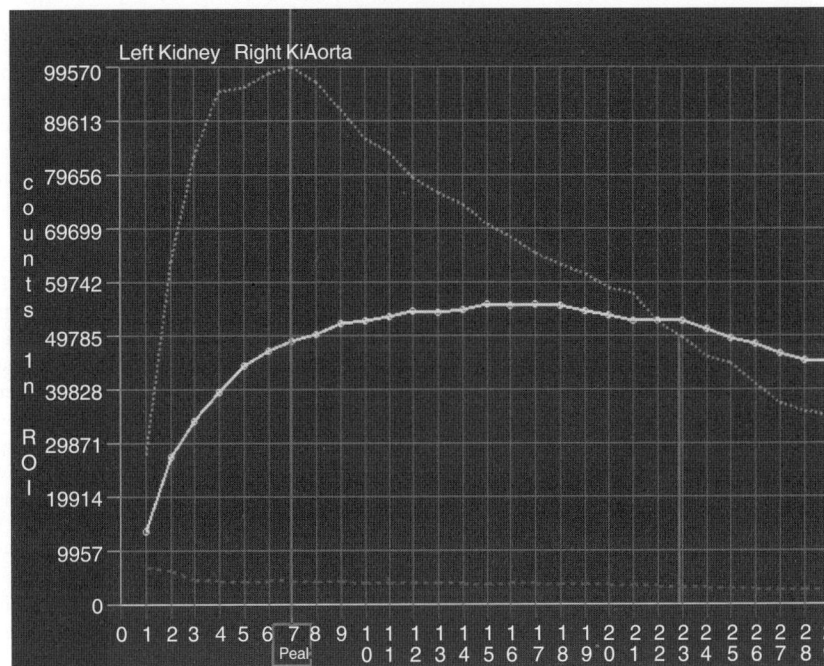

Figure 116-3 Renogram showing left-sided obstruction. Note that both kidneys take up the tracer. On the right side, this is followed by an excretion of the tracer, whereas on the left the tracer remains at peak value.

with a scintillation counter (Figure 116-3). This test provides functional information via demonstration of decreased excretion in the obstructed kidney. The sensitivity of the test may be enhanced by administering a loop diuretic prior to the scan. The increased urine flow may unmask an occult obstruction. Isotope renography may be used if obstruction is suspected clinically but hydronephrosis is absent, or to diagnose a nonobstructive cause of hydronephrosis. In this case, excretion will be normal despite the presence of the hydronephrosis. Isotope renography does not provide anatomic information.

INTRAVENOUS UROGRAPHY

Intravenous urography (IVU), in which the collecting system is imaged after the administration of intravenous (IV) contrast, used to be the study of choice for patients with acute flank pain. The need to administer nephrotoxic IV contrast and the delay in obtaining information render IVU less attractive than a CT scan.[32]

RETROGRADE PYELOGRAPHY

CT scanning and US have largely superseded retrograde pyelography for the diagnosis of obstruction. Retrograde pyelography may be indicated when obstruction is highly suspected on clinical grounds, the US is negative for hydronephrosis, and the patient is unable to receive IV contrast.[1]

Pathophysiology of Obstruction

Urinary tract obstruction may cause intrinsic kidney dysfunction. The most important effects are changes in renal blood flow, increased tubular hydrostatic pressure (as a result of increased ureteral pressure), and development of fibrosis in long-standing obstruction. Specific tubular derangements in sodium, water, potassium, acid, and divalent cation handling occur as well.

CHANGES IN RENAL BLOOD FLOW AND TUBULAR HYDROSTATIC PRESSURE

Over the last 3 decades, various animal models have demonstrated the pattern of renal blood flow and tubular hydrostatic pressure over time with obstruction. The initial renal response to obstruction follows a triphasic pattern.[35] During the first 2 hours of obstruction, there is an initial increase in both renal blood flow and ureteral pressure. This is followed by a brief (2-3 hour) period in which renal blood flow declines due to increased afferent arteriolar resistance, yet ureteral pressures continue to rise. Ultimately the decrease in renal blood flow leads to a decrease in ureteral pressure, with the pressure returning to normal levels by 10 to 12 hours after obstruction.[35] Unresolved obstruction will lead to persistent afferent arteriolar constriction and a sustained decrease in both renal blood flow and glomerular filtration rate (GFR).

The mediators of the hemodynamic responses are still under investigation. Prostaglandins may be involved in the initial vasodilation and increased blood flow, as this can be prevented with the prostaglandin inhibitor, indomethacin.[36] The subsequent vasoconstriction is thought to be due to a decrease in available nitric oxide resulting from decreased nitric oxide synthetase substrate.[35] In support of this theory are animal studies showing that the decrease in renal blood flow and GFR after obstruction may be attenuated with the administration of L-arginine, a nitric oxide precursor.[37] The renin-angiotensin system, in particular angiotensin II (AT II), has also been implicated as an important mediator of renal vasoconstriction during obstruction.[38] Identification of these mediators may result in future treatment strategies for patients with urinary tract obstruction.

CHANGE IN GLOMERULAR FILTRATION RATE

The change in GFR during obstruction is directly related to changes in tubular hydrostatic pressure and renal blood flow. GFR is determined by the interaction of Starling's forces between the glomerular capillary and the tubules. In the initial response to obstruction, GFR may decrease due to increasing tubular hydrostatic pressure, although the increased renal blood flow may attenuate this somewhat. Over time, however, the tubular hydrostatic pressure normalizes, and the decrease in renal blood flow becomes the main mechanism for the decreased GFR.

TUBULAR ATROPHY AND FIBROSIS

As with all long-standing kidney diseases, prolonged obstruction is associated with the development of tubular atrophy and interstitial fibrosis. Fibrosis results from an imbalance between extracellular matrix deposition and degradation. In urinary tract obstruction, there is simultaneous overproduction of profibrotic and underproduction of antifibrotic agents. Prominent among the former is AT II. In addition to its vasoconstrictive properties, AT II also has many profibrotic actions, including up-regulation of several other profibrotic mediators such as transforming growth factor beta-1 (TGF-β_1), tumor necrosis factor alpha (TNF-α), and nuclear factor kappa B (NFκB).[39] Conversely, the activities of metalloproteinases and plasminogen activating inhibitor-1, both antifibrotic, are decreased during obstruction.[38,39]

The tubular atrophy and loss of renal mass seen with obstruction are mainly due to apoptosis, which may begin as early as 4 days after obstruction.[39] Many mediators are involved including, potentially, AT II.[39] Given the importance of the renin-angiotensin system in promoting renal injury after obstruction, antagonizing AT II would appear to be a viable strategy to attenuate injury. Although human data are lacking, animal data show benefit, provided the intervention is done after renal development is complete.[38]

TUBULAR FUNCTION

Tubular responses to unilateral or bilateral obstruction differ, with bilateral obstruction (or unilateral obstruction in a patient with a solitary kidney) being much more severe and having more important clinical implications. The following discussion will be limited to bilateral obstruction. Urinary tract obstruction impairs all aspects of renal tubular function including the ability to transport sodium, potassium, and hydrogen and to regulate urine concentration.

SODIUM REABSORPTION

Upon release of a bilateral obstruction, sodium excretion increases five to nine times that of normal.[40] Because the GFR is also decreased due to the obstruction, fractional excretion of sodium may be 20 times higher than normal.[40] Clinically, this failure of sodium reabsorption may manifest as hypovolemia.

Animal studies have provided some insights as to the mechanisms of the abnormal sodium handling. Sodium reabsorption in the kidney is accomplished by various apical membrane transporters, which are coupled to the basolateral sodium-potassium ATPase. Many of these transporters, including the sodium/proton exchanger, sodium-phosphate cotransporter, sodium-potassium-2 chloride cotransporter, and the thiazide-sensitive cotransporter are down-regulated during and after release of obstruction.[41] Recent studies suggest that the amiloride-sensitive epithelial sodium channel may be down-regulated as well.[42] In addition to the down-regulation of transporters, up-regulation of atrial natriuretic peptide, a potent stimulus for sodium excretion, has been demonstrated during and after release of bilateral obstruction.[43]

RENAL WATER HANDLING

Several mechanisms render the kidneys unable to either concentrate or dilute urine after release of an obstruction. Both urinary concentration and dilution require function of the sodium transporters. In the case of urinary concentration, the sodium-potassium-2 chloride cotransporter is required to establish the medullary concentration gradient needed for osmotic water movement out of the collecting tubule. Dilution requires removal of solute in both the loop of Henle and distal convoluted tubule via the sodium-potassium-2 chloride cotransporter and the thiazide-sensitive cotransporter, respectively. Osmotic diuresis due to retained solutes may also lead to an inability to conserve water.

In addition to the effects of abnormal sodium reabsorption on water metabolism in the postobstructed kidney, animal data have demonstrated a direct role of antidiuretic hormone in the concentrating defect as well. Many studies have shown a down-regulation of aquaporins in the obstructed kidney,[44-47] which may persist for weeks, accompanied by a long-term defect in urinary concentration.[44] Clinically, this inability to conserve water may manifest as nephrogenic diabetes insipidus and hypernatremia.

ACID-BASE AND POTASSIUM BALANCE

Obstruction may be associated with an inability to excrete acid. Acid-base balance is accomplished by reclamation of filtered bicarbonate and excretion of acid, either as titratable acidity (buffering of hydrogen ions by phosphates, sulfates, and other buffers) or by ammonium excretion. Clinically, obstructed or postobstruction patients may have a hyperkalemic, hyperchloremic metabolic acidosis. Although this may be due solely to the decreased GFR, some patients have persistent metabolic abnormalities long after the release of obstruction and stabilization of GFR.[48] Human data reveal several pathophysiologic mechanisms. The majority of patients studied had a distal renal tubular acidosis in which systemic acidosis did not lower the urinary pH below 5.5.[48] Abnormalities in sodium transport in the distal nephron (see earlier) may render this tubular segment unable to generate the lumen negative transepithelial difference needed for proton excretion—a so-called voltage-dependent defect.[49] This voltage defect also leads to potassium retention and clinically apparent hyperkalemia. Other patients were able to acidify their urine to a pH of below 5.5. These patients had low plasma levels of aldosterone with subsequent hyperkalemia—a typical type IV renal tubular acidosis (RTA).[48] The underlying mechanism in this case is decreased ammoniagenesis, most likely due to the hyperkalemia, although the hypoaldosteronism may also contribute.[49] Patients with a type IV RTA retain the ability to excrete acid (via titratable acidity) and usually have a mild, self-limited acidosis, whereas those with a distal RTA cannot excrete acid, and the resultant acidosis may be severe.

Recent animal studies have demonstrated down-regulation of key renal acid-base transporters in urinary tract obstruction, including the cortical and medullary sodium hydrogen exchanger and several basolateral sodium-bicarbonate transporters.[50]

POSTOBSTRUCTIVE DIURESIS

Release of a bilateral obstruction (or unilateral obstruction of a solitary kidney) may lead to a profound diuresis. Several of the mechanisms have already been described. Defects in sodium and water handling predispose to large urinary losses of both. The osmotic load of retained solutes also contributes. Much of the diuresis is appropriate, however, in that previously retained salt and water must be excreted. Typically, a postobstructive diuresis is mild, transient, and requires no treatment. Often the degree and duration of this diuresis is worsened by overzealous saline administration in the face of a large, but potentially appropriate, urine output.

Clinical manifestations of a postobstructive diuresis which mandate treatment include volume depletion and hypernatremia (which may be managed by administration of isoosmotic and hypoosmotic fluid, respectively). Careful attention to potassium, magnesium, phosphorus, and calcium levels is warranted as well.

OTHER TUBULAR FUNCTIONS

After release of bilateral obstruction, phosphorus excretion rises proportionally to sodium excretion.[40] This may be mediated by a decrease in the number of proximal sodium phosphate cotransporters.[41] Magnesium excretion also rises, likely from decreased absorption in the thick ascending loop of Henle, due to a decrease in transepithelial voltage difference created by the decreased sodium-potassium-2 chloride cotransporter activity.[40] Calcium handling after obstruction is unclear and differs depending upon species studied.[40]

▨ Treatment

Management of obstructive uropathy depends on the location, severity, symptomatology, and etiology of obstruction, as well as the presence of concomitant factors such as infection or a decline in kidney function. The clinical scenario guides timing and whether initial management should be conservative or aimed at reestablishing patency of the urinary tract. A chronic asymptomatic partial obstruction does not need emergent release, whereas an acute, complete obstruction accompanied by infection, pain, or evidence of kidney dysfunction does.

Lower tract obstruction may be relieved simply by placing a urethral catheter, with subsequent evaluation by a urologist for definitive treatment. Upper urinary tract obstructions may be managed either with percutaneously inserted nephrostomy tubes or via retrograde (i.e., via cytoscope) ureteral stenting. As is the case with lower tract obstruction, subsequent urologic input for specific therapy for upper tract disease is indicated.

Factors which may cause or exacerbate obstruction, such as constipation or the use of medications associated with urinary retention, should be addressed. Other supportive measures such as antibiotics and IV hydration should be instituted if clinically warranted. The metabolic abnormalities of kidney failure, particularly hyperkalemia, should be addressed. If needed, dialysis should not be withheld while awaiting decompressive therapy.

Should the obstruction be chronic and the kidney deemed nonfunctional, it may be appropriate to proceed with nephrectomy if there is persistent pain or unresolved infection. This decision requires an estimate of the likelihood of recovery of kidney function.

Recovery of Kidney Function

Whether or not an obstructed kidney will regain function is of paramount importance to the clinician and may dictate whether aggressive interventions are indicated, or if the affected kidney should be removed. Unfortunately, data addressing this question, particularly human data, are scant. Currently there are no methods available which reliability predict kidney recovery after relief of an obstruction,[40] although one recent study found that a GFR of less than 10 mL/min in the obstructed kidney and abnormal renal perfusion (determined via isotope renography) predicted poor recovery in patients with unilateral ureteral occlusion.[51]

Animal studies demonstrate that the likelihood of renal recovery diminishes with longer duration of obstruction.[40] Even with recovery of GFR, there may be ongoing injury and progressive long-term kidney damage after release of obstruction, likely due to interstitial fibrosis associated with prolonged urinary tract obstruction.[52] In humans, the cutoff point at which renal function is unlikely to return has not been determined, and partial recovery has been seen even after months of obstruction,[53] suggesting that all obstructions be relieved and followed by serial determinations of kidney function. If desired, a kidney biopsy may be done to assess the degree of interstitial fibrosis and provide prognostic information.

KEY POINTS

1. Urinary tract obstruction is relatively common. It should be considered in all cases of unexplained acute kidney injury.

2. The causes of urinary tract obstruction are diverse and may be due to pathology anywhere from the renal tubules to the tip of the urethra. A common classification scheme divides urinary tract obstruction into upper (from the renal tubules to the ureteral-vesicular junction) and lower urinary tract (between the bladder and the urethra) pathology. Upper and lower urinary tract obstruction typically have a different constellation of signs and symptoms, and the treatment of these disorders is different.

3. Urinary tract obstruction may also be divided into intrinsic (due to pathology within the urinary tract itself) and extrinsic (compression of the urinary tract due to pathology in a different organ system) and congenital or acquired causes. Intrinsic causes may either be intraluminal or intramural.

4. The clinical presentation of urinary tract obstruction is varied. Upper urinary tract obstruction may present as renal colic with or without hematuria, whereas lower tract obstruction may present with lower urinary tract symptoms such as frequency, urgency, nocturia, hesitancy, and incomplete emptying. Urinary tract obstruction may also be completely asymptomatic and discovered only after finding an elevated blood urea nitrogen (BUN) and creatinine in the serum.

5. The presence of urine output does not exclude the diagnosis of urinary tract obstruction. Obstruction may present with any degree of urine output; the classic presentation of acute anuria is uncommon.

6. There are no specific laboratory findings which suggest obstruction. Patterns that may be seen include acute or chronic kidney disease with associated hyperphosphatemia, hypocalcemia, and anemia or a hyperchloremic metabolic acidosis with or without hyperkalemia. Urine findings may mimic prerenal azotemia early on, with low urinary sodium and a fractional excretion of sodium less than 1%; typically this is not seen in a chronic obstruction. Alternatively, the laboratory values may be completely normal.

7. Renal ultrasound is very specific in detecting obstruction. False-positive findings may be seen in cases of increased urinary flow or with vesicoureteral reflux. Computed tomography has become the imaging modality of choice for suspected nephrolithiasis.

8. Renal tubular function is altered in urinary tract obstruction. Tubular dysfunction may manifest as sodium wasting, abnormal water handling resulting in a nephrogenic diabetes insipidus, and derangements in acid-base balance resulting in an acidosis with or without hyperkalemia.

9. Release of bilateral obstruction (or unilateral obstruction of a solitary functioning kidney) may result in a postobstructive diuresis. The diuresis may be due to tubular dysfunction or an appropriate response to retention of nitrogenous waste products. Overzealous saline administration may prolong or even drive the diuresis.

10. Treatment of obstruction consists of addressing life-threatening complications such as hyperkalemia and gram-negative sepsis. Next, one must decide whether and how quickly the urinary system should be decompressed. A workup to determine and treat the underlying causes should be done in conjunction with a urologist.

11. Data regarding recovery of renal function are inconclusive. There is no imaging test that will predict whether renal function will return. Typically, recovery is dependent on the duration of obstruction; however, recovery has been observed even in patients who were dialysis dependent for months.

ANNOTATED REFERENCES

Shokeir AA. Renal colic: new concepts related to pathophysiology, diagnosis and treatment. Curr Opin Urol 2002;12:263-9.
This is an excellent overall review to the approach of renal colic. Newer data regarding pathophysiology, diagnosis, and treatment are reviewed. The article provides a rational approach to imaging in this disorder, focusing on the newer imaging modalities.

Fowler K, Locken J, Duchesne J, Willamson M. US for detecting renal calculi with nonenhanced CT as a reference standard. Radiology 2002;222:109-13.
This study examined the utility of ultrasound for diagnosing renal calculi as compared with a nonenhanced CT. The study found a sensitivity of 24% and a specificity of 90% for the detection of renal stones by ultrasound. Further, ultrasound failed to identify 73% of stones less than 3 cm. The authors concluded that ultrasound was of limited value in diagnosing nephrolithiasis compared with nonenhanced CT scanning.

Vaughan JED, Marion D, Poppas DP, Felsen D. Pathophysiology of unilateral ureteral obstruction: studies from Charlottesville to New York. J Urol 2004;172:2563-9.
This study provides an excellent overview of the changes in renal tubular function during obstruction. The authors provide data implicating up-regulation of the renal renin-angiotensin-aldosterone system, as well as the role of nitric oxide deficiency. The mechanisms of fibrosis are discussed, and the authors present current and future strategies to prevent the development and progression of kidney disease due to obstructive uropathy.

Chevalier R, Thornhill B, Forbes M, Kiley S. Mechanisms of renal injury and progression of renal disease in congenital obstructive nephropathy. Pediatr Nephrol 2010;25:687-97.
This articles reviews the cellular and molecular mechanisms responsible for the progressive kidney injury associated with obstruction. Pertinent cytokines and growth factors as well as mediators of renal injury are discussed. The authors discuss current and future strategies for preventing this injury.

Li C, Wang W, Kwon T-H, Knepper MA, Nielsen S, Frokiaer J. Altered expression of major renal Na transporters in rats with bilateral ureteral obstruction and release of obstruction. Am J Physiol Renal Physiol 2003;285:F889-901.
This article provides the molecular basis for the salt wasting observed after relief of bilateral obstruction. Levels of expression of renal sodium transporters were examined in rats after 24 hours of bilateral ureteral obstruction and at days 3 and 14 after relief of the obstruction. This article demonstrates the down-regulation of essentially all transporters during obstruction and the rates at which transporter function begins to normalize.

REFERENCES

Access the complete reference list online at http://www.expertconsult.com.

117

Contrast-Induced Nephropathy

M. KHALED SHAMSEDDIN | BRENDAN BARRETT

The use of intravascular iodinated radiocontrast media is very prevalent. After injection of these contrast agents, a mild transient kidney function impairment can be detected by sensitive tests.[1] However, clinically important kidney injury, known as *contrast-induced nephropathy* (CIN) or *contrast-induced acute kidney injury* (CIAKI), is less common, especially with normal preexisting kidney function.

CIN is usually defined as an acute kidney function impairment within 72 hours of intravascular injection of iodinated radiocontrast media, in the absence of other etiology. For research purposes, CIN is commonly defined as a 25% increase or an absolute increase in serum creatinine of 0.5 mg/dL (44 µmol/L) relative to precontrast values. Acute kidney injury (AKI) markers such as serum cystatin C, urinary neutrophil gelatinase-associated lipocalin (NGAL), or interleukin (IL)-18 will possibly be used in upcoming studies of CIN and may predict later CIN-associated morbidity and mortality.[1]

Awareness of the nephrotoxicity of contrast and the factors predisposing to it have improved over time to the point that clinicians may now overestimate the risk associated with some specific medical conditions.[2] However, the increasing use of radiographic contrast media, possibly combined with increasing age and comorbidity of the treated population, contribute to the continuing importance of contrast nephropathy. In reality, given the mild and transient nature of the AKI in most CIN cases, it is the association with later more momentous clinical adverse events that drives current interest in preventing CIN.

Epidemiology

The exact incidence of CIN is not clear, ranging from 1% to 30%. This variability is due to lack of consistent definitions, variation in patient risk, contrast dose, and likely route of injection (intraarterial versus intravenous [IV]).[2-4]

Typically, about 15% of patients undergoing coronary angiography have serum creatinine rise by more than 25%, but the risk for dialysis is less than 1%.[3] In the recent Cardiac Angiography in Renally Impaired Patients (CARE) Study,[5] CIN defined by serum creatinine rise occurred in 11.1% of the 414 enrolled patients, while smaller increments in creatinine or rise in cystatin C occurred more frequently.[5]

The frequency of similar kidney function impairment after IV contrast injection appears to be many-fold less common than after cardiac angiography.[6,7] In several studies, IV injection of nonionic low-osmolality contrast media (LOCM) in patients with chronic kidney disease was associated with a low risk of CIN.[8]

The fluctuation in serum creatinine due to other causes makes control groups not receiving contrast necessary to truly judge the risk to the kidney from IV contrast. In a small study, Langner et al. found a similar pattern of kidney function in a group having multiple contrast-enhanced studies with IV iodixanol as in a control group receiving no contrast media.[9]

A variety of contrast media are available for use, and certain media are recommended ahead of others if a contrast study is required in a patient at risk for CIN. Contrast media are often classified according to osmolality and as ionic or nonionic (Table 117-1), but these factors are not necessarily the most important in determining nephrotoxicity. High-osmolality contrast agents such as diatrizoate are not commonly used nowadays and were associated with greater risk to the kidney. The relative toxicity of low and iso-osmolal contrast agents is controversial. Recent analyses suggest that CIN incidence may be higher with iohexol

than with other LOCM, but the comparisons were across rather than within studies.[10] A meta-analysis of pooled data from 16 randomized controlled trials (RCTs) including 2727 patients showed that intraarterial injection of the iso-osmolar contrast medium (IOCM), iodixanol, was associated with smaller rises in serum creatinine and lower incidence of CIN relative to low-osmolar contrast media (LOCM) (1.4% versus 3.5%, P = 0.003), especially in chronic kidney disease patients with or without diabetes mellitus (3.5% versus 15.5%, P = 0.003; and 2.8% versus 8.4%, P = 0.001, respectively).[11] Nonetheless, a more recent meta-analysis of pooled data from 3270 patients and 25 trials including some of the above RCTs in addition to 7 new RCTs published within the last 3 years indicated that iodixanol is not associated with a significant decrease in the incidence of CIN compared with LOCM in the general population (relative risk [RR] = 0.80; 95% confidence interval [CI]: 0.61–1.04).[12] Further, in this meta-analysis, iodixanol (IOCM) was less nephrotoxic than iohexol but not noticeably superior to other LOCM.[12] Based on these data, current American Heart Association (AHA) guidelines recommend that either ioxaglate or a low-osmolality medium other than iohexol or ioxaglate be used in cases at risk for CIN.[13]

Risk Factors

The presence or absence of risk factors, especially preexisting kidney function, in addition to the type of imaging procedure are the most relevant predictors of CIN.[3] The risk of dialysis-requiring CIN will increase considerably if precontrast creatinine clearance is less than 47 mL/min (0.78 mL/sec).[3] Diabetes is a major risk factor,[3,14] particularly in patients with diabetic nephropathy.[15] Other factors associated with variable risk for CIAKI are: age older than 75 years, periprocedure volume depletion, heart failure, hypotension, cirrhosis, proteinuria, coadministration of nephrotoxins (e.g., diuretics, nonsteroidal antiinflammatory drugs [NSAIDs]), high doses of contrast, and intraarterial injection. The tolerable contrast dose depends in part on kidney function.[3,16] Exceeding a maximum recommended contrast dose derived from serum creatinine and body weight strongly predicts dialysis-requiring CIN.[4,16] The risk for CIN can be predicted by counting the number of risk factors present[17] or by specific risk prediction models such as that shown in Table 117-2.[18,19]

Pathogenesis

Although debate remains about the exact pathogenesis in humans and the relevance of animal models, pathogenetic considerations inspire most efforts to prevent CIN. In vitro and animal studies suggest CIN results from direct toxic injury to renal tubular cells and medullary ischemic injury secondary to subcorticomedullary congestion.[20,21]

Injection of a contrast agent induces a biphasic renal hemodynamic change, resulting initially in a transient increase and then a more prolonged decrease in global renal blood flow.[21] Cortical vasoconstriction and outer medullary vasodilation and congestion occurred during the hypoperfusion phase.[20] Vasoactive substances including endothelin, vasopressin, prostacyclin, nitric oxide, and adenosine are involved in the cortical vasoconstriction.[22-25]

In humans, the pathogenesis of CIN is still unclear, and there is no specific diagnostic marker for CIN. Contrast may be a contributory rather than a sole cause of AKI in specific cases of CIN. Concomitant

TABLE 117-1	Classification of Iodinated Contrast Media		
Ionicity	**Relative Osmolality**	**Contrast Agent**	**Osmolality (mOsm/kg H₂O)**
Ionic	High osmolality	Diatrizoate Iothalamate Ioxitalimate	1500-1860
Ionic	Low osmolality	Ioxaglate	600
Nonionic	Low osmolality	Iobitridol Iohexol Iomeprol Iopamidol Iopromide Ioversol	521-695
Nonionic	Iso-osmolal	Ioxaglate Iotrolan	290-320

insults may include intravascular volume depletion, surgery, atheroembolic disease, or coadministration of other nephrotoxins (e.g., NSAIDs). The mechanism of cellular injury may also vary by contrast viscosity, dose and concentration, associated ions, concomitant hypoxemia, and oxygen free radicals.[21,26]

Clinical Features and Diagnosis

Patients with CIN are generally asymptomatic but have an acute rise in serum creatinine concentration 24 to 72 hours after administration of the contrast agent. The renal failure is usually nonoliguric, but it may be oliguric, especially if there is significant preexisting renal impairment.[27,28] Serum creatinine level typically peaks at 3 days and returns to baseline within 10 days.[29] Clinically significant deterioration is unlikely if the serum creatinine concentration does not increase by more than 0.5 mg/dL within 24 hours.[30] In a minority of cases, the renal failure is severe enough to require dialysis, or renal function does not recover to precontrast values. To make an unequivocal diagnosis of contrast nephropathy, other potential causes of acute renal failure must be ruled out. Prerenal factors, atheroembolic disease, and other

TABLE 117-2	Risk Prediction Score for Contrast-Induced Nephropathy Following Percutaneous Coronary Intervention	
Risk Factor		**Score**
Systolic blood pressure <80 mm Hg longer than 1 h, requiring inotropes or intraaortic balloon pump (IABP) *within 24 h of procedure*		5
Utilization of intraaortic balloon pump		5
Heart failure (NYHA class III/IV) and/or history of pulmonary edema		5
Age >75 years		4
Hematocrit <39% in males, <36% in females		3
Diabetes		3
Volume of contrast medium		1 for every 100 mL
Serum creatinine level >1.5 mg/dL (133 μmol/L)		4
Estimated GFR (eGFR) <60 mL/min per 1.73 m²		2; 40-59 mL/min/1.73 m² 4; 20-39 mL/min/1.73 m² 6; < 20 mL/min/1.73 m²

eGFR = 186 × (serum creatinine mg/dL)^{-1.154} × age^{-0.203} × (0.742 if female) × (1.21 if black)

Total Risk Score	**Risk of CIN %**	**Risk of Dialysis %**
≤5	7.5	0.04
6-10	14.0	0.12
11-15	26.1	1.09
≥16	57.3	12.6

Adapted from Mehran R, Aymong ED, Nikolsky E, Lasic Z, Iakovou I, Fahy M et al. A simple risk score for prediction of contrast-induced nephropathy after percutaneous coronary intervention: development and initial validation. J Am Coll Cardiol 2004; 44:1393–9.

CIN, contrast-induced nephropathy; *NYHA*, New York Heart Association.

nephrotoxic insults should be excluded. The relatively rapid onset and typical course may help differentiate CIN from other causes of AKI. Urinalysis may be unremarkable or may show granular casts, tubular cells, or proteinuria. Fractional excretion of sodium can be low.[27,29]

Prognosis

Most episodes of CIN are self-limiting and resolve within 10 days, but CIN is consistently associated with increased morbidity, prolonged hospital stay, major adverse cardiac events, and early death.[3,31] In the United States and Europe, CIN is the third leading cause of AKI in hospitalized patients, accounting for 10% of all causes of hospital-acquired renal failure.[32] Less than 1% of CIN cases may require dialysis, and 13% to 50% of such cases may become permanently dialysis dependent.[3,33]

Although the association of CIN with adverse clinical outcomes other than requirement for dialysis has been clearly and consistently shown, it is not yet known whether CIN events are causally linked to early death and adverse cardiovascular events.[5] If in fact CIN is causally related to these later events, efforts to prevent CIN become even more important. However, if CIN does not cause early death or major adverse events, it may be a less important health issue. Future trials using a variety of interventions with different mechanisms of action showing parallel diminution in CIN and adverse events are required to establish some evidence for causality.

Preventive Interventions

As outlined in Box 117-1, the risk of CIN can be reduced by general and specific measures. The first step is to assess the presence of risk factors and indications for use of a contrast agent. Most risk factors

Box 117-1

RECOMMENDATIONS TO REDUCE THE RISK OF CONTRAST-INDUCED NEPHROPATHY

1. Identify patients at risk for contrast-induced nephropathy (CIN), and calculate their total risk score.
2. Assess risk/benefit of the proposed contrast-requiring intervention, and consider alternative not requiring contrast intervention.
3. Assess kidney function by estimated glomerular filtration rate (eGFR) or calculated creatinine clearance prior to contrast, especially in patients at risk for CIN.
4. Modify correctable risk factors, and hold medications that may act as co-nephrotoxins.
5. In high-risk patients receiving intraarterial contrast, consider either a low-osmolar contrast medium (other than iohexol) or an iso-osmolar contrast agent.
6. Use the lowest dose of appropriate contrast medium.
7. In high risk patients, correct hypovolemia. Stop diuretics and consider IV fluid if there is no contraindication. The optimal fluid type and quantity is not clear. Data support the use of either 0.9% saline or isotonic sodium bicarbonate, beginning at least 1 hour prior to contrast injection and continuing for at least 6 hours post injection. Initial rates of 3 mL/kg for 1 hour, followed by 1 mL/kg/h are commonly recommended. The patient should be monitored for signs and symptoms of hypervolemia or pulmonary edema.
8. In high risk patients, consider *N*-acetylcysteine (NAC), particularly if higher doses of contrast media or intraarterial administration is necessary. A total of 4 doses of NAC 1200 mg, orally twice a day starting the day prior to contrast injection, is an acceptable regimen. For emergent procedures, may consider 1200 mg IV as an initial dose followed by above 4 doses.
9. In patients with advanced kidney disease, prophylactic hemofiltration before and after contrast was associated with reduced mortality in one study.
10. In high risk patients, serum creatinine should be rechecked within 24-72 hours post contrast injection.

can be detected with a routine history and physical examination. It is not practical or necessary to measure serum creatinine concentration on every patient before use of a contrast agent, but this should be done in those patients with other risk factors.[34] The following specific prophylactic measures have been studied and should be considered for high-risk patients.

FLUID ADMINISTRATION AND BICARBONATE

Dehydration is one of the risk factors for CIN, so fluid restriction and diuretic use prior to contrast administration should be avoided unless necessary for other reasons. Although hydration is recommended in guidelines to reduce the risk for CIN, the optimal fluid type and regimen remain unclear.[35] Prolonged IV fluid regimens (12 hours before and after contrast injection) are the best supported but are impractical for ambulatory procedures. In a large RCT, isotonic saline was found to be superior to 0.45% saline in patients with preserved kidney function.[36]

In an initial trial that was prematurely terminated, Merten et al. found that alkalinizing the urine using IV isotonic sodium bicarbonate reduced CIN.[37] Since then, several further trials and meta-analyses have been completed. In a recent meta-analysis of 23 published and unpublished trials involving 3563 patients and 396 CIN events, the pooled RR of CIN with isotonic sodium bicarbonate as compared to other fluids was 0.62 (95% CI: 0.45-0.86).[38] However, as in other meta-analyses on this question, there was evidence of both heterogeneity and publication bias, suggesting that the true effect of bicarbonate has yet to be fully established.[38] In an effort to reduce the influence of publication bias, Brar et al. analyzed the protective effects of sodium bicarbonate in three large trials (n = 1145) out of 14 total trials (n = 2290) and reported a non-significant RR of 0.85 (95% CI: 0.63-1.16) without evidence of heterogeneity ($I^2 = 0\%$; $P = 0.89$).[39] Furthermore, several meta-analyses showed no significant effects of sodium bicarbonate on the risk of post-CIN dialysis, heart failure, and total mortality.[38-40]

At this time, it is practical to use either IV isotonic saline or IV isotonic sodium bicarbonate as described by Merten et al.[37] to diminish the risk of CIN. Meanwhile, patients should be observed for signs of volume overload.

N-ACETYLCYSTEINE

In the earliest trial, Tepel et al. showed a significantly lower incidence rate of CIN with N-acetylcysteine (NAC) compared with placebo (CIN occurred in 2% versus 21%; $P = 0.01$).[41] However, the rate of CIN in the placebo group was unexpectedly high. Numerous further trials and meta-analyses have been completed since.

More recent meta-analyses generally find evidence of heterogeneity that is not easily explained.[42,43] In one of these, Gonzales et al. divided the trials into two groups.[42] The first group showed no benefit (RR = 0.87; 95% CI: 0.68-1.12; $P = 0.28$), whereas in the second group which contained relatively early, small, and lower-quality trials, NAC was extremely beneficial (RR = 0.15; 95% CI: 0.07-0.33; $P < 0.0001$). Marenzi showed a dose-dependent effect of NAC on CIN risk after intraarterial contrast injection and a positive effect on in-hospital mortality.[44] This latter finding was recently confirmed in a meta-analysis of 16 RCTs with a total sample size of 1677 patients and no significant heterogeneity ($I^2 = 34\%$; $P = 0.09$).[45] The odds ratio for CIN was 54% lower in patients assigned to high-dose NAC (95% CI: 0.33-0.63).[45]

While there remains uncertainty about the benefit of NAC, and the results of ongoing trials such as the Acetylcysteine for Contrast-Induced Nephropathy Trial (ACT)[46] are pending, the drug appears safe, and it would be reasonable to use it giving at least 1200 mg orally (PO) or IV prior to contrast and repeated 12 hourly for the following 24 hours.

PROPHYLACTIC RENAL REPLACEMENT THERAPY

Lee et al. in a recent trial showed that prophylactic hemodialysis immediately post coronary angiography in patients with baseline creatinine clearance around 13 mL/min lessened the decrease in creatinine clearance on the fourth day post contrast injection (0.4 ± 0.9 versus 2.2 ± 2.8 mL/min/1.73 m²; $P < 0.001$).[47] Additionally, the risk for further or permanent dialysis was also reduced. However, the same benefit was not seen in several other trials, and the procedure carries its own inherent risks.[48-50] Prophylactic hemofiltration before and after contrast, but not post contrast alone, was associated with a lower rate of CIN in patients with advanced kidney disease as reported by Marenzi et al.[51,52] These trials are challenging to interpret insofar as it is hard to judge the effect of contrast on kidney function from trends in serum creatinine in patients undergoing hemofiltration. In-hospital mortality was also lower in those exposed to hemofiltration, but the mechanism by which hemofiltration led to better outcomes is unclear. The invasive nature of both prophylactic dialysis and hemofiltration suggests that these should only be considered in patients with existing advanced kidney disease.

OTHER PHARMACOLOGIC AGENTS

The volume contraction associated with forced diuresis with furosemide, mannitol, dopamine, or a combination of these agents at the time of contrast exposure has been associated with equal or higher rates of CIN when compared to prophylactic fluids alone.[53-56] A recent meta-analysis of three published trials including 251 patients found that forced euvolemic diuresis with furosemide and mannitol was associated with a significant risk of CIN (pooled RR = 2.15; 95% CI: 1.37-3.37; $I^2 = 0\%$).[57]

The vasodilatory effects of calcium channel blockers, dopamine, fenoldopam, atrial natriuretic peptide (ANP), prostaglandin E1, and a nonselective endothelin receptor antagonist failed to reduce the CIN risk compared with fluid hydration in several small trials.[53,58-62] In a more recent trial, the incidence of CIN was significantly lower in the ANP group than in the control group within 48 hours (3.2% versus 11.7%, respectively; $P = 0.015$) and at 1 month ($P = 0.006$) following contrast.[63]

Two small trials using captopril as a prophylactic agent for CIN had conflicting results, and no conclusion can be reached about the efficacy of this approach.[64,65] Similarly, ascorbic acid seemed promising in one small trial[66] but was inferior to NAC in another trial.[67]

Although lipid-lowering drugs such as high-dose simvastatin or probucol failed to show protective effects against CIN,[68,69] a recent trial compared the protective effects of simvastatin 80 mg versus 20 mg on renal function in 228 patients with good kidney function undergoing percutaneous coronary intervention (PCI).[70] The results favored the 80-mg dose, but the differences were not really clinically significant.[70]

Trimetazidine, a cellular antiischemic and antioxidant agent, restrains the cellular and mitochondrial ischemia/reperfusion toxic effects and inhibits the release of oxygen free radicals in various tissues.[71] In a single trial in 82 patients, 72 hours of 20 mg trimetazidine, 3 times daily starting 48 hours prior to coronary angiography together with IV saline, reduced the incidence rate of CIN from 16.6% to 2.5% compared with IV saline alone ($P < 0.05$).[71]

Theophylline and aminophylline antagonize adenosine-mediated vasoconstriction and have been used as a means to prevent CIN. However, the benefit was quite modest, and there was a potential for harm shown in meta-analysis.[72]

▣ Management and Outcome

In most instances, CIN never becomes clinically evident, and renal function returns to baseline. In more severe cases, management is no different than that for acute renal failure of any other cause. Careful control of fluid and electrolyte balance, avoidance of further nephrotoxic insults, attention to nutrition, and surveillance for complications are generally all that is required, although dialysis may be necessary in the occasional patient.[4,73] Prophylactic hemodialysis soon after administration of a contrast agent in patients with high serum creatinine concentrations has had inconsistent effects as previously noted.

Dialysis does not have to be done for routine removal of contrast medium after imaging in previously dialysis-dependent cases.[74]

Conclusion

CIN remains a concern, especially with interventions involving intra-arterial contrast. CIN is not common in the absence of risk factors, and these are generally detectable with a history and physical examination plus or minus determination of a serum creatinine concentration. Because CIN can be associated with other adverse clinical outcomes, preventive measures are advisable, especially with advanced preexisting renal disease when there is a risk the patient may require dialysis. Although CIN or CIAKI is associated with later adverse events, causality has not been proven, and the efficacy of preventive measures directed at CIN in preventing these associated events has not been established. Future research is needed in this area. At this time, the optimal approach to prevent CIN is unclear. Minimizing contrast dose, using either iodixanol or a LOCM other than iohexol, use of isotonic sodium bicarbonate or saline, and possibly NAC are the main components of our approach, which is summarized in Box 117-1. Finally, supportive care is indicated if contrast nephropathy occurs.

KEY POINTS

1. The likelihood of contrast-induced nephropathy (CIN) is largely determined by the presence of risk factors, with preexisting renal impairment with or without diabetes, reduced intravascular volume, and contrast dose being the major ones.

2. The pathogenesis of CIN remains somewhat unclear but seems to involve ischemic and direct toxic injury to renal tubules.

3. Although contrast dye–induced renal dysfunction is often transient, some cases require permanent renal replacement therapy, and mortality is increased, particularly in those requiring dialysis.

4. Management of established cases of CIN remains supportive.

5. Prevention of contrast dye–induced renal injury is important. The need for a contrast agent should be carefully considered and the dose used minimized in those at risk for nephropathy. Deliberate saline or isotonic sodium bicarbonate hydration may be indicated if volume excess is not a problem; *N*-acetylcysteine should also be considered.

ANNOTATED REFERENCES

Heinrich MC, Häberle L, Müller V, Bautz W, Uder M. Nephrotoxicity of iso-osmolar iodixanol compared with nonionic low-osmolar contrast media: meta-analysis of randomized controlled trials. Radiology 2009;250:68-86.
This large meta-analysis shows no major protective effect of IOCM (iodixanol) over LOCM (with the exception of iohexol).

Gruberg L, Mintz GS, Mehran R, Gangas G, Lansky AJ, Kent KM, et al. The prognostic implications of further renal function deterioration within 48 hours of interventional coronary procedures in patients with pre-existent chronic renal insufficiency. J Am Coll Cardiol 2000;36:1542-8.
This study, with others, establishes the overall negative prognostic impact associated with contrast nephropathy, particularly if renal replacement therapy is required.

Thomsen HS, Morcos SK. Members of the Contrast Media Safety Committee of European Society of Urogenital Radiology (ESUR). In which patients should serum creatinine be measured before iodinated contrast medium injection? Eur Radiol 2005;15:749-54.

A simple guideline on serum creatinine measurements prior to iodinated contrast medium administration.

Brar SS, Hiremath S, Dangas G, Mehran R, Brar SK, Leon MB. Sodium bicarbonate for the prevention of contrast-induced acute kidney injury: a systematic review and meta-analysis. Clin J Am Soc Nephrol 2009;4:1584-92.
In an effort to minimize the influence of publication bias on heterogeneity of meta-analyses, this meta-analysis with its subanalysis including three large trials shows no protective effect of sodium bicarbonate hydration relative to saline on CIN.

Marenzi G, Assanelli E, Marana I, Lauri G, Campodonico J, Grazi M, et al. *N*-acetylcysteine and contrast-induced nephropathy in primary angioplasty. N Engl J Med 2006;354:2773-82.
This randomized control trial shows a dose-dependent protective effect of N-acetylcysteine on CIN risk compared with a lower dose of NAC and placebo.

REFERENCES

Access the complete reference list online at http://www.expertconsult.com.

118

Glomerulonephritis and Interstitial Nephritis

CHRISTINA R. KAHL | RONALD J. FALK

Over half of all critically ill patients develop some degree of acute kidney injury (AKI), and nearly 5% require renal replacement therapy (RRT). For those patients with severe AKI requiring. RRT, mortality can be as high as 70%, and up to 30% of surviving patients remain dialysis dependent.[1-6] AKI may be a consequence of prerenal causes resulting in hypoperfusion of the kidneys, intrinsic renal causes, and postrenal or obstructive causes. In critically ill patients, the majority of AKI is related to ischemic or toxic acute tubular injury, which is treated supportively and is often reversible. AKI related to acute glomerulonephritis (GN) and acute interstitial nephritis (AIN) occurs in a smaller percentage of patients, but the incidence may be as high as 20% of all AKI.[7] In addition to supportive care, initiation of correct treatment regimens is paramount for patient and renal survival. The focus in this chapter is on the renal causes of AKI, particularly GN and AIN.

Glomerulonephritis

In GN, patients present with nephritic syndrome characterized by hematuria, proteinuria, AKI, edema, and hypertension.[8] Hematuria may be microscopic or macroscopic, and urine sediment demonstrates dysmorphic red blood cells (RBC) and RBC casts. Urinary protein excretion typically exceeds 1 gram per day, and the degree of proteinuria can be rapidly assessed using a spot urine protein-to-creatinine ratio. In some instances, patients may have nephrotic-range proteinuria (>3 g/d) with associated clinical manifestations including edema, hypoalbuminemia, and hypercholesterolemia. Leukocyturia with or without white blood cell casts may be observed with GN of inflammatory origin.

In renal biopsy series of patients with unexplained AKI, the most common diagnoses included various forms of GN (pauci-immune GN, immunoglobulin [Ig]A nephropathy, postinfectious GN, lupus nephritis, anti–glomerular basement membrane [anti-GBM] disease) and AIN.[7,9-11] Indeed, the third most common cause of end-stage kidney disease (ESKD) in the United States and Europe is GN.[8] Distinguishing the type of GN with renal biopsy is critical for diagnosis as well as assessing the degree of acute versus chronic disease, which helps guide treatment and prognosis.

The most aggressive form of GN is described clinically as *rapidly progressive glomerulonephritis* (RPGN). Rather than a single disease entity, RPGN is the severe form of many of the glomerular diseases that are divided into renal limited etiologies and systemic diseases that involve the kidneys (Table 118-1). RPGN is defined as rapidly declining renal function, progressive oliguria, hematuria, proteinuria, and hypertension.[8] Although many critically ill patients may have hematuria associated with infection or trauma, hematuria and AKI should always prompt consideration of acute GN. Renal ultrasound documents normal renal blood flow and normal to slightly enlarged kidneys. Renal biopsy reveals a high degree of glomerular injury with extensive crescent formation (Figure 118-1). Importantly, the transition from an acute cellular crescent to chronic, irreversible injury may occur rapidly over days. The presentation of a patient with RPGN constitutes a need for prompt diagnosis with early intervention and therapy to interrupt a natural progression to chronic renal failure. In adults, the most common cause of RPGN is pauci-immune GN associated with

antineutrophil cytoplasmic antibodies (ANCA), and other common causes include Goodpasture's syndrome (or anti-GBM disease) and immune-complex disease such as lupus nephritis.[8,12] Immunohistology of the renal biopsy shows pauci-immune staining in ANCA-associated GN, linear IgG staining of the GBM in Goodpasture's syndrome, and immune complex deposition in lupus nephritis, IgA nephropathy, and postinfectious GN.

Pulmonary renal syndrome, characterized by RPGN and diffuse alveolar hemorrhage (DAH), often presents as a medical emergency requiring early aggressive treatment.[13-15] It is associated with high mortality rates and rapid progression to ESKD if left untreated. Admission to the intensive care unit (ICU) and mortality are related to both the disease itself and infection. Patients often present with dyspnea, fever, cough, and hemoptysis, with chest radiography documenting pulmonary infiltrates. It may be difficult to distinguish from pneumonia, especially in patients without hemoptysis. Roughly 30% of patients with DAH do not present with hemoptysis. The presence of renal dysfunction and hematuria in patients presenting with these pulmonary symptoms should raise suspicion for a pulmonary renal syndrome. Although Goodpasture's syndrome was first used in 1958 to describe patients presenting with pulmonary hemorrhage and GN,[16] the most common cause of pulmonary renal syndrome is actually ANCA-associated small-vessel vasculitis.[8] *Goodpasture's syndrome* (also termed *anti-GBM disease*) now refers to the triad of DAH, RPGN, and the presence of anti-GBM antibodies and is the second most common cause of pulmonary renal syndrome. Much less common causes of pulmonary renal syndromes are SLE (systemic lupus erythematosus), thrombotic microangiopathies, and other systemic vasculitides.

A thorough history and physical examination may provide evidence for a systemic vasculitis (e.g., scleritis, purpuric rash, oral or sinus lesions). Bronchoscopy is critical to confirm DAH and evaluate for infection. The gold standard for diagnosis is renal or pulmonary biopsy, but critically ill patients are often high risk for these procedures. The majority of patients have either ANCA-associated small-vessel vasculitis or anti-GBM disease. Because both diseases are treated similarly in the acute setting of RPGN and DAH, appropriate treatment with plasma exchange, corticosteroids, and cyclophosphamide may be initiated rapidly prior to the results of serologic testing.

PAUCI-IMMUNE NECROTIZING GLOMERULONEPHRITIS

Pauci-immune necrotizing GN or ANCA-associated GN may present as a systemic small-vessel vasculitis, pulmonary renal syndrome, or renal limited disease. The spectrum of disease includes microscopic polyangiitis, Wegener's granulomatosis, and Churg Strauss syndrome. Renal biopsy features crescentic GN, fibrinoid necrosis, and an absence of immunoglobulin or complement within the glomeruli by immunohistology. Either anti-myeloperoxidase (MPO) or anti-proteinase 3 (PR3) antibodies are detectable in most patients. However, some patients with characteristic clinical manifestations of these diseases and pauci-immune GN do not have detectable antibodies.

Mortality of untreated disease is roughly 90% at 2 years following disease onset.[17] However, systematic studies of different treatment regimens have led to significant progress in this field and improved patient

TABLE 118-1	Diseases Associated with Rapidly Progressive Glomerulonephritis and Pertinent Laboratory Studies	
Renal Limited		
IgA nephropathy		
Postinfectious glomerulonephritis	Low complement, streptococcal serologies, bacterial cultures	
ANCA-associated glomerulonephritis (pauci-immune glomerulonephritis)	ANCA titers	
Anti-GBM disease (Goodpasture's syndrome)	Anti-GBM antibodies	
Systemic Disorders		
Lupus nephritis	Low complement, ANA, dsDNA antibodies	
ANCA-associated small-vessel vasculitis	ANCA titers	
Anti-GBM disease	Anti-GBM antibodies	
Henoch-Schönlein purpura	None	
Cryoglobulinemic vasculitis	Low complement, cryoglobulins, hepatitis C serologies	

ANCA, antineutrophil cytoplasmic antibodies; *ANA,* antinuclear antibodies; *dsDNA,* double-stranded DNA; *GBM,* glomerular basement membrane; *IgA,* immunoglobulin A.

outcomes.[18] Treatment consists of pulse intravenous (IV) methylprednisolone followed by oral corticosteroids and IV cyclophosphamide.[14,19-21] Even patients who are dialysis dependent on presentation often recover renal function with appropriate treatment. Poor prognostic indicators for patient and renal survival are the presence of DAH, severity of renal injury at diagnosis, degree of glomerular injury, extent of tubulointerstitial lesions on biopsy, and older age.[22-26] Patients with DAH have a high mortality rate, and plasma exchange improves patient survival.[17,27,28] For severe pulmonary disease, a few patients have been successfully treated with ECMO (extracorporeal membrane oxygenation).[29,30] Additionally, patients with severe renal disease have an increased likelihood of renal recovery when treated with plasma exchange.[23,25,31-33] With appropriate treatment, roughly 80% to 90% of patients achieve remission.[17,21,27,34,35] Treatment resistance is more common in females, African Americans, and patients with severe renal disease. Relapse is more common in patients with anti-PR3 antibodies and involvement of the pulmonary and upper respiratory systems. The ANCA-associated small-vessel vasculitides follow a remitting and relapsing course, making long-term monitoring a key component to patient and kidney survival.

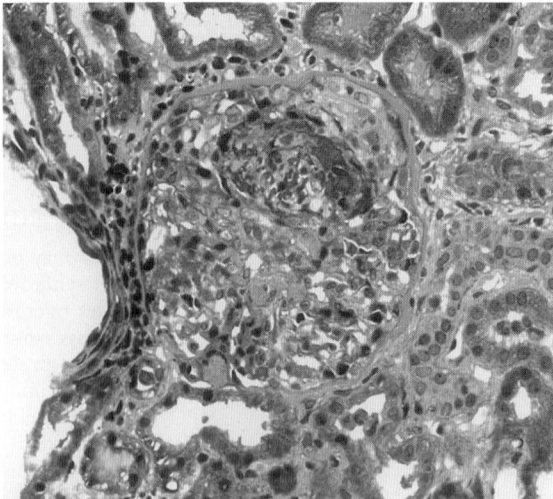

Figure 118-1 Rapidly progressive glomerulonephritis. Cellular crescent is present in glomerulus (4- to 8-o'clock position), with fibrinoid necrosis of the glomerular capillary tuft (×200, trichrome).

ANTI-GLOMERULAR BASEMENT MEMBRANE GLOMERULONEPHRITIS

Goodpasture's syndrome or anti-GBM disease presents as DAH and RPGN with evidence of anti-GBM antibodies on serologic testing. However, roughly 30% to 40% of patients present with renal limited disease without pulmonary involvement. It commonly affects Caucasians in a bimodal age distribution with peaks during the third and sixth decades.[14,36-38] Renal biopsy shows linear deposition of antibodies, most commonly IgG and C3, along the GBM and glomerular crescent formation.

Untreated disease is highly fatal, and death is usually due to pulmonary hemorrhage or infection. Treatment with plasma exchange, cytotoxic agents, and corticosteroids was introduced in the 1970s, resulting in improved patient and renal survival.[39] Plasma exchange is crucial for rapid clearance of anti-GBM antibodies[40] and should be continued daily until antibodies are undetectable.[38] Long-term outcomes are related to the degree of pulmonary compromise and renal dysfunction at presentation. With appropriate treatment, survival rates may exceed 90% for acute disease, but patients requiring RRT on initial presentation have lower survival rates.[37,38,41] For those patients, only a very few recover renal function despite treatment with plasma exchange, corticosteroids, and cyclophosphamide. In contrast, those patients with creatinine (Cr) below 5.7 on presentation demonstrated 100% 1-year patient survival and 95% renal recovery in one study.[37,41] In addition to dialysis dependence and elevated creatinine, predictors of poor renal outcome include oligoanuria, high anti-GBM antibody titers, and high percentage of glomeruli with crescent formation and extensive tubulointerstitial disease on renal biopsy.[36,40,42,43] Although patient and renal survival is generally worse with anti-GBM disease than with ANCA-associated disease, late recurrence of anti-GBM disease is much rarer than recurrence of ANCA-associated disease.[12,38]

Both ANCA-associated vasculitis and anti-GBM disease are rare diseases, and interestingly, a subset of patients actually demonstrates both types of antibodies on serologic studies. Roughly 15% to 30% of patients with ANCA-associated disease also have anti-GBM antibodies, while only 5% to 10% of patients with anti-GBM antibodies also have detectable ANCA titers.[12,37,38,44-46] Although outcome data are limited in this small group of patients, the outcomes of these patients may be better than patients with only anti-GBM antibodies.

LUPUS NEPHRITIS

Lupus nephritis occurs in 40% to 70% of patients with SLE and often occurs in the first 2 years following diagnosis.[47-49] Less than 5% of patients present with RPGN or pulmonary renal syndrome. However, 10% to 20% of patients with lupus nephritis ultimately progress to ESKD. In addition to history and physical examination, evaluation includes analysis of urine sediment (because lupus nephritis may present as nephritic or nephrotic syndrome), assessment of proteinuria, complement levels, and serologies for ANA and anti-dsDNA antibodies. Cellular casts or proteinuria over 0.5 g/d is consistent with the diagnosis of lupus nephritis. Renal biopsy is critical for diagnosis, prognosis, and guiding treatment.

Renal biopsy is used to classify lupus nephritis into six categories: class I (minimal mesangial lupus GN), class II (mesangial proliferative lupus GN), class III (focal proliferative lupus GN), class IV (diffuse proliferative lupus GN), class V (membranous lupus GN), and class VI (advanced sclerosis).[50-52] The most severe classes are the proliferative lesions of lupus nephritis (classes III and IV) and have poor renal survival without aggressive treatment. These classes often present with hematuria, proteinuria, hypertension, and AKI. Patients who present with RPGN are likely to have class IV lupus nephritis on renal biopsy. Sclerosing lupus nephritis is a chronic lesion that carries a poor prognosis.

Treatment of the more severe forms of lupus nephritis includes pulse methylprednisolone followed by oral corticosteroids and IV cyclophosphamide.[48,53-57] Similar to treatment of pauci-immune GN, pulse IV cyclophosphamide is preferred over oral cyclophosphamide. Over 80% of patients respond to treatment.[47,48] Importantly, about 5% to 10% of patients who require RRT initially recover enough renal function to become dialysis independent following treatment.[49] Recent studies suggest that mycophenolate mofetil (MMF) is similar to cyclophosphamide in inducing remission; however, relapse appears more common in patients treated with MMF.[58-62] Induction should be followed by maintenance therapy; the optimal maintenance regimen remains under intense investigation. Options for maintenance include additional cyclophosphamide, azathioprine, and MMF.[48,57,63,64]

Poor prognostic indicators at the beginning of treatment include male gender, African American race, severe hypertension, antiphospholipid syndrome (APS), and delayed initiation of immunosuppressive therapy. Following induction treatment, poor prognostic indicators are failure to achieve remission at 6 months and uncontrolled hypertension.[48,49] Roughly one-third to half of patients will have relapse of disease. In some patients, recurrence of disease may be preceded by falling complement levels and rising anti-dsDNA titers. However, some patients with severe lupus nephritis have negative titers.[47,65] Patients with only partial remission often recur sooner than patients with complete remission, and they are more likely to progress to ESKD.[66] All patients with a history of lupus nephritis should be carefully monitored for recurrence of disease, and repeat renal biopsy is often needed to guide treatment decisions with relapsed disease.

POSTINFECTIOUS GLOMERULONEPHRITIS

Postinfectious glomerulonephritis (PIGN) presents as a classic nephritic syndrome occurring about 1 to 3 weeks after a group A β-hemolytic *Streptococcus* infection.[67-69] It commonly occurs in children following a skin or pharyngeal infection. Although PIGN remains the most common cause of acute nephritic syndrome in the pediatric population in developing countries, the incidence of this disease has declined dramatically in the industrialized world. Children present with a classic nephritic syndrome with hematuria, proteinuria, hypertension, edema, and mild renal impairment. Severe hypertension with encephalopathy and seizures is uncommon and may require admission to the ICU.[69-71] Laboratory findings demonstrate depressed complement levels (CH50 and C3) consistent with activation of the alternate complement cascade; levels return to normal by 8 to 12 weeks. Serologic studies may be used to confirm recent streptococcal infection, particularly with recent pharyngitis.[69,72,73] Renal biopsy demonstrates endocapillary proliferation and granular deposition of immune complexes by immunohistology.[67,72,74-76]

The acute nephritic syndrome usually resolves in 7 days, and the prognosis of children with PIGN is excellent. However, roughly 10% to 20% of children have persistent urinary abnormalities including proteinuria and hematuria.[68,69,73,77-79] Treatment is generally supportive with antihypertensives and diuretics as needed in the acute phase. Active infections should be treated, and prophylactic antibiotics are often indicated in endemic situations and for household contacts in regions with high prevalence of disease.

In contrast to children, outcomes for PIGN in adults in the industrialized world are much worse, particularly for patients with underlying chronic disease.[67,68,80-82] PIGN can be associated with almost any infection, including most streptococcal and staphylococcal strains, gram-negative bacteria, mycobacteria, viruses, fungi, and parasites. Elderly patients often present with AKI, congestive heart failure, and nephrotic-range proteinuria. Up to half of these patients have underlying chronic diseases or risk factors including diabetes mellitus, liver disease or alcoholism, cancer, and IV drug use.[80-83] Some patients demonstrate skin or pharyngeal infections, but many have other infections such as endocarditis and pulmonary infections. Streptococcal and staphylococcal infections account for only half of cases. Treatment consists of supportive care and eradication of infection. Although recent studies of adults with PIGN remain small, one-quarter to one-half of patients have persistent renal dysfunction, and as high as 15% may progress to ESKD.[80-82,84] In one small study, patients with

underlying diabetic nephropathy had an extremely poor prognosis, with 81% progressing to ESKD.[82]

IgA NEPHROPATHY

IgA nephropathy (IgAN) is an extremely common form of GN worldwide. However, IgAN is a renal-limited disease, with only 3% of patients presenting with AKI[85] and most patients diagnosed in the outpatient setting. It commonly presents in the second or third decade of life and affects males more often than females.[86] The majority of patients present with macroscopic or microscopic hematuria. Many patients have episodic hematuria, often associated with a concurrent upper respiratory tract or gastrointestinal infection. Patients may develop hypertension and varying degrees of proteinuria. Crescentic IgAN is associated with nephrotic-range proteinuria, severe hypertension, and rapidly declining renal function.[87] No specific laboratory study to date can establish the diagnosis; renal biopsy is required. The extent of changes by light microscopy is variable, and the diagnosis is based on the demonstration of mesangial IgA deposits by immunohistology.

The long-term prognosis of patients with IgA nephropathy is highly variable, but many patients develop progressive renal failure. Between 15% and 40% of patients reach ESKD within 10 to 20 years of diagnosis.[88,89] No consensus on the optimum treatment of IgAN is available owing to the lack of well-designed controlled trials. Progress is hampered by the fact that renal failure develops slowly over decades, and short clinical trials have limited usefulness.[74,88,90,91] In all patients, hypertension should be aggressively treated with renin-angiotensin blockade. Patients with significant proteinuria and declining renal function may benefit from corticosteroids or immunosuppressive agents. Corticosteroids appear to reduce the risk of progression to ESKD and decrease proteinuria in selected patients.[89,90,92] The small percentage of patients presenting with RPGN and crescentic GN are usually treated with pulse corticosteroids and cyclosphosphamide.[87,88] Predictors of disease progression include renal dysfunction at diagnosis, significant proteinuria, hypertension, and evidence of chronic disease by renal biopsy.[86,88,93,94]

HENOCH-SCHÖNLEIN PURPURA

On renal biopsy, Henoch-Schönlein purpura (HSP) is indistinguishable from IgAN. However, HSP is a systemic disease characterized by a distinct purpuric rash and gastrointestinal involvement. It occurs in children much more commonly than adults. The classic presentation is sudden onset of rash, progressing from nonblanching erythematous macules to urticarial papules to purpura with a symmetrical distribution on the extensor surfaces of the distal extremities and buttocks.[95,96] Children present more frequently with gastrointestinal manifestations and fevers, whereas adults often have more severe renal involvement as well as joint symptoms.[97,98] Renal involvement occurs in roughly one-third of children and two-thirds of adults.[99,100]

Renal involvement in HSP is usually more severe at presentation than IgAN, but most children completely recover.[97,101,102] Estimates of recovery and chronic kidney disease vary widely, but the prognosis for renal recovery is worse in adults. Poor prognostic indicators include renal dysfunction and significant proteinuria at presentation, hypertension, and extensive glomerular disease by renal biopsy.[98,99,102,103] Treatment is primarily supportive care, and trials to date do not support any specific treatment regimen.[104] Corticosteroids may be useful in the short term, but there is no clear evidence that prednisone prevents serious long-term renal disease.[100,105] Recently, two adults with severe systemic manifestations refractory to corticosteroids and immunosuppressive agents were treated with plasmapheresis with subsequent improvement.[106]

THROMBOTIC MICROANGIOPATHIES

Thrombotic microangiopathy (TMA) is characterized by widespread thrombosis of arterioles and capillaries, with intraluminal platelet aggregation and vessel wall thickening.[107-109] The underlying patho-physiologic cause of TMA is endothelial damage due to a variety of insults. The classic diseases associated with TMA are thrombotic thrombocytopenic purpura (TTP) and hemolytic uremic syndrome (HUS), but it may also be seen with catastrophic antiphospholipid syndrome (APS) and scleroderma renal crisis. TMA is also associated with a variety of medications including chemotherapeutic agents, calcineurin inhibitors (cyclosporine and tacrolimus), antiplatelet agents (ticlopidine and clopidogrel), and quinine.[107] The classic pentad of findings in TTP includes microangiopathic hemolytic anemia, thrombocytopenia, neurologic symptoms and signs, impaired renal function, and fevers.[107-109] Neurologic symptoms may dominate, presenting as confusion, headache, seizures, and coma. The renal manifestations are usually more prominent in HUS, and the typical presentation in children includes microangiopathic hemolytic anemia, thrombocytopenia, and AKI. Laboratory hallmarks include microangiopathic hemolytic anemia with schistocytes on peripheral smear, elevated lactate dehydrogenase levels, and thrombocytopenia, with platelets usually less than 60,000.

Remarkable progress has been made in elucidating the molecular basis for TTP and HUS. TTP occurs as familial and acquired forms, and both forms are related to abnormalities in the function of a zinc metalloprotease, ADAMTS 13 (a disintegrin and metalloprotease with thrombospondin type 1 motif 13).[108-110] This protein is involved in the cleavage of von Willebrand factor (vWF), and deficiency of ADAMTS 13 leads to the accumulation of large multimers of vWF which bind platelets, leading to microvascular thrombosis. Familial TTP is associated with mutations of ADAMTS 13 leading to decreased or undetectable activity, and acquired TTP is caused by antibodies which inhibit its activity. Historically, untreated TTP had a mortality rate of over 90%. However, mortality has fallen to 10% to 20% with the advent of treatment using plasma exchange. Familial forms require chronic treatment with fresh frozen plasma or cryosupernatant that contains the active metalloprotease.

Hemolytic uremic syndrome is the most common cause of AKI in children and presents with hemolytic anemia, thrombocytopenia, and AKI.[107,111-113] The classic or diarrheal form of HUS (D+ HUS) occurs most commonly following diarrheal infection with Shiga-like toxin–producing Escherichia coli (SLTEC). The peak incidence occurs in children younger than 5 years of age, and outbreaks often occur in association with E. coli O157:H7. The illness begins with abdominal cramps and nonbloody diarrhea, following by hemorrhagic diarrhea in 70% of patients. Within days, patients develop severe renal failure, anemia, and thrombocytopenia. These children are often critically ill, and roughly one-half to two-thirds of patients require RRT. About 70% of patients will require RBC transfusions, and 25% will have neurologic involvement. Over the last few decades, mortality rates have fallen from roughly 40% to 50% to 3% to 5%, primarily due to aggressive supportive care with red blood cell transfusions and RRT as needed. Numerous therapies for HUS have been investigated without clear benefit, and treatment remains largely supportive. Treatment of the diarrheal illness associated with E. coli O157:H7 with antibiotics is associated with increased risk of developing HUS. Spontaneous resolution occurs 1 to 3 weeks following disease onset, and the majority of patients demonstrate renal recovery. Unfortunately, some children develop ESKD, and up to 40% have long-term sequelae including chronic kidney disease, persistent proteinuria, and hypertension. Non–diarrheal associated HUS occurs in a minority of patients and may be associated with other infections such as Streptococcus pneumoniae.

A small percentage of patients with HUS have sporadic or familial forms. These patients have defects in the alternative complement pathway, and mutations have been described in complement factor H, complement factor I, and membrane cofactor protein.[108-110] Mortality rates are over 50%, and most survivors progress to ESKD. Therapies with fresh frozen plasma, plasma exchange, and monoclonal antibodies targeting the alternative complement pathway are under investigation for treatment of this devastating disease.

A small percentage of patients with antiphospholipid syndrome (APS) present with "catastrophic" APS characterized by acute TMA involving the small vessels of multiple organs.[114] The disease progresses over days to weeks and commonly affects the kidneys, lungs, central nervous system, heart, and skin. The kidney is the most common organ affected, with renal involvement in over 70% of patients. Renal disease manifests as malignant hypertension and AKI, with 25% of patients requiring RRT. Mortality is estimated at 50% of patients, and treatment based on case reports includes anticoagulation, corticosteroids, plasmapheresis, and intravenous immunoglobulin.

Scleroderma renal crisis presents as accelerated hypertension, and AKI and may be accompanied by encephalopathy with seizures or flash pulmonary edema.[115] Roughly 10% of patients develop scleroderma renal crisis, usually occurring within 4 years of disease onset. The risk is greatest with diffuse cutaneous disease, and antecedent treatment with high-dose corticosteroids increases the risk of scleroderma renal crisis.[116,117] Patients demonstrate microangiopathic hemolytic anemia, thrombocytopenia, proteinuria, microscopic hematuria, and marked increases in plasma renin. In the past, untreated disease had a dismal prognosis with less than 10% survival. The use of angiotensin-converting enzyme (ACE) inhibitors has revolutionized treatment; acute mortality rates are now below 25% with appropriate treatment.[115,118,119] About half to two-thirds of patients will require RRT, but half of those patients recover enough renal function to become dialysis independent. Poor outcomes are associated with Cr above 3 at the initiation of ACE inhibitor therapy, poor blood pressure control, male gender, older age, and congestive heart failure. Patients with scleroderma renal crisis who do not require RRT have 90% survival rates at 5 years. In contrast, patients who become dialysis dependent have only 40% survival at 5 years. Early recognition and treatment are critical for both patient and renal outcomes. ACE inhibitors should be initiated rapidly and continued even if patients develop progressive renal failure or require RRT.

Interstitial Nephritis

Acute interstitial nephritis (AIN) demonstrates inflammation of both the renal interstitium and tubules, being more properly described as acute tubulointerstitial nephritis (Figure 118-2). This disorder reflects a hypersensitivity reaction, commonly induced by medications or infections.[120,121] AIN accounts for 2% to 6% of renal biopsies, but the incidence may be as high as 25% in patients with unexplained AKI.[120,122-124] Many critically ill patients are treated with medications commonly associated with AIN, such as antibiotics, proton pump inhibitors, and diuretics (Table 118-2).[125,126] AIN is important to recognize early so that the cause may be identified and the medication discontinued to minimize renal damage.

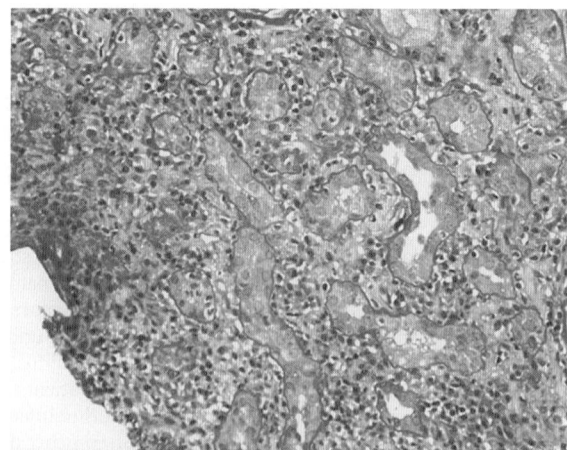

Figure 118-2 Acute interstitial nephritis. Diffuse, predominantly mononuclear cell infiltrate is present within an expanded and mildly edematous interstitium, and periodic acid–Schiff (PAS)-positive tubular basement membranes have wrinkling. Foci of tubulitis are also present (×200, PAS).

TABLE 118-2	Common Medications Associated with Acute Interstitial Nephritis

Antibiotics—penicillins, cephalosporins, sulfonamides
Anticonvulsants – phenytoin, carbamazepine, phenobarbital, valproate
Diuretics—thiazides, furosemide, triamterene
Herbal medications
NSAIDs
Proton-pump inhibitors

The classic example of AIN is described for methicillin. The majority of patients developed fevers, eosinophilia, pyuria, and hematuria a few weeks following exposure. About half of patients developed AKI for a duration of several weeks, followed by full recovery in 90%.[125] Unfortunately, the classic triad of fever, rash, and eosinophilia occurs in only 10% to 15% of patients.[120-122,125] Patients may present with mild renal impairment or severe AKI requiring RRT. Urine sediment may be bland or demonstrate sterile pyuria, white blood cell casts, and hematuria. In most cases, patients have subnephrotic-range proteinuria (<3 grams per day), but two-thirds of patients with NSAID-induced AIN present with nephrotic syndrome.[121,125] Eosinophiluria, based on Wright or Hansel stain, is suggestive of acute AIN but is neither sensitive nor specific for this disorder.[125,127,128] Eosinophiluria is also found in a variety of other disorders including pyelonephritis, cystitis, prostatitis, acute tubular necrosis, and glomerulonephritis.

Drug-induced AIN usually presents a few weeks following initiation of the medication, but it may take months to develop. With removal of the offending agent, the duration of AKI is quite variable from a few weeks to months. Medications account for over two-thirds of AIN, and the remainder of cases are associated with infection and other diseases, particularly autoimmune diseases.[120,121,126] A few cases of acute AIN are associated with Chinese herbal remedies.[129]

The diagnosis of AIN may be difficult, as systemic manifestations may mimic infection. Patients with pyelonephritis often have leukocyturia, hematuria, and mild proteinuria. Urine culture is essential to document infection, and sterile pyuria should prompt consideration of AIN as a diagnosis. AIN may be hard to distinguish from acute tubular injury, particularly in patients with bland urinary sediments. Because the absence of eosinophiluria does not exclude the diagnosis of AIN, a definitive distinction between these disorders on clinical grounds may not be possible. Renal biopsy may be required to provide a precise diagnosis and guide medical therapy.

The initial management of a patient with AIN is largely supportive, with dialysis as indicated. Identification of all candidate etiologic agents, elimination of potentially causative medications, and control of potential infectious causes are fundamental to the control of AIN.[121,125] When replacing medications, it is important to choose medications that are not likely to cross-react with the original agent. The use of corticosteroid therapy remains controversial, and no large randomized trials have thoroughly examined the effectiveness of corticosteroid therapy in AIN.[125,130] One small study in which the majority of patients developed AIN from antibiotics or NSAIDs demonstrated improved renal recovery with early steroid use.[131] Another study demonstrated that the majority of patients improve with medication withdrawal, but those patients who do not respond after a few weeks may subsequently benefit from corticosteroid administration.[132] In another retrospective study in which over 90% of patients had drug-induced AIN and 60% of patients received corticosteroids, there was no difference in renal outcomes.[123] Recently, MMF has been used successfully in patients who did not initially respond to corticosteroids.[133] Early improvement of renal impairment and patchy infiltrates on biopsy are prognostic indicators for improved renal outcomes.[121,134] Poor prognostic indicators include advanced age, prolonged renal impairment, and degree of chronic tubulointerstitial changes on renal biopsy. Roughly 30% to 40% of patients will have some degree of long-term renal impairment.[121,125,126]

KEY POINTS

1. Many underlying causes for acute kidney injury (AKI) due to intrinsic renal disease are reversible. Because the transition of active glomerular lesions to irreversible scar occurs rapidly, prompt diagnosis and early intervention are crucial.

2. Pulmonary renal syndromes constitute a medical emergency. Studies demonstrate that early aggressive treatment improves patient and renal survival.

3. Detailed histories and physical exams are important for distinguishing renal-limited disease from systemic diseases.

4. Initial evaluation should include basic chemistries, evaluation of urine sediment, complete blood counts with peripheral blood smear review, assessment for proteinuria, and renal ultrasound.

5. Serum complement levels are important tools in distinguishing causes of glomerulonephritis (GN): (a) normal serum complement (IgA nephropathy, Henoch-Schönlein purpura (HSP), pauci-immune necrotizing GN, and Goodpasture's syndrome) and (b) depressed serum complement (postinfectious GN and lupus nephritis).

6. Depending on the clinical scenario, additional evaluations may include antineutrophil cytoplasmic antibodies (ANCA), anti–glomerular basement membrane (GBM) antibodies, antinuclear antibodies (ANA), anti–double stranded DNA (dsDNA) antibodies, serologies for streptococcal infection, viral serologies, and bacterial cultures.

7. The gold standard for diagnosis of glomerulonephritis remains renal biopsy. However, critically ill patients are often at increased risk for complications, and it may be necessary to proceed with treatment in the absence of biopsy in certain situations.

8. Treatment of drug-induced acute tubulointerstitial nephritis (AIN) begins with discontinuation of the causative agent. Subsequent use of a causative agent may result in prolonged renal failure.

ANNOTATED REFERENCES

Appel GB, Contreras G, Dooley MA, Ginzler EM, Isenberg D, Jayne D, et al. Mycophenolate mofetil versus cyclophosphamide for induction treatment of lupus nephritis. J Am Soc Nephrol 2009;20:1103-12.
This randomized controlled trial of IV cyclophosphamide versus mycophenolate mofetil in the treatment of lupus nephritis (classes III to V) demonstrates similar response rates in both treatment groups.

De Groot K, Harper L, Jayne DR, Florez Suarez LF, Gregorini G, Gross WL, et al. Pulse versus daily oral cyclophosphamide for induction of remission in antineutrophil cytoplasmic antibody-associated vasculitis: a randomized trial. Ann Intern Med 2009;150:670-80.
This randomized controlled trial of IV pulse cyclosphosphamide versus daily oral cyclosphosphamide in ANCA-associated vasculitis demonstrates no difference in remission among the two groups.

Levy JB, Turner AN, Rees AJ, Pusey CD. Long-term outcome of anti-glomerular basement membrane antibody disease treated with plasma exchange and immunosuppression. Ann Intern Med 2001; 134:1033-42.
Retrospective review of patients with anti-GBM disease, with emphasis on renal function at presentation and patient outcomes.

Nasr SH, Markowitz GS, Stokes MB, Said SM, Valeri AM, D'Agati VD. Acute postinfectious glomerulonephritis in the modern era: experience with 86 adults and review of the literature. Medicine (Baltimore) 2008;87:21-32.
Review of cases of biopsy-proven PIGN in adults and demonstration of very poor renal outcomes in patients with diabetic glomerulosclerosis and PIGN.

Schwarz A, Krause PH, Kunzendorf U, Keller F, Distler A. The outcome of acute interstitial nephritis: risk factors for the transition from acute to chronic interstitial nephritis. Clin Nephrol 2000;54:179-90.
This study analyzes risk factors important in the development of chronic renal insufficiency following acute tubulointerstitial nephritis.

Steen VD, Medsger TA Jr. Long-term outcomes of scleroderma renal crisis. Ann Intern Med 2000; 133:600-3.
This study evaluates the long-term outcomes of patients with scleroderma renal crisis, with emphasis on renal outcomes.

REFERENCES

Access the complete reference list online at http://www.expertconsult.com.

Infectious Diseases

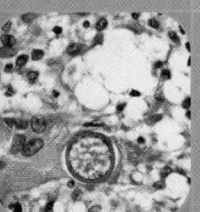

Antimicrobials in Chemotherapy Strategy

DOUGLAS N. FISH

Infections are frequently suspected or documented in critically ill patients. Patients are often admitted to the intensive care unit (ICU) for treatment of community-acquired or hospital-acquired infections, whereas many other patients require treatment for nosocomial infections acquired during their ICU stay. Although patients in ICUs represent only 8% to 15% of hospital admissions in the United States,[1] these patients suffer a disproportionately high rate of infectious complications and are exposed to very high rates of antimicrobial use.[1-3] The importance of antimicrobial drugs in the modern management of critically ill patients with a variety of bacterial, fungal, and viral infections can scarcely be understated. However, despite the availability of improved diagnostic techniques and a wide variety of potent, highly effective antimicrobials, the prevention and appropriate treatment of infections in ICU patients remain a formidable challenge to the clinician.

Antimicrobial Resistance in the ICU

The continuing emergence of antimicrobial resistance in ICUs is a major factor in the appropriate selection and use of antimicrobials in the critical care setting. It has been estimated that 50% to 60% of all nosocomial infections occurring each year in the United States are caused by antimicrobial-resistant strains of bacteria.[3,4] The overall incidence of infections due to antibiotic-resistant pathogens, changes in the epidemiology of infections caused by specific pathogens, and increasing resistance to even the most potent broad-spectrum agents make the selection of appropriate antimicrobial therapy extremely challenging in many institutions.[1-4] The difficulties in selecting antimicrobial therapy are particularly acute in ICUs because of the higher prevalence of antimicrobial resistance in these areas compared with other non-ICU settings.[1,5-8]

A number of factors are associated with high rates of antimicrobial resistance in the ICU. Chief among these is the heavy use of antimicrobial agents in critically ill patients. A number of studies have identified a close association between antimicrobial use and the subsequent development of antibiotic resistance.[9-19] Whereas use of antibiotics is associated with the emergence of resistance during therapy, previous exposure to antibiotics is also a well-established risk factor for antimicrobial resistance.[1-3,8] The higher severity of illness found among ICU patients is also related to several other risk factors for antimicrobial resistance, including the presence of invasive devices such as endotracheal tubes and intravascular and urinary catheters, prolonged length of hospital stay, immune suppression, and malnutrition.[1,2,4,5,8-19] The increasing prevalence of antimicrobial-resistant pathogens among residents in long-term care facilities is also an increasingly important source for resistant bacteria in ICUs.[1-5,8,20] Finally, antimicrobial-resistant pathogens are easily cross-transmitted among patients in ICUs, owing to poor adherence of hospital personnel to appropriate infection prevention techniques, contamination of equipment, and frequent overcrowding of patients.[1-5,8] All of these various factors combine to make ICUs the epicenter of antimicrobial resistance in hospitalized patients.[1,5]

Increased antimicrobial resistance has been observed among both gram-positive and gram-negative bacteria as well as among certain fungi, particularly *Candida* species. Table 119-1 summarizes important trends in increasing resistance in the United States among selected pathogens and drug classes.[1,3,4,21] Much of the changing epidemiology

of infection in the ICU has centered around the emergence of gram-positive organisms as predominant pathogens in the critically ill patient. Surveillance programs such as the National Healthcare Safety Network [NHSN], which incorporates the former National Nosocomial Infection Surveillance (NNIS) System sponsored by the Centers for Disease Control and Prevention, have repeatedly documented impressive increases in antimicrobial resistance among pathogens such as methicillin-resistant *Staphylococcus aureus* (MRSA), vancomycin-resistant enterococci (VRE), and multidrug-resistant *Streptococcus pneumoniae*.[1-3,20]

Rates of MRSA and methicillin-resistant coagulase-negative staphylococci have continued to steadily increase over the past decade and are most commonly associated with central catheter-associated bloodstream and wound infections,[1-3,5,7,8] whereas MRSA has also been increasingly documented as a frequent pathogen in ventilator-associated pneumonias as well as skin/soft tissue and other infections.[1,21-23] Although MRSA has been traditionally regarded as a hospital-acquired pathogen, this bacteria has also emerged as a common cause of community-acquired infections[1,24,25]; approximately 30% to 40% of all MRSA isolates found in hospitals are now actually community acquired.[26] The increase in methicillin resistance among staphylococci has led to a heavy reliance on vancomycin as a drug of choice for infections due to these pathogens and is perhaps related to the dramatic increase in the number of infections caused by VRE among ICU patients. High-level penicillin resistance among *S. pneumoniae* is approximately 20% to 30% in most geographic areas.[27-29] Additionally, penicillin-resistant pneumococci tend to be multidrug resistant; 25% to 30% of *S. pneumoniae* have decreased susceptibility to macrolide antibiotics, and rates of resistance to several other drug classes including sulfonamides, tetracyclines, and cephalosporins have also increased.[27-29] Although the prevalence of fluoroquinolone resistance among *S. pneumoniae* is still very low (<1%),[27-29] there is still significant concern regarding excessive use of fluoroquinolones and the potential for significant resistance in the future.[27-30]

Antimicrobial resistance continues to be a problem of major importance among gram-negative bacilli. Of particular concern is the rapid spread of resistance mediated by extended-spectrum β-lactamases (ESBLs) among organisms such as *Escherichia coli* and *Klebsiella pneumoniae*. Organisms that produce ESBLs are usually resistant to multiple antimicrobials, including third- (e.g., ceftriaxone, ceftazidime) and fourth-generation (e.g., cefepime) cephalosporins and aztreonam, and are also associated with high rates of resistance to aminoglycosides and fluoroquinolones.[31-34] The increase in ESBL-mediated resistance is reflected in rates of *E. coli* and *K. pneumoniae* resistance to third-generation cephalosporins, as shown in Table 119-1. Antimicrobial resistance among *Pseudomonas aeruginosa* is also alarming in that nearly all major drug classes are currently being affected; nearly 10% of *P. aeruginosa* isolates are now resistant to multiple drug classes, including cephalosporins, carbapenems, aminoglycosides, and/or fluoroquinolones.* Multidrug resistance is also very common (approximately 30% of isolates) among strains of *Acinetobacter baumanii*.[4,35] Fluoroquinolone resistance is being increasingly reported among organisms such as *E. coli* that were previously considered to be extremely susceptible to this class of drugs.[1-4,36] Antimicrobial

---

*References 1, 4, 16, 20, 35, and 36.

TABLE 119-1	Trends in Antimicrobial Resistance Among Selected Nosocomial Pathogens from ICU Patients in the United States, 1998-2002 and 2006-2007		
Pathogen	Pooled Resistance Rate, 1998-2004	Resistance Rate, 2006-2007	Percent Change, 1998-2002 to 2006-07
Vancomycin-resistant enterococci	13.9	33.3	139%
Methicillin-resistant *Staphylococcus aureus*	52.9	56.2	6%
Methicillin-resistant coagulase-negative staphylococci	76.6	NR	—
Fluoroquinolone-resistant *Escherichia coli**	7.3	25.3	246%
3GC-resistant *E. coli**	1.3	6.0	362%
3GC-resistant *Klebsiella pneumoniae**	6.2	16.8	171%
Imipenem-resistant *Pseudomonas aeruginosa*	19.1	25.3	32%
Fluoroquinolone-resistant *P. aeruginosa*	34.8	30.7	−9%
3GC-resistant *P. aeruginosa*	17.5	13.8	−21%
3GC-resistant *Enterobacter* species	27.7	NR	—
Imipenem-resistant *Acinetobacter baumannii**	12.1	33.2	174%

*Rates reflect nonsusceptibility (resistant and intermediate susceptibility).
3GC, third-generation cephalosporin (cefotaxime, ceftriaxone, or ceftazidime).

resistance among gram-negative organisms such as *P. aeruginosa* has been of great concern in the ICU setting for many years, but increasing resistance among previously susceptible organisms and the involvement of multiple drug classes clearly indicates that the problem continues to grow worse. An additional troubling development in recent years is the detection of *K. pneumoniae* carbapenemase (KPC) enzymes which, as the name implies, confer resistance to a broad range of β-lactam-type antibiotics including the carbapenems.[37] The increase in ESBL-producing strains and other multidrug-resistant pathogens has led to a heavy reliance on the carbapenems for treatment of gram-negative infections. Although KPC-producing strains are still relatively uncommon, their rapid spread through many geographic areas has led to serious concerns regarding the loss of carbapenems as reliable agents for empirical or "definitive" (i.e., based on culture and susceptibility information) treatment of many infections in ICU patients.[37]

Candida albicans is now the fourth most common pathogen associated with nosocomial infections in critically ill patients in the United States. While *C. albicans* is associated with approximately 7% of all nosocomial infections, it is the second most common cause of nosocomial urinary tract infections (15% of infections), the third most common cause of central line–associated bloodstream infections (6% of infections), and fourth most common cause of all nosocomial bloodstream infections.[1,2] Resistance to antifungal agents among *Candida* species is now a significant problem in many hospitals, with fluconazole resistance being reported in up to 10% of *C. albicans* isolates from bloodstream infections.[38-40] Because susceptibility testing for *Candida* species is not routinely performed in most hospitals, the true scope of resistance among *C. albicans* and other strains is not well characterized and may in fact be higher than currently assumed. It is well documented, however, that the relative frequency of fungal infections with *Candida glabrata*, *Candida krusei*, and other strains with decreased susceptibility to azole antifungals is increasing among certain populations, such as the critically ill and patients with hematologic malignancies.[38-40] The increased proportion of non-*albicans* strains of *Candida* is particularly problematic because it has often led to the use of non-azole type agents such as the echinocandins for empirical therapy of patients at high risk for *Candida* infections.[38-40]

Infections caused by antimicrobial-resistant bacteria have been demonstrated to be associated with higher mortality rates, longer length of ICU and hospital stays, and higher medical costs.[41-44] Antimicrobial-resistant strains of bacteria have been demonstrated to express virulence factors that may be different from those expressed by antimicrobial-susceptible strains; this may explain some of the increased mortality associated with these infections.[6,7,37,44] However, increased mortality associated with infections caused by resistant bacteria may also be explained by the increased likelihood that patients will receive inadequate antimicrobial treatment. Inadequate antimicrobial therapy, defined as the use of drugs with poor in vitro activity against the infecting pathogen and/or improper dosing of drugs, has

been demonstrated in numerous studies to be significantly associated with increased mortality and other measures of poor patient outcomes.[45-54] Treatment with inadequate antimicrobial therapy is particularly problematic during the initial empirical treatment of infections when specific pathogens and antibiotic susceptibility information are not yet known.[45,47,51,53,54] It is logical to assume that selection of adequate empirical therapy becomes more difficult as the organisms become more resistant to antimicrobial therapy, and it has in fact been demonstrated in clinical studies that most inadequate treatment of nosocomial infections in the ICU is related to the presence of pathogens that are resistant to the selected antibiotics.[46,48,51-53] Furthermore, it has been shown in patients with nosocomial pneumonia that changing to more appropriate antibiotics when culture and susceptibility results became available (typically 48–72 hours after initiating therapy) did not significantly lower mortality rates compared with patients who received inadequate antibiotics for the entire duration of therapy.[45] The importance of antimicrobial resistance in terms of antimicrobial selection and patient outcomes is thus difficult to overstate.

Strategies to Reduce Antimicrobial Resistance

Various strategies have been recommended to decrease problems of resistance through improved use of antimicrobials. These strategies include the use of antimicrobial protocols and guidelines, hospital formulary-based antimicrobial restrictions, scheduled antimicrobial rotation or "cycling," improved techniques for detection and/or diagnosis of infections, improved dosing of antimicrobials based on pharmacokinetic and pharmacodynamic concepts, use of combination antimicrobial therapy, decreased duration of antimicrobial therapy, and early involvement of infectious diseases specialists in the management of infected patients.[55] All of these various strategies fall within the realm of "antimicrobial stewardship," a process for collectively improving the overall use of antimicrobials through many different means.[56]

Among these various strategies, the roles of antimicrobial restrictions and antimicrobial cycling are two particularly controversial issues. Hospital formulary–driven restriction of specific drugs or drug classes is a common method of controlling antimicrobial use within an institution. Formulary-based restrictions have historically been used to control drug costs; they may also reduce rates of adverse effects of high-risk agents.[56] Antimicrobial restrictions are also used in an attempt to either decrease overall emergence of antimicrobial resistance within an institution or to control acute outbreaks of resistance affecting specific drugs and pathogens.[56-59] The effectiveness of antimicrobial restrictions in reducing overall levels of resistance has not been consistently demonstrated. Indeed, it can be argued that antimicrobial restrictions cause intense selective pressure from a small number of agents and may actually promote the emergence of resistance rather than preventing it.[60] Antibiotic restrictions that are instituted in response to specific outbreaks of antibiotic-resistant infections, together with appropriate infection control measures, have been shown to successfully manage specific resistance problems.[56-59] However, it has also been shown that restriction of a drug in response to a resistance issue may in turn cause other resistance problems affecting other drugs.[60] This phenomenon is sometimes referred to as "squeezing the balloon" because the enforcement of antimicrobial restrictions leads to new selective pressures that may effectively solve the original problem but cause the development of new resistance issues.[61] A classic example involved restriction of ceftazidime and increased use of imipenem in response to an outbreak of ceftazidime-resistant *K. pneumoniae*. Although ceftazidime resistance among *K. pneumoniae* isolates was effectively decreased by 44%, the rates of imipenem-resistant *P. aeruginosa* significantly increased by 69%.[60] Although antimicrobial restrictions may be effective in reducing drug costs and limiting specific outbreaks of resistant infections, the emphasis must clearly be on appropriate and rational drug use rather than relying on such restrictions to overcome resistance problems.

Antibiotic cycling, in which a specific drug or an entire antibiotic class is periodically withdrawn from clinical use and replaced with a different drug or class, has been investigated as a means of decreasing resistance by limiting narrow selective pressures and exposing organisms to a wide variety of different antimicrobials over time.[62-65]

Although initial studies were promising and demonstrated reduced antimicrobial resistance as well as decreased incidence of certain nosocomial infections and reduced patient mortality,[62-65] these studies have not been consistent in the overall effectiveness of the antibiotic cycling strategy. In addition, a number of important questions concerning antibiotic cycling have not been adequately addressed by previous studies. These questions include which specific agents or classes are most appropriate to cycle, whether agents or classes of drugs should be cycled in a specific order, how often to change drugs within the scheduled cycle, and whether the potential effectiveness of antimicrobial cycling is maintained over long periods of time.[62-65] Further research is clearly needed to answer these and other relevant questions, and cycling is currently not widely accepted as an effective means of improving infection-related patient outcomes and reducing resistance.

Principles of Appropriate Antimicrobial Use

Whereas many of the issues regarding antimicrobial use in critically ill patients are currently centered on issues related to antimicrobial resistance, adherence to basic principles of appropriate drug use is still crucial in overall optimization of drug therapy (Table 119-2).

TABLE 119-2 Basic Principles of Appropriate Antimicrobial Use in Critically Ill Patients

1. Establish definitive diagnosis before initiating antimicrobials.
   a. Perform comprehensive clinical evaluation.
   b. Perform appropriate diagnostic tests.
   c. Obtain appropriate specimens for culture and susceptibility testing.
   d. Evaluate patient for noninfectious sources of fever.
2. Initiate appropriate empirical antimicrobial therapy.
   a. Consider known/probable site of infection and most likely pathogens.
   b. Consider colonization versus infection when evaluating culture results.
   c. Consider rates of antimicrobial resistance among potential pathogens.
   d. Consider need for combination antimicrobial therapy versus monotherapy.
   e. Initial therapy should be broad spectrum, parenteral, and at appropriately aggressive doses.
      (1) Consider pharmacokinetic properties of potentially used agents and potential alterations.
      (2) Consider pharmacodynamic properties of potentially used agents.
      (3) Consider age, organ dysfunction, and site of infection when determining proper dose.
      (4) Consider potential drug-related adverse effects and toxicities.
      (5) Consider potentially relevant drug/drug or drug/disease state interactions.
      (6) Consider use of less expensive agents when appropriate.
3. Change to appropriate definitive drug therapy when possible.
   a. Monitor culture and susceptibility test results.
   b. Spectrum of antimicrobial activity of selected agents should be as narrow as possible when pathogen(s) is/are known.
   c. Consider need for combination antimicrobial therapy versus monotherapy.
   d. Therapy should be at appropriately aggressive doses.
      (1) Consider pharmacokinetic properties of potentially used agents and potential alterations.
      (2) Consider pharmacodynamic properties of potentially used agents.
      (3) Consider age, organ dysfunction, and site of infection when determining proper dose.
      (4) Consider potential drug-related adverse effects and toxicities.
      (5) Consider potentially relevant drug/drug or drug/disease state interactions.
      (6) Consider use of less expensive agents when appropriate.
4. Consider use of oral antimicrobials when appropriate.
   a. Patients clinically respond to parenteral therapy.
   b. Patients have functional gastrointestinal tracts.
   c. Suitable oral alternatives to parenteral therapy are available.
5. Perform careful patient monitoring for duration of antimicrobial therapy.
   a. Evaluate for clinical resolution of signs and symptoms and evidence of response to therapy.
   b. Evaluate for changes in organ function that may require change in drug-dosing regimen.
   c. Monitor serum drug concentrations when appropriate.
   d. Evaluate for drug-related adverse effects and toxicities.
   e. Evaluate for potential adverse drug interactions.
6. Carefully reassess patients who appear to be failing antimicrobial therapy.
   a. Evaluate patient for unidentified or new sources/sites of infection or superinfection.
   b. Obtain additional specimens for culture and susceptibility testing.
   c. Evaluate drug regimen for proper spectrum of activity against known or presumed pathogens.
   d. Consider emergence of antibiotic resistance among certain pathogens (e.g., *Pseudomonas aeruginosa*).
   e. Evaluate drug regimen for proper dosing of individual antimicrobial agents.
   f. Consider pharmacokinetic and pharmacodynamic properties of agents and potential need for increased daily doses or alternative dosing methods.
7. Limit duration of therapy when possible.
   a. Short courses are desired over long courses in patients who have promptly responded to antimicrobial therapy.
   b. In patients with no documented infection/pathogens, discontinue antimicrobials after appropriate course of therapy and assess continued need for treatment.

DIAGNOSTIC ISSUES

Establishing a definitive diagnosis of infection is paramount to the appropriate selection and use of antimicrobials. Once infection is suspected in the ICU patient, a comprehensive workup must be performed to identify the site of infection. The microbial causes of various ICU infections are reasonably predictable once the actual site of infection is known; appropriate drug selection thus properly begins with identification of a known or suspected site of infection. Unfortunately, the site of infection is often unable to be identified with any certainty; studies in septic patients have shown that no source of infection is identified in up to 30% to 40% of patients.[53,66] Modern ICU practitioners have access to a wide range of invasive and noninvasive diagnostic techniques, and these should be employed when appropriate. However, the institution of antimicrobial therapy should not be unnecessarily delayed for the sake of performing exhaustive diagnostic tests. Although not yet in common use, polymerase chain reaction (PCR) and other molecular-based laboratory methods may offer the potential to improve detection of causative pathogens and facilitate the early initiation of appropriate antimicrobial therapy.[67,68]

Gram stain of appropriate specimens from potential sites of infection should also be utilized to help determine appropriate empirical or antimicrobial therapy. Although the yield of useful information from Gram stains is usually not high in critically ill patients, performing this test is nevertheless of value for those patients in whom causative pathogens are identified.[45,67,68] Gram stains from specimens obtained from certain sites such as the respiratory tract and wounds should be interpreted with caution, owing to high rates of colonization with nonpathogenic organisms, particularly in patients who have already been hospitalized for several days. Studies have clearly demonstrated the high frequency and rapid time course of microbial colonization of ICU patients.[69-71] Classic studies demonstrated that rates of colonization of the oropharynx and bronchi of critically ill patients with gram-negative organisms reached 45% and 65% within 5 days after ICU admission, respectively, and over 90% at both sites by day 10.[72] These patients also become highly colonized with gram-positive cocci and particularly yeast soon after ICU admission.

Great care must be taken to differentiate colonizing organisms from true pathogens when evaluating Gram stain and culture results from nonsterile areas of the body or areas that may become colonized after the placement of foreign devices such as catheters (e.g., urinary tract and respiratory tract). Colonization is often distinguished on the basis of Gram stain results showing multiple morphologic types of bacteria or the absence of clinically relevant signs and symptoms of infection despite the presence of microbial growth. However, in critically ill patients, colonization is often extremely difficult to distinguish from true infection and antimicrobials are initiated based on a presumptive diagnosis.

Clinicians must keep in mind that there are numerous sources of fever in critically ill patients that are not associated with infection (Table 119-3). The occurrence of new fever in an ICU patient should prompt a thorough evaluation of noninfectious sources for the fever before initiation of antimicrobial therapy. Patients who have been started on antimicrobial therapy and have persistent fever despite the resolution of other signs and symptoms of infection should also be evaluated for noninfectious sources of fever.

SELECTION OF EMPIRICAL DRUG THERAPY

Initial selection of adequate drug therapy is of vital importance in optimizing outcomes of antimicrobial use in critically ill patients. Selection of inadequate therapy has been demonstrated in numerous clinical studies to be associated with increased patient mortality,[45-54] and the risk of inadequate therapy is often directly related to rates of antimicrobial resistance in certain pathogens.[46,48,51-53] A number of factors are therefore important to consider when choosing initial empirical therapy. These considerations should include suspected site(s) of infection and corresponding potential pathogens, rates of

TABLE 119-3	Noninfectious Sources of Fever in Critically Ill Patients

Hemorrhage

Central nervous system
Gastrointestinal
Intraarticular
Pulmonary
Retroperitoneal

Inflammatory Conditions

Atelectasis
Blood product transfusion
Cholecystitis
Collagen vascular diseases:
   Systemic lupus erythematosus
   Rheumatoid arthritis
Gout and pseudogout
Ischemic bowel
Pericarditis
Postoperative fever
Postpericardiotomy syndrome
Trauma
Vasculitis:
   Cerebral angiitis
   Temporal arteritis
   Lymphomatoid granulomatosis
   Cholesterol embolism
   Drug-induced vasculitis
   Giant cell arteritis
   Henoch-Schönlein purpura
   Polyarteritis nodosa
   Radiation arteriopathy
   Wegener's granulomatosis

Medications

Allergic reactions
Idiopathic drug fever

Metabolic Conditions

Adrenal insufficiency
Alcohol withdrawal
Heat stroke/exhaustion
Hyperthyroidism
Malignant hyperthermia
Neuroleptic malignant syndrome
Seizures

Neoplasms

Colorectal carcinoma
Hepatoma
Hepatic metastases
Leukemia
Lymphoma
Renal cell carcinoma

Thromboembolism

Deep venous thrombosis
Dissecting aortic aneurysm
Graft/venous access thrombosis
Myocardial infarction
Pulmonary embolism
Thrombophlebitis
Thrombotic thrombocytopenia purpura

resistance of these pathogens to potentially used drugs, a patient's prior exposure to antimicrobial therapy that may potentially increase the likelihood of antimicrobial resistance, and the results of any pertinent prior diagnostic tests. A reasonable understanding of the pharmacology, pharmacokinetics, pharmacodynamics, potential toxicities, potential drug interactions, and appropriate dosing of individual antimicrobials is also important in the selection of a specific agent once the type of drug to be used has been decided on. These drug-specific considerations are discussed in more detail later in this chapter. In general, empirical antimicrobial regimens for critically ill patients should be aggressive, that is, sufficiently broad spectrum in pharmacologic activity to cover the most likely (rather than all possible) pathogens, initiated promptly, and given in relatively high doses when the presence of any significant renal or hepatic dysfunction is considered.

Clinicians should be familiar with patterns and rates of resistance of key pathogens involved in both community-acquired and nosocomial infections. Resistance rates for pathogens occurring in community-acquired infections may be very different from those same types of pathogens causing nosocomial infections.[1] For example, *E. coli* causing community-acquired urinary tract infections may have a rate of resistance to ciprofloxacin of 1% to 2%, whereas *E. coli* associated with nosocomial urinary tract infections may display resistance to ciprofloxacin in greater than 10% to 15% of strains.[73,74] Likewise, *S. aureus* associated with community-acquired infections is usually susceptible to methicillin, whereas the rate of MRSA is now 60% to 70% in many hospitals in the United States.[1,3] Information concerning rates of antimicrobial resistance in the outside community is often not as readily available as information concerning institutional susceptibilities, but ICU practitioners should nevertheless be familiar with resistance rates in both settings in order to choose appropriate antibiotics. Although antibiograms summarizing drug susceptibilities of key pathogens are available in most institutions, clinicians should recognize that published susceptibilities often do not differentiate between ICU and non-ICU isolates. It is well recognized that resistance rates are often much higher among isolates obtained from patients in ICUs where antimicrobial use is heaviest and more risk factors for resistance (e.g., higher severity of illness, invasive devices, immune suppression) are present.[1,2,4,5,8-19] It is also known that susceptibilities often differ markedly among different types of ICUs (e.g., medical, surgical, burn, trauma) owing to patients with varying risk factors and potential differences in the types and amounts of antimicrobials used in each of these areas.[2,3] When such information is available, ICU practitioners must be aware of any important differences between unit-specific drug susceptibilities and resistance rates for the institution as a whole. Appropriate use of such information can lead to more effective drug selection and enhance the provision of adequate drug therapy.[75]

DEFINITIVE DRUG SELECTION

When the results of culture and susceptibility tests are available, clinicians must utilize this information to reassess and make appropriate changes to empirical drug regimens. Antimicrobial regimens should be selected that provide suitable activity against identified pathogens while at the same time using the fewest required number of drugs, narrowing the spectrum of antimicrobial activity as much as possible, minimizing the risk of drug-related toxicities, and minimizing the cost of drug therapy. It is common for patients to be treated empirically for the entire duration of therapy because of an inability to identify the site(s) of infection, negative culture results, cultures suspected to be positive for colonizing organisms rather than pathogens, or other reasons. However, rational antimicrobial therapy dictates that culture and susceptibility information must be utilized in the selection of more definitive antimicrobial therapy when such information is available and felt to be reliable. It is inappropriate to continue empirically selected drug regimens simply because the patient is clinically responding to present therapy and the clinician is unwilling to make a change of any kind.

COMBINATION THERAPY

Combinations of drugs are often recommended and used in both empirical and definitive antimicrobial regimens as a means of increasing the spectrum of pharmacologic activity, providing potentially additive or synergistic activity against selected organisms such as *P. aeruginosa*, improving clinical efficacy, and minimizing the potential for emergence of resistance during therapy.[76-83] Combination regimens are also associated with the potential disadvantages of increased drug-related toxicities and increased drug costs. Although combination therapy is considered standard practice for certain specific infections, such as some types of endocarditis,[84] the efficacy of combination therapy has not been well proven in respect to its presumed advantages. Whereas combinations of drugs may increase the overall spectrum of activity compared with the same drugs used alone, single agents such as carbapenems (imipenem/cilastatin and meropenem) and piperacillin/tazobactam provide very broad ranges of pharmacologic activity that

includes gram-negative (including *P. aeruginosa*), gram-positive, and anaerobic bacteria. A number of older studies concerning the treatment of sepsis showed that monotherapy with ceftazidime, cefepime, or carbapenems is similar in efficacy to combination regimens (77%–93% and 76%–94% clinical response rates, respectively), with no differences in the development of resistance during therapy.[79] However, a more recent study found that because of the current spectrum of pathogens and frequent antimicrobial resistance encountered in contemporary ICU practice, the use of combination therapy was associated with significantly higher rates of adequate antibiotic therapy and improved survival in gram-negative sepsis.[80] Recent studies have also shown that the use of combination regimens for empirical treatment of ventilator-associated pneumonia may lead to improved patient outcomes in those patients proven to be infected specifically with multidrug-resistant pathogens such as *P. aeruginosa* and *Acinetobacter*.[81,82] Although it is most appropriate to use antimicrobials with a narrow spectrum of activity whenever possible, monotherapy during empirical treatment may not be feasible in many institutions in which high rates of antimicrobial resistance are present among common pathogens such *P. aeruginosa* and *S. aureus*. As previously discussed, the selection of adequate empirical antimicrobial regimens is becoming more difficult as bacteria become more resistant; the routine use of monotherapy regimens is very difficult in many institutions from this standpoint. In institutions with high antibiotic resistance rates and/or high rates of infection with multidrug-resistant organisms, the best strategy seems to be use of combination regimens for empirical therapy until pathogen susceptibilities are known, followed by rapid narrowing or "de-escalation" of therapy to a suitable monotherapy regimen when possible.

Aside from considerations regarding empirical antimicrobial regimens, combination regimens are appropriately used in the treatment of mixed infections caused by aerobic and anaerobic bacteria, gram-negative and gram-positive bacteria, and/or bacteria and fungi. In these situations it is often more appropriate to select two or more agents with focused activity against known pathogens rather than treat with an excessively broad-spectrum single agent. Combination regimens are also often recommended in the treatment of systemic infections caused by certain gram-negative organisms such as *P. aeruginosa*, *Acinetobacter* species, *Enterobacter* species, and *Serratia marcescens*, as well as severe staphylococcal and enterococcal infections to achieve the potential benefits of antibiotic synergy, improved efficacy, and decreased resistance.[79] Although some studies indicate that combination regimens for gram-negative pathogens such as *P. aeruginosa* are no more efficacious than monotherapy with newer agents such as cefepime and the carbapenems,[79,81-83] use of combination regimens will likely remain controversial and based largely on clinical preference. The use of combination regimens is, however, often recommended for critically ill patients with neutropenia or other conditions that cause them to be severely immunocompromised.[85,86]

DRUG DOSAGE AND ADMINISTRATION

Antimicrobials are selected based primarily on their pharmacologic activity against presumed or documented pathogens. However, because of the severity and high risk of morbidity and mortality associated with infections in critically ill patients, particular consideration must be given to other pharmacologic properties as well. Optimization of antimicrobial therapy requires that drugs be dosed in a manner that maximizes their pharmacologic activity while minimizing the risk of adverse effects and toxicities. Special consideration should be given to antimicrobial mechanisms of action, pharmacokinetics and pharmacodynamics, routes of administration, potential adverse effects, and potential drug interactions.

Mechanisms of Action

Because infections in critically ill patients are often severe and fulminant, it is theoretically most desirable to use antimicrobials that are "cidal" rather than "static" (i.e., merely inhibiting growth). The use of bactericidal agents has not specifically been shown to be superior to bacteriostatic agents in ICU patients. However, alterations in immune function that inherently accompany critical illness and the otherwise immunocompromised state of many ICU patients as the result of neutropenia, immunosuppressive diseases, or use of immunosuppressive drugs make it prudent to use antimicrobials that quickly reduce the antimicrobial burden at the site of infection and potentially result in more rapid eradication of pathogens through their bactericidal actions. β-Lactams, aminoglycosides, fluoroquinolones, vancomycin, daptomycin, metronidazole, and amphotericin B are examples of "cidal" antimicrobials commonly used for the treatment of ICU infections.

Pharmacokinetic Considerations

Pharmacokinetic properties that should be specifically considered in critically ill patients include distribution to various tissues and fluids, and routes of metabolism and excretion.[87] The ability of a drug to penetrate to the site of infection in sufficient quantities to have activity against a pathogen is crucial for achieving clinical and microbiologic efficacy. Although the distributional characteristics of antimicrobials are often only specifically considered in the treatment of central nervous system or bone infections, good penetration to tissues and fluids present at the site of infection is a necessary consideration when selecting agents for any infection in ICU patients. Routes of drug metabolism and elimination are also important pharmacokinetic properties because of the prevalence of acute and chronic organ failures in most critically ill populations. Severe organ dysfunction, particularly of the liver or kidneys, should prompt clinicians to select agents that do not rely on that organ for metabolism or excretion from the body to avoid excessive drug accumulation and increased potential for unacceptable drug toxicities. Clinicians should also be mindful of the fact that some common antimicrobials (e.g., ceftriaxone, ciprofloxacin) are dependent on both the liver and kidneys for metabolism and excretion, and their use may be particularly problematic in patients with dysfunction of both of these organ systems. Practitioners must be familiar with the pharmacokinetic properties of commonly used antimicrobials to use them in the most efficacious and safe manner.[87]

Pharmacodynamic Considerations

Pharmacodynamics is the discipline that attempts to define and apply the relationships between concentrations of a drug and its pharmacologic effects (both desirable and undesirable).[88-90] Although both the pharmacologic activity of an agent and its pharmacokinetic disposition are important considerations in drug selection and dosing, it is the combination of these two properties that is critical to achieving optimal outcomes during treatment of infections. The pharmacologic activities of antibacterial drugs are commonly defined by their minimal inhibitory concentration (MIC) as determined by in vitro testing. The MIC is the minimal concentration required to inhibit the growth of a target organism; highly active agents are associated with low MICs— that is, only low concentrations are required to inhibit bacterial growth, whereas agents with poor activity are associated with high MICs for the organism in question. It is logical that even extremely active agents with very low MICs will not be efficacious against a pathogen if the drug does not reach the site of infection in sufficient quantity; likewise, agents with relatively poor activity and higher MICs may be just as clinically efficacious if they are able to achieve high drug concentrations at the site of infection. Pharmacodynamic considerations combine MIC-defined pharmacologic activity and pharmacokinetic properties of a drug to make predictions regarding the drug's probable efficacy in the treatment of a given type of infection. Models of infection have allowed antibacterial drugs to be broadly classified into two major categories: concentration-dependent agents and time-dependent (concentration-independent) agents.[88-90]

Concentration-dependent agents, particularly aminoglycosides and fluoroquinolones, exert bactericidal activities when drug concentrations are well above the MIC of the organism; the higher the ratio of drug concentration at the site of infection to the MIC, the more rapid and/or complete the bacterial killing becomes. Previous studies have established that important pharmacodynamic predictors of clinical

efficacy of concentration-dependent agents include the ratio of maximum serum concentration divided by the MIC (C_{max}/MIC) and the ratio of the 24-hour area under the serum concentration-versus-time curve divided by the MIC (AUC_{0-24}/MIC).[88-94] Although the ratios required to achieve maximal effects are not exactly known, in vitro and in vivo studies indicate that C_{max}/MIC ratios of at least 10 to 12 and, for the fluoroquinolones, AUC_{0-24}/MIC ratios of 30 to 50 for gram-positive and 125 to 250 for gram-negative organisms are required for optimal clinical and microbiologic outcomes as well as for the prevention of antimicrobial resistance.[88-94] Both C_{max}/MIC and AUC_{0-24}/MIC ratios appear to be important determinants of clinical and microbiologic outcomes, although it is less clear which of these parameters is most predictive of drug efficacy because they are closely linked by the pharmacokinetic properties of the drugs.

Time-dependent killing agents only exert antimicrobial effects when their concentrations at the site of infection are higher than the MIC of the pathogen; the so-called time above MIC (T>MIC) thus becomes the pharmacodynamic parameter of interest for these drugs.[88-90] Important time-dependent agents common in ICU practice include the penicillins, cephalosporins, carbapenems, clindamycin, and the macrolides. Studies indicate that T>MIC should be at least 40% to 50% of the dosing interval, although it has also been suggested that achieving T>MIC for 100% of the dosing interval may be desirable for optimal outcome.[88-90] These studies have also suggested that both the AUC_{0-24}/MIC as well as the T>MIC are important predictors of clinical efficacy and the risk of the development of microbial resistance.[88-90]

Because patients in the ICU are frequently infected with serious nosocomial pathogens that display decreased susceptibilities to antimicrobials and are prone to developing resistance with inadequate therapy, failure to properly dose antimicrobial agents predisposes patients to clinical and microbiologic failure. The appropriate consideration of pharmacodynamic principles in the treatment of infection in critically ill patients enables clinicians to select dosing regimens that will maximize the potential effectiveness of the specific agent. Thus, aminoglycosides and fluoroquinolones (concentration-dependent drugs) should be used in relatively high doses that facilitate their distribution into infected tissues and achieve concentrations many-fold higher than the MIC of pathogens. Direct application of these pharmacodynamic principles has resulted in the common use of extended-interval dosing (also referred to as *once-daily* or *single-daily dosing*) of aminoglycosides, in which these drugs are administered in single doses of 6 to 9 mg/kg rather than smaller divided doses,[91,92,95-97] as well as the use of increased daily doses of fluoroquinolones (ciprofloxacin and levofloxacin) for severe infections such as nosocomial pneumonia and complicated skin and skin structure infections.[98] Likewise, β-lactam antibiotics such as the penicillins and cephalosporins are best given as several smaller divided doses administered intermittently throughout the day, or even as a continuous infusion of drug to maintain high concentrations of drug over long periods of time. Thus, β-lactams are usually administered every 4 to 12 hours depending on achievable serum concentrations and the serum half-life of the specific agent.

The severity of infections encountered in the ICU population and the need for adequate C_{max}/MIC and AUC_{0-24}/MIC ratios are important considerations in severely ill patients. However, there is still much to learn regarding the direct application of pharmacodynamic principles to the routine care of critically ill patients. Although it is assumed that serum concentrations of most drugs are related to their concentrations in various tissues, the use of serum C_{max}/MIC and AUC_{0-24}/MIC ratios does not always accurately predict tissue concentrations of drugs. A particularly important limitation of pharmacodynamic principles in the routine care of ICU patients is that they have not been thoroughly clinically validated in critically ill populations. Numerous studies have demonstrated that the pharmacokinetics of antimicrobials are often significantly altered in critical illness and that there is a high degree of interpatient (and even intrapatient) variability in this population.[91,99-104] Distribution of antimicrobials to infected tissues may also be affected by hemodynamic instability and regional or local changes in perfusion of various organs and tissues. The difficult combination of severe illness, pharmacokinetic variability, and life-threatening infections involving potentially drug-resistant pathogens makes the ICU population a difficult one in which to optimize drug therapy through appropriate application of pharmacodynamic principles. However, it is also only through the use of these principles that optimization of antimicrobial therapy is likely to be achieved in any consistent manner.

Dosing

Because of the severity of infections encountered in critically ill patients and because of the variability in pharmacokinetics, tissue penetration, and other important factors relating to efficacy of antimicrobials, the general recommendation for antimicrobials in ICU patients is to use high, aggressive doses. Use of high doses potentially compensates for pharmacokinetic variability that may be present and ensures that patients are receiving enough drug to successfully achieve pharmacodynamic goals of antimicrobial use. However, use of high doses also puts patients at higher risk of drug-related adverse effects and toxicities, again partially owing to pharmacokinetic variability in drug distribution and elimination. Although drug dosing should be aggressive, it must also be based on appropriate clinical considerations involving relevant issues such as drug toxicities, presence of renal or hepatic dysfunction that may lead to drug accumulation, the presumed site of infection and the ability of the drug to achieve adequate concentrations in that site, and susceptibilities of presumed or documented pathogens to the drugs in question.

Route of Administration

For initial therapy for serious infections, antimicrobials should generally be administered by the intravenous route to avoid any problems of drug absorption related to gut malperfusion and to ensure rapid, adequate serum and tissue concentrations. However, although drugs are usually given intravenously at the initiation of therapy, drugs with good oral bioavailability may be effectively switched to oral formulations once patients are stable and responding to therapy. A number of drugs including levofloxacin, linezolid, and fluconazole have oral bioavailabilities approaching 100%; such agents may be administered orally without any apparent loss of therapeutic efficacy and with substantial cost savings.[99,105] Oral antibiotics are an option for many hospitalized patients, including those in the ICU, and should be considered when patients have responded favorably to initial parenteral regimens and are able to take oral medications.[99,105]

Adverse Effects and Toxicities

Critically ill patients have higher rates of adverse effects from drugs compared to the general population of non-ICU patients. This is attributable to several factors, including the frequent presence of renal and/or hepatic dysfunction that may lead to excessive accumulation and excessively high concentrations of drugs, administration of many concurrent medications that may have overlapping adverse effect profiles or additive toxicities, and underlying illness that makes the patients more predisposed to adverse effects such as central nervous system or renal toxicities. Clinicians must carefully evaluate patients for any predisposing conditions potentially associated with increased risk of drug toxicities, and either use high-risk antimicrobials with caution or avoid them altogether. A common example of this concept is the use of aminoglycosides. The overall incidence of aminoglycoside-induced nephrotoxicity is approximately 10% or less, compared with rates of 16% to 36% in the critically ill.[91,92,95,106] Although they may be effectively used in ICU patients, aminoglycosides must be carefully dosed and monitored to decrease the risk of toxicities. Alternatively, many clinicians would choose an agent such as a fluoroquinolone that may be used as part of combination regimens as alternatives to aminoglycosides and do not have the risk of nephrotoxicity. Clinicians must be familiar with the safety profiles of the various antimicrobials they commonly use and apply appropriate benefit-versus-risk considerations when selecting agents for a specific patient. The use of multidisciplinary teams in the ICU has also been associated with a substantially decreased incidence of adverse effects in critically ill patients.[107-110]

Drug Interactions

Patients in ICUs are often managed with large numbers of drugs. With polypharmacy being the rule rather than the exception, clinicians must be alert to the potential for adverse drug interactions.[111] Drug interactions involving delayed or decreased absorption of orally administered agents and metabolic interactions involving inhibition of hepatic enzyme systems (e.g., azole antifungals, macrolides) are among the most common types of interactions likely to be seen in this population and should be avoided whenever possible. Drug–disease state interactions involving antimicrobials and increased risk of adverse effects should also be considered and prospectively monitored.[111]

DURATION OF ANTIMICROBIAL THERAPY

The appropriate duration of antimicrobial therapy for most infectious processes has been poorly studied. Beyond community-acquired urinary tract infections, endocarditis, and a handful of other infections, the appropriate duration of treatment for most infections remains incompletely defined. This is particularly true in critically ill patients wherein relatively few studies have specifically examined the appropriate duration of antibiotic therapy for various infections. The general tendency has been to treat severe infections for long periods of time on the assumption that long courses of antimicrobials are required to provide good clinical efficacy, reduce the probability of treatment failure or relapse, and prevent the emergence of resistance due to the incomplete eradication of pathogens. However, long durations of therapy may themselves contribute to the development of resistance by subjecting endogenous or colonizing bacterial flora to unnecessary antimicrobial exposure. Long durations of treatment may also increase the risk of drug-related toxicities and add unnecessary treatment costs. Available studies, although few, have shown that shorter courses of antimicrobial therapy (e.g., 8 days versus 15 days for ventilator-associated pneumonia) are equal or superior in efficacy to longer courses and may be associated with a decreased incidence of superinfections and decreased antimicrobial use, drug costs, adverse effects, and antimicrobial resistance.[112-114] Despite the potential advantages of shorter treatment durations, the decision to discontinue antimicrobial use in seriously ill patients is often very difficult to make on clinical grounds. Clinical response to antimicrobial therapy may be masked by underlying illnesses or concurrent drugs, and critically ill patients may not always manifest an association between successful treatment of an infection and rapid improvement in clinical signs and symptoms.[115] Until additional research is able to better define optimal treatment durations for specific types of infections in ICU populations, the decision to discontinue therapy will largely rest on the clinical judgment of the ICU practitioner. Nevertheless, clinicians must remain cognizant of the desirability of limiting antimicrobial treatment durations and seek to de-escalate (i.e., reduce the number of drugs used in treatment or discontinue antibiotics altogether) whenever appropriate.

MONITORING RESPONSE TO ANTIMICROBIALS

The appropriate use of antimicrobials in any population requires careful monitoring of patients for clinical response and adverse effects. This is particularly important in critically ill patients, owing to the potential for a number of events that may indicate the need to modify drug selection or drug-dosing regimens to improve the probability of successful treatment, enhance patient safety, and decrease drug costs and antimicrobial resistance. Such events include inadequate initial drug selection, the availability of culture and susceptibility test results that may influence subsequent drug selection, emergence of bacterial resistance during therapy, rapidly changing organ function that would influence drug dosing, drug-related adverse effects and toxicities, and the occurrence of superinfection. Serum concentrations of drugs, particularly aminoglycosides, should be monitored to guide appropriate drug dosing.

Clinicians should be mindful that failure of patients to promptly respond to antimicrobial therapy does not necessarily imply that the patient is receiving inadequate therapy. Critically ill patients are often slow to respond to therapy because of severity of the infection, concomitant disease states, immunosuppression, advanced age, and a number of other patient-specific factors.[115] Thus, patients who are not clearly showing signs of clinical improvement within 24 to 48 hours after initiating antibiotics may merely require additional time to respond and do not necessarily require the modification of antimicrobial regimens. In addition, many noninfectious sources of fever are present in ICU patients and may confound assessment of a patient's response to therapy. The finding of a persistent fever while other clinical signs and symptoms are improving should thus prompt clinicians to carefully assess patients for other noninfectious sources of fever or failure to respond. Finally, it must be recognized that not every patient treated in the ICU will recover from their infection, and failure to respond does not mean that antimicrobial therapy is inadequate. Whether failure to respond to therapy is in fact related to inadequate drug therapy can only be discerned through careful patient monitoring and assessment. However, even with the most conscientious ongoing assessment, this is often a very difficult distinction to make. Appropriate management of patients who are initially unresponsive to antimicrobial therapy is one of the most challenging dilemmas in the treatment of infections in the ICU.

Protocols and Guidelines for Use of Antimicrobials

The use of prescribing guidelines and protocols, often electronically based or embedded into computerized clinical care systems (e.g., computerized physician order entry, or CPOE), has been shown to effectively improve overall antimicrobial appropriateness,[116-118] decrease the incidence of adverse drug effects,[119] avoid unnecessary antimicrobial use,[118,120,121] reduce or stabilize bacterial resistance rates,[61,121] reduce drug costs,[117,120,121] and improve mortality and other outcomes.[122-124] The use of guidelines for the treatment of ventilator-associated pneumonia in ICU patients has also been associated with increased initial administration of adequate antimicrobial therapy and decreased durations of antibiotic therapy.[116,117] Although using clinical guidelines and protocols has been demonstrated to produce a number of favorable results, the implementation of such tools is often difficult because they are perceived as being too restrictive on clinical decision making by individual practitioners. Properly prepared guidelines are multidisciplinary in their preparation and implementation, involve key physicians in their development to make them practical and promote support from other practitioners, and are tailored to the individual institution. Although numerous established guidelines are available in the literature and elsewhere, they must be adapted to each institution and based on specific needs and practice patterns. Guidelines and protocols must also involve intensive education of all affected parties, physicians and non-physicians alike; this education must precede implementation and must also be ongoing to optimize guideline use. Finally, practitioners involved in use of the guidelines must be regularly updated regarding benefits already achieved and areas for continued improvement. Guidelines and protocols that are based on these principles are more likely to be successful and achieve the potential benefits associated with their use.

KEY POINTS

1. The continuing emergence of antimicrobial resistance in ICUs is a major factor in the appropriate selection and use of antimicrobials in critically ill patients.

2. Inadequate antimicrobial therapy, defined as the use of drugs with poor in vitro activity against infecting pathogens and/or improper dosing of drugs, has been demonstrated in numerous studies to be significantly associated with increased mortality and other measures of poor patient outcome.

3. Hospital formulary-based antimicrobial restrictions may be effective in reducing drug costs and limiting specific outbreaks of resistant infections; however, appropriate drug use must be based on basic principles of rational antimicrobial use rather than relying on such restrictions to prevent or overcome resistance problems.

4. Although establishment of a definitive diagnosis of infection is paramount to the appropriate selection and use of antimicrobials, the actual site of infection and specific pathogens are never identified in many critically ill patients.

5. Patients who have a new fever, or who have previously been started on antimicrobial therapy and have persistent fever despite the resolution of other signs and symptoms of infection, should also be evaluated for noninfectious sources of fever before continuing or instituting unnecessary antimicrobial therapy.

6. The initial selection of adequate empirical drug therapy is of vital importance in optimizing outcomes of antimicrobial use in critically ill patients.

7. Empirical antimicrobial regimens for critically ill patients should be sufficiently broad spectrum in pharmacologic activity to cover the most likely pathogens, initiated promptly, and given in relatively high doses to optimize the provision of adequate and aggressive therapy.

8. Clinicians must utilize the results of culture and susceptibility tests when available to reassess and make appropriate changes to empirical drug regimens.

9. Antimicrobial regimens selected for either empirical or definitive therapy should provide suitable activity against suspected or known pathogens while at the same time using the fewest required number of drugs, narrowing the spectrum of antimicrobial activity as much as possible, minimizing the risk of drug-related toxicities, and minimizing the cost of drug therapy.

10. Combination antimicrobial regimens are most appropriately used in the treatment of mixed infections or to provide adequate empirical therapy in institutions with high rates of antimicrobial resistance; the benefits of using combination therapy for documented infections with difficult pathogens such as *Pseudomonas aeruginosa* have not been well documented.

11. Basic knowledge and understanding of pharmacokinetic and pharmacodynamic properties of antimicrobials are necessary to achieve the most effective and safe use of antimicrobials in critically ill patients.

12. Although most antimicrobial use in critically ill patients should be administered by the intravenous route, oral therapy may also be administered in selected patients and should be considered when appropriate.

13. Limited studies have shown that shorter courses of antimicrobial therapy, such as 8 days versus 15 days for ventilator-associated pneumonia, may be equal in efficacy to longer courses of therapy and may be associated with a decreased incidence of superinfections and decreased antimicrobial use, drug costs, adverse effects, and antimicrobial resistance.

14. Careful monitoring of antimicrobial use is required in all critically ill patients and should include evaluation of clinical response to therapy, changes in organ function that may necessitate changes in the dosing regimen, occurrence of drug-related adverse effects and toxicities, evaluation for adverse drug interactions, and monitoring of serum drug concentrations when appropriate.

ANNOTATED REFERENCES

Chastre J, Wolff M, Fagon J-Y, et al. Comparison of 8 vs 15 days of antibiotic therapy for ventilator-associated pneumonia in adults: a randomized trial. JAMA 2003;290:2588-98.

This prospective, randomized, double-blind, multicenter trial evaluated whether an 8-day course of antimicrobial therapy was as effective as a 15-day course in the treatment of ventilator-associated pneumonia. The shorter duration of treatment was associated with equal clinical efficacy as measured by mortality, recurrent infections, and ICU length of stay and was also associated with a statistically significant reduction in multidrug-resistant pathogens among those patients who experienced recurrence of pulmonary infection.

Kollef MH, Sherman G, Ward S, et al. Inadequate antimicrobial treatment of infections: a risk factor for hospital mortality among critically ill patients. Chest 1999;115:462-74.

This prospective cohort study evaluated the relationship between inadequate antimicrobial treatment of infection and hospital mortality in 2000 consecutive patients admitted to the medical or surgical intensive care units. Inadequate treatment of infection was demonstrated to be an important determinant of hospital mortality and other poor patient outcomes, and administration of inadequate therapy in both community-acquired and nosocomial infections was shown to be most commonly related to infection with pathogens associated with high rates of antimicrobial resistance.

Luna CM, Vujacich P, Niederman MS, et al. Impact of BAL data on the therapy and outcome of ventilator-associated pneumonia. Chest 1997;111:676-85.

This prospective observational study evaluated the impact of antibiotic selection on outcomes of patients with ventilator-associated pneumonia and determined the impact of bronchoalveolar lavage (BAL) on these outcomes. Although mortality rates were significantly reduced when adequate empirical therapy was administered before BAL, mortality was not reduced compared with patients receiving no therapy or who continued inadequate therapy if adequate therapy was not achieved until after BAL was performed or results were known.

Heyland DK, Dodek P, Muscedere J, et al. Randomized trial of combination versus monotherapy for the empiric treatment of suspected ventilator-associated pneumonia. Crit Care Med 2008;36:737-44.

This prospective, randomized, multicenter trial examined the combination of meropenem plus ciprofloxacin versus ciprofloxacin alone in the empirical treatment of ventilator-associated pneumonia in 740 patients and found no overall differences in mortality or secondary outcomes. However, in the subset of patients infected with Pseudomonas, Acinetobacter, and multidrug-resistant gram-negative bacilli, combination therapy was associated with a statistically significant increased rate of adequate initial antibiotic therapy as well as trends toward higher microbiological eradication rates, shorter durations of ICU and hospital length of stay, and reductions in ICU and hospital mortality.

U.S. Department of Public Health and Human Services, Public Health Service. National Nosocomial Infections Surveillance (NNIS) System Report, data summary from January 1992-June 2003, issued August 2003. Am J Infect Control 2003;31:481-98.

This latest report from the Centers for Disease Control and Prevention summarizes data related to antimicrobial use and resistance in intensive care units in the United States. Data regarding sites of infections and pathogen prevalence, infection rates, standardized measures of antibiotic utilization, and trends in antimicrobial resistance among key pathogens are presented.

Craig WA. Pharmacokinetic/pharmacodynamic parameters: Rationale for antibacterial dosing of mice and men. Clin Infect Dis 1998;26:1-12.

Although now somewhat dated, this article remains a classic summary of pertinent pharmacokinetic and pharmacodynamic properties of commonly used antibiotics. Written by one of the earliest and still most preeminent researchers in this area, this article provides an excellent overview of basic pharmacodynamic principles.

Pea F, Viale P, Furlanut M. Antimicrobial therapy in critically ill patients: a review of pathophysiological conditions responsible for altered disposition and pharmacokinetic variability. Clin Pharmacokinet 2005;44:1009-34.

This article provides an excellent overview of antimicrobial pharmacokinetic alterations and the physiologic alterations found in critically ill patients which may account for those changes. Although quite extensive, the article provides practical recommendations for how to predict pharmacokinetic changes and empirically alter antimicrobial dosing regimens.

REFERENCES

Access the complete reference list online at http://www.expertconsult.com.

Beta-Lactam Drugs

STEVEN J. MARTIN

The β-lactam antibiotics are the most commonly prescribed antibiotics in the critical care setting. Their individual microbiological spectra and relative safety have made them first-line therapy for prophylaxis and treatment of infection. From the oldest (penicillin) to the newest (doripenem) agents, β-lactams continue to be useful for the myriad infectious complications of critical illness. Table 120-1 lists the parenteral β-lactam antibiotics commonly used in the intensive care unit (ICU).

The β-lactam compounds share a similar mechanism of action, mechanisms of resistance, pharmacodynamic properties, and many common adverse effects. However, each individual class of β-lactam has unique microbiological spectrums, and each of the agents has unique pharmacokinetic properties.

Mechanism of Action

β-Lactam antibiotics are similar in that each contains a β-lactam ring in addition to other pharmacologically active side chains stemming from this central structure. Side chain manipulation is largely responsible for both spectrum of activity and stability against enzymatic degradation, pharmacokinetics, and adverse effects. β-Lactam antibiotics inhibit bacterial wall synthesis by binding to penicillin-binding proteins (PBPs). These PBPs are transpeptidases, carboxypeptidases, and endopeptidases involved in the structure and function of the cell wall.[1,2] The cell wall is made up of a peptidoglycan consisting of long polysaccharide chains of *N*-acetylglucosamine and *N*-acetylmuramic acid cross-linked by shorter peptide chains.[3] There are three stages to peptidoglycan formation, including accumulation of peptidoglycan precursors in the cytoplasm, linkage of precursor products in a long polymer, followed by cross-linking by transpeptidation. β-Lactams inhibit this final transpeptidation step.

Transpeptidation cross-links adjacent sugar chains via their pentapeptides. Peptidoglycan transglycosylase and D-alanyl-D-alanine transpeptidase are responsible for this activity. β-Lactams inhibit D-alanyl-D-alanine transpeptidase activity by acetylation, forming stable esters with the open lactam ring attached to the enzyme's active site. The propensity of D-alanyl-D-alanine trans- and carboxypeptidase to form stable bonds with β-lactams provides these enzymes with their collective name of *penicillin-binding proteins* (PBPs).[3] PBPs lie on the outer side of the cytoplasmic membrane in gram-positive bacteria and are shielded only by the peptidoglycan and outer capsule. In gram-negative bacteria, most β-lactams must cross the outer membrane via porin channels to reach PBPs. Entry through the porin channels is determined by size, charge, and hydrophobicity.

Bacterial killing and clinical efficacy for β-lactam antibiotics is associated with the percent of time during the dosing interval that the drug concentration is above the minimum inhibitory concentration (MIC). Maximal killing occurs when the antibiotic concentration is maintained at 4 to 5 times the MIC. Carbapenems have faster killing rates than penicillins; cephalosporins have the slowest killing rates of the β-lactam class.[4] Therefore, percentages for time above the MIC required for bacterial killing are highest for the cephalosporins and lowest for the carbapenems.[4] Near-maximal bactericidal effect is typically observed when the free drug serum concentration exceeds the MIC for 60% to 70% of the dosing interval for cephalosporins, 50% for penicillins, and 40% for carbapenems. In vitro data in an experimental *Pseudomonas aeruginosa* aortic endocarditis model in rabbits suggested that bacterial resistance to β-lactams may develop if the antibiotic concentration falls below the MIC for more than half the dosing interval.[4]

All intravenous (IV) β-lactam antibiotics are recommended to be given in several daily intervals. Administering a β-lactam agent as an infusion for longer than the conventional 30- to 60-minute infusion produces a lower peak concentration of the drug while maintaining a serum drug concentration in excess of the pathogen MIC for a longer period of time. Continuous infusion of these agents is also an attractive administration method to maintain serum drug concentrations above the MIC. Several clinical trials have validated the use of extended infusion and continuous infusion β-lactams in the critically ill, and institutions may institute these administration methods to improve outcomes and reduce daily drug costs.[5-10]

β-Lactams are commonly used in antibiotic combinations that may include an aminoglycoside, a fluoroquinolone, a macrolide, or another β-lactam. Combination therapy is used empirically to broaden the spectrum of activity or minimize the likelihood of resistance. In documented infection with a known organism, combination therapy may be used to provide synergistic bacterial killing in an attempt to rapidly and thoroughly eradicate the pathogen. For combinations of aminoglycosides and β-lactams, there are ample in vitro data to substantiate the potential synergistic bactericidal activity of the drugs in combination. These data are not clear for β-lactam/fluoroquinolone combinations, and there are theoretical concerns about antagonistic interactions with this combination as well as combinations of two β-lactam agents.

Mechanisms of Resistance

Bacteria resist the cytotoxic activity of the β-lactams by modifying the normal PBPs, bypassing the normal PBPs, reducing the permeability of drug through the outer membrane (gram-negative bacteria), actively removing drug from the cell through the efflux pump mechanism, and producing β-lactamases. PBP modification and bypassing of normal PBPs are the most important mechanisms of resistance in gram-positive cocci, but β-lactamases are important mechanisms of antibiotic resistance in gram-negative bacteria.[11]

Alteration of PBPs, including decreased expression of PBPs and structural modifications to the PBPs to decrease antibiotic binding affinity, are seen in both gram-positive and gram-negative bacteria.[11] In gram-positive bacteria, altered PBPs occur commonly in *Streptococcus pneumoniae*, *Enterococcus faecium*, and *Staphylococcus aureus*. Genes encoding these PBP changes in *S. pneumoniae* contain segments from several different organisms, including the viridans streptococci.[12] In *S. aureus* and *E. faecium*, novel PBPs may be inducible through exposure to certain antibiotics.[13,14] These novel PBPs have a low affinity for β-lactam antibiotics. PBP alterations are best illustrated in methicillin-resistant *S. aureus* (MRSA). Methicillin resistance occurs through the actions of the *mecA* gene that encodes PBP2′ (PBP2a). MRSA produces PBP2′ as a fifth PBP in addition to the four PBPs found in all *S. aureus* strains.[15] β-Lactam antibiotics have very low affinity for PBP2′, so the enzyme's function continues even in the presence of β-lactams.

Gram-negative bacteria, including *Neisseria meningitides*, *Haemophilus influenzae*, and *Escherichia coli*, also produce altered PBPs.[11,16-19] Imipenem resistance due to altered PBPs has been reported in *P. aeruginosa*, *Acinetobacter baumannii*, and *Proteus mirabilis*, although this

TABLE 120-1	Beta-Lactam Antibiotics

Natural Penicillins

Penicillin GK

Penicillinase-Resistant Penicillins

Methicillin
Nafcillin
Oxacillin

Aminopenicillins

Ampicillin
Ampicillin/clavulanate

Anti-Pseudomonal Penicillins

Carboxypenicillins:
  Carbenicillin
  Ticarcillin
  Ticarcillin/clavulanate
Ureidopenicillins and piperazine penicillins:
  Azlocillin
  Mezlocillin
  Piperacillin
  Piperacillin/tazobactam

Cephalosporins

First generation:
  Cefazolin
Second generation:
  Cefoxitin
  Cefotetan
  Cefuroxime
Third generation:
  Cefoperazone
  Cefotaxime
  Ceftazidime
  Ceftriaxone
  Ceftizoxime
Fourth generation:
  Cefepime
  Ceftobiprole*

Carbapenems

Imipenem/cilastatin
Meropenem
Ertapenem

Monobactams

Aztreonam

*This drug is not yet approved by the FDA and has not been designated a fourth-generation agent.

PBP alteration is not the primary mechanism responsible for most imipenem resistance.[20-22]

β-Lactamase production is largely responsible for β-lactam antibiotic resistance among gram-negative bacteria in the critical care setting. β-Lactamase hydrolyzes the β-lactam ring structure within the antibiotic molecule, rendering the drug inactive. Most β-lactamases function by a serine ester hydrolysis mechanism, but a few use a zinc ion to attack the β-lactam ring.[11] β-Lactamase can be chromosomal (inherent within the chromosome of the organism) or can be encoded by plasmids or transposons, which are mobile genetic elements that can carry genes for resistance mechanisms. β-Lactamase production may be constitutive or inducible, and β-lactam antibiotics vary in their ability to induce β-lactamase production.[23,24] Penicillin G, ampicillin, cefoxitin, imipenem, clavulanate, and first-generation cephalosporins are strong β-lactamase inducers.[24] Third-generation cephalosporins, ureidopenicillins, aztreonam, and semisynthetic penicillinase-stable penicillins are weak β-lactamase inducers.[24]

Some measure of β-lactamase stability can be achieved through addition to the β-lactam ring of a substituent that hinders hydrolysis.[25] For example, the semisynthetic penicillinase-stable drugs such as oxacillin and nafcillin remain active against methicillin-susceptible S. aureus because of this ring structure manipulation. β-Lactamase stability has been difficult to achieve in compounds with activity against gram-negative bacteria and may be due to the periplasmic location of β-lactamase in the gram-negative cell structure.[11] Antibiotics including the β-lactams have difficulty accessing the gram-negative cell wall owing to the presence of an outer membrane. Porins within the membrane permit limited access through to the peptidoglycan layer of the cell, but the periplasmic space between the membrane and peptidoglycan layer allows β-lactamase to overwhelm the limited concentrations of drug that enter.

Third-generation cephalosporins have activity against β-lactamase-producing Enterobacteriaceae because they do not induce enzyme synthesis. However, these drugs may select spontaneous "derepressed" mutants that constitutively produce β-lactamase.[11] Emergence of derepressed mutants of Enterobacter spp. during third-generation cephalosporin therapy may be significant, particularly in pneumonia and bacteremia.[26] Through this selective pressure, organisms have developed that overproduce their chromosomal AmpC (class C) β-lactamase.[27] This type of β-lactamase is broad spectrum and inactivates most cephalosporins and aztreonam. AmpC resistance has been demonstrated in many clinically important gram-negative bacteria, including Acinetobacter spp., Citrobacter freundii, Enterobacter spp., E. coli, Morganella morganii, P. aeruginosa, and Serratia marcescens.[26,27] AmpC β-lactamase is not inhibited by β-lactamase inhibitors such as clavulanic acid, sulbactam, or tazobactam.[27] Unfortunately, these chromosomal AmpC β-lactamases have been found on plasmids worldwide, suggesting that this broad-spectrum class of enzymes may be spread much more readily in clinical settings.[27]

Enterobacter spp. are intrinsically resistant to aminopenicillins, cefazolin, and cefoxitin due to production of constitutive chromosomal AmpC β-lactamases, which hydrolyze third-generation or expanded spectrum cephalosporins, and are resistant to inhibition by clavulanate or other β-lactamase inhibitors.[26] β-Lactam antibiotic exposure drives AmpC-mediated resistance, leading to development of resistance to third-generation cephalosporins and mutations that may result in permanent enzyme hyperproduction. Exposure of Enterobacter organisms to third-generation cephalosporins may select for mutant strains associated with hyperproduction of AmpC β-lactamase.[26]

Other plasmid-mediated β-lactamases with more limited hydrolytic capacity have been found in Klebsiella pneumoniae, E. coli, Enterobacter spp., and other common Enterobacteriaceae. These so-called extended-spectrum β-lactamases (ESBL) are active against the oxyiminocephalosporins and aztreonam but not 7-α-methoxycephalosporins (cefoxitin, cefotetan) and are blocked by clavulanic acid, sulbactam, and tazobactam.[28] There are numerous reports of outbreaks of ESBL-producing Klebsiella and Enterobacter infections in ICUs.[28,29-35] Most organisms producing AmpC and ESBL enzymes remain susceptible to carbapenems such as imipenem. However, β-lactamase that uses zinc as an active site for β-lactam hydrolysis is able to hydrolyze carbapenems along with every other β-lactam presently available.[36] Carbapenemases found in Enterobacteriaceae can be either metallo-β-lactamases, expanded-spectrum oxacillinases, or clavulanic acid–inhibited β-lactamases. The most concerning carbapenemases prevalent worldwide today are the K. pneumoniae carbapenemase (KPC) enzymes, a group of mostly plasmid-encoded enzymes from K. pneumoniae. Klebsiella pneumoniae carbapenemase enzymes hydrolyze all β-lactam antibiotics including penicillins, cephalosporins, and aztreonam, although cephamycins and ceftazidime are weakly hydrolyzed.[37] The KPC enzymes may be mistaken for extended-spectrum β-lactamases (ESBLs), since they also hydrolyze expanded-spectrum cephalosporins, but unlike extended-spectrum β-lactamases, they also weakly hydrolyze carbapenems. The hydrolytic activity of KPC enzymes is not sufficient to produce resistance against carbapenems, but increases in MICs can occur.

To achieve full resistance to carbapenems, organisms must also exhibit impaired outer-membrane permeability. Clavulanic acid and tazobactam are not clinically effective against carbapenemase. Klebsiella pneumoniae carbapenemase-producing isolates are also often resistant to fluoroquinolones, aminoglycosides, and sulfamethoxazole/trimethoprim. Amikacin, gentamicin, colistin, and tigecycline typically retain activity against these enzymes. Combination therapies may be an alternative based on in vitro data, but clinical data supporting such recommendations are lacking.

TABLE 120-2 Microbiological Activity of Beta-Lactam Antibiotics Against Aerobic Gram-Positive Bacteria*

Antibiotic	Gram-Positive Bacteria					
	Staphylococcus aureus (Methicillin Susceptible)	Coagulase-Negative Staphylococci	Streptococcus pneumoniae	Viridans Streptococci	Enterococcus faecalis	Enterococcus faecium
Penicillin G			67.7% (3632)[38]	75.4% (680)[38]		
Oxacillin	100% (6826)[38]	23.9% (3283)[38]				
Ampicillin					100% (1401)[39]	26.6%[1] (203)[39] 0%[2] (640)[39]
Cefuroxime			77.3% (21,605)[40]			
Cefotaxime			89.4% (341)[41]	87.8% (47)[42]		
Ceftazidime	96.5% (6826)[38]	31.6% (3283)[38]				
Ceftriaxone	99.6% (6826)[38]	47.1% (3283)[38]	97.5% (3632)[38]	91.6% (680)[38]		
Cefepime	>99.9% (6826)[38]	76.2% (3283)[38]	96.3% (3632)[38]	91.3% (680)[38]		
Imipenem	>99.9% (6826)[38]	79.9% (3283)[38]	83.1% (3632)[38]	96% (47)[42]		

*Percent susceptible by CLSI[37] interpretation (no. of isolates tested). When possible, data represent North American isolates from large national susceptibility databases.
[1]Vancomycin-susceptible E. faecium.
[2]Vancomycin-non-susceptible E. faecium.

TABLE 120-3 Microbiological Activity of Beta-Lactam Antibiotics Against Aerobic Gram-Negative Bacteria*

Antibiotic	Gram-Negative Bacteria								
	Acinetobacter spp.	Citrobacter spp.	Enterobacter spp.	Escherichia coli	Haemophilus influenzae	Klebsiella spp.	Proteus spp.	Pseudomonas aeruginosa	Serratia spp.
Ampicillin/ sulbactam	50.4% (879)[38]	59.5% (237)[38]	30.2% (1373)[38]	54.5% (4938)[38]	100% (929)[38]	86% (246)[67]	83.3% (420)[38]		9.3% (557)[38]
Ticarcillin/ clavulanate	33.9% (879)[38]				92.9% (986)[43-45]			69.1% (2239)[38]	
Piperacillin/ tazobactam	37.5% (879)[38]	83.1% (237)[38]	76.4% (1373)[38]	94.3% (4938)[38]	100% (929)[38]	94.9% (3754)[43,44,46,47]	99.3% (420)[38]	84.8% (420)[38]	89.0% (557)[38]
Cefazolin				88.8% (663)[43,48]		87.3% (71)[43]			
Cefotetan				99% (511)[49]		93.2% (449)[44,49]			96% (47)[49]
Cefoxitin				94.4% (663)[43]		86.1% (274)[43,44]			
Cefuroxime				92.9% (98)[43]					
Ceftazidime	34.8% (879)[38]	75.9% (237)[38]	71.1% (1373)[38]	95.0% (4938)[38]	100% (371)[44,49]	95.6% (3288)[43,44,46,50]	98.3% (420)[38]	75.5% (420)[38]	95.2% (557)[38]
Ceftriaxone		75.1% (237)[38]	71.7% (1373)[38]	93.4% (4938)[38]	100% (929)[38]	97.4% (4000)[43,44,46,47,51]	92.4% (420)[38]		90.5% (557)[38]
Cefepime	44.1% (879)[38]	98.3% (237)[38]	93.4% (1373)[38]	96.0% (4938)[38]	100% (929)[38]		94.3% (420)[38]	79.4% (420)[38]	97.5% (557)[38]
Doripenem	73.4% (289)[52]	99.8% (514)[52]	99.2% (508)[52] All E. cloacae	99.8% (1772)[52]		99.6% (1227)[52]	99.2% (636)[52]	88.3% (875)[52]	98.7% (372)[52]
Imipenem	72.4% (879)[38]	99.6% (237)[38]	98.4% (1373)[38]	100% (4938)[38]	100% (929)[38]	94.5% (416)[53]	99.8% (420)[38]	75.8% (420)[38]	99.8% (557)[38]
Meropenem	69.1% (879)[38]	100% (237)[38]	98.9% (1373)[38]	100% (4938)[38]	100% (929)[38]	94.2% (416)[53]	100% (420)[38]	80.9% (420)[38]	94.1% (557)[38]
Aztreonam	34.6% (404)[49,50]	83% (66)[49]	81% (1655)[43,46]	97.7% (1174)[43,48,49]	95.8% (371)[44,49]	95.3% (3288)[44,46,49,54]	96% (81)[49]	65.7% (420)[38]	94% (47)[49]

*Percent susceptible by CLSI[37] interpretation (no. of isolates tested). When possible, data represent North American isolates from large national susceptibility databases.

Penicillins

The microbiological activity of the penicillins is shown in Tables 120-2 to 120-4. Natural penicillins are most active against non-β-lactamase-producing gram-positive aerobic and anaerobic bacteria as well as selected gram-negative cocci such as *Neisseria* spp. Penicillin G is effectively the only natural penicillin used in the critical care setting. Gram-positive bacteria inhibited by natural penicillins are generally more susceptible to these penicillins than to semisynthetic penicillins. Penicillin and ampicillin remain the drugs of choice for enterococcal infections, but resistance to ampicillin among enterococcal isolates in North America is nearly 20%.[60] Semisynthetic penicillins (oxacillin, nafcillin) are the agents of choice for penicillin-resistant *S. aureus* and *Staphylococcus epidermidis*, because penicillins exhibit faster bactericidal activity and improved clinical outcomes when compared with vancomycin.[61,62] Semisynthetic penicillins should be reserved for staphylococcal infections, even though they are active against streptococci. Methicillin is seldom used because of an associated higher incidence of interstitial nephritis than oxacillin or nafcillin. Nafcillin and oxacillin have similar antistaphylococcal activity and can be used interchangeably for this indication.

TABLE 120-4 Microbiological Activity of Beta-Lactam Antibiotics Against Anaerobic Gram-Positive and Gram-Negative Bacteria*

Antibiotic	Gram-Negative and Gram-Positive Bacteria		
	Peptostreptococcus	Fusobacterium	Bacteroides fragilis
Ampicillin/ sulbactam	98.3% (116)[56,57]	100% (22)[57]	95.5% (198)[58]
Piperacillin/ tazobactam	100% (61)[57,59]	100% (83)[57,59]	99.0% (198)[58]
Cefotetan	100% (12)[59]	100% (11)[59]	64.6% (961)[56]
Cefoxitin	100% (61)[57,59]	100% (33)[57,59]	96.0% (198)[58]
Imipenem	100% (21)[57,59]	100% (33)[57,59]	99.0% (198)[58]
Meropenem	100% (49)[57]	100% (22)[57]	98.5% (198)[58]
Ertapenem	100% (49)[57]	100% (22)[57]	98.0% (198)[58]
Doripenem			98.5% (198)[58]

*Percent susceptible by CLSI[55] interpretation (no. of isolates tested). When possible, data represent North American isolates from large, national susceptibility databases.

Ampicillin possesses the same spectrum as penicillin G and is active against gram-negative cocci and members of the family Enterobacteriaceae. Ampicillin alone is seldom used any longer in critical care settings, because β-lactamase production is common for almost all Enterobacteriaceae and staphylococci. With the addition of sulbactam to ampicillin, activity is regained against most organisms within these categories. Use of the antipseudomonal penicillins is increasingly limited to ticarcillin/clavulanate and piperacillin/tazobactam, owing to the prevalence of β-lactamase and the poor activity of these agents against this enzymatic activity. Carbenicillin and ticarcillin are less active than piperacillin against streptococci, enterococci, *Haemophilus* spp., and *P. aeruginosa*. Ticarcillin and piperacillin have good clinical activity against both gram-positive and gram-negative anaerobes, including *Bacteroides fragilis, Fusobacterium,* and *Prevotella* spp.. Mezlocillin and azlocillin have similar activity to piperacillin against *P. aeruginosa*, but the lack of a β-lactamase inhibitor combination has dramatically reduced the use of either of these compounds in North America.

The pharmacokinetics of the penicillins and their dosing guidelines and administration are shown in Table 120-5. The pharmacokinetics of these agents has not been well investigated in critically ill patients, so extrapolation from healthy volunteers and less acutely ill patients is required. When penicillin was first available in the 1940s, the drug was administered as a continuous infusion to treat bacterial endocarditis. Nearly 70 years later, there is a resurgence of interest in using a continuous infusion or extended infusion of a β-lactam to improve bacterial killing activity and reduce development of resistance.

Piperacillin has been well studied (with and without tazobactam) as a continuous infusion. Several studies have demonstrated improved clinical cure rates and reduced overall drug exposure and drug costs compared to traditional intermittent 30- to 60-minute infusions.[63] Patients with ventilator-associated pneumonia (VAP) caused by gram-negative pathogens with MICs of 8 to 16 μg/mL demonstrated higher probability of clinical cure when piperacillin-tazobactam was administered by continuous compared with intermittent infusion.[64]

In a study of 194 seriously ill patients with *P. aeruginosa* infection, the use of piperacillin/tazobactam in an extended infusion period (4-hour infusion with doses administered every 8 hours) demonstrated reduced 14-day mortality for patients with high Acute Physiology and Chronic Health Evaluation [APACHE] II scores (>17) when compared to conventional 30-minute infusions (12.2% versus 31.6%; $P < 0.04$).[65] Extended infusion may offer some advantages over continuous infusion. A continuous infusion requires a dedicated IV line or lumen of a catheter. This is not always practical in the critically ill, especially for patients who have limited IV access, patients who require multiple daily infusions, or in situations where drug compatibility concerns may occur. An extended infusion provides a period of time in which the IV line is available. For either administration method, intensive nursing attention is required to make sure the drug is delivered properly.

Oxacillin and nafcillin are inactivated largely by the liver, with some biliary secretion and the remaining drug eliminated unchanged through the kidneys. Ampicillin also undergoes some liver metabolism and biliary excretion, but about 75% of an IV dose is excreted unchanged in the urine. IV ampicillin/sulbactam is administered in a 2 : 1 ratio. Sulbactam is principally excreted unchanged in the urine. Ticarcillin undergoes some metabolism in the liver, and small amounts of drug are secreted into the bile. Significantly more piperacillin is excreted into the bile, with some minor drug inactivation in the liver. The pharmacokinetics of piperacillin and mezlocillin are dose dependent, with nonproportional increases in serum concentration with increasing dosage. This occurs because of saturation of liver and biliary transformation pathways. Clavulanic acid undergoes approximately 50% elimination in the urine as unchanged drug, with 50%

TABLE 120-5	Pharmacokinetics of Beta-Lactam Antibiotics*				
Antibiotic	*Adult Dose†*	*Peak Serum Concentration*	*Renal Elimination*	*Half-life (h)*	*Dosing Alteration for Renal Dysfunction*
Penicillin G	2-3 million units q 4-6 h	20 μg/mL	90%	0.5	CrCl 10-50 mL/min: 50% of dose or full dose q 8-12 h CrCl <10 mL/min: 50% of dose or full dose at q 12-18 h Post HD: 2 million units Post CV/VH: 2 million units
Oxacillin	1 g q 4-6 h	52-63 μg/mL	50%	0.5-0.7	CrCl <10 mL/min: 1 g q 12 h Post HD, CVVH: none
Nafcillin	1 g q 4 h	20 μg/mL	35%	0.5-1	Not necessary
Ampicillin/sulbactam	1.5-3 g q 6 h	40-71 μg/mL (after 1.5 g)	75-85%	1	CrCl 15-29 mL/min: q 12 h CrCl 5-14 mL/min: q 24 h Post HD: 1.5 g Post CVVH: 3 g
Ticarcillin/clavulanate	3.1 g q 4-6 h	330 μg/mL	60-70%	1.1	CrCl 30-60 mL/min: 2 g q 4 h CrCl 10-30 mL/min: 2 g q 8 h CrCl <10 mL/min: 2 g q 12 h Post HD: 3.1 g Post CVVH: 3.1 g
Piperacillin/tazobactam	2.25-4.5 g q 6 h	298 μg/mL (after 4.5 g)	68%	0.7-1.2	CrCl 40-60 mL/min: 3.75 g q 6 h CrCl 10-39 mL/min: 2.25 g q 6 h CrCl <10 mL/min: 2.25 g q 8 h Post HD: 2.25 g Post CVVH: 4.5 g
Cefazolin	1 g q 8 h	185 μg/mL	80%	1.8	CrCl ≤35 mL/min: 500 mg q 12 h CrCl <10 mL/min: 500 μg q 18-24 h Post HD: 500 mg Post CVVH: 1 g
Cefotetan	2-3 g q 12 h	230 μg/mL	80%	3.5	CrCl 40-60 mL/min: 1 g q 12 h CrCl 10-40 mL/min: 1 g q 24 h CrCl <10 mL/min: 1 g q 48 h Post HD: 1 g Post CVVH: 2 g
Cefoxitin	2 g q 4-6 h	150 μg/mL	80%	0.8	CrCl 40-60 mL/min: 1 g q 8 h CrCl 10-40 mL/min: 1 g q 12 h CrCl <10 mL/min: 1 g q 24 h Post HD: 1 g Post CVVH: 2 g

Continued on following page

TABLE 120-5	Pharmacokinetics of Beta-Lactam Antibiotics—cont'd				
Antibiotic	*Adult Dose†*	*Peak Serum Concentration*	*Renal Elimination*	*Half-life (h)*	*Dosing Alteration for Renal Dysfunction*
Cefuroxime	1.5 g q 8 h	100 μg/mL	90%	1.3	CrCl 10-20 mL/min: 750 mg q 12 h CrCl <10 mL/min: 750 mg q 24 h Post HD: 750 mg Post CVVH: 1.5 g
Ceftazidime	1-2 g q 8 h	160 μg/mL	90%	1.8	CrCl 30-50 mL/min: 1 g q 12 h CrCl 15-30 mL/min: 1 g q 24 h CrCl 5-15 mL/min: 500 mg q 24 h CrCl <5 mL/min: 500 mg q 48 h Post HD: 1 g Post CVVH: 2 g
Ceftriaxone	1-2 g q 24 h	123 μg/mL	40-50%	8	Not necessary Post CVVH: 1-2 g
Cefepime	1-2 g q 8-12 h	130 μg/mL	85%	2.1	CrCl 10-30 mL/min: 1 g q 12 h CrCl <10 mL/min: 1 g q 24 h Post HD: 1 g Post CVVH: 2 g
Imipenem	500 mg to 1 g q 6-8 h	21-50 μg/mL (after 500 mg)	70%	1	CrCl 10-30: 500 mg q 12 h CrCl <10 mL/min: 250 mg q 12 h Post HD: 250 mg Post CVVH: 500 mg
Meropenem	1 g q 8 h	49 μg/mL	70%	1	CrCl 25-50 mL/min: 1 g q 12 h CrCl 10-25 mL/min: 500 mg q 12 h CrCl <10 mL/min: 500 mg q 24 h Post HD 500 mg Post CVVH: 1 g
Ertapenem	1 g q 24 h	155 μg/mL	80%	4	CrCl <30 mL/min: 500 mg q 24 h Post HD: 150 mg
Doripenem	500 mg q 8 h	23 μg/mL	70%	1	CrCl ≥30 to ≤50 mL/min: 250 mg q 8 h CrCl ≥10 to ≤30 mL/min: 250 mg q 12 h

*Data compiled from package insert information.
†All administration is intravenous; dosing is for serious, life-threatening infections.
CrCl, Creatinine clearance; HD, hemodialysis; CVVH, continuous venovenous hemofiltration.

metabolism. Tazobactam is mainly eliminated unchanged in the urine, with some biliary secretion and liver metabolism.

The most common adverse event with the penicillins is hypersensitivity reaction. The most frequent clinical presentations of such hypersensitivity reactions are maculopapular or urticarial rashes and angioedema, but severe reactions such as anaphylaxis can also occur. The avoidance of β-lactams based only on the clinical history may exclude the use of several effective and cost-effective agents. Clinical data in over 500 cases suggest that patients who report penicillin allergies are unlikely to experience hypersensitivity reactions if penicillin skin testing is negative.[66] Although some critically ill patients may be anergic, Arroliga and associates demonstrated that 106 of 117 ICU patients with a history of nonanaphylactic penicillin allergy responded to histamine control as part of a penicillin skin testing protocol, and 105 (90%) tested negative for penicillin reaction.[67,68] Cross-reactivity between penicillins and cephalosporins has been reported at anywhere between 0.1% and 10%.[69] The true rate is probably closer to 1%.[69] In most allergic reactions to cephalosporins, the side chain on the β-lactam ring is responsible for the hypersensitivity response.[70] Because older cephalosporins have side chains similar to penicillin and may have contained penicillin contaminants, the rates of cross-reactivity reported with early use of the cephalosporins were high.[70] Cross-reactivity between penicillin and carbapenems is low, but this may reflect the low underlying rate of reaction with rechallenge of penicillin rather than a lack of cross-reactivity. Aztreonam is unlikely to elicit a reaction in penicillin-allergic individuals, owing to the unique side chain structure on the monobactam chemical.

Robinson and associates have published an approach to the treatment of patients with a possible or probable β-lactam allergy.[70] For patients with a history suggestive of hypersensitivity to β-lactams, such as urticarial rash, pruritus, angioedema, hyperperistalsis, bronchospasm, hypotension, or arrhythmia, a penicillin skin test should be performed before initiating therapy. If the test is negative, β-lactam

therapy can be started. Patients who react to the test should avoid β-lactams or undergo desensitization.

Penicillin is rarely used in the ICU except for treatment of meningococcal meningitis, tertiary syphilis, streptococcal endocarditis, or streptococcal necrotizing fasciitis. The semisynthetic penicillins are indicated for nonurinary methicillin-susceptible staphylococcal infections. Ampicillin/sulbactam is useful for a variety of infections in the critically ill, including urinary tract infections, community-acquired respiratory tract infections, meningitis, endocarditis, biliary infections, skin and skin structure infections, and intraabdominal infections. Piperacillin/tazobactam and ticarcillin/clavulanate are workhorse agents for many infections that arise in the critically ill, including pneumonia, bacteremia, urinary and biliary tract infections, intraabdominal infections, and skin and skin structure infections. These agents can be used alone, but growing resistance problems dictate that empirical combination therapy with aminoglycosides or fluoroquinolones may be optimal until culture data are available. Piperacillin/tazobactam has maintained activity against *P. aeruginosa* in recent years, but trends toward slightly decreased susceptibility have been noted across the United States.[71]

Cephalosporins

The microbiological activity of the cephalosporins is shown in Tables 120-2 to 120-4. Only parenteral cephalosporins are useful in the critical care setting, because higher serum and tissue concentrations are required for serious infections, and these can be achieved only through parenteral administration. The cephalosporins can be divided into generations based on their microbiological activity. Cefazolin is effectively the only parenteral first-generation cephalosporin in general use, although cephapirin and cephradine are also marketed in North America. Cefazolin has activity against methicillin-susceptible *S. aureus* and coagulase-negative staphylococci but may be susceptible to staphylococcal β-lactamase. Cefazolin is also active against most streptococci, but all cephalosporins lack clinically useful activity against the enterococci. Cefazolin activity against gram-negative bacteria is limited to *Moraxella catarrhalis*, *E. coli*, *P. mirabilis*, *K. pneumoniae*, *Salmonella* spp., and *Shigella* spp.

The second-generation cephalosporins may be divided by their anaerobic activity, with cefoxitin and cefotetan (cephamycins) active against most gram-negative anaerobic organisms, including *Prevotella* spp., *Fusobacterium* spp., and *B. fragilis*. Cephamycins have less gram-positive potency than the first-generation cephalosporins but increased activity against Enterobacteriaceae, such as *M. morganii*, *Proteus vulgaris*, *Providencia* spp., and *S. marcescens*. Cefoxitin is a potent inducer of chromosomally mediated β-lactamases.[72] True parenteral second-generation cephalosporins include cefonicid and cefuroxime. Cefuroxime is stable to most β-lactamases produced by gram-negative bacilli and is more active against methicillin-susceptible staphylococci and streptococci than is cefazolin. Cefuroxime has good potency against *H. influenzae* and is effective against most typical community-acquired respiratory tract pathogens.

Third-generation parenteral cephalosporins include cefoperazone, cefotaxime, ceftazidime, ceftizoxime, and ceftriaxone. These agents have expanded potency against gram-negative bacilli and *S. pneumoniae*. Third-generation cephalosporins may be divided by their antipseudomonal activity, with cefoperazone and ceftazidime having clinically useful potency against *P. aeruginosa*. Cefoperazone possesses a methylthiotetrazole side chain that causes hypoprothrombinemia; this problem limits cefoperazone use in the critically ill who may be predisposed to bleeding due to underlying disease. Ceftazidime has the greatest potency of the third-generation agents against *S. aureus*. Third-generation cephalosporins have excellent clinical activity against the Enterobacteriaceae but lack activity against enterococci, MRSA, *Listeria monocytogenes*, *Stenotrophomonas maltophilia*, and many *Acinetobacter* spp. Third-generation cephalosporins may be hydrolyzed by ESBL-producing Enterobacteriaceae such as *Klebsiella*, *Enterobacter*, and *E. coli*.

Cefepime, touted as a fourth-generation cephalosporin, has the same activity as the third-generation agents, but it has variable stability to ESBLs and is comparatively stable to AmpC β-lactamases. It could be useful in the treatment of *Enterobacter* infections which constitutively produce AmpC β-lactamase, but ESBL-producing *Enterobacter* spp., particularly *Enterobacter cloacae*, have been identified in the United States. Thus, not all resistance to later-generation cephalosporins in *E. cloacae* may be the result of hyperproduction of AmpC β-lactamases, and ESBL-producing strains of *E. cloacae* may be resistant to cefepime as well as to third-generation cephalosporins. Carbapenems are also active against *Enterobacter* spp., and are alternatives to cefepime.

Eradication of ESBL-producing organisms with standard cefepime regimens (1-2 g every 12 hours) is low due to the higher MICs of these bacteria. Cefepime pharmacodynamic exposure (time above MIC [T>MIC]) was determined for 18 patients with ESBL and non-ESBL infections using a published population pharmacokinetic model.[73] Eradication was 80% when T>MIC was 50%, compared with 0% when T>MIC was less than 50% ($P < 0.05$), regardless of ESBL-production. Since median cefepime MICs for ESBL-producing isolates are generally several-fold higher than non-ESBL-producing isolates, higher doses of 4 to 6 grams administered IV as a continuous infusion, or 2 grams IV every 6 to 8 hours with a 4-hour infusion, are required to optimize therapy against ESBL-producing organisms that still retain cefepime susceptibility. It is important to note that critically ill patients, such as after trauma, may have an increased glomerular filtration rate or increased apparent volume of distribution, making the ability to optimize the time exceeding the MIC less likely.

Ceftobiprole is an investigational agent and the first of a new generation of cephalosporins with activity against MRSA. Potential applications for compounds such as ceftobiprole may include many infections commonly observed in critically ill patients. Ceftobiprole is an extended-spectrum β-lactam with in vitro activity against many gram-positive, gram-negative, and anaerobic bacteria.[74,75] Ceftobiprole's MRSA activity is due to its strong affinity for PBP2a and PBP2x, which are responsible for resistance in staphylococci and streptococci, respectively.[74] Its activity against gram-positive bacteria includes *S. aureus* (methicillin-resistant, vancomycin-intermediate, and resistant strains), methicillin-resistant *S. epidermidis*, penicillin-susceptible and -resistant *S. pneumoniae*, and *Enterococcus* (ampicillin-susceptible *E. faecalis* and *E. faecium* as well as vancomycin-resistant *E. faecalis*).[74-76] Studies have reported that ceftobiprole has a MIC for methicillin-susceptible *S. aureus* ranging from less than 0.12 to 1 μg/mL (MIC required to kill 90% of organisms [MIC90], 0.5 μg/mL) and for MRSA ranging from 0.25 to 4 μg/mL (MIC90, 1 μg/mL).[77]

The pharmacokinetics of the cephalosporins and their dosing guidelines and administration are shown in Table 120-5. Most cephalosporins have short half-lives and undergo extensive renal elimination. Cefoperazone and ceftriaxone, with significant biliary excretion, do not require dosing adjustments in renal dysfunction. The half-life of cefotaxime is not significantly increased in patients with renal failure; however, its active metabolite, desacetylcefotaxime, accumulates significantly, and thus dosing adjustments are required.

Pharmacokinetics in the critically ill have been studied for ceftazidime, ceftriaxone, and cefepime. Ceftazidime volume of distribution (V_D) and terminal half-life were increased in critically ill patients without renal dysfunction.[78,79] Ceftazidime area under the concentration-time curve (AUC) was increased 1.8-fold, clearance was increased 1.3-fold, V_D was increased 4.1-fold, and half-life was increased from 1.8 hours to 4.75 hours.[80] This expansion of the V_D may lead to inadequate serum concentrations throughout the dosing interval with intermittent bolus dosing.[80] Continuous infusion of ceftazidime, 60 mg/kg/d, in trauma patients was shown to maintain serum concentrations at well above the MIC90 for most ICU pathogens.[5] Continuous infusion of ceftazidime, 3 g/d, has been effective in treating nosocomial pneumonia, and the dose of drug administered is typically less than that required for intermittent bolus dosing.[78]

Ceftriaxone clearance in critically ill patients correlates to the degree of glomerular filtration function and is typically halved, even in patients with normal renal function.[54] Vd is also increased by up to 90% in the critically ill, possibly resulting in suboptimal serum concentrations with daily dosing of 2 g.[54] Cefepime V_D is also expanded in the critically ill, with a delay in renal clearance resulting in serum trough concentrations below the MIC50 for many *P. aeruginosa* isolates with 2-g, every-12-hour dosing.[81] Pharmacokinetic modeling suggests that shorter dosing intervals, such as 1 g every 4 hours, extended infusions (over 3-4 hours), or continuous infusion could be used to improve serum trough concentrations.[81]

Continuous infusion of cefuroxime has also been studied in critically ill patients after coronary artery bypass grafting.[82] A continuous infusion of 3 g over 24 hours provided serum concentrations above the MIC for common ICU pathogens throughout the 24-hour dosing interval and prevented sternal wound infection in the 54 patients studied.[82]

Cefepime has been studied in adult critical care patients with ventilator-associated pneumonia. Thirty two patients treated with high-dose cefepime (2 g every 8 hours [3-h infusion] or a renal function-adjusted equivalent dose) were studied. The likelihood of 2 g every 8 hours (3-hour infusion) achieving free drug concentrations above the MIC for 50% of the dosing interval were 91.8%, 78.1%, and 50.3% for MICs of 8, 16, and 32 μg/mL, respectively.[83] A recent study suggested that maintaining a T>MIC of 100% for cefepime or ceftazidime is associated with significantly greater clinical cure (82% versus 33%; $P < 0.002$) and bacteriologic eradication (97% versus 44%; $P < 0.001$) in patients with severe infections.[84]

Cephalosporins are generally well tolerated and cause minimal adverse effects. Agents with the methylthiotetrazole (MTT) side chain may cause hypoprothrombinemia via inhibition of synthesis and absorption of vitamin K and competitive inhibition of vitamin K–dependent clotting factors. Agents possessing the MTT side chain are cefamandole (no longer available), cefoperazone, cefotetan, and cefmetazole. Use of these agents may require vitamin K supplementation. The MTT side chain has also been associated with a disulfiram-like reaction.

Carbapenems and Monobactams

The carbapenems have a broad antibacterial spectrum of activity, including most aerobic and anaerobic gram-positive and gram-negative bacteria. They are useful for the treatment of infection due to gram-negative bacteria resistant to other antibiotics or to streamline complex polypharmacy. The microbiological activity of the carbapenems is shown in Tables 120-2 to 120-4.

Aztreonam, a monobactam, has broad aerobic gram-negative activity but lacks gram-positive activity or efficacy against anaerobes. Carbapenems are not active against MRSA. Imipenem and doripenem have clinically useful potency against most enterococci, but meropenem and ertapenem have significantly less activity against these bacteria. Doripenem is active against MRSA, but breakpoints have not been established against this organism. Against 22,389 oxacillin-susceptible *S. aureus* isolates, doripenem inhibited 100% of all strains at ≤4 mcg/ml.[85] Against 16,515 MRSA isolates, doripenem inhibited 59.3% at ≤4 µg/mL, and 69.3% at ≤8 µg/mL.[85]

Meropenem and ertapenem are less active against gram-positive aerobic bacteria than are imipenem and doripenem. Ertapenem, meropenem, and doripenem are more active than imipenem against Enterobacteriaceae. Doripenem has more potent activity against *P. aeruginosa* than any other carbapenem. Imipenem and meropenem have similar activity against *P. aeruginosa* and *Acinetobacter* spp., but ertapenem has no activity against important nonfermenting gram-negative rods, including *P. aeruginosa*, *S. maltophilia*, and *Acinetobacter* spp. Aztreonam generally has activity against *P. aeruginosa*, but ceftazidime is usually twice as active.[86] The carbapenems have potent activity against gram-positive and gram-negative anaerobic bacteria (see Table 120-4).

Carbapenems are generally stable against most β-lactamases; however, metalloenzymes that can hydrolyze the carbapenem ring are increasing in the ICU setting.[87] The most concerning carbapenemases prevalent worldwide today are the KPC enzymes, a group of mostly plasmid-encoded enzymes from *K. pneumoniae*. *Klebsiella pneumoniae* carbapenemase enzymes hydrolyze all β-lactam antibiotics including penicillins, cephalosporins, and aztreonam, although cephamycins and ceftazidime are weakly hydrolyzed. The KPC enzymes may be mistaken for ESBLs, since they also hydrolyze expanded-spectrum cephalosporins, but unlike extended spectrum β-lactamases, they also weakly hydrolyze carbapenems. The hydrolytic activity of KPC enzymes is not sufficient enough to produce resistance against carbapenems, but increases in MICs can occur. To achieve full resistance to carbapenems, organisms must also exhibit impaired outer membrane permeability. Carbapenems are stable to ESBLs, but aztreonam is not. Carbapenems are also affected by multidrug efflux pumps and porin channel changes, particularly in *P. aeruginosa*. Imipenem is not affected by the common efflux pump mediated by MexA-MexB-OprM.[88] However, imipenem readily selects resistant mutants of *P. aeruginosa* that lack a crucial porin channel (OprD) necessary for bacterial permeability to carbapenems but not other β-lactamase drugs.[88] Loss of this porin channel produces imipenem MICs for *P. aeruginosa* of 8 to 32 mg/mL, conferring clinical resistance.[88] Meropenem is recognized and ejected by the Mex-B-mediated efflux pump, as well as being affected by the loss of the OprD porin channel.[88] Although either mechanism produces a threefold rise in meropenem MICs, neither mutation alone produces clinical resistance to meropenem. Rather, the combination of resistance mechanisms is required to preclude meropenem's clinical effectiveness.

The pharmacokinetics of the carbapenems and aztreonam are shown in Table 120-5. Ertapenem is highly protein bound and has a 4-hour half-life, compared with 1 hour for doripenem, imipenem, and meropenem. Consequently, it is administered once daily. In critically ill patients, imipenem, meropenem, and doripenem have an expanded V_D and prolonged half-life.[89-91] Similar changes were observed for critically ill patients receiving aztreonam.[89] These data suggest that trough concentrations of carbapenems and aztreonam may be low in critically ill patients, and aggressive dosing may be warranted to minimize treatment failure and drug resistance. For carbapenems, extended infusions (2-6 hours) of intermittent dosing may also be advantageous. When MICs are low, either intermittent or extended-infusion dosing strategies may be effective. However, with higher MICs, as are often observed in ICU-related infections, extended infusion dosing may be advantageous. A recent large clinical trial supported this concept, with clinical cure rates for doripenem administered as a 4-hour infusion greater than for imipenem administered as a 30-minute infusion in patients with *P. aeruginosa* infections (16/20 [80%] versus 6/14 [42.9%], respectively).[92]

Continuous infusion of meropenem has been studied in the critically ill and produced steady-state serum concentrations well above the MIC90 for most common ICU pathogens, including *P. aeruginosa*. As with the cephalosporins, a lower dosage is required when administering the carbapenems by continuous infusion than by intermittent injection. Carbapenems and aztreonam are eliminated principally by the kidney, and dosage adjustment is necessary in renal dysfunction.

Imipenem is metabolized extensively by renal dehydropeptidase-1 (DHP-1), producing nephrotoxic metabolites that can produce proximal tubular necrosis. Cilastatin is a competitive inhibitor of DHP-1 that results in protection against the toxic metabolites of imipenem and increases the imipenem urine delivery to approximately 70%.[93] Doripenem, meropenem, and ertapenem do not require cilastatin coadministration. Imipenem has proconvulsive activity when administered in higher doses (4 g/d) or to patients with significant renal dysfunction in whom the drug may accumulate.

The carbapenems are used in the critical care setting for management of drug-resistant bacterial infections and in situations where broad-spectrum empirical therapy is necessary. There are insufficient data to conclude that the carbapenems are interchangeable. Imipenem and doripenem have the broadest spectrum of activity, but the potential for adverse effects in the ICU population may limit imipenem use. Ertapenem will probably be reserved for use in non–critical care settings. Aztreonam is effective for gram-negative bacterial infections and has been used in place of aminoglycosides when renal toxicity is a concern. However, increasing gram-negative resistance to aztreonam and attractive alternatives such as the third-generation cephalosporins and the fluoroquinolones have relegated aztreonam to a second- or third-line choice for many infections.

KEY POINTS

1. β-Lactamase is largely responsible for bacterial resistance to the β-lactam antibiotics. Drugs that are stable to β-lactamase enzymatic activity, such as the carbapenems and cefepime, are most reliable in institutions where significant β-lactam resistance has occurred.

2. Penicillin allergy is commonly reported, but true anaphylaxis is rare. Cross-reactivity among the other β-lactam antibiotics is also low, and prudent consideration should be given to the type of reaction and response to skin testing before eliminating the β-lactams from consideration.

3. In some institutions, extended-spectrum β-lactamases have rendered most third-generation cephalosporins unreliable for the treatment of *Klebsiella* and *Enterobacter* infections. Alternatives include cefepime or carbapenems.

4. Extended infusion of some β-lactams may improve pharmacodynamic parameters to enhance organism eradication, reduce resistance, and improve clinical outcomes.

ANNOTATED REFERENCES

Lodise TP, Lomaestro BM, Drusano GL. Application of antimicrobial pharmacodynamic concepts into clinical practice: focus on beta-lactam antibiotics: insights from the Society of Infectious Diseases Pharmacists. Pharmacotherapy 2006;26:1320-32.

This paper provides a thorough review of the pharmacokinetic principles and pharmacodynamic applications of various administration concepts for β-lactam antibiotics. Use of these techniques in clinical practice is described.

Ramphal R, Ambrose PG. Extended-spectrum beta-lactamases and clinical outcomes: current data. Clin Infect Dis 2006;42:S164-72.

Extended-spectrum β-lactamase (ESBL)-producing gram-negative bacteria are an important source of nosocomial infection in critically ill patients. This paper explores the literature on this topic, describes divergent views of the effect of ESBL carriage on morbidity and mortality, and suggests that ESBL production may have its most marked effect on ceftazidime. Strategies to overcome ESBL resistance are outlined.

Roberts JA, Webb S, Paterson D, Ho KM, Lipman J. A systematic review on clinical benefits of continuous administration of beta-lactam antibiotics. Crit Care Med 2009;37:2071-8.

A meta-analysis of 14 randomized clinical trials including 846 patients was analyzed to determine the clinical benefits of extended infusion or continuous infusion of β-lactam antibiotics. This paper provides an excellent reference of the trials of continuous and extended-infusion β-lactams.

Livermore DM. Of *Pseudomonas*, porins, pumps and carbapenems. J Antimicrob Chemother 2001; 47:247-50.

This is an excellent review of the mechanism of resistance for Pseudomonas aeruginosa against the carbapenems and compares resistance to imipenem to that of meropenem.

Robinson JL, Hameed T, Carr S. Practical aspects of choosing an antibiotic for patients with a reported allergy to an antibiotic. Clin Infect Dis 2002;35:26-31.

Penicillin or other β-lactam allergy is a common occurrence in clinical medicine. This paper provides a nuts-and-bolts approach to the use of antimicrobial therapy to which the patient may be allergic.

REFERENCES

Access the complete reference list online at http://www.expertconsult.com.

121

Aminoglycosides

ROSE JUNG

Aminoglycosides remain important but underutilized antibacterials in combating infections in critically ill patients. Most of the aminoglycoside use in intensive care units (ICUs) consists of additive or synergistic roles with penicillins or cephalosporins against serious infections caused by aerobic gram-negative bacilli or gram-positive cocci. Fortunately, the prevalence of bacterial resistance against the aminoglycosides has remained relatively low.

Concentration-dependent bactericidal activity, post-antibiotic effects, and synergism with β-lactam compounds are clear advantages of aminoglycosides. However, their usefulness has been limited by the potential for nephrotoxicity, ototoxicity, and rarely, neuromuscular blockade. As the mechanisms of activity and toxicities are better elucidated, the potential for adverse events may be reduced by modifying dosing strategies, avoiding risk factors, and using shorter durations of therapy. In addition, the cost of these agents is low in comparison to other antibacterials with similar spectra of activity and efficacy. Consequently, aminoglycosides remain valuable weapons against infections in the ICU, especially in the era of increasing resistance to other commonly used antibacterials.

Although the aminoglycoside family includes a variety of agents that have a wide spectrum of activity, this chapter focuses on the three most commonly prescribed antibacterials of this class, gentamicin, tobramycin, and amikacin and their clinical utility in combating gram-negative bacilli and gram-positive cocci infections in the ICU.

Mechanism of Action

The mechanisms of bactericidal activity of aminoglycosides are not completely understood. In gram-negative bacteria, binding to and subsequent alteration of the cell envelope in addition to interaction with ribosomes, that causes inhibition of protein synthesis, may contribute to their bactericidal activity. Aminoglycosides are cations that bind passively to negatively charged portions of the outer membranes of gram-negative bacilli and competitively displace cell wall Mg^{2+} and Ca^{2+} that link lipopolysaccharide molecules.[1,2] The result is a rearrangement of the cell envelope and subsequent formation of transient holes in the cell wall, which interrupts normal permeability function of the bacteria.[3,4] In gram-positive bacteria, aminoglycoside uptake is decreased because of thicker outer cell wall membranes, and thus higher minimum inhibitory concentrations (MIC) are reported with these organisms.

Aminoglycosides are transported slowly across the cytoplasmic membrane via an energy-dependent process; this is the rate-limiting step in the drug action.[5,6] The transmembrane electrical potential correlates to the uptake and antibacterial effect. This energy-dependent transport mechanism is impaired in an anaerobic environment, conditions of low pH, and high osmolality. Thus in certain clinical settings such as in infections involving abscesses, aminoglycoside transport is reduced and may not be as effective.

Once across the cell membrane, aminoglycosides are trapped inside bacteria, leading to high intracellular concentration of the drug. Subsequently, aminoglycosides bind to the 16S rRNA of 30S subunits of ribosomes.[7] This aminoglycoside-ribosome interaction causes termination and miscoding of protein synthesis, with subsequent bacterial cell death.

Spectrum of Activity

Aminoglycosides have a broad spectrum of activity against microorganisms, including gram-negative and gram-positive bacteria, mycobacteria, and protozoa. Among aerobic and facultative gram-negative bacilli, most aminoglycosides are active against Enterobacteriaceae (*Escherichia coli*, *Proteus mirabilis*, *Klebsiella* spp., *Morganella* spp., *Citrobacter* spp., *Serratia* spp., and *Enterobacter* spp.), *Pseudomonas* spp., and *Acinetobacter* spp. Resistance of clinical isolates to aminoglycosides varies with organism, patient population and their comorbidities, and local or regional usage patterns. According to the analyses of the Surveillance Network Database from 1998 to 2001, the susceptibility rates to aminoglycosides was higher against Enterobacteriaceae than nonfermentative organisms such as *Pseudomonas* and *Acinetobacter* spp.[8] In addition, susceptibility to amikacin was higher than to gentamicin against species of Enterobacteriaceae, *Pseudomonas*, and *Acinetobacter*.[9] Among ICU patients, the susceptibility of Enterobacteriaceae to gentamicin was 91.8% and amikacin was 98.5%.[9] The susceptibility of *Pseudomonas aeruginosa* was 78.5% and 93.9% for gentamicin and amikacin, respectively. Against *Acinetobacter baumannii*, the susceptibility was 58.2% and 82.7%, respectively.[8] For Enterobacteriaceae and *P. aeruginosa*, both gentamicin and amikacin susceptibility rates were similar among ICU and non-ICU patients or slightly better in non-ICU patients. However, among *A. baumannii* isolates, the susceptibility rates among non-ICU patients were lower than those reported for ICU patients (43.6% versus 58.2% for gentamicin and 77.2% versus 82.8% for amikacin).[8]

Since 2001, analyses of other databases indicate consistent but marginal decreases in susceptibility to aminoglycosides in comparison to other antibacterials in the United States. In 2008, a U.S. surveillance study encompassing 15 medical centers reported tobramycin susceptibility rates of 88.4% among Enterobacteriaceae, 89.1% among *P. aeruginosa*, and 59.1% in *Acinetobacter* spp.[10] In 2007, a surveillance study of isolates from mostly North American sites but also including information from Europe, Asia, Latin America, Africa, and the Middle East reported susceptibility to amikacin of better than 95% among Enterobacteriaceae isolates, 92.3% among *P. aeruginosa*, and 69.6% among *A. baumannii* isolates.[11] In comparison to the United States, the susceptibility to aminoglycosides against *P. aeruginosa* in Europe and Latin was lower. A surveillance study conducted in 2007 showed tobramycin susceptibility rates among *P. aeruginosa* isolates of 92% in North America, 77% in the European Union, and 63.8% in Latin America.[12] A European surveillance study reported tobramycin susceptibility of 74.2% among *P. aeruginosa* isolates in 2007,[13] and the International Nosocomial Infection Control Consortium (INICC) surveillance study from 2003 to 2008 reported an amikacin resistance rate of 31% among *P. aeruginosa* isolates collected from ICU patients from 25 countries in Latin America, Asia, Africa, and Europe.[14]

Aminoglycosides are active against methicillin-susceptible *Staphylococcus aureus*. For other gram-positive pathogens such as methicillin-resistant *S. aureus* (MRSA), *Streptococcus* spp., and *Enterococcus* spp., aminoglycosides are used in a limited fashion to provide synergistic activity with β-lactam antibiotics. In *Enterococcus* spp., the synergism is only observed in organisms that display low-level gentamicin resistance (4-250 μg/mL).[15] A poor active transport of drug due to anaerobic metabolism and the thick cell wall is thought to be responsible for this low-level resistance. Synergism is achieved in these organisms because gentamicin uptake is enhanced when combined with β-lactam antibiotics. *Enterococci* may acquire one or more of the following resistance mechanisms to demonstrate high-level resistance: alteration of the target site, interference with drug permeability, or enzyme inactivation of drug.[16] In organisms with high-level resistance, synergistic activity of gentamicin is not observed. In high-level gentamicin resistance, it may be worthwhile to test for high-level streptomycin resistance. High-level gentamicin and streptomycin resistance is considered with MIC ≥ 500 μg/mL and MIC ≥ 2000 μg/mL, respectively.

Rates of high-level gentamicin resistance in *Enterococcus* spp. varies markedly among institutions, but the nationwide prevalence is estimated at 30% to 60%.[15] High-level resistance is low in *Enterococcus faecalis*, which is responsible for approximately 60% of nosocomial enterococcal bloodstream infections. However, this type of resistance is observed in greater than 50% of *Enterococcus faecium*, which causes approximately 20% of nosocomial enterococcal bloodstream infections.

Aminoglycosides have activity against less common ICU pathogens. Streptomycin has greatest activity against *Mycobacterium tuberculosis* and *Yersinia pestis*.[17,18] Both streptomycin and gentamicin have been reported to be effective in *Francisella tularensis* infection.[19] Amikacin has the best activity among aminoglycosides against *Mycobacterium avium-intracellulare*. Spectinomycin is useful in treating *Neisseria gonorrhoeae* infection.[20] Paromomycin has been used against intestinal parasites.[21]

Mechanisms of Resistance

Bacterial resistance to aminoglycosides is achieved through multiple mechanisms. These include modification of the ribosomal target, enzymatic modification, decreased antibiotic uptake, and efflux of antibiotics. Mutations at the ribosomal (16S rRNA) binding sites results in resistance to aminoglycosides. This mechanism has not been detected in most clinical isolates, except for *Mycobacterium tuberculosis* against streptomycin.[22]

The most common mechanism of resistance for aminoglycosides is inactivation by aminoglycoside-modifying enzymes. The exposed hydroxyl and amino groups of aminoglycosides are subject to structural modification and loss of antimicrobial activity by enzymes from both gram-positive and gram-negative bacteria.[23] There are three types of enzymes which transfer a functional group to the aminoglycoside structure: (1) aminoglycoside nucleotidyltransferases (ANT) that transfer nucleotide triphosphates; (2) aminoglycoside acetyltransferases (AAC) that transfer the acetyl group from acetyl-CoA; and (3) aminoglycoside phosphotransferases (APH) that transfer the phosphoryl group from ATP.[23,24] Once the structure of aminoglycosides has been modified, they bind poorly to ribosomes, and this then results in high-level resistance. Genes encoding aminoglycoside-modifying enzymes are usually found on extrachromosomal bacterial plasmids and transposons within the periplasmic space. Thus, they can be easily transferred from bacteria to bacteria.[25] Amikacin is the aminoglycoside most stable to these enzymatic effects because it has fewer sites for enzymatic attack.

Resistance can also be developed by preventing penetration of the drug through the outer bacterial cell membrane or by preventing active transport through the cytoplasmic membrane.[26] Chromosomal mutations that alter transmembrane electrical potential may down-regulate aminoglycoside uptake into the bacterial cell after the first aminoglycoside exposure. This temporary disruption of the energy-dependent phase of aminoglycoside uptake is called *adaptive resistance* and lasts for several hours. Extended-interval aminoglycoside dosing may allow this effect to reverse, owing to the higher peak serum concentration (C_{max})/MIC ratios achieved. Aminoglycoside exposure may also select for subpopulations of bacteria with active efflux pumps resulting in low-level resistance. The efflux pump, MexXY, in *P. aeruginosa* is involved in resistance to many antibacterials including aminoglycosides.[27]

Pharmacokinetics

All the aminoglycosides have similar pharmacokinetic properties. The distribution from the vascular to the extravascular space occurs rapidly within 15 to 30 minutes post infusion.[28] Aminoglycosides are primarily excreted by glomerular filtration.[29] Thus, dosage adjustments are based on creatinine clearance (CrCl). In patients with normal renal function, the half-lives of all aminoglycosides range from 1.5 to 3.5 hours. The half-life is shortened in febrile illnesses and prolonged in any condition that decreases renal function. More than 90% of a parenterally administered dose is recovered in urine unchanged during the first 24 hours. The remainder is slowly recycled into the tubular lumen, where accumulation of the drug causes nephrotoxicity.[30]

Aminoglycoside concentrations are generally low in infected secretions and tissues such as respiratory secretions, pleural fluid, cerebrospinal fluid, and aqueous humor. High drug concentrations are found in the proximal tubular cells of the renal cortex, which is thought to correlate with the nephrotoxic potential of aminoglycosides.[30]

Pharmacodynamics

Pharmacodynamic principles associated with aminoglycosides include concentration-dependent bactericidal activity, post-antibiotic effect (PAE), and synergism with other cell wall–active agents.[31] Aminoglycosides are rapidly bactericidal, and their rate and extent of bacterial killing increases as the antibiotic concentration is increased. Exposure of bacteria to a single 24-hour aminoglycoside dose with the associated high peak drug concentration results in faster and a greater extent of bactericidal activity than that noted for the same total dose administered in divided doses.[32] In 236 patients with gram-negative infections, attainment of a C_{max}/MIC ratio of 10 and 12 exhibited a response rate of 80% or higher.[33] Another study of 78 patients with gram-negative nosocomial pneumonia suggested that achieving C_{max}/MIC ratio ≥ 10 within the first 48 hours of therapy had a 90% probability of temperature and leukocyte count resolution by day 7.[34]

PAE is a persistent suppression of bacterial growth after short antimicrobial exposure.[35] The higher the peak aminoglycoside concentration, the longer the PAE. In vitro, the aminoglycosides consistently demonstrate a PAE that varies from 1 to 3 hours for *P. aeruginosa* and 0.9 to 2.0 hours for Enterobacteriaceae. A PAE is also demonstrated for *S. aureus*.[36]

Synergy is frequently reported in vitro with a combination of an aminoglycoside and a cell wall–active antimicrobial (e.g., penicillin, cephalosporin, carbapenem, monobactam, glycopeptide).[37] Synergy is noted when significantly greater effect with two drugs is observed compared to that anticipated based on the effect of each individual drug. Enhanced aminoglycoside uptake in the presence of a cell wall–active drug has been demonstrated with *Streptococcus* spp., *Enterococcus* spp., *S. aureus*, and *P. aeruginosa*. Two meta-analyses have evaluated synergism in vivo by comparing the efficacy of monotherapy with a β-lactam antibiotics and combination therapy with a β-lactam antibiotic plus an aminoglycoside.[38,39] All-cause mortality was comparable in both groups in sepsis and in suspected ventilator-associated pneumonia. This lack of synergism observed in patients may be due to the poor quality of pooled studies, such as lack of blinding, analysis not based on intention to treat, and unspecified follow-up period. The studies included in these meta-analyses also reported high susceptibility to both β-lactam antibiotics and aminoglycosides (≥90% susceptibility) among gram-negative pathogens and included very few patients with multidrug resistant pathogens such as *P. aeruginosa* and *A. baumannii*. Therefore, it is yet to be determined if the synergism observed in vitro between a β-lactam antibiotic and an aminoglycoside translates into survival advantage in patients. However, resistance among gram-negative pathogens is increasing, especially among *P. aeruginosa*, and combination therapy of β-lactam antibiotics and aminoglycosides offers broader coverage in ICU patients than combination with fluoroquinolones.[40] In the future, a high percentage of adequate empirical therapy with aminoglycosides may translate into improved survival in patients infected with multidrug-resistant pathogens.

Adverse Events

The most common adverse event with aminoglycosides is nephrotoxicity. The reported incidence of this complication ranges from 5% to 25%.[41,42] The variability results from differences in the definition of nephrotoxicity, the tests used to measure renal function, and the clinical setting in which the drugs were administered. In general, a decrease in the glomerular filtration rate is small, with most patients experiencing a nonoliguric decline in CrCl. Recovery occurs upon discontinuation of the drug, and progression to dialysis-dependent oliguric or anuric renal failure is rare.

Risk factors for aminoglycoside toxicity include older age, preexisting renal disease, diabetes, frequent dosing interval, treatment lasting longer than 4 days, and concurrent nephrotoxic drugs (vancomycin, amphotericin B, furosemide, clindamycin, piperacillin, cephalosporins, methoxyflurane, foscarnet, and intravenous [IV] radiocontrast agents).[42,43] In addition, ICU patients are at increased risk due to hypotension or contracted intravascular volume from volume depletion or diuretic therapy.[43] Minimizing use in patients with risk factors for nephrotoxicity and using extended-interval dosing of aminoglycosides are recommended to reduce toxicity.

Aminoglycosides may cause cochlear and vestibular damage.[41] Ototoxicity may be a result of irreversible damage to the sensory hair cells of the organ of Corti and reduction of cochlear ganglion cells due to accumulation of drug. Streptomycin and gentamicin are thought to be primarily vestibulotoxic, whereas amikacin, neomycin, and kanamycin are primarily cochleotoxic.[44] The incidence of cochlear toxicity is estimated to be 3% to 14%. Toxicity may manifest unilaterally or bilaterally. The true incidence of vestibular toxicity in patients is very difficult to determine because symptoms are masked by compensatory mechanisms (visual and proprioceptive clues) over time. Clinical manifestations include dizziness, ataxia, and/or nystagmus.

The risk factors for ototoxicity include inherited susceptibility, age of the patient, drug dosage, renal function, and additive effects of other ototoxic agents (loop diuretics).[42] When aminoglycoside therapy is indicated, the risk of ototoxicity can be minimized by shortening the duration of therapy as clinically appropriate and by periodic assessments of renal function to avoid accumulation of drug. High-frequency audiometric testing may aid in early diagnosis and prevention of progressive damage in patients receiving more than 4 days of therapy.

The most life-threatening adverse reaction to aminoglycosides, although very rare, is neuromuscular blockade.[45] Blockade results from inhibition of the presynaptic release of acetylcholine and blockage of postsynaptic receptor sites of acetylcholine. The resulting clinical manifestations include muscle weakness, respiratory depression with apnea, flaccid paralysis, and dilated pupils. Suppression of deep tendon reflexes may be variable. Risk factors include a diagnosis of myasthenia gravis, hypomagnesemia, severe hypocalcemia, and concomitant administration of a neuromuscular blocking agent. A rapid rise in serum drug concentration due to short duration of IV administration may also be a risk factor. Aminoglycosides are usually administered IV over 15 to 30 minutes, but the dosing may extend to 30 to 60 minutes for large doses to reduce the risk of neuromuscular blockade.

Drug Interaction

Aminoglycosides interact chemically with β-lactam antibiotics such as the antipseudomonal penicillins (e.g., carbenicillin, ticarcillin, piperacillin, mezlocillin, and azlocillin).[46,47] This interaction results in a nucleophilic opening of the β-lactam ring, with acylation of an amino group of the aminoglycoside and mutual loss of antibacterial activity. When patients with renal failure were concomitantly administered an aminoglycoside and an antipseudomonal penicillin, the serum aminoglycoside concentration was reduced by 10% to 20%. Thus, the administration of these drugs should be separated by at least 1 hour.

Extended-Interval Dosing Versus Multiple Daily Dosing

The aminoglycosides are licensed to be administered multiple times per day based on a patient's renal function. With normal renal function (CrCl ≥ 80 mL/min), empirical maintenance doses for gentamicin and tobramycin range from 1.2 to 1.5 mg/kg every 8 hours, and for amikacin, 7.5 mg/kg every 8 to 12 hours, in patients with gram-negative infections.[48] Dose reduction and/or dosing interval prolongation may be necessary in those with renal dysfunction and in patients with advanced age (Table 121-1). Higher dosages or shorter intervals may be required in neonates, in burn patients with serious pseudomonal infections, or in patients with cystic fibrosis. In patients with gram-positive infections such as infective endocarditis, a synergistic effect is achieved with gentamicin 1 mg/kg IV every 8 hours. This dosage in normal renal function will achieve a peak concentration of 3 μg/mL and a trough concentration of less than 0.5 μg/mL. Dosage adjustment may be necessary in those with renal dysfunction.

A dosing strategy frequently referred to as *extended-interval aminoglycoside dosing* (EIAD) has been used widely in non-ICU patients since its introduction in 1980s. EIAD employs a large bolus dose over an extended period to achieve high serum concentrations to produce rapid bactericidal effect and undetectable trough concentrations at the

TABLE 121-1	Recommended Dosing Regimens for Selected Aminoglycosides Based on Renal Function						
				Recommended Regimen			
Aminoglycoside	*Indication*	DOSE	CrCl ≥ 60 mL/min	CrCl = 40-60 mL/min	CrCl = 20-40 mL/min	CrCl < 20 mL/min OR HD
Traditional Dosing						
Gentamicin	Pneumonia or other severe infections	1.5-2.5 mg/kg	Every 8 hours	Every 12 hours	Every 24 hours	Redose based on trough levels < 1 μg/mL
	Synergy	1 mg/kg	Every 8 hours	Every 12 hours	Every 24 hours	Redose based on trough levels < 1 μg/mL
Tobramycin	Pneumonia or other severe infections	1.5-2.5 mg/kg	Every 8 hours	Every 12 hours	Every 24 hours	Redose based on trough levels < 1 μg/mL
Amikacin	Pneumonia or other severe infections	5-7.5 mg/kg	Every 8 hours	Every 12 hours	Every 24 hours	Redose based on trough levels < 5 μg/mL
Once-Daily or Extended-Interval Dosing						
Gentamicin	Pneumonia or other severe infections	7 mg/kg	Every 24 hours	Every 36 hours	Every 48 hours	Redose based on trough levels < 1 μg/mL
Tobramycin	Pneumonia or other severe infections	7 mg/kg	Every 24 hours	Every 36 hours	Every 48 hours	Redose based on trough levels < 1 μg/mL
Amikacin	Pneumonia or other severe infections	15 mg/kg	Every 24 hours	Every 36 hours	Every 48 hours	Redose based on trough levels < 1 μg/mL

CrCl, creatinine clearance; *HD,* hemodialysis.

end of the dosing interval to reduce accumulation of drugs, limiting nephrotoxicity.[48] Based on improved patient outcome and decreased selection of resistant organisms, targets of EIAD are a peak concentration of 20 mg/L or a C_{max}/MIC of 10. Since reduced risk for nephrotoxicity and ototoxicity has been observed in patients receiving EIAD with at least 4 hours of drug-free period, concentrations of less than 0.5 mg/L for 4 hours at the end of the dosing interval are also recommended. During this time, the regimen relies on PAE to provide therapeutic effect.

Numerous clinical studies of EIAD have been evaluated in patients with bacteremia, intraabdominal infections, urinary tract infections, pelvic infections, cystic fibrosis, and febrile neutropenia.[49-51] Unfortunately, none of these studies specifically examined efficacy and safety in critically ill patients, thereby limiting its application in the ICU. Because of the altered pharmacokinetics of aminoglycosides in critically ill patients, previous studies have reported low probability of achieving pharmacodynamic targets in such patients.[52] The mean volume of distribution in critically ill patients ranges from 0.3 to 0.4 L/kg. However, in surgical and trauma patients in the ICU, a volume of distribution of up to 0.8 L/kg has been reported.[53,54] Since the C_{max}/MIC ratio is directly affected by a large volume of distribution, the ratio in critically ill patients is expected to be less than optimal. In addition, several studies reported that critically ill patients had drug-free intervals ranging from 6 to 9 hours at the end of the dosing interval.[55] Since such drug-free intervals exceed the PAE observed for most organisms in vitro, this dosing strategy may not effectively inhibit regrowth of surviving organisms. Finally, a poor correlation between estimated CrCl and aminoglycosides has been documented in ICU patients.[56] This variability in drug clearance may be secondary to unstable renal function, malnutrition, hemodynamic instability, and use of drugs such as vasopressors, diuretics, and other nephrotoxic drugs.

A recommended empirical dose in adults with serious gram-negative infections and normal renal function is 7 mg/kg/d for gentamicin or tobramycin and 15 mg/kg for amikacin. The dosing interval may have to be prolonged if a patient's calculated CrCl is below 60 mL/min. In those patients with normal renal function or in surgical or trauma patients, the dosing interval may need to be shortened to every 12 hours. Serum monitoring is necessary to recommend an optimal dosing regimen in critically ill patients, especially in those with renal dysfunction and those receiving large quantities of IV fluids.

▓ Serum Concentration Monitoring

Monitoring serum concentrations of aminoglycosides is essential for both efficacy and toxicity. Monitoring schemes are different for the two methods of administering aminoglycosides. For traditional multiple daily dosing regimens, peak concentrations should be checked 30 minutes after the end of an IV infusion. Since the drug is often infused over a 30-minute period, it may be convenient to request the serum sample 1 hour after the start of the drug administration. The desired peak concentration may be different depending on the site of infection. For nosocomial infections involving tissues where aminoglycoside penetration is low (e.g., lower respiratory tract infections), the target peak concentration should range from 8 to 12 mg/L for gentamicin and tobramycin and 25 to 30 mg/L for amikacin. On the other hand, for infections where the drug concentrates heavily (e.g., urinary tract infections), adequate peak concentrations can range from 5 to 8 mg/L for gentamicin and tobramycin and 10 to 20 mg/L for amikacin.

Trough concentration is a good indication of accumulation and therefore a good predictor of nephrotoxicity and ototoxicity. Trough concentrations should be less than 2 mg/L, although less than 1 mg/L is preferred in most critically ill patients. These serum concentrations should be measured during steady state, which is approximately after the third dose in most cases. The frequency of subsequent monitoring of serum drug concentrations will vary among patients (usually once weekly throughout therapy) but should be more frequent in patients with changing renal function or in those with more resistant pathogens.

For EIAD, there are two different methods of determining the optimal regimen. The first and the more well known method uses the Hartford Nomogram.[57] According to this method, serum concentrations are drawn between 6 and 14 hours after the first dose and applied to a nomogram to determine the recommended fixed-dose and dosage interval. Although the use of a nomogram is simpler and less expensive because of the reduced number of serum concentrations evaluated, available studies in critically ill patients indicate that the use of this nomogram did not reliably predict targeted C_{max}/MIC ratio and allowed excessively long drug-free periods at the end of the dosing interval. Instead, in critically ill patients, monitoring of two serum drug concentrations to derive a dosing regimen is recommended. Obtaining a peak concentration at 1 hour after a 1-hour infusion (2 hours after the start of infusion) and another serum concentration between 8 and 18 hours after the end of the infusion will allow adequate determination of a patient-specific regimen. This will allow assessment of peak serum concentration for the targeted C_{max}/MIC ratio and the length of the drug-free interval. Thereafter, in the absence of worsening renal function, periodic trough concentrations should be monitored to ensure adequacy of renal clearance of drug. A high trough concentration is a reflection of impaired renal clearance of drug and indicates the need to adjust the dosage regimen. The targeted peak concentration should be 20 mg/L or a C_{max}/MIC of 10, and trough concentration should be undetectable (<0.5 mg/L) for approximately 4 hours at the end of the dosing interval.

KEY POINTS

1. Most of the aminoglycoside use in intensive care units includes consideration of a synergistic role with β-lactam antibiotics against serious infections caused by aerobic gram-negative bacilli or aerobic gram-positive cocci.

2. Bactericidal activity of the aminoglycosides is believed to be a result of binding to and subsequent alteration of the cell envelope in addition to ribosomal interaction causing inhibition of protein synthesis.

3. Aminoglycosides have a broad spectrum of activity against aerobic gram-negative bacilli, including Enterobacteriaceae (*Escherichia coli*, *Proteus mirabilis*, *Klebsiella* spp., *Morganella* spp., *Citrobacter* spp., *Serratia* spp., and *Enterobacter* spp.), *Pseudomonas* spp., and *Acinetobacter* spp.

4. The prevalence of bacterial resistance against Enterobacteriaceae and *P. aeruginosa* has remained relatively low when compared to other antibacterials.

5. Bacterial resistance to aminoglycosides is achieved through enzymatic modification, modification of the ribosomal target, decreased antibiotic uptake, and efflux of antibiotics.

6. Pharmacodynamic properties of aminoglycosides consist of concentration-dependent bactericidal activity, post-antibiotic effects, and synergism with β-lactam compounds.

7. Aminoglycosides are limited by their potential to cause nephrotoxicity, ototoxicity, and rarely, neuromuscular blockade.

8. Serum concentration monitoring is important for both efficacy and safety.

ANNOTATED REFERENCES

Rea RS, Capitano B, Bies R, et al. Suboptimal aminoglycoside dosing in critically ill patients. Ther Drug Monit 2008;30:674-81.

A retrospective review of 102 MICU patients receiving either gentamicin or tobramycin were evaluated to determine the probability of achieving C_{max}/MIC ratio of ≥ 10. Only 20% and 40% of patients receiving 7 mg/kg of gentamicin and tobramycin, respectively, achieved this ratio. The low probability was thought to be the result of larger volume of distribution in ICU patients.

Paul M, Sibiger I, Grozinsky S, et al. Beta lactam antibiotic monotherapy versus beta lactam-aminoglycoside antibiotic combination therapy for sepsis. Cochrane Database Syst Rev 2006;1:CD003344.

A total of 64 randomized and quasi-randomized trials were included in a meta-analysis to compare any β-lactam monotherapy to any combination of one β-lactam and one aminoglycoside for sepsis. The primary outcome of all-cause mortality was not different between monotherapy and combination therapy groups in studies that compared the same β-lactams (RR 1.01; 95% CI, 0.75-1.35) and in studies that compared different beta lactams (RR 0.85; 95% CI, 0.71-1.01). Nephrotoxicity was significantly more frequent with combination therapy (RR 0.30; 95% CI, 0.23-0.39).

Aarts MW, Hancock JN, Heyland D, et al. Empiric antibiotic therapy for suspected ventilator-associated pneumonia: A systematic review and meta-analysis of randomized trials. Crit Care Med 2008;36: 108-17.

Although a total of 41 randomized controlled trials were included in a meta-analysis to compare monotherapy to combination therapy for the empirical treatment of ventilator-associated pneumonia, only two trials evaluated a combination with an aminoglycoside therapy. In these two trials evaluating meropenem versus ceftazidime plus aminoglycoside, no difference in all-cause mortality was reported (RR 0.73; 95% CI, 0.47-1.18), but treatment failure was lower in the meropenem group (RR 0.70; 95% CI, 0.53-0.93).

Cosgrove SE, Vigliani GA, Campion M, et al. Initial low-dose gentamicin for *Staphylococcus aureus* bacteria and endocarditis is nephrotoxic. Clin Infect Dis 2009;48:713-21.

A secondary analysis of a randomized controlled trial of daptomycin versus vancomycin or antistaphylococcal penicillin plus gentamicin in patients with S. aureus bacteremia and endocarditis was conducted to determine rates of gentamicin-associated nephrotoxicity. All patients receiving standard therapy and patients who are likely to have left-sided endocarditis in the daptomycin group also received the initial 4 days of low-dose gentamicin(1 mg/kg every 8 h, with appropriate dose adjustment). Gentamicin use prior to enrollment in the randomized study were also reviewed. A clinically significant decrease in creatinine clearance (CrCl) was defined as a decrease in CrCl to < 50 mL/min in those with baseline CrCl of ≥ 50 mL/min or a decrease of ≥ 10 mL/min if the baseline was < 50 mL/min. A total of 22% of patients who received versus 8% of patients who did not received initial low-dose gentamicin experienced clinically significant decrease in CrCl. Independent predictors of a clinically significant decrease in CrCl were age ≥ 65 years and receipt of initial low-dose gentamicin.

Oliveira JFP, Silva CA, Barbieri CD, et al. Prevalence and risk factors for aminoglycoside nephrotoxicity in intensive care units. Antimicrob Agents Chemother 2009;53:2887-91.

A total of 360 patients who received gentamicin or amikacin for at least 4 days were evaluated for risk factors for aminoglycoside-associated nephrotoxicity. Aminoglycoside doses were adjusted based on calculated glomerular filtration rate (cGFR). Nephrotoxicity was defined as a decrease in the cGFR of 20% or more from the baseline during aminoglycoside use. A logistic regression revealed that a baseline cGFR of less than 60 mL/min/1.73m², diabetes, treatment with other nephrotoxic agents or iodinated contrast, and hypotension were independently associated with aminoglycoside-associated nephrotoxicity.

Buchholtz K, Larsen CT, Hassager C, Bruun NE. Severity of gentamicin's nephrotoxic effect on patients with infective endocarditis: a prospective observational cohort study of 373 patients. Clin Infect Dis 2009;48:65-71.

A database of infective endocarditis patients from two tertiary university hospitals in Copenhagen, Denmark, was evaluated for gentamicin's nephrotoxic effects. A total of 287 of 373 patients with infective endocarditis received gentamicin therapy that was adjusted according to serum creatinine and trough drug levels. Kidney function was evaluated using estimated endogenous creatinine clearance (EECC). The mean number of days on gentamicin therapy was 17 days (range 1-69). The mean EECC decrease was 8.6%, with a 0.5% decrease noted per day of gentamicin treatment. This decrease in EECC did not correlate to post-discharge mortality. This study did not evaluate the use of other nephrotoxic agents and doses of gentamicin used.

REFERENCES

Access the complete reference list online at http://www.expertconsult.com.

122

Fluoroquinolones

DOUGLAS N. FISH

The fluoroquinolones are synthetically derived, broad-spectrum antibacterial agents designed for both intravenous (IV) and oral administration. Since the introduction of ciprofloxacin in the late 1980s, fluoroquinolones have assumed an important role in the treatment of infections in critically ill patients. Their broad spectrum of antimicrobial activity, favorable safety profiles, and ease of administration have made fluoroquinolones popular choices for both empirical and directed therapies of a wide variety of infectious diseases. However, widespread use of fluoroquinolones has not come without concern regarding appropriate use and development of resistance among certain hospital-acquired pathogens such as *Pseudomonas aeruginosa*. This chapter will briefly review fluoroquinolone pharmacology, antimicrobial activity, safety, and other clinically relevant issues regarding their use and will focus on the three agents most frequently used in the critical care setting: ciprofloxacin, levofloxacin, and moxifloxacin.

Mechanism of Action

DNA gyrase and topoisomerase IV enzymes are thought to be essential for the replication of DNA and partition of replicated chromosomal DNA.[1] DNA gyrase, a tetrameric enzyme consisting of two A and two B subunits, is known to be a primary target of fluoroquinolones in gram-negative bacteria and is the only known enzyme capable of introducing negative super-helical twists into bacterial DNA.[1,2] The two subunits of gyrase are encoded by *gyrA* and *gyrB*, which are also potential sites of mutation and subsequent quinolone resistance.[1,3] Topoisomerase IV seems to be a primary target of many fluoroquinolones in gram-positive bacteria such as *Staphylococcus aureus* and *Streptococcus pneumoniae*.[3,4] Bacterial topoisomerase IV appears to be the principal enzyme that resolves or "decatenates" interlocked daughter DNA circles occurring at the completion of a round of DNA replication, allowing segregation of daughter chromosomes into daughter cells.[1,3,4] Topoisomerase IV, like DNA gyrase, is composed of four subunits, two each of the *parC* and *parE* gene products.

As part of the topoisomerase reaction mechanism, DNA gyrase and topoisomerase IV transiently break the DNA backbone and pass a double strand of DNA through those breaks, thus introducing a negative supercoil into the DNA strand.[1,2] Fluoroquinolone antibiotics have been shown to target DNA gyrase and topoisomerase IV while these enzymes are functionally attached to the DNA strand in the presence of adenosine triphosphate, resulting in a drug/enzyme/DNA complex in which the DNA remains broken.[1,2] Cell death apparently results from release of double-stranded DNA breaks from multiple drug/enzyme/DNA complexes throughout the chromosome.[1,2] This mechanism of action does not in itself explain why the fluoroquinolones kill bacteria so rapidly, and it has been suggested that additional protein synthesis mechanisms involving unidentified "protein factors," interference with the "SOS" response involved in the repair of damaged DNA, dissociation of gyrase subunits, and increased oxidative stress may all play a role in the rapidly bactericidal effects of these drugs.[1,2] Fluoroquinolones have also been noted to substantially decrease the synthesis of proinflammatory cytokines, although the relevance of this finding to their overall pharmacologic activity is unknown.[5]

Antimicrobial Spectrum of Activity

Fluoroquinolones have excellent in vitro activity against a wide range of both gram-positive and gram-negative organisms. Representative activities of fluoroquinolones which are currently available and frequently used in critically ill patients are shown in Table 122-1. The entire fluoroquinolone class displays excellent activity against enteric gram-negative aerobic bacteria as well as *Haemophilus influenzae*, *Moraxella catarrhalis*, and *Neisseria* spp. Gastrointestinal (GI) pathogens such as *Salmonella* spp., *Shigella* spp., and *Campylobacter* spp. are also highly susceptible to fluoroquinolones. Although some differences in relative potency exist between individual drugs as determined by the minimum inhibitory concentration (MIC) for these organisms, little difference in clinical efficacy should be expected in the treatment of infections due to susceptible strains. Activity against *P. aeruginosa* is more variable, however. Ciprofloxacin has traditionally been considered the most active fluoroquinolone against this organism, but data suggest there is little difference between ciprofloxacin and levofloxacin in terms of relative susceptibility of *P. aeruginosa* strains.[6] Ciprofloxacin was active against greater than 95% of *P. aeruginosa* strains when first released to the market in 1987, but by 2001 both ciprofloxacin and levofloxacin were active against only approximately 65% to 80% of strains. Such high levels of resistance (25%-35%) are still seen among *P. aeruginosa* strains.[6-10] Clinically relevant differences between ciprofloxacin and levofloxacin are further minimized when pharmacokinetic and pharmacodynamic properties are considered.[9] Moxifloxacin tends to be the least active of the currently available agents.[6,11-13] Nearly all fluoroquinolones adequately inhibit *P. aeruginosa* at concentrations achieved in the urine.

Activity of the fluoroquinolones against other hospital-acquired pathogens is also highly variable. Levofloxacin tends to be slightly more active against *Acinetobacter* spp., whereas moxifloxacin usually displays the best activity and ciprofloxacin is consistently the least active agent against *Stenotrophomonas maltophilia*.[6,11-13] However, resistance to these latter organisms is quite common, and even agents with the best relative in vitro activity are not reliably clinically effective against many isolates.[6,11-13]

Several studies have reported that fluoroquinolones produce synergistic activity against gram-negative bacilli when used in combination with β-lactam antibiotics.[14,15] These studies primarily evaluated antibiotic synergy against *P. aeruginosa* due to the frequent use of fluoroquinolones in antipseudomonal treatment regimens; ciprofloxacin and levofloxacin have been shown to achieve synergy against 25% to 75% of tested strains. One previous study also demonstrated synergistic in vitro activity against *P. aeruginosa* with the combination of moxifloxacin and either ceftazidime or cefepime[15]; however, additive or synergistic activity with moxifloxacin-containing combinations has not been extensively evaluated against other organisms. The ability of moxifloxacin to produce synergistic activity against *P. aeruginosa* may often be limited by clinically achievable drug concentrations. The use of ciprofloxacin and levofloxacin in combination regimens is most likely to result in synergistic activity, owing to their more potent activity and higher serum concentrations relative to the bacterial MICs.[14,15]

Newer fluoroquinolones have improved activity against gram-positive bacteria relative to older agents such as ciprofloxacin. Moxifloxacin has the best overall activity against staphylococci and streptococci, followed by levofloxacin and more distantly by

TABLE 122-1	Representative in Vitro Antibacterial Activity (MIC90) of Selected Fluoroquinolones		
Organism	Ciprofloxacin (≤1 mg/L)*	Levofloxacin (≤2 mg/L)*	Moxifloxacin (≤2 mg/L)*
Gram-Negative Aerobic Bacteria			
Escherichia coli	≤0.03->4	≤0.03->8	≤0.03->8
Klebsiella pneumoniae	0.25->4	0.5->8	0.13->8
Proteus mirabilis	0.12-2	≤0.05-2	0.05->4
Enterobacter cloacae	0.03-1	0.06-2	0.06-2
Serratia marcescens	>4	>8	>8
Morganella morganii	0.03-0.125	0.06-0.25	0.13-0.5
Citrobacter freundii	0.25-1	0.5-2	1->8
Pseudomonas aeruginosa	>4	>8	>8
Acinetobacter spp.	1->4	0.5->8	0.25->8
Stenotrophomonas maltophilia	>4	>8	>8
Haemophilus influenzae	0.008-0.03	0.008-0.06	≤0.03
Moraxella catarrhalis	0.015-0.25	0.03-0.06	0.06
Gram-Positive Aerobic Bacteria			
Staphylococcus aureus (MS)	0.5-4	0.25-4	0.06-1
Staphylococcus aureus (MR)	>4	>8	>8
Staphylococcus epidermidis (MS)	2	0.5	0.13
Staphylococcus epidermidis (MR)	>4	>8	>8
Streptococcus pneumoniae (PS)	2[†]	1	0.25[†]
Streptococcus pneumoniae (PR)	2[†]	1	0.25[†]
Streptococcus pyogenes	1	1	0.25
Enterococcus faecalis	≥8	>4	8
Enterococcus faecium (VS)	16	8	4
Listeria monocytogenes	1	2	0.5
Atypical Bacteria			
Chlamydia pneumoniae	1	0.25	0.03
Legionella pneumophila	0.12	0.03	0.016
Mycoplasma pneumoniae	1	2	0.06
Anaerobic Bacteria			
Bacteroides fragilis	8	2	1
Bacteroides spp.	32	4	1
Fusobacterium spp.	4	2	1
Clostridium perfringens	4	2	0.25
Clostridium difficile	16	8	2
Peptostreptococcus spp.	4	2	0.25

*Recommended susceptibility breakpoints for staphylococci and Enterobacteriaceae.

[†]Recommended susceptibility breakpoints for testing of trovafloxacin, gatifloxacin, and moxifloxacin versus S. pneumoniae are ≤1 mg/L. No recommended breakpoint exists for ciprofloxacin.

MIC90, minimal inhibitory concentration at which 90% of tested strains are inhibited; MS, methicillin-susceptible; MR, methicillin-resistant; PS, penicillin-susceptible; PR, penicillin-resistant; VS, vancomycin-susceptible.

ciprofloxacin.[12,13] Levofloxacin and moxifloxacin are reliably active against penicillin-susceptible strains of S. pneumoniae; this activity is also retained against strains of S. pneumoniae resistant to other drug classes including penicillins, macrolides, and sulfonamides. Although ciprofloxacin has only moderate activity against methicillin-susceptible S. aureus (MSSA), newer agents have excellent activity against this organism. None of the fluoroquinolones is reliably active against methicillin-resistant S. aureus (MRSA), and rates of fluoroquinolone resistance among MRSA are quite high. Fluoroquinolones as a class also have only moderate activity against enterococci, with great variability seen among the various agents and specific bacterial strains.[11-13] Fluoroquinolones have consistently excellent activity against Listeria monocytogenes.[11-13]

The activity of various fluoroquinolones against anaerobic bacteria is highly variable. Trovafloxacin was the first commercially available fluoroquinolone with clinically relevant anaerobic activity in vitro, as well as proven clinical efficacy for anaerobic infections including complicated intraabdominal infection. Moxifloxacin has in vitro activity against Bacteroides fragilis, Bacteroides group organisms, Fusobacterium spp., Clostridium spp., and other anaerobes that is generally comparable to trovafloxacin.[12,13,16] However, recent data have demonstrated resistance rates in excess of 30% for many clinically important anaerobes, and the appropriateness of moxifloxacin for treatment of serious anaerobic infections is questionable.[16] Neither ciprofloxacin nor levofloxacin have clinically relevant activity against anaerobic bacteria.

Fluoroquinolones are highly active against atypical pathogens including Legionella pneumophila, Chlamydia pneumoniae, and Mycoplasma pneumoniae. Many authorities consider fluoroquinolones to be the drugs of choice for treatment of severe pneumonias caused by atypical pathogens, particularly Legionella, because of their very potent in vitro activity, bactericidal actions, and high serum and intracellular concentrations.

Mechanisms of Fluoroquinolone Resistance

Two basic mechanisms of fluoroquinolone resistance have been identified. One involves alteration of DNA gyrase and topoisomerase IV, whereas the other results in reduced drug accumulation within bacterial cells.[2,17] Plasmid-mediated resistance, once considered quite rare, appears to be spreading rapidly among enteric gram-negative bacilli in certain geographic regions.[18] However, plasmid-mediated resistance is relatively unusual compared with the more typical chromosomally mediated mechanisms of resistance.

Mutations in quinolone-resistance determining regions (QRDR) of topoisomerase enzymes prevent formation of drug/enzyme/DNA complexes, allowing DNA synthesis to occur in the presence of the drugs. Mutations in the genes encoding DNA gyrase (gyrA and gyrB) have been most frequently identified. However, other quinolone-resistant mutations in parC and parE, the genes encoding topoisomerase IV, have also been identified.[1,2,17,19] Resistance to fluoroquinolones appears to arise in a stepwise manner. In some species (e.g., gram-negative bacteria), first-step mutations occur in gyrA and occasionally in gyrB, whereas in other species (e.g., S. aureus, S. pneumoniae) first-step mutations occur in parC and less often in parE.[17,19] First-step mutations usually result in a low-level resistance (≤fourfold increased MIC), whereas additional mutations in either primary or secondary enzyme targets (second-step mutations) result in high-level resistance to drugs at clinically relevant concentrations. Dual gyrA and parC mutations have been described in clinical isolates of S. pneumoniae; however, it is thought that these strains were selected by fluoroquinolones with less potent antipneumococcal activity (e.g., ciprofloxacin).[19-22]

The first efflux system for quinolones was identified in Escherichia coli,[23] whereas the first evidence for actual efflux-mediated quinolone resistance came from the characterization of S. aureus with overexpression of the norA gene product, a protein that mediates efflux.[24] Such efflux may occur in both quinolone-resistant and quinolone-susceptible strains of S. aureus. In some species (e.g., P. aeruginosa), at least two different efflux systems may be present that mediate resistance to multiple other drug classes in addition to fluoroquinolones.[25] Although most efflux proteins appear to be relatively nonspecific multidrug transporters whose substrates include hydrophilic fluoroquinolones as well as monocationic organic compounds, relatively substrate-specific efflux pumps have also been described.[26]

Many other genetic mutations have been described that result in decreased intracellular accumulation of fluoroquinolones and low-level drug resistance. Nearly all these mutations are associated with decreased expression of OmpF, a nonspecific outer membrane porin channel that is a major route of passage of hydrophilic fluoroquinolones through bacterial cellular membranes into the periplasmic space.[27] Although decreased membrane permeability is relatively common and easily induced, this is an unusual mechanism for clinically significant resistance. Strains of S. pneumoniae, E. coli, S. aureus, and P. aeruginosa have been identified that possess both altered outer membrane permeability and gyrA mutations, resulting in high-level resistance to all tested fluoroquinolones.[28,29] Strains of highly ciprofloxacin-resistant Salmonella with both outer membrane protein alterations and expression of efflux pumps have also been described.[30]

Fluoroquinolone resistance among pathogens such as S. aureus and P. aeruginosa has been particularly problematic since the introduction of these agents into clinical use. As fluoroquinolones have become more extensively used in the treatment of respiratory tract infections, reports of increasing resistance among *S. pneumoniae* have focused attention on newly recognized mechanisms of drug action and drug resistance.[19-22] Resistance to fluoroquinolones has tended to emerge rapidly in bacteria with lower intrinsic susceptibility (e.g., *S. aureus*, *P. aeruginosa*, and *Acinetobacter* spp.) because potentially fewer mutational steps are required to confer clinically relevant MIC changes.[26,31,32] However, fluoroquinolone resistance has also been noted to be an increasing problem among gram-negative bacilli such as *Enterobacter* spp., *Klebsiella pneumoniae*, and even *E. coli*, organisms that were originally considered to be highly susceptible to the drugs.[6,8,10] This problem is particularly an issue among isolates from ICUs.[10] Development of resistance is also accelerated by the use of drugs with lower in vitro activity, use of inappropriately low doses to treat infections caused by less susceptible organisms, and treatment of infection at sites where quinolone penetration may be decreased.[31-34] Development of resistance to one fluoroquinolone usually causes decreased susceptibility to all other agents in the class, although clinically relevant resistance may not necessarily occur. Of note, fluoroquinolone use has also been associated with high rates of cross-resistance among drugs of unrelated antibiotic classes such as the carbapenems, cephalosporins, and aminoglycosides.[33-35] Although not well understood, such cross-resistance is probably mediated by up-regulation and/or reduction in multiple efflux pump systems involved in passage of antibiotics through cell membranes and intracellular drug accumulation.[33-35] Although the fluoroquinolones remain highly active and clinically effective against a wide variety of important pathogens found in critically ill patients, increasing resistance is clearly an important issue in the clinical use of these drugs.

Pharmacokinetics

Pharmacokinetic properties of the currently used fluoroquinolones are shown in Table 122-2. Individual agents in the class exhibit distinct differences in properties such as oral bioavailability, half-lives, extent of metabolism, and routes of excretion. However, fluoroquinolones as a whole are characterized by rapid oral absorption and extensive distribution into many fluids and tissues, resulting in concentrations that are well above the MIC for many gram-negative and gram-positive organisms; serum half-lives are sufficiently long to allow once- or twice-daily dosing. Ciprofloxacin and levofloxacin have been most extensively studied in critically ill patients. Although large interpatient variability and some differences in mean parameters were observed compared with normal volunteers, pharmacokinetics of the drugs were generally similar enough to allow the use of normally recommended doses.[36,37]

Certain pharmacokinetic features are of particular importance during use of these drugs in critically ill patients. Limited data suggest that fluoroquinolones are well absorbed after oral administration to critically ill patients, although patients must be carefully selected for clinical stability and absence of GI diseases or processes that may affect drug absorption.[37]

Fluoroquinolones have excellent distribution into many tissues and fluids and often reach concentrations many-fold higher than found in blood. For example, ciprofloxacin achieves tissue-to-serum concentration ratios of approximately 2 in bronchial and lung tissues, 2 in lung tissues, 13 in the kidneys, and up to 30 in the bile.[38] Levofloxacin has been shown to achieve pulmonary epithelial lining fluid–to–plasma and alveolar macrophage–to–plasma ratios of 2.1 to 2.3 and 8.9 to 12.0, respectively, 12 hours after multiple-dose administration of levofloxacin, 500 to 750 mg orally.[39] Such high tissue and fluid levels have important pharmacodynamic implications (see later) and increase the likelihood of successfully treating infections at these sites. In contrast, penetration of the fluoroquinolones into the cerebrospinal fluid is relatively poor and ranges from 20% to 40% of serum concentrations in the absence of inflamed meninges.

Ciprofloxacin and levofloxacin are excreted to a large degree through the kidneys as unmetabolized drug; doses should therefore be appropriately adjusted in the presence of moderate to severe renal dysfunction to avoid unnecessary drug accumulation. In contrast, elimination of moxifloxacin is relatively insensitive to changes in renal function; this drug is highly metabolized, and even severe renal impairment does not influence dosing requirements. Mild to moderate hepatic impairment does not appear to significantly affect the pharmacokinetics of these agents; however, most drugs have not been well studied in patients with severe or end-stage liver disease, and consideration should be given to empirically decreasing the daily dosage of hepatically eliminated drugs. Ciprofloxacin has been shown to undergo compensatory increases in renal clearance in patients with severe liver disease, and no dosage adjustments are required if renal function is normal[40]; however, caution is warranted when dosing ciprofloxacin in patients with both hepatic and renal dysfunction.[38,40]

Pharmacodynamic Considerations

Studies have clearly demonstrated that fluoroquinolones exhibit concentration-dependent bacterial killing.[41-48] A number of studies, including a prospectively developed model of the pharmacodynamic response to levofloxacin during treatment of respiratory tract, skin, and urinary tract infections, have provided evidence that achieving a ratio of fluoroquinolone maximum serum concentrations to the bacterial MIC (C_{max}/MIC ratio) of greater than 10 to 12 appears to be predictive of clinical drug efficacy and successful bacterial eradication.[41-48] The ratio of area under the 24-hour serum concentration time curve to MIC (AUC_{0-24}/MIC) has also been shown in vitro and retrospectively in vivo to be predictive of favorable clinical response and reduced development of resistance.[41-48] Although the optimal AUC_{0-24}/MIC ratio breakpoints are still unclear, favorable AUC_{0-24}/MIC ratios appear to be 125 to 250 for gram-negative organisms and 30 to 50 for *S. pneumoniae*.[41-48] Whether either the C_{max}/MIC ratio or AUC_{0-24}/MIC ratio is superior to the other parameter and which specific ratios are most predictive of drug efficacy remain somewhat controversial; however, the strong relationships between these pharmacodynamic parameters and clinical and microbiological outcomes during fluoroquinolone therapy have been well established.

TABLE 122-2	Summary of Mean Pharmacokinetic Parameters of Fluoroquinolones				
	Ciprofloxacin		Levofloxacin		Moxifloxacin
Parameter	*400 mg IV q 12 h*	*400 mg IV q 8 h**	*500 mg IV q 24 h**	*750 mg IV q 24 h*	*400 mg IV q 24 h*
Peak (mg/L)	4.6	6.5	7.5	12.1	4.2
Volume of distribution (L/kg)	1.2	1.3	1.2	1.3	1.7
Half-life (h)[†]	4.0	3.3	8.0	7.9	14.8
AUC_{0-24} (mg · h/mL)	12.7	46.5	66.1	108	38.0
Renal excretion as unchanged drug (%)	50-70	NR	NR	>95	45

*Data from critically ill ICU patients.
[†]In patients with creatinine clearance > 40-50 mL/min.
AUC$_{0-24}$, area under the 24-hour serum concentration time curve from 0 to 24 hours; *NR*, not reported.

Certain principles of fluoroquinolone pharmacodynamics can be readily applied to appropriate treatment of infections in critically ill patients. Fluoroquinolone pharmacokinetics are somewhat variable in the critically ill, and the drugs are often used as empirical therapy for infections potentially caused by organisms with reduced fluoroquinolone susceptibility (i.e., higher MICs). High doses will thus often be necessary to minimize the importance of variability in both pharmacokinetics and pathogen susceptibilities, and also optimize the concentration-dependent pharmacodynamic properties of the drugs in patients with severe infections. Use of higher doses (e.g., ciprofloxacin, 400 mg IV every 8 hours; levofloxacin, 750 mg IV every 24 hours) are particularly recommended in the treatment of severe infections suspected or documented to be caused by pathogens with intrinsically higher MICs to the drugs (e.g., *P. aeruginosa* and *Acinetobacter* spp.). Fluoroquinolones readily penetrate into most tissues and fluids of the body, but the use of high doses in treating serious infections should also maximize tissue penetration and more reliably achieve adequate drug concentrations at the site of infection. Based on the pharmacodynamic properties of fluoroquinolones, the intensity of dosing and ability to achieve favorable C_{max}/MIC or AUC_{0-24}/MIC ratios should also minimize the development of resistance. However, it should be noted that many pathogens found in critically ill patients (e.g., most of the enteric gram-negative bacilli, MSSA, streptococci) are highly susceptible to fluoroquinolones, and the use of high doses is not necessary to achieve concentrations adequate for the treatment of most infections.

Adverse Effects

With some notable exceptions (e.g., trovafloxacin), fluoroquinolones have generally proven to be a safe and well-tolerated class of drugs. The most common adverse effects associated with fluoroquinolones are GI effects such as nausea, vomiting, and diarrhea (~1% to 5% incidence); rash (<2.5%); and central nervous system (CNS) effects, including headache, dizziness, and sleep disturbances (<1% to 2%). These adverse effects are generally mild and self-limiting and seldom result in discontinuation of fluoroquinolone therapy. With IV preparations, pain and inflammation at the injection site have also been reported.[49-52]

Adverse GI effects of the fluoroquinolones are thought to be caused by a combination of direct GI irritation and CNS-mediated effects; adverse GI effects may still be seen when these drugs are administered IV. *Clostridium difficile*–associated colitis has been associated with fluoroquinolone use in several epidemiological studies, but other studies have not confirmed fluoroquinolone use as a significant risk factor for *C. difficile* infection.[53-56] There was initially some concern that newer fluoroquinolones with enhanced anaerobic activity and GI elimination (e.g., moxifloxacin) may perhaps be associated with an increased risk of *C. difficile*–associated colitis, but whether there is a difference among the various fluoroquinolones, or indeed whether fluoroquinolones in general are truly associated with increased risk of *C. difficile* infection, is still controversial.[53-56]

CNS disturbances caused by fluoroquinolones can be broadly divided into two types: those resulting from direct effects of the drugs on the CNS caused by inhibition of γ-aminobutyric acid (GABA) binding, and those resulting from adverse drug-drug interactions (either pharmacokinetic or pharmacodynamic). Of all the fluoroquinolones, levofloxacin is associated with the lowest incidence of adverse CNS events; however, the occurrence of adverse CNS effects with ciprofloxacin and moxifloxacin is similar and only slightly more frequent than with levofloxacin. Seizures have been only rarely reported during fluoroquinolone therapy and usually occurred in the presence of predisposing factors such as seizure disorder, head trauma, anoxia, metabolic disturbances, or concomitant drug therapy with specific interacting agents (i.e., theophylline).[49-52]

Elevations in serum transaminase, alkaline phosphatase, and/or bilirubin levels have been noted to occur in 2% to 3% of patients receiving fluoroquinolone therapy.[49-52] These liver abnormalities are usually mild, are reversible, and do not necessitate discontinuation of therapy. Although trovafloxacin was associated with clinically significant

hepatotoxicity and acute hepatic failure, currently used fluoroquinolones have been only rarely associated with liver injury.

Fluoroquinolones as a class have been implicated in causing abnormalities of glucose homeostasis.[52] Both hypoglycemia and hyperglycemia have been reported, and patients with preexisting diabetes mellitus or other known glucose abnormalities are apparently at particularly high risk. Glucose abnormalities appeared to occur most commonly with gatifloxacin, and that drug was first restricted in use then removed from the market because of the potentially increased risk. Although other fluoroquinolones have also been associated with glucose abnormalities, the overall risk appears to be quite low. However, glucose levels should be monitored in all acutely ill patients receiving fluoroquinolone therapy, with special care being warranted in elderly patients and those with diabetes mellitus or pre-diabetes.[52]

The potential of fluoroquinolones to cause cardiac toxicity has also been examined; such toxicity manifests as electrocardiographic prolongation of the corrected QT (QTc) interval and arrhythmias including ventricular tachycardia, ventricular fibrillation, and torsades de pointes.[52,57-59] Some controversy exists as to the true risk of cardiac toxicity associated with fluoroquinolones and whether specific agents might be associated with a greater degree of risk. It appears that all currently available fluoroquinolones are capable of causing some degree of QTc prolongation. However, QTc interval prolongation is usually quite minor (mean of <5 to 10 ms, with greatest prolongation usually observed with moxifloxacin), does not predictably occur in all patients exposed to fluoroquinolones, and is of no clinical significance in the vast majority of patients treated with these agents. Patients who may be at particular risk of drug-induced cardiac toxicity and who should be more closely monitored during fluoroquinolone use include those with the following characteristics: advanced age (>60 years), history of significant cardiac disease or previous arrhythmia, presence of electrolyte abnormalities (e.g., potassium, calcium, magnesium), and concomitant use of antiarrhythmic or other drugs known to cause prolongation of the QTc interval.[52,57-59]

Tendonitis and tendon rupture are unusual complications of fluoroquinolone use. A total of only 33 cases associated with ciprofloxacin or levofloxacin had been reported in the medical literature up until 2003.[60] Several studies have subsequently carried out detailed analyses of fluoroquinolone-associated tendonitis and tendon rupture and have confirmed tendinopathies to be uncommon complications of drug use, with an estimated incidence of approximately 1/200,000 treated patients.[52,61] The median duration of drug use before the onset of symptoms is approximately 10 to 14 days. Risk factors for the occurrence of tendinopathy appear to include male sex, age older than 60 years, concurrent corticosteroid use, and presence of renal disease.[52,61]

Drug-Drug Interactions

Concurrent administration of oral fluoroquinolones with multivalent cation-containing products such as aluminum- or magnesium-containing antacids and products containing calcium, iron, or zinc (including multivitamins with minerals) should be avoided. Concomitant use of these agents with a fluoroquinolone invariably results in a marked reduction of oral absorption of the antimicrobial; bioavailability of fluoroquinolones may be reduced as much as 90% owing to the formation of insoluble chelation complexes in the GI tract that inhibit drug absorption.[51,62] Similar changes in oral antibiotic absorption have also been observed with concurrent administration of sucralfate or ferrous sulfate. Effects of enteral feeding formulas on the absorption of fluoroquinolones are variable, but concurrent administration should nevertheless be avoided. Concomitant administration of H$_2$-receptor antagonists and proton-pump inhibitors have no clinically significant effects on the absorption of fluoroquinolones.[51,62]

Ciprofloxacin has been shown to decrease theophylline clearance by a mean of approximately 25% to 30%.[51,62] Levofloxacin and moxifloxacin have no significant effects on theophylline metabolism. Ciprofloxacin was also shown to reduce the clearance of the *R*-enantiomer of

TABLE 122-3	Recommended Dosing Regimens for Selected Fluoroquinolones in Severely Ill Patients			
	Recommended Regimen			
Drug and Indications	*CrCl ≥30 mL/min*	*CrCl<30 mL/min*	*Hemodialysis*	*CVVH/CVVHDF*
Ciprofloxacin				
Nosocomial pneumonia; severe/complicated LRTI, SSSI; febrile neutropenia	400 mg IV q 8 h	200 mg IV q 8 h or 400 mg IV q 12-18 h	400 mg q 24 h	400 mg IV q 24 h
Complicated intraabdominal; other systemic infections of mild/moderate severity	400 mg IV q 12 h	400 mg IV q 24 h	200-400 mg q 24 h	200-400 mg IV q 24 h
Levofloxacin	*CrCl ≥ 50 mL/min*	*CrCl < 50 mL/min*	*Hemodialysis*	*CVVH/CVVHDF*
Nosocomial pneumonia; complicated SSSI	750 mg IV q 24 h	750 mg × 1, then 750 mg q 48 h	500 mg q 48 h	250-500 mg IV q 24 h
Other systemic infections	500 mg q 24 h	500 mg × 1, then 250 mg q 24-48 h	250 mg q 48 h	250 mg IV q 24 h
	750 mg IV q 24 h	750 mg × 1, then 750 mg q 48 h	500 mg q 48 h	250-500 mg IV q 24 h
Moxifloxacin	*Normal/impaired renal function*	*Mild/moderate cirrhosis*	*Hemodialysis*	*CVVH/CVVHDF*
All indications	400 mg IV q 24 h	400 mg IV q 24 h	400 mg IV q 24 h	ND

CrCl, creatinine clearance; *CVVH*, continuous venovenous hemofiltration; *CVVHDF*, continuous venovenous hemodiafiltration; *LRTI*, lower respiratory tract infection; *ND*, no data; *SSSI*, skin/skin structure infection.

warfarin by 15% to 32%; however, the clearance of the *S*-enantiomer, which is more potent and is thought to cause the majority of warfarin's anticoagulant activity, was not affected. Therefore, this interaction was not thought to be clinically significant. No apparent effects on either the *R*- or *S*-warfarin concentrations or prothrombin times were noted during concomitant dosing of levofloxacin or moxifloxacin.[51,62] Although significant pharmacokinetic or pharmacodynamic interactions between the fluoroquinolones and warfarin have not been documented through studies, several anecdotal case reports have described clinically significant interactions between warfarin and fluoroquinolones. Anticoagulation of any patient receiving concomitant fluoroquinolone and warfarin therapy should therefore be closely monitored.

Dosing

Recommendations for dosing of currently available fluoroquinolones are given in Table 122-3. Recommended regimens in the presence of renal or hepatic dysfunction are also given when appropriate and where data are available. Consideration should always be given to the susceptibility of presumed or documented pathogens, site of infection, severity of infection, presence of organ dysfunction, and pharmacodynamic characteristics of fluoroquinolones when choosing an appropriate dosing regimen for a specific patient.

KEY POINTS

1. Fluoroquinolones play an important role in the treatment of infections in critically ill patients, owing to their broad spectrum of antimicrobial activity, favorable safety profiles, and ease of administration.

2. Fluoroquinolones are rapidly bactericidal agents that have a broad spectrum of activity against important gram-positive, gram-negative, and atypical pathogens.

3. Although ciprofloxacin has traditionally been considered the most active fluoroquinolone against *Pseudomonas aeruginosa* and other important gram-negative pathogens, data suggest that there is little difference between ciprofloxacin and levofloxacin in terms of relative susceptibilities or clinical efficacy in the treatment of infections caused by these bacteria.

4. Newer fluoroquinolones, including levofloxacin and moxifloxacin, are more reliably active than ciprofloxacin against penicillin-susceptible or penicillin-resistant strains of *Streptococcus pneumoniae*, methicillin-susceptible *Staphylococcus aureus*, and other gram-positive organisms against which these agents have clinically relevant activity.

5. Resistance to fluoroquinolones has tended to emerge rapidly in bacteria with lower intrinsic susceptibility (e.g., *S. aureus*, *P. aeruginosa*, and *Acinetobacter* spp.); however, fluoroquinolone resistance among isolates from ICUs has also become an increasing problem among gram-negative bacilli such as *Escherichia coli*, *Enterobacter* spp., and *Klebsiella pneumoniae*.

6. Fluoroquinolones as a whole have excellent pharmacokinetic properties and are characterized by rapid oral absorption and extensive distribution into many fluids and tissues, resulting in concentrations that are well above the minimal inhibitory concentration (MIC) for many gram-negative and gram-positive organisms; serum half-lives are sufficiently long to allow once- or twice-daily dosing.

7. High doses of fluoroquinolones are often necessary to minimize the pharmacokinetic variability and optimize the concentration-dependent pharmacodynamic properties of the drugs, particularly in the treatment of severe infections suspected or documented to be caused by gram-negative pathogens with intrinsically higher MICs to the drugs (e.g., *P. aeruginosa* and *Acinetobacter* spp.).

8. Fluoroquinolones have generally proven to be safe and very well tolerated, and most drug-related adverse effects are mild and self-limiting.

9. Although there are differences among the individual drugs in terms of clinically important drug interactions and the clinical relevance of these interactions, fluoroquinolones are associated with drug interactions involving decreased drug absorption and inhibition of hepatic metabolism of drugs such as warfarin and theophylline.

10. Consideration should always be given to the susceptibility of presumed or documented pathogens, site of infection, severity of infection, presence of organ dysfunction, and pharmacodynamic characteristics of fluoroquinolones when choosing an appropriate dosing regimen for a specific critically ill patient.

ANNOTATED REFERENCES

Fish DN. Fluoroquinolone adverse effects and drug interactions. Pharmacotherapy 2001;21:253S-72S.
This review article provides a comprehensive evaluation of incidence and risk factors for fluoroquinolone-associated adverse effects and toxicities. The paper also discusses relevant drug-drug and drug-food interactions and highlights safety differences between individual fluoroquinolone agents.

Neuhauser MM, Weinstein RA, Rydman R, et al. Antibiotic resistance among gram-negative bacilli in US intensive care units: implications for fluoroquinolone use. JAMA 2003;289:885-8.

This study evaluated susceptibilities to 16 commonly used antibiotics among clinical isolates gathered from ICUs throughout the United States during the years 1994 to 2000. Whereas most antibiotics showed an absolute decreased susceptibility of 6% or less during the study period, overall susceptibility to ciprofloxacin decreased by 10% and was statistically associated with increased fluoroquinolone use.

Preston SL, Drusano GL, Berman AL, et al. Pharmacodynamics of levofloxacin: a new paradigm for early clinical trials. JAMA 1998;279:125-9.

This prospective study was one of the first clinical trials in humans to prospectively include a pharmacodynamic evaluation of clinical and microbiological success during fluoroquinolone therapy. As predicted from earlier in vitro and animal models, the ratios of both the maximum serum concentration divided by the pathogen minimum inhibitory concentration (MIC) and the pharmacokinetic area under the serum concentration-versus-time curve divided by the MIC were found to be the significant predictors of clinical and microbiological treatment success.

Rebuck JA, Fish DN, Abraham E. Pharmacokinetics of intravenous and oral levofloxacin in critically ill patients in a medical intensive care unit. Pharmacotherapy 2002;22:1216-25.

This prospective study evaluated the pharmacokinetics of IV and oral levofloxacin in 30 severely ill patients in a medical ICU. The pharmacokinetics of levofloxacin were found to be only slightly altered in comparison to those found in normal volunteers, and the bioavailability of oral levofloxacin was approximately 95%, highlighting the favorable pharmacokinetic and safety profile of this agent in severely ill patients.

Sahm DF, Critchley IA, Kelly LJ, et al. Evaluation of current activities of fluoroquinolones against gram-negative bacilli using centralized in vitro testing and electronic surveillance. Antimicrob Agents Chemother 2001;45:267-74.

This large, prospective surveillance study evaluated compared activities of ciprofloxacin and levofloxacin versus clinical isolates of important gram-negative pathogens. Although ciprofloxacin is often considered to be more active than other fluoroquinolones, levofloxacin was comparable against most strains, including

Pseudomonas aeruginosa, and was actually more active against certain problematic organisms such as Stenotrophomonas maltophilia.

Hidron AI, Edwards JR, Patel J, et al. NHSN annual update: antimicrobial-resistant pathogens associated with healthcare-associated infections: annual summary of data reported to the National Healthcare Safety Network at the Centers for Disease Control and Prevention, 2006-2007. Infect Control Hosp Epidemiol 2008;29:996-1011.

This comprehensive report provides detailed, more current data regarding rates of infection due to antimicrobial-resistant pathogens in various types of patient populations and in various specific types of infections during 2006-2007. Rates of resistance to fluoroquinolones (and other antibiotic classes) among key pathogens are presented, and the serious problem of antimicrobial resistance in clinical practice is clearly illustrated.

Owens RC, Ambrose PG. Antimicrobial safety: focus on fluoroquinolones. Clin Infect Dis 2005; 41:S144-57.

This article is among the most thorough and useful reviews of fluoroquinolone safety currently available. Cardiac toxicity, glucose abnormalities, arthropathy, and other unusual but important safety-related issues pertaining to the fluoroquinolones are discussed in detail, as well as other more common adverse effects of the drugs.

REFERENCES

Access the complete reference list online at http://www.expertconsult.com.

123

Macrolides

DAVID T. BEARDEN

The macrolide class of antibiotics is based on the structure of erythromycin, the prototype natural macrolide isolated from *Streptomyces erythreus*.[1] Commonly the term *macrolide* is expanded to include the azalide, azithromycin. The newly developed ketolides, owing to their similar structural bases, are close members of the macrolide family. There are many macrolides available throughout the world, the most commonly used being erythromycin, clarithromycin, and azithromycin. Roxithromycin is available in Europe and Asia. Telithromycin is the only currently available ketolide.

Mechanism of Action

The macrolides inhibit bacterial protein synthesis by binding to the 50S ribosomal subunit.[2] The advanced macrolides have improved binding to ribosomes compared with erythromycin. Telithromycin, the ketolide, has a similar target site, but its structure allows for enhanced binding, even in the presence of ribosomal mutations.

Mechanisms of Resistance

There are three major mechanisms of bacterial resistance to macrolides: drug efflux, ribosomal mutations, and enzymatic inactivation. Active efflux, mediated by *mef* genes, and ribosomal methylation of the target site, mediated by *erm* genes, are the most clinically important resistance mechanisms.[3] Organisms containing the *mef* gene commonly express low-level resistance that can often be overcome with larger doses of the antibiotic. In contrast, *erm*-containing organisms, expressing phenotypic macrolide-lincosamide-streptogramin B resistance, often express high-level resistance, rendering macrolides clinically ineffective.

Antimicrobial Spectrum of Activity

The macrolides have activity against many classes of bacteria but have only sporadic activity within each of these groups. Their primary microbiologic activity is directed against respiratory and intracellular pathogens (Table 123-1).[3-21]

GRAM-POSITIVE AEROBES

Among the gram-positive aerobes, erythromycin activity is limited to the streptococci with reasonable activity against *Streptococcus pneumoniae*. The advanced macrolides (azithromycin, clarithromycin, roxithromycin) have similar activity against *S. pneumoniae*. The utility of the macrolides against pneumococci is hampered by increasing resistance, commonly coupled with penicillin resistance. A 2001-2004 study from 40 countries reported 37% worldwide erythromycin resistance.[3] In the United States, macrolide-resistant pneumococci are found in up to 35% of isolates.[22] The predominant worldwide resistance mechanism is *ermB*-mediated high-level resistance (58%), but there is considerable international variability. Resistant North American isolates most commonly contain low-level *mefA* resistance, whereas most European and Far East countries report higher levels of *ermB*-containing pathogens. The prevalence of pneumococci expressing both mechanisms simultaneously is increasing.[3]

Resistance mechanisms for macrolides are important, because low-level resistance may possibly be overcome with conventional dosing of the macrolides.[23] Pneumococcal resistance to one macrolide commonly confers resistance to all members of the macrolide class. The ketolides, however, maintain their activity against macrolide-resistant *S. pneumoniae* possessing both *erm*- and *mef*-mediated resistance.[3]

GRAM-NEGATIVE AEROBES

The macrolides, with the exception of erythromycin, and the ketolide, telithromycin, have activity against *Haemophilus influenzae*. The activity of clarithromycin against *H. influenzae* is enhanced in the presence of its active metabolite.[24] The macrolides and ketolide also display activity against *Moraxella catarrhalis*, *Bordetella pertussis*, *Neisseria gonorrhoeae*, and *Neisseria meningitidis*. Clarithromycin has been the most commonly used macrolide against *Helicobacter pylori*, although resistance rates are currently 13% in the United States, with higher rates reported worldwide.[25] The macrolides are largely ineffective against the Enterobacteriaceae and other nosocomial pathogens. Though not directly active, limited auxiliary azithromycin activity has been noted against *Pseudomonas* spp.[26]

MISCELLANEOUS

The macrolides and the ketolide attain high intracellular concentrations and are active against *Legionella* spp., *Chlamydia* spp., and *Mycoplasma pneumoniae*. In vitro activity is also present against *Rickettsia*, *Bartonella*, and *Brucella* spp.,[27-29] as well as *Borrelia burgdorferi*, the agent of Lyme disease.[30] In addition, azithromycin, clarithromycin, and telithromycin have activity against some strains of atypical nontuberculosis mycobacteria, including *Mycobacterium avium* complex.[31-33]

ANAEROBES

The macrolides and the ketolide have poor activity against obligate anaerobes but maintain moderate activity against a variety of oral anaerobes, including *Prevotella* and *Porphyromonas* spp.

Pharmacokinetics

Erythromycin base is acid labile but still adequately absorbed from the gastrointestinal (GI) tract. Food can decrease absorption (Table 123-2).[1,34-42] More stable oral formulations have complexed erythromycin with salts or esters to form erythromycin estolate, stearate, and ethylsuccinate. Erythromycin lactobionate has also been formulated to allow for intravenous (IV) delivery. Peak concentrations are 0.73 μg/mL after 250 mg base orally and 10 μg/mL after 500 mg IV.[1,34] The half-life is 1 to 1.5 hours.[35] Like all macrolides, erythromycin is widely distributed throughout the body, with higher tissue and intracellular concentrations compared with plasma. Erythromycin is not found in the cerebrospinal fluid in normal volunteers, but low levels have been reported in patients with meningitis.[35] Erythromycin is metabolized by cytochrome P450 (CYP) enzymes in the liver and excreted as inactive metabolites, primarily in the feces.

Clarithromycin is well absorbed from the GI tract (bioavailability 52%-55%), with or without food. An IV lactobionate form is available in some countries. A peak concentration of 1.65 to 2.12 mg/mL is obtained after a 500-mg oral dose with a half-life of 3 to 5 hours.[37] Similar pharmacokinetics are observed after dosing with the

TABLE 123-1	Antibacterial Activity of the Macrolides and a Ketolide				

	MIC90 Range (µg/mL)				
Organism	Erythromycin	Clarithromycin	Azithromycin	Roxithromycin	Telithromycin
Gram-Positive Bacteria					
Staphylococcus aureus (MS)[4-6]	>128	>16->128	64	>128	0.06-0.25
Staphylococcus aureus (MR)[4-6]	>128	>16->128	>64	>128	0.5->128
Streptococcus pneumoniae[3,5,7]	32->128	16->64	>64	64	0.12-0.5
Viridans group streptococci[4,6,8,9]	8	>16	>64		0.12
Group A streptococci[5,10]	0.12-2	0.12-0.25	0.5	0.5-1	0.015-0.03
Group B streptococci[4,5,10]	0.03-0.12	0.015-0.06	1	0.06-0.25	0.008-0.06
Gram-Negative Bacteria					
Bordetella pertussis[11,12]	0.06-0.25	0.06	0.06	0.125-0.5	0.03
Haemophilus influenzae[5,13,14]	8	8-16	2	16	2
Moraxella catarrhalis[4-6,10,13,14]	0.06-0.5	0.03-0.25	≤0.06-≤0.25	0.12	0.03-0.12
Neisseria gonorrhoeae[4,5,14]	0.5-1	0.12-1	0.12	0.5	0.03-0.06
Neisseria meningitidis[4,5]	0.25	0.03-0.06		0.25	0.03
Listeria monocytogenes[14]	0.12	0.12	1		
Anaerobes					
Bacteroides fragilis group[15,16]	16->64	2->64	>64	>64	16->64
Clostridium difficile[4,5,15-17]	16->64	4->64	>64	16->64	1->64
Peptostreptococcus spp.[4,5,15-17]	4->128	2->32	>32->64	16-64	0.008-0.12
Prevotella spp.[16,18]	8	1	8	4	0.5-1
Porphyromonas spp.[16,17]	0.125-0.25	0.125	0.5	0.125	0.25
Atypical Pathogens					
Legionella spp.[14,19]	0.5-1	0.12-0.25	0.25-2		0.03
Mycoplasma pneumoniae[20,21]	≤0.004-0.06	≤0.001-0.03	≤0.001-0.03	0.25	0.008

MIC90, minimum inhibitory concentration required to inhibit growth of 90% of organisms; *MR*, methicillin resistant; *MS*, methicillin sensitive.

oral suspension, even in critically ill patients.[43] An extended-release formulation is available that delays the time to peak concentrations, provides similar total drug exposure, and allows for once-daily dosing.[36] Clarithromycin is well distributed throughout the body, with respiratory tract tissue and fluid concentrations 3 to 30 times that of the plasma and alveolar macrophage concentrations 10^2 to 10^3 higher than plasma.[37] Cerebrospinal fluid concentrations are unknown. Hepatic metabolism is the major metabolic pathway and leads to the formation of 14-hydroxy-clarithromycin, an active metabolite with greater activity than the parent compound.[24,37] Clarithromycin is extensively metabolized, with 18.4% and 4.4% of unchanged drug excreted in the urine and feces, respectively, after a 250-mg dose.[37] Dosing changes are required in patients with moderate to severe renal dysfunction.

Azithromycin is 37% bioavailable when administered orally but is also available in an IV formulation.[39,44] Food has little effect on bioavailability. Peak concentrations in the plasma after a 500-mg dose range from 0.4 µg/mL for the oral formulation to 3.6 µg/mL for the IV formulation.[38,39] An extended-release formulation of a single 2-g azithromycin dose shows a similar overall pharmacokinetic profile to standard oral dosing.[40] Azithromycin is unique in its extended half-life of 14 to 40 hours, thus providing low sustained plasma concentrations

that persist after cessation of dosing.[39] Whereas plasma concentrations are very low, azithromycin attains very high concentrations in tissues (100 times plasma) and phagocytes (3000-7000 times plasma).[38] Little to no azithromycin can be recovered from the cerebrospinal fluid, but brain tissue concentrations well exceed those in the serum.[45] Azithromycin is minimally metabolized and largely excreted via the biliary tract into the feces.

Roxithromycin is well absorbed orally, with peak plasma concentrations of 6.6 to 7.9 µg/mL after a 150-mg oral dose, and a half-life of 8.4 to 15.5 hours.[41] Fasting prior to dosing improves absorption. Tissue concentrations exceed those of the plasma. Roxithromycin is metabolized by multiple mechanisms, with the majority of the dose excreted in feces.[41,46]

Telithromycin is 57% bioavailable, with peak plasma concentrations of 1.9 and 2.3 µg/mL after single or multiple 800-mg doses, respectively.[42] The half-life of telithromycin is 7 to 10 hours. Like the macrolides, telithromycin achieves high concentrations in respiratory tissues, alveolar macrophages, and peripheral polymorphonuclear cells. Telithromycin is metabolized by CYP3A4 and non-CYP–related mechanisms. Fecal elimination of metabolites accounts for the majority of the excretion of telithromycin.

TABLE 123-2	Comparative Pharmacokinetics of Macrolides and a Ketolide				

Drug	Normal Dosing	C_{max}	$T_{1/2}$	Absorption with Food
Erythromycin[1,34,35]	250-500 mg PO 4 times daily	0.7 µg/mL	1-1.5 h	Better fasting
	500 mg-1 g IV q 6 h	10 µg/mL		
Clarithromycin[36,37]	250-500 mg PO twice daily	1.6-2.1 µg/mL	3-5 h	No effect
	1000 mg PO once daily (extended release)	2.3-2.6 µg/mL	3-5 h	Better with food
Azithromycin[38-40]	500 mg × 1, followed by 1,250 mg PO once daily	0.4 µg/mL	14-40 h	No effect
	2000 mg PO × 1 (extended release)	0.75 µg/mL		No effect
	500 mg IV once daily	3.6 µg/mL		
Roxithromycin[41]	150 mg PO twice daily	6.6-7.9 µg/mL	8.4-15.5 h	Better fasting
Telithromycin[42]	800 mg PO once daily	1.9-2.3 µg/mL	7-10 h	No effect

C_{max}, maximum plasma concentration of drug; *IV*, intravenous; *PO*, oral; *$T_{1/2}$*, half-life.

Pharmacodynamics

The macrolides and ketolides appear to have time-dependent antibacterial activity that is slowly bactericidal or bacteriostatic.[47,48] The relationship between drug concentration and bacterial effect that best explain drug activity is the free (unbound) drug area under the inhibitory curve (fAUC: MIC).[47,48] Differences in the pharmacokinetics of the individual agents and limited analyses do not allow absolute determination of the best dosing strategy. It should be noted that pharmacodynamic principles for antibacterials have generally been related to plasma concentrations.[49] As noted earlier, the plasma concentrations of the macrolides are usually lower than those of the tissues, where the majority of bacteria reside. Models looking at both epithelial lining fluid (a proxy for lung concentrations) and serum concentrations suggest that increasing bacterial resistance favors telithromycin in its ability to maintain favorable pharmacodynamics.[50]

Immune Modulation

Increasing evidence suggests that antibacterial macrolides have antiinflammatory effects.[51-53] In vitro studies have suggested macrolide effects on a number of cellular mechanisms within human cells.[54] In addition to in vitro and animal models, clinical data suggest that macrolides may have activity in the treatment of inflammatory diseases including cystic fibrosis, diffuse panbronchiolitis, chronic sinusitis, and inflammatory skin diseases.[51,53] Azithromycin has been cautiously recommended for use in cystic fibrosis for its antiinflammatory effects in patients colonized with *Pseudomonas* spp.[55]

Adverse Effects

Gastrointestinal effects (nausea and diarrhea) are the most common adverse events observed with macrolide therapy.[41,56] Erythromycin has the highest level of GI effects.[1] Nausea with erythromycin may occur after IV dosing, as erythromycin is secreted into the GI tract via the bile.[57] The advanced macrolides have a similar incidence of GI adverse events. A review of azithromycin safety data from over 4000 patients treated with the immediate-release formulation reported GI event rates of 4% for diarrhea and 3% for nausea.[58] Gastrointestinal side effects in patients receiving the 2-g extended release azithromycin formulation were higher, with 12% nausea and 4% diarrhea.[59] In 3800 patients receiving immediate-release clarithromycin, similar side-effect rates were observed for nausea (3.8%) and diarrhea (3.0%). Tolerability of the extended-release clarithromycin formulation was similar to those with the immediate-release product.[36] Roxithromycin was reported to have a 4% incidence of side effects in 32,405 patients, with 75% being mild to moderate GI events.[41] From data in clinical trials, GI side effects were reported frequently with telithromycin (10.8% diarrhea, 7.9% nausea), although considerable variability was observed across studies.[56]

More serious events associated with macrolide use include prolongation of the QT interval, with torsades de pointes. In vitro estimations of *HERG* blockade suggest that clarithromycin ≈ roxithromycin > erythromycin.[60] In contrast, erythromycin was found to have a higher proarrhythmic potential than clarithromycin and azithromycin in animal models.[61] Torsades de pointes has been reported in patients receiving macrolides. Sudden cardiac death was observed with greater frequency in patients taking erythromycin than amoxicillin in a large database study.[62] Although the relative ability of the macrolides to cause arrhythmias is difficult to ascertain, arrhythmias associated with clarithromycin use were reported more frequently than with erythromycin.[63]

Severe hepatotoxicity associated with telithromycin was identified through post-marketing surveillance in the United States.[64] Forty-two cases were available for full review, with 5 patients dying or requiring liver transplants. Clinical features included short time to hepatotoxicity (as short as 1-2 days), fever, abdominal pain, and ascites. As a result of this toxicity, telithromycin use has been limited to more severely infected individuals with a careful review of risks and benefits.

Prokinetic Activity

The intestinal prokinetic activity of the macrolides has been used to improve GI mobility. Erythromycin has been shown to improve gastric emptying in a dose-dependent manner.[65] However, concerns have been raised over the potential to increase bacterial resistance with non-antibacterial macrolide use.[66] In a comparative multidose trial in patients with enteral nutrition intolerability, erythromycin provided better results than metoclopramide, with both agents showing efficacy.[67] Optimal use of erythromycin as a prokinetic agent is not yet confirmed.[66-68]

Drug-Drug Interactions

Drug-drug interactions must be evaluated when considering macrolide therapy. The macrolides have variable degrees of inhibition of CYP3A4 and are also substrates of this enzyme. The use of macrolides with other drugs metabolized by CYP3A4 may result in increases in the second drug concentrations. Erythromycin is the most potent inhibitor of CYP3A4, followed by moderate inhibition with clarithromycin and roxithromycin and little to no inhibition by azithromycin.[69] Erythromycin has been implicated in multiple drug interactions, including with benzodiazepines, carbamazepine, cyclosporine, digoxin, HMG-CoA inhibitors, tacrolimus, and theophylline. Case reports of interactions with warfarin have been documented for many of the macrolides.[70] Clarithromycin, although in vitro a less potent inhibitor of CYP3A4, has been associated with a similar scope of clinical interactions.[70] As expected by its limited CYP activity, few clinically important interactions have been reported with roxithromycin and azithromycin.[39,41,70]

The pharmacodynamic interaction between macrolides and other drugs known to increase the QT interval must not be overlooked (see Adverse Effects).

KEY POINTS

1. The spectrum of activity of the macrolides is primarily focused on streptococci and atypical bacteria, with minor gram-negative activity.

2. Two main mechanisms of resistance limit macrolide utility: ribosomal mutations (*erm* related), conferring high levels of resistance, and drug efflux (*mef* related), conferring minor MIC elevations.

3. The pharmacokinetics of macrolides are variable, but all of the macrolides are available orally and attain high intracellular and tissue concentrations.

4. Incomplete data are available to determine the optimal pharmacodynamic principles guiding macrolide activity, but the ratio of the free drug area under the macrolide concentration curve to the minimal inhibitory concentration (fAUC/MIC) appears most promising.

5. Antiinflammatory properties of the macrolides have been described by in vitro and animal experiments.

6. Gastrointestinal disturbances are among the most common adverse effects of macrolides, but the most serious adverse effect is QT-interval prolongation and torsades de pointes.

7. The macrolides are cytochrome P450-3A4 inhibitors (erythromycin > clarithromycin ≈ roxithromycin >> azithromycin) and have the potential to interact with similarly metabolized medications.

ANNOTATED REFERENCES

Jenkins S, Farrell D. Increase in pneumococcus macrolide resistance, United States. Emerg Infect Dis 2009;15:1260-4.
This study presents the current regional and national level data on susceptibilities and minimum inhibitory concentrations for pneumococci. These are important for selection of empirical therapy.

Noreddin A, El-Khatib W, Aolie J, Salem AH, Zhanel GG. Pharmacodynamic target attainment potential of azithromycin, clarithromycin, and telithromycin in serum and epithelial lining fluid of community-acquired pneumonia patients with penicillin-susceptible, intermediate, and resistant *Streptococcus pneumoniae*. Int J Infect Dis 2009;13:483-7.
Simulations of macrolide and ketolide concentrations in both the blood and lung compartments are modeled. These models are used to predict the attainment of favorable pharmacodynamic profiles based on the susceptibilities of pneumococcal isolates.

Shaffer D, Singer S, Korvick J, Honig P. Concomitant risk factors in reports of torsades de pointes associated with macrolide use: review of the United States Food and Drug Administration Adverse Event Reporting System. Clin Infect Dis 2002;35:197-200.
Review of a spontaneous adverse events report provided data on 156 cases of torsades de pointes in patients receiving macrolide antibiotics. Concomitant use of drugs known to increase the QT interval was found in half of the cases. Increased age, female sex, and comorbid diseases were other common risk factors.

Ribeiro C, Hurd H, Wu Y, Martino ME, Jones L, Brighton B, et al. Azithromycin treatment alters gene expression in inflammatory, lipid metabolism, and cell cycle pathways in well-differentiated human airway epithelia. PLoS One 2009;4:e5806.
Using human bronchial epithelial cells, the investigators performed in vitro experiments to outline the effect of azithromycin on gene expression after inflammatory stimulation. This investigation helps outline the wide and variable immunomodulatory effects of azithromycin.

Brinker A, Wassel R, Lyndly J, Serrano J, Avigan M, Lee WM, et al. Telithromycin-associated hepatotoxicity: clinical spectrum and causality assessment of 42 cases. Hepatology 2009;49:250-7.
Forty-two cases of hepatic failure associated with telithromycin use were analyzed for their likely causation with drug therapy. This report solidifies the warnings related to telithromycin use.

REFERENCES

Access the complete reference list online at http://www.expertconsult.com.

124

Agents with Primary Activity Against Gram-Positive Bacteria

DIANE M. CAPPELLETTY

The causes of nosocomial infections have changed in recent years. A 25-year study of nosocomial bacteremia demonstrated a change from *Staphylococcus aureus* and gram-negative bacilli as the predominant pathogens during the 1970s and 1980s to coagulase-negative staphylococci and *Enterococcus*, along with *S. aureus* and *Pseudomonas aeruginosa*, as the most common contemporary pathogens.[1] The EPIC II study in 2007 demonstrated gram-positive organisms were associated with 47% of infections in the ICU.[2] There can also be differences in the predominance of pathogens in different ICUs and different types of nosocomial infections. Nosocomial bacteremias are caused most often by coagulase-negative staphylococci and *S. aureus* in the medical ICU.[3] *S. aureus* is the most common pathogen associated with nosocomial pneumonia and the fourth most common cause of skin and soft-tissue infections.[3] Along with the increase in prevalence of gram-positive cocci in the ICU, staphylococci are becoming multidrug resistant. This chapter addresses gram-positive organisms and resistance issues associated with each of the antimicrobials with activity against these pathogens.

Vancomycin

Vancomycin was discovered in 1956 and marketed in 1958. Early preparations of the drug contained pyrogens and impurities that produced a brownish, muddy appearance that provided vancomycin's nickname, "Mississippi mud." In addition, these pyrogens and impurities caused high fevers, hypotension, severe phlebitis, and possibly nephrotoxicity.[4]

MECHANISMS OF ACTION AND RESISTANCE

Vancomycin inhibits synthesis of the cell wall by binding to the D-alanyl-D-alanine terminus of cell wall precursor units. Vancomycin is slowly bactericidal against dividing organisms except for *Enterococcus* and tolerant staphylococci, against which it is bacteriostatic.[5] In 2006 the Clinical and Laboratory Standards Institute (CLSI) changed the vancomycin breakpoints against *Staphylococcus aureus* from ≤4 µg/mL to ≤2 µg/mL for susceptible strains. Intermediate susceptibility is now 4 to 8 µg/mL, and resistance to vancomycin is ≥16 µg/mL.[6] The U.S. Food and Drug Administration (FDA) adopted these new breakpoints in 2008. The European Committee on Antimicrobial Susceptibility Testing (EUCAST) changed their vancomycin interpretations against *S. aureus* to ≤2 µg/mL as susceptible and >2 µg/mL as resistant. These changes in breakpoints will alter how literature is interpreted with respect to the frequency or prevalence of vancomycin-intermediate or vancomycin-resistant *S. aureus* over the past 30 years.

Five types of resistance for vancomycin have been isolated from enterococci: VanA, VanB, VanC, VanD, and VanE. The VanA phenotype confers high-level resistance to both teicoplanin (minimum inhibitory concentrations [MICs]: 16 to 512 µg/mL) and vancomycin (MICs: 64 to >1000 µg/mL). Vancomycin can induce expression of the VanA gene and has been identified in both *Enterococcus faecium* and *Enterococcus faecalis*. The VanB phenotype has also been identified in both *E. faecium* and *E. faecalis* and confers low-level resistance primarily to vancomycin. VanA, B, D, and E are all transferable to other organisms. In contrast, the VanC phenotypes are endogenous (constitutively produced)

and are components of *Enterococcus gallinarum*, *Enterococcus casseliflavus*, and *Enterococcus flavescens* and confer resistance to vancomycin alone. The VanB gene has been identified in a strain of *Streptococcus bovis*. This gene showed 96% homology with the prototype VanB gene from *E. faecalis V583*, indicating the likelihood of the gene transfer from enterococcus to this strain of *S. bovis*.[7]

Vancomycin-intermediate *S. aureus* using the prior breakpoints of MIC 8 to 16 µg/mL was first reported in 1996 from Japan, and by June 2002, eight cases were confirmed in the United States.[88] Using the new breakpoints, the incidence of vancomycin-intermediate *S. aureus* will increase. In June 2002, the first case of vancomycin-resistant *S. aureus* (MIC > 32 µg/mL) was identified in Michigan, followed in September 2002 by the second case in Pennsylvania.[8,9] No mechanism of resistance has yet been identified from the strains of vancomycin-intermediate *S. aureus*, but the two strains of vancomycin-resistant *S. aureus* both possessed the VanA gene.

Tolerance is another mechanism by which bactericidal activity is decreased. Tolerance can be measured or assessed by two methods: the ratio of minimum bactericidal concentration to minimum inhibitory concentration (MBC:MIC) and time-kill curves. By definition, a MBC:MIC ratio of 32 or greater or less than 99.9% kill after 24 hours incubation in time-kill studies equates to tolerance. Tolerance to vancomycin has been identified in *S. aureus*, *Streptococcus pneumoniae*, and groups C and G streptococci.[10-12]

SPECTRUM OF ACTIVITY

Vancomycin is active primarily against aerobic gram-positive cocci including *Corynebacterium* and methicillin-resistant *S. aureus* (MRSA). The MIC90 against methicillin-susceptible *S. aureus* (MSSA) is 1 µg/mL, and against MRSA it is 1 to 2 µg/mL.[13-15] The incidence of vancomycin-intermediate or vancomycin-resistant *S. aureus* currently is very low and less than 1%. The activity of vancomycin against enterococci varies greatly with the species. *E. faecium* is the most resistant species of enterococci to vancomycin, with the resistant rates ranging from 30% to 90% depending on the institution. For all enterococci the vancomycin resistance rates are 20% to 25%.[16]

Most streptococci are susceptible to vancomycin, although it is considered an agent of last resort against these organisms. Vancomycin has been shown to be inferior to nafcillin or oxacillin for the treatment of MSSA infections. Treatment failures, prolonged treatment, and higher mortality rates have been demonstrated when vancomycin was used to treat MSSA infections compared with nafcillin or oxacillin.[17,18]

Vancomycin is active against anaerobic gram-positive organisms such as *Peptostreptococcus* spp., *Propionibacterium* spp., *Eubacterium* spp., *Bifidobacterium* spp., and most *Clostridium* spp., including *C. difficile*.[19]

PHARMACOKINETICS/PHARMACODYNAMICS

Vancomycin is administered orally and intravenously (IV). The drug is poorly absorbed after oral administration, and the majority of the drug is excreted unchanged in feces. Inflammation of the gastrointestinal tract may result in increased absorption of vancomycin, and measurable serum concentrations might be obtained.[20] Intramuscular injections are extremely painful and should not be used. Distribution of the drug is complete 1 hour after a 1- to 2-hour IV infusion. Vancomycin is approximately 55% bound to plasma proteins. The volume of distribution corrected for weight ranges from 0.4 to 0.9 L/kg.[21-27] Vancomycin does not penetrate well into noninflamed meninges or aqueous humor.[28] Distribution into inflamed meninges is variable, with reported ranges of 1% to 37% of serum concentrations[29,30] and a mean concentration of 15% of serum or approximately 2.5 µg/mL.[31] Penetration into ascitic, pericardial, and synovial fluids is greater than 75% serum concentrations; penetration approximates 50% into pleural fluid, and 30% to 50% into bile.[25] Elimination of vancomycin is 80% to 90% unchanged drug in the urine via glomerular filtration and the remaining via nonrenal elimination. The nonrenal elimination rate in healthy individuals is 40 mL/min, and in chronic renal failure patients it is 6 mL/min.[32] The half-life of the drug increases with decreased renal function; in patients with creatinine clearances (CrCl) greater than 80 mL/min, the half-life is 4 to 6 hours. The pharmacodynamic effect of vancomycin is time-dependent killing or time above the MIC.[33] Therefore, the most important goal of therapy is to maintain a free serum trough concentration above the MIC of the organism. There is no documented correlation between serum peak concentrations and clinical outcomes.

DOSAGE REGIMENS

Oral Administration

Oral administration of vancomycin is only for treating *C. difficile* colitis and is considered second-line therapy for mild/moderate infections and primary therapy for moderate/severe infections. The dose is 125 to 500 mg orally every 6 hours and is not adjusted for renal dysfunction, owing to the poor absorption. Two oral formulations (capsules or liquid) can be used, or the IV solution can be administered orally to treat *C. difficile*. Table 124-1 lists dosing regimens for the antimicrobials discussed in this chapter.

Intravenous Administration in Adults

In nonobese adults with normal renal function, the usual dose of vancomycin is 1 g (~15 mg/kg) every 12 hours. This dose results in peak serum concentrations of 25 to 40 µg/mL 1 hour after completion of the infusion and trough serum concentration of 5 to 15 µg/mL. Dosing should be based on actual body weight. Several dosing guidelines have been developed to accurately and easily dose vancomycin. The most popular methods include the Moellering[23] and Matzke[24] nomograms. These methods use body weight and CrCl to calculate vancomycin dose. The weaknesses of these nomograms include the small number of patients used to develop and evaluate the nomogram and the fixed volume of distribution assumed for all patients (0.9 L/kg). Matzke[24] found that for patients younger than 65 years of age, a volume of distribution of 0.7 L/kg may be more accurate, and for those older than 65, it is 0.9 L/kg. This variance in volume of distribution does affect the reproducibility of these nomograms when applied to different patient populations. The Cockcroft and Gault and modified Cockcroft and Gault methods of estimating CrCl are relatively reliable and accurate methods in patients of normal body mass.[33]

Morbidly obese patients are difficult to dose given the lack of pharmacokinetic studies. Doses of approximately 30 mg/kg/d based on actual body weight should provide a peak serum concentration of 25 to 35 µg/mL. Because CrCl is the best correlate to vancomycin clearance, the most accurate method for estimating CrCl should be used and varies with body mass. CrCl estimations in the obese patient are best predicted by the Salazar-Corcoran method.[34] Young obese patients with no comorbid conditions affecting renal function often require the dosing interval to be more frequent to achieve a trough serum concentration of 5 to 15 µg/mL. This is due to the faster rate of clearance of the drug (2.3-2.5 times higher) in obese compared with nonobese patients.[35,36]

Vancomycin Dosing in Critically Ill Patients

Garaud evaluated critically ill patients and found an average volume of distribution of 0.6 L/kg in patients with CrCl greater than 70 mL/min and 0.4 L/kg with CrCl of 10 to 60 mL/min.[26] Critically ill patients are often receiving medications to improve hemodynamics, such as dopamine, dobutamine, and furosemide. These medications result in increases in renal function and changes in volume status for the patient. In a study designed to assess the impact of such medications on vancomycin pharmacokinetics, two observations were made.[37] First,

TABLE 124-1	Dosages for Agents with Primary Activity Against Gram-Positive Bacteria		
Drug	**Dosage**	**Adverse Effects**	**Considerations**
Vancomycin	Oral (PO) and intravenous (IV) administration Dose based on actual body weight (ABW) PO: 125 mg q 6 h IV: 1 g (~15 mg/kg) q 12 h for average-weight adult IV: For morbidly obese adult, dose on ABW ~15 mg/kg/dose	Red man syndrome: erythema, pruritus, flushing of upper torso Thrombophlebitis Ototoxicity: rare Nephrotoxicity: rare Maculopapular or erythematous rashes	Intramuscular injections painful Poorly absorbed orally Half-life of drug increases with decreased renal function. Moellering and Matzke methods for dosing guidelines For obese patients and patients on dialysis, consider drug clearance.
Teicoplanin	IV administration Moderate infections: 400 mg (6 mg/kg) once followed by maintenance dose 200 mg (3 mg/kg) q 24 h Severe infections: 400-800 mg (6-12 mg/kg) q 12 h for 2-3 doses, followed by 400-800 mg q 24 h	Nephrotoxicity: rare Ototoxicity: rare Hypersensitivity	Special dosage considerations for patients with renal failure, patients on dialysis Compassionate use only in the United States (not FDA approved)
Daptomycin	IV: 4 mg/kg q 24 h for average-weight adult	Transient muscle weakness Myalgia	Contraindicated in pneumonia
Quinupristin/dalfopristin	IV: 7.5 mg/kg q 8-12 h infused over 1 h	Arthralgia Myalgia Infusion-related Nausea, vomiting, diarrhea, rash	
Linezolid	Bioequivalence between PO and IV formulations Moderate infections: 600 mg twice daily Uncomplicated infections: 400 mg twice daily	Reversible myelosuppression Anemia Neutropenia Thrombocytopenia Diarrhea Headache Nausea and vomiting	
Telavancin	IV: 10 mg/kg once daily	Nausea and vomiting Taste perversion Foamy urine	Teratogenic in animal models, further information needed in humans Interferes with common anticoagulation and urine protein dipstick testing

some of the patients required larger total daily doses of vancomycin to achieve therapeutic concentrations than the Moellering nomogram predicted (26.78 + 3.01 mg/kg/d versus 18.95 + 3.41 mg/kg/d). Second, on discontinuation of these medications, the serum trough concentrations increased despite no change in CrCl or body weight. The theory is that these medications enhanced vancomycin clearance by improving renal blood flow and/or interacting with the renal anion transport system, thus increasing glomerular filtration and renal tubular secretion. Therefore, larger doses of vancomycin may be required while on these medications, and smaller doses may be more appropriate on discontinuation of these medications.

Vancomycin Dosing for Patients on Dialysis/Hemofiltration/ Cardiopulmonary Bypass

The percentage of vancomycin removed by low-permeability cellulose hemodialyzers is 4% to 6.9%.[38-40] Therefore, no supplemental vancomycin dosing is required after hemodialysis with these older systems. The removal of vancomycin during intradialytic administration has been studied using three types of cellulose membranes: cellulose acetate (CA), cellulose triacetate (CT), and CA high-performance 210 (CAHP-210). With the CA membranes, 0% to 25% (mean of ~13%) of vancomycin is removed.[38,41] The CT membranes remove 16% to 44% (mean of ~26%) of vancomycin.[38,41] Vancomycin removal during intradialytic administration with the CAHP-210 membranes is 0% to 35%, with a mean of 24%.[42] High-flux synthetic membranes such as polysulfone or polyacrylonitrile remove significantly more vancomycin than do the cellulose membranes, with 30% to 55% and 25% to 40% of vancomycin removed, respectively.[38-40,43-45]

Continuous renal replacement therapy (CRRT) is a low-volume (1-2 L/h) therapy. The most frequently used methods of CRRT are continuous venovenous hemofiltration (CVVH), continuous venovenous hemodialysis (CVVHD), and continuous arteriovenous hemodialysis (CAVHD). Both CVVHD and CAVHD result in a greater total body clearance of vancomycin than does hemofiltration. The clearances achieved with each of these methods vary with blood flow rate, ultrafiltration rate, and the membranes used. The total clearance of vancomycin with CVVHD or CAVHD is 31 to 39 mL/min, and the half-life ranges from 14 to 25 hours.[46-49] Clearance of vancomycin in patients with normal renal function (CrCl > 70 mL/min) and with mild renal dysfunction (CrCl 40-70 mL/min) has been reported to be 88 and 48 mL/min, respectively.[50] High-volume hemofiltration (HVHF), with an ultrafiltration rate of 6 L/h, increases vancomycin clearance to approximately 60 mL/min.[51] Therefore, patients receiving CAVHD or CVVHD should receive vancomycin every 36 to 48 hours, and those undergoing HVHF should receive the drug every 12 to 24 hours.

Cardiopulmonary bypass (CPB) significantly impacts the pharmacokinetic parameters of vancomycin. Immediately after initiating CPB, vancomycin serum concentration decreased by 7 µg/mL (5.7 to 8.4 µg/ mL), which represented approximately a 38% decrease in concentration.[52] Over the next 30 minutes, serum vancomycin concentration may increase 1 to 2 µg/mL but thereafter gradually and steadily decreases.[52] The half-life is not affected by CPB and does not change during the process.

ADVERSE EFFECTS

Common toxicities that have been associated with vancomycin therapy include red man syndrome, thrombophlebitis, ototoxicity, and nephrotoxicity. Evidence establishing a clear relationship between these toxicities and vancomycin peak or trough concentrations or the incidence of these events is limited and contradictory.[4,53-55]

Red man syndrome comprises erythema, pruritus, and flushing of the upper torso and is often associated with too rapid an infusion of the drug. In general, the infusion rate should not exceed 1 g/h. Less frequently, hypotension and angioedema can occur. It is thought that increased histamine release is the cause of this syndrome.[4,54-56] A comparative trial of once-daily versus twice-daily vancomycin found the incidence of this syndrome to be 13.7% and 9.6%, respectively.[54] The effects of red man syndrome can be relieved by antihistamines.[57,58]

Thrombophlebitis is reported in 3% to 23% of patients receiving vancomycin and is more common in patients who receive vancomycin for more than 7 days or have peripheral catheter lines for prolonged durations.[4,54]

Ototoxicity rates range from 0% to 9% in patients receiving vancomycin.[4,54] The definition of ototoxicity ranges from tinnitus to hearing loss. The evidence demonstrating any relationship between ototoxicity and high peak serum concentrations of vancomycin is limited. In cancer patients, only 4 of 19 patients with ototoxicity had elevated serum concentrations of vancomycin, and only 1 had a concentration greater than 80 µg/mL.[4] Others have reported ototoxicity associated with peak serum concentrations of 37.5 to 152 µg/mL.[59,60] A trial comparing once-daily to twice-daily dosing of vancomycin demonstrated more frequent ototoxicity in the twice-daily dosed group (15.6% versus 3.2%), which had a significantly lower peak concentration and similar trough concentration compared to the group receiving daily doses.[54] This lack of correlation between serum concentrations of vancomycin and ototoxicity suggests that the observed toxicity was due to either another drug or to the combination of another drug with vancomycin. In the majority of cases, ototoxicity symptoms disappear within a month of discontinuing vancomycin.

The issue of nephrotoxicity associated with vancomycin is complicated by several confounding factors. The original formulation was very impure, and the impurities were associated with toxicities including nephrotoxicity. In addition, many definitions of nephrotoxicity have been used over the years, different patient populations have been studied, and different doses used, making it difficult to compare one study to another. In general, the rate of nephrotoxicity is 5% to 10% when vancomycin is not administered with other nephrotoxic agents and trough concentrations are less than 10 µg/mL.[54,61,62] Elting and colleagues identified older age, Acute Physiology and Chronic Health Evaluation (APACHE) score greater than 40, and duration of therapy of greater than 14 days to be the best predictors for a patient to develop nephrotoxicity due solely to vancomycin therapy.[4] A number of other studies have found an increased incidence of nephrotoxicity (21%-35%) when vancomycin serum trough concentrations are greater than 10 µg/mL.[62-64] In addition, Lodise demonstrated an increased rate of nephrotoxicity (~35%) when the total daily dose is 4 grams or more compared to total doses less than 4 grams (~11%).[65] Studies have demonstrated higher rates of nephrotoxicity when vancomycin is used in combination with an aminoglycoside compared with either agent alone.[62,66,67] Goetz performed a meta-analysis of eight studies and found the incidence of nephrotoxicity associated with combination therapy was 13% greater than with vancomycin alone and 4% greater than with an aminoglycoside alone.[67]

Other toxicities associated with vancomycin include maculopapular or erythematous rashes (2%-8%)[26,68,75] and anecdotal reports of neutropenia and thrombocytopenia.[68,69]

THERAPEUTIC DRUG MONITORING

Routine monitoring of vancomycin serum concentrations has become a highly debated issue over the years. Those who advocate routine monitoring cite the need to ensure therapeutic concentrations as well as minimize toxicities. To date there is only one trial that compared efficacy and toxicity with high-dose once-daily versus twice-daily dosing of vancomycin; with these dosing regimens, peak serum concentrations were vastly different but trough serum concentrations were similar.[54] The mean peak serum concentrations in the once-daily and twice-daily dosed groups were 42.8 + 16.1 and 27.0 + 9.2 µg/mL, respectively. There were no differences in clinical efficacy, red man syndrome, thrombophlebitis, ototoxicity, and nephrotoxicity between the two groups.

Studies over the past 20 years have shown that peak concentrations of vancomycin are not associated with toxicities or clinical efficacy.

Therefore, monitoring peak serum concentrations only adds to hospital and healthcare system costs and provides no beneficial clinical information. Some studies have demonstrated a correlation of nephrotoxicity to serum trough concentrations ≥ 10 µg/mL, whereas others have not. Given the lack of consensus, it may be prudent to measure serum trough concentrations until more definitive studies are conducted to address this issue.[70]

In patients with end-stage renal disease, the fluorescence polarization immunoassay (FPIA) overestimates vancomycin concentrations.[71] FPIA is the most common method for determining vancomycin concentrations, and when it was compared with the enzyme multiplied immunoassay technique, it was found to produce higher peak serum concentrations by 7 to 11 µg/mL and higher trough concentrations by 4 to 6 µg/mL.

Teicoplanin

Teicoplanin is a glycopeptide antibiotic and is not approved for use in the United States. It is available for use in Europe, some Asian countries, Mexico, New Zealand, and Australia. It has a more favorable adverse-effect profile than vancomycin; however, there is concern over teicoplanin's clinical efficacy in the treatment of severe gram-positive infections.

MECHANISMS OF ACTION AND RESISTANCE

Teicoplanin, like other glycopeptide antibiotics, inhibits synthesis of the cell wall by binding to the D-alanyl-D-alanine terminus of cell wall precursor units. Resistance has been reported in both staphylococci and enterococci. The VanA phenotype confers high-level resistance to both teicoplanin (MIC: 16 to 512 µg/mL) and vancomycin (MIC: 64 to >1000 µg/mL). The VanB phenotype has also been identified in both *E. faecium* and *E. faecalis* and usually confers low-level resistance to vancomycin but not to teicoplanin. This may limit the utility of teicoplanin for some vancomycin-resistant enterococcal infections. Several reports of *S. aureus* resistance developing during therapy with teicoplanin have been reported.[72-74] The mechanism of the resistance was determined in one patient to be constitutive and non-plasmid mediated.[73]

SPECTRUM OF ACTIVITY

Teicoplanin is only active against gram-positive organisms. Activity against MSSA and MRSA is comparable to that of vancomycin. Coagulase-negative staphylococci have a varied pattern of susceptibility to teicoplanin. *Staphylococcus haemolyticus* is the most resistant species to teicoplanin (30%).[75] These isolates are 25% more resistant to teicoplanin than to vancomycin. Against methicillin-resistant coagulase-negative staphylococci, 39% of isolates have teicoplanin MICs greater than 8 µg/mL compared with 1% with vancomycin.[75,76] Teicoplanin is similar in activity to vancomycin against enterococci, although its reliability in treating infections with VanB resistance to vancomycin may be limited. Teicoplanin is active against other aerobic and anaerobic gram-positive organisms such as *Corynebacterium* spp., *Clostridium* spp., including *C. difficile* and *C. perfringens*, *Peptostreptococcus* spp., and *Propionibacterium acnes*.

PHARMACOKINETICS/PHARMACODYNAMICS

Teicoplanin is administered orally and intravenously. The drug is poorly absorbed after oral administration, and approximately 40% of the drug is excreted unchanged in feces. The pharmacokinetic model that best describes the elimination of teicoplanin is triexponential. IV administration of 400 mg (6 mg/kg) should provide a peak serum concentration of 20 to 50 µg/mL attained 1 hour after administration.[77] The volume of distribution is large at 0.9 to 1.41 L/kg, and teicoplanin is 90% to 95% protein bound.[77] Penetration into body fluids and tissues has not been extensively studied. Penetration into noninflamed meninges and fat is poor, but distribution into myocardium and pericardium is good.[78,79] Teicoplanin is primarily eliminated via glomerular filtration, and only 3% is metabolized.[77] The half-life is approximately 150 hours in patients with normal renal function.[77] Because of the long half-life, it takes 14 days to reach steady state. In patients with CrCl of 13 to 25, the half-life was found to be 280 to 667 hours.[80,81]

DOSAGE REGIMENS/THERAPEUTIC DRUG MONITORING

Despite the long half-life in patients with normal renal function, teicoplanin should be administered daily, and the dose is dependent on the severity of infection. For less serious infections involving the urinary tract, skin, soft tissue, and lower respiratory tract, a loading dose of 400 mg (6 mg/kg) × 1 is administered, followed by a maintenance dose of 200 mg (3 mg/kg) every 24 hours. For severe infections such as septicemia, endocarditis, and osteomyelitis, 400 mg of teicoplanin is administered every 12 hours for 3 doses, followed by 400 mg every 24 hours.[77] Although no therapeutic range has been established for teicoplanin, trough concentrations should be at least 10 µg/mL.[77]

Renal Failure/Dialysis

Teicoplanin is not removed by hemodialysis or continuous ambulatory peritoneal dialysis (CAPD).[82,83] The amount removed by CVVHD is dependent on the flow rate but is often minimal.[84,85] Several dosing regimens exist for renal dysfunction, and the simplest method is administering a dose of 6-10 mg/kg every 48 to 72 hours.

ADVERSE EFFECTS

Nephrotoxicity associated with teicoplanin is much lower than with vancomycin. The incidence from published and unpublished studies found the nephrotoxic rate to be 4%.[55] Ototoxic rates with teicoplanin are similar to those with vancomycin.[55] Hypersensitivity reactions are the most common adverse reaction to teicoplanin (2%-15%).[55]

Daptomycin

Daptomycin is a lipopeptide that was first discovered in the 1980s and was approved in 2003 by the FDA for complicated skin and skin structure infections. More recently it was approved for *S. aureus* bloodstream infections, including right-sided endocarditis.

MECHANISMS OF ACTION AND RESISTANCE

Daptomycin has a unique mechanism of action and has been found to inhibit lipoteichoic acid synthesis, owing to binding to the membrane in the presence of calcium.[86,87] Minimal information is available on the mechanism(s) of resistance to daptomycin. Limited in vitro studies have been performed attempting to create daptomycin resistance in the laboratory.[88] Mechanisms of resistance have not been elucidated, and the clinical relevance of in vitro resistance is unknown.

SPECTRUM OF ACTIVITY

Daptomycin's antibacterial activity encompasses most gram-positive bacteria, including vancomycin-resistant isolates and penicillin-resistant pneumococci. The MICs of daptomycin are 8- to 16-fold lower in the presence of calcium. Therefore, all in vitro testing must be supplemented with physiologic concentrations of calcium.[89] The breakpoint for susceptible is ≤1 µg/mL for staphylococci and β-hemolytic streptococci. Given the rare number of isolates not susceptible to daptomycin, a resistant breakpoint has yet to be determined. The MIC90 against MSSA, MRSA, *Staphylococcus epidermidis*, and *Staphylococcus saprophyticus* are all 0.5 µg/mL or less.[89,90] In a recent surveillance study, 7 *S. aureus* and 6 coagulase-negative staphylococci were non-susceptible to daptomycin.[91] Daptomycin also appears active against vancomycin-intermediate and vancomycin-resistant strains of *S. aureus*.[92,93] The breakpoint for susceptible against enterococci is ≤4 µg/mL, and again no resistant breakpoint has been established. Against *E. faecalis* and *E. faecium*, including vancomycin-resistant strains, the MIC90 is 2 µg/mL or less.[89,90] Daptomycin resistance is higher among *E. faecium* than *E. faecalis*.[91] The MIC90 is 0.25 µg/mL against *S. pneumoniae* and β-hemolytic streptococci, and resistance has not been reported with these organisms.[89-91]

PHARMACOKINETICS/PHARMACODYNAMICS

Healthy volunteers who received 6 mg/kg of daptomycin given as either a 30- or 2-minute infusion achieved bioequivalent pharmacokinetic results. The maximum plasma concentration (C_{max}) was about 94 and 88 µg/mL for the 2- and 30-minute infusions, respectively.[94] Daptomycin demonstrates linear kinetics at dosing from 4 to 12 mg/kg, and the half-life is 7 to 9 hours in patients with normal renal function.[95] The drug is 90% to 95% protein bound and is primarily eliminated by the renal route. In patients with CrCl less than 30 mL/min, end-stage renal disease/hemodialysis/peritoneal dialysis, a 4 mg/kg dose should provide a peak serum concentrations around 25 to 30 µg/mL and half-life of about 30 hours.[95]

Daptomycin is rapidly bactericidal and exhibits concentration-dependent killing against gram-positive organisms including enterococci.[86,87] Daptomycin also exhibits a post-antibiotic effect which allows for once daily dosing.[96]

DOSAGE REGIMENS AND THERAPEUTIC MONITORING

For complicated skin and skin structure infections (cSSSIs), dosing of daptomycin is 4 mg/kg every 24 hours. Dosing for bacteremia or right-sided endocarditis is 6 mg/kg every 24 hours.[95]

Renal Failure/Dialysis

In patients with CrCl less than 30 mL/min or undergoing hemodialysis or chronic peritoneal dialysis, the dose should be reduced to 4 mg/kg every 48 hours and 6 mg/kg every 48 hours for bacteremia or endocarditis.[95] In patients undergoing continuous renal replacement therapy (CRRT), the amount of daptomycin removed is dependent upon the type of filter and the flow rates.[97] Dosing recommendations for patients undergoing CRRT are 4 to 6 mg/kg every 48 hours, and there is some speculation that doses may need to be increased to 8 to 10 mg/kg every 48 hours.[98,99]

Dosing in the Setting of Obesity

Two single-dose studies using 4 mg/kg total body weight have been performed in moderately and morbidly obese patients. The C_{max} was increased 25% to 60% compared to normal-weight patients and the area under the curve (AUC) increased 30% to 60% in the obese patients. Half-life was also longer and ranged from 7 to 9 hours; all patients had normal renal function.[100,101] Recommendations are to base daptomycin dosage on total body weight, but difficulties in assessing renal function in obese patients have to be considered when selecting the dosing interval.

Burn Patients

One study evaluated single-dose pharmacokinetics (4 mg/kg) in burn patients and found the C_{max} was 44% lower, with 47% lower AUC and an increase in volume of distribution and clearance.[102] The authors suggest a dose of 10 to 12 mg/kg in burn patients should provide the same drug exposure as 6 mg/kg in healthy volunteers.

ADVERSE EFFECTS

Creatine phosphokinase (CPK) concentrations increased in 2.8% of patients treated with daptomycin in the cSSSI studies and was composed 100% of the MM isoenzyme.[87,95] Elevations in CPK can occur 2 to 3 days before clinical signs or symptoms of myopathy present.[96]

Quinupristin/Dalfopristin

MECHANISMS OF ACTION AND RESISTANCE

Quinupristin/dalfopristin is a streptogramin antibiotic and is a mix of two different streptogramin components from groups A and B. The individual components are bacteriostatic, but the combination is often bactericidal. Each component binds to different sites on the 50S subunit of the ribosome, inhibiting translation of mRNA at the elongation step.[103] The resulting complex of drug and ribosome inhibits protein synthesis.

Streptogramins share similar sites of action with macrolide and lincomycin antibiotics. As a result, mechanisms of resistance are also shared. The most common type of resistance to streptogramins involves the erythromycin resistance methylase *(erm)* genes, termed MLS_B.[104] These genes decrease the binding of antibiotics such as streptogramins group B, erythromycin, and clindamycin by dimethylating a residue on the 23S ribosome. Group A streptogramins are not affected, and the combination often retains its synergistic activity.[104] Enzymatic modification of both components is another mechanism of resistance to the drug.[105,106] The third mechanism involves efflux pumps: one that pumps out both macrolides and streptogramins and one specific for streptogramins.[105,107,108]

SPECTRUM OF ACTIVITY

Quinupristin/dalfopristin is active against a wide variety of gram-positive organisms as well as many anaerobes and oral flora organisms. A MIC of 2 µg/mL or less indicates susceptibility. The MIC90 of most MSSA, MRSA, and coagulase-negative staphylococci is 1 to 2 µg/mL.[14,15,90] Against vancomycin-intermediate and vancomycin-resistant *S. aureus*, the drug is active with MICs of 0.25 to 1 µg/mL.[93,109] Both vancomycin-susceptible and vancomycin-resistant *E. faecium* are susceptible to quinupristin/dalfopristin (MIC90: 1-4 µg/mL); however, *E. faecalis* is resistant to quinupristin/dalfopristin (MIC90: 4-32 µg/mL).[110,111] Against a variety of streptococcal organisms, including penicillin-resistant pneumococci, the MIC90 ranges from 0.5 to 2 µg/mL. Quinupristin/dalfopristin is also active against a variety of other organisms including *Chlamydia* spp., *Mycoplasma pneumoniae*, *Legionella* spp., *Peptostreptococcus* spp., *Fusobacterium* spp., *Prevotella* spp., *Actinomyces* spp., and *Clostridium* spp.

PHARMACOKINETICS/PHARMACODYNAMICS

Quinupristin/dalfopristin infusions should be administered over 1 hour, and the drug is incompatible with saline. In healthy volunteers and in patients undergoing CAPD, the mean peak serum concentration of quinupristin was 2.6 and 2.9 µg/mL, respectively, and for dalfopristin it was 7.1 and 8.5 µg/mL, respectively, following a single 7.5-mg/kg dose.[112] Quinupristin/dalfopristin is hepatically metabolized to several active metabolites, and both the parent components and the metabolites are primarily eliminated via bile into feces.[113] Urinary excretion of quinupristin/dalfopristin and metabolites is 15% to 19%. The mean half-life ranges from 1.2 to 1.5 hours. The drug is 90% protein bound.[114]

Quinupristin/dalfopristin is bactericidal against staphylococci and streptococci, but it is bacteriostatic against *E. faecium*. The pharmacodynamic parameters that best predict efficacy have not been well characterized.

DOSAGE REGIMENS AND THERAPEUTIC MONITORING

The normal dose of quinupristin/dalfopristin is 7.5 mg/kg every 8 to 12 hours and infused over 1 hour. Dosage reduction is likely required in patients with severe liver dysfunction, although specific recommendations are not available.

Renal Failure/Dialysis

Neither hemodialysis nor peritoneal dialysis removes any appreciable amount of quinupristin/dalfopristin.[112,115] Penetration into the peritoneal cavity is negligible in CAPD patients. No dosage adjustment is needed in patients with renal insufficiency or on dialysis.

ADVERSE EFFECTS

Myalgias (6%-7%) and arthralgias (9%-9.5%) are the most severe adverse effects and are often the reason for discontinuation of the drug.[116,117] Elevations in direct and conjugated bilirubin and γ-glutamyl transferase are common. Infusion-related adverse effects occur in 30% to 45% of patients with peripheral lines used for the infusion.[116] The reactions include pain, burning, inflammation, and thrombophlebitis. Other toxicities include nausea, diarrhea, vomiting, and rash.

Linezolid

MECHANISMS OF ACTION AND RESISTANCE

Linezolid is an oxazolidinone antibiotic, a new class of synthetic agents. Linezolid binds to the 50S ribosome and inhibits the binding of mRNA, thereby preventing protein synthesis.[118] Clinical isolates of S. aureus, E. faecium, and E. faecalis resistant to linezolid have been identified but currently are rare. The most common mechanism of resistance is alteration of the 23S rRNA.[119] There are three case reports of vancomycin-resistant E. faecium infections in which the organisms were resistant to linezolid without the patient having any prior exposure to linezolid.[120,121] A second mechanism of resistance has been identified in S. aureus and involves acquisition of the natural resistance gene, cfr.[122,123] The cfr gene confers resistance to chloramphenicol and clindamycin. In animals, this gene is located on a plasmid which could result in propagating the spread of resistance. In humans, the gene has not been identified on a plasmid but rather on the chromosome.[122] These resistance issues, although rare, do raise concern and emphasize the importance of appropriate use of linezolid.

SPECTRUM OF ACTIVITY

Linezolid's breakpoint for susceptibility is ≤4 µg/mL for staphylococci and ≤2 µg/mL for enterococci and streptococci. It is active against both methicillin-susceptible and methicillin-resistant staphylococci. The MIC90 against S. aureus and coagulase-negative staphylococci is 2 and 1 µg/mL, respectively.[124-126] Against vancomycin-intermediate and vancomycin-resistant S. aureus, the drug is active with MICs of 1 to 2 µg/mL.[93,109] Linezolid is equally active against both vancomycin-susceptible and vancomycin-resistant enterococci with an MIC90 of 2 µg/mL.[124,126,127] Against both penicillin-susceptible and penicillin-resistant S. pneumoniae, the MIC90 is 1 µg/mL.[124,126] Linezolid is also active against a variety of other organisms, including Pasteurella multocida, Peptostreptococcus spp., Fusobacterium spp., and Prevotella spp.

PHARMACOKINETICS/PHARMACODYNAMICS

Linezolid is available in both oral and IV formulations. Oral absorption is over 90%, making the oral formulation bioequivalent to the IV formulation. The peak serum concentration and half-life at steady state after 600 mg twice daily were 14 to 18 µg/mL and 5 to 6 hours.[128-130] Linezolid is approximately 30% protein bound and penetrates quickly into bone, fat, and muscle, achieving 50% to 60% of serum concentrations in bone and 90% to 95% in muscle.[131] Elimination of linezolid is 30% renal and 70% metabolized, with essentially no linezolid eliminated in feces as unchanged drug.[130] Linezolid is not an inducer of the cytochrome P450 enzyme system.

Linezolid is bacteriostatic against staphylococci and enterococci and is bactericidal against streptococci. It appears that the pharmacodynamic parameter best modeling the killing activity is the area under the concentration time curve to MIC ratio (AUC/MIC).[132] The AUC/MIC ratio required to produce a bacteriostatic effect varied from 22 to 97 (mean 48) for pneumococci and 39 to 167 (mean 83) for staphylococci. A dosage regimen of 600 mg twice daily achieves these values for organisms with MICs as high as 4 µg/mL.

DOSAGE REGIMENS AND THERAPEUTIC MONITORING

The usual dose of linezolid is 600 mg twice daily, and for uncomplicated skin and skin structure infections, the dose is 400 mg twice daily.

Critically Ill Patients

One small study evaluated the pharmacokinetics of linezolid in critically ill patients when administered as standard intermittent bolus therapy or continuous infusion. Standard bolus therapy resulted in free and total trough concentrations below the breakpoint of 4 µg/mL in all patients, and 50% of patients had free trough concentrations less than 1 µg/mL. Standard bolus therapy resulted in only 40% of patients achieving at least 85% of the dosing interval with free concentrations above a MIC of 2 µg/mL (the most common MIC for pathogens identified in the study) compared to 100% in the continuous infusion group. Achieving the target AUC/MIC ratio of at least 80 occurred in only 62.5% of patients given standard bolus therapy compared with 87.5% of patients receiving continuous infusion.[133] Wide variability in linezolid pharmacokinetic parameters were observed, and continuous infusion may provide an option for optimizing the pharmacodynamic parameters, but further studies are needed to assess the efficacy and safety of continuous infusion.

Renal Failure/Dialysis

Hemodialysis removes approximately 30% of linezolid during a 3- to 4-hour session. However, no dosage adjustment is needed in patients with renal dysfunction or end-stage renal disease.

ADVERSE EFFECTS

Reversible myelosuppression is the most significant adverse effect associated with linezolid therapy. Anemia, neutropenia, and thrombocytopenia have all been reported, and the incidence increases with durations of therapy exceeding 14 days.[134,135] The decrease in hemoglobin when linezolid therapy is greater than 2 weeks is 18% compared with 13% for comparator agents and linezolid therapy less than 2 weeks' duration.[134] The thrombocytopenia rate is 8% with the longer duration of therapy compared with 5% to 6% in all durations of therapy compared with 3% with comparator agents. Rates of neutropenia also increase to about 10% with extended durations of therapy. Complete blood cell counts should be monitored weekly, especially in patients in whom the duration of therapy is likely to exceed 2 weeks.

Linezolid is a reversible nonselective inhibitor of monoamine oxidase; therefore, the potential for interaction with adrenergic and serotonergic agents exists. Several case reports of serotonin syndrome (fever, agitation, tremors, and mental status changes) secondary to an interaction between linezolid and selective serotonin reuptake inhibitors (SSRIs) have been identified.[136-138]

Other adverse reactions to linezolid include diarrhea (8%), headache (7%), nausea and vomiting (6% and 4%), dizziness, rash, fever, constipation (2%), and abnormal liver function tests (1%). Rare but serious reactions include optic or peripheral neuropathy; optic neuropathy tends to be reversible upon discontinuation of linezolid, but peripheral neuropathy tends to be permanent.[139]

Telavancin

Telavancin was approved in 2009 for the treatment of complicated skin and skin structure infections. No pediatric studies have been conducted at this time.

MECHANISMS OF ACTION AND RESISTANCE

Telavancin is a lipoglycopeptide which has a dual mechanism of action. It binds to the D-alanyl-D-alanine terminus of the cell wall precursors as vancomycin does, but additionally it binds to bacterial membranes, resulting in the depolarization and increased permeability of the membrane.[140]

SPECTRUM OF ACTIVITY

Telavancin is active against MSSA, MRSA, coagulase-negative staphylococci, vancomycin-susceptible enterococci, *Streptococcus pyogenes*, *Streptococcus agalactiae*, and *Streptococcus anginosus*. The breakpoint for susceptible against the streptococci is ≤0.12 μg/mL and for staphylococci and enterococci is ≤1 μg/mL. No interpretations for intermediate or resistant exist at this time. Telavancin is active against most anaerobic gram-positive organisms including *C. difficile* and *C. perfringens*.[141] The MIC90 is ≤1 μg/mL for most clostridia, and against most other anaerobic gram-positive cocci and bacilli it is ≤0.5 μg/mL.[141]

PHARMACOKINETICS/PHARMACODYNAMICS

Telavancin demonstrates linear pharmacokinetics over doses of 7.5 to 15 mg/kg. In healthy subjects, doses of 7.5 and 15 mg/kg at steady state resulted in mean C_{max} serum concentrations of 88 and 186 μg/mL and trough concentrations of 6 and 16 μg/mL, respectively.[142] Approximately 70% of telavancin is renally eliminated, and the half-life was dose dependent and ranged from 6 to 7.5 hours.[142] Telavancin is 90% protein bound to albumin and has a volume of distribution of approximately 0.14 L/kg.[143] Telavancin penetrates lung epithelial lining fluid and alveolar macrophages well, and concentrations exceeded 0.5 μg/mL during the entire dosing interval.[144] Penetration into blister fluid is approximately 40% of serum concentrations.[145]

Telavancin exhibits rapid concentration-dependent killing. The pharmacodynamic parameter identified in animal models as the best predictor of efficacy is the AUC/MIC ratio.[146] The minimum AUC/MIC ratio needed to provide a favorable clinical outcome in humans has not yet been identified.

DOSAGE REGIMENS AND THERAPEUTIC MONITORING

For complicated skin and skin structure infections, telavancin is dosed 10 mg/kg IV every 24 hours when CrCl is over 50 mL/min.

Renal Failure/Dialysis

Due to the high urinary elimination of telavancin, dosage reductions are required when the patient's CrCl falls below 50 mL/min. If CrCl is 30 to 50 mL/min, the dose of telavancin is 7.5 mg/kg every 24 hours, and when less than 30 mL/min, the dose is further reduced to 10 mg/kg every 48 hours.[143] In vitro studies evaluated the affect of CRRT on telavancin elimination and found high ultrafiltrate or dialysate rates can remove a significant amount of telavancin, which could require supplemental dosing.[147]

ADVERSE EFFECTS

Telavancin is a pregnancy category C drug with little information available in pregnant women. In three animal species, telavancin was found to have fetal effects including decreased birth weight and increased digit and limb malformations. A serum pregnancy test should be performed in women of childbearing age prior to starting telavancin. There is a pregnancy exposure registry should there be a need to use telavancin in a pregnant woman.[143]

The most common adverse effects associated with telavancin are nausea, vomiting, taste disturbance, and foamy urine.[148-150] Telavancin interferes with urine protein qualitative dipstick tests, and several anticoagulation tests including PT, APTT, INR, and ACT.[143] These tests should be performed when telavancin concentrations are lowest in the bloodstream to minimize the impact on anticoagulation tests.

KEY POINTS

Vancomycin

1. Vancomycin is bactericidal except for *Enterococcus* and tolerant staphylococci, against which it is bacteriostatic. Vancomycin resistance of the VanA phenotype confers high-level resistance to both teicoplanin and vancomycin. Resistance is relatively common within *Enterococcus*. In 2002, this resistance gene was passed to two different *Staphylococcus aureus* isolates and for the first time conferred high-level resistance to vancomycin within the *Staphylococcus* genus.

2. The pharmacodynamic effect of vancomycin is time-dependent killing or time above the minimum inhibitory concentration (MIC). The most important parameter or goal of therapy is to maintain a free serum trough concentration above the MIC of the organism. There is no documented correlation between serum peak concentrations and clinical outcomes.

3. Ototoxicity rates range from 0% to 9%, and these numbers have not changed from initial studies conducted in the 1960s through studies conducted in the 2000s. There is no correlation between serum concentration and ototoxicity. The rate of nephrotoxicity when vancomycin is not administered with other nephrotoxic agents or trough concentrations are less than 10 μg/mL is 5% to 10%. Trough concentrations of more than 10 μg/mL result in nephrotoxicity rates of 20% to 35%.

Daptomycin

1. Approved for bacteremia, right-sided endocarditis, and complicated skin and skin structure infections. It is contraindicated for lung infections, as surfactant breaks down the drug. Creatine phosphokinase concentrations increase 2 to 3 days before clinical manifestation of symptoms and are derived 100% from the MM isoenzyme.

Quinupristin/Dalfopristin

1. This drug is active against vancomycin-resistant *Enterococcus faecium*, methicillin-resistant *S. aureus*, vancomycin-intermediate *S. aureus*, and vancomycin-resistant *S. aureus*. It has no activity against *Enterococcus faecalis*. Myalgias (6%-7%) and arthralgias (9%-9.5%) are the most severe adverse effects and are reasons for discontinuation of the drug.

Linezolid

1. Oral absorption is over 90%, making the oral drug bioequivalent to the intravenous formulation. Linezolid is bacteriostatic against staphylococci and enterococci.

2. Reversible myelosuppression is the most significant adverse effect associated with linezolid therapy. Anemia, neutropenia, and thrombocytopenia have all been reported, and the incidence of these complications increases with duration of therapy exceeding 14 days.

3. Linezolid is a reversible nonselective inhibitor of monoamine oxidase; therefore, the potential for interaction with adrenergic and serotonergic agents exists. Case reports of serotonin syndrome secondary to an interaction between linezolid and selective serotonin reuptake inhibitors have been reported.

Telavancin

1. Telavancin was approved by the FDA in September 2009 for treating complicated skin and skin structure infections. The drug is categorized as pregnancy category C; however, teratogenicity in animals has been observed (digit and limb malformation and decreased birth weight).

2. Telavancin interferes with anticoagulation tests including INR, PT, APTT and ACT. These tests should be performed when telavancin concentrations are lowest in the blood.

ANNOTATED REFERENCES

Gerson SL, Kaplan SL, Bruss JB, Le V, Arellano FM, Hafkin B, et al. Hematologic effects of linezolid: summary of clinical experience. Antimicrob Agents Chemother 2002;46:2723-6.

The clinical trial data are reviewed, and the timeline for development of reversible myelosuppression is presented.

Vincent J, Rello J, Marshall J, Silva E, Anzueto A, Martin C, et al. International study of the prevalence and outcomes of infection in intensive care units. JAMA 2009;302:2323-9.

One-day snapshot of the epidemiology of infections in intensive care units. The type of infection, causative organism, resistance issues, and morbidity and mortality were assessed.

Rybak M, Lomaestro B, Rotschafer JC, Moellering R Jr, Craig W, Billeter M, et al. Therapeutic monitoring of vancomycin in adult patients: a consensus review of the American Society of Health-System Pharmacists, the Infectious Diseases Society of America, and the Society of Infectious Diseases Pharmacists. Am J Health Syst Pharm 2009;66:82-98.

Vancomycin guidelines developed provide the evidence or lack of evidence supporting the dosing, monitoring efficacy, and toxicity of vancomycin therapy. This is the first guideline for the use of vancomycin.

Chakraborty A, Roy S, Loeffler J, Chaves RL. Comparison of the pharmacokinetics, safety and tolerability of daptomycin in healthy adult volunteers following intravenous administration by 30 min infusion or 2 min injection. J Antimicrob Chemother 2009;64:151-8.

A small pharmacokinetic study performed in two different healthy adult populations was conducted to assess the pharmacokinetics and safety of rapid bolus administration of daptomycin. The 2-minute infusion was bioequivalent to the standard 30-minute infusion with regard to C_{max} and AUC. The 2-minute infusion was well tolerated.

Gotfried MH, Shaw JP, Benton BM, Krause KM, Goldberg MR, Kitt MM, et al. Intrapulmonary distribution of intravenous telavancin in healthy subjects and effect of pulmonary surfactant on in vitro activities of telavancin and other antibiotics. Antimicrob Agents Chemother 2008;52:92-7.

Small study in healthy volunteers evaluating the penetration of telavancin into ELF and alveolar macrophages. Over the entire dosing interval, concentrations in the ELF and macrophages was greater than 0.5 µg/mL. Telavancin is stable in the presence of pulmonary surfactant.

REFERENCES

Access the complete reference list online at http://www.expertconsult.com.

Metronidazole and Other Antibiotics for Anaerobic Infections

JESSICA C. NJOKU | JOHN C. ROTSCHAFER | ELIZABETH D. HERMSEN

Metronidazole

Metronidazole [1-(2-hydroxyethyl)-2-methyl-5-nitroimidazole], a nitroimidazole antimicrobial, was introduced in 1960 and quickly became the treatment of choice for *Trichomonas vaginalis*.[1] Initially, metronidazole was regarded as an antiprotozoal agent, proving to be an effective treatment for such infections as trichomoniasis, amebiasis, and giardiasis. The antibacterial activity of metronidazole versus obligate anaerobes was not widely recognized until the 1970s.[2,3] Since then, metronidazole has been used extensively for anaerobic infections such as *Clostridium difficile* infection (CDI) and those involving *Bacteroides* spp.

Because metronidazole has been in use for more than 40 years, a plethora of information exists regarding basic knowledge about this antimicrobial, including the mechanism of action, spectrum of activity, pharmacokinetics, adverse drug effects, and clinical uses. The newest addition to the nitroimidazole antimicrobial class is tinidazole, which was approved by the U.S. Food and Drug Administration (FDA) in 2004.[4] However, this agent is not widely used for infections of a nonparasitic nature, so much of the discussion in the chapter is focused on metronidazole.

MECHANISM OF ACTION

Metronidazole possesses bactericidal activity against obligate anaerobes, although the mechanism of action has not yet been thoroughly elucidated. Metronidazole is a prodrug, requiring intracellular nitroreduction to become active; thus metronidazole in the unchanged form is not pharmacologically active.[1] During the process of reduction, cytotoxic intermediates are formed, and these intermediates are thought to be responsible for killing the cells. The reduction process depends on ongoing energy metabolism but not on ongoing cell multiplication, which translates into activity against both dividing and nondividing cells.[1,4]

SPECTRUM OF ACTIVITY AND CLINICAL USES

Anaerobic bacteria of the *Bacteroides fragilis* group are known to be the most clinically important anaerobic pathogens, owing to their multidrug-resistant nature and the frequency with which they are involved in infectious diseases including polymicrobial infections such as intraabdominal infections, obstetric-gynecologic infections, and diabetic foot infections.[5,6] Nosocomial diarrhea and/or pseudomembranous colitis associated with antibiotic use are frequently caused by *Clostridium difficile*, another clinically important anaerobe.[7] Metronidazole is highly effective against both of these medically relevant anaerobes (Table 125-1). Although metronidazole possesses significant antimicrobial activity against several obligate anaerobes, it is not considered to be clinically active versus aerobic bacteria.[1] Tinidazole has similar spectrum of activity to metronidazole against most anaerobic bacteria, including *B. fragilis* and microaerophilic bacteria such as *Helicobacter pylori* and *Campylobacter* spp., but is only currently approved for the treatment of trichomoniasis, giardiasis, amebiasis, and amebic liver abscess. Other uses outside of these indications are considered experimental.[8]

Clinically, metronidazole has been used successfully to treat anaerobic bacteremia, endocarditis, meningitis, brain abscesses, intraabdominal infections, and mixed aerobic-anaerobic infections, although the addition of an antibiotic effective against aerobic bacteria is necessary for the latter.[2,9-11] Additionally, although without formal FDA approval, metronidazole remains the drug of choice for mild and moderate CDI due to historical and epidemic BI/NAP1/027 strains, owing to excellent oral bioavailability, low potential for selecting for vancomycin-resistant *Enterococcus* (VRE), lack of detectable resistance among BI/NAP/027 strains, and low cost.[12] However, in patients with severe CDI, treatment with metronidazole resulted in a less than optimal response compared to oral vancomycin therapy.[13] Consequently, vancomycin is the preferred agent for severe CDI.[12]

PHARMACOKINETICS

Given orally, metronidazole is almost completely absorbed, with a bioavailability of greater than 90%.[14] In patients with CDI, absorption of oral metronidazole is reduced due to increased bowel emptying causing fecal concentrations to be high, coupled with secretion from plasma into the colon.[15] However, levels decrease rapidly after treatment of CDI is initiated, from 9.3 mg/g in watery stools to 1.2 mg/g in formed stools to an undetectable level once diarrhea has resolved.[15] Intravenous metronidazole is able to maintain high fecal levels in patients with CDI with toxic megacolon or ileus; otherwise, oral metronidazole is recommended.[12,15] Metronidazole is a relatively small molecular entity (molecular weight = 171.16 D) with low protein binding (<20%) and is widely distributed throughout the body.[1] The steady-state volume of distribution in adults is 0.51 to 1.1 L/kg.[13] The elimination half-life of metronidazole is 6 to 8 hours for patients with normal liver function.[1,14] Metronidazole undergoes metabolism in the liver to form five known metabolites, two of which are 1-(2-hydroxyethyl)-2-hydroxymethyl-5-nitroimidazole (the hydroxy metabolite) and 2-methyl-nitroimidazole-1-acetic acid (the acid metabolite). The hydroxy metabolite exhibits 30% to 65% of the anaerobic activity of the parent compound.[14]

ADVERSE REACTIONS

The most common side effects of metronidazole treatment (at standard doses) are gastrointestinal disturbances including mild nausea, a bad/metallic taste in the mouth, and furring of the tongue. More rare adverse reactions to metronidazole include vaginal and/or urethral burning, dark/discolored urine, and neurologic toxicity such as headache, ataxia, vertigo, somnolence, depression, and peripheral neuropathy.[1] Metronidazole is recognized for causing a disulfiram-like reaction with the concurrent ingestion of alcohol. However, a study conducted by Visapää and coworkers found no evidence of disulfiram-like properties of metronidazole when it was given concomitantly with ethanol,[16] and this reaction has also been disputed by others.[17]

PHARMACODYNAMICS

The standard dosing regimen for metronidazole (500-1000 mg q 6-8h) was determined long before pharmacodynamics emerged as a science.

TABLE 125-1	Metronidazole Minimal Inhibitory Concentration and Percent Susceptibility for Various Anaerobes		
Anaerobe (No. of Isolates Tested)		**MIC90 (mg/L)**	**% Susceptible**
Clostridium difficile (186)		2	100
Peptostreptococcus (49)		2	94
Bacteroides fragilis group* (401)		1	100
Prevotella spp. (65)		2	100
Fusobacterium spp. (22)		2	100
Porphyromonas spp. (19)		2	100

Adapted and modified from Drummond LJ, McCoubrey J, Smith DG et al. Changes in sensitivity patterns to selected antibiotics in *Clostridium difficile* in geriatric in-patients over an 18-month period. J Med Microbiol 2003;52:259-63; and from Aldridge KE, Ashcraft D, Cambre K et al. Multicenter survey of the changing in vitro antimicrobial susceptibilities of clinical isolates of *Bacteroides fragilis* group, *Prevotella*, *Fusobacterium*, *Porphyromonas*, and *Peptostreptococcus* species. Antimicrob Agents Chemother 2001;45:1238-43.

*Includes *Bacteroides fragilis, B. distasonis, B. thetaiotaomicron, B. ovatus, B. vulgatus, B. uniformis.*

MIC90, minimum inhibitory concentration that inhibits 90% of organisms.

Metronidazole exhibits concentration-dependent bactericidal activity along with a significant post-antibiotic effect (>3 h).[14,18-20] These factors, in combination with a long half-life and a favorable safety profile, provide a wide corridor to manipulate the metronidazole dose and dosage interval. Much more convenient regimens of larger doses (e.g., 1000-1500 mg) given every 12 hours or once daily are plausible because of the pharmacokinetic and pharmacodynamic (PK/PD) characteristics of this antibiotic.[18,19] PK analyses show that similar and adequate drug exposure is achievable with metronidazole doses of 500 mg every 8 hours, 1000 mg daily, or 1500 mg daily.[19,21] Therefore, from a convenience and cost standpoint, once-daily doses of metronidazole may be adequate when the organism minimum inhibitory concentration (MIC) is less than 2 mg/L.[19,21] Knowledge of pharmacodynamic parameters and utilization of such parameters to appropriately dose patients is of utmost importance in the current era of antimicrobial resistance.

RESISTANCE

With more than 40 years of clinical use, worldwide resistance of anaerobes to metronidazole is estimated to be less than 5%.[22] A recent multicenter study conducted in the United States reported the first confirmed metronidazole-resistant *B. fragilis* isolate (MIC = 64 mg/mL) in 2002.[23] Following this report, additional data collected revealed two more isolates that were metronidazole resistant, one of which was also a *B. fragilis* isolate.[22] This report is the first to document metronidazole resistance among *Bacteroides* spp. and, although negligible, still raises concern, since susceptibility testing is not typically performed on anaerobic cultures. The concern with increasing resistance is not limited to metronidazole alone but includes agents such as ampicillin/sulbactam, clindamycin, and moxifloxacin. Susceptibility of carbapenems, cefoxitin, and piperacillin/tazobactam appears stable.[22]

Four genes (chromosomally borne *nimB* and plasmid-borne *nimA, nimC*, and *nimD*) of *Bacteroides* spp. are commonly associated with metronidazole resistance.[1,11] The suggested mechanism of resistance mediated by these genes is the conversion of the nitro group of metronidazole to an amino group, foregoing the formation of the toxic nitroradicals.[11] Evidence of gene transfer has also been found within different *Bacteroides* spp. and between *Bacteroides* and *Prevotella*.[11]

Diniz and associates exposed *B. fragilis* group species to 4 mg/L of metronidazole and found that exposure to low levels of metronidazole increased both the virulence and the viability of the isolates.[6] Another factor to consider is the supposed protective effect of *Enterococcus faecalis* on *B. fragilis* when exposed to metronidazole.[24] The investigators found that *E. faecalis* was able to negate the bactericidal effect of metronidazole on *B. fragilis*. However, a more recent study could not confirm these findings.[25]

Using a resistance breakpoint of 32 mg/L or higher for metronidazole, Peláez and coworkers, when studying 415 *C. difficile* isolates, found that 6.3% of the isolates were resistant.[26] Another study evaluated the susceptibility patterns of 186 *C. difficile* isolates from a geriatric population.[7] Contrary to the findings of Peláez and associates, no resistance to metronidazole was documented.

Susceptibility testing of anaerobes is usually either not performed or not used to make clinical decisions because of several limiting factors: the slow growth of anaerobes, convolution of the testing method, questions surrounding the appropriate testing media, involvement of multiple organisms in anaerobic infections, and the generally held belief that susceptibility patterns of anaerobes have not changed over the years and remain forseeable.[27] Studies have proven the value and importance of susceptibility testing, showing that appropriate initial therapy is critical to a positive patient outcome[28] and that in vitro susceptibility results reliably predict the clinical outcome of patients.[27] Therefore, clinicians must realize that susceptibility testing of anaerobes is necessary and that the susceptibility patterns have changed over the years.

Other Agents Effective Against Obligate Anaerobes

Several classes of antimicrobials, including some broad-spectrum penicillins, clindamycin, carbapenems, β-lactam/β-lactamase inhibitor combinations, certain cephalosporins, certain quinolones, and glycylcyclines, exhibit activity versus certain anaerobic bacteria.[11] Metronidazole, carbapenems, and piperacillin/tazobactam have proven to be the most reliable agents, whereas clindamycin, moxifloxacin, piperacillin alone, and cephalosporins such as cefotetan and cefoxitin have exhibited significantly decreased susceptibility rates.[5,11,22] In vitro studies of select compounds (Tables 125-2 and 125-3) from the representative class of antibacterials with anaerobic activity showed better than 15% resistance to *B. fragilis* group in the United States as well as in other parts of the world.[11] The species that are worrisome include *Bacteroides ovatus* versus carbapenems, *Bacteroides vulgatus* versus piperacillin/tazobactam, *Bacteroides distasonis* versus ampicillin/sulbactam and cefoxitin, and *Bacteroides ovatus, Bacteroides uniformis*, and *Bacteroides vulgatus* versus moxifloxacin and clindamycin.[22] The newest glycylcycline, tigecycline, has extensive activity against anaerobes, with resistance rates that compare to those of the β-lactam class.[29] The clinical utility of these agents for intraabdominal infections is extensively reviewed in the intraabdominal guidelines by the Infectious Diseases Society of America (IDSA) and the Surgical Infection Society.[30] β-Lactams such as piperacillin/tazobactam and carbapenem monotherapy are reserved for complicated cases of intraabdominal infection, whereas metronidazole is the anaerobic agent of choice for combination therapy with agents devoid of clinically significant anaerobic activity.[30]

BETA-LACTAM ANTIBIOTICS

Some β-lactam antibiotics, including some broad-spectrum penicillins (piperacillin, ticarcillin), β-lactam/β-lactamase inhibitors (piperacillin/tazobactam, ticarcillin/clavulanate, ampicillin/sulbactam, amoxicillin/clavulanate), certain cephalosporins (e.g., cefoxitin, cefotetan), and carbapenems (imipenem, meropenem, ertapenem, doripenem), possess activity versus various anaerobic bacteria.[5,11,22] Because β-lactams are generally regarded as concentration-independent or time-dependent antibiotics, the free drug concentration must remain above the MIC (%fT>MIC) for a certain proportion of the dosing interval. Although several investigators have demonstrated antibacterial activity of β-lactams with percent time free drug fraction is above MIC being as little as 40% of the dosing interval,[18] the pharmacodynamic characteristics of β-lactam antibiotics against anaerobic bacteria have not been well characterized. However, owing to the existing knowledge of β-lactam pharmacodynamics, once-daily regimens are

TABLE 125-2	Antibacterial Activity of Various Antibiotic Agents Against Several Anaerobes		
Anaerobe and Antimicrobial Agent (No. of Isolates Tested)		**MIC90 (mg/L)**	**% Susceptible**
Prevotella spp.[a,b]			
Penicillin G (65)		16	17
Piperacillin/tazobactam (65)		≤0.06	100
Ampicillin/sulbactam (65)		4	100
Cefoxitin (65)		4	100
Doripenem (35)		0.5	100
Ertapenem (35)		0.25	100
Imipenem (65)		0.06	100
Meropenem (65)		0.12	100
Ciprofloxacin (65)		16	35
Clindamycin (65)		4	89.2
Fusobacterium spp.[a,b]			
Penicillin G (22)		0.5	91
Piperacillin/tazobactam (22)		0.12	100
Ampicillin/sulbactam (22)		0.25	100
Cefoxitin (22)		0.5	100
Doripenem (15)		1	100
Ertapenem (15)		1	93
Imipenem (15)		0.12	100
Meropenem (15)		0.5	95
Ciprofloxacin (22)		2	96
Clindamycin (22)		0.12	91
Porphyromonas spp.[a,b]			
Penicillin G (19)		4	79
Piperacillin/tazobactam (19)		1	100
Ampicillin/sulbactam (19)		1	100
Cefoxitin (19)		4	95
Doripenem (20)		0.5	100
Ertapenem (20)		0.5	95
Imipenem (20)		0.12	100
Meropenem (20)		0.5	95
Ciprofloxacin (19)		4	90
Clindamycin (19)		8	90
Peptostreptococcus[a,c]			
Penicillin G (49)		0.5	94
Piperacillin/tazobactam (10)		0.5	100
Ampicillin/sulbactam (10)		2	100
Cefoxitin (10)		1	100
Doripenem (10)		0.125	100
Ertapenem (10)		0.125	100
Imipenem (10)		0.25	100
Meropenem (10)		0.125	100
Moxifloxacin (10)		32	60
Clindamycin (10)		32	80

Adapted and modified from [a]Aldridge KE, Ashcraft D, Cambre K et al. Multicenter survey of the changing in vitro antimicrobial susceptibilities of clinical isolates of *Bacteroides fragilis* group, *Prevotella*, *Fusobacterium*, *Porphyromonas*, and *Peptostreptococcus* species. Antimicrob Agents Chemother 2001;45:1238-43; and from [b]Wexler HM, Engel AE, Glass D, Li C. In vitro activities of doripenem and comparator agents against 364 anaerobic clinical isolates. Antimicrob Agents Chemother 2005;49:4413-7; and from [c]Snyman DR, Jacobus NV, McDermott LA. In vitro activities of doripenem, a new broad-spectrum carbapenem, against recently collected clinical anaerobic isolates, with emphasis on the *Bacteroides fragilis* group. Antimicrob Agents Chemother 2008;52:4492-6.

MIC90, minimum inhibitory concentration that inhibits 90% of organisms.

TABLE 125-3	Antibacterial Activity of Various Antibiotic Agents Against B. fragilis Group Isolates		
Antibiotic Agent (No. of Isolates Tested)		**MIC90 (mg/L)**	**% Susceptible[a]**
Penicillin G (160)[a]		128	0
Piperacillin (384)[a]		128	77
Ticarcillin (137)[a]		128	63
Piperacillin/tazobactam (142)[a]		8	99.3
Ticarcillin/clavulanate (191)[a]		8	96
Ampicillin/sulbactam (382)[a]		8	93
Cefoxitin (515)[a]		32	84
Cefotetan (473)[a]		64	64
Imipenem (378)[a]		1	99.5
Meropenem (127)[a]		0.5	98
Ertapenem (92)[a]		2	94
Doripenem (1351)[b]		0.5	98.7
Clindamycin (1351)[b]		>128	64
Moxifloxacin (1351)[b]		32	59.2
Tigecycline (1351)[b]		8	95.3

Adapted and modified from Alridge KE, Ashcraft D, O'Brien M et al. Bacteremia due to *Bacteroides fragilis* group: distribution of species, β-lactamase production, and antimicrobial susceptibility patterns. Antimicrob Agents Chemother 2003;47:148-53; and from [b]Snydman DR, Jacobus NV, McDermott LA et al. Lessons learned from the anaerobe survey: historical perspective and review of the most recent data (2005-2007). Clin Infect Dis 2010;50:S26-33.

[a]Isolates categorized according to CLSI breakpoints. Nonsusceptible isolates include both intermediate and resistant isolates.

MIC90, minimum inhibitory concentration that inhibits 90% of organisms.

changes in outer membrane permeability, and efflux.[11] Aldridge and associates found the order of activity of cephalosporins-cephamycins against *B. fragilis* group species to be cefoxitin > ceftizoxime > cefotetan = cefotaxime = cefmetazole > ceftriaxone, whereas no isolates were susceptible to penicillin G.[5] Piperacillin and ticarcillin alone exhibited 77% and 63% susceptibility, respectively, whereas piperacillin-tazobactam and ticarcillin-clavulanate showed 99.3% and 96% susceptibility, respectively. Ampicillin-sulbactam, another β-lactam/β-lactamase inhibitor combination, exhibited 93% susceptibility. All carbapenems had favorable activity (see Table 125-3).[5,32] In the study by Snydman et al., a resistance rate of 1.5% was documented for doripenem versus *B. fragilis*, but no resistance was documented for other *Bacteroides* spp. or gram-positive anaerobes, including *Clostridium* spp.[32] These rates were not significantly different compared to the other carbapenem agents. In general, the carbapenem agents maintained excellent activity against the tested clinical anaerobes. In the same study, the susceptibility pattern to piperacillin/tazobactam remained stable, with resistance rates similar to those of carbapenems (0.9%-2.3%); however, this was not the case for ampicillin/sulbactam, which showed an increasing resistance trend, particularly to *B. distasonis* at 20.6%.[22]

CLINDAMYCIN

Clindamycin has been used in clinical practice for many years and exhibits concentration-independent activity against anaerobes. In the first study to establish this pharmacodynamic property, clindamycin was evaluated against *B. fragilis* in an in vitro model.[3] The findings of the study of concentration-independent activity would suggest an alternate dosing regimen than what is currently utilized in practice. Standard dosing for clindamycin ranges from 600 mg every 6 to 8 hours to 900 mg every 8 hours to 1200 mg every 12 hours, but the findings of Klepser and colleagues imply that doses of 300 mg every 8 to 12 hours may be more appropriate. The investigators further confirmed the effectiveness of this dosing regimen (300 mg q 8 to 12 h) against *B. fragilis* by obtaining serum inhibitory and bactericidal titers (SIT, SBT) from the sera of 12 healthy volunteers.[33] The advantages of using a lower total dose include less drug exposure and decreased likelihood of adverse events.

unlikely to be effective. However, when comparing the β-lactams, some agents do have more convenient regimens than others because of differences in their pharmacokinetics (e.g., ertapenem 1000 mg q 24 h versus cefoxitin 1000 mg q 6 to 8 h).

Several β-lactam antibiotics have circumvented much of the resistance among anaerobes, maintaining relatively high susceptibility rates. Aldridge and associates showed that the susceptibility of *Prevotella* spp., *Fusobacterium* spp., *Porphyromonas* spp., and *Peptostreptococcus* was the highest and the most consistent for piperacillin-tazobactam, imipenem, and meropenem (see Table 125-2).[31] In vitro data for doripenem, the newest addition to the carbapenem class, show that its activity mirrors that of meropenem in terms of gram-negative activity, and that of imipenem with respect to gram-positive activity (see Tables 125-2 and 125-3).[32]

Resistance of *B. fragilis* group isolates to β-lactams can be caused by β-lactamase production, alteration in penicillin-binding proteins,

The main concerns with clindamycin are resistance, which based on many reports ranges from 14.3% to 66.7%, and resultant superinfection with *C. difficile*.[7,22] The resistance pattern also appears to increase with time. Serial national susceptibility surveys of *B. fragilis* group initiated in the early 1980s provide a good framework for such trends.[22,23] At study inception, *Bacteroides* spp. had only around 6% resistance rate to clindamycin. By 2004, the resistance rate had increased to 31.6%, and the most recent data for time period 2005-2007 shows a resistance rate as high as 49.2%. Resistance to clindamycin is isolate specific, and the isolates with highest resistance rates are *B. ovatus, B. vulgatus, B. uniformis,* and *B. thetaiotaomicron* at 45.5%, 42.6%, 49.2%, and 39.8%, respectively. Of note, these isolates were among the most frequent clinical isolates (order of frequency: *B. fragilis* [48%] > *B. thetaiotaomicron* [19.3%] > *B. ovatus* [10.3%] > *B. vulgatus* [6%] > *B. uniformis* [4.4%]), highlighting the need for specific pathogen identification and susceptibility testing. Drummond and coworkers examined the susceptibility of 186 *C. difficile* isolates to clindamycin and found that 66.7% of the isolates were resistant and 24.7% were intermediate.[7] Interestingly, Alridge and associates showed that clindamycin-intermediate or clindamycin-resistant isolates are more likely to have decreased susceptibility to other agents.[5] Representative antimicrobial agents tested in the study that are presented in Table 125-3 exhibited further decreased susceptibilities when tested against isolates with decreased clindamycin susceptibility. Metronidazole was the only agent tested that did not show decreased susceptibility when exposed to these isolates.

FLUOROQUINOLONES

The utility of fluoroquinolones for the treatment of mixed aerobic and anaerobic infections is limited by increasing resistance in the *Bacteroides* group and their impact on CDI.[34] The first agent in this class to receive approval for treatment of anaerobic infections was trovafloxacin, which has since been withdrawn from the market. Levofloxacin and ciprofloxacin do not have clinically significant activity against anaerobes.[34] The one fluoroquinolone currently in the market with in vitro potency similar to that of trovafloxacin against a broad spectrum of anaerobic bacteria is moxifloxacin.[34] Limited data exist regarding the pharmacodynamics of fluoroquinolones against anaerobic bacteria. Peterson and colleagues conducted a study to explore whether the AUC/MIC ratio was predictive of quinolone activity versus *B. fragilis*.[35] Interestingly, the investigators found that the quinolones demonstrated concentration-independent activity versus *B. fragilis*, with an AUC/MIC ratio greater than or equal to 44 being predictive of activity. Furthermore, the authors suggest that the potential for the selection of resistant isolates may increase with an AUC/MIC ratio that is less than 44.

Resistance is a major concern with fluoroquinolones and gram-negative anaerobes. One study showed an increase from 0% to 12% fluoroquinolone resistance among *B. fragilis* isolates in just 3 years.[36] Data from another study demonstrated significantly increased moxifloxacin resistance (>30%) among *B. fragilis* group species, with the highest resistance rate among *B. vulgatus* at higher than 50%.[22] Furthermore, the new epidemic strain of *C. difficile* (BI/NAP1/027) is notable for its resistance to fluoroquinolones in addition to a novel mutation (an 18 base pair deletion in its *tcdC* gene) and hyperproduction of toxins A and B as compared to historical strains.[37] The inciting event for the BI/NAP1/027 outbreak is thought to be the over-utilization of fluoroquinolones, which then selected for the fluoroquinolone-resistant BI/NAP1/027 strain.[37] Decreased susceptibility to fluoroquinolones (ciprofloxacin and moxifloxacin) among other anaerobic bacteria is evident from Tables 125-2 and 125-3.

GLYCYLCYCLINE

The newest class of antibiotic with a broad spectrum of activity including anaerobic coverage is the glycylcycline class, with tigecycline

as the representative agent.[29] Tigecycline was approved by the FDA in 2005 for the treatment of skin and skin structure infections and intraabdominal infections. Tigecycline has excellent activity against multidrug resistant (MDR) gram-positive and gram-negative pathogens, atypical bacteria, and anaerobes including *Clostridium* spp., *Fusobacterium* spp., *Prevotella* spp., *Porphyromonas* spp., and *B. fragilis* group. However, it does not have activity against *Pseudomonas aeruginosa, Proteus* spp., *Providencia* spp., or *Morganella morganii* owing to constitutive high expression of tigecycline-specific multidrug efflux pump systems that renders these organisms intrinsically resistant to this agent.[29]

Pharmacokinetic and pharmacodynamic studies show that tigecycline exhibits time-dependent killing properties and prolonged post-antibiotic effects. The pharmacodynamic predictor of in vivo activity is AUC/MIC, which is 7 for anaerobes.[38] The FDA MIC susceptibility breakpoint for tigecycline versus anaerobes is ≤ 4 mg/L; however, typical MICs of *Bacteroides* spp. in in vitro studies ranged from 1 to 8 mg/L. Tigecycline is widely distributed in tissues, achieving only minimal peak serum concentration. Depending on the site of infection, the high tissue binding of tigecycline may be advantageous.[11,38] Conversely, if the infection is endovascular, the concentration of tigecycline in the serum (~1 mg/L) is likely at or below the MIC of the infecting organism, which will impede the effectiveness of the drug.

Several in vitro studies have evaluated the activity of tigecycline versus anaerobic pathogens, specifically the *Bacteroides* spp.[11,22,23,39] In the survey by Snydman and colleagues, tigecycline outperformed clindamycin, linezolid, and moxifloxacin among the non-β-lactam agents.[22,23] However, about 7.2% of the group *Bacteroides* "other" (*B. caccae, B. eggerthii, B. merdae,* and *B. stercoris*) was resistant to tigecycline compared to an average resistance rate of ≤ 5% for other species.[23] Tigecycline also outperformed cefoxitin and ampicillin/sulbactam but was less active than carbapenems and piperacillin/tazobactam among the β-lactam class (see Tables 125-2 and 125-3). Thus, tigecycline may have a role in the treatment of anaerobic infections, particularly when mixed infection with MDR pathogens is suspected in a patient intolerant to preferred regimens.

INVESTIGATIONAL AGENTS

Several investigational agents have shown potential for the treatment of anaerobic infections. Ednie and colleagues found ranbezolid, a new oxazolidinone, to possess significant anaerobic activity.[40] Snydman and associates tested the in vitro activity of NVP-LMB415 against clinical anaerobic isolates. The compound had excellent in vitro activity against all species of *B. fragilis* group isolates, including *B. fragilis* group strains resistant to β-lactams, quinolones, or clindamycin, and exhibited lower MICs than linezolid, tigecycline, and garenoxacin against the strains tested. However, MICs for *Clostridium* spp. were higher than the MICs for other anaerobes.[41] Additionally, DX-619; PTZ601, an intravenous carbapenem; sulopenem, an oral and intravenous carbapenem; and fidaxomicin, a novel macrolide antibiotic for CDI, have demonstrated potential for use in anaerobic infections.[11] Experimental treatments for CDI include tolevamer (a toxin-binding polymer); two poorly orally absorbed antimicrobials, CB-183,315 and ramoplanin; monoclonal antibodies; and a *C. difficile* vaccine.[42] Preliminary data with tolevamer does not show it to be significantly better than metronidazole or oral vancomycin for the treatment of CDI. Nitazoxanide and rifaximin have been used successfully for the treatment of CDI.[43-46] However, according to the CDI treatment guidelines, nitazoxanide should be reserved as alternative therapy, and caution is recommended with use of rifaximin due to emergence of resistance in clinical studies.[12] Tigecycline has been used anecdotally in combination with metronidazole for CDI treatment.[47,48] However, the role of tigecycline in the treatment of CDI is still a matter for debate and was not recognized in the CDI treatment guidelines.[12]

1. Metronidazole, a nitroimidazole antimicrobial, requires intracellular reduction for pharmacologic activity and provides activity against both dividing and nondividing bacterial cells. Metronidazole's activity extends to many obligate anaerobes but not to aerobic bacteria. The newest addition to this class of antibiotics is tinidazole (Tindamax), which shares similar activity to metronidazole.

2. Anaerobes are often involved in mixed infections, which present unique situations for antimicrobial use. The interactions between the different bacteria and the various antibiotics can be difficult to distinguish and/or predict.

3. Standard dosing of metronidazole (500-1000 mg q 6-8h) was established before the emergence of pharmacodynamics. Pharmacodynamics of metronidazole are concentration dependent, with a significant post-antibiotic effect. Data from pharmacodynamic studies suggest that metronidazole can be dosed in larger doses (e.g., 1000-1500 mg) every 12 hours or once daily for an effect similar to the standard regimens.

4. Susceptibility patterns of anaerobes have been changing over the years, and susceptibility to metronidazole cannot be assumed. Although susceptibility testing of anaerobes is difficult, clinicians must realize the importance of performing and analyzing the susceptibility tests.

5. Several β-lactam antibiotics, fluoroquinolones, clindamycin, and tigecycline possess activity against anaerobic organisms. However, resistance is a concern with all of these classes of antibiotics. A few investigational agents have the potential for use in anaerobic infections, but clinical data are needed.

ANNOTATED REFERENCES

Aldridge KE, Ashcraft D, O'Brien M, et al. Bacteremia due to *Bacteroides fragilis* group: distribution of species, beta-lactamase production, and antimicrobial susceptibility patterns. Antimicrob Agents Chemother 2003;47:148-53.
This paper presents susceptibility data on 542 blood isolates of B. fragilis *group tested over a 12-year period. Metronidazole, β-lactam/β-lactamase combinations, and carbapenems were consistently the most active agents. These data show the importance of susceptibility testing of the* B. fragilis *group and serve as a guide in the choice of empirical antimicrobial therapy.*

Lamp KC, Freeman CD, Klutman NE, et al. Pharmacokinetics and pharmacodynamics of the nitroimidazole antimicrobials. Clin Pharmacokinet 1999;36:353-73.
This review presents a comprehensive overview of the pharmacokinetics, pharmacodynamics, and use of metronidazole and nitroimidazole antimicrobials.

Pelaez T, Alcala L, Alonso R, et al. Reassessment of *Clostridium difficile* susceptibility to metronidazole and vancomycin. Antimicrob Agents Chemother 2002;46:1647-50.

C. difficile *is generally assumed to be sensitive to metronidazole and vancomycin. However, this manuscript shows that some isolates are either resistant (6.3% for metronidazole) or have intermediate resistance (3.1% to vancomycin) to these agents.*

Snydman DR, Jacobus NV, McDermott LA, et al. Lessons learned from the anaerobe survey: historical perspective and review of the most recent data (2005-2007). Clin Infect Dis 2010;50:S26-33.
This report affirms the findings of Aldridge and colleagues and documents the first report of metronidazole resistance among Bacteroides *spp. in the United States. Trends in susceptibility testing showed increasing resistance to clindamycin, moxifloxacin, and ampicillin/sulbactam, with relatively stable resistance rates to carbapenems, and piperacillin/tazobactam.*

Wexler HM. *Bacteroides*: the good, the bad, and the nitty-gritty. Clin Microbiol Rev 2007;20:593-621.
A comprehensive review of Bacteroides *with emphasis on virulence, infections in humans, resistance, antianaerobic agents, and susceptibilities.*

REFERENCES

Access the complete reference list online at http://www.expertconsult.com.

126

Prevention and Control of Nosocomial Pneumonia

RICHARD G. WUNDERINK

Preventing pneumonia in the critically ill is a daunting task, and even controlling the incidence is difficult. Despite this, many in the patient safety movement have suggested that nosocomial pneumonia should be a "never" event. While complete prevention of nosocomial pneumonia is unlikely, substantial progress has been made in reducing the incidence.

Pneumonia is the most common nosocomial infection in the intensive care unit (ICU).[1] The frequency of ventilator-associated pneumonia (VAP) varies from 8% to 28%.[2] A large 1-day point prevalence study of pneumonia demonstrated that nearly 10% of ICU patients were being treated for pneumonia.[1] However, rather than overall rates, the incidence per day of mechanical ventilation is a more legitimate description. The National Nosocomial Infection Surveillance program reports VAPs/1000 ventilator days. However, the risk of VAP also does not remain static throughout the duration of ICU stay. The greatest risk is early in the course of mechanical ventilation, dropping from a daily hazard rate of 3.3% at day 5 to a 1.3% rate at day 15.[3] The incidence also varies significantly among different types of ICU patients. Postoperative patients, especially those undergoing cardiothoracic and trauma-related surgery, appear to have the highest rates. Coronary care unit patients appear to have the lowest rates; medical, respiratory, and other surgical patients demonstrate intermediate rates.

The influence of endotracheal intubation is so dominant that ICU-acquired pneumonia is almost synonymous with VAP. Endotracheal intubation increases the rate of nosocomial pneumonia between 3- and 21-fold.[2] Research on hospital-acquired pneumonia has been dominated by VAP, and very little is known about pneumonia in nonintubated ICU patients. Because the effect of nosocomial pneumonia on morbidity and mortality in nonintubated patients is minor compared with that of VAP, concentration on VAP is appropriate.

A distinction should be made between prevention of all nosocomial pneumonia and prevention of life-threatening nosocomial pneumonia. The latter is almost exclusively VAP. The crude mortality rate for VAP ranges from 24% to 76%, with an estimated attributable mortality of 20% to 30%.[2,4] Early-onset VAP (within 5-7 days of intubation) has a minimal effect on mortality if any. The greatest crude and attributable mortality rates are associated with late-onset multidrug resistant (MDR) microorganisms such as *Pseudomonas aeruginosa*, *Acinetobacter* spp., and methicillin-resistant *Staphylococcus aureus* (MRSA). Unfortunately, the most effective and well-documented strategies to prevent pneumonia work predominantly or exclusively in early-onset VAP and therefore have not resulted in a significant improvement in mortality. Conversely, one of the most consistent adverse effects of VAP (including early onset) is a prolonged duration of mechanical ventilation. Because duration of ICU stay is the principal determinant of cost of care, prevention measures may be cost-effective even if they do not result in improved mortality.

Pathogenesis

The key to effective prevention and control strategies is a clear understanding of the underlying pathogenesis of nosocomial pneumonia.

The essence of nosocomial pneumonia pathogenesis involves three basic steps:

1. Colonization of the oropharynx with pathogenic microorganisms
2. Aspiration
3. Overwhelming of the lower respiratory tract's host defense mechanisms

Effective prevention and control measures can be analyzed by their effect on one or more of these steps.

Despite the convenience of this simple analysis, to assume that the pathogenesis of all types of nosocomial pneumonia and VAP is the same would be naive and incorrect. An example is the role of gastric colonization preceding oropharyngeal colonization, the basis for attention to enteral feedings and stress ulcer prophylaxis in VAP prevention. Although possibly an important factor for pneumonia due to Enterobacteriaceae, gastric and enteric colonization has no role in the pathogenesis of *S. aureus* or *P. aeruginosa* pneumonia, the two most common causes of VAP. Conversely, daily chlorhexidine baths did not prevent VAP in a trauma population but did significantly decrease VAP from MRSA.[5] Therefore, prevention strategies should be individualized to the pathogens and mechanisms prevalent in a specific ICU.

COLONIZATION WITH PATHOGENIC MICROORGANISMS

The antecedent event to most nosocomial pneumonias is colonization of the oropharynx with pathogenic bacteria. The oropharynx is not sterile normally, but the character of the normal flora is remarkably constant. A variety of factors alter the normal flora, allowing more pathogenic microorganisms to appear and increase in number.

Time of exposure to these selective forces is a critical issue. Early-onset pneumonia, even early-onset VAP, tends to be caused by less pathogenic microorganisms such as streptococci, *Hemophilus influenzae*, or methicillin-sensitive *S. aureus*. Most of these selective forces are introduced in the hospital environment itself, rather than specifically in the ICU. Therefore, patients who develop pneumonia during the first few days of ICU admission or mechanical ventilation are at risk for MDR pathogens if the ICU admission was preceded by a 3- to 5-day hospital stay. Many of the same factors also operate in skilled-care nursing home facilities, blurring the distinction between hospital- and community-acquired pneumonia, and have led to a new designation of healthcare-associated pneumonia (HCAP).

Previously, colonization of the oropharynx by gram-negative enteric bacilli, generally from the Enterobacteriaceae family, was the major concern. These microorganisms are part of the normal bowel flora. Oropharyngeal colonization occurred by one of two main routes. The first is reflux of bacteria into the stomach from the duodenum, with subsequent gastroesophageal reflux into the esophagus and oropharynx. Colonization and proliferation in the stomach are critical intermediate steps in this pathway. Therefore, many prevention strategies logically target the stomach. The other route is self-inoculation by the fecal-oral route, through contamination of equipment or the hands of healthcare providers or the patient.

S. aureus is now the most common microorganism causing ICU-acquired pneumonia, with *P. aeruginosa* the next most common. In addition, *Acinetobacter* species have become a common cause of VAP in many institutions. None of these three microorganisms has a typical colonization pattern like that of the Enterobacteriaceae. *S. aureus* is a normal colonizer of the skin and the nasopharynx. Antegrade colonization of the oropharynx from the nose, especially with the use of nasogastric tubes in many critically ill patients, can occur quite easily. Similarly, *Acinetobacter* is found on moist body surfaces and in the gingival crevices of patients with poor oral hygiene. *P. aeruginosa* is usually not part of normal bowel flora but is ubiquitous in the environment. One of the unique aspects of *Pseudomonas* VAP is the appearance of tracheal colonization before oropharyngeal colonization.[6] Because colonization of the stomach is not an important intermediary step for these pathogens, prevention measures directed at the stomach are not likely to affect pneumonia caused by these microorganisms. Both MRSA and *Acinetobacter* colonization can be decreased with the use of chlorhexidine whole-body bathing.[5]

Avoidance of Antibiotics

The most important factor that leads to increased colonization of the oropharynx with pathogenic microorganisms is the use of systemic antibiotics, especially broad-spectrum antibiotics.[7] Antibiotic therapy results in alteration of the oropharyngeal flora and gives pathogens a selection advantage. The broader the antibiotic spectrum, the greater the likelihood normal flora will be affected. At the same time, some pathogens are also eliminated. For this reason, antibiotics function more as amplifying agents rather than as true causes of colonization. The pathogenic microorganisms must still reside in the area normally, such as nasopharyngeal carriage of *S. aureus*, or be transferred from other sites including the environment to colonize. Thus pneumonia can still occur despite avoidance of antibiotics. However, the causative microorganisms are more likely to be less virulent pathogens or even normal flora, such as -hemolytic streptococci, and less likely to lead to life-threatening pneumonia.

Diagnostic strategies for fever in the ICU that result in the use of fewer antibiotics have been associated with lower mortality.[8] Shorter courses and fewer antibiotics for documented infections in critically ill patients have also been associated with a decreased risk of superinfection.[9-11] Although avoiding antibiotics may have only a small effect on the risk of developing the first episode of pneumonia, limiting their usage has a major effect on secondary pneumonia and infection-related death in the ICU.

Use of Topical Antibacterial Agents

In contrast to systemic antibiotics, the use of topical antibiotics for the prevention of colonization may be beneficial. In general, strategies rely on controlling pathogenic microorganisms at specific sites, despite the effect on normal flora. Topical agents generally do not have the toxicity of systemic agents, and although the use of topical antibiotics can lead to MDR isolates, the risk may not be as great as with systemic antibiotics.

Selective Digestive Tract Decontamination. By far the most extensively studied and most aggressive form of topical antibiotic strategy to prevent colonization is selective digestive tract decontamination. Although the specific agents used in different studies vary, the major focus is on controlling oropharyngeal colonization by almost sterilizing the bowel. Therefore, the antibiotics used are directed primarily at gram-negative bacilli (usually polymyxin B and an aminoglycoside) and *Candida* (usually amphotericin B). Most regimens include two components—topical antibiotics in the oropharynx, and nonabsorbable antibiotics via a gastric tube. Some also include an initial short course of systemic antibiotics.

Despite more than 40 randomized controlled trials and several meta-analyses,[12-13] the benefit of selective digestive tract decontamination remains unclear. However, several patterns have emerged. Selective digestive tract decontamination fairly consistently decreases the incidence of VAP when systemic antibiotics are used for the first 48 to 72 hours.[14] The rationale for the use of systemic antibiotics is to prevent incipient endogenous infections until sterilization of the bowel

occurs. However, an equivalent benefit has been found with a short course of prophylactic antibiotics alone.[15]

The efficacy of selective digestive tract decontamination in preventing life-threatening late-onset VAP is less clear. Most studies do not demonstrate lower mortality in the treated group, despite lower rates of VAP. Treatment is directed primarily against the Enterobacteriaceae and yeast in the gastrointestinal tract, but because these microorganisms do not cause the majority of cases of VAP in the ICU, its benefit in preventing VAP due to these microorganisms may be diluted by the many cases of pneumonia caused by organisms that are not specifically addressed by the regimen.

The major criticism of selective digestive tract decontamination is the potential for promoting antibiotic resistance. This theoretical risk has not been clearly demonstrated, even in ICUs that have used the regimen for prolonged periods.[14] However, recent data which look at the whole ICU and non-ICU ecosystem suggest this may be an issue.[16] The major determining factor is probably not the selective decontamination, but rather the concomitant systemic antibiotics. If selective digestive tract decontamination truly decreases the incidence of VAP (and possibly other nosocomial infections), the resultant decrease in systemic antibiotic use may cancel out the risk of selecting for resistant isolates.

Because the major benefit of selective digestive tract decontamination appears to be in preventing VAP due to Enterobacteriaceae, this strategy is probably best reserved for patient populations at increased risk for VAP due to these microorganisms. Postsurgical, trauma, and solid organ transplant patients are in this category. In addition, this approach appears to be very effective as part of the management of epidemics of antibiotic-resistant clones.

Topical Oropharyngeal Agents. Controlling colonization of the oropharynx alone has also generated interest. In a randomized controlled trial of open heart surgery patients, use of a chlorhexidine oral rinse lowered the risk of VAP from 9.4% to 2.9%, with the major effect being on gram-negative bacteria.[17-18] This primary finding was accompanied by decreases in all nosocomial infections, fewer nonprophylactic antibiotic prescriptions, and a trend toward lower mortality. Subsequent studies have confirmed the benefit of chlorhexidine topical oral treatments on risk of VAP.[19] One advantage of oral decontamination only is no disruption of the normal bowel flora by treating only the primary area of concern. Conversely, chlorhexidine may not be able to prevent infection with MDR pathogens such as *Pseudomonas* and *Acinetobacter*.[20] Oral decontamination with other agents such as antimicrobial peptides[21] has not been demonstrated to be of benefit.

Aerosolized Antibiotics. The earliest studied form of topical colonization prevention was aerosolized antibiotics. In the early era of mechanical ventilation, daily aerosolized polymyxin B resulted in a dramatic decrease in the rate of gram-negative VAP.[22] Not surprisingly, routine use was soon complicated by the emergence of antibiotic-resistant microorganisms. This issue, combined with a lack of mortality benefit, led to abandonment of this strategy. Recently, aerosolized ceftazidime was not shown to decrease VAP rates in trauma patients, but also did not increase MDR pathogen colonization.[23] A recent variation is to use aerosolized antibiotics for purulent tracheobronchitis, thought to be a precursor to VAP.[24]

Avoidance of Increased Gastric pH

The normally acidic environment of the gastric lumen is extremely effective in preventing colonization with either swallowed oropharyngeal flora or refluxed enteric flora. Several prevention strategies focus on this aspect of prevention of VAP.

Stress Ulcer Prophylaxis

At one time, gastrointestinal bleeding from stress ulceration was a substantial problem in ventilated patients and a major cause of death. Prophylaxis against stress ulceration was thus considered critical for ventilated patients. However, the incidence of stress mucosal ulceration has decreased markedly as a result of better hemodynamic resuscitation, improved ventilatory strategies, and earlier use of enteral nutrition.

The debate regarding optimal gastrointestinal bleeding prophylaxis has therefore evolved over the last few decades. Initially, antacids were found to be inferior to histamine type 2 blockers (H_2 blockers). In addition to increasing gastric pH, antacids increase gastric volume, which is probably an independent risk factor for VAP. Subsequently sucralfate was hypothesized to be superior to H_2 blockers because it did not affect gastric pH and might have intrinsic antibacterial properties. No clear-cut benefit of sucralfate over H_2 blockers in reducing VAP has been found, while a slight but consistent increase in gastrointestinal bleeding has been documented.[25] Proton pump inhibitors are also used frequently despite more limited data.

The major issue is whether stress ulcer prophylaxis is needed at all in most mechanically ventilated patients.[25] The few placebo-controlled trials suggest both H_2 blockers and sucralfate may lead to an increased risk of VAP. Several multivariate analyses found proton pump inhibitors to be associated with increased pneumonia rates, including HAP/VAP,[26] HCAP, and even community-acquired pneumonia. Ironically, use of gastrointestinal prophylaxis is actually encouraged as part of a ventilator/VAP bundle in many institutions. A subgroup of patients at increased risk for gastrointestinal hemorrhage can be identified and patients without these high risk factors may not need prophylaxis.[27]

Enteral Nutrition Strategies

Malnutrition is clearly associated with an increased risk of pneumonia and increased mortality in the critically ill.[28] In addition to classic effects on cell-mediated immunity, an effect specific to pneumonia is increased binding of gram-negative bacilli, including *Pseudomonas*, to epithelial cells.[6]

Enteral administration of nutrition is the preferred route for treating and preventing malnutrition in the critically ill, although parenteral nutrition in high risk patients is preferable to no nutrition.[28] Meta-analysis has suggested that patients can even be fed soon after gastrointestinal surgery.[29-30] However, continuous enteral nutrition infusions may increase both gastric pH and gastric volume and theoretically increase VAP risk. Several multivariate studies have suggested that this potential risk is real.[31-32] A randomized trial found that the risk of VAP was increased with early aggressive feedings compared with low-level enteral nutrition (approximately 20% of goal feeding rate).[33] The lower rate was chosen to avoid atrophy of the microvilli of the enteric mucosa, a potential source of nosocomial infection. The increased risk of VAP was attributed to an increased risk of aspiration, which is also seen in surgical series.[30] Despite this, meta-analyses of early versus delayed enteral nutrition suggest a mortality benefit and probable decreased risk of VAP with early feedings.[34] A balance between potential risks would be early initiation of enteral feeding but avoidance of aggressive infusions that might cause high gastric residuals and gastric distention.

Several strategies have been tried to provide enteral feeding yet prevent increased gastric colonization with pathogenic microorganisms. Theoretically, bolus feedings allow intermittent lowering of the gastric pH, potentially sterilizing the stomach between doses. However, one randomized controlled trial found that bolus feedings did not decrease the risk of VAP, and fewer patients achieved their goal feeding rates.[35] Acidification of enteral feedings not only did not improve VAP rates but also caused adverse consequences from the resultant metabolic acidosis.[36]

Modified Endotracheal Tubes

Attention has recently focused on colonization of the endotracheal tube itself. Many bacteria can adhere to the polyvinyl chloride surface of endotracheal tubes through secretion of a glycocalyx. Protected from systemic antibiotics and host defense mechanisms, microorganisms in this glycocalyx can become a source of re-inoculation of the lower respiratory tract. This mechanism may explain the high recurrent VAP rates, particularly for *Pseudomonas*. Early tracheostomy may also get around this problem,[37] at least temporarily. A silver-impregnated endotracheal tube has been demonstrated to lower the incidence of VAP and delay onset in those who do develop VAP,[21] although cost remains a barrier to routine use. Other treatments of endotracheal tubes may be developed which kill bacteria, prevent glycocalyx, or prevent quorum sensing.

Cross-Infection

The role of cross-contamination in the ICU should never be underestimated. Cross-contamination can cause colonization with specific pathogenic bacteria in a patient who has no other risk factors for that microorganism. In particular, *P. aeruginosa* and MRSA appear to have the greatest potential to cause cross-contamination and subsequent infection.

By far the most important factor in cross-infection is handwashing among caregivers. Multiple studies have documented the poor infection control practices of medical personnel, including physicians and bedside nurses. The risk of poor handwashing increases with the intensity of care needed for an individual patient and with the number of patients per nurse. The use of an alcohol-based, self-drying hand wash appears to be effective and to increase compliance with handwashing.[38-39]

Avoiding cross-contamination via medical equipment is also important. Contaminated equipment is still a major cause of epidemic outbreaks of nosocomial pneumonia. Any clustering of VAP, especially when caused by an unusual agent, should raise this possibility. Respiratory therapy equipment is particularly suspect, and adherence to standards for the sterilization of ventilators, bronchoscopes, and other reusable equipment should be rigorous.

Probably the best strategy is a continuous, multifaceted, multidisciplinary program of infection control.[40] An important component of this program is monitoring VAP rates and providing feedback to individual units on infection rates. Although such a program is costly to develop, the substantial cost benefit of avoiding pneumonia usually justifies the expense.

ASPIRATION

Evidence from a variety of sources documents the importance of aspiration in nosocomial pneumonia, although the definition of aspiration may vary.

Large-Volume Aspiration

Large-volume aspiration is clearly a risk factor in nonintubated ICU patients. Although the aspirated material itself may not be infectious, such as enteral feedings, aspiration of a large bolus clearly predisposes to pneumonia. Large-volume aspiration may result in ARDS, which is by itself associated with an increased risk of VAP. Predisposing factors for this type of aspiration are gastrointestinal, such as protracted vomiting from bowel obstruction or gastrointestinal bleeding, and neurologic, including seizures, induction of anesthesia, and alcohol intoxication.

Appropriate use of endotracheal intubation is actually a protective factor for this type of aspiration. Once large-volume aspiration has occurred, selective use of bronchoscopy to extract solid material that might occlude a bronchus and cause a postobstructive pneumonia is one of the few preventive measures of benefit. Empirical antibiotics, especially prolonged courses, do not clearly prevent pneumonia but do select for more virulent microorganisms.

A form of large-volume aspiration unique to ventilated patients is the inadvertent instillation of ventilator tubing condensate. The condensate in tubing closest to the endotracheal tube frequently contains high levels ($>10^5$ organisms/mL) of pathogenic microorganisms. If this condensate is accidentally spilled back into the patient's tracheobronchial tree, VAP is very likely. This may be one explanation for the increased risk of VAP associated with patient transport out of the ICU.[41]

Small-Volume Aspiration

Aspiration of a smaller volume of secretions is also associated with an increased risk of pneumonia in both intubated and nonintubated patients. Neurologic disease with inability to protect the upper airway is consistently documented as a risk factor for pneumonia. In this situation, aspiration occurs before or in conjunction with endotracheal intubation. The bolus can be either oropharyngeal secretions or gastric secretions. In the former situation, a large inoculum of oropharyngeal flora can reach the lower respiratory tract, and clinical pneumonia usually occurs within 48 to 72 hours.

Prevention of pneumonia from small-volume aspiration is probably best achieved by prophylactic antibiotics. Prospective observational studies have suggested that antibiotics early in the course of mechanical ventilation are associated with a lower incidence of pneumonia.[3,31] However, the best evidence is a prospective randomized trial of short-course cephalosporin prophylaxis (two doses) in patients intubated for nontraumatic coma.[15] The incidence of VAP was only 23% in the prophylaxis group, compared with 66% in the control group that did not receive any antibiotic. The findings of this randomized controlled trial are corroborated by many studies of selective decontamination of the digestive tract which found a decreased incidence of pneumonia only if a short course of systemic antibiotics was included with the topical antibiotics.

Prophylactic antibiotics have clearly been demonstrated to be of benefit only in the initial intubation of patients not previously hospitalized for a significant period. The efficacy of the short course is dependent on the fact that the aspirated bolus contains mainly normal oral flora rather than a high concentration of MDR pathogens. These conditions may apply to patient groups other than those with nontraumatic coma, such as respiratory failure from non-bronchitic exacerbations of chronic obstructive lung disease, but the benefit must still be determined.

This prevention strategy seems to contradict the importance of avoiding unnecessary antibiotics, discussed earlier. One very real risk is that preventing early-onset pneumonia, which does not have an attributable mortality, may increase the risk of more lethal late-onset VAP. Two aspects of this strategy outweigh the potential downside of increased risk of oropharyngeal colonization with more pathogenic bacteria. First, the antibiotics are continued for only 24 hours. Second, the 40% lower risk of pneumonia in patients given prophylaxis avoids a longer course of antibiotics, often with a wider spectrum.

Microaspiration

Microaspiration is by far the most important form of aspiration in endotracheally intubated patients. Oropharyngeal secretions pool above the cuff of the endotracheal tube in most intubated patients. Extremely small volumes of secretions can pass below the cuff during small movements of the endotracheal tube associated with head repositioning, coughing, and other activities. Because oropharyngeal secretions contain 10^6 to 10^{10} colony-forming units per milliliter of secretions, even 0.1 mL of secretions can present a significant challenge to the host defenses of the lower respiratory tract. In addition, the endotracheal tube itself may become colonized with viable bacteria encrusted in the glycocalyx and deposited on the polyvinyl chloride surface of the tube. Subsequent suctioning or other manipulations of the endotracheal tube can reintroduce bacteria into the lower respiratory tract. Simply suctioning the patient prior to repositioning may decrease the rate of VAP. Several other preventive therapies are directed at stopping or limiting this type of aspiration.

Shorter Duration of Endotracheal Intubation

Epidemiologic studies have demonstrated that the risk of VAP is not linear. The greatest risk occurs early, with a 3% per day risk in the first week, 2% per day in the second week, and 1% per day subsequently.[3] In addition, early-onset VAP (within the first 5-7 days of mechanical ventilation) has the lowest attributable mortality.[2,4]

Therefore, the sooner the patient is extubated, the lower the cumulative risk of pneumonia and the lower the risk of lethal nosocomial pneumonia.

Probably the best strategy is avoiding intubation completely. Management of many patients with noninvasive ventilation is now standard practice in most ICUs. However, patients who fail noninvasive ventilation appear to have an increased duration of subsequent endotracheal intubation and thus an increased risk of VAP. Careful selection of candidates for noninvasive ventilation and early abandonment of this treatment in unsuccessful cases are critical to decreasing the pneumonia risk.

Even when patients are intubated, variations in the duration of mechanical ventilation for the same type and severity of critical illness suggest that efforts to shorten this duration are a viable approach to preventing VAP. Several strategies have demonstrated a significant benefit, including daily interruption of sedation[42-43] and daily assessment of ability to wean.[44] The overall benefit is partially attributable in part to lower VAP rates.

The downside of an aggressive extubation strategy is the association between reintubation and increased risk of VAP. Several studies have demonstrated that reintubation increases the risk of VAP threefold.[41,45] The need for reintubation reexposes the patient to the risk of small-volume aspiration discussed earlier. In addition, colonization of the oropharyngeal secretions by pathogenic bacteria is more likely because of the prior episode of intubation. Therefore, although avoiding or shortening the duration of mechanical ventilation is clearly a laudable goal, an increase in the risk of VAP may occur with an overly aggressive approach.

Early Tracheostomy

The benefit of early tracheostomy remains unsettled.[37,46] Tracheostomy has some potential benefits in the prevention of VAP. The glottis is not held open by the endotracheal tube, and the vocal cords can be opposed, decreasing the risk of aspiration significantly. Routine tracheostomy may be one explanation for the leveling off of the incidence of VAP after several weeks of mechanical ventilation. Probably just as important is that the security of a tracheostomy may allow greater mobilization of the patient and a greater amount of time spent in the upright position. Early reports of an increased risk of pneumonia with tracheostomy were compromised by lack of adjustment for prior duration of mechanical ventilation, inaccurate diagnosis (with some tracheostomy site infections classified as pneumonia), and variable surgical techniques. Early tracheostomy performed with the percutaneous dilatational technique may be more beneficial,[37] but more data are needed.

Semirecumbent Positioning

Elegant clinical experiments have demonstrated that the degree of gastroesophageal reflux is significantly greater in supine patients than in semirecumbent patients.[47] Not only was reflux greater, but bowel flora colonized the oropharynx and bronchial tree in 68% of patients ventilated in the supine position, compared with only 32% in the semirecumbent position.

A prospective randomized trial clearly demonstrated that both clinically suspected and microbiologically confirmed cases of VAP were more common in patients ventilated in the supine position (8% of clinically suspected VAPs versus 34% for semirecumbent).[32] Supine body position (odds ratio 6.8) and enteral nutrition (odds ratio 5.7) were both independent risk factors for VAP, with the highest frequency in patients receiving enteral nutrition in the supine position (14 of 28; 50%). This finding suggests that gastric distention, whether caused by feedings or increased gastric secretions, may have an amplifying effect in the supine position.

Avoiding the supine position as much as possible is a simple and effective preventive measure that should be practiced in all ICUs. However, compliance with elevation of the head of the bed to 45 degrees is difficult, and achieving lower degrees of elevation are not associated with decreased VAP rates.[48] In patients who are unable to be placed in the semirecumbent position, continuous lateral rotation with specialized beds may have a beneficial effect.[49]

Avoidance of Ventilator Tubing Manipulation

Several lines of evidence suggest that minimizing the number of manipulations of the ventilator tubing can decrease the incidence of VAP, possibly by decreasing the incidence of small-volume or micro-aspiration. Condensation of exhaled gas in the expiratory limb of the tubing or from humidifiers in the inspiratory limb can become heavily colonized with bacteria. Instillation of this liquid bolus into the patient's airway during manipulation of the tubing or movement of the patient can present a significant bacterial challenge to the lower respiratory tract defenses.

The use of heat and moisture exchangers rather than heater-humidifiers would theoretically alleviate some of this risk. A meta-analysis of eight randomized controlled trials suggested a 30% reduction in VAP rates, especially if the patient was ventilated for more than 7 days.[50] This benefit is partially offset by increased rates of endo-tracheal tube occlusion secondary to inspissated secretions with the use of heat and moisture exchangers. Because the rate of VAP is clearly not increased with heat and moisture exchangers, other considerations determine the frequency of their use, especially cost.

The most consistent evidence that ventilator tube manipulation may increase the risk of VAP is that increasing the interval between changes of the ventilator tubing decreases the incidence of VAP. A series of studies progressively increased the duration of time between changes and found equivalent or less VAP with longer intervals. Most institutions no longer change ventilator tubing unless gross contamination is present.

Transporting patients outside the ICU, usually for diagnostic procedures, has also been associated with an increased risk of VAP.[41] In a prospective study, 24% of patients requiring transport outside of the ICU developed VAP, compared with only 4% of patients who did not. Unfortunately, more than half of ventilated patients required transport at least once. The need for bagging, changing ventilators, moving the patient out of bed, and other aspects of the process all increase the possibility of inadvertent introduction of condensate from the ventilator tubing into the patient. In addition, unintentional extubation is greater when transferring ventilated patients.

Routine chest physiotherapy, even in a high risk neurologic population, does not prevent VAP.[51] However, use of saline instillation when suctioning ventilated patients[52] and suctioning prior to repositioning in bed may decrease VAP risk slightly.

Continuous Aspiration of Subglottic Secretions

A specially modified endotracheal tube allows continuous aspiration of subglottic secretions pooled above the endotracheal tube cuff. This tube has an extra channel with the lumen on the dorsal surface, just above the level of the inflatable cuff. Studies of continuous aspiration of subglottic secretions have variably demonstrated lower VAP rates[53-54] but mainly in early-onset VAP, usually due to *H. influenzae* and strep-tococci. No decrease in VAP due to MDR microorganisms and no mortality differences have been demonstrated. Consistent with this pattern, the benefit is obviated if the patient receives antibiotics early in the course of mechanical ventilation,[55] similar to the benefit of prophylactic antibiotics in early-onset VAP.[15] Pneumonia can also occur if the system malfunctions, usually due to plugging of the lumen or low cuff pressures allowing secretions to drain into the distal trachea rather than collecting above the cuff. These factors and the high cost have limited the use of this modality.

Avoidance of Gastric Overdistention

Unfortunately, even when in the semirecumbent position, many patients still have gastroesophageal reflux and microaspiration when given enteral feedings. The major issue is overdistention of the stomach. The adverse effect of increased gastric volume may cancel out the beneficial effect of bolus feedings on gastric pH, contributing to this strategy's lack of benefit. Two strategies have been studied to address

this problem. The first is use of nasoenteric tubes rather than nasogas-tric tubes. Although this strategy is attractive theoretically, meta-analysis of eleven randomized controlled trials did not show a benefit of postpyloric feeding compared with nasogastric feeding.[56] The major limitation is the difficulty in placing feeding tubes in the small bowel. The second strategy is the use of gastric prokinetic agents such as metoclopramide. An additional benefit is that these agents increase the tone of the lower esophageal sphincter, potentially decreasing the risk of reflux while increasing gastric emptying. Once again, a randomized controlled trial failed to confirm the benefit of using metoclopramide to decrease the risk of VAP.[39] However, the ability of these agents to increase the tolerance of enteral nutrition warrants their continued use, despite no demonstrated effect on VAP.

OVERWHELMING LOWER RESPIRATORY HOST DEFENSES

An underappreciated fact about nosocomial pneumonia is that despite aspiration of oropharyngeal secretions documented to contain patho-genic bacteria, only a minority of colonized patients actually develop pneumonia. In the classic study of Johanson et al., only 23% of patients with gram-negative colonization of the oropharynx subsequently developed pneumonia.[57] Others have shown that quantitative culture levels of microorganisms equivalent to those found in pneumonia can transiently appear in routine non-bronchoscopic bronchoalveolar lavage samples without the subsequent clinical VAP.[58] Thus, the two steps described earlier—colonization by pathogens and aspiration—are necessary but not sufficient causes of nosocomial pneumonia.

The third step in the pathogenesis of nosocomial pneumonia, the overwhelming of lower respiratory tract defenses, is the least studied or understood. One major reason may be that the causes are hetero-geneous and patient dependent, rather than the stereotypical steps of colonization and aspiration. As infection control and patient safety efforts become more effective in limiting these risk factors, the remaining patients who do develop VAP are likely to have significant defects in host immunity.

Patients who develop VAP should generally be considered to have a form of acquired immunosuppression.[59] The more frequent occurrence of other nosocomial infections in patients with VAP supports this concept. In addition, a subgroup of VAP patients develop multiple separate episodes of VAP,[60] suggesting even greater compromise of their lower respiratory tract defenses.

Many of the causes of compromised lower respiratory tract defenses are due to the underlying disease or critical illness precipitating ICU admission and the need for mechanical ventilation. However, several are generic to most ICU patients and may be targets for prevention strategies.

Malnutrition

The overall rate of VAP appears to have decreased since early in the era of mechanical ventilation. Although a variety of factors may explain this finding, one important change is the aggressive use of nutritional support. In addition to increasing the risk of oropharyngeal coloniza-tion, malnutrition blunts many of the inflammatory responses to the bacterial challenge. The need for aggressive early nutrition may be somewhat debatable, but provision of nutrition after 48 hours of mechanical ventilation is clearly the standard of care. Specialized immune-enhancing formulas have not been proven to significantly impact the risk of infection.

Corticosteroids

Systemic corticosteroids have well documented antiinflammatory effects that can clearly influence immune function. The difficulty in determining the effect of corticosteroids on risk of VAP is the compet-ing beneficial effect on other risk factors for VAP. An example is use of corticosteroids may allow earlier extubation of a patient intubated for an exacerbation of asthma, thereby lowering the risk of VAP. This dual effect probably holds true for most cases in which corticosteroids are used acutely for critically ill patients. The potential benefits begin to be outweighed by clear adverse consequences after more prolonged courses.

Transfusions

A common cause of immunosuppression is the use of red blood cell transfusions. This effect of transfusions has been known for several decades and was used therapeutically in pretransplantation management of patients with end-stage renal disease. Because the trigger for red blood cell transfusion varies widely among institutions and even among individual practitioners,[61] a more restrictive transfusion policy may avoid compromising host immunity. Hebert and colleagues demonstrated that a conservative transfusion policy was associated with equivalent mortality to more liberal transfusions in most ICU patients.[62] A more conservative transfusion practice in trauma patients was associated with decreased VAP rates.[63] A complementary policy of routinely using leukoreduction filters with all blood transfusions decreased the incidence of posttransfusion fever as well as overall antibiotic use,[64] potentially decreasing the risk of pneumonia via several mechanisms.

KEY POINTS

1. The influence of endotracheal intubation is so dominant that ICU-acquired pneumonia is almost synonymous with ventilator-associated pneumonia (VAP).

2. A distinction should be made between prevention of all nosocomial pneumonia and prevention of life-threatening nosocomial pneumonia, usually late-onset VAP.

3. The pathogenesis of nosocomial pneumonia can be broken down into three basic steps: colonization of the oropharynx with pathogenic microorganisms, aspiration, and overwhelming of the lower respiratory tract's host defense mechanisms.

4. The most important factor in colonization of the oropharynx with pathogenic microorganisms is the use of systemic antibiotics, especially broad-spectrum antibiotics.

5. The risk of VAP is time dependent, so any maneuver that decreases the duration of mechanical ventilation will decrease pneumonia rates.

6. Avoiding the supine position as much as possible in ventilated patients is a simple and effective preventive measure for nosocomial pneumonia; it should be practiced in all ICUs.

7. Several lines of evidence suggest that minimizing the number of manipulations of the ventilator tubing will decrease the incidence of VAP.

8. Causes of the relative immunocompromised state that allows bacteria to overwhelm local host defenses in the lung are heterogeneous and patient dependent, unlike the stereotypical steps of colonization and aspiration.

ANNOTATED REFERENCES

Drakulovic MB, Torres A, Bauer TT, et al. Supine body position as a risk factor for nosocomial pneumonia in mechanically ventilated patients: A randomised trial. Lancet 1999;354:1851-8.
   This randomized controlled trial of body positioning clearly demonstrated a decreased risk with the semi-recumbent position, providing strong evidence of the role of microaspiration in the pathogenesis of VAP.
Girard TD, Kress JP, Fuchs BD, et al. Efficacy and safety of a paired sedation and ventilator weaning protocol for mechanically ventilated patients in intensive care (Awakening and Breathing Controlled trial): a randomised controlled trial. Lancet 2008;371:126-34.
   The combination of daily awakening from sedation and spontaneous breathing trials resulted in earlier extubation, shorter ICU length of stay, and lower mortality than the group with attempts at spontaneous breathing trials without specified sedation holds.
de Jonge E, Schultz MJ, Spanjaard L, et al. Effects of selective decontamination of digestive tract on mortality and acquisition of resistant bacteria in intensive care: a randomised controlled trial. Lancet 2003;362:1011-16.
   Parent multicenter randomized trial of SDD and selective decontamination of the oropharynx which demonstrated a small mortality benefit. Subsequent published substudies found selection for

cephalosporin resistance by SDD and an increased incidence of infections once patients were transferred to the floor.
Sirvent JM, Torres A, El Ebiary M, et al. Protective effect of intravenously administered cefuroxime against nosocomial pneumonia in patients with structural coma. Am J Respir Crit Care Med 1997;155:1729-34.
   Randomized controlled trial of true prophylactic antibiotic use to prevent VAP in a defined subgroup illustrated the two-edged sword of antibiotics—decreasing the risk of early pneumonia while selecting for more pathogenic microorganisms and possibly increasing the risk of late-onset VAP.
Valles J, Artigas A, Rello J, et al. Continuous aspiration of subglottic secretions in preventing ventilator-associated pneumonia. Ann Intern Med 1995;122:179-86.
   Randomized trial demonstrating the decreased risk of early-onset VAP with a manipulation that decreases the amount of microaspiration. Even if the practical use of continuous aspiration of subglottic secretions is limited, the study illustrated the problem of secretions pooling above the cuff of the endotracheal tube and its role in VAP.

REFERENCES

Access the complete reference list online at http://www.expertconsult.com.

127

Selective Decontamination of the Digestive Tract

ANNE MARIE G.A. DE SMET

Infections acquired in the intensive care unit (ICU) often occur during the treatment of critically ill patients, increasing morbidity, mortality, and health care costs.[1,2] Several studies have suggested that the use of prophylactic antibiotic regimens such as selective decontamination of the digestive tract (SDD)[3-6] and selective oropharyngeal decontamination (SOD) can reduce the incidence of respiratory tract infections in ICU patients.[5,7,8] The SDD approach[9,10] is directed to the prevention of secondary colonization with gram-negative bacteria, *Staphylococcus aureus*, and yeasts through application of nonabsorbable antimicrobial agents in the oropharynx and gastrointestinal tract, preemptive treatment of possible infections due to commensal respiratory tract bacteria through systemic administration of cephalosporins during the patient's first 4 days in the ICU, and maintenance of anaerobic intestinal flora through selective use of antibiotics (administered both topically and systemically) without antianaerobic activity.[10]

Background

The digestive tract has been considered an important source of infections in ICU patients. The intestinal flora is highly diverse and consists primarily of anaerobic bacteria. Intact anaerobic flora is, amongst others, considered an important defense mechanism against intestinal colonization with (potentially) pathogenic microorganisms. The commensal flora of the oropharynx consists of hundreds of bacterial species, including enterococci and anaerobic bacteria, which are replaced by gram-negative bacteria during the first week of hospitalization in the ICU. Gastric acidity usually prevents bacterial overgrowth in the stomach. Yet, in ICU patients, reduced acid production due to underlying diseases, usage of acid-modifying medication (stress ulcer prophylaxis), and intragastric administration of enteral nutrition (with a pH of 6) leads to a gastric environment that favors bacterial growth, especially of gram-negative bacteria.

Anaerobic bacteria grow well on the mucosa of the gut and actively line the epithelium.[11] Disruption of this layer by antibiotics that destroy the anaerobic flora may create a portal of entry for pathogenic microorganisms.

Combinations of nonabsorbable antibiotics have been used to selectively decontaminate the digestive tract and reduce the load of pathogenic aerobic microorganisms while maintaining the anaerobic flora. This concept was first investigated in mice[9] and later developed into an infection prevention strategy for neutropenic leukemia patients, which the investigators called *selective decontamination of the digestive tract*, or SDD.[12,13]

FROM CONCEPT TO PRACTICE IN THE ICU

The earlier experience with SDD in leukemia patients suggested that some infections in ICU patients might have an endogenous source and could be prevented in the same way. After an observational microbiological study among trauma patients during 2 years, an infection classification was proposed (Table 127-1) that included definitions for colonization and the use of SDD for infection prevention in trauma patients in the ICU.[10,14,15] These studies resulted in an SDD regimen consisting of application of nonabsorbable antimicrobial agents in the oropharynx and gastrointestinal tract to prevent acquired colonization with gram-negative bacteria, *Staphylococcus aureus*, and yeasts, in combination with 4 days of intravenous administration of a third-generation cephalosporin to (preemptively) treat incubating respiratory tract infections with gram-positive and gram-negative bacteria. Topical and systemic antibiotics were selected based on their antibacterial spectrum and absence of activity on the anaerobic intestinal flora.[14,15]

Clinical Results

EARLIER STUDIES

The first study with SDD in ICU patients was performed in 63 trauma patients, using a historical control group of 59 trauma patients.[10] This study, because of its design and use of a historical control group, not only triggered many critical comments and editorials but also resulted in additional studies in more heterogeneous ICU patient populations, with different combinations of absorbable and nonabsorbable antibiotics, with or without parenteral antibiotics.[3,16-18] The conflicting results of these clinical trials led to the conclusion that there was insufficient scientific evidence to recommend SDD as a routine infection control measure in ICU patients.[19]

RECENT STUDIES

A single-center prospective, controlled, randomized, unblinded study in 2003 reported significantly lower ICU and hospital-mortality rates (35% and 22%, respectively), shorter length of stay, and a lower incidence of antibiotic resistance in patients with an expected duration of mechanical ventilation of ≥2 days and/or expected length of stay in the ICU of ≥3 days and receiving SDD.[4,20] A subsequent multicenter controlled crossover study using cluster randomization and identical inclusion criteria was performed in the Netherlands that compared SDD with SOD. SOD was included because of the hypothesis that the main effect of SDD—a reduction in the incidence of ventilator-associated pneumonia (VAP)—could be achieved by oropharyngeal decontamination only, without intestinal decontamination and without the routine prophylactic use of systemic antibiotics during the first 4 days of ventilation.[7,8] The results of this Dutch multicenter study with almost 6000 patients showed that compared to the control group, both SDD, SOD, and a control group were associated with an adjusted relative reduction of mortality at day 28 of 13% and 11%, respectively, corresponding with an absolute reduction of 3.5% and 2.9%.[5] Of note, there were several limitations to this study, particularly the fact that the study was not blinded. Because of its unblinded nature, all physicians were aware of the treatment patient participants would receive, and because inclusion was based on several criteria, this created the possibility of selection bias. To minimize the occurrence of selection bias, patient eligibility and inclusion rates were monitored frequently and immediately followed by feedback to the participating investigators. Yet despite the use of these measures next to the objective inclusion criteria, in the end, there were baseline differences between the control and the two intervention groups. Patients in the intervention groups (SDD and SOD) were more frequently intubated, were less likely to be surgical patients, and had a higher baseline APACHE score. Further, SDD patients were older compared to SOD and control patients.[5]

TABLE 127-1	Definitions
Colonization resistance	The strong protective effect of the endogenous anaerobic fraction of the intestinal microflora in resisting colonization by aerobe microorganisms along the alimentary canal. When the anaerobic flora is suppressed, there is an enhanced risk of overgrowth by gram-negative bacteria.
PPM	Potentially pathogenic microorganisms
SDD	*Selective decontamination of the digestive tract* is the selective elimination of PPM from the oral and intestinal flora by topical nonabsorbable antibiotics.
SOD	*Selective oropharyngeal decontamination* is the selective elimination of PPM from the oral flora by topical nonabsorbable antibiotics.
Primary endogenous infections	Caused by PPM with which the oropharynx and/or digestive tract of the patient was colonized at admission. These PPM are part of the "normal" flora of the patient.
Secondary endogenous infections	Caused by PPM with which the oropharynx and/or digestive tract of the patient was not colonized at admission but acquired during ICU stay
Exogenous infections	Caused by PPM not present at admission and developing without preceding colonization
Colonization	Presence of the same species of PPM in an organ system for more than 3 days (≥2 positive cultures) without signs of infection

A Cochrane meta-analysis was published in 2009 on the effects of topical antibiotics (with or without systemic antibiotics) and its effects on mortality and the incidence of respiratory tract infections (RTI).[6] This meta-analysis included 36 trials with a total of 6914 patients (without the previously mentioned Dutch multicenter study for the reasons described). The authors concluded that:

1. In trials comparing a combination of topical and systemic antibiotics to control, there was a significant reduction in both RTIs (16 studies, OR 0.28, 95% CI 0.20-0.38) and mortality (17 studies, OR 0.75, 95% CI 0.65-0.87).
2. In trials comparing topical antibiotics alone to control, or comparing topical plus systemic to systemic alone, there was a significant reduction in RTIs (17 studies, OR 0.44, 95% CI 0.31-0.63) but not in mortality (19 studies, OR 0.97, 95% CI 0.82-1.16).

This last conclusion contrasts the results of the Dutch multicenter trial which showed a significant reduction in mortality by using topical antibiotics in the oropharynx only.[5]

In Table 127-2 the "what, when, and why" of the different parts of the SDD regimen as it is used in the latest studies is listed.

TABLE 127-2	Selective Decontamination of the Digestive Tract Regimen	
What	**When**	**Why**
Baseline		
Oropharyngeal application of 0.5 g of a paste containing polymyxin E, tobramycin, and amphotericin B, each in a 2% concentration*	4 times daily until ICU discharge	Selective decontamination of the oropharynx
Administration of 10 mL of a suspension containing 100 mg polymyxin E, 80 mg tobramycin, and 500 mg amphotericin B via the nasogastric tube	4 times daily until ICU discharge	Selective decontamination of the gut from stomach to rectum
Cefotaxime 1 g intravenously during the first 4 days of study (or other third-generation cephalosporins)	4 times daily during the first 4 days	Preemptive treatment of primary endogenous infections
Avoidance of (systemic) antibiotics which might impair the colonization resistance (i.e., with antianaerobic activity)	During treatment with SDD, until ICU discharge	Avoidance of penicillins, carbapenems, etc. No addition of antibiotics for patients with colonization without clinical signs suggestive for infection
Cultures of endotracheal* aspirates, oropharyngeal* and rectal swabs	On admission and surveillance cultures twice weekly	Determination of colonization pattern at admission and during treatment, including monitoring of effectiveness of SDD Detection of infection
Oropharyngeal care*	4 times daily using sterile water or chlorhexidine† mouthwash, preceding application of oropharyngeal paste; includes brushing of teeth twice daily Clean visually contaminated oropharyngeal cavity with swab moistened with 1.5% hydrogen peroxide	Cleansing of mouth and teeth Removing residue of paste Preparing mouth for (next) application of paste
Use of normal hygiene guidelines*	Always	Preventing transmission of pathogens in the patient Prevention of (exogenous) cross-contamination and infections from and to other patients Control of outbreak
Modifications for Patients with:		
Tracheostomy*	0.5 g of paste applied around the tracheostomy 4 times daily	Selective decontamination of the oropharynx
Duodenal tube or jejunostomy	Divide the 10 mL of suspension into 5 mL suspension via the gastric tube and 5 mL via the duodenal tube or jejunostomy	Selective decontamination of the gut from stomach to rectum
Colostoma or ileostoma	SDD suppositories (containing 100 mg polymyxin E, 40 mg tobramycin, and 500 mg amphotericin B) twice daily in the distal part of the gut	Selective decontamination of the gut from stomach to rectum
Documented cephalosporin allergy	Cefotaxime can be replaced by ciprofloxacin (twice daily 400 mg).	Avoidance of allergic reaction
Modifications for Patients with Persistent Respiratory Tract Colonization with Yeasts or Gram-Negative Bacteria		
If a surveillance culture (>48 h after admission culture) of the throat yields yeasts and/or gram-negative bacteria*	Increase application of oropharyngeal paste to 8 times daily until 2 surveillance cultures are negative.	Decolonization
If a sputum surveillance (>48 h after admission culture) culture yields yeasts*	Nebulize 5 mL (5 mg) amphotericin B 4 times daily until 2 sputum cultures are negative.	Decolonization
If a sputum surveillance culture (>48 h after admission culture) yields gram-negative bacteria*	Nebulize 5 mL (80 mg) polymyxin E 4 times daily until 2 sputum cultures are negative.	Decolonization

*The SOD regimen from de Smet AM, Kluytmans JA, Cooper BS et al. Decontamination of the digestive tract and oropharynx in intensive care patients. N Engl J Med 2009;360: 20-31.

†Chlorhexidine was not used in the Dutch SDD-SOD trial. (N Engl J Med 2009;360:20-31).

Microbiological Effects of Selective Decontamination

DECONTAMINATING EFFECT

There are few recent studies which describe the results of the decontaminating effect of SDD. The Dutch multicenter trial showed that the proportions of SDD patients colonized with gram-negative bacteria isolated from rectal swabs decreased from 56% at day 3 to 25% at day 8 and 15% at day 14. Oropharyngeal colonization rates with gram-negative bacteria decreased from 18% at day 2, to 4% at day 8 among SDD patients. The same trial showed a comparable decrease in oropharyngeal colonization rates with gram-negative bacteria in SOD patients from 20% at day 2 to 7% at day 8.[5] These results were comparable to those reported in other studies.[10,21,22]

The positive effects of SDD (and SOD) on respiratory tract colonization and infection have been described extensively.[4,6-8] The Dutch multicenter trial showed significantly lower incidences of ICU-acquired bacteremia during SOD and SDD for *S. aureus*, glucose-nonfermenting gram-negative rods (mainly *Pseudomonas aeruginosa*), and Enterobacteriaceae, as compared to controls. Patients receiving SDD had lower incidences of ICU-acquired bacteremia with Enterobacteriaceae than those receiving SOD. The incidence of ICU-acquired candidemia was lower in the SDD group compared to either SOD or control groups.[5]

EMERGENCE AND SELECTION OF ANTIBIOTIC RESISTANCE IN GRAM-NEGATIVE AND GRAM-POSITIVE MICROORGANISMS DURING SELECTIVE DECONTAMINATION

Enhanced selection of antibiotic-resistant microorganisms has been considered an important threat of SDD and SOD.[23] Consistent use of surveillance cultures as part of SDD and SOD protocols makes it possible to assess the efficacy of enteral decontamination as well as detect emergence of antibiotic-resistant pathogens early.

Gram-Negative Microorganisms

Several studies showed an overall decrease of antibiotic-resistant gram-negative microorganisms in patients receiving SDD, including a significant beneficial effect on colonization with resistant gram-negative bacteria such as *P. aeruginosa* resistant to ceftazidime, imipenem, and ciprofloxacin and other aerobic gram negatives resistant to imipenem, ciprofloxacin, and tobramycin.[4,18] Patients receiving SDD during the Dutch multicenter trial had lower incidences of ICU-acquired candidemia, bacteremia with Enterobacteriaceae, and bacteremia with highly resistant microorganisms (HRMO; according to Dutch guidelines[24]) than those receiving SOD.[25] The incidence of candidemia and bacteremia caused by HRMO were low in this study, so whether this difference will translate into a difference in clinical outcome between both interventions depends on the overall incidence of candidemia and bacteremia caused by HRMO, the appropriateness of empirical antimicrobial therapy in such patients, and the attributable effects of such events on outcome and length of stay. These findings do not support the concern that use of topical antibiotics, with or without systemic prophylaxis with third-generation cephalosporins, increases prevalence levels of antibiotic resistance in gram-negative bacteria. Further studies are needed to distinguish the effects of the individual components of SDD.

Gram-Positive Microorganisms

Methicillin-resistant *S. aureus* (MRSA) and vancomycin-resistant *Enterococcus* (VRE) are highly prevalent in ICUs in many countries, unlike the Netherlands where the last two major studies have been carried out. It is generally considered that the use of topical antibiotics for SDD or SOD is contraindicated in such settings, as such regimens may increase colonization and infection rates with these bacteria. Yet, few data are available on the effects of SDD or SOD in settings with high levels of MRSA. In one study, a shift toward gram-positive organisms was detected after the introduction of SDD in trauma patients that included an outbreak and increased carriage rates with MRSA 2 years after the introduction of SDD.[26,27] This was successfully addressed by implementation of control measures.[26] To prevent infections with MRSA, some investigators add vancomycin to the SOD or SDD regimen.[7,28] When applied topically, vancomycin will not be absorbed and will reach high concentrations in the intestinal tract. In a Spanish burn unit, SDD with topical vancomycin was associated with improved patient outcome and lower colonization rates with MRSA.[28] A disadvantage of such an approach will be the selection of VRE in ICUs where both pathogens are prevalent.

The results of the Dutch study indicated that both SDD and SOD were associated with higher rates of acquired respiratory tract colonization but not with higher bacteremia rates caused by enterococci. In ICU patients, enterococci will colonize all body sites (especially the skin) and contaminate the inanimate environment. Enterococci have become among the most frequent causes of hospital-acquired infections worldwide, and the proportion of infections caused by ampicillin-resistant enterococci (ARE) has increased substantially in Western countries, including the Netherlands.[29] In the United States, approximately 35% of all ICU-acquired bacteremias caused by enterococci are due to VRE. The clinical relevance of ARE and VRE infections is unclear.

Widespread use of topical vancomycin in units with high levels of MRSA will enhance the selective pressure for VRE. This should be carefully balanced against the benefits of SDD or SOD with vancomycin. In the United States, ICUs with high levels of MRSA frequently also have high endemic levels of VRE. In such settings, addition of oropharyngeal chlorhexidine oral washings and/or chlorhexidine body washings may help in controlling spread and bloodstream infections caused by VRE and MRSA.[30,31] Chlorhexidine is a bacteriostatic and bactericidal chemical antiseptic with effects on both gram-positive and, to a lesser extent, gram-negative bacteria. Several studies and meta-analyses addressing the use of oropharyngeal chlorhexidine demonstrated a significant reduction in pneumonia, but so far none have shown a significant reduction in mortality. New studies combining several infection-prevention measures using topical antibiotics combined with topical application of agents such as chlorhexidine should be performed, preferably in surroundings with a high incidence of gram-positive multiresistant bacteria.

ECOLOGICAL EFFECTS

During the Dutch multicenter study, surveillance cultures from the respiratory and intestinal tract were obtained each month on a fixed day from all patients present in the ICU, regardless of whether they were included in the study.[5] These 18 point-prevalence studies in 13 ICUs allowed an analysis of the effects of SDD and SOD on the bacterial ecology in these ICUs together. Effects of SDD (during periods of 6 months) and of SDD/SOD (combined during periods of 12 months) on intestinal and respiratory tract carriage with gram-negative bacteria were determined by comparing results from consecutive point-prevalence surveys using intervention to consecutive point-prevalence data in the pre- and postintervention periods.[32] The average proportions of patients colonized with ceftazidime, tobramycin, or ciprofloxacin-resistant gram-negative bacteria in the intestinal tract decreased during the use of SDD in the ICU and increased again after discontinuation. During combined SDD/SOD, resistance levels in the respiratory tract were low ($\leq$6%) for all three antibiotics but seemed to increase gradually, with a significant increase only for ceftazidime resistance (P <0.05). After discontinuation of SDD/SOD, the resistance levels increased to levels of 10% or higher. Obviously, both SDD and SOD have marked ecological effects, particularly in the intestinal and respiratory tract for SDD and in the respiratory tract for SOD. Df note, some of these patients were only briefly in the ICU and the incidence of resistance in other hospital wards was unknown. An increasing incidence of resistance in the participating hospitals might have influenced these results. Yet the observed increase of ceftazidime resistance during SDD/SOD is of concern. Nevertheless, the ecological effects (i.e., lowest resistance levels during interventions) corroborate the positive effects of SOD and SDD on antibiotic resistance in individual patients.[4,25] Larger and longer longitudinal studies are needed to determine the long-term effects of SOD and SDD on antibiotic resistance, with special attention to the changes in antibiotic resistance among gram-negative bacteria.

OTHER ISSUES

Effectiveness of SDD in Specific Patient Groups

There is some evidence that SDD might not be equally effective in all patient groups. In one meta-analysis, increased efficacy of SDD was observed in surgical patients.[17]

In a post hoc subgroup analysis of the Dutch multicenter study, different effects of SDD and SOD were found for surgical and nonsurgical patients.[25] Compared to control, SDD was equally effective in reducing 28-day mortality in surgical and nonsurgical patients, but with significant reductions in duration of mechanical ventilation, ICU stay, and hospital stay among surgical patients. On the other hand, SOD appeared to be even more effective in reducing mortality in nonsurgical patients but was not associated with reduction in day-28 mortality in surgical patients, nor in duration of mechanical ventilation or ICU or hospital stay. These findings suggest that surgical patients benefit from the addition of the enteric and/or systemic component of the SDD regimen. These results should be considered as hypothesis generating; further studies are needed to confirm such observations. If confirmed, they may help elucidate the mechanisms of the protective action of SDD and SOD in specific groups of ICU patients.

Hospital-Acquired Infections After Treatment with SOD and SDD

In the SDD study by De Jonge et al., the relative risk reduction in ICU mortality of 35% decreased to 22% at hospital discharge.[4] Triggered by these findings, it was hypothesized that this reduction in survival benefit after ICU discharge might have been related to an increased incidence of hospital-acquired infections (HAI) in patients who had received SDD in the ICU. Nested within the multicenter SDD-SOD trial, the incidence of HAI was prospectively monitored during the first 14 days after ICU discharge in all patients transferred to regular wards in two university hospitals.[33] Most HAI were respiratory tract infections, with similar incidence and similar duration of infection in all three posttreatment study groups. The incidence of bloodstream infections was also similar in the three posttreatment groups, but time until infection tended to be longer in the post-SOD and post-SDD groups compared to the postcontrol group. On the other hand, the incidence of surgical site infections (SSI) seemed to increase in the postintervention groups. The proportion of patients developing post-ICU HAI in the post-SOD and post-SDD periods combined tended to be higher than during the postcontrol period, though this did not reach statistical significance. Considering the low rates of HAI, the overall low mortality rates after ICU discharge, and the low prevalence of infections among those who succumbed after ICU discharge, the hypothesis that discontinuation of SDD and SOD post ICU increases the infection rate and thus affects clinical outcome could not be supported.[33]

Antibiotic Use

No formal cost/benefit evaluations of the use of SDD or SOD have been performed. De Jonge evaluated the total costs of antibiotics, topical and systemic, which were 11% lower in the SDD group compared to the control group. This was primarily due to the decrease in the use of antibiotics such as ciprofloxacin, ceftazidime, imipenem, and antifungal treatment.[4] These results were confirmed by the multicenter study, with (compared to control) a decrease of 12% and 10% in the use of daily defined doses of systemic antibiotics in SDD and SOD, respectively.[5]

Adverse Events

Three patients are reported who suffered from accumulation of the buccally applied oral SDD/SOD oral paste to large clots which caused obstruction in the esophagus or jejunum. This complication can be prevented by regular and appropriate oral care.[34]

KEY POINTS

1. Selective decontamination of the digestive tract (SDD) improves survival in ICU patients.

2. SDD lowers the incidence of bacteremia, candidemia, and respiratory tract infection (RTI).

3. SDD lowers the use of systemic antibiotics.

4. There is no evidence to support the concern that the use of topical antibiotics with or without systemic prophylaxis increases the prevalence of antibiotic resistance to gram-negative bacteria. On short term (0.5-2 yrs) SDD reduces antibiotic resistance to gram-negative bacteria.

5. Selective oropharyngeal decontamination (SOD) has comparable effects in reducing RTI, bacteremia (although significantly less compared to SDD), use of systemic antibiotics, and mortality. Whether SOD has positive effects similar to those associated with SDD on the emergence of antibiotic resistance in gram-negative microorganisms remains to be determined.

6. Further research is needed to assess SDD and SOD in surroundings with high antibiotic resistance levels and in combination with other topical agents such as chlorhexidine.

ANNOTATED REFERENCES

Stoutenbeek CP, van Saene HKF, Miranda DR, Zandstra DF. The effect of selective decontamination of the digestive tract on colonization and infection rate in multiple trauma patients. Intensive Care Med 1984;10:185-92.
  First study on SDD in ICU patients. Good description and overview of theoretical background.
Liberati A, D'Amico R, Pifferi S, Torri V, Brazzi L, Parmelli E. Antibiotic prophylaxis to reduce respiratory tract infections and mortality in adults receiving intensive care. The Cochrane Library 2009, Issue 4. Available at http://www.thecochranelibrary.com.
  State of the art and very recent meta-analysis. Provides a very good and thorough overview on the studies on SDD, concluding that a combination of topical and systemic antibiotics caused a significant reduction of RTIs (16 studies, OR 0.28) and mortality (17 studies, OR 0.75) compared to control. Comparing topical antibiotics alone to control, or comparing topical plus systemic to systemic alone, there was a significant reduction in RTIs (17 studies, OR 0.44) but not in mortality (19 studies, OR 0.97).
de Jonge E, Schultz M, Spanjaard L, et al. Effects of selective decontamination of the digestive tract on mortality and acquisition of resistant bacteria in intensive care: a randomised controlled trial. Lancet 2003;362:1011-16.
  Prospective, randomized, controlled, single-center study on SDD in 934 ICU patients with an expected length of stay more than 72 hours and/or expected duration of mechanical ventilation more than 48 hours.

The most important finding was a remarkable relative reduction of ICU mortality of 34.7% for patients treated in the SDD ward. For these patients, the relative reduction of hospital mortality was 22.6%. In addition, SDD-treated patients had a shorter duration of ventilation, and total antibiotic costs were less for these patients. Furthermore, isolation of antibiotic-resistant gram-negative bacteria occurred more frequently among non-SDD patients.
de Smet AM, Kluytmans JA, Cooper BS, et al. Decontamination of the digestive tract and oropharynx in intensive care patients. N Engl J Med 2009;360:20-31.
  First multicenter cluster-randomized trial which compared SDD with SOD and control in groups of 2000 patients each. Both interventions significantly improved survival (absolute mortality reduction of 3.5% and 2.9%, respectively) and decreased the rate of bacteremia (ORs SDD versus control, 044; SOD versus control, 0.68; SDD versus SOD, 0.65).
Bergmans DC, Bonten MJ, Gaillard CA, et al. Prevention of ventilator-associated pneumonia by oral decontamination: a prospective, randomized, double-blind, placebo-controlled study. Am J Respir Crit Care Med 2001;164:382-8.
  Prospective randomized double-blind placebo-controlled study on oropharyngeal decontamination which showed prevention of acquired oropharyngeal colonization and significantly lower incidence of VAP, albeit not associated with shorter durations of ventilation or ICU stay or better survival.

REFERENCES

Access the complete reference list online at http://www.expertconsult.com.

128

Vascular Catheter–Related Infections

SCOTT NORWOOD | ALAN D. COOK

Catheter-related bloodstream infection (CRBSI) is the third leading device-related infection among U.S. hospitals and ambulatory surgical centers in the United States participating in the National Healthcare Safety Network (NHSN) that report to the Centers for Disease Control and Prevention (CDC).[1] In the 2009 report, 14,332 primary bloodstream infections over 7.4 million catheter days (1.93 infections per 1000 catheter days) were identified. This infection rate ranks third in magnitude behind catheter-associated urinary tract infections and ventilator-associated pneumonias.[1] CRBSI ranks second worldwide only to ventilator-associated pneumonia.[2] The estimates in both of these reports are limited to only central venous catheter (CVC) infections. However, peripheral venous catheters, more permanent cuffed and tunneled catheters, arterial catheters, and peripherally inserted central catheters (PICC) also have associated bloodstream infection rates.[3-4]

The cost of CRBSI in terms of morbidity is significant to both the patient and the healthcare provider. The impact on resource utilization was summarized by Dimick et al., who conducted a prospective cohort study among surgical ICU patients at a large tertiary care center. A single CRBSI increased hospital costs by $56,167 and hospital length of stay by 22 days.[5] The increased mortality of CRBSI was estimated in a meta-analysis by Siempos et al. He analyzed eight different studies that included 2540 ICU patients and determined the relative risk of mortality to be 1.57.[6] In a mixed cohort of 2201 medical and surgical patients hospitalized in 15 French ICUs, CRBSI was associated with an estimated excess mortality of 11.5% to 20%.[7]

Because of the burden of mortality to patient populations and the increased costs to payers, CRBSI was included in the list of eight hospital-acquired conditions, the so-called "never events." By inclusion as a "never event," the Centers for Medicare and Medicaid Services (CMS) are prohibited by Congress from reimbursing hospitals for charges associated with these conditions after October 1, 2008.[8] Thus, prevention of CRBSI has attracted substantial attention from multiple stakeholders in the healthcare industry.

This chapter will clarify some commonly used terms associated with CRBSI, discuss various pathogenic theories, analyze patient- and hospital-related risk factors, discuss available diagnostic techniques, and review the existing data on infections associated with the most commonly employed types of vascular catheters.

■ Definitions

Clinicians and researchers historically have used different definitions for vascular catheter–related infections. Infections can be linked to peripheral, central, venous, and arterial catheters. These catheters can further be designated as permanent, short-term, or long-term. The clinical presentation of a catheter-related infection can be designated as either local (site inflammation, purulent drainage, tenderness) or systemic (bacteremia with or without systemic sepsis). Although it is certain that inanimate objects do not become "infected," there is strong evidence to suggest that bacteria may be able to live and multiply on catheter surfaces, possibly deriving nutrients from catheter polymers, the deposited glycocalyx of certain bacterial species, and other nonviable bacteria.[9,10] Earlier clinical investigations used erroneous descriptions and definitions for catheter contamination, colonization, and infection. These different definitions have led to confusion and incorrect interpretations by previous investigators.[11] This is further complicated by confusion regarding subtle differences between surveillance definitions by the NHSN[1] and clinical definitions. The commonly accepted clinical definitions have been previously published[11,12]:

Catheter-related bloodstream infection (CRBSI): a bacteremia or fungemia in a patient with an intravascular catheter with at least one positive blood culture obtained from a peripheral vein and clinical manifestations of infection (i.e., fever, chills, and/or hypotension) with no apparent source for the bacteremia except the catheter. One of the following culture techniques should be used: (1) a positive semiquantitative (>15 colony-forming units [CFUs]/catheter segment) or (2) quantitative (>10^3 CFUs/catheter segment) culture whereby the same organism is isolated from the catheter segment and peripheral blood; (3) simultaneous quantitative blood cultures with greater than 5:1 ratio (CVC versus peripheral catheter), (4) differential positivity time (greater than 2-hour period between the initiation of growth of organisms in culture from a qualitative peripheral blood culture when compared with a simultaneously collected CVC culture).[13]

Localized catheter colonization: significant growth of a microorganism in a semiquantitative or quantitative culture of the catheter tip, subcutaneous segment of the catheter, or the catheter hub (see Diagnostic Techniques), without evidence of systemic infection.

Microbiological exit site infection: exudate at the catheter exit site yields bacterial or fungal growth on a standard qualitative culture with or without concomitant bloodstream infection.

Clinical exit site infection: tenderness, erythema or site induration greater than 2 cm from the catheter exit site, with or without other signs or symptoms of infection.

Tunnel infection: tenderness, erythema, and/or induration greater than 2 cm from the catheter exit site, along the subcutaneous tract of a tunneled catheter.

Pocket infection: purulent fluid in the subcutaneous pocket of a totally implanted intravascular device that might or might not be associated with spontaneous rupture and drainage or necrosis of the overlying skin, in the absence of concomitant bacteremia.

Infusate-related bloodstream infection: concordant growth of the same organism from the infusate and blood cultures (preferably percutaneously obtained), with no other identifiable source of infection.

It is important to understand that both microbiological and clinical exit site infections, tunnel infections, and pocket infections, when accompanied by a positive blood culture, will be classified as a CRBSI for hospital surveillance purposes.[1,11,12]

Culture of drainage around a catheter insertion site may in some situations be helpful in that a positive bacterial culture result assists in confirming the presence of an exit site infection. It is important to also understand that values of 15 CFUs or less for semiquantitative and 10^3 CFUs or less for quantitative cultures may be regarded as a negative culture, a contaminant, or an insignificant infection that does not require treatment in the absence of a confirmatory blood culture. Insertion site manifestations of inflammation are neither sensitive nor specific for diagnosing CRBSI or catheter colonization. Immunosuppressed patients may manifest local signs of inflammation, and other patient groups may develop intense local insertion site inflammation without associated CRBSI.[14]

Pathogenesis

Microbial colonization and biofilm formation on intravascular catheters are universal, occurring soon after catheter insertion.[9,10,15] The final determinate of whether colonization progresses to clinical infection is multifactorial. A variety of host factors, catheter composition, and the interaction between microorganisms and the catheter surface may all contribute to the ultimate development of CRBSI.

There are four established routes for catheter contamination leading to CRBSI:

1. Microorganisms migrate from the skin at the insertion site into the subcutaneous tract along the external surface of the catheter and ultimately gain access to the distal intravascular catheter segment.[16] This is the most common mechanism for developing infection of short-term non-cuffed non-tunneled central venous catheters.
2. Microorganisms gain access to the catheter through the hubs or ports of the vascular device. The most common sources for contamination are the hands of healthcare workers or the infusion of minimally contaminated fluids (contaminated at the bedside) or attachment of contaminated tubing. This route of infection is more commonly identified in patients with long-term tunneled catheters (Hickman, Broviac, Groshong) or mediports.[16] Bacteria can be introduced via one or more hubs from frequent manipulations. As the biofilm grows, bacteria migrate into the inner luminal surface and gain access to the venous circulation. In low-flow regions, the biofilm attachment is weaker and breaks more easily, allowing entry of bacteria into the venous circulation.[16]
3. Remote infections may produce bacteremia and hematogenously seed an intravascular device. Although this scenario is plausible, hematogenous catheter seeding is considered a rare cause of CRBSI.[16]
4. Infusate contamination is a rare fourth mechanism for development of CRBSI. Parenteral nutrition solutions, lipid emulsions and heparin flush solutions can support bacterial and fungal growth, but the risk from infusate contamination today is considered very low.[17,18]

Following insertion, the intravascular portion of the catheter is quickly coated with a thrombin layer covering both the external and internal surfaces. Thrombin contains a number of proteins including fibronectin, thrombospondin, and laminin which create an adhesive surface on the catheter that promotes adherence of microbial pathogens. Multiple species of *Staphylococcus epidermidis*, *Staphylococcus aureus*, *Candida albicans*, and various gram-negative organisms are all capable of adhering to catheter surfaces.[19] A mature biofilm can shield organisms from antibiotics at 10 to 1000 times the concentration required to kill planktonic bacteria.[20]

This helps explain why the commonly reported pathogens for hospital-acquired bloodstream infections remain coagulase-negative staphylococci (*Staphylococcus epidermidis*), *Staphylococcus aureus*, enterococci, and *Candida* species.[20] Gram-negative bacilli account for approximately 20% of CRBSIs reported.[20,21]

Risk Factors

A number of factors potentiate the risk for CRBSI. These are generally similar to the same factors that increase the risk for any hospital-acquired infection. Extremes of age (i.e., pediatric, elderly), immunodeficiency, chronic disease states, remote infection sites, and heavy colonization of the skin with bacteria or fungi may all increase the risk. Alterations in skin integrity (psoriasis, burns) also increase risk. Whereas patient-related factors cannot be significantly modified during an acute illness, they must be considered when developing catheter maintenance protocols. Penel et al. identified age younger than 10 years, difficulties with catheter insertion, and the need for total parenteral nutrition as significant risk factors for intravascular device–related infections.[22]

In contradistinction to patient-related risk factors, many hospital-related risk factors can be significantly modified, and prevention protocols are designed to focus on these risks.[22,23] A number of interventions have been proposed by the CDC to assist in the prevention of CRBSI.[24,25] Implementation of educational programs for hospital personnel regarding proper insertion and maintenance of intravascular catheters and appropriate preventive control measures should reduce infection rates. A number of other interventions and measures are also recommended collectively as the "central line bundle." These recommended procedures and interventions are: hand washing, using full sterile-barrier precautions during insertion of central venous catheters, preparing the insertion skin site with chlorhexidine, avoiding the femoral site if possible, and removing central venous catheters as soon as possible when no longer needed.[23] In a large multicenter trial involving 108 intensive care units (ICUs), a central line bundle was initiated to determine its effect on reduction of catheter-related bloodstream infections. Implementing these strategies reduced the mean rate of CRBSI from 7.7 to 1.4 per 1000 catheter-days at 16 to 18 months follow-up ($P < 0.002$).[26] This large multicenter study provided evidence that the guidelines recommended by the CDC[24,25] are indeed beneficial in reducing CRBSI rates. Others have suggested that the act of prospective surveillance alone without any specific intervention to reduce CRBSI will also have a beneficial result in decreasing infection rates.[27]

Although the number of catheter manipulations and the experience of the individual performing the catheter insertion may be risk factors, these often cannot be changed or controlled for the individual patient at risk. The need for total parenteral nutrition, the area within the hospital where the insertion is performed, and the number of catheter lumens have all been associated with increased risk for catheter-related infection.[28] Cutdowns should be avoided whenever possible because of the historically high incidence of catheter-related complications.[29] The most common risk factors for catheter colonization and CRBSI that can be successfully altered are separately discussed.

ANATOMIC INSERTION SITE

An early study by Mermel showed that the use of the internal jugular site, particularly for pulmonary artery catheters, is a significant risk factor for catheter-related infection.[30] This may be related to the closer proximity of oropharyngeal secretions, greater catheter motion from neck movement, and greater difficulty in maintaining a sterile occlusive dressing.[30] However, it is still recommended that the internal jugular or the femoral vein site be used over the subclavian vein site for short-term hemodialysis catheters to reduce the risk of subsequent subclavian vein stenosis.[24,25]

The femoral site is also more likely to become heavily colonized and thus is also at higher risk for CRBSI. Merrer et al. in a randomized controlled clinical trial involving eight different ICUs identified a threefold higher incidence of clinical sepsis (with or without bloodstream infection) and a tenfold increase in thrombotic complications when femoral catheters were compared to subclavian catheters.[31]

Data collected in our own center suggest that colonization rates for femoral sites, even with the use of chlorhexidine and silver sulfadiazine-bonded catheters, are significantly higher than for subclavian or internal jugular catheter sites.[32]

DURATION OF CATHETER USE

Bacterial colonization of catheter surfaces begins shortly after insertion and is directly proportional to the length of time a catheter remains in place. The risk of CRBSI increases over time. Nonetheless, the optimal timing of catheter removal remains uncertain. The risk of an individual catheter causing CRBSI is low if inserted under optimal sterile conditions and removed within 4 to 7 days. However, critically ill patients typically require venous access for prolonged periods, and the timing of catheter removal must be weighed against clinical necessity. Central venous catheters and pulmonary artery catheters do not have predetermined lifespans.[33]

Recommendations and guidelines for catheter exchange may be used to minimize CRBSI and to prolong site use on the basis of existing published data. However, it is important to realize that CRBSI risk factors are multifactorial and that global recommendations for catheter maintenance or removal may not be applicable to the individual patient. Generally, catheters should be removed (1) when they are no longer needed, or (2) if CRBSI is suspected clinically and appropriate cultures confirm clinical suspicions (see Diagnostic Techniques). Individual hospitals, individual ICUs, and in certain situations individual practitioners should study their catheter infection rates to develop specific guidelines appropriate to their practice patterns and environment. Rates of CRBSI per 1000 catheters-days can be calculated and compared with published standards.[1,2,24,25]

Diagnostic Techniques

The clinical diagnosis of CRBSI is often inaccurate, leading to premature catheter removal. Assuming that appropriate sterile technique during insertion and appropriate site care have been followed, the presence of entry-site inflammation is neither sensitive nor specific for CRBSI.[14] Qualitative broth cultures collected through the CVC are generally discouraged for determining CRBSI for short-term, nontunneled catheters. The positive predictive value of blood cultures obtained through the catheter is significantly less than from a peripheral venipuncture,[34,35] and additional cultures are usually necessary to make the definitive diagnosis. However, a negative culture from either a peripheral venipuncture or a CVC has excellent negative predictive value, and cultures obtained through the catheter are frequently performed to rule out CRBSI.[35]

The unreliability of clinical diagnosis and qualitative blood cultures has led to a variety of microbiological diagnostic techniques. These can be categorized into diagnostic methods that require catheter removal and catheter-sparing diagnostic methods. Because each method has advantages and disadvantages, some investigators have suggested that simply performing peripheral blood cultures and clinical evaluation may be all that is necessary and cost-effective. Clinical diagnosis alone and qualitative blood cultures will both significantly overestimate the rate of CRBSI and should generally be avoided.

DIAGNOSTIC TECHNIQUES REQUIRING REMOVAL OF THE CENTRAL VENOUS CATHETER

Quantitative Catheter Cultures

This type of culture involves flushing, sonicating, or vortexing the catheter segment with broth. This is designed to retrieve organisms from both the internal and external catheter surface. This technique is particularly useful for catheters in situ for more than 7 days.[11] In this situation, intraluminal spread from the hub is the most likely mechanism for catheter colonization. Therefore, obtaining a culture from both the internal and external surface should be more sensitive and specific. A culture yielding over 10^3 CFU is diagnostic for CRBSI if accompanied by the appropriate clinical diagnosis, a positive peripheral blood culture with the same organism, and no other likely source for the infection. A meta-analysis conducted by Safdar in 2005 showed that the pooled sensitivity and specificity for this culture technique was 83% and 87% respectively.[36]

Semiquantitative Catheter Culture

The semiquantitative (roll-plate) technique developed by Maki and colleagues remains the most common diagnostic technique for determining catheter-related infection.[37] A 5-cm segment (either catheter tip or intracutaneous segment) is rolled across a blood-agar plate in a reproducible, defined manner. In the original study, a positive result was defined as more than 15 CFUs per plate, although most of the culture-positive catheters in the original study yielded confluent growth.[37] A positive catheter segment culture result (>15 CFUs) resulted in a 16% risk of CRBSI. This technique is probably most accurate for catheters that are removed within the first 7 days.[36] It may

become less sensitive for more long-term catheters, because this technique does not culture the internal lumen. A recent meta-analysis of 19 studies using the semiquantitative catheter culture technique identified an overall sensitivity of 85% and specificity of 82%.[36]

CENTRAL VENOUS CATHETER–SPARING DIAGNOSTIC TECHNIQUES

A number of techniques have been developed as an alternative for diagnosing CRBSI in patients for whom catheter removal is undesirable because of limited vascular access.[11]

Paired Device–Collected Quantitative Blood Cultures

This technique involves obtaining quantitative cultures of paired blood samples—one obtained through the central venous catheter hub and the other from a peripheral venipuncture site. The samples should be obtained less than 10 minutes apart using the same blood volume for each culture. Central venous catheter cultures yielding a colony count at least fivefold greater than the colony count obtained from the peripheral venipuncture sample is considered predictive of CRBSI.[11,38] This technique is used more frequently for long-term tunneled catheters. A comparative meta-analysis of various diagnostic methods reviewed 7 studies utilizing the differential quantitative blood culture method. The overall pooled sensitivity was 75% to 93%, and the specificity was 97% to 100%.[36]

Differential Time to Positivity for Central Venous Catheter versus Peripheral Blood Cultures

This method makes use of continuous blood culture monitoring for positivity.[11] Radiometric methods are utilized comparing the differential time to positivity for qualitative cultures of blood samples drawn from the catheter and from a peripheral vein. This test is based on the hypothesis that the time to positivity of a culture is closely related to the inoculum size of the microorganisms. The difference between the time required for culture positivity in simultaneously drawn samples of catheter blood and peripheral blood are measured. Raad determined that the cutoff time for positivity was 120 minutes.[39] A subsequent meta-analysis revealed an overall sensitivity of 85% and a specificity of 81%.[36]

Catheter and Site Maintenance

Skin preparation before insertion and appropriate site and catheter maintenance are crucial factors in preventing CRBSI. The long-term maintenance of catheters and insertion sites has been extensively studied, including the type and frequency of dressing changes, intravenous (IV) tubing changes, skin antiseptics, topical ointments, antibiotic lock solutions, and guidewire exchange to diagnose or prevent infection. Great care should be taken in preparing the insertion site, practicing sterile precautions during catheter insertion, and maintaining sterility in the day-to-day use of the catheter. All members of the multidisciplinary patient care team, including physicians, nurses, nursing assistants, technicians, and pharmacists, should be educated about the critical importance of hand hygiene, standards of catheter care, and the aseptic preparation of infusate solutions. Hospital-wide and ICU policies should be regularly reviewed and reinforced with all team members to maintain an environment of conscientious patient safety.

ADJUNCTS TO CATHETER AND SITE MAINTENANCE

Several trials have compared various antiseptic solutions' efficacy in preventing CRBSI. Parienti et al. randomized 223 catheters to either a 10% aqueous povidone-iodine solution or a 5% povidone-iodine solution in 70% ethanol.[40] They observed that the ethanol-based solution was associated with a lower catheter colonization rate and a longer time to catheter colonization compared to the aqueous solution. However, the rates of catheter-related bacteremia were similar in both groups.[40] Mimoz et al. compared 5% povidone-iodine in 70% ethanol to a solution of 0.25% chlorhexidine gluconate, 0.025% benzalkonium chloride, and 4% benzylic alcohol.[41] A total of 538 catheters were randomized, with 481 of these providing evaluable culture results. The solutions were used for skin preparation and then as a single application during subsequent dressing changes. There was a 50% decrease in the incidence of catheter colonization and a trend toward lower rates of CRBSI in the chlorhexidine group.[41] Other studies have focused on trials of chlorhexidine-impregnated dressing materials as a strategy to decrease CRBSI. A meta-analysis of eight studies was conducted by Ho et al.[42] The chlorhexidine-impregnated dressing demonstrated an odds ratio (OR) for catheter or exit site bacterial colonization of 0.47, $P < 0.001$. Like other investigators, they observed a trend towards reduction in CRBSI. Interestingly, they estimated that the dressings would have to be used on 142 catheters, with a total cost of $532.50, to prevent one episode of CRBSI.[42] It is noteworthy that although the studies cited here achieved impressive reductions in colonization, none demonstrated significant reduction in CRBSI. Thus, dressing materials alone are not sufficient to realize decreases in CRBSI rates.

Timsit et al. performed a prospective randomized multicenter study in 2009 comparing standard catheter dressings and site care to a chlorhexidine gluconate–impregnated sponge dressing to determine the effect on catheter colonization and the incidence of major catheter-related infection (defined as either catheter-related clinical sepsis without bloodstream infection or catheter-related bloodstream infection).[43] This study also randomized patients to receive dressing changes at either 3 or 7 days. The novel chlorhexidine dressing reduced catheter colonization from 15.8/1000 catheter-days to 6.3/1000 catheter-days (hazard ratio 0.36, 0.28–0.46, $P < .001$). Similar hazard risk reduction was identified for both major catheter-related infection (1.4/1000 catheter-days versus 0.6/1000 catheter-days) and CRBSI (1.3/1000 catheter-days versus 0.4/1000 catheter-days). It should be mentioned that almost 50% of the catheters studied were arterial catheters. Also, the majority of the catheter sites required more frequent dressing changes before the 3- or 7-day time periods expired. The authors concluded that 117 catheters would require management with the chlorhexidine gluconate–impregnated sponges to prevent one major catheter-related infection.[43] Use of these dressings with central venous catheters and arterial catheters in the ICU reduced the risk of infection even when background infection rates were low. Reducing the frequency of changing unsoiled adherent dressings from every 3 days to every 7 days modestly decreased the total number of dressing changes and appeared to be safe.[43]

Investigation to find other effective adjuncts to CRBSI prevention has extended into use of antimicrobials as flush (or lock) solutions. Safdar and Maki published a meta-analysis of seven prospective, randomized trials comparing vancomycin-heparin to heparin alone as lock solutions for prevention of CRBSI. The study cohorts included patients with cancer, those requiring parenteral nutrition, and critically ill neonates. The vancomycin-heparin lock solution was associated with an odds reduction of 0.49 for CRBSI compared to heparin alone.[44] When vancomycin was used as a true lock solution, it conferred a greater benefit, with an OR of 0.34. The authors concluded that this strategy warranted consideration for high-risk patients requiring central access.[44] Other antibiotic-based solutions have been tested in various populations, with similarly impressive reductions in CRBSI rates.[45]

In addition to evaluating topical application of antimicrobial solutions and lock solutions, investigators have tested various strategies of catheter replacement as a means to reduce CRBSI by decreasing prolonged exposure to any individual catheter. Both new-site replacement and guidewire exchange protocols have been examined. Cook et al. systematically reviewed the literature consisting of 12 relevant trials of catheter replacement over a guidewire versus new-site placement.[46] They observed that new-site placement presented a higher risk of mechanical complications compared to guidewire exchange. However, guidewire exchange, regardless of whether the patient was suspected of having an infection, was associated with trends toward higher rates of catheter site infection and CRBSI. Additionally, exchanging catheters routinely every 3 days, either by new-site placement or by guidewire exchange, was not effective in reducing CRBSI compared to exchange on an as-needed basis. They concluded that if guidewire exchange is necessary, meticulous sterile technique is required.[46]

SUGGESTED METHOD FOR GUIDEWIRE EXCHANGE

The following procedure of guidewire exchange is recommended:

1. Guidewire exchange begins with a complete sterilization of the external portion of the exiting catheter before the guidewire is placed. All IV tubing, including parenteral nutrition tubing, is carefully separated from the catheter hubs and replaced with sterile caps or plugs. The separated IV tubing tips are also sterilely protected until they are reconnected to the new catheter or preferably replaced with new tubing.
2. Sterile disposable gowns and gloves are worn by personnel performing the procedure, along with surgical hats and masks, and a sterile field for the necessary equipment is prepared on a bedside table.
3. The distal ports of the catheter to be exchanged are placed on a sterile paper or cloth towel barrier (usually provided in the new catheter kit), and the insertion site, along with a 10-cm circumferential area of skin and the entire external portion of the catheter from insertion site to capped hubs, is scrubbed for 5 minutes with 10×10-cm gauze pads soaked in 4% chlorhexidine skin cleanser. The most important aspect of this preparation is that chlorhexidine be allowed to remain in contact with the skin and the entire external portion of the catheter for at least 5 minutes.
4. After this scrub, the excess soap is carefully removed from the area with dry 10×10-cm gauze pads, and the skin sutures securing the catheter are removed with a No. 11 disposable scalpel.
5. The operator then exchanges sterile surgical gloves, and the entire area is widely draped with six sterile cloth surgical towels or other large commercially available sterile barriers, with the distal catheter hubs being carefully and sterilely removed from the previous paper or cloth towel barrier to the new widely draped sterile barrier.
6. A sterile guidewire is carefully inserted through the distal port of the catheter after removal of the cap, with care taken that the wire does not touch the external portion of the hub.
7. The old catheter is carefully removed, with care taken to avoid contact with the surrounding skin.
8. Appropriate culture specimens are then obtained by amputating the 5-cm intracutaneous segment and the 5-cm distal tip of the removed catheter. This can be done with a sterile disposable suture removal kit (containing disposable forceps and scissors). The segments are placed into two separate culturettes following removal of the cotton-tipped swab, and the tip of the culturette is manually crushed to release the inner preservative. The two culturettes are labeled appropriately and transported immediately to the microbiology laboratory for semiquantitative or quantitative cultures.
9. The portion of the guidewire protruding from the skin is then cleaned with 4% chlorhexidine. Before handling the new catheter, it is best to change to a third pair of sterile gloves. A new catheter is then placed over the guidewire into the proper anatomic position.
10. The catheter is sutured into place after the guidewire is removed.

A chest radiograph is generally not required after guidewire exchange.

For CVCs (16-30 cm in length), both the tip and the intracutaneous 5-cm segments from the removed catheter are sent for semiquantitative or quantitative culture. For PA catheters and introducers, the 5-cm tip of the PA catheter and the 5-cm intracutaneous segment of the catheter introducer are sent in separate culturettes for semiquantitative or quantitative culture.

Whereas strategies aimed at reducing CRBSI are traditionally focused on isolated technical interventions, there is accumulating evidence that systems-based interventions are also very effective in improving patient outcomes. Common themes in the various systems-based strategies are education of nursing and physician staff in evidence-based practices of hand hygiene and catheter site preparation. Additionally, these interventions should employ ongoing compliance and CRBSI surveillance and feedback to the teams with observed compliance and CRBSI event rates. By utilizing evidence-based practices, monitoring compliance and CRBSI rates, and updating the care teams concerning their progress, an environment of conscientious quality improvement and patient safety is created. Several investigators have studied this type of intervention and realized 50% to greater than 70% reductions in CRBSI rates across various critical care settings.[47-49] It is clear that individual technical innovations offer the means to decrease CRBSI rates. However, initiating a multimodal approach that incorporates evidence-based practices, team education, results tracking, and feedback may offer the most robust and sustainable improvements in patient outcomes.

Infection Risks of Specific Catheters

Previously we have discussed CRBSI as a uniform phenomenon without distinguishing the specific burden of risk associated with specific catheters. Each type of catheter carries an associated degree of risk for CRBSI. Many investigators have focused on individual catheter types when reporting these risks. Maki et al. conducted a meta-analysis of 200 published prospective studies encompassing 65,105 intravascular catheters ranging from peripheral IV catheters to left ventricular assist devices. The pooled mean CRBSI rates vary from 0.1/1000 catheter-days observed in subcutaneous venous ports to 9.0/1000 catheter-days reported for venous cutdowns.[4] In the following sections, we will discuss the most commonly used catheters and their associated CRBSI infection risks.

MULTIPLE-LUMEN CENTRAL VENOUS CATHETERS

Zürcher et al. conducted a meta-analysis of five published reports from randomized controlled trials to test whether the number of catheter lumens influenced catheter colonization and CRBSI. The authors observed a statistically significant difference in the CRBSI rate between single and multiple-lumen catheters. The multiple-lumen catheters were associated with an 8.4% rate of CRBSI, while single-lumen catheter rates were 3.1%.[50] The report is limited because the number of infections per 1000 catheter-days is not reported. Lorente et al. conducted a prospective study of all patients admitted to a 24-bed ICU in Spain. They observed an overall CRBSI rate of 2.79/1000 catheter-days. Data were analyzed by anatomic site. Femoral, jugular, and subclavian sites were analyzed, with the CRBSI risk decreasing in that order.[51] Maki et al. observed a range of CRBSI for short-term, noncuffed central venous catheters from 1.2 to 4.8/1000 catheter-days.[4]

ARTERIAL CATHETERS

Arterial catheterization for hemodynamic monitoring is a common procedure in the ICU. The anatomic sites used for arterial access include the radial artery (the site most commonly used), brachial, dorsalis pedis, axillary, and femoral arteries. Lorente et al. prospectively observed 2018 ICU patients over 3 years to analyze the incidence of CRBSI according to different access sites. The overall incidence of CRBSI for arterial catheters in their study was 0.59/1000 catheter-days. They observed no infections in the brachial and dorsalis pedis sites, although these sites combined accounted for less than 10% of the total number of catheters included in the study. The incidence of CRBSI was 0.25/1000 catheter-days for the radial site and 1.92/1000 catheter-days for the femoral site. They concluded that using the femoral site increases the risk of arterial catheter-related infection.[3] The incidence rates for arterial CRBSI noted by Lorente was lower than the pooled

mean of 1.7/1000 catheter-days published in the meta-analysis by Maki et al.[4] Of note, the study by Lorente was published in 2006, the same year as the review by Maki, and was not included in Maki's report.

LONG-TERM CENTRAL VENOUS CATHETERS

Although seldom used in the acute critical care setting, catheters for long-term central venous access in both the inpatient and outpatient setting are frequently employed for total parenteral nutrition and chemotherapy. In cancer patients, the catheters most frequently used have been long-dwelling tunneled devices (Hickman, Broviac, Groshong).[52] These catheters allow for long-term IV therapy without the need for frequent catheter exchanges. Darouiche et al. conducted a randomized controlled trial comparing antimicrobial-impregnated, non-tunneled, long-term central venous catheters to nonimpregnated tunneled catheters in terms of rates of catheter colonization and CRBSI. Their study included 312 catheters. They observed no significant difference in CRBSI rates between the two types of catheters.[53] The tunneled catheters were associated with 1.43/1000 catheter-days, whereas the impregnated catheters had a rate of 0.36/1000 catheter-days, $P = 0.13$.[53] In the meta-analysis by Maki et al. the CRBSI rate for long-term cuffed and tunneled central venous and hemodialysis catheters was 1.6/1000 catheter-days. The rate for subcutaneous ports was 0.1/1000 catheter-days.[4]

The rates of colonization per 1000 catheter-days observed in Darouiche's study were 7.9 for antimicrobial-impregnated catheters and 6.3 for tunneled catheters. These rates were not significantly different, $P=0.46$.[53]

PERIPHERALLY INSERTED CENTRAL VENOUS CATHETERS

Peripherally inserted central venous catheters (PICCs) have become a standard approach to securing long-term IV access for patients in both the inpatient and outpatient settings. PICCs are regarded as durable and associated with easier insertion and removal compared to long-term central venous catheters. Despite the ease of placement and removal, PICCs are no less vulnerable to CRBSI than other forms of vascular access. Safdar and Maki prospectively studied patients from two randomized trials assessing the efficacy of chlorhexidine-impregnated sponge dressings and chlorhexidine for cutaneous antisepsis. In total, 115 patients had 251 PICCs placed for a mean duration of catheterization of 11.3 days. A CRBSI rate of 3.5/1000 catheter-days was observed in this cohort. It is important to note that the CRBSI rate was calculated from the pooled control groups of both trials.[54] A lower rate of CRBSI was observed by Walshe et al., who prospectively followed 351 patients with PICC lines over a 1-year period. A CRBSI rate of 2.46/1000 catheter-days including 19 primary and 7 secondary bloodstream infections were found in this cohort.[55]

Table 128-1 from Maki et al.[4] lists rates of intravascular device–related bloodstream infection caused by various types of devices used for vascular access.

Adjuncts To Prevent CRBSI

Central venous catheters should be removed as soon as possible and when no longer medically necessary. Hand hygiene, use of the subclavian vein site when possible, preparation with chlorhexidine-based solutions, and maximal sterile barrier precautions during catheter insertion are all important in reducing CRBSI risk. In addition to these recommendations, a number of other technological advances may be indicated.

ANTISEPTIC-IMPREGNATED AND ANTIBIOTIC-IMPREGNATED CATHETERS

Central venous catheters impregnated with various antiseptic and antibiotic agents are now commonly used to reduce the frequency of CRBSI. There are conflicting studies in the literature concerning

TABLE 128-1	Rates of Intravascular Device–Related Bloodstream Infection Caused by Various Types of Devices Used for Vascular Access							
					Rates of IVD-Related Bloodstream Infection			
					Per 100 Devices		Per 1000 IVD Days	
Device	No. of Studies	No. of Catheters	No. of IVD (d)	No. of BSIs	Pooled Mean	95% CI	Pooled Mean	95% CI
Peripheral IV Catheters								
Plastic catheters	110	10,910	28,720	13	0.1	0.1-0.2	0.5	0.2-0.7
Steel needles	1	148	350	3	2.0	0.0-4.3	8.6	0.0-18.2
Venous cutdown	1	27	111	1	3.7	0.0-10.8	9.0	0.0-26.6
Midline catheters	3	514	9251	2	0.4	0.0-0.9	0.2	0.0-0.5
Arterial catheters for hemodynamic monitoring	14	4366	21,397	37	0.8	0.6-1.1	1.7	1.2-2.3
Peripherally Inserted Central Catheters								
Inpatient and outpatient	15	3566	105,839	112	3.1	2.6-3.7	1.1	0.9-1.3
Inpatient	6	625	7137	15	2.4	1.2-3.6	2.1	1.0-3.2
Outpatient	9	2813	98,702	97	3.5	2.8-4.1	1.0	0.8-1.2
Short-Term Noncuffed Central Venous Catheters								
Nonmedicated								
Non-tunneled	79	20,226	322,283	883	4.4	4.1-4.6	2.7	2.6-2.9
Tunneled	9	741	20,065	35	4.7	3.2-6.2	1.7	1.2-2.3
Medicated								
Chlorhexidine-silver sulfadiazine	18	3367	54,054	89	2.6	2.1-3.2	1.6	1.3-2.0
Minocycline-rifampin	3	690	5797	7	1.0	0.3-1.8	1.2	0.3-2.1
Silver impregnated	2	154	1689	8	5.2	1.7-8.7	4.7	1.5-8.0
Silver iontophoretic	2	396	4796	16	4.0	2.1-6.0	3.3	1.7-5.0
Benzalkonium chloride	1	277	2493	12	4.3	1.9-6.7	4.8	2.1-7.5
Pulmonary artery catheters	13	2057	8143	30	1.5	0.9-2.0	3.7	2.4-5.0
Hemodialysis Catheters								
Temporary, noncuffed	16	3066	51,840	246	8.0	7.0-9.0	4.8	4.2-5.3
Long-term, cuffed and tunneled	16	2806	373,563	596	21.2	19.7-22.8	1.6	1.5-1.7
Cuffed and tunneled central venous catheters	29	4512	622,535	1013	22.5	21.2-23.7	1.6	1.5-1.7
Subcutaneous Venous Ports								
Central	14	3007	983,480	81	3.6	2.9-4.3	0.1	0.0-0.1
Peripheral	3	579	162,203	23	4.0	2.4-5.6	0.1	0.1-0.2
Intraaortic balloon pumps	1	101	414	3	3.0	0.0-6.3	7.3	0.0-15.4
Left ventricular assist devices	3	157	19,653	41	26.1	19.2-33.0	2.1	1.5-2.7

Data from Maki DG, Kluger DM, Crnich CJ. The risk of bloodstream infection in adults with different intravascular devices: a systematic review of 200 published prospective studies. Mayo Clin Proc 2006;81:1159–71. Reproduced with permission from the publisher.

BSI, bloodstream infection; *CI*, confidence interval; *IV*, intravenous; *IVD*, intravascular device.

whether or not such catheters are cost-effective.[56-59] Among the most commonly used antiseptic impregnated catheters is one in which both the inner and outer lumens are bonded with silver sulfadiazine and chlorhexidine antiseptics. Both silver sulfadiazine and chlorhexidine possess broad-spectrum antimicrobial properties, and the two agents exhibit a synergistic activity, reducing the risk of the emergence of resistant strains of bacteria.[56,60] Reports of hypersensitivity to chlorhexidine have emerged as its use has become more commonplace.[61]

In the late 1990s, polyurethane CVCs impregnated with minocycline and rifampin on both the internal and external surfaces were developed.[62] Initial concerns that widespread use of surface antibiotics for preventing CRBSI may contribute to the emergence of antibiotic-resistant organisms have not been identified.[63,64]

Recommendations

The following recommendations are based on the studies reviewed in this chapter and published CDC guidelines.[24,25] These guidelines are currently in revision, and the reader is encouraged to refer to the CDC website for any updates.

Physicians in critical care units are encouraged to study their own patient populations to determine the incidence of significant catheter colonization and CRBSI and to develop appropriate guidelines for catheter exchange and site maintenance. On the basis of currently available information, peripheral arterial catheters, CVCs, and PA catheters do not require "routine" exchange either to a different site or over a guidewire. Although the risk of colonization and bacteremia increases with time, the optimal time for catheter removal is not known for peripheral arterial catheters, central venous catheters, and pulmonary artery catheters. Routine catheter exchange in critically ill patients does not alter infection risks.

Recommendations for short-term catheter placement are outlined in Table 128-2. Any catheter (peripheral or central) that is placed under less than ideal conditions should be treated as a potential source of infection. Generally, such a catheter should be removed and a new catheter inserted at a different site if catheterization is needed for longer than 48 hours. Ideal conditions for catheter insertion include:

- Use of sterile disposable surgical gowns, masks, hats, and gloves
- Careful preparation of the skin site with a chlorhexidine solution
- Wide draping of the area to create an adequate sterile field

The subclavian site is preferred over the internal jugular or femoral site for long-term (>72 hours) catheter use because of the higher colonization rates associated with neck and groin insertion sites. The only exception to this rule is for short-term hemodialysis catheters. In this situation, the internal jugular vein or femoral vein is preferred because of the risk for developing subclavian vein stenosis.

The indication for removal of a non-tunneled central venous catheter is the presence of an unexplained bacteremia. In the critical care setting, fever is an unreliable indicator of CRBSI. The authors think that guidewire exchange *using the strict protocol described in this chapter* is an acceptable alternative to placing a catheter at a different site, particularly in patients with difficult or compromised venous access. The most recent CDC guidelines discourage this practice[24,25] because 20% to 25% of catheters removed for suspected infection yield positive semiquantitative culture results. Despite these culture results, less than 10% of catheters removed are associated with CRBSI.

In our experience, antiseptic-impregnated central venous and pulmonary artery catheter introducers allow for prolonged catheter use without significantly increasing the risk of CRBSI over time. Individual institutions and critical care units should review their infection rates and catheter insertion practices to determine whether this readily available technology is cost-effective for their patients.

TABLE 128-2	Recommendations for Short-Term Catheter Placement		
Catheter Type	Preferred Anatomic Site(s) (in Order of Preference)	Frequency of Catheter Exchange	Guidewire Exchange an Option?
Peripheral venous catheter	Upper extremity[†]	72-96 h[†]	No
Emergency peripheral venous catheter*	Upper extremity[†]	24-48 h[†]	No
CVC (single-lumen or multiple-lumen)	Subclavian[†‡] Internal jugular Femoral	Routine replacement not recommended[†‡] Routine replacement not recommended[†‡] Remove within 72 h[‡]	Yes[‡] Yes[‡] Yes[‡]
Peripherally inserted CVC	Upper extremity	Routine replacement not recommended[†]	No
PA catheter and PA catheter introducer	Subclavian[†‡] Internal jugular	Routine replacement not recommended[†‡] Routine replacement not recommended[†‡]	Yes[‡] Yes[‡]
Short-term hemodialysis	Internal jugular Femoral Subclavian	Routine replacement not recommended[†‡] Routine replacement not recommended[†‡] Routine replacement not recommended[†‡]	No recommendation[†] No recommendation[†] No recommendation[†]
Peripheral arterial catheters	Radial[‡] Femoral Axillary	Routine replacement not recommended[†‡] Routine replacement not recommended	Yes[‡] No[‡] No[‡]

*Catheter inserted under emergency conditions in which sterile preparation may have been less than optimal.
[†]Healthcare Infection Control Practices Advisory Committee guidelines. (Data from O'Grady NP et al. Am J Infect Control 2002;30:477.[25])
[‡]Author's recommendation.
CVC, central venous catheter; *PA*, pulmonary artery.

KEY POINTS

1. Catheter-related bloodstream infection (CRBSI) is the third most common nosocomial infection in the United States.

2. A variety of factors including the patient "host," catheter composition, and microorganism/catheter surface interactions contribute to the ultimate development of CRBSI.

3. Although the risk of colonization and bacteremia increases with time, the optimal time for catheter removal is not known for peripheral arterial, central venous, and pulmonary artery catheters.

4. The clinical diagnosis of a catheter infection that requires treatment by catheter removal, antibiotics, or both, is insensitive and nonspecific.

5. Various quantitative catheter culture techniques have been developed to distinguish true infection from colonization; in general, qualitative blood cultures obtained through the catheter should not routinely be used.

6. Skin preparation before insertion and appropriate site maintenance are crucial factors in preventing CRBSI.

7. Existing studies support the general guideline that central venous, pulmonary artery, and peripheral arterial catheters should not be routinely changed at specific intervals to prevent infection.

8. Antiseptic and antibiotic impregnation of catheter surfaces may be helpful in reducing catheter colonization and CRBSI.

9. All members of the multidisciplinary patient care team should be educated about the critical importance of hand hygiene, standards of care, and aseptic preparation of infusate solutions to maintain an environment of conscientious patient safety.

ANNOTATED REFERENCES

Edwards JR, Peterson KD, Mu Y, et al. National Healthcare Safety Network (NHSN) report: data summary for 2006 through 2008, issued December 2009. Am J Infect Control 2009;37:783-805.
This important paper should be read by anyone who wants to understand the mechanisms of hospital infection surveillance and its implications. It is important to understand that surveillance data have subtle differences compared to specific hospital infection data, particularly when reviewing catheter-related bloodstream infections.

Maki DG, Kluger DM, Crnich CJ. The risk of bloodstream infection in adults with different intravascular devices: a systematic review of 200 published prospective studies. Mayo Clin Proc 2006;81:1159-71.
This is an excellent review article of all the current laboratory methods for diagnosing catheter-related bloodstream infections.

Donlan RM, Costerton JW. Biofilms: survival mechanisms of clinically relevant microorganisms. Clin Microbiol Rev 2002;15:167-93.
This paper gives an excellent review of the pathophysiology involved with biofilm formation. It gives insight into why certain organisms are difficult to treat without removal of the catheter.

Mermel LA, Farr BM, Sheretz RJ, et al. Guidelines for the management of intravascular catheter-related infections. Clin Infect Dis 2001;32:1249-72.

This paper was written by acknowledged experts in the field and provides concise and well-written guidelines for managing and preventing catheter-related infections.

Safdar N, Maki DG. The pathogenesis of catheter-related bloodstream infection with non-cuffed short-term central venous catheter. Intensive Care Med 2004;30:62-7.
This article provides a concise review of the four mechanisms of the pathogenesis of CRBSI.

Raad II, Hanna HA. Intravascular catheter-related infections: new horizons and recent advances. Arch Intern Med 2002;162:871-8.
This is an excellent review article covering pathogenesis, treatment, and diagnostic techniques for catheter-related infections.

O'Grady NP, Alexander M, Dellinger EP, Gerberding JL, Heard SO, Maki DG, et al. Guidelines for the prevention of intravascular catheter-related infections. Centers for Disease Control and Prevention. MMWR Recomm Rep 2002;51:1-29.
An exhaustive and comprehensive review of catheter-related infections by a multidisciplinary panel of recognized experts. The guidelines are currently being revised by the CDC to incorporate new scientific data and clinical recommendations.

REFERENCES

Access the complete reference list online at http://www.expertconsult.com.

129

Pathophysiology of Sepsis and Multiple Organ Dysfunction

KONRAD REINHART | FRANK BLOOS

Pathophysiology of Sepsis

The term *sepsis* is derived from a Greek word meaning "putrid." It was believed that putrefaction of a wound was caused by contact with air and that death occurred when the process of putrefaction reached the blood (septicemia). In the 19th century, the concept of infection as a cause of sepsis was introduced by the Austrian obstetrician, Ignaz Philipp Semmelweis and the English surgeon, Joseph Lister. From then on, the term *sepsis* was closely connected to bacterial infection. However, as the understanding of human immune physiology improved, the importance of the host response to infection in the pathophysiology of sepsis was recognized.

Sepsis has been defined as an invasion of microorganisms or their toxins into the bloodstream, together with the host response to this invasion.[1] Thus, the pathophysiology of sepsis combines the impact of infection with the host response of generalized inflammation, which finally leads to multiorgan dysfunction and death. This definition has been extended by the addition of several terms to more carefully describe the disease and its pathophysiology (Table 129-1). The American College of Chest Physicians/Society of Critical Care Medicine (ACCP/SCCM) Consensus Conference defined sepsis as a systemic inflammatory response syndrome (SIRS) caused by infection.[2] More recently it has been recognized that SIRS is counteracted by a hypoinflammatory state that also plays an important role in the further development of organ dysfunction.[3]

Sepsis is characterized by loss of hemostatic balance and endothelial dysfunction, which in turn severely compromise the cardiocirculatory system as well as intracellular homeostasis. Cellular hypoxia and apoptosis (programmed cell death) then contribute to organ dysfunction and death. The network of organ systems affected by sepsis is depicted in Figure 129-1.

MICROBIOLOGICAL STIMULUS

By definition, *infection* is a fundamental part of the pathophysiology of sepsis. Any microorganism able to induce infection in humans may be complicated by sepsis. Bacteria as well as fungi, parasites, and to a lesser degree viruses can trigger the mechanisms that lead to sepsis. Although SIRS is the final common pathway of this process, the signal transduction pathway from infection to complex host response differs with the microbiological stimuli. Induction of an innate immune response is triggered by specific microbial molecules (e.g., bacterial wall components, exotoxins, bacterial DNA, viral RNA) called *pathogen-associated molecular patterns* (PAMPs). *Damage-associated molecular patterns* (DAMPs) are the noninfectious equivalents to PAMPs. DAMPs are released after cellular injury of the host (i.e., trauma) and can also induce the innate immune response.[4]

The presence of PAMPs is sensed by recognition molecules called *pattern-recognition proteins* (PRR), which are able to initiate a host response. These proteins may be categorized into secreted, transmembrane, and cytosolic PRRs. The Toll-like receptors (TLRs) represent the membrane PRRs. Eleven different TLRs have been discovered in mammals, whereas TLR-11 is not expressed in humans (Table 129-2). Retinoic acid-inducible gene I (RIG-I)–like receptors (RLRs) and the nucleotide-binding domain and leucine-rich repeat-containing receptors (NLRs) are cytosolic PRRs. RLRs recognize viral RNA and some

double-stranded DNA. NLRs represent a large family of intracellular sensors that can detect pathogens and stress signals. NLRs detect microbiological products such as peptidoglycans and other degradation products of microorganisms as well as stress-related substances.[5,6]

Gram-Negative Sepsis

In gram-negative bacteremia, initiation of the immune response is mediated primarily by lipopolysaccharide (LPS), a bacterial cell wall product. In plasma, LPS is bound to the LPS binding protein (LBP). Bound LPS is transported to the opsonic receptor, CD14, which is located on several cell membranes including on monocytes.[7] A soluble form of CD14 interacts with CD14-negative cells (e.g., dendritic cells). However, CD14 alone cannot explain the actions of LPS, because CD14 does not have an intracellular tail.

Another binding site of LPS is the transmembranous receptor, TLR4, which exists in combination with the accessory protein, MD2.[8] The binding of LPS to CD14 and TLR4 induces, via other molecules, activation of the transcription factor, nuclear factor kappa-B (NF-κB). Activated NF-κB migrates into the nucleus where it binds to and activates gene promoters, resulting in the transcription and expression of genes for cytokines and other proinflammatory mediators.[9] In monocytes, LPS also induces cytokine transcription via the triggering receptor expressed on myeloid cells-1 and the myeloid DAP12-associated lectin.[10] Intracellular pattern-recognition proteins in monocytes for LPS have recently been identified as another pathway of cytokine expression and include nucleotide-binding oligomerization domain 1 and 2 as LPS binding sites.[11]

Gram-Positive Sepsis

During the last decade, gram-positive bacteria have gained greater importance as causative organisms for sepsis.[12] Gram-positive bacteria lack endotoxin and are recognized by cell wall components such as peptidoglycans and released bacterial toxins (exotoxins). Recently, lipoteichoic acid (LTA), a component of the cell wall in all gram-positive bacteria, has been recognized as the main pattern for recognition of gram-positive bacteria.[13] TLR2 has been identified as the only pattern-recognition protein for gram-positive bacteria.[14] The relationship between LTA and TLR2 is not completely clarified. Although LTA clearly interacts with TLR2, TLR2 is not a specific receptor for LTA, because TLR2 can recognize several other components of gram-positive bacteria.[15] Gram-positive and gram-negative sepsis are indistinguishable clinically, suggesting a similar pathway of signal transduction. Indeed, peptidoglycans and LTA stimulate the release of tumor necrosis factor alpha (TNF-α), interleukin (IL)-6, and IL-10. It has been speculated that CD14 is also involved in the signaling of gram-positive infections.

Some exotoxins cause a special type of septic shock called the *toxic shock syndrome* (TSS). TSS may be caused by the exotoxin, TSS toxin-1, staphylococcal enterotoxins from *Staphylococcus aureus*, or streptococcal pyogenic exotoxins.[16] These toxins are capable of acting as so-called superantigens which deploy their effects via the T-cell antigen receptor (TCR). The TCR consists of five variable elements: Vβ, Dβ, Jβ, Vα, and Jα. Conventionally, the T cell is activated if the major histocompatibility complex (MHC) of an antigen-presenting cell matches all five elements. Thus, T cells are activated by proper antigen contact only. This results in the stimulation of about 1 in 10,000 T cells. However, a

TABLE 129-1	Definitions
Term	*Definition*
Bacteremia	Presence of viable bacteria in the blood
Systemic inflammatory response syndrome (SIRS)	Generalized hyperinflammatory response to several impacts
Sepsis	SIRS caused by infection
Severe sepsis	Sepsis associated with organ dysfunction
Septic shock	Sepsis associated with arterial hypotension

Data from ACCP/SCCM Consensus Conference Committee. Definition for sepsis and organ failure and guidelines for the use of innovative therapies in sepsis. Crit Care Med 1992;20:864–74.

TABLE 129-2	Human Toll-Like Receptors and Their Natural Ligands	
TLR Type	*Related Pathogen-Associated Molecular Pattern*	*Location*
TLR1 (via TLR2)	Bacterial products such as tri-acyl lipopeptides	Cell surface
TLR2	Gram-positive bacterial products, including peptidoglycans; some virus-related proteins	Cell surface
TLR3	Viral double-stranded RNA	Endosomal
TLR4	Endotoxin, other bacterial products, some fungal products	Cell surface
TLR5	Flagellin	Cell surface
TLR6 (via TLR2)	Some bacterial products	Cell surface
TLR7	Single-stranded RNA	Endosomal
TLR8	Viral single-stranded RNA	Endosomal
TLR9	Viral and bacterial DNA	Endosomal
TLR10	Unknown	

TLR, Toll-like receptor.

superantigen such as TSS toxin-1 works as a bridge between the MHC and the Vβ chain of the TCR only (Figure 129-2).[17] Because T-cell activation now occurs independently of a match between the MHC and TCR, about 20% of the entire T-cell pool may be activated at once. Besides further T-cell proliferation, T-cell activation causes the release of several cytokines (i.e., interferon gamma [IFN-γ], IL-2, TNF-α) from T cells, as well as IL-1β and TNF-α from macrophages. Thus, the presence of superantigens results in a release of cytokines similar to gram-negative sepsis. It is assumed that actions other than cytokine production may be responsible for actions of superantigens in TSS; for example, superantigens may amplify the effects of LPS.

Other Microbiological Stimuli of Sepsis

Sepsis can also be induced by fungi, viruses, and parasites. Signal transduction by nonbacterial products, however, is not as well characterized as bacterial sepsis. In part, this may be due to the fact that induction of cytokine release differs markedly not only among different microorganisms but also among species. Nevertheless, the release

of proinflammatory mediators has been demonstrated during infections with nonbacterial infections such as *Candida albicans*[18] and *Plasmodium falciparum.*[19] The signal transduction in viral infections is complicated by the fact that viruses can interfere with TNF-related cytokine release to avoid the host's antiviral activities.[20] Pattern recognition of viruses occurs mainly via endosomal TLR receptors which detect single- and double-stranded RNA or DNA (see Table 129-2).

THE IMMUNE RESPONSE IN SEPSIS

The cytokines TNF-α and IL-1β are released by activated macrophages and CD4 T cells within the first hour after infection. These primary

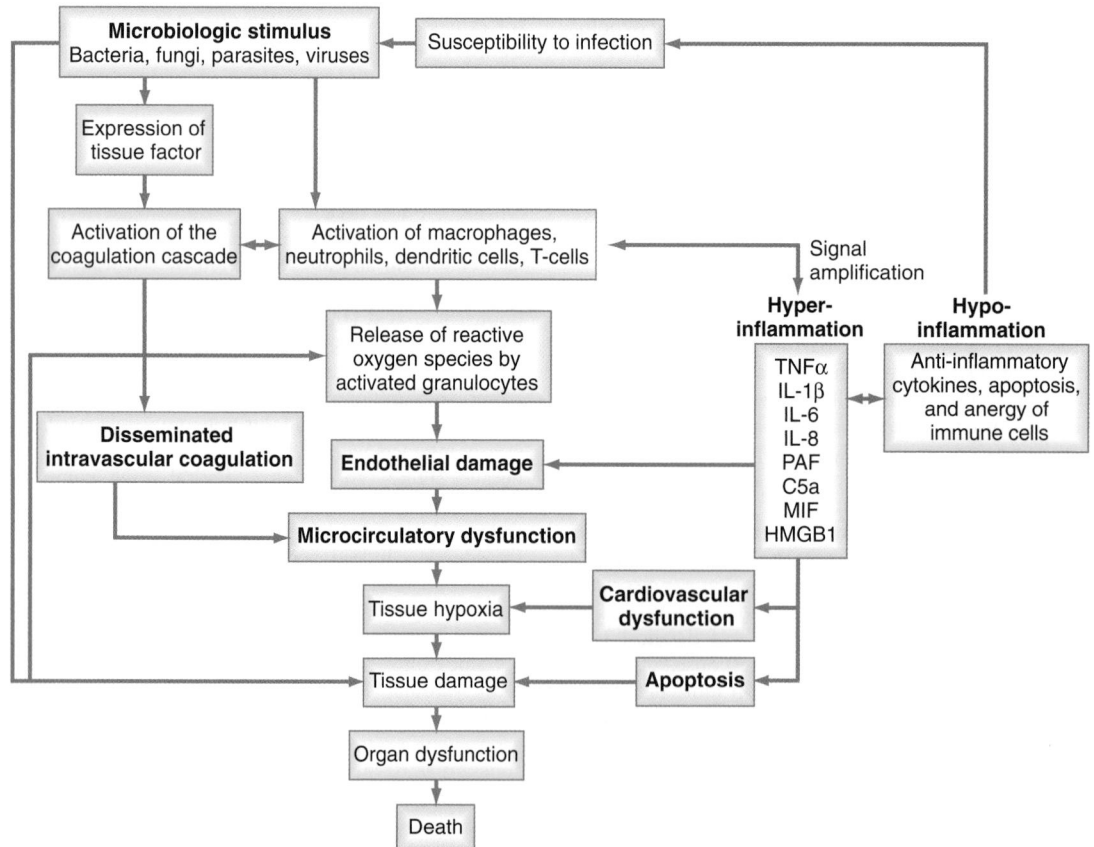

Figure 129-1　Pathophysiology of sepsis. HMGB, high-mobility group B protein; IL, interleukin; MIF, migration inhibitory factor; PAF, platelet-activating factor; TNF, tumor necrosis factor.

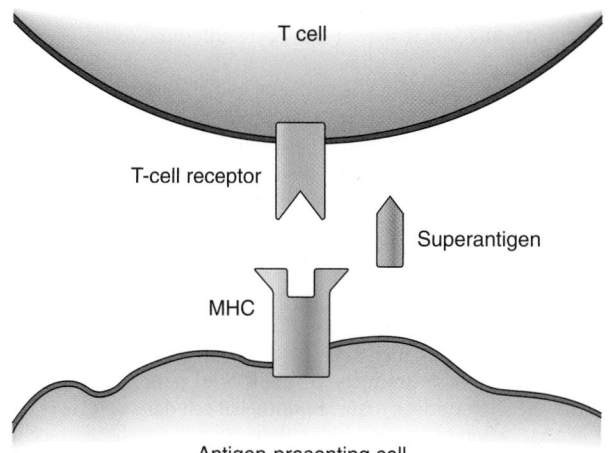

Figure 129-2 Pathophysiology of superantigen action. Superantigens work as a bridge between the T-cell receptor and the class 2 major histocompatibility complex (MHC) molecules.

mediators induce the release of several secondary mediators that amplify inflammation (Table 129-3). An important step in signal amplification is activation of the complement system. Besides being activated by antigen-antibody complexes, the complement system may be stimulated by bacterial surface sugars and endotoxin. The complement fragment C5a, a cleavage product of the complement cascade, is a strong chemoattractant. C5a appears about 2 hours after the initiation of sepsis and stimulates macrophages to further produce proinflammatory mediators. Another mediator that amplifies the immune response is macrophage migration inhibitory factor (MIF), which is produced by T cells, macrophages, monocytes, and pituitary cells in response to an infectious stimulus. MIF appears about 8 hours after the onset of sepsis and activates T cells and macrophages to produce proinflammatory mediators. About 24 hours after the initiation of sepsis, levels of high-mobility group box 1 (HMGB1) protein increase and appear to play a role in endotoxin-related sepsis. HMGB1 is a nuclear binding protein that, among other things, is capable of activating NF-κB. As a rather late mediator in sepsis, it is produced by macrophages and neutrophils and stimulates phagocytic cells.[21]

Normally, the inflammatory process is well balanced and is necessary for the host to overcome the infectious impact. However, under certain conditions, the amplification process of inflammation is not limited to the site of infection and becomes generalized. As noted

earlier, this phenomenon has been called the *systemic inflammatory response syndrome,* or SIRS. SIRS is not restricted to infectious stimuli; it is present in a variety of other conditions such as pancreatitis, burns, multiple trauma, and in patients undergoing heart surgery with cardiopulmonary bypass.

It is not completely understood why inflammation becomes generalized in some patients but stays localized in others. Genetic variants of cytokines may play a role in this issue. Single nucleotide polymorphisms (SNPs) are single-base changes in the DNA which do not cause obvious changes in the function of the respective cytokine. However, SNPs in some cytokines are associated with a worse outcome from septic shock or an increased risk for developing sepsis.[22-24] Among several others, such variants have been described in TNF-α, IL-6, and CD14.[25] However, results from these studies are difficult to interpret because of contradictory results and differences in populations of different ethnicities.

The immune response in sepsis does not involve only proinflammatory mediators. As in many other physiologic processes, the organism produces inhibitors to control certain reactions. Proinflammatory mediators are counteracted by antiinflammatory molecules such as IL-4 and IL-10 because CD4 T cells can switch from the production of inflammatory cytokines (type 1 helper T cells [T_H1]) to the production of antiinflammatory cytokines (type 2 helper T cells [T_H2]). Soluble TNF receptors and IL-1 receptor antagonists (IL-1Ra) are released to inhibit the actions of TNF and IL-1 in their roles as primary mediators of sepsis. T cells, neutrophils, and macrophages also may become unresponsive to infectious stimuli (anergy).[26] Another mechanism of the antiinflammatory response is the onset of apoptosis, a genetically programmed autodestructive release of proteases that induces cell death. In sepsis, enhanced apoptosis causes loss of immune effector cells, including CD4 and CD8 T cells, B cells, and dendritic cells.[27] Absolute lymphocyte counts are significantly decreased in patients with sepsis.[28] Further, apoptotic cells impair the function of surviving immune cells.[29]

Results from animal studies suggest that the autonomic nervous system is also involved in suppression of cytokine release during sepsis. In the experimental setting, vagal stimulation can inhibit TNF expression. It is hypothesized that an inflammatory reflex, with the afferent vagal nerve sensing cytokine release and an efferent immunosuppressing cholinergic arm, exists.[30] The importance of such a reflex in humans merits further investigation.

The antiinflammatory response in sepsis has been termed the *compensatory antiinflammatory response syndrome* (CARS).[3] It has been suggested that the first response to infection is hyperinflammation, which is followed by a hypoimmune state. From there, recovery would be possible, but the prolonged inability to eradicate microorganisms might result in the death of the patient.[31] However, serum levels of antiinflammatory cytokines are increased in parallel with the increase of proinflammatory mediators.[32,33] Thus, diminished inflammation develops at the same time as the process of hyperinflammation. Although the persistence of high levels of antiinflammatory mediators may contribute to mortality in septic patients, the clinical role of change between hyperinflammatory and hypoinflammatory states remains unclear.

LOSS OF HEMOSTATIC BALANCE

Under normal conditions, the vascular luminal surface has anticoagulant properties. Tissue factor is a 4.5-kD protein that is bound to cell membranes which are normally not in contact with blood. Expression of tissue factor mainly depends on release of IL-6.[34,35] Tissue factor expression occurs on mononuclear cells, but endothelial cells, polymorphonuclear cells, and other cell types may be additional sources. The expression of tissue factor induces intravascular thrombin formation initiated by the extrinsic coagulation pathway. Because this process is not restricted to a local area, it is called *disseminated intravascular coagulation* (DIC); DIC causes a consumption of coagulation factors.

Physiologically, excessive coagulation is counteracted by several natural anticoagulants including antithrombin, the thrombomodulin/

TABLE 129-3	Macrophage Mediators Involved in the Pathogenesis of Sepsis
Mediator	**Typical Effects**
Cytokines: IL-1, IL-6, IL-12, IL-15, IL-18, TNF, MIF, HMGB1, IL-10	Activate neutrophils, lymphocytes, and vascular endothelium; up-regulate cellular adhesion molecules; induce prostaglandins, nitric oxide synthase, and acute-phase proteins; induce fever IL-10 is predominantly a negative regulator of these effects.
Chemokines: IL-8, MIP-1α, MIP-1β, MCP-1, MCP-3	Mobilize and activate inflammatory cells, especially neutrophils; activate macrophages
Lipid mediators: platelet-activating factor, prostaglandins, leukotrienes, thromboxane, tissue factor	Activate vascular endothelium; regulate vascular tone; activate extrinsic coagulation cascade
Oxygen radicals: superoxide and hydroxyl radicals, nitric oxide	Antimicrobial properties; regulation of vascular tone

HMGB, high-mobility group B protein; IL, interleukin; MCP, monocyte chemoattractant protein; MIF, migration inhibitory factor; MIP, macrophage inflammatory protein; TNF, tumor necrosis factor.
Data from Cohen J. The immunopathogenesis of sepsis. Nature 2002;420:885-91.

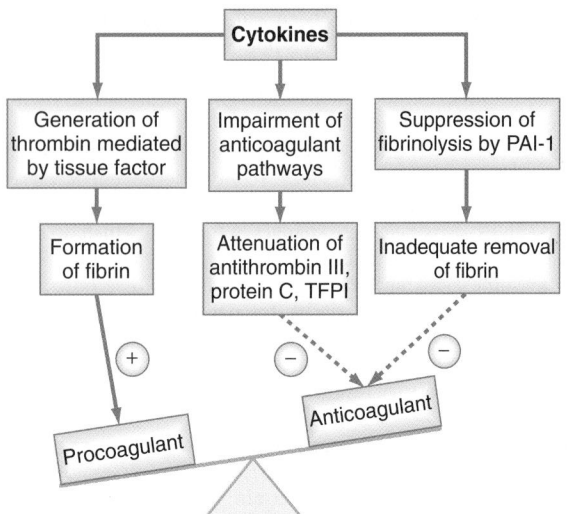

Figure 129-3 Shift of hemostatic balance toward a procoagulant state in sepsis. PAI, plasminogen activator inhibitor; TFPI, tissue factor pathway inhibitor. (*Modified from Levi M, Ten Cate H. Disseminated intravascular coagulation. N Engl J Med 1999;341:586–92.*)

protein C/protein S system, and tissue factor pathway inhibitor. In addition to the activation of tissue factor-dependent thrombin generation, anticoagulant function is attenuated in sepsis. Patients with sepsis demonstrate reduced levels of protein C and antithrombin due to consumption and reduced synthesis.[36] Thus, the physiologic balance between procoagulant and anticoagulant substances is altered in sepsis as there is a shift of the hemostatic balance toward a procoagulant state (Figure 129-3).

Besides its anticoagulant actions, the protein C pathway is an important link between coagulation and inflammation, because activated protein C has antiinflammatory properties. Protein S can bind to receptors that mediate an antiinflammatory regulatory loop of dendritic cell and monocyte inflammatory function. Thrombomodulin has been described to prevent excessive complement activation.[37] Thus, there is considerable cross-talk between inflammation and coagulation which is impaired in sepsis as a result of depletion of the thrombomodulin/protein C/protein S system. There is also evidence that antithrombin blunts activation of several cytokines, suggesting that low antithrombin levels also affect the relationship between coagulation and inflammation.[38]

ENDOTHELIAL DYSFUNCTION

Besides separating blood from tissue, endothelial cells have multiple physiologic functions involving the regulation of vascular tone, coagulation, and immune response.

The endothelium produces several vasoactive mediators, including nitric oxide (NO), prostacyclins, and endothelin. NO is a potent vasodilator produced by NO synthase (NOS) from the amino acid, L-arginine. NO directly relaxes the vessel's smooth muscle. There are two different forms of endothelial NOS: the constitutional form (cNOS) and the inducible form (iNOS). Physiologically, cNOS—also referred to as *endothelial NOS* (eNOS)—produces only small amounts of NO, and iNOS is expressed at low levels.[39] In sepsis, iNOS expression is stimulated by cytokines such as IL-1β and TNF-α.[40] This is followed by massive NO production and profound vasodilatation. Whether increased activity of cNOS also plays a role in sepsis is currently a matter of debate.

During inflammation, endothelial cells express adhesion molecules on their surface, which causes the adherence of leukocytes. These adhesion molecules include endothelial leukocyte adhesion molecule-1, intracellular adhesion molecule-1, and vascular cell adhesion molecule-1. Endothelial leukocyte adhesion molecule-1 is a selectin that mediates the initial step of leukocyte adhesion, followed by leukocyte rolling along the endothelial surface. The leukocyte finally migrates through the endothelial layer into the tissue, mediated by intracellular adhesion molecule-1 and vascular cell adhesion molecule-1 expression on both endothelial cells and leukocytes.[41]

Migration of leukocytes into the tissue is a physiologic mechanism to move immune cells to the site of infection. However, in generalized inflammation such as in sepsis, endothelial cells in several organs remote from the site of infection express adhesion molecules, inducing a generalized rolling and sticking of circulating leukocytes to the vascular surface. Adherence to endothelial cells activates leukocytes and induces a respiratory burst.[42] The respiratory burst involves the release of cytotoxic substances such as elastase, myeloperoxidase, and reactive oxygen species. These products are capable of damaging endothelial cells and the surrounding tissue. Endothelial cell damage causes capillary leakage whereby intravascular fluid penetrates the extracellular space, leading to tissue edema.

Endothelial cells have an anticoagulant surface produced by the expression of heparan sulfate on the cell membrane, release of plasminogen activator, and production of protein C. However, sepsis shifts the hemostatic balance toward a procoagulatory state. Endothelial cells share in this process by expressing tissue factor (see the previous section, Loss of Hemostatic Balance).

CARDIAC AND CIRCULATORY DYSFUNCTION

Sepsis is frequently complicated by organ dysfunction and shock. Shock occurs when the cardiovascular system is unable to transport sufficient amounts of oxygen to the tissues. In fact, sepsis compromises all levels of the cardiovascular system, resulting in cardiac dysfunction, vascular dysregulation, and microcirculatory damage. Impairment of the cardiovascular system causes a characteristic hemodynamic pattern that in cases of adequate fluid loading and the absence of severe preexisting cardiac dysfunction, consists of a high cardiac output, arterial hypotension, and low systemic oxygen (O_2) extraction. In early sepsis, O_2 consumption is increased owing to higher metabolic needs (i.e., tachypnea, fever, increased cardiac work, increased rate of protein synthesis), further compromising the relationship between O_2 supply and demand (Figure 129-4). The hepatic and splanchnic region is markedly affected by these changes associated with sepsis. Hepatosplanchnic O_2 uptake increases markedly during fever and bacteremia.[43]

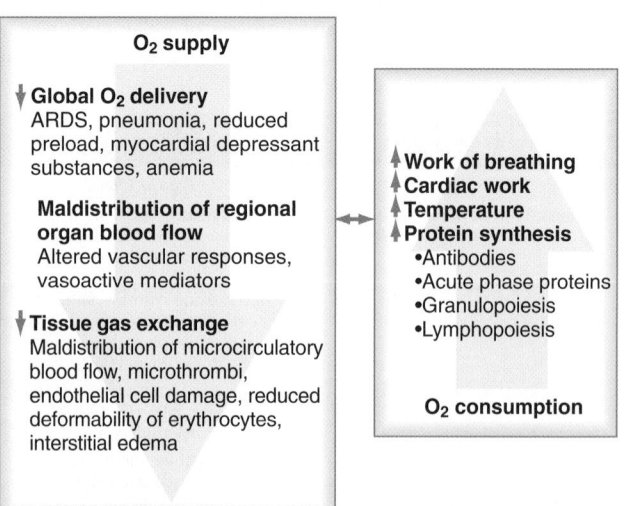

Figure 129-4 The cardiocirculatory system of a septic patient is altered on systemic, regional, and microregional levels. At the same time, sepsis increases O_2 consumption, further deteriorating the O_2 supply/demand relationship. ARDS, acute respiratory distress syndrome.

Cardiac Dysfunction

In experimental septic shock, myocardial contractility is compromised shortly after the induction of sepsis.[44] This finding is confirmed in septic patients when a reduced ejection fraction is observed by echocardiography, especially in patients with elevated troponin levels.[45] The drop in myocardial contractility is accompanied by diastolic dilatation of the left ventricle, which causes the left ventricular end-diastolic volume to rise. This mechanism allows the heart to maintain a sufficient stroke volume despite impaired contractility. Clinically, a rightward shift of the Frank-Starling curve occurs. Thus, compared with healthy humans, patients with sepsis require greater cardiac filling pressures to maintain a similar stroke volume.[46] Septic patients without compensatory left ventricular dilatation have a significantly greater risk of death.[47] Cardiac dysfunction is reversible if the patient recovers from sepsis.

The presence of myocardial depressant substances was initially proposed in the 1980s because the serum of septic patients was able to suppress the contractility of rat myocytes in vitro.[48,49] Cytokines induce increased activation of iNOS, with subsequent enhanced NO production. NO affects myocytes in several ways: NO stimulates guanylate cyclase, and its product, $3',5'$-cyclic guanosine monophosphate, interferes with intracellular myocardial calcium metabolism. This includes a reduction in calcium's affinity to the contractile apparatus and inhibition of the α-adrenergic-mediated increase in the slow inward calcium current. NO may directly damage myocardial cells by the formation of peroxynitrite via combination with superoxide ions. Peroxynitrite deploys toxic effects on many intracellular molecules by means of oxidation.[50]

Sepsis is associated with alterations of regional and microregional blood flow, which results in a mismatch between regional O_2 supply and demand and, subsequently, multiple organ dysfunction. It was therefore hypothesized that the heart shares in this type of injury. Although there were hints from experimental work that the coronary circulatory reserve is altered in sepsis,[51,52] clinical studies did not show a compromised coronary blood flow.[53,54] However, more recently it was demonstrated that patients with sepsis show elevated serum levels of troponin.[55] Elevated troponin values are associated with a higher incidence of regional wall motion abnormalities and death.

Vascular Dysfunction and Hypovolemia

In cardiogenic or hypovolemic shock, vasoconstriction is a common mechanism to avoid arterial hypotension. In sepsis, however, profound arterial vasodilatation occurs. Endothelial cells play an important role in the regulation of vascular tone because they release several vasoactive substances such as NO and endothelin. Sepsis shifts the balance of these substances toward a vasodilatory state by uncontrolled NO production, as discussed earlier. Severe arterial hypotension due to profound systemic vasodilatation is one of the characteristic hemodynamic features of sepsis. The mechanism by which NO induces vasodilatation is complex. Important pathways in which NO participates include the activation of potassium channels and hyperpolarization of the plasma membrane of smooth muscle cells. These mechanisms in turn inhibit the actions of vasopressors such as norepinephrine and angiotensin II, so that vasoconstriction does not occur despite high serum concentrations of these substances.[56]

Endothelial cells regulate vascular tone not only to maintain systemic blood pressure but also to control blood flow to single organs. Several mechanisms to preserve organ blood flow are impaired in sepsis. For example, there is a loss of coupling between the hepatic artery flow and the portal blood flow in endotoxic shock.[50] Similarly, the coronary circulatory reserve necessary to quickly adjust myocardial O_2 supply based on changes in myocardial O_2 requirements is reduced in sepsis.[57] The autoregulation of perfusion of the intestinal mucosa is also depressed in experimental models of sepsis.[58]

Hypovolemia is another characteristic of sepsis. Sepsis is accompanied by the development of significant tissue edema. The underlying mechanism is capillary leakage, which is another effect of endothelial damage.[59] This leakage also allows for the extravasation of albumin,[60] which reduces the intravascular oncotic pressure. Under conditions of capillary leakage, the Starling forces cannot counteract the development of tissue edema or reduce existing edema. Because endothelial damage affects all parts of the capillary network throughout the body, large amounts of intravascular fluid are shifted into the extravascular space.

Microcirculatory Dysfunction

Severe sepsis and septic shock may be associated with high lactate levels and metabolic acidosis despite a low systemic O_2 extraction. These signs of tissue hypoxia, which may be observed despite adequate fluid resuscitation, are interpreted as microcirculatory failure. Some parts of the microcirculation are extremely sensitive to physiologic stress, including hypoxia or ischemia. These areas are referred to as *weak microcirculatory units*.[61,62]

An increase in the number of weak microcirculatory units—and therefore increased microcirculatory shunting—is thought to play a major role in the O_2 extraction deficit in sepsis. This hypothesis has been confirmed in experimental sepsis. By using intravital microscopy, an increased number of capillaries with lack of flow was observed in septic animals.[63] More recently, capillary red blood cell oxygenation was measured in vivo by a spectrophotometric functional imaging system.[64] In the presence of sepsis, an increased proportion of perfused capillaries showed very high red blood cell velocities. These high-flow capillaries were interpreted as microcirculatory shunts. The remaining capillaries with normal flow had a fivefold increase in O_2 extraction. However, this increase in O_2 extraction was insufficient to maintain O_2 supply to all regions, given the number of capillaries without flow.

Several factors may be responsible for microcirculatory shunting in sepsis. The underlying mechanism is the hindrance of blood flow by microvascular obstruction, which has several causes: (1) the onset of intravascular coagulation due to a shift to a procoagulant state causes the development of microthrombi; (2) activation and damage of endothelial cells lead to endothelial cell swelling, narrowing the capillary lumen; (3) activated leukocytes hinder red blood cell flow by rolling and sticking to endothelial cells; and (4) red blood cells have reduced deformability in sepsis, which causes them to be captured in capillaries.[65]

Although there is good evidence from experimental work supporting the hypothesis of microcirculatory dysfunction in sepsis, there is considerable debate whether the O_2 extraction deficit is due to a derangement of intracellular metabolic pathways rather than to microcirculatory dysfunction.[63] Some capillaries are able to increase their O_2 extraction,[66] which argues against this hypothesis. However, the assessment of tissue oxygenation on the cellular level is problematic, even in the experimental setting. Currently it is thought that microcirculatory dysfunction shares in the development of tissue hypoxia in sepsis. Clinically this hypothesis is supported by the finding that early resuscitation guided by central venous O_2 saturation improves survival in these patients.[67]

ENDOCRINE DYSFUNCTION

As depicted in Table 129-4, critical illness is associated with alterations in several endocrine functions. It is not clear whether these changes represent a physiologic response to critical illness or reflect a complex picture of endocrine dysfunction that needs diagnostic and treatment strategies. In sepsis, adrenal insufficiency and vasopressin deficiency might contribute to the loss of vasomotor control. However, current studies do not support treatment of endocrine dysfunction in severe sepsis or septic shock.

Adrenal Insufficiency

Adrenal corticosteroids are involved in several physiologic pathways in the human body, including maintenance of vascular tone, vascular permeability, and distribution of total body water. In the clinical setting, corticosteroids also augment the effects of vasopressors.[68]

TABLE 129-4	Changes in Hormone Concentrations in Critically Ill Patients	
Hormone	*Acute Critical Illness*	*Prolonged Critical Illness*
Catecholamines	++	+
Cortisol	++	+
Adrenocorticotropic hormone	Ø +	Ø −
Growth hormone	Ø −	−
Thyroid hormones	Ø −	−
Thyroid-stimulating hormone	Ø −	−
Androgen hormones	−	−
Prolactin	−	Unknown

Data from Ligtenberg JJ, Girbes AR, Beentjes JA et al. Hormones in the critically ill patient: to intervene or not to intervene? Intensive Care Med 2001;27:1567–77.

Under normal conditions, corticosteroids are secreted by the adrenal cortex in a diurnal pattern. Corticosteroid secretion is tightly controlled by a feedback mechanism involving the hypothalamic-pituitary-adrenal axis. However, several mechanisms may impair the physiologic stress response of the hypothalamic-pituitary-adrenal axis in critically ill patients (Figure 129-5), resulting in an inadequate increase of serum cortisol levels. This condition is referred to as *relative adrenal insufficiency*.[69]

The concept of relative adrenal insufficiency as a clinically relevant condition is a matter of debate. It has been demonstrated that an inadequate rise of cortisol after the corticotropin stimulation test is associated with increased mortality in patients with septic shock.[70] However, most studies measured total cortisol levels, which are reduced due to hypoalbuminemia, while the concentrations of free cortisol may be adequate.[71] Administration of low-dose corticosteroids does not affect survival from septic shock.[72]

Vasopressin Deficiency

Vasopressin is excreted from the neurohypophysis in response to arterial hypotension or hypovolemia. Because septic shock is characterized by both arterial hypotension and hypovolemia, one would expect plasma vasopressin levels to be high; however, they are low in patients with septic shock[73] and do not adequately respond when arterial hypotension occurs.[74] Indeed, the administration of vasopressin or analogs can quickly restore blood pressure in these patients.[75] Inadequate vasopressin levels may be caused by depression of the baroreflex, increased

metabolism of vasopressin, and depletion of vasopressin stores in the pituitary gland.

Vasopressin is metabolized by plasma vasopressinase and by renal and hepatic clearance. Increased vasopressin metabolism seems unlikely in sepsis, because renal and hepatic functions are often compromised in this setting, and there is no evidence of increased vasopressinase activity in this disease. Depression of the baroreflex may play a role in vasopressin depletion. The baroreflex is mediated by sympathetic stimulation, and there is some evidence that sympathetic function might be impaired in sepsis.[76] Depletion of pituitary vasopressin stores was found by magnetic resonance imaging in a case series of three septic shock patients with low plasma vasopressin levels.[77] The clinical relevance of the low vasopressin response to septic shock remains unclear, except in a subgroup with less severe septic shock, because administration of low-dose vasopressin was not associated with better survival.[78]

Insulin Deficiency

Hyperglycemia is a common feature in critically ill patients, such as those with severe sepsis or septic shock, and is caused by the endocrine response to stress. This includes activation of the hypothalamic-pituitary-adrenal axis, with the release of cortisol. Additionally, secretion of epinephrine, glucagon, and growth hormone is increased. All these hormones counteract effects of insulin. Besides the endocrine stress response, several cytokines additionally increase insulin resistance by inhibiting intracellular pathways normally activated by the insulin receptor.[79] There is also evidence that pancreatic insulin secretion is impaired in sepsis.[80,81]

Endocrine stress response, insulin resistance, and impaired insulin secretion are responsible for the hyperglycemic state of patients with sepsis. Besides hyperglycemia, insulin deficiency may also be unfavorable in sepsis, since insulin has several beneficial effects such as potent antiinflammatory and anabolic actions. However, insulin administration to achieve normal glucose levels is not supported by clinical trials; the risk of hypoglycemia seems to outweigh any possible beneficial effects of insulin.[82,83]

Pathophysiology of Multiorgan Dysfunction

Multiorgan dysfunction is the parallel or sequential failure of at least two organs. It is a frequent complication of sepsis. Clinically, multiorgan dysfunction is termed the *multiple organ dysfunction syndrome* (MODS). MODS can involve any organ of a critically ill patient, even

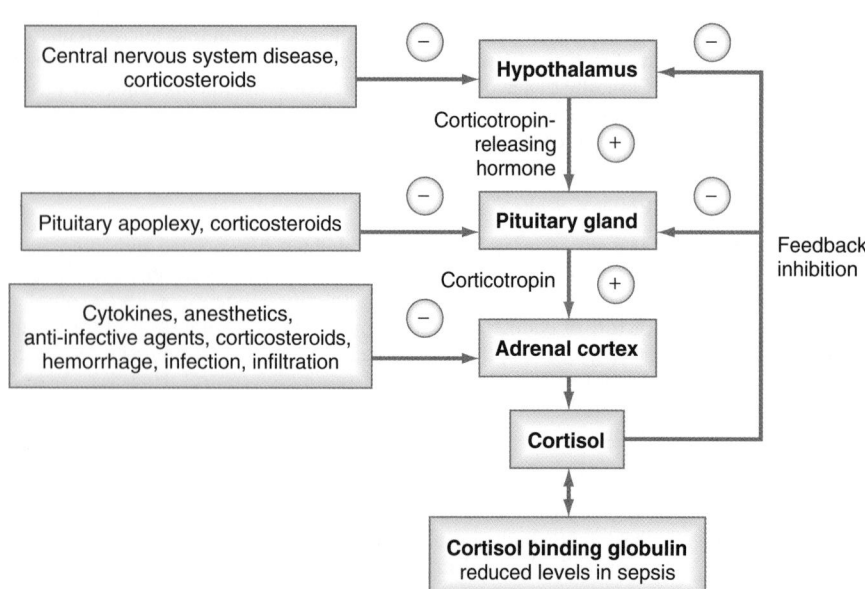

Figure 129-5 Hypothalamic-pituitary-adrenal axis. Physiologic control of cortisol release and its feedback mechanism are illustrated. This axis may be impaired on all levels in critically ill patients. +, stimulation; −, inhibition. *(Modified from Cooper MS, Stewart PM. Corticosteroid insufficiency in acutely ill patients. N Engl J Med 2003;348:727-34.)*

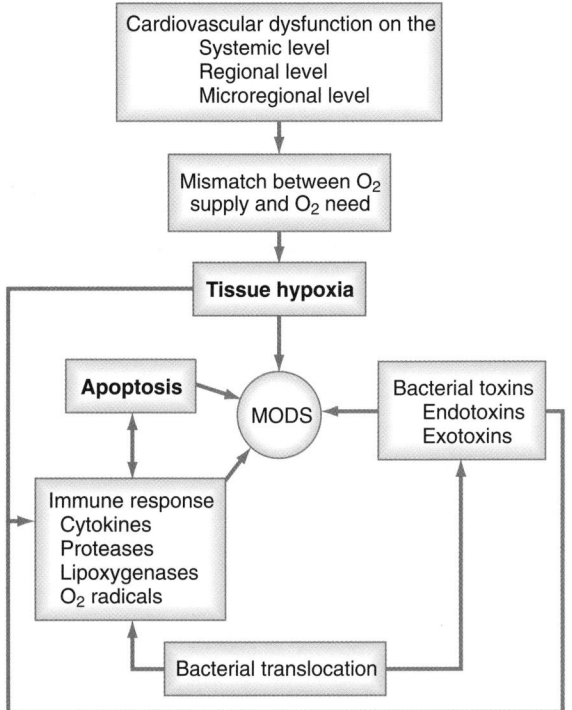

Figure 129-6 Pathophysiology of multiple organ dysfunction syndrome (MODS).

a remote organ that was not originally affected by the underlying disease. The development of MODS significantly contributes to ICU mortality. Scoring systems such as the Sequential Organ Failure Assessment (SOFA) or the Multiorgan Dysfunction Score, which assess the severity of MODS, correlate well with mortality.[4]

Some major components of the pathophysiology of MODS are depicted in Figure 129-6. The development of MODS includes a complicated network of inter- and intracellular actions. Inflammation seems to be a major trigger for the induction of the processes that lead to MODS. Both infectious and noninfectious stimuli may be responsible for activation of the innate immune response. As previously discussed, PAMPs activate the immune response and induce complex metabolic and circulatory changes in the host. Correspondingly, cellular trauma causes the release of DAMPs such as mitochondrial peptides and mitochondrial DNA into the circulation. DAMPs may induce systemic inflammation similar to sepsis.[84]

Because MODS can involve a variety of pathologic changes, different concepts of the pathophysiology of MODS have been generated (Table 129-5).[2,85] Cellular dysfunction due to tissue hypoxia is likely an important factor in the onset of MODS. However, other factors also play a role, including the onset of programmed cell death (apoptosis) and the direct toxic effects of substances such as endotoxin and reactive oxygen species. The development of SIRS does not require the presence of infection; severe trauma, burns, pancreatitis, and cardiac surgery with cardiopulmonary bypass are also associated with SIRS and increase the risk for MODS.[86]

TISSUE HYPOXIA

As discussed previously, the host response to infection severely impairs the cardiovascular system through the development of cardiac dysfunction, systemic and regional vascular dysregulation, and microcirculatory damage. Systemic hemodynamics can be restored by measures such as fluid resuscitation or treatment with catecholamines. However, no clinically available measures allow for a differential diagnosis of regional or microregional disturbances of blood flow, nor are therapies available to specifically address such disturbances. Thus, microcirculatory

dysfunction and maldistribution of regional blood flow will persist or even progress if the underlying disease (e.g., sepsis) cannot be treated successfully. Tissue hypoxia may therefore be present even though treatment goals for adequate systemic hemodynamics have been achieved.

Tissue hypoxia is difficult to assess in a critically ill patient. It is therefore uncertain whether tissue hypoxia plays a leading role in organ dysfunction, because other mechanisms such as apoptosis have been identified as well.[87] In addition, it has been suggested that disturbance of mitochondrial O_2 utilization rather than tissue hypoxia is the motor of organ dysfunction. This hypothesis is supported by the observation that depletion of enzymes of the respiratory chain is associated with the development of MODS in septic patients.[66] Nevertheless, data are available that demonstrate the importance of tissue oxygenation in the development of MODS. For example, when central venous O_2 saturation was used to guide aggressive treatment to maintain O_2 delivery, there was a significant reduction in mortality,[88] supporting the concept of tissue hypoxia as an important mechanism in MODS. Likewise, patients with early lactate clearance have less severe organ dysfunction and improved outcome.[89]

APOPTOSIS

Apoptosis is a physiologic mechanism whereby activation of a specific intracellular program induces cell death. Apoptosis is therefore a regulatory process for the proliferation and differentiation of cells. However, pathologic activation of apoptosis seems to be involved in the pathogenesis of MODS. Apoptosis is induced by a cascade system through either an extrinsic (receptor-dependent) or an intrinsic (receptor-independent) pathway. The extrinsic pathway is activated by the so-called death receptor superfamily, consisting of receptors such as the Fas receptor (CD95) or the TNF receptor. Thus, cytokines are able to induce apoptosis. The intrinsic pathway may be induced by DNA damage. The process of apoptosis is mediated by an enzymatic cascade system in which active caspase-3 is the executioner protein that finally starts apoptosis. The receptors of the extrinsic pathway mediate the activation of procaspase-8 to active caspase-8 via several signaling proteins (Figure 129-7). The intrinsic pathway works by altering the mitochondrial membrane potential through the signal protein, p53, which mediates the activation of caspase-9. Both active caspase-8 and active caspase-9 activate the final common step in the apoptosis pathway (caspase-3).[90]

The extent to which apoptosis-related cell death contributes to the development of MODS is difficult to assess because this process has been investigated primarily in the experimental setting. However, apoptosis of intestinal epithelial cells has been shown in trauma

TABLE 129-5	Conceptual Models of Multiple Organ Dysfunction
Pathologic Process	*Manifestation*
Uncontrolled infection	Persistent infection, nosocomial acquired infection, endotoxemia
Systemic inflammation	Cytokinemia (particularly IL-6, IL-8, TNF), leukocytosis, increased capillary permeability
Immune paralysis	Nosocomial infection, increased antiinflammatory cytokine levels (IL-10), decreased HLA-DR expression; shift from type 1 to type 2 helper T-cells
Tissue hypoxia	Increased lactate, low central venous O_2 saturation
Microvascular coagulopathy and endothelial dysfunction	Increased procoagulant activity, decreased anticoagulant activity (antithrombin III ↓, protein C ↓), high levels of fibrin derivatives, increased von Willebrand factor, soluble thrombomodulin, increased capillary permeability
Dysregulated apoptosis	Increased epithelial and lymphoid apoptosis, decreased neutrophil apoptosis
Gut-liver axis	Increased infection with gut organisms, endotoxemia, Kupffer cell activation

HLA, human leukocyte antigen; IL, interleukin; TNF, tumor necrosis factor.
Modified from Marshall JC. Inflammation, coagulopathy, and the pathogenesis of multiple organ dysfunction syndrome. Crit Care Med 2001;29:S99-106.

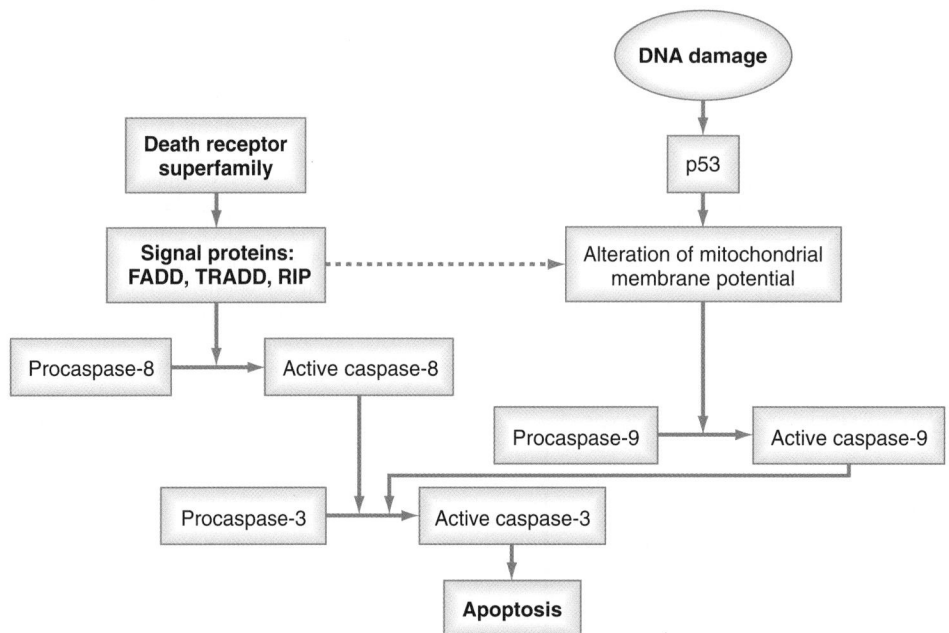

Figure 129-7   Extrinsic and intrinsic signaling process for apoptosis. FADD, Fas-associated death domain protein; RIP, receptor interacting protein; TRADD, TNF receptor 1–associated death protein. (*Modified from Lydon A, Martyn JA. Apoptosis in critical illness. Int Anesthesiol Clin 2003;41:65-77.*)

patients shortly after injury.[91] The importance of increased apoptosis in the clinical setting warrants further elucidation.

THE "TWO-HIT" THEORY

Any severe impact to the human body such as a traumatic or surgical injury or prolonged shock can directly induce the development of organ dysfunction. Possible mechanisms include ischemia, reperfusion injury, or immediate tissue destruction due to trauma. Such an event is called a "first hit." This first hit may be severe enough to induce SIRS, with all the consequences to the cardiocirculatory system and cellular functions mentioned earlier.

Even if the first hit does not induce a primary MODS, a "second hit" such as an infectious insult (e.g., pneumonia or bacteremia due to catheter infection) could further activate an immune system that is already primed by the first hit. The "two-hit" theory hypothesizes that a second (or third) insult amplifies the inflammatory response to the first hit in such a way that SIRS occurs. If these events are followed by multiple organ dysfunction, the term *secondary MODS* is used.

The two-hit theory has been criticized for being somewhat arbitrary, because the differentiation between primary and secondary MODS is not always possible in the clinical setting.[92] However, our current understanding of the inflammatory response to injury supports the concept of priming. Neutrophils are known to produce greater amounts of reactive oxygen species and have increased adhesion properties after they have been exposed to proinflammatory mediators. It has been demonstrated, at least in vitro, that priming followed by activation of neutrophils increases the extent of endothelial damage.

KEY POINTS

Pathophysiology of Sepsis

1. Sepsis is induced by an invasion of microorganisms or their toxins into the bloodstream, together with the host response to this invasion.

2. Any infection may be complicated by sepsis.

3. The innate immune system recognizes specific molecular patterns associated with microorganisms called *pathogen-associated molecular patterns* (PAMPs) that include cell wall products, exotoxins, bacterial DNA, and viral RNA.

4. The host's innate immune system senses the presence of microbial molecules by specific receptors called *pattern-recognition proteins* (PRP), such as Toll-like receptors.

5. An excessive inflammatory response early in sepsis is counteracted by an antiinflammatory response, which may then result in hypoinflammation.

6. Hemostatic balance is shifted to a procoagulant state in sepsis due to activation of tissue factor and attenuation of natural anticoagulants.

7. Sepsis causes endothelial dysfunction.

8. Cardiac dysfunction in sepsis is mainly due to intramyocardial nitric oxide production and perhaps cardiac ischemia resulting in left ventricular diastolic dilatation and a rightward shift of the Frank-Starling curve.

9. Capillary leakage causes a large amount of intravascular fluid to be shifted into the extravascular space resulting in significant hypovolemia.

10. Sepsis is accompanied by profound arterial hypotension due to massive endothelial nitric oxide production.

11. Microcirculatory dysfunction associated with sepsis is a result of intravascular coagulation, endothelial cell swelling, activated leukocytes, and stiff red blood cells.

Pathophysiology of Multiorgan Dysfunction

1. *Multiorgan dysfunction* refers to the parallel or sequential failure of at least two organs.

2. Tissue hypoxia is an important cofactor in the development of multiorgan dysfunction.

3. Cytokine-induced apoptosis (programmed cell death) contributes to organ dysfunction.

4. Dysfunction of a single organ may affect the integrity of other organs.

ANNOTATED REFERENCES

Cohen J. The immunopathogenesis of sepsis. Nature 2002;420:885-91.

Cohen provides a general overview of the complicated pathways involved in the pathophysiology of sepsis.

van der Poll T, Opal SM. Host pathogen interaction in sepsis. Lancet Infect Dis 2008:8:32-43.

Another excellent review describing the complex pathways involved from pathogen detection to the innate immune response.

Hotchkiss RS, Nicholson DW. Apoptosis and caspases regulate death and inflammation in sepsis. Nat Rev Immunol 2006;6:813-22.

This review describes the pathways of apoptosis and how this affects the immune system in sepsis. Apoptosis may be a future target of pharmaceutical interventions, and perspectives are explained in this article.

Levi M, van der Poll T. Inflammation and coagulation. Crit Care Med 2010;38:S26-34.

The interaction between inflammation and coagulation has been identified as a potential target in the therapy of septic shock. This review article provides an overview of the pathophysiologic pathways involved.

Cunnion RE, Parrillo JE. Myocardial dysfunction in sepsis. Crit Care Clin 1989;5:99-117.

Although written years ago, this article thoroughly describes the phenomenon of cardiomyopathy in patients with severe sepsis or septic shock.

Landry DW, Oliver JA. The pathogenesis of vasodilatory shock. N Engl J Med 2001;345:588-95.

This review article describes the biochemical pathways that induce profound vasodilatation as it occurs in septic shock.

Trzeciak S, Rivers EP. Clinical manifestations of disordered microcirculatory perfusion in severe sepsis. Crit Care 2005;9:S20-6.

This review describes the pathophysiology of microcirculatory dysfunctions in sepsis and how biochemistry and hemodynamic monitoring reflect these changes. A short overview is given on how vasodilator agents might have beneficial effects in conditions with altered microcirculation.

Marshall JC. Inflammation, coagulopathy, and the pathogenesis of multiple organ dysfunction syndrome. Crit Care Med 2001;29:S99-106.

Marshall provides an overview of the proposed mechanism of multiple organ dysfunction. This supplement also contains several interesting articles about the interactions among inflammation, coagulation, and the endothelium.

REFERENCES

Access the complete reference list online at http://www.expertconsult.com.

130

Septic Shock

JEAN-LOUIS VINCENT

Incidence

Septic shock is the form of acute circulatory shock that occurs secondary to severe infection. The incidence of severe sepsis and septic shock is rising, partly related to medical progress that allows individuals to survive longer, resulting in increased numbers of older, debilitated, or immunocompromised patients passing through the intensive care unit (ICU). Some 10% to 15% of ICU patients develop septic shock at one time or another, and the mortality rate is 50% to 60%.[1] Somewhat lower mortality rates have been reported in some trials evaluating the effects of new therapeutic interventions,[2] but such studies include a number of exclusion criteria that are often associated with high mortality rates—cirrhosis, immunosuppression, and "do-not-resuscitate orders," for example—so it is perhaps not surprising that mortality rates are lower in these therapeutic trials than in "real life."

Etiology of Septic Shock

The organisms involved in severe sepsis and septic shock are most often bacterial. While in the past gram-negative organisms were most commonly implicated, increasingly gram-positive organisms are isolated, such that roughly similar numbers of gram-positive and gram-negative organisms are now involved.[1] Septic shock can also be caused by a fungal or parasitic infection. In a third of patients, no infectious agent is identified.[1] About half of infections are nosocomial in origin. Although an infection can arise anywhere, the lung is presently the most common source of infection (40%), followed by the abdomen (20%), indwelling venous and arterial catheters and primary bacteremias (15%), and the urinary tract (10%).[1]

Pathophysiology of Septic Shock

The pathophysiology of septic shock is complex and covered in detail in Chapter 129 (Reinhart & Bloos). Essentially, the systemic sepsis response starts with recognition of an invading organism or its toxins. Among the bacterial factors, one of the best-known toxins is lipopolysaccharide (LPS), which is part of the outer gram-negative bacterial membrane, but other bacterial-derived factors include lipoteichoic acid and peptidoglycan. In certain cases, essentially infections involving *Staphylococcus aureus* or β-hemolytic group A *Streptococcus*, the formation of superantigens results in toxic shock syndrome.

The early humoral response involves the complement and contact (kinin-kallikrein) systems. Immune cells, principally monocytes/macrophages and polymorphonuclear neutrophils (PMN), are not only able to recognize pathogenic agents and their products so they can phagocytose and destroy them, but also release a series of mediators which can themselves activate other cells. Among the cell membrane receptors implicated in the recognition of pathogenic agents are the so-called Toll-like receptors (TLR), a family of 10 members. Of these, TLR4 is the receptor for LPS; TLR2 for a number of products from gram-positive bacteria such as peptidoglycans, mycobacteria, and yeasts; and TLR9 for bacterial DNA.[3] In response to cellular stimulation, intracellular signaling is activated, resulting largely in activation of transcriptional factors, including nuclear factor kappa B (NF-κB), which in turn are responsible for initiation of proinflammatory reactions. A number of cytokines, two of the key players being tumor necrosis factor alpha (TNF-α) and interleukin (IL)-1 that interact synergistically, are released by macrophages and other cells. TNF-α and IL-1 are particularly important proinflammatory cytokines whose administration in animals can reproduce all the features of septic shock including hypotension and development of multiple organ failure. A host of secondary mediators including lipid mediators, oxygen free radicals, proteases, and arachidonic acid metabolites are also released by macrophages, PMNs, and other cells. Vasodilator substances such as nitric oxide (NO) and prostaglandins are released by endothelial cells and are responsible for the early hemodynamic changes of sepsis. NO in particular is a powerful vasodilator acting on vascular smooth muscle. Increased NO production is essentially due to induction of inducible NO synthase (iNOS) by proinflammatory cytokines. The formation of large quantities of NO can also have secondary toxic effects on cells. NO can block mitochondrial respiration, directly via inhibition of cytochrome a,a3 and by reaction with superoxide radicals, resulting in the production of peroxynitrite, which inhibits various phases of mitochondrial respiration.[4] These effects result in depletion of cellular adenosine triphosphate (ATP) and potentially severe detrimental effects on cell function. It is important to note that the inflammatory response also causes release of vasoconstrictor substances including thromboxane and endothelins.

Other effects of the inflammatory reaction that accompanies septic shock include expression of adhesion molecules on vascular endothelium and circulating cells (platelets, PMNs, and monocytes), allowing adhesion of activated leukocytes and their migration into subendothelial tissues. Alterations in intercellular endothelial junctions result in increased capillary permeability and generalized edema. Alterations of coagulation and fibrinolysis complete the picture, with proinflammatory mediators creating a procoagulant state. Briefly, activation of tissue factor on the surface of various cells, particularly monocytes and endothelial cells, initiates the coagulation system.[5] In addition, sepsis causes a significant reduction in plasma levels of natural anticoagulants such as protein C, protein S, and antithrombin by reducing their synthesis, increasing their consumption, and increasing their clearance. Thrombolysis is also stimulated with an increase in levels of plasminogen activator inhibitor (PAI-1). The net result is a balance in favor of procoagulant processes, often leading to disseminated intravascular coagulation (DIC) and participating in the microcirculatory disorder that leads to multiple organ failure and death in many patients with severe sepsis.

During the sepsis response, antiinflammatory mediators including IL-4 and IL-10 are also released, which limit the effects of the proinflammatory mediators and can lead to a state of relative immunosuppression, sometimes called immunoparalysis.[6]

Classification

Following recommendations from the Sepsis Conference,[7] patients with septic shock may be classified according to the letters *PIRO*:

P = PREDISPOSING FACTORS

Each patient has specific characteristics. For example, an individual receiving long-term immunosuppressant therapy requires a different approach than someone who was previously healthy. Factors associated with lifestyle, such as alcoholism, may influence the course of septic shock.[8] Patient age and gender may also be important. Increasingly, genetics are being considered, and studies are discovering which genetic factors can influence the development of and survival from severe sepsis. In particular, a polymorphism of the TNF-α promoter gene has been associated with increased risk of sepsis.[9] Multiple other polymorphisms that may influence the response of the host to pathogenic organisms have been described, including for IL-1 receptor antagonist (IL-1ra), TLR2, and IL-6.[10] Improved understanding of these aspects should help better direct therapeutic strategies.

I = INFECTIOUS INSULT

This refers to the specific characteristics of the infection, that is, the agent or pathogen involved (e.g., gram-positive versus gram-negative, bacteria versus fungus),[11] the source of the sepsis (e.g., urinary tract versus respiratory tract),[12] and the degree of extension of the infection (e.g., pneumonia confined to one lobe of one lung versus generalized bilateral lung involvement, appendicitis versus generalized peritonitis). All these factors can influence the severity of the sepsis response and the patient's likely response to therapy.

R = HOST RESPONSE

This refers to the factors involved in the inflammatory response of the host to the infection, assessed largely by the presence or absence of the signs and symptoms of sepsis (e.g., degree of elevation of white blood cell count, CRP, procalcitonin). Each patient mounts a different response dependent on various factors including those previously discussed, and a patient's response will vary with their clinical course and treatment.[13]

O = ORGAN DYSFUNCTION

This refers to the degree of organ dysfunction related to sepsis and can be evaluated using various scoring systems, including the SOFA (sequential organ failure assessment) score,[14] which uses objective, readily available measures to quantify the dysfunction of six organ systems (Table 130-1). Dysfunction of each organ is rated according to a scale (0 [normal function] to 4 [organ failure]), and individual scores can then be summed to provide a total. Individual organ function as well as a composite score can thus be followed during the course of disease and treatment.

▨ Clinical Presentation

It has been suggested that sepsis progresses in a continuum through severe sepsis to septic shock, but in the clinical situation, such a progression is not always so clear-cut or constant, and it is difficult to predict which patients are going to develop septic shock and when. Septic shock can develop very abruptly, without evidence of signs of sepsis in the preceding hours.

Septic shock is characterized by the persistence of severe arterial hypotension despite adequate fluid resuscitation, and the presence of perfusion abnormalities manifest by oliguria, reduced peripheral perfusion, and altered mental status. Septic shock is typically associated with hyperlactatemia (blood lactate concentrations above 2 mEq/L).

One may anticipate that patients with septic shock will have fever, hyperleukocytosis, and other typical features of sepsis, but unfortunately this is not always true. Fever may be an important clue, but moderate fever can be found in other types of shock. More importantly, fever is often absent in septic shock; in fact, hypothermia may be present in 15% to 20% of cases, and this symptom is associated with higher mortality rates.[15] Hyperleukocytosis is also nonspecific and can be found in other types of circulatory failure. Likewise, lactic acidosis, a hallmark of all types of circulatory failure, is usually compensated by hyperventilation, so tachypnea is not specific for septic shock. Similarly, tachycardia can be the result of the circulatory alterations associated with any type of shock.

A more typical characteristic of septic shock is the hyperkinetic pattern characterized by high cardiac output. Although such a hemodynamic pattern is not entirely specific—it can be found in other inflammatory states such as polytrauma or pancreatitis or even anaphylactic shock—it should alert the attending physician to a likely diagnosis of septic shock.

▨ Hemodynamic Changes

The inflammatory reaction causes intense vasodilation that increases vascular capacity and results in a fall in arterial blood pressure. Hypovolemia due to fluid loss (e.g., diarrhea, vomiting, sweating) and to alterations in capillary permeability contributes to hypotension, and reduced myocardial contractility can further aggravate the hemodynamic situation, although it is completely reversible when the septic shock resolves. The pathophysiology of the reduced myocardial contractility includes alterations in endothelial function, alterations in β-adrenergic receptors, and alterations in myocardial calcium metabolism. These effects are caused largely by sepsis mediators such as TNF-α and IL-1, oxygen free radicals, platelet activating factor (PAF), and NO, which all have negative inotropic effects.

In less severe cases, such as severe sepsis without shock, arterial hypotension can be corrected by fluid administration. In more severe cases, even if there is a partial response to fluid repletion, the

TABLE 130-1	The Sequential Organ Failure Assessment Score				
SOFA Score	*0*	*1*	*2*	*3*	*4*
Respiration					
Pao_2/FIo_2, mm Hg	>400	≤400	≤300	≤200 with respiratory support	≤100 with respiratory support
Coagulation					
Platelets × $10^3/mm^3$	>150	≤150	≤100	≤50	≤20
Liver					
Bilirubin, mg/dL (µmol/L)	<1.2 (<20)	1.2-1.9 (20-32)	2.0-5.9 (33-101)	6.0-11.9 (102-204)	>12.0 (>204)
Cardiovascular					
Hypotension	No hypotension	MAP <70 mmHg	Dopamine ≤5 *or* dobutamine (any dose)*	Dopamine >5 *or* epinephrine ≤0.1 *or* norepinephrine ≤0.1*	Dopamine >15 *or* epinephrine >0.1 *or* norepinephrine >0.1*
Central Nervous System					
Glasgow Coma Score	15	13-14	10-12	6-9	<6
Renal					
Creatinine, mg/dL (µmol/L) *or* urine output	<1.2 (<110)	1.2-1.9 (110-170)	2.0-3.4 (171-299)	3.5-4.9 (300-440) *or* <500 mL/d	>5.0 (>440) *or* <200 mL/d

Data from Vincent JL, de Mendonca A, Cantraine F et al. Use of the SOFA score to assess the incidence of organ dysfunction/failure in intensive care units. Results of a multicenter, prospective study. Crit Care Med 1988;26:1793-800.

*Adrenergic agents administered for at least 1 hour (doses given are in µg/kg/min).

persistence of hypotension requires the use of vasopressor agents. This differentiates severe sepsis from septic shock and indicates a very serious condition, as acute circulatory failure (shock) systematically causes dysfunction of other organs.

After vascular filling as a result of volume resuscitation, the hemodynamic status in septic shock is characterized by a fall in vascular tone associated with reduced systemic vascular resistance (SVR) and a raised cardiac output. In addition, reduced myocardial contractility causes a fall in the ventricular ejection fraction. Ejection volume, and particularly cardiac output, may be maintained by an increase in diastolic volumes. Hence, there is myocardial depression or dysfunction without any true cardiac failure (which would be associated with reduced cardiac output).

Monitoring

Any patient with septic shock requires monitoring with an arterial catheter to enable reliable and continuous assessment of arterial pressure. Changes in systolic and pulse pressure in mechanically ventilated patients during the respiratory cycle may also indicate a greater likelihood of response to a fluid challenge.[16] The arterial catheter also facilitates blood sampling, notably for blood gas analysis.

INVASIVE VERSUS LESS-INVASIVE MONITORING

The role of the pulmonary artery catheter (PAC) in critically ill patients has been questioned.[17] However, although no study has conclusively demonstrated positive effects of this type of monitoring on outcome,[18-20] information obtained from the PAC may help in guiding patient management.[21] The PAC is useful not only for monitoring pulmonary artery occlusion pressure (PAOP) and cardiac output but also allows assessment of mixed venous oxygen saturation (Svo_2), a highly useful parameter because a fall in Svo_2 is generally associated with inadequate oxygen transport. Importantly, the PAC is not necessary in all patients but is likely to be of use in complex cases, particularly in patients with concomitant cardiopulmonary disease.

Less-invasive monitoring techniques are increasingly being used. Echocardiography can provide useful additional information, largely to visualize the degree of ventricular filling and ejection volume. However, echocardiography requires an experienced operator, gives no information on the adequacy of cardiac output for the patient's needs, and is difficult to perform continuously, so information is intermittent. Other less-invasive methods of monitoring cardiac output include PiCCO, LidCO, transesophageal Doppler techniques, and even bioimpedance or bioreactance techniques.[22] However, measurement of cardiac output in isolation is not very helpful in most critically ill patients.

BLOOD LACTATE LEVELS

Blood lactate level is an important biological variable in determining the adequacy of perfusion and oxygenation. Normal blood lactate level is around 1 mEq/L, and hyperlactatemia becomes pathological above 2 mEq/L. Although in other forms of circulatory shock, hyperlactatemia is due to cellular hypoxia, in septic shock additional mechanisms may play an important role in raising blood lactate levels. In sepsis, blood lactate levels may be raised by an increase in cellular metabolism, by inhibition of pyruvate dehydrogenase, and by reduced clearance. Repeated measurements enable one to assess the efficacy of treatment and have a predictive value superior to derived oxygenation parameters.[23] The evolution of blood lactate levels enables a global evaluation of the state of the shock, although in view of the relatively slow rate of change, blood lactate levels cannot be used to guide resuscitation.

PERIPHERAL PERFUSION PARAMETERS

Measurement of the gastric intramucosal pH (pHi) or its derivatives (mucosal Pco_2 or the difference between the mucosal and arterial Pco_2

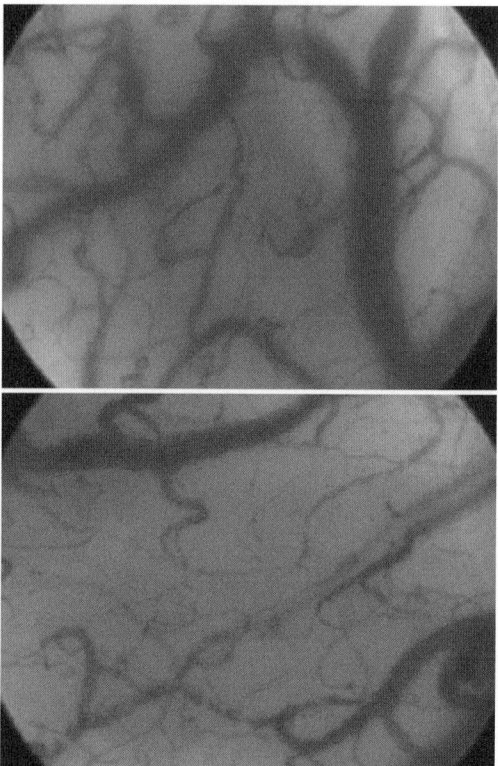

Figure 130-1 Representative examples of sublingual microvasculature in a healthy volunteer *(top panel)* and in a patient with septic shock *(lower panel)*. Note decrease in density of small vessels in sepsis. *(From De Backer D, Creteur J, Preiser JC et al. Microvascular blood flow is altered in patients with sepsis. Am J Respir Crit Care Med 2002;166:98–104 with permission.)*

[the Pco_2 gap]) is considered to reflect splanchnic perfusion and hence provide an idea of the adequacy of regional oxygenation. However, these techniques may be influenced by technical considerations, including the influence of gastric acid and enteral nutrition, and are not used clinically.

Other techniques for monitoring peripheral perfusion have been developed. While the sublingual region is not one that would immediately seem to be of most interest, it is easily accessible, and using techniques of orthogonal polarization spectral (OPS) or sidestream darkfield (SDF) imaging, heterogeneity of microcirculatory flow and reduced perfused vessel density and proportion of perfused vessels can be observed (Figure 130-1) and quantified in patients with sepsis.[24,25] Moreover, the impact of therapeutic interventions on such changes can be monitored,[26,27] opening the possibility that monitoring the microcirculation could be used to guide treatment.

Near-infrared spectroscopy (NIRS) is a technique that uses the differential absorption properties of oxygenated and deoxygenated hemoglobin to evaluate tissue oxygenation (Sto_2). Analysis of changes in Sto_2 during a circulatory stress test, such as a brief episode of forearm ischemia (venous or arterial occlusion), may be more useful to quantify sepsis-induced microvascular dysfunction than an isolated Sto_2 value.[28]

Although these techniques have demonstrated clearly the presence of alterations in the microcirculation in patients with severe sepsis, which are associated with prognosis,[29,30] further research is needed to fully evaluate the relevance of these values to early resuscitation and care of critically ill patients.

Management

Management of the patient with septic shock involves three inseparable components: treatment of the infection, cardiovascular resuscitation, and immunomodulation (Figure 130-2). Detailed guidelines for

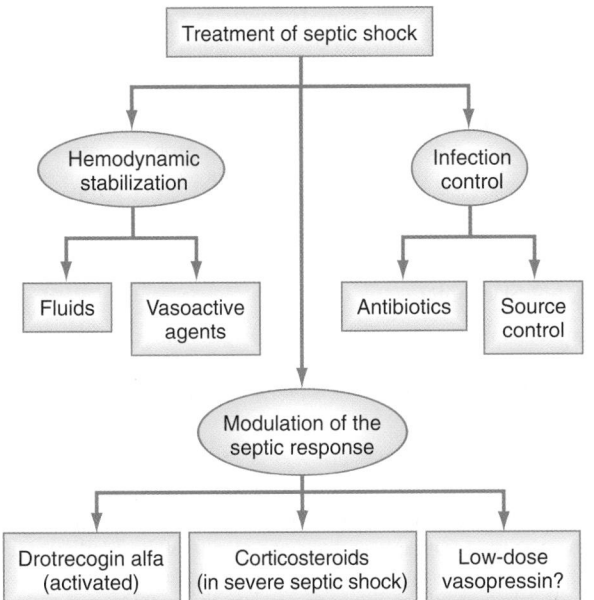

Figure 130-2 The three aspects of treatment of septic shock.

the management of patients with severe sepsis or septic shock have been published.[31]

CONTROL OF INFECTION

Infection must be treated effectively and rapidly. Antibiotics must be started quickly and must cover all likely organisms. The choice of antibiotics may depend on local microbiological flora and resistance patterns. Often the microorganism(s) responsible for sepsis in an individual patient is not known for sure, and empirical broad-spectrum antibiotics must be given to ensure adequate coverage. Such empirical therapy must then be modified as soon as possible as microbiology culture results become available.

In addition to antibiotic treatment, any focus of infection must be removed or drained, by emergency surgery if necessary. If no source is identified, a systematic search should be made based on the "big five": lungs, abdomen, urine, wounds, and catheters.

CARDIOVASCULAR RESUSCITATION

The VIP ruse proposed by Weil and Shubin[32] should be followed. Each patient is in fact a VIP, but the letters refer here to *Ventilation, Infusion,* and *Pump.*

V = Ventilation

All patients with septic shock must be generously oxygenated with the aim of correcting any hypoxemia, regardless of whether it is due to inadequate cardiac output, pulmonary edema, or pulmonary disease. Severe cases need endotracheal intubation and mechanical ventilation. Noninvasive ventilation is not recommended in such hemodynamically unstable patients. Even though it may represent a temporary support rather than a treatment per se, mechanical ventilation allows not only an improvement in gaseous exchange but also has beneficial hemodynamic effects, notably by reducing the oxygen requirement of the respiratory muscles.

I = Infusion

Septic shock is accompanied by absolute and relative hypovolemia, the result of various mechanisms:

- External losses, which may be obvious, such as vomiting and diarrhea, or less apparent, such as sweating

- Internal losses via an increase in capillary permeability with development of edema and sometimes liquid effusions (peritoneal, pleural effusion)
- Increase in plasma volume associated with arterial and venous dilatation

Hypovolemia needs to be corrected rapidly, as it causes hemodynamic instability both at the level of cardiac output and in terms of peripheral perfusion.

Assessment of an adequate volume state is essentially clinical: restoration of arterial pressure, improvement of cutaneous perfusion, improved urine output, and improved mental state. The central venous pressure (CVP) can be a useful guide, but it is not possible to define in advance the CVP level that should be reached in any individual patient. However, monitoring CVP or PAOP is essential to limit the risk of pulmonary edema. In fluid replacement, it is preferable to use a fluid challenge technique in which filling pressures are measured at regular intervals during fluid administration (Table 130-2).[33] If a PAC is in place, it is recommended that fluid replacement be given until cardiac output reaches a plateau and further fluid causes no further increase in cardiac output.

There has been considerable debate as to which fluid should be used in sepsis, but it is the quantity of fluid rather than the type of fluid per se that is of greatest importance. Because of their propensity for leakage into the extravascular space, greater volumes of crystalloids are needed to achieve the same effect as colloid,[34] thus potentially increasing the risk of edema, but colloids are more expensive and carry their own risks. In particular, there has been considerable controversy about the use of albumin in critically ill patients, but a large multicenter study performed in Australasia (the SAFE study)[35] showed that albumin administration was not associated with worse outcomes.

P = Pump (Vasoactive Agents)

If fluid administration alone is unable to restore an adequate perfusion pressure, vasoactive agents are required. Catecholamines are preferred for their rapid action and efficacy and their short half-lives. Adrenergic agents stimulate β_1- (positive inotropes), β_2- (essentially vasodilators and bronchodilators), and α-receptors (essentially vasoconstrictors) to varying degrees. Dopamine also stimulates dopaminergic receptors, causing vasodilation primarily in the splanchnic and renal regions, but the clinical relevance of this effect is uncertain.

Dopamine was often recommended as the first-line drug for its mixed β- and α-adrenergic effects. However, a recent randomized controlled study showed no differences in mortality rates in patients with shock treated with dopamine or norepinephrine as first-line vasopressor, but dopamine use was associated with increased adverse effects, notably arrhythmias.[36] Norepinephrine is, therefore, the preferred first-line vasopressor in patients with septic shock. Epinephrine should *not* be used as a first-line vasopressor in septic shock; it can have deleterious effects on the splanchnic circulation.[37] Dobutamine is often added to vasopressor therapy, particularly when using norepinephrine, to increase cardiac output by its positive inotropic effects.

IMMUNOMODULATION

Clinical trials assessing drugs that limit the effects of proinflammatory cytokines such as TNF-α (anti-TNF antibodies, TNF receptors) and IL-1 (IL-1 receptor antagonist inhibitors) have not given convincing

TABLE 130-2	The Fluid Challenge Technique	
Define	**Example**
The type of fluid	Ringer's lactate
The rate of infusion	500 mL in 20 min
The goal	Mean arterial pressure >75 mm Hg
The limits	Central venous pressure 16 mm Hg

results of beneficial effects of these agents on outcome, probably largely because such cytokines have multiple effects, beneficial as well harmful.

The link between coagulation and inflammation led to the suggestion that some of the key coagulation proteins may have beneficial effects in sepsis. Administration of activated protein C (drotrecogin alfa [activated]) early in severe sepsis or septic shock reduced mortality[2] and morbidity.[38] In addition to its anticoagulation effects, activated protein C has important antiinflammatory effects, can influence cell signaling, and has antiapoptotic effects,[39] which may help explain why it has been shown to have beneficial effects in sepsis while other anticoagulants (antithrombin, tissue factor pathway inhibitor) have not. Drotrecogin alfa (activated) is indicated in patients with severe sepsis (sepsis associated with organ dysfunction) at a dose of 24 µg/kg/h via a continuous intravenous (IV) perfusion for 96 hours. It has not been shown to be effective in patients with less severe sepsis[40] or in children[41] and should not be used in patients who have recently undergone a surgical procedure.[40] Drotrecogin alfa (activated) administration is associated with an increased risk of hemorrhage,[42] such that it is contraindicated in patients with a high risk of bleeding. Infusions should be stopped 2 hours prior to any surgical intervention but may be restarted 12 hours after major interventions or sooner for more minor procedures if hemostasis is assured. The high costs of the drug may also limit its use, although its cost-effective profile is similar to many other accepted ICU therapies.[43]

The administration of steroids for patients with sepsis was proposed many years ago, but at the large doses studied (about 30 mg/kg of methylprednisolone) was never shown to have a beneficial effect on survival. More recently, the concept of relative adrenal insufficiency, based on the response to an ACTH test, reawakened interest in steroids, and moderate doses of corticosteroids (50 mg hydrocortisone IV every 6 hours) in patients with septic shock were shown to restore the activity of vascular adrenergic receptors, without excessive immunosuppressive effects, thus improving hemodynamic status and reducing mortality.[44] Although initially it was recommended that this treatment strategy be guided by an ACTH test, this has now been abandoned because of difficulties with the interpretation of such tests.[31] Moreover, a recent multicenter study failed to confirm the beneficial effects of moderate dose corticosteroids in patients with less severe sepsis.[45] Interestingly, a recent post hoc analysis of a large multicenter trial suggested that administration of low-dose vasopressin in combination with corticosteroids was associated with improved mortality rates and reduced organ dysfunction compared to the combination of norepinephrine and vasopressin.[46]

The treatment of fever is controversial. Increased body temperature increases oxygen requirements, but the increased cellular metabolism may form part of the body's natural defense. Animal studies have suggested that control of fever may be detrimental,[47] and the release of heat shock proteins in fever may have important protective effects.[48] A multicenter study in patients with severe sepsis reported that ibuprofen, a cyclooxygenase inhibitor, was well tolerated but did not reduce mortality.[49]

High-flow hemofiltration techniques can remove a range of bacterial products and mediators but are not without risk, notably because this process can remove beneficial products such as hormones and medications, including antibiotics, as well as potentially harmful substances.[50] Clinical studies have provided conflicting data regarding the effects of these techniques on outcomes.[51,52]

NUTRITIONAL SUPPORT

Malnutrition can prolong the course of sepsis and increase the risk of complications. In considering nutritional support in patients with septic shock, several factors should be remembered:

- The enteral route is preferable to the parenteral route.
- Enteral nutrition should probably not be started during the initial phase of resuscitation. Although studies are limited, increasing the oxygen requirements of the gut is probably unwise in the acute circulatory shock situation. However, as soon as the patient has achieved a degree of hemodynamic stability (after a maximum of 24-48 hours), enteral nutrition should be started.
- Careful control of blood glucose levels is recommended. Control of blood glucose has been shown to be associated with improved outcomes,[53] but hypoglycemia can be a problem with very strict blood glucose protocols. A suggested target glucose concentration is, therefore, 110 to 150 mg/dL.[31,54] Variability in glucose levels should also be avoided.[54,55]

ORGAN SUPPORT

Organ dysfunction can involve any organ and can be quantified using the SOFA score (see Table 130-1). Techniques for individual organ support are covered in separate chapters, but an overview is given here.

Respiratory Alterations

Respiratory failure is a common complication of sepsis and is characterized by hypoxemia associated with the presence of bilateral infiltrates on chest radiograph, with no evidence of left hear failure (normal PAOP). The diagnosis of acute respiratory distress syndrome (ARDS) is made when the Pao_2/Fio_2 ratio is less than 200 mm Hg; the less severe form, acute lung injury (ALI), is defined as a Pao_2/Fio_2 less than 300 mm Hg.[56]

When starting a patient on mechanical ventilation, several factors need particular attention:

- Worsening of arterial hypotension when starting mechanical ventilation suggests the presence of hypovolemia due to a reduction in venous return (and hence in cardiac output) when intrathoracic pressures are increased.
- Tidal volume should be limited, not only for hemodynamic reasons but to avoid a major inflammatory reaction. In patients with ALI, mortality was reduced in patients given tidal volumes of 6 mL/min as opposed to 12 mL/kg.[57]
- Sedation must be avoided whenever possible. Administration of sedative drugs and analgesics should be titrated with respect to the needs of the individual patient. Reduced administration of sedative agents can shorten duration of mechanical ventilation and ICU stay.[58,59]

Renal Alterations

Sepsis is the leading cause of acute renal failure in the ICU.[60] Renal function can worsen as a result of circulatory changes associated with vasoconstriction of the afferent arteries and reduced glomerular filtration rate. In addition, management of the patient with sepsis often involves the administration of nephrotoxic agents—for example, certain medicines or contrast agents for radiologic examinations.

Unfortunately, there is no prophylactic approach to renal failure other than to try and maintain adequate renal perfusion and overall volume state. Administration of low (renal)-dose dopamine is ineffective at preventing renal failure,[61] and diuretics may be harmful.[62]

Renal replacement therapy is frequently necessary in septic patients. In septic shock, continuous venovenous techniques, with or without dialysis, are generally preferred over intermittent techniques to facilitate control of fluid balance.

Coagulation Alterations

Alterations in coagulation parameters occur with high frequency in septic patients, even if they do not meet all the criteria of DIC. A low platelet count is common in sepsis and may be associated with a prolonged prothrombin time and activated partial thromboplastin time. Increased D-dimer levels are present in almost all patients with septic shock, so D-dimer measurements are not very helpful. Treatment of these alterations revolves primarily around the cause, and there is no indication for heparin therapy. In severe cases associated with significant bleeding, fresh frozen plasma or platelet infusions may be indicated.

Hepatic Alterations

Circulatory shock of any cause frequently results in the elevation of liver-associated enzymes, but the contribution of various organs (e.g., muscles) to increased enzyme levels is difficult to quantify. Often there is a rise in bilirubin after several days, without evidence of hemolysis, major hematomas, or biliary pathology. Supplementary examinations such as ultrasound may be indicated to exclude any associated biliary pathology.

Cerebral Function Alterations

Circulatory shock is typically accompanied by an alteration of intellectual function, initially manifested as confusion without real coma and reversible with resolution of shock. Cerebral alterations can be prolonged, and the patient is then said to have septic encephalopathy. The exact cause of the encephalopathy is unclear, although various mediators of sepsis have been implicated. Investigations are of little use except to exclude other causes. The electroencephalogram (EEG) generally shows a slow diffuse slowing, whereas cerebral computed tomography (CT) and cerebrospinal fluid examination are normal.[63]

Conclusion

Optimal treatment of a patient with septic shock requires a rapid and effective management plan with the assistance of the full ICU team. Infection control and achieving hemodynamic stability must be tackled simultaneously. Treatment of severe sepsis per se is currently limited to activated protein C and perhaps moderate doses of corticosteroids.

Other interventions are currently undergoing clinical trials, with the hope that they will improve the microcirculatory changes of sepsis or beneficially modulate the host response. A better characterization of patients with septic shock—for example, by using the PIRO system—is necessary to appropriately titrate therapeutic interventions to the individual patient.

KEY POINTS

1. Septic shock affects 10% to 15% of ICU patients and has a mortality rate of 50% to 60%.

2. Septic shock is most commonly caused by a bacterial infection, although fungi, viruses, and parasites can all be implicated. The most common source of infection is the lung, followed by the abdomen.

3. Patients with sepsis can be classified according to their predisposing factors, the nature of the infection, degree of immune response, and associated organ dysfunction.

4. Septic shock is defined as severe sepsis (i.e., sepsis with organ dysfunction) with persistent arterial hypotension despite adequate fluid resuscitation, in the presence of perfusion abnormalities manifest by oliguria, reduced peripheral perfusion, and/or altered mental status.

5. Blood lactate levels are typically raised in septic shock, and persistently raised levels are a poor prognostic sign.

6. Management of septic shock includes infection control, hemodynamic stabilization, and immunomodulation.

ANNOTATED REFERENCES

Bernard GR, Vincent JL, Laterre PF, et al. Efficacy and safety of recombinant human activated protein C for severe sepsis. N Engl J Med 2001;344:699-709.
   Landmark study, as it was the first phase III study to show beneficial effect of an immunomodulatory agent on survival from severe sepsis and septic shock.
De Backer D, Biston P, Devriendt J, et al. Comparison of dopamine and norepinephrine in the treatment of shock. N Engl J Med 2010;362:779-89.
   Important randomized study demonstrating similar mortality rates with use of dopamine or norepinephrine as first-line vasopressor in shock, but increased complication rates with dopamine.
Dellinger RP, Levy MM, Carlet JM, et al. Surviving Sepsis Campaign: international guidelines for management of severe sepsis and septic shock: 2008. Crit Care Med 2008;36:296-327.

Evidence-based guidelines on all aspects of the management of patients with severe sepsis and septic shock.
Levy MM, Fink MP, Marshall JC, et al. 2001 SCCM/ESICM/ACCP/ATS/SIS International Sepsis Definitions Conference. Crit Care Med 2003;31:1250-6.
   Important report of the Sepsis Definitions Conference and introducing the PIRO concept.
Sprung CL, Annane D, Keh D, et al. Hydrocortisone therapy for patients with septic shock. N Engl J Med 2008;358:111-24.
   Study demonstrating no beneficial effect of corticosteroids in patients with septic shock.

REFERENCES

Access the complete reference list online at http://www.expertconsult.com.

131

Sepsis and Multiple Organ System Failure in Children

JOSEPH CARCILLO | JAN A. HAZELZET

Definitions of Sepsis, Severe Sepsis, Septic Shock, and Multiple Organ Failure

The 2001 International Sepsis Definitions Conference[1] centered discussion on whether *sepsis* should continue to be defined as systemic inflammatory response syndrome plus infection or infection plus systemic inflammatory response syndrome plus signs of organ dysfunction. It was agreed that the definitions of severe sepsis remain intact. Most pediatric literature defines inclusion criteria for *sepsis* as hyperthermia or hypothermia, tachycardia (may be absent in the hypothermic patient), evidence of infection, and at least one of the following signs of new-onset organ dysfunction: altered mental status, hypoxemia, bounding pulses, or increased lactate. *Severe sepsis* is uniformly defined as sepsis and organ failure determined by various organ failure scores.[2-5] *Septic shock* has been defined as infection with hypothermia or hyperthermia, tachycardia (may be absent with hypothermia), and altered mental status in the presence of at least one, but usually more than one, of the following: decreased peripheral pulses compared with central pulses prolonged greater than 2 seconds (cold shock) or flash capillary refill (warm shock), mottled or cool extremities (cold shock), and decreased urine output (<1 mL/kg/h). Hypotension is observed in late decompensated shock.[6]

The American College of Critical Care Medicine[6] further defines shock according to response to therapy as fluid-refractory/dopamine-resistant, catecholamine-resistant, and refractory shock. *Multiple organ failure* is defined as more than one organ failure. The greater the number of concomitant organ failures, the greater the risk of mortality. Multiple organ failure generally is observed in septic shock patients who receive delayed resuscitation or inadequate source control therapies (inadequate nidus removal or ineffective antibiotic regimen). Multiple organ failure also is observed in patients with septic shock who have an underlying primary or acquired immunodeficiency that prevents timely eradication of infection and resolution of inflammation.

Changing Outcomes and Epidemiology

The mortality rate in neonatal and pediatric severe sepsis has improved from 97% in 1963 to 9% in 1999, to 4% in 2003.[7-13] Previously healthy children have better outcomes than children with chronic illness. The randomized controlled trial of bactericidal permeability-increasing protein[14] for children with purpura fulminans/presumed meningococcal septic shock showed 10% mortality rates in the placebo groups. The reported outcomes in children with septic shock when using therapeutic approaches similar to those recommended in the 2002 American College of Critical Care Medicine *Clinical Practice Parameters for Hemodynamic Support of Pediatric and Neonatal Patients in Septic Shock*[6] show a decreasing tendency. In children with meningococcal septic shock in the United Kingdom, a 5% mortality rate was reported,[15] and in the Netherlands a decreasing mortality was shown in the same patient group.[16] A single-center study in the United States reported a 10% mortality rate.[17] The investigators observed 0% mortality in previously healthy children but a 15% mortality rate in children with chronic illness (for the most part cancer patients). All of these children died with multiple organ failure. Ngo and colleagues[18] observed a 0%

mortality rate in a randomized Dengue shock fluid resuscitation trial. The US KIDS database showed a 4.2% severe sepsis mortality overall, with 2% in the previously healthy and 8% in the chronically ill child.[13]

Although outcomes are improving, the burden of newborn and pediatric sepsis is increasing in the United States. More children die with severe sepsis than die with cancer, with an estimated yearly healthcare cost of $4 billion in the United States for patients with this condition.[12] Half are newborns, with most of these having low birth weight.[9] Half of children with severe sepsis have underlying chronic illness. Neurologic and cardiovascular chronic illness is most common in infants with severe sepsis and cancer, whereas immune deficiency is most common in children with severe sepsis. Medical advances have affected etiology and epidemiology. In 1990, Jacobs and coworkers[19] reported that the most common causes of septic shock in children were, in descending order, *Haemophilus influenzae* b, *Neisseria meningitidis*, and *Streptococcus pneumoniae*. The 1995 and 1999 U.S. estimates suggest a change. *H. influenzae* type b is all but nonexistent, *N. meningitidis* is prevalent in only a few regions of the United States, and group B *Streptococcus* is decreasing. The more recent use of *S. pneumoniae* vaccine is reducing the incidence of this infection. The Canadian government has implemented nationwide immunization in children younger than age 2 years for *N. meningitidis* serotype C.[20] The most prevalent causes of severe sepsis and septic shock in the United States now seem to be staphylococcal and fungal infections.[12] Methicillin-resistant *Staphylococcus aureus* (MRSA) is an emerging disease. Influenza vaccines are now universal for both endemic and pandemic forms (H1N1).

Pathophysiology and Developmental Effects

MOLECULAR PATHOGENESIS

Controlled Inflammation with Eradication of Infection

Endotoxin, mannose, and other glycoprotein moieties on the cell walls of yeast and fungi, superantigens, toxins associated with some gram-positive bacteria, mycobacteria, and viruses, also called *pathogen-associated molecular patterns*, activate the innate immune system after recognition by pathogen recognition receptors. The innate immune system comprises polymorphonuclear neutrophils, monocytes, and macrophages, in part through Toll-like receptors, CD14 receptors (endotoxin), and other costimulatory molecules. These innate immune cells internalize microorganisms and kill them. Monocytes and macrophages present processed antigens from these killed microorganisms to circulating T lymphocytes and coordinate the adaptive immune response. This second wave of immune response includes B-cell activation and antibody production and generation of cytotoxic T cells and natural killer cells (particularly in viral and fungal infection). Opsonization with antibodies allows more efficient recognition, killing, and clearing of microorganisms by resident macrophages in the reticuloendothelial system.[21,22]

The activated inflammatory cells also initiate a series of biochemical cascades that result in phospholipase A$_2$, platelet-activating factor, cyclooxygenase, complement, and cytokine release that orchestrate an efficient and controlled inflammatory/immune response. The cytokines, tumor necrosis factor (TNF) and interleukin (IL)-1β, synergistically interact to promote positive feedback cascades that result in fever and vasodilation. These cytokines stimulate the production of many important effector molecules, including proinflammatory cytokines (e.g., IL-6, IL-8, and interferon-[IFN]-γ), which promote immune cell-mediated killing and antiinflammatory cytokines (e.g., soluble TNF receptor, IL-1 receptor antagonist protein, IL-4, and IL-10), which turn off the immune response when the infection has been cleared. These cytokines also stimulate nitric oxide (NO) production, which leads to vasodilation. NO also combines with superoxide radicals to form peroxynitrite radicals (ONOO⁻), which participate in intracellular killing of microorganisms. Cytokines also increase expression of endothelial-derived adhesion molecules, including E-selectin, which facilitates white blood cell rolling, and intercellular adhesion molecule and vascular adhesion molecule, which facilitate white blood cell adhesion and diapedesis. This activity guides activated inflammatory cells to the site of infection. The cytokines also induce a change in the endothelium to a prothrombotic and antifibrinolytic state. Expression of thrombomodulin is possibly decreased, and expression of the prothrombotic molecule tissue factor and the antifibrinolytic molecule plasminogen activator inhibitor-1 (PAI-1) is increased. The ensuing thrombus "walls off" the infection and allows vascular remodeling until antiinflammatory cytokines turn off the proinflammatory cytokine response and restore the antithrombotic profibrinolytic milieu after infection is cleared.

Uncontrolled Inflammation and Persistent Infection Lead to Septic Shock and Multiple Organ Failure

If the controlled activated immune cell response is ineffective in killing the infectious agent and clearing antigen, inflammation is uncontrolled, and systemic organ injury ensues. Increased TNF and NO production in cardiac cells and circulating myocardial depressant substances can lead to cardiac dysfunction and cardiovascular collapse. Peroxynitrite can cause DNA damage, and subsequent polyadenosyl ribose synthase (PARS) activation depletes cells of oxidized nicotinamide adenine dinucleotide and adenosine triphosphate (ATP), leading to secondary energy failure. Thrombosis and antifibrinolysis becomes systemic. Antithrombotic molecules, including protein C and antithrombin III, are consumed, and ongoing systemic release of tissue factor and PAI-1 results in unremitting thrombosis. At some point, consumption of procoagulant factors leads to a precarious state in which thrombosis is accompanied by bleeding because there are insufficient clotting factors. The antiinflammatory response also becomes deleterious. IL-10 induces a T_H2 response and reduces the ability of monocytes/macrophages to kill infection. Overactivated immune cells also release Fas and Fas ligand. Circulating Fas prevents activated immune cell apoptosis and ensures ongoing inflammation, and Fas ligand can induce liver injury. In patients with natural killer (NK) cell dysfunction, activated immune cell death is further hampered. Ineffective and unresolving inflammation leads to systemic organ failure.

CLINICAL PATHOLOGIC CORRELATES

On the basis of in vivo biochemical analyses and autopsy histology, several forms of multiple organ failure could be characterized.[23-26] *Thrombocytopenia-associated multiple organ failure* (platelet count <100,000/μL or a 50% decrease in platelet count from baseline) was attributable to purpura fulminans and disseminated intravascular coagulation (DIC) with increased tissue factor activity in vivo and fibrin thrombi at autopsy in only 20% of patients. Of these patients, 80% showed thrombotic thrombocytopenic purpura pathophysiology with increased thrombogenic ultra-large von Willebrand factor multimers, absent von Willebrand factor cleaving protease (ADAMTS 13), increased PAI-1 activity in vivo, and platelet/fibrin thrombi at autopsy.

Sequential or liver dysfunction–associated multiple organ failure (shock/acute respiratory distress syndrome followed sequentially by liver and renal failure) was associated with viral sepsis and lymphoproliferative disease. These patients were found to have unremitting Epstein-Barr virus infection, with lymphocyte Fas ligand–mediated destruction of liver and high circulating Fas and Fas ligand levels. This syndrome is also found in patients with defects in NK cell activity. Absent NK cell activity is found in primary hemophagocytic lymphohistiocytosis (HLH), and decreased NK cell activity in secondary HLH. NK cells are responsible for killing viruses and stopping lymphoproliferation.

Unresolving multiple organ failure with prolonged monocyte deactivation (monocyte HLA-DR expression <30% or ex vivo TNF response to lipopolysaccharide <200 pg/mL for >5 days) was associated with secondary bacterial, fungal, or herpesvirus family infection. These patients had elevated IL-10 and IL-6 levels. Patients who died had infection at autopsy.

Lymphoid depletion syndrome (lymphocyte depletion of lymph nodes and spleen) was found at autopsy. All of these children had fungal, bacterial, or herpesvirus family infection at the time of death. Risk factors (odds ratio >10) for this process included lymphocytopenia (<1000/mm³) or hypoprolactinemia or both for more than 7 days. Phagocytosis of these apoptotic bodies by monocytes/macrophages leads to immunoparalysis.

These clinical pathologic correlates support the following hypotheses: (1) uncontrolled inflammation contributes to organ failure after septic shock; (2) uncontrolled inflammation contributes to systemic thrombosis; (3) uncontrolled inflammation leads to adrenal dysfunction not only through thrombosis but also potentially through NO-mediated inhibition of cytochrome P450 activity; and (4) uncontrolled inflammation is commonly associated with uneradicated infection. It is likely that genetic and environmental factors can increase an individual patient's risk for systemic thrombosis and uneradicated infection.

COAGULATION SYSTEM

As is generally accepted and explained in many reviews, coagulation and fibrinolysis are an integrative part of the immune system.[27] There are important physiologic differences in the hemostatic system in children compared with adults. The decreased levels of several crucial coagulants and increased levels of α2-macroglobulin may contribute in part to the lower risk of thrombotic events in childhood during physiologic conditions.[28,29] In pathologic conditions, these physiologic differences might lead to an earlier exhaustion of coagulation factors and DIC in infants and young children.[30] ADAMTS 13 is also decreased in infancy, therefore there may be an increased susceptibility to systemic fibrin and platelet thrombosis The coagulation system is a marker of organ dysfunction in sepsis. It is associated with subsequent endothelium activation and systemic clotting and finally antifibrinolysis.

CARDIOVASCULAR SYSTEM

Ceneviva and associates[31] found that in contrast to adults, who predominantly have high-cardiac-output/low-vascular-resistance shock, children with fluid-refractory/inotropic-resistant shock have varied hemodynamic states, including low cardiac output/high systemic vascular resistance (60%), low cardiac output/low vascular resistance (20%), and high cardiac output/low vascular resistance (20%), which can change with time and depend on age. In contrast to adults, death from shock is most commonly associated with progressive cardiac failure, not vascular failure. Infants and children frequently are insensitive to dopamine or dobutamine and respond to epinephrine (cold shock) or norepinephrine (warm shock).[31-33] Newborns are different as well. Adults can double their heart rate to improve cardiac output, but newborns cannot. Newborns, although tachycardic, depend on increased vascular tone to maintain blood pressure. Persistent pulmonary hypertension and right ventricular failure also complicate newborn septic shock.[34,35]

Predisposing Factors and Prevention Strategies

Environmental and genetic factors associated with reduced immune function predispose children to the development of sepsis and septic shock. These factors include age (prematurity, neonate, and age < 1 year), cancer and immunosuppressive chemotherapeutic agents, transplantation and immunosuppressive agents, primary immunodeficiency disorders (e.g., hypocomplementemia, hypogammaglobulinemia, chronic granulomatous disease), acquired immunodeficiency disorders (neutropenia, lymphocytopenia, monocyte deactivation), and malnutrition. Prolonged use of invasive catheters, muscle relaxants, and broad-spectrum antibiotics also predispose to infection.

Among the community-acquired causes of sepsis, *N. meningitidis* has a diverse clinical picture, ranging from a self-limiting bacteremia to meningitis to a severe rapidly fatal sepsis. After invasion of the bloodstream by the bacteria, three main cascade pathways are activated: the complement system, the inflammatory response, and the coagulation and fibrinolysis pathway. These pathways do not act independently but are able to interact with each other. Genetic polymorphisms among components of these pathways have been shown to be involved in the susceptibility, severity, and outcome of meningococcal disease. Knowledge of genetic variations associated with susceptibility to and severity of meningococcal infection has been reviewed.[36]

Complement deficiencies and defects in sensing or opsonophagocytic pathways, such as the rare Toll-like receptor 4 single nucleotide polymorphisms and combinations of inefficient variants of Fcγ-receptors, seem to have the most important role in genetically established susceptibility. The most recent and largest study on susceptibility is a genome-wide analysis of DNA from 1600 children with meningococcal sepsis. This study showed the significant influence of genetic variants in the complement factor H in the susceptibility.[37] Effect on severity has repeatedly been reported for FcγRIIa and PAI-1 polymorphisms. Angiotensin-converting enzyme is associated with a proinflammatory response. The absence of a 284-base pair marker in the angiotensin-converting enzyme gene (D allele) is associated with higher circulating angiotensin-converting enzyme activity compared with the presence of this marker (I allele). The DD genotype is associated with increased disease severity, and although not significant, a twofold increase in mortality rate has been reported. Outcome effects have been confirmed for single nucleotide polymorphisms in properdin deficiencies, PAI-1 and combination of the −511C/T single nucleotide polymorphisms in IL-1β, and +2018C/T single nucleotide polymorphisms in IL RN. Conflicting results are reported for the effect of the −308G/A promoter polymorphism in TNF. These differences may reflect discrepancies in group definitions among studies or the influence of additional single nucleotide polymorphisms in the TNF promoter, which can form haplotypes representing different cytokine production capacity. For several single-nucleotide polymorphisms, the potential effect on susceptibility, severity, or outcome has not yet been confirmed in an independent study.

The hallmark of pediatric medicine is prevention. Public health programs that reduce prematurity could be expected to have the greatest impact on the incidence of sepsis. The use of group B streptococcal prophylaxis in at-risk mothers has reduced the incidence of septic shock in premature and term infants. Immunization programs for diphtheria, pertussis, tetanus, measles, mumps, rubella, *H. influenzae* type b, *S. pneumoniae*, *N. meningitidis* (type C for infants and type C, A, and Y for college students), and influenza all effectively reduce the incidence of sepsis in newborns and children. The primary immunodeficiency initiative is an important physician education program. Children with frequent pneumonia, sinus infections, or skin infections can benefit from early immunodeficiency workups, including quantitative immunoglobulins, complement levels, nitroblue toluene testing of polymorphonuclear neutrophil function, and antibody titer response to immunization. Early identification of these children can lead to use of therapies that reduce the incidence of sepsis.

Diagnostic Approach and Scoring Systems

Several prognostic factors have been related to severity and nonsurvival, as follows:

- Increased levels of endotoxin, cytokines, lactate, PAI-1, adhesion molecules, procalcitonin, elastase, troponin, and adrenocorticotropic hormone
- Decreased levels of C-reactive protein (or increased), glucose, fibrinogen, coagulation factors, protein C, ADAMTS 13,* leukocytes, and platelets
- Many scoring systems in use are specific for pediatric patients, including pediatric risk of mortality[38] and pediatric organ failure,[5] and specific for certain categories of patients, including Rotterdam score,[39] Glasgow Meningococcal Septicaemia Prognostic Score,[40] DIC,[41,42] PELOD,[43] and adapted adult scores (e.g., organ failure score).[44]

Therapy

EARLY RECOGNITION AND GOAL-DIRECTED THERAPY TO IMPROVE OUTCOME

Early recognition, adequate resuscitation, appropriate therapeutic response, removal of the nidus of infection, and effective antibiotic therapy are crucial to optimal outcome.[45,46] In June 2007, the American College of Critical Care Medicine published its evidence-based *Clinical Practice Parameters for Hemodynamic Support of Newborns and Children with Septic Shock*, based in part on the concept that early recognition and resuscitation improve outcome (Figure 131-1). The major new recommendations include the use of inotropes through a peripheral intravenous (IV) or intraosseous catheter until a central catheter is available, and administration of antibiotics in the first hour.

IMMEDIATE RESUSCITATION (FIRST HOUR)

Airway and Breathing

Newborns and children usually have an adequate airway, but mechanical ventilation is required in 80% in shock. Intubation should be performed according to pediatric advanced life support and Neonatal Resuscitation Program guidelines on the basis of clinical diagnosis of respiratory distress or hemodynamic instability, not blood gas analysis. Volume resuscitation and the use of the non–cardiac depressant drug ketamine as an induction agent are recommended to prevent worsening positive-pressure ventilation–associated hypotension. It is clinical practice to intubate pediatric patients in an early stage of the disease, generally when they need more than 60 mL/kg of fluid resuscitation.[15]

Volume Resuscitation

Virtually all children with shock require aggressive volume resuscitation[10,47,48]; this should be given as 20 mL/kg boluses of normal saline or colloid as IV pushes to a total of 60 mL/kg in the first 10 to 20 minutes. If the liver edge becomes palpable, rales are heard, or the perfusion pressure (mean arterial pressure—central venous pressure) narrows, more fluid is not advised. Some children have required 200 mL/kg in the first hour. Many clinicians use crystalloid as the first fluid and follow with colloid if this is unsuccessful. Serum glucose should be checked because hypoglycemia can have devastating neurologic consequences. Glucose should be administered rapidly in this condition.

Cardiovascular Therapy

Children in shock can present with low cardiac output and high systemic vascular resistance, high cardiac output and low systemic vascular resistance, or low cardiac output and low systemic vascular resistance.[31] Depending on which situation exists, inotropic support should be started in the case of fluid-refractory shock or a combination of an inotrope with a vasopressor or a vasodilator. Dopamine or

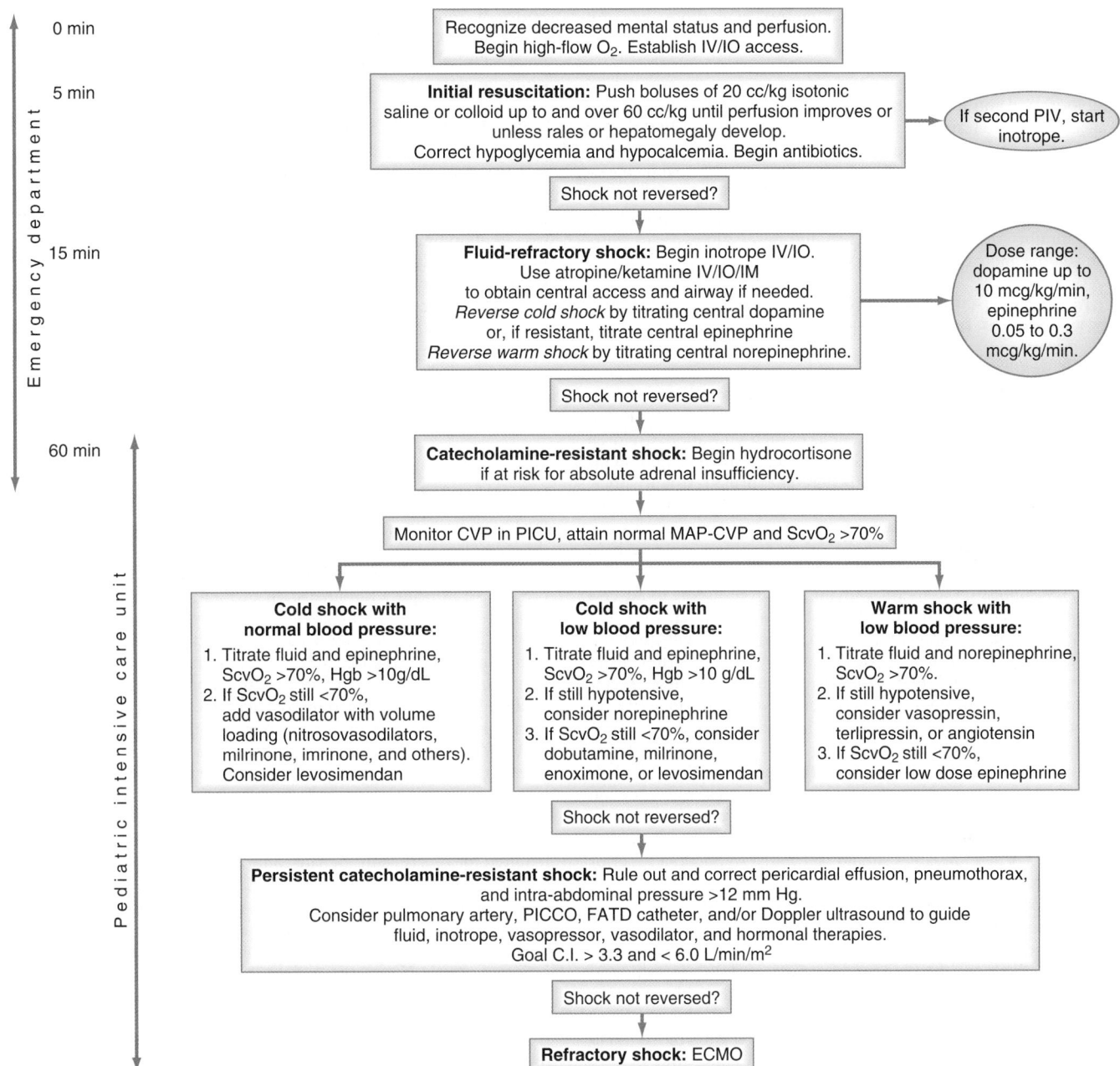

Figure 131-1 Clinical practice parameters for hemodynamic support of newborns and children with septic shock. This evidence-based treatment algorithm is based on early recognition and resuscitation to improve outcome. ACTH, adrenocorticotropic hormone; APLS/PALS, advanced pediatric life support/pediatric advanced life support; CI, cardiac index; CVP, central venous pressure; ECMO, extracorporeal membrane oxygenation; MAP, mean arterial pressure; PDE, phosphodiesterase; PICU, pediatric intensive care unit; ScvO₂, central venous oxygen saturation; PICCO, pulse index contour cardiac output; FATD, femoral artery thermodilution. *(From Brierly J, Carcillo JA, Choong J, Cornell T, Decaen A, Deymann A et al. Clinical practice parameters for hemodynamic support of pediatric and neonatal septic shock: 2007 update from the American College of Critical Care Medicine. Crit Care Med 2009;37:666-88.)*

dobutamine is probably the first choice of support for a pediatric patient with hypotension refractory to fluid resuscitation. The choice of vasoactive agent is determined by the clinical examination. Dobutamine-refractory or dopamine-refractory shock often can be reversed with epinephrine or norepinephrine infusion.[31] Pediatric patients requiring inotropic support are in a state of low cardiac output, not high cardiac output. The use of vasodilators can reverse shock in pediatric patients who remain hypodynamic with a high systemic vascular resistance state, despite fluid resuscitation and implementation of inotropic support. Nitrosovasodilators (nitroprusside or nitroglycerin have a short half-life) are used as first-line therapy for children with epinephrine-resistant low cardiac output and elevated systemic vascular resistance shock.

Adrenal Insufficiency

Lack of response to epinephrine (cold shock) or norepinephrine (warm shock) can be caused by adrenal insufficiency or thyroid deficiency.[49-51] Children at risk for this condition (e.g., purpura fulminans, prior steroid exposure, central nervous system disease) should be treated with hydrocortisone. The proper dose has been poorly investigated and ranges from a stress dose (2 mg/kg) to a shock dose (50 mg/kg of hydrocortisone) followed by the same dose over 24 hours.

Which dose is better in catecholamine-resistant shock has not been determined.

Antibiotics

Antibiotics and antifungal therapies should be administered according to age, setting, and resistance patterns (empirical therapy) after proper cultures have been performed. The emergence of resistant organisms mandates that antibiotics be specific to regional practice. Some investigators advocate antibiotic cycling in the ICU.[52] Although survival from sepsis and septic shock can occur only if the infection is eradicated, administration of antibiotics should never supersede or postpone volume and cardiovascular resuscitation.

STABILIZATION OF SEPSIS AND SEPTIC SHOCK (AFTER FIRST HOUR OF RESUSCITATION)

Cardiovascular

The first hour of resuscitation is directed toward restoration of normal perfusion pressure; however, ensuing therapies should be directed toward obtaining normal central venous oxygen saturation. Children with persistent warm shock can respond to more volume and norepinephrine. In selected children with norepinephrine-resistant shock, vasopressin (at physiologic dose) or angiotensin can bypass alpha receptor desensitization and restore vascular tone; however, this can increase afterload and decrease cardiac output.[53-55] In a large study in pediatric patients with vasodilatory shock (majority being post cardiac surgery), vasopressin was useful, with limitations regarding its adverse effects on the renal system and platelet counts.[56] Children with cold shock and normal blood pressure respond to afterload reduction and volume loading.[31,56] When pediatric patients remain in a normotensive low-cardiac-output and high-vascular-resistance state despite epinephrine and nitrosovasodilator therapy, the use of milrinone (if liver dysfunction is present) or amrinone (if renal dysfunction is present) should be strongly considered.[57] These type III phosphodiesterase inhibitors can bypass β-adrenergic receptor desensitization.[57-59] Children with cold shock and hypotension are most worrisome. They can respond to more volume and epinephrine. Neonates and children with pulmonary hypertension and right ventricular failure can respond to inhaled NO.[60] These therapies should be titrated to obtain a superior vena cava oxygen saturation above 70%.[61]

Extracorporeal membrane oxygenation is an effective therapy in refractory neonatal shock (80% survival) and should be considered as a possible therapy in refractory pediatric shock (50% survival).[62,63] This success is likely due to the fact that refractory shock in newborns and children is usually cardiac, not vascular, failure. Adults with refractory shock from Hantavirus (a low-cardiac-output/high-vascular-resistance state) have similar extracorporeal membrane oxygenation outcomes to newborns with refractory shock.[64]

Respiratory

Lung "protection" ventilation strategies reduced mortality rates in adults with acute respiratory distress syndrome (many who had sepsis).[65] Effective tidal volumes of 6 mL/kg are a reasonable compromise when ventilating septic children with acute respiratory distress syndrome. Positive end-expiratory pressure protects against volutrauma by maintaining functional residual capacity and optimal compliance. Optimal positive end-expiratory pressure can be determined using partial pressure of oxygen in arterial blood–to–inspired oxygen fraction ratio or compliance.

Renal Failure

Renal failure occurs if ischemia continues for greater than 60 minutes, thrombosis prevents perfusion, or myoglobin and uric acid obstruct tubular flow. During the first 60 minutes of ischemia, the neurohormonal system releases aldosterone, angiotensin, and antidiuretic hormone (vasopressin), which prevent natriuresis and diuresis; this manifests clinically with oliguria. Rapid resuscitation reverses ischemia and, because 20% of blood flow goes to renal perfusion, manifests as

return of urine output greater than 1 mL/kg/h. If ischemia lasts more than 1 hour, ATP depletion causes epithelial cells to separate from and obstruct tubules, leading to tubulo-obstructive renal failure (also called *acute tubular necrosis*). Tubular regeneration requires 6 weeks to 3 months.

Blood flow to the kidney is autoregulated by preglomerular and postglomerular constriction and dilation. The ability of the preglomerular arterioles to dilate is impaired during endotoxemia and cirrhosis. Blood flow to the kidney depends on perfusion pressure (measured as mean arterial pressure—central venous pressure or, in the case of abdominal compartment syndrome, mean arterial pressure—intraabdominal pressure) in children with sepsis.[66] Perfusion pressure should be maintained with volume, inotropes, and in some cases vasopressor therapies. Creatinine clearance should be measured daily to assess function. Diuretics are recommended to prevent fluid overload. Patients with myoglobinuria or uric aciduria should be treated with mannitol, alkalinization, and allopurinol (uric aciduria). Severe oliguria or anuria despite diuretics should be managed with daily or continuous hemofiltration/hemodialysis or peritoneal dialysis.

PURPURA FULMINANS AND DISSEMINATED INTRAVASCULAR COAGULATION

DIC is recognized clinically as a prolonged prothrombin time/partial thromboplastin time, reduced fibrinogen, increased fibrin degradation products or D-dimers and thrombocytopenia.[41,42] When patients present with purpura fulminans/DIC, with genetic proclivity (thrombophilias), or with rapidly growing organisms (meningococcus), the process is deadly unless reversed. Tissue factor is exposed by endothelial injury and released into the bloodstream. If tissue factor is unmatched by tissue factor pathway inhibitor, it activates factor VII–mediated coagulation. Ongoing coagulation consumes clotting factors (including fibrinogen), antithrombotic factors (antithrombin III and protein C), and platelets; this leads to a state of massive clotting and bleeding. Therapeutic strategies must restore a homeostatic milieu by removing or inhibiting tissue factor activity and replacing anticoagulant factors, procoagulant factors, and platelets. If systemic clotting is limb-threatening or life-threatening, fibrinolytic therapies may be required for reperfusion. Debate continues on whether specific therapies (e.g., antithrombin III, protein C, heparin, activated protein C, tissue plasminogen activator), nonspecific therapies (fresh frozen plasma and platelet replacement or plasma exchange), or a combination of both (plasma exchange plus antithrombin III, protein C, or activated protein C with tissue plasminogen activator added for limb-threatening or life-threatening thrombosis) is best. An activated protein C trial initiated in pediatric septic shock, in which patients at risk of bleeding (low platelet counts) or receiving heparin-based continuous venovenous hemofiltration were excluded, showed no benefit of treatment compared to placebo.[67] Some investigators think that patients with meningococcemia cannot activate protein C,[68] whereas others have shown that these children can activate protein C.[68] So far there is no evidence for benefit of either product. Studies using intensive plasma exchange therapy appears to be of possible benefit because plasma exchange reverses both fibrin and platelet-vWF multimer-mediated thrombosis.[69-71]

NUTRITION, ELECTROLYTES, ENDOCRINE, AND METABOLISM

It is debated whether one should feed patients enterally when in shock; however, there is agreement the enteral route is best when shock resolves. Total parenteral nutrition should be considered in patients not tolerating enteral feeds and "calories given" directed to "calories expended" if a metabolic monitor is available. If a monitor is not available, calorie needs can be overestimated when using classic formulas in critically ill children. Hypoglycemia should be rigorously avoided and treated. Hypoglycemia is associated with devastating neurologic outcomes. Strict control of hyperglycemia with insulin infusion substantially reduced mortality in a pediatric ICU by reducing deaths from multiple-organ dysfunction syndrome/multiple organ failure.[72] In general, infants are at risk for developing hypoglycemia when they depend on IV fluids; a glucose intake of 4 to 6 mg/kg/min or maintenance fluid intake with glucose 10% and sodium chloride 0.45% is advised.

IMMUNE MODULATION

Children who cannot kill invading organisms die from sepsis. Primary and acquired immunodeficiency states must be treated. Children with chronic granulomatous disease require white blood cell transfusions and interferon. Patients with hypogammaglobulinemia require treatment with IV immunoglobulin. Granulocyte-macrophage colony-stimulating factor was shown in a randomized controlled trial to improve survival in newborn neutropenic septic shock.[73,74] Transplant and nontransplant patients who develop septic shock while receiving immune suppression die unless the immune suppressants are rapidly tapered. Polyclonal IV immunoglobulin has been reported to reduce mortality rate and is a promising adjuvant in the treatment of sepsis and septic shock. All the trials have been small in children, however, and the totality of the evidence is insufficient to support a robust conclusion of benefit. Adjunctive therapy with monoclonal IV immunoglobulin is experimental.[75]

DRUG DOSING

Decreased cytochrome P450 activity not only is manifest in impaired steroid synthesis, but also impaired drug metabolism is present in children with sepsis, septic shock, or multiple organ failure.[23] Patients with multiple organ failure are at particular risk of toxicity with drugs that are metabolized by the cytochrome P450 system. Renal function also is impaired. Creatinine clearance–directed drug dosing of renally eliminated drugs is necessary in these patients. Drugs should be administered according to pharmacodynamic and pharmacokinetic goals.

Multicenter Randomized Controlled Trials for Pediatric Septic Shock

Two studies were completed examining the role of endotoxin-neutralizing therapies in children with presumed meningococcal purpura fulminans/shock. Derkx and colleagues[76] reported a 25% reduction in mortality rate with the HA-1A antibody, and Giroir and others[14,77] reported a 25% reduction in mortality rate with rhBPI. Both studies were underpowered. Nadel repeated the Activated Protein C trial in children with septic shock and observed no benefit of DrotAA in children with severe sepsis; serious bleeding events were similar between groups and the overall safety profile acceptable, except in

children younger than 60 days.[78] It is unknown whether this was due to developmental differences or greater use of plasma products in children compared to adults. deOliveira and colleagues observed a greater than threefold reduction in mortality when using ACCM-PALS therapies directed to RA/SVC or RA/IVC oxygen saturations over 70%.[61] The intervention arm received more fluids, blood, and inotrope/vasodilators than the nonintervention arm. In two trials, neither vasopressin nor terlipressin were effective in improving outcomes in refractory vasodilated shock.[79-80]

KEY POINTS

1. The mortality of severe sepsis in neonatal and pediatric patients has improved from 97% in 1963 to 9% in 1999 to about 4% in 2003. Previously healthy children have better outcomes than children with chronic illness.

2. Although outcomes are improving, the burden of newborn and pediatric sepsis is increasing in the United States. More children die with severe sepsis than die with cancer, with an estimated yearly healthcare cost of $4 billion in the United States for patients with this condition.

3. The physiologic differences in coagulation and fibrinolysis between adults and children might lead to an earlier exhaustion of coagulation factors and disseminated intravascular coagulation in infants and young children.

4. In contrast to adults, death from shock in children is most commonly associated with progressive cardiac failure, not vascular failure. Pediatric patients have low cardiac output/high systemic vascular resistance (60%), low cardiac output/low vascular resistance (20%), or high cardiac output/low vascular resistance (20%).

5. Genetic polymorphisms in components of the inflammatory pathways have been shown to be involved in the susceptibility, severity, and outcome of pediatric sepsis.

6. The American College of Critical Care Medicine published in 2007 evidence-based *Clinical Practice Parameters for Hemodynamic Support of Newborns and Children with Septic Shock*, based in part on the concept that early recognition and resuscitation improve outcome.

7. The moment of intubation should be estimated on the basis of clinical diagnosis of respiratory distress or hemodynamic instability, not on blood gas analysis.

8. Virtually all children with shock require aggressive volume resuscitation; this should be given as 20 mL/kg boluses of normal saline or colloid as intravenous push to a total of 60 mL/kg in the first 10 to 20 minutes unless hepatomegaly or rales develop.

9. Patients with multiple organ failure are at particular risk of toxicity with drugs that are metabolized by the cytochrome P450 system.

ANNOTATED REFERENCES

Carcillo JA, Fields AI. American College of Critical Care Medicine Task Force Committee Members. Clinical practice parameters for hemodynamic support of pediatric and neonatal patients in septic shock. Crit Care Med 2002;30:1365-78.
Evidence-based guidelines for the treatment of sepsis in neonates and pediatric patients are presented.
Emonts M, Hazelzet JA, de Groot R, Hermans PW. Host genetic determinants of *Neisseria meningitidis* infections. Lancet Infect Dis 2003;3:565-77.
This is a review of the genetic polymorphisms and mutations known so far to be involved in the inflammatory process in meningococcal sepsis.
Leteurtre S, Martinot A, Duhamel A, Gauvin F, Grandbastien B, Nam TV, et al. Development of a pediatric multiple organ dysfunction score: use of two strategies. Med Decis Making 1999;19:399-410.

This article describes an organ failure score useful in pediatric sepsis. The score is practical for use in daily practice.
Pollard AJ, Britto J, Nadel S, DeMunter C, Habibi P, Levin M. Emergency management of meningococcal disease. Arch Dis Child 1999;80:290-6.
An overview of the acute treatment of pediatric meningococcal sepsis is presented.
Watson RS, Carcillo JA, Linde-Zwirble WT, Clermont G, Lidicker J, Angus DC. The epidemiology of severe sepsis in children in the United States. Am J Respir Crit Care Med 2003;167:695-701.
This is the first large overview of this size concerning epidemiology of pediatric sepsis in the United States.

REFERENCES

Access the complete reference list online at http://www.expertconsult.com.

132

Acute Bloodstream Infection

WALTER ZINGG | PHILIPPE EGGIMANN | DIDIER PITTET

Acute bloodstream infection, which may be primary or secondary and community-acquired or nosocomial, is one of the most severe forms of infection. Frequently observed among immunocompromised and critically ill patients, bloodstream infection is rarely asymptomatic and may be associated with multiple organ failure.[1-3]

Definitions

The term *bloodstream infection* includes all forms of confirmed or unconfirmed bacteremia and fungemia. Acute bloodstream infections should be distinguished from *septicemia*, *clinical sepsis*, and *sepsis*, which refer to clinical syndromes. Definitions are summarized in Table 132-1.

Epidemiology

The epidemiology of bloodstream infection varies according to its source. Bloodstream infections represented 12% of all nosocomial infections reported in 10,038 patients from 1417 intensive care units (ICUs) in the European Prevalence of Infection in Intensive Care (EPIC) study,[4] and similar data were found in other clinical studies.[5] A worldwide prevalence study among 1265 ICUs (EPIC 2) reported bloodstream infections representing 15% of all healthcare-associated infections among 1265 participating ICUs from 75 countries.[6] Almost half of all positive blood cultures obtained in a hospital are due to nosocomial bloodstream infections.[7] Of these, most are primary and associated with central catheters.[8]

Most surveillance systems today such as the U.S. National Healthcare Safety Network (NHSN), the German Krankenhaus Infektions Surveillance System (KISS), or the International Nosocomial Infection Control Consortium (INICC) focus on catheter-associated, laboratory-confirmed, primary bloodstream infections, with reporting of bloodstream infections as episodes per 1000 device-days. Surveillance of clinical sepsis has been mostly abandoned because the definition of this infection leaves much room for interpretation and is resource demanding.[8] The exception to this rule are studies among neonates; as blood cultures are often unreliable in this population.[9] However, even among adults, clinical sepsis may represent up to two-thirds of central line–associated bloodstream infections (CLABSI), but focusing on microbiologically documented bloodstream infections on the other hand may underestimate true CLABSI rates.[8]

Most community-acquired bloodstream infections are secondary and due to documented infections such as pneumonia and urinary tract or soft-tissue infections (Table 132-2).[10-13] Similar to nosocomial bloodstream infections, many primary bloodstream infections are associated with intravascular access devices.[14-16]

The incidence of bloodstream infection in various patient populations is presented in Table 132-3.[10,13,14,17-29] The large observed differences may be related to variable definitions and reporting systems. Thus, comparisons and benchmarking should be done with caution.[30,31]

Microbiology

The distribution of microorganisms causing bloodstream infections varies according to source, age category (neonates, children, adults), and resources available for healthcare (Table 132-4).* In most institutions,

a shift in predominant organisms from gram-negative bacilli to gram-positive cocci has been observed over the past 2 decades.[11,15,28] However, in countries with limited resources, gram-negative pathogens and, among these, non-fermentative organisms such as *Pseudomonas* spp. and *Acinetobacter* spp., are still predominant.[34-38] The predominance of non-fermentative organisms may be ascribed to contamination of infusates and thus to breaches in basic infection control procedures.[35,42] Such breaches are likely due to the multiple use of infusates or single-use vials and a lack of respect of aseptic conditions. The shift towards gram-positive cocci seen in high-resource countries is largely due to the use of intravascular devices and the fact that the proportion of patients with risk factors such as neutropenia, solid organ and bone marrow transplantation, or the use of immunosuppressive agents has increased. The current high density of medical facilities and unrestricted access to medical care for the majority of the population in most developed countries have played major roles in the prescription of antibiotics very early in the course of most infections. In addition, the widespread use of broad-spectrum antibiotics, either for therapy or surgical prophylaxis, may be partially responsible for the increase in the relative proportions of coagulase-negative staphylococci (CoNS) and enterococci. The proportion of *Candida* spp., especially infections with non-*albicans* spp., has considerably increased in many institutions, although recent studies suggest a trend toward fewer *Candida* infections, at least in North America.[43,44] Prolonged treatments with multiple antibiotics, the use of intravascular devices, total parenteral nutrition, and prolonged neutropenia in patients with cancer have been identified as independent risk factors in this context.[45-52]

CoNS are the most common pathogens isolated from blood cultures, especially in primary bloodstream infections.[7] Often considered contaminants, the detection of CoNS may not always be harmless; associated mortality up to 18% has been reported.[7] In contrast, mortality from *Staphylococcus aureus* bloodstream infection ranges between 13% and 25%, with higher rates for nosocomial than for community-acquired infection.[53,54] Detection of *S. aureus* on catheter tips is a predictor for subsequent bacteremia, even in the absence of clinical signs and negative blood cultures at the time of catheter removal.[55-57] Likewise, bloodstream infections due to *Candida* spp. have a poor prognosis. Mortality with this microorganism ranges between 15% and 55%, especially when antifungal treatment is delayed by 3 or more days.[45,58] An important shift in the epidemiology of *Candida* bloodstream infections has occurred over the past decades, with decreasing infections due to *Candida albicans*, but increasing numbers of infections due to non-*albicans* isolates. In particular, fungemia due to *Candida glabrata* has increased.[59] The emergence of this species presents clinical problems insofar as it is often resistant to fluconazole.[60]

Impact

Patients with bloodstream infections are at risk for increased mortality.[16,18] A meta-analysis by Siempos and colleagues found attributable mortality rates for CLABSI between 2% and 35%.[61] Nosocomial bloodstream infections and, in this context CLABSI in particular, are associated with increased morbidity, prolonged length of hospital stay, and resource utilization in almost all groups of patients studied (Table 132-5).† Attributable costs and length of stay among neonates depend largely on the birthweight category, with extremely

---

*References 10, 13-15, 17, 18, 23-25, 28, and 32-41.

†References 1, 10, 12-14, 17, 18, and 61-70.

TABLE 132-1 Definitions of Bloodstream Infection

Type of Bloodstream Infection	Criteria
Positive blood culture	Recognized pathogens* identified from one or more blood cultures and not related to an infection at another body site
Laboratory-confirmed bloodstream infection	Positive blood culture with at least one of the following signs or symptoms: fever (>100.4°F [38°C]) or hypothermia (<98.6°F [37°C]); chills; low blood pressure (systolic blood pressure ≤ 90 mm Hg or a decrease > 40 mm Hg from baseline)
Primary	Laboratory-confirmed bloodstream infection or clinical sepsis occurring without a documented distal source of infection, including those resulting from catheter-related or catheter-associated infections
Secondary	Laboratory-confirmed bloodstream infection occurring in the presence of another documented site of infection
Catheter-associated	Primary bloodstream infection and presence of an intravascular access device
Catheter-related	Laboratory-confirmed bloodstream infection in a patient with an intravascular access device and at least one positive blood culture obtained from a peripheral vein, clinical manifestations of infection (fever, chills, hypotension), and no apparent source of bloodstream infection except for vascular access plus one of the following: positive semiquantitative culture (>15 CFU/catheter segment) with the same organism,[103] positive quantitative culture (>10³ CFU/catheter segment) with the same organism,[104] simultaneous quantitative blood cultures with a ≥ 5:1 ratio CVC versus peripheral,[105] and differential period of CVC culture versus peripheral blood culture positivity of > 2 h[106]

*One of the following: common skin contaminant (diphtheroids, *Bacillus* spp., *Propionibacterium* spp., coagulase-negative staphylococci, or micrococci) cultured from two or more blood cultures drawn on separate occasions; common skin contaminant cultured from one or more blood cultures from a patient with vascular access, and the physician institutes appropriate antimicrobial therapy; positive antigen test on blood *and* signs and symptoms with positive laboratory results not related to infection at another site.

CFU, colony-forming unit; *CVC,* central venous catheter.

TABLE 132-2 Sources of Bloodstream Infection

Author	No. of Cases	Primary (%)*	Secondary (%)	Urinary (%)	Abdominal (%)	Pulmonary (%)	Skin/Soft Tissue (%)	Bone/ Joint (%)	Cardiovascular (%)	CNS (%)	Other (%)
Hospital-Wide, Community-Acquired											
Valles et al.[13]	339	25	75	20	20	21	ND	ND	4	ND	10
Hospital-Wide, Nosocomial											
Pittet et al.[16]	1745	62	38	7	2	11	10	ND	ND	ND	8
ICU, Community-Acquired and Nosocomial											
Pittet et al.[12]	176	21	79	6	31	28	ND	ND	ND	2	12
Hugonnet et al.[11]	196	47	53	4	15	29	ND	ND	ND	1	4
ICU, Nosocomial											
Valles et al.[13]	590	65	35	6	6	18	2	ND	ND	ND	3
Brun-Buisson[18]	111	55	45	ND	ND	ND	ND	ND	ND	ND	ND
Pittet & Wenzel[15]	3464	59	41	8	ND	12	10	ND	ND	ND	ND

*Catheter-related or of unknown origin.

ICU, intensive care unit; *CNS,* central nervous system; *ND,* not done.

TABLE 132-3 Incidence of Bloodstream Infection in Differing Populations

Author	No. of Hospitals	Type of Hospital	Type of Infection	Per 1000 Admissions or Discharges	Per 1000 Patient-Days
Hospital-Wide Series					
Brun-Buisson et al.[10]	24	Any	Nosocomial	4.4 (4.0-4.9)	—
Banerjee et al.[22]	124	Community	Nosocomial	1.3	—
Banerjee et al.[22]	124	University	Nosocomial	6.5	—
Pittet & Wenzel[15]	1	University	Nosocomial	13.2	1.5
ICU Series					
Valles et al.[17]	30 Mixed	Any	Community	10.2	—
Luzzaro et al.[32]	16 Mixed	Any	Any*	6.8	—
Richards et al.[28]	205 Mixed	Any	Nosocomial	7.5	2.4
Legras et al.[29]	5 Mixed	Any	Nosocomial	—	4.1
Brun-Buisson[18]	15 Mixed	Any	Nosocomial	50.4	4.5
Kollef et al.[20]	1 Mixed	University	Nosocomial	—	9.6
Valles et al.[17]	30 Mixed	Any	Nosocomial	36.0	—
Richards et al.[23]	112 Medical	Any	Nosocomial	16.3	4.1
Richards et al.[24]	61 Pediatric	Any	Nosocomial	14.6	3.7
Raymond & Aujard[25]	20 Pediatric	Any	Nosocomial	—	3.4
Gastmeier et al.[26]	72 Pediatric	Any	Nosocomial	—	2.1
Gilio et al.[27]	1 Pediatric	University	Nosocomial	—	1.5
Pittet & Wenzel[15]	1 Surgical	University	Nosocomial	26.7	—
Richards et al.[19]	93 coronary	Any	Nosocomial	—	1.8

*Both community-acquired and nosocomial infections were reported together.

TABLE 132-4	Microbiology of Bloodstream Infections											
Author	Year of Publication	No. of Organisms	CoNS (%)	S. aureus (%)	S. pneumoniae (%)	Enterococci (%)	Other GPC (%)	E. coli (%)	Enterobacter (%)	P. aeruginosa (%)	Other GNB (%)	Yeasts (%)
Community-Acquired												
Luzzaro et al.[32]	2002	1031	5	19	10	6	12	42	3	4	7	2
Valles et al.[13]	2003	339	3	15	18	3	5	28	2	3	22	1
Nosocomial												
Pittet & Wenzel[15]	1995	3464	26	16	NR	4	12	12	6	9	8	7
Valles et al.[17]	1997	511	28	20	NR	6	3	6	10	9	15	5
Edmond et al.[2]	1999	10617	32	16	NR	11	1	6	7	4	16	8
Richards et al.[23]	1999	2971	36	13	NR	16	NR	3	6	3	11	12
Richards et al.[24]	1999	1887	40	9	6	NR	1	3	5	5	21	10
Renaud et al.[18]	2001	111	18	14	NR	7	5	NR	25	NR	15	7
Richards et al.[28]	2000	4394	40	12	11	NR	7	2	7	4	5	12
Luzzaro et al.[32]	2002	1478	13	23	1	9	12	15	8	9	11	9
Nonindustrialized Countries, Nosocomial												
Pawar[40]	2004	17	6	12	NR	NR	NR	47	6	NR	18	12
Almuneef[107]	2006	73	14	7	NR	10	1	4	10	11	35	8
Moreno[37]	2006	126	10	37	NR	NR	NR	NR	NR	6	45	2
Girao[36]	2008	1286	12	27	NR	8	NR	NR	7	9	30	6
Macias[35]	2010	108	10	14	NR	4	1	NR	8	23	35	5
Rosenthal[34]	2010	5433	NR	14	NR	2	NR	11	NR	46	26	NR

CoNS, coagulase-negative staphylococci; *E. coli, Escherichia coli*; *GNB*, gram-negative bacilli; *GPC*, gram-positive cocci; *NR*, not reported; *P. aeruginosa, Pseudomonas aeruginosa*; *S. aureus, Staphylococcus aureus*; *S. pneumoniae, Streptococcus pneumoniae*.

low-birthweight infants generating more expense than very low to normal-birthweight infants.[71] Interestingly, mortality from secondary bloodstream infections is higher compared to primary bloodstream infections (29%-45% versus 18%-29%, respectively). Furthermore, mortality from CLABSI is lower than mortality from other primary bloodstream infections (15%-26% versus 18%-29%, respectively).[16,18] Although the reason for this difference is unclear, delayed antibiotic therapy for community-acquired bloodstream infections and serious comorbidity in the context of secondary bloodstream infections may partially explain such trends.

Microbiological factors have been found to be important in the context of mortality among patients with nosocomial bloodstream infection, even after adjustment for major confounders intrinsic to patients' underlying conditions.[16] Pathogens that are independently

TABLE 132-5	Impact of Nosocomial Bloodstream Infection in Critically Ill Patients								
					Mortality (%)		Attributable		
Author	Study Population	Year of Publication	Study Period	No. of Cases	Crude	Attributable	LOS (Days)	Costs (US$)[#]	
Community-Acquired									
Valles et al.[13]	ICU	2003	1998	339	43	32	NA	NA	
Community-Acquired and Nosocomial									
Pittet et al.[12]	ICU	1996	1984-88	176	35	NA	NA	NA	
Brun-Buisson et al.[10]	ICU	1996	1993	832	55	NA	NA	NA	
Hugonnet et al.[11]	ICU	2003	1994-97	369	35-37	NA	NA	NA	
Nosocomial									
Forgacs et al.[64]	ICU	1986	1971-85	468	61	NA	NA	NA	
Smith et al.[65]	ICU[†]	1991	1986-89	34	82	30	NA	NA	
Rello et al.[66]	ICU[†]	1994	1990-92	111	65	35[‡]	NA	NA	
Pittet et al.[1]	ICU[†]	1994	1988-90	86	50	35	8.0	40,000	
Pittet & Wenzel[67]	ICU, catheter-associated	1994	1988-90	20	45	25	6.5	29,000	
Valles et al.[17]	ICU	1997	1993	590	42	19	NA	NA	
Soufir et al.[62]	ICU, catheter-associated	1999	1990-95	38	50	29	NA	NA	
Di Giovine et al.[68]	ICU[ǁ]	1999	1994-96	68	35	4[¶]	10.0	35,000	
Rello et al.[69]	ICU, catheter-related	2000	1992-99	49	22	13[¶]	20.0	4000	
Renaud & Brun-Buisson[18]	ICU	2001	1998	96	52	35	5.5	NA	
Renaud & Brun-Buisson[18]	ICU[ǁ]	2001	1998	28	50	2	8.0	NA	
Renaud & Brun-Buisson[18]	ICU, catheter-related	2001	1998	26	39	12[¶]	14.0[¶]	NA	
Dimick et al.[70]	ICU, catheter-related	2001	1998-99	17	56	35[‡]	20.0	71,443*	
Rosenthal et al.[108]	ICU, catheter-associated	2003	1998-02	142	54	24	11*	4,888	
Payne et al.[71]	Neonatal ICU	2004	1998-99	553	NA	NA	4-7**	5875-12,480**	
Blot et al.[109]	ICU	2005	1992-02	176	28	2	8*	14,268	
Elward et al.[110]	Pediatric ICU	2005	1999-00	57	NA	NA	NA	39,219	
Warren et al.[111]	ICU, catheter-associated	2006	1998-00	41	51	23	19*	11,971	
Higuera et al.[112]	ICU, catheter-associated	2007	2002-03	55	42	20	6*	11,591	

*ICU days.
[†]Includes both primary and secondary bloodstream infections.
[‡]Attributable mortality was determined by a simple comparison with the crude mortality of all patients who did not develop a bloodstream infection.
[§]*Acinetobacter baumannii* nosocomial bloodstream infections only.
[ǁ]Includes primary bloodstream infections after exclusion of catheter-related infections.
[¶]Differences are nonsignificant.
[#]Based on billing database.
**Depending on the birth weight category.
LOS, Length of stay, *NA*, not available.

associated with mortality are *Candida* spp. and *Pseudomonas aeruginosa*. CoNS are less associated with mortality compared to other pathogens, although these pathogens are isolated most frequently.[16]

General Principles of Management

When patients are suspected to have bacteremia or fungemia, blood cultures are performed. The clinical threshold to draw blood cultures should be low, and such testing is often justified in the presence of isolated fever. This may explain why only 10% to 15% of blood cultures performed turn positive. Even in the presence of systemic inflammatory response syndrome, blood cultures are negative in 40% to 60% of cases[13]; however, severe sepsis and septic shock are associated with increased morbidity, mortality, and end-organ dysfunction.[72] Accordingly, when sepsis is suspected, it is generally not possible to wait for results of blood cultures, and empirical antimicrobial treatment is prescribed in most cases (Figure 132-1). Owing to the low quality of blood culture sampling, the situation among neonates is even more pronounced. In one study, only 46% of blood cultures obtained from neonates contained an adequate blood volume, and only 35% were adequate submissions on the basis of collection into the correct blood culture bottle type.[9] The overall positive yield of blood cultures was low, and cultures with adequate blood volume were more likely to be positive than those with inadequate blood volumes (5.3% versus 2.1%). The quality of blood culture sampling is better among older children. Of all positive cultures, 32% were contaminants, and 68% grew significant pathogens. However, only 35% of the contaminant cultures had adequate weight-adjusted blood volume, while this rate was 60% in the true bacteremia group ($P < 0.001$).[73] Thus, inappropriate blood culture sampling is more likely to produce pseudobacteremia than correct sampling.

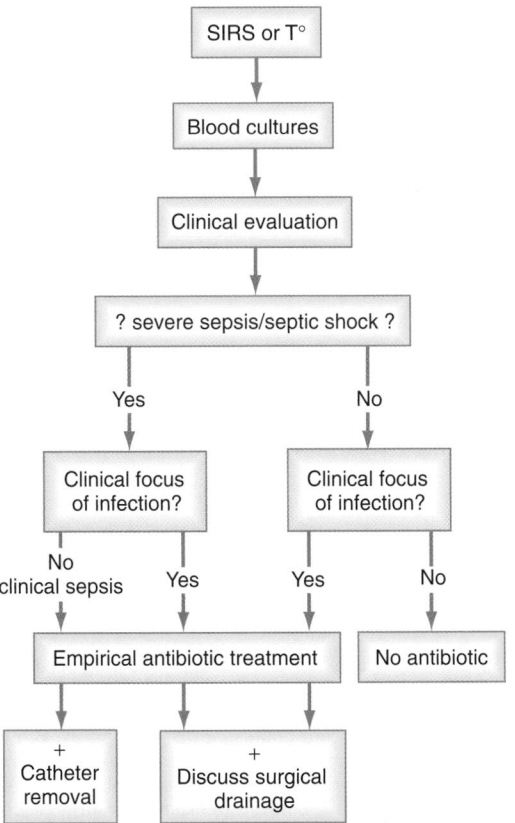

Figure 132-1 Management of a patient with suspected acute bloodstream infection. SIRS, systemic inflammatory response syndrome; T°, >100.4°F (38°C).

The management of bloodstream infection should combine early antimicrobial treatment and the active search for a source of infection that might require specific therapeutic measures for eradication or therapy (Figure 132-2). It has been repeatedly shown that either delayed or inappropriate antibiotic treatment is associated with higher mortality rates.[11,20,74-76] Similar results were observed for candidemia, where mortality was significantly higher when antifungal therapy was delayed.[58,77,78] Conversely in some studies, inappropriate antibiotic treatment was not found to be a risk factor for developing septic shock in patients with positive blood cultures,[13] but the mortality of those requiring inotropic drugs was significantly higher—85% versus 75% and 58% versus 24%, respectively.

The choice of antibiotics to start empirical therapy should be based on knowledge of the local epidemiology, susceptibility of pathogens, and source of the infection. A multidisciplinary approach, including close collaboration between the physician in charge of the patient, the infectious disease specialist, and the microbiology laboratory, is of paramount importance. Such collaboration improves the accuracy of empirical therapy. Once susceptibility testing from microorganisms identified from blood cultures has been obtained, antibiotic treatment should be adjusted accordingly. In some conditions, pathogens identified from other body sites also have to be considered for treatment. In addition to antimicrobial therapy, specific measures such as drainage of abscesses, adequate surgical management of peritonitis, and removal of infected prosthetic material are necessary to control the infection. Procalcitonin-based deescalation of antibiotic therapy has been reported to reduce exposure to antibiotics by almost 30%.[79-81]

In the case of primary bloodstream infection or sepsis, central lines should be removed if in place at time of infection. Catheter retention may result in a several-fold increase in risk for recurrence of bloodstream infection. However, recent data suggest that antibiotic locks in addition to systemic antibiotic therapy can be used as a salvage strategy if CLABSI involves long-term catheters, signs of exit site or tunnel infection are absent, and blood cultures reveal the presence of CoNS or enterococci.[82,83] Removal of the catheter is mandatory in severe or complicated infections, in the presence of shock, in case of recurrent bloodstream infection, and when microorganisms such as *S. aureus*, gram-negative bacilli or *Candida* spp. are isolated.[84] Relapse, continuous fever, or bacteremia despite catheter removal requires an active search for complications such as metastatic abscess, septic thrombophlebitis, or endocarditis. Following the completion of antimicrobial therapy, careful follow-up is mandatory owing to the frequent occurrence of late complications.[85,86] Recovery of *S. aureus* on a catheter tip may suggest the initiation of therapy even in the absence of clinical signs and negative blood cultures.[55]

Prevention

As for any other infection, prevention of bloodstream infection relies on strict respect for the basic rules of hygiene, particularly hand hygiene practices.[87-89] It has been shown that improved hand hygiene and good work organization prevents transmission of pathogens.[90] For prevention of device-associated infections, there is good evidence that multimodal strategies combining procedural and technical interventions are effective.[91-95] Procedural interventions include introducing standardized written procedures for catheter insertion and catheter care. Technical interventions include using chlorhexidine for skin antisepsis; devices (catheters, connectors, sponges) impregnated with chlorhexidine, chlorhexidine/silver sulfadiazine, silver, and antibiotics; using closed rather than open systems; and using lock solutions with agents such as taurolidine, citrate, EDTA, and ethanol. Alcohol-based, chlorhexidine-containing skin antiseptics have now become the standard of care. Use of a chlorhexidine-impregnated sponge was found effective in two randomized controlled trials.[96,97] Interestingly, daily bathing with a chlorhexidine-containing solution in the ICU was found effective in reducing bacteremia due to vancomycin-resistant enterococci (VRE) as well as VRE-colonization and methicillin-resistant *S. aureus* (MRSA) acquisition.[98] Two meta-analyses show that products impregnated with

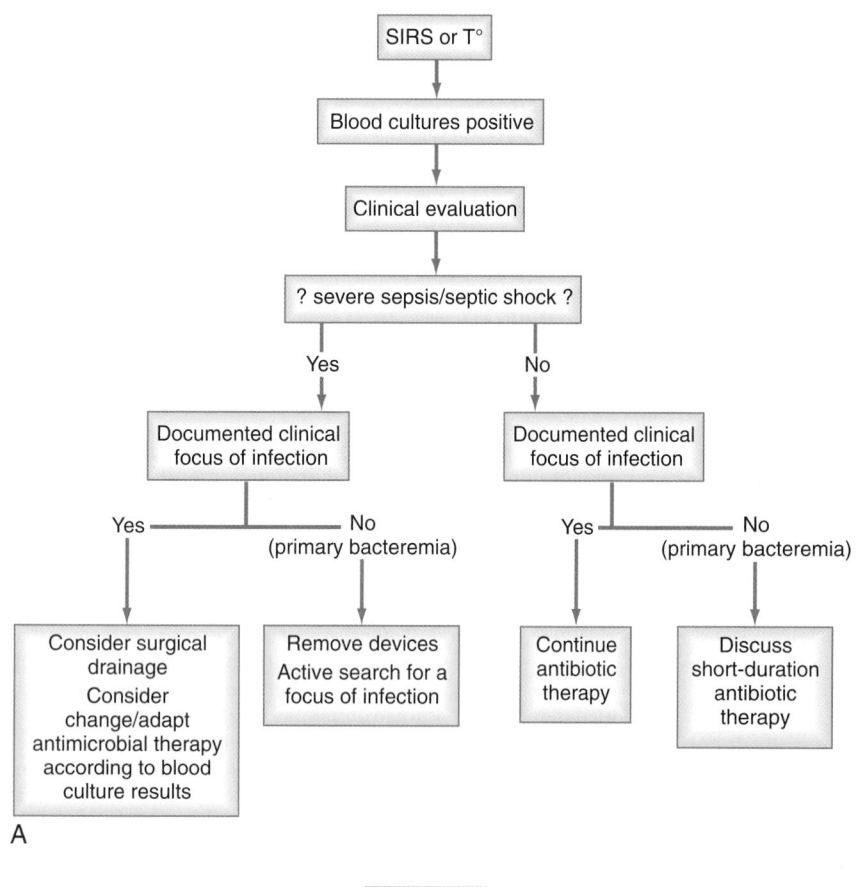

A

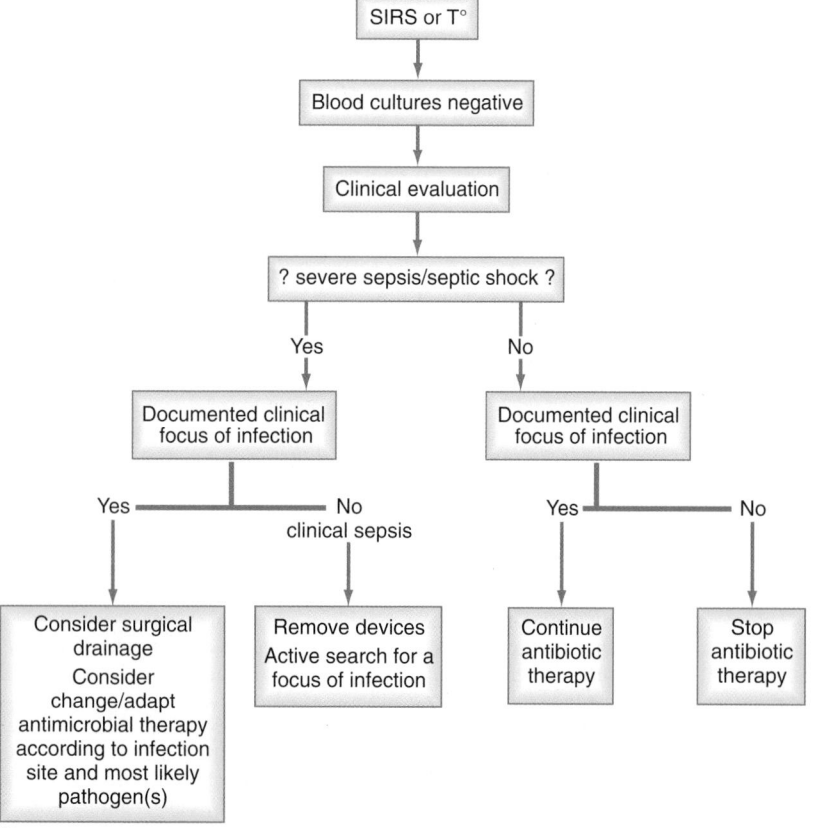

B

Figure 132-2 **Workup following results of blood cultures. A,** Evaluation of a patient treated for suspected acute bacteremia in the presence of a positive blood culture at 48 to 72 hours. **B,** Evaluation of a patient treated for suspected acute bacteremia in the presence of a negative blood culture at 48 to 72 hours. SIRS, systemic inflammatory response syndrome; T°, >100.4°F (38°C).

chlorhexidine/silver sulfadiazine are effective in reducing catheter colonization but not CLABSI; rifampicin/minocycline-coated catheters are effective in reducing both catheter colonization and CLABSI.[99,100] Most studies with central venous catheters are conducted in the ICU, including catheters with a relatively short dwell time. For longer insertion times, there are no data about the efficacy of antibiotic-coated devices, and there is evidence that chlorhexidine/silver sulfadiazine–coated catheters are ineffective.[101] The efficacy of lock solutions remains undetermined at present, although some studies show promising results.[102] Educational programs or global preventive strategies based on strict application of specific preventive measures and careful control of all factors associated with infection have been shown to be very effective in reducing infection rates. Specific devices such as antiseptic- or antibiotic-coated catheters or chlorhexidine-impregnated sponges are considered to be of advantage when procedural interventions are already successfully in place.[96]

KEY POINTS

1. A large proportion of all clinical forms of sepsis and most cases associated with multiple organ failure are related to acute bloodstream infections. These entities are responsible for significant mortality, morbidity, additional length of hospital stay, and resource utilization in almost all groups of patients studied.

2. In most institutions in high-resource countries, a shift in predominant organisms from gram-negative bacilli to gram-positive cocci has occurred over the past 2 decades, whereas gram-negative organisms are still predominant in countries with limited resources. This may be due to the fact that a large proportion of these infections are associated with the presence of intravascular medical devices, known to be colonized by microorganisms from the skin flora. Basically the same is true for countries with limited resources; however, breaches in basic infection control procedures may favor infections with nonfermentative pathogens.

3. Blood cultures are negative in at least 40% to 60% of episodes of severe sepsis and septic shock, and this proportion is even more important among neonates, but these conditions are associated with increased morbidity, mortality, and end-organ dysfunction even when blood cultures are negative.

4. Delayed or inappropriate antibiotic therapy of acute bloodstream infection is associated with significantly higher mortality. Accordingly, empirical antimicrobial treatment based on the most likely source and local resistance patterns should be prescribed while awaiting blood culture results.

5. Prevention of acute nosocomial bloodstream infection relies on strict adherence to the basic rules of hygiene, particularly hand hygiene practices and correct insertion and handling of intravascular devices.

ANNOTATED REFERENCES

Hugonnet S, Harbarth S, Ferrière K, Ricou B, Suter P, Pittet D. Bacteremic sepsis in intensive care: temporal trends in incidence, organ dysfunction, and prognosis. Crit Care Med 2003;31:390-4.
This study compared two cohorts of patients with bacteremic sepsis in the same surgical ICU during two separate periods (1984-1988 and 1994-1997). The incidence increased significantly from 3.2 to 4.3 per 100 admissions, with a comparable 28-day case fatality of 35% and 37%, respectively. The frequency of primary bacteremia increased from 21% to 47%, paralleled by an increase in the frequency of gram-positive microorganisms. The proportion of patients with at least one organ dysfunction increased from 69% to 80%. For both cohorts, the two strongest predictors of mortality remained the APACHE II score at the onset of sepsis and the number of evolving organ dysfunctions.

Pittet D, Tarara D, Wenzel RP. Nosocomial bloodstream infection in critically ill patients: excess length of stay, extra costs, and attributable mortality. JAMA 1994;271:1598-601.
This study revealed the dramatic impact of nosocomial bloodstream infection in critically ill patients. A pairwise-matched (1:1) case-control study of critically ill surgical patients who developed nosocomial bloodstream infections showed that the crude mortality rates in cases and controls were 50% and 15%, respectively, corresponding to an attributable mortality of 35%. The extra hospital and ICU length of stay attributable to bloodstream infection was 24 and 8 days, respectively. Extra costs attributable to the infection averaged $40,000 per survivor.

Nobre V, Harbarth S, Grafs JD, Rohner P, Pugin J. Use of procalcitonin to shorten antibiotic treatment duration in septic patients. Am J Respir Crit Care Med 2008;177:498-505.
In this prospective single-center study, an algorithm based on serial measurements of procalcitonin allowed the reduction of antibiotic therapy duration by 3.5 days in patients with severe sepsis and septic shock. Antibiotics were stopped when procalcitonin levels decreased 90% or more from the initial value at day 3 (if baseline levels were 1 mg/L) or at day 5 (if baseline PCT levels were >1 mg/L). Mortality and recurrence of primary infections were similar between intervention and control groups.

Timsit JF, Schwebel C, Bouadma L, Geffroy A, Garrouste-Orgeas M, Pease S, et al. Chlorhexidine-impregnated sponges and less frequent dressing changes for prevention of catheter-related infections in critically ill adults. JAMA 2009;301:1231-41.
In this French multicenter randomized controlled trial, a chlorhexidine-containing sponge which can be placed around the catheter at the insertion site reduced central line–associated bloodstream infections from 1.4 episodes per 1000 catheter-days to 0.6 episodes per 1000 catheter-days. This well-conducted study confirmed existing promising, but not conclusive, results. Based on the results of this study, the use of a chlorhexidine dressing is now recommended in catheter care.

REFERENCES

Access the complete reference list online at http://www.expertconsult.com.

Infections of the Urogenital Tract

FLORIAN M.E. WAGENLEHNER | KURT G. NABER

Infections in the intensive care unit (ICU) contribute significantly to patient morbidity. Depending on the type of ICU, nosocomial infections may account for 70% of infections.[1] Nosocomial infections of the urogenital tract are frequent and sometimes underestimated in the ICU.[2]

Definition

Urinary tract infection can be the primary cause for admission to the ICU or can be acquired after intensive care procedures. Because patients are frequently sedated in the ICU, clinical diagnosis of urinary tract infection (UTI) is often difficult. Nevertheless, UTI is an important cause of morbidity and antibiotic resistance in the ICU. Complicated UTI is a very heterogeneous entity, with a common pattern of the following factors[3,4]:

- Anatomic, structural, or functional alterations of the urinary tract which significantly impede urodynamic properties (e.g., stents, urine transport disturbances, instrumentation of the urinary tract, stones, tumors, neurologic disorders)
- Impaired renal function due to parenchymal diseases or prerenal, intrarenal, or postrenal nephropathies (e.g., acute and chronic renal insufficiencies, cardiac insufficiency)
- Accompanying diseases impairing the patient's immune status (e.g., diabetes mellitus, liver insufficiency, use of immunosuppressive agents such as corticosteroids, AIDS, hypothermia)

Etiology

Causative pathogens of UTI are almost exclusively bacteria and yeast. Viral pathogens are only found in patients with severe immunosuppression, such as after bone marrow transplantation. High antibiotic pressure and special circumstances in the ICU modulate the microbial spectrum. *Escherichia coli* is the most frequent pathogen but occurs less frequently than in uncomplicated community-acquired UTI. Other Enterobacteriaceae may also be uropathogens (e.g., *Klebsiella, Proteus, Enterobacter, Serratia, Citrobacter,* or *Morganella* species). Nonfermenters such as *Pseudomonas aeruginosa*, gram-positive cocci such as staphylococci and enterococci, and *Candida* species may also play an important role (Table 133-1). The microbial spectrum is likely to differ over time and from one institution to the next. To follow the spectrum and development of antibiotic resistance, each ICU has to update its own analyses.

Epidemiology

The Extended Prevalence of Infection in Intensive Care (EPIC II) study[1] revealed that 51% of patients were infected on the study day, and 71% of all patients were receiving antibiotics. The total occurrence of the most frequent types of ICU-acquired infection were respiratory tract infections 63.5%, abdominal infections 19.6%, bloodstream infections 15.1%, and renal or urinary tract infections in 14.3%.[1] The true incidence of UTI, however, may be even higher if meticulously looked for. In a prospective study specifically evaluating nosocomial UTI, nosocomial UTIs accounted for 28% of the nosocomial infections, lower respiratory tract infections for 21%, pneumonia for 12%, and bloodstream infections for 11%. The rates of urinary catheter–associated UTIs varied between 4.2% (symptomatic UTI) and 14.0%

(asymptomatic UTI), which shows that asymptomatic bacteriuria is frequent in ICU patients, although symptoms of UTIs in intensive care patients are frequently difficult to assess.[2] In the one-day point prevalence study in urological patients in Europe (PEP/PEAP study) asymptomatic bacteriuria accounted for 29% of nosocomial UTIs, followed by cystitis (26%), pyelonephritis (21%), and urosepsis (12%),[5] showing that nosocomial UTI is present with high frequency in certain patient groups.

Urinary tract infections in the ICU are divided into two groups:

1. UTIs with nonurologic complicating causes: diabetes mellitus, renal insufficiency, immunodeficiency, infectious foci contiguous to the urogenital tract, or trauma patients
2. UTIs with urologic complicating causes: renal transplantation, neurogenic bladder dysfunction, procedures in the urogenital tract, urinary stones or foreign bodies in the urogenital tract

In UTI with primary nonurologic complicating causes, antimicrobial therapy is generally sufficient. However, in UTI with primary urologic causes, the complicating factors must be identified and treated. In such cases, antimicrobial therapy is only one component of the treatment.

URINARY TRACT INFECTIONS WITH NONUROLOGIC COMPLICATING CAUSES

Individuals with diabetes are at higher risk for urinary tract infection.[6] Increased susceptibility in patients with diabetes is positively associated with increased duration and severity of diabetes as a result of impaired granulocyte function, decreased excretion of Tamm-Horsfall protein, low interleukin (IL)-6 and IL-8 levels in the urine that lead to lower "cidality" of the urine, and altered microflora in the genital region. In addition, diabetic cystopathy and nephropathy may be complicating factors in the urinary tract. In addition to antibiotics, treatment must address the metabolic situation. In pyelonephritis, usually a switch to insulin or to insulin-analogous therapy is necessary.

Immunosuppression is generally associated with increased risk of UTI. Patients with leukopenia (<1000/µL) show a higher rate of febrile UTIs and bacteremia due to UTI.[4] Symptoms and findings in these patients frequently are not diagnostic. Febrile episodes, however, are due to infections in approximately 60% of cases.

Pathogens may be translocated into the urinary tract from contiguous infectious foci (e.g., appendicitis, sigmoid diverticulitis, translocation by ileus). Symptoms and localization of pain can be misleading and may delay diagnosis. Operations or trauma may cause hypothermia, tissue hypoxia, and hemodynamic alterations that produce kidney dysfunction and impaired mucosal perfusion. The use of latex catheters in these critical situations (e.g., operations with heart-lung machine) can also lead to urethral strictures. Silicone catheters or suprapubic catheters are recommended in these patients.[7] Suprapubic catheters cannot prevent UTI. They can, however, lower the rate of UTI from 40% to 18%.[8]

URINARY TRACT INFECTIONS WITH UROLOGIC COMPLICATING CAUSES

Patients show a high risk to develop bacteriuria after renal transplantation, threatening clinical outcomes for both the patient and transplant. Early infections (up to 3 months after transplantation) are differentiated from late infections (more than 3 months after transplantation).

TABLE 133-1	Bacterial Spectrum of Nosocomial Uropathogens (≥2%) from Distinct Surveillance Studies				
Name of Study	**SENTRY (60)**	**SENTRY (60)**	**SENTRY (60)**	**ESGNI-003 (61)**	**PEP-Study (37)**
Regions of the world	North America	Latin America	Europe	Europe	Europe
Year of surveillance	2000	2000	2000	2000	2003
Type of surveillance	Longitudinal	Longitudinal	Longitudinal	Cross-section	Cross-section
Origin of samples	Microbiology laboratories	Microbiology laboratories	Microbiology laboratories	Different departments in the hospital	Urology departments
Number of pathogens	n = 1466	n = 531	n = 783	n = 607	n = 320
Species, %					
Escherichia coli	43%	60%	46%	36%	35%
Klebsiella spp.	12%	12%	9%	8%	10%
Pseudomonas spp.	7%	6%	9%	7%	13%
Proteus spp.	6%	7%	10%	8%	7%
Enterobacter spp.	3%	4%	4%	4%	3%
Citrobacter spp.	4%	2%	2%	2%	n.r.
Enterococcus spp.	16%	4%	13%	16%	9%
Staphylococcus spp.	6%	3%	3%	4%	4%
Resistance Rates of Antibiotics, %					
Ampicillin	59%[e]	62%[e]	65%[e]	66%[a]	51%
Ampicillin + BLI	31%[e]	36%[e]	36%[e]	29%[a]	30%
TMP/SMZ	43%[e]	38%[e]	48%[e]	32%[a]	45%
Ciprofloxacin	29%[e]	32%[e]	29%[e]	17%[b]	34%
Gentamicin	n.r.	n.r.	n.r.	18%	34%
Ceftazidime	n.r.	n.r.	n.r.	13%[c]	17%
Amikacin	n.r.	n.r.	n.r.	19%[c]	14%
Piperacillin/tazobactam	n.r.	n.r.	n.r.	n.r.	15%
Imipenem	n.r.	n.r.	n.r.	14%[c]	7%
Vancomycin	n.r.	n.r.	n.r.	1%[d]	n.r.

[a], gram-negative bacteria excluding *Pseudomonas aeruginosa*; [b], gram-negative bacteria; [c], *P. aeruginosa*; [d], enterococci.; [e], *E. coli, Klebsiella* spp., *P. aeruginosa*, enterococci.
BLI, β-lactam inhibitor; *n.r.*, not reported; *TMP-SMZ*, trimethoprim-sulfamethoxazole.

Early infections may present with no symptoms. In this phase, occult bacteremia (60% of bacteremias after renal transplantation originate from the urinary tract), allograft dysfunction, and recurrent UTI after antibiotic therapy are frequently seen.[4] The newer immunosuppressive agents are associated with a lower incidence of rejection but a higher risk of late infection. In particular, mycophenolate mofetil is associated with an increasing incidence of UTI and with infections caused by cytomegalovirus.[4] Infection can induce graft failure by the direct effect of cytokines and free radicals or reactivation of cytomegalovirus infection. It can be very difficult to distinguish rejection from infection.[4] Patients must also be investigated for a surgical complication.

UTIs caused by *Candida* species are frequently asymptomatic. There is, however, a risk of obstructive fungal balls leading to candidemia or invasion of the anastomosis in renal transplant recipients. Asymptomatic candiduria should therefore be treated in these patients.[4] Urine transport disturbances (e.g., from obstructive ureteral stone) require specific urologic therapy such as percutaneous nephrostomy or stenting. In the case of bladder obstruction, an indwelling urinary catheter (suprapubic or transurethral) will be the primary therapy in the ICU. Long-term indwelling catheters (more than 30 days) are associated with a selected microbial spectrum of difficult-to-treat uropathogens (e.g., *Providencia* spp., *Proteus* spp., *Pseudomonas* spp.).[9] After initiation of antimicrobial therapy, the catheter should be exchanged to remove biofilm material.

Pathophysiology

UTIs generally occur from organisms invading the urinary tract via the urethra. Pathogens originate from endogenous or exogenous nosocomial flora. Hematogenous spread to the urinary tract is rare.

In uncomplicated UTI, pathogens need to have very specific virulence factors enabling them to initiate an infection after invasion of the urinary tract. The medical conditions of an ICU patient may weaken physiologic barriers and defenses, thus facilitating entry of pathogens. In addition, the nosocomial environment in the ICU, including antibiotic pressure and decreased supply of oxygen or nutrients (e.g., iron) to tissues, can select pathogens with specific resistance patterns. A general adaptation strategy is the formation of hypermutator strains, which show 100- to 1000-fold increased mutation frequencies, enabling the pathogens to rapidly adapt to challenging environments and to thus develop effective mechanisms for antibiotic resistance.[10,11]

An important mechanism contributing to UTI is the formation of biofilms, associated with the increased number of biomaterials used in medical practice. Biofilm infections develop not only around foreign bodies such as urinary catheters or stents but also in urinary stones, scar or necrotic tissue, obstructive uropathies, or even chronic bacterial prostatitis. Biofilm has been defined as an accumulation of microorganisms and their extracellular products, forming a structured community on a surface. The formation of biofilm generally consists of three steps:

1. Deposition of a host conditioning film
2. Attachment of microorganisms followed by microbial adhesion and anchorage to the surface by exopolymer production
3. Growth, multiplication, and dissemination of the organisms

The basic structural unit of a biofilm is a microcolony—that is, a discrete matrix-enclosed community consisting of bacteria of one or more species. The biofilm is usually built up of three layers[12,13]:

1. Linking film that attaches to the surface of a tissue or biomaterial
2. Base film of compact microorganisms
3. Surface film as an outer layer where planktonic organisms can be released to float freely and spread on the surface

Bacteria within the biofilms differ both in behavior and in phenotypic form from the planktonic, free-floating bacteria. The failure of antimicrobial agents to treat biofilms has been attributed to a variety of mechanisms:

- Organisms encapsulated in the biofilm grow more slowly than the planktonic ones, probably because the encapsulated bacteria have a decreased nutrient and oxygen supply, leading to a decreased metabolic rate and antimicrobial susceptibility. This may select a less susceptible genotype, forming a resistant population. Furthermore, antimicrobial binding proteins are poorly expressed in these slow-growing bacteria.
- The biofilm matrix itself delays or impedes the diffusion of antibiotic molecules into the deeper layer of the film (extrinsic resistance).

- Bacteria within the biofilm are phenotypically so different from their planktonic counterparts that antimicrobial agents fail to eradicate them. Bacteria within a biofilm activate many genes that alter the cell envelope and molecular targets by altering the susceptibility to antimicrobial agents (intrinsic resistance). These phenotypic changes are likely to play a more important role in the development of antimicrobial resistance than the external resistance (biofilm matrix, glycocalyx).
- Bacteria within a biofilm can sense the external environment, communicate with each other, and transfer genetic information and plasmids within biofilms.
- Bacteria in biofilms can usually survive antibacterial concentrations 100 to 150 times higher than needed to kill planktonic bacteria of the same species.[14]

Antimicrobial treatment can be effective only in "young" biofilms (<24 hours). At present, combination therapy with fluoroquinolones and macrolides or fosfomycin seems to be the most effective against biofilm infections. During an acute febrile phase of a biofilm infection, antimicrobial therapy is essential and can be effective because the planktonic bacteria are responsible for the febrile reactions and not the bacteria covered in the biofilm. However, to eradicate pathogens from biofilm, the biofilm itself has to be removed (e.g., catheter change, extraction of infectious stones).

Diagnosis

MEDICAL HISTORY AND PHYSICAL EXAMINATION

Sedated intubated patients often are difficult to evaluate regarding their signs and symptoms of UTI. The patient or a family member should be asked about previous episodes of UTI as well as urologic diseases (e.g., stones, tumors) or operations.

The physical examination should include inspection and palpation of the costophrenic area, lower abdomen, pubic region, inguinal lymph nodes, genitals, and a digital transvaginal or transrectal examination. Ultrasound is an important diagnostic device, and its use should be frequently considered because of the close proximity of the urogenital organs to the intestine, spleen, liver, pancreas, gallbladder, ovary, or uterus.

URINARY EXAMINATIONS

Urine specimens in ICU patients are almost exclusively collected from catheters. Because urine from catheters has to be collected into a closed system, the urine specimen should be taken from the puncture site at the catheter after disinfection, without opening the closed system. There are different complementary methods for laboratory examination of the urine specimen.

Dipstick Test

The dipstick test is done with undiluted urine and investigates the following infection-related parameters[15]:

- pH; an alkaline urine (pH >8.0) points to urease-producing organisms such as *Proteus* or *Providencia* and is associated with magnesium-ammonium-phosphate stones.
- Nitrate; most enterobacteria harbor a nitrate reductase that reduces nitrate to nitrite. Some common uropathogens such as *Enterococcus* and *Staphylococcus* lack nitrate reductase and will therefore not be detected using this parameter, whatever their urinary concentration. Positive detection of nitrate requires its inclusion in the patient's diet.
- Leukocytes (positive leukocyte esterase); granulocytes are the most frequently detected leukocytes in the urine of UTI patients. Macrophages appear fairly often in patients with UTI, but their significance remains unknown.
- Erythrocytes (positive hemoglobin); hematuria remains a major sign of urinary tract and renal disease.
- Specific gravity/osmolality (degree of urine dilution)

TABLE 133-2	Standard Values for Urine in Counting Chamber and Field of Vision		
		Erythrocytes	*Leukocytes*
Uncentrifuged urine (chamber counting)		<10/mL	<10/mL

Data from European Urinalysis Guidelines, 2000.

- Protein; total protein in urine is a mixture of high- and low-molecular-weight plasma proteins from the kidney and urinary tract or bacteria.
- Glucose (metabolic condition of the patient)

Microscopy

There are two possibilities of microscopic evaluation[15]:

1. Chamber counting of uncentrifuged urine (standard values for urine shown in Table 133-2)
2. Urinary sediment findings; at least 10 fields of vision at 400× magnification are counted, and the mean value of particles is registered. However, centrifugation methods are never quantitative in counting erythrocytes and leukocytes because of variable loss during centrifugation.

Microbiology

To differentiate contamination in urine from significant bacteriuria, quantitative microbiology is needed. The microbial count has to be interpreted in relation to the urinary dilution.

CLINICAL DIAGNOSIS

To survey and compare infection rates in different institutions, UTIs should be classified according to widely accepted definitions, such as the definitions of the U.S. Centers for Disease Control and Prevention (CDC). The CDC/National Healthcare Safety Network (NHSN) definitions[16] stratify health care associated UTIs into symptomatic, asymptomatic, and other infections of the urinary tract. To be of value in determining a nosocomial infection, the urine specimens must be obtained aseptically using an appropriate technique such as clean catch collection, bladder catheterization, or suprapubic aspiration.

Therapy

GENERAL PRINCIPLES

Not all bacteriuric patients in the ICU need to be treated. Asymptomatic bacteriuria in general does not have to be treated.[17] Therapy should only be started in patients with significant symptoms and morbidity and in whom asymptomatic bacteriuria may be deleterious (e.g., before traumatizing intervention of the urinary tract and in pregnant women). In the ICU, indications for treatment of asymptomatic UTI might include some other circumstances such as renal transplant, severe diabetes mellitus, or severe immunosuppression. In complicated UTI, antibiotic therapy can only be successful when the complicating factors can be eliminated or urodynamic functions restored. Treatment of complicated UTI therefore comprises adequate antibiotic treatment and successful urologic intervention.

ANTIBIOTIC THERAPY

For therapy of complicated UTI, antibiotics must possess appropriate pharmacodynamic and pharmacokinetic prerequisites: high renal unmetabolized clearance with good antibacterial activity, both in acidic and alkaline urine. Moreover, microbial resistance patterns must be considered in the choice of antibiotics. Increasing antibiotic resistance, especially amongst enterobacteria, makes prudent antibiotic treatment more and more difficult. The increasing appearance of quinolone-resistant and extended-spectrum β-lactamase (ESBL)-forming enterobacteria will inevitably lead to increased use of

TABLE 133-3	Division and Dosage of Distinct Antibiotics Recommended for Treatment of Urinary Tract Infections		
		Dosage	
Antibiotic Group	**Substance**	**Oral**	**IV**
Aminopenicillin + BLI	Ampicillin/sulbactam	0.750 g twice daily	0.75-3 g 3 times daily
	Amoxicillin/clavulanic acid	1 g twice daily *or* 0.625 g 3 times daily	1.2-2.2 g 3 times daily
Acylureidopenicillin + BLI	Piperacillin/tazobactam	—	2.5-4.5 g 3 times daily
	Piperacillin/Combactam	—	5 g 3 times daily
Cephalosporin Gr. 1	Cephalexin	Prophylaxis only	—
Cephalosporin Gr. 2	Cefuroxime axetil	500 mg twice daily	
	Cefuroxime	—	0.75-1.5 g 3 times daily
	Cefotiam	—	1-2 g 2-3 times daily
Cephalosporin Gr. 3	Cefpodoxime proxetil	200 mg twice daily	—
	Ceftibuten	200-400 mg daily	—
Cephalosporin Gr. 3a	Cefotaxime	—	1-2 g 2-3 times daily
	Ceftriaxone	—	1-2 g daily
Cephalosporin Gr. 3b	Ceftazidime	—	1-2 g 2-3 times daily
Cephalosporin Gr. 4	Cefepime	—	2 g twice daily
Carbapenem Gr. 1	Imipenem	—	0.5-1 g q 6-8 h
	Meropenem	—	0.5-1 g 3 times daily
	Doripenem	—	0.5 g 3 times daily
Carbapenem Gr. 2	Ertapenem	—	1 g daily
Fluoroquinolone Gr. 2	Ciprofloxacin	500-750 mg twice daily	400 mg twice daily
	Ciprofloxacin XR	1000 mg daily	—
Fluoroquinolone Gr. 3	Levofloxacin	500-750 mg daily	500 mg daily
Antimycotic Group			
Azole derivatives	Fluconazole	400-800 mg daily	400-800 mg daily
	Voriconazole	4-6 mg/kg BW daily	4-6 mg/kg BW daily
Pyrimidine analog	Flucytosine		100-150 mg/kg BW 4 times daily
Echinocandin	Caspofungin		50-70 mg daily

Data from Grabe M, Bishop MC, Bjerklund-Johansen TE, Botto H, Cek M, Lobel B et al. Guidelines on urological infections. In: European Association of Urology guidelines. Arnhem, The Netherlands: European Association of Urology 2009; p. 1-110.

BLI, β-lactam inhibitor; *BW*, body weight, *IV*, intravenous.

carbapenems in the empirical treatment, thus increasing the antibiotic pressure on these highly potent antibiotics. To diminish the selection pressure for resistant pathogens, antibiotics from different classes should be used.

Multiple antimicrobial agents are available for therapy for complicated UTI (Table 133-3): second- or third-generation cephalosporins, broad-spectrum penicillins with β-lactamase inhibitors, monobactams, and carbapenems. For empirical therapy for severe UTI, broad-spectrum antibiotics should be used (e.g., broad-spectrum penicillins with β-lactamase inhibitors, third-generation cephalosporins, fluoroquinolones, or carbapenems). Synergism with aminoglycosides, which inhibit protein synthesis and thus block the forming of toxins or virulence factors, might be useful for initial therapy, but side effects have to be considered.

Candiduria is a common problem in ICUs. It may represent harmless colonization, but it can also be an early sign of systemic candidosis.[18] A second urine culture after exchanging the urethral catheter can rule out contamination. In the critically ill patient, systemic therapy for *Candida* species should be started according to susceptibility testing or species differentiation (see Table 133-3). Complicating factors such as diabetes mellitus or urologic abnormalities should be treated concomitantly. Systemic antimycotic therapy is preferred to local instillation therapy because of the potentially systemic nature of candiduria in ICU patients.

UROLOGIC THERAPY

Urologic operative therapy of complicated UTI is divided into acute therapy and delayed drainage therapy. The primary aim of acute therapy is improved urinary flow, with minimal patient contamination by infected urine. In primary therapy, catheters, stents, or drains are frequently used. Delayed drainage therapy of the urinary tract (e.g., lithotomy, prostatic resection, ureter reimplantation) is frequently performed after days or weeks of stabilization.

PROPHYLAXIS OF CATHETER-ASSOCIATED URINARY TRACT INFECTIONS

Some 80% to 90% of nosocomial UTIs are associated with urinary catheters or instrumentation of the urinary tract. The best prophylaxis is to avoid a catheter or, if catheterization is necessary, to minimize catheter duration. Various techniques have been used to avoid catheter-related infections.

Silver coating of catheters may exert a bactericidal effect, but the concentration of free silver ions must be high, whereas the exposure to albumin and chloride ions has to be low, because silver-chloride complexes can precipitate.[19] Heparin-coated catheters also demonstrate promising results. Suprapubic catheterization can initially decrease the rate of UTI from 40% to 18%, because the proximity to the anal region as well as the irritation of the urethral mucosa with ensuing mucopurulent discharge are avoided.[8] Urinary drainage should be performed with a closed system that should not be opened either for emptying or for urinary sampling. The sites used for urinary sampling must be adequately sterilized. A rigid vertical, ventilated, drop chamber should be available to prevent encrustation.[20] General hygienic procedures such as aseptic catheter insertion, wearing of disposable gloves, and hygienic hand disinfection to prevent cross-contamination or cross-infection are mandatory. International consensus recommendations for the use of urinary catheters to prevent healthcare-associated infections have been recently described.[21]

RECOMMENDED EVIDENCE-BASED MEASUREMENTS FOR PREVENTING CATHETER-ASSOCIATED URINARY TRACT INFECTIONS

The primary methodologies for preventing catheter-associated UTIs[21] include:

- Limiting unnecessary catheterization and discontinuation of the catheter as early as possible

- Policies and procedures for recommended catheter insertion indications, insertion and maintenance techniques, discontinuation strategies, and replacement indications should be developed and closely followed.
- Alternatives to indwelling urethral catheterization should be considered, such as condom catheterization, intermittent catheterization, or suprapubic catheterization, although data are insufficient to recommend one over the other.
- Closed catheter drainage systems should be used.
- Most other measures for prevention of catheter-associated UTI, such as prophylaxis with systemic antimicrobials, methenamine salts, cranberry products, enhanced meatal care, and catheter irrigation with either antimicrobials or saline, are not recommended.[21]
- It is also unclear whether routine catheter changes reduce the risk for catheter-associated bacteriuria or UTI.

Special Clinical Issues

INFECTIONS OF THE UPPER URINARY TRACT AND CONTIGUOUS ORGANS

Pyelonephritis

The high osmolality of the renal medulla has a negative effect on leukocyte function. For that reason, the interstitium of the renal medulla is much more affected in pyelonephritis than the cortex is. Clinical symptoms are unilateral or bilateral flank pain, painful micturition, dysuria, and fever (>38°C). Focal nephritis is limited to one or more renal lobules, comparable to lobular pneumonia. Ultrasonographic findings are of a circumscribed lesion with interrupted echoes that break through the normal cortex/medulla organization. Computed tomography (CT) scan shows typical wedge-shaped, poorly limited areas of diminished sonographic density. As differential diagnoses, renal abscess, tumor, and renal infarction must be taken into account. Emphysematous pyelonephritis characteristically shows gas formation in the renal parenchyma and perirenal space. Diabetes mellitus or obstructive renal disease are predisposing factors. The most frequently isolated organisms are *E. coli*, *Klebsiella pneumoniae*, and *Enterobacter cloacae*. Fermentation of glucose in Enterobacteriaceae occurs via two different metabolic pathways: mixed acid fermentation and the butylene glycol pathway. Organisms of the *Klebsiella-Enterobacter-Hafnia-Serratia* group, and to a lesser extent *E. coli*, use the butylene glycol pathway and produce copious amounts of CO_2, which appears clinically as gas formation.[22] Aggravated by diminished tissue perfusion, the contralateral side is often affected as well.

Renal and Perirenal Abscess

Clinical symptoms are rigors, fever, back or abdominal pain, flank tenderness, mass lesion and redness of the flank, and protection of upper lumbar and paraspinal muscles. Respiratory insufficiency, hemodynamic instability, or reflectory paralytic ileus occurs frequently. Frequent signs of renal abscess formation are fever and leukocytosis for more than 72 hours, despite antibiotic therapy. Urinary culture may be negative in 14% to 20%.[23] Frequently isolated organisms are *E. coli*, *K. pneumoniae*, *Proteus* spp., and *Staphylococcus aureus* from hematogenous spread. Caudad, the fascial limitations are open, and the perirenal fat is in close contact with the pelvic fat tissue. A perinephritic abscess may therefore point to groin or perivesical tissue or to the contralateral side, thus penetrating the peritoneum. Inflammation of flank, thigh, back, buttocks, and lower abdomen may occur. Because of late diagnosis, the mortality can be as high as 57%. Blood cultures are positive in 10% to 40%, and urinary cultures are positive in 50% to 80%.[24]

INFECTIONS OF THE LOWER URINARY TRACT AND CONTIGUOUS ORGANS

Cystitis

Cystitis is frequently limited to the bladder mucosa and hence shows no systemic signs or symptoms. An ascending infection can, however,

clinically result. Cystitis in the ICU is almost exclusively catheter associated and can cause hematuria. Spontaneous elimination is frequently found after removal of the indwelling catheter, but less frequently in elderly patients.[4]

Epididymitis/Orchitis

Epididymitis in the ICU usually is an ascending infection and can also involve the testis as well. Possible causes are subvesical obstruction, transurethral resection of the prostate, or an indwelling transurethral urinary catheter, in which case the pathogens are identical with the pathogens in the urine. Of note, epididymitis is frequently involved in urogenital tuberculosis. Orchitis with the formation of a sterile hydrocele can appear in the course of polyserositis or cardiac failure and may point to a generalized systemic disease.

Cavernitis

Cavernitis of the penis is a rare phlegmonous infection of the cavernous bodies. Possible causes are indwelling transurethral urinary catheters, penile operations, autoinjection for erectile dysfunction, pelvic operations, or trauma. Pathogens may represent skin flora or uropathogens. Treatment consists of suprapubic catheterization, broad-spectrum antibiotic therapy and, if needed, operative débridement.

Acute Prostatitis and Prostatic Abscess

Acute prostatitis and prostatic abscess are bacterial infections of the prostate gland. The bacterial spectrum consists of 53% to 80% *E. coli* and other enterobacteria, 19% gram-positive bacteria, and 17% anaerobic bacteria.[25] In regions with a high incidence of *Neisseria gonorrhoeae*, the prostate may be involved. Symptoms are high fever, rigors, dysuria, urinary retention, and perineal pain. Rectal palpation reveals an enlarged, tender prostate. Prostate massage is contraindicated. In acute prostatitis, the pathogens are usually detected in urine. However, the urine may be sterile in prostatic abscess formation. Therapy consists of a combination of antibiotic therapy with broad-spectrum antibiotics, as well as insertion of a suprapubic catheter. In the case of a prostatic abscess, urologic drainage is necessary.[25]

Fournier's Gangrene

Fournier's gangrene is a necrotizing fasciitis of the dartos and Colles fascias. It is mainly seen in men in the fourth to seventh decade but also occurs in women or the newborn. Causes are operations or trauma in the genital or perineal region, including microlesions, or infectious processes from the rectal or urethral areas. Important predisposing factors are diabetes mellitus, liver insufficiency, chronic alcoholism, hematologic diseases, or malnutrition. Patient-related predictors of mortality are increasing age, increased Charlson comorbidity index, preexisting conditions such as congestive heart failure, renal failure or coagulopathy, and hospital admission via transfer.[26] Fatality rates nowadays were 7.5% in one large study.[27] The infectious process follows anatomically preformed spaces. The superficial perineal fascia is fixed dorsally at the transverse deep perineal muscle and laterally at the iliac bone and merges ventrally in the superficial abdominal fascia. Hence, a ventrally open and craniodorsally and laterally closed space is formed (Colles space) that facilitates the spread of infection. In contrast to gas gangrene, the fascial borders are respected in Fournier's gangrene. A mixed bacterial flora is seen, consisting of gram-positive cocci, enterobacteria, and anaerobic bacteria. The released toxins facilitate platelet aggregation and activation of complement, which in conjunction with the release of heparinase by anaerobic bacteria, leads to small vessel thrombosis and tissue necrosis. The destruction of tissue enhances the potential of acute renal failure. Fournier's gangrene is a rapidly progressing infection leading to septic shock if not treated in time.

Therapy for Fournier's gangrene consists of immediate operative débridement followed by subsequent operations until the infectious process has been controlled. A suprapubic catheter is advisable, and a colostomy may have to be performed in cases in which fecal contamination of the wound is inevitable. Combination of antibiotic therapy with broad-spectrum β-lactam antibiotics, fluoroquinolones, and clindamycin is recommended.

UROSEPSIS

In 20% to 30% of all septic patients, the initial infectious focus is in the urogenital tract. The most frequent causes for urosepsis are obstructive diseases of the urinary tract such as ureteral stones, anomalies, stenosis, or tumor. Effective treatment eliminates the infectious focus and improves organ perfusion.

Immediately after microbiological sampling of urine and blood, empirical broad-spectrum antibiotic therapy should be started parenterally. Adequate initial (e.g., in the first hour) antibiotic therapy ensures improved outcome in septic shock.[28,29] Inappropriate antimicrobial therapy in severe UTI is linked to a higher mortality rate,[30] as it has been shown with other infections as well.[31,32] Empirical antibiotic therapy therefore needs to follow rules[33] which are based upon the expected bacterial spectrum, institutional-specific resistance rates, specific pharmacokinetic and pharmacodynamic factors in UTI, and individual patient characteristics.

The bacterial spectrum in urosepsis predominantly consists of enterobacteria such as *E. coli*, *Proteus* spp., *Enterobacter* and *Klebsiella* spp., non-fermenting organisms such as *P. aeruginosa*, and also grampositive organisms.[34-36] *Candida* spp. and *Pseudomonas* spp. occur as causative agents in urosepsis mainly if host defense is impaired.[37] Patients with candiduria also show frequently invasive candidiasis and candidemia.[38,39] Candiduria at any time in an ICU is associated with higher mortality rates (OR, 2.86).[39] Viruses are not common causes of urosepsis.

Although urosepsis is a systemic disease, the activity of an antibiotic at the site of the infection is critical. A variety of studies show that inflammatory mediators such as IL-6, CXC chemokines, endotoxin, or HMGB1 are produced and released in the urinary tract.[40-43] Therefore predominantly antimicrobial substances with a high activity in the urogenital tract are recommended.[44,45]

The increasing antibiotic resistance rates of pathogens causing urosepsis significantly diminish the choice of antibiotics available for adequate empirical initial treatment in urosepsis. In particular, the increasing rates of Enterobacteriaceae producing ESBL pose clinically relevant problems.[46-48] Other recent developments of concern include increased rates of fluoroquinolone-resistant enterobacteria and vancomycin-resistant enterococci.[49,50] There are no specific pharmacokinetic/pharmacodynamic parameters yet available for the treatment of uroseptic patients.

Correct dosing in urosepsis has to consider the altered systemic and especially renal pathophysiology that exists in patients with urosepsis. Sepsis and the treatment thereof result in higher clearances of antibacterial drugs.[51] The increased volume of distribution as a result of peripheral edema in sepsis will lead to underexposure, especially of hydrophilic antimicrobials such as β-lactams and aminoglycosides, which exhibit a volume of distribution mainly restricted to the extracellular space.[52] Urosepsis may also cause multiple organ dysfunction such as hepatic or renal dysfunction, resulting in decreased clearance of antibacterial drugs. Increased dosing is therefore necessary. As β-lactams are time-dependent antibacterials, optimal administration would be by continuous infusion. In one study, an area under the antibiotic concentration time curve (AUIC) ≥ 250 and time over the minimal inhibitory concentration (T > MIC) = 100% has been

associated with treatment success.[53] Fluoroquinolones, on the other hand, display largely concentration-dependent activity. The volume of distribution of fluoroquinolones in sepsis is not greatly influenced by fluid shifts, and therefore no alterations of standard doses are necessary unless renal dysfunction occurs.[51]

Depending on local susceptibility patterns, a third-generation cephalosporin such as piperacillin in combination with a β-lactamase inhibitor (BLI) or carbapenem may be appropriate for empirical treatment.[4,53-57] In areas with a high (>10%) rate of Enterobacteriaceae producing ESBL, initial treatment with a carbapenem might be advisable.[54-58] Aminoglycosides as monotherapy might be an alternative; however, the data supporting monotherapy in uroseptic patients are not sufficient.[59] In case of candiduria with signs of sepsis, antifungal treatment is recommended.[38,39]

KEY POINTS

1. Complicated urinary tract infection (UTI) is a very heterogeneous entity with a common pattern of complicating factors.

2. The bacterial spectrum of complicated UTI is much broader than in uncomplicated UTI, comprising a variety of gram-negative and gram-positive pathogens and among these, frequently multiresistant pathogens.

3. UTIs are frequent in ICUs. It would be pragmatic to stratify UTIs into those with nonurologic complicating causes, in which antimicrobial therapy is the primary therapy, and those with urologic complicating causes, in which the complicating urologic anomaly has to be effectively treated.

4. Pathogens of nosocomial complicated UTIs may be characterized by certain properties such as adaptation strategies to changing environments (i.e., hypermutator strains) or propensity to biofilm formation.

5. The diagnosis of UTI is based on medical history and thorough physical examination, including bedside ultrasound as well as investigations of urine (dipstick test, microscopy, and microbiology). For clinical diagnosis, general accepted criteria should be employed. Symptomatic UTIs in ICU patients are especially difficult to evaluate.

6. Not all bacteriuric patients in ICUs need to be treated. Therapy should, however, be started in those with significant symptoms and morbidity, and in those, even asymptomatic bacteriuria may be deleterious. Management of complicated UTI comprises adequate antibiotic therapy and successful treatment of complicating factors.

7. Prophylaxis of UTI is important. However, the percentage of infections that can be prevented is not known. Important points in prophylaxis encompass training of staff, hygiene measures, type of catheter and drainage, and patient care.

8. Special clinical pictures of UTI and infections of contiguous organs are seen in the ICU. UTIs of the upper urinary tract are distinguished from those of the lower urinary tract and infections of the male adnexal glands and fasciitis of the perineum and scrotum. All these pictures can potentially merge into urosepsis if the UTI is not treated adequately. The urogenital tract is the source for sepsis in 20% to 30% of cases.

ANNOTATED REFERENCES

Goto T, Nakame Y, Nishida M, Ohi Y. Bacterial biofilms and catheters in experimental urinary tract infection. Int J Antimicrob Agents 1999;11:227-31.
An experimental setup to study the antibiotic susceptibility of pathogens in biofilm. Fluoroquinolones, and perhaps macrolides, have advantageous effects in the treatment of biofilm infections.

Grabe M, Bishop MC, Bjerklund-Johansen TE, Botto H, Cek M, Lobel B, et al. Guidelines on urological infections. In: European Association of Urology guidelines. Arnhem, The Netherlands: European Association of Urology; 2009. p. 1-110.

This is the extensive version of the UTI Guidelines elaborated by the Urinary Tract Infection Working Group of the Health Care Office of the European Association of Urology (ESIU). The topics include classification, diagnosis, treatment, and follow-up of uncomplicated UTI, UTI in children, UTI in diabetes mellitus, renal insufficiency, renal transplant recipients and immunosuppression, complicated UTI due to urological disorders, sepsis syndrome, urosepsis, urethritis, prostatitis, epididymitis, orchitis, and principles of perioperative prophylaxis in urology.

Hooton TM, Bradley SF, Cardenas DD, Colgan R, Geerlings SE, Rice JC, et al. Diagnosis, prevention, and treatment of catheter-associated urinary tract infection in adults: 2009 International Clinical Practice Guidelines from the Infectious Diseases Society of America. Clin Infect Dis 2010; 50:625-63.

These international guidelines deal with diagnosis, prevention, and treatment of catheter-associated urinary tract infection in adults, the most frequent cause for UTI in the intensive care units.

Oliver A, Cantón R, Campo P, et al. High frequency of hypermutable *Pseudomonas aeruginosa* in cystic fibrosis lung infection. Science 2000;288:1251-3.

This study elucidates an excellent model for the special propensities of nosocomial pathogens. There were 36.7% of patients with cystic fibrosis who harbored P. aeruginosa isolates with 100- to 1000-fold increased mutation rates, thus enabling them to rapidly adapt to changing environmental needs.

Vincent JL, Rello J, Marshall J, Silva E, Anzueto A, Martin CD, et al. International study of the prevalence and outcomes of infection in intensive care units. JAMA 2009;302:2323-9.

This multicenter 1-day prevalence study on 1265 ICUs in 75 countries investigated 14,414 patients; 51% were infected on the study day. The ICU mortality rate of infected patients was more than twice that of noninfected patients. Therefore, infection control in critically ill patients is important.

REFERENCES

Access the complete reference list online at http://www.expertconsult.com.

134

Central Nervous System Infections

KAREN C. BLOCH

Central nervous system (CNS) infections represent life-threatening conditions that frequently require treatment in a critical care unit. These infections may be challenging to recognize, as numerous noninfectious conditions may mimic CNS infection. For example, a necrotic brain tumor may be clinically and radiologically indistinguishable from a brain abscess. Even when an infectious syndrome is suspected, it may take several days before a specific microorganism is identified, necessitating use of broad empirical therapy directed against the most likely pathogens based on clinical, epidemiologic, and demographic clues. Pharmacologic considerations in selecting appropriate antimicrobials include the ability of the agent to cross the blood-brain barrier and achieve bacteriocidal levels at the site of infection. Clinical outcomes associated with CNS infections are directly related to the rapidity with which appropriate medical or surgical interventions are able to be provided, adding urgency to the diagnostic and therapeutic evaluation.

Infections of the meninges can be subclassified by the acuity of onset of symptoms. Bacterial infections almost exclusively cause acute meningitis syndrome, characterized by rapid (<48 hours) progression of fever, headache, and meningismus. In contrast, the subacute meningitis syndrome, frequently due to viruses, fungi, or mycobacteria, is more slowly evolving, with symptoms developing over several days to weeks (Table 134-1). The following sections outline approaches to acute meningitis and subacute CNS infection syndromes. These approaches prioritize the competing needs of obtaining a precise etiologic diagnosis versus instituting early antimicrobial therapy.

Bacterial Meningitis

ANATOMY

Bacterial meningitis is a pyogenic infection of the cerebral ventricles and the subarachnoid space, with bacteria usually confined to the nutrient-rich cerebrospinal fluid (CSF). CSF is formed in the choroid plexus of the ventricles, flows into the subarachnoid space at the cisterna magna and around the cerebral hemispheres, and is reabsorbed by the arachnoid villi (Figure 134-1). In adults, CSF is produced at a rate of approximately 500 mL/day, yet the CSF space averages only 140 mL in volume, consistent with rapid production and reabsorption. The cerebral and spinal subarachnoid spaces connect at the cisterna magna. Flow through the spinal subarachnoid space is of variable velocity and direction.

There are numerous potential and actual spaces among the layers of the meninges (Figure 134-2). Meningitis involves the actual space (i.e., the subarachnoid space), which consists of multiple interconnected compartments. The small size of the foramina of Luschka and Magendie allows unidirectional caudal flow toward the cisterna magna, where the CSF then moves either cephalad or into the spinal canal. This compartmentalization has implications for therapy, because the movement of medications and infectious agents depends on the rate and direction of CSF flow. A blockage at any of these levels may restrict entry of antibiotics into sites of ongoing infection.

Infectious agents can invade the CSF by at least three routes (Table 134-2). First, the vascular structures of the choroid plexus and pia and the vessels that traverse the subarachnoid space may serve as conduits during systemic bacteremia. A second less common route is direct invasion across the protective meninges. Physical disruption of

the dura by trauma or surgery allows direct invasion of the subarachnoid space and should be considered in patients with a history of CSF leakage or rhinorrhea. Emissary veins provide another pathway for bacteria to spread from contiguous foci into the subarachnoid space. These veins traverse the skull and dura, directly connecting the soft tissues of the head and neck with the venous system of the brain and meninges, including the arachnoid villi. Although blood in the emissary veins usually flows away from the brain, the CNS veins and dural sinuses do not contain valves, and retrograde flow of bacteria is possible. Rarely, organisms may reach the ventricles or subarachnoid space from within the neural tissue; for example, rupture of a brain abscess into the ventricles may have disastrous effects.

PATHOPHYSIOLOGY

Neural damage occurs as a direct result of the host inflammatory response. The unique anatomy and composition of the CSF-filled compartments, combined with a paucity of host immunologic defenses, create a microenvironment that allows the persistence and proliferation of microorganisms.[1] Polymorphonuclear leukocytes are not normal inhabitants of the CSF, and mobilization of these phagocytic cells is delayed during the early stages of infection. Similarly, the concentration of immunoglobulin in CSF is significantly less than that in serum, limiting the effectiveness of humoral immunity. Most important, complement, which plays a critical role in chemotaxis, phagocytosis, and intracellular killing, is virtually absent from normal CSF. Once in the CSF, bacteria induce leukocyte migration into the subarachnoid space, resulting in occlusion of cortical blood vessels, damage to nerve roots that traverse the subarachnoid space (see Figure 134-2), and impaired CSF flow (see Figure 134-1). Clinically, this manifests as cranial or spinal nerve dysfunction and hydrocephalus. Activation of leukocytes leads to an inflammatory cascade, with the release of cytokines, oxidants, and proteolytic enzymes. At the cellular level, this chain of events produces disruption of the blood-brain barrier and impaired cerebrovascular autoregulation.[4] Increased intracranial pressure may result in transtentorial herniation or tissue hypoxia due to decreased tissue perfusion.

CLINICAL COURSE

Acute Meningitis Syndrome

Early recognition and therapy of acute meningitis syndrome are essential to minimize morbidity and mortality. The initial manifestation of the illness may be subtle, with a low-grade headache or fever. However, once meningeal symptoms (vomiting, severe headache, stiff neck) develop, the clinical course is dramatic. Patients appear "toxic," and higher integrative functions may deteriorate rapidly. The classic clinical triad associated with bacterial meningitis, fever, neck stiffness, and altered mental status is present in only 44% of cases.[6] A rash is highly suggestive of meningococcal infections; however, skin lesions are noted in only 64% of meningitis cases due to this organism.[7] Other common signs and symptoms include headache and nausea. In the elderly, recognition of acute bacterial meningitis may be delayed by the absence of suggestive clinical findings. Nuchal rigidity, vomiting, and headache are significantly less frequently noted in the elderly; in contrast, seizures are present in 26% of patients ≥65 years of age.[10] In addition, the elderly have a higher incidence of noninfectious conditions that may

TABLE 134-1	Causes of Acute and Subacute Central Nervous System Infection Syndromes

Acute Meningitis Syndrome

Rapid onset (<24-48 h) of fever, headache, or meningismus, with early cognitive impairment

Common

Pyogenic meningitis (pneumococcal, meningococcal, *Listeria*, other)

Uncommon

Viral encephalitis (especially herpes simplex), subarachnoid bleed, brain abscess (with rupture)

Rare

Viral meningitis, granulomatous meningitis (cryptococcal, mycobacterial), carcinomatous meningitis, brain tumor

Subacute Central Nervous System Infection Syndrome

Subacute onset (>24-48 h) of fever, headache, or meningismus, with no or gradual cognitive impairment

Common

Viral meningitis, viral encephalitis, rickettsial infection

Uncommon

Brain abscess, brain tumor, granulomatous meningitis

Rare

Cerebrovascular accident, carcinomatous meningitis

mimic acute meningitis syndrome (e.g., subarachnoid bleeding and malignancies involving the CNS) complicating the initial evaluation.

Acute meningitis syndrome represents an infectious disease emergency. Baseline predictors of adverse outcome in adults include advanced age, tachycardia (heart rate >120 beats/min), low Glasgow Coma Scale score, cranial nerve palsies, CSF WBC count less than 1000/mm^3, and presence of gram-positive cocci on CSF Gram stain.[8] This latter variable reflects the higher mortality associated with pneumococcal meningitis. Despite the availability of antibiotics active against all common causes of acute bacterial meningitis, in adults the overall mortality remains approximately 20%.[6] A delay in antibiotic therapy increases the risk of an adverse outcome, particularly when progressive neurologic impairment occurs before receiving therapy.[9] For this reason, recently published guidelines recommend the administration of empirical antibiotics to patients with a presumptive diagnosis of bacterial meningitis as soon as possible after presentation (Figure 134-3).[5]

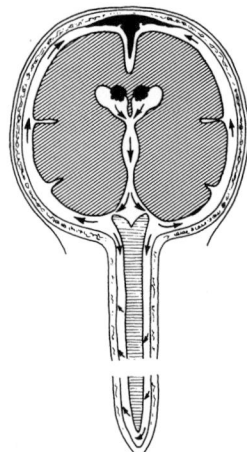

Figure 134-1 Cerebrospinal fluid (CSF) flow within the central nervous system. CSF that forms at the choroid plexus of the cerebral ventricles rapidly enters the subarachnoid space at the foramina of Luschka and Magendie. From the cisterna magna, an organized flow of CSF occurs around the convexities of the brain to the arachnoid villi. There are multiple pathways of bidirectional flow around the spinal cord.

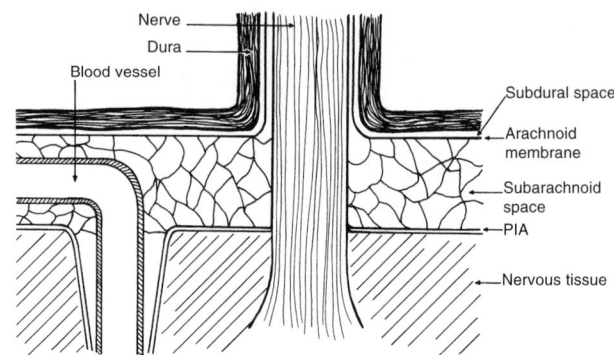

Figure 134-2 This diagram of the potential and actual spaces between the layers of the meninges shows the relationship of blood vessels and nerve roots to the subarachnoid space.

Coupled with the need for urgent treatment is the need for urgent diagnosis. Identification of a pathogen allows the clinician to tailor the antibiotic regimen based on susceptibility patterns, and has prognostic and therapeutic implications. However, situations arise when lumbar puncture is unavoidably delayed. This may be due to anatomic factors that make lumbar puncture technically difficult or the need to perform neuroimaging studies to exclude a contraindication to lumbar puncture. If a significant delay in obtaining CSF is anticipated, antibiotics should be given immediately after peripheral blood cultures are obtained. The yield of CSF culture decreases within as little as 15 minutes following administration of antibiotics.[11] Nevertheless, the risk of delaying treatment outweighs the need to make a microbiological diagnosis. Despite the inhibitory effect of prior antibiotics on bacterial culture and Gram stain, the absolute neutrophil count and neutrophilic pleocytosis remain suggestive of bacterial meningitis,[12,13] and a full course of empirical therapy should be completed if CSF parameters are consistent with this diagnosis.

Historically, the perceived risk (and legal consequences) of uncal herniation following lumbar puncture in the presence of an intracranial mass lesion led to the ubiquitous use of neuroimaging. More recently, studies have challenged this practice, citing the potential deleterious effect of computed tomography (CT) scan–related delays in the initiation of therapy or the compromising effect of premature sterilization of CSF cultures.[9,11,16] Even among patients with an abnormal CT scan, only a minority of cases have radiographic findings precluding lumbar puncture.[14] For this reason, guidelines suggest that neuroimaging prior to lumbar puncture should be reserved for patients with compromised immune systems (e.g., human immunodeficiency

TABLE 134-2	Routes by Which Bacteria May Enter the Subarachnoid Space

Vascular (Blood-Brain Barrier)

Mostly likely pathogens: pneumococci, meningococci, *Listeria, Escherichia coli* (neonates), group B streptococci (neonates), *Haemophilus influenzae*
Choroid plexus: may be common site of invasion for *H. influenzae*
Meningeal blood vessels: throughout the subarachnoid space; may be usual route for pneumococci
Arachnoid villi: possible route of invasion, located between the sagittal sinus and subarachnoid space

Transdural

Most likely pathogens: pneumococci, gram-negative enteric bacilli, staphylococci (including coagulase-negative), *H. influenzae*
Surgery: including ventriculoatrial or ventriculoperitoneal shunts
Trauma: especially when cribriform plate or petrous bone is fractured
Parameningeal infective focus: including sinusitis, mastoiditis, otitis, or osteomyelitis; emissary veins may serve as conduit
Congenital defects: including myelomeningocele and spinal dermal sinus

Transparenchymal

Mostly likely pathogens: anaerobic bacteria, enteric gram-negative bacilli
Occurs when brain abscess ruptures directly into ventricles or subarachnoid space

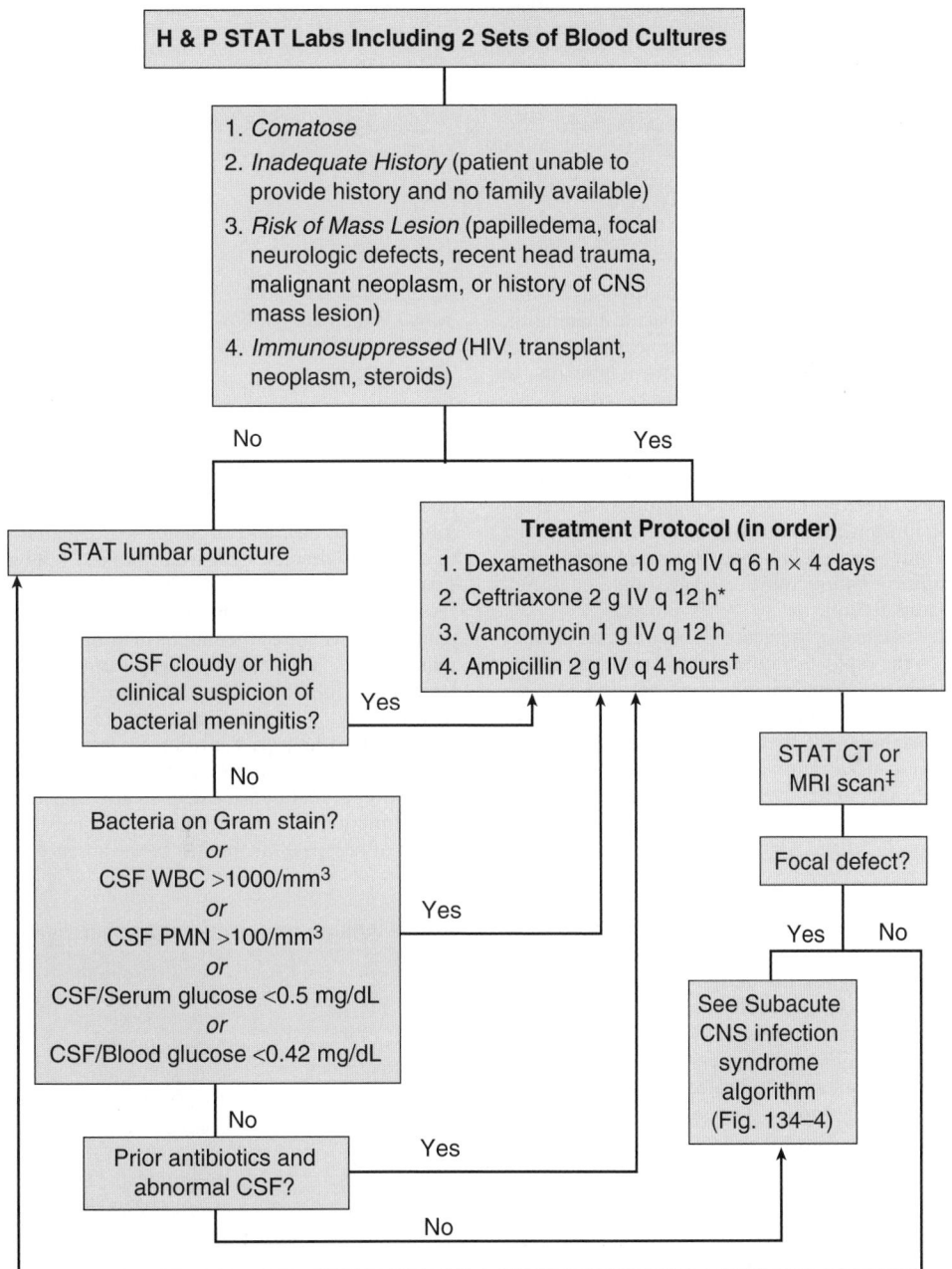

Figure 134-3 Algorithm for management of adult patients with acute meningitis syndrome. *For severe cephalosporin allergy, consider meropenem or moxifloxacin. †Ampicillin is indicated if there is a history of alcoholism, organ transplant, malignancy, pregnancy, or age older than 50 years. For penicillin-allergic patients, an alternative is trimethoprim-sulfamethoxazole. ‡Consider magnetic resonance imaging (MRI) if the patient is known or suspected to have human immunodeficiency virus (HIV), if it can be obtained rapidly. *CNS*, central nervous system; *CSF*, cerebrospinal fluid; *CT*, computed tomography; *H&P*, history and physical examination; *PMN*, polymorphonuclear leukocyte; *WBC*, white blood cell.

virus [HIV] infection, use of immunosuppressive medications, or organ transplantation), history of an intracranial mass lesion, abnormal level of consciousness, papilledema, or focal neurologic deficit.[5] In the absence of one of these features, the recommendation is to proceed directly to lumbar puncture, followed by immediate administration of empirical antibiotics.[5]

Subacute Central Nervous System Infection Syndrome

Febrile illness associated with a somewhat more gradual progression of signs and symptoms of CNS involvement represents the subacute meningitis syndrome. Headache can be mild to severe, and neck stiffness can be minimum or marked. However, patients with this syndrome are typically oriented and clinically stable at the onset of illness,

TABLE 134-3	Empirical Antimicrobial Therapy for Adult Patients with Presumed Bacterial Meningitis		
Site of Acquisition	*Predisposition*	*Organism(s)*	*Antimicrobial Agent(s)*
Community			
	Age 16-50 years	*Streptococcus pneumoniae* *Neisseria meningitidis*	Vancomycin plus 3rd-generation cephalosporin*
	T-cell deficiency	*S. pneumoniae, N. meningitidis* *Listeria monocytogenes*	Vancomycin plus 3rd-generation cephalosporin* *plus* ampicillin
	Age > 50 years	*S. pneumoniae, N. meningitidis* *L. monocytogenes*	Vancomycin plus 3rd-generation cephalosporin* *plus* ampicillin
Nosocomial			
		Staphylococcal species Gram-negative bacilli (including *Pseudomonas aeruginosa*)	Vancomycin plus 4th-generation cephalosporin[†] *or* meropenem

*Ceftriaxone or cefotaxime.
[†]Cefepime, ceftazidime.

with a gradual progression of neurologic symptoms (>24-48 hours). Although bacterial infection may rarely cause subacute meningitis, most cases are due to other pathogens or noninfectious factors.

Herpes simplex encephalitis, brain abscess, and meningitis due to fungi, mycobacteria, fastidious bacteria (e.g., *Rickettsia rickettsii, Treponema pallidum)*, or viruses all produce fever, worsening headache, and progressive impairment of higher integrative functions. On occasion, carcinomatous meningitis, brain tumor, and subarachnoid bleeding cause similar findings (see Table 134-1). To avoid inappropriate therapy and unnecessary hospitalization, the decision to institute antimicrobial therapy should be carefully weighed. However, if pyogenic meningitis is still a possibility, empirical antimicrobial therapy should be begun, as outlined in the previous section.

The first priority when managing subacute CNS syndrome is rapid diagnosis (as opposed to the rapid-therapy approach to acute meningitis syndrome). With this syndrome, the physician has time to carefully evaluate the patient and relevant laboratory data (Figure 134-4). Peripheral blood granulocytosis (>10,000/mm^3), CSF cell counts over 1000/mm^3, CSF protein concentration over 100 mg/dL, and CSF glucose concentrations below 40 mg/dL favor a bacterial cause, and these patients should be given empirical antibiotics for acute meningitis syndrome until a specific diagnosis is made or bacterial cultures return negative.

If history and physical examination suggest a space-occupying lesion, lumbar puncture and even antimicrobial therapy can be safely delayed pending results of emergent head CT or magnetic resonance imaging (MRI). However, if significant delays are likely, empirical therapy should be given. Other causes of subacute CNS infection syndrome are discussed later (see Brain Abscess and Viral Infections of the Central Nervous System).

Additional diagnostic studies may be indicated for subacute infections. Serologic testing for HIV should be performed, because the spectrum of infectious agents is much broader among HIV-infected individuals. Testing for enteroviruses (CSF polymerase chain reaction [PCR] or viral culture), *Cryptococcus* (cryptococcal antigen), neurosyphilis (VDRL), mycobacterial infection (culture or PCR of CSF), herpes simplex virus (CSF PCR), tickborne infections *(Ehrlichia, Rickettsia,* Lyme disease), and arboviral encephalitides (West Nile virus) should be individualized based on patient characteristics, severity of illness, knowledge of local pathogens, and season. Despite intensive diagnostic testing, a pathogen is identified in only two-thirds of patients with subacute meningitis syndrome.[17]

EPIDEMIOLOGY

The epidemiology of bacterial meningitis has evolved in the last twenty years. The incidence of bacterial meningitis in the pediatric population has decreased markedly in the United States following the widespread use of conjugate vaccines active against *Haemophilus influenzae* type B, *Neisseria meningitidis, and Streptococcus pneumoniae.*[18]Conversely, the incidence of nosocomial bacterial meningitis caused by resistant strains

of Enterobacteriaceae, *Pseudomonas aeruginosa*, and *Staphylococcus aureus* is increasing following surgery or instrumentation of the CNS.[2]

THERAPY

Antibiotics

The choice of empirical antibiotics is based on knowledge of the likely causative agents, which vary based on host characteristics (e.g., age, immunocompromise), site of acquisition (nosocomial versus community acquired), and local resistance patterns. Recommendations for empirical therapy are listed in Table 134-3, with dosages commonly used for the treatment of CNS infections listed in Table 134-4.[3,5] Pneumococci and meningococci remain the most common causes of community-acquired meningitis in immunocompetent adults younger than 50 years.[3] In the last decade, pneumococci that are intermediately (minimum inhibitory concentration [MIC] >0.12 to 1 µg/mL) or highly (MIC >2 µg/mL) resistant to penicillin have emerged as important pathogens. Penicillin-resistant pneumococci are typically multidrug resistant; however, many isolates remain sensitive to third-generation cephalosporins, and all are susceptible to vancomycin.

Antimicrobial therapy should be directed against the most common causes of bacterial meningitis. In the absence of a positive CSF Gram

TABLE 134-4	Antimicrobial Dosages for Central Nervous System Infections	
Drug	*Dosage (by Total Body Weight)*	*Usual Dosage (for 70-kg Adult)*
Acyclovir	10 mg/kg IV q 8 h	700 mg IV q 8 h
Ampicillin	30 mg/kg IV q 4 h	2 g IV q 4 h
Cefotaxime	30 mg/kg IV q 6 h	2 g IV q 6 h
Ceftazidime	30 mg/kg IV q 8 h	2 g IV q 8 h
Cefepime	30 mg/kg IV q 8 h	2 g IV q 8 h
Ceftriaxone	30 mg/kg IV q 12 h	2 g IV q 12 h
Meropenem	40 mg/kg IV q 8 h*	2 g IV q 8 h
Metronidazole	7.5 mg/kg IV q 6 h	500 mg IV q 6 h
Nafcillin	30 mg/kg IV q 4 h	2 g IV q 4 h
Penicillin G	60,000-70,000 units/ kg IV q 4 h	4 million units IV q 4 h
Tobramycin or gentamicin[†]	2 mg/kg IV load, then 1.7 mg/kg q 8 h[‡]	140 mg IV load, then 120 mg IV q 8 h[‡]
Intrathecal	0.1 mg/kg/d	5-10 mg/d
Intraventricular	0.1 mg/kg/d	5-10 mg/d
Trimethoprim-sulfamethoxazole	5 mg/kg IV q 6 h	350 mg IV q 6 h[§]
Vancomycin	15 mg/kg IV q 6 h	500 mg IV q 6 h[‡] or 1 g IV q 12 h

*Pediatric dosage. Adults should receive usual dosage.
[†]Regardless of which aminoglycoside is used, only preservative-free preparations should be used.
[‡]Adjust dosage based on serum levels.
[§]Dosage indicates trimethoprim component.

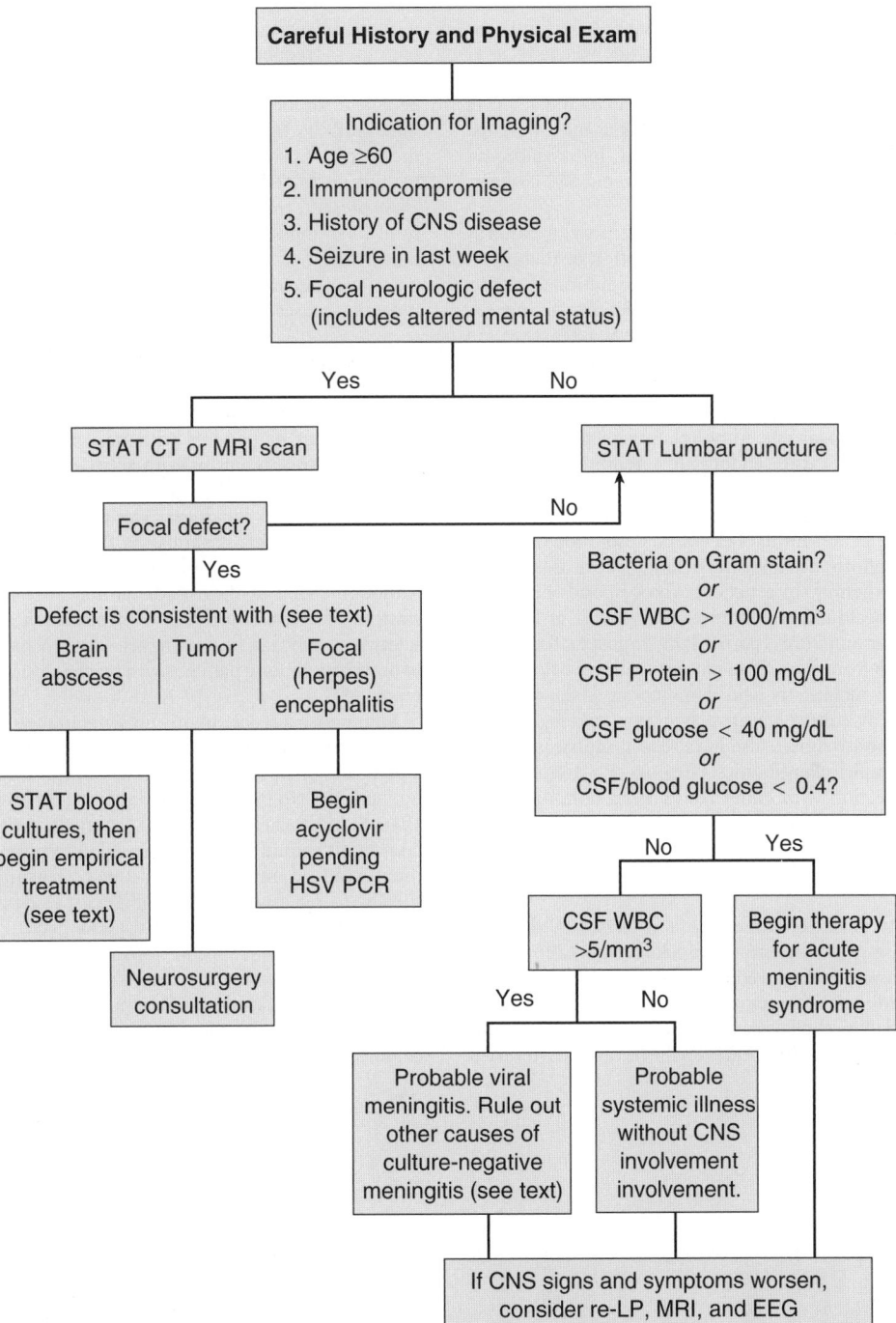

Management of Adults with Subacute CNS Infection Syndrome
(Subacute illness—3-7 days—with moderate fever and worsening headache;
often with progressive impairment of higher integrative function and/or focal defects.)

Careful History and Physical Exam

Indication for Imaging?
1. Age ≥60
2. Immunocompromise
3. History of CNS disease
4. Seizure in last week
5. Focal neurologic defect
   (includes altered mental status)

Yes — STAT CT or MRI scan
No — STAT Lumbar puncture

Focal defect?
No → STAT Lumbar puncture
Yes ↓

Defect is consistent with (see text)
Brain abscess | Tumor | Focal (herpes) encephalitis

STAT blood cultures, then begin empirical treatment (see text)

Begin acyclovir pending HSV PCR

Neurosurgery consultation

Bacteria on Gram stain?
or
CSF WBC > 1000/mm³
or
CSF Protein > 100 mg/dL
or
CSF glucose < 40 mg/dL
or
CSF/blood glucose < 0.4?

No — CSF WBC >5/mm³
Yes — Begin therapy for acute meningitis syndrome

CSF WBC >5/mm³
Yes — Probable viral meningitis. Rule out other causes of culture-negative meningitis (see text)
No — Probable systemic illness without CNS involvement involvement.

If CNS signs and symptoms worsen, consider re-LP, MRI, and EEG

Figure 134-4 Algorithm for the management of patients with subacute central nervous system (CNS) infection syndrome. CSF, cerebrospinal fluid; CT, computed tomography; EEG, electroencephalogram; HSV, herpes simplex virus; LP, lumbar puncture; MRI, magnetic resonance imaging; PCR, polymerase chain reaction; WBC, white blood cell.

stain, initial therapy for adults with community-acquired meningitis should include a third-generation cephalosporin such as cefotaxime or ceftriaxone, as well as vancomycin. Vancomycin should never be used alone as initial therapy because of its marginal CNS penetration and lack of activity against gram-negative organisms. Empirical ampicillin therapy for *Listeria monocytogenes* should be added for adults aged

50 years or older or for patients with T-cell immunocompromise (e.g., on chronic steroid therapy), pregnant women, or patients with significant use of alcohol.[3,5] If the CSF Gram stain shows gram-positive rods suggestive of *Listeria*, intravenous (IV) gentamicin should be added. For patients intolerant of penicillins, trimethoprim-sulfamethoxazole is an acceptable alternative for treatment of *Listeria* meningitis.

In contrast to community-acquired meningitis, organisms causing nosocomial meningitis reflect the highly resistant strains endemic to the hospital. Empirical therapy for patients suspected to have nosocomial meningitis must therefore be directed against staphylococcal species (both coagulase-positive and coagulase-negative strains) and multidrug-resistant strains of gram-negative bacilli, including *P. aeruginosa* and *Acinetobacter baumannii* (see Figure 134-3). Empirical treatment in this population should therefore include vancomycin as well as an antipseudomonal cephalosporin (ceftazidime or cefepime) or carbapenem. Imipenem is active against *Pseudomonas* and achieves therapeutic levels in the CSF; however, because this agent lowers the seizure threshold, it is relatively contraindicated for meningitis. Meropenem, a related carbapenem, is less epileptogenic and is therefore preferred for this indication.[19]

Initial antibiotic choices can be refined when sensitivity patterns become available, typically in 2 to 3 days. The duration of therapy in bacterial meningitis varies with the pathogen and the clinical response. Although there have been few randomized studies evaluating the optimal duration of therapy, 7 days of treatment for *H. influenzae* and *N. meningitidis* meningitis is typically sufficient,[20] whereas *S. pneumoniae* requires 10 to 14 days of therapy.[5,17] Adults with pneumococcal meningitis may have predisposing infections including pneumonia, sinusitis, otitis, or rarely endocarditis. Although therapy for meningitis usually treats the primary cause, endocarditis requires prolonged therapy with bactericidal antibiotics.

For all causes of bacterial meningitis, abnormalities of the CSF (high protein and cell counts) persist for days to weeks. Resolution of symptoms (e.g., fever, leukocytosis, meningismus) should serve as adequate evidence of successful therapy. In a patient who responds poorly to 48 hours of therapy, repeat lumbar puncture and head CT or MRI are indicated. Repeat lumbar puncture is particularly important for detecting clearance of bacteria from the CSF in patients with cephalosporin-resistant pneumococcal meningitis who demonstrate a slow clinical response.[19] Patients with culture-negative pyogenic meningitis and suboptimal clinical response should also have repeat lumbar puncture to ensure response to empirical antibiotics. Ongoing or worsening CSF parameters suggest infection with either resistant bacteria or with a pathogen more typically associated with subacute meningitis syndrome (see Table 134-1).

Corticosteroids

Much of the morbidity of bacterial meningitis is caused by the host inflammatory response. Corticosteroids block inflammation, and animal studies have shown an improvement in outcome when corticosteroids are given as adjuvant therapy with antibiotics. A number of randomized controlled clinical trials have evaluated the use of steroids in patients with bacterial meningitis; however, the findings have varied based on the population studied. A large meta-analysis found use of adjuvant corticosteroids significantly decreased mortality as well as sequelae, including hearing loss and neurologic debility.[21] Age stratification showed the survival benefits were restricted to adults, where the reduction in hearing loss was only seen among children. This may reflect the divergent microbiology among this age group; the decrease in mortality was restricted to patients with *S. pneumoniae*, a pathogen seen more frequently in adults, while the decrease in hearing loss was only found in patients with *H. influenzae*, who were almost exclusively pediatric. A more recent meta-analysis of individual patient data by the same authors failed to find a protective effect with adjunctive dexamethasone.[22] Theoretical concerns regarding use of corticosteroids include decreased penetration of vancomycin across the meninges.

At present, treatment guidelines recommend adjuvant dexamethasone (0.15 mg/kg IV every 6 hours for 2-4 days) be given concomitantly with the first dose of antibiotics for adult patients with suspected or proven pneumococcal meningitis.[5] Whether steroids are beneficial for other causes of bacterial meningitis remains unknown.

COMPLICATIONS

Systemic complications are frequent in acute bacterial meningitis. Forty percent of patients with pneumococcal meningitis have concomitant sepsis, typically from an extra-CNS infection such as pneumonia. Less commonly, sepsis represents seeding of the bloodstream from the infected meninges. The approach to sepsis associated with bacterial meningitis is similar to that in any patient in the intensive care unit (ICU): protection of the airway and hemodynamic support. Although many of these patients may meet the criteria for administration of activated protein C (drotrecogin alfa), limited data on its safety and efficacy in meningitis exist. Increased risk of intracranial hemorrhage among patients with severe sepsis and meningitis has been reported.[23]

Meningococcal meningitis presents unique public health and infection control challenges. This diagnosis is suggested by the presence of a petechial or purpuric rash; however, this finding is neither sensitive nor specific.[7] To prevent secondary cases of meningococcal meningitis among healthcare workers, all patients with presumed bacterial meningitis should initially be placed in respiratory isolation to prevent the spread of infection by droplet transmission.[25] Complications specific to meningococcal meningitis include purpura fulminans and necrotizing vasculitis leading to skin necrosis and digital gangrene (Figure 134-5). Nonspecific complications associated with meningococcal as well as other forms of meningitis include adrenal insufficiency due to infarction (Waterhouse-Friderichsen syndrome), renal failure (due to acute tubular necrosis in the setting of hypotension), deafness, hydrocephalus, and cognitive impairment.

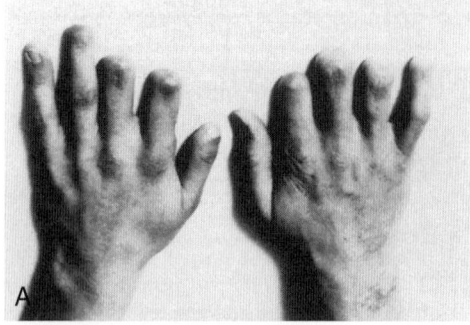
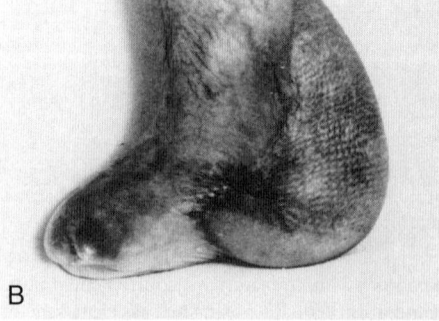

Figure 134-5   Extremities—hands **(A)** and foot **(B)**—of a 14-year-old boy observed by two physicians as his petechial rash progressed to "bruises" (purpura fulminans). Purpura were not recognized as the hallmarks of *Neisseria meningitidis*–induced sepsis. In addition to the loss of extremities from the necrotizing vasculitis of meningococcemia, the patient rapidly developed signs and symptoms characteristic of the acute meningitis syndrome.

TABLE 134-5	Differential Diagnosis of Central Nervous System Infection and Tumor			
	Brain Abscess	Bacterial Meningitis	Herpetic Encephalitis	Brain Tumor
History				
Headache	Severe, often focal	Severe, generalized	Mild to severe	Absent to severe
Focal defect	Often	Occasional	Occasional	Often
Progression	Days to weeks	Hours to days	Days	Days to months
Physical Examination				
Fever/degree	Variable	>90%	>90%	Rare
Early focal signs	Often	Occasional	Occasional	Often
Pressure signs	Often	Rare	Occasional	Often
Extra-CNS infection	Often	Often	No	No
CT or MRI Scan				
Focal	Always*	No	Often	Always
Ring effect/onset	Often/late†	No	No	Often/early

*May be negative or nonspecific during first 48 hours of illness.
†Development of abscess wall may be delayed by steroid therapy.
CT, computed tomography; MRI, magnetic resonance imaging.

Brain Abscess

Pyogenic brain abscess is a localized suppurative infection of parenchymal CNS tissue and may involve any region of the CNS from the cerebral cortex to the conus medullaris. Differentiating brain abscess from other CNS infections or brain tumors may be challenging, as there is significant overlap in the clinical and radiologic presentation (Table 134-5). Even with a combined medical and surgical approach, mortality is significant. Rapid progression of symptoms and impaired mental status at presentation are predictors of an adverse outcome, with rupture of the abscess into the ventricle almost uniformly fatal.[26]

PATHOPHYSIOLOGY

A brain abscess begins as a localized area of parenchymal inflammation (cerebritis) which evolves to necrosis and frank suppuration. The initial stage, characterized by vascular congestion, petechial hemorrhage, cerebral edema, and tissue softening, is demonstrable by MRI even before CT changes are evident. As cerebritis progresses, CT findings become abnormal, revealing a capsule-like hyperemic zone surrounding the area of inflammation. In time, liquefaction results in frank abscess formation. As the abscess matures, a dense capsule is formed. In relatively avascular areas such as the cerebral white matter of the brain, capsule formation is delayed, and these sites have higher rates of spontaneous rupture.

In the preantibiotic era, brain abscesses arose from extension of infection from contiguous foci (middle ear, mastoids, sinuses). With the availability of antibiotics, however, such complications have become less common. An increasing number of cases are due to distant foci of infection[27] or are associated with local seeding following neurosurgery or trauma.[15] Abscesses arising from hematogenous seeding tend to develop in the distribution of the middle cerebral artery. Brain abscesses associated with endocarditis are rare but, when present, are often multiple and small. Filtration of bacteria by the pulmonary vasculature protects the brain from hematogenous seeding. Therefore, when cardiac shunts or pulmonary arteriovenous fistulas are present, the risk of brain abscess is increased. In as many as a third of patients, there is no obvious source of infection.

The etiologic pathogen for brain abscesses differs according to the route of infection. Abscesses that arise from contiguous sites are frequently polymicrobial. In contrast, brain abscesses associated with hematogenous spread are usually due to a single pathogen. Infections following neurosurgery reflect nosocomial flora and often include multidrug-resistant organisms such as methicillin-resistant *S. aureus* (MRSA) or multidrug-resistant *A. baumannii*. The bacteria most often isolated from brain abscess include Enterobacteriaceae, streptococci, staphylococci, and pneumococci.[27] Fastidious bacteria such as *Nocardia*, fungi such as *Aspergillus*, and even protozoa such as *Toxoplasma* can also be etiologic agents, particularly in immunosuppressed patients.

CLINICAL COURSE

The variable signs and symptoms of brain abscess relate to variations in location, size, and rapidity of development. At one extreme, the course may span weeks, with few constitutional symptoms. In this setting, signs and symptoms of a space-occupying lesion predominate, and neoplasm is the primary diagnostic concern. In contrast, a previously asymptomatic brain abscess may rupture into the subarachnoid space, causing death within hours. The differential diagnosis in this setting includes an acute cerebrovascular event and pyogenic meningitis. However, brain abscess usually progresses subacutely over 7 to 14 days. Classic symptoms include headache, low-grade fever, and focal neurologic signs. Occasionally, a patient has no symptoms referable to the CNS, and fever may be absent in as many as 50% of cases.

Lumbar puncture is contraindicated if there is evidence of a space-occupying lesion with significant associated edema. When CSF is available, it may demonstrate increased white blood cells and protein and normal or decreased glucose. CSF culture adds little diagnostic information, as organisms are identified in only 10% of cases. CNS complications of brain abscess relate to both tissue inflammation and increased intracranial pressure from a space-occupying lesion. Nonspecific complications common to all critically ill patients include aspiration and gastrointestinal bleeding. Specific complications include focal neurologic defects, altered mental status, or seizures. Although signs and symptoms related to increased intracranial pressure help localize the infection to the brain, these findings do not differentiate infection from other intracerebral mass lesions. When surrounding edema is excessive, aggressive therapy with corticosteroids is warranted.

IMAGING

MRI is superior to CT in assessing brain abscesses, as the latter may miss small lesions or those localized to the brainstem or cerebellum. Neuroimaging plays a role in both diagnosis and in monitoring for response to therapy. Changes in lesion size after the institution of therapy can be closely monitored from week to week. An expanding abscess may be aggressively drained, or conversely, a stable or shrinking abscess can be assiduously observed.

Maturation of a brain abscess is associated with encapsulation, and this is suggested by ring enhancement on CT or MRI. Misinterpretation can occur, particularly when the abscess is in the white matter, where decreased vascularity may result in delayed encapsulation with minimal ring enhancement. Similarly, steroid therapy may decrease local inflammation, resulting in resolution of ring enhancement. Ring enhancement is not specific for bacterial abscesses and may be seen with other infections or brain tumors.

THERAPY

In general, a combination approach of antimicrobials coupled with surgical drainage remains the standard approach for management of pyogenic brain abscesses. Choice of antimicrobials should be guided by culture results, given the diversity of potential pathogens and the need for prolonged therapy (e.g., 6-8 weeks). Because of the difficulty in getting therapeutic concentrations of antibiotics across the blood-brain barrier, additional pharmacologic considerations include CNS penetration and parenteral administration. Empirical therapy should be begun while awaiting culture results and should be guided by the likely microbiology based on the origin of the infection. In cases in which the source is unknown or metastatic spread from a distant focus is likely, empirical therapy with vancomycin, metronidazole, and a third-generation cephalosporin is suggested.[15] An antipseudomonal cephalosporin should be substituted for the third-generation cephalosporin for postoperative infections or for an abscess arising from an otogenic site. Neurosurgical aspiration is invaluable in identifying specific pathogens, and sensitivity testing is crucial for narrowing therapy. Fungal and mycobacterial cultures should be obtained on all aspirates. Positive cultures from blood or extra-CNS suppurative foci occasionally establish a presumptive etiologic agent. Ancillary testing for a culture-negative brain abscess includes HIV serology, serum cryptococcal antigen, and toxoplasmosis titers.

In selected cases, brain abscesses can be treated with antimicrobials alone, particularly when the causative agent is known and the lesion measures less than 2.5 cm.[28] Medical management without drainage may be necessary when the lesion is inaccessible or surgical intervention poses unacceptable risks. However, open or stereotactic drainage is indicated when (1) cultures of extra-CNS sites do not yield a pathogen, (2) deterioration from increased intracranial pressure occurs, and (3) there is no radiographic improvement on medical therapy. Patients treated without drainage may require a longer duration (e.g., 12 weeks) of parenteral antibiotics and should be followed closely for clinical and radiographic improvement. Steroids should be reserved for cases in which significant edema is present.

Viral Infections of the Central Nervous System

Depending on the anatomic site of infection, viruses may cause a clinical syndrome of meningitis, encephalitis, or myelitis. Acute viral meningitis is characterized by meningeal irritation, CSF lymphocytic pleocytosis, and a self-limited clinical course. Myelitis implies infection of the spinal cord and may be present in isolation (e.g., poliovirus infection) or as part of an overlap syndrome of encephalomyelitis (e.g., acute flaccid paralysis associated with West Nile virus encephalitis). The hallmark of viral encephalitis is alteration in cognition lasting 24 hours or more. Personality changes may occur, with irritability and inability to concentrate. Patients may also develop fever, headache, nausea, and vomiting. As a result of parenchymal involvement, CNS function may deteriorate over several days; confusion, lethargy, somnolence, coma, and seizures are common. Meningismus is variably present with viral encephalitis.

PATHOPHYSIOLOGY

Most viral infections of the CNS occur through hematogenous spread.[29] The virus may initially traverse mucous membranes (e.g., enteroviruses) or be inoculated into subcutaneous tissue (e.g., arboviruses). After local replication within extraneural tissues, sustained viremia occurs. Alternatively, the virus may gain access to the CNS by direct neuronal invasion, as occurs when rabies virus spreads retrograde along peripheral nerves into the CNS. The olfactory tracts may provide a route of entry for herpes simplex virus type 1.

Individual viruses demonstrate affinities for different anatomic areas of the CNS. Enteroviruses and mumps viruses usually infect the ependyma and tissues of the subarachnoid space, producing meningeal irritation. In contrast, arboviruses and rabies viruses almost always involve the parenchyma and cause encephalitis. In older children and adults, herpes simplex virus type 1 characteristically causes temporal lobe encephalitis, whereas herpes simplex virus type 2 more typically causes meningitis. Such affinities are not absolute. For example, enteroviruses may on rare occasions cause encephalitis.

ACUTE VIRAL MENINGITIS

Although many viruses cause meningitis, in clinical practice, the specific pathogen is rarely identified. In most cases, extensive diagnostic evaluation is not indicated; viral meningitis is typically a self-limited syndrome and does not require treatment. Epidemiologic studies suggest that enteroviruses are the most common cause of viral meningitis[17,30] and are particularly prevalent in children and young adults. Other viral causes of meningitis include arboviruses (see Viral Encephalitis), herpes simplex virus type 2, acute HIV infection, and lymphocytic choriomeningitis virus.

At the time of presentation, it may be difficult to differentiate viral meningitis from other forms of culture-negative meningitis that may be more aggressive or require directed therapy. The differential diagnosis for culture-negative or aseptic meningitis includes tickborne infections such as *Ehrlichia* or *Rickettsia*, secondary syphilis, mycobacterial or fungal infections, irritation from a parameningeal focus, and partially treated bacterial infections (see Figure 134-3). Signs and symptoms of viral and bacterial meningitis are indistinguishable. CSF findings suggestive of a viral cause include lymphocytic pleocytosis (typically with a total white blood cell count <1000), normal glucose, and normal to slightly elevated protein. Management is supportive, with fluid repletion for significant dehydration and pain control the mainstays of care. Meningeal symptoms usually resolve in the first 2 weeks, but malaise may be prolonged.

VIRAL ENCEPHALITIS

A host of viral agents infect the parenchyma of the brain or spinal cord to produce encephalitis or myelitis, respectively; however, despite intensive investigation, in the majority of cases, no organism is identified.[24,31,32] Viral encephalitis is typically an acute febrile illness associated with headache, an altered level of consciousness disproportionate to systemic illness, behavioral or speech disturbances, and focal neurologic signs such as seizures or hemiparesis. In contrast, viral myelitis causes hemiparesis or hemiplegia but spares higher integrative functions. Overlap syndromes of encephalomyelitis can occur.

Viral encephalitis is caused by acute invasion of brain parenchyma. Clinically, viral encephalitis must be differentiated from acute disseminated encephalomyelitis (ADEM), an autoimmune phenomenon that typically occurs 5 to 21 days after a viral respiratory or gastrointestinal illness. MRI in ADEM reveals enhancing multifocal white matter lesions suggestive of demyelination.[33] Neuroimaging to distinguish these entities is important because ADEM responds to high-dose steroids. With the exception of herpes simplex encephalitis (see later), management of viral encephalitides revolves around supportive care and control of seizures.[24] Despite the lack of specific antiviral treatments, thorough evaluation is important to direct public health interventions (e.g., mosquito eradication for West Nile virus or other arboviruses) or provide prognostic information (e.g., rabies).

HERPES SIMPLEX ENCEPHALITIS

Herpes simplex encephalitis (HSE) is the most common cause of sporadic encephalitis in the United States. The mortality of untreated HSE exceeds 70%; however, timely administration of acyclovir has been shown to significantly improve survival. While clinical, laboratory, or radiographic findings may be suggestive of HSE, no combination of presenting features is sufficiently sensitive, and empirical acyclovir should be given to all patients with encephalitis until definitive diagnostic studies are completed.[24]

Common signs and symptoms of HSE include fever, personality change, and dysphasia. Hemiparesis and seizures occur in approximately 40% of cases.[34,35] Without treatment, progressive obtundation occurs. CSF typically exhibits a lymphocytic pleocytosis, but this is nonspecific. Suggestive findings include temporal lobe localization on neuroimaging studies, with MRI being superior to CT, and periodic lateralizing epileptiform discharges (PLEDS) on the electroencephalogram. Definitive diagnosis requires detection of herpes simplex in the brain or spinal fluid. PCR on CSF, a noninvasive test with a sensitivity greater than 95%, is now considered the gold standard for diagnosis.[36] Empirical acyclovir can usually be discontinued if the PCR is negative, although there have been reports of false-negative results early in the course of the disease.[37] For PCR-confirmed cases, acyclovir therapy should be continued for a minimum of 14 days, with treatment extended to 21 days if the CSF remains PCR-positive at the end of treatment.[38]

Central Nervous System Infection and the AIDS Patient

CNS dysfunction is common in patients with HIV, found in as many as half of all infected patients during the course of the infection.[45] Neuroimaging followed by lumbar puncture is indicated for any patient with acquired immunodeficiency syndrome (AIDS) who has significant headache or altered mental status, even when CNS symptoms do not dominate the picture. In addition to the standard diagnostic studies, CSF analysis in HIV/AIDS patients should include cytology, cryptococcal antigen, VDRL (for syphilis), and PCR for herpes viruses, JC virus, and *Mycobacterium tuberculosis*.[45]

This sequential approach to evaluation is recommended because mass lesions, including toxoplasmosis, lymphoma, and progressive multifocal leukoencephalopathy, are common. Ring-enhancing lesions on CT or MRI are suggestive of the first two entities, whereas focal white matter disease favors the last. Positive serologic testing for *Toxoplasma gondii* or the presence of multiple mass lesions increases the likelihood of CNS toxoplasmosis, and if either of these is present, empirical therapy for toxoplasmosis should be begun.[39] Single-photon emission tomography (SPECT) imaging may be useful in differentiating lymphoma from infection for mass lesions ≥2cm[46]; however, definitive diagnosis requires tissue analysis. Surgical intervention is typically reserved for cases with signs of impending herniation or lack of radiographic response after 2 weeks of empirical therapy for toxoplasmosis.

Cryptococcal meningitis is also common in AIDS and typically presents as a slowly progressive syndrome marked by fever and headaches. Diagnosis of this infection can be made by either serum or CSF cryptococcal antigen testing, both of which have sensitivity greater than 90%. CSF testing provides additional important prognostic and therapeutic information, and an opening pressure should be obtained at the time of lumbar puncture. Treatment recommendations include induction therapy with amphotericin B and flucytosine for at least 2 weeks, followed by consolidation therapy with fluconazole.[40]

Paradural Abscess

The epidural space is between the dura and the bony structures of the skull and vertebral column; the subdural space is between the subarachnoid membrane and the dura (see Figure 134-2). Unlike the subarachnoid space, the paradural tissues are only potential spaces, with the arachnoid membrane and the dura limiting the spread of infection across their surfaces. Although subdural abscesses are more common within the cranium, and epidural abscesses are more common within the vertebral column, the causes, pathophysiology, and therapies are similar. These abscesses usually develop from a contiguous infection, surgery, or trauma.

CRANIAL PARADURAL ABSCESS

In the skull, the epidural tissues are dense, and abscess formation is unusual. The subarachnoid membrane is less adherent to the dura, making the subdural space the more likely site of infection. Intracranial paradural abscesses tend to evolve rapidly, often producing irreversible damage to underlying neural structures. Antibiotics alone are inadequate, and neurosurgical drainage remains the mainstay of therapy. MRI has greatly aided in the rapid localization and management of intracranial paradural abscesses.

Cranial epidural abscesses most commonly occur adjacent to the frontal sinus, but untreated, infection can spread into the subdural or even parenchyma. Disease may be due to trauma, but most commonly

is a complication of sinusitis, which is reflected in the microbiology of cranial epidural abscesses.[47] Treatment requires emergent surgical drainage followed by antibiotics tailored against the bacteria cultured intraoperatively.

Cranial subdural empyema may be clinically indistinguishable from a brain abscess. Subdural abscess is usually associated with infection of the paranasal sinuses and, less commonly, the ears or mastoids.[41] Trauma, surgical intervention, or hematogenous spread are responsible for the remaining cases. Organisms common to sinusitis, including streptococci, pneumococci, *Haemophilus*, anaerobes, and staphylococci, cause most infections. Gram-negative enteric bacilli may be associated with middle ear and mastoid infections. As with cranial epidural abscess, surgical drainage is crucial for treatment, followed by prolonged antibiotics.[47]

SPINAL PARADURAL ABSCESS

Spinal epidural abscess typically present with localized spinal pain, with fever present in less than 50% of cases.[42-43] Cognition generally remains intact; systemic manifestations are rarely severe enough to cause cortical dysfunction. Symptoms usually progress through four clinical phases: spinal ache, nerve root pain, radicular weakness, and paralysis. The triad of back pain, fever, and progressive neurologic deficits strongly suggests this syndrome; however, the presence of any of these signs or symptoms should raise concern for the diagnosis.

Diagnosis hinges on visualization of a collection in the epidural space (Figure 134-6). The diagnostic study of choice is MRI, which defines cord compression and the presence and extent of abscess, identifies drainable paraspinal fluid collections, and detects concomitant vertebral osteomyelitis. Other procedures such as myelography and CT scanning may be used if MRI cannot be performed.

S. aureus accounts for more than two-thirds of cases of epidural abscess.[42,44] Although most cases are community acquired, an increasing number are due to spinal instrumentation (surgery or nerve block), and nosocomial flora such as MRSA or *Pseudomonas* may be causative in this population. Other risk factors for spinal epidural abscess include IV drug use, diabetes mellitus, trauma, and comorbid conditions such as malignancy or alcohol use.[42] Empirical therapy is directed against the most likely organisms and typically includes vancomycin and an antipseudomonal agent such as cefepime. Therapy should be refined once cultures confirm a causative pathogen.

Emergency neurosurgical intervention is considered mandatory for spinal paradural abscess if there is clinical evidence of cord compression. In a few selected cases, patients may be successfully treated with antibiotics alone. Nonsurgical management might be considered if a pathogen is identified by peripheral blood cultures or by needle biopsy; if the patient is neurologically intact and there is no progression of neurologic findings (e.g., weakness) on frequent examination; if pain improves with treatment; and if fever, peripheral white blood cell count, and sedimentation rate all decline on therapy. Unfortunately, some patients treated conservatively develop sudden neurologic impairment even weeks into conservative therapy, and retrospective data suggest a combined medical and surgical approach is associated with improved outcomes.[42] Progressive weakness mandates the need for immediate MRI and neurosurgical consultation, because decompression within 24 hours offers the best chance of neurologic recovery.[44]

Sepsis Syndrome with Central Nervous System Involvement

In the sepsis syndrome, an acutely ill patient develops CNS dysfunction late in the course of the illness, typically in the setting of multiorgan system failure. Altered mental status, attributable to hypotension and hypoperfusion, ranges from confusion to obtundation. Seizures may occur due to metabolic abnormalities, ischemia, or hemorrhage. In

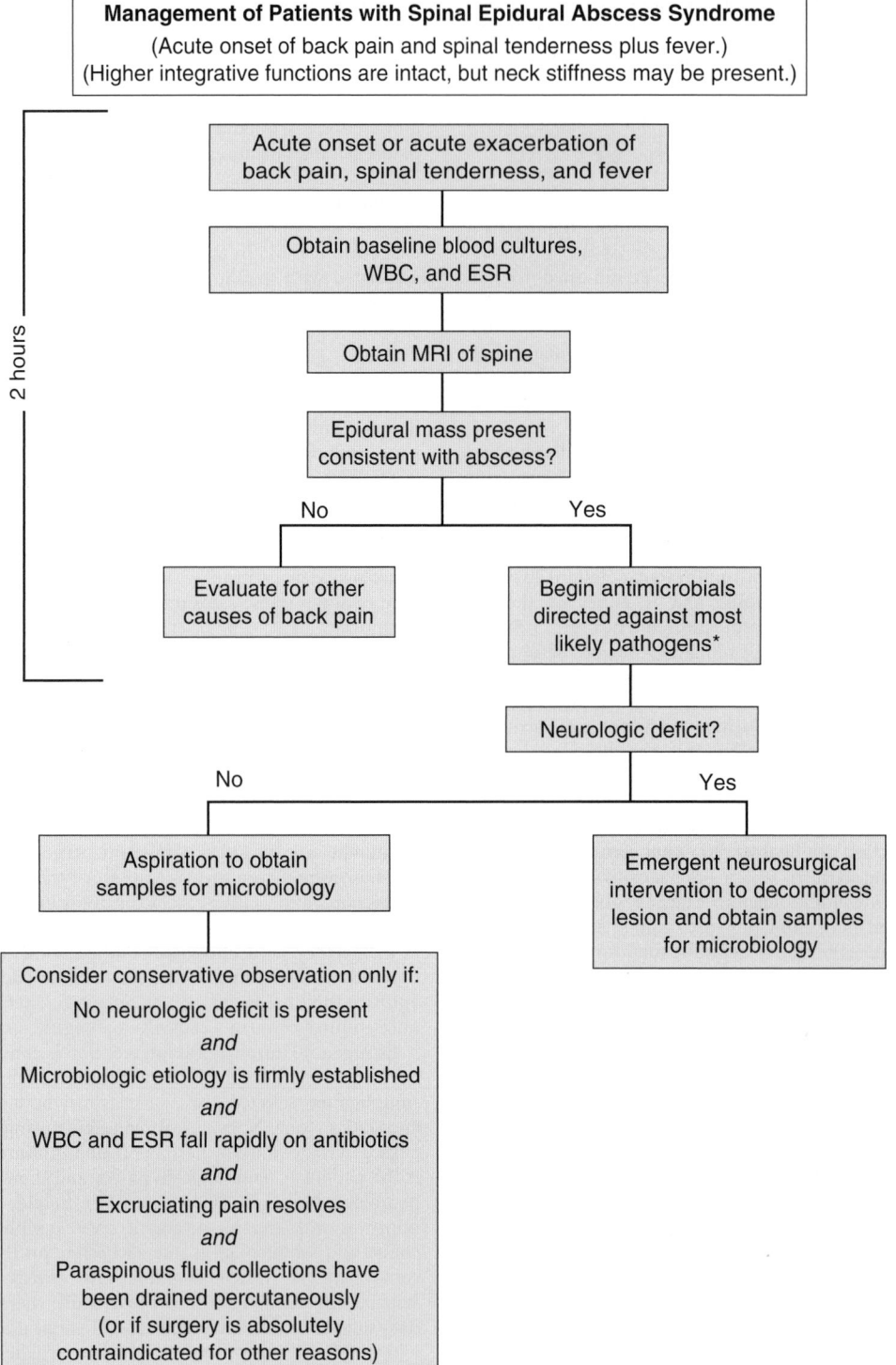

Figure 134-6 Algorithm for the management of patients with the spinal epidural abscess syndrome. If magnetic resonance imaging (MRI) cannot be performed, myelography, high-contrast computed tomography (CT), or CT-myelography may be an acceptable alternative to localize an epidural abscess. *If abscess drainage can be performed promptly, antimicrobial drugs may be withheld until specimens for microbial analysis are obtained. WBC, white blood cell; ESR, erythrocyte sedimentation rate.

treating such patients, general supportive measures take precedence over CNS concerns. After a brief assessment, general life-support measures should correct hypotension, hypoxia, and anuria. As soon as they are easily accessible, body fluid specimens are obtained for culture, and broad-spectrum antimicrobials should be administered. At this point, a careful history should be taken and physical examination performed.

The patient is treated as outlined for subacute CNS infection syndrome (see Figure 134-4). Delays in directly assessing the CNS are justifiable only when the history is adequate to document that a clear-cut systemic illness preceded the onset of CNS symptoms and signs. Otherwise, a more aggressive use of lumbar puncture and CT or MRI is warranted (see Figures 134-3 and 134-4).

Conclusions

Acute infection of the CNS requires rapid therapeutic intervention. Because the four major syndromes of CNS infection (acute meningitis syndrome, subacute CNS infection syndrome (which includes brain abscess, viral meningitis and encephalitis), spinal epidural abscess, and sepsis syndrome) differ in their signs and symptoms, as well as in the approach to definitive diagnosis and therapy, it is important to distinguish among them. Moreover, diverse infectious and noninfectious causes may produce similar CNS syndromes. For therapy to be maximally effective, it must be instituted within minutes to hours of the initial evaluation. Thus, in the practice of critical care medicine involving CNS disease, the goal remains rapid institution of empirical therapy for treatable infectious syndromes while efficiently working to identify the specific disease process.

KEY POINTS

Bacterial Meningitis

1. Fever, headache, and meningismus are the classic presenting signs and symptoms of bacterial meningitis; however, absence of any one (or all) of these features may be seen.

2. Neuroimaging studies should precede lumbar puncture in the presence of papilledema, focal findings on neurologic examination, immunocompromise (human immunodeficiency virus [HIV] infection, malignancy, or transplant), seizures in the week prior to presentation, or coma.

3. Empirical antibiotic therapy should begin as soon as possible after appropriate cultures have been obtained; these can be modified later based on results of cerebrospinal fluid (CSF) Gram stain and culture.

4. Patients with negative cultures and limited clinical response after 48 hours of therapy should undergo repeat lumbar puncture and head computed tomography (CT) or magnetic resonance imaging (MRI) scans.

5. Corticosteroid treatment in adults is controversial, but initial combination therapy with dexamethasone and antibiotics has been associated with improved outcomes in patients with pneumococcal meningitis.

Brain Abscess

1. MRI is superior to CT for imaging brain abscesses, especially in the early stages of infection.

2. Microbiology of brain abscesses is dependent on the route of infection; abscesses spreading from a contiguous focus are frequently polymicrobial.

3. Treatment of brain abscesses typically requires prolonged administration of antibiotics tailored to culture results.

Viral Encephalitis

1. An infectious cause of encephalitis is found in less than 50% of cases.

2. Herpes simplex virus (HSV) must be included in the differential diagnosis of all cases of encephalitis, as this infection has a high morbidity and mortality unless treated with acyclovir. Herpes simplex encephalitis typically presents with temporal lobe lesions on MRI, and HSV polymerase chain reaction of CSF is more than 95% sensitive for diagnosis.

Central Nervous System Infection in HIV-Infected Patients

1. HIV-infected patients are at risk for a number of opportunistic infections. Because many of these cause mass lesions, CT or MRI should be performed before lumbar puncture.

2. Ring-enhancing lesions seen on neuroimaging are most frequently due to either toxoplasmosis or lymphoma. In patients with positive *Toxoplasma* serology, empirical treatment for 2 weeks is indicated; brain biopsy should be performed in patients with lack of radiographic improvement.

3. Cryptococcal meningitis can be rapidly diagnosed by the detection of cryptococcal antigen in either the serum or the CSF.

Epidural Abscess

1. Epidural infections typically present initially with back pain and fever, with progressive neurologic impairment. Diagnosis is confirmed by MRI.

2. In the presence of impaired neurologic function, surgical drainage is imperative; there is little chance of recovery if symptoms have been present for more than 24 hours before decompression. Empirical antibiotics to cover staphylococci and enteric gram-negative rods should be continued until culture results are available.

ANNOTATED REFERENCES

Tunkel AR, Hartman BJ, Kaplan SL, et al. Practice guidelines for the management of bacterial meningitis. Clin Infect Dis 2004;39:1267-84.

This paper provides clinicians with evidence-based recommendations regarding the diagnosis and treatment of bacterial meningitis. It also provides guidance regarding controversies in this syndrome, such as which patients require neuroimaging prior to lumbar puncture and which patients benefit from adjunctive dexamethasone therapy. The specific antimicrobial recommendations outlined in the paper are considered the current gold standard for treatment of patients with this condition.

Van de Beek D, de Gans J, Spanjaard L, et al. Clinical features and prognostic factors in adults with bacterial meningitis. N Engl J Med 2004;251:1849-59.

This prospective cohort study performed between 1998 and 2002 identified 696 adult patients with community-acquired bacterial meningitis. The authors confirmed that S. pneumoniae and N. meningitides remain the most common pathogens, even in the era of conjugate vaccination for these organisms. The overall mortality from this infection remains significant at 21% and was highest for the subgroup with pneumococcal meningitis. Other risk factors for an unfavorable outcome included advanced age, a contiguous source of infection (sinusitis or otitis), depressed consciousness, bacteremia, thrombocytopenia, and a relatively low CSF WBC count.

Tunkel AR, Glaser CA, Bloch KC, et al. The management of encephalitis: clinical practice guidelines by the Infectious Diseases Society of America. Clin Infect Dis 2008;47:303-27.

Similar to the meningitis guidelines, this paper serves as a reference for clinicians evaluating patients with meningoencephalitis. The paper gives evidence-based recommendations on the optimal diagnostic evaluation and therapy for patients with this life-threatening disorder. Detailed discussion of the specific pathogens causing encephalitis is provided.

Glaser CA, Honarmand S, Anderson LJ, et al. Beyond viruses: clinical profiles and etiologies associated with encephalitis. Clin Infect Dis 2006;43:1565-77.

This prospective study included diagnostic testing on 1570 patients with a clinical diagnosis of encephalitis. An infectious etiology was documented in 16% of cases, with viruses accounting for almost 70% of these cases. A noninfectious etiology was ultimately identified in 8% of cases. In 13% of cases, evidence of extra-CNS infection with a pathogen not classically associated with CNS infection was identified, but causality was not established. Overall, almost two-thirds of cases remained undiagnosed despite extensive laboratory evaluation.

Curry WT, Hoh BL, Amin-Hanjani S, et al. Spinal epidural abscess: clinical presentation, management and outcome. Surg Neurol 2005;63:364-71.

These authors retrospectively reviewed the institutional experience with spinal epidural abscess over a 5-year period. They identified 48 patients with this diagnosis. Almost 50% of the patients initially treated with antibiotic therapy alone ultimately required delayed surgical intervention. Patients treated medically had significantly poorer outcomes than those treated with a combined medical and surgical approach.

REFERENCES

Access the complete reference list online at http://www.expertconsult.com.

135

Infections of Skin, Muscle, and Soft Tissue

DAVID CLAY EVANS | STEVEN M. STEINBERG

Infections of skin, soft tissue, and muscle include a broad range of diseases from those originating in the skin (impetigo, ecthyma, erysipelas, pyoderma), superficial fascia (embolic ulcers, cellulitis), fascia cleft, and deep fascia (necrotizing fasciitis) to muscle (myonecrosis). In this chapter, we focus on infections of skin, soft tissue, and muscle that are commonly encountered in intensive care units (ICUs) and are often severe and potentially life threatening. These infections include necrotizing soft-tissue infections (NSTIs), soft-tissue infections of the neck and head, and infectious complications of bites, burns, and pressure ulcers.

▣ Necrotizing Soft-Tissue Infections

NSTIs represent a spectrum of infectious processes that are extensive and rapidly progressive. Based on the depth of skin and soft-tissue involvement, NSTIs are divided into three categories: necrotizing cellulitis, necrotizing fasciitis, and myonecrosis. Table 135-1 shows the classification of NSTIs. The sine qua non of these infections is necrosis of subcutaneous tissue, fascia, and muscle, with widespread undermining of the skin. The lack of anatomic boundaries and the fact that the infection is deep to the skin helps account for the severity of the infection as well as the frequent delay in its recognition. The trunk, extremities, and perineum are the most common sites of NSTIs, but other anatomic sites may be involved. For example, intraabdominal abscess, bowel perforation, and pancreatitis can present as necrotizing infection of the abdominal wall or extend into the thigh along the psoas muscle.[1,2] Similarly, cervical fasciitis due to dental or neck abscess can extend to the mediastinum.

Many different descriptive terms and eponyms have been used to describe NSTIs. The most common infections encountered in ICU patients are postoperative progressive bacterial synergistic gangrene, clostridial cellulitis, synergistic gangrene, necrotizing fasciitis, Fournier's gangrene, gas gangrene, and Meleney's synergistic gangrene. Although the terminology and depth of infection may be different, the severity and emergent need for surgical intervention are common to all varieties of these infections.

PATHOGENESIS

Pathophysiologic factors involved in the development and progression of NSTIs are host resistance, bacterial pathogens involved, and local barrier factors.

Host Resistance

As shown in Table 135-2, individuals who are immunocompromised or have chronic diseases are more likely to develop necrotizing skin and soft-tissue infections than those without such medical problems.

Bacterial Pathogens

There are specific bacteria that are more likely than others to cause NSTIs, as shown in Table 135-1. Although necrotizing cellulitis and fasciitis may be caused by a single bacterial pathogen such as group A Streptococcus, Vibrio spp., or zygomycetes, about 80% of necrotizing cellulitis or fasciitis results from polymicrobial infections with synergistic facultative aerobes and anaerobic gas-forming organisms. An

average of 4.4 organisms are isolated from polymicrobial necrotizing infections.[3] The former includes gram-positive and gram-negative aerobes such as Streptococcus pyogenes, Staphylococcus aureus, Enterococcus faecalis, Escherichia coli, or Pseudomonas aeruginosa, and the latter includes Clostridium perfringens, Bacteroides fragilis, and Peptostreptococcus.[4] Certain predisposing conditions can be correlated with specific bacteria—for example, trauma with Clostridium spp., diabetes mellitus with Bacteroides spp., S. aureus, and Enterobacteriaceae, and immunosuppression with Pseudomonas spp. and Enterobacteriaceae.[5]

Traditionally, gas gangrene is synonymous with clostridial infection, and gas in the soft tissue is thought to be a grave finding. The majority of gas-producing infections do not involve Clostridium spp. but are instead necrotizing infections due to other bacterial pathogens. Many bacteria, especially facultative gram-negative bacilli (e.g., E. coli), produce insoluble gases such as hydrogen, nitrogen, and methane whenever they are forced to use anaerobic metabolism. Thus, the presence of crepitus in a soft-tissue infection on physical examination or radiographs implies anaerobic metabolism and existence of an NSTI.

Local Barrier Failure

Most serious soft-tissue infections require some degree of tissue injury and break in the skin to establish infection. The break in the skin may be due to a surgical incision or trauma; it may be related to large wounds or very small ones. The tissue injury may be due to either blunt or penetrating trauma of any kind. However, in a significant percentage of cases, it is difficult to find evidence of a break in the skin or soft-tissue trauma.

CLINICAL MANIFESTATIONS AND DIAGNOSIS

The critical aspect of diagnosing NSTIs is maintaining a high index of suspicion, which allows for early recognition of the nonlocalized necrotizing nature of the infection and the need for surgical intervention. Although necrotizing cellulitis and fasciitis may occur after significant tissue trauma or a relatively trivial injury, up to 40% of NSTIs have no identifiable cause. NSTIs with identifiable barrier failure are more likely to be polymicrobial and are easier to diagnose than the more virulent infections caused by a single organism. In necrotizing cellulitis, gas is invariably found in the skin, but the fascia and deep muscle are spared. Early clinical findings are similar to those of common wound infections, including local edema (89%), erythema (30%), fever (71%), and local cutaneous anesthesia (27%) due to cutaneous nerve necrosis.[6] These are followed by gangrenous skin changes with rapid extension beyond the borders of the original infection. Synergistic polymicrobial necrotizing fasciitis is characterized by "dishwater pus." Patients usually have high fever, but no obvious source of clinical infection can be detected. Pain in the area of infection is usually out of proportion to the physical findings. As the infection progresses, patients develop shock and multiple organ failure. Mortality rates are high, with necrotizing fasciitis being fatal in 23.5% of cases.[7]

Clostridial myonecrosis typically develops within 12 to 24 hours after a traumatic event or closure of a deep contaminated wound. Recurrent gas gangrene caused by C. perfringens has been described in individuals with nonpenetrating injuries at sites of previous clostridial

TABLE 135-1	Classification of Necrotizing Skin, Soft-Tissue, and Muscle Infections	
Disease	*Bacteriology*	*Comments*
Necrotizing Cellulitis		
Clostridial cellulitis	*Clostridium perfringens*	Local trauma, recent surgery; fascial/deep muscle spared
Nonclostridial cellulitis	Mixed: *Escherichia coli, Enterobacter, Peptostreptococcus* spp., *Bacteroides fragilis*	Diabetes mellitus predisposes; produces foul odor
Meleney's synergistic gangrene	*Staphylococcus aureus*, microaerophilic streptococci	Rare infection; postoperative; slowly expanding, indolent, ulceration in superficial fascia
Synergistic necrotizing cellulitis	Mixed aerobic and anaerobic, including *B. fragilis, Peptostreptococcus* spp.	Diabetes mellitus predisposes; variant of necrotizing fasciitis type I; involves skin, muscle, fat, and fascia
Necrotizing Fasciitis		
Type I	Mixed aerobic and anaerobic; staphylococci, *B. fragilis, E. coli*, group A streptococci, *Peptostreptococcus* spp., *Prevotella, Porphyromonas* spp., *Clostridium* spp.	Usually requires a breach in the mucous membrane layer either through surgery or penetrating injuries or from chronic medical conditions such as diabetes, peripheral vascular disease, malignancy, and anal fissures
Type II	Group A streptococci	Increasing in frequency and severity since 1985; very high mortality; often begins at site of nonpenetrating minor trauma such as a bruise or muscle strain but often no identified precursor. Predisposing factors: blunt/penetrating trauma, varicella (chickenpox), intravenous drug abuse, surgical procedures, childbirth, NSAID use
Myonecrosis		
Clostridial myonecrosis	*Clostridium* spp.	Predisposing factors: deep/penetrating injury, bowel and biliary tract surgery, improperly performed abortion and retained placenta, prolonged rupture of the membranes, and intrauterine fetal demise or missed abortion in postpartum patients. Recurrent gas gangrene occurs at sites of previous gas gangrene.
Streptococcal myonecrosis	Streptococci	
Special Type of Necrotizing Soft-Tissue Infection		
Fournier's gangrene	Polymicrobial, with *E. coli* the predominant aerobe and *Bacteroides* the predominant anaerobe. Other microflora: *Proteus, Staphylococcus, Enterococcus*, aerobic and anaerobic *Streptococcus, Pseudomonas, Klebsiella*, and *Clostridium*	Necrosis of the scrotum or perineum that starts with scrotal pain and erythema and rapidly spreads onto anterior abdominal wall and gluteal muscle. It is more often seen in diabetics and can be associated with trauma.

myonecrosis, where spores of *C. perfringens* remain quiescent in tissue and then germinate when minor trauma provides conditions suitable for growth. Patients present with the triad of severe pain, tachycardia out of proportion to fever, and crepitus in the soft tissue. Once overt gangrene with edema and bronze, purplish, or brown discoloration with bullae and watery discharge occur, the disease is at an advanced stage. Gram stain of the exudate shows gram-positive rods occasionally accompanied by other flora. In contrast, streptococcal myonecrosis usually develops over 2 to 4 days after trauma or closure of a wound. The onset is not as rapid, patients do not appear as sick, pain is not as severe, and gas formation is not as obvious as in those with clostridial myonecrosis.

MANAGEMENT

Initial management of NSTIs involves aggressive fluid resuscitation, appropriate broad-spectrum parenteral antibiotics, and most importantly, expedient and radical surgical débridement. Other adjunctive therapies such as hyperbaric oxygen and immunoglobulin have been used, but their efficacy has not been as well established.

TABLE 135-2	Factors Predisposing to Necrotizing Soft-Tissue Infections

Human, animal, or insect bites
Contaminated or dirty surgical procedures
Diabetes mellitus
Long-term corticosteroid use
Malignancy
Trauma/burns
Intravenous drug abuse
Chronic alcoholism
Malnutrition
HIV infection/AIDS
Cirrhosis
Peripheral vascular diseases
Chronic renal failure

Antibiotics

For type I necrotizing fasciitis (mixed aerobic and anaerobic), antibiotic treatment should be guided initially on results of the Gram stain. Early empirical treatment should be initiated with extended-spectrum penicillins (e.g., ampicillin-sulbactam, piperacillin-tazobactam, ticarcillin-clavulanic acid) or carbapenem antibiotics (e.g., imipenem-cilastatin). If there is a suspicion that resistant coliforms might be participating, such as in patients who have been hospitalized or who have been treated with antibiotics recently or where there is suspicion of rectal or intestinal involvement, a third-generation cephalosporin, aminoglycoside, or aztreonam combined with either clindamycin or metronidazole may be used. For those patients with severe cases or in whom clostridia are suspected, clindamycin in addition to penicillin is useful for inhibiting toxin production. The incidence of both community- and hospital-acquired methicillin-resistant *S. aureus* (MRSA) is increasing, and consideration of anti-MRSA treatment should be based on patient history and local resistance patterns. Nosocomial infections should be empirically treated.

Although there are no data from clinical trials establishing the benefit of combined therapy in type II necrotizing fasciitis (group A streptococci), penicillin G combined with clindamycin is the antibiotic therapy of choice. Clindamycin, but not metronidazole, is recommended not for its antianaerobic properties but because of its additional activity against gram-positive organisms, including specific inhibition of toxin production.[8] Cefotaxime and ceftriaxone are acceptable alternatives. For patients allergic to penicillin, vancomycin is the recommended treatment.

Surgical Intervention

Early surgical débridement is critical in the management of NSTIs. Aggressive surgical excision of all involved tissue with a margin of normal-appearing tissue is mandatory. All necrotic tissue should be excised back to healthy bleeding margins. Additional incisions parallel to cutaneous nerves and blood vessels may be used to assess fascial

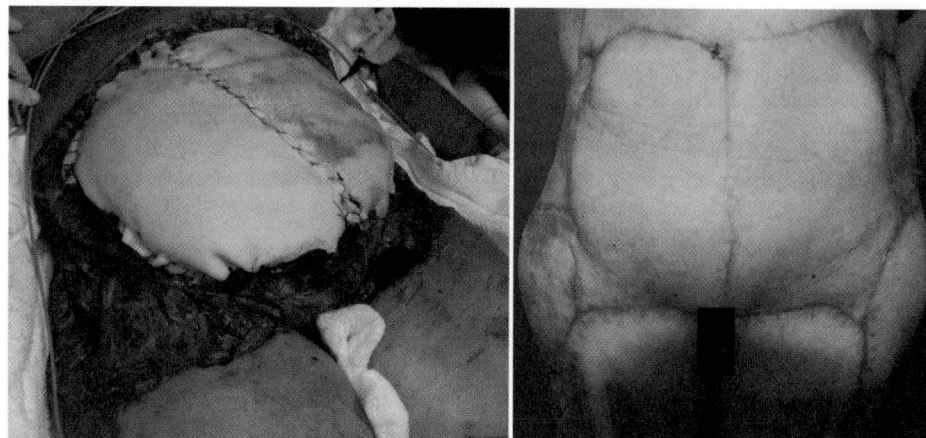

Figure 135-1   Necrotizing fasciitis of the abdominal wall after extensive débridement and application of porcine dermal collagen implant for temporary abdominal closure *(left)* and after healing of anterolateral thigh flaps to reconstruct the abdominal wall *(right)*.

viability without elevating the skin. The wound should be frequently reexamined for viability of tissue and repeat operative débridement is frequently required. Aggressive fascial débridement of abdominal surgical wounds may necessitate the use of prosthetic material to replace an abdominal wall defect, as depicted in Figure 135-1. In Fournier's gangrene and perineal/perirectal NSTI, a colostomy for fecal diversion may be necessary to keep the wound clean. The testes generally survive because their blood supply is usually spared, but they may need to be temporarily implanted in the soft tissue of the medial thighs if the scrotum must be débrided. On rare occasion, NSTI of the extremities may require amputation.

Myonecrosis or gas gangrene requires radical débridement to viable muscle. When this process involves the extremities, control of the infection is more easily achieved, although as mentioned previously, amputation may be necessary. In contrast, clostridial myonecrosis involving the trunk may present some very difficult therapeutic decisions because the removal of nonviable tissue may leave the peritoneal or thoracic cavities open and their contents exposed. Temporary coverage with prosthetic materials may be necessary. Trunk infections are therefore associated with a grim prognosis.

Adjunctive Therapy

Hyperbaric Oxygen.   The use of hyperbaric oxygen (HBO) in NSTIs is controversial. Although there are no randomized prospective studies of HBO in these infections, in vitro data and reviews of clinical series seem to show beneficial effects of HBO when combined with antibiotics and surgical débridement in the management of clostridial infection.[9,10] Hyperbaric oxygen is toxic to clostridia and inhibits bacterial growth, blocks production of alpha toxin, and preserves marginally perfused tissue. Debate also exists about the use of HBO for nonclostridial necrotizing skin and soft-tissue infection. In one report, the addition of HBO to the surgical and antimicrobial treatment of nonclostridial necrotizing fasciitis significantly reduced mortality and the need for débridement.[9]

Intravenous Immunoglobulin.   Intravenous immunoglobulin (IVIG) has been administered to patients with streptococcal and staphylococcal toxic shock syndrome and may be efficacious in the treatment of this toxin-mediated disorder. Some studies have demonstrated IVIG has some beneficial effect in the treatment of NSTIs, theoretically owing to its neutralization of circulating clostridial toxins and streptococcal superantigens.[11] However, a large multicenter retrospective cohort study of children with streptococcal toxic shock syndrome showed no improvement in outcomes with administration of IVIG.[12] There is no clear consensus at this time regarding the efficacy of IVIG.

Important Soft-Tissue Infections of the Head and Neck

LUDWIG'S ANGINA

In 1836, German physician Wilhelm Frederick von Ludwig described five patients with gangrenous induration of the connective tissues of the neck that progressed rapidly to involve the tissues covering the muscles between the larynx and the floor of the mouth.[13] Ludwig's angina is a potentially life-threatening, rapidly progressive, diffuse "woody" or brawny cellulitis of the submandibular and sublingual spaces that occurs most often in young adults with dental infections.

Pathogenesis

In adults, 50% to 80% of cases of Ludwig's angina are caused by dental caries, and the disease has a mortality rate of 5% to 10%.[14] Submandibular and sublingual spaces freely communicate, and with involvement of the deep cervical fascia, infection may spread rapidly, with grave consequences. Extension along the carotid sheath or the retropharyngeal space can cause mediastinitis.[15] Infection is commonly caused by oral cavity anaerobes such as *Fusobacterium*, anaerobic streptococci, *Bacteroides*, spirochetes, and hemolytic *Streptococcus* organisms, although the infection may be mixed with *Staphylococcus* and *Streptococcus*, *Klebsiella*, or a combination of aerobic or anaerobic organisms.[16] The presence of anaerobes commonly accounts for the occurrence of gas in the tissues.

Clinical Manifestations

The patient is febrile and complains of severe neck pain and swelling, odynophagia, dysphagia, drooling, and leaning forward to maximize the airway diameter. Patients usually have a recent history of dental work, obviously poor dental hygiene, or deep neck abscess.

Examination may reveal a tender, symmetrical, and indurated swelling, sometimes with palpable crepitus in the submandibular area. The tongue may be swollen or displaced upward and backward, and the mouth is held open because of the lingual swelling. The presence of stridor, dyspnea, decreased air movement, or cyanosis suggests airway compromise. The appearance of significant asymmetry of the submandibular area is an ominous sign because it may represent an extension of the inflammation to the parapharyngeal space.

Radiographic views of the teeth may indicate the source of infection, and lateral views of the neck will demonstrate soft-tissue swelling around the airway and possibly submandibular gas. Computed tomography (CT) of the neck may be recommended to determine the extent of inflammation.

The diagnosis of Ludwig's angina is usually made clinically according to three criteria: (1) presence of cellulitis with little or no pus in both submandibular and sublingual spaces; (2) presence of gangrene with serosanguineous putrid fluid; and (3) rapidly spreading cellulitis in connective tissue, fascia, and muscles, without glandular tissue and lymphatic involvement.[17]

Management

Control of Airway. Progression from the first findings of symptoms to asphyxia may occur rapidly over several minutes to a few hours. Therefore, airway protection is a critical component of initial management. Stridor, tachypnea, dyspnea, inability to handle secretions, and agitation are all indicative of impending airway loss. In the past, the standard of care for Ludwig's angina was early emergency intubation or tracheostomy to protect the airway. However, this practice has been gradually abandoned. Recent data show that most cases can be managed initially by close observation in a critical care unit and intravenous antibiotics.[18] If an artificial airway is required, flexible fiberoptic-guided nasotracheal intubation is the preferred method of airway control. Tracheostomy, under local anesthesia and performed through the cellulitis, is still the most widely recommended means of obtaining a surgical airway.

Antibiotics and Other Pharmacotherapy. Penicillin and clindamycin are the antibiotics of choice for treating Ludwig's angina. Ampicillin-sulbactam, metronidazole and penicillin, imipenem-cilastatin, piperacillin-tazobactam, and second- and third-generation cephalosporins (i.e., cefoxitin, cefotaxime) are other reasonable choices for treating the obligate anaerobes that are most commonly encountered in this infection. Coverage for MRSA may be required based on patient and local factors.

Corticosteroids have been used empirically to treat airway edema. The value of corticosteroids in the setting of Ludwig's angina is unclear, and they probably are not indicated.[19]

Surgical Intervention. Surgical débridement may only moderately improve the airway. Surgical incision and drainage was the therapy of choice in the preantibiotic era. Unless antibiotic therapy is significantly delayed, it is unlikely pus will be identified, because pus collections develop relatively late. With the exception of dental extraction, surgery is reserved for those patients who do not respond to medical therapy and those with crepitus and purulent collections.[20] Any patient requiring surgical intervention should have an artificial airway in place before neck exploration. The location of abscesses should be identified using CT or magnetic resonance imaging (MRI). Infection localized above the carina is usually addressed by cervical incision, but infection below the carina requires additional surgical drainage of the mediastinum.[21]

ACUTE EPIGLOTTITIS

Acute epiglottitis is a rare, potentially life-threatening bacterial infection causing inflammation and edema of the epiglottis, aryepiglottic folds, and surrounding tissues. Before the era of *Haemophilus influenzae* vaccine, epiglottitis used to be a primarily pediatric infection. However, in recent years, the infection has become primarily an adult disease.

Pathogenesis

Invading bacteria cause inflammation and edema of the epiglottis, aryepiglottic fold, and surrounding tissues. These structures then may protrude downward and over the glottic opening, causing airway obstruction. In the past, most of the cases (50%-70%) were caused by *H. influenzae* B (HIB).[22] However, at the present time, other bacteria including group A β-hemolytic *Streptococcus*, *S. aureus*, and *Streptococcus pneumoniae* have become more common, and more patients present with epiglottic abscess.

Clinical Manifestations and Management

Early signs of epiglottitis include hoarseness, dysphagia, odynophagia, and a sore throat (present in 94% of patients).[23] Some authors advocate direct or indirect laryngoscopy on adult patients without respiratory distress; it is safe to perform such procedures in the operating room or ICU, where both the equipment and personnel required for emergency intubation are at hand. The most common misdiagnosis is streptococcal pharyngitis. Patients who can maintain their airway and adequate oxygenation should be closely observed in an ICU where definitive airway management can be achieved in a controlled fashion. Corticosteroids, racemic epinephrine, and heliox can be considered for initial management, but their role is unresolved. Dyspnea and stridor indicate impending airway obstruction, and emergency airway control should be established. Flexible fiberoptic laryngoscopy is usually used during intubation because it provides direct visualization of the airway while serving as a guide for intubation.

The third-generation cephalosporins, cefotaxime and ceftriaxone, are the antibiotics of choice for acute epiglottitis. These antibiotics are usually effective against *H. influenzae*, streptococci, and staphylococci. A number of other antibiotics including cefuroxime, ampicillin-sulbactam, piperacillin-tazobactam, ticarcillin-clavulanic acid, and levofloxacin are also effective in epiglottitis.

Infections of Bite Wounds

It is estimated that 4.7 million dog bites, 400,000 cat bites, and 250,000 human bites occur in the United States annually. In addition to bites, exposure to mouth flora can also occur in clenched-fist injuries and finger or thumb sucking, The incidence of infection after cat bites can be more than 50%, and infection after dog or human bite wounds can be 15% to 20%. Wild animal bites also are a potential source of serious infection. Although the majority of patients with bite wounds do not seek medical attention, some bite wounds can become disasters, leading to severe infections and sepsis that result in loss of limb function or even require amputation. Although many of these wounds may look innocuous initially, they may lead to serious infections (i.e., NSTIs) and sepsis. Complications also include lymphangitis, septic arthritis, tenosynovitis, and osteomyelitis.

PATHOGENESIS

The microbiology of bite wounds generally is polymicrobial, reflecting the aerobic and anaerobic microbiology of the oral flora of the biter and the skin of the victim, as well as the environment.

Soft-tissue infections caused by human mouth flora are usually due to a mixture of pathogens.[24] It has been reported that the human mouth hosts 42 different species of bacterial flora, of which aerobes (*Eikenella corrodens*, *Staphylococcus*, *Streptococcus*, and *Corynebacterium* spp.) are the most common isolates from infected bite wounds.[25] *E. corrodens* is a slow-growing, gram-negative bacillus frequently associated with chronic infection and abscess formation in human bites. Commonly isolated anaerobes include *Bacteroides* and *Peptostreptococcus* spp.

As in human bites, polymicrobial infections are frequently encountered in animal bites. Whereas almost any oral flora isolate is a potential pathogen, *Pasteurella multocida* is the most prevalent organism found in 50% of dog bite wounds and 70% of cat bite wound infections.[26,27] *S. aureus*, α-, β-, and δ-hemolytic streptococci, gram-negative organisms, and anaerobic microorganisms that are usually part of the normal mouth flora of animals also have all been isolated.

MANAGEMENT

Management goals for bite wounds are to prevent or appropriately treat infection and minimize soft-tissue deformity. For domestic animal bites, unless the animal is suspected of having rabies, rabies prophylaxis is not necessary. Many wild animals including skunks, raccoons, foxes, and bats should be considered rabid unless proved otherwise, and a bite by such an animal should result in rabies prophylaxis. Tetanus immunization status must also be determined, and if not up to date, tetanus toxoid should be administered. Tetanus immune globulin should also be considered for those victims whose last tetanus booster was more than 10 years before the bite injury. Radiography is indicated if there are any concerns that deep structures are at risk. These include hand wounds, deep punctures, and crushing bites, especially those over joints.

Meticulous wound care is the cornerstone of human or animal bite wound management. Copious irrigation of the wound decreases the incidence of wound infection. Careful débridement of devitalized tissue, particulate matter, and clot is also necessary to reduce the infection risk and improve the cosmetic result. Puncture wounds and dog bite injuries of the hand should not be closely primarily. Other wounds with extensive crush injuries or those requiring extensive débridement can be approximated and be closed by delayed primary or secondary intention.

Cultures of clinically uninfected wounds are not indicated. However, it is recommended that cultures be performed in infected wounds that are not improving despite apparently adequate antibiotic treatment. In bite victims, prophylactic broad-spectrum antibiotics are recommended for patients with high-risk bites but are only of proven benefit in human bites.[28] The high-risk factors for infection include human bites, wounds of the hand, foot, face, scalp, and perineum, puncture wounds, crush wounds that cannot be débrided, bites over vital structures (artery, nerve, or joint), patient age older than 50 years, or patients who are immunosuppressed.[29] In most patients, amoxicillin-clavulanic acid is the preferred antibiotic. Alternatives include moxifloxacin, amoxicillin, doxycycline, and cefuroxime. In human bites, amoxicillin-clavulanic acid will cover E. corrodens as well as most other oral flora and is the recommended antibiotic. Other options include second- or third-generation cephalosporins, quinolones, or doxycycline. In patients who are allergic to penicillin, trimethoprim-sulfamethoxazole is an alternative for both dog and cat bites, whereas quinolones or erythromycin may be used for human bites.

Patients who require inpatient care for complex wounds, systemic toxicity, established infection, or suspicion of musculoskeletal, neurologic, or vascular involvement, or patients who are at very high risk of invasive infection (e.g., immunosuppression), should be treated with parenteral antibiotics, irrigation, and débridement with cultures.[30] Consultation with a hand surgeon should be considered in those with hand wounds, because the risk of severe infection of bite wounds on a hand is higher than other sites.

Infections of Burn Wounds

Burn wound infection/sepsis is one of the most common causes of death in burn patients. It is estimated that more than 100,000 of the 2.5 million burned patients in the United States require hospital admission, and 12,000 patients die per year.[31] The highest risk of bacterial invasion from skin flora into the eschar occurs 5 to 7 days after burn. Mechanisms of burn wound infection include breakdown of the natural cutaneous barrier, compromised host defenses, and exposure to pathogenic and opportunistic bacteria. The surface of a burn contains a large amount of necrotic tissue and protein-rich wound exudate, so it provides an excellent growth medium for surface bacteria, leading to bacterial colonization and invasion. Burns are also associated with an immunocompromised status. The percentage of total body surface area (TBSA) burned and the duration of hospitalization correlate well with the incidence of wound infections.[32] The predisposing factors for development of burn wound infection are listed in Table 135-3.

PATHOGENESIS

After thermal injury, all burn wounds become contaminated with microorganisms, either from the patient's endogenous flora or from resident microorganisms in the burn unit. This colonization is initially

TABLE 135-3	Predisposing Factors for Burn Wound Infections
Burn wound greater than 30% total body surface area
Full-thickness burn
Extremes in patient age
Preexisting diseases: immunosuppression, diabetes mellitus, vascular insufficiency
Virulence and antibiotic resistance of colonizing pathogens
Failure of skin graft
Prolonged open burn wound
Improper initial burn wound care

without clinical significance. However, surface-colonizing bacteria can penetrate the avascular eschar and proliferate beneath the eschar at the viable/nonviable tissue interface. When host defense mechanisms are compromised, bacteria can break this barrier and spread systemically, resulting in bacteremia and sepsis.

The most common organisms found in burn wound infections are bacteria, and 70% to 90% are endogenous to the patient. Bacterial organisms can also be acquired by cross-infection, principally from the hands of healthcare professionals. Before the era of penicillin, streptococci and staphylococci were the predominant pathogens. Since the 1950s, P. aeruginosa has become the most important species.[33] Other important bacterial species include S. aureus, group A Streptococcus, Enterobacter cloacae, E. faecalis, Klebsiella spp., and Acinetobacter spp.[34] Fungi, especially Candida albicans and Aspergillus spp., and viruses (herpesvirus) are also pathogens that can be isolated from infected burn wounds.[35]

CLINICAL MANIFESTATIONS AND DIAGNOSIS

Successful treatment of burn wound infections largely depends on early detection of infection. Burn wound infection is difficult to diagnose on the basis of clinical signs and symptoms, because burn-induced inflammatory responses (e.g., fever, leukocytosis) are indistinguishable from those of infection. The local signs of infection may be absent, minimal, or late. Diagnosis is generally based on a combination of clinical signs that indicate sepsis (e.g., fever, leukocytosis, organ dysfunction, hyperdynamic state) and the results of surveillance cultures. Any of the findings listed in Table 135-4 should raise suspicion of burn wound infection.[36] The practice of culturing the burn wound surface does not accurately predict progressive bacterial colonization or incipient burn wound sepsis. Qualitative and quantitative correlations are poor between flora on the surface of the burn wound and bacterial colonization and invasion of the deep layers of the eschar. It has been reported that biopsy of the wound with quantitative cultures of greater than 10^5 CFU per gram of tissue is an accurate indicator of invasive burn would infection.[37] When bacterial invasion to viable tissue is detected, excision of the infected wound is important, and systemic antibiotics are indicated.

MANAGEMENT

Prevention of Burn Wound Infections

Systemic antibiotic prophylaxis is not routinely administered to burn patients admitted to the hospital, because the unexcised burn wound does not lead to significant bacteremia.[38] Frequent wound dressing

TABLE 135-4	Clinical Signs Suggestive of Burn Wound Infection
Progression of second-degree to third-degree burn injury
Increased pain, erythema, color changes
Unexpected change in appearance or depth of wound
Unexpected rapid eschar separation
Metastatic septic lesion in unburned tissue
Systemic signs of sepsis

changes with evaluation of the burn wound and surrounding tissue allow for early detection and therapy of cellulitis. In many burn units in the United States, early excision and grafting of burn wounds has become the standard of care. *Early excision* is defined as the staged excision of all deep partial- and full-thickness burns by the third to seventh postburn day. The philosophy of early burn wound excision has resulted in improved survival in patients with TBSA burns greater than 30% to 40%, shorter hospital length of stay, lower costs of hospital care, and fewer painful dressing changes. If for some reason such as hemodynamic instability or severe respiratory failure, the patient cannot undergo early excision and coverage, surveillance wound cultures should be performed several times per week to diagnose burn wound infection early. In addition, strict antiseptic measures such as handwashing, barrier isolation, and equipment and room cleaning decrease the incidence of wound infection.

Topical antimicrobials are commonly used in burn patients. Their use has substantially decreased the incidence of conversion of partial-thickness to full-thickness wounds by local infection, and thereby has reduced mortality associated with burn wound infection. In addition, these agents may prolong the sterility of the full-thickness burn wound. However, they have not eliminated the need for aggressive removal of necrotic tissue and closure of the wound with autografts. The commonly used topical agents are listed in Table 135-5. According to an international survey, silver sulfadiazine is the topical agent of choice for partial- to full-thickness burn wounds.[39] Nanocrystalline silver mesh dressings that adhere for a week have reduced the discomfort of dressing changes and allow more outpatient care of partial-thickness burn wounds.[40]

TREATMENT OF BURN WOUND INFECTIONS

Antibiotics

Systemic antibiotics are not used prophylactically in patients with burn wounds.[41] Instead, they should be reserved for use in cases of known or suspected invasive infection. As long as bacterial culture results are available, antibiotics with the narrowest spectrum of activity should be used to minimize the development of resistant organisms. Recommendations for empirical therapy are based on the length of time since the burn was sustained, previous administration of antibiotics to the patient, and knowledge of likely pathogens and the local antibiogram. Combination of multiple antibiotics for a single infection is only used when bacteremia persists in the face of therapeutic doses of a single antibiotic. Inappropriate use of multiple antibiotics does not decrease mortality. Instead, it promotes overgrowth of resistant pathogens such as *Candida* spp., enterococci, and multiple antibiotic-resistant species.

Surgical Intervention

Invasive bacterial or fungal burn wound infections are treated with surgical excision to the level of viable tissue. Early burn wound excision significantly reduces bacterial colonization and reduces the risk of invasive burn wound infection. Patients who undergo topical treatment and delayed burn wound excision exhibit greater bacterial colonization and increased rates of infection.[42] Wounds that can be excised completely should be covered with an allograft or autograft. If complete débridement is not possible, topical antimicrobials should be applied and the wound reexamined within 24 hours for possible repeat débridement.

Infections of Pressure Ulcers

Pressure ulcers are caused by localized tissue necrosis and infection due to prolonged compression between a bony prominence and an external surface. Pressure ulcers in ICU patients occur primarily in patients with impaired mobility due to injury, weakness, sedation, or use of paralytic agents. Pressure ulcers result in significant morbidity in critically ill patients. Although infection of decubitus ulcers is high in the nursing home setting and in spinal cord injury patients, it is an uncommon cause of infection or sepsis in ICU patients.[43] Pressure ulcers may pose a risk to other hospitalized patients by serving as a reservoir for resistant organisms such as MRSA, vancomycin-resistant enterococci, and multiply-resistant gram-negative bacilli.

PATHOGENESIS AND CLASSIFICATION

Risk factors for pressure ulcers in patients in ICUs are essentially the same as for those on a general hospital floor. They include limited physical activity, impaired sensory perception, poor nutritional status, chronic disorders (e.g., diabetes mellitus, cardiovascular disease, and cerebrovascular accident), impaired circulation, low serum hemoglobin concentration, and increased blood urea nitrogen and serum creatinine concentrations.[44] Also, a number of infectious complications have been implicated in the development of pressure ulcers. In order of frequency, these are local infection, cellulitis of surrounding tissue, contiguous osteomyelitis, and bacteremia.[45]

TABLE 135-5	Commonly Used Topical Agents in Burn Wounds		
Agent	*Advantage*	*Dose*	*Precaution*
Silver sulfadiazine	Useful in prevention of infections from second- or third-degree burns. Bactericidal activity against many gram-positive and gram-negative bacteria; also effective against yeast.	Apply to open wounds twice or three times daily.	Does not penetrate eschar. Neutropenia. Caution in glucose-6-phosphate dehydrogenase deficiency.
Mafenide acetate cream and solution	Topical. Diffuses into the eschar and is highly effective against gram-negative organisms, including *Pseudomonas* spp.	Apply cream to open wounds twice or three times daily. Soaks with solution must be kept moist.	Pain/burning may occur. Metabolic acidosis due to inhibition of carbonic anhydrase (especially with cream).
Silver nitrate (0.5%)	Silver ion has broad-spectrum antibacterial activity but does not penetrate burn wound eschar; therefore, it is most effective when applied early.	Apply topically to wound to a thickness of approximately 1.5 mm daily or twice daily as moistened dressings.	Not for internal use. Stains wound and everything else. Does not penetrate eschar. Hyponatremia.
Nanocrystalline silver mesh dressings	Dressings coated with nanocrystalline silver with broadest-spectrum activity covering gram-negative organisms including *Pseudomonas*, gram-positive bacilli, methicillin-resistant *Staphylococcus aureus*, and vancomycin-resistant enterococcus. Good eschar penetration.	Apply to affected area, and monitor for adherence. If silver dressing is adherent, leave in place for 7-10 days. Some dressings should be kept moist.	Limited toxicity issues. Adherence is poor in wounds with significant exudates.
Mupirocin	Active against a wide variety of gram-positive bacteria, including MRSA. Also active against certain gram-negative bacteria. Exerts activity by binding to bacterial isoleucyl transfer RNA-synthetase. Good for face.	Apply to affected areas three times a day and cover with gauze dressing.	Prolonged use may result in growth of resistant organisms; do not use on very large wounds where polyethylene glycol absorption is possible (especially in patients with moderate renal failure).

TABLE 135-6	National Pressure Ulcer Advisory Panel Classification of Pressure Ulcers
Staging	*Description*
I	Intact skin with non-blanchable redness of a localized area usually over a bony prominence. Darkly pigmented skin may not have visible blanching; its color may differ from the surrounding area. The area may be painful, firm, soft, warmer or cooler as compared to adjacent tissue.
II	Partial-thickness loss of dermis presenting as a shallow open ulcer with a red pink wound bed, without slough. May also present as an intact or open/ruptured serum-filled blister.
III	Full-thickness skin loss. Subcutaneous fat may be visible, but bone, tendon, or muscle are not exposed. Slough may be present but does not obscure the depth of tissue loss. May include undermining and tunneling.
IV	Full-thickness tissue loss with exposed bone, tendon, or muscle. Slough or eschar may be present on some parts of the wound bed. Often include undermining and tunneling.

Several different classification systems have been developed to describe the extent of pressure ulcers. Table 135-6 shows the most commonly used system promulgated by the National Pressure Ulcer Advisory Panel.[46]

Infections of pressure ulcers are usually polymicrobial. Aerobes commonly recovered include staphylococci (including MRSA), enterococci, *Proteus mirabilis*, *E. coli*, and *Pseudomonas* spp. Anaerobic *Peptostreptococcus*, *Bacteroides fragilis*, and *Clostridium* spp. are also found in these infections. Pressure ulcers are a major reservoir of MRSA. Making an accurate microbiological diagnosis is usually impractical and difficult because all pressure ulcers are colonized with microorganisms, and a superficial culture will not distinguish between colonizing and infecting organisms. If it is necessary to determine the microbiology accurately, it is more appropriate to perform deep-tissue biopsy or direct a needle through intact skin and aspirate a specimen for bacterial culture from the margin of the ulcer.

MANAGEMENT

There are many different approaches to the treatment of pressure ulcers; however, none has been shown to be more effective than any other. Prevention of decubitus ulcers, including pressure relief with support surfaces and repositioning, appropriate nutrition, and skin moisturizers, is the best prophylactic treatment.[47] Once the ulcer has been established and infection is present, débridement of necrotic and marginally viable tissue is absolutely necessary to obtain healing. Topical agents such as povidone-iodine, hydrogen peroxide, and others have been widely used, but there is no difference in terms of outcome among these agents. Proper use of occlusive dressings such as balsam Peru/trypsin/castor oil preparations increases patient comfort, enhances healing, decreases the possibility of infection, saves time, and reduces costs.[48] Topical antimicrobial agents have not been shown to be effective. Systemic antibiotic therapy should be reserved for infected ulcers. Skin grafting of clean wounds, if the underlying cause of the pressure ulcer has been removed, is an accepted method of treatment and has been shown to be effective. However, adequate treatment frequently requires much more complex therapies, including tissue flaps and sometimes even amputation to effect wound closure. Treatment of recalcitrant wounds can be difficult and costly. Several newer therapeutic strategies include alginates, a variety of wound dressings, and growth factor therapies (e.g. platelet-derived growth factor). Cultured and tissue-engineered skin substitutes have emerged and are in varying degrees of clinical evaluation.[49]

A variety of empirical antibiotic regimens have been suggested for patients with pressure ulcer–associated cellulitis, osteomyelitis, or bacteremia. In general, any regimen active against the majority of organisms likely to be causal is appropriate. Although advanced inanition is the most common cause of failure of these lesions to heal, osteomyelitis has to be ruled out by physical examination and radiograph. If osteomyelitis is present, a more extended course of therapy is required and, frequently, amputation.

Mechanical therapies aimed at healing decubitus ulcers include removal of all necrotic and undermined tissues and some strategy to relieve the pressure that caused the ulcer.[50] Once dead tissue has been débrided, the ulcer may be covered with a negative-pressure wound therapy sponge, a moist dressing, or an engineered skin substitute. Studies have shown that these dressings are cost-effective in treating chronic wounds.[51] However, before such local therapy is chosen, it is very important that infection be controlled and that the patient is in good nutritional balance.

KEY POINTS

1. Soft-tissue infections include infections of the skin, subcutaneous tissue, and muscle. They are commonly encountered in ICUs and are often severe and potentially life threatening.

2. Most serious soft-tissue infections require some degree of tissue injury and break in the skin to establish infection. The break in the skin may be due to a surgical incision or trauma; it may be related to large wounds or very small ones. Tissue injury may be due to either blunt or penetrating trauma of any kind.

3. Initial management of necrotizing soft-tissue infections (NSTIs) involves physiologic support, aggressive fluid resuscitation, appropriate broad-spectrum parenteral antibiotics, and most importantly, expedient and radical surgical débridement. Other adjunctive therapies such as hyperbaric oxygen and immunoglobulin may be used, but their efficacy has not been as well established.

4. Topical antimicrobial agents are commonly used in burn patients. Their use has substantially decreased the incidence of conversion of partial-thickness to full-thickness wounds by local infection and thereby has reduced mortality associated with burn wound infection. Systemic antibiotics are not used prophylactically in burn patients.

5. Pressure ulcers in ICU patients occur primarily in patients with impaired mobility due to injury, weakness, sedation, or use of paralytic agents. Pressure ulcers are almost entirely preventable, and measures to prevent development of decubitus ulcers, including pressure relief and appropriate nutrition, should be taken in all patients felt to be at risk.

ANNOTATED REFERENCES

Brook I. Management of human and animal bite wound infection: an overview. Curr Infect Dis Rep 2009;11:389-95.

This article reviewed 60 publications on bite wound infections and described the microbiology, diagnosis, and management of human and animal bite wound infections. The author pointed out that hand wounds present a special problem because 30% or more become infected.

Cumming J, Purdue GF, Hunt JL, et al. Objective estimates of the incidence and consequences of multiple organ dysfunction and sepsis after burn trauma. J Trauma 2001;50:510-15.

In this prospective study, a total of 85 patients with ≥ 20% total body surface area burns admitted to a single center were prospectively enrolled over 1 year. The study revealed that severe multiple organ dysfunction and severe sepsis/septic shock are both related to burn size, age, and male sex and to the length of ICU stay and duration of ventilatory support.

Elliot D, Kufera JA, Myers RA. The microbiology of necrotizing soft tissue infections. Am J Surg 2000;179:361-6.

This retrospective study reviewed charts of 182 patients with NSTIs in a 100-bed level I trauma center. The authors reported that NSTIs are frequently polymicrobial, and the most common organisms are, in order, Bacteroides spp., Escherichia coli, and other gram-negative rods.

Gibbs S, van den Hoogenband HM, Kirtschig G, et al. Autologous full-thickness skin substitute for healing chronic wounds. Br J Dermatol 2006;155:267-74.

This case series describes application of cultured and tissue-engineered skin substitutes derived from healthy skin biopsy in 14 patients with chronic leg ulcers, with excellent results. The entire process including molecular biology and manufacture of the skin substitute as well as results and histology is well presented. Tissue-engineered skin substitutes are increasingly utilized in chronic wounds and severe burns.

May AK, Stafford RE, Bulger EM, et al. Treatment of complicated skin and soft tissue infections. Surg Infect (Larchmt) 2009;10:467-99.

This consensus document presents guidelines developed by the Surgical Infection Society for the treatment of complicated and necrotizing skin and soft-tissue infections. It includes 344 comprehensive references and a complete overview of the current literature.

Reddy M, Gill SS, Rochon PA. Preventing pressure ulcers: a systematic review. JAMA 2006;296:974-84.

Fifty-nine randomized controlled trials are assessed in this systematic review. Pressure relief with specialized support surfaces and frequent repositioning, improved nutrition, and sacral skin moisturization all contribute to prevention of pressure ulcers.

Shah SS, Hall M, Srivastava R, et al. Intravenous immunoglobulin in children with streptococcal toxic shock syndrome. Clin Infect Dis 2009;49:1369-76.

Intravenous immunoglobulin was shown to increase hospital costs but not improve outcomes in a sophisticated and well-executed retrospective multicenter cohort study of children with toxic shock syndrome. The study was underpowered to detect improvements in mortality but is otherwise a high-quality contribution to the vast literature surrounding a therapy with uncertain indications and outcomes.

Wang C, Schwaitzberg S, Berliner E, et al. Hyperbaric oxygen for treating wounds: a systematic review of the literature. Arch Surg 2003;138:272-9.

This is a meta-analysis of the use of HBO for wound care and clinical outcomes on 57 studies, including randomized controlled trials, cohorts, and case series that reported original data. The studies suggest that HBO may be helpful as an adjunctive therapy for gas gangrene, chronic non-healing diabetic wounds, compromised skin grafts, osteoradionecrosis, and soft-tissue radionecrosis, but there is insufficient evidence to determine the timing for HBO and whether patients will benefit.

REFERENCES

Access the complete reference list online at http://www.expertconsult.com.

136

Head and Neck Infections

JEREMY D. GRADON

Infections of the head and neck range in severity from minor to life threatening. The intensivist is called upon to manage such patients either when they are critically ill or when airway compromise has occurred or is imminent. Besides airway management and control of sepsis, the intensivist must also be aware of the local anatomy and relevant microbiology. This knowledge will help guide the choice of antimicrobial agents as well as allow the clinician to anticipate the potential for spread of infection to related anatomic spaces and subsequent complications.

Normal Head and Neck Flora

Huge numbers of bacteria reside in the oral cavity in health, with the bacterial load exceeding 10^{11}/mL in the gingival crevices of patients with teeth.[1] The main bacterial species are anaerobes including *Bacteroides, Fusobacterium, Prevotella,* and *Peptostreptococcus.* Other common oral inhabitants include *Streptococcus mutans, Staphylococcus aureus, Actinomyces* spp., and *Eikenella corrodens.* Pharyngeal colonization and subsequent infection with organisms such as *Streptococcus pneumoniae, Neisseria meningitidis,* and *Streptococcus pyogenes* may also occur.

In acute illness, an additional modifying factor is the decreased production of oral mucosal fibronectin. This is of relevance to the clinician because fibronectin in normal physiologic amounts will preferentially bind gram-positive bacteria (such as *S. mutans*); however, when the production of fibronectin is decreased, there is rapid colonization of the oral cavity with gram-negative organisms, including species such as *Pseudomonas aeruginosa.*[2] These gram-negative organisms may then participate in head and neck infections of oral or odontogenic origin, necessitating broad nosocomial-type gram-negative antibiotic coverage when the patient has been recently hospitalized or acquired the infection in the intensive care unit (ICU).

Sites of Deep Head and Neck Infection

Serious infection of the head and neck can involve the following general anatomic areas:

- Sinus
- Pharynx
- Epiglottis
- Retropharyngeal space
- Submandibular space (Ludwig's angina)
- Lateral pharyngeal space (anterior and posterior)
- Internal jugular vein (Lemierre syndrome)

Some of these anatomic areas are connected via actual or potential spaces. Thus infection beginning in one space may spread rapidly to involve others, with potential resultant damage or destruction of vital structures. Such connections are discussed in the following sections, and differentiating features are highlighted in Table 136-1.

Clinical Syndromes

SINUSITIS

Acute bacterial sinusitis accounts for a high proportion of physician visits in the primary care setting.[5] In the ICU, patients who are critically ill, with nasogastric tubes or endotracheal or nasotracheal tubes in

place, may develop acute sinusitis caused by resistant nosocomial organisms (e.g., methicillin-resistant *S. aureus* [MRSA], *P. aeruginosa*) and anaerobes.[3] Treatment involves the use of broad-spectrum antimicrobial agents (Table 136-2) and close collaboration with an otolaryngologist to determine if drainage is needed. In addition, application of topical vasoconstrictors and steroids to the nasal mucosa is often recommended to help the sinus secretions drain.

Complications of nosocomial sinusitis are related to the local anatomy. Spread via the diploic veins can result in meningitis, brain abscess, contiguous osteomyelitis, or cavernous sinus thrombosis. Spread from the ethmoid sinuses can result in frontal lobe brain abscesses, whereas sphenoid sinus infection can spread to involve the surrounding pituitary gland, optic chiasm, internal carotid artery, cavernous sinus, or temporal lobe of the brain.[1]

In patients with diabetic ketoacidosis, high-dose steroid treatment, severe neutropenia, or history of desferrioxamine treatment, rhinocerebral mucormycosis or aspergillosis can develop. This infection can be rapidly fatal if the underlying problem cannot be corrected. The general teaching has been that high-dose antifungal therapy (see Table 136-2) plus extensive surgery is always required for any hope of survival. However, the need for major surgery in all cases has come into question recently.[4] Close collaboration with appropriate surgeons and infectious disease colleagues is required in such cases.

PHARYNGEAL INFECTIONS

Life-threatening pharyngeal infections include acute anaerobic pharyngitis (Vincent's angina) caused by a combination of oral anaerobes and spirochetes. The clinical manifestations of this entity in the critically ill host include acute ulcerations and necrosis of the oral mucosa and gums. Secondary bacteremia with sepsis syndrome can complicate matters. Treatment involves adequate oral débridement and administration of antibiotics with both aerobic and anaerobic activity (see Table 136-2).[1]

Quinsy (peritonsillar abscess) can complicate prior tonsillitis and is most common among young adults. Presenting symptoms include fever, pharyngeal pain, and unilateral pharyngeal swelling. If not adequately drained, the infection can spread into the lateral pharyngeal space, which was the commonest cause of mortality due to quinsy in preantibiotic days. Infection with anaerobes can result in a higher rate of recurrence of quinsy.[5] *Fusobacterium necrophorum* is currently the most commonly encountered organism in peritonsillar abscesses in Denmark.[6]

Diphtheria is now rare thanks to mass vaccination. It presents as a sharply demarcated adherent dark gray nasal or pharyngeal membrane. Clinical illness is due to release of a bacterial toxin that inhibits translocase (via inhibition of elongation factor 2). Myocardial dysfunction and central nervous system toxin-mediated injury may occur late, but fulminant infections can be complicated by death from acute respiratory obstruction or circulatory failure (bull-neck diphtheria).[1] Culture of the organism (*Corynebacterium diphtheriae*) requires the use of specific Loeffler medium.

EPIGLOTTITIS

Acute epiglottitis is primarily a disease of children who have not received the *Haemophilus influenzae* type b (Hib) vaccine and is thus

TABLE 136-1	Differentiating Features of Deep Neck Infections
Space	**Clinical Features***
Submandibular space ("Ludwig's angina")	Woody submental induration, protruding swollen/necrotic tongue, no trismus, rotted lower molars commonly present
Lateral pharyngeal space (anterior)	Fever, toxicity, trismus, neck swelling
Lateral pharyngeal space (posterior)	No trismus, no swelling (unless ipsilateral parotid is involved), cranial nerve IX-XII palsies, Horner's syndrome, carotid artery erosion
Retropharyngeal space (retropharynx)	Neck stiffness, decreased neck range of motion, soft-tissue bulging of posterior pharyngeal wall, sore throat, dysphagia, dyspnea
Retropharyngeal space ("danger space")	Mediastinal or pleural involvement
Retropharyngeal space (prevertebral)	Neck stiffness, decreased neck range of motion, cervical instability, possible spread along length of vertebral column
Jugular vein septic thrombophlebitis (Lemierre syndrome)	Sore throat, swollen tender neck, dyspnea, chest pain, septic arthritis

*Fever and signs of systemic toxicity are common to all.

rare at present.[7] Acute epiglottitis presents as an acute febrile illness usually of less than 12 hours duration, with the child characteristically sitting forward, drooling saliva, and taking shallow and apprehensive breaths (deeper breathing draws the epiglottis over the airway and produces obstruction). The diagnosis is made clinically, although lateral neck radiography (if the child is stable enough to go for x-ray) characteristically shows enlargement of the epiglottis 30% to 57% of the time. Attempts to visualize the classically described edematous cherry red epiglottis directly may precipitate acute airway obstruction and should not be attempted unless the ability to secure an airway immediately is certain. Blood and epiglottis cultures usually grow *H. influenzae* type b. However, since the introduction of mass vaccination against *H. influenzae* type b, the incidence of infection with non–type b strains is increasing.[7]

Antibiotic options for epiglottitis are outlined in Table 136-2. There is no clear consensus on the role of exogenous corticosteroids to decrease epiglottic edema. Rifampin prophylaxis should be administered for 4 days to close household and hospital contacts of patients (especially those younger than 4 years) with invasive *H. influenzae* type b disease.

RETROPHARYNGEAL INFECTIONS

The area situated between the pharynx anteriorly and the vertebrae posteriorly constitutes the retropharyngeal space, which begins behind the pharynx and ends at the junction of the cervical and thoracic vertebrae (see Table 136-1). The space is subdivided into several distinct anatomic spaces (retropharyngeal, prevertebral, "danger space"), some of which may provide the means of spread of infection from the initial retropharyngeal area to distant sites.[8]

Located between the prevertebral space posteriorly and the retropharyngeal space anteriorly is a potential space called the *danger space*, which connects the base of the skull with the posterior mediastinum and diaphragm. Infection may spread unimpeded within in this space. In addition, infection occurring between the vertebrae and the prevertebral fascia may spread along the length of the vertebral column.

Infections of the retropharynx occur either as:
- Primary infections
- Secondary to extension posteriorly from the pharynx or anteriorly from infected cervical vertebrae
- Via hematogenous spread

Clinically, retropharyngeal infections present with acute fever, systemic toxicity, sore throat, neck stiffness, dysphagia, and dyspnea. Airway obstruction may occur as a consequence of anterior bulging of the pharyngeal wall with supraglottic compression.

Prevertebral infections usually involve the cervical vertebrae and present with neck pain and stiffness and prevertebral soft-tissue swelling. Rarely, instability or destruction of the cervical vertebrae may develop, with death due to acute spinal cord compression.

Danger-space infection is suspected when pleural or mediastinal infection or pain complicates a retropharyngeal infection.[8] Mediastinitis secondary to danger-space infection is generally fulminant with pleural extension and a high mortality rate. Rarely, mediastinal infections, such as may occur after coronary artery bypass graft surgery, may spread upwards through the danger space and present in the retropharynx.

The bacteriology of retropharyngeal infections is that of mixed aerobic/anaerobic oral bacteria. In the critically ill host with nosocomial infection, colonization of the oropharynx with resistant pathogens will necessitate modification of antimicrobial coverage. The imaging techniques needed include plain lateral neck x-rays that will show loss of normal cervical lordosis as well as thickening of the retrotracheal area (usually < 22 mm) or of the prevertebral fascia (usually < 7 mm). Bedside ultrasonography may provide information regarding the presence or absence of drainable collections, but if the patient is

TABLE 136-2	Therapeutic Options for Sinusitis, Pharyngitis, Epiglottitis	
Syndrome	**Likely Flora**	**Antibiotic Options***
Sinusitis (community-acquired)	*Haemophilus influenzae, Streptococcus pneumoniae, Staphylococcus aureus*	• Ampicillin-sulbactam (3 g IV q 6 h) • Levofloxacin (500 mg IV q 24 h) *or* moxifloxacin (400 mg IV q 24 h) • Levofloxacin (500 mg IV q 24 h) *plus* clindamycin (300-900 mg IV q 8 h) *or* moxifloxacin (400 mg IV q 24 h)
Sinusitis (ICU-acquired)	*Pseudomonas aeruginosa* *Escherichia coli* and related coliforms Methicillin-resistant *S. aureus* (MRSA)	• Ceftazidime (2 g IV q 8 h) *or* piperacillin-tazobactam (3.375 g IV q 4 h) *plus* an aminoglycoside, *plus* vancomycin (1 g IV q 12 h)
Sinusitis (fungal)	*Aspergillus* spp. *Mucorales* spp.	• Amphotericin B (1-1.5 mg/kg/d IV) • Liposomal amphotericin B (5-10 mg/kg/d IV) • Voriconazole (6 mg/kg q 12 h × 2 doses, then 4 mg/kg q 12 h) • Caspofungin (70 mg IV day 1, then 50 mg/d IV) • Itraconazole (200 mg IV q 12 h × 4 doses, then 200 mg/d IV)
Pharyngitis	*Corynebacterium diphtheriae* Epstein-Barr virus (with airway compromise)	• IV penicillin or erythromycin • PLUS diphtheria antitoxin • No antiviral therapy effective • IV steroids
Epiglottitis	*H. influenzae* type b *Streptococcus pyogenes* (group A strep)	• Ceftriaxone (1-2 g IV q 24 h) • Ampicillin-sulbactam (3 g IV q 6 h) • Rifampin prophylaxis (600 mg orally q 24 h) for close contacts for 4 days

*Antibiotic choices listed are **examples**, since for most infections, multiple different antibiotics are effective, and individual choice will be influenced by patient factors (allergies, etc.), local hospital bacterial resistance rates, and microbiological culture results.

TABLE 136-3	Therapeutic Options for Deep Neck Infections	
Syndrome	**Likely Flora**	**Therapeutic Options***
Submandibular space infection (community-acquired)	Anaerobes, streptococci, *Staphylococcus aureus*	• Ampicillin-sulbactam (3 g IV q 6 h) • Ceftriaxone (1-2 g IV q 24 h) *plus* clindamycin (300-900 mg IV q 8 h) *or* metronidazole (500 mg IV q 6 h) • Ertapenem (1 g IV q day)
Submandibular space infection (hospital/ICU-acquired)	*Pseudomonas aeruginosa* Methicillin-resistant *S. aureus* (MRSA) Anaerobes	• Imipenem (500 mg IV q 6 h) *or* piperacillin-tazobactam (3.375 g IV q 4 h) *plus* vancomycin (1 g IV q 12 h)[15]
Retropharyngeal space infection	Anaerobes, streptococci, *S. aureus*	• Ampicillin-sulbactam (3 g IV q 6 h) • Ceftriaxone (1-2 g IV q 24 h) *plus* clindamycin (300-900 mg IV q 8 h) *or* metronidazole (500 mg IV q 6 h) • Ertapenem (1 g IV q day)
Lateral pharyngeal space infection	Anaerobes, streptococci, *S. aureus*	• Ampicillin-sulbactam (3 g IV q 6 h) • Ceftriaxone (1-2 g IV q 24 h) *plus* clindamycin (300-900 mg IV q 8 h) *or* metronidazole (500 mg IV q 6 h) • Ertapenem (1 g IV q day)
Internal jugular vein septic thrombophlebitis	*Fusobacterium necrophorum*	• Metronidazole (500 mg IV q 6 h) • Clindamycin (300-900 mg IV q 8 h) • Ampicillin-sulbactam (3 g IV q 6 h)

*Antibiotic choices listed are **examples**, since for most infections, multiple different antibiotics are effective, and individual choice will be influenced by patient factors (allergies, concurrent medications, etc.), local hospital bacterial resistance rates, and microbiological culture results.

stable enough to go to the radiology suite, computed tomography (CT) or magnetic resonance imaging (MRI) scans provide the best definition studies. Close collaboration with appropriate surgical colleagues is necessary for successful management.[8] Therapy is outlined in Table 136-3. On occasion, nonbacterial processes such as Kawasaki disease can mimic retropharyngeal abscesses.[9]

SUBMANDIBULAR SPACE INFECTION (LUDWIG'S ANGINA)

The submandibular space is contained between the mucous membranes of the floor of the mouth superiorly and the muscle and fascia attachments of the hyoid bone inferiorly. The most common route of infection into this space is via infected lower molar teeth, and infection is more common in persons with underlying diabetes, neutropenia, or systemic lupus erythematosus.

Clinical presentation of submandibular space infection is that of an acutely ill patient with mouth pain, dysphagia, drooling of saliva, stiff neck, and fever. The submandibular tissues are "woody," not fluctuant, and true drainable collections are uncommon. The tongue may be swollen and displaced upwards against the palate and also protrude out of the mouth. Trismus is not present; however if the infection spreads to the lateral pharyngeal space, trismus may occur. Unrecognized lateral pharyngeal space involvement may be complicated by subsequent spread to the retropharyngeal space. Late complications of Ludwig's angina include death from airway obstruction, aspiration pneumonia, carotid artery erosion, and tongue necrosis.[10]

Lateral neck x-rays will demonstrate edema of the submandibular soft tissues. Pockets of gas may be seen if gas-forming organisms are involved. CT scanning is most helpful diagnostically. However, attention must be paid to having qualified staff accompany the patient to the CT scanner in case acute airway obstruction develops. Should airway protection be needed, tracheotomy or cricothyroidotomy is advocated because of the risk of inducing acute airway obstruction with routine "blind" nasal or oral intubation. The infection is commonly polymicrobial, and appropriate antibiotic therapy options are described in Table 136-3. In approximately 50% of cases, surgical drainage is required. In addition, causative rotted molar teeth (if present) should be removed.[10]

LATERAL PHARYNGEAL SPACE INFECTIONS

Infection of the lateral pharyngeal space is one of the most common deep neck infections encountered. In a review of 110 deep neck infections in adults seen at an academic medical center over a 10-year period, infections of the lateral pharyngeal space accounted for 55%.[10] In contrast, in children such infections are rare, with peritonsillar infection (quinsy) being the most common deep neck infection.

The lateral pharyngeal space is cone shaped, extending from the sphenoid bone down to the hyoid bone. Posteriorly it is bound by the prevertebral fascia (that separates it from the retropharyngeal space) and anteriorly by the buccinator and superior constrictor muscles. The parotid gland communicates with this space. The styloid process divides the space into an anterior compartment (containing fat, lymph nodes and muscle) and a posterior compartment (containing the carotid artery, cranial nerves IX-XII, and the cervical sympathetic trunk).

Common precipitating causes of lateral pharyngeal space infection include dental disease (33%), injection drug use (inserting needles directly into the space; 20%), local trauma (9%) and tonsillitis (4%). Patients frequently have underlying diabetes or human immunodeficiency virus (HIV) infection.

Clinically, anterior lateral pharyngeal space infections present with fever, pain, trismus, and systemic toxicity. Turning the head to the opposite side causes increased pain due to stretching of the ipsilateral sternocleidomastoid muscle.

Infection of the posterior lateral pharyngeal space presents differently from infections involving the anterior pharyngeal space. Common symptoms include fever, systemic toxicity, and parotid swelling. Trismus and external swelling do not occur. Involvement of local vital structures can occur, including carotid artery erosion or clot, septic thrombophlebitis of the internal jugular vein, cranial nerve IX-XII palsies, or Horner's syndrome.

Therapy involves urgent surgical intervention to drain purulent material and prevent spread of infection to the retropharyngeal space or erosion of the carotid artery. The choice of antibiotics for this frequently polymicrobial infection is shown in Table 136-3.

DESCENDING NECROTIZING MEDIASTINITIS

Rapid downward spread of deep neck infections can result in the development of necrotizing soft-tissue infections of the chest wall and mediastinum. A recent study of 45 such cases collected over a 12-year period demonstrated that they tended to develop as a complication of dental or deep neck polymicrobial infections, affecting persons aged 40 to 60 years most commonly. Mixed aerobic/anaerobic flora was the rule, and risk factors included alcoholism and diabetes mellitus. Mortality was around 15% to 20%.[8]

INTERNAL JUGULAR VEIN SEPTIC THROMBOPHLEBITIS (LEMIERRE SYNDROME)

Septic thrombophlebitis of the internal jugular vein is known as *Lemierre syndrome.* It is a relatively rare entity usually caused by infection with the anaerobe *Fusobacterium necrophorum*, a normal inhabitant of the human gingival crevice. Latest theories on the pathogenesis of this infection indicate that the first stage of infection is pharyngitis in approximately 87% of cases. Recent data suggest that *F. necrophorum* causes pharyngitis in young adults aged 15 to 24 years as frequently as *Streptococcus pyogenes.*[6] This is then followed by invasion of the lateral pharyngeal space, with development of septic thrombophlebitis of the internal jugular vein.[11] Subsequently, bloodborne infection develops, with the classic findings of septic pulmonary emboli or cavitating pneumonia and septic arthritis. Other precipitating factors include mastoiditis, lateral pharyngeal space infection, or trauma to the internal jugular vein.

Clinically, Lemierre syndrome begins with fever and sore throat. When internal jugular vein involvement develops, patients complain of a swollen and/or tender neck, which is thus a warning sign of danger in a patient with recent pharyngitis. Dyspnea and pleuritic chest pain indicate pulmonary involvement.

Early diagnosis is critical to minimize the risk of infectious metastatic complications requiring surgical intervention or drainage. Blood cultures should be promptly obtained and empirical antianaerobic bacterial coverage begun. Radiologic diagnosis is made most reliably by CT scanning, although bedside ultrasound examination of the internal jugular vein can be useful in the critically ill patient who cannot leave the ICU. If the infection occurs secondary to mastoiditis, it is necessary to rule out intracerebral vein thrombosis by MRI scanning.

Antibiotic choices are outlined in Table 136-3. There are no firm data to support or refute the use of anticoagulants in Lemierre syndrome.[12] In addition, surgical ligation or excision of the internal jugular vein for uncontrollable sepsis was necessary in approximately 8% of cases in a recently published series of cases.[12] MRSA has recently been shown to cause Lemierre syndrome, especially in injection drug users or patients with the infection developing as a complication of venous cannulation.[14]

Conclusions

The intensivist will frequently be asked to assist in the care of patients with serious deep neck infections. Critical issues encountered include protection of the airway, sepsis management, and the potential for erosion of the infection into surrounding vital structures in the neck. Such infections are frequently polymicrobial in nature, and thus broad-spectrum antibiotics with both aerobic and anaerobic coverage should be chosen.

Common issues to be decided for each patient individually include:
- The safety of performing an intraoral examination, for fear of precipitating acute airway obstruction.
- The safety of sending a patient out of the ICU for studies such as CT scanning. Although patients may appear stable initially, they are at risk for sudden development of acute airway obstruction and thus should always be accompanied by a team capable of securing an airway when they travel out of the ICU for tests or procedures.
- The need for and timing of possible surgical intervention. Early close collaboration with otolaryngologists, head and neck surgeons, neurosurgeons, or vascular surgeons is critical for successful management of these complex and frequently critically ill patients.

ANNOTATED REFERENCES

Bilal M, Cleveland KO, Gelfand MS. Community-acquired methicillin-resistant *Staphylococcus aureus* and Lemierre syndrome. Am J Med Sci 2009;338:326-7.
A case report highlighting what is being seen more commonly in the community, namely the increasing role of MRSA in invasive head and neck infections.

Centor RM. Expand the pharyngitis paradigm for adolescents and young adults. Ann Intern Med 2009; 151:812-15.
A discussion of the role of preceding pharyngitis in the subsequent development of Lemierre syndrome in light of data suggesting that Fusobacterium necrophorum causes about 10% of cases of acute pharyngitis in young adults.

Chow AW. Infections of the oral cavity, neck, and head. In: Mandell GL, Bennett JE, Dolin R, editors. Principles and practice of infectious diseases. 7th ed. Philadelphia: Saunders; 2009, Chapter 60.
A comprehensive discussion of the latest thoughts on the pathophysiology and management of deep neck space infections. Numerous anatomic diagrams are provided, as is discussion of pathways of spread of such infections from one anatomic site to another.

Gavriel H, Vaiman M, Kessler A, Eviatar E. Microbiology of peritonsillar abscess as an indication for tonsillectomy. Medicine (Baltimore) 2008;87:33-6.
A study of 469 patients with peritonsillar abscesses showing that patients with predominant growth of anaerobes from peritonsillar abscess aspirates were at higher risk of recurrent abscess formation compared to patients from whom aerobes were the main isolates cultured—suggesting a role for prophylactic tonsillectomy earlier in such patients.

Klug TE, Rusan M, Fuursted K, Ovesen T. *Fusobacterium necrophorum*: most prevalent pathogen in peritonsillar abscess in Denmark. Clin Infect Dis 2009;49:1467-72.
A study of 847 patients with peritonsillar abscess. Cultures of the abscesses grew pure growth of F. necrophorum in 23%, as compared with group A streptococci from "only" 17%.

O'Grady NP, Barie PS, Bartlett JG, et al. Guidelines for evaluation of new fever in critically ill adult patients: 2008 update from the American College of Critical Care Medicine and the Infectious Diseases Society of America. Crit Care Med 2008;36:1330-49.
Expert guidelines on evaluation of fever in critically ill patients. The section on sinusitis (pp. 1340-1341) suggests CT scanning and sinus aspiration as necessary steps for the more critically ill patient.

Ridder GJ, Maier W, Kinzer S, et al. Descending necrotizing mediastinitis. Contemporary trends in etiology, diagnosis, management and outcome. Ann Surg 2010;251:528-34.
A review of 45 patients with necrotizing chest and mediastinal infections seen over 12 years in one medical center. The source of infection was usually pharyngeal, dental, or deep neck infection. With aggressive diagnostic efforts and multidisciplinary management, a survival rate of 85% was achieved.

Rybak M, Lomaestro B, Rotschafer JC, et al. Therapeutic monitoring of vancomycin in adult patients: a consensus review of the American Society of Health-System Pharmacists, the Infectious Diseases Society of America and the Society of Infectious Diseases Pharmacists. Am J Health Syst Pharm 2009; 66:82-98.
A consensus statement suggesting that vancomycin is a concentration-independent killer of gram-positive organisms. The trough level to aim for is suggested to be 15 to 20 μg/mL. If the MIC of S. aureus to vancomycin is >2 μg/mL, it is suggested that an alternate agent other than vancomycin be used for MRSA coverage for theoretical pharmacologic reasons.

Walsh TJ, Anaissie EJ, Denning DW. Treatment of aspergillosis: clinical practice guidelines of the Infectious Diseases Society of America. Clin Infect Dis 2008;46:327-60.
Expert guidelines for the very difficult-to-manage invasive Aspergillus-infected patient, including a thoughtful discussion on the role and feasibility of surgery in the critically ill patient with sinus involvement with Aspergillus (pp. 343-344).

REFERENCES

Access the complete reference list online at http://www.expertconsult.com.

Infections in the Immunocompromised Patient

YOSHIRO HAYASHI | DAVID L. PATERSON

Many immunocompromised patients are managed in intensive care units (ICUs) every year, with infection being a leading cause of ICU admission. Common examples of such infections include community-acquired pneumonia, bacteremia, and central nervous system (CNS) infections. The incidence of infections acquired by immunocompromised patients during ICU admissions is also significant.[1] Mortality for certain infections in immunocompromised patients exceeds 50%.[2] Early diagnosis, initiation of appropriate antimicrobial and supportive therapy, and reduction in immunosuppression where possible can improve outcome significantly.

Commonly Encountered Immunocompromising Conditions

Immunocompromise can be broadly defined as a state in which the response of the host to a foreign antigen is subnormal. Immunocompromise could be congenital (primary) or acquired. Congenital immunodeficiencies are now much less common than acquired immunodeficiencies. In general, congenital immunodeficiency is observed more frequently in patients in pediatric ICUs than in adult ICUs. Patients with congenital immunodeficiencies usually have repeated infections, especially infections affecting the sinuses and lower respiratory tract. Congenital immunodeficiencies are usually "pure" in that the defects in host response to foreign antigens are usually specific and well defined. For example, Bruton's X-linked agammaglobulinemia is associated with a defect in the normal maturation process of immunoglobulin-producing B cells. As a result, mature circulating B cells, plasma cells, and serum immunoglobulin are absent. The patient is susceptible to organisms normally dealt with by immunoglobulin, such as *Streptococcus pneumoniae* and *Haemophilus influenzae*. Other congenital immunodeficiency syndromes are listed in Table 137-1.

Most immunocompromised patients managed in adult ICUs have acquired immunocompromise. Although the response of host defenses in the elderly, diabetics, and alcoholics is compromised, this chapter deals primarily with four categories of immunocompromised patients: (1) patients receiving chemotherapy for hematologic malignancies and solid tumors; (2) patients receiving immunosuppressive therapy in the context of solid-organ transplantation; (3) patients receiving corticosteroids, methotrexate, monoclonal antibodies to tumor necrosis factor, and other disease-modifying agents for rheumatoid arthritis, Crohn's disease, and autoimmune disorders; and (4) patients with human immunodeficiency virus (HIV) infection.

HEMATOLOGIC MALIGNANCIES AND SOLID TUMORS

Prolonged neutropenia from chemotherapy has a significant risk of bacterial and fungal infection. Classically, gram-negative organisms such as *Pseudomonas aeruginosa* and fungal organisms such as *Aspergillus* species have been associated with severe neutropenia. It has long been known that the severity and duration of neutropenia influence the risk of infection.[3] It also has been well established that aggressive chemotherapy and radiotherapy for Hodgkin's disease coupled with splenectomy significantly impairs humoral defense against encapsulated organisms such as *S. pneumoniae, H. influenzae,* and *Neisseria meningitidis.*[4] Transplantation is associated with a risk of graft-versus-host disease (GVHD). Prophylaxis and treatment for GVHD may involve use of drugs such as cyclosporine or tacrolimus plus corticosteroids. Cyclosporine and tacrolimus inhibit calcineurin, an enzyme important in the lymphocyte activation cascade. Corticosteroids also affect lymphocyte function and depress functions of activated macrophages. As a result, patients receiving therapy for GVHD may be prone to fungal, viral, and mycobacterial infections.

SOLID-ORGAN TRANSPLANTATION

Solid-organ transplant recipients are uniquely susceptible to infection.[5] They undergo significant surgery, breaching the defenses provided by the skin. They remain in ICUs for prolonged periods, requiring intravenous access and mechanical ventilation—here, cutaneous and pulmonary barriers to infection are breached. Finally, solid-organ transplant recipients receive immunosuppressive therapy to prevent graft rejection. Commonly used immunosuppressive medications are listed in Table 137-2. Immunosuppressive regimens are in a constant state of flux—more recent trends have been toward aggressive "pretreatment" immediately before transplantation, coupled with decreased immunosuppression in the posttransplant period.[6]

In the early posttransplant period, transplant recipients are susceptible to nosocomially acquired bacterial infections such as pneumonia, catheter-related bloodstream infection associated with general ICU care, and wound and intraabdominal infections associated with surgical procedures. Opportunistic infections may be acquired from the organ graft; cytomegalovirus (CMV) is the most pertinent example,[7] but a wide variety of infections (e.g., rabies, histoplasmosis, tuberculosis, West Nile virus) have been acquired from grafts. Solid-organ transplant recipients, by virtue of their iatrogenic immunosuppression, also are susceptible to reactivation of latent infection (e.g., CMV infection, tuberculosis, histoplasmosis) or to infections acquired through the hospital environment (e.g., aspergillosis, legionellosis, tuberculosis).

RHEUMATOID ARTHRITIS AND AUTOIMMUNE DISORDERS

Therapy for rheumatoid arthritis and other autoimmune disorders may be with simple analgesics or nonsteroidal antiinflammatory drugs (NSAIDs). Drugs with the potential to cause significant immunocompromise are also frequently used. Classically, therapy has been with corticosteroids or disease-modifying antirheumatic drugs such as azathioprine, cyclosporine, penicillamine, gold salts, hydroxychloroquine, leflunomide, methotrexate, or sulfasalazine. The effects of corticosteroids, azathioprine, and cyclosporine on host defenses have been noted previously (see Table 137-2). Methotrexate reversibly inhibits dihydrofolate reductase and interferes with DNA synthesis, repair, and cellular replication. In addition to its use in rheumatoid arthritis, it also can be used as an antineoplastic agent. Methotrexate can cause significant neutropenia. Low-dose methotrexate is generally less likely to increase infection risk in patients with rheumatoid arthritis.[8,9]

TABLE 137-1	Congenital (Primary) Causes of Immunodeficiency	

Condition (Immunodeficiency)	Organisms with Increased Tendency to Cause Infection in This Condition
T-lymphocyte Deficiencies	
DiGeorge syndrome (thymic aplasia with reduced CD4 and CD3 cells)	Viruses (especially HSV and measles), sometimes *Pneumocystis jirovecii*, fungi, or gram-negative bacteria
Purine nucleoside phosphorylase deficiency (marked T-cell depletion)	*P. jirovecii* and viruses
B-lymphocyte Deficiencies	
Bruton's X-linked agammaglobulinemia (absence of B cells, plasma cells, and antibody)	*Haemophilus influenzae, Streptococcus pneumoniae, Staphylococcus aureus, Pseudomonas aeruginosa, P. jirovecii* (after first 4-6 months of life when maternal antibody has been consumed)
Selective IgG subclass deficiencies	Variable
Selective IgA deficiency	*S. pneumoniae, H. influenzae*
Hyper-IgM immunodeficiency (elevated IgM but reduced IgG and IgA)	*S. pneumoniae, H. influenzae, P. jirovecii* (rarely)
Mixed T- and B-lymphocyte Deficiencies	
Common variable immunodeficiency (leads to various B-cell activation or differentiation defects and gradual deterioration of T-cell number and function)	*S. pneumoniae, H. influenzae*, CMV, VZV, *P. jirovecii*
Severe combined immunodeficiency (severe reduction in IgG and absence of T cells)	*P. jirovecii*, viruses, *Legionella*
Wiskott-Aldrich syndrome (decreased T-cell number and function, low IgM, occasionally low IgG)	*S. pneumoniae, H. influenzae*, HSV, *P. jirovecii*
Ataxia-telangiectasia (decreased T-cell number and function; IgA, IgE, IgG$_2$, and IgG$_4$ deficiency)	*S. aureus, S. pneumoniae, H. influenzae*
Disorders of Complement	
C3 deficiency (congenital absence of C3 or consumption of C3 due to deficiency of C3b inactivator)	*S. pneumoniae, H. influenzae*, enteric gram-negative bacilli
Phagocyte Defects	
Chronic granulomatous disease (defect in NADPH oxidase in phagocytic cells)	*S. aureus, Escherichia coli, Klebsiella pneumoniae, Enterobacter cloacae, S. marcescens, P. aeruginosa, Aspergillus*
Chédiak-Higashi syndrome (impaired microbicidal activity of phagocytes)	*S. aureus, H. influenzae, Aspergillus*
Kostmann syndrome, Shwachman-Diamond syndrome, cyclic neutropenia (low neutrophil count)	*S. aureus*, enteric gram-negative bacilli, *P. aeruginosa*

CMV, Cytomegalovirus; *HSV*, herpes simplex virus; *Ig*, immunoglobulin; *NADPH*, nicotinamide adenine dinucleotide phosphate; *VZV*, varicella-zoster virus.

A variety of anticytokine agents have become available for rheumatoid arthritis (Table 137-3). Use of these drugs also has been reported in treatment of Behçet's disease, Crohn's disease, GVHD, hairy cell leukemia, psoriasis, pyoderma gangrenosum, sarcoidosis, and ulcerative colitis. Considerable attention has been paid to the possibility of tuberculosis developing after treatment with such agents.[10] The risk is sufficiently high that it is recommended that tuberculin skin testing or interferon gamma (IFN-γ) release assays be performed to detect latent tuberculosis before the initiation of anticytokine agents. Invasive infections with *Histoplasma, Candida, Pneumocystis jirovecii, Aspergillus, Cryptococcus, Nocardia, Salmonella, Listeria, Brucella, Bartonella*, nontuberculous mycobacteria, *Leishmania*, and *Toxoplasma* have also been reported associated with the use of these medications.[11-14] As is the case with transplant-associated immunocompromise, these infections may be reactivation of latent infection or new acquisition of organisms through environmental exposure.

HUMAN IMMUNODEFICIENCY VIRUS INFECTION

HIV infection remains a relatively common infection, but acquired immunodeficiency syndrome (AIDS) has become less frequently encountered in ICUs since the advent of highly active antiretroviral therapy. A decline in CD4 counts creates a predisposition to *P. jirovecii* pneumonia, mycobacterial infection, fungal infection (e.g., cryptococcal meningitis), and viral infection (e.g., CMV infection). Many patients with HIV infection are co-infected with hepatitis C virus, and as a result, liver failure is now a relatively common reason for ICU

TABLE 137-2	Immunosuppressive Drugs Used in Solid-Organ Transplantation and Their Mechanisms of Activity
Immunosuppressive	**Mode of Action**
Corticosteroids	Negative regulation of cytokine gene expression
Azathioprine	Inhibits DNA and RNA synthesis; inhibits T- and B-cell function
Cyclosporine	Calcineurin inhibitor; inhibits cytokine expression
Tacrolimus	Calcineurin inhibitor; inhibits cytokine expression
Sirolimus (rapamycin)	Prevents translation of mRNAs encoding cell cycle regulators
Mycophenolate mofetil	Blocks purine biosynthesis; inhibits T- and B-cell proliferation
Polyclonal antilymphocyte	Lymphocyte depletion antibodies (e.g., Atgam, Thymoglobulin)
Muromonab-CD3 (OKT3)	Anti-CD3 monoclonal antibody
Alemtuzumab (Campath)	Anti-CD52 monoclonal antibody
Daclizumab, basiliximab	Anti-CD25 monoclonal antibody

TABLE 137-3	Commonly Used Anticytokines for Management of Rheumatoid Arthritis	
Drug	**Mechanism of Action**	**FDA-Approved Indications**
Adalimumab (Humira)	Recombinant, fully human anti-TNF monoclonal antibody	Ankylosing spondylitis Crohn's disease Psoriatic arthritis Rheumatoid arthritis
Anakinra (Kineret)	Recombinant human interleukin-1 receptor antagonist	Rheumatoid arthritis
Etanercept (Enbrel)	TNF receptor p75 Fc fusion protein	Ankylosing spondylitis Juvenile rheumatoid arthritis Plaque psoriasis Psoriatic arthritis Rheumatoid arthritis
Infliximab (Remicade)	Chimeric monoclonal antibody to TNF	Ankylosing spondylitis Crohn's disease Psoriatic arthritis Plaque psoriasis Rheumatoid arthritis Ulcerative colitis
Tocilizumab (Actemra)	IL-6 receptor–inhibiting monoclonal antibody	Rheumatoid arthritis

FDA, U.S. Food and Drug Administration; *IL-6*, interleukin 6; *TNF*, tumor necrosis factor.

admission in HIV-infected patients. In some centers, liver transplantation is performed in HIV-infected patients with hepatitis virus–induced liver diseases.[15,16]

General Diagnostic Approach to Immunocompromised Patients with Severe Infections

Immunocompromised patients are a heterogeneous group. The infections commonly encountered by a patient with neutropenia as a consequence of chemotherapy may be different from infections observed in a patient with rheumatoid arthritis who is receiving infliximab. Even within a particular category, different renal transplantation recipients, for example, may have a different degree of immunocompromise and a different susceptibility to infection. In solid-organ transplant recipients, the "net state of immunosuppression" (i.e., the cumulative burden of immunosuppression with a special weighting toward recent T-cell ablative therapy) influences the risk of infection. A renal transplant recipient who is receiving tacrolimus monotherapy twice per week would be less susceptible to opportunistic infection than a patient with recent acute cellular rejection treated with OKT3 or alemtuzumab. There have been more recent attempts to quantify immune function in solid-organ transplant recipients,[17] although it has not yet been definitively proved that such tests predict infection risk. In contrast, with HIV infection, CD4 lymphocyte count and HIV RNA quantification ("viral load") predict risk of infection.[18] Patients with CD4 counts greater than 500 are unlikely to be infected with an opportunistic pathogen. Patients with CD4 counts of 200 to 500 may be infected with organisms such as *Mycobacterium tuberculosis*, but they are unlikely to be infected with opportunistic pathogens such as CMV or *Mycobacterium avium* complex. Patients with CD4 counts less than 200 have an increased risk of a wide variety of opportunistic infections.

Specific environmental exposures may be potentially important for immunocompromised patients. A travel history to the deserts of the southwestern United States and northern Mexico may increase the likelihood that an immunocompromised patient has coccidioidomycosis.[19] Histoplasmosis is endemic in the Ohio River valley.[20] Alternatively, there may be environmental risks within the ICU. Outbreaks of invasive pulmonary aspergillosis have been linked to construction activity within the hospital. Outbreaks of legionellosis may be waterborne.[21] It is possible that many fungal and bacterial infections may also be waterborne.[22,23] Tuberculosis transmission has been well described in ICUs caring for transplant recipients or HIV-infected patients.[24] The net state of immunosuppression must be considered in the context of recent environmental exposures.

Although elements of history taking and physical examination may narrow the differential diagnosis of the causative agent of infection in immunocompromised patients, some of the "rules" applied to diagnosis in immunocompetent patients do not apply. Caution must be exercised in use of the diagnostic principle that follows Occam's razor: "entities are not to be multiplied without necessity." In an immunocompetent patient, given all the patient's symptoms, signs, and noninvasive laboratory test results, one unifying diagnosis usually explains all. In contrast, immunocompromised patients may have more than one infection at any given time. A neutropenic patient may have bacterial pneumonia and invasive pulmonary aspergillosis simultaneously, whereas an immunocompromised patient with HIV infection may have *P. jirovecii* pneumonia and pulmonary infiltrates due to human herpesvirus-8 (HHV-8) infection (Kaposi sarcoma).

The potential for multiple diagnoses underscores the need for early invasive testing in immunocompromised patients with severe infection. Patients with unexplained severe community-acquired pneumonia may be best managed by early bronchoalveolar lavage performed before antimicrobial therapy has commenced. Bronchoalveolar lavage could be sent for Gram stain, Ziehl-Neelsen stain, modified acid-fast stain, calcofluor stain, direct fluorescent antibody tests, polymerase chain reaction (PCR), and cytologic analysis to enable rapid diagnosis of infection with bacteria, mycobacteria, *Nocardia*, fungi, *Legionella*, CMV, community-acquired respiratory viruses, and *P. jirovecii*. The bronchoalveolar lavage should be inoculated onto solid media, and molecular diagnostic testing should be used as appropriate. An outline of the diagnostic approach in immunocompromised patients is given in Box 137-1.

Box 137-1

DIAGNOSTIC APPROACH FOR SEVERE INFECTIONS IN IMMUNOCOMPROMISED PATIENTS

History Taking and Review of Prior Records
Likely degree of immunocompromise:
  Recent CD4 lymphocyte count and HIV viral load
  Time since transplantation
  Recent acute cellular rejection or GVHD and treatment thereof
  Current or recent receipt of immunosuppressive medications
  Current or recent receipt of antiretroviral medications
Prophylaxis against opportunistic infections:
  Receipt of antimicrobial prophylaxis against *Pneumocystis jirovecii*, HSV, or CMV
  Vaccination status (pneumococcus, influenza, *Neisseria meningitidis*)
Family history:
  Personal or family history of tuberculosis or chickenpox
Potential environmental exposures:
  Travel history to southwestern United States
  Exposure to hospital construction activity (aspergillosis)
  Exposure to hospital water supply (legionellosis, aspergillosis)
  Exposure to patients with tuberculosis or chickenpox
  Donor and recipient serostatus for CMV or *Toxoplasma gondii*

Physical Examination
Skin:
  Presence of cutaneous nodules consistent with cryptococcosis or nocardiosis
  Presence of cutaneous manifestations of GVHD
  Kaposi sarcoma
  Line insertion site erythema or pus
  Peripheral embolic phenomena
  Scars consistent with prior surgery
Mouth and other mucous membranes:
  Presence of candidiasis
Respiratory system:
  Presence of signs of focal versus multilobar pneumonia
Cardiovascular system:
  Murmurs, prosthetic heart sounds
Abdominal examination:
  Signs of peritonitis
  Hepatomegaly or splenomegaly
  Tenderness of renal allograft
Neurologic examination:
  Nuchal rigidity
  Cranial nerve signs

Noninvasive Laboratory Tests
White blood cell count and differential
Blood and urine cultures
Serum cryptococcal antigen
Serum galactomannan antigen (aspergillosis)
Serum and urine *Histoplasma* antigen
Urinary *Legionella* antigen

Invasive Laboratory Tests
Bronchoalveolar lavage
Pleural fluid aspiration
Upper gastrointestinal endoscopy
Colonoscopy
Biopsy of liver, kidney, bone marrow

CMV, cytomegalovirus; GVHD, graft-versus-host disease; HIV, human immunodeficiency virus; HSV, herpes simplex virus.

TABLE 137-4	Host Defenses Against Respiratory Infections and How They Are Affected in Immunocompromised Patients		
Location	**Host Defense**		**Defect**
Upper airway	Filtration		Endotracheal intubation
	Mucociliary apparatus		CF, cigarette smoking
	Cough		Impaired consciousness
Lower airway (nonspecific)	Alveolar macrophages		Immunosuppressive medication, corticosteroids
	Polymorphonuclear leukocytes		Corticosteroids, malnutrition, chemotherapy, malignancies
Lower airway (specific)	B lymphocytes		Hypogammaglobulinemia, CLL, MM
	T lymphocytes		AIDS, malignancies, immunosuppressants

AIDS, acquired immunodeficiency syndrome; *CLL,* chronic lymphocytic leukemia; *CF,* cystic fibrosis; *MM,* multiple myeloma.

Major Manifestations of Infection in Immunocompromised Patients

The organism causing infection in an individual immunocompromised patient sometimes can be inferred by the specific host defect in immunologic defense or the specific clinical manifestation. In most circumstances, the differential diagnosis is too broad, however, for definitive clinical diagnosis.

PULMONARY INFECTION

Pneumonia is a significant cause of morbidity and mortality in immunocompromised patients. In contrast to the normal host, the impaired responsiveness of the immune system means that the disease presents in unusual ways, which may lead to challenges in establishing a diagnosis.

Infectious microorganisms usually gain access to the respiratory tract through inhalation, although hematogenous spread sometimes may occur. Mechanical defenses remove the bulk of potentially harmful agents from the lungs (Table 137-4). Inhaled particles greater than 10 μm in diameter usually become trapped in the upper airways or are removed by coughing or mucociliary clearance. Most bacteria range from 0.5 to 2 μm in size and are able to reach the terminal airways/alveoli and potentially cause infection. In the alveoli, the alveolar macrophages are the first line of defense. Subsequently an inflammatory response consisting of polymorphonuclear neutrophils is important. Finally, specific T-cell and B-cell immune responses are essential for successful defense against many pathogens.

As noted earlier, although it may be possible to pinpoint a major immunologic deficiency, most immunocompromised individuals have an assortment of deficiencies in host defense working together. An organ transplant recipient may be intubated, have multiple intravenous lines, be diabetic, and be on corticosteroids and tacrolimus. All these factors contribute to the overall degree of immunity, each paving the way for its peculiar array of susceptibilities to pulmonary infection. In solid-organ transplant recipients, specific causes of pulmonary infection are most frequent at certain times post transplantation (Table 137-5). In a similar manner, specific causes of pulmonary infection are more frequent at different CD4 lymphocyte counts for patients with HIV infection (Table 137-6).

A normal chest radiograph does not rule out pulmonary infection in immunocompromised patients. Additionally, although some diseases have suggestive radiologic findings (e.g., apical cavitations in tuberculosis), most radiographic findings have to be interpreted in the light of all other data available. Frequently, computed tomography (CT) is required (e.g., evaluation of pulmonary nodules). Pulmonary nodules have a broad differential diagnosis in immunocompromised patients, including infections due to fungi (especially *Cryptococcus neoformans, Coccidioides immitis,* and *Aspergillus fumigatus*), *Nocardia,*

TABLE 137-5	Occurrence of Pulmonary Infection After Solid-Organ Transplantation Stratified by Time from Transplantation
Time After Transplant (mo)	**Organism**
<1	Nosocomial bacteria (e.g., MRSA, ESBL-producing Enterobacteriaceae, *Pseudomonas aeruginosa, Acinetobacter baumannii*) *Legionella* spp. Respiratory viruses (e.g., influenza virus, parainfluenza virus, RSV, adenovirus, rhinovirus, human metapneumovirus) *Aspergillus* spp.
1-6	Nosocomial bacteria (if still mechanically ventilated) *Legionella* spp. *Nocardia* spp.[†] *Mycobacterium tuberculosis* Herpesviruses (e.g., HSV, VZV, CMV)[‡] Respiratory viruses (e.g., influenza virus, parainfluenza virus, RSV, adenovirus, rhinovirus, human metapneumovirus) *Pneumocystis jirovecii*[†] *Cryptococcus neoformans* *Aspergillus* spp. *Coccidioides* spp. *Histoplasma* spp.
>6	Bacteria associated with community acquired pneumonia (e.g., *Streptococcus pneumoniae, Haemophilus influenzae, Legionella* spp., *Mycoplasma pneumoniae*) *Nocardia* spp.*[†] *Rhodococcus equi** *Mycobacterium tuberculosis* Atypical mycobacterium *Aspergillus* spp.* Zygomycetes* *Cryptococcus neoformans**

*These organisms should be considered when immune-suppression is still substantial.
[†]These organisms are less likely in patients on prophylactic cotrimoxazole.
[‡]These viruses are less likely in patients on prophylactic ganciclovir or valganciclovir.
CMV, cytomegalovirus; *ESBL,* extended-spectrum β-lactamase; *HSV,* herpes simplex virus; *MRSA,* methicillin-resistant *Staphylococcus aureus; RSV,* respiratory syncytial virus; *VZV,* varicella-zoster virus.

mycobacteria, *Rhodococcus equi,* and *Bartonella.* Additionally, carcinomas and posttransplant lymphoproliferative disorders may present with pulmonary nodules. The differential diagnosis of cavitary lesions includes mycobacteria, invasive pulmonary aspergillosis, legionellosis, and infection with *R. equi.* As noted earlier, the broad differential diagnosis of pulmonary infection in immunocompromised patients mandates early and aggressive diagnostic strategies such as bronchoscopy with bronchoalveolar lavage sent for a comprehensive battery of microbiologic investigations.

CENTRAL NERVOUS SYSTEM INFECTIONS

Most infectious agents reach the CNS via hematogenous dissemination from an extraneural site. Exceptions include retrograde propagation of infected thrombi within emissary veins, spread along olfactory nerves,

TABLE 137-6	Etiology of Pulmonary Infections in Patients Infected with Human Immunodeficiency Virus, Stratified by CD4 Lymphocyte Count			
	CD4 Count (Cells/mm³)			
	>500	**200-500**	**50-200**	**<50**
Organism	*Streptococcus pneumoniae*	*S. pneumoniae*	*Pneumocystis jirovecii*	*P. jirovecii*
	Haemophilus influenzae	*H. influenzae*	*Mycobacterium tuberculosis*	*Cryptococcus*
		M. tuberculosis	*Cryptococcus*	CMV MAC *Aspergillus*

CMV, cytomegalovirus; *MAC, Mycobacterium avium* complex.

and spread from a contiguous focus of infection. The blood-brain barrier presents a natural and efficient barrier to hematogenous infection. The function of the blood-brain barrier in immunocompromised patients has not been well studied. It is well known, however, that when CNS infection is established, immune defenses (even in immunologically competent hosts) are inadequate to control the infection. Local opsonization is deficient within the brain. In animal models of bacterial brain abscess, corticosteroid administration led to a reduction in macrophage and glial response, with an increased number of viable bacteria in the abscess.[25]

Bacterial meningitis due to *N. meningitidis* is relatively uncommon in immunocompromised patients, except if they have undergone splenectomy. In contrast, pneumococcal meningitis seems to occur with increased frequency in patients who have undergone stem cell transplantation[26-28] and in patients with HIV infection.[29,30] Meningitis due to *Listeria monocytogenes* is classically associated with immunocompromise, reflecting the need for adequate T-cell function and IFN-γ production to kill this intercellular pathogen.[31] In addition to meningitis, *Listeria* infection may be associated with brain abscess, particularly that occurring in the brainstem.[32,33] Enteric bacteria (e.g., *Escherichia coli*) are rare causes of bacterial meningitis in immunocompromised patients. A classic association exists, however, between meningitis with such organisms and disseminated infection with *Strongyloides stercoralis*.[34,35] In the presence of immunosuppression (e.g., large doses of corticosteroids), *Strongyloides* can migrate from the gastrointestinal (GI) tract to the CNS, carrying enteric bacterial flora into the CNS. Mortality is high without prompt recognition and treatment. *Nocardia* and mycobacteria must also be considered in the differential diagnosis of CNS infections in immunocompromised patients; diagnostic samples should be sent for inoculation onto appropriate media for isolation of these organisms.[36-38]

Fungal infection of the CNS may cause meningitis or space-occupying lesions. Cryptococcal meningitis is associated with advanced HIV infection (CD4 lymphocyte count < 100/mm^3) but also can occur in transplanted patients.[39] The presentation is usually subacute, although dangerous elevations in intracranial pressure sometimes are observed. Space-occupying lesions in the brain may occur with disseminated mold infections. These infections usually arise in the lung, but dissemination to the brain is part of multiorgan spread. Mortality is extremely high. Any of the pathogenic molds[40,41] such as *Aspergillus*,[2] zygomycetes,[42,43] *Scedosporium*,[44] or *Fusarium*[45] can undergo dissemination to the brain. The dimorphic fungi (e.g., *Histoplasma*, *Coccidioides*) also may disseminate from the lung, causing infection of the CNS. Zygomycetes also may be associated with frequently fatal infection arising within the nose or sinuses (rhinocerebral mucormycosis).[42,43]

The most common protozoal pathogen to affect the CNS is *Toxoplasma gondii*. The classic association is between *T. gondii* infection and advanced HIV infection, although cases have been reported associated with other forms of immunocompromise.[46-48] Amebic encephalitis has been reported occasionally in conjunction with advanced HIV infection or organ transplantation.[49]

A variety of viruses can cause CNS infections in immunocompromised patients. Perhaps as a result of the widespread use of antiherpesvirus prophylaxis in many immunocompromised populations, herpes simplex virus (HSV) encephalitis is rare.[50] Some of the newer herpesviruses, such as human herpesvirus-6 (HHV-6), have been associated with neurologic infection in transplant recipients.[51-53] Lack of diagnostic capabilities for these viruses may partially explain their apparent infrequency. CMV meningoencephalitis is well described in patients with advanced HIV infection[54] and occasionally has been reported in transplant recipients.[55] Disseminated infection with varicella-zoster virus (VZV) in immunocompromised patients also may result in CNS infection. West Nile virus may be acquired from transplanted organs or blood transfusions and is associated with a significant meningoencephalitis in transplant recipients.[56,57] Table 137-7 summarizes agents capable of causing CNS infections in an immunocompromised host.

TABLE 137-7	Central Nervous System Infections in the Immunocompromised Host	
Etiologic Agent	*Special Considerations*
Meningitis	
Streptococcus pneumoniae	Especially in HIV-infected individuals
Listeria monocytogenes	Predilection for brainstem
Enteric bacteria	Associated with disseminated *Strongyloides* infection
Cryptococcus neoformans	Rapid diagnosis by cryptococcal antigen or India ink stain
Mycobacterium tuberculosis	Consider PCR for rapid diagnosis
Meningoencephalitis	
HSV	Rare in immunocompromised patients
HHV-6	May be associated with lack of CSF pleocytosis
VZV	Skin lesions yield diagnosis
West Nile virus	Transmitted via transplanted organ or blood
Space-Occupying Lesions	
Nocardia	Pulmonary lesions usually also present
Toxoplasma gondii	Especially in HIV-infected individuals
Fungi	Pulmonary lesions usually also present

CSF, cerebrospinal fluid; *HHV-6*, human herpesvirus-6; *HIV*, human immunodeficiency virus; *HSV*, herpes simplex virus; *PCR*, polymerase chain reaction; *VZV*, varicella-zoster virus.

The wide variety of organisms that could be responsible for CNS infection presents a need for a broadly based diagnostic workup before empirical therapy is begun. If cerebrospinal fluid (CSF) is collected, it should be sent for Gram stain and Ziehl-Neelsen stain for rapid diagnosis of bacterial and mycobacterial infections. PCR can be applied to the diagnosis of most viral infections such as HSV, CMV, and VZV. Cryptococcal antigens can be detected rapidly in CSF, enabling a rapid diagnosis of this form of meningitis, but for patients with space-occupying lesions of the brain, collection of CSF may not be possible. Aspiration may be performed in some circumstances. Before invasive diagnostic testing of the brain is performed, however, the patient's skin is examined for lesions (such as may occur with cryptococcosis or nocardiosis), and the lungs are carefully reviewed by CT. Because most CNS lesions arise from infection in other parts of the body, a diagnosis may often be made more easily by microbiological sampling of these body sites.

GASTROINTESTINAL INFECTIONS

Severe GI infections in immunocompromised patients may occasionally warrant ICU admission because of dehydration or visceral perforation. As with respiratory and CNS infections, the differential diagnosis is usually broad, and a precise diagnosis rarely can be made based on clinical suspicion only. Immunocompromised patients have an increased predisposition to GI infections, depending on the type and degree of immunocompromise and exposure to certain pathogens.

The most commonly involved organisms in the etiology of infective esophagitis or gastritis are *Candida*, CMV, and HSV, although a variety of other organisms (e.g., mycobacteria, zygomycetes) occasionally are implicated. Candidal esophagitis is a common opportunistic infection in patients with AIDS. Rates of about 13.3 events of candidal esophagitis per 100 person-years occur in HIV-infected patients with CD4 counts less than 300/mm^3.[58] A study of renal transplant patients in the United States showed that esophageal candidiasis is the most common fungal infection in these patients, making up 22% of all fungal infections.[59] Other predisposing factors for severe esophageal candidiasis include broad-spectrum antibiotic therapy, steroid therapy, cancer chemotherapy, diabetes mellitus, cutaneous burns, radiotherapy, and hematologic stem cell transplant. Although *Candida albicans* is the most frequently diagnosed organism, there is an increase of other species, including *Candida krusei* and *Candida glabrata*—this is notable because of the increase in resistance to fluconazole in these species. Finally, as noted previously, patients with immunocompromise may have a combination of pathogens causing infection at any one time. Upper GI endoscopy with biopsy is the gold standard for making the diagnosis.

Diarrhea is a common problem in immunocompromised patients with multifactorial etiologies. It may lead to diagnosis of immunosuppression in a previously undiagnosed patient when an opportunistic pathogen is found and appropriately investigated. Severe complications such as malabsorption leading to malnutrition, dehydration, and wasting can occur. Occasionally, intestinal perforation may result from GI infection. In an immunosuppressed patient, it is important to differentiate diarrhea due to opportunistic infections from diarrhea due to neoplasms, GVHD, drugs, and other therapeutic agents. GVHD accounts for more diarrhea in blood and bone marrow transplant patients than infective organisms.[60] In these patients, organisms that cause mild self-limiting disease in the normal host may cause severe and life-threatening infections.[60]

Prolonged use of multiple antibiotics in high doses predisposes patients to colonization with *Clostridium difficile* and development of pseudomembranous colitis. Antibiotic prophylaxis to prevent *P. jirovecii* pneumonia or spontaneous bacterial peritonitis has been associated with *C. difficile*. In addition to the classic antibiotic risk factors of clindamycin or cephalosporin use, fluoroquinolones may predispose to epidemic strains of *C. difficile* (BI/NAP1/027 strain).[61] Enteric bacterial pathogens such as *Salmonella* occur at increased frequency in immunocompromised patients, especially HIV-infected individuals. In some regions of Africa, nontyphoidal *Salmonella* infections are among the most common causes of bacteremia.[62] Severe *Salmonella* infections may be associated with intestinal perforation. *Shigella*, *Campylobacter jejuni*, *E. coli* (enterotoxigenic, enteroadherent, and enteroaggregative), and *Yersinia* species are other bacterial causes of diarrhea, although less commonly associated with bacteremia.

Protozoal infections are seen more commonly in HIV-infected patients than other immunocompromised groups. At CD4 counts less than 200 cells/mm³, patients with HIV infection may present with unusual protozoa (e.g., *Cryptosporidium* and *Microsporidium*). Occasionally these pathogens are also seen in transplant recipients.[63,64] Such pathogens are not detected on routine microscopic examination for ova, cysts, and parasites. Special stains and microbiological techniques are needed. Routine examination usually detects *Giardia lamblia*, *Entamoeba histolytica*, and other more common pathogenic protozoa.

CMV can cause significant colitis in all immunocompromised populations. CMV colitis may occur in the absence of systemic evidence of infection (i.e., PCR on peripheral blood may be negative[65,66]). Intestinal biopsy may be required to make the diagnosis. CMV intestinal infection may present with diarrhea but may have more profound presentations such as intestinal perforation.[67,68]

Finally, mycobacterial infections such as tuberculosis occasionally can be associated with colitis.[69] *M. avium* complex can be grown readily from the feces of patients with HIV infection and CD4 counts of less than 50/mm³, but it is not always the cause of diarrhea in such patients.

Therapeutic Difficulties in Immunocompromised Patients

EMPIRICAL THERAPY

The choice of empirical antimicrobial therapy is often difficult in immunocompromised patients because of the broad differential diagnosis involved. As emphasized earlier, management of infection in an immunocompromised patient can be simplified by narrowing the differential diagnosis by thorough history taking, review of prior medical records, and careful physical examination. Aggressive early diagnostic maneuvers before beginning empirical antimicrobial therapy can enable a definitive diagnosis to be made. Failure to collect specimens before beginning empirical therapy can lead to prolonged, expensive, and unnecessary therapy.

Empirical antibiotic therapy in suspected bacterial infections should be tailored to the individual patient to maximize the chance that the therapy is microbiologically adequate. There is a clear link between microbiologically adequate empirical therapy and successful outcome from infections in the ICU.[70] In settings such as severe pneumonia in the immunocompromised patient, empirical regimens comprising vancomycin, ciprofloxacin, meropenem, amphotericin (or voriconazole), ganciclovir, and trimethoprim/sulfamethoxazole may be necessary to cover potentially lethal infection with methicillin-resistant *Staphylococcus aureus*, *P. aeruginosa*, *Legionella*, fungi, CMV, and *P. jirovecii*. There is no established role for combination empirical therapy with antifungal agents. The decision to start empirical mycobacterial therapy is never an easy one. In general, we only advise it when there is a risk factor for tuberculosis. Empirical therapy for disseminated *Strongyloides* infection may have a place in immunocompromised patients coming from an endemic area and with the classic presentation of disseminated infection.

Immunocompromised patients presenting with acute meningitis should receive treatment that covers *S. pneumoniae* and *L. monocytogenes*. The combination of vancomycin, ampicillin, and ceftriaxone may be necessary (vancomycin and ceftriaxone for multidrug-resistant *S. pneumoniae* and ampicillin for *Listeria*). The combination of amphotericin and 5-flucytosine is recommended empirically for meningitis in which antigen testing or India ink stain of CSF reveals encapsulated fungi consistent with *C. neoformans*. Immunocompromised patients with space-occupying lesions of the brain can be treated empirically with an antifungal drug (amphotericin or voriconazole) if suspicion of disseminated fungal infection is high, although nocardiosis, toxoplasmosis, or mycobacterial infection would not be covered without specific therapy.

For immunocompromised patients with severe diarrhea requiring ICU admission, empirical treatment with metronidazole or oral vancomycin (for *C. difficile*) and ganciclovir (for CMV) may be given after fecal samples have been collected. Colonic biopsy may be necessary if it can be safely performed. For immunocompromised patients with intestinal perforation, antibiotic coverage against gut flora (i.e., treatment of peritonitis) plus treatment of the most likely causes of perforation (e.g., ganciclovir for CMV) may be chosen.

PATHOGEN-DIRECTED THERAPY

The importance of appropriate specimen collection is that empirical therapy can be streamlined (de-escalated) if cultures or other diagnostic tests are positive. With immunocompromised patients, antimicrobial therapy often is complicated by drug interactions or adverse reactions. Transplant recipients taking calcineurin inhibitors (e.g., cyclosporine or tacrolimus) or HIV-infected patients taking protease inhibitors are most at risk because these drugs may be metabolized by the cytochrome P450 system.[71,72] Significant interactions may occur between rifampin, macrolide antibiotics, azole antifungal drugs, and the calcineurin inhibitors.[72] Aggressive treatment of infections in immunocompromised hosts (e.g., with amphotericin, pentamidine, or foscarnet) may be associated with renal dysfunction, compounding the nephrotoxic effects of the calcineurin inhibitors. Antimicrobial agents such as linezolid or ganciclovir frequently cause neutropenia, potentially adding further host defense defects.

Conclusion

Infection is likely to be one of the most significant problems an immunocompromised patient faces. These patients may present with severe infection or acquire infection while critically ill for other reasons. Prevention of infection in the ICU is of primary importance. Pneumonia can be readily prevented by many strategies. Ventilator-associated pneumonia may be prevented by a bundle of interventions.[73] Aspiration of subglottic secretions and selective digestive tract decontamination, while supported by some trials, are still controversial. Opportunistic pneumonia with *P. jirovecii* can be prevented by use of prophylaxis with trimethoprim/sulfamethoxazole, dapsone, or nebulized pentamidine. Environmental exposure to *Legionella* and

Aspergillus spp. can be prevented by ensuring water purification techniques (e.g., copper-silver ionization) and by preventing exposure of patients to construction activity. Infections due to pathogens transmitted human to human, such as *M. tuberculosis*, can be prevented by isolation precautions.

Many extrapulmonary infections can also be prevented. CMV infection can be prevented by universal prophylaxis with ganciclovir, valganciclovir, valacyclovir, or a preemptive approach using serial PCR of peripheral blood.[74,75] A similar preemptive approach may be useful in preventing aspergillosis by monitoring peripheral blood for the galactomannan antigen, although this remains controversial.[76,77] *C. difficile* infection is difficult to prevent because there is a clear need for antibiotic therapy for immunocompromised patients with infection. The increasing incidence, severity, and high rate of recurrence of *C. difficile* infection has become a significant problem.[78] A recent randomized controlled study demonstrated that the addition of monoclonal antibodies against *C. difficile* toxins to antibiotic agents significantly reduced the recurrence of *C. difficile* infection, even among patients with the epidemic BI/NAP1/027 strain.[79] Finally, attention to classic infection control practices such as appropriate immunizations,[80-82] hand hygiene, and contact isolation is paramount in immunocompromised patients.

KEY POINTS

1. The degree of immunocompromise in a patient is a guide to the likelihood of particular opportunistic infections and may be indicated by the type and timing of immunosuppressive therapy and, in human immunodeficiency virus (HIV)-infected patients, by the CD4 lymphocyte count and viral load.

2. Environmental exposures can be important predictors of infection type. Travel history and exposure to *Mycobacterium tuberculosis*, *Aspergillus*, or *Legionella* are important considerations.

3. The differential diagnosis of opportunistic lung infection in immunocompromised hosts is so broad that bronchoscopy with bronchoalveolar lavage, before antimicrobial therapy, is highly desirable.

4. Central nervous system (CNS) lesions in immunocompromised hosts are often the result of disseminated infection. Careful examination of the skin, with biopsy of suspicious lesions, and computed tomography of the lungs may obviate the need for brain biopsy.

5. Antimicrobial therapy in immunocompromised hosts is beset by difficulties with drug interactions and adverse effects. Increased frequency of monitoring of immunosuppressive drug levels is essential.

ANNOTATED REFERENCES

Fishman JA. Infection in solid-organ transplant recipients. N Engl J Med 2007;357:2601-14.
This review article is suitable to comprehensively understand management of infections associated with solid-organ transplantation. It describes clinical problems related to the use of solid-organ transplants, potential drug interactions with medications commonly used in the ICU, and controversies surrounding the use of antiretroviral therapy in the ICU.

Huang L, Quartin A, Jones D, Havlir DV. Intensive care of patients with HIV infection. N Engl J Med 2006;355:173-81.
Antiretroviral therapy has changed the long-term prognosis and clinical spectrum of diseases in patients with HIV infection who are admitted to the ICU.

Keane J, Gershon S, Wise RP, et al. Tuberculosis associated with infliximab, a tumor necrosis factor-α neutralizing agent. N Engl J Med 2001;345:1098-104.
Although patients with rheumatoid arthritis may become immunocompromised by way of therapy with corticosteroids or methotrexate, the development of anticytokine agents for this condition has opened the way for a new range of opportunistic infections in this patient population. This study showed that tuberculosis occurs with increased frequency in patients receiving infliximab.

Kotton CN, Kumar D, Caliendo AM, et al. International consensus guidelines on the management of CMV in solid organ transplantation. Transplantation 2010;89:779-95.
CMV is one of the most common infections after solid-organ transplantation, resulting in significant morbidity and mortality. However, management of CMV varies considerably among transplant centers. This evidence and expert opinion-based guidelines include topics on diagnostics, immunology, prevention, treatment, resistance, and pediatrics.

Kowalski R, Post D, Schneider MC, et al. Immune cell function testing: an adjunct to therapeutic drug monitoring in transplant patient management. Clin Transplant 2003;17:77-88.
The degree of immunocompromise and the subsequent risk of infection in transplant recipients have been difficult to quantify. This study examined the utility of an in vitro immune cell function assay as a means of quantifying global immune response in transplant recipients.

REFERENCES

Access the complete reference list online at http://www.expertconsult.com.

138

Infectious Endocarditis

ANASTASIA ANTONIADOU | HELEN GIAMARELLOU

Infectious endocarditis (IE) is a rare disease with an incidence of 3 to 10 episodes per 100,000 person-years, varying between countries and increasing dramatically with age. It is presently classified by mode of acquisition (healthcare-associated IE [nosocomial and non-nosocomial], community acquired, and IE in intravenous drug users [IVDU]), by localization as left- or right-sided prosthetic or native valve IE, or as device related (e.g., pacemaker or cardioverter defibrillator). The new classification of *healthcare-associated infectious endocarditis* (HAIE) includes patients hospitalized for more than 48 hours before symptoms of IE develop (previously called *nosocomial IE* [NIE]) or patients with symptoms less than 48 hours after admission but with extensive healthcare contact defined as: (1) home-based nursing or IV therapy, hemodialysis, or IV chemotherapy fewer than 30 days before onset of IE symptoms, (2) hospitalization fewer than 90 days before onset of IE, or (3) residency in a nursing home or a long-term care facility. The definition of HAIE applies both to native (NVE) and prosthetic valve endocarditis (PVE). Early prosthetic valve endocarditis (now defined as presenting <1 year post surgery) has a portion included in the HAIE definition.[1]

HAIE was estimated to have occured in 0.8 of 10,000 hospital admissions and is often diagnosed late during hospitalization (39 ± 25 days).[2] When compared with the 2.5 million cases (at least) of nosocomial infections occurring per year in the United States, the overall incidence of HAIE seems low,[2] but the associated morbidity and high mortality renders HAIE of great importance for the clinician. The current in-hospital mortality rate for patients with IE is 15% to 20%, with 1-year mortality approaching 40%.[3]

Healthcare-Associated Native Valve Endocarditis

During the past decade, 14% to 25% of all cases of IE have been considered nosocomial. It is, however, expected that the incidence will increase in the future because of (1) an increase in the incidence of nosocomial bacteremia, (2) improvement in survival of immunocompromised patients, (3) the steady increase in the number of ICU beds admitting seriously ill patients worldwide, and (4) the improved survival rate of elderly patients in whom degenerative heart disease and/or prosthetic valves are more frequently encountered.[2] The current understanding of HAIE has been based primarily on retrospective studies with small sample size. New data emerged from the International Collaboration on Endocarditis Prospective Cohort Study (ICE-PCS) from 61 medical centers in 28 countries.[4] From this database, as defined by the modified Duke criteria, native valve IE in patients without IV drug abuse was recognized in 1622 patients. Of these patients, 1065 had community-acquired infection, and 557 (34%) had healthcare-associated native valve endocarditis (HANVE), consistent with the contemporary high incidence of healthcare-associated infection.[5] Almost half of these infections were acquired outside of the hospital, a result consistent with previous reports of healthcare-associated bacteremia. Compared with patients with community-acquired IE, patients with HANVE more often have comorbid conditions such as diabetes mellitus, cancer, or long-term immunosuppressive therapy. Fever is the most common presenting feature, but physical signs of IE present more rarely in HANVE, suggesting a more acute course. Non-nosocomial acquisition of HANVE is most often dependent on hemodialysis or an

intravascular catheter (54%), while patients with nosocomial acquisition more often have preexisting valvular disease or undergo a nondental invasive medical procedure. The mitral valve is most frequently involved, followed by the tricuspid and aortic valve.[4]

Staphylococci (both *Staphylococcus aureus* and coagulase-negative strains) represent the major pathogens in HAIE. *S. aureus* is responsible for 52% to 57% of HAIE episodes, 91% of which have an intravascular device as the most probable source of bacteremia.[2] In the ICE-PCS study, *S. aureus* was the most common pathogen in HANVE, among which 47% was methicillin-resistant *S. aureus* (MRSA).[4] The second most common bacteria was enterococci (15%), followed by coagulase-negative strains of staphylococci (13%). MRSA is more prevalent in hospital-acquired infections (57% versus 41% of HANVE acquired outside the hospital).[4] Among coagulase-negative strains of staphylococci, *Staphylococcus lugdunensis* deserves attention because it behaves like *S. aureus* with high virulence, has a 50% probability of complicated infection when isolated in blood, and an aggressive course when it is the cause of IE.[6]

Gram-negative bacilli are rare causes of HANVE despite the fact that they cause lethal bacteremias in hospitals, probably as a result of their decreased ability to adhere to heart valves and susceptibility to bactericidal action of serum.[2,7] Fungal infectious endocarditis is a rare infection, comprising in total less than 10% of IE cases, with a mortality rate ranging from 36% to 50%. However, increased frequency of fungal endocarditis has been observed in recent years, attributed to the increasing use of vascular lines, as well as to noncardiac surgery and increased numbers of immunocompromised patients.[8] The fungi most commonly associated with endocarditis are *Candida albicans*, non-*albicans* species of *Candida*, *Aspergillus* spp., and *Histoplasma capsulatum*. In the past decade, the incidence of *Candida parapsilosis* HAIE has increased and is attributed to (1) frequent colonization by this organism of the skin and subungual area, (2) ability of the pathogen to proliferate in glucose-containing solutions (hyperalimentation), (3) ability of the organism to adhere to synthetic material because of slime production, and (4) contamination of intravascular pressure monitoring devices.[2]

In contradistinction to *Candida* spp., in which blood cultures in cases of IE are positive in 83% to 95% of cases, blood cultures are positive in only 11% or less of patients with *Aspergillus* spp. In cases of *Curvularia*, *Penicillium*, and *Phycomyces* infection, blood cultures are usually 100% negative. In cases in which *Coccidioides immitis*, *Cryptococcus neoformans*, *Rhodotorula*, and *Saccharomyces cerevisiae* are involved, blood cultures are usually positive if properly collected.[2,8]

In cases of fungal endocarditis, prolonged symptoms before hospitalization and embolization of major arteries are classic findings. However, diagnosis is delayed or missed in 82% of patients.[8,9] For fungal endocarditis to be diagnosed early, it should be considered in the differential diagnosis and echocardiography performed, which then demonstrates large, bulky vegetations. Peripheral blood cultures should be obtained and accessible embolic specimens subjected to histologic examination.[9,10]

HANVE has higher mortality compared to community-acquired IE (25% versus 13%). In HANVE, factors recognized to be independently associated with increased risk of death are increased age (>60), diabetes, *S. aureus* infection, paravalvular abscess, stroke, heart failure, and new conduction abnormality. Cardiac surgery during the IE episode is found to be associated with lower mortality.[4] Therefore, in addition to appropriate antimicrobial therapy, early surgical intervention is often mandatory. In fungal endocarditis, removal of the infected valve is indicated, followed by postsurgical prophylaxis with oral azoles for 2 or more years and prolonged surveillance to detect relapses.[9,10]

Special consideration should be given to chronic hemodialysis (HD) patients, in whom IE is significantly more common (16-18 times) and causes greater morbidity and mortality. In this group of patients, IE is the second leading cause of death after cardiovascular disease, and it has been proposed to be added as a fifth category in classification by acquisition.[11,12] In the ICE-PCS study, 63% of HANVE were HD patients.[4] S. aureus was the pathogen in 75% to 80% of cases, half of which were MRSA. Fever may not be present, and blood cultures may less often be positive, complicating diagnosis by the Duke criteria. Mortality remains high: 30% during the first month, about 65% during the first year, and reaching more than 70% if cardiac surgery is indicated. Age older than 65, diabetes as the cause of renal failure, mitral involvement, large vegetations, septic emboli, and infections due to MRSA or VRE have been identified as risk factors for mortality.[11]

For methicillin-sensitive S. aureus (MSSA), antistaphylococcal penicillins should be the treatment of choice, whereas in cases of MRSA with minimum inhibitory concentration (MIC) over 1 mg/L to vancomycin, antimicrobial choices include daptomycin and linezolid.[1] If vancomycin is indicated, drug levels should be followed, with trough levels of 25 to 30 mg/L required for efficacy.[13]

Healthcare-Associated Prosthetic Valve Endocarditis

PVE accounts for 9.5% to 20% of all cases of IE, with mortality rates ranging between 25% and 60%.[14] It is a distinct and important form of IE because more than 100,000 artificial heart valves are implanted annually in the United States, and eradicating infection on foreign material is a major therapeutic challenge which as a rule necessitates their surgical removal.[14]

It has been reported that "early" PVE (within 1 year of implantation) is found less often with porcine than mechanical valves, whereas it is almost absent from homografts. However, studies with long-term follow-up have suggested that no significant differences exist in the incidence of PVE related to the valve type.[14] As noted, PVE has been classified as *early* or *late*, with the former occurring within 12 months of implantation.[1] Contamination of prosthetic valves during this early period occurs either directly at the time of implantation by a break in sterile surgical techniques or via transient episodes of bacteremia, emanating mostly from infected intravascular catheters and wound or skin infections while the patient is still hospitalized, therefore representing a real nosocomial infection.[14] In the early postoperative period, the sewn ring and the valve annulus are not yet endothelialized and are therefore a site of thrombus formation and a target for adherence of bacteria. Transient bacteremia can seed these thrombi and incite infection, leading to the formation of large vegetations that may cause functional obstruction or incompetence. As the infection advances, abscesses, fistulas, and progressive annular destruction may further complicate the underlying process, causing conduction blocks, mycotic aortic aneurysms, and even purulent pericarditis.[14]

PVE may manifest as an indolent illness with low-grade fever and immune-mediated manifestations or as a fulminant acute febrile disease with hypotension. When early PVE is caused by S. aureus, the clinical picture is accompanied in more than 40% of cases by central nervous system (CNS) and intracardiac complications and a subsequent mortality ranging from 42% to 85%.[15] The microbiology of PVE is shown in Table 138-1. In the ICE-PCS study, 556 definite cases of PVE were found among 2670 cases of IE (20%), with 36.5% being healthcare-associated prosthetic valve endocarditis (HAPVE) and 70% acquired in the hospital.[16] Of the cases of PVE, 71% were diagnosed during the first year post surgery and the majority after day 60 (median on day 84). In 43% of HAPVE, an intravascular device was in place. S. aureus was the most common pathogen in PVE, with higher incidence in cases with HAPVE (34% and 13.3% MRSA), followed by coagulase-negative staphylococci.[16]

TABLE 138-1	Etiology of Prosthetic Valve Endocarditis Versus Nosocomial Native Valve Endocarditis			
	Native Valve Endocarditis		**Prosthetic Valve Endocarditis**	
	Healthcare Associated	*Community Acquired*	*Early (<12 mo)*	*Late (>12 mo)*
Streptococcus species	8%	28%	3.8%	20%
Enterococcus species	15%	9%	7.5%	12.7%
Staphylococcus aureus	45%	20%	36%	18%
MRSA	47%	12%	19%	3.3%
Coagulase-negative *Staphylococcus*	13%	6%	17%	19.9%
Gram-negative bacilli*			3%	1.2%
HACEK*			0%	2.1%
Fungi*			9.4%	3.3%
Culture negative	5%	11%	11.2%	12.4%

Modified from Benito N, Miró JM, de Lazzari E et al. Health care–associated native valve endocarditis: importance of non-nosocomial acquisition. Ann Intern Med 2009;150:586-94; and from Wolff M, Witchitz S, Chastang C et al. Prosthetic valve endocarditis in the ICU: prognostic factors of overall survival in a series of 122 cases and consequences for treatment decision. Chest 1995;108:688-94.

*Rare; approximately 2% among all cases of native valve endocarditis.
HACEK, *Haemophilus* spp. (*H. parainfluenzae, H. aphrophilus, H. paraphrophilus*), *Actinobacillus actinomycetemcomitans, Cardiobacterium hominis, Eikenella corrodens, Kingella* spp.; MRSA, methicillin-resistant *Staphylococcus aureus*.

Recent progress in transesophageal echocardiography (TEE), by applying a high-resolution biplane or multiplane transducer, has enhanced the diagnostic approach to PVE. Studies have demonstrated that the sensitivity of TEE in the diagnosis of PVE ranges from 90% to 100% versus 40% to 63% with transthoracic echocardiography (TTE).[17,18]

The Duke criteria have been used effectively to diagnose PVE, particularly when TEE is used to supplement non-diagnostic TTE.[1]

Mortality in PVE is still substantial, being higher in early PVE (77%) than in late-onset infection (42%). The leading causes of death in early PVE are septic shock (36%), congestive heart failure (29%), and renal failure (21%).[2,19,20] In the ICE-PCS study, overall mortality for PVE was 22.8%, with the mortality from HAPVE being higher at 30.5%. Other factors related to increased risk of death were older age, S. aureus as the pathogen, and complications such as heart failure, stroke, intracardiac abscess, and persistent bacteremia.[16] The survival rate with medical therapy alone in cases of moderate to severe chronic cardiac failure due to prosthesis dysfunction is almost nil. However, valve replacement in this group plus antimicrobial therapy will achieve a survival rate of 44% to 64%.[21] It is noteworthy that PVE recurs in only 6% to 15% of patients who are operated on with active bacterial invasive infection. After surgery for removal of the infected prosthetic valve, antibiotics should be continued for at least 6 weeks.[14]

Infective Endocarditis in the ICU

Few studies have focused on IE acquired or admitted in the ICU. The most recent studies to report on ICU-IE are those of Mourvillier et al.[22] and Saydain et al.[23] Confirming the high morbidity and mortality rates for this subset of patients requiring ICU admission, Mourvillier et al. reported 228 patients admitted to the ICU with IE. In that study, 36% of patients had PVE, with S. aureus as the predominant pathogen. The overall mortality was 45%, and factors strongly associated with outcome included septic shock, cerebral emboli, immunocompromised state, and cardiac surgery. Most complications occurred early during the course of IE. Surgical treatment appeared to improve in-hospital outcome.[22] Saydain et al. reported 33 patients with IVDU-IE requiring admission in the ICU because of severe sepsis or septic shock (36%), respiratory failure (33%), or neurologic deterioration (18%). S. aureus was found in 94% of cases, while 15% were polymicrobial. Of the patients, 45% had septic emboli. In-hospital mortality was 27%, and the risk of death increased with a history of previous IE and a high APACHE

II score.[23] Gouëllo and associates[24] examined 4416 ICU hospitalized patients during a 6-year period (1992-1997) and described 22 patients with ICU-IE defined by the Duke criteria, among which 16 were acquired in the ICU. The prevalence was 5 cases per 1000 admissions. The time elapsed between admission in the ICU and subsequent diagnosis for ICU-IE was generally quite prolonged (range, 11 to 100 days; mean, 39 ± 25 days). In 21 of the 22 cases, IE was the consequence of bacteremia related to a medical or surgical procedure; *S. aureus* was the causal organism for IE in 77% of patients, and *P. aeruginosa*, *Streptococcus* spp., and *Candida* spp. were also isolated. All patients were febrile. In only 9 of the 22 patients was a new murmur found, whereas in 2 and 1, respectively, embolic events and cardiac failure were observed.[24]

The expected classic clinical features of IE are often not present in ICU patients. For instance, central nervous system (CNS) signs due to sedation may be blunted, and manifestations of renal failure are usually attributed to septic multiple organ dysfunction syndrome.

Because the risk of HAIE is proportionally increased with the duration of hospitalization, the diagnosis of IE should always be suspected in the presence of fever of unknown origin with positive blood cultures after a prolonged stay in the ICU. The latter suspicion is strengthened in patients with prosthetic valves, in those undergoing procedures that may damage the right side of the heart, and whenever bacteremia lasts for more than 72 hours after catheter removal and/or positive blood cultures persist 3 days after starting appropriate antimicrobials.[25]

In several studies, the diagnostic value of echocardiography in the diagnosis of IE and particularly of the transesophageal view has been pointed out.[17] In case of a negative TEE, if clinical suspicion is high, a second examination has been advocated.[1] It should be noted that TEE provides an advantageous acoustic window in mechanically ventilated patients in comparison to TTE, where visualization may be poor. Significant complications such as bronchospasm, hypoxemia, angina pectoris, pharyngeal bleeding, vomiting, and hematemesis have been reported in fewer than 4% of ventilated patients subjected to TEE.[26]

HAIE in the ICU requires prompt initiation of antimicrobial therapy and cardiosurgical evaluation, keeping in mind that mortality increases sharply with *S. aureus* as a pathogen, with age, and with the origin of the infection (i.e., ICU-acquired versus community acquired). Of note, treatment duration of catheter-related staphylococcal (*S. aureus*) bacteremia aiming to treat successfully any seeded valve—as occurs in 23% of the cases—should never be shorter than 2 weeks, and echocardiography should be performed before treatment discontinuation. Otherwise, a treatment duration of 4 weeks has been recommended.[27]

Prophylaxis of HAIE, especially in ICU patients, mandates (1) IV access and intravascular procedures to be performed with aseptic care, (2) IV and intraarterial catheters to remain in place for as brief a duration as possible, and (3) tunnelization, although a controversial issue, to be considered either as an immediate approach for temporary dialysis catheters or as a systemic procedure if the catheter has been or will be in place for more than 4 days.[28] Antimicrobial prophylaxis is not justified before performing TEE.[1]

KEY POINTS

1. ICU infectious endocarditis (ICU-IE) shares overlapping characteristics with healthcare-associated infectious endocarditis (HAIE) and is either acquired in the ICU or is an emergency necessitating critical care. *HAIE is defined as IE occurring 48 hours or more after admission to the hospital or earlier but is related to extensive healthcare contact (hemodialysis, hospitalization in the previous 90 days, home-based therapy, or residency in a nursing home or long-term care facility). It is characterized by a low incidence but high morbidity and mortality.*

2. HAIE can involve either native valves (NVE) or prosthetic valves (PVE). Mitral involvement is most often encountered, and medical/surgical interventions and instrumentation (e.g., intravascular devices, pacemakers) are the usual risk factors.

3. Major pathogens in HAIE (90%) include staphylococci (*S. aureus*, with increasing rates of MRSA, and *Enterococcus* spp. as the second most common pathogen).

4. Mortality of HAIE is higher in the elderly, in patients with *S. aureus* and fungal endocarditis, and in patients with complications (heart failure, stroke, intracardiac abscess, persistent bacteremia). Early surgical intervention is mandatory and may improve in-hospital outcome.

5. Fungal endocarditis is rare, presenting as a complication of intravascular instrumentation or surgery or in the context of an immunocompromised state. *Candida* is the most common fungal causative agent. Delayed diagnosis, major embolic phenomena, and large vegetations are the rule. Combined surgical and medical treatment of long duration is needed to ameliorate the high (>50%) mortality rate.

6. Prosthetic valve–associated endocarditis (PVE) is classified as early (<1 year) or late, with approximately 70% of the cases being early and healthcare acquired. *S. aureus* is the predominating pathogen and is an independent factor for increased risk of death.

7. Transesophageal echocardiography (TEE) has enhanced our diagnostic approach in HAIE (NVE or PVE), especially when the Duke diagnostic clinical criteria are effectively used.

8. ICU-acquired infectious endocarditis has a low but increasing incidence. It appears long after admission and is related to medical or surgical procedures and devices, with *S. aureus* being the predominating pathogen. Prolonged fever may be the only clinical feature, and TEE is a sensitive tool for effective diagnosis. Patients with IE requiring critical care present with early and serious complications and have a high overall mortality (45%).

9. The diagnosis of HAIE requires a high degree of suspicion and should prompt early initiation of antimicrobial therapy and evaluation for early valve replacement as soon as this is indicated (by complication or pathogen type).

ANNOTATED REFERENCES

Task Force on the Prevention, Diagnosis, and Treatment of Infective Endocarditis of the European Society of Cardiology (ESC). Guidelines on the prevention, diagnosis, and treatment of infective endocarditis. Eur Heart J 2009;30:2369-413.
Comprehensive review gathering all recent evidence-based knowledge and guidelines (for Europe) about diagnosis, treatment, and prevention of IE.

Giamarellou H. Nosocomial cardiac infections. J Hosp Infect 2002;50:91-105.
This comprehensive review of nosocomial infectious endocarditis includes risk factors, microbiology, types of infection, diagnosis, treatment, and prophylaxis.

Benito N, Miró JM, de Lazzari E, et al. Health care–associated native valve endocarditis: importance of non-nosocomial acquisition. Ann Intern Med 2009;150:586-94.
Contemporary data about HAIE from the biggest multinational database on infectious endocarditis.

Wang A, Athan E, Pappas EA, et al. Contemporary clinical profile and outcome of prosthetic valve endocarditis. JAMA 2007;297:1354-61.
The most recent data about PVE from the biggest multinational database in infectious endocarditis.

Nucifora G, Badano LP, Viale P, et al. Infective endocarditis in chronic haemodialysis patients: an increasing clinical challenge. Eur Heart J 2007;28:2307-12.
The most common HAIE acquired outside hospitals merits special attention because of some unique characteristics.

Mourvillier B, Trouillet JL, Timsit JF, et al. Infective endocarditis in the intensive care unit: clinical spectrum and prognostic factors in 228 consecutive patients. Intensive Care Med 2004;30:2046-52.
Large retrospective study revealing the profile and prognosis of IE patients admitted to the ICU.

Saydain G, Singh J, Dalal B, et al. Outcome of patients with injection drug use–associated endocarditis admitted to an intensive care unit. J Crit Care 2010;25:248-53.
A small but unique retrospective series of IE in IVDU patients admitted to an ICU.

Gouëllo JP, Asfar P, Brenet O, et al. Nosocomial endocarditis in the intensive care unit: an analysis of 22 cases. Crit Care Med 2000;28:377-81.
A prospective cohort study of clinical features, microbiology, diagnosis, and outcome of infectious endocarditis acquired in an ICU. Retrospective analysis of ICU patients with prosthetic valve endocarditis, including prognostic factors and treatment outcome.

REFERENCES

Access the complete reference list online at http://www.expertconsult.com.

139

Fungal Infections

PAUL O. GUBBINS

Medical advances continue to improve the prognosis of patients with cancer and other immunodeficiencies. In the past 50 years, the field of transplantation has greatly impacted the management of patients with cancer, renal, cardiac, and liver diseases. Moreover, advances in neonatology continue to increase the survival of premature infants. Undoubtedly these advances have benefited society greatly, but they have also fueled the emergence of systemic mycoses. *Candida* species first appeared as significant nosocomial pathogens approximately 30 years ago.[1] For 2 decades, infections due to these pathogens increased dramatically. With the establishment of the National Healthcare Safety Network (NHSN) in 2005, several Centers for Disease Control and Prevention (CDC) surveillance systems, including the Nosocomial Infections Surveillance System (NNIS), were phased out. The NHSN provides broader surveillance data of healthcare-associated infections than the NNIS, thus the results of the two systems are not exactly comparable. Although the surveillance methods have changed, the trends have not. NHSN pathogen distribution data for 2006-2007 were comparable to that of the NNIS reports from 1986-1999.[2]

Fungal infections among critically ill patients are primarily due to *Candida* spp. However, infections caused by other opportunistic fungal pathogens including *Aspergillus*, *Fusarium*, *Cryptococcus neoformans*, and agents of zygomycosis also occur in select critically ill populations (e.g., solid-organ transplant [SOT], hematopoietic stem cell recipients, and acquired immunodeficiency syndrome [AIDS] patients). Moreover, primary or endemic mycosis caused by *Blastomyces dermatitidis*, *Histoplasma capsulatum*, and *Coccidioides immitis* can cause severe disseminated infection in immunocompetent or compromised hosts.

Fungal infections are generally more prevalent in ICUs than on the general medical wards.[3] The importance of effective preventive measures against systemic mycosis is widely appreciated in critically ill oncology patients or hematopoietic stem cell transplant (HSCT) recipients. As our understanding of these infections in the general intensive care unit (ICU) setting continues to improve, so too does the ability to institute appropriate preventive measures. In the past decade, the development of agents possessing either a different mode or broader spectrum of activity, less toxicity, or a reduced propensity to interact with other drugs has increased the number of available systemic antifungal agents. Consequently, clinicians can now tailor antifungal therapy to specific patients. Moreover, our understanding of antifungal pharmacodynamics is developing, and methods to measure antifungal susceptibility are improving.

Fungal Infections in the Critically Ill

CANDIDA INFECTIONS IN THE ICU

Epidemiology

Candida albicans remains the fourth most common pathogen of healthcare-associated infections, and only coagulase-negative staphylococci, *Staphylococcus aureus*, and enterococci are more common.[2] *Candida* spp. have consistently caused a substantial disease burden for at least the past decade. ICUs have a higher incidence of *Candida* bloodstream infections (BSIs) than medical and surgical wards.[3] Although prior data had suggested the frequency of *Candida* BSIs among ICU patients in the United States had declined, estimates from national secondary databases and population-based studies suggest the

disease burden may be shifting from the ICU to the general hospital population.[1]

C. albicans remains the most common invasive *Candida* spp. worldwide.[4] However, decreasing trends in the isolation of this species over time have been observed in the ICU and non-ICU setting.[4,5] An increased prevalence of *C. albicans* and *Candida parapsilosis* among neonatal ICU patients and an increasing prevalence of *Candida glabrata* infections among adults has been widely appreciated.[1,4,5] *C. albicans* is responsible for approximately 45% of episodes of candidemia.[6] The incidence of infection due to a particular *Candida* sp. varies considerably by the clinical service on which the patient is hospitalized. However, in general, *C. albicans* is the primary fungal pathogen in the ICU setting and is followed by *C. glabrata*, *C. parapsilosis*, *Candida tropicalis*, *Candida krusei*, and other *Candida* spp. (i.e., *Candida guilliermondii*, *Candida lusitaniae*, etc.).[6] This rank order varies little across infection site, but it may vary with age.[1,4-6] Surveillance data have noted that candidemia in neonatal ICUs is predominantly due to *C. albicans* and *C. parapsilosis* and rarely due to *C. glabrata* or other *Candida* spp.[1,4-6] Surveillance studies have demonstrated that BSI due to *C. albicans* occurs less frequently with increasing age.[1,4-6] In contrast, *C. glabrata* is rarely isolated among infants and children but is more frequently found with increasing patient age.[1,4-6]

C. albicans is part of the normal flora of the gastrointestinal tract. Infections including BSIs caused by most *Candida* spp., particularly *C. albicans*, arise endogenously from the gastrointestinal mucosa, skin, and urinary tract.[7] Invasive *Candida* infections occur when alteration of endogenous flora leads to overgrowth of yeast which, in the presence compromised skin or gastrointestinal mucosa integrity, translocates from its commensal environment to the bloodstream.[7] *Candida* spp., including *C. albicans*, may be transmitted exogenously in ICU settings.[8,9] Exogenous transmission of non-*albicans Candida* spp. through indirect contact with the ICU environment occurs commonly.[8] For example, *C. parapsilosis* is an exogenous pathogen known for its ability to form biofilms on catheters and inert devices. *C. parapsilosis* persists in the nosocomial environment.[10] Moreover, it is spread throughout the hospital through hand carriage by healthcare workers.[10] Therefore, colonization with this pathogen is not a prerequisite for infection.[10]

Mortality

Candida BSIs are often difficult to detect. Symptomatically, BSIs due to *Candida* spp. are indistinguishable from BSIs of bacterial etiology. *Candida* spp. are cleared from the blood very efficiently by several organs, particularly the liver, and blood cultures yield positive results in only 50% of patients with hematogenously disseminated candidiasis. However, the ability of automated blood culture systems to recover *Candida* spp. has continued to improve. For example, in a simulated candidemia study, *Candida* spp. were isolated in 74% (479/648) of blood culture bottles.[11] However, isolation rates were highest in aerobic blood and mycology culture bottles (98% [211/216] and 97% [210/216], respectively) but lowest in anaerobic culture bottles (27% [58/216]).[11] The ability to detect growth improved as inoculum size increased.[11] Although the time to detect growth varied with *Candida* spp., most species were detected within 24 to 48 hours. Growth was detected faster in aerobic and mycology culture bottles than in anaerobic bottles. These data and other studies demonstrated the improved ability of current technology to detect simulated or clinical candidemia due to most common and uncommon *Candida* pathogens in aerobic cultures.[11,12]

Even with improved ability to recover *Candida* spp. from the blood, *Candida* BSIs carry a relatively poor prognosis. *Candida* spp. isolated from the blood have consistently been identified as an independent predictor of mortality.[13-15] The overall attributable mortality of nosocomial BSIs among critically ill patients is 35%.[16] This mortality rate for nosocomial BSIs in the ICU setting is comparable to the mortality rate associated with BSIs due to *Candida* spp. Historically, the estimated crude mortality rate associated with *Candida* BSIs hospital-wide and in the ICU setting has ranged from 35% to 69%, while the estimated attributable mortality has been 38%.[14,17]

Recent estimates suggest that the attributable mortality due to candidemia and other forms of invasive candidiasis ranges from 10% to approximately 50%.[1] Moreover, data demonstrate that despite the advent of potent and safer anti-*Candida* antifungal therapy, the risk mortality associated with candidemia has essentially remained unchanged for at least 2 decades.[19,20] Inadequate treatment may be a reason why mortality has not improved despite the availability of potent and safe antifungal therapy. Inadequate therapy resulting from delays in administration, treatment with an agent to which the organism is resistant, inadequate dosing or treatment duration, or failure to recognize and treat candidemia all contribute to the mortality associated with *Candida* BSI.[21-27] In particular, it is increasingly clear that delaying initiation of adequate antifungal therapy even 12 to 48 hours is independently associated with mortality in candidemia patients.[22,23,26,28,29]

Candidemia produces significant morbidity and adds as much as a month to the length of hospital stay.[1,7] Given the severity of illness associated with this infection, the added length of stay utilizes significant healthcare resources. Considering the incidence of candidemia in the United States alone, it is not surprising that the estimated annual healthcare costs associated with this infection easily exceed $1 billion.[20]

Risk Factors

Among critically ill patients, risk factors for *Candida* infections are well described.[30,31] Broad-spectrum antimicrobial use, colonization, indwelling vascular catheters, and hemodialysis have been consistently identified as independent risk factors for *Candida* BSIs.[14] In most ICU settings, many of these risk factors are commonly present and unavoidable. The ICU itself provides an ideal environment for transmission of *Candida* spp. among patients, thus it is not surprising that prolonged ICU stay has been identified as an independent risk factor.[32] A study using validated risk factors in a simulated ICU population demonstrated that in the presence of multiple risk factors, the probability of infection increases exponentially.[32] For example, in a hypothetical critical care unit, if a patient had prior exposure to 4 antibiotic classes, the calculated risk of candidemia for that patient would range from 5% to 35%, depending on the overall baseline candidemia rate in the ICU, varying between 1% and 5%. However, if that same hypothetical patient subsequently had *Candida* spp. cultured from another (nonbloodstream) anatomic site, the calculated risk would increase substantially to 40% to 80%.[32] Given how common many of the risk factors (such as indwelling catheters, antibiotics, immunosuppressants, and TPN) are in the ICU, these data illustrate the need to accurately predict or identify patients who truly are at risk so that therapy can be instituted as early as possible.

The risk factors for non–*C. albicans* and *C. albicans* BSIs are similar, and the probability of a patient having either infection cannot be differentiated based on clinical characteristics alone.[30,31] Several studies have developed prediction rules to stratify patients at increased risk for developing invasive infections with either *C. albicans* or non-*albicans Candida* spp. in hopes of providing guidance for clinical decision making to prevent candidemia in the ICU. These prediction rules are based upon retrospective studies and assess the combination of ICU length of stay, prior *Candida* colonization, and other host risks.[33-36] While these systems demonstrate risk stratification is possible, they are somewhat complicated to apply, and some have questioned the practicality of certain components of individual prediction rules.[31,37] Using the database from a large prospective multicenter Spanish study in which fungal colonization was assessed weekly along with other potential risk factors, León and colleagues developed the "*Candida* Score" based upon four independent risk factors: multifocal *Candida* spp. colonization, surgery upon ICU admission, severe sepsis, and total parenteral nutrition (TPN). The score, obtained by adding the statistical weight of each risk factor, has a cutoff value of 2.5, providing a sensitivity of 81% and specificity of 74% for identifying patients with current or future candidal infection. Patients with a score greater than 2.5 were more than 7 times as likely to have proven infection as patients with a *Candida* Score up to 2.5.[35] A prospective multicenter observational study demonstrated that a *Candida* Score ≥3 discriminated between colonization and invasive candidiasis in non-neutropenic ICU patients colonized with *Candida* spp., with a minimum length of ICU stay of 7 days.[37] These data lend credence to the idea of using the *Candida* Score for guiding the start of empirical antifungal therapy in the ICU. However, even though the *Candida* Score is promising, the clinical utility of such prediction rules in establishing the benefit of targeted antifungal prophylaxis remains to be established in prospective studies.[38]

OPPORTUNISTIC FUNGAL INFECTIONS IN IMMUNOCOMPROMISED CRITICALLY ILL PATIENTS

Invasive Aspergillosis in Critically Ill Patients with Hematologic Malignancies

In contrast to *Candida* spp., the burden of infection due to *Aspergillus* spp. is small.[1] National hospital discharge data from the 1990s through 2003 reveal that there are approximately 10,000 aspergillosis-related hospitalizations annually in the United States.[1] Nonetheless, *Aspergillus* spp. cause infection in critically ill populations immunocompromised by burns, cytotoxic chemotherapy, prolonged corticosteroid therapy, malignancy, leukemia, SOT or HSCT, and other congenital or acquired immunodeficiencies. *Aspergillus* spp. are ubiquitous environmental molds. While several hundred species of *Aspergillus* have been described, relatively few are known to cause disease in humans. Most *Aspergillus* infections are acquired exogenously via inhalation. In the absence of an effective immune response, airborne conidia invade sinus or lung vasculature. Although the lung is the most common site of invasive aspergillosis, *Aspergillus* spp. also demonstrate tropism for cutaneous, central nervous system (CNS), and cardiac vasculature.

The incidence of invasive aspergillosis in immunocompromised patients varies among specific populations.[39] Among patients with hematologic malignancies, those with acute myelogenous leukemia have the highest incidence of invasive aspergillosis. For more than a decade the incidence of invasive aspergillosis in this population remained stable (5%-6%).[40] However, advances in diagnosis (i.e., galactomannan assay, high-resolution computed tomography [CT] scan) have improved the ability to confirm cases that would previously been labeled as "suspected" invasive aspergillosis, and thus the incidence of this infection in patients with leukemia has risen significantly (12.7%).[40] Like patients with leukemia, patients undergoing HSCT are at high risk for invasive aspergillosis. The incidence of invasive aspergillosis varies depending on transplant type but not type of conditioning regimen (myeloablative versus non-myeloablative).[39] The incidence is higher among allogeneic HSCT recipients than among autologous HSCT recipients.[39] In the HSCT population, whether the incidence of invasive aspergillosis is truly increasing or decreasing is difficult to ascertain, because the rate of autopsy continues to decline.[41] The incidence of invasive aspergillosis among SOT is highest among lung transplant recipients and lowest among renal transplant recipients.[39] Patients receiving HSCT or SOT can develop invasive aspergillosis shortly (within 40 days) after transplantation, but typically it occurs late post HSCT (>40-100 days) or SOT (>90 days).[42-45]

In patients with acute leukemia or in HSCT recipients, prolonged neutropenia after cytotoxic chemotherapy or HSCT is the primary risk for early invasive aspergillosis. Risk factors associated with invasive aspergillosis in HSCT and SOT recipients vary with time after the transplant. However, in general, risks early in the transplant process are related to transplant related factors (underlying disease, neutropenia, type of transplant), biological factors (hyperglycemia, iron overload), and extrinsic factors (excluding spores from the environment, air filtration). In contrast, risks for invasive aspergillosis occurring later in the transplant process include transplant complications (acute GVHD (grade ≥ 3) and high-dose corticosteroid therapy.[43]

Lesions associated with invasive pulmonary aspergillosis evolve over a period of weeks. CT findings, especially the "halo sign," are strongly suggestive of invasive aspergillosis and infection from other angioinvasive fungi in immunocompromised patients. Moreover, this finding is associated with significantly improved response and survival if antifungal therapy is initiated shortly upon detection of this sign of infection.[46] The combination of radiologic and clinical data may help in the differential diagnosis of fungal disease.

Recent diagnostic efforts have focused on detecting non–culture-based serum markers (e.g., galactomannan test, 1,3-β-D-glucan, polymerase chain reaction [PCR]). Galactomannan is a cell wall constituent of *Aspergillus* spp. that can be detected in the serum during invasive infection. The test is specific for invasive aspergillosis and is commercially available as a sandwich enzyme immunoassay (ELISA) that detects circulating galactomannan. The values from this test have been shown to strongly correlate with the clinical outcome of patients with invasive aspergillosis.[47-49] Because 1,3-β-D-glucan is a cell-wall component of many fungal pathogens, it can be detected by colorimetric detection assays. Although the test is highly sensitive, the presence of 1,3-β-D-glucan in the serum is not specific for any fungi. Using both of these non–culture-based serum markers may improve the ability to diagnose invasive aspergillosis in high-risk populations and could lead to earlier diagnosis or improved monitoring of the success of antifungal therapy.[50,51] The combination of radiologic, serologic, and clinical data may ultimately improve the diagnosis of invasive aspergillosis and speed up initiation of appropriate antifungal therapy.

Miscellaneous Pathogens in Critically Ill Patients with Hematologic Malignancies

Candida and *Aspergillus* spp. are the primary fungal pathogens in critically ill patients with hematologic malignancies. However, other pathogens such as *Fusarium* spp., *Pseudallescheria* spp., and the zygomycetes are increasing in frequency.[7] Each of these less common organisms has characteristic clinical characteristics or tissue tropism. In addition, they are often less susceptible than *Aspergillus* spp. to systemic antifungal agents. Consequently, infections due to these pathogens are associated with high mortality. Of these, the zygomycetes (which cause mucormycosis) are the most common among critically ill patients, particularly in a surgical ICU. These angioinvasive pathogens are acquired through inhalation and produce a necrotic infection. Rhinocerebral and paranasal infections are common manifestations of zygomycetes. Common risks are diabetic ketoacidosis, immunosuppression, organ transplantation, skin damage, and a prolonged ICU stay. Data suggest that exposure to voriconazole prophylaxis to prevent invasive aspergillosis in certain immunosuppressed populations (i.e., HSCT recipients) may be a risk factor for zygomycosis.[52]

CRYPTOCOCCOSIS, HISTOPLASMOSIS, BLASTOMYCOSIS, AND COCCIDIOIDOMYCOSIS IN CRITICALLY ILL PATIENTS

Cryptococcus neoformans, *Histoplasma capsulatum* var. *capsulatum*, *Blastomyces dermatitidis*, and *Coccidioides immitis* are not common pathogens in the ICU setting. These organisms can cause infection in patients with intact immune function. However, with the exception of *B. dermatitidis*, severe infections due to these pathogens are more common among critically ill immunocompromised populations, particularly those with AIDS and SOT recipients. Cryptococcosis is the third most common invasive fungal infection among SOT recipients.[7]

C. neoformans is a ubiquitous encapsulated yeast isolated from diverse environmental sources (i.e., soil, trees and plant material, and droppings from pigeons). This pathogen is primarily acquired by inhalation. In the lung, the organism elicits a cell-mediated response involving neutrophils, monocytes, and macrophages. The cryptococcal polysaccharide capsule, an important virulence factor, facilitates laboratory identification and recognition by host cell-mediated immune response and possesses immunosuppressive properties. The advent of AIDS significantly altered the incidence of cryptococcosis. Before the AIDS epidemic, cryptococcosis was an uncommon disease in the United States, but since then, the majority of cases have been associated with HIV infection. The prevalence of cryptococcosis in HIV in the United States has declined with the widespread use of fluconazole and highly active antiretroviral therapy to treat HIV infection. Cryptococcosis still produces significant acute mortality, but overall long-term outcomes have improved dramatically in the past 2 decades.[53] Mortality among HIV-infected patients and SOT recipients is similar and is estimated to be approximately 15% to 20%.[53-55]

Among critically ill immunosuppressed populations, cryptococcal infections typically involve the CNS. However, non-HIV cases may have only extra-CNS (i.e., skin, soft tissue, or osteoarticular) manifestations. The onset of this infection may be acute or gradual, and patients often present with nonspecific complaints. When the disease manifests as subacute meningitis or meningoencephalitis, classic meningeal findings such as photophobia or nuchal rigidity may be absent.

In cases of cryptococcal meningitis, characteristic cerebrospinal fluid (CSF) findings may be present; however, CSF leukocyte count can be low, and CSF protein and glucose values may be normal. Therefore, CSF analysis for cryptococcal antigen and culture of the organism are required to diagnose cryptococcal meningitis. Detection of the organism by India ink stain is highly specific but associated with low sensitivity (=50%). Determination of serum cryptococcal antigen using latex agglutination is a highly sensitive (≈99%) and specific test, and therefore it is an important component of the diagnosis of cryptococcal disease. In patients with cryptococcal meningitis, particularly those with AIDS, the serum cryptococcal antigen is usually positive, and usually titers are very high (i.e., >1:2048). Detection of antigen in the CSF strongly suggests infection, but in HIV-infected patients, false-negative results can occur in up to 10%, even in the presence of positive cultures. The definitive diagnosis of cryptococcal infection requires a positive culture for *C. neoformans*.

Histoplasmosis (caused by *H. capsulatum* var. *capsulatum*), blastomycosis (*B. dermatitidis*), and coccidioidomycosis (*C. immitis*) are the major endemic mycoses found in North America. Infections by these pathogens are reported primarily in distinct geographic areas, but owing to population mobility, they can be reported throughout the United States. *H. capsulatum* is endemically distributed primarily in the Mississippi and Ohio River valleys, *B. dermatitidis* is found primarily in the south central United States, the Mississippi and Ohio River valleys, and in certain regions of Illinois and Wisconsin. *C. immitis* is found primarily in the arid southwest regions of the United States. Infection with all these pathogens is acquired via inhalation. Overall, hospitalization is required in an estimated 4.6 and 28.7 cases per million children and adults, respectively.[56] Nationwide, endemic mycoses require substantial healthcare resources to manage and produce significant crude mortality rates in children and adults (5% and 7%, respectively).[56] The severity of histoplasmosis depends on host immune function and the extent of exposure, particularly in the immunocompetent host. Hematogenous dissemination from the lungs occurs in all infected patients, but in immunocompetent hosts, it is controlled by the reticular endothelial system. However, among elderly hosts or those with cell-mediated immune disorders (e.g., HIV infection), progressive disseminated infection readily occurs. After inhalation, *B. dermatitidis* can disseminate from the lungs to other organs as the yeast form. The primary pneumonia is often undetected and resolves without sequelae. Endogenous reactivation in the lungs, skin, or bones is often the first sign of infection.

C. immitis requires the inhalation of only a few arthroconidia to produce primary coccidioidomycosis. Like the other endemic mycoses, in the majority of patients, primary coccidioidomycosis typically manifests as an asymptomatic pulmonary disease. However, it can also manifest as an acute respiratory illness, chronic progressive pneumonia, pulmonary nodules and cavities, extrapulmonary nonmeningeal disease, and meningitis.[57]

Among critically ill patients, histoplasmosis manifests as either chronic pulmonary histoplasmosis or progressive disseminated (extrapulmonary) histoplasmosis. Chronic or cavitary pulmonary histoplasmosis occurs in middle-aged and elderly patients with underlying lung disease that compromises the ability of nonspecific host defenses to effectively clear the organism.

Progressive disseminated histoplasmosis occurs in healthy or critically ill immunocompromised hosts, but it is more common and severe in the latter population (i.e., patients with malignancies or HIV infection). The infection can disseminate to a variety of organs including the reticuloendothelial system, oropharyngeal and gastrointestinal mucosa, skin, adrenal glands, and kidneys.

Clinical manifestations of blastomycosis can mimic many other diseases, such as TB and cancer, but typically occurs as an asymptomatic infection, acute or chronic pneumonia, or disseminated (extrapulmonary) disease.[58] Extrapulmonary blastomycosis typically afflicts the skin, bones, and genitourinary system.[58] Cutaneous lesions are the most common skin manifestations of this disease.[58] Extrapulmonary (disseminated) coccidioidomycosis afflicts 1% to 5% of all patients infected with *C. immitis*, and is deadly if not treated properly. Even with appropriate treatment chronic infection is common.[57]

Systemic Antifungal Agents

AMPHOTERICIN B FORMULATIONS

Amphotericin B Deoxycholate

Amphotericin B deoxycholate (AmB-d), a polyene antifungal agent, disrupts biological membranes, thereby increasing their permeability. AmB-d also stimulates the release of cytokines, which causes arteriolar vasoconstriction in the renal vasculature.[59]

Pharmacology and Pharmacokinetics. The majority (70%) of an administered AmB-d dose is recovered from the urine and feces over a 7-day period; approximately 30% of the administered dose remains in the body a week after dosing.[60]

Overview of Toxicity. AmB-d infusion-related reactions, including hypotension, fever, rigors, and chills, occur in approximately 70% of patients.[61] These reactions occur early in therapy and often subside with time. Pretreatment regimens consisting of diphenhydramine, acetaminophen, meperidine, and hydrocortisone may be used to prevent infusion-related reactions. The efficacy of these regimens is unclear, so their routine use is discouraged until the reactions occur, after which pretreatment regimens should be employed with subsequent dosing.[61] Although common and noxious, infusion-related reactions rarely cause early termination of AmB-d therapy or interfere with the use of other medications.

AmB-d also produces dose-related toxicities, including nephrotoxicity, azotemia, renal tubular acidosis, electrolyte imbalance, cardiac arrhythmias, and anemia.[59] AmB-d–induced nephrotoxicity is the most common dose-related toxicity.[62] In the ICU this toxicity often limits the use of AmB-d or interferes with the ability to use other medicines. Saline hydration before dosing can reduce the incidence of AmB-d–induced nephrotoxicity, but in the ICU setting, the utility of saline hydration may be limited by fluid restriction employed to manage the fluid status of critically ill patients.

Lipid Amphotericin B Formulations

Amphotericin B lipid complex (ABLC), amphotericin B colloidal dispersion (ABCD), and liposomal amphotericin B (LAmB) are lipid AmB formulations that in many centers have supplanted the use of AmB-d. They all retain the activity of AmB-d but have significantly less associated nephrotoxicity than the parent drug.[62]

Pharmacokinetic Comparisons of Lipid Amphotericin B Formulations. The lipid AmB formulations differ in physicochemical properties and composition. These differences produce subtle differences in their pharmacokinetic behavior that may ultimately prove to be clinically significant. The disposition and activity of these formulations in human tissue is poorly characterized. However, animal data indicate that high serum concentrations may influence the delivery of lipid AmB formulations to certain infection sites such as the CNS and lungs.[63]

Toxicity Comparisons of Lipid Amphotericin B Formulations. Compared with AmB-d, the lipid formulations have significantly less associated nephrotoxicity.[62] The formulations differ in the incidence of infusion-related reactions and other adverse events associated with AmB-d infusion.[64,65] These reactions typically do not result in early termination of therapy.[64,66] Observational safety comparisons between ABLC and LAmB suggest the two formulations have a similar nephrotoxicity profile, but prospective comparative data suggest LAmB may be somewhat less nephrotoxic than ABLC.[62,67] There are few data comparing the safety of lipid AmB formulations to the triazole antifungal agents in critically ill patients. Given the safety of triazoles, it is unlikely the lipid AmB formulations will prove to be any safer.

AZOLE ANTIFUNGAL AGENTS

Fluconazole, Itraconazole, Voriconazole, Posaconazole

The systemic azoles exert a fungistatic effect by dose-dependent inhibition of cytochrome P450 (CYP)-dependent 14α-demethylase, the enzyme necessary for the conversion of lanosterol to ergosterol, leading to the depletion of ergosterol, the essential sterol of the fungal cell wall, an event that ultimately compromises cell wall integrity. The degree of inhibition varies among the different azole agents, which accounts for differences in spectrum of activity.

Pharmacology and Pharmacokinetics. The triazoles differ subtly in chemical properties, which form the basis of the pharmacokinetic differences between the agents and the propensity of this class to interact with other medications. Such properties can limit the use of these agents, particularly itraconazole and posaconazole in the ICU setting. For example, the lack of an intravenous (IV) formulation often precludes the use of posaconazole and itraconazole in critically ill patients.

Several studies have examined fluconazole pharmacokinetics in critically ill patients.[68-70] In surgical ICU patients, fluconazole clearance correlates with creatinine clearance (CrCl), and its volume of distribution correlates with body weight.[69] In addition, fluconazole volume of distribution is greater in this population than in healthy volunteers.[69] The fluconazole half-life is markedly prolonged in surgical ICU patients.[69] In patients with severe renal dysfunction (CrCl <30 mL/min), some recommend dosage reductions of 50%,[69] but such reductions should be made cautiously and take into account the infecting pathogen in patients receiving fluconazole via enteral feeding tubes.[69] Data suggest that the systemic availability of fluconazole is relatively unaffected by administration via enteral feeding tubes. However, serum concentrations obtained with standard doses administered via an enteral feeding tube may not be adequate to treat *C. glabrata* infections.[68] Moreover, in critically ill abdominal trauma patients with and without abdominal wall closure, IV fluconazole may be warranted because the bioavailability of enterally dosed fluconazole in these patients is highly variable.[70]

Itraconazole is a highly lipophilic weak base and practically insoluble in water. It is available as a capsule and as an oral solution formulated in hydroxypropyl-β-cyclodextrin (HP-βCD). The IV solution was removed from the U.S. market in 2008; however, this dosage form may be available in other countries. Slow and erratic absorption of the capsule form precludes its use in critically ill ICU patients. HP-βCD enhances itraconazole solubility and improves its oral systemic availability. HP-βCD is poorly absorbed from the gastrointestinal tract, stimulates gastrointestinal secretion and propulsion, and causes diarrhea.

Under fasting conditions in healthy adults, itraconazole is rapidly absorbed from the oral solution, and compared to the capsule there is less interpatient and intrapatient variability in serum concentrations.[71] After IV administration, renal elimination of itraconazole is negligible, but HP-βCD is renally eliminated (80%-90%). IV itraconazole was contraindicated in cases of significant renal impairment (CrCl ≤ 30 mL/min) because of concerns over the renal accumulation of HP-βCD.

Voriconazole is a derivative of fluconazole with limited aqueous solubility and improved antifungal activity. It is available in IV and oral formulations. IV voriconazole contains sulfobutyl ether β-cyclodextrin (SBECD) as a solubilizing agent. There are few data on how critically ill patients handle voriconazole. In healthy volunteers, voriconazole exhibits good oral availability and wide tissue distribution, with hepatic metabolism and renal excretion of metabolites.[72] In patients with moderate to severe renal function, SBECD accumulates, and it is recommended that oral dosing be used in patients with a CrCl less than 50 mL/min.[73] Oral dosing in critically ill patients is often not possible, therefore how SBECD is handled in critically patients on dialysis has been examined. A small study observed accumulation of SBECD in three patients during hemodialysis. No toxicity due to accumulation of SBECD was observed, and the accumulated dose values were lower but comparable with those used in previous toxicity studies with animals.[73] Nonetheless, if possible, use of IV voriconazole in patients on hemodialysis should be avoided. Data demonstrate that voriconazole achieves adequate CSF concentrations.[72]

Posaconazole is available as oral suspension and exhibits linear pharmacokinetics with dosages between 50 and 800 mg/d. However, absorption is saturated at doses exceeding 800 mg/d.[74] Posaconazole absorption is influenced by gastric pH and is optimal under acidic conditions.[75] There are no data describing the disposition of posaconazole in critically ill ICU patients. However, posaconazole absorption and exposure are maximized by dividing the total daily dose 4 times daily rather than administering it as a single dose.[75,76] Posaconazole absorption and exposure are also enhanced by administration with or shortly after a meal. In the ICU it is often impractical to give posaconazole with or shortly after a meal, but absorption and exposure are also enhanced by administering the drug with a liquid nutritional supplement.[75,77,78] Although posaconazole binds extensively (>95%) to plasma proteins, its large estimated volume of distribution suggests that it distributes widely throughout the body, but there are few data describing its penetration into the CSF.[79] Posaconazole is primarily eliminated in feces and urine as unchanged drug.[80]

Overview of Toxicity. The azoles are a relatively safe class of drugs and are associated with few serious adverse effects. The advent of fluconazole and subsequent agents greatly improved the safety of this class. All the azoles are associated with gastrointestinal intolerance, transient transaminitis, hepatic toxicity, rashes, and dizziness. Nausea, vomiting, and diarrhea commonly occur with all agents in this class, particularly with oral itraconazole solution. These effects are usually observed with high doses of the azoles, but rarely are they severe enough to warrant discontinuation of therapy. All azoles may produce significant elevations in transaminases. Patients experiencing azole-associated transaminase abnormalities are asymptomatic, but these increases can on rare occasions evolve into fatal drug-induced hepatitis. The azoles can also produce allergic skin rashes that are generally mild and subside with discontinuation of the drug.

Fluconazole is perhaps the safest azole, and doses four to five times in excess of the recommended daily dose have been well tolerated. Adverse effects with itraconazole occur frequently and often may necessitate discontinuation of therapy.[81] Although adverse effects associated with itraconazole are common, they are rarely life threatening, and symptoms typically abate when the drug is stopped or the dose is reduced.[81] In addition to the adverse effects seen with other azoles, voriconazole produces transient visual disturbances in approximately 30% of patients, which rarely lead to discontinuation of therapy.[82] These visual disturbances are acute and include changes in color discrimination, blurred vision, photophobia, and the appearance of bright spots.[82] To date, the common adverse effects associated with posaconazole use have been similar to those observed with the other agents in the class (i.e., gastrointestinal, transient transaminase abnormalities).

Azole Drug Interactions. Drug interactions occur primarily in the intestine, liver, and kidneys by a variety of mechanisms. In the intestine they can occur as a result of changes in pH, complex formation with ions, or interference with transport and enzymatic processes involved in gut wall (i.e., presystemic) drug metabolism. In the liver, drug interactions can occur because of interference with drug-metabolizing enzymes. Drug interactions in the kidney can occur through interference with glomerular filtration, through active tubular excretion, or by other mechanisms. The azoles are one of the few drug classes that can cause or be involved in drug interactions at all of these anatomic sites by one or more of the above mechanisms. Drug interactions involving the azoles have been extensively reviewed.[83] Several of the drug-drug interactions involving the azoles occur class wide. Therefore, when using the azoles, the clinician must be aware of the many drug-drug interactions, both real and potential, associated with this class.

Interactions involving the azoles result because of their physicochemical properties. All azoles are somewhat lipophilic and thus undergo CYP-mediated metabolism. The azoles all inhibit one or more CYP enzymes. Of the four azoles reviewed here, only itraconazole appears to interact significantly with P-glycoprotein (P-gp), which is a transport protein involved in drug distribution.[83] Fluconazole is not affected by agents that increase gastric pH, but its potential to cause CYP-mediated interactions is more than that suggested by in vitro studies. CYP-mediated interactions involving fluconazole are often dose dependent and can involve drugs metabolized by CYP3A4 (e.g., midazolam, rifampin, phenytoin) and CYP2C9 (e.g., warfarin).[83] Because of its linear and predictable pharmacokinetic properties, these interactions may sometimes be avoided or managed by using the lowest effective fluconazole dose.

Itraconazole is subject to pH-based interactions and interactions involving CYP3A4 and P-gp. Drugs that can interact with itraconazole include agents that increase gastric pH (e.g., protonics) and lipophilic CYP3A4 (e.g., HMG-CoA reductase inhibitors, benzodiazepines, immunosuppressive agents), and/or P-gp substrates (e.g., digoxin) with poor oral availability.[83] Voriconazole is not affected by agents that increase gastric pH. However, CYP-mediated interactions involving voriconazole can involve drugs metabolized by CYP3A4 (e.g., midazolam, rifampin, phenytoin), CYP2C9 (e.g., warfarin), or CYP2C19 (e.g., omeprazole).[83] Approximately 17% of a posaconazole dose undergoes biotransformation.[84] Unlike other azoles, posaconazole is only minimally (2%) metabolized by CYP; instead its metabolites are glucuronide conjugates formed via uridine diphosphate glucuronosyltransferase (UGT) pathways.[84,85] Although posaconazole is minimally metabolized by CYP, it inhibits hepatic CYP3A4.[86] Like the other azoles, the most clinically significant interactions associated with posaconazole involve benzodiazepines (oral midazolam), calcineurin inhibitors (cyclosporine, tacrolimus), other immunosuppressive agents (sirolimus), and phenytoin.[83] With more widespread use of posaconazole, the list of medications it interacts with will likely grow. Drug interactions involving the azoles that are relevant to the ICU setting are summarized in Table 139-1.

TABLE 139-1	Drug Interactions Involving Azoles in the ICU Setting				
	Fluconazole	*Itraconazole*	*Voriconazole*	*Posaconazole*	*Comments*
CYP Inducers					
Rifamycins	+	+	+	+	
Phenytoin	+	+	+	+	Significantly ↓s azole concentration
Phenobarbital	X	+	X	X	Significantly ↓s azole concentration
Carbamazepine	X	+	X	X	Significantly ↓s azole concentration
Benzodiazepines and Anxiolytics					
Midazolam	+	+	+	+	Effect of midazolam ↑'d by triazoles
Triazolam	+	+	X	X	Effect of midazolam ↑'d by triazoles
Diazepam	+	+	+	X	Effect of midazolam ↑'d by triazoles
Immunosuppressants					
Cyclosporine	+	+	+	+	Triazoles ↑ calcineurin exposure, troughs
Tacrolimus	+	+	+	+	Triazoles ↑ calcineurin exposure, troughs
Sirolimus	+	+	+	+	Triazoles ↑ calcineurin exposure, troughs
Gastric pH Modifiers					
H_2 Antagonists	−	+	X	X	Significantly ↓s itraconazole concentration
Antacids	X	+	X	−	Significantly ↓s itraconazole concentration
PPIs	X	+	X	+	Significantly ↓s itraconazole and posaconazole concentration

KEY: (+) = interaction documented by clinical study or case series; (−) = no interaction documented by clinical study; X = no published data. PPI, proton pump inhibitor.

Emergence of Resistance and the Selective Pressure of Azoles. Azole resistance in *Candida* has been widely observed for fluconazole and *C. albicans*; however, resistance to other azoles among other *Candida* spp. has been reported and studied. There is concern that resistance to the azoles, particularly among *C. glabrata,* may be related to the widespread use of fluconazole, but this hypothesis has proven difficult to confirm.

ECHINOCANDIN ANTIFUNGAL AGENTS

Caspofungin, Micafungin, Anidulafungin

Pharmacology and Pharmacokinetics. The echinocandins are generally fungicidal and disrupt cell wall synthesis by inhibiting 1,3-β-D-glucan synthase. The echinocandins are active against *Aspergillus* and *Candida* spp. In addition, their spectrum of activity extends to *Pneumocystis carinii*. These agents have little or no activity against *H. capsulatum, B. dermatitidis,* or *C. neoformans.* The echinocandins are large lipopeptide compounds and thus cannot be formulated for oral dosing. The individual echinocandins all demonstrate linear pharmacokinetic behavior. However, each agent differs slightly in how it distributes throughout the body and how it is metabolized or degraded. These differences, though, are not clinically significant. The echinocandins are not appreciably metabolized by the cytochrome P450 enzyme system; but their interactions with drug transport proteins remain to be elucidated.

Caspofungin binds extensively to plasma proteins (primarily albumin). Caspofungin distribution is multiphasic; initially it distributes to plasma and extracellular fluid before being actively transported slowly into the liver and other tissues via organic anion transport proteins.[83] The prolonged elimination half-life (8-13 hours) of caspofungin is due in part to this slow multiphasic distribution.[83] Caspofungin is slowly metabolized in the liver via *N*-acetylation and peptide hydrolysis to inactive metabolites, which are then excreted in bile and feces.[87] Compared with healthy subjects, caspofungin average serum concentrations 24 hours after administration vary greatly and are elevated in surgical ICU patients.[88] Body weight and hypoalbuminemia were found to be prognostic factors responsible for these increased caspofungin concentrations.[88] The clinical significance of such findings is unclear. Dosage adjustment is not required in patients with impaired renal function, but the dose should be reduced by 50% in patients with significant hepatic impairment.[89] Micafungin distribution and metabolism are not fully understood. Following IV administration, micafungin binds extensively to albumin, but the significance of this interaction on drug activity is unclear.[90] Micafungin is hepatically metabolized to several metabolites, and it is predominately eliminated as parent drug and metabolite(s) in feces.[90]

Anidulafungin distribution and metabolism are not fully understood. Of all the other echinocandins, anidulafungin binds the least to plasma proteins; has a larger volume of distribution and achieves lower peak (C_{max}) serum concentrations.[91] Anidulafungin is not hepatically metabolized, but rather in the plasma it undergoes slow nonenzymatic chemical degradation to an inactive peptide breakdown product, which likely undergoes further enzymatic degradation and is excreted in feces and bile.[91] The majority of an anidulafungin dose is excreted in feces or urine as unchanged drug.[91]

Toxicity and Drug Interactions. In general, caspofungin is well tolerated but is associated with nonspecific (i.e., fever, headache, nausea, phlebitis, rash, elevated hepatic enzymes) adverse effects which are generally mild and rarely cause early discontinuation of therapy. Similarly, caspofungin has low potential to interact with other drugs. Clinically insignificant interactions with the cyclosporine, tacrolimus, have been reported, but their clinical significance is unclear.[83]

PYRIMIDINE ANTIFUNGAL AGENTS (5-FLUOROCYTOSINE)

Pharmacokinetics and Toxicity

5-Fluorocytosine (5-FC) is a fluorinated pyrimidine related to 5-fluorouracil, and it is the only agent in this therapeutic class. This antimycotic possesses a narrow spectrum of activity and is often associated with significant toxicity. Moreover, when used as monotherapy, resistance develops rapidly. Orally, 5-FC is nearly completely absorbed and distributes to total body water. Hepatic metabolism and protein binding of 5-FC are negligible. Nearly all of a dose is renally excreted as unchanged drug, and renal clearance is highly correlated with creatinine clearance (CrCl). Reductions in CrCl prolong the half-life of 5-FC.

Myelosuppression is the primary toxicity associated with 5-FC. In addition, 5-FC can cause significant rash, nausea, vomiting, diarrhea, and liver dysfunction. Flucytosine toxicity is associated with elevated drug concentrations and often occurs in the presence of renal dysfunction. Because 5-FC is primarily used in combination with AmB, the effects of renal dysfunction on 5-FC pharmacokinetics and the subsequent risk of toxicity cannot be ignored.

Dosing and Therapeutic Drug Monitoring

Therapeutic drug monitoring for 5-FC is beneficial. Ideally, 5-FC serum concentrations should be maintained between 25 to 100 µg/mL to minimize toxicity and avoid the emergence of resistance. There are several nomograms for dosing 5-FC based on CrCl in patients with renal dysfunction. However, the nomograms are based on serum creatinine measurements; thus, they should be used only with chronic renal dysfunction. In addition, the nomographs should be utilized cautiously in elderly patients. During therapy, any necessary dosage adjustments should be made on the basis of plasma concentrations. Use of lower 5-FC doses (75-100 mg/kg/d) to minimize toxicity has been advocated. In vitro data suggest antifungal efficacy would not be compromised by such dosing.

In Vitro Susceptibility Testing of Systemic Antifungal Agents

In vitro susceptibility testing of *Candida* spp. is now widely accepted. Standardized broth microdilution and disk diffusion methods developed by the Clinical and Laboratory Standards Institute (CLSI) for in vitro susceptibility testing of *Candida* spp. are reproducible and accurate. Interpretative breakpoints for *Candida* spp. exist for fluconazole, itraconazole, voriconazole, 5-FC, and the echinocandins but do not exist for amphotericin B formulations or posaconazole. Although interpretive breakpoints for AmB in the treatment of *Candida* spp. have not been established, minimum inhibitory concentrations (MICs) for most isolates of *Candida* are ≤1 µg/mL. In addition, resistance to AmB formulations among the most commonly isolated species is unusual. In contrast to *Candida* spp., in vitro susceptibility testing of *C. neoformans* is not routinely performed, because primary resistance to first-line antifungal drugs (5-FC, AmB, fluconazole) is not currently a significant clinical problem, and the susceptibility testing methods and interpretive breakpoints for *Cryptococcus* spp. against any antifungal are not validated.[92] Validated broth microdilution methods for in vitro susceptibility testing methods of *Aspergillus* spp. for the azoles and AmB have been developed, but interpretive breakpoints for these agents have not been established.[93] Validated agar-based disk diffusion methods and commercial kits (Etest) are available and may be reliable methods for determining susceptibilities for *Aspergillus* spp.[93] Although broth microdilution methods for susceptibility testing for *Aspergillus* spp. for the echinocandins exist, the MIC is not the ideal measure of drug activity for this class of agents.[93]

Treatment of Fungal Infections in the Critically Ill

CANDIDIASIS IN THE ICU

There are many options for empirical therapy of fungal infections in the ICU, including the AmB formulations, fluconazole, itraconazole, voriconazole, posaconazole, caspofungin, micafungin, and anidulafungin. For many years, the poor prognosis associated with systemic candidiasis has fueled widespread use of antifungal agents, particularly fluconazole, in ICU patients with or without an established source of fungal infection.

The paradigms of preventive antimycotic therapy are prophylaxis and "preemptive therapy" (sometimes referred to as *empirical therapy*). Prophylaxis is generally initiated in a population in anticipation of certain risk factors, regardless of whether they ever manifest. There are few data to justify the use of this paradigm in the ICU setting, where concerns regarding selection of resistant fungal pathogens with indiscriminate antifungal use persist.[94] Moreover, the risk for invasive candidiasis is not the same for all ICU patients, and some risk factors evolve during an ICU stay. Therefore, universal institution of antifungal prophylaxis in the general ICU population is generally discouraged

in favor of a more targeted approach selectively directed toward those patients at the highest risk.[94,95]

Preemptive therapy is the administration of antifungal treatment before the occurrence of a septic syndrome in patients with several risk factors for infection and evidence of significant *Candida* colonization.[94] Historically, AmB-d was the sole option for prevention or treatment of candidiasis in the ICU setting. However, the risk of nephrotoxicity and the advent of safe and effective alternatives such as the echinocandins have diminished its use in the ICU.

Prophylaxis

Most studies of prophylactic antifungal use in the ICU setting have evaluated fluconazole. A placebo-controlled study for the prevention of intraabdominal *Candida* infections in a selected group of high-risk abdominal surgical patients showed that daily fluconazole (400 mg) significantly reduced the incidence of invasive candidiasis.[96] This study included patients who had recurrent gastrointestinal perforations or anastomotic leakages; therefore, they were at very high risk of developing intraabdominal candidiasis. The patients in this study had moderate acuity (APACHE II score 13), but prophylactic fluconazole prevented *Candida* colonization and dissemination of *Candida* spp. Similar to experiences with HSCT recipients, this study illustrates that when the prophylactic paradigm is selectively applied it may benefit specific patient populations. This has also been shown in the HSCT population.[96] Similar results were obtained in critically ill surgical patients staying in ICU longer than 3 days.[68,97] However, these results should be interpreted cautiously. This was a single-center study, and true to the paradigm, patient selection was somewhat subjective and based on an anticipated ICU stay of 3 or more days and the clinician's experience. Therefore, the results may not be widely generalizable. Others have also prospectively studied prophylactic fluconazole and shown an advantage for low-dose IV fluconazole (100 mg/d) in reducing *Candida* colonization and candidemia, with no effect on either invasive candidiasis or overall mortality.[98] In this double-blind randomized placebo-controlled study, all patients received selective digestive decontamination. The incidence of *Candida* infections, particularly candidemia, was significantly less in the fluconazole-treated patients.

Using these three studies and others that included ketoconazole or nonabsorbable antifungal agents, three meta-analyses have attempted to provide further insight into the role of antifungal prophylaxis in critically ill patients, but with disparate results. One analysis concluded that prophylactic fluconazole administration to prevent mycoses in surgical ICU patients successfully decreased the rate of fungal infections, but it did not improve survival.[99] Conversely, a second analysis demonstrated that antifungal prophylaxis indeed reduced the risk of candidemia and resulted in a reduction of overall mortality and attributable mortality (31% and 79%, respectively).[100] The third and perhaps most rigorous meta-analysis demonstrated that antifungal prophylaxis in non-neutropenic critically ill patients reduces proven invasive fungal infections by approximately half and total mortality by approximately one-quarter.[95] Although the analyses had slightly differing results, all concluded that if antifungal prophylaxis is employed, it should be done so selectively and targeted toward those patients at high risk of developing infection.[95,99,100] Thus, what the prophylactic studies have highlighted is the need to identify high-risk patients for preemptive therapy.

Preemptive Therapy

There are few randomized prospective data addressing preemptive therapy. Nonetheless, in the absence of mechanisms to identify patients who would most benefit by preemptive antifungal therapies, this strategy shares similar drawbacks to the prophylactic strategy. However, a growing body of data clearly demonstrate the importance of early institution of antifungal therapy in the adult ICU.* There are a number

---

*References, 22, 23, 26, 28, 29, and 101.

TABLE 139-2	Summary of Recommended Antifungal Therapy for Aspergillosis and Candidiasis in the ICU Setting	
Infection	*Recommended Treatment*	*Alternative Treatment*
Aspergillosis		
Invasive pulmonary aspergillosis therapy	VCZ, 6 mg/kg IV q 12 h for 1 day, followed by 4 mg/kg q 12 h; oral dose is 200 mg q 12 h	L-AmB, 3-5 mg/kg/d IV; ABLC, 5 mg/kg/d IV; caspofungin, 70 mg IV on day 1, and 50 mg/d IV thereafter
Empirical and preemptive antifungal therapy	L-AmB, 3 mg/kg/d IV; *or* Caspofungin, 70 mg IV on day 1, and 50 mg/d IV thereafter; *or* ITZ, 200 mg daily IV, or 200 mg BID; *or* VCZ, 6 mg/kg IV q 12 h for 1 day, followed by 3 mg/kg IV q 12 h; oral dosage is 200 mg q 12 h	
Prophylaxis invasive aspergillosis	PCZ, 200 mg q 8 h in patients with GVHD and neutropenic patients with AML or MDS	ITZ, 200 mg q 12 h IV for 2 days, then 200 mg q 24 h IV; *or* ITZ, 200 mg PO q 12 h; micafungin (50 mg/d)
Invasive Candidiasis (Candidemia)		
Treatment (non-neutropenic)	FCZ, 800 mg (12 mg/kg) loading dose, then 400 mg (6 mg/kg) daily; *or* an echinocandin* (for moderate-severe infection in patients with azole exposure)	LF-AmB, 3-5 mg/kg/d; *or* AmB-d, 0.5-1 mg/kg/d; *or* VCZ, 400 mg (6 mg/kg) BID for 2 doses, then 200 mg (3 mg/kg) BID
Treatment (neutropenic)	An echinocandin* or LF-AmB, 3-5 mg/kg/d (VCZ can be used when additional mold coverage is desired; removal of intravascular catheter is advised but is debatable.)	FCZ, 800 mg (12 mg/kg) loading dose, then 400 mg (6 mg/kg) daily; *or* VCZ, 400 mg (6 mg/kg) BID for 2 doses, then 200 mg (3 mg/kg) BID
Suspected candidiasis treated with empirical antifungal therapy (non-neutropenic patients)	Treat as above for candidemia. An echinocandin* or fluconazole is preferred (for patients with moderate/severe infection or recent azole exposure, an echinocandin* is preferred).	LF-AmB, 3-5 mg/kg/d; *or* AmB-d, 0.5-1 mg/kg/d
Suspected candidiasis treated with empiric antifungal therapy (neutropenic patients)	LF-AmB, 3-5 mg/kg/d; *or* Caspofungin,* 70-mg loading dose, then 50 mg/d; *or* VCZ, 400 mg (6 mg/kg) BID for 2 doses, then 200 mg (3 mg/kg) BID	FCZ, 800 mg (12 mg/kg) loading dose, then 400 mg (6 mg/kg) daily; *or* ITZ, 200 mg (3 mg/kg) BID
Prophylaxis		
Neutropenic (HSCT)	FCZ, 400 mg/d while patients are at high risk	

Adapted from Mora-Duarte J, Betts R, Rotstein C et al. Comparison of caspofungin and amphotericin B for invasive candidiasis. N Engl J Med 2002;347:2020-2029; Pappas PG, Kaufman CA, Andes D et al. Clinical practice guidelines for the management of candidiasis: 2009 update by the Infectious Diseases Society of America. Clin Infect Dis 2009;48:503-35; and Walsh TJ, Anaissie EJ, Denning DW et al. Treatment of aspergillosis: clinical practice guidelines of the Infectious Diseases Society of America. Clin Infect Dis 2008;46:327-60.

ABLC, amphotericin B lipid complex; *AmB-d*, amphotericin B deoxycholate; *AML*, acute myeloid leukemia; *BID*, twice daily; *FCZ*, fluconazole; *GVHD*, graft-versus-host disease; *HSCT*, hematopoietic stem cell transplant; *ITZ*, itraconazole; *L-AmB*, liposomal amphotericin B; *LF-AmB*, any marketed lipid amphotericin B formulation; *MDS*, myelodysplastic syndromes; *PCZ*, posaconazole; *VCZ*, voriconazole.

*Monitor for persistence; in vitro susceptibilities reveal caspofungin MICs for *Candida parapsilosis* higher than other *Candida* spp., and results of clinical trial demonstrated caspofungin to be effective in treatment of *C. parapsilosis* fungemia, but persistent cultures are common.

of predictive rules of varying complexity described in the literature. All of the studies have produced different predictive algorithms; few have been prospectively validated.[37] While the methods are improving, published methods have yet to be widely applied in ICU patients as part of routine practice Moreover, there are few data describing the outcomes associated with preemptive therapy instituted based upon a predictive rule. One small study assessed the use of a scoring system to identify high-risk patients and demonstrated that fluconazole significantly decreased the incidence of invasive candidiasis in patients with a corrected colonization index (CCI) of ≥0.5.[102] Another prospective study to assess whether preemptive antifungal therapy in high-risk ICU patients (CCI ≥ 0.4) would reduce invasive candidiasis demonstrated a significant decrease in the incidence of surgical ICU–acquired invasive candidiasis with preemptive therapy compared to historical controls.[103] However, to generate the CCI, required weekly surveillance cultures at multiple anatomic sites in all ICU patients is necessary. This method is not practical for most ICUs, and it is doubtful that the CCI could be used with similar success without routine surveillance cultures.[31]

With the exception of fluconazole, there are few prospective data assessing the efficacy of other antifungal agents as preemptive therapy in the ICU. Administering itraconazole capsules through feeding and nasogastric tubes, as used in ICU patients, is difficult. Although the oral solution solves this problem, there are few data assessing its effectiveness in preventing or treating systemic candidiasis. Furthermore, the use of itraconazole in critically ill patients is also limited by a significant drug-drug interaction profile with agents commonly used in the ICU. Comparative studies assessing the efficacy of voriconazole or posaconazole, micafungin, or anidulafungin in preventing candidiasis in the ICU setting are lacking.

A prospective randomized double-blind study demonstrated that caspofungin is at least as effective as AmB-d for the treatment of invasive candidiasis.[104] However, that study included ICU and non-ICU patients and assessed primary treatment of invasive candidiasis, not preemptive therapy. Lipid AmB formulations have lowered the risk of nephrotoxicity associated with AmB, but there are no data regarding their use in the ICU setting. The results of studies assessing these formulations as empirical or salvage therapy in immunocompromised hosts should not be extrapolated to the general ICU setting.

A cost analysis has illustrated the potential benefit of preemptive therapy. According to this analysis of empirical therapy, caspofungin is the most effective strategy for ICU patients, but its high cost made it less cost-effective than empirical fluconazole.[105] The analysis also demonstrated that empirical AmB and the lipid AmB formulations were the least effective strategies, largely because of drug toxicities.[105] The authors concluded that empirical fluconazole should reduce mortality at an acceptable cost.[105] Similar to other decision model analyses, this study also recognized that in low-risk ICU patients, even empirical strategies are not justified.

The recommended antifungal therapy for candidiasis in the ICU setting is summarized in Table 139-2.[106]

INVASIVE ASPERGILLOSIS AND OTHER OPPORTUNISTIC MYCOSES IN BONE MARROW TRANSPLANTATION

Fever and neutropenia are common among critically ill immunocompromised individuals with hematologic malignancies. Although fever can be due to many causes, these patients, and particularly HSCT recipients, are at risk of developing systemic mycosis due to *Candida* or *Aspergillus* spp. Owing to the difficulty in diagnosing infections due to these pathogens, antifungal prophylaxis is standard in HSCT patients. Fluconazole has been shown to decrease the incidence of invasive infections with *Candida* spp. and is widely used in the prophylactic paradigm.[96] As stated previously, invasive aspergillosis occurs relatively late after transplantation. Therefore, persistently febrile HSCT recipients should be treated empirically with antifungal agents with activity against molds, particularly *Aspergillus* spp.

For many years "high-dose" AmB-d was employed as standard empirical therapy of invasive aspergillosis, but within the last decade, based upon data from a randomized trial that compared voriconazole to AmB and suggested superiority with the azole, voriconazole has been considered the gold-standard therapy of documented and suspected aspergillosis.[107] Although voriconazole is considered an initial option for prophylactic therapy, the choice of therapy may vary based upon the individual's organ function. Voriconazole may not be ideal in cases where liver disease is present or if the patient is being treated with concomitant medicines that interact with this azole. Similarly, the presence of reduced renal function may preclude the use of lipid AmB formulations. The other azoles are not appropriate as preemptive therapy in HSCT. Fluconazole lacks activity against molds. Itraconazole has activity against *Aspergillus* spp., but as discussed previously, the capsule dosage form is not suitable for many critically ill patients and produces erratic blood levels. The oral solution of itraconazole is not well tolerated and is commonly associated with diarrhea. If available, IV itraconazole solution suffers the same drawback as lipid AmB formulations in patients with diminished renal function. Lastly, posaconazole is only available as an oral liquid, and it requires food and multiple daily dosing to optimize serum concentrations. These characteristics preclude its use in patients who experience vomiting, diarrhea, decreased appetite, and mucositis related to their cytotoxic chemotherapy.

With their lack of toxicity and low propensity for drug-drug interactions, the echinocandins are promising agents for empirical therapy of invasive aspergillosis in critically ill patients. However, their lack of cidal activity, and the lack of prospective data assessing their use in this population leads many to consider them only as a secondary option. Recommended antifungal therapy for the treatment of aspergillosis in the ICU setting is summarized in Table 139-2.[108]

CRYPTOCOCCOSIS, HISTOPLASMOSIS, AND BLASTOMYCOSIS

Although cryptococcosis, histoplasmosis, blastomycosis, and coccidioidomycosis are not considered nosocomial mycoses, patients with severe infections may require intensive care. The treatment of cryptococcosis, particularly that in the CNS, evolved from a series of classic clinical trials. Current guidelines base their recommendations on the best data available to address unresolved questions surrounding treatment of this infection. Recommended antifungal therapy for treatment of cryptococcosis in the ICU setting is summarized in Table 139-3.[92]

Management of Increased ICP in CNS Cryptococcosis

Elevations in ICP occur in more than half of patients with cryptococcal meningitis and contribute significantly to the morbidity and mortality associated with this infection.[92] There are much less data on treatment of HIV-negative patients with acute elevated ICP with regard to

TABLE 139-3	Summary of Recommended Antifungal Therapy for Cryptococcosis and Endemic Mycoses in the ICU Setting	
Infection	*Recommended Treatment(s)*	*Alternative Treatment*
Cryptococcosis		
CNS infection (HIV infected)	Induction: AmB, 0.7-1 mg/kg + 5-FC, 100 mg/kg/d for 2 wk; *or* L-AmB, 3-4 mg/kg/d; *or* ABLC, 5 mg/kg/d + 5-FC (100 mg/kg/d) for 2 wk Consolidation: FCZ, 400 mg/d for 8 wk	AmB-d + FCZ FCZ + 5-FC
CNS infection (transplant recipient)	Induction therapy: L-AmB, 3-4 mg/kg/d; *or* ABLC, 5 mg/kg/d + 5-FC, 100 mg/kg/d for 2 wk Consolidation therapy: FCZ, 400-800 mg/d for 8 wk Maintenance therapy: FCZ, 200-400 mg/d for 6 mo-1 y	L-AmB, 6 mg/kg/d; *or* ABLC, 5 mg/kg/d for 4-6 wk
CNS infection (non-HIV, non-transplant recipient)	Induction: AmB-d, 0.7-1 mg/kg/d + 5-FC, 100 mg/kg/d for ≥ 4 wk; *or* AmB-d, 0.7-1 mg/kg/d for ≥ 6 wk; *or* L-AmB, 3-4 mg/kg/d; *or* ABLC, 5 mg/kg/d + 5-FC, if possible ≥ 4 wk; *or* AmB-d, 0.7 mg/kg/d + 5-FC, 100 mg/kg/d for 2 wk Consolidation therapy: FCZ, 400-800 mg/d for 8 wk Maintenance therapy: FCZ, 200 mg/d for 6 mo-1 y	
Histoplasmosis		
Acute pulmonary (moderately severe-severe)	LF-AmB, 3-5 mg/kg/d; *or* AmB, 0.7-1 mg/d for 1-2 wk, then ITZ, 200 mg BID to finish 12 wk*	
Progressive disseminated histoplasmosis (moderately severe to severe)	L-AmB, 3 mg/kg daily; *or* ABLC, 5 mg/kg daily; *or* AmB-d, 0.7-1 mg/kg/d for 1-2 wk; followed by ITZ, 200 mg BID for at least 1 y	
Blastomycosis		
Pulmonary (moderately severe to severe)	L-AmB, 3-5 mg/kg/d; *or* AmB-d, 0.7-1 mg/kg/d for 1-2 wk; followed by ITZ, 200 mg BID for 6-12 mo	
Extrapulmonary (Disseminated)		
CNS	L-AmB, 5 mg/kg/d for 4-6 wk is preferred; followed by an oral azole for at least 1 y	
Non-CNS (moderately severe to severe)	L-AmB, 3-5 mg/kg/d; *or* AmB-d, 0.7-1 mg/kg/d for 1-2 wk; followed by ITZ, 200 mg BID for 12 mo	

Adapted from Perfect JR, Dismukes WE, Dromer F, et al. Clinical practice guidelines for the management of cryptococcal disease: 2010 update by the Infectious Diseases Society of America. Clin Infect Dis 2010;50:291-322; Wheat LJ, Freifield AG, Kleiman MB et al. Clinical practice guidelines for the management of patients with histoplasmosis: 2007 update by the Infectious Diseases Society of America. Clin Infect Dis 2007;45:807-25; and Chapman SW, Dismukes WE, Proia LA et al. Clinical practice guidelines for the management of blastomycosis: 2008 update by the Infectious Diseases Society of America. Clin Infect Dis 2008;46:1801-12.

*Consider corticosteroids 60 mg × 2 wk.

ABLC, amphotericin B lipid complex; *AmB-d,* amphotericin B deoxycholate; *BID,* twice daily; *CNS,* central nervous system; *5-FC,* 5-fluorocytosine; *FCZ,* fluconazole; *HIV,* human immunodeficiency virus; *ITZ,* itraconazole; *L-AmB,* liposomal amphotericin B; *LF-AmB,* any marketed lipid amphotericin B formulation.

recommendations of pressure control. Therefore, ICP management may be underutilized in the management of non-HIV-infected patients with CNS cryptococcosis. Persistent elevations in ICP should be managed by sequential lumbar punctures.[92] If necessary, more invasive procedures, including insertion of a lumbar drain or placement of a ventriculoperitoneal shunt, should be performed.[92] The frequency with which sequential lumbar punctures are performed depends on the initial opening pressure and symptoms. For patients with elevated baseline opening pressure, lumbar puncture should be done to reduce the pressure 50% and performed daily to maintain the ICP in the normal range.[92]

Serum and CSF antigen titers are important in establishing the presumptive diagnosis and assessing the prognosis of CNS infection. The test measures cryptococcal polysaccharide capsule antigens but does not differentiate viable from nonviable organism. Therefore, once therapy is started, treatment decisions should not be based on antigen test results.[92] A reduction in antigen titers during therapy is desired, but treatment decisions should be based on culture results.

Treatment of Histoplasmosis in Critically Ill Patients

Although there are no comparative studies, the efficacy of individual antimycotics for therapy of chronic and disseminated histoplasmosis has been well documented. AmB-d and itraconazole have proven efficacy. The efficacy of 6 weeks to 4 months of AmB-d therapy for chronic infection is approximately 75%; however, relapse is common. The efficacy of itraconazole ranges from 75% to 85% but, as is the case for AmB-d, relapse may be common. In vitro susceptibility of *H. capsulatum* to fluconazole is poor, and generally it is not used to treat this infection. Voriconazole and posaconazole are likely effective in the treatment of histoplasmosis, but data assessing their safety or efficacy as treatment for this infection are lacking.

The efficacy of AmB-d for therapy for disseminated histoplasmosis among immunocompetent patients is 70% to 90%. Therefore, AmB-d is recommended initially in severely ill patients. In a small study, all patients responded to itraconazole, 200 to 400 mg daily.[109] Once an adequate response is noted to AmB-d, therapy can be switched to itraconazole.[109] Few data exist concerning the efficacy of the lipid AmB formulations as therapy for disseminated histoplasmosis in immunocompetent patients. Recommended antifungal therapy for treatment of histoplasmosis in the ICU setting is summarized in Table 139-3.[109]

Treatment of Disseminated (Extrapulmonary) Blastomycosis in the Critically Ill

Disseminated blastomycosis and diffuse pulmonary infection are both associated with significant mortality. Treatment of these infections produces cure rates ranging from 85% to 90%, and the effective agents cause little associated toxicity.[110] The optimal duration of therapy for the treatment of blastomycosis with existing antifungal agents is unknown and has been empirically derived from noncomparative studies and clinical experience. In cases of life-threatening infections or extrapulmonary disease and in patients who are severely immunocompromised or have already failed therapy with an azole, the risk of relapse is high.[110] Therefore, the duration of therapy is lengthy to prevent relapse. Patients can be switched to safer azole therapy when significant improvement is observed.[110] Pharmacologic treatment of blastomycosis in the ICU setting is summarized in Table 139-3.[110]

Conclusions

Systemic mycoses are now widespread in critically ill patients. Specifically in the ICU setting, *Candida* spp. are a common cause of nosocomial BSIs. There are many risks associated with the ICU environment or the patients' underlying disease states that predispose them to infections with these pathogens. In addition, historically, because of the high mortality associated with BSIs caused by *C. albicans*, this species has been the primary fungal pathogen of concern. Although the epidemiology of *Candida* isolates in the ICU continues to shift, whether the changing epidemiology is a consequence of injudicious antifungal use is a matter of speculation and debate. Nonetheless, the steady increase in BSIs due to *C. glabrata*, a species with reduced susceptibility to antifungal therapy, is concerning. Furthermore, select populations of critically ill patients are at risk of developing life-threatening infections due to non-*Candida* spp. of fungi such as *Aspergillus* spp., *Fusarium*, and the zygomycetes. These pathogens are angioinvasive and often respond poorly to antifungal therapy. The endemic mycoses (e.g., histoplasmosis, blastomycosis, coccidioidomycosis) are not typically a concern in the ICU setting, but patients with severe infections due to *B. dermatitidis*, *H. capsulatum*, or *C. immitis* will often require intensive care.

Methods to perform antifungal susceptibility tests on a variety of pathogens, particularly *Candida* spp., are becoming routine in clinical practice. There is improved understanding of antifungal resistance and the pharmacodynamic actions of antifungal drugs. This understanding may ultimately lead to more rational use of antifungal agents and perhaps improved outcomes in infected patients. The advent of additional safer agents means that the available drugs differ sufficiently in terms of toxicity and potential for drug-drug interactions that clinicians have the luxury of choice when tailoring antifungal therapy to a specific patient.

KEY POINTS

Overview

1. Generally, fungal infections are more prevalent in ICUs than on the general medical wards. Although *Candida* spp. are the most commonly isolated fungi in critically ill patients, infections caused by other opportunistic fungal pathogens (i.e., *Aspergillus*, *Cryptococcus neoformans*, *Fusarium*, and agents of zygomycosis) are also a concern in selected critically ill populations.

2. New antifungal agents differ in mode and spectrum of activity, toxicity, and propensity to interact with other drugs. Consequently, antifungal therapy can now be tailored to the specific needs of the patient.

Fungal Infections in the Critically Ill

1. *C. albicans* is the primary fungal pathogen in the ICU setting, but the prevalence of a given species may vary with age. For example, candidemia among neonates is predominantly due to *C. albicans* and *C. parapsilosis* and rarely due to *C. glabrata* or other *Candida* spp. In adults, *C. glabrata* and *C. albicans* predominate.

2. Age differences in the isolation of specific species may have important repercussions for infection control, dosing, and selection of antifungal agents in older critically ill patients.

3. Bloodstream infections (BSIs) due to *C. glabrata* have continually become more prevalent.

4. In the ICU, *Candida* BSIs are common and difficult to detect, and consequently they carry a relatively poor prognosis. Although isolation techniques have improved, the attributable mortality rate associated with *Candida* BSIs is 35%, and *Candida* spp. are the only BSI pathogens that are an independent predictor of mortality. In surviving patients, candidemia adds approximately 1 month to the length of hospital stay.

5. Critically ill patients with hematologic malignancies are at high risk for infections due to *Candida* and *Aspergillus* spp. Infections due to these pathogens are associated with high mortality.

Systemic Antifungal Agents

1. Amphotericin B deoxycholate (AmB-d) possesses a broad spectrum of activity and a long history of use with little acquired resistance, but its toxicity is significant, and it is potentially costly. In low doses for short courses, this agent is tolerable.

2. Lipid amphotericin B formulations are safer than amphotericin B deoxycholate, but their cost may limit their use.

3. Triazoles (azoles) possess a broad spectrum of activity and are relatively safe, but they interact with a vast array of drugs that are commonly used in ICU populations.

4. Echinocandins are safe and interact with few drugs, but their spectrum of activity is limited to primarily *Candida* and *Aspergillus* spp.

Treatment of Fungal Infections in the Critically Ill

1. The paradigms of preventive antimycotic therapy are prophylaxis and "preemptive therapy" (also known as *empirical therapy*). There are few data to support the prophylaxis paradigm in the ICU setting. *Preemptive therapy* (empirical therapy) is the administration of antifungal treatment before the appearance of sepsis syndrome in patients with risk factors for infection and evidence of significant *Candida* colonization.

2. Studies have demonstrated that general prophylaxis in the ICU is not warranted, that high-risk patients must be identified, and that preemptive fluconazole is likely to be a cost-effective strategy in the ICU. Most studies have focused on the prophylaxis paradigm and demonstrate prophylaxis must be targeted toward high-risk patients. A growing body of evidence shows that early antifungal therapy improves outcome. Methods to identify high-risk ICU patients are improving but still often lack practicality. A prospective randomized double-blind study demonstrates that caspofungin is at least as effective as AmB-d for the treatment of invasive candidiasis. Cost-effective analysis predicts caspofungin therapy as the most effective strategy for ICU patients, but effectiveness is outweighed by its cost. Therefore, empirical fluconazole appears preferable to reduce mortality at an acceptable cost.

3. Despite the increased number of antifungal agents, choices for preemptive therapy are still limited.

4. The treatment of CNS cryptococcosis evolved from a series of classic clinical trials. Elevations in intracranial pressure (ICP) occur in greater than 50% of patients and contribute significantly to the morbidity and mortality of this infection. Therefore, in addition to antifungal therapy, elevations in ICP should be managed by sequential lumbar punctures. Serum and cerebrospinal fluid antigen titers aid in the presumptive diagnosis and assessing the prognosis of infection. A reduction in antigen titers during therapy is desired, but treatment decisions should be based on culture results.

ANNOTATED REFERENCES

Wey SB, Mori M, Pfaller MA, et al. Risk factors for hospital-acquired candidemia: a matched case-control study. Arch Intern Med 1989;149:2349-53.
   This study was one of the first rigorous epidemiologic assessments of the risk factors that predispose patients to candidemia. Established risk factors have been borne out on subsequent analyses.
Pittet D, Li Ning, Woolson RF, Wenzel RP. Microbiological factors influencing the outcome of nosocomial bloodstream infections: A 6-year validated, population-based model. Clin Infect Dis 1997;24:1068-78.
   This article provides compelling data concerning the importance of Candida *spp. as bloodstream pathogens, as well as data regarding the crude and attributable mortality rates of Candida BSIs in the hospital. The study demonstrates that of all the microbial causes of BSIs, only* Candida *spp. are an independent predictor of mortality due to BSI.*
Pelz RK, Hendix CW, Swoboda SM, et al. Double-blind placebo-controlled trial of fluconazole to prevent candidal infections in critically ill surgical patients. Ann Surg 2001;233:542-48.
   This study was perhaps the largest and most well-controlled trial to evaluate the prophylactic use of enteral fluconazole to prevent invasive candidal infections in critically ill surgical patients. After controlling for confounding variables, this study demonstrated a 55% reduction in the risk of fungal infection among patients treated with fluconazole. Based on these data, it was concluded that enteral fluconazole safely and effectively decreased the incidence of fungal infections in high-risk critically ill surgical patients.
Garey KW, Rege M, Pai MP, et al. Time to initiation of fluconazole therapy impacts mortality in patients with candidemia: a multi-institutional study. Clin Infect Dis 2006;43:25-31.
   Inadequate antimicrobial treatment is an independent determinant of hospital mortality, and in companion publications this group demonstrated the most common causes of inappropriate therapy for fungal BSIs are

omission of initial empirical therapy and incorrect dosing of fluconazole. In this work, the authors link inadequate therapy to mortality. They demonstrate that delays in initiation of therapy of more than 24 hours were independently associated with mortality in candidemia patients. The rate of development of newer and more potent antifungal agents is tailing off. Thus, this work, which has been subsequently corroborated, illustrated that current antifungal agents, if used properly, can perhaps help reduce mortality more than realized to date. In addition, it calls attention to the need to focus on early appropriate therapy as a strategy to reduce the significant mortality associated with candidemia.
Golan Y, Wolf MP, Pauker SG, et al. Empirical anti-*Candida* therapy among selected patients in the intensive care unit: a cost-effectiveness analysis. Ann Intern Med 2005;143:857-69.
   *Few studies have prospectively evaluated antifungal prophylaxis, and meta-analyses of these studies all produce slightly different conclusions. However, the meta-analyses all agree that in the ICU, targeted empirical therapy directed at targeted high-risk ICU patients is probably a better strategy than general prophylaxis. However, even fewer studies have prospectively evaluated empirical therapy directed at targeted high-risk ICU patients. This study provides a decision analytic model to evaluate the cost-effectiveness of empirical anti-*Candida *therapy given to high-risk patients in the ICU, defined as those with altered temperature (fever or hypothermia) or unexplained hypotension despite 3 days of antibacterial therapy in the ICU. In doing so, they identify that although empirical caspofungin is the most effective strategy, it does not reduce mortality at an acceptable cost. On the other hand, empirical amphotericin B regardless of formulation was the least effective strategy, owing to drug toxicity. Thus, the most effective strategy was empirical fluconazole, because it reduced mortality at an acceptable cost.*

REFERENCES

Access the complete reference list online at http://www.expertconsult.com.

140

Influenza

STEVEN M. OPAL | ANAND KUMAR

Influenza is a zoonosis indigenous to waterfowl, with periodic introduction of the virus into humans and other mammals. The consequences of host species transfer from birds to humans can be devastating, with substantial mortality rates and rapid transmission by the respiratory route with global pandemic potential. The fate of influenza virus infection in human populations depends upon the viral virulence properties, immunologic differences from previous influenza outbreaks, fitness of the virus for replication and dissemination within humans, and status of the host immune defenses.[1]

In the winter months, severe disease in individual patients is usually limited to those with vulnerabilities in host defenses, including the very young, the very old, and individuals with immunodeficiency or underlying cardiopulmonary disease. The annual incidence rate varies each season depending upon the degree of antigenic "drift" (point mutations in coding regions of genes for major surface antigens) from one year to the next. However, influenza pandemics can occur following an antigenic "shift" (i.e., whole-scale reassortment of the influenza virus genome, with the expression of entirely new antigenic components), and these novel influenza hybrid viruses circulate throughout the entire susceptible global population. This set of events occurred in 2009 with the novel swine influenza virus strain where everyone, including healthy young people, became susceptible to this novel influenza infection and its complications.[2]

Even in a typical year between pandemics, influenza viruses account for the deaths of hundreds of thousands of people worldwide and exact billions of dollars from society in terms of morbidity and lost productivity. Recent estimates from the United States indicate that at least 610,660 life-years are lost, with 3.1 million hospital days, 31.4 million outpatient visits, and $10.4 billion in direct medical costs annually from influenza alone. The staggering amount expended for influenza care is $16.3 billion in projected lost earnings and an estimated total cost burden (including lost-life years) amounting to $87.1 billion.[3] The total costs to society during a pandemic year such as 2009 are even higher and likely incalculable. The costs of intensive care services required for managing the most severely ill influenza victims alone are enormous.[2]

Pathogenicity of Influenza Viruses

Influenza virus is a single-stranded RNA virus of the family Orthomyxoviridae It affects birds and mammals and includes three genuses: influenza virus A, B, and C, based upon their matrix proteins.[1,4] Influenza A virus is typically the most virulent, has pandemic potential, and leads to the most severe disease. Based upon the antibody response to two major antigenic proteins on the outside of virus, hemagglutinin (HA) and neuraminidase (NA), influenza A is subdivided into different serotypes including: H1N1 (responsible for Spanish flu in 1918, in addition to the 2009 flu pandemic); H2N2 (Asian flu of 1957); H3N2 (Hong Kong flu of 1968); H5N1 (the avian flu, often sited as the most recent pandemic threat), and a number of others currently less relevant to humans (H7N7, H1N2, H9N2, H7N2, H7N3, H10N7). The two other forms of influenza include B (which almost exclusively infects humans but is less common) and C (affecting humans, dogs, and pigs), which only rarely cause severe illness and epidemics in humans.[5]

A notable characteristic of influenza virus is the genomic structure consisting of eight separate single-strand segments, each encoding a single major protein to complete the synthesis of the mature virus. The RNA-based genome provides a high background mutation rate and gives the virus genetic plasticity. The multiple genome segments provide the substrate for reassortment of large sequences of RNA and permit hybrid viruses to form in hosts infected simultaneously by more than one virus strain. These events lead to whole-scale recombination of entirely novel hybrid viruses with new antigenic constituents (antigenic shift). As an example, the novel swine-origin influenza A/Mexico City/4/2009 (H1N1) outbreak strain was a quadruple-reassorted virus derived from gene segments originating from ducks, Eurasian swine, North American swine, and human-adapted influenza virus.[6]

Avian-adapted viruses can occasionally be transmitted to mammals, causing outbreaks in animals or giving rise to disease in human pandemics. The pig is an important "mixing vessel" host in shuttling avian influenza viruses to humans, as they can carry both avian and human influenza viruses.[1] Porcine mucous membranes express a mixture of sialic acid–coated glycopeptides linked in a favorable conformation to bind both avian and human-adapted viruses. This is vitally important in the biology of influenza viruses, as the initial event in influenza infection is interaction of the hemagglutinin receptor to binding sites on host epithelial tissues. Avian species express $\alpha2,3$-linked sialic acid–galactose disaccharides on their epithelial surfaces, and avian-adapted influenza preferentially binds to this linkage pattern. Human upper respiratory airways primarily express $\alpha2,6$-linked sialyl-galactose surface receptors, and seasonal influenza strains in humans bind readily only to $\alpha2,6$ linkages. Pigs, in contrast, normally express both $\alpha2,3$- and $\alpha2,6$-linked disaccharides on their mucous membranes, facilitating the opportunity for dual infections with avian- and human-adapted viruses.[1,6,7]

The lower airways and alveolar pneumocytes of humans actually express $\alpha2,3$-linked sialylated glycopeptides, and viruses that bind efficiently to $\alpha2,3$ linkages can cause severe pneumonia if deposited into the distal airways. Most seasonal influenza strains bind preferentially to $\alpha2,6$-linked disaccharide hemagglutinin (HA) binding sites found in human upper airways. This usually leads to high transmission frequency by the airborne droplet nuclei deposited upon the upper airways, but a low risk of primary influenza pneumonia.[8] The avian strain of H5N1 preferentially binds to $\alpha2,3$ linkages and therefore is poorly transmissible from person to person, but it has the potential to cause severe pneumonia if delivered to the lower airways. Poultry workers in Asia in close proximity to infected livestock can occasionally receive enough viruses deposited into the distal airways to cause severe influenza pneumonia with a high mortality rate (60% to 70%).[9,10]

One of the explanations for the severity of the 1918 pandemic of H1N1 influenza was its HA that could bind with high affinity to both $\alpha2,6$- and 2,3-linked sialyl-galactose moieties.[11,12] The result of this unusual HA binding affinity was a highly transmissible virus with the capacity to replicate and cause severe disease in the lower airways. Disturbingly, the hemagglutinin of the 2009 outbreak strain of novel swine origin also bound with high affinity to both $\alpha2,6$ and $\alpha2,3$ linkages. Fortunately, influenza A Mexico City 4/2009 (H1N1) virus lacked the full complement of other known virulence factors of the influenza virus (Table 140-1), resulting an overall low case-fatality rate (<0.1 %). A further mitigating factor against mortality in older populations during the 2009 outbreak was the presence of already-existing memory cells with B-cell and T-cell epitope recognition sites in humans born

TABLE 140-1 Pathogenicity Traits and Virulence Factors of Influenza Viruses

Viral Trait	Mechanism of Virulence	Comments
Epitope variations on HA and NA	Immune escape from recognition by pre-existing antibodies within the population from previous virus exposure	Antigenic drift (point mutations) leads to epidemics; antigenic shift (reassorted viral genomes) leads to pandemics
Cleavability of HA	HA undergoes proteolysis by host-derived proteases before receptor binding	Readily cleaved HA is associated with avid binding and disease severity
Binding preference of HA	α2,3-linked sialic acid receptor in alveoli and α2,6 linkage in upper airways	Viruses that bind to the α2,3 linkage or both α2,3 and α2,6 are more virulent
HA:NA ratio	NA cleaves sialic acid on glycopeptides on epithelium (binding site for HA)	Optimal ratio of NA and HA activity needed for high replication and release
NS-1	This nonstructural protein inhibits host-derived interferons.	Mutation or truncated variants are associated with loss of virulence.
PB1-F2	This peptide targets virus trafficking to mitochondria and induces apoptosis.	Mutations or truncated forms of PB1-F2 associated with loss of virulence
NA inhibitor resistance	H274Y mutation blocks NA inhibitor binding site and oseltamivir activity	Commonly seen mutation is seasonal H1N1 but rare in the 2009 outbreak strain
M2 inhibitor resistance	S31N mutation blocks activity of amantidine	Now commonplace in both H3N2 and H1N1
PB2 temperature range	Polymerase activity at lower (mammals) and higher (avian) temperature	Broad Pol temperature range aids transfer from bird to human hosts

H274Y, histidine substitution for tyrosine at amino acid at position 274; *HA*, hemagglutinin; *M*, matrix protein; *NA*, neuraminidase; *NS-1*, nonstructural protein; *PB*, polymerase basic; *Pol*, polymerase; *S31N*, serine substitution for asparagine at amino acid position 31.

before the early 1950s, induced by H1N1 viruses circulating in the first half of the 20th century.[13]

Clinical Manifestations and Complications of Influenza

Classical seasonal influenza in adults is typified by a 4- to 5-day period of sudden-onset fever, chills, upper respiratory tract symptoms, headache, muscle pain, and weakness. Rhinitis is relatively uncommon and diarrhea is more common with influenza than with most rhinovirus upper respiratory tract infections. Severe complications and death can occur, especially in infants, the elderly, and individuals with chronic medical conditions. Among the most severe complications are primary influenza pneumonia and secondary bacterial infection leading to respiratory failure.[14,15] Influenza can also cause central nervous system, cardiac, skeletal muscle, kidney, and hepatic complications.[5,15] Underlying pulmonary disease is a frequent risk factor, occurring in 18% of patients, most commonly asthma (7%), followed by neurologic disease (12%), hematologic or oncologic (9.9%), and cardiac conditions (4.6%).[16] However, approximately half of those hospitalized (rates ranging from 1-5/1000) for influenza are otherwise healthy.[14-16]

In the absence of a pandemic, 11% to 19% of patients hospitalized with laboratory-confirmed influenza require treatment in the intensive care unit (ICU).[15] The mean duration of mechanical ventilation is approximately 5 days; the sickest patients require treatment with advanced techniques for the treatment of hypoxemia, such as high-frequency oscillatory ventilation (HFOV), extracorporeal membrane oxygenation (ECMO), prone positioning, and nitric oxide. These patients have an attendant increase in length of stay, duration of ventilation, and mortality.[14,16,17]

An estimated 50 to 100 million people died during the 1918 pandemic. Death followed from aggressive secondary bronchopneumonia, influenza-related lung disease with associated hypoxemia, and cardiac collapse.[18,19] During the 1918 pandemic, there was unexplained excess influenza mortality in persons 20 to 40 years of age. This mortality increase may have been due to limited native immunity and/or a vigorous immune response directed against the virus in healthy young persons.[18] Today the high mortality rate observed in the 1918 pandemic would almost certainly be reduced because of the availability of ICUs, vaccines, antibacterial agents, and antiviral medications. However, the cost would be a dramatic increase in critical care admissions and length of stay, assuming that this surge capacity is available. Long-stay ICU patients have significantly higher critical care and hospital mortality rates compared to short-stay patients, occupy a disproportionate number of critical care bed-days,[4] and consume even greater resources.[8] Sophisticated ICU care is often unavailable in developing countries today, and the case-fatality rates in these countries will probably be regrettably similar to the 1918 pandemic.[20]

Influenza A 2009 H1N1-Related Epidemiology and Clinical Manifestations

Since March 2009, influenza A 2009 H1N1 has spread from Mexico to virtually all countries of the world. By September 27, 2009, there were over 340,000 cases with 4100 deaths worldwide.[7,21] The World Health Organization issued the first phase 6 pandemic alert of the century, anticipating substantial influenza transmission and related disease. Over the period of June to September 2009, there were dramatic spikes in H1N1-related disease in Australia, New Zealand, and South America that breached the capacity for ICU care in some regions. In Australian provinces, approximately 5% of the population developed H1N1-related illness, 0.3% of infected patients were hospitalized, and 20% of hospitalized patients required ICU care.[22] In the Northern Hemisphere, an early and severe influenza outbreak occurred that was blunted in part by widespread deployment of an effective inactivated monovalent influenza vaccine program.[23]

The events that transpired in Canada were illustrative of the influenza situation in much of the Northern Hemisphere in 2009. Among 168 critically ill Canadian patients with influenza A 2009 H1N1, the mean age has been 32 years, with a possible predilection for more severe disease in women (67% of patients).[24] Pregnant women in particular suffered from a disproportionate high level of influenza disease severity.[25,26] Nosocomial transmission was the mechanism of acquisition in approximately 10% of patients. Hospital-acquired transmission to healthcare workers occurred early in the outbreak, but healthcare-related infection occurred at a low incidence rate once the pandemic was recognized and appropriate infection-control safeguards were instituted. One or more comorbidities were observed in nearly all patients, most commonly chronic lung disease such as asthma, chronic obstructive pulmonary disease, bronchopulmonary dysplasia (41%), obesity (33%, mean body mass index of 34.6 kg/m²), hypertension (24%), history of smoking (23%), and diabetes (21%). Similar clinical findings and predisposing illnesses were reported in other regions of the world during the 2009 outbreak.[21,22,27,28] Serious comorbid illness was observed in only 30% of patients. Notably, aboriginal Canadians have thus far been over-represented (26% of patients). A summary of clinical risk factors and comorbidities associated with severe influenza complications is found in Table 140-2.

The most common specific symptoms with influenza A 2009 H1N1 have included fever and respiratory symptoms in greater than 90% of patients, and less commonly weakness and myalgias. Several severe clinical syndromes associated with influenza A 2009 H1N1 infection may be seen, including:

- Rapidly progressive diffuse pneumonitis associated with severe, refractory hypoxemia in relatively healthy teens or adults and in immunocompromised patients

TABLE 140-2	Prognostic Indicators and Risk Factors for Severe Influenza Complications
Risk Factors and Comorbidities	**Comments**
Age <5 years	Children < 2 years and those with chronic cardiopulmonary disease at greatest risk
Age >65 years	Poor vaccine response, poor host response to influenza infection
Chronic cardiopulmonary diseases	COPD, asthma, congestive heart failure
Metabolic disease and chronic liver disease	Diabetes mellitus and cirrhosis increase the risk of influenza complications.
Chronic neurologic illness	Neurocognitive and neuromuscular diseases associated with increased complications
Pregnancy	Particularly women in the third trimester
Obesity	BMI >35 kg/m² increased the risk of influenza complications in the 2009 outbreak.
Hemoglobinopathy	Sickle cell disease patients at increased risk
Immunosuppression	Glucocorticoids, chemotherapy, HIV transplant recipients at increased risk
Children receiving salicylates	Increased risk of Reye syndrome
Aboriginal populations, poverty, poor access to healthcare services	Delayed treatment associated with increased risk of influenza complications
Secondary bacterial pneumonia	Bacterial pneumonia associated with longer ICU and hospital stays with more nosocomial complications and a greater mortality rate

- Decompensation of chronic underlying disease in those patients with serious comorbidities including congestive heart failure, chronic renal failure, end-stage liver disease, poorly controlled diabetes, or immune compromise
- Acute and prolonged exacerbation of chronic obstructive pulmonary disease and asthma in those with preexisting disease
- Bacterial pneumonia, frequently with gram-positive pathogens including *Streptococcus pneumoniae, Staphylococcus aureus,* and group A streptococci, and superinfection on a background of mild or severe influenza A 2009 H1N1 infection
- Bronchiolitis and croup in infants and young children, which frequently required hospitalization but not ICU care

The typical clinical syndrome requiring ICU care among all age groups appeared to be a diffuse bilateral four-quadrant pneumonitis that was often rapidly progressive. This process accounted for over 80% of ICU admissions in Canada and elsewhere and often necessitated advanced ventilatory/oxygenation modalities including HFOV, inhaled nitric oxide, and/or ECMO therapy.[24,29,30]

Patients who subsequently developed critical illness generally presented to the hospital within 4 days of symptom onset and required ICU admission within 1 day of hospital presentation for bilateral pulmonary infiltrates and hypoxic respiratory failure. The mean Acute Physiology and Chronic Health Evaluation (APACHE) II score was 20. Notable laboratory findings have included elevated creatine kinase levels and normal white blood cell counts. Concomitant presenting conditions included possible bacterial pneumonia (32.1%), hypotension requiring vasopressors (13.7%), and asthma or chronic obstructive pulmonary disease exacerbation (13.7%).

Over 80% of patients with H1N1-related acute lung injury (ALI) received mechanical ventilation; very few patients were successfully managed with noninvasive ventilation strategies alone. Oxygenation support included high concentrations of inspired oxygen (mean admission Pao_2/Fio_2 147 mmHg), positive end-expiratory pressure (PEEP), frequent use of HFOV (12%), nitric oxide (14%), neuromuscular blockade (30%), prone ventilation (5%), and occasionally ECMO (7%). Medical therapies included neuraminidase inhibitors (90.5%), antibacterial agents (98.8%), and, despite uncertain efficacy, corticosteroids (50.6%).[24]

Secondary bacterial pneumonia following ICU admission was found in 24% of cases, most commonly due to *S. aureus* and *S. pneumoniae*. The frequency of secondary bacterial infection was difficult to accurately determine owing to the widespread use of empirical antibacterial therapy in influenza patients with rapidly progressive respiratory failure. Overall mortality among critically ill patients at 90 days was 17.3% (similar to that reported from Australia).[22] The median duration of ventilation was 12 days. The most common cause of death was severe acute respiratory distress syndrome (ARDS) and hypoxemia, complications thereof, secondary infection, sepsis, or multiorgan dysfunction syndrome. Characteristic radiographic changes of severe primary influenza pneumonia are shown in Figure 140-1, A and B.

Lung pathology in fatally infected patients who underwent autopsy examination revealed a diffuse alveolar filling process, often with early

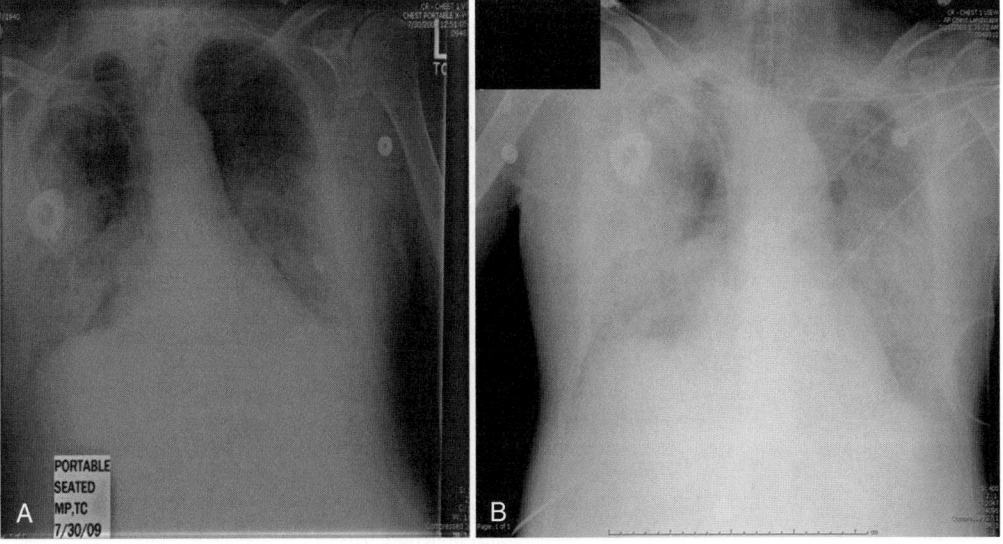

Figure 140-1 **A,** Chest radiograph of a 70-year-old male with B-cell lymphoma and hypogammaglobulinemia, with primary influenza pneumonia at the time of his ICU admission. Note Port-a-Cath in right anterior chest wall and diffuse pulmonary infiltrates, most prominently seen in both lower lung fields. **B,** Chest radiograph of same patient 3 days later; note diffuse alveolar filling process associated with profound hypoxemia. The patient expired despite oseltamivir and ventilatory support, with severe hypotension and acute kidney injury.

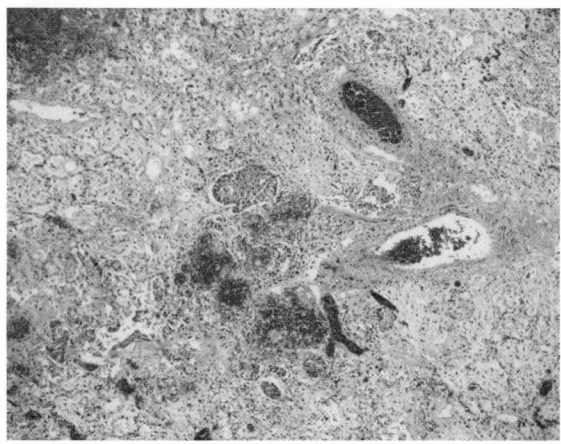

Figure 140-2   Lung pathology of fatal case of primary influenza pneumonia in previously healthy 20-year-old woman. Note diffuse alveolar filling, squamous metaplasia, lymphocytic infiltrates, focal hemorrhage, loss of ventilatable lung tissue. *(Figure courtesy David Horn, MD.)*

hyaline membrane formation that was sometimes accompanied by focal areas of hemorrhage. The alveolar lining was usually thickened, with evidence of lymphocytic infiltrates and early organization with fibrosis. A typical lung tissue section of a patient with fatal influenza pneumonia is seen in Figure 140-2. Lung tissue in deaths occurring early in the presentation of influenza pneumonia often revealed diffuse immunohistochemical evidence of viral infection and intraalveolar hemorrhage.

In children, the median age of hospitalized patients was 5.0 years (range 1 month to 17 years); 54.4% were female, and the mean PRISM III score was 9.[14-16,24] One or more chronic comorbid illnesses were observed in 70.2% of patients: lung disease (44%), neurologic diseases (19%), immune suppression or immunodeficiency (16%), history of prematurity (9%), and congenital heart disease (7%). Mechanical ventilation was used in 68% of children admitted to ICU, and the median duration of ventilation was 6 days (range 0-67).

Clinical and Laboratory Diagnosis

Significant difficulties with definitive virologic diagnosis existed in the early phase of the 2009 influenza outbreak that were partially rectified as the pandemic unfolded. Fever and upper respiratory symptoms were present in almost all patients who progressed to critical illness. However, shortness of breath, a symptom not typical of uncomplicated influenza virus infection, was likely suggestive of severe disease. Other clinical signs noted in patients with severe disease have included hemoptysis, frothy pink sputum, and purulent sputum with diffuse lung crackles. Percutaneous oximetric assessment of oxygenation or arterial blood gas evaluation of Po_2 should be performed when assessing a patient with suspected severe influenza. Relative hypoxia should trigger further assessment including a chest radiograph. Laboratory findings typically found at presentation with severe disease include normal or low-normal leukocyte counts and elevated creatine kinase[22,24,28] (Figure 140-3).

Early laboratory diagnosis of influenza infection is greatly facilitated by the use of reverse transcriptase–polymerase chain reaction (RT-PCR) methodology. This assay should be employed when available in the evaluation of a patient with suspected severe influenza. Immunofluorescent techniques, enzyme-linked immunoassays, and other rapid

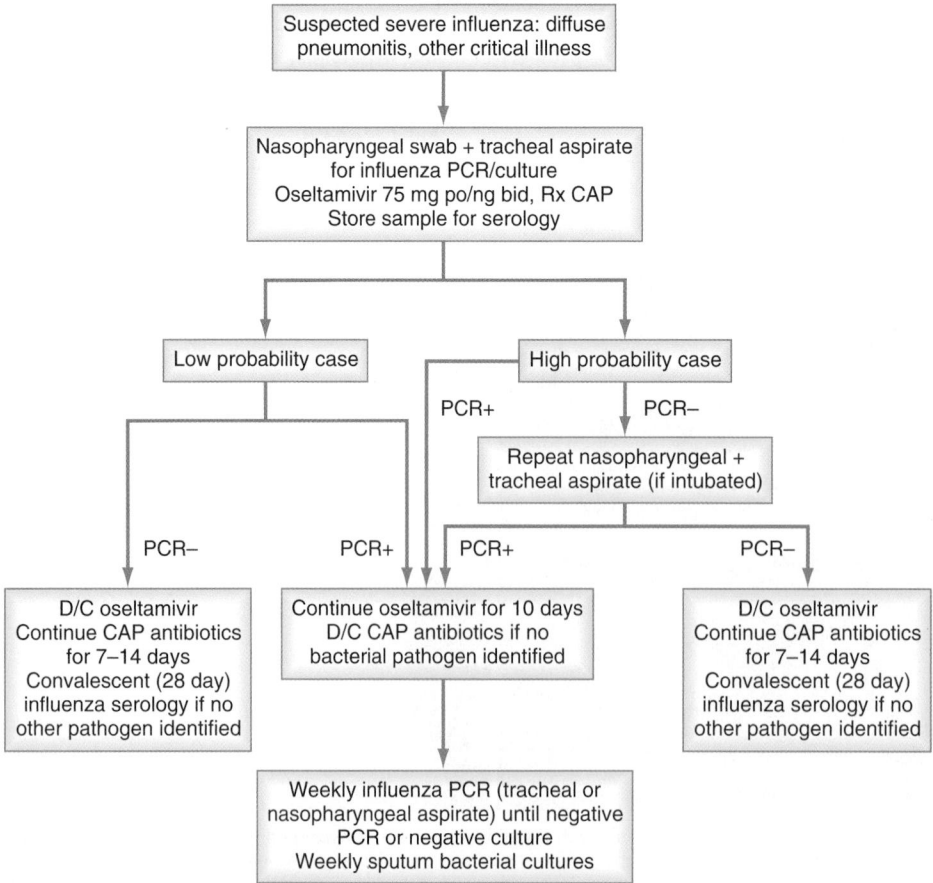

Figure 140-3   Suggested algorithm in the workup and management of suspected severe influenza pneumonia in the critical care unit.

diagnostic tests of clinical specimens often lack diagnostic sensitivity.[31,32] Viral cultures require up to 1 week for processing. Whereas RT-PCR is the preferred definitive diagnostic technique and has very high sensitivity, the adequacy of the clinical specimen is essential. Standard nasopharyngeal swab samples are adequate but can be falsely negative. Nasopharyngeal samples should be repeated in 48 to 72 hours if diagnostic suspicion remains. Paired nasopharyngeal and tracheal aspirates are useful for RT-PCR in intubated patients and may increase the diagnostic yield in critically ill patients.

Supportive Care

Almost all patients with severe infection in the ICU setting will have deficits in oxygenation and subsequently require ventilatory support.[22,24,33] Shock and renal failure can occur during therapy as a consequence of efforts to optimize oxygenation though diuresis coupled with high intrathoracic pressures and limited venous return.[24,28] Other important but less frequently seen disorders at presentation may include encephalitis (with or without obtundation or seizure activity), cardiac injury (myocarditis, pericarditis, conduction defects), and rhabdomyolysis.[17]

Most critically ill patients with severe influenza will manifest evidence of ARDS; supportive care for severe hypoxemia with diffuse pulmonary disease and supplemental oxygenation and ventilation assistance is required.[24] During pandemic periods, patients are often relatively young compared with non-pandemic years, and much greater numbers can be expected to be in need of ventilatory support than during a usual flu season.[18,22,24,29,30]

Primary influenza pneumonia is unusual in that patients often display a relative insensitivity to usual measures of oxygenation assistance with PEEP. Controlled ventilation with attention to a lung-protective strategy,[34] in combination with appropriate sedation and judicious use of neuromuscular blockade, is appropriate. Avoidance of volume overload (and judicious diuresis) may also be associated with reduced duration of ventilation and length of stay in ICU for most patients with ALI and ARDS, and this strategy should be attempted for patients with influenza.[30,35] Other ventilation measures (despite unproven benefit in other forms of ARDS) that might improve oxygenation for individual patients have included prone positioning and inhaled nitric oxide.[36,37] HFOV is currently being evaluated as a rescue therapy for patients with severe ARDS in randomized controlled trials[38] and might be an option in patients with influenza-related refractory hypoxemia. ECMO remains a controversial option to manage severe respiratory failure in influenza-associated ALI in adults.[29,30,39] Clinicians in Australia similarly recommend consideration of ECMO for refractory hypoxemia in influenza infection.[40] HFOV and ECMO might be considered as a salvage therapy in centers familiar with these modalities in desperately ill patients.

Antiviral Therapy

In severely ill patients with suspected influenza, early initiation of antiviral therapy should be based upon clinical presentation and epidemiologic data and not delayed pending laboratory confirmation.[22,24,41] Various influenza strains are circulating throughout the world, and susceptibility to currently available antiviral agents is strain specific. The 2009 H1N1 swine influenza variant was resistant to amantidine but sensitive to neuraminidase inhibitors including oseltamivir and zanamivir.[42] Oseltamivir-resistant strains were isolated during the 2009 H1N1 influenza A pandemic but fortunately were uncommon.[43] In contrast, the seasonal H1N1 influenza A strains circulating in 2008 and onwards are almost uniformly resistant to oseltamivir, yet many remain susceptible to zanamivir.[44-46] At this time, only an oral form of oseltamivir and an inhaled form of zanamivir are available for use.

Initiation of antiviral therapy within 48 hours of onset of symptoms of seasonal influenza is associated with a 1-day or greater reduction in duration of symptoms in ambulatory patients.[44,47] Oseltamivir therapy may reduce the risk of secondary bacterial superinfection.[48] Early therapy of severe influenza A 2009 H1N1 infections requiring ICU support with neuraminidase inhibitors contributed to improved outcomes.[49]

Little data are available to guide the optimal dose or duration of therapy for antiviral agents. Severe influenza infections, including those caused by the 2009 H1N1 strain, can represent a systemic in addition to a pulmonary infection,[50] favoring the use of a systemic rather than an inhaled antiviral agent. Despite concerns over inadequate gastrointestinal absorption of oseltamivir among critically ill patients, published studies indicate comparable blood levels in ICU patients as compared with normal volunteers.[51] Available evidence suggests that an oseltamivir dose of 75 mg twice daily is adequate; higher doses might be indicated and are the current subject of ongoing clinical trials.

Viral shedding can be prolonged in hospitalized patients with seasonal or pandemic influenza. In one study, approximately one-third of patients continued to shed live virus at least 1 week after symptom onset.[52] Neuraminidase-inhibitor therapy for longer than 5 days has been used in outbreak situations and in immunocompromised patients known to shed virus for prolonged periods, but formal recommendations on optimal duration are lacking.[30] The intravenous neuraminidase inhibitor, peramivir, is available on a compassionate basis for emergency use in severe influenza pneumonia. The recommended dose is 600 mg of peramivir intravenously once daily for 5 days.[53]

Adjunctive Pharmacologic Therapy

Several potential adjunctive immunomodulatory or antiviral therapies for treatment of severe influenza exist. Convalescent serum/plasma or hyperimmune globulin derived from patients who have recovered from influenza has been used for many decades. A series of studies were performed using convalescent plasma/serum during the 1918 pandemic and have recently undergone a meta-analysis showing that early, but not late, administration of such products may be associated with a significant survival benefit.[54] In addition, several case series suggest the possibility that similar therapy may be of use in severe influenza A/H5N1 infection.[55,56]

High-dose corticosteroid therapy has been advocated for a variety of infectious and inflammatory conditions.[57] Corticosteroids have been useful as adjunctive therapy to suppress inflammatory responses in certain serious infections including severe influenza pneumonia. The uncertain benefits and known risks of corticosteroids in the presence of ongoing infection warrant caution before employing this strategy in primary influenza pneumonia. The use of glucocorticoid therapy for influenza is best limited to randomized clinical trial protocols rather than uncontrolled use. Similarly, a wide variety of immunomodulator agents are commercially available and might have salutary effects in selected patients (e.g., statins, peroxisome proliferator activated receptor alpha and gamma [PPARα, PPARγ] agonists, resveratrol). Many of these agents are readily available at low cost in developing countries and should be studied in controlled clinical trials in patients with severe influenza pneumonia.[58]

Secondary Bacterial Pneumonia

Available evidence indicates that the majority of deaths from the 1918 pandemic occurred as a consequence of secondary bacterial infection.[18,19] Similarly, a substantial number of the deaths from the 1957 and 1968 pandemics were caused by bacterial co- or superinfection. The common pathogens in all series have been *S. pneumoniae*, group A streptococci, *S. aureus*, and *Haemophilus influenzae*. Given the frequency of secondary bacterial infection, clinicians should have a low threshold for considering antibiotic coverage against these commonly observed pathogens.

Secondary bacterial pneumonia as a complication of viral pneumonia takes two forms: mixed viral/bacterial pneumonia and postinfluenza pneumonia during the convalescent phase of influenza.

Postinfluenza pneumonia is generally attributable to damaged airways and poor mucociliary clearance mechanisms following severe influenza pneumonia.[18] The early mixed form of bacterial pneumonia during ongoing viral replication in the airways is more complex, with possible synergism between the bacterial and viral pathogens. Apoptosis of pneumocytes induced by the viral PB1-F2 protein facilitates pneumococcal growth in lung tissue.[59] Pneumococci bind to epithelial surfaces more readily if sialic acids have been cleaved by neuraminidase.[60] Viral neuraminidase from influenza virus has been found to promote pneumococcal adhesion in lung tissues and increase lethality in experimental pneumococcal pneumonia.[61] Early institution of effective antiviral agents with neuraminidase inhibitors might serve to decrease virus replication and decrease the risk for secondary pneumonia.[48]

Infection Control in the ICU

Patients with suspected influenza should be managed using droplet precautions by healthcare professionals, who should wear a standard surgical tie mask. There are different recommendations as to which face mask is optimal and whether N95 masks or similar personal respirators might be preferable to surgical tie masks. A recent study found limited to no additional protection of N95 masks in comparison to surgical masks, yet many still advocate their use during cough-inducing procedures when treating patients with influenza.[62] Vaccines, when available against circulating strains of influenza, should be mandatory for all healthcare workers unless specific contraindications exist. Healthcare workers should also consider appropriate gloves when likely to have contact with body fluids or to touch contaminated surfaces, and they should wear gowns during procedures and patient care activities where clothing might be contaminated. Protective eyewear is recommended when providing direct care in close proximity to the patient.[63] Patients with suspected influenza should be in single patient rooms, if available, during the initial phase of hospital admission. If clinical demand exceeds the availability of such quarters, then cohorting of patients with influenza in common areas may be necessary. Influenza patients who must be transported outside of the room should wear a mask if tolerated, or when necessary, an oxygen delivery system that limits the spread of aerosols.

With respect to infection prevention and control related to mode of ventilatory assistance, there is circumstantial evidence from the SARS (severe acute respiratory syndrome) epidemic that noninvasive ventilation and HFOV may promote excess aerosolization of viral-laden particles and place surrounding patients and staff at risk. Limited evidence suggests that the process of endotracheal intubation, especially in an uncontrolled setting, may be associated with increased risk of acquiring infection; however, this risk is mitigated if adequate personal protective equipment is worn.[64,65] HFOV circuits should be equipped with microbial filters and a scavenger system to the exhalation port to limit aerosol generation.

Global Critical Care Collaboration

A working group composed of members from the international critical care community formed the International Forum for Acute Care Trialists (InFACT) to aid with global collaborative research in critical care.[66] For the 2009 H1N1 pandemic, the InFACT group focused on developing a case report form as a reference for generating an international "minimal clinical dataset" through collaboration with members of global critical care societies. This web-entry case report form system was available to clinicians around the world to contribute patient-based data in a manner that can be analyzed in real time and help inform decision makers and clinicians during the outbreak. InFACT also supports large, simple, investigator-initiated interventional studies in many countries. The impact of the InFACT initiative will only be determined over time, but this is an important global critical care attempt to more efficiently and more inclusively improve the care of critically ill patients.

ANNOTATED REFERENCES

Molinari NA, Ortega-Sanchez IR, Messonnier ML, Thompson WW, Wortley PM, Weintraub E, et al. The annual impact of seasonal influenza in the US: measuring disease burden and costs. Vaccine 2007;25:5086-96.
This paper presents a careful analysis of the direct costs to society in medical expenditures for the care of patients with influenza in one season throughout the United States. The costs are exceedingly high and argue strongly in favor of widespread use of annual influenza vaccines as a cost-savings measure.

Kumar A, Zyrychanski R, Pinto R, Cook DJ, Marshall J, Lacroix J, et al. Critically ill patients with 2009 influenza A (H1N1) infection in Canada. JAMA 2009;302:1872-79.
This report provides a detailed and valuable review of the impact of influenza upon critical care services and the relative values of various support measures in managing critically ill patients during an outbreak of pandemic influenza A (H1N1) in 2009.

Novel Swine-Origin Influenza A (H1N1) Virus Investigation Team. Emergence of a novel swine-origin influenza A (H1N1) virus in humans. N Eng J Med 2009;360:2605-15.
This paper traces the fundamental virology, evolution, and epidemic behavior of the novel influenza A strain that caused a worldwide pandemic in 2009.

Moscona A. Global transmission of oseltamivir-resistant influenza. N Engl J Med 2009;360:953-6.
This report defines the molecular mechanisms responsible for development of resistance to the neuraminidase-inhibitor antiviral agents against influenza and explains why this is a major problem for oseltamivir rather than for a related antiviral agent, zanamivir.

Garten RJ, Davis CT, Russell CA, Shu B, Lindstrom S, Balish A, et al. Antigenic and genetic characteristics of swine-origin 2009 A(H1N1) influenza viruses circulating in humans. Science 2009;325:197-201.
This paper provides the molecular details about the novel swine-origin quadruple reassorted influenza A H1N1 pandemic strain of 2009 and how it escapes immune clearance preexisting antibodies against currently circulating H1N1 strains. The virus possesses rapid human-to-human transmission potential but lacks many important virulence properties of many previous pandemic influenza viruses. These features explain its high transmissibility but rather low mortality rate.

Gamblin SJ, Haire LF, Russell RJ, Stevens DJ, Xiao B, Ha Y, et al. The structure and receptor binding properties of the 1918 influenza hemagglutinin. Science 2004;303:1838-42.
This structural immunology paper analyzes the unique ability of the 1918 hemagglutinin to bind equally well to the α2,3-linked sialic acid–galactose moieties covering avian epithelial surfaces and to the α2,6-linked sialic acids typically found on human epithelial surface glycopeptides.

Harper SA, Bradley JS, Englund JA, File TM, Gravenstein S, Hayden F, et al. Seasonal influenza in adults and children–diagnosis, treatment, chemoprophylaxis and institutional outbreak management: clinical practice guidelines of the Infectious Disease Society of America. Clin Infect Dis 2009;48:1003-32.
This paper provides a useful review of the current existing evidence in support of a variety of diagnostic, therapeutic, and infection-control measures that are instituted when managing patients with influenza. This up-to-date guideline is a practical guide to optimal care of influenza in individual patients and in institutions during an outbreak.

REFERENCES

Access the complete reference list online at http://www.expertconsult.com.

141

Human Immunodeficiency Virus Infection

M. PATRICIA GEORGE | ALISON MORRIS

Many changes have occurred in the overall management and prognosis of patients with human immunodeficiency virus (HIV). Management of HIV-infected patients early in the acquired immunodeficiency syndrome (AIDS) epidemic was based largely on the diagnosis and treatment of opportunistic infections and neoplasms. Because these disorders were diagnosed late in the course of HIV infection, treatment often yielded poor results. In 1987, the first antiretroviral medication, zidovudine, became available and was followed by other nucleoside analogs.[1-2] In concert with chemoprophylaxis for opportunistic infections, these agents offered the first hope that HIV infection could be slowed. As time has passed, other classes of medications have been developed to combat HIV. With the discovery of protease inhibitors and the use of combination antiretroviral therapy (ART), there has been dramatic improvement in the morbidity and mortality of patients infected with HIV.[3] These combinations of medications can result in prolonged suppression of HIV viral RNA levels and sustained increases in CD4 cell counts.

Changes in the clinical characteristics and survival of those patients with HIV admitted to an intensive care unit (ICU) have occurred since the widespread introduction of combination ART in 1996. Unfortunately, not all patients have been able to benefit from antiretroviral therapy. Those not known to be HIV-infected, those without access to medications, and those not responding to antiretroviral therapy may still present with AIDS-associated opportunistic infections and neoplasms.[4] In this chapter, we discuss recent trends in the epidemiology and survival of HIV-infected patients admitted to an ICU. Because *Pneumocystis carinii* pneumonia (PCP) remains a leading cause of respiratory failure in HIV-infected patients and still carries a high mortality rate in the ICU, we will also discuss diagnostic approaches and therapy for PCP. Finally, we will examine problems unique to the ICU care of HIV-infected patients, particularly those related to combination ART.

Intensive Care Trends Among HIV-Infected Patients

EPIDEMIOLOGY

Both the epidemiology of ICU admissions and views of the utility of ICU care for HIV-infected patients have undergone several shifts during the course of the AIDS epidemic. In the beginning of the epidemic, most patients with HIV infection admitted to the ICU had PCP, and survival was poor.[5] ICU admission was often considered futile. Over the course of the epidemic, bacterial pneumonia, sepsis, and non–HIV-associated diagnoses have become increasingly common, although PCP remains an important cause of ICU admission, with high mortality in certain groups of patients. With the widespread availability of combination ART, there have been continued changes in ICU mortality and epidemiology so that ICU care is again indicated for most patients. Unfortunately, with reports of antiretroviral resistance and transmission of multidrug-resistant HIV, ICU trends may shift again, with an increase in opportunistic infections and poor outcomes.[6-8]

The most extensive series documenting ICU epidemiology has come from San Francisco General Hospital where researchers have tracked the trends in ICU diagnoses, admissions, and survival throughout the different eras of the AIDS epidemic. During era I (1981-1985), overall

hospital mortality for those admitted to an ICU was 69%, and median survival was only 7 months.[5] The number of ICU admissions peaked in 1984 and then decreased despite rising numbers of hospital admissions for AIDS patients. This decrease in ICU admissions was attributed to both physicians' and patients' views of ICU care as futile. In era II (1986-1988), mortality decreased, largely as a result of the use of adjunctive corticosteroids for PCP, which was still the leading cause of ICU admission.[9] Era III (1989-1991) actually saw an increase in mortality rates for PCP, likely from a bias away from withholding or withdrawing care.[10] In era IV (1992-1995), rates of ICU admission remained stable, and overall mortality was 36.9%, a significant improvement from era I.[11]

Era V, or the era of combination ART (1996-1999), brought about significant changes in both mortality and admission rates.[12] The number of ICU admissions decreased significantly from an average of 111 per year in era IV to 88.5 per year in era V, and survival rate increased to 71%. Respiratory failure was still the most common cause of ICU admission (40.7% of diagnoses), but PCP only accounted for 10.7% of admissions compared with 17.6% in era IV. Admission demographics of patients reflected national trends in the HIV epidemic. During previous eras, the majority of patients were white homosexual men.[11] During era V, African-Americans accounted for 44.6% of persons admitted to the ICU, and women and intravenous (IV) drug users were also more commonly admitted. During era VI (2000-2004), survival was about 69% over the entire period, with survival ratios increasing yearly during that time period from 58% in 2000 to 75% in 2004 ($P = 0.001$).[13] In addition, while PCP was the most common cause of respiratory failure in patients not on ART, obstructive airways disease was the most common cause of respiratory failure among patients on ART.[13]

Exact mortality and admission rates are different in different centers, but overall trends of decreasing mortality and changes in the spectrum of diagnoses related to HIV remain similar. A recent French study described the etiology and outcome of acute respiratory failure in HIV-infected patients from 1996 to 2000. Overall survival was 80% in this series.[14] In a British study examining 102 patients between 1999 and 2005, ICU and hospital discharge rates in HIV-infected patients were 77% and 68%, respectively, and no different than non–HIV-infected patients.[15] A study in Brazil of all HIV-infected ICU patients admitted between 1996 and 2006 found an ICU mortality of 55% and a 6-month mortality of 69%, and the authors postulated that their higher mortality rate was due to differences in patient characteristics and ICU access in their country.[28]

In most series, respiratory failure remains the leading cause of ICU admission in HIV-infected patients, although the percentage of respiratory admissions has declined. PCP accounted for as many as 62% of all ICU admissions in the early days of the epidemic and was by far the most common cause of respiratory failure.[5] Since the advent of ART, bacterial pneumonia has become more common, although PCP still accounts for many cases of respiratory failure.[13-16] In the ART era, Casolino reported an increase in ICU admissions for severe sepsis, often associated with respiratory failure ($P = 0.03$).[17] HIV-infected patients with bacterial pneumonia are more likely to become bacteremic, and mortality may be as high as 68% in this setting.[18] Non–AIDS-related diagnoses such as myocardial infarction, airways obstruction, and trauma are becoming more common during the current era of ART, as are ART-associated diagnoses.

In addition to respiratory failure, other comorbid conditions associated with HIV infection may be seen on admission to the ICU. These include cardiac disease, end-stage liver disease, and HIV-related renal disease. Combination ART has been associated with metabolic syndrome, dyslipidemias, and increased risk of myocardial infarction.[19-21] End-stage liver disease due to viral hepatis and HIV co-infection is a significant nonrespiratory problem seen in HIV-infected patients admitted to the ICU. Due to similar mechanisms of infection, chronic hepatitis B virus (HBV) has been reported in 10% and chronic hepatitis C virus (HCV) in 25% of HIV-infected individuals.[22] It is not clear whether HIV alters the course of HBV infection; however, HIV is a known risk factor for the accelerated progression of HCV to cirrhosis.[23] In addition to hepatotoxicity from hepatitis co-infection, many antiretrovirals can also elevate transaminase levels.[24] Finally, end-stage renal disease (ESRD) secondary to HIV is also a common complication. Although the prevalence has also decreased with the development of combination ART, it remains a significant problem, especially in HIV-infected African Americans, who are at higher risk of developing HIV-associated nephropathy with progression to ESRD.[25,26] Other risk factors for progression of chronic kidney disease include comorbidities such as hypertension, diabetes, HCV co-infection, and ART.[27]

PROGNOSTIC FACTORS

Clinicians and patients making decisions regarding the utility of care should understand risk factors for ICU mortality among HIV-infected patients. Studies have shown that there are several key factors that influence mortality, and these factors seem not to have changed over the years. Multivariate analysis of the cohort from era V at San Francisco General Hospital demonstrated that mechanical ventilation or a diagnosis of PCP predicted a higher mortality rate, whereas admission for a non–AIDS-associated diagnosis, an albumin level greater than 2.6 g/dL, and an Acute Physiology and Chronic Health Evaluation (APACHE) II score less than 13 all were associated with an increase in survival to hospital discharge.[12] These factors—particularly mechanical ventilation, vasopressor use, serum albumin, and PCP—had been known to influence mortality before the ART era as well.[11,14,17] In the cohort from era VI at San Francisco General Hospital, lack of invasive mechanical ventilation and albumin level were associated with improved survival to hospital discharge.[13] A recent study found that a CD4 cell count below 50 cells/μL is associated with ICU mortality and sepsis, and APACHE score above 19, need for mechanical ventilation during the first 24 hours of ICU admission, and year of ICU admission were associated with 6-month mortality.[28] Other long-term mortality predictors include an AIDS diagnosis before admission or first AIDS-defining condition.[17]

Intensive Care Trends in *Pneumocystis* Pneumonia

Because PCP has historically been the most common cause of respiratory failure in AIDS patients and the most common reason for ICU admission, more is known about the outcome of intensive care for AIDS patients with PCP than for any HIV-infected group. Mortality for PCP in the ICU, particularly for patients requiring mechanical ventilation, has been high throughout the course of the AIDS epidemic, but there have been some improvements. In the 1980s, HIV patients with PCP who required intensive care had a mortality rate as high as 81%, and mortality for patients requiring mechanical ventilation was 87%.[5] The introduction of adjunctive corticosteroids in the mid-1980s improved mortality for PCP-associated respiratory failure to approximately 60%.[9,29,30]

Mortality due to PCP has continued to decline in the era of combination ART. In a study of 59 consecutive patients admitted to the ICU, Miller and colleagues reported a 71% mortality prior to mid-1996, which decreased to 34% thereafter ($P = 0.008$).[31] In addition to year of diagnosis, risk factors associated with death also included age (odds

ratio [OR], 19.76; 95% confidence interval [CI], 1.74-224.34; $P = 0.016$) and mechanical ventilation and/or pneumothorax (OR, 5.18; 95% CI, 1.16-23.15; $P = 0.031$). In another large cohort study, Walzer and colleagues performed a retrospective study of HIV-infected adults admitted to the hospital with confirmed PCP between 1985 and 2006 and reported an overall mortality of 13.5%.[32] Risk factors associated with mortality included age 50 years or older, prior history of PCP, low hemoglobin level, Pao$_2$ less than 8.0 kPa on admission, pulmonary Kaposi sarcoma, and presence of a medical comorbidity. This study excluded complications subsequent to admission such as need for mechanical ventilation, pneumothorax, ICU admission, and treatment failure.[32]

Although there has been improvement in PCP survival in the era of combination ART, a diagnosis of PCP still remains a risk factor for overall mortality.[13,33] In a retrospective cohort study of 148 consecutive HIV-infected adults admitted to the ICU with respiratory failure, PCP was associated with increased risk of in-hospital mortality (OR, 3.19; 95% CI, 1.15-8.89; $P = 0.029$).[33]

DIAGNOSIS AND TREATMENT OF *PNEUMOCYSTIS* PNEUMONIA

Clinical Presentation

Although the number of cases of PCP has decreased, it remains a leading cause of respiratory failure among HIV-infected patients. PCP most commonly occurs in patients with CD4 cell counts below 200 cells/μL, and the risk of PCP increases exponentially as the CD4 cell count decreases below that level.[34,35] The clinical presentation of PCP ranges from the subtle to the fulminant. Most patients have most or all of the following symptoms and signs: fever, tachypnea, dyspnea with a nonproductive cough, and a chest examination that is normal or has a few dry rales.[36,37] In the HIV-infected patient, symptoms have generally been present for days to weeks before the diagnosis is made. Many patients may not be known to be HIV-infected. Recent studies have shown that approximately two-thirds of patients admitted to the ICU with PCP are unaware they are infected with HIV,[31,32] so clinicians must remember to include PCP in their differential of respiratory failure, even in those patients not known to have HIV.

Severe PCP is often similar in presentation and pathogenesis to acute respiratory distress syndrome (ARDS). The organism appears to cause a widespread capillary leak, and the chest radiograph usually resembles that in ARDS, with diffuse bilateral interstitial infiltrates. Less commonly, PCP results in focal airspace consolidation. Infiltrates are occasionally unilateral or asymmetrical, and the pattern seen (interstitial and nodular) is more suggestive of the diagnosis than the distribution of the abnormalities.[38] Finally, about 10% to 15% of patients who prove to have PCP initially have normal chest radiographs.[39,40]

Diagnosis

Although PCP may have a typical clinical and radiographic presentation, definitive diagnosis is encouraged, particularly in those who are critically ill. Many respiratory diseases in HIV have overlapping presentations, and prompt initiation of appropriate therapy is important to prevent clinical deterioration and avoid unnecessary drug side effects. The diagnosis of PCP is made when the organism is identified in the pulmonary secretions of a patient with a compatible clinical presentation. PCP may be diagnosed by examination of induced sputum, which has a sensitivity of 79% and a negative predictive value of 61% in experienced hands.[41] The usefulness of sputum induction is often limited because many hospitals may not be experienced in performing the test, and sputum induction is generally not tolerated in patients with respiratory distress.

When the sputum examination is negative or when it is not possible to obtain induced sputum, bronchoscopy with bronchoalveolar lavage (BAL) is the procedure of choice, with a sensitivity of over 90% for diagnosis of PCP in an HIV-infected individual and even greater yield

TABLE 141-1	Treatment Regimens for Severe *Pneumocystis* Pneumonia in Decreasing Order of Preference	
Agent	**Dose**	**Side Effects**
Trimethoprim-sulfamethoxazole	trimethoprim, 15-20 mg/kg/d, with sulfamethoxazole, 75-100 mg/kg/d IV, divided q 6-8 h	Rash, nausea, bone marrow suppression, hyponatremia, hyperkalemia, nephrotoxicity, transaminitis
Pentamidine isethionate	3-4 mg/kg/d IV	Nausea, hypotension, hypoglycemia or hyperglycemia, pancreatitis, bone marrow suppression, nephrotoxicity
Clindamycin-primaquine	clindamycin, 900 mg IV q 8 h; primaquine, 30 mg PO daily	Nausea, diarrhea, rash, hemolytic anemia, methemoglobinemia, leukopenia
Adjunctive therapy:		
Prednisone if Pao₂ <70 mm Hg or alveolar-arterial gradient >35 mm Hg	40 mg PO q 12 h for 5 days, 40 mg PO daily for 5 days, 20 mg PO daily for 11 days	Hyperglycemia, psychosis

when bilateral sampling is performed.[42,43] Bronchoscopy with BAL should be performed as early as possible in undiagnosed patients. Although the addition of transbronchial biopsy generally adds little to the yield of lavage in the diagnosis of HIV-associated PCP, it can be helpful in HIV-infected patients with other pulmonary processes.[44] Transbronchial biopsy is thus a reasonable initial invasive study when the probability of PCP is low and the risks associated with the procedure are acceptable; it is a useful follow-up test when the BAL fails to demonstrate PCP.

Treatment

A summary of treatment regimens in decreasing order of preference is given in Table 141-1. The treatment of choice for moderate to severe PCP is IV trimethoprim-sulfamethoxazole (TMP-SMX).[37] In a retrospective study of 1122 patients with PCP, comparison of 3-month survival rates between TMP-SMX, clindamycin-primaquine and IV pentamidine were 85%, 81%, and 76% (P = 0.09), respectively.[45] The TMP-SMX should be administered at a total daily dose of 15 to 20 mg/kg of trimethoprim and 75 to 100 mg/kg of sulfamethoxazole divided into 3 or 4 doses per day; recommended duration of therapy is 21 days.[37] Approximately 25% of patients will have therapy-limiting toxicity from TMP-SMX, with most severe toxicities occurring between days 6 and 10 of treatment.[46-49] Side effects of TMP-SMX include nausea, rash, bone marrow suppression, hyponatremia, hyperkalemia, renal dysfunction, and transaminitis.

Intravenous pentamidine isethionate is an effective alternative for therapy in patients who cannot tolerate TMP-SMX or have failed treatment.[37] Although this agent has been reported to have success rates equivalent to TMP-SMX, some studies have found that it is somewhat less efficacious.[45,50-52] The recommended daily dose of pentamidine is 3 to 4 mg/kg administered over 1 hour. Pentamidine has a high rate of serious toxicity that includes nausea, hypotension, pancreatitis, hypoglycemia and hyperglycemia, bone marrow suppression, and nephrotoxicity. Because pentamidine is toxic to the pancreatic islet cells, initial hypoglycemia from a surge of insulin release followed by hyperglycemia from inadequate insulin may be seen, and the patient may progress to chronic diabetes mellitus. Adverse reactions may be seen in as many as 50% of patients treated with pentamidine.

Second-line therapy may be used if first-line therapies prove to be ineffective or have unacceptable side effects. Because treatment of PCP is often accompanied by an initial worsening, treatment failure should not be diagnosed before 4 to 8 days of therapy. If TMP-SMX has been the first-line agent, IV pentamidine or the combination of IV clindamycin with oral primaquine may be substituted. Recent studies

of second-line regimens found that TMP-SMX and clindamycin-primaquine had equivalent success rates, but response to pentamidine was significantly lower.[45,53] These studies included both ICU and non-ICU patients, and the lower response rate seen with pentamidine may have resulted from in an increased tendency to use IV pentamidine in ICU patients, because oral absorption of primaquine may be poor in this population.

The most profound improvement in PCP mortality has occurred with the introduction of adjunctive corticosteroids.[9,29,30] In a meta-analysis of six randomized controlled trials comparing adjunctive corticosteroids to standard care in HIV-infected patients with PCP, risk ratios for overall mortality were 0.54 (95% CI, 0.38-0.79) at 1 month and 0.67 (95% CI, 0.49-0.93) at 3 to 4 months in favor of corticosteroids. In patients undergoing mechanical ventilation, corticosteroids were also associated with an improved outcome (risk ratio of 0.37; 95% CI, 0.20-0.70).[54] It is recommended that patients with PCP and either a Pao₂ in room air of less than 70 mm Hg or an alveolar-arterial oxygen gradient greater than 35 mm Hg receive corticosteroids to reduce mortality.[37] Corticosteroid therapy should be administered within 72 hours of initiating anti-*Pneumocystis* therapy, even if the diagnosis has not yet been established, because corticosteroids act to decrease the inflammation seen during the first few days of treatment. The recommended regimen is oral prednisone, 40 mg, given twice daily for 5 days, followed by 40 mg once daily for 5 days, then 20 mg daily for 11 days. For those patients unable to take oral medications, IV methylprednisolone may be substituted at 75% of the prednisone dose.[37]

Treatment Failure

Clinical deterioration is commonly seen 3 to 5 days after initiation of treatment. Patients may experience worsening respiratory status with decreases in arterial oxygenation. These symptoms are likely due to an inflammatory response to dead or dying organisms that may increase capillary permeability and pulmonary edema formation. This edema formation may be inadvertently worsened by administration of excessive IV fluids.

Given that patients' conditions may deteriorate and that symptoms may be prolonged, it is difficult to determine when a treatment regimen is failing and should be abandoned for an alternative. Whether treatment failure is more likely in patients with previous prophylaxis use is unknown, but *Pneumocystis* has been shown to develop genetic mutations with exposure to sulfa- or sulfone-containing medications such as TMP-SMX and dapsone.[55,56] The relationship of these mutations to outcome is still controversial.[57-60] In general, treatment should be continued for 4 to 8 days before considering changing to a different agent.[37] It is also important to investigate alternative diagnoses that may be responsible for the patient's symptoms. Other causes of pneumonia including other opportunistic pathogens and nosocomial organisms should be considered when treatment appears to be failing. Patients with PCP are also at increased risk of pulmonary edema, which may explain worsening respiratory status with increasing radiographic infiltrates. Alternative diagnoses should be pursued with chest computed tomography (CT), sputum cultures, or echocardiography as clinically indicated. Repeat bronchoscopy is helpful to diagnose agents other than PCP, but is not useful in determining whether PCP treatment is failing, because *Pneumocystis* may persist in the bronchoalveolar lavage fluid for several weeks.[61]

Ventilation of the Patient with PCP

The physiology of severe PCP resembles that of ARDS, and patients with PCP are at high risk for developing barotrauma and pneumothoraces, often heralding a fatal outcome. Low tidal volume ventilation per ARDSNet protocol has been shown to be associated with decreased mortality in HIV-infected patients with acute lung injury (OR, 0.76 per 1 mL/kg decrease; 95% CI, 0.58-0.99, P = 0.043).[33,62] Similar to non–HIV-infected patients with acute lung injury (ALI), low tidal volume ventilation is becoming the standard of care in HIV-infected patients with ALI from PCP or other causes. Noninvasive positive-pressure ventilation (NIPPV) has been studied in PCP and has been found to lower the rate of intubation, decrease the incidence of pneumothorax, and improve ICU survival.[63] Use of NIPPV would be a reasonable first-line ventilation mode in patients with PCP and respiratory distress who can tolerate this form of ventilation and who can protect their airway.

Combination Antiretroviral Therapy and the ICU

LACTIC ACIDOSIS

With the increasing use of combination ART, ICU physicians need to be familiar with some of the life-threatening side effects that can occur with these medications. The syndrome of severe hepatic steatosis and lactic acidosis was first described in the 1990s.[64,65] The syndrome is most commonly associated with nucleoside reverse transcriptase inhibitors (NRTIs), particularly didanosine and stavudine, and results from mitochondrial toxicity of these agents.[66,67] The incidence of hyperlactatemia in patients taking NRTIs has been reported as high as 227 cases per 1000 person-years.[68] Symptomatic lactic acidosis in HIV-infected patients taking NRTIs ranges from 1 to 25.2 cases per 1000 patient-years, and mortality rates may be as high as 77%.[69] Risk factors for development of hyperlactatemia include older age, drug regimens containing stavudine or combined stavudine-didanosine, use of buprenorphine, creatinine clearance less than 70 mL/min, and nadir CD4 cell count less than 250 cells/μL.[70,71] A case-control study indicated that female sex and obesity were also risk factors for stavudine-related lactic acidosis.[70]

Patients often present with abdominal pain, nausea, and vomiting and may have myalgias or peripheral neuropathies. Serum lactate levels are elevated, and hepatic steatosis and elevation of transaminases occur frequently. Often, cessation of the ART results in resolution of the syndrome; however, some patients can progress to life-threatening organ failure. An initial lactate level above 9 mmol/L seems to be associated with a higher risk of death, and some authors believe that a level greater than 5 mmol/L should be considered life threatening.[72,73]

In patients presenting with mild lactic acidosis, the offending agent should be switched to a safer alternative (e.g., abacavir, tenofovir, lamivudine, emtricitabine). Lactate levels should be closely monitored after changing the NRTI. For severe lactate acidosis, ART should be discontinued, and supportive care should be administered.[24] Although data regarding treatment outcomes are not extensive, treatment should be started in those patients with a lactate level above 5 mmol/L. Treatment with riboflavin, thiamine, and L-carnitine has reversed toxicity in some case reports.[24,72-75] One recommended regimen is to administer 50 mg of riboflavin daily with 50 mg/kg of L-carnitine and 100 mg of thiamine until the lactic acidosis resolves. The exact length of treatment and the lactate level above which treatment is unlikely to succeed remain unclear.

IMMUNE RECONSTITUTION

The immune reconstitution inflammatory syndrome (IRIS) leads to paradoxical worsening of an infection shortly after initiation of ART. This syndrome results from improvement in the immune system and a renewed inflammatory response directed against infectious agents.[76] Although this syndrome has been reported to occur in diseases such as tuberculosis, cytomegalovirus (CMV), and *Mycobacterium avium* complex, it usually results only in a symptomatic worsening of these conditions.[76-78] A recent meta-analysis of 54 cohort studies of patients who developed IRIS found that IRIS occurred in 16.1% (95% CI, 11.1-22.9) of all patients and was associated with a 4.5% (95% CI, 2.1-8.6) mortality.[79] There have been case reports of paradoxical worsening occurring during PCP, with patients experiencing increasing respiratory distress and hypoxemia and some requiring mechanical ventilation.[80-82] All patients subsequently recovered, and there seemed to be some benefit from continuing or reintroducing corticosteroids.[82] Patients admitted to the ICU with a presumed paradoxical worsening

of PCP should receive corticosteroids, and appropriate testing should be performed to rule out other infections or respiratory disorders causing clinical worsening.

ADMINISTRATION OF ANTIRETROVIRAL THERAPY IN THE ICU

The question of whether to continue or initiate ART while HIV-infected patients are in the ICU is an unresolved issue in critical care. Traditionally, antiretroviral regimens have been discontinued while patients are in intensive care, and clinicians have been reluctant to initiate ART in this population. Many issues relating to the use of ART exist in the ICU, including possible poor gastric absorption of antiretroviral medications, the potential for drug interactions and side effects, and concern about patient compliance in continuing ART after discharge. There is also concern that initiating ART in a patient with borderline respiratory status might lead to respiratory failure through paradoxical worsening and immune reconstitution.

ART therapy is complicated in the ICU. Only zidovudine is available in an IV form. Other agents that are available as liquids and therefore could be administered via a feeding tube are listed in Box 141-1. If physicians choose to administer ART to an ICU patient, they need to be particularly aware of possible side effects including renal toxicity and hepatotoxicity, pancreatitis, and lactic acidosis. Many common ICU medications such as benzodiazepines, fluconazole, pentamidine, and amiodarone may have dangerous interactions or altered metabolism when given with antiretrovirals. Medications may also affect the serum levels of antiretrovirals, resulting either in toxic or subtherapeutic concentrations. Consultation with a specialist familiar with the many antiretroviral regimens is advised.

It is currently unclear whether the mortality benefits of ART administration in ICU patients outweigh the risks and difficulties. Although not limited to critically ill patients, results from a recent randomized controlled trial compared deferring therapy to initiating ART within 14 days of starting therapy for an AIDS-related opportunistic infection or serious bacterial infection; early ART resulted in decreased progression of AIDS or death compared to deferred therapy (OR, 0.51; 95% CI, 0.27-0.94).[83] In a retrospective cohort study of 278 HIV-infected patients admitted to the ICU in Sao Paolo from 1996 through 2006, Croda and colleagues found beginning ART during the ICU stay was associated with reduced 6-month mortality, significantly less than patients not on ART while in the ICU (hazard ratio, 0.55; 95% CI, 0.31-0.98; P = 0.004).[28] Survival was worse in those who were previously on ART and had it stopped while in intensive care; however, use

---

Box 141-1

LIST OF ANTIRETROVIRAL AGENTS AVAILABLE IN NON–PILL FORM

Protease Inhibitors
Amprenavir
Fosamprenavir
Lopinavir/ritonavir
Nelfinavir
Ritonavir
Tipranavir

Nucleoside Reverse Transcriptase Inhibitors
Abacavir
Didanosine
Emtricitabine
Lamivudine
Stavudine
Zidovudine (also intravenous)

Non-nucleoside Reverse Transcriptase Inhibitor
Nevirapine

Fusion Inhibitor
Enfuviritide (subcutaneous injection)

of ART in the ICU was associated with adverse events in 18% of patients. Morris and colleagues studied patients with PCP admitted to the ICU during the era of ART. They found that mortality among patients who did not receive ART was 63%, whereas those patients either receiving ART at time of admission or started on ART in the ICU had a mortality rate of only 25%.[84] There have been several reports of improved cumulative survival (e.g., months to years post ICU discharge) among ICU survivors started on ART.[17,33,85-87] Other studies, however, have not found that starting ART in the ICU improves ICU or in-hospital survival.[31,87] One study of HIV-infected patients with respiratory failure found a trend toward worse outcome in those receiving ART in the ICU (30% mortality in those on ART versus 15% in those not on ART, $P = 0.07$).[14]

Given the lack of consensus guidelines for whether and when to initiate combination ART in the ICU, the decision to do so must be made on a case-by-case basis. A useful treatment strategy was described by Huang and colleagues.[88] In patients who are known to be HIV-positive and are already receiving combination ART, combination ART should be continued if the viral load is undetectable and there are no contraindications to continuing the drugs (e.g., drug toxicities, resistance, IRIS, difficulty in delivery or drug absorption). If the patient has a contraindication to ART, the entire regimen should be held so as not to foster resistance, and an HIV specialist should be consulted. In patients who are known to be HIV positive but are not on ART, or who are diagnosed with HIV on their ICU admission, consideration should be given to starting combination ART if the condition is an AIDS-associated condition, and an HIV specialist should be consulted. If the condition is not AIDS-associated, and CD4 count is greater than 200 cells, ART should probably be deferred until after the patient is discharged from the ICU, unless their ICU course is prolonged. The importance of consultation with an HIV specialist in these ART treatment decisions cannot be overemphasized.

Metabolic Abnormalities in the ICU

METABOLIC COMPLICATIONS OF ANTIRETROVIRAL THERAPY

Many drugs included in ART regimens have adverse effects on the metabolism of lipids and glucose. Patients treated with these drugs commonly develop metabolic abnormalities including hyperlipidemia, hypercholesterolemia, glucose intolerance, and diabetes.[89-91] Conditions such as cardiovascular disease, dyslipidemia, insulin resistance, and osteoporosis seem to be associated with ART, and protease inhibitors have been specifically associated with an increased relative risk of myocardial infarction (MI).[19,20,92] The HIV Outpatient Study (HOPS) found that risk of MI increased among those using protease inhibitors (OR for MI = 7.1).[93] In the landmark multicenter prospective study of 23,468 patients, the Data Collection on Adverse Events of Anti-HIV Drugs (DAD) study group reported that combination ART was independently associated with a 26 percent relative increase in the rate of MI per year of exposure in the first 4 to 6 years of use.[20] In a follow-up study, the group showed that exposure to protease inhibitors was associated with increased risk of MI, likely related to dyslipidemia.[19] More recent studies have reported that the nucleoside reverse transcriptase inhibitors, abacavir and didanosine, are also associated with increased risk of cardiovascular disease,[94,95] but not all studies support this association. A cohort of over 36,000 HIV-infected patients followed from 1993 to 2001 demonstrated no relationship between use of antiretroviral medications and cerebrovascular or cardiovascular events, but follow-up may have been too short to detect an effect.[96] In general, HIV-infected patients admitted to the ICU with cardiac disease should be treated as the non–HIV-infected population, with interventions including cardiac artery bypass grafting as indicated. Data show that short-term outcome is equivalent, although HIV-infected patients have a higher long-term risk of requiring revascularization.[97] As HIV-infected patients live longer due to ART, clinicians can expect to see problems such as cardiac disease more frequently as the HIV-infected population ages.

ADRENAL INSUFFICIENCY

Adrenal insufficiency is an important syndrome in the ICU that is more common among HIV-infected patients. The adrenal glands of patients with HIV may be damaged by infections such as CMV, neoplasms such as lymphoma, and drugs such as ketoconazole and rifampin.[98-100] At its most severe, adrenal insufficiency can present as refractory hypotension and may lead to death if not recognized. Marik and colleagues studied adrenal function in 28 critically ill HIV-infected patients. In this study, depending on the criteria used, the rate of adrenal insufficiency varied from 7% to 75%.[101] Evidence of CMV infection was more common among the patients with adrenal insufficiency. Clinicians should have a high degree of suspicion for adrenal insufficiency in HIV-infected patients, particularly in those with CMV, and should consider adrenocorticotropic hormone stimulation testing. Patients with septic shock or early ARDS should be empirically treated for adrenal insufficiency according to American College of Critical Care Medicine guidelines.[102]

Conclusion

The outlook for ICU patients with HIV has improved dramatically since the beginning of the AIDS epidemic. Physicians caring for HIV-infected patients in the ICU need an understanding of both the HIV-associated and the non–HIV-associated conditions that can affect these patients. Knowledge of antiretroviral therapies and their side effects is also important because these therapies may lead directly to patients' ICU admissions and impact their morbidity and mortality. It is hoped that information will become available to guide clinicians in use of ART in the ICU, and survival will continue to improve.

KEY POINTS

1. Intensive care survival of HIV-infected patients has improved over the course of the AIDS epidemic, and ICU care is now indicated for most patients.

2. Non–AIDS-related diagnoses have become more common since the introduction of combination antiretroviral therapy (ART), although many patients admitted to the ICU may not be receiving this therapy.

3. Mortality from *Pneumocystis* pneumonia (PCP) can still be high, particularly if patients develop a pneumothorax while on mechanical ventilation.

4. Clinicians should have a high suspicion for PCP, because many patients will not be aware that they are HIV-infected before ICU admission.

5. Early bronchoscopy with bronchoalveolar lavage should be performed in patients with pneumonia who do not have a definitive microbiological diagnosis.

6. Trimethoprim-sulfamethoxazole is the treatment of choice for PCP, and corticosteroids should be given to those meeting established criteria.

7. Fatal lactic acidosis can develop as a result of antiretroviral medications. Treatment consists of drug discontinuation and supportive care. Administration of riboflavin, thiamine, and L-carnitine may be beneficial.

8. Immune reconstitution syndrome after initiating ART can occasionally lead to respiratory failure, particularly in patients with PCP.

9. Administration of ART in the ICU is difficult, may lead to viral resistance, and is associated with many side effects and drug interactions; however, the association of ART use with mortality remains unclear.

10. Adrenal insufficiency is more common in HIV-infected patients and should be suspected in patients with hypotension.

ANNOTATED REFERENCES

Barbier F, Coquet I, Legriel S, et al. Etiologies and outcome of acute respiratory failure in HIV-infected patients. Intensive Care Med 2009;35:1678-86.

A retrospective study of 147 HIV-infected patients admitted to an ICU for acute respiratory failure (ARF) between 1996 and 2006, describing the etiologies of respiratory failure in this cohort. The most common cause of ARF was bacterial pneumonia (n = 74), followed by Pneumocystis jirovecii pneumonia (PCP; n = 52), other opportunistic infections (n = 19), and noninfectious pulmonary disease (n = 33). Two or more causes were identified in 33 patients. The 43 patients on ART more frequently had bacterial pneumonia and less frequently had opportunistic infections (P = 0.02). Noninvasive ventilation was needed in 49 patients and endotracheal intubation in 42. Hospital mortality was 19.7%. Factors independently associated with mortality were mechanical ventilation (OR, 8.48; P < 0.0001), vasopressor use (OR, 4.48; P = 0.03), time from hospital admission to ICU admission (OR, 1.05 per day; P = 0.01), and number of causes (OR, 3.19; P = 0.02). HIV-related variables (CD4 count, viral load, and ART) were not associated with mortality.

Casolino E, Wolff M, Ravaud P, et al. Impact of HAART advent on admission patterns and survival in HIV-infected patients admitted to an intensive care unit. AIDS 2004;18:1429-33.

This prospective observational cohort study of 426 HIV-infected patients admitted to an ICU between 1995 to 1999 examined ICU epidemiology and survival. The incidence of sepsis increased while AIDS-related admissions decreased. Overall ICU survival was 77%, and cumulative survival rates after ICU discharge were 85.3% and 70.8% after 1 year and 2 years, respectively. While ICU survival was dependent on the non–HIV-associated prognostic indicators (SAPS II score > 40, Omega score > 75, and mechanical ventilation), long-term survival was associated with HIV disease stage and availability of combination antiretroviral therapy.

Davis JL, Morris A, Kallet RH, et al. Low tidal volume ventilation is associated with reduced mortality in HIV-infected patients with acute lung injury. Thorax 2008;11:988-93.

This retrospective cohort study compared ventilator strategies in 148 HIV-infected patients with respiratory failure before and after the introduction of low tidal volume ventilation in 2000. Among all those with acute lung injury, lower tidal volume was associated with decreased mortality (adjusted OR, 0.76 per 1-mL/kg decrease; 95% CI, 0.58-0.99; P = 0.043). This study supports the use of low tidal volume ventilation strategy in HIV-infected patients with acute lung injury and respiratory failure.

Dickson SJ, Batson S, Copas AJ, et al. Survival of HIV-infected patients in the intensive care unit in the era of highly active antiretroviral therapy. Thorax 2007;62:964-8.

This retrospective study of 102 HIV-infected patients admitted to the ICU between January 1999 and December 2005 reported an overall ICU and hospital survival of 77% and 68%, respectively. Factors predicting survival to ICU discharge included hemoglobin, CD4 cell count, APACHE II score, and mechanical ventilation. Use of combination ART was not associated with survival. Outcomes for HIV-infected patients were comparable to general medical patients.

Muller M, Wandel S, Colebunders R, et al. Immune reconstitution inflammatory syndrome in patients starting antiretroviral therapy for HIV infection: a systematic review and meta-analysis. Lancet Infect Dis 2010;10:251-61.

A systematic review and meta-analysis describing the prevalence of IRIS in patients with different opportunistic infections. The overall prevalence of IRIS was 16.1% (11.1-22.9) in unselected patients starting ART, and 4.5% (2.1-8.6) of patients with any type of IRIS died. Meta-regression analyses showed that the risk of IRIS is associated with CD4 cell count at the start of ART, with a high risk in patients with fewer than 50 cells per μL. Occurrence of IRIS might therefore be reduced by initiation of ART before immunodeficiency becomes advanced.

Powell K, Davis JL, Morris AM, et al. Survival for patients with HIV admitted to the ICU continues to improve in the current era of combination antiretroviral therapy. Chest 2009;135:11-7.

Sixth in a series of articles from San Francisco General Hospital documenting ICU epidemiology and mortality of HIV-infected patients throughout the course of the AIDS epidemic. In the most recent era of combination antiretroviral therapy, respiratory failure remained the most common indication for ICU admission (42% overall). The proportion of patients with respiratory failure decreased each year from 52% to 34% (P = 0.02), and hospital survival ratios significantly increased during the 5-year period (P = 0.001). ART use at ICU admission was not associated with survival, but it was associated with higher CD4 cell counts, lower plasma HIV RNA levels, higher serum albumin levels, and lower proportions with AIDS-associated ICU admission diagnoses and with Pneumocystis pneumonia.

Walzer PD, Evans HE, Copas AJ, et al. Early predictors of mortality from Pneumocystis jirovecii pneumonia in HIV-infected patients: 1985-2006. Clin Infect Dis 2008;46:625-33.

This study is the largest retrospective study to date of 494 consecutive patients with 547 episodes of laboratory-confirmed PCP and identified risk factors for mortality on or soon after admission. Overall mortality was 13.5%. Multivariate analysis identified factors associated with risk of death, including increasing patient age (adjusted odds ratio [AOR], 1.54; 95% CI, 1.11-2.23; P = .011), subsequent episode of PCP (AOR, 2.27; 95% CI, 1.14-4.52; P = .019), low hemoglobin level at hospital admission (AOR, 0.70; 95% CI, 0.60-0.83; P < .001), low partial pressure of oxygen breathing room air at hospital admission (AOR, 0.70; 95% CI, 0.60-0.81; P < .001), presence of medical comorbidity (AOR, 3.93; 95% CI, 1.77-8.72; P = .001), and pulmonary Kaposi sarcoma (AOR, 6.95; 95% CI, 2.26-21.37; P = .001). Patients with a first episode of PCP were sicker (mean partial pressure of oxygen at admission ± standard deviation, 9.3 ± 2.0 kPa) than those with a second or third episode of PCP (mean partial pressure of oxygen at admission ± standard deviation, 9.9 ± 1.9 kPa; P = .008), but mortality among patients with a first episode of PCP (12.5%) was lower than mortality among patients with subsequent episodes of PCP (22.5%) (P = .019). While mortality decreased in the ART era, no patient was receiving highly active antiretroviral therapy before presentation with PCP, and none began highly active antiretroviral therapy during treatment of PCP; thus the trend towards improved outcome after June 1996 occurred in the absence of highly active antiretroviral therapy.

Zalopa A, Andersen J, Powderly W, et al. Early antiretroviral therapy reduces AIDS progression/death in individuals with acute opportunistic infections: a multicenter randomized strategy trial. PLoS One 2009;4:e5575.

Randomized strategy trial of "early ART" given within 14 days of starting treatment for an acute opportunistic infection (OI) versus "deferred ART" given after OI treatment was completed. There was no statistically significant difference in primary outcomes at 48 weeks (death/AIDS progression or HIV progression with complete or incomplete viral suppression), but the early ART arm did have fewer AIDS progression/deaths (hazard ratio [HR] 0.51; 95% CI, 0.27-0.94) and a longer time to AIDS progression/death (stratified HR 0.53; 95% CI, 0.30-0.92). The early ART arm also had a shorter time to achieving a CD4 count over 50 cells/mL (P < 0.001) and no increase in adverse events.

REFERENCES

Access the complete reference list online at http://www.expertconsult.com.

142

Tuberculosis

EDWARD D. CHAN | MARINKA KARTALIJA

Epidemiology

The World Health Organization (WHO) estimates that one-third of the world's population is latently infected with *Mycobacterium tuberculosis*.[1] From this pool, approximately 9 million active tuberculosis (TB) cases emerge annually, resulting in 2 million deaths and making TB the second leading cause of death by an infectious agent worldwide.[2] The vast majority of TB cases (95%) occur in the developing world. Incidence rates exceed 300 cases per 100,000 persons throughout sub-Saharan Africa, the Indonesian and Philippine archipelagos, Afghanistan, Bolivia, and Peru.[1,3] Areas with the most cases per year include densely populated India (2 million cases per year) and China (1.3 million cases per year).

In the United States, the TB rate continues to decline, with 3.8 new cases per 100,000 reported in 2009, the lowest rate recorded since national reporting began in 1953. Foreign-born persons and racial/ethnic minorities continue to bear a disproportionate burden of TB disease in the United States. In 2008, the TB rate within the foreign-born population in the United States was 10 times higher than in U.S.-born persons.[4] TB rates among Hispanics and blacks were nearly eight times higher than among non-Hispanic whites, and rates among Asians were nearly 23 times higher than among non-Hispanic whites. Among U.S.-born racial and ethnic groups, the greatest racial disparity in TB rates was seen in the black population, who are seven times more likely to develop active TB than U.S.-born whites. Other groups at increased risk for active TB include prisoners, the homeless, and human immunodeficiency virus (HIV)-positive individuals.

The acquired immunodeficiency syndrome (AIDS) epidemic has contributed significantly to the rise in TB cases worldwide, with about 1.5 million individuals with active TB per year co-infected with HIV. HIV increases the risk of developing TB by 20.6-fold in countries where the prevalence of HIV is more than 1% in the general population.[5] Co-infection with HIV contributes significantly to TB-related mortality.

The Serious Problem of Highly Drug-Resistant Tuberculosis

Drug-susceptible TB is readily curable provided adherence to medications is followed. However, drug-resistant TB requires a significantly longer course of antibiotics coupled with second-line agents that often are accompanied by difficult-to-tolerate side effects. More importantly, highly drug-resistant TB is associated with significant increase in morbidity and mortality. In the early 1990s, substantial levels of drug resistance began emerging in urban parts of the United States.[6] Although the incidence of drug-resistant TB has diminished in the United States, it is increasingly problematic in many parts of the world.[7]

Multidrug-resistant TB (MDR-TB) is defined as resistance to two of the most powerful first-line anti-TB drugs, isoniazid (INH) and rifampin (RIF). Isolates that are resistant to multiple other combinations of anti-TB drugs but not to INH or RIF are not classified as MDR-TB. It is estimated that of the 9 million new cases of TB per year in the world, 500,000 are due to MDR-TB. Whereas drug-resistant TB is increasing at an alarming rate worldwide, particularly in India and China, prevalence in the United States decreased between 1991 and

2006 from 3.5% to 1.1%.[8] MDR-TB disproportionately affects foreign-born individuals, accounting for 0.4% of TB cases occurring in U.S.-born persons and 1.3% in foreign-born individuals.[9]

Extensively drug-resistant tuberculosis (XDR-TB) is defined as resistance to INH, RIF, any fluoroquinolone, and to a second-line injectable (amikacin, kanamycin, or capreomycin). XDR-TB has emerged with a wide geographic distribution, including the United States, and is associated with worse treatment outcomes than MDR-TB, especially in those co-infected with HIV.[7,10-15]

Tuberculosis in the Intensive Care Unit

TB patients requiring intensive care unit (ICU) care represent 1% to 3% of all patients with active TB. Most studies of TB patients requiring ICU admission are retrospective and frequently include a disproportionate number of HIV-positive individuals. TB should be considered in the differential diagnosis of critically ill patients, particularly in foreign-born individuals who emigrated from countries with a high prevalence of TB. With the increased use of tumor necrosis factor alpha (TNF-α) antagonists and other immunosuppressive agents, ICU physicians are more likely to encounter patients with non-classical features of TB. In this chapter, selected critical care issues in TB are discussed. Some disease forms, such as renal and peritoneal TB, are omitted because they are less likely to be seen in the ICU.

Pulmonary Tuberculosis

Pulmonary disease is by far the most common manifestation of active TB and of TB requiring ICU admission. Pulmonary disease may be due to a primary infection or to reactivation disease.

Primary infection occurs following airborne implantation of tubercle bacilli into the lungs. *M. tuberculosis* spreads from the lungs to hilar lymph nodes, and then throughout the bloodstream (Figure 142-1). Although primary infection is usually asymptomatic in adults, it can present with fever, hilar adenopathy, lung infiltrates, pleural effusions, and even severe pulmonary disease that may mimic viral or bacterial pneumonia, which may delay the diagnosis of TB. In severely immunocompromised patients, primary TB may be aggressive and become disseminated. Pleural TB is usually a manifestation of primary TB, although it may also occur with reactivation disease. Pleural TB can present as pleuritis or empyema. Pleural biopsy specimens are more likely to yield positive cultures than pleural fluid.

Most cases of active TB are due to reactivation of latent TB infection (LTBI). Active TB develops in about 10% of immunocompetent individuals with LTBI and tends to occur within the first 2 years of the initial infection. Typically, reactivation TB is a subacute fibrocavitary pneumonia involving the upper lobes and/or superior segments of the lower lobes. However, reactivation TB can involve any organ system and can present in a fulminant fashion with respiratory failure.[16]

There are some common clinical characteristics of TB patients who require ICU care. In a study of 58 ICU patients with confirmed TB, 22 (37.9%) required mechanical ventilation, and 15 (25.9%) died in the hospital.[17] The factors independently associated with mortality were acute renal failure, need for mechanical ventilation, chronic pancreatitis, sepsis, acute respiratory distress syndrome (ARDS), and nosocomial pneumonia.[17] Both primary and reactivation TB can cause bilateral alveolar infiltrates, hypoxic respiratory failure, and ARDS.[16,18]

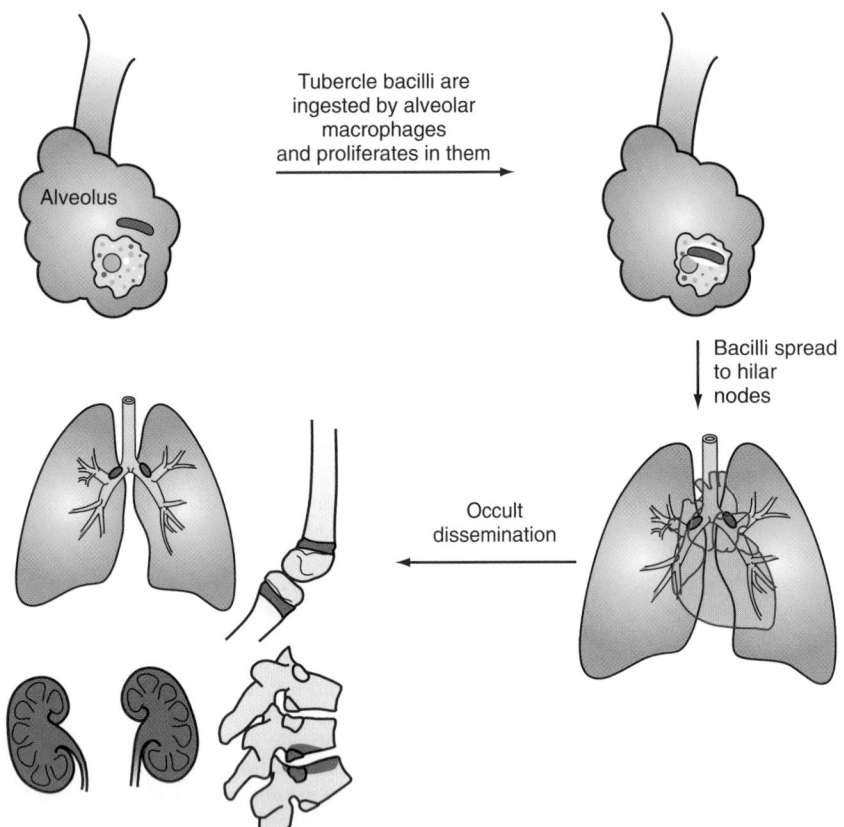

Tubercle bacilli are ingested by alveolar macrophages and proliferates in them

Alveolus

Bacilli spread to hilar nodes

Occult dissemination

Figure 142-1 Representation of a primary infection of TB and occult dissemination. Largely asymptomatic, dissemination of *M. tuberculosis* following primary infection occurs when infected mononuclear cells migrate throughout the body, particularly to lung apices, kidneys, bone growth plates, and vertebrae, resulting in latent infection.

In another study of patients hospitalized with pulmonary TB, six factors were shown to be associated with respiratory failure or death: lymphopenia, advanced age, concomitant smear-positive extrapulmonary TB, alcoholism, a high percentage of neutrophils on the peripheral white blood cell count, and lack of radiographic cavitation.[19] Laboratory findings of anemia and hypoalbuminemia have been shown to be predictors for death in patients with respiratory failure due to TB.[20] However, these findings are not specific to TB and commonly present in the critically ill.

Consolidation is the most frequent radiographic pattern of patients with pulmonary TB who are admitted to the ICU.[21] Because this radiographic pattern is highly nonspecific, chest x-rays are often unhelpful in raising the suspicion for TB. Consolidation on initial chest radiograph has also been shown to be a strong independent risk factor for in-hospital mortality.[22] One possible reason for this is a delay in the diagnosis; clinicians may be more prone to favor a diagnosis of nontuberculous pneumonia in the absence of cavitation or miliary pattern. Another is that consolidation may be an indication of a suboptimal immune response to the infection. Pulmonary gangrene, which carries a mortality of up to 75%, can ensue when rapid progression of infiltrate causes vascular damage and death of lung tissue.[23] Other life-threatening complications of pulmonary TB include hemoptysis, spontaneous pneumothoraces, bronchopleural fistulas, and empyema. Not unexpectedly, delayed recognition and treatment of nosocomial pneumonia complicating TB in patients requiring mechanical ventilation has a significant adverse effect on survival.[24]

Perhaps the best safeguard to prevent missing a diagnosis of pulmonary or disseminated TB in the critically ill is to maintain a high index of suspicion of it in at-risk individuals (e.g., foreign-born or immunosuppressed patients). Studies have shown that the presence of diffuse infiltrates consistent with ARDS and acute respiratory failure may cause physicians to inappropriately dismiss the diagnosis of TB.[25-27]

Older individuals (≥65 years) or patients with AIDS may also have delayed diagnosis of TB, due in part to atypical presentations.[28,29]

Hospital mortality has been reported to be 60% for patients with respiratory failure due to pulmonary TB.[22] Hence, despite being a relatively rare cause of respiratory failure in ICU patients, pulmonary TB carries a poor prognosis. Early recognition of the infection is essential to reduce mortality and prevent nosocomial spread of *M. tuberculosis*.[27]

Disseminated Tuberculosis

Disseminated, or "miliary," TB is more likely to occur in the very young and very old and in patients with underlying diseases such as HIV. It may result from either primary or reactivation TB. Disseminated TB typically presents subacutely with symptoms present for days to months, but it can manifest fulminantly with septic shock and multiorgan failure.[30] Typical presenting signs and symptoms include fever, malaise, weight loss, dyspnea, and hypoxia.

The chest radiograph (Figure 142-2, *A*) and computed tomography (CT) scan (see Figure 142-2, *B*) show a typical miliary pattern manifested by a profusion of diffuse small (<2 mm) nodules that resemble the size and uniformity of millet seeds (see Figure 142-2, *C*). In some cases of disseminated disease, the chest radiograph may appear normal. Virtually any organ may be involved, including the adrenals, brain, meninges, liver, pancreas, eyes, urinary tract, and skin. Bone marrow involvement by TB commonly manifests with anemia, leukemoid reaction, and thrombocytosis. The diagnosis of miliary TB can be difficult. If disseminated TB is suspected, sputum smears should be obtained even if lung disease is not apparent. Biopsy and culture of affected tissue(s), such as the bone marrow, are often required. Culture of blood, urine, and/or stool may be positive, especially in HIV-positive patients.[30]

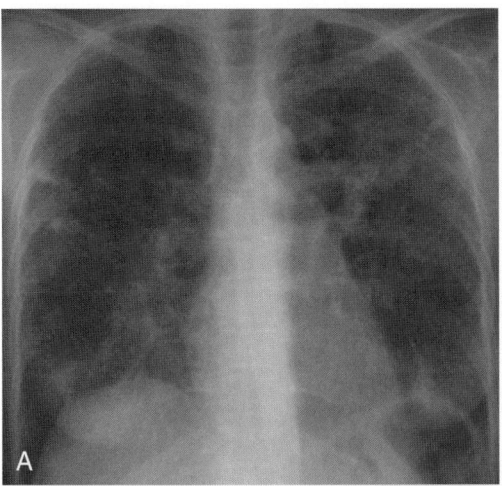
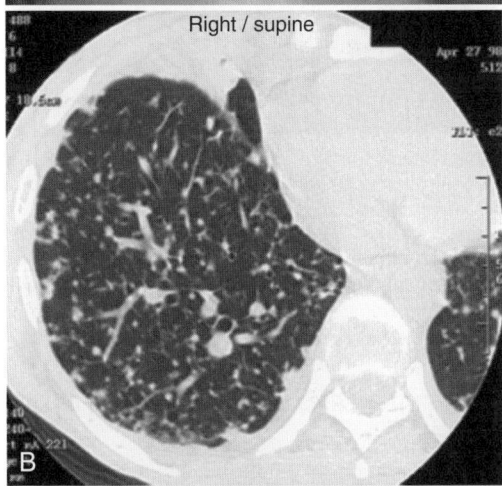
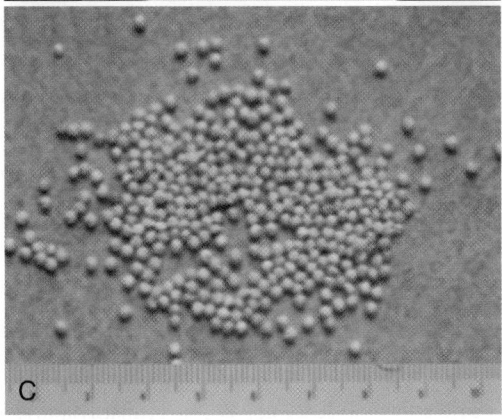

Figure 142-2 Miliary TB. A, Chest radiograph of patient with miliary TB. **B,** Chest computed tomography (CT) scan of same patient. Both show characteristically small (<2 mm) nodules thought to resemble millet seeds **(C).** Note that millet seeds are about 2 mm in diameter.

Neurologic Tuberculosis

TUBERCULOUS MENINGITIS

TB meningitis is rare in developed countries, with approximately 300 to 400 cases in the United States each year. It occurs via rupture of a subependymal tubercle that has seeded and formed during primary infection or disseminated disease. Individuals at high risk for TB meningitis include very young children with primary TB and older patients with immunodeficiency disorders such as HIV. Most patients with TB

meningitis will have no known history of TB, but evidence of extrameningeal disease (e.g., pulmonary, urinary, etc.) can be found in about half of these patients.[31,32] The tuberculin skin test is positive in only about 50% of patients with TB meningitis.

TB meningitis is typically a subacute disease. In one review of 58 cases, symptoms were present for 1 day to 9 months, with a median of 10 days prior to diagnosis.[31] A prodromal phase of low-grade fever, malaise, headache, dizziness, vomiting, and/or personality changes may persist for 2 to 3 weeks before the patient presents for medical care. Typical findings at presentation include severe headache, altered mental status, stroke, hydrocephalus, and cranial neuropathies. These clinical features are the result of basilar meningeal fibrosis and vascular inflammation.[33] Classic features of bacterial meningitis such as stiff neck and fever may be absent. When allowed to progress, coma and seizures may ensue.

The diagnosis of TB meningitis can be difficult and may be based only on clinical findings without definitive microbiological proof. Certain clinical characteristics such as longer duration of symptoms (>6 days), moderate cerebrospinal fluid (CSF) pleocytosis, and the presence of focal deficits increase the probability of TB meningitis.[34,35] Characteristic CSF findings of TB meningitis include:

- Leukocytosis with predominance of lymphocytes. White blood cell counts are usually between 100 and 500 cells/μL. Lower white blood cell counts and neutrophil predominance may be seen very early in the course of disease.
- Elevated protein levels, usually between 100 and 500 mg/dL
- Low glucose, typically less than 45 mg/dL

CSF samples should be sent for acid-fast smears, but this is associated with low sensitivity (<20%). Large volumes (10-15 mL) from several daily lumbar punctures are often needed for a microbiological diagnosis. Sensitivity is increased if four spinal taps are performed. Culture can take weeks and is also associated with low sensitivity. Stereotactic biopsy can be performed if tissue samples are needed. Mycobacterial antigens by enzyme-linked immunosorbent assay (ELISA) or radioimmunoassay have been detected in the CSF of patients with TB meningitis.[36]

Recent meta-analysis calculated that commercial nucleic acid amplification (NAA) assays used for the diagnosis of TB meningitis were 56% sensitive and 98% specific.[37,38] Unfortunately, considerable variability in sensitivity and specificity among tests from different laboratories makes it more difficult to interpret results. Most studies conclude that commercial NAA tests can confirm TB meningitis but cannot rule it out.[39] Thus a negative test neither excludes the diagnosis nor obviates the need for continued empirical therapy if the clinical suspicion is high. Comparisons of NAA and microscopy/culture using large volumes of CSF have indicated that the sensitivity of microscopy was similar to NAA for the diagnosis of TB meningitis, and repeated testing gave the highest diagnostic yield.[40] The sensitivity of CSF microscopy and culture falls rapidly after the start of treatment, whereas mycobacterial DNA may remain detectable within the CSF up to a month after the start of treatment.[41]

Magnetic resonance imaging (MRI) often reveals basilar meningeal enhancement (Figure 142-3) and/or hydrocephalus.[32] Hypodensities due to cerebral infarcts, and ring or nodular enhancing lesions can also be seen. MRI is superior to CT for evaluating the brainstem and the extent of lesions.

The outcome of TB meningitis is improved by timely treatment. Thus empirical treatment is warranted when risk factors and clinical features are suggestive of this diagnosis, even before microbiological confirmation. Chemotherapy for TB meningitis follows the model of short-course chemotherapy for pulmonary TB—an induction phase followed by a continuation phase. But unlike pulmonary TB, the optimal drug regimen and duration of each phase of treatment are not clearly established. INH and RIF remain the most essential drugs. INH penetrates the CSF freely and has potent early bactericidal activity.[42-44] RIF penetrates the CSF less well (maximum concentrations around 30% of plasma), but the high mortality from RIF-resistant TB meningitis has confirmed its central role in the treatment

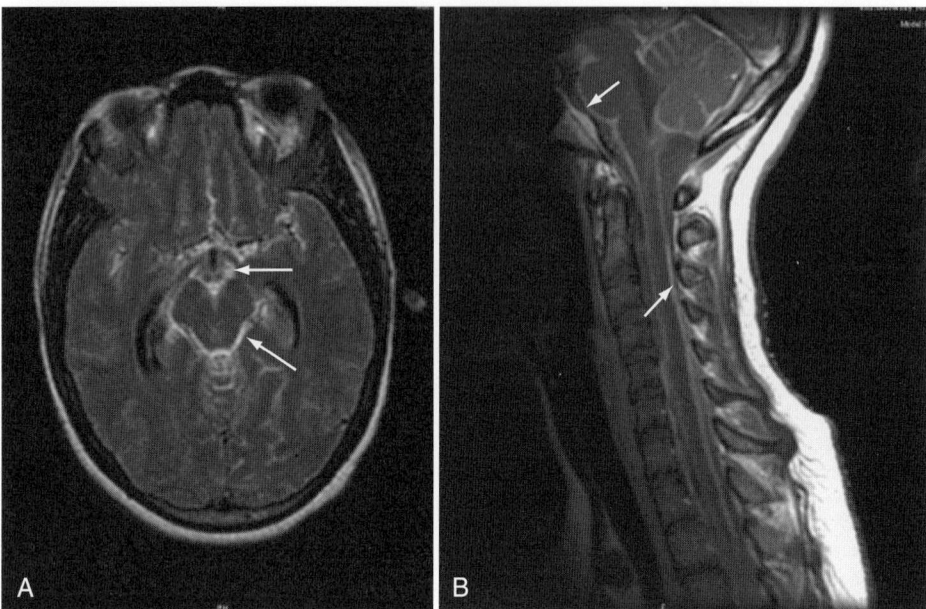

Figure 142-3 **Tuberculous meningitis. A,** T$_1$-weighted transverse magnetic resonance image (MRI) of the brain. **B,** Sagittal MRI of base of brain and spinal cord in patient with tuberculous meningitis. Note enhanced meninges (arrows) in basilar regions of brain, brainstem, and spinal cord.

of CNS disease.[45] INH, RIF, and pyrazinamide are considered mandatory at the beginning of TB meningitis treatment, and some centers use all three drugs for the duration of therapy.[46] There are no data from controlled trials to guide choice of the fourth drug. Most authorities recommend either streptomycin or ethambutol, although neither penetrates the CSF well in the absence of inflammation, and both can produce significant adverse reactions. Therapy should be continued for 9 to 12 months.

Adjunctive corticosteroid treatment of TB meningitis has been recommended for more than 50 years, but there has been long-standing concern that corticosteroids may reduce the penetration of anti-TB drugs into the CNS.[33] A recent Cochrane systematic review and meta-analysis of 7 randomized controlled trials involving 1140 participants (with 411 deaths) concluded that corticosteroids improved outcome in HIV-negative children and adults with TB meningitis, but the benefit in HIV infected individuals remains uncertain.[47] The results were heavily influenced by a study performed in 545 Vietnamese adults with TB meningitis which observed that treatment with dexamethasone was associated with a significantly reduced risk of death.[48] However, there was no demonstrable improvement in the combined endpoint of death or severe disability at 9-month follow-up. The survival benefit associated with corticosteroid therapy may have been due in part to a reduction in severe adverse events (9.5% versus 16%), particularly hepatitis, that necessitated changes in anti-TB drug regimens. No mortality benefit from dexamethasone was evident in 98 HIV-infected patients included in the study.[48]

Because there are no controlled trials comparing different corticosteroid regimens, the choice should be based on those found to be effective in published trials. One recommended regimen for adults is dexamethasone, 12 mg a day for 3 weeks, followed by gradual taper over the next 3 weeks.[49] In the large study from Vietnam, patients with mild disease received intravenous (IV) dexamethasone, 0.3 mg/kg/d × 1 week, 0.2 mg/kg/d × 1 week, and then 4 weeks of tapering oral therapy.[48] For patients with more severe TB meningitis, IV dexamethasone was given for 4 weeks (1 week each of 0.4 mg/kg/d, 0.3 mg/kg/d, 0.2 mg/kg/d, and 0.1 mg/kg/d), followed by 4 weeks of tapering oral dexamethasone therapy.[48]

Prognosis of TB meningitis largely depends on neurologic status at the time of presentation and time to treatment initiation. Most patients will die in 5 to 8 weeks if not treated. Various case series indicate a mortality rate between 7% and 65% in developed countries and up to

69% in underdeveloped areas.[31,32,50] Neurologic sequelae occur in up to 50% of survivors.[50] Mortality risk is highest in those with comorbidities, severe neurologic involvement on admission, rapid progression of disease, and being elderly.

OTHER CENTRAL NERVOUS SYSTEM MANIFESTATIONS OF TUBERCULOSIS

Other CNS manifestations of TB include brain abscesses, intracranial tuberculomas, vasculitis, radiculomyelitis, and spinal arachnoiditis. These can occur in conjunction with TB meningitis but are less likely to be seen as isolated findings in the ICU. Intracranial tuberculomas are more common among pediatric patients, especially infants, and can occur in any region of the brain. They result from hematogenous spread of TB. Tuberculous radiculomyelitis is a paradoxical reaction to the treatment of TB meningitis and may respond to corticosteroids. Signs and symptoms include subacute paraparesis, radicular pain, bladder disturbance, and paralysis.[51]

Cardiovascular Tuberculosis

TUBERCULOUS PERICARDITIS

Pericarditis is an uncommon but important manifestation of TB. In countries with a low incidence of TB, it is primarily a disease of the elderly and those with HIV, but it should be in the differential diagnosis of any patient with pericarditis and/or pericardial effusion. TB pericarditis can result from local spread from the lungs, tracheobronchial tree, lymph nodes, or adjacent bones, or by disseminated infection. The onset is usually insidious. Presenting signs and symptoms can be nonspecific (fever, dyspnea, weight loss) and/or more specific to the pericardium, such as the characteristic chest pains of pericarditis. Large hemorrhagic effusions may develop, resulting in cardiac tamponade. Pericardial inflammation and thickening may eventually cause a constrictive pericarditis. The presence of both pericardial effusion and constrictive pericarditis is physiologically characterized by continued elevation of diastolic pressure after pericardiocentesis. Such a finding should raise suspicion for TB pericarditis.

The diagnosis of TB pericarditis can be difficult to prove. Culture of pericardial fluid is positive in only 30% of cases, and pericardial biopsy has a yield of approximately 60%. Biopsy of the pericardium may reveal granulomatous changes consistent with TB or stains positive for acid-fast bacteria. The presence of elevated adenosine deaminase levels in the pericardial fluid has been shown to indicate TB pericarditis, but confirmation is needed.[52] PCR holds promise as a more sensitive test in diagnosis of TB pericarditis.[53] Many individuals are treated empirically for TB pericarditis based on clinical suspicion, positive tuberculin skin test, imaging studies, and exudative pericardial fluid with high protein and mononuclear white count. Treatment involves standard four-drug regimens as for other manifestations of TB. Prednisone, 60 mg a day, tapered over 11 weeks, is sometimes used in addition to anti-TB therapy, and has been shown to reduce the need for operative intervention.[54] Pericardiectomy is sometimes necessary in the treatment of refractory or recurrent disease.

OTHER CARDIOVASCULAR MANIFESTATIONS OF TUBERCULOSIS

In addition to the pericardium, TB may also affect the myocardium, endocardium, and epicardium (coronary arteries). These disorders are very rare. TB myocarditis occurs via direct spread from pericardium or mediastinal lymph nodes or from disseminated disease.[55] Endocardial involvement may manifest as endocarditis or as mural thrombi with entrapped *M. tuberculosis*. TB may also affect the coronary arteries, resulting in coronary arteritis with granulomatous inflammation of the arterial wall and obliterative intimal fibrosis.[56]

The aorta may be affected by TB, causing aortitis, aortointestinal fistula formation, or rupture.[57,58] The pathogenesis of aortitis includes septic embolization from endocarditis, seeding of a preexisting aneurysm from bacteremia, or extension from a contiguous site of infection. Signs and symptoms include fever, abdominal or back pain, and a palpable abdominal mass. Blood cultures are positive for *M. tuberculosis* in about 15% of cases. CT findings include air in the aortic wall, periaortic nodularity, saccular aneurysm in a noncalcified aorta, and rapidly increasing aortic diameter. Primary mycotic aneurysm of the aorta may be a sequela of chronic tuberculous aortitis.[59,60]

Tuberculosis in HIV-Positive Patients

HIV is the most important host risk factor for active TB.[61] In many developing countries, TB is the most common opportunistic infection associated with HIV. The estimated annual risk for active TB among persons with LTBI in the general population is 12.9 per 1000 person-years. In contrast, rates of progression to active TB among HIV-infected persons with LTBI range from 35 to 162 per 1000 person-years. Because TB may be an initial manifestation of HIV infection, all patients with TB should be tested for HIV. The WHO estimates that TB causes death in 13% of persons with AIDS.[62]

The mechanism of increased TB susceptibility in HIV positive persons is incompletely understood. Unlike other AIDS-related opportunistic infections, CD4+ count is not always a reliable predictor of increased risk for TB disease. Alveolar macrophages (AM) are important components of an effective immune response to TB,[63] and AM apoptosis represents a critical host defense mechanism that promotes *M. tuberculosis* elimination. In this context, one possible reason HIV increases susceptibility to TB is that HIV-infected AM have a reduced apoptotic response to *M. tuberculosis* compared to AM from healthy individuals.[64,65]

When the CD4+ count is above 350 cells/μL, pulmonary TB in AIDS patients is more likely to present with typical chest radiograph findings of upper lobe fibrocavitary disease.[66] However, as the CD4+ count decreases, pulmonary TB tends to manifest with more atypical radiographic manifestations such as mediastinal adenopathy, diffuse miliary or nodular infiltrates, focal lower zone infiltrates, and lack of cavitation. Extrapulmonary TB is more common among HIV-positive patients, occurring in up to 70% of patients. Disease involving the lymph nodes is especially common. Other extrapulmonary manifestations include miliary disease, TB sepsis, and CNS disease.[28] Empirical treatment may be necessary before the diagnosis is confirmed. If rapid

diagnosis is needed, NAA tests can be used, although these tests are more accurate in smear-positive cases.

After initiating highly-active antiretroviral therapy (HAART) in severely immunosuppressed patients, those with subclinical or recently diagnosed TB may display a paradoxical reaction, where there is an apparent clinical worsening of TB while on appropriate anti-TB treatment.[67-69] This phenomenon, also known by the more descriptive name of *immune reconstitution inflammatory syndrome* (IRIS), can manifest as early as 7 days after starting HAART. Signs and symptoms include fever, weight loss, and evidence of local inflammatory reactions such as lymphadenitis and worsening pulmonary disease such as increased pulmonary consolidation, nodules, and effusions. Histologically, a vigorous suppurative and necrotizing granulomatous reaction occurs, with or without caseation; cultures of infected material are almost invariably positive.

Treatment of TB in patients with HIV is similar to that in HIV-negative patients but is often complicated by drug interactions between TB medications and antiretrovirals.[70] The protease inhibitors (PIs) and non-nucleoside reverse transcriptase inhibitors (NNRTIs) can either induce or inhibit activity of the P450-3A (CYP3A) system. RIF can increase activity of CYP3A, leading to decreased levels of several antiretrovirals. Rifabutin is a less potent inducer of the CYP3A system and is associated with less drug-drug interactions, but dose adjustments may be needed. Despite these potential drug interactions, a RIF-based regimen should be used whenever possible. Patients with liver disease such as hepatitis C may be at increased risk for drug-induced hepatotoxicity. Another treatment issue in HIV-TB co-infection is that patients may fail to properly absorb the anti-TB drugs, which may increase the risk of treatment failure, relapses, and acquired drug resistance.[71]

Because of increased risk of RIF resistance, patients with HIV should *not* receive once weekly INH-rifapentine in the continuation phase of treatment. Twice-weekly INH-RIF or INH-rifabutin should be avoided when the CD4+ cell count is less than 100/μL. Treating drug-susceptible pulmonary TB in HIV-positive individuals for 9 months rather than the standard 6 months is associated with lower relapse rates.[72,73] Recommendations regarding treatment of TB in HIV patients are frequently revised as new drugs and information become available. The following websites can assist with treatment decisions and information on drug-drug interactions:

- http://www.cdc.gov/tb/publications/guidelines/TB_HIV_Drugs/default.htm
- http://www.medscape.com/updates/quickguide
- http://www.nationaltbcenter.edu/

If a patient develops IRIS while on HAART, it is generally recommended that HIV therapy be continued during TB treatment whenever possible, because IRIS is usually self-limited. However, more severe IRIS may require addition of corticosteroids and/or temporary discontinuation of HAART. In patients who are not already on HAART, it is usually advisable to delay HIV treatment for at least 4 to 8 weeks after TB therapy is initiated.

Tuberculosis and Immunomodulatory Therapies

TNF-α plays a central role in the pathogenesis to various inflammatory disorders and in the pathophysiologic response to many infections. TNF-α is produced predominantly by macrophages and lymphocytes and is active both as a membrane-bound and soluble protein.[74,75] In several animal models, TNF-α plays an essential part in the host defense to TB.[76] One mechanism by which TNF-α potentiates host defense is by its ability to induce apoptosis of infected cells. Macrophage apoptosis helps to contain *M. tuberculosis* by maintaining granuloma integrity, increasing efficiency of antigen presentation, and promoting killing of intracellular *M. tuberculosis*.[77] Administration of antibodies neutralizing TNF-α resulted in reactivation of TB in a mouse model.[78] Interruption of the normal TNF-α controlled response to TB reduces apoptosis, disrupts granuloma integrity, and predisposes to disseminated infection.

TNF-α antagonists are increasingly used for the treatment of various chronic inflammatory disorders. Currently licensed TNF-α antagonists fall into two main types: monoclonal neutralizing anti-TNF-α antibodies and soluble p75 subunits of the TNF-α receptor (TNFα-R). The soluble TNFα-Rs antagonize TNF-α function by acting as decoys to bind TNF-α. Three monoclonal anti-TNF-α antibodies (infliximab, adalimumab, and certolizumab pegol) and two TNFα-Rs (etanercept and abatacept) are in clinical use. Patients treated with TNF-α blockers have a TB incidence rate of 1.17 per 1000 patient-years, 12.2 times that of the general population.[79] Almost all of these cases are due to reactivation of LTBI.

Important differences have emerged among the TNF-α antagonists in regard to the risks of reactivation TB. Consistently, the excess risk is associated with infliximab and adalimumab rather than etanercept. For example, compared with etanercept, infliximab is associated with a two- to sevenfold greater risk of TB, shorter time to TB onset (17 versus 48 weeks), and a higher proportion of TB cases with disseminated or extrapulmonary disease (25 versus 10%).[80,81] It is not entirely clear why the neutralizing antibodies to TNF-α put people at greater risk of reactivation TB than soluble TNF-α receptors. Possible reasons include a longer duration of action of infliximab and adalimumab and their ability to bind to membrane-bound TNF-α with greater affinity than etanercept.[74] As a result, infliximab can induce death in T cells that express the membrane-bound TNF-α, whereas etanercept cannot. In addition, anti-TNF-α antibodies can inhibit T-cell activation and interferon gamma (IFN-γ) production, whereas etanercept cannot. Thus the pharmacokinetic and biological differences between the two main types of TNF-α antagonists may account for the greater susceptibility to intracellular pathogens with the use of the anti-TNF-α antibodies.[74,82]

Antagonists to other inflammatory cytokines are also being used in the management of patients with rheumatologic and inflammatory disorders. Interleukin 1 (IL-1) receptor antagonist (IL-1Ra) is the naturally occurring protein that prevents the action of IL-1 and IL-1β by competitively binding to IL-1R. Anakinra is a recombinant human form of IL-1Ra. In a case report, anakinra was associated with reactivation TB.[83]

Diagnosis of Tuberculosis

When TB is suspected, the first diagnostic test should be microscopic examination and culture for mycobacteria of relevant body fluids or tissues. Several specimens are often required, especially for CNS disease.

Patients with suspected pulmonary TB should be placed in respiratory isolation until three sputa are collected, separated by at least 8 hours between samples, for acid-fast bacteria (AFB) and culture. Because patients with extrapulmonary disease may also have occult pulmonary disease, it is generally recommended that sputum smears be sent on these patients regardless of chest radiographic findings.

Because acid-fast smear does not differentiate between *M. tuberculosis* and non-tuberculous mycobacteria, culture is used to confirm species and determine drug susceptibility. Simultaneous culture on both liquid and solid media is recommended. Liquid medium such as the newer BACTEC system allows growth of the organism in about 14 days, whereas growth takes 3 to 6 weeks on solid media (Lowenstein-Jensen or Middlebrook 7H11). Once sufficient growth is obtained, species identification can be obtained via conventional biochemical tests or more rapid tests such as nucleic acid probes, high-performance liquid chromatography (HPLC), the NAP test (*p*-nitro-acetylamino-β-hydroxypropiophenone), or molecular tests. Only experienced laboratories should complete susceptibility testing on culture-positive specimens. Molecular fingerprinting by restriction fragment length polymorphism (RFLP) can be used to distinguish strain types when laboratory contamination is suspected.

Although rapid and inexpensive, acid-fast smear microscopy is limited by its poor sensitivity (~50% sensitivity in culture-confirmed

pulmonary TB cases) and suboptimal specificity (50%-80%) in settings where nontuberculous mycobacteria are commonly isolated.[84-86] NAA testing has become a routine procedure in many settings, because NAA tests can reliably detect *M. tuberculosis* in specimens 1 or more weeks earlier than culture.[85] Because of the increasing use of NAA tests and the potential impact on patient care and public health, the Centers for Disease Control and Prevention (CDC) and the Association of Public Health Laboratories (APHL) made recommendations for using NAA tests for laboratory confirmation of TB. CDC recommends that NAA testing be performed on at least one respiratory specimen from each patient in whom a diagnosis of TB is being considered but has not yet been established, and for whom the test result would alter case management or TB control activities.[87,88]

Treatment of Tuberculosis

Standard treatment of adults with drug-susceptible TB is a three- or four-drug regimen for at least 6 months.[89,90] The typical course of therapy for drug-susceptible disease is 2 months of INH, RIF, pyrazinamide (PZA), and ethambutol (EMB) (initial phase), followed by 4 months of INH and RIF (continuation phase) (Tables 142-1 and 142-2). A 9- to 12-month regimen is suggested for TB meningitis, for pulmonary TB that is slow to respond to therapy (e.g., those with cavitary lesions and persistent sputum culture positivity even after 2 months of an appropriate four-drug regimen), or when PZA is not used in the induction regimen. EMB can be discontinued when drug susceptibility studies show sensitivity to INH and RIF. Streptomycin (SM) can be used instead of EMB if resistance is unlikely or susceptibility is shown. The continuation phase can be daily therapy, twice-weekly therapy, or thrice-weekly therapy for drug-susceptible TB (see Table 142-1). See the HIV section for details of treating TB in HIV-positive patients. Specific guidelines including information on first- and second-line agents have been published by the CDC.[91]

When MDR-TB is suspected or confirmed, additional drugs that may be used include amikacin, a fluoroquinolone (levofloxacin, moxifloxacin), capreomycin, ethionamide, cycloserine, and/or para-aminosalicylic acid. Local public health departments should be contacted to meet reporting requirements and will usually be responsible for treatment monitoring. Directly observed therapy (DOT) should be implemented whenever possible. Patients with MDR-TB require DOT and longer therapy (generally 18 months of treatment after the last negative sputum culture). Surgical resection after 2 to 3 months of treatment may improve outcome.[91]

Parenteral therapy may be required in ICU patients and is recommended for patients with fulminant disease (Table 142-3). INH and RIF are available in parenteral forms; EMB and PZA are not. Other active medications available for IV use include the aminoglycosides, fluoroquinolones, and capreomycin. In patients with renal failure, dose

TABLE 142-1	Current Regimens for Treatment of Drug-Susceptible Tuberculosis	
Regimen	*Initial Phase*	*Continuation Phase*
Daily or 5 days per week*	8 weeks of INH, RIF, PZA, ± EMB	18 weeks of INH and RIF
Intermittent†	(a) 2 weeks of daily INH, RIF, PZA, and EMB (or SM); then 6 weeks of INH, RIF, PZA, EMB BIW or TIW	18 weeks of INH and RIF BIW
	(b) 8 weeks of thrice-weekly INH, RIF, PZA, and EMB (or SM)	18 weeks of INH and RIF TIW

*The daily regimen is employed when patients self-administer their drugs. There is enough redundancy that if patients miss some of their doses, the outcome will remain acceptable.

†The intermittent regimens are intended for directly-observed therapy (DOT). Regimen (a) entails a total of 62 doses and has yielded over 95% success rates for the past 22 years in Denver, Colorado.[97] Regimen (b) involves 78 doses and has also resulted in success rates of approximately 95% in Hong Kong, where it is the standard regimen.[98]

BIW, twice weekly; *EMB*, ethambutol; *INH*, isoniazid; *PZA*, pyrazinamide; *RIF*, rifampin; *SM*, streptomycin; *TIW*, thrice weekly.

TABLE 142-2	Dosages of First-Line Anti-Tuberculosis Drugs (in Adults) and Major Adverse Effects		
Drug	**Daily Dosage**	**Twice- or Thrice-Weekly Dosage**	**Adverse Effects**
Isoniazid	5 mg/kg oral (max: 300 mg)	900 mg BIW 600 mg TIW	Hepatitis, peripheral neuritis, drug-induced lupus, seizures, and hypersensitivity with rash and fever. Drug interactions with dilantin and disulfiram. Pyridoxine can decrease neurotoxicity.
Rifampin	10 mg/kg oral (max: 600 mg)	10 mg/kg 600 mg BIW 600 mg TIW	Orange body secretions, flulike syndrome, hepatitis, pruritus, thrombocytopenia, nausea, anorexia, diarrhea, renal failure, and **multiple drug interactions**
Rifabutin*	10 mg/kg oral (max: 300 mg)	5 mg/kg	Neutropenia, uveitis, hepatotoxicity, orange discoloration of body fluids
Rifapentine†	10 mg/kg *once WEEKLY* (max: 600 mg)		Similar to rifampin
Pyrazinamide	15-30 mg/kg oral (max: 2 g)	30-35 mg/kg	Hyperuricemia, hepatitis, rash, nausea, and anorexia
Ethambutol	25 mg/kg initial 2 months, then 15 mg/kg oral	50 mg/kg BIW 30 mg/kg TIW	Optic neuritis and gastrointestinal discomfort

*Rifabutin and rifapentine are considered first-line agents when intolerance to rifampin precludes its use or concerning drug interactions exist.

†Rifapentine is only used in once-weekly dose in HIV-negative patients with noncavitary and uncomplicated disease. It is not approved for use in children.

BIW, twice weekly; *TIW,* thrice weekly.

TABLE 142-3	Selected Parenteral Medications Used in Treating Tuberculosis[91]	
Medication	**Preparation**	**Initial Dosage in Adults (Maximum Dosage)**
Isoniazid	PO, IV, IM	5 mg/kg/d (300 mg)
Rifampin	PO, IV	10 mg/kg/d (600 mg)
Streptomycin	IV, IM	10-15 mg/kg/d or 750-1000 mg/d
Amikacin	IV, IM	Same as above
Kanamycin	IV, IM	Same as above
Capreomycin	IV, IM	Same as above
p-Aminosalicylic acid⁻	PO, IV	8-12 g/d in 2 or 3 doses
Levofloxacin	PO, IV	500-1000 mg/d
Moxifloxacin	PO, IV	400 mg/d

Notes: Table shows routine daily dosing. Dosages may differ in children and in patients in intermittent therapy. Persons over age 59 should receive the lower dose for aminoglycosides (750 mg).

IM, intramuscular; IV, intravenous, PO, oral.

Risk to Healthcare Workers

An awareness that caring for TB patients poses a risk to healthcare workers (HCWs) did not emerge until the 1950s and 1960s when studies established that *M. tuberculosis* infection was transmitted by the airborne route.[93] However, occupational transmission received little attention until numerous outbreaks of TB and MDR-TB occurred in U.S. and European hospitals in the late 1980s and early 1990s.[94] At that time, more than 20 HCWs became ill with MDR-TB, and at least 10 died.[95] Hundreds of HCWs may be latently infected with MDR-TB and thus represent a relatively large reservoir of individuals at risk for future reactivation MDR-TB.

Pulmonologists are at higher risk for occupational exposure to TB compared to other medical specialists. Atypical presentations of TB can put providers at increased risk when TB is not suspected and proper precautions are not taken.[96] Bronchoscopy requires close contact with patients and provokes coughing, which likely contributes to the tuberculin skin test conversion rate of 11% among pulmonary fellows.[96] DMF-HEPA respirators should be used when performing bronchoscopy on patients with known or suspected TB.[96]

In HCWs with negative tuberculin skin test reactions who undergo repeat testing, an increase in reaction size of more than 10 mm within a period of 2 years should be considered a skin test conversion indicative of recent infection with *M. tuberculosis*. Because tuberculin skin test conversion typically occurs 3 to 8 weeks after primary infection, skin testing should be performed at least 3 weeks following exposure.

HCWs with potential exposure should be monitored for symptoms and, unless known to have a positive tuberculin skin test at baseline, skin testing or an IFN-γ release assay should be performed as soon as possible after the exposure to establish a baseline. If initial screening is negative, testing should be repeated 8 to 10 weeks following exposure and, if found to be positive, treatment for LTBI is recommended.

adjustments are required for those taking EMB, PZA, cycloserine, an aminoglycoside, capreomycin, or a fluoroquinolone. INH and PZA should probably be withheld in the setting of severe liver failure. An expert in the treatment of TB should be consulted when treating the complicated ICU patient or those with MDR-TB.

Corticosteroids are generally recommended in the treatment of several TB conditions, including TB meningitis and pericarditis, as discussed above.[92] Their role in patients with respiratory failure due to TB and in patients with severe AIDS-associated TB has not been proven, but many have used corticosteroids for these conditions. Typical therapy includes prednisone, 40 to 80 mg per day, tapered over a few weeks.

ANNOTATED REFERENCES

Chan ED, Strand MJ, Iseman MD. Treatment outcomes in extensively resistant tuberculosis. N Engl J Med 2008;359:657-9.
This study compared the outcomes of MDR-TB versus XDR-TB patients at a referral hospital in the United States. Odds ratios for long-term treatment success was 21.1 (MDR-TB versus XDR-TB). The hazard ratio of death from TB was 7.9 (XDR-TB versus MDR-TB). Despite aggressive treatment, XDR-TB was associated with significantly poorer long-term outcome and survival than MDR-TB.

Thwaites GE, Nguyen DB, Nguyen HD, Hoang TQ, Do TT, Nguyen TC, et al. Dexamethasone for the treatment of tuberculous meningitis in adolescents and adults. N Engl J Med 2004;351:1741-51.
This is a prospective randomized placebo-controlled trial of adjunctive dexamethasone in 545 patients over 14 years of age with tuberculous meningitis in two hospitals in Vietnam. The results showed that adjunctive treatment with dexamethasone reduced mortality, but there was no demonstrable improvement in the combined endpoint of death or severe disability after 9 months.

Erbes R, Oettel K, Raffenberg M, Mauch H, Schmidt-Ioanas M, Lode H. Characteristics and outcome of patients with active pulmonary tuberculosis requiring intensive care. Eur Respir J 2006;27:1223-8.
Retrospective study from Germany looking at 58 TB patients admitted to ICU. The in-hospital mortality was 15 of 58 (25.9%); 13 (22.4%) patients died in the ICU. The factors independently associated with

mortality were acute renal failure, need for mechanical ventilation, chronic pancreatitis, sepsis, acute respiratory distress syndrome, and nosocomial pneumonia.

Tubach F, Salmon D, Ravaud P, Allanore Y, Goupille P, Bréban M, et al. Risk of tuberculosis is higher with anti-tumor necrosis factor monoclonal antibody therapy than with soluble tumor necrosis factor receptor therapy: the three-year prospective French Research Axed on Tolerance of Biotherapies registry. Arthritis Rheum 2009;60:1884-94.
This is a case-control study investigating the risk of newly diagnosed TB associated with the use of anti-TNF-α agents. Authors identified 69 cases of TB in patients treated for various inflammatory diseases with infliximab (n = 36), adalimumab (n = 28), and etanercept (n = 5). In the case-control analysis, exposure to infliximab or adalimumab versus etanercept was an independent risk factor for TB (odds ratio [OR], 13.3; 95% CI, 2.6-69.0; and OR, 17.1; 95% CI, 3.6-80.6, respectively).

Nahid P, Gonzalez LC, Rudoy I, de Jong BC, Unger A, Kawamura LM, et al. Treatment outcomes of patients with HIV and tuberculosis. Am J Respir Crit Care Med 2007;175:1199-206.
The optimal length of tuberculosis treatment in patients co-infected with HIV is unknown. HIV-infected patients who received a 6-month rifamycin-based course of tuberculosis treatment or who received intermittent therapy had a higher relapse rate than HIV-infected subjects who received longer therapy or daily therapy, respectively. Standard 6-month therapy may be insufficient to prevent relapse in patients with HIV.

REFERENCES

Access the complete reference list online at http://www.expertconsult.com.

143

Malaria and Other Tropical Infections in the Intensive Care Unit

MONICA DHAND | DANIEL G. BAUSCH

Although the spectrum of possible "tropical" infections in a patient with exposures overseas may initially seem daunting, a detailed history of the travel itinerary, activities, and exposures can often significantly narrow the differential diagnosis (Table 143-1). This must include more than simply recording the countries to which the patient traveled. Exposures of a business traveler staying at hotels and dining in fine restaurants in a major city may differ drastically from those of a student back-packing through rural areas of the same country. General knowledge of the diseases endemic in a given area and their incubation periods and drug resistance patterns is vital (Figure 143-1 and Table 143-2). In addition, most "non-tropical" infections are also common in developing countries. Thus, although the differential diagnosis must be expanded to include tropical pathogens, common illnesses seen in developing as well as industrialized countries must be considered.

Patients prone to tropical infections can be divided into three groups: (1) nonimmune persons who have no history of exposure to tropical pathogens, primarily tourists and young children, regardless of geographic origin, after the waning of maternal antibodies (around age 6 months); (2) immune or semi-immune persons residing in tropical countries who are repeatedly exposed; (3) those originally from tropical countries but now residing elsewhere who, in the absence of continued exposure, have waning immunity. The degree of immunity may exert profound effects on the presentation and severity of illness. For example, a returning traveler may develop severe malaria at a relatively low parasitemic load, whearas a resident of sub-Saharan Africa with the same degree of parasitemia may be asymptomatic. Genetic differences in susceptibility may also exist, such as resistance to *Plasmodium vivax* in blacks due to the absence of Duffy factor, which serves as the receptor, or the relative protection from severe malaria of any species afforded to those carrying the sickle cell trait.[1,2,3]

In returning travelers, knowledge of pre-travel vaccinations as well as prescribed and taken chemoprophylaxis (which often turn out not to be the same) is imperative. Nevertheless, these preventive measures do not confer 100% protection and should not be used to completely discard a given entity from the differential diagnosis. Both physicians and patients frequently err in the prescribing of and adherence to appropriate prophylactic regimens.[4,5] Chemotherapy, complete or partial, may prolong the incubation period or alter the presentation of the illness. Those initially from tropical countries are often less likely to seek pre-travel medical advice before making a visit home and also often have considerably more exposures to tropical pathogens during their visit than do short-term travelers from industrialized countries.[6]

People living in resource-poor tropical countries may be more likely to have complicating health problems but less likely to have them previously diagnosed or controlled. Underlying diabetes, hypertension, malnutrition, chronic anemia, intestinal parasites, tuberculosis, HIV, or hepatitis virus infection may be discovered at the time of the acute illness.[7] Infection with multiple tropical pathogens is common in those living in endemic areas. Thus the finding of a given pathogen cannot automatically be assumed to be the cause of the patient's current illness.

Epidemiology

Malaria parasites are spread to humans by the bite of anopheline mosquitoes. Four species of *Plasmodia* commonly cause malaria in humans: *Plasmodium falciparum*, *P. vivax*, *Plasmodium ovale*, and *Plasmodium malariae* (see Table 143-2). A fifth species, *Plasmodium knowlesi*, is a zoonotic parasite of monkeys recently found to also cause disease in humans with exposure in forests of Southeast Asia.[8,9] Furthermore, recent evidence suggests that there may be distinct species of *P. vivax*.[10]

Malaria is the most common serious infection in most tropical countries as well as in returning travelers, and it should therefore be considered in any patient reporting travel in malaria-endemic areas or with exposure to unscreened blood products ("transfusion malaria") or blood-contaminated needles. Increased travel and immigration over the past several decades have resulted in increases in imported malaria in most industrialized countries.[11,12] The risk of acquiring *P. falciparum*, the cause of most severe disease, is highest for those traveling to sub-Saharan Africa and New Guinea, moderate in India, and comparatively low in Southeast Asia and Latin America.[13,14] Malaria is occasionally reported in individuals without reported travel, usually resulting from the carriage of malaria-infected passengers (who may be asymptomatic) or anopheline mosquitoes on aircraft arriving from endemic areas.[15] The parasite may then be secondarily transmitted by anopheline mosquitoes endemic in some industrialized countries, including the United States.

Pathophysiology

P. falciparum accounts for the vast majority of severe malaria because of (1) its ability to infect red blood cells (RBCs) of all ages, resulting in overwhelming parasitemia (up to 70% of RBCs); (2) its induction of adherence of parasitized RBCs to the microvascular wall, with consequent obstruction; (3) its induction of severe metabolic derangements directly through glucose consumption and lactate production and indirectly through the induction of cytokines; and (4) the high prevalence of chloroquine resistance to *P. falciparum* in many parts of the world (see Table 143-2). Nonimmune persons and pregnant women are at greatest risk. Human genetic as well as parasite strain differences probably play roles in the ultimate course of any given malaria infection.

Unlike the other species of malaria, *P. falciparum* causes decreased RBC deformability and the production of small protrusions or "knobs" on parasitized RBC membranes that mediate their adhesion to the venular endothelium (Figure 143-2). The rupture of schizont-stage parasites exposes glycosylphosphatidylinositol anchors on the parasite and RBC surface that induce macrophages and other inflammatory cells to release a host of inflammatory mediators including tumor necrosis factor alpha (TNF-α), interleukin-1, TNF-β, and various kinins and reactive nitrogen intermediates.[16-18] These cytokines play a role in up-regulation and activation of endothelial adhesion molecules such as ICAM-1 and E-selectin, enhancing cytoadherence

Text continued on page 1086.

TABLE 143-1	Some Tropical Diseases Which May Merit Management in an Intensive Care Unit*			
Disease and Organism	**Distinguishing Clinical Features**	**Incubation Period**	**Geographic Distribution**	**Mode of Transmission and Typical Risk Factors**
Nonspecific Febrile Syndromes				
African trypanosomiasis, hemolymphatic stage (*Trypanosoma brucei gambiense* and *T.b. rhodesiense*)	Lymphadenopathy, HSM, edema, rash, 30% have history of chancre, rarely DIC and thrombocytopenia	3-21 days	Sub-Saharan Africa	Tsetse fly bite; Camping, safari
Babesiosis (*Babesia* spp.)	Hemolytic anemia, HSM	3-28 days	North America, Europe, sporadic cases worldwide	Tick bite, blood transfusion (rare); especially severe in asplenic persons
Brucellosis (*Brucella* spp.)	Subacute presentation over weeks/months, HSM, weight loss, may involve large bones, joints, spine	2-8 weeks	Worldwide, especially Mediterranean, Middle East, and Latin America	Ingestion of contaminated dairy products; respiratory, skin, or conjunctival inoculation from contact with farm animals; abattoir workers, butchers, farmers
Candidiasis, disseminated (*Candida* spp.)	May involved any organ; skin or mucosal lesions not always present	1-4 weeks	Worldwide	Usually in IH or after administration of long-term antibiotics or maintenance of indwelling catheters
Cat scratch disease (*Bartonella henselae*)	Papule or eschar at site of inoculation, regional lymphadenopathy, fever may be mild, may progress to CNS involvement or endocarditis	1-2 weeks	Worldwide	Cat scratch or bite, severe disease most often seen in IH
Coccidioidomycosis (*Coccidioides immitis*)	May see pneumonia with cavities, meningeal, skin, and bone involvement, eosinophilia	1-4 weeks, often RD† in IH	Desert areas of the Americas	Inhalation of spores from soil; disseminated disease more common in Filipinos, blacks, Hispanics, IH, and in pregnancy
Echinococcal cyst, leak, or rupture (*Echinococcus* spp.)	Allergic symptoms: urticaria, pruritus, anaphylaxis	Years	Worldwide	Ingestion of eggs in feces of infected carnivores such as dogs and wolves; raising of domestic livestock
Ehrlichiosis (*Ehrlichia* spp.)	Rash (<50%), leukopenia, thrombocytopenia, HSM; may progress to GI, renal, pulmonary, or CNS involvement	7-21 days	Sporadic foci worldwide	Tick bite; camping, safari
Histoplasmosis, disseminated (*Histoplasma capsulatum*)	Mucocutaneous lesions, lymphadenopathy, HSM, DIC; any organ may be involved	1-4 weeks, usually RD	Tropics worldwide	Inhalation of spores from soil; severe disease usually IH
Leptospirosis (*Leptospira* spp.)	Icterus, jaundice, conjunctival suffusion, rash, HSM; may be biphasic; may develop hepato-renal syndrome, CNS involvement, or pulmonary disease with hemorrhage	2-20 days	Worldwide	Contaminated urine of many types of small mammals, either directly or through soil or standing water; hunting, military exercises
Malaria (*Plasmodium falciparum, P. vivax, P. ovale, P. malariae,* and *P. knowlesi*)	See text	See Table 143-2	See Figure 143-1 and Table 143-2	Mosquito bite, transfusion
Measles	Conjunctivitis, coryza, cough, rash, Koplik spots	5-14 days	Worldwide	Person-to-person via aerosol
Melioidosis (*Burkholderia pseudomallei*)	May develop pneumonia or local suppurative infection, shock (especially if IH)	2-21 days	Southeast Asia (especially Thailand), Australia, sporadic foci in tropics worldwide	Exposure to contaminated soil or infected animals, person-to-person (rare), often IH
Monkeypox (monkeypox virus)	Diffuse vesicular rash resembling chicken pox but involving palms and soles, lymphadenopathy	3-21 days	Central and West Africa	Person-to-person as well as from exposure to infected small mammals and monkeys; exotic pets; rule out smallpox/bioterrorism
Mycobacterium avium-intracellulare, disseminated	Usually subacute, HSM, weight loss	Months-years	Worldwide	Environmental organism causing opportunistic infection in IH
Oroya fever (*Bartonella bacilliformis*)	Acute anemia, jaundice, HSM, lymphadenopathy	2-3 weeks	Peru, Ecuador, and Colombia	Sandfly bite; hiking, camping
Paracoccidioidomycosis (*Paracoccidioides brasiliensis*)	May involve lungs, bones, skin, lymph nodes, adrenal glands, or mucous membranes	1-4 weeks, often RD	Tropical America	Inhalation of spores from soil; more severe in IH
Penicilliosis (*Penicilliosis marneffei*)	Mucocutaneous lesions, HSM, lymphadenopathy, may have skeletal or pulmonary involvement	Unknown, probably >1 week	Southeast Asia	Reservoir unknown most often IH
Plague (*Yersinia pestis*)	Localized tender lymphadenitis ("bubo"), pneumonia, shock	2-8 days	Worldwide	Flea bite or person-to-person; areas of heavy rat infestations, R/O bioterrorism
Q fever (*Coxiella burnetii*)	HSM; may develop pneumonia, endocarditis, hepatitis, osteomyelitis, or neurologic abnormalities	2-29 days	Worldwide	Inhalation of organism from products of infected livestock or pets, especially birth products but also milk, urine, and feces; farmers, ranchers
Rat bite fever (*Spirillum minor* or *Streptobacillus moniliformis*)	Peripheral rash, sometimes with desquamation, polyarthritis in *S. moniliformis,* eschar or ulcer at site of bite in *S. minor*	2-28 days	Worldwide, especially Asia and North America	Bite of rat or other animal that preys on rats; ingestion of food contaminated by rat
Relapsing fever (*Borrelia* spp.)	Recrudescent fever pattern, HSM, petechiae, epistaxis, neurologic abnormalities	4-18 days	Worldwide (especially East Africa)	Body louse (*B. recurrentis*) or tick bite (various *Borrelia* species); conditions of poor hygiene, outdoor exposures, refugee camps, camping, safari

Continued on following page

TABLE 143-1	Some Tropical Diseases Which May Merit Management in an Intensive Care Unit* (Continued)			
Disease and Organism	**Distinguishing Clinical Features**	**Incubation Period**	**Geographic Distribution**	**Mode of Transmission and Typical Risk Factors**
Rickettsiosis, spotted fever group (*Rickettsia rickettsii, R. conorii, R. africae, R. australis, R. sibirica, R. japonica, R. honei,* and *R. akari*)	Peripheral skin rash, eschar at site of tick bite may be seen ("tache noire"), may progress to GI, renal, pulmonary, or CNS involvement	7-14 days	Worldwide (with circumscribed distributions of each specific organism)	Tick bite (mite for *R. akari*); camping, safari
Rickettsiosis, typhus group (*Rickettsia prowazekii, R. typhi,* and *R. felis*)	Centripetal rash (~50%), no eschar	7-14 days	Worldwide, especially cold climates	Feces from infected louse (*R. prowazekii*) or flea (*R. typhi* and *R. felis*) rubbed into broken skin; crowding, poor hygiene, abundant rodents, refugee camps, flea-infested cats
Scarlet fever (group A *Streptococcus pyogenes*)	Pharyngitis, "sandpaper" rash, cervical adenopathy	1-4 days	Worldwide	Person-to-person via aerosolization/droplets
Schistosomiasis, Katayama fever (*Schistosoma* spp., especially *S. japonicum*)	Lymphadenopathy, HSM, eosinophilia	1-2 months	Africa, Asia, Caribbean, Middle East, South America, Caribbean	Skin penetration of cercaria; swimming or bathing in contaminated water
Scrub typhus (*Orientia tsutsugamushi*)	Centripetal rash, conjunctival suffusion, lymphadenopathy, eschar at site of chigger bite (~50%), hearing loss in one-third of cases	6-18 days	Asia, Australia, Pacific Islands	Chigger bite; outdoor rural or suburban exposures
Strongyloidiasis, disseminated (*Strongyloides stercoralis*)	Abdominal pain and distension, shock, pulmonary and CNS involvement common	2-3 weeks; may be maintained via autoinfection for decades	Tropics worldwide	Skin contact with contaminated soil; miliary exercises; dissemination may occur in IH (AIDS, steroid treatment)
Toxic shock syndrome (*Staphylococcus aureus,* group A *S. pyogenes*)	Rash, extremity or abdominal pain, skin desquamation, soft-tissue infection (70%)	2-10 days	Worldwide	Wound or vaginal colonization with toxin-producing bacteria; history of minor trauma (often without break in skin), previous surgery, or varicella infection; staphylococcal syndrome often associated with menses
Trench fever (*Bartonella quintana*)	Rash, HSM, shin pain, may develop endocarditis and angioma-like lesions	1-2 weeks	Worldwide	Body louse bite; areas of crowding or poor sanitation, more severe in IH
Trichinellosis (*Trichinella* spp.)	Diarrhea followed by myalgias, periorbital edema, eosinophilia, may involve heart or CNS	7-30 days	Worldwide	Ingestion of contaminated meat, including pork (*T. spiralis*), wild boar, horse, bear, and walrus
Tularemia, typhoidal form (*Francisella tularensis*)	Pulse-temperature dissociation, diarrhea (~40%); may develop pneumonia	1-21 days	Sporadic foci worldwide, mostly Northern Hemisphere	Tick or fly bite or direct exposure to small mammals; hunting, camping, military exercises; R/O bioterrorism
Typhoid fever (*Salmonella typhi*)	Pulse-temperature dissociation, abdominal pain, rash, intestinal perforation and bleeding, HSM, 10% with extra-intestinal manifestations	8-28 days	Worldwide	Fecal-oral
Vibrio infection, nonepidemic type (*Vibrio vulnificus*)	Bullous skin lesions, DIC, thrombocytopenia, GI bleeding, shock	1-2 days	Worldwide	Contaminated salt water or seafood; severe disease mostly in IH, history of alcoholism, liver disease
Viral hemorrhagic fever (dengue, yellow fever, Ebola, Marburg, Lassa, Junin, Machupo, and Rift Valley fever viruses, many others)	Capillary leak syndrome; may or may not exhibit frank hemorrhage, GI hemorrhage, shock	3-21 days, depending upon specific virus	Select areas worldwide	Depending on specific virus: exposure to rodent excreta, infected non-human primates, person-to-person, tick or mosquito bite, some unknown; R/O bioterrorism
Viral hepatitis (hepatitis A, B, C, D, and E; Epstein-Barr virus; cytomegalovirus; others)	HSM, light-colored stools, dark urine, jaundice	2 weeks-5 months, depending on specific organism	Worldwide	Fecal-oral or ingestion of seafood from contaminated sea beds (hepatitis A, E); percutaneous (blood exposure), sexual, or mother-to-child transmission (hepatitis B, C, D); hepatitis D requires co-infection with hepatitis B virus
Visceral leishmaniasis (*Leishmania* spp.)	Weight loss, HSM, neutropenia	Months-years	Tropics worldwide, especially Indian sub-continent, Middle East, and North Africa	Sandfly bite; military exercises, outdoor exposures
Gastrointestinal Syndromes				
Amebic dysentery (*Entamoeba histolytica,* rarely other amebae)	Abdominal pain and diarrhea, sometimes bloody, minority may develop ameboma, toxic megacolon, peritonitis, or abscesses in solid organs (usually liver)	2-4 weeks (usually longer for solid organ involvement)	Worldwide	Fecal-oral; may be transmitted through anal sex
Anthrax, gastrointestinal or oropharyngeal (*Bacillus anthracis*)	Abdominal pain and bloody diarrhea, neck swelling, pharyngitis, mucosal lesions, shock	2-10 days	Worldwide	Ingestion of spores; exposure to domestic animals or animal byproducts; R/O bioterrorism

| TABLE 143-1 | Some Tropical Diseases Which May Merit Management in an Intensive Care Unit* (Continued) | | | | |

Disease and Organism	Distinguishing Clinical Features	Incubation Period	Geographic Distribution	Mode of Transmission and Typical Risk Factors
Ascending cholangitis (*Clonorchis sinensis* and *Opisthorchis* spp.)	May be recurrent and accompanied by pancreatitis	Months-years	Asia, former USSR	Ingestion of raw infected freshwater fish; sushi consumption
Bacterial dysentery (*Shigella* spp., *Campylobacter* spp., invasive and hemorrhagic *Escherichia coli*, non-*typhi Salmonella* spp., *Vibrio parahaemolyticus*, others)	Abdominal pain and diarrhea, sometimes bloody	10 hours-7 days, depending on specific organism	Worldwide	Fecal-oral
Cholera (*Vibrio cholerae*)	Copious "rice water" diarrhea, abdominal pain, severe hypovolemia, fever minimal or absent	1-3 days	Tropics worldwide	Contaminated water or food, especially seafood; ceviche consumption
Clostridial gastroenteritis (*Clostridium difficile*)	Abdominal pain and diarrhea, sometimes with mucus or blood, toxic megacolon	~1 week to months	Worldwide	Alteration of GI flora through previous antibiotic administration and/or GI manipulation
Eosinophilic gastroenteritis (*Angiostrongylus costaricensis*)	Mimics appendicitis or inflamed Meckel's diverticulum, right lower quadrant abdominal pain and mass, eosinophilia	Estimated 3-4 weeks	Latin America	Ingestion of larvae in undercooked mollusks, crustaceans, or frogs
Hemolytic uremic syndrome (*Escherichia coli* O157:H7)	Bloody diarrhea followed by hemolysis and renal failure	2-5 days	Worldwide	Ingestion of poorly cooked meat, fecal-oral
Neurologic Syndromes				
African trypanosomiasis, meningoencephalitic stage (*Trypanosoma brucei gambiense* and *T.b. rhodesiense*)	Headache, HSM, cervical lymphadenopathy, somnolence, change in mental status, extrapyramidal and cerebellar signs	Months-years	Sub-Saharan Africa	Tsetse fly bite; camping, safari
Antiretroviral syndrome (human immunodeficiency virus-1)	Usually asymptomatic or mild flulike illness, meningoencephalitis occurs rarely	2-4 weeks	Worldwide	Sexual transmission or percutaneous blood exposure; unprotected sex, IV drug use
Arboviral encephalitides (eastern equine, Japanese encephalitis, West Nile, Murray Valley encephalitis, St. Louis encephalitis, and Venezuelan equine encephalitis viruses, many others)	Encephalitis, focal neurologic deficits, seizures, change in mental status	3-21 days	Sporadic foci worldwide	Mosquito bite, seasonal
Bacterial meningitis (*Neisseria meningitides*, *Streptococcus pneumoniae*, *Haemophilus influenza* type B, *Listeria monocytogenes*, others)	Petechiae, ecchymoses, and bleeding suggest *N. meningitides*	2-10 days, depending on specific organism	Worldwide; *N. meningitides* more frequent in African "meningitis belt"	Person-to-person, asymptomatic carrier states, seasonal fluctuations
Botulism (*Clostridium botulinum*)	Bilateral cranial nerve deficits with symmetric descending weakness, fever absent	1-3 days	Worldwide	Toxin ingestion or wound contamination; home-canned foods, soil contamination
Brain abscess (various bacteria, fungi, and parasites)	Focal neurologic signs	Days-months, depending on specific organism	Worldwide	Varies with infecting organism
Cryptococcosis (*Cryptococcus neoformans*)	Mild meningitis with low-grade fever, nonfocal neurologic exam, sometimes seizures or pulmonary involvement	1-4 weeks	Worldwide	Inhalation of spores from soil and bird and bat excreta; usually IH
Eosinophilic meningitis (*Angiostrongylus cantonensis*)	Headache, meningitis, sometimes cranial nerve involvement, fever minimal	1-7 days	Southeast Asia, South Pacific, sporadic foci worldwide	Ingestion of larvae in undercooked mollusks, crustaceans, or frogs
Gnathostomiasis (*Gnathostoma* spp.)	Migratory skin and subcutaneous swellings, epigastric pain and vomiting, eosinophilia, may invade any organ, especially CNS	Weeks-years	Southeast Asia, with sporadic cases from Central and South America	Consumption of raw freshwater fish, frogs, snakes, crustaceans, or poultry; sushi consumption
Herpes encephalitis (various herpesviruses)	Encephalitis, focal neurologic deficits, seizures, change in mental status, may show vesicular eruption	2-20 days, depending on specific virus	Worldwide; herpes B virus via monkey exposure in Asia and North Africa (wild monkeys) or captive monkeys worldwide	Person-to-person, often more severe in IH; herpes B virus via bite or other exposure to monkeys of the genus *Macaca*; person-to-person transmission reported; researchers, animal handlers
Mucormycosis (various fungi from the order Mucorales)	CNS infiltration with loss of consciousness, black exudate around mucous membranes of face, pulmonary infiltrates	1-7 days	Worldwide	Inhalation of spores from soil, traumatic inoculation of wound; usually IH (diabetes mellitus or steroid use)
Neurocysticercosis (*Taenia soleum*)	Seizures, headache, change in mental status, muscle pain	Years	Worldwide, especially Latin America and India	Ingestion of cysticerci in contaminated pork; areas where pigs roam freely

Continued on following page

TABLE 143-1	Some Tropical Diseases Which May Merit Management in an Intensive Care Unit* (Continued)

Disease and Organism	Distinguishing Clinical Features	Incubation Period	Geographic Distribution	Mode of Transmission and Typical Risk Factors
Paragonimiasis, cerebral (*Paragonimus* spp.)	Meningoencephalitis, often accompanied by pulmonary disease	Years	Sporadic foci worldwide, especially East Asia, Peru, Ecuador, West Africa	Ingestion of raw infected crustaceans; sushi consumption
Poliomyelitis (poliovirus)	Acute flaccid paralysis, meningeal signs, muscle pain	9-12 days	Sporadic foci in Africa, Asia, and eastern Mediterranean	Fecal-oral
Primary amebic meningoencephalitis (*Naegleria fowleri*)	Fulminant meningoencephalitis	3-7 days	Sporadic foci worldwide	Entry of trophozoite through the nose; swimming in contaminated fresh warm water; hot springs
Rabies (rabies virus)	Change in mental status, autonomic instability, photophobia, aerophobia, paralysis	20-90 days	Worldwide	Animal bite or bat exposure; spelunking, caring for injured animals
Schistosomiasis, CNS (*Schistosoma* spp.)	Encephalopathy, meningoencephalitis, transverse myelitis, seizures	Weeks-months	Africa, Asia, Caribbean, Middle East, South America, Caribbean	Skin penetration of cercaria; swimming or bathing in contaminated water
Tetanus (*Clostridium tetani*)	Diffuse muscle spasms, opisthotonos, trismus, autonomic dysfunction	3-21 days	Worldwide	Soil contamination of wound, commonly involves umbilical stump in neonates
Tickborne encephalitis (tickborne encephalitis virus)	Encephalitis, focal neurologic deficits, seizures	7-14 days	Central and East Asia, Europe, North Africa, North America	Tick bite
Toxoplasmosis, cerebral (*Toxoplasma gondii*)	Meningoencephalitis, HSM, focal neurologic deficits, seizures, change in mental status	Usually RD	Worldwide	Ingestion of cysts in undercooked meat or oocysts from exposure to cat feces; usually IH
Variant Creutzfeldt-Jacob disease (prion)	Change in mental status, myoclonus, spasticity, rigidity, extrapyramidal and cerebellar signs and symptoms, occasionally seizures	Months-years	United Kingdom, with sporadic cases elsewhere in Europe, Canada, and United States	Recipients of cadaveric transplants or injections of biomedical products derived from infected patients, contaminated surgical apparatuses, person-to-person(?), ingestion of contaminated beef or lamb(?)
Visceral larva migrans (*Toxocara canis*)	Cough, wheezing, HSM, eosinophilia; may develop CNS or other solid organ involvement	Weeks-years	Worldwide	Ingestion of eggs in puppy feces
Pulmonary Syndromes				
Anthrax, inhalation (*Bacillus anthracis*)	Pulmonary infiltrates with widened mediastinum, shock, CNS involvement	2-60 days	Worldwide	Inhalation of spores, exposure to domestic animals or animal by-products; R/O bioterrorism
Aspergillosis (*Aspergillus* spp.)	Pulmonary "fungus ball," (aspergilloma), transient infiltrates and allergic symptoms in allergic bronchopulmonary aspergillosis	1-4 weeks	Worldwide	Inhalation of spores from soil
Bacterial pneumonia (*Streptococcus pneumoniae, Legionella pneumophila, Mycoplasma pneumoniae, Haemophilus influenza, Chlamydia* spp., others)	Extrapulmonary findings frequent in Legionnaire's disease and psittacosis	2-21 days, depending on specific organism	Worldwide	Person-to-person spread; Legionnaire's disease associated with colonized air/water systems; psittacosis associated with bird exposure
Blastomycosis (*Blastomyces dermatitidis*)	Subacute pneumonia; bone, skin, and GU tract involvement	1-4 weeks, usually RD	Sporadic foci worldwide	Inhalation of spores from soil
Diphtheria (*Corynebacterium diphtheriae*)	Low-grade fever, cough, pharyngitis, oropharyngeal membrane, neck swelling, mucosal bleeding, myocarditis, polyneuritis	3-7 days	Worldwide, especially temperate areas	Person-to-person through respiratory route as well as breaks in the skin
Eosinophilic pneumonia (various parasites, helminthes and filaria)	Eosinophilia, asthma-like condition, elevated IgE	Days-weeks, depending on specific organism	Worldwide, depending on specific organism	Lung passage of larvae or adult helminthes, mosquito bite (filaria), filarial disease occurs primarily in those living in endemic areas with continued exposure
Hantavirus pulmonary syndrome (various hantaviruses)	ARDS, thrombocytopenia, leukocytosis, hemoconcentration, circulating immunoblasts	1-5 weeks	Americas	Contaminated rodent urine or feces; outdoor exposures
Pertussis (*Bordetella pertussis*)	Low-grade fever, coryza, rhinorrhea, paroxysmal dry cough	5-21 days	Worldwide	Person-to-person; adults vaccinated as children are susceptible to milder disease
Pneumocystosis (*Pneumocystis jiroveci*)	Dyspnea, dry cough, hypoxemia, often only mild findings on pulmonary auscultation and CXR	Usually RD	Worldwide	Inhalation; usually IH
Tuberculosis (*Mycobacterium tuberculosis*)	Upper lobes infiltrates and cavities; miliary TB, meningitis, and GU involvement all also common	Usually RD	Worldwide	Person-to-person via aerosol/droplet; increased frequency and likelihood of extrapulmonary involvement in IH
Tularemia, pneumonic form (*Francisella tularensis*)	Pulse-temperature dissociation, diarrhea (~40%)	1-21 days	Sporadic foci worldwide, mostly Northern Hemisphere	Tick or fly bite, or direct exposure to small mammals; hunting, camping, military exercises, R/O bioterrorism

TABLE 143-1	Some Tropical Diseases Which May Merit Management in an Intensive Care Unit* (Continued)			
Disease and Organism	*Distinguishing Clinical Features*	*Incubation Period*	*Geographic Distribution*	*Mode of Transmission and Typical Risk Factors*
Viral pneumonia (influenza, parainfluenza, respiratory syncytial, and SARS coronavirus, many others)	May be complicated by bacterial suprainfection	Days-weeks, depending on specific organism	Worldwide, depending on specific organism	Person-to-person spread as well as zoonotic, depending on specific virus; contact with farms or live-animal markets, birds, or pigs (zoonotic influenzas); civet cats suspected to be a reservoir of SARS coronavirus
Localized Infections				
Mycetoma (various fungi and bacteria)	Chronic swollen limb with nodules, sinus tracts, drainage of pus and "grains"	Weeks-months	Tropics worldwide	Traumatic implantation of organism into skin; soil exposure
Necrotizing fasciitis (group A *S. pyogenes*, *Clostridia* spp., *S. aureus*)	Rapid progression of edema, erythema, tenderness, bullae, necrosis, and gangrene	~24 hours	Worldwide	Posttraumatic or surgical

*Only diseases which typically have acute or subacute presentations and may cause severe disease are included. Diseases are classified by the most typical associated severe syndrome. In practice, significant variation may exist.

†Initial infection is usually asymptomatic or mild. Reactivation with severe disease may occur years later, usually in immunocompromised hosts.

ARDS, acute respiratory distress syndrome; *CNS*, central nervous system; *CXR*, chest x-ray; *DIC*, disseminated intravascular coagulopathy; *GI*, gastrointestinal; *GU*, genitourinary; *HSM*, hepatosplenomegaly; *IH*, immunocompromised host; *IV*, intravenous; *RD*, reactivation disease; *R/O*, rule out; *TB*, tuberculosis.

Figure 143-1 Malaria-endemic countries in the Western and Eastern Hemispheres. The risk of malaria may vary within specific regions of each country. (*From Health information for international travel 2010. Atlanta: Centers for Disease Control and Prevention; 2010. Available at: http://wwwnc.cdc.gov/travel/yellowbook/2010/chapter-2/malaria.aspx.*)

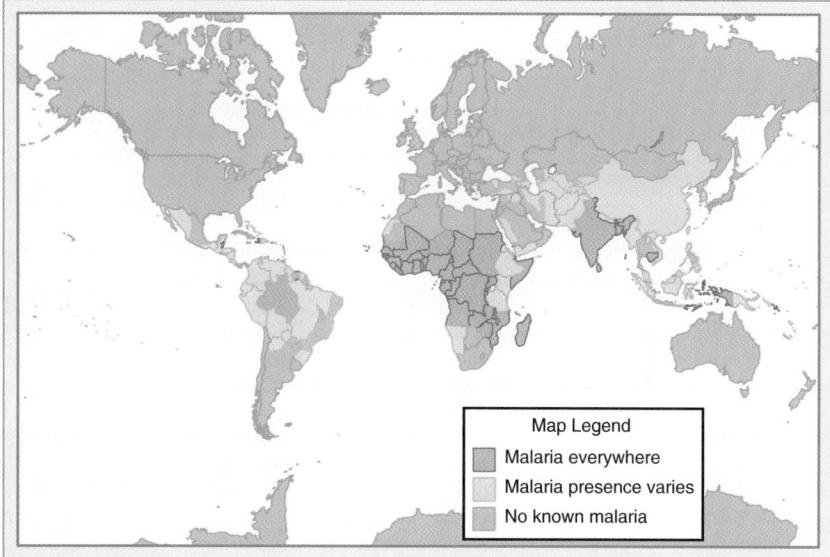

Map Legend
- Malaria everywhere
- Malaria presence varies
- No known malaria

TABLE 143-2	Features of the Five Species of Malaria Known to Cause Disease in Humans				
	Plasmodium falciparum	*Plasmodium vivax*	*Plasmodium ovale*	*Plasmodium malariae*	*Plasmodium knowlesi*
Incubation period (days)	6-25	8-27	8-27	16-40	12
Asexual cycle (hours)	48 (tertian)	48 (tertian)	48 (tertian)	72 (quartan)	24 (tertian)
Relapse	No	Yes*	Yes*	No†	No
Chloroquine resistance	Yes‡	Rare§	No	No‖	No
Characteristic on thin blood film	Rings predominate, multiply infected RBCs, high parasitemia, rings with thread-like cytoplasm, double nuclei, banana-shaped gametocytes	Enlarged RBCs, Schüffner's dots, trophozoite cytoplasm ameboid, 12-24 merozoites in mature schizont	Oval RBCs with fringed edges, Schüffner's dots, trophozoites cytoplasm compact, 6-16 merozoites in mature schizont	Trophozoite cytoplasm compact (band forms), 6-12 merozoites in mature schizont, RBC unchanged	Similar to *P. malariae*, 8-10 merozoites in mature schizont, often in rosette pattern with central clump of pigment

*Relapses may appear months to years after initial infection due to dormant hypnozoites in the liver.

†Although relapse does not occur, *P. malariae* can produce persistent infections that remain below detectable limits in the blood for 20 to 30 years or more.

‡*P. falciparum* resistance to sulfadoxine/pyrimethamine, mefloquine, halofantrine, and artemisinin have also been reported in some areas, along with partial resistance to quinine and quinidine.[102-104]

§*P. vivax* resistance to chloroquine now reported in some areas of southeast Asia, Oceania, and South America.[105-116]

‖Chloroquine-resistant *P. malariae* has also been reported in south Sumatra, Indonesia.[117]

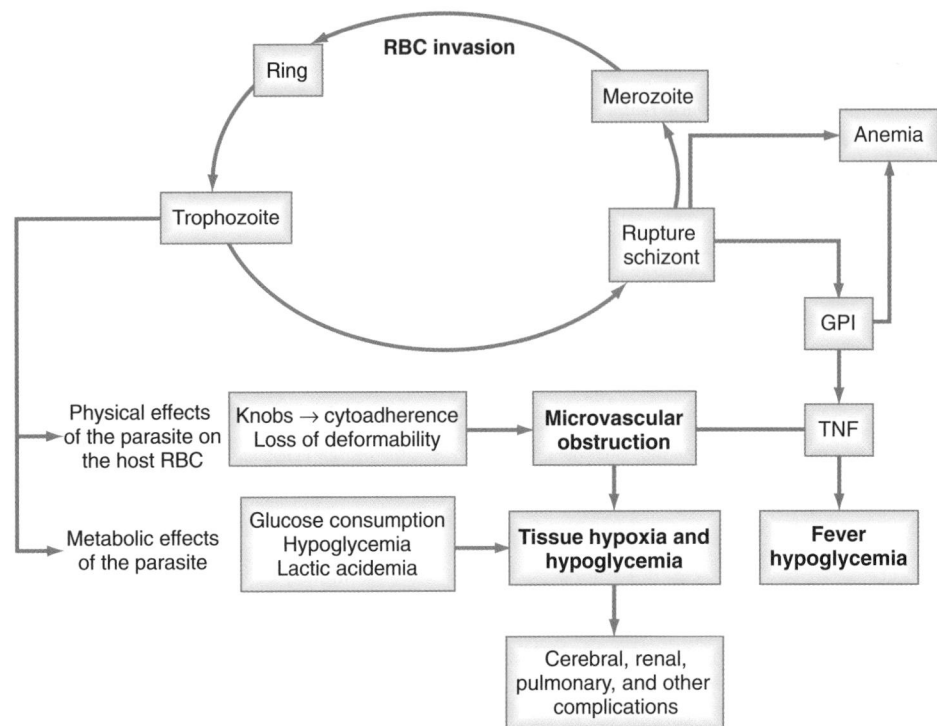

Figure 143-2 Pathogenesis of severe and complicated *Plasmodium falciparum* malaria. GPI, glycosylphosphatidylinositol; RBC, red blood cell; TNF, tumor necrosis factor. *(Modified from Krogstad D. Plasmodium species (malaria). In: Mandell GL, Bennett JE, Dolin R, editors. Principles and practice of infectious diseases. 5th ed. Philadelphia: Churchill Livingstone; 2000).*

of parasitized cells as well as mediating pathologic processes such as hypoglycemia, lactic acidemia, shock, gut mucosal damage, and increased permeability and neutrophil aggregation in the lung. The sum total of this cascade is sequestration of parasitized RBCs in the microvasculature where they are not only sheltered from removal but cause sluggish flow and obstruction, resulting in impaired oxygen delivery and organ dysfunction.[16,19] The most profound effects are usually on the cerebral capillaries, although a host of tissues may be affected, including the kidney, liver, spleen, placenta, intestine, lung, bone marrow, heart, and retina. Histopathologic changes are usually minimal, but ring hemorrhages and perivascular infiltrates sometimes develop at the sites of obstructed vessels, perhaps facilitated by thrombocytopenia due to splenic sequestration of platelets. Although subendocardial and epicardial hemorrhages have been noted at autopsy, myocarditis does not occur, and primary cardiac events are relatively rare in malaria.

Clinical Presentation

Malaria infections are classified broadly into three clinical categories: (1) *asymptomatic parasitemia*, which generally does not require treatment; (2) *uncomplicated malaria*, defined as parasitemia and fever without evidence of end-organ damage or other signs of severe disease (these patients may often be treated as outpatients with oral antimalarials); and (3) *severe and complicated malaria*, defined as parasitemia and the presence of vital organ damage or other signs of severe disease. Patients with severe and complicated malaria require hospitalization, often in an intensive care unit (ICU), and parenteral antimalarials. This third category is the focus of this chapter.

Malaria classically produces three stages of symptoms which progress over an 8- to 12-hour period, comprising a "paroxysm." These correspond and are attributable to the period of schizont rupture and appearance of ring forms (merozoites) in the blood, accompanied by the release of numerous host inflammatory mediators. The paroxysm classically begins suddenly with a "cold stage" in which the patient experiences rigors and chills, often accompanied by headache, nausea, and vomiting. Intense peripheral vasoconstriction may result in pale, goose-pimpled skin and cyanosis of the lips and nail beds. Within a few hours, the "hot stage" ensues, with high fever, flushed skin, throbbing headache, and palpitations. The paroxysm concludes with the "defervescent stage," consisting of a drenching sweat and resolution of the fever. The exhausted patient often then sleeps. Clinical deterioration with *P. falciparum* usually appears 3 to 7 days after onset of fever.

Although a classic periodicity is described for the different malaria species (see Table 143-2), this occurs only when the infection has persisted untreated long enough to allow for synchronization of schizont rupture. Furthermore, schizont rupture tends to be asynchronous in *P. falciparum* and in most primary infections of any plasmodium species. Therefore, malaria may often result in persistently spiking fevers difficult to distinguish from fever produced by many other infections. The absence of a classic paroxysm and periodicity therefore should not be used to exclude the diagnosis. Paroxysms may be accompanied by cough, sore throat, myalgias, back pain, postural hypotension, abdominal pain, nausea, vomiting, diarrhea, and weakness. These are more common in children and may lead to misdiagnoses. Rash and lymphadenopathy are not typical of malaria and suggest another diagnosis.

SEVERE AND COMPLICATED MALARIA

Although all species of malaria may produce severe consequences in a debilitated patient, potentially fatal malaria which merits attention in an ICU can be grouped into three categories: (1) severe complications of *P. falciparum* in nonimmune children and adults, responsible for the vast majority of severe disease worldwide (Table 143-3); (2) splenic rupture, which occurs most frequently with *P. vivax*; and (3) chronic nephrotic syndrome due to immune-complex nephritis associated with *P. malariae*, usually seen in children and often complicated by overwhelming bacterial infection. There is emerging evidence that

TABLE 143-3	Clinical and Laboratory Features That Classify a Patient as Suffering from Severe *Plasmodium falciparum* Malaria According to the World Health Organization

Clinical Features

Impaired consciousness or unarousable coma
Prostration (generalized weakness so that the patient is unable walk or sit up without assistance)
Failure to feed
Multiple convulsions (more than two episodes in 24 hours)
Deep breathing/respiratory distress (acidotic breathing)
Circulatory collapse or shock (systolic blood pressure <70 mm Hg in adults and <50 mm Hg in children)
Clinical jaundice plus evidence of other vital organ dysfunction
Hemoglobinuria
Abnormal spontaneous bleeding
Pulmonary edema (radiologic evidence)

Laboratory Findings

Hypoglycemia (blood glucose <2.2 mmol/L or <40 mg/dL)
Metabolic acidosis (plasma bicarbonate <15 mmol/L)
Severe normocytic anemia (hemoglobin <5 g/dL, packed cell volume <15%)
Hemoglobinuria
Hyperparasitemia (>2% or 100,000/μL in low-intensity transmission areas or > 5% or 250,000/μL in areas of high stable malaria transmission intensity)
Hyperlactatemia (lactate >5 mmol/L)
Renal impairment (serum creatinine >265 μmol/L).

Modified from Guidelines for the treatment of malaria 2010. Geneva: World Health Organization; 2010. Available at: http://whqlibdoc.who.int/publications/2010/9789241547925_eng.pdf.

P. knowlesi can also cause severe fatal malaria and should be treated in an ICU setting.[8]

CEREBRAL MALARIA

This is the most frequent severe complication of plasmodium infection, accounting for most fatalities as well as chronic sequelae. It is most frequent in children of 3 to 5 years of age. Strictly defined, *cerebral malaria* implies unarousable coma due to *P. falciparum*.[20,21] Hyperpyrexia and febrile convulsions in young children may produce transiently altered mental status without true involvement of the cerebral microvasculature and thus technically do not constitute cerebral malaria. However, in clinical practice, seizures or persistent changes in sensorium which cannot be attributed to other disease processes should be considered cerebral malaria until proven otherwise. Although cerebral malaria is classically attributed to cytoadhesion and microvascular obstruction in the brain, other ongoing processes including hypoglycemia, metabolic acidosis, and impaired oxygenation due to anemia and pulmonary edema likely contribute.

The altered sensorium of cerebral malaria may develop gradually within a few days of onset of illness or manifest as persistent coma after a generalized convulsion. Compared to adults, children with cerebral malaria have a shorter history of fever before progressing to coma (average about 2 days). The most common neurologic picture is of a symmetrical upper motor neuron lesion with hypertonia, hyperreflexia, clonus, absent abdominal reflexes, and extensor Babinski responses. Hypotonia and acute cerebellar ataxia are sometimes seen as well, especially in India and Sri Lanka. There is usually a diffuse symmetric encephalopathy, sometimes with signs of frontal lobe release such as a pout reflex or bruxism. There is usually no grasp reflex, and the gag reflex is normally maintained. Both decorticate as well as decerebrate posturing may occur.[21] Meningismus, opisthotonos, and disconjugate gaze are frequently seen. Nystagmus and a sixth nerve palsy are rare. Pupils are usually symmetric with intact pupillary, corneal, oculocephalic, and oculovestibular reflexes. Photophobia, severe neck rigidity, and papilledema are almost never seen.

Convulsions may occur in up to 50% of cases of cerebral malaria. As a child ages above 3 to 4 years, seizures become more likely to represent cerebral malaria rather than febrile convulsions.[22] Although generalized seizures are classically reported, partial motor seizures, with or without secondary generalization, may occur.[20] Although often showing only diffuse cortical dysfunction, EEG studies may sometimes reveal underlying status epilepticus even when it is not clinically evident.[21]

PULMONARY EDEMA AND ACUTE RESPIRATORY DISTRESS SYNDROME

Pulmonary edema, which may progress to acute lung injury (ALI) and acute respiratory distress syndrome (ARDS), is frequent and typically the most lethal of the complications of malaria. Recent evidence suggests that the mechanism may involve acute pulmonary hypertension precipitated by nitric oxide consumption by free plasma hemoglobin released from intravascular hemolysis.[Janka et al., in press] Endothelial injury leading to increased alveolar permeability and noncardiogenic pulmonary edema may also contribute. Interstitial edema and inflammatory cell infiltrates are seen at autopsy, but sequestration of parasitized RBCs in the lung is uncommon.[23] Pulmonary complications occur in 5% to 30% of patients with severe malaria, especially pregnant women, nonimmune persons, and patients already suffering from other complications.[23] The onset may be any time during the course of illness, even if the patient appears to be improving and parasitemia has decreased. Symptoms include dyspnea and cough, with rapid progression to hypoxia and respiratory distress.

ANEMIA AND HEMATOLOGIC PERTURBATIONS

Although some degree of anemia is common in all types of malaria, severe anemia (hemoglobin less than 5 g/100 mL) occurs almost exclusively with *P. falciparum* infections, owing to their high parasitemias. It is most common and often severe in pregnant women and young children (<1 year), in whom it may be the presenting sign.[24] In addition to the acute hemolytic destruction of parasitized RBCs, the more chronic processes of removal of parasitized cells from circulation by the spleen and cytokine inhibition of erythropoiesis may contribute.[25] Nonimmune subjects may develop anemia within days after infection, whereas anemia usually develops more slowly in those who are semi-immune. The degree of anemia generally correlates with bilirubin level and level of parasitemia. It may be exacerbated by underlying glucose-6-phosphate dehydrogenase (G6PD) deficiency in the setting of administration of oxidant antimalarial drugs (e.g., quinine, sulfadoxine) and iron-deficiency anemia due to malnutrition. Significant jaundice and hemoglobinuria may result. Thrombocytopenia, although frequent, is not usually associated with bleeding or correlated with disease severity. Disseminated intravascular coagulation (DIC) is seen in less than 10% of severe cases.

ACUTE RENAL FAILURE

Acute renal failure (ARF) is seen in about 30% of adult patients with cerebral malaria but is uncommon in children. For unclear reasons, ARF is rare in semi-immune persons. ARF is usually due to acute tubular necrosis, is oliguric in nature (<400 mL urine/24 h for adults), and is most often reversible. Renal ischemia due to hypovolemia, renal vasoconstriction, microvascular obstruction, and pigment nephropathy from hemolysis may all contribute. Electrolyte abnormalities such as hyponatremia, hypocalcemia (usually related to albumin loss), hypophosphatemia, and metabolic acidemia, as well as fluid overload with pulmonary edema, may result.

Blackwater fever refers to a severe syndrome characterized by low or absent parasitemia, intravascular hemolysis, hemoglobinuria, and ARF. It is classically seen in people of northern European descent chronically exposed to *P. falciparum* and irregularly taking the quinoline antimalarial drugs, quinine or quinidine, which together are known as the *cinchona alkaloids*. The syndrome virtually disappeared after 1950 when chloroquine superseded quinine. However, it is now said to be resurgent, albeit with lower mortality, in relation to mounting chloroquine resistance and consequent increased use of quinine and the newer quinolines, such as mefloquine and halofantrine.[26]

HYPOGLYCEMIA, LACTIC ACIDOSIS, AND OTHER METABOLIC PERTURBATIONS

Severe metabolic derangements are frequent, especially in pregnant women and young children. Although sometimes asymptomatic in pregnancy, hypoglycemia often causes impaired consciousness, extensor posturing, and convulsions and may be confused with cerebral malaria. In addition to direct glucose consumption by the malaria parasite, decreased oral intake, depletion of liver glycogen, cytokine inhibition of gluconeogenesis, and insulin release stimulated by quinine or quinidine may contribute to hypoglycemia. Serum insulin levels are low, and lactate, alanine, and counter-regulatory hormones are appropriately elevated. Although rarely clinically significant, mild hepatocellular damage may occur and be manifested by elevated hepatic transaminases and jaundice. At least theoretically, such hepatic dysfunction could result in impaired metabolic clearance of antimalarial medications and lactate and deficits in the production of coagulation factors and albumin.

SHOCK AND BACTERIAL AND OTHER SUPRAINFECTION

So-called *algid malaria*, referring to hypotension and shock, may resemble and indeed sometimes be due to gram-negative sepsis from impaired flow in intestinal capillaries, with resultant mucosal erosion. Non-typhoidal salmonella septicemia is specifically associated with *P. falciparum.*[27] Algid malaria is often seen in the setting of hyperparasitemia, with concomitant hypoglycemia and lactic acidemia, and may progress to multiorgan system failure and death. As with most malaria complications, severe hemodynamic derangements are most often seen in nonimmune persons.[28] Whether bacteria are isolated or not, a classic septic shock picture is typical, with elevated cardiac index and decreased systemic vascular resistance.[29] Hemodynamic decompensation due to splenic rupture may mimic algid malaria.

A host of other infectious complications, including aspiration pneumonia and parvovirus infection, may be related to *falciparum* malaria. Malaria occurs with increasing frequency and severity in those who are human immunodeficiency virus (HIV) infected, especially during pregnancy, and can also transiently up-regulate HIV replication.[30-34] An association between severe malaria infection and hepatitis B surface antigen carriage has also been noted.[35]

TROPICAL SPLENOMEGALY AND SPLENIC RUPTURE

Splenomegaly is common in infection with all species of malaria. The *tropical splenomegaly syndrome*, also sometimes termed *hyperreactive malarial syndrome* (HMS), refers to a condition of massive splenomegaly, high titers of total serum IgM and malaria-specific antibodies, and scanty or absent parasitemia. It is seen in individuals with a history of residence in an endemic area and can be associated with any malaria species. Host genetic factors appear to play a role.[36]

Unlike virtually all the other complications of malaria that are most often associated with *P. falciparum*, acute splenic complications occur most commonly in *P. vivax*, especially with the first infection. Although the term *spontaneous splenic rupture* has traditionally been used, in reality a range of hematomas or tears of varying severity may occur. The rupture or tear usually occurs 2 to 3 months after infection, presumably due to increased intrasplenic tension, often precipitated by trauma of varying degrees or mechanical ventilation.[37] Over-eager examiners have been suggested to play a role, although no cases of clear palpation-induced rupture have been reported. Fever, tachycardia, vomiting, prostration, abdominal pain or guarding, tender splenomegaly, hypovolemia, and rapidly worsening anemia are common presenting features. Abdominal pain may be localized or diffuse, mild or severe. Shock may ensue. Diaphragmatic irritation after rupture may cause referred pain to the left shoulder, supraclavicular, or scapular regions ("Kehr's sign"). This is present in about one-half of cases and is said to have good specificity for rupture.

MALARIA IN PREGNANCY AND CHILDREN

In addition to being more susceptible to infection, malaria is particularly dangerous in pregnant women and their fetuses, with increased risk of pulmonary edema, hypoglycemia, severe anemia, premature delivery, low birth weight, and maternal and fetal death. Malaria parasites can often be found in the placenta and may impair oxygen and nutrient transport to the fetus. Disease is most severe in primiparae, especially if nonimmune. In contrast, women from endemic areas are usually asymptomatic, with the exception of the effects of anemia, again more severe in primiparae. Congenital malaria is rare except in those infants born to nonimmune mothers.[38]

Diagnosis

CLINICAL

Malaria often presents with nonspecific signs and symptoms, so making a clinical diagnosis may be difficult. Although almost all patients have a history of fever, they may frequently be afebrile at the time of examination.[39] Physicians in industrialized countries who are unfamiliar with the disease may not initially include malaria in the differential diagnosis. Delayed diagnosis is frequent and associated with a poor outcome.[6,40] Although patients with other species of malaria parasite may not present for months or even years after infection, the vast majority of those with *P. falciparum* will present within 6 months of exposure.[4] The differential diagnosis includes most febrile illnesses found in the tropics (see Table 143-1). Babesiosis may present both clinically and microscopically similar to malaria in patients without travel to malaria-endemic areas. Cerebral malaria must be distinguished from bacterial meningitis, the viral meningoencephalitides, metabolic coma, and intoxications by lumbar puncture.[41] In cerebral malaria, the cerebrospinal fluid (CSF) opening pressure is usually normal, although a few lymphocytes and moderate elevation of protein may be seen. High CSF lactate and low glucose indicate a poor prognosis.

CONVENTIONAL MICROSCOPY

Laboratory diagnosis has traditionally been made via the examination of thick and thin Giemsa-stained smears. Thick smears are more sensitive in diagnosing malaria, whereas thin smears allow identification of the specific parasite. Either smear can be used to quantify the level of parasitemia, but thick smears are theoretically more sensitive for this purpose.[42,43] Simultaneous infections with multiple strains of *P. falciparum* are common in some areas of sub-Saharan Africa and also may occur with *P. vivax* in Southeast Asia and Latin America.[44,45] Blood obtained by pricking a fingertip or earlobe is preferred because parasite densities are higher in these capillary-rich areas, although blood obtained by venipuncture collected in heparin or EDTA anticoagulant-coated tubes is acceptable if used shortly after being drawn (to prevent alteration in the morphology of white blood cells and malaria parasites).[46] Smears should be taken as soon as the diagnosis of malaria is considered, without waiting for manifestation of a classic paroxysm. Parasitemia may be undetectable in the early stages of the illness, in those with partial immunity, and in those who have previously self-administered antimalarials, a common practice in malaria-endemic areas.[47] Levels of parasitemia may fluctuate over time, necessitating repeated smears for diagnosis. Furthermore, *P. falciparum*–parasitized red blood cells may be sequestered in the deep capillaries of the spleen, liver, and bone marrow. Although a blood film is unlikely to be falsely negative in a patient with severe disease, negative smears should not prevent prompt administration of antimalarial therapy if the diagnosis is strongly suspected.[14] Conversely, asymptomatic parasitemia is common in children from endemic areas, and thus a positive smear does not necessarily signify a clinical case under these circumstances.

Considerable expertise at reading malaria smears may be necessary to detect and distinguish the parasites (see Table 143-2). The most important point is to distinguish *P. falciparum*, with its concomitant risk of severe complications, from the other plasmodia. Superimposed platelets, particles of stain, pits in the slide, RBC inclusions such as Howell-Jolly bodies and those seen in siderocytes, and other intracellular pathogens such as *Bartonella* and *Babesia* must be distinguished from malaria parasites. Furthermore, alterations in parasite morphology may occur related to strain variation, drug pressure, and blood collection method.

NEWER LABORATORY METHODS

Various new diagnostic techniques for malaria have been developed in recent years, including microscopy with fluorescent stains, dipstick antigen detection, DNA probes, polymerase chain reaction (PCR) assays, and automated blood cell analysis.[42,43,48-52] Use of one of these new diagnostic modalities should be considered when a high suspicion of malaria remains despite repeatedly negative blood smears, especially if the microscopist has limited experience with reading malaria smears.[43] Each technique has unique advantages and disadvantages, but the sensitivity and specificity for *P. falciparum* is generally similar or better than conventional microscopy. Because of its greater sensitivity (as low as 5 parasites/µL), PCR may be a particularly valuable tool in nonimmune persons. PCR also allows evaluation for possible infection with multiple malaria strains and determination of drug resistance. The U.S. Food and Drug Administration (FDA) recently approved a rapid diagnostic test—the BinaxNOW malaria test (Binax/Alere Inc., Scarborough, Maine)—that detects the HRP-2 protein of *P. falciparum* as well as an aldolase common to all plasmodia, with sensitivities of 100% and 97%, respectively.[42] However, the sensitivity of this and other dipstick antigen tests is diminished when the parasitemia is less than 100 parasites/µL. Furthermore, the HRP-2 protein may persist in the bloodstream and give a false-positive test result for up to 4 weeks after successful treatment of malaria. Hence, it is still important to confirm the rapid diagnostic test with microscopy when possible.

IMAGING

Computed tomography (CT) or magnetic resonance imaging (MRI) scanning of the abdomen is the usual diagnostic modality when splenic rupture is considered, although ultrasonography, arteriography, bleeding scans, or exploratory laparotomy may sometimes be needed. Findings such as increased brain volume and occasionally brain swelling have been noted in CT and MRI studies in cerebral malaria, but these tests are generally unhelpful clinically and are indicated only to rule out suspected mass lesions when the diagnosis of cerebral malaria is uncertain.[53]

◼ Clinical Management

INDICATIONS FOR ADMISSION TO THE INTENSIVE CARE UNIT AND GENERAL MANAGEMENT

Features that indicate severe disease meriting admission to an ICU and urgent IV therapy are noted in Table 143-3. In these critically ill patients, chloroquine-resistant *P. falciparum* should be assumed until proven otherwise. As per routine ICU management, the patient's breathing and circulatory status should first be rapidly assessed, the airway secured, and the neurologic status scored on the Glasgow Coma Scale or other appropriate scoring system.[54] For patients in profound shock, blood cultures should be drawn and broad-spectrum antibiotics begun unless the diagnosis of severe malaria has already been confirmed or if bacterial suprainfection is suspected. Unconscious patients should have a lumbar puncture to rule out bacterial meningitis.

Careful attention to fluid balance is imperative, especially considering the very poor prognosis once pulmonary edema or ARDS develops. Measurements of urine output and daily weights should be routinely performed. Monitoring of central venous pressure should be considered in delicate cases, such as those with respiratory distress or compromised renal function. Considering that the prognosis associated with pulmonary failure is considerably poorer than that of ARF, some authors recommend early use of inotropes rather than excessive fluids in the setting of hypotension, although a beneficial effect on the overall hemodynamic profile has yet to be conclusively demonstrated.[39,55] Dialysis is indicated for ARF and may aid not only through improved fluid balance and control of acidemia but also via removal of circulating cytokine mediators of inflammation. Although observations are limited, the quinolines appear not to be dialyzed.[56] Cautious transfusion of packed cells is usually indicated when the hematocrit falls below 20%. In addition to improved oxygen transport, blood transfusion may reduce the parasite load and cytokine mediators of inflammation.[39,57] Concurrent administration of diuretics or low-dose dopamine may be warranted to avoid fluid overload.

Increasing respiratory distress may indicate the onset of ALI or ARDS. Arterial blood gas measurements may reveal hypoxemia, and chest x-rays bilateral infiltrates. Supplemental oxygen and mechanical ventilation may be required. In accordance with the NIH ARDS Network Trial, lung-protective ventilation, with tidal volume of 6 mL/kg predicted body weight and plateau pressures less than 30 cm H_2O are indicated for improved survival.[23] Extracorporeal oxygenation has also been employed.[58] Metabolic acidosis should be treated by improving pulmonary gas exchange, correcting hypovolemia and hypoglycemia, and treating associated septicemia. Blood glucose should be checked frequently, especially in pregnant patients, and 50% dextrose administered when needed. Results of studies on the efficacy of continuous IV infusion of 5% dextrose have been mixed.[59,60] Quinoline-induced hypoglycemia may be prevented by administering somatostatin analogs followed by glucagons.[61] Acute seizures may be treated with benzodiazepines or paraldehyde, and prolonged seizures terminated with phenytoin.[21] However, prophylactic anticonvulsants are not recommended and may be harmful.[54] Although the risk of bleeding is low, aspirin should be avoided in the presence of thrombocytopenia. Many patients with splenic rupture can be managed conservatively with supportive therapy, although splenectomy may be necessary.[36]

In late pregnancy, fetal monitoring should be begun prior to initiation of quinoline therapy so that the effects of the disease can be distinguished from those of drug toxicity. Early obstetric intervention should be considered for the benefit of both mother and fetus. Although fetal distress is usually the result of placental insufficiency, it may sometimes be related to high maternal temperature and hypoglycemia. Thus these parameters should be carefully monitored and treated accordingly. Fluid balance is particularly crucial in pregnant patients; the sudden increase in peripheral vascular resistance postpartum may precipitate pulmonary edema. In young children prone to febrile convulsions, extra efforts should be made to control fever by the use of acetaminophen, cooling blankets, and baths.

ANTIMALARIAL CHEMOTHERAPY

Because delay of therapy is associated with increased mortality, empirical parental treatment should be implemented immediately in all suspected cases of severe malaria after obtaining appropriate blood specimens. Infection with chloroquine-resistant *P. falciparum* should be assumed unless specifically ruled out. Treatment regimens for severe *P. falciparum* are also effective for the more infrequent cases of severe malaria due to other species.

Two classes of medicines are indicated for parenteral treatment: the artemisinin derivatives (artesunate, artemether, and others) and the cinchona alkaloids (Table 143-4). Randomized trials in Southeast Asia show artesunate to be superior to quinine for severe malaria in adults, although there is currently insufficient evidence to support this conclusion in children.[54,62] Despite its use throughout much of the world, in the United States, intravenous (IV) artesunate has "investigational new drug" status and is only available through request to the Centers for Disease Control and Prevention (CDC).[63,64] Because IV quinine is also

TABLE 143-4	Treatment Guidelines for Severe *Plasmodium falciparum* Malaria	
Drug	**Dose**	**Comments**
Artemisinin Compound Regimens*		

Artesunate	2.4 mg/kg IV daily × 3 days, followed by one of the following:
	1. Doxycycline, 100 mg PO BID × 7 days
	2. Clindamycin, 20 mg base/kg/d PO, divided TID × 7 days
	3. Atovaquone/proguanil:
	— Adults: 4 adult tabs PO daily × 7 days
	— Children: PO daily × 7 days as follows:
	    5-8 kg: 2 pediatric tabs
	    9-10 kg: 3 pediatric tabs
	    11-20 kg: 1 adult tab
	    21-30 kg: 2 adult tabs
	    31-40 kg: 3 adult tabs
	    >40 kg: 4 adult tabs
	1. Mefloquine:
	— Adults: 684 mg base (=750 mg salt) PO as initial dose, followed by 456 mg base (=500 mg salt) PO given 6-12 hours later (total dose = 1250 mg salt)
	— Children: 13.7 mg base/kg (=15 mg salt/kg) PO as initial dose, followed by 9.1 mg base/kg (=10 mg salt/kg) PO 6-12 hours later (total dose = 25 mg salt/kg)
		Artesunate has "investigational new drug" status in the United States and is only available on request to the CDC (770-488-7788). Eligibility requirements include inability to take oral medications, high levels of parasitemia, clinical evidence of severe malaria, intolerance of or contraindication to quinidine, failure of quinidine therapy, and lack of rapid access to quinidine.[64] Where available, artesunate rectal suppositories (10 mg/kg) may be used in children < 5 years of age if IV or IM administration is not possible. Doxycycline is contraindicated in children < 8 years of age and in pregnancy. Atovaquone/proguanil is packaged in the United States in fixed-dose combination tablets of 250 mg atovaquone/100 mg proguanil for adults and 62.5 mg atovaquone/25 mg proguanil for children. Safety of atovaquone/proguanil in pregnancy has not been established.

Cinchona Alkaloid Regimens		
Quinine dihydrochloride	20 mg salt/kg IV or IM on admission, then 10 mg/kg q 8 h. Can be given IM if IV administration is not possible. One of the following drugs should also be given concurrently: 1. Doxycycline as above. If patient unable to take PO, give 100 mg IV q 12 h and switch to PO when possible. Avoid rapid IV administration. 2. Clindamycin as above. If patient unable to take PO, give 10 mg base/kg loading dose IV followed by 5 mg base/kg IV q 8 h and switch to PO when possible. Avoid rapid IV administration.	The infusion rate of IV quinine should be rate controlled and not exceed 5 mg salt/kg/h. The drug is usually diluted in 5% dextrose and infused over 4 hours. IV quinine is not available in the United States. When administering IM, the dose should be split and diluted to a concentration of 60-100 mg/kg delivered to each thigh. Reduce the quinine dose by one-third after 48 hours in patients with severe renal and/or hepatic dysfunction. Doxycycline is contraindicated in children <8 years old and in pregnancy.
Quinidine gluconate	6.25 mg base/kg (=10 mg salt/kg) IV on admission, then 0.0125 mg base/kg/min (=0.02 mg salt/kg/min) continuous infusion. An alternative regimen is 15 mg base/kg (=24 mg salt/kg) loading dose IV infused over 4 hours, followed by 7.5 mg base/kg (=12 mg salt/kg) infused over 4 hours q 8 h, starting 8 hours after the loading dose. A second drug should be given concurrently as listed above for quinine.	The loading dose should be omitted if the patient received >40 mg/kg quinine in the preceding 48 hours or mefloquine in the previous 12 hours. Reduce the dose by one-third after 48 hours in patients with severe renal and/or hepatic dysfunction. Quinidine should be given for 7 days in infections in southeast Asia and 3 days in Africa or South America.

*Various other artemisinin combined therapy regimens are in use around the world depending upon drug availability, national policy, and personal preference, including artesunate plus amodiaquine, artemether plus lumefantrine, dihydroartemisinin plus piperaquine.

unavailable in the United States, quinidine gluconate is often used.[65] Cinchona alkaloids may also be considered for first-line treatment of patients infected in Southeast Asia, where resistance to artemisinin compounds has been documented, or if the patient has already received but not responded to an artemisinin-based therapy.[66,67]

According to CDC recommendations, the patient should receive at least 24 hours of parenteral therapy with quinidine gluconate even if there is immediate dramatic improvement.[64] After 24 hours, patients may be transitioned to oral quinine only if they are able to tolerate oral medications and the parasite density is less than 1%. The IV quinidine/oral quinine treatment course is 7 days total if malaria was contracted in Southeast Asia and 3 days if in South America or Africa.

The patient should be given a 7-day oral course of second drug in addition to the IV artesunate or IV quinidine/oral quinine therapy (see Table 143-3). Artemisinin compounds should be followed by oral doxycycline, clindamycin, atovaquone/proguanil, or mefloquine, whereas either doxycycline or clindamycin are given concurrently with the cinchona alkaloids. Doxycycline is preferred to other tetracyclines because it can be given once daily and does not accumulate in renal failure. Mefloquine should be avoided if the patient presented initially with impaired consciousness; an increased incidence of neuropsychiatric complications associated with mefloquine following cerebral malaria has been documented. Chloroquine is no longer recommended for the treatment of severe malaria because of widespread resistance. Intramuscular sulfadoxine/pyrimethamine is no longer recommended.

Adverse Effects of Therapy

Side effects associated with artemisinin compounds are infrequent and generally mild and include abdominal pain, diarrhea, contact dermatitis, decreases in reticulocyte and neutrophil counts, and elevated hepatic transaminases.[68] Severe allergic reactions and cerebellar dysfunction have been rarely reported.[69]

Side effects of quinine and quinidine, known as *cinchonism*, are common and typically include nausea, vomiting, headache, dysphoria, vasodilation, tinnitus, and changes in auditory and visual acuity. These alterations are dose related and reversible. Less common side effects include rash, urticaria, angioedema of the face, pruritus, agranulocytosis, hepatitis, blackwater fever, and psychiatric disorders. Overdoses are associated with depressed respiration, circulatory collapse, and CNS alterations including seizures and coma, which may be difficult to distinguish from cerebral malaria.[70] Simultaneous use of two quinolines or retreatment with the same quinoline within a short period of time may predispose to severe side effects.[71] The cinchona alkaloids are metabolized in the liver and excreted in the urine. Monitoring blood levels is recommended for persons with impaired renal or hepatic function, and dose reduction is necessary in those with severe renal impairment. Quinine metabolism appears to be decreased in children with kwashiorkor but increased in those with marasmus.[72]

Although rarely clinically significant, prolongation of the electrocardiographic QT interval with IV quinoline therapy is common.[73] Severe conduction abnormalities may occur along with hypotension, blindness, and deafness.[54,63,64,73] Dysrhythmias and hypotension may also result from overly rapid infusion. Coma may result when serum quinoline levels exceed 20 mg/L. Cardiac monitoring should be performed with IV quinoline use, especially with quinidine, which although more potent against the malaria parasite is also generally more toxic.[73] Infusion rates of quinidine should be decreased if the QT interval increases by more than 25% of its baseline level.

Quinoline-induced stimulation of insulin release may elicit significant hypoglycemia, especially in pregnancy.[60,74] Hypophosphatemia may also be precipitated by both quinoline and IV dextrose, causing

CNS dysfunction.[39] Levels of digoxin, mefloquine, neuromuscular blocking agents, and oral anticoagulants may all be increased with quinoline administration. Quinine can cause hemolysis in patients with G6PD deficiency. Because of their curare-like effect on skeletal muscle, quinolines are contraindicated in patients with myasthenia gravis.

Atovaquone/proguanil is usually well tolerated. Gastrointestinal symptoms, skin rash, headache, insomnia, and (rarely) hematologic and renal effects have been reported, especially at high levels.[75,76]

ANCILLARY THERAPIES

Various ancillary therapies have been proposed for severe malaria. In most cases, controlled data are not available to judge their efficacy. Exchange transfusion and erythrocytapheresis have been employed with apparent benefit in cases of severe disease with high parasitemia (>15%) and should be considered in such situations, especially if the patient's condition is worsening despite adequate chemotherapy.[77-80] The rationale for this form of therapy is based on (1) rapid reduction in parasite load; (2) removal of toxic substances; and (3) reducing microcirculatory sludging.[77] In some studies, iron chelators such as desferrioxamine have been demonstrated to hasten malaria parasite clearance and shorten the duration of cerebral malaria coma.[81,82] Proposed mechanisms include depriving the parasite of necessary iron, enhancing the T-helper immune response, and protecting against iron-mediated peroxidant cerebral tissue damage.[58] Antioxidants such as pentoxifylline and inhaled nitric oxide have been used, but attempts to attenuate the immune response in malaria have generally met with mixed results.[83-85] Monoclonal antibodies directed against TNF-α had no impact on mortality and may increase morbidity (neurologic sequelae), probably reflecting the participation of multiple cytokines in the pathogenesis of severe and complicated malaria.[86,87] Dichloroacetate to counter lactic acidosis is also under study.[88] Corticosteroids are detrimental in severe malaria and should not be used.[89]

LABORATORY MONITORING

Findings in severe malaria may include profound hemolytic anemia and thrombocytopenia, leukocytosis with a left shift (although milder cases may show leukopenia), prolonged coagulation times (with increased fibrin split products and diminished fibrinogen reflecting DIC), hyponatremia, hypoalbuminemia, hypophosphatemia, hypoglycemia, lactic acidemia, and elevated hepatic enzymes, LDH, bilirubin, BUN, and creatinine. Urinalysis may reveal proteinuria, RBCs and RBC casts, and hemoglobinuria. Coagulation defects and thrombocytopenia often correlate with the degree of parasitemia. The level of parasitemia should be monitored via blood smear every 12 hours after initiation of therapy. A decrease of 75% should be noted within 48 hours. If this does not occur, drug resistance should be suspected, and the regimen should be changed accordingly (see Table 143-4).

▨ Prognosis

Case fatality rates in severe malaria range from 2% to 50%.[20,21,90-92] Factors which correlate with a poor prognosis include the infecting species and resistance profile, CNS involvement, pulmonary edema, hypoglycemia, lactic acidosis, renal failure, severe anemia, younger age, pregnancy, and treatment in a rural health facility as opposed to an ICU.[39,93-100] There is a semiquantitative relationship between level of parasitemia and risk of death, especially in nonimmune patients. Although less than 10% of adults with cerebral malaria have persistent neurologic sequelae, this number may be as high as 40% in children, especially if associated with hypoglycemia.[59,90] Commonly seen sequelae include psychosis, hemiparesis, cerebellar ataxia, and extrapyramidal rigidity.[20,21] Children who survive without obvious neurologic sequelae appear to then develop normally neuropsychologically.[101] A postmalarial neurologic syndrome, usually associated with mefloquine use, of an acute confusional state, psychosis, convulsions, and tremors has been described but is usually self-limited.[21]

ACKNOWLEDGMENTS

The authors thank Andrew Bennett, Jenna Iberg, Frederique Jacquerioz, Emily Jentes, Donald Krogstad, Nikki Maxwell, Corina Monagin, Laura Morgan, Obinna Nnedu, Christina Styron, Torrey Theall, and Kent Wagoner for their advice and assistance preparing the manuscript.

KEY POINTS

1. A detailed history of the patient's travel itinerary, activities and exposures, and any pre-travel prophylaxis, as well as general knowledge of the prevalent diseases and their incubation periods and drug-resistance patterns in the region of travel are imperative when evaluating patients with exposures overseas.

2. Most "non-tropical" infections are also common in developing countries and thus need to be considered.

3. Assessing the patient's immune status based on history of exposure to tropical pathogens is essential in directing the diagnostic workup and management.

4. Infection with multiple tropical pathogens is common in those living in endemic areas.

Uncomplicated Malaria

1. Malaria is the most common serious infection in most tropical countries, as well as in returning travelers, and therefore should be considered in any patient reporting travel in malaria-endemic areas or exposure to unscreened blood products ("transfusion malaria") or blood-contaminated needles.

2. Malaria classically produces a three-stage "paroxysm" progressing over an 8- to 12-hour period, consisting of rigors and chills ("cold stage"), followed by fever ("hot stage"), followed by sweating with resolution of all symptoms ("defervescent stage"). In practice, neither the classic paroxysm nor the periodicity is invariably seen.

Severe and Complicated Malaria

1. The overwhelming majority of severe and complicated malaria is due to *Plasmodium falciparum* in nonimmune children, adults, and pregnant women.

2. The risk of acquiring *P. falciparum* is highest for those traveling to sub-Saharan Africa and New Guinea, moderate in India, and comparatively low in Southeast Asia and Latin America.

3. The most frequent severe complication is cerebral malaria, mostly seen in children and manifesting as coma, convulsions, changes in sensorium, or focal neurologic signs. Other severe complications include severe anemia, hypoglycemia, lactic acidosis, acute renal failure, pulmonary edema, acute respiratory distress syndrome, shock, and bacterial suprainfection.

4. Potentially severe complications due to non-*falciparum* malaria include splenic rupture (*Plasmodium vivax*) and chronic nephrotic syndrome (*Plasmodium malariae*).

Diagnosis

1. Malaria often presents with nonspecific signs and symptoms, and the differential diagnosis is broad, so making a clinical diagnosis may be difficult.

2. The vast majority of those with *P. falciparum* will present within 6 months of exposure.

3. Laboratory diagnosis is traditionally made through microscopy of thick and thin Giemsa-stained smears. Low or fluctuating parasitemias or altered parasite morphology may complicate diagnosis, especially with an inexperienced microscopist. Asymptomatic parasitemia is common in children from endemic areas.

4. Various new diagnostic techniques for malaria have been developed in recent years, with sensitivities and specificities for *P. falciparum* generally similar or better than conventional microscopy. Use of one of these new modalities should be considered when the diagnosis of malaria is unclear.

5. Radiographic imaging of the abdomen is indicated when splenic rupture is suspected.

Clinical Management

1. Patients with evidence of severe or complicated malaria should be assumed to have chloroquine-resistant *P. falciparum* and admitted to the intensive care unit for aggressive supportive care and urgent antimalarial drug therapy. Therapy should consist of intravenous administration of either an artemisinin compound (e.g., artesunate) followed by oral doxycycline, clindamycin, atovaquone-proguanil, or mefloquine; or a cinchona alkaloid (quinine or quinidine) given together with doxycycline or clindamycin.

2. Artemisinin compounds are usually well tolerated. Side effects with cinchona alkaloid therapy are frequent, but are usually mild, dose related, and reversible.

3. Ancillary therapies proposed for severe malaria include exchange transfusion, erythrocytapheresis, iron chelation, antioxidants, monoclonal antibodies, and dichloroacetate. In most cases, insufficient controlled data are available upon which to judge their efficacy.

4. Many patients with splenic rupture can be managed conservatively with supportive therapy, although splenectomy may be necessary.

5. The hemoglobin/hematocrit, electrolytes, platelet count, glucose, lactate, arterial blood gas, BUN/creatinine, liver function and coagulation enzymes, and the level of parasitemia in response to therapy should be monitored closely.

6. Case fatality rates in severe malaria range from 2% to 50%.

ANNOTATED REFERENCES

Cox-Singh J, Davis TM, Lee KS, Shamsu SS, et al. *Plasmodium knowlesi* malaria in humans is widely distributed and potentially life threatening. Clin Infect Dis 2008;46:165-71.

P. knowlesi has been misdiagnosed as P. malariae in humans until recent years. In this study, 960 blood samples from hospitalized malaria patients and 54 archival blood samples previously diagnosed as P. malariae in Malaysian Borneo, in addition to 5 archival samples from Peninsular Malaysia, were subjected to nested PCR. P. knowlesi was detected in 27.7% of samples from hospitalized patients, 83.7% of archival samples in Borneo, and 100% of samples from Peninsular Malaysia. Since P. knowlesi is frequently misdiagnosed and has been implicated in severe disease, all patients with P. malariae contracted in Southeast Asia should be treated as for severe falciparum malaria.

Griffith KS, Lewis LS, Mali S, Parise ME. Treatment of malaria in the United States: a systematic review. JAMA 2007;297:2264-77.

This systematic review explores the evidence for management of both uncomplicated and severe malaria to provide clinicians with practical recommendations for the diagnosis and treatment of malaria in the United States.

Mishra SK, Newton C. Diagnosis and management of the neurological complications of falciparum malaria. Nat Rev Neurol 2009;5:189-98.

This review article summarizes the pathogenesis, symptoms, and sequelae of the neurologic complications of falciparum malaria. First-line and adjuvant therapies are also discussed.

Mohan A, Sharma SK, Bollineni S. Acute lung injury and acute respiratory distress syndrome in malaria. J Vector Borne Dis 2008;45:179-93.

The acute respiratory distress syndrome is a dangerous complication of severe falciparum malaria. Mechanisms of pathogenesis are proposed but not well understood. This review article details the difficult management of fluid balance and mechanical ventilation in the setting of respiratory compromise in severe malaria.

Stauffer WM, Cartwright CP, Olson DA, et al. Diagnostic performance of rapid diagnostic tests versus blood smears for malaria in US clinical practice. Clin Infect Dis 2009;49:908-13.

The diagnosis of malaria is difficult in countries where few cases are seen, and clinicians and laboratorians are thus unfamiliar with the disease. This prospective study of 852 blood samples compared testing by standard thick and thin smears with a rapid antigen capture assay. The rapid diagnostic test's sensitivity was 97% and 100% for all malaria and P. falciparum, respectively, compared to 85% and 88% by Giemsa thick blood smear. Rapid diagnostic tests are recommended, especially for inexperienced microbiologists.

REFERENCES

Access the complete reference list online at http://www.expertconsult.com.

144

Rickettsial Diseases

DIANA F. FLORESCU | ANDRE C. KALIL

Proteobacteria are small gram-negative obligate intracellular organisms that can be divided into two classes: Alphaproteobacteria including *Rickettsiaceae* (genus *Rickettsia*) and *Anaplasmataceae* (with four genera: *Ehrlichia*, *Anaplasma*, *Neorickettsia*, and *Wolbachia*), and Gammaproteobacteria that include *Coxiellaceae* (genus *Coxiella*).[1]

The *Rickettsia* genus is divided into the spotted fever group (SFG), which comprises about 15 different species of human pathogens, the typhus group, and the scrub typhus group.[2] The spotted fever group includes arthropod-borne diseases and comprises mainly *Rickettsia rickettsii*, the agent of Rocky Mountain spotted fever, and *Rickettsia conorii*, the agent of Mediterranean spotted fever.[2] The typhus group comprises *Rickettsia prowazekii*, causing louse-borne epidemic typhus, and *Rickettsia typhi*, the agent of the fleaborne murine typhus. The scrub typhus group includes *Orientia tsutsugamushi*, a mite-borne disease.[2] Part of the clinical manifestations and sequelae associated with most human rickettsioses are due to the bacteria's affinity for the blood vessels' endothelium, leading to damage to the vascular endothelium, triggering vascular inflammation, and compromising vascular permeability.[3,4] Exceptions are *Rickettsia akari* and *O. tsutsugamushi*, which invade and multiply in the monocytic cells.[4]

Ehrlichioses are zoonoses increasingly recognized as human pathogens. The human pathogens of this family, depending on the causative species, invade various target cells of the hematopoietic and lymphoreticular systems.[4] *Coxiella burnetii*, the agent of Q fever, infects many mammal species, including humans. The clinical presentation and evolution of Q fever seem to be related to host immune response, especially to tumor necrosis factor (TNF)-α and IL-10 production by stimulated monocytes.[4,5] The ability of macrophages to kill the organisms and the clinical presentation of infection seem to depend on the immune status of the patient.[4]

Rickettsial Diseases

SPOTTED FEVER GROUP

Rickettsia rickettsii is the causative agent of Rocky Mountain spotted fever (RMSF), an arthropod-borne disease, transmitted by *Dermacentor* ticks.[2,6,7] RMSF occurs mainly in rural and suburban locations throughout North America, Central America, and parts of South America (Colombia, Bolivia, Brazil).[8] The disease is highly seasonal, with the highest incidence during late spring and summer months.[8] After a 2- to 14-day incubation period, patients typically develop fever, myalgia, and severe headaches.[4] The inoculation eschar is rarely found. The major diagnostic sign, the petechial rash (Figure 144-1), usually appears 3 to 5 days after the onset of fever, although older patients and black patients might not develop the rash.[4,9] The rash is usually first noted around the wrists and ankles, and then involves the palms and soles, with centripetal progression.[4,8,9] Because *R. rickettsii* produces small-vessel injury, patients can present with other symptoms such as seizures, focal neurologic deficits, transient deafness, meningoencephalitis, gastrointestinal symptoms (abdominal pain and tenderness mimicking acute abdomen), myocarditis, pericarditis, and pneumonia.[4,8] Despite widespread endothelial damage and microangiopathic thrombosis in some cases, fulminant disseminated intravascular coagulopathy (DIC) is rarely seen.[8] However, fulminant RMSF has been associated with older age, black males with glucose-6-phosphate dehydrogenase (G6PD) deficiency, and possibly with alcoholism.[4]

Rickettsia conorii is the causative agent of several infections designated by geographic names and differentiated by serologic techniques: Marseilles fever, Mediterranean spotted fever (boutonneuse fever), Kenya tick typhus, Israeli tick typhus, Astrakhan spotted fever, and Indian tick typhus.[4,10] Several serotypes merit mention:
- *R. conorii sensu stricto* is the etiologic agent for Mediterranean spotted fever, a disease transmitted by the dog tick, *Rhipicephalus sanguineus*.[2] Most cases originate from the Mediterranean area during the warm months. The classic presentation is a patient with fever, rash, and a single eschar ("tache noir") at the site of the arthropod bite.[4,10] Up to 99% of patients develop a papular rash. The natural evolution of the illness is 12 to 20 days, with extremely low associated mortality (<1%) and no sequelae.[10] Severe cases have been described and are due to diffuse vascular infections and injury complicated by renal, cardiac, and neurologic manifestations.[10] The risk factors associated with poor outcome are older age, G6PD deficiency, alcoholism, immunocompromised status, diabetes, heart failure, respiratory insufficiency, prior prescription of an inappropriate antibiotic, and delayed treatment.[10]
- *R. conorii* serotype Israel, the causative agent of Israeli spotted fever, also transmitted by *R. sanguineus*, is found in Israel, Portugal, and Sicily.[4] Clinical presentation and complications of the disease are similar to Mediterranean spotted fever. However, the eschar is less frequently observed, and the evolution is milder.[2]
- *R. conorii* serotype Astrakhan, the causative agent for Astrakhan fever, is transmitted by *Rhipicephalus pumilio*. The disease, mainly observed in Astrakhan, is very similar to Mediterranean spotted fever, but the eschar is rarely observed, and the severity is mild.[2]
- *R. conorii* serotype Indian, the etiologic agent of Indian tick typhus, is transmitted by *R. sanguineus*. The disease has been described in India.[11] Clinical presentation is relatively similar to Mediterranean spotted fever and mild to moderate in severity; the eschar is rarely seen, and the rash is often purpuric.[11]

Rickettsia akari, the etiologic agent of rickettsialpox or smallpox rickettsia, is transmitted by *Allodermanyssus sanguineus*.[2] One week after a mite bite, a vesicle appears, then dries and leaves a black eschar (Figure 144-2). The typical presentation of a patient with rickettsialpox is fever, papular or vesicular rash, and eschar.[12] The rash does not involve the palms and soles; tender lymphadenopathy is commonly found on physical examination.[12,13]

Rickettsia africae, transmitted in sub-Saharan Africa and West Indies by *Amblyomma* ticks, causes African tick bite fever.[14] The disease is described mainly in people who hunted or traveled in a bushy area in southern Africa.[14] In a high proportion of cases, several inoculation eschars (Figure 144-3) can be seen; patients often have lymphadenitis in the regions that drain the eschars.[14] One week after the tick bite, 46% of patients develop fever, headache, myalgia, and a rash, which can be vesicular.[14] The evolution is much milder than Mediterranean spotted fever.[14]

Rickettsia parkeri infection, transmitted by *Amblyomma maculatum*, has been recently documented in the eastern coastal states of the United States.[15] Patients present approximately 1 week after a tick bite with fever, myalgia, malaise, headache, and a maculopapular eruption that may involve the palms or soles; an eschar can be found in the majority of cases.[15] *R. parkeri* infection seems to be a milder illness than RMSF.[15]

Rickettsia slovaca causes tickborne lymphadenopathy, also known as *TIBOLA*, a disease common in Europe and transmitted by

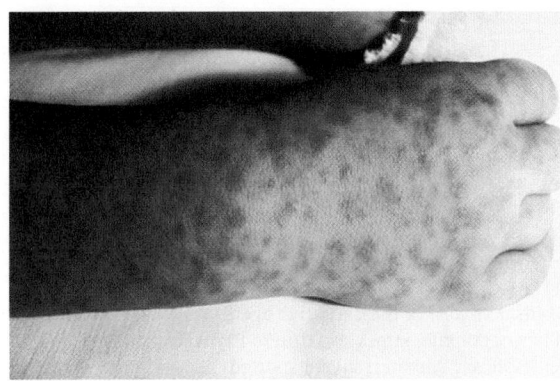

Figure 144-1 Child's right hand and wrist displaying the characteristic spotted rash of Rocky Mountain spotted fever. *(Courtesy Public Health Image Library, Centers for Disease Control and Prevention.)*

Dermacentor marginatus ticks during winter and early spring.[2,6,16-18] This disease is more prevalent in children and women; it is characterized by the presence of an eschar in the scalp and enlarged, tender, draining lymph nodes.[16,18] Fever and rash are rarely observed. Post-infectious asthenia and residual alopecia at the site of the tick bite have been reported.[16,18]

Rickettsia helvetica has been isolated from *Ixodes ricinus* ticks in many European and Asian countries.[19,20] The disease can be mild or self-limited with associated fever, headache, and myalgia, or it can have a more severe clinical presentation.[17,19-21] Cases of fever without rash or eschar have also been reported.[19]

Rickettsia aeschlimannii has been isolated from *Hyalomma marginatum* in Africa, Corsica, and Spain and is responsible for a disease similar to Mediterranean spotted fever.[22]

Rickettsia australis, the etiologic agent of Queensland tick typhus, is transmitted by *Ixodes holocyclus* in Australia.[2,23] Patients present with a rash (which can be vesicular), an inoculation eschar, and regional lymphadenopathy.[23] The evolution is mild.[23]

Rickettsia honei causes Flinders Island spotted fever, found in continental eastern Australia and probably in Thailand.[2,6,24] It is a febrile illness associated with an erythematous rash and headache; an eschar is found in 25% of patients, whereas regional adenopathy occurs in 55% of patients.[2,6] *R. honei* subsp. *marmionii*, or *R. marmionii*, has more recently been described to cause an acute febrile illness associated with headache, myalgia, arthralgia, cough, maculopapular or petechial rash, pharyngitis, eschar, and adjacent lymphadenopathy.[25,26] It has also been associated with chronic illness, but it is unclear whether the bacteria are responsible for any of the chronic symptoms or whether they are just a marker of increased immunosuppression.[26]

Rickettsia japonica causes Japanese or Oriental spotted fever, and it is transmitted by *Haemaphysalis longicornis* and *Dermacentor taiwanensis* in Japan and in eastern China.[27-29] Patients present with fever, headache, inoculation eschar, adjacent adenopathy, and a maculopapular rash.[2,6,30] Meningoencephalitis and even fulminant cases complicated by DIC and death have been reported.[27-31]

Rickettsia sibirica, the agent of Siberian tick typhus, is transmitted by *Dermacentor marginatus* and *Haemaphysalis concinna*.[4,32] The disease has been described in Siberia and China.[4] After 1 week of incubation, an ulcerated necrotic lesion appears at the inoculation site, often accompanied by regional lymphadenopathy.

Rickettsia mongolotimonae, related to *R. sibirica*, is transmitted by the *Hyalomma asiaticum* tick in Mongolia, sub-Saharan Africa, and southern Europe.[33-35] The main clinical manifestation is lymphangitis associated with an inoculation eschar and satellite lymphadenopathy.[33-35] Patients present with fever, severe headache, and a discrete rash.[33-36]

Rickettsia felis causes fleaborne spotted fever and is transmitted by the cat flea, *Ctenocephalides felis*; it has been documented worldwide.[4,21] The disease is characterized by fever, maculopapular rash, and headache.[37-39] Eschar and gastrointestinal and neurologic signs are not common.[39]

TYPHUS GROUP

Rickettsia typhi, the agent of murine typhus or endemic typhus, is transmitted through scratching contaminated pruritic lesions after rat flea bites.[2,40] Murine typhus has been diagnosed worldwide and is prevalent in tropical and subtropical seaboard regions.[41] After 1 to 2 weeks' incubation, the disease abruptly begins with fever, nausea, myalgias, arthralgias, and headache.[42-45] Gastrointestinal symptoms and a maculopapular rash that starts on the trunk, spreads peripherally, and spares the palms and soles develop later in the course of the disease.[42,45] A third of patients can develop respiratory symptoms.[4] Neurologic symptoms can be present, ranging from confusion and stupor to seizures and coma in severe forms.[4] Severe forms of disease are described in males of African descent with G6PD deficiency and in the elderly, especially when the diagnosis is delayed; such patients can present with central nervous system abnormalities, pulmonary compromise, as well as hepatic and renal dysfunction.[42,45] Splenic rupture has been reported with acute infection, patients presenting with acute abdomen.[46-48] Prognosis is usually favorable, with a low fatality rate.[45]

Rickettsia prowazekii, the etiologic agent of epidemic typhus or exanthematic typhus, is transmitted by the human body louse, *Pediculus humanus corporis* (Figure 144-4).[2,40,49] The human body louse lives in clothes and multiplies rapidly when cold weather and lack of hygiene allow (during war, in poor countries, and in the homeless population

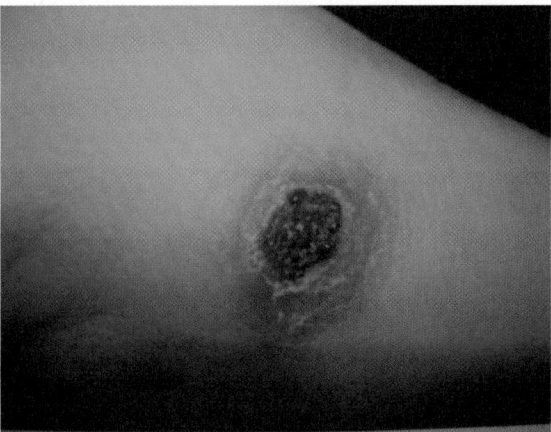

Figure 144-2 Rickettsialpox early lesion. *(Courtesy Dr. Daniel Caplivski, Division of Infectious Diseases, Mount Sinai School of Medicine.)*

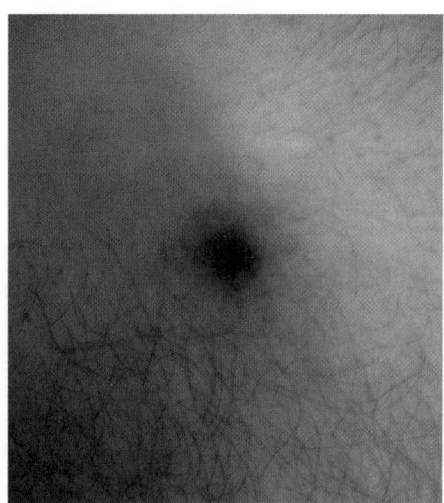

Figure 144-3 Eschar (tache noir) in a patient with *Rickettsia africae*. *(Courtesy Dr. Daniel Caplivski, Division of Infectious Diseases, Mount Sinai School of Medicine.)*

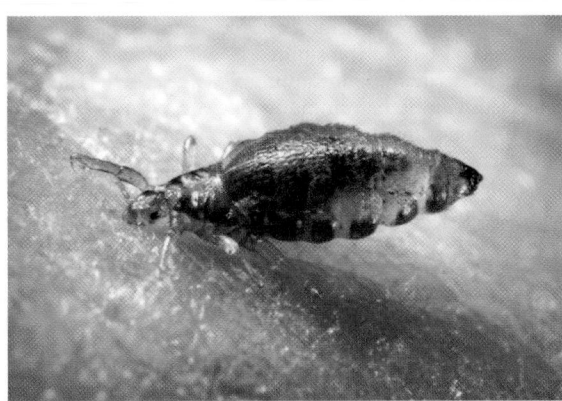

Figure 144-4 Body louse, *Pediculus humanus* var. *corporis*, as it was obtaining a blood-meal from a human host. *(Courtesy Public Health Image Library, Centers for Disease Control and Prevention).*

in developed countries).[40,49] This bacterium is a potential warfare agent and has been classified in category B of biological agents by the Centers for Disease Control and Prevention (CDC).[50] The disease begins abruptly with fever and headache.[51] The presence of myalgia, arthralgia, and constitutional symptoms are variable.[51] In more than one-third of patients, the rash can be macular, petechial, and even purpuric; the lesions are distributed mostly on the trunk and may spread centrifugally to involve the extremities; rarely, lesions are found on the soft palate and conjunctiva, but not on the face, palms, and soles; eschars are absent.[51] Neurologic involvement such as delirium, stupor, confusion, and even coma is common.[51] Brill-Zinsser disease, a milder form of typhus, is diagnosed during the convalescent period if the bacteria is not completely eradicated and infection persists subclinically.[51,52] It is frequently underdiagnosed because the rash as well as a history of recent exposure can be lacking.[51,52] The prognosis is good.

Orientia tsutsugamushi causes scrub typhus, or tsutsugamushi disease; it is transmitted by the bite of mite larvae.[40] The disease occurs in Japan, eastern Australia, eastern Russia, China, and the Indian subcontinent, mainly in autumn and spring.[53] Approximately 1 week after the bite, patients present with fever, headaches, and myalgias.[54] An eschar may be observed in 50% of patients and is often associated with adjacent lymphadenopathy.[54] The rash is macular, faint, and transient and can be missed.[4] Neurologic symptoms are relatively common and vary from confusion to delirium and coma.[54] Severe forms can progress to septic shock.[55] Relapses can occur and are less severe than the first episode.[55]

DIAGNOSIS

The leukocyte count can be within normal limits, but a leukopenia can be observed.[56] Thrombocytopenia can occur and may be marked in severe cases. Anemia can also be present, especially when hemolysis is observed (frequently in patients with G6PD deficiency).[56] Coagulopathy, with decrease in clotting factors (including fibrinogen) and prolonged coagulation times, may contribute to bleeding. C-reactive protein and hepatic enzyme levels can be increased.[56] Hyponatremia and hypocalcemia, as well as increased lactate dehydrogenase and creatine phosphokinase levels, usually reflect the severity of the disease and organ involvement.[56]

The diagnosis of rickettsioses is based on serology.[57] Rickettsial antibodies can be detected by several serologic tests which have different sensitivities and specificities: complement fixation,[58] indirect hemagglutination,[59] latex agglutination,[60] enzyme-linked immunosorbent assay (ELISA),[61] immunoperoxidase assay,[62] and immunofluorescence assay (IFA).[63] Not all serologic tests differentiate between immunoglobulins (ig)IgG and IgM or are specific enough for the diagnosis of different spotted fever–group *Rickettsiae*.[64] IFA is regarded as the gold standard for serologic diagnosis of rickettsial infections; its sensitivity and specificity are highest among the diagnostic methodologies, and

it is able to differentiate between IgG and IgM.[60,64-66] Two sera samples should be tested because the early serum is often negative. A cutoff value of 1/64 for total immunoglobulins and 1/32 for specific IgM is usually required for the diagnosis.[64] Cross-reactive antibodies have been observed with infections caused by *Ehrlichia*, *Bartonella*, *Legionella*, and *Proteus*. A cross-adsorption test is used to discriminate cross-reacting antibodies between two or more antigens, but the technique is limited by the large amount of antigen needed.[64] Western immunoblot assay is the most specific and sensitive serologic assay and is used for epidemiologic purposes and confirmation of serologic diagnoses obtained by conventional tests.[64]

In skin biopsies, preferably from petechial lesions and eschar, the bacteria can be detected before seroconversion occurs. Skin biopsies can also be used for retrospective diagnosis.[2,64] Immunofluorescence and immunoperoxidase techniques can be performed on frozen or fixed samples as well as on paraffin-embedded material.[64]

Skin biopsy specimens, peripheral white blood cells, or suspected arthropods may be used for polymerase chain reaction (PCR) diagnosis. PCR is a highly useful tool for the diagnosis of rickettsioses, but the sensitivity of the usual PCR amplification with clinical specimens seems to be variable.[67] In an effort to improve rickettsial DNA detection and to avoid false-positive results, a new technique called suicide PCR has been introduced that is more sensitive and specific than traditional methods.[67]

The isolation of rickettsiae can be performed from human samples (decanted plasma or skin biopsies, ideally from the eschar) and from arthropods.[64] Culture is restricted to specialized laboratories with biohazard and cell culture facilities. Usually, culture of rickettsiae takes 3 to 7 days.[64] This technique is fundamental for the identification of new rickettsial pathogens.

TREATMENT

Doxycycline is the treatment of choice for rickettsioses.[68] It can be prescribed in adults and children,[69] but not in pregnant women and patients with allergy to tetracycline or related antibiotics. The fever typically subsides within 1 or 2 days after treatment is started; clinical improvement might be slower in complicated cases or critically ill patients, especially if they have multiple organ dysfunction.[70] The treatment should be given orally, except in patients with gastric intolerance or coma, for whom it should be administered intravenously (IV).[4] A single treatment of 200 mg of doxycycline in one day is sufficient for most of the rickettsioses (but not RMSF).[4] For RMSF, scrub typhus, or the severe form of spotted fever, treatment duration is usually longer, and the recommendation is to continue doxycycline, 100 mg twice daily for 2 to 3 days after the patient becomes afebrile and until evidence of clinical improvement is noted, usually at least 7 days.[4,70] The pediatric dose of doxycycline is 2.2 mg/kg body weight per dose administered twice daily (orally or IV) for children weighing less than 100 lbs (45.4 kg).[70] *R. akari* and *R. prowazekii* infections are treated with doxycycline, 200 mg daily for 7 days, or with chloramphenicol as alternative treatment.[4] Chloramphenicol, 50-75 mg/kg/d for 10 days, is the only available alternative to doxycycline in pregnant women and allergic patients.[68] Chloramphenicol is available only in an IV form in the United States. Erythromycin has been used with success for murine typhus in several cases.[44,71] Rifampin (600-900 mg daily) and azithromycin (500 mg daily) are alternative treatment for scrub typhus and can also be prescribed during pregnancy.[72]

Severely ill patients must be treated in intensive care units (ICUs). Fluid administration should be carefully monitored. Anemia and coagulation abnormalities should be corrected. Mechanical ventilation can be required in cases of respiratory distress. Hemodialysis may be required in patients with renal insufficiency. Antiepileptic drugs should be given to treat seizures. In cases of gangrene, amputation is sometimes necessary. Glucocorticoids have not proven beneficial.[73]

There is no current vaccination for rickettsial diseases, and prevention is based on the avoidance of tick, flea, and body lice bites.[4] Lice are fragile, so changing and boiling clothes is effective. Repellents and/

or protective garments can also be used. After possible exposure, ticks can be removed by forceps followed by skin disinfection.[4]

Ehrlichioses

Human monocytic ehrlichiosis (HME) is caused by *Ehrlichia chaffeensis*, which is transmitted by *Amblyomma americanum*, the Lone Star tick, and possibly by other ticks.[74,75] This disease has only been described in the United States, mainly in rural and suburban areas, from April to September.[40,76] After spreading through lymphatics and blood vessels, the bacteria can be observed in the macrophages and monocytes (Figure 144-5).[77,78] The clinical picture of HME varies from mild to severe in immunocompetent patients, whereas in immunocompromised patients the disease tends to be more severe.[79-83] After 1 week incubation, patients present with fever, chills, headache, myalgia, and malaise.[79-83] Respiratory and gastrointestinal symptoms are present less frequently.[79-83] The rash is observed in approximately a third of adults and in up to 66% of children.[74,80,81] The rash involves the extremities, trunk, face and (rarely) the palms and soles; it typically occurs later in the course of disease and can be maculopapular, petechial, or diffusely erythematous.[84-86] Severe complications that require ICU admission include acute lung injury with severe hypoxemia, seizures, meningoencephalitis, coagulopathy, acute renal insufficiency, myocardial failure, septic shock, and coma.[79-83] The prognosis of HME depends on age, immune status, and early antibiotic treatment.[4,79-83]

Human granulocytic ehrlichiosis (HGE) is due to *Anaplasma phagocytophila*, which is transmitted by *Ixodes scapularis* ticks in New England and the North Central United States and by the western blacklegged tick, *Ixodes pacificus*, in northern California.[40,56,74,76] The disease is observed in the United States and Europe from spring to fall. In the United States, the geographical distribution overlaps with that of Lyme disease and babesiosis because of the shared *Ixodes* tick vector[74]; up to 36% of patients with positive serology for *A. phagocytophila* also have positive serology for *Borrelia burgdorferi* (Lyme disease) or *Babesia microti* (babesiosis).[87,88] After a 5- to 21-day incubation period, patients develop nonspecific manifestations including fever, chills, headache, and myalgias.[89-92] Rash is rarely observed in HGE in comparison to HME.[74,93] Most cases are mild, even self-limited, but serious manifestations with fatal outcome have been described.[79,94] Severe cases have been described in the elderly, patients on immunosuppressive therapy, and those with chronic inflammatory illnesses or underlying malignancy.[79,92,94]

Canine granulocytic ehrlichiosis (CGE) is due to *Ehrlichia ewingii*, an uncultured bacterium transmitted by *Amblyomma americanum*.[74] The disease occurs in immunocompromised hosts in the United States, those infected with human immunodeficiency virus (HIV), or those receiving immunosuppressive drugs.[74,82] Patients present with fever, chills, headache, myalgia, and arthralgia.[56,76] Rash is rare in patients with *E. ewingii* infection; however, it is more common in children.[74,93]

Canine monocytic ehrlichiosis is caused by *Ehrlichia canis*, which is transmitted by *R. sanguineus*. In 1996, a single case of infection was reported in an asymptomatic man from Venezuela who owned an infected dog.[95] In 1991, an immunohistology examination identified an organism antigenically related to *E. canis* in tissues from a patient who died of ehrlichiosis.[77] This pathogen should be considered a potential etiologic agent in compatible human illness in endemic areas.

Sennetsu neoehrlichiosis is due to *Neorickettsia sennetsu*. In 1953, one case was described in Japan. The bacterium was isolated from the blood, bone marrow, and lymph node of a 25-year-old man who had a mononucleosis-like disease with fever, headaches, myalgia, and anorexia.[96] Sennetsu neorickettsiosis is probably underdiagnosed in southeastern Asia, as shown by the high seroprevalence in febrile patients (14%-15%) and healthy persons (17%) in Laos and in febrile patients (3%) in Thailand.[97]

Panola Mountain *Ehrlichia* and *Ehrlichia ruminantium* have recently been associated with human infections.[98,99]

DIAGNOSIS

Leukopenia (up to 53% of cases), thrombocytopenia (up to 94% of cases), and mildly elevated hepatic enzymes are described in ehrlichioses.[74,76] Diagnosis by identification of morulae (intracellular inclusion formed by clusters of bacteria) is the most rapid diagnostic method during the first week of infection, but such inclusions are rarely seen in neutrophils of patients with HGE and CGE and are even less frequent in monocytes and macrophages of patients with HME (see Figure 144-5).[92] Indirect immunofluorescence antibody assay is a more sensitive diagnosis and is based on acute and convalescent serologic examination, with a fourfold rise in specific antibody titers being diagnostic.[76,92,100,101] High titers (≥640) by indirect fluorescence antibody assay are also diagnostic for recent infection.[101] Cross-reactivity among various species prevents definitive identification of the etiologic agent only by serology. Rapid detection and identification of *Ehrlichia* spp. by PCR amplification may also be performed on blood samples.[101] This test is available from the CDC, state health laboratories, and research and commercial laboratories.[74]

TREATMENT

Antibiotic therapy should be started if ehrlichiosis infection is suspected, before laboratory diagnosis has been confirmed.

The dosage (orally or IV) for doxycycline is 100 mg twice daily for adults and 2.2 mg/kg body weight per dose twice daily for children weighing less than 100 lbs. (45.4 kg).[74] The fever usually subsides within 1 to 2 days after treatment initiation; patients with more severe illness might require a longer time before clinical improvement is noted.[74] The optimal duration of therapy is unclear, but it is currently recommended to treat HME for at least 3 days after fever resolution and until evidence of clinical improvement, which is usually for 5 to 7 days.[74] Severe or complicated cases might require longer treatment courses.[74] Patients with HGA should be treated with doxycycline for 10 to 14 days to provide appropriate length of therapy for possible co-infection with *Borrelia burdogferii*.[74,92] Chloramphenicol may not be effective for ehrlichioses.[74] Patients with mild illness due to HGA who cannot take doxycycline because of drug allergy or pregnancy can be treated with rifampin for 7 to 10 days (300 mg twice daily for adults and 10 mg/kg twice daily for children, to a maximum 300 mg per dose). Patients co-infected with *Borrelia burgdorferi* should also be treated with amoxicillin or cefuroxime.[92] Persistence of fever for more than 2 days after initiation of doxycycline suggests the need to look for

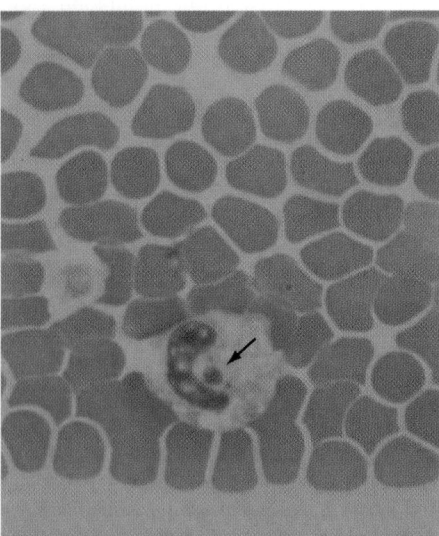

Figure 144-5   White blood cells infected with the agent of human granulocytic ehrlichiosis (*Anaplasma phagocytophila*). (Courtesy Dr. Daniel Caplivski, Division of Infectious Diseases, Mount Sinai School of Medicine.)

an alternative diagnosis or that the patient is co-infected with *Babesia microti*.[92] Prevention relies on limiting exposure to tick habitats, inspection of the body for ticks after being in areas potentially infested, and removing attached ticks immediately.[74] For patients who have had recent tick bites but are not ill, preventive antibiotic therapy for rickettsial infection is not indicated.[74]

Q Fever

Q fever is caused by *Coxiella burnetii* and occurs worldwide except in New Zealand; humans are incidental hosts, developing an acute or chronic infection.[102] The reservoir of this bacterium includes mammals, birds, and ticks.[102] Humans are usually infected by aerosol from amniotic fluid, placenta, contaminated wool, or less frequently, by milk products.[103] *C. burnetii* is a potential warfare agent and classified in category B of biological agents by the CDC.[50] *C. burnetii* is a strict intracellular bacterium that has characteristic antigenic variations (called *phase variation*).[104] After exposure to contaminated aerosols or products, up to 60% of patients develop asymptomatic infection diagnosed by seroconversion; 38% of cases will have self-limited disease, and only 2% necessitate hospitalization and diagnostic workup; about 0.5% of patients develop chronic Q fever.[103,105,106]

Patients with acute Q fever may present with a variety of symptoms that include flulike illness, pneumonia (mainly in elderly or immunocompromised patients), or acute hepatitis (mainly in younger patients).[105,106] Complications associated with acute Q fever are rare and may include aseptic lymphocytic meningitis, encephalitis, encephalomyelitis, polyradiculopathy, seizures, pericarditis, myocarditis with congestive heart failure, and respiratory failure with acute respiratory distress syndrome.[105] Patients infrequently present with cutaneous manifestations such as maculopapular or purpuric rash and erythema nodosum.[105] Less common manifestations of acute Q fever include hemolytic anemia, thyroiditis, gastroenteritis, pancreatitis, lymphadenopathy, splenic rupture, proliferative glomerulonephritis, orchitis, and epididymitis.[105] Post–Q fever chronic fatigue syndrome has also been described, and in England has been characterized by fatigue, sweats, and dyspnea on effort, while in Australia it is characterized by painful lymphadenopathy, myalgia, and arthralgia.[105,107,108] In pregnant women with or without symptoms, Q fever compromises the pregnancy and can be responsible for abortion, oligoamnios, fetal death, or prematurity.[109]

Pregnant women, patients with cardiac abnormalities, and immunocompromised patients are at risk to progress to chronic infection.[104,105,109] *Chronic Q fever* is defined as an infection that persists more than 6 months, with recurrent fever being the most common manifestation.[105] Aneurysm or prosthetic valve infections carry a poor prognosis.[105] Patients with Q fever endocarditis have chronic low-grade fever, progressive deterioration of valve function, and progressive heart failure; vegetations are rarely observed on echocardiography.[105] If not diagnosed, the disease progressively worsens, and complications include cerebral emboli, hepatosplenomegaly, and glomerulonephritis.[103,105] Cases of chronic osteomyelitis and cirrhosis have been also reported.[105]

DIAGNOSIS

Thrombocytopenia, leucopenia, abnormal liver function tests, and elevated sedimentation rate are frequently reported.[103,105] Immunologic abnormalities including elevated cryoglobulins, rheumatoid factor, anticardiolipin, and antiphospholipid antibodies may be observed, especially during chronic infection.[105] Diagnosis is primarily based on serology, with the most commonly used method being the IFA with the test of phase I and phase II antigens.[103] Patients seroconvert 14 days after development of symptoms.[105,110] Acute Q fever is diagnosed when IgM phase II antigen titers are ≥50, IgG phase II antigen titers are ≥200, seroconversion occurs, or a fourfold increase of phase II antigen can be documented.[103,105] Chronic Q fever is diagnosed when IgG to phase I antigens titer is at least 800 or IgA to phase I antigens titer is ≥ 100.[105] Serology is also useful for following the clinical course of patients with acute infection and underlying disease and in those with chronic Q

fever undergoing treatment.[4] The other diagnostic tools are direct detection by cell culture performed in a specialized laboratory with biohazard facilities, PCR, or immunochemistry of the involved tissue (cardiac valve, liver, or blood samples).[103] Liver or lymph node biopsy shows nonspecific granulomas characterized by a vacuole containing the bacteria and surrounded by a fibrinoid ring.[103,105,110]

TREATMENT

Acute Q fever can be a self-limited disease, and only symptomatic patients warrant treatment.[102] In a randomized trial, tetracycline was proven to shorten fever duration.[111] No clinical trials have been performed to determine the adequate length of therapy for acute Q fever; however, it is recommended to prescribe doxycycline (200 mg/d) for 3 weeks or 1 week after fever resolution.[103,105] In cases with central nervous system involvement, fluoroquinolones are the drugs of choice.[105,111] The new macrolides look promising for treatment of Q fever, but clinical data are limited.[112-115] In patients with a valvular abnormality, it is recommended to treat acute Q fever with doxycycline (200 mg/d) and hydroxychloroquine (600 mg/d) for 12 months.[116] In patients with *Coxiella* endocarditis, the recommended treatment is doxycycline (200 mg/d) and hydroxychloroquine (600 mg/d) for at least 18 months; IgG and IgA to phase I antigens titers should be monitored to assess the response to treatment, especially during the first year.[103,105] In patients with Q fever hepatitis with slow regression of symptoms, clinical benefit has been described with the addition of prednisone to the antibiotic therapy; prednisone could be considered in patients who do not become afebrile after 3 days of antibiotic therapy and should be started at 40 mg for 48 hours, then tapered to 20 mg for 48 hours, and then 10 mg for an additional 48 hours.[103] In pregnant women, cotrimoxazole (sulfamethoxazole 1600/trimethoprim 320 mg/d) should be started and continued throughout the pregnancy to decrease the risk of infection of the placenta and obstetric complications.[105,109] A vaccine is available in Australia.[117] Prevention of Q fever is based on veterinary control of the disease in animals.[105]

KEY POINTS

1. Three families of diseases are grouped under the name *rickettsial diseases*: diseases caused by bacteria belonging to the *Rickettsia* genus, ehrlichioses, and Q fever.

2. The *Rickettsia* genus is divided into the spotted fever group, which comprises about 15 different species of human pathogens, and the typhus group.

3. The spotted fever group causes arthropod-borne diseases.

4. The main symptoms that may be observed during spotted fever rickettsial diseases include fever, a rash, headache, an inoculation black eschar at the site of the arthropod bite, and lymphadenopathy.

5. Human monocytic ehrlichiosis (HME) has only been described in the United States.

6. Human granulocytic ehrlichiosis (HGE) is observed in the United States and Europe.

7. The onset of ehrlichiosis, especially HME, can be rapid and potentially fatal. Antibiotic therapy should be started if ehrlichiosis infection is suspected, before laboratory diagnosis has been confirmed.

8. *Coxiella burnetii*, the agent of Q fever, can cause acute and chronic disease. An acute primary infection may be followed by a chronic disease in the presence of predisposing factors, such as cardiac valve damage or immunocompromised state.

9. The diagnosis of rickettsial diseases is based on serology, although polymerase chain reaction (PCR) can also be helpful.

10. Doxycycline is the treatment of choice for rickettsial diseases. It could be prescribed in adults and in children but not in pregnant women and allergic patients.

ANNOTATED REFERENCES

Chapman AS, Bakken JS, Folk SM, Paddock CD, Bloch KC, Krusell A, et al, Tickborne Rickettsial Diseases Working Group, CDC. Diagnosis and management of tickborne rickettsial diseases: Rocky Mountain spotted fever, ehrlichioses, and anaplasmosis—United States: a practical guide for physicians and other health-care and public health professionals. MMWR Recomm Rep 2006;55:1-27
This report will assist clinicians in recognizing epidemiologic features and clinical manifestations of tickborne rickettsial diseases; developing a differential diagnosis; understanding that doxycycline is the treatment of choice for both adults and children and that early empirical antibiotic therapy can prevent severe morbidity and death; and reporting suspected or confirmed cases to local public health authorities to assist them with control measures and public health education efforts.

Wormser GP, Dattwyler RJ, Shapiro ED, Halperin JJ, Steere AC, Klempner MS, et al. The clinical assessment, treatment, and prevention of Lyme disease, human granulocytic anaplasmosis, and babesiosis: clinical practice guidelines by the Infectious Diseases Society of America. Clin Infect Dis 2006;43:1089-134.
This article presents updated evidence-based guidelines for the management of human granulocytic anaplasmosis.

Schutze GE, Buckingham SC, Marshall GS, Woods CR, Jackson MA, Patterson LE, et al, Tick-borne Infections in Children Study (TICS) Group. Human monocytic ehrlichiosis in children. Pediatr Infect Dis J 2007;26:475-9.
This study allows clinicians to better understand the epidemiology and natural history, clinical manifestations, role of therapy, prognostic indicators for outcome, and the long-term progression of ehrlichiosis.

Paddock CD, Finley RW, Wright CS, Robinson HN, Schrodt BJ, Lane CC, et al. *Rickettsia parkeri* rickettsiosis and its clinical distinction from Rocky Mountain spotted fever. Clin Infect Dis 2008;4:1188-96.
This article summarizes the clinical and epidemiologic features of infections with R. parkeri, a recently identified spotted fever in the United States, and comments on distinctions between R. parkeri rickettsiosis and other U.S. rickettsioses.

Mandell GL, Bennett JE, Dolin R, editors. Mandell, Douglas, and Bennett's principles and practice of infectious diseases. 7th ed. Philadelphia: Churchill Livingstone; 2009. p. 2495-538.
This is the reference book for infectious diseases specialists; it has a more comprehensive review of all diseases described in this chapter.

REFERENCES

Access the complete reference list online at http://www.expertconsult.com.

145

Acute Viral Syndromes

YOSHIRO HAYASHI I DAVID L. PATERSON

Acute infections with viruses produce a variety of clinical manifestations with a wide spectrum of clinical severity. Viral upper respiratory tract infections in immunocompetent hosts are usually trivial, although they may be life threatening and associated with subsequent lower respiratory tract infection and disseminated disease in immunocompromised hosts. Viral infections can affect virtually every organ system of the body.

Vesicular Rash

POXVIRUSES INCLUDING SMALLPOX AND MONKEYPOX

Poxviruses are double-stranded DNA viruses that are relevant because of concerns regarding possible bioterrorism with smallpox.[1,2] Additionally, outbreaks of monkeypox infection in humans have been detected, albeit rarely.[3] The poxviruses and their major clinical manifestations are listed in Table 145-1. In general, a common feature of poxviruses is that they cause vesicular skin eruptions.

Smallpox

The last case of endemic smallpox occurred in Somalia in 1977, and eradication of the disease was declared in 1980.[4] The virus (variola) has been maintained in some laboratories—the last known case of laboratory-acquired smallpox occurred in the United Kingdom in 1978. In part as a result of this accident, the number of laboratories that retained the virus was reduced from 76 to just 2. These laboratories are at the Centers for Disease Control and Prevention (CDC) in Atlanta in the United States and the Vektor Institute in Novosibirsk, Russia. It is not known if all other laboratories destroyed their stocks of virus—therefore, the potential exists for a deliberate release of variola as an act of bioterrorism.[1,5]

The incubation period for smallpox is 7 to 17 days (mean 10-12).[4] A prodromal phase which consists of abrupt onset of severe headache, backache, and fever occurs. The fever often reaches 40°C, but then subsides. The rash then begins; initial lesions are small, red macules, which over 2 to 3 days become macular then vesicular. The lesions commence on the face and extremities, then cover the entire body including palms and soles of feet. The lesions subsequently may umbilicate and crust.

The rash of smallpox could be confused with monkeypox, generalized vaccinia and eczema vaccinatum, chickenpox, coxsackievirus infection, herpes simplex virus (HSV) infection (especially eczema herpeticum), rickettsialpox, insect bites, drug eruptions, and acne. A classic feature of smallpox is that the lesions are all at the same stage of development. In contrast, with chickenpox, individual lesions are present at different stages. With chickenpox, fever occurs with the onset of the rash.

It is well known that smallpox is associated with significant mortality; however it is not clear what the likelihood of mortality would be in patients who receive good supportive care, such as exists in modern intensive care units (ICUs). There are many reasons for the mortality associated with smallpox. Substantial amounts of fluid and protein can be lost by febrile persons with numerous weeping lesions. In some patients, death may occur before the appearance of any rash, since this prodromal period is associated with significant viremia. A hemorrhagic form of smallpox also is associated with high mortality.[4] Encephalitis occurs in fewer than 1% of patients infected. Secondary

bacterial infections of the skin lesions may occur and are heralded by a second temperature spike.[4] Although cough is not usually a prominent symptom of smallpox, secondary bacterial pneumonia may occur, particularly in patients with severe disease.

The CDC recommends an algorithmic approach to the diagnosis of smallpox (this is described in detail at http://www.bt.cdc.gov/agent/smallpox). Patients can be subdivided into low-risk, moderate-risk, and high-risk groups depending on a variety of variables (Boxes 145-1 and 145-2). Patients at low or moderate risk for smallpox should undergo polymerase chain reaction (PCR) testing of the skin lesion for varicella-zoster virus (VZV) infection, HSV, plus enterovirus. Patients at moderate risk should undergo consultation by infectious diseases or dermatology specialists. Electron microscopy should be performed if PCR for these viruses is negative. If rapid testing for VZV and HSV is negative for a moderate-risk patient, the adequacy of specimen collection should be confirmed. If there is ongoing clinical suspicion for smallpox, local and state health departments should be consulted. For patients at high risk for smallpox, all testing should be performed at the CDC. This testing should include variola real-time PCR, *Orthopoxvirus* real-time PCR, and nonvariola *Orthopoxvirus* real-time PCR, in addition to tests for VZV, HSV, and enteroviruses.

There is no approved treatment for smallpox.[4] Prevention of secondary cases is crucial. A suspected case of smallpox should be managed in a negative-pressure room. Additionally, strict respiratory and contact isolation is essential (detailed instructions are available at http://www.bt.cdc.gov/agent/smallpox).[4]

Vaccinia

Vaccinia is the poxvirus used in smallpox immunization. Primary vaccination results in a vesicle at the site of vaccination, usually within 3 to 5 days. This vesicle becomes pustular or is surrounded by induration or congestion 6 to 8 days after vaccination. Rarely, a generalized rash characterized by multiple small, vesicular lesions occurs. Occasionally, severe complications result from smallpox vaccination. If vaccinia is administered to a person with an immunologic deficiency, progressive necrosis at the site of vaccination may occur (vaccinia necrosum). Secondarily, lesions may spread to other parts of the body. Such cases may be fatal. Patients with eczema may develop dissemination of vaccinia virus in the abnormal skin, leading to a generalized rash (eczema vaccinatum or Kaposi varicelliform eruption). Vaccinia immunoglobulin (0.6 mL/kg every 24 hours) can be prescribed for disseminated infection.

Encephalitis due to vaccinia may occur 1 to 2 weeks after vaccination and is associated with a mortality of 10% to 30%. Myocardial infarction, pericarditis, myocarditis, and dilated cardiomyopathy have been observed after smallpox vaccination. In 2003, 37,901 potential bioterrorism first responders received smallpox vaccine in the United States. There were 822 reports of adverse events; 100 of 822 were serious, resulting in 85 hospitalizations, 2 permanent disabilities, 10 life-threatening illnesses, and 3 deaths. Among the 100 serious adverse events, 21 cases were myocarditis and/or pericarditis, 10 cases were ischemic cardiac events, 2 cases were generalized vaccinia, and 1 case was postvaccinial encephalitis. Serious adverse events were more common among older revaccinees than in younger first-time recipients.[6]

From December 2002 to January 2004, the U.S. Department of Defense vaccinated 578,286 military personnel with vaccinia.[6] Thirty

TABLE 145-1	Common Clinical Manifestations of Poxviruses
Virus	**Clinical Manifestations**
Variola (smallpox)	Diffuse vesicular rash; systemic disease
Monkeypox	Vesicular rash
Vaccinia (cowpox)	Vesicular rash; postinfectious encephalitis
Parapoxvirus	Orf (localized vesicular lesion)
Molluscipoxvirus	Molluscum contagiosum
Tanapox virus	Vesicular rash

cases of suspected contact transfer of vaccinia were reported.[6] *Contact transfer* is the spread of vaccinia from a recipient of the smallpox vaccine to another person. This spread occurs because the live virus used in the vaccine is present on the skin at the site of the vaccination. Spread of the virus to other parts of the body (autoinoculation) also can occur via the same mechanism. No cases of vaccinia necrosum or eczema vaccinatum were observed in the people with contact transfer of the virus.

Monkeypox

Monkeypox was first recognized in 1958 as a disease of primates. The disease subsequently was recognized in rodents. Beginning in 1970, cases in humans were reported in central Africa.[7] In 2003, cases occurred in the United States in residents of the Midwest who had contact with imported prairie dogs.[3] Patients developed vesicular skin lesions and fever/sweats. Although case-fatality rates of 4% to 22% have been observed in outbreaks of the infection in Africa, none of the 11 patients in the American outbreak died.[3]

HERPESVIRUSES

HSV, VZV, and herpes B virus all are capable of causing vesicular skin rash and other systemic manifestations of disease. The herpesviruses are large, enveloped DNA viruses that exhibit lifelong latent infection.[8,9] The eight known human herpesviruses are HSV types 1 and 2; VZV; cytomegalovirus (CMV); human herpesvirus (HHV) types 6, 7, and 8; and Epstein-Barr virus (EBV).

Herpes Simplex Virus

HSV infections are found worldwide. Characteristically, HSV-1 is associated with orolabial disease, and HSV-2 is associated with genital infection, although this is not a rigid distinction. Primary infections (first infections with HSV-1 or HSV-2) are usually associated with mucosal lesions and systemic signs and symptoms. Mucosal and cutaneous lesions are vesicular and usually localized, although disseminated infection may occur rarely. Patients with atopic eczema or severe burns may develop extensive infections.

Primary HSV infection may have severe complications. Aseptic meningitis may occur and is more common with HSV-2. Meningeal symptoms usually start 3 to 12 days after the onset of genital lesions. Transverse myelitis and autonomic nervous system dysfunction also may occur in conjunction with primary genital HSV infection. HSV encephalitis in adults usually is not associated with primary infection. Potentially, reactivation of latent HSV-1 infection in trigeminal or autonomic nerve roots may be associated with extension of virus into the central nervous system (CNS) via the enervation of the middle cranial fossa. Occasionally, patients with primary HSV infection develop hepatitis, pneumonia, or thrombocytopenia.

By virtue of the establishment of latency, HSV-1 or HSV-2 may reactivate. HSV reactivations may be less severe than primary infections. In immunocompromised hosts, however, reactivation of HSV-1 or HSV-2 may be associated with disseminated infection or severe local esophagitis, hepatitis, or pneumonia. Neonatal herpes, occurring in an infant of a mother with primary or reactivation infection at the time of delivery, carries a high risk of disseminated fatal infection.

HSV-1 encephalitis is frequently seen in the ICU and is characterized by confusion or coma accompanied by a cerebrospinal fluid (CSF) lymphocytosis. Magnetic resonance imaging (MRI) of the brain may show temporal lobe lesions. Testing of CSF by PCR for HSV-1 is typically positive.

Diagnosis of HSV-1 or HSV-2 infection causing a vesicular skin lesion can be suspected clinically by the presence of multiple vesicular lesions on an erythematous base, occurring in the orolabial or anogenital areas. A precise diagnosis can be established easily by use of PCR on scrapings from lesions. Results can be available within hours of specimen collection.

Varicella-Zoster Virus

Primary VZV infection causes chickenpox, whereas reactivation infection causes shingles (zoster). Chickenpox is characterized by multiple vesicular lesions, whereas shingles is characterized by a unilateral vesicular eruption with a dermatomal distribution. Immunocompromised patients with shingles may develop disseminated cutaneous infection that may resemble chickenpox.

Chickenpox usually is associated with fever, constitutional symptoms, and a vesicular skin rash. Most skin lesions are small vesicular lesions with an erythematous base. Successive crops of lesions occur over 2 to 4 days, so lesions at all stages from fresh vesicles to crusted lesions are present simultaneously.

Secondary bacterial infection of vesicular lesions is relatively common, with infection involving *Staphylococcus aureus* and *Streptococcus pyogenes* being most common. One manifestation of secondary bacterial infection is the occurrence of fever after the fever associated with onset of chickenpox has subsided. Severe infection with toxic shock syndrome may result.[10,11]

Box 145-1

CRITERIA FOR THE SUSPICION OF SMALLPOX IN PATIENTS WITH ACUTE GENERALIZED VESICULAR OR PUSTULAR RASH

Major Smallpox Criteria
Febrile prodrome:
>101°F, 1-4 days before rash onset
With headache, backache, or abdominal pain
Firm, deep-seated, well-circumscribed vesicles/pustules
Lesions in the same stage of development in any one area of the body

Minor Smallpox Criteria
Centrifugal distribution
First lesions in the pharynx, oral mucosa
Patient appears "toxic"
Slow evolution of the rash:
1-2 days each stage: macule, papule, vesicle
Lesions on palms and soles

Box 145-2

CATEGORIZATION OF RISK OF SMALLPOX FROM CLINICAL CRITERIA*

High Risk of Smallpox
Febrile prodrome *and*
Classic smallpox lesion *and*
Lesions in the same stage of development

Moderate Risk of Smallpox
Febrile prodrome *and* one other *major* smallpox criterion *or*
Febrile prodrome *and* four or more minor smallpox criteria

Low Risk of Smallpox
No febrile prodrome *or*
Febrile prodrome *and* fewer than four minor smallpox criteria

*The major and minor criteria are listed in Box 145-1.

Chickenpox is associated with pneumonia in 1 in 400 cases of infection.[12,13] A larger proportion of people may have some pulmonary involvement, but it is typically asymptomatic. Pregnant women and immunocompromised patients are at high risk of life-threatening pneumonia. Chickenpox pneumonia is generally manifested by cough and shortness of breath 3 to 5 days after the onset of the rash. Chest radiography typically shows a reticulonodular infiltrate. Respiratory failure may occur.

Neurologic complications of chickenpox include encephalitis, acute cerebellar ataxia (one in about 4,000 cases),[14] and cerebral angiitis. Encephalitis due to VZV is less common than pneumonia but nevertheless may be life threatening. The typical manifestation is onset of headaches followed by depression in level of consciousness occurring in an adult within 2 weeks of chickenpox. Acute cerebellar ataxia is more common in children 1 to 3 weeks after the onset of chickenpox. Ataxia and slurred speech may occur, but usually with complete resolution.

As with HSV infections, the rash of chickenpox or shingles can usually be diagnosed confidently on clinical grounds or confirmed by PCR of scrapings of a skin lesion. PCR can also be performed on CSF to diagnose VZV encephalitis.[14]

Herpes B Virus (Cercopithecine herpesvirus 1)

Herpes B virus (*Cercopithecine herpesvirus* 1) infection is a relatively benign disease of monkeys. However, herpes B virus infection of humans, usually occurring from monkey bites or scratches, is a severe and potentially fatal disease. Monkeys of the *Macaca* genus (rhesus and cynomolgus monkeys) are considered highest risk. An incubation period of 2 to 14 days usually is observed after the bite or scratch. Initial symptoms are nonspecific but include fever, malaise, and headache. A cluster of small vesicles may occur at the bite site. A severe encephalomyelitis may ensue, with death occurring in days. In the United States, only one reference laboratory is equipped to identify the virus. Prompt and exhaustive cleaning of wounds, followed by early initiation of acyclovir or valacyclovir, may prevent the occurrence of severe disease. Additional information with contacts is available at http://www.cdc.gov/niosh/docs/99-100/.[15,16]

Fever in Immunocompromised Patients

Numerous viruses can cause fever as a presenting symptom. In the absence of specific manifestations such as pneumonia or encephalitis, viral infections are rarely life threatening. The onset of fever in immunocompromised individuals may, however, be the harbinger of severe overwhelming viral infection.

CYTOMEGALOVIRUS

CMV infection is a classic cause of severe infection in immunocompromised hosts, especially transplant recipients and patients with human immunodeficiency virus (HIV) infection.[17-19] Infection can be primary or due to reactivation. The risk of end-organ CMV infection depends on the degree of immunosuppression and whether infection is primary or reactivation. For solid-organ transplant recipients, there is a significant risk of primary infection in patients who were seronegative for CMV before transplantation and received an organ from a seropositive donor.[17,19]

The organs commonly affected by CMV infection include the esophagus, colon, retina, and lungs. Virtually any organ can be infected, however, including the CNS. Some patients present with a syndrome of fever, malaise, and hematologic abnormalities, without specific end-organ abnormalities.

Given the high risk of CMV infection in solid-organ transplant recipients, strategies should be employed to prevent CMV infection.[17,20,21] Two options are prophylaxis or preemptive therapy. *Prophylaxis* implies the administration of preventive therapy to all persons at risk.[17] In contrast, *preemptive* therapy is the administration of antiviral therapy only to persons at highest risk, as determined by a positive result on a regularly monitored blood test for CMV infection.[17] Such therapy is given even if the patient is asymptomatic. Detection of CMV by PCR is used most often for early detection of CMV infection.

EPSTEIN-BARR VIRUS

Primary EBV infection may be associated with fever, malaise, and hematologic abnormalities in immunocompromised patients (and also in some immunocompetent individuals). EBV infection can be associated with development of malignancies such as posttransplant lymphoproliferative disorder.[22-24] In some transplant populations, regular quantitative monitoring of EBV in peripheral blood by PCR is performed to determine the risk of significant EBV infection.[25]

HUMAN HERPESVIRUS 6

HHV-6 is a ubiquitous viral infection that usually occurs in infancy. Primary HHV-6 infection and possibly reactivation infection in immunocompromised patients can be associated with serious disease.[26,27] HHV-6 seems to have neurotropism—in addition to fever, HHV-6 infection may be associated with confusion, coma, and seizures.[28,29] Occasionally, CSF examination is normal apart from increased protein and the finding of HHV-6 by PCR.

HUMAN HERPESVIRUS 8

HHV-8 is associated with Kaposi sarcoma, primary effusion lymphoma, and Castleman syndrome.[30,31] It may be transmitted via the organ allograft in solid-organ transplantation. Primary infection in immunosuppressed patients may be associated with high fever, thrombocytopenia and other severe cytopenias, and mental state abnormalities.[32] Detection of HHV-8 by PCR in whole blood can establish the diagnosis.

WEST NILE VIRUS

In the 1990s, West Nile virus infection was detected in North America for the first time.[33,34] Although many cases of infection were directly from the vector of infection (mosquitoes), other cases were via blood transfusion or organ allograft.[35,36] West Nile virus exhibits neurotropism; infected patients may have confusion and headache in addition to fever and other more general symptoms.

ADENOVIRUS

Adenoviruses have a myriad of presentations in immunocompetent and immunocompromised hosts. Adenovirus infection in immunocompetent individuals rarely is associated with severe disease.[37] Although adenovirus infection in immunocompromised hosts may have trivial manifestations, severe disease certainly may occur. In recipients of hematologic stem cell transplantation, adenovirus may cause interstitial pneumonitis, hepatitis including ascending cholangiohepatitis, hemorrhagic cystitis, nephritis, hemorrhagic colitis, CNS disease, and disseminated disease.[37] In the solid-organ transplant recipient, the primary site of adenovirus disease is usually related to the transplanted organ. Clinical manifestations of adenovirus infections described in solid-organ transplantations include pneumonia, hepatitis, nephritis, hemorrhagic cystitis, enteritis, and disseminated disease.[37] Adenovirus infection in patients with HIV may cause pneumonia, hepatitis, meningoencephalitis, nephritis, and gastrointestinal and disseminated disease.[37]

POLYOMAVIRUSES

The most commonly encountered polyomaviruses are JC virus and BK virus. JC virus may be associated with progressive multifocal leukoencephalopathy, a progressive and ultimately fatal neurologic disease occurring in profoundly immunosuppressed individuals, such as patients with advanced HIV infection. BK virus is associated most commonly with renal infection in renal transplant recipients.[38] This infection is usually not accompanied by systemic manifestations such as fever. Infected patients have steadily rising serum creatinine. This presentation may be mistaken for acute rejection. Treatment with augmented immunosuppression is contraindicated, however, in patients with BK virus-associated nephropathy. Instead, immunosuppression should be minimized.

Viral Hemorrhagic Fevers

Hemorrhagic fevers may be due to Filoviridae, Bunyaviridae, Arenaviridae, or Flaviviridae. Dengue hemorrhagic fever is not discussed in this chapter because it is reviewed in detail elsewhere in this book.

MARBURG AND EBOLA VIRUS HEMORRHAGIC FEVERS

Marburg virus and Ebola virus are members of the *Filovirus* genus. Marburg virus appears to have originated in Uganda and western Kenya, where it infected monkeys and subsequently humans. *Marburg* refers to a town in Germany where monkeys from Uganda infected medical researchers, who subsequently infected hospital staff. The major subtypes of Ebola virus have occurred in central Africa. An additional subtype (Reston) was discovered in Reston, Virginia, among infected monkeys imported from the Philippines.[39] The source of this infection has not been definitively determined.

Marburg and Ebola virus infections have an incubation period of 5 to 10 days and begin with the abrupt onset of fever, myalgia, and headache. Somnolence and delirium usually follow. Most patients have abdominal pain and diarrhea. Many have a maculopapular rash on the trunk. Hemorrhagic manifestations such as bleeding around needle puncture sites and from the mucous membranes become prominent. Most patients have significant thrombocytopenia, leukopenia, and elevated transaminase levels. Viral culture, serology, and PCR have all been used to establish the diagnosis. At present, management is purely supportive. Additionally, strict contact isolation precautions are necessary.

HANTA FEVER AND CRIMEAN-CONGO HEMORRHAGIC FEVER

Hantavirus and Crimean-Congo hemorrhagic fever (CCHF) virus (CCHFV) are from the Bunyaviridae family of viruses. Hantaviruses cause hemorrhagic fever with renal syndrome (HFRS) and hantavirus pulmonary syndrome (HPS). There are several human pathogenic strains of hantavirus. The subtypes Hantaan, Dobrava, and Seoul cause moderate to severe HFRS in Asia and Europe, whereas Puumala causes a mild form of HFRS.[40] Unlike other Bunyaviridae, hantaviruses do not appear to have an arthropod vector and are usually transmitted via aerosols of urine-contaminated rodent urine or feces. The incubation period is typically 2 weeks. Initially, patients develop fever, headache, dizziness, blurred vision, abdominal pain, and back pain. Petechiae may be evident on the palate and the trunk; most patients have significant thrombocytopenia. After 4 to 7 days, significant hypotension can occur. In patients who survive, oliguria and mucosal hemorrhage occur, followed by polyuria. Sin Nombre virus and Andes virus caused HPS in North America and South America, respectively.[40]

CCHF is a severe hemorrhagic fever with a mortality rate of 3% to 30%; it has been described in parts of Africa, Asia, eastern Europe, and the Middle East.[41] It has the most extensive geographic distribution of medically important tickborne viral diseases. CCHF occurs through tick (*Hyalomma* spp.) bites, by contact with blood or tissues from viremic livestock, and after contact with a patient with CCHF during the acute phase of infection.[41] Patients have severe thrombocytopenia, disseminated intravascular coagulation, and extensive bleeding, with increased levels of liver enzymes, creatinine phosphokinase, and lactate

dehydrogenase. Diagnosis is made by enzyme-linked immunoassay (ELISA) and PCR. The clinical course of CCHF is composed of an incubation period (3-7 days), a prehemorrhagic period (3-7 days) characterized by flulike symptoms, a hemorrhagic period (2-3 days), and a convalescence period. Supportive therapy is the most essential part of the management of CCHF. Ribavirin (30 mg/kg as an initial dose, then 15 mg/kg 6-hourly for 4 days, then 7.5 mg/kg 8-hourly for 6 days) is the recommended antiviral agent for severe CCHF, although its mechanism of action is unknown.[41]

LASSA FEVER AND SOUTH AMERICAN HEMORRHAGIC FEVERS

Lassa fever and South American hemorrhagic fevers are due to the Arenaviridae. Lassa fever occurs in West Africa. South American hemorrhagic fevers occur in Argentina, Bolivia, and Venezuela. Lassa fever is transmitted via rodents, but subsequent nosocomial transmission has been extensive. Many cases of Lassa fever are only mildly symptomatic. Some patients develop high fever, pharyngitis, and retrosternal chest pain accompanied by significant mucosal bleeding. Hypotension, renal failure, and pulmonary edema may follow. Serology can be used to establish the diagnosis, but the virus also is isolated easily from the blood during the first week of illness, when viremia is often striking. Ribavirin use has been associated with a decrease in mortality.[42]

South American hemorrhagic fevers (Argentine, Bolivian, and Venezuelan) usually present with unremitting fever accompanied by a variety of nonspecific symptoms. Petechiae are often present on the palate and the skin, especially the axilla; mucosal bleeding may result. Pulmonary edema may occur. Management is extremely difficult owing to the combination of hypotension and refractory pulmonary edema. The diagnosis can be established by serologic tests. No specific therapy is available.

2009 Pandemic Influenza A and Avian Influenza A

The rapid dramatic increase in the frequency of severe illness due to 2009 influenza A (H1N1) has affected intensive care facilities around the world.[43-45] Suggested risk factors for severe illness associated with 2009 H1N1 infection include age (<5 years or ≥65 years), pregnancy, chronic cardiovascular conditions, chronic lung disorders, diabetes, immunosuppression, morbid obesity, hemoglobinopathy, chronic renal disease, chronic hepatic disease, and long history of smoking.[46] Therapy with a neuraminidase inhibitor (e.g., oseltamivir, zanamivir) is especially important for patients with such risk factors, as well as pregnant women. Epidemiologic studies estimated the case-fatality ratio to be 0.05% to 0.5%.[47] However, as more than three-quarters of cases of the 2009 influenza A (H1N1) pandemic occurred in persons younger than 30 (with a peak in the group aged 10-19 years), years of life lost are estimated to be 3 to 5 times higher than for typical seasonal influenza, and of the same order as the 1968 pandemic.[47]

Avian influenza A (H5N1) virus remains a cause for concern. The first human case of influenza A (H5N1) virus infection was documented in Hong Kong in 1997.[48] Since reemergence in 2003, it has caused human cases in 15 countries (e.g., China, Egypt, Indonesia, Iraq, Nigeria, Thailand, Turkey, Viet Nam) around the world.[49-53] The cumulative number of cases of avian influenza A (H5N1) virus infections reported to WHO as of 8 June 2010 was 499, with 295 subsequent deaths representing a mortality rate of approximately 60% (http://www.who.int/csr/disease/avian_influenza/country/en/). Although it has limited ability for human-to-human transmission, the continued circulation of influenza A (H5N1) virus increases the possibility of the reassortment of this virus with other circulating human influenza A viruses and increases the threat of a global influenza pandemic.[50]

Hendra and Nipah Viruses

These paramyxoviruses have been associated with deaths due to encephalitis or an acute pulmonary syndrome in Australia (Hendra virus) and Malaysia, Singapore, India, and Bangladesh (Nipah virus). The reservoir for these closely related viruses appears to be fruit bats. Viral transmission appears to occur from bats to horses (Hendra virus) or pigs (Nipah virus). Humans exposed to ill horses or pigs have developed fatal infection. In Bangladesh, nosocomial transmission of Nipah virus may have occurred.

Other Acute Viral Syndromes

Many viruses can cause aseptic meningitis, encephalitis, pneumonia, or hepatitis. These viruses are summarized in Tables 145-2, 145-3, and 145-4.

Antiviral Drugs

Since the advent of HIV infection, there has been an increase in development of drugs active against viruses. This section describes the currently available antiviral drugs, with the exception of drugs for HIV and viral hepatitis.

ACYCLOVIR

Acyclovir is a deoxyguanosine analog that inhibits viral DNA polymerase. When incorporated into viral DNA, it acts as a chain terminator. Acyclovir has its greatest clinical utility against HSV-1, HSV-2, and VZV. It has some activity against CMV, but it is far inferior to ganciclovir for infections with this virus. Acyclovir-resistant HSV has been well described, whereas acyclovir-resistant VZV is rare. Acyclovir is available in oral and intravenous (IV) forms. It penetrates the CSF reasonably well, and CSF levels are about 50% of plasma levels.[43] Dosing for acute mucosal HSV infections is 200 mg, 5 times a day, administered orally; and for VZV infections is 800 mg, 5 times a day, administered orally. In HSV encephalitis, the usual dose is 10 mg/kg given IV every 8 hours. Dose reduction is required in the presence of renal dysfunction. In the absence of appropriate reduction in dosage for renal dysfunction, neurotoxicity is observed, usually manifesting as confusion, hallucinations, and occurrence of tremor. As acyclovir can cause crystalline nephropathy, patients receiving the drug should be well hydrated.

VALACYCLOVIR

Because the bioavailability of orally administered acyclovir is low, valacyclovir (the L-valyl ester prodrug of acyclovir) was developed. It is usually administered twice daily for HSV infections and three times daily for VZV infections. Valacyclovir is also used for prevention of CMV disease in renal transplant recipients.[54]

FAMCICLOVIR

Famciclovir lacks antiviral activity but is the prodrug of penciclovir, which is active against HSV and VZV. Similar to acyclovir, penciclovir is an inhibitor of viral DNA synthesis. In general, acyclovir-resistant strains also are resistant to penciclovir. Dose adjustment of famciclovir is needed in renal insufficiency.

GANCICLOVIR

Similar to acyclovir, ganciclovir is a deoxyguanosine analog. It has activity against HSV and VZV. Its primary use has been in the treatment or prevention of CMV infections. Ganciclovir acts by inhibiting viral DNA polymerases. Patients with end-organ disease due to CMV are treated initially with ganciclovir, 5 mg/kg IV every 12 hours. Alterations in dose and frequency are required in patients with renal dysfunction. Typically, maintenance therapy is given at a reduced frequency (e.g., once per day) in patients who have received 2 to 3 weeks of induction therapy. Myelosuppression is the major toxicity of ganciclovir. Neutropenia typically begins to occur in the second week of ganciclovir therapy. Regular monitoring of hematologic parameters is mandatory for patients receiving ganciclovir. CNS abnormalities such as headache and confusion have been well described in patients receiving ganciclovir. In addition to an IV preparation, ganciclovir is available in an orally administered form. This form may be useful in prophylaxis against CMV infection.[17] Ganciclovir also can be administered into the eye via an ocular implant.[55,56] Ganciclovir is less active against acyclovir-resistant HSV strains than against acyclovir-susceptible strains. Resistance of CMV to ganciclovir has been well described, and mutations

TABLE 145-2	Viruses That Cause Aseptic Meningitis or Encephalitis
Virus	**Important Clinical Features**
Enteroviruses	Common cause of aseptic meningitis; rapid diagnosis available via PCR of CSF
HSV	In adults usually due to reactivation; rapid diagnosis available via PCR of CSF
VZV	Uncommonly may cause encephalitis after chickenpox
HHV-6	Causes encephalitis in transplant recipients
JK virus	Causes progressive multifocal leukoencephalopathy
Japanese encephalitis	Endemic in parts of Asia
St. Louis encephalitis	Outbreaks have occurred in all U.S. states
West Nile virus	Now common in U.S. and Canada
Tickborne encephalitis	Several foci of infection
Nipah virus	Zoonosis occurring in Malaysia, Singapore, India, and Bangladesh
Hendra virus	Zoonosis occurring in Australia
Rabies virus	Well-known zoonosis
California encephalitis	La Crosse virus is responsible for most cases
Human immunodeficiency virus	May cause acute encephalitis

CSF, cerebrospinal fluid; *HSV*, herpes simplex virus; *HHV-6*, human herpesvirus 6; *PCR*, polymerase chain reaction; *VZV*, varicella-zoster virus.

TABLE 145-3	Viruses That Cause Pneumonia
Virus	**Important Clinical Features**
Respiratory syncytial virus	Common cause of infection in infants
Influenza	Well-known cause of respiratory infection
Parainfluenza virus	Croup and pneumonia
Measles virus	Leading cause of pneumonia in children in underdeveloped nations
Coronaviruses	Severe acute respiratory syndrome
CMV	Important cause of pneumonia in immunosuppressed hosts
VZV	Pneumonia can complicate chickenpox
Adenovirus	Ubiquitous virus; severe pneumonia in immunosuppressed hosts
Hantavirus	Severe pneumonia in immunocompetent hosts
Hendra virus	Zoonosis in Australia

CMV, cytomegalovirus; *VZV*, varicella-zoster virus.

TABLE 145-4	Viruses That Cause Hepatitis
Virus	**Important Clinical Features**
Hepatitis A virus	Fecal-oral transmission
Hepatitis B virus	Parenteral, sexual, vertical transmission
Hepatitis C virus	Parenteral transmission
Hepatitis D virus	Requires coinfection with hepatitis B
Hepatitis E virus	Fecal-oral transmission

on the *UL97* phosphotransferase gene are generally associated with ganciclovir resistance.[17,57] Risk factors for ganciclovir resistance include prolonged exposure to ganciclovir (usually several months), ongoing active viral replication due to severe immunosuppression, lack of prior CMV immunity, and inadequate antiviral drug delivery with oral ganciclovir.[17]

VALGANCICLOVIR

The oral bioavailability of ganciclovir is poor. Valganciclovir, a prodrug of ganciclovir, can be used to enhance bioavailability. Valganciclovir is widely used as prophylaxis against CMV infection.[17] However, a meta-analysis demonstrated that valganciclovir for CMV prevention in solid-organ transplant patients had no superior efficacy and significantly higher risk of absolute neutropenia, CMV late-onset disease, and CMV tissue-invasive disease compared to other standard therapies (e.g., valacyclovir, ganciclovir).[58] A recent study has suggested the safety and efficacy of valganciclovir for preemptive therapy and treatment of CMV disease in solid-organ transplant recipients.[59]

FOSCARNET

Foscarnet is used most frequently in patients with CMV infection refractory to or intolerant of ganciclovir. Foscarnet also has activity against HSV and VZV, including acyclovir-resistant and ganciclovir-resistant strains. Although foscarnet and ganciclovir may have synergistic activity against CMV, there is no proven usefulness of combination therapy.[60] Use of the combination of ganciclovir and foscarnet is associated with greater toxicity than use of ganciclovir alone.[60] Foscarnet is available in an IV formulation only. Toxicity is common with foscarnet. Nephrotoxicity is a major dose-limiting side effect. Electrolyte abnormalities also are common, especially hypocalcemia, hypophosphatemia, hypomagnesemia, hypokalemia, and hypocalcemia, which may be symptomatic. Foscarnet may produce painful genital ulcerations; saline loading may diminish the likelihood of nephrotoxicity or genital ulceration.

CIDOFOVIR

Cidofovir is a nucleotide analog that is active against many herpesviruses and other DNA viruses, including polyomaviruses, poxviruses, and adenovirus. It is active against acyclovir-resistant and ganciclovir-resistant HSV and CMV. Cidofovir is administered IV once a week or once every 2 weeks. Its use is accompanied by high rates of nephrotoxicity. Neutropenia occurs in 20% of patients receiving this drug.

RIBAVIRIN

Ribavirin has found wide use as part of combination therapy for hepatitis C virus infection, but it is discussed here in the context of its use against other viruses. In vitro, ribavirin has activity against a wide range of DNA and RNA viruses. Ribavirin (aerosolized) is approved by the U.S. Food and Drug Administration (FDA) for the treatment of bronchiolitis and pneumonia due to respiratory syncytial virus. It has been used systemically in the treatment of some hemorrhagic fevers. Systemic ribavirin administration is associated with hemolytic anemia. Use of aerosolized ribavirin is controversial because of the drug's teratogenicity. Healthcare worker exposure to the drug potentially may occur when the drug is used in conjunction with mechanical ventilation, and use of aerosol containment systems is recommended.

ANTI-INFLUENZA DRUGS

Amantadine, rimantadine, zanamivir, and oseltamivir are used as treatment of influenza and for postexposure prophylaxis. Amantadine and rimantadine are active only against influenza A virus, whereas zanamivir and oseltamivir are active against influenza A and B viruses. In patients who have not received reduced doses of amantadine or rimantadine in the setting of renal dysfunction, serious neurotoxic reactions (including confusion and seizures) have been observed. Extensive experience with oseltamivir has been gained in recent years, and the drug has been found to be generally safe.

IV formulations of zanamivir or peramivir are now available on a compassionate-use basis for treating seriously ill patients, and peramivir was recently authorized for emergency use in hospitalized patients in the United States and licensed for use in Japan.[46] The efficacy of IV peramivir appeared to be similar to that of oseltamivir for seasonal influenza, but peramivir is less active for oseltamivir-resistant viruses than for oseltamivir-susceptible viruses. Thus IV zanamivir is the preferred option for seriously ill patients with suspected or documented oseltamivir resistance.[46]

KEY POINTS

1. For a generalized vesicular rash, scraping the base of the lesion and using polymerase chain reaction (PCR) to detect herpesviruses can assist in the rapid diagnosis of chickenpox or disseminated herpesvirus infections.

2. Cytomegalovirus (CMV) infection should be rapidly excluded as a cause of fever in an immunocompromised patient by way of detection of CMV DNA in peripheral blood by use of PCR.

3. Travelers from Africa, Asia, or South America who present with thrombocytopenia and fever should be assessed for the viruses that cause hemorrhagic fevers. Strict contact isolation should be considered.

4. Herpes simplex virus (HSV), varicella-zoster virus (VZV), and enteroviruses can be detected by PCR of cerebrospinal fluid, enabling a rapid diagnosis.

5. Dosage adjustment is necessary for most commonly used antiviral agents in patients with renal dysfunction. Failure to adjust dosage may lead to adverse effects such as neurotoxicity.

ANNOTATED REFERENCES

Breman JG, Henderson DA. Diagnosis and management of smallpox. N Engl J Med 2002;346:1300-8.
  Many textbooks have progressively diminished their coverage of smallpox since the 1970s. This review article fills in the gaps.
Ergönül Ö. Crimean-Congo haemorrhagic fever. Lancet Infect Dis 2006;203-14.
  Crimean-Congo hemorrhagic fever (CCHF) has a high mortality rate and the most extensive geographic distribution of medically important tickborne viral diseases. This review article comprehensively describes the epidemiology, virology, and ecology of CCHF virus and clinical issues of CCHF.
Luppi M, Barozzi P, Schulz TF, et al. Bone marrow failure associated with human herpesvirus 8 infection after transplantation. N Engl J Med 2000;343:1378-85.
  Occurrence of significant viral syndromes after organ transplantation may be associated with primary infection transmitted via the graft or reactivation of prior infection. In this study, HHV-8 infection occurred after renal transplantation and was associated with severe pancytopenia.

Reed KD, Melski JW, Graham MB, et al. The detection of monkeypox in humans in the western hemisphere. N Engl J Med 2004;350:342-50.
  There are numerous more recent examples of viral syndromes moving out of their traditional geographic locations. One is the occurrence of monkeypox in the United States.
Writing Committee of the WHO Consultation on Clinical Aspects of Pandemic Influenza. Clinical aspects of pandemic 2009 influenza A (H1N1) virus infection. N Engl J Med 2010;362:1708-19.
  In 2009, the first influenza pandemic in the 21st century occurred. This article reviews virologic, epidemiologic, and clinical data on 2009 H1N1 virus infections and summarizes key issues for clinicians.

REFERENCES

Access the complete reference list online at http://www.expertconsult.com.

146 *Clostridium difficile* Colitis

JOHN G. BARTLETT

Antibiotic-associated colitis was recognized soon after antibiotics were introduced in the 1940s, but the cause was not known until 1978 with the original reports of the role of *Clostridium difficile* as the putative agent in nearly all cases of antibiotic-associated pseudomembranous colitis and 10% to 15% of those with uncomplicated antibiotic-associated diarrhea.[1] Subsequent work has identified the pathophysiology, epidemiology, diagnostic methods, and treatment for this condition. The major challenges continue to be prevention and the management of patients with advanced disease, particularly those with ileus.

Etiology

C. difficile causes a spectrum of enteric complications of antibiotic use ranging from nuisance diarrhea to severe and sometimes life-threatening pseudomembranous colitis. There are occasional cases of antibiotic-associated colitis due to other pathogens (*Staphylococcus aureus*, *Klebsiella oxytoca*, enterotoxin-producing strains of *Clostridium perfringens* or *Salmonella*), but most cases are either due to *C. difficile* or are enigmatic.[2]

Pathophysiology

There are six relevant issues:

1. Colonization with *C. difficile:* this organism is found in the colonic flora of 2% to 3% of healthy adults and 20% to 30% of hospitalized patients.[3]
2. Toxin production: *C. difficile* produces two toxins, designated toxin A and toxin B.[5] Early studies implicated toxin A as the major cause of enteric toxin based on animal studies that showed florid colitis with injection of toxin A into bowel loops, but more recent studies establish that toxin B is critical for clinical expression.[5] Most strains of *C. difficile* produce both toxins, but about 1% to 2% produce only toxin B.[6]
3. Antibiotic exposure: this is the most important identifiable risk and presumably reflects the impact of the inducing agent on the colonic flora, establishing the opportunity for *C. difficile* to convert from the spore form to the vegetative form, with replication and toxin production. Virtually every antibiotic with an antibacterial spectrum has been implicated, but the most frequent are clindamycin and broad-spectrum cephalosporins. In current practice, fluoroquinolones account for the majority of cases, presumably reflecting their enormous usage rates.[4] Particularly important in recent years is the NAP-1 strain which is associated with fluoroquinolone use (see 5 below).
4. Epidemiology: *C. difficile* is relatively infrequent in ambulatory persons, but rates of colonization and disease are much higher as a result of exposure to the hospital environment.[3] *C. difficile* now represents an important and potentially lethal nosocomial pathogen. Nursing homes are another setting in which there is clustering of vulnerable patients with high rates of antibiotic use where *C. difficile* may be endemic or epidemic.[6] In the period 2001-2006, the NAP-1 strain emerged as an important epidemic agent of *C. difficile* in Canada, the United States, and Europe.[4,6] This strain appears to be particularly virulent, with increased toxin production, mortality, treatment failure, and relapses.

5. Age: there is increasing susceptibility to the development of *C. difficile* colitis with age, possibly due to immunosenescence.
6. Immunologic susceptibility: many patients harbor toxigenic strains of *C. difficile*, with no clinical expression despite extensive antibiotic exposure. One reason for this paradox is the apparent immune protection due to the presence of neutralizing antibody to toxins A and B. This observation accounts for the increasing interest in monoclonal antibodies to toxins A and B for treatment and vaccines for prevention.[7]

Clinical Signs and Symptoms

The typical presentation of *Clostridium difficile* infection (CDI) is watery diarrhea associated with cramps.[2] Other common features are fecal leukocytes, endoscopy showing PMC or colitis, characteristic changes on computed tomography (CT) (thickened bowel restricted to the colon, often associated with ascites), fever, hypoalbuminemia, and leukocytosis, sometimes with a leukemoid reaction. Nearly all cases of CDI are associated with diarrhea, but occasional postoperative patients will not have this owing to ileus. The laboratory clue that best predicts this diagnosis and its severity is the white blood cell (WBC) count. The average is about 15,000 cells/mL, but it may be much higher with counts over 20,000 or even 50,000 cells/mL. This strongly supports the CDI diagnosis and predicts severe disease.[8]

Diagnosis

The diagnosis is based on detection of the *C. difficile* (culture, EIA for glutamine dehydrogenase or polymerase chain reaction [PCR] for toxigenic *C. difficile*) or its toxins, designated toxin A and toxin B (enzyme immunoassay [EIA] for toxins A + B, or cytotoxin assay). Relative merits are shown in Table 146-1.

Treatment

Most important to treatment of CDI is discontinuing the implicated antibiotic. If there is a need for antibiotic treatment, select a drug that is unlikely to cause CDI (narrow-spectrum β-lactams, macrolides, aminoglycosides, antistaphylococcal drugs, tetracyclines; Table 146-2). The two favored drugs for treatment of CDI are metronidazole and vancomycin, both given by mouth.[1,6,7] Metronidazole is often preferred because it is less expensive. Earlier studies showed it to work as well as vancomycin, but more recent trials show oral vancomycin is superior to metronidazole in seriously ill patients,[8] defined as having a WBC over 15,000 cells/mL or elevated creatinine to 1.5 × baseline.[6] Other markers of serious disease are albumin less than 2 mg/dL, admission to the ICU for CDI, pseudomembranous colitis (PMC) on endoscopy, or pancolitis on CT scan.[9] Vancomycin is superior to metronidazole owing to pharmacology.[8] All *C. difficile* are in the colon, so the challenge is getting an active drug to the colonic lumen. Vancomycin is not absorbed, so it all goes to the colon when given orally; metronidazole given orally is nearly completely absorbed, so it gets to the colon primarily through an inflamed colonic mucosa. Most patients improve with resolution of diarrhea in 3 to 5 days.[1,7] Patients who are seriously ill (megacolon, septic shock, WBC >30,000/mL, lactate >5) and fail to respond to standard treatment should be considered for colectomy.[9]

TABLE
146-1 **Diagnostic Tests for *Clostridium difficile* Infection**

Test	What Detected	Time	Assessment
Culture	*Clostridium difficile**	3-4 days	Nonspecific; not used in United States
Culture-toxin	Toxigenic *C. difficile**	3-4 days	Test for toxin after culture for clostridia; moderate use in Europe
Cytotoxin	Toxin B	2-3 days	Formerly gold standard, but costly and rarely used now
EIA toxin A & B	Toxin A and B	Hours	Most-used test in United States, but not sensitive
EIA GDH	*C. difficile*	Hours	Detects *C. difficile* but not specific; good screening test
Toxin B gene	Toxigenic *C. difficile**	Hours	Detects toxigenic *C. difficile*; sensitive

*About 50% to 60% of *C. difficile* strains produce toxin.

The major indications are failure to respond to standard medical management and colonic perforation.

Prevention

Prevention of *C. difficile* includes: (1) surveillance to detect epidemics, (2) methods to prevent transmission of *C. difficile*, and (3) strategies to prevent unnecessary exposure to antibiotics, especially those most likely to induce CDI. For surveillance purposes, a rate of more than 4-10/10,000 patient days or 3-8/1000 admissions is regarded as excessive.[6,10] For prevention of horizontal transmission, the key preventive measures are hand hygiene (use of soap and water in epidemics), barrier precautions, use of private rooms or cohorting of case patients until diarrhea resolves, and disinfection of environmental surfaces using sporicidal agents such as chlorine-containing agents. For hand hygiene, it is noted that soap and water in place of alcohol-based hygiene is recommended only in *C. difficile* epidemics. Patients with CDI should have their own commode and room (or be cohorted) until diarrhea resolves. The decision to stop barrier precautions or for patient transfer should not be based on stool studies for *C. difficile*, since there is no test to determine response to treatment. Avoidance of unnecessary antibiotic use with antibiotic stewardship programs is an important general practice principle but is especially important in controlling this complication. With epidemics as described by surveillance rates, it is important to define the associated antimicrobials. Published reports indicate control of epidemics through restraining or eliminating use of clindamycin, cefotaxime, or fluoroquinolones when these agents were implicated.[6] Identification of the serotype of the

TABLE
146-2 **Treatment of *Clostridium difficile* Infection**

Category	Characteristics	Treatment Recommendations
Mild-moderate	WBC ≤ 15,000/mL and creatinine < 1.5 × baseline	Metronidazole 500 mg PO 3×/d × 10-14 days
Severe	WBC > 15,000/mL or creatinine > 1.5 × baseline	Vancomycin, 125 mg 4×/d PO × 10-12 days
Severe and complicated	Hypotension, shock, ileus or megacolon	Vancomycin, 500 mg PO 4×/d by NG tube or by rectum, *plus* Metronidazole 500 mg IV q 8 h
First relapse Second relapse		As above Vancomycin, standard dose, then taper and/or pulse

Adapted from Cohen SH, Gerding DN, Johnson S, Kelly CP, Loo VG et al. Clinical practice guidelines for *Clostridium difficile* infection in adults: 2010 update by the Society for Healthcare Epidemiology of America (SHEA) and the Infectious Diseases Society of America (IDSA). Infect Control Hosp Epidemiol 2010;31:431-55.
PO, per os (orally); *NG,* nasogastric; *WBC,* white blood cell.

implicated strain (e.g., NAP-1) may facilitate epidemiologic investigations in outbreaks. However, this requires stool culture for *C. difficile*, which most hospital labs do not usually do, and referral of the strain to a reference lab for serotyping.

Complications

The major complications of *C. difficile* for the intensivist are toxic megacolon and sepsis.[1,6,9] Toxic megacolon poses two problems: first is the severity of this complication per se, but also important is the inability to deliver vancomycin to the site of infection. Methods to deal with toxic megacolon are included in Table 146-2. For rectal instillations, the vancomycin is diluted with saline and delivered by enema, with a goal to get it to the right colon. Some patients will be severely ill with signs of sepsis, but bacteremia with enteric bacteria is rare, and *C. difficile* bacteremia as a complication of CDI has not been reported. *C. difficile* perforation has been reported as a complication of megacolon but is unusual. Most seriously ill patients respond to standard management of sepsis, with particular attention to rehydration, while attempting to control disease with oral vancomycin and IV metronidazole.

Conclusion

C. difficile has emerged as a major nosocomial pathogen that is usually associated with antibiotic use, may cause a devastating colitis, is usually detected with the standard stool assay, and usually responds rapidly to the combination of discontinuing the implicated antibiotic, with the addition of oral vancomycin or metronidazole. Important issues for the intensivist are (1) that this is a nosocomial pathogen that requires understanding the management guidelines for the CDI patient who is critically ill and (2) the need for implementing careful infection-control procedures in all cases.

KEY POINTS

1. Most cases of antibiotic-associated diarrhea are caused by *C. difficile* or are enigmatic.

2. Major complications of *C. difficile*-associated infection (CDI) are severe disease with ileus or toxic megacolon, sepsis, and relapsing disease.

3. Risks for CDI are advanced age, exposure to antibiotics, and being in a hospital or chronic care facility. Antibiotics with the greatest risk are fluoroquinolones, broad-spectrum β-lactams, and clindamycin.

4. The preferred diagnostic tests for *C. difficile* infection are PCR to detect toxigenic *C. difficile* or a combination test with screening for *C. difficile* by EIA to detect glutamine dehydrogenase and testing for toxin. The EIA test for toxin lacks sensitivity.

5. The usual treatment is to (a) discontinue the implicated antibiotic, (b) treat with oral metronidazole or vancomycin, and (c) maintain contact precautions to avoid nosocomial spread.

6. The NAP-1 strain became epidemic in North America and Europe in the early 2000s. This strain is promoted by fluoroquinolone use and causes severe disease, contributing to the increasing rates of CDI and lethal CDI.

7. The intensivist is likely to see CDI as a common complication of antibiotic use in seriously ill patients; treatment is straightforward if the diagnosis is considered.

8. The intensivist may also selectively see the complicated case, with critical disease indicated by a leukemoid reaction, renal failure, sepsis, ileus, or megacolon. These patients may require IV metronidazole, rectal vancomycin, and consideration of colectomy.

ANNOTATED REFERENCES

Bartlett JG. Narrative review: the new epidemic of *Clostridium difficile*-associated enteric disease. Ann Intern Med 2006;145:758-64.
A review of CDI including the recent developments with the NAP-1 strain.

Bartlett JG. Clinical practice. Antibiotic-associated diarrhea. N Engl J Med 2002;346:334-9.
Review of antibiotic-associated diarrhea—its cause and management. Note that CDI accounts for only 15% to 20% of cases.

McFarland LV, Mulligan ME, Kwok RY, Stamm WE. Nosocomial acquisition of *Clostridium difficile* infection. N Engl J Med 1989;320:204-10.
This is a classic paper showing that stool carriage rates of C. difficile in outpatients is only 1% to 2%, but the risk for acquisition increases to 25% to 30% with hospitalization.

McDonald LC, Killgore GE, Thompson A, Owens RC Jr, Kazakova SV, et al. An epidemic, toxin gene-variant strain of *Clostridium difficile*. N Engl J Med 2005;353:2433-41.
There has been recognition of an epidemic of CDI in North America and Europe starting in the period 2000-04. This is commonly attributed to the NAP-1 strain that causes more disease, more serious disease, disease that is often refractory to therapy, and disease likely to relapse.

Lyras D, O'Connor JR, Howarth PM, Sambol SP, Carter GP, et al. Toxin B is essential for virulence of *Clostridium difficile*. Nature 2009;458:1176-9.
The role of toxin B as an essential component of the pathophysiology of CDI.

Cohen SH, Gerding DN, Johnson S, Kelly CP, Loo VG, et al. Clinical practice guidelines for *Clostridium difficile* infection in adults: 2010 update by the Society for Healthcare Epidemiology of America (SHEA) and the Infectious Diseases Society of America (IDSA). Infect Control Hosp Epidemiol 2010; 31:431-55.
The 2010 guidelines for management of CDI. This is the basis for recommendations given here for treatment and infection control.

Lowy I, Molrine DC, Leav BA, Blair BM, Baxter R. Treatment with monoclonal antibodies against *Clostridium difficile* toxins. N Engl J Med 2010;362:197-205.
This report showed humanized monoclonal antibodies to C. difficile toxins A and B protected against relapse. This provides further evidence for an important role in humoral response as an important factor in protection against CDI.

Zar FA, Bakkanagari SR, Moorthi KM, Davis MB. A comparison of vancomycin and metronidazole for the treatment of *Clostridium difficile*-associated diarrhea, stratified by disease severity. Clin Infect Dis 2007;45:302-7.
A therapeutic trial that showed metronidazole and oral vancomycin were comparable for mild disease, but vancomycin was clearly superior for serious disease.

Lamontagne F, Labbé AC, Haeck O, Lesur O, Lalancette M, et al. Impact of emergency colectomy on survival of patients with fulminant *Clostridium difficile* colitis during an epidemic caused by a hyper-virulent strain. Ann Surg 2007;133:718-20.
A large experience with severe CDI is reviewed showing risks for lethal outcome, including a WBC over 50,000, age older than 75 years, immunosuppression, and serum lactate above 5. In this series, colectomy was associated with a substantial benefit, but the reported experience shows an operative mortality rate ranging from 25% to 75%.

McDonald LC, Coignard B, Dubberke E, Song X, Horan T, et al. Recommendations for surveillance of *Clostridium difficile*-associated disease. Infect Control Hosp Epidemiol 2007;28:140-5.
Recommendations for surveillance for CDI to determine if rates are excessive compared to national norms. Excessive rates imply the need to impose stringent infection control and possibly antibiotic restrictions.

REFERENCES

Access the complete reference list online at http://www.expertconsult.com.

147

Tetanus

C. LOUISE THWAITES | LAM M. YEN

Tetanus is caused by toxin from the bacterium *Clostridium tetani* and is characterized by muscle rigidity, spasms, and disturbance of the autonomic nervous system.

Epidemiology

Tetanus is now rare in the Western world, with only 28 cases in the United States in 2007,[1] but it is still a common problem in developing countries, where 80% of cases occur in Africa and Southeast Asia. Immunization programs targeting infants and pregnant women have coincided with a decline in the incidence of tetanus over recent years, but the estimated global incidence remains high, with an estimated 290,000 people dying from the disease in 2006.[2] In developing countries, neonatal deaths account for a large proportion of cases, and maternal and neonatal tetanus are responsible for an estimated 180,000 deaths/year (Figure 147-1).[3] In developed countries, the elderly are particularly at risk, owing to missed boosters and reduced antibody levels.[4] Drug users are also at risk from injection site contamination, especially those using subcutaneous administration methods. Up to 18% of infections in the United States occur in injecting drug users.

Pathophysiology

Tetanus is caused by a potent neurotoxin from the gram-positive bacterium, *C. tetani* (Figure 147-2). *C. tetani* is a ubiquitous organism capable of surviving in the environment as highly resistant spores and has been isolated from soil, street dust, and human and animal feces.[5] Once in a suitable anaerobic environment, these spores germinate, the bacteria multiply, and toxin is released. The most common sources of infection are minor lacerations to the limbs or the umbilical stump in neonates (Figure 147-3).[6] In 20% of cases, no source of infection can be found.[7] More unusual entry sites include dental infection, ear piercing, unsterile surgery, or injections.

Tetanus toxin is preferentially taken up by motor nerves, either locally or after circulation in the bloodstream. It enters the nerve and is transported by a specific component of the neuronal retrograde transportation system up the axon. It crosses the synapse and enters the γ-aminobutyric acid (GABA) G presynaptic nerve terminal.[8] The toxin is a zinc-dependent endopeptidase and cleaves vesicle-associated membrane protein II (VAMP II, or synaptobrevin) at a single peptide bond. This molecule is essential for synaptic release of neurotransmitters, and cleavage disrupts synaptic transmission. The toxin preferentially affects the GABA inhibitory interneurons afferent to motor nerves in the spinal cord and brainstem. By preventing inhibitory discharge, unrestricted motor nerve activity occurs, resulting in the increased muscle tone and spasms characteristic of tetanus. In severe forms of tetanus, the autonomic nervous system is also affected, perhaps as a result of toxin action within the brainstem, giving rise to marked cardiovascular instability.[9,10]

Clinical Features

Two main forms of tetanus exist. The majority of tetanus cases are generalized, affecting all muscle groups. However, a milder form—localized tetanus—also exists, affecting muscle groups in the immediate vicinity of a wound. A subgroup of localized tetanus—cephalic

tetanus—is also recognized and is associated with a higher mortality,[11] perhaps owing to early laryngospasm or autonomic disturbance resulting from brainstem involvement. Cephalic tetanus is often associated with lower motor neuron palsies affecting the third or seventh cranial nerves (Figure 147-4). Localized tetanus of any variety may progress to the generalized form.

After infection, a period of time known as the *incubation period* elapses before symptoms arise; this period is usually between 4 and 14 days. Initial symptoms include muscle stiffness, with muscle groups with short neuronal pathways affected first; hence, trismus and back pain are present in most cases on admission. Involvement of the facial and pharyngeal muscles produce the characteristic "risus sardonicus" and dysphagia (Figure 147-5). Increased tone in the muscles of the trunk results in opisthotonus. Muscle groups adjacent to the initial site of infection are often particularly severely affected, producing an asymmetric picture.

The time from the first symptom to the first spasm is termed the *period of onset*. Both the period of onset and incubation period have prognostic significance, with shorter times being associated with more severe disease (<48 hours for period of onset and <7 days for incubation period).[12] Spasms may be spontaneous but can also be provoked by physical or emotional stimuli. Laryngospasm can occur early in the disease process, often in isolation, resulting in acute upper airway obstruction. Respiration may also be affected by spasms involving the chest muscles. Without facilities for mechanical ventilation, respiratory failure due to muscle spasm is the most common cause of death.[5] Hypoxia is common in tetanus,[13] either due to spasms or difficulties clearing the copious bronchial secretions and aspiration.

Muscle spasms are usually most severe during the first and second weeks of illness but may persist for 3 to 4 weeks, after which rigidity may remain for several more weeks. In severe tetanus, autonomic disturbance usually appears during the second week. Signs of sympathetic overactivity usually predominate, evident as periods of tachycardia and hypertension. Severe tetanus is associated with a hyperkinetic circulation, particularly if muscle spasms are poorly controlled.[14] Changes in blood pressure are mainly due to changes in systemic vascular resistance, with little alteration in the cardiac index.[15] Circulating catecholamines, in particular epinephrine, are increased in patients with tetanus compared to others with similar-severity critical illness.[16]

Acute renal failure is a recognized complication of tetanus, with dehydration, rhabdomyolysis due to spasms, and autonomic disturbance all contributing.[17,18] Other complications include tendon avulsions, vertebral fractures secondary to muscle spasm, gastrointestinal bleeding, venous thrombosis, and thromboembolism (Table 147-1).[19]

Diagnosis

Diagnosis is clinical, based on history and examination findings. Strychnine, a glycine agonist, may give rise to a similar clinical picture, but muscle tone is usually normal between spasms. Urinary or plasma measurement of strychnine will exclude this as a cause. Because abdominal muscle rigidity is often an early sign, the disease may mimic an acute abdomen. Other differential diagnoses include orofacial infections causing trismus, dystonic drug reactions, or hysteria. Culture of *C. tetani* from a wound is difficult, and a positive culture is supportive of the diagnosis but not confirmatory.

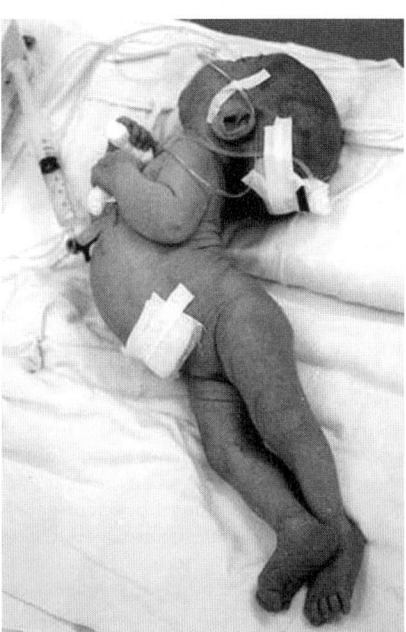

Figure 147-1 Neonatal tetanus.

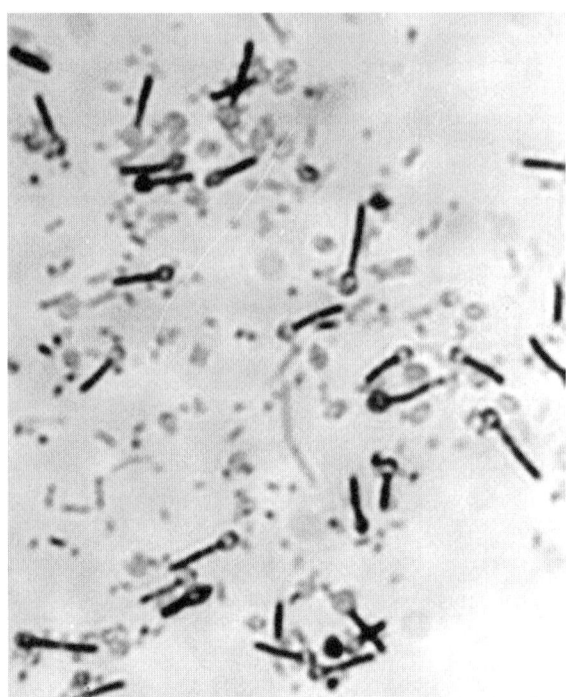

Figure 147-2 *Clostridium tetani*: a gram-positive bacillus with terminal spores. *(Courtesy J. Campbell, Oxford University Clinical Research Unit, Hospital for Tropical Diseases, Ho Chi Minh City, Vietnam.)*

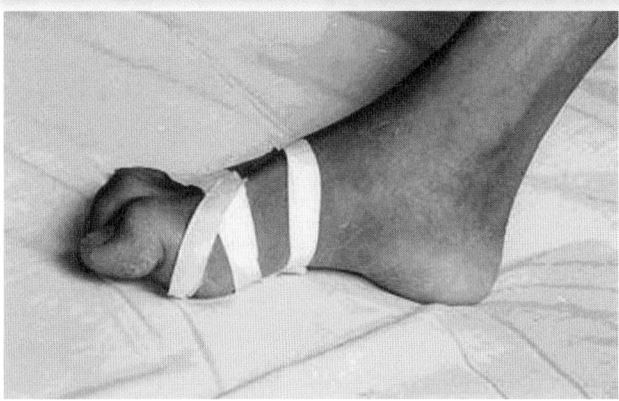

Figure 147-3 Lacerations to the feet are the most common focus of *Clostridium tetani* infection. Note clawing of toes secondary to increased tone in surrounding muscles.

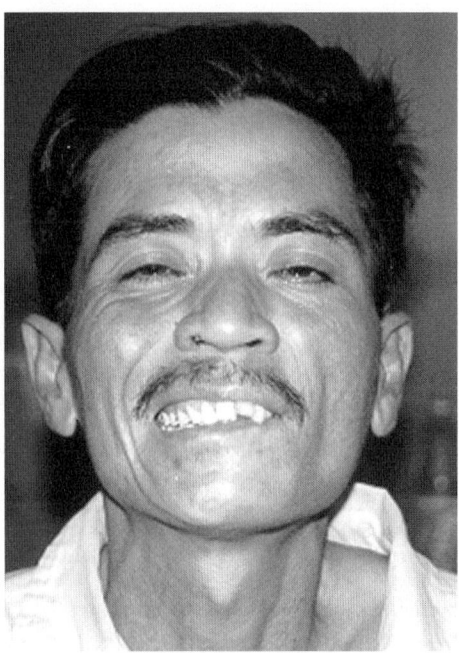

Figure 147-4 Cephalic tetanus associated with lower motor neuron palsy of seventh cranial nerve on left side of face.

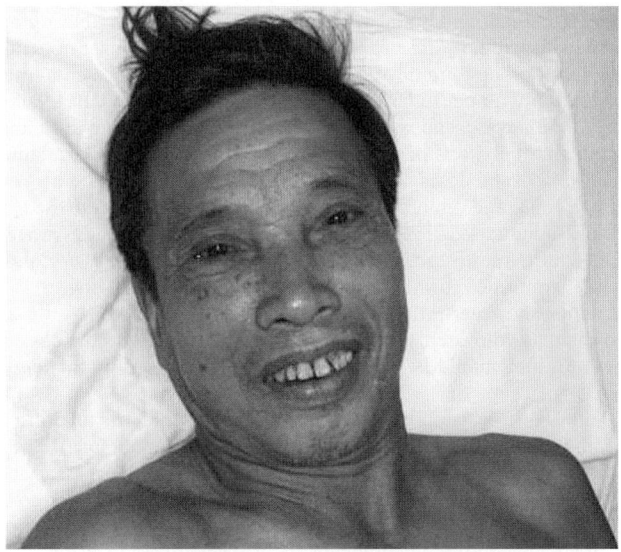

Figure 147-5 Facial muscle involvement in tetanus, producing characteristic "risus sardonicus."

TABLE 147-1	Complications of Tetanus
System	*Complication*
Cardiovascular	Hyper/hypotension Tachy/bradycardia Arrhythmias Ischemia Venous thrombosis/thromboembolism
Respiratory	Type I and type II respiratory failure Acute respiratory distress syndrome (ARDS) Aspiration pneumonia Ventilator-associated pneumonia
Other	Acute renal failure Gastrointestinal bleeding Sepsis Vertebral fractures Bed sores

Management

Tetanus patients should be nursed in a quiet environment and all stimuli minimized. To prevent further toxin release, wounds should be cleaned and débrided of any necrotic material and antibiotics given. Metronidazole (400 mg/kg rectally or 500 mg/kg intravenously [IV] every 6 hours for 7 days) is the antibiotic of choice, although penicillin (100,000-200,000 units/kg/d) remains the standard therapy throughout most of the world.

Antitoxin should be administered to neutralize any unbound toxin. Standard therapy is human immune globulin (HIG) (3000-6000 International Units intramuscularly as a single dose (or if unavailable, equine antitoxin, 500 units/kg). However, a recent meta-analysis and a randomized controlled trial have indicated intrathecal administration of 50 to 1500 International Units of human immune globulin may result in better outcome.[20] Tetanus infection does not result in immunity; therefore, all patients should be actively immunized with a full primary immunization course.

Further management consists of supportive care until the effects of the bound toxin wear off. The evidence base for most of the treatments listed in the discussion that follows is limited. Many older therapies have never been subjected to trials, although their use is now routine. Small case series and case reports exist describing the use of newer agents, but few randomized controlled trials have been published.

Airway management is a priority in tetanus. Generalized muscle spasm, laryngospasm, aspiration, or large doses of sedatives may all impair respiration, and airway compromise should be anticipated. Tracheostomy is the preferred means of securing the airway, although endotracheal intubation is acceptable as an initial measure. Copious bronchial secretions are produced in tetanus, and patients need frequent suctioning to remove secretions.

Sedation with benzodiazepines is the standard therapy for tetanus; they inhibit endogenous antagonists of $GABA_A$ receptors and may counteract the effects of tetanus toxin. IV diazepam or midazolam is usually used, and doses up to 200 mg/d are frequently required.[21] Phenobarbitone and chlorpromazine have historically been used to provide adjunct sedation, and their use may be beneficial in patients with autonomic disturbance. Alternatively, if spasms are not sufficiently controlled using benzodiazepines, nondepolarizing muscle relaxants and intermittent positive-pressure ventilation (IPPV) are indicated. Cardiovascularly inert drugs should be used if possible, and pancuronium should be avoided owing to its sympathomimetic side effects.[22]

Autonomic instability is difficult to treat. Rapid fluctuations in blood pressure mean drugs with short half-lives are desirable. The use of beta-blockers is controversial because their use has been associated with episodes of profound hypotension.[23] Esmolol may confer some advantage in this setting, but little data have been published to support its use. Conventional therapy consists of heavy sedation using high-dose benzodiazepines, morphine, and/or chlorpromazine.[24] Other treatments reported include clonidine and epidural bupivacaine, but data supporting their use are limited.[25] In addition to hypertension, hypotensive episodes may also occur, and if they are unresponsive to volume expansion, inotropes are required.

Recent interest has focused on the use of IV magnesium sulfate to control spasms and treat autonomic dysfunction, either as an adjunct to sedation or as a first-line agent. Doses of 1 to 3 g/h have been used to achieve serum concentrations of 2 to 4 mmol/L. A case series of 40 patients used magnesium as a first-line therapy in place of benzodiazepines[26] and reported adequate spasm control in 38 of 40 patients, with 17 of the 24 patients aged younger than 60 years avoiding IPPV. However, these results were not born out by a larger randomized controlled trial of 195 patients which found that ventilation rates did not differ between those receiving magnesium (serum concentrations 2-4 mmol/L) and placebo, although requirements for nondepolarizing neuromuscular blocking agents and other sedatives was reduced.[27] Concerns still exist regarding the safety of magnesium in sites without facilities for mechanical ventilation, and on the basis of published data, its routine use in this setting cannot yet be endorsed.

Patients with severe tetanus often require 2 or 3 weeks of mechanical ventilation until spasms subside, and nosocomial infection, particularly pneumonia, is an important problem. In one series, the incidence of ventilator-associated pneumonia in tetanus patients was reported to be 52.6%, with autonomic disturbance an independent risk factor (RR, 31.65; 95% CI, 2.68-373.74).[28]

Outcome

Outcome in tetanus depends on the severity of the disease and the facilities available for treatment. Adverse prognostic factors are given in Table 147-2. If the disease is not treated, mortality from tetanus is greater than 60% and higher in neonates. Even with treatment, adult mortality rates of 10% to 45% are reported, and up to 65% in neonates.[3,6,29] Few studies have been performed investigating the long-term effects of tetanus on patients who survive, but it appears that recovery is complete in most, although some persistent electroencephalographic abnormalities and difficulties in balance, speech, and memory have been reported.[30,31]

TABLE 147-2	Adverse Prognostic Features in Tetanus
Age	*<7 Days, Premature Birth, or >70 Years*
Incubation period	<7 days (<6 days in neonate)
Period of onset	<48 hours
Portal of entry	Umbilicus, uterus, burns, open fractures, postoperative, intramuscular injections
Spasms	Present
Temperature	>38.5°C
Heart rate	>140 beats/min (adult) >150 beats/min (neonate)

From Thwaites CL, Yen LM, Glover C et al. Predicting the clinical outcome of tetanus: the tetanus severity score. Trop Med Int Health 2006;11:279-87; and from Vakil BJ. Table ronde: propositions pour une classification internationale. In: 4th International Conference on Tetanus, Dakar, 1975, p. 3349-67.

KEY POINTS

1. Tetanus is rare in the developed world, although much of the population is vulnerable, owing to insufficient protective antibody levels. Even in the developed world, mortality from severe disease is high.

2. The disease is caused by a toxin produced by the gram-positive bacterium, *Clostridium tetani*. The toxin inhibits GABA neuronal discharge. It principally affects the motor nervous system, producing muscle spasms. In severe cases, the autonomic nervous

system is also involved, resulting in marked cardiovascular instability.

3. The disease has a characteristic natural history. Initial symptoms of stiffness give way to muscle spasms, which are maximal during the second week of illness. Autonomic disturbance is seen during the second and third weeks.

4. Poor prognosis is associated with a short incubation period and rapid onset of symptoms.

5. Initial treatment consists of wound cleaning and débridement. Antitoxin (human immune globulin, HIG) and antibiotics (metronidazole or penicillin) should be given.

6. Spasms are initially treated with benzodiazepines. Severe spasms require paralysis with nondepolarizing neuromuscular blocking agents or magnesium sulfate. Tracheostomy is the preferred means of securing the airway.

7. Little evidence exists to guide treatment of autonomic disturbance. High doses of benzodiazepines, morphine, short-acting beta-blockers, clonidine, and magnesium have all been used. Inotropes may be required in cases of hypotension.

8. Disease does not confer immunity; therefore, all patients require active immunization with three doses of tetanus toxoid.

ANNOTATED REFERENCES

Caleo M, Schiavo G. Central effects of tetanus and botulinum neurotoxins. Toxicon 2009;54:593-9.
  Detailed description of actions of tetanus toxin and pathophysiology of tetanus.
Roper MH, Vandelaer JH, Gasse FL. Maternal and neonatal tetanus. Lancet 2007;370:1947-59.
  Report of global epidemiology and public health initiatives.
Miranda-Filho Dde B, Ximenes RA, Barone AA, Vaz VL, Vieira AG, Albuquerque VM. Randomised controlled trial of tetanus treatment with antitetanus immunoglobulin by the intrathecal or intramuscular route. BMJ 2004;328:615-7.
  Trial of 120 patients with tetanus in ICU reporting that patients given intrathecal HIG suffered less severe tetanus, shorter hospital stay, and shorter duration of mechanical ventilation than those treated with intramuscular antitoxin.

Brunelte GW, Kozarsky PE, Magill AJ, et al. CDC yellow book. CDC Health Information for International Travel 2010. Atlanta: Centers for Disease Control and Prevention; 2010.
  Current recommendations for travelers and immunization schedules.
Thwaites CL, Yen LM, Loan HT, et al. Magnesium sulphate for the treatment of severe tetanus: a randomised controlled trial. Lancet 2006;368:1436-43.
  Randomized controlled trial of 195 adult patients reporting improved cardiovascular stability and reduced requirements for sedatives and muscle relaxants in those treated with magnesium.

REFERENCES

Access the complete reference list online at http://www.expertconsult.com.

148

Botulism

VERN C. JUEL | THOMAS P. BLECK

Botulism is the neuroparalytic disorder resulting from intoxication with exotoxins produced by *Clostridium botulinum* and several other strains of clostridia. *C. botulinum* are spore-forming obligate anaerobic bacilli[1] whose heat-resistant spores are widely distributed in soil and marine sediment throughout the world.[2] The term *botulism* is derived from the Latin word for "sausage," *botulus*. Botulism initially was recognized as sausage poisoning in Europe in the early 19th century. Kerner, a German health official, characterized the relationship between sausage ingestion and paralysis in 230 people in 1820.[3] The toxin and the bacterium were initially demonstrated by Van Ermengem[4] in his study of an epidemic of foodborne botulism following raw ham consumption at a Belgian funeral music festival in 1895. In addition to foodborne botulism after ingestion of preformed toxin, forms of botulism owing to in vivo toxin production subsequently were recognized, including wound botulism in 1943,[5] infant botulism in 1976,[6,7] and adult intestinal botulism in 1986.[8] Inhalational botulism has been identified only in a single outbreak in humans[9] but has received more recent attention related to the potential for aerosolized toxin used as a biological weapon.[10]

Toxin Characteristics

Seven distinct serotypes of botulinum toxin, A through G, are defined by the absence of cross-neutralization with antitoxin.[11] Human disease is produced by types A, B, E, and rarely F toxin, whereas types C and D produce disease in birds and mammals.[12] Type G has been implicated in human disease only rarely.[12,13] Neurotoxigenic strains of *Clostridium baratii* may produce type F toxin,[14,15] and some strains of *Clostridium butyricum* may produce type E toxin.[16]

Botulinum toxins are 150-kD polypeptides that are converted during bacterial lysis by proteases into an active form consisting of a 50-kD light chain and a 100-kD heavy chain joined by a disulfide bond.[17] After absorption into the systemic circulation, the carboxy-terminal domain of the heavy chain facilitates binding of the toxin to polysialoganglioside receptors on neuronal membranes, whereas the amino-terminal domain of the heavy chain mediates translocation of the toxin into motor or autonomic neurons.[18,19] The light chain is a zinc endopeptidase that cleaves a toxin-specific location of one or more of the *SNARE* (*soluble N-ethylmaleimide-sensitive fusion associated protein receptor*) proteins mediating the docking and fusion of acetylcholine vesicles with the presynaptic membrane at the neuromuscular junction, in autonomic ganglia, and in parasympathetic nerve terminals.[20] SNARE proteins, SNAP-25 (synaptosomal-associated protein of 25 kD) and syntaxin, are associated with the presynaptic membrane, whereas synaptobrevin or vesicle-associated membrane protein (VAMP) is located on the synaptic vesicle membrane. SNAP-25 is cleaved by types A, C, and E toxins, and syntaxin is cleaved by type C toxin.[21-23] Synaptobrevin is cleaved by types B, D, F, and G and tetanus toxins.[24-26] After cleavage of SNARE proteins by botulinum toxin, the release of acetylcholine is permanently halted at affected synapses. Recovery from botulism occurs when the presynaptic neuron sprouts another nerve terminal to reform the cholinergic synapse.[27-29] The original synapse remains intact, however, and over a period of months becomes functional again. After this occurs, the new synapse is pruned.

Botulinum toxin is considered to be the most toxic substance by weight,[30] with a lethal dose in humans estimated to be approximately 1 ng/kg of type A toxin.[31] By extrapolation from primate studies,[32] the lethal dose of type A toxin for a 70-kg man is estimated to be 70 μg by mouth, 0.70 to 0.90 μg by inhalation, and 0.09 to 0.15 μg by intramuscular or intravenous routes.[33] In contrast to the heat-resistant spores of *C. botulinum*, the toxins are heat labile and are inactivated by heating to 85°C for at least 5 minutes.[34]

Forms of Human Botulism

FOODBORNE BOTULISM

Ingestion of contaminated food, with absorption of toxin from the duodenum and jejunum, causes foodborne botulism. Because several individuals may be exposed to a single contaminated food source, foodborne botulism often presents in outbreaks. The average annual number of foodborne botulism cases in the United States between 1973 and 1998 was 24 (range 14-94),[35] with an average of 9.4 outbreaks a year between 1950 and 1996.[12] The most frequently implicated foods include home-canned vegetables, fruits, and fish.[12] Failure to use a proper combination of heat, pressure, and time to kill spores during home canning, particularly with low-acid (pH > 5) foods, may permit survival and germination of spores.[36] Although restaurant and commercially prepared foods are responsible for fewer outbreaks (7% from 1950-1996),[12] nearly half of foodborne cases may arise from these sources.[37] Fish preparation using fermentation among Alaskan natives is responsible for a large fraction of the total cases (29% from 1973-1998).[12]

Foodborne botulism due to type A toxin is most common in the United States, constituting 45% of outbreaks compared with 36% of outbreaks due to type E and 13% due to type B toxin during the period 1990 to 1996. Type F foodborne outbreaks are rare in the United States.[12] The geographic distribution of foodborne botulism outbreaks mirrors the type of spores residing in soil. Type A spores predominate in the western United States, and type B spores predominate in the northeastern and central United States.[38,39] Type E spores are found in marine life and sediments.[40,41] In a corresponding fashion, during the period 1950 to 1996, 86% of the type A outbreaks occurred west of the Mississippi River, whereas 61% of the type B outbreaks were from eastern states. Marine products have been implicated in 91% of type E outbreaks.[12]

Signs and symptoms of foodborne botulism generally develop within 12 to 36 hours of ingestion of contaminated food, with the acuity and severity of illness related to the amount of toxin absorbed. In general, a symmetrical, descending paralysis with multiple cranial neuropathies evolves rapidly in the absence of fever or altered sensorium. In foodborne botulism, initial symptoms are often gastrointestinal (GI) and include nausea, vomiting, diarrhea, and abdominal cramping, which may be due to ingestion of other bacterial metabolites along with botulinum toxin in contaminated food.[42] Parasympathetic dysfunction may present early with dry mouth and blurred vision associated with dilated, poorly reactive pupils. Diplopia often develops secondary to extraocular muscle weakness with paretic, disconjugate eye movements. With paralysis of bulbar muscles, patients may exhibit flaccid dysarthria, chewing difficulty, and dysphagia. The upper extremities, trunk, and lower extremities may become paretic in a descending fashion. Autonomic dysfunction may manifest as GI dysmotility, orthostatic hypotension, altered resting pulse, urinary retention, or hypothermia.[43]

Respiratory compromise may occur secondary to a combination of upper airway obstruction from weak oropharyngeal muscles and diaphragmatic weakness. Requirements for mechanical ventilation are more prolonged for patients with type A disease (mean 58 days) compared with patients with type B disease (mean 26 days).[44] The clinical findings related to intoxication with various types of botulinum toxin are varied (Table 148-1), with type A disease causing more frequent extraocular and bulbar muscle weakness, and type B and E disease causing relatively more pupillary and autonomic dysfunction.[45-47]

With improvements in respiratory care, the case-fatality rate has diminished from 60% during 1899 to 1949 to 12.5% during 1950 to 1996.[12] The fatality risk for the index case in an outbreak is 25%, with a 4% fatality risk for subsequent cases after recognition of an outbreak.[48] Because of the potential for exposure of other individuals to a contaminated food source and for additional cases accumulating from previous exposure, every case of suspected foodborne botulism should be reported to local and state public health authorities.

WOUND BOTULISM

Wound botulism results from in vivo toxin production in abscessed and devitalized wounds.[49] In the event of contamination by spores, these wounds provide an ideal anaerobic environment for spore germination and local colonization by *C. botulinum* with absorption of toxin into systemic circulation. In contrast to the rapid onset of botulism in foodborne disease with ingestion of preformed toxin, the incubation period for wound botulism is 7 days (range 4-14 days).[50] Single cases occur in isolation with a case-fatality rate of approximately 15%.[51] Before 1980, wound botulism was a rare disorder generally associated with deep wounds containing avascular areas. Between 1943 and 1985, 33 cases were reported in the United States.[12] During the period 1986 through 1996, 78 cases of wound botulism were reported in the United States, most related to subcutaneous injection or "skin popping" of black tar heroin.[12,52] Wound botulism due to sinusitis after repeated cocaine inhalation also has been observed.[53] The neurologic signs and symptoms are virtually identical to foodborne disease except for the absence of prodromal GI symptoms.[12] When present, fever is related to the wound infection.[54] The diagnosis should be suspected in patients with a drug-injection history and without known exposure to a contaminated food source.[55]

INTESTINAL BOTULISM

Infant Intestinal Botulism

Infant and adult intestinal botulism result from the ingestion of *C. botulinum* spores that germinate, colonize the large intestine, and produce botulinum toxin in vivo.[6] Infant intestinal botulism is now recognized as the most common form of botulism in the United States, with approximately 100 cases reported annually. About half of the cases relate to type A toxin, and the other half to type B intoxication.[12] Most individual cases occur sporadically, although rare unexplained clusters are reported.[56-58] Since the recognition of infant intestinal botulism in 1976, nearly half of the reported cases have occurred in California. The geographic distribution of infant botulism is unexplained, with the highest incidence rates observed in Delaware, Hawaii, Utah, and California.[12] The average age of onset is 13 weeks, and most cases occur before 6 months, although some cases have occurred at 15 months of age.[12]

Ingestion of ambient *C. botulinum* spores, distributed widely in soils and dust, is thought to represent the primary route of exposure.[56] Honey is also a source of spores and has been implicated as a significant risk for infant intestinal botulism.[59-61] In an animal model of infant intestinal botulism, mice between 7 and 13 days old proved susceptible to intestinal colonization with *C. botulinum* after intragastric injection of spores.[62] Epidemiologic studies suggest a parallel peak human susceptibility to intestinal colonization by *C. botulinum* between 2 and 4 months of age.[63] This susceptibility appears related to the intestinal flora in the immature infant GI tract. The resident flora are influenced by an infant's food sources,[64] although the potential significance of breastfeeding versus formula feeding as a risk for infant intestinal botulism is unresolved.[65]

A clinical spectrum of disease exists, with some infants exhibiting relatively mild and limited disease involving several days of constipation, poor feeding, and lethargy, and other infants developing acute tetraparesis and respiratory failure.[65] In classic cases, constipation is often the initial symptom, followed by lethargy, poor feeding, and weak cry. Examination reveals hypotonia with head lag, ptosis, reduced facial expression, and reduced gag, suck, and swallow reflexes. Deep tendon reflexes are reduced or absent. Extraocular movements are often paretic, and pupils may be large and poorly reactive. In one series, more than half of the patients were intubated and mechanically ventilated, usually following loss of protective upper airway reflexes.[66] Although the course is variable, most hospitalized infants reach maximal paralysis at approximately 1 to 2 weeks after hospitalization and begin to improve after 1 to 3 weeks.[65] In California between 1976 and 1991, the average length of hospitalization was 4.9 weeks. A longer length of stay was documented for type A cases (5.7 weeks) compared with type B cases (3.6 weeks), suggesting that type A intoxication causes more severe disease.[65] The case-fatality rate is less than 1% in hospitalized patients in the United States.[56]

TABLE 148-1	Symptoms and Signs in Human Botulism Types A, B, and E		
	Type A (%)	Type B (%)	Type E (%)
Neurologic Symptoms			
Dysphagia	96	97	82
Dry mouth	83	100	93
Diplopia	90	92	39
Dysarthria	100	69	50
Upper extremity weakness	86	64	NA
Lower extremity weakness	76	64	NA
Blurred vision	100	42	91
Dyspnea	91	34	88
Paresthesias	20	12	NA
Gastrointestinal Symptoms			
Constipation	73	73	52
Nausea	73	57	84
Vomiting	70	50	96
Abdominal cramping	33	46	NA
Diarrhea	35	8	39
Other Symptoms			
Fatigue	92	69	84
Sore throat	75	39	38
Dizziness	86	30	63
Neurologic Findings			
Ptosis	96	55	46
Reduced gag reflex	81	54	NA
External ophthalmoparesis	87	46	NA
Facial weakness	84	48	NA
Tongue weakness	91	31	66
Pupils fixed or dilated	33	56	75
Nystagmus	44	4	NA
Upper extremity weakness	91	62	NA
Lower extremity weakness	82	59	NA
Ataxia	24	13	NA
DTRs reduced or absent	54	29	NA
DTRs hyperactive	12	0	NA
Initial mental status:			
Alert	88	93	27
Lethargic	4	4	73
Obtunded	8	4	0

Adapted from Bleck TP. *Clostridium botulinum* (botulism). In: Mandell GL, Bennett JE, Dolin R, editors. Principles and practice of infectious diseases. 5th ed. Philadelphia: Churchill Livingstone; 2000, p. 2543-8. Data from references 45, 46, and 47.

DTRs, deep tendon reflexes; *NA*, not available.

Adult Intestinal Botulism

Children and adults also may be susceptible to intestinal colonization and in vivo toxin production by *C. botulinum*, *C. baratii*, or *C. butyricum* when the gastric barrier is compromised and the intestinal flora are altered.[8,15,67,68] Previously classified by the Centers for Disease Control and Prevention (CDC) as "botulism of undetermined origin," adult intestinal botulism has occurred in the setting of intestinal surgery, gastric achlorhydria, broad-spectrum antibiotic treatment, and inflammatory bowel disease.[69-71] Although adult intestinal botulism is uncommon (10 cases reported between 1986 and 1996),[71] it is probably underdiagnosed.

INHALATIONAL BOTULISM

Inhalational botulism does not occur in nature but is the result of an attempt to use the toxin in aerosolized form as a bioweapon.[10] The three documented human cases were reported from Germany in 1962, when botulinum toxin type A became accidentally reaerosolized during disposal of laboratory animals.[9] These patients initially developed dysphagia on day 3 after exposure and exhibited tonic pupils, paretic eye movements, dysarthria, and diffuse weakness by day 4. In animal experiments, monkeys became symptomatic 12 to 18 hours after exposure to aerosolized toxin, with descending paralysis and death in some animals.[72] Aerosolized botulinum toxin was released by the Japanese religious cult, Aum Shinrikyo, on several occasions in the 1990s in Japan, although the attacks were not known to have produced human illness.[10] By the time of the 1991 Persian Gulf War, the state of Iraq had produced large quantities of concentrated botulinum toxin which were loaded onto weapons for military use but never deployed.[73]

Release of aerosolized toxin has the potential to produce a botulism outbreak. The features of such an outbreak that might suggest a deliberate release of toxin[10] include: numerous cases within an outbreak (the mean number of cases in foodborne outbreaks has averaged 2.5 for many years)[12]; toxin types within an outbreak that rarely cause natural disease (type C, D, F, G, or E not related to marine sources); outbreaks with a common geographic factor without a common dietary exposure; and multiple simultaneous outbreaks.[74]

IATROGENIC OR INADVERTENT BOTULISM

The therapeutic use of botulinum toxin for dystonia, spasticity, hyperhidrosis, sialorrhea, and other conditions occasionally has resulted in inadvertent paresis of nearby noninjected muscles, such as dysphagia in neck muscle injections for cervical dystonia[75] and jaw dislocation after parotid injections for sialorrhea in amyotrophic lateral sclerosis.[76] Although there are rare reports of paretic muscles distant to the site of injection,[77,78] it has been estimated that healthy patients would require a 10-fold toxin overdosing to develop systemic symptoms.[79] Nevertheless, single-fiber electromyography studies showed abnormal neuromuscular transmission in muscles distant to botulinum toxin injections.[80-82] Patients with underlying neuromuscular disorders seem to be predisposed to developing generalized weakness after therapeutic intramuscular botulinum toxin injections.[83-85] Systemic autonomic dysfunction also has been noted after therapeutic injections of type B toxin.[86]

Diagnosis

The diagnosis of botulism is primarily clinical, with the use of laboratory techniques initially to exclude other diagnoses. Currently the confirmation of a diagnosis of botulism and the identification of the toxin type takes several days. Recommendations for specimen acquisition and diagnostic testing change over time; the most current recommendations are available at http://www.bt.cdc.gov/agent/botulism/lab-testing.asp.

DIFFERENTIAL DIAGNOSIS

The differential diagnosis for botulism includes Guillain-Barré syndrome and its variants, particularly Miller-Fisher syndrome and polyneuritis cranialis. Classic Guillain-Barré syndrome generally occurs with limb weakness and sensory disturbances and is readily distinguished from botulism. Patients with polyneuritis cranialis who exhibit extraocular and bulbar muscle weakness may be difficult to distinguish clinically from botulism in the early phases of illness. Despite prominent extraocular muscle weakness and areflexia in Miller-Fisher syndrome, the presence of limb ataxia helps to distinguish it from botulism.

Myasthenia gravis also commonly produces weakness of extraocular and bulbar muscles, but the temporal course of the weakness is often fluctuating, with diurnal variation and improvement with rest or acetylcholinesterase medications. In contrast to botulism, myasthenia gravis does not affect autonomic function in general or pupillary function in particular. The presence of acetylcholine receptor antibodies is extremely specific for myasthenia gravis. Lambert-Eaton myasthenic syndrome often is associated with a neuroendocrine carcinoma of the lung and the presence of voltage-gated calcium channel antibodies. Although the symptoms and findings may be similar to botulism, the degree of bulbar paralysis is not as marked, and the clinical course is rarely acute or rapidly progressive.

Tick paralysis produces an acute flaccid paralysis due to neurotoxins of ixodid ticks. A meticulous physical examination of the scalp and intertriginous regions should be performed for an attached tick. Acute brainstem lesions, including strokes, may also be diagnostic considerations, particularly if consciousness is impaired. In suspected infant botulism, the differential diagnosis includes sepsis, meningoencephalitis, Werdnig-Hoffmann disease, congenital myasthenia gravis, and metabolic disorders.

ELECTRODIAGNOSTIC STUDIES

Electrodiagnostic studies may confirm the presence of a presynaptic neuromuscular junctional disorder and strongly suggest the diagnosis of botulism or may support an alternative diagnosis. In botulism, sensory nerve conduction studies should be normal, and no evidence for segmental demyelination on motor nerve conduction studies (e.g., prolonged F latencies, conduction block, temporal dispersion) should be observed to suggest Guillain-Barré syndrome. Compound muscle action potential amplitudes commonly are reduced in clinically affected muscles.[87] The more affected muscles are often proximal ones, however, and routine motor nerve conduction studies recorded in intrinsic hand or foot muscles may fail to detect this nonspecific abnormality. In contrast with myasthenia gravis[88] and Lambert-Eaton myasthenic syndrome,[89] low-frequency (2-3 Hz) repetitive nerve stimulation studies in botulism rarely show a decremental response in terms of reduced amplitude and area of the compound muscle action potential elicited by stimulating a motor nerve.[87]

The characteristic finding in a presynaptic neuromuscular junctional disorder such as botulism is postexercise facilitation or posttetanic facilitation with high-frequency (20-50 Hz) repetitive nerve stimulation. Although Lambert-Eaton myasthenic syndrome and botulism share this finding, posttetanic facilitation may be less prominent[90] and more sustained[91] in botulism. Proximal muscles also may exhibit a comparatively greater degree of facilitation in botulism.[90] Posttetanic facilitation may be more common in type B botulism compared with type A disease.[92]

Needle electromyography may reveal low-amplitude, short-duration motor unit potentials with an unstable firing pattern, although this nonspecific finding may be observed in many motor unit disorders.[90] Positive sharp waves and fibrillation potentials also are observed in about half of cases.[93]

Single-fiber electromyography uses statistical analysis of muscle fiber action potentials generated by the same motor neuron to evaluate neuromuscular transmission. It is the most sensitive diagnostic test for detecting abnormal neuromuscular transmission, although it cannot distinguish reliably between presynaptic neuromuscular disorders. In botulism, it is more sensitive than repetitive nerve stimulation studies for showing neuromuscular junctional pathology.[94-96]

MOUSE BIOASSAY

Confirmatory testing for botulism currently involves a mouse bioassay, which is available only through the CDC and several state laboratories. In the mouse bioassay, mice are inoculated with type-specific antisera and patient serum or extracts from samples of body fluids or suspicious foodstuffs. In a positive mouse bioassay, all the mice die except those receiving the antisera matching the botulinum toxin type present in the patient or food specimens. Test results are generally available within 1 or 2 days after inoculation.[10] Details regarding specimen preparation and handling are available online.[12] Specimen samples in suspected cases of foodborne botulism should include serum, feces, gastric aspirates, vomitus, and foods suspected to be contaminated. In wound botulism, serum, feces, exudate, débrided tissue, and wound swab samples should be examined. In intestinal botulism, serum and feces should be sampled.[12] To obtain an adequate fecal sample, particularly in infant botulism where constipation is common, an enema using sterile, non-bacteriostatic water may be necessary. In addition to administering extracts to mice, the samples are anaerobically cultured, and the culture isolates are evaluated using the mouse bioassay.

Mass spectroscopy for detection and characterization of botulinum toxins is emerging as a valuable diagnostic technique.[97] Molecular diagnostic techniques are under development and should eventually replace older techniques.

🔬 Management

All cases of suspected botulism should be reported to the hospital epidemiologist or infection control officer and to local or state health departments and the CDC for cases in the United States. This reporting is essential to coordinate laboratory testing and shipment of antitoxin and to initiate investigation of the toxin source.[10] Patients with suspected or confirmed botulism should be monitored carefully in an intensive care unit (ICU), with particular attention to their ability to protect the upper airway. Many patients require intubation and mechanical ventilation. Purgatives or activated charcoal may be useful if there is suspicion of residual contaminated food in the GI tract.[54] The use of antibiotics that impair neuromuscular transmission should be avoided, particularly aminoglycosides and macrolides.[98,99]

Botulinum antitoxins may reduce the duration and severity of neurologic dysfunction associated with botulism if administered early in the course of disease. The effect of antitoxin is limited to circulating toxin, and the paralytic effects of previously bound and internalized toxin are not reversed by antitoxin.[48,65] Four types of antitoxin currently are available in the United States: (1) a licensed bivalent (A, B) human antiserum for infant botulism, (2) a licensed bivalent (A, B) equine antiserum, (3) an investigational monovalent (E) equine antiserum, and (4) an investigational heptavalent (A, B, C, D, E, F, G) antiserum.[100]

BOTULISM IMMUNE GLOBULIN INTRAVENOUS (HUMAN)

Botulism immune globulin intravenous (BIG-IV) is a licensed, bivalent human antiserum (type A, B) available for treatment of infant botulism. A 5-year randomized, double-blinded, placebo-controlled treatment trial demonstrated the safety and efficacy of botulism immune globulin intravenous in infant botulism. The mean length of hospital stay was significantly reduced in patients receiving BIG-IV (from 5.5 weeks to 2.5 weeks).[65] BIG-IV was officially licensed by the U.S. Food and Drug Administration (FDA) in October 2003 for treatment of infant botulism types A and B under

the proprietary name of BabyBIG. BIG-IV is available through the California Department of Health Services (24-hour telephone number: 510-231-7600). Current information on infant botulism treatment is available at http://www.infantbotulism.org.

SEROTHERAPY

A heptavalent despeciated equine antitoxin (H-BAT) is available from the U.S. Centers for Disease Control and Prevention, and is essentially devoid of serum sickness risk. H-BAT is available through state health departments; more information is available at http://www.cdc.gov/laboratory/drugservice/formulary.html#ia. and through http://www.infantbotulism.org/general/babybig.php.

PENTAVALENT TOXOID

An investigational pentavalent toxoid (type A, B, C, D, E) for preexposure prophylaxis is available for military personnel and laboratory workers. A primary series of immunizations is given at 0, 2, and 12 weeks, followed by a 1-year booster.[100,101] Because it induces immunity over several months, the toxoid is not appropriate for postexposure prophylaxis.[10]

KEY POINTS

1. Botulinum toxins are zinc endopeptidases that cleave specific sites of proteins mediating the release of acetylcholine at the neuromuscular junction in autonomic ganglia and in parasympathetic nerve terminals.

2. Foodborne botulism is caused by the ingestion of preformed toxin from contaminated food sources. Foodborne disease may present in outbreaks involving multiple individuals.

3. Intestinal botulism is caused by ingestion of clostridial spores in susceptible individuals, with colonization of the intestinal tract and in vivo toxin production.

4. Wound botulism is due to clostridial colonization of individuals with devitalized tissues and subsequent in vivo toxin production. Subcutaneous injection of illicit drugs, particularly black tar heroin, is responsible for a recent increase in cases.

5. Inhalational botulism from aerosolized toxin causes a neuroparalytic syndrome indistinguishable from the other forms of human botulism.

6. Outbreaks due to deliberate release of toxin may be characterized by numerous cases, rare toxin types, a common geographic factor without a common dietary exposure, and multiple simultaneous outbreaks.

7. The cardinal clinical features of botulism include a symmetrical descending paralysis and multiple cranial neuropathies evolving rapidly in the absence of fever or altered sensorium. In foodborne disease, initial symptoms may include nausea, vomiting, diarrhea, and abdominal cramping. In infant intestinal botulism, the initial symptom is often constipation.

8. Differential diagnosis of botulism includes Guillain-Barré syndrome and its variants, myasthenia gravis, Lambert-Eaton myasthenic syndrome, tick paralysis, and acute brainstem lesions. For infant intestinal botulism, the differential diagnosis includes sepsis, meningoencephalitis, Werdnig-Hoffmann disease, congenital myasthenia gravis, and metabolic disorders.

9. Electrodiagnostic studies may help to support the diagnosis, although the findings may not be specific. The mouse bioassay is the confirmatory test for botulism.

10. Airway protection and ventilatory support are the main issues for supportive care.

11. Antitoxin may shorten the course of the disease when administered early to bind circulating toxin.

ANNOTATED REFERENCES

Arnon SS. Infant botulism. In: Feigin RD, Cherry JD, editors. Textbook of pediatric infectious diseases. 5th ed. Philadelphia: Saunders; 2004. p. 1758-66.
This chapter summarizes the known pathophysiology of infant intestinal botulism and contemporary treatment guidelines.

Arnon SS, Schechter R, Inglesby TV, et al. Botulinum toxin as a biological weapon: medical and public health management. JAMA 2001;285:1059-70.
This consensus report by the Working Group on Civilian Biodefense reviews the clinical and laboratory findings, differential diagnosis, and treatment recommendations for the various forms of human botulism. The features of a botulism outbreak suggesting a deliberate release of toxin are highlighted.

Centers for Disease Control and Prevention. Botulism in the United States, 1899-1996: handbook for epidemiologists, clinicians, and laboratory workers. Atlanta: Centers for Disease Control and Prevention; 1998.

Available at: http://www.cdc.gov/ncidod/dbmd/diseaseinfo/botulism.pdf. This comprehensive work provides contemporary epidemiologic information relating to all forms of human botulism and detailed information relating to laboratory confirmation and specimen preparation and handling.

Hughes JM, Blumenthal JR, Merson MH, et al. Clinical features of types A and B foodborne botulism. Ann Intern Med 1981;95:442-5.
This classic series delineates the clinical symptoms and findings in a large series of patients with the most common toxin types in human foodborne botulism.

REFERENCES

Access the complete reference list online at http://www.expertconsult.com.

149

Dengue

TRAN TINH HIEN | JEREMY FARRAR

Millions of individuals across the tropical and subtropical world become infected with dengue viruses every year. A small percentage of individuals infected with dengue develop overt clinical illness, and an even smaller percentage develops severe dengue. With the enormous shift to urban living, increase in tourism, business-related travel, and global deployment of military and international nongovernmental organizations in recent decades, dengue cases have been seen more frequently outside endemic areas. The daytime biting habits of the *Aedes* mosquito and the urban environment visited by most international travelers make it all but impossible to avoid exposure (bed nets offer only limited protection). There is no vaccine or prophylaxis available. Dengue infections in travelers are monitored by TropNetEurop (www.tropneteurope/dengue) and in the United States by the Centers for Disease Control and Prevention (CDC; www.cdc.gov/dengue). Most infections in travelers (78%) manifest after short holidays or business-related travel to South and Southeast Asia and the Americas.[1,2] There have been major epidemics in West Africa in recent years.[2]

Of the many clinical features associated with dengue infections, from the standpoint of threat to life and clinical intervention, the most important is increased vascular permeability leading to dengue shock syndrome (DSS). Children are particularly prone to the development of shock, probably because of age-related differences in capillary fragility that may make them more susceptible than adults to capillary leak syndrome.[3]

Epidemiology

Dengue is the most widely distributed mosquito-borne viral infection of humans, affecting an estimated 100 million people worldwide each year, with 40% (2.5 billion) of the world's population estimated to be at risk of infection.[4] It is endemic in parts of Asia and the Americas and has been reported increasingly from many tropical countries in recent years.[4,5] It is now classified by the World Health Organization (WHO) into *dengue fever* and *severe dengue* (Box 149-1). The most important feature of severe dengue is increased capillary permeability, leading to DSS (Figure 149-1). It is among the leading causes of hospitalization in Asia during the rainy season, with 500,000 cases reported annually to the WHO. When shock becomes established, mortality rates of 12% to 40% have been reported, although this can be less than 1% when patients are looked after by experienced clinical teams.

The dengue virus is a single-stranded, positive sense RNA virus of approximately 11 kb in length and encodes 3 structural and 7 nonstructural genes.[6] It is a member of the *Flavivirus* genus, which also includes yellow fever, Japanese encephalitis, West Nile virus, and hepatitis C virus.[7] There is considerable genetic diversity in the dengue virus family, with four serotypes (Den-I, Den-II, Den-III, and Den-IV), all of which may produce a nonspecific febrile illness, dengue fever, or may result in the more severe manifestation of severe dengue.

The dengue viruses are transmitted from viremic individuals to susceptible hosts by mosquitoes of the subgenus *Stegomyia*; the major global vector is *Aedes aegypti*, although other species may be more important in restricted geographic areas. *A. aegypti* lays individual eggs in the damp walls of artificial and natural water containers, and these eggs can remain viable for months. The adult mosquito is strongly anthropophilic, prefers resting in sheltered dark areas inside houses, and has a diurnal feeding pattern, usually peaking in the midmorning and late afternoon. The female usually feeds twice during a single gonotrophic cycle, and the average life span is 8 to 14 days.

Pathophysiology

Severe dengue is characterized by increased vascular permeability and plasma leakage, thrombocytopenia, and hemorrhage (see Figure 149-1). Vascular permeability is the most important parameter determining the severity of dengue, and the plasma leak that occurs can precipitate DSS through circulatory failure (reduced pulse pressure and hypotension).[5] The capillary leak predisposes to pulmonary edema, pleural effusion, ascites, intravascular compromise, and hemoconcentration. Dengue is characterized by only mild hemorrhage, as indicated by spontaneous petechiae and a positive tourniquet test, whereas in severe dengue, mucosal bleeding (including that associated with peptic ulceration and menorrhagia) and other clinically important manifestations of hemorrhage can be present. These are usually associated with prolonged shock.

The most widely cited hypothesis to explain the vascular leak and hemorrhage associated with dengue is increased viral replication due to enhanced infection of monocytes in the presence of preexisting antidengue antibodies at subneutralizing levels, leading to antibody-dependent immune enhancement.[8] This observation, which has strong epidemiologic and in vitro experimental evidence to support it, argues that in asymptomatic dengue infection, the moderate viremia is controlled. The host immune system develops long-lasting immunity to the serotype of the infecting strain and short-lived cross-protection against heterologous serotypes. After a few months, the levels of cross-protective antibodies directed against the heterologous serotypes fall below neutralizing levels, however, and from this stage onward infection with a second heterologous strain may result in increased viral uptake via Fcγ receptors into monocytes and enhanced viral replication. Severe disease has been reported during primary infections, however, and not all secondary infections lead to severe disease, so other theories (viral and host genetic factors) have been suggested to explain the complex epidemiologic and immunopathogenetic features.[9-12]

Clinical Features

Dengue fever is a mild, self-limited febrile episode that is commonly associated with a rash. It usually begins with fever, respiratory symptoms (sore throat, coryza, cough), anorexia, nausea, vomiting, diarrhea, and headache. Back pain, myalgias, arthralgias, and conjunctivitis also may occur. The initial fever usually resolves within 1 week, and a few days later a generalized morbilliform or maculopapular rash may develop. Fever may return with the rash. As noted, dengue is now classified into dengue and severe dengue by the WHO (see Box 149-1). These two groups form part of a continuous spectrum of severity, with the most important clinical features of severe dengue being capillary permeability leading to DSS (see Figure 149-1). Other complications include severe mucosal (and less commonly, intracerebral and pulmonary hemorrhage) bleeding, pleural

WORLD HEALTH ORGANIZATION CASE CLASSIFICATION 2009

Dengue

Acute febrile illness, live in or travel to endemic region, with two or more of the following:

Headache and/or retro-orbital pain

Nausea and/or vomiting

Rash

Aches and pains

Tourniquet test positive

Leukopenia

Any warning signs (abdominal pain, persistent vomiting, fluid accumulation, mucosal bleeding, lethargy, liver enlargement, increase in hematocrit, falling platelet count with laboratory confirmation)

Severe Dengue Including Dengue Shock Syndrome

Severe capillary permeability and plasma leakage leading to dengue shock syndrome

Fluid accumulation and respiratory distress

Severe bleeding

Severe organ involvement (liver, CNS, heart, kidneys, and others)

---

effusions, encephalopathy, pneumonia, and liver dysfunction. The differential diagnosis is extensive and varies depending on where the patient is seen, but would include malaria, typhoid, leptospirosis, scrub and murine typhus, septicemia, other viral hemorrhagic fevers (e.g., Ebola, Lassa fever), chikungunya, West Nile fever, o'nyong-nyong fever, and Rift Valley fever (usually without a rash).

A pulse pressure of less than 20 mm Hg is one of the earliest manifestations of shock and usually occurs before the onset of systolic hypotension. The mainstay of treatment is prompt but careful fluid resuscitation. If appropriate volume resuscitation is instituted at an early stage, shock is usually reversible; in certain severe cases and in patients who are inappropriately resuscitated, patients may progress to irreversible shock and death. Careful clinical judgment is required throughout the patient's stay in the hospital to maintain an effective circulation while assiduously avoiding fluid overload. During the critical phase of illness, regular review (every 15-30 minutes) of vital signs—pulse rate, blood pressure (BP), respiratory rate (RR), and peripheral temperature—as well as measurement of hematocrit (Hct) at least every 2 hours (more frequently if very severe or unstable).[13,14,15] It is imperative that these measurements be made, the patients assessed, and the treatment modified in light of the clinical situation and results. Ideally the Hct should be measured on the ward (or the results be made available immediately). Dengue has a very dynamic clinical progression, and it is not acceptable to define therapy on the basis of blood results taken hours earlier. For patients with DSS, the WHO recommends immediate volume replacement with isotonic crystalloid solutions, followed by the use of plasma or colloid solutions, specifically dextrans, for profound or continuing shock.[4]

Thrombocytopenia is a very common feature in dengue, and platelet function is abnormal. Mild prolongation of the prothrombin and partial thromboplastin times with reduced fibrinogen levels is common, but fibrin degradation products have not been found to be elevated to a degree consistent with classic disseminated intravascular coagulation (DIC). Patients with DSS have significant abnormalities in all the major pathways of the coagulation cascade.[16]

Diagnosis

Classic dengue illness can be an easy diagnosis to make in endemic regions with experienced clinical staff and a high prior probability that a febrile illness with rash and thrombocytopenia is caused by dengue. Most of the symptoms and signs accompanying dengue infection are common to many febrile illnesses, with few features that reliably discriminate dengue, especially at early stages.[17,18] The differential diagnosis invariably is large; it is region, country, and season specific. The differential diagnosis includes measles, rubella, enterovirus, influenza, typhoid, chikungunya, scarlet fever, malaria, leptospirosis, hepatitis A, rickettsiosis, bacterial sepsis, Hanta virus infection, viral hemorrhagic fevers (including Ebola, Lassa fever), West Nile virus, o'nyong-nyong fever, and Rift Valley fever (usually without a rash). Because of the variation in clinical findings and the multiplicity of possible causative agents, the descriptive term *dengue-like disease* may be used until the clinical picture becomes clearer or the laboratory provides a specific diagnosis (Figure 149-2).

Proof of a dengue infection depends on confirmatory RT-PCR, dengue serology, specific dengue NS1 antigen detection, or viral isolation if available. Serologic confirmation of acute dengue infection relies on the demonstration of specific immunoglobulin (Ig)M and IgG antibodies against dengue in the serum of patients. Dengue virus RNA also can be amplified by reverse transcriptase nested polymerase chain reaction (RT-PCR) from serum.[19] Viral isolation is performed by culturing the patient's serum with *Aedes albopictus* C6/36 cell monolayers. Virus infection of C6/36 cells is confirmed by immunofluorescent assay using a flavivirus-specific monoclonal antibody.

Management

Although there are currently no specific drugs for dengue, effective treatment is based primarily on judicious fluid management (Figure 149-3). Prompt restoration of circulating plasma volume is the cornerstone of therapy for patients with DSS. For uncomplicated dengue fever, less aggressive oral or parenteral fluid therapy frequently is indicated. This section focuses on the management of DSS; the management of unusual complications such as dengue encephalopathy or fulminant hepatitis is not addressed, as the management of these complications is similar to standard treatment protocols.

Patients admitted with established DSS should be cared for in an intensive care unit (ICU) staffed by experienced medical and nursing

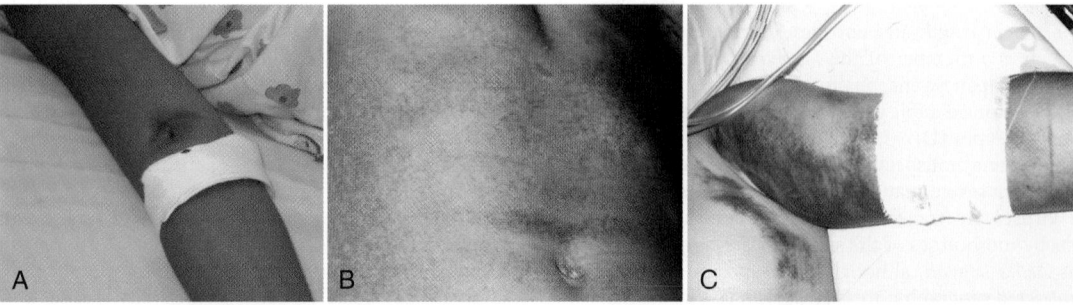

Figure 149-1 Acute skin manifestations of dengue. **A,** Characteristic minor bleeding near injection sites. **B,** Rash in established dengue shock syndrome. **C,** Severe bleeding following IV injection. Staff should press after IV injections for five minutes to ensure bleeding stops.

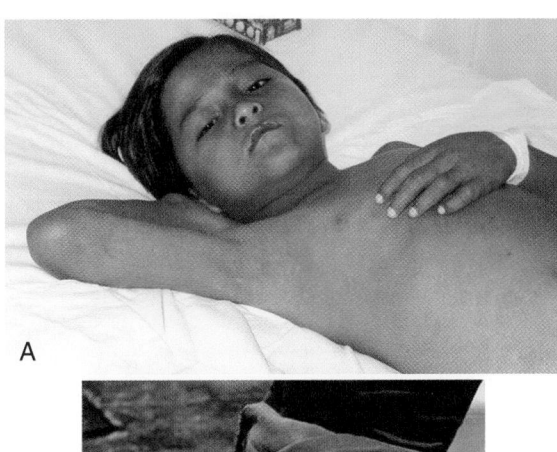

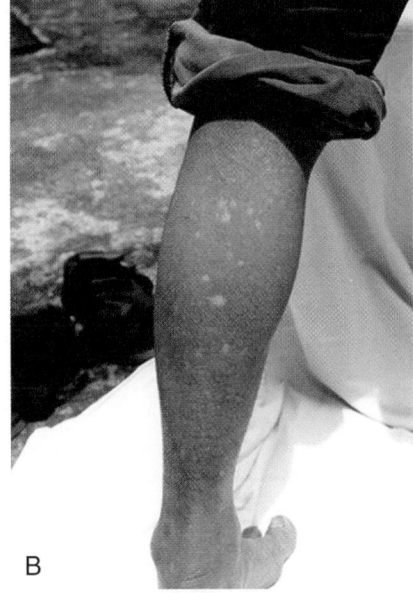

Figure 149-2 Characteristic skin manifestations in convalescent dengue. **A,** Early convalescent macular diffuse rash occurring in the first week after recovery. **B,** Typical convalescent rash with "islands of white in a sea of red."

personnel. Immediate restoration of a stable and effective circulation with parenteral fluid therapy is the primary aim of treatment. Extreme care is needed to balance the requirement for intravenous (IV) fluid to maintain plasma volume against the inherent risk of leakage of the administered fluid into the interstitial space. The leaked fluid may contribute to the development of pleural effusions, ascites, and respiratory compromise, and the potential downward spiral toward multiorgan failure, DIC, and death. Patients with the most severe capillary leak syndrome and most at risk of multiorgan dysfunction also are the patients most in need of the most aggressive circulatory support. Correctly balancing fluid resuscitation and ongoing capillary leak is the most difficult issue in caring for patients with DSS.

Rapid clinical assessment of cardiovascular status (pulse, BP, peripheral perfusion, urine output, and mental state) determines initial management. The results of basic laboratory investigations including Hct (preferably available on the ward) and platelet count are useful, but initiation of treatment must not be delayed pending their availability. Detailed examination should be carried out when resuscitation is in progress. The following features are commonly associated with severe disease and a complicated clinical course:

- Unrecordable pulse and BP with poor peripheral perfusion
- Narrow pulse pressure (<10 mm Hg) with poor peripheral perfusion
- Compromised cerebral perfusion (lethargy, irritability, drowsiness, or restlessness)

- Presentation with shock early in the course of the disease (before day 4 of fever)
- Age younger than 1 year. Severe dengue occurs infrequently in infants, but special care must be taken with fluid management in this age group. In infants, fluid accounts for a greater proportion of body weight, and minimal daily requirements are correspondingly greater; cardiovascular and renal function still are developing, and there is less reserve to cope with disturbance; finally, capillary beds are intrinsically more permeable than the capillary beds of older children or adults. All infants must be treated as high-risk patients and warrant early intervention with very careful resuscitation and intensive monitoring.
- Marked elevation or rapid increase of Hct
- Pleural effusions or ascites at the time of presentation with shock. Large volumes of intrathoracic or intraabdominal fluid must be present to be clinically detectable, implying either recent onset of catastrophic leak or a steady loss of fluid over a longer period before the development of hemodynamic compromise.

After an initial rapid assessment, resuscitation with parenteral fluids should be started immediately. Reliable IV access must be secured as soon as possible; rarely, in patients with profound shock, a venous cutdown or insertion of an intraosseous line may be necessary. All patients with shock or respiratory compromise should receive oxygen by facemask or nasal cannulae. A regular schedule of clinical observations (pulse, BP, RR) at least every 30 to 60 minutes should be instituted, along with a detailed record of all fluid intake and output. The Hct should be measured every 2 hours for the first 6 hours, and thereafter every 4 to 6 hours until the patient is stable.

SEVERE DENGUE INCLUDING DENGUE SHOCK SYNDROME

For most patients with DSS, resuscitation should be started with an isotonic crystalloid solution (physiologic saline, Ringer's lactate, or Ringer's acetate) at a rate of 15 to 20 mL/kg over 1 hour. If the patient's clinical condition has stabilized after this time (wider pulse pressure, stable pulse rate, warm peripheries, stable Hct), the rate of fluid administration may be reduced to 10 mL/kg/h for 2 hours, then gradually reduced to maintenance levels over the next 6 to 8 hours. A suitable schedule might be as follows: 10 mL/kg/h for 2 hours, 7.5 mL/kg/h for 2 hours, 5 mL/kg/h for 4 hours, then 2 to 3 mL/kg/h for 24 to 36 hours. For most patients, IV therapy can be stopped at this time, provided that the clinical condition has been stable for 24 hours.[4]

If there is evidence of ongoing cardiovascular compromise after the first hour of treatment (no improvement in pulse pressure or pulse rate, persisting peripheral shutdown, rising Hct), colloid solution (6% dextran 70 or 6% starch solution) should be substituted for the crystalloid solution at an initial rate of 10 to 20 mL/kg over 1 hour. Hyperoncotic preparations such as 10% dextran have been implicated in the development of renal failure when used in hypovolemic patients and should be avoided. If large volumes of colloid are infused, regular assessment of the coagulation profile is required.

Frequent observation of vital signs, mental state, and urine output, as well as serial Hct measurements, are used to assess the response to treatment. After initial resuscitation, most patients can be managed successfully with isotonic crystalloid fluid until the reabsorptive phase of the illness begins around day 6 to 7. If there are further episodes of cardiovascular decompensation after the initial episode, supplementary treatment with small infusions of 5 to 10 mL/kg of colloid may be required.

Patients with no recordable pulse or BP must be managed more vigorously. Patients in shock require colloid therapy (6% dextran 70 or 6% starch solution) immediately. Despite initial hemodynamic instability, most patients improve with aggressive volume replacement and can be managed subsequently as outlined earlier. Central venous pressure monitoring provides useful information to direct fluid therapy, but insertion of lines should be carried out only by experienced personnel and with careful attention to the coagulation state.

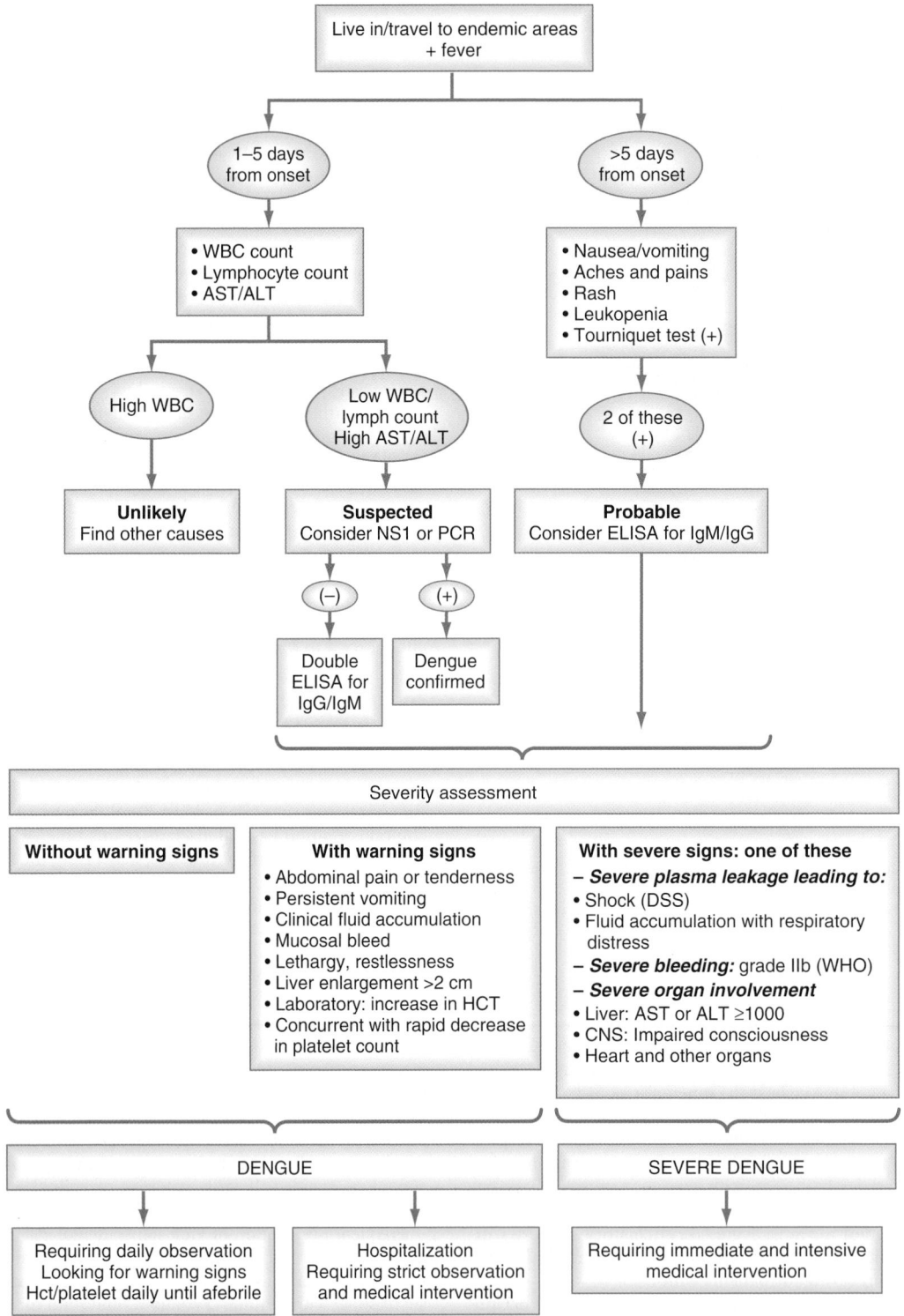

Figure 149-3 Clinical algorithm for a child with dengue infection. AST/ALT aspartate aminotransferase/alanine aminotransferase; BP, blood pressure; BUN, blood urea nitrogen; CR, cardiac rhythm; CVP, central venous pressure; DIC, disseminated intravascular coagulation; DSS, dengue shock syndrome; ELISA, enzyme-linked immunosorbent assay; GI, gastrointestinal; GU, genitourinary; Hct, hematocrit; HR, heart rate; Ig, immunoglobulin; ORS, oral rehydration solution; PCR, polymerase chain reaction; PEEP, positive end-expiratory pressure; PR, pulse rate; RR, respiratory rate; WBC, white blood cell; WHO, World Health Organization.

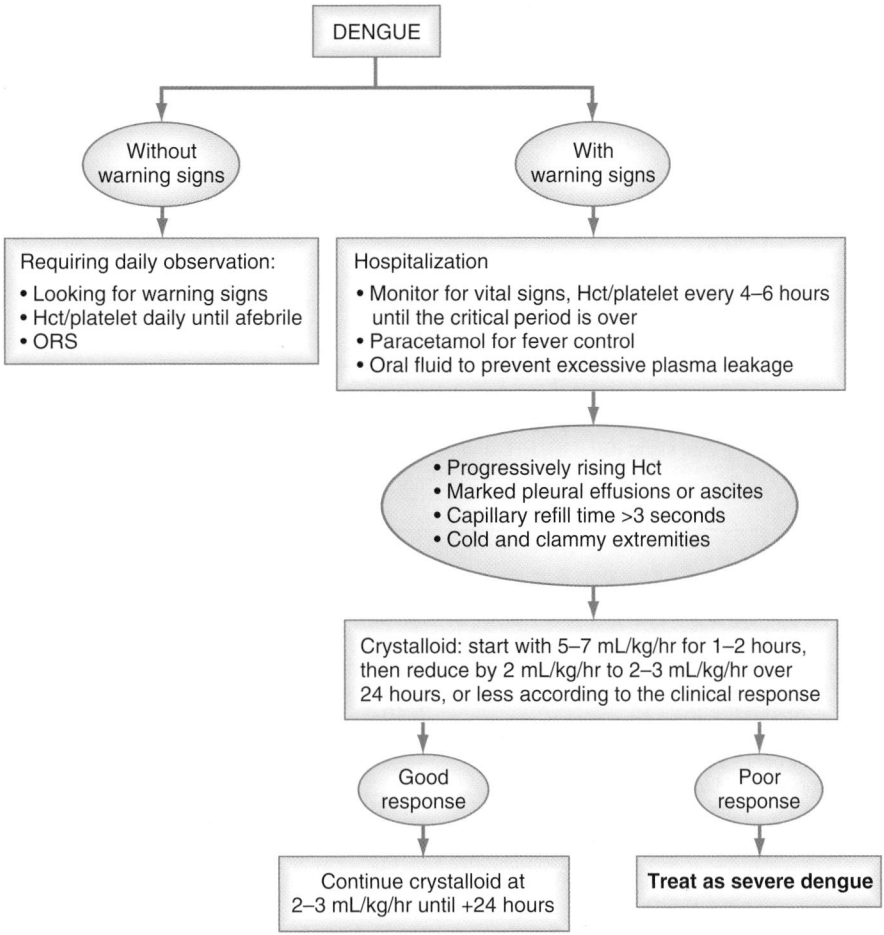

Figure 149-3, Cont'd. *Continued*

Inotropic support may be required in addition to volume support. Significant pleural effusions and respiratory compromise are likely to develop, and pleural and ascitic drainage and artificial ventilation may prove to be necessary. Metabolic and electrolyte derangements are common in these critically ill patients and should be actively sought and treated.

BLOOD TRANSFUSION

Blood transfusion is indicated only for patients with major bleeding and should be undertaken with extreme care because of the problem of fluid overload. In patients with DSS, major bleeding is almost always associated with severe or prolonged shock and is usually from the gastrointestinal tract or vagina. Severe mucosal bleeding appears to be more common in adult patients. Underlying causes include profound thrombocytopenia in combination with gastritis or stress ulceration. Internal bleeding may not become apparent for many hours until the first melena stool is passed. Blood transfusion should be considered in all patients who fail to improve clinically after appropriate fluid resuscitation, particularly if the Hct is stable or unexpectedly falling. (<35% Hematocrit and persistent shock). Platelet concentrates and fresh frozen plasma also can be helpful but are effective only for a few hours, and routine platelet transfusions are not indicated.[20]

Steroids are not recommended in the management of severe dengue; the evidence for this comes from a series of small trials performed in the 1970s and 1980s. The total number of patients with severe dengue randomized to steroids (each study used a different form of steroid in varying doses, and not all studies were controlled) in the international literature is 150 in 5 published studies.[21-25] Most of these reported no benefit in the small number of patients investigated, although one trial reported a remarkable reduction in mortality.[21] The evidence from these five studies would not now be considered sufficiently robust on which to base a global recommendation.

Clinically significant fluid overload develops in several situations associated with dengue infection and circulatory failure. Echocardiograms may help to determine cardiac function and output in patients who have persistent shock. Most commonly, it follows either administration of IV fluid in excessive amounts or too rapidly to patients with moderate capillary leak or continued parenteral fluid therapy when leak has resolved and the reabsorptive phase of the disease has begun. Rarely, it may be seen in patients with catastrophic capillary leak for whom support of circulation is not possible without administration of large volumes of fluid. Finally, fluid overload may occur in patients with underlying chronic diseases, particularly cardiac or renal disorders. Careful attention to treatment guidelines and frequent reassessment of the patient should help limit the occurrence of iatrogenic fluid overload, whereas early identification of the rare patient with catastrophic leak or severe underlying disease may allow preemptive intervention before significant respiratory compromise occurs.

Early signs of respiratory compromise include tachypnea and evidence of ascites and pleural effusions. Pulmonary edema, cyanosis, and respiratory failure are late manifestations. In addition, severe fluid overload may compromise cardiac function, resulting in hypotension and circulatory failure. Measurement of central venous pressure is helpful in differentiating between hemodynamic instability resulting from severe volume overload and instability caused by inadequate treatment of the underlying hypovolemia. However, great caution should be taken with use of CVP catheters in dengue and should only be inserted by experienced clinicians and with careful attention to post insertion bleeding at the site. They should be removed as soon as possible.

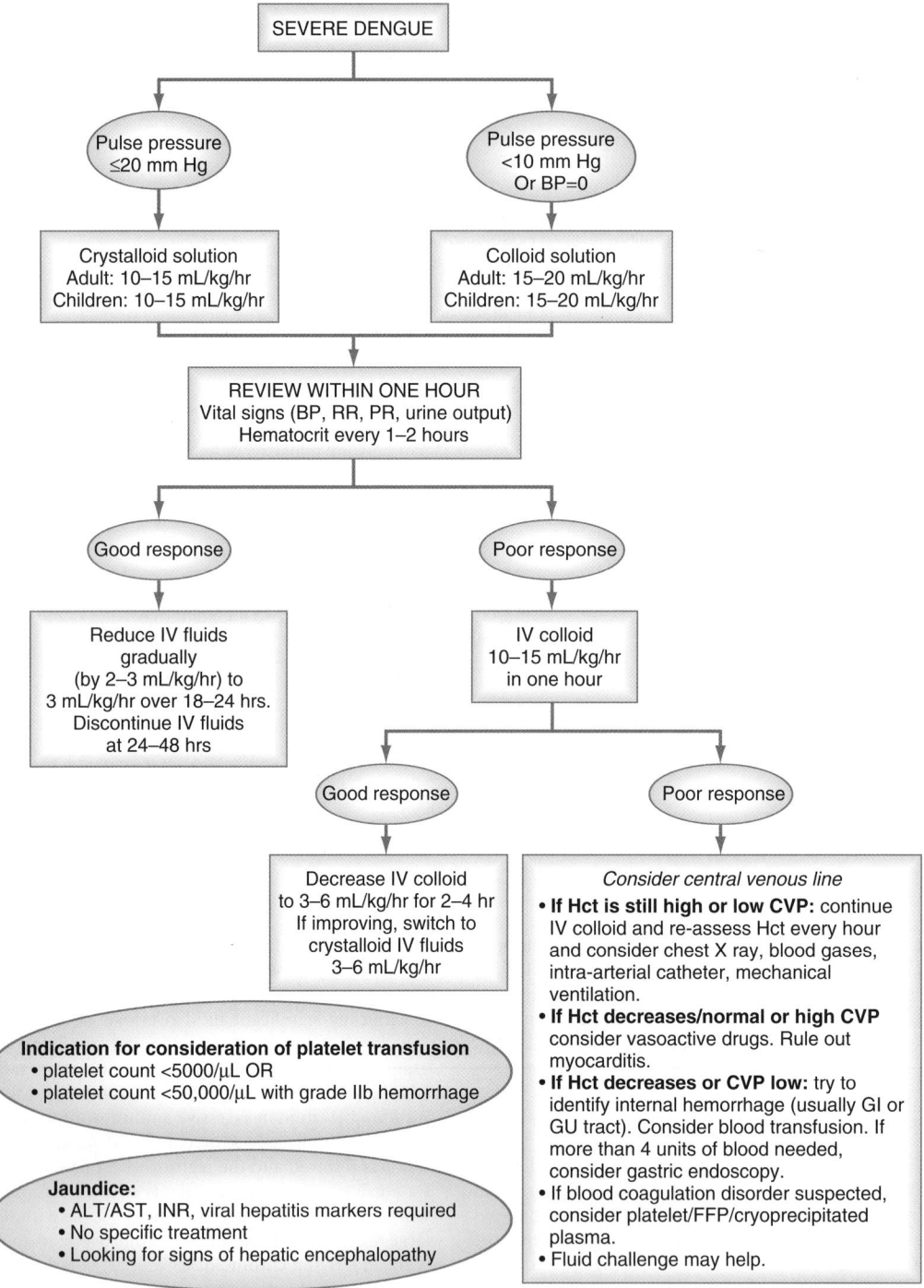

Figure 149-3, Cont'd.

■ Conclusion

Over the past 40 years, the incidence of dengue infections, particularly the more severe forms including DSS, has increased dramatically, and dengue is now one of the most common reasons for hospital admission in Asia and the Americas during the rainy seasons. The mortality rate for patients admitted with established DSS is 1% to 5%, even with the best available care. Again, the most important clinical feature of dengue is increased vascular permeability leading to DSS. Infants and young children are particularly prone to the development of shock, and adults are at increased risk of bleeding. Prompt but judicious fluid resuscitation in DSS is the most important therapeutic intervention. Regular clinical assessment of patients is essential. Dengue has a very dynamic clinical progression, and it is unacceptable to guide therapy on the basis of blood results taken hours earlier. It is imperative that frequent measurements be made, patients be continuously assessed, and treatment be modified in light of the clinical situation and results. Ideally the Hct should be measured on the ward (or the results made available immediately). Overzealous resuscitation in the presence of ongoing capillary leak must be avoided.

KEY POINTS

1. Dengue is the most widely distributed mosquito-borne viral infection of humans, affecting an estimated 100 million people worldwide each year, with 40% (2.5 billion) of the world's population estimated to be at risk for infection. Dengue should be considered in any patient with fever, particularly if there is a recent travel history to endemic regions.

2. Dengue severity exists as a continuous spectrum of dengue through to severe dengue. Of the many clinical features associated with severe dengue, from the standpoint of threat to life and guiding clinical intervention, the most important is increased vascular permeability leading to the dengue shock syndrome (DSS).

3. During the critical phase of illness, regular review (every 15-30 minutes) of vital signs—pulse rate, blood pressure, respiratory rate, peripheral temperature—and hematocrit at least every 2 hours is essential.

4. The mainstay of treatment is prompt, vigorous, but judicious fluid resuscitation. If appropriate volume resuscitation is instituted at an early stage, shock is usually reversible. Careful clinical judgment is required throughout the patient's stay in the hospital to maintain an effective circulation while assiduously avoiding fluid overload.

ANNOTATED REFERENCES

Hales S, de Wet N, Maindonald J, Woodward A. Potential effect of population and climate changes on global distribution of dengue fever: an empirical model. Lancet 2002;360:830-4.
There is clear evidence that the world's climate is changing. There has been much interest in the impact this change will have on the distribution of diseases, particularly vector-borne diseases. Projections for the future spread of dengue using conservative predictions of changes in humidity and population suggest that 4.1 billion people (44% of the world's population) will be at risk for dengue by 2055.

Gubler DJ. Cities spawn epidemic dengue viruses. Nat Med 2004;10:129-30.
An excellent review of one of the main drivers of the spread of dengue, global urbanization and travel.

Halstead SB. Pathogenesis of dengue: challenges to molecular biology. Science 1988;239:476-81.
This remains the best overview of the hypothesis of antibody-dependent enhancement. Dengue viruses replicate in cells of mononuclear phagocyte lineage, and subneutralizing concentrations of dengue antibody enhance dengue virus infection in these cells. This antibody-dependent enhancement of infection regulates dengue disease in humans, although disease severity also may be controlled genetically, possibly by permitting and restricting the growth of virus in monocytes.

Cummings DA, Iamsirithaworn S, Lessler JT, McDermott A, Prasanthong R, Nisalak A, et al. The impact of the demographic transition on dengue in Thailand: insights from a statistical analysis and mathematical modeling. PLoS Med 2009;6:e1000139. Epub 2009 Sep 1.
There is increasing and welcome integration and application of mathematics and modeling in dengue. This paper seeks to understand the rapidly changing and increasing age spectrum of patients with dengue in Southeast Asia. Recent demographic change reducing the force of infection is leading to a shift in the pattern of the age of patients with dengue. This has very important implications for many aspects of dengue, planning of clinical services, public health, vaccines, and therapeutics.

Wills BA, Nguyen MD, Ha TL, Dong TH, Tran TN, Le TT, et al. Comparison of three fluid solutions for resuscitation in dengue shock syndrome. N Engl J Med 2005;353:877-89.
The largest clinical trial of fluid resuscitation in DSS is reported. Initial resuscitation with Ringer's lactate is indicated for children with moderately severe DSS. Dextran 70 and 6% hydroxyethyl starch performed similarly in children with severe shock, but given the adverse reactions associated with the use of dextran, starch may be the best option. Further randomized controlled trials of treatment of dengue are needed. Clinical trials in dengue have been neglected.

REFERENCES

Access the complete reference list online at http://www.expertconsult.com.

Hematology/Oncology

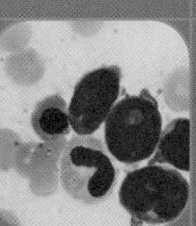

150

Anemia and Red Blood Cell Transfusion in Critically Ill Patients

PAUL C. HÉBERT | ALAN TINMOUTH

Anemia is a common problem in critically ill patients admitted to intensive care units (ICUs).[1] Indeed, in a recent cross-sectional study, 29% of patients had a hemoglobin concentration below normal values, and 37% required a red blood cell (RBC) transfusion.[2] Allogeneic RBC transfusions are complex biological products prepared from individual blood donations and are unique in many respects when compared with other health interventions. Decisions concerning the use of RBC transfusion in the treatment of anemia and hemorrhage require a clear understanding of the risks and benefits of both the condition and its treatment. Although we have developed a much clearer appreciation of the infectious and immunomodulatory risks of RBC transfusion over the past 2 decades, the risks of anemia in many clinical settings and the benefits of RBC transfusion are still inadequately characterized. We presume that the most significant risk associated with anemia is the harm resulting from the decrease in oxygen-carrying capacity and plasma volume. Development of adverse health consequences from anemia will in part depend on the capacity of the individual patient to compensate for these changes. The benefit of transfusion refers to the capacity of RBCs to correct these risks and possibly provide additional benefits such as increasing oxygen delivery to supranormal ranges. Such a framework highlights the concept of tradeoffs of risks and benefits. With the exception of patients who refuse blood for religious reasons, it is impossible outside a randomized clinical trial to distinguish clearly between these competing risks and benefits to patients.

Natural History of Uncorrected Anemia

Numerous laboratory experiments indicate that extreme hemodilution is well tolerated in healthy animals. Animals subjected to acute hemodilution tolerate decreasing hemoglobin concentrations down to 50 to 30 g/L, with ischemic electrocardiographic changes and depressed ventricular function, respectively, occurring at these levels of hemoglobin concentration.[3] However, acute hemodilution is less well tolerated in experimental animal models of coronary stenosis, with ischemic electrocardiographic changes and depressed cardiac function occurring at hemoglobin concentrations between 70 and 100 g/L. Human data regarding the limits of anemia tolerance are inadequate and often conflicting. Leung et al.[4] found electrocardiographic changes that may have been indicative of myocardial ischemia in 3 of 55 conscious resting volunteers subjected to acute isovolemic hemodilution to a hemoglobin concentration of 50 g/L.

While providing insight into the human physiologic response to acute anemia, the experimental data mentioned are of limited applicability to the perioperative setting, where many of the factors that influence oxygen consumption—muscle activity, body temperature, heart rate, sympathetic activity, metabolic state—are altered. Instead we need to determine the risk of withholding RBC transfusions in the perioperative setting. From a systematic review completed for the Canadian Guidelines on Red cells, Hébert and associates[5] identified numerous reports of severe anemia being well tolerated in surgical patients.[6,7] Additional reports or case series[8,9-11] describe successful outcomes in patients with chronic anemia due to renal failure. Finally, descriptive studies in patients refusing red blood cell transfusion[12-14,15] and from regions experiencing limited blood

supplies[16,17] have demonstrated that patients can survive surgical interventions with hemoglobin levels as low as 45 g/L.

In examining some of these studies in more detail, there appears to be an association between preoperative hemoglobin concentrations, intraoperative estimated blood loss, and postoperative mortality.[13,14] Indeed, there were no reported deaths in more than 100 patients undergoing major elective surgery when preoperative hemoglobin concentrations were above 80 g/L and the estimated blood loss was less than 500 mL. In a single-center series of 542 Jehovah's Witness patients undergoing a cardiac surgical procedure, the overall mortality rate was 10.7%; only 2.2% of the deaths observed were considered to be a direct consequence of anemia. More recently, Viele and Weiskopf[7] identified 134 Jehovah's Witness patients with a hemoglobin concentration less than 80 g/L or a hematocrit below 24% who were treated for various medical and surgical conditions without the use of blood or blood components. There were 50 reported deaths, 23 of which were attributed primarily or exclusively to anemia (defined as deaths with hemoglobin concentration < 50 g/L). For those patients who died of their anemia, 60% were older than 50 years. However, in 27 survivors with hemoglobin concentration below 50 g/L, 65% were younger than 50. Although publication bias must be kept in mind in examining these data, young healthy patients may survive without transfusion at hemoglobin concentrations in the range of 50 g/L. From these data, it is clear that extreme anemia is often tolerated in the perioperative setting but also appears to increase the risk of death. However, these observations should not be interpreted as support for a restrictive or conservative transfusion strategy, especially because most of the literature related to tolerance of anemia has not explored patient characteristics that predispose patients to adverse outcomes from moderate to severe anemia.

Anemia in High-Risk Groups

A number of risk factors for adverse outcomes associated with anemia have been identified in clinical practice guidelines[18-20] and reviews.[21-23] Anemia is thought to be less tolerated in older patients, in the severely ill, and in patients with clinical conditions such as coronary, cerebrovascular, or respiratory disease. However, the clinical evidence confirming that these factors are independently associated with an increased risk of adverse outcome is lacking. One small case-control study following high-risk vascular surgery suggests an increase in postoperative cardiac events with increasing severity of anemia.[24] In perioperative[25] and critically ill patients,[26] two large cohort studies have documented that increasing degrees of anemia were associated with a disproportionate increase in mortality rate in the subgroup of patients with cardiac disease. In 1958 Jehovah's Witness patients,[25] the adjusted odds of death increased from 2.3 (95% confidence interval [CI], 1.4-4.0) to 12.3 (95% CI, 2.5-62.1) as preoperative hemoglobin concentrations declined from the range of 100 to 109 g/L to the range of 60 to 69 g/L in patients with cardiac disease (Figure 150-1). There was no significant increase in mortality in noncardiac patients with comparable levels of anemia. In a separate study of critically ill patients,[26] those with cardiac disease and hemoglobin concentrations less than 95 g/L also had a trend toward an increased mortality rate (55% versus 42%; $P = .09$) as compared with anemic patients with other diagnoses.

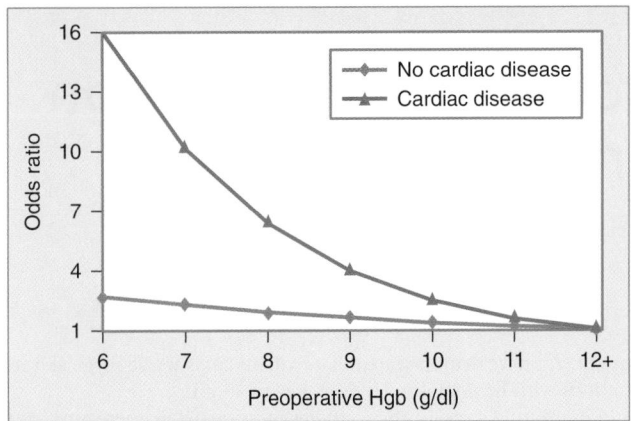

Figure 150-1 Adjusted odds ratio for mortality by cardiovascular disease and preoperative hemoglobin (Hgb). *(Adapted from Carson JL, Spence RK, Poses RM, Bonavita G. Severity of anemia and operative mortality and morbidity. Lancet 1988;1:727-9.)*

Although both cohort studies were retrospective in nature and may not have controlled for a number of important confounders, the evidence suggests that anemia increases the risk of death in patients with significant cardiac disease.

Severity of illness also appears to be a risk factor in critically ill patients.[13,26] Two retrospective studies document that degree of blood loss contributes to perioperative mortality.[13,26] However, there are no studies examining the independent contributions of age, cerebrovascular disease, and respiratory disease to an increased mortality risk in anemic patients. This relationship may well be complex, given that age and cerebrovascular disease are risk factors associated with coronary artery disease. Smoking-related respiratory diseases may have similar associations to cardiac disease. Therefore, the association between anemia and increased rates of adverse outcomes in these patients can best be described as speculative at this time.

Risks and Benefits of Transfusion

Five large observational studies that were specifically designed to compare clinical outcomes at varying hemoglobin concentrations in transfused and nontransfused patients have been conducted in various clinical settings. In the first of these, Hébert and colleagues[26] used a combined retrospective and prospective cohort design to examine 4470 critically ill patients admitted to 6 Canadian tertiary-level ICUs during 1993. After controlling for disease severity, there remained a trend toward increased mortality when hemoglobin concentrations were less than 95 g/L in patients with cardiac diagnoses (ischemic heart disease, arrhythmia, cardiac arrest, or cardiac and vascular surgical procedures). Furthermore, analysis of a subgroup of 202 patients with anemia, an Acute Physiology and Chronic Health Evaluation (APACHE) II score above 20, and a cardiac diagnosis revealed that transfusion of 1 to 3 units or 4 to 6 units of RBCs was associated with a significantly lower mortality rate as compared with those patients who did not receive a transfusion (55% [no transfusions] versus 35% [1-3 units] or 32% [4-6 units]; $P = .01$).

Wu et al.[27] retrospectively studied Medicare records of 78,974 patients older than age 65 who were hospitalized with a primary diagnosis of acute myocardial infarction. The authors then categorized patients according to their admitting hematocrit. Although anemia, defined in the study as a hematocrit less than 39%, was present in nearly half the patients, only 3680 patients received an RBC transfusion. Lower admission hematocrit values were associated with increased 30-day mortality rate, with a mortality rate approaching 50% among patients with a hematocrit of 27% or lower who did

not receive an RBC transfusion. Unfortunately, this study had no data on nadir hemoglobins and their relationship to mortality. Interestingly, RBC transfusion was associated with a reduction in 30-day mortality for patients who received at least one RBC transfusion if their admitting hematocrit was less than 33%, whereas RBC transfusion was associated with increased 30-day mortality for patients whose admitting hematocrit values were 36.1% or higher. These associations were present even when adjustments were made for clinical patient factors including APACHE II scores, location of myocardial infarction, and presence of congestive heart failure; as well as treatment factors including use of reperfusion therapies, aspirin, and β-adrenergic blockade.

In the only study exclusively focusing on the perioperative period, Carson and associates[28] attempted to determine the effect of perioperative transfusion on 30- and 90-day postoperative mortality with a retrospective cohort study involving 8787 patients with hip fractures undergoing repair between 1983 and 1993 in 20 different U.S. hospitals. This was a large, high-risk, elderly (median age 80.3 years) population with extensive coexisting disease and with an overall 30-day mortality rate of 4.6%. A total of 3699 patients (42%) received a perioperative transfusion within 7 days of the surgical repair. After controlling for trigger hemoglobin concentrations, cardiovascular disease, and other risk factors for death, the results suggested that patients who had hemoglobin concentrations as low as 80 g/L and did not receive transfusion were no more likely to die than those with similar hemoglobin concentration levels who received a transfusion. (With hemoglobin concentrations less than 80 g/L, nearly all patients received a transfusion, so investigators were unable to draw conclusions about the effect of transfusion at these lower hemoglobin concentrations levels.) However, as the authors point out, despite the large sample size, inadequate power may still explain the inability to detect a reduction in mortality related to transfusion, and they estimated that the study would need to be 10 times larger to detect a 10% difference in 30-day mortality with 80% power.

Vincent et al.[29] completed a prospective observational cross-sectional study involving 3534 patients admitted to 146 western European ICUs during a 2-week period in November 1999. Of these patients, 37% received an RBC transfusion during their ICU admission, with the overall transfusion rate increasing to 41.6% over a 28-day period. For those patients who received a transfusion, the mean pretransfusion hemoglobin concentration was 84 ± 13 g/L. In an effort to control for confounding factors created by illness severity and the need for transfusion, these investigators used a strategy of matching transfused and nontransfused patients based on their propensity to receive a transfusion, thereby defining two well-balanced groups (516 patients in each group) to determine the influence of RBC transfusions on mortality. Using this approach, the associated risk of death was increased instead of decreased by 33% for patients who received a transfusion compared to similar patients who did not receive blood. However, as pointed out in the accompanying editorial,[30] the results may have differed if the propensity scores were derived separately for categories of pretransfusion hemoglobin concentrations (e.g., <80, 80-100, and >100 g/L) instead of hemoglobin concentrations at ICU admission. For example, if one were to consider groups of patients with a pretransfusion hemoglobin concentration of less than 60 g/L, it is unlikely that the observed 33% increase in mortality would hold true, or blood transfusion would never be recommended.

Corwin and colleagues completed a similar prospective observational study evaluating 4486 patients admitted to 284 U.S. ICUs from August 2000 to April 2001. Overall, 44% patients were transfused RBCs, and the mean nadir hemoglobin was 8.6 ± 1.7 g/L. This study used logistic regression to evaluate the effects of transfusion on mortality. RBC transfusions of 1 to 2 units, 3 to 4 units, and more than 4 units were associated with increased odds ratio (OR) for mortality of 1.48 (95% CI, 1.07-2.05; $P = 0.018$), 2.62 (95% CI, 1.80-3.81; $P < 0.001$), and 4.01 (95% CI, 2.74-5.87; $P < 0.001$), respectively. Baseline hemoglobin levels were not significant in the logistic regression model, but a nadir hemoglobin below 9 g/L was associated with

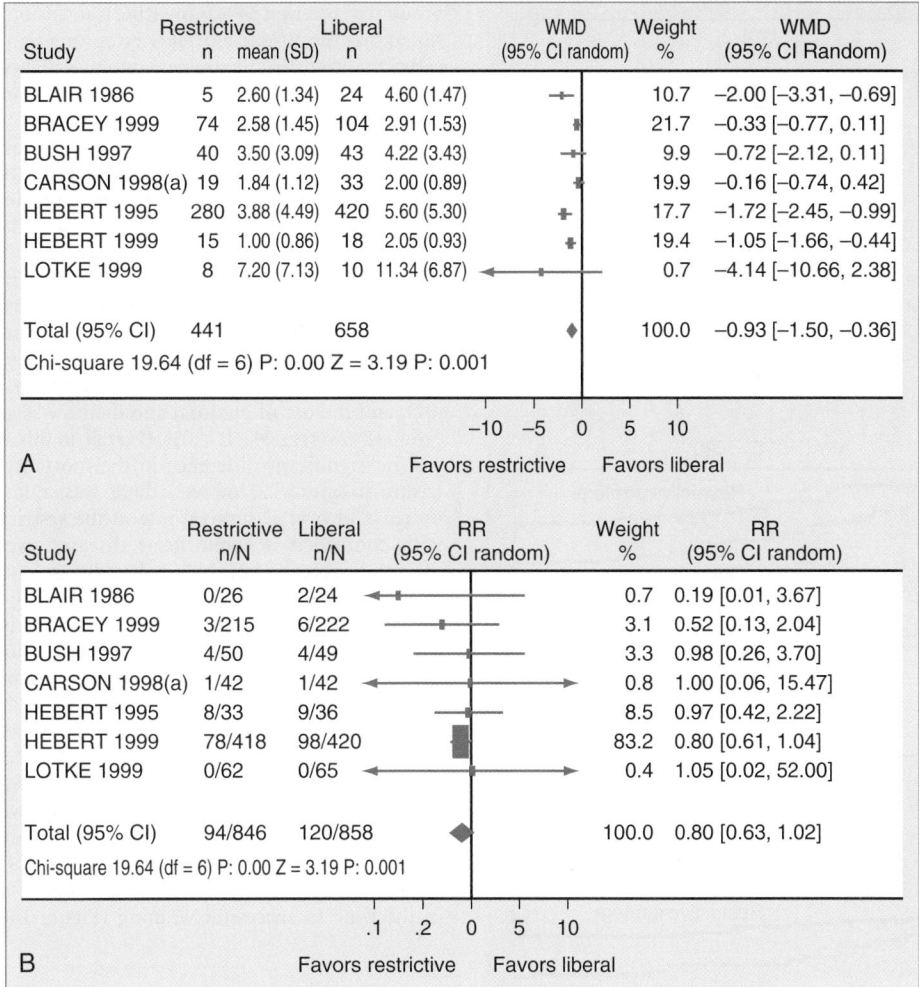

Study	Restrictive n	mean (SD)	Liberal n		WMD (95% CI random)	Weight %	WMD (95% CI Random)
BLAIR 1986	5	2.60 (1.34)	24	4.60 (1.47)		10.7	−2.00 [−3.31, −0.69]
BRACEY 1999	74	2.58 (1.45)	104	2.91 (1.53)		21.7	−0.33 [−0.77, 0.11]
BUSH 1997	40	3.50 (3.09)	43	4.22 (3.43)		9.9	−0.72 [−2.12, 0.11]
CARSON 1998(a)	19	1.84 (1.12)	33	2.00 (0.89)		19.9	−0.16 [−0.74, 0.42]
HEBERT 1995	280	3.88 (4.49)	420	5.60 (5.30)		17.7	−1.72 [−2.45, −0.99]
HEBERT 1999	15	1.00 (0.86)	18	2.05 (0.93)		19.4	−1.05 [−1.66, −0.44]
LOTKE 1999	8	7.20 (7.13)	10	11.34 (6.87)		0.7	−4.14 [−10.66, 2.38]
Total (95% CI)	441		658			100.0	−0.93 [−1.50, −0.36]
Chi-square 19.64 (df = 6) P: 0.00 Z = 3.19 P: 0.001							

−10 −5 0 5 10

A Favors restrictive   Favors liberal

Study	Restrictive n/N	Liberal n/N	RR (95% CI random)	Weight %	RR (95% CI random)
BLAIR 1986	0/26	2/24		0.7	0.19 [0.01, 3.67]
BRACEY 1999	3/215	6/222		3.1	0.52 [0.13, 2.04]
BUSH 1997	4/50	4/49		3.3	0.98 [0.26, 3.70]
CARSON 1998(a)	1/42	1/42		0.8	1.00 [0.06, 15.47]
HEBERT 1995	8/33	9/36		8.5	0.97 [0.42, 2.22]
HEBERT 1999	78/418	98/420		83.2	0.80 [0.61, 1.04]
LOTKE 1999	0/62	0/65		0.4	1.05 [0.02, 52.00]
Total (95% CI)	94/846	120/858		100.0	0.80 [0.63, 1.02]
Chi-square 19.64 (df = 6) P: 0.00 Z = 3.19 P: 0.001					

.1 .2 0 5 10

B Favors restrictive   Favors liberal

Figure 150-2 Effect of restrictive transfusion triggers on the use of allogeneic blood transfusion. **A,** Number of red cell units transfused. **B,** Proportion transfused/receiving red cells. (*Adapted from Carson JL, Hill S, Carless P et al. Transfusion triggers a systematic review of the literature. Trans Med Rev 2002;16:187-99.*)
WMD, Weighted mean difference.

increased mortality (nadir hemoglobin < 8 g/L: OR, 1.49; 95% CI, 1.13-1.95; $P = 0.004$; and nadir hemoglobin 8 to < 9 g/L: OR, 1.54; 95% CI, 1.12-2.12; $P = 0.009$). A second analysis using propensity scores matched 1059 transfused patients on a 1:1 basis with non-transfused patients based on baseline characteristics associated with a likelihood of receiving transfusions. The transfused patients had an adjusted mortality ratio of 1.65 (95% CI, 1.35-2.03; $P < 0.001$).

Numerous observational studies have examined the relationship between RBC transfusions and morbidity and mortality in critically ill patients. These studies have been recently summarized in a systematic review by Marik and Corwin[31]; 45 studies (including the previous 4 studies) involving 272,596 trauma, surgery, cardiac, and ICU patients were identified. Overall, 42 studies showed an increase in at least one of the outcomes of interest. Of the 18 studies that reported the relationship between RBC transfusions and mortality, 17 found an association between RBC transfusion and mortality, with a pooled OR of 1.7; 95% CI, 1.4-1.9. While these findings suggest that the risks associated with RBC transfusion may outweigh the benefits, the authors suggest caution in interpreting these data. Multivariate analysis was used in many of the observational studies to control for other clinical variables, but it is not possible to control for all factors, especially the fact that blood transfusion itself is a marker for severity of illness. The complex interrelationship between disease severity, number of transfusions, and degree of anemia may result in a spurious association reported between increased mortality risk and anemia or RBC transfusion. Thus, randomized controlled trials are required to

definitively determine the relationship between RBC transfusions and mortality.

Unfortunately, as evidenced by a recent systematic review, there is a paucity of clinical trials comparing restrictive to liberal transfusion studies to examine the efficacy of RBC transfusion. Carson et al.[32] (Figure 150-2) were able to identify only 10 randomized clinical trials of adequate methodological quality in which different RBC transfusion triggers were evaluated. Included were a total of 1780 surgery, trauma, and ICU patients enrolled in trials conducted over the past 40 years. The transfusion triggers evaluated in these trials varied between 70 and 100 g/L. Data on mortality or hospital length of stay were available in only 6 of these trials. Conservative (low hemoglobin) transfusion triggers were not associated with an increase in mortality rate; on average, the rate of mortality was one-fifth lower (relative risk [RR], 0.80; 95% CI, 0.63-1.02) with conservative as compared with liberal transfusion triggers. Likewise, cardiac morbidity and length of hospital stay did not appear to be adversely affected by the lower rate of RBC transfusions. There were insufficient data on potentially relevant clinical outcomes such as stroke, thromboembolism, multiorgan failure, delirium, infection, and delayed wound healing to perform any pooled analysis. The Carson review[28] stated there were insufficient data to address the full range of risks and benefits associated with different transfusion thresholds, particularly in patients with coexisting disease. They also noted that their meta-analysis was dominated by a single trial: the Transfusion Requirements in Critical Care (TRICC) trial,[33] which enrolled 838 patients and was the only individual trial identified

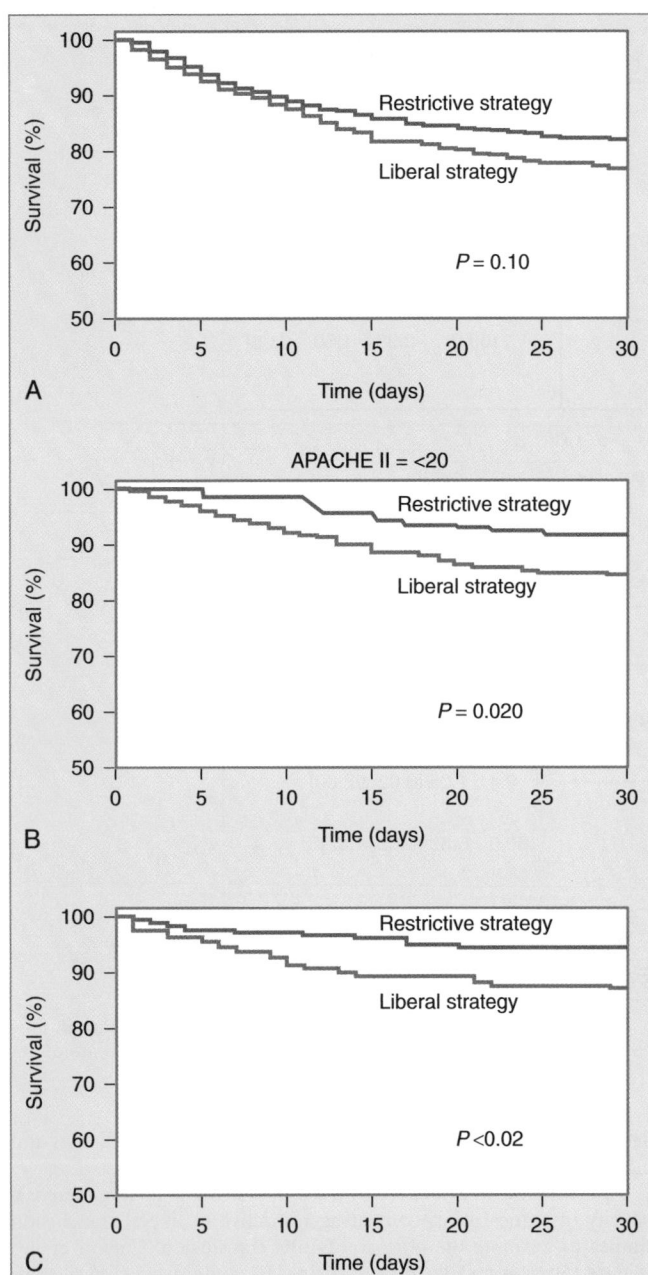

Figure 150-3 ICU survival over 30 days in study patients in restrictive and liberal allogeneic RBC transfusion strategy groups. **A,** Kaplan-Meier survival curves for all patients in both study groups. There is a trend toward lower mortality in patients in the restrictive group *(red line)* as compared to the liberal group *(purple line)* (*P* = .10). **B,** In the subgroup with an APACHE II score less than 20, fewer patients died in the restrictive group than in the liberal group (*P* = .02). **C,** There were also significant differences in survival among groups in the subgroup with ages less than 55 years (*P* = .02). *(Adapted from Hébert PC, Wells G, Blajchmann MA et al. A multicentre, randomized, controlled trial of transfusion requirements in critical care. N Engl J Med 1999;340:409-17.)*

that was adequately powered to evaluate the impact of different transfusion strategies on mortality and morbidity.

The TRICC Study[33] documented an overall non-significant trend toward decreased 30-day mortality (18.7 versus 23.3%; *P* = .11) and significant decreases in mortality among patients who were less acutely ill (8.7 versus 16.1%; *P* = .03) in the group treated using a hemoglobin transfusion trigger of 70 g/L compared with a more liberally transfused

group that received 54% more RBC transfusions. The investigators also noted that the 30-day mortality rates were significantly lower with the restrictive transfusion strategy among patients who were less acutely ill (APACHE II scores less than 20) and among patients who were younger than 55 years of age (Figure 150-3).

A number of additional questions arose from the TRICC trial. The investigators were particularly interested in the risks and benefits of anemia and transfusion in patients with cardiovascular disease and in patients attempting to wean from mechanical ventilation. In the first of these subgroup analyses,[34] 357 patients (43%) were identified with cardiovascular disease. Of these, 160 had been in the restrictive RBC transfusion group and 197 in the liberal transfusion group. The two groups were fairly equally balanced with regard to baseline characteristics and concurrent therapies, with a few exceptions: there was less frequent diuretic use in the restrictive group (43% versus 58%; *P* < .01), and the use of epidural anesthetics was greater in the restrictive group (8% versus 2%; *P* < .01). Overall, in this subgroup analysis, there was no significant difference in the mortality rate between the two treatment groups. However, there was a non-significant (*P* = .3) decrease in overall survival rate in the restrictive group for patients with confirmed ischemic heart disease, severe peripheral vascular disease, or severe comorbid cardiac disease.

The subgroup analysis of patients receiving mechanical ventilation was limited to 713 (85% of the 838 patients in the TRICC trial who required invasive mechanical ventilatory support).[35] Of these, 357 had been in the restrictive RBC transfusion group and 356 in the liberal group. The mean duration of mechanical ventilation was 8.3 ± 8.1 days in the restrictive group and 8.8 ± 8.7 days in the liberal group (*P* = .48). Ventilator-free days were 17.5 ± 10.9 and 16.1 ± 11.4 in the restrictive and liberal RBC transfusion groups, respectively (*P* = .09); 82% of the patients in the restrictive transfusion group were considered successfully weaned and extubated for at least 24 hours, compared with 78% in the liberal group (*P* = .19). Among the 219 patients who required mechanical ventilation for more than 7 days, there were no differences in the time to successful weaning (Figure 150-4). The independent

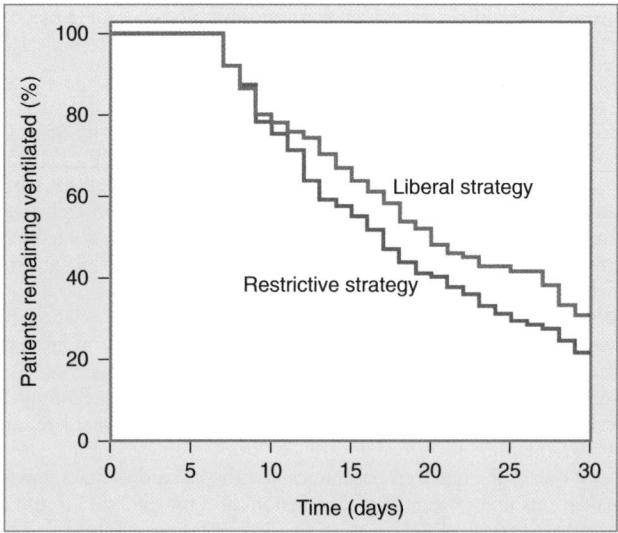

Figure 150-4 Time remaining on mechanical ventilation in 283 patients requiring mechanical ventilation for more than 1 week. Time to successful weaning from mechanical ventilation is illustrated using Kaplan-Meier survival curves in patients who required mechanical ventilation for more than 1 week. Weaning success is defined as remaining off mechanical ventilation once extubated during the 30 days of observation. Red line = restrictive group; purple line = liberal group. Survival curves were not statistically different when compared using a log rank test (*P* = .08). *(Adapted from Hébert PC, Blajchmann MA, Cook DJ et al. Do blood transfusions improve outcomes related to mechanical ventilation? Chest 2001;119:1850-7.)*

effects of RBC transfusions and hemoglobin concentration were also examined. Each additional transfusion was associated with an increased duration of mechanical ventilation (RR, 1.10; 95% CI, 1.14-1.06; P < .01) after adjusting for the effect of age, APACHE II score, and comorbid illnesses. Hemoglobin concentrations did not influence the duration of mechanical ventilation (RR, 0.99; 95% CI, 1.01-0.98; P = .45). Complications including pulmonary edema and acute respiratory distress syndrome (ARDS) were increased in patients in the liberal strategy group.

Recently, two other large randomized clinical trials have compared liberal and restrictive transfusion strategies in different populations. Lacroix and colleagues[36] undertook a non-inferiority trial comparing a restrictive (7.0 g/L) and a liberal (9.5 g/L) transfusion threshold in 648 pediatric ICU patients. There were no differences in new or progressive multiple-organ dysfunction (12% in both groups; absolute RR, 0.4%; 95% CI, −4.6 to 5.4) or the number of deaths (14 in each group).

Results from the recently completed FOCUS trial have also been reported. Carson et al. (Carson, ASH annual meeting 2010) randomized 2016 patients with a history or risk factors for cardiovascular disease who underwent surgery for hip fracture to symptomatic RBC transfusion (permitted if hemoglobin < 8 g/L) or a transfusion threshold of 10 g/L. The percentage of patients who were dead or unable to walk without assistance were identical in the two groups (35%), and there were no differences in 60-day mortality (OR, 1.19; 99% CI, 0.76-1.86).

Even though three large randomized controlled trials have been completed, a number of questions remain to be answered. One of the most important questions is why the liberal RBC transfusion strategy failed to improve 30-day mortality rate and rates of organ failure in critically ill patients. It is conceivable that the greater number of allogeneic RBC units in the liberal group significantly depressed host immune responses[35,37] or resulted in altered microcirculatory flow as a consequence of prolonged storage times.

Subsequent to the publication of the TRICC trial, a study by Rivers et al.[38] documented that the use of early goal-directed care based on a mixed central venous saturation (Scvo$_2$) decreased mortality from 46.5% in the control group to 30.5% in the goal-directed therapy group (P = .009). As one of the many interventions in patients with early septic shock, hematocrits were increased to greater than 30% if the Scvo$_2$ fell to less than 70%. As a consequence of goal-directed therapy, 64% of patients, compared to 18.5% of the control group, received RBC transfusions (P < .0001). The significant differences in patient populations studied by Rivers and colleagues and the TRICC trial may account for the apparently conflicting results between the studies. Results from the early goal-directed therapy study should be reproduced and better understood. In the interim, they highlight the need for further studies in subpopulations of critically ill patients.

Alternatives to Transfusion

Numerous strategies have been explored and are recommended to decrease or to eliminate the need for blood transfusions during major surgery and critical illness. Some are relatively benign, but others carry their own risks that must be weighed against the administration of RBCs. Alternatives include decreasing the use of medications that result in perioperative bleeding (e.g., nonsteroidal antiinflammatory drugs and acetylsalicylic acid), avoidance of unnecessary phlebotomy, use of blood conservation strategies (e.g., pediatric test tubes and arterial catheter reinfusion setups), medications to decrease blood loss (e.g., antifibrinolytic agents), and medications to increase hemoglobin production. In addition to a restrictive transfusion strategy, the two most useful approaches to decreasing RBC transfusions in critically ill patients appear to be blood conservation techniques such as decreased phlebotomies and erythropoietin therapy. Other therapeutic strategies are better suited to patients undergoing high-risk surgical procedures.

Decreased RBC production is one of the causes of anemia observed in the critically ill. Indeed, critical illness is characterized by blunted erythropoietin production and response.[39] This blunted erythropoietin response observed in critically ill patients appears to result from inhibition of the erythropoietin gene by inflammatory mediators.[40,41] It has also been shown that these same inflammatory cytokines directly inhibit RBC production by the bone marrow and may produce distinct abnormalities of iron metabolism.[42,43] In patients with multiple organ failure, recombinant human erythropoietin therapy (600 units/kg) has been shown to stimulate erythropoiesis.[44] Similarly, in a small randomized placebo-controlled trial (160 patients), therapy with recombinant human erythropoietin resulted in an almost 50% reduction in RBC transfusions compared to patients treated with a placebo.[45] Erythropoietin was given at a dose of 300 units/kg daily for 5 days followed by every-other-day dosing until ICU discharge. Despite receiving fewer RBC transfusions, patients in the recombinant human erythropoietin group had a significantly greater increase in hematocrit.

Recently the efficacy of recombinant human erythropoietin in critically ill patients was evaluated in two similar large randomized controlled trials involving a total of 2762 patients.[46,47] In the first trial, recombinant human erythropoietin was given weekly at a dose of 40,000 units. All patients received three weekly doses, and patients who remained in the ICU on study day 21 received a fourth dose. Treatment with recombinant human erythropoietin resulted in a 10% reduction in the number of patients receiving any RBC transfusions. The authors reported a 60.4% rate of transfusions following randomization in the placebo group, as compared with 50.5% in the recombinant human erythropoietin group (OR, 0.67; 95% CI, 0.54-0.83; P < .0004) and a 20% reduction in the total number of RBC units transfused in patients receiving recombinant human erythropoietin (P < .001). All clinical outcomes including mortality rates, rates of organ failure, and lengths of stay in the ICU and the hospital were comparable between groups (all P values > .05). A second large trial in 1460 critically ill patients randomly allocated patients to receive either 40,000 units/wk versus a placebo for a maximum of 3 weeks. This confirmatory trial did not find a significant decrease in mortality (OR, 0.72; 95% CI, 0.51-1.02). A systematic review incorporating results from 9 trials in 3326 critically ill patients documented a decrease in transfusions without affecting mortality rates (OR, 0.86; 95% CI, 0.71-1.05).[48] These studies and the systematic review[45-49] demonstrate that recombinant human erythropoietin therapy in critically ill patients can decrease in RBC transfusions and increase hemoglobin levels. This is consistent with the hypothesis that the anemia in critically ill patients is similar to the anemia of patients with chronic disease and is characterized at least in part by a relative erythropoietin deficiency.[50] However, given the high costs of erythropoietin and the lack of clinical benefit demonstrated in the randomized controlled trial, its use is not recommended as a blood conservation strategy in routine practice.

Conclusions

Despite the frequent use of RBC transfusions, only three large randomized trials have examined RBC administration in postoperative and critically ill patients. Together, they consistently document that a restrictive transfusion strategy is safe and minimizes red cell use in critically ill adults and children as well as postoperative patients. However, there is insufficient evidence in early septic shock or in patients with a myocardial infarction or acute coronary syndromes. In addition, most transfusion practice guidelines published prior to completion of the TRICC trial[32-34] are now dated and warrant expert opinion by solid evidence in diverse clinical settings. Still, high-quality clinical evidence is not yet available for many decisions related to RBC transfusions. In terms of alternatives, human recombinant erythropoietin should not be widely used in critically ill patients. We anticipate that risks and benefits of red cells and alternatives will be better elucidated in the coming years.

Recommendations

1. Adopt a transfusion threshold of 70 g/L in volume-resuscitated critically ill patients, including patients with a history of coronary artery disease and septic shock after initial resuscitation.

2. Similar recommendations would hold in critically ill children and in postoperative patients.

3. Aim to maintain patients' hemoglobin concentration between 70 and 90 g/L.

4. Transfuse 1 RBC unit at a time, and measure after every transfusion.

5. Insufficient evidence does not allow for specific recommendations in patients with acute coronary syndromes (acute myocardial infarction and unstable angina) and patients with early septic shock.

6. Erythropoietin is not recommended in critically ill patients without another indication for its use (such as chronic renal failure).

KEY POINTS

1. Anemia has an incidence ranging from 29% to 37% in critically ill patients.

2. Patients with ischemic heart disease may be at increased risk of adverse clinical consequences if also anemic.

3. Restrictive transfusion strategies decrease the need for red blood cell transfusions without adverse clinical consequences.

4. Further studies are required in patients with acute coronary syndromes and early septic shock.

ANNOTATED REFERENCES

Corwin HL, Krantz SB. Anemia of the critically ill: "acute" anemia of chronic disease. Crit Care Med 2000;28:3098-9.
  Good review article.
Napolitano LM, Corwin HL. Efficacy of red blood cell transfusion in the critically ill. Crit Care Clin 2004;20:255-68.
  This article evaluates the literature on the efficacy of RBC transfusions in the critically ill. It concludes the RBC transfusion does not improve tissue oxygen consumption consistently in critically ill patients; it is not associated with improvements in clinical outcome and may result in worse outcomes in some patients. Specific factors that identify patients who will improve from RBC transfusion are difficult to identify, and lack of efficacy of RBC transfusion likely is related to storage time, increased endothelial adherence of stored RBCs, nitric oxide binding by free hemoglobin in stored blood, donor leukocytes, host inflammatory response, and reduced red cell deformability. Taken together, these studies generally support conservative RBC transfusion strategies in critical care to reduce the risk of transfusion-related adverse effects.

REFERENCES

Access the complete reference list online at http://www.expertconsult.com.

151 Blood Component Therapies

JAMES P. ISBISTER

Blood component therapy has had a central role in the development and practice of numerous medical advances, especially in modern surgery. It is only in more recent years that blood transfusion is no longer regarded as essential for a wide range of medical and surgical conditions. It is now possible for most uncomplicated major surgery to be conducted without allogeneic blood component therapy.[1] *Blood component transfusion* is generally supportive therapy for the correction of one or more hematologic deficiencies until the basic disease process can be controlled or corrected. Appropriate attention to accurate diagnosis of the hematopoietic deficiency and consideration of the range of therapeutic options available and their potential hazards are essential before accepting blood component therapy as indicated.[2]

Blood component therapy and its immediate endpoints are part of a medical management process. Although appropriate endpoints may be achieved in terms of measurable parameters or immediate clinical response, the clinician needs evidence that these traditional surrogate endpoints are relevant and correlate with a beneficial final clinical outcome for the patient. The human immunodeficiency virus (HIV) crisis shocked clinical medicine into a realization that there were many transfusion practices exposing patients to potential hazards without evidence for identifiable short-term or long-term benefits.

Evidence-based medicine is increasingly influencing the practice of transfusion medicine. In many areas of transfusion medicine, evidence from prospective randomized trials is not available, and the clinician must base therapy on a good understanding of the problem in terms of pathophysiology and indicators of severity. Transfusion medicine decision making can be difficult, and there is ongoing debate regarding the indications for various allogeneic blood components. Unnecessary allogeneic transfusion can be avoided or minimized by giving attention to the clinical time frame, hematologic defect, alternatives, and knowledge about blood components and the potential hazards. There have been considerable advances in minimizing allogeneic transfusion and the development of "transfusion alternatives." The concept of transfusion alternatives can be challenged as inappropriate, as most of the so-called alternatives are indeed optimal patient management. Emphasis away from the blood component to a focus on the patient's blood (i.e., patient blood management) is the new paradigm. In managing a patient's oxygen-carrying capacity, a three-pillar approach—optimizing red cell mass, minimizing blood loss, and tolerating anemia in the short term—results in avoidance of allogeneic transfusion in most uncomplicated elective surgical cases. This can be achieved by identifying patients at high bleeding risk, giving attention to surgical and anesthetic techniques (e.g., controlled hypotension, hypothermia prevention, reduction of venous pressure at operative site), and using pharmacologic agents to minimize blood loss. Autologous methodologies including perioperative hemodilution, blood salvage, fibrin glue, and platelet fibrin gel all may have a part to play.

Guidelines for Blood Component Therapy

The following is a brief summary of the guidelines for use of commonly available blood components. An evidence-based approach to blood component transfusion has resulted in many long-standing transfusion dogmas being challenged and better guidelines for their use being developed for safe, effective clinical practice. Figure 151-1

illustrates the general approach to the decision to transfuse blood components, with the emphasis on patient blood management and how blood component therapy fits into the bigger picture.[1]

RED BLOOD CELL CONCENTRATES

Appropriate and inappropriate use of red blood cell (RBC) transfusions in acute medicine has received considerable attention in recent years; however, identifying the benefits of RBC transfusion in many circumstances has been difficult.[2-3] The question of the lowest safe hematocrit continues to receive considerable attention. Pushing any aspect of a system to its limits risks "sailing close to the wind" and may be appropriate in some situations but potentially hazardous in others. In an otherwise stable patient, the transfusion of RBC concentrates is likely to be inappropriate when the hemoglobin level is above 100 g/L. Their use may be appropriate when hemoglobin is in the range 70 to 100 g/L if there are other defects in the oxygen transport system. The decision to transfuse should be supported by the need to relieve clinical signs and symptoms of impaired oxygen transport and to prevent morbidity and mortality, ultimately to improve clinical outcomes. The transfusion of RBC concentrates is likely to be appropriate when hemoglobin is less than 70 g/L and the anemia is not reversible with specific therapy in the short term, but lower levels may be acceptable in patients who are asymptomatic, especially in the younger age group.

PLATELET CONCENTRATES

Platelet transfusions may benefit patients with platelet deficiency or dysfunction, and there are some general recommendations for their use.[4] Prophylactic transfusion of platelet concentrates is indicated in patients with bone marrow failure when the platelet count is (1) less than 10×10^9/L and there are no associated risk factors for bleeding or (2) less than 20×10^9/L in the presence of additional risk factors. However, recent evidence suggests lower levels may be tolerated if there is no clinical evidence of hemostatic failure.

In patients undergoing surgery or invasive procedures, the platelet count should be maintained at greater than 50×10^9/L. In patients with qualitative defects in platelet function, platelet count is not a reliable indicator for transfusion, and transfusion decisions and monitoring of efficacy should be based on the setting and clinical features.

Platelet transfusions are indicated in hemorrhaging patients in whom thrombocytopenia is secondary to marrow failure and is considered a contributory factor to the bleeding. In massively hemorrhaging patients, platelet transfusions in conjunction with correcting plasma coagulation factor deficits are indicated when the platelet count is less than 50×10^9/L or less than 100×10^9/L in the presence of diffuse microvascular bleeding. The transfusion of platelet concentrates is not generally considered appropriate when thrombocytopenia is due to immune-mediated destruction, in patients with thrombotic thrombocytopenic purpura and hemolytic uremic syndrome, or in uncomplicated cardiac bypass surgery.

FRESH FROZEN PLASMA AND CRYOPRECIPITATE

Fresh frozen plasma is widely used, but there are limited specific indications for its use, and there is a dearth of evidence for efficacy in many clinical settings.[5-6] The use of fresh frozen plasma may be

1133

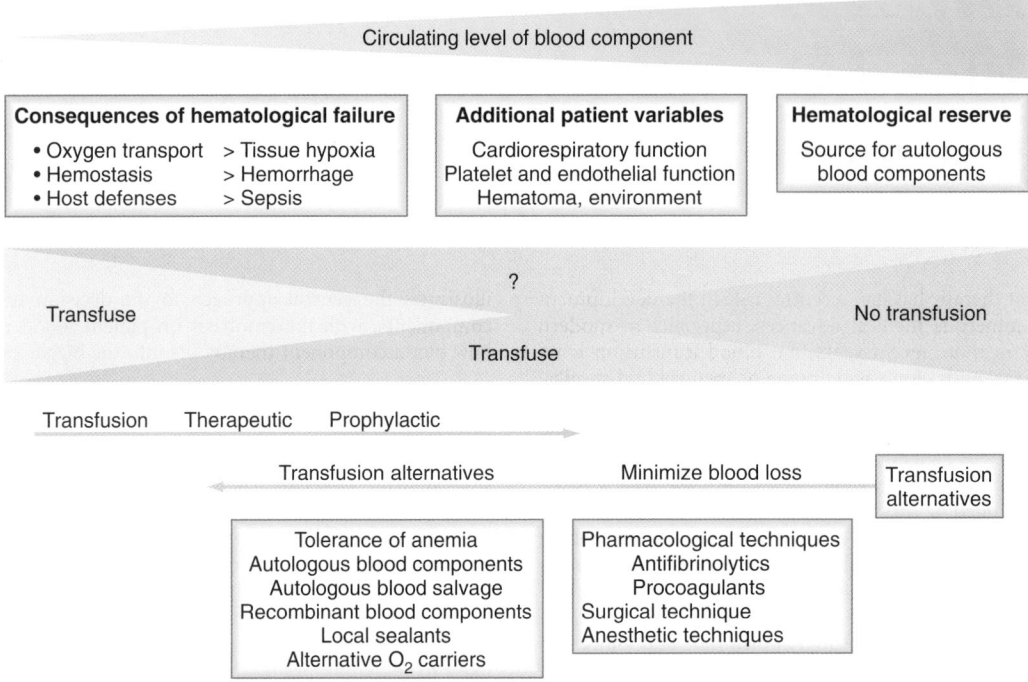

Figure 151-1 Overview of blood management and where blood component therapy may be appropriate.

appropriate in patients with a coagulopathy who are bleeding or at risk for bleeding when a specific therapy or factor concentrates are not appropriate or unavailable. Fresh frozen plasma generally is indicated in hemorrhaging patients for replacement of labile plasma coagulation factors (e.g., massive transfusion, cardiac bypass, liver disease, or acute disseminated intravascular coagulation [DIC]). Fresh frozen plasma is rarely indicated in vitamin K deficiency or reversal of warfarin therapy, because concentrates are now generally available.[7] The use of fresh frozen plasma generally is not considered appropriate in cases of hypovolemia, in plasma exchange procedures (unless post-exchange invasive procedures are planned), or in treatment of immunodeficiency states.

Compatibility tests before transfusion are not necessary, but plasma should be ABO group compatible with the patient's RBCs, and volume transfused depends on the clinical situation and patient size. As a guide, initial dosing of 10 to 15 mL/kg is recommended, and efficacy should be monitored by laboratory tests of coagulation function.

Cryoprecipitate is prepared by thawing fresh frozen plasma between 1°C and 6°C and recovering the precipitate, which is refrozen. The component contains factor VIII, fibrinogen, factor XIII, von Willebrand factor, and fibronectin and is principally indicated for fibrinogen deficiency or dysfibrinogenemia when there is clinical bleeding, invasive procedures, trauma, or acute DIC. The role for cryoprecipitate will diminish as fibrinogen concentrates become increasingly used for hypofibrinogenemic states. Cryoprecipitate should not be used for the treatment of hemophilia or von Willebrand disease unless factor concentrates are unavailable.

PLASMA-DERIVED PRODUCTS

A wide range of highly purified plasma-derived blood products is available for use in numerous clinical conditions. It is beyond the scope of this chapter to discuss their use in detail; Table 151-1 summarizes commonly used fresh and plasma-derived blood products. Fibrinogen concentrate instead of cryoprecipitate is having an increasing role in the management of hypofibrinogenemic states, depending on local availability.

RECOMBINANT BLOOD PRODUCTS

Development and introduction of recombinant blood components continues to be one of the most exciting advances in transfusion medicine. Recombinant growth factors (cytokines) such as erythropoietin and granulocyte stimulating factors have had a major impact on managing anemia and neutropenia. There are further promising recombinant cytokines in development that could have a role in countless clinical conditions, especially as antiinflammatory and tissue-protecting agents. Recombinant hemostatic factors have improved the management of hemophilia, and recent expansion of clinical indications for the use of recombinant activated factor VII (factor VIIa)— beyond treating hemophiliac patients with coagulation factor inhibitors—is having an impact on management of a range of hemostatic disorders.[8] Because factor VIIa is dependent on tissue factor, which is usually available in limited quantities within the circulation, its clinical use is generally regarded safe from a thrombosis-inducing point of view, and its use is now being recommended as a "panhemostatic agent." Factor VIIa initiates the extrinsic coagulation pathway only when complexed to tissue factor at sites of injury. It may have a role in a wide range of hemostatic disorders (e.g., massive blood transfusion, liver disease, uremia, severe thrombocytopenia, and platelet disorders). It has been difficult to establish a sound evidence base outside the hemophilia setting for the use of rVIIa, with most experience being observational and anecdotal. Randomized controlled trial results have shown a significant reduction in transfusion requirements but could not demonstrate a reduction in mortality. There is also an increased risk of thromboembolism.

BLOOD SUBSTITUTES

Efforts have been ongoing for many years to develop substitutes for RBCs and platelets, but results have been disappointing, and safety concerns have plagued clinical development. The development of substitutes for cellular blood components has also been slow, and as their introduction into clinical medicine remains in the research phase, the reader is referred to reviews for further information.

TABLE 151-1	Blood Products
Blood Product	**Main Indications**
Whole blood*	Rarely indicated in acute hemorrhage if other blood products are unavailable
Red blood cell concentrates*	Hemorrhage and anemia
Leukocyte-depleted blood*	In patients having febrile reactions, to avoid leukocyte immunization in selected patients (especially patients with hematologic malignancy). Universal prestorage leukodepletion is more widely used and has the added benefit of minimizing storage lesions.
Platelet concentrates*	Thrombocytopenia due to marrow hypoplasia or platelet functional defect
Granulocyte concentrates*	Occasionally in patients with sepsis associated with profound and prolonged neutropenia secondary to marrow suppression
Fresh frozen plasma*	Specific or multiple plasma protein deficiencies (especially coagulation)
Cryoprecipitate*	Hypofibrinogenemia and rarely in factor VIII and von Willebrand disease, when concentrates are unavailable
4% or 5% albumin solutions†	Plasma volume expansion. Use is controversial, and the role of albumin solutions in critically ill patients remains under deliberation.[30]
Concentrated albumin†	Severe hypoalbuminemic states with complicating hypovolemia
Concentrate of coagulation factors II, VII, IX, and X†	Vitamin K–dependent factor II, IX, and X deficiency and reversal of oral vitamin K antagonists[31]
Specific factor concentrates†	Factor VIII and IX concentrates have an established role in management of hemophilia, but others are in the process of establishing their clinical efficacy and indications. Fibrinogen concentrates for hypofibrinogenemia and dysfibrinogenemia[32] Antithrombin concentrates are available for thrombophilia due to antithrombin deficiency and are increasingly recommended in other disorders in which antithrombin may be depleted (e.g., DIC, MODS).[31]
Gamma globulin†	Generally used intravenously for replacement in hypogammaglobulinemia or in high dosage in autoimmune disorders[33]
Specific immune gamma globulins†	Rhesus prophylaxis, specific infection prophylaxis (e.g., tetanus, zoster, hepatitis B)

*Fresh products.
†Fractionated plasma products.
DIC, disseminated intravascular coagulation; *MODS*, multiorgan dysfunction syndrome.

Transfusion Management of Massive Acute Hemorrhage

In recent years there has been a reappraisal of guidelines for the use of blood components in acutely hemorrhaging patients. Guidelines are more focused on managing critical bleeding and avoiding the massive transfusion coagulopathy quagmire in which a patient spirals down into the "triad of death": coagulopathy, acidosis, and hypothermia. Advances in patient retrieval, resuscitation protocols, techniques for rapid and real-time diagnosis, trauma teams, and early "damage-control" surgery have improved the management of acutely hemorrhaging patients. There is also greater attention and research being directed toward the nature of clear fluids and the importance of plasma viscosity, colloid oncotic pressure, and functional capillary density. Patients are now surviving increasingly larger volumes of blood transfusion, but sepsis, acute lung injury, and multiorgan failure remain challenges. Immediate lifesaving blood transfusion is increasingly being recognized as an independent risk factor for delayed morbidity and mortality.

Transfusion can be minimized with tolerance of hypotension until hemorrhage is controlled and acceptance of lower hemoglobin levels.

The immediate posttransfusion function of stored red cells and hemoglobin in delivering oxygen to microcirculation and in oxygen unloading is also being questioned, with the storage age of RBCs possibly being associated with poorer clinical outcomes.[9] Recent animal data point to the immediate clinical benefit of transfused red cells in treating hypovolemic shock relating more to reconstitution of the macrocirculation, with potentially adverse effects on the functional capillary density in the microcirculation.

A protocol approach to blood component therapy has generally not been recommended. However, this remains a controversial issue, with advocates for up-front protocol component therapy with red cell and hemostatic components, especially fresh frozen plasma with or without cryoprecipitate. With better understanding of coagulopathy in the critical hemorrhage setting and the importance of hypofibrinogenemia and hyperfibrinolysis, there is a reanalysis of the approach to blood component therapy. Failure of hemostasis is common in acutely bleeding patients and may be complex and multifactorial. Accumulating evidence supports the view that the pathophysiology of coagulopathy, when occurring in the context of critical hemorrhage, should be viewed as related to the primary insult or initiating event. A secondary coagulopathy may compound the problem in the resuscitated patient, such as massive stored blood transfusion, hemodilution, hypothermia, and continuing tissue hypoxia.[10-11] The primary mechanisms of coagulopathy relating to the initiating event may relate to trauma, hypoxia, pregnancy, sepsis, envenomation, or antithrombotic agents.[12-13] In all circumstances there is activation or inhibition of some aspect of the hemostatic system, and therapy is better informed if these varied mechanisms are better understood. Frequently, complex tests are required for definitive diagnosis, but the urgency of the situation cannot always wait for the results, and therapy may be initiated on clinical evidence with minimal laboratory information.

Many trauma patients have coagulopathy at presentation related to hypovolemic shock and not consumption or dilution. Recent evidence indicates that activation of the protein C system and hypofibrinogenemia due to secondary hyperfibrinolysis are important.[14] Except when severe clotting test abnormalities are present, hemostatic laboratory parameters correlate poorly with clinical evidence of hemostatic failure. In the massively transfused patient, thrombocytopenia and impaired platelet function are the most consistent significant hematologic abnormalities, correction of which may be associated with control of microvascular bleeding. A problem with standard screening tests of coagulation function is they do not provide information about the formation of the hemostatic plug, its size, structure, or stability. Global tests of hemostatic plug formation and stability such as thromboelastography, thrombin generation tests, and clot waveform analysis in which changes in light transmission in routine activated partial thromboplastin time (APTT) are measured are of increasing use. With ongoing bleeding with associated microvascular oozing, various approaches may be taken. Having ensured that all identifiable hemostatic defects have been corrected, questions then arise as to the role of fresh blood and, more recently, recombinant activated factor VII.

Hazards of Allogeneic Transfusion

It cannot be overemphasized that allogeneic blood transfusion is a tissue transplant that is probably associated with the greatest range of potential hazards of any medical intervention and should only be used in circumstances in which there is good evidence that clinical outcomes will be improved.[15-16]

The pathophysiology of transfusion reactions can be divided broadly into three categories:

1. Reactions may occur due to *immunologic differences* between the donor and recipient, resulting in varying degrees of blood component incompatibility. In general, for a reaction to occur, the recipient needs to have been previously immunized to a cellular or plasma antigen.[17]
2. A wide range of *infectious agents* may be transmitted by allogeneic blood component therapy.

3. *Alterations in blood products due to preservation and storage* may result in quantitative or qualitative deficiencies in the blood components that reduce transfusion efficacy and expose the patient to potentially adverse consequences from substances that accumulated during storage (Table 151-2).

In terms of causation of an adverse clinical event, the possible role of transfusion can be classified broadly into three categories on the basis of probability (Figure 151-2):

1. *Definite—unifactorial.* The well-understood and well-reported hazards of transfusion (i.e., immunologic, technical, infectious) are generally unifactorial, with a 1:1 well-understood deterministic causal relationship between the blood component transfused (usually a specific individual unit) and the adverse consequence for the patient. ABO blood group incompatibility, transfusion-related infection transmission, transfusion-associated graft-versus-host disease, and transfusion-related lung injury due to donor leukoagglutinins are examples in this category.

2. *Probable—oligofactorial.* Some adverse consequences of transfusion result from interaction with other insults, pathophysiology, or host factors, but the contribution of the transfusion usually can be specifically identified in a deterministic manner. Fever, allergic reactions, hypotensive reactions, pulmonary edema, some cases of transfusion-related lung injury, hyperbilirubinemia, and cytomegalovirus transmission are examples of this category.

3. *Possible—multifactorial.* Transfusion may contribute to a complication or poor clinical outcome. In these circumstances, a causal implication for transfusion is probabilistic (i.e., a risk factor), and it is not necessarily the major factor. Transfusion-induced immunomodulation and the clinical consequences of storage lesions fall into this category. The role of transfusion contributing to adverse clinical outcomes can only be identified from observational studies using powerful multifactorial statistical analysis, although some supportive evidence is available from a limited number of randomized controlled clinical trials.[17] Potential adverse clinical consequences of the storage lesions fall into this group, with product preparation method, dosage, and age of blood component being relevant.[9] Prevention of complications from the storage lesion and immunomodulation focus on the quality of preservation and minimizing transfusion rather than elimination of the risk, as is the case with ABO incompatibility or HIV.

TABLE 151-2	Red Blood Cell Storage Lesions and Possible Clinical Consequences
Storage Lesion	*Potential Clinical Consequences*
Alterations in red blood cell structure and function:	
ATP depletion	Echinospherocyte formation, increased osmotic fragility, impaired RBC deformability with adverse effects on oxygen transport and delivery
Microvesiculation and loss of membrane lipid, lipid peroxidation and hemolysis, and irreversible damaged RBCs	Reduced RBC viability and cell death Hyperbilirubinemia, LDH, increased serum iron, free radical generation (?), hyperkalemia
Reduced 2,3-DPG	Increased hemoglobin affinity for oxygen and impaired unloading
Decreased CD47 antigen (integrin-associated protein) expression	Reduced posttransfusion survival due to premature clearance post transfusion
RBC adhesion to endothelial cells	Adverse effects on microcirculatory hemodynamics
Storage temperature	Hypothermia unless pretransfusion warming
Additives:	
Citrate	Hypocalcemia, acid-base imbalance, initial acidosis alkalosis
Glucose	Hyperglycemia
Sodium	Hypernatremia
Cytokines: IL-1, IL-6, IL-8, TNF	Fever, hypotension, flushing
Enzymes: myeloperoxidase, elastase, arginase, secretory phospholipase A₂	Transfusion-related immunomodulation, neutrophilia
Reactive proteins: defensins, annexin, soluble HLA, Fas ligand, soluble endothelial cell growth factor, and others	Proinflammatory, potential "priming" for ARDS, TRALI, and MODS
Histamine and kinin accumulation	Hypotension, anxiety, flushing, pain syndromes, proinflammatory
Microaggregates and procoagulants	Blockade of reticuloendothelial system Risk factor for development of ARDS, MODS, TRALI Activation of hemostasis > DIC (?), VTE (?), arterial thrombotic events (?)

ARDS, acute respiratory distress syndrome; *ATP,* adenosine triphosphate; *DIC,* disseminated intravascular coagulation; *2,3-DPG,* 2,3-diphosphoglycerate; *HLA,* human leukocyte antigen; *IL,* interleukin; *LDH,* lactate dehydrogenase; *MODS,* multiorgan dysfunction syndrome; *RBC,* red blood cell; *TNF,* tumor necrosis factor; *TRALI,* transfusion-related acute lung injury; *VTE,* venous thromboembolism.

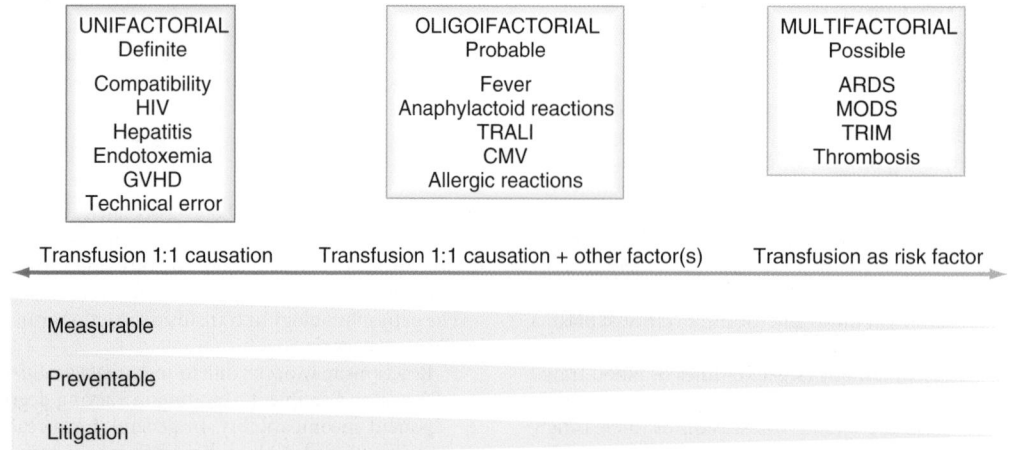

Figure 151-2 Hazards of allogeneic blood transfusion. ARDS, acute respiratory distress syndrome; CMV, cytomegalovirus; GVHD, graft-versus-host disease; HIV, human immmunodeficiency virus; MODS, multiorgan dysfunction syndrome; TRALI, transfusion-related acute lung injury; TRIM, transfusion-related immunomodulation.

HEMOLYTIC TRANSFUSION REACTIONS

Most severe acute hemolytic transfusion reactions usually have an identifiable and avoidable cause and result from an error at some point along the compatibility chain, most commonly incorrect patient identification. ABO incompatibility is the most common potentially fatal complication of blood transfusion, and meticulous attention to patient and sample identification is crucial. Various strategies are advocated to eliminate the possibility of ABO incompatibility, including bar coding, vein-to-vein patient identification, bedside compatibility testing, and double patient sample collection. All of these strategies have problems, however, and the human factor remains important.

Most delayed hemolytic reactions are also immune in nature and usually cannot be prevented because the blood is serologically compatible at the time of transfusion. The clinician should always be on the outlook for the possibility of hemolytic episodes in critically ill patients, however, because these are commonly due to reactions to blood transfusion or medications.

Clinical features of hemolytic transfusion reactions are as follows:
- *Initial symptoms and signs*: classic symptoms and signs of an acute hemolytic transfusion reaction include apprehension, flushing, pain (e.g., infusion site, headache, chest, lumbosacral, and abdominal), nausea, vomiting, rigors, hypotension, and circulatory collapse. In unconscious or anesthetized patients, these symptoms are unlikely to be noted.
- *Hemostatic failure*: coagulopathy due to DIC may be a feature, resulting in generalized hemostatic failure with hemorrhage and oozing from multiple sites. Because the responsible transfusion is likely to have been administered for hemorrhage, increasing severity of local bleeding may be the first clue to an incompatible transfusion, especially if the patient is under anesthesia.
- *Oliguria and renal impairment*: renal failure may complicate a hemolytic transfusion reaction, and early recognition and prevention are crucial. If circulating volume and urinary output are rapidly restored, established renal failure is unlikely to develop. Death from acute renal failure directly caused by an incompatible blood transfusion is preventable. It is likely to occur only if expeditious action is not taken or there are complicating clinical problems.
- *Anemia and jaundice*: a severe hemolytic transfusion reaction may be suspected from the development of jaundice or anemia.

ALLERGIC AND ANAPHYLACTOID REACTIONS

Noncellular blood (plasma and plasma derivatives) components rarely are considered to be a major cause for adverse reactions to transfusion therapy, but considering the complexity of plasma and component preparation processes, a broad range of potential adverse effects is possible.[18] Plasma reactions may be related to immunologic differences between the donor and the recipient; either the component is antigenic to the recipient or the plasma contains an antibody reacting with a recipient antigen. There may be physicochemical characteristics of the plasma component such as temperature, additives, alterations due to preparative processes, and accumulation of metabolites or cellular release products on storage. Clinical severity may range from minor urticarial reactions or flushing to fulminant cardiorespiratory collapse and death. Many such reactions are probably true anaphylaxis, but in others, mechanisms have been less clear, and the term *anaphylactoid* has been used.

Immunologic reactions to normal components of plasma may occur in two ways. First, plasma proteins may contain epitopes different from those on the recipient's functionally identical plasma proteins (e.g., anti-immunoglobulin A [IgA] antibodies). Second, there may be antibodies in the donor plasma that react with cellular components of the recipient's blood cells or plasma proteins (e.g., transfusion-related lung injury).

Various contaminants in donor plasma or plasma components related to the fractionation process may be implicated in some reactions. Processing of plasma and its freezing may lead to activation of some of the proteolytic systems. Of particular importance in this respect are the complement and kinin/kininogen systems. If these systems are activated, there may be generation of vasoactive substances and anaphylotoxins. Subjective sensations (that may be missed in an unconscious patient) and hypotension occurring during rapid infusion of a hypovolemic patient may be misinterpreted as further volume loss. Histamine levels may be increased in stored blood components, and histamine levels may correlate with nonfebrile, nonhemolytic transfusion reactions.

TRANSFUSION-RELATED ACUTE LUNG INJURY

Transfusion-related acute lung injury (TRALI) is a potentially severe complication of blood transfusion, characterized by acute respiratory distress arising within hours of a transfusion. Most patients who are well resuscitated improve within 48 hours and usually make a full recovery. The pathophysiology of TRALI is classically due to the presence of leukoagglutinating or human leukocyte antigen (HLA)-specific antibodies in the plasma of the donor of the implicated components. When complement is activated, C5a promotes neutrophil aggregation and sequestration in the lung microvasculature, causing endothelial damage. The concept of TRALI has been expanded to embrace a broader spectrum of acute lung injury after transfusion to include cases of posttransfusion lung injury in which other mechanisms may be responsible (e.g., anaphylactic reactions, cytokine reactions, platelet reactions, granulocyte transfusions, blood storage lesion).[18] The patient's lungs may be "primed" by other pathologic factors such as shock and sepsis, and transfusion becomes an additional risk factor.[19]

POSTTRANSFUSION PURPURA

Posttransfusion purpura is a potentially life-threatening complication of transfusion in which platelet-specific alloantibodies develop at 5 to 10 days, with the patient developing severe thrombocytopenia. Paradoxically, in contrast to other immunologically mediated transfusion reactions, the patient's own platelets are destroyed during the immunologic reaction. Early recognition of this rare complication, which typically occurs in women, is essential to minimize morbidity and mortality. Platelet transfusions are usually ineffective even if crossmatch compatible, and high-dose intravenous immunoglobulin (2 g/kg given over 2-5 days) is the recommended treatment.

TRANSFUSION-ASSOCIATED GRAFT-VERSUS-HOST DISEASE

Transfusion-associated graft-versus-host disease is due to infusion of immunocompetent lymphocytes, precipitating an immunologic reaction against the host tissues. It is most commonly observed in immunocompromised patients but also may be seen in recipients of directed blood donation from first-degree relatives. This response is also occasionally seen when donor and recipient are not related; homozygosity for HLA haplotypes for which the recipient is heterozygous is responsible. Transfusion-associated graft-versus-host disease is generally a devastating and fatal condition, with onset of the syndrome 2 to 4 weeks after allogeneic transfusion. Presenting signs and symptoms are fever, liver function test abnormalities, profuse watery diarrhea, erythematous skin rash, and progressive marrow failure.[20]

TRANSFUSION-RELATED IMMUNOMODULATION

Transfusion-related immunomodulation (TRIM) is an evolving and complex area of research and new knowledge.[21] Leukocytes seem to be the main blood component responsible for the immunomodulatory effects of transfusion. Space does not permit detailed analysis; however, it is likely that prestorage leukodepletion minimizes the effects. Allogeneic transfusion has been shown to be an independent risk factor for postoperative infection, with many infections being distant from the wound site, suggesting a systemic reduction in host resistance. Immunomodulation also may be responsible for increased cancer recurrence rates after surgery, but this remains controversial. The possible role of TRIM in the association between allogeneic blood transfusion and poorer clinical outcomes is discussed later.

FEVER

The term *nonhemolytic febrile transfusion reaction* defines an acute complication of blood transfusion characterized by fever with or without chills and rigors. These reactions are generally not life threatening, but they cause discomfort, involve the use of medications, and employ resources of medical, nursing, and laboratory personnel. The effects of rigors and pyrexia in critically ill patients are concerning, and temperatures above 38°C should not be ignored. Most febrile reactions are due to immunologic reactions against one or more of the transfused cellular or plasma components, usually leukocytes. The use of leukocyte-depleted blood products minimizes the likelihood of nonhemolytic febrile transfusion reaction.

TRANSFUSION-TRANSMITTED INFECTIONS

Transfusion-related infections have received much attention, and their recognition has been a driving force behind many changed blood donation and processing policies. The reader is referred to recent reviews of transfusion-transmitted infections.[16,21-23]

BACTERIAL CONTAMINATION

Bacterial contamination of stored blood can cause fulminant endotoxic shock. In recent years, the storage of platelets at room temperature has made this blood component particularly susceptible to bacterial contamination.[24] The clinical features of transfusion-related endotoxic shock in a nonanesthetized patient include violent chills, fever, tachycardia, and vascular collapse with prominent nausea, vomiting, and diarrhea. Anesthetized patients may have delayed onset of symptoms, and in patients who are already febrile and on antibiotics, diagnosis can be elusive or missed.

BLOOD STORAGE LESIONS AND POTENTIAL CLINICAL CONSEQUENCES

Blood is altered from the moment of its initial collection and subsequent storage. Physical and biochemical characteristics may be of particular importance when large volumes are infused rapidly. Warming of all rapid blood transfusions should minimize the possibility of hypothermia. Patients receiving massive blood component therapy are likely to be seriously ill and have multiple problems. Potential adverse effects must be considered in conjunction with the injuries and multiorgan dysfunction. It is not always possible to define complications caused or aggravated by massive blood transfusion.

The storage lesions progressively increase until the time of expiry, and the extent of these changes is determined by the specific blood component, preservative medium, container, storage time, and storage conditions.[25] Storage results in quantitative or qualitative deficiencies (or both) in blood components, which may reduce the efficacy of a transfusion. Quantitative deficiencies may result in reduced RBC survival, failure to achieve anticipated endpoints, and excessive donor exposure, increasing immunization and infection risks. Qualitative deficiency includes decreased membrane flexibility and increased adhesion to endothelium, which may impair microcirculatory hemodynamics. Reduced 2,3-diphospho-glycerate decreases hemoglobin oxygen affinity, impairing oxygen unloading.

In parallel with these storage changes is an accumulation of degenerate material (e.g., microaggregates and procoagulant material), release of vasoactive agents, cytokine generation, and hemolysis (Figure 151-3). Many of the changes occurring during storage are related to the presence of leukocytes (especially granulocytes) and can be minimized by prestorage leukoreduction. The clinical significance of storage lesions continues to be debated. In some cases, the effects are widely accepted; in others, further studies are needed. There is evidence that the storage lesion is clinically significant in several respects.[26] Transfusion may result in significant increases in unconjugated bilirubin and lactic dehydrogenase, neutrophilia, and saturation of serum iron. The transfusion of biologically active lipids in stored blood may be associated with development of acute lung injury in patients with predisposing conditions. Blood transfusion has been shown to be an independent risk factor for development of postinjury multiorgan failure and acute

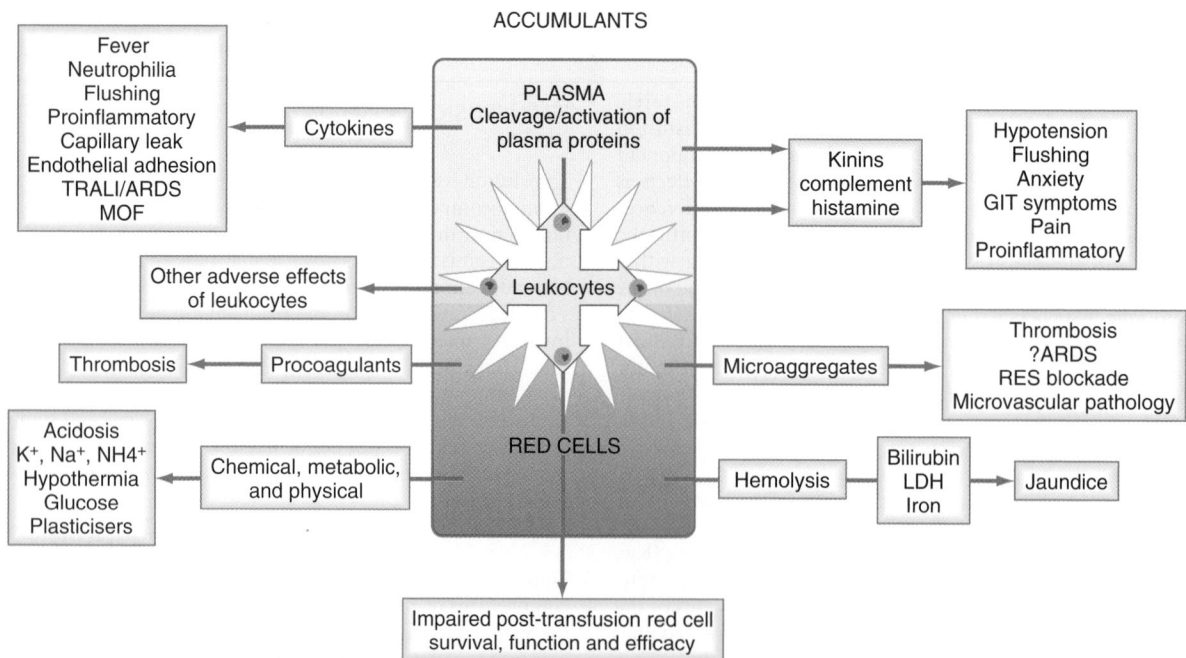

Figure 151-3   Red blood cell storage lesions. ARDS, acute respiratory distress syndrome; GIT, gastrointestinal tract; LDH, lactate dehydrogenase; MOF, multiple organ failure; RES, reticuloendothelial system; TRALI, transfusion-related acute lung injury.

respiratory distress syndrome, and this relationship may be stronger with the age of the transfused blood. There is an increased rate of infection associated with transfusion of old blood after severe injury, suggesting that transfusion-related immunomodulation may not be related only to allogeneic transfusion but contributed to by the storage lesion. In some studies, transfusion of stored blood older than 15 days in trauma patients was a predictor of a greater likelihood of admission to the intensive care unit (ICU) and predicted a prolonged length of ICU stay. Further information about the storage lesion and the possible clinical implications is summarized in Table 151-2.

The commonly recognized potential hazards of rapid blood transfusion are as follows:

- *Citrate toxicity*: a patient responds to citrate infusion by the removal of citrate and mobilization of ionized calcium. Citrate is metabolized by the Krebs cycle in nucleated cells, especially the liver. A marked elevation in citrate concentration is seen with transfusions of greater than 500 mL in 5 minutes; the citrate level rapidly falls when infusion is slowed. Citrate metabolism is impaired by hypotension, hypovolemia, hypothermia, and liver disease, and toxicity may be potentiated by alkalosis, hyperkalemia, hypothermia, and cardiac disease. There are many potential consequences of citrate-induced depression of ionized calcium, but a warm, well-perfused adult patient with normal liver function can tolerate a unit of blood every 5 minutes without requiring calcium replacement.

- *Acid-base and electrolyte changes*: transfusion of stored blood presents a patient with an appreciable acid load, which may be of particular importance if there is a preexisting metabolic acidosis. The acidity of stored blood is mainly due to the citric acid of the anticoagulant and the lactic acid generated during storage. Their intermediary metabolites are metabolized rapidly with adequate tissue perfusion, and citrate is metabolized into bicarbonate, ultimately resulting in metabolic alkalosis. Routine use of sodium bicarbonate is unnecessary, and acid-base abnormalities should be corrected only in the context of the clinical situation. The acid-base status of the recipient is more important and predominantly dependent on tissue perfusion. Although controversial, it is unlikely that the high serum potassium levels in stored blood have pathologic effects in adults, except in the presence of acute renal failure. In contrast, hypokalemia may be a problem 24 hours after massive transfusion as the transfused cells correct their electrolyte composition and potassium returns into the cells. The sodium content of whole blood and fresh frozen plasma is higher than normal blood levels, owing to sodium citrate. This fact should be taken into account when large volumes of plasma are being infused into patients who have disordered salt and water handling (e.g., renal, liver, or cardiac disease).

HYPERBILIRUBINEMIA

Hyperbilirubinemia is common after massive blood transfusion, because a significant proportion of RBCs transfused (30% if aged blood is used) may not survive, and the resulting bilirubin load causes varying degrees of hyperbilirubinemia. If the patient has been hypovolemic and shocked, biliary transport functions may be impaired, particularly in the presence of sepsis or multiorgan dysfunction. An important rate-limiting step in bilirubin transport is the energy-requiring process of transporting conjugated bilirubin from the hepatocyte to the biliary canaliculus. Bilirubin from destroyed transfused RBCs may be conjugated, but delayed excretion may lead to conjugated hyperbilirubinemia. A hemolytic transfusion reaction and resorbing hematoma also have to be considered as possible causes of hyperbilirubinemia.

ALLOGENEIC TRANSFUSION AS AN INDEPENDENT RISK FACTOR FOR POORER CLINICAL OUTCOMES

In recent years, experimental and clinical studies have identified blood transfusion as an independent risk factor for morbidity and mortality

as well as increased admission rates to ICUs, increased length of hospital stay, and additional costs. The implication of RBC transfusion as part of the problem rather than optimal therapy has challenged long-held views about the safety of allogeneic blood transfusion. It has always been assumed that blood transfusion can only be of *benefit* to the bleeding or anemic patient, with immunologic and infection transfusion hazards well understood and minimized. There is thus increasing evidence that TRIM and the transfusion effects of storage lesions may be responsible for poorer clinical outcomes in a range of clinical settings.[27-28] There is also an association of transfusion with a higher incidence of venous thromboembolism.[29] The case for this association between blood transfusion and poorer outcomes is strengthening, and evidence for the efficacy of many transfusions is being reassessed, as are studies supporting restrictive red cell transfusion policies as not jeopardizing clinical outcomes. Until these concerns are resolved, a precautionary approach should be adopted, with avoidance or minimization of allogeneic transfusion and the use of appropriate patient blood conservation techniques whenever possible.

Basic Immunohematology

RBC serology is a highly specialized area of knowledge, and it is not possible to expect clinicians to have more than a basic working knowledge essential for patient safety. This section summarizes core knowledge for the clinician.

SALINE AGGLUTINATION

Safe RBC transfusion has revolved around the traditional serologic technique of saline agglutination. A saline suspension of RBCs is mixed with serum and observed for agglutination. Saline agglutination is used for ABO blood grouping and is one of the techniques for compatibility testing of donor blood.

DIRECT AND INDIRECT ANTIGLOBULIN TEST

In RBC serology, the antiglobulin test (Coombs test) is used to detect IgG immunoglobulins or complement components. The direct antiglobulin test (DAT) detects immunoglobulin or complement components present on the surface of the RBCs circulating in the patient. The result is positive in autoimmune hemolytic anemia and hemolytic disease of the newborn and during a hemolytic transfusion reaction. The indirect antiglobulin test (IAT) detects the presence of nonagglutinating antibodies in the patient's plasma, usually IgG type. Antibody screening for atypical antibodies and pretransfusion compatibility testing are the main applications of the IAT.

REGULAR AND IRREGULAR (ATYPICAL) ANTIBODIES

The regular alloantibodies (isoagglutinins) of the ABO system are naturally occurring agglutinins present in all ABO types (except AB), depending on the ABO group. Group O people have anti-A and anti-B isoagglutinins, group A people have anti-B, and group B people have anti-A. Group A cells cause the most common and most dangerous ABO-incompatible hemolytic reactions. Atypical antibodies are not normally present in the plasma but may be found in some people as naturally occurring antibodies or immune antibodies. Immune antibodies result from previous exposure due to blood transfusion or pregnancy. Naturally occurring antibodies more frequently react by saline agglutination, and although they may be stimulated by transfusion, they usually are of minimal clinical significance. In contrast, many of the immune atypical antibodies are of major clinical significance, and their recognition is the raison d'être for pretransfusion compatibility testing and antenatal antibody screening. Most clinically significant immune atypical antibodies are detected by the IAT. Blood group antigens vary widely in frequency and immunogenicity The D antigen of the Rhesus (Rh) blood group system is common and highly immunogenic. When an Rh-negative (i.e., D-negative) patient is exposed to D-positive blood, there is a high likelihood of forming an anti-D antibody. For this reason, the D antigen is taken into account when providing blood for transfusion, in contrast to the numerous other RBC antigens that are less common or less immunogenic. Beyond the Rh (D), and sometimes the Kell (K) blood group antigens, it is not practical or necessary to take notice of other blood group antigens unless an atypical antibody is detected during antibody screening procedures.

ANTIBODY SCREEN

On receipt of a blood sample by the transfusion service, the RBCs are ABO and Rh D typed, and the serum is screened for atypical antibodies. This screen consists of testing the patient's serum with group O screening cells. The screening panel consists of RBCs obtained usually from two group O donors containing all common RBC antigens occurring with a frequency of greater than approximately 2% in the community. If an atypical antibody is detected on the antibody screen, further serologic investigations are done to identify the specificity of the antibody. These investigations are time consuming and when possible should be carried out electively.

CROSSMATCH (COMPATIBILITY TEST)

The crossmatch is the final compatibility test between the donor cells and the patient's serum. The crossmatch test tends to be overemphasized to the detriment of the antibody screen. With sophisticated knowledge of serology, the emphasis in the supply of compatible blood is now concentrated on the steps before the final compatibility crossmatch.

TYPE AND SCREEN SYSTEM

As precompatibility testing has assumed the major role in the selection of blood for transfusion, there has been a rethinking of policies relating to the supply of blood for elective transfusions. Whenever elective surgery is planned for a patient who is likely to require blood transfusion, the transfusion service must receive a clotted blood sample well before the anticipated time of surgery. Precompatibility testing should be carried out during routine working hours when facilities are geared for large workloads and enough staff are available to handle all contingencies.

PROVISION OF BLOOD IN EMERGENCIES

When quick clinical and laboratory decisions are made under conditions of stress, it is frequently difficult for all involved personnel to appreciate the difficulties of others. The decision to give uncrossmatched or partially crossmatched blood or to wait for crossmatch-compatible blood is not easy, and certain basic serologic considerations may clarify for the clinician some of the problems faced by the serologist. Depending on the degree of urgency and extent of previous knowledge about the patient's RBC serology, blood can be provided with varying degrees of safety. When a patient is exsanguinating and likely to die, however, giving ABO-compatible, uncrossmatched blood, especially if the antibody screen is negative, is safe and appropriate therapy.

UNIVERSAL DONOR GROUP O BLOOD

Group O blood under normal circumstances is ABO compatible with all recipients. The transfusions should be given as RBC concentrates screened for high-titer A or B hemolysins and used only in extreme emergencies. If the recipient is of childbearing age, every attempt should be made to give Rh D-negative blood until the patient's blood group is known.

ABO GROUP-SPECIFIC BLOOD

Transfusion of blood of the correct ABO type circumvents the isoagglutinin problems alluded to earlier. Simple as this approach may seem, its safety depends on meticulous attention to grouping. Previous blood group information such as a "bracelet" group or "unofficial" group written in the patient's records may be incorrect, and there may be considerable risk if blood is administered on the basis of this information alone.

SALINE-COMPATIBLE BLOOD

Administration of saline-compatible blood is, for practical purposes, administration of ABO group-specific blood.

KEY POINTS

1. An evidence-based approach to blood component transfusion has resulted in many long-standing transfusion dogmas assuming clinical efficacy of the labile allogeneic blood components (red cell, platelets, and fresh frozen plasma) in improving clinical outcomes.

2. The decision to transfuse red blood cell concentrates should be supported by the need to relieve clinical signs and symptoms of impaired oxygen transport and to prevent morbidity and mortality, with the aim of improving clinical outcomes.

3. Allogeneic blood transfusion may be an independent risk factor for adverse clinical outcomes.

4. The development of clinical practice guidelines for the use of blood components should focus on patient blood management, and transfusion of allogeneic blood should no longer be the default decision in the context of clinical uncertainty.

5. The classic symptoms and signs of an acute hemolytic transfusion reaction include apprehension, flushing, pain (e.g., infusion site, headache, chest, lumbosacral, abdominal), nausea, vomiting, rigors, hypotension, and circulatory collapse.

6. A clinician needs a basic working knowledge of red blood cell serology to ensure patient safety.

ANNOTATED REFERENCES

Isbister JP. Decision making in perioperative transfusion. Transfus Apher Sci 2002;27:19-28.
This paper reviews in detail the transfusion decision-making process, overviewing all the interacting factors meriting consideration when assessing the need for transfusion of blood components.

Thomson A, Farmer S, Hofmann A, Isbister J, Shander A. Patient blood management—a new paradigm for transfusion medicine? Vox Sang ISBT Science Series 2009;4:423-35.
This article reviews patient blood management, describing the evolution of transfusion medicine from a product focus to a problem-based patient focus.

Ganter MT, Pittet JF. New insights into acute coagulopathy in trauma patients. Best Pract Res Clin Anaesthesiol 2010;24:15-25.
This paper is a good and well-referenced review of recent research that has improved our understanding of coagulopathies in trauma patients.

Zubair AC. Clinical impact of blood storage lesions. Am J Hematol 2010;85:117-22.
With increasing concern about blood storage lesions, storage age of blood, and clinical consequences, this article provides the reader with a succinct and well-referenced review.

Buddeberg F, Schimmer BB, Spahn DR. Transfusion-transmissible infections and transfusion-related immunomodulation. Best Pract Res Clin Anaesthesiol 2008;22:503-17.
As mentioned in the text, space has not permitted discussion of transfusion-transmitted infections. Basic information is available in this review, with significant references.

Marik PE, Corwin HL. Efficacy of red blood cell transfusion in the critically ill: a systematic review of the literature. Crit Care Med 2008;36:1-8.
This review is a good summary of recent evidence supporting the case that for ICU, trauma, and surgical patients, red blood cell transfusions are associated with increased morbidity and mortality.

REFERENCES

Access the complete reference list online at http://www.expertconsult.com.

152

Management of Neutropenic Cancer Patients

MICHAËL DARMON | ÉLIE AZOULAY

Among patients with chemotherapy-induced neutropenia, 1% to 5% experience toxic side effects or infections and benefit from intensive care unit (ICU) management.[1] The outlook for cancer patients requiring ICU admission has long been considered dismal. Several recent studies have shown improved ICU outcomes in the overall population of patients with hematologic malignancies,[2-6] highlighting that it is no longer relevant to deny ICU admission to patients with neutropenia or after autologous bone marrow transplantation.[7,8-13]

Several factors have contributed to improving the survival of neutropenic cancer patients admitted to the ICU:

- Better selection of patients likely to benefit from ICU admission has been achieved via close cooperation between oncologists and intensivists.[2] Selection is based on clinical status of the patient and available treatment options for the malignancy. By working together, oncologists and intensivists can arrange for early ICU admission, before multiple organ failure develops.
- Overall survival has improved in recent years in patients with hematologic or solid malignancies. The reasons include the introduction of new treatments,[14-16] advances in the management of treatment side effects,[17,18] and development of new ways to use existing treatments.
- Advances have been made in the life-supporting treatments used to manage cancer patients in the ICU. Two studies have established the benefits of noninvasive mechanical ventilation, which was independently associated with better survival in patients requiring respiratory support.[3,19] Survival rates in patients with septic shock have climbed steadily over the years.[20] The diagnostic benefits provided by widespread use of bronchoalveolar lavage or noninvasive diagnostic strategies in ICU patients with acute respiratory failure[21] have improved survival of cancer patients in this setting.[22-24]

The prognosis of these neutropenic patients is determined by the number of organ failures at ICU admission. The proliferative potential and other characteristics of the underlying malignancy seem to have a far smaller impact on survival.[25-27] The general severity scores (Simplified Acute Physiology Score II and Acute Physiology and Chronic Health Evaluation II)[28] are of limited assistance for several reasons:

1. They are intended for evaluating patient groups and do not perform well in the individual patient.
2. Although they have been validated in cancer patients, their calibration and discrimination for predicting survival are poor in this subset of patients.
3. The prognosis in cancer patients admitted to the ICU is not related to physiologic variables, but rather to organ failures and organ support therapies that may be best described by organ failure scores. The number of organ failures at ICU admission and, to an even greater extent, the time course of organ failures during the first few ICU days govern the chances for survival.[7,29]

Finally, although bone marrow transplantation has been associated with a poor prognosis in many studies,[10,30,31] these studies failed to separate autologous from allogeneic bone marrow transplant recipients or bone marrow transplant recipients from patients given "peripheral" hematopoietic stem cells (i.e., cells collected after mobilization out of the marrow). Allogeneic bone marrow transplant recipients who require ICU management have extremely high mortality rates,[32,33] and mortality is highest when the need for life-supporting treatment arises late after the transplantation procedure.[31] Allogeneic bone marrow transplantation differs from autologous bone marrow transplantation in important ways, including the risk of graft-versus-host disease and the intensity of the immunosuppressive treatment required for this complication.

Management of Neutropenic Cancer Patients in the Intensive Care Unit

IMMUNODEFICIENCY

Vulnerability to infections occurs in cancer patients for several reasons. Neutropenia diminishes the ability to fight against infectious agents. Neutrophil counts less than $1000/mm^3$ are associated with a significant risk of infection, and the lower the count, the greater the risk.[34] Infections are far more likely to occur when counts fall below $500/mm^3$, and risk is even greater at neutrophil counts less than $100/mm^3$. The duration of neutropenia also influences the rate and the severity of infections.[35]

Qualitative abnormalities in the functions of neutrophils, phagocytes, and lymphocytes contribute to the susceptibility of cancer patients to infection. An increased risk of infection by intracellular agents occurs in patients with hairy cell leukemia or T-cell acute lymphoblastic leukemia and in association with specific treatment agents.

FEVER

Probabilistic antibiotic therapy should be given routinely if a fever develops. The antibiotics should be active against gram-positive cocci (e.g., streptococci infecting mucositis lesions or staphylococci in intravascular catheters) and gram-negative rods (enterobacteria or *Pseudomonas aeruginosa*) (Table 152-1). The Infectious Diseases Society of America (IDSA) has updated its recommendations.[36] A good first-line regimen in an ICU patient with prolonged neutropenia (as often occurs in hematologic malignancies) is a penicillin that is active against *P. aeruginosa* and gram-positive cocci, given either alone or in combination with an aminoglycoside or a fluoroquinolone active against *P. aeruginosa*. Although not given routinely, vancomycin is usually added. Indeed, many neutropenic ICU patients meet IDSA criteria for introducing a glycopeptide, including suspected catheter-associated infection, methicillin-resistant *Staphylococcus aureus* colonization, gram-positive cocci in blood cultures before identification of the organism, shock, and two situations associated with infection by gram-positive cocci—grade III or IV mucositis and abrupt body temperature elevation to greater than 40°C.[36] Fluconazole, 400 mg/d, as prophylactic treatment of fungal infections has been found to be beneficial only in allogeneic bone marrow transplant recipients.[18] After 5 to 7 days with febrile neutropenia, the risk of fungal infection (not only with *Candida* but also with *Aspergillus*) is sufficiently high to warrant

TABLE 152-1	Clinical Sepsis with Bacterial Identification in the Saint-Louis Hospital Cohort*					
	All (59), n (%)	*Pulmonary Infection, n (%)*	*Bacteremia, n (%)*	*Gastrointestinal Infection, n (%)*	*CNS Infection, n (%)*	*Urinary Tract Infection, n (%)*
Gram negative	27 (45.8%)	11/27 (40.7%)	10/27 (37%)	3/27 (11.1%)	1/27 (3.7%)	1/27 (3.7%)
Klebsiella spp.	2 (3.4%)	0	0	0	1	1
Escherichia coli	11 (18.7%)	4	5	2	0	0
Proteus spp.	1 (1.7%)	1	0	0	0	0
Pseudomonas aeruginosa	10 (16.9%)	5	5	0	0	0
Enterobacter spp.	1 (1.7%)	1	0	0	0	0
Acinetobacter spp.	1 (1.7%)	0	0	1	0	0
Stenotrophomonas maltophilia	1 (1.7%)	0	0	0	0	0
Gram positive	21 (35.6%)	12/21 (57.1%)	8/21 (38.1%)	1/21 (4.8%)	1/21 (4.8%)	**0**
Staphylococcus spp.	10 (16.9%)	4	6	0	0	0
Corynebacterium spp.	1 (1.7%)	1	0	0	0	0
Streptococcus spp.	4 (6.8%)	2	1	0	0	0
Streptococcus pneumoniae	3 (5.1%)	2	0	0	1	0
Enterococcus spp.	2 (3.4%)	1	1	0	0	0
Clostridium difficile	1 (1.7%)	0	0	1	0	0
Miscellaneous	11 (18.6%)	10/11 (90.1%)	**0**	**0**	1/11 (8.9%)	**0**
Aspergillus	7 (11.8%)	7	0	0	0	0
Histoplasma capsulatum	1 (1.7%)	1	0	0	0	0
Epstein-Barr virus	1 (1.7%)	0	0	0	1	0
Cytomegalovirus	1 (1.7%)	1	0	0	0	0
Respiratory syncytial virus	1 (1.7%)	1	0	0	0	0
		33/59 (55.9%)	18/59 (30.5%)	4/59 (6.8%)	3/59 (5.1%)	1/59 (1.7%)

*Among 82 neutropenic patients with sepsis, 59 bacterial identifications were documented in 55 patients.
CNS, central nervous system.

routine antifungal therapy in combination with antibacterial agents. In our ICU, we use amphotericin B as the first-line drug. Finally, the need for antiviral agents or trimethoprim-sulfamethoxazole should be evaluated on a case-by-case basis according to patient-related factors and the clinical picture.[36] Initiation of treatment for herpesvirus infection should be considered in all patients with grade III or IV mucositis.

When the organism is recovered and identified, antimicrobial therapy should be adjusted accordingly. ICU patients whose body temperature returns to normal on the third treatment day but who have negative tests for causative organisms should continue to receive antibiotics until their blood cell counts return to normal.[36]

The source of infection should be looked for on chest radiographs, blood cultures, urine sediment and cultures, and stool cultures with tests for *Clostridium difficile* in patients with diarrhea or a high risk of infection with this agent (including patients with hematologic disease). The Herpes Consensus PCR (polymerase chain reaction) test and a serum *Aspergillus* antigen assay should be done once or twice a week in patients who have been neutropenic for longer than 1 week.

Hematopoietic Growth Factors

Among available hematopoietic growth factors, granulocyte colony-stimulating factor (G-CSF) is the most widely used in patients with hematologic or solid malignancies. G-CSF increases neutrophil counts and enhances neutrophil functions. In non-ICU patients, G-CSF has been shown to decrease the duration of neutropenia, reducing the rate of serious infections.[37,38] G-CSF also decreased mortality related to bone marrow transplantation complications[39] or dose-intensive chemotherapy.[40]

Intensivists and hematologists place considerable emphasis on correcting neutropenia. However, neutropenia recovery during the ICU stay was not associated with better survival in a study conducted at our institution.[13] For instance, G-CSF therapy that was associated with more rapid recovery from neutropenia did not contribute to increased survival. Nevertheless, using a statistical model appropriate for the time dependency of neutropenia recovery contradicted two earlier studies in which G-CSF provided no benefit in ICU patients (Table 152-2).[41,42] G-CSF should be given to all neutropenic ICU patients in

TABLE 152-2	Comparison of Studies Evaluating Impact of Colony-Stimulating Factors on Outcome of Neutropenic Patients in the ICU					
	Bouchama et al.[41]		*Gruson et al.*[42]		*Darmon et al.*[13]	
Year	1999		2000		2001	
Method	Case-control		Cohort		Cohort	
Multivariate analysis	No		No		Yes*	
	With CSF	*Without CSF*	*With CSF*	*Without CSF*	*With CSF*	*Without CSF*
No. patients	30	30	28/33	33	53	49
Day of fever	Unknown	Unknown	103	72†	Unknown	Unknown
NR (%)	36.6	33.37	25	33.3	71.2	57.2†
Time before NR (days)	7.8 (±1.4)	5.7 (±1.3)	14 (±2.5)	13 (±3.5)	11 (6.7-16.5)	8 (2-16)
ICU survival (%)	23	10	18	18	55	61.5†

*Two models of multivariate analyses were compared, logistic regression and Cox model, in which neutropenia recovery was introduced as a time-dependent variable. In both models, 30-day mortality was the outcome variable of interest.
†P < .05.
CSF, cerebrospinal fluid; *NR*, neutropenia recovery.

whom neutropenia recovery can be expected within 7 days.[43] Examination of a bone marrow smear may be more accurate for predicting the time to neutropenia recovery but is not performed routinely in patients given standard chemotherapy regimens. A bone marrow smear may be useful, however, after dose-intensive chemotherapy with bone marrow transplantation or after the first induction course for leukemia. G-CSF can stimulate the leukemic clone in patients receiving induction chemotherapy for acute leukemia and is contraindicated in this setting.

In contrast, G-CSF is given to nearly every patient with Hodgkin's or non-Hodgkin's lymphoma. Close monitoring is needed in patients with respiratory symptoms or lung infiltrates, as respiratory failure may get worse at time of recovery from leukopenia. It is imperative that G-CSF be discontinued as soon as bone marrow function improves (neutrophils > 500/mm^3).[44] G-CSF can be given intravenously or subcutaneously; in the ICU, the intravenous route is simplest. Dosages recommended for adults are 10 µg/kg/d for filgrastim and 150 µg/m^2/d for lenograstim; however, the optimal dosages in ICU patients have not been determined. The drug is given as a single injection daily. No dosage adjustment is required in patients with kidney dysfunction. Blood cell counts should be obtained daily, and the G-CSF should be stopped as soon as the leukocyte count increases to greater than 1000/mm^3 or the neutrophil count increases to greater than 500/mm^3.

ISOLATION MODALITIES

Protective isolation involves reducing the patient's exposure to potentially infective microorganisms via geographic and technical measures (routine use of nonsterile gloves, gown, head covering, mask, and in some cases, overshoes). Because the gut lumen is a reservoir for bacteria that can cause bacteremia, selective digestive decontamination (SDD) is often added to isolation measures. In our ICU, we use oral colimycin capsules and oral amphotericin B. Efficacy data on these regimens come from old and methodologically flawed studies that often produced conflicting results. No data are available on neutropenic ICU patients. Finally, there is a paucity of studies comparing isolation measures. A combination of geographic isolation with air filtering (laminar flow or high-efficiency particulate-arresting filters), technical isolation (usually involving use of a mask, head covering, and gown, although variations exist across studies), and SDD have been found to decrease the mortality rate or the infection rate in many prospective and retrospective studies.[45] Although the optimal modalities for protective isolation and their usefulness in the ICU have not been determined, a reasonable approach to the management of neutropenic ICU patients is maximal protective isolation, including geographic isolation with air filtration, technical isolation with at least a mask and gown, and SDD.

Specific Organ Failures

ACUTE RESPIRATORY FAILURE

Together with circulatory shock, acute respiratory failure is the most common organ failure leading to ICU admission of neutropenic patients.[20] In these patients, acute respiratory failure often stems from a combination of factors that may be closely intertwined, such as infection and cardiogenic edema or alveolar hemorrhage. The causes of acute respiratory failure in cancer patients can be divided into infectious and noninfectious categories. At least three distinctive features characterize them:

1. In contradistinction to patients with human immunodeficiency virus-related conditions, only 50% of cancer patients derive diagnostic benefit from bronchoscopy with bronchoalveolar lavage (BAL), and the proportion is even smaller in case of neutropenia, bone marrow transplant, or mechanical ventilation.
2. Chances of survival are better when the cause is identified (allowing adjustments in management), a finding that has prompted BAL studies in patients managed with noninvasive mechanical ventilation or a laryngeal mask.[24]

3. Noninvasive diagnostic tools are being developed (e.g., antigen assays in serum and urine and PCR testing for viruses) and, when incorporated into current diagnostic strategies, should enable the noninvasive diagnosis of opportunistic pneumonia,[21] obviating the need for bronchoscopy and protecting the patient from the morbidity associated with this procedure.

SEPTIC SHOCK

Survival rates in cancer patients with septic shock have increased over the years.[7] Earlier treatment is one component. There is a need for studies evaluating the impact of new management strategies in these patients, who were excluded from large multicenter randomized studies.[46-48]

MACROPHAGE ACTIVATION SYNDROME

Lymphohistiocytic activation syndrome is another name for macrophage activation syndrome, which may develop in a neutropenic patient or cause neutropenia. Multiple organ failure with vasoplegic shock may occur.[49] Fever, thrombocytopenia, and hepatosplenomegaly are almost universally present. Other manifestations include low counts of other cell lines, cholestasis with jaundice, high serum levels of ferritin and triglycerides, and low serum albumin and fibrinogen. Bone marrow smear findings are typical, with activated macrophages phagocytizing platelets, erythrocytes, and leukocytes, although false-positive results are encountered occasionally. Corticosteroids and etoposide are the mainstays of treatment and should be considered on an emergency basis.[50]

TYPHLITIS OR NEUTROPENIA-ASSOCIATED ENTEROCOLITIS

Typhlitis occurs chiefly after intensive chemotherapy and manifests as any combination of abdominal pain, fever, and diarrhea.[34,51] The protean nature of the manifestations raises diagnostic challenges. Typhlitis is probably a multifactorial condition related to chemotherapy-induced colonic mucosal damage, thrombopenia-related bleeding within the colonic wall, and bowel colonization by pathogenic microorganisms.[51] Complications include bacteremia (28%-82% of cases), gastrointestinal bleeding (65% of cases), and gastrointestinal perforation (5%-10%).[52] Ultrasonography or computed tomography (CT) of the gastrointestinal tract confirms the diagnosis and evaluates the severity of the disease. CT may show pneumoperitoneum or colonic pneumatosis, indicating severe parietal damage with imminent perforation. Bowel-wall thickening on ultrasound scan confirms the diagnosis.[53] In a retrospective study, bowel-wall thickening was significantly associated with a high mortality rate (29% versus 0%), especially when the bowel wall was thicker than 10 mm.[54] Conservative treatment should be used if possible, but surgery is required in patients with life-threatening gastrointestinal bleeding, perforation, or uncontrolled sepsis.[52] A diagnosis of typhlitis requires prior elimination of other abdominal conditions, most notably classic surgical conditions and pseudomembranous colitis.[52]

ACUTE TUMOR LYSIS SYNDROME

Although the onset usually precedes the development of neutropenia by several days, the two problems of acute tumor lysis syndrome and neutropenia are frequently interrelated. The risk of tumor lysis syndrome varies with the tumor burden and with the nature and intensity of induction chemotherapy. Neutropenia develops soon afterward. Although a detailed description of tumor lysis syndrome is beyond the scope of this chapter, five key words come to mind: *Hyperuricemia* stems from the metabolism and lysis of tumor cells and can cause precipitates to form within the renal tubules if the urine is acidic. The administration of recombinant *urate oxidases* (rasburicase) completely prevents this problem, obviating the need for alkalinization.[55]

Hyperphosphatemia is an absolute contraindication to alkalinization (the risk being nephrocalcinosis related to precipitation) but can be controlled by hyperhydration and *renal support therapy. Dehydration* is almost always present and requires volume repletion with nonalkaline isotonic solutions.

Conclusion

The last years have seen improvements in the survival of cancer patients managed in the ICU. Neutropenia no longer indicates a poor prognosis. The type and number of organ failures at ICU admission and their time course during the first few days are the main determinants of survival. The potential benefits of early ICU admission need to be evaluated. Similarly, rather than routine denial of ICU admission, neutropenic patients should be allowed a *therapeutic trial*, in which high-intensity management (with no treatment limitations) is provided for a few days; the prognosis is then reappraised based on the course of the organ failures to determine whether further aggressive treatment is warranted.

KEY POINTS

1. Patient selection for ICU admission is based on the clinical status and the available treatment options for the malignancy. Oncologists and intensivists should cooperate for early ICU admission before multiple organ failure develops.

2. The number of organ failures at ICU admission is the cornerstone of the prognostic evaluation in neutropenic patients. Together with circulatory shock, acute respiratory failure is the most common organ failure leading to ICU admission of neutropenic patients.

3. Neutropenia diminishes the ability to fight against infectious agents. The lower the neutrophil count, the greater the risk of infection. Infections are far more likely to occur when the count declines to less than 500/mm^3. Duration of neutropenia also influences the rate and severity of infections.

4. Probabilistic antibiotic therapy should be given routinely if fever develops. The antibiotics should be active against gram-positive cocci and gram-negative rods. When the organism is recovered and identified, antimicrobial therapy should be adjusted accordingly.

ANNOTATED REFERENCES

Brenner H. Long-term survival rates of cancer patients achieved by the end of the 20th century: a period analysis. Lancet 2002;360:1131-5.
Analysis of the Surveillance, Epidemiology, and End Results Database of the United States National Cancer Institute over a 25-year period. This study confirms the improvement in long-term survival rates of cancer patients and gives an estimation of 5-year, 10-year, 15-year, and 20-year relative survival rates for many types of cancer.

Darmon M, Azoulay E, Alberti C, et al. Impact of neutropenia duration on short-term mortality in neutropenic critically ill cancer patients. Intensive Care Med 2002;28:1775-80.
This study confirms that organ failure, not disease progression or neutropenia duration, affects 30-day mortality of neutropenic critically ill cancer patients.

Hughes WT, Armstrong D, Bodey GP, et al. 2002 Guidelines for the use of antimicrobial agents in neutropenic patients with cancer. Clin Infect Dis 2002;34:730-51.

This article prepared by the Infectious Diseases Society of America (IDSA) Fever and Neutropenia Guidelines Panel updates the guidelines published in 1997 by the IDSA.

Larche J, Azoulay E, Fieux F, et al. Improved survival of critically ill cancer patients with septic shock. Intensive Care Med 2003;29:1688-95.
Study demonstrating an improvement of the 30-day survival of critically ill cancer patients with septic shock over time.

Massion PB, Dive AM, Doyen C, et al. Prognosis of hematologic malignancies does not predict intensive care unit mortality. Crit Care Med 2002;30:2260-70.
Observational study over a 10-year period concluding that severity of the underlying hematologic malignancies does not influence ICU or hospital mortality of critically ill cancer patients but may affect 6-month mortality.

REFERENCES

Access the complete reference list online at http://www.expertconsult.com.

153

Venous Thromboembolism in Medical-Surgical Critically Ill Patients

DEBORAH J. COOK | MARK A. CROWTHER

Venous thromboembolism (VTE) is a common complication of serious illness, conferring considerable morbidity and mortality in hospitalized patients. Patients with deep vein thrombosis (DVT) are at risk of subsequently developing pulmonary embolism, which may be fatal if untreated. Approximately 90% of cases of pulmonary embolism are believed to arise in the lower limbs,[1] so DVT can be viewed as an important precursor to more serious disease. Most clinical research on VTE in the intensive care unit (ICU) is focused on DVT, and it will be the major focus of this chapter.

In the ICU, patients with DVT are significantly more likely to have pulmonary embolism[2] and a longer duration of mechanical ventilation ($P = .02$), ICU stay ($P = .005$), and hospitalization ($P < .001$) than patients without DVT.[3] Clinically unsuspected DVT and pulmonary embolism are found frequently at autopsy in critically ill patients.[4-6]

Increased attention has focused on the risk factors, prevalence, incidence, clinical importance, and prevention of VTE in critically ill patients in the ICU. Concerns have arisen for several reasons:

1. ICU patients have multiple predispositions to VTE, including acute severe inflammatory conditions that affect the coagulation cascade and major and minor surgical procedures.[7-9]
2. Critically ill patients rarely can communicate their symptoms, sharply curtailing any possibility that patient self-reported symptoms would prompt intensivists to pursue the diagnosis of VTE.
3. The physical examination is devalued in the high-technology critical care environment, and patients with acute VTE may not manifest cardinal signs seen in non-critically ill patients, making detection of VTE using clinical skills infrequent.
4. The clinical consequences of VTE may be more serious in the ICU because of the decreased cardiorespiratory reserve of critically ill patients, which makes it less likely they would tolerate pulmonary embolism, which in healthy patients would not lead to clinical sequelae.[10]
5. When screening ultrasound studies are conducted in heterogeneous ICU patients, DVT is frequently diagnosed despite its infrequent clinical detection.[11]

Prophylaxis against VTE was rated the number-one patient safety initiative for hospitalized patients in the U.S. Agency for Health Care Policy Research Evidence Report and Technology Assessment document.[12] Juxtaposed against the foregoing is the invisibility of medical-surgical critically ill patients in publications such as the National Institutes of Health Consensus Conference on Prevention of Venous Thrombosis and Pulmonary Embolism,[13] the European Consensus Statement on Prevention of Venous Thromboembolism,[14] the Thromboembolic Risk Factors Consensus Conference,[15] the Fifth American College of Chest Physicians Antithrombotic Consensus Conference,[16] and the American Thoracic Society Clinical Practice Guideline on Diagnosis of Venous Thromboembolism.[17] An editorial in 1998 stated that the medical-surgical ICU was "the last frontier for prophylaxis."[18]

Risk Factors for Venous Thromboembolism in Medical-Surgical ICU Patients

Established risk factors for VTE can be classified broadly under the framework of stasis, vascular injury, and congenital and acquired hypercoagulable states. This section presents evidence categorizing risk factors as conventional clinical risk factors, congenital hypercoagulable states, and acquired hypercoagulable states based on thrombophilic markers.

CLINICAL RISK FACTORS

One conceptualization of risk factors for VTE in the ICU is to consider ICU admitting diagnosis as a risk factor. Medical-surgical ICU patients are at higher risk of VTE than general medical or surgical patients cared for on the ward, but at lower risk than other subgroups of critically ill patients such as trauma victims or neurosurgical patients (Figure 153-1). In the largest prospective cohort study using venographic diagnosis, of 716 trauma patients who did not receive prophylaxis, 201 (58%) had DVT between days 14 and 21, one-third of which were in the proximal venous circulation (and likely of clinical significance).[19] Of these 201 patients, only 3 patients had symptoms of DVT. Among neurosurgical patients in three cohort studies using radioactive iodine leg scanning, the DVT rate was 35% without prophylaxis; in 7 randomized clinical trials that included a nonprophylaxis arm, the pooled incidence of DVT was 22%.[7] Patients with acute spinal cord injury have been evaluated in 4 randomized trials and 6 cohort studies, 5 of which did not use prophylaxis.[7] Four studies using either radioactive iodine fibrinogen or impedance plethysmography identified DVT in 39% to 90% of patients. In the single study using the reference standard for the diagnosis of DVT, which is ascending venography, 81% of the subgroup of trauma patients with spinal cord injury had DVT.[19]

Another conceptualization of risk factors for VTE in the ICU is to consider patient characteristics, events, and exposures that increase the risk of VTE. Critically ill patients have an increased risk of VTE due acute and chronic illnesses, immobility propagated by sedatives and paralytic drugs, and thrombin-generating invasive procedures. Observational studies in medical-surgical ICU patients have identified VTE risk factors[11,20] including patient demographics (e.g., female sex), prior VTE events (i.e., personal history of VTE), morbidity (e.g., malignancy), ICU procedures (e.g., central venous catheters), treatments (e.g., mechanical ventilation), and VTE prophylaxis (i.e., decreasing risk). Inferences about many of these risk factors are limited by small sample sizes and infrequent use of multiple logistic regression to rigorously evaluate baseline and time-dependent risk factors.

Studies large enough to perform multivariate analysis are most helpful.[2,3,21,22] In a prospective cohort study of patients ventilated for

POPULATIONS AT RISK OF VENOUS THROMBOSIS

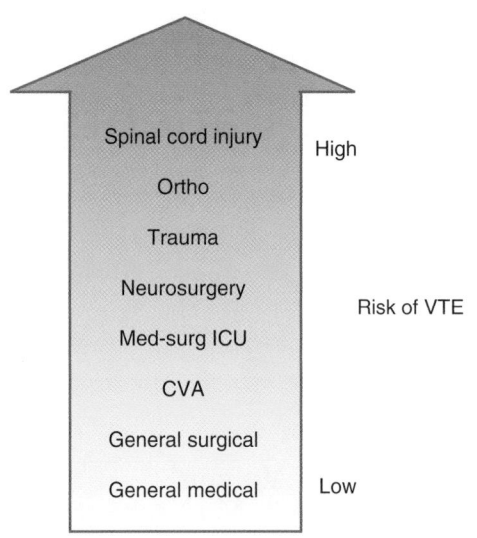

Figure 153-1   Underlying population risk of venous thromboembolism (VTE) in hospitalized patients. Medical-surgical ICU patients have a midrange risk of VTE, higher than ward patients with medical or surgical problems and lower than patients with spinal cord injury or trauma. CVA, cerebrovascular accident.

at least 1 week, the only independent risk factor for VTE was central venous catheterization; each day the catheter was in place was associated with a relative risk (RR) increase of 1.04.[2] In another prospective cohort study,[3] we enrolled consecutive medical-surgical patients 18 years of age or older expected to be in the ICU for 72 hours or more. Exclusion criteria were an admitting diagnosis of trauma, orthopedic surgery, pregnancy, and life-support withdrawal. We performed bilateral lower extremity compression ultrasound within 48 hours of ICU admission, then twice weekly thereafter or if VTE was clinically suspected. Thromboprophylaxis was protocol-directed and universal using unfractionated heparin. We recorded DVT risk factors at baseline and daily, using multivariate regression analysis to determine independent predictors. Patients were followed to hospital discharge. Among 261 patients with a mean Acute Physiology, Age, and Chronic Health Evaluation (APACHE) II score of 26, we identified four independent risk factors for ICU-acquired DVT: personal or family history of VTE (hazard ratio, 3.9; 95% confidence interval [CI], 1.5-10), end-stage renal failure (hazard ratio, 3.7; 95% CI, 1.3-11.2), platelet transfusion (hazard ratio, 3.2; 95% CI 1.2-8.5), and vasopressor use (hazard ratio, 2.8; 95% CI 1.1-7.2).

CONGENITAL HYPERCOAGULABLE STATES

A growing number of epidemiologic studies have highlighted how inherited and acquired abnormalities in the coagulation system predispose to VTE. Activated protein C resistance due to factor V Leiden (found in 5% of the population) is the most common hereditary biochemical defect that predisposes to venous thrombosis, followed by the prothrombin 20210A regulatory sequence mutation, found in 2%.[23-25] Although the impact of these prothrombotic states on the risk of VTE is confounded by the use of prophylactic anticoagulants, there is some evidence that these states increase the risk of first DVT in patients in high-risk clinical situations. Lowe and colleagues,[26] in a large prospective cohort study of patients undergoing elective hip replacement, found in a univariate analysis that patients with the factor V Leiden mutation had an increased risk of postoperative venous thrombosis. No large-scale studies have yet reported on the incremental risk of DVT in high-risk situations for patients with factor V Leiden, but it is known that the prothrombin gene mutation predicts DVT in otherwise

healthy outpatients (odds ratio [OR], 2.8).[27] Additional but less common inherited hypercoagulable states include deficiencies of antithrombin, protein C, and protein S, each of which is a naturally occurring anticoagulant protein. The ORs for venous thrombosis are 8.1 to 13.7 for antithrombin deficiency, 7.3 to 11.9 for protein C deficiency, and 8.5 to 10 for protein S deficiency.[28-30] Antiphospholipid antibodies including the lupus anticoagulant and anticardiolipin antibody are strong predictors of first and recurrent venous thrombosis. Elevations in the levels of homocysteine and coagulation factors VIII, IX, and XI also predispose to VTE in other settings.[31-35]

In the observational study described earlier, we evaluated the frequency and clinical importance of thrombophilia markers at the time of ICU admission and during the ICU stay.[36] To examine whether baseline markers of activation of the coagulation system and known thrombophilic risk factors predicted the development of DVT, a comprehensive battery of tests was done at the time of enrollment, including activated protein C ratio (with confirmation of factor V Leiden where appropriate), protein C level, protein S level, antithrombin level, anticardiolipin antibody titer, and screening and confirmatory assays for the lupus anticoagulant. The receiver operating curves for four baseline coagulation tests at the time of ICU admission showed areas under the curve for each of the activated protein C ratio, antithrombin, protein C, and protein S tests that were not significantly different than 50%; that is, the presence of these abnormalities did predict the presence of DVT at the time of ICU admission. Tests with areas under the curve of 0.75 to 0.80 represent moderate diagnostic power. Baseline coagulation tests also were not useful predictors of DVT developing during the ICU stay.

ACQUIRED HYPERCOAGULABLE STATES

Coagulation abnormalities acquired in the ICU have received considerable attention. Acquired thrombophilic markers associated with thrombosis include lupus anticoagulant, anticardiolipin antibody, and increased levels of homocysteine. In critically ill patients, acquired reductions in the levels of antithrombin, protein C, and protein S due to consumption may be common, and it is possible these deficiencies are associated with a high risk of VTE and other complications of ICU stay including death. The relationship between the inflammatory and coagulation cascades has been the focus of intense discussion in the sepsis literature.[37] Longitudinal studies have shown that protein C levels in sepsis are inversely correlated with mortality.[38] A randomized trial of recombinant activated protein C in 1690 patients with systematic inflammation and organ dysfunction showed a decrease in 28-day mortality from 30.8% to 24.7% (number needed to treat, 16).[39] Approximately 80% of patients had protein C deficiency on entry into the trial, highlighting the prevalence of this acquired thrombophilic marker. The efficacy of recombinant activated protein C was the same, however, in patients with and without protein C deficiency. In another large randomized trial of antithrombin administration in patients with sepsis, antithrombin levels were less than 60% of normal functional levels in more than 50% of patients, but antithrombin administration did not decrease mortality.[40]

In the study of DVT incidence described earlier,[3] we also evaluated whether quantitative D-dimer tests at the time of ICU admission and during ICU stay[41] were associated with DVT. At the time of enrollment, twice weekly during the ICU stay, and at the time of any suspected venous thromboembolic events, patients had a battery of D-dimer tests, including whole-blood SimpliRed D-dimer tests, and five D-dimer assays performed using D-dimer Plus, IL test DD, MDA-DD, Sigma DD, and Biopool. For the five quantitative baseline D-dimer tests in relation to DVT detected at the time of ICU admission, the areas under the curve for each of D-dimer Plus ($P = .01$), MDA-DD ($P = .002$), and Sigma DD ($P = .054$) were significantly different from .50. The receiver operating curves for time-dependent quantitative D-dimer tests and DVT developing during the ICU stay did not differ from 50%, indicating that D-dimer tests are not useful for predicting the development of VTE in the ICU.

SUMMARY

Venous thromboembolism is a multicausal disease.[42] In considering clinical risk factors, it is useful to classify them into risk factors that are *fixed*, such as admitting diagnoses, and risk factors that are *modifiable*, such as invasive procedures. Modifiable risk factors can form the basis of VTE prevention strategies. Studies to analyze the relative contributions of congenital and acquired thrombophilia markers suggest that these markers are not useful for screening or diagnostic purposes in the ICU.

Heightened awareness of risk factors for VTE has at least four consequences: first, increased attention to the problem of VTE in the ICU; second, known risk factors could be used to risk-stratify patients and identify those who should have limited exposure to other VTE risk factors (e.g., minimal sedation and short periods of central venous catheterization); third, high-risk patients may be considered for intensified VTE prevention (e.g., low-molecular-weight heparin [LMWH] prophylaxis); and fourth, high-risk patients may warrant surveillance screening with lower-limb ultrasound.

◼ Prevalence and Incidence

The incidence of VTE in the ICU depends on whether the events are clinically diagnosed or detected by screening methods. Venous thromboembolism rates observed in usual clinical practice are much lower than rates observed during systematic screening, because the former primarily represent diagnoses prompted by signs or symptoms. For example, 10%[43] to 100%[11,44] of proximal DVTs found by ultrasound screening were clinically unsuspected. In this section, we report the incidence of VTE in critically ill patients based on studies using systematic screening methods for case identification.

Understanding DVT rates requires distinguishing events diagnosed at the time of ICU admission (prevalence at a point in time) from the events that develop over the course of critical illness (incidence over the ICU stay). Cross-sectional studies at the time of admission to a medical ICU[45] and surgical ICU[44] suggest a 10% prevalence of DVT diagnosed by screening compression ultrasonography. As mentioned earlier in the section on risk factors, however, the prevalence of DVT on admission to any ICU is influenced heavily by the case mix of patients.

The risk of DVT developing over the ICU stay was established in three longitudinal studies using systematic screening.[11,43,46] Among ICU patients not receiving prophylaxis, 76% of whom were mechanically ventilated, radioactive iodine fibrinogen scanning for 3 to 6 days identified DVT in 3 of 34 (9%) patients.[46] Using Doppler ultrasound twice weekly then at 1 week after ICU discharge in 100 medical patients expected to stay more than 48 hours—70% of whom were ventilated—DVT was diagnosed in 32% of 100 patients receiving no prophylaxis, in 40% of patients receiving unfractionated heparin, and in 33% of patients who received mechanical prophylaxis.[11] In a third study of 102 medical-surgical ICU patients undergoing duplex ultrasound during days 4 to 7 and as clinically indicated,[43] DVT rates were 25%, 19%, and 7% in patients receiving no prophylaxis, mechanical prevention, and unfractionated heparin.

Earlier studies suggest that the prevalence of proximal DVT on admission to a medical-surgical ICU is estimated to be 10%, and the incidence of DVT developing over the ICU stay based on systematic screening ranges from 9% to 40%. Two of these studies performed surveillance for approximately 1 week,[43,46] however, and one study used radioactive iodine fibrinogen scanning for detection,[46] which likely underestimated the risk of ICU-acquired DVT. No studies used systematic screening for pulmonary embolism, and the true incidence of pulmonary embolism is not known.

More recent studies suggest a lower rate of VTE in medical-surgical ICU studies, partly due to the administration of thromboprophylaxis. In a single-center cohort of 239 medical ICU patients who did not undergo systematic screening ultrasound, 44 (18.4%) patients had lower-extremity DVT.[47] Ibrahim et al.,[2] in a cohort study involving

twice-weekly upper- and lower-extremity ultrasound screening, found a 26.6% incidence of DVT. Among 261 patients with a mean APACHE II score of 25.5 (±8.4), the prevalence of DVT was 2.7% (95% CI, 1.1-5.5) on ICU admission, and the incidence was 9.8% (95% CI, 6.5-14.2) over the ICU stay.[3]

SUMMARY

The risk of DVT is highest for acute spinal cord injury patients, followed by trauma, neurosurgery, and medical-surgical ICU patients. From observational studies and randomized trials, it can be concluded that critically ill patients have an incidence of DVT that is dependent on whether the event is detected by screening, the diagnostic test method used, and the type of prophylaxis. Specifically, DVT rates are higher among patients undergoing screening compared with patients who have clinically detected events; among patients undergoing venography compared with patients undergoing compression ultrasound or leg scanning; and among patients not receiving prophylaxis compared with patients who receive it.

◼ Diagnosis

A helpful constellation of signs and symptoms in a mathematically derived and validated clinical model has been developed and validated for its prediction of DVT in outpatients.[48] Diagnosing DVT in the ICU is more challenging, however. Symptoms rarely are elicited from mechanically ventilated patients, most of whom receive sedation and analgesia, rendering the notion of symptomatic DVT unhelpful in this setting. Compounding the problem is the fact that physical examination of the lower extremities may be devalued in the high-technology ICU environment compared with cardiopulmonary monitoring. In a survey of Canadian ICU directors, respondents stated that physical examination did not yield information that was helpful in the diagnosis of DVT.[49]

The reference standard for DVT remains ascending contrast lower limb venography, despite its widespread replacement by ultrasonography. Venography can reliably detect all clinically important forms of DVT—calf thrombosis, thrombosis in the pelvis, and thrombosis of the muscular veins of the thigh, for example—none of which are reliably detected by ultrasonography. Despite its utility, venography rarely is performed in practice in the ICU. In a Canadian ICU directors' survey, the use of venography to detect thrombosis was reported rarely (56%) or never (9%).[49] Concern about transporting potentially unstable patients to the radiology department,[50] the invasive nature of the test, and the risk of contrast dye–induced nephropathy[51] may contribute to the aversion to venography in this setting; however, it is also possible that many intensivists are unaware of the limitations of ultrasonography for diagnosing DVT. Studies conducted in the 1980s cited contrast nephropathy as the third leading cause of new-onset renal failure in hospitalized patients.[52] Although currently employed nonionic contrast media are associated with a lower rate of nephrotoxicity than ionic contrast media,[53] the volume of contrast administered remains an independent predictor of nephrotoxicity.[54] Additional risk factors for acquired renal insufficiency in medical ICU patients include common problems such as sepsis, volume depletion, mechanical ventilation, and surgery.[55] The high rate of renal dysfunction in critically ill patients with normal serum creatinine is concerning, and even mild renal insufficiency in these patients is associated with increased attributable mortality. For patients undergoing venography, intravenous fluid loading before and after the contrast dye and acetylcysteine, 600 mg twice daily by nasogastric tube the day before and the day after the procedure, reduce the rate of contrast-induced nephropathy, as shown in a randomized trial.[56]

The test properties of lower-extremity bilateral Doppler ultrasound in medical-surgical ICU patients have not been determined. A meta-analysis reported a pooled sensitivity of Doppler ultrasound for proximal DVT in symptomatic patients of 97% (95% CI, 96%-98%) and in asymptomatic patients of 62% (95% CI, 53%-71%).[57] Ultrasound is more insensitive for distal DVT (pooled sensitivity for symptomatic patients, 73% [95% CI, 54%-93%] and asymptomatic patients, 53% [95% CI, 32%-74%]). Symptomatic outpatients with suspected DVT and serially negative screening ultrasound studies have a 1% likelihood of subsequently developing a DVT or pulmonary embolism, suggesting that serially negative ultrasound studies safely and effectively rule out clinically important DVT.[58-60] It is unclear, however, to what extent serially negative ultrasound studies in medical-surgical ICU patients indicate the absence of DVT. Finally, ultrasound also inaccurately diagnoses some patients with DVT who do not have DVT by venogram, highlighting the false-positive rate of ultrasonography. Robinson and colleagues[61] performed ultrasonography and contrast venography in a large group of asymptomatic patients at the time of hospital discharge after joint replacement surgery; in this study, 6 of 19 positive compression ultrasound studies were not confirmed by venography.

Despite the advantages of using ultrasonography to diagnose DVT in the ICU, it is associated with a false-positive and false-negative rate that is not yet clearly established in the critical care setting. Nevertheless, bilateral lower-extremity ultrasound is the most widely used diagnostic test for DVT, according to VTE researchers in the medical-surgical ICU[11,43-46] and according to a survey of radiologists from the United Kingdom.[62] A recent review referred to ultrasonography as the imaging procedure of choice for the diagnosis of DVT.[63] The American College of Radiology cited bilateral lower-extremity ultrasound as the most appropriate test for DVT.[64] Finally, bilateral lower-limb ultrasound is also the most feasible diagnostic test in the ICU. An ultrasound diagnosis of DVT requires non-compressibility of one or more lower-limb venous segments, including (1) the trifurcation of the deep calves, (2) distal popliteal, (3) proximal popliteal, (4) distal femoral, (5) mid-femoral, and (6) common femoral veins.

There is no diagnostic test for DVT that is highly accurate and feasible in the ICU population for daily practice. Nevertheless, Doppler ultrasound is the most widely accepted DVT diagnostic test. Because the likelihood of embolization from undiagnosed, untreated proximal DVT is high, strategies that screen for proximal DVT in these critically ill patients have the potential to reduce the risk of pulmonary embolism and its cardiopulmonary consequences through early treatment. Universal screening for DVT with ultrasonography cannot be recommended currently, however.[44,65] Development of a reliable screening test for VTE in critically ill patients should be a high clinical priority because it is possible that the most widely used screening test today (ultrasonography) has an unacceptably high rate of false-positive tests. A false-positive ultrasound study is likely to lead to unneeded anticoagulant therapy (with its attendant risks).

Thromboprophylaxis

Only 4 published randomized trials have tested DVT prophylaxis in medical-surgical ICU patients.[66,67] One double-blind, single-center trial allocated 119 medical-surgical ICU patients at least 40 years old to unfractionated heparin, 5000 units twice daily, or placebo subcutaneous injections.[66] Using serial fibrinogen leg scanning for 5 days, the rate of DVT was 13% in the unfractionated heparin group and 29% in the placebo group (RR, 0.45; P < .05). Rates of bleeding and pulmonary embolism were not reported. In a more recent multicenter trial by Fraisse et al.,[67] 223 patients with an acute exacerbation of chronic obstructive pulmonary disease requiring mechanical ventilation for at least 2 days were allocated to the LMWH, nadroparin, 3800 or 5700 International Units once daily, or placebo. Patients were screened with weekly duplex ultrasound studies and on clinical suspicion of DVT; venography was attempted in all patients. The rate of DVT was 16% in the nadroparin group and 28% in the placebo group (RR, 0.67; P < .05). A similar number of patients bled in each group (25 versus 18 patients, P = .18). Although patients were not screened for pulmonary embolism, no patients developed pulmonary embolism during the trial.

A third trial among critically ill patients scheduled to undergo major elective surgery compared unfractionated heparin, 5000 International

Units twice daily, with LMWH enoxaparin, 40 mg once daily. Each patient was evaluated postoperatively clinically and confirmed by Doppler study for development of DVT. Among 156 patients completing the protocol, there was similar efficacy of unfractionated heparin as compared with LMWH in the prevention of DVT (2 patients [2.66%] versus 1 [1.23%], P = 0.51). There was no difference in the incidence of major complications between groups. However, minor hemorrhagic complications such as wound hematoma and surgical site bleeding were significantly more in the heparin group as compared with the LMWH group. Overall, 18 patients (24%) had bleeding either from the gastrointestinal tract or from incision site or tracheostomy site in the unfractionated heparin group, whereas 8 patients (9.87%) developed wound hematoma or gastrointestinal bleeding in the LMWH group (P = 0.01).[68]

A fourth study, Xigris and Prophylactic Heparin Evaluation in Severe Sepsis (XPRESS), was a randomized, double-blind, placebo-controlled trial of prophylactic heparin in patients with severe sepsis and higher disease severity who were treated with drotrecogin alfa (activated; DAA).[69] A recent report focused on how patients were randomized to unfractionated heparin, LMWH, or placebo during the DAA infusion period. All patients underwent ultrasonography between days 4 and 6; 1935 patients were included, and before enrollment approximately half were given no form of prophylaxis. By day 6, 5% of patients developed a VTE, and the rate of VTE did not vary based on type of heparin administered. The vast majority of VTE detected by day 6 were clinically silent. Of factors analyzed, history of VTE was the only variable independently associated with development of a VTE (OR, 3.66; 95% CI, 1.77-7.56; P = 0.005).[70]

A fifth trial outside the ICU setting but of some relevance to the ICU enrolled acutely ill medical patients hospitalized with heart failure, respiratory failure not requiring mechanical ventilation, or one of the following if associated with an additional VTE risk factor: infection without septic shock, musculoskeletal disorder, or inflammatory bowel disease.[71] Patients were excluded if they required intubation, had a coagulopathy, or had serum creatinine greater than 150 μmol/L. Patients were randomized to receive daily subcutaneous LMWH enoxaparin, 40 mg or 20 mg, or placebo for 6 to 14 days. Patients had venography between days 6 and 14 or as clinically indicated. Ultrasonography was performed if venography was not feasible. Of 1102 randomized patients, 236 were not included in the main analysis (because the venogram could not be evaluated [n = 72], was technically unfeasible [n = 12], was not performed [n = 4], was not performed at the investigators' discretion [n = 58]; the patient refused [n = 62]; or the patient died [n = 28]). Among the remaining 866 patients, the DVT rate was 6% in patients receiving enoxaparin, 40 mg, compared with 15% among patients receiving either enoxaparin, 20 mg, or placebo (RR, 0.37). Major hemorrhage developed in 12, 4, and 7 patients (P = not significant). Clinically suspected and objectively confirmed pulmonary embolism developed in one patient in the low-dose enoxaparin group and three patients in the placebo group, although pulmonary embolism events were not evaluated per protocol. The fact that these patients, although requiring medical admission to the hospital, were not critically ill limits the generalizability of these findings to the critical care setting. Nonpharmacologic approaches such as pneumatic compression devices and antiembolic stockings, although widely used, have not been evaluated in medical-surgical ICU patients, and their effectiveness must be extrapolated from other settings.

SUMMARY

Only four randomized trials evaluating VTE prophylaxis in the ICU have been published. One trial of medical-surgical patients showed that unfractionated heparin is better than no prevention (the number of patients who needed to receive prophylaxis with 5000 units twice daily of subcutaneous unfractionated heparin to prevent one DVT was four).[66] The second trial of exclusively ventilated chronic obstructive pulmonary disease patients showed that nadroparin is better than no prevention (the number of patients who needed to receive prophylaxis with weight-adjusted LMWH to prevent one DVT was eight).[71] Two trials compared unfractionated heparin with LMWH for VTE prophylaxis in medical-surgical ICU patients, but they were underpowered and inconclusive.[68,70] In contrast, in trauma patients, LMWH is clearly superior to unfractionated heparin based on randomized trials.[72]

Thromboprophylaxis Compliance

Several prospective single-center usage reviews of VTE prophylaxis provide evidence about practice patterns. Prophylaxis was prescribed in 33% of 152 medical ICU patients in one study[73] and 61% of 100 medical ICU patients in another.[11] In contrast, in a medical-surgical ICU in which a clinical practice guideline was in place, VTE prophylaxis was prescribed for 86% of 209 patients.[74] In another study of medical-surgical ICU patients, after excluding patients receiving therapeutic anticoagulation and for whom heparin was contraindicated, 63% of 96 patients received unfractionated heparin thromboprophylaxis.[20]

In a 1-day cross-sectional multicenter usage review of Canadian surgical ICU patients whose procedure was no more than 1 week earlier, unfractionated heparin was used predominantly.[75] We considered a range of patients, including those with an admission diagnosis of hemorrhage and the potential for immediate postoperative bleeding, to highlight the dual risks of thrombosis and bleeding. Two methods of VTE prophylaxis were prescribed for 20 of 89 (22.5%) patients. Prophylaxis with unfractionated heparin or LMWH was significantly less likely for postoperative ICU patients requiring mechanical ventilation compared with patients weaned from mechanical ventilation later in their ICU course (OR, 0.36; $P = .03$). Use of intermittent pneumatic compression devices was significantly associated with current hemorrhage (OR, 13.5; $P = .021$) and risk of future hemorrhage (OR, 19.3; $P = .001$).

In a 1-day bi-national cross-sectional usage review of medical ICU patients in France and Canada,[76] we found that among 1222 patients (65% of whom were mechanically ventilated), heparin VTE prophylaxis was administered similarly to 63.9% of patients between the two countries. Excluding patients with contraindications to heparin and patients receiving therapeutic anticoagulation, 91.7% of medical ICU patients appropriately received either unfractionated heparin or LMWH prophylaxis. Independent predictors of any type of heparin prophylaxis were invasive mechanical ventilation (OR, 2.4; 95% CI, 1.4-4.3]) and obesity (OR, 3.1; 95% CI, 1.1-8.8). LMWH was less likely to be prescribed for patients with renal failure (OR, 0.1; 95% CI, 0.0009-0.9) or receiving antiembolic stockings (OR, 0.4; 95% CI, 0.1-0.9) and much more likely to be prescribed in French ICUs (OR, 9.2; 95% CI, 5-16.9). However, among patients receiving LMWH, high doses were more likely to be prescribed in Canadian ICUs (OR, 8.7; 95% CI, 2-37.6). Patients who were pregnant or postpartum (OR, 7.7;

95% CI, 1.3-44.3), had neurologic failure (OR, 2.1; 95% CI, 1.3-3.4), or were Canadian (OR, 3; 95% CI, 2.1-4.4) were most likely to receive mechanical VTE prophylaxis (with antiembolic stockings or pneumatic compression devices), whereas patients who already were receiving heparin were less likely to receive mechanical prophylaxis (OR, 0.5; 95% CI, 0.3-0.7).

SUMMARY

Use of effective VTE prophylaxis ranges widely. One inference from the health services research describing practice patterns is that insufficient attention is paid to VTE prevention in the critical care setting. When deciding on the type and intensity of prophylaxis, clinicians seem to risk-stratify such that patients with a greater number of VTE risk factors are more likely to receive more intensive prophylaxis than patients with fewer risk factors. The variety of prophylactic approaches used highlights the diverse and dynamic competing risks of bleeding and thrombosis in heterogeneous ICU patients, underscoring population-based and individual risk-to-benefit ratios and delineating the need for large definitive studies to guide prophylaxis. VTE prevention methods should be individualized based on current and potential risks of bleeding and thrombosis. More randomized trials of VTE prophylaxis in medical-surgical critically ill medical patients would better inform practice. These trials should be followed up with effective implementation strategies designed to change clinician behavior and improve patient outcomes.[77]

KEY POINTS

1. Venous thromboembolism (VTE) is a multicausal disease, and critically ill medical-surgical patients have many baseline and time-dependent VTE risk factors.

2. The true frequency of deep vein thrombosis (DVT) and pulmonary embolism in critically ill patients is unclear but likely to be substantial.

3. Unrecognized VTE is likely to be associated with significant complications including death, prolonged need for ventilation, and prolonged hospital and ICU stay.

4. The test of choice for the diagnosis of DVT in the ICU is compression ultrasonography; it is easy to perform at the patient's bedside and has been shown in symptomatic outpatients to be sensitive and specific for acute DVT.

5. Large randomized clinical trials are required to determine which types of thromboprophylaxis are most effective and cost-effective in medical-surgical ICU patients. Results of these trials would need active implementation strategies to ensure they are used appropriately and safely in practice and individualized according to each patient's thrombosis and bleeding risks.

ANNOTATED REFERENCES

AHCRQ evidence report/technology assessment: prevention of venous thromboembolism after injury. Rockville, MD: Agency for Health Care Research and Quality; 2002.
  This is a comprehensive review of thromboprophylaxis and clinical recommendations relevant to the ICU.
Attia J, Ray JG, Cook DJ, et al. Deep vein thrombosis and its prevention in critically ill patients. Arch Intern Med 2001;161:1268-79.
  This is a comprehensive systematic review of the incidence of VTE and thromboprophylaxis randomized trials in several types of ICU patients (medical-surgical, trauma, neurosurgical, and spinal cord injury patients).
Ibrahim EH, Iregui M, Prentice D, et al. Deep vein thrombosis during prolonged mechanical ventilation despite prophylaxis. Crit Care Med 2002;30:771-4.

This is a well-conducted cohort study involving ultrasound screening for DVT in ICU patients; incidence and risk factor data are established.
Kearon CJ, Julian JA, Newman TE, et al. Noninvasive diagnosis of deep vein thrombosis. McMaster Diagnostic Imaging Practice Guidelines Initiative. Ann Intern Med 1998;128:663-7.
  This is a systematic review of the properties of ultrasonography for the diagnosis of DVT.
Lacherade JC, Cook DJ, Heyland DK, et al. French and Canadian ICU Directors Groups. Prevention of venous thromboembolism (VTE) in critically ill medical patients: a Franco-Canadian cross-sectional study. J Crit Care 2003;18:228-37.
  This is a Franco-Canadian survey of thromboprophylaxis patterns in medical ICU patients.

REFERENCES

Access the complete reference list online at http://www.expertconsult.com.

154

Hematologic Malignancies in the Intensive Care Unit

DELPHINE MOREAU | ÉLIE AZOULAY | BENOIT SCHLEMMER

With the rapid improvement in chemotherapy, targeted therapy, and supportive care of hematology patients, almost all hematologic malignancies in children and adults are potentially curable with chemotherapy, either alone or in combination with immunotherapy or radiotherapy and sometimes bone marrow transplantation. If the malignancy is not curable, prolonged remission with acceptable quality of life is achievable for most patients. Nevertheless, delay in treatment of some aggressive malignancies can greatly jeopardize the chances of recovery for some acutely ill patients. In addition, intensivists may be confronted with unusual presentations of hematologic emergencies which they must learn to manage adequately.

Emergency Management of Hematologic Malignancies in the Intensive Care Unit

EMERGENCY DIAGNOSIS

Emergency diagnosis of a hematologic malignancy is rarely necessary, and most patients with suspected or confirmed hematologic malignancies can be admitted directly to the hematology unit with simple supportive care (e.g., management of febrile neutropenia, transfusion if appropriate). Indeed, the specific care of patients diagnosed with acute leukemias or aggressive lymphomas should always be left to highly trained hematologists. For most of these patients, emergency initiation of induction chemotherapy is not required; chemotherapy can easily be delayed for 1 day or longer until an attending hematologist and cytologist can be reached and the necessary samples can be drawn and adequately processed.

In rare cases, patients present with life-threatening complications when no attending hematologist is available. Especially for leukemias, one should always try to obtain the following blood and marrow samples to allow for a precise diagnosis (i.e., cytologic characterization of the myeloid or lymphoid lineage, precise subtyping, and immunocytometric studies):

- 15 to 30 mL of peripheral blood (depending on leukocytosis) in heparinized tubes for molecular biology and flow cytometry studies (stored at room temperature)
- Bone marrow smears obtained by sternal or iliac aspiration, air-dried, and stored at room temperature (four to six slides) for cytology and immunohistochemistry studies
- Whenever possible, 1 mL of bone marrow aspirate (heparinized tube) for molecular biology and flow cytometry studies and another 1 mL for karyotyping (growth can be obtained even for some samples stored overnight at room temperature)
- If pleural or peritoneal effusions or cerebrospinal fluid are accessible, or emergency pericardial drainage is performed, a few milliliters of the fluid, stored at room temperature in heparinized tubes. If superficial lymph nodes are present, a fine-needle aspiration for cytologic examination of smears whenever possible.

CLINICAL SITUATIONS REQUIRING URGENT CHEMOTHERAPY

A small number of patients are admitted directly to ICUs with life-threatening complications[1] and require emergency chemotherapy because of specific organ involvement and respiratory, kidney, neurologic, or liver injury. In these cases, chemotherapy must be initiated in the ICU along with the hematologist consultant. From the intensivist's point of view, emergency chemotherapy may be indicated in seven main clinical situations, independent of the absolute circulating blast counts:

1. Cerebral leukostasis, which should be suspected in the presence of any alteration of consciousness, even a simple slowing down of cognitive functions, once an emergency computed tomography (CT) scan has ruled out an intracranial hemorrhage. Platelet count must be kept as high as possible using large platelet transfusions, disseminated intravascular coagulation (DIC) controlled by urgent chemotherapy, and every effort made to avoid blood transfusion so as to lower viscosity and maintain adequate hydration.

2. Pulmonary leukostasis (generally observed in hyperleukocytotic leukemias) with circulating blast counts greater than 50,000/mm^3 for acute myeloid leukemia (AML) or greater than 100,000/mm^3 by definition for acute lymphoid leukemia (ALL). However, symptomatic leukostasis is very rare in ALL, even for greatly elevated blasts counts, because of the smaller size and higher plasticity of these blasts.

3. Leukemic infiltration of the lungs, which is different from leukostasis, can occur with low blast counts and is often associated with AML4 or 5. These patients should be admitted to the ICU early in the course of their induction, because rapid deterioration of hematosis is frequent, both spontaneously and after initiation of chemotherapy.[2]

4. Central nervous system (CNS) involvement suspected on the basis of clinical signs such as focal deficits, seizures, or any degree of alteration of consciousness.[3] Here again, intracranial hemorrhage must first be ruled out by a CT scan.

5. Bulky mediastinal involvement with vascular compression (superior vena cava syndrome) or tracheobronchial repercussion, especially as seen in T-cell ALL

6. Threatening DIC with low fibrinogen levels and a prolonged prothrombin time

7. Severe hemophagocytic syndrome with failure of one or more organs. The choice of cytoreductive regimen depends on the type of malignancy, which is not always precisely known on arrival of the patient in the ICU. For acute leukemias, efforts should be made to characterize the lineage (ALL or AML) before treatment is initiated, but if lineage cannot be determined, a non-lineage-specific cytotoxic regimen should be chosen. Intensivists can, therefore, be confronted with five main situations, depending on

whether the lineage diagnosis has been established: ALL, AML, promyelocytic leukemia (AML3), acute leukemia of unknown lineage, non-Hodgkin's lymphoma (NHL), and very rarely, Hodgkin's disease (HD).

Emergency Chemotherapy in Leukemias

ACUTE LYMPHOBLASTIC LEUKEMIA

Classic induction therapy is based on a 7-day course of steroids alone, followed by a combination of prednisone, vincristine, and an anthracycline (daunorubicin in most studies), with or without the addition of cyclophosphamide.[4-6] In cases of compressive emergency or high tumor burden, progressive steroid therapy should be prescribed first (beginning with 0.5 mg/kg prednisone for the first dose); patients with high tumor burden should be carefully monitored because they can rapidly develop a severe acute tumor lysis syndrome (ATLS).[7-10]

The steroid dose should be increased to 1 mg/kg/d of prednisolone (or equivalent), 8 to 12 hours after the first dose, in the absence of an uncontrolled ATLS. If ATLS is present, half-dose steroids should be used until metabolic control is regained; in severe ATLS, the second steroid dose could even be postponed. In most cases of ALL, steroids alone will be able to halt the rising white blood cell (WBC) count or initiate the reduction of bulky mediastinal tumors. On day 2 or 3, full-dose vincristine (1 mg/m² of body surface, with a maximum dose of 2 mg/d) and daunorubicin (30 to 60 mg/m², or equivalent anthracycline) should be added; combination with other drugs will be decided by a hematologist according to local protocols.

For patients with increasing or stagnating WBC counts or without biological indicators of tumor response for lymphomas (especially increasing lactate dehydrogenase [LDH] levels) after two full doses of steroids, emergency adjunction of vincristine with or without daunorubicin as early as day 2 is required.

ACUTE PROMYELOCYTIC LEUKEMIA

The main complication of acute promyelocytic leukemia (APL) is DIC, with early mortality essentially related to hemorrhages located in the CNS.[11] Nevertheless, although leukostasis in APL is almost never a problem because these patients are usually pancytopenic, their leukemia should be considered (and treated) as hyperleukocytic APL as soon as the WBC count is higher than 5000/mm³. "Variant" type AML3 can be misleading, because patients are not always cytopenic, but they can display true hyperleukocytosis, sometimes greater than 100,000 cells/mm³.

Although APL is remarkably sensitive to anthracyclines, emergency treatment of APL with severe coagulation disorder now relies on early administration of all-*trans*-retinoic acid (ATRA).[12,13] There is no indication for progressive dosing of this drug, which should be prescribed immediately at 45 mg/m²/d in two oral doses taken at 12-hour intervals. Initial worsening of the DIC is the rule, and patients should receive abundant transfusion support to ensure a platelet count above 50,000/mm³ and at least 1.5 g/L of fibrinogen at all times. ATRA is available only in sealed, thick-walled, hardly soluble capsules that contain an oil-based solution. No parenteral form is available. Therefore, administration of ATRA is problematic through nasogastric tubes in mechanically ventilated patients; there is currently no other way than piercing the capsule, emptying its content, and carefully resuspending it in oil to allow injection into a gastric tube.

In hyperleukocytic APL, immediate coadministration of ATRA with daunorubicin is required, starting with half the usual dose (20 to 25 mg/m²/d) for at least 4 days, because transient exacerbation of DIC is almost universal.

ACUTE MYELOID LEUKEMIA OTHER THAN PROMYELOCYTIC LEUKEMIA

Urgent induction is derived from the classic reference treatment, a combination of 3 days of an anthracycline (classically daunorubicin, but idarubicin is one of the many possible alternatives) with 7 days of cytarabine.[4,14] The difference is that the scheme of administration is progressive: daunorubicin should be administered alone and at half the usual dose (20-25 mg/m²/d for a total of 6 days, equivalent to the 3 days of the standard full-dose regimen) before the continuous infusion of cytarabine (200 mg/m²/d for 7 days) is started on day 3 or 4.

ACUTE LEUKEMIA OF UNDETERMINED LINEAGE

In cases in which the lineage cannot be determined (e.g., no specialized cytologist on duty, poorly differentiated leukemia requiring complementary immunohistochemical study) and the patient requires urgent chemotherapy, then daunorubicin should be chosen because of its activity on all types of blasts (AML or ALL). In contrast, empirical steroid therapy could be efficient in ALL but not in AML. The scheme of administration would again be half doses of daunorubicin (20-25 mg/m²/d), and the priority should be to have blood or marrow smears reviewed as soon as possible by a trained cytologist so as to get at least the lineage determination within 24 hours. Chemotherapy can then be adjusted accordingly.

SPECIFIC PRECAUTIONS FOR LEUKEMIC PULMONARY INFILTRATION

Acute respiratory failure revealing a leukemia is rare, but intensivists should be aware that respiratory failure with bilateral consolidation can reveal nonhyperleukocytic monocytic leukemias (AML5).[2] This condition should be recognized promptly because it appears to be associated with a high risk of rapid respiratory deterioration after initiation of chemotherapy. However, this should not be viewed as a hopeless complication of a rapidly fatal disease. On the contrary, these patients should receive early invasive or noninvasive ventilatory support and immediate chemotherapy, even if they are not hyperleukocytic and their respiratory impairment is still moderate. The induction treatment is based on low-dose daunorubicin alone (20-25 mg/m²/d) for 2 to 3 days, followed by the introduction of cytarabine. Aggressive supportive care should be initiated in case of respiratory deterioration, because in our experience, 50% of these patients can survive these difficult inductions. It should be noted that blood gas analysis is useless in hyperleukocytic leukemia, since activated blast cells consume oxygen, so oxygen tension rapidly decreases in the syringe.

THE ROLE OF LEUKAPHERESIS

Therapeutic leukapheresis has been reported to be of benefit for patients with AML who have high WBC counts, and it is routinely used in some centers for acute hyperleukocytic leukemia.[15] However, controversial data have been published, and the results suggest that despite a potential reduction in early mortality, there is no overall improvement in long-term survival.[16-18] Optimal supportive care based on hyperhydration, hypouricemic drugs, and prompt induction yields similar results, whether preceded or not by a single oral dose of 2 to 4 g of hydroxyurea, without the complications inherent to the leukapheresis procedure. Based on currently available literature and the fact that this technique is not available 24 hours a day or during weekends in most centers, we cannot recommend its use for unstable ICU patients, and chemotherapy-based cytoreduction protocols should be the first choice. In our experience, leukapheresis should be reserved for failure to decrease blast cells in the presence of clinical symptoms of leukostasis.

Emergency Treatment of Non-Hodgkin's Lymphomas

Emergency initiation of chemotherapy in non-Hodgkin's lymphomas (NHLs) can be necessary in the following clinical situations[1]:

1. Massive pleural or pulmonary involvement compromising hematosis
2. Bulky mediastinal tumor with compression of trachea or main bronchi
3. Poorly tolerated superior vena cava syndrome
4. CNS localization with alteration of consciousness
5. Spinal cord compression
6. Airway compromise in cases of pharyngeal localization
7. Pericardial or cardiac involvement
8. Occlusive syndrome in massive abdominal tumors
9. NHL-related severe hemophagocytic syndrome

In these cases, initiation of chemotherapy may be required before exhaustive assessment of the disease has been completed, or even before definitive typing of the lymphoma has been established, thus complicating the therapeutic choices.[19] Nevertheless, most of these life-threatening complications occur in the setting of aggressive large-cell lymphomas, and the important point is not to choose the optimal protocol for a specific NHL but to be efficient in ensuring survival with limited toxicity in these patients with compromised respiratory, cardiac, renal, or hepatic functions.

All of these patients should receive adequate preventive treatment for ATLS, and they should be closely monitored for the occurrence of this syndrome during the first 3 days.[7-9]

BURKITT'S LYMPHOMAS

The risk of an overwhelming ATLS is so high in patients with Burkitt's lymphomas that steroids alone should be administered first and in increasing doses. Most protocols recommend that known or suspected Burkitt's lymphomas with high tumor burden be treated with a cytoreductive course of chemotherapy before full-dose chemotherapy is administered.[20-23] The consensual choice is to deliver a first initial dose of 0.25 to 0.5 mg/kg of methylprednisolone, with the following dose administered 8 to 12 hours later if no uncontrolled metabolic disorder related to an ATLS is observed. In "steroid responders," lysis will be obvious on biological criteria, especially the elevation of LDH, even in the absence of an obvious ATLS. Dosing should then be increased to 1 mg/kg/d on day 2, before infusion of one dose of vincristine and one dose of cyclophosphamide (dosing specified below) on day 2 or 3, depending on the response to steroids. If no sign of lysis occurs after two doses of steroids (as revealed by stable LDH levels), the addition of one dose of vincristine is usually sufficient to initiate a spectacular response. The cyclophosphamide dose is delivered on the following day if the ATLS is controlled. We recommend prophylactic hemodialysis in patients without kidney injury but with hyperphosphatemia before any chemotherapy of steroid therapy. Indeed, if the use of rasburicase has dramatically decreased the risk for uratic nephropathy, nephrocalcinosis remains a potential complication that can be prevented only by lowering blood phosphate levels.

THREATENING NON-BURKITT'S, NON-HODGKIN'S LYMPHOMAS

With the exception of confirmed or suspected Burkitt's lymphomas (which require smaller doses of steroids on day 1), treatment of bulky NHLs should be started with steroids at 1 mg/kg/d of methylprednisolone or equivalent on day 1 and completed as early as day 2 with vincristine (1 mg/m^2 once, maximum total dose 2 mg, in the absence of severe preexisting peripheral neuropathy) and cyclophosphamide (500-700 mg/m^2) on day 2 in the absence of uncontrolled ATLS.[20-22]

Whether bulky or not, NHLs with immediate life-threatening localization can require that all three drugs be infused on day 1, but intensivists should then be aware of the increased risk of uncontrolled ATLS, which may require extrarenal replacement.

CENTRAL NERVOUS SYSTEM INVOLVEMENT

Patients with NHL of the CNS who display focal deficits, alterations of the level of consciousness, or seizures should receive emergency steroid therapy with at least 2 mg/kg/d of methylprednisolone or equivalent. Optimal dosing is controversial in the literature, and doses ranging from 2 to 4 mg/kg/d can be considered appropriate. Administration of high-dose methotrexate, a key drug in the treatment of CNS NHL, is not necessary in an emergency situation and requires normal renal and liver functions.[3,24]

Emergency Treatment of Hodgkin's Disease

Emergency chemotherapy is a rare necessity in HD, but life-threatening mediastinal or cardiac involvement is possible, compromising oxygenation or hemodynamic stability. Nevertheless, one should remember that HD is a slow-responding tumor, so no spectacular reduction of tumor burden should be expected within 24 or 48 hours after the initiation of chemotherapy, and decisions regarding supportive care should take into account this parameter.

HD is not a steroid-sensitive disease, no single drug is rapidly efficient, and no recommendation is available in the literature regarding urgent cytoreduction in HD. Therefore, if a decision for emergency chemotherapy is made, a standard combination may be recommended: bleomycin, 10 units/m^2; vinblastine, 6 mg/m^2; doxorubicin, 25 mg/m^2; and dacarbazine, 375 mg/m^2—all administered on day 1 in the absence of cardiac or pulmonary contraindications.[25-27]

Blastic Meningitis

Although prophylactic intrathecal chemotherapy is required in all patients with ALL or hyperleukocytic AML, very few patients require urgent intrathecal chemotherapy (coma, seizures, cauda equina syndromes).[3] Therefore, specialized consultation should always be obtained before administering any intrathecal chemotherapy, even in the presence of highly suggestive symptoms such as peripheral radicular pains or deficits or hyposensitivity or dysesthesia of the chin (infiltration of the dental nerve). In addition, lumbar puncture, even for exploratory purposes, is contraindicated in patients with hyperleukocytosis, to prevent any seeding of the cerebrospinal fluid with blasts during the procedure, and in those patients with marked DIC. Moreover, intensivists should be aware that some cases of ATLS have been described after therapeutic lumbar punctures.

Nevertheless, if the indication of an emergency intrathecal treatment is confirmed, samples of cerebrospinal fluid should always be drawn for biochemical, cytologic, and bacteriologic examination before the chemotherapeutic agents are injected (usually a combination of 15 mg cytarabine, 15 mg methotrexate, and 40 mg conservative free methylprednisolone or equivalent).

Organ Failures Related To Hemophagocytic Syndrome

Severe hemophagocytic syndrome is now well recognized as a common presenting feature in NHL and HD.[28-30] In many cases, organ failures are related to the intensity of the histiocytic activation and not to the invasiveness of the lymphoma itself, which can have a very low tumor burden, making the etiologic diagnosis all the more difficult. The clinical course of these patients is generally fulminant, especially once ICU admission is required.[31,32] The clinical presentation is confounding—it precisely mimics septic shock with fever, chills, vasoplegic shock, acute respiratory distress syndrome, and oliguric renal failure—but severe pancytopenia, high blood transfusion requirements, organomegaly, lymph node enlargement, and hepatic dysfunction several days or weeks before the occurrence of this pseudoseptic shock should suggest

DIAGNOSTIC CRITERIA FOR HEMOPHAGOCYTIC LYMPHOHISTIOCYTOSIS*

Diagnosis of hemophagocytic lymphohistiocytosis (HLH) can be established by fulfilling five of the eight following criteria:

Clinical Criteria
Fever (>7 days)
Spleen enlargement

Laboratory Criteria
Bicytopenia without marrow hypoplasia, including:
  Hemoglobin <9 g/L
  Platelet count <100 × 10^9 mm^3
  Neutrophil count <1 × 10^9 mm^3
Hypertriglyceridemia (>3 mmol/L fasting value) and/or
  hypofibrinogenemia (<1.5 g/L)
Hyperferritinemia (>500 μg/L)
Low/absent natural killer cell activity
Increased soluble CD25 levels (>2400 U/mL)

Histologic Criteria
Hemophagocytosis

Adapted from Janka GE. Hemophagocytic lymphohistiocytosis. Hematology 2005;10:104-7.
*As established in the HLH 2004 protocol of the Histiocyte Society.

the diagnosis of severe hemophagocytic syndrome.[33] Biological features such as elevated serum ferritin and hypertriglyceridemia are precious but inconstant markers of the disease, and the identification of hemophagocytosis on marrow smears or in lymph node or hepatic biopsy samples sometimes requires an experienced cytologist. The 2004 criteria for the diagnosis of hemophagocytic lymphohistiocytosis are listed in Box 154-1.[33]

If sufficient clinical and biological elements are highly suggestive of the diagnosis, treatment should be promptly administered to allow emergency control of cytokine-induced organ failures. Treatment of the underlying lymphoma itself can be postponed for 2 or 3 days if the diagnosis is not yet confirmed, until urgent processing and reading of smears or biopsies have been conducted. No randomized trial of chemotherapy has been conducted in lymphoma-related hemophagocytic syndrome, so no consensus is available in the literature regarding the optimal strategy. However, etoposide-based regimens seem to be the most appropriate choice for these high-risk patients,[33,34] frequently in combination with steroids. Based on case reports and our experience, administration of 150 to 200 mg of etoposide, depending on the severity of the renal and hepatic failures, combined with 1 to 2 mg/kg/d of methylprednisolone, is rapidly effective in most cases (within 12-48 hours). The effect is only transient, and recurrence of the initial symptoms is the rule within 6 to 10 days in the absence of a specific treatment of the lymphoma, which should be started by a hematologist as soon as the lymphoma has been identified. If an aggressive NHL is highly suspected on preliminary results of smears (lymph node, marrow, or pleural effusion), a nonspecific cytoreductive combination of steroid, vincristine, and cyclophosphamide can be administered while awaiting the definitive results of the cytologic, histologic, and immunochemistry techniques.

Management of Disseminated Intravascular Coagulation

DIC is a common and serious complication of hematologic malignancies, but most of the time the bleeding is only moderately threatening, with mainly mucosal and cutaneous hemorrhagic manifestations.[35] In fact, DIC is often triggered by the initiation of chemotherapy in several types of ALLs and AMLs (AML4, AML5, and to a lesser extent AML1). However, severe forms of coagulation disorders are typically observed as a presenting symptom in untreated acute promyelocytic leukemias (APL or AML3), frequently combining DIC and a severe

hyperfibrinolytic state.[13,36] Optimal treatment includes both symptomatic measures to reduce the risk of life-threatening hemorrhage (in the CNS but also in lungs and gastrointestinal tract) and specific treatment of the leukemia.

Supportive care is essential in DIC and should include repeated platelet transfusions to reach a minimum platelet count greater than 50,000/mm^3 permanently; correction of the prothrombin time and of hypofibrinogenemia with fresh frozen plasma (2-4 units to start with) to ensure a prothrombin time less than 2.5 times normal; and a fibrinogen level greater than 1 g/L before the start of the treatment.[37] The use of low-dose unfractionated heparin (100 International Units/kg/d) is controversial, requires platelet counts permanently superior to 50,000/mm^3, and cannot be recommended for patients with active bleeding.[12,36,38,39] Its prescription in DIC with thrombotic tendencies should be discussed according to local protocols. As soon as appropriate transfusion support is initiated, chemotherapy should be started, always with progressive dosing, to reduce the leukemic load as quickly as possible. Transient worsening of DIC is common and justifies intensification of transfusions as required by biological and clinical manifestations.

In DIC caused by hematologic malignancies, the use of antithrombin III cannot be recommended based on currently available data, with the exception of severe DICs occurring after infusion of L-asparaginase.[40-42] In uncontrolled and life-threatening bleeding in nonhematology patients, the adjunctive use of recombinant factor VIIa has yielded some response, but this treatment has never been evaluated in the peculiar case of hematologic malignancies, and further well-designed evaluation of this molecule in severe malignancy-related DIC is needed to recommend its use in hematology patients.[43-47]

Multiple Myeloma and Other Causes of Hyperviscosity Syndromes

Severe infectious complications and metabolic emergencies (e.g., hypercalcemia, acute renal failure) can lead myeloma patients to the ICU, and these conditions are detailed elsewhere in this text. Myeloma patients can also present with severe organ failures early in the course of their disease. Intensivists should not be discouraged from admitting these patients to the ICU if the disease is not refractory and the patient is in poor condition, because prognosis in the ICU has improved over the years and can justify their admission.[48] Hyperviscosity syndrome is one specific complication that can initially require ICU admission.

Hyperviscosity syndromes may be encountered in multiple myeloma and Waldenström's macroglobulinemia, symptomatic forms being more common in the latter.[49,50] Clinical manifestations are mainly neurologic (headaches, alteration or slowdown of cognitive function, stupor, even coma, and rarely seizures), ocular (visual impairment, papillary edema with dilated retinal veins, retinal hemorrhages), and excessive bleeding (mainly mucosal, cutaneous, and retinal). Emergency management is directed at rapidly decreasing blood viscosity through plasmapheresis, which leads to rapid alleviation of the initial symptoms. Long-term management, whether based on high-dose steroids or chemotherapy, is aimed at reducing production of monoclonal immunoglobulin and can be postponed until a hematologist consultant has been reached. Plasmapheresis is the only therapeutic option with immediate efficacy[51,52]; it consists of the exchange of 1 to 1.5 plasma volumes (5 L maximum), with 100% replacement by 4% human albumin solution. Plasmapheresis should preferably be conducted by a trained hemapheresis team using specifically designed machines. If no such team is available, plasmapheresis can be performed by intensivists on several machines designed for ICU continuous renal replacement (e.g., Spectra-Cobe, Prisma-Hospal), equipped with plasma exchange kits. The rate of plasma exchange is then lower, but these devices allow easy exchange of 1 plasma volume, with standard anticoagulation of the filter (whereas "classic" plasmapheresis is generally performed with citrate anticoagulation). The hemodynamic tolerance is usually correct, even if most patients require volume expansion because of a moderate hypotension after 60% or 70% of the plasma exchange (due to rapid removal of the osmotically active paraprotein).

1. Short-term survival after critical care illness has improved understanding of organ dysfunction. Classic predictors of mortality are no longer relevant, and the usual triage criteria for ICU admission are unreliable.

2. Early admission to the ICU for cancer patients is recommended.

3. In difficult cases, an ICU trial (typically 3 days) should be considered before making a final decision.

4. Attempts should be made to find a balance between noninvasive treatments and quick application of optimal therapies.

5. Close collaboration must be developed between intensivists and hematologists/oncologists in the global management of cancer patients.

ANNOTATED REFERENCES

Azoulay E, Fieux F, Moreau D, et al. Acute monocytic leukemia presenting as acute respiratory failure. Am J Respir Crit Care Med 2003;167:1-5.
This is a recent report of pulmonary leukemic infiltration with acute respiratory failure as a presenting feature in 20 patients with acute monocytic leukemia. Intensivists should be aware of both its rapid progression after initiation of chemotherapy and its potential reversibility with adequate ICU management.

Barbui T, Finazzi G, Falanga A. The impact of all-*trans*-retinoic acid on the coagulopathy of acute promyelocytic leukemia. Blood 1998;91:3093-102.
A comprehensive review of DIC in APL, the interactions between ATRA and the hemostatic system, and the impact of ATRA on the early hemorrhagic events in the treatment of APL.

Giles FJ, Shen Y, Kantarjian HM, et al. Leukapheresis reduces early mortality in patients with acute myeloid leukemia with high white blood cell counts but does not improve long-term survival. Leuk Lymphoma 2001;45:67-73.
One of the only randomized trials testing early leukapheresis in hyper-hyperleukocytic patients with acute leukemia, it demonstrated the absence of benefit on long-term survival. These patients should, therefore, be treated urgently with chemotherapy, without wasting time organizing leukapheresis or transfer to a medical center performing leukapheresis.

Lister A, Abrey LE, Sandlund JT. Central nervous system lymphoma. Hematology Am Soc Hematol Educ Program 2002:283-96.
This is a complete and meticulous review of up-to-date management of all types of CNS involvement in lymphoma (primary CNS lymphoma, blastic meningitis, secondary CNS lymphoma).

Patte C, Sakiroglu O, Sommelet D. European experience in the treatment of hyperuricemia. Semin Hematol 2001;38:9-12.
This study, comparing the rate of dialysis required for ATLS-related renal failure, demonstrated the superiority of urate oxidase over allopurinol in preventing acute tumor lysis during the induction chemotherapy of diseases with high tumor burden.

REFERENCES

Access the complete reference list online at http://www.expertconsult.com.

155

Hematopoietic Stem Cell Transplantation Patient

SANJAY CHAWLA | LOUIS P. VOIGT | JEFFREY S. GROEGER

Bone marrow transplantation was developed as a treatment for hematologic malignances in the early 1970s. Since peripheral blood stem cells or umbilical cord blood can be used as sources of donor stem cells, the term *bone marrow transplantation* has been replaced by the more inclusive *hematopoietic stem cell transplantation* (HSCT). The use of peripheral blood stem cells provides a shorter duration of neutropenia and more rapid hematopoietic reconstitution, which may reduce some of the infectious and bleeding complications.[1] Worldwide in 2006, approximately 50,000 to 60,000 patients received an HSCT. Of these, peripheral blood was the most common source in adults. Approximately 45% of all allogeneic transplants were from unrelated donors. Between 2003 and 2007, 10% of HSCT recipients were older than 60 years. Given that the indications for HSCT are increasing, older patients receiving an HSCT will likely increase as well. The most common indications for HSCT in general are multiple myeloma and lymphoma, while acute myeloid leukemia is the most common reason for allogeneic HSCT.[2] HSCT has also been used as a treatment for aplastic anemia and hemoglobinopathies as well as cancers of the breast, ovaries, and testicles.

The immune system fully recovers over a period of several months; rapidity is dependent on the type of transplant (autologous or allogeneic) as well as source of stem cells, with peripheral blood generally being the earliest, and umbilical cord blood being the longest. Other factors that impact on immune reconstitution include age of the recipient, conditioning regimen (myeloablative versus non-myeloablative), graft-versus-host disease (GVHD) status, use of immunosuppressive medications, and donor's age and gender.[3]

Immune reconstitution occurs in three rough timeframes. Phase I (preengraftment) occurs between days 0 and 30, and host risk factors for infection and includes prolonged neutropenia and disruption in mucocutaneous barriers due to mucositis or vascular access devices. Phase II (early postengraftment) occurs from days 30 to 100, at which time cell-mediated immunity is impaired. Pathogens including cytomegalovirus (CMV), *Pneumocystis jirovecii* (formerly *Pneumocystis carinii*), and *Aspergillus* spp. are the predominant causes of infection. Phase III (late postengraftment) occurs beyond 100 days and is of particular risk for allogeneic patients with chronic GVHD or alternative donors (matched unrelated, umbilical cord blood, or mismatched related donor) because of impaired function of the reticuloendothelial system as well as cell-mediated and humoral defects. Patients are at risk for infection from encapsulated bacteria, gram-negative bacilli, CMV, varicella-zoster virus (VZV), and Epstein-Barr virus (EBV).[4] Over the following year, there is further gradual reconstitution.

Various series have reported rates of intensive care unit (ICU) admission ranging from 5% to as high as 55%, with lower rates in autologous HSCT.[5] In one study of umbilical cord blood recipients, 57% required ICU admission, which was most likely to be predicted by the preparative regimen, while a higher number of infused nucleated cells appeared to be protective from ICU transfer.[6] Complications of HSCT that require ICU care develop in up to 40% and often involves the lung.[7,8] Respiratory manifestations account for up to 58% of ICU admissions of HSCT recipients,[5] and almost half of those require mechanical ventilation. Certain pulmonary complications are unique to the HSCT patient, including cumulative lung damage from repeated chemotherapy and radiation, pulmonary infections from immunosuppression, and lung manifestations of the underlying hematologic disease.[9] Other reasons for ICU admission include septic shock, hypotension, mucositis, cardiac dysfunction, neurologic complications, bleeding, and hepatic veno-occlusive disease.[7,10] Less common primary reasons for ICU admission include seizures, intracranial or gastrointestinal bleeding, or renal failure.[5]

Risk factors for ICU admission include conditioning with total body irradiation, posttransplant immunosuppression, visceral organ toxicity, and GVHD.[11] A number of risk factors for mechanical ventilation per se have been identified, including older age, hematologic disease in relapse at the time of transplantation, and receipt of a mismatched HSCT graft.[12] The complications that may result in critical illness are shown in Boxes 155-1 and 155-2. Space does not permit in-depth discussion of all these issues, so this chapter will focus on the pulmonary complications of HSCT and discuss bronchoscopy, hepatic veno-occlusive disease, outcomes, prognosis, and triage.

Pulmonary Infections

Pulmonary complications can occur in up to 50% of patients undergoing HSCT[13]; they are more frequent in recipients of allogeneic or matched unrelated transplants than in those receiving autologous transplants. Pneumonia that develops during the first 100 days after HSCT is usually caused by gram-negative enteric bacilli (see Box 155-1). As the immune system recovers and the patient spends less time in the hospital, this pattern changes, and gram-positive organisms become more common. CMV infection used to be a major cause of pulmonary morbidity and mortality in the HSCT population. The introduction of CMV antigen surveillance and the use of preemptive treatment with ganciclovir have reduced the incidence of CMV pneumonitis to less than 10%.[14] The incidence of *P. jirovecii* pneumonia in the HSCT population has also been reduced to about 2% with effective use of antibiotic prophylaxis.[15]

Despite these advances, prevention and treatment of invasive fungal infection remains a serious problem in this population. Invasive pulmonary aspergillosis remains the leading cause of infectious death in recipients of allogeneic or matched unrelated transplants,[16] despite the development of newer antifungal agents such as caspofungin and voriconazole.[17,18] The role of combination antifungal therapy remains unclear, owing to the lack of a well-controlled prospective trial. However, expert consensus recognizes the role of this strategy as salvage therapy in which case agents of different classes should be used.[19]

Additionally, the recently described human metapneumovirus has been reported to cause mild to severe respiratory disease in HSCT recipients. Infections can occur as early as at the time of transplantation up to 4 years later and most commonly occurs in the late winter or early spring months.[20,21] The immunocompromised HSCT population is also vulnerable to outbreaks of pneumonia from *Legionella pneumophila*[22] and respiratory syncytial virus.

COMPLICATIONS OF HEMATOPOIETIC STEM CELL TRANSPLANTATION THAT MAY LEAD TO INTENSIVE CARE

Infection
Bacterial:
  Escherichia coli, Pseudomonas, Klebsiella, Acinetobacter,
    Staphylococcus spp., *Enterococcus, Streptococcus,*
    Clostridium spp.
Viral:
  Herpesvirus
  Varicella-zoster virus
  Influenza, parainfluenza, adenovirus, respiratory syncytial virus
  Cytomegalovirus
Fungal:
  Candida spp.
  Aspergillus spp.
Protozoal:
  Toxoplasma
  Pneumocystis jirovecii

Cardiac Complications
Cardiogenic pulmonary edema
Arrhythmias
Pericardial effusion
Myocarditis

Neurologic Complications
Seizures
Encephalopathy
Polyneuropathy
Intracranial hemorrhage
Subarachnoid hemorrhage

Pulmonary Complications
Noncardiogenic pulmonary edema
Acute respiratory distress syndrome
Idiopathic pneumonia syndrome
Diffuse alveolar hemorrhage syndrome
Peri-engraftment respiratory distress syndrome (PERDS)
Infectious pneumonia
Aspiration pneumonia
Bronchiolitis obliterans/airflow obstruction
Delayed pulmonary toxicity syndrome
Pleural effusions
Interstitial fibrosis

Gastrointestinal Complications
Mucositis
Diarrhea
Drug-induced hepatotoxicity
Hepatic veno-occlusive disease
Pancreatitis

Renal Complications
Drug toxicity
Hepatorenal syndrome

Graft-versus-Host Disease
Acute
Chronic

Noninfectious Pulmonary Disease

Noninfectious pulmonary complications are an important cause of critical illness in HSCT recipients. It is important to keep in mind that infectious and noninfectious pulmonary complications may occur contemporaneously.

Acute adverse reactions can occur during stem cell infusions and range from benign symptoms such as nausea, vomiting, asymptomatic hypotension, and arrhythmias to more serious complications such as cerebrovascular ischemia, malignant cardiac arrhythmias, acute renal failure, and sudden death.[23-27] The causes and mechanisms are unclear,

but recipient age, dimethylsulfoxide (DMSO) concentration, and content of non-mononuclear cells in the stem cell mixture, as well as histamine and other byproducts of cell lysis, have been implicated.[27,28] Infusion of DMSO-washed stem cells under cardiac monitoring or in the ICU is occasionally advocated for high-risk patients. However, the administration of antihistaminic agents and close observation in the ICU does not mitigate the risks of significant adverse reactions, because the pathophysiology is likely multifactorial. Treatment is often supportive.

Respiratory failure that develops within days after transplantation may be caused by cardiogenic pulmonary edema. There is usually a brisk response to aggressive treatment, and intubation and mechanical ventilation can sometimes be avoided. Pulmonary edema causing respiratory failure in the HSCT recipient is a positive predictor of survival in those requiring mechanical ventilation.[29] The large volumes of intravenous (IV) fluids and blood products used during HSCT can increase the circulating blood volume. Additionally, cyclophosphamide is commonly used in the preparative regimen and may cause acute cardiac toxicity.[30] Findings that suggest cardiogenic pulmonary edema include diffuse pulmonary infiltrates, a rapid response to diuretics, and reduced left ventricular ejection fraction on echocardiogram. The risk/benefit ratio of hemodynamic monitoring with a pulmonary artery catheter in this setting is not clear. These subjects often have a signifi-

TIMELINE OF COMPLICATIONS AFTER HEMATOPOIETIC STEM CELL TRANSPLANTATION

Preengraftment Complications (Days 0-30)
Regimen-related toxicity:
  Mucositis
  Hemorrhagic cystitis
  Hypervolemia
Cardiogenic pulmonary edema
Peri-engraftment respiratory distress syndrome (PERDS)
Diffuse alveolar hemorrhage
Idiopathic pneumonia syndrome
Veno-occlusive disease
Drug toxicity
Graft failure
Infections:
  Coagulase-negative *Staphylococcus* spp., methicillin-resistant
    Staphylococcus aureus
  Gram-negative bacilli
  Candida and *Aspergillus*
  Herpes simplex virus, adenovirus, influenza virus, respiratory
    syncytial virus

Immediate Postengraftment Complications (Days 30-100)
Acute graft-versus-host disease (GVHD)
Idiopathic pneumonia syndrome
Diffuse alveolar hemorrhage
Infections:
  Bacterial infections that occur during early phase
  Encapsulated bacteria
  Fungi, including *Aspergillus*
  Viruses, including cytomegalovirus, respiratory viruses
  Pneumocystis jirovecii

Late Postengraftment Complications (Beyond Day 100)
Chronic GVHD
Bronchiolitis obliterans
Airflow obstruction
Disease relapse
Infections:
  Encapsulated bacteria
  Gram-negative bacilli
  Nocardia
  Aspergillus
  Cytomegalovirus, varicella-zoster virus, Epstein-Barr virus
  P. jirovecii

cant bleeding diathesis in addition to leukopenia, increasing the risk of hemorrhage and infection with catheter use.

Diffuse alveolar hemorrhage (DAH) occurs in 1% to 5% of autologous and 3% to 7% of allogeneic HSCT recipients.[31] Injury to the pulmonary endothelial lining from high-dose chemotherapy and radiation, as well as various infections, play a role in the pathogenesis. Although infection can lead to alveolar hemorrhage, the term DAH in HSCT recipients should be solely used for noninfectious alveolar hemorrhage.[32] Old age, severe oral mucositis, acute GVHD, intensive pretransplantation chemotherapy, total body irradiation, and allogeneic stem cells are important risks factors.[31,33] Symptoms such as cough, dyspnea, and fevers are frequent, whereas hemoptysis is rare.[32] Anemia and pulmonary infiltrates on chest radiographs are usually present. Diagnostic criteria include diffuse multilobar infiltrates, high Pao_2/Fio_2 ratio or widened alveolar-arterial gradient, absence of any identifiable infection, and progressively bloodier return on bronchoalveolar lavage (BAL), while cytology confirms hemosiderin-laden macrophages.[32] Treatment is challenging, with cohort studies reporting variable success rates with high-dose steroids.[34] In the past decade, reports of intrapulmonary and IV human recombinant activated factor VIIa and IV aminocaproic acid have resulted in apparent control of active bleeding, but such success did not translate into improved outcomes.[35-37] Mortality rates of 30% to 90% have been reported, particularly when DAH is associated with respiratory failure requiring mechanical ventilation or multiorgan failure.[38,39] Relapse is occasional and portends a higher mortality rate.[34]

The term *idiopathic pneumonia syndrome* (IPS) refers to a diffuse interstitial pneumonia with evidence of widespread alveolar injury and absence of lower respiratory tract infection in an HSCT patient.[40] Additional features include abnormal pulmonary physiology and multilobar infiltrates on chest radiography or chest computed tomography (CT). The incidence of IPS is about 7%, and it occurs at a median time of 21 days after HSCT.[41] Although there is no difference in incidence between autologous and allogeneic HSCT recipients, significant risk factors have been identified in allogeneic transplantation and include an underlying diagnosis other than leukemia, grade 4 acute GVHD, and CMV-seropositive donor status.[41] Other potential risk factors include exposure to pretransplantation radiation, busulfan, and cyclophosphamide.[42-44] These data suggest that IPS may be caused by cumulative damage to the lung from chemotherapy, radiation, and GVHD. Almost 70% require mechanical ventilation for respiratory failure. The hospital mortality rate is above 70%, and respiratory failure leading to death occurs in 62% of patients with IPS.[41] It is important to differentiate IPS from the other syndromes outlined in this section that may also manifest with bilateral pulmonary infiltrates.[41] Treatment is mainly supportive, and even with aggressive care, the prognosis remains poor.[41,45] Limited data have suggested high clinical response rates and improved short-term survival with a combination of etanercept and corticosteroids.[46]

The peri-engraftment respiratory distress syndrome (PERDS) is a well-recognized noninfectious complication of HSCT and occurs between 5 days before and 5 days after the onset of neutrophil production. Symptomatology includes rash, fevers, dyspnea, and occasional weight gain associated with severe hypoxemia and bilateral pulmonary infiltrates.[47,48] Endothelial cell damage and cytokine production are the proposed mechanisms of this syndrome. Other possibilities such as acute GVHD, infectious pneumonitis, IPS, and DAH must be ruled out. The diagnosis relies on a high index of suspicion, particularly when the workup for infectious etiologies is negative. Bronchoscopy and BAL are often necessary to rule out DAH and other infectious and noninfectious pulmonary complications. Steroids and supportive care often result in rapid recovery. PERDS has been identified as a marker of increased posttransplantation mortality.[48]

Bronchoscopy

Several observational and prospective studies have established the safety and diagnostic utility of flexible fiberoptic bronchoscopy in the evaluation of the HSCT recipients who developed focal or diffuse pulmonary infiltrates associated with respiratory insufficiency/failure.[49-51] The diagnostic yield of bronchoscopy and BAL ranges from 63% in earlier studies to about 42% to 47% in more recent studies. Indeed, recipients of HSCT tend to be on prophylactic antimicrobials; when they develop apparent sepsis syndrome and/or pulmonary infiltrates, initiation of an empirical antimicrobial regimen is rather prompt. Such strategies may explain the perceived reduction in the diagnostic yield of bronchoscopy. Although bronchoscopy can lead to radical modification in treatment in up to two-thirds of HSCT recipients, it has no impact on survival.[52-54] The addition of transbronchial biopsy provides specific information in less than 10% of cases.[55] Allogeneic HSCT recipients are three times more likely to undergo bronchoscopy than autologous patients because of greater need for immunosuppression and GVHD prophylaxis/treatment and higher risk of infectious pulmonary complications.[52] Diffuse alveolar hemorrhage and pulmonary infections are the most frequent diagnoses obtained by bronchoscopy, followed by IPS, bronchiolitis obliterans with or without organizing pneumonia, and radiation-induced lung injury.[54,56]

Bronchoscopy can be associated with significant complications such as acute respiratory failure, pneumothoraces, epistaxis, pulmonary bleeding, and even sudden death.[50] The use of noninvasive positive pressure ventilation (NIPPV) delivered by face mask and by laryngeal mask airway (LMA) may partially mitigate these risks. Bronchoscopy with BAL via facemask, helmet, or LMA appears to be a safe alternative to intubation in immunocompromised patients.[57-59] HSCT recipients who require mechanical ventilation are also at risk of hemodynamic instability and worsening hypoxemia/ARDS when they received sedative and narcotic agents during BAL.

The decision to perform fiberoptic bronchoscopy in the HSCT patient with pulmonary disease can be difficult. The risk/benefit ratio of the procedure must be carefully analyzed in this vulnerable population. Severe hypoxemia is a contraindication to fiberoptic bronchoscopy in the nonintubated HSCT patient, and the risk of elective intubation for fiberoptic bronchoscopy must be balanced against the benefits of empirical treatment. Overall, careful patient selection is the most efficient method to minimize the risks of complications related to bronchoscopy.

Sepsis

HSCT recipients have a number of risk factors for infection and septic shock, including immunosuppression, mucositis from preparative regimens, and the use of long-term indwelling catheters for vascular access. There is a temporal pattern to some of the infections, as shown in Box 155-2. Some of the more common organisms isolated are gram-positive cocci, gram-negative enteric bacilli, *Candida* spp., and *Aspergillus* spp. Infection with CMV and herpesviruses also occurs. Impaired host defenses in the HSCT patient may prevent localization of infection, and as a result, septic shock may develop. Septic shock is the admitting diagnosis in about 18% of HSCT patients transferred to the ICU, and the diagnosis of septic shock is made in about 60% of all HSCT patients receiving ICU care.[60,61] HSCT patients with septic shock require vasopressor support in most cases and may progress to multisystem organ failure. The prognosis of septic shock in the HSCT patient is poor, and the 30-day mortality rate after ICU admission exceeded 80% in one recent study.[60] The need for more than 4 hours of vasopressor support has been shown to increase mortality among mechanically ventilated HSCT patients.[10] Empirical antibiotics and antifungal agents, along with blood products, form an important part of the management of critical illness in the HSCT patient. To date, there has been no randomized controlled trial evaluating the efficacy and safety of recombinant human activated protein C in the treatment of sepsis in the HSCT population.[62]

Hepatic Veno-Occlusive Disease

Veno-occlusive disease (VOD) is the most common cause of liver failure in HSCT patients and has also been referred to as *sinusoidal obstruction syndrome* (SOS), because sinusoidal obstruction is prominent on pathology. The mean incidence is 13.7% (0%-62.5%) in all HSCT recipients and has increased over time.[63] The diagnosis should be suspected if jaundice, painful hepatomegaly, ascites, fluid retention, and weight gain develop within the first 4 weeks after HSCT, although it can occur later.[64] As the liver fails, encephalopathy, coagulopathy, bleeding, fluid retention, and renal failure may develop and result in critical illness. The spectrum of disease ranges from mild reversible disease to a severe syndrome associated with multiorgan failure (MOF). The overall mortality in severe VOD is 84.3%, which increases to almost 100% at 100 days after HSCT and is most commonly due to MOF.[63,65,66] A number of risk factors have been identified, including receipt of an allogeneic transplant, abnormal liver function tests before transplantation, high-dose chemotherapy, and previous abdominal radiation.[66]

Right upper quadrant ultrasonography with color Doppler typically shows hepatomegaly, ascites, and reversal of blood flow through the hepatic vein. Liver biopsy, although uncommonly performed, should be considered if the differential diagnosis includes acute GVHD or drug toxicity and may change therapeutic plans. Treatment of VOD is mainly supportive, with careful fluid balance, preservation of renal function, and judicious diuresis for management of ascites. Thrombolytic agents and heparin have been used but have a success rate of less than 30% with a high risk of bleeding.[67] Defibrotide is an oligonucleotide with local antithrombotic, antiischemic and antiinflammatory effects. In a dose-finding trial, defibrotide was shown to be effective in 46% of patients with severe VOD, achieving clinical remission and 42% alive at 100 days after HSCT.[64]

Supportive Care

Advances have been made in regard to overall HSCT care as well as ICU management, and recent trials that have shown improved outcomes in critically ill patients are generally applicable to HSCT patients. Strategies such as NIPPV, low tidal volumes for ALI/ARDS, early goal-directed therapy, and glycemic control should be utilized when appropriate.[11]

NIPPV has been shown to be effective in immunocompromised patients with hypoxemic respiratory failure. In a small prospective randomized study of 52 neutropenic patients with hypoxemia and pulmonary infiltrates, the use of intermittent NIPPV was associated with a lower intubation rate, fewer serious complications, and improved ICU and hospital survival, compared with spontaneous breathing and supplemental oxygen alone.[68] Only 17 (33%) of the subjects enrolled in this study had undergone HSCT. Sources of bias included patient selection and the inability to blind the study. NIPPV may be useful in the HSCT population, but mucositis and severe GVHD of the oropharynx are complications that may interfere with NIPPV. In general, it is important to not delay intubation if the patient does not improve with NIPPV.

As a result of the conditioning regimen, pancytopenia is expected, and neutropenia is a major factor for the development of infectious complications in the early posttransplant phase. Even with the use of prophylactic antibiotics and colony stimulating factors (CSF), infection due bacteria or fungi are common in this population. Granulocyte-CSF (G-CSF) can enhance granulocyte function by increasing production of superoxide radicals, phagocytosis, and cytotoxicity. Granulocyte transfusions have been used in neutropenic septic patients, but a Cochrane review concluded that the available evidence could neither refute nor support this practice. A possible survival benefit was suggested with doses of greater than 1×10^{10} granulocytes, but further investigation is required.[69]

Outcomes, Prognostication, and Triage

Initial studies on outcomes of HSCT patients generally reported an overall poor outcome for those requiring ICU care. An early report on mechanical ventilation use in HSCT found that only 3% survived 6 months beyond ICU admission[12]; however, more recent data found

that up to 10% were alive at 6 months. Overall hospital survival has also improved to 20% to 32.5% for those requiring mechanical ventilation[70-72] and 95% for those who did not need it.[72] However, the overall hospital and 30-day mortality for critically ill HSCT recipients remains high at 74%.[5] Patients who require more than 4 hours of vasopressor support and have two other organ failures (e.g., serum bilirubin >4 mg/dL and serum creatinine >2 mg/dL), have a mortality rate of almost 100%.[10,60,61,70] There are conflicting data on any association between ICU outcome and the timing of ICU admission after transplantation.[10,29,60] Data demonstrating a survival benefit to early posttransplantation admission have not been reproducible. The need for endotracheal intubation to manage respiratory failure and the need for more than 15 days of mechanical ventilation have been associated with a survival rate of less than 5%.[7,10,29,73,74]

Attributed mortality in allogeneic HSCT is most commonly due to disease relapse, followed by infection, GVHD, and organ toxicity.[2] Prognostic factors that influence outcomes of critically ill HSCT patients include age, coexisting comorbidities, and functional status. Severity of illness as measured by ICU scoring systems have generally underestimated actual mortality rates even if they account for immunosuppression, hematologic malignancy, or metastatic neoplasm.[5,7,61] Additionally, the models do not take into account unique features such as GVHD or prior chemotherapy, and none have been evaluated specifically in predicting mortality of HSCT recipients. The utility of the Acute Physiology and Chronic Health Evaluation II (APACHE II) scoring system in the HSCT population is unclear, but there is evidence that a score higher than 45 is associated with poor survival.[7,61] One study has suggested that APACHE III scores better predict ICU mortality.[60]

A pragmatic approach to deciding when to admit an HSCT patient to the ICU would employ providing full supportive care during the engraftment process, especially for those patients with isolated or limited organ failure.[71] An ongoing need for mechanical ventilation, vasopressors, and multiple organ support generally portends a poor prognosis, particularly if hepatic failure, renal failure, or active GVHD is present.[71,75] Such conditions would warrant a reassessment of goals after a defined period of supportive treatment.[11,76]

Patients who consent to receive an HSCT are hopeful and are making a commitment to proceed with a complex procedure that has inherent risks. Prior to developing critical illness, a great deal of effort is made in preparation, evaluation, and donor search. Intensivists are not part of the discussion that occurs during this period and therefore cannot offer their perspective until a patient is admitted to the ICU. Once the need for ICU care becomes evident, there has been a deep investment in that patient's care as well as desire to control the underlying problem that required transplantation. Nevertheless, the critical care team should work closely with the transplant team to ensure that uniform and clear communication occurs with the patient and families. As such, both teams must be able to agree to specific endpoints during the patient's critical illness. One study looking at a 72-hour interval of ICU care found that continued presence of respiratory failure as well as degree (Pao_2/Fio_2 <250), BUN over 40 mg/dL, and urinary output of less than 150 mL for any 8-hour period portended a worse prognosis. When combined with clinical judgment, these parameters could help guide discussions about goals of care.[76] Additionally, the presence of respiratory failure requiring mechanical ventilation with combined hepatic and renal dysfunction was highly predictive of death.[75] HSCT recipients with acute lung injury requiring mechanical ventilation who had a prolonged need for vasopressors or sustained hepatic and renal failure had a mortality rate of almost 100%.[10] By reevaluating the ICU course with objective data and clinical judgment, discussions of end-of-life care should be jointly reviewed with the family.

The Future

The field of stem cell transplantation is evolving. The development of reduced-intensity (nonmyeloablative) conditioning regimens rely on a graft-versus-tumor effect to control residual disease, rather than high-dose chemotherapy and its attendant toxicity. As a result, transplantation in older patients with more comorbid illnesses can be feasible.[77] Other strategies for the future include focused therapies to reduce the incidence of GVHD such as cytokine blockade or modified T cells, more specific HLA typing, increased use of umbilical cord blood, or possibly embryonic stem cells.[78-81] Additionally, indications for transplantation may expand to nononcologic conditions such as sickle cell disease and hemoglobinopathies or inborn errors of metabolism.

KEY POINTS

1. Effective prophylaxis and screening have reduced the incidence of opportunistic infections among patients undergoing hematopoietic stem cell transplantation (HSCT). Invasive fungal disease remains an important problem and is difficult to both prevent and treat.

2. Engraftment syndrome, diffuse alveolar hemorrhage, and idiopathic pneumonia syndrome are all characterized by diffuse multilobar infiltrates, a widened alveolar-arterial gradient, and the absence of any identifiable infection. These syndromes may be related, but they have to be distinguished clinically because they have different outcomes.

3. The safety and diagnostic utility of fiberoptic bronchoscopy in stable HSCT patients has been established. Bronchoscopy findings can result in a change in management in up to two-thirds of cases. In HSCT patients with worsening respiratory failure, bronchoscopy must be undertaken with caution because the procedure can precipitate the need for mechanical ventilation.

4. HSCT patients who require prolonged mechanical ventilation and vasopressor support and have evidence of other organ failure tend to have a very high mortality rate.

5. End-of-life care in the critically ill HSCT patient remains complex and challenging.

6. The use of nonmyeloablative conditioning and umbilical cord stem cells is increasing. These alternative regimens and stem cells are broadening the scope, indications, and complications.

ANNOTATED REFERENCES

Afessa B, Tefferi A, Litzow MR, et al. Diffuse alveolar hemorrhage in hematopoietic stem cell transplant recipients. Am J Respir Crit Care Med 2002;166:641-5.
This clinical commentary provides a broad review of DAH in the HSCT population, including pathogenesis, clinical findings, differential diagnosis, and treatment.
Patel NR, Lee PS, Kim JH, et al. The influence of diagnostic bronchoscopy on clinical outcomes comparing adult autologous and allogeneic bone marrow transplant patients. Chest 2005;127:1388-96.
This retrospective review studied the diagnostic yield and management impact of fiberoptic bronchoscopy as well as transbronchial biopsy in both autologous and allogeneic HSCT. The study confirmed findings of prior reports that while additional information was yielded and may have led to changes in management, in-hospital mortality was unchanged in both groups.
Hilbert G, Gruson D, Vargas F, et al. Noninvasive ventilation in immunosuppressed patients with pulmonary infiltrates, fever, and acute respiratory failure. N Engl J Med 2001;344:481-7.
This was a prospective randomized trial of intermittent noninvasive ventilation compared with standard treatment (supplemental oxygen without ventilatory support) in the immunosuppressed population.

Fifty-two subjects with pulmonary infiltrates, fever, and hypoxemic acute respiratory failure were studied. Early initiation of noninvasive ventilation was associated with significant reductions in the rates of endotracheal intubation and serious complications and an improved likelihood of survival to hospital discharge. The study included only 17 HSCT subjects, limiting its generalizability.
Rubenfeld GD, Crawford SW. Withdrawing life support from mechanically ventilated recipients of bone marrow transplants: a case for evidence-based guidelines. Ann Intern Med 1996;125:625-33.
This nested case-control study evaluated the prognostic factors associated with increased mortality in mechanically ventilated HSCT patients. The authors developed guidelines to help medical decision making in the critically ill HSCT patient.
Capizzi SA, Kumar S, Huneke NE, et al. Peri-engraftment respiratory distress syndrome during autologous hematopoietic stem cell transplantation. Bone Marrow Transplant 2001;27:1299-303.
This 10-year retrospective series describes one center's experience of PERDS, including incidence, BAL findings, treatment, and outcomes.

REFERENCES

Access the complete reference list online at http://www.expertconsult.com.

156

Organ Toxicity of Cancer Chemotherapy

AMÉLIE SEGUIN | VIRGINIE LEMIALE | ANNE-SOPHIE MOREAU | MICHAËL DARMON |
ADELINE MAX | LIONEL KARLIN | ÉLIE AZOULAY

Substantial improvements in survival rates among cancer patients admitted to the intensive care unit (ICU) have been achieved over the last decade.[1] Three factors have contributed to these advances: (1) better patient selection, following reports in the 1980s of dismal outcomes[2,3] and ensuing recommendations that ICU admission be denied in many situations involving cancer patients[4-6]; (2) improved overall survival of cancer patients,[7] owing to therapeutic innovations and measures to prevent infections and drug toxicity; and (3) recent advances in ICU management of acute respiratory failure[1,8] and septic shock.[9]

Today, hospital mortality among cancer patients admitted to the ICU is approximately 50%, which is not higher than in other patient groups (e.g., chronic obstructive pulmonary disease, chronic heart failure, pancreatitis, extensive burns, etc.). In addition, characteristics such as neutropenia, autologous bone marrow transplantation, or progression of malignancy no longer predict mortality.[10-12] New treatments such as granulocyte colony-stimulating factor (G-CSF) shorten the duration of bone marrow failure,[13,14] thereby diminishing the risk of treatment-related infection, and medications that have limited toxicity can achieve remissions in patients initially considered as having relentlessly progressive disease.[15-17] As a result of these major therapeutic advances, the number of cancer patients referred for ICU admission is increasing steadily, with infection and treatment-related toxicity being the most common reasons.[18]

Intensivists are aware that further progress in diagnostic, prophylactic, and therapeutic strategies used in the ICU should provide additional survival gains in these patients. Better knowledge of the adverse effects of cancer chemotherapy would help intensivists recognize drug toxicity earlier in patients admitted with suggestive symptoms; administer specific treatments if available; and anticipate, prevent, or treat toxic effects of medications started in the ICU.

This chapter focuses on the main toxic effects of cancer chemotherapy. It is written for intensivists who are called on to care for cancer patients with chemotherapy-related toxicity affecting the lungs, heart, metabolism, kidneys, nervous system, and bone marrow.

Pulmonary Toxicity

Many anticancer agents can cause lung disease, usually with radiographic infiltrates. Lung toxicity may be life-threatening. Extrinsic evidence of causality varies widely. Abundant documentation of lung toxicity is available in the literature for some drugs such as bleomycin, whereas only anecdotal case reports have been published for others. Consequently, the diagnostic strategy should follow the rules that apply to all drug-induced lung disorders:

1. Rule out pulmonary edema due to congestive heart failure.
2. Rule out lung infection due to an opportunistic or nonopportunistic organism (consider toxicity as a diagnosis of exclusion).
3. Rule out lung infiltration by cancer cells.
4. Check that the time from chemotherapy administration to respiratory symptom onset matches cases reported in the literature (see, e.g., www.pneumotox.com), and determine whether the respiratory symptoms recur with each chemotherapy course (rechallenge).
5. Check that the clinical manifestations and laboratory test abnormalities are consistent with lung toxicity induced by the suspected drug (intrinsic evidence of causality).
6. Determine whether the symptoms resolve after the drug is stopped and glucocorticoids are given (if applicable).

When seeking to establish the diagnosis, intrinsic evidence should continuously be confronted with extrinsic evidence to ensure optimal selection of diagnostic investigations. Surgical or transbronchial biopsy is rarely appropriate but may deserve consideration if there is no response to treatment (drug discontinuation and glucocorticoid therapy) or if there is a strong suspicion of lung infection despite negative bronchoscopic bronchoalveolar lavage (B-BAL) findings.

BLEOMYCIN-INDUCED LUNG TOXICITY

Bleomycin is a glycopeptide antibiotic that has been used since the 1970s in a wide range of solid tumors (lung cancer, esophageal cancer, head and neck cancer, germ-cell tumors of the ovary and testis, Kaposi sarcoma) as well as Hodgkin's disease and non-Hodgkin's lymphoma. Bleomycin lung toxicity occurs in 2% to 46% of patients.[19,20] Pneumonitis with diffuse infiltrates and fibrosis is the most typical manifestation, and it has a fatal outcome in 1% to 3% of cases.[19,20] Mean time to onset is 4 months after bleomycin administration, but some cases can develop up to 10 years after completion of bleomycin treatment.[21,22] Earlier lung toxicity is less common and is responsible for clinical and radiographic manifestations reminiscent of bronchiolitis obliterans or hypersensitivity pneumonitis.[20]

Available knowledge of the pathophysiology of bleomycin-induced lung toxicity stems mainly from animal models. Skin and lungs are main targets because of the lack of bleomycin-inactivating hydrolase in these organs.[20] By increasing free radicals, bleomycin induces endothelial damage, nuclear factor-kappa B (NF-κB) stimulation, then proinflammatory and profibrosis cytokines such as tumor necrosis factor α (TNF-α), interleukin (IL)-1β and IL-18, and transforming growth factor β (TGF-β).[23,24] Subsequently, there is an influx of inflammatory cells and fibroblasts, and progression to lung fibrosis can occur.[20]

Established risk factors include the cumulative dose of bleomycin, although the toxic amount varies across patients, without any consensual threshold for toxicity but rather a linear relation between the bleomycin dose and the incidence of lung toxicity.[20] Renal failure seems to be the most important risk factor for predicting lung toxicity, with a significant association between diffusing capacity of the lung for carbon monoxide (DLCO) and creatinine clearance.[19] Other risk factors for bleomycin-induced lung fibrosis include age older than 70 years, tobacco use, concomitant radiation therapy to the chest, bolus administration, oxygen exposure (often during or after surgery), and concomitant use of G-CSF or other cancer chemotherapy agents exhibiting lung toxicity.[19,20,25]

A dry cough, dyspnea on exertion and then at rest, tachypnea, fever, and cyanosis are the earliest symptoms.[20] Fine, crackling rales are heard over both lung bases, and later in the course, rhonchi or a friction rub may be found. Infiltrates in both lung bases are typically seen on the chest radiograph, and progression to diffuse interstitial fibrosis may occur.[20] However, asymmetric or more focal images are seen. Computed tomography shows earlier changes consisting of subpleural linear and nodular opacities in the lung bases that may suggest lung metastases.[26] Blood gas measurements show hypoxemia and hypocapnia, and lung function testing discloses a restrictive defect with decreases in vital capacity and in the DLCO.[20] The diagnosis is often one of exclusion when lung metastases and infections are eliminated. No real pathognomonic histologic finding exists. The most characteristic lesions are interstitial inflammatory cell infiltration and fibrosis and squamous metaplasia of bronchiolar epithelium.[19,20]

To decrease the risk of bleomycin-induced lung toxicity, the total dose should be determined according to the patient's risk-factor profile, the objective being to find the best compromise between minimizing toxicity and optimizing the anticancer effect. Suggested prophylactic agents include anti-TNF-α and anti-TGF-β antibodies, IL-1 receptor antagonists, and antioxidants such as dexrazoxane, pentoxifylline, amifostine, and diallyl sulfide.[20,24] Curative treatment starts with discontinuation of all chemotherapy agents known to cause lung toxicity and with respiratory function support. Infection must be ruled out. Glucocorticoid therapy in a dose of 60 to 100 mg/d of methylprednisolone is usually given, although compelling proof of efficacy is lacking. This practice is warranted given the possibility of bronchiolitis obliterans–organizing pneumonia or hypersensitivity pneumonitis, both of which respond to glucocorticoid therapy.[20] In survivors, the symptoms resolve completely, and respiratory function returns to normal.[20]

METHOTREXATE PNEUMONITIS

Methotrexate (MTX) is a cytotoxic agent belonging to the antimetabolite class. It blocks purine synthesis by inhibiting dihydrofolate reductase. Methotrexate is not only used in various solid tumors and hematologic malignancies but also in nonmalignant diseases such as rheumatoid arthritis and severe psoriasis. Acute or subacute pneumonitis simulating an infection, usually with interstitial involvement, occurs in 1% to 7% of patients receiving MTX.[27] It may occur even at low doses.[28] Toxicity mechanisms include up-regulation of the p38 MAPK pathway and inflammatory cytokines such as IL-1β and IL-8.[29] The symptoms may develop gradually over several weeks or months and include dyspnea, dry cough, crackling rales, and less often, fever and headaches. Extrapulmonary manifestations may include erosive mucositis, rash, and hepatic cytolysis.[27] Peripheral blood eosinophil counts are moderately and transiently elevated. Hypoxemia, a restrictive defect, and a decrease in DLCO are typically found. BAL fluid contains an abundance of cells, with a predominance of lymphocytes; the CD4/CD8 ratio varies, most notably with the time from MTX administration to respiratory symptom onset.[30] Lung biopsy, use of which is declining, shows lymphocytic infiltration of the interstitial tissue and, rarely but distinctively, granulomas in areas of type II pneumocyte hyperplasia[27] with a variable degree of lung fibrosis.

OTHER ANTICANCER AGENTS WITH LUNG TOXICITY

The purine analog, fludarabine, is an antimetabolite used mainly to treat advanced chronic lymphocytic leukemia and selected cases of low-grade lymphoma. Lung toxicity occurs in 8% of patients. Differential diagnosis with opportunistic infection includes *Pneumocystis jirovecii* pneumonia. A favorable outcome is the rule after discontinuation of fludarabine and systemic glucocorticoid therapy.

Gemcitabine is an antimetabolite used to treat solid tumors and hematologic malignancies. Although the bone marrow is the main target of gemcitabine toxicity (with at times profound myelosuppression), pulmonary toxicity occurs in 10% to 42% of patients.[31] Age older than 65 years, previous lung disease, chest radiation, and concomitant treatment with another agent (especially bleomycin in Hodgkin's disease) are risk factors. There are two clinical variants: (1) infusion-related reactions, usually mild, characterized by dyspnea or bronchospasm within hours of infusion and by favorable outcome with corticosteroids[32]; and (2) gemcitabine-induced pneumonitis characterized by pulmonary edema at the time of a capillary leak syndrome,

diffuse alveolar damage, or alveolar hemorrhage.[32] Dyspnea, fever, pulmonary infiltrates, and cough are the main symptoms.[31] Although the mortality can reach 37%, great improvement can be obtained with corticosteroids.[31,32]

Cytarabine, an agent similar to gemcitabine, has a longer history of use in acute myelogenous leukemia in combination with anthracyclines. Respiratory failure of variable severity develops in 12% to 20% of patients within 2 weeks of cytarabine initiation.[33] Noncardiogenic pulmonary edema and organized pneumonia are described, with favorable outcome under corticosteroids. However, differential diagnosis with infection, leukemic infiltrates, or heart failure is often difficult.[33,34]

Tyrosine kinase inhibitors are generally well tolerated. Imatinib, the main treatment for chronic myeloid leukemia (CML), is also effective in gastrointestinal stromal tumors. It frequently induces edema and weight gain. Dyspnea and cough, observed in up to 14% of treated patients, are often attributed to pulmonary edema and pleural effusion.[32] However, interstitial pneumonitis, alveolar hemorrhage, or pulmonary fibrosis can also occur (0.2% and 1.3% of grade 3 and 4 in the chronic phase of CML). Inhibition of platelet-derived growth factor (PDGF) is one of the mechanisms. Corticosteroid therapy can be effective.[35] This lung toxicity is also described with some epidermal growth factor (EGF) inhibitors used in solid neoplasm.[32]

Prognosis of acute promyelocytic leukemia (APL) dramatically improved until introduction of all-*trans*-retinoic acid (ATRA). However, differentiation syndrome (DS), also known as *retinoic acid syndrome*, can be a life-threatening complication of this molecule. In the most recent study, it occurs in 25% of patients, with a severe form in 50% of them.[36] Unexplained fever, weight gain greater than 5 kg, edema, dyspnea, interstitial pulmonary infiltrates, pleuropericardial effusion, unexplained hypotension, and renal failure are the main diagnosis criteria. High white blood cell count greater than 5×10^9/L and abnormal creatinine level are risk factors. Dexamethasone is used to prevent and treat this syndrome. Mortality in severe forms is 11%.[36]

Finally, a few cases of interstitial pneumonitis have been reported with carmustine, cyclophosphamide, melphalan, procarbazine, chlorambucil, mitomycin, vinblastine, etoposide, hydroxyurea, taxanes, alkylating agents, platin derivatives, rapamycin analogs, and monoclonal antibodies to EGFR.[32] An exhaustive list of drugs potentially responsible for lung toxicity and the corresponding clinical presentations can be found online at http://www.pneumotox.com.

◼ Cardiac Toxicity

Anthracyclines are the main culprits of cardiac toxicity. Evidence of cardiac toxicity for other agents (taxanes, antimetabolites, alkylating agents, and spindle poisons) is limited to anecdotal case reports.[37]

ANTHRACYCLINE-INDUCED CARDIAC TOXICITY

The anthracycline class—which includes doxorubicin, daunorubicin, epirubicin, idarubicin, and mitoxantrone—plays a major role in the treatment of many solid tumors (breast cancer, esophageal cancer, osteosarcomas) and hematologic malignancies (Hodgkin's disease, non-Hodgkin's lymphoma, acute leukemia). Anthracycline-induced myocardial toxicity can be life threatening or dose limiting, thereby affecting the prognosis of the disease by precluding optimal anticancer treatment.[38]

Anthracyclines induce cell death of dividing cells via inhibition of topoisomerase-2, intercalation to nucleus DNA, and production of free radicals.[39] The myocardium is vulnerable to free radicals because antioxidant enzyme activity is weaker in myocytes than in other tissues (e.g., liver, kidney). The cumulative anthracycline dose is the main risk factor for cardiac toxicity (1%-5%, up to 550 mg/m²; 30% at 600 mg/m²; 50% at 1g/m²) with individual variation.[40] Other risk factors include female gender, age at either end of the lifespan, black race, and Down's syndrome.[38] Opinions are divided regarding the roles of prior radiation therapy to the chest, lymphoma, preexisting heart disease, and a preexisting decrease in the left ventricular ejection fraction.[38,41]

Two clinical presentations can be distinguished based on the timing of symptoms relative to anthracycline therapy—acute cardiotoxicity and chronic cardiotoxicity, which may be early (subacute) or delayed.

Acute cardiotoxicity manifests as an acute myocarditis, namely a rapid deterioration in cardiac function during or within 1 week after the administration of anthracycline therapy, usually with reversal of the abnormalities after discontinuation of the drug.[38] Ventricular or supraventricular rhythm disorders are common. Congestive heart failure with or without cardiogenic shock is the most common clinical presentation, although myocarditis or pericarditis may also occur.[41] Adjustments in chemotherapy regimens have noticeably reduced the rate of acute cardiac toxicity, which now occurs in fewer than 1% of patients.[41]

Chronic cardiotoxicity is far more common. The subacute form is characterized by irreversible dilated cardiomyopathy within 1 year after anthracycline discontinuation.[42-44] The delayed form develops insidiously after more than 1 year and runs a slowly progressive course.[42-44] Long-term follow-up studies allow better evaluation of the prevalence of subclinical cardiotoxicity after anthracycline doses between 450 and 550 mg/m^2. It can reach 27.6%, with a median follow-up of 8 years, and the risk of cardiac failure clearly increases over time.[40,45]

Patients develop systolic or diastolic dysfunction indistinguishable from heart failure due to other causes. Coronary artery disease is rare,[45] so electrocardiographic (ECG) changes are nonspecific and include sinus tachycardia, flat T waves, QT prolongation, and low amplitudes. Ventricular tachycardia and supraventricular rhythm disorders have been reported in patients with acute cardiac toxicity.[41] B-type natriuretic peptide (BNP) is under study but not validated.[40] Echocardiography with tissue Doppler studies is the most widely used noninvasive and sensitive tool for monitoring and early detection of anthracycline cardiomyopathy.[38,40,41] Diastolic dysfunction is often the earlier sign. However, myocardial scintigraphy with technetium-99m may be more informative than transthoracic echocardiography, notably in obese patients. Dobutamine stress echocardiography has also been suggested as a diagnostic tool.[46] Finally, myocardial biopsy is an invasive diagnostic method whose sensitivity and specificity are controversial. Histologic analysis shows myofibril loss, dilation of the sarcoplasmic reticulum, and intracytoplasmic vacuoles in myocytes.[41]

In these immunocompromised patients, even with a history of anthracycline therapy and evidence of cardiac dysfunction, shock should prompt investigations for sepsis. A diagnosis of congestive heart failure can be accepted only if fluid depletion induces full normalization of respiratory function. B-BAL is mandatory in doubtful cases.

Curative Treatment

Standard treatment for congestive heart failure should be given, and anthracycline and other potentially cardiotoxic agents should be stopped, bearing in mind the negative consequences of this action on the chances of recovery from the malignant disease. Administration of an inotropic agent may be required in cases of acute cardiotoxicity. In chronic cardiotoxicity, angiotensin-converting enzyme inhibitors, diuretics, digitalis, and beta-blockers are valuable. Heart transplantation has been used in patients with delayed cardiotoxicity and no evidence of active cancer.

Preventive Treatment

The mainstay of prevention is routine evaluation of cardiac function (measurement of left ventricular ejection fraction by echocardiography or cardiac scintigraphy) before starting anthracycline therapy. The anthracycline doses should be selected according to the patient's riskfactor profile and the results of cardiac function evaluation. Close monitoring and in some cases cardioprotective therapy should be considered. Cardiac function should be tested at regular intervals throughout anthracycline therapy.

Epirubicin and idarubicin may be less likely to induce cardiotoxicity than the other anthracyclines. Continuous administration over several hours also seems to reduce the cardiotoxicity of anthracyclines. Available cardioprotective agents include dexrazoxane, an antioxidant that chelates iron.[47] Finally, liposomal encapsulation of anthracyclines reduces their cardiotoxicity without altering their anticancer effects.[48]

CARDIAC TOXICITY OF OTHER ANTICANCER AGENTS

Drugs of the taxane class, most notably paclitaxel, given in combination with anthracyclines are effective in the treatment of breast cancer. However, cardiotoxicity occurs in more than 20% of patients treated with this combination.[49]

Furthermore, cardiotoxicity has been reported with high-dose 5-fluorouracil (5-FU) and with cyclophosphamide, cisplatin, and vincristine. The clinical presentation may be congestive heart failure, pericarditis or pancarditis, or supraventricular or ventricular rhythm disorders. These severe manifestations are fairly uncommon, and the cardiac abnormalities are usually reversible.

◼ Hematologic Toxicity

In addition to the myelosuppressive effects expected with all anticancer agents, alterations in hemostasis, impairments in cell-mediated immunity, and second leukemia or myelodysplasia can occur in patients with a history of chemotherapy for cancer (Table 156-1).

MYELOSUPPRESSION

Myelosuppression is virtually unavoidable but usually reversible. The mechanism of action of the anticancer agent (i.e., the cell cycle phase affected by the drug) determines which cell lines are affected and governs the severity of marrow toxicity. For instance, nitrosoureas and mitomycin selectively destroy stem cells, causing severe and in some cases irreversible myelosuppression. In contrast, myelotoxicity is less marked with drugs that act more selectively on a specific cell-cycle phase, such as vincristine, bleomycin, and cisplatin. Table 156-2 recapitulates the severity of myelosuppression seen with various agents.

The severity of myelosuppression varies also with patient-dependent factors such as age, extent of bone marrow invasion by tumor, prior treatments (radiation therapy and/or chemotherapy associated with myelofibrosis), and nutritional status. The World Health Organization has suggested a scheme for classifying the severity of myelosuppression based on peripheral blood cell counts, as shown in Table 156-3.

Infection, anemia, and bleeding are the main complications of myelosuppression. Whereas febrile neutropenia has been associated with 90% mortality in the absence of antimicrobial therapy,[50] mortality among neutropenic inpatients is now less than 10% in hematology wards and 50% in ICUs.[11] This improved survival can be ascribed to the development of recommendations for the diagnosis, prophylaxis, and treatment of infections in neutropenic patients,[51,52] improved knowledge of the pharmacokinetics and toxicity of anticancer agents, and introduction of medications with greater efficacy in fungal infections.[53,54] Shortened duration of neutropenia may be obtained with injection of G-CSF[13,14] or injection of mobilized peripheral stem cells (autologous or allogeneic). Bone marrow transplantation is followed by approximately 3 weeks of myelosuppression.

Anemia induced by chemotherapy requires transfusion of packed red blood cells but sometimes can be minimized by regular injections of erythropoietin.[55] Finally, careful attention should be given at all times to correcting nutritional deficiencies, particularly deficiencies of folic acid, iron, and vitamin B$_{12}$.

No consensus exists about the amount of platelet transfusion necessary to avoid bleeding. Dose above 1.1×10^{11} platelets per square meter of body-surface area when platelet count is 10,000/mm^3 or lower does not decrease the incidence of bleeding.[56] In our practice, situations such as diffuse alveolar hemorrhage require a platelet count above 50,000/mm^3.

TABLE 156-1	Hematologic Toxicity of Cancer Chemotherapy Agents		
Toxic Effect	*Anticancer Agents*	*Diagnostic Findings*	*Treatments*
Anemia	Methotrexate, 5-FU, cytarabine, 6-mercaptopurine	Macrocytic anemia with normal levels of vitamin B_{12} and folate	Erythropoietin, blood transfusion
Thrombocytopenia	Nitrosoureas Gemtuzumab ozogamicin	Onset 4 to 6 weeks after chemotherapy	Transfusions
Marrow hypoplasia	Nitrosoureas, anthracyclines, busulfan	Anemia, thrombocytopenia, leukoneutropenia; nadir between 6 and 15 days after chemotherapy	Transfusions, erythropoietin, growth factors (G-CSF), stem cell reinjection
Thrombotic microangiopathy	Gemcitabine, mitomycin C	Mechanical hemolysis (anemia, profound haptoglobin decrease, negative Coombs test, schizocytes), high levels of LDH and free bilirubin, thrombocytopenia, renal failure	VIP transfusion, plasmapheresis, glucocorticoids, aspirin, dialysis
Hemostasis disorders	L-Asparaginase	Decreased PT, increased APTT; decreased fibrinogen, AT III, and plasminogen	Symptomatic: VIP transfusion, injection of AT III
	Thalidomide	Thromboembolic events	
Induced leukemia	Alkylating agents, nitrosoureas, etoposide, methotrexate, anthracyclines	AML 2 to 10 years after initial chemotherapy; complex karyotype abnormalities	
Impaired cell-mediated immunity	2-CdA (cladribine [Leustatin]), fludarabine (Fludara), pentostatin (Nipent), anti-CD52 (alemtuzumab [Campath])	Lymphopenia, opportunistic infections	Prophylaxis for *Pneumocystis jirovecii* infection

AML, acute myeloid leukemia; *APTT,* activated partial thromboplastin time; *AT III,* antithrombin III; *5-FU,* 5-fluorouracil; *G-CSF,* granulocyte colony-stimulating factor; *LDH,* lactate dehydrogenase; *PT,* prothrombin time; *VIP,* virus-inactivated plasma.

HEMOSTASIS DISORDERS

L-Asparaginase is widely used to treat acute lymphoblastic leukemia (ALL). Produced from strains of *Escherichia coli*, L-asparaginase hydrolyzes asparagine, an amino acid required by cells for protein synthesis. However, L-asparaginase causes a global decrease in protein synthesis, notably in clotting factors. This leads to low levels of fibrinogen, prothrombin, antithrombin (AT), plasminogen, and factors IX and X, so activated partial thromboplastin time (APTT) is increased.[57] If the alterations in hemostasis are severe, thromboembolic events (pulmonary embolism, stroke, and cerebral vein thrombosis) are more frequent than bleeding episodes and are reported in up to 15% of adults.[58]

Prevention includes detection of inherited thrombophilia, monitoring of fibrinogen and AT levels, and AT substitution without consensual scheme. Otherwise, the administration of a pegylated form of asparaginase is preferred at present because it has fewer thromboembolic complications.[58] Thromboembolism treatment should consider risks and benefits of anticoagulation.[57]

Thalidomide, used in multiple myeloma treatment, has immunomodulatory and anti-angiogenic effects. When combined with dexamethasone or doxorubicin, but not as monotherapy, it increases the risk of venous thromboembolic events (VTE). Incidence is usually around 15% but can reach 58% with doxorubicin.[59] Pulmonary embolisms are not specifically reported in all studies but occur in about 7% of patients treated with thalidomide and dexamethasone, versus less than 2% in those treated with dexamethasone only.[60] These complications are usually observed during the 2 months after beginning therapy.

IMPAIRED CELL-MEDIATED IMMUNITY

Lymphocyte depletion occurs with 2-CdA, fludarabine, pentostatin, and the recently introduced monoclonal antibody to CD52, alemtuzumab (Campath). Lymphodepletion can be profound and promotes the development of opportunistic infections. Prophylactic treatment is mandatory, most notably to prevent *P. jirovecii* infection.

Neurologic Toxicity

Neurologic adverse effects of anticancer agents are both common and severe (Table 156-4). They may preclude administration of optimal chemotherapy, thereby compromising the chances for recovery. Both peripheral and central components of the nervous system may be affected. The diagnosis is one of exclusion; infections, trauma, and infiltration by malignant cells should be ruled out first.[61]

CONSEQUENCES OF INTRATHECAL INJECTIONS

Transient aseptic meningitis occurs within a few hours after intrathecal injection of anticancer agents in about 30% of cases. Introduction of a pathogen during the injection should be ruled out. Meningeal symptoms and fever develop in about 60% of cases. The incidence of this acute complication has decreased with concomitant intrathecal injection of dexamethasone.

Other complications are less common but usually severe. Spinal cord lesions manifested by motor deficit and cauda equina syndrome develop some weeks after injection, with a median of 10 days. Both MTX and aracytine are incriminated. Risk factors for MTX toxicity are

TABLE 156-2	Severity of Myelosuppression Seen with Various Chemotherapy Agents	
Mild	*Moderate*	*Severe*
Cisplatin	Antipurine	Anthracycline
Bleomycin	Podophyllin	Nitrogen mustard
Vinca alkaloids	Alkylating agents	Antifolates
	Hydroxyurea	Antipyrimidines
	Mitomycin Procarbazine	Nitrosoureas (carmustine, lomustine)
		Busulfan
		Dacarbazine

TABLE 156-3	World Health Organization Scheme for Classifying Severity of Myelosuppression			
Toxicity Grade	Hemoglobin (g/dL)	Leukocytes (×1000)	Neutrophils (×1000)	Platelets (×1000)
0	Normal	Normal	Normal	Normal
1	9.5-10.9	3-4.5	1.5-1.9	75-100
2	8-9.4	2-2.9	1-1.4	50-74
3	6-7.9	1-1.9	0.5-0.9	25-49
4	4-5.9	0.5-0.9	0.1-0.4	<25
5	Death	Death	Death	Death

TABLE 156-4	Neurologic Toxicity of Cancer Chemotherapy Agents		
Toxic Effect	*Drugs*	*Diagnostic Findings*	*Treatments*
Encephalopathies (headache, confusion, seizures)	BiCNU, cisplatin, cytarabine, 5-FU, ifosfamide, asparaginase, methotrexate, procarbazine	—	—
Cerebellar syndrome	Cytarabine, 5-FU	Clinical, imaging studies	—
Myelopathy (paraplegia, cauda equina syndrome)	Intrathecal methotrexate, cytarabine, thiotepa	—	—
Peripheral neuropathy	Vincristine, platinum derivatives and taxanes, thalidomide, bortezomib	Clinical, electrophysiologic testing	Prevention: glutathione, amifostine for cisplatin; pain control
Stroke and cerebral vein thrombosis	Asparaginase, high-dose methotrexate, BiCNU, or cisplatin by intracarotid injection	Clinical, imaging (CT, MRI)	—
Ototoxicity	Cisplatin	Audiogram	Amifostine, glutathione
SIADH	Vincristine	Low serum sodium	—
Cranial nerve involvement	Vincristine (nerves IV, V, and VI), ifosfamide	—	—
Aseptic meningitis	Intrathecal methotrexate and cytarabine	Spinal tap	—
Leukoencephalitis	Methotrexate	MRI	Hydration, folinic acid rescue therapy
Ophthalmologic involvement	Cisplatin, vincristine	Transient cortical blindness, retrobulbar optic neuropathy, retinal involvement, extraocular nerve palsy	Glutathione IV, amifostine

BiCNU, carmustine; *CT,* computed tomography; *5-FU,* 5-fluorouracil; *MRI,* magnetic resonance imaging; *SIADH,* syndrome of inappropriate secretion of antidiuretic hormone.

cumulative dose, high MTX levels in the cerebrospinal fluid, and concomitant radiation therapy.[62] High dose and the liposomal form of aracytine lead to more toxicity by prolonging release of aracytine, but neurotoxicity occurs above all when both drugs are associated.[63] Magnetic resonance imaging eliminates epidural compression or cord infiltration and shows multiple foci of atrophy and demyelination selectively affecting the periventricular white matter and the centrum semiovale, ventricular dilation, and calcifications. Recovery is poor, often with bowel and urinary incontinence. No treatment exists. Folate supplementation may decrease MTX toxicity when patients receive concomitant systemic MTX therapy or display renal failure.[63]

PERIPHERAL NEUROPATHIES

Chemotherapy-induced peripheral neuropathy (CIPN) is a major dose-limiting side effect of many drugs including taxanes, vinca alkaloids, platinum compounds, and newer agents such as thalidomide and bortezomib. Incidence is variable and can be influenced by age, alcohol abuse, diabetes mellitus, liver or renal dysfunction, dose intensity, cumulative dose, and concomitant administration of several neurotoxic agents. Distal sensory peripheral neuropathy with neuropathic pain and paresthesias is the most common presentation but is not specific. Some motor losses are also described (Table 156-5). CIPN may appear from the first chemotherapy infusion or later. Symptoms can resolve totally or partially with interruption of treatment or dose reduction, but severe impairment can persist. Treatment continuation should consider the relative prognosis of CIPN and cancer, drug importance for cancer control, and quality of life impairments due to neuropathy.[64]

More precisely, paclitaxel is the main taxane associated with CIPN (significant neuropathy in up to 10% of cases), especially when used with a platinum compound. Vincristine, the most neurotoxic among vinca alkaloids, can produce CIPN in up to 75% of patients with a cumulative dose over 10 mg/m². It leads to severe autonomic dysfunction associated with peripheral sensorimotor loss. Cisplatin and oxaliplatin, two platinum derivatives, are more toxic than carboplatin, but cisplatin is also a better antitumor agent. The incidence of CIPN is close to 50%, whatever the grade. Except this typical form, acute reversible neuropathy is observed in 80% of patients who received oxaliplatin. Distal paresthesia and pain develop within a few hours to days of infusion and resolve spontaneously.[64]

CIPN is observed in over half of patients treated with thalidomide, and the risk increases greatly after 6 months on therapy. A recent trial reported a grade 3 and 4 neurotoxicity in 3.4% of patients.[60] Lenalidomide, an analog of thalidomide, has less neurotoxicity. Finally, bortezomib, a proteasome inhibitor, can lead to 35% of CIPN, with some degree of motor loss in a third of cases.[64]

No specific treatment exists. Calcium and magnesium infusion can attenuate the development of CIPN after oxaliplatin treatment, but there is some controversy about consequences on antitumor effect. Many other drugs are promising but need larger studies.[64,65]

CENTRAL NERVOUS SYSTEM TOXICITY

Most anticancer agents are high-molecular-weight or water-soluble compounds that do not cross the blood-brain barrier. Central nervous system toxicity is therefore uncommon with intravenous chemotherapy but may occur with high doses of some compounds (MTX, cytarabine). Cerebellar syndrome has been reported with cytarabine (cytosine arabinoside) and 5-FU (particularly in patients with dihydropyrimidine dehydrogenase deficiency). High-dose cisplatin can cause encephalopathy (headache, behavioral or personality disorders, confusion, drowsiness, seizures, and coma); concomitant optic nerve involvement may occur (Table 156-6). Ifosfamide is responsible for

TABLE 156-5	Classification of Toxic Neuropathy		
Toxicity Grade	*Deep Tendon Reflexes*	*Paresthesia*	*Transit*
0	Normal	Absent	Normal
1	Decreased	Present	Irregular
2	Absent	Severe	Constipation
3	Absent	Painful	Subobstruction
4	Paralysis	Autonomic disorders	Obstruction
5	Death	Death	Death

TABLE 156-6	Classification of Encephalopathy According to Severity	
Severity Grade	*Description*	
0	No symptoms	
1	Agitation, drowsiness	
2	Bedridden	
3	Requires treatment	
4	Coma, manic episode, suicidal behavior	
5	Death	

TABLE 156-7	Renal and Urologic Toxicity of Cancer Chemotherapy Agents		
Toxic Effect	*Drugs*	*Diagnostic Findings*	*Treatments*
Chronic renal failure (cumulative dose)	Carmustine, semustine, streptozocin, platin derivatives, ifosfamide, pentostatin	Renal biopsy	Discontinuation of the anticancer agent
Acute renal failure	Methotrexate, platin derivatives, ifosfamide	—	Hyperhydration, urine alkalinization with methotrexate
Glomerular disease	Carmustine, semustine, streptozocin	—	—
Tubular disease	Cisplatin, carboplatin, ifosfamide, methotrexate, cytarabine, streptozocin	Hypophosphatemia, hypokalemia, hypomagnesemia, hypouricemia, metabolic acidosis, glucosuria, aminoaciduria	Hyperhydration, magnesium supplementation, avoid other nephrotoxic drugs, urine alkalinization with methotrexate
Hemorrhagic cystitis	Ifosfamide, cyclophosphamide	—	Hyperhydration, mesna
Dysuria, hematuria	Methotrexate, pentostatin	—	Appropriate hydration

reversible non–dose-dependent neuropsychiatric disorders including visual or auditory hallucinations, a dreamlike state, confusion, personality disorders, and anxiety. Seizures or coma may occur. Extrapyramidal manifestations with myoclonus and spasticity are classic manifestations of ifosfamide neurotoxicity. Among patients treated with MTX in doses greater than 1 g/m^2, 15% experience spontaneously reversible encephalopathy, which must be differentiated from leukoencephalopathy with irreversible chronic pseudo dementia. L-Asparaginase treatment causes encephalopathy in 15% to 60% of patients. Fludarabine is associated with neurotoxicity in 15% of patients. It is dose dependent and can be prevented by using low doses (25 mg/m^3, 5 days per month).[66]

CRANIAL NERVE INVOLVEMENT

Vincristine is responsible for involvement of the fourth, fifth, and sixth cranial nerves, facial palsy, laryngeal nerve palsy, and transient cortical blindness. Hearing loss is common with cisplatin; this effect is dose dependent and can be irreversible, with loss of ciliated cochlear cells.

Urologic and Renal Toxicity

Many factors can cause renal dysfunction in patients receiving anticancer chemotherapy,[67] including radiation-induced nephritis, tumor lysis syndrome, hyperuricemia, hyperphosphatemia, hypercalcemia, lysozymuria, thrombotic microangiopathy, disseminated intravascular coagulation, infiltration by cancer cells, amyloidosis, and renal consequences of obstructive uropathy. Exacerbation of renal dysfunction can occur with nephrotoxic agents (e.g., aminoglycosides, antifungal agents, antiviral agents, iodine).

A number of anticancer agents can cause renal failure (Table 156-7). This effect is dose limiting and therefore compromises the chances of recovery from the malignancy. In addition to renal failure, tubular disease or, more rarely, glomerular disease or thrombotic microangiopathy may occur with some agents. The distal urinary tract may be affected by ifosfamide or cyclophosphamide.

The World Health Organization has developed a grading system for chemotherapy-related renal failure, based on urine output and serum creatinine levels, as shown in Table 156-8.

TABLE 156-8	World Health Organization Grading System for Chemotherapy-Related Renal Failure	
Grade	*Urine Output*	*Creatinine (μmol/L, mg/dL)*
0	Normal	Normal
1	Transient decrease	115-180, 13-20
2	Diuretic agents	181-354, 20-40
3	High-dose diuretic agents	355-530, 40-60
4	Dialysis	531-800, 60-90
5	Death	—

RENAL FAILURE

Methotrexate nephrotoxicity occurs with high doses (>1 g/m^2).[68] Whereas several toxicities are due to its antimetabolite action, the underlying mechanism of nephrotoxicity involves precipitation of MTX and its even less soluble metabolite, 7-hydroxymethotrexate, within the renal tubules.[68,69] Acute renal failure enhances other toxic effects by delaying MTX elimination. Tubule precipitation is more likely to occur at acid pH, so it is important to maintain high urine output and alkaline urine. Folinic acid is given to antagonize the other side effects of MTX. With optimal management, the incidence of renal failure has decreased from 10% to 2%, with less than 1% grade 3 or 4 and a mortality close to 4%.[68,70] Coadministration of several drugs, notably antibiotics, promotes this toxicity.[71] When renal failure occurs, hydration and folinic acid administration are increased based on plasma MTX concentration, so daily monitoring is essential. Hemodialysis decreases plasma MTX concentration, but a marked rebound can occur after the procedure, so it is not recommended. The carboxypeptidase G can metabolize MTX to its inactive metabolite and seems to be effective but is not routinely used.[68,70,72]

With platin derivatives, nephrotoxicity is common, dose dependent, and potentially irreversible. In non-small-cell lung cancer, platinum-based chemotherapy triples the risk of nephrotoxicity.[73] Cisplatin nephrotoxicity is reported in up to 40% of patients.[74] This toxicity is the main dose-limiting adverse effect of these agents.[75] Cisplatin, the main platinum salt, induces tubular injury with minimal proteinuria, polyuria, and potentially severe hypomagnesemia. Secondary hypokaliemia, hypocalcemia, and tubular acidosis are observed. If a renal biopsy is performed, histologic analysis shows tubular dilation, epithelial cell necrosis, interstitial edema and fibrosis, and thinning of the tubular basement membrane. Prevention of tubular injury and acute renal failure includes generous hydration. It is also essential to adjust the doses of cisplatin according this renal function. Diuretics are not advised. Magnesium supplementation is often necessary.[74] Carboplatin and oxaliplatin are less toxic, moreover, since high doses can be adjusted for renal function.[76] However, in some cases, they are less effective against cancer than cisplatin.

Prolonged ifosfamide therapy can rarely result in progressive renal failure and damage the proximal tubules. The suspected mechanism is inhibition of the Na$^+$/H$^+$ pump and impairment of the sodium-dependent transporters of glucose, phosphate, and L-alanine by two ifosfamide metabolites, chloroacetaldehyde and 4-OH-ifosfamide. Risk factors for ifosfamide-induced tubulopathy include a cumulative dose greater than 45 g/m^2, age younger than 5 years, a history of cisplatin therapy, and a preexisting renal dysfunction of any cause.[67,77,78]

THROMBOTIC MICROANGIOPATHY

Chemotherapy-induced thrombotic microangiopathy is manifested by atypical hemolytic uremic syndrome (aHUS), usually with thrombocytopenia, mechanical hemolytic anemia (with schizocytes and negative Coombs test), elevated blood pressure, proteinuria, hematuria, and acute renal failure. Peripheral edema and neurologic signs can occur. It is often difficult to separate the respective roles of chemotherapy and underlying cancer. The incidence ranges from 3% to 13% for either malignancy-induced or chemotherapy-induced aHUS.[79] The first cases were described after mitomycin C. A few cases have been reported in patients treated with gemcitabine, CCNU (lomustine), and platin derivatives; combinations such as daunorubicin/cytarabine or bleomycin/cisplatin have also been reported to cause thrombotic microangiopathy.[80]

Chemotherapy-induced thrombotic microangiopathy occurs after several months of treatment (up to 24 months with gemcitabine). Pathogenesis is unclear, but endothelial injury seems to be a central feature. Direct endothelial damage is described.[79] ADAMTS 13 activity is not always tested but is usually not decreased. Management of these aHUS is not well established. Discontinuation of the treatment involved and blood pressure control are the first step. Then virus-inactivated plasma transfusions, plasmapheresis, or glucocorticoid therapy can be proposed, but no study is able to determine their efficacy.[81] Prognosis is poor, with a mortality rate of 40% to 90% despite discontinuation of treatment. This prognosis is determined as much by underlying disease as by aHUS.[79]

HEMORRHAGIC CYSTITIS

Hemorrhagic cystitis is a common adverse effect with the alkylating agents, cyclophosphamide and ifosfamide.[82,83] Degradation of oxazaphosphorine in the kidneys produces acrolein, which has direct toxic effects on the bladder mucosa.[82,83] Prevention relies on appropriate saline hydration and administration of mesna,[84,85] which binds to acrolein, producing a stable, water-soluble thioester that is promptly eliminated. Mesna has no curative effects.[85] If cystitis occurs despite preventive measures, a double-lumen urinary catheter should be inserted for continuous bladder irrigation until the bleeding stops completely.[83]

▓ Digestive Toxicity

LIVER TOXICITY

Many antineoplastic drugs have potential liver toxicity. Alcoholism, malnutrition, hepatic neoplasm or metastases, infection, or other toxic medicines are risk factors for this toxicity, above all when chemotherapy doses are not adjusted according to baseline liver function. Several injuries are described. Hepatitis, characterized by cytolysis and sometimes by liver failure, can be observed with many antineoplastic drugs such as alkylating agents, nitrosoureas, platinum derivatives, antimetabolites. Cholestasis is also nonspecific and can occur with many drugs. Fibrosis and chronic hepatitis is rare and mainly described with methotrexate.[86] For all these toxicities, drug discontinuation is the best treatment.

Veno-occlusive disease, also called *sinusoidal obstruction syndrome*, is a rare complication that can lead to organ dysfunction. Risk factors are treatment by cyclophosphamide, busulfan, gemtuzumab ozogamicin, sirolimus, and total body irradiation, so patients with stem cell transplantation ongoing are particularly exposed. Incidence is around 10% to 15% after stem cell transplantation within 70% of severe cases. Patients develop painful hepatomegaly, ascites, weight gain, and increase in bilirubin levels. Mortality can reach 100% when multiple organ failure appears.[87] Management consists in supportive care including renal replacement therapy. Few effective treatment or prevention options exist apart from defibrotide.[88]

PANCREATITIS

Acute pancreatitis occurs in up to 18% of patients treated for acute lymphoblastic leukemia (ALL). The main drug involved is L-asparaginase, followed by cytarabine and corticosteroids. Mortality is higher in these patients, among others by impairment of ALL management.[89]

GUT TOXICITY

Neutropenic enterocolitis or typhlitis is the consequence of direct toxicity to bowel mucosa and microbial invasion of this mucosa during immunosuppression. It can be secondary to high-dose chemotherapy for acute leukemia or lymphoma, especially in cases of cytarabine administration. The incidence is unknown but may reach 46% (in an autopsy study) and can be fatal.[90] Diagnosis and management are difficult. Surgery is limited by the presence of cytopenia.[91]

▓ Metabolic Toxicity

Metabolic disorders in patients receiving cancer chemotherapy fall into two groups: disorders related directly to the tumor (e.g., urinary tract compression, spontaneous lysis, syndrome of inappropriate secretion of antidiuretic hormone [SIADH]) and disorders related to anticancer agents (e.g., drug-induced tumor lysis, electrolyte disturbances).[92] Hyponatremia (related chiefly to SIADH) is the main source of clinical symptoms.[93] SIADH can be observed with spindle poisons (vincristine, vinblastine, and more rarely, vinorelbine),[94,95] alkylating agents such as cyclophosphamide melphalan, and more rarely, chlorambucil and thiotepa.[92,93] Cisplatin is associated with hyponatremia related to SIADH or tubular wasting in 4% to 10% of patients. However, a diagnosis of chemotherapy-induced SIADH requires the exclusion of other causes including paraneoplastic syndromes, central nervous system disorders, lung infections, and SIADH induced by other drugs.

KEY POINTS

1. Hospital mortality among cancer patients admitted to the ICU is up to 50%, which is quite similar to some other diseases.

2. Diagnostic strategy for chemotherapy toxicity should follow the rules that apply to all drug toxicity.

Pulmonary Toxicity

- Bleomycin toxicity occurs in 2% to 46% of patients, the lung being the main target.

- Methotrexate causes acute or subacute pneumonitis simulating an infection, usually with interstitial involvement, in 1% to 7% of patients.

- Fludarabine causes lung toxicity in 8% of patients.

- Gemcitabine use causes pulmonary toxicity in 10% to 42% of patients.

- Cytarabine initiation causes respiratory involvement of variable severity within 2 weeks in 12% to 20% of patients.

Cardiac Toxicity

- Anthracyclines (doxorubicin, daunorubicin, epirubicin, idarubicin, and mitoxantrone) are mostly responsible for cardiac toxicity.

- Drugs of the taxane class, most notably paclitaxel, given in combination with anthracyclines, leads to cardiotoxicity in more than 20% of patients.

Hematologic Toxicity

- Severity of myelosuppression varies with mechanism of action of the anticancer agent and patient-dependent factors.

- L-Asparaginase and thalidomide are associated with hemostasis disorders such as thrombo-embolic events.

Neurologic Toxicity

- Peripheral nervous system toxicity is associated with vinca alkaloids, platin derivatives, taxanes, thalidomide, and bortezomib.

- Central nervous system toxicity is associated with high doses of methotrexate, cytarabine, and intrathecal injection. Every effort must be made to rule out infectious involvement.

Urologic and Renal Toxicity

- Acute renal failure and tubulopathy occur chiefly with high doses of methotrexate or with platin derivatives.

- Hemorrhagic cystitis is a common adverse effect with cyclophosphamide and ifosfamide.

Metabolic Toxicity

- Spindle poisons can cause SIADH, often with concomitant peripheral neuropathy and intestinal ileus.

GI Toxicity

- Veno-occlusive disease is associated with cyclophosphamide, busulfan, gemtuzumab ozogamicin, and sirolimus.

- L-Asparaginase can lead to acute pancreatitis.

- Neutropenic enterocolitis occurs in up to 46% of patients.

ANNOTATED REFERENCES

Kintzel PE. Anticancer drug-induced kidney disorders. Drug Saf 2001;24:19-38.
    Renal toxicity of chemotherapy and physiopathologic explanations.
Lewis C. A review of the use of chemoprotectants in cancer chemotherapy. Drug Saf 1994;11:153-62.
    The interest of chemoprotectants in oncohematology.
Singal PK, Iliskovic N. Doxorubicin-induced cardiomyopathy. N Engl J Med 1998;339:900-5.
    Diagnostic procedures of doxorubicin-induced cardiomyopathy.

Sleijfer S. Bleomycin-induced pneumonitis. Chest 2001;120:617-24.
    Clinical features, pathogenesis, risk factors, and treatment of bleomycin-induced pneumonitis.
Verstappen CC, Heimans JJ, Hoekman K, Postma TJ. Neurotoxic complications of chemotherapy in patients with cancer: clinical signs and optimal management. Drugs 2003;63:1549-63.
    Recent review of neurologic toxicity of chemotherapy.

REFERENCES

Access the complete reference list online at http://www.expertconsult.com.

Hematology and Oncology in Children

GUILLAUME EMERIAUD | JACQUES LACROIX

This chapter is an overview of the main hematologic and oncologic problems that can be observed in the pediatric intensive care unit (PICU). Differences between critically ill children and adults are emphasized.

Hematology

ANEMIA

A normal decrease in the hemoglobin (Hb) level is observed during the first weeks of life because of a limited release of erythropoietin. For this reason, the normal range of Hb concentration changes with age: 18.5 ± 2.0 g/dL (mean $\pm$ 2 standard deviations) during the first week of life, 11.5 ± 1.2 g/dL at 2 months, 12.0 ± 0.7 g/dL at 12 months, 13.5 ± 1.0 g/dL at 9 years, and 14.0 ± 1.0 g/dL after 12 years of age.[1] Based on these ranges, anemia is observed in 33% of patients on admission to PICU, and an additional 41% become anemic during their PICU stay.[2]

The small total blood volume of neonates and children (e.g., about 240 mL in a 3-kg patient) makes blood loss from phlebotomy or procedures a major cause of anemia in PICU.[2] Other causes include hemorrhage, hemolysis (immunologic, infectious, microangiopathic, or toxic), and decreased production (invasion of the bone marrow, side effect of therapy, nutritional deficiency, blunted production of erythropoietin in response to hypoxia).[3] Causes quite specific to pediatric practice include congenital anemias (e.g., sickle cell disease, thalassemia, Blackfan-Diamond disease), glucose-6-phosphate dehydrogenase deficiency, and metabolic disorders. Sickle cell disease merits specific comment.

Sickle Cell Disease

Many types of abnormal Hb are observed in sickle cell disease. However, only Hb SS (homozygous sickle cell Hb), Hb SC, and Hb S-β-thalassemia can cause severe clinical problems. Hypoxemia, acidosis, polycythemia, infection, and a high proportion of abnormal Hb concentration are the main risk factors for sickle cell disease complications. The following sickle cell crises can be life threatening: acute chest syndrome, stroke, acute splenic sequestration, aplastic crisis, and infection. General management always includes optimization of oxygenation, adequate analgesia, and treatment of the precipitating cause of the crisis.[4] Hyperhydration is also recommended in most instances, but fluid requirements must be adapted with caution in patients with respiratory symptoms or pulmonary hypertension. Red blood cell (RBC) transfusion is a cornerstone of therapy, aiming to decrease abnormal Hb while maintaining hematocrit below 35%. An exchange transfusion should be considered in severe cases, especially in acute chest syndrome or stroke.

Acute chest syndrome is a leading cause of morbidity and mortality in sickle cell disease.[5,6] It is defined by the development of a new pulmonary alveolar infiltrate involving at least one complete lung segment, accompanied by fever, chest pain, tachypnea, cough, and hypoxia. Severe forms are analogous to acute respiratory distress syndrome. Acute chest syndrome results from intricate mechanisms including pulmonary infection (mostly by atypical bacteria and virus), fat embolization, and local vaso-occlusion.[6] Perturbation of nitric oxide metabolism[7] and hypercoagulability have also been demonstrated.[6] Growing evidence suggests that pulmonary hypertension play a crucial role

during sickle cell disease evolution, which may lead to abrupt severe right heart failure.[6] Besides general management and empirical antibiotic therapy, covering atypical bacteria and *Streptococcus pneumoniae*, incentive spirometry is encouraged. Mechanical ventilation may be required to improve oxygenation; noninvasive ventilation can be successful.[8] Owing to disturbance of nitric oxide metabolism, inhaled nitric oxide has been used in small trials or case reports, but its efficacy remains to be validated.[9]

Stroke must be considered in patients with sudden onset of neurologic symptoms. Specific management includes an urgent exchange transfusion and careful attention to neurologic worsening. Intracranial pressure monitoring can be helpful in severe stroke.

During acute splenic sequestration crisis, the blood volume retained in the spleen may lead to severe hypovolemic shock. An acute reduction of Hb concentration of 2 g/dL or more, with no other cause of blood loss, is considered diagnostic. Aplastic crisis can also cause an acute and severe anemia, usually during a viral infection, particularly with parvovirus B19. The half-life of RBCs is severely shortened in patients with sickle cell diseases, and a compensatory increase of RBC production occurs. During aplastic crisis, the reticulocyte count falls, causing rapid development of severe anemia. Mortality rates associated with both sequestration and aplastic crises are significant, and these conditions must be treated aggressively with volume administration and RBC transfusion.

Sickle cell disease can cause a functional asplenia with increased susceptibility to severe bacterial infections, especially with encapsulated organisms. An infection should therefore be suspected early and treated aggressively in patients with sickle cell disease.

Preventive measures must also be used if possible. In particular, patients with sickle cell disease should be monitored in the PICU after significant surgery—the goals being to prevent dehydration and hypoxemia, provide optimal analgesia, and maintain the hematocrit between 30% and 35%.

Red Blood Cell Transfusion

The management of anemia in critically ill patients is discussed in Chapters 19 and 150; this includes prevention of blood loss, transfusion of blood products, and administration of folic acid and iron. Prophylactic erythropoietin use has not been evaluated in large pediatric trials, but its utility appears questionable insofar as most RBC transfusions are received during the first few days after admission.[2,10]

The risks and benefits of RBC transfusion are not similar in adults and children. Necrotizing enterocolitis in neonates[11] or erythrocyte alloimmunization in young girls (up to 8% of patients)[12] are significant problems in pediatric patients. RBC transfusion to neonates increases the ratio of adult to fetal Hb, which decreases the affinity of blood for oxygen.[13] Nevertheless, RBCs improve oxygen transport in critically ill children,[14-17] although the improvement in clinically significant outcomes remains to be determined. Large variation in transfusion practice was observed among pediatric intensivists,[18,19] reflecting the unidentified Hb threshold with the best risk/benefit ratio in critically ill children. Maintaining Hb above 5.0 g/dL in hospitalized pediatric patients decreases the risk of death.[20,21] In a large randomized clinical trial enrolling 637 patients in 19 PICUs, Lacroix et al.[22] demonstrated that a transfusion strategy to maintain Hb above 7 g/dL was as safe as a strategy to maintain Hb above 9.5 g/dL in stable critically ill children. While the number of transfusions was much lower in the restrictive transfusion group, no difference was observed in mortality rate or occurrence of new organ dysfunction.[22] These findings were not different in three planned a priori subgroup analyses of patients in sepsis,[23] in postsurgical patients,[24] or in patients admitted following cardiac surgery.[25] These data and the cohesiveness of all subgroup analyses strongly support limiting RBC transfusion to patients with Hb below 7.0 g/dL in stable conditions. More data are required to identify a threshold in patients with cardiorespiratory instability.

In pediatric patients, packed RBCs should be administered on a unit-by-unit basis to limit exposure to multiple donors. Packed RBCs are available in half-units (standard division) or in small units of 75 mL (Pedipak) for young children. Packed RBC units must be warmed to 37°C for infants or if the transfused volume exceeds 30% of blood volume.

Transfusion in the neonatal period, in children with immunodeficiency, or transfusion using blood donated by family members are situations at higher risk of transfusion-associated graft-versus-host disease[26]; irradiated packed RBCs should be used in these conditions.

HEMORRHAGIC DISORDERS

Disseminated intravascular coagulation (DIC) is the most frequent hemorrhagic disorder observed in the PICU. Its causes, pathophysiology, and treatment are similar to those in adults (see Chapter 21), even though purpura fulminans is more frequent in the PICU.

Severe hemorrhage can be caused by congenital deficiencies of coagulation factors, as in hemophilia A (factor VIII), hemophilia B (factor IX), or factor VII deficiency. Massive RBC transfusion is a frequent cause of coagulation factor deficiency, which should be anticipated and prevented. Acquired (dietary, antibiotics) vitamin K deficiency can also cause severe bleeding, especially in the neonatal period.

Thrombocytopenia in critically ill patients is related most often to sepsis, DIC, multiple organ dysfunction syndrome, or is drug-induced (see Chapter 20). Heparin-induced thrombocytopenia must also be considered. Immune-mediated thrombocytopenia in newborns can be secondary to alloimmunization or maternal disease (e.g., maternal lupus erythematosus). Idiopathic thrombocytopenic purpura is frequent in children, but it rarely causes severe bleeding. Patients with hemolytic uremic syndrome and thrombotic thrombocytopenic purpura mostly require PICU admission because of renal failure or central nervous system involvement, but significant hemorrhage can occur. In these conditions, platelet transfusion can accelerate microangiopathy and should therefore be avoided unless a significant bleeding is present.

THROMBOSIS AND EMBOLI

Elsewhere in this book, there are chapters on pulmonary emboli (Chapter 62), thromboembolic diseases (Chapter 153), and their prophylaxis. Most thromboses observed in pediatric critically ill patients are acquired during the PICU stay. Catheter-related thrombosis is common, appearing rapidly after catheter insertion.[27] Heparin-coated catheters may prevent catheter-related thrombosis,[28] but their cost/benefit ratio and the risk of heparin-induced thrombopenia remains to be determined. DIC, allergy to heparin, prothrombic states (e.g., G20210A prothrombin gene mutation, factor V Leiden, anticardiolipin antibody, antithrombin III, or protein C deficiency), and blood flow stasis are common risk factors for thrombosis in children. The incidence of deep vein thrombosis is lower with peripherally inserted central catheters (PICC lines) than with centrally inserted catheters.[29]

Cerebral venous sinus thrombosis and renal vein thrombosis are more frequent in children than in adults. Symptoms of cerebral venous sinus thrombosis include seizures, headache, coma, paresis, cranial nerve palsies, and increased intracranial pressure. Head and neck infections, connective tissue disorders, or prothrombic states are frequently associated.[30] Symptoms of neonatal renal vein thrombosis are acute renal insufficiency, hematuria, and hypernephrosis.

IMMUNODEFICIENCY

A significant proportion of critically ill children are immunodeficient. Most cases of acquired immunodeficiency are caused by chemotherapy and immunosuppressive drugs, but any severe condition such as severe head trauma, sepsis, or burns can induce immunodeficiency. Congenital immunodeficiencies are also frequent in PICU. For example, a high prevalence of DiGeorge syndrome is observed among patients with congenital heart disease. As in adults, immunocompromised patients have an increased risk of contracting infections with unusual pathogens, in unusual sites, and with increased severity.

▣ Oncology

The initial presentation of an undiagnosed cancer can occasionally represent an acute emergency requiring critical care, but in most cases, children with cancer are admitted to PICU owing to a complication of the malignancy or its treatment. Any organ or system can be involved. This section gives a brief overview of the most frequent cancers seen in critically ill children and describes the most frequent causes of system dysfunction encountered in such patients. Finally, some ethical considerations specific to these patients are presented.

CANCER IN CHILDREN

The most frequent cancers in children are leukemias, lymphomas, neuroblastoma, Wilms' tumor, central nervous system solid tumors, bone tumors, and soft-tissue cancers. Cancer patients may need a stay in a PICU for the following reasons: (1) need for close monitoring during or after a high-risk procedure, (2) life-threatening complications of a cancer (e.g., compression of airways), or (3) therapy-related complications. The prognosis of the patients in the first group is usually good. Most of the discussion in the subsequent sections involves the two other presentations.

Respiratory System

Causes of respiratory dysfunction in cancer patients include those observed in patients without cancer (see Chapters 58 and 72). However, many specific diseases merit comments.

Primary lung malignancy is rare in children (histiocytosis), but leukemia, lymphoma, and metastases (neuroblastoma, bone cancer, Wilms' tumor) can invade the lungs. Airways can be obstructed, particularly by anterior mediastinal masses. In this situation, mostly observed in lymphomas, a rapid cardiorespiratory failure can be precipitated by a sedation or anesthesia. Such maneuvers should therefore be strictly avoided until the treatment induces regression of the compression.

Pediatric cancer patients frequently develop acute respiratory failure resulting from infections due to unusual pathogens and from noninfectious mechanisms: pulmonary edema, local treatment toxicity, graft-versus-host disease, bronchiolitis obliterans, alveolar hemorrhage. Invasive investigations should be discussed, such as bronchoalveolar lavage or lung biopsy, because identification of an atypical pathogen or a noninfectious cause can facilitate management. However, the risk of severe complications (death, barotrauma, hemorrhage) is high in the most severe patients,[31,32] and empirical treatment is frequently considered in the absence of diagnostic maneuvers.

Noninvasive mechanical ventilation is an effective means of preventing endotracheal intubation in pediatric immunocompromised patients with acute respiratory failure.[33] Patients who require intubation and invasive ventilation have a higher risk of death[33,34]; a lung-protective strategy should be applied (see Chapter 58).

Cardiovascular System

All types of shock can be observed in patients with malignancy, but sepsis is the leading cause of shock in pediatric cancer patients (see Chapter 130). Hemodynamic failure can also result from heart obstruction (e.g., mass in the auricula), extrinsic compression, pericardial effusion (inflammatory, hemorrhagic, or septic), infection or inflammation of cardiac structures (endocarditis, myocarditis, pericarditis), fibrotic restrictive myocarditis, or dysrhythmia induced by cardiac electrical system inflammation. Congestive heart failure may also be caused by chemotherapy, especially anthracycline and cyclophosphamide.

Arterial hypertension is a frequent side effect of cancer treatment. Severe hypertensive crisis can also result from malignant synthesis of sympathic mediators (neuroblastoma, Wilms' tumor, and pheochromocytoma).

Neurologic System

Causes of seizures include mass effect, metastasis, infection, vasculitis, thrombosis, hemorrhage, adverse reaction to therapy, hyponatremia, hypocalcemia, and hypertensive crisis.

Intracranial hypertension can be caused by infection, hemorrhage, a volume-expanding tumor, or hydrocephalus due to an infratentorial tumor blocking spinal fluid flux.

Meningitis can be caused by the cancer itself or by an infectious process. Unusual organisms may be involved, such as *Cryptococcus neoformans*, *Toxoplasma gondii*, *Listeria monocytogenes*, and gram-negative rods.

Coma or paralysis can result from cerebral or spinal cord compression, ischemia, hemorrhage, or radiotherapy side effects. Opsoclonus, raccoon eyes, and Horner's syndrome are suggestive of a neuroblastoma.

Digestive System

Stress gastritis, peptic ulcer, and upper gastrointestinal bleeding are frequent in the PICU in children with cancer. Bleeding from a digestive cancer is rare in children. Epstein-Barr virus, herpes simplex virus, or cytomegalovirus can cause hemorrhagic necrosis of the gastrointestinal tract and severe bleeding. *Candida* esophagitis is another cause of bleeding.

Typhlitis is an inflammation of the caecum and surrounding tissue, reported in 10% of leukemic patients at postmortem examination.[35] Usual clinical signs of abdominal inflammation can be absent in neutropenic patients; therefore, typhlitis must be feared in all patients with suspicion of infection. Abdominal computed tomography is a good diagnostic test for this condition. Secondary sepsis or bleeding is the usual cause of death.

Diarrhea is also frequent in this population. *Clostridium difficile* colitis must be suspected in patients who have recently received antibiotics (see Chapter 146). Gastroenteritis may be caused by unusual organisms such as *Cryptosporidium*.

Hepatic dysfunction can be caused by viral infection, drug toxicity (methotrexate), or veno-occlusive disease resulting from chemotherapy or radiation therapy. Severe hepatic veno-occlusive disease has a high mortality rate and should be aggressively managed. Treatment includes reduction of weight gain (diuretics, close fluid and electrolytes monitoring) and appropriate nutrition. Thrombolytic therapy or anticoagulation (antithrombin III) have been proposed but need to be evaluated.[36] Defibrotide also seems to be a promising adjunctive therapy which is under evaluation.[37,38]

Most cases of pancreatitis result from cytotoxic reactions to chemotherapy.

Renal System

Cancer-related causes of acute renal failure include chemotherapy (e.g., cyclosporine, methotrexate), obstruction of the urinary tract by a tumor, radiation nephritis, invasion of the kidneys (leukemia, lymphoma), or multiple organ dysfunction syndrome. Acute tumor lysis syndrome can cause an acute renal insufficiency, but prevention is usually effective.

Metabolic Problems

Electrolyte disorders are frequently observed. These disorders are discussed in Parts 1 and 6 of the text.

Lactic acidosis in critically ill patients is usually a consequence of cardiovascular dysfunction, sepsis, or multiple organ dysfunction. However, cancer with rapid and large turnover of malignant cells (e.g., leukemia, lymphoma) can be associated with lactic acidosis.[39,40]

Craniopharyngioma, some types of histiocytosis, and intracranial metastases can cause panhypopituitarism.

Anorexia, nausea, and vomiting are extremely frequent in this population, and malnutrition must be aggressively prevented. Enteral feeding should be attempted, but it is frequently limited by intolerance or abdominal complications. Therefore, parenteral nutrition is frequently required.

Fasting hypoglycemia is relatively frequent in this population. Severe hypoglycemia can also be the consequence of an insulinoma. Hyperglycemia is also frequent, and insulin therapy may be indicated to avoid limitation of caloric intake.

Steroids are part of many therapeutic protocols. Secondary adrenal insufficiency may appear if steroid treatment is inadvertently suspended.

Hematologic Problems

The proportion of cancer patients receiving chemotherapy who present with a significant hemorrhage is about 10%.[41] Hemorrhagic risk is the consequence of multiple mechanisms: coagulopathy, thrombocytopenia, and treatment-induced tissue fragility.

Thrombosis is also a concern. Many cancers are associated with a hypercoagulable state. DIC, heparin-induced thrombocytopenia, and catheter-related thrombosis are frequent.

Bone marrow failure is extremely frequent in patients with cancer. It is an expected side effect of cytotoxic and radiation therapies, but it can also result from the cancer itself, infection, and many other causes. A reactive hemophagocytic syndrome can also occur in patients with severe multiple organ dysfunction syndrome.[42]

The risk of infections particularly increases if the neutrophil count is lower than 1000/mm³. Various colony-stimulating factors (CSFs) such as granulocyte-macrophage CSF, granulocyte CSF, and macrophage-granulocyte inducer are frequently used to shorten neutropenia. However, the usefulness of these treatments on the number of transfusions required, incidence of infection, and survival rate remains to be established.[43,44]

Infectious Problems

Children with cancer must always be considered immunodeficient. Community-acquired pneumonia (Chapter 66), nosocomial pneumonia (Chapter 67), infections in the immunocompromised patient (Chapters 68 and 137), vascular catheter–related infections (Chapter 128), and prevention as well as control of nosocomial infection (Chapter 126) are of considerable importance in these patients.

Many symptoms anticipated in normal patients are attenuated in immunocompromised patients; an infection should therefore always be suspected early and checked for carefully. Aggressive empirical antibiotic treatment must be initiated as soon as an infection is suspected, and association with antifungal or antiviral agents should be discussed promptly.

OUTCOME AND ETHICAL CONSIDERATIONS

The current consensus among PICU caregivers is that intensive care is inappropriate if the chance of short-term survival is poor because the patient is in the late stage of a chronic disease.[45,46] However, over the last 2 decades, the outcomes of cancer patients requiring intensive care has largely improved (Table 157-1).[47] Oncologic patients admitted to PICU for severe sepsis have a survival rate similar to patients without cancer.[48,49] The mortality rate remains high when the admission cause is acute respiratory failure, but more than half of patients will survive. The mortality risk is higher in patients with a history of hematopoietic stem cell transplant.[47] Various scores or indicators of severity at admission have been correlated with mortality, but no index is powerful enough to permit a decision on the futility of a PICU admission if the

TABLE 157-1	Outcomes of Patients Admitted to the Pediatric Intensive Care Unit with Malignancy or Hematopoietic Stem Cell Transplant		
Admission Cause	*First Author (Ref. No.)*	*Years of Admissions*	*Survival Rate*
Patients with acute respiratory failure	Tamburro[47]	2002-2004	61%
	Van Gestel[52]	1999-2007	58%
	Kache[55]	2000-2004	59%
	Hagen[56]	1990-1999	41%
	Jacobe[57]	1994-1998	42%
Patients with severe sepsis or septic shock	Pound[48]	1994-2005	84%
	Fiser[49]	1990-2002	83%

oncologic disease itself is controlled. Usually these patients should be admitted to PICU, and full efforts should be made in support of a curative goal. However, it is important to reevaluate the survival possibility after a few days of this "ICU trial,"[50] because mortality is highly correlated with the number of persistent organ dysfunctions after several days,[50-53] and the goal of care may sometimes be redirected to comfort care.

End-of-life decisions (see Chapter 217) about patients with cancer or bone marrow transplant must be addressed by a multidisciplinary team including the patient when capable, family members, nurses, oncologists, and intensivists. It must be based on the chance of recovery from the acute disease, chance of survival from the underlying disease, quality of life before the acute problem, and the wishes of the patient and parents.[54]

KEY POINTS

1. Anemia occurs in 74% of critically ill children.

2. Phlebotomy is a major cause of anemia in children, which should be minimized.

3. Five types of events can be life threatening in sickle cell disease: acute chest syndrome, stroke, acute splenic sequestration, aplastic crisis, and infection.

4. A red blood cell (RBC) transfusion must be given to critically ill children who present with a hemoglobin (Hb) concentration lower than 5 g/dL.

5. In critically ill patients without cardiorespiratory instability, a conservative strategy aiming at giving RBC transfusion only when Hb falls below 7 g/dL is safe.

6. Disseminated intravascular coagulation is the most frequent hemorrhagic disorder observed in the pediatric intensive care unit (PICU).

7. Catheter-related thrombosis is common in the PICU.

8. An acute oncologic emergency can be the initial presentation of an undiagnosed cancer, or it can be the consequence of a complication of the malignancy or its treatment.

9. Many system dysfunctions observed in critically ill children with malignancy are attributable to side effects of chemotherapy and radiation therapy.

10. The majority of children with cancer or hematopoietic stem cell transplant admitted to PICU survive. A trial of intensive care should be proposed in most cases. However, the persistence of multiple organ failure after a few days of intensive care is associated with high mortality, and a multidisciplinary team should reassess if the aggressive support appears unwarranted or futile.

ANNOTATED REFERENCES

Bateman ST, Lacroix J, Boven K, et al. Anemia, blood loss and blood transfusion in North American children in the intensive care unit. Am J Respir Crit Care Med 2008;178:26-33.
  This paper describes the importance of anemia prevalence in pediatric critical care patients. The main causes of anemia are highlighted, and in particular the importance of blood draws.
Lacroix J, Hébert PC, Hutchison JH, et al. Transfusion strategies for patients in pediatric intensive care units. N Engl J Med 2007;356:1609-19.
  This article reports on the large multicenter randomized trial that established the non-inferiority of a restrictive strategy for RBC transfusions which supports avoidance of transfusion when Hb is above 7 g/dL in stable pediatric critically ill patients.
Jenkins TL. Sickle cell anemia in the pediatric intensive care unit: novel approaches for managing life-threatening complications. AACN Clin Issues 2002;13:154-68.

This paper reviews the main complications of sickle cell disease observed in the PICU, with a particular highlight on recent advances in pathophysiology and therapy.
Piastra M, De Luca D, Pietrini D, et al. Noninvasive pressure-support ventilation in immunocompromised children with ARDS: a feasibility study. Intensive Care Med 2009;35:1420-7.
  This paper suggests that noninvasive ventilation permits avoidance of tracheal intubation in a large proportion of immunocompromised children with acute respiratory failure.
Tamburro RF, Barfield RC, Shaffer ML, et al. Changes in outcomes (1996-2004) for pediatric oncology and hematopoietic stem cell transplant patients requiring invasive mechanical ventilation. Pediatr Crit Care Med 2008;9:270-7.
  This paper reports the improvement observed in outcomes of pediatric critically ill patients with cancer during recent years and characterizes some risk factors for mortality.

REFERENCES

Access the complete reference list online at http://www.expertconsult.com.

Obstetrics

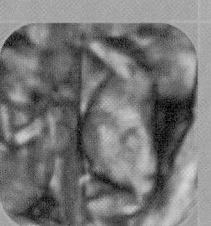

158

Cardiovascular and Endocrinologic Changes Associated with Pregnancy

MARIE R. BALDISSERI

Fundamental to the management of a critically ill pregnant woman is a thorough knowledge of the physiologic changes that occur during gestation and immediately after delivery. Clinicians must have a clear understanding of the extent of these changes, which occur in all pregnant women, to appropriately treat the critically ill patient whose additional pathology complicates the altered metabolic homeostasis and hemodynamics of the normal pregnant state. It is important to recognize that these physiologic changes add a level of complexity to diagnosis and management in the critically ill pregnant woman. The normal physiologic changes of pregnancy may alter the presentation of a disease process or illness during pregnancy, as well as alter interpretation of clinical and diagnostic examination findings in the pregnant woman. Subsequently, the endpoints of treatment can be significantly different than those for nonpregnant patients.

Some of the physiologic changes associated with pregnancy occur early in the normal course of gestation, whereas others occur during the middle or later stages. To render the most effective care of critically ill pregnant patients, the clinician must be aware of the timing of important physiologic changes. They affect almost all organ systems to varying degrees, depending in part on the gestational age of the fetus. Hemodynamic, metabolic, hormonal, and structural changes all occur during pregnancy and allow for the natural growth and development of the fetus. The pregnant woman adapts remarkably well to these changes, as does the fetus, allowing the two to coexist without harm to the other. However, if the pregnant woman is ill, either from a preexisting underlying disease process or from a new process that occurs during the pregnancy, the normal physiologic adaptive mechanisms of pregnancy can be insufficient to maintain the normal healthy union between mother and fetus. Depending on the severity of the underlying process or new illness, the hemodynamic ramifications to the pregnant woman and her fetus can be devastating and life threatening.

Cardiovascular Changes in Pregnancy

Cardiovascular and blood volume changes are among some of the more dramatic changes that occur in pregnancy (Table 158-1). These changes are primarily adaptive mechanisms, allowing the pregnant woman to accommodate her additional metabolic needs as well as those of the fetus during gestation and immediately after delivery. Cardiac output is significantly increased during pregnancy by as much as 50% compared with nonpregnant values. Cardiac output is further increased in twin pregnancies and multiple gestations.[1,2] The dramatic rise in cardiac output is seen as early as the first 6 to 8 weeks of pregnancy. After the 10th week, cardiac output is increased by 1 to 1.5 L/min and reaches a maximum value by approximately the 20th to 24th week of gestation. The early increase in cardiac output is primarily due to a significant increase in stroke volume. However, stroke volume decreases as the pregnancy advances because of aortocaval compression by the uterus and the pressure of the fetal presenting part on the common iliac vein. Caval compression occurs because the large, gravid uterus rests on the vena cava, effectively decreasing venous return to the heart and therefore decreasing ventricular preload. In the latter half of pregnancy, a progressive increase in the maternal heart rate by 15

to 20 beats/min is primarily responsible for maintaining the elevated cardiac output. The additional increase in cardiac output before labor and delivery is caused by a further increase in heart rate. Resting cardiac output either is maintained or decreases slightly as term approaches.[3]

INFLUENCE OF BODY POSITION

Venous return is further compromised with changes in body position, particularly if the pregnant patient is supine. As a result, cardiac output can be diminished by as much as 25% to 30%. The effects of changes in body position are most obvious in the latter half of pregnancy when the fetal size and gravid uterus can effectively tamponade the vena cava. This phenomenon is exaggerated in women with poorly developed venous collaterals. With compression of the vena cava in the supine position, these women exhibit signs of severe hypoperfusion (hypotension and bradycardia), a phenomenon described as the *supine hypotensive syndrome of pregnancy*.[4] Symptoms quickly resolve after the patient is repositioned to the left lateral recumbent position.[4] Cardiac output can decrease by 30% to 40% in patients with this syndrome. This vasovagal phenomenon underscores the influence of maternal body position on the hemodynamic alterations occurring in pregnancy.

Hemodynamic changes associated with a decrease in preload and, subsequently, a reduced cardiac output are less pronounced when the gravid uterus is minimally compressing the vena cava. This is optimally achieved by maintaining the pregnant woman with more than 20 weeks gestation in the full left lateral position whenever she is recumbent. Alternatives to this position, less optimal than the left lateral position but preferable to the supine position, are a left lateral tilt to 15 degrees or manual displacement of the gravid uterus. The latter maneuver of left uterine displacement can be performed by manually moving the uterus away from the midline to the left side when the patient is supine. This maneuver is particularly useful when performing cardiac compressions in a pregnant patient. In the supine position, the gravid uterus, which accounts for as much as 10% of the cardiac output, hinders successful resuscitation because of its adverse effects on intrathoracic pressure and venous return. Although hemodynamics are optimized in the left lateral position, it is difficult to achieve optimal chest compressions with the patient tilted all the way into the left lateral decubitus position. Acceptable alternatives are to perform cardiac compressions with the patient supine but with concurrent manual displacement of the uterus to the other side; it is also satisfactory to place a wedge under the right hip of the patient.[5,6]

OXYGEN CONSUMPTION AND VENTRICULAR PERFORMANCE

As cardiac output progressively increases, maternal oxygen consumption also increases. However, the increase in cardiac output is seen earlier than the rise in maternal oxygen consumption. Accordingly, the arteriovenous oxygen difference actually narrows early in pregnancy. The arteriovenous oxygen difference widens at the end of gestation. By

TABLE 158-1	Normal Hemodynamic Changes During Pregnancy		
Physiologic Parameter	*Term Pregnancy*	*Labor and Delivery*	*Postpartum*
Cardiac output	Increases 30%-50%	Increases 50%	Increases 60%-80% within 15-20 min
Blood volume	Increases 30%-50%	Additional 300-500 mL with each contraction	Decreases to baseline
Heart rate	Increases by 15-20 beats/min	Increase depends on stress and pain relief	Decreases to baseline
Blood pressure	Decreases by 5-10 mm Hg in midpregnancy	Increase depends on stress and pain relief	Decreases to baseline
Systemic vascular resistance	Decreases	Increases	Decreases to baseline
Oxygen consumption	Increases by 20%	Increases with stress of labor and delivery	Decreases to baseline
Red blood cell mass	Increases by 15-20%	—	—

term, there is a 20% increase in maternal oxygen consumption, mostly as a result of the increase in metabolic needs of the fetus. The increase in oxygen consumption is also a result of the increased work of ventilation during pregnancy, the increase in myocardial oxygen demand, and the increase in renal oxygen consumption. Oxygen extraction also gradually increases throughout gestation. The increase in cardiac output is probably the result of a combination of factors including increased uterine blood flow, increased maternal circulating blood volume (and hence ventricular preload), and possibly estrogen- and prolactin-induced augmentation of myocardial contractility. Ventricular dynamics are improved during pregnancy as a direct result of the action of steroid hormones on the pregnant myocardium. In animal models, estrogens have been shown to increase cardiac output and decrease peripheral vascular resistance.[7] Echocardiographic studies performed in healthy pregnant women have demonstrated a decrease in the pre-ejection period of left ventricular systole but an increase in the left ventricular end-diastolic dimension.[8-10] It may be that a combination of improved myocardial contractility and increased ventricular diastolic area may be responsible for increases in cardiac output during normal pregnancy.[11]

HEMODYNAMIC CHANGES DURING LABOR AND DELIVERY

Although cardiac output remains relatively constant in the latter half of pregnancy, there is a significant increase during active labor and immediately after delivery. With each uterine contraction, cardiac output dramatically increases as an additional 300 to 500 mL of maternal blood volume from the uterus is returned to the heart. Cardiac output can rise to 50% greater than normal when the pregnant woman is pushing in the second stage of labor. The amount of blood returned to the heart is accentuated in the supine position. When the pregnant patient is supine, uterine contractions can cause a 25% increase in cardiac output, a 15% decrease in maternal heart rate, and a 30% to 35% increase in stroke volume. In the lateral recumbent position, the hemodynamic changes associated with uterine contractions are less pronounced; cardiac output and stroke volume may rise by only 6% to 7%, and there may be only a small change in maternal heart rate. Cardiac output may be preferentially diverted to the heart if there is partial obstruction of the abdominal aorta by the uterus during contraction.

The hemodynamic changes seen during labor and delivery are influenced by anesthetic and analgesic techniques. The increase in cardiac output is less if caudal anesthesia is used.[12,13] Within the first 20 to 30 minutes after delivery of the fetus and placenta, there is an even greater increase in cardiac output, because blood is no longer diverted to the uteroplacental vascular bed. Approximately 500 mL is redirected to the maternal circulation in the so-called autotransfusion effect of pregnancy. This effect can cause cardiac output to increase by 60% to 80% after aortocaval compression is removed and blood volume is increased. Most of the physiologic changes of pregnancy resolve and revert to normal within several days after delivery. Cardiac output returns to normal within 2 weeks to 3 months after delivery as sodium and water balances normalize.

BLOOD VOLUME CHANGES

The changes in maternal blood volume during pregnancy are dramatic. Plasma volume increases by 30% to 50% by the end of gestation. This value is increased in the multigravida patient compared with primigravidas, but the exact mechanism responsible for this effect is unclear. The increase in blood volume can be as high as 70% with twin pregnancies. An increase of 10% to 15% in blood volume is seen as early as the seventh week of gestation. Blood volume is maximal at 30 to 34 weeks, after which the value plateaus until term.[14] Ventricular filling pressures do not increase despite the large increases in plasma volume.[15] This is most likely the result of concurrent decreases in systemic and pulmonary vascular resistance.

The increase in blood volume is a striking adaptive mechanism that permits additional blood flow to the uterus and other maternal organs, in particular the kidneys. Uterine blood flow increases to 100 mL/min by the end of the first trimester and reaches 1200 mL/min at term. Both sodium and water retention contribute to the increase in plasma volume. Total body water increases by approximately 6.5 to 8 L. Most of this increase is seen in the extracellular space and is preferentially distributed in the lower extremities. The total increase in body water includes approximately 3.5 L of amniotic fluid, placental fluid, and water in the fetus. The maternal blood volume increases by 1 to 2 L. Red blood cell (RBC) mass accounts for only 300 to 400 mL of the increase in total blood volume.

Plasma renin and aldosterone levels are elevated during pregnancy despite expansion of the maternal blood volume. Activation of the renin-angiotensin-aldosterone system may result from the concomitant decrease in peripheral vascular resistance and the increase in vascular capacitance seen as early as the first 6 weeks of pregnancy.[2] Both estrogens and progesterone increase aldosterone levels, increasing sodium and water retention.[16] At 12 weeks of gestation, atrial natriuretic peptide levels also increase, most likely in response to the increase in plasma volume.

The increase in blood volume is an adaptive mechanism that provides some level of protection for the inevitable blood loss that accompanies delivery of the fetus and placenta. Average blood loss during vaginal delivery is 500 mL; average blood loss during cesarean delivery is approximately 1000 mL. Although providing some degree of protection from peripartum blood loss, the increased plasma volume associated with pregnancy also can lull the clinician into a false sense of security. A pregnant woman can lose up to 35% of her blood volume before the usual signs of hypovolemia and acute hemorrhage are obvious. Although the pregnant woman may appear to have stable vital signs up to this point, the fetus may be severely compromised and deprived of adequate maternal blood flow. Tachycardia, hypotension, and other signs of hemodynamic instability are late manifestations of a significant deficit in maternal blood volume.

PHYSIOLOGIC ANEMIA OF PREGNANCY

Accompanying the increase in blood volume is an increase in RBC mass stimulated by increased circulating levels of erythropoietin. The RBC mass increases during the second trimester and continues to increase progressively throughout the pregnancy. However, the increase of 15% to 20% in RBC mass is disproportionate to the 30% to 50% increase in blood volume. As a result, the hematocrit decreases, resulting in the "physiologic hemodilutional anemia" of pregnancy. Hemodilution is most notable during the 30th to 34th gestational weeks. The hemoglobin concentration can decrease by as much as 9%. In the second trimester, the hemoglobin level can decrease to 11 to 12 g/100 mL, compared with the normal nonpregnant value of 13 to 14 g/100 mL. The decrease in blood viscosity associated with the anemia of pregnancy allows for decreased resistance to blood flow and facilitates placental perfusion. The hematocrit decreases until the end of the second trimester but increases later in the pregnancy, when the increase in RBC mass is proportionate to the increase in plasma volume. The hematocrit stabilizes at that point or even increases slightly as term approaches.

The degree of change in RBC mass during pregnancy depends in part on whether iron is supplemented. With the increase in RBC mass, there is a need for additional iron to prevent the development of iron-deficiency anemia. Maternal requirements for iron can increase to 5 to 6 mg/d. The fetus uses iron from maternal stores to prevent fetal anemia, but the presence of significant maternal iron-deficiency anemia has been shown to result in a higher incidence of fetal complications, including preterm labor and late spontaneous abortions.[17]

RENAL BLOOD FLOW DURING PREGNANCY

Under the influence of circulating hormones, there is a preferential redistribution of blood flow to the uterus, breast, and kidneys during pregnancy. Each kidney increases in length and weight, and the renal pelvis and ureters dilate. The glomerular filtration rate (GFR) increases by 50%, and renal blood flow increases by 25% to 50%. Changes in GFR and renal blood flow occur by the sixth week of gestation. The increase in renal blood flow plateaus early in pregnancy and remains unchanged or decreases slightly as term is approached. Urine flow and sodium excretion are increased and are influenced by position, especially in late pregnancy. Flow rates and the sodium excretion rate are significantly higher in the lateral recumbent position compared with the supine position. Concentrations of serum creatinine and blood urea nitrogen are reduced proportionately to the increase in GFR. Glycosuria may also occur during pregnancy as a result of the increase in GFR and impaired tubular reabsorption of glucose.

CHANGES IN BLOOD PRESSURE AND VASCULAR SYSTEM

Arterial blood pressure decreases as early as the sixth week of pregnancy; the lowest diastolic pressures are recorded during the second trimester. By the eighth week of gestation, diastolic blood pressure decreases by approximately by 10%. Diastolic pressure reaches a nadir at 16 to 24 weeks and is typically 5 to 10 mm Hg less than normal. After the 16th gestational week, blood pressure progressively increases and is back to baseline by term. With the increase in venous return associated with uterine contractions and the additional factors of pain, anxiety, and stress during labor and delivery, an increase in blood pressure usually occurs during this time. The decrease in blood pressure during pregnancy is associated with a significant decrease in peripheral vascular resistance. The decrease in arteriolar tone is influenced by several factors, including hormonal changes that induce vasodilatation and lack of responsiveness to the pressor effect of angiotensin II.[18] There is evidence for blood vessel remodeling in pregnancy, leading to increased venous compliance.[19,20] During pregnancy, circulating levels of numerous endogenous procoagulant and anticoagulant proteins change, leading to a hypercoagulable state. As a consequence, the risk of venous thrombosis increases during pregnancy. The reported incidence is 0.7 cases per 1000 women, and this rate increases threefold to fourfold in the postpartum period.[21]

The treatment of choice for severe hypotension resulting from acute hemorrhage, sepsis, or other critical illness during pregnancy is (ideally) aggressive fluid resuscitation. However, in cases of fluid-unresponsive hypotension, vasopressors must be used to prevent detrimental consequences to both the mother and fetus as a result of inadequate uterine blood flow secondary to hypotension. Most vasopressors increase maternal blood pressure at the expense of fetal blood flow, inducing vasoconstriction of the uterine vessels. There are few human studies of these agents in pregnant women. However, animal studies animals indicate that ephedrine and dopamine increase uterine blood flow to the uteroplacental circulation while at the same time increasing maternal blood pressure.[22]

STRUCTURAL REMODELING OF THE HEART

The heart is dramatically remodeled during the first few weeks of pregnancy. There is enlargement of all four chambers. The valvular annular diameters increase, as does the thickness of the left ventricular wall. End-diastolic volume increases, although end-diastolic pressure remains unchanged.[10,20] Chamber enlargement, particularly of the left atrium, may be a predisposing factor for supraventricular and atrial arrhythmias. Nonspecific ST-T wave changes may also be found in asymptomatic pregnant woman.

As the uterus enlarges and the diaphragm elevates, the heart is rotated upward and to the left. The apical impulse on physical examination is heard best over the fourth intercostal space, lateral to the midclavicular line. Left axis deviation is seen on the electrocardiogram as a result of the rotation of the heart. Because of the displacement of the heart, pregnant women may appear to have cardiomegaly on the chest radiograph. In addition, lung markings may be more prominent, suggesting vascular congestion. These changes can be similar to those seen in patients with heart disease. Even in women with no underlying cardiac pathology, the normal physiologic changes of pregnancy can result in signs and symptoms that are difficult to differentiate from those associated with cardiac disease. Symptoms such as fatigue, decreased exercise tolerance, peripheral edema, palpitations, chest pain, dyspnea, and orthopnea are common complaints as pregnancy advances.

New murmurs often appear during pregnancy. Systolic flow murmurs and a third heart sound are common but are soft. Mild pulmonic and tricuspid regurgitation occurs in more than 90% of healthy pregnant woman.[23,24] One-third of pregnant women have evidence of clinically insignificant mitral regurgitation. Diastolic, pansystolic, and late systolic murmurs are rare in normal pregnancy and may indicate underlying heart disease. Bruits originating from the internal mammary artery and venous hums with diastolic components are common during pregnancy. These findings can initially confuse the diagnosis of a more serious underlying cardiac illness.

CARDIAC DISEASE AND PREGNANCY

In women with significant cardiac pathology, the hemodynamic aberrations associated with pregnancy can be life threatening. The incidence of significant cardiac disease in pregnancy is less than 2% but is increasing.[25,26] Advances in medical therapy and in cardiac surgery have allowed female cardiac patients to survive to childbearing age and to have successful term pregnancies.[27] For women with severe cardiac problems such as pulmonary hypertension, Eisenmenger's syndrome, severe mitral stenosis, or Marfan syndrome (in which the risk of aortic dissection is high during pregnancy), the physiologic changes of pregnancy can increase both maternal and fetal morbidity and mortality by transiently or permanently worsening the underlying heart disease.[28] Increases in blood volume, stroke volume, cardiac output, and heart rate and the decrease in systemic vascular resistance are poorly tolerated by pregnant women with severe underlying cardiac disease. Maternal mortality is less than 1% for patients with less severe cardiac problems, but it increases to 50% if pregnancy is associated with the presence of underlying primary pulmonary hypertension or cyanotic disorders such as Eisenmenger's syndrome.[29,30]

Approximately 90% of pregnant women with cardiac disease are rated as New York Heart Association (NYHA) functional class I or class II. These patients tolerate the hemodynamic changes of pregnancy and can be managed well with medical therapy, although the incidence of heart failure and arrhythmias tends to be higher in this group of patients.[31] The 10% of pregnant patients with NYHA functional class III or IV heart disease account for 85% of cardiac deaths.[32] Fetal morbidity and mortality are increased in these patients, and there is a higher incidence of prematurity, miscarriage, and intrauterine growth retardation.[33] Cardiac telemetry, fetal monitoring, and hemodynamic monitoring are usually necessary for these high-risk patients during labor and delivery and, because of the large changes in intravascular volume after delivery, during the first few postpartum days.

Endocrine and Metabolic Changes in Pregnancy

There are numerous endocrine and metabolic alterations during pregnancy, many of which are directly attributable to hormonal signals originating from the fetoplacental unit. Maternal adaptations to hormonal changes that occur during pregnancy directly influence the growth and development of the fetus and placenta. In pregnancy, there is also a change in the normal hormonal feedback mechanisms that control the synthesis and release of hormones. As with cardiac disease, the presentation of endocrine and metabolic disorders may be difficult to differentiate from the normal hypermetabolic state of pregnancy.

HYPOTHALAMIC AND PITUITARY ALTERATIONS

As in the nonpregnant state, the hypothalamic-pituitary axis is responsible for regulating many aspects of metabolism. Circulating levels of most of the releasing hormones of the hypothalamus increase during pregnancy because of increased production by the placenta rather than increased production and release by the hypothalamus. The target organ of the hypothalamus, the pituitary gland, undergoes remarkable structural and metabolic changes in pregnancy. Its size increases almost threefold secondary to estrogen stimulation. Gonadotropin and growth hormone production decrease during pregnancy. However, synthesis of ACTH, prolactin, and thyroid-stimulating hormone (TSH) increases.

Free and bound cortisol levels are increased in pregnancy, even though circulating ACTH concentrations are elevated. These changes suggest that the normal negative feedback loop between ACTH and cortisol concentrations is altered in the pregnant state.[34] Free plasma cortisol concentrations may be two to three times higher than normal at term. Diurnal variation of cortisol is blunted but maintained throughout pregnancy. The clinical signs of weakness, peripheral edema, glucose intolerance, and weight gain associated with Cushing's disease are sometimes difficult to differentiate from the clinical features of normal gestation. The symptoms of Cushing's disease are exacerbated by pregnancy but often resolve after delivery. Improved outcomes are seen with surgical therapy intrapartum, if pituitary or adrenal tumors are discovered during the course of the pregnancy.[35,28] In normal pregnancy, cortisol release may not be suppressed with a low intravenous dose (1 mg) of dexamethasone. An 8-mg dose of dexamethasone is usually needed to suppress cortisol secretion if a tumor is present. In patients with occult adrenal insufficiency, a life-threatening adrenal crisis may be precipitated by the stress of labor and delivery. During pregnancy, the signs and symptoms may be vague and nonspecific, but with the stress of labor, these symptoms are exaggerated. The clinical diagnosis is made in conjunction with laboratory evidence of a low cortisol level or even a low-normal level and no increase in the plasma cortisol concentration with an ACTH stimulation test. Immediate treatment with stress doses of hydrocortisone is indicated in these patients.

In preparation for lactation, circulating prolactin levels progressively increase to about 10 times normal during the course of pregnancy, secondary to stimulation of the anterior pituitary by placental estrogens and progesterone. The dramatic increase in plasma prolactin concentration may lead to an increase in size of preexisting pituitary adenomas larger than 1 cm.[36] Symptoms resulting from an increase in prolactin secretion usually subside within 6 weeks after delivery if the patient is not breastfeeding.

TSH secretion is transiently decreased in the first trimester, but circulating TSH concentrations are usually increased by term. Circulating levels of thyroxine (T_4) and triiodothyronine (T_3) increase as a result of a twofold estrogen-stimulated increase in the synthesis of thyroxine-binding globulin. Levels of free (dialyzable) T_4 and free T_3 are unchanged. The thyroid gland does not increase in size, despite the increase in production of thyroid hormones. Pregnant women who obtain sufficient dietary iodine (more than 200 µg daily) have no untoward complications from the changes in thyroid function.[37,38]

Posterior pituitary hormones are altered in pregnancy. Circulating oxytocin levels increase, but the vasopressin concentration remains essentially unchanged. Plasma osmolality decreases by 5 to 10 mOsm/kg, suggesting that the threshold for secretion of vasopressin decreases during gestation. Although vasopressin levels remain unchanged, some women develop transient diabetes insipidus during pregnancy.[39]

CHANGES IN GLUCOSE METABOLISM

Early in pregnancy, glucose metabolism is influenced primarily by increased levels of estrogens and progesterone, which induce pancreatic β-cell hyperplasia and increased insulin secretion. Glucose metabolism is primarily controlled by placental hormones later in the pregnancy in response to the increased nutritional and metabolic demands of the fetus. Circulating glucose and insulin levels fluctuate widely depending on the nutritional state of the mother. Morning fasting levels of glucose can decrease to less than 55 mg/dL. Fasting blood glucose levels decrease by 10% to 20% because of increased peripheral glucose utilization, decreased hepatic glucose production, and increased consumption of glucose by the fetus.

Pregnant women with diabetes mellitus experience more hypoglycemic episodes in the first trimester, because hepatic gluconeogenesis is decreased during this period. Insulin secretion increases during pregnancy. There is a relative state of insulin resistance, as evidenced by postprandial maternal hyperglycemia.[40] Normally, women adapt to the state of relative insulin resistance during pregnancy. However, those women with marginal pancreatic reserve or preexisting insulin resistance due to obesity may not produce sufficient insulin, leading to the development of gestational diabetes mellitus. Pregnant women with preexisting diabetes mellitus require as much as 30% more insulin than before pregnancy. There is a close correlation between maternal blood glucose levels and glucose uptake and utilization by the fetus, because glucose crosses the placental barrier. Poor maternal glucose control worsens fetal morbidity. For patients with preexisting insulin-dependent diabetes mellitus, fetal and neonatal mortality rates have decreased significantly, from 65% to between 2% and 5%, as a result of implementing strict metabolic glucose control with insulin.[41]

Lipid metabolism is accelerated in pregnancy, and the circulating concentrations of triglycerides and cholesterol increase. Increased production of triglycerides allows for maternal consumption while sparing glucose for use by the fetus.[42] Lipolysis is stimulated in adipose tissue, and there is a release of glycerol and fatty acids that decreases maternal glucose utilization, additionally sparing glucose for the fetus.

KEY POINTS

1. Normal pregnancy is associated with numerous physiologic changes that affect almost all maternal organ systems.

2. Hemodynamic, metabolic, hormonal, and structural changes that occur during pregnancy are adaptive mechanisms for maintaining a healthy homeostasis between the mother and the fetus.

3. Maternal hemodynamic alterations and poor fetal outcome can occur if the physiologic adaptive mechanisms are insufficient to maintain the normal homeostasis between the mother and the fetus.

4. The physiologic changes occur at different stages throughout the pregnancy.

5. The normal physiologic changes of pregnancy may alter the presentation of a maternal disease process, confound the diagnosis, or alter the endpoints of treatment.

6. Cardiac output is increased significantly, up to 50% above prepartum values, by the 24th week of gestation. The value then plateaus until term. During labor and delivery, cardiac output is further increased with uterine contractions and the "auto-transfusion" effect of increased preload after delivery of the fetus and placenta.

7. The increase in cardiac output early in pregnancy is primarily caused by an increase in blood volume. Later in pregnancy, an increase in the heart rate by 15 to 20 beats/min is mainly responsible for the increase in cardiac output. Improved myocardial contractility may account in part for an improvement in cardiac output in pregnancy.

8. Maternal body position directly affects cardiac output and stroke volume. In the supine position, the gravid uterus causes aortocaval compression and decreased preload. An extreme manifestation of this effect is the "supine hypotensive syndrome" of pregnancy.

9. After the 20th week of gestation, pregnant women should not be placed supine but rather in the left lateral recumbent position, which maximizes maternal hemodynamics. During cardiac resuscitation, the pregnant patient should be placed in this position, or manually displace the uterus to the left.

10. Left ventricular end-diastolic volume is increased during pregnancy, but filling pressures are relatively unchanged; this may reflect the decrease in afterload caused by a decrease in systemic and pulmonary vascular resistance.

11. Blood volume increases by 30% to 50% by the end of gestation. However, red blood cell mass increases by only 15% to 20%, creating the "physiologic anemia" of pregnancy.

12. A pregnant woman can lose up to 35% of her blood volume before tachycardia and hypotension occur as a result of acute hemorrhage or severe hypovolemia.

13. Blood flow is increased to many organs during pregnancy, especially to the breasts, uterus, and kidneys. Renal blood flow increases by 25% to 50%, and the glomerular filtration rate increases by up to 50%, with a decrease in the plasma creatinine and blood urea nitrogen concentrations.

14. A decrease in the diastolic blood pressure by 10% is seen in the second trimester, secondary to the decrease in systemic vascular resistance. By the end of pregnancy, blood pressure levels should increase to prepartum values.

15. Blood vessel remodeling and changes in the coagulation system during pregnancy, including an increase in most clotting factors, makes the pregnant woman hypercoagulable and more susceptible to venous thromboembolism throughout pregnancy and in the postpartum period.

16. Remodeling of the heart causes enlargement of all four chambers. The pregnant woman may be more susceptible to supraventricular and atrial arrhythmias because of left atrial enlargement.

17. Systolic ejection murmurs and a third heart sound can commonly be heard during pregnancy. Diastolic, pansystolic, and late systolic murmurs should prompt the clinician to look for an underlying cardiac problem.

18. Pregnant patients with mild to moderate cardiac disease usually tolerate the hemodynamic changes of pregnancy. Those patients with pulmonary hypertension and right-to-left shunts have mortality rates as high as 50%.

19. There are numerous endocrine and metabolic alterations during pregnancy that primarily affect the hypothalamus, pituitary, and adrenal glands. As with cardiac disease, the presentation of a patient with endocrine and metabolic disorders may be difficult to differentiate from the normal hypermetabolic state of pregnancy.

20. Both corticotropin (ACTH) and cortisol levels are elevated in pregnancy. Cushing's syndrome can be exacerbated by pregnancy. Acute adrenal crisis may be precipitated by the stress of labor and delivery. The treatment is immediate glucocorticoid administration.

21. In preparation for lactation, prolactin levels are increased 10-fold throughout the pregnancy as a result of estrogen and progesterone stimulation. This increase in prolactin may increase the size of pituitary adenomas and precipitate symptoms during the pregnancy.

22. Thyroid hormones are increased during pregnancy as a result of increased synthesis of thyroxine-binding globulin. Free levels are unchanged. Despite the complex thyroidal changes that occur during pregnancy, pregnant women have no untoward complications if their daily iodine intake is sufficient.

23. Transient diabetes insipidus can develop during pregnancy, secondary to a state of vasopressin resistance.

24. Large fluctuations in glucose and insulin levels are seen in pregnancy, depending on the nutritional state of the mother. Fasting glucose levels can decrease by 10% to 20%.

25. During pregnancy, there is increased insulin secretion, with a relative state of insulin resistance.

26. Obese women with insulin resistance and women with marginal pancreatic reserve can develop gestational diabetes mellitus.

27. Fetal and neonatal mortality rates are low if strict metabolic glucose control with insulin therapy is maintained.

28. Maternal lipid metabolism is increased during pregnancy, allowing for increased glucose utilization by the fetus.

ANNOTATED REFERENCES

2005 American Heart Association Guidelines for cardiopulmonary resuscitation and emergency cardiovascular care. Part 10:8: cardiac arrest associated with pregnancy. Circulation 2005;112:IV-150.

Recommendations and guidelines for CPR and ACLS drug administration in pregnancy are presented by the AHA. Evidence extrapolated from peri-arrest resuscitation scenarios indicated that ultrasound assessment undertaken by trained rescuers may help to identify intraabdominal hemorrhage as a cause of cardiac arrest in pregnancy in the hospital setting. Clinicians are advised to identify common and reversible causes of cardiac arrest in pregnancy during the resuscitation attempts. The use of abdominal ultrasound by a skilled operator should be considered in detecting pregnancy and possible causes of cardiac arrest in pregnancy, but this should not delay other treatments.

Clark SL, Cotton DB, Lee W, et al. Central hemodynamic assessment of normal term pregnancy. Am J Obstet Gynecol 1989;161:1439.

This landmark paper presents central hemodynamic data obtained with the use of a pulmonary artery catheter during pregnancy and after delivery. Ten primigravidas patients in late pregnancy (between the 36th and 38th weeks of gestation) underwent pulmonary artery catheter and arterial catheter placement. These same patients were restudied with a pulmonary artery catheter at 11 to 13 weeks after delivery. All measurements were performed with the patient in the left lateral recumbent position. The authors found significant decreases in systemic vascular resistance, pulmonary vascular resistance, colloid oncotic pressure, and colloid oncotic pressure-pulmonary capillary wedge pressure gradient in the third-trimester measurements (P <.05). A significant rise in cardiac output and heart rate was seen in all patients before delivery (P <.05). No significant changes in pulmonary capillary wedge pressure, central venous pressure, left ventricular stroke work index, or mean arterial pressure were found. Although blood volume and preload are elevated in pregnancy and end-diastolic volume increases, there were no substantial increases in the filling pressures of the heart as measured by the pulmonary artery catheter, suggesting a decrease in afterload with the decrease in the systemic and pulmonary vascular resistance.

Snow V, Qaseem A, Barry P, et al. Management of venous thromboembolism: a clinical practice guideline from the American College of Physicians and the American Academy of Family Physicians. Ann Intern Med 2007;146:204.

Recommendation 4: There is insufficient evidence to make specific recommendations for types of anticoagulation management of VTE in pregnant women. During pregnancy, women have a fivefold increased risk for VTE compared with nonpregnant women. Clinicians should avoid vitamin K antagonists in pregnant women, because these drugs cross the placenta and are associated with embryopathy between 6 and 12 weeks' gestation, as well as fetal bleeding (including intracranial hemorrhage) at delivery. Neither LMWH nor unfractionated heparin crosses the placenta, and neither is associated with embryopathy or fetal bleeding.

Burt CC, Durbridge J. Management of cardiac disease in pregnancy. Contin Educ Anaesth Crit Care Pain 2009;9:44.

This article is an excellent review of cardiac disease in pregnancy, focusing on the different causes of cardiac disease and their management in pregnancy. Cardiac disease is the most common cause of mortality in pregnancy and may present with cardiovascular decompensation during pregnancy, at the time of delivery, or immediately postpartum. The goals of therapy are: early risk assessment, optimization, regular monitoring for deterioration, planning of delivery, and surveillance for deterioration in the immediate postpartum period. Vaginal delivery with low-dose regional analgesia and careful fluid management is the preferred method of delivery and cesarean section deliveries should be reserved for obstetric indications.

Van De Velde M, De Buck F. Anesthesia for non-obstetric surgery in the pregnant patient. Minerva Anestesiol 2007;73:235-40.

Surgery during pregnancy is relatively common. This review of the literature focuses on relevant issues such as maternal safety during nonobstetric surgery in pregnancy, teratogenicity of anesthetic drugs, avoidance of fetal asphyxia, prevention of preterm labor, the safety of laparoscopy, and the need to monitor the fetal heart rate and will finally give a practical approach to manage these patients.

REFERENCES

Access the complete reference list online at http://www.expertconsult.com.

159

Hypertensive Disorders in Pregnancy

MARIE R. BALDISSERI

Hypertensive disorders associated with pregnancy are not uncommon, occurring in approximately 7% of pregnancies. Guidelines from the Society of Obstetricians and Gynecologists have classified hypertension of pregnancy into two categories: preexisting or gestational with preeclampsia superimposed on either gestational or preexisting chronic hypertension.[1] The National High Blood Pressure Education Working Group on High Blood Pressure in Pregnancy classified hypertension as: (1) chronic hypertension, (2) preeclampsia-eclampsia, (3) preeclampsia superimposed on chronic hypertension, and (4) gestational hypertension which is transient during pregnancy or chronic hypertension identified in the latter half of pregnancy.[2] Gestational hypertension including preeclampsia occurs de novo after 20 weeks of gestation. Chronic hypertension will either be preexisting before the pregnancy or manifest earlier than the 20th week of gestation. Chronic hypertension is present in up to 22% of women of childbearing age. Approximately 1% of pregnancies are complicated by chronic hypertension, 5% to 6% by gestational hypertension, and 1% to 2% of all pregnancies are associated with preeclampsia. Preeclampsia occurs in 20% to 25% of women with preexisting chronic hypertension.

Chronic hypertension is seen more commonly in women older than 35 years of age. Preeclampsia is also seen more frequently in the older parturient but also in younger women of less than 18 years of age. Predisposing factors for the development of hypertension and/or preeclampsia during pregnancy include a family history of hypertension or preeclampsia, preexisting diabetes mellitus, black race, obesity (BMI ≥ 30), vascular or renal disorders, primigravid state, preeclampsia with a previous pregnancy, migraine history, and multiple gestational pregnancies.[3] Smoking during pregnancy may actually decrease the incidence of hypertension and preeclampsia during pregnancy, although this is controversial.[4] Hypertensive disorders in pregnancy are a significant leading cause of maternal mortality and morbidity, particularly when preeclampsia is superimposed on preexisting chronic hypertension. A pregnancy-related mortality of 15.7% was reported as a result of hypertensive disorders in the United States from 1991 to 1999.[5]

Blood Pressure Measurements in Pregnancy

The definition of hypertension during pregnancy has been controversial in the past. *Hypertension* is now most commonly defined as a blood pressure (BP) greater than 140/90 mm Hg. Recently there has been a general consensus that the degree of increase in systolic (SBPs) and diastolic blood pressures (DBPs) may actually be more important than the baseline values. Many authors now agree that significant hypertension in pregnancy is defined by an increase of at least 30 mm Hg in the SBP and an increase in the DBP of at least 15 mm Hg. Treatment of a DBP greater than 110 mm Hg or a SBP greater than 160 mm Hg is advocated because of the increase in maternal complications with this degree of hypertension.[6]

Sustained (rather than transient) increases in BP are the key risk factor; accordingly, BP should be measured on at least two separate occasions. BP measurements should be made in a standardized fashion (e.g., with the patient sitting in the same position) at each evaluation. Measurements in the upper arm in the recumbent position may give falsely low values because of aortal and caval compression by the gravid uterus. BP is best recorded with the patient in the sitting position or in the inferior arm in the lateral recumbent position. Many automated

blood pressure cuffs are accurate during pregnancy but may underestimate blood pressure measurements in preeclamptic women. Manual BP readings are best suited for this group.

Physiologic Changes in Pregnancy

Essential to the management of hypertension in pregnancy is an understanding of the normal physiologic changes in cardiac output, vasomotor tone, and systemic BP that occur. During pregnancy, cardiac output increases by 30% to 40% in the second trimester, peaking at about the 24th week of gestation. The increase in cardiac output during the first two trimesters of pregnancy is primarily caused by increased maternal blood volume. Cardiac output plateaus for the remainder of the pregnancy until labor. An increase in cardiac output is seen with each uterine contraction. Cardiac output increases again during the immediate postpartum period after delivery of the fetus and the placenta. It is during this period that cardiac output is highest due to the so-called autotransfusion effect (see Chapter 158).

Systemic vascular resistance and consequently BP decrease during the second trimester. Increased synthesis of vasodilating prostaglandins may play a role in the regulation of BP and uterine blood flow in pregnancy. In normal pregnancy, vascular resistance is determined by a proper balance of the effects of vasoconstricting factors and vasodilating factors, including prostaglandins. This balance may be disturbed in hypertensive states, owing to inadequate prostaglandin synthesis. In pregnancy-related hypertensive states, there is a paradoxical increase in the systemic vascular resistance, compared with pregnancy without hypertension. It is noteworthy that all patients with newly acquired or preexisting hypertension in pregnancy have a relative decrease in DBP during the second trimester, reflecting a relative decrease in systemic vascular resistance. Indeed, BP normalizes during the second trimester in some patients with preexisting hypertension.

Causes of Hypertension in Pregnancy

There are multiple causes of hypertension during pregnancy (Box 159-1). The most common hypertensive states are gestational hypertension without the presence of proteinuria, essential chronic hypertension, and preeclampsia (gestational hypertension with significant proteinuria). This classification is clinically useful to the practitioner, but the risk from systemic hypertension is significant for all three conditions, regardless of the specific cause of high BP. Hypertension during pregnancy is associated with an increased risk of death for both mother and fetus. Severe maternal hypertension during pregnancy is associated with placental abruption and intrauterine growth retardation.[7]

Preeclampsia is defined as primarily diastolic hypertension that occurs transiently during the pregnancy, usually manifesting after the 20th gestational week, and resolves within 1 to 2 months after delivery. Women who develop preeclampsia have a high rate of recurrence of hypertension with subsequent pregnancies and often develop chronic hypertension at a later time.

Essential chronic hypertension (i.e., hypertension that was present before the pregnancy, whether diagnosed or undiagnosed) persists in the postpartum period and accounts for approximately one-third of all cases of hypertension during pregnancy. Essential chronic hypertension may manifest during the first 20 weeks of pregnancy. Women who develop hypertension without proteinuria in the last trimester of pregnancy may have essential hypertension, either unmasked or

CAUSES OF HYPERTENSION IN PREGNANCY

Pregnancy-induced hypertension (gestational hypertension without proteinuria)
Essential hypertension
Preeclampsia (gestational hypertension with proteinuria)
Primary aldosteronism (Conn's syndrome)
Renal artery stenosis
Coarctation of the aorta
Pheochromocytoma
Cushing's syndrome

precipitated by the pregnancy. In these cases of de novo presentation of hypertension, care must be exercised to rule out other non–pregnancy-related causes of hypertension such as renal artery stenosis, polycystic kidneys, glomerular or interstitial renal disease, pheochromocytoma, coarctation of the aorta, primary aldosteronism, Cushing's syndrome, hyperthyroidism, and hyperparathyroidism. Previously undiagnosed essential chronic hypertension is a consideration, particularly in older multiparous women. As the age of parturients has increased, the incidence of essential hypertension in pregnant women has also increased. For some patients, the initial diagnosis of hypertension may be made during a routine prenatal visit with an obstetrician. For some patients, this prenatal visit is their first encounter with a physician as an adult. Essential hypertension should be suspected if there is a family history of hypertension, diabetes, or obesity. If there is a suspicion of preexisting essential hypertension, cardiac echocardiography should be performed to evaluate for left ventricular hypertrophy, which would suggest that hypertension has been a problem for an extended period. If extremes of BP are avoided with treatment, there is no significant worsening of maternal and perinatal outcomes for pregnant patients with essential hypertension. Complications related to intrapartum hypertension, such as placenta previa, placental abruption, and preeclampsia, are less likely with judicious treatment of elevated BP. Patients with essential hypertension have not been shown to have a higher incidence of preeclampsia, particularly if BP is well controlled. In general, mortality and morbidity are not increased in patients with uncomplicated mild chronic hypertension However, morbidity and mortality are both increased in those patients with severe uncontrolled hypertension, and this is further complicated by superimposed preeclampsia.[8]

Pathology of Preeclampsia

Preeclampsia is a pregnancy-related multisystem disease process that usually occurs after the 32nd week of gestation. Systemic hypertension and significant proteinuria (0.3 g or greater in a 24-hour urine collection) are invariably present. Clinical onset is usually characterized by rapid weight gain associated with generalized edema, followed by onset of hypertension or proteinuria or both. The incidence of preeclampsia in the United States is 5% to 7%. The highest frequency occurs in young primigravidas, and the second highest incidence is in older multiparous women, a group that has a higher maternal mortality rate than the young primigravidas. The incidence is higher in patients with preexisting hypertension or renal vascular disease, and the symptoms may present earlier than the 32nd gestational week in these patients. Diastolic hypertension is most often seen in association with preeclampsia. It is less common to record SBP values greater than 160 mm Hg. If the SBP is greater than 200 mm Hg, the clinician should consider the possibility of underlying essential hypertension, which may be superimposed on the preeclamptic state. Because preeclampsia is a multisystem disease process, it may imitate or mask other pathologic conditions, and a thorough investigation to rule out other coexisting pathologies should be carried out.[9] Familial prevalence of preeclampsia has been reported.[10,11] In some cases, preeclampsia manifests 1 to 7 days after delivery.[12,13] Most commonly, if preeclampsia is present in the postpartum period, it manifests as the

HELLP syndrome, a severe variant of the preeclamptic spectrum of diseases.[14] This syndrome always includes some, if not all, of the following features: microangiopathic hemolytic anemia (H), elevated liver enzymes (EL), and low platelets (LP). The syndrome can develop without substantial BP changes or with no significant changes compared with BP readings taken during the pregnancy.

A significant elevation of the BP in the second trimester is associated with an increased risk of preeclampsia later in the pregnancy.[15] One-third of pregnant women with mean arterial pressures greater than 90 mm Hg in the second trimester develop preeclampsia later during pregnancy. Only 2% of women with mean arterial pressures less than 90 mm Hg develop preeclampsia. Relatively mild hypertension early in pregnancy, which might be ignored in nonpregnant patients, should not be overlooked or dismissed in the parturient. As many as 25% of all pregnant women have slightly elevated BPs in the last month of pregnancy, but the incidence of preeclampsia is also highest during this period. Accordingly, clinicians must remain vigilant when faced with new-onset hypertension and look for other signs and symptoms that might suggest the presence of the preeclamptic syndrome.

The exact pathogenesis of preeclampsia is still unknown, although it is believed to be related to endothelial cell injury and dysfunction that occurs in most maternal organs as a result of toxic substances released from a poorly perfused placenta. Genetic and immunologic factors also have been implicated in the pathogenesis of preeclampsia.[16,17] The generalized vasospasm that occurs in preeclampsia is responsible for many of the organ-specific signs and symptoms seen in this multisystem disease. Widespread vasospasm is associated with increased circulating levels of vasoconstrictors, increased sensitivity to angiotensin II, and decreased levels of vasodilators. An imbalance in circulating angiogenic factors is emerging as a prominent mechanism that mediates endothelial dysfunction and the clinical signs and symptoms of preeclampsia.[18] There is an imbalance in the ratio of prostacyclin to thromboxane production that contributes to the pathogenesis of preeclampsia, although preeclampsia is not simply a state of prostacyclin deficiency. This idea has prompted studies of low-dose aspirin to prevent development of preeclampsia. Duley et al. reviewed 59 trials involving 37,560 women that examined the use of antiplatelet agents in preeclampsia. Antiplatelet agents including low-dose aspirin showed moderate benefits when used for prevention of preeclampsia and its consequences, decreasing preterm births, fetal and neonatal deaths, and small-for-gestational age babies. However, they recommended that further information would be required to assess which women are most likely to benefit, when treatment is best started, and at what dose.[19] The maternal organs most affected in preeclampsia are the kidneys, brain, liver, and hematologic system. Despite a lack of understanding of the exact pathogenesis of preeclampsia, significant improvements in identification of the disease, monitoring, and management of these complex cases has improved perinatal and maternal morbidity and mortality. If vasospasm affects the uteroplacental bed, the incidence of intrauterine growth retardation, stillbirths, and neonatal deaths increases.[20]

Peripheral edema is a common symptom and complaint of pregnant women that cannot be ignored, because it may herald the onset of preeclampsia. The majority of women with preeclampsia present with generalized edema, and significant weight gain is the first symptom. However, since peripheral edema is a ubiquitous symptom during pregnancy, it is no longer considered a hallmark trait of preeclampsia. Preeclampsia is often manifested initially by peripheral edema that is usually accompanied by a gradual increase in BP. Sodium retention is partly responsible for edema formation and hypertension. In normal pregnancy, the glomerular filtration rate increases by as much as 50%. There is a concomitant increase in sodium reabsorption by the renal tubules and a 60% to 80% increase in renal blood flow. Renal blood flow increases because of the increase in cardiac output and a decrease in renal vascular resistance. In preeclampsia, sodium retention is caused by a decrease in the glomerular filtration rate, possibly resulting from vasospasm of the renal vasculature, commonly seen in preeclampsia. Renin and aldosterone secretion decrease in patients with preeclampsia, probably as a result of extracellular volume expansion and associated edema. The exact cause of the decreased activity of these factors is unknown, but it may be related to decreased renal prostaglandin synthesis, increased systemic BP, or expansion of extracellular volume. In spite of the decreased levels of renin and aldosterone, sensitivity to angiotensin II is increased, a factor that may play a role in the pathogenesis of hypertension in preeclampsia.[21] Vascular maladaptation with increased vasomotor tone, endothelial dysfunction, and increased sensitivity to angiotensin II and norepinephrine in preeclampsia may be explained on the basis of angiotensin II-mediated mechanisms. Although sodium retention occurs in preeclampsia, blood volume actually can be diminished compared with that in normotensive pregnant patients.[22] Plasma volume contracts as extracellular fluid is preferentially shifted from the vascular space to the interstitium. However, the decrease in plasma volume does not indicate volume depletion in patients with preeclampsia. In contrast to hypovolemic patients, cardiac output is increased and central venous and pulmonary capillary wedge pressures are normal to high in patients with preeclampsia.[23] These data guide the management of preeclampsia, because efforts should be directed to BP control rather than injudicious volume resuscitation.

Hyperuricemia in preeclampsia occurs at least in part because of decreased renal excretion of uric acid. However, the development of hyperuricemia frequently predates increases in serum blood urea nitrogen and creatinine, suggesting that other mechanisms are involved as well. Hyperuricemia has been used as a marker of severity of preeclampsia, and it is a risk factor for fetal mortality.[24]

Clinical Presentation of Preeclampsia

Severity of illness is defined as mild, moderate, or severe depending on the presenting signs and symptoms and associated comorbidities. Because of the multisystem nature of the process, preeclampsia may manifest with a wide spectrum of organ-specific abnormalities in addition to the general findings of edema, hypertension, and proteinuria. Because the pathologic abnormalities associated with preeclampsia are not necessarily secondary to hypertension, the severity of preeclampsia does not always correlate with the degree of BP elevation.[15] BP elevations are classified as mild, moderate, or severe. Hypertension in preeclampsia may result from increases in systemic vascular resistance and cardiac output.

In mild preeclampsia, SBP is 130 to 140 mm Hg and DBP is 80 to 95 mm Hg. Peripheral edema is minimal, and there are no associated visual or cerebral symptoms. In moderately severe preeclampsia, the SBP may increase to as high as 150 to 160 mm Hg, and the DBP can be as high as 110 mm Hg. An increase in SBP of 25 mm Hg or more and an increase in DBP of 15 mm Hg or more suggests the presence of moderate to severe preeclampsia. Peripheral edema, hyperreflexia, and visual symptoms are present with moderately severe preeclampsia. In severe forms of preeclampsia, the SBP is greater than 160 mm Hg, and the DBP is 110 mm Hg or greater. In severe preeclampsia, there are signs of multiple organ system involvement. Pulmonary, cardiac, renal, and neurologic disturbances may be present. Severe renal involvement in preeclampsia leads to glomeruloendotheliosis, which manifests as marked proteinuria (excretion of greater than 5 g protein daily). Oliguria (urine output less than 500 mL/day) is also common, and the serum creatinine concentration is usually greater than 1.6 mg/dL. Acute renal failure is relatively rare, although clinical evidence of renal involvement in preeclampsia significantly increases perinatal mortality.[25] Hepatic involvement is manifested by epigastric or right upper quadrant pain with elevated circulating levels of bilirubin and transaminases. Severe preeclampsia itself is the commonest cause of hepatic tenderness and liver dysfunction in pregnancy.[26] Severe hepatic pathology can result in subcapsular hematomas and lacerations that may require surgical intervention. Neurologic changes may include persistent headaches, visual disturbances, focal neurologic deficits, and severe hyperreflexia with or without clonus. Computed tomography of the brain may show cerebral edema, especially in the occipital region.

Severe preeclampsia associated with central nervous system irritability, manifesting as generalized tonic-clonic seizures not caused by other cerebral pathology, is defined as *eclampsia*.[27] Eclampsia can occur without significant hypertension or proteinuria. Cardiovascular and respiratory changes can manifest as pulmonary edema, resulting from iatrogenic fluid overload, acute systolic left ventricular failure, or diastolic left ventricular dysfunction secondary to chronic essential hypertension. Pulmonary edema may also result from increased capillary permeability or from a decrease in colloid osmotic pressure that occurs to some extent during normal pregnancy but can be accentuated by preeclampsia.[28] Hematologic disturbances consist of thrombocytopenia, disseminated intravascular coagulation, and hemolysis.

It is unknown whether preeclampsia leads to persistent chronic hypertension after delivery, although it seems that this is unlikely. Nevertheless, an episode of preeclampsia may identify a subgroup of women with increased risk for eventual development of essential hypertension at a later time. In a recent study, women with preeclampsia had an increased risk of cardiovascular disease death later in life, independent of other measured risk factors.[29] These findings reinforced previously reported recommendations that a history of preeclampsia should be used to target women at risk for cardiovascular disease. Debate continues as to whether the presence of preeclampsia or the duration of the disease process may be responsible for influencing factors that later lead to the development of essential hypertension. Women who develop preeclampsia superimposed on previously undiagnosed essential hypertension or underlying renal disease are predisposed to the later development of essential hypertension.

Other Causes of Hypertension in Pregnancy

Some of the less common causes of hypertension are listed in Box 159-1.

Primary aldosteronism in pregnant women has been reported but is uncommon. The treatment of hypertension in these patients is directed toward medical management during the pregnancy and postpartum operative intervention if an adenoma is present.

Renal artery stenosis can be associated with preeclampsia. Medical therapy with antihypertensive agents is recommended. Although ideal therapy for these patients would include angiotensin-converting enzyme (ACE) inhibitors, these agents are contraindicated during pregnancy, and other alternatives must be employed.[30]

Coarctation of the aorta is a rare cause of hypertension. It may be previously undiagnosed and then initially diagnosed during a patient's first pregnancy. It can be associated with preeclampsia. The greatest risk to these patients is aortic rupture due to cystic medial necrosis of the aortic wall. This risk is amplified because the normal physiologic changes of pregnancy place further stresses on the abnormal aorta. Increases in BP, cardiac output, and the strain of labor with contractions can increase this risk. Aggressive medical management with antihypertensive medications, including β-adrenergic blockers, improves outcome in these high-risk patients.

Pheochromocytoma is a rare cause of hypertension, but patients have a poor outcome if the tumor is not diagnosed and treated. These patients can present with nausea, vomiting, profuse diaphoresis, severe headache, generalized weakness, palpitations, and seizures. The immediate causes of sudden death are secondary to pulmonary edema, cerebral hemorrhage, and cardiovascular collapse. Because of the risk of significant morbidity and mortality to both mother and fetus, it was previously recommended that immediate surgical intervention be carried out during pregnancy. Currently, most experts advocate medical therapy with α- and β-adrenergic blockade during pregnancy and tumor removal after delivery.

General Treatment Principles

The benefits of a well-balanced low-salt diet and exercise have been shown to decrease the incidence and severity of hypertension. Bennett conducted a retrospective analysis of women who had prior bariatric surgery before becoming pregnant. These patients had lower rates of hypertensive disorders in subsequent pregnancies.[31] Previously, some experts were concerned that aggressive management of hypertension in pregnancy might be detrimental, perhaps because hypertension improved uterine blood flow. These concerns appear to be unfounded, because later studies showed that uterine blood flow either increases or shows no change after hypertension is controlled. Nevertheless, caution must be exercised to ensure that treatment of hypertension during pregnancy does not induce hypotension, which adversely affects maternal hemodynamics and compromises fetal well-being. There is significant correlation between maternal BP control and fetal morbidity, and evidence now suggests that antihypertensive treatment for severe hypertension results in improved perinatal outcome. The development of mild hypertension or preeclampsia at or near term is associated with minimal maternal and neonatal complications. However, the onset of severe gestational hypertension and/or severe preeclampsia early in gestation is associated with significant maternal and perinatal complications.[32] General recommendations for management and monitoring of hypertension in pregnant patients include stabilization and treatment of acute changes in BP. Specific goal-directed therapy is indicated for various organ system abnormalities that may be present, particularly in those patients with moderate to severe preeclampsia. If proteinuria is not present and there is no suspicion of preeclampsia, conservative management on an outpatient basis is usually adequate. Immediate hospitalization with bed rest is recommended for patients presenting with proteinuria if there is a high index of suspicion for the diagnosis of preeclampsia.

Antihypertensive Drug Therapy

There is now an extensive pharmaceutical armamentarium available for the treatment of hypertension in pregnancy. In 1979, the U.S. Food and Drug Administration (FDA) established categories for all drugs with potential and real adverse effects on the fetus.[33] Although helpful to the clinician, these categories most often do not reflect current scientific knowledge regarding specific teratogenic effects of the drugs.[34]

The FDA categories are listed in Table 159-1. Most antihypertensive drugs used during pregnancy are classified as category C. Thiazide diuretics, prazosin, and α-methyldopa are designated as category A; metoprolol is a category B agent. Because most antihypertensive drugs are used later in pregnancy, the potential teratogenic effects of these drugs are usually not of concern. However, if treatment is initiated for patients with preexisting essential hypertension or early onset gestational hypertension, teratogenic effects must be considered when choosing antihypertensive drugs. It may be necessary to change

TABLE 159-1	FDA Categories of Fetal Drug Toxicities
Category	**Description**
A	Controlled studies in pregnant women have not demonstrated any risk to the fetus in the first trimester. These drugs are considered to be relatively safe for use during pregnancy.
B	No known specific risks are associated with use of the drug in pregnancy, but controlled human studies are lacking. If adverse effects were shown in animal reproduction studies, these were not confirmed in controlled human trials.
C	Studies in women and animals are not available, or studies in animals have revealed adverse effects on the fetus. Most new drugs fall into this category. These drugs should be given only if the potential benefit justifies the potential risk to the fetus.
D	These drugs have shown a definite fetal risk in controlled human trials. However, their use may be necessary during pregnancy, and a risk-benefit assessment needs to be considered for the use of these agents.
X	These drugs have shown a definite risk to the fetus, and their use is contraindicated because the potential risks to the fetus outweigh the potential benefits.

FDA, U.S. Food and Drug Administration.

antihypertensive therapy early in pregnancy, if the patient is taking drugs that could increase the risks of fetal abnormalities.

The goal of hypertensive therapy in pregnancy is prevention of maternal complications such as intracerebral hemorrhage, stroke, and decompensated heart failure. There are no convincing data to determine the optimal BP goal with drug therapy. There is disagreement concerning the proper normal values for BP during pregnancy, but most agree that acute treatment is mandated (1) if the SBP is greater than 160 mm Hg or the DBP is 110 mm Hg or greater or (2) if the SBP is more than 30 mm Hg greater than the baseline value or the DBP is more than 15 mm Hg greater than baseline. If acute and urgent drug therapy management is required, some patients may need to be hospitalized, depending on their compliance with drug therapy and the urgency of lowering the BP based on concomitant organ system involvement. For patients presenting with SBP 140 mm Hg or higher and DBP 90 mm Hg or higher, urgent drug therapy should be implemented if there is concurrent evidence of symptoms, underlying essential hypertension, or end-organ involvement. If the patient presents after the 24th gestational week and fetal viability is ascertained, both cardiac and fetal telemetry may be required. For patients presenting with SBP less than 140 mm Hg and DBP less than 90 mm Hg and no evidence of significant proteinuria, management and treatment can be provided on an outpatient basis, with frequent office visits and close maternal and fetal assessments. If the hypertension is refractory to standard therapy, hypertension worsens despite adequate drug therapy, or the suspicion of preeclampsia arises, then immediate hospitalization is recommended.

Conservative drug therapy is advocated for moderately severe preeclampsia, but the treatment of choice for severe preeclampsia and associated end-organ involvement is immediate delivery of the fetus. Delay in delivery for patients with severe preeclampsia and end-organ involvement can result in serious maternal and fetal complications. If the fetus is of mature gestational age, factors influencing the decision to deliver are dependent on progression of the disease process, assessment of fetal lung maturity, and status of the cervix. Conservative management of preeclamptic patients at a gestational age less than 24 weeks is associated with serious maternal complications, and termination of the pregnancy should be considered. For patients at 28 to 32 weeks of gestation, conservative management with vigilant monitoring and assessment should be performed in a hospital setting. There is not enough evidence from the limited trials performed to recommend either early delivery or expectant care for women with severe preeclampsia before 34 weeks of pregnancy.[35]

During pregnancy, the clinician must decide when to use antihypertensive medications and what level of BP to target. The choice of antihypertensive agents is more limited in pregnancy, since not all available antihypertensive drugs have been adequately evaluated in pregnant women, and some agents are contraindicated.[36] A first-line drug still used today in the pregnant patient, although less commonly in the general populace, is oral α-methyldopa, a central α_2-adrenergic agonist. Historically this has been a first-line drug of choice for many obstetricians over the years, and there has been little evidence to convince them otherwise. The starting dose is 250 mg orally 2 to 3 times a day for the first 48 hours of treatment. Dosing can be increased every 2 days until the desired BP level is achieved. The maximum daily dose is 4 g. β-Adrenergic blocker therapy with oral labetalol, a combined α- and β-adrenergic antagonist, has become popular as a single-agent antihypertensive. The recommended initial dose is 100 mg orally twice daily. The dose can be increased as indicated, either semiweekly or weekly. The maintenance dose is usually 200 to 400 mg administered twice daily. The benefits of β-adrenergic blockade make this an attractive drug for parturients with underlying chronic essential hypertension and possible cardiac and vascular involvement. Diuretics also may be used, although care must be exercised to prevent excessive fluid losses, which can exacerbate the decrease in blood volume associated with preeclampsia. As mentioned previously, ACE inhibitors and angiotensin II receptor antagonists should be avoided intrapartum because these agents can increase perinatal morbidity and mortality.

For acute and emergent drug therapy for severe hypertension, intravenous (IV) antihypertensive drugs should be used; IV infusions are particularly attractive because they provide rapid control of BP and can be titrated easily. Intravenous hydralazine, a direct arteriolar vasodilator, remains the standard for many obstetricians, although other drugs may be preferable since hydralazine may decrease BP precipitously.[37] Excessive lowering of BP is a particular problem when hydralazine is administered to preeclamptic patients with contracted blood volume. If hydralazine is used, it should be given as 5- to 10-mg IV boluses every 15 to 30 minutes until BP is controlled. Onset of the hypotensive effect is 10 to 20 minutes, and duration of action is about 8 hours. Infusions of hydralazine are difficult to titrate and may be associated with increased incidence of fetal distress.

Intravenous labetalol, a nonselective β- and α-adrenergic receptor blocker, is also commonly used for the acute management of hypertension. Labetalol rapidly decreases BP but not at the expense of uteroplacental blood flow. Labetalol crosses the placenta but rarely causes significant neonatal bradycardia. An initial IV bolus of 10 or 20 mg should be given, followed by boluses of 40 to 80 mg at 10- to 15-minute intervals as needed to control hypertension. Labetalol also can be given by continuous IV infusion; the usual dose is 1 to 4 mg/min. Contraindications to the use of labetalol are the same as those for other β-adrenergic antagonists, notably heart block and acute asthma.

Sodium nitroprusside is a potent arterial and venous vasodilator that quickly decreases the BP. Rapid titration with a continuous IV infusion can be instituted starting at a dose of 0.25 to 0.5 µg/kg/min and adjusted every few minutes and titrated to effect. Invasive arterial monitoring is often recommended in conjunction with its use. As with all potent vasodilators, care must be taken when using sodium nitroprusside, because patients with volume depletion may be particularly sensitive to its effects. Despite a paucity of data, concern regarding the risks of fetal cyanide toxicity prompts some practitioners to avoid using this drug in pregnant patients. Careful attention to dosing and duration of use should minimize the risk of toxicity.

Other less frequently used agents include IV nitroglycerin, oral clonidine, and β-adrenergic blockers other than labetalol. Intravenous nitroglycerin is easily titrated and is especially attractive for the management of patients with pulmonary edema. However, its antihypertensive potency is somewhat limited. Oral clonidine, a centrally acting α₂-adrenergic agonist, is an effective antihypertensive drug, but concerns about the risk of rebound hypertension after cessation limit its use.

There remains considerable debate concerning the use of β-adrenergic blockers in pregnancy because of the potential risks of fetal bradycardia and a decrease in perfusion to the uteroplacental bed. Beta-blockers have been used during pregnancy without evidence of teratogenic effects. Although there is limited experience, they are considered as indicated in pregnant women with hypertension, mitral stenosis with pulmonary hypertension, coarctation of the aorta, ischemic heart disease, supraventricular and ventricular arrhythmias, and can be continued during delivery.[2,38,39] Esmolol has been used widely for heart rate control in pregnancy, but its efficacy is limited as an antihypertensive agent.

Antihypertensive drugs commonly used during pregnancy are listed in Table 159-2.

TABLE 159-2	Antihypertensive Drugs Commonly Used in Pregnancy	
Type	**Agents**
Oral	α-Methyldopa
	Labetalol
	Clonidine
	Diuretics
Parenteral	Labetalol
	Hydralazine
	Sodium nitroprusside
	Nitroglycerin

Management of Hypertension During Labor and Delivery

Management of hypertension during labor and delivery is directed toward avoiding acute and maternal complications. Antihypertensive drug therapy with judicious use of IV fluids is of paramount importance to avoid unnecessary complications. Postpartum monitoring is advocated for high-risk, chronically hypertensive patients. Hypertension associated with preeclampsia usually resolves spontaneously within a few weeks after delivery. These patients are at risk for development of acute complications such as hypertensive encephalopathy, pulmonary edema, and acute renal failure. The choice of antihypertensive medications or the doses used may have to be adjusted after delivery. Minute amounts of all antihypertensive agents are found in breast milk. Although limited data are available, adverse perinatal effects have not been observed with the more commonly used drugs such as α-methyldopa, hydralazine, and the various α-adrenergic blockers.

KEY POINTS

1. Hypertensive disorders associated with pregnancy are not uncommon and can either predate the pregnancy or be precipitated or unmasked by the pregnancy.

2. Women with a prenatal history of diabetes mellitus, renal disease, vascular disease, or a family history of hypertension are predisposed to developing hypertension during pregnancy.

3. Treatment is recommended if the systolic blood pressures (SBPs) are 160 mm Hg or higher, or the diastolic blood pressures (DBPs) are 110 mm Hg or higher, or with lower BPs if the patient is symptomatic.

4. BP measurements should be consistently taken in either the sitting position or in the inferior arm in the lateral recumbent position with each evaluation.

5. Cardiac output and blood volume are dramatically increased during pregnancy, and there is a decrease in systemic vascular resistance, particularly during the second trimester. DBP is lowest during the second trimester.

6. Elevated BPs caused by essential hypertension may transiently improve during the second trimester of pregnancy.

7. Consistently elevated SBPs greater than 200 mm Hg should prompt the practitioner to consider undiagnosed chronic hypertension or some of the less common causes of hypertension such as primary aldosteronism, renal artery stenosis, or pheochromocytoma.

8. Preeclampsia most often appears after the 32nd week of gestation and resolves with delivery of the fetus.

9. Preeclampsia can be superimposed on chronic hypertension.

10. Preeclampsia may initially present after delivery as the HELLP syndrome (hemolysis, elevated liver enzymes, and low platelets).

11. Hypertension with BP elevation of 140/90 mm Hg or higher and proteinuria are the principal characteristics of preeclampsia. Edema is no longer a criterion for preeclampsia.

12. Preeclampsia is a multisystem disease. Severe preeclampsia manifests with signs and symptoms of end-organ involvement.

13. The antihypertensive drugs most frequently used in pregnancy have not been associated with significant fetal abnormalities.

14. First-line antihypertensive drugs for moderate hypertension are oral α-methyldopa and oral labetalol.

15. Parenteral antihypertensive agents are used for more severe elevations of BP. The agents most commonly employed are labetalol, hydralazine, and sodium nitroprusside.

16. Caution should be exercised with the administration of hydralazine, particularly in patients with decreased plasma volume.

17. Most forms of gestational hypertension resolve in the postpartum period.

ANNOTATED REFERENCES

Magee L, Cham C, Waterman EJ, et al. Hydralazine for treatment of severe hypertension in pregnancy: meta-analysis. BMJ 2003;327:955.

A meta-analysis was performed to review outcomes in randomized controlled trials published between 1966 and 2002 that compared hydralazine with other antihypertensive agents for severe hypertension in pregnancy. In 13 trials comparing hydralazine with either nifedipine or labetalol, hydralazine was an effective antihypertensive drug for severe hypertension but was associated with an increased incidence of maternal hypotension, cesarean section, placental abruption, oliguria, adverse effects on fetal heart rate, and lower Apgar scores.

Sibai B, Dekker G, Kupferminc M. Pre-eclampsia. Lancet 2005;359:785.

This is a comprehensive review of preeclampsia with information on epidemiology, pathogenesis, and different treatment modalities. Maternal and perinatal outcomes are also discussed. The authors reviewed findings on the diagnosis and risk factors of preeclampsia and the present status of its prediction, prevention, and management.

AACE Hypertension Task Force. American Association of Clinical Endocrinologists medical guidelines for clinical practice for the diagnosis and treatment of hypertension. Endocr Pract 2006;12:193.

In 2006, the American Association of Clinical Endocrinologists (AACE) proposed guidelines for the diagnosis and treatment of hypertension, focusing on identifying and managing hypertension relating to or coinciding with endocrinopathies. These guidelines are based on positive data from randomized clinical trials. They recommended diuretics, beta-blockers, angiotensin-converting enzyme inhibitors (ACEIs), angiotensin receptor blockers (ARBs), and calcium channel blockers (CCBs) for treating hypertension in patients, particularly those with diabetes mellitus.

Magee LA, Helewa M, Moutquin J-M, et al. Diagnosis, evaluation, and management of the hypertensive disorders of pregnancy. J Obstet Gynaecol Can 2008;30:S1.

These guidelines from the Society of Obstetricians and Gynecologists are a comprehensive review of the different manifestations of hypertension during pregnancy. The guidelines focus on classification, pathophysiologic features, and management of the hypertensive disorders of pregnancy. The authors classified hypertension of pregnancy into two categories, preexisting or gestational with preeclampsia superimposed on either gestational or preexisting chronic hypertension. Through a combination of evidence-based medicine and consensus, this report updates contemporary approaches to hypertension control during pregnancy.

Seely EW, Maxwell C. Chronic hypertension in pregnancy. Circulation 2007;115:e188-e190.

This review describes chronic hypertension during pregnancy. It further describes the complications of chronic hypertension during pregnancy and how chronic hypertension affects both maternal and fetal outcomes.

REFERENCES

Access the complete reference list online at http://www.expertconsult.com.

160

Acute Pulmonary Complications in Pregnancy

CORNELIA R. GRAVES

During pregnancy, the respiratory system undergoes a number of changes and is subject to functional and anatomic stresses. The critical care provider must remember these changes to appropriately care for the maternal-fetal unit. Although the need for ventilatory support is rare in pregnancy, respiratory insufficiency is still the most common indication in pregnancy for admission to a critical care unit. In this chapter, the unique physiologic changes that occur during pregnancy are addressed, and guidance is provided to the critical care specialist who may encounter pregnancies that are complicated by acute pulmonary complications.

Pulmonary Physiology in Pregnancy

A number of physiologic changes affect respiration during pregnancy. Normal pregnancy is associated with a 20% increase in oxygen consumption and a 15% increase in metabolic rate. During the first trimester, minute ventilation is increased while respiratory rate remains the same. Although one might assume that lung volume during pregnancy would decrease owing to the rise in the maternal diaphragm, tidal volume (V_T) is actually increased by 40% over baseline values. The increase in V_T is thought to be due to the increase in circulating progesterone that affects the respiratory center.[1] Arterial blood gas measurements reflect a respiratory alkalosis that is compensated by a metabolic acidosis that results in a relatively normal pH. $Paco_2$ usually ranges from 28 to 32 mm Hg. Functional residual capacity (FRC), residual volume, and total lung volume are decreased near term. Because of this decrease, respiratory distress occurs more rapidly in the gravid than in the nongravid state. The function of the large airways as measured by forced expiratory volume at 1 second (FEV_1), and peak expiratory flow rate (PEFR) is essentially unchanged throughout pregnancy.[2]

Colloid osmotic pressure is decreased by 20%. This change in hydrostatic pressure results in a propensity for the pregnant patient to develop cardiogenic and noncardiogenic pulmonary edema.

Dyspnea on exertion is common, especially in the third trimester of pregnancy, making diagnosis of respiratory problems more difficult than in the nongravid state.

Figure 160-1 illustrates the graphic relationship of pulmonary changes.

Asthma

EPIDEMIOLOGY

Asthma is one of the most common pulmonary problems in pregnant women; recent studies report that approximately 8% are affected.[3] The disease is characterized by hyperactive airways leading to episodic bronchoconstriction. The role of inflammatory mediators in the pathogenesis of asthma has become apparent in recent years, leading to earlier use of inflammatory medications in the treatment of exacerbations.

The cause of asthma is unknown; however, it has been observed that its prevalence in the general population is increasing.

EFFECTS OF ASTHMA ON PREGNANCY

Asthma may be triggered by environmental allergens, medications, especially aspirin or nonsteroidal antiinflammatory drugs (NSAIDs), or stress.[4] Most exacerbations are marked by cough, wheezing, and dyspnea. Rapid therapeutic intervention at the time of an exacerbation is imperative to prevent impaired maternal and fetal oxygenation, because uncontrolled asthma can increase maternal morbidity. In several studies, even after controlling for confounding variables, adverse pregnancy outcomes are more pronounced in patients with asthma. These include low birth weight, preeclampsia, preterm birth, and stillbirth.[5,6]

Whereas historical data have shown an increase in perinatal death and low birth weight,[7] Fitzsimmons and colleagues observed low birth weight in only those patients treated for status asthmaticus.[8] In addition, Schatz and colleagues noted that intrauterine growth restriction was directly related to lung function as measured by FEV_1.[9]

EFFECT OF PREGNANCY ON ASTHMA

Numerous studies have observed that the course of asthma may be affected by pregnancy. Gluck et al. found that on average, asthma improved in 36% of women during pregnancy, remained unchanged in 41%, and worsened in 23%.[10] Schatz et al., in an analysis of 366 pregnancies in which patient status was followed by objective criteria, found that asthma improved in 28%, remained unchanged in 33%, and worsened in 35%. Fifty-nine percent of the patients had similar asthma control in successive pregnancies.[11]

Fetal sex may influence asthma in pregnancy. In one study, mothers who gave birth to boys were more likely to report improved asthma symptoms.[12] Dodds and colleagues also found that the use of medications to treat asthma was less common in mothers of boys.[13] While a number of hypotheses have been proposed, including alterations in progesterone and the role of leukotrienes, changes in not one of these mediators can explain the varied course of the pregnant asthmatic.[14]

MANAGEMENT

The National Asthma Education and Prevention Program (NAEP) issued specific guidelines regarding asthma treatment. In 1993, the Working Group on Asthma and Pregnancy established criteria for diagnosis and treatment in the gravid population (Figure 160-2).[15]

The goals of treatment during pregnancy are to control exacerbation and prevent status asthmaticus, thereby reducing maternal and fetal hypoxemia. The initial step in treatment involves monitoring pulmonary function, and FEV_1 is the single best measure. Physical examination and chest radiography are poor measures of disease severity. A portable hand-held peak flowmeter gives a quick, accurate assessment by measuring the PEFR. Most authorities believe that airways remain essentially unchanged throughout pregnancy; therefore, every patient with asthma should be given a peak flowmeter and be educated in its use. The patient should obtain a baseline PEFR during a quiescent period. The severity of disease is determined by the occurrences of

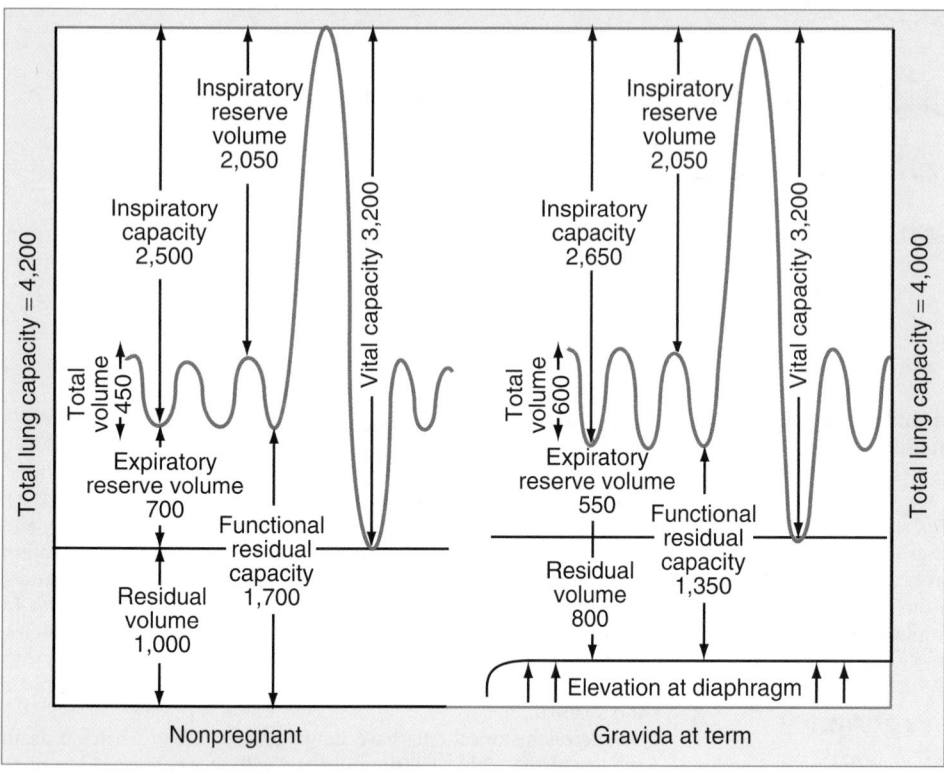

Figure 160-1 Respiratory changes in pregnancy.

exacerbations and the changes in FEV$_1$ and PEFR. The PEFR can be used as a guide to refer the patient for emergency care.

Pharmacologic therapy is the mainstay of asthma treatment. Most drugs used in the treatment of asthma are thought to be safe in pregnancy. Inhaled β-agonists are the most frequently used in asthma treatment. A prospective study of inhaled β-agonists in 259 pregnancies showed no change in the rate of congenital malformation, perinatal mortality, low birth weight, or complications of pregnancy.[16] There is

little role for the use of oral β-agonists, which may have more adverse systemic symptoms and are no more effective than inhaled drugs.

Inhaled corticosteroid therapy remains the mainstay of antiinflammatory treatment of asthma. Corticosteroids have also been advocated as first-line therapy in patients with mild asthma.[17] Studies have demonstrated that with asthma, those taking an inhaled corticosteroid were four times less likely than their nontreated counterparts to suffer an exacerbation.[18] Another randomized study noted that there was a 55% reduction in readmission rates for acute asthma in patients using inhaled beclomethasone.[19] Inhaled corticosteroids can increase the effectiveness of β-adrenergic agents by inducing the formation of new β receptors. Because beclomethasone is the most studied of the inhaled corticosteroids in pregnancy, it is recommended as first-line therapy.[15] However, if patients are well controlled on other corticosteroid preparations, it is suggested they be continued on their current medication, because all inhaled corticosteroids are labeled by the U.S. Food and Drug Administration (FDA) as pregnancy class C. Other antiinflammatory medications used in the treatment of asthma (e.g., cromolyn sodium and nedocromil sodium) appear to be less effective than inhaled corticosteroids in reducing asthma symptoms.

Systemic corticosteroids should be reserved for the periodic treatment of acute asthma exacerbations. Chronic oral corticosteroid therapy may increase the risks of gestational diabetes mellitus, preterm labor, low-birthweight infants, and preeclampsia; however, it is evident that the benefits of controlled severe asthma outweigh the potential risks to the mother and fetus.

Intravenous corticosteroids have no increased benefits over oral corticosteroids in the treatment of acute exacerbations.[20] Methylprednisolone, hydrocortisone, and prednisone are safe for use in pregnancy, unlike betamethasone or dexamethasone, because very little active drug crosses the placenta.

Leukotriene pathway moderators have been shown to improve pulmonary function, as measured by FEV$_1$.[21] Zafirlukast and montelukast are rated FDA category B; however, there is little experience with these drugs in pregnancy, and their role is undetermined.

The treatment of asthma requires patient education to provide optimization in the preconceptional period and during the pregnancy to

---

Offer all pregnant and postpartum women (at least 2 weeks after delivery) the influenza vaccine

H1N1 and standard vaccine---nasal mist is contraindicated

↓

Chemoprophylaxis should be offered to women who have a history of close contact

| Oseltamivir (Tamiflu) 75-mg capsule once per day for 10 days | Zanamivir (Relenza) Two 5-mg inhalations (10 mg total) once per day for 10 days |

↓

Early treatment for women with symptoms

| Oseltamivir (Tamiflu) 75-mg capsule twice daily for 5 days | Zanamivir (Relenza) Two 5-mg inhalations (10 mg total) twice per day for 5 days |

↓

Admission with observation for patients with severe illness

Figure 160-2 Treatment during pregnancy.

TREATMENT OF ASTHMA IN PREGNANCY

Mild Asthma
Characterized by FEV_1 or PEFR ≥80%
Brief (<1 hour) exacerbations
Treatment: inhaled β_2-agonist

Moderate Asthma
Characterized by FEV_1 or PEFR range from 60% to 80%
Exacerbations more than twice per week; exacerbations may last
   for several days, and occasional emergency care needed
Treatment: inhaled corticosteroids and inhaled β_2-agonist

Severe Asthma
Characterized by FEV_1 or PEFR <60% of baseline
Continuous symptoms, limited activity, frequent exacerbations
   and nocturnal symptoms, occasional hospitalization and
   emergency treatment needed
Treatment: inhaled corticosteroids, inhaled β_2-agonist, sustained-
   release theophylline; oral corticosteroid taper for active
   symptoms

provide optimum outcome. Box 160-1 offers a suggested schematic for the treatment of asthma in pregnancy.

STATUS ASTHMATICUS

Status asthmaticus is a rare complication in pregnancy. Diagnosis is established by a Pao_2 of less than 70 mm Hg, a $Paco_2$ of greater than or equal to 35 mm Hg, or a measured expiratory flow of less than 25% of expected. Because of impending respiratory failure, these patients should be managed in a critical care unit. Aggressive treatment of status asthmaticus is mandatory to protect the mother and fetus. Maternal mortality may be as high as 7% and fetal mortality as high as 11% despite adequate treatment. Epinephrine is not contraindicated in pregnancy during a respiratory emergency. Criteria for intubation in the gravida with status asthmaticus include (1) inability to maintain Pao_2 of greater than 60 mm Hg despite supplemental oxygen; (2) inability to maintain a Pco_2 of less than 40 mm Hg; (3) evidence of maternal exhaustion, with worsening acidosis (pH < 7.2) despite intensive bronchodilator therapy; and (4) altered maternal consciousness.[15]

When traditional treatment proves to be ineffective, a number of therapies have been reported beneficial. The use of a helium-oxygen mixture that has been reported to be effective in nonpregnant studies has been used safely in pregnancy.[22]

Pulmonary Edema

Pulmonary edema can be divided into two categories during pregnancy. *Cardiogenic pulmonary edema* is the result of high intravascular pressures creating a hydrostatic pressure gradient that results in extravasation of fluid into lung tissues despite the integrity of the normal lung microcirculation. *Noncardiogenic pulmonary edema* is the result of a leaky pulmonary capillary bed despite normal intravascular pressures. During pregnancy, the distinction between these two types of edema may be blurred owing to disease states that exacerbate the hypo-oncotic state of pregnancy.

ETIOLOGY

There are a number of causes of pulmonary edema in pregnancy. Some are pathologic in their process, others are due to idiopathic causes. One of the most common associations with pulmonary edema during pregnancy is hypertensive disease. In patients with hypertensive disease, pulmonary edema may be cardiogenic due to fluid overload or left ventricular dysfunction, or noncardiogenic due to decreased oncotic pressure.

Another common cause of pulmonary edema in pregnancy is tocolytic therapy. Most cases described have resulted from the intravenous use of beta sympathomimetics. The use of magnesium sulfate therapy as well as the use of corticosteroids in association with tocolysis for preterm labor has been shown to exacerbate the condition. The incidence of edema is increased in multiple gestations and in patients with subclinical infection.

Other causes of acute pulmonary edema in pregnancy include amniotic fluid embolism, aspiration, and the need for massive transfusion after hemorrhage.[23]

TREATMENT

The treatment of pulmonary edema during pregnancy depends on its etiology. Determination of the cause is best obtained by the use of pulmonary artery catheterization and measurement of pulmonary capillary wedge pressure. Although all patients may not require this intervention, it is recommended in patients in whom the clinical picture may be unclear (e.g., those with hypertensive disease) and in those who do not respond to standard diuretic therapy.

For patients who do not improve rapidly with diuretic therapy, intubation and ventilation with positive pressure is recommended. In addition to the use of diuretic therapy, reduction of preload and afterload may be achieved by the use of vasodilators such as nitrates, hydralazine, or calcium channel blockers. All are safe for use in pregnancy.

Box 160-2 offers a guide for treatment of patients with pulmonary edema.

Acute Respiratory Distress Syndrome

ETIOLOGY

The causes of acute respiratory distress syndrome (ARDS)[24-27] in pregnancy include preeclampsia, sepsis, aspiration, pyelonephritis, intrauterine infections, acute fatty liver of pregnancy, and amniotic fluid embolism.[28] In a review of 83 cases of ARDS associated with pregnancy, it was noted that among the causes of ARDS, 35 cases were attributed to uniquely obstetric conditions.[29] In addition, it was noted that varicella pneumonia and pyelonephritis were associated with ARDS. These conditions rarely trigger ARDS in immunocompetent adults. De Vaciana et al. pointed out that development of lung injury in pregnancy correlates with known physiologic changes including increased blood volume, decreased colloid osmotic pressure, and an unchanged critical lung closing volume despite a diminished FRC.[30]

MANAGEMENT

Management of ARDS includes diagnosis, maternal stabilization, fetal monitoring, investigation and treatment of underlying causes, and in many cases, evaluation for delivery.[29]

Maternal stabilization includes intubation for mechanical ventilation if necessary. The clinician should consider intubation sooner

TREATMENT IN PATIENTS WITH PULMONARY EDEMA

1. Determine the etiology, stop fluids, tocolysis, etc.
2. Treat with a diuretic (the author prefers furosemide in increments of 10-20 mg IV push).
3. Consider the use of morphine sulfate for patient comfort, 1-2 mg IV push q 2-3 h.
4. Proceed with hemodynamic monitoring if the patient does not rapidly respond to the above measures.
5. Consider intubation and mechanical ventilation with positive pressure for those patients with noncardiogenic pulmonary edema and those patients with cardiogenic pulmonary edema who need further support.

rather than later in the presence of respiratory deterioration, keeping in mind that decreased FRC exacerbates respiratory distress.

Contemporary thinking regarding the treatment of ARDS has found that a lung-protective ventilator strategy is the first therapy that has been found to improve outcomes in ARDS. It has been noted in numerous studies that decreasing the V_T from the standard of 12 mL/kg to 6 mL/kg or less and peak inspiratory pressures to less than 30 cm H_2O from 50 cm H_2O have resulted in decreased morbidity and mortality in patients with ARDS.[31] There has been much discussion in the literature concerning permissive hypercapnia and its use in preventing lung injury. However, there have been no controlled studies in pregnancy, and it is the opinion of the author that increasing $Paco_2$ in the pregnant patient should be undertaken with caution.

Judicious use of fluids is important in the management of ARDS. Although some authors have advocated the use of fluid restriction, the clinician must consider the volume-dependent status of pregnancy. It is recommended that fluid management be carefully guided by the use of hemodynamic monitoring.

Whereas oxygenation is important, it should be noted that oxygen should be used at the lowest concentration possible because it is toxic to lung tissue in high doses. The goal of therapy is to keep the $Sao_2 \geq 95\%$.

A number of other methods have been discussed in the treatment of ARDS, including inhaled nitric oxide, prostacyclin, surfactant, and inverse ratio ventilation. Currently these modalities cannot be recommended, because they have not been shown to decrease morbidity and mortality. Other trials considering prone ventilation and corticosteroids in late ARDS appear promising but have not been proven in large prospective randomized trials.[32-34]

Fetal surveillance during ARDS may be more difficult because drugs used to sedate the mother can affect fetal heart rate and variability. Sedatives, anxiolytics, hypnotics, and nondepolarizing agents are not contraindicated in pregnancy. In addition, preterm contractions and labor may present a problem due to maternal hypoxemia. The clinician is cautioned against starting tocolytic therapy before achieving adequate maternal oxygenation. If tocolysis in needed, β-agonists such as terbutaline should be avoided because of the risk of increased pulmonary capillary permeability and increased demands on cardiac load. Magnesium sulfate is not strictly contraindicated but also may increase pulmonary capillary permeability. The use of NSAIDs may be the best choice for tocolysis because they have been proven to improve ARDS in animal models.[29] Consultation with a maternal-fetal specialist is recommended to assist the intensivist in caring for these complex patients.

The timing of delivery of the patient with ARDS is a question that must be addressed by the clinician. Some authors advocate delivery after maternal stabilization, citing the possible "therapeutic effect" of delivery. Whitty and colleagues failed to demonstrate any significant benefit to delivery.[33] It is this author's opinion that delivery should be considered on a case-by-case basis, carefully weighing the risk/benefit ratio to the mother and fetus.

Box 160-3 represents a reasonable management scheme for the patient with ARDS.

Embolism

Because of the hypercoagulable changes in the coagulation cascade associated with pregnancy, there is an increased risk of venous thromboembolism. It has been estimated that clinically symptomatic pregnancy-related venous thromboembolism occurs in 1 to 2 per 1000 pregnancies. Maternal age (>40 years) and ethnic and genetic factors may increase this risk. Postpartum thromboembolism is three to five times more common than antepartum thrombotic events. Cesarean section confers a risk of 3 to 16 times that of a vaginal delivery.

Clinical signs of a pulmonary embolism include unexplained tachycardia, dyspnea, diaphoresis, and a nonproductive cough. The workup for a suspected pulmonary embolism should include normal laboratory studies (arterial blood gases) and an electrocardiogram in conjunction with radiographic testing.[35] Pregnancy should not prevent

---

Box 160-3

MANAGEMENT OF THE PATIENT WITH ARDS

1. Evaluate the patient in respiratory distress; calculate Pao_2/Fio_2 ratio; consider intubation if ≤200 mm Hg. The PEEP or CPAP mask is not recommended in pregnancy, owing to the high risk of aspiration.
2. Set tidal volume at 8 to 9 mL/kg to prevent increased peak pressures. Given recent evidence, aim to keep peak pressures less than 40 cm H_2O.
3. Use PEEP starting at 5 to 8 cm H_2O to assist in recruiting alveoli.
4. Aim to keep Fio_2 less than 60%; keep Sao_2 greater than or equal to 95%.
5. Use a pulmonary artery catheter to assist in fluid management and to guide hemodynamic parameters.
6. Consider the use of tocolysis only after the patient has been adequately hydrated and oxygenated.
7. Consider delivery if indicated for obstetric conditions or if continuing the pregnancy has no clear benefit.

ARDS, acute respiratory distress syndrome; CPAP, continuous positive airway pressure; PEEP, positive end-expiratory pressure.

---

obtaining appropriate radiographic studies. In patients with a high clinical index of suspicion for thromboembolic phenomena, definitive diagnosis is imperative (Box 160-4). Ventilation-perfusion scans are recommended as the first diagnostic test. Spiral computed tomography has replaced ventilation-perfusion scanning in many centers as an initial test. Pulmonary angiography is still the gold standard for offering definitive diagnosis. All of the aforementioned tests use less than the 5 rads of radiation exposure that has been associated with fetal teratogenesis. The use of an abdominal shield further decreases fetal exposure.

D-dimer may not be useful for the diagnosis of thromboembolism during pregnancy because it may be elevated in the absence of a thrombus. Heparin is the anticoagulant of choice in the antepartum patient. Unfractionated or low-molecular-weight heparin can be used. Neither of these drugs cross the placenta, owing to the size of the drug molecule. Patients on low-molecular-weight heparin should be monitored with factor Xa levels to ensure a therapeutic level.

Warfarin may be used in the second and third trimesters in patients in whom heparin therapy may be contraindicated. It is the anticoagulant of choice in the postpartum period and is compatible with breastfeeding.

The goals of therapy during the antepartum and postpartum period (6-8 weeks post delivery) should be an activated partial thromboplastin time (APTT) of 2.0 to 2.5, a factor Xa level of 0.6 to 1.1, or an International Normalized Ratio (INR) of 2.5 to 3.0.

Amniotic fluid embolism is a rare phenomenon that may initially present as severe respiratory distress. Risk factors include rapid labor, multiple gestation, polyhydramnios, and uterine rupture. Patients with amniotic fluid embolism usually have symptoms of acute respiratory

---

Box 160-4

TREATMENT OF PULMONARY EMBOLISM IN PREGNANCY

1. Begin therapy immediately based on strong clinical suspicion while awaiting complete diagnostic workup.
2. Establish the diagnosis with appropriate diagnostic imaging test.
3. Maintain maternal and fetal oxygenation.
4. Administer intravenous heparin and maintain full anticoagulation for 7 to 10 days prior to changing to subcutaneous injections (antepartum) or warfarin (postpartum). Oral anticoagulation should be continued 6 to 8 weeks after delivery.
5. Keep International Normalized Ratio, activated partial thromboplastin time, or factor Xa level in therapeutic range.

distress, cardiovascular collapse, and profound disseminated intravascular coagulation. Treatment is supportive; however, maternal mortality may be as high as 80%.

Pneumonia

Concern over the H1N1 virus has reinforced the seriousness of influenza infection in pregnant patients. Historical data show that during an influenza pandemic, mortality rates among pregnant women are unusually high. Neuzil et al. noted that even during a normal season, compared to their postpartum counterparts, pregnant women were more likely to be hospitalized.[36] The risk of hospitalization was highest in the third trimester, with women nearly 5 times more likely to be hospitalized than the postpartum control group. Influenza-related morbidity occurs in 10.5 of 10,000 pregnant women, compared to a rate of 1.91 of 10,000 in nonpregnant controls. Influenza pneumonia mortality in pregnancy has been noted to range from 12.5% to 42.1%.[38]

Contemporary management of influenza infection in pregnancy includes the use of antiviral medications for preventing and treating the disease. Amantadine and rimantadine have been shown to be effective in shortening the course and duration of disease in influenza A and influenza B. Recently, oseltamivir (Tamiflu) and Zanamivir (Relenza) has been recommended for prevention of influenza infection. Current Centers for Disease Control and Prevention (CDC) guidelines recommend that treatment be initiated for pregnant women (including patients until 2 weeks postpartum) with documented exposure to influenza virus and those patients who present with symptoms in the first 48 hours of illness, regardless of gestational age. Medication should be started at the first sign of symptoms; awaiting confirmation of the diagnosis and delaying therapy could result in rapid progression of disease. In the 2009 flu season, 6% of deaths were in pregnant women, even though only 1% of the population is pregnant at any given time. Data suggest that the use of antiviral medications can significantly reduce perinatal morbidity and mortality. Since 1995, the CDC has recommended that all pregnant women receive influenza immunizations. There has been some discussion regarding the use of thimerosal, which is used in the standard influenza vaccine; most authorities feel that the thimerosal-free vaccine when available is preferable. It is the opinion of the author that all pregnant patients who present with respiratory symptoms after exposure to viral illness should be hospitalized for observation.[37-39] Changes in maternal respiratory physiology during pregnancy can make progression from mild respiratory distress to respiratory distress rapid and unpredictable[36] (see Figure 160-1).

Conclusion

Because of the rare need for mechanical ventilation, there are no randomized controlled trials to determine the treatment modalities that are most effective in pregnancy. A retrospective study noted a maternal mortality rate of 14% and a fetal mortality of 11% in patients who required mechanical ventilation during pregnancy. The critical care specialist, perinatologist, anesthesiologist, and other members of the healthcare team should work closely to provide coordinated care. Understanding of the physiologic changes during pregnancy combined with aggressive treatment of early pathologic changes will assist in providing improved management in gravid patients with potentially lethal pulmonary complications.

KEY POINTS

Pregnancy

1. Tidal volume (V_T) is increased during pregnancy; however, functional residual capacity (FRC) is decreased.

2. A normal arterial blood gas determination in pregnancy reflects a compensated respiratory alkalosis.

3. Respiratory distress occurs more rapidly in the gravid patient, owing to changes in pulmonary physiology.

Asthma in Pregnancy

1. The treatment of asthma in pregnancy does not differ significantly from treatment in the nongravid state.

2. Because FEV_1 does not change during pregnancy, a peak flowmeter is a useful tool in monitoring patients with asthma.

3. A $PaCO_2$ of greater than 35 mm Hg in the setting of severe asthma represents respiratory distress in the gravid patient.

Acute Respiratory Distress Syndrome in Pregnancy

1. Caution should be used when considering treatment for preterm labor in patients requiring respiratory support. Correction of oxygenation is usually more effective than pharmacologic therapy.

2. The need for mechanical ventilatory support does not mandate delivery of the fetus. Most studies do not report significant maternal improvement after delivery.

3. Sedatives, hypnotic drugs, anxiolytic agents, and nondepolarizing neuromuscular blockade agents are not contraindicated in pregnancy.

Embolism in Pregnancy

1. Pregnancy is a hypercoagulable state that increases the risk of thromboembolic phenomena.

2. Radiographic studies should not be avoided in the gravid patient with respiratory compromise.

3. Anticoagulation therapy is not contraindicated in pregnancy; however, warfarin is contraindicated for use in the first trimester.

4. Amniotic fluid embolism occurs in about 1 in 80,000 pregnancies. It is associated with significant maternal morbidity and mortality.

Pneumonia in Pregnancy

1. Pneumonia during pregnancy is the third most common cause of indirect obstetrical death.

2. Misdiagnosis may occur in up to 20% of pregnant patients.

3. Care should be taken to carefully evaluate pregnant patients with influenza for acute respiratory symptoms.

4. Prompt pharmacologic treatment for influenza is safe during pregnancy and is recommended by the CDC.

ANNOTATED REFERENCES

Cole DE, Taylor TL, McCullough DM, Shoff CT, Derdak S. Acute respiratory distress syndrome in pregnancy. Crit Care Med 2005;33:S269-78.
This is one of only a few reviews in the obstetrical literature evaluating ARDS and its effect on pregnancy.
Jenkins TM, Troiano NH, Graves CR, et al. Mechanical ventilation in an obstetric population: characteristics and delivery rates. Am J Obstet Gynecol 2003;188:549-52.
One of only a few studies that evaluate characteristics of patients who receive mechanical ventilation during pregnancy, this retrospective review evaluates 51 women admitted during pregnancy for mechanical ventilation. Fetal and maternal morbidity and mortality are discussed.
Schatz M, Dombrowski MP. Asthma in pregnancy. N Engl J Med 2009;360:182-9.
An excellent review article that evaluates asthma, pregnancy, and considerations for treatment.

Tomlinson MW, Caruthers TJ, Whitty JE, Gonik B. Does delivery improve maternal condition in the respiratory-compromised gravida? Obstet Gynecol 1998;91:108-11.
A retrospective review is presented of 10 pregnant patients requiring mechanical ventilation. Outcome variables are reviewed, including respiratory improvement after delivery. This is the only study to look at maternal improvement as a primary outcome.
Robertson L, Greer I. Thromboembolism in pregnancy. Curr Opin Obstet Gynecol 2005;17:113-6.
Provides a current summary regarding the treatment of venous thromboembolism during pregnancy.
Graves CR. Pneumonia in pregnancy. Clin Obstet Gynecol 2010;53:329-36.
Recent review of pneumonia in pregnancy, including guidelines for treatment of influenza during pregnancy.

REFERENCES

Access the complete reference list online at http://www.expertconsult.com.

161

Postpartum Hemorrhage

MARIE R. BALDISSERI

Definition

The commonly accepted definition of *postpartum hemorrhage* (PPH) is excessive and life-threatening bleeding after 20 weeks of gestation, which occurs at the time of delivery of the fetus or placenta. Primary PPH is excessive blood loss within 24 hours of delivery. Secondary PPH is any abnormal or excessive bleeding that occurs between 24 hours and 12 weeks after delivery. Most commonly, bleeding occurs in the third stage of labor, which refers to the time between delivery of the fetus and delivery of the placenta after its separation and expulsion from the uterus. Defining excessive bleeding is somewhat problematic because it can be difficult to determine the exact amount of blood loss, and clinicians tend to underestimate blood loss. With a normal vaginal delivery, blood loss is typically 500 mL or less; after a normal cesarean section, it is usually 800 to 1000 mL. Blood loss greater than these amounts has been used to define PPH. However, uncomplicated vaginal and cesarean deliveries can occasionally occur with greater amounts of blood loss but without hemodynamic compromise. Therefore, a more comprehensive definition of PPH is bleeding (regardless of the volume of shed blood) that is severe enough to cause hemodynamic compromise.

A decrease in hematocrit greater than 10% as a diagnostic criterion has also been widely accepted as a definition of postpartum hemorrhage. The hematocrit level initially may be in the low-normal to normal range despite excessive bleeding, because hematocrit does not change quickly in response to rapid hemorrhage. The hematocrit is also determined in part by the volume of infused resuscitation fluid. Because the parturient's blood volume is increased by 30% to 50%, she may not manifest signs of tachycardia and hypotension until blood loss exceeds 1500 mL. If the patient is hemodynamically unstable but the amount of blood visualized externally is relatively insignificant, occult sites of internal bleeding should be suspected immediately.

Incidence and Mortality

Maternal mortality has significantly decreased over the past 50 years in developed countries, in part because of improvements in obstetric care. According to the National Center for Health Statistics of the Centers for Disease Control and Prevention (CDC), in 2006 the national maternal mortality rate was 13.3 deaths per 100,000 live births.[1] Mortality rates are significantly higher for African American and Asian or Pacific Island women compared with Caucasian women.[2,3] According to a study by the CDC of pregnancy-related mortality in the U.S. between 1991 and 1997, the leading causes of maternal death are hemorrhage, hypertensive disorders, pulmonary and amniotic fluid emboli, infections, and preexisting chronic conditions (such as cardiovascular disease).[2]

Obstetric hemorrhage is the world's leading cause of maternal mortality, causing 24% of maternal deaths or an estimated 127,000 maternal deaths annually. Postpartum hemorrhage is the most common type of obstetric hemorrhage and accounts for the majority of the 14 million cases of obstetric hemorrhage that occur each year.[2] In developing countries, PPH may cause up to 60% of all maternal deaths.[3]

Pathophysiology

At term, blood flow to the uterus and placenta increases to 600 to 1200 mL/min, accounting for 10% of the maternal cardiac output. To stem the flow of blood and provide immediate hemostasis after delivery of the fetus, the uterus begins to contract. Myometrial contraction is the primary mechanism for both placental separation and hemostasis. The myometrial muscle fibers of the uterus contract and simultaneously retract, causing compression and occlusion of the blood vessels. Uterine atony results when this adaptive mechanism fails and the myometrial fibers are unable to contract and retract normally. Excessive bleeding from the uterus and lower genital tract from many causes, including lacerations, placental anomalies, and trauma, is directly related to the increase in blood flow to the uterus and placenta. At term, there is a physiologic increase in the circulating concentrations of various clotting factors. This adaptive response also helps control the bleeding that is a normal consequence of delivery. However, these factors are overwhelmed by the excessive bleeding of PPH.

Presentation

PPH often manifests as brisk and excessive flow of blood from the vagina. This finding is easily observed on physical examination. If the placenta has been delivered, blood can be seen at the vaginal entrance. Maternal hemodynamics may be unaltered initially. If the bleeding is left untreated, typical presenting signs of hypovolemic shock (i.e., tachycardia, tachypnea, and hypotension) become apparent. Bonnar described the symptoms related to PPH in relation to the amount of blood loss (Table 161-1).[4] However, the signs and symptoms of hemorrhagic shock may not occur immediately and may extend over a longer period of time if shed blood is sequestered in the uterus. Occult bleeding occurs most frequently with retained placental fragments, uterine atony, and concealed hematomas in the pelvis, perineum, or retroperitoneal space. Occult hemorrhage in the uterus or hematomas should be suspected in patients who are in the third stage of labor with hemodynamic instability but little or no evidence of external bleeding. Signs and symptoms of excessive bleeding also may be delayed because of the relative hypervolemic state of the patient and by the position of the patient after delivery with the legs elevated in stirrups.

Causes of Postpartum Hemorrhage

Obtaining a detailed antenatal history is important in helping to determine a possible cause of PPH. A history of prior bleeding episodes associated with heavy menses or with dental or surgical procedures should raise the possibility of an underlying coagulation or bleeding disorder. Significant predisposing risk factors for the development of PPH include previous episodes of PPH, multiparity, and multiple fetuses. Women with a prior history of PPH can have up to a 15% risk of recurrence with subsequent pregnancies.[5] Risk factors associated with the development of PPH are listed in Box 161-1. Early recognition of these risk factors may aid in the diagnosis and subsequently in the management of PPH. A randomized controlled trial (RCT) comparing oxytocin administration before and after delivery of the placenta found that birth weight, labor induction with augmentation, chorioamnionitis, use of magnesium sulfate infusions, and previous episodes of PPH increased the risk of developing PPH.[6] However, a significant number of patients with PPH have no obvious predisposing factors.

Potential causes of PPH are listed in Box 161-2. The most frequent cause of PPH is uterine atony after delivery of either the fetus or placenta. Bleeding is from the uterine vessels or from the placental site of

TABLE 161-1	Presentation of Symptoms in Postpartum Hemorrhage	
% Blood Loss (mL)	**Systolic Blood Pressure (mm Hg)**	**Signs and Symptoms**
10-15 (500-1000)	Normal	Tachycardia, palpitations, dizziness
15-25 (1000-1500)	Low-normal	Tachycardia, weakness, diaphoresis
25-35 (1500-2000)	70-80	Restlessness, pallor, oliguria
35-45 (2000-3000)	50-70	Collapse, air hunger, anuria

implantation if the placenta has been delivered. The incidence of uterine atony is approximately 1 in 20 deliveries. Uterine atony can lead to rapid and severe PPH. Overdistention of the uterus secondary to multiple gestation, fetal macrosomia, or polyhydramnios is a major predisposing risk factor for the development of uterine atony. Other predisposing factors are retained placenta, chorioamnionitis, uterine structural abnormalities, and muscle fatigue after prolonged or stimulated labor. General anesthesia, particularly with halogenated anesthetics, and magnesium sulfate infusions can inhibit effective uterine contractions and lead to uterine atony. The diagnosis of uterine atony is a clinical diagnosis made by assessing the tone of the uterus and its size by manually palpating the uterus externally. Bimanual examination of the uterus also can be performed to diagnose uterine atony. A boggy uterus associated with heavy vaginal bleeding or with an appreciable increase in the size of the uterus is diagnostic of uterine atony. The size of the uterus may be larger than normal due to accumulated blood within.

Lacerations of the lower genital tract are the second most frequent cause of PPH. Lacerations of the vagina and cervix can result from a number of causes. These lesions occur most commonly as a result of prolonged or tumultuous labor, particularly with uterine hyperstimulation with oxytocic agents. Nevertheless, lacerations can occur spontaneously as well. They are seen in deliveries associated with instrumentation, such as forceps deliveries, or with extrauterine or intrauterine manipulations of the fetus. Attempts to remove the placenta or placental fragments manually or with instrumentation can lead to traumatic lesions or hematomas. Excessive vaginal bleeding or traumatic hematomas can result from these lacerations. Careful examination with palpation of the vagina and cervix may reveal the presence of lacerations.

Retention of placental fragments or the entire placenta can lead to severe and life-threatening hemorrhage, which may be immediate or delayed depending on the extent of accumulated blood in the uterus. The most common definition of retention of the placenta in utero for more than 30 to 60 minutes after delivery of the fetus. Retained placenta is more likely to occur with a preterm gestation of less than 24 weeks. Placental abnormalities (i.e., placenta accreta, placenta increta,

and placenta percreta) have been associated with retained placenta and failure of complete separation of the placenta from the uterus. Placenta accreta occurs when a portion or the entire surface of the placenta is abnormally attached to the uterus. Where placenta accreta is present, the failure of the placenta to separate normally from the uterus after delivery is accompanied by severe postpartum hemorrhage. Placenta increta involves actual invasion of the uterus by the placenta. If the placenta has been delivered, it is imperative to closely examine the placenta to look for missing fragments, a finding that suggests retained placental tissue.

Another less frequent cause of PPH is uterine rupture. Rupture is more common in patients with prior cesarean incisions and in those with any prior operative procedures of the uterus (e.g., intrauterine device placement, laparoscopy, hysteroscopy). Uterine rupture may manifest with severe and acute abdominal pain and hemodynamic instability, but there may not be significant bleeding initially. Uterine inversion is relatively uncommon but may be associated with blood losses of up to 2 L.

A defect in hemostasis resulting from an underlying coagulopathy should be considered if the uterus is contracting normally and manual exploration has excluded either placental retention or uterine rupture. Disseminated intravascular coagulation (DIC) associated with placental abruption (premature separation of a normally implanted placenta), the HELLP syndrome (hemolysis, elevated liver enzymes, and low platelets), intrauterine fetal death, acute fatty liver of pregnancy, sepsis, or amniotic fluid embolism may precipitate PPH. The incidence of severe DIC associated with PPH is estimated at 0.1% of pregnancies.[7]

Amniotic fluid embolism syndrome (AFES) is a catastrophic condition that can occur either during the pregnancy or after the delivery. AFES manifests with acute respiratory failure, cardiogenic shock, and/or DIC.[8] As many as 80% of these patients develop DIC, and in some, DIC is the major clinical abnormality. Oozing from intravenous (IV) or skin puncture sites, mucosal surfaces, or surgical sites should raise the suspicion of DIC; confirmation of the diagnosis is made by laboratory coagulation studies. Although the coagulation profile is unlikely to be abnormal with acute postpartum bleeding in the absence of DIC, coagulation parameters are clearly abnormal in the presence of DIC regardless of the cause. In late pregnancy, the circulating fibrinogen level usually is two to three times the normal prenatal value, but fibrinogen concentration is dramatically decreased if DIC is present. Preexisting or pregnancy-acquired disorders of coagulation are relatively infrequent causes of significant PPH.

Diagnostic Studies

Although the diagnosis is obvious with significant and excessive bleeding after delivery, not all patients present with immediate bleeding, because of hematoma formation or accumulations in the interior of the uterus. Bedside ultrasonography can be used for the detection of clots, hematomas, and retained placental products. For patients who are at high for risk for development of PPH, periodic ultrasound examinations during pregnancy can offer invaluable information concerning the extent and progression of placental disease. Angiography with selective arterial embolization can be used both diagnostically and

---

Box 161-1

PREDISPOSING RISK FACTORS FOR POSTPARTUM HEMORRHAGE

Previous postpartum hemorrhage
Prolonged third stage of labor
Augmented or stimulated labor
Multiple gestation
Multiparity
Coagulation abnormalities
Cervical, vaginal, or perineal lacerations
Preeclampsia
Arrest of descent of the fetus
Mediolateral episiotomy
Nulliparity
Polyhydramnios
Maternal hypotension
Asian or Hispanic ethnicity

Box 161-2

CAUSES OF POSTPARTUM HEMORRHAGE

Uterine atony
Cervical or vaginal lacerations
Retention of placental fragments
Placental anomalies
Traumatic hematomas of the perineum or pelvis
Coagulation disorders
Uterine rupture
Uterine inversion

therapeutically. Bleeding sites can be visualized and embolized simultaneously. For evaluation of a proven or suspected case of PPH, the following laboratory studies are almost always indicated: complete blood count with platelet count, coagulation studies with prothrombin and activated partial thromboplastin times, fibrinogen, and D-dimer level. With acute hemorrhage, the measurements of hemoglobin concentration and hematocrit may be of limited use.

Prevention

There has been much controversy concerning the preferred methods of managing the third stage of labor in terms of decreasing bleeding complications. The debate concerns active versus expectant management. Expectant management consists of waiting for separation and expulsion of the placenta, with minimal intervention except for gentle fundal massage. Active management of the third stage of labor involves three components. The first consists of administering a uterotonic drug, usually oxytocin, immediately after delivery of the fetus to promote contraction of the uterus and subsequent expulsion of the placenta. The second maneuver consists of gentle traction on the umbilical cord after the uterus is well contracted and then using countertraction against the uterine fundus.[9] The third maneuver is uterine massage after delivery of the placenta. The two modalities were compared in five randomized, controlled trials in a Cochrane meta-analysis of studies enrolling more than 6000 women. A 60% decrease in PPH was associated with active management of the third stage of labor.[10]

General Treatment Measures

Many deaths associated with PPH may have resulted because clinicians underestimated the extent of blood loss and failed to provide rapid and aggressive resuscitation with fluids and blood products. Several authors have suggested the use of specific management protocols for the care of patients with PPH.[4,11,12] These guidelines can expedite rapid diagnosis and management of obstetric hemorrhage. A general assessment of the patient, evaluation of vital signs, a detailed physical examination, and a review of the obstetrical delivery details are all necessary for the clinician to formulate a comprehensive evaluation and critique of the situation. The general treatment measures for PPH are the same as those for any patient with acute hemorrhage (Box 161-3). Oxygen should be administered routinely. At least two large-caliber IV lines should be placed immediately. Central venous access is usually unnecessary unless peripheral access cannot be obtained quickly. Aggressive volume resuscitation should be instituted immediately, because this intervention can be life saving in patients with ongoing bleeding and hemodynamic instability. Either normal saline or lactated Ringer's solution is the preferred fluid for aggressive resuscitation. Isotonic electrolyte solutions provide transient intravascular volume expansion. Monitoring of changes in blood pressure, heart rate, and pulse pressure can help the clinician to determine the amount of blood loss, particularly in cases in which bleeding is internal (Table 161-2).

General guidelines for fluid resuscitation of patients with hemorrhagic shock are based on the "3:1" rule. This recommendation derives from the empirical observation that patients require about 300 mL of crystalloid fluid replacement for every 100 mL of blood loss. This rule

TABLE 161-2	Therapeutic Response to Initial Fluid Resuscitation	
Response	*Description*	*Follow-up Treatment*
Rapid response	<20% of blood volume lost	No additional fluids or blood are needed.
Transient response	20%-40% of blood volume lost; responds to initial fluid bolus but later has worsening vital signs	Continue fluids and consider blood transfusions.
Minimal or no response	Ongoing severe hemorrhage with >40% blood volume lost	Continue aggressive fluid and blood product replacements.

must be applied in the context of the clinical scenario. Applied blindly, this guideline can result in either excessive or inadequate volume resuscitation. Patients with expanding hematomas or areas of concealed active bleeding have hypotension out of proportion to the obvious blood loss and require resuscitation in excess of the 3:1 recommendation. In contrast, patients with ongoing blood losses that are being replaced with blood transfusions typically require less electrolyte fluid replacement. Although initial fluid resuscitation is critical, caution should be exercised to prevent abdominal compartment syndrome that may occur when more than 10 liters of fluids are administered. Red blood cell transfusions to replace ongoing blood loss remain the mainstay of fluid replacement.

Blood transfusions usually are necessary for patients with severe ongoing PPH. Healthy pregnant patients usually do not require transfusion if blood loss is 2000 mL or less. However, if blood loss is greater than 2 L or there is ongoing hemorrhage and hemodynamic instability, transfusion can be life saving. Crossmatched packed red blood cells or type-specific blood can be infused rapidly using a blood warming device in cases of severe ongoing hemorrhage (Box 161-4). Recombinant activated factor VII (rFVIIa) has been recommended in cases of refractory postpartum hemorrhage that has not responded to medical measures including blood product administration.[13] Although supported by few and uncontrolled studies, the available data suggest a potential role of rFVIIa in the management of severe PPH prior to performing a definitive hysterectomy.

Manual external uterine massage should be performed immediately to stimulate uterine contractions and express clots if uterine atony is suspected or confirmed. If the uterus does not respond to vigorous manual external massage and the rapid administration of oxytocin, bimanual massage with one hand on the uterus and the other hand placed anterior to the cervix in the vagina should be performed. Aggressive uterine manipulation can result in uterine inversion. Direct pressure should be maintained over visible perineal, vaginal, or cervical

---

Box 161-3

GENERAL TREATMENT MEASURES FOR POSTPARTUM HEMORRHAGE

Oxygen administration
Gentle massage of the uterine fundus
Placement of large-caliber intravenous catheters for rapid and aggressive fluid resuscitation with isotonic solutions using the "3:1" rule
Blood product administration depending on the extent of bleeding and coagulation abnormalities

---

Box 161-4

BLOOD PRODUCT REPLACEMENT

Crossmatched blood
Type-specific or "saline crossmatched" blood
Compatible ABO and Rh blood types
Rh-negative blood is preferable.
Warm the blood, if possible, especially if the rate of infusion is >100 mL/min or if the total volume transfused is high; cold blood is associated with an increased incidence of arrhythmias and paradoxical hypotension.
Administer calcium if blood is transfused rapidly at >100 mL/min because of binding of calcium by anticoagulants in banked blood.
Give 6-10 units fresh frozen plasma (FFP) for every 10 units of packed red blood cell (PRBC) transfusions.
Give 10-12 units of platelets if the platelet count decreases to <50 × 10^9/L.
Cryoprecipitate can be given to replace fibrinogen in addition to the FFP.
Consider 60-120 μg/kg intravenous bolus injection of recombinant activated factor VII (rFVIIa).

TABLE 161-3	Dosing Regimens for Oxytocic Drugs
Drugs	*Regimens*
Oxytocin (Pitocin)	5-unit IV bolus Add 20-40 units oxytocin to 1 L of fluids. 10 units intramyometrially
Methylergonovine (Methergine)	0.2 mg IM every 2-4 h
Ergonovine (Ergotrate Maleate)	100-125 µg IM or intramyometrially every 2-4 h 200-250 µg IM Total dose 1.25 mg
Carboprost (Hemabate)	250 µg IM or intramyometrially every 15-90 min Total dose 2 mg
Misoprostol	800 µg PR or 800 µg of sublingual misoprostol

IM, intramuscular; *IV,* intravenous; *PR,* per rectum.

lacerations. These general treatment measures can control excessive bleeding and even stop the hemorrhage in a significant proportion of patients.

Specific Treatment Measures

Oxytocic (uterotonic) drugs administered IV, intramuscularly, or intramyometrially are used to stimulate the uterus by producing rhythmic contractions and control the degree of hemorrhage. Dosing regimens for oxytocic drugs are listed in Table 161-3.

Oxytocin (Pitocin) remains first-line therapy for most obstetricians. Prophylactic oxytocin, given either before or after placental delivery, decreases the incidence of PPH up to 40%.[14] It is also used prophylactically after delivery of the fetus but before delivery of the placenta to decrease the duration of the third stage of labor and the amount of blood loss. In an RCT, the incidence of PPH was similar regardless of whether oxytocin was given before or after placental delivery.[6] Additionally, the incidence of retained placenta was similar for patients treated with oxytocin before or after delivery of the placenta. Oxytocin should be used with caution in patients with hyperactive uterine contractions or hypertension, because the pressor effect of sympathomimetic drugs can increase if they are used with oxytocin.

Methylergonovine (Methergine) is now considered second-line therapy. It is a direct uterotonic agent that reduces uterine bleeding and shortens the third stage of labor. Hypertension is a relative contraindication for the use of Methergine. Carboprost tromethamine (Hemabate), a synthetic prostaglandin similar to prostaglandin $F_{2\alpha}$ but with a longer duration, produces myometrial contractions that induce hemostasis at the placentation site, reducing postpartum bleeding. It is used in some centers as a second-line uterotonic agent. Asthma is a relative contraindication to the use of carboprost. Carboprost has been shown to be as effective in decreasing PPH refractory to oxytocin and ergonovine. Misoprostol, prostaglandin E_1, causes uterine contractions, and rectal administration of this drug has been shown to be useful in refractory PPH. Although oxytocin is considered the standard of care for treating postpartum hemorrhage, it is not always viable nor available, particularly in resource-poor clinical settings, because of refrigeration requirements and the need for IV administration. In a large randomized prospective trial, the efficacy and acceptability of 800 µg of sublingual misoprostol was compared to 40 International Units of IV oxytocin to control postpartum bleeding.[15] The primary endpoints were cessation of active bleeding within 20 minutes and additional blood loss of 300 mL or more after treatment. The findings suggested that sublingual misoprostol is a viable alternative to 40 International Units of IV oxytocin for treatment of primary postpartum hemorrhage after oxytocin prophylaxis during the third stage of labor. Misoprostol stopped bleeding as rapidly as oxytocin and with a similar quantity of additional blood loss.

The practice of uterine packing to control bleeding remains somewhat controversial. Although this practice had been abandoned for many years, it has recently resurged as an effective method for tamponade of bleeding from the uterus. Opponents of this practice argue that significant amounts of blood may be sequestered behind the uterine packing and that infection risks are increased. The packing can conceal the actual amount of bleeding, leading to gross underestimation of the extent of hemorrhage. The packing usually is removed in 24 to 36 hours. Uterine packing has been proposed as a temporizing maneuver to stop or decrease PPH before surgery or selective arteriography. Balloon occlusion catheters also have been used in the treatment of PPH.[16] Placement of a Sengstaken-Blakemore tube also has been used for control of bleeding.[17]

If there is a suspicion of retained placenta, examination of the uterus is both diagnostic and therapeutic. The uterus must be explored digitally and retained placental fragments removed either manually or with instruments. Because this procedure can be difficult and quite painful, it may be necessary to use regional or general anesthesia to obtain optimal visualization and manipulation of the uterus. Administration of oxytocic drugs should continue during manual extraction of placental fragments. Administration of broad-spectrum antibiotics has been recommended whenever there is manipulation or instrumentation of the uterus.

Compression of the abdominal aorta against the vertebral column, which can be achieved by pressing a fist on the abdomen cephalad to the umbilicus, can be a lifesaving temporizing maneuver to control hemorrhage before surgery in the presence of fulminant bleeding with severe hemodynamic compromise. If there is persistent and significant bleeding despite the therapeutic measures described, consideration should be given to arteriography with selective arterial embolization. This procedure requires the expertise of an interventional radiologist and may not be readily available in many hospitals. Successful embolization of the bleeding sites can be accomplished, obviating the need for surgical intervention.[18] Fertility can be preserved with this procedure.[19] Prophylactic placement of embolectomy catheters in patients at high risk for PPH to minimize the procedural delay in the presence of active bleeding has also been utilized in some centers. If embolization is unsuccessful, balloon catheter occlusion of the hypogastric and iliac arteries has been successfully performed as a temporizing measure before surgery.[20-22] Complications are minimal, and post-procedural fever appears to be the most common complication of the procedure.

Surgical Therapy

Surgical therapy is reserved for cases not amenable to medical therapy. Patients with ongoing hemorrhage despite aggressive medical therapy are candidates for operation. Surgery is the treatment of choice for uterine rupture. Lacerations, if visible, are directly repaired and oversewn. Lacerations high in the vaginal vault or in the cervix may require operative repair, primarily for improved visualization of the lesions. Hematomas of the lower genital tract are incised and drained. Arterial embolization of vaginal and vulvar lesions has been used. Hematomas of the broad ligament and in the retroperitoneal space are often managed conservatively if there is only minimal further expansion of the hematoma, but surgical exploration or embolization is mandated if additional significant bleeding occurs. Radiographic imaging with computed tomography, magnetic resonance imaging, and/or ultrasonography is a useful adjunct to monitor the expansion of these hematomas.

Ligation of the uterine, ovarian, or internal iliac (hypogastric) arteries can be performed. The uterine arteries provide 90% of uterine blood flow. Ligation of these arteries can often control bleeding with success rates of up to 92% and a complication rate of 1%.[23] If hemostasis is not achieved with uterine artery ligation, the ovarian and internal iliac arteries can be ligated as well. Ligation of the internal iliac arteries is technically more difficult, and success rates range from 40% to 100%.[23-24] Ligation of the internal iliac arteries usually is done only if ligation of the uterine and ovarian arteries has proved unsuccessful in halting bleeding.

Uterine compression sutures running through the full thickness of both uterine walls (posterior as well as anterior) have recently been described for surgical management of atonic PPH.[25-27] The different uterine suture techniques have proved to be valuable and safe alternatives to hysterectomy in the control of massive PPH. In contrast, hysterectomy remains the definitive surgical therapy to control bleeding. Hysterectomy is required if bleeding continues despite ligation of the internal iliac arteries. Subtotal or total hysterectomy is curative in PPH. In cases of uterine rupture, it is the only surgical option, and nonsurgical modalities are only temporizing measures until the patient can be brought to the operating room. In developed countries, the incidence of postpartum emergent hysterectomy is approximately 1 in 2000 deliveries. Rossi et al. reviewed 24 articles that included 981 cases of emergency postpartum hysterectomy. They found women at highest risk of emergency hysterectomy are those who are multiparous, had a cesarean delivery in either a previous or the present pregnancy, or had abnormal placentation.[28]

Complications

Serious morbidity may follow postpartum hemorrhage. Complications from postpartum bleeding include hematologic abnormalities such as DIC and dilutional coagulopathy from massive fluid resuscitation and/or massive transfusion (greater than 10 units of packed red blood cells). Dilutional coagulopathy occurs when more than 80% of the original blood volume has been replaced. Life-threatening complications of hemorrhagic shock, including renal failure and liver failure, acute respiratory distress syndrome (ARDS), and pituitary necrosis (Sheehan's syndrome), can occur. Sheehan's syndrome can result from severe PPH that causes permanent hypopituitarism from avascular necrosis of the pituitary gland.[29]

Prognosis

The prognosis of PPH depends on many factors, some of which are directly related to prompt diagnosis and treatment. The cause of bleeding, the duration of bleeding, and the extent of bleeding all affect the likelihood of a good outcome.

KEY POINTS

1. *Postpartum hemorrhage* (PPH) is defined as excessive bleeding after a vaginal or cesarean delivery that can be associated with hemodynamic instability if the bleeding is severe.

2. The usual signs of tachycardia and hypotension associated with severe bleeding may not manifest early because of the relative hypervolemic state of pregnancy or in cases of concealed hematomas with ongoing blood losses.

3. PPH is the leading cause of maternal death worldwide and one of the major causes of death in the United States, along with embolism, infection, and hypertensive disorders of pregnancy.

4. Massive blood loss can occur from the uterus because of the significant physiologic increase in blood flow to the uterus at term.

5. Occult bleeding occurs most frequently with retained placental fragments, uterine atony, and concealed hematomas in the pelvis, perineum, or retroperitoneal space.

6. Women with a prior history of PPH have a 10% risk of recurrence with a subsequent pregnancy.

7. Many women have predisposing factors leading to the development of PPH. Antenatal identification of potential predisposing factors allows for close monitoring of the high-risk patient.

8. The most frequent cause of PPH is uterine atony, which occurs in 1 of every 20 deliveries. Risk factors for uterine atony include overdistention of the uterus, retained placenta, uterine muscle fatigue, and use of halogenated anesthetic agents.

9. The diagnosis of uterine atony is made clinically by palpation of a boggy and enlarged uterus.

10. The second most frequent cause of PPH is lacerations of the lower genital tract that occur as a result of traumatic labor or spontaneously.

11. Manual exploration of the uterus confirms the diagnosis of retained placental fragments. Placental retention is most commonly associated with several types of placental anomalies.

12. Disseminated intravascular coagulation (DIC) is associated with placental abruption, the HELLP syndrome (hemolysis, elevated liver enzymes, and low platelets), acute fatty liver of pregnancy, intrauterine fetal death, sepsis, and amniotic fluid embolism.

13. Amniotic fluid embolism syndrome usually manifests as sudden and acute respiratory failure, cardiogenic shock, and DIC.

14. In the United States, most obstetricians practice expectant management of the third stage of labor, allowing for spontaneous delivery of the placenta. Active management of the third stage of labor involves fundal massage, use of an oxytocic drug, and gentle traction on the umbilical cord, with countertraction of the uterus to facilitate delivery of the placenta.

15. General treatment measures include aggressive and early fluid resuscitation while investigating the potential source of the bleeding. Higher maternal mortality rates are seen when blood losses are underestimated and treatment is delayed.

16. Patients with ongoing severe bleeding, blood losses greater than 2 L, or hemodynamic compromise require blood transfusions in addition to volume resuscitation.

17. Specific treatment modalities include administration of oxytocic drugs, uterine packing, tamponade procedures with arterial balloon occlusion, and selective arterial embolization.

18. Surgical therapy is reserved for cases of uterine atony and after all other modalities have failed. Uterine, ovarian, and iliac artery ligations and uterine compression sutures have been successful in controlling bleeding.

19. Total or partial hysterectomy is the definitive surgical procedure. Uterine rupture necessitates a hysterectomy.

20. Complications from PPH are the same as those of hemorrhagic shock, with risk of multiple organ failure, acute respiratory distress syndrome, dilutional coagulopathy, and Sheehan's syndrome.

21. Sheehan's syndrome results from severe PPH and manifests as severe hypopituitarism.

22. The prognosis of PPH depends on the cause of the bleeding, its extent and duration, and the speed of diagnosis and treatment.

ANNOTATED REFERENCES

ACOG Practice Bulletin. Clinical management guidelines for obstetrician-gynecologists. Number 76, October 2006: postpartum hemorrhage. Obstet Gynecol 2006;108:1039.
The ACOG (American College of Obstetricians and Gynecologists) Practice Bulletins provide obstetricians and gynecologists with current information on established diagnostic techniques and clinical management guidelines for a wide variety of clinical scenarios and various disease processes, including review of the etiology, evaluation, and management of postpartum hemorrhage.

Quinones JN, Uxer JB, Gogle J, et al. Clinical evaluation during postpartum hemorrhage. Clin Obstet Gynecol 2010;53:157.
This review describes an etiology-based approach to clinical evaluation of postpartum hemorrhage and a suggested system process that allows for a multidisciplinary, timely, and appropriate evaluation of the patient with postpartum hemorrhage. These guidelines can expedite rapid diagnosis and management of obstetric hemorrhage. A general assessment of the patient, evaluation of vital signs, a detailed physical

examination, and a review of the obstetrical delivery details are all necessary for the clinician to formulate a comprehensive evaluation and critique of the situation.

Berg CJ, Chang J, Callaghan W, et al. Pregnancy-related mortality in the United States, 1991-1997. Obstet Gynecol 2003;10:289.
The objective of this epidemiologic study, using data from the Pregnancy-Related Mortality Surveillance System of the CDC, was to examine the trends of risk factors and causes for maternal mortality and to identify patients at high risk for death. Since 1979, the CDC and ACOG have collected information on all maternal deaths in the United States. Results showed that maternal death rates, which had been decreasing annually after 1979, began to increase from 1987 to 1990. The three leading causes of maternal death were hemorrhage, embolism, and hypertensive disorders of pregnancy. The number of deaths due to hemorrhage and anesthesia complications has decreased, but deaths associated with heart disease and infection have increased.

Jackson KW Jr, Allbert JR, Schemmer GK, et al. A randomized controlled trial comparing oxytocin administration before and after placental delivery in the prevention of postpartum hemorrhage. Am J Obstet Gynecol 2001;185:873.

The objective of this RCT was to determine the optimal time to administer oxytocin in the third stage of labor. Previous studies had shown a decreased incidence of PPH when prophylactic oxytocin was given after fetal or placental delivery. However, opponents of this practice are concerned about the potential risk of retained placental parts. In this study, 1486 patients were randomly assigned to receive oxytocin either at presentation of the fetal anterior shoulder or with delivery of the placenta. The authors found no difference in frequency of PPH or in duration of the third stage of labor when oxytocin was given before or after delivery of the placenta. There was no increase in the incidence of retained placenta among those patients who received oxytocin after delivery of the fetus but before delivery of the placenta. Their final recommendation was to proceed with active management of the third stage of labor with controlled cord traction until the placenta is removed. Oxytocin can be given either before or after placental delivery to facilitate uterine contractions.

Rossi AC, Lee RH, Chmait RH. Emergency postpartum hysterectomy for uncontrolled postpartum bleeding: a systematic review. Obstet Gynecol 2010;115:637.

The objective of this review was to describe factors leading to and outcomes after emergency postpartum hysterectomy for uncontrolled postpartum hemorrhage. PubMed, MEDLINE, EMBASE, and Cochrane Library databases were used for the search up to August 2009. Twenty-four articles that included 981 cases of emergency postpartum hysterectomy were reviewed. Their findings showed that women at highest risk of emergency hysterectomy are those who are multiparous, had a cesarean delivery in either a previous or the present pregnancy, or had abnormal placentation.

REFERENCES

Access the complete reference list online at http://www.expertconsult.com.

162

Trauma in the Gravid Patient

SAMUEL A. TISHERMAN | GRETA PIPER

Trauma is the most common nonobstetric cause of death in pregnant women, accounting for 46% of maternal deaths.[1] In the United States, 5% to 7% of all pregnancies are complicated by some form of traumatic injury.[2] The most common mechanisms of blunt trauma are motor vehicle accidents (55%-70%), assaults (11%-21%) and falls (9%-22%).[3,4] Penetrating trauma and burns are less common in most communities. The risk of trauma to the fetus increases as pregnancy progresses and the size of the uterus and fetus increases. The most common causes of fetal death are maternal hemorrhagic shock, abruptio placentae, and uterine rupture. A common maternal injury that results in fetal death is pelvic fracture, frequently leading to fetal skull fracture and intracranial injury. However, even relatively minor injuries to the mother can be devastating to the unborn child.[5]

The major causes of death from trauma (i.e., head injury and hemorrhage) are similar in gravid and nongravid patients. Patterns of injury are generally the same, based upon mechanism of injury. Hepatic and splenic injuries remain common, though gastrointestinal injuries are less common as the pregnancy progresses and the uterus enlarges.[6]

The outcome from trauma for the mother and fetus is dependent upon multiple factors, including gestational age of the fetus and the mechanism and severity of injury. The largest contributor to fetal mortality is gestational age less than 28 weeks.[5] Scorpio et al.[7] found in gravid victims of mostly blunt trauma (80% motor vehicle crashes) that injury severity score and admission serum bicarbonate level were the only independent factors that predicted fetal demise. The serum bicarbonate or base deficit may be important markers of occult hypoperfusion in trauma victims, though serum bicarbonate is normally decreased late in pregnancy. El Kady et al.[5] and Schiff et al.[8] reported that while the actual injury severity score was not predictive of fetal outcomes, maternal and fetal mortality were highest with internal injuries to the thorax, abdomen, and pelvis. The critical factor for the fetus is the extent to which trauma disrupts normal uterine and fetal physiology. Fetal demise occurs in up to 80% of gravid patients who develop hemorrhagic shock. In addition, however, even minor injuries to the mother can result in abruptio placentae or fetal demise.[5] In one study of interpersonal violence as a cause of trauma in pregnancy, 5 of 8 women with fetal losses had no apparent physical injury.[9]

Any female patient of child-bearing potential could be pregnant at the time of injury. Screening (beta-human choriogonadotropin) should therefore be routine during the initial assessment of the patient. Recognition that a "second" patient is present is essential for the care of both mother and fetus. Optimal management of the pregnant trauma victim is the best way to optimize outcome for the fetus: "save the mother, save the fetus." To manage the gravid patient, the traumatologist or intensivist must have an understanding of fetal and maternal physiology, as well as the specific complications of trauma that are unique to these patients. Early obstetric consultation should be obtained. If delivery of a viable fetus is imminent, neonatology consultation may also be needed.

Fetal Physiology

During the first week after conception, the conceptus has not yet implanted in the uterus, making it relatively resistant to injury. Soon thereafter, the blastocyst begins implantation and the placenta begins to develop. The embryo attaches to the uterus via anchoring villi. The placenta is not as elastic as the myometrium, potentially leading to shear stresses and disruption of these villi (particularly if intraamniotic fluid pressure is increased) when force is applied to the uterus. The resulting abruptio placentae rapidly leads to fetal hypoxemia, acidosis, and death.

On the positive side, amniotic fluid is a cushion for the fetus, but the fetus may still suffer injury as a result of rapid compression, deceleration, or contrecoup injury. Late in pregnancy, however, the head of the fetus is typically in the pelvis. Pelvic fractures may lead to fetal skull fracture and brain injury.[4]

Adequate oxygen delivery to the fetus is critical during pregnancy. Blood flow to the uterus decreases proportionally as maternal systemic blood pressure decreases. In addition, as the mother becomes hypovolemic, peripheral vasoconstriction can further decrease uterine circulation. The placenta is exquisitely sensitive to catecholamines. The ability of the fetus to withstand changes in uterine blood flow and/or oxygenation is variable. The fetus can redistribute blood flow to the most vulnerable organs, the brain and heart, but this response (the "diving reflex") is limited. Decreased placental blood flow quickly leads to fetal distress.

Anatomic and Physiologic Changes Associated with Pregnancy

The gravid patient undergoes a multitude of anatomic and physiologic changes to accommodate the developing fetus. Theses changes have a significant impact upon anatomic injury patterns and the response to injury.

From a respiratory standpoint, maternal tidal volume increases by as much as 40%, causing respiratory alkalosis. Renal compensation maintains a normal arterial pH. The diaphragms are elevated, decreasing functional residual capacity and risking intraabdominal placement of chest tubes. The gravid patient has little respiratory reserve and desaturates quickly.

From a cardiovascular standpoint, heart rate increases by 15 to 20 beats per minute by the third trimester. During the second trimester, both systolic and diastolic blood pressure decrease by about 15 mm Hg, then increase to normal levels during the third trimester. By the 10th week of pregnancy, cardiac output increases by 1 to 1.5 L/min due to increased plasma volume and decreased peripheral resistance.

Maternal blood volume increases by nearly 50% by 28 weeks. Red cell mass does not increase proportionally, leading to the "anemia of pregnancy." Normal hematocrit late in pregnancy is 31% to 35%. A mild leukocytosis (up to 18,000 cells/mL) occurs during the second trimester. Coagulation factors and fibrinogen levels increase while plasminogen activator levels decrease during pregnancy, leading to an increased risk of thromboembolism. Trauma to the gravid uterus can lead to release of thromboplastic factors (e.g., amniotic fluid) which can cause disseminated intravascular coagulation (DIC). Serum albumin levels decrease to 2.2 to 2.8 gm/dL.

Decreased gastric motility and cephalad displacement of the abdominal contents predispose women to gastroesophageal reflux and aspiration. Gallbladder function is also impaired, increasing risk of stone formation.

The abdominal examination of gravid women is complicated by cephalad displacement of the abdominal contents by the enlarging uterus. The urinary bladder is displaced upward out of the pelvis, and the ureters become dilated after the 10th week of gestation.

During pregnancy, the uterus increases in size from 70 to 1100 g, taking on an intraabdominal position after 12 weeks, increasing risk of direct trauma. At 20 weeks, the fundus reaches the umbilicus. By 34 to 36 weeks, it reaches the costal margin. Uterine blood flow increases to 10 times normal. One of the most important consequences of the anatomic changes during the latter half of pregnancy is that the uterus can occlude the inferior vena cava when the patient is in the supine position (supine hypotension syndrome), leading to hypotension from decreased venous return. Positioning the patient with the right side of the torso elevated can increase cardiac output by up to 25%. The pelvis of the gravid female has relaxed ligaments, causing gait instability and risk of falls. In addition, venous engorgement in the pelvis increases risk of severe hemorrhage.

From an endocrine standpoint, the hormones of pregnancy (placental lactogen, progesterone, estrogen, parathormone, and calcitonin) lead to insulin resistance and diabetes of pregnancy, decreased lower esophageal sphincter pressure, decreased gastric emptying, and increased calcium absorption. The pituitary gland is increased in size by 135% with increased blood flow demands. Hemorrhagic shock can lead to necrosis of the gland and pituitary insufficiency (Sheehan's syndrome). Preeclampsia (triad of hypertension, proteinuria, and peripheral edema) can increase risk of intracranial hemorrhage or seizures. Subsequent neurologic findings may mimic head injury.

Initial Assessment and Resuscitation

Optimal care of the mother will maximize the chances for survival of the fetus. Resuscitation of the gravid patient should follow guidelines for the nongravid patient. Given the exquisite sensitivity of the placenta and fetus to hypoperfusion and hypoxemia, supplemental oxygen and intravenous fluids should be administered early, even before extrication if possible, particularly since the latter may be delayed by anatomic factors. There is no indication for fetal assessment in the field. Use of the pneumatic antishock garment for stabilization of fractures or control of hemorrhage is contraindicated because the resulting increase in intraabdominal pressure can further decrease venous return in the gravid patient.

Prehospital protocols and interhospital transfer arrangements must account for management of a pregnant trauma victim. The optimal receiving facility should have obstetric and neonatology consultants available, even if it is not the closest trauma center.

The airway of the gravid patient is at risk because of the tendency toward gastroesophageal reflux and aspiration. In addition, the vocal cords are frequently edematous. Ventilation of the gravid patient late in pregnancy may be impeded by the enlarged uterus and cephalad positioning of the abdominal contents. Functional residual capacity may be significantly reduced, leading to more rapid decompensation, particularly with chest trauma.

Because of the increased blood volume late in pregnancy, the mother may not show signs of hypovolemia, given the same blood loss (up to 1500 mL) as a nongravid patient. Uterine perfusion, however, may still be compromised. Uterine blood flow may decrease by up to 30% before the mother demonstrates clinical signs of shock. Aggressive volume replacement is necessary to assure adequate uterine blood flow. Blood transfusions should be administered per standard guidelines, but the mother's Rh-antigen status must be considered. If it is unknown, Rh-negative blood should be administered. Invasive hemodynamic monitoring should be considered early during resuscitation to assure adequate volume resuscitation.

To prevent the supine hypotensive syndrome, beyond 20 weeks of gestation, patients should be placed in the left lateral decubitus position to relieve the pressure of the uterus from the inferior vena cava. The uterus can also be manually displaced to the left. If the patient is immobilized on a long board before spinal injury is ruled out, the entire board can be tilted 15 degrees with a wedge. Vasopressors, which are very rarely indicated in trauma patients, should be avoided unless absolutely necessary because of the risk of decreasing uterine blood flow.

In addition to the standard initial assessment, evaluation of the gravid trauma patient should include a focused history and physical examination related to the pregnancy. The obstetric history should include the date of last menstrual period, expected date of delivery, date of first fetal movement, and status of current and previous pregnancies. The physical examination should include measurement of fundal height. Fetal age can be estimated as 1 week for each centimeter fundal height above the symphysis pubis. The abdominal examination should assess uterine tenderness and consistency, presence or absence of contractions, and determination of fetal position and movement. Pelvic examination should evaluate the presence of blood or amniotic fluid, cervical effacement, dilation, and fetal station. Amniotic fluid can be identified using Nitrazine paper to detect pH. A pH of 7 to 7.5 suggests the presence of amniotic fluid. Vaginal bleeding may indicate abruptio placentae. The Kleihauer-Betke (KB) test is used after maternal injury to identify fetal blood in the maternal circulation. When fetomaternal hemorrhage is present, additional doses of Rho(D) immunoglobulin may be given.[10] Examination of the fetus beyond 20 weeks should include auscultation of fetal heart tones. Normal range is 120 to 160 bpm.

Standard laboratory tests should be obtained, including a pregnancy test. In addition, coagulation studies, including fibrinogen level, should be checked since DIC can occur during pregnancy from release of thromboplastic substances from abruptio placentae or amniotic fluid embolism. Treatment may include urgent delivery of the fetus and blood component therapy.

RADIOGRAPHIC STUDIES

Evaluation of the trauma victim invariably involves multiple radiographic studies. Concern for fetal radiation exposure should not prevent clinicians from obtaining studies needed for optimal care of the mother, though duplication of radiographic studies should be avoided.

The effect of radiation during development of the embryo and fetus is dependent upon dose and timing. Previously it was felt that any radiation very early in development of the embryo would be injurious. More recent findings, however, suggest that this is not the case, and that the fetus is most sensitive to the effects at 8 to 15 weeks when brain development is maximum.[11] Radiation can be teratogenic and can retard growth or cause postnatal neoplasia, but the risk is low after 15 weeks gestation when organogenesis is nearly complete.

Mann et al.[12] stratified risk of adverse effects of radiation for diagnostic studies. Less than 10 mGy (equivalent to 1 rad) was considered low risk, 10 to 250 mGy as intermediate risk, and over 250 mGy as high risk. In general, a single exposure for a plain radiograph results in an exposure of 2 mGy, whereas computed tomography (CT) may lead to an exposure of 5 mGy per slice and fluoroscopy as much as 10 mGy per minute. Exposure in the low category carries minimal risk of mutations. Though the risk of childhood cancers may be increased, the resultant risk remains less than 0.1%. In the intermediate category, specifically above 150 mGy, teratogenic effects may be seen. In the high category, the risk of teratogenic or carcinogenic effects increases significantly, perhaps to 2% to 3% above that of the normal population.

The greatest exposure to the fetus occurs when it is in the direct beam of the radiograph. To minimize exposure, the lower abdomen and pelvis of the gravid patient can be shielded with lead. Typical radiation exposure for the shielded fetus during a maternal chest radiograph is less than 0.01 mGy. In contrast, a pelvic CT scan for which the fetus cannot be shielded is 20 to 80 mGy.[13] The exact efficacy of shielding with lead during these examinations is unclear.

BLUNT TRAUMA

Radiographic evaluation of the gravid blunt trauma victim should begin with the standard chest and pelvis radiographs. Beyond this, additional studies should be chosen based on the findings on physical examination, potential benefit to the mother, and risk to the fetus. If there are acceptable choices for evaluation, the one that entails the least radiation exposure to the fetus should be utilized. For example, one could use ultrasound or diagnostic peritoneal lavage (DPL) instead of CT to evaluate the abdomen, although the latter should be performed if necessary. The focused abdominal sonogram for trauma (FAST) should be utilized in the gravid patient just as in other trauma patients, except that superior displacement of abdominal organs by the uterus should be considered for probe placement. DPL should be performed above the umbilicus. On the other hand, if given a choice between radiographic embolization of bleeding from a splenic injury versus laparotomy, the laparotomy may be the more appropriate choice. Weighing the risks and benefits of radiographic studies is complex. Decisions should be made by the most senior physician involved in the care of the patient.

PENETRATING TRAUMA

As gestation progresses, the uterus becomes the most likely organ to be injured. The uterus and amniotic fluid can slow the velocity of missiles, decreasing potential injury to the mother, though not protecting the fetus very well. Approximately 60% to 70% of gunshot wounds to the pregnant abdomen result in fetal injury, with a subsequent fetal mortality of subsequently 40% to 65%.[14] Penetrating trauma to the upper abdomen frequently involves multiple loops of bowel, which are compressed above the enlarged uterus, leading to complex injuries. Management of gravid patients with entry wounds below the fundus of the uterus is controversial. Although immediate laparotomy is indicated for most nongravid victims of penetrating abdominal trauma, particularly gunshot wounds, this is not the universal standard in the gravid patient. Nonoperative management can be employed if maternal vital signs and fetal heart rate tracings remain normal, suggesting no evidence of maternal or fetal compromise or intraabdominal hemorrhage.[2] Radiographic determination of bullet location may be helpful. Intrauterine bullets may be observed. If laparotomy is performed, all bowel should be carefully explored and wounds repaired. Wounds to the uterus should also be closed. Antibiotics for gram-positive cocci and clostridia should be given as soon as possible.[15] Also, tetanus prophylaxis is safe in pregnancy, and the indications for use in penetrating trauma patients are the same for pregnant and nonpregnant patients.

OPERATIVE PROCEDURES

Operative intervention in the gravid patient should be based upon standard indications for nongravid patients. There is no reason for delay. Anesthetic management using inhalational agents and neuromuscular blockade is considered safe. Local anesthetics should be used with caution, as they may cross the placenta. The uterus should be handled carefully without using excessive traction in order to protect fetal perfusion via the uterine arteries. In damage-control laparotomies, the abdomen can be left open in both gravid and nongravid patients who are predisposed to the development of abdominal compartment syndrome.

MEDICATIONS

Medications frequently have different effects on the gravid patient and the fetus compared to normal, nongravid females. Table 162-1 lists commonly used medications and the current recommendations regarding their use during pregnancy. Because not all medications, particularly newer ones, have been extensively tested in pregnant women, all medications should be administered with some caution in the gravid patient.

MONITORING

Monitoring of fetal cardiac activity and maternal uterine activity (cardiotocographic monitoring) is indicated if the fetus has reached the point of viability if delivered. Since this complication can occur shortly after injury, monitoring should begin as soon as possible. Almost all patients who develop abruptio placentae have frequent uterine contractions (>8 per hour) during the first few hours after trauma; this is the most frequent finding with abruption. Continuous monitoring of the fetal heart beat can detect fetal distress quickly. Normal fetal heart rate is 120 to 160 beats/min. Signs of fetal distress include an abnormal baseline fetal heart rate, absence of normal accelerations and beat-to-beat variability, and repetitive decelerations. The duration of monitoring is somewhat controversial. Although delayed abruption has been reported,[16,17] these patients were not monitored immediately after injury. Monitoring is clearly recommended for gravid patients with frequent uterine activity (>5 contractions per hour), abdominal or uterine tenderness, vaginal bleeding, rupture of amniotic membranes,

TABLE 162-1	Medications and Pregnancy		
Category	*Safe*	*Use with Caution*	*Contraindicated*
Analgesics		Narcotics (fetal respiratory depression) Nonsteroidal antiinflammatory drugs (prostaglandin inhibition) Acetaminophen (safe for short-term use; liver toxicity)	Aspirin (prolonged labor and increased bleeding, intrauterine growth retardation)
Anesthesia	Inhalational anesthetics Neuromuscular blockers	Local anesthetics (cross placenta)	
Antibiotics	Penicillins Cephalosporins Erythromycin Clindamycin	Aminoglycosides (fetal ototoxicity) Sulfonamides (neonatal kernicterus) Quinolones (insufficient data) Metronidazole (insufficient data; carcinogen in rats) Azithromycin (insufficient data)	Chloramphenicol (bone marrow suppression) Tetracyclines (inhibit fetal bone growth) Fluconazole (teratogenic)
Anticoagulants	Heparin Low-molecular-weight heparins		Warfarin (crosses placenta)
Anticonvulsants		Benzodiazepines (fetal respiratory depression) Barbiturates (fetal respiratory depression)	Phenytoin (teratogenic) Valproic acid (congenital malformations, fetal hyperbilirubinemia, neural tube defects)
Antiemetics	Metoclopramide Prochlorperazine Ondansetron	Promethazine (fetal respiratory depression) Droperidol (insufficient data; increased mortality in rats) Trimethobenzamide (limited risk of teratogenicity)	
Gastric protection	Sucralfate Lansoprazole Pantoprazole	Histamine-2 blockers (insufficient data)	
Sedatives		Propofol (fetal depression) Haloperidol (limb malformations, cardiac anomalies)	Benzodiazepines (floppy baby syndrome, withdrawal syndrome)
Vasopressors	Dobutamine	Dopamine, norepinephrine (increased uterine vascular resistance)	
Other		Hydrocortisone (low birthweight, cataracts, cleft palate)	

or hypotension. Some have suggested that patients who are asymptomatic should be observed for at least 4 to 6 hours because approximately 80% of abruptions will occur during this interval.[18] Fetal monitoring throughout a 24-hour observation admission may be performed, though the utility of continuous fetal monitoring beyond this point is limited.

The utility of ultrasound of the pelvis during initial management of the gravid patient is less clear. It is less accurate than cardiotocographic monitoring for detecting abruptio placentae or fetal distress, with a sensitivity of less than 50%.[19] When a CT scan is performed on a pregnant trauma patient to look for abdominal or pelvic injuries, Manriquez et al. found that placental injuries could be diagnosed with 86% sensitivity and 98% specificity.[20] On the other hand, ultrasound can also establish gestational age, determine fetal well-being if the cardiac monitoring is equivocal, verify presence or absence of fetal cardiac activity, and estimate the volume of amniotic fluid if rupture of membranes is suspected. Early obstetric consultation is critical so that if fetal distress occurs, rapid intervention, including Cesarean section, can proceed. Neonatology consultation may also be indicated.

Specific Complications of Pregnancy

FETOMATERNAL HEMORRHAGE

Following trauma, fetal blood can cross the placenta and enter the maternal circulation. This occurs in 10% to 30% of pregnant trauma patients.[15] The volume can be approximated by measuring the ratio of fetal to maternal red blood cells in the maternal circulation with the Kleihauer-Betke (KB) test. Complications include Rh sensitization of the mother, neonatal anemia, cardiac arrhythmias in the fetus, and fetal death from exsanguination. Maternal sensitization may be prevented by administration of Rho(D) immune globulin. Because the KB test may not be sensitive enough to detect the amount of fetal hemoglobin that can sensitize the mother, administration of Rho(D) immune globulin is indicated in almost all Rh-negative mothers unless the injury is relatively minor and far removed from the uterus. In addition, positive KB tests should be repeated in 24 to 48 hours to follow the progression of fetomaternal hemorrhage.[18]

Abruptio Placentae

The most common cause of fetal death with maternal survival is abruptio placentae, which can occur after minor trauma, particularly late in pregnancy. Patients present with abdominal pain, vaginal bleeding, premature rupture of membranes with leakage of amniotic fluid, uterine tenderness and rigidity, expanding fundal height, and maternal shock. Fetal distress may rapidly follow. If the fetus is viable, Cesarean section may be necessary.

AMNIOTIC FLUID EMBOLISM

Trauma to the uterus can result in embolization of amniotic fluid into the maternal circulation, causing a consumptive coagulopathy. Treatment consists of delivery of the fetus and transfusion of platelets and clotting factors, including fibrinogen.

PREMATURE LABOR

Premature uterine contractions associated with cervical dilatation and effacement (i.e., signs of premature labor) are common after trauma. A positive KB test may be one of the most predictive factors for premature labor.[18] Fortunately, premature labor is usually self-limited, but some patients require tocolytics. Evidence of abruptio placentae is a contraindication to tocolytic therapy.

UTERINE RUPTURE

Direct trauma to the uterus can result in rupture, which almost always leads to fetal death and significantly increases risk of maternal death

(usually from concomitant injuries). Typical findings include abdominal pain and tenderness with peritoneal signs. If the fetus is out of the uterus, it may lie in a transverse or oblique position. Fetal body parts may be palpable, although the uterine fundus may not be. Fortunately, uterine rupture only occurs in the most seriously injured patients and remains rare.

FETAL DEMISE

If fetal demise occurs, labor usually begins within 48 hours. If it does not, induction or Cesarean delivery are indicated, as well as observation for evidence of DIC.

CESAREAN SECTION

Depending upon the potential for viability based on fetal age, the indications for urgent Cesarean section in gravid trauma victims include fetal distress, abruptio placentae, uterine rupture, and fetal malposition with premature labor. Possible maternal factors include inadequate exposure for control of other injuries and DIC.

CARDIAC ARREST

During resuscitation, standard algorithms should be applied initially. The uterus can be manually displaced toward the left side, off the inferior vena cava. Optimizing cardiac output and perfusion of the uterus via left thoracotomy and open cardiac massage along with emergency Cesarean section should be considered. By the time the mother has suffered a cardiac arrest from trauma, the fetus has already suffered severe hypoxia. Cesarean delivery may be indicated if the fetus is thought to be viable and the procedure can be performed within 5 minutes of the loss of pulse in the mother.[2] If fetal vital signs persist, delivery may be performed after 5 minutes, though survival becomes less likely as time passes. Cardiopulmonary resuscitation must be continued until delivery is accomplished. Delivery has also been reported to allow successful maternal resuscitation. Decision to proceed with postmortem delivery must be made quickly by the traumatologist and obstetrician; hemostasis and antisepsis become secondary issues. Perimortem Cesarean delivery is performed via a midline incision through all layers of the uterus. Neonatologists must be available.

MATERNAL HEAD TRAUMA

Continuing life support in gravid patients with severe head trauma but viable fetuses is controversial. Brain-dead patients have been sustained long enough for safe delivery of the fetus.[21] Consultation with obstetricians and ethicists is essential.

Prevention

Risk factors for maternal trauma include age younger than 25 years, African American or Hispanic race, low socioeconomic status, use of illicit drugs or alcohol, noncompliance with proper seatbelt use, and domestic violence.

Ikossi et al. revealed that 19.6% of pregnancy-related trauma was associated with illicit drug use, and 12.9% involved alcohol.[22] Education about the risks of drug and alcohol use during pregnancy is needed for all women, especially those in high-risk situations.

Proper seat belt use improves survival after motor vehicle crashes by preventing ejection from the vehicle. According to the National Highway Traffic Safety Administration, the lap belt should cross over the bony pelvis as low as possible under the pregnant belly, with the shoulder belt between the breasts and away from the neck.[15] The shoulder belt can help dissipate the force of deceleration and prevent severe flexion at the waist. Although standard seat belt and shoulder harnesses were not specifically designed for the gravid patient, it is estimated that up to 50% of fetal losses following motor vehicle collisions could be prevented if seat belts are used correctly.[23]

Violent trauma is a major cause of maternal and fetal death that is most likely quite under-reported.[15,18] Approximately 17% to 32% of gravid trauma patients have reported being injured by another person, and up to 60% of these are repeated cases of domestic violence.[3] Factors that should raise concern about domestic violence include injuries inconsistent with the history, diminished self-image, depression, history of self-abuse or suicide attempts, substance abuse, self-blame for injuries, and frequent visits. One should also be concerned if the partner insists upon being present for the examination and monopolizes the conversation. Physicians have a responsibility to identify these injuries and document them with the appropriate authorities.

Summary

Initial assessment and resuscitation of the gravid trauma patient should follow standard trauma management guidelines, recognizing that maternal respiratory reserve may be limited and that the fetus may be compromised even if the mother looks well resuscitated. Maternal and fetal physiology should be kept in mind. Specific complications related to pregnancy should be sought. A viable fetus should be monitored. Early obstetric consultation is needed. Radiographic studies necessary for optimal care of the mother should be obtained. "Save the mother, save the fetus."

KEY POINTS

1. Optimal care for the mother provides the best care for the fetus: "save the mother, save the fetus."

2. Initial assessment and resuscitation of the gravid patient should follow standard protocols including radiographic studies, with few exceptions.

3. Early fetal monitoring and obstetric consultation is critical if the fetus has reached the point of potential viability.

ANNOTATED REFERENCES

Sosa ME. The pregnant patient in the intensive care unit: collaborative care to ensure safety and prevent injury. J Perinat Neonatal Nurs 2008;22:33-8.
This review examines the management of the pregnant trauma patient from the nursing perspective, with emphasis on coordination of care of the pregnant trauma patient in the ICU.
Pearlman MD, Tintinalli JE, Lorenz RP. Blunt trauma during pregnancy. N Engl J Med 1990;23:1609-13.
This classic paper reviews fetal physiology and the anatomic and physiologic changes that occur in the gravid patient. The authors then review the initial assessment of the gravid trauma victim from the perspective of the obstetrician, with emphasis on issues that directly impact upon the fetus.
Cusick SS, Tibbles CD. Trauma in pregnancy. Emerg Med Clin North Am 2007;25:861-72.
This review examines the management of the pregnant trauma patient from the emergency medicine perspective, with emphasis on management prehospital and in the emergency department.

Weiss HB, Songer T, Fabio A. Fetal deaths related to maternal injury. JAMA 2001;286:1863-8.
This study was a retrospective review of fetal deaths related to maternal injury from the death registries from 16 states. A better understanding of the mechanisms of injury based on this data should help target prevention programs.
Brent RL. Saving lives and changing family histories: appropriate counseling of pregnant women and men and women of reproductive age, concerning the risk of diagnostic radiation exposures during and before pregnancy. Am J Obstet Gynecol 2009;200:4-24.
From the perspective of the trauma surgeon, this paper provides detailed background information to assist the clinician with an honest discussion with a patient or family regarding the risks of radiologic tests in trauma patients.

REFERENCES

Access the complete reference list online at http://www.expertconsult.com.

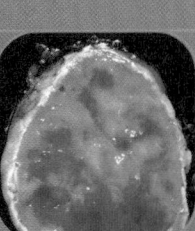

Endocrine

163

Hyperglycemic Comas

P. VERNON VAN HEERDEN

Diabetic ketoacidosis (DKA) and hyperosmolar nonketotic hyperglycemia syndrome (HNHS) are life-threatening syndromes caused by metabolic derangement associated with diabetes mellitus, both insulin dependent (type 1) and non–insulin dependent (type 2). Although a distinction is made in the definitions of the two syndromes, there is much commonality between them, with up to 30% of presentations having features of both syndromes. DKA is approximately three times as common as HNHS in patients presenting with hyperglycemic syndromes.[1] Although the metabolic derangement seen in DKA and HNHS is extreme, the death rate associated with these syndromes is low with appropriate and meticulous therapy. Surveys of patients presenting with hyperglycemic syndromes have found an overall mortality rate of less than 5% associated with DKA and 15% associated with HNHS.[1,2] Most deaths are not caused by the metabolic derangement but occur as a result of coexisting disease (e.g., myocardial infarction), sepsis (particularly pneumonia), or less frequently, the management methods employed.[2]

Hyperglycemic Syndromes

DIABETIC KETOACIDOSIS

DKA is a syndrome of hyperglycemia (blood glucose >13.8 mmol/L), metabolic acidosis (pH <7.30, serum bicarbonate <18 mmol/L, anion gap >10), ketosis, and severe volume depletion. DKA occurs mainly in insulin-dependent diabetics, and severe insulin deficiency is the hallmark of this syndrome. Raised serum levels of stress hormones (glucagon, catecholamines, cortisol, and growth hormone) are also a feature. The hyperglycemia results in a glucose load in the glomerular filtrate that overwhelms the reabsorptive capacity of the renal tubules, resulting in an osmotic diuresis with fluid and electrolyte depletion. Ketone bodies contribute to this osmotic diuretic effect. The lack of insulin causes unfettered lipolysis and formation of ketoacids.

DKA has an incidence of approximately 8.6% in diabetics[2] and occurs in a younger age group (mean age, 33 years) compared with DKA-HNHS (44 years) or HNHS (69 years).[1] Precipitating factors associated with the development of DKA include[3-5]:

- Lack of insulin, either relative or absolute:
  Newly diagnosed or undiagnosed insulin-dependent diabetes
  Noncompliance with treatment or inadequate treatment in diagnosed diabetes
  Dietary mismanagement
- Physical stressors:
  Acute infective illness (e.g., pneumonia, cholecystitis, urinary tract infection)
  Myocardial infarction
  Systemic inflammatory syndromes (e.g., pancreatitis)
  Medication interactions or mismanagement
  Glucocorticoid, phenytoin, inotropic or diuretic therapy
- Postsurgical management
- Substance abuse

Although there are many "stressors" in the intensive care unit (ICU) environment that could potentially cause or predispose to DKA (e.g., sepsis, altered caloric intake, use of total parenteral nutrition, catecholamine use), new development of DKA in the ICU is not common, presumably because of the high level of vigilance in this environment.

Presenting clinical features of DKA reflect the underlying metabolic derangements of dehydration, ketosis, and metabolic acidosis and include:

- Thirst and polyuria
- Tachycardia and hypotension
- Reduced skin turgor
- Dry mucous membranes
- Kussmaul respiration and ketotic fetor
- Evidence of infection/inflammation (e.g., fever)
- Altered mental state (discussed in detail later)

Laboratory tests supporting the diagnosis of DKA commonly reveal the following:

- Hyperglycemia
- Spurious hyponatremia if hyperglycemia is severe
- Preserved or high levels of serum potassium (reflecting acid-base status and not the severe total body depletion of potassium that is present)
- Variable levels of serum magnesium, calcium, and phosphate (although these are usually low or are revealed to be low on commencement of therapy)
- Hyperosmolality
- Metabolic acidosis with low pH, low serum bicarbonate, raised anion gap, and raised serum ketone levels and a compensatory hypocapnia
- Elevated serum urea and creatinine levels
- Elevated serum ketone levels, as measured by the concentrations of β-hydroxybutyrate and acetoacetone

HYPEROSMOLAR NONKETOTIC HYPERGLYCEMIA SYNDROME

The defining features of HNHS include hyperglycemia (blood glucose level >33.3 mmol/L), acidemia (pH <7.3, bicarbonate >15), dehydration, and hyperosmolality (serum osmolality >320) without ketoacidosis. The main differentiation from DKA appears to be the presence of at least some insulin (i.e., relative rather than absolute lack of insulin), more variable levels of stress hormones or counter-regulatory hormones, and the fact that renal dysfunction is commonly present. Renal dysfunction and impaired tubular function result in less capacity to deal with high solute and osmotic loads. This, together with impaired water intake, may result in severe dehydration.

As mentioned earlier, HNHS is less common than DKA, occurs in an older age group, and has a higher mortality rate. Mortality may be associated with missed diagnosis (especially if the patient's mental state is impaired), comorbidity, or delayed or inappropriate therapy.

For HNHS, particularly in elderly patients, the precipitating factors (in addition to those listed for DKA above) commonly feature:

- Mental obtundation, dementia, or physical impairment limiting access to water (e.g., previous cerebrovascular accident)
- Severe dehydration
- Renal dysfunction
- Inappropriate diuretic use

Laboratory test results are similar to those listed for DKA but differ somewhat in degree, in that:

- Serum glucose levels are usually higher.
- Serum sodium levels may be normal (inappropriately so for the degree of hyperglycemia).

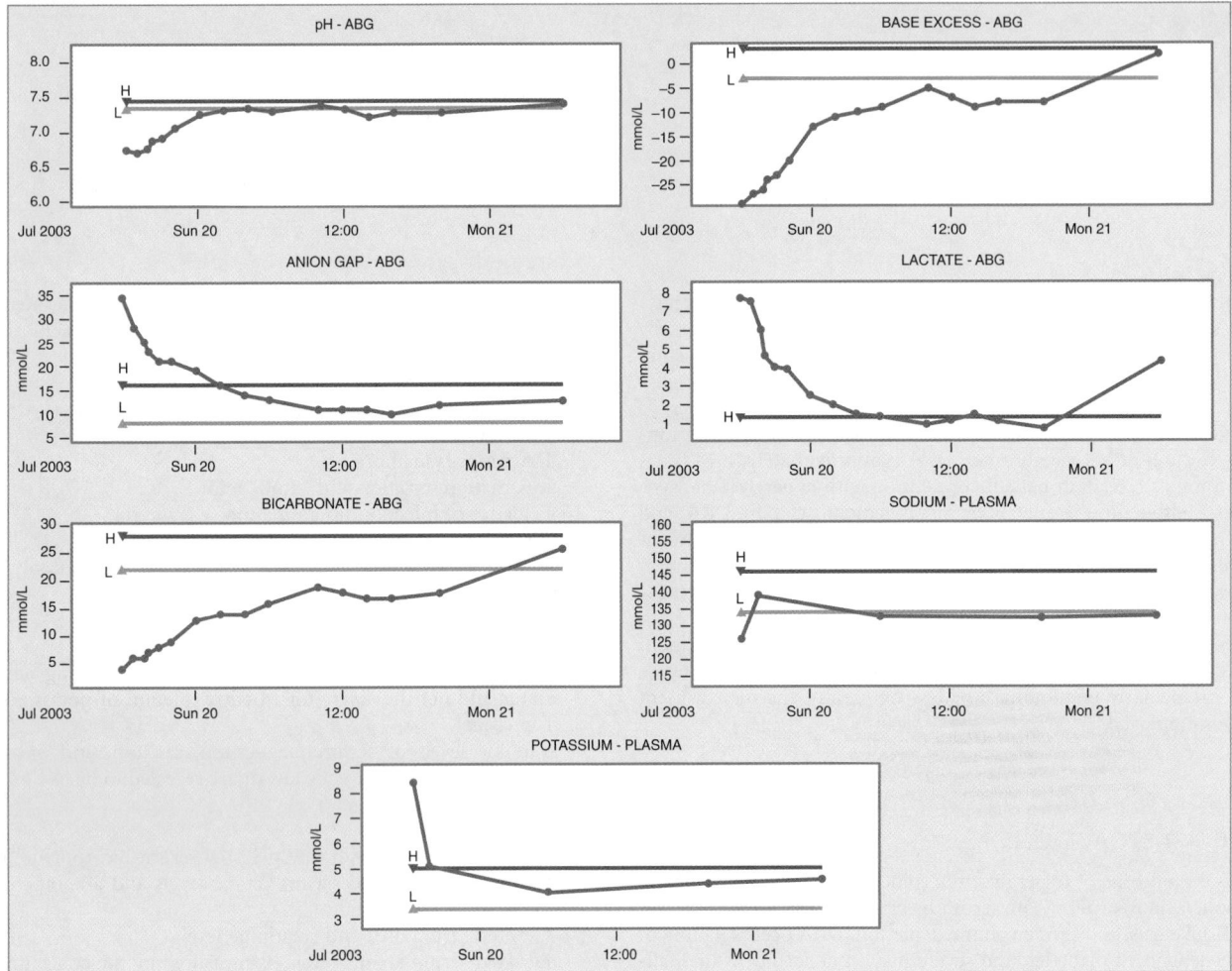

Figure 163-1 Trends in metabolic parameters monitored during treatment of diabetic ketoacidosis. ABG, arterial blood gases.

- Markers of renal dysfunction are worse.
- Hyperosmolality is more marked.
- Metabolic acidosis is not as severe.
- Normal anion gap and serum ketone levels are present.

METABOLIC DERANGEMENTS IN HYPERGLYCEMIC SYNDROMES

The main metabolic derangements that result in morbidity and must be urgently addressed in the management of both DKA and HNHS are severe dehydration, insulin deficit, electrolyte depletion, and metabolic acidosis. These are discussed in detail in Chapters 12 and 18.

Severe dehydration is estimated to be a water deficit in the range of 100 to 200 mL/kg.[4] Although there is no consensus on the ideal approach to fluid management in these patients, prompt restoration of the circulation with isotonic fluid (e.g., normal saline or preferably compound sodium lactate solution), followed by more moderate replacement of the water deficit using hypotonic fluid, are the underlying principles.

The insulin deficit should be treated initially with intravenous soluble insulin to produce normal blood glucose levels within 12 to 24 hours. More rapid correction may predispose to cerebral edema.

Electrolyte depletion is treated by appropriate replacement of sodium, potassium, magnesium, calcium, and chloride, as indicated by frequent laboratory testing during the early phase after presentation.

Metabolic acidosis rarely requires specific therapy and corrects with volume expansion and insulin therapy. Bicarbonate therapy is controversial but currently is not advocated, regardless of the presenting pH, because of the possibilities of exacerbation of hypokalemia, intracellular acidosis, reduced myocardial contractility, and reduced tissue oxygenation.

Figure 163-1 shows serial measurements taken from a typical patient with DKA on presentation and during his treatment in the ICU.

Therapy may be complicated if there is severe comorbidity such as acute or acute-on-chronic renal failure or severe congestive heart failure, and in the patient who requires complex postsurgical care. In all cases, treatment of hyperglycemic syndromes should occur in an appropriate ICU environment with adequate monitoring and meticulous attention to detail to avoid the neurologic sequelae associated with these syndromes.

◼ Neurologic Sequelae of the Hyperglycemic Syndromes

Neurologic sequelae of the hyperglycemic syndromes are not uncommon. They may occur before presentation (and may in fact be the precipitating cause), during the period of severe metabolic derangement, or after apparently uneventful correction of the hyperglycemic syndrome. The following sections describe recognized neurologic sequelae associated with the hyperglycemic syndromes.

ALTERED MENTAL STATE

Patients who present with DKA or HNHS commonly have an altered mental state, which may range from delirium to coma. Often the patient is very unwell and as a consequence is stuporous and uncommunicative, requiring continual prompting to elicit responses to questioning. This condition rapidly improves after rehydration, correction of the hyperglycemia, and correction of acidemia if present, provided there is no underlying neurologic disease. Occasionally, a patient is completely unresponsive, even to painful stimuli, and requires management appropriate to the unconscious patient during treatment of the hyperglycemic syndrome (see later discussion). Clinically, there is no good correlation between blood glucose level, osmolality or pH, and the presenting mental state, which appears to be more a function of the patient's general health, comorbidities, precipitating cause, and duration of the hyperglycemic syndrome before presentation.

Clinical features of the comatose patient include all the features of the hyperglycemic syndrome and in addition, reduced level of consciousness as determined by the Glasgow Coma Scale (GCS), reactive pupils, variable reflex responses (due to the possibility of diabetic peripheral nerve disease), and occasional lateralizing motor signs. The presence of lateralizing signs and lack of improvement in level of consciousness with correction of the metabolic derangement mandate further investigations such as urgent computed tomographic (CT) scanning of the brain or toxicology screening for sedative or illicit drugs.

Less commonly, the main feature of altered mental state is delirium. Delirium is marked by features of disorientation and psychomotor agitation. Delusions and hallucinations may also be manifested, particularly if drug intoxication has been a precipitant of the hyperglycemic episode. These patients can be very difficult to manage, presenting a danger to themselves and to their caregivers (e.g., pulling out venous or monitoring lines, refusing to cooperate with treatment regimens). Adequate sedation with either minor or major tranquilizers may be necessary to allow treatment to proceed smoothly.

CEREBRAL EDEMA

Rapid correction of hyperglycemia and hyperosmolality is associated with the development of cerebral edema in patients with hyperglycemic syndromes. The mechanism of how the cerebral edema arises is unclear.[6-8] The edema might be due to an effect of pH on the Na^+/K^+ exchange pump causing entry of sodium and water into brain cells, osmotic or inflammatory disruption of the blood-brain barrier, or accumulation of osmotically active solutes ("pseudo-osmoles") such as amino acids, polyols, and trimethylamines as an adaptation to the hyperosmolar environment. Other theories of the mechanism of cerebral edema include paradoxical central nervous system acidosis or a left shift in the oxygen-hemoglobin dissociation curve that reduces tissue oxygenation.

The use of isotonic rather than hypotonic solutions for rehydration and avoidance of a too-rapid correction of hyperglycemia appear to offer some protection against the development of cerebral edema. Cerebral edema is more common after treatment of DKA than after treatment of HNHS. Cerebral edema is also more common in newly diagnosed diabetics and in young patients.

Cerebral edema after treatment for a hyperglycemic syndrome usually manifests as prolongation of the altered mental state seen on presentation or new development of an altered mental state with features as described previously. In adults, the signs and symptoms may be very subtle and abate over the course of a few days. Usually no specific therapy is required besides good supportive care. Rarely, cerebral edema can produce focal and permanent neurologic damage.[9] Cerebral edema associated with DKA in children is a much more serious condition with a considerable mortality.[6,8] Urgent treatment of severe cerebral edema relies on intravenous osmotherapy (e.g., mannitol) in the first instance, followed by steroids and loop diuretics as second-line therapy.

FOCAL NEUROLOGIC DEFICITS ASSOCIATED WITH HYPERGLYCEMIC SYNDROMES

There are isolated reports in the literature describing focal neurologic damage in patients with hyperglycemic syndromes. Most commonly, cerebrovascular accidents (CVA), particularly hemorrhagic and thrombotic types, have been associated with HNHS. This is not surprising, because CVA may be the precipitating factor for the development of HNHS in diabetic patients, and the hyperosmolar state in both DKA and HNHS may predispose to thrombotic CVA. Intracerebral venous thrombosis has also been reported[10] and has a poor outlook.

CVA may result in neurologic deficit evident on presentation, but often the final clinical picture is obscured by the altered mental state and only becomes clear after treatment of the hyperglycemic syndrome. The high incidence of neurologic signs and symptoms in diabetics may make the detection of new neurodeficits difficult. Many of the focal neurologic signs seen in these patients, particularly those with HNHS, disappear after treatment of the hyperglycemic syndrome. This may represent unmasking of focal areas of cerebrovascular insufficiency by the dehydration.[5]

Focal neurologic damage may also occur as a result of fluid and electrolyte shifts produced during treatment of the hyperglycemic syndromes (e.g., putaminal hemorrhage,[9] lateral pontine and extrapontine myelinolysis[11]). In patients who are treated for prolonged periods in the ICU for complications related to their episode of hyperglycemic syndrome, critical illness polyneuropathy is also a possibility.

Adequate investigation of a residual or new focal neurologic deficit is mandated. This may include CT scanning, magnetic resonance imaging (MRI), and nerve conduction studies.

COGNITIVE IMPAIRMENT AFTER HYPERGLYCEMIC SYNDROMES

Cognitive impairment may occur after hyperglycemic syndrome. This impairment may be gross and clinically apparent (more common in elderly patients) or very subtle (e.g., poor concentration, loss of memory). It may be associated with focal or global neurologic deficit, as described previously, or it may be apparent in the presence of a structurally normal brain. Most cognitive impairment that is not caused by structural brain damage improves with time. Sensory evoked potentials have shown promise as a sensitive test to detect subclinical brain dysfunction in patients with severe DKA.[12]

SEIZURES ASSOCIATED WITH HYPERGLYCEMIC SYNDROMES

Focal and generalized seizures are common in patients with hyperglycemic syndromes and may be resistant to treatment with the usual anticonvulsant agents.[5] Epilepsia partialis continua, an unusual form of seizure typified by abnormal MRI signal intensity in the precentral gyrus, can occur in DKA or HNHS.[13]

PAIN ASSOCIATED WITH HYPERGLYCEMIC SYNDROMES

Pain may be a prominent clinical feature of patients with hyperglycemic syndromes. Pain, often neuropathic in origin, may be so severe as to mimic the acute surgical abdomen. Pleuritic chest pain and headache are also common. Proper evaluation of pain is very difficult in the patient with emergent hyperglycemic syndrome. Frequent clinical evaluation, while addressing the main pillars of therapy (fluid and electrolyte replacement and insulin therapy) is important to detect early the true surgical cause of pain. Pain caused by the hyperglycemic syndrome itself usually diminishes with time and appropriate treatment, whereas other pathologic causes of pain may not. To complicate matters, chronic pain syndromes are also common in diabetics. A careful history is essential to differentiate the known ("old") pain from the new pain.

HYPERGLYCEMIA AND POOR NEUROLOGIC OUTCOME AFTER HEAD INJURIES AND CEREBROVASCULAR ACCIDENTS

Hyperglycemic syndromes are possible in diabetics who have suffered head injury or CVA. In these patients, it is vital to regain control of metabolic function and provide adequate resuscitation to prevent secondary neurologic damage. Both hypovolemia and hyperglycemia have been shown to contribute to poorer neurologic outcomes.

▣ Clinical Approach to the Obtunded Hyperglycemic Patient in the Intensive Care Unit

The clinical approach to the obtunded hyperglycemic patient presenting to the ICU requires strict attention to the principles of management of the patient with a depressed level of consciousness, together with management of the underlying hyperglycemic syndrome.

DIAGNOSIS

Metabolic derangement is a differential diagnosis for all obtunded patients, even those who present with a much more graphic confounding diagnosis such as traumatic brain injury, because such injuries may be the result of an altered mental state associated with a hyperglycemic syndrome, or they may be the precipitating cause of a hyperglycemic syndrome. The usual clinical pathway of careful history, clinical examination, and appropriate laboratory testing will reveal the underlying hyperglycemic syndrome. Once the hyperglycemic syndrome is detected, the precipitating cause for DKA or HNHS should also be carefully sought. In particular, blood, sputum, and urine cultures should be taken early, and a chest radiograph may reveal pneumonia. If the initial tests do not reveal a source of sepsis, a more extensive series of tests for sepsis (e.g., cerebrospinal fluid examination) may be deferred until the metabolic state has been improved. Similarly, extensive neuroradiologic testing (CT or MRI) can usually wait until the patient has been appropriately resuscitated and treated. Because many of the neurologic signs resolve with the acute treatment, unnecessary testing is thereby avoided.

Specific diagnostic tests that are useful in the diagnosis and management of DKA or HNHS in the obtunded patient include:

- Blood glucose level and glycated hemoglobin (HbA_{1c}) concentration
- Arterial blood gas analysis, including bicarbonate level and anion gap
- Serum urea and electrolytes
- Serum osmolality (calculated and measured)
- Serum magnesium, calcium, and phosphate levels
- Full blood count
- Serum ketone levels, if available

MANAGEMENT PRINCIPLES

Treatment must be provided in a safe environment, preferably in an ICU, with adequate monitoring of the cardiovascular system (blood pressure, heart rate, electrocardiographic parameters) and the respiratory system (pulse oximetry and serial blood gas measurements). More invasive monitoring techniques such as central venous or pulmonary arterial catheterization should be reserved for patients with severe comorbidities (e.g., renal or cardiac failure). Catheterization of the urinary bladder provides a sample for culture as well as a monitor of urine flow. Treatment for DKA or HNHS (as described earlier and in detail elsewhere) must be promptly initiated:

- Fluid resuscitation is vital.
- Insulin therapy is mandatory.
- Electrolyte replacement (particularly potassium and to a lesser extent magnesium and calcium) is important. Phosphate

replacement is controversial, but routine supplementation is currently not advocated.[3]
- Airway protection is a priority, including proper posturing, placement of a nasogastric tube to avoid gastric distention and aspiration of gastric contents, and intubation of the trachea if necessary.
- Sedation of the delirious patient with either minor or major tranquilizers may be necessary to allow treatment to proceed. The major tranquilizers are probably safer because they present a lower risk of respiratory depression.
- Monitoring response to these therapeutic measures should be charted either manually or electronically on a suitable bedside chart so that trends may be viewed as treatment proceeds.
- Serial laboratory testing is necessary at a frequency that allows timely adjustment in fluid, electrolyte, and insulin therapy (e.g., hourly or more often to begin with, with a decreasing frequency as the patient improves). Arterial cannulation is helpful in providing access for serial blood sampling. Access to a "stat" laboratory or good laboratory service is essential.
- Treatment of the precipitating cause of the hyperglycemic syndrome, if one has been identified, should be initiated. This may involve, for example, antibiotic therapy for known or suspected sepsis or withholding of precipitating drugs.
- Serial clinical examinations should be performed, as well as investigation and treatment of new problems that arise or neurologic problems that are not resolving. This may include imaging of the brain by CT or MRI to delineate cerebral edema or focal neurologic pathology or treatment of complications seen with variable frequency in patients with hyperglycemic syndromes, such as acute respiratory distress syndrome (ARDS), gastric distention, rhabdomyolysis, and thrombotic episodes.
- Treatment of comorbidities (e.g., renal replacement therapy for acute or acute-on-chronic renal failure, treatment of acute myocardial ischemia) is also important. This may prove challenging, and the requirements may be diametrically opposed to those necessary for treatment of the hyperglycemic syndrome. For example, high-dose catecholamine therapy for cardiogenic shock after myocardial infarction may worsen insulin resistance.

COMPLICATIONS OF TREATMENT

Complications of the treatment itself must also be dealt with and may include:

- Hypokalemia—monitoring and necessary potassium supplementation should be provided long before there is a risk of cardiac arrhythmia.
- Hypoglycemia due to overenthusiastic insulin therapy—avoided by adequate blood glucose level monitoring.
- Hyperchloremic metabolic acidosis due to loss of bicarbonate precursors (ketones) in the urine and use of chloride-containing solutions such as normal saline for resuscitation—reduced by using compound sodium lactate solution for resuscitation and 0.45% saline for subsequent rehydration.
- Hypophosphatemia is also common and should be corrected along with other deficient electrolytes.
- Fluid overload
- Cerebral edema—described previously

ONGOING CARE

Once the patient is stable and has been adequately resuscitated and metabolic control has been reestablished, arrangements should be made for the smooth transition of care to an endocrinologist familiar with the chronic care of diabetic patients. This may be facilitated by the institution of enteral feeding and conversion from short-acting intravenous insulin to longer-acting subcutaneous insulin before handover. Ongoing care of the patient must address preventable precipitating factors (e.g., prompt treatment of septic foci, compliance with diabetic treatment regimens).[3]

KEY POINTS

1. Diabetic ketoacidosis (DKA) and hyperosmolar nonketotic hyperglycemia syndrome (HNHS) are life-threatening syndromes with a 6.2% overall mortality rate. The mortality rate for DKA is less than 5%, and for HNHS it is approximately 15%.

2. DKA is a syndrome of hyperglycemia, metabolic acidosis, ketosis, and severe volume depletion. Severe insulin deficiency is the hallmark of this syndrome. Fluid and electrolyte depletion is a major component of the pathophysiology, as is unfettered lipolysis which leads to the formation of ketoacids.

3. Precipitating factors for DKA include lack of insulin (either relative or absolute), physical stressors (including infections), post-surgical management, and substance abuse. Presenting clinical features of DKA include dehydration, ketosis, and metabolic acidosis. Laboratory tests usually show hyperglycemia, spurious hyponatremia, hyperosmolality, metabolic acidosis, elevated serum urea and creatinine levels, and elevated serum ketone levels.

4. Defining features of HNHS include hyperglycemia, dehydration, and hyperosmolality, but without ketoacidosis, indicating the presence of at least some insulin. HNHS is usually associated with a degree of renal dysfunction and impaired water intake.

5. Clinical features of HNHS that differentiate it from DKA are that it is less common than DKA, occurs in an older age group, and has a higher mortality rate; that hyperosmolality may be severe, but metabolic acidosis is not as severe; and that normal anion gap and normal serum ketone levels are present. Precipitating factors for HNHS include mental obtundation, severe dehydration, renal dysfunction, and inappropriate diuretic use. Main metabolic derangements of HNHS are severe dehydration, relative insulin deficit, electrolyte depletion, and metabolic acidosis.

6. Neurologic sequelae of the hyperglycemic syndromes include altered mental state, cerebral edema, focal neurologic deficits, cognitive impairment, post-hyperglycemic syndrome, seizures, and pain associated with hyperglycemic syndromes.

7. Diagnosis of hyperglycemic syndrome includes high clinical index of suspicion in the target population group, metabolic derangement on laboratory testing, hyperglycemia, and usually identification of a precipitating cause. Neuroradiologic testing may be required to exclude focal neurologic pathology (e.g., subdural hemorrhage), and specific diagnostic tests may be required to determine the exact type of metabolic acidosis (e.g., lactic acidosis versus ketoacidosis), identify the precipitating cause of the hyperglycemic syndrome, or exclude differential diagnoses.

8. The principles of management of hyperglycemic syndrome are as follows:
   - Treat the patient in a safe environment.
   - Institute treatment promptly, even if it means delaying precise diagnosis.
   - Airway protection and volume resuscitation are priorities.
   - Sedation of the delirious patient may be required to allow treatment to proceed safely.
   - Monitoring is important and is tailored to the severity of illness of the patient.
   - Serial laboratory testing is essential to guide therapy.
   - Treatment of the precipitating cause is important.
   - Serial clinical examinations and investigations allow more accurate therapy.
   - Treatment of comorbidities (e.g., severe ischemic heart disease) must not be overlooked in the critically ill patient.

9. Complications of treatment must be anticipated and dealt with expeditiously and may include hypokalemia, hypoglycemia, hyperchloremic metabolic acidosis, fluid overload, and cerebral edema.

ANNOTATED REFERENCES

Kearney T, Dang C. Diabetic and endocrine emergencies. Postgrad Med J 2007;83:79-86.
   A good overview of endocrine emergencies that puts the two conditions of DKA and hyperglycemic hyperosmolar states in overall perspective with regard to endocrine clinical emergencies.
Chiasson J, Aris-Jilwan N, Belanger R, et al. Diagnosis and treatment of diabetic ketoacidosis and the hyperglycemic hyperosmolar state. CMAJ 2003;168:859-66.
   This paper provides an excellent review of DKA and the hyperglycemic hyperosmolar states. Insulin deficiency and raised counterregulatory hormone levels are the major underlying abnormalities. Clinical observations (dehydration and raised blood sugar levels) and simple confirmatory laboratory tests (pH, serum bicarbonate, and serum osmolality) are all that are required to make the diagnosis.

Kitabachi AE, Umpierrez GE, Murphy MB, et al. Management of hyperglycemic crisis in patients with diabetes. Diabetes Care 2001;24:131-53.
   This review article discusses in depth the precipitating causes, pathogenesis, and management of diabetic comas and provides clear treatment algorithms.
MacIsaac RJ, Lee LY, McNeil KJ, et al. Influence of age on the presentation and outcome of acidotic and hyperosmolar diabetic emergencies. Intern Med J 2002;32:379-85.
   This review of diabetic presentations to an Australian tertiary hospital showed that a combination of ketoacidosis and hyperosmolality was present in 30% of admissions for diabetic hyperglycemic emergencies.

REFERENCES

Access the complete reference list online at http://www.expertconsult.com.

164

Hyperglycemia and Blood Glucose Control

DIETER MESOTTEN | GREET VAN DEN BERGHE

Altered Glucose Regulation in Stress

At the end of the 19th century, Claude Bernard described the link between acute trauma and the development of hyperglycemia irrespective of underlying diabetes. It was considered to be an adaptive stress response ensuring adequate glucose supply to the obligatory glucose-consuming neurons, phagocytes, and reparative cells.[1,2] Stress-induced hyperglycemia is evoked by integrated hormonal, cytokine, and nervous "counter-regulatory" signals on glucose metabolic pathways. Essentially, the hyperglycemia is due to insulin resistance in the liver and skeletal muscle. Hepatic insulin resistance leads to increased hepatic gluconeogenesis and glucose output.[3] Decreased glycogen synthesis and a shift from insulin-dependent to non–insulin-dependent glucose uptake characterize skeletal muscle insulin resistance.[4]

In the acute phase of critical illness, it is assumed that increased levels of glucagon, cortisol, and growth hormone jointly increase hepatic gluconeogenesis. In addition, the catecholamines epinephrine and norepinephrine, released in response to acute injury, promote hepatic glycogenolysis. The cytokines interleukin (IL)-1, IL-6, and tumor necrosis factor (TNF) may directly or indirectly enhance both of these hyperglycemic responses.[5]

The important exercise-stimulated glucose uptake in skeletal muscle totally disappears because of the immobilization of the critically ill patient. Insulin-dependent glucose uptake is hampered also through a combined inhibition of glucose transporter-4 (GLUT-4) and glycogen synthase activity.[6,7] Although some studies have shown decreased glucose oxidation[8] through pyruvate produced by glycolysis, others have demonstrated an opposite effect during critical illness.[9] The decrease in insulin-dependent glucose uptake in skeletal muscle is completely offset by a strong increase in total body glucose uptake, of which the mononuclear phagocyte system in liver, spleen, and ileum are the main receivers.[10] However, in skeletal muscle, non–insulin-dependent glucose uptake is also increased by increased expression of GLUT-1.[11,12] The overall increased peripheral glucose uptake[13] in light of hyperglycemia underscores the pivotal role of increased hepatic glucose production during critical illness, which cannot be suppressed by exogenous glucose.[14]

The position of adipose tissue in the regulation of glucose metabolism during critical illness has been neglected. Nevertheless, in diabetes mellitus, adipose tissue strongly modulates insulin resistance, as it is regarded as an insulin-dependent glucose uptake organ. Recent studies have now revealed that during critical illness, adipose tissue undergoes major changes.[15] Possibly stimulated by illness-induced macrophage infiltration, adipocytes become more numerous and smaller and have an increased expression of the non–insulin-dependent glucose transporters, GLUT-1 and GLUT-3. The levels of GLUT-4 remain unaltered. As such, adipose tissue seems reprogrammed during critical illness to facilitate glucose uptake independent of circulating insulin levels.

Hyperglycemia in Critically Ill Patients

In a normal individual, blood glucose levels are tightly regulated within the narrow range of 60 to 140 mg/dL (3.3-7.7 mmol/L), both in fed and fasted states. Diabetic hyperglycemia is defined by the World Health Organization (WHO) as a fasting blood glucose concentration of 126 mg/dL (7 mmol/L) or higher and fed blood glucose levels higher than 200 mg/dL (11.1 mmol/L). In their 2006 guidelines, the WHO functionally defined *normoglycemia* as the glucose level associated with low risk of developing diabetes or cardiovascular disease. Unlike the diagnostic criteria for diabetes mellitus, no clear guidelines have been set for defining hyperglycemia in a critically ill patient. This explains the wide variations in the reported prevalence of hyperglycemia in critically ill patients.

However, stress hyperglycemia is also associated with adverse outcome in several critically ill patient populations. More precisely, a large cohort study of over 66,000 critically ill patients revealed a J-curved relationship between on-admission blood glucose level and the risk of mortality, with the nadir between 100 and 150 mg/dL (5.6-8.3 mmol/L).[16] In patients with an acute coronary syndrome, a similar association has been observed, with the lowest risk of mortality at blood glucose levels between 80 and 100 mg/dL (4.4-5.5 mmol/L).[17-20] Importantly, in patients with established diabetes mellitus prior to critical illness or an acute coronary syndrome, the relationship between hyperglycemia and mortality is significantly blunted and somewhat shifted to the higher blood glucose[17] (Figure 164-1).

Until recently, it was considered state of the art to tolerate blood glucose levels up to 220 mg/dL (12 mmol/L) in fed critically ill patients. It was even suggested that this moderate hyperglycemia in critically ill patients was beneficial for organs such as the brain and the blood cells which rely solely on glucose for their energy supply and do not require insulin for glucose uptake. Motivation for treatment of blood glucose levels higher than 12 mmol/L was primarily the occurrence of hyperglycemia-induced osmotic diuresis and fluid shifts. Also, from the diabetes literature it was known that uncontrolled and pronounced hyperglycemia predisposes to infectious complications.[21] In patients with known diabetes mellitus, usually more attention was paid to blood glucose levels and consequently more strictly controlled. This approach contrasts—in hindsight—with the blunting of the J-shaped relation between glycemia and mortality risk. Observational studies have also revealed that hyperglycemia in patients with established diabetes mellitus gives an at least threefold higher risk of mortality compared to patients with known diabetes.[22]

Maintenance of Normoglycemia in the Intensive Care Unit

THE LEUVEN STUDIES

In 2001, a large prospective, randomized, controlled trial (RCT) was the first to challenge the classic dogma of beneficial stress hyperglycemia.[23] It examined the effect of tight glycemic control (TGC) with intensive insulin therapy on mortality and morbidity of critically ill patients. Over a 1-year period, 1548 mechanically ventilated patients admitted to the intensive care unit (ICU), predominantly after extensive or complicated surgery or trauma, were randomly allocated to either intensive insulin therapy with blood glucose levels kept tightly between 80 and 110 mg/dL (4.5-6.1 mmol/L) or the conventional approach, which recommended insulin therapy only if blood glucose

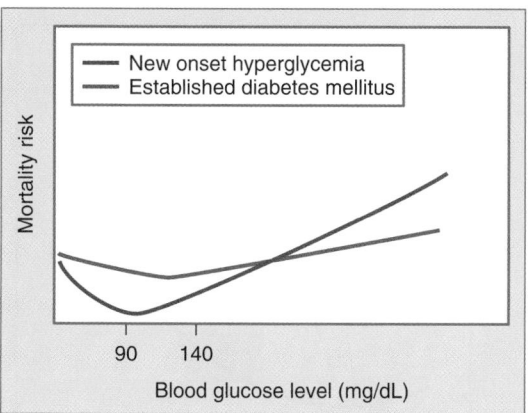

Figure 164-1 J-shaped association between blood glucose levels and mortality risk in critically ill patients. In patients without diabetes mellitus, hyperglycemia shows an almost linear relationship with mortality risk. Hypoglycemia is associated with an even steeper increase in mortality risk. Normoglycemia during critical illness conveys the lowest risk of dying. In patients with established diabetes, the J-shaped curve is significantly flattened out.

levels exceeded 12 mmol/L. The intervention of TGC comprised accurate arterial blood glucose measurements by a blood gas analyzer and a reliable continuous infusion of insulin exclusively via a central venous line, using an accurate syringe-driven infusion pump. The fine insulin dose adaptations were performed by trained bedside nurses and based on a guideline which requires a high level of intuitive and anticipating decision making. In this study, patients were kept in a nonfasting state at all times. Dextrose 20% was administered on the first day (192 g glucose over 24 hours or 768 kcal/d). Thereafter, enteral nutrition was started, with the daily amount progressively increased as tolerated. When enteral nutrition was insufficient, early supplemental parenteral nutrition was given, resulting in administration on average of 1100 nonprotein kcal/d.

Intensive insulin therapy, resulting in the administration of on average 1100 nonprotein kcal/d, lowered ICU mortality from 8% to 4.6% (absolute risk reduction [ARR] 3.4%) and in-hospital mortality from 10.9% to 7.2% (ARR 3.7%). The effect occurred particularly in the population with prolonged critical illness, among whom mortality was reduced from 20.2% to 10.6%. Even patients in the conventional insulin treatment schedule with only moderate hyperglycemia (110-150 mg/dL) showed higher mortality compared with patients in the strict glycemic control schedule.[24] Intensive insulin therapy also had a major effect on morbidity. It decreased the duration of ventilatory support and ICU stay, reduced the need for blood transfusions, and lowered the incidence of bloodstream infections and excessive inflammation. Even more striking, intensive insulin therapy caused a highly significant decrease in the development of critical illness polyneuropathy and acute kidney failure.

Subsequently, the effect of TGC was tested in a medical ICU setting by the same group.[25] The difference in in-hospital mortality, 40.0% in the control group and 37.3% in the intervention group, was not statistically significant in an intention-to-treat analysis of the 1200 included patients. However, in patients who stayed in the ICU for 3 or more days, in-hospital mortality was reduced from 52.5% to 43.0% by TGC. Intensive insulin therapy also reduced morbidity (incidence of acute kidney failure, weaning of the ventilator, ICU/hospital stay) but not as strikingly as in the surgical study. This was in part explained by a larger fraction of patients in medical ICUs who were admitted with established organ damage, possibly reducing the opportunity of prevention by glucose lowering.[26] The fact that intensive insulin therapy to normal-for-age blood glucose targets in mainly postoperative pediatric critically ill patients did reduce mortality by an ARR of 3% may further corroborate this finding.[27]

The downside of TGC has been the increase in the incidence of hypoglycemia (blood glucose levels < 40 mg/dL [<2.2 mmol/L]) despite improving patient outcome. In the Leuven studies, 5.1% (surgical ICU), 18.7% (medical ICU), and 25% (pediatric ICU) of patients randomized to TGC experienced at least one episode of hypoglycemia. To date, long-term follow-up studies to gauge the impact of brief hypoglycemia on neurocognitive function have been lacking. In addition, it is possible that fluctuations in glucose levels such as those induced by insulin therapy based on inaccurate glycemic monitoring, or by overcorrection of hypoglycemia, may be more deleterious that hypoglycemia by itself. Such aspects remain to be investigated in great detail.

THE INITIAL REPEAT STUDIES

Two European multicenter studies designed to assess whether intensive insulin therapy exerts benefit, with mortality as the primary endpoint, failed to reproduce the Leuven findings. The VISEP (*V*olume substitution and *I*nsulin therapy in severe *SEP*sis) (N = 537) trial was designed as a four-arm study to assess the difference between two choices of fluid resuscitation (10% pentastarch versus modified Ringer's lactate) and the efficacy and safety of intensive insulin therapy in patients with severe sepsis and septic shock.[28] In this study, blood glucose targets comparable to the Leuven studies were set out for the intervention (80-110 mg/L) and control (180-200 mg/dL) groups. Likewise, the insulin administration and blood glucose measurements had been standardized. Nevertheless, the insulin arm of the study was stopped early after 488 patients had been included, because the rate of hypoglycemia (12.1%) in the intensive insulin therapy group was considered unacceptably high and may be associated with higher mortality. Then at the first planned interim analysis, the fluid resuscitation arm of the study was also suspended because of increased risk of organ failure in the 10% pentastarch arm. The primary endpoint, 90-day mortality, was 39.7% in the intensive versus 35.4% in the conventional treatment arm.

The GLUCONTROL multicenter RCT (N=1101) investigated whether tight glycemic control (80 and 110 mg/dL) with intensive insulin therapy versus an intermediate target for blood glucose (140-180 mg/dL [7.8-10.0 mmol/L]) improves survival in a mixed population of critically ill patients.[29] This study was also stopped early because the target glycemic control was not reached and the incidence of hypoglycemia was 9.8%. ICU mortality did not differ between the intensive insulin therapy group (17.2%) and the control group (15.3%).

Two single-center studies in a mixed medical/surgical ICU population, both smaller than the Leuven studies, followed and were unable to reproduce a significant mortality benefit.[30,31] In contrast, a number of small RCTs in selected subpopulations, mostly focusing on morbidity as primary endpoint, as well as several larger implementation studies revealed improved outcome as did the Leuven studies.[32-35]

NICE-SUGAR

All the described studies were in fact statistically underpowered to detect a reasonable mortality difference. To address this issue, the NICE-SUGAR (*N*ormoglycemia in *I*ntensive *C*are *E*valuation and *S*urvival *U*sing *G*lucose *A*lgorithm *R*egulation) included 6100 patients over 41 participating centers.[36] This study compared a blood glucose target of below 108 mg/dL (<6.0 mmol/L) versus "usual care," which meant an intermediate blood glucose target of 140 to 180 mg/dL (8 to 10 mmol/L). Owing to the results from the Leuven studies, clinicians had become aware of the negative impact of hyperglycemia, so tolerating higher glucose levels was considered unacceptable or even unethical by clinicians and investigators. The aim of NICE-SUGAR, therefore, was to assess whether further lowering blood glucose levels to less than 108 mg/dL (<6.0 mmol/L) in a broad context of clinical practice in ICUs, predominantly located in Australia and New-Zealand, and using the normal daily clinical practice tools available would exert additional benefit. Contrary to expectations, NICE-SUGAR revealed that targeting 108 mg/dL with insulin *increased* 90-day mortality from 24.9% to 27.5% as compared with the 140 to 180 mg/dL (8-10 mmol/L) glucose target. Excess deaths were attributed to cardiovascular causes.

COIITSS

Patients with septic shock requiring administration of glucocorticoids are faced with a high mortality risk; the severity of illness and glucocorticoid treatment make hyperglycemia common. Therefore, this would be an optimal population in whom to study whether TGC could reduce mortality. In the Corticosteroids and Intensive Insulin Therapy for Septic Shock (COIITSS) multicenter study, 509 patients were randomized to either intensive insulin therapy aiming for blood glucose levels between 80 and 110 mg/dL or to conventional insulin therapy.[37] In the latter group, an intermediate target was used, as the physicians were recommended to follow the 2004 Surviving Sepsis Campaign Guidelines (blood glucose levels < 150 mg/dL [8.3 mmol/L]). Hospital mortality in the intensive insulin therapy group (45.9%) did not differ from the conventional group (42.9%). Poor separation of the blood glucose levels between the study groups and the small size of the study may have made it hard to detect any treatment effect of TGC.

META-ANALYSES

Nowadays, practice guidelines ideally are based on systematic reviews and meta-analyses. The two most recent meta-analyses showed that in critically ill adult patients, TGC did not significantly reduce hospital mortality but is associated with an increased risk of hypoglycemia.[38,39] However, TGC may be beneficial to patients admitted to a surgical ICU.

Critical Appraisal of the Evidence for Tight Glycemic Control in the ICU

Given that the effect of controlling blood glucose levels during critical illness ranges from benefit, to no effect, to potentially harmful, most clinicians are now in agreement that blood glucose levels do in fact play a role in patient outcome. The pre-2001 era where blood glucose levels were hardly measured in critically ill patients has passed forever. However, discrepancies in the study results have made it difficult to make strong recommendations. Likewise, consensus statements on glycemic management of hospitalized patients by the American Association of Clinical Endocrinologists and the American Diabetes Association have changed significantly over the last years.[40] While the 2004 and 2006 statements recommended stricter targets for glycemic management in the ICU, in 2009 it was advised that the starting threshold for intravenous insulin therapy in the ICU should be 180 mg/dL (10 mmol/L). And once started, blood glucose levels should be maintained between 140 and 180 mg/dL (7.8-10 mmol/L). Somewhat lower levels may be appropriate in selected patient populations. Targets below 110 mg/dL (<6.1 mmol/L) are not recommended.

Still, more can be learned from the differences between the Leuven proof-of-concept studies and the subsequent repeat trials.[41] First, "normoglycemia" was compared with distinct "control" targets (140-180 mg/dL or 8-10 mmol/L in NICE-SUGAR and GLUCONTROL; 180-215 mg/dL or 10-12 mmol/L in Leuven), making the studies fundamentally different. The control group in the Leuven studies reflected the assumption of hyperglycemia as a potentially beneficial adaptation. Hence, a "do-not-touch" approach unless glucose exceeded the renal threshold of 215 mg/dL was used in this group. In contrast, the NICE-SUGAR trial was executed in the "flatter" part of the observational glycemia-mortality risk curve, with 70% of the patients in the control group receiving insulin treatment to target an intermediate blood glucose level of 140 to 180 mg/dL (8-10 mmol/L) (Figure 164-2).[16-19] The control group in NICE-SUGAR, as a result of the changed usual care, already could have benefited from reducing blood glucose as compared with the control group in Leuven. The lower observed mortality than the carefully documented expected mortality (24.9% versus

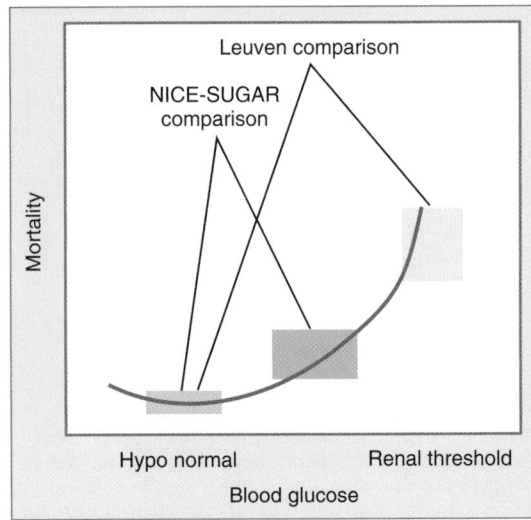

Figure 164-2 Comparing tight glycemic control with "usual care" strongly depends on mortality risk in the control group. In the Leuven proof-of-concept studies, tight glycemic control was compared with the usual care of tolerating hyperglycemia up to the renal threshold (215 mg/dL). The control group in the NICE-SUGAR trial targeted intermediate blood glucose levels (145-180 mg/dL).

30%, respectively) in the NICE-SUGAR control group may indeed suggest that there was already such a benefit in the control group.

Second, the level of therapy compliance, in this case the degree of success in reaching and maintaining the preset target range for glucose in the intervention group, as well as the degree of overlap with the control group, varied greatly between the studies. The methodological aspects of glucose measurement and the level of expertise of the nursing team with blood glucose control in the Leuven studies may have played a key role. In the Leuven studies, 70% of the patients in the intervention group were on average in target,[42] whereas this was much less than 50% in NICE-SUGAR and in several of the other repeat studies. This could be important, as a recent meta-analysis suggested that studies that actually managed to adequately achieve the blood glucose target showed a reduced mortality, whereas studies that did not succeed in reaching the target reported no benefit or even increased mortality.[38,43] Maintaining normoglycemia may be more feasible in patients after surgical critical illness than in those with medical illnesses.

Third, a requirement for safe insulin dose adjusting to reach and maintain normoglycemia is a standardized, accurate glucose measurement technology. In NICE-SUGAR, a variety of glucose meters were allowed, whereas most of them have recently been shown to be unsuitable for this purpose.[44] Accuracy of certain glucometers has been shown to be extremely poor in the ICU setting, and the wide error goes in the opposite direction for the low and high glucose ranges, making it impossible to use them for targeting a very narrow glucose range.[45,46] In addition, varying sampling sites (arterial, venous, and capillary) were accepted in the context of routine clinical practice, and these too have led to erroneous results for blood glucose.[47] Inaccuracy of glucose measurement may have misguided the insulin titration and thereby induced (undetected) hypoglycemia and large blood glucose fluctuations. Avoiding highly variable blood glucose levels requires experience and thus has a learning curve, which is inherent with complex interventions.

Fourth, feeding strategies differed in the major studies. The substantially higher amounts of parenteral nutrition in the Leuven studies, although still on average below normal caloric requirements, may have increased the severity of stress-induced hyperglycemia, and thus the intervention may have been in part directed to counteract this side effect of parenteral nutrition. In NICE-SUGAR, feeding relied almost exclusively on the enteral route (80 kcal intravenous glucose on the first day; on average a total of 880 kcal/d), whereas in Leuven, early parenteral nutrition (768 kcal on the first day) supplemented insufficient enteral feeding, resulting in an average 1100 kcal/d for adult patients. Insulin treatment in a nutritionally deprived state early in the disease course, as in NICE-SUGAR as a result of their feeding guidelines, may have been deleterious by evoking a global substrate deficit via insulin-induced counteracting of proteolysis, lipolysis, glycogenolysis, and gluconeogenesis, which could be vital in starvation.

Fifth, in a setting where hyperglycemia is triggered by surgery or trauma, the equivalent of acute ischemia/reperfusion, the delay between onset of hyperglycemia and the start of glycemic control is short. In contrast, when ICU patients already suffered from chronic illness prior to ICU admission and hyperglycemia was present for a longer time, adaptive changes to protect the cells against elevated extracellular glucose may have been induced such that acute lowering of blood glucose may be harmful. Alternatively, the time window for prevention of toxicity may have passed and irreversible damage done.[48] Such a mechanism was suggested by the pooled analysis of the two Leuven trials[42] and by the different results of RCTs on glucose control in patients with type 2 diabetes.[49-54]

Finally, insulin therapy induces shift of potassium from the extracellular to the intracellular compartment. This may induce hypokalemia and hypokalemia-induced arrhythmias. By using arterial blood and an accurate point-of-care blood gas analyzer for glucose monitoring with each blood glucose check, potassium levels can be measured and corrected when needed.

All these differences may have contributed to the different outcomes in different studies. It has become clear that results from single-center, proof-of-concept studies cannot simply be repeated in large multicenter effectiveness trials, certainly when studying the effects of a complex intervention which is too often incompletely implemented in the repeat studies.[55] Hence, in reality, such studies did not investigate the same intervention as the proof-of-concept study.

Biological Rationale for Tight Glycemic Control

Research using human material, animal models, and in vitro systems has unraveled potential mechanistic explanations for the beneficial effects of TGC (Table 164-1). As in diabetes mellitus, insulinization to lower blood glucose levels exerts its effects on a wide array of biological pathways. Striving for metabolic control and inhibiting excess inflammation and mitochondrial damage seem of chief importance. Further molecular biology research will not only be essential to fine-tune TGC

TABLE 164-1	Studies of Biological Effects of Tight Glycemic Control Also Point to Its Potential Benefit		
Pathway	*Critical Illness*	*Effect IIT*	*References*
Insulin Resistance and Glucose Uptake			
Circulating insulin	Transient ↑, then ↓	Transient ↑	56, 57
Circulating C-peptide	Transient ↑, then ↓	↓	56
Circulating adiponectin (insulin-sensitizing hormone)	↓	↑	56, 58
Liver			
Insulin signaling	↓	=	56
Gluconeogenesis (phosphoenolpyruvate carboxykinase mRNA)	↑	=	59
Cytokines, growth hormone, glucagon, cortisol	↑ in acute phase	≈ , ↑ , ? , ↓	57, 60-62
Glucose uptake and glycogen synthesis (glucokinase mRNA)		=	63
Insulin-like growth factor binding protein-1 mRNA and circulating levels	↑	=	59
Skeletal Muscle			
Insulin signaling	↓	↑	56
Glucose transporter-4	↓	↑	63
Hexokinase-II	↓	↑	63
Cellular Energy Provision			
Microcirculation	↓		
Endothelial activation, endothelium-mediated vasorelaxation	↑, ↓	↓, ↑	60, 64
Perfusion and oxygen supply	↓	=	65, 66
Endothelial nitric oxide synthase, inducible nitric oxide synthase	↓, ↑	=, ↓	60, 67
Endogenous nitric oxide synthase inhibitor asymmetric dimethylarginine	↑	↓	67-69
Mitochondrial function	↓	↑	65, 70, 71
Toxic glucose metabolites compromising mitochondrial function (dicarbonyls)	↑	↓	70
Oxidative stress	↑	↓	70
Inflammation, Innate Immunity, Coagulation			
C-reactive protein	↑	↓	27, 72, 73
Cytokines	↑	≈	57, 60
Mannose-binding lectin	↑	↓	73
Monocyte phagocytosis and oxidative burst	↓	↑	64, 72
Coagulation	abnormal	=	57
Fibrinolysis	↑	=, ↑	57, 74
Anabolism			
Skeletal muscle protein content	↓	(↑)	71
Insulin-like growth factor-1	↓	↓	61
Myocardial Function			
Myocardial contractility	↓	↑	64
Myocardial damage	↑	↓	27
Bile and Lipid Abnormalities			
Hypertriglyceridemia	↑	↓	63, 75
Free fatty acids	↑	↓	75
HDL and LDL cholesterol	↓	↑	63
Cholestatic liver dysfunction and biliary sludge	↑	↓	76
Glucose and triglyceride storage in adipose tissue	↑	=	15
Adipocyte size	↓	=	15
Macrophage infiltration in adipose tissue	↑	↓	15

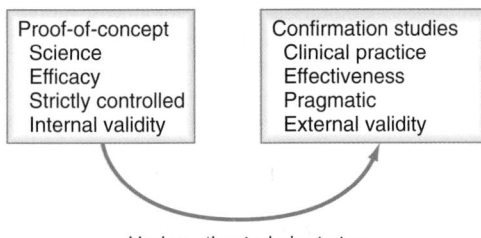

Figure 164-3 Difference between proof-of-concept studies and confirmation studies. Proof-of-concept studies are driven by the specific question of whether a certain intervention may work (efficacy). The intervention is tested in a highly controlled setting to minimize confounding factors, resulting in high internal validity. In contrast, confirmation studies wonder whether this intervention would work in clinical practice (effectiveness). Potential confounders are allowed to test the generalizability and pragmatic character of the intervention (external validity). When testing complex interventions, these differences between proof-of-concept and confirmation studies in aim and setup are often underestimated.

with other metabolic treatment strategies, it will also contribute to the quest to explain the potential harm of glucose lowering in critical illness.

IMPLICATIONS FOR DAILY PRACTICE

The failure to repeat the results from well-controlled, meticulously executed, proof-of-concept studies in large pragmatic confirmation trials has indicated that the TGC is not yet ready to be broadly implemented in every ICU across the globe (Figure 164-3). This does not undermine the scientific validity of the benefits of TGC in critically ill patients. Blood glucose levels should be normalized as much as safely possible without causing a too-rapid lowering of blood glucose, without an increase in the incidence of hypoglycemia, and without large blood glucose fluctuations. Therefore it is advisable to gradually tighten glycemic control under diligent monitoring of the safety aspects. Nevertheless, three conditions should always be met:

1. Accurate and frequent blood glucose measurements as a reliable invasive, continuous glucose sensor is not yet available. Capillary blood samples are unreliable in the ICU and should never be used. Blood glucose measurements on on-site blood gas analyzers are currently the preferred devices. However, the use of a single handheld blood glucose meter with an acceptable error range and using arterial blood may be an alternative.
2. Continuous intravenous insulin administration using accurate syringe pumps

3. Thorough training of ICU healthcare providers (i.e., physicians and nurses) in the execution of the complex intervention of TGC. This stimulates intuitive and anticipating decision making, as computer algorithms to assist in TGC still have to show their benefit on patient outcome.

Conclusion

The discrepancy in study quality and results do not permit clear-cut, evidence-based recommendations for one optimal blood glucose target in heterogeneous ICU populations and settings. One could recommend keeping blood glucose levels between 80 and 130 mg/dL (4.4-7.2 mmol/L). A broader target range would partially compensate for the inaccuracies of handheld blood glucose meters and allow more inexperienced ICU teams to implement targeted glycemic control. Trying to steer blood glucose levels within a narrow range without proper measurement devices and experience may cause large blood glucose variations and hypoglycemia. Therefore, frequent and reliable measurements of blood glucose remain mandatory.

KEY POINTS

1. "Stress hyperglycemia" results from the interplay of an increased hepatic glucose output and a decreased insulin-dependent glucose uptake in skeletal muscle. Adipose tissue seems to shift from insulin-dependent to insulin-independent glucose uptake.

2. Stress hyperglycemia was once regarded as a beneficial response. Nevertheless, large observational studies showed a J-shaped association between blood glucose levels and mortality risk in critically ill patients. In patients with established diabetes mellitus, this relationship is significantly blunted. As such, new-onset hyperglycemia is associated with a higher mortality risk than hyperglycemia in patients with diabetes mellitus.

3. In 2001, a large proof-of-concept study challenged the classic dogma that so-called stress hyperglycemia up to 12 mmol/L (220 mg/dL) is a beneficial response in nondiabetic patients. Glycemic control at less than 6.1 mmol/L (110 mg/dL) with exogenous insulin reduced mortality and morbidity among critically ill patients in a surgical ICU.

4. Two other single-center studies from the Leuven investigators showed similar effects of tight glycemic control in medical and pediatric ICU patients. However, several repeat studies could not confirm the beneficial effects of tight glycemic control. The NICE-SUGAR multicenter trial even showed an increased mortality risk by tight glycemic control.

5. Differences in patient populations, blood glucose control in the "usual care" group, nutritional strategies, and methodology of blood glucose measurements may all have contributed to the variability in the treatment effect of tight glycemic control.

ANNOTATED REFERENCES

Mizock BA. Alterations in fuel metabolism in critical illness: hyperglycaemia. Best Pract Res Clin Endocrinol Metab 2001;15:533-51.
   This article gives a concise overview of the changes in the carbohydrate mechanism during critical illness.
Van den Berghe G, Wouters P, Weekers F, et al. Intensive insulin therapy in critically ill patients. N Engl J Med 2001;345:1359-67.
   This paper reported on the first large (N = 1548) prospective, randomized, controlled single-center study showing that insulin-titrated maintenance of normoglycemia (less than 110 mg/dL) during intensive care improves outcome of (surgical) ICU patients.
NICE-SUGAR Study Investigators, Finfer S, Chittock DR, Su SY, Blair D, Foster DA, Dhingra V, et al. Intensive versus conventional glucose control in critically ill patients. N Engl J Med 2009;360: 1283-97.

This manuscript reports on the increased mortality risk of tight glycemic control (<110 mg/dL) in comparison with an intermediate blood glucose target (140-180 mg/dL) during critical illness in a large (N = 6100) multicenter trial.
Van den Berghe G, Schetz M, Vlasselaers D, Hermans G, Wilmer A, Bouillon R, et al. Clinical review: intensive insulin therapy in critically ill patients: NICE-SUGAR or Leuven blood glucose target? J Clin Endocrinol Metab 2009;94:3163-70.
   This article gives insight on the potential causes why tight glycemic control had different treatment effects in repeat studies in contrast to the proof-of-concept studies.

REFERENCES

Access the complete reference list online at http://www.expertconsult.com.

165

Adrenal Insufficiency

HERWIG GERLACH

The adrenal gland is an important endocrine organ that supports the human organism's reaction to factors threatening the integrity of the body, either acutely or in a more chronic/adaptive manner. During the stress response, the central nervous system (CNS) induces activation of both the sympathoadrenergic system (by release of catecholamines) and the hypothalamic-pituitary (HPA) axis (by release of steroid hormones, glucocorticoids and mineralocorticoids), with the target of maintaining homeostasis by influencing metabolic, cardiovascular, immunologic, and endocrine functions. In this context, the adrenal gland plays the key role, combining the location for synthesis and expression of catecholamines, glucocorticoids (GC), androgenic hormones, and factors of the renin-angiotensin-aldosterone (RAA) system. Acute and chronic inflammatory diseases include stimulation of the HPA axis by the immune system, thereby leading to morphologic and functional changes, especially of the adrenal cortex. This phenomenon has been described for acute infectious diseases as well as for other forms of severe sepsis and septic shock.

Over 50 years ago, the seminal observation was made that administering an adrenal cortical steroid extract to a patient with progressive, active rheumatoid arthritis stopped the disease. This soon led to the development of synthetic adrenal cortical steroids, which gained a remarkable reputation in the treatment of a wide range of inflammatory and autoimmune disorders. However, it soon became apparent that this efficacy did not come without a cost in terms of potentially serious adverse effects. In patients with severe sepsis and septic shock, negative results of trials with high doses of glucocorticoids evoked skepticism over the years. Meanwhile, two large trials revealed contradictory results with low doses of corticosteroids in patients with septic shock. Hence, there is still controversy about which patients profit best from this therapy and how to define and evaluate adrenal gland disorders. This chapter will review recent data and focus on the clinical relevance of adrenal insufficiency in critical care.

Historical Review

"The unknown function of the adrenal gland safeguards this organ against annoying questions in medical science."
— Hyrtl, *Textbook of Anatomy*, 19th Century

In 1564, the Roman anatomist, Bartholomeus Eustachius (1520-1570), discovered the adrenal gland as "glandulae quae renibus incumbent"—glands with an unknown function. Multiple hypotheses on its possible role were posited over centuries, such as that by the anatomist Adrianus Spigelius (1570-1625), who described the adrenal gland as the "upholstering space holder" between kidney and diaphragm. In 1855, Thomas Addison (1793-1860) first described a phenomenon wherein the only pathologic finding in some deceased patients was a morphologic destruction of the adrenal gland. He concluded that this organ must have a crucial function, and he called the syndrome *Morbus Addison* (Addison's disease). One year later, Brown-Séquard confirmed his hypothesis after performing a series of bilateral adrenalectomies in cats, demonstrating that these endocrine glands were necessary for life. Addison's conclusions, however, were not accepted, and even 2 years after his death, the famous pathologist, Rudolf Virchow, declared that he had never heard such an illogical statement.

In the 19th and early 20th century, several key findings were made. In 1856, von Koelliker described the anatomic division of the adrenal gland into cortex and medulla; and in 1903, Biedl confirmed that the adrenal cortex is the essential part. In 1894, epinephrine (adrenaline) was isolated from the adrenal medulla as the first hormone. Its chemical structure was described 3 years later, and in 1901, epinephrine was synthesized. In patients with Addison's disease, however, the administration of epinephrine had no success, whereas the use of an animal extract of the adrenal cortex was life saving. Purification techniques were rapidly improved, and the resulting "Cortin" was the first-choice drug for treatment of Addison's disease until the middle of the 20th century. Three independent groups of biochemists (Kendall, Winterstein, and Reichstein) successfully isolated 17-hydroxy-11-dehydrocorticosterone (later called *cortisone*) from the adrenal cortex; the physiologic compound, cortisol, was first described by Reichstein in 1937. The extraction of cortisone, however, remained arduous and uneconomical. Bovine adrenal glands of more than 20,000 animals were necessary to produce 1 kg of cortisone. The first synthesis and pharmaceutical preparation of cortisone was described in 1947 by an industrial company. Until that time, cortisone was only used in patients with Addison's disease.

In the same decade, Hench and Kendall, two rheumatologists at the Mayo Clinic, found that in patients with different forms of rheumatism, the symptoms showed temporary remissions during pregnancy and inflammatory diseases like hepatitis. They speculated that this might be due to a general stimulation of the endocrine system and concluded that the use of cortisone might be beneficial in patients with acute rheumatoid arthritis. In September 1948, a female bedridden patient with severe and painful rheumatism that was resistant to all standard therapies at the time was the first documented case of cortisone treatment for inflammatory disease. After 3 days, the patient was able to stand up; 1 week later, she left the clinic without pain and on her own feet. Retrospectively, the speculations regarding pregnancy and hepatitis were obviously wrong, but the antiinflammatory character of cortisone was a key finding in pharmaceutical research. In contrast to Selye, who described cortisone as a crucial promoter of the physiologic stress response, the aforementioned finding that the adrenal gland cortex is the location for endogenous production of cortisone, an important inhibitor of stress and inflammation, has been confirmed. In 1950, Kendall, Hench, and Reichstein received the Nobel Prize in Medicine for their historical findings on the physiologic role of the adrenal gland.[1-4]

Anatomy of the Adrenal Gland

The two paired adrenal glands are located in the retroperitoneal soft tissue near the top of each kidney. In neonates, the adrenal glands are relatively large (approximately one-third of the kidney's size) compared with other organs. In the postnatal period, the cortex portion shrinks, leading not only to a relatively but also an absolutely smaller size of the organ. In adults, each adrenal gland weighs 4 to 5 g, has a flat form with a sagittal diameter of less than 1 cm, a transverse diameter of 3 cm, and a crani-caudal diameter of 4 to 5 cm. The right gland has a triangle/pyramid-like shape, whereas the left organ is shaped like a half-moon. The adrenal gland is composed of two embryologically distinct tissues. The adrenal cortex develops during the 5th week of gestation from a clump of mesodermal cells within the urogenital ridge known as the *adrenal primordium*. Later, during the 12th week of gestation, the adrenal medulla develops from neuroectodermal cells of the embryonic neural tube. In the fetal period, the cortex surrounds the medullar cells, resulting in the typical "sandwich" structure, consisting of a flat grey medulla with a yellow cortex.

The circulatory supply, with a flow rate of about 5 mL per minute, is maintained by up to 50 arterial branches from the aorta, renal arteries, and inferior phrenic arteries for each adrenal gland. Blood flow is directed from the capsule into the subcapsular arteriolar plexus through the cortex towards the medulla, where a single vein drains the blood entering the vena cava or the renal vein, respectively. A direct blood supply to the medulla is maintained by medullary arteries.

The adrenal cortex receives afferent and efferent innervation. Direct contact of nerve terminals with adrenocortical cells has been suggested, and chemoreceptors and baroreceptors present in the adrenal cortex infer efferent innervation. Diurnal variation in cortisol secretion and compensatory adrenal hypertrophy are influenced by adrenal innervation. Splanchnic nerve innervation has an effect in regulating adrenal steroid release. The adrenal medulla secretes the catecholamines, epinephrine and norepinephrine, that affect blood pressure, heart rate, sweating, and other activities also regulated by the sympathetic nervous system. The adrenal cortex is divided into three layers: (1) the zona glomerulosa, just under the capsule, (2) the zona fasciculata, the middle layer, and (3) the zona reticularis, the innermost net-like patterned area with reticular veins draining into medullary capillaries. The zona glomerulosa exclusively produces the mineralocorticoid, aldosterone; the zonae fasciculate and reticularis produce glucocorticoids and androgens.[5]

Physiology of the Hypothalamic-Pituitary-Adrenal Axis

The adrenal glands are part of a complex system that produces interacting hormones to maintain physiologic integrity, especially during the stress response.[6,7] This system, the *hypothalamic-pituitary-adrenal (HPA) axis*, includes the hypothalamic region which produces corticotropin-releasing hormone (CRH), triggering the pituitary gland. The pituitary gland is composed of two major structures: the adenohypophysis (anterior pituitary) and neurohypophysis (posterior pituitary). The anterior pituitary is responsible for the secretion of corticotropin (adrenocorticotropic hormone [ACTH]), thyroid-stimulating hormone (TSH), growth hormone (GH), β-lipotropin, endorphins, prolactin, luteinizing hormone (LH), and follicle-stimulating hormone (FSH). The posterior pituitary secretes vasopressin (antidiuretic hormone [ADH]) and oxytocin. Corticotropin regulates the production of corticosteroids by the adrenal glands. Hypothalamic neurons receive input from many areas within the CNS; they integrate these inputs and initiate an output to the anterior pituitary via the median eminence. The median eminence secretes releasing hormones into a hypophyseal portal network of capillaries that connect the median eminence with the pituitary hormones.

The anterior pituitary gland secretes corticotropin (ACTH) under stimulation from hypothalamic CRH. ACTH in turn stimulates the synthesis and release of glucocorticoids, mineralocorticoids, and androgenic steroids from the adrenal gland. In terms of a feedback loop, ACTH release is inhibited by glucocorticoids, which act on both the pituitary corticotropic cells and hypothalamic neurons. ACTH is also released during stress, independent of the circulating serum cortisol level. CRH, vasopressin, and norepinephrine act synergistically to increase ACTH release during stress. Endorphinergic pathways also play a role in ACTH regulation. Acute administration of morphine stimulates release of ACTH, while chronic administration blocks ACTH secretion. ACTH and cortisol are secreted normally in a diurnal pattern, with lowest concentrations between 10 PM and 2 AM and highest levels around 8 AM. From a practical point of view, it is important to know about rhythms, because inadequate assessment of endocrine function

must take into account the variability of hormone levels in the blood. Samples obtained at different times can provide useful dynamic information regarding hypothalamic-pituitary-adrenal function. Loss of diurnal rhythm may indicate hypothalamic dysfunction.

The HPA axis is stimulated not only by physical or psychic stress but also by peptides like ADH and cytokines. Thus, the HPA axis plays an important role during infections and immunologic disorders.[8,9] By interaction with the renin-angiotensin-aldosterone system (RAAS) regulating fluid and salt balance, synthesis of androgens (e.g., dehydroepiandrosterone) with possible impact on immunomodulation, and the sympathoadrenergic system, the HPA axis is probably the most important organ of stress response. Stimulation of the immune system by infections induces the release of proinflammatory cytokines like tumor necrosis factor alpha (TNF-α), interleukin (IL)-1β, or IL-6. Following a cascade, these cytokines stimulate both the hypothalamus and the anterior pituitary gland, which finally leads to the release of glucocorticoids. IL-6 is also able to induce steroid release directly from the adrenal gland. The adequate increase of glucocorticoid levels during inflammation is a crucial factor for appropriate stress response. In acute infections, this release maintains metabolic and energy integrity. If the process is chronic, the HPA axis develops an adaptation which induces typical clinical manifestations such as hypercatabolic states, hyperglycemia, and suppression of androgens and growth and thyroid hormones. These changes, however, may increase the risk for secondary infections. Increased cortisol levels suppress higher regulatory levels of the HPA axis in terms of a negative feedback loop. Hence, after major surgery or during sepsis and septic shock, high cortisol and low ACTH levels are detectable.[10,11] Even the infusion of dexamethasone or CRH is not able to suppress increased cortisol levels in these patients.[12,13] This phenomenon leads to the question of how cortisol release is induced. Several investigations demonstrated that adrenal cortisol synthesis in critically ill patients is not regulated by ACTH, but by paracrine pathways via endothelin, atrial natriuretic peptide (ANP), or cytokines like IL-6.[14-16] IL-6 directly induces the adrenal cortex to release cortisol, which in chronic courses, can worsen the prognosis.[17]

Cellular Response to Adrenocortical Hormones and Related Drugs

Cortisol, the major free circulating adrenocortical hormone, is a hydrophobic hormone; being a steroid, it circulates bound to protein. Complexed cortisol-binding globulin (CBG, or transcortin) accounts for about 95% of circulating cortisol, but only the free form is biologically active. Its plasma half-life is 60 to 120 minutes. Cortisol is metabolized by hydroxylation in the liver, and the metabolites are excreted in urine. Steroid hormones enter the cytoplasm of cells where they combine with a receptor protein. Metabolic, immunologic, and hemodynamic responses to adrenocortical steroid hormones are regulated in a very complex manner that includes transactivation, transrepression, posttranscriptional/translational regulation, and nongenomic effects. The immediate nongenomic effects of steroid hormones were primarily attributed to mineralocorticoids (aldosterone). Rapid activation of the sodium-proton exchanger, increase of intracellular Ca^{++}, and activation of second messenger pathways were described.[18,19] A randomized trial in patients during cardiac catheterization revealed that within minutes after aldosterone injection, cardiac index and arterial pressure increased significantly for 10 minutes and returned to baseline afterwards.[20] Interestingly, the genomic effects of aldosterone seemed to be mediated by binding to glucocorticoid (GC) receptors and not to mineralocorticoid receptors.[21] There is evidence that GC, like cortisol, also modulates immune functions by rapid nongenomic effects via nonspecific interactions with cellular membranes and specific binding to membrane-bound GC receptors (GR).[22] Nonspecific membrane effects have been demonstrated for inhibition of sodium and calcium cycling across plasma membranes by impairing Na^+/K^+-ATPase and Ca^{++}-ATPase. Moreover, the rapid activation of lipocortin-1

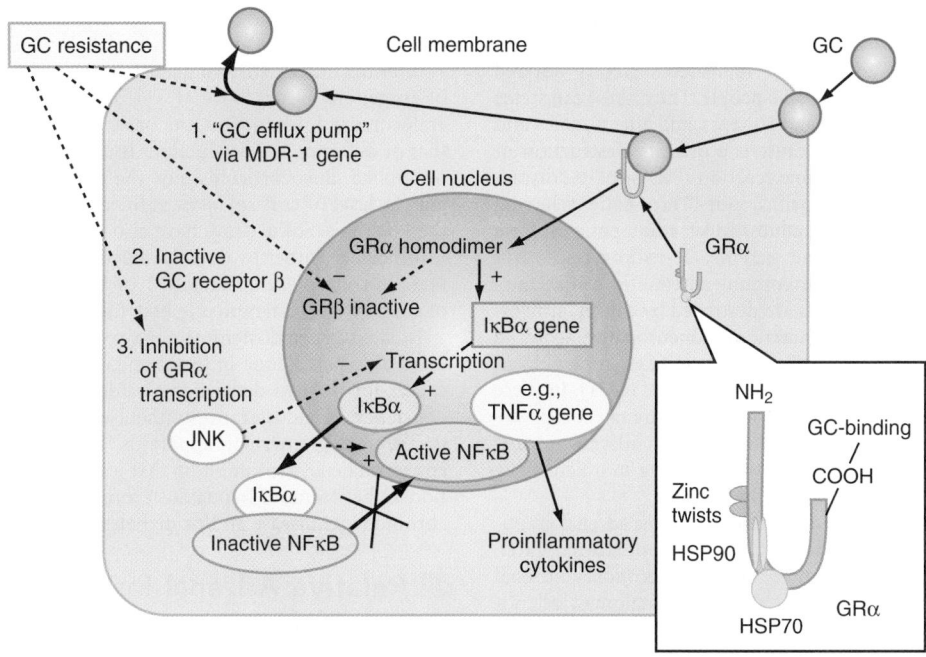

Figure 165-1 **Cellular mechanisms of glucocorticoid effects** *(right)* **and glucocorticoid resistance** *(left)*. After passive transport through the cell membrane, glucocorticoids (GC) bind to the intracellular GC receptor alpha (GRα), which is sequestered in the cytoplasm, bound to the heat-shock protein (HSP) complex that comprises chaperone molecules HSP70 and HSP90. Binding of GC to GRα allows formation of a homodimer which is transported into the nucleus. GR-mediated transcription induces inhibitor kappa B alpha (IκBα), which binds to and inhibits nuclear factor kappa B (NF-κB). Thus, GC inhibits the NF-κB-mediated synthesis of proinflammatory cytokines like tumor necrosis factor alpha (TNFα). Impaired GC sensitivity (GC resistance) includes three major pathways *(dotted arrows)*: (1) decreased cytoplasmatic GC concentrations secondary to increased P-glycoprotein-mediated efflux of GC due to overexpression of the MDR-1 gene; (2) increased expression of a truncated splice variant of the GR which is unable to transactivate GC-sensitive genes (GRβ); and (3) activation of proinflammatory mediators via upstream kinases (JNK), which can directly inhibit GR transcription activity. GC, glucocorticoids; GR, glucocorticoid receptor; HSP, heat shock protein; JNK, c-Jun N-terminal kinase; MDR-1, multidrug resistance gene 1.

and inhibition of arachidonic acid release after GC was independent from GR translocation. Finally, high-sensitivity immunofluorescence staining revealed membrane-bound GR on circulating B lymphocytes and monocytes.[22]

The multiple mechanisms by which GCs modulate cellular responses include mainly genomic pathways.[23-25] Nongenomic effects are thought to account for immediate immune effects of high doses of GC, whereas membrane-bound receptors probably mediate low-dose GC effects. The classic model is that GCs bind to the cytoplasmic ligand-regulated GC receptor alpha (GRα), which is an inactive multiprotein complex consisting of two heat shock proteins (hsp90) acting as molecular chaperones and other proteins (Figure 165-1). Upon GC binding to GRα, conformational change causes dissociation of hsp90, with subsequent nuclear translocation of GRα homodimers, binding of GRα to GC response elements (GRE) of DNA, and transcription of responsive genes (transactivation) such as lipocortin-1 and β₂-adrenoreceptors. Alternatively, GRα may bind to negative GRE (nGRE) and repress transcription of genes (transrepression) such as pro-opiomelanocortin (POMC). More importantly, transrepression without direct binding of GRα to GRE by protein-protein interactions of GRα with transcription factors, nuclear factor kappa B (NF-κB) and AP-1, has been recognized as a key step by which GC suppress inflammation,[26] inhibiting synthesis of TNF-α, IL-1β, IL-2, IL-6, IL-8, inducible nitric oxide synthase (iNOS), cyclooxygenase (COX)-2, cell adhesion molecules, and growth factors, and promoting apoptosis.[27] In addition, NF-κB repression may be mediated by GC-induced up-regulation of the cytoplasmic NF-κB inhibitor, IκBα (see Figure 165-1) which prevents translocation of NF-κB.[28] Clinical investigations provide support for the presence of endogenous GC inadequacy in the control of inflammation and peripheral GC resistance.[29] With GC treatment, the intracellular relations between the NF-κB and GRα signaling pathways change from an initial NF-κB-driven and

GRα-resistant state to a GRα-sensitive one. However, data are conflicting and probably do not explain early (<2 hours) suppressive effects of GC but may account for the longer-term dampening effect of GC on inflammatory processes.[23]

Besides transcriptional regulation, posttranscriptional, translational, or posttranslational processes have been described for GC-induced modulation of COX-2, TNF-α, GM-CSF, IL-1β, IL-6, IL-8, and interferon gamma (IFN-γ).[23] Furthermore, GCs act at multiple levels to regulate iNOS expression by decreased iNOS gene transcription and mRNA stability; reduced translation and increased degradation of the iNOS protein by the cysteine protease, calpain[30]; limitation of the availability of the NOS cofactor, tetrahydrobiopterin; reduced transmembranous transport and de novo synthesis of the NOS substrate, L-arginine; and lipocortin-1-induced inhibition of iNOS.[31,32] Together, these complex mechanisms result in the considerable effect of GC to inhibit inflammation and to stabilize hemodynamics. Finally, GC receptors have been found in nearly every nucleated cell in the body, and since each cell type has its own expression of GC effect, it follows that GCs have many effects in the body, which is equally true of endogenously produced GC hormones or exogenously administered GC medications. Both increase hepatic production of glucose and glycogen and decrease peripheral use of glucose. Steroids also affect fat and protein metabolism. They increase lipolysis both directly and indirectly by elevating free fatty acid levels in the plasma and enhancing any tendency to ketosis. GCs further stimulate peripheral protein metabolism, using the amino acid products as gluconeogenic precursors.

■ Definitions of Adrenal Insufficiency

Adrenal glands may stop functioning when the HPA axis fails to produce sufficient amounts of the appropriate hormones. *Primary adrenal insufficiency* is defined by the inability of the adrenal gland to produce steroid hormones even when the stimulus by the pituitary gland via corticotropin is adequate or increased. Primary adrenal insufficiency affects 4 to 6 out of 100,000 people. The disease can strike at any age, with a peak between 30 and 50 years, and affects males and females about equally. In 70%, the cause is a primary destruction of the adrenal glands by an autoimmune reaction ("classical" Addison's disease or autoimmune adrenalitis), with about 40% of patients having a history of associated endocrinopathies. Most adult patients have antibodies against the steroidogenic enzyme, 21-hydroxylase,[33] but their role in the pathogenesis of autoimmune adrenalitis is uncertain. In the other 30%, the adrenal glands are destroyed by cancer, amyloidosis, antiphospholipid syndrome, adrenomyeloneuropathy, acquired immunodeficiency syndrome (AIDS), infections (e.g., tuberculosis, cytomegaly, fungi), or other identifiable diseases (Box 165-1). In these cases, the typical morphologic changes of the adrenal cortex are atrophy, inflammation, and/or necrosis. In primary adrenal insufficiency, the whole adrenal cortex is involved, resulting in a deficiency of GCs, mineralocorticoids, and adrenal androgenes.[34,35]

Secondary adrenal insufficiency is characterized by adrenal hypofunction due to the lack of pituitary ACTH or hypothalamic CRH. Diseases of the anterior pituitary that can cause secondary adrenal insufficiency include neoplasms (e.g., craniopharyngiomas, adenomas), infarction (e.g., Sheehan's syndrome, trauma), granulomatous disease (e.g., tuberculosis, sarcoidosis), hypophysectomy, and infection.[36] Causes also include hypothalamic dysfunction, such as after irradiation or surgical interventions (see Box 165-1). Because aldosterone secretion is more dependent on angiotensin II than on ACTH, aldosterone deficiency is not a problem in secondary adrenal insufficiency. Selective aldosterone deficiency can occur as a result of depressed renin secretion and angiotensin II formation.[34] Rare patients have an isolated deficiency of CRH,[37] and lymphocytic hypophysitis with subsequent adrenal insufficiency was described in women.[38] These disorders may lead to an isolated ACTH deficiency.[34]

The so-called *tertiary adrenal insufficiency*, which is often summarized together with secondary forms, commonly occurs after withdrawal of exogenous GCs. Many of these patients do well during normal activities but are unable to mount an appropriate GC response to stress. This effect depends on the dose and duration of treatment and varies greatly from person to person. It should be anticipated in any patient who has been receiving more than 30 mg of hydrocortisone per day (or 7.5 mg of prednisolone or 0.75 mg of dexamethasone per day) for more than 3 weeks.[35] If supraphysiologic doses of GCs have been administered to a patient for more than 1 to 2 weeks, the drug should be tapered to allow for adrenal gland recovery. It may take 6 to 12 months for the adrenal glands to recover fully after prolonged use of exogenous GCs.[39] Since ACTH is not a major determinant of mineralocorticoid production, the basic deficit in adrenal insufficiency is that of deficient GC production. It is important that neither the dose of applied glucocorticoids, nor the time of treatment, nor the basal plasma level of cortisol allow sufficient assessment of the function of the HPA axis. Some drugs have also been described to induce adrenal insufficiency, either by directly affecting adrenocortical steroid release (e.g., fluconazole, etomidate)[40,41] or by enhanced hepatic metabolism of cortisol (e.g., rifampicin, phenytoin).[35]

Isolated hypoaldosteronism is very rare and should be suspected in cases of hyperkalemia in the absence of renal insufficiency. The main causes for isolated deficiency of aldosterone secretion are congenital deficiency of aldosterone synthetase, hyporeninemia due to defects in the juxtaglomerular apparatus, or treatment with angiotensin-converting enzyme inhibitors that lead to loss of angiotensin stimulation. Other forms of hypoaldosteronism usually occur in patients with chronic renal disease and/or diabetes mellitus.

Relative Adrenal Insufficiency

The aforementioned forms of adrenal insufficiency which lead to an absolute deficiency of steroids are rare in critically ill patients (0%-3%).[42] They are mostly characterized by morphologic changes of the HPA axis. To reflect the notion that subnormal adrenal corticosteroid production during acute severe illness can also occur without obvious structural defects in the HPA axis, deficiency syndromes due to a dysregulation have been termed *functional adrenal insufficiency*.[43] Functional adrenal insufficiency can develop during the course of an illness and is usually transient.[35] Decreased levels of GCs are registered much more often; these levels might be sufficient in normal subjects but are too low for stress situations, owing to higher need, and are associated with a worse outcome.[44] This led to the concept of *relative adrenal insufficiency* (RAI). The major cause for RAI is inadequate synthesis of cortisol due to cellular dysfunction. Hence, in contrast to absolute adrenal insufficiency, the morphologic changes in RAI may be minor, sometimes characterized by cellular hyperplasia within the adrenal cortex. This is often combined with peripheral GC resistance of the target cells, which is caused by inflammatory events and aggravates the clinical course, although the absolute cortisol serum levels might be normal.[45] In septic shock, RAI may be due to impaired pituitary corticotropin release, attenuated adrenal response to corticotropin, and reduced cortisol synthesis (Figure 165-2).[35,46,47] In addition, cortisol transport capacity to effect sites may be reduced, and response to cortisol may be impaired at the tissue level by cytokines modulating GC receptor affinity to cortisol and/or GC response elements.[48,49] In clinical trials, it was demonstrated that prolonged treatment of systemic inflammation in patients with severe acute respiratory distress syndrome (ARDS) with methylprednisolone can improve the decreased GC response by increasing the GC receptor affinity and reducing the NF-κB-mediated DNA binding and transcription of proinflammatory cytokines.[29] Thus, if RAI can be identified, treatment with supplemental corticosteroids may be of benefit.[35] Prevalence of RAI in the critically ill varied from 0% to 77% with different definitions, cutoff values, study populations, and adrenal function tests[34,35,46,50,51] and may be as high as 50% to 75 % in severe septic shock.[52]

Evaluation of Adrenal Insufficiency

In clinical practice, assessment of adrenal function is difficult, especially in critically ill patients, since the diurnal rhythm is lost. Values indicating normal adrenocortical function are listed in Box 165-2. Normally, serum cortisol concentrations in the morning (8 AM) of less than 3 μg/dL (80 nmol/L) are strongly suggestive of absolute adrenal insufficiency,[53] while values below 10 μg/dL (275 nmol/L) make the diagnosis likely. Basal urinary cortisol and 17-hydroxycorticosteroid

---

Box 165-1

ETIOLOGY OF ADRENAL INSUFFICIENCY

Primary Adrenal Insufficiency
- Autoimmune adrenalitis (Morbus Addison), often with concomitant endocrinopathies
- Hemorrhage (trauma, anticoagulants)
- Infarction, thrombosis
- Tumors
- Infections (tuberculosis, cytomegaly, fungi, AIDS)
- Amyloidosis, hemochromatosis, sarcoidosis
- Congenital hyper- or hypoplasias
- Congenital ACTH resistance
- Adrenomyeloneuropathy

Secondary Adrenal Insufficiency (Lesions of Pituitary and/or Hypothalamic Regions)
- Tumors
- Hemorrhages, apoplexy
- Infections, inflammations
- Autoimmune lesions
- Trauma, surgery
- Radiation
- Congenital syndromes (e.g., familial CBG deficiency)

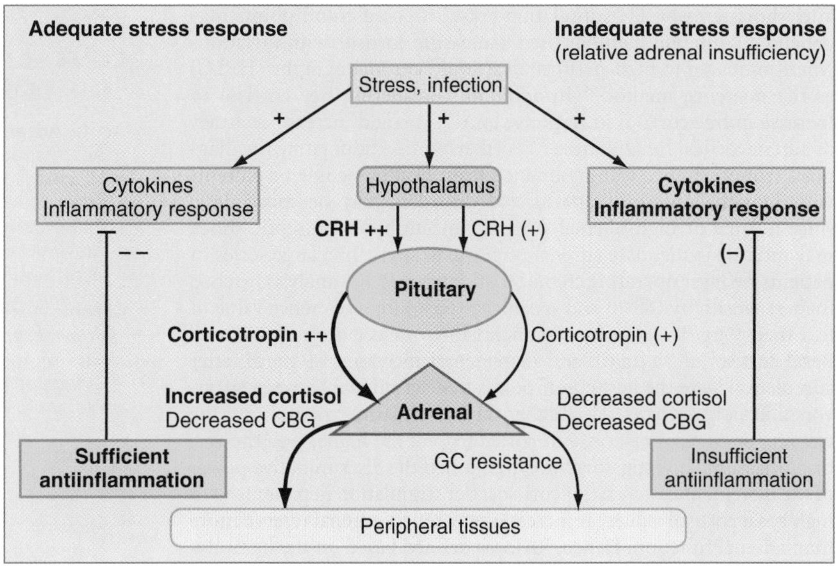

Figure 165-2 Concept of relative adrenal insufficiency (RAI). Unlike in adequate stress response *(left)*, RAI may occur when causal or additional factors impair the function of the hypothalamic-pituitary-adrenal (HPA) axis. This may be due to microcirculatory failure, additional drugs like antibiotics, anesthetic drugs, infections, long-term use of steroids, or hemorrhages. Impaired HPA axis function results in insufficient antiinflammatory response and increased inflammatory response. Plus (+) denotes activation; minus (–), inhibition. CRH, corticotropin-releasing hormone; CBG, cortisol-binding globulin; GC, glucocorticoids.

excretion is low in patients with severe adrenal insufficiency but may be low-normal in patients with partial adrenal insufficiency. Generally, baseline urinary measurements are not recommended for the diagnosis of adrenal insufficiency. To differentiate between primary, secondary, and tertiary adrenal insufficiency in cases of low cortisol, it is recommended to measure plasma ACTH concentrations simultaneously. Inappropriately low serum cortisol concentrations in association with increased ACTH concentrations are suggestive of primary adrenal insufficiency, whereas the combination of low cortisol and ACTH concentrations indicates secondary or tertiary disease. This, however, should be confirmed by stimulation of the adrenal gland with exogenous ACTH. In secondary or tertiary adrenal insufficiency, the adrenal glands release cortisol, whereas in primary adrenal insufficiency, the adrenal glands are partially or completely destroyed and do not respond to ACTH.

ACTH stimulation tests usually consist of administering 250 μg (40 International Units) of ACTH (so-called high-dose ACTH stimulation test). For long-term stimulation tests, which are preferred for differentiating between secondary and tertiary adrenal insufficiency, 250 μg of ACTH are infused either over 8 hours or over 2 days.[54] Serum cortisol and 24-hour urinary cortisol and 17-hydroxycorticosteroid (17-OHCS) concentrations are determined before and after the infusion. This test may be helpful in distinguishing primary from secondary/tertiary adrenal insufficiency. In primary adrenal insufficiency, there is no or a minimal response of plasma or urinary cortisol and urinary 17-OHCS. Increases of these values in the 2 to 3 days of the test are indicative of a secondary/tertiary cause of adrenal insufficiency. In normal subjects, the 24-hour urinary 17-OHCS excretion increases 3- to 5-fold above baseline. Serum cortisol concentrations reach 20 μg/dL (550 nmol/L) at 30 to 60 min and exceed 25 μg/dL (690 nmol/L) at 6 to 8 hours post initiation of the infusion. Today this is not very often used, because clinical manifestations of adrenal insufficiency combined with basal cortisol levels, short-term ACTH stimulation tests, and CRH tests (see later) usually provide sufficient information.

Box 165-2

VALUES INDICATING NORMAL ADRENOCORTICAL FUNCTION

- Plasma cortisol (7-8 AM): 5-25 μg/dL (135-700 nmol/L)
- Plasma ACTH (7-8 AM): <70 pg/mL
- Urine excretion rate of free cortisol: 20-90 μg/d
- Urine excretion rate of 17-hydroxycorticosteroid (17-OHCS): 4-10 mg/d

A short-term stimulation test with 250 μg ACTH, mostly used for patients who are not critically ill, determines basal serum cortisol levels and the induced-response concentration 30 and 60 minutes after intravenous (IV) administration of ACTH. The advantage of the high-dose test is that pharmacologic plasma ACTH concentrations can be achieved by either IV or intramuscular injection.[55] This way of application, however, may be too high to identify mild cases of secondary adrenal insufficiency or chronic deficiencies.[56] Furthermore, it should not be used when acute secondary adrenal insufficiency (e.g., Sheehan's syndrome) is presumed, since it takes several days for the adrenal cortex to atrophy, and it will still be capable of responding to ACTH stimulation normally. In these cases, a low-dose ACTH test or an insulin-induced hypoglycemia may be required to confirm the diagnosis.[57,58] A rise in serum cortisol concentration after 30 or 60 minutes to a peak of 18 to 20 μg/dL (500 to 550 nmol/L) or more is considered a normal response to a high-dose ACTH stimulation test and excludes the diagnosis of primary adrenal insufficiency and almost all cases of secondary adrenal insufficiency except those of recent onset.[59-61]

To further differentiate between secondary and tertiary adrenal insufficiency, laboratory investigations may be augmented by a CRH stimulation test. In both conditions, cortisol levels are low at baseline and remain low after CRH. In patients with secondary adrenal insufficiency, there is little or no ACTH response, whereas in patients with tertiary disease, there is an exaggerated and prolonged response of ACTH to CRH stimulation which is not followed by an appropriate cortisol response.[62,63] Formerly, the HPA axis was also tested by a stimulated hypoglycemia test. After administering 0.1 units of insulin per kilogram bodyweight, inducing a hypoglycemic state of less than 40 mg/dL serum glucose, an intact HPA axis induces a serum cortisol concentration of more than 20 μg/dL. Nowadays, this procedure is considered obsolete because of the high risk of hypoglycemia.

In critically ill patients, primary causes of absolute or relative adrenal insufficiencies are multiple and often undetectable if no specific hypothesis exists. Volume-resistant septic shock or any other form of life-threatening hypotension with increasing need for catecholamines should give reason to evaluate adrenal function. Formerly, a serum cortisol value less than 20 μg/dL was suggestive for the diagnosis. Meanwhile, it is acknowledged that several factors complicate investigations of the HPA axis in patients with critical illness. A short-term ACTH stimulation test may be performed in critically ill patients suspected of having adrenal insufficiency. However, in most patients, RAI will be present, especially in patients with severe sepsis and septic shock. A clear definition of RAI is still missing, and the pathophysiology is rather complex, which makes it difficult to define clear cutoffs for both basal serum cortisol concentrations and incremental increases after short-term ACTH stimulation tests. Proposed cutoff points may depend on different methods used to measure cortisol, with variations when compared to high-performance liquid chromatography (HPLC) as the reference method.[64] In addition, considering free cortisol or increase in free cortisol in response to ACTH could increase accuracy of adrenocortical function tests.[48] Furthermore, extrapolating the diagnosis from reference values obtained from healthy people or patients with hypothalamic-pituitary-adrenal disorders may be misleading, since normal or high-normal cortisol concentrations in septic shock may indicate inadequate adrenal response to stress. In a large series of patients, receiver operating characteristic curve (ROC) analysis reached highest sensitivity (68%) and specificity (65%) for a reference value of less than 9 µg/dL (incremental increase) to detect nonresponders.[52] Basal cortisol of 34 µg/dL and incremental increase of 9 µg/dL after stimulation were the best cutoff points to discriminate between survivors and nonsurvivors. The higher the basal plasma cortisol and the weaker the cortisol response to corticotropin, the higher was the risk of death. Some investigators have questioned the discriminative power of the incremental increase of cortisol after stimulation in patients with high basal cortisol values, as increases may reflect adrenal reserve more than adrenal function. Hence, RAI was defined based on the hemodynamic response when a randomly measured cortisol was less than 25 µg/dL.[46]

Routine use of the low ACTH stimulation test in critically ill patients cannot be recommended at present, although the low-dose test is preferred in patients with secondary or tertiary adrenal insufficiency.[65] After stimulation with 250 µg ACTH, circulating corticotropin concentrations are 40 to 200 pg/mL during stress but may be as high as 60,000 pg/mL.[35] Stimulation of the adrenal gland with low doses of ACTH (1 µg) was shown to increase sensitivity and specificity to detect adrenal insufficiency in patients with hypothalamic-pituitary-adrenal disorders who respond normally to traditional high-dose stimulation.[35,66-69] The test is performed by measuring serum cortisol concentrations immediately before and 30 minutes after IV injection of ACTH in a dose of 1 µg (160 mIU) per 1.73 m² body surface.[34] This dose stimulates maximal adrenocortical secretion up to 30 minutes post injection, and in normal subjects results in a peak plasma ACTH concentration about twice that of insulin-induced hypoglycemia.[70] A value of 18 µg/dL (500 nmol/L) or more at any time during the test is indicative of normal adrenal function. The advantage of this test is that it can detect partial adrenal insufficiency that may be missed by the standard high-dose test.[57,58]

Using the 1-µg ACTH stimulation test to more precisely uncover patients with RAI in septic shock has been proposed, but the 1-µg stimulation test has not been well validated in critically ill patients and patients with septic shock.[34,35] In addition, studies evaluating low-dose and high-dose ACTH stimulation tests in septic shock may have been flawed by methodological problems. At present, using the 1-µg ACTH stimulation test cannot be recommended routinely until further data from well-designed randomized studies in septic shock patients are available. The current recommendation is to use a three-level therapeutic guide for evaluating RAI in critically ill patients, especially those with septic shock. Patients with a random basal cortisol below 15 µg/dL will likely profit from low-dose corticosteroid therapy, whereas corticosteroid replacement is unlikely to be helpful when basal cortisol is above 34 µg/dL. When a random basal cortisol value is between 15 and 34 µg/dL, adrenocortical stimulation with 250 µg ACTH should discriminate responders (incremental increase ≥ 9 µg/dL) from nonresponders (<9 µg/dL). However, it has been pointed out that no cutoff values will be entirely reliable.[35]

Clinical Symptoms

About 25% of patients with adrenal insufficiency present with adrenocortical crisis.[34] The symptoms are nonspecific and include sudden dizziness, weakness, dehydration, hypotension, and shock (Box 165-3). In many cases, the clinical picture may be indistinguishable from shock due to loss of intravascular fluid volume. Other features such as

---

Box 165-3

CLINICAL MANIFESTATIONS OF ADRENAL INSUFFICIENCY

Acute Adrenal Insufficiency
- Acute apathy
- Nausea, vomiting
- Fever
- Acute dehydration, tachycardia
- Craving for salt
- Hypotension, shock

Chronic Adrenal Insufficiency
- Weakness, fatigue
- Lack of appetite
- Orthostatic hypotension
- Weight loss, anorexia
- Hyperpigmentation (only in primary Addison's disease due to increased ACTH)
- Vitiligo
- Nonspecific gastrointestinal symptoms (diarrhea, nausea, abdominal pain)
- Nonspecific pain (myalgia, arthralgia, headaches)
- Nonspecific psychological symptoms (depression, lack of concentration, confusion, psychosis)
- Hypoglycemia
- Hyponatremia
- Hyperkalemia
- Acidosis, prerenal azotemia
- Lymphocytosis, eosinophilia

---

anorexia, nausea, vomiting, diarrhea, abdominal pain, and delirium may be present, but they are also common in patients with other acute illness. Hence, these symptoms may not be helpful in establishing the diagnosis of adrenal insufficiency and are often misleading. Hypoglycemia is rare in acute adrenal insufficiency but more common in secondary adrenal insufficiency; it is a common manifestation in children and thin women with the disorder. Especially in patients in the intensive care unit (ICU), it remains extremely difficult to recognize an acute, absolute adrenal insufficiency based on clinical symptoms. However, if the diagnosis is missed, the patient will probably die, so the threshold for laboratory investigations in cases of unexplained catecholamine-resistant hypotension should be low. It is important to be mindful that the onset of an acute adrenocortical crisis is not necessarily an acute beginning of the underlying disease itself. The preceding course is often gradual and may go undetected until an acute illness, stress, trauma, pregnancy, or other conditions precipitate adrenal crisis.[34,71]

In most cases, primary adrenal insufficiency is the underlying disorder. Typical symptoms such as hyperpigmentation, scanty axillary and pubic hair, hyponatremia, or hyperkalemia may be diagnosed in the acutely ill patient. Adrenal crisis can occur in patients receiving appropriate doses of GCs if their mineralocorticoid requirements are not met.[72] After spontaneous events (e.g., hemorrhage, myocardial infarction, adrenal vein thrombosis), these signs are absent. If an acute adrenal crisis is suspected, a blood sample should be obtained to confirm the diagnosis. The main clinical problem is hypotension and shock due to acute mineralocorticoid deficiency. This is one reason for the fact that an acute adrenal crisis after secondary adrenal insufficiency is not so typical. However, GC deficiency may also contribute to hypotension by decreasing vascular responsiveness to angiotensin II, norepinephrine, and other vasoconstrictive hormones, reducing the synthesis of renin substrate and increasing production and effects of prostacyclin and other vasodilatory hormones.[73,74] Finally, panhypopituitarism may be associated with symptoms, owing not only to lack of corticotropin but also TSH, gonadotropin, and growth hormone.

In chronic adrenal insufficiency, the major clinical features (see Box 165-3) may be detected but may also be absent if adrenal gland insufficiency develops over a prolonged period of time. There is a stage characterized by normal basal steroid secretion but an inability to respond to stress. Hence, the patient may be asymptomatic. In other cases, there may also be signs and symptoms suggestive of other hormone deficiency such as decreased thyroid and gonadal function. Independent from the underlying cause, the most common clinical manifestations are general malaise, fatigue, weakness, anorexia, weight loss, nausea, vomiting, abdominal pain, arthralgia, postural syncope, diarrhea that may alternate with constipation, hypotension, electrolyte abnormalities (hyponatremia, hyperkalemia, metabolic acidosis), decreased axillary and pubic hair, and loss of libido and amenorrhea in women.[34,71]

In primary adrenal insufficiency, hyperpigmentation and autoimmune manifestations (vitiligo) are typically due to increased ACTH concentrations, whereas this is not seen in secondary or tertiary adrenal insufficiency. Soon after the disease develops, the skin becomes dark, which may appear to be tanning but appears on both sun-exposed and nonexposed areas. Black freckles develop on the forehead, face, and shoulders; a bluish-black discoloration may develop around the lips, mouth, rectum, scrotum, or vagina. Another specific symptom of primary adrenal insufficiency is a craving for salt.[35] Typical laboratory abnormalities are hyponatremia, hyperkalemia, acidosis, slightly elevated creatinine concentrations, mild normocytic anemia, and rarely, hypercalcemia.[35]

In secondary adrenal insufficiency, since production of mineralocorticoids by the zona glomerulosa is mostly preserved, dehydration and hyperkalemia are not present, and hypotension is less prominent than in primary disease. Especially in the early stages, the onset of chronic adrenal insufficiency is often insidious, and the diagnosis may be difficult. Some patients initially present with gastrointestinal symptoms such as nausea, vomiting, diarrhea, and abdominal cramps.[35,75] In other patients, the disease is misdiagnosed as depression or anorexia nervosa.[76,77] Hyponatremia and increased intravascular volume may be the result of "inappropriate" increase in vasopressin secretion. Decreased libido and potency as well as amenorrhea may occur. Hypoglycemia is more common in secondary adrenal insufficiency, possibly due to concomitant growth hormone insufficiency, and in isolated ACTH deficiency. Clinical manifestations of a pituitary or hypothalamic tumor, such as symptoms and signs of deficiency of other anterior pituitary hormones, headache, or visual field defects, may also be present.[34,71] Finally, in young patients suspected of having adrenal insufficiency, delayed growth and puberty would point to the presence of hypothalamic-pituitary disease, as would headaches, visual disturbances, or diabetes insipidus in patients of any age.[35,36] Laboratory screening in patients with chronic adrenal insufficiency usually reveals hyponatremia, hypoglycemia, lymphocytosis, and eosinophilia.[35]

Therapeutic Strategies

Treatment of adrenal insufficiency involves eradication of the precipitating cause (e.g., tumor, infection) and hormone replacement. In acutely ill patients, if the diagnosis of adrenal crisis is suspected but not known, blood should be obtained for measurement of cortisol concentrations, followed by the administration of 250 µg of ACTH in patients with unknown history. Therapy should be started immediately while awaiting results of testing.[78] Dexamethasone (1 mg every 6 hours) may be given as the initial GC replacement, since it does not cross-react with cortisol in the plasma while adrenal testing is being performed. Patients are usually treated with IV fluids in the form of isotonic saline to restore intravascular volume and replace urinary salt losses. Dextrose infusion may be added to prevent hypoglycemia. Hydrocortisone (100 mg IV bolus or over 30 min, followed by continuous infusion of 10 mg/h, or 50 mg every 4 hours, or 75 to 100 mg every 6 hours, resulting in a total daily dose of 240-300 mg hydrocortisone) is frequently given for hormonal replacement.[34,78] However, equivalent GC doses of methylprednisolone or dexamethasone may also be used. Typically, mineralocorticoid replacement therapy is not required in adrenal crisis so long as the patient is receiving isotonic

saline. Prophylactic use of antibiotics is not beneficial, but specific infections should be treated aggressively with appropriate antibiotic therapy.

Once the patient is stable, or in cases of chronic adrenal insufficiency, GCs can be tapered to maintenance doses. Long-term replacement doses consist of hydrocortisone, 30 mg/d, with two-thirds (20 mg) given in the morning and one-third (10 mg) given at night; or prednisone, 7.5 mg in a similar regimen (5 and 2.5 mg, respectively). The daily dose may be decreased to 20 or 15 mg of hydrocortisone as long as the patient's well-being and physical strength are not reduced.[34] The goal should be to use the smallest dose that relieves the patient's symptoms, in order to prevent weight gain and osteoporosis.[34,78,79] If the patient continues to experience weakness or other symptoms of GC deficiency, the dose can be increased. Excessive GC therapy should be avoided so as to minimize complications of this therapy. In addition, a mineralocorticoid effect is provided with fludrocortisone (50-100 µg PO daily) to prevent sodium loss, intravascular volume depletion, and hyperkalemia, especially when the dose of hydrocortisone decreases below 100 mg/d. Therapy can be guided by monitoring blood pressure, serum potassium, and plasma renin activity, which should be in the upper normal range.[34,61] Clinical response, however, is the best indicator of adequacy of replacement. The optimal dosage of mineralocorticoids remains stable over long periods. Excessive mineralocorticoid replacement may cause congestive heart failure, alkalosis, hypokalemia, or hypertension. Patients receiving prednisone or dexamethasone may require higher doses of fludrocortisone to lower their plasma renin activity to the upper normal range, whereas patients receiving hydrocortisone, which has some mineralocorticoid activity, may require lower doses. The mineralocorticoid dose may have to be increased in the summer, particularly if patients are exposed to temperatures above 29°C (85°F). In cases of isolated hypoaldosteronism, treatment includes liberal sodium intake and daily administration of fludrocortisone. In patients with secondary adrenal insufficiency due to panhypopituitarism, replacement with other hormones may also be necessary. In women, the adrenal cortex is the primary source of androgen in the form of dehydroepiandrosterone and dehydroepiandrosterone sulfate. Although the physiologic role of these androgens in women has not been fully elucidated, their replacement is being increasingly considered in the treatment of adrenal insufficiency.[80,81]

Once the patient is stable and on maintenance doses of steroids, ACTH testing can be repeated to document adrenal recovery. Patients with primary adrenal insufficiency require lifelong GC and mineralocorticoid replacement therapy and should carry a card containing information on current therapy, as well as some type of MedicAlert bracelet or necklace with recommendations for treatment in emergency situations. One of the important aspects of the management of chronic primary adrenal insufficiency is patient and family education. Patients should understand the reason for lifelong replacement therapy, the need to increase the dose of GCs during minor or major stress, and how to inject hydrocortisone, methylprednisolone, or dexamethasone in emergencies. Patients should also have supplies of dexamethasone sodium phosphate and should be educated about how and when to administer them. The survival rate for patients with chronic primary adrenal insufficiency has gone from 2 years or less before the availability of steroid replacement to that of the normal population now that GCs are readily available. In acute adrenal insufficiency, prompt recognition and treatment usually result in a favorable outcome, provided the underlying disease process can be treated.

Glucocorticoid Replacement in Patients with Septic Shock

In patients with severe sepsis and septic shock, the individual clinical course is extremely varied. The impact of the primary disease, as well as immunologic factors (cytokines), affect the HPA axis, and functional testing is aggravated. In contrast to the early phase of septic shock, adrenal cortisol release may recover, thus leading to RAI with absolute steroid levels around or even above normal range.[82] In refractory septic shock, prevalence of RAI may be as high as 50% to 75%.[52] Furthermore, dynamic testing is not always available in ICUs, which makes it difficult for the physician considering hormone replacement therapy, because decisions have to be made within hours in severe forms of septic shock to improve prognosis. Rationale for the use of high-dose GCs in infection, sepsis, and shock can be attributed to well-defined antiinflammatory and hemodynamic effects recognized for decades. Proposed mechanisms of protection include improvement of hemodynamic, metabolic, endocrine, and phagocytic functions, resulting in maintenance of normal morphologic-functional status of tissues including brain, liver, heart, kidneys, and adrenals.[83] In addition, GCs were recognized to inhibit key features of inflammation: endothelial cell activation and damage, capillary leakage, granulocyte activation, adhesion and aggregation, complement activation, and formation and release of eicosanoid metabolites, oxygen radicals, and lysosomal enzymes.[84-89]

However, only in one long-term prospective study in humans receiving high doses of methylprednisolone (30-60 mg/kg) or dexamethasone (2-4 mg/kg), including 179 bacteremic septic shock patients over a period of 8 years, were experimental results confirmed and mortality reduced from 38% to 10%.[90] Evidence from another study suggested that prolongation of treatment might have been beneficial, since shock reversal and improved survival occurred after bolus GC application in an early time window but vanished after several days.[91] Two meta-analyses included 9 and 10 randomized trials, respectively, of patients with severe sepsis and septic shock who received up to 42 g of hydrocortisone equivalent or more; both concluded that high doses of corticosteroids were ineffective[92] or harmful.[93] This was confirmed by a large randomized trial in 1987.[94] Patients with proven gram-negative infections probably benefited more from GCs.[92] In one analysis, studies with the highest quality demonstrated worse outcomes with corticosteroids.[93] High-dose GCs were associated with increased risk of secondary infections, mortality,[93] and increased incidence of renal and hepatic dysfunction.[95] Taken together, these results suggest that high-dose GCs failed to be effective in septic shock in the long run, most probably owing to immune system breakdown.

Similar to studies of high-dose GC treatment, numerous randomized controlled trials with low-dose corticosteroids in patients with septic shock also confirmed shock reversal and reduction of vasopressor support within few days after initiation of therapy in most patients.[96-101] In a crossover study, mean arterial pressure and systemic vascular resistance increased during low-dose hydrocortisone treatment, and heart rate, cardiac index, and norepinephrine requirement decreased significantly.[102] All effects were reversible with cessation of hydrocortisone. Some studies indicate that corticosteroid-induced increase of sensitivity to norepinephrine is more pronounced in patients with RAI than in patients without RAI.[46,101] There are multiple potential mechanisms by which corticosteroids may modulate vascular tone. Considerable evidence confirms that cytokine-induced formation of nitric oxide (NO) plays a central role in vasodilation, catecholamine resistance, maldistribution of blood flow, and mitochondrial and organ dysfunction, and that the amount of NO production correlates with shock severity and outcome.[103,104] In a crossover trial, norepinephrine requirement could be reduced by low-dose hydrocortisone in nearly all patients within 1 to 2 days. Hydrocortisone treatment also induced a significant and prolonged decline of nitrite/nitrate levels, which significantly correlated with reduction of norepinephrine requirement during hydrocortisone infusion.[102] Considering the complex genomic and nongenomic actions of corticosteroids described earlier, it is probable that NO is not the only target. However, inhibition of NO synthesis by hydrocortisone at least contributes to shock reversal.

It is recognized that GCs modulate the stress response in a very complex manner that includes not only antiinflammatory and immunosuppressive actions to protect the host from overwhelming inflammation, but also immune-enhancing effects.[27] The final effect of corticosteroids may be dependent on multiple factors such as the dose,

type of cell or tissue, time point of action, and the balance of proinflammatory and antiinflammatory cofactors. Markers of the inflammatory response, antiinflammatory response, granulocyte, monocyte, and endothelial activation, antigen-presenting capacity, and innate immune response were investigated in septic shock patients.[102] Hydrocortisone significantly attenuated inflammatory and antiinflammatory responses as well as granulocyte, monocyte, and endothelial activation. Monocyte HLA-DR expression was depressed, but receptor downregulation was limited and followed by a rebound increase after drug withdrawal.[102] One could thus conclude that the immune effects of low-dose hydrocortisone treatment in septic shock may be characterized as immunomodulatory rather than immunosuppressive. Attenuation of a broad spectrum of the inflammatory response without causing severe immunosuppression might be a promising therapeutic approach, which goes far beyond hemodynamic stabilization.

Although data on outcome in septic shock patients after low-dose corticosteroid treatment are limited, up to 300 mg hydrocortisone per day may improve survival. In most trials with low-dose corticosteroids,[96-100] 28-day all-cause mortality was reduced, whereas in high-dose trials, there was no significant effect. In a multicenter trial in 300 patients with severe volume and catecholamine-refractory septic shock, survival time was significantly increased in patients with RAI but not in responders to ACTH.[97] Similar results were obtained for ICU and hospital mortality, but not for 1-year follow-up. Significant increases of serious adverse events during treatment with low-dose hydrocortisone have not been reported. The incidence of gastrointestinal bleeding, superinfections, or hyperglycemia has not been different in patients treated with corticosteroids or placebo, and wound infections were even less frequent in patients treated with low-dose hydrocortisone.[97] These findings were not confirmed by another large randomized trial, the Corticosteroid Therapy of Septic Shock (CORTICUS) trial[105] which, however, used different inclusion criteria. Only patients who were successfully resuscitated by volume therapy plus applied vasopressor were included.[105] These contradictory results led the Surviving Sepsis Campaign to redefine their guidelines in 2008,[106] recommending the use of low-dose GCs only for patients who are not responding adequately to volume plus vasopressor therapy—that is, those who are still hypotensive.[106]

Treatment with low-dose hydrocortisone may induce an increase of sodium levels within a few days, and hypernatremia with values over 155 mmol/L have been reported during prolonged treatment.[100] Nevertheless, the indication for low-dose corticosteroids should be weighed against possible risks, and treatment should be limited to the duration of volume- and vasopressor-restrictive hypotension.

Dosing of hydrocortisone in septic shock is similar to adrenal crisis (100 mg initial bolus, followed by 200-300 mg per day), and the dose should be tapered when the patient stabilizes. Hydrocortisone should be preferred, although a comparative study of different corticosteroids has not been performed in septic shock, since most experience of low-dose corticosteroid treatment in septic shock was derived from studies using hydrocortisone (see earlier). Furthermore, hydrocortisone is the synthetic equivalent to the physiologic final active compound, cortisol, so treatment with hydrocortisone directly replaces cortisol independently from metabolic transformation. Finally, in contrast to dexamethasone, hydrocortisone has intrinsic mineralocorticoid activity. A recent randomized trial demonstrated that the addition of oral fludrocortisone to low-dose hydrocortisone has no benefit in septic shock patients.[107] It has not been established whether a weight-adjusted regimen (e.g., 0.18 mg/kg/h)[56] of continuous hydrocortisone infusion is superior to a fixed regimen; moreover, a comparative study of bolus versus infusion regimens has not been performed so far. Patients should be weaned from low-dose hydrocortisone over several days to avoid hemodynamic and immunologic rebound effects. In patients with septic shock, abrupt cessation of low-dose hydrocortisone was followed by significant reversal of many hemodynamic and immunologic effects observed during corticosteroid therapy, even after a short treatment period of 3 days.[102] Adrenal function tests with 250 μg ACTH can be performed in patients with septic shock; however, at present it cannot be recommended to exclude responders or patients with high random cortisol values from low-dose corticosteroid therapy.[35] When basal serum cortisol concentrations are less than 15 μg/dL in septic shock, low-dose hydrocortisone replacement is recommended; levels of over 34 μg/dL are considered sufficient. Between 15 and 34 μg/dL, an incremental increase of less than 9 μg/dL serum cortisol makes relative adrenal insufficiency likely, and therapy may be considered according to the clinical state.[35] Other recommendations prefer a randomly assigned cutoff level of below 25 μg/dL serum cortisol.[46] The routine use of the low ACTH stimulation test (1 μg ACTH) cannot be recommended at present until further data from well-designed randomized studies in septic shock patients are available. Most importantly, it has to be realized that all the aforementioned studies were performed in patients with catecholamine-resistant septic shock. So far there are no data justifying the use of low-dose steroids in patients with sepsis and severe sepsis. Significant effects on outcome have been observed only in patients with systolic blood pressure below 90 mm Hg despite vasopressor therapy.[97] It is not yet known whether low-dose corticosteroids are also effective in patients with less severe shock. Sufficient data on the dose-response characteristics of GCs in septic patients are still lacking, and the current recommended strategy using 200 to 300 mg hydrocortisone per day is based on empirical recommendations; further investigations are needed.

Further Implications for Anesthesia and Critical Care

Surgical stress increases serum cortisol levels five- to sixfold postoperatively, with return to normal at 24 hours unless stress continues. Patients who have received GCs equivalent to 30 mg/d cortisol for longer than 3 weeks may have impairment in this stress response, and steroid supplementation should be considered. However, short-term treatment of heterogeneous groups of patients with critical illness is controversial, and supraphysiologic doses of GCs are not beneficial and may even be harmful.[108] Hence, outside the situations in which benefit has been proved, supraphysiologic doses of GCs (e.g., 30 mg methyl-prednisolone per kilogram of body weight per day) in patients with critical illness are not indicated. Some successful indications, however, have been described: in patients with unresolving ARDS, pharmacologic doses (2 mg methylprednisolone/kg/d) reduced mortality and improved organ function.[29] Furthermore, early treatment with dexamethasone may decrease morbidity in bacterial meningitis,[109,110] although a recent meta-analysis was less enthusiastic.[111] The positive effects of steroid treatment on tissue-specific resistance to GCs have already been described. However, despite the frequent suggestion that unexplained intraoperative hypotension and even death reflect unrecognized hypocortisolism, there is no evidence that primary adrenal insufficiency is a likely explanation for this response.

Patients with known chronic adrenal insufficiency must be advised to double or triple the dose of hydrocortisone temporarily whenever they have any febrile illness or injury.[34] In stressful situations or during major surgery, trauma, burns, or medical illness, high doses of GCs up to 10 times the daily production are required to avoid an adrenal crisis, although no data from randomized trials are available. A continuous infusion of 10 mg of hydrocortisone per hour or the equivalent amount of dexamethasone or prednisolone eliminates the possibility of GC deficiency. This dose can be halved the second postoperative day, and the maintenance dosage can be resumed the third postoperative day. However, it is important that with regard to possible detrimental effects and the possibility of decreased resistance to infections, this treatment should not be used for prolonged periods in the absence of evidence of corticosteroid insufficiency. General perioperative management should include avoidance of etomidate as an anesthetic drug (selection of other drugs and muscle relaxants is not influenced by the presence of treated hypocortisolism), infusion of sodium-containing fluids, minimal doses of any anesthetic drugs to avoid increased sensitivity to drug-induced myocardial depression, invasive monitoring of

hemodynamics, glucose, and electrolytes, and decreased initial doses of muscle relaxant, monitoring the effect using a peripheral nerve stimulator. Especially when acute adrenal insufficiency has been detected in a critically ill patient with a previously unknown disorder, thorough diagnostics are demanded even after improvement.

Observations suggest that control of cortisol secretion in response to stress is more complex than originally thought. Interactions between corticotropin-releasing factor (CRF), vasoactive intestinal polypeptide, arginine vasopressin, catecholamines, and other hormones in the control of cortisol secretion have been described.[112] α_2-Adrenergic receptor antagonists (e.g., clonidine), which are widely used in ICUs, may suppress the cortisol response to surgical stress. On the other hand, increases in intracranial pressure stimulate cortisol release without increasing ACTH levels, and adrenalectomy but not adrenal demedullation increased the permeability of brain tissue to macromolecules.[113] Further evidence also suggests that white blood cells may release ACTH-like peptides that can stimulate adrenal gland secretion of cortisol, and that primary adrenal insufficiency is associated with increases in serum levels of angiotensin-converting enzyme.[114]

There are multiple interactions between drugs and the HPA axis that have to be considered if absolute or relative adrenal insufficiency is suspected. Moreover, in patients with hepatic dysfunction, GC doses should be tapered, especially when using prednisone, since hydroxylation to the active component needs considerable metabolic capacity. Special attention is required in the concomitant use of GCs with other drugs, because of potential interactions and because some drugs may affect the metabolism of steroids, which may lead to a decreased or increased GC effect on their target tissues.[115,116] Glucocorticoids decrease blood levels of aspirin, coumarin anticoagulants, isoniazid, insulin, and oral hypoglycemic agents, whereas cyclophosphamide and cyclosporine levels may be increased. Inversely, antacids, carbamazepine, cholestyramine, colestipol, ephedrine, mitotane, phenobarbitone, phenytoin, and rifampicin decrease GC blood concentrations, whereas they are increased by cyclosporine, erythromycin, oral contraceptives, and troleandomycin. Furthermore, the combination of exogenous GC administration and amphotericin B, digitalis glycosides, and potassium-depleting diuretics may induce or worsen hypokalemia, warranting frequent monitoring of potassium levels. Finally, the general risk for immunosuppression by GCs precludes any use of vaccines from live attenuated viruses to avoid severe generalized infections.[115,116]

Conclusions

Underproduction of adrenal hormones can lead to serious illness. Glucocorticoids play a critical permissive role in intermediary metabolism, are counter-regulatory in relation to insulin, modulate inflammatory and immune responses, and optimize cardiovascular and central nervous system function. Therefore, diseases with a primary adreno-cortical dysfunction or those leading to secondary adrenal insufficiency may have severe sequelae, which often are life threatening. The concept of relative adrenal insufficiency in critically ill patients with functional disorders of the HPA axis has gained attention during recent years. Especially in patients with severe sepsis and septic shock, this phenomenon is suspected of having a major impact on severity of illness and prognosis. Both absolute adrenal insufficiency and RAI should be diagnosed by using adequate laboratory investigations. In most cases, testing the basal level of cortisol, combined with a short-term stimulation test with 250 μg ACTH, can identify the disease. In patients with critical illnesses, however, it continues to be difficult to diagnose RAI.

In cases of severe volume- and catecholamine-resistant shock with suspected adrenal crisis, immediate replacement therapy is indicated. If the diagnosis is questionable, dexamethasone should be administered to allow functional diagnostics. Once the diagnosis is made, hydrocortisone is the preferred drug, since it provides both gluco- and mineralocorticoid effects. After stabilization, the dose of GCs should be tapered down to a total of 20 to 35 mg hydrocortisone per day or equivalent analogs. The fundamental role of GCs in the stress response to infection, and increasing knowledge of the antiinflammatory and immunosuppressive pharmacodynamic profile, have been the rationale for its use in sepsis trials for decades. Timing, dosage, and duration of GC administration were adapted to different disease pathophysiologic models and had a major impact on outcome. Randomized controlled trials of high-dose GCs failed to improve outcome, leading to skepticism and avoidance of any GCs in septic patients by most ICU physicians over the years, with the exception of some special indications. However, recent randomized controlled trials with low doses of hydrocortisone in septic shock evoked a corticosteroid renaissance. Based on current data, an incremental increase of less than 9 μg/dL after a 250-μg ACTH stimulation test may be used in patients with severe septic shock to determine relative adrenal insufficiency, although this is still under discussion. Meanwhile, prolonged treatment of septic shock with low doses of corticosteroids is considered a therapeutic option to promote shock reversal if the patient does not respond to volume replacement and vasopressor therapy.

KEY POINTS

1. The definition of adrenal insufficiency is based on the inability of the adrenal gland to produce adrenocortical steroid hormones.

2. Three major regulatory influences affect the hypothalamic-pituitary-adrenal (HPA) axis and lead to secretion of corticotropin (ACTH) as the main stimulatory factor for the adrenal cortex to release its hormonal products are circadian diurnal rhythms, stress, and feedback from free cortisol levels in blood and body fluids.

3. Each occurrence of physical or emotional stress leads to an immediate, significant, and possibly continual increase of ACTH and cortisol excretion. This is typically paralleled by loss of the circadian rhythm. The response to stress is proportional to the intensity of the stimulus.

4. The main cause for *primary adrenal insufficiency* (70%-80%) is an autoimmune disorder that induces morphologic destruction of more than 90% of the adrenal cortex. The result is a critically decreased synthesis of steroids, with typical clinical manifestations.

5. In contrast, *secondary adrenal insufficiency* is characterized by reduced stimulation of the intact adrenal gland due to low ACTH levels (hypothalamic-pituitary insufficiency), which also results in reduced cortisol levels.

6. *Tertiary adrenal insufficiency* is caused by long-term treatment with steroid hormones, which induces a feedback inhibition of the hypothalamic-pituitary-adrenal (HPA) axis.

7. The definition of *relative adrenal insufficiency* (RAI) in critically ill patients is based on plasma cortisol levels. The critical threshold is a basal cortisol level of 18 to 25 μg/mL without preceding stimulation. Whereas absolute adrenal insufficiency is rare in critical care medicine, RAI has received considerable attention.

8. Clinical manifestations of adrenal insufficiency are usually nonspecific and include weakness, anorexia, orthostatic hypotension, and general gastrointestinal symptoms. Typical signs for primary forms are hyperpigmentation due to increased ACTH levels, vitiligo in cases of autoimmune disorders, and hyperkalemia. Secondary forms cause milder symptoms due to maintained mineralocorticoid effects.

9. Evaluation of adrenal insufficiency generally includes measurement of basal serum cortisol concentrations as well as the incremental increase after stimulation with ACTH. Mostly, a high-dose test (250 μg ACTH) is preferred, which uses 30- and 60-minute cortisol levels after stimulation. Long-term tests or low doses (1 μg ACTH) are only used for special indications. Basal values of less than 3 μg/dL serum cortisol indicate severe, absolute hypocortisolism warranting immediate intervention. In critically ill patients, basal cortisol levels of less than 18-25 μg/mL have been recommended as an indication for low-dose replacement therapy.

10. Acute adrenal insufficiency (Addisonian crisis) requires immediate intervention. Establishing intravenous access, infusion of saline, monitoring serum glucose, and administering dexamethasone after drawing a blood sample may be life saving. ACTH stimulation tests should be used for diagnosis. Once the results after stimulation are known, hydrocortisone therapy is preferred for its mineralocorticoid effects.

11. Chronic adrenal insufficiency may require long-term replacement therapy with gluco- and mineralocorticoids (for primary forms). Any physical or emotional stress must be considered as possibly harmful, with the need for 3 to 10 times increased doses of glucocorticoids.

12. In patients with septic shock who are not adequately responding to volume and vasopressor therapy, replacement with low-dose hydrocortisone (200-300 mg/d) seems to provide benefit, although optimal dosing and timing has yet to be established. A preliminary ACTH test in these patients is no longer recommended.

ANNOTATED REFERENCES

Annane D, Bellissant E, Bollaert PE, Briegel J, Confalonieri M, De Gaudio R, et al. Corticosteroids in the treatment of severe sepsis and septic shock in adults: a systematic review. JAMA 2009;301: 2362-75.
This review presents the current concepts of pathophysiology, diagnosis, and treatment of corticosteroid insufficiency in acutely ill patients.
Liberman AC, Druker J, Garcia FA, Holsboer F, Arzt E. Intracellular molecular signaling. Basis for specificity to glucocorticoid anti-inflammatory actions. Ann N Y Acad Sci 2009;1153:6-13.
This paper is an important publication on the cellular pathways of glucocorticoid response. It demonstrates how steroids inhibit NF-κB, which represents a key pathway of inflammatory diseases.
Loriaux DL, Fleseriu M. Relative adrenal insufficiency. Curr Opin Endocrinol Diabetes Obes 2009;16:392-400.
This review demonstrates that the phenomenon of relative adrenal insufficiency has a crucial impact on outcome in critically ill patients.
Keh D, Boehnke T, Weber-Carstens S, Schulz C, Ahlers O, Bercker S, et al. Immunologic and hemodynamic effects of "low-dose" hydrocortisone in septic shock: a double-blind, randomized, placebo-controlled, crossover study. Am J Respir Crit Care Med 2003;167:512-20.

The authors performed a randomized trial in patients with septic shock, using a crossover design which demonstrated that (1) hemodynamic stabilization by low-dose steroids is paralleled by reduced synthesis of endogenous nitric oxide, (2) low-dose hydrocortisone modulates rather than suppresses immunologic functions, and (3) rapid withdrawal of steroids induces rebound phenomena with impairment of the clinical course.
Annane D, Sebille V, Charpentier C, Bollaert PE, Francois B, Korach JM, et al. Effect of treatment with low doses of hydrocortisone and fludrocortisone on mortality in patients with septic shock. JAMA 2002;288:862-71.
This is the first multicenter clinical trial which was able to demonstrate that low-dose hydrocortisone combined with fludrocortisone reduces mortality in patients with severe volume- and vasopressor-restrictive septic shock.
Sprung CL, Annane D, Keh D, Moreno R, Singer M, Freivogel K, et al. CORTICUS Study Group. Hydrocortisone therapy for patients with septic shock. N Engl J Med 2008;358:111-24.
In contrast to the aforementioned study, this randomized trial did not show any benefit of low-dose hydrocortisone therapy in septic shock; however, these patients were responsive to vasopressor therapy, which underlines the relevance of thorough patient selection.

REFERENCES

Access the complete reference list online at http://www.expertconsult.com.

166

Thyroid Gland Disorders

ANGELA M. LEUNG | ALAN P. FARWELL

Thyroid storm and myxedema coma are life-threatening emergencies that represent the extreme ends of the spectrum of thyroid dysfunction in the decompensated patient. Their presentation is usually dramatic and is often precipitated by a nonthyroidal-related illness or event. Recognition of these disorders requires a high degree of clinical suspicion, because thyroid function abnormalities, as well as other biochemical parameters, do not differ significantly from uncomplicated thyrotoxicosis and hypothyroidism. As thyroid storm and myxedema coma are clinical diagnoses, measurement of serum thyroid hormones serve as confirmatory tests in the appropriate setting.

In contrast to these dramatic clinical presentations, critical illness also causes multiple nonspecific alterations in thyroid hormone concentrations in patients without intrinsic thyroid dysfunction that relate to the severity of the illness. Since a wide variety of illnesses tend to result in the same changes in serum thyroid hormones, such alterations in thyroid hormone indexes have been termed the *sick euthyroid syndrome*. The differentiation between patients with the sick euthyroid syndrome and those with intrinsic thyroid disease is a frequent diagnostic challenge in the intensive care unit (ICU).

This chapter will review normal thyroid physiology, the changes in thyroid hormone metabolism seen with critical illness, and the evaluation of thyroid function in critically ill patients. Finally, diagnosis and management of the sick euthyroid syndrome, thyroid storm, and myxedema coma will be reviewed.

◼ Normal Thyroid Hormone Economy

REGULATION

Synthesis and secretion of thyroid hormone is under the control of the anterior pituitary hormone, thyrotropin (or thyroid-stimulating hormone [TSH]). Following a classic negative feedback system, TSH secretion increases when serum thyroid hormone levels fall and decreases when they rise (Figure 166-1). TSH secretion is also under the regulation of the hypothalamic hormone, thyrotropin-releasing hormone (TRH). The negative feedback of thyroid hormone is targeted mainly at the pituitary level but likely affects TRH release from the hypothalamus as well. In addition, input from higher cortical centers can affect hypothalamic TRH secretion.

Under the influence of TSH, the thyroid gland synthesizes and releases thyroid hormone. Thyroxine (T_4, 65% iodine by weight) is the principal secretory product of the thyroid gland, comprising about 90% of secreted thyroid hormone under normal conditions.[1] Whereas T_4 may have direct actions in some tissues, it primarily functions as a hormone precursor that is metabolized in peripheral tissues to the transcriptionally active 3,5,3′-triiodothyronine (T_3, 59% iodine by weight).

METABOLIC PATHWAYS

The major pathway of metabolism of T_4 is by sequential monodeiodination.[2] At least three deiodinases, each with its unique expression in different organs, catalyze the deiodination reactions involved in the metabolism of T_4. Removal of the 5′-, or outer ring, iodine by type I iodothyronine 5′-deiodinase (D1) or type II iodothyronine 5′-deiodinase (D2) is the "activating" metabolic pathway leading to formation of T_3. Removal of the inner ring, or 5-, iodine by type III iodothyronine deiodinase D3 is the "inactivating" pathway producing

the metabolically inactive hormone, 3,3′,5′-triiodothyronine (reverse T_3, rT_3). D1 is found most abundantly in the liver, kidneys, and thyroid. It is up-regulated in hyperthyroidism and down-regulated in hypothyroidism. D2 is found primarily in the brain, pituitary, and skeletal muscle and is down-regulated in hyperthyroidism and up-regulated in hypothyroidism. D3 is expressed primarily in the brain, in skin, and in placental and chorionic membranes. The actions of D3 also include inactivation of T_3 to form T_2, another inactive metabolite. Under normal conditions, about 41% of T_4 is converted to T_3, about 38% is converted to rT_3, and about 21% is metabolized via other pathways, such as conjugation in the liver and excretion in bile.[4,5]

T_3 is the metabolically active thyroid hormone and exerts its actions via binding to chromatin-bound nuclear receptors and regulating gene transcription in responsive tissues.[3] Important in understanding the alterations in circulating thyroid hormone levels seen in critical illness is the fact that only around 10% of circulating T_3 is secreted directly by the thyroid gland while more than 80% of T_3 is derived from conversion of T_4 in peripheral tissues.[1,2] Thus, factors that affect peripheral T_4-to-T_3 conversion will have significant effects on circulating T_3 levels. Serum levels of T_3 are approximately 100-fold less than those of T_4, and like T_4, T_3 is metabolized by deiodination to form diiodothyronine (T_2) and by conjugation in the liver. The half-lives of circulating T_4 and T_3 are 5 to 8 days and 1.3 to 3 days, respectively.[4]

SERUM BINDING PROTEINS

Both T_4 and T_3 circulate in the serum as hormones bound to several proteins synthesized by the liver.[5] Thyroid-binding globulin (TBG) is the predominant transport protein and binds roughly 80% of the circulating serum thyroid hormones. The affinity of T_4 for TBG is about 10-fold greater than that of T_3 and is part of the reason circulating T_4 levels are higher than T_3 levels. Other serum binding proteins include transthyretin,[6] which binds some 15% of T_4 but little if any T_3, and albumin, which has a low affinity but a very large binding capacity for T_4 and T_3. Overall, 99.97% of circulating T_4 and 99.7% of circulating T_3 is bound to plasma proteins.

FREE HORMONE CONCEPT

Essential to an understanding of the regulation of thyroid function and the alterations of circulating thyroid hormones seen in critical illness is the "free hormone" concept, which is that only the unbound hormone has any metabolic activity. Under regulation by the pituitary, overall thyroid function is affected when there are any changes in free hormone concentrations. Changes in either the concentrations of binding proteins or the binding affinity of thyroid hormone to the serum binding proteins have significant effects on total serum hormone levels, owing to the high degree of binding of T_4 and T_3 to these proteins. Despite these changes, this does not necessarily translate into thyroid dysfunction.

◼ Thyroid Hormone Economy in Critical Illness

Widespread changes in thyroid hormone economy in the critically ill patient occur as a result of (1) alterations in peripheral metabolism of

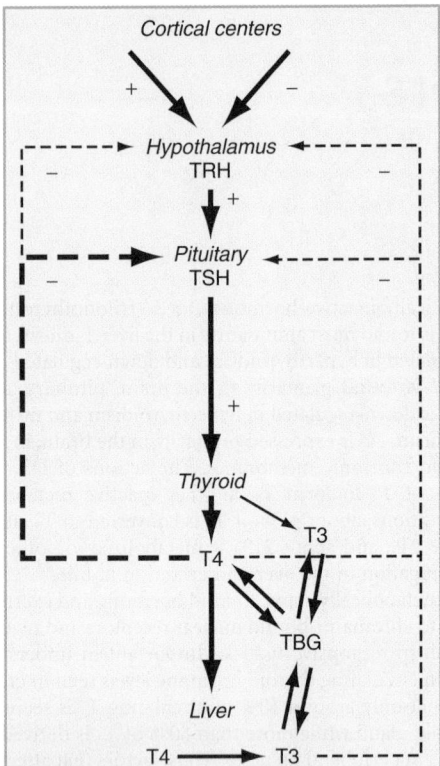

Figure 166-1   Diagram of the hypothalamic-pituitary-thyroid axis. Inhibitory effect of T_4 and T_3 on TSH secretion is shown by dashed line and minus sign, and stimulatory effects of TRH on TSH secretion and TSH on thyroid secretion are shown by solid lines and plus signs. T_4 and T_3 may also have an inhibitory effect on TRH secretion.

thyroid hormones, (2) alterations in TSH regulation, and (3) alterations in the binding of thyroid hormone to TBG.

PERIPHERAL METABOLIC PATHWAYS

One of the initial alterations in thyroid hormone metabolism in acute illness is the acute inhibition of D1, resulting in the impairment of T_4-to-T_3 conversion in peripheral tissues.[7] D1 is inhibited by a wide variety of factors, including acute illness (Box 166-1),[2] resulting in the acute decrease in T_3 production in critically ill patients. In contrast, inner ring deiodination by D3 may be increased by acute illness, resulting in increased levels of rT_3.[8] Additionally, because rT_3 is subsequently deiodinated by D1, degradation of rT_3 decreases, and levels of this inactive hormone rise in proportion to the fall in T_3 levels. Finally,

Box 166-1

FACTORS THAT INHIBIT TYPE 1 5'-DEIODINASE ACTIVITY

Acute and chronic illness
Caloric deprivation
Malnutrition
Glucocorticoids
β-Adrenergic blocking drugs (e.g., propranolol)
Oral cholecystographic agents (e.g., iopanoic acid, sodium ipodate)
Amiodarone
Propylthiouracil
Fatty acids
Fetal/neonatal period
Selenium deficiency
Hepatic disease

there is impaired transport of T_4 to peripheral tissues such as the liver and kidney, where much of the circulating T_3 is produced, further contributing to the decrease in production of T_3.[9]

THYROTROPIN REGULATION

Serum TSH levels are usually normal early in acute illness.[10] Decreased TRH secretion due to inhibitory signals from higher cortical centers, impaired TRH metabolism,[11] the alteration of pulsatile TSH,[12] and the decrease or absence of a nocturnal TSH surge[12,13] may all further lower TSH levels. Serum levels of leptin, the ob gene product that has been shown to vary directly with thyroid hormone levels,[14] also falls as illness progresses[15] and hypothalamic TRH secretion falls, which in turn leads to lowered TSH levels.[16]

The decrease of hypothalamic TRH gene expression in animal models is, however, not associated with increased serum T_4 and T_3 levels.[17] Finally, certain thyroid hormone metabolites that are increased during acute nonthyroidal illness may play a role in the inhibition of TSH and TRH secretion.[18]

Common medications used in the treatment of the critically ill patient may also have inhibitory effects on serum TSH levels (Box 166-2). Van den Berghe et al.[19] reported that intravenous (IV) administration of dopamine for as short a time as 15 to 21 hours can acutely decrease TSH levels, and its withdrawal results in a 10-fold increase in serum TSH levels. In one study, children who received dopamine infusions during a pediatric ICU admission for meningococcal sepsis had lower TSH levels than those who did not.[20,21] Increased levels of glucocorticoids, whether from endogenous or exogenous sources, also have direct inhibitory effects on TSH secretion.

SERUM BINDING PROTEINS

The affinity of thyroid hormones binding to transport proteins and the concentrations of serum binding proteins are altered with acute illness (Table 166-1). Serum levels of transthyretin and albumin decrease, especially during prolonged illness, malnutrition, and in high catabolic states. TBG levels may be increased, as seen with liver dysfunction and human immunodeficiency virus (HIV) infection, or decreased, as seen with severe or prolonged illness.[5] TBG may also be rapidly degraded by protease cleavage during cardiac bypass, thereby partially explaining the rapid fall of serum T_3 levels in patients undergoing cardiac surgery.[22]

Box 166-2

FACTORS THAT DECREASE THYROTROPIN SECRETION

Acute and chronic Illness
Adrenergic agonists
Caloric restriction
Carbamazepine
Clofibrate
Cyproheptadine
Dopamine and dopamine agonists
Endogenous depression
Glucocorticoids
IGF-1
Metergoline
Methysergide
Opiates
Phenytoin
Phentolamine
Pimozide
Somatostatin
Serotonin
Surgical stress
Thyroid hormone metabolites

IGF, insulin-like growth factor.

TABLE 166-1	Factors That Alter Binding of T_4 to Thyroid-Binding Globulin	
	Increase Binding	*Decrease Binding*
Drugs	Estrogens	Glucocorticoids
	Methadone	Androgens
	Clofibrate	L-Asparaginase
	5-Fluorouracil	Salicylates
	Heroin	Mefenamic acid
	Tamoxifen	Antiseizure medications (phenytoin, Tegretol)
	Raloxifene	Furosemide
		Heparin
		Anabolic steroids
Systemic Factors	Liver disease	Inherited
	Porphyria	Acute illness
	HIV infection	Nonesterified free fatty acids (NEFAs)
	Inherited	

An acquired binding defect of T_4 to TBG is commonly seen in patients with critical illness. This is thought to result from the release of some as yet unidentified factor from injured tissues that has the characteristics of unsaturated nonesterified fatty acids (NEFA),[23] which also inhibit T_4-to-T_3 conversion.[24] In systemically ill patients, NEFA levels rise in parallel with the severity of the illness,[25] and drugs such as heparin stimulate the generation of NEFA.[26] Many drugs including high-dose furosemide, antiseizure medications, and salicylates also alter binding of T_4 to TBG. The alterations in serum binding proteins in critical illness make estimating free hormone concentrations difficult (see later).

Evaluation of Thyroid Function in the Critically Ill Patient

DIAGNOSTIC TESTS

Thyrotropin Assays

Abnormal thyroid function tests have been reported in 20% to 40% of acutely ill patients, more than 80% of whom have no intrinsic thyroid dysfunction after resolution of the illness.[27-29] In a study of 1580 hospitalized patients, only 24% of patients with suppressed TSH values (TSH < assay limit of detection) and 50% of patients with TSH values over 20 mU/L were found to have thyroid disease.[27,28] More importantly, none of the patients with subnormal but detectable TSH values and only 14% of patients with elevated TSH values less than 20 mU/L were subsequently diagnosed with intrinsic thyroid dysfunction. The development of sensitive third-generation TSH assays have led to small improvements in discerning between overt hyperthyroidism and nonthyroidal illness.[27] Overall, however, while a normal TSH level has a high predictive value of normal thyroid function, an abnormal TSH value alone is not helpful in evaluating thyroid function in the critically ill patient.

Serum T_4 and T_3 Concentrations

Measurement of free thyroid hormone concentrations in the patient with nonthyroidal illness is fraught with difficulty.[30] The gold standard for determination of free hormone levels is equilibrium dialysis. However, this technique is labor intensive and time consuming and thus is rarely used. The most commonly available laboratory tests of thyroid hormone concentrations, the free T_4 index, free T_4, and free T_3, are measured by analog methods which represent estimates of the free hormone concentration and are therefore subject to inaccuracies.[31,32]

The free T_4 index is determined by multiplying the total T_4 concentration by the T_3 or T_4 resin uptake, which is an inverse estimate of serum TBG concentrations.[32] Recent developments have allowed the measurement of free T_4 levels by the analog method, a less expensive alternative to the free T_4 index,[33] but the two tests are likely comparably accurate.[34] In a healthy population, there is a close correlation between the free T_4 index and free T_4 levels. In the critically ill patient, this association is no longer seen, mainly because of difficulties in estimating TBG binding with resin uptake tests. In spite of this, the sensitivity of the free T_4 index in a large study of hospitalized patients was 92.3%, compared to 90.7% for the sensitive TSH test.[27]

Serum T_3 concentrations are affected to the greatest degree by alterations in thyroid hormone economy resulting from acute illness. Therefore, there is no indication for routine measurement of serum T_3 levels in the initial evaluation of thyroid function in the critically ill patient. This test should only be obtained if thyrotoxicosis is clinically suspected in the presence of a suppressed sensitive TSH and elevated (or high normal) free T_4 index or free T_4 values. The total T_3 assay is preferable to the free T_3 (analog) assay, owing to the variability between laboratories with the latter test.[32]

Although some investigators have reported that serum rT_3 levels are a significant prognostic indicator of mortality in the ICU,[35] rT_3 levels are generally unreliable and should not be used to distinguish between intrinsic thyroid dysfunction and nonthyroidal illness.[36]

Serum Thyroid Autoantibodies

Autoantibodies to thyroglobulin and thyroid peroxidase (TPO), two intrinsic thyroid proteins, are commonly ordered tests.[32] Significant titers of either or both of these antibodies indicate the presence of autoimmune thyroid disease, but the presence of thyroid autoantibodies alone does not necessary indicate thyroid dysfunction, as they are present in approximately 12% to 26% of the general population.[37] Thyroid autoantibodies do, however, add to the sensitivity of abnormal TSH and FTI values in diagnosing known intrinsic thyroid disease.[27,28]

Imaging Studies

Imaging studies are rarely essential to the diagnosis of thyroid disorders in the critically ill patient. Occasionally, functional analysis of the thyroid gland using the radioisotope, iodine-123 (^{123}I), may be useful in the patient with suspected thyrotoxicosis and equivocal laboratory tests. However, these studies are labor intensive, and managing the underlying acute illness often overshadows the benefits of obtaining these studies. Anatomic studies such as ultrasound, isotopic imaging, computed tomography (CT), and magnetic resonance imaging (MRI) are useful in the evaluation of thyroid nodules and goiter, but these conditions rarely are the cause of acute illness; as such, these studies are not usually helpful in the critically ill patient.

DIAGNOSIS

Routine screening of an ICU population for the presence of thyroid dysfunction is not recommended because of the high prevalence of abnormal thyroid function tests and low prevalence of true thyroid dysfunction. When thyroid function tests are ordered in a hospitalized patient, it should only be done if there is a high clinical index of suspicion for thyroid dysfunction. Whenever possible, it is best to defer evaluation of the thyroid-pituitary axis until the patient has recovered from the acute illness. Because every test of thyroid hormone function can be altered in the critically ill patient, no single test can definitively rule in or rule out the presence of intrinsic thyroid dysfunction.

If there is a high clinical suspicion for intrinsic thyroid dysfunction in the critically ill patient, reasonable initial tests would include either free T_4 index or free T_4 and TSH measurements. Assessment of these values in the context of the duration, severity, and stage of illness of the patient will allow the correct diagnosis in most patients. For example, a mildly elevated TSH coupled with a low free T_4 index or free T_4 is more likely to indicate primary hypothyroidism early in an acute illness, as opposed to the same values obtained during the recovery phase of the illness. Similarly, the combination of an elevated TSH and low-normal free T_4 index or free T_4 is more likely to indicate thyroid dysfunction in the hypothermic, bradycardic patient than the tachycardic, normothermic individual. If both the free T_4 index or free T_4 and TSH are normal, thyroid dysfunction is effectively eliminated as a significant contributing factor to the clinical picture. If the diagnosis is still unclear, measurement of thyroid antibodies is helpful as a marker of intrinsic thyroid disease and increases the sensitivity of both the free T_4 index or free T_4 and the TSH. Only in the case of a suppressed TSH and a mid- to high-normal free T_4 index or free T_4 are measurement of serum T_3 levels indicated.

Sick Euthyroid Syndrome

As discussed earlier, critical illness causes multiple nonspecific alterations in thyroid hormone concentrations in patients without intrinsic thyroid dysfunction that relate to the severity of the illness.[18,38,39] One author has postulated that sick euthyroid syndrome may be a compensatory mechanism in response to the oxidative stress of acute illness.[40] Whatever the underlying cause, these alterations in thyroid hormone parameters represent a continuum of changes that depends on the severity of the illness and can be categorized into several distinct stages (Figure 166-2).[18] The wide spectrum of changes observed often results from the differing points in the course of the illness when the thyroid function tests were obtained. Importantly, these changes are rarely isolated and often associated with alterations of other endocrine systems, such as decreases in serum gonadotropin and sex hormone concentrations[41] and increases in serum ACTH and cortisol levels.[42] Thus, the sick euthyroid syndrome should not be viewed as an isolated pathologic event but as part of a coordinated systemic reaction to illness involving both the immune and endocrine systems.

LOW T₃ STATE

Common to all of the abnormalities in thyroid hormone concentrations seen in critically ill patients is a substantial depression of serum T_3 levels, which can occur as early as 24 hours after the onset of illness. Over half of patients admitted to the medical service will demonstrate depressed serum T_3 concentrations.[27,28] Development of the low T_3 state arises from impairment of peripheral T_4-to-T_3 conversion through inhibition of type 1 deiodinase (discussed earlier). This results in marked reduction of T_3 production and rT_3 degradation,[43] thereby leading to reciprocal changes in serum T_3 and serum rT_3 concentrations. Low T_3 levels are also found in peripheral tissues.[35] Thyroid hormone receptor expression is also decreased in acute nonthyroidal illness,[44] possibly in response to the decrease in tissue T_3 levels.

HIGH T₄ STATE

Serum T_4 levels may be elevated early in acute illness due to either the acute inhibition of type 1 deiodinase or increased TBG levels. This is seen most often in the elderly and in patients with psychiatric disorders. As the duration of illness increases, non-deiodinative pathways of T_4 degradation increase serum T_4 levels to the normal range.[28]

LOW T₄ STATE

As the severity and duration of the illness increases, serum total T_4 levels decrease into the subnormal range. Contributors to this decrease in serum T_4 levels are (1) a decrease in the binding of T_4 to serum carrier proteins, (2) a decrease in serum TSH levels, leading to decreased thyroidal production of T_4, and (3) an increase in non-deiodinative pathways of T_4 metabolism. The decline in serum T_4 levels correlates with prognosis in the ICU, with mortality increasing as serum T_4 levels drop below 4 µg/dL and approaching 80% in patients with serum T_4 levels below 2 µg/dL.[45-47] Despite marked decreases in serum total T_4 and T_3 levels in the critically ill patient, free hormone levels have been reported to be normal or even elevated,[30,31] providing a possible explanation for why most patients appear eumetabolic despite thyroid hormone levels in the hypothyroid range. Thus, the low T_4 state is unlikely to be a result of a hormone-deficient state and is probably more of a marker of multisystem failure in these critically ill patients.

RECOVERY STATE

As acute illness resolves, so do the alterations in thyroid hormone concentrations. This stage may be prolonged and is characterized by modest increases in serum TSH levels.[48] Full recovery with restoration of thyroid hormone levels to the normal range may require several weeks[49] or months after hospital discharge.[27] One study reported that 35 of 40 patients with nonthyroidal illness after coronary artery bypass grafting were able to regain normal thyroid function 6 months after surgery.[50]

TREATMENT OF THE SICK EUTHYROID SYNDROME

The question of whether the sick euthyroid syndrome in critically ill patients represents pathologic alterations in thyroid function that negatively impact these patients or simply reflects the multisystem failure (i.e., respiratory, cardiac, renal, hepatic failure) that occurs in critically ill patients is still debatable.[51-54] What is not debatable is that thyroid hormone replacement therapy has not been shown to be of benefit in the vast majority of these patients in the published studies to date (Box 166-3).[54] Evidence does suggest a beneficial effect of liothyronine (L-T_3) on increasing organs available for harvest from brain-dead organ donors. While L-T_3 appears to slightly improve hemodynamic and neurohumoral parameters in patients with

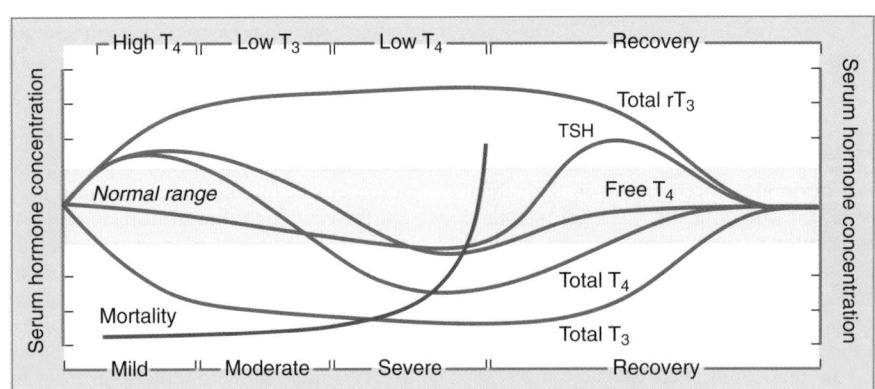

Figure 166-2 Alterations in thyroid hormone concentrations with critical illness. Schematic representation of the continuum of changes in serum thyroid hormone concentrations in patients with nonthyroidal illness. Alterations become more pronounced with increasing severity of illness, and return to normal range as illness subsides and patient recovers. A rapidly rising mortality accompanies the fall in total and free T_4 concentrations. rT_3, reverse triiodothyronine (3,3',5'-triiodothyronine); T_3, 3,5,3'-triiodothyronine; TSH, thyroid-stimulating hormone (thyrotropin). (*From Farwell AF. Sick euthyroid syndrome in the intensive care unit. In: Irwin RS, Rippe JM, editors. Intensive care medicine. 5th ed. Philadelphia: Lippincott Williams & Wilkins; 2003.*)

SUMMARY OF CLINICAL TRIALS ON THE EFFECTS OF TREATMENT OF SICK EUTHYROID SYNDROME WITH THYROID HORMONE*

Starvation/Undernutrition
- L-T_3 treatment results in increased protein breakdown and increased nitrogen excretion in fasting normal and obese patients.

General ICU Patients
- No benefit of L-T_4 on general medical patients, patients with acute renal failure, or renal transplant
- No benefit of L-T_3 on burn patients

Premature Infants
- No benefit of L-T_4 on developmental indices of premature infants at 26-28 weeks gestation
- Possible beneficial effect of L-T_4 on infants of at 25-26 weeks gestation but possible deleterious effects on infants of 27-30 weeks gestation
- No benefit of L-T_3
- Meta-analysis shows no significant effects of thyroid hormone treatment of premature infants.

Cardiac Surgery Patients
- Small studies suggest improved hemodynamic parameters with L-T_3.
- Large trials show no benefit of L-T_3 noted in patients undergoing cardiac bypass.
- Possible improvement in hemodynamic parameters and hospital stay with L-T_3 in children undergoing cardiac surgery

Cardiac Donors
- Variable results (helpful to no benefit) on the effects of L-T_3 in preserving function of normal hearts in brain-dead cardiac donors prior to transplantation
- Possible benefits of L-T_3 in improving function of impaired hearts prior to transplant, potentially increasing the pool of organs available for transplantation
- Consensus conferences recommend the use of L-T_3 as part of the hormonal resuscitation in donors whose cardiac ejection fraction is <45%.

Congestive Heart Failure
- Small uncontrolled study suggested short-term L-T_4 therapy increased cardiac output and functional capacity and decreased systemic vascular resistance.
- Improved hemodynamic parameters and neurohumoral profiles with short-term intravenous L-T_3 infusion, possibly requiring supraphysiologic concentrations

*Refer to Reference 54 for detailed citations.

congestive heart failure, these benefits may represent a pharmacologic effect of T_3 rather than a physiologic replacement hormonal effect. Further, the studies involving patients with congestive heart failure are more remarkable for a lack of deleterious effect of L-T_3 treatment then for any sustained clinical benefit. However, future studies do appear to be warranted in this patient population. At the present time, in the absence of any clinical evidence of hypothyroidism, there does not appear to be any compelling evidence for the use of thyroid hormone therapy in any patient with decreased thyroid hormone parameters due to the sick euthyroid syndrome.

Thyroid Storm

Thyroid storm is an acute, life-threatening complication of hyperthyroidism and represents the extreme manifestation of the disease.[55-57] Historically, thyroid storm was frequently associated with surgery for hyperthyroidism and approached an incidence of 10% in some series, depending upon the diagnostic criteria employed. Currently, because of better recognition of the disease and improved perioperative management, thyroid storm is rare, accounting for less than 2% of all hospital admissions related to thyrotoxicosis.[58] Most often, thyroid storm is precipitated by an intercurrent medical problem in untreated or partially treated hyperthyroid patients.[55-57] The diagnosis of thyroid storm is a clinical one; there are no distinctive laboratory features, and thyroid hormone concentrations are similar to those observed in uncomplicated thyrotoxicosis. Although the cause of the rapid clinical decompensation is unknown, a sudden inhibition of thyroid hormone binding to plasma proteins by the precipitating factor, causing a rise in free hormone concentrations in the already elevated free hormone pool, may play a role in the pathogenesis of thyroid storm.[59]

CLINICAL MANIFESTATIONS

Thyroid storm is primarily a clinical diagnosis; as such, the varying incidence of this disorder in patient series likely results from how strict the diagnostic criteria employed are. Clinical features are similar to those of thyrotoxicosis but more exaggerated (Box 166-4). Cardinal features of thyroid storm include fever (temperature usually > 38.5°C), tachycardia out of proportion to the fever, and mental status changes.[60] Tachyarrhythmias, especially atrial fibrillation in the elderly, are common. Nausea, vomiting, diarrhea, agitation, and delirium are frequent presentations. Vascular collapse and shock due to dehydration and cardiac decompensation are poor prognostic signs, as is the presence of jaundice.[61] Multiorgan failure has been reported.[62] Coma and death may ensue in up to 20% of patients, frequently due to cardiac arrhythmias, congestive heart failure, hyperthermia, or the precipitating illness.[63]

Most patients display the classic signs of Graves disease, the most common cause of thyrotoxicosis, with ophthalmopathy and a diffusely enlarged goiter as the usual manifestations.[56] Thyroid storm has also been associated with toxic nodular goiters. In the elderly, atypical signs and symptoms may include severe myopathy, profound weight loss, apathy, and a minimally enlarged goiter.[64]

PRECIPITATING FACTORS

In the past, thyroid storm was frequently associated with surgery for hyperthyroidism (Box 166-5), with symptoms beginning a few hours after thyroidectomy in patients prepared for surgery with potassium iodide alone. Most of these cases occurred in patients who were not appropriately prepared for surgery by current standards. Certain clinical and socioeconomic factors have also been suggested to be associated with complicated hyperthyroidism, including the lack of insurance, age younger than 30 or older than 50 , and serum T_4 concentrations greater than twice the upper limit of normal.[65] Because of better recognition of the disease, preoperative treatment with thionamides to deplete the gland of thyroid hormone prior to surgery, and improved perioperative management with β-blockade, thyroid storm now is rarely a postoperative complication of thyroid surgery.

CLINICAL FEATURES OF THYROID STORM

Fever (as high as 105.8°F)
Tachycardia/tachyarrhythmias
Mental status changes
Delirium/agitation
Congestive heart failure
Tremor
Nausea and vomiting
Diarrhea
Sweating
Vasodilatation
Dehydration
Hepatomegaly
Splenomegaly
Jaundice

PRECIPITATING FACTORS FOR THYROID STORM

Surgery:
  Thyroidal
  Nonthyroidal
Infections:
  Pneumonia
  Upper respiratory
  Enteric
  Other
Stress
Trauma
Diabetic ketoacidosis
Labor
Cardiac disease
Iodinated intravenous contrast agents
Radioactive iodine (^{131}I) therapy

Currently, thyroid storm appears most commonly following infection, causing the thyrotoxic state to decompensate.[56] Pneumonia, upper respiratory tract infections, and enteric infections are common precipitating infections. Other precipitating factors include stress, trauma, nonthyroidal surgery, diabetic ketoacidosis, labor, heart disease, and iodinated contrast studies in the unrecognized or partially treated hyperthyroid patient.[66-69] Iatrogenic thyroid storm has been reported due to thyroid hormone overdose.[70,71] Thyroid storm occurring after ^{131}I therapy is extremely rare,[72-74] especially considering the frequency of the use of radioiodine in the definitive treatment of hyperthyroidism. When reported, radioiodine-induced thyroid storm usually occurs if there was no pretreatment with antithyroid drugs.[72]

DIAGNOSIS

As mentioned earlier, the diagnosis of thyroid storm is a clinical one. To emphasize this point, Wartofsky et al.[55] developed a modified Acute Physiology and Chronic Health Evaluation (APACHE) score with criteria including temperature, central nervous system effects, gastrointestinal effects, cardiovascular effects, and precipitant history to assist in the diagnosis. There are no distinct laboratory abnormalities outside of elevated thyroid hormone concentrations, which are similar to those found in uncomplicated thyrotoxicosis. Serum T_3 concentrations are often elevated to a greater degree than serum T_4 concentrations, owing to the preferential secretion of T_3 in the hyperthyroid gland.[56] There is little correlation between the degree of elevation of thyroid hormones and the presentation of thyroid storm. Serum TSH concentrations are typically undetectable; however, because of the influence of nonthyroidal illness on TSH secretion (see earlier), a low TSH by itself is insufficient to make a diagnosis of thyroid storm. Serum T_4 and T_3 concentrations in the normal range, regardless of the TSH concentration, effectively eliminate thyroid storm as a tenable diagnosis.

Abnormal liver function tests are common. Hypocalcemia may be observed secondary to increased osteoclast-mediated bone resorption in the hyperthyroid patient. Hematocrit concentrations may be elevated due to volume contraction, and leukocytosis is common even in the absence of infection.

The differential diagnosis of thyroid storm includes sepsis, neuroleptic malignant syndrome, malignant hyperthermia, and acute mania with lethal catatonia, all of which can precipitate thyroid storm in the appropriate setting. Clues to the diagnosis of thyroid storm are a history of thyroid disease, history of iodine ingestion, and the presence of a goiter or stigmata of Graves disease. Clearly the physician must have a high clinical index of suspicion for thyroid storm, as therapy must be instituted before the return of thyroid function tests in most cases.

TREATMENT

It should be emphasized that a thyroid storm is a major medical emergency that must be treated in an ICU.[55-57] Therapy can divided into two major categories (Box 166-6): (1) *thyroid-directed treatment* aimed at decreasing thyroid hormone production, conversion, and secretion and blocking the peripheral manifestations of thyroid hormone; and (2) *supportive treatment* aimed at controlling the fever, stabilizing the cardiovascular system, and managing the precipitating cause.

Thyroid-Directed Treatment

Prompt inhibition of thyroid hormone synthesis and secretion is essential. Antithyroid drugs are given in large doses to both inhibit synthesis of thyroid hormones and block the uptake of iodine. Propylthiouracil (PTU) is preferred over methimazole, given its greater efficacy when used in large doses, in reducing T_3 levels during severe hyperthyroidism (by inhibition of type 1 deiodinase), and impairing peripheral conversion of T_4 to T_3.[75] However, since other more powerful inhibitors of type 1 deiodinase are usually part of the therapeutic regimen in thyroid storm, the main beneficial effects of PTU are its inhibition of iodide uptake and hormone synthesis. PTU and methimazole can be administered by nasogastric tube or rectally if necessary.[76] Neither of these preparations is available for parenteral administration, although a protocol has been reported for the reconstitution of methimazole to be given IV.[77]

TREATMENT OF THYROID STORM

Thyroid-Directed Therapy
Direct:
  Inhibition of thyroid hormone synthesis:
    Propylthiouracil: 800 mg PO/PR first dose, then 200-300 mg
      PO/PR q 8 h, or
    Methimazole: 80 mg PO/PR first dose, then 40-80 mg PO/PR
      q 12 h
  Block release of thyroid hormones from the gland:
    Telepaque (iopanoic acid): 1 g PO once daily (if available), or
    SSKI: 5 drops PO q 8 h, or
    Lugol's solution: 10 drops PO q 8 h, or
    Lithium: 800-1200 mg PO once daily; achieve serum lithium
      levels 0.5-1.5 mEq/L
Adjunctive:
  Block T_4-to-T_3 conversion:
    Telepaque (iopanoic acid)
    Corticosteroids: dexamethasone, 1-2 mg PO/IV q 6 h
    Propylthiouracil
    Most beta-blockers: propranolol, 40-80 mg PO q 6 h
  Remove thyroid hormones from circulation:
    Cholestyramine: 4 g PO q 6 h, or
    Colestipol: 20-30 mg PO once daily, or
    Plasmapheresis, or
    Peritoneal dialysis

Supportive Therapy
Hyperthermia:
  IV fluids
  Antipyretics
  Cooling blanket
Hemodynamic:
  β-Adrenergic blocking drugs:
    Propranolol: 1 mg IV/min to a total dose of 10 mg, then
      40-80 mg PO q 6 h, or
    Esmolol: 500 mg/kg/min IV, then 50-100 mg/kg/min, or
    Metoprolol: 100-400 mg PO q 12 h, or
    Atenolol: 50-100 mg PO daily
Other:
  Vasopressors
  Digoxin
Etiologic:
  Treatment of underlying illness(es)
Other:
  Anxiolytics (once mental status clears)

IV, intravenous; PO, orally; PR, rectally.

Iodides, the most effective drugs to block release of thyroid hormone from the thyroid gland, should be used only after antithyroid drugs have been administered. Monotherapy with iodides will actually increase the synthesis of new thyroid hormones and markedly worsen the hyperthyroidism when the gland escapes from the initial iodide-induced blockade of hormone secretion (acute Wolf-Chaikoff effect).[78] Previously, the iodide preparation of choice was the radiographic contrast dye, iopanoic acid (Telepaque), because of its high iodine content (0.6 mg iodine/g dose) and the ability for the drug to directly inhibit type 1 deiodinase and thus block T_4-to-T_3 conversion.[2] However, this drug is largely unavailable worldwide. Lugol's solution or saturated solution of potassium iodide (SSKI) are currently the main source of therapeutic iodides.[79,80] It is important to realize that use of iodides preclude the use of radioactive iodine as a definitive therapy for hyperthyroidism for several months. Lithium has also been reported to be effective in inhibiting thyroid hormone release to a similar degree as iodides.

High-dose dexamethasone is recommended as supportive therapy, both as an inhibitor of T_4-to-T_3 conversion and as management of possible coexistent adrenal insufficiency. β-Adrenergic blockers, specifically propranolol, are also weak inhibitors of T_4-to-T_3 conversion, although their main beneficial effect is on heart rate control.[81] Orally administered ion-exchange resin (colestipol or cholestyramine) can trap hormone in the intestine and prevent recirculation.[82,83] Plasmapheresis, peritoneal dialysis, and charcoal hemoperfusion have also been used in severe cases.[84]

Supportive Treatment

Simultaneously with antithyroid-directed therapy, treatment aimed at cooling the patient down to a reasonable temperature and providing hemodynamic support should be instituted. IV fluids, antipyretics, and cooling blankets all are effective. β-Adrenergic blockers such as propranolol (oral or IV) and esmolol (IV) are given for heart rate control. Calcium channel blockers may be used to control tachyarrhythmias. Anxiolytics are frequently helpful once the patient's mental status improves. Finally, treatment of the underlying precipitating illness is essential to survival in thyroid storm.

LONG-TERM THERAPY

Once the acute phase of thyroid storm is controlled, antithyroid drug therapy should be continued until euthyroidism is achieved, while the adjunctive therapy can be discontinued. Definitive therapeutic options for hyperthyroidism include radioactive iodine (after a few months to allow excretion of the excess iodides used during the acute management of thyroid storm) and surgery.[85-87] Long-term (1-2 years) treatment with antithyroid drugs in hopes of achieving a remission is an option for the patient with Graves disease,[88] although this is best achieved using methimazole because of the concern of the rare complication of severe liver injury with PTU.[89]

Myxedema Coma

Myxedema coma is a rare syndrome that represents the extreme expression of severe long-standing hypothyroidism.[57,90,91] It is a medical emergency, and even with early diagnosis and treatment, the mortality can be as high as 60%.[92] The name is somewhat of a misnomer, as actual coma is rare.[90] The syndrome includes decompensated hypothyroidism, central nervous system impairment, and cardiovascular compromise. Myxedema coma occurs most often in the elderly and during the winter months; in one series, 9 of 11 cases of myxedema coma were admitted in late fall or winter. As with thyroid storm, myxedema coma is usually caused by a precipitating event in the untreated or partially treated hypothyroid patient.

CLINICAL MANIFESTATIONS

The cardinal features of myxedema coma are: (1) hypothermia, which can be profound, (2) altered mental status, (3) cardiovascular

---

Box 166-7

CLINICAL FEATURES OF MYXEDEMA COMA

Mental obtundation
Hypothermia
Bradycardia
Hypotension
Coarse, dry skin
Myxedema facies
Hypoglycemia
Atonic gastrointestinal tract
Atonic bladder
Pleural, pericardial, and peritoneal effusions

depression, and (4) a precipitating cause(s) (Box 166-7). The severely hypothyroid patient essentially becomes poikilothermic due to disordered thermoregulation. This is the reason many cases occur in the winter months. Body temperatures as low as 23.3°C have been reported; thus, rectal temperatures are essential to making the diagnosis. Excessive lethargy and sleepiness may have been present for weeks to months, often interfering with meals. Decreased consciousness has been found to be an important adverse prognostic indicator for mortality.[93] Rarely, psychosis and delirium have been reported. Bradycardia and hypotension may be profound, and the respiratory rate is often depressed. Since intrinsic hypothyroidism by itself is insufficient to produce the clinical syndrome of myxedema coma, a precipitating cause must be assumed to be present.[90]

In addition to the noted features, most patients have the physical features of severe hypothyroidism,[91] including macroglossia, delayed reflexes, dry, rough skin and myxedematous facies, which results from periorbital edema, pallor, hypercarotinemia, and patchy hair loss. Hypotonia of the gastrointestinal tract is common and often so severe as to suggest an obstructive lesion.[94] Urinary retention due to a hypotonic bladder is related but less frequent. Pleural, pericardial, and peritoneal effusions may be present. Severe airway obstruction has been reported.[95]

PRECIPITATING FACTORS

As mentioned, cold stress is a common precipitant to myxedema coma (Box 166-8). Other common precipitating factors include pulmonary and urinary tract infections, cerebrovascular accidents, trauma, surgery, congestive heart failure, and intravascular volume loss from acute or chronic gastrointestinal bleeding or overuse of diuretics.[57,90,91] The clinical course of lethargy proceeding to stupor and then coma is

Box 166-8

PRECIPITATING FACTORS OF MYXEDEMA COMA

Cold stress
Infection:
  Pneumonia
  Urinary tract
  Other
Stroke
Congestive heart failure
Trauma
Burns
Surgery
Intravascular volume contraction:
  Gastrointestinal blood loss
  Diuretic use
CNS-active drugs:
  Analgesics/narcotics
  Sedatives/hypnotics
  Tranquilizers
  Anesthetic agents

CNS, central nervous system.

often hastened by drugs, especially sedatives, narcotics, antidepressants, and tranquilizers.[96] Indeed, many cases of myxedema coma have occurred in the undiagnosed hypothyroid patient who has been hospitalized for other medical problems.

DIAGNOSIS

Like the diagnosis of thyroid storm, myxedema coma is a clinical diagnosis. Elderly patients may present with particularly subtle findings.[97] Even though rare, the diagnosis of myxedema coma should be considered in any hypothermic, obtunded patient. Medical history in these patients, including a prior history of hypothyroidism, may only be able to be confirmed from other sources. Friends, relatives, and acquaintances might have noted increasing lethargy, complaints of cold intolerance, and changes in the voice. Clues to the diagnosis include an outdated container of L-T$_4$ discovered with the patient's belongings, which suggests that he or she has been remiss in taking medication. The medical record may also indicate thyroid hormone use, previous referral to treatment with radioactive iodine, or a history of thyroidectomy. Finally, the physical exam finding of a thyroidectomy scar should raise suspicion as to the diagnosis.

Because more than 95% of cases of myxedema coma are due to primary hypothyroidism,[57,90,91] the laboratory findings include an elevated serum TSH and low or undetectable total and free serum T$_4$ concentrations. These thyroid hormone abnormalities are similar to those in uncomplicated overt hypothyroidism. In the patient with central hypothyroidism, the diagnosis of myxedema coma may be very difficult, as serum TSH concentrations will be normal or low. However, other symptoms of pituitary dysfunction are usually present in these rare patients.

Dilutional hyponatremia is common and may be severe. Elevated creatine kinase concentrations, sometimes markedly so, are encountered frequently and may misdirect the clinical picture towards cardiac ischemia.[98,99] However, the MB fraction in most of these cases is normal, and an electrocardiogram (ECG) often demonstrates low voltage and loss of T waves that is characteristic of severe hypothyroidism. Elevated lactate dehydrogenase (LDH) concentrations, acidosis, and anemia are common findings. Lumbar puncture reveals increased opening pressure and high protein content in the cerebrospinal fluid.

Few of the signs and symptoms discussed are unique to myxedema coma. Protein-calorie malnutrition, sepsis, hypoglycemia, and exposure to certain drugs and toxins, as well as cold exposure can cause severe hypothermia. Hypotension and hypoventilation, other cardinal features of myxedema coma, occur in other disease states. Furthermore, low thyroid hormone concentrations may be seen in the critically ill patient with nonthyroidal illness (see earlier). As with thyroid storm, the physician must have a high clinical index of suspicion for myxedema coma, because therapy must be instituted before the availability of thyroid function tests results in most cases.

TREATMENT

Treatment of myxedema coma is a medical emergency and should be managed in an ICU setting. The mainstays of therapy are: supportive care with ventilatory and hemodynamic support, rewarming, correction of hyponatremia and hypoglycemia, treatment of the precipitating incident, and administration of thyroid hormone (Box 166-9).[57,90,91] Sedatives, hypnotics, narcotics, and anesthetics must be minimized or avoided altogether because of their extended duration of action and exacerbation of obtundation in the hypothyroid patient.

Hypothermia is one of the hallmarks of myxedema coma, and its severity may be underestimated if the thermometer used does not register below 30°C. At core temperatures below 28°C, ventricular fibrillation is a significant life-threatening risk. Despite its gravity, the management of the hypothermia of myxedema coma differs from the treatment of exposure-induced hypothermia in euthyroid subjects. In myxedema coma, the patient should be kept in a warm room and covered with blankets. Active heating should be avoided, since it

---

Box 166-9

TREATMENT OF MYXEDEMA COMA

Supportive
Assisted ventilation
Hemodynamic support
Passive rewarming for hypothermia
Intravenous glucose for hypoglycemia
Water restriction or hypertonic saline for severe hyponatremia
Hydrocortisone IV (100 mg q 8 h)
Treatment of precipitating factor(s)
Avoidance of all CNS-acting medications

Thyroid Hormone Replacement
L-T$_4$: 200-300 µg loading dose IV, up to 500 µg IV in the first 24 h
and/or
L-T$_3$: 12.5 µg IV q 6 h

CNS, central nervous system; IV, intravenous.

---

increases oxygen consumption and promotes peripheral vasodilation and circulatory collapse. Active heating is recommended only for situations of severe hypothermia where ventricular fibrillation is an immediate threat. In these cases, the rate of rewarming should not exceed 0.5°C per hour, and the core temperature should be raised to approximately 31°C.[57,90,91]

Because of a 5% to 10% incidence of coexisting adrenal insufficiency in patients with myxedema coma,[100] IV steroids (i.e., hydrocortisone, 100 mg IV every 8 hours) are indicated before initiating T$_4$ therapy. Parenteral administration of thyroid hormone is necessary owing to uncertain absorption through the gut.[101-103] A reasonable approach is an initial IV loading dose of 200 to 300 µg L-T$_4$. If there is inadequate improvement in the state of consciousness, blood pressure, or core temperature during the first 6 to 12 hours after administration, another dose of L-T$_4$ should be given to bring the total dose during the first 24 hours to 0.5 mg. This should be followed by 50 to 100 µg IV every 24 hours until the patient is stabilized. Alternatively, in the most severe cases, some clinicians recommend using L-T$_3$ at a dosage of 12.5 to 25 µg IV every 6 hours until the patient is stable and conscious. Caution must be used to avoid overstimulation of the cardiovascular system. Once stable, the patient should be switched to L-T$_4$. The dose of thyroid hormone should be adjusted on the basis of hemodynamic stability, the presence of coexisting cardiac disease, and the degree of electrolyte imbalance.[104]

Although myxedema coma is associated with a high mortality, which may be as high as 60%,[92,105] survival can be maximized by correcting the secondary metabolic disturbances and reversing the hypothyroid state in a sustained but gradual fashion, since an effort to correct hypothyroidism too rapidly may completely negate the beneficial effects of the initial treatment.

LONG-TERM THERAPY

Once the patient with myxedema coma is clinically stable, thyroid hormone replacement can be switched to oral L-T$_4$. The dose of L-T$_4$ should be adjusted over the ensuing weeks and months to achieve serum T$_4$ and TSH concentrations in the normal range.

▓ Summary

In summary, thyroid storm and myxedema coma are medical emergencies, diagnosed by their clinical presentation and confirmed by serum thyroid function tests. The interpretation of thyroid function tests in the ICU patient outside of these dramatic presentations is often fraught with difficulty. Identifying those patients with intrinsic thyroid dysfunction must take into consideration both the clinical assessment of the patient and the duration and severity of the illness. Whenever possible, it is best to defer evaluation of thyroid function until the patient has recovered from the critical illness.

ANNOTATED REFERENCES

Midgley JE. Direct and indirect free thyroxine assay methods: theory and practice. Clin Chem 2001;47:1353-63.

The current clinically available tests that report "free" T_4 and T_3 levels actually only estimate the free fraction and as such may not accurately reflect hormone levels in critically ill patients. This paper reviews the methodology used to measure these hormones and points out the potential pitfalls in interpreting results.

Hennemann G, Krenning EP. The kinetics of thyroid hormone transporters and their role in non-thyroidal illness and starvation. Best Pract Res Clin Endocrinol Metab 2007;21:323-38.

A major new field in the understanding of thyroid hormone metabolism has been the identification of thyroid hormone transporters. This important paper reviews current data regarding the function of thyroid hormone transporters in the sick euthyroid syndrome.

Plikat K, Langgartner J, Buettner R, Bollheimer LC, Woenckhaus U, Scholmerich J, et al. Frequency and outcome of patients with nonthyroidal illness syndrome in a medical intensive care unit. Metabolism 2007;56:239-44.

This paper provides an in-depth review of the mortality associated with the sick euthyroid syndrome.

Farwell AP. Thyroid hormone therapy is not indicated in the majority of patients with the sick euthyroid syndrome. Endocr Pract 2008;14:1180-7.

This paper reviews all the evidence currently available on treatment of the sick euthyroid syndrome with thyroid hormone.

Nayak B, Burman K. Thyrotoxicosis and thyroid storm. Endocrinol Metab Clin North Am 2006;35:663-86.

This is the most recent review of thyroid storm.

Wartofsky L. Myxedema coma. Endocrinol Metab Clin North Am 2006;35:687-98.

This is the most recent review of myxedema coma.

Dutta P, Bhansali A, Masoodi SR, Bhadada S, Sharma N, Rajput R. Predictors of outcome in myxoedema coma: a study from a tertiary care centre. Crit Care 2008;12:R1.

This important study updates the mortality risk of myxedema coma and provides evidence that the route of administration of thyroid hormone in this life-threatening emergency does not affect outcome.

REFERENCES

Access the complete reference list online at http://www.expertconsult.com.

167

Diabetes Insipidus

SERGE BRIMIOULLE

Diabetes insipidus is a disorder of water metabolism associated with polyuria, urine hypotonicity, and hypernatremia.[1-3] The quantitative criteria include urine output greater than 200 mL/h or 3 mL/kg/h, urine osmolality less than 150 mOsm/kg, and plasma sodium greater than 145 mEq/L. If urine osmolality measurement is not available, hypotonicity can be assessed from a urine specific gravity less than 1.005.

Central Diabetes Insipidus

Neurogenic or central diabetes insipidus is characterized by a lack of antidiuretic hormone (ADH) that may result from any injury to the anterior hypothalamus, pituitary stalk, or posterior pituitary gland. In acute critically ill patients, the most common causes of diabetes insipidus are surgery for pituitary tumors, cerebral trauma, intracranial hypertension, and brain death (Box 167-1). Diabetes insipidus also may occur as a complication of bacterial meningitis or encephalitis, vascular aneurysm or thrombosis, drug administration, or alcohol intoxication. Injuries to the hypothalamus most often yield permanent diabetes insipidus because ADH is synthesized in the hypothalamus itself. Injuries to the pituitary stalk and neurohypophysis more commonly cause transient diabetes insipidus, because hypothalamic ADH secretion can be effective even in the absence of anatomic pathways to the normal site of release. Chronic diabetes insipidus in critically ill patients generally results from tumors of the pituitary region and from the sequelae of cerebral trauma.

Clinical Picture

In complete hypothalamic or pituitary injuries, diabetes insipidus generally develops 6 to 24 hours after the injury, because previously released ADH remains circulating this long. Patients with untreated diabetes insipidus usually develop urine outputs of 10 to 15 L/d. When the thirst mechanism is preserved, it is activated as soon as osmolality or volemia decreases. If the patient remains conscious and is given free access to water, he or she may be able to drink large amounts and compensate for the urine losses. In other cases, the large amounts of dilute urine rapidly result in dehydration with hypovolemia and hypotension and in hypernatremia with neurologic deterioration. It is important that diabetes insipidus be recognized and treated rapidly, especially in comatose or uncommunicative patients. In patients with partial diabetes insipidus, the onset of polyuria may be delayed, and the volume of urine may be lower. Nevertheless, if urine is hypoosmolar and the diabetes insipidus is not treated, dehydration and hypernatremia finally occur and cause symptoms.

Clinical signs of hypernatremia usually appear only when the plasma sodium concentration increases to greater than 155 to 160 mEq/L or plasma osmolality increases to greater than 330 mOsm/kg.[4] Signs may appear sooner if hypernatremia is associated with other metabolic disorders, particularly with disorders that also increase plasma osmolality. Symptoms mainly include confusion and lethargy. Severe hypernatremia results in coma and sometimes seizures. Acute and severe dehydration and hypernatremia may lead to cerebral shrinkage, sometimes associated with subdural or intraparenchymal hemorrhages.

Clinical signs of dehydration include blood volume depletion and hypotension in the most severe cases. Biological markers of dehydration are usually absent in intensive care unit (ICU) patients with

central diabetes insipidus, because the urine loss begins abruptly and commonly reaches more than 1 L/h. The free water deficit can be estimated by the following formula:

$$\text{Deficit (L)} = \text{body weight (kg)} \times 0.6 \times (\text{Na}^+ - 140)/\text{Na}^+$$

The formula assumes that only free water has been lost and that sodium stores are normal. Most often, some sodium has been lost together with additional water, and the total water deficit is even higher than that estimated from the formula. A moderate level of hypernatremia (e.g., 155 mEq) already is associated with a free water deficit of more than 4 L and a total water deficit that may be much higher if sodium has been lost.

Differential Diagnosis

The differential diagnosis of polyuria includes diuretic drug intake, hyperglycemia, fluid overload, and fluid mobilization. The search for diuretic administration should include not only conventional diuretics but also mannitol and iodinated contrast agents. Administration of diuretics may not be evident when these substances have been given before admission to the ICU (e.g., in another hospital before patient transfer; in an ambulance during transfer; or in the operating room during neurosurgery, trauma surgery, or vascular surgery). Preventive administration of furosemide and mannitol is given routinely in some neurosurgical procedures and may result in marked polyuria during and after the operation. Hyperglycemia-induced osmotic diuresis is common, can be suspected from polyuria or from hyperglycemia, and is confirmed or ruled out by the presence or absence of glucosuria. Hypervolemia resulting from fluid overload or unmasked by discontinuation of sustained positive-pressure ventilation may increase urine output to greater than 5 L/day for several days in patients with normal renal function. Mobilization of edema during recovery from disease or surgery also can result in sustained polyuria. In all these conditions, however, urine remains close to isotonic (osmolality ≈300 mOsm/kg). Abundant intake of hypotonic fluid can cause polyuria and urine hypotonicity but does not result in hypernatremia if renal function is normal. The observation of decreased urine output after ADH administration is not diagnostic of diabetes insipidus, because ADH can reduce urine output and increase urine osmolality in all conditions except nephrogenic diabetes insipidus.

Treatment

Management of diabetes insipidus includes two components: (1) reduction of excessive urine output and (2) correction of water deficit (Box 167-2). The polyuria of central diabetes insipidus is treated effectively by vasopressin (ADH) or by its synthetic analog, desmopressin acetate (DDAVP [1-deamino-8-D-arginine vasopressin]).[5-7] As indicated by its multiple names, vasopressin not only has antidiuretic but also vasoconstrictive and oxytocic effects, whereas desmopressin essentially retains the antidiuretic action. The effects of aqueous vasopressin (4-10 units subcutaneously or intramuscularly) on diuresis begin rapidly but last for only a few hours. Vasopressin must be repeated every 4 to 6 hours, and it has been recommended only for diagnostic purposes or in acute conditions (e.g., trauma) in which the diabetes insipidus might be transient. The effects of vasopressin tannate in oil emulsion (2-5 units intramuscularly) last 48 to

CAUSES OF DIABETES INSIPIDUS

Central
Congenital anomalies: corpus callosum agenesis, cleft palate
Granulomatous disease: sarcoidosis, tuberculosis, Wegener's disease
Histiocytosis
Sickle cell disease
Idiopathic: autoimmune
Tumors: suprasellar, infrasellar, aneurysms
Infection: meningitis, encephalitis
Head trauma, neurosurgery, brain death

Nephrogenic
Congenital disease
Renal disease: obstructive uropathy, reflux nephropathy, cystic disease, electrolyte disorders
Renal involvement in systemic disease: sarcoidosis, amyloidosis, sickle cell disease
Drugs: phenytoin, aminoglycosides, amphotericin, antivirals, demeclocycline, lithium

96 hours, but the preparation requires close attention to warming and mixing the suspension before injection. Vasopressin tannate was once standard therapy in patients with central diabetes insipidus, but now it has been abandoned in favor of desmopressin. Where still available, vasopressin tannate may be used in patients who are refractory to desmopressin or who experience significant side effects of the drug. Desmopressin has prolonged effects (8-20 hours) and is appropriate for intravenous (IV), subcutaneous, and intranasal routes. Lypressin is another ADH analog that is appropriate for intranasal use, but its effectiveness is limited by its duration of action of only 4 to 6 hours. Desmopressin is known to increase factor VIII and von Willebrand factor levels and is sometimes used for this purpose in patients with coagulation disorders and in surgical procedures associated with significant bleeding; however its efficacy in the absence of von Willebrand syndrome is doubtful. In the ICU and for acute central diabetes insipidus, desmopressin is initially given as 10 to 20 µg intranasally and repeated every 30 to 60 minutes until urine output is reduced to less than 100 mL/h. The initial dose required to maintain a normal urine volume ranges from 10 to 60 µg in most patients. The total appropriate dose is repeated when urine output again increases to greater than 200 mL/h (i.e., after 8-24 hours). The dosage must be reduced if urine output is excessively decreased. Systematic administration is not recommended because most cases of diabetes insipidus seen in ICUs are associated with acute events and may be incomplete or intermittent or both. The subcutaneous route is seldom used, because absorption may be erratic in vasoconstricted patients and an IV line is virtually always available in ICU patients. Desmopressin is injected IV when the intranasal route is not available (i.e., in cases of rhinorrhea and facial trauma). The required initial dose ranges from 2 to 20 µg and is given as repeated 2- to 4-µg boluses.

Vasopressin therapy can be associated with arterial hypertension, myocardial infarction, mesenteric infarction, peripheric ischemia, and uterine cramps. Vasopressin tannate may cause allergic reactions ranging from urticaria to anaphylaxis and sterile abscesses at sites of

MANAGEMENT OF DIABETES INSIPIDUS

Control polyuria with DDAVP or vasopressin.
Calculate and replace free water loss.
Monitor and replace urine losses hourly.
Monitor plasma electrolytes and adapt therapy every 4 hours.

DDAVP, 1-deamino-8-D-arginine vasopressin.

injection. Desmopressin may interfere with anticoagulant drugs and cause hypercoagulability. When given in excess, all these antidiuretic agents can result in oliguria, hyponatremia, and water intoxication. The severity of diabetes insipidus may vary over time, even in patients with chronic diabetes insipidus, and some patients with chronic diabetes insipidus who are used to drinking large amounts of water may continue to do so even if urine output is limited by a diuretic drug.

Patients with acute diabetes insipidus should receive a sufficient amount of water to match urine output until the polyuria is controlled and to correct the deficit of free water that already exists at the time of diagnosis. If the gastrointestinal system is functional, water can be infused at rates of 1 to 2 L/h through a gastric tube. Otherwise, isotonic dextrose should be infused IV in appropriate amounts (hypotonic dextrose administration can be obtained by infusing equal amounts of water and isotonic dextrose in a central vein, but this procedure has been associated with vascular injuries). Practically, the dedicated gastric or IV infusion rate is adjusted at least hourly to match the urine output of the last equivalent period. Additional water is provided to correct the initial water deficit over a few hours. Plasma electrolytes should be monitored every 4 hours until a normal natremia is restored and stabilized. Blood glucose must be monitored closely and hyperglycemia treated aggressively using IV insulin. Failure to control hyperglycemia may be associated with osmotic diuresis due to glucosuria and superimpose an equivalent of diabetes mellitus on the already present diabetes insipidus.

Nephrogenic Diabetes Insipidus

Nephrogenic diabetes insipidus is characterized by the inability of the renal parenchyma to concentrate urine in response to ADH.[7-9] The disorder is seldom diagnosed in the ICU and is usually more severe when it is congenital. Hereditary forms generally result from mutations to the AVP-2 receptors or AQP-2 water channels. Acquired forms are due to vasopressin resistance of the distal tubule and collecting duct, or to markedly reduced renal concentrating capacity. Most of them are attributed to electrolyte disturbances and lithium therapy, but many other drugs have been implicated. Nephrogenic diabetes insipidus may be treated with a low-sodium, low-protein regimen that reduces the solute load, thiazide diuretics that induce a mild volume depletion and help reduce urine volume to acceptable values, and nonsteroidal anti-inflammatory drugs such as indomethacin that inhibit prostaglandin synthesis.

KEY POINTS

1. Diabetes insipidus is characterized by polyuria, urine hypotonicity, and hypernatremia.

2. Central diabetes insipidus results from a lack of antidiuretic hormone (ADH); nephrogenic diabetes insipidus results from renal insensitivity to ADH.

3. In the ICU, diabetes insipidus is caused mainly by pituitary surgery, trauma, and brain death.

4. Clinical signs are dehydration and hypernatremia.

5. ICU patients generally are unable to compensate for excessive urine losses by drinking.

6. Differential diagnosis includes administration of diuretics, mannitol, and iodinated agents.

7. Polyuria is controlled with desmopressin, 10 to 20 µg intranasally or 2 to 4 µg intravenously.

8. Water deficit is corrected with enteral water or intravenous 5% dextrose in water.

9. Diuresis should be monitored hourly, and ongoing urinary losses should be compensated.

ANNOTATED REFERENCES

Verbalis JG. Diabetes insipidus. Rev Endocr Metab Disord 2003;4:177-85.
A general review on diabetes insipidus.

Maghnie M. Diabetes insipidus. Horm Res 2003;59:42-54.
A general review that focuses on etiology and clinical and radiologic features.

Bagshaw SM, Towsend DR. Disorders of sodium and water balance in hospitalized patients. Can J Anesth 2009;56:151-67
A review on sodium and water disorders that includes an extended discussion on the etiology and management of diabetes insipidus.

Sands JM, Bichet DG. Nephrogenic diabetes insipidus. Ann Intern Med 2006;144:186-94.
A updated review of nephrogenic diabetes insipidus.

Garofeanu CG, Weir M, Rosas-Arellano MP, Henson G, Garg AX, Clark WF. Causes of reversible nephrogenic diabetes insipidus: a systematic review. Am J Kidney Dis 2005;45:626-37.
A review of the many causes of acquired nephrogenic diabetes insipidus.

REFERENCES

Access the complete reference list online at http://www.expertconsult.com.

168

Endocrine and Metabolic Crises in the Pediatric Intensive Care Unit

ANDREW C. ARGENT

Increasing numbers of endocrine and metabolic conditions are being recognized, and the number of children in treatment programs for them is increasing. Although improved screening programs and therapy may decrease the number of children requiring critical care for these conditions, it is likely they will be recognized in increasing numbers of critically ill children for the foreseeable future. There is also increasing awareness of the significance of metabolic changes such has hypo- and hyperglycemia in the pediatric intensive care unit (PICU).[1] General principles of PICU management apply to patients with endocrine and metabolic crises (Table 168-1).[2,3] Crises may cause damage with long-term sequelae for the child and family; however, they also present unique diagnostic opportunities. The intensivist has a particular responsibility to:

- Be aware of endocrine and metabolic problems.
- Consider them in the differential diagnosis of particular clinical syndromes.
- Perform appropriate clinical and biochemical investigations.
- Seek advice from specialists in the clinical and laboratory diagnosis and management of the conditions.
- Consider the implications of metabolic and endocrine problems for the family of the affected child.[4]
- Support the development of structures for the comprehensive management of metabolic problems from infancy through adulthood.[5]

Abnormalities of glucose control are relatively common in the PICU, but with the possible exception of diabetes mellitus, endocrine and metabolic crises are uncommon, and most intensivists do not see sufficient case numbers to become expert at managing these disorders. It is crucial to manage children with suspected or proven endocrine or metabolic crises in conjunction with specialist teams. The laboratory investigation of inborn errors of metabolism may be complex, and there are relatively few laboratories worldwide that have the capacity to fully elucidate most of the inborn errors of metabolism. Close cooperation with specialist laboratory centers is essential for accurate diagnosis and management.

A particular problem of endocrine and metabolic crises is that laboratory investigation of specific conditions may take time while patients require urgent therapeutic intervention. Because it may not always be possible to follow algorithms of investigation, a reasonable approach is to collect all relevant specimens immediately,[6] store them appropriately, and liaise with laboratory services to use the specimens in a logical and cost-effective manner to confirm the diagnosis.

Endocrine Crises

Endocrine crises present in a limited number of ways that include abnormalities of glucose control, fluid and electrolyte balance, and blood pressure control. Management of these crises consists of identifying the problem, investigating the cause, and correcting the abnormality directly or managing the underlying problem. This section provides a clinical overview of pediatric endocrine crises; detailed pathophysiology is discussed in other chapters.

ABNORMALITIES OF GLUCOSE CONTROL

Abnormalities of glucose control, including diabetic ketoacidosis, are the most common endocrine crises encountered in the PICU. Hypoglycemia and hyperglycemia are associated with increased mortality[1,7] in sick children and may be part of a wide variety of disease processes. Measurement of blood glucose is part of the initial biochemical evaluation of any sick child, particularly if a depressed level of consciousness or shock is present. When an abnormal glucose level has been identified, it must be addressed and levels be remeasured at appropriate intervals until the problem has been resolved. The situation is further complicated by technical issues in the measurement of blood glucose,[8,9] with differences between blood and plasma glucose level (glucose concentration in plasma is approximately 11% higher than whole blood because of the higher water content in plasma, but this may be affected by anemia or polycythemia); differences between arterial, venous, and capillary glucose levels (which may also vary depending on clinical context),[8] and potentially significant differences between measurement techniques.[9] A particular concern is that in general, inaccuracies increase at lower glucose levels.[9] Generally, central laboratory devices are taken as the standard, although there is increasing utilization (and convenience) of point-of-care devices.

Hypoglycemia

Hypoglycemia may be associated with devastating damage to the brain and requires immediate attention. In general, a diagnosis of hypoglycemia depends on the presence of symptoms and a low blood glucose level, and resolution of symptoms on correction of the low glucose level. Unfortunately, symptoms of hypoglycemia are relatively nonspecific, ranging from lethargy, poor feeding, hypotonia, and "jitteriness" to convulsions, apneic episodes, cardiovascular collapse, and sudden infant death syndrome (SIDS). Hypoglycemia may be hidden in the complex of critical illness, particularly if patients are deeply sedated and paralyzed. In addition, some diabetic patients have reduced awareness of hypoglycemia.[10] Thus, regular monitoring of blood glucose is an important component of the management of any critically ill child.

Hypoglycemia immediately following birth may be common, but there are considerable controversies in the definition of hypoglycemia in this period.[11-13] Table 168-2 lists an approach to hypoglycemia immediately following birth.

Symptomatic hypoglycemia occurs more frequently during the neonatal period than in any other period of childhood. Infants at particular risk include infants with poor hepatic glycogen stores (e.g., preterm or small-for-gestational-age infants); poor glucose intake (e.g., preterm or ill infants); and hyperinsulinism, either primary or secondary to high intrauterine glucose levels (e.g., infants of diabetic mothers).[14] Hypoglycemia also may be a feature of perinatal illness including asphyxia, polycythemia, hypothermia, septicemia, and respiratory distress syndrome. Much less common causes include growth hormone[15] or adrenal insufficiency,[16] inborn errors of metabolism, and glucagon insufficiency. Drugs administered to the mother during pregnancy, including oral hypoglycemic agents, also must be considered.

TABLE 168-1	Principles of Management of Metabolic and Endocrine Crises	
Principle	*Specifics of Conditions*	
Airway management	Many patients have depressed level of consciousness, and airway management is essential to prevent complications.	
Breathing support	Acidotic patients may make huge respiratory effort; ventilatory support may help decrease the metabolic demands on these patients. Although administration of sodium bicarbonate may help to settle some of the acidosis-related symptoms such as hyperventilation, bicarbonate may aggravate some problems seen in conjunction with urea cycle defects. Give bicarbonate only if the plasma bicarbonate <10 mmol/L, and then only half correct deficits.	
Circulatory support	Ensure adequate circulating volume; this may be a particular issue if there has been excessive fluid loss from vomiting or diarrhea.	
Disability	Control seizures using anticonvulsant agents. Administer pyridoxine if possibility of pyridoxine dependency.	
Dialysis to remove toxins where necessary	Hemodialysis is the most efficient means of removing toxins such as ammonia and leucine. Hemofiltration is less efficient but may be more applicable in critically ill children. Peritoneal dialysis is slower but has the advantage of ease of initiation.[1] In some conditions, it may be possible to remove toxins by stimulating alternative pathways of metabolism.	
Ensure that glucose is maintained in the normal range	A normal glucose level should be maintained at all times. Excessive administration of glucose in the mitochondrial energy chain problem may exacerbate lactic acidosis. Also, attempt to provide an adequate energy supply (may use medium-chain fatty acids where appropriate). Minimize energy demands on patient.	
Fluids	In general, provide 1.5× normal fluid maintenance requirements to accelerate excretion of water-soluble toxins. In the context of encephalopathy (MSUD or urea cycle defects), be careful to avoid overhydration, which may contribute to development of cerebral edema.	
Feeds	If there is accumulation of a product, this needs to be eliminated from the diet (e.g., fructose, galactose). Start with protein-free diet, but do not continue beyond 2 days, because the catabolic state also creates problems. If diagnosis not identified, need gradual reintroduction of feeds and nutrition. If there is deficiency of any nutrient (e.g., carnitine, which may have a primary or a secondary deficiency), supplement that nutrient. Ensure there is an adequate energy source along a metabolic route that is functional. Provide specific vitamin therapy where indicated.	
Family support and information	The diagnosis of an inborn error of metabolism has major implications for families, and considerable support is required.[2]	
Treat *infection*	Infections are an important component of pediatric ICU presentation of inborn errors of metabolism. Some conditions such as galactosemia are related to specific infections such as *Escherichia coli*. Other conditions are related to pyogenic infections because of neutropenia. Children who are in a poor nutritional or metabolic state are more susceptible to infection. Intercurrent infections may be the precipitating factor for metabolic decompensation.	
Investigations	A wide variety of investigations are relevant to inborn errors of metabolism. Biochemical testing on a range of body fluids and on tissues is fundamental to accurate diagnosis of the problem. Biochemical tests may range from simple screening tests to more complex tests on tissue culture. Imaging techniques such as CT, MRI, magnetic resonance spectroscopy, and echocardiography may be relevant. Functional tests such as EEG, ECG, and EMG may be useful in diagnosis. Increasingly, genetic diagnosis is available if children have recognized genetic mutations.	
Monitor response to therapy	Clinical monitoring is essential. Biochemical monitoring of the appropriate metabolites is essential to ensure that metabolic control is established.	

CT, computed tomography; *ECG*, electrocardiogram; *EEG*, electroencephalogram; *EMG*, electromyogram; *ICU*, intensive care unit; *MRI*, magnetic resonance imaging.

In childhood, hypoglycemia may result from inadequate glucose intake (prolonged starvation, malabsorption); defects in glycogenolysis (glycogen storage disorders) or gluconeogenesis (fructose-1,6-diphosphatase deficiency, ethanol intoxication, Jamaican vomiting sickness, etc.), fatty acid oxidation disorders and defects in ketogenesis, deficiency of gluconeogenic hormones (e.g., adrenalin, corticosteroids, glucagons, growth hormone, thyroid hormone), excessive insulin secretion (hyperinsulinism), and a variety of specific disorders including abnormalities of amino acid metabolism.[17]

TABLE 168-2	At-Risk Infants for Whom Routine Monitoring of Blood Glucose Is Recommended

Associated with Changes in Maternal Metabolism

Intrapartum administration of glucose
Drug treatment:
  Terbutaline, ritodrine, propranolol
  Oral hypoglycemic agents
Diabetes in pregnancy/infant of diabetic mother

Associated with Neonatal Problems

Idiopathic condition or failure to adapt
Perinatal hypoxia-ischemia
Infection
Hypothermia
Hyperviscosity
Erythroblastosis fetalis, fetal hydrops
Other:
  Iatrogenic causes
  Congenital cardiac malformations

Intrauterine Growth Restriction

Hyperinsulinism

Endocrine Disorders

Inborn Errors of Metabolism

From Cornblath M, Hawdon JM, Williams AF et al. Controversies regarding definition of neonatal hypoglycemia: suggested operational thresholds. Pediatrics. 2000;105:1141-5.

The amount of glucose required to achieve normoglycemia and the duration of fast that can be endured without the development of hypoglycemia may assist in identifying a likely cause. Transient hypoglycemia that can be reversed with normal infusion rates of glucose (4-6 mg/kg/min) and does not recur is unlikely to be associated with an endocrine problem. Hyperinsulinemia is associated with rapid development of hypoglycemia and high glucose requirements (>6-8 mg/kg/min to >15-20 mg/kg/min). Hypoglycemia associated with adrenal insufficiency, growth hormone deficiency, and hypothyroidism tends to occur after several hours of fasting, is associated with ketosis, and can be reversed with normal infusion rates of glucose. Fatty acid oxidation defects are associated with hypoglycemia after a fast of some hours.

As soon as hypoglycemia is noted, specimens should be collected immediately for appropriate tests (Table 168-3). Treatment of hypoglycemia with intravenous (IV) glucose should be initiated promptly. An initial bolus dose of 0.5 g/kg of glucose (may need 0.5-2 g/kg in neonates) should be given as a 10% or 25% (in older children) dextrose solution, followed by an ongoing infusion of glucose at a rate of 4 to 8 mg/kg/min. The concentration of the ongoing infusion depends on the fluid requirements of the child and the availability of central venous access (for higher concentrations). Glucagon may be given at a dose of 0.1 to 0.3 mg/kg (IV or intramuscularly [IM]) but is unlikely to be effective in patients with low glycogen stores, glycogen storage disorders, or hepatic dysfunction. Hydrocortisone at a dose of 5 mg/kg every 12 hours may be useful in some patients. Diazoxide and IV octreotide decrease insulin release and may be useful in the management of hyperinsulinemia.

If non–glucose-reducing substances are present in the urine, galactosemia, hereditary fructose intolerance, or tyrosinemia should be considered. In the absence of reducing substances, low urinary ketones with hypoglycemia suggest hyperinsulinism or defects of fatty acid oxidation. The latter can be distinguished from hyperinsulinemia by

TABLE 168-3	Investigation of Hypoglycemia
Blood glucose	Measurement of glucose using blood from capillary specimens and using test strips may be unreliable (particularly in poorly perfused patients or patients with high hematocrit); where possible, low glucose levels should be confirmed using laboratory assays on venous or arterial blood.
Actual glucose intake	Hypoglycemia in the presence of normal glucose intake or after brief fast suggests hyperinsulinism. Hypoglycemia after hours of fasting is associated with fatty acid oxidation defects and endocrine insufficiency.
Non–glucose-reducing substances in the urine	Particularly in neonates and probably not relevant in older children. If present in the urine, consider galactosemia, hereditary fructose intolerance, or tyrosinemia.
Serum and urinary ketones	Low ketones suggest hyperinsulinism or fatty acid oxidation problem.
Serum free fatty acids	Free fatty acids are low in hyperinsulinism but high in fatty acid oxidation defect.
Serum insulin (and C peptide), cortisol, glucagon, growth hormone, and thyroid levels	Normal serum insulin in the presence of hypoglycemia is evidence of hyperinsulinism. C peptide may be necessary to ascertain whether exogenous insulin was administered. Release of C peptide may not be as pulsatile as that of insulin.
Serum ammonia	To recognize hyperinsulinism/hyperammonemia syndrome
Urinary organic acids and serum amino acids	To diagnose fatty acid oxidation defects (urinary organic acids). Aminoacidopathies such as MSUD, propionic acidemia, isovaleric acidemia, methylmalonic acidemia, and tyrosinemia may also present with hypoglycemia.
Total and free carnitine with acylcarnitine profile	To recognize primary and secondary deficiency of carnitine and fatty acid oxidation defects

the presence of high serum free fatty acids. Assays of insulin levels can confirm the diagnosis of hyperinsulinism.

Abnormalities of growth hormone, cortisol, or thyroid hormone typically are associated with high urinary ketones, the absence of hepatomegaly, and increased lactate. Hypoglycemia also may occur as a complication of insulin therapy for diabetes mellitus. Patients with diabetes mellitus may have inadequate responses to hypoglycemia.

Neonates. In the neonatal period, glucose is not the only energy source from oxidative metabolism in the brain, and alternative energy sources such as ketones may be used.[11] In fact, breast-fed babies routinely have lower glucose levels and higher ketone levels than formula-fed infants. Recent reviews have highlighted that "there is inadequate information in the literature to define any one value of glucose below which irreparable hypoglycemic injury to the central nervous system occurs, at any one time or for any defined period of time, in a population of infants or in any given infant."[18] However, there is evidence that hypoglycemic injury is more likely to occur at very low levels of glucose (20-25 mg/dL [1.1-1.4 mmol/L]) and if hypoglycemia is prolonged, is the consequence of hyperinsulinemia (when alternative energy sources for the brain may be very limited), and in the presence of other potential injuries.[18,19]

A suggested approach to hypoglycemia in the neonatal period is shown in Figure 168-1. Although the threshold for treatment in the asymptomatic neonate is 25 to 30 mg/dL (1.1-1.4 mmol/L), the recommended levels during treatment are above 45 mg/dL (2.5 mmol/L).

Although the exact definition of hypoglycemia in children is controversial, a minimal level of 2.6 mmol/L or greater should be maintained to ensure normal neural function.[12,20,21] It probably is safer to maintain a level of greater than 3.5 mmol/L. Because there are multiple causes for hypoglycemia, and symptoms may not be due to the hypoglycemia alone, it is essential to identify the cause.

Hypoglycemia is associated with severe illness. A wide range of illnesses including infections,[22] cyanotic and acyanotic congenital heart disease, and cardiomyopathy/myocarditis have been associated with

hypoglycemia. Hepatic failure from infection, toxin ingestion, or drug reactions may be associated with severe hypoglycemia, and Reye syndrome classically presents with hypoglycemia. Toxins such as salicylates and ethanol also may cause hypoglycemia. Hypoglycemia has been linked with increased mortality from malaria,[23-26] gastroenteritis,[27] and acute bacterial meningitis[28] among other conditions. Hypoglycemia also has been described as a complication of therapy for leukemia with mercaptopurine and methotrexate.[29,30] Although severe illness or sepsis may be an adequate explanation for hypoglycemia, a diagnosis of sepsis should not exclude the possibility of an endocrine or metabolic crisis.

Hyperinsulinemic Hypoglycemia. Hyperinsulinism is the most common cause of persistent or recurrent hypoglycemia in infancy.[31-33] Hyperinsulinism may be secondary to risk factors in the perinatal period (associated with high maternal glucose levels,[34] rhesus incompatibility, intrauterine growth retardation,[35] and perinatal asphyxia[36]) but may also be congenital[37,38] or associated with Beckwith-Weidemann syndrome and some other developmental syndromes.[33]

Although most patients with hyperinsulinemic hypoglycemia present in the neonatal period, first presentation may be during infancy and occasionally during childhood,[39] when the condition may be more likely to respond to medical therapy. Neonates with hypoglycemia may have the macrosomia typical of infants of diabetic mothers, but hyperinsulinemic hypoglycemia may occur in apparently normal infants of normal or low birth weight. Hypertrophic cardiomyopathy and hepatomegaly may be seen[31] in affected infants. The characteristic features of hyperinsulinism include hypoglycemia with glucose requirements of greater than 6 to 8 mg/kg/min to maintain normoglycemia, absence of ketonemia and ketonuria, low plasma free fatty acids and branch chain amino acids, detectable insulin at the time of hypoglycemia, and response to glucagon administration.[31] The combination of hypoglycemia with low free fatty acids and absence of ketonemia is responsible for the potentially devastating effects of this condition on the brain, as it is deprived of both normal and alternate substrates.[32]

Hyperinsulinemic hypoglycemia with hyperammonemia (previously called *leucine-sensitive hypoglycemia)* is well described[40,41] and is attributed to mutations in the gene for glutamate dehydrogenase. Patients generally respond well to therapy with diazoxide, and consumption of extra carbohydrate before protein meals may help ameliorate symptoms. Special low-leucine milks are available.

Congenital hyperinsulinemic hypoglycemia is caused by abnormalities in genes controlling the secretion of insulin by the beta cells of the pancreas, with abnormalities described in seven genes.[32]

Initial stabilization therapy consists of glucose infusions to achieve normoglycemia. Because there may be extremely high glucose requirements and any cessation of infusion may be associated with severe hypoglycemia, it is essential to ensure that secure vascular access is *always* available, and central venous access may be required. Glucagon (0.5-1 mg/kg as an emergency dose IM or by IV bolus; alternatively, subcutaneously or as an IV infusion of 1-20 µg/kg/h) must always be available and can be used as short-term, emergency therapy to maintain normoglycemia if there are problems with vascular access. Administration of glucagon may be associated with rebound hypoglycemia, and frequent glucose monitoring must be continued. Octreotide (5-30 µg/kg/day subcutaneously or as an IV infusion) may also be given together with glucagon, but this drug may be associated with an increased risk of enterocolitis. As soon as normoglycemia has been achieved, the child should be transported to a center with specific expertise in the management of hyperinsulinemia. Great care must be taken to ensure that hypoglycemia does not occur during transport.

The aim of further management is to confirm the diagnosis and ensure normoglycemia (keep glucose levels > 3.5 mmol/L in view of low alternative sources of energy) without the ongoing use of glucose infusions. Glucose polymers can be added to the diet to provide an enteral source of glucose, but care must be taken to limit the osmolar load on the gut, particularly in premature infants.

Clinically, hyperinsulinemic hypoglycemic patients may be categorized by their response to diazoxide (5-20 mg/kg/d in 2-3 divided

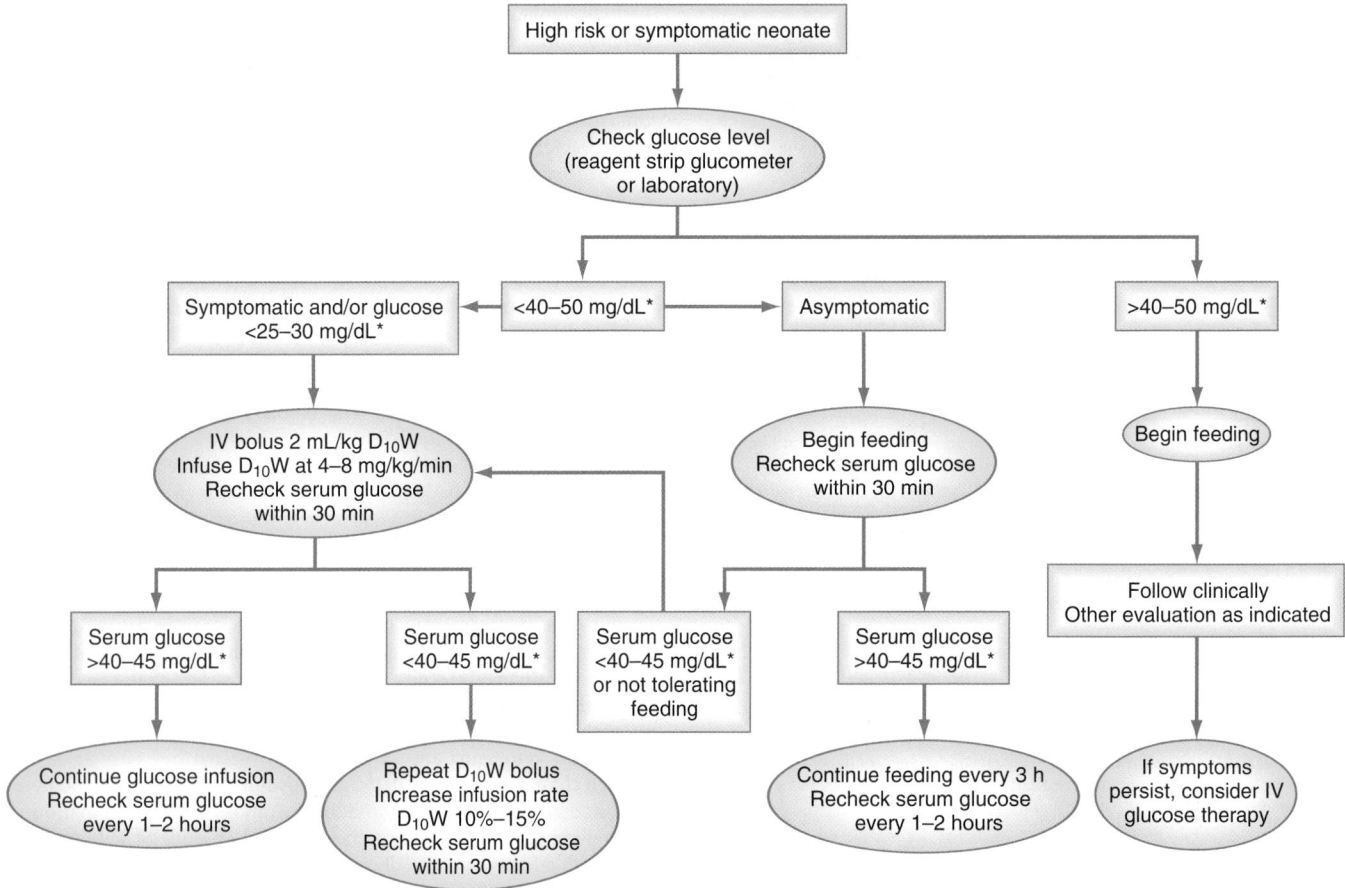

Figure 168-1   A suggested approach to management of the neonate with low glucose. *(From Rozance PJ, Hay WW. Hypoglycemia in newborn infants: features associated with adverse outcomes. Biol Neonate 2006;90:74-86.)*

doses), with most responding. Exceptions include those with congenital hyperinsulinemia related to focal hyperinsulinemia and those with diffuse hyperinsulinemia related to inactivating mutations in *ABCC8* and *KCNJ11*. Unfortunately, diazoxide may predispose to fluid retention, and use must be carefully monitored. Chlorothiazide (7-10 mg/kg/day in 2 divided doses) may be added (particularly in neonates).[32] Nifedipine (0.25-2.5 mg/kg/d in 3 divided doses) may also be useful in some patients.[42]

A suggested approach to ongoing diagnosis and management is outlined in Figure 168-2, showing a marked change from previous practice. In those patients who are responsive to diazoxide, that will remain the basis of therapy. In those with no response to diazoxide, genetic testing (for homozygous or compound heterozygous mutations in *ABCC8* and *KCNJ11*), followed by fluorine-18 (^{18}F)-dopa positron emission tomography (PET) scanning for those with potentially focal pancreatic lesions will enable identification of those who may benefit from resection of the pancreas. Pancreatic islets cells take up L-3, 4-dihydroxyphenylalanine (L-dopa), where it is converted to dopamine by dopa-decarboxylase. Uptake of the positron-emitting tracer ^{18}F-dopa PET is increased in beta cells with a high rate of insulin synthesis and secretion provides visualization of the focal lesion.[43-46] Patients with focal lesions should respond to partial pancreatectomy, which may be done laparoscopically.[47,48] Diffuse disease that is unresponsive to diazoxide therapy will require a near-total pancreatectomy and may be associated with a high incidence of both endocrine and exocrine problems.[49]

Close long-term follow up will be required in all these patients, and there may be significant neurologic and psychological problems to be dealt with.[49]

Ketotic Hypoglycemia.   Although ketotic hypoglycemia ("accelerated starvation") is probably the most common cause of hypoglycemia in previously healthy children,[50] it is unlikely to present in the PICU. This condition usually affects children aged 6 months to 8 years, and the clinical features include ketosis, severe nausea, and hypoglycemia, usually occurring in the morning after a moderate fast. Treatment consists of ensuring that there is an adequate and regular intake of glucose, particularly during intercurrent infections. Urinary ketones may act as a warning signal, because the ketosis usually precedes the onset of hypoglycemia by several hours.

Adrenal Insufficiency.   Adrenal insufficiency after high-dose inhaled corticosteroid therapy has presented with hypoglycemia[51-54] and should be considered if there is a past history of inhaled steroid use (particularly fluticasone).[53,55] Adrenal insufficiency also may occur after adrenal bleeds (e.g., after meningococcal septicemia or difficult delivery), as part of adrenal disease (e.g., congenital adrenal hyperplasia or hypoplasia) in which ambiguous genitalia may (or may not) be a pointer in females, or as part of hypopituitarism (e.g., congenital, after craniopharyngioma, or after cranial irradiation[56]). Some patients with primary adrenal insufficiency may present with hypoglycemia, particularly during acute illnesses.[16,57] Adrenoleukodystrophy should be considered as part of the etiologic diagnosis in any male patient with Addison's disease (pigmentation may be a clue) and should be tested for by measurement of very-long-chain fatty acids.[58,57]

There has been considerable interest in adrenocorticoid deficiency in children with critical illness and particularly acute severe sepsis (see Chapter 131).[59-63] Currently, supplementary steroids are recommended for children with acute severe sepsis and catecholamine resistant

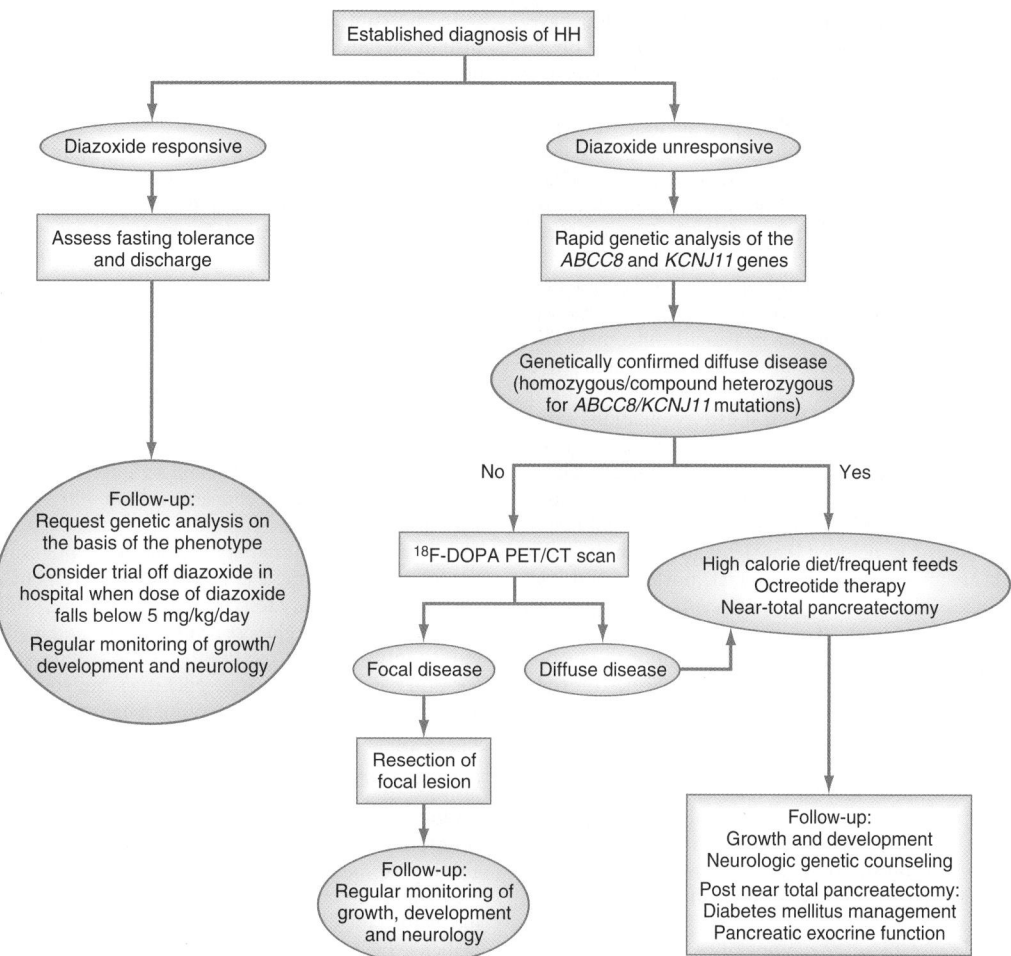

Figure 168-2 Flow chart outlining the management cascade of neonates with hyperinsulinemic hypoglycemia (HH). Clinically, HH can be classified into diazoxide-responsive and diazoxide-unresponsive disease. A fluorine-18 L-3, 4-dihydroxyphenylalanine positron emission tomography (^{18}F-dopa PET) scan is currently only indicated in neonates who are unresponsive to diazoxide and do not have genetically confirmed diffuse disease. *(From Kapoor RR, Flanagan SE, James C, Shield J, Ellard S, Hussain K. Hyperinsulinaemic hypoglycaemia. Arch Dis Child 2009;94:450-7.)*

shock,[64,65] but there are not clear definitions for either adrenal insufficiency or catecholamine resistance, nor are there firm recommendations for the dose of adrenal replacement therapy.

Adrenocorticoid deficiency also has been shown in preterm infants.[66] A randomized controlled study of "stress" dose hydrocortisone therapy in hypotensive very low-birthweight infants showed that steroids were effective in treating refractory hypotension.[67]

Congenital adrenal hyperplasia is associated rarely with hypoglycemia. Female patients are usually diagnosed early in life as a result of virilization, whereas male patients tend to present later. Patients with the salt-losing form of congenital adrenal hyperplasia present with hyponatremic dehydration and shock, usually associated with hyperkalemia. Because patients with salt-wasting 21-hydroxylase deficiency also may have catecholamine deficiency, shock may be a significant feature. Diagnosis is based on the clinical picture, typical electrolyte pattern, hypoaldosteronism, and hyperreninemia.[68] Long-term treatment consists of hydrocortisone (to suppress excess secretion of corticotropin-releasing hormone and corticotropin), 10 to 20 mg/m^2 of body surface area per day in three divided doses, although larger doses may be required during adrenal crises, together with mineralocorticoid replacement (0.1-0.2 mg of fludrocortisone daily) and sodium chloride supplementation. Little is known about the dose of hydrocortisone required during critical illness, although Charmandari et al.[69] showed that when 6-hourly bolus doses of 15 mg/m^2 of hydrocortisone are given, high immediate serum levels are achieved, followed by rapid decline to undetectable levels by 4 hours after administration.

These authors postulated that continuous infusion of hydrocortisone may be more appropriate in critical illness.

Growth Hormone Deficiency. In the neonatal period, growth hormone deficiency presents with hypoglycemia (possibly with seizures), prolonged jaundice, and in boys, micropenis and undescended testes. Growth failure becomes apparent only toward the end of the first year of life. In later childhood, growth failure is a more common presentation, and hypoglycemia rarely occurs[56] unless associated with adrenocorticotropic hormone deficiency.

Hyperglycemia Other Than Diabetes Mellitus

Hyperglycemia is relatively common in the PICU.[70] In a retrospective study of 948 nondiabetic patients admitted to the PICU, there was a high prevalence of hyperglycemia, with 70.4% of patients having a glucose value above 120 mg/dL, 44.5% above 150 mg/dL, and 22.3% above 200 mg/dL within 10 days of admission. A 2.5-fold increased risk of dying was seen if the maximum glucose obtained within 24 hours of admission was over 150 mg/dL and a 5.68-fold increased risk if the maximum glucose obtained within 10 days of admission to the PICU was over 120 mg/dL.[71] However, that study was retrospective and not corrected for severity of illness. In addition, ascertainment bias was present,[72] so the study could not really provide insight in terms of causality or the potential impact of therapy.[73]

Hyperglycemia is common in a wide variety of conditions including bronchiolitis,[74] sepsis, hemolytic uremic syndrome,[75] tetanus,[76] and toxin ingestion (e.g., theophylline poisoning[77]). Other studies have confirmed that high glucose levels are not only common in the PICU population but are associated with increased mortality and/or morbidity in a wide variety of conditions.[78-81]

Iatrogenic causes of hyperglycemia in the PICU include resuscitation using glucose-containing fluids, parenteral nutrition or high load of administered glucose, and high-dose corticosteroid therapy. Continuing hyperglycemia may also be an indication of ongoing stress or undiagnosed type 1 diabetes and should prompt the clinician to investigate further.

An initial report from an adult surgical unit (predominantly cardiac)[82] provided evidence that "tight" control of glucose levels was associated with a significant improvement in patient outcomes. The same group studied a cohort of patients in a medical ICU, and there was no difference in mortality between groups.[83] There have been numerous studies in a variety of adult critical care populations since that time, with positive effects of tight glucose control noted on cholestasis,[84] renal function,[85] neurologic and neuromuscular complications,[86,87] and endothelial function.[88] Unfortunately, there have also been increased reports of iatrogenic hypoglycemia, and a recent meta-analysis of studies in adults[89] concluded that tight glucose control was not associated with an improvement in hospital mortality and was associated with an increased incidence of hypoglycemia. Subsequently, a large randomized controlled trial (RCT) of adult patients compared "tight" (81-108 mg/dL or 4.5-6.0 mmol/L) with "conventional" glucose control (target of ≤180 mg/dL or ≤10.0 mmol/L). The 90-day mortality was higher in the group on tight glucose control, and subgroup analysis showed that the outcomes favored conventional control in all groups except trauma patients and patients on steroids.

Pediatricians have been more cautious in their approach to control of hyperglycemia, but a number of protocols for PICU management of hyperglycemia have been implemented and reported.[90,91] An RCT of protocols for tight glucose control in the PICU showed no difference between a paper-based protocol and a computerized decision support tool.[92]

In a study of glycemic control in 177 postoperative cardiac patients,[93] there was no difference in glucose levels on day 1 between survivors and nonsurvivors, but the 5-day mean peak glucose levels were significantly higher in nonsurvivors. Insulin usage was higher in the nonsurvivors, and nonsurvivors had more hypoglycemic events. The authors speculated that targeting a more permissive glucose level of 90-140 mg/dL (5-7.7 mmol/L) might be associated with both improved outcomes and reduced risk of hypoglycemia. In a retrospective review of 100 postoperative cardiac patients, there was high incidence of hyperglycemia (and an association with higher severity of illness), and implementation of a pediatric glycemic control protocol had a low incidence of hypoglycemia.[79]

A prospective RCT of 700 critically ill children (317 infants and 383 children) admitted to PICU[94] randomized patients to targeted blood glucose levels (throughout PICU stay) of 2.8 to 4.4 mmol/L in infants and 3.9 to 5.6 mmol/L in children, with insulin infusion throughout PICU stay (intensive group [n=349]) or to insulin infusion only to prevent blood glucose from exceeding 11.9 mmol/L (conventional group [n=351]). Mean blood glucose concentrations were lower in the intensive group than in the conventional group, and hypoglycemia (glucose ≤2.2 mmol/L) occurred in 87 (25%) patients in the intensive group ($P < 0.0001$) versus 5 (1%) patients in the conventional group. Severe hypoglycemia (blood glucose less than 117 mmol/L) occurred in 17 (5%) of the intensive group versus 3 (1%) of the conventional group ($P=0.001$). Duration of PICU stay was reduced in the intensively treated group (5.51 days [95% CI, 4.65-6.37] versus 6.15 days [95% CI, 5.25-7.05]; $P=0.017$). The number of patients with stay in PICU longer than the median was 132 (38%) in the intensive group versus 165 (47%) in the conventional group ($P=0.013$). Nine (3%) patients died in the intensively treated group versus 20 (6%) in the conventional group ($P = 0.038$). There is ongoing debate about appropriate targets for glucose, optimization of protocols, balance of nutrient and glucose intake versus insulin therapy, and the like.

In the context of major burns there is also some evidence that insulin therapy to maintain lower blood glucose levels may be associated with improvements in metabolism.[95]

A recent review[96] concluded:

Hence, efficacy and safety of intensive insulin therapy may be affected by patient-related and ICU setting-related variables. Therefore, no single optimal blood glucose target range for ICU patients can be advocated. It appears safe not to embark on targeting "age-normal" levels in PICUs that are not equipped to accurately and frequently measure blood glucose, and have not acquired extensive experience with intravenous insulin administration using a customized guideline. A simple fallback position could be to control blood glucose levels as close to normal as possible without evoking unacceptable blood glucose fluctuations, hypoglycemia, and hypokalemia.

Pediatricians have been reluctant to implement tight glucose control in PICU because of concerns about the deleterious effects of hypoglycemia.[97,98]

A recent review of hyperglycemia in the preterm infant[99] suggested the following pragmatic approach to management: confirm hyperglycemia with laboratory test; treat any underlying problem such as sepsis, stress, etc.; calculate glucose infusion rates, and if above 12 mg/kg/min, reduce infusion rate; treat with insulin if glucose is over 10 mmol/L (or other symptoms such as polyuria), but start cautiously with very low doses; finally, if hyperglycemia persists, consider other diagnoses such as diabetes.

Diabetes Mellitus

Children with diabetes mellitus have a higher mortality than healthy children,[100,101] with standardized mortality ratios of 2.15[102] to 4.2,[103] although some deaths are not directly related to diabetes. The highest mortality is in children aged 1 to 4 years, in whom the standardized mortality ratios may be 9.2[104] to 13.7.[105] Most deaths attributable to diabetes mellitus occur as a consequence of diabetic ketoacidosis (DKA) or hyperglycemia, with the remainder attributable to hypoglycemia.[104] Diabetic ketoacidosis is relatively common at the time of first presentation, particularly in younger children,[106] in whom diagnosis may be delayed. Although the incidence of type 1 diabetes mellitus has been increasing in many parts of the world, the hospitalization rate for DKA in established and new cases of type 1 diabetes mellitus has not increased in Canada and Europe since the 1990s[107,108] because of earlier diagnosis and safer ambulatory management with the help of a multidisciplinary team.

The mortality rate in the developed world for DKA ranges from 0.15% to 0.31%[109] but may be far higher in other settings.[110] The most common cause of death among patients with DKA is cerebral edema. Other causes of death in DKA include electrolyte disturbances, hypoglycemia, pulmonary edema, rhabdomyolysis, infections (including mucormycosis), and thrombosis. The management of DKA in childhood has been extensively reviewed elsewhere,[109,111,112] with current recommendations.

Cerebral Edema in Diabetic Ketoacidosis. In affluent countries, symptomatic cerebral edema occurs in 0.5% to 1% of pediatric DKA episodes,[113] with risks being higher in young children and previously undiagnosed diabetics. Mortality is high (21%-24%), and 15% to 26% of survivors will have permanent morbidity (including pituitary insufficiency).[113]

The exact mechanisms of cerebral edema in DKA are not clear,[114] although some imaging studies suggest that cerebral edema may be related to vasogenic factors rather than osmotic factors.[115] Cerebral hyperemia has also been demonstrated as part of abnormal autoregulation.[116,117] Factors that have been associated with the development of cerebral edema include the administration of bicarbonate, a higher plasma urea, arterial partial pressure of carbon dioxide (Pco_2),[118,119] and a smaller increase in plasma sodium concentration during therapy.[120] However, a recent systematic review[121] of the literature concluded that there was no clear evidence that treatment was related to the development of cerebral edema. Cerebral ischemia and reperfusion injury have also been considered.[122] Cerebral edema may be present before therapy for DKA in 5% of cases, although most cases develop 4 to 12 hours after initiation of therapy.[118,123] The clinical signs of cerebral edema in DKA are variable and include headache, deterioration in level of consciousness, inappropriate slowing of pulse rate, and increased blood pressure. However, children with no clinical signs of cerebral edema have been documented to have brain swelling,[124] and a significant proportion of children have disrupted memory function following episodes of DKA.[125]

Adverse outcomes have been associated with greater neurologic depression at the time of diagnosis, high initial serum urea nitrogen,[118,126] and intubation with hyperventilation to a P_{CO_2} less than 22 mm Hg.[126,127]

Although the biochemical derangements of hyperglycemia, metabolic acidosis with ketosis, and electrolyte abnormalities are the most obvious problems in DKA, significant derangements in other systems have been documented, including plasma tryptophan levels,[128] thiamine levels,[129] cytokine[130] and lymphocyte responses,[130] and coagulation abnormalities.[130] There is little doubt that DKA is associated with a thrombotic state[131] and an increased incidence of cerebrovascular accidents, and care should be taken about the use of femoral central venous access because this may have a higher than usual complication rate in these patients.[132] A reported case of myocardial infarction related to DKA[133] may be a complication of the thrombotic state. Although myocardial function is generally normal in DKA, myocarditis[134] has been noted in occasional case reports, whereas pulmonary edema may be more common than previously recognized.[135] Prolongation of the QTc interval may be common in DKA (it correlates with ketosis), and careful cardiac monitoring is essential.[136]

Principles of Management. Management of DKA should be coordinated by an experienced diabetes team. The biochemical criteria for the diagnosis of DKA include a serum glucose concentration above 11 mmol/L (~200 mg/dL), ketonemia and ketonuria, and acidosis with venous pH below 7.3, or serum bicarbonate level below 15 mEq/L.[112] The severity of DKA is defined by the level of acidosis, with mild having venous pH less than 7.3 (or bicarbonate <15 mmol/L); moderate, pH less than 7.2 (or bicarbonate <10 mmol/L); and severe, pH less than 7.1 (or bicarbonate <5 mmol/L).[112] Children with severe DKA should be managed in a specialized diabetic unit or in the PICU.

Baseline Assessment. An admission weight should be obtained if at all possible, and future therapy should be based on this weight. Blood samples should be taken for the following investigations: serum or plasma glucose, electrolytes (including bicarbonate or total carbon dioxide), blood urea nitrogen, creatinine, osmolality, venous (or arterial in critically ill patient) pH, P_{CO_2}, calcium, phosphorus, and magnesium concentrations (if possible), HbA_{1c}, hemoglobin and hematocrit or complete blood count. Measurement of blood β-hydroxybutyrate concentration, if available, is useful to confirm ketoacidosis and may be used to monitor the response to treatment.[137-140] Urine specimens should be analyzed for ketones. Electrocardiograms may be useful if delays are expected in getting potassium results.

Fluid Management. The objectives of fluid and electrolyte replacement therapy are restoration of circulating volume, replacement of sodium and body fluid deficit, improved renal function with enhanced clearance of glucose and ketones from the blood, and minimization of risk of cerebral edema.[112] There is a wide range in the amount and rate of fluid and electrolyte loss in patients presenting with DKA (depending on the rate of onset and duration of symptoms, the severity of vomiting or diarrhea or both, and the fluid ingested by the patient).[112] There is a wide range of intravascular status ranging from normovolemia to severe hypovolemia (uncommon). Clinical assessment of dehydration is notoriously inaccurate, and there is an unpredictable rate of ongoing fluid loss related to the osmotic diuresis. In the (unusual) presence of hypovolemic shock, it is reasonable to infuse 0.9% saline

using aliquots of 5 to 10 mL/kg until an acceptable blood pressure is obtained.[141] Typically, 10 to 20 mL/kg needs to be infused over 1 to 2 hours.[109] Ringer's lactate may be a reasonable alternative, because administration of large volumes of 0.9% saline has been associated with the development of hyperchloremic acidosis. There is no evidence to support the use of colloid solutions.

Thereafter the acceptable principles are that hypovolemia, rapid changes in plasma osmolality, and large volumes of sodium uptake should be avoided. Fluid therapy should be calculated to achieve rehydration over 48 hours.[109,112,113] Careful monitoring of fluid balance is essential to ensure that patients are neither losing excessive fluid (via osmotic diuresis) nor gaining excessive fluid. Fluid with a tonicity less than that of 0.45% saline should not be used, and a positive balance of around 6 mmol of sodium chloride per kilogram over 24 hours should be regarded as the upper limit.[141] The rate of fluid infusion rarely exceeds 1.5 to 2 times the usual daily requirement.

Despite the fact that almost all patients with DKA are potassium depleted, serum potassium levels frequently are increased at presentation. With initiation of insulin therapy and correction of acidosis, there is rapid intracellular movement of potassium, and careful monitoring of potassium levels is essential. As soon as potassium levels are less than 5.5 mEq/L, 30 to 40 mEq/L of potassium should be added to the fluid infusions, and 0.5 to 1 mEq/kg/h of potassium may be required to correct potassium deficits. Potassium may be given as chloride or phosphate. Although severe hypophosphatemia is relatively common,[142] and symptomatic hypophosphatemia has been reported,[143] there is no evidence that phosphate administration is routinely necessary in the management of DKA, and the clinical effects of severe hypophosphatemia rarely are seen in DKA. Theoretically, phosphate administration may reduce insulin resistance and depletion of adenosine triphosphate and have positive effects on 2,3-diphosphoglycerate.[144] Administration of potassium phosphate helps decrease the chloride load given to patients with DKA. Potassium phosphate may be used safely,[145] provided that calcium levels are monitored carefully.[146,147] Glucose must be added to the infusion of fluids when the glucose levels are 14 to 17 mmol/L to avoid hypoglycemia.

Bicarbonate. The use of bicarbonate in DKA is extremely limited. Many studies have shown no clinical benefit from its administration.[148-150] More recently, bicarbonate administration has been associated with the development of cerebral edema. It should not be given routinely, not in bolus form, and possibly only in patients who have a pH of less than 6.9 despite appropriate correction of intravascular volume and ongoing adequate insulin therapy.

Insulin Therapy. Intravenous insulin should be provided as a continuous low-dose infusion starting at 0.1 unit/kg/h about 1 to 2 hours after starting fluid replacement. If there is no response to insulin therapy, the infusion should be reviewed for technical problems (incorrect preparation, adhesion of insulin to infusion tubing), and the patient should be reviewed for ongoing hypovolemia or uncontrolled sepsis. There is no place for a bolus of IV insulin or an initial loading dose, other than in the management of life-threatening hyperkalemia. The insulin infusion should be continued until ketoacidosis is resolved and the patient is fully conscious and retaining solid food.

Treat Underlying Cause. In previously undiagnosed patients, the cause of DKA is insulin deficiency. Even in previously diagnosed patients, most episodes of DKA probably are related to insulin omission or treatment error, although children 3 years old or younger are more likely to have a bacterial infection.[151] If infection is suspected as the precipitating cause of DKA, aggressive therapy with antibiotics and drainage of any pus should be instituted. Routine prophylactic antibiotic therapy is not indicated in DKA.

Monitoring. Although some patients are hypovolemic on presentation, there is little evidence that invasive hemodynamic monitoring is necessary. Careful monitoring of sodium levels is essential because smaller changes in serum sodium with therapy have been associated with development of cerebral edema.[118] Hyperlipidemia may decrease the aqueous phase of serum and artificially reduce sodium levels; this can be corrected using the following formula[152]:

$$[\text{True sodium}](\text{mEq/L}) = [\text{reported sodium (mEq/L)}] \times [0.021 \times [\text{triglycerides (mg/dL)}] + 0.994])$$

The osmotic load of glucose also decreases serum sodium levels, with a decrease in sodium concentration of approximately 1.6 to 1.8 mEq/L per 100 mg/dL increase in glucose[153] (alternatively, Corrected sodium = measured Na + 2([plasma glucose − 5.6]/5.6) (mmol/L). The expectation is that with decreasing levels of hyperglycemia and hyperlipidemia, sodium levels should increase. This increase may be offset, however, by urinary losses of sodium secondary to osmotic diuresis. Careful and frequent monitoring of potassium and glucose levels is essential. If phosphate is being administered, calcium levels should be monitored. Regular acid-base monitoring is required.

Monitoring of end-tidal Pco_2[154] or transcutaneous Pco_2[155] could be used as a noninvasive method for continuous monitoring of response to therapy for DKA. The only proviso (as pointed out by the authors and in an accompanying editorial[156]) is that any changes in respiratory drive or efficiency of the respiratory system may mask changes in acid-base that otherwise might be reflected by capnometry.

Investigations for Possible Cerebral Edema in Diabetic Ketoacidosis. Although cerebral edema is the most common cause of depressed level of consciousness in DKA, there are other causes that are amenable to alternative therapy, including cerebral venous thrombosis[157] and acute hydrocephalus.[158] Other abnormalities such as brain infarction[159] and extrapontine myelinolysis[160] have been shown. Computed tomography (CT) of patients with a depressed level of consciousness may be recommended to exclude other treatable pathology. Because the risks are relatively low, however, excluding other pathology must be balanced against the risks associated with moving ill patients to the radiology suite.

Mannitol has been used for the management of cerebral edema[161] (0.25-1 g/kg over 20 minutes), although there are no controlled studies. Hypertonic saline (5-10 mL/kg of 3% saline) may be an alternative to mannitol.[162] Hyperventilation after intubation for cerebral edema may be associated with worse outcomes.[126]

Despite improvements in the management of DKA, it remains a serious illness with significant morbidity and mortality. In addition to improving management of the condition, strong focus must be brought to ensure that the condition is avoided where possible and diagnosed and treated promptly when it occurs.

Thyroid Insufficiency

Neonates exposed to large amounts of iodine in iodine-containing antiseptics may develop transient hypothyroidism[163-167] (also called the *Wolff-Chaikoff effect)* as a result of transcutaneous absorption of iodine. This condition also has been shown in infants undergoing cardiac catheterization and cardiac surgery.[168] Care should be taken to limit the exposure of infants to iodine-containing agents. Triiodothyronine supplementation may be considered in children who have been exposed to significant amounts of iodine before or during a critical illness.

The sick euthyroid syndrome has been well documented in the PICU, particularly in patients undergoing cardiac surgery. The subject has been reviewed elsewhere.[169] Although there may be benefit to some children from triiodothyronine supplementation after cardiac surgery,[170-172] there is no established role for triiodothyronine supplementation after cardiac surgery.[173]

Children with Down syndrome have a high incidence of hypothyroidism.[174,175] Attention should be paid to the possible need for triiodothyronine supplementation in critically ill children with Down syndrome.

▣ Metabolic Crises

EPIDEMIOLOGY

Population data on inborn errors of metabolism suggest that there is a minimal incidence of 35 to 40 per 100,000 live births[176,177] in countries such as Canada or Italy, while the incidence may be as high as 150 per 100,000 live births in other countries.[178] In addition, some conditions have a particularly high incidence in particular population groups (e.g., maple syrup urine disease has an incidence of 568 per 100,000 births in the Mennonite community in Pennsylvania). Inborn errors of metabolism have a diverse presentation and are part of the differential diagnosis of many children admitted to the PICU with acute illness. Until more recently, only conditions such as phenylketonuria and galactosemia had been identified at birth using screening programs. With increasing availability of technology such as tandem mass spectrometry, screening of other inborn errors of metabolism (including fatty acid oxidation abnormalities and aminoacidopathies) has been introduced in some parts of the world,[179-182] and this potentially may decrease the number of children presenting with acute metabolic decompensation.

There is evidence that SIDS may be related to inborn errors of metabolism in at least 1% of cases,[183,184] and inborn errors of metabolism must be considered as part of the differential diagnosis of any infant who presents to the PICU or neonatal ICU after a near-SIDS episode. A family history of SIDS also should raise the possibility of inborn errors of metabolism in siblings presenting to the PICU with acute illness.

Although there are a bewildering number of inborn errors of metabolism, many are amenable to therapy, and screening may be performed using relatively simple tests. Patients with incurable conditions may derive considerable relief of suffering from diagnosis and appropriate therapy. Even when a condition is not amenable to therapy, it is important to make a diagnosis to facilitate counseling for the family involved and prevent unnecessary suffering in future children. Long-term management of most inborn errors of metabolism requires a team approach including metabolic experts, dietitians, geneticists, biochemists, and social workers to elucidate the exact nature of the problem, provide appropriate therapy and therapeutic plans, and give genetic and family counseling. Although many screening tests for inborn errors of metabolism can be done in most diagnostic laboratories, the specialized tests required to identify the exact nature of an inborn error of metabolism can be done at relatively few laboratories. Despite the complexity of inborn errors of metabolism, there are principles germane to the management of all children who are admitted to a PICU, and these should apply (see Table 168-1).

WHEN TO CONSIDER AN INBORN ERROR OF METABOLISM IN THE PEDIATRIC INTENSIVE CARE UNIT

Inborn errors of metabolism may be classified into diagnostically useful groups[185]: (1) disorders that give rise to intoxication (e.g., organic acidemias and urea cycle defects); (2) disorders involving energy metabolism (e.g., fatty acid oxidation defects and respiratory chain defects); (3) disorders involving complex molecules in which symptoms are permanent, progressive, and independent of intercurrent events (e.g., peroxisomal disorders, lysosomal disorders, and congenital defects of glycosylation); and (4) those disorders that present with seizures (particularly in the neonatal period). The conditions most likely to present acutely in the PICU are conditions involving intoxication and energy metabolism. There is overlap, however, between all of these groups in terms of clinical presentation. There also may be considerable variation in the clinical presentation of conditions that have the same underlying genetic abnormality; this may apply even within families.

Although the clinical features of an inborn error of metabolism may be related primarily to the accumulation of a toxic metabolite, the condition may be complicated by the relative deficiency of another compound or increased stress put on other metabolic pathways by the primary problem.[186] Management may involve limiting the intake of potentially toxic substances, increasing the removal of toxic substances, supplementation of deficient substances, and supplementation of other metabolic pathways that are being stressed.

Inborn errors of metabolism should be considered as part of the differential diagnosis of any child or infant who presents with a severe

TABLE 168-4	Factors That Should Alert the Intensivist to the Possibility of an Inborn Error of Metabolism

History

General	Population group with high incidence of inborn errors of metabolism
	Consanguinity of parents
	Previous history of apparent SIDS or childhood deaths in the family
	Presence of dysmorphic features associated with inborn error of metabolism
During pregnancy	Previous history multiple spontaneous abortions
	Hyperemesis may be associated with fat oxidation disorders,[240] as may frank hepatic symptoms such as acute fatty liver of pregnancy or the more severe HELLP syndrome (hemolysis, liver enzymes, low platelets).
In neonatal period	Deterioration after apparently being normal at birth, particularly if Apgar scores and early neonatal period were normal
	Earliest signs of inborn error of metabolism in the neonatal period may include lethargy and poor feeding, which may progress rapidly to obvious depressed level of consciousness.
	Depressed level of consciousness without obvious explanation
	Vomiting is an unusual clinical feature of illness in neonates and is strongly associated with inborn errors of metabolism.
	Strange odors
In childhood	Previous history of being "sickly" with episodes of intermittent vomiting
	Previous hospital admissions (even for apparent respiratory symptoms as this may be acidosis)
	Unusual dietary preferences by the child
	Onset of virtually any organ dysfunction (liver, heart, renal, etc.) may be related to inborn error.

Examination

General in neonatal period	Dysmorphic features that may be associated with inborn errors of metabolism
	Strange odors
	Neurologic signs in inborn errors of metabolism tend to include increased tone and abnormal movements, in contrast to the features of sepsis, which usually is associated with decreased tone.
In childhood	Acute or intermittent ataxia is a common feature of inborn errors of metabolism in children.

SIDS, sudden infant death syndrome.

illness, particularly during the neonatal period.[185] Acute symptoms that are particularly associated with inborn errors of metabolism include encephalopathy (acute or acute on chronic), intractable seizures, hepatic failure, cardiomyopathy, metabolic acidosis, and hypoglycemia (Table 168-4). Family history of SIDS or of previous childhood deaths may suggest an inborn error of metabolism. Particular attention should be paid to the identification of specific risk factors for the differential diagnoses, including drug exposure, prolonged rupture of membranes, and perinatal asphyxial episodes.

CLINICAL PRESENTATIONS OF INBORN ERRORS OF METABOLISM

Intractable Seizures

Seizures (in isolation) are an uncommon presentation of inborn errors of metabolism and, with the exception of the pyridoxine-dependent seizures, tend to be associated with other clinical and metabolic abnormalities. In neonates or some infants presenting with intractable seizures, (particularly if associated with grimacing and abnormal eye movements), pyridoxine-dependent seizures (PDS),[187] pyridoxine phosphate oxidase deficiency (PNPO) hypophosphatasia, and folinic acid–responsive seizures[188] should be considered. The clinical diagnosis of both PDS and PNPO depends on demonstration that seizure control

is dependent on continuous pharmacologic doses of pyridoxine or pyridoxal-5′-phosphate, respectively. However, it has recently been shown that detection of elevated levels of α-amino-adipic semialdehyde in blood, urine, or cerebrospinal fluid (CSF), along with the demonstration of mutations in the *ALDH7A1* (antiquitin) gene, confirm a diagnosis of PDE[189]; whereas an abnormal pattern of CSF catecholamine and indole amine metabolite levels, together with elevated CSF plasma glycine and threonine concentrations and urinary vanillactic acid excretion are characteristic but not uniformly present in PNPO.[190,191] It has also been shown that patients with folinic acid–dependent seizures have the same mutation in the antiquitin gene.[188] There is a considerable range in clinical presentation, and pyridoxine-dependent seizures probably should be considered in any infant up to age 18 months presenting with seizures.

Patients with defects in transport of glucose across the blood-brain barrier associated with mutations in the *GLUT1* gene may present with seizures. The only clue is the presence of low CSF glucose in the presence of normal blood glucose. Patients may improve on a ketogenic diet.[192]

Inborn errors of metabolism that may present with seizures associated with lactic acidosis include biotinidase deficiency, disorders of mitochondrial energy metabolism (including pyruvate dehydrogenase deficiency and mitochondrial electron transport chain defects), and peroxisomal and storage disorders.

Biotinidase deficiency (an autosomal recessively inherited disorder of biotin recycling—estimated incidence of biotinidase deficiency is about 1 in 60,000[193]) can be ameliorated or prevented by administering pharmacologic doses of the vitamin biotin (5-20 mg daily independent of age). A large proportion of cases present with seizures and hypotonia, associated with failure to thrive, and rash or alopecia. Some 50% of cases have ataxia, developmental delay, and eye problems (conjunctivitis and optic atrophy), with more than 75% developing hearing loss. There is a considerable variation in clinical presentation, even within affected families,[194] with features ranging from mild episodes of seizure and ataxia to severe metabolic failure and death. Onset of symptoms may occur at any time from the neonatal period through to adulthood. Untreated individuals may have ketoacidosis, lactic acidosis, and/or hyperammonemia, with a wide range of other metabolic anomalies.[194] Diagnosis can be made from analysis of organic acids in urine, whereas an enzyme assay can be done on blood. Guidelines for testing have recently been published.[194]

Intractable tonic/clonic seizures also may be a feature of molybdenum cofactor deficiency.[195,196] This condition presents in early infancy with seizures, encephalopathy in the absence of metabolic acidosis, hypoglycemia or hyperammonemia, and failure to thrive. Imaging of the brain initially shows cerebral edema, which may progress to cerebral atrophy. There are typical imaging findings.[197] Clinical features, CT findings, and neuropathology may be similar to that seen in severe hypoxic-ischemic brain injury.[198,199] Lens dislocation may be a clinical feature.[200] Uric acid levels are low, whereas urinary amino acid analysis shows increased *S*-sulfocysteine. Sulfite may be demonstrated on fresh urine specimens. Electrospray tandem mass spectrometry of urine or urine-soaked filter paper may facilitate rapid diagnosis.[201] Seizures may be part of the clinical presentation of many other disorders, including seizures with lactic acidosis (Leigh disease; mitochondrial encephalopathy lactic acidosis and strokelike episodes [MELAS]; mitochondrial encephalopathy with ragged red fibers [MERRF]), GM_2 gangliosidosis, and peroxisomal disorders. Other clinical features predominate in these conditions and should direct investigation.

Investigation and Management. In infants presenting primarily with intractable seizures, investigations should include measurement of blood glucose, blood acid-base status, blood lactic acid (in association with pyruvate levels), CSF glucose, lactic acid and pyruvic acid levels, urinary organic acids, and sulfite. CT and magnetic resonance imaging (MRI) help diagnose disorders of abnormal accumulation of metabolites and exclude structural brain problems that are responsible for symptoms. Treatment focuses on control of the airway and respiration, together with control of seizures. Pyridoxine or biotin should be administered early in appropriate doses if indicated.

Encephalopathy

The onset of acute encephalopathy always constitutes a medical emergency, and the cause must be elucidated as rapidly as possible. The differential diagnosis includes trauma, infection, intracranial space-occupying lesions, toxin ingestion, acute hepatic failure or Reye syndrome, intracranial vascular problems (including thrombosis, hemorrhage, and embolic phenomena), and seizure disorders. There is often a strong tendency to attribute neurologic symptoms to hypoglycemia or hypocalcemia, but because these may be associated with inborn errors of metabolism, it is vital to consider an inborn error of metabolism as part of the cause of the hypoglycemia.

The inborn errors of metabolism that present with acute encephalopathy vary with age. In the neonatal period, the common inborn errors of metabolism include urea cycle defects (with hyperammonemia), maple syrup urine disease, nonketotic hyperglycinemia, and organic acidopathies.[202] All of these conditions, with the exception of nonketotic hyperglycinemia, also may present during childhood. During childhood, the common inborn errors of metabolism presenting with acute encephalopathy include fatty acid oxidation defects and maple syrup urine disease.

Investigation. The specimens that normally would be collected for diagnosis of sepsis should be collected, including blood culture, hemoglobin, white blood cell count (including differential), and platelets. Serum electrolytes should be checked, including sodium, potassium, calcium, phosphate, and magnesium. Liver function tests are essential because acute hepatic failure may cause acute encephalopathy, and the liver may be affected by inborn errors of metabolism. Specimens for testing for inborn errors of metabolism must be collected at the time

of presentation, because this may provide the best opportunity for diagnosis (Table 168-5).

Blood Glucose Levels. The reader is referred to the earlier discussion of the approach to hypoglycemia. Hypoglycemia may be a particular feature of fatty acid oxidation defects and organic acidurias. Immediate correction of hypoglycemia is an essential element of treatment.

Plasma Ammonia Levels. Plasma ammonia levels should be checked in all children, especially neonates with unexplained depressed level of consciousness, particularly if there is hypotonia and apnea (see section on hyperammonemia for management and investigation). Treatment of severe hyperammonemia is an emergency.

Liver Function Tests. Reye syndrome is part of the differential diagnosis of acute encephalopathy, but fatty acid oxidation defects such as medium-chain acyl-CoA dehydrogenase deficiency, carnitine deficiency (usually with associated myopathy), and far less frequently, long-chain acyl-CoA dehydrogenase deficiency and short-chain acyl-CoA dehydrogenase deficiency, may present with encephalopathy (usually in the neonatal period).

Blood Gas Analysis. Arterial blood gas analysis should be performed, with particular attention to the presence of metabolic acidosis and calculation of the anion gap (this should be corrected for the presence of hypoalbuminemia).[203-205]

Blood Lactate Levels. Blood lactate levels may be increased in many situations but typically are very elevated in mitochondrial electron transport chain defects.

Plasma Carnitine. Levels of carnitine may be substantially decreased in organic acidurias and fatty acid oxidation defects. Analysis of acylcarnitine and amino acid profile may help to make the diagnosis of isovaleric aciduria, methylmalonic aciduria, and propionic acidemia.

Quantitative Amino Acid Analysis. Quantitative amino acid analysis is necessary to identify the aminoacidopathies. This test is not

TABLE 168-5	Specimen Collection for Inborn Errors of Metabolism		
Substance	**Tests**	**Comments on Technique**	**Conditions Identified**
Urine	Detecting odors	Urine odors are best identified from urine drying on filter papers or from urine that has been kept in a closed container at room temperature for a while.	MSUD (smell of maple syrup; some describe this as burnt sugar[133]) Isovaleric acidemia (sweaty feet odor) 3-methylcrotonyl glycinuria (catlike)
Urine (screening tests)	Ketones		Urinary ketones are rare in neonates and are almost diagnostic of an inborn error of metabolism in a neonate.
	Dinitrophenylhydrazine		Strongly positive with MSUD, PKU, or in ketoacidosis
	Ferric chloride		Green color with PKU; other colors may occur with other conditions
	Merckoquant 10013 Sulfit test	Urine specimen must be fresh because sulfite oxidizes rapidly at room temperature.	Molybdenum cofactor deficiency
	Reducing substances		Galactosemia
Urine	Measurement of organic acids and amino acids	Specimen collected and frozen at −20°C	All aminoacidemias and organic acidurias
	Measurement of acylcarnitines and acylglycines	Can increase the sensitivity of these tests by the use of loading dose of levocarnitine, 100 mg/kg orally	Many fatty acid oxidation defects
Blood	Anion gap	Correct for hypoalbuminemia	Screen to identify generally unmeasured anions
	Tandem mass spectrometry	Collected as blood on filter paper	All fatty acid oxidation defects, many of the aminoacidemias Abnormalities of the carnitine pathways
	Galactose-1-phosphate uridyltransferase	Collected as blood on filter paper	Galactosemia
	Estimation of ammonia, lactate, pyruvate, and ketoacids	All of these substances may be unstable; must collect on ice and transport immediately to laboratory	Aminoacidopathies, urea cycle defects
	Genetic studies	Before blood transfusion	All problems with identified genetic abnormalities Enzyme defects, organelle defects
Skin, liver, muscle, and endocardial biopsy	Fibroblast culture, enzyme identification, identification of abnormal collections and organelles		

MSUD, maple syrup urine disease; *PKU,* phenylketonuria.

always available, and results may take some time. Screening tests on the urine may point in the direction of certain conditions.

Urinary and Blood Ketones. Ketones are unusual in the neonatal period but tend to be a feature of maple syrup urine disease and propionic, isovaleric, and methylmalonic acidemia. Quantitative determination of blood ketones (acetoacetate using urine ketone strips or β-hydroxybutyrate by specific blood strip) may be a useful bedside screen.

Urinary Organic Acids. Urinary organic acids are abnormal in maple syrup urine disease, organic aciduria, and fatty acid oxidation defects.

Management. The principles of therapy are as follows:
1. Maintain airway control and breathing.
2. Maintain circulation.
3. Treat underlying or associated sepsis.
4. Remove toxic compounds.
5. Ensure an appropriate energy source for the body.
6. Provide any specific therapy that is available.

The toxic compounds that potentially can be removed include ammonia and leucine (see details subsequently).

SPECIFIC INBORN ERRORS OF METABOLISM

Maple Syrup Urine Disease

If there is no acidosis and the ammonia is not increased, maple syrup urine disease (MSUD) should be considered. Patients typically are not dehydrated, are not acidotic, have no hyperammonemia, and have no hematologic abnormalities. Cerebral edema is a feature of maple syrup urine disease within the neonatal period and during later presentations.

The urine may smell like maple syrup, but the smell is also similar to that of burned sugar.[202] The urine smell may be difficult to detect in the first few days of life, then may be detected on diapers that have been allowed to dry.[206] Urine tests for ketones are usually strongly positive, and dinitrophenylhydrazine is usually positive, although both tests may be negative before 3 days of age.[206] Tandem mass spectrometry is the quickest and most efficient screening test in neonates. Leucine levels can be checked rapidly on whole-blood filter paper specimens, or quantitative amino acid analysis should be done on plasma or serum. Principles of management have been to remove leucine using dialysis and to reduce the production of leucine by dietary manipulation. Hemodialysis has been shown to decrease leucine levels rapidly,[207] particularly if used in conjunction with dietary therapy. Previously, exchange transfusion, peritoneal dialysis, and hemofiltration were reported to decrease leucine levels. Morton and colleagues[206] have used a protocol consisting of total caloric intake of 120 to 140 kcal/kg/d, with lipid forming 40% to 50% of calories; 3 to 4 g/kg/d of protein as essential and nonessential amino acids, with 80 to 120 mg/kg/d each of isoleucine and valine and 250 mg/kg/d each of glutamine and alanine, with tyrosine, histidine, and threonine supplemented to normalize plasma amino acid ratios; careful attention to sodium balance to ensure that serum sodium is kept at greater than 140 mEq/L; and hyperosmolar therapy if cerebral edema develops. This protocol produces decreases in leucine equal to that seen after dialysis. Recent studies suggest that norleucine may have a place in reducing brain injury in patients with MSUD.[208]

Isovaleric Aciduria, Methylmalonic Aciduria, and Propionic Acidemia

Isovaleric aciduria, methylmalonic aciduria, and propionic acidemia may present in the neonatal period with encephalopathy hyperammonemia, ketoacidosis (occasionally hyperammonemia may induce a respiratory alkalosis), moderate lactic acidosis, and hypocalcemia. The smell associated with isovaleric aciduria may be distinctive ("sweaty feet"). Blood glucose levels may be variable from hypoglycemia to hyperglycemia. Dehydration is a feature of the clinical presentation, partly related to vomiting and poor intake and partly related to poor

renal concentrating ability. One-third of patients may present later in life.

Strokelike episodes are a feature of isovaleric aciduria, methylmalonic aciduria, and propionic acidemia in later life, although there may be a wide range of neurologic presentations including hypotonia and developmental delay. Extrapyramidal signs related to infarction of the basal ganglia may be a feature of methylmalonic aciduria and propionic acidemia. Neutropenia, thrombocytopenia, and anemia are common in the neonatal presentation, whereas neutropenia also may be a feature of a later presentation. Sepsis may be a significant component of clinical exacerbations, particularly in propionic acidemia. Pancreatitis has been reported to be associated with these disorders.[209] Cardiomyopathy also may develop, particularly during metabolic decompensation.[210] Isovaleric aciduria, propionic acidemia, and methylmalonic aciduria are diagnosed by the organic acid profiles, and tandem mass spectroscopy may be useful by looking at the acylcarnitine profiles.

Patients presenting in the neonatal period with encephalopathy require treatment with limitation of protein intake (this requires varied adjustment to a diet with appropriate amino acid profile), removal of toxin (exchange transfusion may be useful; methylmalonic aciduria can be cleared renally if adequate fluid volumes are given), ensuring normal glucose levels, promoting anabolism, and management of sepsis. Some patients with methylmalonic aciduria may respond to therapy with hydroxycobalamin, and this should be given for several days to assess response. Supplemental glycine should be given to patients with isovaleric aciduria, and carnitine supplementation is useful for all. Some patients with propionic acidemia may benefit from metronidazole to decrease propionate metabolites from the bowel.

Nonketotic Hyperglycinemia

Nonketotic hyperglycinemia presents in early infancy with severe encephalopathy in the absence of acidosis, ketosis, hypoglycemia, hyperammonemia, or any other clinical abnormalities. Although the outcome is almost invariably poor, there have been more recent descriptions of transient neonatal hyperglycinemia.[211] There also is an association of abnormality of the corpus callosum with nonketotic hyperglycinemia.[212] Diagnosis is confirmed by the presence of high CSF glycine. The enzyme defect can be confirmed on a liver biopsy specimen.[213,214] Sodium benzoate may be helpful in therapy, possibly in combination with imipramine.[215]

HYPOGLYCEMIA AND INBORN ERRORS OF METABOLISM

The reader is referred to the section on endocrine crises for an approach to hypoglycemia. In hyperinsulinemia, the hypoglycemia typically develops soon after the intake of a feed, whereas patients with defects in fatty acid oxidation tend to be able to tolerate fasts of 4 to 8 hours. In hyperinsulinemia, it often is difficult to provide adequate amounts of glucose to correct the hypoglycemia (may require >12 mg/kg/min together with glucagon to control the hypoglycemia). In defects of gluconeogenesis, the hypoglycemia is relatively easy to control but usually does not respond to glucagon administration. In hereditary fructose intolerance, the onset of hypoglycemia is concurrent with the introduction of sucrose (source of fructose) into the diet. Although hypoglycemia may occur in association with sepsis, many inborn errors of metabolism are associated with sepsis (e.g., direct association with *Escherichia coli* and galactosemia, sepsis as precipitant of crisis, or ill health from inborn error of metabolism causing increased risk of sepsis) and should be considered diagnostically even if sepsis is proven.

Investigation and Management

If the glucose level is low, a venous specimen of blood should be collected immediately for laboratory glucose estimation (because bedside measuring techniques may be inaccurate at low levels of glucose). The clinician should give 0.5 g/kg of 10% to 25% dextrose in water (diluted with water for injection) promptly as a bolus IV followed by administration of 4 to 8 mg/kg/min of glucose. The glucose level should be reviewed within 30 minutes. The rate of glucose infusion may need to be increased, and high requirements suggest hyperinsulinemia.

Urine for Reducing Substances. Glucose should be excluded, but in the setting of hypoglycemia, this is unlikely unless there have been substantial doses of glucose given. If reducing substances are positive, this suggests galactosemia, hereditary fructosemia, or tyrosinemia.

Urinary Ketones. If urinary ketones are positive, the clinician should assess for urinary and plasma organic acids and quantitative amino acids. High urinary ketones in the presence of hepatomegaly suggest glycogen storage disease type 1, fructose-1,6-diphosphatase (FDPase) deficiency, or β-ketothiolase deficiency.[216] In the last-mentioned condition, lactate levels are normal, whereas they are increased in glycogen storage disease type 1 and FDPase deficiency. In the absence of hepatomegaly, high ketones suggest ketotic hypoglycemia or deficiencies of growth hormone or glucocorticoids.

Plasma Free Fatty Acids. If plasma free fatty acids are elevated, the patient is likely to have a fatty acid oxidation defect, but if they are low, hyperinsulinemia is more likely.

Lactate Levels. Lactic acidosis in association with hypoglycemia is characteristic of defects of gluconeogenesis such as glycogen storage diseases.

Urinary Organic Acids, Plasma Amino Acids, and Ammonia Levels. Urinary organic acids, plasma amino acids, and ammonia levels should be measured, because hypoglycemia may be a feature of abnormalities of all these systems.

Specific Conditions Associated with Hypoglycemia

Galactosemia. Please see the section on hepatitis. Hypoglycemia may be a prominent feature of galactosemia, whereas hepatitis may be a more common presentation.

Hereditary Fructose Intolerance. Hereditary fructose intolerance is characterized by the onset of severe vomiting and hypoglycemia after the ingestion of fructose or sucrose.

Glycogen Storage Disease Type 1. Glycogen storage disease type 1 may present in the neonatal period with hypoglycemia which may be mild or easily controlled. However, the patients present later with hepatomegaly and lactic acidosis. Characteristically, the hypoglycemia does not respond to therapy with glucagon.

Fatty Acid Oxidation Defects. Fatty acids are metabolized primarily via β-oxidation in the mitochondria and to a lesser extent in the peroxisomes (β-oxidation) and the microsomes (ω-oxidation). Defects in the mitochondrial oxidation of free fatty acid result in the accumulation of fatty acid oxidation products, which may be responsible for encephalopathy, hepatocellular dysfunction, and cardiac arrhythmias, which are a potentially fatal complication of fatty acid oxidation defects. Defects in fatty acid oxidation also may result in failure to meet the energy requirements of tissues such as skeletal muscles or cardiac muscles, resulting in myopathy or cardiomyopathy.

Many studies have suggested that fatty acid oxidation defects may be an important cause of SIDS. Fatty acid oxidation defects are an important cause of cardiomyopathy.[217]

Medium-chain acyl-CoA deficiency is the most common of the fatty acid oxidation defects and most frequently presents with a Reye-like episode, with acute or recurrent Reye-like episodes with vomiting, encephalopathy hypoglycemia, and hyperammonemia. Cardiomyopathy never occurs in medium-chain acyl-CoA deficiency. Cardiomyopathy is a more common presentation of carnitine deficiency and long-chain acyl-CoA dehydrogenase deficiency.

Diagnosis is based on the clinical features described earlier: tolerance of 8 to 24 hours of fasting, high plasma free fatty acid levels, normal to low ketone levels, increased urinary organic acids (C-6 to C-10 dicarboxylic acids), and low plasma carnitine levels. The abnormal findings may not be present between acute exacerbations, and it is crucial to collect specimens during the acute illness. Urine specimens must be collected; blood can be collected on filter paper for tandem mass spectrometry (these assays may be abnormal while the child is well). Specific mutation analysis is available for the most common medium-chain acyl-CoA deficiency. Treatment consists of supplying adequate glucose, supplementing carnitine, and providing symptomatic support.

HYPERAMMONEMIA

Transient hyperammonemia may occur in preterm infants in so-called transient hyperammonemia of the newborn, which is not associated with an inborn error of metabolism. Aggressive therapy may be associated with completely normal outcome. Hyperammonemia results in a marked encephalopathy, although patients typically are more hypotonic than in other metabolic encephalopathies and may develop a respiratory alkalosis, which is uncommon in other encephalopathies.

Primary hyperammonemia occurs in the urea cycle defects, but a secondary hyperammonemia may occur in defects of fatty acid oxidation or organic acidemia. Hyperammonemia also may be a consequence of acute hepatic failure (e.g., with acute viral infection; toxin ingestion; and drug reactions, particularly antituberculosis drugs).

Investigation

Ammonia is potentially toxic, and therapy must be instituted urgently to remove ammonia. It is crucial to collect appropriate diagnostic specimens at the time of presentation because it may be difficult to establish a diagnosis when dialysis and other therapy have been instituted. The following tests enable an approach to diagnosis.[218]

Plasma Ammonium Levels. Hyperammonemia with levels of greater than 250 μmol/L typically are associated with urea cycle defects or transient hyperammonemia of the newborn.

Arterial Blood Gas Analysis. Hyperammonemia with urea cycle defects and transient hyperammonemia of the newborn are not associated with acidosis. Patients often may have a respiratory alkalosis. A metabolic acidosis is more likely to be associated with organic acidopathies.

Tests of the Urea Cycle. Tests of the urea cycle include plasma citrulline, urinary argininosuccinic acid synthetase, and urinary orotic acid.

Amino Acids. Quantitative amino acids may be difficult to interpret but help with diagnosis of conditions such as methylmalonic aciduria, isovaleric aciduria, and propionic acidemia.

Carnitine Levels and Acylcarnitine Analysis. Carnitine and the acylcarnitines may be affected as part of the aminoacidemias.

Management

Principles of management for hyperammonemia consist of the following:

1. Provide IV glucose and lipid to decrease ammonia production from endogenous protein breakdown.
2. Administer arginine (L-arginine hydrochloride, 600 mg/kg IV over 1 hour, followed by 2 to 4 mmol/kg/24 h in 4 divided doses).
3. Administer sodium benzoate (250 mg/kg IV followed by 250 mg/kg/d in 4 divided doses) and sodium phenylacetate (250 mg/kg IV immediately followed by 250 mg/kg/24 h in 4 divided doses).
4. Dialyze to remove excessive ammonia. Hemodialysis is the most efficient means to remove ammonia, hemofiltration is the next option (and may be particularly useful in neonates who are too unstable to tolerate hemodialysis), and finally peritoneal dialysis

may be used. Exchange transfusion has been performed but is relatively inefficient at removal of ammonia.

METABOLIC ACIDOSIS

Metabolic acidosis can occur in many ways. It may be related to inadequate excretion of acid via the kidneys (e.g., proximal and distal renal tubular acidosis) or excessive production of acid in the body. In the case of inadequate excretion of acid from the kidneys, the pH of the urine almost always is inappropriately high. In addition, there is no anion gap. In the context of excessive acid production, there is an excessive anion gap.

The most common acids related to an increased anion gap are lactic acid and ketoacids, such as acetoacetate and 3-butyrobutyrate. All the organic acidopathies and aminoacidopathies may be associated with an increased anion gap, however. A variety of inborn errors of metabolism may be associated with proximal renal tubular acidosis, particularly cystinosis and Lowe syndrome.

Acid also may be produced by bacterial overgrowth in the bowel and absorbed, as occurs in D-lactic acidosis.[219] D-Lactic acid is not detected by routine blood tests for lactic acid, which employ a lactic dehydrogenase, but is detected by urinary assays for organic acids. These patients present with acidosis with increased anion gap.

Patients with organic acidemias rarely present with metabolic acidosis as a primary feature of the illness, and the rest of the clinical presentation frequently provides clues as to the appropriate line of investigation. Investigation of organic acids remains an important component of the investigation of any patient, however, with unexplained metabolic acidosis.

Lactic Acidosis

Lactic acidosis is associated with inadequate oxygenation of tissues, as occurs in hypoxemia or in shock. In this situation, treatment consists of ensuring adequate oxygen content of blood and appropriate cardiac output.

So-called primary lactic acidosis occurs in the absence of hypoxemia and shock. Lactate accumulates either as a consequence of increased production of lactate or because of inadequate clearance and metabolism of lactate (primarily in the liver). Accumulation of lactate may occur without the development of acidosis, depending on the compensatory mechanisms. Many patients with congenital lactic acidosis have increased lactate levels with no acidosis between episodes of exacerbation, although episodes of exacerbation usually are associated with severe lactic acidosis.

Congenital lactic acidoses are variable in presentation, ranging from severe neonatal lactic acidosis with generally poor prognosis to children with milder defects and other children with syndromes such as the MELAS and MERRF syndromes and Leigh disease. In many of these conditions, the lactic acidosis is completely or partially overshadowed by the other clinical features of the conditions. Not all children with defects of mitochondrial energy metabolism have elevated levels.

Lactate production may be caused by increased glycolysis (e.g., glycogen storage disease type 1, hereditary fructose intolerance) or by decreased oxidation of pyruvate. Oxidation of pyruvate can be limited by many conditions, including the following:

1. Pyruvate dehydrogenase complex deficiency
2. Primary pyruvate carboxylase or holocarboxylase deficiency (this is related to biotin/biotinidase deficiency)
3. Electron transport chain defects (associated with increased lactate pyruvate ratios in blood and CSF)

The clinical course of pyruvate dehydrogenase deficiency may be extremely variable, and diagnosis is confirmed by studies of enzyme activity in cultured fibroblasts. The lactic acidosis in pyruvate dehydrogenase deficiency can be ameliorated by a ketogenic diet,[220] although many factors must be considered before embarking on this diet, including its protein content, particularly if there is associated renal failure, and the long-term problems of ketogenic diets.[221] Dichloroacetic acid may be helpful in some cases.[222] Many cases have been reported

in which thiamine was associated with clinical improvement, although high levels may be required.[223]

Lactic acidosis occurs in all of the conditions affecting the metabolism of pyruvate through the tricarboxylic acid cycle. Abnormalities include pyruvate dehydrogenase deficiency and mitochondrial energy cycle defects. The mitochondrial energy cycle problems frequently are associated with persistent lactic acidosis, myopathy, failure to thrive, psychomotor retardation, and seizures. Other symptoms that may be present in mitochondrial energy conditions in children include antenatal problems,[224] cardiomyopathy[225-227] and cardiac arrhythmias,[225] sensorineural hearing loss,[228] stroke and abnormalities of central respiratory drive,[229] and diabetes mellitus.[230]

Acquired defects in mitochondrial function have been associated with severe lactic acidosis in adults and children on antiretroviral therapy.[231] Lactic acidosis also may be a secondary phenomenon of defects of organic acid metabolism, including 3-hydroxy-3-methylglutaryl-CoA lyase deficiency, propionic acidemia, and methylmalonic acidemia.

Ketoacidosis

Primary defects in ketone use are rare but include β-ketothiolase deficiency, which may respond rapidly to administration of IV glucose. Ketoacidosis is a common feature of many of the organic acidemias, including MSUD, methylmalonic acidemia, propionic acidemia, and isovaleric aciduria. Investigation of patients with ketoacidosis should include measurement of urinary organic acids.

CARDIOMYOPATHY

A wide variety of inborn errors of metabolism may present with cardiomyopathy or cardiac arrhythmias. In most of these conditions, other clinical problems and symptoms predominate (e.g., in glycogen storage disease, organic acidopathies), and the cardiomyopathy is just part of an overall picture. In these situations, the diagnosis is assisted by the associations.

A few conditions may present with cardiac problems apparently in isolation. In the differential diagnosis of myocarditis/cardiomyopathy, many conditions need to be excluded, including carnitine deficiency, trifunctional protein defects, or isolated long-chain 3-hydroxyacyl-CoA dehydrogenase deficiency. In the latter two conditions, urinary organic acid analysis *at the time of the acute illness* shows the presence of medium-chain and long-chain dicarboxylic acids. At least one form of very-long-chain acyl-CoA dehydrogenase deficiency can present as an acute cardiomyopathy. For all these conditions, measurement of acylcarnitines using tandem mass spectrometry allows diagnosis. Diagnosis is confirmed using enzyme activity in cultured fibroblasts. At least one case report[232] shows that substantial clinical improvement can be achieved by elimination of long-chain fatty acids from the diet (replacing with medium-chain fatty acids). Many of the disorders of the mitochondrial energy chain have poor myocardial function as a component of their multiple symptoms, but echocardiography may be needed to show more subtle features of poor contractility.

HEPATOPATHOLOGY

Inborn errors of metabolism can affect the liver in a variety of ways. Patients may present with symptoms ranging from acute hepatic failure to hepatomegaly to chronic hepatitis to cirrhosis. The hepatic dysfunction may present in apparent isolation or in association with cardiac, cerebral, muscle, and renal disease. The presentations of "hepatitis" may be virtually indistinguishable from the presentation of acute viral hepatitis or toxin ingestion.

In one study of infants presenting to a transplant service in acute hepatic failure, inborn errors of metabolism were responsible for the hepatic failure in 42.5% of the patients. Of these patients, 35% had hepatorenal tyrosinemia, whereas 50% had mitochondrial abnormalities. Hereditary fructose intolerance and galactosemia together were present in less than 9% of patients.[233]

Hepatorenal tyrosinemia may present in the neonatal period as acute hepatic failure. It is difficult to distinguish from acute viral hepatitis, because plasma amino acid levels may be similar in both situations. Alpha-fetoprotein levels may be substantially elevated in hepatorenal tyrosinemia and may be a distinguishing feature. The coagulopathy tends to be relatively severe in hepatorenal tyrosinemia, and coagulopathy may be the only presenting feature of hepatorenal tyrosinemia.[234] Patients tend to have moderate to severe anemia. The response to treatment with 2-(2-nitro-4-triflu-oromethylbenzoyl)-1,3-cyclohexandion (NTBC) may be dramatic.[235-238]

Galactosemia is characterized by the development of hypoglycemia in the neonatal period in association with jaundice (initially unconjugated, but subsequently conjugated), marked increase in transaminase levels, some abnormality of coagulation, and moderate hypoalbuminemia. Severe cerebral edema occasionally may be a dominant feature. Management has been reviewed elsewhere.[239] There is a close association with *Escherichia coli* septicemia, and any infant presenting with *E. coli* septicemia should be investigated for galactosemia. Galactosuria clears rapidly if feeds are stopped. A screening test is available on blood collected on filter paper (semiquantitative measure of galactose-1-phosphate uridyltransferase). The diagnosis can be confirmed on a quantitative measurement of galactose-1-phosphate uridyltransferase. Wilson's disease may present as acute hepatitis, but rarely before age 5 years.

KEY POINTS

1. Although endocrine and metabolic conditions are individually rare, collectively they constitute a significant cause of pathology in the pediatric intensive care unit (PICU).

2. PICU admission is a crucial opportunity to identify endocrine problems and inborn errors of metabolism.

3. Hyperglycemia and hypoglycemia are important metabolic abnormalities and require both an etiologic diagnosis and management. A cause for hypoglycemia or hyperglycemia always must be identified.

4. Inborn errors of metabolism always must be considered as part of the differential diagnosis of critical illness, particularly in young infants.

5. Appropriate specimens should be collected at the time of the acute illness, and thereafter the clinician should consult with a specialist laboratory for diagnostic routes.

6. Specialist teams should be consulted early in the course of the illness, because few intensivists develop expertise in the management of inborn errors of metabolism.

7. A multidisciplinary team approach is essential to successful care for affected children.

ANNOTATED REFERENCES

Boles RG, Buck EA, Blitzer MG, et al. Retrospective biochemical screening of fatty acid oxidation disorders in post-mortem livers of 418 cases of sudden death in the first year of life. J Pediatr 1998;132:924-33.
The authors devised a biochemical protocol for evaluation of frozen postmortem liver specimens for defects of fatty acid oxidation. On review of specimens from 418 cases of sudden death in the first year of life, the authors were able to identify 14 cases that closely matched the biochemical profiles seen in fatty acid oxidation defects. No cases of death due to abuse or accidents tested positive. Of deaths that had been classified as infectious, 20% showed multiple abnormalities in the liver specimens, suggesting that fatty acid oxidation defects should be considered as part of the differential diagnosis of sudden or unexpected death, even when an infectious agent has been identified.

Dunger DB, Sperling MA, Acerini CL, et al. ESPE/LWPES consensus statement on DKA in children and adolescents. Arch Dis Child 2004;89:188-94.
This is an extensive evidence-based review of acute DKA in children and adolescents. Consensus guidelines are presented with appropriate references for the management of acute DKA in children and adolescents.

Durand P, Debray D, Mandel R, et al. Acute liver failure in infancy: A 14-year experience of a pediatric liver transplantation center. J Pediatr 2001;139:871-6.
This article presents a 14-year review of 80 infants (children <1 year old) admitted to the pediatric hepatology unit or ICU of a French hospital with acute liver failure (defined as prothrombin time >17 seconds and factor V plasma levels <50% of normal). Acute liver failure was a result of inherited metabolic disorders in

42.5% of cases, including mitochondrial respiratory chain disorders, type 1 hereditary tyrosinemia, and urea cycle defects.

Marcin JP, Glaser N, Barnett P, et al. Factors associated with adverse outcomes in children with DKA-related cerebral edema. J Pediatr 2002;141:793-7.
This is a retrospective study of 61 children (≤18 years old) from 10 U.S. pediatric centers admitted between 1982 and 1997 with DKA and cerebral edema. Only 59% survived without neurologic sequelae, and 28% died or survived in a vegetative state. Intubation with hyperventilation was associated with adverse outcome after adjustment for confounding variables. Poor outcome also was associated with greater neurologic depression at the time of diagnosis and a higher initial serum urea nitrogen concentration.

Morton DH, Strauss KA, Robinson DL, et al. Diagnosis and treatment of maple syrup disease: a study of 36 patients. Pediatrics 2002;109:999-1008.
This article evaluates an approach to the diagnosis and treatment of MSUD. Eighteen neonates were diagnosed as having MSUD between 12 and 24 hours of age using amino acid analysis of plasma or whole blood collected on filter paper. No infant identified before 3 days of age and treated with the protocol became ill during the neonatal period. A further 18 neonates who were intoxicated at the time of diagnosis responded rapidly to the management protocol without the need for dialysis or hemoperfusion. Follow-up of the 36 infants over more than 219 patient-years showed generally good metabolic control, with good developmental outcome. A management protocol is presented.

REFERENCES

Access the complete reference list online at http://www.expertconsult.com.

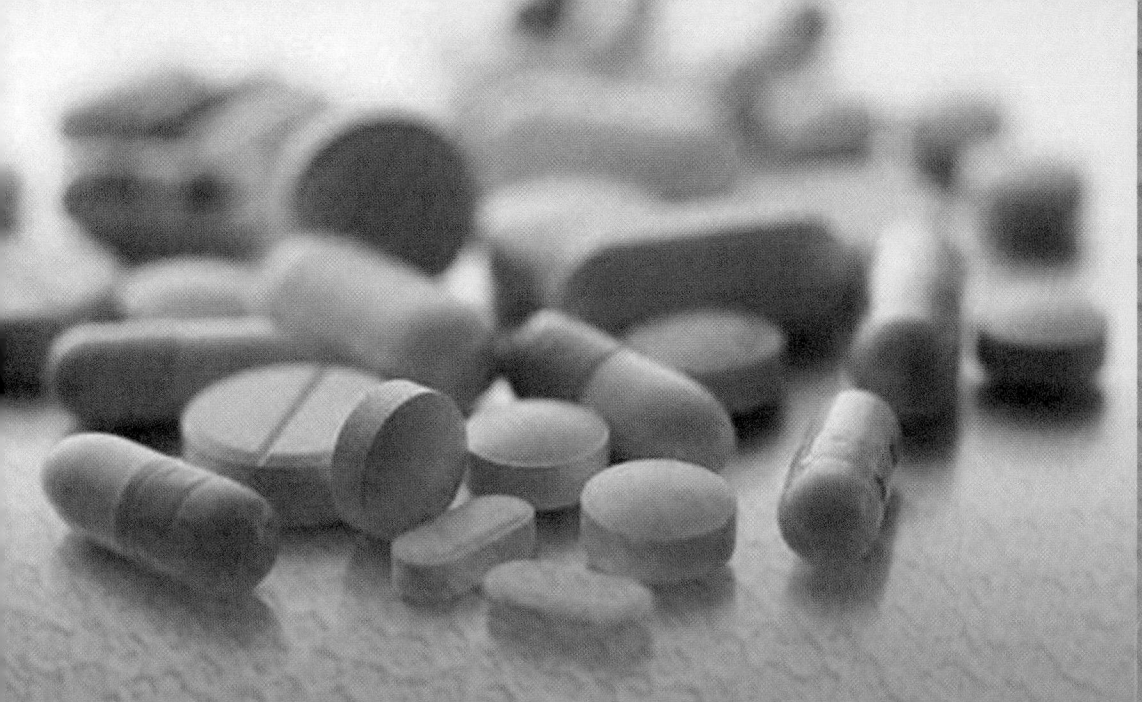

Pharmacology/ Toxicology

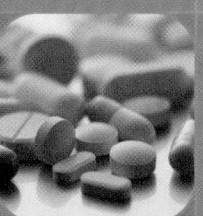

169

General Principles of Pharmacokinetics and Pharmacodynamics

RICHARD C. BRUNDAGE | HENRY J. MANN

Critically ill patients admitted to intensive care units (ICUs) suffer from a variety of physiologic insults that accompany their severe illness. These insults, combined with the rapidly changing physiologic status of the patient, can make appropriate drug dosing a challenging problem for the clinician. An understanding of the pharmacokinetic implications of these physiologic changes and their subsequent effect on pharmacodynamics is required to properly treat critically ill patients. This chapter reviews the basic principles of pharmacokinetics and pharmacodynamics with an emphasis on how they might be affected by critical illness.

Pharmacokinetics and *pharmacodynamics* describe, respectively, the amount of drug in the body at a given time and the pharmacologic effects caused by the drug.[1] Pharmacokinetics describes the movement of a drug into, within, and out of the body over time, whereas pharmacodynamics explains the effects the drug has on the body that result in a clinical response. A general understanding of pharmacokinetic parameters such as clearance, volume of distribution, half-life, steady state, and absorption, along with pharmacodynamic principles such as receptor theory, potency, affinity, tolerance, and minimum effective concentration greatly enhances the clinician's ability to make informed choices in the treatment of the critically ill patient.

General Principles of Pharmacokinetics

Clearance, volume of distribution, half-life, and bioavailability are four pharmacokinetic parameters that allow the clinician to better estimate dosing requirements. If the concentration of a drug in an easily assessable sampled fluid (e.g., plasma, urine, saliva) correlates well with the pharmacologic response (therapeutic or toxic) to the drug, then the application of pharmacokinetics in dosing is likely to be beneficial.[2] Usually the concentration of a drug cannot be measured at the exact site of action (e.g., a receptor on the cell surface), so it is necessary that there be a predictable relationship between the concentration that is measurable and the concentration at the site of the effect.[3,4] These concentrations do not have to be equal, but they should reflect a similar direction and magnitude of change over time (Figure 169-1).

Measurement of the relationship between drug concentration and therapeutic or toxic response in a large number of patients allows development of a therapeutic range or target concentration for that drug (Figure 169-2).[5-10] Table 169-1 lists a number of drugs commonly used in the ICU for which therapeutic ranges have been established and for which therapeutic drug monitoring is often recommended.[11,12] Critically ill patients have a multitude of host factors (e.g., hemodynamic status, decreased organ function, nutritional status, concurrent disease states) that increase the likelihood that individualized drug dosing based on individualized pharmacokinetic assessment will be beneficial (Figure 169-3).[13-16] There can be gender-related differences in both pharmacokinetic and pharmacodynamic responses.[17-19] Individual chapters in this text are devoted to many of these agents and their adjustments for dosage in patients with renal or hepatic failure.

PHARMACOKINETIC MODELS

The pharmacokinetic concepts of clearance, volume of distribution, half-life, and bioavailability are based on physiologic principles.[20]

The physiologic processes governing these concepts are enormously complex, and many simplifying assumptions must be made before the mathematics describing drug concentrations become tractable. Although sophisticated computer modeling approaches are available in research settings, most of the clinically useful pharmacokinetic equations are based on one- or two-compartment models (Figure 169-4).[21]

The simplest model and the most basic equations describe the one-compartment model. When the drug enters the compartment, it is assumed to be instantaneously and completely mixed in a given volume of distribution (V) resulting in a uniform concentration throughout the compartment. The parameter K is the first-order rate constant that reflects the usual situation of elimination being a first-order linear process. The drug is assumed to enter the compartment instantaneously in the case of an intravenous bolus dose. If the dosage is administered through oral or intramuscular routes, entry into the compartment is assumed to occur at a rate defined by a first-order absorption rate constant (Ka). Entry into the compartment is assumed to occur at a rate described by a zero-order rate constant (Ro) if the drug is administered by constant intravenous infusion. *Bioavailability* (F) is defined as the fraction of the administered dose that reaches the systemic circulation.

Clearance (CL) is a primary parameter that can be physiologically associated with a particular organ in the body such as the liver or kidney. Clearance can be calculated according to the equation CL = K × V, leading to the impression that CL is a function of the parameters K and V. However, this arrangement of the equation is not correct from a physiologic point of view. CL and V are both primary parameters, and K is a secondary parameter. The first-order rate is determined by changes in either CL or V, and the equation is correctly written: K = CL/V.

Half-life ($t_{1/2}$) is a useful measure of how quickly a drug is eliminated from the body, and it is related to the first-order elimination rate constant:

$$t_{1/2} = \frac{ln(2)}{K} = \frac{0.693}{K}$$

Specifically, $t_{1/2}$ defines the length of time it takes for the drug concentration to decrease by one-half. In a linear pharmacokinetic system with first-order elimination, the $t_{1/2}$ is a constant, and it takes the same amount of time for the concentration to fall from 100 to 50 arbitrary units as it does to decline from 50 to 25 arbitrary units (Figure 169-5).

The single-compartment model allows concentration at any point in time to be calculated using the following equation:

$$C2 = C1 \times exp^{-K \times \Delta t}$$

where Δt is the time elapsed between the measurement of two concentrations, C1 and C2. It is the properties of this equation that give rise to the familiar exponentially decreasing concentration-time curve, which becomes linear when plotted on semilog coordinates.

The human body is not a single well-stirred compartment, and it is amazing that such a simple mathematical model can be so useful in the clinical setting. If the body is conceptualized as consisting of individual tissues and organs, the same mathematical treatment can be applied. The concept of the volume of distribution has to be somewhat

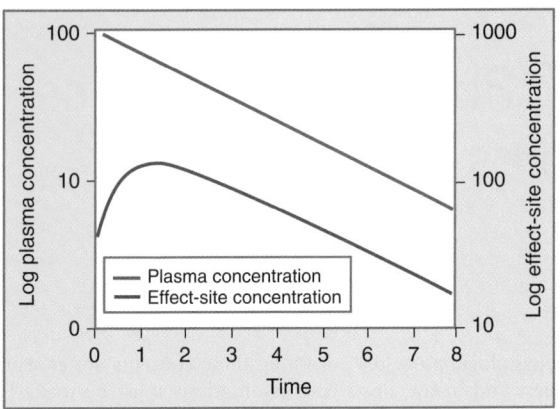

Figure 169-1 For concentration monitoring to be useful, there must be a strong relationship between concentration of the drug measured in an easily accessible fluid and concentration at the effect site. Concentration at the effect site may be less, more, or equal to concentration in the sampled fluid.

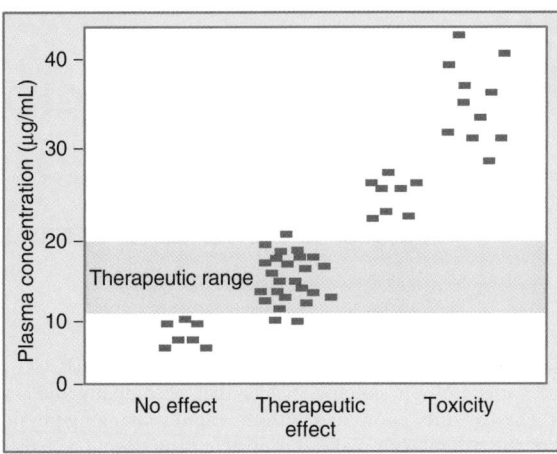

Figure 169-2 Therapeutic range represents the concentration at which a desired effect is likely to occur in most patients and an adverse or toxic effect is rare. If such a range cannot be established, concentration monitoring for the drug is not likely to be of benefit. Therapeutic range is often established by dose-ranging studies during phase 2 drug development and confirmed during the phase 3 trial.

modified to recognize not only the physical size of the organ or tissue, but also the fact that drugs accumulate to differing degrees in different tissue spaces.[22,23] For example, lipophilic drugs have a high affinity for adipose tissue, and this property is reflected by a large partition coefficient (R). The time constant associated with each tissue is a function of the rate of blood flow to that tissue (Q), the physical volume of the tissue (V_T), and the partition coefficient. The time constant determines the rate at which equilibrium is reached. As a result, it is possible to construct a set of exponential equations with a time constant unique to each tissue:

$$\exp^{-[Q/(V \times R)] \times t}$$

There is a branch of pharmacokinetics known as *physiologically based pharmacokinetic modeling* that uses blood flows, organ volumes, and partition coefficients to characterize concentration-time profiles.[24-27] According to this approach for pharmacokinetic modeling, each tissue space ultimately contributes to the venous pool (Figure 169-6). However, the overall shape of the concentration-time profile in the venous blood is controlled not by the number of tissue spaces or their effective volumes, but by their time constants. Tissues with similar time constants, $Q/(V \times R)$, produce similar drug profiles in their venous outflows and appear as a single exponent in pooled venous blood. Practically speaking, many tissues and organs reach equilibrium over similar time frames, and often no more than two distinct time constants

are observed. Therefore, this situation can be described adequately by a two-compartment model, characterized by a rapidly distributing central compartment and a more slowly equilibrating peripheral compartment (Figure 169-7). The equation describing the concentration-time profile for the two-compartment model is:

$$C = A \times \exp^{-\alpha \times t} + B \times \exp^{-\beta \times t}$$

The distinguishing feature of this biexponential equation is that when it is plotted on semilog coordinates, the concentrations are the sum of two distinct straight lines. Hence, there are two half-lives. One is known as the *terminal* or *β half-life*, and the other is the *rapid distribution* or *α half-life*. Once the rapid distribution exponential becomes negligible in the equation, all that remains is the slower

TABLE 169-1	Therapeutic Ranges of Drugs Commonly Used in Critical Care
Drug	*Therapeutic Range*
Amikacin	Trough < 5 µg/mL Peak < 30 µg/mL
Cyclosporine	Whole blood, 150 ng/mL
Digoxin	0.50-2.0 ng/mL
Gentamicin*	Trough < 2 µg/mL Peak < 10 µg/mL
Lidocaine	1.5-5 µg/mL
Phenytoin	10-20 µg/mL
Quinidine	2-5 µg/mL
Theophylline	10-20 µg/mL
Tobramycin*	Trough < 2 µg/mL Peak < 10 µg/mL
Vancomycin†	Trough < 5 µg/mL Peak < 30 µg/mL

*Once daily aminoglycoside dosing may result in different therapeutic ranges.
†Vancomycin concentrations are currently focusing on higher peak concentrations, and practice varies considerably between sites.

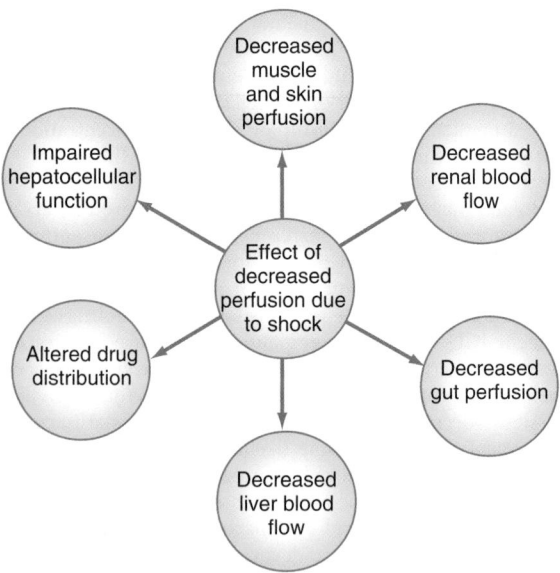

Figure 169-3 Example of interacting factors that determine the effect seen after administration of a single drug dose in an individual patient in the intensive care unit. A patient experiencing shock has decreased drug clearance by the liver and kidney; slowed absorption of oral, intramuscular, or topical medications; and a highly variable volume of distribution based on fluid status.

ONE-COMPARTMENT MODEL

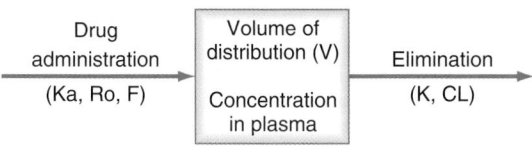

TWO-COMPARTMENT MODEL

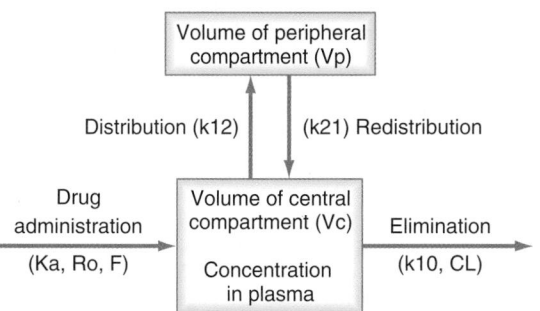

Figure 169-4   In the simplest pharmacokinetic model, the body is treated as a single compartment into which drug is delivered and eliminated. The resulting concentration in the compartment defines the apparent volume of distribution. Most drugs follow the more complicated two-compartment model, which assumes a distribution phase between the central or plasma compartment and the tissue. See text for explanation of terms.

exponential term, and the concentration-time profile resembles that for a single-compartment drug. Consequently, the equation:

$$C2 = C1 \times \exp^{-\beta \times \Delta t}$$

in which β replaces K, can still be used to predict concentrations, as long as both C1 and C2 are in the postdistributive phase. This sum-of-exponentials approach can be extended to three-compartment or even more complex models, but it is difficult to obtain all the concentrations needed to characterize each exponent.

CLEARANCE

Clearance (CL) is a primary pharmacokinetic parameter that measures the ability of the body to eliminate a drug.[28,29] It is often stated that

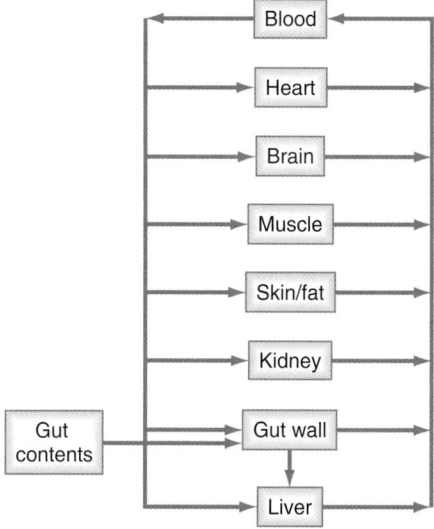

Figure 169-6   Physiologically based models allow individual characterization of drug distribution or clearance for each organ or tissue and also describe the mixed volume effects seen when sampling from blood.

clearance is the volume of blood (plasma) that is completely cleared of drug per unit time. Although this is one way to define clearance, it does not capture the relationship between drug clearance (mL/min) and the rate of drug elimination (mg/h). In pharmacokinetics, the general concept of clearance is defined as the rate of elimination relative to the concentration. In a first-order pharmacokinetic system, the rate of elimination is proportional to the drug concentration, and clearance is this proportionality constant:

$$\text{Rate of elimination} = \text{CL} \times \text{concentration}$$

Clearance is clinically useful because it can be related directly to the organ of elimination. We can talk about renal clearance, hepatic clearance, or biliary clearance, and the sum of each of the individual clearances is the total body clearance.[30,31] The immediate clinical consequence is the ability to adjust doses in response to changes in specific organ function. For example, a patient with developing renal failure is likely

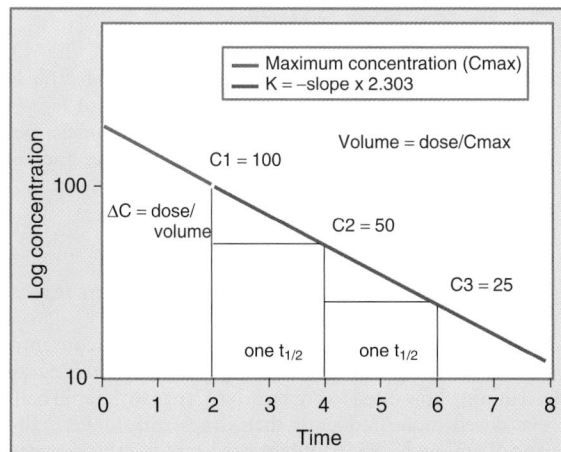

Figure 169-5   Log concentration-time curve for a one-compartment model after intravenous administration, illustrating volume of distribution, elimination rate constant (K), and half-life ($t_{1/2}$). C1, C2, and C3 are measured drug concentrations.

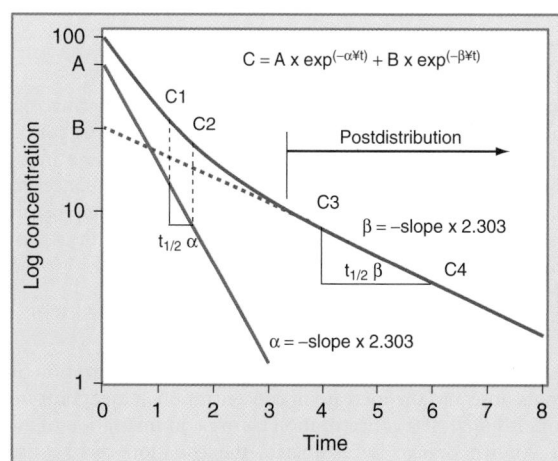

Figure 169-7   Log concentration-time curve for a two-compartment model after intravenous push administration, illustrating a distribution period (α) and postdistribution period (β). Concentrations at C1 and C2 are reflective of both distribution and elimination processes, whereas concentrations at C3 and C4 are primarily affected by elimination processes (clearance).

to require a reduction of the dose of a drug that is eliminated by the kidney, but not necessarily a reduction of the dose of a drug that is eliminated by the liver.[32] If the clearance of a drug is known to be 50% renal and 50% hepatic, and renal function is decreased by 50%, it is necessary to reduce the dose by only 25% to maintain the same concentration.

The primary clinical utility of clearance is that it is the single pharmacokinetic parameter that determines overall drug exposure. The area under the curve (AUC) on a plot of drug concentration as a function of time is often taken as a measure of drug exposure, and it is determined from the dose and clearance (CL):

$$AUC = \frac{Dose}{CL}$$

This relationship is also observed when the steady-state concentration is considered as the measure of drug exposure. During a continuous intravenous infusion, the steady-state concentration (Css) is solely a function of the infusion rate (Ro) and the clearance (CL):

$$Css = \frac{Ro}{CL}$$

Notice that Css is not a function of the volume of distribution. As counterintuitive as it may seem, doubling the volume of distribution will not result in a halving of Css. The important point to keep in mind is that *the equation is predicting the concentration at steady state.* During a constant infusion at steady state, the rapid doubling of the volume of distribution will only *transiently* decrease the concentration by half. If the infusion rate remains unchanged, the concentration will return to the same steady-state concentration, as long as clearance remains unchanged.

The same principle applies to intermittent intravenous or oral dosing as well as continuous infusion. With intermittent dosing, drug concentrations go up and come down during each dosing interval. The average concentration at steady state (Css, avg) is a time-averaged concentration (i.e., the mean of *all* concentrations during the dosing interval); as in the case of a constant infusion, it is a function of clearance and the dosing rate. In the case of oral administration, the dosing rate becomes slightly more complicated, in that it is a function of the dose administered (D), the dosing interval (τ), and bioavailability (F):

$$Css, avg = \frac{F \times D/\tau}{CL}$$

As before, overall drug exposure is not influenced by volume of distribution, but it does change in proportion to changes in clearance or the dosing rate, through changes in F, D, or τ.

VOLUME OF DISTRIBUTION

The volume of distribution (V) is another primary pharmacokinetic parameter that is useful in determining the change in drug concentration for a given dose.[33] After an intravenous bolus dose in a one-compartment pharmacokinetic model, the change in concentration (ΔC) between Cmax and the concentration immediately before the dose is administered is a function of the dose (D) and the volume of distribution (V):

$$\Delta C = \frac{D}{V}$$

This equation is useful for predicting both the concentration after a first bolus dose and the increase in concentration at any point in time after a bolus dose. If a concentration before administration of a bolus dose is known or can be estimated, the equation can be used to predict the increase in concentration after the dose is administered (see Figure 169-5). It is important to recognize that the calculated value of ΔC must be added onto the pre-dose concentration to estimate the Cmax after the bolus dose. This equation is also useful for estimating the dose needed to reach a given concentration. If it is known that the volume of distribution is 0.45 L/kg, and a Cmax of 10 mg/L is desired

after the loading dose, the dose is estimated to be 10 mg/L × 0.45 L/kg = 4.5 mg/kg. It is not necessary to have a steady-state condition to use this equation, a fact that makes it very useful in critical care.

The value for volume of distribution does not necessarily coincide with any particular physiologic space. The veracity of this statement becomes readily apparent when one considers a drug such as digoxin which has a volume of distribution of approximately 440 L. Clearly, a volume of distribution of that magnitude cannot have a relationship to any physiologic space in a standard-sized human. For this reason, the term *apparent volume of distribution* is often used.

The concept of volume of distribution gets more confusing when more than one compartment is needed to describe the pharmacokinetics of a drug. Mathematically, the volume of distribution is a hypothetical volume that is needed to relate the amount of drug in the body to a measured concentration in a fluid (usually plasma). Unlike the one-compartment model, wherein all of the drug in the body is regarded as being in a single compartment until it is eliminated, drug also circulates through additional compartments in a multicompartment model. In this situation, the volume of distribution must increase as drug distributes to other compartments until pseudodistribution equilibrium among all compartments is reached. Technically, an infinite number of volumes of distribution are observed as this equilibration process occurs, but only three are commonly defined. The *volume of distribution of the central compartment* (Vc) is the volume of the usual sampling compartment; it is always the smallest volume term. Immediately after administration of an intravenous bolus, all added drug is in the central compartment, and Vc can be used to calculate a change in concentration.

The volume of distribution increases over time until a *distribution equilibrium* is reached among all compartments. This is the largest value for the volume of distribution. The fact that distribution equilibrium has occurred can be determined from a log-concentration versus time plot (see Figure 169-7). The curve becomes log-linear when the rate of drug entry into each peripheral compartment equals the rate of exit from each compartment. Because it is often calculated using the clearance and the β or terminal elimination half-life, this volume is often called V_β:

$$V_\beta = \frac{CL}{\beta}$$

The third commonly used volume term is the *steady-state volume of distribution* (Vss). It is the sum of the volumes of all the compartments in the model. If a drug were infused to steady state, Vss would be the proportionality constant relating the steady-state concentration to the total amount of drug in the body. Practically speaking, Vss is not often used in individualizing drug dosing.

HALF-LIFE

The *half-life* ($t_{1/2}$) is a pharmacokinetic parameter defined as the length of time it takes to reduce the drug concentration by half (see Figure 169-5).[33] The half-life is referred to as a *secondary parameter* because it is a function of the two primary parameters, clearance and volume of distribution:

$$t_{1/2} = \frac{ln(2) \times V}{CL} = \frac{0.693 \times V}{CL}$$

A change in either clearance or volume of distribution results in a proportional change in half-life.

Because the half-life characterizes how rapidly concentration decreases over time, the primary clinical application for this parameter is for determining how often to dose a drug. Drugs with rapid half-lives have to be dosed more frequently than drugs with longer half-lives. The dosing of aminoglycoside antibiotics exemplifies this concept. The half-life for an aminoglycoside is relatively short in patients with good renal function (high clearance), and the drug may have to be dosed every 6 hours. In patients with poor renal function, the half-life is relatively longer, and dosing may be prolonged to 12- or 24-hour intervals to maintain appropriate peak and trough concentrations. In the critical care patient, the development of renal failure can significantly change aminoglycoside clearance, and the accompanying change in drug half-life will necessitate a change in dosing interval.

In a one-compartment system with constant clearance and volume of distribution, drug half-life also is constant. However, in a multicompartment model, the volume of distribution increases over time as drug equilibrates into tissue compartments until V_β is reached. According to the previous equation, the half-life also increases over time and eventually reaches a maximum at $t_{1/2}\beta$ (see Figure 169-7).

In multicompartment models, there is usually one half-life of interest for each compartment. These half-lives are derived from the hybrid time constants associated with each compartment. In a two-compartment model, these two exponentials are typically called α and β and are arbitrarily termed the *rapid* and *slow exponents*, respectively. These time constants give rise to the rapid or distribution $t_{1/2}\alpha$ and the slower or terminal $t_{1/2}\beta$. One useful way to think about distribution half-lives is analogous to the standard way of thinking about any half-life. In the one-compartment model, it takes five half-lives for 97% of the drug to be eliminated from the body. The situation is similar for each exponent, but the interpretation is that it takes five distribution half-lives for that exponent to become negligible in the sum of exponentials equation. In other words, it takes five α half-lives before the rapid distribution phase is completed, and the remaining concentration-time profile reflects the elimination or β phase.

Most drugs have a rapid distribution phase that could be detected if concentrations were measured frequently enough. Aminoglycosides again are a good illustrative example of this concept, because they have a rapid, although not instantaneous, distribution phase (Figure 169-8). With a distribution phase half-life of 5 to 10 minutes, it would take approximately 25 to 50 minutes before the log-linear elimination phase could be observed. It is this distribution process that is the basis for the recommendation to wait approximately 1 hour after the end of an infusion before sampling blood to measure the aminoglycoside concentration. If a blood sample is obtained before this time, the drug still will be in the distribution phase, and the concentration measured will lead to underestimation of the drug half-life. In addition, slowly equilibrating compartments have been demonstrated when aminoglycoside concentrations are measured during washout.[34] Aminoglycosides are

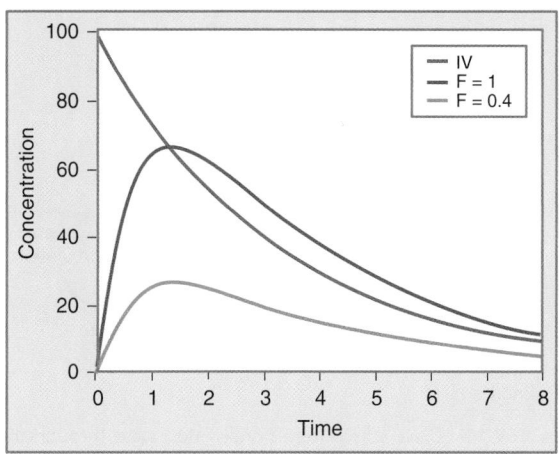

Figure 169-9 Bioavailability is determined relative to the area under the concentration-time curve (AUC) after intravenous (IV) administration of drug. An extravascular (e.g., intramuscular, oral, rectal) dose that is 100% absorbed (F = 1) has complete bioavailability (i.e., the extravascular AUC equals the intravenous AUC). A drug dose with 40% bioavailability (F = 0.4) would result in 40% of the drug exposure relative to an intravenous dose.

usually dosed frequently enough so that the slowly equilibrating compartment is not detected.

BIOAVAILABILITY

The extent of drug absorption, termed *bioavailability* (F), is generally referenced to the amount of drug available systemically when the drug is given intravenously. This parameter is determined by comparing the AUC of the drug given by intravenous administration to that of the same drug given by another route (Figure 169-9). The bioavailability of a drug given via the intravenous route is regarded as being 100% (i.e., F = 1.0), and other routes of administration (e.g., oral dosing, intramuscular injection) often have a reduced bioavailability (e.g., F = 0.8, or 80% bioavailability). A number of drug-related and patient-related factors determine bioavailability. In essence, however, F is a function of the degree of absorption and the amount of drug metabolized or eliminated before entering the systemic circulation (first-pass effect).[35] Drugs with low bioavailability either cannot be administered by any route other than the intravenous one (e.g., sodium nitroprusside, dobutamine) or require higher doses when given via the oral route compared with the intravenous route (e.g., furosemide, morphine, propranolol). Alternative routes of administration (e.g., rectal, topical, subcutaneous injection, intramuscular injection) are occasionally used in critically ill patients, owing to poor oral bioavailability. These routes all suffer from problems with delayed or poorly predictable serum concentrations. Vasoconstriction, hypoperfusion, edema, gastric suctioning, ileus, diarrhea, and enhanced gastrointestinal motility are all common problems in critically ill patients that can further adversely affect bioavailability.

The *first-pass effect* (Figure 169-10) refers to the elimination of drug that is absorbed orally but then is metabolized by enzymes in the gut wall or in the liver before reaching the systemic circulation. As a drug is absorbed and passes through the gut wall, it can be acted upon by transport proteins (primarily P-glycoprotein) that actively pump drug molecules back into the lumen of the gastrointestinal tract.[36-40] All drug molecules that are not pumped out enter the hepatic circulation and are subject to metabolism in the liver before their first opportunity to be presented to the systemic circulation.[41] Drugs that have a high hepatic extraction ratio (i.e., are very efficiently removed by the liver) are most likely to show decreased bioavailability due to this first-pass effect; conversely, the bioavailability of these drugs increases if liver dysfunction decreases the hepatic extraction ratio.

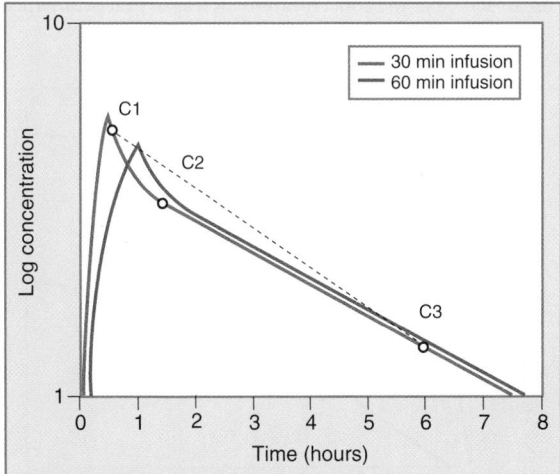

Figure 169-8 If an aminoglycoside (tobramycin) is administered by intravenous infusion over 30 minutes, the peak concentration will be higher than with infusion over 60 minutes, but the total area under the curve will be the same. If therapeutic drug monitoring occurs and a sample is taken during the distribution phase (C1) and paired with a concentration obtained during the postdistribution phase (C2 or C3), the calculated half-life will be shorter than if two samples from the postdistribution phase (e.g., C2 and C3) are paired together.

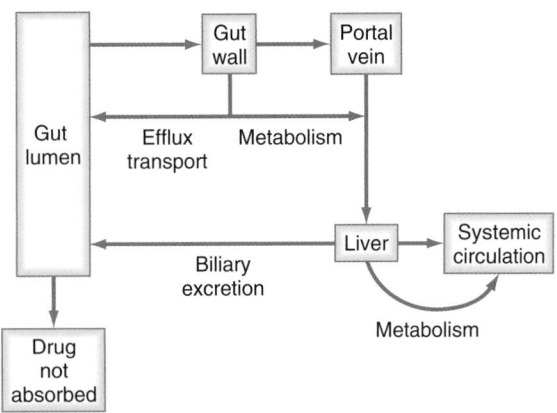

Figure 169-10 Drug administered orally must pass through the gut wall and through the liver before becoming available in the systemic circulation. Drug transporters and metabolism in the gut wall, combined with metabolism during the first pass through the liver, can result in significant decreases in bioavailability.

STEADY STATE

After an infusion is started, drug concentrations increase and eventually reach a concentration that does not change over time (Figure 169-11).[42] At this point, the amount of drug entering the body is equal to the amount leaving it during a given period of time, and steady-state conditions apply. During intermittent dosing, drug concentrations accumulate over time, and eventually a steady state is attained. Drug concentrations increase as more drug is administered or absorbed and decrease during elimination, but the concentration profile over each interval resembles all the other profiles during steady state (Figure 169-12). In the clinical setting, measurement of drug concentration is often delayed for a period equal to five half-lives, because at that point the concentration will reflect 97% of the final steady-state concentration.

🔲 Pharmacodynamics

Pharmacodynamics is the study of the relationship between the concentration of a drug and its pharmacologic effect.[2] Pharmacodynamic models are routinely employed during drug development, where they are used to determine drug-dosing regimens. These models can become quite complex, particularly if they are mechanism-based models.

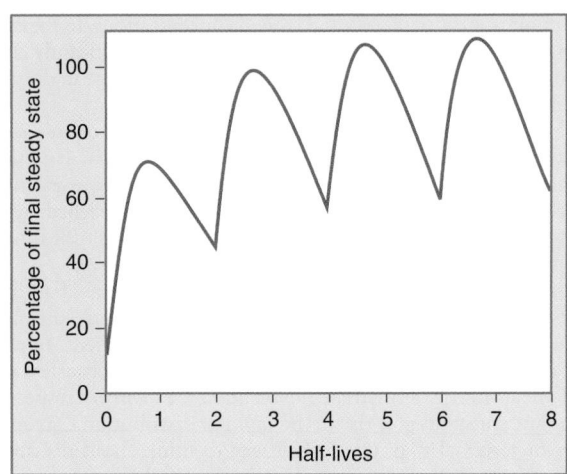

Figure 169-12 With intermittent dosing (oral, intravenous, or intramuscular), concentration profiles also approach a steady state wherein peak and trough concentrations during a given cycle are reproducible in the next cycle.

Although a pharmacodynamic model can involve many linked mathematical submodels, this is not the type of model that is likely to be useful in a clinical setting. The principles underpinning the relatively simple Emax model are often adequate.[43] Mathematically, the equation relating effect and concentration can be described with the Emax equation:

$$\text{Effect} = \frac{\text{Emax} \times \text{concentration}}{\text{EC50} + \text{concentration}}$$

Graphically, this equation has a hyperbolic shape (Figure 169-13). The parameters of this model are the Emax and the EC50. Emax represents the maximal effect attainable due to the drug. The EC50 is the concentration at which half the maximal effect is observed; it is a measure of drug potency. An important feature of this plot reaffirms the intuitive notion that increasing the dose of the drug to higher and higher amounts does not increase the effect of the drug proportionately; eventually, the effect of the drug begins to reach a plateau. In essence, the law of diminishing returns applies: continually smaller increases in effect are observed as the concentration increases. Practically speaking,

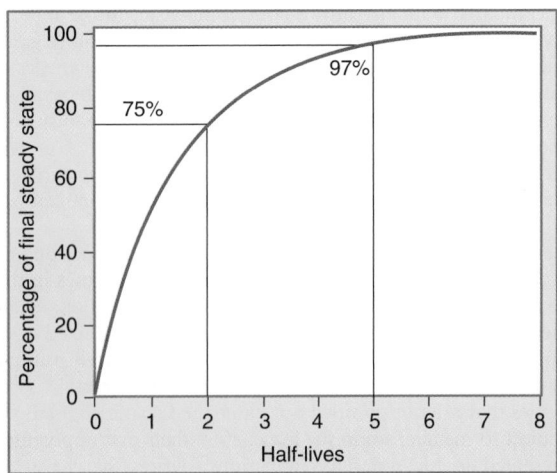

Figure 169-11 Concentrations exponentially approach a steady-state value during a constant infusion in a one-compartment model. After five half-lives of a drug, its concentration is at 97% of the final steady-state value.

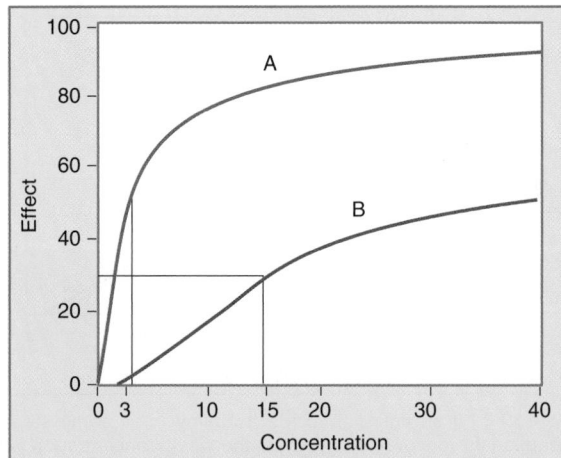

Figure 169-13 The Emax pharmacodynamic model illustrates that when drug concentrations exceed the concentration at which half the maximal effect is expected (EC50), there is a decreasing return in terms of effect as the dose is further increased. Drug A has a lower EC50 (3) than drug B (15) and is said to be more potent than drug B.

if the drug concentration is expected to be at the EC50 or lower, increasing the dose will produce a meaningful increase in effect. However, if the concentration exceeds the EC50, increasing the dose may not be warranted, because only small increases in effect may be expected, and the increased concentrations may place the patient at risk for development of adverse (i.e., off-target) drug-related effects.

Several modifications of the basic Emax model are found in the literature. For example, a baseline can be added to the model, the drug may actually be responsible for inhibiting a given effect, the effect can be re-parameterized as a percentage change from baseline, or a sigmoidicity term may be added to create an S-shape in the functional relationship. The same basic features of the plot will be observed. In the absence of drug (i.e., when the concentration equals zero), there will be no effect due to the drug. At the other extreme, there will be a maximal effect that can be elicited by the drug. As concentrations increase beyond EC50, the change in effect due to the drug begins to reach a plateau.

Another point to consider is that time does not appear in the effect model. The concentrations are explicitly defined as steady-state concentrations, and the effect resulting from a given concentration is considered to be a steady-state effect. This model applies when drug in the plasma rapidly equilibrates with drug at the site of action, and there is no indirect mechanism between the concentration at the site of effect and the effect. The more common situation is that the effect lags somewhat behind the concentration (Figure 169-14). If concentrations are going up and coming down over time, as would be expected with an intermittent intravenous or oral dosing schedule, the effect is also expected to go up and down over time, but the time frames may not exactly coincide. For example, the plasma concentration might peak at 1 hour and the effect might peak several hours later. There is a mismatch or disequilibrium between concentration and effect, and a plot of effect versus concentration, with the points connected in time order, yields a hysteresis loop (Figure 169-15). It can be seen that for any given concentration, there are two levels of effect, one on the upswing of the concentration-time curve and the other on the downswing. Both empirical and mechanistic pharmacodynamic modeling approaches have been developed to allow for this disequilibrium. Although the modeling of effect-time curves is achievable, and these models are useful in predicting effects with various dosing regimens, their routine use in clinical settings has been limited.

The pharmacodynamic effects noted with a given drug result from the drug's interaction with receptors and the resultant activation or inhibition of effects mediated by that receptor. These effects may be either the therapeutic action desired or a toxic effect that is unwanted.

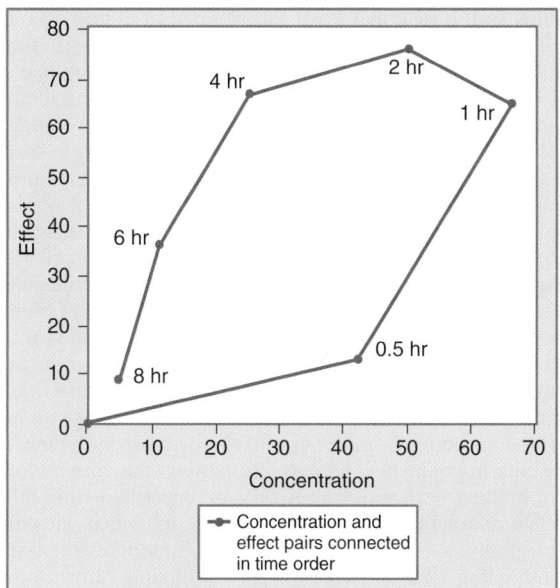

Figure 169-15 A counterclockwise hysteresis loop occurs when an effect at a given concentration is less at an early point in time but strengthens at the same concentration later in time. This may be caused by an active metabolite, increased sensitization to the drug, or the need for a distribution period from the sampled fluid to the effect site. The opposite can occur (i.e., a clockwise hysteresis loop) if a given effect decreases over time, as in the development of tolerance to the drug.

Generally it is assumed that the intensity of effect produced by the drug is a function of the quantity of drug at the receptor site, whereas relative potency results from varying degrees of selectivity for the receptor and the receptor's affinity for binding the drug. More potent drugs elicit a given effect at lower concentrations than less potent drugs.

Drugs that stimulate a response from the receptor are *agonists*, and those that inhibit a response from the receptor are *antagonists*. Because antagonists have no effect of their own at the receptor, the net effect depends on both the concentration of the antagonist and that of the agonist that is blocked. The relative concentration of the agonist compared with the antagonist primarily determines the effect observed when an antagonist is competitive for the same binding site as the molecule or drug that stimulates the receptor. Irreversible antagonists, however, either bind with very strong affinity to the receptor so they cannot be displaced or bind to another site on the substrate that interferes with binding at the receptor. The effect of irreversible antagonists is independent of the agonist's concentration and results in a decrease in the maximal effect of the agonist. The duration of effect for irreversible antagonists is determined by the rate of turnover for the receptor.

Tolerance to a drug is seen when the response at a given dose decreases. This may be a result of receptor down-regulation (decreased number or sensitivity of receptors) or enzyme induction (increased metabolism). Cross-tolerance, as is commonly seen with opioids, occurs when similar drugs act on the same receptor.

PROTEIN BINDING

Many drugs are bound to plasma proteins, and the terms *bound drug concentration* (Cb), *unbound* (or *free*) *drug concentration* (Cu), *total* (bound plus unbound) *drug concentration* (Ctot), and *unbound* (or *free*) *fraction* (fu) are frequently used:

$$Ctot = Cu + Cb$$

$$fu = \frac{Cu}{Ctot}$$

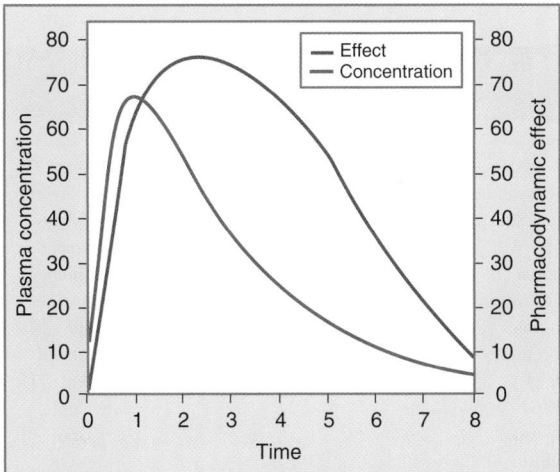

Figure 169-14 Pharmacodynamic effects often lag behind the matching pharmacokinetic model. In this instance, maximum concentration in blood occurs at 1 hour, whereas maximal drug effect occurs between 2 and 3 hours.

Intuitively, it is clear that when a drug is displaced from its binding sites in the plasma, the increase in unbound drug concentration can lead to adverse reactions. A series of scientific papers published in the mid-1960s set this direction for interpretation of the clinical implications of protein binding. In a study of the interaction between warfarin and phenylbutazone, it was shown that phenylbutazone increases plasma warfarin concentration and also increases prothrombin time.[44] In addition, warfarin binding was studied in vitro, and it was clearly shown that phenylbutazone displaces warfarin from binding sites. It was concluded that phenylbutazone potentiates the action of warfarin in vivo by displacing warfarin from its binding to plasma albumin, causing more warfarin to be available to specific sites of biological action. Although it may have been intuitive to relate the in vivo and in vitro observations in a cause-and-effect manner, change in protein binding is not the correct explanation for the drug interaction. It is now known that the drug interaction is mediated through an inhibition of the metabolic clearance of warfarin by phenylbutazone.[45]

The pharmacokinetic concepts concerning the implications of protein binding were reviewed in 2002 by Benet and Hoener.[46] The mathematical approach is not repeated here, but when one employs physiologically based models for clearance, volume of distribution, and protein binding, changes in plasma protein binding can be shown to have little clinical relevance. These clearance concepts illustrate that physiologic parameters (intrinsic clearance, organ blood flow, and protein binding) have an impact on some pharmacokinetic parameters, and these changes result in changes to the shape of the plasma-concentration time profiles. However, these effects do not necessarily translate into clinically relevant changes in effective concentrations. To better understand this concept, the relationship between drug exposure and pharmacodynamic effect must be considered.

One of the more useful measures of exposure is the AUC. When talking about pharmacologic effects, some statement is usually made that effect is related to the unbound concentration. This extrapolates directly to say that the unbound AUC (AUCu) is what is important in determining drug effect.

$$AUCu = fu \times AUC = fu \times F \times \frac{Dose}{CL}$$

where *fu* is the fraction unbound, *F* is the bioavailability, and *CL* is the clearance.

After standard well-stirred model assumptions are made regarding high- and low-clearance drugs, something quite interesting occurs when the appropriate equations for clearance and bioavailability are substituted into the equation for AUCu. For all drugs administered orally and eliminated hepatically, the *fu* term cancels out of the equation. Overall unbound drug exposure is not a function of fu at steady-state, and there should be no changes in pharmacologic effect with changes in protein binding. Similarly, it can be seen that the AUCu for all drugs with low extraction ratios—whether administered orally or by the intravenous route, and whether eliminated by the liver or nonhepatically—is not a function of fu after the appropriate substitutions are made. Again, changes in protein binding will not result in changes in the steady-state exposure to the unbound drug. It is important to emphasize that *AUCu* refers to the AUC based on unbound concentrations. The AUC based on total concentrations, AUCtot, is calculated from this equation: AUCtot = AUCu/fu. If the protein binding of a drug changes such that fu is doubled, AUCtot will be halved, and AUCu will remain the same. The expression for AUCu retains a term for protein binding for all high-clearance drugs administered by the intravenous route (regardless of clearance method) and for high-clearance drugs administered orally that are eliminated by extrahepatic pathways.

To address this issue, Benet and Hoener reviewed pharmacokinetic data on 456 drugs from the literature (Table 169-2). No orally administered drug which has a high elimination ratio and is cleared nonhepatically met the criterion for significant (>70%) protein binding. Only 25 (5%) of the 456 drugs had high extraction ratios, were not administered by the oral route, and met the criterion for which protein

binding may influence drug exposure. However, many of these 25 agents are routinely used in critical care (Table 169-3).

In critically ill patients, protein concentrations can change over time. This is particularly true of the acute-phase reactant, α_1-acid glycoprotein (AAG). In addition, some patients (e.g., those undergoing dialysis or those with cachexia) have altered protein binding.[47,48] Although it might seem intuitive to automatically adjust drug doses in response to changes in protein binding, the information in Table 169-2 should be considered. The extent of protein binding, route of administration, route of elimination, and extraction ratio of the drug all should be considered when determining whether a change in binding is likely to result in a change in effect.[49,50]

As a final note on protein binding, care must be taken when evaluating drug concentrations in patients with altered protein binding. Consider the case of phenytoin. The percentage of unbound drug is typically 10% but is approximately doubled (to about 20%) in patients receiving hemodialysis (Table 169-4). If phenytoin were administered as a standard dose to all patients, there would not be a problem; phenytoin is a low-clearance drug, and protein binding should not influence overall unbound exposure whether the drug is administered orally or intravenously. However, phenytoin concentrations are often obtained for the purposes of therapeutic drug monitoring, and efforts are made to achieve circulating levels within the commonly accepted therapeutic range of 10 to 20 mg/L. In patients with normal protein binding, this drug level equates to an unbound therapeutic range of 1 to 2 mg/L. However, in patients with a higher percentage of unbound drug, say 20%, the desired unbound concentration is still 1 to 2 mg/L, but the corresponding total concentration is approximately halved. In

TABLE 169-2	Circumstances in Which Changes in Protein Binding Will Affect Unbound AUC	
	Low-Extraction-Ratio Drugs	*High-Extraction-Ratio Drugs*
IV Administration		
Hepatic clearance	No	Yes*
Nonhepatic clearance	No	Yes*
Oral Administration		
Hepatic clearance	No	No
Nonhepatic clearance	No	Yes†

*Only 25 of the 456 drugs reviewed met the criteria.
†None of the 456 drugs reviewed met the criteria.
AUC, area under the concentration-time curve; IV, intravenous.

TABLE 169-3	25 Drugs for Which Changes in Protein Binding May Influence Clinical Drug Exposure After Intravenous or Intramuscular Administration*	
Alfentanil		Itraconazole
Amitriptyline		Lidocaine
Buprenorphine		Methylprednisolone
Chlorpromazine		Midazolam
Cocaine		Milrinone
Diltiazem		Nicardipine
Diphenhydramine		Pentamidine
Doxorubicin		Propofol
Erythromycin		Propranolol
Fentanyl		Remifentanil
Gold sodium thiomalate		Sufentanil
Haloperidol		Verapamil
Idarubicin		

*Criteria for selection included > 70% protein binding and hepatic clearance > 6.0 mL/min/kg or nonhepatic extraction ratio clearance ≥ 0.28 × renal blood flow (>4.8 mL/min/kg).
Modified from Benet LZ, Hoener BA. Changes in plasma protein binding have little clinical relevance. Clin Pharmacol Ther 2002;71:115-21.

	TABLE 169-4	Effect of Decreased Protein Binding on Bound and Unbound Concentrations of Phenytoin		

	Concentrations of Phenytoin at Therapeutic Range (mg/L)		*Result of Erroneous Increase in Phenytoin Dose in Patient with Decreased Protein Binding**
Concentration	*Typical Patient*	*Patient with Protein Binding Decreased by 50%*	
Total (Ctot)	20	10	20
Unbound (Cu)	2 (10%)	2 (20%)	4 (20%)
Bound (Cb)	18	8	16

*Because of the altered protein binding, Ctot is less when Cu is in the therapeutic range (i.e., 2 mg/L). During therapeutic drug monitoring, it is the Ctot that is measured. If the decreased protein binding is not taken into account and the phenytoin dose is increased to achieve a Ctot of 20 mg/L, the actual Cu will be 4 mg/L, twice the desired therapeutic range, and toxic effects could ensue.

such cases, if the dose of phenytoin is increased to bring the total concentration into the therapeutic range, toxicities may be observed because the unbound concentration will be approximately twice the desired value.

Nonlinear Pharmacokinetics

The application of pharmacokinetics to therapeutic drug monitoring becomes considerably more difficult with drugs that exhibit nonlinearities. With linear pharmacokinetics, parameters are stable over time and across concentrations. Doubling of the dose results in doubling of the concentration, and a given dose provides the same AUC regardless of the dosing history, even when the dose in question is the first dose. *Nonlinear pharmacokinetics* is a term used when the principle of superposition no longer holds. An increase in dose may result in an increase in concentration that is more than or less than proportional, or it may result in clearance changes over time (Figure 169-16). There are several common types of nonlinearities that occur in the clinical setting.[51]

Phenytoin is the classic example for nonlinear elimination. Increases in a phenytoin dose can result in greater than proportional increases in concentration. In any pharmacokinetic system, clearance (CL) is defined as the rate of elimination relative to the concentration (C). Hence, an instantaneous rate of elimination can be defined as follows:

$$\text{Rate of elimination} = \text{CL} \times \text{C}$$

In a linear elimination process, clearance is constant, and doubling the concentration doubles the rate of elimination. In the case of phenytoin with nonlinear elimination, the rate of elimination does not increase in proportion to the concentration, and clearance is not a constant. The nonlinear elimination of phenytoin occurs because the metabolic

pathway responsible for the elimination of the drug is saturable. The enzyme system has a maximum rate of metabolism that can be approached at therapeutic concentrations of phenytoin. These principles can be better understood by considering the rate of elimination described by the Michaelis-Menten equation (Figure 169-17). It has two parameters, the *maximum rate of elimination* (Vmax) and the *concentration that results in one-half the maximum rate* (Km):

$$\text{Rate of elimination} = \frac{\text{Vmax} \times \text{C}}{\text{Km} + \text{C}}$$

Although the parameters Vmax and Km are constant, it can be seen that clearance is a function of concentration (C). The clearance of a drug decreases as the concentration increases:

$$\text{CL} = \frac{\text{Rate of elimination}}{\text{C}} = \frac{\text{Vmax}}{\text{Km} + \text{C}}$$

Although enzyme systems do have maximal rates, the usual concentrations of drug attained in the clinical setting produce rates of elimination that are far below the maximal rate of the enzyme. In the last equation, if C is considerably lower than Km (i.e., negligible), then the quantity, Vmax ÷ (Km + C), is minimally influenced by concentration, and clearance becomes a constant. Therefore, even though many drugs are metabolized by hepatic enzymes, few drugs of clinical interest display detectable nonlinear elimination.

At steady state, the amount of drug eliminated every day must equal the dose taken, so the elimination rate equals the dosing rate. The equation for the steady-state concentration (Css) is:

$$\text{Css} = \frac{\text{Dosing rate} \times \text{Km}}{\text{Vmax} - \text{Dosing rate}}$$

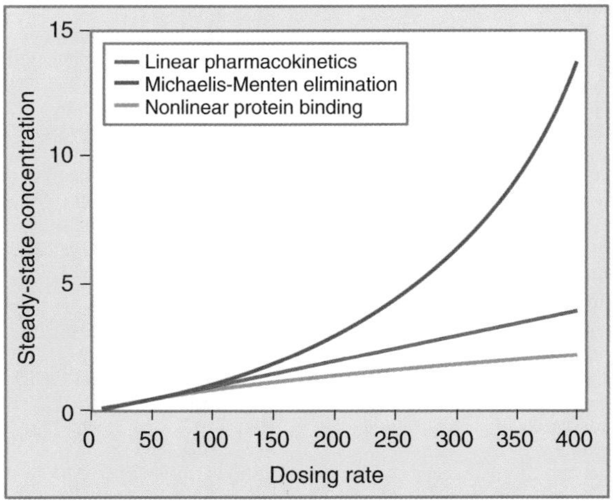

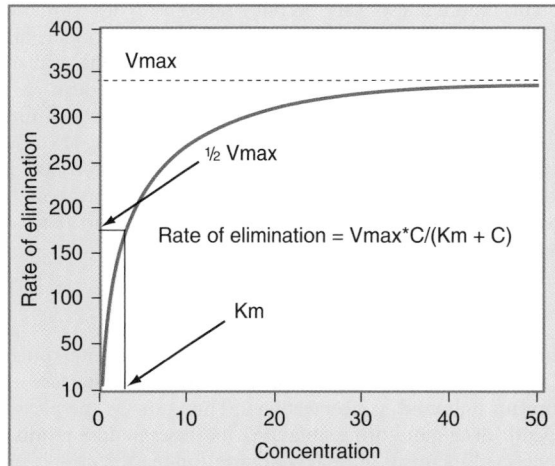

Figure 169-16 Drugs with nonlinear characteristics often can be predictable within a given dose range but then exhibit disproportionate increases or decreases in concentration as doses are increased further.

Figure 169-17 The Michaelis-Menten model demonstrates elimination as a nonlinear function of concentration, with characteristics including a maximum rate of elimination (Vmax) and a concentration at which one-half of the maximum rate of elimination occurs (Km).

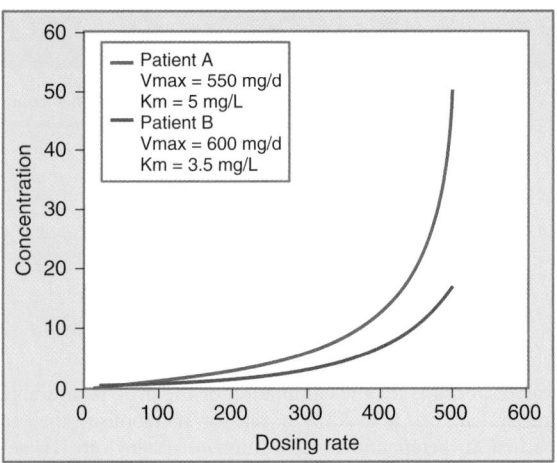

Figure 169-18   The same phenytoin dose increase can result in very different steady-state concentrations in patients with differing Vmax and Km parameters. Patient A is likely to have controlled seizures at doses of 350 to 400 mg/d, whereas seizures in patient B would not be controlled in this dose range.

This equation shows that an increase in dosing rate produces a greater than proportional increase in the steady-state concentration. Furthermore, if the dosing rate exceeds Vmax, a steady-state concentration will never be attained. The nonlinear relationship between phenytoin dosing rate and steady-state concentration can be seen for two patients with different Vmax and Km parameters (Figure 169-18). It is easy to understand the difficulties clinicians can encounter when adjusting doses for a drug such as phenytoin which displays nonlinear elimination kinetics. A dose increase that provides a nearly proportional increase in concentration in one patient could produce a much greater concentration in another. These two curves would be straight lines for drugs that displayed linear pharmacokinetics.

Another type of nonlinearity is time-dependent pharmacokinetics. The classic example in this category is the ability of carbamazepine to induce its own metabolism.[52] This autoinduction causes the clearance of carbamazepine to increase over time. It is important to gradually increase the dose of carbamazepine during the first few weeks of therapy up to the expected maintenance dose so as to avoid toxicities related to elevated concentrations.

Protein binding also can become saturable with some drugs. Intuitively, one might think that saturation of protein binding would result in higher unbound drug concentrations available to exert desirable effects and toxicities, but it must be kept in mind that the organs responsible for drug clearance are eliminating unbound drug. Therefore, unless the clearance of a drug also changes, the steady-state unbound concentration will remain constant in the face of saturable protein binding. The total concentration (Ctot) is a function of the unbound concentration (Cu) and the fraction unbound (fu):

$$Ctot = \frac{Cu}{fu}$$

The fraction unbound does increase at higher unbound concentrations, with the result that total concentrations do not increase in proportion to unbound concentrations. This can be perplexing in therapeutic drug monitoring situations. Increases in dose produce less than expected increases in total concentration. As the dose is pushed higher to reach therapeutic concentrations based on total concentration, toxicities may be observed, because saturable binding causes the unbound concentration to be greater than expected.

■ Alterations in the Elderly

The number of people over 65 years of age is increasing in the United States and in many European countries, and this growth in the elderly population will result in an even greater percentage of ICU beds occupied by older patients. Compared with younger patients, elderly patients typically are taking more drugs, have more underlying organ dysfunction (hepatic, renal, central nervous system), are more likely to be malnourished and to have altered protein binding on this basis, and have reduced or increased responses to some medications.[53] These age-related changes further complicate management of the superimposed critical illness because of large variations among individuals with respect to disposition of drugs (Figure 169-19).

Elderly patients may have a decreased rate of drug absorption, although the total amount of drug absorbed is usually unchanged. As the body ages, the percentage of body mass that is fat increases. This change results in greater distribution of lipophilic drugs into fat, leading to longer half-lives for certain classes of drugs such as anesthetics, barbiturates, and benzodiazepines. Clearance of many drugs is decreased in the elderly, because the hepatic and renal function decreases with increasing age (Table 169-5). These changes can lead to a greater incidence of toxicity because metabolites associated with adverse effects can accumulate. Overall, the same careful attention to dosing required for all critically ill patients must be extended to the elderly. Drugs should be stopped as soon as possible, and dosage increases should be applied cautiously.

■ Pharmacogenomics

The responses to drugs can vary widely among individuals within a population, and pharmacogenetic differences have been identified that help explain some of this variability. *Pharmacogenomics* is the term applied to the study of the expression and regulation of genes that effect drug response. It was initially reported in the 1960s that the *N*-acetylation pathway of isoniazid metabolism was under genetic control. Based upon these findings, individuals could be classified as being rapid or slow acetylators. Some of the more commonly known genetic polymorphisms that affect pharmacokinetics are related to various enzymes belonging to the cytochrome P450 family.

It is now recognized that genetic variants exist in drug transporters that influence the distribution of drugs into tissue spaces. Research in

TABLE 169-5	Effects of Aging on Clearance of Some Oxidized and Conjugated Drugs		
Drug	*Effect*	*Reference*	
Oxidized			
Chlordiazepoxide	↓↓	Am J Psychiatry 1977;134:559	
Desmethyldiazepam	↓↓	Br J Clin Pharmacol 1979;7:119	
Erythromycin	↓↓	Eur J Clin Pharmacol 1990;39:161	
Haloperidol	↓↓	Neuropsychobiology 1996;33:12	
Midazolam	↓↓	Biochem Pharmacol 1992;44:275	
Nicardipine	↓↓	Am Heart J 1989;117:256	
Nifedipine	↓↓	Br J Clin Pharmacol 1988;25:297	
Phenytoin (free)	↓↓	Clin Pharmacokinet 1981;6:389	
Propranolol	—	Br J Clin Pharmacol 1979;7:49	
Theophylline	↓↓	Eur J Clin Pharmacol 1989;36:29	
Verapamil	↓↓	Acta Med Scand 1984;681(Suppl):25	
Conjugated			
Acetaminophen	↓	Br J Clin Pharmacol 1990;30:634	
Lamotrigine	↓	J Pharm Med 1991;1:121	
Lidocaine	↓↓	J Cardiovasc Pharmacol 1983;5:1093	
Lorazepam	↓	Clin Pharmacol Ther 1979;26:103	
Metronidazole	—	Hum Exp Toxicol 1990;9:155	
Morphine	↓	Age Ageing 1989;18:258	
Oxazepam	—	Clin Pharmacol Ther 1981;30:805	

—, no effect; ↓, minor effect; ↓↓, significant effect.
Modified from Woodhouse K, Wynne HA. Age-related changes in hepatic function: implications for drug therapy. Drugs Aging 1992;2:243.

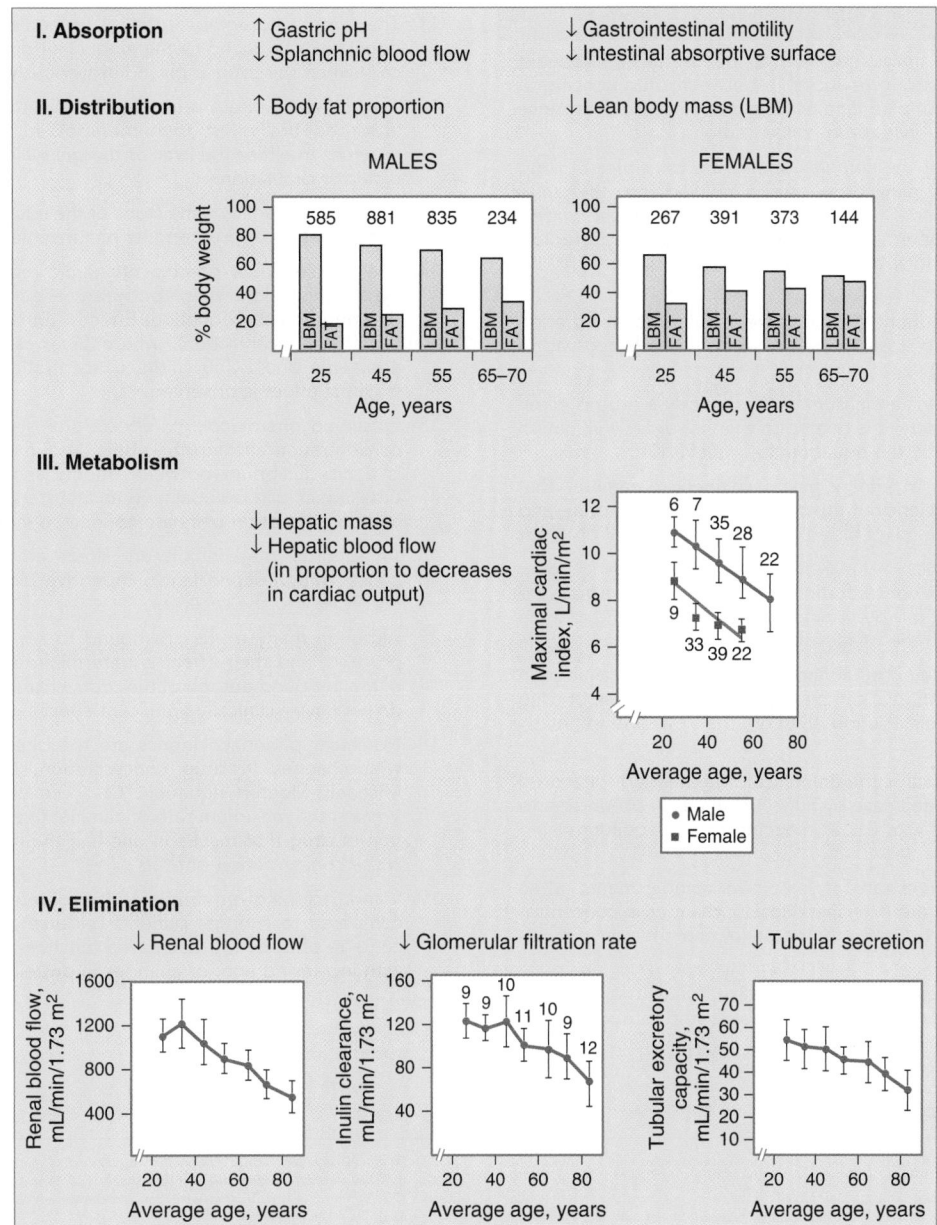

Figure 169-19 Physiologic changes with aging that may affect drug distribution are reflected. (*From Evans WE, Schentag JJ, editors. Applied pharmacokinetics: principles of therapeutic drug monitoring. 3rd ed. Vancouver, WA: Applied Therapeutics; 1992, p. 919-43.*)

this area increased dramatically following the recognition that overexpression of the multidrug-resistance protein, MDR-1, in tumor cells led to a loss of drug effect. This class of efflux proteins functions to pump drugs out of cells and is responsible for reducing drug concentrations in tissues such as the brain, testes, gastrointestinal tract, and biliary tree. There is evidence that the expression of some of these transporters is under genetic control. Concentrations of digoxin reportedly are elevated in patients with low MDR-1 expression.[54]

Drug effects are often mediated through direct receptor proteins, or proteins that influence control of the cell cycle or signal transduction cascades. Polymorphisms in the expression of these proteins could result in pharmacodynamic differences. For example, a polymorphism has been linked to increased down-regulation of the β_2-adrenergic receptor when patients are treated with a β-agonist for amelioration of the symptoms of asthma.[55] Genetic polymorphisms leading to altered drug sensitivity also have been identified in angiotensin-

converting enzyme, the angiotensin II T1 receptor, and the sulfonylurea receptor.[56]

Mapping the human genome holds enormous potential for improving our understanding of variations among individuals with regard to responses to drug therapy. The pharmaceutical industry is embracing DNA arrays, high-throughput screening, and bioinformatics in the drug development process. It is conceivable that drugs will be specifically developed for patients with a genetic predisposition to a particular disease, and drug doses will be identified for subgroups of patients with particular genetic polymorphisms. Pharmacogenomics is a field that is clearly in its infancy, but it is quite likely to alter the manner whereby drugs are selected and dosed. However, the full clinical relevance of polymorphisms that effect pharmacokinetics and pharmacodynamic processes is not known. At present, there are no clinical instances that clearly mandate genotyping prior to the selection of a drug or a dosing regimen.

KEY POINTS

1. Pharmacokinetic analysis is likely to be useful in treatment when there is a strong relationship between drug concentration in an easily sampled fluid and the pharmacologic response associated with a given drug concentration.

2. Although many of the complex underlying principles of drug distribution and elimination are simplified by the one-compartment model, this paradigm is the most widely employed for patient care, because it successfully predicts future concentrations of drugs with sufficient accuracy to be clinically useful.

3. Volume of distribution (V) reflects the resulting concentration from a given drug dose and is not directly associated with a physiologic space.

4. Drug half-life ($t_{1/2}$) is a measure of how quickly a drug is eliminated from the body; it is related to the first-order elimination rate constant (K) by the equation: $t_{1/2} = 0.693/K$.

5. Clearance (CL) is a primary pharmacokinetic parameter that describes the efficiency of the body in eliminating a drug, and is given by the volume of blood completely cleared of drug per unit time.

6. The area under the concentration-time curve (AUC) is a measure of drug exposure; it is determined by the dose of drug and the clearance through the relationship: $AUC = Dose/CL$.

7. In a one-compartment pharmacokinetic model, the change in drug concentration (ΔC) can be predicted by the dose of drug and volume of distribution through the relationship: $\Delta C = Dose/V$.

8. Half-life ($t_{1/2}$) measures the amount of time needed for a drug concentration to decrease by 50%; it changes in proportion to changes in either V or CL, as reflected by the equation: $t_{1/2} = 0.693 \times V/CL$.

9. Most drugs demonstrate at least two compartments when pharmacokinetics are examined closely; changes in concentration reflect a short distribution phase (α) and a longer elimination phase (β).

10. After five half-lives of either α (the distribution $t_{1/2}$) or β (the elimination $t_{1/2}$), a drug will be 97% distributed throughout the body or eliminated from the body.

11. The extent of drug absorption is termed *bioavailability* (F); it is generally referenced to the amount of drug available systemically when the drug is given intravenously.

12. The *first-pass effect* refers to the elimination of drug that is absorbed orally but then metabolized and/or secreted by enzymes in either the liver or the gut wall before reaching the systemic circulation.

13. Pharmacodynamics is the study of the relationship between the concentration of drug and its pharmacologic effect.

14. The simple Emax pharmacodynamic model demonstrates a hyperbolic relationship between effect and dose that is described by the equation: Effect = (Emax × concentration) ÷ (EC50 + concentration), where Emax is the maximal effect attainable and EC50 is the concentration at which half the maximal effect is observed.

15. Observed pharmacologic effects often lag behind the serum concentration eliciting the effect, and in some instances there is a disequilibrium between effects and concentration over time, which can be observed as a hysteresis loop when effect and concentration pairs are connected in a time order.

16. Antagonists may inhibit an effect at a receptor through concentration-dependent competitive blocking or by binding irreversibly to the receptor.

17. Although many drugs are bound to some extent by plasma proteins, and their effect is determined by the concentration of the unbound portion of the drug, changes in protein binding do not have a clinically significant effect in most clinical patients.

18. Nonlinear pharmacokinetics are exhibited when CL changes with changes in drug concentration, as reflected by the Michaelis-Menten equation, $CL = Vmax/(Km + C)$, wherein *Vmax* is the maximum rate of elimination, *Km* is the concentration of drug that results in one-half the maximum rate, and *C* is the concentration of drug.

19. V and CL for a given drug are often different in elderly patients compared to younger patients because of differences in percentage of body fat, decreased function of the kidney or liver with increasing age, or changes in protein binding.

ANNOTATED REFERENCES

Benet LZ, Hoener B. Changes in plasma protein binding have little clinical relevance. Clin Pharmacol Ther 2002;71:115-21.
This manuscript systematically presents the rationale behind the statement that changes in protein binding have little clinical relevance. The physiology and mathematics needed to understand the rationale are presented in an easily understood fashion.
De Paepe P, Belpaire FM, Buylaert WA. Pharmacokinetic and pharmacodynamic considerations when treating patients with sepsis and septic shock. Clin Pharmacokinet 2002;41:1135-51.
This review article details the pharmacokinetic changes observed during sepsis and septic shock. It provides a good discussion of the relationships between drug clearance and organ function.
Gibaldi M, Perrier D. Pharmacokinetics. 2nd ed. New York: Marcel Dekker; 1982.

This text provides detailed coverage of the mathematical aspects of pharmacokinetics. Most of the equations used in clinical pharmacokinetics, and their derivations, are presented.
Renton KW. Alteration of drug biotransformation and elimination during infection and inflammation. Pharmacol Ther 2001;92:147-63.
This review describes the relationship between cytochrome P450 expression and inflammation. Mechanisms of cytochrome P450 regulation and the impact of cytokines on drug metabolism are presented.
Schulz M, Schmoldt A. Therapeutic and toxic blood concentrations of more than 800 drugs and other xenobiotics. Pharmazie 2003;58:447-74.
This is an excellent reference article that contains an exhaustive compilation of drugs with their therapeutic, toxic, and fatal concentration ranges. The article also provides half-lives and references for each drug.

REFERENCES

Access the complete reference list online at http://www.expertconsult.com.

170 Poisoning: Overview of Approaches for Evaluation and Treatment

DONNA SEGER

▓ Gastrointestinal Decontamination

The theory of gastric decontamination (GID) is that removal of toxins from the stomach (where absorption is poor) before they move into the small bowel (where absorption is more rapid) decreases the toxicity of the poisoning. Because of controversies regarding the role of gut decontamination, senior toxicologists from the American Academy of Clinical Toxicology and the European Association of Poison Centres and Clinical Toxicologists (EAPCCT) agreed to collaborate on the production of Position Statements on GID treatments. These statements, published in 1997, are systematically developed guidelines founded on a criteria-based critical review of all relevant scientific literature.[1] The Position Statements were updated in 2004. GID Position Statement summaries are presented in this chapter.

IPECAC

Ipecac is a prepared form of the *Cephaelis acuminata* or *Cephaelis ipecacuanha* plants. Vomiting within 30 minutes after administration is caused by local irritation of the gastric mucosa. Vomiting after 30 minutes is centrally induced.[2]

Position Statement

Syrup of ipecac should not be administered routinely for the management of poisoned patients. In experimental studies, the amount of marker removed by ipecac treatment was highly variable and diminished with time. There is no evidence from clinical studies that ipecac improves outcome for poisoned patients, and its routine administration should be abandoned.[3]

GASTRIC LAVAGE

For gastric lavage, a large-bore (36F-40F) orogastric tube is passed, after which small volumes (200-300 mL) of liquid are alternately administered and aspirated. Endotracheal intubation should precede this procedure in comatose patients. An oral airway prevents biting of the tube. The amount of stomach contents removed via this procedure is highly variable and decreases with time.[4-6] The procedure can actually push stomach contents into the intestine.[7] Contraindications include loss of protective airway reflexes (unless the patient is endotracheally intubated), ingestion of a corrosive substance or a hydrocarbon, gastrointestinal pathology, and other medical conditions that could be worsened by the use of lavage. Complications of the procedure include aspiration, laryngospasm, hypoxia, hypercapnia, mechanical injury, and fluid and electrolyte imbalances in children.[8]

Position Statement

Gastric lavage should not be employed routinely in the management of poisoned patients. It should not be considered unless the patient has ingested a potentially life-threatening amount of a poison and the procedure can be undertaken within 60 minutes after ingestion. Even then, clinical benefit has not been confirmed in controlled studies.[8]

SINGLE-DOSE ACTIVATED CHARCOAL

Activated charcoal is made when coconut shells, peat, wood, or other materials undergo controlled pyrolysis and are subsequently activated by heating in steam or air at high temperatures. Activation creates multiple internal pores and the small particle size necessary for adsorption. The particles have a large surface area and are capable of adsorbing poisons with varying affinities. Although in vitro studies demonstrate adsorption of many drugs to activated charcoal, animal studies reveal variable reductions in the systemic uptake of marker substances.[9] Volunteer and clinical studies have not demonstrated that single-dose administration of activated charcoal improves outcome. Contraindications to the administration of activated charcoal include decreased level of consciousness and unprotected airway, ingestion of caustic substances or hydrocarbons, gastrointestinal pathology, and medical conditions that could be further compromised by the administration of activated charcoal. Complications include aspiration and direct administration of charcoal into the lung.[10]

Because activated charcoal is an inert substance, it is thought that lung injury after aspiration of activated charcoal is caused by gastric contents. Aspiration of gastric contents causes neutrophils to release neutrophil elastase, which increases pulmonary vascular permeability.[11] In comparison, intratracheal administration of activated charcoal does not increase elastase in the bronchoalveolar fluid.[12] Activated charcoal can activate alveolar macrophages, which are a potent source of oxygen radicals, proteases, and other inflammatory mediators. Charcoal also causes obstruction of small distal airways Overdistention of alveolar segments in areas not occluded by charcoal leads to volutrauma in those areas, which increases microvascular permeability.[13] Although case reports reveal long-term pulmonary pathology after aspiration or instillation of activated charcoal,[14,15] the true incidence of chronic problems after charcoal aspiration is unknown.

Position Statement

Single-dose activated charcoal should not be administered routinely in the management of poisoned patients. The effectiveness of charcoal decreases with time; the greatest benefit is obtained within the first hour after ingestion. Administration of activated charcoal may be considered if a patient has ingested a potentially toxic amount of poison (that is known to be adsorbed to charcoal) not longer than 1 hour before treatment. There is no evidence that the administration of activated charcoal improves outcome.[10,16]

CATHARTICS

Position Statement

Administration of a cathartic alone has no role in the management of poisoned patients. Routine use of a cathartic in combination with activated charcoal is not endorsed.[17]

WHOLE-BOWEL IRRIGATION

Whole-bowel irrigation consists of administration through a nasogastric tube of an osmotically balanced, polyethylene glycol–based electrolyte solution to decontaminate the entire gastrointestinal tract by physically expelling intraluminal contents. As much as 1500 to 2000 mL/h can be administered to an awake patient. Negotiations to let the patient attempt to drink the solution only cause delay, because patients are unable to drink at a constant rate. Contraindications include bowel pathology, unprotected or compromised airway, hemodynamic instability, and intractable vomiting. Complications are nausea, vomiting, and abdominal cramps.[18]

Position Statement

Whole-bowel irrigation should not be used routinely in the poisoned patient. Whole-bowel irrigation should be considered for potentially toxic ingestions of sustained-release or enteric-coated drugs. There are insufficient data to support or exclude the use of whole-bowel irrigation for toxic ingestions of lithium, iron, lead, zinc, or packets of illicit drugs.[18]

CLINICAL IMPLICATIONS OF GASTROINTESTINAL DECONTAMINATION

There is no role for syrup of ipecac in the hospital setting. Gastric lavage may be considered for obtunded patients if it can be instituted within one hour after the ingestion. Single-dose activated charcoal should not be routinely administered to patients with mild to moderate degrees of poisoning. Whole-bowel irrigation should be considered for awake patients within the first hours after ingestion of a sustained-release preparation, ionic compounds (e.g., lithium), or packets of illicit drugs.

These guidelines refer to the routine management of poisoned patients. Cellular toxins require special consideration. The physician should always call the Poison Center (1-800-222-1222 in the United States) to discuss a patient with a potentially life-threatening ingestion.

◼ Enhanced Elimination

MULTIPLE-DOSE ACTIVATED CHARCOAL

Multiple-dose activated charcoal is the repeated oral administration of activated charcoal to enhance drug elimination. If the drug concentration in the gut is lower than that in the blood, the drug will passively diffuse back into the gut. The concentration gradient, intestinal surface area, permeability, and blood flow determine the degree of passive diffusion. As the drug passes continuously into the gut, it is adsorbed onto the charcoal particles, a process called *gastrointestinal dialysis*. Multiple-dose activated charcoal also interrupts the enterohepatic and enterogastric circulation of drugs. Drugs with a prolonged elimination half-life, a small volume of distribution (less than 1 L/kg), and little protein binding are the most amenable to this sort of management.[19]

The initial dose of charcoal is 50 to 100 g, and this treatment is followed every 1, 2, or 4 hours by a dose equivalent to 12.5 g/h. More frequent, smaller doses may prevent vomiting. Addition of a cathartic (e.g., sorbitol) can be considered for the initial one or two doses. Continuous use of a cathartic can cause diarrhea and fluid and electrolyte imbalances. Multiple-dose activated charcoal can be continued until the patient improves clinically. Contraindications include an unprotected airway, intestinal obstruction, and an anatomically abnormal gastrointestinal tract. Complications include bowel obstruction and vomiting with subsequent aspiration.[19]

Position Statement

Multiple-dose activated charcoal should be considered if a patient has ingested a life-threatening amount of carbamazepine, dapsone, phenobarbital, quinine, or theophylline. With all of these drugs, data confirm enhanced elimination, although no controlled studies have demonstrated clinical benefit.[19]

URINARY ALKALINIZATION

Urinary alkalinization is the administration of intravenous (IV) sodium bicarbonate to produce urine with a pH ≥ 7.5. The objective of treatment is pH manipulation, not forced diuresis. Hypokalemia is the most common complication. Alkalemia also can occur.[20]

Position Statement

Urinary alkalinization should be considered as first-line treatment in patients with moderately severe salicylate poisoning who do not meet the criteria for hemodialysis. Urinary alkalinization also should be considered for patients with severe poisoning due to 2,4-dichlorophenoxyacetic acid or mecoprop (MCPP) poisoning. Urinary alkalinization is not recommended as first-line treatment for cases of phenobarbital poisoning, because multiple-dose activated charcoal is superior.[20]

◼ Selected Antidotes

Stabilization of the patient always should precede administration of antidote(s). The effects of the toxin can outlast the effects of the administered antidote. Patients receiving antidotes should be observed in a critical care setting.

DEXTROSE

Up to 8% of patients with altered mental status are hypoglycemic.[21] Hypoglycemia can be a result of drug or toxin exposure, nutritional deprivation, or a medical complication (e.g., sepsis, hyperthermia). Glucose should be checked at the bedside for all patients with altered mental status.

NALOXONE

Endogenous and exogenous opiates produce their effects by binding at one or more opiate receptors. Naloxone, nalmefene, and naltrexone are competitive opioid antagonists that bind at the mu (μ), kappa (κ), and delta (δ) receptors and competitively prevent the binding of endogenous and exogenous opiates at these receptors. The duration of action of naloxone is 15 to 90 minutes. Its clinical effects depend on the dose and route of naloxone administration as well as the dose and rate of elimination of the opiate agonist. Naloxone can be administered by IV, intramuscular, intratracheal, or sublingual routes. After IV administration, naloxone rapidly enters the central nervous system (CNS). In patients with opiate poisoning, consciousness is restored and respiration improves within 1 to 2 minutes. Meiosis, inhibition of baroreceptor reflexes, laryngospasm, and decreased gastrointestinal motility are also reversed.[22]

Certain nonopiate drugs can cause release of endogenous opiates, contributing to CNS and respiratory depression as well as hypotension. Alternatively, nonopiate drugs and naloxone can compete for an unidentified nonopiate receptor that contributes to CNS depression and hypotension. Naloxone can reverse the toxicity caused by drugs that are not opioids, such as clonidine, angiotensin-converting enzyme inhibitors, and sodium valproate. Naloxone should be administered to all patients with altered mental status or coma of unknown cause. Opiate-dependent patients should receive only small doses in an effort to prevent rapid withdrawal. If a patient is not opiate dependent, a reasonable starting dose is 2 mg, increasing to 10 mg (in increments) if there is no response. Large doses of naloxone may be necessary to reverse the effects of nonopiate drugs or of opiate drugs with high affinity for the δ and κ opiate receptors.

If respiratory depression returns, the initial dose of naloxone may have to be repeated or a constant infusion of naloxone initiated. The starting dose for a constant infusion of naloxone is hourly administration of about one-half to two-thirds of the bolus dose that reversed the opiate effects. If withdrawal is precipitated, it is short lived and not life threatening. Complications of naloxone administration are very rare.[23]

FLUMAZENIL

Flumazenil competitively antagonizes the pharmacologic effects of drugs that act on the benzodiazepine receptor (e.g., all drugs in the benzodiazepine class). Receptor occupancy follows the law of mass action, and antagonism is dose dependent. The duration of action of flumazenil is variable and depends on the type of benzodiazepine ingested, relative doses of agonist and antagonist, presence of ongoing benzodiazepine absorption, and relative receptor binding affinities. Flumazenil also antagonizes the sedative effects of drugs other than benzodiazepines, such as zolpidem (Ambien), cannabis, ethanol, promethazine, chlorzoxazone, and carisoprodol. These drugs may have differing affinities for the γ-aminobutyric acid A (GABA$_A$) receptor, implying that the dose of flumazenil required to reverse the effects depends on the affinity of the specific drug for the receptor.[24]

Flumazenil is safe and effective for reversing conscious sedation after short procedures such as endoscopy. This safety has been generalized to imply that flumazenil also is safe for patients with a multidrug overdose and that reversal of benzodiazepine-induced sedation prevents morbidity from procedures such as endotracheal intubation or computed tomography. However, many patients have experienced single or multiple seizures after flumazenil administration. Status epilepticus has been precipitated, leading to death. The data are insufficient to determine whether morbidity or mortality is increased as a result of flumazenil-precipitated seizures.[25,26]

Flumazenil administration can precipitate seizures in patients with an overdose who have ingested both a benzodiazepine and a proconvulsant drug or just a pro-convulsant drug. Flumazenil also can precipitate seizures in patients who have a history of seizures, chronic benzodiazepine ingestion, or head injury. Identification of patients at risk for seizures is difficult.[27] Before administering flumazenil to a patient with an ingestion, it is reasonable to first obtain an electrocardiogram (to rule out exposure to pro-convulsant tricyclic antidepressants) and a urine drug screen. Re-sedation occurs after 18 to 120 minutes in approximately half of patients awakened by flumazenil. Therefore, either continuous IV infusion or observation for a number of hours is required.[28]

Administration of flumazenil to patients with an overdose should be limited to the following situations: iatrogenic overdose with known patient history, obtundation in a toddler secondary to ingestion of benzodiazepine, and reversal of a paradoxical response to benzodiazepine.

PHYSOSTIGMINE

Physostigmine inhibits acetylcholinesterase, the enzyme responsible for the metabolism of acetylcholine (ACH). ACH is an endogenous neurotransmitter that mediates action by binding to muscarinic and nicotinic receptors. Accumulation of ACH stimulates cholinergic nerve endings. In the poisoned patient, physostigmine is most frequently administered to treat anticholinergic toxicity. Clinical signs of anticholinergic toxicity are recognized by the mnemonic, "Blind as a bat, Red as a beet, Hot as a hare, Dry as a bone, Mad as a hatter." Physostigmine administration should be considered if life-threatening clinical signs of anticholinergic peripheral effects (hypertension, tachycardia, and seizures) or central effects (painful psychosis) are present. However, it is extremely difficult to balance cholinergic and anticholinergic forces. Complications of cholinergic crises (caused by excessive doses of physostigmine) include hypertension, arrhythmia, asystole, bronchorrhea, bronchoconstriction, seizures, and status epilepticus. Contraindications to physostigmine administration include reactive airway disease, peripheral vascular disease, intestinal or bladder obstruction, and treatment with a depolarizing neuromuscular blocking agent (e.g., succinylcholine). An acceptable dose of physostigmine is 2 mg IV over 10 minutes. This drug should be administered in the presence of a physician because of the potential for precipitation of life-threatening cholinergic effects.[29]

◼ Hypotension in the Poisoned Patient

Hypotension in the poisoned patient is most frequently caused by receptor blockade, drug-induced myocardial depression, or drug-induced vasodilatation. Clinicians reflexively initially treat hypotension by infusing IV fluids; however, unless the poisoned patient is hypovolemic, large volumes of fluid can predispose patients to the development of acute respiratory failure.

Catecholamines are the pressors of choice for treatment of hypotension in most intensive care unit (ICU) patients who are older, chronically ill, or acutely ill from an infectious process. The causative factors in sepsis-induced vasodilation and myocardial depression/ischemia are different from the factors that cause drug-induced vasodilation, myocardial depression, or ischemia. Treatment approaches must address the cause of the hypotension and not assume that all hypotensive patients should be treated in a similar manner.

Poisoned patients who are young and healthy respond to hypotension with an outpouring of endogenous catecholamines. Adrenergic receptors are sensitive in young patients. Administration of exogenous catecholamines is unlikely to be of much benefit, because catecholamine receptors are already maximally stimulated by endogenous catecholamines. Agents that must be considered for the treatment of hypotension in the poisoned patient are sodium bicarbonate (for a sodium channel-blocking agent), glucagon, and insulin/glucose.

GLUCAGON

The cardiovascular effects of glucagon are mediated by myocardial glucagon receptors which are catecholamine independent. Stimulation activates adenylate cyclase, leading to increased intracellular levels of the second messenger, cyclic adenosine monophosphate (cAMP). This cyclic nucleotide increases myocardial calcium uptake. Both the slope of phase zero of the action potential and the conduction velocity through the atrioventricular node are increased. Glucagon increases heart rate and stroke volume, thereby increasing cardiac output. After IV administration, augmented inotropy is seen within 1 to 3 minutes, with a peak effect in 5 to 7 minutes.[30]

Glucagon should be considered early in the treatment of hypotensive poisoned patients. Treatment regimens vary. An acceptable regimen is 10 mg of glucagon given over 10 minutes (rapid administration causes vomiting), followed by 1 to 3 mg/h. If the patient wretches, the hourly dose of glucagon should be decreased. Elderly patients may be more sensitive to the emetic effects of the drug.

INSULIN AND GLUCOSE

Insulin improves contractility in anoxic rat hearts and improves cardiac index after cardiopulmonary bypass surgery. During drug-induced shock, insulin shifts myocardial fatty acid oxidation to carbohydrate oxidation, which increases contractility, left ventricular pressure, and rate of change of developed pressure. Enhanced fatty acid oxidation, such as occurs after epinephrine administration, transiently increases contractility at the expense of increased myocardial oxygen consumption.[31]

In hypotensive poisoned patients, a reasonable dose of insulin is 10 units of regular insulin and 50 mL of 50% dextrose solution. These priming doses should be followed by infusion of 6 units of insulin per hour, with concurrent administration of sufficient glucose to maintain euglycemia. Hourly serum glucose checks are mandatory because hypoglycemia occurs frequently.

Cardiac Arrhythmias

ICU treatment regimens assume that a diseased heart is the cause of most cardiac arrhythmias. This assumption is invalid in poisoned patients. Treatment of the arrhythmia must take into consideration the pharmacology of the toxin causing the arrhythmia.

Acute Renal Failure

In poisoned patients, acute renal failure (ARF) is most frequently the result of a decrease in extracellular fluid volume and renal hypoperfusion caused by drug- or chemical-induced vasodilation, drug-induced myocardial depression, or rhabdomyolysis. Attempts to prevent ARF are important because there is no specific therapy once ARF is established. Studies evaluating the efficacy of low-dose dopamine (0.5-3.0 mg/kg/min) in preventing ARF have not demonstrated any benefit, but the patient populations in these studies consisted of critically ill patients with established ARF or at high risk for developing ARF.[32] The efficacy of administration of low-dose dopamine after periods of hypotension in poisoned patients who typically are younger and without chronic disease has not been evaluated. When dopamine is administered to normal human subjects, there is a dose-dependent increase in renal blood flow, sodium excretion, and glomerular filtration rate.[33] Low-dose dopamine also limits adenosine triphosphate (ATP) utilization and oxygen requirements in nephron segments at risk for ischemia.[34] Although there are no studies regarding the efficacy of low-dose dopamine in cases of drug-induced hypotension, one may consider administration in previously healthy poisoned patients who have adequate vascular volume and remain oliguric or anuric despite maximal diuretic therapy.

Seizures

Blood pH can be as low as 7.17 at 30 minutes and 7.20 at 60 minutes after resolution of a 30- to 60-second seizure.[35] Acidosis decreases cardiac output, oxygen extraction, and left ventricular end-diastolic pressure and impairs myocardial contractility. If a patient has ingested a cardiotoxic drug (e.g., a tricyclic antidepressant) that causes significant myocardial depression, the consequences of acidosis can increase the toxicity of the drug. Ictal increases in plasma epinephrine levels can add to the potential risk for cardiac arrhythmias. Additionally, airway reflexes are inhibited postictally, which adds to the potential for aspiration.[36]

Whether seizures increase morbidity and mortality in poisoned patients is difficult to ascertain. Deaths of poisoned patients who sustain seizures are usually attributed to the toxicity of the drug. Because of the number of variables, it is impossible to know whether the risk for mortality is influenced by the presence of convulsions. Accordingly, the physician should take an aggressive approach toward terminating seizures in poisoned patients. Benzodiazepines are the drugs of choice to quickly terminate seizures, because they are lipophilic and rapidly enter the CNS.

Mechanical Ventilation and Extubation

Endotracheal intubation is commonly indicated for the management of poisoned patients on the basis of respiratory depression or impaired protective airway reflexes or both. As the drug is metabolized, its effects abate, and the patient's sensorium improves. The patient may become alert slowly or very suddenly. The patient should be extubated if ability to protect the airway is evident and ventilation is adequate for 15 to 60 minutes with minimal respiratory support (e.g., 5 cm H_2O positive end-expiratory pressure and 5 cm H_2O pressure support). Unnecessary or excessive administration of sedatives or anxiolytics in an attempt to make the patient more comfortable can delay weaning from mechanical ventilation and extubation and increase the risk for complications.

Toxicology Laboratory

Urine drug screens are usually obtained in poisoned patients; however, there is no standardized screen. Interpretation of urine drug screen results depends on the clinician's knowledge of which toxins have been screened and whether confirmatory testing (ideally performed by a different analytic method) will follow. The length of time required to receive results varies among hospitals. Quantitative serum drug testing is done when quantitation of a toxin is clinically relevant, as is the case for acetaminophen, anticonvulsant agents, salicylates, digoxin, ethanol, ethylene glycol, methanol, iron, lithium, and theophylline. The clinician caring for the poisoned patient should discuss drug testing with the analytic toxicologist so that the results of testing can be appropriately interpreted. The clinical value of analytic toxicology testing depends on the clinician's ability to understand and interpret the results.

KEY POINTS

1. The theory of gastric decontamination is that removal of toxins from the stomach (where absorption is poor) before they move into the small bowel (where absorption is more rapid) decreases the toxicity of the poisoning.

2. Stabilization of the patient should always precede administration of antidote(s). The effects of the toxin can outlast the effects of the administered antidote. Patients receiving antidotes should be observed in a critical care setting.

3. Treating hypotensive, poisoned patients with large volumes of intravenous fluids can increase the risk for acute respiratory failure.

4. Efforts to prevent development of acute renal failure (ARF) in the poisoned patient are important because there is no specific therapy once ARF is established.

5. An aggressive approach should be taken toward terminating seizures in the poisoned patient. Benzodiazepines are the drugs of choice to quickly terminate seizures, because they are lipophilic and rapidly enter the central nervous system (CNS).

6. The clinical value of analytic toxicology testing depends on the clinician's ability to understand and interpret the results.

ANNOTATED REFERENCES

Arnold TC, Willis BH, Xiao F. Aspiration of activated charcoal elicits an increase in lung microvascular permeability. J Toxicol Clin Toxicol 1999;37:9-16.
The capillary filtration coefficient, a measure of lung microvascular permeability, was determined in rat lungs before and after intratracheal instillation of activated charcoal. There was a marked increase in permeability in those lungs exposed to activated charcoal.

Bateman DN. Gastric decontamination—a view for the millennium. J Accid Emerg Med 1999;16:84-6.
Management of overdose patients should be modified in light of position papers on GI decontamination.

Clarke SFJ, Dargan PI, Jones AL. Naloxone in opioid poisoning: walking the tightrope. Emerg Med J 2005;22:612-16.
Recommendations are made for naloxone administration in acute opiate intoxication and overdose.

Holger JS, Engebretsen KM, Obetz CL, et al. A comparison of vasopressin and glucagon in beta-blocker-induced toxicity. Clin Toxicol 2006;44:45-51.
In a pig model of beta-blocker toxicity, there was no difference in survival between vasopressin and glucagon.

Marques I, Gomes E, de Oliveira J. Treatment of calcium channel blocker intoxication with insulin infusion: case report and literature review. Resuscitation 2003;57:211-3.

An elderly lady overdosed on diltiazem. Multiple pressors were administered for hypotension, but hemodynamic stability was not achieved until insulin and glucose were administered.

Mathieu-Nolf M, Babe MA, Coquelle-Couplet V, et al. Flumazenil use in an emergency department: a survey. Clin Toxicol 2001;39:15-20.
This survey reported on 29 patients who received flumazenil in the emergency department. Subsequent expert review considered that flumazenil was indicated in only 18 of these patients. Of the remaining 11 patients, a severe complication occurred in 1. There was no difference in outcome measures between those patients who received flumazenil and those who did not.

Merigian K, Glaho K. Single-dose oral activated charcoal in the treatment of the self-poisoned patient: a prospective, randomized controlled trial. Am J Ther 2002;9:301-8.
A total of 1479 patients with overdose were randomly assigned to receive or not receive activated charcoal. Gastric emptying was not performed. There were no differences between the two groups in length of intubation time, length of hospital stay, or complication rate.

Orringer DE, Eustace JC, Wunsch CD, Gardner LB. Natural history of lactic acidosis after grand mal seizures. N Engl J Med 1977;15:796-9.
This classic article demonstrated that significant acidosis can occur for up to 1 hour after a single 30- to 60-second seizure.

Pond SM, Lewis-Driver DJ, Williams GM, et al. Gastric emptying in acute overdose: a prospective randomized controlled trial. Med J Aust 1995;163:345-9.

This was a randomized study of gastric emptying versus no gastric emptying. A total of 342 patients underwent lavage or no gastric lavage before administration of charcoal. There were no significant differences between the two groups in incidence of clinical deterioration or improvement during the first 6 hours. However, only 55 patients presented within 1 hour, of whom just 14 were not lavaged.

Sauvadet A, Rohn T, Pecker F, et al. Arachidonic acid drives mini-glucagon action in cardiac cells. J Biol Chem 1997;272:12437-45.

Glucagon triggers release of arachidonic acid (AA) and is then processed by cardiac cells into a terminal fragment mini-glucagon which is an essential component of the contractile positive inotropic effect. AA and cAMP are both second messengers.

REFERENCES

Access the complete reference list online at http://www.expertconsult.com.

Ethanol, Methanol, and Ethylene Glycol

JAMES A. KRUSE

Ethanol Intoxication

Ethanol, also known as *ethyl alcohol* or *grain alcohol*, is one of many compounds chemically classified as alcohols, but it is the only one legitimately contained in alcoholic beverages. It is a clear, colorless liquid with a pleasant odor and a burning taste, found in fermented alcoholic beverages. Ethanol also finds wide use in laboratories and in industry as a solvent and synthetic precursor, in pharmaceutical manufacturing as a vehicle for certain medicines (e.g., cough syrups, some intravenous [IV] drugs), and in numerous toiletries including mouthwashes, colognes, and cosmetics. It also serves as a component in various commercially available cleaning agents and paint removers, in which case it is usually *denatured*, that is, intentionally rendered unfit for consumption, usually to comply with governmental regulations. Some versions of the alternative motor vehicle fuel known as *gasohol* consist of a mixture of gasoline and ethanol.

The ethanol content of alcoholic beverages varies widely, but typical concentrations range from 40% to 55% (volume/volume) in whiskey and related distilled spirits, 10% to 15% in table wines, and 4% to 6% in most beers. The ethanol concentration in distilled spirits is traditionally listed in terms of *proof*. In the United States, this expression represents twice the percentage concentration; for example, 80 proof is equivalent to 40% ethanol by volume.

Ethanol is rapidly absorbed by the gastrointestinal tract and distributed throughout body water.[1] The blood ethanol concentration (in mg/dL) resulting from a one-time dose can be estimated from the volume (in mL) of ingested alcoholic beverage, the fractional concentration of ethanol (by volume) in the beverage, and body weight (in kg), by the following equation:

$$\text{Blood ethanol concentration} = \frac{\text{Volume ingested} \times \text{Ethanol concentration} \times 79}{0.6 \times \text{Body weight}}$$

The denominator coefficient is the fraction of body weight representing total body water volume, approximating the volume of distribution for ethanol, about 0.6 L/kg. The numerator coefficient converts volume units to weight units based on the density of ethanol (0.79 g/mL) and converts the resultant concentration units from g/L to mg/dL. Accordingly, each 1 ounce of 100 proof whiskey, 12 ounces of beer, or 4 ounces of a typical table wine consumed by a 70-kg man theoretically should raise the blood ethanol concentration by approximately 30 mg/dL. Given that ingestion of ethanol-containing beverages commonly occurs over time and metabolism is ongoing, this prediction formula tends to overestimate peak blood ethanol levels.

METABOLISM

Between 2% and 10% of ingested ethanol is excreted intact by the kidneys and lungs, but the major fraction is metabolized by hepatic alcohol dehydrogenase (ADH) to acetaldehyde by the following reaction[2]:

$$\underset{\text{Ethanol}}{CH_3CH_2\text{-}OH} + NAD^+ \xrightarrow{ADH} NADH + H^+ + \underset{\text{Acetaldehyde}}{CH_3 - \overset{\overset{O}{\|}}{C} - H}$$

At high blood ethanol levels, a particular isoform of the hepatic microsomal cytochrome P450 enzyme (CYP2E1) provides an additional, albeit normally minor, oxidative pathway for ethanol metabolism:

$$\underset{\text{Ethanol}}{CH_3CH_2\text{-}OH} + NADPH + H^+ + O_2 \xrightarrow{CYP2E1} NADP^+ + \underset{\text{Acetaldehyde}}{CH_3 - \overset{\overset{O}{\|}}{C} - H} + 2H_2O$$

This alternative pathway is inducible with chronic ethanol exposure. Minor amounts of ethanol can also be metabolized by peroxisomal catalase:

$$\underset{\text{Ethanol}}{CH_3CH_2\text{-}OH} + H_2O_2 \xrightarrow{Catalase} \underset{\text{Acetaldehyde}}{CH_3 - \overset{\overset{O}{\|}}{C} - H} + 2H_2O$$

Acetaldehyde produced by any of the preceding reactions is converted by hepatic acetaldehyde dehydrogenase (ALDH) to acetate:

$$\underset{\text{Acetaldehyde}}{CH_3 - \overset{\overset{O}{\|}}{C} - H} + NAD^+ + H_2O \xrightarrow{ALDH} NADH + 2H^+ + \underset{\text{Acetate}}{CH_3 - \overset{\overset{O}{\|}}{C} - O^-}$$

Acetate can then enter the tricarboxylic acid cycle and ultimately be metabolized to carbon dioxide (CO_2) and water. Polymorphisms in the dehydrogenase enzymes can result in increased production rates or diminished metabolic clearance of acetaldehyde. As a consequence, some individuals experience marked vasodilation, facial flushing, tachycardia, and other unpleasant symptoms after ethanol consumption because of the effects of excessive acetaldehyde accumulation. Alleles leading to this reaction are particularly prevalent in persons of Chinese or Japanese descent but are uncommon in Caucasians.[2]

Metabolic conversion of ethanol to acetaldehyde and acetate by dehydrogenases raises the ratio of reduced nicotinamide adenine dinucleotide (NADH) relative to its oxidized form (NAD$^+$). This change in intracellular redox state favors conversion of pyruvate to lactate by lactate dehydrogenase (LDH) and can thereby raise the blood lactate concentration:

$$CH_3\text{-}\overset{\overset{O}{\|}}{C}\text{-}\overset{\overset{O}{\|}}{C}\text{-}O^- + NADH + H^+ \xrightarrow{\ LDH\ } NAD^+$$
Pyruvate

$$+ CH_3 - \overset{\overset{HO}{|}}{CH} - \overset{\overset{O}{\|}}{C} - O^-$$
Lactate

The resulting increase in blood lactate level is usually small, however, and the presence of lactic acidosis should prompt consideration of an alternative cause such as circulatory shock or seizures.[3]

Ethanol elimination generally follows zero-order kinetics, with elimination rates of 5 to 10 g/h in nonhabituated subjects, approximately corresponding to a fall in blood ethanol concentration of 10 to 25 mg/dL/h. This rate can more than double in individuals who are chronically habituated to high doses of ethanol.

CLINICAL MANIFESTATIONS

Excessive chronic ingestion of ethanol plays a causative role in a number of important diseases such as cirrhosis, hepatitis, pancreatitis, cardiomyopathy, and malignancies. Ethanol use can result in gastrointestinal hemorrhage by several mechanisms including gastritis, ulcers, esophageal varices, and Mallory-Weiss tears.

Acute intoxication can induce cardiac dysrhythmias, particularly atrial fibrillation. As denoted by the descriptive sobriquet, "holiday heart syndrome," this phenomenon frequently occurs during an alcoholic binge. A variety of neurologic abnormalities are associated with chronic alcoholism, including Wernicke-Korsakoff syndrome, chronic cerebellar ataxia, Marchiafava-Bignami syndrome, and central pontine myelinolysis.[4] Wernicke encephalopathy can manifest as lethargy, confusion, truncal ataxia, nystagmus, and ophthalmoplegia, whereas Korsakoff dementia manifests as retentive memory impairment, confabulation, and learning deficits.[5]

Acutely, ethanol has well-known, dose-dependent inebriating and sedating effects (Table 171-1), although remarkable variability in this relationship is observed in some individuals.[4] These central nervous system (CNS) effects appear to be at least partly caused by interference with N-methyl-D-aspartate receptor and perhaps γ-aminobutyric acid receptor function.[4,6,7] The cognitive, behavioral, perceptual, and psychomotor effects of ethanol intoxication play a causative role in a substantial proportion of deaths and injuries involving motor vehicle–related trauma, accidental drownings, residential fires, homicides, and suicides. The legal driving threshold for blood ethanol concentration is 80 mg/dL in the United States for operators aged 21 years or older. Tachycardia, mydriasis, diaphoresis, hypotension, and hypothermia can occur in cases of marked intoxication. Blood ethanol concentrations of approximately 350 mg/dL have been associated with fatal outcomes, although many patients have survived much higher levels, including one subject who reportedly survived a level of 1500 mg/dL.[8]

LABORATORY MANIFESTATIONS

Blood ethanol concentration correlates at least approximately with the manifestations of intoxication (see Table 171-1). In chronic alcoholic subjects, a blood ethanol concentration below 250 mg/dL is an unlikely explanation for alterations in consciousness and should prompt a search for an alternative cause.[8] Numerous other blood test abnormalities can be seen in intoxicated subjects, particularly in patients with chronic ethanol abuse: hyponatremia, hypokalemia, hypomagnesemia, hypophosphatemia, hypoglycemia, thrombocytopenia, and coagulopathy. Elevated activities of various circulating enzymes including amylase, lipase, creatine phosphokinase, transaminases, and γ-glutamyl transpeptidase, can occur as a reflection of alcohol-induced

TABLE 171-1	Relationship Between Blood Ethanol Concentration and Clinical Manifestations*	
Blood Ethanol Concentration (mg/dL)	**Clinical Manifestations**
<30	Little demonstrable effect
30-50	Mild euphoria, minimal central nervous system effects, subjective sensation of cutaneous warmth
50-80	Relaxation, jocularity, gregariousness, cutaneous flushing, prolongation of reaction time
80-100	Statutory intoxication in many jurisdictions
100-200	Loquacity, animation, exuberance, exaggerated emotional responses, uninhibited behavior, impaired judgment
200-300	Sedation interrupted by periods of boisterous or antisocial behavior, nausea, emesis, dysarthria, horizontal nystagmus, impaired visual pursuit, diplopia, ataxia
300-400	Unstable station and gait, incoherent speech, somnolence, impairment of protective airway reflexes, incontinence, obtundation, stupor
>400	Coma, loss of protective reflexes, respiratory depression, death

*This information serves only as an imperfect guide, because considerable variability and overlap is possible, and individuals with chronic heavy ethanol exposure often develop learned tolerance.

pancreatitis, rhabdomyolysis, hepatitis, or cirrhosis. The latter can also result in hyperbilirubinemia and hypoalbuminemia.

TREATMENT

In the absence of associated illness or injury (Table 171-2), mild to moderate intoxication requires no special treatment other than abstinence and a period of observation. Regardless of the degree of intoxication, withdrawal precautions are recommended for chronic imbibers, particularly those with a history of heavy chronic use or alcohol withdrawal manifestations. The treatment of severe ethanol intoxication is largely supportive. As with any patient who presents to the hospital in an unconscious state, initial empirical treatment should include IV thiamine, dextrose, and naloxone, once adequate airway, ventilation, and perfusion are ensured. Gastric lavage and activated charcoal administration are of dubious value for hastening removal of ethanol from the body.[9-12]

The unconscious, stuporous, or delirious patient with ethanol intoxication can present a diagnostic challenge. Historical information is often lacking or inadequate, and the physical examination can be

TABLE 171-2	Concomitant or Complicating Disorders Associated with Alcohol Intoxication or Withdrawal	
Alcoholic hepatitis	Hypoglycemia
Aspiration pneumonitis	Hypothermia
Circulatory shock (due to dehydration or hemorrhage)	Infections (e.g., pneumonia, meningitis)
Cirrhosis	Intracranial hemorrhage (e.g., subdural hematoma)
Coagulopathy	Pancreatitis
Dehydration	Peripheral neuropathy
Drug overdose or other toxic ingestion	Psychosis
Electrolyte derangements	Rhabdomyolysis
Gastrointestinal hemorrhage (due to gastritis, peptic ulcer disease, esophageal varices, hemorrhoids, or Mallory-Weiss tear)	Seizures Sepsis
Head injury	Thrombocytopenia
Heat stroke	Vitamin deficiency (folate, thiamine, other B vitamins)
Hepatic encephalopathy	Wernicke-Korsakoff syndrome

compromised by lack of cooperation. A central concern is that another disorder may be present in lieu of or in addition to ethanol intoxication. The other disorder may be chiefly responsible for the alteration in consciousness or may require specific urgent treatment. For example, inebriated subjects are at high risk for trauma (e.g., battery, falls, motor vehicle accidents) and therefore should be evaluated for physical injuries. Subdural hematoma is a particular concern, and any findings or suspicion of head injury should prompt cranial imaging by computed tomography. Chronic ethanol abuse also predisposes to infection, particularly aspiration pneumonia. Pneumococcal or *Listeria* meningitis, although not as common, is a consideration in the intoxicated patient with an altered sensorium, fever, and other compatible findings. Additional potentially confounding problems include concomitant toxic ingestions or drug overdoses, psychiatric disorders, alcohol withdrawal, and in patients with advanced cirrhosis, hepatic encephalopathy or spontaneous bacterial peritonitis.

A thorough evaluation for common associated illnesses and injuries should include physical and laboratory examinations for evidence of head, neck, and somatic trauma, rhabdomyolysis, pancreatitis, hepatic dysfunction, coagulopathy, blood dyscrasias, and fluid and electrolyte derangements. Accordingly, routine laboratory testing should include a complete blood count, prothrombin and partial thromboplastin times, serum assays for electrolytes (including sodium, potassium, chloride, total CO_2 content, magnesium, and phosphorus), glucose, liver and kidney function tests, and amylase, lipase, transaminases, and creatine phosphokinase activities. Screening for alternative or concomitant intoxications or overdoses is occasionally fruitful.[13] Identification of metabolic acidosis should prompt investigation for alcoholic ketoacidosis, lactic acidosis, renal failure, and relevant toxic ingestions, particularly methanol and ethylene glycol. Microbiological cultures are indicated if there are signs of serious infection.

Intravenous thiamine and a multivitamin preparation containing folate are routinely administered to hospitalized patients with alcohol intoxication or withdrawal. Parenteral thiamine (50 or 100 mg) is given during the initial phase of management, regardless of the level of sensorium, to prevent or treat Wernicke-Korsakoff syndrome.[5]

Hydration is necessary in some intoxicated patients. Dextrose-containing saline solutions are usually the fluid of choice to correct dehydration and prevent hypoglycemia. Dextrose administration is traditionally preceded by thiamine dosing. Patients with hypoglycemia require rapid IV injection of dextrose followed by a continuous dextrose infusion titrated to the results of frequent serial blood glucose tests. Hypokalemia, hypomagnesemia, and hypophosphatemia should be corrected with the use of appropriate oral or parenteral supplementation. Patients with anemia may require further investigation for gastrointestinal hemorrhage. Patients requiring admission to an intensive care unit (ICU) should have a chest radiograph as well as electrocardiographic evaluation.

Oxygenation may be assessed either by pulse oximetry or by arterial blood gas analysis, and supplemental oxygen should be provided as necessary. Administration of vitamin K, fresh frozen plasma, or platelet transfusions may be necessary if there is gastrointestinal or other hemorrhage and coagulopathy or severe thrombocytopenia. The level of consciousness should be monitored periodically. Hemodialysis has been employed and is effective at removing ethanol from the body, but in general, this modality poses greater risks than simply providing supportive care and allowing physiologic ethanol elimination. Its use might be warranted in rare cases of profound life-threatening ethanol intoxication, or if there are other reasons for dialysis.[14,15]

Alcoholic Ketoacidosis

Alcoholic ketoacidosis (AKA) is an uncommon metabolic disturbance that occurs in a small proportion of chronic ethanol abusers for unclear reasons. Although the degree of acidosis can sometimes be severe, the disorder usually has a benign hospital course so long as IV dextrose and fluids are provided. Morbidity results chiefly from associated complications of alcohol abuse.

METABOLISM

Although the precise metabolic mechanisms that lead to the development of AKA are incompletely understood, several mechanisms appear to be operative. Abnormal insulin and counterregulatory hormone levels occur,[16] but the disorder is distinct from simple starvation and diabetes mellitus. Ethanol results in inhibition of gluconeogenesis and depletion of glycogen stores, leading to low glucose availability, particularly when coupled with fasting. Hypoglycemia causes release of epinephrine, cortisol, and growth hormone, as well as decreased insulin production; these are all factors that favor ketone synthesis. Ethanol metabolism results in a surfeit of acetate and NADH, which promotes lactate and ketone production. Marked ketonemia results in acidosis and ketonuria. The latter causes osmotic diuresis, intravascular volume depletion, and electrolyte losses. Thus, starvation, dehydration, excessive acetate production, an altered redox state, hormonal imbalances, and perhaps genetic predisposition are all potentially involved.[17]

The so-called ketone bodies that accumulate in all forms of endogenous ketoacidosis are acetone, β-hydroxybutyrate, and acetoacetate. Acetone is only a minor product produced by decarboxylation of acetoacetate, either spontaneously or catalyzed by acetoacetate decarboxylase (AAD):

$$CH_3\text{-}\underset{O}{\underset{\|}{C}}\text{-}CH_2\text{-}\underset{O}{\underset{\|}{C}}\text{-}O^- + H^+ \xrightarrow{AAD} CH_3\text{-}\underset{O}{\underset{\|}{C}}\text{-}CH_3 + CO_2$$

Acetoacetate   Acetone

Acetone is excreted in the breath and urine, where it may be detected by physical examination or urinalysis, respectively. β-Hydroxybutyrate and acetoacetate are interconvertible by the enzyme β-hydroxybutyrate dehydrogenase (βHD), and the two compounds normally exist in equilibrium:

$$CH_3\text{-}\underset{OH}{\underset{|}{CH}}\text{-}CH_2\text{-}\underset{O}{\underset{\|}{C}}\text{-}O^- + NAD^+ \underset{\beta HD}{\rightleftharpoons} NADH + H^+$$

β-Hydroxybutyrate

$$+ CH_3\text{-}\underset{O}{\underset{\|}{C}}\text{-}CH_2\text{-}\underset{O}{\underset{\|}{C}}\text{-}O^-$$

Acetoacetate

In both AKA and diabetic ketoacidosis (DKA), β-hydroxybutyrate is quantitatively the more important molecule. However, the ratio of β-hydroxybutyrate to acetoacetate tends to be higher in AKA (typically 5:1 but sometimes exceeding 10:1),[18] compared with DKA (typically 3:1).

CLINICAL MANIFESTATIONS

AKA characteristically develops 24 to 72 hours after an alcoholic debauch as the blood ethanol concentration is declining, during which time the subject ceases ethanol consumption and has little or no caloric intake. Gastrointestinal symptoms predominate and include anorexia, nausea, epigastric pain, and vomiting.[19,20] The subject usually has a temporary aversion to food and alcoholic beverages and complains of malaise. On physical examination, there is a clear sensorium in most cases. The odor of acetone may be detectable on the subject's breath. Tachypnea or Kussmaul respirations may be evident if there is marked acidemia. Tachycardia and other signs of volume depletion may be apparent. In some cases, manifestations of underlying cirrhosis (e.g., jaundice, ascites, ecchymoses, hemorrhoids) or other disorders commonly associated with chronic alcohol abuse (see Table 171-2) may be present.

LABORATORY MANIFESTATIONS

The key laboratory findings in AKA are metabolic acidosis, ketonemia, and ketonuria in the presence of a normal, low, or mildly elevated blood glucose concentration. Ethanol may be detectable in the blood, but it is not a requirement for the diagnosis and is frequently not detectable by the time the patient presents to the hospital. If the acidosis is clinically significant, elevation of the serum anion gap is expected. Other causes of metabolic acidosis must be excluded. Simple starvation can cause mild ketoacidosis, but with simple starvation the serum total CO_2 content or bicarbonate concentration generally remains above 18 mmol/L. DKA and renal failure are readily excluded by routine blood glucose and creatinine measurements. Lactic acidosis may be suggested by the associated clinical setting (e.g., seizures, hypotension), but it should be excluded by direct assay. Mild degrees of hyperlactatemia can occur in AKA, but concentrations greater than 3 mmol/L should prompt consideration of occult hypoperfusion, seizures, or another cause. Occult toxic ingestions also require exclusion, particularly ingestions of methanol, ethylene glycol, and salicylate intoxication.[15,21-24] Ingestion of exogenous acetone or isopropanol can cause marked ketosis due to acetonemia, but in isolation these intoxications are not associated with anion gap elevation or metabolic acidosis unless the poisoning is severe enough to cause seizures or circulatory shock, thereby resulting in lactic acidosis.

The high ratio of β-hydroxybutyrate to acetoacetate seen in AKA has clinical relevance when interpreting laboratory tests. A common assay for ketone bodies uses the semiquantitative nitroprusside reaction. Nitroprusside reacts colorimetrically with acetone and acetoacetate but not with β-hydroxybutyrate. As a result, and in comparison with DKA, the degree of ketonemia detectable in AKA is often disproportionately low relative to the degree of metabolic acidosis present. Therefore, severe metabolic acidosis due to DKA is typically associated with marked levels of ketosis, whereas severe acidemia in AKA may appear to be associated with only mild to moderate ketosis by nitroprusside-based testing. In milder cases of AKA, those associated with a mild degree of metabolic acidosis in which the acidosis is due mostly to elevation of β-hydroxybutyrate, the acetoacetate and acetone levels may not be sufficiently elevated to yield detectable ketosis by the nitroprusside test.

Because vomiting and dehydration are frequent manifestations in AKA, metabolic alkalosis can complicate the acid-base derangement. The combination of metabolic acidosis (from ketoacidosis) and metabolic alkalosis (from vomiting and volume contraction) can result in arterial pH and blood gas values that underestimate the severity of one or both of these metabolic disturbances. For example, mild metabolic alkalosis can be obscured by the presence of moderate or severe metabolic acidosis. Rarely, both metabolic processes are present and of approximately equal severity. In this situation, blood pH and bicarbonate concentration can be within normal limits despite the acid-base disturbances.[23] Or, the metabolic alkalosis can predominate and obscure the acidosis. The serum anion gap can aid in detecting these situations. An abnormally high anion gap suggests metabolic acidosis even if no acid-base disorder is evident by arterial blood gas analysis. In the face of a wide serum anion gap, the quotient of the delta anion gap (i.e., the subject's anion gap minus the average normal anion gap) divided by the delta bicarbonate (i.e., the average normal bicarbonate concentration minus the subject's blood bicarbonate concentration) should equal unity in organic metabolic acidoses if there is no metabolic alkalosis.[25] A quotient well above unity (e.g., >1.2) is evidence of concomitant metabolic alkalosis.

TREATMENT

Alternative explanations for the metabolic acidosis should be promptly excluded.[24] As in acute alcohol intoxication, the initial assessment should focus on identifying relevant alternative, underlying, or complicating illnesses or injuries that may require specific urgent therapy. Although patients with AKA sometimes have severe metabolic acidemia, the acid-base disturbance usually responds rapidly to IV hydration and ample dextrose administration.[17] Rapid infusion of 50 mL of 50% dextrose is indicated if hypoglycemia is identified. Five percent dextrose in normal saline is infused IV, at a high rate initially, to correct any hypovolemia or hypoglycemia and provide substrate for metabolic correction of the ketoacidosis. Thereafter, dextrose-containing normal or half-normal saline can be substituted at a high maintenance infusion rate, titrated to ongoing fluid losses. Ample dextrose administration is key to reversing the metabolic acidosis. The blood glucose concentration should be monitored frequently to allow detection of recurrent hypoglycemia or any intolerance to the provided glucose load.

In addition to specific tests related to acid-base imbalances, the same screening laboratory studies listed for acute alcohol intoxication should be evaluated. Serial acid-base and serum electrolyte testing is performed to monitor the response of the acidosis to treatment and to monitor for specific electrolyte abnormalities. Sodium bicarbonate and insulin are rarely if ever necessary. Potassium, magnesium, or phosphorus supplementation is provided if a deficiency is found by blood testing. Thiamine and multivitamins are indicated routinely. Because vomiting is common, the patient should be given nothing by mouth initially. Gastric intubation may be indicated if there is recent or ongoing vomiting, evidence of pancreatitis, or suspicion of gastrointestinal hemorrhage. Ethanol withdrawal precautions are observed.

▣ Ethanol Withdrawal

Ethanol withdrawal is common among hospitalized patients, either as a primary reason for admission or as a development during hospitalization for some other illness or injury. It is a potentially fatal syndrome that occurs after abrupt discontinuation of ethanol in individuals who regularly consume ethanol-containing beverages. Although in most cases it occurs after complete abstinence, it can also occur in the face of ongoing ethanol consumption if the level of ethanol intake is substantially decreased. The pathophysiology is incompletely understood but probably involves changes in neurotransmitter levels and alterations in neurotransmitter receptor function, as well as elevated circulating catecholamine levels.[6,7,26,27] A number of disorders should be of particular consideration in the differential diagnosis of alcohol withdrawal (see Table 171-2). The mortality rate associated with advanced stages of alcohol withdrawal can exceed 15%.[28,29]

CLINICAL MANIFESTATIONS

The syndrome is traditionally classified into four stages, although the stages do not always follow the indicated sequence, and not every patient develops every stage.[29] The time of development of each stage is also quite variable, and overlaps can occur. A typical temporal sequence is described.

The first stage occurs 6 to 24 hours or more after the last drink or after a somewhat longer period of markedly decreased ethanol intake. Manifestations include anxiety, restlessness, decreased attention, tremulousness, insomnia, and craving for alcoholic beverages. Stage 2, which occurs about 24 hours after the onset of abstinence, is characterized by hallucinations, misperceptions, irritability, and vivid dreams.[30] Hallucinations may be auditory, but more often they are visual or tactile. Formication, the delusional sensation of insects crawling on the skin, and vivid or threatening visual hallucinations are particularly common. During this stage, the patient may appear otherwise lucid or somewhat confused, hypervigilant, and easily startled or misled. In stage 3, which commonly occurs 7 to 48 hours after cessation of drinking, seizures occur, usually of the grand mal variety.[4] The seizures classically manifest as a cluster of brief tonic-clonic convulsions, at one time referred to as "rum fits." They are more likely to occur in subjects with a history of repeated withdrawal episodes.[32] A relatively lucid interval ranging from hours to 2 or 3 days is sometimes seen between stages 3 and 4. Stage 4 manifests 2 to 6 days or more after initiation of abstinence and consists of a global confusional state associated with signs of neuronal excitation and severe autonomic hyperactivity. Vernacular usage notwithstanding, the term *delirium tremens* specifically refers to stage 4 of withdrawal. Only a small minority of individuals with alcohol withdrawal develop delirium tremens. Tremors, hallucinations, and seizures are common during this stage. As is characteristic of delirium in general, the degree of confusion and disorientation can wax and wane. Hyperadrenergic manifestations may include diaphoresis, flushing, mydriasis, tachycardia, hypertension, and low-grade fever.[4]

LABORATORY MANIFESTATIONS

There are no specific laboratory manifestations of ethanol withdrawal. Laboratory abnormalities are a reflection of any concomitant or underlying disorders such as cirrhosis, coagulopathy, gastrointestinal bleeding, infection, pancreatitis, or aspiration pneumonitis. Electrolyte disorders are common, particularly hypokalemia, hypomagnesemia, and hypophosphatemia. Serum creatine phosphokinase activity should be evaluated because rhabdomyolysis is a common complicating problem and if severe can lead to renal failure or compartment syndrome.

TREATMENT

Early-stage withdrawal with mild symptoms does not generally require treatment in an ICU setting. Full-blown delirium tremens, on the other hand, often requires more vigilant monitoring than can be provided on many general medical or surgical units. Comorbid conditions that should prompt special consideration for ICU admission include acute coronary syndromes, congestive heart failure, severe sepsis, acute gastrointestinal bleeding, pancreatitis, hepatic failure, spontaneous bacterial peritonitis, hypothermia, and hyperthermia. Other factors to consider include advanced age, renal failure, severe electrolyte deficiencies, marked rhabdomyolysis, symptomatic hypoglycemia, recurrent or prolonged seizures, cardiac dysrhythmias, hypotension, and respiratory or airway compromise.

Initial steps in management include ensuring that a patent airway is present and that ventilation, oxygenation, and perfusion are adequate; establishing IV access; and excluding serious coexisting or complicating disorders. Subsequent treatment focuses mainly on judiciously titrated sedation and vigilant monitoring for progression of the syndrome or development of complications. All patients with alcohol withdrawal are given prophylactic multivitamin supplements including parenteral thiamine and folate, and fluid deficits and electrolyte deficiencies are corrected.[33] Routine administration of magnesium sulfate in the absence of hypomagnesemia has not been shown to be beneficial.[34,35] Prophylaxis against deep vein thrombosis is recommended.

A calm, nonthreatening, protective environment with frequent verbal orientation and reassurance is provided to allay anxiety and fear and to minimize agitation. This approach may suffice in milder cases, but more advanced withdrawal necessitates pharmacologic intervention. The principle underlying this pharmacotherapy is that administration of a cross-tolerant agent to achieve light to moderate sedation will ameliorate the severe manifestations of withdrawal (including autonomic and psychomotor hyperactivity), provide subjective relief, protect the patient from self-harm, and allow specific therapeutic interventions until spontaneous recovery occurs.

The agent of choice is a benzodiazepine given orally in milder cases or IV in more severe withdrawal states.[30,33,36-38] Limited evidence suggests that symptom-triggered dosing is superior to fixed-schedule benzodiazepine dosing.[39] Individualized dosing requires the expert judgment of an experienced clinician, but practicality often necessitates substitution of protocol-driven dosing schemes. These typically use a quantitative assessment scale such as the Revised Clinical Institute Withdrawal Assessment Scale for Alcohol to score the degree of withdrawal manifestations.[40,41] Lorazepam can be administered IV in incremental doses, starting with 1 or 2 mg, followed by intermittent (e.g., every 2-6 hours) IV dosing or a continuous IV infusion (e.g.,

initiated at 1 mg/h and titrated to effect).[29,42] Alternatively, midazolam can be employed, beginning with 2 to 4 mg by IV injection, followed by 2 mg/h by continuous IV infusion, which may be titrated to effect. Diazepam is another option, given initially in titrated doses of 5 to 10 mg at intervals as frequent as every 10 minutes if necessary until a calm but awake level of consciousness is achieved. Subsequent dosing at 5 to 20 mg every 4 to 6 hours is typically required with this agent. Prolonged administration of diazepam can lead to prolonged duration of sedation due to accumulation of the parent drug and an active metabolite, both of which have long half-lives. This effect is less likely to occur with lorazepam.

Oral benzodiazepines have been employed commonly in mild cases of withdrawal that do not require IV sedation.[30,31] These agents also can be used in more serious cases after the severe manifestations have abated and parenteral benzodiazepines are no longer required. Typical oral chlordiazepoxide dosage is 25 to 100 mg every 6 to 12 hours. Intramuscular administration is sometimes employed, but it entails a less predictable dose-response due to erratic absorption, and there is the potential for a depot effect.

Other sedative-hypnotic drugs can be effective but are not considered first-line therapeutic agents.[33,36] Barbiturates have a long history of successful use. The most commonly used agent is phenobarbital, which can be difficult to titrate because of its long duration of action. The shorter-acting barbiturate, pentobarbital, also has been employed. Oral ethanol and, in the past, paraldehyde have been used but have been discouraged, in part because of the risks of aspiration and gastric irritation, but also because their use can be interpreted as reinforcing the acceptability of using alcoholic beverages, either in general or for treatment of withdrawal symptoms. The latter criticism has also been directed at the use of ethanol administered IV for this purpose. A randomized trial examining IV ethanol administration for alcohol withdrawal prophylaxis in trauma ICU patients found no advantage compared to benzodiazepine management.[43] Propofol is effective, but it is not a first-line agent and is not recommended unless an endotracheal tube is in place and mechanical ventilation is used.[29] Regardless of the specific sedative agent employed, appropriate dose titration is crucial. The goal is to ameliorate the manifestations of withdrawal without causing excessive sedation. Sedation should be titrated with the use of an objective sedation scale such as the Ramsay Sedation Scale,[44] the Riker Sedation-Agitation Scale,[45] or the Richmond Agitation-Sedation Scale.[46] The goal should be to achieve a calm awake state or, if that is not feasible, a state of light somnolence from which the patient can easily be aroused and is able to respond verbally.

Clonidine may be administered if hyperautonomic symptoms are prominent.[47-49] Typical oral dosing is 0.1 to 0.2 mg every 6 to 12 hours. β-Adrenergic receptor blockers are not recommended for routine use, but barring contraindications, they may be considered in selected cases as adjunctive agents for controlling severe hyperadrenergic manifestations. Haloperidol and other neuroleptic agents are not routinely used, because they can lower the threshold for seizures. In selected cases, haloperidol may be used in conjunction with benzodiazepines for marked agitation or hallucinations, but this agent or similar drugs should probably not be used as monotherapy.[36]

Seizure precautions should be instituted for all patients in withdrawal. Withdrawal seizures are managed primarily with benzodiazepines, which usually are effective at the doses used for sedation.[42] In refractory cases, higher doses may be necessary but may necessitate endotracheal intubation and mechanical ventilation. Concomitant use of other anticonvulsants also can be considered. Barbiturates may be used for this purpose, but phenytoin is usually ineffective unless the seizures are due to a specific cause other than alcohol withdrawal, such as underlying epilepsy or a complicating acute disorder of the CNS (e.g., meningitis, head trauma).[33,50,51] In such cases, phenytoin is usually the anticonvulsant of choice. A variety of other anticonvulsant and sedative drugs have been studied for potential use in treating alcohol withdrawal, including valproic acid, baclofen, γ-hydroxybutyrate, gabapentin, oxcarbazepine, and carbamazepine. However, data on safety and efficacy are limited, particularly for hospitalized patients and those with comorbid illness.[52-59]

Once severe manifestations have been controlled with parenteral sedation for a period of at least 24 hours, tapering of the dose can be attempted. If tapering of sedation is tolerated, further gradual tapering is attempted, with the goal of substituting oral for parenteral benzodiazepine administration. This process typically takes up to several days, but there is substantial variability.

Methanol Intoxication

Methanol, also known as *wood alcohol*, is a clear, colorless liquid having a faint alcoholic odor. It is widely used in laboratories and industry as a solvent and synthetic precursor. It is also a constituent or vehicle in numerous commercially available products for residential use (Box 171-1).[15] Methanol is also used as a denaturant to intentionally render ethanol unfit for consumption. The minimum lethal dose of methanol is highly variable, reportedly ranging from less than 10 mL to more than 500 mL. This variability may result from multiple factors including the degree of concomitant ethanol intoxication, the presence of folate deficiency, and perhaps other factors.

More than 2000 cases of methanol exposure, most of which are accidental, are reported annually by the American Association of Poison Control Centers.[60,61-63] Intentional ingestion can represent a suicidal gesture or attempt, but it more commonly occurs among desperate alcoholics who have no access to ethanol-containing beverages and are either unaware or heedless of the risks of consuming methanol. There are individual cases of surreptitious poisoning in which an individual prepares a small volume of an alcoholic drink intentionally laced with methanol with malice aforethought for the intended victim. More often, malicious intent is absent, and the goal is simply illicit production of a small or large volume of alcoholic beverage, with methanol used because of its availability or under a mistaken notion that it will serve as a more potent but still potable inebriant. Sharing or black-market distribution of these illicit concoctions has resulted in periodic epidemics of methanol intoxication, sometimes involving hundreds of unwitting subjects.[64-68] There are also rare reports of dermal or inhalational exposure causing intoxication, but most cases involve oral ingestion.[69]

METABOLISM

Other than its inebriant and mucosal irritant effects, methanol per se is nontoxic. However, it is metabolized slowly to formaldehyde:

$$CH_3-OH + NAD^+ \xrightarrow{\text{ALDH}} NADH + H\overset{\overset{\textstyle O}{\|}}{-}C\text{-}H + H^+$$

Methanol   Formaldehyde

and then rapidly to formic acid, depicted here as its dissociation products, formate and a hydrogen ion[70]:

$$H\overset{\overset{\textstyle O}{\|}}{-}C\text{-}H + NAD^+ \xrightarrow{\text{ALDH}} NADH + H\overset{\overset{\textstyle O}{\|}}{-}C\text{-}O^- + 2H^+$$

Formaldehyde   Formate

Formic acid production can result in metabolic acidosis. Independent of the acidosis, formic acid inhibits cytochrome oxidase and has direct neurotoxic effects, particularly affecting the retina and optic nerves.[68,71-76] Small amounts of methanol are present as congeners in fermented alcoholic beverages.[77] Small amounts are also formed during the metabolism of certain fruits and vegetables and by metabolism of the artificial sweetener, aspartame.[78,79] However, the quantity of methanol available or formed from these sources is small, and there are enzyme systems present in the body that can convert these small amounts of formate to harmless CO_2 (Figure 171-1). The large amounts of formate produced in serious cases of methanol intoxication overwhelm these enzymes, resulting in toxic accumulation of formate. Certain nonhuman mammalian species have enzymes with much higher activity for metabolism of formate; even large quantities of methanol are nontoxic to these species. Methanol ingested by these species is still converted to formaldehyde and formate, but these toxins are rapidly metabolized to CO_2 so that significant formate accumulation does not occur. The enzymes that convert formate to CO_2 require folinic acid, the activated form of folic acid, as an obligate cofactor.[70]

CLINICAL MANIFESTATIONS

Like ethanol, methanol has dose-dependent sedating and inebriating effects that manifest shortly after ingestion, but methanol is less potent in this regard. Both alcohols also have similar gastrointestinal irritant effects that can provoke nausea, vomiting, abdominal pain, gastritis, hematemesis, and pancreatitis, although methanol may be more potent in this regard. Methanol ingestion can lead to additional CNS manifestations that are not observed with ethanol intoxication, which can sometimes provide helpful clinical clues in cases of occult methanol intoxication.[66,68] These more specific manifestations are caused by formate, the end product of methanol metabolism. There is a characteristic delay, usually 12 to 24 hours, between ingestion and development of these manifestations, and this delay is attributable to the relatively slow conversion of methanol to formaldehyde. Delayed CNS manifestations can include cerebral edema, seizures, signs of meningeal irritation, and cerebral infarction (particularly infarction of basal ganglia).[80] However, the most specific clinical findings are ocular and range from mildly blurred vision to visual field defects or tunnel vision to complete and sometimes permanent blindness.[66,68] Other possible ocular manifestations include scotomata, scintillations, papilledema, and loss of pupillary light reflexes. Most survivors recover visual function, but permanent visual deficits occur in as many as a third of patients with serious intoxication. If the metabolic acidosis is severe, it can result in Kussmaul respirations and dyspnea. In the most severe cases of poisoning, profound acidosis, respiratory failure, and circulatory shock intervene. Severe global brain injury and brain death can also occur.

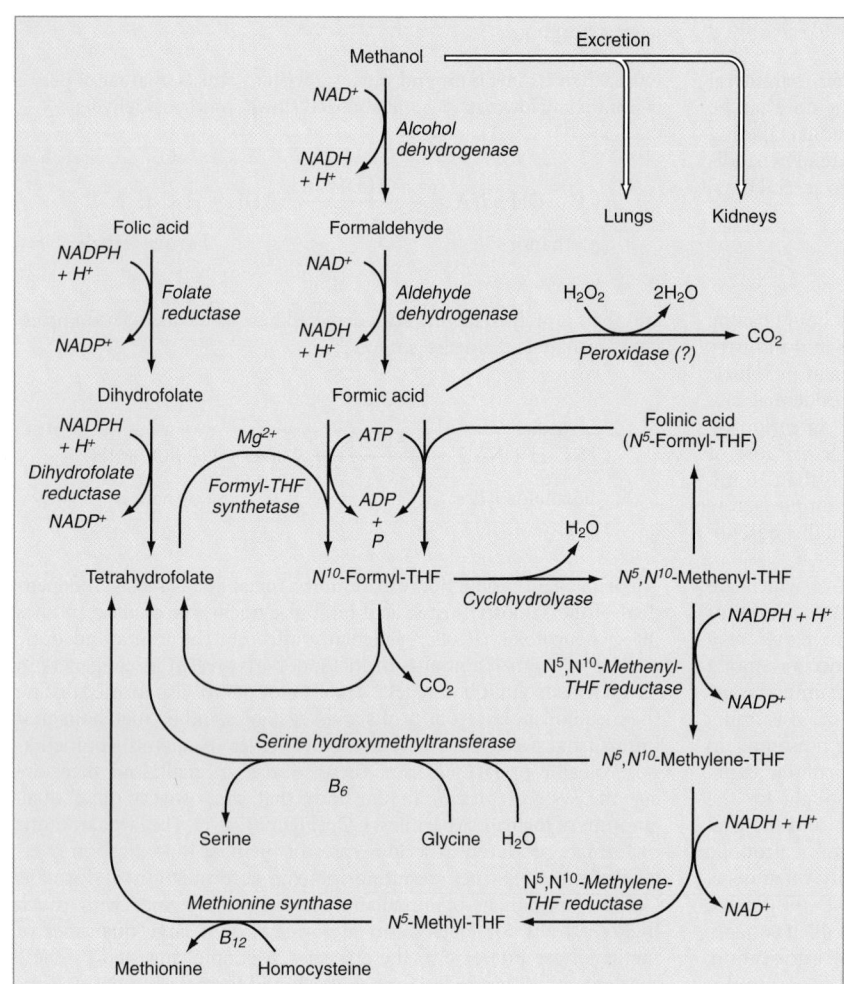

Figure 171-1 Metabolic pathways involved in methanol metabolism, showing the role of folate derivatives as enzymatic cofactors operative in the elimination of formic acid. ADP, adenosine diphosphate; ATP, adenosine triphosphate; NAD^+ and NADH, oxidized and reduced forms of nicotinamide adenine dinucleotide, respectively; $NADP^+$ and NADPH, oxidized and reduced forms of nicotinamide adenine dinucleotide phosphate, respectively; THF, tetrahydrofolate. (*Adapted from Kruse JA. Methanol poisoning. Intensive Care Med 1992;18:391-7, with permission.*)

If the patient offers historical information detailing an obvious toxic ingestion, the diagnosis of methanol intoxication is straightforward. Confirmatory diagnostic studies can be obtained and treatment initiated. In other cases, the diagnosis is not straightforward. Some poisoned patients may be unable to provide any history because of stupor or coma. Alert patients may be unaware that the alcoholic beverages they were provided were adulterated. Others may be alert and aware that they ingested a toxic substance but unwilling to provide the necessary history because of fear of social stigmatization or legal recrimination or as a manifestation of irrational or sociopathic behavior.

The presence of methanol may be detectable on the intoxicated patient's breath, but the agent's subtle odor can be difficult to appreciate and may be confused with ethanol. As a corollary, if a patient who appears inebriated has no breath odor of any type of alcohol, suspicion should be raised of methanol or a related toxic ingestion. In some cases, a faint odor reminiscent of formalin may be noticeable on the patient's breath. The obvious presence of ethanol on the breath does not exclude the possibility of methanol ingestion; co-ingestions involving these two alcohols are frequent.

LABORATORY MANIFESTATIONS

The clinical laboratory can be helpful by providing clues to the diagnosis in cases of occult intoxication and by corroborating cases with a clear history of methanol ingestion. The serum total CO_2 content may be abnormally low as a consequence of metabolic acidosis due to formic acid production. The dissociation product of formic acid, formate, is negatively charged, and can widen the serum anion gap. Arterial blood gas analysis can corroborate the presence of metabolic acidosis. Metabolic acidosis associated with a wide serum anion gap has a limited number of causes, the most common of which are lactic acidosis, ketoacidosis, and renal failure.[23,24] These other causes of wide-gap metabolic acidosis are easily excluded by measuring the concentrations in blood of lactate, ketones, glucose, and creatinine. Certain toxins (e.g., propylene glycol) can result in lactic acidosis by direct metabolic conversion of the parent compound to lactate. More commonly, lactic acidosis can occur in association with any toxic exposure or drug overdose that causes seizures or circulatory shock (e.g., iron, isoniazid). The metabolic acidosis seen in methanol intoxication is mainly due to formic acid formation but can also be due in part to lactic acidosis secondary to these other mechanisms. Analogous to ethanol metabolism, conversion of methanol to formaldehyde and formic acid leads to a reducing environment in cells, which tends to increase lactate concentration. By inhibiting cytochromes, formate also may interfere with normal aerobic metabolism and lead to an increase in anaerobic glycolysis with resulting lactic acidosis. Therefore, hyperlactatemia does not exclude methanol poisoning. A few other toxic agents besides methanol, notably ethylene glycol and salicylates, can directly cause a wide anion gap metabolic acidosis. Although measurement of plasma formate concentration would seem to be a rational method to confirm the diagnosis of methanol poisoning, this assay is rarely available in hospital laboratories.[81]

Life-threatening methanol poisoning can result in profound metabolic acidosis which sometimes is refractory to large doses of sodium bicarbonate. However, even with severe methanol exposure, metabolic acidosis may be absent if testing is performed within a few hours after the ingestion.[81] In these cases, the plasma methanol level may be very high, but the slow rate of its metabolism has not allowed for appreciable conversion to formic acid. Therefore, in the presence of a compatible history for toxic alcohol ingestion, the absence of a wide anion gap or hypobicarbonatemia should not be regarded as excluding the possibility of methanol poisoning.

A potentially useful screening test for recognition of methanol exposure early in its course is the serum osmolality gap. Serum osmolality is determined by the concentration of osmotically active solutes, or *osmoles*.[82,83] Osmotic activity is directly proportional to the osmole concentration of a solution, which is directly proportional to the mass concentration of the solute and inversely proportional to the solute's molecular weight. Therefore, to have an appreciable effect on osmolality, a solute must be present at relatively high mass concentration and have a relatively low molecular weight. For example, albumin is present at relatively large mass concentrations in serum, normally averaging about 4000 mg/dL, in comparison with urea, which normally averages only about 10 mg/dL. However, albumin has a far higher molecular weight (approximately 69,000 daltons, compared with 60 daltons for urea), making its osmolar concentration less than 1 mOsm/L. The elemental ions sodium and chloride are present in appreciable mass concentration, and their atomic weight is comparatively low (23 and 35 daltons, respectively), making them quantitatively important serum osmoles. Therefore, total serum osmolality normally comprises sodium, low atomic or molecular weight anions, plus urea and glucose; although many other osmoles are present in serum, their collective contribution is comparatively small. Based on these principles, serum osmolality may be estimated by the following formula[83]:

$$\text{Estimated serum osmolality} = 2 \times \text{Na} + \frac{\text{SUN}}{2.8} + \frac{\text{Glucose}}{18}$$

where the serum sodium concentration (Na) is given in mmol/L, and the serum urea nitrogen (SUN) and serum glucose concentrations are in mg/dL. The divisors, 2.8 and 18, are necessary to convert the conventional units of mg/dL to mmol/L. They are based on the molecular weights of the respective compounds.

Because ethanol is osmotically active and may be present in the blood in relatively high concentrations, the formula may be expanded to include a term for ethanol:

$$\text{Estimated serum osmolality} = 2 \times \text{Na} + \frac{\text{SUN}}{2.8} + \frac{\text{Glucose}}{18} + \frac{\text{Ethanol}}{4.6}$$

Here, the units for ethanol are mg/dL, and the divisor is based on the molecular weight of ethanol, 46 daltons. These millimolar concentration units technically provide an estimate of serum *osmolarity*; however, for practical purposes, they can be equated to millimolal units and designated *osmolality* (i.e., milliosmoles per kilogram of water). Just as ethanol can appreciably affect serum osmolality, so too can methanol.[84,85] The serum osmolality may be estimated from the formula shown and compared with a more direct measurement of serum osmolality; the difference between the two results affords a method for detecting and crudely quantifying the concentration of exogenous osmoles such as methanol. This is accomplished by means of the following formula:

$$\text{Osmole gap} = \text{Measured osmolality} - \text{Estimated osmolality}$$

Measured serum osmolality is determined in most clinical chemistry laboratories by analysis of the freezing point of the sample. Freezing point represents a colligative property of solutions that is depressed in proportion to osmolality, regardless of the chemical nature of the osmoles. This method, therefore, allows an empirical assessment of osmolality. The normal serum osmole gap is typically less than 10 mOsm/kg H$_2$O with this formula. Appreciable elevation of the osmole gap suggests the presence of an exogenous osmole (e.g., methanol). The only toxins that can appreciably affect the osmole gap are those that have a low molecular weight and can accumulate in relatively high concentration in the blood. A number of other exogenous compounds besides methanol meet these criteria, including ethylene glycol, acetone, isopropanol, propylene glycol, and acetonitrile, all of which have been reported to increase osmolality and the osmole gap.[15,23,82,83]

The constellation of laboratory findings that includes metabolic acidosis along with abnormal widening of both the serum anion gap and the serum osmole gap provides presumptive or corroborative evidence of methanol (or ethylene glycol) poisoning in compatible clinical settings. However, the serum osmole gap is not foolproof, and it has important limitations. False-positive results have been described in cases of circulatory shock, DKA or AKA, the hyperglycemic nonketotic dehydration syndrome, chronic renal failure, and multiple organ system failure.[83] False-negative results can occur if the ingestion involved a small but still potentially lethal volume of methanol. When assessing the serum osmole gap, it is important to ensure that all relevant measurements are made from the same serum specimen to minimize variability due to temporal changes in individual analyte concentrations. Some clinical chemistry laboratories assay serum osmolality by the dew point or vapor pressure method. For technical reasons, this method yields spuriously low osmolality readings in the presence of ethanol, methanol, and other volatile alcohols, and therefore it should not be used to assess the osmole gap.[83]

Methanol assays are available in many clinical chemistry laboratories and provide a direct assessment of methanol concentration in serum samples. This test is not definitive, because patients who present late after methanol intake may have metabolized much or all of the ingested alcohol, although the toxic byproducts may be present in appreciable concentration.[86] The delay between ingestion and presentation represents another factor that may explain the wide range of blood methanol concentrations reportedly associated with fatal outcome.[87] Methanol assay results should be interpreted in conjunction with assessments of acid-base status, serum anion gap, and serum osmole gap, as well as the history and clinical findings.

TREATMENT

As with any toxic ingestion, the patient's airway and ventilation must be immediately assessed and, if necessary, adequate support provided. Circulatory shock is treated with fluid resuscitation, inotropic support, and vasopressor agents, as appropriate. Whether the patient is initially unstable or not, close monitoring of vital signs, cardiopulmonary status, and neurologic status is indicated. Vomiting should not be induced because of the risk of aspiration and the lack of demonstrable benefit. Gastric lavage is unlikely to be of value unless the patient presents within 1 hour after ingestion. Activated charcoal is also of dubious benefit unless there is a concomitant toxic ingestant.[9,10,12,88-93] However, co-intoxication with another drug or toxin should be considered routinely. Accordingly, naloxone should be administered if the subject is unconscious. Blood and urine samples should be obtained for toxicologic screening. As in acute ethanol intoxication, complicating and occult underlying comorbid disorders must be considered (see Table 171-2).

Specimens should also be obtained for diagnostic laboratory tests. However, because specific toxicologic identification is not available on site at all hospital laboratories, antidotal therapy should not be delayed if there is an obvious history of methanol ingestion.[8,70,93,94] Even if "stat" testing is available, methanol intoxication may not be considered in occult cases until routine laboratory test results are obtained and reveal unexplained metabolic acidosis. In such cases, the preliminary laboratory test results in conjunction with a compatible setting and perhaps physical findings may allow a presumptive diagnosis to be made and antidotal treatment to be initiated. Treatment predicated on the presumptive diagnosis can be stopped if further studies convincingly argue against methanol intoxication. Symptomatic poisoned patients require ICU admission for frequent monitoring of vital signs and level of consciousness and to provide specific antidotal treatment, which consists of ethanol or fomepizole administration, hemodialysis, and folate administration.

Ethanol has been the conventional form of antidotal pharmacotherapy for methanol intoxication. The principle is that the enzymes, alcohol dehydrogenase and aldehyde dehydrogenase, have higher affinity for ethanol than for methanol, and ethanol thereby serves as an effective competitive inhibitor.[95-98] As a result, conversion of methanol to formaldehyde and formate is significantly slowed in the presence of ethanol, allowing methanol to be excreted by the kidneys and lungs, and by hemodialysis if that modality is employed. If inhibition is incomplete, the body may be able to safely eliminate the much smaller amounts of formaldehyde and formate that are metabolically produced from the methanol. Indications for ethanol therapy include a serum methanol concentration greater than 20 mg/dL or a history or strong clinical suspicion of methanol ingestion in conjunction with either an elevated osmole gap or evidence of metabolic acidosis (e.g., arterial blood pH < 7.30 and bicarbonate < 20 mmol/L).

Ethanol can be given orally, by gastric instillation, or by vein. Oral dosing can be considered in mild cases if the patient is completely alert and is accustomed to drinking liquor. The solution is usually prepared from commercially available liquor, available in many hospital formularies, and diluted to a final concentration of 20% ethanol. Even with dilution, subjects who are uninitiated to drinking this quantity of ethanol over a short interval are unlikely to avoid vomiting. Vomiting increases the risk of aspiration, particularly when coupled with the sedating effects of the administered ethanol and the potential CNS effects of the ingested methanol. For these reasons, IV ethanol administration is usually preferred over the oral route. Intravenous administration of ethanol can be accomplished with the use of a sterile solution of either 5% or 10% (volume/volume) ethanol in 5% (weight/volume) dextrose. These solutions are markedly hyperosmolar (approximately 2000 mOsm/kg H_2O for 10% ethanol in 5% dextrose and water), and therefore must be administered through a central venous catheter.

A loading dose is given so as to rapidly effect maximal enzyme inhibition. The goal is to achieve a serum ethanol level of 100 to 150 mg/dL. Based on the volume of distribution of ethanol (0.6-0.7 L/kg in men, slightly less in women and elderly subjects, and less in obese subjects) and a target serum ethanol concentration of 100 mg/dL, the necessary loading dose is theoretically 600 mg/kg in terms of absolute ethanol. Given the specific gravity of absolute ethanol (0.79), this is equivalent to a dose of 0.76 mL/kg in terms of absolute ethanol. Absolute (i.e., 100%) ethanol is unlikely to be available in a hospital formulary. Oral loading can be accomplished using 100 proof liquor, which is 50% ethanol by volume (equivalent to 40 g/dL), at a dose of 1.5 mL/kg. Alternatively, IV loading using a 5% (volume/volume) solution of ethanol in dextrose and water (i.e., an ethanol concentration of 4 g/dL by weight/volume) would require 15 mL/kg, typically administered over 1 hour. The dosing calculations described frequently underestimate the ethanol dose necessary to achieve the target level. Loading doses of 700 mg/kg given IV, or even higher doses if given orally, are more likely to achieve the goal initially.[1] If the patient's current ethanol concentration is already at or above the targeted level due to co-ingestion of ethanol, no ethanol loading dose is required. A proportionately lower loading dose is used in patients with a preexisting subtherapeutic blood ethanol concentration.

Maintenance dosing is required to maintain the targeted blood ethanol concentration. For patients with little or no history of ethanol exposure, the average required maintenance dose has been estimated to be about 70 mg/kg/h, in terms of absolute ethanol. For oral dosing with 100 proof liquor, this is equivalent to 0.18 mL/kg/h. Hourly oral maintenance doses are necessary and should be diluted to 20% to minimize epigastric pain and emesis. Using IV maintenance dosing, a continuous infusion of 5% ethanol solution is administered at 1.8 mL/kg/h. Subjects who consume ethanol chronically on a regular basis metabolize ethanol at considerably higher rates and therefore require higher maintenance doses. The necessary maintenance dose in such cases depends on the individual's exposure history, but it can be 2 to 3 times higher than the cited dose, or even higher in some cases. If hemodialysis is used during ethanol therapy, it will effectively remove ethanol from the body. Therefore, the maintenance ethanol dose has to be increased, often doubled or tripled, during dialysis. Accurate prediction of the required ethanol dosing in individual cases is not possible, and maintenance of the desired therapeutic ethanol

concentration can be challenging. Serial serum ethanol levels are obtained every 1 to 2 hours to allow the ethanol dosing to be titrated, striving to maintain a serum ethanol level between 100 and 150 mg/dL. Lower serum ethanol concentrations risk incomplete inhibition and toxicity from the products of methanol metabolism. The risks with higher levels are sedation, inebriation, and impairment of protective airway reflexes. Treatment is continued until serum methanol levels are less than 20 mg/dL. Intravenous ethanol therapy can entail large fluid volumes to achieve and maintain the desired blood ethanol level; for this reason, attention to fluid balance is important.

Fomepizole (4-methylpyrazole) is a newer therapeutic alternative to ethanol.[99-102] The indications for fomepizole use are the same as for ethanol therapy. Like ethanol, fomepizole inhibits alcohol dehydrogenase, but it is considerably more costly than ethanol. Nevertheless, fomepizole has supplanted ethanol at many centers, owing to its advantage of being easier to dose and titrate and because it has no sedative effects. Frequent serial blood ethanol assays are avoided. Compared with oral dosing of ethanol, there is no risk of nausea, vomiting, gastritis, or abdominal pain with fomepizole. Compared with IV ethanol administration, there is less risk of overhydration.

Fomepizole is given IV as a loading dose of 15 mg/kg, followed by 10 mg/kg every 12 hours for 4 doses and then 15 mg/kg every 12 hours until the serum methanol concentration is less than 20 mg/dL. Each dose is infused over 30 minutes. Dosing is altered if hemodialysis is employed. If dialysis is initiated, the next slated dose is given immediately if 6 hours or longer has elapsed since the last dose, but no dose is given if it has been less than 6 hours since the last dose. During ongoing hemodialysis, fomepizole is dosed at intervals of 4 hours. At termination of hemodialysis, if less than 1 hour has elapsed since the last dose, no fomepizole is administered; if 1 to 3 hours has elapsed between the last dose and the end of dialysis, half of the next scheduled fomepizole dose is administered; and if more than 3 hours has elapsed, the next scheduled fomepizole dose is given at the end of hemodialysis. Subsequent fomepizole dosing after hemodialysis is every 12 hours.

Severe methanol poisoning can be associated with profound metabolic acidosis in some cases. Traditionally, sodium bicarbonate was a staple part of the treatment for most causes of metabolic acidosis, but lack of demonstrable efficacy has tempered its routine use, particularly in the treatment of lactic acidosis and DKA. There are laboratory animal data and anecdotal clinical reports ascribing benefit to bicarbonate administration in cases of alcohol or glycol poisoning. Specifically, administration of bicarbonate is claimed to be capable of reversing ocular manifestations and lowering mortality, but controlled clinical trials are lacking. There is also evidence that undissociated formic acid is more toxic than the dissociation product, formate; increasing the extracellular fluid pH favors conversion of formic acid to formate.[103] Given the potential severity of the acidosis and the likely benefit of alkali therapy, sodium bicarbonate is recommended for subjects with an arterial pH less than 7.30, although intentional alkalemia is not advocated.

Ethanol and fomepizole minimize conversion of methanol to its toxic metabolites, but these forms of pharmacotherapy do not hasten elimination of methanol from the body. Methanol is excreted by the kidneys and lungs, but only slowly. Hemodialysis can effectively and more rapidly remove methanol and its toxic metabolites from the body. Charcoal or resin hemoperfusion techniques are not effective, and peritoneal dialysis is recommended only if hemodialysis is not available. Hemodialysis is recommended as a supplement to ethanol or fomepizole in patients with serious degrees of methanol intoxication. Serious intoxication is defined by the presence of metabolic acidosis, a serum methanol level above 50 mg/dL, any type of subjective or objective ocular findings, or other findings that indicate severe poisoning. Hemodialysis also is recommended if there is renal impairment. As previously noted, fomepizole and ethanol dosing must be altered during hemodialysis. Methods have been described to incorporate ethanol into the dialysate to facilitate maintaining therapeutic ethanol levels during hemodialysis.[104] The endpoint for dialysis is a serum methanol level less than 20 mg/dL and normalization of the anion gap, indicating clearance of formate. Direct measurement of plasma formate would be a logical method of monitoring if rapid assays were available.

In humans and certain nonhuman primates, formate is only slowly metabolized, allowing the development of acidosis and ocular pathology if substantial amounts of methanol are ingested. Monkeys given large doses of folinic or folic acid before or after methanol administration had lower formate levels and less toxicity than control animals.[105] Based on these and other experimental data, large doses of folic or folinic acid are recommended in clinical methanol poisoning. Typical recommendations are to administer 50 mg of folinic or folic acid IV every 4 to 6 hours. Folic acid must be reduced to tetrahydrofolate before it can serve as a cofactor for metabolizing formate. Folinic acid does not require reduction and therefore is the preferred form of the vitamin when available.

Ethylene Glycol Intoxication

Ethylene glycol is a clear, colorless, almost odorless, sweet-tasting, viscous liquid that is commonly used as the main constituent in most formulations of permanent automotive antifreeze. It also finds use in a variety of commercially available automotive fluids and paint products (Box 171-2), and it is used industrially as a solvent and synthetic precursor. Like methanol, it is occasionally ingested, either intentionally as an ethanol substitute or accidentally. More than 5000 cases of ethylene glycol exposure have been reported annually by the American Association of Poison Control Centers in recent years.[60,61,62] Based on limited anecdotal data, the lethal dose in humans has been estimated at 1 to 2 mL/kg, but there are case reports of fatalities after lower doses and survival after higher doses.

Box 171-2

COMMON COMMERCIAL PRODUCTS THAT MAY CONTAIN ETHYLENE GLYCOL

"Permanent" antifreeze
Paints and lacquers
Polishes and detergents
Inks
Cosmetics
Hydraulic brake fluids
Solar collector fluids
Car wash fluids

Data from Kruse JA. Methanol, ethylene glycol, and related intoxications. In: Carlson RW, Geheb MA, editors. Principles and Practice of Medical Intensive Care. Philadelphia: Saunders; 1993, p. 1716, with permission.

METABOLISM

The metabolism of ethylene glycol is more complicated than that of methanol.[106,107] As with methanol, the parent compound is only minimally toxic, but its metabolites are very toxic. Also, in common with methanol, the initial step in metabolism is catalyzed by alcohol dehydrogenase (Figure 171-2). The action of alcohol dehydrogenases converts ethylene glycol to glycoaldehyde, which can be converted further to glyoxal. Both glycoaldehyde and glyoxal are metabolized first to glycolic acid, then more slowly to glyoxylic acid, and finally to oxalic acid. Glycoaldehyde and glyoxylate have demonstrable nephrotoxicity in isolated rodent renal tubular segments, whereas glycolate, oxalate, and ethylene glycol do not.[108] Glycolate and probably some of the other

---

Figure 171-2 Metabolic pathways involved in ethylene glycol metabolism, with schematic morphologies of representative urinary crystals. LDH, lactate dehydrogenase; THF, tetrahydrofolate. (*Adapted from Kruse JA. Ethylene glycol intoxication. J Intensive Care Med 1992;7:234-43, with permission.*)

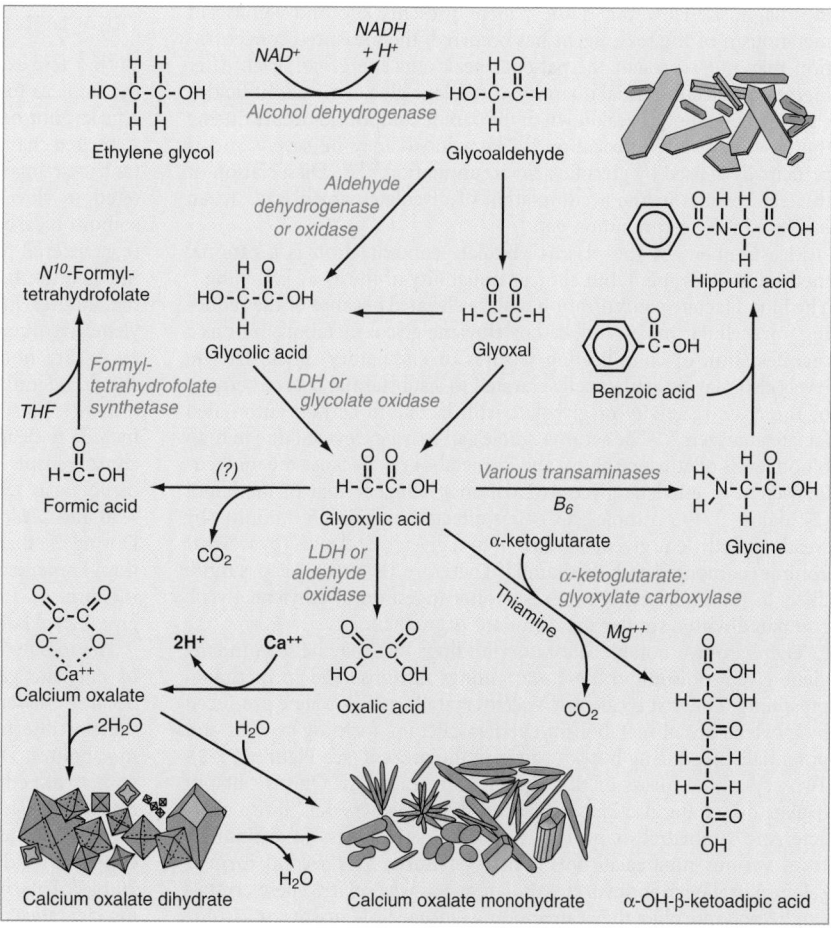

metabolites are also neurotoxic. Oxalic acid can precipitate as calcium oxalate crystals within various tissues, including notably the renal parenchyma and tubules.

CLINICAL MANIFESTATIONS

The initial effects involve the CNS and typically manifest within 30 minutes to 12 hours after ingestion.[15] The CNS manifestations of ethylene glycol poisoning can range from effects that are similar to those seen with acute ethanol intoxication, such as excitement, confusion, disorientation, and ataxia, to signs of CNS depression, such as lethargy, stupor, or coma. Nausea, vomiting, myoclonus, and seizures also can occur. Cranial nerve deficits including nystagmus, ophthalmoplegia, facial palsy, dysarthria, and dysphagia have been reported. There are also rare case reports of pupillary abnormalities and changes in visual acuity, but these findings are not characteristic; if they do occur, they may be the result of co-ingestion of methanol. Classically, the second phase manifests 12 to 24 hours after ingestion and consists of cardiorespiratory effects which may include dyspnea and a Kussmaul respiratory pattern secondary to metabolic acidosis or pulmonary edema. The latter can result in frank respiratory failure necessitating endotracheal intubation and mechanical ventilation. Tachycardia, hypotension, frank circulatory shock, coma, and death also can occur during this phase. The third phase, which usually takes 1 to 3 days to manifest, consists of renal failure, either oliguric or nonoliguric, due to acute tubular necrosis. Flank pain also can occur. The time course of each phase of intoxication is variable, and overlap is frequent.

LABORATORY MANIFESTATIONS

Laboratory findings are similar to those seen in methanol poisoning. Detection of ethylene glycol in serum provides definitive evidence of the diagnosis. However, if the patient presents late and significant metabolism of the toxic agent has occurred, the measured concentration may not represent the patient's peak ethylene glycol level. After ingestion of a substantial quantity of ethylene glycol, metabolic acidosis due to metabolic breakdown of the parent compound occurs during the first phase of intoxication.[86] The acidosis may be severe and is principally caused by glycolic acid accumulation.[109-112] Dissociation of this acid results in the accumulation of glycolate, which leads to an increase in the serum anion gap.

Measurement of the plasma glycolate concentration is a rational method of assessment, but clinical availability of the assay is lacking.[81] The blood lactate concentration may be elevated because of the reducing intracellular milieu induced by ethylene glycol metabolism or as a manifestation of complicating seizures or circulatory shock. Lactate levels also may be artifactually elevated to a substantial degree because of the cross-reactivity of glycolate with lactate in certain automated lactate analyzers.[113] The serum osmole gap may be elevated due to high blood levels of ethylene glycol and its metabolites. Because the molecular weight of ethylene glycol (62 daltons) is higher that of methanol (32 daltons), the osmole gap is less affected by a given amount (by weight) of ethylene glycol ingested or by a given blood level (by weight/volume) compared with methanol.[84] Therefore, the osmole gap is more likely to yield a false-negative result after ingestion of ethylene glycol, compared with a similar mass amount of methanol.

There are two notable laboratory findings that may be seen in ethylene glycol poisoning; these are findings not observed in methanol poisoning. The first is calcium oxalate crystalluria.[114] Oxalate produced by ethylene glycol metabolism chelates calcium, forming crystals and potentially producing hypocalcemia in the process (see Figure 171-2). Two crystalline forms of this organic salt can occur. One is calcium oxalate dihydrate, also known as *weddellite*. These crystals have a characteristic octahedral shape, making them relatively easy to distinguish from various nonoxalate forms of crystalluria. The second form is calcium oxalate monohydrate, also known as *whewellite*. These crystals can be polymorphic; they can appear as monoclinic prisms or assume

a needle-like, dumbbell-shaped, ovoid, or hempseed-like appearance. Hippurate crystalluria also has been described, but it can be difficult to morphologically discriminate hippurate from some forms of whewellite by light microscopy.[106] The finding of oxalate crystalluria corroborates the diagnosis; however, these crystals occasionally can be seen in the urine in the absence of ethylene glycol exposure, so their presence is not proof of glycol poisoning. On the other hand, because crystalluria does not uniformly occur after ethylene glycol ingestion, its absence does not exclude the diagnosis.

The other potential finding is fluorescence of the urine on exposure to ultraviolet radiation.[115,116] This finding is present when the ingested formulation of ethylene glycol contains fluorescein, a fluorescent dye added to many automotive antifreeze solutions to facilitate identification of cooling system leaks and to mitigate accidental confusion with potable liquids. The fluorescein is excreted in the urine and fluoresces yellow-green on exposure to ultraviolet light, such as from a Wood's lamp (commonly used in emergency departments and ophthalmology clinics to detect corneal lesions after topical application of fluorescein to the eye). False-positive results have been described due to other fluorescent substances in urine (e.g., carotene, carbamazepine, niacin, benzodiazepine metabolites) and from certain types of glass or plastic specimen containers that have a high degree of native fluorescence.[115,117] False-negative results may occur if more than 4 hours has elapsed since the ingestion—that is, sufficient time for the fluorescein to be excreted, at least by some individuals. A false-negative result is obviously expected if the ingested ethylene glycol formulation did not contain fluorescein or involved a small volume. False-negative results can occur if the urine pH is less than 4.5, but this may be circumvented by urine pH testing followed by upward titration of the specimen's pH if necessary. Owing to interfering factors and the limited ability of untrained examiners to detect fluorescence, clinical decision making should not hinge on this test in isolation.[118]

TREATMENT

With a few exceptions, the treatment of ethylene glycol poisoning is the same as for methanol intoxication. Gastric lavage may have some efficacy, but only if it is performed within 1 hour after the ingestion. Activated charcoal is not effective unless there is an amenable concomitant toxic ingestion.[12,119] Ethanol[98,120,121] or fomepizole[99-102] is administered to slow the conversion of the glycol to toxic intermediates; sodium bicarbonate is given if there is significant metabolic acidosis (e.g., arterial pH < 7.30); and hemodialysis is used in cases of serious intoxication to speed elimination of the parent compound and toxic metabolites. Ethanol or fomepizole is recommended if the serum ethylene glycol concentration is above 20 mg/dL. However, ethylene glycol assays are not available at all institutions, and inhibitor treatment should be initiated while awaiting definitive identification of the glycol if there is presumptive evidence of intoxication.[8,94,106] This evidence can include a clear history of recent ethylene glycol ingestion or strong clinical suspicion of ingestion in conjunction with either an elevated osmole gap, evidence of metabolic acidosis (e.g., arterial blood pH < 7.30 and bicarbonate < 20 mmol/L), or oxalate crystals in the urine. Dosing of ethanol and fomepizole is the same as for methanol intoxication. Fomepizole can be recommended over ethanol if the sensorium is depressed. Inhibitor treatment is continued until the serum ethylene glycol level falls below 20 mg/dL.

Hemodialysis can be even more important for the treatment of cases of ethylene glycol poisoning than it is for methanol intoxication, because ethylene glycol ingestion can result in severe renal dysfunction, thereby interfering with excretion of the compound and its toxic metabolites. Dialysis is conventionally recommended for all patients with serum ethylene glycol levels over 50 mg/dL. Hemodialysis is indicated for all patients with renal dysfunction and for patients with metabolic acidosis or other toxic manifestations. The conventional endpoint for dialysis is a serum ethylene glycol concentration less than 20 mg/dL in conjunction with normalization of the anion gap, indicating clearance of toxic metabolites.

Although there is some evidence that formic acid may be produced as a minor product of ethylene glycol metabolism, it probably does not play a significant role in the pathophysiology of this form of poisoning. Therefore, folate administration has not been routinely recommended. However, there is more convincing evidence that glyoxylate may be metabolized to nontoxic products by enzyme systems that rely on other vitamin cofactors, specifically pyridoxine (vitamin B_6) and thiamine (see Figure 171-2). Providing supplements of pyridoxine (e.g., 50 mg IV every 6 hours) and thiamine (e.g., 100 mg IV every 6 hours) could hasten elimination of toxic intermediates, although evidence of efficacy is quite limited.[106] Given the low toxicity of these vitamins, both are recommended. Magnesium is a necessary cofactor for the enzymatic degradation of glyoxylate, and supplemental magnesium should be given if there is hypomagnesemia.

Routine IV administration of calcium salts was advocated at one time as a therapeutic means of lowering oxalate levels in body fluids in cases of ethylene glycol poisoning. However, precipitation of calcium oxalate in vital organs is probably more likely to have harmful effects. Therefore, routine therapeutic administration of calcium to correct hypocalcemia is no longer advised unless the hypocalcemia is severe enough to cause manifestations.

KEY POINTS

1. Critically ill patients with ethanol intoxication or withdrawal should routinely receive intravenous (IV) thiamine, a multivitamin preparation, and unless hyperglycemic, dextrose.

2. The primary drug of choice for treating severe ethanol withdrawal is an IV benzodiazepine titrated to achieve a calm awake state or, if necessary, light somnolence from which the patient can easily be aroused.

3. Low or undetectable plasma ethanol concentrations are commonly observed in patients presenting with alcoholic ketoacidosis.

4. Indications for therapeutic ethanol or fomepizole administration include plasma concentrations of methanol or ethylene glycol exceeding 20 mg/dL or a history or strong clinical suspicion of ingestion of either of these toxins in conjunction with either an elevated osmole gap or metabolic acidosis.

5. Hemodialysis is indicated in methanol or ethylene glycol exposure accompanied by ocular findings, metabolic acidosis, impaired renal function, or plasma concentrations exceeding 50 mg/dL.

ANNOTATED REFERENCES

Amato L, Minozzi S, Vecchi S, et al. Benzodiazepines for alcohol withdrawal. Cochrane Database Syst Rev 2010;3:CD005063.
This systematic review of 64 studies found that benzodiazepines have a protective benefit against alcohol withdrawal symptoms, particularly seizures.

Barceloux DG, Bond GR, Krenzelok EP, et al. American Academy of Clinical Toxicology practice guidelines on the treatment of methanol poisoning. J Toxicol Clin Toxicol 2002;40:415-46.
An expert panel provides an extensive review covering the epidemiology, mechanisms of toxicity, clinical and laboratory manifestations, and detailed practice guidelines pertaining to methanol intoxication.

Brent J, McMartin K, Phillips S, et al. Fomepizole for the treatment of ethylene glycol poisoning. N Engl J Med 1999;340:832-8.
This multicenter open-label study of fomepizole use in patients with ethylene glycol intoxication demonstrated decreases in urinary oxalate, plasma ethylene glycol, and plasma glycolate concentrations after initiation of fomepizole therapy.

Kruse JA, Cadnapaphornchai P. The serum osmole gap. J Crit Care 1994;9:185-97.
This comprehensive review covers the underlying principles, derivation, clinical utility, and interpretation of the serum osmole gap. The review includes important caveats regarding factors that can lead to false-negative and false-positive findings.

Winter ML, Ellis MD, Snodgrass WR. Urine fluorescence using a Wood's lamp to detect the antifreeze additive sodium fluorescein: a qualitative adjunctive test in suspected ethylene glycol ingestions. Ann Emerg Med 1990;19:663-7.
This study involving healthy volunteers who ingested sodium fluorescein documents the potential usefulness of exposing urine samples to ultraviolet radiation as a simple means of identifying occult toxic exposure to ethylene glycol–based automotive antifreeze. Various pitfalls and limitations of the technique are described.

REFERENCES

Access the complete reference list online at http://www.expertconsult.com.

172

Anticonvulsants

MAREK A. MIRSKI

The treatment of seizures in the intensive care unit (ICU) involves two distinct elements: (1) acute termination of all clinical and electrographic seizure activity and (2) prevention of further seizures. Many seizures manifest as a single, self-limiting episode that alerts the ICU team to a metabolic or structural abnormality. Correcting the underlying pathology and initiating prophylaxis may prevent recurrence of the seizure(s). Thus, there are instances in the ICU when acute treatment of the seizure is not necessary. Prophylaxis against recurrence may not be warranted if the precipitating factors have been eliminated. However, owing to the potential for refractory seizures, it is common to place a patient in the ICU on seizure prophylaxis once a seizure has been documented. To optimally treat patients in the ICU who have seizures or are at risk for seizures, the risks and benefits of the anticonvulsant must be assessed prior to initiation of therapy.

Anticonvulsants: General ICU Concerns

An ideal anticonvulsant for use in the ICU would have the following properties: the drug can be administered intravenously (IV); the drug does not irritate veins; the drug is lipophilic, enabling excellent penetration into the central nervous system (CNS); the drug does not cause sedation; the drug provides prolonged protection against seizures; the drug does not cause side effects and is not toxic; the metabolites of the drug are biologically inactive; and the drug (and its metabolites) are cleared via mechanisms that are not dependent upon normal hepatic or renal function. From a review of our drug armamentarium, it is obvious that none of the currently available anticonvulsants meet all of these criteria.

Specific anticonvulsant medications are selected based on several considerations such as the type of seizure activity being treated, the periodicity of the seizure activity, and the need for acute or emergency therapy versus chronic seizure prophylaxis. In the ICU, additional concerns arise secondary to the common observance of drug-induced side effects. Both idiosyncratic and dose-dependent complications can occur. Various factors are implicated in the development of anticonvulsant toxicity. The following are common metabolic and pharmacodynamic features of anticonvulsants that are important concerns in ICU practice.

PROTEIN BINDING

Drugs such as phenytoin, carbamazepine, and valproic acid are extensively protein bound, but only the unbound drug in the plasma is biologically active. Critically ill patients are often catabolic and have abnormally low circulating protein levels; thus, the concentration of unbound drug can be greater than anticipated despite a total serum (or plasma) drug level that is within the normal target range for the medication.[1] Patients with hepatic and/or renal dysfunction are prone to discordance between total and unbound (free) serum levels. Routine monitoring of free drug levels is expensive but warranted in these patients. Unfortunately, most hospital laboratories routinely offer unbound serum levels for only one commonly used anticonvulsant, phenytoin.

SEDATION AND COGNITIVE IMPAIRMENT

Sedation and cognitive impairment are the two most common *dose-dependent* side effects of anticonvulsants. These side effects commonly occur even when the drugs are administered so as to achieve therapeutic concentrations. These side effects are most common in vulnerable patients such as the elderly and the seriously ill. Clinically significant alterations in level of consciousness or cognition can be seen with the use of phenobarbital, primidone, phenytoin, and topiramate.

METABOLIC DERANGEMENTS

Hyponatremia has been reported in patients who have been treated with carbamazepine, oxcarbazepine, and (rarely) other anticonvulsants. Anticonvulsant-induced hyponatremia has been attributed to the syndrome of inappropriate antidiuretic hormone (SIADH) (Table 172-1). Selected subgroups of patients are more at risk for anticonvulsant-induced hyponatremia, including elderly persons, menstruating women, patients who require administration of large fluid volumes, patients with renal failure, postoperative patients, and patients who are concurrently receiving other medications associated with hyponatremia.[2]

DRUG FEVER

Development of a fever coincident with initiation of an anticonvulsant in the ICU setting complicates patient management and is a serious potential concern. Drug fever is a particularly common occurrence with the two agents, phenytoin and fosphenytoin, but can occur with other anticonvulsants as well.[1] Peripheral eosinophilia supports the diagnosis. However, it is frequently the case that the diagnosis of drug-induced fever is firmly established only when hyperthermia resolves after an alternative anticonvulsant is substituted for the original agent.

ALTERATION IN NEUROLOGIC EXAMINATION

The toxic side effects of phenytoin or carbamazepine can promote development of ataxia. Valproic acid can induce tremors. Carbamazepine toxicity can present in a biphasic fashion (i.e., acutely and subacutely) as a consequence of increasing levels of a toxic metabolite.[1]

RENAL DISEASE

Clearance of anticonvulsants can be significantly reduced when the glomerular filtration rate (GFR) falls below 10 mL/min. The clearance of phenobarbital and carbamazepine are not greatly affected by low GFR, but the clearance of phenytoin and valproic acid can be affected by changes in renal function. The higher protein binding exhibited by these latter agents makes measurement of the free levels of these drugs a better guide for dosage adjustments.[1] Hemodialysis does not affect circulating phenytoin levels to a large extent, but renal replacement therapy can markedly affect serum levels of phenobarbital.

TABLE 172-1	Medications Associated with SIADH	
Barbiturates		Haloperidol
Carbamazepine		Chlorpropamide
Oxcarbazepine		Thioridazine
Thiazides		Imipramine
Vincristine		MAO inhibitors
Cyclophosphamide		Bromocriptine
General anesthetics		Oxytocin
Nicotine		Acetamides
Clofibrate		Tolbutamide
Nonsteroidal antiinflammatory drugs		

Adapted from Asconape J. Some common issues in the use of antiepileptic drugs. Semin Neurol 2002;22:27.

TABLE 172-2	Metabolic Pathways of Anticonvulsant Drugs		
CYP 1A2	*CYP 2C9*	*CYP 2C19*	*CYP 3A4*
Carbamazepine*	Phenytoin	Phenytoin*	Carbamazepine
	Phenobarbital	Diazepam	Tiagabine
	Valproate*	Lacosamide*	Zonisamide
			Ethosuximide
			Felbamate

*Minor metabolic pathway.
Adapted from Asconape J. Some common issues in the use of antiepileptic drugs. Semin Neurol 2002;22:27.

DRUG INTERACTIONS

Many anticonvulsants can affect metabolism and or protein binding of other agents. Phenytoin, carbamazepine, and phenobarbital are all potent inducers of the hepatic P450 enzyme systems (Tables 172-2 and 172-3), and treatment with these anticonvulsants can affect the circulating concentrations of other medications (Tables 172-4 and 172-5) including concomitantly administered anticonvulsant drugs (see Table 172-5). Phenytoin can reduce the plasma concentrations of carbamazepine and valproic acid, whereas interaction with phenobarbital is variable. Phenytoin decreases the effectiveness of warfarin and theophylline. Valproic acid inhibits the metabolism of phenobarbital and carbamazepine (including its 10,11-epoxide metabolite), which can result in increased serum levels. Carbamazepine increases the hepatic

TABLE 172-3	Anticonvulsant Induction of Hepatic Metabolic Enzymes	
Inducers	*Inhibitors*	*No or Minimal Effect*
Carbamazepine	Valproate	Gabapentin
Phenytoin	Felbamate	Lamotrigine
Phenobarbital		Topiramate
Primidone		Tiagabine
		Oxcarbazepine
		Levetiracetam
		Zonisamide

Adapted from Asconape J. Some common issues in the use of antiepileptic drugs. Semin Neurol 2002;22:27.

metabolism of diazepam and valproic acid. Phenobarbital results in decreased circulating levels of warfarin, theophylline, and cimetidine.[3] Cimetidine, amiodarone, isoniazid (INH), and chlorpromazine all decrease hepatic metabolism of many drugs including phenytoin (Table 172-6). Drugs that commonly decrease circulating phenytoin levels include digoxin, cyclosporine, corticosteroids, warfarin, and theophylline. Aluminum hydroxide, magnesium hydroxide, and calcium-containing antacids decrease the absorption of enterally administered phenytoin. Some of the newer anticonvulsants such as levetiracetam and lacosamide are excreted via the kidneys for the most part, and their circulating levels are unaffected by hepatic metabolism. In addition, drug-drug interactions are not a major concern with these newer agents, and they do not affect the levels of other anticonvulsants.

IDIOSYNCRATIC REACTIONS

Hypersensitivity reactions are common with phenytoin and carbamazepine and can be manifested by fever, rash, and/or eosinophilia.[1] Drugs associated with a high risk for the development of rash include phenytoin, phenobarbital, primidone, lamotrigine, carbamazepine, oxcarbazepine, and zonisamide[4] (Table 172-7). Transient leukopenia and thrombocytopenia are commonly seen with carbamazepine and valproate. Other less common drug-related effects include hepatic failure, pancreatitis (valproic acid), agranulocytosis, aplastic anemia, megaloblastic anemia (phenytoin), Stevens-Johnson syndrome, and lupus-like syndromes. Although rare, severe hepatic dysfunction secondary to formation of a toxic metabolite can occur with valproic acid therapy. This potentially fatal reaction most often occurs in children younger than 2 years of age who are also receiving aspirin and other drugs for control of seizures.

TABLE 172-4	Alterations in Drug Plasma Levels with Combination Anticonvulsant Use					
		Effect on Plasma Levels of Primary Agents				
Added Drug	*% Bound*	*Phenytoin*	*Phenobarbital*	*Carbamazepine*	*Valproic Acid*	*Benzodiazepines*
Phenytoin	90		Variable	↓	↓	
Phenobarbital	45	↑ then ↓		Variable	↓	↓
Carbamazepine	75	Variable	Variable	↓	↓	↓
Valproic acid	90	↓ but ↑ in free levels	↑	Variable or ↑ in 10,11 epoxide		↑
Benzodiazepines		↓	Variable		Variable	

% Bound: percentage serum protein bound.

TABLE 172-5	Effects of Anticonvulsant Drugs on Commonly Used Medications				
	Effect on Plasma Levels or Clinical Effectiveness of Primary Agents				
Added Drug	*Warfarin*	*Theophylline*	*Corticosteroids*	*Haloperidol*	*Lithium*
Phenytoin	↓	↓	↓		
Phenobarbital	↓	↓	↓	↓	↑

↓, decrease; ↑, increase.

TABLE 172-6	Common Drug Interactions of Anticonvulsants	
Phenytoin and Carbamazepine		
Added Drug	*Phenytoin*	*Carbamazepine*
Salicylates	↑	
Erythromycin		↑↑
Chloramphenicol	↑	
Trimethoprim	↑	
Isoniazid	↑	↑
Propoxyphene	↑	↑
Amiodarone	↑	
Diltiazem, verapamil		↑
Cimetidine	↑	↑
Ethanol	↓	
Rifampin	↓	
Digitoxin	↓	
Cyclosporine	↓	
Warfarin	↓	
Theophylline	↓	
Glucocorticoids	↓	

↓, decrease in plasma levels; ↑, increase in plasma levels.

MANAGEMENT OF ANTICONVULSANT TOXICITY

Management of patients suffering from severe toxicity requires comprehensive supportive therapy including airway management, hemodynamic support, and oral administration of activated charcoal. Charcoal has been especially useful for managing cases of acute valproate acid intoxication.[5] In cases of valproic acid or carbamazepine poisoning, concurrent hemoperfusion and hemodialysis to enhance elimination of the anticonvulsant can be useful when patients are hemodynamically unstable and the clinical condition is worsening despite aggressive supportive care.[6]

Specific Anticonvulsant Properties by Class

BENZODIAZEPINES

For immediate therapy, benzodiazepines are still considered first-line treatment for most seizures. These drugs are highly lipophilic, are potent γ-aminobutyric acid (GABA)-activated agonists, and serve to improve local inhibition of signal transmission. The most commonly used benzodiazepines in the ICU are diazepam, lorazepam, and midazolam. In the case of hepatic failure, oxazepam may be preferred because it is the only benzodiazepine not metabolized by the liver.[7]

There are instances where short-acting benzodiazepines (e.g., midazolam or diazepam) may be preferable; anticonvulsants that offer prolonged sedation may interfere with reliable neurologic assessment and management. When such concerns exist, it may be preferable to initiate treatment of seizures using a short-acting benzodiazepine,

TABLE 172-7	Antiepileptic Drugs and Risk of Skin Rash
High Risk	*Low Risk*
Phenytoin	Valproate
Phenobarbital	Topiramate
Primidone	Gabapentin
Carbamazepine	Tiagabine
Oxcarbazepine	Levetiracetam
Lamotrigine	Lacosamide
Zonisamide	

Data from Asconape J. Some common issues in the use of antiepileptic drugs: Semin Neurol 2002;22:27.

followed immediately by a loading dose of a less-sedating medication such as phenytoin or other maintenance anticonvulsant.

If the seizure(s) have not been controlled following therapeutic doses of benzodiazepines, treatment with additional medications is warranted. Tachyphylaxis rapidly develops with the use of benzodiazepines, and these agents are not indicated for prophylaxis or maintenance therapy. Common secondary agents which are efficacious in the acute setting and are available for IV administration include phenytoin, fosphenytoin, carbamazepine, and valproic acid. Levetiracetam and lacosamide are newly developed agents that can be administered IV and are often used as second-line agents in the setting of uncontrolled seizures in the ICU.

DIAZEPAM

Diazepam (Valium) has been available for many years, and most clinicians have considerable experience with this drug. Its use has been declining in recent years due to the availability of more effective agents such as midazolam and lorazepam. Following administration, the highly lipophilic drug, diazepam, rapidly redistributes from plasma into tissue. Because of this, the anticonvulsant duration is just a few minutes. Diazepam is not water soluble and requires emulsification with a vehicle (propylene glycol) for IV administration. Diazepam can induce phlebitis and should be administered slowly and preferably into a large vein.

Dosing

Adults: oral, 2-10 mg, 2 to 4 times per day; IV, 2 to 4 mg, may repeat in 3 to 4 hours if needed.

In status epilepticus: IV, 5 to 10 mg every 10 to 20 minutes, up to 30 mg in an 8-hour period.

Elderly: oral absorption is more reliable than IM; consider dosage reduction.[8,9]

Hepatic impairment: reduce the dose by 50% in patients with cirrhosis, and avoid in patients with severe or acute liver disease.

Renal impairment: diazepam is not dialyzable; supplemental dosing is not necessary.

Forms available: rectal gel, 5 mg/mL (15 mg, 20 mg); injection solution, 5 mg/mL; oral solution, 5 mg/mL (30 mL); tablet (2 mg, 5 mg, 10 mg).

Mechanism(s) of action: diazepam binds to $GABA_A$ receptors, resulting in opening of the chloride channel, leading to hyperpolarization and inhibition of neuronal firing.

Pharmacokinetics

Oral absorption: 85-100%.

Distribution: 98% protein bound.

Elimination: half-life parent drug 20 to 50 hours; active major metabolite (desmethyldiazepam) 50 to 100 hours.

Metabolism: hepatic.

Drug interactions: theophylline can antagonize the effects of benzodiazepines. Oral contraceptives can decrease the clearance of benzodiazepines. Benzodiazepines can interfere with the therapeutic effects of levodopa. Additive sedative effects and/or respiratory depression can occur with ethanol, barbiturates, and narcotic analgesics. Potential hepatic P450 enzyme induction exists with phenobarbital, phenytoin, carbamazepine, rifampin, and rifabutin.[1,3,10]

Adverse reactions/toxicities: hypotension, drowsiness, ataxia, paradoxical excitement or rage, memory impairment, rash, decrease in respiratory rate, and frank apnea all can occur following administration of diazepam. All benzodiazepines are associated with dependence and/or withdrawal symptoms on discontinuation or reduction in dose following prolonged dosing.[11] Acute withdrawal symptoms including seizures can be precipitated when the drug is discontinued or the dosage is reduced. Withdrawal reactions including seizures can occur following administration of the GABA antagonist, flumazenil.[12]

Contraindications: narrow angle glaucoma, pregnancy.

MIDAZOLAM

When a short-acting benzodiazepine is needed, most clinicians now employ midazolam instead of diazepam. Midazolam is highly lipophilic, and the onset of its effects occur very rapidly following IV administration.[13] Midazolam is marketed as a water-soluble prodrug. Following IV administration, the drug is transformed into a lipophilic compound by virtue of rapid closure of the diazepine ring. Thus the drug is less irritating to veins than diazepam.

Dosing

Adults: IV initial dose is 0.5 to 2 mg; no more than 2.5 mg should be administered over a period of 2 minutes. A total dose of more than 5 mg is generally not required. Maintenance is approximately 25% of the dose needed to reach the sedative effect. Consider a decrease in dosage by 30% if narcotics or other CNS depressants are administered concurrently.

Elderly: consider a dosage reduction based on altered kinetics[14] and sensitivity.

Hepatic impairment: reduce dose by 50% in patients with cirrhosis and avoid in severe/acute liver disease.

Renal impairment: midazolam is not dialyzable; supplemental dosing is not necessary.

Forms available: injection solution, 1 mg/mL (2 mL, 5 mL, 10 mL) and 5 mg/mL (1 mL, 2 mL, 5 mL, 10 mL); syrup, 2 mg/mL (118 mL); tablet (2 mg, 5 mg, 10 mg).

Mechanism(s) of action: midazolam binds to GABA$_A$ receptors, resulting in the opening of the chloride channel, with resultant hyperpolarization and inhibition of neuronal firing.

Pharmacokinetics

Absorption: bioavailability 45%.
Distribution: 0.8 to 2.5 L/kg; 95% protein bound.
Elimination: half-life parent drug 1 to 4 hours.
Metabolism: midazolam is hepatically metabolized, yielding biotransformation into two active metabolites: alpha-hydroxymidazolam (60% potency) and alpha-hydroxymidazolam glucuronide (10% potency). Less than 1% of the drug is excreted unchanged in the urine, the excreted compounds being glucuronide-conjugated metabolites.[13]
Drug interactions: same as with diazepam.
Adverse reactions/toxicities: same as diazepam.
Contraindications: narrow angle glaucoma, pregnancy.

LORAZEPAM

Lorazepam is the least lipid-soluble agent among the three commonly used benzodiazepines. As a consequence, the pharmacologic effects of lorazepam are delayed in onset and prolonged in duration.[15] Lorazepam is ideally suited for acute therapy, together with longer prophylaxis against recurrence of seizures. In a 5-year randomized double-blind multicenter trial of four IV regimens for the treatment of generalized status epilepticus, Treiman et al. found that treatment with lorazepam (0.1 mg/kg) was successful in 64.9% of patients and significantly superior to phenytoin ($P = 0.002$) in a pairwise comparison.[16] It is important to note that lorazepam's longer duration of action can adversely impact the neurologic examination for several hours, potentially complicating medical management.

Dosing

Adults: oral, 1 to 2 mg every 30 to 60 minutes for tranquilization of agitated patient; IV, 2 to 4 mg, may repeat in 3 to 4 hours if needed.
In status epilepticus: IV, 4 to 8 mg given over 2 to 5 minutes; also can dose 0.1 mg/kg. May be given intramuscularly (IM) with little discomfort.
Elderly: consider a dosage reduction.
Hepatic impairment: reduce dose by 50% in patients with cirrhosis, and avoid in severe/acute liver disease.

Renal impairment: lorazepam is not dialyzable; supplemental dosing is not necessary. Large doses of the polyethylene glycol emulsion may induce nephrotoxicity.[17]
Forms available: injection solution, 2 mg/mL (30 mL); tablet (0.5 mg, 1 mg, 2 mg).
Mechanism(s) of action: binds to GABA$_A$ receptors, resulting in opening of the GABA chloride channel, with resultant hyperpolarization and inhibition of neuronal firing.

Pharmacokinetics

Absorption: rapid in the CNS.
Distribution: 85% protein bound; V_d 1.3 L/kg in adults.
Elimination: hepatic metabolism followed by renal excretion.
Metabolism: hepatic to inactive compounds. Metabolism of lorazepam is inhibited by valproic acid. Drug half-life is 12.9 hours (adults), 15.9 hours (elderly), or 32 to 70 hours (end-stage renal disease).
Drug interactions: same as for diazepam.
Adverse reactions/toxicities: similar to diazepam. Additionally, lorazepam's use in higher doses and in infusions has been associated with development of lactic acidosis, hyperosmolar coma, and/or reversible nephrotoxicity due to the presence of the solvents, propylene glycol and polyethylene,[17] in the IV formulation of the drug.
Contraindications: narrow angle glaucoma, pregnancy.

PHENYTOIN

Phenytoin has been and remains the drug most commonly used in the ICU for prophylaxis against seizures. Several reasons for the continued popularity of phenytoin include its ease of administration, its availability in formulations suitable for either IV or enteral administration, its relative safety (severe toxic reactions are uncommon), and its efficacy against many seizure syndromes that occur in the ICU setting, including status epilepticus. Temkin et al. reported that prophylactic administration of phenytoin decreased the incidence of seizures during the first week following traumatic head injury by 73% compared to placebo.[18] In light of its non-GABA-agonist action, phenytoin is not particularly effective against most drug-induced convulsions, especially those triggered by β-lactam antibiotics. Phenytoin is indicated for use against generalized tonic/clonic seizures and focal and complex-partial seizures. Phenytoin also is indicated for prevention of seizures following head trauma or elective neurosurgical procedures.

Dosing

Adults: for seizure prophylaxis or initial therapy to combat seizures, the loading dose is 15 to 20 mg/kg IV; oral (PO) loading doses should be administered as 3 divided doses every 2 hours. For IV administration, the drug should be given at a rate of less than 50 mg/min, because the glycol-based vehicle can induce hypotension and/or heart block. The maintenance dose of 5 to 6 mg/kg/d PO can be given all at once or in divided doses.
Elderly: administration rate should be decreased owing to increased likelihood of hypotension and/or heart block (e.g., rate of administration = 20 mg/min).
Hepatic impairment: phenytoin should be used with caution, as there is decreased clearance of the drug in patients with cirrhosis. Monitoring of liver function tests and free phenytoin levels is advocated.
Renal impairment: in patients with renal insufficiency, interpretation of total levels is difficult, since the free fraction is altered (increased) due to the reduction of plasma protein concentration. Monitoring of free serum levels is recommended.
Forms available: capsule (30 mg, 100 mg, 200 mg, 300 mg); injection (50 mg/mL; 2 mL, 5 mL); oral suspension (125 mg/5 mL; 240 mL); chewable tablet (50 mg).
Mechanism of action: its mechanism is not entirely clear, although it blocks sodium channels, which reduces neuronal excitation.

Pharmacokinetics

Absorption: phenytoin is slowly absorbed orally, and uptake from the gastrointestinal tract is even less reliable when the drug is given concurrently with enteric tube feedings. Thus, tube feedings should be discontinued for 2 hours prior to and 2 hours after each enteral dose. The bioavailability of phenytoin is form dependent; reference range 10 to 20 µg/mL total; free levels 0.1 to 0.2 µg/mL. Free drug levels should be monitored in physiologic states associated with decreased circulating albumin concentrations (e.g., burns, head injury,[19] hepatic cirrhosis, nephrotic syndrome, pregnancy, cystic fibrosis), and in patients with hepatic and/or renal failure.

Distribution: V_d is 0.6 to 0.7 L/kg; 90% to 95% protein bound.

Elimination: hepatically metabolized; phenytoin is excreted in the urine as glucuronides, with a half-life of approximately 22 hours.

Metabolism: hepatic metabolism; phenytoin follows dose-dependent capacity-limited (Michaelis-Menten) pharmacokinetics. Thus, serum and free levels may abruptly increase once capacity for metabolism is exceeded (zero-order kinetics).

Drug interactions: as isolated phenomena, phenytoin can enhance the hepatotoxic potential of acetaminophen, blunt the diuretic effect of furosemide, increase the metabolism of HMG-CoA reductase inhibitors, decrease the duration of effect of neuromuscular blocking agents, and reduce the metabolism of thyroid hormones.[3,10] Antacids can decrease absorption of phenytoin, whereas amiodarone can increase circulating concentrations. The sedative effects of phenytoin can be additive with other CNS depressants.

As a known inducing agent for hepatic metabolism, phenytoin increases the clearance of corticosteroids and many anticonvulsants (barbiturates, carbamazepine, ethosuximide, felbamate, lamotrigine, tiagabine, topiramate, and zonisamide).[3] Thus, anticonvulsant polypharmacy can be frustrated by the addition of phenytoin. However, phenytoin does not affect gabapentin or levetiracetam levels. As would be expected, circulating levels of phenytoin can be decreased by concomitant use of other "hepatic enzyme inducers" (e.g., barbiturates, carbamazepine, chronic ethanol, dexamethasone, rifampin). Because it can precipitate acute attacks, use of phenytoin should be avoided if possible in patients with hepatic forms of porphyria.

In contrast, inhibitors of the hepatic enzymes, CYP28/C9 (e.g., amiodarone, cimetidine, fluvoxamine, some nonsteroidal antiinflammatory drugs, metronidazole, ritonavir, sulfonamides, troglitazone, valproic acid) and CYP2C19 (e.g., felbamate, fluconazole, fluoxetine, fluvoxamine, omeprazole) can increase circulating phenytoin levels.[4]

Adverse reactions/toxicities: phenytoin is associated with thrombophlebitis and toxic epidermal necrolysis.[20,21] Administration of the drug can induce hypotension, bradycardia, and bundle branch block, especially if the drug is administered rapidly (>50 mg/min). A phenytoin-induced rash is quite common (20%).[4] Hyperglycemia, leukopenia, and thrombocytopenia are reported complications of therapy with phenytoin. Skin necrosis related to extravasation of phenytoin can occur at the site for IV infusion of the drug. For this reason, fosphenytoin is a preferable agent, particularly when completely reliable venous access is unavailable. Small veins can develop phlebitis and cause transient discomfort during infusion even if no extravasation occurs.

Side effects: with long-term use of phenytoin include gingival hypertrophy, cerebellar atrophy, coarsening of facial features, osteoporosis, vitamin D deficiency, and peripheral neuropathy.[1,4,10] In high doses or concentrations, administration of phenytoin can be associated with nystagmus, diplopia, ataxia, slurred speech, drowsiness, and coma.

FOSPHENYTOIN

Fosphenytoin (Cerebyx) is a phosphate ester prodrug of phenytoin. It is highly water soluble. When administered parenterally (IV or IM), fosphenytoin is rapidly metabolized into phenytoin. It can be infused up to three times faster than phenytoin (i.e., maximal rate of infusion, 150 mg/min).[22] The times to peak effect are similar for phenytoin and fosphenytoin, because enzymatic conversion of the prodrug occurs rapidly. Kugler et al. suggested that fosphenytoin and phenytoin are likely to control status epilepticus with similar rapidity.[23] The benefits of fosphenytoin compared to phenytoin are faster safe rate of administration and lower likelihood for certain adverse effects (e.g., hypotension, phlebitis, and soft-tissue injury from extravasation). Although fosphenytoin is more expensive than phenytoin, the costs associated with treating complications from the use of IV phenytoin can be substantially greater; accordingly, fosphenytoin may be advantageous on a pharmaco-economic basis.[20]

Dosing

Although a different drug from phenytoin when initially administered, the dosage of fosphenytoin is always described in phenytoin equivalents (PE). Because fosphenytoin is water soluble, it can be administered safely IM, whereas phenytoin cannot.[24]

Adults: for acute management and in prophylaxis, 15 to 20 mg/kg IV administered at 100 to 150 mg/min.[22] Maintenance dose is 4 to 6 mg/kg/d IV or IM; oral phenytoin is 90% bioavailable, as compared to 100% bioavailability using IV and IM preparations, so a higher dosage may be necessary when converting from IV or IM to PO. Therapeutic range is the same as the therapeutic range for phenytoin: 10 to 20 µg/mL.

Elderly: the geriatric population may be more sensitive to hypotension and sedation associated with higher infusion rates.

Hepatic impairment: phenytoin clearance can be markedly reduced in cirrhosis; free phenytoin levels should be monitored.

Renal impairment: free phenytoin levels should be monitored closely. Phenytoin is not significantly dialyzed.

Forms available: injection solution 75 mg/mL (equivalent to phenytoin sodium 50 mg/mL).

Mechanism of action: fosphenytoin is the diphosphate ester salt of phenytoin, which acts as a water soluble prodrug of phenytoin. Following administration, plasma esterases convert fosphenytoin to phosphate, formaldehyde, and phenytoin as the active moiety. Phenytoin acts as a sodium channel blocker to reduce neuronal excitability.

Pharmacokinetics

Absorption: the rise in serum concentration of fosphenytoin may be faster compared to phenytoin when administered IV, because of the higher maximal recommended infusion rate for the prodrug (150 mg/min versus 50 mg/min, respectively). However, owing to the necessary biotransformation (conversion to phenytoin after IV administration is approximately 15 minutes), the resulting time-to-peak serum levels of phenytoin are similar for the two agents.[22] Bioavailability of each approaches 100%.

Distribution: 95% to 99% of fosphenytoin is bound to albumin. During IV administration, fosphenytoin can displace phenytoin and increase free fraction (up to 30% unbound) during the period required for conversion of fosphenytoin to phenytoin. The half-life of fosphenytoin is 12 to 29 hours.

Elimination: fosphenytoin is excreted in the urine as an inactive metabolite.

Metabolism: fosphenytoin is converted via hydrolysis to phenytoin. See Phenytoin for further metabolism.

Drug interactions: see Phenytoin monograph.

Adverse reactions/toxicities: most important with IV use of fosphenytoin (or phenytoin) are cardiovascular collapse and/or CNS depression. Paresthesias and pruritus are more common with fosphenytoin than phenytoin and occur more often with IV than IM administration.[4,10] The drug is contraindicated for patients with sinus bradycardia, sinoatrial block, second- or third-degree atrioventricular (AV) block, or Stokes-Adams syndrome. As with phenytoin, it is important to monitor hematologic and liver function tests. Other side effects include gingival hyperplasia, gynecomastia, bone marrow suppression, and vermian cerebellar atrophy.[4,10] Venous irritation is less common with fosphenytoin compared to phenytoin.[25]

Contraindications: pregnancy category D.

CARBAMAZEPINE

Carbamazepine (Tegretol) is indicated for partial seizures with complex symptomatology (psychomotor, temporal lobe), generalized tonic/clonic (grand mal) seizures, and mixed seizure patterns. The drug is not available for IV administration and is rarely used for acute termination of seizures or as standard prophylaxis in the ICU. When using carbamazepine, it is recommended (see later) to monitor complete blood count, reticulocyte count, serum iron concentration, liver function tests, urinalysis, serum electrolytes, serum drug levels, and thyroid function tests.

Dosing

Adults: typically carbamazepine is dosed as 200 mg twice or thrice daily, then increased by 200 mg/d at weekly intervals until therapeutic levels are achieved. The usual therapeutic dose is 800 to 1200 mg/d in 3 to 4 divided doses. Dosage must be adjusted according to the patient's response and serum concentrations (therapeutic range is 4-12 μg/mL).[26]

Elderly: lower doses are typically used in the elderly: 100 mg 1 to 2 times per day. The typical dose is 400 to 1000 mg/d.

Hepatic impairment: carbamazepine is hepatically metabolized to an epoxide intermediate, which itself has an appreciable anticonvulsant action.

Renal impairment: in renal impairment, if GFR is less than 10 mL/min, administer 75% of typical dose.

Forms available: capsule, extended release (200 mg, 300 mg); oral suspension, 100 mg/5 mL; tablet, 200 mg; chewable tablet, 100 mg; extended-release tablet, 100 mg, 200 mg, 400 mg.

Mechanism of action: like phenytoin, carbamazepine acts as a sodium channel blocker. It also stimulates release of antidiuretic hormone (ADH) and is chemically related to the tricyclic antidepressants.

Pharmacokinetics

Absorption: orally administered doses of carbamazepine are slowly absorbed, and the time to peak circulating concentration is 4 to 8 hours. Bioavailability approximates 85%.

Distribution: V_d of carbamazepine is 1 to 2 L/kg in adults; 75% to 90% of the drug is protein bound.[26]

Elimination: carbamazepine is excreted in the urine.

Metabolism: carbamazepine is hepatically metabolized to an active epoxide metabolite; half-life is 8 to 60 hours.[27]

Drug interactions: oral carbamazepine suspension should not be administered at the same time as other liquid medicinal agents, as it can form a precipitate when combined with chlorpromazine or thioridazine. Barbiturates, benzodiazepines, and phenytoin can decrease plasma carbamazepine levels, owing to induction of hepatic metabolism.[3,10] Conversely, isoniazid, felbamate, danazol, diltiazem, and verapamil can increase plasma carbamazepine levels. Carbamazepine itself can increase the metabolism of warfarin, valproic acid, tricyclic antidepressants (particularly selective serotonin reuptake inhibitors [SSRIs]), thyroxine, theophylline, oral contraceptives, methadone, doxycycline, corticosteroids, calcium channel blockers (except diltiazem and verapamil), cyclosporine, tacrolimus, and ethosuximide.[10]

Adverse reactions/toxicities: like phenytoin, carbamazepine can induce AV block and other dysrhythmias.[28] Carbamazepine can promote sedation, dizziness, ataxia, and rash, although less commonly than phenytoin. Severe hyponatremia secondary to SIADH is a relatively common adverse effect of carbamazepine.[2] Nausea, aplastic anemia, agranulocytosis, thrombocytopenia, bone marrow suppression, and hepatic failure all have been reported. Pregnancy category D.

Contraindications: carbamazepine should not be used concurrently with monoamine oxidase (MAO) inhibitors and should be administered with caution to patients with hepatic, renal, or hematologic disease. Caution should be exercised in patients with increased intraocular pressure, as carbamazepine has mild anticholinergic activity.

VALPROIC ACID

Valproic acid is indicated as monotherapy and as adjunctive therapy in the treatment of almost all seizures types, including complex partial seizures, absence seizures, generalized tonic/clonic seizures, myoclonic seizures, and other partial seizures. In two European studies, IV valproate was shown to be effective for the treatment of refractory status epilepticus.[29,30] Because of the recent availability of an IV formulation, valproic acid is now used relatively commonly in the ICU setting and as a treatment for acute seizures including status epilepticus.

Dosing

Adults: usual oral adult dose of valproic acid is 10 to 15 mg/kg/d in 3 divided doses, increased by 5 to 10 mg/kg/d at weekly intervals until therapeutic levels are achieved. Maintenance dose is 30 to 60 mg/kg/d. Sustained-release valproic acid (Depakote ER) is usually given once daily. Conversion to ER may require an increase in the dose by 20%. The IV dose is 15 to 20 mg/kg, with an IV infusion rate limit of 20 mg/min.

Elderly: dosing of valproic acid is approximately the same as the adult dosing recommendation.

Hepatic impairment: dosage reduction is necessary with hepatic failure, as the clearance of valproic acid is decreased in patients with impaired liver funciton.[1,31] Decreased plasma albumin concentration in hepatic disease is associated with a 2- to 2.6-fold increase in the unbound fraction of the drug. Therefore, free concentrations of valproate can be elevated even when the total concentration of drug is within the therapeutic range.

Renal impairment: when GFR is less than 10 mL/min, clearance of unbound in valproic acid is reduced by 27%. Hemodialysis reduces circulating valproic acid concentrations by 20%. Because valproic acid is highly protein bound, dialysis is not very effective for clearing the drug.

Forms available: capsule, 250 mg; capsule/sprinkles, 125 mg; injection, 100 mg/mL (5 mL), syrup, 250 mg/5 mL (5 mL, 480 mL); tablet, *delayed* release (125 mg, 250 mg, 500 mg); tablet, *extended* release (250 mg, 500 mg).

Mechanism of action: current data suggest that valproic acid increases the availability of GABA. Alternatively, the drug may enhance the action of GABA. Valproic acid also is thought to act on thalamic (T-type) calcium channels as an inhibitor, and it also may cause sodium channel blockade and enhanced potassium channel conductance.

Pharmacokinetics

Absorption: enteric forms of valproic acid are rapidly and nearly completely absorbed from the GI tract. Peak plasma concentrations are observed 1 to 4 hours following ingestion. Therapeutic serum concentrations are 50 to 125 μg/mL.

Distribution: valproic acid is 80% to 90% protein bound. Hence, at usual concentrations or dosing, the V_d is only slightly greater than plasma volume.

Elimination: valproic acid is excreted in urine following hepatic metabolism. Less than 3% of the anticonvulsant is excreted unchanged in the urine, and it is eliminated by first-order kinetics. The half-life of valproic acid is 9 to 16 hours.

Metabolism: valproic acid is metabolized extensively by the liver via glucuronic acid conjugation and mitochondrial β and ω

oxidation to produce multiple metabolites, some of which are biologically active.

Drug interactions: serum levels of valproic acid can be reduced by acyclovir, whereas lamotrigine and phenytoin can induce metabolism of the drug.[3,10] Valproic acid can increase circulating diazepam, lamotrigine, and carbamazepine concentrations.[32] Macrolide antibiotics and nimodipine can decrease metabolism of valproic acid. Metabolism of phenobarbital is inhibited by valproic acid.

Adverse reactions/toxicities: potential side effects of valproic acid include somnolence, dizziness, insomnia, alopecia, pancreatitis,[33] thrombocytopenia, tremor, weight gain, rash, bone marrow suppression,[34] decreased carnitine, hyperammonemia, and SIADH. Additionally, the anticonvulsant has been reported to cause frank hepatic failure. Developmentally, neural tube defects are a recognized toxicity. Valproic acid can stimulate the replication of human immunodeficiency virus (HIV) and cytomegalovirus (CMV) in infected patients.

Acute valproic acid intoxication induces mild to moderate lethargy at lower doses and coma or fatal cerebral edema at higher, more toxic doses.[35] In contrast to either phenytoin or carbamazepine, nystagmus, dysarthria, and ataxia are rarely noted following valproic acid overdose. Valproic acid can increase serum ammonia levels through interaction with carnitine. In the management of valproic acid intoxication, naloxone occasionally is effective for reversing symptoms.

Contraindications: pregnancy, urea cycle disorders, hepatic dysfunction.

PROPOFOL

Typically used for induction and/or maintenance of anesthesia, propofol occasionally is used for the acute termination of seizures and for treatment of status epilepticus. Propofol is not a true "anticonvulsant," as seizures are terminated only by virtue of the induction of general anesthesia. The drug must be used in association with continuous cardiac and blood pressure monitoring, and the patient prepared for mechanical ventilation.

Dosing

Adults: dosage of propofol must be individualized based on total body weight and titrated to desired effect. When given as a continuous infusion, the initial sedation dose is usually 1.2 mg/kg/h (20 µg/kg/min). However, for cessation of seizures, a dose yielding a general anesthetic state (or a flat or "burst-suppression" electroencephalogram [EEG]) is required, and this dose is in the range of 7.2 to 14 mg/kg/h (120-240 µg/kg/min).[36] The infusion rate can be increased by 1 to 2 mg/kg/h every 5 to 10 minutes until the desired sedation level or EEG correlate is achieved.

Elderly: doses of propofol should be reduced for elderly patients, as less drug is required to promote EEG silence or burst suppression.

Hepatic impairment: propofol is hepatically metabolized, and metabolic intermediates may be toxic. Such intermediates may accumulate during low-flow states (e.g., due to low cardiac output).

Renal impairment: propofol is hepatically metabolized, and the conjugated drug is excreted in urine.

Forms available: propofol comes as an emulsion (10 or 20 mg/mL); contains sodium metabisulfite, egg lecithin, soybean oil, and EDTA.

Mechanism of action: the mechanism of this drug appears to be similar to that for ultra short-acting barbiturates. Propofol is a GABA receptor agonist. It is a phenolic compound with general anesthetic properties. It is, however, structurally unrelated to the barbiturates, opioids, or benzodiazepines.

Pharmacokinetics

Absorption: onset of action of propofol is extremely rapid; one "arm-brain circulation time," 10 to 15 seconds.[37]

Distribution: the drug is highly lipophilic and has a large V_d of 2 to 10 L/kg. Propofol is 97% to 99% protein bound while in plasma.

Elimination: duration of action is approximately 3 to 5 minutes after a single bolus. It is excreted in the urine (88% as metabolites, 40% as the glucuronide metabolite). Clearance of propofol is 20 to 30 mL/kg/min, which exceeds liver blood flow.[37] There is some evidence to suggest extrahepatic sites of propofol metabolism to account for the rapid clearance of the drug.

Metabolism: propofol is metabolized in the liver (and possibly additional sites) to water-soluble sulfate and glucuronide conjugates.

Drug interactions: propofol can potentiate the neuromuscular blockade of vecuronium.[36]

Adverse reactions/toxicities: common side effects include burning discomfort at the injection site, hypotension, and apnea. Propofol can promote respiratory acidosis as patients are weaned from mechanical ventilation. The use of propofol may have more severe cardiovascular consequences in patients with severe cardiac disease (ejection fraction < 50%). The emulsion promoted development of hypozincemia due to the chelating action of the additive, ethylenediaminetetraacetate (EDTA). Because the drug is insoluble in aqueous solvents, it is formulated as an emulsion that is a potential growth medium for bacteria.[38] Thus, EDTA is added as a bacteriostatic agent, but the risk of contamination with bacteria remains a concern. Strict aseptic technique must be observed with its use, and IV delivery lines should be changed routinely.

A "propofol infusion syndrome" has been described, and common clinical features can include hyperkalemia, hepatomegaly, lipemia, metabolic acidosis, myocardial failure, and rhabdomyolysis.[39] This syndrome was initially described in children who were cared for in an ICU for prolonged periods, using high doses of propofol for sedation.[40-42] Propofol-induced lactic acidosis and myocardial dysfunction also can occur in adults.[39] Administration of propofol in the ICU should be restricted to doses ≤ 5 mg/kg/h, and infusion of propofol for the purpose of sedating critically ill adults should be limited to 48 hours, especially if high (general anesthesia level) doses are being used.

Contraindications: propofol is relatively contraindicated in patients with increased intracranial pressure (ICP) or in patients with hyperlipidemia or sepsis. Due to the emulsion base, patients who are allergic to egg whites also should not be given this drug. Pregnancy category is B. For seizure control, propofol is absolutely contraindicated in nonintubated patients, because induction of general anesthesia is required to terminate seizure activity.

PHENOBARBITAL

Phenobarbital remains a mainstay of anticonvulsant therapy. As a potent GABA agonist, phenobarbital is an effective anticonvulsant against a broad range of seizure types, The drug is used most commonly to treat or prevent generalized motor seizures. A favorable feature is its relative lack of serious toxic effects. Additional desirable characteristics of the drug which recommend it for use in the ICU include its broad efficacy, its availability for IV administration, ability to titrate the dose of the drug to burst suppression on the EEG,[43-45] and ease of transition to PO dosing if desired. Its chief negative attributes include its long half-life and its tendency to induce hepatic enzyme expression.

Dosing

Adults: oral, 30 to 120 mg/d in 2 to 3 divided doses; in status epilepticus, loading dose is 15 to 18 mg/kg IV.[45] Anticonvulsant maintenance dose ranges between 1 and 3 mg/kg/d in divided doses.

Elderly: phenobarbital is not recommended for use in the elderly, although in the outpatient setting, the drug is often used in this population of patients.

Hepatic impairment: metabolism of phenobarbital is primarily hepatic, so increased side effects can occur in patients with severe liver disease. One should monitor plasma levels and liver function tests to estimate clearance of this already long-acting agent.

Renal impairment: when GFR is less than 10 mL/min, phenobarbital should be administered every 12 to 16 hours. Phenobarbital, unlike phenytoin, is substantively (20%-50%) cleared during hemodialysis.

Forms available: elixir, 20 mg/5 mL; injection, 60 mg/mL, 130 mg/mL; tablet, 15 mg, 30 mg, 32 mg, 60 mg, 65 mg, 100 mg.

Mechanism of action: classic and potent GABA agonist at the barbiturate locus of the GABA receptor site of the chloride channel.

Pharmacokinetics

Absorption: oral absorption is rapid and almost complete (70%-90%). Time to peak plasma concentration is 1 to 6 hours following an oral dose and approximately 30 minutes after IV administration. Serum reference range is 20 to 40 μg/mL.

Distribution: phenobarbital is 20% to 45% protein bound, which is less than the case for many other anticonvulsants.

Elimination: half-life in adults is 37 to 73 hours. Hepatic metabolites are excreted in urine, and 20% to 50% of the drug is excreted unchanged in urine.

Metabolism: phenobarbital is chemically modified by the liver via hydroxylation and glucuronide conjugation.

Drug interactions: barbiturates are enzyme inducers and thus can reduce the half-life of many agents, as well as increase toxicity of those drugs having toxic intermediates as a result of hepatic metabolism.[1,10] Thus, barbiturates can enhance the hepatotoxicity of acetaminophen. Phenobarbital increases the metabolism of antiarrhythmics (disopyramide, propafenone, and quinidine), anticonvulsants (ethosuximide, lamotrigine, phenytoin, tiagabine, topiramate, and zonisamide, but not levetiracetam or gabapentin), beta-blockers, calcium channel blockers, chloramphenicol, cimetidine, corticosteroids, cyclosporine, doxycycline, estrogens, furosemide, methadone, oral contraceptives, tricyclic antidepressants, and warfarin.[3,10] Conversely, the metabolism of barbiturates is inhibited by MAO inhibitors and valproic acid. Barbiturates can decrease vitamin D levels.

Adverse reactions/toxicities: phenobarbital, like all barbiturates, retards cerebral excitation and can lead to cognitive dysfunction, sedation, lethargy, ataxia, nystagmus, and (in large doses) coma and respiratory depression.[43-45] Although uncommon, hematologic disturbances can occur and include agranulocytosis, thrombocytopenia, and megaloblastic anemia.[1] Administration of activated charcoal and hemoperfusion are therapeutic interventions which have been implemented in cases of acute massive phenobarbital poisoning.[46-48]

Contraindications: since barbiturates have a significant impact on hepatic function, these drugs should be used with caution or not at all in patients with hepatic impairment. Phenobarbital should not be given to patients with porphyria. When phenobarbital is given in large doses, such as to arrest active seizures, respiratory depression is a major concern, and airway protection is commonly required. Phenobarbital is not suggested for use during pregnancy, but considering that all anticonvulsants fall into this category, it appears no worse than other agents. Indeed, concerns related to promotion of neural tube defects and other malformations, which are associated with other agents, may be less of a concern with phenobarbital.

NEWER ANTICONVULSANTS

Several newer anticonvulsants have been introduced into the market during the past 15 years. However, the lack of available IV preparations severely limits their use in treating seizures in the ICU. The agents typically used are initiated when enteral therapy is suitable. Some studies have demonstrated that the oral preparations of some of these agents can still be of some benefit. Topiramate tablets, for example, have been administered when crushed to a powder and mixed with water and administered via nasogastric tube and have been shown to be effective in refractory status epilepticus. Agents like gabapentin, lamotrigine, topiramate, and vigabatrin are often considered more suitable for adjunctive therapy than for monotherapy. Lamotrigine is the only agent approved for monotherapy, but gabapentin and oxcarbazepine also soon may have such an indication.[8,49]

Gabapentin and vigabatrin are excreted unchanged in the urine and are useful for treating patients with hepatic failure. In patients with renal failure, vigabatrin, gabapentin, and topiramate should be used cautiously and in reduced dosages. The pharmacokinetics of tiagabine are not affected by either renal or hepatic dysfunction. The possibility of drug interaction is important to know as well. Combination therapy with lamotrigine and carbamazepine can increase the risk of carbamazepine-induced toxic effects. Other anticonvulsant drugs have little effect on gabapentin; it also has no substantial influence on the pharmacokinetics and serum concentrations of other seizure medications.[8,49]

LEVETIRACETAM (KEPPRA)

Levetiracetam is currently recommended for use as adjunctive therapy against partial-onset seizures. There is, nonetheless, increasing interest in this drug for use in the ICU setting because of its very low toxicity and relatively low tendency to promote drug-drug interactions. It is now available in an IV preparation and is frequently used to aid in the treatment of new-onset seizures.

Dosing

Adults: agent is available in both PO and IV preparations; dosing is typically 500 to 1500 mg twice daily, with a maximal recommended dose of 3000 mg/d. Higher doses have been used, however. It can be loaded in dosing equal to 500 mg, 1000 mg, or 1500 mg; this can be done orally or with IV dosing.

Elderly: no major changes in dosing have been recommended.

Hepatic impairment: no adjustment for hepatic impairment is required.

Renal impairment: the following is recommended:
GFR above 80 mL/min: 500 to 1500 mg twice daily
GFR 50 to 80 mL/min: 500 to 1000 mg twice daily
GFR 30 to 50 mL/min 250 to 750 mg twice daily
GFR less than 30 mL/min 250 to 500 mg twice daily
Patients with end-stage renal failure and receiving hemodialysis should be treated with 500 to 1000 mg daily, plus a supplemental dose of 250 to 500 mg after each dialysis session. Approximately 50% of levetiracetam is removed during standard hemodialysis.

Forms available: levetiracetam is available in PO form (tablet [250 mg, 500 mg, 750 mg]) and as an IV preparation in prepackaged doses of 500 mg/250 mL.

Mechanism of action: the mechanism for anticonvulsant action of this drug is unknown.

Pharmacokinetics

Absorption: following PO ingestion, absorption is both rapid and complete. Time to peak effect is 1 hour, with 100% bioavailability.

Distribution: levetiracetam is less than 10% protein bound.

Elimination: the drug has a half-life of approximately 6 to 8 hours and is excreted essentially unchanged in urine.

Metabolism: the drug is not extensively metabolized.

Drug Interactions: no significant drug interactions have been reported.

Adverse Reactions/Toxicities: although relatively free of side effects, somnolence, weakness, ataxia, and dizziness can occur. Behavioral abnormalities have been reported, although rarely. There is some evidence linking levetiracetam with bone marrow suppression.[4]

Contraindications: pregnancy category C.

LACOSAMIDE (VIMPAT)

Lacosamide (previously known as *harkoseride*) is indicated as adjunctive treatment for partial-onset seizures. It comes in both a PO and IV formulation and is hence an alternative agent for those patients unable to take oral preparations.[50]

Dosing

Adults: initial oral dosing recommendation is 100 to 200 mg twice daily and a maximal dose of 600 mg/d.

Elderly: there is only limited age-dependent variability in sensitivity and dose delivery.[51]

Hepatic impairment: Lacosamide is methylated via the cytochrome P450 enzyme, CYP2C19 prior to renal excretion. In the presence of hepatic dysfunction, the drug is renally excreted in polarized (20%) and unmetabolized (40%) forms.[52,53]

Renal impairment: dose reductions may be necessary based on the patient's creatinine clearance.

Forms available: lacosamide is available in tablets (50 mg, 100 mg, 150 mg, 200 mg) and IV formulations (200 mg in 250 mL D_5W).

Mechanism of action: lacosamide is a slow inactivator of voltage-gated sodium channels.

Pharmacokinetics

Absorption: the drug is completely absorbed after oral administration.

Distribution: lacosamide is absorbed into the blood with less than 15% binding to proteins in plasma.

Elimination: drug half-life is 13 hours, and peak concentration occurs at 1 to 4 hours. The drug is renally excreted.

Metabolism: there is no appreciable drug metabolism.

Drug interactions: lacosamide does not effect plasma concentrations of anticonvulsants such as carbamazepine (or its epoxide metabolite, levetiracetam), oxcarbazepine MHD (10-monohydroxy metabolite of oxcarbazepine), lamotrigine, topiramate, valproate, phenytoin, or other drugs such as metformin, digoxin, oral contraceptives, or omeprazole.[52,53] Also, carbamazepine, valproic acid, metformin, digoxin, oral contraceptives, and omeprazole do not effect plasma concentrations of lacosamide.

Adverse reactions/toxicities: although the drug is usually very well tolerated, lacosamide can induce dizziness, headache, nausea, diplopia, vomiting, blurred vision, somnolence, ataxia, or fatigue.

Contraindications: cardiogenic syncope and arrhythmias. A slight prolongation of the P-R interval has been observed. It should be avoided in pregnancy if possible.

GABAPENTIN (NEURONTIN)

Gabapentin is indicated as adjunctive treatment for partial-onset seizures. It is also widely prescribed for the treatment of neurogenic or neuropathic pain.

Dosing

Adults: only the oral dose is available, and initial dosing recommendations are 300 mg thrice daily, with a maximum dose of 3600 mg/d.

Elderly: dose reductions may be necessary for gabapentin, based on age-related decreases in renal function.

Hepatic impairment: no dosage adjustment is required.

Renal impairment: dose reductions may be necessary based on the patient's creatinine clearance. Supplemental dosing is commonly administered following hemodialysis.

Forms available: gabapentin is available in capsule (100 mg, 300 mg, 400 mg), elixir (250 mg/5 mL), and tablet (600 mg, 800 mg) forms.

Mechanism of action: exact mechanism of action remains unknown. It appears not to interact with GABA receptors.

Pharmacokinetics

Absorption: the drug is incompletely absorbed (50%-60%).

Distribution: gabapentin's V_d is only 0.6 to 0.8 L/kg, and protein binding is minimal.

Elimination: the drug's half-life is 5 to 6 hours, and it is renally excreted.

Metabolism: there is no appreciable drug metabolism.

Drug interactions: the interactions of gabapentin with other agents are not as complex as they are with phenytoin, valproic acid, or phenobarbital. By the same token, gabapentin is not as "clean" as levetiracetam in terms of the potential for drug-drug interactions. Antacids reduce the bioavailability of enteral gabapentin by 20%.[4] Thus, gabapentin should be taken at least 2 hours after antacid administration. Cimetidine can decrease the clearance of gabapentin. Serum concentrations of gabapentin have been shown to increase with concurrent morphine use. Although phenytoin serum concentrations can be increased by gabapentin, valproic acid, carbamazepine, and phenobarbital do not seem to be affected by this drug.[3,4,10]

Adverse reactions/toxicities: although it is usually very well tolerated, gabapentin can induce somnolence, dizziness, ataxia, fatigue, peripheral edema, pruritus, nausea and vomiting, leukopenia, and tremor.[4]

Contraindications: pregnancy category C.

ANNOTATED REFERENCES

Dreifuss FE. Toxic effects of drugs used in the ICU. Anticonvulsant agents. Crit Care Clin 1991; 7:521-32.

This is an excellent review of the most common anticonvulsants used in the ICU. Despite its age, the information remains highly useful, especially in light of the fact that most medications used for the treatment of seizures in the ICU setting are the older, IV-available preparations (except valproic acid, which is more recent).

Cramer JA, Fisher R, Ben-Menachem E, et al. New antiepileptic drugs: comparison of key clinical trials. Epilepsia 1999;40:590-600.

A good review of data accrued from clinical trials of five new antiepileptic drugs (AEDs). The efficacy in reducing seizures and self-reported adverse events are incorporated here as a basis of selection among new AEDs. Drawbacks to use of these data also are demonstrated.

Treiman DM, Meyers PD, Walton NY, et al. A comparison of four treatments for generalized convulsive status epilepticus. Veterans Affairs Status Epilepticus Cooperative Study Group. N Engl J Med 1998;339:792-8.

This represents the largest controlled drug trial (384 patients) for the treatment of status epilepticus: a 5-year randomized, double blind, multicenter trial of four IV regimens: diazepam followed by phenytoin, lorazepam, phenobarbital, and phenytoin. The study concluded that lorazepam was superior to phenytoin alone (P < 0.02), and phenobarbital and phenytoin/diazepam were similar in efficacy to lorazepam.

Mirski MA, Williams MA, Hanley DF. Prolonged pentobarbital and phenobarbitone coma for refractory generalized status epilepticus. Crit Care Med 1995;23:400-4.

A case report of a particularly difficult and refractory case of status epilepticus that describes the difficulties of adequacy of control and treatment with the adverse actions of the anticonvulsant therapeutics. Included are clearly presented problematic issues relating to hepatic enzyme induction, polypharmacy, induced "burst-suppression" coma, hemodynamic and respiratory decompensation, and emergence with control of the primary seizure state. This describes the longest duration of barbiturate coma for the treatment of seizures that has been reported, 53 days, with good outcome.

Varelas P, Mirski MA. Seizures in the ICU. J Neurosurg Anesthesiol 2001;13:163-75.

A recent comprehensive review of seizures occurring in the ICU setting; it includes etiology of seizures (including a review of the ICU iatrogenic causes), diagnosis algorithm, and treatment. Numerous tables of anticonvulsant drug mechanisms, toxicity, and drug-drug interactions are included.

Asconape J. Some common issues in the use of antiepileptic drugs. Semin Neurol 2002;22:27-39.

In this article, several common clinical situations in the management of patients with epilepsy are presented in the form of case studies. These cases illustrate current aspects of the use of the anticonvulsants and will give some guidelines to help the treating physician in the increasingly complex process of seizure therapy.

REFERENCE

Access the complete reference list online at http://www.expertconsult.com.

173

Calcium Channel Blocker Toxicity

DANIEL E. BROOKS | KENNETH D. KATZ

Calcium channel blockers (CCBs), also referred to as *calcium entry blocking agents* or *calcium antagonists*, are commonly used in the treatment of angina, hypertension, and headache disorders. Their use is complicated by adverse side effects, iatrogenic errors, and intentional overdoses. Significant morbidity and mortality can occur after accidental or intentional poisoning. In 2008, the American Association of Poison Control Centers recorded 10,398 human exposures to CCBs and 60 deaths. As a group, cardiovascular drugs including CCBs were responsible for more than 91,000 human exposures and 238 deaths.[1]

Pharmacology

CCBs are classified into five groups based on structure or functional activity. The first group, exemplified by the T-channel blocker mibefradil, is unique because these agents antagonize T-type calcium channels. The other four groups all antagonize L-type calcium channels and are divided based on structural differences. These groups include the phenylalkylamines (e.g., verapamil), benzothiazepine (diltiazem), dihydropyridines (e.g., nifedipine and the synthetic agent, clevidipine), and diarylaminopropylamine ether (bepridil). Their mechanism of action involves inhibition of calcium influx through voltage-dependent L-type calcium channels.[2,3,4] This inhibition results in decreased intracellular calcium concentration, relaxation of vascular smooth muscle, decreased systemic vascular resistance, and inhibition of intracardiac nodal excitation.[3,5] Some CCBs, particularly verapamil, have higher binding affinity for myocardial calcium channels, resulting in sinoatrial and atrioventricular nodal inhibiton.[3,6]

The most commonly used CCBs (verapamil, diltiazem, and nifedipine) are well absorbed, highly protein bound at therapeutic concentrations, and undergo a variable amount of first-pass metabolism following oral administration.[7,8] There is variability in volumes of distribution (V_d). For example, the V_d for verapamil is 5.3 L/kg, whereas the V_d for nifedipine is 0.8 L/kg. These characteristics (high protein binding and large V_d) suggest limited utility of hemodialysis for toxicity. After absorption, CCBs are hepatically metabolized by saturable enzymes to metabolites with variable activity.[7,9-11] Therapeutic half-lives range from less than two hours to longer than 60 hours. After massive ingestion or in patients with congestive heart failure or hepatic dysfunction, decreased metabolism leads to increased concentrations of active compounds and prolonged half-lives.[12-15] Patients with decreased hepatic perfusion or function may experience decreased elimination of CCBs.[10,16]

All CCBs are pregnancy category C drugs and have been associated with teratogenic and embryocidal effects in animal studies. After therapeutic use, CCBs can be recovered from breast milk and exposed offspring, but the effects of these drugs on neonates require further investigation.[17-20]

Clinical Manifestations of Toxicity

The potentially life-threatening effects of CCB intoxication are related to alterations in the function of the cardiovascular system. The most common clinical manifestations are sinus bradycardia, hypotension, and shock. Clinical effects may vary in mild to moderate poisoning, depending on the specific medication. Toxic doses of phenylalkylamines or benzothiazepines commonly cause bradycardia and hypotension secondary to the negative inotropic and chronotropic effects

of these drugs.[21,22] Toxic doses of dihydropyridines, however, may result in hypotension with reflex tachycardia because of the affinity of these agents for the peripheral vasculature.[21,22] In massive overdoses, specificity is lost, and all CCBs can cause bradycardia, depressed cardiac contractility, and cardiovascular collapse.[22] Furthermore, cardiovascular compromise may be compounded by ingestion of other cardiovascular toxins, in addition to underlying patient comorbidities. Of note, sustained-release preparations can cause delayed-onset toxicity as late as 12 hours or longer after ingestion.[2,21]

Pulmonary toxicity from CCB poisoning includes both cardiogenic and noncardiogenic pulmonary edema secondary to several purported mechanisms: negative chronotropy, excessive fluid resuscitation, increased capillary permeability secondary to drug effects, and increased sympathetic discharge in response to shock.[23]

Neurologic manifestations include myoclonus, dizziness, syncope, focal deficits, and seizures. These neurologic findings are most likely related to central nervous system hypoperfusion.[22,24] Gastrointestinal symptoms due to toxic doses of CCBs are nonspecific and include nausea and vomiting.[22] CCB toxicity with ensuing shock can cause diffuse organ dysfunction, such as acute kidney injury, secondary to poor tissue perfusion.

Metabolic derangements can include hypokalemia and hyperglycemia. Abnormally high circulating glucose levels are due to calcium channel antagonism in the pancreatic beta islet cells, which inhibits insulin release.[25] Metabolic acidosis can be caused by poor tissue perfusion and mitochondrial dehydrogenase inhibition.[26]

Differential Diagnosis

The most common agents in the differential diagnosis of CCB poisoning are β-adrenergic antagonists, cardiac glycosides, imidazolines, class 1a and 1c antidysrhythmics, cyanide, organophosphates, and late tricyclic antidepressants.[22,27] Also included in the differential diagnosis of CCB poisoning are nontoxicologic entities such as acute coronary syndromes, hyperkalemia, myxedema coma, hypothermia, and sepsis.

Diagnostic Testing

The diagnosis of CCB poisoning is based predominately on history and physical examination. Both routine and comprehensive drug screening assays routinely miss CCBs.[28] Although there are no specific laboratory tests available to diagnose CCB poisoning, some laboratory studies should be obtained to aid clinical management.

A 12-lead electrocardiogram should be obtained to define the cardiac rhythm and intervals. Arterial or venous blood gas measurements offer rapid assessment of tissue perfusion, acid-base status, and critical electrolytes. Chest radiography can demonstrate cardiac size and pulmonary edema. Serum electrolytes and markers of renal function should be measured. Serum calcium levels are neither affected by CCBs nor routinely helpful, but serial levels may be necessary for patients treated with parenteral calcium. Echocardiography may help management decisions based on fluid status, global function, and chamber sizes.

Serum levels of cardioactive medications with established therapeutic concentrations (e.g., digoxin) should be obtained for patients with a suggestive history or physical examination.

Treatment

Gastric decontamination plays a limited role in the vast majority of acute poisonings, including CCB poisoning. A single dose of activated charcoal, without a cathartic, may be administered within one hour after ingestion if the patient is willing to drink. Insertion of a nasogastric tube solely for the purpose of charcoal administration is not recommended.[29] Whole-bowel irrigation also has been used following the ingestion of sustained-release CCBs but is not routinely indicated.[30,31]

Treatment of the patient poisoned by CCBs focuses on early recognition of shock and aggressive cardiovascular support. Endotracheal intubation and mechanical ventilation are indicated to ensure adequate oxygenation and ventilation if any of the following are present: obtunded mental status, poor airway protective mechanisms, hypoxemia, or arterial hypotension. A low threshold should be used to initiate invasive monitoring techniques (arterial, central venous, or pulmonary arterial catheters) for both administration of treatments and assessment of clinical responses. All symptomatic patients should have a bladder catheter placed to accurately monitor urinary output.

Treatment of patients with CCB toxicity should generally be guided by the degree of end-organ dysfunction (e.g., mental status, cardiac output, urine output) and not solely by blood pressure. For example, a bradycardic patient with normal mental status, normal blood pressure, and no demonstrable acidosis or renal dysfunction may not require further treatment unless clinical deterioration ensues.

Treatment of symptomatic bradycardia includes atropine, external or internal pacing, parenteral calcium, glucagon, vasopressors, and even extracorporeal hemodynamic support. No treatment has been studied in randomized controlled human studies, and their use is based on animal data and/or human case reports. Severely poisoned patients typically require several concomitant therapies to achieve cardiovascular stabilization.

Intravenous (IV) fluids should be administered to hypotensive patients to improve blood pressure and tissue perfusion. In adults, 2 L of lactated Ringer's or normal saline solution should be given. Care should be maintained not to administer excessive volumes of crystalloid solutions to patients poisoned by CCBs because of the risk of pulmonary edema.[23]

Atropine has limited utility in reversing bradycardia, but it may be administered on an emergency basis while other therapies are being prepared.[22,32]

External or internal pacemaker therapy may be attempted to ameliorate symptomatic bradycardia. If capture is achieved, the heart rate should be set at 60 bpm. The target systolic blood pressure should be 90 to 100 mm Hg in order to ensure adequate tissue perfusion. However, pacemaker therapy is often ineffective in sustaining hemodynamic improvement.[22,32]

Administration of parenteral calcium salts may occasionally augment heart rate and blood pressure in the face of CCB poisoning.[32] Calcium chloride contains approximately three times the amount of calcium as the gluconate salt and is the preferred agent.[33] Slow boluses of one to three g of calcium chloride may be given, and a continuous infusion of two to six g/h may be initiated if a response is noted.[34,35] Serum ionized calcium levels should be monitored during parenteral calcium infusions and maintained at approximately 2 to 3 mmol/L.[22,33] If digoxin toxicity is suspected, use of parenteral calcium salts should be avoided; use of digoxin antibodies should be considered.[22]

Although more commonly associated with β-adrenergic antagonist poisoning, IV glucagon may offer another treatment modality. Intravenous glucagon activates adenyl cyclase, leading to increased intracellular levels of the second messenger, cyclic adenosine monophosphate (cAMP). In cardiac myocytes, increased levels of cAMP lead to improvements in cardiac contractility and rate.[21,36] Intravenous boluses of glucagon (2-10 mg) may be administered; if hemodynamics improve, glucagon should be infused at the effective IV mg dose per hour. Side effects of glucagon administration include nausea, vomiting, and hyperglycemia.[22,37]

Although several vasoactive medications have been advocated for the treatment of CCB toxicity, there is no one agent that is clearly optimal. Norepinephrine, dopamine, epinephrine, isoproterenol, amrinone, and aminophylline all have demonstrated efficacy. In general, patients with severe CCB poisoning should receive a pressor titrated to achieve a perfusing blood pressure. In the face of significant hypotension, the choice of vasopressor should be based on the preexisting heart rate. For example, if the patient is hypotensive with reflex tachycardia, an α-adrenergic agonist should be employed. Norepinephrine or epinephrine are reasonable first-line agents, based on the patient's presenting heart rate, blood pressure, and pharmacologic properties.

Four novel therapies for CCB toxicity are insulin/dextrose infusion, hypertonic saline, 4-aminopyridine, and lipid emulsion. The use of an insulin/dextrose infusion (high insulin–euglycemia treatment [HIE] therapy) may correct the state of hypoinsulinemia and impaired cellular glucose uptake found in CCB poisoning.[25] The underlying mechanism of HIE may involve altered myocardial metabolism. Under normal physiologic conditions, the heart preferentially utilizes fatty acids for energy production. However, when drug-induced cardiac dysfunction is present, carbohydrates are used for myocardial energy requirements.[38,39] Despite a lack of concensus, a reasonable starting regimen can be found in Table 173-1. Potassium and glucose concentrations should be monitored closely; blood glucose levels and hemodynamic response will dictate changes in insulin or glucose administration.[3,40,41] Although animal data and human case reports

TABLE 173-1	Pharmaceutical Interventions After Calcium Channel Blocker Toxicity	
Drug	**Dose**	**Goal**
Activated charcoal	1-2 g/kg orally (max. 100 g)	Decreased systemic absorption (give within 1 hour after ingestion)
Whole-bowel irrigation	500-2000 mL/h until clear rectal effluent	Decreased system absorption (use after contacting a poison control center)
IV fluids	2 L of NS or lactated Ringer's solution	Correct dehydration; increased BP and perfusion
Calcium chloride	1 ampule IV over 2 min	Increased HR and SVR
Atropine	0.5-1 mg IV every 3 min (max. 3 mg)	Increased HR and CO
Glucagon	5-10 mg bolus, then 2-10 mg/h infusion	Titrate for increased SVR
Isoproterenol	Initiate at 2 mg/min	Titrate for increased CO
Epinephrine	Initiate at 2 µg/min	Titrate for increased SVR
Norepinephrine	Initiate at 0.5 mg/min	Titrate for increased SVR
Insulin (euglycemia)	1 unit/kg regular insulin IV bolus, then 0.5-1 unit/kg/h. Co-administer 25 g of dextrose if blood glucose is <200 mg/dL.	Titrate for increased CO; closely monitor blood glucose and potassium levels.
Lipid fat emulsion	1-1.5 mL/kg (20% lipid emulsion) IV over 2 min. Can repeat if no effect in 5 min. If effective, start a drip at 0.25 mL/kg/min for 60 min.	Recovery of cardiac output
Ventricular pacing	Achieve ventricular capture at 50-60 bpm	Increased HR and CO
Intraaortic balloon pump	Consult cardiologist	Refractory to all other interventions
Cardiopulmonary bypass	Consult cardiothoracic surgeon	Refractory to all other interventions

BP, blood pressure; *CO*, cardiac output; *HR*, heart rate; *IV*, intravenous; *SVR*, systemic vascular resistance.

describing the use of HIE are increasing, it is not recommended as a first-line agent.[26,41-45]

Hypertonic saline has been studied only in animals as a potential treatment for verapamil poisoning. The proposed mechanism involves increasing the pH around the calcium channel and reversing potential verapamil-induced sodium channel blockade.[46] The drug 4-aminopyridine blocks the outward rectifying potassium channel, allowing more calcium to enter the myocardial cell.[22] This drug has demonstrated success in animal models and in a single verapamil-poisoned patient receiving hemodialysis.[47]

Lipid emulsion (Intralipid) infusion has been used for the treatment of several lipophilic drug-induced toxicities, including verapamil.[48-51] The mechanism of action involves the IV administration of lipids (fat emulsion) that reduce the V_d of lipophilic drugs (e.g., verapamil). By serving as a "sink" for lipophilic drugs, these lipid microspheres bind to intravascular drug and keep it from reaching target tissues. This mechanism suggests that the optimal effect would occur if the lipids are administered very soon after the exposure when a large percentage of the drug is still in the intravascular space.

The use of any experimental therapies, particularly as a first-line approach, cannot be recommended. Before routine use is warranted, further investigation is needed. In terms of CCB toxicity, lipid emulsion therapy should be reserved for verapamil exposures only.

Treatment endpoints are maintenance of oxygenation, heart rate, and blood pressure to sustain adequate tissue perfusion. Continuous monitoring of hemodynamic parameters, mentation, urine output, and acid-base status are paramount and will help guide effective therapy. Patients who remain in a state of cardiovascular collapse despite aggressive resuscitation may be candidates for extracorporeal blood pressure support using cardiopulmonary bypass or intraaortic balloon pump.[21,52]

Table 173-1 presents a summary of pharmaceutical interventions after CCB toxicity.

Patient Monitoring and Disposition

Patients should be monitored in a high-acuity setting for evidence of cardiovascular instability for at least six hours after an acute ingestion of a regular-release CCB. Medical stability requires normal mentation and physical examination, and hemodynamics, as well as excluding other ingestions. Patients who have ingested toxic amounts of a sustained-released CCB formulation should be monitored for 24 hours because of the risk of delayed symptoms. Patients who develop any evidence of cardiovascular instability should be admitted to an intensive care unit.

After recovery from significant toxicity, asymptomatic patients should be observed closely for an additional 24 hours. As expected, a psychiatrist should evaluate all patients with a history or suspicion of intentional ingestion prior to ultimate disposition.

Conclusions

CCBs hold the potential for causing severe or delayed hemodynamic instability. Appropriate evaluation and monitoring of asymptomatic patients, as well as aggressive interventions in those patients with cardiovascular collapse, ensures optimal patient outcomes. Clinicians should initiate catecholamine infusions early in hypotensive patients who fail to respond to moderate fluid resuscitation. Consultation with a regional poison control center (telephone 800-222-1222 in the United States or find online at www.eapect.org in Europe) or a medical toxicologist can offer insights into underlying pathophysiology and assistance with patient management.

KEY POINTS

1. An accurate history of ingestion is critical for guiding treatment of the toxicology patient. Attempts should be made to determine whether other substances have been ingested. Family, witnesses, or other health care personnel (EMS, ED) may offer relevant information.

2. Patients can rapidly deteriorate after a toxic ingestion of a calcium channel blocker (CCB) and require at least 6 hours of high-acuity monitoring after an acute ingestion of an immediate-release formulation. Patients who have ingested a sustained-release medication and those with evidence of hemodynamic instability require admission and continuous cardiac monitoring.

3. Gastric decontamination has very limited utility after ingestion of any toxic substance, including CCBs. The routine use of ipecac, gastric lavage, or cathartics is not recommended. The use of activated charcoal is recommended only if treatment is initiated within 1 hour after ingestion and continued airway protection can be ensured. The use of whole-bowel irrigation should be discussed with a medical toxicologist.

4. After the development of cardiovascular shock, the mainstay of therapy involves the use of vasopressors to maintain adequate perfusion. Atropine, calcium, and excessive volumes of intravenous fluids have only limited utility. Novel therapies such as high-dose insulin and Intralipid may be beneficial and should be discussed with a medical toxicologist.

5. Invasive hemodynamic monitoring should be instituted quickly in patients severely poisoned by CCBs and should be continued until resolution of cardiovascular instability.

6. Pulmonary edema can accompany severe poisoning by CCBs, especially after excessive fluid resuscitation. Physicians should maintain a high clinical suspicion throughout the peri-resuscitation and extubation periods.

7. Optimal treatment for individual poisoned patients depends on exact information and unique factors. Consultation with a regional poison control center (800-222-1222) or a medical toxicologist will ensure optimal patient management.

ANNOTATED REFERENCES

Albertson TE, Dawson A, Latorre F, et al. TOX-ACLS: toxicologic-oriented advanced cardiac life support. Ann Emerg Med 2001;37:S78-90.
    A consortium of medical toxicologists and emergency physicians reviews the medical literature in an attempt to provide evidence-based recommendations for treatment of the acutely poisoned toxicology patient. The uses of both calcium salts and insulin/dextrose in CCB toxicity are critically discussed.
Kerns W. Management of β-adrenergic blocker and calcium channel antagonist toxicity. Emerg Med Clin North Am 2007;25:309-31.
    This article provides an overview of management options and goals for CCB (and beta-blocker) toxicity. Underlying pathophysiology is briefly covered.
Salhanick SD, Shannon MW. Management of calcium channel antagonist overdose. Drug Saf 2003;26:65-79.

This article provides a detailed review of calcium channels and treatment options. We do not support their reliance on early initiation of insulin and euglycemia as optimal treatment.
Lheureux P, Zahor S, Gris M, et al. Bench-to-bedside review: hyperinsulinemia/euglycemia therapy in the management of overdose of calcium-channel blockers. Crit Care 2006;10:212.
    This article provides a detailed description and history of insulin and euglycemia for the treatment of CCB toxicity.
Jamaty C, Bailey B, Larocque A, et al. Lipid emulsions in the treatment of acute poisoning: a systematic review of the human and animal studies. Clin Toxicol (Phila) 2010;48:1-27.
    A comprehensive review of the use of lipid emulsion for acute poisonings. All relevant research on this topic is included or reviewed.

REFERENCE

Access the complete reference list online at http://www.expertconsult.com.

174

Drug Therapy in Renal Failure

RIMA A. MOHAMMAD | GREGORY A. ESCHENAUER | GARY R. MATZKE

The incidence of acute kidney injury or insufficiency (AKI) in the intensive care unit (ICU) ranges from 5.9% to 25%, depending on how AKI is defined.[1] Renal replacement therapy is required for 4.3% of all critically ill patients and up to 72.5% of patients with AKI.[2] In-hospital mortality in ICU patients ranges from 5% to 10% in those with no renal dysfunction, 9% to 27% at risk of renal dysfunction, 11% to 30% with AKI, and 26% to 40% with overt kidney failure.[3] Critically ill patients with chronic kidney disease (CKD) have poorer outcomes than patients with normal renal function on admission, and the presence of CKD is a significant predictor of hospital mortality in Acute Physiology, Age, and Chronic Health Evaluation (APACHE) III score tools.[4,5] Renal insufficiency, whether acute or chronic, alters the absorption, distribution, metabolism, and elimination of many pharmacotherapeutic agents used in the treatment of critically ill patients. In this chapter, the drugs affected are tabulated, and the mechanisms responsible for the changes in disposition are discussed. A general construct for the individualization of drug therapy in patients with CKD or AKI is presented, along with dosage guidelines for the most commonly used ICU medications. Finally, the influence of continuous and intermittent renal replacement therapy on drug clearance is discussed, and dosage guidelines are tabulated for selected drugs for patients with severe CKD or AKI.

Quantitation of Renal Function

Accurate assessment of renal function in critically ill patients is imperative. Serial estimates or measurements of renal function routinely are recommended to guide individualization of drug dosage regimens to optimize clinical outcomes. The calculation of creatinine clearance (CL_{cr}) from a timed urine collection with creatinine measurement in serum and urine has been the standard clinical measure of renal function for decades. Urine is difficult to collect accurately in the ICU. Furthermore, many commonly used medications interfere with measurement of creatinine, especially when colorimetric assay methods such as the Jaffé method are used. Thus, measurement of CL_{cr} by this approach is not always the best way to assess glomerular filtration rate (GFR).[6,7] The administration of radioactive (^{125}I iothalamate, ^{51}Cr-EDTA, or technetium-99m DTPA) or nonradioactive (aminoglycosides, iohexol, iothalamate, and inulin) markers of GFR, although scientifically sound, is clinically impractical because intravenous (IV) or subcutaneous (SQ) administration of the marker and the collection of multiple timed blood and urine collections make the procedures expensive and difficult to perform.

Estimation of CL_{cr} or GFR requires only routinely collected laboratory and demographic data and is inexpensive and clinically feasible. The Cockcroft and Gault (C-G) method for estimation of CL_{cr}[8] and the Modification of Diet in Renal Disease (MDRD) method for estimation of GFR[9] correlate well with CL_{cr} and GFR measurements in individuals with stable renal function.[9] These methods lose their predictive performance, however, in patients with liver disease,[10-12] unstable renal function,[6,13,14] estimated GFR above 60 mL/min,[15] or obesity.[16,17] In critically ill patients with AKI, both MDRD and C-G overestimate estimated GFR by 33% and 80%, respectively.[18] Finally, although several methods for CL_{cr} estimation in patients with unstable renal function have been proposed,[7] as well as equations for "adjusted" weights (for use in the C-G equation) in the obese,[16,17] the accuracy of these methods has not been rigorously assessed, and at present their use cannot be recommended.

There is considerable controversy at this time regarding whether the C-G or MDRD equation should be utilized to guide drug dosing adjustments in patients with CKD. The MDRD equation was developed to estimate GFR in patients with CKD.[15] However, renal dosing recommendations for currently approved drugs are predominantly (>95%) based on relationships between drug clearance and CL_{cr} estimated by the C-G equation.[19] The literature now suggests that the two equations cannot be utilized interchangeably, as several studies have shown that the use of the MDRD equation results in discordant dosing recommendations (compared to dosing based on C-G) in up to 40% of patients.[19-21] Complicating these comparisons even further is another problem: several versions of the MDRD equation (and most recently, an equation called *Chronic Kidney Disease Epidemiology Collaboration* [CKD-EPI]) have been reported since the publication of the original formula.[22] As such, clinicians should continue to utilize CL_{cr} estimated by C-G for drug dosing.[23]

Altered Drug Disposition in Critically Ill Patients with Renal Insufficiency

EFFECT ON DRUG ABSORPTION

Absorption of drugs from the gastrointestinal (GI) tract is rarely altered in patients with CKD or AKI. Systemic availability of some drugs (i.e., some β-adrenergic blockers, dextropropoxyphene, and dihydrocodeine) is increased in CKD patients as a result of a decrease in metabolism during the drug's first pass through the GI tract and liver.[24,25] Some orally administered drugs that are extensively metabolized before reaching the systemic circulation may have increased bioavailability, but this phenomenon has been documented for relatively few drugs.[26,27]

EFFECT ON DRUG DISTRIBUTION

The volume of distribution of several drugs is increased significantly in patients with AKI or severe CKD.[25,28-30] Increases may result from fluid overload, decreased protein binding, or altered tissue binding (Table 174-1). The volume of distribution of only a few drugs is decreased in patients with CKD, and the mechanism proposed for this change is a reduction in tissue binding. Digoxin and pindolol are two prime examples, and for both of these drugs, a significant relationship exists between the decrease in distribution volume and CL_{cr}.[29,30]

EFFECT ON DRUG METABOLISM

Preliminary human data suggest a differential effect of CKD on cytochrome P450 (CYP) enzyme activity: the activities of CYP2C19 and CYP3A4 are reduced, whereas the activities of CYP2D6 and CYP2E1 are not affected.[29,30] This differential effect on individual enzymes may help explain some of the conflicting data regarding changes in drug metabolism in the presence of severe CKD.

Reduction of nonrenal clearance of several drugs reported in patients with severe CKD supports the premise that alterations in hepatic cytochrome P450 enzyme expression and/or activity is responsible (Table 174-2).[25,28-30] Prediction of the effect of CKD on metabolism of a particular drug is difficult even for drugs within the same pharmacologic class.[29,30] Patients with CKD exhibit reductions in nonrenal clearance and alterations in bioavailability of predominantly

TABLE 174-1	Effect of End-Stage Renal Disease on Volume of Distribution (L/kg) of Selected Drugs Used in the ICU*		
Drug	*Normal*	*ESRD*	*Change from Normal*
Increased			
Amikacin	0.20	0.29	45%
Cefazolin	0.13	0.16	31%
Cefoxitin	0.16	0.26	63%
Ceftriaxone	0.28	0.48	71%
Dicloxacillin	0.08	0.18	125%
Doripenem	0.25	0.47	88%
Erythromycin	0.57	1.09	91%
Furosemide	0.11	0.18	64%
Gentamicin	0.20	0.32	60%
Isoniazid	0.60	0.80	33%
Phenytoin	0.64	1.40	119%
Trimethoprim	1.36	1.83	35%
Vancomycin	0.64	0.85	33%
Decreased			
Chloramphenicol	0.87	0.60	−31%
Digoxin	7.30	4.0	−45%
Ethambutol	3.70	1.60	−57%

*A change of ±25% was considered to be clinically significant.
ESRD, end-stage renal disease.
Data from references 25, 28-30, and 46-48.

hepatically metabolized drugs which are generally proportional to the reductions in GFR.

Critically ill patients with AKI have been noted to have higher residual nonrenal clearance for three drugs—imipenem, meropenem, and vancomycin—than patients with CKD who have similar CL_{cr}.[31] This difference may be the result of less exposure to or accumulation of uremic waste products that alter hepatic function. Because patients with AKI may have a higher nonrenal clearance than patients with CKD, the resultant plasma concentrations will be lower than expected and possibly subtherapeutic if classic CKD-derived dosage guidelines are followed. Thus for these agents, initial dosing should be adjusted upward, and only after 7 to 10 days of persistent AKI do the dosing guidelines derived from CKD subjects likely become applicable.

EFFECT ON RENAL EXCRETION

Renal clearance is the composite of GFR, renal tubular secretion, and reabsorption: renal clearance = (GFR × f_u) + (renal tubular secretion − renal reabsorption), where f_u is the fraction of the drug unbound to plasma proteins. An acute or chronic progressive reduction in GFR decreases renal clearance; historically, drug dosage guidelines for patients with AKI or CKD have been based on this phenomenon. The contribution of a reduction in renal clearance to the degree of change in the total body clearance of a drug is highly dependent, however, on the fraction of the dose eliminated unchanged by the normal kidney,

TABLE 174-2	Effect of End-Stage Renal Disease on Nonrenal Clearance of Selected Drugs Used in the ICU	
Decreased		
Acyclovir	Erythromycin	Nitrendipine
Aztreonam	Imipenem	Procainamide
Bufuralol	Isoniazid	Propranolol
Cefotaxime	Ketorolac	Quinapril
Ceftriaxone	Metoclopramide	Vancomycin
Cilastatin	Morphine	Verapamil
Ciprofloxacin	Nicardipine	Warfarin
Doripenem	Nimodipine	
Increased		
Bumetanide	Fosinopril	Phenytoin
Cefpiramide	Nifedipine	Sulfadimidine
Unchanged		
Acetaminophen	Insulin	Nisoldipine
Chloramphenicol	Lidocaine	Pentobarbital
Clonidine	Metoprolol	Theophylline

Data from references 25, 28-30.

the intrarenal pathways for drug elimination and transport, and the degree of functional impairment of each of these pathways.[29,30]

Drug elimination by GFR occurs by diffusion, but renal tubular secretion and renal reabsorption are bidirectional processes that involve carrier-mediated renal transport systems and passive diffusion. The important renal transport systems involved in the renal tubular excretion of multiple compounds include the organic anionic (i.e., ampicillin, cefazolin, and furosemide), organic cationic (i.e., famotidine, trimethoprim, and dopamine), nucleoside (i.e., zidovudine), and P-glycoprotein transporters (i.e., digoxin and steroids).[32,33] Accordingly, the clearance of drugs that are extensively renally secreted (renal clearance > 300 mL/min) may be reduced significantly by drug interactions (i.e., probenecid with β-lactam antibiotics) and/or impaired function of one or more of the renal transporter systems. For example, AKI due to ischemia or toxicants results in a significant impairment in the function of renal solute carrier (SLC) 22A organic ion transporters, compounding the effects of decreased GFR on drug clearance.[34]

Strategies for Drug Therapy Individualization

Secondary references such as the *American Hospital Formulary Service Drug Information*,[35] *Drug Prescribing in Renal Failure* by Aronoff and colleagues,[36] and *Goodman and Gilman's The Pharmacological Basis of Therapeutics*[37] are excellent sources from which one can acquire information on the pharmacokinetic characteristics of drugs in subjects with normal renal as well as impaired renal function. However, these references often do not provide the explicit relationships of kinetic parameters with CL_{cr} or GFR. In addition, since the references employ different definitions of renal impairment and utilize varying methodologies for deriving recommendations, drug dosing recommendations occasionally differ significantly.[38] This section provides a practical approach for drug dosage individualization in critically ill patients with AKI or CKD and patients receiving continuous renal replacement therapy (CRRT) or intermittent hemodialysis (IHD). Basic pharmacokinetic principles (see Chapter 169) combined with the disposition properties of a particular drug and a quantitative measure of the patient's degree of renal function enable the clinician to design an individualized therapeutic regimen.

If the relationship of a drug's total body clearance with CL_{cr} or GFR is not known, one can estimate the patient's total body clearance, provided that the fraction of the drug that is eliminated renally unchanged (f_e) in subjects with normal renal function is known. The following approach makes six assumptions: (1) the volume of distribution is unchanged, (2) the change in total body clearance is proportional to CL_{cr}, (3) renal disease does not alter the drug's metabolism, (4) metabolites, if formed, are inactive and nontoxic, (5) the drug obeys first-order (linear) kinetic principles, and (6) the drug's pharmacokinetics can be described adequately by a one-compartment model. If these assumptions are valid, the kinetic parameter/dosage adjustment factor (Q) can be calculated as Q = 1 − (f_e [1 − KF]), where *KF* is the ratio of the patient's CL_{cr} to an assumed normal value of 120 mL/min. The estimated total body clearance (CL_{PT}) can be calculated as follows: CL_{PT} = CL_{normT} × Q, where CL_{normT} is the value in patients with normal renal function (i.e., patients with a CL_{cr} of ≥ 120 mL/min). The elimination rate constant of the drug can be calculated as the quotient of the estimated total body clearance and volume of distribution. When these three key kinetic parameters are estimated, the individualized dosage regimen can be calculated as described in Chapter 169.

The optimal dosage regimen for an ICU patient with AKI or CKD depends on the desired goal. If there is a significant relationship between maximal plasma concentration and clinical response[39,40] (i.e., aminoglycosides) or toxicity[40,41] (i.e., quinidine, phenobarbital, and phenytoin), the dose and dosing interval may have to be modified. If the dosing interval is increased, the maximal plasma concentration and minimal plasma concentration are similar to values in individuals with

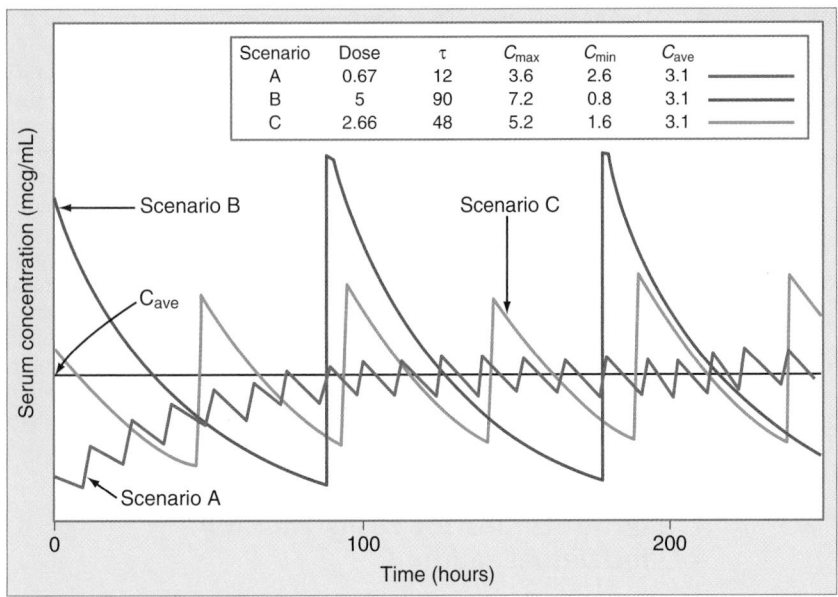

Scenario	Dose	τ	C_{max}	C_{min}	C_{ave}
A	0.67	12	3.6	2.6	3.1
B	5	90	7.2	0.8	3.1
C	2.66	48	5.2	1.6	3.1

Figure 174-1 Although the average steady-state concentrations (C_{ave}) are identical, the concentration-time profile would be markedly different if one changes the dose and maintains the dosing interval constant (scenario A) versus changing the dosing interval and maintaining the dose constant (scenario B) or changing both (scenario C). C_{max}, maximal concentration; C_{min}, minimal concentration. (From Matzke GR, Frye RF. Drug therapy individualization for patients with renal insufficiency. Adapted from Dipiro JT, Talbert RL, Yee GC et al., editors. Pharmacotherapy: a pathophysiologic approach. 7th ed. New York: McGraw Hill; 2008, p. 833-44. Copyright McGraw Hill.)

normal renal function, but the desired target concentrations may not be precisely attained. In this case, consultation with a clinical pharmacist/pharmacologist may be warranted to facilitate the design of a revised dosage regimen. If no specific target values for maximal plasma concentration or minimal plasma concentration have been reported, attaining the same average steady-state concentration may be appropriate (i.e., cephalosporins). This goal can be achieved by decreasing the dose ($D_{PT} = D_{NORM} \times Q$) or prolonging the dosing interval (τ) ($\tau_{PT} = \tau_{NORM} \div Q$).* If the dose is reduced while the dosing interval remains unchanged, the maximal plasma concentration becomes lower and the minimal plasma concentration higher (Figure 174-1). This dosage adjustment method, if taken to the extreme, results in maintenance of the desired average steady-state concentration by continuous infusion of a parenteral product. These principles have been used to derive dosage recommendations for commonly used drugs in the ICU for patients with mild, moderate, and severe kidney injury (Table 174-3).

IMPACT OF RENAL REPLACEMENT THERAPY

Removal of a drug from the systemic circulation by renal replacement therapy involves several processes: movement from the blood across the dialyzer/hemofilter membrane and into the dialysate/ultrafiltrate and potentially adsorption on the membrane. Passive diffusion (i.e., movement from an area of higher concentration [blood] to one of lower concentration [dialysate]) is the primary mode of drug removal. The renal replacement therapy clearance tends to increase when there is an increase in the surface area of the dialyzer/hemofilter, blood and dialysate/ultrafiltrate flow rate, or duration of the treatment. Convective transport and clearance, which represent the simultaneous movement of drug within ultrafiltered plasma water, must be considered if ultrafiltration is a significant component of the renal replacement therapy prescription. Renal replacement therapy clearance is higher for drugs that are water soluble, have a low molecular weight, have minimal to no binding to plasma proteins, and have a small volume of distribution.

CONTINUOUS RENAL REPLACEMENT THERAPY

The three most commonly used forms of CRRT are continuous venovenous hemofiltration (CVVH), continuous venovenous

hemodialysis (CVVHD), and continuous venovenous hemodiafiltration (CVVHDF). During CVVH, drugs are removed primarily by convection/ultrafiltration.[42] The clearance of a drug is a function of the permeability of the hemofilter, which is called the *sieving coefficient*, and the ultrafiltrate flow rate. The sieving coefficient can be approximated by dividing the concentration of the drug in the ultrafiltrate (C_{uf}) by the concentration in the plasma entering the hemofilter (C_a): sieving coefficient = C_{uf}/C_a. The sieving coefficient is often approximated by the fraction unbound to plasma proteins (f_u) because plasma concentrations of the drug of interest may not be readily available. The clearance by CVVH can be estimated as ultrafiltrate flow rate × f_u. Drug clearance by CVVHDF can be estimated, provided that the blood flow rate is over 100 mL/min and dialysate flow rate is less than 33 mL/min, as (ultrafiltrate flow rate + dialysate flow rate) × (f_u or sieving coefficient). If ultrafiltrate flow rate is negligible (<3 mL/min), as is often the case with CVVHD, CVVHD clearance can be estimated as the product of dialysate flow rate and f_u or sieving coefficient.

Individualization of therapy for a patient receiving CRRT depends on the patient's residual renal function and clearance of the drug by the mode of CRRT the patient is receiving. The patient's residual drug clearance can be predicted based on the CL_{cr} and the relationship between total body clearance of the drug and CL_{cr} as described previously. The CRRT type (CVVH, CVVHD, or CVVHDF) and recommended initial dosage regimens of selected drugs that are used frequently in ICU patients receiving CRRT are listed in Table 174-4.[43,44] In cases in which specific data on drug clearance are not available and the patient receiving CRRT is functionally anuric (i.e., urine output is <300 mL/d), drug dosing can be initiated at a level consistent with the individual having a CL_{cr} of 30 to 50 mL/min, if their ultrafiltration/dialysate or ultrafiltrate flow rate is 2 L/h or greater.

HEMODIALYSIS

Drug-related factors that influence hemodialyzability include the molecular weight, protein binding, and volume of distribution of a drug.[25] The dialysis prescription factors include the composition of the dialyzer, surface area, and blood and dialysate flow rates. The semisynthetic and synthetic dialyzers used in high-flux hemodialysis have the largest ultrafiltration rates and more closely mimic the filtration characteristics of the human kidney. These dialyzers allow the passage of most drugs that have a molecular weight of ≤15,000 D.[45] High-molecular-weight drugs such as vancomycin are significantly cleared by this mode of dialysis, and the clearance of many smaller drugs is significantly increased, as reviewed by Matzke.[46] In order to obtain

---

*D_{PT} = dose for the patient; D_{NORM} = dose for the patient with normal function.

| TABLE 174-3 | Dosing Guidelines for Drugs Commonly Used in the ICU by Patients with Renal Insufficiency |

Drug	Volume of Distribution (L/kg)	Plasma Protein Binding (%)	Percent Excreted Unchanged in Urine	Regimen for Normal Renal Function	Method	Glomerular Filtration Rate (mL/min)[1]		
						30-50	10-30	<10
Acetazolamide	0.2	70-90	100	250 mg q 6-12 h	IDI	q 6 h	q 12 h	Avoid (ineffective)
Acyclovir (IV)	0.7	15-30	40-70	5-10 mg/kg q 8 h	DD and IDI	5-10 mg/kg q 12	5-10 mg/kg q 24 h	2.5-5 mg/kg q 24 h
Amiodarone (oral)	60 (18-148)	96	<5	Ventricular arrhythmia: 800-1600 mg load, then 400-800 mg q 24 h	NC	100%	100%	100%
Amphotericin B	4	90	5-10	20-50 mg	IDI	q 24 h	q 24 h	q 24-36 h
Amphotericin B lipid complex	1.7-3.9	90	<1	5 mg/kg q 24 h	NC	100%	100%	100%
Ampicillin	0.31	0.17-20	60-90	0.5-2 g q 4-6 h	IDI	q 6-8 h	q 8-12 h	q 12 h
Ampicillin/ sulbactam				1.5-3 g q 6 h	IDI	q 8 h	q 12 h	q 24 h
Atracurium	0.1-0.4	40-50	0	0.4-0.5 mg/kg IV bolus, then 0.08-0.1 mg/kg IV q 15-25 min as needed	NC	100%	100%	100%
Azithromycin	18	8-50	6-12	250-500 mg q 24 h	NC	100%	100%	100%
Aztreonam	0.5-1	45-60	75	1-2 g q 6-8 h	DD[2]	100%	50%	25%
Bumetanide	0.2-0.5	94-96	45	0.5-2 mg q 8-12 h	NC	100%	100%	100%
Caspofungin	0.14	97	1-9	70 mg, then 50 mg q 24 h	NC	100%	100%	100%
Cefazolin	0.13-0.22	80	75-95	1-2 g q 8 h	DD and IDI	q 8 h	0.5-1 g q 12 h	0.5-1 g q 24 h
Cefepime	0.3	16	85	2 g q 8-12 h	DD and IDI	2 g q 12-24 h	1-2 g q 24 h	500 mg-1 g q 24 h
Ceftazidime	0.28-0.4	17	60-85	1-2 g q 8 h	IDI	q 12 h	q 24 h	q 48 h
Ceftriaxone	0.12-0.18	90	30-65	1 g q 24 h	NC	100%	100%	100%
Ciprofloxacin (IV)	2.5	20-40	50-70	400 mg q 8-12 h	IDI	q 8-12 h	q 24 h	Q24 h
Clindamycin (IV)	0.6-1.2	60-95	10	600-900 mg q 8 h	NC	100%	100%	100%
Daptomycin	0.1	92	78	4-6 mg/kg q 24 h	IDI	q 24 h	q 48 h	q 48 h
Dexmedetomidine	1.33	94	0	Individualize 1 µg/kg load, then 0.2-0.7 µg/kg/h	NC	100%	100%	100%
Digoxin	4-7	20-25	76-85	Indication dependent; 1-1.5 mg oral/IV load, 0.125-0.5 mg oral or 0.125-0.25 mg IV maintenance	DD and IDI	100% load, 25-75% q 36 h	100% load, 25-75% q 36 h	50% load, 10-25% q 48 h
Diltiazem	5.3	77-93	<5	IV infusion: 5-10 mg/h Oral (regular): 30 mg q 6-8 h	NC	100%	100%	100%
Doripenem	0.24	8	70	500 mg q 8 h	DD and IDI	250 mg q 8 h	250 mg q 12 h	250 mg q 12 h
Enalaprilat	1-2.4	50-60	>90	1.25-5 mg q 6 h	DD	100%	50%	50%
Enoxaparin	0.06	ND	43	Indication dependent	DD	100%	50%	50%
Ertapenem	0.11	85-95	38	1 g q 24 h	DD	100%	50%	50%
Etomidate	2-4.5	76	2	0.2-0.6 mg/kg	NC	100%	100%	100%
Famotidine	1.1-1.4	15-20	65-80	20-40 mg q 24 h	DD or IDI	50% or q 36-48 h	50% or q 36-48 h	50% or q 36-48 h
Fenoldopam (IV)	0.6-0.7	85-90	4	0.05-0.1 µg/kg/min	NC	100%	100%	100%
Fentanyl	3-8	80-86	≤10	Individualize	DD	75%	75%	50%
Fluconazole	0.7	12	70	200-800 mg q 24 h	DD	50%	50%	50%
Fondaparinux	0.1	>94 (ATIII)	77	Prophylaxis: 2.5 mg q 24 h Treatment: 5-10 mg q 24 h	DD	60% (use caution)	Avoid	Avoid
Furosemide	0.2	91-99	60-90	Individualize	NC	100%	100%	100%
Gabapentin	0.7	<3	90	300-600 mg q 8 h	DD and IDI	200-700 mg q 12 h	200-700 mg q 24 h	100-300 mg q 24 h
Ganciclovir	0.47	ND	90-100	2.5-5 mg/kg q 12-24 h	DD and IDI	1.25-2.5 mg/kg q 24 h	0.625-1.25 mg/kg q 24 h	0.625-1.25 mg/kg q 48 h
Hydralazine (oral)	0.5-0.9	87	25	25-50 mg q 6 h	IDI	q 8 h	q 8 h	q 8-16 h
Hydrocortisone (IV)	ND	90	<1	100 mg q 8 h	NC	100%	100%	100%
Imipenem[3]	0.17-0.3	13-21	20-70	0.5 g q 6 h	DD and IDI	0.5 g q 8 h	0.5 g q 12 h	0.25 g q 12 h
Insulin	0.15	5	None	Variable	DD	75%	75%	50%
Labetalol (oral)	5.1-9.4	50	5	200-400 mg twice daily	NC	100%	100%	100%

Continued on following page

TABLE 174-3	Dosing Guidelines for Drugs Commonly Used in the ICU by Patients with Renal Insufficiency (Continued)							
			Percent			Glomerular Filtration Rate (mL/min)[1]		
Drug	Volume of Distribution (L/kg)	Plasma Protein Binding (%)	Excreted Unchanged in Urine	Regimen for Normal Renal Function	Method	30-50	10-30	<10
Lansoprazole	0.39	>97	<1	15-60 mg q 24 h	NC	100%	100%	100%
Lepirudin	~0.2	ND	35	0.2 mg/kg IV bolus (only for perceived life- or limb-threatening thrombosis), 0.1 mg/kg/h IV infusion	DD	See note[4]	See note[4]	See note[4]
Levetiracetam (oral immediate release)	0.7	<10	66	500-1500 mg q 12 h	DD	250-750 mg q 12 h	250-500 mg q 12 h	500-1000 mg q 24 h
Levofloxacin	1.1-1.5	24-38	67-87	500-750 mg q 24 h	DD and IDI	100% q 48 h	250-500 mg q 48 h	250-500 mg q 48 h
Linezolid	0.93	30	30	600 mg q 12 h	NC	100%	100%	100%
Lorazepam	1.3	85-91	0	Variable	NC	100%	100%	100%
Meropenem	0.35	2	65	1 g q 8 h	DD and IDI	1 g q 12 h	500 mg q 12 h	500 mg q 24 h
Methylprednisolone	1.2-1.5	40-60	<10	Variable	NC	100%	100%	100%
Metoclopramide	3.5	30	10-22	10-20 mg IV/IM q 4-6 h as needed	DD	75%	75%	50%
Metoprolol (oral)	5.6	12	<5	25-200 mg q 12 h	NC	100%	100%	100%
Metronidazole	0.25-0.85	20	20	7.5 mg/kg q 8 h	DD	100%	100%	50%
Micafungin	0.39	99	<15%	50-150 mg q 24 h	NC	100%	100%	100%
Midazolam	1-6.6	95	0	Individualize	DD	100%	100%	50%
Milrinone	0.3-0.5	70	85	50 μg/kg IV, then 0.375-0.75 μg/kg/min IV infusion	DD	See note[5]	See note[5]	See note[5]
Morphine	1-6	20-36	2-12	2-20 mg q 4 h Variable (IV/IM/SQ/oral)	DD	75%	75%	50%
Moxifloxacin	2-3.5	40	20	400 mg q 24 h	NC	100%	100%	100%
Nafcillin	0.35	85	35	1-2 g q 4-6 h	NC	100%	100%	100%
Nicardipine	8.3	>95	0	5-15 mg/h IV infusion	NC	100%	100%	100%
Nitroprusside	0.2	0	0	0.3-3 μg/kg/min IV infusion (max. 10 μg/kg/min)	DD	100% (use caution)[6]	100% (use caution)[6]	Avoid
Omeprazole	0.34-0.37	95-96	<5	20-60 mg q 24 h	NC	100%	100%	100%
Ondansetron	2.2-2.5	70-76	5	4-8 mg IV q 6-12 h	NC	100%	100%	100%
Pantoprazole	0.2-0.3	98	0	40-80 mg IV/oral q 12 h or 80 mg IV bolus, then 8 mg/h IV infusion	NC	100%	100%	100%
Penicillin G	0.3-0.42	50	60-85	1-4 million units q 4-6 h	DD	100%	100%	50%
Phenytoin	0.5-1	90	2	300-400 mg q 24 h	NC	100%	100%	100%
Piperacillin[7]	0.2-0.3	30	75-90	4 g q 6 h	IDI	q 8 h	q 8 h	q 12 h
Piperacillin/ tazobactam[7]				3.375-4.5 g q 6 h		2.25-3.375 g q 6 h	2.25-3.375 g q 6 h	2.25 g q 6-8 h
Propofol	60	97-99	0.3	0.5-1 mg/kg IV bolus or 0.3-3 mg/kg/h IV infusion	NC	100%	100%	100%
Rocuronium	0.26	30	33	Variable 0.45-1.2 mg/kg IV bolus, then 0.1-0.2 mg/kg IV as needed or 0.01-0.012 mg/kg/min IV infusion	NC	100%	100%	100%
Ranitidine	1.04-4.1	15	30-70	150-300 mg oral q 24 h or 50 mg IV q 6-8 h	DD and IDI	150 mg oral q 12-24 h; 50 mg IV q 12-24 h	150 mg oral q 12-24 h; 50 mg IV q 12-24 h	150 mg oral q 12-24 h; 50 mg IV q 12-24 h
Tigecycline	7-9	71-89	22	100 mg; then 50 mg q 12 h	NC	100%	100%	100%
Tobramycin[8]	0.22-0.33	<5	95	5-7 mg/kg q 24 h	DD and IDI	5-7 mg/kg q 36-48 h	See note[8]	See note[8]
Trimethoprim/ sulfamethoxazole (IV)[9]	1-2.2/0.28-0.38	30-70/50	40-70/70	2.5-5 mg/kg q 6-12 h	IDI	q 6-12 h	q 12-24 h	q 24 h
Vancomycin[10]	0.6-0.9	30-50	90-100	15-20 mg/kg q 8-12 h	IDI	q 24 h	See note[10]	See note[10]
Vasopressin	ND	ND	5-10	Variable; septic shock: 0.01-0.04 units/min IV infusion	NC	100%	100%	100%

						Glomerular Filtration Rate (mL/min)[1]		
	TABLE 174-3	**Dosing Guidelines for Drugs Commonly Used in the ICU by Patients with Renal Insufficiency (Continued)**						
Drug	**Volume of Distribution (L/kg)**	**Plasma Protein Binding (%)**	**Percent Excreted Unchanged in Urine**	**Regimen for Normal Renal Function**	**Method**	**30-50**	**10-30**	**<10**
Vecuronium	0.2-0.4	60-80	25	0.08-0.1 mg/kg load, then 0.01-0.015 mg/kg q 12-15 min	NC	100%[11]	100%[11]	100%[11]
Voriconazole	4.6	58	<2%	4-6 mg/kg q 12 h	NC	100%	100%	100%

[1]The range following glomerular filtration rate (GFR) indicates the use of the dose that corresponds to that range of GFR in patients not on dialysis.

[2]When DD method is employed, the reduced maintenance dose should be preceded by the administration of the standard (loading) dose for a patient with normal renal function.

[3]Seizures in end-stage renal disease.

[4]Dosed based on serum creatinine (S_{cr}). S_{cr} 1.02-1.58: 0.05 mg/kg/h IV infusion; S_{cr} 1.58-4.52: 0.01 mg/kg/h IV infusion; S_{cr} > 4.52: 0.005 mg/kg/h IV infusion.

[5]IV infusion dosed based on creatinine clearance (CL_{cr} [mL/min/1.73 m^2]). CL_{cr} 50: 0.43 µg/kg/min; CL_{cr} 40: 0.38 µg/kg/min; CL_{cr} 30: 0.33 µg/kg/min; CL_{cr} 20: 0.28 µg/kg/min; CL_{cr} 10: 0.23 µg/kg/min; CL_{cr} 5: 0.2 µg/kg/min.

[6]Use caution in patients with kidney injury, and monitor thiocyanate levels to ensure levels < 10 mg/dL.

[7]First dosage modification should be made at a GFR of ≤ 40 mL/min. Second dosage modification should be made at a GFR of < 20 mL/min.

[8]Dosing of aminoglycosides in critically ill patients should be individualized based on pharmacokinetic monitoring. Patients with glomerular filtration rates ≤ 30 mL/min should not receive "extended- interval" (i.e., 7 mg/kg)" empirical doses. Rather, loading doses ≤ 5 mg/kg should be administered.

[9]Dosed based on trimethoprim component.

[10]A vancomycin loading dose of 25-30 mg/kg (based on actual body weight) should be considered for all patients. In patients with a GFR ≤ 30 mL/min, subsequent doses of 15-20 mg/kg should be given when the serum concentration falls below 10 mg/L or 20 mg/L (depending on the site of infection and MIC of organism).

[11]Use lowest physiologically effective dose in patients with kidney injury.

DD, dose reduction method—the percent of the dose for normal renal function to be given at the interval for normal renal function is listed; IDI, increase dose interval method—the interval to be used with the dose for normal renal function is listed; DD and IDI, adjustment of dose and interval; ND, no data; NC, no change.

Data from references 35, 36, 49-56.

therapeutic plasma concentrations, patients receiving high-flux dialysis often require larger drug doses than the doses recommended in most references.

Quantification of the impact of hemodialysis on drug disposition can be calculated in several ways, and this contributes to the variability of values in the literature.[25] The difference between the half-life during dialysis and the half-life of the drug when the patient is off dialysis provides a crude guide to the impact of dialysis. The half-life during dialysis may not be interpretable in AKI patients because declining plasma drug concentrations during dialysis represent elimination by the patient, which may be considerable. The most accurate means of assessing the effect of hemodialysis is to calculate the dialyzer clearance of the drug.[25] Because drug concentrations generally are determined in plasma, the calculation of plasma clearance by the dialyzer (CL^p_D) can be calculated as: $CL^p_D = Q_p ([A_p - V_p]/A_p)$, where A_p is the concentration of drug in plasma going into the dialyzer, V_p is the concentration of drug in the plasma leaving the dialyzer, and Q_p is plasma flow, which equals blood flow through the dialyzer (1 hematocrit). This method accounts for clearance due to diffusion, convection, and adsorption to the dialyzer. The recovery clearance (CL^r_D) approach also has been used for the determination of dialyzer clearance: $CL^r_D = R/AUC_{0-t}$, where R is the total amount of drug recovered unchanged in the dialysate and AUC_{0-t} is the area under the predialyzer plasma concentration-time curve during hemodialysis.[25] This method yields lower clearance values than the previous method if there is a significant degree of binding of the drug to the dialyzer. If adsorption contributes minimally to clearance, the two methods are likely to correlate well.

Drug-dosage regimen individualization can be accomplished by using values of dialyzer clearance, volume of distribution, or half-life during dialysis from the literature. Because clearance terms are additive, the total clearance during dialysis can be calculated as the sum of the patient's residual total body clearance and dialyzer clearance. The half-life during the period between dialysis treatments can be calculated using an estimate of the drug's distribution volume: half-life = $(CL_{PT} + CL_D)/V_D$, where CL_{PT} is the patient's residual total body clearance, CL_D is dialyzer clearance, and V_D is volume of distribution.

Because there is marked variability among dialyzers in the clearance of some drugs, it is recommended that dialyzer clearance data for a cellulose dialyzer-drug pair not be extrapolated directly to a synthetic dialyzer. If there are no data regarding high-flux dialysis for a given drug, one should anticipate that the dialyzer clearance by the synthetic dialyzer will be 60% to 100% greater than that of the cellulose dialyzer. If there are no published data on dialyzer clearance, or reference sources do not identify the dialyzer that was used, prospective plasma concentration monitoring is recommended to guide therapy. Table 174-4 lists initial dosage recommendations for several drugs commonly administered to patients in the ICU.

Summary

The clearance of hundreds of drugs is reduced in critically ill patients, especially patients with AKI or CKD. The impact of renal replacement therapy can increase significantly the clearance of many of these agents and necessitate the generation of a revised dosage regimen if one hopes to achieve the desired therapeutic outcomes. The principles in this chapter and the tabulated pharmacokinetic data provide a construct from which clinicians can initiate this process.

KEY POINTS

1. The calculation of creatinine clearance (CL_{cr}) from a timed urine collection with creatinine measurement in serum and urine has been the standard clinical measure of renal function for decades.

2. Clearance of hundreds of drugs is reduced in critically ill patients, especially patients with acute kidney injury or insufficiency (AKI) or chronic kidney disease (CKD).

3. Volume of distribution of several drugs is increased significantly in patients with AKI or CKD, typically as a result of fluid overload, decreased protein binding, or altered tissue binding.

4. Individualization of therapy for a patient receiving continuous renal replacement therapy (CRRT) depends on the patient's residual renal function and clearance of the drug by the mode of CRRT the patient is receiving.

TABLE 174-4	Dosing Guidelines for Drugs Commonly Used in the ICU by Patients Receiving CVVH/CVVHD/CVVHDF/IHD*				
Drug[a]	Loading Dose	CVVH[b,c] Maintenance Dose	CVVHD[b] Maintenance Dose	CVVHDF[b] Maintenance Dose	IHD Dosing[d]
Acyclovir	None	HSV: 5-7.5 mg/kg q 24 h HSV encephalitis/VZV: 5-7.5 mg/kg q 24 h	Same Same	Same Same[e]	HSV: 2.5-3.375 mg/kg q 24 h HSV encephalitis/VZV: 5-7.5 mg/kg q 24 h
Amikacin	10 mg/kg	7.5 mg/kg q 24-48 h[f]	Same	Same	5-7.5 mg/kg q 48-72 h[g]
Amphotericin B	None	0.5-1 mg/kg q 24 h	Same	Same	Same
Amphotericin B lipid	None	3-5 mg/kg q 24 h	Same	Same	Same
Ampicillin	2 g	1-2 g q 8-12 h	1-2 g q 8 h	1-2 g q 6-8 h	1-2 g q 12-24 h
Ampicillin sulbactam	3 g	1.5-3 g q 8-12 h	1.5-3 g q 8 h	1.5-3 g q 6-8 h	1.5-3 g q 12-24 h
Azithromycin	None	250-500 mg q 24 h	Same	Same	Same
Aztreonam	2 g	1-2 g q 12 h	1 g q 8 h, or 2 g q 12 h[h]	1 g q 8 h, or 2 g q 12 h[h]	500 mg 12 h
Caspofungin	70 mg	50 mg q 24 h	Same	Same	Same
Cefazolin	2 g	1-2 g q 12 h	1 g q 8 h, or 2 g q 12 h[h]	1 g q 8 h, or 2 g q 12 h[h]	500-1000 mg q 24 h[i]
Cefepime	2 g	1-2 g q 12 h	1 g q 8 h, or 2 g q 12 h[h,j]	1 g q 8 h, or 2 g q 12 h[h,j]	500-1000 mg q 24 h[i]
Cefotaxime	None	1-2 g q 8-12 h	1-2 g q 8 h	1-2 g q 6-8 h	1-2 g q 24 h
Ceftazidime	2 g	1-2 g q 12 h	1 g q 8 h, or 2 g q 12 h[h,j]	1 g q 8 h, or 2 g q 12 h[h,j,k]	500-1000 mg q 24 h[i]
Ceftriaxone	2 g	1-2 g q 12-24 h	Same	Same	1-2 g q 24 h
Ciprofloxacin	None	200-400 mg q 12-24 h	400 mg q 12-24 h	400 mg q 12 h	200-400 mg q 24 h
Clindamycin	None	600-900 mg q 8 h	Same	Same	Same
Colistin	None	2.5 mg/kg q 48 h[l]	Same[l]	Same[l,m]	1.5 mg/kg q 24-48 h
Daptomycin	None	4-6 mg/kg q 48 h	Same	Same	4-6 mg/kg q 48-72 h[n]
Digoxin	1-1.5 mg oral/IV	25-75% usual MD q 36 h	Same	Same	Load 0.5-0.75 mg oral/IV, 10-25% usual MD q 48 h
Doxycycline	None	100 mg q 12 h	Same	Same	Same
Enalaprilat	None	75-100% usual MD	Same	Same	0.625 mg q 6 h (after HD if blood pressure level warrants)
Famotidine	None	10-20 mg q 24 h, or 20-40 mg q 36-48 h	Same	Same	10-20 mg q 24 h, or 20-40 mg q 36-48 h (after HD)
Fluconazole	400-800 mg	200-800 mg q 24 h	400-800 mg q 12 h[o]	800 mg q 24 h[p]	200-800 mg q 48 h
Gabapentin	None	200-700 mg q 24 h	Same	Same	Load 300-400 mg, then 200-300 mg TIW (after HD)
Ganciclovir (CMV infection)	None	I = 2.5 mg/kg q 24 h MD = 1.25 mg/kg q 24 h	I = 2.5 mg/kg q 12 h MD = 2.5 mg/kg q 24 h	Same Same	I = 1.25 mg/kg q 48-72 h MD = 0.625 mg/kg q 48-72 h
Gentamicin:	2-3 mg/kg				2-3 mg/kg load × 1, then
Mild UTI/synergy		1 mg/kg q 24-36 h (redose when Cp < 1 mg/L)			1 mg/kg q 48-72 h[q]
Moderate-severe UTI		1-1.5 mg/kg q 24-36 h (redose when Cp < 1.5-2 mg/L)			1-1.5 mg/kg q 48-72 h[q]
Systemic GNR infection		1.5-2.5 mg/kg q 24-48 h (redose when Cp < 3-5 mg/L)			1.5-2 mg/kg q 48-72 h[q]
Hydralazine (oral)	None	25-50 mg q 8 h	Same	Same	ND
Imipenem	1 g	500 mg q 8 h[r]	500 mg q 6-8 h[r]	500 mg q 6 h[r]	250-500 mg q 12 h
Itraconazole	None	200 mg q 12 h × 4 doses, then 200 mg daily	Same	Same	Same
Levetiracetam	None	250-750 mg q 12 h	Same	Same	500-1000 mg q 24 h and 250-500 mg TIW (after HD)
Levofloxacin	500-750 mg	250 mg q 24 h	250-500 mg q 24 h	250-750 mg q 24 h	250-500 mg q 48 h
Linezolid	None	600 mg q 12 h	Same	Same	Same
Meropenem	1 g	0.5-1 g q 12 h[s]	0.5-1 g q 8-12 h[s]	Same[s,t]	500 mg q 24 h
Metoclopramide	None	75% usual MD	Same	Same	5-10 mg IV/IM q 4-6 h PRN
Metronidazole	None	250-500 mg q 6-12 h[u]	Same	Same	250-500 mg q 8-12 h[u]
Micafungin	None	100-150 mg q 24 h (treatment); 50 mg q 24 h (prophylaxis)	Same	Same	Same
Moxifloxacin	None	400 mg q 24 h	Same	Same	Same
Nafcillin	None	2 g q 4-6 h	Same	Same	Same
Penicillin G	4 MU	2 MU q 4-6 h	2-3 MU q 4-6 h	2-4 MU q 4-6 h	Normal dose load × 1, then 25%-50% normal dose q 4-6 h, or 50%-100% normal dose q 8-12 h[v]
Piperacillin- tazobactam	None	2.25-3.375 g q 6-8 h	2.25-3.375 g q 6 h	3.375 g q 6 h	2.25 g q 8-12 h
Ranitidine	None	150 mg oral q 12-24 h; 50 mg IV q 12-24 h	Same	Same	150 mg oral q 24 h; 50 mg IV q 24 h (after HD)
Rifampin	None	300-600 mg q 12-24 h[u]	Same	Same	Same
Ticarcillin- clavulanate	3.1 g	2 g q 6-8 h	3.1 g q 6-8 h	3.1 g q 6 h	2 g q 12 h[w]
Tigecycline	100 mg	50 mg q 12 h	Same	Same	Same

TABLE 174-4	Dosing Guidelines for Drugs Commonly Used in the ICU by Patients Receiving CVVH/CVVHD/CVVHDF/IHD (Continued)				
Drug[a]	Loading Dose	CVVH[b,c] Maintenance Dose	CVVHD[b] Maintenance Dose	CVVHDF[b] Maintenance Dose	IHD Dosing[d]
Tobramycin	2-3 mg/kg	GNR infection: 1.5-2.5 mg/kg q 24-48 h (see gentamicin for redosing)	Same	Same	Same as gentamicin
TMP-SMX	None	2.5-7.5 mg/kg (TMP) q 12 h[u]	Same	Same[x]	2.5-10 mg/kg (TMP)/d or 5-20 mg/kg TIW (after HD)[u]
Vancomycin	15-25 mg/kg	10-15 mg/kg q 24-48 h[y,z,aa]	10-15 mg/kg q 24 h[y,z,bb]	7.5-10 mg/kg q 12 h[y,z]	Load 15-25 mg/kg on day 1, then give 5-10 mg/kg after HD[y,cc]
Voriconazole	400 mg po q 12 h × 2[cc]	200 mg po q 12 h[dd]	Same	Same	Same

*Data are mean or range.

a. Doses are based on the provided references and the authors' opinions; however, should not replace clinical judgment.

b. All CRRT doses assume ultrafiltration and dialysis flow rates of 1-2 L/h, intravenous administration and minimal residual renal function. Dosing ranges are provided to accommodate for differences in ultrafiltration and dialysis flow rates, patient size, severity and site of infection, MIC of infecting pathogen(s), level of intrinsic renal function and immune status, among other factors.

c. Note that clearance of antimicrobials by CVVH depends on the CVVH filtration rate, primarily for antimicrobials with low PBC and V_d and provide dosing recommendations for aztreonam, cefazolin, cefotaxime, ceftazidime, imipenem, and piperacillin for CVVH filtration rates of 1-4 L/h.

d. Hemodialysis assumes TIW regimen and patient received full dialysis session (use clinical judgment); dose *after* dialysis on days of dialysis for q 24-72 h dosing. Doses assume critically ill patients with serious infections receiving standard IHD. Extended daily dialysis (EDD) may require larger doses than standard IHD.

e. 10 mg/kg q 12 h may be needed for encephalitis/VZV among patients receiving CVVHDF.

f. For severe GNR infections, target peak = 15-30 mg/L; redose when Cp < 10 mg/L.

g. Redose when pre-HD levels (Cp) < 10 mg/L; redose when post-HD levels (Cp) < 6-8 mg/L.

h. Doses of 1 g IV q 8 h results in similar steady state Cp as 2 g IV q 12 h; however, is more cost-effective.

i. Dose after dialysis on dialysis days. As an alternative, dose 1-2 g IV q 48-72 h post dialysis.

j. Doses of 2 g IV q 8 h may be needed for GNR pathogens with a MIC ≥ 4 mg/L.

k. Recommend dosing ceftazidime, 3 g IV, as a continuous infusion over 24 h after 2-g load to maintain Cp ≥ 4 × MIC for all susceptible pathogens in CVVHDF.

l. Drug clearance is highly dependent on the method of renal replacement, filter type, flow rate, site of infection, MIC of infecting pathogen(s), etc. For example, 2.5 mg/kg IV q 24 h may be required in patients receiving CVVHD with deep-seated infections and/or highly resistant GNR pathogens. Appropriate dosing requires close monitoring of pharmacologic response, signs of adverse reactions due to drug accumulation, as well as drug levels in relation to target trough (if appropriate).

m. Recommend dosing colistin up to 2.5 mg/kg IV q 12 h in patients receiving CVVHDF to achieve adequate Cp for highly resistant GNR pathogens.

n. Note that dosing daptomycin, 4-6 mg/kg IV q 48 h, in CRRT and SLEDD, respectively, may result in significant underdosing. Consider dosing 4-6 mg/kg IV q 24 h (or 8 mg/kg IV q 48 h) for critically ill patients receiving CRRT with deep-seated infections or those not responding to standard dosing. Therapeutic drug monitoring and/or more frequent creatine kinase serum levels may be warranted if dosing is increased.

o. Recommend dosing fluconazole, 800 mg daily, in CVVHF if the dialysate flow rate is ≥2 L/h and/or treating fungi with relative triazole resistance (i.e., *Candida glabrata*).

p. Recommend dosing fluconazole, 500-600 mg IV q 12 h, in CVVHDF.

q. Need for gentamicin redosing is primarily dependent on the clinical indication and availability of gentamicin levels (Cp), including reported values and timing (i.e., pre- vs. post-HD). Consider redosing gentamicin for pre-HD levels <1 mg/L (mild UTI and synergy), <1.5-2 mg/L (moderate-severe UTI) and <3-5 mg/L (severe GNR infection). Consider redosing gentamicin for post-HD levels <1 mg/L (UTI and synergy) and <2 mg/L (severe GNR infection).

r. Note imipenem doses of 500 mg IV q 8-12 h appear to achieve adequate Cp needed to treat most GNR pathogens with MIC ≤2 mg/L in patients receiving CRRT, however they recommend dosing imipenem 500 mg IV q6h to achieve adequate Cp for pathogens with higher MIC (MIC = 4-8 mg/L) or for deep-seated infections in patients receiving CRRT.

s. Consider dosing meropenem, 500 mg q 8 h or 1 g q 12 h, in CVVH; and 500 mg q 6-8 h or 1 g q 8-12 h in CVVHD(F).

t. Recommend dosing meropenem, 750 mg IV q 8 h or 1500 mg IV q 12 h in CVVHDF to optimize pharmacodynamic target attainment.

u. Dosing regimen is highly dependent on clinical indication (i.e., trichomoniasis vs. *Clostridium difficile* colitis for metronidazole; tuberculosis vs. infective endocarditis for rifampin; and cystitis vs. *Pneumocystis jiroveci* pneumonia for TMP-SMX).

v. Mild-moderate infections: 0.5-1 MU IV q 4-6 h or 1-2 MU IV q 8-12 h; neurosyphilis, endocarditis, or serious infections: doses up to 2 million units IV q 4-6 h; dose after HD on days of dialysis or supplement with 500,000 units after dialysis.

w. A supplemental dose of 3.1 g is recommended post dialysis. As an alternative, consider dosing 2 g IV q 8 h without a supplemental dose for deep-seated infections.

x. Doses up to 10 mg/kg IV q 12 h may be required for critically ill patients with *P. jiroveci* pneumonia receiving CVVHDF.

y. Recommended vancomycin doses and need for redosing must be individualized, as they are dependent on a number of variables including reported and targeted vancomycin concentrations.

z. Consider redosing vancomycin for Cp <10-15 mg/L for CRRT.

aa. Doses of vancomycin typically ranges from 500-1500 mg IV q 24-48 h among patients receiving CVVH to achieve desired Cp; however doses may have to be increased to achieve target vancomycin Cp of 15-20 mg/L (i.e., *Staphylococcus aureus* deep-seated infections).

bb. 7.5 mg/kg IV q 12 h may be required among patients receiving CVVHD to achieve desired Cp.

cc. Consider redosing vancomycin for pre-HD Cp as follows: <10 mg/L, give 1000 mg after HD; <10-25 mg/L, give 500-750 mg after HD; >25 mg/L, hold vancomycin. Consider redosing vancomycin 500-1000 mg for post-HD Cp <10-15 mg/L; however, recommended doses and need for redosing are dependent on reported and targeted vancomycin concentrations, utilization of high- vs. low-flux filters, among other factors.

dd. Oral therapy preferred to prevent accumulation of cyclodextran vehicle; bioavailability > 95%.

CMV, cytomegalovirus; Cp, plasma drug concentration(s); CRRT, continuous renal replacement therapy; CVVH, continuous venovenous hemofiltration; CVVHD, continuous venovenous hemodialysis; CVVHDF, continuous venovenous hemodiafiltration; GFR, glomerular filtration rate; GNR, gram-negative rods; GPC, gram-positive cocci; HD, hemodialysis; HSV, herpes simplex virus; I, induction dosing; IHD, intermittent hemodialysis; MD, maintenance dosing; MIC, minimum inhibitory concentration; MU, million units; ND, no data; SLEDD, slow extended daily dialysis; TIW, three times weekly; TMP-SMX, trimethoprim-sulfamethoxazole; UTI, urinary tract infection; VZV, varicella zoster virus.

Table adapted from Heintz BH, Matzke GR, Dager WE. Antimicrobial dosing concepts and recommendations for critically ill adult patients receiving continuous renal replacement therapy or intermittent hemodialysis. Pharmacotherapy 2009;29:562-77. Data from references 36, 43, 44, and 49.

ANNOTATED REFERENCES

Heintz BH, Matzke GR, Dager WE. Antimicrobial dosing concepts and recommendations for critically ill adult patients receiving continuous renal replacement therapy or intermittent hemodialysis. Pharmacotherapy 2009;29:562-77.

This review discusses the impact of CKD and AKI on antimicrobial drug pharmacokinetic and pharmacodynamic properties and provides recommendations for drug dosing in patients receiving CRRT and IHD.

Aronoff GR, Bennett WM, Berns JS, et al. Drug prescribing in renal failure: dosing guidelines for adults and children. 5th ed. Philadelphia: American College of Physicians; 2007.

This has been the premier clinical reference source for dosage recommendations for adults and children with reduced renal function. This edition included dosing guidelines for individuals receiving various modalities of dialysis (i.e., CRRT, IHD, and peritoneal dialysis). Although it is not designed to precisely individualize therapy such that desired target plasma drug concentrations are achieved, it remains a sound and reliable tool for initiating drug therapy in critically ill patients.

Levey AS, Greene T, Kusek JW, Beck GJ. A simplified equation to predict glomerular filtration rate from serum creatinine. J Am Soc Nephrol 2000;11:A0828.

The authors refined their earlier equation to predict GFR from serum creatinine concentration and other factors. It was initially developed by stepwise regression of the results from 1070 of the patients enrolled in the baseline period of the MDRD Study. The simplified equation provided a more accurate estimate of GFR than measured CL_{cr} or other commonly used equations. It demonstrated accuracy similar to the full equation. This approach has now become the "accepted" method to evaluate renal function in patients with CKD.

Matzke GR. Status of hemodialysis of drugs in 2002. J Pharm Practice 2002;15:405-18.

This review article addresses drug dialyzability in a quantitative fashion and outlines the key hemodialysis procedure variables that affect drug removal/dialyzer clearance. It also provides a conceptual framework for the individualization of drug therapy for patients receiving acute or chronic hemodialysis. Drug dosage regimen guidelines are presented for initiation of drug therapy with many medications commonly utilized for the dialysis-dependent patient; 43 commonly utilized medications, the majority of which are classically considered to be dialyzable, were reviewed. For 60% of these agents, the data were derived from studies conducted with dialyzers that are no longer commercially available. Data for 17 drugs that were evaluated with new, currently available dialyzers as well as those that are no longer commercially available revealed that the clearance by the dialyzer increased by as much as 3- to 10-fold. The dosage regimens of many drugs for dialysis patients are thus antiquated and likely will result in an excessively conservative approach to therapy.

Churchwell MD, Mueller BA. Drug dosing during continuous renal replacement therapy. Semin Dial 2009;22:185-8.

Although drug dosing in CRRT may appear uncomplicated (slow, constant removal of drug that can be approximated by assessing dialysate and/or ultrafiltrate flow rates), there are numerous other factors which may significantly affect drug clearance. This review summarizes these lesser known factors, illustrates the dearth of literature assessing drug dosing in CRRT, and advises clinicians to remain skeptical and vigilant when recommending doses.

Nolin TD. Altered nonrenal drug clearance in ESRD. Curr Opin Nephrol Hypertens 2008;17:555-9.

This review summarizes data available regarding the effect of CKD on drug metabolism and renal drug transport. Knowledge of the impact and nature of these alterations associated with kidney disease may facilitate the individualization of medication management in patient populations.

REFERENCE

Access the complete reference list online at http://www.expertconsult.com.

175 Antidepressant Drug Overdose

JOHN W. KREIT

Major depressive disorder (MDD) is a common and extremely important disease. The most recent national survey found a prevalence of 6.6% during the preceding 12 months and estimated that 16.2% of Americans will experience MDD during their lifetime.[1] The treatment of MDD underwent a major revolution in the 1950s and 1960s with the introduction of the tricyclic antidepressants (TCAs) and monoamine oxidase inhibitors (MAOIs). Subsequently, the development of the so-called selective serotonin reuptake inhibitors (SSRIs) and serotonin and norepinephrine reuptake inhibitors (SNRIs) allowed effective treatment of depression without most of the side effects and toxicity associated with the older classes of medications. This favorable side-effect profile has led to a fundamental shift away from the use of TCAs and MAOIs and has dramatically increased the number of patients taking antidepressant medications.

Since they are used to treat MDD, it is not surprising that antidepressants have always figured prominently on the list of drugs used during intentional self-poisonings. According to data published by the American Association of Poison Control Centers, antidepressants have been the third most commonly ingested class of medications, after analgesics and sedatives/hypnotics/antipsychotics, for the past 15 years.[2-4] As the use of TCAs and MAOIs has declined, so have the number of fatalities associated with these overdoses. In 1998, antidepressants were associated with almost 20% of fatal drug ingestions, but by 2008, this number had dropped to 8%.[2,3] Despite this dramatic decrease, antidepressants remain the third most common cause of fatal drug ingestions.[2]

Classification

As shown in Table 175-1, the most commonly used classification scheme divides antidepressant medications into tricyclic antidepressants, monoamine oxidase inhibitors, selective serotonin reuptake inhibitors, serotonin and norepinephrine reuptake inhibitors, and a miscellaneous group of drugs referred to as *atypical antidepressants*.[5-7] This classification is suboptimal from a pharmacologic standpoint because it mixes structural (TCA) and functional (e.g., SSRI, MAOI) drug characteristics. In addition, as discussed later, functional characteristics can vary markedly among the drugs in each category, and significant overlap can occur between categories. Nevertheless, this classification scheme does provide a framework for discussing the pharmacology, clinical manifestations, and management of antidepressant overdose.

Pharmacology

Before describing the pharmacology of the antidepressant drugs, it is important to review the release, reuptake, and metabolism of serotonin (5-hydroxytryptamine [5-HT]) and norepinephrine (NE), two monoamine neurotransmitters that are believed to play a major role in the pathogenesis of depression. As illustrated in Figure 175-1, 5-HT and NE are each synthesized by specific neurons and packaged into vesicles in the presynaptic nerve terminal. An action potential causes these vesicles to fuse with the nerve membrane, thereby releasing 5-HT or NE into the synaptic cleft. After release, these neurotransmitters bind to specific postsynaptic receptors. Seven serotonin receptor families (designated 5-HT$_1$, 5-HT$_2$, and so forth) have been identified, and many contain more than one receptor subtype (e.g., 5-HT$_{1A}$, 5-HT$_{1B}$).[8] Each family and each receptor subtype appears to have specific functions and distributions throughout the body, although all are present in the central nervous system (CNS). NE binds to two major families

of postsynaptic receptors termed α and β, and each has two major subtypes, referred to as α_1, α_2, β_1, and β_2. After release, the actions of 5-HT and NE are terminated primarily by active reuptake into the presynaptic neuron by amine-specific transporters. There, they are either repackaged into vesicles for future release or inactivated by the mitochondrial-bound enzyme, monoamine oxidase (MAO). MAO has the important role of inactivating a wide variety of monoamines and is found in the brain, gastrointestinal (GI) tract, and liver as well as other organs and tissues. There are two enzyme subtypes. MAO-A primarily functions to inactivate 5-HT, NE, and tyramine, whereas dopamine, phenylethylamine, tyramine, and tryptamine are the major substrates of MAO-B.[8]

PHARMACOLOGIC ACTIONS

Most antidepressant medications act to increase the extraneuronal concentrations of serotonin and/or norepinephrine in the CNS. The TCAs, SSRIs, and SNRIs do this by inactivating specific transporters in the presynaptic neuron, thereby preventing the reuptake of these biogenic amines from the synaptic cleft. As shown in Table 175-2, the TCAs have a wide range of potencies and specificities for the 5-HT and NE transporters.[5,9] For example, desipramine is the most potent inhibitor of NE reuptake, whereas clomipramine is the most effective serotonin reuptake blocker. The SSRIs, although much more specific, also demonstrate variable potency for transporter blockade.[5,10-13] The SNRIs inhibit both 5-HT and NE reuptake, but with the exception of duloxetine have relatively low potency.[5,14,15] At present, it is not clear that differences in drug selectivity translate into differences in efficacy, and differences in potency are largely eliminated through dosage adjustments.

MAOIs prevent the breakdown of 5-HT and NE after reuptake has occurred.[16] The antidepressant effect of these drugs requires the inhibition of MAO-A and is presumed to result from increased concentrations of 5-HT and NE in the brain. Most MAOIs, including isocarboxazid, phenelzine, and tranylcypromine, irreversibly inactivate both MAO-A and MAO-B. Recently, several new drugs which selectively and reversibly inactivate MAO-A have been developed. The most widely studied of these drugs, moclobemide, has been approved for use in several European countries but is not yet available in the United States.

The so-called atypical antidepressants act through a variety of different mechanisms.[6,7,17] Bupropion primarily inhibits the reuptake of dopamine by blocking specific presynaptic transporters. Mirtazapine is a potent central α-adrenergic agonist that promotes the release of both serotonin and norepinephrine. It also acts as an antagonist at 5-HT$_2$ and 5-HT$_3$ receptors. Reboxetine is a selective inhibitor of NE reuptake. Nefazodone and trazodone act primarily by blocking 5-HT$_{2A}$ receptors.

In addition to their therapeutic effects, many of the antidepressant drugs also have a variety of undesirable properties. As shown in Table 175-3, many of them block α_1-adrenergic, cholinergic, and/or histamine (H$_1$) receptors.[5-15] The TCAs are the most potent antagonists of all three receptor types, although the atypical antidepressants, mirtazapine, nefazodone, and trazodone, also block H$_1$ and/or α_1-adrenergic receptors. In general, the SSRIs and SNRIs have little or no effect on these receptors. The TCAs also block fast inward sodium channels on myocardial cells, which is analogous to the effect of type I antiarrhythmic drugs.

TABLE 175-1	Classification of Antidepressant Medications	
Generic Name		*Brand Name*
Tricyclic Antidepressants		
Amitriptyline		Elavil
Amoxapine		Asendin
Clomipramine		Anafranil
Desipramine		Norpramin
Doxepin		Adapin, Sinequan
Imipramine		Tofranil
Maprotiline		Ludiomil
Nortriptyline		Pamelor
Protriptyline		Vivactil
Trimipramine		Surmontil
Monoamine Oxidase Inhibitors		
Isocarboxazid		Marplan
Phenelzine		Nardil
Tranylcypromine		Parnate
Moclobemide		Manerix
Selective Serotonin Reuptake Inhibitors		
Citalopram		Celexa
Escitalopram		Lexapro
Fluoxetine		Prozac
Fluvoxamine		Luvox
Paroxetine		Paxil
Sertraline		Zoloft
Serotonin and Norepinephrine Reuptake Inhibitors		
Venlafaxine		Effexor
Desvenlafaxine		Pristiq
Duloxetine		Cymbalta
Milnacipran		Savella
Atypical Antidepressants		
Bupropion		Wellbutrin
Mirtazapine		Remeron
Reboxetine		Edronax
Nefazodone		Serzone
Trazodone		Desyrel

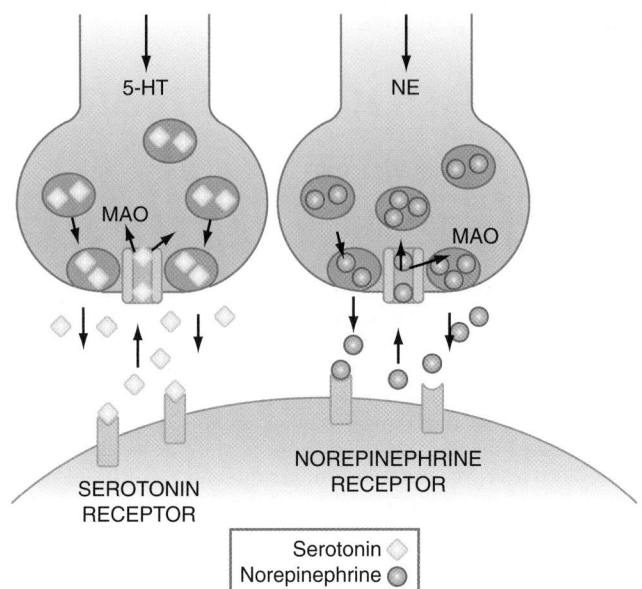

Figure 175-1 Serotonin (5-HT) and norepinephrine (NE) are released into the synaptic cleft and bind to specific post-synaptic receptors. Their effects are terminated by active reuptake into the pre-synaptic neuron by amine-specific transporters. There, they are either repackaged into vesicles or inactivated by monoamine oxidase (MAO).

ABSORPTION, DISTRIBUTION, METABOLISM, AND EXCRETION

In general, all antidepressants are well absorbed after oral administration, and peak plasma concentrations are usually achieved within several hours. Once absorbed, the TCAs in particular become tightly bound to plasma proteins and have a large volume of distribution. The MAOIs are metabolized primarily by hepatic acetylation, and the rate at which this process occurs varies widely among the population. Inactivation of the TCAs, SSRIs, SNRIs, and atypical antidepressants occurs largely via hepatic CYP450 enzymes, and the final byproduct is excreted in the urine. This means that coadministration of these drugs or use of another medication that inhibits CYP450 function may lead to significant drug toxicity.[5,9,18]

The duration of action of the antidepressants depends on the clearance rate of the parent compound as well as that of any active metabolites. Except for moclobemide, which is reversible and short acting, irreversible enzyme inactivation by the MAOIs causes their effects to last up to 2 weeks after these drugs have been ingested. In general, the other antidepressant drugs have half-lives in the range of 20 to 40 hours.[5] Exceptions are fluoxetine, and its active metabolite norfluoxetine, which have half-lives of about 2 and 10 days, respectively; and venlafaxine and nefazodone, which have half-lives of approximately 5 and 3 hours, respectively.[5] Because it takes approximately five half-lives for complete drug elimination to occur, most of the antidepressants can have prolonged effects after a toxic ingestion.

Toxicology

The symptoms and signs that accompany an overdose, the severity and duration of toxicity, and even specific therapeutic strategies can be predicted based on a knowledge of the pharmacologic actions of each of the antidepressant drugs. Because of their potent antagonistic effects at cholinergic, adrenergic, and histaminic receptors and their ability to

block sodium channels in the myocardium, TCAs are the most likely class of antidepressant drugs to cause major morbidity or death when taken in overdose.[19] Not surprisingly, significant morbidity and mortality are very uncommon following ingestion of the SSRIs and SNRIs, which lack these properties.[19] MAOIs and the atypical antidepressants have an intermediate toxicity profile.

TRICYCLIC ANTIDEPRESSANTS

Clinical Features

The manifestations of TCA overdose are caused by the receptor and sodium channel blocking properties of these drugs.[19,20] Patients typically present with symptoms and signs of an anticholinergic syn-

TABLE 175-2	Potencies of Antidepressants for Blocking Neurotransmitter Reuptake	
Drug	*Norepinephrine (NE)*	*Serotonin (5-HT)*
Tricyclic Antidepressants		
Desipramine	+++++	++
Protriptyline	++++	++
Nortriptyline	+++	+
Amoxapine	++	+
Doxepin	++	+
Clomipramine	+	+++++
Imipramine	+	++++
Amitriptyline	+	++
Selective Serotonin Reuptake Inhibitors		
Paroxetine	+	+++++
Sertraline	±	++++
Escitalopram	—	++++
Citalopram	—	+++
Fluoxetine	±	+++
Fluvoxamine	—	++
Serotonin and Norepinephrine Reuptake Inhibitors		
Duloxetine	+++	+++++
Venlafaxine	±	+
Desvenlafaxine	+	++
Milnacipran	+	+

Potency increases progressively from ± to +++++. —, no effect.

	Receptors Blocked		
TABLE 175-3 Potencies of Antidepressants as Receptor Antagonists			
Drug	*Cholinergic*	*Histamine (H_1)*	*Adrenergic (α_1)*
Tricyclic Antidepressants			
Amitriptyline	+++++	++++	++++
Protriptyline	+++++	++	++
Clomipramine	+++++	+++	+++
Doxepin	++++	+++++	++++
Imipramine	++++	++	++++
Nortriptyline	+++	++++	+++
Desipramine	++	+	++
Selective Serotonin Reuptake Inhibitors			
Paroxetine	+++	—	—
Fluoxetine	+	—	—
Sertraline	+	—	±
Citalopram	+	—	—
Escitalopram	—	—	—
Fluvoxamine	—	—	—
Serotonin and Norepinephrine Reuptake Inhibitors			
Venlafaxine	—	—	—
Desvenlafaxine	—	—	—
Duloxetine	—	—	—
Milnacipran	—	—	—
Atypical Antidepressants			
Bupropion	—	—	—
Mirtazapine	±	+++++	±
Reboxetine	—	±	—
Nefazodone	—	+++	++++
Trazodone	—	+	++++

Drug potency increases progressively from ± to +++++. —, no effect.

drome, or toxidrome, which may include mydriasis, dry mouth, slowed intestinal peristalsis or ileus, urinary retention, fever, flushing, sinus tachycardia, CNS depression that ranges from lethargy to coma, respiratory depression, and seizures. Blockade of α_1-adrenergic receptors causes vasodilation, which decreases preload and vascular resistance and can lead to hypotension. Through their direct toxic effect on the myocardium, TCA overdose may slow depolarization and lead to prolongation of the QRS and QT intervals, heart block, and ventricular arrhythmias. Inhibition of the sodium current may also lead to decreases in myocardial contractility, stroke volume, and cardiac output. Hypotension can result from vasodilation, impaired contractility, or both. The life-threatening complications of TCA overdose, therefore, are ventricular arrhythmias, advanced heart block, shock, stupor and coma, respiratory depression, and recurrent generalized seizures.

Diagnosis and Initial Evaluation

The diagnosis of TCA overdose should be strongly suspected in any patient who presents with an anticholinergic toxidrome, especially if the electrocardiogram (ECG) demonstrates characteristic changes. Qualitative urine immunoassays for TCAs may be used to increase the level of suspicion, but they do not distinguish therapeutic from toxic ingestions, and they have relatively low specificity owing to cross-reactivity with other drugs including phenothiazines and diphenhydramine.[21] Quantitative serum assays can be used to confirm a toxic ingestion, but long turnaround times often limit their clinical usefulness.

Patients with a suspected or known TCA ingestion must be frequently assessed for the development of major complications. The physical examination should focus on detecting hypotension, tissue hypoperfusion, altered level of consciousness, respiratory depression, and ileus. A 12-lead ECG must be obtained to detect conduction disturbances and arrhythmias, and continuous ECG monitoring is required. Arterial blood gas measurements can be useful for detecting or confirming respiratory depression and acidemia.

Since TCA overdose causes major morbidity and death in a relatively small proportion of patients, there has been a great deal of interest in identifying factors that can accurately predict major toxicity. Most studies have focused on ECG measurements and the serum drug concentration. Over the past 30 years, limb-lead QRS duration greater than 100 msec, a QTc greater than 430 msec, and a terminal 40-msec frontal plane QRS axis (T40) between 130 and 270 degrees all have been reported to predict future seizures, ventricular arrhythmias, and death, although the sensitivity and specificity of each has varied considerably.[22-24] Similarly, an initial or maximum drug concentration greater than 1000 ng/mL has been found to have very good, fair, or poor prognostic value, depending on the study.[22-26] A meta-analysis published in 2004 found that all four of these parameters have equally poor sensitivity and specificity for predicting seizures, ventricular arrhythmias, or death.[27] On the other hand, QRS duration and serum concentration were found to have low negative likelihood ratios, indicating that these criteria can be used to predict the absence of future toxicity.[27]

Management

Prevention of Absorption. Activated charcoal is an inert, nonspecific adsorbent that irreversibly binds most drugs and toxins, including tricyclic antidepressants. Many studies in volunteers have shown that charcoal administration has a time-dependent effect on drug absorption. For example, after a single dose of nortriptyline, activated charcoal given at 30 minutes, 2 hours, or 4 hours reduced the peak serum concentration by 77%, 37%, and 19%, respectively.[28] Despite its proven ability to reduce drug absorption, the efficacy of single-dose charcoal cannot be assessed because of the lack of satisfactorily designed clinical trials. The only prospective randomized placebo-controlled trial of single-dose charcoal in TCA-poisoned patients found no differences in clinical outcome or the rate of fall of drug concentrations.[29] Aspiration appears to be the main complication of charcoal administration and is quite common. In their most recent position paper, the American Academy of Clinical Toxicology recommended that the administration of activated charcoal be *considered* only in patients who present within 1 hour of a potentially toxic ingestion.[30]

Although gastric lavage has been used in the initial management of most drug intoxications, there is virtually no evidence to support its use. In most poisoned patients, including those who have ingested TCAs, gastric lavage fails to significantly reduce drug absorption.[31] Furthermore, several randomized trials comparing lavage plus activated charcoal with activated charcoal alone have failed to show an improvement in patient outcome.[32-35] A number of serious risks of the procedure also have been well documented, including aspiration, cardiac arrhythmias, and esophageal perforation. Based on a thorough review of the literature, the American Academy of Clinical Toxicology has stated that "gastric lavage should not be employed routinely, if ever, in the management of poisoned patients."[36]

Enhancement of Drug Elimination. Repeated doses of activated charcoal can increase drug clearance by interrupting enterohepatic circulation and by reducing the concentration of free drug in the intestinal lumen, thereby creating a diffusion gradient from the blood (a process referred to as *gastrointestinal dialysis*). Although multiple doses of activated charcoal increase the clearance of several drugs including carbamazepine, phenobarbital, and theophylline, studies examining TCA clearance in volunteer subjects have yielded inconclusive and often conflicting results, and no studies have examined this therapy in poisoned patients.[37] For this reason, and because multiple-dose charcoal has been reported to cause intestinal obstruction, this therapy is not recommended for patients with TCA intoxication.[37]

Hemodialysis and charcoal hemoperfusion would be expected to be ineffective in removing TCAs and their active metabolites, because avid tissue and plasma protein binding leaves only a small fraction of free drug available for diffusion or adsorption. Although beneficial effects have been reported,[38,39] based on these pharmacokinetic considerations, extracorporeal therapy is not recommended for patients with TCA poisoning.[20]

Sodium Bicarbonate. Several controlled trials in animals and case reports and case series in humans have demonstrated that administration of sodium bicarbonate is often effective in shortening the QRS interval, terminating ventricular arrhythmias, and increasing blood pressure after TCA overdose.[40] Three potential mechanisms for these beneficial effects have been proposed.[40] First, alkalinization of the serum increases protein binding, thereby reducing the concentration of free drug. Second, by causing drug ionization, alkalinization may reduce the affinity of TCAs for the myocardial sodium channel receptor. Third, an increase in the serum sodium concentration may overcome sodium channel blockade. This final mechanism may explain why hypertonic saline has been reported to reverse cardiac toxicity in some animal studies and in case reports in humans.[41] It may also explain the observation that hyperventilation appears to be less effective than sodium bicarbonate administration.[40] Based on this information, it is currently recommended that patients with evidence of cardiac toxicity (i.e., QRS or QT prolongation, ventricular arrhythmias, heart block, hypotension) receive sodium bicarbonate with the goal of achieving and maintaining an arterial pH of 7.50 to 7.55.[42,43]

Treatment of Specific Complications

Arrhythmias. Ventricular tachycardia and fibrillation accompanying TCA overdose are often refractory to drug therapy, and treatment should focus on the administration of sodium bicarbonate and the correction of acidemia, hypoxemia, and electrolyte abnormalities.[43] Antiarrhythmic drugs categorized as class Ia (e.g., procainamide), Ic (e.g., flecainide, propafenone), and III (e.g., amiodarone, sotalol) are not only ineffective but also should be avoided because they, like the TCAs, can prolong depolarization. Case series have described the successful use of lidocaine,[44] phenytoin,[45,46] and magnesium sulfate[47] in patients with refractory ventricular arrhythmias.

Hypotension. Because TCA-induced hypotension may result from vasodilation, impaired cardiac contractility, or both, right heart catheterization is often useful in determining the predominant cause and the most appropriate therapy. Arterial and venous dilation resulting from α_1-adrenergic blockade cause a drop in systemic vascular resistance (SVR) and ventricular preload which are most effectively treated with volume resuscitation, followed if necessary by the use of one or more vasopressors. Norepinephrine may be more effective than dopamine in this setting,[48] and high-dose glucagon has also been reported to be beneficial.[49] On the other hand, impaired myocardial contractility leads to a fall in cardiac output and a compensatory rise in SVR and responds best to dobutamine and afterload reduction. Sodium bicarbonate administration may be effective in improving hypotension, regardless of the underlying cause.

Seizures. The treatment of seizures induced by TCA overdose does not differ from that of other seizure disorders. Status epilepticus is a medical emergency that must be quickly and effectively treated to prevent anoxic brain injury.

Clinical Course and Monitoring

Patients with TCA overdose can become critically ill very rapidly, even when initial symptoms or signs are minimal.[50] However, patients who develop major signs of toxicity (coma, seizures, respiratory depression, hypotension, ventricular arrhythmias) almost invariably do so within 6 hours of presentation, and almost all deaths occur within the first 16 hours.[50] The maximum QRS duration also typically occurs within the first 6 hours[22] and usually returns to normal within 12 to 18 hours.[51] Patients rarely develop seizures or ventricular dysrhythmias after the QRS interval has decreased to less than 0.10 second.[22,51] Based on this information, patients should be admitted to an intensive care unit (ICU) if they have signs of toxicity or QRS prolongation, or if they have been monitored for less than 6 hours in the emergency department. Patients should be transferred from the ICU only after their QRS interval has returned to normal.

REUPTAKE INHIBITORS

Clinical Features

The SSRIs and SNRIs have a much more favorable side-effect profile than the TCAs, and overdoses are usually associated with little significant toxicity.[19,52,53] The most common manifestations are lethargy, diaphoresis, nausea and vomiting, sinus tachycardia, and tremor.[19] Seizures, cardiac conduction disturbances (including QRS and QTc prolongation), and atrial and ventricular arrhythmias are very uncommon but are most likely to occur after venlafaxine or citalopram ingestion.[7,19,54,55] Mortality is also quite uncommon and in most reported cases has been associated with co-ingestion of other psychotropic agents, benzodiazepines, opiates, or alcohol.[2,52,53]

Another uncommon but potentially serious toxic manifestation of the SSRIs and SNRIs is a constellation of symptoms and signs referred to as *serotonin syndrome*.[56] This disorder results from excessive stimulation of central and peripheral serotonin receptors and is characterized by the triad of altered mentation, autonomic dysfunction, and neuromuscular hyperactivity. Symptoms and signs range from mild to very severe and include delirium, diaphoresis, diarrhea, hyperthermia, tremor, hyperreflexia, clonus, and muscular rigidity. Laboratory findings are variable and nonspecific and may include leukocytosis and elevations of creatine phosphokinase and the hepatic transaminases. When it occurs, the serotonin syndrome usually develops within 6 hours following self-poisoning.[56]

Management

The treatment of SSRI and SNRI overdose is primarily supportive.[53] As discussed earlier, gastric lavage is virtually never indicated, and single-dose activated charcoal should be considered only when patients present with major signs of toxicity within 1 hour of drug ingestion. Because major morbidity and mortality usually result from the effects of other medications, efforts must be made to identify all co-ingested substances.

Treatment of serotonin syndrome is also largely supportive, and usually the most important intervention is to identify and discontinue all serotonergic drugs.[56] Serotonin syndrome usually has a benign course, and symptoms and signs typically resolve within 24 hours of onset. Occasionally, however, severe complications occur and require specific therapy; these include marked hyperthermia, rhabdomyolysis, disseminated intravascular coagulation, renal failure, and acute respiratory distress syndrome. Limited data suggest that the serotonin receptor (5-HT$_{2A}$) antagonist, cyproheptadine, may be useful in severe cases.[57]

MONOAMINE OXIDASE INHIBITORS

The symptoms and signs that accompany MAOI overdose are believed to result primarily from a hyperadrenergic state produced by the inability to metabolize and inactivate NE in the central and peripheral nervous systems. Overdose with the irreversible MAOIs is commonly accompanied by life-threatening toxicity, and the mortality rate is similar to that of TCA ingestion.[2,7,58] Clinical manifestations, which may be delayed for up to 24 hours, include mydriasis, flushing, diaphoresis, tachycardia, hypertension, hyperthermia, muscular rigidity, agitation, delirium, and seizures.[59,60] Hypotension may occur later in the course, probably as the result of depletion of NE stores. Since MAOIs act to increase serotonin levels in the brain, overdose may also precipitate the serotonin syndrome.

Patients with MAOI overdose should receive activated charcoal if they present within 1 hour after drug ingestion.[30] Severe hypertension is best controlled with sodium nitroprusside, and hypotension usually responds well to NE.[56,58,59] Dopamine acts largely by releasing stored NE and should be avoided because it may either worsen the hyperadrenergic state or be ineffective due to endogenous NE depletion.[59,60] Hyperthermia may be severe and require evaporative cooling techniques. Muscle rigidity usually responds to benzodiazepines but may require the use of neuromuscular blockade.[56,59,60] Seizures typically respond to benzodiazepines, phenytoin, and phenobarbital.

ATYPICAL ANTIDEPRESSANTS

Relatively little is known about the consequences of overdose with the atypical antidepressants. It is recognized, however, that bupropion has the greatest toxicity.[7,19] The most common manifestations of bupropion overdose are neurologic, and delirium and recurrent seizures are common. Cardiac complications including QRS and QT_C prolongation and ventricular arrhythmias have been reported.[7,61] Mirtazapine, reboxetine, nefazodone, and trazodone appear to produce relatively little toxicity following self-poisoning, and CNS depression is the most commonly reported effect.[7,17,19,62-64]

KEY POINTS

1. Antidepressants are the third most common cause of overdose-related death.

2. Antidepressants can be divided into five categories: tricyclic antidepressants (TCAs), monoamine oxidase inhibitors (MAOIs), selective serotonin reuptake inhibitors (SSRIs), serotonin and norepinephrine reuptake inhibitors (SNRIs), and the "atypical" antidepressants.

3. Most antidepressant medications act to increase the extraneuronal concentration of both serotonin (5-HT) and norepinephrine (NE). TCAs, SSRIs, and SNRIs prevent the reuptake of these neurotransmitters by inactivating specific transporters in the presynaptic neuron. MAOIs prevent the breakdown of 5-HT and NE after reuptake has occurred.

4. The clinical manifestations of TCA overdose are largely caused by antagonism at α_1-adrenergic, cholinergic, and histamine receptors and direct blockade of sodium channels in the His-Purkinje system and ventricular myocardium. Patients typically present with a cholinergic toxidrome that may be complicated by ventricular arrhythmias, impaired cardiac conduction and contractility, hypotension, seizures, and respiratory failure.

5. MAOI overdose is usually accompanied by mydriasis, flushing, diaphoresis, tachycardia, and hypertension and may cause severe hyperthermia, muscular rigidity, delirium, and seizures.

6. Unlike TCA and MAOI overdose, SSRI and SNRI ingestion is usually accompanied by little significant toxicity, although seizures, cardiac conduction disturbances, atrial and ventricular arrhythmias, and serotonin syndrome may occur.

7. Treatment of antidepressant drug overdose is largely supportive. Single-dose activated charcoal may be considered in patients who present within 1 hour of a potentially toxic ingestion. Gastric lavage is virtually never indicated. Patients with TCA overdose who have signs of cardiac toxicity (i.e., QRS or QT prolongation, ventricular arrhythmias, heart block, hypotension) should receive intravenous sodium bicarbonate, with the goal of achieving and maintaining an arterial pH of 7.50 to 7.55.

ANNOTATED REFERENCES

Gillman PK. Tricyclic antidepressant pharmacology and therapeutic drug interactions updated. Br J Pharmacol 2007;151:737-48.
 This is the most complete and most recent review of the pharmacology of the tricyclic antidepressants.
Richelson E. Pharmacology of antidepressants. Mayo Clin Proc 2001;76:511-27.
 This is an authoritative and comprehensive review of the absorption, elimination, and pharmacologic actions of the antidepressants.
Krishnan KR. Revisiting monoamine oxidase inhibitors. J Clin Psychiatry 2007;68(S8):35-41.
 This article provides an excellent overview of the pharmacology and clinical use of the MAO inhibitors.
Woolf AD, Erdman AR, Nelson LS, et al. Tricyclic antidepressant poisoning: an evidence-based consensus guideline for out-of-hospital management. Clin Toxicol 2007;45:203-33.

Although it focuses on prehospital management, this article contains a great deal of well-referenced information regarding TCA overdose.
Blackman K, Brown SG, Wilkes GJ. Plasma alkalinization for tricyclic antidepressant toxicity: a systematic review. Emerg Med 2001;13:204-10.
 This article reviews the mechanisms of action and therapeutic effects of sodium bicarbonate administration in patients with severe TCA toxicity.
Boyer EW, Shannon M. The serotonin syndrome. N Engl J Med 2005;352:1112-20.
 This is the most recent authoritative review of serotonin syndrome.
Buckley NA, Faunce TA. Atypical antidepressants in overdose. Drug Saf 2003;26:539-51.
 This is the best review of the pharmacology and toxicology of the atypical antidepressants.

REFERENCES

Access the complete reference list online at http://www.expertconsult.com.

176

Clinical Use of Immunosuppressants

KRISTINE S. SCHONDER | ROBERT J. WEBER | JOHN J. FUNG | THOMAS E. STARZL

Advances in molecular biology and immunology have provided for greater understanding of the mechanisms involved in allograft rejection. Many of the key pathways of organ rejection are targeted by today's growing armamentarium of immunosuppressive drugs, and a vast array of immunosuppressive combinations has dramatically decreased the incidence of acute allograft rejection. However, very little ground has been gained with respect to the impact of chronic allograft rejection on long-term allograft survival. Furthermore, with long-term use, the relative nonselectivity of current immunosuppressants can lead to development of malignancies and opportunistic infections. As we continue to explore different combinations of immunosuppressants and new immunosuppressive pathways, our comprehension of the immune system will grow, and we can help patients come closer to true allograft acceptance.

Basic Principles of Immunosuppression

Optimal *immunosuppression* as it relates to transplantation is defined as the level of drug therapy that achieves graft acceptance with least suppression of systemic immunity. By optimizing immunosuppressive therapy, systemic toxicity (i.e., infection and malignancy) and other side effects can be minimized, albeit not entirely eliminated. Because monitoring of blood levels and titration of immunosuppression on this basis is possible with only a few agents in practice, oversuppression or undersuppression almost invariably becomes apparent only in retrospect. Recently, monitoring CD3+ cell counts has provided an alternative means of measuring the degree of immunosuppression.

Current immunosuppression protocols typically use multiple drugs, each directed at a discrete site in the T-cell activation cascade.[1] Most immunosuppressive regimens combine drugs, often with differing modes of action and toxicities, allowing lower doses of each drug. Transplantation immunosuppression can be (1) *pharmacologic*, consisting of drugs such as corticosteroids, cytokine suppressive agents, and cell cycle inhibitors, or (2) *biological*, consisting of monoclonal and polyclonal antilymphocyte antibodies and anticytokine receptor antibodies.[2]

The combination of cyclosporine or tacrolimus with a corticosteroid forms the backbone of most maintenance immunosuppressive regimens being used today. An antiproliferative agent also may be added. In general, the early postoperative period calls for the greatest degree of immunosuppression. As time goes on, many patients can maintain graft function with smaller doses of immunosuppressive agents.

If acute cellular rejection occurs, it is common to treat it with a brief course of high doses of corticosteroids, antilymphocyte antibodies, or both. Generally, high doses of a corticosteroid are used initially to reverse the acute attack on the allograft. Antilymphocyte antibody therapy with monoclonal or polyclonal antibodies is used for more severe rejection or if corticosteroid therapy fails.

Induction therapy, also called *prophylactic therapy*, refers to the use of antilymphocyte antibodies immediately after transplantation. This practice is based on the theory that early incapacitation of the immune system may reduce the likelihood of subsequent rejection. Claimed benefits are delayed onset of acute rejection, fewer episodes of rejection, and no significant increase in infectious complications.[3,4] The related concept of *sequential therapy* was introduced in response to the significant renal toxicity of cyclosporine observed in recipients of liver, heart, and kidney transplants. The practice is to use antibody therapy for the first 1 to 2 weeks after transplantation—the period in which

renal injury is most likely to occur from a variety of insults. Cyclosporine therapy is not used during this period but is started later. The impact of this strategy on long-term renal function is much less clear.

This early intensification of immunosuppression is not universally accepted. Some experts voice concern because of the well-known association between antilymphocyte antibody therapy (and immunosuppression in general) and infection and malignancy.[5,6] Others describe no benefit, greater expense,[7] or the successful use of regimens that avoid induction altogether.[8] Intermediate strategies involve the use of induction only in high-risk patients or the use of just one dose of an antilymphocyte agent, followed by early evaluation of renal function.

Although some patients can tolerate complete withdrawal of immunosuppressive therapy without exhibiting rejection,[3] it is best done as a protocol-based strategy with patients under strict supervision. The current general approach is to minimize long-term immunosuppression. Various withdrawal protocols target individual components of the immunosuppressive regimen (e.g., corticosteroids, calcineurin inhibitors) in an attempt to decrease serious complications of immunosuppression—namely, infection, malignancy, and renal dysfunction.

Overview of Transplantation Immunobiology

Antigen specificity is determined by an antigen-binding unit on the surface of the T cell called the *T-cell receptor* (TCR). The specificity and diversity of the TCR binding site result from variations in its amino acid composition among different T cells. The gene sequence coding for the TCR rearranges during development in the thymus such that each T cell has a different TCR binding specificity. The result is a complex system that enables lymphocytes to discriminate between "self" and "nonself" or foreign antigens.

Once inside tissues or the circulation of the body, foreign antigens are presented to lymphocytes by antigen-presenting cells (APCs), epitomized by dendritic cells. APCs phagocytose foreign proteins and cleave them enzymatically into small peptides that are 8 to 12 amino acids in length. These peptides are loaded onto a class of specialized carrier molecules known as *major histocompatibility complex* (MHC) molecules. The MHC molecule carries the peptide fragment to the cell surface, where it is displayed to T cells in the host's lymphoid organs. Thus, there are three essential requirements for the adaptive immune response known as *rejection*: (1) the presence of an antigen fragment or protein (a ligand) at the cell surface of the APC, (2) a receptor that recognizes the ligand, and (3) activation of T cells.

The migration pattern of the antigen also is a critical factor. The only mobile antigens in solid organ transplantation are "passenger leukocytes" of donor bone marrow origin that are present in the graft. After transplantation of the solid organ, these white blood cells migrate promptly and preferentially to host lymphoid organs.[9-11] These organs or organized heterotopic lymphoid collections provide the unique architectural structure and cellular milieu wherein factors necessary for progression from an immunogenic environment to a tolerogenic environment are present in abundance. These factors include cytokines, other molecules, cell-cell proximity, and homing mechanisms that ensure an efficient response to the antigen.[12] In the lymphoid organs, dendritic cells and other APCs that have captured and processed the antigen present the peptide fragment of the antigen to antigen-specific TCRs in the context of their upregulated host MHC peptide.

The efferent (effector) phase begins with the secretion of interleukin (IL)-2, or T-cell growth factor) and interferon alpha (IFN-α) by activated lymphocytes. The antigen-specific immune activation and clonal expansion is aborted unless there is upregulation by the APCs of "accessory" cell-bound (co-stimulatory) molecules that sustain accelerated production of IL-2 and foster the secretion of numerous other cytokines (e.g., IL-1, IL-6, IL-9, IL-10, IFNs, tumor necrosis factor alpha [TNF-α, TNF-β]) and growth factors (granulocyte colony-stimulating factor [G-CSF] and granulocyte-macrophage colony-stimulating factor [GM-CSF]).[13] The sequential nature of the response amplification has been obscured by use of the term *co-stimulatory* to describe the accessory molecules, implying that the afferent and early effector phases are simultaneous.

The TCR is a cell-surface molecule that associates with accessory molecules including CD3, and either CD4 or CD8. The TCR-CD3 complex interacts with the peptide fragment carried by the MHC molecule of the APC. This complex is stabilized by the CD4 or CD8 molecule of the T cell. This interaction produces the signal that initiates activation of the T cell, leading to proliferation of a T-cell clone that recognizes the particular antigen fragments of the foreign protein. The basis for MHC-restricted antigen recognition requires antigen presentation by APCs bearing an MHC molecule specific to the host.

Antigen-directed proliferation of T-cell clones is absolutely essential for an effective immune response. The response is driven by a positive feedback loop. T cells that recognize antigen make the potent growth factor, IL-2, and simultaneously become responsive to IL-2 by expressing the IL-2 receptor. This dual synthesis allows the cells to stimulate their own proliferation, as well as the proliferation of other T cells. Lymphocytes recirculate at a rate of 1% to 2% per hour, migrating through all tissues of the body. Specialized cell-surface "homing" molecules on T lymphocytes mediate attachment to targeted alien tissues, with a special avidity for the endothelial cells of an allograft's vessels.

During an ongoing immune response, proliferating T cells recruit many other cell types and immune mechanisms into action. Cytokines and chemokines can attract and activate other leukocytes. For example, cytokines produced by CD4-positive helper T cells attract macrophages and CD8-bearing cytotoxic lymphocytes into rejecting allografts.[14] These cytokines also trigger macrophage activation and CD8+ T-lymphocyte cell maturation. The resulting multicellular tissue infiltration has traditionally been referred to as a *delayed-type hypersensitivity response*. Cytokines released by helper T cells also are responsible for the activation of B cells and thus, indirectly, for the majority of antibody production. Cytokines also upregulate expression of both MHC molecules on tissues and adhesion molecules on endothelium. These events aid in the entry and accumulation of leukocytes. Finally, cytokines activate distant organ responses such as the hepatic acute-phase response, production of phagocytes in the bone marrow, and the hypothalamic-pituitary axis, producing the systemic signs of inflammation.

Once the antigen is consumed or removed, the process downregulates. If antigen removal is incomplete, continuously sensitized ("memory") T cells remain and contribute to a stronger secondary response on rechallenge with the same antigen. However, in some instances, if the antigen cannot be eliminated, the immune response can become exhausted and T cells deleted by mechanisms that are not fully understood but include Fas ligand-mediated apoptosis. Exhaustion-deletion in the first weeks or months after transplantation is never complete, but it can be maintained in a stable state by small numbers of persistent donor leukocytes.

Molecular insights regarding IL-2 gene transcription and the structure of the IL-2 receptor (IL-2R) have led to IL-2R-targeted therapy. As molecular knowledge has advanced, investigators have gained greater understanding of the workings of many immunosuppressants. New strategies guided by this knowledge have resulted in attempts to develop site-directed immunosuppression. Virtually every known step of the immune process can be targeted, and many new drugs are now in various stages of evolution.

Specific Agents

CORTICOSTEROIDS

Corticosteroids are extensively used in brief courses at high doses for the reversal of acute rejection episodes. These drugs are also used extensively in clinical immunosuppressive protocols for both induction and maintenance phases.[15] Five glucocorticosteroids are commonly used in transplantation: hydrocortisone, prednisone, prednisolone, methylprednisolone, and dexamethasone.

Because hydrocortisone has the greatest mineralocorticoid activity per unit of glucocorticoid activity, its routine application in transplantation is relatively limited. The other four agents have more glucocorticoid activity in proportion to their mineralocorticoid activity.

Prednisone has an oral bioavailability of about 80%, and it is metabolized in the liver to its active form, prednisolone. Oral prednisolone has a bioavailability of 100%. The serum half-life of both prednisone and methylprednisolone is 2 to 3 hours.[16] The oral bioavailability of dexamethasone is 61%, and this drug has a half-life of 2 hours.[17] However, the clinical activity of corticosteroids (i.e., suppression of cytokine production) persists for 24 hours or longer. In other words, the half-life for biological activity is much longer than the circulating half-life.

There is no universally accepted fixed dosing regimen for corticosteroids. Rather, the dose is often dictated by local protocols. A preoperative dose of 250 to 1000 mg of methylprednisolone may be given, followed by 20 to 200 mg/d during the first week. Acute rejection may be treated with 1 to 3 large doses—250 to 1000 mg of methylprednisolone—or by a regimen starting at 200 mg/d of oral prednisone and tapering to baseline maintenance doses over 3 to 6 days. There is evidence that doses lower than those traditionally used can be equally effective. In combination regimens, steroid doses often can be reduced to 5 or 10 mg/d or less and perhaps given every other day.

Corticosteroids have broad effects on many cell types. These agents interfere with the production of IL-1 and IL-2, blocking the early steps of T-cell activation. Other pharmacologic effects related to immune function include:

1. Antagonism of inflammatory mechanisms by stabilization of leukocyte lysosomal membranes, reduction in capillary permeability, and inhibition of histamine release and inhibition of activation of the kinin and complement systems
2. Drastic reduction of lymphocyte trafficking and circulating immunoglobulin levels and reduction in the number of neutrophils and eosinophils
3. Inhibition of leukocyte adhesion to endothelium

Prednisone and prednisolone have much less mineralocorticoid effect than the naturally occurring glucocorticoids do; however, sodium retention, edema, hypertension, potassium loss, and hypokalemic alkalosis can be seen with prolonged use of these drugs. Suppression of the pituitary-adrenal axis can be seen with all corticosteroids, but the magnitude of this effect varies among patients. Acute adrenal insufficiency can develop unexpectedly if patients are stressed, even as long as 12 months after corticosteroids are withdrawn.

The adverse effects of corticosteroids are numerous and cause considerable morbidity. An increased incidence of serious infections is well documented. Impaired fibroblast growth and collagen synthesis contribute to poor wound healing. Hence, surgical wounds and anastomoses are at increased risk for dehiscence, and gastrointestinal ulcers tend to heal slowly, leading to increased risks of perforation and rebleeding. Spontaneous ulceration of the gastrointestinal tract occurs in approximately 2% of patients taking steroids. Because signs of inflammation are suppressed, the diagnosis of intraabdominal infection and peritonitis can be significantly delayed, sometimes with disastrous consequences.

Corticosteroids impair glucose tolerance, often dramatically. For patients receiving large doses of corticosteroids, it often is best to use sliding-scale insulin regimens to ensure adequate control of blood sugar levels. Some patients require long-term therapy with oral hypoglycemic agents or insulin to maintain adequate glucose control.

Central nervous system effects such as euphoria and mood swings are well known. These adverse effects are generally dose dependent and are seen most frequently early in the postoperative period or with therapy for acute rejection episodes when higher doses of steroids are used. Central nervous system effects are usually self-limited and do not require treatment.

Long-term use of corticosteroids can cause bone demineralization and lead to osteoporosis. Atherosclerosis may be accelerated. Prolonged administration of glucocorticoids is associated with increased incidence of cataracts and elevated intraocular pressure (glaucoma). Soft-tissue and dermal changes (e.g., fat redistribution, skin atrophy, "moon face," striae) produce the characteristic cushingoid appearance.

To minimize development of adverse sequelae, most immunosuppressive protocols attempt to reduce the dose of corticosteroids over time to physiologic levels (equivalent to 5 mg/d or less of prednisone). However, corticosteroid doses must be reduced carefully to minimize side effects while maintaining adequate immunosuppression to prevent acute rejection of the allograft.

CYTOKINE INHIBITORS

Before the introduction of cyclosporine, immunosuppression protocols relied heavily on corticosteroids and cytotoxic drugs. These regimens had the disadvantage of producing broad suppression of the immune and inflammatory cascades. Cyclosporine introduced a new era of immunosuppression because it provided potent, relatively specific, and noncytotoxic suppression of T-cell activation.

Cyclosporine

Cyclosporine is a lipophilic cyclic polypeptide with 11 amino acids and a molecular weight of 1202. On entering the T cell, cyclosporine binds to cyclophilin, a cytoplasmic immunophilin protein. The cyclosporine-cyclophilin complex inhibits the activity of calcineurin, which in turn inhibits transcription of several genes including those encoding IL-2, IL-3, IL-4, GM-CSF, IFN-γ, and TNF-α. One key action that results from blockade of calcineurin is inhibition of signaling via nuclear factor of activated T cells (NF-AT), which regulates activation of the IL-2 gene; this effect ultimately prevents synthesis of IL-2.[18] Inhibition of the synthesis of IL-2, a potent T-cell growth factor, is the crucial activity of cyclosporine.

Cyclosporine is insoluble in water and therefore must be dissolved in an organic solvent. There currently exist two formulations: cyclosporine (Sandimmune [Novartis Pharmaceuticals, East Hanover, New Jersey]) and cyclosporine for microemulsion (cyclosporine, modified; Neoral [Novartis Pharmaceuticals] and Gengraf [Abbott Laboratories, North Chicago, Illinois]). The microemulsion formulation substantially increases cyclosporine absorption; the overall time to peak cyclosporine concentration is reduced, the peak concentration is higher, and the area under the curve (AUC) is increased. The lipophilicity of the conventional cyclosporine formulation is responsible for its variable bioavailability

Oral bioavailability is about 30%, but there is much individual variability (range 10%-60%). Absorption in the small intestine decreases with bowel dysfunction or reduced bile flow.[19] The volume of distribution of cyclosporine is large and variable. The drug is metabolized in the liver via cytochrome P450 (CYP) 3A4 enzymes. It also is a substrate for the P-glycoprotein efflux pump. The mean terminal half-life with normal liver function is 19 hours. The microemulsion formulation of cyclosporine has superior pharmacokinetics, does not require bile excretion for its bioavailability, and is better dispersed and absorbed compared to conventional/toxicosporine. The relative bioavailability of the microemulsion formulation is approximately 60%.[20]

TABLE 176-1	Drugs That Alter Cyclosporine and Tacrolimus Concentrations	
Increase	**Decrease**
Diltiazem	Rifampin
Nicardipine	Carbamazepine
Verapamil	Phenobarbital
Fluconazole	Phenytoin
Itraconazole	Ticlopidine
Ketoconazole	Nafcillin
Clarithromycin	
Erythromycin	
Methylprednisolone (in large doses)	
Bromocriptine	
Danazol	
Protease inhibitors	

The total AUC is increased by 30% compared with the conventional formulation.[21]

At least 17 cyclosporine metabolites have been identified, and a few of them are immunosuppressive, although considerably less so than the parent compound. The half-life of cyclosporine increases with hepatic failure and is changed significantly by coadministration of a large number of other drugs that can increase or decrease serum levels by induction or competitive inhibition of P450 (Table 176-1).[22] For all these reasons, it is essential that cyclosporine levels be monitored regularly and dosage adjusted accordingly.

Monitoring cyclosporine levels is not straightforward. Different results are obtained when cyclosporine concentrations in blood or plasma are determined by radioimmunoassay or by high-pressure liquid chromatography (HPLC). Neither method is clearly superior, and there are no universally accepted blood levels; target levels vary widely from center to center. Desired levels in serum or plasma as measured by radioimmunoassay[23] are 150 to 250 ng/mL at the time of transplantation, tapering to 50 to 100 ng/mL after 3 to 6 months. If the drug is measured in whole blood by HPLC, desired levels are 100 to 300 ng/mL initially, tapering to 80 to 200 ng/mL.

Recent literature suggests that AUC values and peak concentrations measured 2 hours after dosing (C_2) are more sensitive predictors of cyclosporine effects and may be better parameters to guide therapeutic monitoring of the microemulsion formulation of cyclosporine. Decreased bioavailability of cyclosporine has been correlated with acute rejection.[24] The first 4 hours after administration of a dose of cyclosporine represents the period of greatest variability in cyclosporine absorption.[25] Limited sampling techniques consisting of 2 to 5 blood samples drawn within the first 4 hours after cyclosporine administration are used to determine the AUC. AUC values greater than 4400 μg/L/h correlate well with a low incidence of allograft rejection.[24,26] One study compared the correlation between the trough concentration, C_2, and the occurrence of rejection and concluded that trough concentrations lack predictive value; however, acute rejection did not occur in patients with C_2 values above 1200 μg/L.[27] Because of the convenience of a single blood sample compared with the multiple blood samples necessary for AUC measurements, C_2 monitoring is becoming a preferred way to adjust cyclosporine dosing. C_2 levels should range between 1.5 and 2.0 μg/mL for the first few months after transplantation and should be reduced to 0.8 μg/mL after 6 to 12 months of therapy.[26,28]

The typical daily intravenous (IV) dose of cyclosporine is 4 to 5 mg/kg. This amount can be given in two divided doses, each being delivered over 2 to 6 hours. Alternatively, some prefer to use a slow continuous infusion over 24 hours. The changeover to oral dosing usually requires a dose 3 times higher, or about 12 to 15 mg/kg/d. Oral cyclosporine should be administered every 12 hours. After 1 to 2 weeks, the dosage can be slowly tapered once equilibration within body fat stores occurs. In many patients, the dose is tapered to as low as 3 mg/kg/d by 6 months after transplantation. Liver transplant recipients who have a

T tube which diverts some bile flow require higher oral doses because of decreased absorption. Pediatric patients eliminate cyclosporine faster than adults, and they require larger doses, typically about 5 to 6 mg/kg/d IV and 14 to 18 mg/kg/d orally. Some pediatric patients require doses up to 50% to 100% larger than adult doses.

Several adverse effects can occur early after initiation of cyclosporine therapy. Acute nephrotoxicity and hypertension are major problems. The mechanisms responsible for these adverse effects are controversial.[29,30] Nephrotoxicity may be the result of cyclosporine-induced afferent arteriolar vasoconstriction that results in part from an imbalance between the production of prostaglandin E_2, a vasodilator, and that of thromboxane A_2, a vasoconstrictor.[31,32] Other possible factors include endothelin-1-induced vasoconstriction and impaired nitric oxide production.[33] Cyclosporine-induced nephrotoxicity is transient and reversible with a decrease in dosage or discontinuation of the drug.[34] The incidence of nephrotoxicity varies from approximately 25% to 38%.[35]

Neurotoxicity associated with cyclosporine ranges from minor toxicity, manifesting as tremors, to severe complications such as seizures or encephalopathy.[36] Tremors caused by cyclosporine are common (prevalence 10%-55%) and may improve over time without a change in therapy. The causal association between seizures and encephalopathy is often unclear.[36] Several reports have detailed a rare syndrome characterized by confusion and cortical blindness in both liver and bone marrow transplantation patients. Hypomagnesemia and hypocholesterolemia are believed to be risk factors for cyclosporine-induced neurotoxicity.[29]

Hypertension occurs frequently and usually begins within weeks after commencement of cyclosporine therapy. The incidence of hypertension varies widely in different patient populations, ranging from 10% to 80%.[35] It is hypothesized[37] that hypertension is caused by cyclosporine-induced vasoconstriction in the renal or systemic circulation or both, perhaps as a result of antagonism of endothelium-derived relaxation factors or increased synthesis of endothelin-1, a vasoconstrictor. Hypertension responds to sodium restriction and is best managed with diuretics or calcium channel blockers.[30]

Cyclosporine is diabetogenic, although analysis of this effect is confounded by the frequent concomitant use of steroids with cyclosporine. Other metabolic effects of cyclosporine include hypochloremic alkalosis and changes in serum concentrations of potassium, magnesium, prolactin, and testosterone. Hepatotoxicity, manifested by cholestatic jaundice, is common,[29] but intrahepatic cholestasis often resolves if the dose of cyclosporine is reduced. Connective tissue side effects of cyclosporine are common and can be distressing to the patient because of the cosmetic manifestations. These changes include hirsutism (seen within 2-4 weeks in 20%-45% of patients receiving cyclosporine), gingival hyperplasia (in 4%-16% of patients), and coarsening of facial features.[38] Long-term administration of cyclosporine is associated with irreversible nephrotoxicity. The incidence of this serious side effect is estimated to be 15% to 40%.[39] The pathologic lesion resembles nephrosclerosis.[40]

Tacrolimus

Tacrolimus (FK-506; Prograf [Fujisawa Healthcare, Deerfield, Illinois]) is a macrolide antibiotic with immunosuppressive activity produced by the fungus *Streptomyces tsukubaensis*. It is approved by the U.S. Food and Drug Administration (FDA) for heart, liver, and kidney transplant recipients. It is also used extensively in small bowel, pancreas, and lung transplantation. The molecular structure of tacrolimus is unrelated to that of cyclosporine, and the two drugs have different cytosolic binding sites.[41,42] Tacrolimus binds to the immunophilin called *FK-binding protein-12* (FKBP12).[43] Like the cyclosporine-cyclophilin complex, the tacrolimus-FKBP12 complex binds to and inhibits the activity of calcineurin. As is the case with cyclosporine, inhibition of calcineurin by tacrolimus blocks transcription of several genes including those encoding IL-2, IL-3, IL-4, GM-CSF, IFN-γ, and TNF-α. The effect of tacrolimus on TNF-β expression differs from that induced by cyclosporine. Tacrolimus-mediated inhibition of TNF-β expression may play a role

in reducing chronic rejection,[43] although no clinical difference has been noted between the two drugs. Like cyclosporine, inhibition of calcineurin disrupts signaling via NF-AT, ultimately inhibiting synthesis of the potent T-cell growth factor, IL-2; this is the key pharmacologic effect of tacrolimus. The immunosuppressive effects of tacrolimus also may involve other pathways that activate T cells.[44]

Tacrolimus is highly lipophilic and must be dissolved in an organic solvent. Oral bioavailability is highly variable and poor, reportedly ranging from 6% to 56%, with a mean of 25%.[45] The gastrointestinal absorption of tacrolimus, compared with that of cyclosporine, is less dependent on bile flow.[46] Tacrolimus is extensively bound to erythrocytes because of the high concentration of FKBP12 found in the red blood cells. Like cyclosporine, tacrolimus is metabolized in the liver via the cytochrome P450 enzyme system, primarily by CYP3A4, although other enzymes have been reported to be involved as well.[47] Tacrolimus metabolism, like that of cyclosporine, can be significantly altered by liver dysfunction or coadministration of other drugs that induce or competitively inhibit P450; these effects can decrease or increase circulating levels of tacrolimus (see Table 176-1). Tacrolimus is a substrate for the P-glycoprotein efflux pump. The mean terminal half-life of tacrolimus is 12 hours. At least 15 metabolites of tacrolimus have been identified[43]; some of these have as much as 10% of the immunosuppressive activity of the parent compound.[47]

Therapeutic monitoring of circulating tacrolimus concentrations is essential for preventing toxicity while maintaining adequate immunosuppression. Plasma and whole-blood trough concentrations correlate with AUC as well as clinical outcomes and toxicities.[48] Because of the extensive binding of tacrolimus to erythrocytes, whole-blood tacrolimus concentrations are 10 to 30 times higher than the corresponding plasma concentrations.[47] The most commonly used tacrolimus assay is the microparticulate enzyme immunoassay, although HPLC and enzyme-linked immunosorbent assays are also readily available.[49] The therapeutic range for tacrolimus levels in whole blood is 5 to 20 ng/mL. Plasma tacrolimus levels should be maintained between 0.5 and 2 ng/mL.

The typical IV dose of tacrolimus is 0.05 to 0.1 mg/kg/d. The drug should be administered as a slow continuous infusion over 24 hours. Oral doses are generally 3 to 4 times higher than IV doses and range from 0.1 to 0.2 mg/kg/d, administered in 2 divided doses every 12 hours. Maintenance doses of tacrolimus range from 0.0125 to 0.5 mg/kg/d owing to variability among patients with respect to absorption of the drug and requirements for immunosuppression.[47] No decrease in tacrolimus dose is needed when the T tube is clamped after liver transplantation. Because tacrolimus clearance is faster in pediatric patients, larger doses may be required in children compared with adults.[47] Pediatric IV doses range from 0.03 to 0.05 mg/kg/d, and pediatric oral doses range from 0.15 to 0.3 mg/kg/d in divided doses.

Tacrolimus has a potential advantage over cyclosporine because of its ability to reverse ongoing acute rejection.[50-53] Experience with tacrolimus was first gained when the drug was used as rescue therapy in liver and kidney transplantation.[54-56] Today, tacrolimus is used as a primary immunosuppressive agent for all types of solid-organ transplants.

The toxicity profile for tacrolimus is similar to that of cyclosporine, perhaps because they have a similar mechanism of action (i.e., calcineurin inhibition). As experience has been gained with tacrolimus, it is clear that many of the toxic side effects are dose related and are best managed by reducing the dose. Acute nephrotoxicity induced by tacrolimus is dose related. The incidence of this adverse effect is not clearly defined in the literature, but it is similar to that of cyclosporine and most likely results from afferent arteriolar vasoconstriction. Nephrotoxicity resolves after the dose of tacrolimus is reduced or the drug is discontinued. As with cyclosporine, irreversible renal injury can occur after prolonged therapy with tacrolimus.[57]

Neurotoxicity is the most commonly reported adverse effect of tacrolimus. The reported incidence ranges from 3.6% to 32%.[58] This side effect can range from mild toxicity such as tremors, headaches, paresthesias, and insomnia to severe complications including encephalopathy, coma, seizures, and psychosis. Usually, neurotoxicity associated with tacrolimus responds to a reduction of the dose, but idiosyncratic reactions may require discontinuation of the drug.

The potential for tacrolimus to induce a diabetic state is similar to that for cyclosporine.[59,60] Increased fasting glucose levels and the development of overt diabetes mellitus are associated with elevated tacrolimus concentrations (>15 ng/mL), acute rejection, and higher body mass index.[61] Tacrolimus-induced diabetes mellitus is reversible.[62]

Hyperkalemia and hypomagnesemia are commonly noted in patients receiving tacrolimus. Acute hyperkalemia can be managed with standard approaches including administration of insulin and glucose and sodium bicarbonate or a cation exchange agent (sodium polystyrene sulfonate). Chronic hyperkalemia may require therapy with fludrocortisone acetate to increase renal potassium excretion. Hypomagnesemia often requires magnesium replacement to avoid complications.

The incidences of hypertension and hyperlipidemia associated with tacrolimus therapy appear to be lower than those reported with cyclosporine.[63-66] This more favorable adverse-effect profile has been reported to translate into a decrease in the number of cardiovascular complications in patients treated with tacrolimus compared to cyclosporine.[66]

Tacrolimus is not associated with the connective-tissue side effects seen with cyclosporine, so cosmetic problems are not seen. Alopecia can be problematic for patients receiving tacrolimus, but this problem is reversible and usually does not require dosage adjustments.[67]

CELL CYCLE INHIBITORS

The precise mechanism of immunosuppression mediated by cytotoxic drugs is unknown; however, the negative effect of these agents on the proliferation of lymphocytes is believed to inhibit generation of antigen-specific T-cell clones. As one might expect, an increased risk of malignancies with the long-term use of these agents is a concern.

Azathioprine

Azathioprine (AZA; Imuran [Prometheus Laboratories, Greenville, North Carolina]), a thio analog of the purine, adenine, inhibits purine metabolism. The parent drug is inactive but is rapidly converted to 6-mercaptopurine (6-MP) in red blood cells and subsequently to 6-thioinosine monophosphate, a purine analog, in vivo.[68] Both the de novo and salvage pathways of purine synthesis are inhibited by azathioprine. 6-Thioguanine nucleotides interfere with DNA and RNA synthesis, rendering cells unable to function properly and allowing strand breaks in chromosomes. Azathioprine is most toxic to proliferating cells that are making new DNA.

Azathioprine can be used in maintenance immunosuppressive regimens; it has no usefulness for the treatment of acute rejection episodes.[69] The oral bioavailability of azathioprine is approximately 40%. Metabolism of 6-MP involves catabolism by xanthine oxidase in the liver and gut to inactive metabolites that are excreted by the kidneys. The 6-thioguanine nucleotides have a very long tissue half-life (approximately 13 days), permitting azathioprine to be administered by once-daily dosing. The inactive end metabolite is 6-thiouric acid, which is excreted by the kidneys. With congenital deficiency of the enzyme, thiopurine methyltransferase (incidence 1 in 300 patients), or with renal failure, accumulation of 6-thioguanine nucleotides causes increased toxicity.

The starting dose for azathioprine is 3 to 5 mg/kg once daily. The drug can be given IV at half the dose for brief periods. The typical maintenance oral dosage after transplantation is 2 to 3 mg/kg daily. Tapering of the dose to 1 to 2 mg/kg/d is often possible over time. In combination regimens, azathioprine can be reduced to as low as 0.25 to 0.5 mg/kg/d.

Dose-limiting myelosuppression usually occurs 1 to 2 weeks into therapy. Pancytopenia and thrombocytopenia with megaloblastic anemia is the pattern usually seen. White blood cell counts lower than 3000 cells/mm³ warrant dose reduction or discontinuation of the drug.

As with other antiproliferative drugs, nausea, vomiting, and hair loss may occur. Hepatic injury can occur in two patterns. One form is reversible hepatitis. The other form is rare but serious hepatic veno-occlusive disease, which can cause irreversible liver damage. Azathioprine therapy also has been associated with pancreatitis. Because of concerns about hepatotoxicity and pancreatitis, some transplantation experts questioned the value of azathioprine for immunosuppression.[70,71] Hypersensitivity to azathioprine has been reported to cause a variety of manifestations; diagnosis of these disorders is based largely on clinical findings.

Allopurinol inhibits xanthene oxidase, one of the enzymes involved in degradation of azathioprine metabolites, thereby increasing the toxicity of the parent compound. Accordingly, if therapy with allopurinol is indicated, this agent should be added cautiously to an immunosuppressive regimen containing azathioprine. If allopurinol must be used, the dose of azathioprine should be reduced by more than 50%.

Mycophenolate Mofetil

Mycophenolate mofetil (MMF; CellCept [Roche Laboratories, Nutley, New Jersey]) is a prodrug of mycophenolic acid (MPA). MPA noncompetitively inhibits inosine monophosphate dehydrogenase (IMPDH), a key enzyme that regulates the purine nucleotide de novo synthesis pathway.[72] T and B lymphocytes are dependent on IMPDH and the de novo pathway for purine synthesis during proliferation. Other cell types including granulocytes, red blood cells, platelets and tissue cells use both the de novo and the salvage pathways for purine synthesis.[73] For this reason, MPA is more selective for T and B lymphocytes than azathioprine, which results in a more favorable adverse effect profile. MPA also may induce apoptosis in activated T cells, and it may interfere with expression of adhesion molecules in leukocytes and lymphocyte recruitment.[74]

Mycophenolate mofetil is rapidly absorbed after oral administration and undergoes rapid first-pass metabolism in the liver to MPA, the active form of the drug. The bioavailability of MPA is 94%.[72] Maximum concentrations of MPA are reached approximately one hour after oral administration.[75] MPA binds to plasma albumin, and free MPA levels can be altered by fluctuations in albumin levels or other medications that compete for albumin binding. Metabolism of MPA occurs by glucuronidation in the liver and renal tubular cells, primarily to an inactive compound, mycophenolic acid glucuronide (MPAG), which is eliminated by the kidneys,[72] and to a second acylglucuronide (M-2) which has in vitro activity.[76]

The dose of mycophenolate needed to prevent rejection in kidney and liver transplant recipients is 2 g/d. Cardiac transplant recipients generally require higher levels of immunosuppression and should receive 3 g/d. The total daily dose should be administered over two dosing intervals. Patients who are unable to tolerate twice-daily dosing may benefit from separation of the total daily dose into three or four dosing intervals.

The need for therapeutic monitoring of MPA levels remains controversial. Currently, two assays are available: HPLC and an enzyme-multiplied immunoassay technique (EMIT). HPLC can measure both MPA and metabolite concentrations and is sensitive enough to measure free MPA concentrations.[77] The active metabolite of MPA, M-2, cross-reacts with the EMIT assay, resulting in higher measured concentrations. A correlation between acute rejection and both total MPA AUC and trough MPA concentrations determined by HPLC has been demonstrated.[78] Acute rejection is predicted better by trough levels than by the AUC. However, the risk of adverse effects correlates better with the dose of MPA than with circulating MPA concentrations.[79] The therapeutic range for total MPA AUC is 30 to 60 mg × h/L.[78] MPA trough levels should be maintained between 1 and 3.5 mg/L.[77] Another monitoring strategy is measurement of the early peak concentration (30 minutes after oral dose [C_{30}]).[80] Further studies are necessary to determine the most appropriate strategy for therapeutic monitoring of MPA.

The most common adverse effects of mycophenolate mofetil are gastrointestinal. Mild effects include nausea, vomiting, diarrhea, constipation, and dyspepsia. Severe complications including cholecystitis, large bowel perforation, and pancreatitis are rare and have not been definitively related to treatment with MPA. Mild gastrointestinal effects usually are transient. Prolonged symptoms can be managed by either reducing the dose of MPA or increasing the number of dosing intervals from twice daily to three or four times daily.[81]

Hematologic adverse effects are rare and manifest as bone marrow suppression. The most commonly reported features are leukopenia and anemia, but the side-effect profile also can include thrombocytopenia and pancytopenia. The onset of myelosuppression typically occurs within the first six months after starting MPA therapy and may be dose related. Resolution occurs within one week after stopping the drug in most cases.[72]

Infections are frequently cited as adverse effects of MPA, but they are a complication of immunosuppression in general. The reported incidence of opportunistic infections was increased in patients receiving MPA in addition to cyclosporine and prednisone compared with those receiving cyclosporine and prednisone alone[81,82]; however, no difference was reported when the MPA-containing regimen was compared with cyclosporine, prednisone, and azathioprine.[83] Nephrotoxicity and hepatotoxicity have not been reported with MPA.

MPA is effective maintenance therapy for prevention of acute rejection of solid organ allografts in combination with other immunosuppressive agents such as corticosteroids and cyclosporine[83-84] or tacrolimus.[85] MPA has been used to treat acute rejection of renal transplants[86] and, in refractory rejection, to reduce the use of antilymphocyte therapy.[87] In addition, MPA has been used as rescue therapy for acute and chronic rejection of cardiac transplants.[88] Recent studies have shown promise in combining MPA with sirolimus to eliminate the need for calcineurin inhibitors, thereby reducing the potential for nephrotoxicity.[89,90]

Sirolimus and Everolimus

Sirolimus (rapamycin, rapa; Rapamune [Wyeth Laboratories, Philadelphia, Pennsylvania]) is a macrolide antibiotic that is structurally related to tacrolimus. Like tacrolimus, sirolimus binds to FKBP12, but sirolimus does not inhibit calcineurin or block cytokine gene transcription in T cells; rather, sirolimus inhibits the mammalian targets of rapamycin (mTOR), leading to cell cycle arrest. By blocking mTOR, sirolimus inhibits the cellular response to IL-2 and inhibits progression of the cell cycle, thereby prohibiting T-cell proliferation.[91]

Sirolimus is insoluble in water and must be dissolved in an organic solvent. It has poor bioavailability (15%). Maximum concentrations are reached within 2 hours after oral administration.[92] Because of its high lipophilicity, sirolimus readily enters cells, producing a large volume of distribution. Sirolimus binds extensively to erythrocytes (95%) because of their high FKBP12 content; minimal binding occurs with other plasma proteins.[93] Like cyclosporine and tacrolimus, sirolimus is metabolized primarily in the liver by CYP3A4. Sirolimus is also a substrate for the P-glycoprotein efflux pump. O-demethylation and hydroxylation produce several metabolites. The metabolites of sirolimus have less than 10% of the immunosuppressive activity of the parent compound and are excreted via the bile into feces.[91]

Hepatic metabolism by CYP3A4 enzymes creates the potential for significant changes in the half-life of sirolimus if other drugs affecting these enzymes are also administered. These changes can decrease or increase serum levels by induction or competitive inhibition of P450. Many of the same drugs that alter cyclosporine and tacrolimus levels can also alter sirolimus levels (see Table 176-1). Coadministration of sirolimus with cyclosporine significantly increases the AUC and trough concentrations for sirolimus. Likewise, sirolimus also significantly increases the AUC and trough concentrations for cyclosporine. To minimize the interaction and potential toxicities of the two drugs, sirolimus administration should be separated from cyclosporine administration by 4 hours.[94]

Its long half-life of approximately 60 hours[95] makes sirolimus suitable for once-daily dosing. The two pivotal trials that led to the FDA approval of sirolimus capitalized on the interaction that occurs with coadministration of cyclosporine and sirolimus. These studies demonstrated a reduction of acute rejection episodes in kidney transplant recipients when sirolimus was given using either of two fixed dosing regimens: a 6-mg loading dose followed by 2 mg daily, or a 15-mg loading dose followed by 5 mg daily.[96,97] These results suggest that therapeutic drug monitoring is unnecessary, but clinical experience indicates that sirolimus therapy is optimized when doses are based on blood concentrations, particularly if sirolimus is used in the absence of cyclosporine synergy.[98]

Therapeutic monitoring of sirolimus should be based on whole-blood concentrations, because large amounts of the drug are sequestered in erythrocytes, resulting in undetectable concentrations in plasma.[99] HPLC with mass spectroscopy and ultraviolet detection are the most commonly used methods to measure sirolimus concentrations. A correlation between the trough level and the AUC for sirolimus has been established.[100,101] Furthermore, there is a strong correlation between the rate and severity of acute rejection and low trough levels, as well as between the occurrence of adverse effects and high trough levels. The therapeutic range is 5 to 15 ng/mL.[101] A microparticle enzyme immunoassay has been developed[102] and may be beneficial for analyzing multiple samples with more rapid turnaround.[103] Frequent monitoring of sirolimus levels is unwarranted because of the long half-life of the drug. Sirolimus levels should be evaluated 5 to 7 days after initiation of therapy or a dose change, to allow sufficient time for drug levels to reach steady state.[100]

The adverse-effect profile of sirolimus is different from that of other immunosuppressants. Unlike cyclosporine and tacrolimus, sirolimus rarely causes nephrotoxicity or neurotoxicity. Dose-dependent myelosuppression can be seen after initiation of sirolimus therapy. Thrombocytopenia commonly manifests within the first two weeks of therapy but improves with continued treatment. Leukopenia and anemia may also manifest shortly after initiation of therapy, but they are transient.[103] Thrombocytopenia and leukopenia are related to sirolimus trough concentrations above 15 ng/mL.[101]

Hyperlipidemia is commonly seen in patients receiving sirolimus; the findings are hypercholesterolemia and hypertriglyceridemia. This effect has been reported in virtually all clinical trials.[91] Peak levels of total cholesterol and triglycerides are dose related and usually are reached within three months after initiation of sirolimus, but the levels decrease after one year.[103] Both changes are reversible with dose reduction or discontinuation.[92] The cause of sirolimus-associated hyperlipidemia is thought to be overproduction of lipoproteins or inhibition of hepatic lipoprotein lipase, leading to decreased lipolysis.[103] Use of antihyperlipidemic agents such as the 3-hydroxy-3-methylglutaryl coenzyme A (HMG-CoA) reductase inhibitors is effective for treating hyperlipidemia in patients receiving sirolimus. Analysis of cholesterol values after 1 year of sirolimus therapy in the Framingham Model indicates that sirolimus should cause only a modest increase in the incidence of ischemic heart disease in kidney transplant recipients (2 to 3 new cases per 1000 persons per year).[103] Therefore, treatment with sirolimus should have only a minimal impact on the risk for cardiovascular disease. It has been proposed that the decreased incidence of hyperlipidemia associated with tacrolimus compared with cyclosporine may lessen the frequency and severity of hyperlipidemia in transplant recipients who receive tacrolimus- and sirolimus-based immunosuppressive therapy.[103]

Mouth ulcers have been reported with sirolimus; they appear to be more pronounced with the liquid formulation and may be dose related. Other adverse effects reported with sirolimus include elevated liver enzymes, lymphocele formation, hypertension, rash, acne, diarrhea, and arthralgia.

Sirolimus is effective as maintenance therapy for preventing acute rejection of solid-organ allografts, in combination with corticosteroids and cyclosporine[96,97] or tacrolimus.[105] It also is effective in steroid-withdrawal regimens[106] or to spare cyclosporine in an attempt to minimize nephrotoxicity associated with this agent.[107,108] It is speculated that sirolimus may reduce the potential for chronic rejection by inhibiting growth factor–mediated cell proliferation and intimal hyperplasia associated with chronic rejection,[103] but longer follow-up is necessary to prove this theory.

Everolimus (Zortress [USA] and Certican [Europe and other countries]) is the 42-O-(2-hydroxyethyl) derivative of sirolimus. The mechanism of action of everolimus as an mTOR inhibitor is similar to sirolimus. The FDA approved everolimus for prevention of organ transplant rejection prophylaxis on April 22, 2010. The half-life of everolimus is shorter than that of sirolimus (28 hours versus 62 hours)[5] and reaches stable therapeutic blood concentrations more quickly. Everolimus in combination with cyclosporine and corticosteroids is indicated for prevention of acute rejection in adult heart transplant recipients. Everolimus can be recommended for most heart transplant recipients, although there are certain subgroups who might derive particular benefit from the antiproliferative effects of the drug. These subgroups include patients at high risk of developing cardiac allograft vasculopathy or nephrotoxicity induced by calcineurin inhibitors or posttransplant malignancies.[104] In combination with cyclosporine and corticosteroids, everolimus should be started as soon as possible at a dose of 0.75 mg every 12 hours; patients with mild to moderate liver dysfunction require much lower doses, often less than half the standard dose. Plasma levels of everolimus should be monitored. The therapeutic level is 3 to 8 ng/mL.[104] Frequently reported adverse effects of everolimus include hyperlipidemia and peripheral edema. Less common but potentially very serious adverse effects include angioedema and proteinuria, especially in renal transplant recipients.[104]

BIOLOGICAL AGENTS

Antithymocyte Globulin

Antilymphocyte antibodies such as antilymphocytic globulin (ALG) were first produced by immunization of animals against purified lymphocyte preparations, resulting in multispecific polyclonal antibodies. Antibodies that cross-reacted with other cellular molecules in blood were then removed by extensive adsorption to blood components. Because of variability among immunized animals, substantial amounts of ALG were pooled to produce a more homogeneous preparation.

Antibodies to surface molecules on lymphocytes interfere with lymphocyte function in the immune response by several possible mechanisms. Lymphocytes are removed from the circulation rapidly after treatment with antilymphocyte antibodies. In addition, lymphocytes are phenotypically and functionally altered. Thymocytes, unactivated lymphocytes, and T and B lymphoblasts are used to produce the equine polyclonal antibody, antithymocyte globulin (ATG; Atgam [Pharmacia & Upjohn, Kalamazoo, Michigan]). A newer rabbit preparation, RATG (Thymoglobulin [SangStat Medical Corporation, Fremont, California]), is less immunogenic and may have other advantages over the equine preparation. B lymphocytes are targeted to a lesser extent with RATG than with equine ATG,[109] helping to some extent to preserve infection-induced antibody production. Furthermore, CD4+ T lymphocytes are the predominant target of RATG,[110] and this agent has lesser effects on other leukocytes compared to equine ATG. RATG-induced lymphocytopenia persists for a much longer time than with former antilymphocyte preparations. Surface molecules that serve as binding sites for RATG include the T-cell antigens, CD6, CD16, CD18, CD38, CD40, and CD58, among others. The result is inhibition of cellular function of other cell lines including monocytes, thymocytes, natural killer cells, leukocytes, and dendritic cells.

Equine ATG is administered in a single daily dose (10-15 mg/kg). The dose of RATG, which is more potent, is 1 to 1.5 mg/kg given as a single daily dose. Therapy for acute rejection usually is continued for 7 to 14 days. Induction therapy with polyclonal antibodies typically uses the same doses for 5 to 10 days of therapy. Polyclonal preparations cause a high incidence of febrile reactions with the first few doses. Antihistamines (usually diphenhydramine, 50 mg), antipyretics (i.e., acetaminophen, 650 mg), and corticosteroids are given as premedications.

Because of the lack of specificity of polyclonal antibodies, therapeutic drug monitoring generally is not useful. In addition, fixed weight-based dosing regimens reduce the need for drug concentration monitoring. Some advocate monitoring the number of CD3+ lymphocytes with flow cytometry as a gauge of immunosuppressive effect.

The effects of ATG on other cell types is the basis for adverse effects associated with these preparations. The most troublesome adverse effect is myelosuppression, manifested by leukopenia, anemia, and thrombocytopenia. These effects are dose related and can be managed by decreasing the dose or discontinuing the drug.

As described previously, the first few doses of ATG preparations are often accompanied by fever, which can be ameliorated with the use of appropriate premedications. Other adverse effects include anaphylactic reactions, hypotension, urticaria, and serum sickness, particularly with equine ATG. After approval of RATG, use of equine ATG declined considerably because of the better side-effect profile of RATG and its increased efficacy in reducing acute rejection[111] and preventing rejection as part of induction therapy.[112]

The efficacy of ATGs in reversing solid-organ allograft rejection has been well established. ATGs are frequently reserved for steroid-resistant allograft rejections. Prospective controlled studies have demonstrated equal or superior efficacy for both equine and rabbit ATG in preventing rejection as induction therapy, compared with OKT3.[113,114] High doses of RATG are also being used in T cell–depleting regimens to induce tolerance and allow for monotherapy after transplantation, with subsequent weaning of immunosuppression.[115]

Anti-CD3 Monoclonal Antibody

Efforts to increase the potency and decrease the variability of ALGs led to development of single-specificity monoclonal antibodies. The first of these products was muromonab CD3 (OKT3; Orthoclone OKT3 [OrthoBiotech Products, Raritan, New Jersey]). OKT3 is a purified murine-derived monoclonal antibody directed at the ε chain of the CD3 receptor[116] which is found on all mature human T cells.[117] After administration, OKT3 binds to the CD3 receptor, opsonizing the cells and promoting their rapid removal from the circulation.[117,118]

Elimination of OKT3 occurs in two phases and is principally linked to T-cell binding. The first phase is elimination associated with rapid removal of the T cells bound to OKT3. The second slower phase occurs days after initiation of therapy. The overall half-life for the agent is 18 hours.[118]

Dosing for OKT3 uses a fixed regimen of 5 mg/d for 10 to 14 days for treatment of acute rejection. Prophylactic induction regimens use the same dose for 7 to 10 days. After the first one or two doses, proinflammatory cytokines are released by opsonized lymphocytes, leading to clinical findings reminiscent of severe sepsis.[118] This "first-dose effect" frequently is associated with fever, chills, tachycardia, nausea, vomiting, diarrhea, bronchospasm, pulmonary edema, and elevation or depression of blood pressure. These effects can be ameliorated if the patient is pretreated with a 1-g IV bolus of methylprednisolone 15 to 60 minutes before OKT3 infusion.[119] Premedication often also includes antihistamines, diphenhydramine, and acetaminophen. Anaphylaxis occurs in fewer than 1% of patients; nonetheless, a skin test or test dose is recommended before OKT3 therapy is initiated.

The murine nature of the drug leads to anti-mouse immunoglobulin antibody formation. Individuals vary in the amount of endogenous antibody (directed against the mouse antibody) they form. This antibody production can be decreased by continuing other immunosuppressive treatments during monoclonal antibody administration. Human antimurine OKT3 antibodies usually peak after 1 to 2 weeks of therapy and can decrease the efficacy of future courses of therapy.[118] Repeat treatment with OKT3 is still successful in many cases if larger doses of antibody are used for subsequent courses. Patients who produce very high antibody titers, probably about 5% to 20% of those receiving OKT3, fail to respond to subsequent doses of the drug even when the dose is increased. Some advocate monitoring CD3+ T-cell counts with flow cytometry for patients receiving OKT3. If CD3+ cells reach 10%, it is recommended either that the dose of OKT3 be increased (to as much as 15 mg/d) or that treatment be discontinued. Others suggest monitoring anti-OKT3 antibody titers.

As described previously, OKT3 therapy produces a first-dose response that manifests within 45 to 60 minutes and must be managed with premedication. Because of the risk of severe pulmonary edema, fluid status should be evaluated if patients weigh more than 2% more than their usual body weight, and diuresis should be considered before proceeding with OKT3 therapy.

Septic meningitis also has been described as an early complication of OKT3 therapy, manifesting 2 to 7 days after initiation of OKT3. The common symptoms are fever, headache, and photophobia. The phenomenon appears to be self-limited and may be related to the release of cytokines early after OKT3 administration.

The potent suppression of T-lymphocyte populations is associated with an increased incidence of viral infections and lymphoproliferative disorders. It is not clear whether antibody therapy is worse in this regard than other approaches for achieving immunosuppression. Some evidence suggests that problems arise because antibodies are used for too long a time or too late in the course of resistant rejection, when the immunosuppression burden is already high.

The efficacy of OKT3 for treatment of acute rejection and induction strategies is well documented. However, OKT3 use has declined with the availability of better-tolerated antithymocyte preparations (i.e., RATG) that do not induce antibody production against the drug. OKT3 is often reserved as therapy for acute rejection that is resistant to steroids or other antilymphocyte preparations.

Anti-Interleukin-2 Receptor Monoclonal Antibodies

T-cell activation is characterized by the expression of IL-2 and high-affinity IL-2R by T cells. IL-2 exerts its effects on T lymphocytes by binding to the IL-2R. By binding to the α subunit of the IL-2R on activated T cells, anti-IL-2R antibodies inhibit IL-2-mediated T-cell activation and proliferation. Two anti-IL-2R monoclonal antibodies are currently available, daclizumab (Zenapax [Hoffman-LaRoche, Nutley, New Jersey]) and basiliximab (Simulect [Novartis Pharmaceuticals]). The important differences between the two drugs relate to the structure of the antibodies and the dosing strategies for each.

Daclizumab is a unique hybrid monoclonal antibody in which the variable region (binding site for the IL-2R) is murine, but the remainder of the immunoglobulin molecule is human (immunoglobulin G_1). Only 10% of the hybrid molecule is of murine origin. As a result, antibody formation directed against the drug is decreased (e.g., in comparison with OKT3) and half-life is prolonged. Basiliximab is a chimeric anti-IL-2R antibody with a mechanism of action that is the same as daclizumab. In this monoclonal antibody, murine immunoglobulin amino acid sequences represent an even smaller fraction of the protein than is the case for daclizumab.

Dosing strategies for anti-IL-2R monoclonal antibodies begin with administration of the first dose, before transplantation. A dose of 1 mg/kg of daclizumab is administered IV, and this dose is repeated every 14 days for a total of 5 doses. Newer dosing strategies use higher doses (2 mg/kg), or abbreviated schedules of 2 or 3 total doses, or both.[120] A 20-mg/kg dose of basiliximab is administered IV before transplantation, and this dose is repeated once more on day 4.

Anti-IL-2R monoclonal antibodies are effective in preventing acute rejection after transplantation. However, these agents are ineffective for reversing acute cellular rejection. Both drugs are well tolerated, with no differences in adverse effects reported in clinical trials between the drugs and placebo. Daclizumab and basiliximab have the reported beneficial effects of reducing delayed graft function and delaying calcineurin inhibitor use (to decrease nephrotoxicity).[121,122]

Anti-CD52 Monoclonal Antibody

CD52 is a surface marker found on mature T and B lymphocytes. It also is found to varying degrees on monocytes, macrophages, granulocytes, and natural killer cells. Alemtuzumab (Campath [ILEX Pharmaceuticals, San Antonio, Texas]) is a humanized monoclonal antibody directed at the CD52 antigen that causes complete lympholysis, resulting in significant T-cell depletion. Experience with alemtuzumab suggests that lower degrees of immunosuppression are needed after T-cell depletion following alemtuzumab infusion. Reports indicate that only single-drug therapy, usually with a calcineurin inhibitor (cyclosporine or tacrolimus) or sirolimus, is necessary after patients receive induc-

tion therapy with alemtuzumab.[123-125] Alemtuzumab also has been successfully used to treat acute rejection episodes.[126,127]

The dose of alemtuzumab administered in transplantation is 30 mg IV. Significant adverse effects are noted with administration of alemtuzumab, notably rigors, hypotension, fever, shortness of breath, bronchospasms, and chills. Premedication with diphenhydramine, acetaminophen, and corticosteroids is required before alemtuzumab administration to minimize the infusion-related effects. Other adverse effects noted after alemtuzumab therapy include neutropenia, anemia, thrombocytopenia, and pancytopenia.

Rituximab

Rituximab (Rituxan) monoclonal chimeric human-murine anti-CD20 antibody was first approved in the United States for the treatment of refractory or relapsed B-cell lymphomas. Rituximab eliminates B cells by complement-dependent cytotoxicity and antibody-dependent cellular toxicity. In relation to organ transplantation, rituximab has been used to treat posttransplant lymphoproliferative disease, decrease presentation to blood group or HLA antigens, and treat antibody-mediated rejection. Recently, Clatworthy et al.[128] reported that there was a significantly higher incidence of acute cellular rejection episodes in patients treated with rituximab, whereas Tyden et al.[129] reported that the number of cellular rejection episodes in patients treated with rituximab was exceptionally low. For desensitization to blood group or HLA antigens, rituximab typically is administered as a single dose (200 mg, 300 mg, or 500 mg) within 7 days before transplantation, and administration of the antibody often is combined with three or four plasmapheresis sessions prior to transplantation to remove anti-HLA and/or anti–blood type antibodies.[130]

KEY POINTS

1. Allograft rejection is mediated primarily by the T cell in response to the presence of an antigen which is processed by antigen-presenting cells (APC) and carried on the major histocompatibility complex (MHC) molecules to the T cell.

2. The T-cell receptor (TCR), in conjunction with accessory molecules such as CD3, CD4, and CD8, interacts with the antigen fragment on the MHC molecule and produces the growth factor, interleukin 2 (IL-2), to activate and stimulate proliferation of the T cell.

3. During allograft rejection, cytokines attract various cells into rejecting allografts, stimulate the production of antibodies, and produce inflammation.

4. Effective immunosuppressive protocols combine multiple drugs targeted at different sites of the T-cell activation cascade.

5. Corticosteroids block the early steps of T-cell activation; they are used in tapering doses during the induction and maintenance phases of immunosuppressive protocols and in high, brief doses for the reversal of acute rejection episodes.

6. The backbone of immunosuppressive protocols are the calcineurin inhibitors, cyclosporine and tacrolimus, which inhibit IL-2 production and subsequent T-cell activation and proliferation.

7. Azathioprine and mycophenolate mofetil inhibit purine synthesis, thereby disrupting the cell cycle and T-cell proliferation.

8. Sirolimus blocks the cellular response to IL-2 and inhibits progression of the cell cycle, inhibiting T-cell proliferation.

9. Antithymocyte globulin and monoclonal antibodies are potent cytotoxic compounds that cause rapid, profound, and prolonged T-cell depletion; they are effectively used to reverse acute rejection episodes or as induction therapy before transplantation.

10. Drug concentration monitoring is necessary to maximize efficacy in preventing allograft rejection while minimizing the potential for significant adverse effects. Monitoring aids in the management of drug interactions, particularly with cyclosporine, tacrolimus, and sirolimus therapy.

ANNOTATED REFERENCES

Bullingham RES, Nicholls AJ, Kamm BR. Clinical pharmacokinetics of mycophenolate mofetil. Clin Pharmacokinet 1998;34:429-55.

The pharmacokinetics of mycophenolate mofetil is emphasized in this article, with an overview of the mechanism of action and pharmacodynamic properties of the drug. Clinical monitoring and the correlation of plasma concentrations with adverse and immunosuppressive effects are highlighted.

Denton MD, Magee CC, Sayegh MH. Immunosuppressive strategies in transplantation. Lancet 1999;353:1083-131.

This article provides a thorough review of the mechanisms of allograft rejection and the rationale for selection of agents directed at specific targets in the immune cascade. Various approaches to immunosuppression in transplantation are highlighted, as well as specific agents used and novel agents currently under investigation.

Dunn CJ, Wagstaff AJ, Perry CM, et al. Cyclosporine: an updated review of the pharmacokinetic properties, clinical efficacy and tolerability of a microemulsion-based formulation (Neoral) in organ transplantation. Drugs 2001;61:1957-2016.

This article provides in-depth review of the pharmacokinetic properties of cyclosporine and its use in various solid-organ transplants. In addition to novel approaches to clinical monitoring of cyclosporine, comparisons with other immunosuppressive agents in solid-organ transplantation is discussed.

Kahan BD, Camardo JS. Rapamycin: clinical results and future opportunities. Transplantation 2001;72:1181-93.

This article provides a review of the pharmacology and pharmacodynamics of sirolimus and its role in solid-organ transplantation. Adverse effects, clinical efficacy, and therapeutic monitoring are addressed, as well as immunosuppressive strategies with sirolimus-based therapy.

Scott LJ, McKeage K, Keam SJ, Plosker GL. Tacrolimus: a further update of its use in the management of organ transplantation. Drugs 2003;63:1247-97.

An extensive review of the pharmacokinetic and pharmacokinetic properties of tacrolimus and its use in various solid-organ transplants is presented, with emphasis on the use of tacrolimus for immunosuppressive strategies. Therapeutic efficacy, adverse effects, and its place in therapy are addressed.

REFERENCES

Access the complete reference list online at http://www.expertconsult.com.

Digitalis

MARK A. MUNGER | PRZEMYSŁAW B. RADWAŃSKI | BENJAMIN W. VAN TASSELL

Therapeutic Indications

Digoxin is indicated for the treatment of mild to moderate congestive heart failure (CHF) and for the control of ventricular response rates in patients with chronic atrial fibrillation.[1] Digoxin improves left ventricular ejection fraction, improves exercise tolerance, ameliorates CHF-related symptoms, and decreases CHF-related hospitalizations and emergency care. But treatment with digoxin has not been shown to improve survival in patients with systolic left ventricular dysfunction.[2-4] However, digoxin is not indicated as primary treatment for stabilization of acutely decompensated heart failure.[5]

In the critical care setting, digoxin may be used to treat atrial arrhythmias, predominantly atrial fibrillation.[6] In *chronic atrial fibrillation*, digoxin is useful for controlling the ventricular rate in patients with left ventricular systolic dysfunction.[5] Rate control occurs in a linear dose-response fashion over a range of digoxin doses from 0.25 to 0.75 mg/d for adults,[1] but the drug may not consistently control ventricular rate in dysfunctional states associated with increased sympathetic tone, such as exercise- or emotional stress–induced tachycardia.[6-9] In *acute atrial fibrillation*, digoxin provides effective ventricular rate control and represents a useful therapy for rate control, especially if left ventricular function is compromised.[1,10] The agent does not restore normal sinus rhythm, although occasionally atrial fibrillation spontaneously resolves during initial therapy.[5]

Mechanism of Action

Digoxin is a cardiac glycoside with specific effects on the myocardium. Inhibition of the sodium/potassium–adenosine triphosphatase (Na^+/K^+-ATPase) pump increases intracellular sodium concentration and subsequently increases intracellular calcium concentration by stimulation of sodium-calcium exchange.[1,11] The pharmacologic effects of digoxin include increased force of systolic contraction (i.e., positive inotropic activity); decreased activation of the sympathetic nervous system and renin-angiotensin system (neurohormonal deactivating effect); sensitization of arterial baroreceptor nerve endings, which then normalizes the reflex vasodilation response to cardiac unloading; and decreased heart rate and conduction velocity within the atrioventricular (AV) node (vagomimetic effect). Neurohormonal effects occur at low dosages, independent of inotropic effects. Hemodynamic improvement is observed in CHF related to both the inotropic and neurohormonal effects of digoxin. The vagal effects of digoxin result in slowed conduction and prolongation of AV node refractoriness, which slows the ventricular response in patients with atrial fibrillation. The overall response to digoxin is an increase in cardiac output and reduction in pulmonary artery pressure, systemic vascular resistance, plasma norepinephrine level, and pulmonary capillary wedge pressure. Minimal changes in blood pressure occur with initiation of therapy.[1,12-13]

Pharmacokinetics

Intravenous (IV) preparations are 100% bioavailable, whereas most oral formulations provide only 60% to 80% bioavailability.[1] Capsules containing liquid have increased bioavailability, being about 90% to 100% of the IV formulation. Therefore, dosing considerations are important when switching between oral and IV preparations. Digoxin absorption occurs primarily in the small intestine. When some digoxin oral preparations are taken after meals, the rate of absorption is slowed, but the total amount of digoxin absorbed remains unchanged.[1] Impaired absorption after oral administration can occur if intestinal function is impaired, although partial gastrectomy or jejunoileal bypass does not affect absorption to an appreciable extent.[1,14-15]

The distribution phase of digoxin metabolism is prolonged after oral or IV administration. For patients started on oral therapy, the onset of action occurs within 0.5 to 2 hours, and peak effects are seen within 6 to 8 hours.[1] After IV administration, onset occurs in 5 to 30 minutes, and peak effect is observed within 1 to 5 hours.[16] This delay in pharmacologic effect may be undesirable in the setting of acute atrial fibrillation. Pharmacologic effects typically persist for 3 to 4 days after withdrawal of digoxin therapy.

Approximately 20% to 30% of digoxin is protein bound in patients with normal renal function or uremia.[1] Digoxin is extensively bound to multiple tissues, particularly to Na^+/K^+-ATPase in cardiac and skeletal muscle, and demonstrates a large volume of distribution, which averages 6 to 7 L/kg of total body weight in patients with normal renal function. A decrease in the volume of distribution occurs in patients with renal dysfunction or dialysis.

With normal renal function, the elimination half-life is 36 to 48 hours. Elimination is prolonged in patients with renal dysfunction, being about 3.5 to 5 days in anuric patients.[11] Metabolism occurs primarily in the liver, but the drug also is metabolized by bacteria within the large intestine after oral administration.[1] Excretion of digoxin is predominantly in the urine as unchanged drug. The drug is cleared by glomerular filtration and active tubular secretion. Small amounts are excreted in bile and feces. Approximately 30% of the total digoxin load in the body is eliminated daily in patients with normal renal function. The metabolism and excretion of digoxin is not appreciably altered in patients with liver disease if normal renal function is present. Importantly, increased urinary output does not result in enhanced elimination of digoxin, because elimination is dependent on age, gender, and serum creatinine. Estimations of creatinine clearance (CrCl) in milliliters per minute can be calculated from the patient's age (in years) and the serum creatinine concentration (in mg/dL) by the modified Cockcroft and Gault equation:

$$CrCl = [140 - age/(serum\ creatinine)]$$

This is the value for a male patient; for a female, multiply the result by 0.85. Given the CrCl, estimates of daily digoxin elimination can be made by the following equation:

$$Daily\ percentage\ of\ digoxin\ eliminated = 14 + [CrCl \div 5]$$

Dosing Recommendations

GENERAL CONSIDERATIONS

Lean body mass should be used to calculate the appropriate digoxin dosage for adult patients in intensive care units (ICUs), because no appreciable amount of digoxin is distributed to body fat.[17] Age, renal function, and weight all have to be considered when calculating both loading and maintenance doses for initiation of digoxin therapy.[18] Digoxin dosages in the pediatric population must be carefully titrated, especially in neonates. For children from infancy to age 10 years, substantially higher dosing is necessary in comparison with adult patients (see later discussion). In addition, concomitant medications (discussed later) may influence serum digoxin levels and should be considered when initiating therapy.

INITIAL LOADING DOSE

Recent literature does not support initial bolus dosing for patients with CHF.[18] If deemed appropriate, a daily dose of 8 to 12 µg/kg is suggested for adult patients in heart failure who are in normal sinus rhythm. Adult patients with CHF may receive initial dosing (62.5 to 250 mg/day), based on ideal body weight and kidney function.[19] In the acute setting, administering an initial loading dose is recommended for management of supraventricular tachyarrhythmias. Determining lean body weight (LBW in kilograms) is necessary for calculating digoxin loading and maintenance dosing. Appropriate dosing weight can be calculated from the following equations:

For a male patient,

$$LBW = 50 + [(2.3)(\text{number of inches tall over 5 feet})]$$

or

$$LBW = [(0.9)(\text{height in centimeters})] - 88$$

For a female patient,

$$LBW = 45.5 + [(2.3)(\text{number of inches tall over 5 feet})]$$

or

$$LBW = [(0.9)(\text{height in centimeters})] - 92$$

An initial IV loading dose for adults of 10 to 15 µg/kg based on LBW is necessary for adequate ventricular rate control in the setting of atrial fibrillation or atrial flutter. Patients with impaired renal function and those older than 70 years of age require lower initial loading doses; a 50% dose reduction is recommended. Typically, the loading dose is administered as approximately half of the total dose immediately (maximum of 500 µg administration at one time), followed in 6 to 8 hours by 25% of the total dose, with the remaining 25% given after another 6 to 8 hours.[18] For example, a loading dose of 1000 µg should be administered as a 500-µg IV bolus, followed by 250 µg IV every 6 hours for 2 doses. To prevent toxicity, a thorough clinical evaluation of the ICU patient should be completed before additional bolus doses are given during the loading dose phase of therapy.

MAINTENANCE DOSING

If the initial loading dose of digoxin successfully controls the ventricular response of a supraventricular arrhythmia, a maintenance dose should be initiated.[18] The maintenance dose is also determined by renal function and the patient's LBW. The maintenance dose needed by patients not previously receiving digoxin therapy can be estimated from the loading dose and the percentage of drug eliminated each day as follows:

$$\text{Maintenance dose (in µg)} = \text{Loading dose (in µg)} \times \text{Amount eliminated daily}$$

Typical IV maintenance dosages range from 125 to 250 µg/day for patients with adequate renal function. Occasionally patients require higher dosages to maintain ventricular rate control. In patients with significantly impaired renal function (CrCl < 10 mL/min), dosages of less than 125 µg/day are necessary to prevent toxicity. Digoxin in these patients is commonly administered as 125 µg every other day.

Patients who are switched from IV to oral therapy must have dosage adjustments made as necessary.[18] If changing from IV therapy to oral tablets or elixir, the digoxin dosage should be increased by approximately 20% to 25%. However, no dosage adjustment is needed if the oral therapy uses liquid-filled capsules. For example, 100 µg of the IV product is approximately equivalent to 100 µg of the liquid-filled capsules (Lanoxicaps) or 125 µg of the tablet (Digitek, Lanoxin) or the elixir formulation.

Special Populations

THYROID DYSFUNCTION

Thyroid dysfunction results in an altered pharmacodynamic profile. Hypothyroid patients require decreased digoxin dosages compared to euthyroid ICU patients.[14,15,18] Hyperthyroid patients commonly need increased digoxin dosages, potentially secondary to increased resistance to digoxin therapy. Alterations in absorption, tissue distribution, renal excretion, and sensitivity of digitalis receptors in patients with thyroid disease have been proposed as mechanisms to explain altered serum digoxin concentrations.[14,15]

ELECTROLYTE DISTURBANCES

Hypokalemia enhances the effects of digoxin by increasing the cardiac effects due to depletion of intracellular potassium.[18] Hypomagnesemia requires larger digoxin doses for rate control in the setting of atrial fibrillation.[18] Repletion of potassium and magnesium to adequate levels should be completed before initiation of digoxin therapy to prevent potential proarrhythmic effects. Significant hypercalcemia may enhance digoxin toxicity.[18]

HEART DISEASE

For patients with coronary artery disease, cor pulmonale, or extensive myocardial damage including previous myocardial infarction, a reduction of digoxin dosage may be necessary.[18] Digoxin has been reported to increase mortality in patients with acute ischemic syndromes,[20,21] although more recent data do not support this idea.[16] The increase in sensitivity to digoxin based on underlying cardiac disease mandates caution and careful patient monitoring.

GENDER

When used to treat heart failure and decreased left ventricular function, digoxin was found to have different effects on all-cause mortality in men compared to women.[22] Specifically, digoxin was associated with increased all-cause mortality among women in a population with heart failure and depressed left ventricular systolic function.[22] The impact of gender on the pharmacologic effects of digoxin used to treat supraventricular arrhythmias is currently unknown, and dosage adjustments are not recommended on the basis of gender at this time.

PREGNANCY

Digoxin is a category C medication and should be considered for pregnant patients only if the benefits clearly outweigh the risks, and no alternative is available. The impact in terms of fetal harm or reproductive capacity is unknown.[1]

RENAL DYSFUNCTION

The kinetic parameters of digoxin are severely altered in patients with impaired renal function. The elimination half-life is prolonged, and clearance is impaired. In addition, volume of distribution is decreased. The degree of dosage adjustment needed to maintain therapeutic drug levels correlates with the degree of renal insufficiency. Dosage adjustment is necessary to prevent toxicity, because digoxin is primarily excreted by the kidney. Digoxin is not removed to any appreciable extent by either peritoneal dialysis or hemodialysis. The pharmacokinetics of digoxin have not been studied during continuous renal replacement therapy.

PEDIATRICS

Individualized dosing is extremely important in pediatric patients. In newborns, a reduction in renal clearance of digoxin is observed, necessitating dosage adjustments, especially in premature infants.[18] Divided daily dosing is often necessary in infants and those younger than 10 years of age. The elixir formulation is especially suitable for the pediatric population. Loading dosages of the pediatric elixir differ based on age: 20 to 30 µg/kg for premature infants, 25 to 35 µg/kg for full-term newborns, and 35 to 60 µg/kg for children younger than 2 years of age. For children aged 2 to 5 years, oral loading doses of 30 to 40 µg/kg are appropriate, and for those aged 5 to 10 years, the oral loading dose is 20 to 35 µg/kg. Children older than 10 years of age require 10 to 15 µg/kg initially. Maintenance doses for pediatric patients are approximately 25% of the oral loading dose necessary to achieve the optimal therapeutic effect. If IV therapy is necessary, the dose is approximately 80% of the total oral elixir requirement.

Therapeutic Monitoring

Measurements of digoxin concentration are useful in certain situations to assist in evaluating the effects of the drug on the disease state being treated and to avoid toxicity.[18] For treatment of supraventricular tachyarrhythmias, the usual therapeutic range for serum digoxin concentration is 1 to 2 ng/mL. However, patients can require serum concentrations as great as 3 ng/mL. The concentration is correlated with effectiveness or toxicity in a particular patient. The same level that is toxic in one patient may be therapeutic in another. Therefore, dose titration should be based on the heart rate and signs or symptoms of toxicity rather than the absolute digoxin concentration.

Evidence to support the use of serum concentrations to ensure efficacy in the treatment of heart failure is lacking. Lower digoxin concentrations (0.5-0.8 ng/mL) appear to provide equal or superior efficacy and avoid toxicity. Gheorghiade et al.[23] found that exercise time, heart failure scores, heart rate, and neurohormonal findings were similar among patients with serum digoxin concentrations of 0.67 ± 0.22 ng/mL compared to those at 1.22 ± 0.35 ng/mL. Mean concentrations of 0.8 ng/mL provided a reduction in rate of hospitalizations and worsening heart failure.[4,24] Rathore et al.[25] demonstrated that patients with digoxin concentrations of 0.5 to 0.8 ng/mL had a reduction in absolute mortality rate of 6.3% compared with patients who received placebo. However, no reduction in mortality was observed for patients with concentrations of 0.9 to 1.1 ng/mL compared to the placebo group, and an increase in mortality was found for patients with levels of 1.2 ng/mL or greater.

Measurements of serum digoxin concentrations may be particularly useful when kinetic parameters are changing.[18] For example, in patients with improving or declining renal function or in situations in which a drug interaction could decrease absorption or digoxin clearance, monitoring levels is helpful. Digoxin concentrations can be obtained periodically to detect excessive drug levels and prevent toxicity.

Proper timing of digoxin measurements is critical. Although digoxin is found in the plasma compartment within a brief period after administration, the medication distributes slowly into the heart and other tissues.[26] Because the heart is the site of action, digoxin concentrations measured less than 4 hours after IV administration or 6 hours after oral administration are misleading. The optimal time to measure digoxin levels is 12 to 24 hours after administration. For patients with normal renal function, digoxin concentrations do not reach steady state for 7 to 10 days in the absence of a loading dose. As renal function declines, clearance of digoxin is impaired, and the time to reach steady state is prolonged. In patients with end-stage renal failure, this duration is extended to 15 to 20 days. Levels obtained before the drug has reached steady state can be useful to prevent toxicity or assess a trend. However, these concentrations do not reflect the maximum concentration at steady state.

Contraindications

Contraindications to the use of digoxin include ventricular fibrillation and hypersensitivity to digoxin or digitalis compounds.[1] The risk of digoxin toxicity is higher in patients with preexisting sinus node disease or incomplete AV block, in those with an accessory AV pathway (Wolff-Parkinson-White syndrome), and in those who have heart failure with preserved left ventricular systolic function (isolated diastolic dysfunction). Patients with sinus node disease can develop severe sinus bradycardia or sinoatrial block. An advanced or complete AV block may develop in individuals with a previously incomplete block. The use of digoxin in patients with an accessory AV pathway may result in increased frequency of anterograde conduction via the accessory pathway, with a rapid ventricular response or atrial fibrillation. Individuals with restrictive cardiomyopathy, constrictive pericarditis, amyloid heart disease, or acute cor pulmonale are particularly susceptible to digoxin toxicity.[1] Digoxin therapy can adversely affect patients with idiopathic hypertrophic subaortic stenosis by causing further obstruction to outflow.

Drug-Drug and Drug-Assay Interactions

Digoxin is a substrate of P-glycoprotein,[27-33] while amiodarone,[27] verapamil,[28] quinidine,[29,30] clarithromycin,[31] itraconazole,[32] and cyclosporin A[33] are potent inhibitors of P-glycoprotein. P-glycoprotein is encoded by the multidrug-resistance (MDR1) gene and is found in kidney, liver, colon, jejunum, adrenal glands, blood-brain barrier, placenta, and testis.[28] The role of P-glycoprotein in the body appears to be to act as an ATP-dependent efflux pump.

Within 5 to 7 days after institution of amiodarone therapy in patients receiving digoxin, amiodarone inhibits P-glycoprotein function in kidneys and liver, resulting in a decrease in both renal and nonrenal clearance of digoxin.[7,18,34] Renal and nonrenal clearance of digoxin also decreases with concurrent administration of verapamil, resulting in a 70% to 100% increase in serum digoxin concentration.[7,18] Although not as extensively studied, a decrease in digoxin clearance also may occur with concomitant administration of diltiazem.[35] Administration of digoxin plus verapamil or digoxin plus diltiazem should be avoided by selecting an alternative agent to the aforementioned calcium channel blockers. Quinidine decreases renal and nonrenal clearance of digoxin and increases the rate and extent of digoxin absorption. If amiodarone, verapamil, or quinidine is administered to a patient taking digoxin, the digoxin dose should be decreased by 50%, and serum digoxin concentrations should be monitored closely.

With the administration of clarithromycin, the oral bioavailability of digoxin increases and nonglomerular renal clearance of digoxin decreases.[31] This results in a 1.8-fold increase in digoxin concentration. By inhibiting P-glycoprotein, itraconazole decreases the renal clearance of digoxin by approximately 20%, increases oral bioavailability by 30%, and results in a twofold increase in digoxin serum concentrations.[32] Renal excretion of digoxin is also inhibited by administration of cyclosporine.[33] Serum digoxin concentrations should be monitored closely when clarithromycin, itraconazole, or cyclosporine therapy is started in a patient receiving digoxin.

In patients with severe heart failure, captopril causes a 1.6-fold increase in peak digoxin concentrations.[36] This effect may not occur in patients with New York Heart Association class II or III heart failure. The mechanism of the interaction is unknown; however, it may be caused by a decrease in glomerular filtration and tubular secretion of digoxin.

Spironolactone decreases renal[37] and nonrenal[7,18] clearance of digoxin. In addition, spironolactone and canrenone, a metabolite of spironolactone, cross-react with several of the assays used to monitor digoxin concentrations.[38,39] An increase in the apparent digoxin concentration was observed when the drug was assayed by fluorescence polarization immunoassay (FPIA), aca,[38] or Elecsys 2020.[39] In contrast, a decrease in the apparent concentration occurred when the microparticle enzyme immunoassay (MEIA),[38] AxSYM MEIA II,[39] IMx MEIA II,[39] or Dimension Systems[39] were used to measure digoxin levels. Spironolactone did not appear to interact with the chemiluminescent assay (CLIA),[38] EMIT 2000,[39] Tina Quant,[39] or Vitros slides.[39] Interference with the MEIA and FPIA assays was eliminated when free concentrations were measured.[38] Digoxin concentrations should be monitored more frequently after starting spironolactone to avoid accumulation of the medication; also, CLIA, EMIT 2000, Tina Quant, Vitros slides, or free levels should be used to accurately measure digoxin concentrations.

There are multiple medications that decrease the bioavailability of digoxin and result in lower serum concentrations.[7,18] Cholestyramine, colestipol, kaolin-pectin, and oral antacids decrease the absorption of oral digoxin by binding digoxin in the gastrointestinal tract. These medications should be administered at least 2 hours apart to prevent this effect. Metoclopramide decreases the absorption of digoxin tablets by increasing gastrointestinal motility The administration of digoxin capsules instead of tablets in patients receiving metoclopramide is suggested to avoid this reaction. Absorption of digoxin is lowered by the concurrent administration of neomycin or sulfasalazine. This interaction should be avoided; however, if a patient needs to receive both medications, the doses should be spaced by approximately 2 hours.

Patients receiving levothyroxine and digoxin should have close monitoring of thyroid hormone levels and digoxin concentrations. Hyperthyroidism was shown to decrease digoxin levels by increasing the volume of the central compartment.[40] In contrast, hypothyroidism may have no effect or may cause an increase in the digoxin concentration.[40,41]

Rifampin administration induces intestinal P-glycoprotein activity.[42] This results in a decrease in digoxin oral bioavailability by approximately 30%, with no apparent change in digoxin renal clearance. Because of the decrease in bioavailability, maximum plasma digoxin concentrations are reduced by 58%.

Adverse Effects

Numerous cardiac arrhythmias may result from digoxin toxicity.[7,34] Some predisposing factors for digoxin toxicity include hypokalemia along with hypercalcemia, renal insufficiency, and hypothyroidism. Cardiac effects can manifest as an increase in vagal tone, causing sinus bradycardia. In the early phase of an overdose or in acute toxicity, bradycardia is likely to respond to atropine administration. However, atropine may be ineffective in later phases of acute poisoning. Frequent premature ventricular complexes are another electrocardiographic manifestation of early-phase digoxin toxicity. These phenomena are believed to be due to spontaneous calcium release from calcium-overloaded sarcoplasmic reticulum (SR),[43] which is brought upon by cytosolic calcium accumulation secondary to channeling of sodium efflux away from Na^+/K^+-ATPase and toward the sodium-calcium exchanger. These frequent premature ventricular complexes can degenerate to bigeminal activity and subsequent bidirectional ventricular tachycardia. Such ventricular arrhythmias, along with complete heart block and ventricular fibrillation, are indicative of the late stages of digoxin toxicity.

Noncardiac digoxin toxicities include gastrointestinal effects (anorexia, nausea, vomiting, diarrhea, abdominal pain), central nervous system abnormalities, and hyperkalemia.[1,7] Possible central nervous system effects include lethargy, confusion, weakness, headache, delirium, psychosis, transient amblyopia, photophobia, blurred vision, scotomata, photopsia, decreased visual activity, and color irregularities such as yellow-green or red-green halos around lights. Hyperkalemia results from excessive blockade of the Na^+/K^+-ATPase pump and is an index for outcome. Acute manifestations of digoxin toxicity are often more severe than chronic adverse effects.

Treatment of Digoxin Toxicity

The treatment of digoxin toxicity includes several steps which vary based on the acuteness of the situation. In acute overdoses, prevention of further absorption using activated charcoal should be instituted.[44] Syrup of ipecac, insertion of a gastric tube, and gastric lavage should be avoided, because vomiting induced by these methods intensifies vagal tone.

Supportive care is required to manage electrolyte disturbances and dysrhythmias.[34,44,45] Hyperkalemia should be treated by standard approaches. Sodium polystyrene sulfonate (Kayexalate) may remove potassium, and if hyperkalemia is severe, digoxin immune Fab should be administered (see next section). Caution should be used in administering both digoxin immune Fab and sodium polystyrene sulfonate, because hypokalemia may occur.

In the case of life-threatening arrhythmias, digoxin immune Fab should be administered.[34,44] If administration of digoxin immune Fab is delayed or treatment is needed until the onset of the effect of this agent, advanced cardiac life support (ACLS) protocols should be followed.

DIGOXIN IMMUNE FAB

The digoxin immune Fab (ovine) products available in the United States are Digibind and DigiFab. The products are developed by immunizing sheep with a digoxin analog and then isolating the digoxin-specific Fab fragments from ovine blood.[46,47] Digoxin immune Fab is used for the treatment of acute and chronic life-threatening digoxin toxicity or overdose. In addition, digoxin immune Fab is used to bind other digitalis glycosides.[44] Digoxin binds to digoxin immune Fab with a higher affinity compared to its sodium pump receptors. Once formed, the Fab-digoxin complex is eliminated by the kidneys and the reticuloendothelial system.

Based on an in vivo kinetic study of healthy volunteers, Digibind and DigiFab result in similar reductions in free serum digoxin concentrations.[48] Resolution of gastrointestinal symptoms occurs within minutes after beginning a bolus infusion.[49,50] Within 30 to 60 minutes, hyperkalemia secondary to skeletal muscle Na^+/K^+-ATPase inhibition starts to resolve, and electrocardiogram abnormalities cease. This effect can last for several days, requiring the complex and the drug to be cleared renally,[46,47] particularly since digoxin immune Fab is not removed by hemodialysis.

Each vial contains 38 mg (Digibind) or 40 mg (DigiFab) of digoxin immune Fab and binds approximately 0.5 mg of digoxin.[46,47] Adult and pediatric patients who acutely ingest an unknown amount of digoxin or other digitalis glycoside should receive 20 vials of either product. Pediatric patients should be closely monitored for volume overload. Administration of all 20 vials at once is likely to result in a faster onset of action but may increase the risk of an allergic reaction. Alternatively, 10 vials may be administered with careful observation of the patient, after which 10 additional vials may be given if clinically indicated.

Adults exhibiting toxicity due to chronic dosing of digoxin and for whom a digoxin level is unavailable should be given 6 vials of either product.[46,47] One vial should be sufficient for infants and children weighing 20 kg or less.

If an individual acutely ingests a known amount of digoxin, the dose is based on the estimated total body load (in milligrams) for digoxin capsules or digitoxin:

$$\text{Total body load} = (\text{Number of capsules ingested}) \times (\text{Dose of capsules}) \times 0.8$$

If tablets instead of capsules were ingested, the number of vials needed can then be calculated:

$$\text{Number of vials needed} = (\text{Total body load}) \div 0.5 \text{ mg of digoxin/vial}$$

Calculation of the digoxin immune Fab dose can also be based on the steady-state digoxin concentration.[46,47] Concentrations obtained in an acute overdose may be misleading and may result in underdosing, because digoxin can continue to be absorbed via the gastrointestinal tract. Calculation of the number of vials of Fab product required for an adult patient who is experiencing digoxin toxicity is based on the serum digoxin level (in ng/mL) and the patient's weight in kilograms as follows:

$$\text{Number of vials} = (\text{Serum digoxin concentration}) \times (\text{Weight}) \div 100$$

For digitoxin, the calculation is as follows:

Number of vials = (Serum digitoxin concentration) × (Weight) ÷ 1000

For infants and children who require small doses of digoxin immune Fab, the vial may be reconstituted to provide a 1 mg/mL concentration by adding 34 mL of sterile sodium chloride to a vial of Digibind, or 36 mL to a vial of DigiFab.

The rate of administration has varied in clinical trials and case reports. Doses are typically given as a bolus over 15 to 30 minutes.[50-52] Schaumann and colleagues[53] evaluated the kinetics of digoxin immune Fab in 17 patients with acute overdose. They concluded that a bolus dose of 160 mg (4 vials) over 30 minutes, followed by an infusion of 0.5 mg/minute over 8 hours, optimally binds digoxin as it rediffuses into the blood from the tissues. Patients experiencing rebound toxicity 8 to 12 hours after the initiation of treatment could be given 0.1 mg/min.

There are no known contraindications to the use of digoxin immune Fab.[46,47] However, allergic reactions and anaphylactic reactions have occurred. Patients at a higher risk for experiencing allergic reactions are those who are allergic to papain, chymopapain, other papaya extracts, pineapple enzyme bromelain, dust mites, or latex. Because the drug is an animal product, individuals who are allergic to sheep or wool are at higher risk. In addition, patients who have previously received digoxin immune Fab are at an increased risk. However, skin testing has not been shown to be useful and results in delay of therapy.

Patients must be closely monitored for significant decreases in potassium concentrations, as well as for deterioration secondary to the withdrawal of an inotropic agent in patients with low cardiac output states.[46,47] There is a theoretical risk of development of antibodies to the drug; however, this occurrence has not been reported.

After acute digoxin administration, rebound of free digoxin concentrations was observed 8 to 24 hours after initiation of Fab therapy.[48,53] The cause of this phenomenon is not entirely clear. Proposed mechanisms include a release of free digoxin by metabolic degradation of the Fab-digoxin complex[46] and rediffusion of free digoxin from the tissues into the serum.[53] Patients should be observed closely for indications of a rebound effect. However, monitoring of total serum concentrations is of little utility, because immune Fab interacts with most assay methods. Free digoxin concentrations in ultrafiltration samples provide the most accurate results.[54]

KEY POINTS

1. Initial loading doses of intravenous digoxin for new-onset atrial fibrillation, approximately 10 μg/kg over a 24-hour period based on lean body weight, should be administered to adequately control ventricular rate in most patients.

2. Patients with impaired renal function and elderly patients commonly require 50% less digoxin than other ICU patients.

3. The therapeutic range for circulating digoxin concentration when the drug is used to control supraventricular tachyarrhythmias is 1 to 2 ng/mL; the therapeutic range for heart failure is 0.5 to 0.8 ng/mL.

4. Adverse effects of digitalis include nausea, vomiting, diarrhea, visual disturbances, confusion, hyperkalemia, and cardiac arrhythmias.

5. An increase in digoxin concentration may occur with concomitant administration of amiodarone, verapamil, quinidine, spironolactone, clarithromycin, itraconazole, or captopril.

6. A decrease in digoxin concentration may occur with concomitant administration of cholestyramine, colestipol, kaolin-pectin, oral antacids, metoclopramide, neomycin, sulfasalazine, levothyroxine, or rifampin.

7. Digoxin toxicity should be treated by administering activated charcoal to prevent further absorption of the drug and infusing digoxin immune Fab to bind the drug once absorption has occurred. Supportive care with advanced cardiac life support protocols and treatment of hyperkalemia along with magnesium supplementation also should be undertaken.

ANNOTATED REFERENCES

The Digitalis Investigation Group. The effect of digoxin on mortality and morbidity in patients with heart failure. N Engl J Med 1997;336:525-33.
The Digitalis Investigation Group (DIG) trial was a multicenter randomized study that included patients with an ejection fraction of 45% or less. No difference in mortality was found between the group of patients receiving digoxin and those receiving placebo. There were statistically significant decreases in overall hospitalizations and heart failure–related hospitalizations.

Packer M, Gheorghiade M, Young JB, et al. Withdrawal of digoxin from patients with chronic heart failure treated with angiotensin-converting-enzyme inhibitors. RADIANCE Study. N Engl J Med 1993;329:1-7.
Patients with New York Heart Association class II or III heart failure and ejection fraction of 35% or less were randomly assigned to continue digoxin or change to placebo. Compared to the digoxin group, the placebo group had worsening heart failure, decreased functional capacity, decreased quality-of-life scores, and decreased ejection fraction.

Rathore SS, Curtis JP, Wang Y, et al. Association of serum digoxin concentration and outcomes in patients with heart failure. JAMA 2003;289:871-8.
This post hoc analysis of men in the DIG trial found that the mortality rate of patients with serum digoxin concentrations between 0.5 and 0.8 ng/mL was lower than that of patients receiving placebo. The mortality rate in the group of patients with serum concentrations between 0.9 and 1.1 ng/mL was not different from that in the placebo group. Those patients with a serum concentration of 1.2 ng/mL or greater had a higher mortality rate than patients in the placebo group.

Rathore SS, Wang Y, Krumholz HM. Sex-based differences in the effect of digoxin for the treatment of heart failure. N Engl J Med 2002;347:1403-11.
This post hoc subgroup analysis of the DIG trial found in a multivariate analysis that men who received digoxin had a slight reduction in risk of death, compared with men who received placebo. However, there was a significantly increased risk of death for women in the digoxin group, compared with women in the placebo group.

Rich MW, McSherry F, Williford WO, et al. Effect of age on mortality, hospitalizations and response to digoxin in patients with heart failure: the DIG study. J Am Coll Cardiol 2001;38:806-13.
This subanalysis of the DIG study stratified patients with chronic heart failure by age. The reduction in all-cause admissions, heart failure–related admissions, and heart failure–related deaths found in the original study was independent of age.

REFERENCES

Access the complete reference list online at http://www.expertconsult.com.

178

Heavy Metals

DANIEL E. RUSYNIAK | ANNA ARROYO | BLAKE FROBERG | BRENT FURBEE

As a species, humans are highly dependent on heavy metals. In fact, their abundance in nature and their chemical properties make our very existence possible. Because they are reactive and form complexes with other elements or compounds such as oxygen, sulfur, and chlorine, metal-containing enzymes play key roles in a number of normal physiologic processes (e.g., oxygen transport and defense against redox stress). In addition, the use of metal tools was the crucial step for Man's advancement out of the Stone Age and into the Bronze and Iron Ages. Today we use metals in an ever-increasing number of industrial processes and will likely continue to do so for the remainder of our existence. Therefore, it should not be surprising that along with the benefits conferred upon us by heavy metals, there have been a number of problems. Entering our bodies by way of food, drink, and the air we breathe, a variety of metals (and metalloids) can disrupt numerous physiologic processes. Years of chronic low-level exposure to some metals can lead to a variety of problems, including cancer, dermatologic conditions, hypertension, and renal dysfunction. On the other hand, acute or subacute exposure to high concentrations of some heavy metals (or metalloids) can cause immediate life-threatening disorders. Successful treatment of these disorders requires knowledgeable critical care physicians. In this chapter we will review the clinical presentations and treatments of the heavy metal poisonings that are most likely to require intensive care management, notably intoxication caused by arsenic, mercury, lead, and thallium.

Arsenic

BACKGROUND

Enormous achievements and incredible misfortune mark arsenic's history. Dating back to 400 BC, Greek and Roman physicians included arsenic in their medical armamentarium.[1] Today, arsenic continues to be found in treatments offered by practitioners of Indian folk medicine and traditional Chinese medicine.[2,3] In addition, in Western medicine, arsenic trioxide (Trisenox) and melarsoprol are used to treat promyelocytic leukemia[4] and late-stage African trypanosomiasis.[5]

Arsenic's therapeutic usefulness is based on its ability to poison cells, and it is best known as a poison. While arsenic has been noted to produce a garlic odor and possess a characteristically sweet flavor, most arsenical compounds have no perceptible smell or taste.[6] This has made the detection of arsenic difficult when employed as a homicidal agent. Historically, this has afforded arsenic the illustrious title of "Poison of Kings and the King of Poisons."[7]

TOXICITY

Environmental arsenic comes from both natural (volcanic eruption, water runoff) and manmade sources (mining, smelting, combustion of fossil fuels, and pesticide use).[7,8] Food, predominantly seafood, represents the principal route for human exposure; however, rice, mushrooms, and poultry also contribute to exposure.[6] Alternative sources include air and water, particularly in Bangladesh where tube-wells supply millions with arsenic-contaminated drinking water.[9] In the United States, the average person consumes 50 μg of arsenic daily, with inorganic arsenic accounting for 3.5 μg of this total. Certain occupations such as metal working, electronics manufacturing, and glass manufacturing also increase arsenic exposure.[6]

Arsenic is found in nature in several different forms: combined with carbon and other elements in organic compounds, in inorganic compounds, in gaseous compounds, and in the nontoxic elemental form. Arsenobetaine, an organic arsenic compound found in fish and shellfish, possesses a low risk for human toxicity.[6] Inorganic arsenicals, found as trivalent (As^{3+}, arsenite, more toxic) or pentavalent (As^{5+}, arsenate, less toxic) compounds, account for the majority of human toxicity. Arsenite compounds exhibit high affinity for binding to proteins, whereas the majority of arsenate compounds remain unbound. Weak protein binding allows arsenate compounds to be freely excreted. Protein-bound arsenite functions as both a storage depot and a target action site.[10] Alternating hepatic reduction and methylation reactions convert inorganic arsenic to an organic form. This transformation detoxifies the parent compound but also increases arsenic's carcinogenicity.[7,10,11]

The mechanism accounting for arsenic's ability to disrupt cellular function, and that which results in acute toxicity, differs depending on the form of arsenic responsible for the exposure. By disrupting the activity of key enzymes by binding to critical sulfhydryl groups, arsenite impairs both oxidative phosphorylation and gluconeogenesis. Especially important in this regard is arsenite's ability to inhibit the enzyme, pyruvate dehydrogenase (PDH), which catalyzes the first and rate-limiting step in the tricarboxylic acid (TCA) cycle. Inhibition of PDH hinders the production of acetyl-CoA from pyruvate, limiting cellular ATP production. In addition, arsenate can substitute for phosphate and become incorporated into arsenate analogs of glucose-6-phosphate, 6-phosphogluconate, and adenosine triphosphate (ATP).[6,12,13] These arsenate analogs are less stable than their phosphate-containing counterparts, and their formation can lead to uncoupling of oxidative phosphorylation.[6,13-16]

Arsine gas (AsH_3) is released when many arsenic-containing compounds come in contact with an acid or when metallic arsenic comes into contact with water. Workers involved with lead plating, soldering, etching, smelting, and galvanizing are at risk for exposure to arsine gas.[17] Being colorless and nonirritating, arsine gas is particularly difficult to detect following industrial exposure. As with arsenic, arsine gas has been noted to possess a slight garlic odor; also like arsenic, however, arsine's odor is not always detectable.[18]

Exposure to arsine causes acute hemolysis. The exact mechanism for this hemolysis is not completely understood and is likely multifactorial, involving both binding of arsine to hemoglobin and perhaps inhibition of sulfhydryl-containing enzymes.[19-22] One complication of arsine exposure is acute renal failure. Arsine-induced renal failure most likely is secondary to direct nephrotoxic effects of arsine as well as the renal toxicity caused by the release of hemoglobin from lysed red blood cells.[23] Although chronic renal dysfunction has been described after arsine exposure, recovery is possible.[22,24]

CLINICAL PRESENTATION

A patient's clinical presentation after arsenic exposure is influenced by four factors: the arsenic species, the amount, the route, and the duration of exposure. In addition, the symptoms of acute arsenic toxicity differ depending on whether exposure was oral or inhalational. Gastrointestinal symptoms are a reliable finding in cases of acute arsenic poisoning. Shortly after exposure, patients typically experience abdominal discomfort, nausea, emesis, and profuse diarrhea.[7,25,26] Severe gastroenteritis and hemorrhage may develop. Furthermore, arsenic induces capillary dilation, third-spacing of fluid, ventricular arrhythmias, and cardiomyopathy. Collectively these changes can result in pulmonary edema, hypotension, congestive heart failure, and shock.[7,20] Cardiac abnormalities following arsenic exposure can include QTc prolongation, T-wave abnormalities, second-degree heart block, QRS widening, nonconducted P-waves, nonsustained ventricular tachycardia, torsades de pointes, complete heart block, asystole, pericardial effusion, and serositis.[27-31] Cardiac conduction abnormalities have been described following therapeutic use of arsenic trioxide. These conduction abnormalities may be a consequence of arsenic trioxide–induced electrolyte abnormalities (hypokalemia or hypomagnesemia).[29] Alternatively, these changes in cardiac conduction might reflect the cardiotoxic effects of other cancer chemotherapeutic agents. Additionally, arsenic-induced blockade of I_{Kr} and I_{Ks} channels with activation of I_{K-ATP} channels has been demonstrated.[32] The variability seen in arsenic-induced QTc prolongation likely occurs secondary to the combined effects of this activation and blockade.

Neurologic symptoms are also associated with arsenic toxicity and typically include altered mental status and confusion.[20,25] Seizures have been linked to arsenic-induced arrhythmias,[27,33] and if related to hypoxemia may signal a terminal stage in cases of arsenic poisoning. While typically delayed 2 to 8 weeks after exposure, peripheral neuropathy from large arsenic exposures sometimes can become apparent within a few hours.[7,34] Patients describe pain, numbness, and paresthesias in a "stocking/glove" sort of distribution.[20,25,35] The symmetric sensorimotor neuropathy seen following arsenic exposure can be misdiagnosed as Guillain-Barré.[7,35] Marked abnormalities in sensory and mixed nerve conduction in conjunction with moderate motor conduction abnormalities can be seen on electrophysiologic testing. These results are consistent with axonal degeneration, which is also apparent histologically in nerve biopsies.[36]

Symptoms of chronic arsenic toxicity differ from those of acute toxicity. Patients demonstrate hematologic abnormalities including pancytopenia, anemia, and macrocytosis. Dermal manifestations include Mees lines (transverse white striae on the fingernails), hyperkeratotic extremity lesions, and hyperpigmented melanosis. Gastrointestinal symptoms as well as liver disease are also described.[7,26,37,38] Additionally, patients may note a metallic taste.[7,38,39]

Inhalational exposure to arsenic in the form of arsine gas produces symptoms that differ from those seen with oral arsenic exposure. Classically, exposure is characterized by the development of a triad of symptoms: abdominal pain, hematuria, and jaundice. Within 2 to 24 hours of exposure, patients develop headache, malaise, abdominal discomfort, nausea, and emesis. The variability in the onset of symptoms is influenced by the duration of exposure and the concentration of the gas.[17] Hemolysis with subsequent gross hematuria and renal failure often follow. Additionally, patients may develop scleral icterus and a bronze skin discoloration.[17,24] As with exposure to other arsenic compounds, exposure to arsine gas can lead to development of peripheral neuropathy.[40]

DIAGNOSIS

The potential for arsenic toxicity can be determined by combining the patient's clinical presentation with the likelihood of exposure. Blood and urine testing can confirm the diagnosis. Blood arsenic clearance occurs in three phases: Phase 1 takes place 2 to 3 hours following intravenous (IV) administration and is associated with a half-life ($t_{1/2}$) of about 2 hours; phase 2 occurs 3 hours to 7 days following administration and is associated with a $t_{1/2}$ of about 27 hours; and phase 3 occurs 10 or more days following administration and is associated with a $t_{1/2}$ of about 230 hours.[41] Arsenic is rapidly cleared from the blood during phases 1 and 2; thus, the reliability of blood arsenic testing is limited to the early stages of acute toxicity.[33] Following IV administration of radioactive arsenic, urinary recovery has been demonstrated at 18% to 30% after 1 hour, 36% to 56% at 4 hours, 57% to 90% by 9 days, and 96.6% by 18 days.[41] A positive urine arsenic level should be followed up by arsenic speciation to distinguish nontoxic organic

arsenic (commonly found in seafood) from the toxic inorganic form. A random urine arsenic level greater than 50 µg/L, or a 24-hour urine sample demonstrating more than 100 µg of arsenic, can confirm the diagnosis of acute arsenic toxicity. However, this diagnosis should be questioned if there is a history of recent seafood ingestion or the sample was not collected in a metal-free container. Hair and nail samples may be used to confirm exposure when chronic toxicity is suspected.[7] Hair testing can also be performed to estimate an approximate exposure date based on the rate of hair growth (0.4 mm/d) and the distance of the root from the arsenic peak.[42] Additionally, an electrocardiogram (ECG) should be obtained in cases of potential arsenic toxicity; T-wave abnormalities, QTc prolongation, and torsades de pointes have been described following arsenic exposure.[27,31]

Following possible exposure to arsine gas, laboratory evaluation should include complete blood count, measurement of circulating lactate dehydrogenase and other liver enzyme concentrations, measurement of serum bilirubin concentration, Coombs testing, and monitoring of serum electrolyte levels and renal function. Patients will demonstrate a Coombs-negative hemolytic anemia with elevated circulating lactate dehydrogenase, aspartate aminotransferase, alanine aminotransferase, and bilirubin levels, renal dysfunction, and subsequent hyperkalemia. Hemoglobinuria, albuminuria, and occasional erythrocyte and hemoglobin tubular casts are commonly seen on urinalysis. A peripheral blood smear can show signs of red blood cell damage including erythrocyte fragments, basophilic stippling, anisocytosis, poikilocytosis, and Heinz bodies.[17,18,22,43] Methemoglobinemia also has been described.[43]

TREATMENT

Initial treatment of arsenic toxicity must include prevention of further exposure to the poison, careful monitoring of the cardiovascular system, and judicious repletion of intravascular fluid deficits. Hyperkalemia, which can be clinically significant, should be treated. Despite a lack of supporting data, gastric lavage and administration of activated charcoal should be considered following oral exposure to a large of dose of arsenic in an attempt to limit absorption of the toxic compound(s).[7] Patients presenting with renal failure following arsenic exposure may need renal replacement therapy until renal function recovers.[44] Additionally, patients demonstrating ECG abnormalities, particularly QTc prolongation, should have close monitoring of their electrolytes, with replacement as indicated. Antiarrhythmic therapy should be instituted as needed.

Chelators are an additional treatment to be considered. Dimercaprol, a parenteral chelating agent which functions intracellularly as well as extracellularly, is the first line of therapy for patients experiencing abdominal symptoms following acute arsenic exposure.[33] Dimercaprol should be administered intramuscularly (IM) at doses of 3 to 4 mg/kg every 4 to 12 hours.[20] In cases of subacute or chronic exposure when the patient can take oral medications, succimer (DMSA or 2,3-dimercaptosuccinic acid) is the chelator of choice. Succimer should be administered orally (10 mg/kg every 8 hours for 5 days). Following the initial 5 days of administration, succimer dosing is adjusted to every 12 hours.[33] Clinical course determines the duration of chelator therapy.[20] Urinary arsenic levels can be used to calibrate duration of treatment, with therapy being discontinued when 24-hour urinary arsenic levels are below 50 µg/L.[33] Despite its recommended use, succimer has not consistently demonstrated increased urinary arsenic excretion following administration, and neuropathy can progress despite therapy.[25,42] Succimer is not currently approved by the U.S. Food and Drug Administration (FDA) for treatment of arsenic toxicity.[45]

Treatment of arsine gas exposure represents a special circumstance. As with other forms of arsenic exposure, initial therapy requires elimination of the source. Caution should be taken to prevent additional casualties as first responders enter the exposure site. Since arsine toxicity is associated with hemolysis, exchange transfusion can be used to replenish red blood cell mass and remove both the toxic complexes formed from the arsine/hemoglobin interaction as well as the released hemoglobin pigment.[40,46] Patients with renal failure should receive renal replacement therapy as indicated by clinical findings.[17,18] The use of chelation therapy to treat patients acutely poisoned by arsine is controversial and may not affect the clinical course.[18]

Mercury

BACKGROUND

Mercury is a naturally occurring metal found in elemental, inorganic salt, and organic forms. The use of mercury dates back to before 1500 BC. Throughout history, mercury has been employed as a cosmetic component, decoration, and even medicine. Mercury is also a natural part of our atmosphere, with 30,000 to 50,000 tons degassing from the earth's surface annually; human activity adds another 20,000 tons each year.[47] Toxicity from mercury can occur as a result of occupational, environmental, or medical exposure. Each year, mercury exposure accounts for over 6000 cases of toxicity reported to U.S. poison centers.[48] The dose, length of exposure, and form of mercury can cause wide variation in the clinical presentation and ultimate outcome.[49-52]

TOXICITY

Elemental mercury can be found in barometers, dental amalgams, electronics, thermostats, thermometers, and batteries. It is also found in some folk remedies. Elemental mercury is a liquid at room temperature. Even without heating, elemental mercury releases sufficient mercury in the gas phase to cause toxicity. Most problems from elemental mercury are the result of vapor inhalation, with nearly 80% of inhaled vapor being absorbed by the alveoli and transferred into circulating red blood cells. Most absorbed mercury is converted to its divalent (mercuric) form, thus decreasing its lipid solubility. If the patient is exposed to a very high dose of mercury vapor, a small amount of gaseous mercury can remain in the bloodstream, leading to penetration of the blood-brain barrier and central nervous system (CNS) injury.[8] By comparison, the gastrointestinal tract takes up less than 2% of ingested elemental mercury[53]; however, in patients with mucosal disruption, transmucosal absorption of mercury can be markedly increased.[54] Absorption of mercury across intact skin is minimal,[55] but subcutaneous injection can cause an increase in urinary mercury concentrations. Intravenous injection of mercury can cause both mercury toxicity and mechanical obstruction of pulmonary blood flow.[56,57] Elimination of inhaled vapor is via the urinary tract, and the elimination $t_{1/2}$ of absorbed elemental mercury is about 60 days.[56] Elemental mercury when orally ingested is typically nontoxic owing to minimal absorption across intact gastric and intestinal mucosa.[58]

Elemental mercury primarily targets the lungs and brain, but the poison also can cause renal and gastrointestinal injury.[5,14,15] By forming complexes with sulfhydryl groups, mercury interferes with protein and nucleic acid synthesis, protein phosphorylation, and calcium homeostasis. It can also cause oxidant stress via this mechanism.[59,60] Inhaled mercury vapor has a corrosive effect on the lungs and is capable of producing acute inflammation of the bronchi and bronchioles. This may result in a fatal interstitial pneumonitis.[60]

Depending upon the dose and length of exposure, symptoms of poisoning caused by elemental mercury can vary widely. Onset of chills, gastrointestinal distress, cough, weakness, and dyspnea can occur within hours of an acute exposure, and in severe cases can result in adult respiratory distress syndrome and renal failure. On the other hand, it can take weeks or months before symptoms become apparent in some cases of chronic elemental mercury exposure. Commonly attributed to a viral illness, symptoms from chronic elemental mercury exposure are nonspecific and include gastrointestinal upset, anorexia, abdominal pain, headache, dry mouth, and myalgia. Chronic exposure to either elemental or inorganic mercury, however, also can result in a recognizable syndrome called *acrodynia*. Also known as *pink disease*,

Feer syndrome, or *Feer-Swift disease*, acrodynia is a complex of symptoms including the following:

Anorexia
Decreased muscle tone
Erythematous gingiva
Pruritus
Erythematous palms and soles
Diaphoresis
Hypertension
Tachycardia
Insomnia
Oral ulcers
Loose teeth
Weakness

Elemental mercury poisoning can be misdiagnosed as pheochromocytoma. This can occur as mercury inactivates the coenzyme, S-adenosylmethionine, which inhibits catechol-O-methyltransferase (COMT). As a result, catecholamine breakdown decreases and adrenergic symptoms such as hypertension and diaphoresis develop.[18-20] A constellation of personality changes in affected individuals has come to be known as *erethism*. The symptoms include the following[61]:

Confusion
Hallucinations
Decreased libido
Irritability
Depression
Lethargy
Drowsiness
Manic-depressive disorder
Emotional lability
Memory loss
Psychomotor impairment
Suicidal ideation
Shyness

There has been a reported association between mercury exposure, erethism, and the development of parkinsonism[61-63]; however, the evidence for this association comes from only two studies[64,65] and two case reports.[21,22]

Inorganic mercury is most commonly found in nature as cinnabar (mercury [II] sulfide). In humans, however, exposure to inorganic mercury compounds comes from germicides, pesticides, and mercury-containing antiseptics.[61] Of interest, there have been several recent reports of inorganic mercury intoxication due to the use of skin-lightening beauty creams.[66,67] Inorganic mercury can be absorbed through the skin, via the lungs, and via the gastrointestinal tract. In blood, inorganic mercury has a $t_{1/2}$ of about 24 to 40 hours, and clearance of mercury by the kidneys is responsible for the toxic effects on the distal portion of the proximal convoluted tubules.[68,69]

More corrosive to the gut than elemental mercury,[61,70] ingestion of mercury salts commonly causes nausea, vomiting, abdominal pain, and hematemesis. Ingestion of relatively large doses of mercury salts can lead to colitis with necrosis and mucosal sloughing, resulting in massive fluid losses.[14,29,30]

Along with gastrointestinal symptoms, the other notable acute effect of inorganic mercury is development of acute renal failure. Potentially reversible, renal injury can occur within hours to days of an acute exposure.[71,72] Membranous glomerulonephritis and nephrotic syndrome also may occur after chronic exposure. Termination of exposure may lead to resolution of nephrotic syndrome.[50,73]

With prolonged skin exposure, gray-brown hyperpigmentation of skin folds of the neck and face can occur. Used as an analgesic for teething in the 19th century, dental application of calomel (mercuric chloride) can cause loose teeth, blue discoloration of the gingiva, and systemic toxicity.[14,31] As with elemental mercury, acrodynia and erethism have been reported with inorganic mercury exposure.[50,61]

Organic mercury compounds are found in fungicides, antiseptics such as merthiolate and mercurochrome, preservatives including thimerosal, and as a contaminant of predatory fish including tuna and swordfish. As much as 90% of ingested organic mercury is absorbed by the gastrointestinal tract.[74] Pulmonary absorption of organic compounds such as methylmercury vapor, approaches 80%, depending on particle size. Absorption across intact skin also can occur.[47] Methylmercury readily crosses the blood-brain barrier, achieving CNS levels that are three to six times those in blood.[75]

Perhaps the best-known mass poisonings of mercury involved methylmercury. During the 1950s and 1960s, a chemical company in the Japanese fishing village of Minamata dumped wastewater containing mercury into Hyakken Harbor on Minamata Bay. Aquatic organisms converted the inorganic waste to an organic form (methylmercury) that was then passed up the food chain. The mercury eventually was concentrated in larger fish, which were then consumed by residents of the area.[76] Over time, more than 2265 patients developed ataxia, sensory disturbances, constriction of visual fields, dysarthria, auditory disturbances, and tremor. Children exposed in utero developed congenital Minamata disease, which was characterized by seizures, spasticity, deafness, and severe mental deficiency.[77] All these children had mental retardation, cerebellar ataxia, limb deformities, primitive reflexes, and dysarthria. Hypersalivation and chorea were seen in 95% and microcephaly in 60% of affected children.[77-79]

In a second event in 1971, 6500 Iraqis suffered symptoms similar to the Minamata patients after eating bread baked with flour made from grain intended for use as seed. The grain had been treated with a fungicide containing methylmercury.[80]

These two events demonstrated that organic mercury targets the CNS and that fetal brain tissue is more susceptible than the adult brain to the toxic effects of organic mercury. Postmortem findings have shown damage to gray matter of the cerebral and cerebellar cortex. The temporal cortex and calcarine region of the occipital lobe are most affected.[81,82] Pathologic changes in adults and children include cortical atrophy, hypoplasia of the corpus callosum, hypoplasia of the granular cell layer of the cerebellum, and demyelination of the pyramidal tracts.[78]

DIAGNOSTIC TESTS

Following exposure to elemental or inorganic mercury, whole-blood mercury concentrations are elevated for only 2 or 3 days and then rapidly decrease. Mercury detection beyond that point is better done by 24-hour urine testing. Reference ranges for whole blood can vary somewhat among laboratories but usually fall between 0 and 10 ng/mL. As is the case for testing for other metals, care should be taken to follow the instructions for sample collection provided by the reference laboratory. Such information is usually available online. Heparin-containing collection tubes should be avoided unless otherwise specified. Measurement of mercury is usually performed by atomic absorption spectroscopy (AAS) or inductively coupled plasma mass spectroscopy (ICP-MS).

Urine testing (24-hour collection) is most useful for confirming exposure/toxicity to either elemental or inorganic mercury. Collection containers are frequently washed with nitric acid, but laboratory practices may vary. Specimens should be refrigerated to decrease bacterial reduction of mercury to volatile elemental mercury.[83] Samples should not be collected within 48 hours of gadolinium administration (as with magnetic resonance imaging) or within 72 hours of consuming predatory fish (e.g., tuna or swordfish).

Urine concentrations in excess of 50 ng/mL are considered elevated, although reference ranges vary, and there is no exact threshold for determination of toxicity. Some laboratories also report the concentration in µg/gm creatinine along with a reference range. Treatment with chelating agents frequently increases mercury excretion. Results of such tests should *not* be applied to reference ranges for nonchelated specimens.

Because approximately 90% of methylmercury is bound to red blood cells[74] and very little is excreted via the kidneys, the preferred test to determine organic mercury is a whole-blood mercury level. While most persons have whole-blood mercury concentrations of less than 6 ng/mL, diets rich in predatory fish can elevate levels to 200 ng/mL or higher.[84] For that reason, patients should avoid consumption of fish for at least 72 hours prior to blood testing.

Caution is advised in the use of either blood or urine concentrations of mercury as the sole determinant of toxicity. The diagnosis of mercury poisoning should be based upon history and physical findings in conjunction with blood and/or urine testing.

TREATMENT

The first and most important step in treatment of mercury toxicity is to avoid further exposure of the patient to the toxin.[50,61,85,86] Whereas removal of clothing and decontamination of skin may be helpful, gastrointestinal and pulmonary decontamination are of little use. Chelation is often considered the cornerstone of therapy, although the benefit remains somewhat controversial. Chelating agents bind metal ions to form a complex that can be excreted, thereby reducing the body burden of the offending metal. Dimercaptosuccinic acid (DMSA, Chemet, Succimer) is currently the favored agent. Because DMSA is available only in an oral form, dimercaprol (British antilewisite [BAL]) is used in patients unable to take oral medications. D-penicillamine is an alternate but less effective choice. Chelation therapy may take several months to eliminate the body burden of heavy metal, and clear evidence for long-term benefit is lacking.[86,87] Patients with renal failure may require renal replacement therapy. Aggressive fluid replacement may be necessary to correct large losses of fluid from the gastrointestinal tract, particularly in cases of inorganic mercury exposure.

Lead

BACKGROUND

Mined by the ancient Egyptians, Phoenicians, Greeks, and Romans, lead and its toxicity have had a long, storied history. There is evidence that some of the leaders of ancient Rome suffered neurotoxicity and sterility due to lead poisoning.[88] In 1763, Benjamin Franklin described abdominal pain and peripheral neuropathy associated with lead poisoning.[89] With the onset of the Industrial Revolution, lead increasingly was used in machinery and manufacturing. In the United States in the 20th century, lead-containing paint and leaded gasoline became prominent sources of lead exposure in the population. It was not until 1978 that residential use of lead-based paint was banned. Leaded gasoline was not banned until the 1990s.[88] With the recognition of lead toxicity and its removal from households and many industrial processes, the incidence of cases of lead poisoning has steadily declined since the 1970s.[90,91] Nevertheless, lead products—both new and old—continue to be sources of exposure and toxicity.

TOXICITY

Lead exists in both inorganic and organic forms. Inorganic forms include lead oxide, silicate, carbonate, sulfide, and nitrate; organic forms, formerly added to gasoline, include tetraethyl and tetramethyl lead.

Lead is still used in a variety of products. It is sometimes found in paints, plumbing pipes, gasoline, solder, batteries, bullets, toys, moonshine, traditional folk remedies, curtain weights, necklace charms, and food containers. Today the most common source of exposure is from lead-based paints and lead-contaminated soils.[92,93] Many occupations including battery plant worker, metal welder, painter, construction worker, lead miner, firing range worker, glass blower, and ship builder increase the risk of lead exposure.

In the pediatric population, the most common route of exposure is ingestion, especially among children between the ages of 18 and 36 months. Compared to adults, children are also more prone to toxicity from lead ingestion because of increased gastrointestinal absorption of lead, immaturity of the blood-brain barrier, ongoing development of organ systems, and frequent concomitant iron deficiency.[94]

Inhalational exposure is the most common cause of lead exposure in adults. Exposure to lead among adults is often related to occupational exposure or exposure from a hobby. Ingestion of lead-contaminated moonshine also has resulted in "outbreaks" of adult lead poisoning.[95,96]

Lead interferes with numerous enzymatic pathways, including those that utilize sulfhydryl-containing enzymes, calcium, zinc, and iron. Within the CNS, lead poisoning can increase the permeability of the blood-brain barrier, resulting in increased intracranial fluid and pressure. Lead also has been shown to increase the spontaneous firing of neurons which utilize acetylcholine, dopamine, or γ-aminobutyric acid (GABA) as neurotransmitters within the CNS. This change in neuronal signaling can result in the erroneous enhancement of unnecessary neural pathways and destruction of necessary neural pathways. Children are particularly susceptible to this effect from lead poisoning, because the peak of fortification and elimination of neural pathways occurs around 2 years of age.[94,97]

Lead inhibits several enzymes necessary for the synthesis of heme. These enzymes include aminolevulinic acid (ALA) synthetase, δ-ALA dehydratase, coproporphyrinogen decarboxylase, and ferrochelatase. By interfering with erythrocyte membrane formation, lead poisoning shortens the lifespan of erythrocytes.[98,99] Basophilic stippling is sometimes seen with lead toxicity and is a result of the inhibition of pyrimidine-5-nucleotidase.[100] Hematologic consequences of lead poisoning can be compounded by poor nutritional status, especially iron deficiency.[101]

Lead is deposited in the proximal tubules of the kidney as a lead-protein complex, where it can interfere with mitochondrial function. In animal models, exposure to high doses of lead results in renal failure with the nonspecific findings of tubular atrophy, interstitial fibrosis, and glomerular sclerosis.[102]

Chronic lead exposure has been associated with hypertension. Lead can affect vascular smooth muscle by decreasing Na^+/K^+-ATPase function, resulting in increased calcium-mediated contractility. Lead also can increase protein kinase C activity, further altering vascular smooth muscle activity.[103]

The $t_{1/2}$ of lead in blood is 4 to 6 weeks. However, in bone, which is the main reservoir for lead in the body, the $t_{1/2}$ is considerably longer, ranging from 5 to 19 years.[104] This lead depot in bone can be mobilized and consequently reexpose vital tissues to lead during times of increased bone turnover such as growth spurts, pregnancy, and after fractures.[105] In the pediatric population, lead causes increased density of metaphyses through increased calcification of the bone metaphysis.[106] These "lead lines" on radiographs may be the first manifestation of chronic lead exposure in children.

CLINICAL PRESENTATION

The clinical presentation of lead poisoning can be quite variable. Although measurement of blood lead concentration can make the diagnosis of lead poisoning, numerous other factors can contribute to the clinical symptoms seen, including patient age, length of exposure, nutritional status, genetic factors, environmental factors, and underlying medical problems.

In the pediatric population, lead-induced encephalopathy is the most critical presentation of plumbism. The peak incidence occurs between 18 and 36 months of age. Typically patients with encephalopathy caused by lead have circulating levels ≥70 μg/dL. The reverse is not true, however. Patients with circulating lead levels ≥70 μg/dL do not always have encephalopathy and may have no symptoms at all. Patients with lead encephalopathy may present with coma, seizures, failure to meet developmental milestones, ataxia, visual changes, and lethargy. Patients with acute-on-chronic or acute lead ingestion are more likely to present with severe neurologic symptoms. Children with blood lead levels between 50 and 100 μg/dL can have more subtle neurologic signs including irritability, hyperactivity, and developmental delay.[94,97] There is continued controversy regarding the effects of chronic low-level lead exposure and neurodevelopment, particularly with blood lead levels less than 10 μg/dL.[107-109]

Adults also can present with encephalopathy after lead poisoning. Brain edema, coma, seizures, and lethargy are potential symptoms when blood lead levels are over 150 μg/dL. Personality changes, insomnia, and memory deficiencies have been reported with levels above 80 μg/dL, and less obvious symptoms such as mood changes can occur with levels in the 40 to 70 μg/dL range.[91,110,111] Another neurologic sign, often described with plumbism, is predominantly motor neuropathy with clinical signs of foot and wrist drop. This neuropathy can be seen with blood lead levels as low as 40 μg/dL and is more common with long-term exposure in adults and in children with sickle cell disease.[112]

Lead poisoning can cause gastrointestinal symptoms including abdominal pain, anorexia, vomiting, pancreatitis, and hepatotoxicity.[91]

The anemia of plumbism typically does not cause clinical symptoms requiring hospitalization, but anemia can serve as a clue to the diagnosis in patients with signs of other organ system damage after lead poisoning. Lead poisoning can cause normocytic or microcytic anemia. Decreased red cell mass is generally seen in children with blood lead levels higher than 40 μg/dL and in adults with levels above 50 μg/dL.[99] Basophilic stippling is sometimes observed in cases of plumbism but also has been described with arsenic poisoning, other disease states, and in healthy individuals.[100]

Chronic lead exposure has been associated with nephrotoxicity.[102] Adult plumbism can cause renal changes consistent with a Fanconi-like syndrome characterized by aminoaciduria, phosphaturia, and glycosuria. Another complication of renal toxicity from lead is decreased uric acid clearance, leading to flares of gout aptly named "saturnine gout."

Hypertension has been associated with chronic lead poisoning, although the strength of this association is controversial.[113,114]

Poisoning as a result of exposure to organic lead compounds primarily results in neurologic and gastrointestinal symptoms; hematologic toxicity is not always present. The neurologic sequelae of organic lead intoxication can include personality changes, hallucinations, lethargy, and coma.[115] Patients with organic lead poisoning also can exhibit nausea and vomiting as well as liver or kidney damage.

DIAGNOSIS

The best laboratory test to confirm lead exposure is measurement of lead concentration in a whole-blood sample obtained by venipuncture. This test should be sent to the laboratory in a lead-free tube. Blood lead levels are less useful in cases of organic lead toxicity, as they do not correlate well with expected neurotoxicity. A disadvantage to sending a whole-blood lead level is that most laboratories are unable to report results the same day the sample is received. Capillary blood lead levels can be used as a screening test, but they are less reliable than whole-blood levels and may be falsely elevated if contaminated with lead on the skin.[116] Protoporphyrin levels in red blood cells are elevated when heme synthesis is inhibited, as occurs in cases of lead poisoning. However, elevated protoporphyrin levels are also observed in other conditions, such as iron deficiency, sickle cell disease, and vanadium toxicity. Elevated protoporphyrin is more likely to occur in chronic plumbism than with acute lead exposure.[117] A laboratory test that detects urine lead concentration after a dose of $CaNa_2EDTA$ is available but has limited clinical utility and would not be used to guide management. A test that utilizes x-ray fluorescence to determine lead burden in bone is available in some research centers but would not be useful in the acutely ill patient.[118]

Supportive laboratory data that can assist with diagnosis and treatment include a complete blood count with differential white blood cell count and peripheral smear, a comprehensive metabolic panel, and a urinalysis. Other laboratory tests should be ordered according to findings on history and physical examination. If lumbar puncture is being considered, computed tomography (CT) of the head should be reviewed first to look for signs of cerebral edema.

Radiographic imaging may help the clinician determine the etiology and proper treatment of a patient with lead poisoning. A head CT scan should be obtained in anyone with CNS findings and evidence of lead exposure. A reported finding on head CT in patients with lead encephalopathy is evidence of cerebral edema. Anyone with an elevated lead level from an undetermined source should have an abdominal radiograph to look for ingested lead objects. Long-bone radiographs of children with plumbism may show increased densities at the metaphyses (lead lines). Lead lines are a nonspecific finding and can also be seen with bismuth, phosphate, and fluoride toxicity.[106]

TREATMENT

Many sources offer treatment recommendations for lead toxicity, based on blood lead levels and symptoms. Two widely used sources are the Centers for Disease Control and Prevention (CDC) recommendations for pediatric lead toxicity and the Occupational Safety and Health Administration (OSHA) recommendations for adult occupational lead exposure.

An important intervention in the treatment of lead toxicity is removal of the source of exposure. This often requires changes in the patient's living environment or occupation. The source of lead may also require direct medical intervention for removal. Patients who have ingested smaller lead objects may benefit from polyethylene glycol administration; radiographs should be followed to make sure this treatment is effective. A surgeon or gastroenterologist may have to become involved to remove larger lead objects found in the gastrointestinal tract.[119] Lead bullets, especially ones that are in contact with synovial fluid, should be surgically removed.[120]

Children with blood lead levels greater than 69 μg/dL or who have symptoms of plumbism should be hospitalized and started on parenteral chelation therapy. Pediatric patients with levels between 45 and 69 μg/dL who are asymptomatic should receive oral chelation therapy. Children who are asymptomatic and have blood lead levels below 45 μg/dL do not require chelation therapy. This recommendation is based on results from a double-blind randomized clinical trial that showed no benefit from chelation therapy among children with lead levels equal to 20 to 44 μg/dL.[122] The local health department should be notified to help with environmental measures and prevention education with any child with a blood lead level above 20 μg/dL or a child with more than one level equal to 15 to 19 μg/dL.[121] The effectiveness of environmental cleanup and educational initiatives recently has come under question after the publication of a Cochrane review that indicated that 12 published studies have not shown a clear benefit to these interventions.[123]

Adults with severe symptoms such as lead-induced encephalopathy or with blood lead levels over 100 μg/dL should be admitted to the hospital and started on parenteral chelation therapy. Oral chelation therapy is recommended for adults with mild symptoms or levels equal to 70 to 100 μg/dL. In general, chelation is unnecessary for adults who are asymptomatic and have levels below 70 μg/dL.[91]

Standard management of symptoms should be applied to the patient with severe symptoms from lead toxicity. Control of cerebral edema may include hyperventilation assisted by mechanical ventilation, infusion of mannitol, and administration of corticosteroids, as well as neurosurgical consultation. Vomiting and dehydration should be managed with antiemetics and proper IV fluid administration.

In the United States, there are several options for lead chelation: edetate calcium disodium, dimercaprol, and succimer. Edetate calcium disodium is a parenteral chelator approved by the FDA for lead toxicity in all age groups. It is widely available and can be administered IV or IM. The recommended IV dose in adults for severe lead poisoning is 1 to 1.5 g/m^2/d infused over 8 to 12 hours for a total of 5 days; after 2 days, a repeat 5-day course can be administered if indicated. The recommended pediatric IV dose for severe lead poisoning is 1 to 1.5 g/m^2/d divided into equal doses infused every 8 or 12 hours; an additional 5-day course can be given after 2 days if needed. Serious side effects of treatment with edetate calcium disodium include fever, hypersensitivity immune reactions, hypotension, nephrotoxicity, and thrombophlebitis. Patients with renal failure are at greater risk for toxicity from edetate calcium disodium, and in these patients the dose

may have to be adjusted or an alternative chelator selected. Because edetate calcium disodium can increase intracranial pressure in patients with cerebral edema, the manufacturer recommends using the IM route, or alternatively using the IV route with a slow infusion rate in these cases. Edetate calcium disodium can exacerbate symptoms when given as the sole chelator to patients with high blood lead levels[124]; therefore, dimercaprol should be given in conjunction with edetate calcium disodium inpatients with symptomatic lead poisoning. Edetate disodium without calcium should never be used because of the risk of fatal hypocalcemia.[125,126]

Another FDA-approved chelator for lead toxicity is dimercaprol. It is administered by deep IM injection. In severe plumbism, dimercaprol is administered at a dose of 4 mg/kg IM every 4 hours for 2 to 7 days in both pediatric and adult patients. For mild lead poisoning, the recommended dose is 4 mg/kg IM for the first dose followed by 3 mg/kg IM every 4 hours for 2 to 7 days. Adverse reactions with dimercaprol are common and include fever, hypertension, tachycardia, and injection-site abscesses. Dimercaprol is administered in a peanut oil vehicle and should be avoided in patients with peanut allergies.[127]

Succimer is an oral chelator that is FDA approved for lead poisoning. The recommendation for pediatric dosing of succimer is 10 mg/kg/dose every 8 hours for 5 days, followed by 10 mg/kg/dose every 12 hours for 14 days. Succimer is not officially approved for adults, but similar doses to those approved in children have been used. Adverse reactions to succimer include neutropenia, hemolytic anemia, and transient elevations in circulating liver transaminase levels.[128]

There are other lead toxicity treatment options available that are not approved by the FDA, not as widely studied, or not available within the United States. Penicillamine is not approved by the FDA for lead poisoning and should only be considered in cases of serious lead poisoning when the use of other chelators was associated with unacceptable side effects. Penicillamine itself can cause a life-threatening side effect, agranulocytosis, and can also can be associated with serious dermatologic and renal complications.[129] Exchange transfusions have been used in conjunction with chelation in rare cases of neonatal plumbism. Unithiol is a chelator available for oral or parenteral administration that is used mainly in Europe. Side effects include fever and allergic dermatologic reactions, as well as hypotension with the IV formulation.[130]

Thallium

BACKGROUND

Discovered at a time when new techniques in spectrochemical analysis led to a race among scientists to discover the next element in the periodic table,[131] thallium has had a notorious past. Shortly after discovery of the element in 1861 by Sir Edmund Crookes, the toxicity of thallium salts was recognized.[132] One of the earliest recognized manifestations of thallium toxicity was hair loss; this discovery led to the use of thallium as a depilatory agent.[133] It was the use of thallium compounds to treat ringworm in children that first led to medical reports of systemic toxicity. After several reported deaths, thallium as a therapeutic agent was largely abandoned.[134] Although not effective as a medical treatment, the recognized toxicity of thallium, along with its lack of taste and odor, led to its widespread use as a rodenticide. Although effective, its toxicity to unsuspecting children and pets eventually resulted in it being pulled from the U.S. marketplace.[135] Its only clinical use today is as a radiocontrast agent for cardiac disease, where it is used in an extremely low, nontoxic concentrations.[136] Today, cases of thallium poisoning typically are the result of its malicious use. Because of its toxicity, ease of administration, and difficulty in detection, thallium has long been an agent of choice among those seeking to harm themselves or others.[137] Despite its difficulty in detection, a clinician knowledgeable in the early signs and symptoms of thallium poisoning can improve their patients' outcomes by instituting early antidotal therapy.

TOXICITY

Similar to other metals, it is not the elemental form but rather the salts of thallium that are toxic. As a constituent of the earth's crust, thallium is found throughout the environment. In addition, thallium is emitted from the combustion of coal and in the process of iron smelting.[138] Despite its widespread environmental distribution, the majority of clinical problems resulting from thallium are the result of suicide or homicide attempts. Its salts are tasteless, odorless, water soluble, and completely and rapidly absorbed by the gastrointestinal tract. In animal studies, thallium concentrations in urine and feces can be measured within 1 hour of oral administration.[139] Once absorbed, thallium is widely distributed throughout the body, where it interferes with activities of several critical metabolic enzymes. Because its charge and atomic radius are similar to the potassium ion, thallous ion interferes with K+-dependent enzymatic processes, including those catalyzed by pyruvate kinase and Na+/K+-ATPase.[135] It is this similarity of thallous ion and potassium ion that makes thallium a useful radionuclide for cardiac stress testing. Along with interfering with potassium-dependent processes, thallium also inhibits sulfhydryl-containing enzymes such as pyruvate dehydrogenase.[135] The inhibition of potassium- and sulfhydryl-dependent enzymes results in impaired cellular energy production, which if severe enough, leads to cell death.[135] Unlike other metals, the primary route of elimination for thallium is not renal but rather fecal, a result of enterohepatic circulation.[139]

ACUTE CLINICAL PRESENTATION

After a toxic exposure to thallium, the earliest reliable finding is the development of a rapidly progressive painful peripheral neuropathy. Beginning typically within 2 or 3 days of exposure, symptoms begin in the feet.[140] If the dose is large enough, symptoms can also involve or progress to involve the hands. The neuropathic pain resulting from thallium is often described as a "pins-and-needles" sensation and is commonly excruciating to the point where even the weight of a bedsheet is intolerable.[141] In severe cases, the neuropathy can be misdiagnosed as Guillain-Barré syndrome. This diagnostic confusion is prompted by absent or diminished deep tendon reflexes in cases of thallium poisoning[142,143] and symptoms that can rapidly ascend from the lower extremities to involve the respiratory muscles, necessitating in some cases the need for mechanical ventilation.[141] A relatively unique feature of thallium's neurotoxicity is that along with involvement of peripheral nerves, the cranial nerves also can be affected. All of the cranial nerves can be involved, but those innervating the eye (II, III, IV, VI) are the most commonly affected.[144,145] In addition, CNS findings are also commonly seen in cases of severe thallium poisoning and can manifest as hallucinations, insomnia, acute psychosis, or coma.[133,144]

The best-known complication of thallium poisoning is alopecia, which begins around 5 to 14 days after exposure to the toxin.[133] By 3 to 4 weeks, near-total body alopecia including loss of axillary, pubic, and the lateral eyebrow hair can be apparent.[146] The medial part of the eyebrow is typically spared, as its hairs are typically in a resting phase.[147] The exact cause of alopecia is unknown, but it is likely that interruption of keratin synthesis and/or metabolism in the hair matrix is responsible.[146] While alopecia is the most recognizable feature of thallium poisoning, patients can die before it develops, making early diagnosis of thallium poisoning challenging. In addition, peripheral neuropathy can occur in mild cases, without the development of hair loss.[148] In addition to hair changes, other cutaneous manifestations of thallium poisoning can include acneform and eczematous skin eruptions.[146]

Along with the neurologic and dermatologic manifestations of thallium toxicity, other less specific findings are also commonly reported. In some cases, the earliest symptoms of thallium poisoning are abdominal pain, vomiting, and diarrhea. Over days to weeks, constipation or obstipation may develop.[133,147] Compared to arsenic poisoning, the gastrointestinal symptoms associated with thallium exposure are not

as severe and do not dominate the early clinical picture. Other nonspecific manifestations of thallium poisoning include myalgia, pleuritic chest pain, insomnia, hypertension, nonspecific ST-T wave ECG changes, bradycardia, tachycardia, hypotension, acute respiratory distress syndrome, acute hepatitis, delayed development of nail dystrophy (Mees lines), and acute and chronic neuropsychiatric manifestations.[143,148-152]

DIAGNOSTIC TESTS

Because many of the initial features of thallium poisoning are nonspecific, and few clinicians see many if any cases in their career, making the early diagnosis of thallium poisoning can be difficult.[148] However, by being familiar with its most common clinical presentation and obtaining some readily available neurologic and clinical examination findings, diagnosis is possible early in the course of the illness when treatment is most likely to benefit the patient.

Neuropathy is universally present in severe cases of thallium poisoning, so nerve conduction studies may be helpful in diagnosing patients.[148] Although the findings are not specific and may be normal early in the clinical course, electromyogram findings indicative of sensorimotor axonopathy in the setting of rapidly progressive symptoms should prompt consideration of acute thallium poisoning. Once the diagnosis of thallium poisoning is part of the differential diagnosis, visualizing a pulled hair from the patient under a low-powered light microscope and finding markedly darkened hair roots should prompt immediate chelation therapy (Figure 178-1).[147,148] Blackened hair roots after thallium poisoning are secondary to accumulated gaseous inclusions.[146] Darkened roots can be seen as early as 4 days after poisoning,[147] and in cases of repeated poisoning, it is possible to observe several bands.[147] The highest percentage of darkened roots is seen in hairs pulled from the scalp (95%), followed by hairs from the chest and legs (50% to 60%), and less commonly from eyebrows and eyelids (30%).[147] The absence of darkened hair roots in persons with other signs of thallium poisoning should not dissuade clinicians from beginning treatment.

Although clinical features and hair examination may prompt treatment for a presumptive diagnosis of thallium poisoning, the definitive diagnosis requires analytic confirmation of elevated concentrations of thallium in urine or hair. A 24-hour urine specimen is considered the gold standard for laboratory confirmation of thallium poisoning. In most unexposed persons, the thallium concentration in urine should be less than the lower limit for detection. Nevertheless, depending on

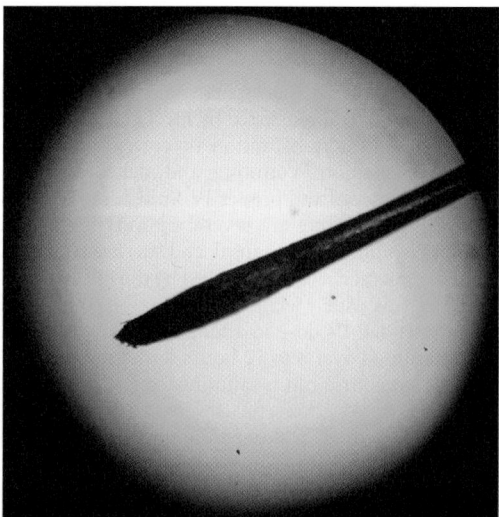

Figure 178-1 Darkened hair root of a thallium-poisoned patient seen under low-power light microscopy.

occupational and environmental exposure, levels ≤20 μg/specimen can be considered normal. Analysis hair of hair samples is not thought to be as reliable as urinalysis, but it has been shown to correlate with concentrations in 24-hour urine specimens.[148] In patients with exposure to thallium many days or weeks prior to obtaining specimens, analyzing samples of hair and nails may be the only means to confirm the diagnosis. Hair levels below 15 ng/g are generally considered normal.[135]

TREATMENT

Once thallium poisoning is suspected or recognized, treatment should focus on decreasing circulating thallium concentrations. As mentioned previously, thallium undergoes enterohepatic circulation. The most effective agent for treating thallium poisoning is Prussian blue, a brightly colored hexacyanoferrate compound $(Fe_4[Fe(CN)_6]_3)$. The unabsorbed and insoluble complex binds thallium in the gut, thereby increasing fecal elimination. The FDA has approved Prussian blue, sold under the brand name Radiogardase, for treatment of both cesium and thallium poisoning. The recommended dose of Prussian blue is 3 g orally 3 times a day for adults. For children (2-12 years), the dose is 1 g 3 times a day. Numerous studies in animals demonstrate Prussian blue's effectiveness for preventing mortality from thallium poisoning.[144] Although the very nature of thallium poisoning makes a human clinical trial impossible, case reports support the safety and efficacy of Prussian blue.[140,149,153] Treatment is generally recommended until 24-hour urine thallium concentrations fall below 0.5 mg/24 h.[140] Although Prussian blue contains cyanide complexes, in vitro studies suggest that the small amounts of cyanide released are clinically insignificant.[154] Adverse events related to the use of Prussian blue have not been reported.[153]

Not all hospitals stock Prussian blue in the pharmacy, so until a supply arrives, alternative treatments may be required. Activated charcoal binds thallium[155,156] and has been used to treat cases of thallium poisoining.[148,157] Although there are no specific dose recommendations, 50 g of charcoal twice a day has been used.[148] Because thallium can promote constipation, the use of charcoal suspended in sorbitol is recommended.

Although thallium is binds sulfhydryl-containing compounds,[135] studies in animals indicate that sulfhydryl-containing chelators such as BAL, D-penicillamine, DMSA, and DMPS either provide no benefit or actually increase toxicity,[156,158-160] possibly by increasing the concentration of thallium within the CNS.[159]

Hemodialysis has been used in cases of thallium poisoning. Commonly employed along with potassium supplementation, it is unclear if the amount of thallium removed results in any clinical benefit.[140,141,144,161,162] For critically ill patients with thallium toxicity, hemodialysis may be justified.

ANNOTATED REFERENCES

Agency for Toxic Substances and Disease Registry. Toxicological profile for arsenic. Atlanta: U.S. Department of Health and Human Services, Public Health Service; 2007.
　In-depth description of arsenic toxicity, including sections geared towards patient education. It can be accessed at http://www.atsdr.cdc.gov/toxprofiles/tp2.html.
Clarkson TW, Magos L. The toxicology of mercury and its chemical compounds. Crit Rev Toxicol 2006;36:609-62. Comment in: Crit Rev Toxicol 2007;37:537-49; discussion 551-2.
　An in-depth and comprehensive review of the toxicity of the various forms of mercury, including a detailed review of the health risks of environmental exposure.
American Academy of Pediatrics Committee on Environmental Health. Lead exposure in children: prevention, detection, and management. Pediatrics 2005;116(4):1036-46.
　A comprehensive review of pediatric lead poisoning, including treatment recommendations.

Rogan WJ, Dietrich KN, Ware JH, et al; Treatment of Lead-Exposed Children Trial Group. The effect of chelation therapy with succimer on neuropsychological development in children exposed to lead. N Engl J Med 2001;344:1421-6.
　A randomized double-blind placebo-controlled trail that showed no benefit in neuropsychological outcome with chelation in children with blood lead levels between 20 and 44 μg/dL.
Hoffman RS. Thallium toxicity and the role of Prussian blue in therapy. Toxicol Rev 2003;22:29-40.
　An excellent and well-researched review on the toxicity of thallium and its treatment.

REFERENCES

Access the complete reference list online at http://www.expertconsult.com.

179

Hydrocarbons

KAPIL SHARMA | KURT C. KLEINSCHMIDT

Hydrocarbons are a diverse array of chemicals composed exclusively of hydrogen and carbon atoms. Some hydrocarbon derivatives such as various halogenated hydrocarbons also contain other elements. They are ubiquitous in daily life and include plant and animal fats, alcohols, solvents, natural gas, petroleum derivates, and a host of industrial chemicals (Table 179-1). Many exist in complex mixtures. This chapter focuses on the toxicity of petroleum distillates, which represents several hundred compounds arising from crude oil.[1]

Chemistry

Hydrocarbons can be categorized based on their chemical structures. Aliphatics are straight-chain and branched-chain hydrocarbons. Mixtures like gasoline and kerosene are primarily composed of aliphatics. Alicyclic hydrocarbons are carbon chains in a ring structure that chemically react similarly to aliphatics. Olefins are hydrocarbons containing carbon-carbon double bonds, and acetylenes contain triple bonds.

The physical properties of hydrocarbons depend primarily on the length of the carbon chain. Methane, ethane, propane, and butane have chains that are 1, 2, 3, and 4 carbons long, respectively, and exist as gases at standard temperature and pressure. Hydrocarbons with chains containing 5 to 20 carbon atoms exist as liquids, and those containing more than 20 carbon atoms exist as semisolids or solids.

Aromatic hydrocarbons have a benzene ring as their base structure. The addition of various side chains results in the formation of toluene, xylene, and other aromatics. Polyaromatics are composed of multiple benzene rings. Aromatic structures form the basis for many biochemically active molecules such as amphetamines, catecholamines, and salicylates.

Halogenated hydrocarbons are hydrocarbons with fluorine, chlorine, bromine, or iodine substitutions. Medicinal uses for halogenated hydrocarbons include anesthetics such as halothane, propellants for inhalers, and chloral hydrate for sedation. Refrigerants such as Freon are mixtures of halogenated hydrocarbons (Figure 179-1).[2]

Epidemiology

The Toxic Exposures Surveillance System database maintained by the American Academy of Poison Control Centers reported 46,357 hydrocarbon exposures and 11 deaths in 2008. Eighty-seven percent of all exposures were unintentional or accidental, and 31% occurred among patients younger than 6 years of age.[3] The number of hydrocarbon-related calls made by the public or healthcare providers to poison centers over the past decade are decreasing.[4] This number certainly underrepresents the actual number of annual exposures.

Determining the incidence of chronic exposures is even more difficult. A 1993 World Health Organization report estimated that 238,000 U.S. workers annually were exposed to benzene.[5] Petrochemical workers, rubber workers, shoe manufacturers, and printers all have workplace exposures to benzene,[6] but second-hand cigarette smoke, products from gasoline combustion, and industrial emissions expose virtually everyone to benzene, at least occasionally.[7,8] Because of its known tendency to promote development of hematologic malignancies, benzene has been extensively studied in terms of its toxic effects. Many other hydrocarbons are encountered in daily life, and the effects of low-level exposures to these compounds are unclear. More than 1 million workers are exposed annually to kerosene and its byproducts.[9] Toluene is present in the air in most urban and suburban environments at concentrations up to 6.6 parts per billion (ppb), and it can be found in higher concentrations in soil and water.[10]

Intentional abuse of inhaled hydrocarbons is a particularly dangerous form of hydrocarbon exposure. In 2007, 13.3% of high school students reported inhalant abuse.[11] Among delinquent youth, 38.5% reported inhalant abuse, and 28.3% of inhalant abusers met DSM-IV dependence criteria.[12,13] Determining the epidemiology of inhalant abuse is difficult because of the poor reliability of self-reported data and the wide availability of inhalants.[14] The use of inhalants as a "gateway drug" is concerning because of the potential for more serious drug abuse later in life.[15] Among students, the highest rates of abuse occur in women, Hispanics, and people in rural communities.[16]

Depending on the type of chemical abused, inhalants are generally categorized as gases, nitrates, solvents, or aerosols.[17] Gases are compressed hydrocarbons such as refrigerants, propane, butane, and inhalational anesthetics. Nitrates, or "poppers," are used as smooth-muscle relaxants to heighten sexual experiences. Solvents are a diverse group of liquids with relatively high vapor pressures and include glues, fuels, paint thinners, and the liquid in felt-tip markers. Aerosols are hydrocarbon-based propellants found in spray bottles. These bottles contain both a gas propellant and a solvent, either of which may be abused. Inverting the can and activating the nozzle selectively releases the gas propellant. Once the gas is released, puncturing the can yields access to the liquid solvent.

Differing methods of inhalant abuse include sniffing, snorting, huffing, and bagging. *Sniffing* is the passive inhalation of gaseous fumes from a container; *snorting* refers to insufflation of liquid hydrocarbons into the nasal passageways; *huffing* is the inhalation of fumes from a rag soaked in solvent; and *bagging* is the inhalation of fumes from a solvent placed into a paper or plastic bag.[18,19]

General Management

Management of hydrocarbon toxicity depends upon the route of exposure (Table 179-2). Hydrocarbon ingestion without aspiration typically results in mild symptoms. Hydrocarbons are gastric irritants, and 35% to 51% of patients will spontaneously vomit.[20-23] Hemorrhagic gastritis following ingestion has been reported.[24] If aspiration does not occur, the outcome from ingestion of a hydrocarbon is usually good, especially if respiratory symptoms are absent for 6 to 8 hours and the chest radiograph is normal.[3,20-23,25,26]

Given that hydrocarbon toxicity primarily results from pulmonary aspiration, gastric lavage and induced emesis with ipecac should be avoided.[26-28] Lavage, spontaneous emesis, and ipecac all increase the risk for hydrocarbon aspiration with subsequent pneumonitis.[20,22,26,29] However, it is appropriate to perform gastric lavage or induce emesis when the ingested hydrocarbon is known to cause systemic toxicities, the volume of hydrocarbon ingested is very large, or the hydrocarbon has been ingested along with one or more other dangerous substances.[28] Activated charcoal fails to adsorb most hydrocarbons, and its use is not routinely recommended.[30,31] Material Safety Data Sheets (MSDS), the Micromedex database, or poison control centers can help identify hydrocarbons that warrant decontamination efforts.

Nonspecific Symptoms of Aspiration

Fever and leukocytosis are common after hydrocarbon aspiration. Fever occurs in up to 73% of ingestions and 93% of intentional

TABLE 179-1	Common Household Products Containing Hydrocarbons		
Adhesives	Car waxes	Cement	Lighter fluid
Kerosene	Lacquers	Mineral oil	Lamp oil
Paint thinner	Petroleum jelly	Pine oil	Furniture polish
Turpentine	Stain removers	Wax	Varnish

TABLE 179-2	Selected Hydrocarbon Toxicities
Agent	***Toxicity***
Pentachlorophenol	Oxidative phosphorylation uncoupler
Formaldehyde	Irritant, respiratory sensitizer, allergen
Diisocyanates	Respiratory sensitizer, allergen
Perchloroethylene (PERC)	Central nervous system depression, cardiac sensitization
Bromomethane	Severe neurotoxicity
Hydrazine-containing fuel	Seizures, pyridoxine depletion

aspirations.[20,23,27,32] Approximately 30% of patients with fever are otherwise asymptomatic.[22,23] In one study, fever resolved after 24 hours in 41% of patients; 5% of patients had persistent fever lasting longer than 5 days.[27] Another study found that fever resolved after an average of 1.25 days.[33] Heating or burning hydrocarbons results in the production of many airborne molecules. Inhalation of these molecules can result in a prolonged fever referred to as *polymer fume fever*.[34,35] One study of patients with hydrocarbon ingestion found leukocytosis in 75% of those with clinical pneumonia, versus only 32% in those without pneumonia. Both groups had a similar percentage of patients with a left shift on the differential white blood cell count.[23]

Pulmonary Toxicity

Aspiration of hydrocarbons results in a lipoid pneumonia. Chronic ingestion of hydrocarbons among patients with gastroesophageal reflux disease can result in slowly developing symptoms.[36,37] Intravenous injection of hydrocarbons can result in a lipoid pneumonia or vascular hydrocarbon emboli.[38-41] A case of lipoid pneumonia due to dermal absorption of hydrocarbons in a patient with severe psoriasis was reported.[42] This patient suffered from severe psoriasis and applied large amounts of petroleum jelly to her skin for 10 days prior to evidence of lipoid pneumonia. Some halogenated hydrocarbons such as trichloroethylene are mucosal irritants which can induce caustic pneumonitis.[43-45] Respiratory tract sensitization and reactive airway disease can occur following repeated exposure to certain hydrocarbons.[46-51] Rarely, the irritant effects of some hydrocarbons can result in upper airway injury and obstruction.[52]

Gastrointestinal absorption plays a minor role in toxicity. Experimental canine and primate models in which esophageal ligation was performed prior to instillation of kerosene by gastrostomy failed to demonstrate pulmonary injury in any of the animals.[25,53,54] However, small doses of hydrocarbons administered intratracheally resulted in severe pulmonary toxicity.[55-58]

Aspiration occurs with the inhalation of a hydrocarbon that exists as a liquid under ambient conditions of temperature and pressure. The risk for pulmonary toxicity is determined in part by the physical properties of liquid hydrocarbons, including surface tension, viscosity, and volatility.[59,60] *Surface tension* refers to the cohesion of molecules generated by van der Waals forces. Materials with low surface tension tend to spread over an area, and therefore these substances are more likely to be aspirated. *Viscosity* measures the resistance of a fluid to flow. Liquids with low viscosity are more likely to be aspirated.[61] *Volatility* refers to the tendency of a liquid to vaporize into a gaseous state. Volatile hydrocarbons are more lipid soluble and more easily disrupt surfactant layers and/or cell membranes, thereby predisposing to toxicity.[61,62] However, hydrocarbons that exist as gases in ambient conditions cannot be aspirated and do not cause lipoid pneumonia. An example is propane, a gas that is purchased as a compressed liquid but which volatilizes completely and rapidly upon return to normal atmospheric pressure. The clinical effects of these gases result from hypoxia and central nervous system (CNS) depression.[63-65] European regulation of

the allowable viscosity, volatility, and surface tension of lamp oils has not led to an appreciable decline in the incidence of patients developing lipoid pneumonia.[66]

Multiple mechanisms of pulmonary injury occur in hydrocarbon aspiration. Microscopic findings include thick hyaline membranes in air spaces, capillary distension, vascular thrombosis, intraalveolar hemorrhage, hyperemia, neutrophilic or lymphocytic alveolitis, and bronchial necrosis.[37,67,68] The most characteristic finding is the presence of lipid-laden macrophages.[67] Foreign body granulomas or "parafinomas" following aspiration have been reported.[70,71] Bronchoalveolar lavage (BAL) reveals thick or greasy fluid. Oil red O staining of the fluid can confirm the presence of exogenous lipids, and polymorphonuclear exudates or hemorrhagic secretions can be present.[38,72,73] Animal models reveal an early exudative phase characterized by the presence of red blood cells, macrophages, and edema fluid in alveolar airspaces along with diminished lung compliance. This early phase is followed by a secondary phase of proliferative bronchiolitis.[68,74] Disruption of the pulmonary surfactant layer from hydrocarbons exacerbates ventilation/perfusion mismatching and decreases pulmonary compliance.[75,76]

The diagnosis of hydrocarbon aspiration is usually suggested by the history. Coughing, gagging, or choking following ingestion of hydrocarbons portends the development of pulmonary injury, although nearly a third of patients with early symptoms do not develop significant toxicity.[22,23,77] Hypoxemia, respiratory distress, and physical examination evidence of pneumonia develop rapidly, although delayed onset of these symptoms has been reported.[32,78] Lung function studies reveal a restrictive or obstructive pattern.[37] In cases of respiratory distress where it is unknown if hydrocarbon aspiration occurred, bronchoalveolar lavage or lung biopsy can be diagnostic. Uncommon complications of aspiration include the development of pneumatoceles, cavitary lesions, abscesses, lung necrosis, bronchopleural fistula, pneumothorax or empyema.[23,71,79-82]

Radiographic findings are variable. Ninety percent of patients with pulmonary symptoms have abnormal radiographs on arrival, and nearly all develop abnormalities by 6 hours.[22] Interestingly, chest radiograph abnormalities in the absence of respiratory symptoms are common. Fifty percent of asymptomatic patients have abnormal chest radiographs, and of these patients with abnormal roentgenographic findings, only 5% go on to develop significant toxicity.[22,27] Chest radiographs can reveal areas of consolidation, atelectasis, fibrosis, ground-glass opacities, or pleural effusions.[23,37,83] Bibasilar interstitial or right lobar findings are the most common and can develop within an hour of aspiration.[20,23,27] Computerized tomography (CT) reveals airspace consolidation with areas of low attenuation and air bronchograms. Ground-glass opacities, airspace nodules, and/or crazed paving patterns can be seen.[84,85] Areas of fat attenuation within pulmonary opacities can be diagnostic, although inflammatory infiltrates can mask this

Figure 179-1 Sample Hydrocarbons.

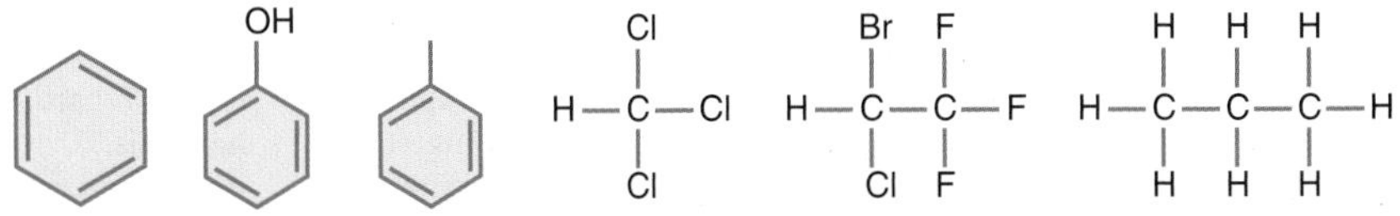

Benzene   Phenol   Toluene   Chloroform   Halothane   Propane

finding.[37,83] Magnetic resonance imaging (MRI) reveals T_1 hyperintensities consistent with, though not specific for, lipid content.[86,87] Chemical shift MR with opposed-phase imaging is sensitive for detecting lipids and can provide a specific test for lipoid pneumonia if available.[88] Positron emission tomography (PET) scanning of a patient suspected to have a malignancy but later found to have exogenous lipoid pneumonia revealed a high standard uptake value.[89]

There are limited data on outcomes following hydrocarbon aspiration. A follow-up of 17 children 8 to 14 years after exposure found that 82% had one or more pulmonary function abnormalities.[90] A separate study found normal pulmonary function in 3 children exposed 8 to 10 years earlier.[91] A retrospective review of 44 adult patients with chronic lipoid pneumonia found that 21% developed complications including pulmonary fibrosis, recurrent infections in the region of injury, and *Aspergillus*-related diseases.[37]

MANAGEMENT OF PULMONARY TOXICITY

Management of hydrocarbon aspiration focuses on respiratory support. β-Adrenergic agonists are indicated for treatment of bronchospasm.[67] Ventilation with high levels of positive end-expiratory pressure and recruitment maneuvers can improve gas exchange.[38] High-frequency percussive ventilation resulted in significant clinical improvement in a patient who deteriorated after multiple modes of ventilation had failed, and mobilized a large amount of thick oily secretions.[92] Clinical improvement has been reported with high-frequency oscillation or high-frequency jet ventilation[93-95] and extracorporeal membrane oxygenation.[96]

Therapy with corticosteroids remains controversial because human data are limited. A double-blind placebo-controlled trial of 71 children with hydrocarbon poisoning did not reveal any difference between treatment groups.[33] There are many case reports with variable outcomes following both oral and inhaled corticosteroid use.[37,68,72,97-99] Various animal models have shown no difference in outcome[100-102] or worsened outcome due to increased infectious complications.[103]

Aspiration and the subsequent presence of pneumonia, fever, radiographic findings, and leukocytosis make antibiotic use common, but no controlled human data demonstrate the value of antibiotics. Various animal models have shown no difference in rates of infection when prophylactic antibiotics were given.[100,101,103] Given the limitations in data, the authors feel that routine administration of antibiotics is not supported by the literature. We recommend antibiotics only for patients with persistent fever lasting longer than 24 hours, patients with peripheral white blood cell count higher than 20,000 cells/μL, or patients with deteriorating clinical status after 24 hours.

Many additional therapies have been used for lipoid pneumonia. Surfactant therapy for acute respiratory distress syndrome (ARDS) is controversial, but there are reports of successful use of this strategy in cases of hydrocarbon aspiration.[75,104,105] An ovine hydrocarbon aspiration model found 100% survival with surfactant therapy versus 25% survival with saline, although all animals were sacrificed at 6 hours.[106] A patient with prolonged respiratory compromise underwent lung lavage on hospital day 49. Polysorbate 80 in Ringer's lactate was used until the effluent was clear of lipid, followed by surfactant instillation. This resulted in clinical and lung aeration improvements.[107] Nitric oxide along with high-frequency oscillatory ventilation was used successfully in a pediatric patient.[94] A rabbit model using partial liquid ventilation and inhaled nitric oxide showed improvements in gas exchange.[108] Animal models of hyperbaric oxygen demonstrated transient improvement in oxygenation followed by rapid decline.[100]

Nervous System Toxicity

CNS effects vary depending on the route and intent of exposure. Among those with hydrocarbon aspiration secondary to ingestion, one-third have signs of CNS toxicity ranging from drowsiness to stupor and seizures. In this setting, the presence of CNS symptoms correlates strongly with the development of fever, hypoxemia, and

pneumonitis.[23] Intentional hydrocarbon inhalation produces euphoric effects that mimic ethanol inebriation. Symptoms include mydriasis, nystagmus, hallucinations, increased libido, and delirium. Severe or prolonged exposures can result in tremors, seizures, and hypoxic encephalopathy.[109-112] These effects usually resolve within a few hours, although prolonged symptoms can occur in some cases.[113]

The neurophysiologic effects of inhalants are not completely understood. Inhalation leads to CNS depression via enhanced γ-aminobutyric acid (GABA)-mediated neurotransmission, antagonism of N-methyl-D-aspartic acid receptors, inhibition of normal cell-cell signaling, and enhanced serotonergic transmission.[115-119] The release of dopamine reinforces abuse patterns.[120] Chronic abusers develop tolerance to these effects and may increase the amount inhaled to compensate.[111,121] Because of physical dependence, chronic users can develop inhalant withdrawal symptoms such as craving, irritability, and insomnia.[122] Baclofen and lamotrigine have been advocated as treatments for inhalant withdrawal syndromes.[123,124]

Chronic exposure to solvents, whether intentional or unintentional, can cause a broad spectrum of CNS disorders. Initial symptoms are nonspecific and include memory difficulties, fatigue, loss of concentration, and personality changes that can be reversible.[114,125-127] Continued exposure leads to an irreversible leukoencephalopathy that can present as cerebellar ataxia, parkinsonism, encephalopathy, convulsions, and/or deficits in higher functioning.[112,128,129] MRI reveals changes in the basal ganglia and thalamus along with cortical and cerebellar atrophy.[112,128,130,131] Single photon emission computerized tomography (SPECT) findings have demonstrated prominent abnormalities with areas of hypoperfusion and hyperperfusion.[132] Many hydrocarbons are associated with the development of peripheral neuropathy, most notably n-hexane and methyl-n-butyl ketone.[126,133-135]

Cardiac Toxicity

Sudden sniffing death refers to cardiac arrest following the inhalation of volatile hydrocarbons, especially halogenated derivatives.[63,64,136,137] Ingestion or inhalation of halogenated hydrocarbons can cause dysrhythmias that persist for days.[138] Sixty-four percent of inhalant-related deaths result from arrhythmias, and most of the remainder result from hypoxia and/or hypercapnia.[65,139] Toluene has been shown to prolong the QT interval and inhibit cardiac sodium currents.[140,141] Electrophysiologic studies on animals identified concentration-dependent suppression of spontaneous pacemaker activity, resulting in asystole, though some animals developed ventricular tachydysrhythmias. Cardiotoxicity worsens in the setting of acidosis or hypoxemia,[142-144] and toxicity persists for hours after exposure.[144] Autopsy findings are usually nonspecific,[65] although myocardial fibrosis induced by hydrocarbon abuse can increase the risk of dysrhythmias.[145] Coronary artery spasm and infarction contribute to toxicity.[146,147] The myocardium may be sensitized to catecholamines following inhalant abuse, and thus sudden excitation or exercise can trigger ventricular dysrhythmias.[148,149] Administration of epinephrine worsened inhalant-induced cardiotoxicity in a canine model.[150] Therefore the management of cases of hydrocarbon-induced toxicity should eschew the use of epinephrine or other adrenergic agonists.[137] β-Adrenergic blockers can blunt myocardial sensitization and have been used successfully in the treatment of ventricular dysrhythmias secondary to hydrocarbon toxicity.[138] Amiodarone and lidocaine also have been used successfully to terminate ventricular arrhythmias.[137,151]

Hepatotoxicity

Hepatitis and liver failure can occur following hydrocarbon exposure.[152,153] Halogenated hydrocarbons are particularly dangerous in this regard, whereas most other hydrocarbons induce only a mild hepatitis.[154-156] Carbon tetrachloride is a prototypical example; it induces centrilobular liver necrosis via cytochrome 2E1 metabolism in a manner similar to the way acetaminophen induces hepatocellular damage.[157-159] Chloroform, 1,1,1-trichloroethane, and other halogenated hydrocarbons can cause significant hepatic injury.[160-162] Treatment with *N*-acetylcysteine has provided hepatoprotection in animal models and in case reports of human exposure.[160,161,163] Although data are limited regarding the use of *N*-acetylcysteine therapy in patients exposed to hepatotoxic hydrocarbons, it should be used because of its low cost and wide safety profile.

Renal Effects

Both halogenated and nonhalogenated hydrocarbons can cause acute renal failure.[164-166] Acute tubular injury is primarily responsible,[164,167] although interstitial nephritis has been reported.[168] Chronic exposure can lead to a slow decline in renal function via progressive tubular injury.[169,170] Albuminuria can be a useful marker to gauge renal injury in chronic exposures.[171]

Toluene inhalation is notorious for inducing a renal tubular acidosis-like syndrome and ureteral calculi; in addition, toluene can cause direct kidney injury and acute renal failure.[172-175] Toluene is metabolized first to benzoic acid and then to hippuric acid, which can be measured in the blood or urine to confirm recent exposure.[176] Acutely, toluene abusers can present with a widened anion gap due to the formation of the unmeasured anions, benzoate and hippurate.[175] However, chronic use can result in a renal tubular acidosis-like syndrome, and patients can present with life-threatening hypokalemia and resultant muscle weakness or paresis.[177] Hippurate-induced acidification of the glomerular filtrate disrupts the normal pH gradient and prevents the distal tubule from excreting hydrogen ions in exchange for potassium ions. Thus, potassium excretion increases along with retention of endogenous hydrogen ions. This combination results in development of hyperchloremic metabolic acidosis with profound hypokalemia and hypophosphatemia.[174,178,179] A serum potassium concentration as low as 0.8 meq/L, which required infusion of 260 mEq potassium over 6 hours, has been reported.[180] Total body stores are depleted, and supplementation with hundreds of mEq of potassium may be required.[178] Treatment includes hydration and repletion of electrolytes; hemodialysis may be required for reversing severe hypokalemia.[181] Prognosis is good, and most patients recover completely.[177]

An unusual toxin is nitromethane, which is commonly found in model engine fuel along with methanol in a 50:50 mixture. Nitromethane interferes with laboratory assays for creatinine, and the presence of nitromethane in samples can yield falsely elevated results.[182-184] Management of concurrent methanol poisoning or renal disease is challenging in the setting of this laboratory interference.

Hematologic Effects

Hydrocarbons can cause many acute hematologic abnormalities. Hemolysis occasionally follows hydrocarbon ingestion.[185,186] Most cases are mild and do not require treatment, although red cell transfusion and exchange transfusion rarely are required.[187,188] Naphthalene found in some mothballs can induce profound and prolonged hemolysis.[189] Methemoglobinemia has been reported following hydrocarbon ingestion, usually with agents containing nitro side groups.[190,191] Methylene chloride and methylene iodide are slowly metabolized to carbon monoxide and cause prolonged carbon monoxide poisoning.[192,193] Aplastic anemia can result from exposure to high concentrations of benzene, typically following chronic occupational exposures.[194]

Dermatologic Effects

Hydrocarbon skin exposure typically results in a mild irritant dermatitis that can be treated by cleansing the area with soap and water to remove residual hydrocarbons, followed by lotion application.[195] However, prolonged exposure over a few hours can lead to chemical burns complicated by blistering and partial or full-thickness skin necrosis.[196] Allergic contact dermatitis can occur in patients with

TABLE 179-3	Known Human Hydrocarbon Carcinogens*	
Agent	*Cancer*
Benzene	Acute myelogenous leukemia
Vinyl chloride	Hepatic angiosarcoma
Formaldehyde	Nasal cancer
Mineral oils	Squamous cell carcinomas
Coal tar pitch	Skin cancer
Ortho-toluidine	Bladder cancer

From the International Agency for Research on Cancer, World Health Organization. Available at: http://monographs.iarc.fr/ENG/Classification/index.php.

chronic exposures.[195,197] Ingestion of chlorobenzenes such as dioxins causes specific lesions known as *chloracne*.[198] Compressed hydrocarbons can cause cold burns due to the endothermic reaction that occurs during rapid vaporization.[199] Hot tar or asphalt can cause prolonged burning. Application of a petroleum-based solvent or antibiotic ointment facilitates tar removal.[200,201] High-pressure hydrocarbon injection injuries, especially to the hand, can result in severe disability and warrant immediate surgical consultation.[202]

Carcinogenicity

In 1775, Percivall Pott noted that chimney sweeps commonly develop testicular cancer, and this association was later found to result from exposure to polyaromatic hydrocarbons.[203] Since then, many hydrocarbon-induced cancers have been discovered, and this problem is a matter of significant public concern owing to the ubiquitous exposure to hydrocarbon products. Various organizations categorize the carcinogenicity of chemicals, including hydrocarbon products. Among these organizations are the National Toxicology Program (NTP) under the U.S. Department of Health and Human Services and the International Agency for Research on Cancer (IARC) under the World Health Organization. IARC divides chemicals into 5 groups; group 1 consists of 107 known human carcinogens (Table 179-3),[204] group 2A consists of 58 probable human carcinogens, group 2B consists of 249 possible human carcinogens, group 3 consists of 512 unclassified carcinogens, and group 4 consists of 1 chemical that is probably not carcinogenic.[205] Thus many thousands of chemicals remain unstudied.

Conclusion

Hydrocarbons are ubiquitous in the environment. Fortunately most exposures are benign, and few patients require treatment. However, all clinicians should be aware of the potential for serious injury. Clinicians should be prepared to manage lipoid pneumonia in these patients, and must be aware of the potential for serious systemic toxicity with some agents.

KEY POINTS

1. Hydrocarbons are ubiquitous in the environment and vary markedly based on their properties.

2. Most hydrocarbon ingestions are benign. Serious toxicity usually develops from inadvertent aspiration of hydrocarbons.

3. Gastric lavage, induced emesis, and activated charcoal are contraindicated in the management of most ingestions.

4. Transient fever, leukocytosis, and abnormal chest radiographs in the absence of significant illness are common.

5. Pulmonary management focuses on aggressive respiratory support. No evidence exists to support the empirical administration of corticosteroids or antibiotics.

6. Central nervous system depression following aspiration or intentional inhalant abuse is common.

7. *Sudden sniffing death* results from cardiac catecholamine sensitization in the setting of inhalant abuse. Epinephrine and β-adrenergic agonists should be avoided.

8. Toluene abuse can lead to renal tubular acidosis and profound hypokalemia.

9. Fulminant liver necrosis can occur with exposure to some halogenated hydrocarbons. Treatment with *N*-acetylcysteine is hepatoprotective.

10. Poison control centers can aid with identification and management of dangerous hydrocarbon exposures.

ANNOTATED REFERENCES

Anas N. Criteria for hospitalizing children who have ingested products containing hydrocarbons. JAMA 1981;246:840-3.

This was a large retrospective study analyzing the records of 950 children who ingested hydrocarbon products. Data collected included incidence of vomiting, fever, chest radiograph abnormalities, duration of hospitalization, and hospital course. Discharge of asymptomatic patients with normal chest radiographs 6 hours after ingestion is advocated based on these data.

Press E. Co-operative Kerosene Poisoning Study. Evaluation of gastric lavage and other factors in the treatment of accidental ingestion of petroleum distillate products. Pediatrics 1962;29:648-74.

This multicenter study assessed gastric lavage in 760 children who ingested hydrocarbon products. Extensive information regarding technique of lavage, demographics of patients, clinical manifestations, and hospital course was obtained. The study concluded that gastric lavage offered no benefit to patients.

Lifshitz M, Sofer S, Gorodischer R. Hydrocarbon poisoning in children: a 5-year retrospective study. Wilderness Environ Med 2003;14:78-82.

This trial retrospectively analyzed the records of 274 children admitted for hydrocarbon ingestion at a single institution. This represents the largest review of children with significant symptoms following hydrocarbon

ingestion. Data regarding radiographic findings, leukocytosis, clinical manifestations, and hospital course were provided.

Marks M. Adrenocorticosteroid treatment of hydrocarbon pneumonia in children: a cooperative study. J Pediatr 1972;81:366-9.

This trial used a double-blind, randomized controlled trial to assess corticosteroid treatment in 89 children with hydrocarbon aspiration. Children received either methylprednisolone or placebo. Information regarding clinical symptoms, hospital course, and inpatient hospital days were obtained. Administration of corticosteroids did not provide any benefit compared with placebo.

Carlisle EJ, Donnelly SM, Vasuvattakul S, Kamel S, Tobe S, Halperin ML. Glue-sniffing and distal renal tubular acidosis: sticking to the facts. J Am Soc Nephrol 1991;1:1019-27.

This paper is a case report of a distal renal tubular acidosis-like syndrome in a chronic toluene abuser. It includes a very detailed discussion and investigation into the metabolic abnormalities caused by toluene abuse and provides evidence for toluene's likely mechanism of action in creating these abnormalities.

REFERENCES

Access the complete reference list online at http://www.expertconsult.com.

180

Lithium

RASHEED A. BALOGUN | MARK D. OKUSA

Lithium as a pharmacologic agent for the treatment of mania was introduced by Cade in 1949.[1] The U.S. Food and Drug Administration (FDA) approved the use of lithium salts for treatment of mania in 1970 and for maintenance therapy of bipolar disorder in 1974.[2-6] Despite the frequent occurrence of lithium intoxication, this drug continues to be used because of its effectiveness when used alone or in combination with other drugs and possibly newer indications.[7-18,19]

The incidence of acute lithium intoxication is not known, but it has been increasing owing to the drug's more frequent use and known narrow therapeutic index.[20,21] The number of cases of toxicologic exposure to lithium reported to poison control centers in the United States grew from 5474 cases in 2004 to 6492 in 2008.[20,22] Ingested lithium is excreted mainly unchanged in the urine, and chronic kidney disease is a major factor that can increase the risk of toxicity even when the drug is used as prescribed.[23,21] Lithium toxicity typically occurs in one of three main settings: acute ingestion of a large dose (e.g., suicide attempt) in a patient not previously taking the drug, acute overdose in a patient chronically on the drug (frequently unintentional), or more commonly, chronic toxicity from accumulation of the drug during prescribed maintenance therapy.[24] The latter problem can be avoided by a thorough understanding of conditions and drug interactions that increase the risk of lithium toxicity.[24] Asymptomatic chronic lithium-induced diabetes insipidus is not acutely life threatening and is not within the scope of this chapter.[25]

Acute lithium intoxication causes multisystem dysfunction and irreversible neurologic deficits; it was reported fatal in 9% to 25% of patients.[26,27] Early detection and treatment are critical to improve outcomes, and reported fatality rates have decreased considerably.[22] This chapter emphasizes the pharmacology and physiology of lithium that underlie its toxicity and provides physicians with the foundation to effectively treat lithium intoxication.[21,24]

Pharmacology

Lithium is a monovalent cation and, like sodium, potassium, rubidium, and cesium, a group IA alkali metal. Lithium shares some characteristics with sodium and potassium; however, differences in ionic radii among lithium (0.60 Å), sodium (0.95 Å), and potassium (1.33 Å) are responsible for the pharmacologic effects of lithium (lithium has no known physiologic role).[23,28-30] For example, unlike sodium and potassium, only a small gradient for lithium can be maintained across biological membranes.

Lithium is usually administered as lithium carbonate or, less commonly, lithium citrate. In adults, the typical dose is 900 to 1800 mg/d in 3 to 4 divided doses (sustained-release preparations available). Lower doses are recommended in children and the elderly, and variations in pharmacodynamics of the drug, even in adults, make it necessary for the correct dose for each individual to be established by the clinician.[31,32] A dose of 300 mg lithium carbonate contains 8.12 mEq lithium ion. After oral administration, lithium is readily absorbed, with complete absorption occurring at approximately 8 hours and peak levels at 1 to 2 hours for the standard-release dosage forms or 4 to 5 hours after ingestion for the sustained-release forms.[21] Lithium is not protein bound; it distributes freely in total body water and accumulates in various tissues, with the exception of cerebrospinal fluid. In the steady state, the volume of distribution for lithium is 0.7 to 0.9 L/kg (Table 180-1). Lithium concentration in cerebrospinal fluid is 40% of the plasma level[21,33] as a result of transport of lithium out of the

cerebrospinal fluid by brain capillary endothelium, arachnoid membrane, or both.[34]

Historically, the therapeutic level of lithium was considered to be between 0.7 and 1.2 mEq/L, but clinicians are now targeting a level of 0.6 to 0.8 mEq/L, because toxicity is associated with levels above 1.5 mEq/L. The plasma elimination half-life of a single dose is between 18 and 36 hours.[21] Elimination takes longer in the elderly; in these patients, the half-life can be as long as 36 hours.[35] Elimination half-life also varies with duration of therapy[36]; it may be considerably longer in patients who have been treated with lithium for a long time. The longer half-life is caused by intracellular accumulation and inhibition of lithium efflux after chronic lithium therapy. Thus it is important to know that lithium has a very narrow therapeutic index, and the patient's age and duration of therapy may affect elimination half-life.

Approximately 95% of a single dose of lithium is excreted unchanged in the urine; only trace amounts are found in feces.[37] Lithium is not bound to proteins and therefore is freely filtered by the glomerulus; 80% of the filtered load of lithium is reabsorbed, and 20% is excreted in urine.[38] Renal lithium clearance in normal individuals is 10 to 40 mL/min[38-40]; the fractional lithium clearance is estimated to be 0.17 to 0.29.[38,40,41]

Because lithium clearance is proportional to the glomerular filtration rate (GFR), factors affecting the GFR have significant influence on the clearance of lithium. Substantial reductions in lithium dosage must be made in patients with chronic kidney disease. Furthermore, alterations in the proximal reabsorption of lithium can alter the fractional excretion of lithium without significantly affecting GFR. This characteristic of renal lithium handling has important therapeutic implications. Drugs known to inhibit proximal reabsorption of lithium can increase the fractional excretion of lithium and thereby increase lithium removal. Diuretics that alter proximal reabsorption of sodium (e.g., acetazolamide, aminophylline, urea) increase fractional excretion of lithium,[38] whereas other diuretics (e.g., thiazides, ethacrynic acid, spironolactone) act distal to the proximal tubule and have no effect on fractional excretion of lithium.[41] These results suggest that the primary site of lithium reabsorption is in the proximal tubule.

Lithium Toxicity

Patients with lithium intoxication exhibit a variety of clinical manifestations. The severity of symptoms frequently is proportional to the degree of elevation of serum lithium levels.[42] However, symptoms do not always correlate with lithium levels, because symptoms of toxicity have occurred at therapeutic levels[28,30,43-45] and minimal symptoms have resulted from high levels.[28,46] In general, however, serum lithium levels of 1.5 to 2.5 mEq/L at 12 hours after the last dose of lithium usually are accompanied by slight or moderate symptoms of intoxication, values of 2.5 to 3.5 mEq/L should be regarded as serious, and values greater than 3.5 mEq/L are life threatening.[28]

The patient's history often reveals associated conditions predisposing to lithium toxicity (Box 180-1). Factors that predispose to toxicity include advanced age,[47] schizophrenia, preexisting brain damage,[48] and rapid rise of serum concentration after an acute overdose. Other conditions such as diarrhea, vomiting, inadequate fluid therapy after surgery, diuretics, and volume depletion are associated with states of sodium depletion. Because sodium balance affects the clearance of lithium,[38,49-51] decreased dietary sodium intake[52-55] and chronic therapy with furosemide or a thiazide diuretic[51,56-61] are situations associated

TABLE 180-1	Pharmacology of Lithium	
Parameter	**Value**	
Molecule	Monovalent cation; radius 0.6 Å; weight 7 D	
Dose (adult)	900-1800 mg/d in 3-4 doses (less in sustained-release form)	
Therapeutic serum level	0.7-1.2 mEq/L (Some clinicians now aim for 0.6-0.8 mEq/L, especially when used in combination with other agents.)	
Toxic levels	>1.5 mEq/L (narrow therapeutic index)	
Bioavailability	>95%	
Volume of distribution	0.7-0.9 L/kg in steady state	
Half-life	12-27 hours after single dose (longer with chronic therapy, chronic kidney disease, and in elderly patients)	
Time to peak plasma level	2-4 hours after ingestion	
Elimination	Primarily renal; excreted unchanged in urine	

TABLE 180-2	Known Drug Interactions of Lithium	
Drug		**Effect on Serum Lithium Levels**
Diuretics:		
Thiazides		Increase
Loop diuretics		Decrease
Osmotic diuretics		Decrease
Potassium sparing		Decrease
Methyl xanthine		Decrease
Acetazolamide		Decrease
Angiotensin-converting enzyme inhibitors		Increase
Angiotensin receptor blockers		Increase
Phenothiazines		Increase
Nonsteroidal antiinflammatory drugs:		
Indomethacin		Increase
Ibuprofen		Increase
Mefenamic acid		Increase
Naproxen		Increase
Sulindac		None
Aspirin		None
Cyclooxygenase II inhibitors		Increase
Tetracycline		Increase
Cyclosporine		Increase
Fluoroquinolones		Increase

Modified from references 125-128.

with lithium intoxication. These conditions often result in a vicious circle that potentiates lithium toxicity (Figure 180-1).

A number of drugs are associated with acute lithium toxicity (Table 180-2). Lithium toxicity has been reported with the concomitant use of nonsteroidal antiinflammatory drugs (NSAIDs), including cyclooxygenase II inhibitors.[62-76] Patients with congestive heart failure and volume depletion who depend on endogenous prostaglandin synthesis to maintain renal blood flow and GFR are more susceptible to lithium toxicity when they take NSAIDs. In these patients, prostaglandin synthesis inhibition by NSAIDs can markedly reduce GFR and lithium clearance, causing significant lithium toxicity. Long-acting angiotensin-converting enzyme inhibitors[77] and angiotensin receptor blockers[78-85] decrease GFR and fractional excretion of lithium,[38] thereby predisposing patients to lithium toxicity.

CLINICAL FEATURES OF LITHIUM TOXICITY

Patients with lithium toxicity present with a variety of clinical manifestations (Box 180-2). Neurologic symptoms are predominant.[27]

Box 180-1

FACTORS PREDISPOSING TO LITHIUM TOXICITY

Infection
Volume depletion
Gastroenteritis
Overdose (e.g., suicide attempt)
Chronic kidney disease
Surgery
Decreased effective arterial volume:
    Congestive heart failure
    Cirrhosis
    Nephrosis
Drugs:
    Nonsteroidal antiinflammatory drugs
    Diuretics
    Tetracycline
    Cyclosporine
Decreased dietary sodium intake
Anorexia

Box 180-2

CLINICAL MANIFESTATIONS OF LITHIUM INTOXICATION

Central Nervous System
State of consciousness (confusion to coma)
Cerebellar symptoms:
    Dysarthria
    Ataxia
    Nystagmus
    Tremor
Basal ganglia:
    Choreiform movements
    Parkinson-like movements
Seizures
Death

Gastrointestinal
Nausea/vomiting
Bloating

Cardiac
Syncope

Renal
Polyuria
Polydipsia
Renal insufficiency

Neuromuscular
Peripheral neuropathy
Myopathy

Endocrine
Hypothermia
Hyperthermia

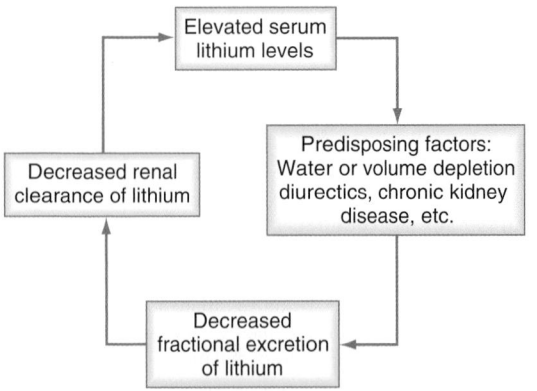

Figure 180-1 Vicious circle of lithium toxicity.

Central nervous system symptoms often develop gradually, starting initially with confusion and progressing to impaired consciousness, coma,[27,86] and occasionally death.[87] Cerebellar manifestations are often prominent and can include dysarthria,[88] truncal ataxia, broad-based ataxic gait, nystagmus, and varying degrees of incoordination. Other central nervous system manifestations of lithium intoxication are seizures[86-90] and involvement of the basal ganglia, as suggested by choreiform movements[48,91,92] and Parkinson's disease–like movements.[93]

Gastrointestinal side effects of lithium therapy include gastric irritation, epigastric bloating, abdominal pain, nausea, vomiting, and diarrhea.[94] Although these are common findings, gastrointestinal complaints are not prominent manifestations of lithium intoxication.[27]

Electrocardiographic changes are frequently associated with lithium therapy.[94] Lithium intoxication can be associated with transient ST-segment depression or inverted T waves in leads V_{4-6}.[27] Although electrocardiographic changes are common, cardiac symptoms are rarely manifestations of lithium intoxication. Sinus node dysfunction has been reported to be a consequence of lithium intoxication leading to syncope.[95,96]

Polyuria and polydipsia are frequent side effects of lithium therapy; they are estimated to occur in 20% to 70% of patients.[3] The concentrating defect may develop not only in patients who are overtly toxic but also in those with therapeutic levels.[3] Polyuria may lead to volume depletion and decrease the fractional excretion of lithium. The mechanisms responsible for lithium-induced polyuria were summarized by Singer[3]; they include primary polydipsia, central diabetes insipidus, and nephrogenic diabetes insipidus.

Other less common manifestations of lithium intoxication are hyperthermia,[97] hypothermia,[98] peripheral neuropathy,[99,100] myopathy,[101] and severe leukopenia.[102]

TREATMENT

The initial management of lithium intoxication is determined by the degree of intoxication (serum level), a history of acute versus chronic lithium exposure, the clinical symptoms, and the adequacy of renal function.[103] As noted in Table 180-2, patients present with a variety of clinical manifestations, from chronic lithium therapy to acute overdose. Those who appear to have severe impairment of consciousness require airway protection and admission to an intensive care unit. Activated charcoal is an ineffective gastrointestinal decontaminant in lithium overdose because it does not absorb strongly ionized chemicals. In contrast, polyethylene glycol (CoLyte, GoLYTELY) has been shown to be effective in acute lithium intoxication.[104] Sodium polystyrene sulphonate has been used only in cases of chronic stable lithium toxicity with serum levels of no more than 2.3 mEq/L.[105]

Volume status should be assessed because significant volume depletion can occur as a result of urinary concentrating defects. Many of these patients have volume-responsive decreases in renal function.[27] Therefore, fluid resuscitation is critical in the initial management. Administration of large volumes of isotonic saline should be done carefully because severe hypernatremia has been associated with such fluid management.[27,42,92,106,107] After fluid resuscitation, efforts to enhance lithium removal are the next step. Various modalities for lithium removal are listed in Table 180-3. The efficacy of each modality in removing lithium can be assessed by comparing lithium clearance values. Because there are no controlled studies of lithium clearance during intoxication, the following data on lithium clearance rely heavily on case reports.

In normal individuals, renal lithium clearance is about 10 to 40 mL/min.[38-40] Hansen and Amdisen[27] reported that renal lithium clearance is 0.9 to 18.4 mL/min in patients with lithium intoxication. Of the 23 patients studied by these authors, only 5 had normal renal function (i.e., creatinine clearance > 78 mL/min). Therefore, in patients with lithium intoxication, the ability to remove lithium by renal excretion can be limited by poor renal function.

Because 80% of lithium is reabsorbed in the proximal tubule, factors that decrease proximal lithium reabsorption can increase lithium

TABLE 180-3	Lithium Removal	
Mode		Lithium Clearance (mL/min)
Renal excretion		10-40
Forced diuresis		0.9-39
Peritoneal dialysis		9-15
Hemodialysis (blood flow, 126-250 mL/min)		70-170
Continuous renal replacement therapies		Variable, about 20.5

clearance, enabling enhanced lithium removal during states of intoxication. Because sodium balance alters the clearance of lithium,[49-51,108] forced diuresis with isotonic saline has been used as a treatment of lithium intoxication. Because consistent therapeutic benefits have not been achieved with forced diuresis[27,109] and because of the potential for hypernatremia, forced diuresis is not recommended for severe lithium intoxication.[27,35] However, if lithium clearance is impaired as a result of volume contraction, administration of isotonic saline may increase lithium clearance transiently.

The effects of various agents on the clearance of lithium have been studied in humans challenged with a single dose of lithium.[38] Whereas water loading, furosemide, thiazide diuretics, ethacrynic acid, ammonium chloride, and spironolactone did not increase clearance of lithium, sodium bicarbonate, acetazolamide, urea, and aminophylline were effective. Clinical studies employing these agents for lithium removal during intoxication have not been reported.

Peritoneal dialysis is another means of lithium removal. Wilson and coworkers,[110] using 2-L exchanges per hour, attained clearances of 13 to 15 mL/min. Similar results were achieved by O'Connor and Gleeson,[109] who reported lithium clearances of 9 mL/min with frequent 2-L exchanges. Although peritoneal dialysis is no more efficient in removing lithium than forced diuresis, it avoids problems associated with intravenous administration of large volumes of isotonic saline.

Conventional hemodialysis remains the mainstay of therapy in severe lithium intoxication.[111] The decision to use hemodialysis (or other extracorporeal therapies) should be made by the nephrologist in consultation with the intensivist and not be expected to come from the poison control centers, because specific factors other than serum lithium levels are not always evident to staff at the local poison control center.[112]

Lithium is one of the most readily dialyzable toxins because of its small atomic weight and negligible protein binding. Several reports indicate lithium clearances between 70 and 170 mL/min with hemodialysis.[27,113,114] Because lithium clearance is almost proportional to blood flow, increasing the blood flow to more than 300 mL/min can further enhance clearance. Table 180-3 compares lithium clearance by various modalities, showing the superiority of hemodialysis to other traditional methods.

The duration of hemodialysis should be guided by serial measurements of serum lithium levels. When levels approach therapeutic range, dialysis may be terminated; however, subsequent hemodialysis may be necessary because serum levels may rise after termination of hemodialysis.[27,103,114] This rebound effect occurs as a result of continued absorption of lithium from the gastrointestinal tract, delayed release from long-acting preparations, and redistribution of lithium from intracellular stores.[103] Although serum lithium clearance has been reported to range from 70 to 170 mL/min,[110,113] the extraction or clearance of lithium from intracellular stores, as reflected by red blood cell clearance, is only 10 to 13 mL/min.[113] This slower extraction of lithium from intracellular stores contributes to the rebound effect.

Continuous renal replacement therapy (e.g., continuous arteriovenous hemodiafiltration, continuous venovenous hemofiltration) has been used either as an alternative to conventional hemodialysis or in addition to conventional hemodialysis.[111,115-119] The combination of conventional hemodialysis followed by continuous renal replacement therapy is very useful for preventing the rebound phenomenon.[103,111,116,117]

MANAGEMENT OF LITHIUM INTOXICATION

Oral airway protection in those patients with severe impairment of consciousness

Volume resuscitation

Whole-bowel irrigation with polyethylene glycol (CoLyte, GoLYTELY) to prevent continued absorption of lithium

Lithium removal:

Serum lithium level > 3.5-4 mEq/L—Most patients require hemodialysis.[111,118,119]

Serum lithium levels 2-4 mEq/L—Unstable patients and patients with severe neurologic signs (seizures, stupor, coma) require hemodialysis.[27]

Serum lithium levels 1.5-2.5 mEq/L—Fluid therapy or forced diuresis treatment should be recommended only for patients with early signs of lithium intoxication and normal renal function, and when it is certain that serum lithium has been elevated for only a few days and not higher than 2.5 mEq/L. Dialysis should be instituted if a serum lithium concentration of 1 mEq/L is not reached within 30 hr.[27]

Box 180-3 summarizes the management of lithium intoxication. Initially, the degree of consciousness and volume status should be assessed. The airway should be protected if necessary, and isotonic saline should be administered for volume repletion. After these critical maneuvers, management should focus on lithium removal. The method of lithium removal is determined by the degree of elevation of the serum lithium concentration, severity of symptoms, and duration of intoxication. Although each patient should be evaluated individually, rough guidelines with rational therapeutic options can be derived from knowledge of the pharmacokinetics of lithium removal. For those patients with minimal symptoms, normal renal function, and mild elevation of serum lithium levels (<2.5 mEq/L), intravenous hydration may be adequate. Urinary electrolytes should be evaluated as a guide to the type of replacement fluid used. This approach avoids hypernatremia, which commonly occurs with forced diuresis. For severe lithium intoxication, hemodialysis is clearly superior to other modalities. Peritoneal dialysis or continuous arteriovenous hemofiltration may be used if hemodialysis is unavailable.

PROGNOSIS

The number of cases of lithium exposure reported to poison control centers in the United States grew to 6492 by 2008, and of these cases, 0.06% died and 2.2% had debilitating outcomes.[20,22] In acute lithium intoxication, the outcome is generally favorable; most patients exhibit reversible neurologic deficits.[20,22,27] However, long-lasting neurologic sequelae may occur.[20,22,120-124] Permanent neurologic changes appear to stem primarily from cerebellar deficits. Prominent manifestations include ataxic scanning articulation, gait and truncal ataxia, inability to perform heel-to-shin and finger-to-nose maneuvers, bilateral adiadochokinesia, nystagmus, hypertonic musculature, short-term memory deficits, and dementia. Concomitant therapy with neuroleptics, associated multisystem organ failure, and alcohol abuse have clouded interpretation of the literature.

KEY POINTS

1. Lithium carbonate (and other salts of lithium) are used widely in the treatment of bipolar disorder and other conditions. Cases of lithium intoxication are common because of the narrow therapeutic index of the drug and various other factors that increase risk of toxicity. Lithium toxicity can occur even when the drug is used as prescribed.

2. In adults, the typical dose is 900 to 1800 mg/d in 3 to 4 divided doses. The time to peak plasma level is 2 to 4 hours after ingestion, and excretion is primarily renal (excreted unchanged in urine). The therapeutic level of lithium is 0.7 to 1.2 mEq/L, and the toxic level is greater than 1.5 mEq/L (narrow therapeutic index).

3. Predisposing factors leading to acute lithium intoxication include chronic kidney disease, surgery, drug interactions, dehydration, and volume depletion.

4. Patients present with a variety of clinical manifestations, which are mainly neurologic. Confusion, seizures, and impaired consciousness leading to coma can occur. Cerebellar manifestations include dysarthria, truncal ataxia, broad-based ataxic gait, nystagmus, and varying degrees of incoordination. Electrocardiographic changes occur frequently with lithium intoxication; examples include transient ST-segment depression and inverted T waves in V_{4-6}.

5. Treatment of acute lithium intoxication depends on serum level and renal function. The usual medical measures to support the airway and circulatory system, common to all intoxications, also apply here. For a serum lithium level greater than 3.5 to 4 mEq/L, most patients require hemodialysis; for patients who have levels between 2 and 4 mEq/L accompanied by clinical instability and severe neurologic signs (e.g., seizures, stupor, coma), hemodialysis is required. For those with serum lithium levels between 1.5 and 2.5 mEq/L, intravenous fluid therapy or forced diuresis treatment should be recommended only if the patient has early signs of lithium intoxication and normal renal function, and it is certain the serum lithium concentration has been elevated for only a few days and not above 2.5 mEq/L. Dialysis should be instituted in all patients if a serum lithium concentration less than 1 mEq/L is not reached within 30 hours.

6. With adequate recognition and treatment, most patients can have a full recovery. Late presentation, delayed treatment, or inadequate treatment may lead to irreversible neurologic deficits or death.

ANNOTATED REFERENCES

Grandjean EM, Aubry JM. Lithium: updated human knowledge using an evidence-based approach. Part II. Clinical pharmacology and therapeutic monitoring. CNS Drugs 2009;23:331-49.

This is an extensive review of data concerning the pharmacokinetics of lithium in different patient cohorts including those with chronic kidney disease and pregnant and breast-feeding women.

Waring WS. Management of lithium toxicity. Toxicol Rev 2006;25:221-30.

This is a review of various extracorporeal therapeutic modalities available to enhance total body clearance of lithium in cases of acute or acute-on-chronic lithium toxicity. It discusses the pros and cons of conventional hemodialysis compared to continuous arteriovenous hemodiafiltration and continuous venovenous hemodiafiltration to increase lithium clearance.

Watson WA, Litovitz TL, Rodgers GC Jr, Klein-Schwartz W, Reid N, Youniss J, et al. 2004 Annual report of the American Association of Poison Control Centers Toxic Exposure Surveillance System. Am J Emerg Med 2005;23:589-666.

This is the annual report of the American Association of poison control centers that shows more than 5400 reported cases of exposure to lithium in United States during 2004. More than 4200 of these were treated in a healthcare facility, with major debilitating outcomes in 286 patients and mortality in 9.

Meyer RJ, Flynn JT, Brophy PD, et al. Hemodialysis followed by continuous hemofiltration for treatment of lithium intoxication in children. Am J Kidney Dis 2001;37:1044-7.

This is an early report of the use of continuous venovenous hemodiafiltration after conventional hemodialysis to treat acute lithium intoxication in two adolescent patients; the continuous clearance of lithium prevented the rebound phenomenon.

Okusa MD, Crystal LJT. Clinical manifestations and management of acute lithium intoxication. Am J Med 1994;97:383-9.

This is an extensive review of the clinical presentation and treatment of acute lithium toxicity, with emphasis on the pharmacology of lithium and comparison of various extracorporeal treatment modalities.

REFERENCES

Access the complete reference list online at http://www.expertconsult.com.

181

Theophylline and Other Methylxanthines

KEITH M. OLSEN

The methylxanthines, theophylline and its water-soluble derivative, aminophylline (theophylline ethylenediamine), have been used in the treatment of acute and chronic asthma for decades. Clinical studies suggest that theophylline offers minimal additional benefit to inhaled bronchodilators and results in a greater frequency of adverse events. Some data propose that theophylline may have a role in the treatment of acute asthma in critically ill patients with impending respiratory failure and in the treatment of severe acute exacerbations of chronic obstructive pulmonary disease (COPD). However, the 2007 National Heart Lung and Blood Institute guidelines on the management of asthma recommends not using methylxanthines in the emergency department and strongly discourages their routine use in hospitalized patients.[1] Theophylline's role in the treatment of pediatric patients also remains controversial. Caffeine, also a methylxanthine and metabolic derivative of theophylline, is indicated in the prevention of neonatal apnea and is a commonly used agent in the neonatal intensive care unit (ICU).

Pharmacology

MECHANISMS OF ACTION

Theophylline has been available for more than 60 years. Thousands of research papers have been written about this drug, and it has been studied in more than 1800 clinical trials. Nevertheless, the specific pharmacologic actions of theophylline in airway disease are not completely known or understood. With the application of new research techniques, the molecular mechanisms responsible for the pharmacologic effects of theophylline are slowly emerging. Theophylline has bronchodilator properties, antiinflammatory effects, and extrapulmonary actions. Bronchodilation is caused by weak, nonselective inhibition of phosphodiesterases 3 and 4 (PDE3, PDE4), which increases the intracellular concentration of cyclic adenosine monophosphate (cAMP).[2] As a consequence, calcium and potassium channels are modulated, leading to relaxation of airway smooth muscle cells. The result is bronchodilation, although the magnitude of the effect is small compared with that induced by β_2-adrenergic agonists. In addition, theophylline may have beneficial airway effects on mucociliary clearance by increasing ciliary beat frequency.[3,4]

Theophylline also appears to have antiinflammatory effects in patients with asthma and COPD.[2,5] The antiinflammatory mechanisms appear to be quite diverse and are related to inhibition of PDE isoenzymes in inflammatory cells, adenosine receptor antagonism, promotion of interleukin (IL)-10 release, inhibition of apoptosis, and inhibition of tumor necrosis factor (TNF) secretion, among other effects.[6] Evidence for the antiinflammatory effects of theophylline includes reduction in CD4+ T lymphocytes in airways exposed to allergens, reduction in neutrophil influx in patients with nocturnal asthma, and reduction in the number of eosinophils in bronchoalveolar lavage (BAL) samples obtained from patients with attacks of severe asthma.[7,8] In subjects with COPD, theophylline reduces total neutrophil count and neutrophil chemotactic responses. The antiinflammatory effects of theophylline are observed when circulating levels of the drug are at the lower end of the therapeutic range, suggesting that lower doses may be beneficial in some patients.[2,9,10]

Theophylline possesses extrapulmonary effects including promotion of diuresis and a poorly understood action on respiratory muscles.[2,11,12] Some investigators have demonstrated increased diaphragmatic muscle contractility and reversal of fatigue. The clinical application of these latter effects remains controversial.

PHARMACOKINETICS AND PHARMACODYNAMICS

Theophylline is regarded as having a narrow therapeutic window, and toxicity develops when therapeutic serum concentrations are exceeded by only a relatively small margin. Benefits and risks are related to the serum concentration, which is a function of the dose and clearance of theophylline in individual patients. Because theophylline exhibits a dose-response relationship, drug-drug interactions, and variable pharmacokinetics among critically ill subjects, only clinicians who are experienced with dosing and adjustment of infusions should use it. If theophylline is administered intravenously (IV), there usually is a lag of 15 to 60 minutes between achievement of therapeutic serum concentrations and detection of pulmonary airway responses.[13,14] The relationship between the serum concentration of theophylline and bronchodilation, as measured by improvement in forced expiratory volume over 1 second (FEV_1), is linear. FEV_1 improves by 2% for each 1 mg/L increase in serum theophylline concentration.[13-15] When the drug concentration approaches 20 mg/L, the potential benefit of increased bronchodilation is minimal and must be weighed against the possibility of unwanted adverse events. In 1997, an expert panel report from the National Institutes of Health (NIH) describing guidelines for diagnosis and treatment of asthma reduced the recommended theophylline therapeutic serum concentrations from between 5 and 20 mg/L to between 5 and 15 mg/L.[15,16-18] Few data are available to support the use of serum concentrations above 15 mg/L. Some patients with impending respiratory failure may benefit from serum concentrations approaching 15 mg/L, but the benefit of pulmonary improvement in relation to the risk of adverse events should be carefully considered before maximizing the therapeutic serum concentration. Antiinflammatory properties, prevention of neonatal apnea, and diaphragmatic contractility are seen at concentrations below 10 mg/L.[2,19,20]

Theophylline distributes readily into fat tissue in both adults and children (mean volume of distribution 0.45 L/kg). Therefore, total body weight should be used for calculating loading doses and initial IV infusion rates. Morbidly obese patients who exceed ideal body weight by more than 50% may be the exception[20]; the initial dose should be approached with extreme caution in this patient population. All methylxanthines are eliminated by hepatic metabolism; renal elimination accounts for up to 10% to 15% of the overall excretion in adults.[20] Neonates have less developed hepatic metabolism, and renal elimination may approach 50%.[20] The primary route of metabolism is mediated via the cytochrome P450 system, and the CYP1A2 microenzyme is the most important pathway for theophylline metabolism.[21] Less than 10% of theophylline is metabolized to caffeine; however, neonates eliminate caffeine in a more predictable fashion, and this agent maybe used in place of theophylline for preventing apnea. Theophylline's half-life varies widely (3.4-30 hours), depending on age and underlying physiologic factors. Numerous factors affect the metabolic clearance of theophylline in critically ill patients; variations within and among patients of 25% or more have been observed.[21-23] Factors that influence the activity of hepatic enzyme function involved in theophylline clearance—gender, age, obesity, diet, and history of tobacco use, for example—may influence metabolism and serum concentrations. Concomitant conditions found in ICU patients that may significantly alter theophylline clearance are listed in Table 181-1. Other drugs that

TABLE 181-1	Physiologic and Environmental Factors That Affect Clearance of Methylxanthines in Critically Ill Patients	
Factor	*Effect on Clearance*
Hepatic insufficiency	Decreased
Congestive heart failure	Decreased
Fever	Decreased
Age	Decreased
Tobacco/marijuana use	Increased
Congestive heart failure	Decreased
Infection	Decreased or no change
Hypothyroid or hyperthyroid disease	Decreased or increased
Cystic fibrosis	Increased
Hypoxemia	No change or decrease
Viral illness	Decrease

either inhibit or stimulate CYP1A2 activity can alter clearance of theophylline and lead to life-threatening adverse events secondary to toxic levels of the drug. Agents known to affect theophylline clearance are outlined in Table 181-2.[23] Clinicians should be vigilant regarding these drug-drug and drug-disease interactions that significantly alter theophylline clearance. Newer drugs used in ICU patients are not routinely assessed for their impact on theophylline clearance, so periodic review of new agents and their impact on CYP1A2 metabolism is also vital. Recognition of these factors is essential to minimize toxicity and maximize efficacy. Careful therapeutic monitoring of serum levels is strongly recommended.[24,25]

Clinical Utility

ACUTE SEVERE ASTHMA

Adult asthmatics with an acute exacerbation are frequently admitted to the hospital after evaluation in the emergency department (ED). These patients are routinely treated with supplemental oxygen, short-acting inhaled or nebulized β_2-adrenergic agonists, nebulized ipratropium, and IV glucocorticoids. Routine use of oral or IV aminophylline or theophylline in the management of acute severe asthma has been replaced by use of high doses of short-acting β_2-adrenergic agonists. The 2007 NIH expert guidelines for management of hospitalized adult patients with severe asthma do not include theophylline as a routine treatment option.[1,26,27] β_2-Adrenergic agonists offer a better safety profile and appear to have equal or greater efficacy. In the emergency department, oral or IV theophylline or aminophylline demonstrated no additional benefit over optimal-dosed short-acting β_2-adrenergic agonists (SABA) but did increase adverse events.[28] Additionally, this meta-analysis failed to demonstrate a benefit of either aminophylline or theophylline in hospitalized patients. However, patients who received IV aminophylline demonstrated an 8% to 9% improvement in predicted FEV_1. The difference in FEV_1 was primarily related to one study, but improvement in airway function did not result in improved outcomes (shortening of ICU length of stay or reduction of symptoms).[29] Patients who received theophylline had a significantly greater number of adverse events and required discontinuation of therapy more often compared to the SABA group.

TABLE 181-2	Drugs That Significantly Alter Theophylline Clearance	
Decrease Clearance	*Increase Clearance*
Erythromycin/clarithromycin	Phenobarbital
Diltiazem/verapamil	Phenytoin
Cimetidine	Rifampin
Ciprofloxacin	Ketamine
Propranolol and other β-adrenergic blockers	Isoproterenol
Ticlopidine	Allopurinol
	Methotrexate
	Propafenone

In a second meta-analysis, addition of aminophylline to other therapies in acute asthma offered little additional efficacy, resulted in higher morbidity related to adverse events, and required more intense monitoring of serum concentrations and meticulous dose adjustments.[30] More recently, the Cochrane Database and others[31,32] concluded that aminophylline does not appear to confer additional benefit. Intravenous theophylline or aminophylline should be considered only in adult asthmatics with severe exacerbations who are not responding to other treatment modalities, and in patients with impending respiratory failure.

The role of methylxanthines in the management of acute severe asthma in pediatric patients remains controversial.[33,34] At least seven clinical trials published in the 1990s, all with small sample sizes (range 21-42 subjects), showed no significant benefit when theophylline was added to nebulized albuterol and glucocorticoids in hospitalized patients aged 2 to 18 years.[31,32,35-40] Most of these studies targeted a theophylline serum concentration of 10 to 20 mg/L and used improvement in a clinical score or FEV_1 as the primary readout.[33] Two small trials (21 and 23 patients) demonstrated improvement in FEV_1 and clinical symptom score when theophylline was added to albuterol and either hydrocortisone or methylprednisolone.[41,42] Two larger randomized trials (163 and 47 patients) evaluated IV aminophylline in pediatric patients with severe acute asthma that was unresponsive to glucocorticoids and nebulized albuterol. Both studies demonstrated improvements in FEV_1 and clinical score, but treatment with aminophylline did not reduce hospital length of stay.[43,44] A recent Cochran meta-analysis confirmed these earlier findings.[45] Addition of theophylline to other therapies in adult or pediatric patients with exacerbations of severe asthma should be weighed carefully, considering the potential benefits, toxicities, and need for intensive therapeutic drug monitoring.

SEVERE EXACERBATION OF CHRONIC OBSTRUCTIVE PULMONARY DISEASE

As in severe acute asthma, routine use of IV methylxanthines in severe exacerbation of COPD is not supported by large randomized clinical trials.[46] However, several studies have documented the benefits of using two bronchodilators simultaneously.[47,48] The combination usually consists of a β_2-adrenergic agonist and an anticholinergic drug (e.g., ipratropium). In acute severe exacerbations that require hospitalization, these agents should be continued at the highest doses tolerated. If an inadequate response is observed, addition of IV aminophylline or theophylline should be considered.[49] Patients receiving oral theophylline on presentation to the ED demonstrated deterioration when theophylline was withdrawn.[48] A study that evaluated 143 patients receiving care in the ED demonstrated a trend toward decreased hospitalization rate when aminophylline was added to the treatment regimen.[48] These patients did not demonstrate improvement in FEV_1 but may have been aided by the antiinflammatory effects of the drug and by drug-induced improvements in diaphragmatic muscle strength. A study of 80 patients with nonacidotic exacerbations of COPD were evaluated in a prospective trial following randomization to either IV aminophylline therapy or no aminophylline. The primary endpoint was improvement of FEV_1 over the first 5 days of admission to the hospital. Although a difference was demonstrated in acid-base balance, there was no difference in the primary endpoint or secondary endpoint of improvement in clinical course.[50] Unlike acute severe asthma, addition of theophylline to the regimen of a COPD patient has been shown to improve lung volumes and inspiratory muscle function, but the potential for adverse events is higher, and the benefits must be weighed against the possible risk of toxicities.

OTHER CLINICAL USES

Theophylline has been demonstrated to increase diaphragmatic muscle strength in healthy volunteers. Increased respiratory muscle strength may benefit some patients who are on the verge of needing mechanical ventilation, or it may help wean patients from mechanical ventilation.[1]

However, this effect has not been evaluated in a prospective randomized clinical trial. Theophylline at therapeutic serum concentrations increases mucociliary clearance in mechanically ventilated ICU patients, but its routine use is discouraged because of the availability of agents with lower incidences of toxicity.[49] Finally, theophylline and caffeine have been used for preventing apnea in the neonatal ICU.[50-54]

Adverse Events

Methylxanthines are nonspecific inhibitors of PDE subsets, which results in a wide range of adverse events.[54] Systemic adverse events and theophylline serum concentrations are directly related.[54-56] When the serum concentration is 10 mg/L or less, adverse events are minimal but may include nausea, vomiting, and diarrhea.[57] When the serum concentration is above 10 mg/L, patients often experience tachycardia, tremors, and metabolic abnormalities (electrolytes and glucose). Although these adverse events are generally well tolerated in the outpatient setting, significant morbidity may occur in critically ill patients. An older but historically significant study evaluated IV aminophylline in 48 critically ill patients with COPD. Using standard infusion rates resulted in highly variable serum concentrations that ranged from 7 to 52 mg/L (mean 21.9 mg/L), with the concentration strongly correlated to toxicity in 18 patients.[58]

Management of Acute Toxicity

Despite the declining use of oral theophylline, acute intoxication remains a cause of morbidity and mortality. A review of a clinical toxicology database of U.S. poison control centers from 2008 found 369 total exposures, including 230 single exposures to either aminophylline or theophyllilne.[59] At least 158 of 197 documented episodes of toxicity were unintentional. A total of 118 episodes required treatment in a healthcare facility, and 59 were classified as either moderate or major toxicities. Significant toxicity can occur if the serum theophylline concentration is greater than 25 mg/L.[57] Serum concentrations can impart some diagnostic and prognostic information and further define the level of intervention required, regardless of whether the overdose was intentional or unintentional.[60] Clinical responses to acute theophylline overdose can be classified into neurologic, cardiovascular, and metabolic categories.[61,62] Cardiac toxicity, the most common acute manifestation, is evident by the appearance of tachycardia and arrhythmias. Profound hypotension and cardiovascular collapse have been reported with serum concentrations above 50 mg/L.[57,62] Seizures are rare unless the serum concentration is over 80 mg/L.[57,61] Severe metabolic abnormalities including hypokalemia, hypomagnesemia, hypercalcemia, and hyperglycemia are common and can complicate treatment of cardiovascular and neurologic adverse events.[56,61,62] Even at nontoxic doses, clinicians often fail to recognize the impact of theophylline on metabolic disturbances.[63]

On initial presentation, standard acute overdose therapy should be applied. Initial gastric lavage may be useful. Multidose administration of activated charcoal enhances elimination because theophylline undergoes significant enterohepatic recirculation. If the patient presents with an overdose following ingestion of a sustained-release theophylline formulation, there can be a delay before the appearance of major toxicities. Seizures should be treated with benzodiazepines; if they are refractory, phenobarbital may be effective. Phenytoin can worsen theophylline-induced seizures and should be avoided.[64] Supraventricular arrhythmias and tachycardia may be managed with β-adrenergic blockers or calcium antagonists, and hypotension with fluids that expand vascular volume.[61,65,66] β-Adrenergic blockers should be used cautiously in patients with underlying COPD or asthma. Ventricular arrhythmias are managed with lidocaine and other standard agents.

In a study of 356 patients with theophylline serum concentrations over 30 mg/L, the most notable finding was tolerance of extremely high theophylline concentrations without development of major toxicity.[57] Despite these data, when life-threatening conditions such as refractory seizures, hypotension, or arrhythmias are present or the serum concentration is above 80 mg/L, hemodialysis or hemoperfusion with charcoal should be initiated.[51] Institutions that cannot provide charcoal hemoperfusion should institute continuous venovenous hemofiltration, because this intervention results in rapid reduction of theophylline serum concentration and is an acceptable alternative.[66] Important developments in hemodialysis including high-flux, high-efficiency membranes and albumin dialysis using a molecular adsorbent recirculating system offer possibilities for removing of highly protein-bound drugs such as theophylline.[67,68] Theophylline serum concentration should be monitored every 2 hours until declining values are confirmed.

Summary

A narrow therapeutic index, frequent toxicities, drug-drug interactions, and complicated dosing issues make the use of methylxanthines problematic in the acute care setting. Potential benefits should be weighed against the risks. Clinicians who are unfamiliar with the dosing of theophylline should consider consulting other experts before initiating therapy.

KEY POINTS

1. Methylxanthines demonstrate highly variable clearance that is dependent on age and physiologic factors such as liver function that may increase or decrease serum concentrations.

2. Administration and dosing of intravenous methylxanthine infusions is complex and should be performed only by clinicians with experience.

3. Adverse events are minor at serum concentrations less than 10 mg/L, but concentrations exceeding this value may result in life-threatening arrhythmias, seizures, electrolyte disturbances, and hyperglycemia.

4. For patients experiencing life-threatening adverse events, charcoal hemoperfusion is the preferred elimination method. If it is unavailable, clinicians should consider continuous venovenous hemofiltration.

ANNOTATED REFERENCES

Expert panel report 3: guidelines for the diagnosis and management of asthma (EPR-3 2007). NIH Publication No. 07-4051. Bethesda, MD: U.S. Department of Health and Human Services; National Institutes of Health; National Heart, Lung, and Blood Institute; National Asthma Education and Prevention Program; 2007.
This paper updates the comprehensive evidence-based approach to diagnosis and management of asthma based on the currently available science.
Bach PB, Brown C, Gelfand BA, McCrory DC. Management of acute exacerbations of chronic obstructive pulmonary disease: a summary and appraisal of published evidence. Ann Intern Med 2001; 134:600-20.
This paper critically reviews the available data on diagnostic evaluation, risk stratification, and therapeutic management of patients with acute exacerbations of COPD.
Global initiative for chronic obstructive lung disease (updated 2009). Available at: www.goldcopd.org. Accessed 6-22-2010.

These updated guidelines on obstructive lung disease are derived from a consensus expert panel. They are directed toward evidence-documented treatment and provide recommendations for management of various stages and scenarios of obstructive lung disease.
Shannon M. Life-threatening events after theophylline overdose: a 10-year prospective analysis. Arch Intern Med 1999;159:989-94.
This longitudinal cohort study of 356 patients with theophylline overdose identifies major adverse events, their incidence, and their significance after serum concentrations greater than 30 mg/L.
Wrenn K, Slovis CM, Murphy F, Greenberg RS. Aminophylline therapy for acute bronchospastic disease in the emergency room. Ann Intern Med 1991;115:241-7.
This study randomly assigned 135 COPD patients presenting to the ED to receive either IV aminophylline or placebo. Aminophylline appeared to decrease hospital admissions by threefold compared to placebo.

REFERENCES

Access the complete reference list online at http://www.expertconsult.com.

182

Antipsychotics

MARK DERSHWITZ

Pharmacology of Antipsychotics

The broad class of medications used to treat psychoses is of interest to intensivists for two reasons. First, some of these medications are useful in the management of agitated or delirious patients in the intensive care unit (ICU). Second, intensivists may need to care for patients with accidental or deliberate overdose of such medications, either alone or in combination with other medications.

The antipsychotics can be divided into three categories based on their chemical structure and receptor-binding activities: phenothiazines, butyrophenones, and atypical antipsychotics. The prototypical antipsychotic agent in the phenothiazine class is chlorpromazine (Thorazine). Its pharmacology is discussed in detail in this chapter and then compared with that of the newer antipsychotic agents.[1] The structures of some commonly used antipsychotics are shown in Figure 182-1.

In terms of the number of neurotransmitter systems with which it interacts, chlorpromazine is one of the "dirtiest" drugs in pharmacology. It is a competitive antagonist at the dopamine (D_2), muscarinic, cholinergic, histamine (H_1), α-adrenoceptor, and serotonin ($5\text{-}HT_2$) receptors. It is believed that its primary antipsychotic effect results from dopaminergic blockade, whereas many (but certainly not all) of its adverse effects result from blockade of cholinergic (sedation, dry mouth) and α-adrenoceptor (orthostatic hypotension) receptors. The relative propensities of some of the antipsychotics to cause sedation, extrapyramidal effects, and hypotension are listed in Table 182-1.

When chlorpromazine is given to a "normal" individual, behavior is diminished and responses to stimuli are fewer, slower, and smaller in magnitude. If it is given in high doses, a catatonic state is induced, although consciousness and memory are preserved. In fact, when the drug wears off, individuals can describe in great detail how bad it made them feel, although they are most unlikely to complain of the dysphoria while it is occurring. This pattern is in distinct contrast to the benzodiazepines, which often produce anterograde amnesia.

When chlorpromazine is given to psychotic patients, there usually is improvement in the thought disorder. In patients with schizophrenia, delusions and hallucinations become less pronounced or disappear, and thinking becomes more orderly. Even if some hallucinations remain, the patient is far more likely to recognize them as unreal.

Because of the wide prevalence of dopaminergic neurons in the central nervous system (CNS), chlorpromazine has widespread effects. The specific areas of the brain responsible for the antipsychotic effects remain obscure. Chlorpromazine lowers the seizure threshold and must be used with caution in persons who are prone to seizures. Because dopamine is released by the hypothalamus to inhibit prolactin secretion by the pituitary, chlorpromazine causes an increase in prolactin secretion. Chlorpromazine exerts its antiemetic effect by blocking dopamine receptors in the chemoreceptor trigger zone.

Blockade of dopamine receptors in the basal ganglia leads to extrapyramidal effects: akathisia, dystonia, rigidity, and tardive dyskinesia. *Akathisia* is an uncomfortable inability to sit still. Patients feel the need to be in constant motion and may appear to be agitated (although they are not). The acute dystonic signs are usually manifested as uncomfortable (and embarrassing) contractions of the muscles of the face and neck. The rigidity that occurs may be clinically indistinguishable from that of Parkinson's disease. All of these effects occur early in the course of treatment with chlorpromazine and are dose related. In addition,

they are readily treated with anticholinergic medications such as benztropine or diphenhydramine (see later discussion).

Tardive dyskinesia may occur after prolonged therapy with chlorpromazine (although it rarely occurs very early after starting treatment with the drug). It is characterized by involuntary repetitive stereotyped movements, usually of the face, such as lip smacking, eye blinking, grimacing, or tongue protruding. Paradoxically, the dyskinetic movements may be suppressed by increasing the dose of chlorpromazine. Tardive dyskinesia is often permanent, persisting after the discontinuation of chlorpromazine.

Neuroleptic malignant syndrome is a rare complication of chlorpromazine therapy and is characterized by hyperthermia (as a result of generalized muscle contracture), stupor, and metabolic abnormalities such as myoglobinemia and elevation of plasma creatine kinase concentration. It resembles malignant hyperthermia, which is a rare adverse reaction to certain anesthetic medications. Treatment of neuroleptic malignant syndrome is discussed later in this chapter.

Because chlorpromazine also blocks muscarinic and α-adrenoceptors, many of its other adverse effects are readily predicted: orthostatic hypotension, nasal stuffiness, dry mouth, blurred vision, and urinary retention. Chlorpromazine (and many other phenothiazines) can cause jaundice. Tolerance does not develop to the antipsychotic effects of chlorpromazine, although tolerance to the sedative effects does occur over a period of a few weeks.

There are many other antipsychotic medications whose effects differ from those of chlorpromazine, primarily on the basis of different degrees of blockade of the various receptor types. In general, medications with greater anticholinergic effects are more sedating and less likely to cause extrapyramidal effects. They also tend to cause more orthostatic hypotension due to α-adrenoceptor blockade. Conversely, those medications with lesser anticholinergic effects tend to be much more potent dopaminergic antagonists and are less sedating, cause less orthostatic hypotension, and are more likely to produce extrapyramidal effects.

Other phenothiazines in common use include thioridazine (Mellaril), trifluoperazine (Stelazine), and fluphenazine (Prolixin). Thioridazine has greater sedating and hypotensive effects than chlorpromazine while causing many fewer extrapyramidal reactions. Trifluoperazine and fluphenazine are less sedating, cause fewer hypotensive effects, and are more likely to cause extrapyramidal reactions than chlorpromazine.

All phenothiazine antipsychotics have antiemetic activity. For reasons related more to brand differentiation than pharmacology, prochlorperazine (Compazine) is marketed as an antiemetic. Its pharmacology is very similar to that of chlorpromazine. It is available in a multitude of preparations to make administration convenient: tablets, liquid, suppository, and injection.

Haloperidol (Haldol) is in the butyrophenone class. It causes little sedation or hypotension and has high incidence of extrapyramidal effects. Because of its decreased propensity to cause hypotension, especially in hypovolemic patients, haloperidol is the most commonly used antipsychotic in the ICU for the management of delirium or agitation (see Chapter 2). Droperidol (Inapsine) is pharmacologically very similar to haloperidol and is commonly used by anesthesiologists as an antiemetic.

The atypical antipsychotics are "atypical" in that they have less (or no) antagonistic activity at dopaminergic and cholinergic receptors. Their antipsychotic activity is thought to be due to blockade of

1342

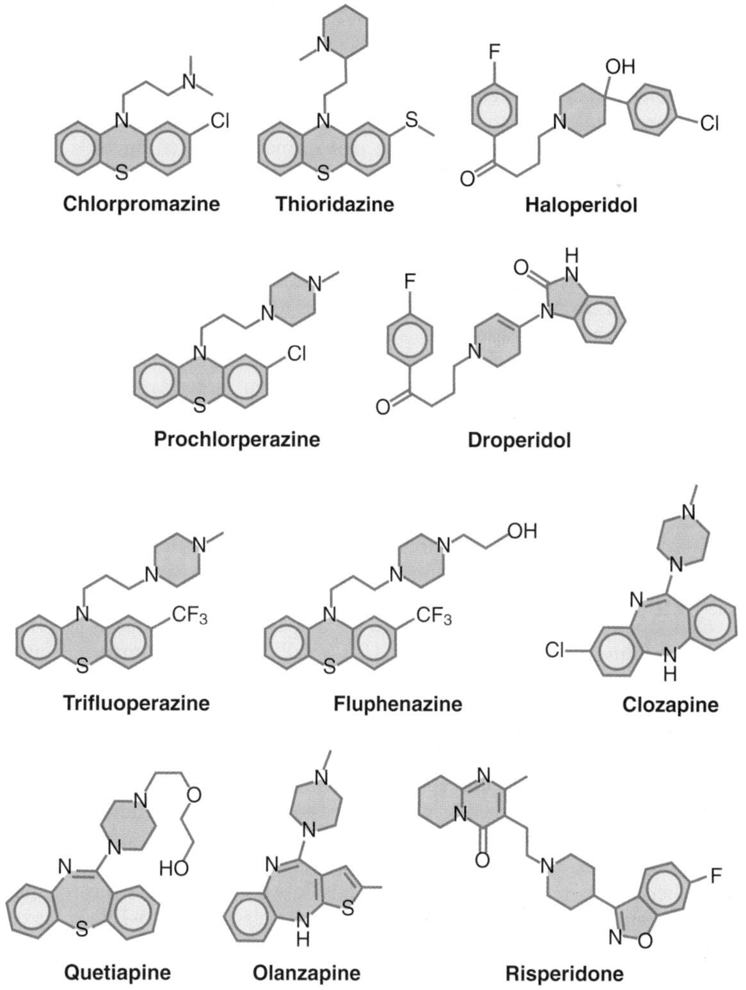

Figure 182-1 Structures of the antipsychotics discussed in this chapter.

5-hydroxytryptamine 2 (5-HT$_2$) receptors. Because they are also potent α-adrenoceptor antagonists, orthostatic hypotension is a common problem. However, extrapyramidal effects are much rarer than with any of the older antipsychotic agents. Drugs in this class include clozapine (Clozaril), olanzapine (Zyprexa), quetiapine (Seroquel),

ziprasidone (Geodon), risperidone (Risperdal), and aripiprazole (Abilify). Clozapine can cause agranulocytosis and seizures; regular monitoring of the white blood cell count is necessary in patients taking the drug. Aripiprazole is an "atypical" atypical antipsychotic in that it is a partial agonist at dopamine D$_2$, 5-HT$_{1A}$, and 5-HT$_{2A}$ receptors. It is minimally sedating and produces little hypotension and few extrapyramidal effects.

For emergency management of agitation, delirium, or acute psychosis, haloperidol may be given intravenously (IV) or intramuscularly (IM), or chlorpromazine, olanzapine, or ziprasidone may be given IM. Chlorpromazine should rarely be given IV because of its profound vasodilating effect, which is especially pronounced in hypovolemic patients.

Use of Antipsychotics in the Intensive Care Unit

The most common indication for use of antipsychotic medications in the ICU is for treatment of agitation or delirium. Haloperidol is the usual drug of choice for this indication because of intensivists' familiarity with it and because of its substantial safety record.[2]

If the need to begin treatment is not urgent, and if gastrointestinal absorption is expected to be reliable, oral haloperidol may be used at a beginning dose of 0.5 to 1 mg and repeated as needed. As the duration of therapy increases, the interval between doses also increases because the terminal half-life of haloperidol is about 1 day in normal persons and may be prolonged in critically ill persons. In the urgent management of severe agitation, the IV (or less desirably, the IM) route

TABLE 182-1 Adverse Effects of Some Antipsychotic Medications

Medication	Sedation	Extrapyramidal Effects	Hypotension
Phenothiazines			
Chlorpromazine	+++	++	+++
Thioridazine	+++	+	+++
Trifluoperazine	+	+++	+
Fluphenazine	+	++++	+
Prochlorperazine	+++	++	+++
Butyrophenones			
Haloperidol	+	++++	+
Droperidol	+	++++	+
Atypical Antipsychotics			
Clozapine	+++	0	+++
Olanzapine	+	+	++
Quetiapine	+++	0	++
Risperidone	++	++	+++
Aripiprazole	0/+	0/+	0/+
Ziprasidone	++	0/+	+

0, no effect; increasingly strong effects are indicated by the number of + symbols.
Adapted from Baldessarini RJ, Tarazi FI. Pharmacotherapy of psychosis and mania. In: Brunton LL, Lazo JS, Parker KL, editors. Goodman and Gilman's the pharmacological basis of therapeutics. 11th ed. New York: McGraw-Hill; 2006.

may be used. A reasonable starting dose is 2.5 to 5 mg; if an inadequate response is obtained, additional escalating doses (e.g., twice the previously administered dose) may be given every 5 to 10 minutes. Once reasonable efficacy has been achieved, the last administered dose may then be repeated every 4 to 6 hours. Some critically ill patients require hundreds of milligrams daily for the management of agitation or delirium. One alternative to frequent administration of bolus injections of haloperidol is administration of haloperidol by continuous infusion. This method may provide better control of delirium and agitation in some patients and decrease the nursing effort required to prevent self-inflicted injuries.[3] After steady-state blood concentrations of haloperidol are approached, days are required for the effects to wane after stopping administration.

Chlorpromazine is usually a less desirable alternative in this scenario because of its tendency to cause hypotension secondary to α-adrenoceptor blockade. Hypotension caused by chlorpromazine is especially pronounced after IV administration, and if the drug must be given by this route, the injection should be made very slowly. In comparison to haloperidol, chlorpromazine is also significantly more sedating, which might be an attractive side effect. In general, addition of a sedative such as a benzodiazepine or propofol to a haloperidol regimen provides superior sedation and control of delirium with fewer hemodynamic effects.

Olanzapine recently has been studied in comparison with haloperidol for treatment of delirium in the ICU.[2] Overall efficacy was comparable with either medication, and there were fewer extrapyramidal effects with olanzapine.

All phenothiazine and butyrophenone antipsychotic agents have antiemetic activity by virtue of their ability to block the dopamine receptor in the chemoreceptor trigger zone. Antiemetic doses are much lower than usual antipsychotic doses. The most extensively studied antiemetic antipsychotic drug is droperidol. The usual antiemetic dose is 1.25 mg given 2 to 3 times daily. This dose rarely causes sedation or any other adverse effects. If droperidol at this dose does not relieve the emetic symptoms, an antiemetic from a different class (e.g., a 5-HT$_3$ antagonist) should be given.

MANAGEMENT OF ADVERSE EFFECTS

The extrapyramidal effects of antipsychotics are uncomfortable but rarely hazardous. The exception is an unusual presentation of acute dystonia manifested as airway compromise. If administration of an anticholinergic agent does not provide rapid relief, paralysis and intubation are required to maintain airway integrity.

For treatment of extrapyramidal effects caused by an antipsychotic drug, a centrally acting anticholinergic is given, usually IV. The usual doses are 1 to 2 mg of benztropine (Cogentin) or 25 to 50 mg of diphenhydramine (Benadryl). Diphenhydramine causes more sedation than benztropine, which may or may not be advantageous in a particular patient. Because the extrapyramidal effects are dose related, decreasing the subsequent dose may lessen the likelihood of recurrence. Alternatively, changing to a different medication with fewer inherent extrapyramidal effects is also an option (see Table 182-1). However, such a change in therapy is likely to result in greater hypotensive effects from the antipsychotic medication, a factor that must be considered in critically ill patients.

Neuroleptic malignant syndrome is a rare and occasionally fatal constellation of symptoms which can include catatonia, stupor, rigidity, hyperthermia, autonomic instability, and rhabdomyolysis, leading to myoglobinemia and elevated circulating levels of creatine kinase. The syndrome is commonly associated with the more potent antipsychotics (e.g., haloperidol), and dopaminergic blockade is thought to be the initial underlying mechanism. However, all atypical antipsychotics have been associated with neuroleptic malignant syndrome.

Treatment requires supportive measures such as cessation of the antipsychotic medication, active cooling, and maintenance of blood pressure and urine output. The efficacy of additional pharmacologic therapy is controversial.[4] The dopaminergic agonists, amantadine (Symmetrel) and bromocriptine (Parlodel), and dantrolene (Dantrium), a muscle relaxant with an intracellular mechanism of action that is also used to treat malignant hyperthermia, are commonly administered. However, it is unclear whether these agents convey benefits beyond supportive therapy.

Most phenothiazine and butyrophenone antipsychotics are thought to increase the incidence of torsades de pointes, a form of ventricular tachycardia that can deteriorate into ventricular fibrillation.[5] Cases of torsades de pointes have also been ascribed to therapy with atypical antipsychotics, although the incidence is much lower. Torsades de pointes is usually, but not always, preceded by an increase in the corrected QT interval (QTc) on the electrocardiogram (ECG). QTc prolongation is a known dose-related effect and is common during therapy with thioridazine, chlorpromazine, haloperidol, and droperidol. Torsades de pointes is more likely when the QTc is lengthened beyond 500 msec or when it is prolonged 60 msec or more beyond its usual baseline value. Discontinuation of the antipsychotic agent decreases QTc and the associated risk of torsades de pointes.

Hypotension due to α-adrenoceptor blockade often accompanies therapy with phenothiazines and atypical antipsychotics. The degree of hypotension may be exaggerated in persons with coexisting hypovolemia and those who are receiving therapy with β-adrenoceptor antagonists, because the efferent limb of the barostatic reflex is blocked. Infusion of phenylephrine (Neo-Synephrine), a pure α-adrenoceptor agonist, restores blood pressure without producing other cardiovascular perturbations.

The seizure threshold may be lowered by antipsychotic medications, especially chlorpromazine and clozapine.[6] However, because the effect is dose dependent, large doses of other antipsychotics also have been associated with seizures, both in persons with a known preexisting seizure disorder and in persons with no prior history. The approach to treatment of an antipsychotic-related seizure is similar to that used with other drug-induced or idiopathic seizures: initial measures to maintain airway patency, along with administration of supplemental oxygen, an anticonvulsant medication (e.g., diazepam [Valium]) if the seizure does not terminate spontaneously, and withdrawal or decrease in the dose of the offending medication (if known).

Management of Antipsychotic Overdose

Patients may accidentally or deliberately administer an overdose of an antipsychotic, either alone or in combination with other medications or alcohol. Such patients may require admission to an ICU. In contrast to other classes of medications that are active in the CNS (e.g., tricyclic antidepressants, barbiturates, opioids), all of the antipsychotics have a high therapeutic index (in terms of lethality), and deaths due to overdose are quite rare.[7] When deaths have occurred after overdoses in persons who were found alive and transported to a hospital, the most common cause has been aspiration pneumonitis.

Treatment of overdose in the ICU is supportive. If the patient is comatose and unable to protect the airway, tracheal intubation should be performed, and the endotracheal tube should be kept in place until consciousness returns. Hypotension is treated with IV fluid administration, and infusion of the α-adrenoceptor agonist, phenylephrine, may be added if there is an inadequate response to fluids alone. Because of the possibility of torsades de pointes or other ventricular dysrhythmias, ECG monitoring is continued until the blood concentration of the medication is predicted (or demonstrated) to be subtherapeutic. There is no demonstrated efficacy (and there is certainly a potential for toxicity) associated with administering potassium or magnesium to persons with a prolonged QTc. Seizures that do not resolve spontaneously may be treated with diazepam as described earlier. Extrapyramidal symptoms are treated with diphenhydramine or benztropine as described earlier. Delirium from excessive central cholinergic blockade should respond to administration of physostigmine (Antilirium), 1 to 2 mg IV. Because antipsychotics have large volumes of distribution and a high degree of protein binding, dialysis has little efficacy in decreasing the blood concentration.

KEY POINTS

1. Among the phenothiazines and butyrophenones, there is generally an inverse relationship between the degree of sedation and the propensity to cause hypotension on the one hand, and the likelihood of causing extrapyramidal effects on the other.

2. Atypical antipsychotics tend to cause little to no extrapyramidal effects. They tend to be sedating and are likely to cause hypotension.

3. Haloperidol is the primary medication used in the ICU for managing agitation or delirium. The initial dose is usually low but may be escalated over a short period to control symptoms. An infusion of haloperidol may be used in persons with symptoms that are particularly difficult to manage.

4. Antipsychotic-induced extrapyramidal effects and hypotension are treated with specific pharmacologic agents. Other adverse effects of the antipsychotics usually are managed supportively or by discontinuation of the medication or both.

5. Deliberate or accidental overdose of antipsychotics rarely leads to death. Appropriate care of patients who have overdosed is generally supportive.

ANNOTATED REFERENCES

Baldessarini RJ, Tarazi FI. Pharmacotherapy of psychosis and mania. In: Brunton LL, Lazo JS, Parker KL, editors. Goodman and Gilman's the pharmacological basis of therapeutics. 11th ed. New York: McGraw-Hill; 2006.

  This is a detailed and comprehensive consideration of the pharmacology of antipsychotic medications, from which the initial section of this chapter was drawn.

Burns MJ. The pharmacology and toxicology of atypical antipsychotic agents. Clin Toxicol 2001;39:1-14.

  This is a detailed and comprehensive review of atypical antipsychotic agents, including their adverse effects, management, and treatment of overdose.

Morandi A, Jackson JC, Ely EW. Delirium in the intensive care unit. Int Rev Psychiatry 2009;21:43-58.

  This is a detailed and comprehensive review of the risk factors and treatment of critically ill patients with delirium.

Smith FA, Wittmann CW, Stern TA. Medical complications of psychiatric treatment. Crit Care Clin 2008;24:635-56.

  This is a detailed review of the adverse effects of psychoactive medications in critically ill patients including neuroleptic malignant syndrome, extrapyramidal effects, and cardiac dysrhythmias.

REFERENCES

Access the complete reference list online at http://www.expertconsult.com.

183

Nonsteroidal Antiinflammatory Agents

KEITH M. OLSEN

Nonsteroidal antiinflammatory drugs (NSAIDs) have important clinical uses in selected critically ill patients for treatment of pain and inflammatory states or reduction of fever.[1-3] However, drugs in this class can cause serious side effects and/or affect other medications used concomitantly. The pharmacologic characteristics of NSAIDs related to cyclooxygenase-1 (COX-1) and COX-2 enzyme inhibition may result in severe gastrointestinal, cardiovascular, and renal side effects.[4-8] Two highly COX-2-selective agents have been withdrawn from the market as a result of toxicity.[9] Patient characteristics and differences in NSAID toxicity profiles are important for the judicious use of NSAIDs in the critically ill patient.

NSAID Pharmacodynamics

NSAIDs include aspirin, indomethacin, ibuprofen, naproxen, diclofenac, and a product which is relatively more selective for the COX-2 isoform of cyclooxygenase (i.e., celecoxib). All NSAIDs have analgesic, antiinflammatory, and antipyretic properties. NSAIDs belong to a number of chemical families including acetic acids, oxicams, propionic acids, salicylates, fenamates, furanones and coxibs (Table 183-1). All NSAIDs are weakly acidic chemical compounds and share similarities in pharmacokinetic properties.[10] Their absorption is primarily in the large surface area of the small intestine as well as in the stomach.[10] Gastrointestinal absorption of NSAIDs occurs rapidly, usually within 15 to 30 minutes. Different product formulations, including enteric-coated and delayed-release preparations, decrease gastric emptying, and altered gastric transit time can delay drug absorption and time to peak effect.[11] For example, 4 to 6 hours is required for peak absorption of enteric-coated products.[11] After absorption, NSAIDs are more than 90% bound to albumin, which influences their distribution and drug-drug interaction potential. Hypoalbuminemia (e.g., due to alcoholic liver disease) can result in greater unbound drug and increased risk for NSAID-related adverse events.[11]

NSAIDs are primarily eliminated by renal and biliary excretion.[12] The elimination half-lives of NSAIDs vary from 0.25 to 86 hours, which accounts for differences in dosing schedules (see Table 183-1).[11] Factors that delay NSAID clearance increase their potential for adverse reactions. Reduced renal function prolongs NSAID half-life, and the dose should be lowered proportionally in patients with impaired kidney function.[10,12] Some NSAIDs are hepatically metabolized to both active and inactive metabolites, primarily through the cytochrome P450 enzymes, glucuronidase enzymes, or both.[10,13] Nabumetone and sulindac are prodrugs and require metabolism by the liver to generate pharmacologically active metabolites.[10] Moderate to severe liver disease impairs NSAID metabolism, increasing the potential for NSAID toxicity. With advanced age, the hepatic clearance of diclofenac, etodolac, flurbiprofen, ibuprofen, indomethacin, meloxicam, nabumetone, naproxen, oxaprozin, piroxicam, and sulindac is slower because of decreased hepatic phase I oxidative, reductive, and hydrolytic catalytic reactions.[10]

NSAIDs have a number of physiologic effects, although their principal action is inhibition of the cyclooxygenase enzyme.[1,2] COX is responsible for the production of prostaglandins (PG) and thromboxanes (TX), which are derived from arachidonic acid, an unsaturated fatty acid present in all body cell membranes. PGs and TXs mediate normal homeostatic functions of the upper gastrointestinal tract, kidneys, endothelium, vascular smooth muscle, and platelets, among other tissues and organs. PG and TX are critical in the inflammatory response because of their influences on vascular permeability, platelet function, and immune reactions. These autocoids are involved in both peripheral and central pain processing and have a role in fever production.[14,15]

As noted earlier, there are two isoforms of the COX enzyme: COX-1 and COX-2. Although the COX enzymes are coded on two separate genes, they share 63% structural homogeneity, have similar mechanisms of action, and produce identical compounds from arachidonic acid.[14-17] Expression and regulation of COX-1 and COX-2 differ in various organs and tissues; however, their physiologic effects are overlapping.[2,14,15,18] Differences in the structural configurations of COX-1 and COX-2 enzyme side chains determine whether a particular NSAID will inhibit the enzyme. Isoform nonselective NSAIDs (e.g., naproxen, ibuprofen) inhibit both COX-1 and COX-2, thereby decreasing production of PGs involved in both homeostatic and inflammatory actions. The COX-2-selective agent, celecoxib, is 50-fold more active against COX-2 than COX-1 and therefore exerts actions primarily in inflammatory processes.[18,19] Both COX-1 and COX-2 are involved in pain processing.

Differences in COX-1 and COX-2 inhibition allow for comparisons of drug effect.[6] Nonselective NSAIDs exert one of three kinetic models for inhibiting COX-1 and COX-2: (1) rapid, reversible binding (e.g., ibuprofen); (2) rapid, lower-affinity reversible binding followed by time-dependent, higher-affinity, slowly reversible binding (e.g., indomethacin); or (3) rapid, irreversible binding followed by covalent modification (e.g., aspirin). Aspirin is the only NSAID that covalently modifies both COX enzymes, thereby resulting in permanent inhibition of both isoforms.[20] COX-2-selective inhibitors act on COX-2 by a time-dependent, slowly reversible mechanism. They also can affect COX-1 by a freely reversible and competitive mechanism. The result of this two-stage process by COX-2-selective agents is maximal inhibition of COX-2 with minimal inhibition of COX-1.[16,17,21]

The biochemical selectivity of NSAIDs is related to the in vitro drug concentration necessary to inhibit COX-2 activity completely and COX-1 activity by 50%.[2,15] Data from clinical trials demonstrating a decreased incidence of gastrointestinal toxicity and an absence of platelet inhibition with COX-2-selective versus nonselective agents have been the clinical parameters used to distinguish among the various agents.[2]

COX converts arachidonic acid to the inactive precursor, PGG_2, and then PGH_2. PGH_2 is metabolized in various tissues to physiologically active products including PGI_2, PGE_2, and TXA_2. The concentration of different PGs determine their biological effects on tissues. PGs exert their effects by activating cell-membrane receptors of the superfamily of G protein–coupled receptors.[1] PGI_2 has important regulatory effects on renal blood flow, gastric mucosa, uterine smooth muscle, and bronchial smooth muscle. PGI_2 also inhibits platelet aggregation. PGE_2 is an abundant PG with important regulatory effects on fever and on the reproductive, gastrointestinal, neuroendocrine, and immune systems.[22] PGE_2 is present at sites of inflammation as a potent vasodilator in acute and chronic inflammatory diseases and in tissue injury. PGE_2 also can promote labor and dysmenorrhea.[22] TXA_2 promotes platelet aggregation and vasoconstriction. TXA_2 is released with tissue injury and plays a role in cellular responses to inflammation.[22]

PGs produced by COX-1 are primarily involved in maintaining the protective gastrointestinal mucosal barrier in the stomach and intestines, modulating intrarenal hemodynamics, influencing platelet function (especially aggregation), and regulating vascular homeostasis. For

TABLE 183-1	Characteristics of Commonly Prescribed NSAIDs			
	Dose*		Pharmacokinetics	
Generic Name (Trade Name)	**Available Dosages (mg)**	**Common Dosing Intervals**	**Drug Metabolism**	**Elimination Half-Life (Hours)**
Nonselective NSAIDs				
Acetic Acid Group				
Diclofenac DR	25	BID-TID	Oxidation	1-2
(*Voltaren*)	50	QD-BID		
Diclofenac XR	75			
(*Voltaren XR*)	100			
Etodolac	200	BID-TID	Oxidation, conjugation	7
(*Lodine*)	300	QD		
Etodolac XL	400			
(*Lodine XL*)	500			
	400			
	500			
	600			
Ketorolac IM, IV injection	30	QD-QID	Conjugation	2.5-8.5
(*generic*)				
Indomethacin	25	BID-TID	Oxidation, conjugation	4.5-6
(*Indocin*)	50	QD-BID		
Indomethacin SR	75			
(*Indocin SR*)				
Nabumetone	500	QD-BID	Oxidation	22-30
(*Relafen*)	750			
Sulindac	150	BID	Oxidation, reduction	16
(*Clinoril*)	200			
Tolmetin	400	TID	Conjugation	5
(*Tolectin*)	600			
Oxicam Group				
Meloxicam	7.5	QD	Oxidation	13-20
(*Mobic*)	15			
Piroxicam	10	QD	Oxidation	30-86
(*Feldene*)	20			
Propionic Acid Group				
Fenoprofen	200	TID-QID	Glucuronidation	3
(*Nalfon*)	300			
Flurbiprofen	50	BID-QID	Oxidation	3-6
(*Ocufen*)	100			
Ibuprofen	400	TID-QID	Oxidation	2-2.5
(*Motrin*)	600			
	800			
Ketoprofen	50	TID-QID	Conjugation	2-4
	75	QD		3-7
Ketoprofen CR	100			
	150			
	200			
Naproxen	250	BID	Conjugation, oxidation	12-15
(*Naprosyn*)	375	QD		
(*Naprelan*)	500			
	375			
	500			
Oxaprozin (*Daypro*)	600	QD-BID	Oxidation, conjugation	50-60
Salicylate				
Aspirin	81	QD	Hydrolysis, conjugation, glucuronidation	0.25-0.5
(*Ecotrin, Ascriptin*)	325	BID-QID		
Choline magnesium	500	BID-TID		
	500			
Trisalicylate	750		Conjugation	2-12
(*Trilisate*)	1000			
Cyclooxygenase-2 Agents				
Coxib Group				
Celecoxib	100	QD-BID	Conjugation	11-16
(*Celebrex*)	200			

*A dosage range exists for each NSAID that must be individualized depending on patient characteristics and disease mechanism.

CR, Controlled release; *DR*, delayed release; *IM*, intramuscular; *IV*, intravenous; *NSAID*, nonsteroidal antiinflammatory drug; *QD*, once a day; *BID*, twice a day; *TID*, three times a day; *QID*, four times a day; *XR*, extended release.

Data from references 9-11.

example, PGs produced by COX-1 provide gastric protection by reducing gastric acid secretion, stimulating mucus secretion, and promoting gastric mucosa vasodilation. Kidney function is affected by the localization of COX-1 in the collecting ducts and renal vasculature. COX-1 converts PGH_2 to TXA_2, which promotes platelet aggregation. Although the major role of COX-1 is homeostasis, COX-1 may contribute to PG production in certain inflammatory reactions, including those in the synovia of inflamed joints and atherosclerotic plaques.[14,15,18]

The primary role of COX-2 is in inflammatory reactions that result in PG production by fibroblasts, macrophages, endothelial cells, and synoviocytes. This enzyme is also important in pain and fever mechanisms.[16] Certain other tissues express COX-2, especially the cortical macula densa, medullary interstitial cells, and the kidney vasculature.[15] Small amounts of COX-2 are also found in the small intestine, ovary, uterus, bone, and brain.[14,16] Because COX-2 expression is regulated by growth factors, its role in wound repair is under investigation.[17]

Clinical Implications and Uses of NSAIDs in Critically Ill Patients

Although NSAIDs have important analgesic, antiinflammatory, and antipyretic activity, their role in critically ill patients should be limited, owing to their potential for toxic side effects.[23] In clinical trials, all nonselective and COX-2-selective NSAIDs in equipotent doses have demonstrated similar efficacy in relieving pain, inflammation, and fever.[24-26] However, there is significant variability in the clinical effects of NSAIDs within and among patients, with approximately 70% to 80% of individuals responding to any particular agent.[25] Lack of response to one NSAID does not preclude benefit from another.[25] Differences in NSAIDs may be related to COX-1 and COX-2 inhibitory pharmacodynamics, because no definite clinical characteristics have been identified in nonresponders compared to responders.[10,20] In contrast, toxicity profiles of nonselective and COX-2-selective agents have a defined relationship to the degree of COX-1 and COX-2 inhibition, especially for the development of gastrointestinal adverse events or antiplatelet effects.

MANAGEMENT OF PAIN AND INFLAMMATION

Pain management is a key issue for critical care clinicians. Although morphine is the primary analgesic of choice among critically ill patients with pain, NSAIDS may have a role in selected patients.[26] Pain is initiated by activation of tissue nociceptors in various disease states by mechanical, thermal, and chemical stimuli. Surgical trauma and other forms of tissue injury induce expression of COX-2, and to a lesser extent COX-1, resulting in generation of PGs, especially PGE_2.[27-29] PGs sensitize A-δ and C primary afferent sensory nerve fibers that carry impulses to the dorsal horn of the spinal cord. Glutamate, substance P, and other mediators along with PGs are involved in dorsal horn pain processing.[30] By inhibiting PGs at these different levels of the pain matrix, NSAIDs can have important effects on pain processing. For example, NSAIDs reduce PG-mediated protein kinase A phosphorylation of sodium channels in nociceptor terminals.

SURGICAL PAIN

Inadequate postoperative pain control has been associated with increased morbidity, increased length of stay, and increased costs for intensive care unit (ICU) patients.[31,32] Opioids are commonly prescribed for surgical and trauma pain and other acute pain states, but adverse events such as nausea and vomiting, drowsiness, and respiratory depression may limit their use in some patients and prolong postoperative recovery and increase costs.[31] NSAIDs are effective in combination with other analgesics in managing the acute pain of tissue injury.[33] For example, the use of NSAIDs in orthopedic and other types of surgeries including knee arthroscopy, hip replacement, spinal surgery, and gynecologic laparoscopy decreases postoperative opioid requirements.[24,26,34-38] In addition, NSAID therapy alone can provide effective postoperative pain relief.[31,38,39] However, because of the potential for adverse reactions (e.g., gastrointestinal toxicity, platelet inhibition with increased bleeding risk, renal dysfunction), especially with hypovolemia, NSAIDs should be used cautiously in the management of postoperative pain.[24,31,39] Although COX-2-selective inhibitors are equally effective in pain relief as nonselective NSAIDs, they should be used cautiously in the ICU owing to their potential for cardiac and gastrointestinal toxicity.[39] Recent studies of the use of COX-2-selective inhibitors in orthopedic and gynecologic surgeries demonstrated significant reductions in opioid consumption, decreased postoperative opioid side effects including nausea and vomiting, and improved

subjectively.[24,28,40,41] In addition, preoperative use of COX-2-selective agents in knee arthroscopy, compared with postoperative use, can delay the time to first analgesic request and decrease total opioid consumption.[35] The clinical impact of NSAID therapy on wound and bone healing after surgery is unclear.[42,43] NSAIDs, especially indomethacin, have been used perioperatively to reduce heterotopic bone formation after acetabular fracture surgery.[44] Recent data from animal and human trials suggest that NSAIDs may impair bone healing after fractures because of the role of PGs in osteogenesis.[42,43,45]

Ketorolac is currently the only injectable NSAID available in the United States. Clinical studies comparing injectable ketorolac with morphine in managing postoperative pain after orthopedic, gynecologic, and major abdominal procedures have shown similar efficacy but slower onset of action with ketorolac.[46] Combination therapy with ketorolac and morphine may provide analgesic benefit compared with morphine alone and reduce total morphine consumption.[47] However, use of ketorolac in acute pain states is now limited because of postmarketing reports of toxicity including peptic ulcers, gastrointestinal bleeding, and renal insufficiency.[46] In addition, dosing adjustments are necessary for patients with renal dysfunction and elderly patients, and duration of therapy never should exceed 5 days.[48]

REGIONAL INFLAMMATORY STATES

The antiinflammatory properties of NSAIDs are beneficial in specific acute disease states affecting critically ill patients, including systemic and regional rheumatic disorders and localized inflammatory conditions such as pleuropericarditis. PGs, especially PGI_2 and PGE_2, are induced by interleukin (IL)-1, IL-6, and IL-8. These PGs are important mediators of inflammatory reactions; they influence vascular reactivity and increase vascular permeability.[22]

Rheumatic diseases such as rheumatoid arthritis and systemic lupus erythematosus (SLE) present therapeutic challenges to the critical care clinician. Concerns about the role of NSAIDs in causation of certain acute problems, especially gastrointestinal bleeding and fluid retention, have arisen. NSAIDs are an important component of the therapeutic regimen for the synovitis of inflammatory arthritis and for serositis involving pleural or pericardial membranes.[48,49] Discontinuation of NSAID therapy can result in a significant increase in synovitis. The antiinflammatory effects of NSAIDs often require higher doses than those needed for a chronic analgesic response. No significant differences in effectiveness in suppressing inflammation have been demonstrated among the various nonselective and COX-2-selective agents.[24,25,50] Acute crystal-induced arthritis such as gout and pseudo-gout, although uncommon, still occasionally present in critically ill patients. Inflammation in response to uric acid and calcium pyrophosphate dihydrate crystals, respectively, is induced by immune mediators such as PGs, cytokines, bradykinin, and leukotrienes, which produce capillary dilation, neutrophil migration, and pain stimulation. NSAIDs, especially indomethacin, have been shown to be beneficial in acute crystal-induced arthritis.[51] Aspirin should not be used for gout because it influences renal tubular uric acid excretion, thereby causing fluctuations in serum uric acid levels, potentially aggravating acute gouty arthritis. Because all NSAIDs except ketorolac are administered only orally and can be toxic, their use is limited in the critical care setting. Alternative treatments for crystal-induced arthritis include corticosteroids and colchicine for gout.

Occasionally, acutely ill patients require NSAID therapy for their antiinflammatory and analgesic properties because of concurrent regional musculoskeletal disorders such as shoulder or elbow tendonitis or back problems.[52] Finally, NSAIDs have been used to treat pleuropericarditis of nonrheumatic origin, including viral serositis and postmyocardial infarction syndrome.

CARDIOVASCULAR PROTECTION

Abnormalities within the cardiovascular system are frequently present in critically ill patients. Because PGs play pathophysiologic roles in coagulation and inflammatory mechanisms involved in cardiovascular diseases, NSAIDs, especially aspirin, have an important therapeutic role. TXA_2, synthesized by platelets, is produced by COX-1 (together with another enzyme, thromboxane synthase); it promotes platelet aggregation on abnormal vascular endothelium and in areas of vascular stasis, leading to thrombosis. All nonselective NSAIDs inhibit COX-1; however, only aspirin does so irreversibly through acetylation.[53] The U.S. Preventive Services Taskforce Report strongly recommended the use of aspirin in adult patients who are at risk for coronary heart disease.[54] Practice guidelines recommend the use of low-dose aspirin (81-325 mg/d) for high-risk patients (i.e., 5% risk within 5 years) to reduce cardiovascular events including nonfatal myocardial infarction, fatal coronary heart disease, and nonhemorrhagic stroke.[53,55] For those individuals with a lower risk of having a coronary heart disease event, the benefit was negated by the toxic effects of aspirin, including gastrointestinal events and hemorrhagic stroke. An update of the evidence from the U.S. Preventive Task Force was published in 2009.[55] Following a systematic review of randomized clinical trials, the authors concluded that aspirin reduces the risk of coronary vascular disease (CVD) in adults without a history of CVD.[55] Critical care clinicians should consider using aspirin for patients at risk for CVD; however, the risks must be weighed against the benefits because of the increased risk for gastrointestinal bleeding events.[55]

Although other nonselective NSAIDs reversibly inhibit the COX-1 enzyme in platelets, they have not been demonstrated to reduce cardiac events and currently should not be used for primary or secondary prevention of vascular disease. COX-2-selective agents do not have demonstrated cardiovascular benefits.[56]

Aspirin has been compared with adjusted-dose warfarin for the prevention of stroke in atrial fibrillation. The 8th American College of Chest Physicians (ACCP) Consensus Conference on Antithrombotic Therapy recommended that drug selection in atrial fibrillation be based on risk likelihood: adjusted-dose warfarin for patients with a high risk of stroke, aspirin or adjusted-dose warfarin for those with a moderate risk; and aspirin for those with a low risk.[53] The risk for stroke is increased by a history of prior stroke, systemic embolus, hypertension, poor left ventricular systolic function, age older than 75 years, rheumatic mitral valvular disease, or a prosthetic heart valve.[53] Although both adjusted-dose warfarin and aspirin confer significant stroke reduction in the case of atrial fibrillation, their concomitant use does not impart greater benefit, and increased side effects do occur.[53]

Aspirin therapy, alone or in combination with dipyridamole, can delay progression of established arterial occlusive disease in patients with chronic lower-extremity arterial insufficiency.[53] Low-dose aspirin is beneficial in preventing morbidity and mortality from stroke and myocardial infarction in patients with peripheral arterial disease.[53,57,58] In addition, low-dose aspirin is used as prophylaxis and treatment for ischemic cerebrovascular disease, alone and in combination with dipyridamole, and has been demonstrated to reduce the risk of stroke in individuals with transient ischemic attacks or completed ischemic strokes due to thrombosis.[53]

FEVER

The mechanisms of fever involve either peripheral release of pyrogenic cytokines (IL-1, IL-6, tumor necrosis factor [TNF], and interferon [IFN]-α) from monocytes and macrophages or the presence of circulating endotoxins which stimulate central production of PGE_2 via COX-2 in vascular endothelial cells. PGE_2 targets hypothalamic thermoregulatory neurons.[59-61] Knockout mice lacking the COX-2 enzyme are unable to mount a fever when exposed to exogenous pyrogens.[59,60] The COX-1 enzyme is not involved in thermal regulatory control.[59]

Aspirin has long been recognized as an effective antipyretic agent, and it is the gold standard with which acetaminophen and other NSAIDs are compared. Studies evaluating the antipyretic properties of NSAIDs are primarily from the pediatric literature. A meta-analysis of adult fever trials has not been possible because of differences in patient populations, NSAID dosing schedules, and outcome measures.

However, studies in adults have shown equal or superior antipyretic efficacy of NSAIDs compared with acetaminophen.[60] NSAIDs are more effective in reducing fevers associated with cancer than those caused by infection, although the mechanism is unclear.[60] Duration of action of various NSAIDs in fever is related to drug half-life and drug concentration in the hypothalamus, a parameter determined by drug transport across the blood-brain barrier.[59] There are limited data evaluating clinical use of COX-2-selective agents for fever, but a beneficial effect has been demonstrated.[62,63,64] Toxicities of the various nonselective NSAIDs limit their clinical utility compared with acetaminophen, especially in critically ill patients.[60,65]

SEPTIC SHOCK

Ibuprofen and other NSAIDs have some physiologic effects in sepsis, although they do not reduce morbidity and mortality in septic shock, except possibly in patients with hypothermia.[66,67] A prospective randomized trial evaluated the impact of ibuprofen on organ failure and mortality in 455 patients with sepsis syndrome.[67] Significant improvements in temperature, heart rate, oxygen consumption, and lactic acidosis were noted, but there was no reduction in organ failure or 30-day mortality compared with standard care. The Surviving Sepsis Campaign guidelines do not list NSAIDs as a treatment option for septic shock.[68]

Toxicity of NSAIDs

GASTROINTESTINAL TOXICITY

PGs play a critical role in maintenance of the gastrointestinal mucosal barrier. Beneficial effects include maintenance of epithelial mucus secretion, mucosal blood flow, bicarbonate secretion, and epithelial proliferation. These protective mechanisms may be altered by NSAID-mediated inhibition of PG synthesis and local mucosal damage by the acidic NSAID compounds.[69] The spectrum of gastrointestinal injury includes mucosal irritation and ulceration in the stomach and small intestine, with bleeding and perforation.

There are limited data available regarding the gastrointestinal toxicity of NSAIDs in critically ill patients. However, serious gastrointestinal complications including ulceration, perforation, and bleeding occur in 1% to 2% of short-term NSAID users and in 2% to 5% of patients on chronic NSAID therapy.[70] A prospective observational trial conducted over a 19-week period identified admissions to a medical ICU related to adverse drug reactions (ADR). Bleeding secondary to both nonselective and selective NSAIDS, aspirin, and clopidogrel were the most common ADR admission diagnoses.[71] Gastrointestinal lesions related to NSAIDs frequently are asymptomatic. For example, approximately 40% of patients with endoscopically proven gastritis do not have symptoms.[70,72] Other studies confirm the occurrence of NSAID-induced gastrointestinal toxicities, although reported incidences vary depending on the characteristics of the study population and the evaluation tools used.[73-75]

The Arthritis, Rheumatism, and Aging Medical Information System (ARAMIS) prospectively evaluated outcomes including adverse effects from NSAID therapy in more than 36,000 patients with osteoarthritis or rheumatoid arthritis from 17 centers in the United States and Canada, accounting for more than 300,000 patient-years.[70] Based on this study population, it was calculated that more than 16,000 NSAID-related deaths could occur yearly in the United States, a number similar to the death rate for leukemia and exceeding the rates for malignant melanoma and asthma.[70] The CADEUS (COX-2 inhibitors and NSAIDs: description of users) study of 23,535 coxib and 22,919 traditional NSAIDs (tNSAIDs) identified hospitalizations for gastrointestinal and cardiovascular events.[76] There were only 21 hospitalizations for gastrointestinal events, 12 in the coxib cohort and nine in the tNSAID cohort. The rates of gastrointestinal events of 0.39 per 100 patients were considerably lower than observed in older randomized clinical trials and may reflect the increased use of prophylactic proton pump inhibitors in at-risk patients.

When a critically ill patient is prescribed either nonselective or COX-2-selective therapy, evaluation of their gastrointestinal toxicity profile is essential. In non-ICU patients, evidence-based risk factors for gastrointestinal toxicity with chronic use of nonselective NSAIDs include high doses, age older than 65 years, history of previous upper-gastrointestinal ulcers or upper-gastrointestinal bleeding, and use of corticosteroids and/or oral anticoagulants.[77-81] Data have also implicated cigarette smoking, alcohol use, and *Helicobacter pylori* infection as possible risk factors for nonselective NSAID-related gastrointestinal toxicity.[62,82] Low-dose aspirin increases the occurrence of serious gastrointestinal complications if it is given concomitantly with either nonselective or COX-2-selective NSAIDs because of the COX-1-inhibiting and local effects of the aspirin.

Some individuals on chronic therapy who have an increased risk of developing nonselective NSAID-related gastrointestinal toxicities may benefit from COX-2-selective agents.[76-62] It is unclear whether the risk of gastrointestinal toxicity differs between COX-2 selective and nonselective NSAIDs in critically ill patients. Gastrointestinal toxicity with both nonselective and COX-2-selective agents increases in patients older than 65 years of age; however, COX-2-selective agents pose a lower risk.[62] The Celecoxib Long-Term Arthritis Safety Study (CLASS)[63] and the Vioxx Gastrointestinal Outcomes Research (VIGOR)[64] studies are NSAID safety trials that compared the gastrointestinal side effects of the COX-2-selective agents, celecoxib and rofecoxib, respectively, with those of nonselective NSAIDs.[83,84] The primary outcome endpoints of the CLASS study (ulceration, perforation, and bleeding) were similar for celecoxib compared with ibuprofen or diclofenac, whereas the VIGOR trial showed a statistically significant decrease in primary endpoints (ulceration, perforation, bleeding, and symptomatic ulcers) for rofecoxib compared with naproxen. However, after consideration of symptomatic ulcers was added to the primary analysis of CLASS data, a significantly lower incidence of gastrointestinal toxicity was found with celecoxib. In addition, a subanalysis of CLASS that excluded patients receiving concomitant low-dose aspirin therapy revealed a significantly lower rate of gastrointestinal complications with or without inclusion of symptomatic ulcer in the celecoxib group. However, a U.S. Food and Drug Administration (FDA) report concluded that the CLASS study demonstrated no gastrointestinal advantage with celecoxib and requires gastrointestinal warning labeling similar to that required for nonselective NSAIDs.[85] Differences in study methodology (study duration, subject selection, primary and secondary outcome endpoints), patient population (osteoarthritis and rheumatoid arthritis in CLASS, rheumatoid arthritis in VIGOR), and concomitant therapy (no aspirin in VIGOR) precluded making valid comparisons between the CLASS and VIGOR data. For critically ill patients who are experiencing gastrointestinal problems and taking nonselective or COX-2-selective NSAIDs, proper evaluation of the gastrointestinal tract is imperative and usually requires upper-gastrointestinal endoscopy. Furthermore, additive bleeding risks (e.g., heparin, other anticoagulants) and underlying disease-related factors are often introduced in the critical care setting. The mortality rate for NSAID-induced ulceration and bleeding is approximately 10%.[72] The first step in the management of NSAID-related gastrointestinal ulcers is discontinuation of NSAID therapy.

Pharmacologic treatment options have focused on inhibition of acid secretion and replacement of PG deficiency; these options include proton pump inhibitors (PPIs), histamine-2 receptor antagonists (H$_2$RA), misoprostol, and protective barrier agents.[86-88] Suppression of acid by H$_2$RAs can effectively heal gastric and duodenal ulcers on discontinuation of the NSAID.[88] PPIs markedly suppress acid secretion and are very effective at healing gastric and duodenal ulcers, even if the NSAID is continued.[62,88] PPIs and misoprostol have been shown to be superior to H$_2$RAs for gastric ulcer healing.[62,86,88] However, because misoprostol often is not well tolerated, its role in clinical practice is limited. Comparative studies in non-ICU patients of omeprazole, ranitidine, misoprostol, and sucralfate demonstrated a therapeutic advantage of the PPIs that range from 10% to 40%.[62,88] For NSAID prophylaxis, PPIs are superior to H$_2$RAs in reducing the risk of both gastric and duodenal ulceration.[62,86,88] Although high doses of misoprostol and proton pump inhibitors are effective for preventing NSAID-induced gastric ulcers, misoprostol compliance is poor as a result of gastrointestinal side effects such as nausea and diarrhea.[87,88-90]

Monitoring for bleeding is another important factor in the critical care setting. The effects of aspirin and NSAIDs on fecal occult blood tests have been evaluated. Aspirin in doses less than 325 mg/d does not interfere with fecal occult blood testing and does not have to be discontinued during stool collection.[62,90] Typically, NSAID-induced fecal blood loss is dose dependent and may correlate with the severity of endoscopically detected upper-gastrointestinal lesions.[62,90] Fecal occult blood loss associated with COX-2 inhibitor therapy is reported to be similar to that observed with placebo.[62,90]

CARDIOVASCULAR AND RENAL TOXICITY

All NSAIDs have the potential to aggravate hypertension, congestive heart failure, and edema.[85] The COX-2-selective agents have been linked to serious cardiovascular side effects when compared with nonselective NSAIDs. This has led to withdrawal of rofecoxib and valdecoxib from the U.S. market, and only celecoxib remains.[91] Thromboxane A-2 and prostacyclin (PGI$_2$) are produced from prostaglandins by COX enzymes. TXA$_2$ is expressed most prominently in platelets and leads to enhanced platelet aggregation and vasoconstriction. Conversely, PGI$_2$ is a vasodilator and inhibitor of platelet aggregation. Although the mechanism is not completely understood, the COX-2-selective inhibitors create an imbalance between PGI$_2$ and TXA$_2$ characterized by excessive TXA$_2$-mediated actions. The result is increased vascular tone, platelet aggregation, and vascular smooth muscle proliferation which lead to increased risk of thrombotic events. Not all agents have equal specificity for COX-2 enzymes. Thus, celecoxib is about 10-fold less active than rofecoxib against COX-2 in an in vitro model.[9]

The VIGOR trial[64] reported a significant increase in the incidence of myocardial infarction for rofecoxib compared with naproxen, whereas the CLASS study[63] showed no difference in cardiovascular endpoints between celecoxib and ibuprofen or diclofenac. Differences in methodology between the studies, especially the fact that low-dose aspirin was not permitted in the VIGOR trial, make them difficult to compare. In addition, the antiplatelet effects of the nonselective NSAIDs may have influenced the results. The results of the VIGOR trial were confirmed in the Adenomatous Polyp Prevention on Vioxx (APPROVe) trial.[92] Compared to placebo, rofecoxib was associated with increased cardiovascular events that included myocardial infarction, cerebrovascular events, and other cardiac events (congestive heart failure, pulmonary edema, or cardiac failure). The subsequent events surrounding the withdrawal of rofecoxib from the market have been thoroughly summarized.[93]

Since the VIGOR, CLASS, and APPROVe studies, at least two large randomized trials have demonstrated increased risk of cardiovascular events with celecoxib.[94,95] The Adenoma Prevention with Celecoxib (APC) trial identified an increased risk of myocardial infarction, stroke, and heart failure compared to placebo. Among the 2000 patients enrolled in the trial, cardiovascular events were observed in 2.5% of patients receiving celecoxib compared to 1.9% of those taking a placebo (relative risk [RR], 1.30; 95% confidence interval [CI], 0.65-2.62).[94] A second study evaluating celecoxib, naproxen, or placebo in the Alzheimer Disease Anti-inflammatory Prevention Trial (ADAPT) was stopped early due to increased cardiovascular events.[95] Both celecoxib and naproxen demonstrated a higher incidence of cardiovascular and cerebrovascular events (RR 1.10 and 1.63, respectively). Although none of these trials involved critically ill patients, selective COX-2 inhibitors should be used very cautiously in the ICU. Patients with any risk of cardiovascular disease, or patients taking aspirin or other medications for prevention or treatment of cardiovascular diseases, should not receive a COX-2-selective agent.[92]

Blood pressure elevation has been associated with both nonselective and COX-2-selective agents. Mean blood pressure increases of 3 to 6 mm Hg have been reported with short-term NSAID therapy, especially in patients with preexisting hypertension. Patients with cardiovascular disease, hypertension, renal or hepatic insufficiency, or advanced age should be monitored for fluid retention, which can affect blood pressure during therapy with NSAIDs (including COX-2-selective drugs).[96,97] Data from studies of COX-2-selective agents indicate that there is a similar risk of hypertension, leading to labeling precautions for both COX-2-selective and nonselective NSAIDs.[97,98] In addition, drug-drug interactions of nonselective NSAIDs or COX-2-selective inhibitors with antihypertensive agents including angiotensin-converting enzyme (ACE) inhibitors, β-adrenergic blockers, and diuretics may accentuate NSAID-mediated inhibition of renal PG production, thereby lessening antihypertensive efficacy.[12] Monitoring for hypertension, renal function, and edema is recommended for all patients on NSAID therapy, especially those with the risk factors noted previously.[96]

Both COX-1 and COX-2 are constitutively expressed in the kidney, predisposing to renal problems with either NSAID class. The adverse effects of nonselective NSAIDs and those of COX-2-selective agents on renal function appear to be similar.[98] NSAID-related renal toxicities most commonly include decreased glomerular filtration rate and decreased sodium excretion.[95] The deleterious effects of NSAIDs on renal homeostasis are most pronounced in patients with renal insufficiency and volume depletion. The risk of deleterious effects also is increased in patients with hypertension, congestive heart failure, edema, chronic renal failure, advanced age, or concomitant diuretic therapy.[96,98,83] Less commonly, patients present with NSAID-induced acute interstitial nephritis, which accounts for fewer than 2% of hospital admissions related to drug-induced renal failure.[98] Nephrotic syndrome and papillary necrosis rarely have been associated with chronic NSAID use. Although nephrotic syndrome is generally reversible, papillary necrosis, which occurs most often with NSAID overdose, can result in permanent renal impairment.[96] As with nonselective NSAIDs, the renal adverse effects of COX-2-selective agents tend to occur early in therapy and usually are reversible on discontinuation of the drug.[98,83]

HYPERSENSITIVITY REACTIONS

Hypersensitivity reactions to NSAIDs occur rarely, and they are more common in individuals with nasal polyps or asthma. Allergic reactions including bronchoconstriction, rhinitis, and urticaria have been associated with all nonselective NSAIDs and COX-2-selective inhibitors. Recent data suggest a role of altered COX-2 regulation associated with the aspirin-intolerant asthma/rhinitis syndrome.[84] Because of the potential for cross-reactivity, avoidance of all NSAIDs is recommended in patients with a history of bronchoconstriction or allergic reactions to any NSAID.

Various cutaneous reactions have been described with all NSAIDs, especially skin eruptions of a pustular, acneiform nature that are often pruritic. Cessation of NSAID therapy is usually required. Because of its sulfonamide-like chemical structure, celecoxib should not be used in patients with a history of allergic cutaneous and other hypersensitivity reactions to sulfa drugs.[13,99] Other less common adverse events associated with NSAIDs include hepatic abnormalities with elevated liver function tests, headache, confusion (especially in older individuals), sleep disturbances, and tinnitus. In rare cases, NSAIDs have been implicated in causing aseptic meningitis and, in children, Reye syndrome.[13]

DRUG-DRUG INTERACTIONS

Drug-drug interactions, especially with regard to toxicity, are important considerations when initiating therapy with NSAIDs in the critical care setting or managing treatment in patients who are already taking an NSAID. Drug-drug interactions with NSAID therapy may result from their pharmacodynamic properties (e.g., inhibition of COX and related effects on gastrointestinal mucosa, kidneys, and platelets) or their pharmacokinetic properties (e.g., protein binding, drug metabolism).

Nonselective NSAIDs affect other antiplatelet agents via additive inhibition of platelet aggregation. The result is an increased bleeding risk with the concomitant use of NSAIDs and other antiplatelet agents such as heparin, low-molecular-weight heparin, warfarin, clopidogrel, ticlopidine, lepirudin, and argatroban.[13,100] Similarly, concurrent therapy with drotrecogin-α (activated) and NSAIDs must be undertaken cautiously, especially with aspirin at a dose greater than 650 mg or with other NSAID agents.[101] A COX-2-selective NSAID may be administered concurrently with warfarin with caution and appropriate monitoring.

Significant drug-drug interactions have been documented with use of NSAIDs and lithium. Both nonselective and COX-2-selective NSAIDs decrease lithium clearance and increase serum lithium concentrations by inhibiting renal PG production and altering intrarenal blood flow. Serum lithium levels and the clinical signs and symptoms of bipolar disorder should be evaluated in patients with concomitant NSAID use.[13,100]

Data are conflicting regarding the drug-drug interaction potential of ACE inhibitors and NSAIDs. Mixed results of significant drug interactions have been noted in hypertension, coronary artery disease, and congestive heart failure trials, particularly with doses of aspirin greater than 325 mg/day.[102] In patients with congestive heart failure, ACE inhibitors increase bradykinin production, resulting in increased synthesis of the vasodilating PGs, prostacyclin and PGE_2, which reduces cardiac afterload. By blocking COX and inhibiting the production of PGs, NSAIDs may antagonize the beneficial vasodilatory effects of ACE inhibitors, leading to decreased cardiac output and worsening of heart failure. In addition, concurrent use of ACE inhibitors and NSAIDs may reduce the beneficial effects of renal PGE_2 on sodium excretion produced by ACE inhibitors.

Concurrent administration of digoxin and NSAIDs can decrease renal clearance of digoxin, increase plasma drug concentration, and potentiate digoxin toxicity.[100]

NSAIDs interact with anticonvulsant agents such as phenytoin and valproic acid by displacing the anticonvulsants from their protein-binding sites, which increases the free drug concentration and the potential for anticonvulsant toxicity.[100]

Combination use of corticosteroids and aspirin can increase renal clearance of salicylate and significantly decrease plasma salicylate concentrations. Therefore, a potential for aspirin toxicity exists when tapering high-dose steroids. Appropriate monitoring is warranted, especially for gastrointestinal bleeding, because of increased salicylate concentrations.[100]

◼ Overdose

Despite the common use of NSAIDs in clinical practice, serious acute overdose and adverse sequelae have been reported. The National Poison Data System (NPDS) annual report from the American Association of Poison Control Centers documented 25 deaths due to aspirin and 5 from NSAID overdose in the year 2008.[103] The mechanism of NSAID toxicity in overdose is related to both their acidic nature and their inhibition of PG production.

Prompt recognition and management of NSAID overdose is important. With salicylate overdose, the severity typically depends on the dose ingested and the salicylate concentration that correlates with the degree of acid-base disturbance. Measurement of salicylate serum levels is important in all cases of aspirin overdose to guide management.[103-105] Serum salicylate levels should be measured 4 hours after ingestion and repeated in 2 to 4 hours to determine the peak concentration.[102,103] If the acute ingestion was with an enteric-coated product, salicylate levels should be monitored for 12 hours because of the delay in absorption and time to peak concentration.[104] Generally, salicylate levels of 300 to 600 mg/L are associated with mild toxicity, 600 to 800 mg/L with moderate toxicity, and greater than 800 mg/L with severe toxicity.[103] For nonselective NSAIDs, plasma concentrations are not commonly measured and are less helpful because the half-life of many of these agents is relatively short.[103]

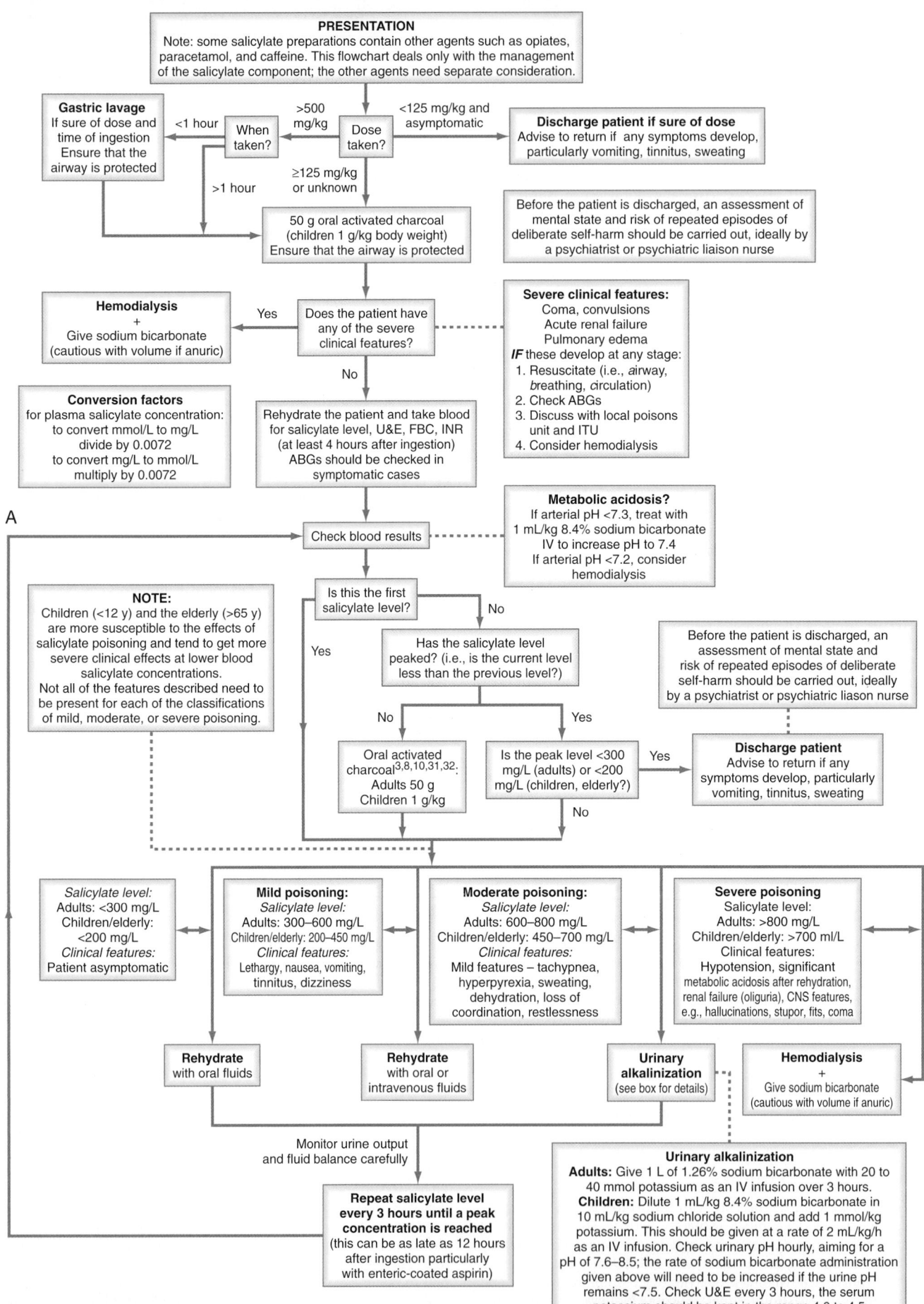

Figure 183-1 Evidence-based flowchart for management of salicylate poisoning. (*From Dargan PI, Wallace CI, Jones AL. An evidence-based flowchart to guide the management of acute salicylate [aspirin] overdose. Emerg Med J 2002;19:206-9, with permission of the BMJ Publishing Group.*)

Although patients with overdoses of aspirin and other NSAIDs may be asymptomatic, depending on the amount ingested, common symptoms include nausea, vomiting, abdominal pain, tinnitus, hearing impairment, and central nervous system (CNS) depression. With higher-dose aspirin ingestion, metabolic acidosis, renal failure, greater CNS changes (e.g., agitation, confusion, coma), and hyperventilation with respiratory alkalosis occur. The presence of acidemia permits more salicylic acid to cross the blood-brain barrier, leading to more severe CNS toxicity.[104] In addition, salicylate toxicity can stimulate the respiratory center, leading to hyperventilation and respiratory alkalosis.[99] With other nonselective NSAID ingestions, symptoms are similar to those occurring with aspirin overdose.[103,105]

There is no antidote for salicylate or NSAID poisoning. Management varies depending on the amount of NSAID ingested and is directed at symptomatic support, prevention of further absorption, and correction of acid-base imbalance.[103,104] Appropriate hydration should be administered in all overdose situations. Although evidence is limited for the benefit of absorption therapy in aspirin overdose, activated charcoal is often administered within 1 hour after aspirin ingestion and repeated hourly for 4 doses until the salicylate level peaks.[78,103,104] Urine alkalinization increases salicylate elimination, especially in adult patients with salicylate levels of 600 to 800 mg/L and in the elderly.[103] Because of the relatively neutral pK_a of salicylic acid, increasing the urine pH from 5 to 8 is associated with a 10- to 20-fold increase in renal salicylate clearance. Infusion of 1 L of sodium bicarbonate (132 mEq/L) over 3 hours is the recommended regimen for urine alkalinization. The circulating potassium level should also be evaluated because of the acidosis. Consideration of potassium replacement is recommended; however, administration of sodium bicarbonate should not be delayed until potassium levels are stabilized.[103,104] In severe cases of aspirin overdose, hemodialysis is effective at removing salicylate and correcting acid-base imbalances and has been shown to reduce morbidity and mortality. Hemodialysis should be considered in patients with salicylate levels greater than 800 mg/L and in the elderly. Hemodialysis also should be considered in patients with metabolic acidosis refractory to treatment, severe and symptomatic CNS toxicity (e.g., coma, convulsions), acute pulmonary edema, or acute renal failure.[103,104] Urinary alkalinization should be continued while hemodialysis is administered. Figure 183-1 provides a treatment algorithm for management of salicylate toxicity.

In non-aspirin NSAID overdose, management is also directed toward supportive care. In addition, activated charcoal is useful if administered within 1 hour after ingestion to patients who took more than 100 mg/kg body weight of ibuprofen or more than 10 tablets of other NSAIDs.[103] If renal insufficiency occurs with the overdose, NSAID accumulation is more pronounced.[105,106] Hepatotoxicity is more commonly seen with diclofenac overdoses, in female patients, in patients older than 50 years of age, and in patients with preexisting autoimmune disease.[105]

Summary

NSAIDs are a class of medications with a variety of pain indications and for fever in selected critically ill patients. In general, NSAIDs should be used judiciously in ICU patients because of the potential for toxic adverse events. The lowest effective dose of the NSAID should be used for the shortest duration indicated. Before initiation of NSAID therapy, the following factors must be considered: diagnosis, patient characteristics, efficacy, side effects, and cost. Appropriate clinical and laboratory follow-up is necessary, especially for patients with changing organ function and those taking other medications known to increase bleeding potential. If a critically ill patient is receiving NSAID therapy at the time of presentation, appropriate monitoring of efficacy and toxicity is essential. When selecting an NSAID, the efficacy profile should be balanced against the toxicity profile and considered together with patient characteristics to provide the most appropriate, safe, and cost-effective therapy.

KEY POINTS

1. Although the pharmacokinetic characteristics of nonsteroidal antiinflammatory drugs (NSAIDs) are similar, pharmacodynamic differences in cyclooxygenase-1 (COX-1) and COX-2 inhibition account for differences in NSAID toxicity.

2. NSAIDs may have a benefit in the management of pain, inflammation, and fever in selected critically ill patients. All nonselective and COX-2-selective NSAIDs exert similar efficacy for these indications.

3. The most common toxicities associated with NSAIDs are gastrointestinal, cardiovascular, and renal and are related primarily to COX inhibition and decreased synthesis of prostaglandins on this basis.

4. When NSAID therapy is initiated in critically ill patients, the risk for toxicity must be considered. A COX-2-selective inhibitor should be used cautiously in patients with underlying cardiovascular disease.

ANNOTATED REFERENCES

Rodriguez LAG, Tolosa LB. Risk of upper gastrointestinal complications among users of traditional NSAIDs and COXIBs in the general population. Gastroenterology 2007;132:498-506.
This nested case control study of a large database identified cases of gastrointestinal complications in patients receiving nonselective NSAIDs or coxibs. The rate of gastrointestinal toxicity was slightly higher with the nonselective NSAIDs. Daily dose and plasma exposure of NSAIDs were the primary risk factors. The use of aspirin concurrently with coxibs negated any benefit over non-select NSAIDs.
Amer M, Bead VR, Bathon J, Blumenthal RS, Edwards DN. Use of nonsteroidal anti-inflammatory drugs in patients with cardiovascular disease. A cautionary tale. Cardiol Rev 2010;18204-12.
This review article is a concise overview of the mechanism, adverse events, and role of NSAIDs in patients with cardiovascular disease. Until further data are available, the authors recommend caution in use of

COX-1 and COX-2 inhibitors for musculoskeletal disorders in patients with existing gastrointestinal or cardiovascular conditions.
Silverstein FE, Faich G, Goldstein JL, et al. Gastrointestinal toxicity with celecoxib vs nonsteroidal antiinflammatory drugs for osteoarthritis and rheumatoid arthritis the CLASS study: a randomized controlled trial. JAMA 2000;284:1247-55.
This prospective, randomized, multicenter study compared the gastrointestinal toxicity (perforation, ulceration, bleeding) of celecoxib with those of ibuprofen and diclofenac. Although there was a trend toward reduction in gastrointestinal endpoints for the primary outcome, a significant reduction in gastrointestinal events was seen with celecoxib for the composite of ulceration, perforation, bleeding, and symptomatic ulcers. Concomitant aspirin use was permitted in this trial.

REFERENCES

Access the complete reference list online at http://www.expertconsult.com.

184

Opioids

NICOLE C. BOUCHARD | LEWIS S. NELSON

History

Few medicines have graced history as have opium and its derivatives. The Sumerians used and cultivated the opium poppy as early as the third millennium BC. Further accounts of its religious and medicinal use are recorded in manuscripts dating back to ancient Egyptian, Greek, and Roman times. Opium is obtained from the opium poppy, *Papaver somniferum*. Incision of the mature seedpod yields opium, a brown saplike gum. Crude opium contains as many as 20 different alkaloids, including approximately 10% morphine and 0.5% codeine.

In 1806, a German pharmacist, Sertürner, isolated the most active alkaloid from opium and named it *morphine*, after Morpheus, the Greek god of dreams. In 1874, heroin was first synthesized from morphine and subsequently marketed as an opioid more potent than morphine and free of abuse potential. The invention of hypodermic needles revolutionized surgery and created a new avenue for abuse. In 1914 in the United States, the landmark Harrison Narcotic Act was passed, prohibiting the nonmedicinal use of opioids. Morphine and related compounds remain essential components of the medical pharmacologic armamentarium but also remain widely abused substances around the world.

Nomenclature

The term *opiate* refers specifically to opioids derived directly from the opium poppy, namely morphine and codeine, whereas the broader term, *opioid*, encompasses a wide range of compounds that display opium-like effects by binding to opioid receptors. The opioids include all of the natural opiates as well as semisynthetic opioids (e.g., oxycodone, heroin) and synthetic opioids (e.g., meperidine, methadone). The term *narcotic* classically has been used in association with illicit drugs of abuse, not necessarily opioids. In the strictest use of the word, "narcotic," derived from the Greek *narcosis*, refers to a drug that induces a somnolent state.

Pharmacology and Receptor Physiology

Opioids act as agonists at opioid receptors at presynaptic and postsynaptic sites in various regions of the brain and spinal cord including the periaqueductal gray area of the brainstem, amygdala, corpus striatum, thalamus, and medulla, as well as the substantia gelatinosa (dorsal/posterior horn) in the spinal cord. Opioid receptors are also found in peripheral tissues at afferent pain neurons, in the smooth muscle of the gastrointestinal (GI) tract, and intraarticularly. Agonism at opioid receptors decreases neurotransmission through pain neurons, both in the periphery and in the spinal cord. Opioid receptor agonism also diminishes the brain's perception of pain. This reduction in nerve transmission occurs through alteration of the release of neurotransmitters such as acetylcholine, norepinephrine, dopamine, serotonin (5-hydroxytryptamine [5-HT]), glutamate, and substance P. Decreased neurotransmission is thought to be secondary to membrane hyperpolarization or decreased release of neurotransmitters from presynaptic vesicles or both.[1]

Three major subtypes of opioid receptors have been identified: mu, delta, and kappa. All these are G protein–coupled receptors and have seven transmembrane helices with significant sequence homology. Opioid receptor agonists and antagonists interact with one or more of these receptors with varying affinities.[1,2] This Greek-derived nomenclature is commonly used by most of the scientific community. In 1996, the International Union of Pharmacology (IUPHAR) recommended a new nomenclature for opioid receptors, having as a goal consistency in naming with other neurotransmitter systems (Table 184-1).[3] The traditional Greek notations are used in this text. Several other new receptor subtypes have been identified. Their clinical significance and classification are unclear at this time.

Pharmacokinetics

ABSORPTION

Most opioids are well absorbed via the subcutaneous (SQ) and intramuscular (IM) routes. Although GI absorption tends to be rapid, the oral bioavailability of many opioids is limited by extensive first-pass hepatic metabolism. After large oral (PO) doses, first-pass metabolism can become saturated, and oral bioavailability can be increased. Codeine and oxycodone are two opioids with very good oral bioavailability. The transdermal application of fentanyl is also used in clinical practice.

DISTRIBUTION

Tissue uptake is variable and depends largely on the drug's lipophilicity. Highly lipophilic compounds such as fentanyl readily penetrate the central nervous system (CNS), the dura of the spinal column, and tissue "reservoirs." Opioids exhibit varying degrees of plasma protein binding and typically have large volumes of distribution. Serum concentrations of opioids should not be used as a gauge of clinical effect, because fat, skeletal muscle, lungs, and viscera act as reservoirs after opioid administration. Redistribution from saturated tissue depots can produce persistent or recurrent sedation after discontinuation of prolonged infusions of certain opioids such as fentanyl.[4]

METABOLISM

Hepatic metabolism of opioids, typically by the P450 cytochromes, CYP3A4 and CYP2D6, can produce metabolites with either greater or lesser activity than the parent compound. For example, codeine is an active antitussive agent but an ineffective analgesic. The metabolism of codeine to morphine by CYP2D6 reduces its antitussive actions but markedly improves its analgesic properties. Morphine and its semisynthetic derivatives are converted to polar glucuronide metabolites, some of which are active. Metabolism of certain opioids also occurs by similar mechanisms in extrahepatic sites, especially the kidneys.

ELIMINATION

Most opioids and their metabolites are cleared by the kidneys and require dosing adjustments in patients with renal failure. Biliary excretion is limited for most opioids.

Clinically Important Effects in the Intensive Care Unit

Analgesia, euphoria, sedation, miosis, and respiratory depression are considered to be the classic opioid effects. In addition, opioids have

TABLE 184-1	Opioid Receptor Subtypes and Their Associated Clinical Effects			
Traditional notation	mu_1	mu_2	delta	$kappa_{1,2,3}$
IUPHAR notation	OP_{3a}	OP_{3b}	OP_1	$OP2_{a,b,c}$
Endogenous ligand	Endorphins	Endorphins	Enkephalins	Dynorphins
Effect	Analgesia (supraspinal and peripheral), sedation, euphoria, urinary retention, miosis, hypothermia	Analgesia (spinal), respiratory depression, bradycardia, physical dependence, gastrointestinal effects, pruritus, growth hormone release	Analgesia (spinal and supraspinal), antitussive effect, modulation of mu receptor function, inhibition of dopamine release	Analgesia (spinal and supraspinal) antitussive effect, psychotomimesis, dysphoria, miosis, diuresis

Data from Dhawan BN, Cesselin F, Raghubir R et al. International Union of Pharmacology. XII. Classification of opioid receptors. Pharmacol Rev 1996;48:567-92.[3]
IUPHAR, International Union of Pharmacology.

many more clinically relevant effects, many of which are not typically relevant in the intensive care unit (ICU) setting; these are summarized by physiologic system in Table 184-2.

ANALGESIA

Opioids are modulators of pain perception both at the level of the CNS and in the periphery. High concentrations of opioid receptors (largely of the mu subtype) are found in areas of the brain that are associated with analgesia. Cortical effects include decreased reception of painful sensory inputs and enhanced inhibitory outflow from the brain to the sensory nuclei of the spinal cord (dorsal root nuclei). In addition, there is decreased neurotransmission from peripheral afferent pain neurons to the spinal cord and from the spinothalamic tract to the brain. The net effect is decreased perception of nociceptive information. Analgesia is mediated by the mu, delta, and kappa opioid receptor subtypes (see Table 184-1). Morphine also appears to be an effective analgesic (via the mu opioid receptor) when administered intraarticularly.[5] Tolerance develops to the analgesic effects with repeated use.

Very low doses of naloxone (e.g., 0.25 µg/kg/h) improve the efficacy of morphine analgesia, whereas at higher doses (1 µg/kg/h), analgesia is obliterated by naloxone. The mechanism of this effect is unclear.[6]

EUPHORIA

The euphoric effects of opioids are typically described as pleasant, floating sensations accompanied by a decrease in anxiety and distress.

TABLE 184-2	Summary of Clinical Effects of Opioids by Physiologic System
System	*Clinical Effect*
Cardiovascular	Hypotension (vasomotor centers and histamine), bradycardia (first or second degree), dysrhythmias (overdose, propoxyphene), QRS prolongation (propoxyphene), QT prolongation (methadone)
Dermatologic	Urticaria, flushing, pruritus (centrally mediated)
Endocrinologic	Reduced release of antidiuretic hormone (controversial), reduced release of gonadotropin
Gastrointestinal	Nausea, vomiting ($5-HT_2$ mediated), delayed gastric emptying, constipation, increased smooth muscle tone (biliary tract, intestinal, pylorus, anal sphincter)
Genitourinary	Urinary retention, ureteral spasm, decreased renal function and renal blood flow, antidiuresis, priapism (neuraxial use)
Immunologic	Mast cell degranulation/histamine release, cytokine stimulation (IL-1), but true allergic reaction is rare
Maternal/fetal	Placental transmission, neonatal blood-brain barrier immature, neonatal respiratory depression and opioid dependence, neonatal withdrawal (seizures)
Musculoskeletal	Truncal/chest wall rigidity and myoclonus (fentanyl derivatives)
Neurologic	Analgesia, euphoria, sedation, psychotomimesis, seizures (meperidine, propoxyphene, tramadol, rarely fentanyl)
Ophthalmic	Miosis, normal or dilated pupils (meperidine, pentazocine, diphenoxylate, propoxyphene, severe systemic hypoxia)
Pulmonary	Respiratory depression, antitussive effect, bronchospasm, pulmonary edema

5-HT, serotonin; *IL,* interleukin.

Not all exogenous opioids induce the same degree of euphoria. Activation of the mu/delta receptor complex in the ventral tegmental area, followed by dopamine release in the mesolimbic system, is most likely responsible for these effects.[7]

The degree of lipophilicity and CNS penetration is directly proportional to the euphoric properties of the opioid. For example, heroin, which enters the CNS with relative ease, is associated with greater euphoria than is the less lipophilic opioid, morphine.[8] Fentanyl produces euphoric effects akin to those of heroin and is occasionally used as an adulterant in illicitly obtained heroin.[9] The apparently enhanced euphoric effect of meperidine may be related to its lipophilicity and its ability to alter serotonergic neurotransmission.

By contrast, pentazocine, an agonist-antagonist opioid (i.e., an agent that is both an agonist at kappa receptors and an antagonist at mu opioid receptors), produces dysphoria and psychotomimesis (psychotic symptoms), an effect that most likely is mediated via $kappa_2$ receptor agonism.[10] Pentazocine also can induce a withdrawal syndrome in opioid-tolerant individuals secondary to its mu opioid receptor antagonist effects. For these reasons, many patients previously exposed to pentazocine will cite allergies to it.

SEDATION

Drowsiness and mental clouding are frequent in opioid-using patients. Different opioids are associated with different degrees of sedation despite equianalgesic dosing. Unlike sedative hypnotics, there is little or no associated amnesia unless the patient has been comatose. Electroencephalograms (EEGs) of opioid-sedated patients usually show slow delta waves that resemble sleep.

RESPIRATORY DEPRESSION

All opioid agonists produce dose-dependent depression of ventilation. At equianalgesic doses, all opioid agonists lead to a similar degree of respiratory depression.[11,12] In the absence of secondary causes, death from opioid overdose is almost exclusively caused by respiratory depression.

Medullary mu_2 receptors are thought to be responsible for the development of respiratory depression. Stimulation of these receptors diminishes chemoreceptor sensitivity to hypercapnia, resulting in loss of hypercarbic ventilatory stimulation.[13] Activation of these receptors also decreases the central response to hypoxia[13] and inhibits the medullary and pontine respiratory centers that regulate the rhythm of breathing.[12] The combination of these effects leads to prolonged pauses between breaths, periodic breathing, hypopnea, bradypnea, and in extreme cases, apnea. It is important to note that the initial manifestation of respiratory depression may be a hypopnea, with or without a decrease in respiratory rate.[12]

Patients do not develop complete tolerance to the respiratory depressant effects of the opioids.[14] For example, patients enrolled in methadone maintenance therapy can experience chronic hypoventilation and hypercapnia.[15] A ceiling effect on respiratory depression exists with partial agonist and agonist-antagonist opioids such as nalbuphine and buprenorphine.

Certain groups of patients are particularly sensitive to the ventilatory depressant effects of opioids. These groups include the elderly, patients with chronically elevated Paco$_2$ (e.g., some patients with chronic obstructive pulmonary disease [COPD]), and patients with a depressed level of consciousness for other reasons. A strong painful stimulus sometimes can transiently overcome or prevent respiratory depression. Similarly, during procedural sedation (e.g., for orthopedic reductions) when pain is relieved, respiratory depression can become apparent. Bronchoconstriction also can occur, most likely as a result of histamine release as well as indirect effects on bronchiolar smooth muscle. Depression of ventilation also can occur in patients receiving neuraxial opioid administration; these effects may be delayed and may be accompanied by respiratory depression (see "Neuraxial Opioids").

SEIZURES

Seizures are rare with therapeutic use of most opioids, the primary exception being tramadol. If seizures occur in the setting of an acute opioid overdose, hypoxia is likely the cause. Seizures are associated with meperidine, propoxyphene, and tramadol toxicity. These drugs are further discussed in a later section. In a mouse model, naloxone antagonized the convulsant effects of propoxyphene, but not those of meperidine or its metabolite, normeperidine.[16] Fentanyl-induced myoclonus can resemble seizure activity, but true seizures are rarely caused by fentanyl.[17]

MUSCULOSKELETAL EFFECTS: TRUNCAL RIGIDITY AND MOVEMENT DISORDERS

Intravenous (IV) administration of opioids has been associated with motor abnormalities ranging from increased tone to overt myoclonus and involving the chest wall and other truncal muscles. This complication is seen when large doses of highly lipophilic opioids such as fentanyl, sufentanil, remifentanil, or alfentanil are administered rapidly by the IV route.[18] Whereas it was previously thought that opioid actions at the level of the spinal cord were responsible for this effect, it now appears that a central dopaminergic effect may be contributory. Both naloxone and neuromuscular blockade can overcome rigidity. Vocal cord spasm, although rare, can cause closure of the vocal cords, leading to difficult bag-valve-mask ventilation. As noted, myoclonic activity resembling seizure activity has been observed in patients after being rapidly infused with large doses of fentanyl.[17] Serotonin syndrome, characterized by coarse tremors, increased muscular tone, myoclonus, agitation, and autonomic instability, has been associated with the use of both meperidine and dextromethorphan in combination with other serotonergic agents.

CARDIOVASCULAR EFFECTS

The peripheral arterial and venous dilation caused by opioids appears to be mediated by both central depression of vasomotor centers and histamine release.[19] Hypotension occurs more frequently in stressed individuals and in those with decreased intravascular volume. Histamine release occurs via non–immunoglobulin (Ig)E-mediated mast cell degranulation.[20] Different opioids produce different degrees of histamine release; for example, meperidine and morphine produce much greater release of histamine than fentanyl and sufentanil.[21] The severity of histamine-mediated responses can be reduced by slowing the rate of infusion, and hypotension can be reduced by optimizing intravascular volume. Use of Trendelenburg position and saline infusion are appropriate initial interventions for opioid-associated hypotension.

Bradycardia is occasionally associated with opioid use and is most often secondary to decreased excitatory stimulation and hypoxia. Primary opioid-induced bradycardia is relatively rare and is thought to be related to increased vagal nerve activity. Morphine also can exert direct slowing effects on the sinoatrial and atrioventricular nodes.

Overall, there are no consistent effects of opioids on cardiac output or the electrocardiogram (ECG). Wide-complex dysrhythmias and impaired contractility are associated with propoxyphene overdose via sodium channel blockade (class Ia antidysrhythmic effect). Illicit opioid use sometimes is associated with cardiac effects secondary to adulterants or co-ingestants; examples are quinine and cocaine ("speedball"). Chronic high-dose methadone use is associated with prolongation of the QT interval.[22]

EFFECTS ON CEREBRAL CIRCULATION

There are minimal effects on cerebral circulation except in the setting of respiratory depression with hypoventilation and increased arterial partial pressure of carbon dioxide (Paco$_2$). Increased Paco$_2$ causes cerebral vasodilatation and increased cerebral blood flow, both of which can increase intracranial pressure. These effects are of importance for the treatment of head injuries or increased intracranial pressure from other causes. In the absence of hypoventilation, opioids actually decrease cerebral blood flow and possibly intracranial pressure.

▧ Specific Agents

Opioids are among the most widely used drugs in clinical practice. A comprehensive knowledge of their effects and therapeutic applications is essential for any intensive care provider. Table 184-3 summarizes specific agents used in clinical practice.

MORPHINE

Morphine is the prototypical opiate. Its pharmacologic effects are primarily caused by binding to the mu opioid receptor and, to a much lesser extent, the delta and kappa opioid receptors. It is a potent analgesic with typical opioid side effects including sedation, respiratory depression, decreased GI motility, nausea and vomiting, histamine release, and miosis. Despite its efficacy, morphine has relatively poor penetration into the CNS, largely because of its low lipid solubility.

The principal pathway of morphine metabolism is via glucuronidation in the liver and kidneys. The active metabolite, morphine-6-glucuronide, is more potent than morphine and is largely excreted via the kidneys. Renal failure can lead to accumulation of this active metabolite, leading to unexpected toxic effects after even low doses.

HEROIN

Heroin, also referred to as *diacetylmorphine*, is a highly lipophilic, semisynthetic opioid produced by acetylation of morphine. Heroin is a prodrug and is devoid of intrinsic opioid effects. It rapidly enters the CNS, where it is deacetylated to the active metabolites, monoacetylmorphine and morphine. Illicit heroin is typically administered by nasal insufflation, SQ injection (i.e., "skin popping"), smoking, or IV injection. The practice of inhaling vapors from heroin heated in aluminum foil is termed "chasing the dragon"; it is associated with a rapidly progressive, irreversible spongiform leukoencephalopathy.[23-25]

HYDROMORPHONE

Hydromorphone is a semisynthetic opioid that acts primarily at the mu receptor. It is a hydrated ketone derivative of morphine. Hydromorphone has become more popular in recent years in the emergency department, in postoperative and outpatient settings, and in the ICU. It is approximately 8 to 10 times more potent than morphine and may be associated with a lower risk of dependence. Hydromorphone also appears to have a better side-effect profile than morphine, as it tends to be associated with less nausea and pruritus.

MEPERIDINE

Meperidine is a synthetic opioid that acts at both mu and kappa receptors. At equianalgesic doses, its side-effect profile is similar to

TABLE 184-3 Summary of Opioids Used in Clinical Practice

Agent	Receptor Effect*	Preparations and Routes of Administration	Typical Doses	Comments
Natural Opioids				
Codeine†	mu > delta, kappa	PO, SQ, IM, IV	Antitussive: 15 mg PO Analgesic: 60-120 mg PO	Mild to moderate pain, antitussive
Morphine (MSIR, MS Contin)	mu ≫ delta, kappa	PO, PR, SQ, IM, IV, SR, NA	IR: 10-30 mg PO q 4 h CR: 30-200 mg PO q 8-12 h 0.1-0.2 mg/kg IM/SQ or slow IV q 4 h PCA: see guidelines elsewhere in this section	Moderate to severe pain, prototype opioid, prolonged effects with CR formulations
Semisynthetic Opioids				
Hydrocodone† (Vicodin, Norco)	mu	PO	2.5-10 mg PO q 4-6 h	Moderate to severe pain
Hydromorphone (Dilaudid)	mu	PO, SQ, PR, IV, NA	2-4 mg PO q 4-6 h or 3 mg PR q 6-8 h 0.5-2 mg IM/SQ or slow IV q 4-6 h	Moderate to severe pain
Oxycodone† (Percocet, OxyContin)	mu	PO	IR: 5 mg PO q 6 h CR: 10-40 mg PO q 12 h	Moderate pain, prolonged effects with CR formulations
Oxymorphone (Numorphan)	mu	SQ, PR, IM, IV	1-1.5 mg IM/SQ q 4-6 h 0.5 mg IV q 4 h	Moderate to severe pain
Synthetic Opioids				
Propoxyphene† (Darvon)	mu, Ia antidysrhythmic	PO	65 mg PO q 4 h	Moderate pain, seizures, dysrhythmias, rhabdomyolysis
Meperidine (Demerol)	mu and kappa, 5-HT	PO, SQ, IM, IV, NA	Analgesia: 50-100 mg IV q 2-4 h Shivering: 25-50 mg IV	Moderate to severe pain, treatment of shivering, seizures, serotonin syndrome
Methadone (Dolophine)	mu	PO, SQ, IM	Analgesia: 2.5-20 mg PO/SQ/IM q 3-4 h MMST: usually 20-200 mg PO daily	Moderate to severe pain; caution with repeat doses; long-acting (>24 h)
Fentanyl (Oralet, Actiq, Duragesic patches, Sublimaze)	mu	PO (lollipop), transdermal, IV, NA	Lollipop: 5-15 μg/kg PO every dose Transdermal: 25-100 μg/h q 72 h Analgesia/procedures: 1-2 μg/kg IV Infusion: 5-50 μg/h IV, titrate	Severe pain, very short-acting (<1 h), truncal rigidity (rapid IV admin), accumulation
Sufentanil	mu	IV, NA	Analgesia: 0.1-0.4 μg/kg IV Anesthesia: 10-30 μg/kg IV Infusion: 0.5 μg/kg/h, titrate	Severe pain, ultra-short-acting, vocal cord closure, favorable hemodynamics
Alfentanil	mu agonist	IV	Infusion: 25 μg/kg/h, titrate	Ultra-short-acting, potent respiratory depression, CYP3A4/5 interactions
Remifentanil	mu agonist	IV	Bolus 0.5-1 μg/kg over 30-60 sec Infusion: 0.1-0.15 μg/kg/min, titrate	Most ultra-short-acting, organ-independent metabolism by esterases; no accumulation
"Nonopioid" Opioids				
Tramadol (Ultram)	weak mu, inhibits NE and 5-HT reuptake	PO, IM, IV	Analgesia: 50-100 mg PO q 4-6 h Shivering: 1 mg/kg IV	Moderate pain, treatment of shivering, seizures
Dextromethorphan ("DM" cough preparations)	NMDA and 5-HT	PO	10-30 mg PO q 4-6 h	Antitussive, other psychoactive effects, poor response to naloxone, serotonin syndrome
Opioid Agonist/Antagonist Opioids				
Buprenorphine‡ (Buprenex, Subutex, Suboxone)	partial mu agonist, kappa antagonist	SL, IM, IV	4-16 mg SL daily 0.3-0.6 mg IM/IV q 6-8 h	Moderate to severe pain, opioid replacement therapy
Butorphanol (Stadol)	kappa agonist, mu antagonist	Intranasal, IM, IV	1-4 mg IM or 0.5-2 mg IV q 3-4 h	Moderate pain
Pentazocine‡ (Talwin)	kappa agonist, mu antagonist	PO, IM, IV	50 mg PO q 3-4 h 30 mg IM/IV q 3-4 h	Moderate pain, dysphoria, opioid withdrawal in tolerant patients
Opioid Antagonists				
Naloxone (Narcan)	mu, kappa, delta antagonist	IM, IV, PO (very limited bioavailability)	Pruritus/analgesia§: 0.25 μg/kg/h IV Antidote: 0.05-2 mg IV q 2-5 min titrate; use very low doses in tolerant patients	Antidote for reversal of opioid effect, continuous infusions for OD with CR opioids or body packer
Naltrexone (Trexan)	mu antagonist	PO	50 mg PO daily	Long-acting (>24 h)
Peripherally Acting Mu-Opioid Receptor Antagonists (PAMORAs)				
Methylnaltrexone (Relistor)	peripheral mu-antagonist	SQ (PO experimental)	0.15-0.3 mg/kg SQ q 48 h (please see package insert for details)	Associated with abdominal cramping, flatulence
Alvimopan (Entereg)	peripheral mu-antagonist	PO	12 mg PO BID (please see package insert for details)	Associated with anemia, hypokalemia, restricted to hospital use

*Agonism unless specified.

†Preparations may also contain acetaminophen or acetylsalicylic acid.

‡May contain naloxone in some oral formulations as a deterrent to parenteral use of the drug.

§For use with continuous infusions of neuraxial opioids or PCA.

CR, controlled release; *5-HT,* serotonin; *IM,* intramuscular; *IV,* intravenous; *IR,* immediate release; *MMST,* methadone maintenance substitution therapy; *NA,* neuraxial; *NE,* norepinephrine; *NMDA,* N-methyl-D-aspartate; *PCA,* patient-controlled analgesia; *PO,* per os; *PR,* per rectum; *SQ,* subcutaneous; *SL,* sublingual; *SR,* sustained release.

morphine's, except meperidine causes more euphoria and pronounced orthostatic hypotension from vasodilation and histamine release.

Of special note is meperidine's extensive hepatic metabolism (90%) to normeperidine, a less potent analgesic eliminated via the kidneys. Normeperidine produces CNS excitation and is associated with myoclonus, delirium, and seizures. Metabolite accumulation occurs primarily in the context of escalating doses and renal failure.[26,27] Meperidine also blocks reuptake of serotonin by presynaptic neurons in the CNS, and by this mechanism may produce serotonin toxicity in patients who are taking monoamine oxidase inhibitors (MAOIs)[28] or other serotonergic drugs (see "Drug Interactions").[29,30] The potential for these side effects, especially seizures, has led to a decline in the popularity of meperidine in many institutions.

Unique ICU uses for meperidine include suppression of shivering in postoperative patients, in patients undergoing therapeutic cooling/hypothermia, and in those receiving blood products or amphotericin. This effect is most likely mediated by changes in the shivering threshold.

FENTANYL, ALFENTANIL, REMIFENTANIL, AND SUFENTANIL

Fentanyl, alfentanil, remifentanil, and sufentanil are synthetic opioids of the 4-anilidopiperidine group. They are metabolized by the liver and subject to bioaccumulation with resultant prolonged clinical effects during continuous infusions.

Around the world, fentanyl is the most widely used of this group of drugs. It has a rapid onset and a short duration of effect and is an important drug for use in the ICU. Fentanyl's peak effect occurs within 6 to 7 minutes after IV administration. Its very short half-life results from rapid distribution into inactive tissues such as fat, lungs, and skeletal muscle. Prolonged infusions or massive doses may lead to accumulation of the drug within these tissue reservoirs, resulting in prolonged duration of effect after discontinuation of the infusion. Lung uptake of up to 75% of a parenteral dose can occur and is often referred to as *first-pass pulmonary uptake*. Fentanyl is associated with fewer cardiovascular effects and histamine release than either morphine or meperidine.[31] It undergoes extensive hepatic metabolism to norfentanyl, an active metabolite eliminated by the kidneys. Prolonged effects can be seen in the elderly and in patients with renal impairment. Fentanyl-associated myoclonus may resemble seizure activity, but EEGs recorded in these patients failed to show seizure activity.[17] Muscle rigidity, particularly of the chest wall, may hamper spontaneous or assisted ventilation. Although this effect can be reversed with naloxone, administration of naloxone simultaneously reduces the analgesic effect of fentanyl.

Sufentanil is a fentanyl analog and 5 to 10 times more potent as an analgesic than fentanyl. Sufentanil offers the advantage of even greater hemodynamic stability, and it is an analgesic of choice in cardiac surgery. Following cessation of a prolonged infusion, persistent sedation is not as prominent with sufentanil as it is with fentanyl. Sufentanil should be considered a practical and appropriate analgesic option for use in selected cases in the ICU.

Alfentanil has the shortest duration of action and the most rapid onset of this group. Alfentanil's unique metabolism by hepatic cytochrome P4503A (CYP3A4 and 5) enzymes render its metabolism variable and unpredictable. Polymorphisms in the genes coding for these cytochromes and inhibition by other drugs, including some macrolide antibiotics, protease inhibitors, and antifungal agents, such as fluconazole, can make its effects less consistent, particularly when administered by prolonged infusion.[32,33]

Remifentanil is an ultra-short-acting mu opioid receptor agonist with a unique pharmacokinetic profile. Though it is a 4-anilidopiperidine like fentanyl, alfentanil, and sufentanil, remifentanil is metabolized directly by nonspecific blood and tissue esterases to remifentanil acid (RA). RA is a relatively inactive metabolite. Remifentanil has a terminal half-life of approximately 10 to 20 minutes and a context-sensitive half-life of 2 to 4 minutes, even following prolonged infusions. Time

to extubation in mechanically ventilated ICU patients is remarkably short after discontinuing remifentanil (15-45 minutes).[34-36] This effect is preserved regardless of the presence of other drugs, disease, or organ failure.[37,38] Despite RA's predominantly renal elimination, and unlike fentanyl and its analogs, renal impairment does not appear to significantly affect time to extubation in patients on continuous infusions of remifentanil.[35-37,39] The properties of organ-independent metabolism, lack of accumulation, and precision and predictability of onset and offset make remifentanil a promising sole agent or combined agent (often with propofol or midazolam) in analgesia-based sedation in ventilated ICU patients.[35-44] As with other opioids, bradycardia, hypotension, muscle rigidity and nausea can occur with remifentanil. Limiting boluses to 0.5 µg/kg is suggested to decrease the incidence of muscle rigidity.[35] Whether remifentanil, like other opioids, can reduce cortisol release—a well-established phenomenon in mechanically ventilated and sedated ICU patients—has yet to be determined.[45] A recent meta-analysis of remifentanil infusions compared to other regimens in mechanically ventilated ICU patients showed no significant benefit on outcomes such as duration of mechanical ventilation, length of stay, or mortality.[36] Remifentanil injections contain glycine and should not be given via neuraxial routes (epidural or intrathecal). Dosing should be based on ideal body weight in obese patients.

METHADONE

Methadone is a synthetic opioid with high oral bioavailability and a prolonged duration of action (>24 hours). Its most common use is in substitution therapy for opioid dependence. It is also used as an analgesic in patients with chronic pain. Methadone is hepatically metabolized to inactive metabolites that undergo urinary and biliary excretion. Overall, its side-effect profile resembles that of morphine, although the (desirable and undesirable) effects of methadone persist for substantially longer. Methadone causes less euphoria and less sedation than other opioids. Tolerance to methadone may require escalating doses when it is used for prolonged periods. Methadone at high doses can prolong the QT interval and increase the risk of torsades de pointes.[22]

BUPRENORPHINE

Buprenorphine is a partial agonist that has 50 times greater affinity for the mu opioid receptor than morphine. It is therefore relatively resistant to antagonism by naloxone and can displace other opioids from mu opioid receptors. It is rarely used as an analgesic but is slowly replacing methadone as the standard agent for substitution therapy in patients with opioid abuse (i.e., Subutex, Suboxone). Because it is a partial mu opioid agonist, there may be less ventilatory depression associated with buprenorphine than with full agonist opioids; a "ceiling effect" exists such that no further respiratory depression occurs beyond a certain dose range. Nevertheless, buprenorphine can still be abused, and particularly when abused in combination with other respiratory depressants, its use can be lethal.

NALOXONE

Naloxone is a pure competitive antagonist at mu, delta, and kappa opioid receptors. It is commonly used in both prehospital and hospital settings to reverse opioid-induced respiratory depression. The typical prehospital dose of naloxone employed by emergency medical service personnel to treat respiratory depression and/or coma is in the range of 0.4 to 2 mg (IM or IV). However, these high doses often precipitate a dramatic and dangerous withdrawal syndrome in tolerant individuals. Vomiting, aspiration, and severe agitation are common with antagonist-precipitated acute withdrawal (see "Opioid Overdose"). Aspiration is a particular risk after use of naloxone in opioid-dependent patients who have nonopioid causes for their depressed level of consciousness. In these patients, naloxone produces vomiting but does not fully awaken the patient, predisposing to aspiration. It appears to be safer and equally effective in most situations to administer 0.04 to

0.05 mg (40-50 µg) IV and titrate upwards at similar doses every 2 to 3 minutes while providing ventilatory support as needed until the desired clinical response is attained.

Some sources recommend the use of low-dose naloxone infusions (0.25 µg/kg/h) to protect against ventilatory depression and decrease symptoms of pruritus, nausea, and vomiting in patients receiving continuous opioid infusions, in addition to augmenting analgesia.[6] In the ICU setting, this approach may benefit patients who are receiving patient-controlled analgesia (PCA) or neuraxial (i.e., epidural or spinal) analgesia.

Of note, orally administered naloxone has very poor bioavailability because of an extensive first-pass effect and therefore produces minimal if any systemic effects. It is included in some oral analgesic preparations as a deterrent to parenteral abuse (see Table 184-3).

METHYLNALTREXONE AND ALVIMOPAN

Methylnaltrexone and alvimopan have been approved recently by the U.S. Food and Drug Administration (FDA) and are members of a new class of drugs: peripherally acting mu opioid receptor antagonists (PAMORAs). In contrast to naloxone, these newly approved drugs do not cross the blood-brain barrier and therefore do not antagonize the central (analgesic) effects of opioids. They act on peripheral opioid receptors only, blocking side effects such as constipation and ileus while preserving centrally mediated analgesia.[46-49] Methylnaltrexone (SQ) is also used for the treatment of opioid-induced constipation in patients with advanced cancer and AIDS.[50-52] It is administered via the SQ route, although experimentally, higher doses of enteric-coated formulations have been effective in increasing GI motility. Alvimopan (PO) has been approved for the treatment of postoperative ileus following bowel resection.[53] PAMORAs, as members of a novel drug class, have led to some realizations concerning the peripheral versus central effects of opioids. It appears that GI motility, pruritus (partly), nausea and vomiting, cough reflex (partly), and urinary retention may be mediated by peripheral opioid receptors. Chronic constipation in patients on chronic methadone maintenance is another area of research.[46-49] Interestingly, effects mediated through activation of peripheral opioid receptors also have been implicated as promoting decreased cellular immunity, increased angiogenesis, increased vascular permeability, and increased bacterial lethality (particularly *Pseudomonas aeruginosa*).[46] These are areas of active research in both the basic science and clinical arenas.

Special Clinical Situations

TOLERANCE, DEPENDENCE, AND WITHDRAWAL

Tolerance and dependence are inevitable features of chronic opioid use. *Tolerance* refers to decreasing effectiveness and the need for higher doses with repeated use, whereas *dependence* refers to the occurrence of withdrawal symptoms on cessation of the drug. Cross-tolerance exists between various opioids but is imperfect. Tolerance usually takes 2 to 3 weeks to develop with analgesic doses of morphine and can occur without dependence. Some mild degree of physical dependence can occur after as brief a period as 48 hours of continuous medication. This consideration is important in the care of patients using PCA devices and symptomatic heroin body packers (individuals who ingests wrapped packets of illicit drugs to transport them).

Although tolerance, dependence, and abuse of opioids for the treatment of pain syndromes can be significant issues in clinical practice, undertreatment in patients with pain for fear of tolerance and dependence is a common mistake made by clinicians. The vast majority of patients can be treated effectively if clinical guidelines for opioid prescription are followed. If tolerance and dependence to opioid analgesics exists, patients may require very large doses to achieve a therapeutic effect. Consultation with a pain management specialist may be warranted for such individuals. Patients on a high-dose chronic methadone regimen are at risk for QT-interval prolongation.

The opioid withdrawal syndrome (OWS) encompasses a consistent cluster of symptoms including initially abdominal cramps, yawning, lacrimation, piloerection, coryza, restlessness, and drug craving and later progressing to nausea, vomiting, and diarrhea. Altered mental status is rarely present in spontaneous OWS but is common in patients with OWS precipitated by administration of an opioid antagonist. Onset and duration of OWS varies with the duration of effect of the implicated opioid. Although it can be extremely distressing to the patient, OWS typically is not life threatening. Exceptions are acute withdrawal precipitated by large doses of an opioid antagonist in dependent individuals and opioid withdrawal in neonates. Treatment options for OWS include supportive care, treatment with antiemetics and clonidine (a centrally acting α₂-agonist that diminishes CNS symptoms), or administration of an opioid agonist, typically methadone. Administration of morphine and/or replacement of the prescribed opioid may be sufficient in a patient who is withdrawing from opioids taken for chronic pain.

OPIOID OVERDOSE

Classic findings in patients with opioid toxidromes are miosis, diminished bowel sounds, CNS depression, and respiratory depression; coma and apnea can be present in extreme cases. The major cause of death in opioid overdose is respiratory depression. Other complications are usually secondary to hypoxia (e.g., seizures, dysrhythmias, brain injury). Many patients with opioid overdose require admission to an ICU for monitoring, medical management, or respiratory support.

Naloxone, administered appropriately to reverse symptoms of respiratory depression, can obviate the need for endotracheal intubation in most cases. For example, for opioid overdoses in opioid-dependent patients (e.g., users of prescription analgesics, heroin, or methadone), a starting dose of 0.05 mg IV is indicated, using ventilatory support and rapid titration to higher doses as necessary. The endpoint of reversal should be adequate respiration, not complete reversal of sedation.[54] High doses of naloxone (e.g., 1 to 2 mg IV) may be used safely in nontolerant individuals. Continuous infusions may be appropriate for patients who have overdosed with long-acting opioids.[55,56] Symptomatic opioid body packers (i.e., people hired to swallow large amounts of tightly wrapped heroin packets and smuggle them across international borders) are likely to require continuous naloxone infusions until the packets are passed or removed.[56] Keeping symptomatic patients awake (with naloxone), administering whole-bowel irrigation using polyethylene glycol/electrolyte lavage solution at 0.5 to 2 L/h, and using a bedside commode can facilitate the patient's passage of the packets. Tolerance and dependence can occur in these patients if "leaking" is protracted. Body packers usually are not opioid users themselves.[56]

There is some suggestion that the catecholamine surge associated with rapid reversal with naloxone in tolerant individuals can precipitate acute lung injury (i.e., acute noncardiogenic pulmonary edema). Dog models of opioid overdose suggest that hypercapnia may worsen the catecholamine release associated with naloxone administration hemodynamics.[57,58] Adequate ventilation to normalize Paco₂ before antagonist administration is suggested to prevent hemodynamic instability. However, no single mechanism is sufficient to explain the development of opioid-associated pulmonary edema, and multiple factors are likely involved. There is an association between naloxone administration and the clinical *diagnosis* of pulmonary edema. The typical clinical presentation is an obtunded patient with profound respiratory depression who awakens either spontaneously or as the result of antagonist administration. In these situations, it is possible that patients with heroin overdose develop acute lung injury as a result of their respiratory depression or apnea, and that naloxone administration merely unmasks the effects of the opioid by restoring spontaneous respirations.[59] This model proposes that hypoxic pulmonary endothelial damage occurs during near-apneic periods. Acute lung injury and/or noncardiogenic pulmonary edema associated with opioid overdose should be treated with standard therapies and supportive care.

If acute withdrawal is precipitated by naloxone, supportive care is recommended. Sedation of an agitated patient experiencing acute withdrawal due to administration of naloxone often leads to even more profound sedation, leading to the necessity for endotracheal intubation once the effects of naloxone wane in 30 to 45 minutes. Withdrawal following naltrexone, a long-acting opioid antagonist, is more complex; some advocate high-dose opioid infusion to overcome the competitive antagonism.[60]

Many illicit drug users "co-ingest" other drugs of abuse such as cocaine (i.e., speedball), amphetamines, and benzodiazepines with opioids. The presence of one or more of these other drugs in the system can complicate the clinical presentation, and their toxic effects may be unmasked after the administration of naloxone. It is important to note that not all opioid-intoxicated patients present with miosis. Severe systemic hypoxia and presence of co-ingestants can produce normal-sized or dilated pupils.

Currently, no role has been established for methylnaltrexone and/or alvimopan in acute overdoses or symptomatic opioid body packers. Their lack of central effects, specifically lack of reversal of CNS and respiratory depression, routes of administration (SQ and PO, respectively), and prolonged duration of effects may limit their appropriateness in such cases.

Acetaminophen and acetylsalicylic acid (ASA) are common ingredients in analgesic combinations, and the presence of these drugs in the serum should be actively sought in any patient with a suicide attempt by overdose.

Consultation with a medical toxicologist or poison control center is strongly recommended for all cases of serious opioid overdose, especially those involving body packers, continuous-release preparations, ECG changes, or severe respiratory depression. Similar consultation is advised when caring for patients with antagonist-precipitated OWS.

DRUG INTERACTIONS

Opioids given in combination with either sedative-hypnotics (e.g., benzodiazepines) or propofol can have a synergistic effect on systemic vascular resistance,[61] level of sedation, and respiratory depression.[61-65]

Meperidine and dextromethorphan are associated with serotonin toxicity. This syndrome typically develops in patients who are simultaneously taking two proserotonergic drugs. Some commonly prescribed proserotonergic drugs include MAOIs, selective serotonin reuptake inhibitors (SSRIs), valproic acid, lithium, clonazepam, and buspirone. Patients taking proserotonergic drugs should not receive meperidine or dextromethorphan.[28-30,66] Morphine, fentanyl, and methadone are not associated with serotonin syndrome.

NEURAXIAL OPIOIDS

The term *neuraxial opioids* refers to administration of opioids into the epidural or subarachnoid space ("spinal"). The use of neuraxial opioids is common in the care of postoperative and traumatized patients in an intensive care setting. To exert their clinical effects, opioids have to diffuse across the dura and gain access to the substantia gelatinosa of the spinal cord. Opioid receptors in the spinal cord are of the mu, delta, and kappa type.

Neuraxial opioids tend to be associated with fewer systemic effects when compared with orally or parenterally administered opioids. Some highly lipophilic opioids (e.g., fentanyl, sufentanil) diffuse into the systemic circulation so quickly that their use in neuraxial analgesia offers little benefit over IV use. For other opioids, especially morphine and meperidine, systemic effects are usually caused by a combination of systemic absorption and cephalad migration of drug into the CNS. Typically, 5 to 10 times the dose used for spinal analgesia is required for epidural analgesia. Care should be taken to avoid inadvertent overdosing, which can occur if doses appropriate for epidural analgesia are injected into the subarachnoid space.

The common side effects of neuraxially administered opioids are pruritus, nausea and vomiting, urinary retention (via inhibition of parasympathetic neurons located in the sacral spinal cord), and ventilatory depression. Although early ventilatory depression rarely occurs, depression occurring within 2 hours after administration most likely represents systemic absorption of a lipid-soluble opioid. Delayed respiratory depression can be seen as long as 6 to 12 hours after neuraxial administration and most likely represents cephalad migration of opioid into the CNS.[67]

In general, neuraxial use of opioids should be considered safe and effective. Care should be taken with their use, because neuraxial opioid administration can cause CNS and systemic side effects. Most side effects respond to parenteral naloxone. The future role for PAMORAs in this setting has yet to be determined.

THE PATIENT WITH PAIN

In the ICU, analgesic requirements can be substantial, and opioids are often chosen because of their efficacy and predictability. Morphine, hydromorphone, fentanyl, sufentanil, and remifentanil are among the most commonly used opioids in the ICU setting. All modes of delivery are associated with systemic side effects. A more complete discussion of analgesia may be found in Chapter 3.

🔹 Summary

Use of opioids in the management of hospitalized and nonhospitalized patients is widespread, as is abuse of opioids in the community. A solid understanding of their physiologic effects in therapeutic and toxic doses is essential for intensive care physicians, especially when treating patients with pain. Withholding or underdosing of opioid analgesics due to fear of tolerance and dependence is not supported by the medical literature and is discouraged. Opioid-tolerant and opioid-dependent patients have different treatment needs, however, and require special attention by the medical staff. Appropriate use of naloxone, a short-acting antagonist, can prevent complications in many cases of opioid toxicity. Buprenorphine, a partial agonist-antagonist, is likely to replace methadone in many outpatient replacement-therapy treatment programs, and physicians need to become familiar with its unique properties. Consultation with a medical toxicologist or poison control center is recommended for managing complicated cases of opioid overdose.

KEY POINTS

1. Most opioids and their metabolites are cleared by the kidneys and require dosing adjustments in patients with renal failure and in the elderly.

2. If tolerance and dependence to opioid analgesics exist, patients may require very large doses to achieve a therapeutic effect. Most patients can be effectively treated if clinical guidelines for opioid prescription are followed.

3. Administration of an appropriate dose of naloxone to reverse symptoms of respiratory depression can avoid the necessity for endotracheal intubation in most cases of opioid toxicity. The suggested doses are 0.05 mg intravenously (IV) rapidly titrated to adequate respirations in opioid-tolerant patients, and 1 to 2 mg IV in nontolerant patients.

4. The empirical use of high-dose (0.4-2 mg) naloxone often precipitates dramatic antagonist-induced withdrawal syndrome in opioid-tolerant patients. This syndrome can be associated with vomiting, aspiration, catecholamine surge, and severe agitation.

5. Opioids can have synergistic effects on central nervous system depression and blood pressure if used in combination with other sedatives.

6. Use of meperidine should be avoided because accumulation of its metabolite is associated with seizures. It is also associated with serotonin syndrome in patients taking proserotoninergic medications.

ANNOTATED REFERENCES

Bailey PL, Egan TD, Stanley TH. Intravenous opioid anesthetics. In: Miller RD, editor. Anesthesia. Vol 1. 5th ed. Philadelphia: Churchill Livingstone; 2000. p. 273-376.

This chapter has an in-depth review of opioid physiology, pharmacodynamics, and pharmacokinetics, as well as concepts and applications that are applicable to both anesthesia and critical care settings.

Chaney MA. Side effects of intrathecal and epidural opioids. Can J Anaesth 1995;42:891-903.

This review is a thorough discussion of side effects that can occur with neuraxial opioid use.

Moss J, Rosow CE. Development of peripheral opioid antagonists' new insights into opioid effects. Mayo Clin Proc 2008;83:1116-30.

This is a thorough review regarding clinical uses and theoretical applications of PAMORAs.

Nelson LS, Olsen D. Opioids. In: Goldfrank LR, Flomenbaum NE, Lewin NA, et al, editors. Goldfrank's toxicologic emergencies. 9th ed. New York: McGraw-Hill; 2010. p. 559-78.

The chapters on opioids and opioid antagonists in this text highlight the management of most forms of opioid overdose and feature detailed information about the toxic effects of opioids and opioids of abuse. Details regarding proper dosing of naloxone and naloxone infusions are featured.

Reisine T. Opiate receptors. Neuropharmacology 1995;34:463-72.

This article is a classic review of opioid receptors and receptor physiology.

Tan JA, Ho KM. Use of remifentanil as a sedative agent in critically ill adult patients: a meta-analysis. Anaesthesia 2009;64:1342-52.

This article provides a good analysis of clinical trials, looking at use of remifentanil versus conventional therapies and clinical outcomes in mechanically ventilated patients in the ICU.

Traub SJ, Hoffman RS, Nelson LS. Body packing: the internal concealment of illicit drugs. N Engl J Med 2003;349:2519-26.

This article is a recent in-depth review of management in opioid body packers.

Wilhem W, Kreuer S. The place for short-acting opioids: special emphasis on remifentanil. Crit Care 2008;12:S5.

This article provides a good review of ultra-short-acting opioids, with an in-depth focus on the use of remifentanil for sedation in mechanically ventilated patients in the ICU.

REFERENCES

Access the complete reference list online at http://www.expertconsult.com.

185

Pesticides and Herbicides

RICK KINGSTON

The U.S. Environmental Protection Agency (EPA) broadly defines a *pesticide* as any substance or mixture of substances intended for preventing, destroying, repelling, or mitigating any pest. These agents are typically further classified according to their chemical, physical, or biological class, or they may also be categorized as acting on either animal or insect pests or undesirable plants. In the context of intended use, the categories of insecticide, herbicide, or rodenticide are also commonly used and often useful for reviewing toxicity profiles of agents most likely to be encountered in critical care medicine.

General Principles of Management

As with a variety of other toxic exposures, the general principles of management for many of the pesticides have changed in recent years. Most notably, these changes have related to gastric decontamination, but there also have been emerging controversies regarding the use of antidotes intended to aid in the treatment of pesticide poisonings, especially those cases involving organophosphate (OP) insecticides.

Methods of gastric decontamination that have been reexamined over the last decade include the use of gastric lavage, activated charcoal, syrup of ipecac, and whole-bowel irrigation.[1] Ipecac largely has been abandoned for routine use in either the prehospital or hospital care setting.[2,3] Its slow onset of action, incomplete return of toxin, and ability to cause emesis in an unconscious or seizing patient render it unacceptable in most cases in which gastric decontamination might be considered a therapeutic option. Furthermore, many of the pesticide products are liquid formulations with hydrocarbon solvents, and this fact further precludes the use of an emetic owing to the risk of aspiration.

Gastric lavage is still a preferred method of decontamination in those substantial ingestion exposures where patients present within 60 minutes of ingestion.[4] Care must be taken to ensure that the patient's airway is protected with a cuffed endotracheal tube. Lavage should be carried out using a large-bore tube with adequate aliquots of water or saline. Since recovery rates may be small, clinicians should evaluate the risk-to-benefit ratio of use for each patient.

Although single-dose administration of activated charcoal has become the empirical treatment of choice for most significant toxic ingestions, its use and ability to improve patient outcomes in pesticide poisoning has not been systematically studied or proven.[5] Furthermore, unless it is administered within the first hour after exposure, even its theoretical benefit may be questioned. Still, potential benefit may warrant its early use, especially with extremely toxic substances such as paraquat and diquat or substantial ingestions of long-acting anticoagulant rodenticides.

Multiple-dose activated charcoal also has been a therapeutic intervention intended to decrease absorption of toxins but, more importantly, enhance elimination of toxins once absorbed. Despite promising results in cases involving selected toxins, there are no data to document effectiveness in poisoning cases involving pesticides.

For those patients in whom activated charcoal may offer potential therapeutic benefit, active bowel sounds must be present, and an appropriate dose must be determined. Adults typically receive 25 to 100 g of charcoal as a mixed aqueous slurry with or without sorbitol as an added cathartic. Children and infants should receive 25 to 50 g or 1 g/kg body weight. Although the addition of sorbitol or other cathartics to activated charcoal has been shown to enhance elimination of certain toxins, their ability to reduce bioavailability or improve patient outcomes after pesticide poisoning has not been demonstrated. Thus, use of a sorbitol-containing activated charcoal preparation is neither indicated nor contraindicated.

Whole-bowel irrigation (WBI) involving the use of large volumes of a polyethylene glycol (PEG)-containing isosmotic solution has also been anecdotally reported to produce positive results in the treatment of poisoning. It is purported to cleanse the gut of toxins by inducing liquid stooling. In dog models, it has been shown to increase the mean total body elimination of paraquat.[6] There have been no systematic controlled clinical studies to demonstrate its effectiveness in humans, and side effects frequently complicate its use and can mask emerging toxin-induced side effects that can confuse the clinical picture.

As many pesticides have hydrocarbon diluents or vehicles, any method of gastric decontamination must be cautiously attempted in only those patients likely to receive the greatest benefit. Hydrocarbon aspiration remains a real concern, and attempts at most forms of gastric decontamination will likely increase the risk of aspiration by either direct or indirect means, including the induction of spontaneous emesis.

Skin decontamination in all substantial dermal exposures remains indicated and should be carried out concomitantly with other life-saving measures. Care should be taken to remove and discard contaminated clothing, consider and avoid contamination of emergency and healthcare personnel, and perform full decontamination of all exposed tissue with copious amounts of soap and water. Note that some agents such as the fungicide, chlorothalonil, or concentrated versions of the herbicide, glyphosate, are corrosive and in cases of ocular exposure may require extensive eye washing and evaluation by an ophthalmologist.

Specific Agents

There are more than 3000 different formulations and 25,000 brand names of pesticides registered with the EPA.[7] A brief list of those categories of agents most likely to be encountered in critical care medicine include the OPs, *N*-methyl carbamates, solid organochlorines, pyrethroids and pyrethrins, chlorophenoxy herbicides, paraquat, diquat, and a limited variety of commonly encountered agents with unique toxicology profiles.

INSECTICIDES

Organophosphates

The primary toxicologic effects of OP insecticides relate to their ability to phosphorylate acetylcholinesterase (AChE), thereby forming an irreversible covalent phosphate linkage with a serine residue at the active site. This inhibition effectively allows unopposed action of acetylcholine at the nerve synapse, resulting in sustained depolarization of the postsynaptic neuron. This action occurs both in the central nervous system (CNS) and at muscarinic sites in the peripheral nervous system, nicotinic sites in the sympathetic and parasympathetic ganglia, and nicotinic sites at the neuromuscular junction. Although OP insecticides registered by the EPA are relatively more selective in acting on insect cholinesterase, they also affect mammalian AChE in the event of excessive exposure.

The rate of spontaneous reactivation of AChE is dependent on the chemical structure of the agent involved. The most commonly encountered agents carry either two methyl or two ethyl ester groups attached to the phosphorus atom. The significance of this structural finding relates to the fact that poisoning with dimethyl agents (e.g., demeton-*S*-methyl, dichlorvos, dimethoate, or malathion) results in rapid and spontaneous reactivation of AChE, whereas poisoning with diethyl agents (e.g., chlorpyrifos, diazinon, or parathion) is associated with slower reactivation of AChE. The differences among the OP insecticides can create therapeutic dilemmas in determining appropriate courses of treatment.[8]

Patients acutely poisoned with OP insecticides present with a range of signs and symptoms, depending on the dose and potency of the agent involved. Significant poisoning exposures result in respiratory failure due to muscle weakness, excessive mucous secretion, and noncardiogenic pulmonary edema, which may be an immediate cause of death. Severe poisoning also can cause neurologic effects including seizures, coma, or delirium, which result from cholinergic input in the midbrain and medulla. Dystonias, choreoathetoid movements, and fasciculations also can be noted.

Varieties of arrhythmias have been reported, including tachyarrhythmias, bradyarrhythmias, and torsades de pointes ventricular tachycardia. Diarrhea and vomiting are almost universally seen in severe poisoning, along with excessive secretions of tears, saliva, and sweat. This constellation of symptoms has given rise to a number of mnemonics to describe the cholinergic excesses, such as DUMBELS (diarrhea, urination, miosis, bronchospasm, emesis, lacrimation, salivation) and SLUDGE (salivation, lacrimation, urination, defecation, emesis).

An intermediate syndrome or type II toxicity also has been described. In this syndrome, patients exhibit paralysis of proximal limb muscles, neck flexor muscles, motor cranial nerves, and respiratory muscles, without significant muscarinic symptoms. These effects are noted 24 to 96 hours after initial signs and symptoms and are thought by some to be a result of initial underdosing with the antidote.[9-12]

Some OPs such as the triaryl phosphates can produce a delayed peripheral neuropathy known as *organophosphate-induced delayed neuropathy* (OPIDN), which manifests 2 to 3 weeks after a single acute poisoning. After abatement of acute cholinergic effects and symptoms associated with the intermediate syndrome (see later), patients with OPIDN develop signs and symptoms including tingling of the extremities, sensory loss, progressive muscle weakness and flaccidity of the distal skeletal muscles of the lower and upper extremities, and ataxia. The mechanisms leading to OPIDN are not fully understood and may not be directly related to inhibition of AChE, since some of the agents involved are poor AChE inhibitors.[13-15]

Diagnosis of OP poisoning typically requires a clinical picture of cholinergic symptoms, onset of symptoms within 12 hours of exposure, a 50% or more reduction of plasma and red blood cell (RBC) cholinesterase below baseline, and clinical improvement of muscarinic signs and symptoms with the administration of atropine.

The most severe cases of poisoning can be rapidly fatal if not aggressively treated. Atropine is the mainstay of treatment, and in some cases extremely large doses (>100 mg/d) may be required to reverse muscarinic symptoms. Critical care clinicians often will be faced with the decision to administer an oxime such as pralidoxime (2-PAM), which regenerates AChE by reversing phosphorylation of the active site on the enzyme before the phosphorylated AChE has undergone aging. Although animal data consistently have shown a positive effect of oxime therapy, a number of authors have questioned their utility, and reviews of the clinical effectiveness of oxime therapy have produced mixed results.[16,17] Still other work has demonstrated a more convincing benefit associated with the use of 2-PAM and provides a rationale for appropriate dosing that includes continuous pralidoxime infusion, as compared to repeated bolus injection.[18] Although various studies have lead the World Health Organization to recommend standard doses of 2-PAM, including an intravenous (IV) bolus of 30 mg/kg as a loading dose followed by infusion of at least 8 mg/kg/h, a modified administration schedule of a 2-g IV bolus dose followed by a continuous infusion of 1 g over an hour for 48 hours demonstrated reduction in both morbidity and mortality of moderately severe cases of acute OP poisoning.[18,19-21]

As such, 2-PAM administration is warranted in moderate to severe poisoning in patients with respiratory compromise, seizures, or coma. Furthermore, 2-PAM is typically used in combination with atropine, as atropine blocks only the effects of acetylcholine at the postsynaptic neuron but does not regenerate AChE.

Animal studies suggest that other new treatment approaches such as alkalinization hold promise in the effective management of OP intoxication, but there is insufficient evidence supporting their role in the routine care of these patients.[22,23] If the patient receives appropriate treatment and survives the first few hours, prognosis is good, even in severe cases of poisoning.

N-Methyl Carbamates

Carbamate insecticides are derivatives of *N*-methyl carbamic acid and share similar toxicologic effects with OP insecticides in that both inhibit AChE. These insecticides differ from the OPs in that they cause a reversible carbamylation of the AChE enzyme. This carbamyl-AChE combination dissociates more readily than the OP phosphoryl-AChE complex, resulting in a shorter duration of clinical effects, a wider range between doses causing clinical effects and fatality, and diminished usefulness of blood cholinesterase measurements.

In cases of serious poisoning, patients demonstrate CNS depression with coma, seizures, and hypotonicity. Nicotinic effects including hypertension and cardiorespiratory depression are also common. Respiratory effects such as dyspnea, bronchospasm, bronchorrhea, and pulmonary edema are also likely to be present.[24]

As in severe cases of OP poisoning, treatment should be based on a high index of suspicion or history suggestive of either OP or carbamate exposure and presence of characteristic symptomatology and should not be delayed pending confirmation by blood cholinesterase testing. Although clinical presentation is quite similar to OP intoxication, seizures as a presenting symptom are uncommon because many carbamates do not cross the blood-brain barrier.

Cholinesterase testing may be of more limited value in carbamate poisoning, depending on the timing of sampling; in vitro regeneration of AChE may render the results unreliable in confirming exposure.[25,26]

Initial treatment of choice is atropine, and as in severe cases of OP poisoning, large doses may be required to reverse symptoms of cholinergic crisis. Although pralidoxime has been suggested to be relatively contraindicated in cases of carbamate poisoning and may serve as an additional competitive inhibitor of AChE, the risk of adverse effects is small in comparison to potential benefit when faced with poisoning from an unknown cholinesterase inhibitor.

Prognosis in cases of carbamate poisoning is typically excellent when treatment is prompt and appropriate, with most cholinergic symptoms resolving within 24 hours. Contrary to OP poisoning, delayed or prolonged symptoms are not expected.

Solid Organochlorines

The use of solid organochlorine compounds as insecticides has been sharply curtailed worldwide in recent years, and almost all EPA registrations for compounds such as aldrin, dieldrin, benzene hexachloride, chlordane, and DDT have been cancelled. The EPA is currently banning endosulfan, leaving dicofol as essentially the last organochlorine compound that is a restricted-use insecticide. Lindane was banned by the EPA for use as a pesticide in 1996 but remains on the market under FDA jurisdiction as a second-line therapy for scabies. Still, a variety of agents remain in other international markets. Although poisoning from banned toxic agents is less likely, occasionally exposures to some residual products occur.

Cases of mild acute poisoning often result in CNS effects including headache, dizziness, nausea, vomiting, incoordination, tremor, and mental confusion. Even in more severe cases of poisoning, neurologic toxicity predominates, with myoclonic jerking progressing to generalized seizures, including status epilepticus.[27,28] Symptoms may progress to coma and respiratory depression, and cardiac irritability may result in arrhythmias.

Confirmation of poisoning is more likely to be made from a strong history of exposure, since laboratory analysis is not routinely available and difficult to interpret. Although severe cases of exposures may demonstrate correspondingly high blood levels, measurable low levels do not necessarily confirm poisoning.

Treatment of severe poisoning is aimed at controlling convulsions and monitoring for respiratory compromise. Atropine, epinephrine, and other adrenergic amines in standard Advanced Cardiac Life Support (ACLS) protocols should be used only if absolutely necessary, as enhanced myocardial irritability predisposes to ventricular fibrillation. Despite the fact that serious and life-threatening effects can occur, especially in instances of intentional ingestion, advances in critical care medicine have significantly reduced the mortality in those patients receiving early and well-managed supportive care.

Pyrethrin/Pyrethroid

Pyrethrins (e.g., jasmolin, cinerin, pyrethrin) are naturally occurring esters of chrysanthemic and pyrethric acid, extracts of the *Chrysanthemum cinerariaefolium* flower. Pyrethroids (e.g., allethrin, bifenthrin, bioresmethrin, cypermethrin, deltamethrin, fenvalerate, permethrin, phenothrin, resmethrin, tetramethrin) are synthetic pyrethrins which have been chemically modified to increase stability in the natural environment. A variety of different types of formulations are used for the control of insects on animals, in the house and garden, and in agriculture. Pyrethroids and pyrethrins interact with sodium channels in peripheral and central nerve cells to prolong the increase in permeability during the action potential excitatory phase of impulse transmission, resulting in failure of the cell to depolarize. In humans, rapid cleavage of the acid/alcohol ester along with oxidation to nontoxic metabolites limits toxicity. Pyrethrins and pyrethroids in their diluted form are poorly absorbed across intact skin and rarely result in toxicity. Despite limited absorption, an additional reason for low toxicity relates to rapid biodegradation by mammalian liver enzymes (ester hydrolysis and oxidation). Pyrethroids are differentiated by the absence (type I) or presence (type II) of an α-cyano group. Type I pyrethroids cause a tremor syndrome, and type II agents demonstrate a choreoathetosis/salivation syndrome.[29] Most human case reports of toxicity involve type II agents. Despite extensive use and frequent exposure, a review of national poison center data revealed that moderate or major adverse effects were relatively rare based on review of 3 consecutive years of data (717 moderate and 23 major outcomes out of 17,873 exposures reported to poison centers nationwide).[30]

Unless significant ingestion of more concentrated type II products occurs, serious toxicity is unlikely. In those few significant exposures, patients must be monitored for the development of neurotoxic effects such as seizures.

Other Agents

A variety of other pest-management agents registered for use in the United States include insecticides, acaricides, and repellents that have pharmacology and toxicology that are distinct from carbamates and OPs. Agents such as boric acid are commonly involved in exposure but may not necessarily result in serious exposures. Exposures to other agents including benzyl benzoate, chlordimeform, chlorobenzilate, and cyhexatin rarely result in significant poisoning. Diethyltoluamide (DEET) is used extensively as an effective insect repellent and rarely results in serious systemic poisoning unless large amounts are ingested. Anticoagulant rodenticides produce predictable and potentially life-threatening anticoagulation and poisoning, and so-called super warfarins produce long-lasting effects requiring weeks of vitamin K_1 therapy to prevent rebound anticoagulation.

HERBICIDES

Chlorophenoxy Herbicides

Chlorophenoxy compounds such as 2,4-dichlorophenoxyacetic acid (2,4-D), MCPA, MCPB, MCPP, and 2-methyl-3,6 dichlorobenzoic acid are some of the most widely used herbicides on the U.S. market today.

Fortunately, as with many herbicides, except for massive suicidal ingestion, severe poisoning is rare. Typical low-level exposures result in moderate irritation to skin and mucous membranes, and inhalations of sprays cause a burning sensation in the nasopharynx and chest. In cases of large deliberate ingestion, severe poisoning involves renal failure, acidosis, electrolyte disturbances, and multiple organ failure. Hyperthermia is also a common feature in significant exposures, possibly a result of uncoupling of oxidative phosphorylation. There are no known antidotes, and management is aimed at controlling organ failure. Forced alkaline diuresis with a high urine flow has been used successfully and has produced clearance values similar to other measures such as hemodialysis.[31,32]

Paraquat

Paraquat and diquat are nonselective dipyridyl contact herbicides. Paraquat is a restricted-use herbicide for most applications, although dilute solutions of 0.276% are available to consumers for spot weed killing. Of all registered herbicides, paraquat exposures are the most serious and potentially life threatening and affect the gastrointestinal tract, kidneys, liver, heart, lungs, and other organs. Ingestion of as little as 10 to 15 mL of a 20% solution is life threatening. Although inhalation toxicity is rare, ingestions result in systemic toxicity, with the lung being the target organ. Both type I and II pneumocytes appear to accumulate paraquat, where biotransformation results in the formation of free radicals, lipid peroxidation, and cell death.[33-35] Concentrated paraquat is also quite corrosive, and prolonged contact may result in erythema, blistering, abrasion, and ulceration.[36,37] Although absorption across intact skin is slow, once the skin is abraded, eroded, or otherwise damaged, much greater absorption can occur.

Ingestions of more concentrated paraquat solutions produce swelling, edema, and painful ulceration of the oral cavity, pharynx, esophagus, stomach, and intestine. Liver injury may be evident from centrizonal hepatocellular injury, with corresponding elevations of circulating concentrations of the enzymes aspartate aminotransferase (AST), alanine aminotransferase (ALT), and lactate dehydrogenase (LDH). Kidney damage is often seen, and evidence of early damage may suggest a grave prognosis, because impaired renal function decreases clearance of paraquat from the body.

Acute poisoning can result in severe pulmonary edema within hours of ingestion, although delayed toxicity, manifested as pulmonary fibrosis, typically results in death 7 to 10 days after exposure. Toxic concentrations of paraquat can accumulate in the lung within hours of exposure, which limits the utility of various methods of decontamination or enhanced elimination. Rough estimates of toxicity suggest that ingestions of less than 20 mg/kg body weight of paraquat typically result in recovery, while ingestions of more than 40 mg/kg body weight result in 100% mortality within 1 to 7 days.[37]

Treatment including gastric decontamination largely has been ineffective, but theoretically, gastric lavage immediately after ingestion may be beneficial; even small returns of the substance may reduce total body burden. Administration of oral adsorbents has been recommended, but there is no conclusive evidence of value. As with gastric lavage, preventing absorption of even small quantities of paraquat may be useful. Agents that are typically recommended include activated charcoal, Robinson's Bentonite, or Robinson's Fuller Earth (adult dose for each is 100-150 g; dose for children is 2 g/kg) via NG tube, with or without a cathartic. In most Western medical facilities, only activated charcoal will be on hand and available for rapid administration.

Diagnosis of paraquat poisoning should be confirmed through qualitative analysis of paraquat in urine, with subsequent quantitative analysis in plasma. Manufacturers of paraquat may be able to aid in obtaining analysis of biological fluids for the presence of paraquat and interpreting results consistent with reported nomograms such as the one provided by Hart et al.[38] Quantitative analysis of plasma concentrations within the first 24 hours can provide an accurate assessment of survival rates. Plasma concentrations in excess of 3 mg/L, regardless of time taken, have been associated with universally fatal outcomes despite aggressive interventions including hemodialysis.

Other treatment considerations focus on organs most likely to be affected, such as the pulmonary and renal systems. Because the presence of oxygen increases free radical formation, use of supplemental oxygen should be restricted if possible.[39,40] Patients should be closely monitored for development of acute respiratory distress syndrome (ARDS) and impending respiratory failure. Varieties of other measures have been employed to increase elimination of paraquat. Although both peritoneal dialysis and hemodialysis have been used, peritoneal dialysis is largely ineffective compared to hemodialysis. Data regarding the benefits of dialysis are still inconclusive. Hemoperfusion for several consecutive days has been the most effective means of paraquat removal, and if used should be started within 24 hours—preferably within 12 hours—of ingestion. Although various antioxidants and free radical scavengers have been postulated to reduce free radical damage, no benefits have been demonstrated in animal studies.

One case reported the use of deferoxamine (100 mg/kg in 24 hours) and continuous infusion of N-acetylcysteine (300 mg/kg/d for 3 weeks) to treat an ingestion of 50 to 60 mL of a 20% solution of paraquat in an adult male.[41] The patient survived without major sequelae. In another case, a 52-year-old male who ingested approximately 50 mL of a solution containing 13% paraquat and 7% diquat subsequently developed ARDS and pulmonary fibrosis. Survival prediction for the corresponding paraquat plasma levels was 30%. Treatment included oral Fuller's earth, forced diuresis, hemofiltration, N-acetylcysteine, methylprednisolone, cyclophosphamide, vitamin E, colchicine, and delayed continuous nitric oxide inhalation. The patient recovered with subsequently normal pulmonary function. The authors were unsure which of the above interventions accounted for the successful outcome, but they were encouraged with the use of nitric oxide.[42] Further data supporting the effectiveness of these modalities are lacking. Ultimately, there is no effective antidote.

Diquat

Diquat is also a dipyridyl compound, similar to but less toxic than paraquat. The lower toxicity may be because diquat is not selectively concentrated in the lungs. Although lung damage to type I pneumocytes does occur, type II pneumocytes are spared, and progressive fibrosis has not been reported.[43,44]

Significant exposures to diquat can result in toxicity to the gastrointestinal tract, brain, and kidneys. Signs and symptoms of CNS toxicity including lethargy, seizures, and coma may be seen.[45,46] Treatment of diquat exposure is similar to treatment of paraquat poisoning, with gastric decontamination and respiratory support, but there are limited studies documenting effectiveness of most therapeutic modalities that have been employed.

KEY POINTS

1. General principles of management for many of the pesticide toxicities have changed in recent years, including decontamination practices involving use of gastric lavage, activated charcoal, and syrup of ipecac, as well as use of antidotes in organophosphorus poisoning.

2. Mnemonics aid clinicians in recognizing the constellation of signs and symptoms associated with organophosphate poisoning and include:
   a. DUMBELS (diarrhea, urination, miosis, bronchospasm, emesis, lacrimation, salivation)
   b. SLUDGE (salivation, lacrimation, urination, defecation, emesis)

3. Severe poisoning from chlorphenoxy herbicides are rare, and management is aimed at supportive care, as there are no known antidotes.

4. Use of high-dose pralidoxime as a continuous infusion has demonstrated decreased morbidity and mortality in moderately severe poisoning caused by organophosphorus compounds.

5. Any ingestion of a concentrated solution of paraquat is potentially life threatening and must be aggressively treated.

ANNOTATED REFERENCES

Pawar KS, Bhoite RR, Pillay CP, Chavan SC, Malshikare DS, Garad SG. Continuous pralidoxime infusion versus repeated bolus injection to treat organophosphorus pesticide poisoning: a randomised controlled trial. Lancet 2006;368:2136-41.
This landmark study addressed the question of both the safety and efficacy of pralidoxime in the treatment of moderately severe poisoning with organophosphorus compounds. In addition to establishing an effective dose and method of administration, the study demonstrated that compared to existing standardized empirical dosing regimens, a high-dose infusion resulted in both decreased morbidity and mortality. Previous to this study, the overall effectiveness of pralidoxime had been debated, since various presumed appropriate dosing models had produced equivocal results. Although challenges related to funding the cost associated with administering the higher-dose regimen remain, its overall effectiveness appears to be less controversial.

American Academy of Pediatrics Committee on Injury, Violence, and Poison Prevention. Poison treatment in the home. American Academy of Pediatrics Committee on Injury, Violence, and Poison Prevention. Pediatrics 2003;112:1182-5.
The AAP states that ipecac should no longer be used routinely as a home treatment strategy for child poisoning and that existing ipecac in the home should be disposed of safety. Recently there has been interest regarding activated charcoal in the home as a poison treatment strategy. After reviewing the evidence, AAP believes that it is premature to recommend the administration of activated charcoal in the home. The first action for a caregiver of a child who may have ingested a toxic substance is to consult the local poison control center. Considering contraindications to ipecac use in poisonings involving pesticides and herbicides, critical care practitioners should be alert to identifying potential prehospital misuse of these decontamination modalities that may otherwise complicate treatment of the pediatric patient.

Bond GR. Home syrup of ipecac use does not reduce emergency department use or improve outcome. Pediatrics 2003;112:1061-4.
The usefulness of syrup of ipecac as a home treatment for poisoning and the need to keep it in the home has been increasingly challenged. This study suggests there is no reduction in resource utilization or improvement in patient outcome from the use of syrup of ipecac at home. Although these data cannot exclude a benefit in a very limited set of poisonings, any benefit remains to be proven. This report, coupled with the fact that there are obvious contraindications to using emetics in cases of pesticide or herbicide poisoning, underscores their lack of benefit in this type of poison exposure.

REFERENCES

Access the complete reference list online at http://www.expertconsult.com.

186

Sedatives and Hypnotics

DEBRA J. SKAAR | CRAIG R. WEINERT

Rationale for Sedative Use in the Intensive Care Unit

Medications are commonly administered to critically ill patients to diminish fundamental activities of the central nervous system (CNS) such as wakefulness, memory, and control of voluntary muscle contraction, and to minimize unpleasant symptoms such as dyspnea, pain, anxiety, and fear. Medications are most often used for these purposes in the management of mechanically ventilated patients; they are more likely to receive sedative-analgesics, and in higher doses, than nonintubated patients.[1] Paradoxically, most intensive care unit (ICU) patients who receive these potent CNS-active medications are not suffering from acute neurologic diagnoses such as stroke, seizure, or infection. Therefore this chapter focuses on sedative use in critically ill patients who may have toxic-metabolic encephalopathy (e.g., delirium) or no CNS abnormalities at all.

The sedative and analgesic drugs commonly administered to ICU patients are derived from five distinct pharmacologic classes: opiates, benzodiazepines (BZDs), isopropylphenol anesthetics, α_2-adrenoreceptor agonists, and dopamine-blocking antipsychotic medications. However, at doses commonly given to critically ill patients, these medications induce relatively similar clinical effects, both desirable and adverse. This problem of drug nonspecificity is compounded by use of imprecise language by caregivers to describe patients' behavior and communicate sedative goals to others.

The expression "sedation" or "sedative medications" encompasses elements of sedation, hypnosis, amnesia, analgesia, and muscle relaxation. These words have discrete but related meanings. *Sedatives* create a state of calmness or lack of excitability without necessarily decreasing awareness. *Hypnotics* and *general anesthetics* induce sleep or, more precisely, create the appearance of sleep by reducing the level of consciousness, arousability, or awareness. *Amnestics* impede new memory formation, whereas *analgesics* reduce the symptom of pain by peripheral or central mechanisms. Excessive skeletal muscle contraction or motor activity is a major manifestation of agitation which, along with level of consciousness, is the primary observable behavior measured by many sedation scales.[2] *Antipsychotics* and *neuroleptics* ameliorate disorganized thinking and inappropriate behavior. Most "sedative" medications have clinical effects in several of these categories. For instance, a drug may have both sedative and hypnotic properties, or both analgesic and hypnotic effects, or antipsychotic and sedative effects. Although no one sedative has a completely specific effect, medications typically have greater effects in one of the categories, and the thoughtful intensivist can prescribe medication combinations that maximize desired effects while minimizing unwanted effects. Importantly, given in higher doses, almost all the medications described in this chapter decrease the level of consciousness and reduce unwanted skeletal muscle activity.

Goals of Sedation for Patients in Intensive Care Units

Table 186-1 lists 15 indications for administration of sedative and analgesic medications to critically ill patients. The clinician should mentally compare the number of possible indications for use of sedative-analgesics in ICU patients with an analogous list for other common ICU medications. For example, antibiotics have two

indications, to prevent or treat infections, and gastric acid–reducing medications have two indications, to prevent or treat gastrointestinal bleeding and improve symptoms of esophageal reflux. Much of the art of sedating ICU patients lies in determining which of the many indications applies to the individual patient on a given day and communicating that rationale to other caregivers.

Epidemiology of Sedative Use in the Intensive Care Unit

Two-thirds of patients requiring mechanical ventilation receive sedative medications.[3,4] International practice surveys show that BZDs or propofol are the most common sedatives selected and are often combined with opioids, although the choice of opioid (e.g., morphine, fentanyl, or sufentanil) varies among countries and institutions. A study of 174 ICUs in 2007 reported that over 50% of ventilated patients received intravenous (IV) sedation: 82% received propofol, 31% received a BZD, and 4% received dexmedetomidine. Intravenous opiates were used more commonly with BZDs (70.1%) than with propofol (23.9%).[5] Continuous infusion therapy was associated with a markedly prolonged duration of mechanical ventilation and longer time to achieve important weaning landmarks.[4,6] In a clinical trial that enrolled patients with adult respiratory distress syndrome, sedatives were administered during 70% of ICU patient-days.[7] Contrary to clinicians' expectations, two studies showed that ventilating patients with small tidal volumes to avoid ventilator-induced lung injury was not associated with an increase in sedative exposure.[8,9] Despite general practice surveys showing widespread use of sedatives, there are hospitals that have successfully managed ventilated patients with a "minimal-to-no-sedation" policy.[10]

What are the clinical consequences of widespread use of potent sedatives? Because there are numerous causes of decreased consciousness in critically ill patients, it is difficult to estimate the independent effect of sedative medications on patients' clinical status. In one study, one-third of subjects were in an unarousable or deeply sedated state, one-third were in a state of moderate to light sedation, and one-third were in an alert and calm state.[11] The correlation between sedation level and amount of sedative medication received during the 8 hours before the assessment was weak ($r = -0.13$ to -0.32) across different medication classes. These results suggest several mutually compatible possibilities: (1) factors (e.g., organ failure-associated encephalopathy) other than medications influence sedation scale measurements, (2) the pharmacologic effects of sedatives accumulate over days rather than hours, and/or (3) dose-response relationships are nonlinear. Another study showed that mechanically ventilated patients were unarousable to tactile stimulation 32% of the time, yet were rated by their nurses as "oversedated" less than 3% of the time.[12]

CONDITIONS REQUIRING SEDATION

Determining the specific reasons for administration of sedative medications is problematic in clinical studies, but the question can be approached by determining the prevalence of the syndromes, symptoms, or behaviors that may lead to sedative intervention. Some 20% to 60% of patients recall having significant pain during their ICU stay.[13-15] Therefore caregivers should consider pain as the most likely cause when patients show signs of distress or agitation. Delirium was

TABLE 186-1	Indications for Administering Sedative-Analgesic Medications to Critically Ill Patients
Indication	**Comment**
Minimize ventilator dyssynchrony	Poor synchrony may lead to hypoxemia and dyspnea and is distressing to caregivers. Ventilator adjustment may improve synchrony without medications.
Reduce dyspnea associated with severe acute respiratory failure	Reducing minute ventilation to avoid barotrauma can cause severe dyspnea. Tachypnea with short expiratory times can lead to increased auto-PEEP and hypotension.
Increase tolerance of intubation	A translaryngeal endotracheal tube can cause pain, gagging, and reflexive biting.
Reduce anxiety	Acute severe illness possibly leading to disability or death may produce unwanted psychological distress.
Reduce recall of ICU symptoms	Recall of distressing symptoms such as severe dyspnea, terror, restraint, or pain can have long-term psychological consequences.[32]
Reduce stress response and oxygen consumption	Reducing unwanted motor activity or respiratory effort can decrease total-body oxygen consumption by 15%.[87]
Reduce elevated intracranial pressure	Coughing, straining, or excessive ventilator dyssynchrony can cause dangerous spikes in intracranial pressure.
Reduce pain	Surgical or traumatic wounds, catheter and tube placement, and immobilization usually cause pain.
Prevent removal of life-support technology	Removal of an endotracheal tube or vascular catheter can cause death within minutes.
Induce sleep	ICU patients often have abnormal chronobiology cycles associated with delirium and impaired immune function. Commonly used sedatives have not been shown to restore normal sleep brainwave patterns.
Increase efficiency of patient care delivery	Constant visual observation and verbal and tactile patient reassurance may not be possible in understaffed units.
Protect caregivers from violent behaviors	Confused patients can violently assault caregivers.
Adjunct during pharmacologic paralysis	Awareness during pharmacologic paralysis is inhumane and can have long-term psychological consequences.
Treat delirium	Antipsychotics may reduce disorganized thought processes or behavior while the underlying cause of the delirium is treated.
Family considerations	Repeatedly observing the distress of a loved one can cause anguish in family members, who may request that additional sedatives be given to the patient.[27]

ICU, intensive care unit; *PEEP*, positive end-expiratory pressure.

objectively diagnosed in 83% of ICU patients at some time during their illness.[16] However, ICU delirium is often hypoactive, manifested as inattention rather than agitation, and therefore may not lead to sedative administration. Because the expected effects of sedative medications can mimic symptoms of delirium (e.g., inattention, confusion, fluctuating level of consciousness), studies that link administration of sedatives such as BZDs to persistent delirium should be interpreted cautiously.[17]

According to one study, agitated behavior, as documented by nursing notes, occurred in 71% of ICU patients, and two-thirds of the episodes were judged as being severe or dangerous. In this study, caregivers often identified three or more factors they believed contributed to the agitated episode.[18] However, another study of mechanically ventilated patients detected agitation in less than 5% of 1833 separate assessments.[11] The low prevalence of agitation in this study may have occurred because agitation was assessed only during a narrow time interval. These results suggest caregivers intervene quickly when patients are agitated, even if the underlying cause or causes are difficult to identify. Caregivers probably respond quickly because agitation is so visibly apparent and is associated with numerous adverse clinical events.

Anxiety during the acute illness is commonly recalled by ICU survivors,[14] although a sample of 192 awake mechanically ventilated ICU patients reported a mean anxiety level during intubation that was only slightly higher than that of nonintubated patients assessed on a general medical-surgical ward.[19] These results imply that caregivers should not assume that all mechanically ventilated patients require treatment with anxiolytic medications.

ICU patients recall sleep disruption as a major problem during their ICU stay. Polysomnograms demonstrated that because of frequent arousals and severely fragmented sleep architecture, only 40% of critically ill patients exhibited even brief periods of normal rapid eye movement (REM) sleep.[20] The other 60% of patients, who also as a group received more sedative medications, showed no evidence of electrophysiologic sleep, but rather had electroencephalograms (EEGs) consistent with diffuse encephalopathy and coma. Sleep deprivation has been associated with a decrease in quality-of-life measures and increased incidence of complications such as neurocognitive dysfunction and delirium.[21] Environmental interventions to improve sleep quality (e.g., noise and light abatement) have not been successful in improving EEG-documented sleep.[22] Pharmacologic interventions such as increasing propofol infusion rates at night can generate a diurnal pattern of patient arousability, but there is no evidence that propofol or any other widely used ICU sedative creates restful physiologic sleep for ICU patients.[23] In a small trial using wrist actigraphy to estimate sleep quality, nighttime administration of melatonin improved sleep in ICU patients with respiratory failure.[24] Newer nonbenzodiazepine hypnotic agents such as zolpidem, zopiclone, and gaboxadol have not been studied in critically ill ICU patients to determine whether they improve disordered sleep or improve outcomes.[21] The rationale for administration of additional sedation at night is often conceptualized as "resting" patients in preparation for weaning trials in the morning. However, there are few data to support this concept, and one study showed that the reintubation rate was greater among patients with lower sedation scores (e.g., greater sedation) during the shift interval before the planned extubation.[11]

Dyspnea is an important symptom to consider, because many ICU patients have respiratory failure requiring mechanical ventilation.[25] Dyspnea is a complex symptom that arises from both acute and chronic cardiopulmonary conditions but also from constraints imposed by mechanical ventilators. Excessively small tidal volumes, short expiratory times, or slow inspiratory flow rates can worsen dyspnea and lead to potentially injurious ventilator dyssynchrony. A ventilatory mode that allows spontaneous respiratory efforts throughout the respiratory cycle was found to decrease sedation requirements in patients with acute respiratory distress syndrome (ARDS).[26] Opiates are considered first-line medications to relieve dyspnea. However, in patients with communication difficulties, caregivers cannot easily determine whether a little dyspnea is causing a lot of anxiety (in which case BZDs are preferred) or a lot of dyspnea is causing a little anxiety (in which case opiates are preferred).[27] ICU personnel may choose to use continuous-infusion opiate therapy for almost all ventilated patients, reasoning that most critically ill patients are dyspneic or in pain or both.[28]

Although detailed investigations are lacking, the severity of respiratory failure is likely positively associated with aggregate dosing of sedatives. However, the number of ICU patient-days with severe respiratory failure (e.g., high positive end-expiratory pressure, high inspired oxygen fraction, prone positioning) represents a minority of all patient ventilator days. For example, among patients with acute respiratory failure due to exacerbation of chronic obstructive pulmonary disease or ARDS, 40% of time on the ventilator was spent in the weaning phase.[29] Similarly, one-third of all ventilated patients examined during a single cross-sectional time point were in the weaning phase.[25] Therefore, as patients' respiratory support requirements lessen, sedation also should be weaned. When patients become more alert, caregivers may have heightened concern for inadvertent removal of life-support technology. Although sedatives or restraints offer no guarantee against "treatment interference,"[30] fewer than 2% of ventilated patients had unexpected extubations that required reintubation.[29]

TABLE 186-2	Opioid Analgesics Recommended for Use in Intensive Care Units				
Drug	Equianalgesic Intravenous Dosage	Half-Life (h)	Elimination Glucuronidation	Active Metabolites	Special Considerations
Morphine sulfate	10 mg Infusion: 0.07-0.5 mg/kg/h	3-7	Reduced in cirrhosis, burns, septic shock, and renal failure	Morphine-3 glucuronide, morphine-6 glucuronides	Histamine release can cause hypotension and cardiovascular instability.
Fentanyl	200 µg Infusion: 0.7-10 µg/kg/h	1.5-6	Oxidation	None	Rigidity is occasionally seen with high doses; preferred for patients with hemodynamic instability, sensitivity to histamine release, or morphine allergy.
Hydromorphone	1.5 mg Infusion: 7-15 µg/kg/h	2-3	Glucuronidation	None	Alternative to fentanyl; oral form available.

Data from Jacobi J, Fraser G, Coursin D et al. Clinical practice guidelines for the sustained use of sedatives and analgesics in the critically ill adult. Crit Care Med 2002;30:119-41.

Sedatives, especially BZDs, may be given to induce anterograde amnesia of the presumably psychologically stressful ICU experience.[31] This indication is supported by results from an observational study of ARDS survivors. In this study, patients who recalled a greater number of traumatic experiences from the period when they were in the ICU were more likely to develop persistent symptoms of posttraumatic stress disorder years later.[32] On the other hand, no one knows the quantity of sedative medication in each class that is required to reliably ensure complete amnesia. In a study of 149 patients, there was no relationship between aggregate sedative dose during mechanical ventilation and patients' recall of the ICU experience 2 months later.[33] In general, intensivists must balance the proven benefits of administering fewer sedative medications (by daily stopping of sedative infusions or use of sedation protocols) against the uncertain adverse effects of unpleasant symptom recall. Indeed, the data suggest that recall of delusional memories (often exacerbated by sedatives) is associated with greater post-ICU psychopathology than is patient recall of unpleasant but real memories.[34]

Pharmacology and Clinical Use of Sedatives Commonly Administered in the Intensive Care Unit

The intensity of sedation required for patients can vary markedly throughout their ICU stay, depending on the course of their disease, the external environment, and the time of day. The ideal sedative possesses a rapid onset of action, is convenient to administer and titrate, produces effective and reproducible sedation to the desired clinical goal, and is free of hemodynamic, cardiac, or respiratory side effects. To simplify extended infusion in the critically ill patient, the ideal sedative also should exhibit linear pharmacokinetics with no clinically significant protein binding or drug interactions. Drug clearance in renal and hepatic impairment should be clearly characterized, and the ideal sedative would not be cleared by dialysis. Finally, the ideal sedative would permit rapid and predictable recovery after discontinuation, with no long-term adverse effects. Although new sedative agents have been added to the armamentarium in recent years, this optimal group of characteristics has yet to be formulated in a single agent. Therapy with more than one drug is often used to optimize sedation in critically ill patients, and some combination of a BZD or propofol with an opioid analgesic is the most commonly employed regimen.[5,35-37]

OPIOID ANALGESICS

Although opioid analgesics are recognized as the drug class most frequently prescribed for pain management, opioids also have a role in management of anxiety. Unrecognized or inadequately treated pain from pathology or ICU procedures can create anxiety in 20% to 60% of patients.[13-15] Patients who are unable to communicate the source of their distress may suffer from persistent pain. For this reason, early and

systematic scrutiny for the presence of pain is crucial to effective management in the visibly anxious ICU patient.

Analgesic agents recommended for use in critically ill patients by the 2002 American College of Chest Physicians/Society of Critical Care Medicine/American Society of Health System Pharmacists Clinical Practice Guidelines[38] (hereafter referred to as the *Practice Guidelines*) are described in Table 186-2. Differences in analgesic potency, response, and recovery time are associated with the pharmacokinetic properties of each drug as well as their mu and kappa receptor-binding affinity in the CNS. In addition to sedation and analgesia, opioids can produce respiratory depression, constipation, urinary retention, nausea, and confusion. Combined use of opioids and BZDs results in synergistic effects that permit dosage reduction, which may reduce adverse effects and drug accumulation. For patients with chronic pain or previous use of opioids, increased dose requirements due to tolerance should be considered. Use of the opioid antagonist, naloxone, as a reversal agent is not recommended routinely after prolonged opioid analgesia because of the risk of withdrawal symptoms and the potential to induce cardiac arrhythmias.[38]

Several analgesics are not recommended for critically ill patients. Meperidine has an active metabolite, normeperidine, which causes CNS excitation associated with delirium and seizures. Because the active metabolite is excreted by the kidneys, patients with renal insufficiency are at high risk for adverse effects. Opioid antagonist-agonists (e.g., nalbuphine, butorphanol, buprenorphine) can reverse the desirable effects of other opiate agents and are not recommended for routine use in the ICU. Nonsteroidal antiinflammatory analgesics offer few advantages for the critically ill and can cause gastrointestinal bleeding, bleeding due to platelet inhibition, and renal insufficiency.[38] Alfentanil, sufentanil, and remifentanil are fentanyl derivatives with higher potency and/or shorter half-lives than fentanyl, but comparative data evaluating these agents for sedation in the ICU are scarce, and the drugs are more expensive than fentanyl.[37,39]

BENZODIAZEPINES

BZDs are widely used as ICU sedatives because they produce anxiolysis and amnesia at lower doses and induce hypnosis at higher doses. BZDs cause anterograde amnesia by blocking the acquisition and encoding of new information and unpleasant experiences. BZDs also exhibit anticonvulsant and muscle relaxant effects that may be desirable in selected ICU patients.

The anxiolytic, amnestic, anticonvulsant, and muscle-relaxing effects of BZDs are mediated through $GABA_A$ binding sites on neuronal γ-aminobutyric acid (GABA) receptors. After binding to the receptor site, BZDs facilitate the GABA-mediated increase in chloride conductance with subsequent membrane hyperpolarization and inhibition of neuronal impulses. The amnestic properties of these drugs correlate with their GABA agonist activity in the limbic system.[40] BZD binding is stereospecific and saturable, and the potency of an individual BZD agent correlates with its receptor affinity. Other ligands act as antagonists (e.g., flumazenil) or inverse agonists. Inverse agonists

TABLE 186-3	Clinical Pharmacology of Selected Sedatives						
Drug	Estimated Comparable Sedative Dose	Onset with Intravenous Administration (min)	Half-Life (h)	Active Metabolites	Intravenous Dose	Infusion Dosage Range	Relative Cost/d*
Diazepam	5 mg	2-5	20-120	Yes	0.03-0.1 mg/kg q 0.5-6 h	—	$-$$
Lorazepam	1 mg	5-20	8-15	None	0.02-0.06 mg/kg q 2-6 h	0.01-0.1 mg/kg/h	$$
Midazolam	2-3 mg	2-5	3-11	Yes	0.02-0.08 mg/kg q 0.5-2 h	0.04-0.2 mg/kg/h	$$
Propofol	50 μg/kg/min	1-2	0.5-1	None	—	5-80 μg/kg/min	$$$
Dexmedetomidine	0.5 μg/kg/h	5-10	2	None	—	0.2-0.7 μg/kg/h	$$$
Haloperidol	—	3-20	18-54	Yes[†]	0.03-0.15 mg/kg q 0.5-6 h	0.04-0.15 mg/kg/h	$$

*Based on 2003 average wholesale price and usual dosages: $, less than $10/d; $$, between $10 and $100/d; $$$, >$100/d.
[†]Associated with extrapyramidal symptoms.

reduce the efficiency of GABA interaction with the receptor, causing CNS stimulation; drugs with these properties are in development.[41] Table 186-3 describes the comparative pharmacology of selected BZDs and other ICU sedatives.

Both acute and chronic tolerance to BZDs (associated with decreased receptor activity) has been described. In ICU patients, acute tolerance can occur after just 24 hours.[41] Paradoxical reactions have also been associated with BZDs, most commonly in the elderly and in patients with a history of preexisting CNS disease, substance abuse, or psychiatric disease. Patients who develop a paradoxical reaction to a BZD should be switched to a medication in another drug class, such as propofol, dexmedetomidine, or haloperidol.

Diazepam is highly lipophilic. This property promotes rapid distribution to the brain and a prompt onset of action (2-5 minutes) when the drug is given IV. Diazepam has a volume of distribution averaging 2.9 L/kg in critically ill patients. Diazepam is highly protein bound and is metabolized by cytochrome P450 (CYP) microsomal enzymes into the active metabolites, oxazepam and desmethyldiazepam. The mean half-life of diazepam is 72 hours, but there is wide interpatient variability. Oxazepam has a half-life of 10 hours and undergoes further conjugation before elimination. Desmethyldiazepam has a half-life between 100 and 200 hours and is eliminated by the kidneys; therefore, sedative effects may be prolonged in patients with renal failure.

A key protein in the primary metabolic pathway for diazepam, the CYP subfamily enzyme, CYP2C19, is genetically polymorphic. Isoenzymes of CYP2C19 that are present in 3% to 5% of Caucasians and African Americans and 12% to 100% of Asian ethnic groups are associated with a significant decrease in diazepam metabolism. Therefore on occasion, a patient treated with diazepam may experience unexpectedly prolonged sedation.[42] Some drugs commonly used in critically ill patients, such as amiodarone, fluconazole, omeprazole, and valproic acid, also inhibit CYP2C19 activity. In contrast, cigarette smoking induces hepatic microsomal enzymes. This effect increases the clearance of diazepam and other BZDs.[43] For these reasons, the clinical response to diazepam is often unpredictable in critically ill patients.

Lorazepam has been a preferred agent for ICU sedation in many critical care units since its approval in 1977; lorazepam is recommended for long-term (>48 hours) ICU sedation in the 2002 Practice Guidelines. Because lorazepam undergoes hepatic glucuronidation to inactive metabolites, its pharmacokinetic parameters are not altered significantly in elderly or critically ill patients, except in those with severe renal or hepatic failure. Lorazepam is the least lipophilic of the injectable BZDs; therefore it crosses the blood-brain barrier slowly, resulting in a delayed onset of action (5-20 minutes) and a longer duration of action, with an elimination half-life of 10 to 20 hours.[44] After chronic dosing, accumulation of lorazepam and prolonged sedation are less likely than with diazepam. Lorazepam is also 5 to 6 times more potent than diazepam, and the amnestic effect of lorazepam has a longer duration than an equivalent diazepam dose. Lorazepam can be given by intramuscular injection.[41]

Lorazepam is formulated in 18% polyethylene glycol (PEG) and 2% benzyl alcohol in propylene glycol (PG) for injection. Although usual lorazepam doses deliver only minute amounts of PEG and PG, long-term sedation with high doses can lead to patients receiving substantial doses of PEG and PG. Both the PEG[45] and the PG[46,47] components of the vehicle have been associated with development of lactic acidosis, hyperosmolar coma, and reversible nephrotoxicity with high doses or lengthy infusions. Although the dosages implicated have not been prospectively defined, lorazepam doses exceeding 18 mg/h for longer than 4 weeks, or 25 mg/h for hours to days, should be avoided.[38] Because of its poor solubility, precipitation can occur when lorazepam is administered by continuous infusion. On the basis of manufacturer information and clinical recommendations, the manufacturer's vial concentration (either 2 or 4 mg/mL) should be diluted 1:1 with 5% dextrose injection in a glass container, *not* in polyvinyl chloride bags.[48]

Midazolam, a short-acting, water-soluble BZD prodrug, is approximately 3 times more potent than diazepam. After self-converting to a lipid-soluble form by closure of the diazepine ring at physiologic pH values in the bloodstream, midazolam rapidly enters the CNS to produce sedation within 2 to 5 minutes. This property makes midazolam ideal for patients who require immediate control of anxiety or agitation.[38] Initial dosages recommended are 2 to 5 mg IV every 5 to 15 minutes. The drug quickly redistributes to peripheral tissues, and effects dissipate if a continuous infusion is not initiated. When infused over days for chronic sedation, the mean elimination half-life of 10 hours may increase to 30 hours as peripheral tissue stores release accumulated midazolam. The pharmacodynamic effects of BZDs often do not correspond well with reported elimination half-lives.[49] In comparing the clinical sedation recovery rate (time to wakefulness) for midazolam versus diazepam, 8 trials reported a faster recovery rate from diazepam, 19 trials reported no difference in sedative recovery time, and only 1 trial demonstrated a faster recovery with midazolam.[38]

Midazolam is metabolized by the CYP3A4 isoenzyme to an active metabolite, α-hydroxymidazolam, which has 60% of the potency of the parent drug. α-Hydroxymidazolam is quickly biotransformed to its conjugated salt, α-hydroxymidazolam glucuronide (10% potency), which does not significantly contribute to the sedative properties of midazolam except when it accumulates in renal failure. Inhibitors of CYP3A4, such as macrolide antibiotics, diltiazem, propofol, and fluconazole, reduce the metabolism of midazolam and prolong its sedative actions.[41] The combined effects of drug interactions, altered protein binding, fluid shifts, altered hepatic metabolism, and renal failure can result in prolonged elimination and an unpredictable time to awakening after discontinuation of midazolam when the drug is used for longer than 48 to 72 hours. For these reasons, the 2002 Practice Guidelines recommend midazolam for short-term use only.[38]

Several randomized controlled studies have compared BZD sedatives in critically ill patients. Two unmasked studies in mixed populations of ICU patients reported no difference between midazolam and lorazepam in time until sedation or in time until return to baseline mental status.[49,50] In contrast, a double-masked randomized comparison of lorazepam versus midazolam, using a target-controlled IV infusion titrated to maintain a moderate level of sedation for 12 to 72 hours, reported a delayed emergence from sedation with lorazepam.[44] Other longer-term studies suggest that lorazepam is easier to titrate to the desired sedation level than midazolam.[51]

Because lorazepam is equally effective and produces less hypotension, it is the BZD recommended in the 2002 Practice Guidelines for most ICU patients; it is administered either by continuous infusion or by intermittent IV dosing (1-4 mg every 2-6 hours).[38]

BZDs, particularly midazolam and diazepam, can cause respiratory depression and hypotension due to vasodilation when administered in large doses. If these effects require rapid reversal, flumazenil may be used to antagonize BZD agonists at the GABA receptor binding site. Flumazenil administered IV in doses of 0.2 to 1 mg reverses the sedative and amnestic effects of BZDs immediately. Flumazenil is metabolized rapidly, with a half-life of 1 hour but a clinical duration of effect often less than 30 minutes; therefore, situations requiring prolonged antagonism may necessitate a continuous flumazenil infusion. Diagnostically, flumazenil has been used to differentiate between BZD-induced unresponsiveness and other forms of CNS pathology. Flumazenil is relatively contraindicated in patients with known BZD dependence and chronic use, because acute withdrawal symptoms and seizures have been reported in these patients.[41]

PROPOFOL AND FOSPROPOFOL

Propofol (2,6-diisopropylphenol) was initially introduced in 1982 as an induction agent for general anesthesia. Over the past 20 years, several other useful indications have been identified for this agent. In addition to being an anxiolytic/sedative/hypnotic, propofol has antiemetic, antipruritic, anticonvulsant, bronchodilatory, muscle relaxant, and possibly antiinflammatory and antiplatelet effects.[52] Propofol has been shown to improve outcome in patients with traumatic brain injury, possibly because of decreases in cerebral metabolism and intracranial pressure.[53] Its anxiolytic properties are thought to result from activation of $GABA_A$ receptors within the CNS. Unlike BZDs, propofol does not exert synergistic sedative effects when administered with opioids, and propofol may not produce an amnestic effect equivalent to that of BZDs.[54] Because of its high lipophilicity and short half-life, propofol has a rapid onset of action (1-2 minutes) and a short duration of action (10-15 minutes). For patients receiving propofol infusions for longer than 72 hours, the wake-up time can extend to 30 to 60 minutes. The pharmacokinetic profile of propofol is best described by a three-compartment model with an elimination half-life of 30 to 60 minutes. Propofol has a volume of distribution of 600 to 800 L, suggesting that the drug is rapidly cleared from the central compartment into fatty tissues, and elimination is not appreciably altered by hepatic or renal failure. For these reasons, an IV infusion of propofol can be predictably titrated from light sedation to a deeper hypnotic state for patients who require varying levels of sedation throughout the day. Simply stopping the infusion can reverse the sedative effects, usually within 1 hour and often within 15 minutes. The 2002 Practice Guidelines recommend propofol as the sedative of choice when rapid awakening is important.[38]

Propofol is a negative inotrope and can cause vasodilation and dose-related hypotension. Patients should be euvolemic before a slow bolus or infusion is administered. Bradycardia and apnea also may occur during bolus administration. When propofol is combined with BZDs or opioids, synergistic cardiovascular and respiratory adverse effects can be seen.

Propofol is available as a 1% oil-in-water emulsion that provides 1.1 kcal/mL from fat. To reduce the possibility of fat overload and hypertriglyceridemia in critically ill patients, the lipid contribution from a propofol infusion should be counted as a calorie source in the daily nutritional plan. Patients receiving propofol infusions for longer than 2 days should have their serum triglycerides monitored.[38]

Reports of infections in patients receiving propofol prompted the addition of 0.005% ethylenediaminetetraacetic acid (EDTA) to retard bacterial growth. A generic propofol formulation (Gensia Sicor Pharmaceuticals, Irvine, California) is also available that contains sodium metabisulfite (0.025%) as a preservative and has a lower pH than the EDTA formulation; individuals who are sensitive to sulfites should not receive this product. Although the U.S. Food and Drug Administration (FDA) considers these products to be bioequivalent and interchangeable (i.e., AB rated), reports suggest that the generic emulsion is less stable physiochemically and more conducive to microbial growth.[40,55] Owing to quality problems with these products, Fresenius Propoven 1% (APP Pharmaceuticals, Schaumburg, Illinois [a company of the Fresenius Kabi Group, Bad Homburg, Germany]) was imported into the United States in 2009 to address a shortage of propofol. Fresenius propofol contains no antimicrobial retardant; each vial is a single-use container that should be discarded after 6 hours. Caregivers should adhere to strict aseptic technique and administer propofol through a dedicated IV line to avoid drug incompatibility problems. Nurses should change the bottles and tubing every 12 hours to minimize the risk of bacterial contamination.[56]

Propofol infusion syndrome (PRIS) is a rare but potentially lethal complication manifested by severe metabolic acidosis, rhabdomyolysis, renal failure, dysrhythmias, and cardiac arrest.[57,58] Because of this risk, propofol is not recommended by the FDA for prolonged sedation of pediatric patients, and it should be used cautiously in adults who develop unexplained metabolic acidosis or cardiac arrhythmias. Caution should be used when propofol is infused for more than 48 hours at dosages above 5 mg/kg/h, particularly in patients with neurologic or inflammatory illnesses.[59] Alternative sedative agents should be considered for patients receiving high-dose propofol and for those who require vasopressors or cardiac inotropes.[38]

Comparing the quality of short-term (<24 hours) sedation of cardiac surgery patients, two trials favored propofol over midazolam, and seven reported no difference. Time to extubation after sedative cessation was shorter for patients receiving propofol than for those receiving midazolam in five of eight studies, but the overall duration of mechanical ventilation was equivalent in six of seven studies. In surgical or mixed medical/surgical ICUs, three of six trials reported that the quality of sedation was better with propofol, whereas the other three trials found no difference. Time to extubation was less with propofol than with midazolam in all studies assessing this endpoint.[60,61] Hypotension was more frequent with propofol.[54,62]

Fourteen surgical or mixed medical/surgical ICU studies have compared the use of sedative drugs for longer than 24 hours. The quality of sedation was comparable between propofol and midazolam in half of the studies. Midazolam was preferred over propofol in one study, and propofol was superior in two studies. In all four trials reporting time to extubation, the group receiving propofol was extubated sooner after sedation cessation than the midazolam group.[54,60,61,63] Therefore, based on the best scientific evidence, propofol is at least as effective as midazolam in sedation quality and is associated with a shorter time to extubation for patients receiving short- or long-term sedation. Propofol is also associated with more hypotension and higher drug costs than midazolam.

Fospropofol (Lusedra) is a water-soluble prodrug of propofol that was recently approved for monitored anesthesia care sedation in adult patients for diagnostic or therapeutic procedures. Because fospropofol is hydrolyzed by circulating alkaline phosphatases to propofol, formaldehyde, and phosphate, its time to onset is prolonged (4-13 minutes). The most common side effects (>20%) reported are paresthesias and pruritus; these adverse effects are seen at all dosage ranges and are thought to be the result of the phosphate ester component. Because clinical experience with fospropofol is limited to studies in relatively healthy patients undergoing colonoscopy or bronchoscopy, the safety and efficacy of long-term infusions in critically ill patients is unknown. Publication of studies in coronary artery surgery and in mechanically ventilated patients may clarify the role of this non–lipid-based sedative-hypnotic agent in the ICU.[64]

CENTRAL α_2-ADRENORECEPTOR AGONISTS

Dexmedetomidine (DEX) is the first selective α_2-adrenoreceptor agonist approved for short-term (less than 24 hours) infusion as a sedative for patients receiving mechanical ventilation. This drug exerts sedative effects via postsynaptic activation of α_2-adrenoreceptors in the CNS and analgesic action by inhibiting norepinephrine release presynaptically. In addition, it inhibits sympathetic activity, thereby decreasing blood pressure and heart rate. DEX is eight times more potent than its relative, clonidine, at stimulating α_2-adrenoreceptors.

DEX offers several advantages as a sedative in the ICU. First, DEX does not cause significant respiratory depression, and it may be the ideal choice for patients nearing extubation who still require light sedation. DEX has a rapid distribution phase (6 minutes) and an elimination half-life of 2 hours. These pharmacokinetic properties permit easy dose titration in response to fluctuating sedative needs. Another advantage is the low level of sedation that can be achieved with DEX. Patients appear comfortably sedated while undisturbed but can easily be awakened.[40] Current research is evaluating the feasibility and benefits of patient-controlled sedation with DEX.[65]

A trial comparing DEX with propofol infusion found equivalent sedation, no difference in arterial pressure, and a similar time interval from cessation of sedation infusion to extubation. Patients in the DEX group required less adjunctive opioid analgesia than patients receiving propofol, and patients receiving DEX were easily aroused for evaluation.[61] Another study also documented a reduction in morphine doses by 50% when patients were treated with DEX.[40] However, in short-term studies of mild to moderate sedation in healthy volunteers, DEX did not demonstrate analgesic effects against heat or electrically generated pain.[66]

Recent comparative studies of DEX versus BZD infusions have identified several advantages to selecting DEX for ICU sedation. The Maximizing Efficacy of Targeted Sedation and Reducing Neurological Dysfunction (MENDS) trial enrolled medical and surgical ICU patients. Patients randomized to DEX exhibited 4 more days alive without delirium and coma than the patients who received lorazepam. The DEX patient group also spent more time at the targeted level of sedation. These benefits were attained with comparable pharmacy, ICU, and hospital costs.[67] In the Safety and Efficacy of Dexmedetomidine Compared with Midazolam (SEDCOM) study, there was no difference between the drugs in time at targeted sedation level, but the DEX-treated patients spent less time on the ventilator and experienced less delirium than patients who received midazolam. In both groups, sedatives were titrated to comparable levels of light sedation.[68]

When amnesia is crucial, DEX should be combined with low doses of a BZD. DEX also has been used successfully to ameliorate the hyperadrenergic state of drug withdrawal following cessation of alcohol, illicit drug, or long-term sedative-analgesic use in the ICU.[69]

Dosage reduction is recommended with hepatic but not renal impairment. Hypotension and/or bradycardia appear to be most frequent in patients with cardiac conduction defects or hypovolemia. Some patients cannot tolerate the 1 µg/kg loading infusion of DEX; for these patients, therapy may be initiated with a maintenance infusion (0.2-0.7 µg/kg/h) that can be titrated to desired effects.

Since delirium is a predictor of mortality and longer hospital stays, DEX may be a better choice for patients who require light to moderate sedation and do not have bradycardia. Reduced incidence and clearing of delirium with DEX compared to GABA agonists suggests DEX may be a preferred agent for sedation when the Practice Guidelines are revised this year.

HALOPERIDOL

Haloperidol, a butyrophenone neuroleptic, is the preferred agent to treat patients with agitated delirium in the ICU, according to the 2002 Practice Guidelines. Neuroleptics antagonize dopamine-mediated neurotransmission in the basal ganglia, ameliorating hallucinations, delusions, and unstructured thought patterns. Haloperidol and other neuroleptic agents also possess sedative effects.

Haloperidol has a fast onset of action (5-20 minutes) and a long half-life (18-54 hours). In the ICU, haloperidol is commonly administered by intermittent IV injection of 2 to 5 mg, followed by repeated doses (sometimes double the previous dose) every 15 to 20 minutes until agitation is controlled. Repeated doses every 4 to 6 hours are usually continued for a few days, after which the drug is tapered as the patient's clinical status permits.

High doses of haloperidol (>400 mg/d) have been associated with QT_C prolongation and an increased risk of ventricular arrhythmias, including torsades de pointes; therefore, patients receiving haloperidol should be electrocardiographically monitored. Extrapyramidal symptoms can occur that require neuroleptic discontinuation and treatment with diphenhydramine or benztropine.[38] Newer atypical antipsychotics (e.g., risperidone, quetiapine, ziprasidone) offer potential safety advantages with fewer cardiovascular and extrapyramidal effects than haloperidol. Further research is needed to make firm recommendations on the comparative efficacy or safety of antipsychotic therapy for delirium.

▣ Optimizing Sedation at the Bedside

For many sedative-analgesic medications used in the ICU, there is a marked variation in the doses needed to achieve a desired clinical effect. This variability may result from altered drug kinetics, changes in receptor density, or unpredictable postreceptor effects. In addition, the intensity of the underlying symptom (e.g., dyspnea, pain) or behavior (e.g., agitation, ventilator dyssynchrony) varies from patient to patient, so most sedative-analgesic medications are titrated to a desired clinical effect. Effective titration requires that caregivers address several concepts. First, providers must identify the unwanted symptom or behavior and exhaust all feasible nonpharmacologic interventions before administering drug therapy. Second, caregivers should use a rating instrument or scale to reliably measure the level or state of the target behavior. Third, providers should agree on the desired level of the symptom or behavior. Fourth, caregivers should realize that the desired level is likely to change over time, and regular reassessment is required.

Most "sedation scales" are observer-rated assessments of level of consciousness and agitation.[2] More comprehensive scales may assess additional domains such as pain, anxiety, or ventilator synchrony, but multidomain instruments can become unwieldy if documentation requirements are excessive. Scales can report domain scores separately or combine two domains in a single choice scale, thereby assuming the activity in one domain precludes activity in the other domain, which is not always the case. For instance, agitation can occur in the presence of decreased level of consciousness. Most consciousness scales use a graded stimulation protocol to obtain a standard patient response such as eye opening. Rating agitation is more ambiguous because patient behaviors (e.g., excessive motor activity, pulling at tubes, striking at staff) are variably graded on intensity, frequency, or probability that the agitation will cause immediate adverse consequences. How "agitated" is an otherwise calm patient who is slowly pulling on his or her endotracheal tube? Sedation scales such as the modified Ramsay sedation scale (RSS), Richmond Agitation and Sedation Scale (RASS), Sedation Agitation Scale (SAS), and Motor Activity and Assessment Scale (MAAS) are similarly constructed and scored, have excellent inter-rater reliability, and have been validated by correlation with other scales, physiologic variables, or medication exposure. The Vancouver Interaction and Calmness Scale (VICS) differs from other sedation scales because it is a summated rating scale that reports two domain scores separately.[70] As such, VICS is more responsive to subtle changes in a patient's condition, but it takes more time to complete. The clinical benefit of documenting or targeting very precisely defined sedation states is unknown and may be impractical. In 15 clinical trials characterized by close attention to achieving and maintaining a predetermined sedation target (usually with the RSS), patients were at the sedation target, on average, only 68% of the time.[61]

Even if sedation effects are reliably measured, determining the optimal sedation state of an ICU patient is based more on clinical opinion than scientific evidence. Titration of medications to achieve a condition such as "lightly asleep but easily arousable" or "calm and cooperative" appears sensible, but a survey of intensivists asked to choose an appropriate sedation level for a patient with severe hypoxemia yielded a remarkably wide range of responses from unresponsive to awake.[71] Sedation targets for clinical trials are also highly variable; in 19 trials using the 6-level RSS, the target sedation level was defined variously as 3, 5, 2-3, 2-4, 2-5, 3-4, or 4-5.[61]

Monitoring cortical electrical activity to indicate sedation intensity has long been a goal of intensivists. Multichannel EEG monitoring is the gold standard for evaluating cortical activity, but interpretation remains predominantly qualitative and requires specialized training. Researchers have developed numerous signal-processing algorithms to convert limited EEG data into simpler quantitative output. The Bispectral Index (BIS) algorithm has been one of the most widely studied and yields a score of 0 (isoelectric, no cortical function) to 100 (fully awake). Initially developed to assess the depth of hypnosis during short-term general anesthesia, BIS is also used to monitor long-term ICU sedation.[72] However, studies have identified problems that have slowed the acceptance of this promising technology. First, spuriously high readings (e.g., readings indicating greater wakefulness than actually exists) can result from muscle activity in nonparalyzed patients.[73,74] Although new electronic filters suppress myographic signals, there can be substantial variability of output even in stable pharmacologically paralyzed patients.[75] Clinicians using BIS should assess trends in BIS output and integrate other clinical data before making an intervention. Second, there is little evidence that BIS monitoring of general ICU patients has advantages over routine sedation assessment using observer-rated scales. BIS technology is superior in specialized situations (e.g., pharmacologically-induced muscle paralysis) when stimulus-response sedation assessment is inadequate. For instance, medicating to a BIS score lower than about 60 makes awareness and recall unlikely. Similarly, sedation scales cannot score below a "floor" level in which patients exhibit no motor response to painful stimuli, but BIS can distinguish between levels of deep sedation. For instance, BIS scores of 55 and 35, respectively, in two patients who both score at the lowest level of a standard sedation scale suggest that the latter patient has greater suppression of cortical activity. If there is no clinical reason for maintaining the patient at 35, sedatives could be decreased to allow the BIS to rise. This process of identifying excessively sedated patients might shorten wake-up time and lead to faster weaning; however, this putative advantage has not yet been demonstrated in large ICU studies. Third, the BIS algorithm was designed to correlate with hypnosis (arousability) and recall, but it is not a pain, dyspnea, or anxiety monitor. Postoperative studies have shown that opiate-induced hypnosis can occur before analgesic effects, and seemingly sedated patients can have significant pain when awakened.[76]

Until recently, clinical research in ICU sedation has focused on investigating changes in acute physiology after medication administration or conducting head-to-head medication trials. Several studies suggest, however, that the method of administering sedatives is as important as the specific drug given to patients. In one study, duration of mechanical ventilation was decreased by more than 50% in ventilated patients who were sedated with a protocol that linked medication dosing to a specified sedation level, compared to patients who were treated without a sedation protocol.[77] The marked decrease in ventilator time was attributable to the protocol, which decreased infusion rates when patients were at target sedation level (RSS 3), thereby minimizing the time during which patients were receiving continuous medication infusions. In another study, a protocol used continuous infusions (midazolam or propofol) but stopped the infusions daily, restarting them (at half the rate) only after patients became awake.[28] Compared with a group that did not have this "stop" intervention, the experimental group used less midazolam but similar amounts of propofol. Nevertheless, in both midazolam and propofol subgroups, the daily interruption of infusions increased the number of days patients were awake, decreased the duration of mechanical ventilation by 2.4 days, and decreased the number of diagnostic tests performed to assess abnormal mental status. Since 2000, numerous studies using randomized or quasi-experimental designs have shown that algorithm-directed

sedation is safe and leads to desirable reductions in ventilator time. These studies also support the view that algorithm-directed sedation often decreases ICU length of stay. Furthermore, when administration of sedatives is carried out using an algorithmic approach, patients are usually more awake yet comfortable. Combining sedative protocols with ventilator weaning protocols gives patients, on average, three extra days alive and off mechanical ventilation compared to patients assigned to non-protocolized sedation.[78]

Patients with prolonged ICU stays may be treated with high doses of sedative-analgesic medications for weeks. There is growing evidence that tolerance to opiates, BZDs, and propofol can develop in less than 1 week and that abstinence or withdrawal symptoms can occur if sedative doses are reduced too rapidly.[79] Withdrawal symptoms of anxiety, agitation, gastrointestinal dysfunction, and tachycardia are nonspecific, and intubated patients have difficulty communicating symptoms to caregivers. Because of the altered pharmacokinetics for many drugs in critically ill patients and the difficulty in identifying withdrawal syndromes, there are few data to guide clinicians for prescribing tapering regimens when withdrawal symptoms are suspected. Logical interventions for patients who have been on prolonged courses of sedative medications include converting continuous infusions to scheduled doses, using longer-acting medications within the same pharmacologic class, reducing the total daily dose by 10% per day, changing the IV route to enteral, and adding an α_2-adrenoreceptor agonist such as clonidine.[80]

Pharmacoeconomics of Sedatives Used in the Intensive Care Unit

Occupied beds in the ICU consume a disproportionate and growing share of hospital resources. It is estimated that pharmaceutical agents account for 10% of the cost of an ICU stay, and 15% of drug expenditures are for sedatives. To promote optimal use of critical care resources, evidence for cost-effectiveness in addition to safety and efficacy must be examined for each sedative. Pharmacoeconomics, the global approach of evaluating the net impact of drug selection on the total cost of delivering health care, determines which therapies offer quality care at an acceptable cost.

New drugs cost more than available generic formulations. One comparison of lorazepam, midazolam, and propofol in critically ill trauma patients found lorazepam to be the best choice for continuous sedation, based on 1995 acquisition costs; however, lorazepam acquisition costs were lower because of an available generic formulation.[81] Because the time to extubation was shorter with propofol than with midazolam, overall costs were lower with propofol in a Spanish study, even though propofol acquisition costs were three times higher than those for midazolam.[63] Other investigators have compared quality of sedation, safety, and costs of propofol versus midazolam during short-to-medium and long-term sedation, with similar results. Propofol provides comparable sedation safety and efficacy at lower healthcare costs due to earlier extubation and shorter ICU stays.[60] Propofol and midazolam are now both available generically at a lower cost.

Economic analysis must consider dynamic pricing of drugs within the United States and throughout the world. Acquisition costs of drugs represent only one piece of the decision-making process. In the analysis of sedative agents, adequacy of sedation, time to extubation, and time to ICU discharge are important endpoints. Preventable adverse drug effects (e.g., delirium) and increased use of diagnostic and therapeutic resources also affect total hospital costs. The SEDCOM study showed that DEX and midazolam are equally effective for attaining the targeted sedation level, but DEX-treated patients spent less time on the ventilator, developed less tachycardia and hypertension, and experienced less delirium.[68] A recent pharmacoeconomic analysis of the SEDCOM study evaluated the post-randomization cost of ICU care and found that sedation with DEX reduced ICU care costs ($9679 in cost savings) compared to sedation with midazolam.[82] Another economic evaluation reported overall lower costs ($6378 in cost savings) and a greater number of ventilator-free days when continuous propofol was used for sedation compared to intermittent lorazepam in the setting of daily sedative interruption.[83] Health-related quality of life and post-ICU long-term consequences of ICU sedation should be incorporated into future pharmacoeconomic analysis.

Implementation of clinical practice guidelines can improve outcomes and lower costs. One institution reduced direct drug costs, ventilator time, and length of stay after implementing interdisciplinary sedation guidelines.[84] The ABC trial that paired spontaneous awakening trials (e.g., daily interruption of sedatives) with spontaneous breathing trials reported better outcomes (fewer ventilator days, earlier discharge from ICU, and lower mortality) with the intensive protocols than standard practice.[78] Evidence-based protocols and practice guidelines should be accompanied by interdisciplinary collaboration and education to ensure that they are positioned as guides, not rigid rules that replace clinical judgment.

Until pharmacoeconomic research provides definitive data on costs and outcomes, the best strategy to optimize sedation at acceptable costs includes selecting a sedative based on current practice guidelines, titrating doses to a patient-specific goal, and frequently reevaluating the defined endpoint with an assessment tool. Scheduled efforts to taper sedative doses or perform daily interruption of therapy (or both), as part of an interdisciplinary sedation plan, may also help optimize sedative outcomes and reduce costs.

Toxic Ingestion of Sedative-Hypnotics

Of the sedative medications discussed in this chapter, BZDs and opiates are most likely to be involved in toxic ingestions, either accidental or intended. Patients with overdoses from either medication class can present with stupor or coma with hypotension (usually mild and responsive to fluid boluses) and hypotonia. Pupil size may be helpful: pupils are pinpoint in cases of opiate ingestion, midsize in cases of BZD toxicity. Toxicity is usually short lived and completely reversible unless complications such as anoxic encephalopathy or aspiration pneumonia occur. General principles of toxic ingestion management are paramount: assume the patient has a polydrug ingestion until conclusive data are obtained; ensure adequate ventilation and airway protection; avoid gastric lavage unless the time of ingestion is very recent; and give activated charcoal for oral ingestions.[85]

Specific antidotes are available for each medication class. Naloxone can be given as both a diagnostic and therapeutic medication. Lack of improvement in level of consciousness or respiratory depression after administration of 10 mg of naloxone (starting with 0.4 mg and giving subsequent doses of 2 mg every few minutes) makes opiate toxicity an unlikely cause of the patient's symptoms. If a response is observed, practitioners should be prepared to administer repeated naloxone boluses every 30 to 60 minutes or to start a continuous infusion at 0.4 to 0.8 mg/h. Occasionally a patient with opiate overdose develops pulmonary edema requiring mechanical ventilation, but the edema usually resolves within a few days without specific treatment.

Flumazenil is a specific antidote for BZD toxicity. A patient's symptoms should improve within a minute after a bolus administration of 0.2 mg and subsequent 0.3-mg doses every 30 seconds. Administration of flumazenil to patients receiving chronic BZD therapy may precipitate an unpleasant acute withdrawal syndrome and (theoretically) increase the risk of seizures.[85] However, no seizures were observed after flumazenil treatment in 110 patients with suspected BZD overdose, including many patients with polydrug ingestions (e.g., co-ingestion of tricyclic antidepressants).[86]

KEY POINTS

1. Unidentified or untreated pain is an important cause of anxiety in critically ill patients.

2. Commonly used sedative medications, in moderate to high doses, lead to comparable changes in patients' level of consciousness and spontaneous muscle activity. Therefore optimal clinical use is determined more by the process of sedation (goal setting, evaluation, and communication) than by prescription of a specific drug.

3. Sedatives may lead to comparable changes in consciousness and muscle activity but differ in their adverse effects, such as prevalence of delirium.

4. Sedatives should be titrated to defined endpoints, with scheduled efforts to taper doses or perform daily interruption of therapy or both.

5. Sedation goals for critically ill patients should frequently be reassessed by a sedation assessment tool acceptable to intensive care practitioners.

6. Implementation of evidence-based guidelines such as a sedation algorithm or protocol to complement clinical judgment improves outcomes in mechanically ventilated patients.

ANNOTATED REFERENCES

Jacobi J, Fraser GL, Coursin DB, et al. Clinical practice guidelines for the sustained use of sedatives and analgesics in the critically ill adult. Crit Care Med 2002;30:119-41.

This is a comprehensive but dated update of the ACCP, SCCM, and ASHP practice guidelines for the optimal use of sedatives and analgesics in critically ill patients, including descriptions of new drugs and grading of the scientific evidence that supports the recommendations.

Kress JP, Pohlman AS, O'Connor MF, Hall JB. Daily interruption of sedative infusions in critically ill patients undergoing mechanical ventilation. N Engl J Med 2000;342:1471-7.

A randomized trial performed in a medical ICU showed that daily awakening of mechanically ventilated patients by interruption of sedative infusions reduced the duration of ventilation, reduced ICU stay, and led to less diagnostic testing compared with no daily awakening. Rates of complications such as unplanned extubations were not different between groups. A follow-up study in these patients showed that patients in the daily awakening group had better psychological adjustment after the ICU experience and less PTSD symptoms.

Sessler CN, Pedram S. Protocolized and target-based sedation and analgesia in the ICU. Crit Care Clin 2009;25:489-513.

Review of the evidence that sedative pharmacotherapy is most effective if it is managed with nurse-driven protocols including frequent assessments of sedation adequacy and scheduled dose reduction.

Girard TD, Kress JP, Fuchs BD, et al. Efficacy and safety of a paired sedation and ventilator weaning protocol for mechanically ventilated patients in intensive care (Awakening and Breathing Controlled trial); a randomized controlled trial. Lancet 2008;371:126-34.

A protocol that paired daily interruption of sedatives with daily spontaneous breathing trials resulted in better patient outcomes (more days alive and off mechanical ventilation) than standard care.

Riker RR, Shehabi Y, Bokesch PM, et al. Dexmedetomidine vs midazolam for sedation of critically ill patients. JAMA 2009;301:489-99.

This study (that incorporated best sedation practices) showed no difference between dexmedetomidine and midazolam in time at target sedation range but reported less time on mechanical ventilation and reduced prevalence of delirium with dexmedetomidine than midazolam.

REFERENCES

Access the complete reference list online at http://www.expertconsult.com.

187

Toxic Inhalants

KURT KLEINSCHMIDT | EVAN SCHWARZ

Toxic inhalants include chemicals used for many reasons in many settings. They differ in structure and produce their effects through various mechanisms. People can be exposed to inhalational toxins in many places, including at home, at work, or in the setting of an industrial accident or terrorist event. This chapter will focus on pulmonary irritants and asphyxiants, but people can be exposed to many other types of inhalants at work.

Many inhalants cause intoxication. Tetrahydrocannabinol is the active ingredient in marijuana and is responsible for hallucinatory effects. Crack cocaine causes a sympathomimetic toxidrome as well as (rarely) hemorrhagic alveolitis. Intoxication from lysergic acid diethylamide (LSD) or phencyclidine (PCP) results in tachycardia, agitation, and hallucinations. Solvents containing hydrocarbons are commonly abused via inhalation. They include paints, glues, hair sprays, deodorants, air fresheners, and lacquers. While patients typically present in an intoxicated state, rarely they can sustain a cardiac arrest. Toluene is a commonly abused solvent. In addition to causing intoxication, users develop metabolic acidosis, severe hypokalemia, and weakness as a result of the hypokalemia.

Exposures to inhalants occur at work. Metalworkers encounter metallic fumes. Zinc oxide and cadmium both cause metal fume fever. Symptoms include fever, fatigue, and shortness of breath. Pulmonary edema from cadmium-containing fumes is very rare. Exterminators are exposed to fumigants including organophosphates and pyrethrins. Organophosphates cause a cholinergic toxidrome that includes bronchorrhea, bronchospasm, and bradycardia. Pyrethrins are associated with allergic reactions and cause symptoms of central nervous system (CNS) dysfunction only at very high doses. Workers in the semiconductor industry are exposed to inorganic hydrides, notably arsine and phosphine. In the past, dry cleaning personnel were exposed to hepatotoxins such as carbon tetrachloride and tetrachloroethylene.

Pulmonary Irritants

The respiratory tract has several anatomic features that prevent injury. Particulates approximately 30 μM in size are trapped on the surface of the nasal turbinates.[1] Nasal hairs filter larger particles, but smaller ones are inhaled into deeper parts of the respiratory tract. The airway surface liquid (ASL) is a thick mucous film that traps particles.[1] As the airway branches into smaller-diameter bronchioles, particles adhere to the respiratory mucosa, further limiting access to the lower respiratory tract. Together, the cilia and ASL form the mucociliary escalator that is responsible for carrying inhaled toxins towards the more proximal airways where they are expelled. Sensory receptors in the upper airways cause a reflexive cough to assist with expulsion.[2]

The extent of injury is determined by the characteristics of the particle and exposure setting. These include particle size, density, shape, duration of exposure, concentration of the inhalant, and water solubility. Particles 0.5 to 3 μM in size are deposited in the distal airways and alveoli.[3] However, smaller particulates are exhaled because they behave like a gas.[3] Inadequate ventilation in confined spaces may lead to higher concentrations of the toxin and more severe injury when exposure occurs.

The irritant's water solubility (Table 187-1) is the primary characteristic that affects the type of injury and likelihood for acute lung injury (ALI). Very hydrophilic (water-soluble) irritants dissolve in the water of the mucosal secretions of the nose and upper airways. Symptoms are unpleasant and occur within seconds. Victims generally escape the exposure, thereby minimizing the risk for injury. Conversely, inability to escape may result in severe injury. Less hydrophilic (i.e., more lipophilic) irritants penetrate deeper into the respiratory tract, injuring the lower airways while sparing the upper airways. As a consequence, victims typically do not experience immediate symptoms and therefore remain in the contaminated area longer, resulting in a more severe injury.[4-5] Damage to the upper and lower airway occurs in prolonged exposures independent of the agent's degree of water solubility.[5] The mechanisms by which irritants damage the respiratory tract vary but include the direct effect of the irritant plus the inflammatory response generated from neutrophils and cytokines. Signs and symptoms include cough, sore throat, dyspnea, chest pain, wheezing, hypoxia, and rales. Rarely, patients have burns involving the skin and eyes.

GENERAL CARE

Most patients exposed to chemicals present with only inhalational injuries, so care should initially focus on airway support and breathing. Bronchodilators are used to treat airway hyperreactivity.[6-7] Endotracheal intubation is sometimes indicated to prevent collapse of the upper airway due to edema[7] or to treat hypoxia. White et al. recommend that a relatively large endotracheal tube be used to intubate patients exposed to highly water-soluble agents to prevent obstruction of the endotracheal tube from mucosal sloughing.[8] If arterial blood gases (ABGs) provide evidence for an acid-base disorder, the median hospital length of stay is longer.[9]

Chemical burns account for only a small percentage of admitted burn patients.[7,10] However, patients with large dermal exposures in addition to the inhalational injury may have significant burns. In these situations, contaminated clothing should be removed and the wounds irrigated.[6-7,10] Ammonia can cause injuries to the skin that result in intraepidermal blisters and necrosis of the dermis, leading to full-thickness tissue loss.[11]

More commonly, patients have ocular injuries. Irritation to the eyes should be treated with copious irrigation. Irrigation may cause additional irritation to the eyes, resulting in confusion as to whether the irritation is due to the irrigation or to remaining irritants. Ocular pH testing can clarify whether additional irrigation is indicated. Irrigation should be continued until the ocular pH is neutral (7.4).[6] The pH strip on a urine dipstick is a readily available way to assess ocular pH. Cycloplegics should be used to decrease pain and prevent morbidity from synechiae.[7] If concern for ocular injury persists, a full examination should be done in consultation with an ophthalmologist.[8]

CORTICOSTEROIDS

Only limited literature exists concerning the value of corticosteroids for adjuvant treatment of inhalant-induced ALI, so consensus and evidence-based recommendations do not exist. Data from animal studies suggest corticosteroids may be beneficial for the treatment of inhalant-induced ALI, but additional research is needed. In a blinded randomized controlled trial of rats exposed to ammonia, corticosteroids were not better than placebo.[12]

Chester et al.[13] published a case report which described two sisters who were simultaneously exposed to chlorine. Both were treated in an emergency department (ED). One of the sisters was admitted to a hospital and treated for 4 days with a corticosteroid. The other sister

TABLE 187-1	Pulmonary Irritants Arranged According to Water Solubility		
High Solubility		*Intermediate*	*Low Solubility*
Ammonia		Chlorine	Phosgene
Chloramines		Hydrogen sulfide	Nitrogen oxides
Hydrochloric acid			Ozone
Hydrofluoric acid			
Sulfur dioxide/sulfuric acid			

was discharged from the ED and did not receive therapy with corticosteroids. At follow-up a year later, the sibling who received corticosteroids had a forced expiratory volume in one second (FEV_1) in the normal range, whereas her sister had an FEV_1 of only 80% to 85% of the predicted value.[13] Multiple authors have discussed using corticosteroids in the treatment of patients with ALI from toxic inhalants,[9,14-18] and one review discouraged the use of these agents because of concerns about unspecified adverse effects.[8]

No randomized controlled trials have investigated corticosteroid treatment of ALI from direct pulmonary inhalants, but there are randomized trials studying the use of corticosteroids for treatment of ALI resulting from all causes.[19-20] A randomized controlled trial by the Acute Respiratory Distress Syndrome (ARDS) Network enrolled 180 patients, including 110 with ALI from direct lung injury.[20] For the most part, these 110 patients had pneumonia and/or aspiration pneumonitis. The number of patients with ALI due to a toxic inhalation was not specified, so it is unclear whether the results of this trial can be generalized to patients with ALI from a toxic inhalation. Another trial also suffered from a similar limitation.[19]

Specific Examples

HIGH WATER SOLUBILITY

Ammonia and Chloramines

Anhydrous ammonia [ammonia (NH_3)] is a colorless gas that is lighter than air at room temperature. It has a very pungent odor which can be detected when the concentration of the gas is ≥ 5 parts per million (ppm).[21] Anhydrous ammonia is the third most abundantly produced chemical in the world, and it has many household and industrial uses.[21] Ammonia was first isolated in its pure gaseous form in 1790, and the first suspected inhalational poisoning was reported in 1841.[7] Ammonia is transported under pressure as a liquid, and it can cause a hypothermic injury when it is decompressed to normal atmospheric pressure. Ammonia is used as a fertilizer, an explosive, and a chemical weapon.[21] It is also used in the production of paper and pulp, in the refrigeration and petroleum industry, and in the production of dyes, plastics, and fibers.[8,16] Accidents and exposures involving ammonia are increasingly common, as this substance is a key intermediate in the illicit production of methamphetamine.[11]

Because of its high water solubility, clinical manifestations of exposure to ammonia gas present immediately. People generally escape the exposure before becoming symptomatic, as the odor threshold of approximately 5 to 50 ppm is much lower than the irritant threshold of 400 ppm.[10,22] However, ammonia is associated with olfactory fatigue,[21] so people may believe they have removed themselves from an exposure when they have not. Ocular injuries are associated with exposures to concentrations ≥ 700 ppm. Exposures to concentrations between 2500 and 4500 ppm can lead to death within 30 minutes, largely due to airway obstruction.[8,21] Concentrations of ammonia ≥ 5000 ppm are rapidly fatal.[7,10,22]

The extent of injury depends upon the duration of exposure, depth of inhalation, gas concentration, and pH of the gas.[11,23] Interestingly, anhydrous ammonia itself is not caustic.[24] When it dissolves in water, such as in the mucous membranes, it forms ammonium hydroxide (NH_4OH), a strong base.[11,21] The dissociation of ammonium hydroxide into hydroxyl ions (see below) also damages tissues and causes liquefaction necrosis.[7,10]

Ammonium hydroxide formation and its dissociation:
$$NH_3 + H_2O \leftrightarrow NH_4OH \leftrightarrow NH_4OH \rightarrow NH_4^+ + OH^-$$

Injury to the mucosa leads to sloughing of the mucosal barrier, formation of cellular debris, edema, hemorrhage, and smooth-muscle contraction. Collectively, these effects of ammonia toxicity can precipitate airway obstruction. In one case report, injury after a massive exposure was so severe the patient required bilateral lung transplantation.[10]

Injuries occur first to the eyes, oropharynx, and upper respiratory tract, owing to ammonia's high water solubility. After prolonged exposure to ammonia or after exposure to a high concentration of the gas, the lower respiratory tract is also injured.[24] Ocular injuries (or their sequelae) include conjunctivitis, ulceration, iritis, cataract formation, blepharospasm, and glaucoma. Ammonia also causes hypoxia when it displaces oxygen in the lower respiratory tract.

Chloramines (see below) are nitrogenous chlorinated compounds. They are very irritating gasses produced when household bleach reacts with ammonia. Symptoms due to exposure to chloramines are typically very mild and occur very quickly, allowing potential victims to escape. However, if there is prolonged exposure or exposure to a high concentration of the gas, the patient can have injuries typical of any highly water-soluble irritant.

Chloramine production:
$$3\ NaOCl + 2\ NH_3 \leftrightarrow NH_2Cl + NHCl_2 + 3\ NaOH.$$
$$\textbf{B,}\ NH_2Cl + H_2O \leftrightarrow HOCl + NH_3$$

INTERMEDIATE WATER SOLUBILITY

Chlorine

Chlorine is a green-yellow gas with a very pungent odor that is twice as dense as air. It was discovered in the 1770s and soon became useful as a commercial agent.[17-18] Its odor can be detected at concentrations as low as 0.2 ppm.[18] Its intermediate solubility in water promotes damage at all levels of the respiratory tract.[25] Exposures to chlorine concentrations greater than 430 ppm have resulted in death.[17] Chlorine causes cellular injury by the generation of oxygen free radicals and oxidation of functional groups in cellular components.[9]

Chlorine has many uses. France and Germany used it as a chemical warfare agent during World War I. Today, people are exposed at home or during industrial accidents. Exposure at home can occur while chlorinating a pool or swimming. Chlorine gas is also produced when bleach containing hypochlorite is mixed with an acid. Industrial uses include water purification, textile and paper bleaching, chemical and plastic manufacturing, and disinfection.[18]

Chlorine gas directly damages the respiratory mucosa when it combines with water to form hypochlorous and hydrochloric acids (see below). Free radicals are formed which propagate an inflammatory response, leading to neutrophil recruitment and cytokine release. Epithelial cell necrosis and increased pulmonary microvascular permeability have been demonstrated in animal models.[26]

Chlorine:
$$Cl_2 + H_2O \rightarrow HCl + HOCl$$

The end result is edema and hemorrhage of the respiratory tract, with bronchiolar mucosal destruction and formation of exudate-filled alveoli. These responses predispose the respiratory tract to bacterial superinfection and ALI. Patients present with inflammation of the conjunctivae and upper respiratory tract, ALI, and respiratory failure. They develop bronchospasm, rales, a sore throat, cough, tachycardia, tachypnea, and hypoxia. Tachycardia is a result of pain, coughing, and hypoxia.

The value of nebulized sodium bicarbonate (NSB) to neutralize hydrochloric acid is debatable,[9] but this therapeutic intervention likely has no adverse effects.[25] The use of NSB is based on the assumption that there is a benefit from neutralization of the acids formed after chlorine exposure.[15,27] The solution for nebulization is prepared by mixing 2 mL of 7.5% sodium bicarbonate with 2 mL of normal saline,[15] or 3 mL of 8.4% sodium bicarbonate with 2 mL of normal saline.[27]

Little data on the use of NSB exist. There are case reports describing rapid and successful improvement in patients after a single NSB treatment.[14-15] No adverse events were reported in a retrospective review of poison center data involving 86 patients treated with NSB.[27] Only 17 of the 86 patients required hospital admission. Among the admitted patients, mean hospital length of stay was 1.4 days. The timing and number of treatments and other adjunctive therapies varied among patients. Although unable to prove its efficacy, the authors concluded that NSB was potentially beneficial.[27] A double-blind study of ED patients concluded that NSB was useful for treating patients with reactive airway dysfunction syndrome (RADS) secondary to chlorine gas exposure.[28] Forty-four patients with RADS who were treated with corticosteroids and β2-agonists were pseudorandomized to receive either NSB or a nebulized placebo. Patients were placed in either the control or treatment group based on an even/odd presentation system (patients numbered 1, 3, 5, etc. were placed into one group, while patients 2, 4, 6, etc. were placed in the other group). To be diagnosed with RADS in this series, patients without preceding disease had to develop pulmonary complaints within 24 hours of a single exposure and have symptoms persist for at least 3 months. The patients who received NSB had significantly higher FEV_1 values.[28]

LOW WATER SOLUBILITY

Phosgene

Phosgene ($COCl_2$ or carbonyl chloride) is a colorless gas that is more dense than air.[29] It was used as a chemical agent during World War I. Today, exposures occur during the synthesis of plastics and industrial materials, from decomposition of chlorinated hydrocarbons, or during the accidental heating of chlorofluorocarbons. The global consumption of phosgene was 5 million metric tons in 2006.[30] Concentrations above 500 ppm/min are associated with fatalities.[31]

Phosgene's odor has been described as similar to that of freshly mown hay. Even with its low odor threshold of 0.4 to 1.5 ppm, people may not remove themselves from an exposure because of its pleasant smell and/or development of olfactory fatigue.[31] These factors combined with its minimal acute irritant effects cause people to suffer prolonged exposures, permitting the gas to enter the lower airways and leading to development of ALI, since dose determines degree of damage.[31]

Phosgene damages the respiratory tract by denaturing proteins and irreversibly disrupting the structure of cellular membranes.[31] It also promotes depletion of glutathione and other endogenous antioxidants.[30-31] Phosgene forms hydrochloric acid (HCl) when it reacts with water in mucous membranes.[29] These pathophysiologic effects result in pulmonary edema and hypoxia.[32]

Symptoms may initially include minor upper respiratory tract irritation. Patients then enter a latent phase and may improve clinically but still have ongoing biochemical injury. This latent phase can last hours; its duration is inversely proportional to the inhaled dose.[31] The latent period is followed by ALI and pulmonary edema.[31] The smell of gas or irritative effects have no prognostic significance,[29,31] so cases of only moderate exposure to phosgene warrant further observation. Patients with a normal chest x-ray and without any signs or symptoms can be discharged after 8 hours of observation.[31] Admitted patients who require endotracheal intubation should be treated with a protective ventilation strategy.[32]

Multiple treatment strategies target the reduction of inflammation produced by phosgene.[31] N-acetylcysteine (NAC), aminophylline, isoproterenol, ibuprofen, and corticosteroids have all been studied in animal models.[33-37] Sciuto et al. tested multiple interventions after exposing rabbits and mice to phosgene.[34] The rabbit model demonstrated improvement in multiple variables including decreased intratracheal pressure, increased cyclic adenosine monophosphate (cAMP) concentration in the lung tissue and decreased leukotriene formation after receiving aminophylline and intratracheal instillation of NAC and

isoproterenol. The 12-hour survival rate was improved in mice exposed to phosgene after treatment with intraperitoneal ibuprofen, although survival at 24 hours was not affected.[34] Others suggest that NAC ameliorates injury by helping to avoid depletion of glutathione.[35-36] In a rabbit model, corticosteroids given 1 hour before exposure to phosgene prevented damage from leukotrienes and other lipoxygenase derived products. Survival was not studied.[33] In a porcine model, treatment with intravenous (IV) methylprednisolone or inhaled budesonide after exposure to phosgene failed to decrease mortality at 24 hours.[37] Borak and Diller suggested treating patients with methylprednisolone (250 mg IV) or NAC (20 mL of a 20% nebulized solution).[31]

ASPHYXIANTS

Inhaled asphyxiants are categorized as either simple or chemical. Simple asphyxiants cause hypoxia by displacing oxygen, thereby decreasing the amount of oxygen reaching the lungs. Common simple asphyxiants include carbon dioxide, methane, nitrogen, hydrogen, and helium.

Chemical asphyxiants disrupt the body's ability to use oxygen by reducing hemoglobin's ability to transport oxygen and/or disrupting the electron transport chain in mitochondria, leading to impaired aerobic respiration and adenosine triphosphate (ATP) formation. Carbon monoxide (CO), cyanide (CN), and hydrogen sulfide (H_2S) are chemical asphyxiants.

Carbon Monoxide

CO is a colorless, odorless gas produced from the incomplete combustion of carbon-containing fuels.[38] Common sources of carbon monoxide include house fires, smoke inhalation, automobile exhaust, indoor heating systems and water heaters, forklifts, electric generators, and Zambonis. CO exposure is the leading cause of mortality from poisoning in the United States, accounting for an estimated 40,000 emergency department visits and 800 to 6000 deaths per year.[39-40] These numbers may be underestimates because of the nonspecific signs and symptoms of CO poisoning.[41]

CO binds hemoglobin, forming carboxyhemoglobin, with an affinity 200 times greater than that of oxygen.[38,40,42-44] The high affinity of CO for hemoglobin interferes with the ability of hemoglobin to bind oxygen and also shifts the oxygen dissociation curve to the left, preventing release of oxygen from hemoglobin in tissues.[43,45-47] CO also binds to other heme-containing proteins.[44-45] CO also disrupts the electron transport chain by binding to cytochrome aa3.[47] By binding to myoglobin,[44] CO reduces oxygen availability in cardiac tissue.[40] CO also increases nitric oxide levels, causing vasodilatation which results in syncope.[40,47] Neurologic injury may be the result of reperfusion injury to the hypoxic tissue.[46]

CO is called the "great imitator," because patients present with nonspecific signs and symptoms including headache, fatigue, malaise, and influenza-like and gastroenteritis-like symptoms.[43] The brain and heart have higher oxygen requirements and are more severely affected by CO-induced cellular hypoxia[46]; patients develop electrocardiographic (ECG) changes, chest pain, myocardial infarction,[43] syncope, and neurologic deficits.[40] Neurologic sequelae are divided into persistent neurologic sequelae (PNS) and delayed neurologic sequelae (DNS).[44] PNS occur at the time of exposure, whereas DNS begin 2 to 40 days after exposure. Fear of these sequelae is the rationale behind hyperbaric oxygen therapy (HBO).

PNS and DNS share the same psychoneurologic symptoms,[48] including aphasia, apraxia, apathy, disorientation, hallucinations, bradykinesia, rigidity, gait disturbances, and personality changes.[47] The incidence of DNS is unknown for two primary reasons: lack of a consistent definition[42] and lack of validated neuropsychometric tests to screen for presence of the syndrome.[40] Current research is focused on finding biomarkers to assess risk for DNS.[49]

Samples of either venous or arterial blood can be used to measure CO levels, because they correlate well in prospective studies.[40-41] A level greater than 2% in nonsmokers or 9% in smokers suggests exposure to exogenous CO.[39,41] Because patients are removed from the exposure and/or receive oxygen prior to the level being obtained, levels may be "falsely" low. Carboxyhemoglobin levels do not correlate well with the patient's clinical presentation or degree of injury, particularly at higher levels.[41,44,47] Patients exposed to CO can have lactic acidosis.[40] Pulse oximeters report falsely elevated hemoglobin saturations, as these devices fail to differentiate between oxygenated hemoglobin and carboxyhemoglobin. Conversely, co-oximetry differentiates between oxyhemoglobin and carboxyhemoglobin. Newer handheld oximetry probes accurately detect carboxyhemoglobin. Low-density bilateral globus pallidus lesions have been reported on head computed tomography (CT). These lesions, which may resolve with time, often develop within a few hours after the injury,[47] but their appearance can be delayed for days.[40]

Placing patients on 100% oxygen lowers the half-life of carboxyhemoglobin from 240 minutes on room air to 80 minutes. Hyperbaric oxygen (HBO) lowers the half-life to approximately 20 minutes.[40]

The use of HBO is controversial.[44,50] Four prospective randomized trials have evaluated its use.[48,50-52] The studies differed with respect to inclusion criteria, outcomes, definition of DNS, and HBO protocols. Of the four, the Weaver et al.[48] and Scheinkestel et al.[50] studies were the only ones that were blinded via the use of sham HBO (chamber was turned "on" and made noise but was not pressurized). The Weaver study is the most methodologically rigorous and well controlled of all the trials but is not above criticism[40]; it included patients with documented exposure to CO and also symptomatic patients thought to be exposed to CO.[48] Patients underwent three treatments within 24 hours; the first at 3 atmospheres absolute (ATA) and the others at 2 ATA. Pregnant patients, patients younger than 16 years of age, moribund patients, and anyone more than 24 hours from exposure were excluded. Weaver et al. concluded that HBO decreased the frequency of cognitive sequelae at 6 weeks and 12 months. The number needed to treat was 5 at 6 weeks.[48] In the Scheinkestel study, the hyperbaric group received HBO once daily at 2.8 ATA for 60 minutes for 3 to 6 days.[50] Except for children and pregnant women, any patient with CO poisoning, regardless of the severity or time since exposure, was included. Patients were assessed with many neuropsychiatric tests at the completion of hyperbaric treatment and 1 month later. All five cases of DNS occurred in the group that received HBO. Also, the normobaric group had fewer abnormal neuropsychiatric tests at the completion of therapy. The authors concluded that HBO did not offer a benefit and may have worsened some outcomes. However, only 46% of patients were followed up at 1 month, weakening the conclusions from this study.[50] Conversely, there was a 97% follow-up rate in the study by Weaver and coworkers.[48]

Two other trials were randomized but not blinded.[51-52] Raphael et al.[52] included 629 patients with accidental inhalation of CO who presented within 12 hours of exposure. Pregnant women were excluded. Patients were stratified on the basis of absence or presence of loss of consciousness (LOC), and treatment groups received one or two treatments with HBO. Follow up at 1 month was carried out using a self-assessment questionnaire. Raphael et al.[52] concluded that HBO might offer some benefit in patients with LOC, but not in patients without LOC. The study by Thom and colleagues[51] enrolled 60 patients who presented within 6 hours of exposure to CO. The subjects were randomized to receive either one session of HBO or normobaric oxygen. Patients with LOC or EKG changes were excluded. Patients receiving HBO had a lower incidence of DNS determined by testing immediately afterwards and at 1 month.[51]

Although controversy exists regarding the indications for HBO, we suggest using the enrollment criteria from the study by Weaver et al.,[48] because this study's methods improved outcomes. Indications, therefore, include neurologic findings (altered mental status, coma, focal deficits, seizures), syncope, pregnancy with carboxyhemoglobin concentration above 15%, cardiovascular compromise (ischemia, infarction, dysrhythmia), metabolic acidosis, concentrations greater than 25% in nonpregnant patients, and extremes of age.[40] The only absolute contraindication is untreated pneumothorax, but relative contraindications include chronic obstructive pulmonary disease, fever, bowel obstruction, and significant upper respiratory tract infection.[40,53]

The most common complication of HBO therapy is barotrauma; however, oxygen toxicity and seizures also have been reported.[40,48,50,53] While in the HBO chamber, the patient cannot receive defibrillation or electrical cardioversion. Also, the treatment team has limited access to the patient. Therefore some patients may be too unstable for HBO. In some cases, logistical challenges or the patient's underlying instability may render the situation so dangerous or so complex that transport to a facility that offers HBO is unfeasible.

Cyanide

Cyanide is one of the most rapidly acting and lethal poisons in existence.[54] Its infamy stems from its use in mass killing by the Nazis during World War II and the mass suicide led by Jim Jones in the 1970s. Other sources of cyanide include food (pits of members of the genus *Prunus*), photographic developer solutions, electroplating solutions, rodenticides, artificial nail remover, and sodium nitroprusside metabolism. Inhalation of smoke from structural fires is the most common source of cyanide exposure in the United States and Western countries.[55-56] Hydrogen cyanide formation from the combustion of carbon- and nitrogen-based materials and abundant plastics, polymers, synthetic fibers, and wools in houses are major contributors.[54-55] Cyanide toxicity also should be suspected in the sudden collapse of a laboratory or industrial worker or an unexplained coma or severe acidosis following a suicide attempt.[57] The clinical effects of cyanide poisoning depend on the dose, duration, and route of exposure.[58]

Cyanide binds to the ferric iron portion of cytochrome oxidase and inhibits it at the cytochrome a3 portion of the mitochondrial electron transport chain.[8,54,58-59] Binding of cyanide to cytochrome oxidase prevents mitochondria from using oxygen, thereby inhibiting aerobic metabolism.[55-56] Clinical manifestations reflect the failure of aerobic respiration.[58] The CNS and heart have high demands for oxygen and are the most susceptible organs to cyanide poisoning.[54] Transient increases in blood pressure, respiratory rate, and heart rate are followed by respiratory depression without cyanosis and cardiovascular collapse.[55] Patients may present with syncope, dilated pupils, or seizures.[59] Other presentations include headache, confusion, lethargy, agitation, and pulmonary edema. Unmetabolized cyanide has a bitter-almond-like odor and is excreted during breathing. However, 50% of the population cannot detect the odor.[55,58]

Hallmark laboratory findings include metabolic acidosis with elevated circulating lactate concentration.[55] In smoke inhalation victims, blood lactate concentration above 10 mmol/L suggests cyanide toxicity.[60] In victims of cyanide poisoning, the oxygen content of venous blood is abnormally high due to inhibition of cellular oxygen utilization.[55,58] The arteriovenous oxygen saturation difference may be less than 10 mmHg, and "arterialization" of venous and capillary blood is responsible for the characteristic cherry-red complexion and bright red retinal veins seen on examination of cyanide poisoning victims.[55,58] Cyanide is an unstable molecule with a short half-life, and blood levels usually are not available from the laboratory in a timely enough fashion to be clinically useful.[59] As such, the diagnosis is difficult to make and requires a high level of suspicion.[61]

There are two specific cyanide treatments available in the United States.[54] The traditional kit available from Eli Lilly and Company contains amyl nitrite, sodium nitrite, and sodium thiosulfate. Amyl nitrite ampules are inhaled to produce a methemoglobinemia. Once IV access is established, sodium nitrite (300 mg) is given IV to induce a methemoglobinemia (methemoglobin concentration = 20%-30%). Cyanide preferentially binds to methemoglobin over hemoglobin, forming cyanomethemoglobin.[62] Administration of nitrites can be detrimental, however, because of the complications associated with methemoglobinemia.[54] These complications include dyspnea, hypotension, acidosis, tachycardia, tachypnea, syncope, and CNS depression. Methemoglobinemia is a problem for patients who have been in a fire, as they may already have a significant carboxyhemoglobinemia[54,56]; thus, deliberate induction of methemoglobinemia results in two hemoglobinopathies at once.[61] Sodium thiosulfate acts as a substrate to convert cyanide to thiocyanate but has a comparatively delayed onset of action.[63] Adult dosing is 12.5 grams IV as a bolus or over half an hour.

Hydroxocobalamin is a precursor of vitamin B_{12} and binds to cyanide to form cyanocobalamin (vitamin B_{12}), which is then renally excreted.[61] Unlike the case with nitrites, hydroxocobalamin has few side effects. It is associated with temporary skin discoloration that can interfere with the accuracy of co-oximetry. A recent review recommends hydroxocobalamin (5 g IV) for empirical treatment of smoke inhalation victims suspected of having cyanide toxicity.[61]

Hydrogen Sulfide

Hydrogen sulfide is a colorless gas with a characteristic "rotten egg" odor.[64] It is a byproduct of human and animal waste and produced by the decay of organic material.[65] Its mechanism of toxicity is through competitive inhibition of the electron transport chain,[66-68] but it also is an irritant.[65, 69]

Hydrogen sulfide's odor is perceived at levels of 3 to 30 ppm,[65] with olfactory paralysis occurring at 100 to 150 ppm.[66-67] Patients present with complaints including headache, weakness, incoordination, cough, dyspnea, and gastrointestinal symptoms.[66] Cyanosis, pulmonary edema, cardiac dysrhythmias, and keratoconjunctivitis are present on examination.[66] If an exposed patient has coins (e.g., dimes or quarters) in his or her pockets during the period when hydrogen sulfide is present in the atmosphere, the coins undergo reaction with the gas and turn black.[67] Diagnosis is based on history, because a clinically useful laboratory test is not readily available.

There may be a role for nitrites and HBO in the treatment of hydrogen sulfide toxicity. The nitrite-induced methemoglobin has a high affinity for hydrogen sulfide and enables cytochrome oxidase to resume aerobic metabolism.[65] Case reports refer to the use of HBO, as it may enhance detoxification of hydrogen sulfide.[64,70] However, there is little supporting evidence for HBO, and its use cannot be recommended enthusiastically until further research is conducted.[64-65,68]

▣ Conclusion

Direct pulmonary irritants and asphyxiants are two types of toxins that cause pulmonary injury. Irritants are classified according to their water solubility, which affects the location of the respiratory tract injury. Care for these patients is mainly supportive; further research is needed to determine whether there is a role for corticosteroids in treatment.

There are simple and chemical asphyxiants. Both CO and cyanide are chemical asphyxiants. Either arterial or venous samples can be used to test for carboxyhemoglobin. For the treatment of CO poisoning, we suggest using the indications in the study by Weaver et al.[48] to determine whether HBO is warranted. Multiple treatments for cyanide poisoning exist including nitrites, sodium thiosulfate, and hydroxocobalamin.

KEY POINTS

1. The degree of water solubility of irritants largely determines which part of the respiratory tract is injured.

2. Agents which are very soluble in water (i.e., very hydrophilic) cause immediate symptoms due to injury of the upper respiratory tract.

3. Agents which are relatively insoluble in water (i.e., lipophilic) produce delayed effects and cause lower respiratory tract injuries such as pulmonary edema.

4. When agents are inhaled at high concentrations or in large amounts, specificity for the location of respiratory tract injury typically is lost.

5. Agreement among experts is lacking regarding the use of steroids for inhalant-induced acute lung injury (ALI).

6. Efficacy data are unclear, but nebulized sodium bicarbonate has been used to treat minor to moderate inhalational injuries from chlorine gas.

7. Simple asphyxiants displace oxygen, whereas chemical asphyxiants impair oxidative respiration by binding hemoglobin or disrupting the mitochondrial electron transport chain.

8. Victims of house fires may be exposed to both cyanide and carbon monoxide. In this situation, physicians should consider avoiding nitrites because production of methemoglobinemia could worsen functional anemia due to the formation of carboxyhemoglobin.

9. Hydroxocobalamin can be used to treat cyanide toxicity instead of the Eli Lilly kit (nitrites and sodium thiosulfate).

10. Patients with elevated carboxyhemoglobin levels may benefit from hyperbaric oxygen therapy to prevent delayed neurologic sequelae (DNS).

ANNOTATED REFERENCES

Weaver LK, Hopkins RO, Chan KJ, et al. Hyperbaric oxygen for acute carbon monoxide poisoning. N Engl J Med 2002;347:1057-67.
Three hyperbaric oxygen treatments within a 24-hour period, compared to a control, reduced the risk of cognitive sequelae 6 weeks and 12 months after acute carbon monoxide poisoning. This contrasts with the Scheinkestel study listed below.

Miller K, Chen A. Acute inhalation injury. Emerg Med Clin North Am 2003;21:533-57.
The lungs can be an efficient means for the absorption of inhaled toxicants, resulting in airway and pulmonary injury or systemic toxicity. Although few specific antidotes exist for inhaled toxicants, the syndrome of acute inhalational injury and clinical therapeutics is linked by common pathways of pathophysiology.

Hall AH, Dart R, Bogdan G. Sodium thiosulfate or hydroxocobalamin for the empiric treatment of cyanide poisoning? Ann Emerg Med 2007;49:806-13.
Based on recent safety and efficacy studies in animals, safety studies in healthy volunteers, and uncontrolled efficacy studies in humans, hydroxocobalamin seems to be an appropriate antidote for empirical treatment of smoke inhalation and other suspected cyanide poisoning for victims in the out-of-hospital setting.

Aslan S, Kandis H, Akgun M, et al. The effect of nebulized NaHCO$_3$ treatment on "RADS" due to chlorine gas inhalation. Inhal Toxicol 2006;18:895-900.
Nebulized sodium bicarbonate has beneficial short-term effects, as measured by PFTs and quality-of-life score, in patients with RADS secondary to chlorine gas exposure.

Sjöblom E, Höjer J, Kulling PEJ, et al. A placebo-controlled experimental study of steroid inhalation therapy in ammonia-induced lung injury. J Toxicol Clin Toxicol 1999;37:59-67.
The major findings in this study were that inhalation of corticosteroids did not improve gas exchange or reduce the airway pressure levels compared to placebo in this animal model.

Scheinkestel CD, Bailey M, Myles PS, et al. Hyperbaric or normobaric oxygen for acute carbon monoxide poisoning: a randomized controlled clinical trial. Med J Aust 1999;170:203-10.
One hyperbaric treatment daily for 3 to 6 days, compared to a control, found no benefit and possible adverse effects. This is in contrast to the Weaver study noted above.

REFERENCES

Access the complete reference list online at http://www.expertconsult.com.

188

Cocaine

JANICE ZIMMERMAN | PHILIP ALAPAT

Cocaine abuse is one of the leading causes of drug-related emergency department visits and hospital admissions. Illicit use of this substance can lead to numerous medical complications, necessitating hospital admission and critical care and yielding significant mortality. Although cocaine use is more prevalent in young adults, complications of cocaine use should also be considered in older individuals.

Cocaine is obtained readily from the *Erythroxylum coca* plant, which is grown primarily in South America. Cocaine is extracted by soaking the leaves in organic solvents, and then precipitating the cocaine hydrochloride salt with the addition of hydrochloric acid. This form of cocaine can be snorted (inhaled through the nose), ingested orally, or intravenously (IV) injected. To smoke cocaine, the hydrochloride salt must be converted to a "free base" by dissolving it in an alkaline solvent. Allowing this product to dry into a rock-like state results in the popular street form of the drug, "crack cocaine." The name comes from the cracking sound produced when this form of the drug is heated.

Testing for cocaine exposure is usually performed with urine assays, but almost any type of biological specimen can be tested. Because cocaine has a short half-life of about 1 hour, the metabolite, benzoylecgonine (half-life of 6 hours), is usually measured. Thus urine testing can usually detect cocaine use for approximately 1 to 2 days after an acute exposure. Chronic cocaine use may cause positive results days to weeks following last use of the drug.[1] There are no other drugs that can yield false-positive test results when benzoylecgonine urine assays are used.[2]

Mechanism of Action

Medicinal use of cocaine has fallen out of favor because other agents that lack potential for abuse and possess the medically useful local anesthetic and vasoconstrictive properties of cocaine have been found. The local anesthetic effects of cocaine occur because of its ability to block voltage-gated sodium channels in the neuronal membrane, resulting in blockade of neural conduction.[3] The vasoconstrictive property of cocaine is mostly due to stimulation of α-adrenergic receptors in arterial wall smooth muscle cells. Increased endothelin-1 and decreased nitric oxide blood concentrations also may contribute to cocaine's vasoconstrictive properties.[4] Two major metabolites of cocaine, benzoylecgonine and ecgonine methyl ester, may persist for over 24 hours and can be associated with delayed or recurrent coronary vasoconstriction.[5,6]

The sympathomimetic activity of cocaine is caused by inhibition of the presynaptic reuptake of biogenic amines including norepinephrine, dopamine, and serotonin. Inhibition of reuptake of these neurotransmitters occurs throughout the body, including the central nervous system (CNS), as cocaine and some of its metabolites readily cross the blood-brain barrier. The resulting systemic effects of cocaine include increased heart rate and blood pressure and diffuse vasoconstriction. The CNS effects include marked euphoria and self-confidence at lower doses and agitation and delirium at higher doses. These CNS effects are most likely due to excessive dopaminergic activity.[2]

The thrombogenic activity of cocaine has been ascribed to increased plasminogen-activator inhibitor activity, increased platelet count, increased platelet activation, and platelet hyperaggregability. Additionally, because circulating elevated concentrations of C-reactive protein, von Willebrand factor, and fibrinogen are seen in cocaine users, it seems likely that the drug induces a proinflammatory state that enhances thrombosis.[4]

Cocaine and ethanol are frequently abused together, which may lead to added detrimental effects. Cocaine in the presence of ethanol is metabolized by the liver into cocaethylene, which has a longer duration of action than cocaine and is more toxic than cocaine or ethanol alone.[3,7] Additionally, ethanol inhibits cocaine metabolism, yielding higher cocaine concentrations.[2]

In addition to the toxic effects of cocaine itself, adulterants that are frequently added to cocaine may cause other undesirable effects. Commonly, talc and cornstarch are used as "fillers." Other potential contaminants include benzocaine, quinine, and more recently, levamisole. Levamisole is an anthelmintic and antineoplastic drug that is not commonly used in humans because of an unacceptably high risk of agranulocytosis. The majority of cocaine tested from the United States is now adulterated with levamisole, and several cases of agranulocytosis have been linked to contaminated cocaine.[8]

Toxicities

CENTRAL NERVOUS SYSTEM

The most significant CNS toxicity associated with cocaine use is stroke; both hemorrhagic and ischemic strokes can occur. Hemorrhagic strokes associated with cocaine use are hypothesized to result from acute elevations of blood pressure, coupled with platelet dysfunction and/or the presence of vascular malformations. The presence of vascular malformations, in particular, was suggested by several reports to be a significant predisposing factor. However, a large retrospective study failed to find a significant association between the presence of vascular malformations and cocaine-induced intracranial hemorrhage. Additionally, there was no predilection for cocaine to affect a particular area of the brain. The study noted that brainstem hemorrhage and intraventricular extension were associated with cocaine use.[9] Ischemic stroke is also thought to be caused by cocaine use and is likely caused by cerebral vasoconstriction, which has been demonstrated experimentally and may be particularly associated with chronic abuse of the drug.[10] Increased thrombogenic activity as described earlier also may play a role, especially with chronic use. All standard stroke care should be provided to patients with stroke related to cocaine use.

Seizures can be induced by acute use of cocaine, as the drug lowers the seizure threshold. Additionally, seizures can be induced by withdrawal of cocaine. Most seizures are self-limiting and usually respond to administration of IV benzodiazepines. Refractory seizure activity may indicate a severe CNS injury or severe hyperthermia.

Hyperthermia can occur with cocaine abuse and may result in death, especially in overdose situations and in hot climates.[11] Cocaine-induced hyperthermia is thought to be related to dysfunction of CNS thermoregulatory centers as well as derangements in regional distribution of blood flow caused by the vasoconstrictor effects of the drug.[3] In addition, most patients present with heat exposure and muscle hyperactivity as contributing causes.[11,12] A syndrome of excited delirium manifested by agitation, paranoia, and psychosis sometimes accompanies hyperthermia. In these cases, body temperature can be markedly elevated (>40.6°C). Patients presenting in this manner often have accompanying complications such as disseminated intravascular coagulation, rhabdomyolysis, and/or renal failure.[13] Other than supportive care and aggressive cooling measures, there are no other standard therapies. Benzodiazepines such as lorazepam (administered IV or intramuscularly) should be used liberally to control agitation and hyperactivity. Haloperidol should be avoided, as this agent can lower the seizure threshold and also itself induce hyperthermia. Evaluation of the agitated cocaine abuser always should include accurate determination of core temperature.

PULMONARY

Pulmonary diseases associated with cocaine use are varied and can range from acute bronchoconstriction to noncardiogenic pulmonary edema to barotrauma. Most reported pulmonary complications have been associated with smoking freebase cocaine. Bronchoconstriction has been shown experimentally to be associated with inhaled cocaine.[14] An increased need for intubation and mechanical ventilation with asthma exacerbations also has been found in cocaine abusers.[15] The term *crack lung* has been used to refer to pulmonary infiltrates related to cocaine use. The pulmonary infiltrates may be transient or associated with significant disease, especially acute respiratory distress syndrome (ARDS).[16] Noncardiogenic pulmonary edema caused by cocaine use is frequently associated with alveolar hemorrhage.[17] Alternatively, hemoptysis can be the only presenting complaint and usually remits with avoidance of further cocaine exposure. Talc in contaminated cocaine has been reported to cause granulomatous lung disease. This entity is primarily associated with IV administration of cocaine, but chronic inhalation of the drug also can produce a similar form of lung disease.[18] Data are lacking to show that administration of corticosteroids is of benefit for addressing pulmonary abnormalities associated with cocaine abuse.

Pneumothorax and pneumomediastinum have also been associated with smoking crack cocaine and are likely caused by coughing triggered by the inhalation of the drug, or particular behaviors such as breath holding which are employed to enhance the desirable effects of the drug. The cause of pneumothorax also may be related to adulterants in the inhaled cocaine.[19] Treatment is usually conservative with supplemental oxygen and serial imaging. Tube thoracostomy is reserved for moderate to large pneumothoraces. The presence of pneumomediastinum by itself is not an indication for hospital or intensive care unit (ICU) admission.

CARDIOVASCULAR

Myocardial ischemia and infarction (acute coronary syndromes [ACS]) related to cocaine use were first reported in 1982.[20] Since then, numerous studies have confirmed that cocaine abuse is an epidemiologically significant cause of myocardial ischemia and infarction and morbidity and mortality on this basis. Chest pain is the most frequent reason for cocaine users to present to emergency departments. Cocaine-induced ACS are not related to the amount of cocaine used, route of administration, or frequency of use. First-time users can develop myocardial infarction (MI).[5] Cocaine-associated myocardial ischemia is likely related to the combination of increased myocardial oxygen demand caused by acute increases in heart rate, blood pressure, and contractility, on the one hand, combined with decreased myocardial oxygen supply caused by coronary vasoconstriction, on the other hand. In addition, coronary artery atherosclerosis can develop prematurely in young cocaine users. In combination with the ability of cocaine to promote a prothrombotic state, cocaine-induced coronary artery disease likely contributes to the risk for ACS among cocaine abusers.[4] Cocaine-associated myocardial ischemia appears to occur most commonly in the first few hours after cocaine exposure; however, delayed infarction can occur several hours to weeks after exposure to the drug. The effects of the metabolites of cocaine (benzoylecgonine and ecgonine methyl ester) are thought to contribute to the delayed presentation.[5]

Diagnosis of cocaine-associated MI should rely on the measurement of cardiac troponin I, as rhabdomyolysis and consequent elevation of total creatine phosphokinase concentrations can otherwise confound diagnosis.[21,22] Diagnosis using electrocardiogram (ECG) is difficult because the majority of patients who present with chest pain associated with cocaine use have ECG abnormalities. Even ST-segment elevation is difficult to interpret in these patients, because an early repolarization pattern is frequently present.[23]

American Heart Association guidelines recommend percutaneous coronary intervention over fibrinolytic therapy for ST-segment elevation MI in the setting of cocaine use. Nitroglycerin and benzodiazepines are advocated as primary therapy aimed at ameliorating the coronary vasoconstriction and the increase in myocardial oxygen demand. Administration of aspirin and heparin is recommended unless contraindicated. Calcium channel blockers may be used in patients unresponsive to nitroglycerin and benzodiazepines.[4] Beta-blockers, including labetalol, were thought to be associated with worse outcomes in patients with recent history of cocaine use. However, this topic provokes considerable controversy, since beta-blocker use was not found to be detrimental in two retrospective studies of patients with a recent history of cocaine use.[24,25] Administration of beta-blockers might be beneficial for selected patients with ACS and a history of cocaine abuse.

Cocaine's ability to block sodium channels yields acute type Ic antiarrhythmic properties including QRS prolongation and a variety of arrhythmias. Sinus tachycardia is the most common abnormal rhythm in cocaine users, and it responds to observation or benzodiazepines. Supraventricular arrhythmias are usually self-limited, but benzodiazepines also may be useful. Ventricular arrhythmias may respond to treatment with sodium bicarbonate, and addition of lidocaine may be necessary.[26] Arrhythmias due to cocaine-associated myocardial ischemia should be treated by correcting the ischemia. As always, treatment of life-threatening arrhythmias should follow Advanced Cardiac Life Support (ACLS) protocols. Aortic dissection is an important consideration when addressing cocaine-associated chest pain. Though many previous reports linked aortic dissection to cocaine use, a large international registry did not confirm the presence of a significant association.[27,28]

MUSCULOSKELETAL

The direct myotoxic effect of cocaine coupled with vasoconstriction-induced muscle ischemia are the likely contributors to rhabdomyolysis induced by cocaine use.[29] In addition, the various adulterants often added to cocaine may worsen the injury. Diagnosis is based on detection of elevated serum creatine phosphokinase (CPK) concentrations. In the absence of hematuria, evaluation for myoglobinuria with urine dipstick testing may aid screening for rhabdomyolysis.[30] It is prudent to consider the possibility of rhabdomyolysis in cocaine abusers with significant agitation or obtundation. Initial CPK concentrations may be normal, and repeat testing after a few hours, especially after volume administration, may identify significant rhabdomyolysis.

Treatment is aimed at preventing renal tubular damage caused by the nephrotoxic effects of myoglobin and some hemoglobin decomposition products. Treatment consists of providing aggressive IV hydration with crystalloid infusion. Recommendations for IV hydration include at least 1 to 2 L as an initial bolus, or achievement of a clinically euvolemic state followed by continuous infusion of 200 to 500 mL/h.[31,32] Recommendations for use of IV bicarbonate, mannitol, and forced diuresis are not supported by available clinical data. Frequent monitoring of electrolytes is imperative, as both the myocyte injury and associated renal injury can contribute to severe electrolyte abnormalities that require immediate intervention. Early acute dialysis may be necessary to treat persistent hyperkalemia.[33]

Other Complications

Ischemic injury due to cocaine also can affect the gastrointestinal (GI) tract. Bowel ischemia, infarction, and perforation have been reported following ingestion, IV injection, or inhalation of cocaine.[34-37] Although most cases of ischemia involve segments of the small bowel, ischemic colitis also can occur.[36,37] Most patients tend to be younger with no predisposing risks for ischemia. Gastroduodenal perforation also has been described.[35] Vasoconstriction and/or thrombosis of mesenteric vessels are proposed mechanisms for bowel ischemia. Patients can present with acute or chronic abdominal pain, and peritoneal signs are often present. Management often includes surgical exploration, but nonoperative approaches with bowel rest and antibiotics may be appropriate in some patients. In some cases, preoperative angiography identified occlusion of celiac or mesenteric vessels that prompted revascularization interventions.[38]

Acute renal injury due to cocaine may be precipitated by rhabdomyolysis, but other etiologic factors can include vasoconstriction or thrombosis of renal vessels, accelerated hypertension, thrombotic microangiopathy, interstitial nephritis and/or glomerulonephritis.[39] Renal infarction should be considered in cocaine users who present with significant persistent abdominal or flank pain that is often accompanied by nausea, vomiting, and fever.[40,41] The right kidney is more commonly involved, based on published reports. Diagnosis is facilitated by imaging and assessment of the renal vasculature. Management of renal infarction due to cocaine includes administration of aspirin, anticoagulation, thrombectomy, if indicated, and supportive care.

The effects of cocaine in pregnant women are similar to the effects of the drug in other groups of patients. In addition, however, cocaine-induced vasoconstriction decreases uterine blood flow and consequently oxygen delivery to the fetus. Obstetrical conditions associated with cocaine use include placental abruption, placenta previa, spontaneous abortion, premature rupture of membranes, and uterine rupture.[42,43] Standard obstetrical management is indicated for these conditions.

Drug Transporters

Cocaine or other illicit drugs are sometimes ingested or inserted into body orifices for the purpose of transport or concealment.[44] Body "stuffers" swallow or otherwise hide small amounts of (wrapped or unwrapped) drug to avoid detection. In this circumstance, toxicity is frequent because the drug is not prepared to limit absorption, usually during passage through the GI tract. Quantities of drug are smaller, so toxicity is usually mild. In contrast, body "packers" swallow larger quantities of drug in packets that are specially prepared to withstand transit through the GI tract.[45] Plain abdominal radiographs often show the location of packets, but a negative result does not rule out body packing. An abdominal computed tomography (CT) scan may be needed to visualize the packets.

Asymptomatic transporters of cocaine packets can be managed conservatively until the packets have been completely evacuated.[45,46] Activated charcoal given every 4 to 6 hours can reduce the lethality of cocaine absorption. Whole-bowel irrigation or mild laxatives such as lactulose may assist with passage of the packets. Surgical intervention is required in patients with clinical manifestations of cocaine toxicity, suspected rupture of packets, or symptoms compatible with GI obstruction or perforation.[45] Patients requiring surgical procedures may have a higher incidence of wound infections.[47,48]

Cocaine Withdrawal

Psychological and biochemical dependency occurs with cocaine use. Withdrawal symptoms are likely related to dopamine deficiency in the CNS after a period of abstinence.[49] Clinical manifestations of withdrawal include depression, fatigue, irritability, insomnia, psychomotor agitation or depression, and craving for more cocaine. Prolonged somnolence ("washout syndrome") can occur after binge use and often leads to extensive evaluations for other etiologies.[50] Patients should be referred for drug counseling.

ANNOTATED REFERENCES

Goldstein RA, DesLauriers C, Burda AM. Cocaine: history, social implications, and toxicity—a review. Dis Mon 2009;55:6-38.
A thorough review of cocaine's uses, abuses, pharmacology, drug interactions, and toxicities.
Knuepfer MM. Cardiovascular disorders associated with cocaine use: myths and truths. Pharmacol Ther 2003;97:181-222.
A review of the various cardiovascular disorders associated with cocaine use.
McCord J, Jneid H, Hollander JE, de Lemos JA, Cercek B, Hsue P, et al. Management of cocaine-associated chest pain and myocardial infarction: a scientific statement from the American Heart Association Acute Cardiac Care Committee of the Council on Clinical Cardiology. Circulation 2008;117:1897-907.
The American Heart Association statement that describes the various cardiology recommendations in the care of patients with cocaine-associated chest pain and myocardial infarction.
Lange RA, Hillis LD. Cardiovascular complications of cocaine use. N Engl J Med 2001;345:351-8.
An important review article that describes the various cardiovascular complications of cocaine use and the scientific understanding of the disease processes.
Martin-Schild S, Albright KC, Hallevi H, Barreto AD, Philip M, Misra V, et al. Intracerebral hemorrhage in cocaine users. Stroke 2010;41:680-4.
A large retrospective study addressing the location, pathology, and outcome of patients with cocaine-associated intracerebral hemorrhage.

REFERENCES

Access the complete reference list online at http://www.expertconsult.com.

189

Methamphetamine, Ecstasy, and Other Street Drugs

JOHN R. RICHARDS | ROBERT W. DERLET

History

The first documented synthesis of methamphetamine, utilizing ephedrine as a substrate, occurred in 1918 in Japan. A closely related compound, d-amphetamine, had been created 20 years earlier in Germany (Figure 189-1). These compounds are not found naturally, although similar substances such as ephedra (ma-huang), cathine, and cathinone have stimulant properties and are extracted from certain plants. Both amphetamine and methamphetamine originally were used in nasal decongestants and bronchial inhalers beginning in the 1930s. A research report in 1937 claimed amphetamine enhanced work output and intellectual performance, and the legal use of amphetamine increased as a result.[1] During this period, amphetamines were noted to reduce impulsive behavior and hyperactivity in children.[2] In 1954, methylphenidate (Ritalin, Concerta, Methylin) was approved for this indication. There are a variety of these drugs with slight differences in chemical structure. For example, Adderall combines dextroamphetamine and amphetamine with d-amphetamine saccharate and d,l-amphetamine aspartate. In the fenethylline (Captagon) molecule, theophylline is covalently linked with amphetamine via an alkyl chain.

Millions of doses of amphetamine and methamphetamine were taken by military personnel of all nations during World War II.[3] Thereafter, surplus supplies entered civilian markets, most notably Japan. Methamphetamine was widely prescribed for depression and obesity, reaching a peak of 31 million prescriptions in the United States in 1967. During this period, production and distribution was largely controlled by motorcycle gangs who hid the drugs in the crankcase of their motorcycles (hence the street name, "crank"). Amphetamines were outlawed after the United States Drug Abuse and Regulation Control Act of 1970. In the 1980s, a concentrated form of methamphetamine, known as "ice," "glass," or "crystal," became popular.[4] Production and trafficking in the United States continues to increase, with significant input from Mexican, Southeast Asian, West African, and European drug cartels. An estimated 12.3 million Americans have tried methamphetamine at least once, and 600,000 are weekly users.[5] The global number of users is estimated to be over 50 million. Methamphetamine is the most prevalent illegally manufactured controlled substance in the United States and worldwide.[6] Abuse of legally prescribed amphetamines represents a new problem among teenagers and young adults.[7]

Pharmacology and Metabolism

Methamphetamine can be ingested orally, snorted, injected, or smoked. It is lipid soluble and crosses the blood-brain barrier readily. Methamphetamine acts primarily on dopaminergic central nervous system (CNS) cells. In small doses, amphetamines cause release of dopamine from the cytoplasmic pool by exchange diffusion at the membrane dopamine uptake transporter locus.[8] Methamphetamine also antagonizes the reuptake of catecholamines by competitive inhibition. As the dose increases, amphetamines diffuse through the presynaptic terminal membrane and bind to the neurotransmitter transporter on the vesicular membrane, resulting in the exchange release of dopamine into the cytoplasm (Figure 189-2). Dopamine is then released into the synapse by reverse transport at the dopamine uptake locus. At even higher doses, methamphetamine diffuses through the cellular and vesicular membranes and alkalinizes the vesicles. This results in dopamine release from the vesicles and delivery into the synapse by reverse transport. Chronic methamphetamine use results in down-regulation of dopamine D1 and D2 receptors.[9]

Increased norepinephrine at the locus ceruleus results in anorectic and locomotor effects. Increased dopamine in the neostriatum results in glutamate release and inhibition of γ-aminobutyric acid (GABA)-ergic neurons.[10] There is evidence that glutamate stimulation contributes significantly to the neurotoxicity of amphetamines.[11] The serotonin transporter exhibits abnormal efflux in response to amphetamines.[12] Elevated serotonin and dopamine levels within the mesolimbic system may cause hallucinations and psychosis. Release of dopamine in the ventral tegmental area is involved in reward and addiction.[13] The rage reaction induced by amphetamines may result from increased release of dopamine in the limbic system.[14]

Metabolism of methamphetamine occurs in the liver. Dealkylation and demethylation are performed by cytochrome P450 isoenzymes. Metabolites include amphetamine, 4-hydroxymethamphetamine, and 4-hydroxyamphetamine, which are also biologically active stimulants.[15] The pharmacokinetics are complex and nonlinear.[16] The biological half-life varies from 6 to 15 hours after a single dose. However, the cellular effects may last for days. Excretion occurs primarily in the urine and is affected by pH. Amphetamines are basic, with a typical pK_a range from 9 to 10, and renal elimination is enhanced with acidic urine. Approximately 60% of an oral dose is eliminated in the urine within the first 24 hours, with about one-third as intact drug and the remainder as metabolites.

Acute Effects

Methamphetamine abusers may present acutely with myriad symptoms including agitation, confusion, tremors, anxiety, hyperthermia, hypertension, tachycardia, and seizures. Less common effects include arrhythmias, cerebral and pulmonary edema, hepatotoxicity, and disseminated intravascular coagulation. Patients may present with atypical chest pain and be at risk for acute coronary syndrome.[17] Compared to cocaine, methamphetamine is less likely to cause myocardial ischemia, as it does not interfere with thromboxane production and platelet aggregation.[18] Severe abdominal pain may be the result of acute mesenteric vasoconstriction. Necrotizing vasculitis is associated with methamphetamine abuse and can involve multiple organ systems.[19] Methamphetamine patients utilize prehospital, emergency department, and hospital resources at a much higher than average rate.[20] Methamphetamine crosses the placenta, and use during pregnancy may result in fetal growth retardation, premature birth, developmental delay in neonates, and cognitive deficits in children.[21]

A dangerous stage of methamphetamine toxicity occurs when an abuser has not slept for days and is irritable and paranoid. This behavior is referred to as "tweaking." The individual craves more methamphetamine, but it is impossible to achieve the original high, causing unpredictable, unstable, and violent behavior.[22] Abusers frequently neglect nutrition and fluid intake during these periods, which can result in rhabdomyolysis when combined with periods of agitation or long periods of inactivity (Figure 189-3).[23] The proliferation of clandestine methamphetamine laboratories has increased the incidence of

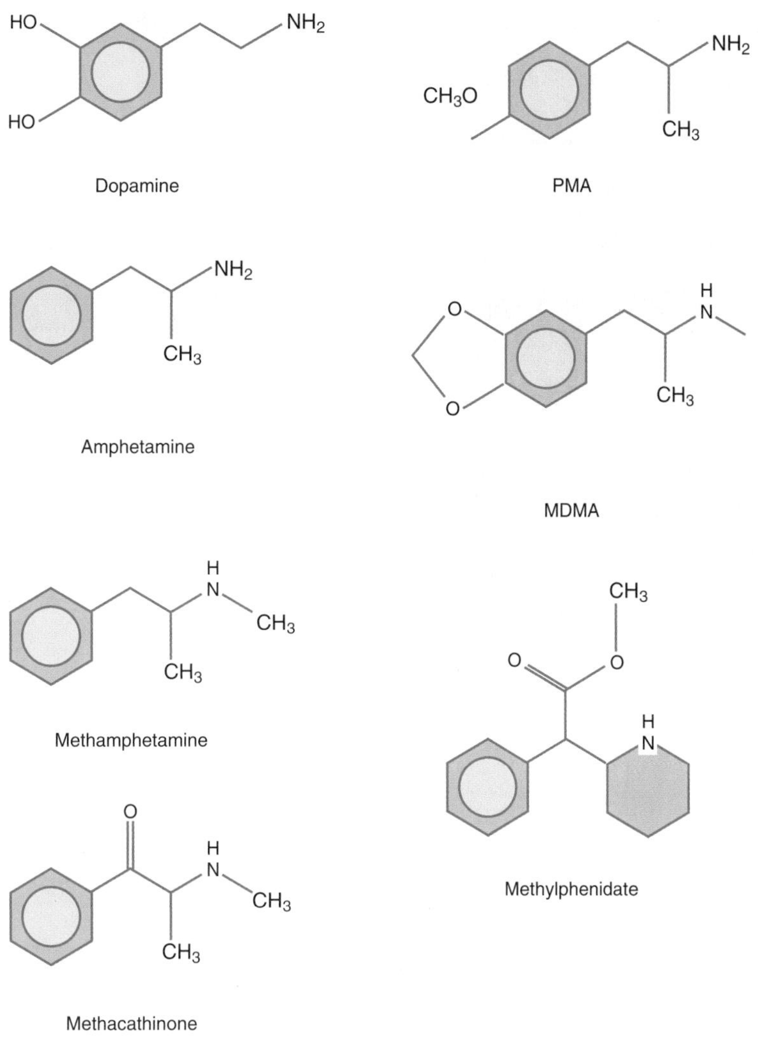

Figure 189-1 Chemical structure of dopamine and related amphetamine derivatives.

chemical and thermal burn injuries.[24] Lead and mercury contamination from illicit production of methamphetamine may result in acute toxicity.[25]

Chronic use of methamphetamine results in numerous harmful and irreversible cellular and end-organ effects. Long-term use has been shown to result in unique patterns of periodontal disease and tooth loss, a condition commonly referred to as "meth mouth" (Figure 189-4); the maxillary teeth tend to be most prominently affected.[26] Chronic users also develop characteristic skin lesions such as prurigo nodularis, also known as "speed bumps," from constant picking and scratching, usually from delusions of parasitosis. Methamphetamine is also neurotoxic to dopaminergic and serotoninergic cells.[27] Chronic users may develop a syndrome similar to Parkinson's disease.[28] Unusual choreoathetoid movements result from increased dopaminergic activity within the striatal area.[29] A magnetic resonance imaging (MRI) study of methamphetamine addicts demonstrated permanent gray-matter deficits of the cingulate, limbic, and paralimbic cortices and white matter hypertrophy, which correlated with memory and mood disorders exhibited by the subjects.[30] Chronic methamphetamine use results in inhibition of tyrosine hydroxylase, deficits in mitochondrial energy production, and neuronal apoptosis from oxidative stress.[31]

Chronic use has been demonstrated to result in cardiomyopathy, congestive heart failure, and accelerated coronary artery disease.[32] Methamphetamine use often results in impulsive behavior, which facilitates transmission of sexually transmitted diseases, viral hepatitis, and human immunodeficiency virus (HIV).[33] Furthermore, for those

injecting the drug, bacterial and foreign-body contamination may result in endocarditis, tetanus, wound botulism, osteomyelitis, and pulmonary and soft-tissue abscesses.[34] Methamphetamine withdrawal syndrome is initially characterized by increased sleep, eating, and dysphoria. This pattern declines into a subacute phase lasting up to 2 weeks.[35] These symptoms, coupled with increased risk-taking behavior, result in a higher incidence of traumatic injuries from motor vehicle accidents, falls, and assaults.[36] Methamphetamine users often exhibit suspicion and paranoia and are rarely forthcoming about the details of their drug use.[37] This pattern includes denial even when presented with a positive toxicology screen or other physical evidence.

Clinical Management

Acute methamphetamine toxicity is a true emergency. Airway, breathing, circulation, and temperature should be assessed, with continuous telemetry monitoring and frequent measurement of blood pressure. For patients with hyperthermia, a rectal thermometer is the most accurate method to trend core temperature. Agitated patients initially should be restrained physically, using a team approach (one person per limb) to protect both the patient and staff from harm. This form of restraint should immediately be followed by chemical restraint, using neuroleptic agents or benzodiazepines. Once adequate sedation has been achieved, physical restraints should be removed as soon as feasible. Neuroleptic agents may have a theoretical advantage over benzodiazepines, as these are CNS dopamine antagonists and may directly counteract the excess levels of dopamine in the CNS which result from

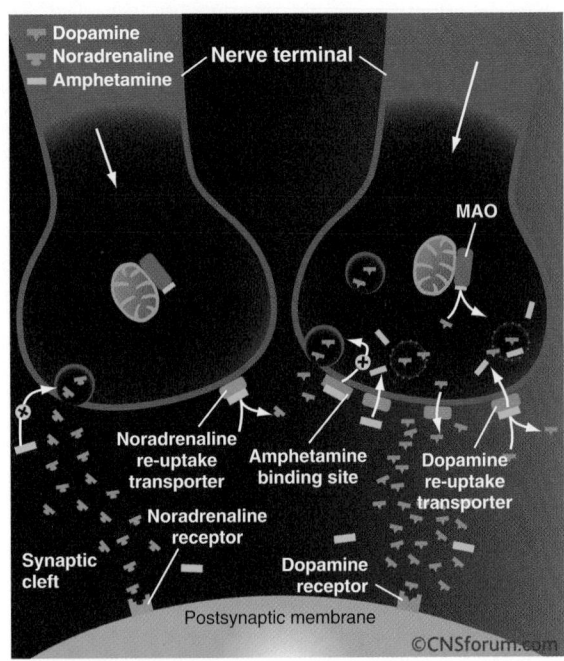

Figure 189-2 Mechanisms of action of high-dose amphetamine on central dopamine and norepinephrine transmission. *(From www.cnsforum.com, with permission.)*

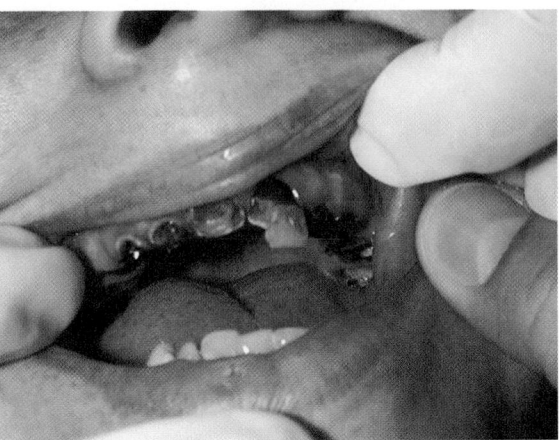

Figure 189-4 Anterior maxillary tooth loss associated with chronic methamphetamine abuse (ungloved finger is the patient's).

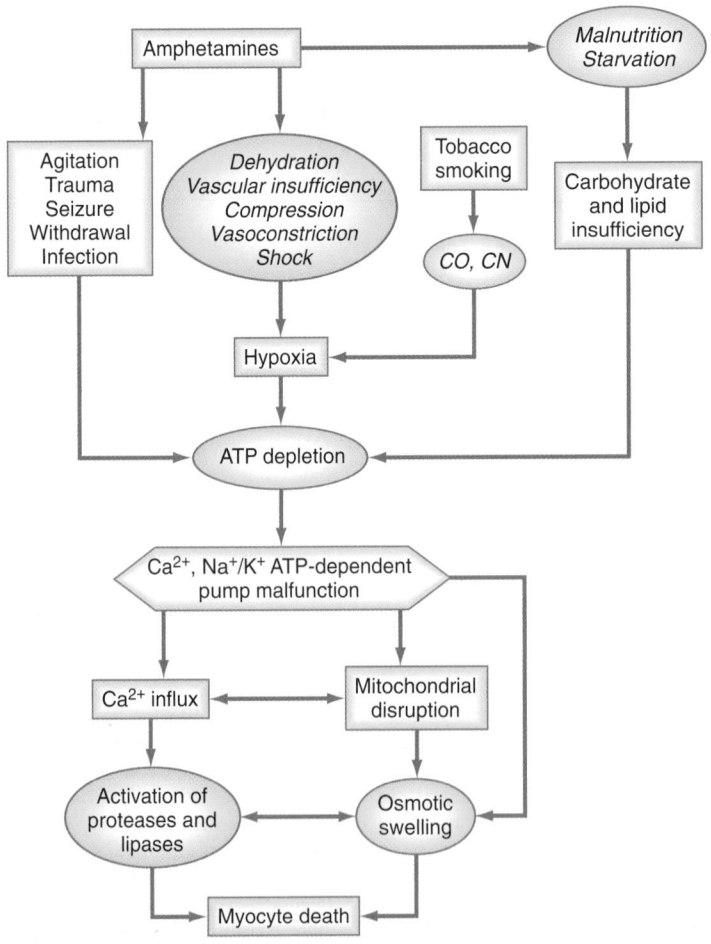

Figure 189-3 Putative relationship between amphetamines and other cofactors with development of rhabdomyolysis.

methamphetamine abuse.[37-41] Furthermore, neuroleptics do not affect respiratory drive, whereas multiple or large doses of benzodiazepines may result in respiratory depression. For benzodiazepines, typical dosages are 5 to 10 mg of diazepam or 1 to 4 mg of lorazepam by intravenous (IV) route.

The authors of a prospective study that compared lorazepam with droperidol for control of agitated methamphetamine users concluded that droperidol was longer acting than lorazepam and required fewer repeat doses to achieve sedation.[37] Droperidol, or the longer-acting agent, haloperidol, may be administered by either the IV or intramuscular route. Typical doses required are 2.5 to 5 mg of droperidol or 5 to 10 mg of haloperidol. Of note, use of the butyrophenones for this particular indication is considered "off-label." Droperidol, however, has been used safely for over 3 decades as an antiemetic, and millions of units have been dispensed; nevertheless, concern for QT-interval prolongation and development of torsades de pointes has resulted in a controversial U.S. Food and Drug Administration (FDA) Black Box warning for doses above 2.5 mg.[42] Haloperidol is not FDA approved for IV use and also has a Black Box warning for use in elderly patients with dementia. Newer antipsychotics such as olanzapine and ziprasidone also may be effective, but they are not FDA approved for IV use and have not been studied in depth for this indication.[43-45] For patients who do not respond to these pharmacologic interventions, rapid-sequence induction using paralytic agents and endotracheal intubation and mechanical ventilation may be required.

Tachycardia and hypertension usually will improve with sedation and hydration. The mixed α- and β-adrenergic antagonist, labetalol, may be used for refractory tachycardia and hypertension. The usual initial dose is 10 to 20 mg IV. Significant hypertension alone may be treated with the α-adrenergic antagonist, phentolamine, or alternatively, hydralazine or sodium nitroprusside. For patients with hyperthermia greater than 40°C, rapid cooling, rehydration, and correction of electrolyte abnormalities is essential. Cooling is safely and easily accomplished by wetting bare skin with a tepid mist and utilizing a fan to promote heat loss from evaporation and convection. Immersion in cold water is impractical and precludes cardiac monitoring, airway support, and other resuscitation maneuvers. Once core body temperature has been reduced to 38°C, external cooling measures should be halted to prevent iatrogenic hypothermia.

Serum chemistry panels should be checked, and circulating levels of creatine phosphokinase should be measured to assess for rhabdomyolysis. Dehydration should be treated with an IV crystalloid solution such as normal saline. Seizures should be controlled with benzodiazepines, and status epilepticus may require administration of phenobarbital, phenytoin, or in extreme cases, general anesthesia for definitive control. For patients who have developed rhabdomyolysis, alkalinization of the urine is important to prevent nephrotoxic precipitation of myoglobin within the renal tubules. Markers of myocardial injury, such as troponin, should be routinely checked in patients with cardiac risk factors. Aspirin and acetaminophen levels always should be included in the chemistry panel of the toxicology patient. Urine toxicology screening tests may be useful as a rapid screen in comatose or uncooperative patients. Activated charcoal should be administered for potential mixed overdoses. Computed tomography (CT) of the brain should be performed to exclude intracranial hemorrhage in comatose patients. In order to obtain this study, patients may require sedation, neuromuscular paralysis, and intubation to achieve imaging without motion artifact. Lumbar puncture also should be considered to detect meningoencephalitis or subarachnoid hemorrhage not visualized on CT.

Amphetamine Derivatives

A large group of drugs have been developed from amphetamine, either by clandestine or legitimate chemists; they include agents with enhanced euphoric and hallucinogenic effects, drugs used for weight loss and attention deficit hyperactivity syndromes, and drugs to overcome narcolepsy or fatigue. These drugs share many of the aforementioned acute or chronic physiologic and toxic effects of methamphetamine.[46]

MDMA, MDA, AND CONGENERS

The first synthesis of 3,4-methylenedioxymethamphetamine (MDMA), alias "Ecstasy," "X," or "Adam," occurred in 1912 by chemists at the German pharmaceutical company, Merck. It was patented in 1914 then shelved. The drug's source compound and longer-acting metabolite, 3,4-methylenedioxyamphetamine (MDA), had been synthesized earlier in 1910, but was marketed decades later for use as a sedative and appetite suppressant in 1960. However, MDMA, MDA, and 5-dimethoxy-4-methylamphetamine (DOM) instead became popular as "love drugs" in the 1960s. In the 1980s, these drugs were used as pharmaceutical adjuncts to psychotherapy and couples' therapy to promote empathy, introspection, and open communication. The use of these drugs in this way was heralded in the press, and widespread public misuse ensued. In 1985, MDMA and related drugs became U.S. Drug Enforcement Agency (DEA) Schedule I compounds. Less commonly available hallucinogenic amphetamine derivatives include methylenedioxyethylamphetamine (MDEA), alias "Eve," 2,5-dimethoxyamphetamine (DMA), 2,4-DMA, 4-bromo-DMA (DOB), propyl-DMA (DPO), p-methoxyamphetamine (PMA), and p-methoxymethylamphetamine (PMMA). The *2C family*, which refers to the two carbon atoms that separate the amine from the phenyl ring, are derivatives of the naturally occurring compound, β-phenethylamine. They contain methoxy groups in positions 2 and 5 of the phenyl ring and a hydrophobic 4-phenyl substituent such as iodine (2C-I), bromine (2C-B), and many others.[47] Their affinity for CNS serotonin receptors has been demonstrated, and these compounds act as mixed agonists/antagonists with resultant hallucinogenic effects. A toxicology study of patients presenting from nightclubs in Ibiza, Spain, revealed a wide range of detected compounds.[48] The most prevalent was MDMA, but others included the aforementioned compounds as well as ketamine and γ-hydroxybutyric acid. Nearly half of the subjects also tested positive for methamphetamine. The most dangerous of these compounds appears to be PMA, alias "Death," with several deaths reported worldwide.[49]

METHCATHINONE

Methcathinone ("Cat") is an amphetamine derivative that appeared on the clandestine market in the United States in the 1990s and is now classified as a DEA Schedule I substance. It is easily synthesized using recipes found on the Internet. Related compounds, cathine and cathinone, are naturally occurring compounds found in the plant, *Cathula edulis* ("khat," "qat," "chat," "jaad"), which is endemic to the Middle East and Africa. The clinical use of khat was described in the 11th century in *Pharmacy and Therapeutic Art*.[50] The fresh leaves or stems are chewed, as the stored product loses activity as it dries.

DERIVATIVES AFFECTING SLEEP

Amphetamine-related agents used for narcolepsy and to increase wakefulness are growing in use. In humans, alteration of CNS dopaminergic transmission affects alertness, performance, and quality of sleep. A case-control study of narcoleptic patients showed that methamphetamine caused a dose-dependent decrease in daytime sleep tendency and improvement in task performance in both narcoleptics and controls.[51] Amphetamine derivatives have been studied most extensively by the military as a countermeasure to fatigue induced by circadian desynchronosis. Modafinil is an amphetamine derivative that enhances wakefulness, vigilance, and memory. It may have effects within the anterior hypothalamus.[52] Its dopamine-releasing action in the nucleus accumbens reward center is weak, and thus its abuse potential is limited. Modafinil is a central α1-adrenergic agonist. It inhibits reuptake of norepinephrine by axon terminals on sleep-promoting neurons of ventrolateral preoptic nucleus and increases excitatory glutamine transmission. This effect in turn reduces GABA transmission. Modafinil is safe and well tolerated and less likely to cause anxiety, agitation, or result in a hypersomnolent rebound effect. It is being studied for attention deficit disorders, Alzheimer's disease, depression, myotonic dystrophy, multiple sclerosis, schizophrenia, cerebral palsy, and memory decline related to aging. In September 2003, the FDA approved modafinil for the additional indications of treating sleep disorders due to shift work and obstructive sleep apnea. Other similar agents include adrafinil and armodafinil.

KEY POINTS

1. Methamphetamine abuse and toxicity is common, cross-cultural, and an increasing problem not only in North America but around the world. People who abuse methamphetamine use prehospital, emergency department, and ICU resources at a much higher level than other patients. They often present with co-ingestions and concomitant blunt or penetrating traumatic injuries.

2. Methamphetamine is lipid soluble and crosses the blood-brain barrier, resulting in release of dopamine from presynaptic cytoplasmic and vesicular storage sites within the central nervous system (CNS). It also blocks reuptake of dopamine. Another indirect action of methamphetamine is to increase levels within the CNS of the neurotransmitters, glutamate and serotonin, and decrease levels of the inhibitory neurotransmitter, γ-aminobutyric acid (GABA).

3. Methamphetamine is metabolized within the liver by cytochrome P450 isoenzymes to amphetamine, 4-hydroxymethamphetamine, and 4-hydroxyamphetamine, which also have stimulant properties. These metabolites are then excreted by the kidneys. The elimination half-life may range from 6 to 15 hours.

4. Signs and symptoms of acute intoxication include agitation, psychosis, pressured speech, headache, chest pain, dyspnea, abdominal pain, hypertension, and tachycardia.

5. Agitation should be rapidly addressed with chemical restraint in the form of benzodiazepines, such as diazepam or lorazepam, or the butyrophenones, haloperidol and droperidol. Tachycardia and hypertension not responding to the aforementioned sedatives should be treated with the mixed α- and β-adrenergic antagonist, labetalol. Dehydration, rhabdomyolysis, and acute renal failure should be identified and treated with infusion of copious amounts of intravenous crystalloid solutions. Hyperthermia should be treated with evaporation and convection.

6. Chronic methamphetamine abuse results in permanent degeneration of CNS neurons, choreoathetoid movement disorders, negative personality changes, accelerated coronary artery disease, cardiomyopathy, periodontal disease, and skin lesions.

ANNOTATED REFERENCES

Cruickshank CC, Dyer KR. A review of the clinical pharmacology of methamphetamine. Addiction 2009;104:1085-99.
  This article is a recent in-depth review of the pharmacology and clinical effects of methamphetamine.
Hall AP, Henry JA. Acute toxic effects of "Ecstasy" (MDMA) and related compounds: overview of pathophysiology and clinical management. Br J Anaesth 2006;96:678-85.
  The authors examine the toxicity of MDMA and similar amphetamine derivatives and describe the clinical management of patients presenting with acute effects from these drugs.
Richards JR, Derlet RW, Duncan DR. Methamphetamine toxicity: treatment with a benzodiazepine versus a butyrophenone. Eur J Emerg Med 1997;4:130-5.

This is the only prospective clinical study to date specifically comparing lorazepam to droperidol for treatment of methamphetamine toxicity in the setting of the emergency department. The authors concluded droperidol was more effective for sedation and required fewer repeat doses.
Shoptaw SJ, Kao U, Ling W. Treatment for amphetamine psychosis. Cochrane Database Syst Rev 2009;(1):CD003026.
  This Cochrane review presents a thorough analysis of all published reports regarding the treatment of amphetamine psychosis.
Yamamoto BK, Moszczynska A, Gudelsky GA. Amphetamine toxicities: classical and emerging mechanisms. Ann N Y Acad Sci 2010;1187:101-21.
  This article examines the myriad toxic effects of methamphetamine and other amphetamine derivatives.

REFERENCES

Access the complete reference list online at http://www.expertconsult.com.

190

Pharmacoeconomics

JOSEPH F. DASTA | SANDRA KANE-GILL

Pharmacoeconomics is a branch of health economics that analyzes the economic impact and cost-effectiveness of pharmaceuticals.[1] This definition has been broadened to include not only the economic costs but also the quality-of-life or humanistic consequences of drug therapy. Evaluation of therapeutic protocols and guidelines also is included in pharmacoeconomic studies.[2] It has been suggested that health economics can help answer two fundamental questions: (1) Is a given therapy (or program) worth using when compared with alternatives? (2) Should a portion of available healthcare resources be allocated to a given therapy or program?[3]

Since the term was first used in 1986, pharmacoeconomics has evolved in complexity and applicability.[2] Although still not required by the U.S. Food and Drug Administration (FDA), clinicians, administrators, and healthcare systems are mandating that economic information be added to the clinical effectiveness information for new therapies before a drug is added to a formulary. The Academy of Managed Care Pharmacy (AMCP) published the *Format for Formulary Submissions*, Version 3.0 as a template pharmaceutical manufacturers can use when submitting drugs for health system review.[4] The goal of these guidelines is to ensure that all new products bring added clinical as well as economic value to the insured population. As such, pharmacoeconomic data can lead to more informed decisions being made about selecting a particular drug for a patient or healthcare system. A recent survey of 540 pharmacy directors revealed that 37% had their staffing budgets reduced in the past 6 months[5]; 56% had to reduce their drug expenditures by 2% to 5%, and 25% reported reductions of 6% to 10%. This can translate into several million dollars cut from drug budgets. Hospital administrators are increasingly focusing on pharmacy costs. Whereas CEOs of hospitals did not rank drug expenditures in their top 20 concerns for 1996, the repeat survey in 2000 yielded drug expenditures as the seventh most important concern.[6] In fact, drug and technology costs were second only to decreased reimbursement, whereas drugs offered the single greatest opportunity for cost savings.

Economics of Health Care in the Intensive Care Unit

One of the catalysts driving the growth of pharmacoeconomics is the staggering cost of health care. In 2009, healthcare spending in the United States increased to a total of $2.6 trillion, and it is projected to be 4.7 trillion in 2019, which would represent 19.3% of the U.S. Gross Domestic Product (GDP).[7] Hospital sector spending in the United States increased 86% in 2009 to $761 billion.

U.S. prescription drug expenditures were $300 billion in 2009, representing a 5% increase from 2008.[8] Data in nonfederal hospitals for 2008 reveal that drug expenditures increased by 2.1% to $27 billion, and injectable drugs accounted for 71% of these expenditures.[8] In 2008, the top 10 therapeutic classes accounted for 73% of hospital drug expenditures, with antineoplastic agents being the highest expenditure at $3.3 billion. The top two individual drugs in 2008 were enoxaparin at $1.1 billion and immune globulin at $868 million.

The cost of drug therapy is complex and comprises multiple components. Table 190-1 summarizes the cost of the drug product versus the cost of complications.[9] It is easy to obtain data on acquisition costs of drugs and materials to prepare and administer drugs. Determining the cost of drug failures or adverse drug events is far more challenging, however, and often is not considered. The estimated annual costs of

drug-related problems in the United States increased from $77.6 billion in 1995 to $155 billion in 2000.[10]

Intensive care units (ICUs) consume significant hospital resources. Quantifying costs attributable to ICU care is complex, since both patients and their costs are constantly being shifted to and from the ICU, and different hospitals use different cost accounting systems. However, the large economic burden of the ICU is out of proportion to the number of ICU beds in the institution. In 2005, 95,000 ICU beds accounted for only 7% of all inpatient beds in the United States yet consumed about 13% of inpatient costs, or $82 billion annually.[11] Furthermore, this figure represents 4% of national health expenditures. The cost of an ICU day is estimated to be three to four times the cost of a ward day and has increased 30% from 2000 to 2005.[12] One study reported that daily ICU costs averaged $3518 during 2000-2005,[12] but a large database of more than 50,000 patients from 252 ICUs revealed a mean ICU cost of $19,725.[13] Daily ICU costs were greatest on day 1 (average $7728), decreased on day 2 (average $3872), and stabilized on day 3 and beyond at approximately $4200 in 2009 dollars. Mechanically ventilated patients had the highest ICU costs; use of a ventilator increased average daily cost by $1800 compared to ICU patients who were not receiving mechanical ventilation. Therapeutic interventions that can reduce ICU length of stay by even 1 day can have a significant impact on total hospital costs, particularly in patients requiring mechanical ventilation. Cost saving initiatives are particularly relevant in this setting, since only 83% of hospital costs are covered for Medicare patients with an ICU admission.[14] This discrepancy can result in a $5.8 billion loss to hospitals when ICU care is required.

Drug costs in the ICU are difficult to quantify because most hospitals are not sufficiently computerized to track these data. In one academic medical center, 15 drugs accounted for more than 50% of drug costs in the ICU.[15] Drug costs in the ICU averaged 38% of the hospital's total drug costs and increased at a higher rate than non-ICU drug costs over the 4-year period studied (12.4% versus 5.9%). Fiscal year 2002 data revealed an ICU drug cost of $312 per day compared with $112 per day outside of the ICU.

Economic Evaluations in Critical Care Medicine

Although any economic analysis could be performed in a critical care environment, some of the more appropriate are cost-effectiveness analysis, cost-benefit analysis, cost minimization analysis, cost utility analysis, and cost of illness.[16] Cost-effectiveness evaluation is discussed in greater depth because it is the most commonly performed and the approach recommended by expert bodies.[17]

Cost-effectiveness analysis is a full economic evaluation because both costs and outcomes are considered. A drug is evaluated on the basis of cost and outcome in reference to a comparator, which is usually the current standard of care. In a cost-effectiveness evaluation, the most preferred therapy has increased effectiveness at decreased cost.

In 1996, the Panel on Cost-Effectiveness in Health and Medicine (PCEHM) published seminal work consisting of guidelines for the conduct and reporting of economic analyses.[18] This work resulted in some key points to consider when employing a cost-effectiveness evaluation, including use of a reference case for comparison, the importance of transparent methods and logic, and consideration of the

TABLE 190-1	Cost of a Drug Versus Cost of a Complication	
Cost of a Drug		**Cost of a Complication**
Acquisition cost		Increased morbidity cost
Associated material preparation and delivery cost		Increased mortality cost
Number of doses per day cost		Increased total cost
Route of administration cost		Increased length of stay
Labor preparation and administration cost		Increased intensity of care
		Decreased patient satisfaction

perspective being evaluated. The PCEHM recommends that the societal perspective is the most comprehensive and considers workforce and familial aspects of illness. The PCEHM recommends using the following steps when designing a cost-effectiveness analysis:

1. The analysis plan should include development of a conceptual model describing the intervention and its effects on health outcomes.
2. The conceptual model should incorporate the schematic of a decision tree wherein all possible treatment outcomes are considered. It should be constructed to represent health effects and should be used to reflect the cascade of cost implications resulting from an intervention. Figure 190-1 depicts a typical decision tree evaluating a new therapy for heart failure.
3. Collecting appropriate data can be the most challenging aspect of a cost-effectiveness evaluation. The researcher can use a variety of resources including experts in the field, published epidemiologic studies, the medical literature, and various cost databases.
4. Computing cost and effectiveness may entail the use of computerized spreadsheets, decision analysis software, or simulation software. Commonly employed methods include Monte Carlo simulation, state-transition models, and decision tree models.

The American Thoracic Society convened a workshop to address the application of the PCEHM guidelines to a critical care environment.[19] A group of experts compiled key considerations for a cost-effectiveness evaluation in the ICU, and details can be reviewed in their report.

Cost utility analysis is a form of cost-effectiveness evaluation that examines the utility or value of an outcome.[16] Patient, family member, provider, or societal preferences can value health outcomes. Cost per quality-adjusted life-year can be measured for alternative therapies by assessing the length of time a patient is in a state of health rated on a scale of 0 to 1, where *0* equals death, and *1* equals perfect health.

Cost minimization assumes equal effectiveness for each alternative and evaluates the impact on an identical outcome. For example, if two ICU sedatives produce the same quality of sedation, but one requires a more labor-intensive administration protocol, a decision maker could apply a cost minimization analysis to determine the preferred, less costly therapy.

Cost-benefit analysis compares the costs and benefits of alternatives. This approach is rarely used in medicine.

Cost-of-illness studies describe the economic burden of a specific condition or disease state and are frequently part of epidemiology studies. This type of analysis may take into consideration the workforce and societal impact of illness, in addition to the financial implications for payers and providers.

The American Recovery and Reinvestment Act of 2009 provided considerable funding for comparative effectiveness research and mandated that the Institute of Medicine (IOM) of the National Academy of Sciences recommend initial national priorities for this research.[20] Its purpose is to compare the ratio of cost to effectiveness of two interventions used for the same condition.[16] These comparisons should be evaluated in the real-world setting and could provide data about which interventions are most effective for patients under specific circumstances.[8] It has been estimated that these data could reduce spending by Medicare and Medicaid by $0.1 billion from 2008 to 2012 and $1.3 billion between 2008 and 2017.

Determining Costs in the Intensive Care Unit

Three approaches frequently are used to assess the economic burden of a disease state: prospective study design, retrospective analysis, and decision modeling.[17] A prospective study gives the investigator an opportunity to measure important variables completely and accurately. Retrospective database analysis reviews data that already have been assembled and has the advantage of being much less costly and time consuming than prospective studies with the ability to review many patients easily.

In retrospective studies, the subjects already are assembled and have been de-identified, baseline measurements have been made, and the follow-up period has occurred. The total direct and indirect costs of a condition can be readily assessed. Total direct costs include the value of all goods, services, and other resources consumed in the provision of an intervention or in dealing with the side effects of the intervention or other current or future consequences linked to the intervention.[21] Indirect costs are the costs that result from a certain therapy or illness, such as lost wages, workforce replacement, or child care that may be necessary.

Patient billing information and summary estimates of department-level expenditures can be used to estimate costs when hospital administrative data are used. At one extreme, hospital charges can be used as a proxy of costs. This approach may be reasonable in a comparative analysis of interventions, assuming that charges per admission are roughly proportional to economic costs per admission. Another approach is to use the department's cost-to-charge ratio, which has been shown to perform accurately when evaluating average costs per diagnosis-related group.[22]

Cost of Intensive Care Unit–Related Conditions

Evaluation of the economic impact of medical conditions is one of several areas of focus since the 1990s in ongoing efforts to decrease overall healthcare spending and identify high-cost diseases to target therapies. More recently, hospital-acquired conditions have received increased attention. Several of these are so-called never events that are not reimbursed by government payers.[23] Representative conditions of the 10 identified areas for 2009 and 2010 include deep venous thrombosis (DVT) or pulmonary embolism (PE) developing after total knee or hip replacements, extreme manifestations of poor glycemic control, and surgical site infections. Recently, a study analyzed the performance of several hundred hospitals for hospital-acquired conditions and their associated additional costs.[24] Top conditions and their associated annual costs were decubitus ulcers ($536,900), DVT and PE ($564,000), and infections ($252,600). Preventing these conditions from

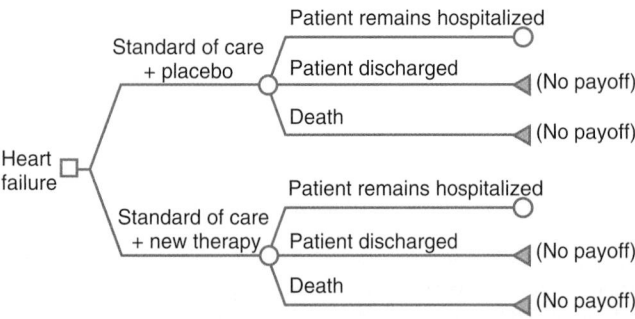

Figure 190-1 Example of a decision tree.

developing could result, for example, in a 200-bed hospital saving $2 million per year.

In this section, we will summarize the data on selected acute care conditions for which information on costs is known. Although the data presented may not be directly from patients in the ICU, the results represent the best data available.

ACUTE CONGESTIVE HEART FAILURE

Among the nearly 5 million Americans with congestive heart failure, the number of hospital discharges has increased by 165% in the past 20 years.[25] Acute congestive heart failure is the reason for at least 20% of hospital admissions in patients older than 65 years of age and the most expensive admission diagnosis, with an estimated $39.2 billion spent in the United States during 2010.[26] In 1998, the cost per admission of a congestive heart failure patient was $5471, and in 2001, hospitals lost on average $1288 per Medicare patient.[27] In fact, one large database study conducted in 2005 revealed 50% of heart failure admissions had costs that exceeded the DRG (diagnosis-related group) payment.[28] More recent data reveal that the mean hospital cost per admission was $21,800 in 2009 dollars, and that 75% of admissions with acute heart failure developed this condition as a secondary diagnosis.[29] As such, the global burden of acute heart failure may be underestimated from these data, since statistics are generated from patients with a primary diagnosis of heart failure.[26]

ACUTE KIDNEY INJURY

Despite considerable information on the clinical effects of acute kidney injury (AKI), there have been only seven studies describing costs associated with this condition.[30] There are substantial differences in methods, such as different definitions of the condition and different definitions of costs. As such, comparisons are difficult. The median hospital costs adjusted to 2008 dollars range from $3300 in patients with uncomplicated AKI to $56,095 from the start of renal replacement therapy to hospital discharge.[30] One study reported that the median postoperative costs of AKI following coronary artery bypass surgery was $44,800 compared to $21,900 in controls in 2009 dollars.[31] Even patients with small increases in serum creatinine postoperatively, namely 1.5 times baseline, had higher postoperative costs ($35,400), whereas patients with the most severe AKI had costs of $62,700 (median value).

INFECTIOUS DISEASES

Healthcare-Acquired Infections

Hospital staffs recognize the importance of preventing infections in patients admitted to their institution. By implementing appropriate procedures and guidelines, hospitals can save on costs associated with these infections. Importantly, the government will not reimburse hospitals if patients develop infections such as catheter-associated urinary tract infections, vascular catheter–associated bloodstream infections, and surgical site infections. The Centers for Disease Control and Prevention (CDC) recently summarized the literature on this topic in a comprehensive published report.[32] They estimate that overall annual direct medical costs of 1.7 million healthcare-associated infections ranged from $28.4 to $33.8 billion, depending on the method used for adjusting to 2007 dollars. They furthermore state that prevention can save $5.7 to $6.8 billion for preventing only 20% of infections. The attributable patient costs are separated by infection site and are shown in Table 190-2. A sample from 69 million hospital discharges between 1998 and 2006 revealed 558,000 identified cases, and costs were adjusted to 2006 dollars.[33] For patients with invasive surgery, the attributable mean length of stay was 11 days with hospital costs of $32,000 for sepsis and 14 days and $46,400 for pneumonia, respectively. The corresponding values for patients without invasive surgery were 6 days and $12,700 for sepsis and 9.7 days and $22,300 for pneumonia,

TABLE 190-2	Average Attributable Costs per Patient of Hospital-Associated Infections by Sites of Infection	
Infection Site	*Low Estimate Adjusted to 2007 Dollars Using CPI-U*	*High Estimate Adjusted to 2007 Dollars Using CPI-U*
Surgical site infection	$11,087	$29,443
Central line–associated bloodstream infection	$6,461	$25,849
Ventilator-associated pneumonia	$14,806	$27,520
Catheter-associated urinary tract infection	$749	$832
*Clostridium difficile–*associated disease	$5,682	$8,090

CPI-U, consumer price index for all urban consumers.

respectively. Another recent evaluation of costs of nosocomial infections[34] reviewed 1.3 million admissions from 55 hospitals; costs were adjusted to 2007 dollars. The 58,000 cases of nosocomial infections had a mean added total hospital cost of $12,200 (95% confidence interval [CI], $4862-$19533). The highest costs were seen in cerebrospinal fluid and respiratory infections.

Ventilator-associated pneumonia (VAP) is a frequent complication of mechanical ventilation in critically ill patients and is associated with a 20% to 54% ICU mortality rate.[35,36] Studies published through 2004 estimated that the cost of VAP ranges from $5365 to $10,062 per patient. One study determined the attributable cost of VAP in a nonteaching U.S. medical center.[37] Compared with noninfected mechanically ventilated patients, patients with VAP had a higher incidence of bacteremia (36% versus 22%), longer ICU length of stay (26 versus 4 days), and greater mortality rate (50% versus 34%). Hospital costs for VAP patients were significantly higher ($70,568 versus $21,620), with a higher proportion of total costs being room, nursing, pharmacy, and respiratory therapy expenses. The cost differences for patients developing early-onset compared to late-onset VAP were $36,822 versus $60,562. The attributable cost of VAP when adjusted for a wide variety of factors was $11,897 (95% CI, $5265-$26,214). Approaches that provide even a small clinical effect can have a significant economic benefit.[35,36]

Additional recent studies have quantified costs of bloodstream infections, colitis due to *Clostridium difficile* infection, catheter-related infections, and severe sepsis.[38-41] A study of catheter-associated bloodstream infections in a medical and surgical ICU at a nonteaching hospital revealed an incidence of 4%, with an attributable total hospital cost of $14,200 in 2009 dollars.[38] The catheter-related infections were associated with an attributable ICU length of stay of 2.4 days. Infections caused by *C. difficile* are a common cause of diarrhea in hospitalized patients, and many of these patients are in ICUs. A review of the literature reveals that the incremental costs in 2008 dollars ranged from $2800 to $4800 for primary infection and $13,600 to $18,000 for recurrent disease.[39] The hospital records of 1.3 million patients revealed 22% of patients had a bloodstream infection.[40] Incremental costs of these patients in 2006 dollars averaged $19,400. When infections occurring after hospital day 7 were excluded, costs were estimated at $20,600.

Severe Sepsis

The incidence of severe sepsis in the United States is estimated to be 751,000 cases per year, and the mortality rate is estimated to be 28.6%, which increases to 38.4% in patients older than 85 years. The average cost per case of severe sepsis in 2009 dollars is $31,100. The estimated annual 2009 cost in the United States is $23.5 billion.[41]

One cautionary note is that the costs of healthcare-associated infections may be overstated due to shortcomings in assessing costs and related outcomes. The authors suggest complete economic evaluations that include changes to all costs and health benefits be performed. Readers are referred to the primary article for more detail on this topic.[42]

VENOUS THROMBOEMBOLISM

Approximately 1 million patients develop venous thromboembolism in the United States, with an annual cost estimated at $3 to $4 billion.[43] Some estimates of the financial consequences of hospitalized patients developing a DVT or PE add $8000 to $14,000 to the bill of general medical ward patients.[44] For patients developing both conditions, additional costs rise to $28,000 per patient. For patients with recurrent disease or readmitted within 1 year, DVT and PE add $11,800 and $14,700, respectively. Hospital stays can be doubled. The Centers for Medicare and Medicaid Services (CMS) in the United States does not reimburse hospitals for the additional costs associated with the development of a DVT or PE. This puts extreme pressures on hospitals to initiate prevention measures, especially in high-risk patients.

DELIRIUM

Annual costs of delirium on the healthcare system are estimated to be between $38 and $152 billion.[45] Some of these costs can be attributed to inpatient care. Delirium has a significant correlation with increased ICU and hospital length of stay.[46] Milbrandt and colleagues were the first to assess the costs of delirium in mechanically ventilated patients.[47] They reported that ICU costs are increased by approximately $10,900 and hospital costs by $17,000 in 2009 dollars for patients who experienced at least one episode of delirium, compared to patients who did not develop delirium. Optimizing approaches to detection of delirium and finding the best strategies to treat this condition could alleviate the economic burden.

MISCELLANEOUS CONDITIONS

There are some additional diseases for which the burden of illness had been estimated. Approximately 74.5 million patients in the United States have hypertension, and the estimated cost associated with this condition in 2010 was $76.6 billion.[26] Approximately 1% of these patients present to emergency departments with acute hypertension.[48] One study evaluated a claims database of patients hospitalized with hypertension as a secondary diagnosis.[49] For the 123,000 admissions with acute hypertension, 13% of total hospital costs were a result of hypertension, which represents $2734 in 2005 dollars. This cost ($3540) was highest for patients with a primary diagnosis of ischemic heart disease. Of interest, the cost attributable to hypertension was still $2254 for patients without ischemic heart disease or cerebrovascular disease, thus documenting the need for cost-effective therapies in these patients. Stroke has a major economic impact, with a prevalence of 6.4 million Americans affected and 795,000 new or recurrent patients per year.[50] The estimated total and indirect medical costs for 2010 were $78 billion.[26] Costs obtained from a database of 8 million admissions for spontaneous intracranial hemorrhage from 1000 hospitals stated that hospital charges increased 61% from 2003 to 2005.[50] The mean hospital charge was $43,200 per patient (adjusted for 2005 dollars), and the aggregate charges in 2005 were $2.9 billion. Finally, a review of 71 studies from 1996-2006 that included the cost of stroke revealed a mean hospital cost of $17,250 ($468-$65,250).[51]

Cost of Pharmacotherapy in Critical Care

ANTIMICROBIALS

Appropriateness of Therapy and Resistance

Antimicrobials are commonly used in the ICU to prevent and treat a wide range of infections.[52] The acquisition cost of an antimicrobial is only one component of the cost associated with use of these agents. In fact, one study revealed that the acquisition cost of gentamicin represented only 33% of the total antimicrobial costs for this drug.[53]

Additional cost drivers associated with antimicrobial use include the treatment of resistant organisms. Methicillin-resistant *Staphylo-*

coccus aureus (MRSA) is increasingly prevalent in ICUs. A review of the literature pertaining to the cost impact of these bacteria revealed three studies.[54] Direct medical costs of MRSA from a database of over 1 million patients with community-acquired infections was $49,300 (adjusted for 2009 dollars). Another study of nosocomial bloodstream infections showed the costs of treating resistant organisms were threefold higher than the costs for treating sensitive organisms. In a study of 188 ICU patients treated for MRSA, the costs (from 2002-2004 data) of initially inappropriate antibiotic therapy was $10,000 greater than the cost of appropriate therapy.[55] The cost difference is thought to be the result of 4 extra days of stay in the ICU required by the patients who received inappropriate therapy. Economic analysis of gram-negative bacterial resistance in the ICU also was reviewed.[56] One study reported that patients with infections caused by antibiotic-resistant Enterobacteriaceae stayed 4 more days in the ICU and had $58,300 more in hospital charges (2009 dollars) than patients with infections caused by drug-sensitive organisms. When patients with resistant *Pseudomonas aeruginosa* infections were compared to patients with drug-sensitive infections, ICU length of stay increased from 1 to 6 days, and charges in 2009 dollars were $13,000 to $32,900 higher. An additional study of healthcare-associated infections caused by resistant gram-negative bacteria reported that the mean hospital cost was $151,500 (range $152-$1,056,000) in 2008 dollars.[57] A univariate analysis of hospital costs showed that the median total cost for patients with infections caused by resistant bacteria was $38,000 higher than for patients with infections caused by susceptible bacteria.

Several studies have evaluated strategies and protocols to minimize the development of resistance to antibiotics and optimize management of septic patients in the ICU to reduce the incidence of resistance and cost of therapy. For example, an educational protocol for nurses and respiratory therapists was developed.[58] This program resulted in a 57% decrease in VAP, with an estimated cost savings in the following 12 months of $425,000. Using a before-and-after study design, Shorr et al. described the economics of a broad-based sepsis protocol based on the Surviving Sepsis Campaign recommendations at their 1200-bed institution.[59,60] The estimated development cost was $5000. The average per-patient total hospital costs in 2005 dollars was approximately $6000, or a total cost difference of $573,000 for the 120 patients studied, despite a higher survival rate in the protocol group. The cost difference was driven by a 35% reduction in ICU costs and a 30% reduction in ward costs following the use of the protocol. A decision analysis was performed to estimate the costs of implementing early goal-directed therapy for severe sepsis and septic shock.[61] Using 2005 dollars, the authors estimated startup costs of $13,000 for the ICU-based strategy, $30,000 for the emergency department (ED)-based strategy, and an annual outlay of $100,113. The estimated annual total cost savings of this protocol for 91 patients was $789,000. In contrast, implementing the early goal-directed therapy for sepsis at one hospital resulted in a mean increase in 2004 total hospital cost of $8800, an increased ICU length of stay, and higher pharmacy costs, largely driven by a lower mortality rate in protocol patients.[62] Further analysis revealed that implementation of this protocol resulted in a cost per quality-adjusted life-year gain of $16,000. This amount is considerably lower than $50,000, a value often used as a threshold for a therapy to be considered cost-effective in medical care.[63] Additionally, protocols that focus on appropriate antimicrobial usage have been shown to have favorable clinical and economic benefits.[64] Antimicrobial stewardship programs include tailoring antimicrobials to the cultured organism following broad-spectrum initial coverage, formulary restriction, guidelines and clinical pathways, decision support systems, and intravenous-to-oral conversion programs. They have demonstrated a 22% to 36% decrease in antimicrobial usage and annual cost savings of $200,000 to $900,000 in addition to reduced mortality and shorter lengths of stay.[64] Whether shorter courses of antibiotics or procalcitonin testing to guide the duration of antibiotic therapy will reduce ICU or hospital costs while maintaining effectiveness remains to be documented.[65,66]

DROTRECOGIN ALFA (ACTIVATED)

A cost-effectiveness analysis of drotrecogin alfa (activated) was conducted in conjunction with a clinical trial of the safety and efficacy of this recombinant protein as an adjuvant treatment for severe sepsis.[67] The acquisition cost of a course of drotrecogin alfa (activated) for a 70-kg patient is approximately $7000. Despite the fact that there were more survivors among patients treated with drotrecogin alfa (activated) compared with placebo, there were no significant differences in costs per patient or resource use, excluding the cost of the drug. The cost per survivor was estimated to be $160,000. Long-term costs and outcomes were modeled, assuming that survivors lived an average of 12.2 years, with utility adjusted to 8.4 quality-adjusted life-years. The cost-effectiveness was $33,000 per life-year saved and the cost per quality-adjusted life-year was $48,800. The cost per quality-adjusted life-year in patients with an APACHE II score greater than 25 was $27,400. Reimbursement for 71 patients with severe sepsis treated with drotrecogin alfa was assessed,[68] and the total treatment cost between December 2001 and December 2003 was $6.3 million, whereas reimbursement was $4.3 million, representing a loss of nearly $2 million, or $28,000 per patient.

SEDATIVES

Although there are many publications on appropriate sedation pharmacotherapy, it is surprising that only a few studies have evaluated the costs associated with treating agitation.[69] In addition to sedative drug acquisition costs, there are costs associated with oversedation, such as prolonged time on the ventilator, and costs of undersedation, such as development of ischemic heart disease, respiratory depression and ileus associated with excessive opioid use, and ineffective treatment of delirium. The economic literature on ICU sedation consists mainly of studies comparing drug acquisition costs between treatments.[69] Two recent studies have evaluated the cost of care associated with various sedatives. One was a decision analysis of a randomized clinical trial of lorazepam versus propofol in adult mechanically ventilated patients, using a daily sedative interruption method.[70] The findings revealed that propofol was cost-effective in 91% of the simulations and resulted in an average total hospital cost saving of $6378 in 2007 dollars and an increase in 3.7 ventilator-free days. Despite the higher cost of propofol, it saved total hospital costs, mainly by reducing time on the ventilator. Finally, a cost minimization analysis was conducted of a randomized clinical trial of dexmedetomidine versus midazolam in adult mechanically ventilated patients.[71] Despite an $1100 higher median acquisition cost for dexmedetomidine compared to midazolam, the total ICU cost in the patients randomized to dexmedetomidine was nearly $10,000 less in 2007 dollars. This cost difference was driven mainly by lower ICU and mechanical ventilator costs. We need studies that capture all costs from study patients, including costs of adverse drug reactions, healthcare provider time using time-motion studies, nursing satisfaction, and a variety of cost-effectiveness ratios.[69]

THROMBOPROPHYLAXIS AND TREATMENT OF DEEP VENOUS THROMBOSIS

In the past, several studies have shown the cost-effectiveness of low-molecular-weight heparins such as enoxaparin compared to unfractionated heparin.[72] More recent economic studies have evaluated the newer agent, fondaparinux. One study used a decision model that evaluated a cohort of 1000 hypothetical patients with DVT treated with either enoxaparin or fondaparinux.[73] Despite biasing the model against fondaparinux, there was a 40% reduction in total costs with use of the newer agent, with drug acquisition costs being the major driver. An incremental cost analysis of a randomized clinical trial of fondaparinux versus enoxaparin for total knee replacement revealed a $1081 total cost savings per venous thrombotic event avoided by using fondaparinux.[72] Also, in medical patients, low-molecular-weight heparins saved $89 per patient in 2004 dollars compared to unfractionated heparin, despite the higher acquisition costs associated with the low-molecular-weight heparin formulations.[72] The data appear to favor low-molecular-weight heparins from both a clinical and economic perspective, compared to unfractionated heparin.

MISCELLANEOUS CONDITIONS

Intensive insulin therapy to maintain tight glycemic control is an important topic for ICUs and can be associated with clinical benefit as long as hypoglycemia can be avoided.[74] The recently published NICE-SUGAR study reported a higher mortality rate in patients randomized to an intensive glucose control group versus conventional therapy.[75] The intensive glucose control group had a higher incidence of hypoglycemia.

One study evaluated costs (in 2004 dollars) in 800 medical/surgical ICU patients in each cohort, using a before-and-after method of tight glucose control compared to usual care.[74] There was a 14% reduction in ICU days following the protocol and a decrease in total hospital costs of $1500 per patient, which translated to a total annualized decrease of $1.3 million. An economic analysis of a randomized clinical trial in surgical ICU patients revealed total ICU costs were 25% lower for patients randomized to intensive insulin therapy.[76] Protocol patients had fewer days requiring mechanical ventilation and a shorter ICU stay. These economic studies apply to the patient population studied. Any economic advantage of intense glucose control should be balanced by the documented effects on mortality.

Although not traditionally considered a drug, blood transfusion also has a variety of components beyond the acquisition cost of blood that add to the total cost of a transfusion. A recent activity-based cost analysis from four hospitals evaluated transfusion-related processes, usage factors, and direct and indirect costs to determine the total transfusion cost.[77] Whereas the average acquisition cost of a unit of red blood cells ranged from $150 to $250, the average total cost per red blood cell unit was $760 (range $522-$1183). Annual costs from the four hospitals in 2007 ranged from $1.6 million to $6 million.

▣ Cost of Adverse Drug Events

Adverse drug event (ADE) detection can be challenging, but it is important because the attributable costs can be substantial.[78,79] Cullen et al.[80] performed the first comparison of patients experiencing an ADE in the ICU to patients experiencing ADEs in general care units. This study had several notable findings: (1) the rate of ADEs was nearly doubled in the ICU compared to a general care unit, because critically ill patients received twice the number of medications; (2) the severity of ADEs was greater in the ICU compared to general care units; and (3) the costs after an ADE occurred were higher in the ICU compared to general care units, although the difference was not statistically significant. The additional costs post ADE in the ICU were approximately $9000 compared to the general care unit after adjusting to 2010 values. Another evaluation in the surgical ICU reported about a 2-day increase in length of stay for patients experiencing an ADE compared to those not having an ADE.[81]

The intravenous route of administration is commonly used for ICU patients. Intravenous administration of drugs can increase the risk and/or severity of ADEs, since the drug immediately enters into the bloodstream, allowing for maximal absorption and relatively quick onset. A study was conducted in three ICUs at an academic institution and two ICUs in a nonacademic institution to evaluate the cost and length of stay associated with intravenous administration–related ADEs.[82] Interestingly, the nonacademic institutions did not demonstrate a difference in the cost or length of stay associated with ADEs compared to controls. The academic institutions had $6691 greater costs (2010 values) and a length of stay 4.8 days longer compared to controls.

Considering the cost of a specific ADE, such as heparin-induced thrombocytopenia (HIT), will provide clinicians a further appreciation for the impact of unintended drug responses. A matched case-control study designed to evaluate the financial impact of HIT reported additional costs ranging between $15,500 and $20,300 (2010 values) and about a 15-day longer length of stay.[83] Although only 22 cases were evaluated, the substantial cost associated with HIT seems apparent. Another evaluation of HIT showed that the cost for patients exposed to unfractionated heparin was significantly greater (by $61,000) compared to HIT in patients exposed to low-molecular-weight heparins.[84] Prevention programs aimed at immediate detection and management of HIT could provide institutional cost savings.

Another example of costly ADEs is opioid-related events.[85] A matched case-control study identified 741 patients experiencing an opioid-related ADE during a 6-year period; these subjects were compared to 10,116 controls. The results were reported according to surgery type. The costs attributable to ADEs ranged from $636 to $990 (2010 values). The ADEs were associated with about a half-day increase in length of stay compared to controls. The patient population selected for this study was surgical patients, but we can imagine the financial impact in critically ill patients that receive high doses and prolonged courses of opioids.

Economic Impact of Critical Care Pharmacists

There have been several studies documenting the clinical and economic impact of pharmacists involved with several areas of patient care, including the ED and ICU.[86-88] For the ICU pharmacist, the literature up to 2003 documented reductions in medication errors, adverse drug events, and reduced rates of VAP.[86] The economic outcomes in 2010 dollars range from annual savings of $34,000 in cost avoidance to $355,000 in reductions of adverse drug events. Using large Medicare databases, more recent studies have compared outcomes from ICUs that have clinical pharmacists to those without clinical pharmacists.[89,90] In patients with infections, institutions with a clinical pharmacist reported lower mortality rates in the ICU, shorter ICU lengths of stay, lower drug charges, and lower Medicare billing charges. In ICU patients with nosocomial-acquired infections from 272 hospitals, the Medicare charges per patient in hospitals with clinical pharmacists was approximately $12,000 less, resulting in over $132 million in reduced total charges for 25,000 patients. In 141,000 patients with thromboembolic or infarction-related events, the presence of an ICU pharmacist was associated with a 37% lower mortality rate and a 15% shorter ICU

length of stay.[90] Average Medicare charges per patient were $3400 lower, resulting in over $215 million in total charges in 2005 dollars. Although these two studies do not prove causal effects, it appears that the presence of a clinical pharmacist is associated with substantial cost savings in patients with common conditions seen in ICU patients.

Conclusion

The ICU is a complex environment associated with extensive drug use. Considering the fiscal constraints on the provision of health care, the ICU is an area where pharmacoeconomic evaluation may be the only way to justify the use of selected drugs. Applying principles of pharmacoeconomics to critical care gives decision makers additional tools to make cost-effective decisions for patient care and for health systems. The economic burden of several conditions seen in the ICU and the costs associated with their treatment are beginning to be understood. The data are less than perfect. Clinicians and administrators rely on existing economic literature to assist with their decisions. The generation of additional cost-effectiveness studies of new and future pharmaceuticals is necessary to make sound decisions. Simply selecting the cheapest therapy or the newest therapy may not be best practice for either patients or society. The ICU clinical pharmacist can provide both clinical and economic input to develop protocols to optimize pharmacotherapy in a cost-effective manner. The intensivist and ICU clinical pharmacist should present data on the cost of care to hospital administrators and show how appropriate drug therapy is not only good for patients but also has a positive economic impact on the hospital or health system.

KEY POINTS

1. Overall healthcare costs continue to rise, with ICUs consuming a third of inpatient costs at a daily cost ranging from $3600 to $4600.

2. Economic evaluations of pharmaceuticals attempt to identify the value of drug therapy from a clinical, economic, or humanistic perspective.

3. Representative expensive ICU-related conditions for which more effective therapy is needed include acute congestive heart failure, acute renal failure, severe sepsis, ventilator-associated pneumonia, catheter-related sepsis, bloodstream infections, venous thromboembolic disease, agitation, delirium, and pain.

ANNOTATED REFERENCES

Drummond MF, Sculpfer MJ, Torrance GW, O'Brien BJ, Stoddart GL. Methods for the economic evaluation of health care programmes. New York: Oxford University Press; 2005.
This book is considered by many to be a classic in the application of economic theory to health care. Because a drug or treatment is evaluated on the basis of cost and outcome in reference to the current standard of care, cost-effectiveness analysis is the most common technique used. The authors conclude that cost-effectiveness analysis is a full economic evaluation because costs and outcomes are considered, and the results from a cost-effectiveness analysis are a crucial component in the decision to allocate limited resources.

Format for formulary submissions (FMCP), Version 3.0. Academy of Managed Care Pharmacy and evidence-based and value-based formulary guidelines. Available at: http://www.amcp.org/amcp.ark?p=0F6E1295. Accessed March 18, 2010.
This reference and website provide guidelines and instructions for developing an evaluation of a drug being submitted for National Formulary consideration status at an institution. It is increasingly used by managed care groups as a way of assessing the clinical and economic benefits of a new drug.

Dasta J, Kim SR, McLaughlin TP, Mody S, Piech CT. Incremental daily cost of mechanical ventilation in patients receiving treatment in an intensive care unit. Crit Care Med 2005;33:1266-71.
The daily cost of an ICU day is estimated from a large database in hospitals with medical, surgical, and trauma ICUs.

Dasta JF, Kane-Gill SL, Pencina M, Shehabi Y, Bokesch P, Riker R. A cost-minimization analysis of dexmedetomidine compared to midazolam for long-term sedation in the intensive care unit. Crit Care Med 2010;38:497-503.
This study is one of a small number of studies comparing ICU costs between two sedative regimens. The type of analysis used is a cost-minimization technique.

Dobesh P. Economic burden of venous thromboembolism in hospitalized patients. Pharmacotherapy 2009;29:943-53.

This is a comprehensive review of the burden of illness of deep venous thrombosis and pulmonary embolism. It also reviews data on cost-effectiveness of thromboprophylaxis, adherence to guidelines, and the role of the clinical pharmacist.

Eber MR, Laxminarayan R, Perencevich EN, Malani A. Clinical and economic outcomes attributable to healthcare-associated sepsis and pneumonia. Arch Intern Med 2010;170:347-53.
A large database is analyzed for the costs attributable to sepsis and pneumonia, and it documents the enormous impact these conditions have on overall healthcare costs.

Halpern NA, Pastores SM. Critical care medicine in the United States 2000-2005: an analysis of bed numbers, occupancy rates, payer mix and costs. Crit Care Med 2010;38:65-71.
This recent analysis of a large database of nonfederal acute care hospitals with critical care medicine beds includes descriptions of occupancy rates, payer mixes, and associated costs.

Zilberberg MD. Understanding cost-effectiveness in the ICU. Semin Respir Crit Care Med 2010;31:13-8.
This article reviews methods for evaluating healthcare costs as they apply to the ICU environment.

Cullen DJ, Sweitzer BJ, Bates DW, Burdick E, Edmondson A, Leape LL. Preventable adverse drug events in hospitalized patients: a comparative study of intensive care units and general care units. Crit Care Med 1997;25:1289-97.
This study is the first to provide an appreciation for the financial impact of ADEs occurring in the ICU, reinforcing the importance of ADE prevention.

Weber RJ, Kane SL, Oriolo VA, et al. Impact of intensive care unit (ICU) drug use on hospital cost: a descriptive analysis, with recommendations for optimizing ICU pharmacotherapy. Crit Care Med 2003;31:S17-24.
This article reviews issues of assessing drug costs in critical care and provides data on drug use and costs at one academic medical center. The unique aspect of this study is that financial information on drugs used while a patient was in the ICU covers 4 years and more than 20,000 patients. This type of analysis can be used as a basis for assessing whether certain expensive drugs are being used appropriately in the ICU.

REFERENCES

Access the complete reference list online at http://www.expertconsult.com.

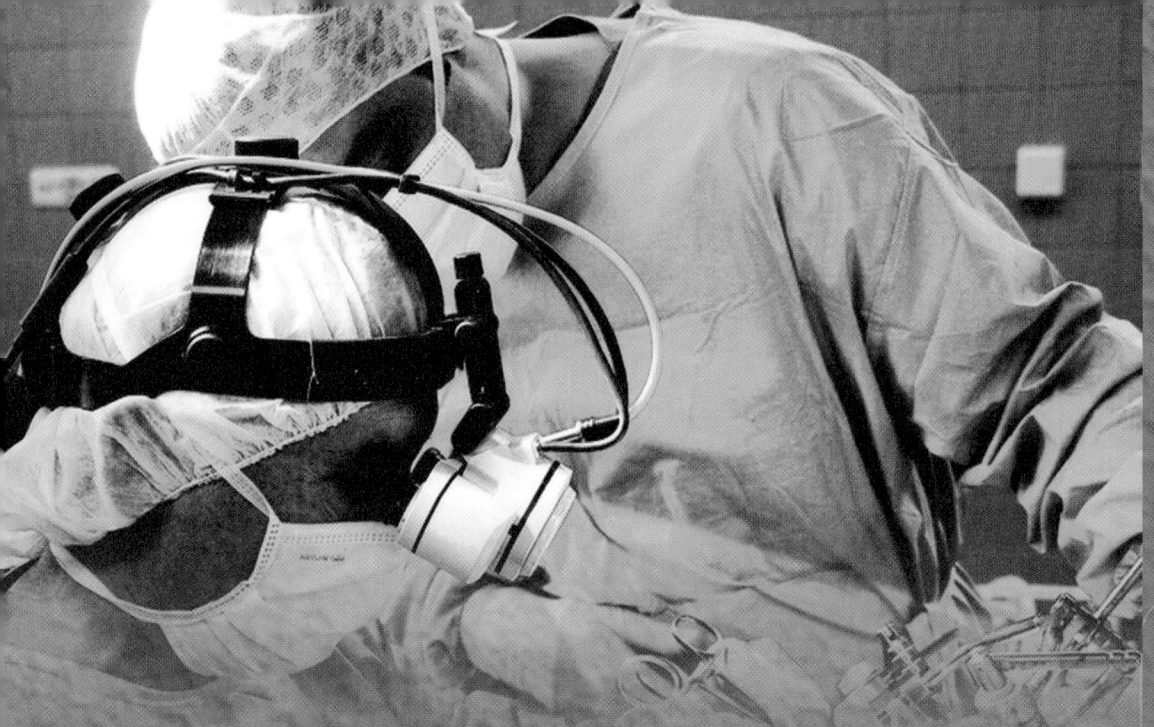

12

Surgery/Trauma

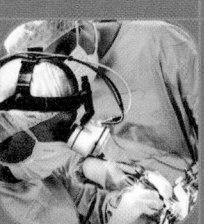

191

Resuscitation of Hypovolemic Shock

JAMES KASIEWICZ | JUAN CARLOS PUYANA

Fluids have been given intravenously (IV) for the management of fluid deficits for more than 100 years. In 1883, the English physiologist Sidney Ringer discovered that calcium-containing tap water was better than distilled water for maintaining the viability of tissues from animals in vitro. The understanding of the circulatory system and the importance of maintaining adequate circulatory volume were realized long ago. Furthermore, the desired elements and their approximate concentrations in IV fluids for plasma substitution have been known for many years.

The first reported IV transfusion occurred in 1492. In a desperate attempt to save a dying pope, blood was transfused from three youngsters, using a vein-to-vein anastomosis. The pope and all three youngsters died. The first known successful animal-to-animal transfusion was carried out in 1667. In 1818, Dr. James Blundell performed the first successful transfusion on a patient suffering from hemorrhage during childbirth. In 1830, the gold-plated steel needle for IV use was invented. In 1831, a paper published by O'Shaughnessy described the need for administering salts and water to cholera victims, an idea that was put into practice by Thomas Latta soon thereafter. During the 1930s, Baxter and Abbott produced the first commercial saline solutions. In the 1950s, plastic IV tubing replaced rubber tubing, and soon thereafter, the central venous approach for venous access was described by a French military surgeon. This approach represented a breakthrough for estimations of the state of hydration (central venous pressure [CVP] measurements) and the need for volume support.

Blalock's fundamental work on shock showed that injury precipitated obligatory local and regional fluid losses, the effects of which could be ameliorated by vigorous restoration of intravascular volume. This concept became a cornerstone to the understanding of the pathophysiology of shock and provided the fundamental rationale for IV therapy for hemorrhage and hypovolemia.

The introduction of blood transfusions as the result of contributions by surgeons during World War I and World War II dramatically changed outcomes in cases of severe hemorrhage. During the Korean War, fluid overload became a common and lethal side effect of resuscitation, owing to a lack of knowledge about how infusates disperse and are eliminated during trauma. Between the Korean War and the Vietnam War, Shires and colleagues described the shifts of fluid and electrolytes into cells after severe hemorrhagic shock. As a consequence, treatment of patients with shock was altered during the Vietnam War, leading to better outcomes and a lower incidence of acute renal failure.

Epidemiology of Severe Hemorrhagic Shock

Traumatic injury is the leading cause of death for individuals younger than 44 years of age in the United States. Overall, trauma results in approximately 150,000 deaths per year, and severe hypovolemia due to hemorrhage is a major factor in nearly half of those deaths. Approximately one-third of trauma deaths occur out of hospital, and exsanguination is a major cause of death occurring within 4 hours of injury. The distribution of battlefield injuries in the Vietnam War showed that 25% of deaths occurred as a result of massive exsanguinations and that the victims were not salvageable. An additional 19% of deaths occurred in cases that were deemed salvageable, and these were the result of torso exsanguinations (10%) and peripheral exsanguinations (19%).

As evidenced recently in the Iraq campaign, the fighting of the future is likely to involve terrorists and guerrilla interdictions and will be fought by small groups of combatants over shorter time periods with smaller numbers of casualties at any point in time. However, because of the likely locations of these conflicts, evacuation by air may be difficult or impossible, as was the case in Somalia in 1993. As a result, immediate and even ongoing treatment of casualties may be significantly extended. Shock and ensuing circulatory failure, therefore, may result from a variety of different trauma scenarios. Therapies used in the field may vary depending on the time frame from injury to medical evacuation, the skills and resources of first responders, and the field site of combatant injury.

Mechanisms of injury and severity of blood loss as well as prehospital interventions vary widely among trauma centers. Preferred fluid resuscitation strategies and optimal blood pressures are still being studied.[1,2] The number of preventable deaths due to hemorrhage are still significant. Definitive control of hemorrhage and resuscitative strategies are the cornerstone of treatment.[3]

Current State of Knowledge About Inadequate or Incomplete Resuscitation in Hemorrhagic and Hypovolemic Shock

Early studies by Wiggers showed that bleeding animals to a shock state followed by reinfusion of blood would not save the animal's life. This phenomenon was termed *irreversible shock*. Clinically, circulatory collapse is the common endpoint of irreversible shock whether it is precipitated by trauma, hemorrhage, or severe hypovolemia.

HEMODYNAMIC PHASES OF IRREVERSIBLE SHOCK

There are four distinct phases of irreversible shock. Phase I is a nonhypotensive period of hemorrhage persisting through a 20% blood volume loss. It is associated with a reduction in cardiac output in the resting individual. In phase II at roughly 20% of blood volume loss, mean arterial pressure decreases due to an inappropriate reduction in sympathetic tone known as *Bezold-Jarisch* or *empty ventricle reflex*. There are variations in the blood volume loss required for this reflex, and in animal models it is modulated by the degree of external stress or pain. Arterial blood pressure stabilizes in phase III as the brain triggers an intense vasoconstriction of all nonessential organs. Blood is diverted to the heart and brain. If hypovolemia is not corrected, an irreversible state of shock in phase IV is entered. During hemorrhage there is also increased adhesion of polymorphonuclear neutrophils leading to leukosequestration in the microcirculation. These processes (decreased cardiac output, vasoconstriction, and leukosequestration) lead to impaired tissue perfusion and eventual death.

CARDIOVASCULAR AND HEMODYNAMIC RESPONSE

Shock is defined as inadequate delivery of O_2 to metabolically active tissues. Failure of O_2 delivery can lead to eventual organ dysfunction and ultimate complete circulatory collapse. Guyton described three major stages describing the mechanisms.[4] First is compensated shock, in which the individual will achieve full recovery with minimal interventions. Regional tissues and organs have different mechanisms to prevent damage. The next stage is decompensated shock. Aggressive resuscitation is required in this stage, or a substantial fraction of individuals will die. There is a poor correlation between changes in cardiac output and systemic blood pressure. Irreversible shock is the last stage. Shock has progressed to the point that all known therapies are inadequate.

NEUROENDOCRINE RESPONSE

Pressure and stretch receptors in the carotid body and aortic arch play a key role in maintaining perfusion to the heart and brain. The nervous system responds immediately to loss of circulating blood volume with sympathetically mediated arteriolar and venous vasoconstriction. Baroreceptors in the carotid bulb and aortic arch sense decreased stretch in the arterial wall. Afferent vagal fibers carry signals that tonically inhibit central processors. A decrease in the effective circulating blood volume or blood pressure causes release of the chronic inhibition imposed by baroreceptors. This message ascends to the nucleus tractus solitarius in the medulla oblongata, resulting in tonic inhibition of heart rate and up-regulation of the sympathetic system.

Acute hypovolemia initiates multiple endocrine responses. The nucleus tractus solitarius signals the hypothalamus to release corticotropin releasing factor and vasopressin. Consequently, corticotropin (ACTH), cortisol, vasopressin, and glucagon levels increase. Glucagon and cortisol are crucial in providing substrate for energy production. Circulating catecholamines inhibit insulin release to increase glucose level. The renin-aldosterone system is stimulated to minimize loss of fluid or salt. Angiotensin II also promotes vasoconstriction. The summation of the neuroendocrine response is to maximize cardiac function, conserve salt and water for the maintenance of circulating blood volume, and provide nutrients and oxygen to the heart and brain.

METABOLIC RESPONSE

If hemorrhage is massive, the compensatory mechanisms designed to spare blood flow to the brain and heart may be overwhelmed, as occurs in cases of irreversible shock. However, if the hemorrhage is controlled or fluid replacement therapy is initiated promptly, the patient may enter a phase described as *compensatory shock*. Recent observations in severely injured patients suggest that continuous monitoring of oxidative metabolism and tissue pH in peripheral organs may be used as indicators of cellular stress and impaired tissue perfusion. Minimally invasive assessment of cellular stress—using interstitial pH, tissue P_{CO_2}, and nicotinamide adenine dinucleotide (NADH) autofluorescence (marker of cellular redox state) as read outs—may reflect anaerobic metabolism and dysoxia. These measurements have been obtained from the gut mucosa, skeletal muscle, subcutaneous tissue, and several other organs. Measurements such as tissue P_{CO_2}, P_{O_2}, and pH in these organs have been correlated with specific measurements of cellular dysfunction specific to those organs.

As a consequence of the stoichiometry of the reactions responsible for the substrate level phosphorylation of adenosine diphosphate (ADP) to form adenosine triphosphate (ATP), anaerobic metabolism is inevitably associated with the net accumulation of protons. Accordingly, determination that tissue pH is not in the acid range should be sufficient to conclude that perfusion (and therefore arterial oxygen content) are sufficient to meet the metabolic demands of the cells, even without knowledge of the actual values for tissue blood flow or oxygen delivery. By the same token, the detection of tissue acidosis should alert the clinician to the possibility that perfusion is inadequate. It seems likely that monitoring tissue P_{CO_2} (tissue capnometry) will play a role in establishing thresholds for and transition points into the metabolic failure associated with circulatory collapse. By eliminating the potentially confounding effects of systemic hypocarbia or hypercarbia, calculating and monitoring the gap between tissue P_{CO_2} and arterial P_{CO_2} may prove to be even more valuable than simply following changes in tissue P_{CO_2}.

Weil et al. described a sublingual P_{CO_2} sensor and demonstrated that changes in sublingual P_{CO_2} are more sensitive to changes in cardiac output and blood pressure than any other parameter currently used to quantify hypoperfusion. Shoemaker et al. described the use of transcutaneous oxygen tension (Pt_{CO_2}) as an early warning signal of tissue hypoxia and transcutaneous carbon dioxide tension (Pt_{CCO_2}) as an early signal of tissue hypoperfusion. These authors proposed the use of transcutaneous sensors for the assessment of Pt_{CO_2} and Pt_{CCO_2} that have been used for years in neonatal medicine as a surrogate measure of arterial blood gases. They showed that compared with survivors, patients who died had significantly lower Pt_{CO_2} and higher Pt_{CCO_2} values, beginning with the early stage of resuscitation. Periods of Pt_{CCO_2} at less than 50 mm Hg for more than 60 minutes or Pt_{CCO_2} at greater than 60 mm Hg for more than 30 minutes were associated with 90% mortality and 100% morbidity.

McKinley and colleagues have demonstrated a correlation between skeletal muscle P_{CO_2}, P_{O_2}, and pH with hemorrhagic shock using fiberoptic sensor technology that allows for continuous monitoring. Both skeletal muscle and gastric mucosa respond similarly to hypotension, and the magnitude of this response is similar for gastric intramucosal pH (pHi) and muscle pH. Skeletal muscle parameters (P_{O_2}, P_{CO_2}, and pH), however, appear to indicate a greater severity of shock and more prolonged recovery than mixed venous measurements or gastric mucosal parameters. Muscle P_{O_2} may also provide information that is comparable to other more elaborate calculations of O_2 delivery and utilization. In one case report, continuous monitoring of skeletal muscle pH, P_{CO_2}, and P_{O_2} was able to detect ongoing hemorrhage of a severely injured trauma patient in the setting of "normal" systemic variables. Although preliminary, these findings suggest that continuous monitoring of skeletal muscle pH and related parameters may provide a minimally invasive and more sensitive way of following the resuscitative effort.

ACUTE INFLAMMATORY RESPONSE

The innate and adaptive immune system is triggered in hypovolemia, hemorrhage, and trauma. When appropriately contained, the immune system can restore the body to healthy function following clearance of the offending agents and appropriate tissue repair. In more severe settings, inflammation is persistent and leads to the detrimental consequences described earlier.

Neutrophils and macrophages react to damaged tissue. Macrophages are present in almost all tissues and can directly detect bacterial lipopolysaccharide through genetically encoded pattern recognition receptors. Adhesion of neutrophils to damaged or dysfunctional endothelium leads to microvascular "plugs" that contribute to progressive hypoperfusion. Additionally, neutrophils reach other capillary beds by detecting specific signals on vascular endothelium and navigate to their target by following chemoattractants. The complement pathway is also activated, triggering further activation of neutrophils and macrophages.

Once activated, neutrophils and macrophages produce and secrete cytokines. Cytokines regulate the activation of neutrophils, macrophages, lymphocytes and other cytokines. Proinflammatory cytokines such as tumor necrosis factor (TNF) and interleukins (IL-1 and IL-6) are produced at various stages of the inflammatory response and promote immune cell activation. Production of these proinflammatory cytokines is counterbalanced by production of antiinflammatory cytokines such as IL-10 and transforming growth factor beta (TGF-β_1) that serve to restore homeostasis and promote tissue repair.

Proinflammatory cytokines also induce macrophages and neutrophils to produce reactive oxygen and nitrogen species such as nitric oxide (NO), superoxide, hydroxyl radical, and hydrogen peroxide, which are directly toxic to tissue. The reactive oxygen species can incite more inflammation and are implicated in the pathology of reperfusion injury. Nitric oxide seems to be especially relevant in irreversible shock. Inducible nitric oxide synthase (iNOS) and its products were found only during the irreversible phase of hemorrhagic shock in rats.

Resuscitative Strategies in Hemorrhagic Shock

The mainstays of therapy in hemorrhagic shock are bleeding control, tissue oxygenation, coagulation support, and maintenance of normothermia.[3] Fluid resuscitation strategies in the prehospital and hospital setting are important.

VASCULAR ACCESS FOR PATIENTS WITH SEVERE HEMORRHAGE

In the trauma patient presenting with multiple serious injuries and hemorrhagic shock, vascular access is necessary. Venous access should never be initiated on an injured limb. When thoracoabdominal injury is suspected, it is prudent to obtain infra-diaphragmatic and supradiaphragmatic access.

Advanced Trauma Life Support (ATLS) guidelines recommend rapid placement of two large-bore (16 gauge or larger) IV catheters. The most suitable veins are at the wrist, on the dorsum of the hand, at the antecubital fossa in the arm, and on the saphenous in the leg. If peripheral IV catheters are unable to be placed, catheters can be placed in the central veins. The femoral vein is the most frequent central vein cannulated. The subclavian vein is another alternative and can be placed safely in experienced hands. The internal jugular vein is rarely used in trauma patients because of the possibility of cervical spine injuries and the need for cervical immobilization with a collar. Patients with absent pulses may need to undergo cutdown to cannulate the femoral vein under direct vision to obtain IV access.

RESUSCITATIVE FLUIDS

Colloids Versus Crystalloids

In the prehospital setting, blood and blood products may not be available, but colloids and isotonic crystalloids are readily available. Randomized controlled trials comparing resuscitation with crystalloids versus colloids showed no survival benefit.[5] A Cochrane Database review concluded that there is no evidence that one colloid solution is more effective or safe than any other.[4] Crystalloids are less expensive than colloids and are recommended as the initial resuscitative fluid.

Hypertonic Saline

Hypertonic saline (7.5% [HS]) resuscitation has been thought of as an attractive option because it rapidly pulls water into the intravascular space owing to its osmotic pressure. A 250-mL bolus of HS has been shown to increase systolic arterial pressure (SAP) in hemorrhagic shock patients.[6] In addition, it is associated with immunomodulatory effects. In a rat model, HS downregulated neutrophil activation, oxidative stress, and proinflammatory mediator production when compared to lactated Ringer's solution.[7] Interestingly, there does not seem to be a difference in bacterial clearance in the peritoneum when comparing the two solutions, suggesting that HS can be safely used in the setting of peritoneal contamination.[8] Given these possible beneficial effects, it has been proposed as a prehospital resuscitative strategy. In fact, it has been used as a prehospital resuscitative fluid, especially in European countries.

However, on March 26, 2009, the National Heart, Lung, and Blood Institute (NHLBI) of the National Institutes of Health (NIH) halted the study by the Resuscitation Outcomes Consortium (ROC) comparing 250 mL of HS, 250 mL of normal saline, and 250 mL of HS with dextran in patients with hemorrhagic shock. There was no significant cumulative difference in 28-day survival in the HS groups versus the normal saline group. In fact, there was a trend toward earlier death in the HS groups. In the United States, normal saline is the recommended prehospital fluid for patients with hemorrhagic shock.

Red Cells

Early identification of severe injuries with the likelihood of hemorrhage should suffice for the trauma team leader to alert the blood bank. Hematocrit levels should not guide the decision for transfusion in acute hemorrhage. Protocols for massive transfusion should be established, and the blood bank should automatically begin preparation of fresh frozen plasma and platelet packs if massive bleeding is anticipated.

Available options are type O-negative, type-specific, typed and screened, or typed and cross-matched packed red blood cells. The initial choice depends on the degree of hemodynamic instability. Type O-negative red cells have no major antigens and can be used safely for patients with any blood type. Unfortunately, only 8% of the population has O-negative blood, and blood bank reserves for O-negative blood are low. O-positive blood can be used in male patients but may be a problem in female Rh-negative patients.

If 50% to 75% of the patient's blood volume has been replaced with type O blood, one should continue to administer type O red cells. Otherwise, the risk of a major cross-match reaction increases, since the patient may have received enough anti-A or anti-B antibodies to precipitate hemolysis if A, B, or AB units are subsequently given. Obtaining type-specific red cells requires 5 to 10 minutes in most institutions.

When blood is typed and screened, the patient's blood group is identified, and the serum is screened for major blood group antibodies. A full cross-match generally requires about 45 minutes and involves mixing donor cells with recipient serum to rule out antigen/antibody reactions.

COAGULATION FACTORS, PLATELETS, AND COAGULOPATHY

Severe bleeding, surgery, and massive transfusion interact synergistically to lead to the lethal triad: hypothermia, acidosis, and coagulopathy. Coagulopathy promotes bleeding and hypotension, which leads to hypothermia and acidosis. Hypothermia and acidosis impair thrombin generation and decrease fibrinogen levels.[9]

Failure of coagulation in trauma is multifactorial and is characterized by the combined presence of coagulation abnormalities resembling disseminated intravascular coagulation (DIC), excessive fibrinolysis (likely caused by to release of tissue plasminogen activator [TPA] from damaged tissues), dilutional coagulopathy due to excessive fluid treatment, and massive transfusion syndrome resulting in dilution of coagulation factors and platelets.[10]

Massive transfusion protocols have been developed and utilized in major trauma centers. Activating the massive transfusion protocol gives a fixed ratio of red cells to plasma to platelets. High plasma- and platelet-to–red cell ratio has been shown to increase survival in retrospective studies.[11] Military data showed an increase in survival with a red cell/plasma ratio approaching 1:1.[12] Civilian trauma centers are increasingly adopting a 1:1:1 ratio for massive transfusion protocols.

USE OF RECOMBINANT ACTIVATED FACTOR VII AS AN ADJUVANT FOR RESUSCITATION IN THE COAGULOPATHIC PATIENT

Patients with diffuse bleeding enter a coagulopathy leading to decreased levels of fibrinogen, factor VIII, and platelets. The low levels of fibrinogen lead to a loose fibrin structure. Low levels of factor XIII, the fibrin-stabilizing factor, decreases the strength of the fibrin clot by limiting the development of complex branching clots.[13] Trauma patients with massive bleeding thus may benefit from recombinant activated factor VII (rFVIIa), because it works to increase thrombin peak, allowing for a stable fibrin plug.

Mechanism of Action

Hemostasis is initiated by the formation of a complex between tissue factor (TF), exposed as a result of a vessel wall injury, and activated factor VII (FVIIa) that is normally present in circulating blood. The TF-FVIIa complex converts factor X into FXa on the TF-bearing cell. FXa then activates prothrombin into thrombin. This limited amount of thrombin activates FVII, FV, FXI, and platelets. Thrombin-activated platelets change shape, resulting in exposure of negatively charged phospholipids which form a template for thrombin generation involving FVIII and FIX. Full thrombin generation is necessary for complete activation of FXIII and thrombin activatable fibrinolytic inhibitor (TAFI) to occur. Furthermore, full thrombin generation is important for the fibrin structure of the hemostatic plug.

The addition of rFVIIa to FVIII- or FIX-deficient plasma has been shown to increase thrombin generation in a cell-based in vitro model. Furthermore, extra rFVIIa was found to normalize fibrin clot permeability in vitro and to tighten the fibrin structure as studied by three-dimensional confocal microscopy. These findings indicate that administration of rFVIIa can compensate for the lack of FVIII and FIX. Accordingly, administration of exogenous rFVIIa has been found to stop bleeding in hemophilia patients and, provided it is given in high enough doses, to allow major surgery to be performed in severe hemophiliacs with inhibitors. Because rFVIIa enhances thrombin generation on already activated platelets, it has been suggested that rFVIIa may also help improve hemostasis in other situations involving impaired thrombin generation, such as platelet disorders (thrombocytopenia and functional platelet defects); the immediate result is an increase in generation of thrombin. Furthermore, exogenous rFVIIa induces hemostasis independently of tissue factor and factors VIII and IX by binding directly to activated platelet surfaces with low affinity to generate thrombin in a dose-dependent manner.

Pharmacology

Intravenous administration of rFVIIa does not induce systemic activation of coagulation. Administration of rFVIIa shortens prothrombin time (PT) and partial thromboplastin time (PTT) but does not affect levels of thrombin, fibrinogen, or platelet count. The half-life of rFVIIa ranges between 1.3 and 2.7 hours, being shorter for children younger than 15 years; however, there is considerable individual variation. Initial work in humans indicates that a dose of 90 to 110μg/kg of rFVIIa (given as a bolus) should be repeated every 2 hours over a 24-hour period. Intervals may be increased thereafter according to the response and severity of bleeding.

Safety

There are case series and reports of thromboembolic events associated with the use of rFVIIa.[14] Tissue factor is expressed under pathologic conditions such as atherosclerosis, sepsis, or cancer, so the risk of thromboembolic complications such as stroke, myocardial infarction, deep venous thrombosis (DVT), and pulmonary embolism (PE) is increased.

Efficacy of rFVIIa in Trauma and Surgery

Martinowitz et al. reported that administration of rFVIIa caused a cessation of diffuse bleeding in seven trauma patients. Advocates for rFVIIa suggest there may be two principal indications for its use: the first on the battlefield or in the prehospital setting before arrival at the trauma setting, and the second at the trauma center as an adjuvant to damage-control management. A retrospective chart review for trauma admissions to a combat support hospital in Iraq indicated that patients receiving rFVIIa early (before transfusion of 8 units of blood) had decreased red blood cell use.[15] In vitro studies demonstrated that administering rFVIIa in mild to moderate hypothermia (31°C-34°C) did not affect ultimate strength, thus suggesting its possible role in hypothermic trauma patients.[16]

ANNOTATED REFERENCES

Johansson PI, Stensballe J. Hemostatic resuscitation for massive bleeding: the paradigm of plasma and platelets—a review of the current literature. Transfusion 2010;50:701-10.
A nice review of 14 retrospective studies looking at the survival and ratios of red cells to blood components.
Bunn F, Trivedi D, Ashraf S. Colloid solutions for fluid resuscitation. Cochrane Database Syst Rev 2008;CD001319.
A good review of randomized and quasi-randomized trials comparing the effects of different colloid solutions in patients needing volume replacement.
Sihler KC, Napolitano LM. Massive transfusion: new insights. Chest 2009;136:1654-67.
A review of massive transfusion strategies and use of hemostatic blood products.
Perel P, Roberts I. Colloids versus crystalloids for fluid resuscitation in critically ill patients. Cochrane Database Syst Rev 2007;CD000567.
A look at randomized controlled trials evaluating the effects of colloids versus crystalloids in the critically ill patient.
Angele MK, Schneider CP, Chaudry IH. Bench-to-bedside review: latest results in hemorrhagic shock. Crit Care 2008;12:218.
This is a review of the latest therapeutic interventions for hemorrhagic shock.

REFERENCES

Access the complete reference list online at http://www.expertconsult.com.

192

Mediastinitis

ROBERT G. JOHNSON

Mediastinitis includes a variety of thoracic infections that occur in the space between the sternum and the spine, above the diaphragm and below the thoracic outlet. Clinically the diagnosis, treatment, and prognosis of these various forms of mediastinitis are determined by their location and etiology. The mediastinum may be divided anatomically into three clinically relevant compartments: anterior (between the posterior sternum and the anterior pericardium), middle (the intrapericardial contents), and posterior (bounded anteriorly by the posterior pericardium and posteriorly by the spine). The pleural cavities are the lateral boundaries for each of these mediastinal spaces. With respect to etiology, mediastinitis may be either primary, arising without prior intervention, or secondary, occurring post intervention. Clinically one can essentially lump the anatomic anterior and middle compartments together, as mediastinitis occurs most commonly in those combined spaces secondarily as a postoperative complication of cardiac operations. Esophageal pathology, primary or secondary to iatrogenic intervention, accounts for the overwhelming majority of mediastinal infections of the posterior compartment. Other more unusual forms of mediastinal infections or inflammation include those that migrate into the mediastinum from adjacent fascially contiguous spaces (most commonly, descending necrotizing mediastinitis of oral origin) and those which are more indolent than acute and are characterized by chronic inflammation and fibrosis. Accordingly, this presentation of the subject will follow these anatomic and etiologic distinctions: acute anterior mediastinitis, acute posterior mediastinitis, and migratory and chronic mediastinal inflammation.

Acute Anterior Mediastinitis

Rarely, acute anterior mediastinitis may occur without antecedent median sternotomy, as reported after traumatic sternal fracture[1] or as a consequence of descending cervical infections (see later), but by far the most common form of acute mediastinitis is that occurring after sternotomy for a cardiac operation. The term *mediastinitis* after cardiac operations should strictly refer to an infection involving the space behind, deep to, the sternum. Post–cardiac surgery infections may more broadly include those that are superficial or subcutaneous "above" the fascia, unassociated with sternal pathology, and those that involve the sternum itself (sternal osteomyelitis or sternitis) without deeper infection. For purposes of the following discussion, we will assume any infection posterior to the sternum is an infection of the anterior mediastinum, including those patients with deep sternal infections, as no impervious anatomic barrier exists between the posterior cortex of the sternum and the space behind it. Deep sternal infection can be considered one end of the spectrum of mediastinitis, with the other being gross pus in the anterior mediastinum and pericardium (deep organ space infection). There are, of course, patients who have sterile sternal dehiscence with no evidence of infection, but this is a diagnosis of exclusion, so that these patients are treated with antibiotics and/or irrigation pending culture results. In patients who have sterile postoperative sternal wound drainage, there is a real opportunity for retrograde infection. Clinically, especially in more obese patients, it is sometimes unclear as to whether one is initially dealing with a superficial problem (anterior to the fascia), a sterile dehiscence, or a deeper infection. More than a small amount of drainage, any sternal instability or evidence of separation (e.g., broken wires on a chest film) suggest at least a sterile dehiscence and the need for reexploration, deep cultures, and appropriate re-closure.

INCIDENCE, PATHOLOGY AND PREVENTION

Even among large well-reported series, the incidence of post–cardiac surgery mediastinitis varies, as noted earlier, due in part to the various definitions of mediastinitis, sternal osteomyelitis, or deep sternal wound infection. On occasion, the diagnosis may be made weeks or months after hospital discharge, and that occurrence may be missed by the institution where the operation was originally performed. Over the past 2 decades, there may be a trend toward lower reported rates of mediastinitis after sternotomy (more large series with <1% incidence), but the reported range remains wide, from 0.24% to 4% of cardiac operations.[2,3,4] Increasingly, as the postoperative length of stay decreases, mediastinal infections are diagnosed days or even months after hospital discharge, with median time to diagnosis variously reported around 10 days after the index cardiac operation.

In October 2008 the Centers for Medicare and Medicaid declared post–cardiac surgery mediastinitis a "preventable condition,"[5] but no existing data manifest it as entirely preventable. Indeed, a number of mostly unmodifiable host factors that increase the risk of post–cardiac surgery mediastinitis have been identified. Among these are diabetes, increased body mass index, older age, renal failure, prolonged preoperative hospitalization, immunosuppression, chronic obstructive pulmonary disease, cigarette smoking, reoperation, preoperative atrial fibrillation, and elevated C-reactive protein.[3,6,7]

In addition to host factors, intraoperative factors influence the risk. An increased incidence of deep sternal wound infection has been associated with bilateral internal mammary use, prolonged operative time, and use of the intraaortic balloon pump.[7] Postoperative management may also influence the risk of mediastinitis; increased glucose levels (>200 mg/dL),[8] reexploration, and prolonged ventilator use are associated with a higher incidence of deep sternal infection.[7] Glucose values as low as ≥130 mg/dL have been linked to such infection in children.[9] Undoubtedly factors such as skin preparation, electrocautery use, glove changes, and attention to a host of other details account for some of the variation in infection rates from surgeon to surgeon and institution to institution. Avoiding sternotomy entirely, as can be done with less chest wall–invasive approaches, appears to drastically reduce or eliminate the risk of mediastinal infection after cardiac operations.[7]

Postoperative tracheostomy is required in some post-sternotomy patients, and many of these have some of the risk factors that are also predictive of deep sternal wound infection. Open tracheostomy for patients with prolonged ventilator dependence, once deferred 2 or more weeks after sternotomy for fear of contaminating the anterior mediastinal space, has not been shown to be associated with an increased incidence of mediastinitis (mean of 5.6 days post cardiac operation).[10] Specifically, the technique of percutaneous tracheostomy has not been associated with subsequent mediastinal infection. This technique may allow an earlier, safer switch from an oral to cervical airway[11] in patients requiring prolonged mechanical ventilation.

Staphylococcal species are the most common organisms seen in patients with post-sternotomy deep wound infection, and these are increasingly methicillin resistant.[12] Coagulase-negative resistant organisms are more common in patients who have prolonged hospitalizations.[13] Gram-negative organisms may be cultured, particularly from diabetics, in patients with gram-negative pneumonia prior to operation, or in those who require reexploration.[14]

The serious consequences of mediastinitis after cardiac operations dictate the use of prophylactic antibiotics as an established practice.

Given the most common organisms causing these infections, a second-generation cephalosporin is still the most accepted prophylaxis. A commonly used regimen would include cephazolin, 2 g, within 1 hour of skin incision, with a second 1-g dose at 3 to 4 hours if the incision remains open. Vancomycin is substituted in patients with penicillin allergy, in deference to the possibility of cross-reactivity, and it may be used routinely for an interval in institutions experiencing an outbreak of resistant staphylococci. The addition of preoperative gram-negative coverage (e.g., gentamicin) is appropriate in such cases, given vancomycin's poor coverage of such organisms.[15] Topical vancomycin has been shown effective in decreasing the incidence of sternal infections, and although used routinely in some practices, the development of resistant staphylococci is a genuine concern.[16] An evidence-based guideline from the Society of Thoracic Surgeons recommends gram-positive prophylaxis for no more than 48 hours, in addition to preoperative nasal mupirocin.[12,15]

DIAGNOSIS

Patients with mediastinitis after sternotomy generally have clinical signs of wound drainage and sternal instability, but neither may be present initially. A spiking fever and an acutely elevated leukocyte count are common. Some patients manifest signs of sepsis with mental status changes and hemodynamic compromise. Mediastinitis can very rarely appear as early as 1 day after operation or as remotely as months after an operation. Rarely, those patients who have an indolent course presenting many months after operation may have isolated deep involvement, tracking down to the aorta and/or involving some artificial material such as a pledget or a braided suture.

The gravity of the diagnosis and variability of clinical signs has encouraged the use of imaging techniques to confirm or refute the possibility of deep sternal or mediastinal infection. Unfortunately, the variable diagnostic accuracy of most of these techniques permits them to be supportive[17] but rarely if ever definitive in the diagnosis of deep infection. This is especially true in the early time frame (<30 days) when the vast majority of patients present. During this time, fluid collections and mediastinal soft-tissue changes are common, if not universal, both being nonspecific for infection.[18] Nuclear studies (^{99m}Tc) have been used in late-presenting indolent cases in an attempt to separate sternal involvement from infections superficial to it.[19] All these imaging studies are, of course, confounded by changes that one can expect following the operative procedure itself. A profile of abnormal cytokine levels has been characterized,[20] with terminal SC5b-9 complement complex concentration being substantially higher in patients with mediastinitis, and having no overlap with values in non-mediastinitis, post–cardiac surgery controls. In difficult to diagnose cases, blind retrosternal, subxiphoid needle aspiration and culture have been variably employed, and aspiration with ultrasound guidance has been reported after cardiac transplantation.[21] A recent small series suggested diagnostic success in patients without classic signs of infection by anteriorly inserting a 22-gauge needle percutaneously and aspirating between the recently closed sternal edges. Cultures and Gram stains were used to establish the presence of infection, with a high degree of specificity and sensitivity.[22]

TREATMENT

While the need for operative treatment in anterior mediastinitis is firmly established, the techniques successfully employed vary greatly. The varied technical approaches are related to the timing of diagnosis (interval since antecedent operation), the depth-extent of infection, and the acuity of the patient. The experience and choice of the treating surgeon is also a factor in the technique used to manage a deep infection. In patients with suspected infection in whom there is drainage and some sternal instability, expeditious reexploration with débridement of the sternal edges and surrounding soft tissues, accompanied by irrigation and drainage may permit sternal re-wiring.[2,23] In patients who are septic, and/or in those with gross retrosternal purulence, a staged approach or immediate tissue coverage may be employed.

If sternal re-closure is elected after débridement an alternative wiring technique, either a variation of the Robicsek[24] weave or a commercially available plate fixation device, is generally used. Cultures obtained at operation dictate the systemic antibiotics ultimately used, but initial coverage may include a second-generation cephalosporin and gram negative coverage until gram stain or culture results are definitive. A variety of irrigation solutions and protocols have been employed in these patients. Diluted antibiotic, povidone iodine, and aqueous acid solutions have been reported.[23,25] The duration of irrigation has varied from three days to a week, while systemic antibiotics are continued, as would be the case for other adult bone infections. Unfortunately, this attempt at primary sternal closure has been reported to require secondary procedures in 20% to 40% of the patients.[26] More recently, one small series[23] employing the single-stage débridement, closure, and irrigation technique had success in 95% of patients so treated.

A two-stage approach involves an interval during which the sternum and skin are left open and a wound vacuum device placed.[27,28] Open management of sternal wounds is associated with a risk of sudden, sometimes fatal, cardiac hemorrhage from exposed grafts, the aorta, or (most frequently) the right ventricle. Needless to say, the risk of death in such patients is very high (>50%).[29,30,31] Given these risks, it has been recommended that close attention be paid to the proximity of the right sternal edge and the right ventricle or grafts. Decreased abrasive contact may be afforded by judicious use of sedation and mechanical ventilation until coverage can be achieved.

Whether used as an initial single-stage procedure or as a secondary procedure, tissue transposition into the anterior mediastinum has dramatically changed the prognosis of this once often fatal complication.[32] Well-vascularized omentum or muscle can be used. Muscle options include rollover of the pectoralis major (detached from its humeral insertion, leaving intact the muscle's origin and blood supply) or rotation and advancement of the pectoralis major (detached from its costal origins and thereby maintaining its lateral blood supply). The rectus abdominis muscle may, depending on the prior use of the ipsilateral mammary artery, be detached distally and rotated on its cephalad attachment into the anterior mediastinal space. The omentum may be based on the right gastroepiploic or mobilized, leaving the gastroepiploic intact. The sternum may be left open with the tissue flap between the remnant edges, or rarely it may be closed over the flap. Either way, closed suction drains are required for the large, mobilized skin flaps and sometimes beneath transposed tissue flap.

The use of omentum versus any specific muscle flap may be dictated by availability (e.g., in patients with prior laparotomies), but when the option exists, the use of omentum has been touted as advantageous over muscle flaps,[33] although it has also been cited as being associated with poorer survival outcome,[34] perhaps related to patient selection. It has also been successfully employed in infections after ascending aortic replacement.[35] Skin coverage over a transposed flap may be accomplished by primary presternal skin reapproximation, split-thickness skin grafting, or, with the rectus muscle, a skin paddle may be transposed as well.

As noted earlier, débrided sternal wounds may be prepared for flap coverage by the use of a closed high-pressure vacuum system in which a polyurethane foam (400-600 μm pore size) is cut to fit the anterior mediastinal space and sealed to the skin permitting a vacuum (negative 75 mm Hg) to be generated over the entire wound surface. The device is changed regularly to avoid tissue ingrowth. Particularly with smaller wounds, the vacuum treatment may obviate the use of flap coverage as the wound heals secondarily, with obliteration of the space over a period of weeks.[36,37]

PROGNOSIS

Although the mortality of mediastinitis has improved dramatically over the past 2.5 decades, the likelihood of death remains high. Early detection with expeditious operative débridement and tissue coverage are the major advances that have allowed that improvement to take place. Still, the acute in-hospital mortality with post-sternotomy mediastinitis reported in larger series has ranged from 12.8% to 47%.[2,38] Patients may die of sepsis or hemorrhage, either as a consequence of direct cardiac injury or secondary to an infected graft or foreign body. More often, death occurs from associated comorbidities or complications, especially an additional infection,[38] that accompany the mediastinal infection. An examination of the predictors for deep sternal infection illuminates the fact that patients who develop this serious complication are more likely to have multiple comorbidities that might limit their survival. Importantly, it is not merely the acute mortality that is elevated in patients with post–cardiac surgery mediastinitis. In studies from the Northern New England Cardiovascular Disease Study Group, adjusting for various comorbidities, the 4-year mortality for patients with a postoperative deep sternal infection was 3 times greater than those without that complication, and this increased all-cause mortality rate persisted with up to 10 years of follow-up. For patients surviving more than 6 months after cardiac operation, the incidence of death was 70% higher than the rate among patients who did not have mediastinal infection.[39]

Posterior Mediastinitis

Acute infections that arise in the posterior mediastinum generally result from disease that may be primary to the esophagus or, more commonly in the United States, secondary to some esophageal intervention. Primarily, esophagitis (e.g., in immunocompromised patients with fungal or viral organisms) may extend through the esophagus, resulting in mediastinitis. Abscess formation, presumably secondary to hematogenous spread, has been reported[40] in a dialysis patient. More commonly, infection of the posterior mediastinum is the result of esophageal instrumentation (scopes, probes, tubes, or dilators), and even esophageal ultrasound-guided needle biopsy may result in abscess.[41] Esophageal perforation (often at the gastric junction) from a swallowed foreign body (e.g., bone or toothpick) has been reported.[42] Esophageal operations may be the source of an infection due to anastomotic disruption, but as transhiatal esophagectomy is increasingly employed for patients with esophageal cancer, its cervical gastropharyngeal anastomosis mostly avoids the consequences of mediastinitis. Still, among patients having an intrathoracic esophagogastric anastomosis, a leak may occur in 4.3% to 8.7% of patients.[43] Traumatic injuries to the trachea, proximal bronchii, or esophagus obviously may result in contamination of this space as well. Other causes of posterior compartment mediastinitis include the classic Boerhaave's syndrome characterized by rupture of the lower esophagus post retching and, more rarely, the erosion of a broncholith from a partially or completely obstructed bronchus.[44]

DIAGNOSIS

Suspicion of posterior mediastinitis should be heightened by any of the mentioned historical factors, and additionally may include prior symptoms of dysphagia. Given a relevant history, the presence of cervical pain and/or chest pain with a high fever would strongly suggest the diagnosis. On examination, supraclavicular crepitus may be identified in patients with upper mediastinal pathology but would generally be absent initially in those with middle or lower esophageal disease. Leukocytosis might be a singular early laboratory abnormality. Depending on the underlying pathology and duration of contamination, sepsis with mental status changes and hypotension may occur. Certainly in some of these patients, the plain chest film reveals a pleural effusion, and more rarely, air may be seen in the retropharyngeal space or other abnormal locations along the length of the mediastinum posterior to the pericardium. Computed tomography (CT) scan with oral Gastrografin is the mainstay for diagnosis and localization, as it can clearly demonstrate any abnormal air or fluid collections along the esophagus

or esophagogastric junction, and water-soluble contrast might diagnose the presence of an esophageal leak. A more indolent subacute presentation might be accompanied by a distinct fluid collection or abscess in the mediastinum. Transesophageal ultrasonography and fine-needle aspiration have been jointly used to diagnose a variety of periesophageal infections,[45] and this bedside technique in critically ill patients likely has improved diagnostic accuracy over standard CT imaging.

TREATMENT

Clearly, some low-grade mediastinitis must occur with any transmural disruption of the esophagus. Stable patients thought likely to have a recent disruption (hours) can have a dilute barium swallow. A *contained* esophageal disruption (usually the result of instrumentation) is manifest by extravasation of contrast that drains rather promptly back into the lumen. Such injuries may be managed successfully by serial clinical evaluation, limited oral intake, antibiotic therapy, and repeat imaging.[46] This may be particularly true in young children.[47] In patients with more frank mediastinal contamination not confined to the local perforation but identified within the first 24 hours, operation with primary repair and drainage is most often indicated.[48,49] If the time since perforation is sufficiently short and the injury sufficiently small, so that local inflammation is limited, primary repair of a disruption— preferably with viable vascularized tissue buttressing—has been successfully employed,[49] even after 24 hours.[50] Success has also been recently reported using covered self-expanding esophageal stents.[51] Image-guided nonoperative drainage with antibiotics has been successfully employed in selected cases where a defined collection or abscess can be identified.

In patients with more extensive local inflammation, those diagnosed more than 24 hours after perforation, and those who are more systemically ill, drainage with or without some esophageal diversion may be employed. A variety of procedures for upper alimentary tract diversion have been described, from simple nasogastric suction to cervical esophagostomy with gastrostomy. If the diagnosis of posterior mediastinal infection is made sufficiently early, prior to the development of sepsis, adequate local drainage and antibiotic therapy are adequate therapy. In such situations, some have advocated resection of the involved esophagus with appropriate diversion and drainage. Alimentary continuity can then be restored after recovery from the mediastinal infection.[48] Continued sepsis and multiple organ failure are the most common cause of death among these patients, and multiple operations to excise necrotic tissue and drain the space are sometimes required before definitive reconstruction.

Migratory and Chronic Mediastinal Inflammation

The mediastinum may be infected secondarily from contiguous acute infections involving adjacent anatomic spaces. Pleural or pulmonary processes may transgress the mediastinal envelope, as may infections of the spine, particularly the vertebral bodies. Mediastinitis has been reported secondary to intraabdominal processes from subdiaphragmatic abscesses[52] to retroperitoneal extension of colonic infections. Perhaps the most dramatic and well described of the migratory mediastinal infections are those that descend from the neck and known as *descending necrosing mediastinitis*. These include those infections that arise as classic Ludwig's angina (odontogenic or nonodontogenic) or from cervical puncture wounds. Gravity and the negative pressure of the thoracic cavity have been cited as reasons for this descent through the pretracheal space into the upper posterior mediastinum. The patients are often young and may have a history of a dental infection. Cervical pain, cellulitis, necrosis, and abscess formation may occur, and a high index of suspicion leading to CT imaging can be diagnostic. Broad-spectrum antibiotics are essential and must be accompanied by cervical and mediastinal drainage directed by the clinical and radiologic findings.[53,54] Drainage may be accomplished in a variety of ways including right thoracotomy, left-sided video-assisted thoracoscopy, or an anterior clamshell incision. The mortality of this condition has historically ranged from 20% to 40% and increases directly with the interval between onset of symptoms and diagnosis. Oropharyngeal cervical infections descending into the mediastinum have been successfully managed with antibiotics and a combination of percutaneous drains and/or videoscopic débridement.[52,55] In any case, aggressive imaging surveillance and a commitment to achieving and maintaining adequate drainage (multiple varied procedures) are necessary to successful management of this relatively rare life-threatening disorder.[56]

Mediastinal fibrosis is a chronic condition that may present precipitously when the process constricts a mediastinal structure compromising its lumen. Pulmonary vein, pulmonary artery,[57] vena caval,[58] and tracheal stenoses have been seen most commonly. The diagnosis is generally established by CT or magnetic resonance imaging (MRI) which reveals a diffusely infiltrating, sometimes calcified, mass. Bronchoscopy may contribute to the diagnosis.[59] The fibrosis is a benign, acellular proliferation of fibrous collagenous tissue which is idiopathic or may be an immunologic sequela of an intervention (e.g., radiofrequency ablation) or infection (mycotic, specifically and most commonly *Histoplasma*).[60,61] Treatment may include steroid therapy[62] and local dilation of stenotic lumina with stents or operation.[63]

ANNOTATED REFERENCES

Prevention of Post–Cardiac Operation Mediastinitis:

Edwards FH, Engelman RM, Houck P, Shahian DM, Bridges CR. The Society of Thoracic Surgeons practice guideline series: antibiotic prophylaxis in cardiac surgery, part I: duration. Ann Thorac Surg 2006;81: 397-404.

Engelman RM, Shahian DM, Shemin R, Guy TS, Bratzler D, Edwards F, et al. The Society of Thoracic Surgeons practice guideline series: antibiotic prophylaxis in cardiac surgery, part II: antibiotic choice. Ann Thorac Surg 2007;83:1569-76.

As post–cardiac operation mediastinitis is the most common manifestation of mediastinitis, and given that the Centers for Medicare and Medicaid Services has determined this to be "preventable" condition, these well-written evidence-based guidelines are essential reading. Indeed, in institutions where cardiac operations are performed, the local implementation of these guidelines will be, or is, a standard of care.

Management of Post–Cardiac Operation Mediastinitis:

Ennker IC, Pietrowski D, Vohringer L, Kojcici B, Albert A, Vogt PM, et al. Surgical debridement, vacuum therapy and pectoralis plasty in poststernotomy mediastinitis. J Plast Reconstr Aesthet Surg 2009;62:1479-83.

Although exploration, sternal débridement, and closure with catheters remains a viable initial technique for these patients, their management has increasingly evolved to include wound vacuum treatment for an interval prior to transposition flap coverage, or as definitive treatment of wounds involving only a segment of sternum, usually inferiorly. This article presents a recent experience that describes the role of wound vacuum therapy as central to the treatment of post–cardiac surgery sternal infections.

Management of Esophageal Perforation:

Abbas G, Schuchert MJ, Pettiford BL, Pennathur A, Landreneau J, Landreneau J, et al. Contemporaneous management of esophageal perforation. Surgery 2009;146:749-55.

Blackmon SH, Santora R, Schwarz P, Barroso A, Dunkin BJ. Utility of removable esophageal covered self-expanding metal stents for leak and fistula management. Ann Thorac Surg 2010;89:931-7.

One might correctly note that the evolution of the treatment of intrathoracic esophageal perforations has not changed much since experiences such as that described by Postlethwait in 1986. The options then, and now, included drainage, repair, diversion and resection, sometimes in combination and/or in sequence. The choice of a management strategy ever requires an assessment of the leak location, extent of infection, and patient condition. The latter two parameters are highly dependent on the timing of diagnosis, the etiology of the disruption, and the pathogen(s) involved. Landreneau's article reflects these considerations in the setting of contemporary imaging, pharmacologic, and technical options.

In contrast to the decades of drainage, repair, diversion, and resection is the more recent ability to much less invasively place a covered self-expanding stent across an area of esophageal disruption. While this affords the opportunity for some leaks to heal without further intervention (perhaps those that previously would have healed with drainage only), it also may temporize, allowing a patient to become a better candidate for any subsequent, more definitive procedure. Blackmon and colleagues describe this technique well in their paper, as well as techniques for dealing with the troubling migration of these devices after placement and prior to closure of the offending defect.

Management of Descending Necrotizing Mediastinitis:

Ridder GJ, Maier W, Kinzer S, Teszler CB, Boedeker CC, Pfeiffer J. Descending necrotizing mediastinitis: contemporary trends in etiology, diagnosis, management, and outcome. Ann Surg 2010;251:528-34.

The rarity of this life-threatening, somewhat protean malady is manifest by this large institution's presentation of 45 cases aggregated over a 12-year period. A corollary of the prior sentence is that as an unusual illness which can present variably and carries a significant risk of death, practitioners who might see such critically ill patients should have a fundamental understanding of DNM. Ridder and colleagues present perhaps the largest extant series of such patients and thus valuable information to those of us who might be confronted with one or two such patients in an entire professional career.

REFERENCES

Access the complete reference list online at http://www.expertconsult.com.

193

Epistaxis

KAREN H. CALHOUN | MINKA SCHOFIELD

Epistaxis is a nosebleed. It ranges from minor blood-tinged mucus when blowing the nose to life-threatening hemorrhage. The focus in this chapter is on prevention, diagnosis, and management of the types of epistaxis that occur commonly in an intensive care unit (ICU) setting. Almost all epistaxis occurs incidentally in patients hospitalized for other reasons, and a significant proportion of ICU nosebleeds are iatrogenic.

Anatomy and Physiology

INTERNAL NASAL ANATOMY

The interior of the nose is divided in half by the bony cartilaginous septum and its mucoperichondrial covering. The septum thus makes up the medial wall of each nasal vault. The floor of the nose is formed by the palatal bone, sloping slightly downward as it goes back. The nasal cavity roof is made up of the sphenoid bone posteriorly, the cribriform plate (ethmoid bone), and the frontal bone anteriorly. Anteroinferiorly, the nostril opens into the nasal vault. The first 8 to 10 mm of nasal lining, going posteriorly from the nostril, is hair-bearing skin. The rest of the nose is lined with respiratory mucosa. The posterior extent of the nasal vault is the choana, or posterior nasal aperture, opening into the nasopharynx.

The most complex nasal anatomy occurs on the lateral wall of each vault, with three bony protrusions, the turbinates, extending into the nasal vault. The inferior turbinate is the biggest, and the superior one, the smallest. The nasolacrimal duct opens into the nasal cavity under the inferior turbinate. The maxillary, anterior ethmoidal, and frontal sinuses drain into the ethmoidal infundibulum, which opens under the middle turbinate. Posterior ethmoidal sinus cells open into the nose under the superior turbinate, and the sphenoidal sinus opens into the nose above and behind the superior turbinate.

VASCULAR ANATOMY

Internal nasal tissue derives blood supply from both the internal and external carotid systems. The internal carotid artery supplies the anterior and posterior ethmoidal arteries via the ophthalmic artery. The external carotid artery supplies the nose via the internal maxillary artery and the facial artery. The sphenopalatine artery (branch of the internal maxillary), the superior labial artery (branch of the facial artery), and the anterior ethmoidal artery (branch of the ophthalmic artery) together supply Kiesselbach's plexus in Little's area of the anteroinferior septal mucosa. This rich vascular supply ensures plentiful bleeding when the mucosa is irritated or breached, resulting in epistaxis.

NASAL PHYSIOLOGY

The nose's primary function is conditioning inspired air and conducting this air into and out of the pharynx. In a normal nose, air is warmed, humidified, and filtered of particulate matter before reaching the nasopharynx. The nose also contains sensor cells for olfaction in the superior nasal vault and improves vocal resonance.

Healthcare Personnel Safety

The patient with epistaxis is often scared, snorting or blowing out blood in attempts to clear the nasal or pharyngeal airway. Blood droplets can be widely and forcefully scattered. Any physician or other healthcare worker caring for a patient with epistaxis must observe Universal Precautions. The caregiver should be gowned and gloved and wear eye protection and a facial mask.

Location of Bleeding

Otolaryngologists refer to nosebleeds as *anterior* or *posterior*. This is both an anatomic and a management differentiation.

Most "spontaneous" bleeding in the anterior half of the nose comes from Kiesselbach's plexus, an area easily seen with a nasal speculum and headlight. This area can be irritated by wiping the nose with a tissue, picking the nose, breathing dry or cold air, or being exposed to environmental factors such as cigarette smoke and other airborne irritants and chemicals. Most spontaneous bleeding in the posterior part of the nose originates from the sphenopalatine artery, often near the posterior end of the inferior turbinate. Iatrogenic bleeding can occur anywhere in the nose where mucosa is traumatized.[1]

Diagnosis

The basic diagnosis of epistaxis sounds easy; epistaxis is present when there is blood coming out of the nose. In the ICU setting, however, with the patient supine and often with diminished alertness, blood from a nasal source may drain under the influence of gravity back into the nasopharynx, pooling there and first being noticed as blood from the mouth. Looking in the nose and nasopharynx of patients bleeding from the mouth may lead to rapid identification of a bleeding source. After determining that bleeding is originating in the nose, the next steps in diagnosis are determining exactly where in the nose the bleeding is coming from, how much bleeding there is, and whether it is tapering off or continuing unabated.

Anterior speculum examination with a good headlight and suction usually permits identification of focal anterior bleeding. The exact site of more posterior bleeding, if intermittent or slow, can be determined with a rigid sinonasal endoscope with gentle suction and irrigation. Topical decongestant/anesthetic spray is instilled into the nose before this examination for control of bleeding and patient comfort.

Sometimes, even with the endoscope, a specific source of bleeding cannot be identified. The two most common causes of this are (1) generalized mucosal ooze in a patient with systemic coagulopathy and (2) copious bleeding that obscures visualization despite irrigation and suctioning.

Treatment

FOCAL ANTERIOR BLEEDING

For spontaneous anterior bleeding from Little's area, pinching the anterior nose firmly between the thumb and finger provides pressure that often controls the bleeding. Firm pressure is applied for 5 minutes without interruption and then is gently released. If bleeding persists, pressure should be applied for an additional 5 minutes. Pressure can be combined with a topical decongestant such as oxymetazoline or Neo-Synephrine to aid in bleeding cessation via vasoconstriction.

If there is a single identifiable anterior source such as a small laceration or varicosity, cautery with a silver nitrate stick or electrocautery may provide permanent cessation. For cautery, additional topical or injected anesthetic will make the patient more comfortable. This can be done by saturating a small cotton ball or pledget with a decongestant mixed with an anesthetic solution such as 4% lidocaine hydrochloride. The cotton ball or pledget should remain inside the anterior nasal cavity for 5 to 10 minutes. If additional anesthesia is needed, lidocaine with epinephrine (commonly 1% lidocaine in 1:200,000 epinephrine) can be injected into the mucosa under direct or endoscopic visualization without causing the patient much discomfort.

If silver nitrate cautery is used, the stick is applied directly to the oozing mucosa, cauterizing only the actively bleeding area. The mucosa touched by silver nitrate becomes black immediately. Once bleeding is well controlled, the mucosal area is gently rinsed with saline solution. If electrocautery is used, the grounding pad (if necessary with the unit) is applied to the patient and the oozing area cauterized. With both techniques, the "dose" of cautery used should be the minimum required to control bleeding, avoiding damage to nearby normal mucosa. A small piece of Gelfoam can be applied to the cauterized area. Antibiotic ointment is applied to the area twice a day for 3 to 5 days. Excessive cauterization should be avoided, since this can lead to inadvertent septal perforation.

A commercially available "pack" can also control anterior bleeding. These packs do not conform as well to the entire shape of the nasal vault in the way packing can and so may be less effective (depending on the exact site of bleeding). They are, however, quicker and easier to place than anterior packing, which is an acquired skill. Nasal tampons such as Merocel (Xomed) are generously coated with surgical lubricant then gently inserted into the nasal cavity dry and compressed. After the tampon is in place, it is expanded with saline to exert pressure on the nasal mucosa.

MIDDLE NOSE: FOCAL OR GENERALIZED OOZE

If bleeding originates slightly more posteriorly but still within the anterior zone, or if there is a generalized mucosal ooze, anterior packing can be used. The nasal cavity is firmly packed with ribbon gauze coated with petroleum jelly or BIP ointment (bismuth subnitrate, iodoform, paraffin). This approach applies pressure from inside the nose against the bleeding mucosa, much as bleeding from a facial laceration is controlled by holding pressure on the bleeding area.

Other options for controlling middle vault bleeding or generalized oozing include variations on anterior packing. The Rhino Rocket (Shippert Medical, Englewood, Colorado) is rolled polyvinyl alcohol foam on a tampon-like inserter. It unfurls when released inside the nose and has a string that remains outside, facilitating later removal. Various balloon nasal tamponades are available as well. Rapid Rhino is a pneumatic tamponade coated with a carboxymethylcellulose fabric, available in varying lengths used to control anterior and posterior epistaxis. It conforms to the nasal cavity better than compressed materials, is easy to insert and remove, and works within minutes.[2]

POSTERIOR BLEEDING: GENERALIZED OR UNIDENTIFIABLE SOURCE

The source of bleeding from the posterior half of the nose is more difficult to visualize. Direct digital pressure, which works well in the anterior nose, is not effective within the posterior bony nasal vault. So if bleeding is significant and sustained, if no nasal endoscope is available, or if blood flow obscures the endoscopic view, posterior/anterior packing is usually the first step.

Posterior bleeding cannot be controlled by anterior packing alone, because it is impossible to apply sufficient pressure. Trying to pack gauze into the posterior part of the nose is like trying to stuff a doughnut hole; as one packs more from the front, the gauze begins to fall out the back (i.e., into the nasopharynx). This is why posterior packing is used for a posterior hemorrhage.

Posterior packing provides a stable platform in the nasopharynx against which the packing inserted from anteriorly can be firmly placed. Traditionally, this is a roll of gauze placed through the mouth and guided into place in the nasopharynx by strings brought out through the nose, which then pull this pack into position and are tied around the columella.

When a patient is endotracheally intubated, firm pharyngeal packing using vaginal gauze can be used as a posterior nasal pack. Other alternatives to a posterior gauze pack include a Foley catheter and various nasal balloon devices. A Foley catheter placed transnasally into the nasopharynx and inflated can provide a similar firm nasopharyngeal platform. The commercially available balloon devices for posterior packing have an extended-length balloon or two balloons that are inflated separately, one for the nasal vault and the other for the nasopharynx.

AFTER PACKING THE NOSE

Even anterior packing of one nostril compromises nasal respiration and blocks sinus drainage into that nasal cavity. Posterior packing that obstructs both nasal cavities places patients at risk for hypoxemia. If seen as outpatients, all patients with posterior packs are admitted to the hospital for bed rest, oxygen supplementation (by face mask or face tent, not nasal cannula), hydration, and antibiotic therapy to prevent development of sinusitis or toxic shock syndrome. In the ICU setting, these supportive therapies should be provided for any patient requiring a nasal pack.

When a posterior gauze pack, Foley catheter, or other posterior packing material is secured at the anterior nares, traction on the columella or ala carries the risk of irritation and necrosis. Careful padding or devising methods of securing the packing are needed to prevent this complication. The key is spreading out the pressure over the columella or ala, rather than having a narrow string crossing these areas. Padding can be provided by folded gauzes, cotton rolls, and so forth. Alternatively, these ties can be attached to another tie that goes across the entire upper lip, over the ears, and behind the head. Umbilical clamps at the nasal openings can also be used to maintain forward pressure on the posterior packs. For a critically ill patient, to maintain pressure, one can also consider suspending the packing material to a halo device or other external fixed point (e.g., trapeze frame, ceiling, intravenous line stands).

GENERALIZED MUCOSAL OOZE

Generalized mucosal oozing is usually due to a systemic clotting problem. In the critical care setting, clotting can be deranged on the basis of a coagulopathy (e.g., secondary to leukemia, an inherited disorder, or anticoagulation medications, disseminated intravascular coagulopathy, posttransfusion coagulopathy) or a systemic illness (e.g., renal or hepatic disease). If the systemic problem is easily correctable (i.e., stopping anticoagulants), nasal packing as described earlier can be used. If, however, the coagulopathy is ongoing, nasal packing can be a self-defeating approach. Although the bleeding stops when the pack is in place, the mucosal microtrauma of pack removal reinitiates bleeding. Use of absorbable hemostatic agents (Gelfoam, Surgicel, Avitene), thrombin-containing products (Floseal, Surgiflo) or fibrin glue can be helpful.[3]

ADDITIONAL TREATMENT OPTIONS

If a bleeding point is identified but is too far posterior to cauterize at the bedside, the patient can be given general anesthesia in the operating suite. Endoscopically guided suction-cautery can be performed as far back as the choana. Sometimes infracture of the inferior turbinate is required to access a posterior bleeding point.

If bleeding is not controlled by packing, or if it recurs after packing is removed, control by arteriography and embolization or surgery is recommended.[4] Surgical options include transnasal sphenopalatine artery ligation, anterior ethmoidal artery ligation, transantral internal maxillary artery ligation, and ligation of the external carotid artery in the neck.[5] In the special case of hereditary hemorrhagic telangiectasia (Osler-Weber-Rendu syndrome), once conservative medical therapies fail, photocoagulation laser or septal mucosal dermoplasty may be required.[6]

Specific Intensive Care Unit Situations

OXYGEN BY NASAL CANNULA

Oxygen supplied by nasal cannula dries the nasal mucosa. The dried mucosa is fragile and bleeds easily. Replacing the oxygen by nasal cannula with humidified oxygen via face mask or face tent will prevent this problem.

Once bleeding has occurred in this situation, the bleeding site can usually be identified on the anterior septum with a nasal speculum and headlight. If the bleeding consists of occasional spotting without active ongoing bleeding, gentle application of petrolatum or antibiotic ointment to this area several times a day will allow the mucosa to heal. If there is active bleeding, chemical or electrical cautery is sometimes needed.

NASAL INTUBATION

The largest cross-sectional diameter in the nasal vault occurs along the floor of the nose, which goes straight back from the nares. The best angle for passing a tube through the nose is found by elevating the nasal tip and passing the tube straight back. For smaller tubes such as nasogastric tubes, lubrication is usually all that is required for smooth passage through the nose.

Nasotracheal intubation is a common cause of epistaxis. Most such bleeding is mild and self-limited. If bleeding occurs during fiberoptic nasal intubation, it can obscure the endoscopic view. Measures that enhance smooth passage of the endotracheal tube through the nose and minimize bleeding include using a topical decongestant on the nasal mucosa before tube passage, generous lubrication of the tube, and thermo-softening of the tube in warmed water. Inspection of the internal nasal passages with a speculum or endoscope allows choosing of the larger side, the one with minimal narrowing by septal deviation, septal spurs, or turbinate hypertrophy. There is some evidence that routinely using the right nostril is associated with a lesser rate of epistaxis.[7] Passage of successively larger soft nasal trumpets can assist with dilating the nasal passage (i.e., compressing the internal soft tissue) before intubation. Traumatic intubation can even result in inadvertent turbinectomy.[8] Aspirin therapy increases the risk of epistaxis occurring with nasotracheal intubation, so being particularly gentle with patients taking aspirin may save having to deal with bleeding.[9]

POSTOPERATIVE EPISTAXIS

Bleeding from the nose occurring after nasal or facial surgery must be reported immediately to the surgeon. Topical decongestants, pressure, cautery, absorbable hemostatic agents, or nasal packing may be required to control such bleeding. Occasionally the patient will need to return to the operating suite for vessel ligation.

MASSIVE FACIAL TRAUMA

The occurrence of multiple facial fractures can cause epistaxis. Usually this type of bleeding ceases with nasal packing. Occasionally a displaced fracture tents open a lacerated vessel, and fracture reduction is required to stop the bleeding. Asch and Rowe forceps are used for this reduction, and a general anesthetic is usually required.

VESSEL PROBLEMS

Rarely, massive epistaxis results from rupture of carotid aneurysms or carotid–cavernous sinus fistulas. Cerebral arteriography and embolization are required to control such bleeding.

Conclusion

Because the nose provides a major route for reaching the digestive tract and the airway, it is almost inevitable that patients hospitalized in the ICU will undergo a procedure or treatment that traumatizes the nasal airway. Measures that can minimize this trauma include gentle technique, good understanding of nasal anatomy, generous use of topical vasoconstrictors, lubricants, and humidified air, and use of the softest acceptable materials for passage through the nasal cavity.

Most epistaxis in the ICU setting is mild and responds to pressure, topical decongestants, fibrin glue, or chemical cautery. Because most ICUs are in tertiary care hospitals with medical specialists readily available, an otolaryngologist should be consulted for assistance in the diagnosis and treatment of epistaxis requiring more intervention.

KEY POINTS

1. Epistaxis ranges from a few flecks of blood in the mucus when blowing the nose to life-threatening hemorrhage.

2. In the ICU setting, with the patient supine and often with diminished alertness, blood from a nasal source may drain under the influence of gravity back into the nasopharynx, pooling there and first being noticed as blood from the mouth.

3. Most epistaxis in the ICU setting is mild and responds to pressure, topical decongestants, fibrin glue, or chemical cautery.

4. It is almost inevitable that patients hospitalized in the ICU will undergo procedures or treatments that traumatize the nasal airway. Measures that can minimize this trauma include:
   a. Gentle technique
   b. Good understanding of nasal anatomy
   c. Generous use of topical vasoconstrictors, lubricants, and humidified air
   d. Use of the softest acceptable materials for passage through the nasal cavity

ANNOTATED REFERENCES

Singer AJ, Blanda M, Cronin K, LoGuidice-Khwaja M, Gulla J, Bradshaw J, et al. Comparison of nasal tampons for the treatment of epistaxis in the emergency department: a randomized controlled trial. Ann Emerg Med 2005;45:134-9.
Both the Rapid Rhino and Rhino Rocket were effective in controlling epistaxis, but the Rapid Rhino was rated by patients as less painful at insertion and removal, rated by physicians as easier to insert, and also had a lower incidence of rebleeding after removal.
Zwank M. Middle turbinectomy as a complication of nasopharyngeal airway placement. Am J Emerg Med 2009;27:513.

A case report of epistaxis as a result of accidental middle turbinate removal during nasopharyngeal airway placement.
Soyka MB, Rufiback K, Huber A, Holzmann D. Is severe epistaxis associated with acetylsalicylic acid intake? Laryngoscope 2010;120:200-7.
"Patients on ASA showed significantly more surgical interventions [for epistaxis], a higher recurrence rate and a larger # of required treatments as well as an increased severity score."

REFERENCES

Access the complete reference list online at http://www.expertconsult.com.

194

Management of the Postoperative Cardiac Surgical Patient

SAJID SHAHUL | DANIEL TALMOR | ALAN LISBON

The first days of care for the cardiac surgery patient present multiple challenges for the intensivist. The intensive care unit (ICU) stay for most of these patients lasts for only 24 to 48 hours, but during this period, life-threatening problems such as low cardiac output (CO), arrhythmias, and coagulopathy may become apparent. After 48 hours in the ICU, the problems encountered by postoperative cardiac surgery patients tend to become more like those experienced by other groups of critically ill patients.

The Cardiac Surgery Patient in the Intensive Care Unit

HISTORY OF CARDIAC SURGERY LINKED TO THE HISTORY OF INTENSIVE CARE

The development of modern cardiac surgery has been intimately related to the development of the ICU. This relationship has worked in both directions. Until the 1950s, cardiac surgery was limited to control of traumatic injuries and the closed repair of valves. Development of the extracorporeal pump oxygenator in 1953 by Gibbon ushered in the era of open-heart surgery.[1] Heart valve replacement then became possible. Subsequently, in the 1960s, coronary artery bypass grafting (CABG) for ischemic heart disease was developed and rapidly popularized.[2]

Several studies have demonstrated that risk-adjusted mortality rates after CABG vary significantly among surgeons and hospitals and that mortality is related both to the number of surgeries performed by each surgeon and the total volume of procedures performed at the hospital.[3-5] For high-risk surgical patients, survival is also related to the characteristics of the ICU care.[6]

THE CHANGING EPIDEMIOLOGY OF CARDIAC SURGERY

Over the last decade, the population of patients treated with cardiac surgery has changed dramatically. Advances in cardiology including reperfusion therapy, angioplasty, stenting, and drug-eluting stents, have obviated the need for surgical approaches to treatment except for particularly complex problems or after failure of other less invasive modalities. In the year 2000, 561,000 patients in the United States underwent percutaneous transluminal coronary angioplasty (PTCA), an increase of 262% relative to 1987. In the same year, 314,000 patients underwent CABG. Multiyear trends, represented in Figure 194-1, show a leveling off and subsequent decrease in the overall number of patients undergoing CABG.[7] The recently developed sirolimus-coated coronary stent has been associated with even better results.[8] Studies comparing the use of stents versus CABG for left main disease have found no significant difference in rates of death or of the composite endpoint of death, Q-wave infarction, or stroke between patients receiving stents and those undergoing CABG. However, stenting, even with drug-eluting stents, was associated with higher rates of target-vessel revascularization than was CABG.[9]

Even as younger patients are being treated with interventional techniques, the elderly are increasingly referred for operation. Although these operations are successful even in most octogenarians, they are associated with increased hospital mortality and longer ICU and hospital stays. It is clear, however, that good results in terms of long-term survival and quality of life are achievable.

ALTERNATIVE TECHNIQUES FOR CARDIAC SURGERY

The increasing age of patients undergoing cardiac surgery and the relatively high incidence of adverse effects related to cardiopulmonary bypass (CPB) in these patients have led to the development of less invasive cardiac surgical techniques. These techniques are intended to decrease postoperative morbidity, reduce hospital length of stay, reduce costs, and hasten recovery of lifestyle (Table 194-1). Three major techniques have been proposed.

Minimally invasive direct coronary artery bypass (MIDCAB) differs from conventional CABG mainly in the type of incision used for access. In place of the conventional median sternotomy, access is obtained via a left or right thoracotomy, a parasternal incision, or a partial sternotomy. The proposed benefit of such an approach is the reduction in morbidity related to median sternotomy. This proposed advantage has not been demonstrated. MIDCAB grafting is a challenging technique and should be performed only in selected patients with favorable coronary anatomy. Both bare metal and drug-eluting stenting have been shown to be inferior to MIDCAB for proximal left anterior descending (LAD) coronary artery lesions, owing to higher reintervention rates with similar results in mortality and morbidity.[4,10]

Off-pump coronary artery bypass (OPCAB) is performed on a beating heart without benefit of CPB. The proposed benefit of this procedure is reduction of morbidity related to hypothermia and CPB. The procedure is undertaken using partial to full heparinization. Extubation may be achieved earlier in these patients because they do not require rewarming and are less coagulopathic. A subset of patients cannot tolerate the extent of retraction of the heart required for the surgery and need to be urgently placed on CPB. These patients may suffer ischemic myocardial injury and require support with inotropes or intraaortic balloon pumping (IABP) during the postoperative period. A retrospective study of 1398 patients showed that use of the OPCAB technique for multivessel myocardial revascularization in high-risk patients significantly reduced the incidence of perioperative myocardial infarction (MI) and other major complications, length of stay in the ICU, and mortality.[11] In a single-center non-randomized registry, the incidence of major cardiac events were similar in OPCAB versus sirolimus-eluting stents in diabetic patients with multivessel disease.[12]

A third method of minimally invasive cardiac surgery is the port-access technique. This operation entails obtaining access for CPB with the use of endovascular catheters. This allows surgery to be performed using CPB via either a left or right thoracotomy. The technique is particularly useful for mitral valve replacement through a right thoracotomy and for redo CABG (avoiding the complications associated with repeat sternotomy). The port-access technique has been shown to be safe and is associated with shorter lengths of stay, reduced transfusion requirements, fewer infections, decreased incidence of renal failure, and less atrial fibrillation when compared with conventional techniques.[13] In outcome data using propensity score analysis for mitral valve repair, minimally invasive repair had similar results to open repair. There was an increase in cross-clamp and bypass times,

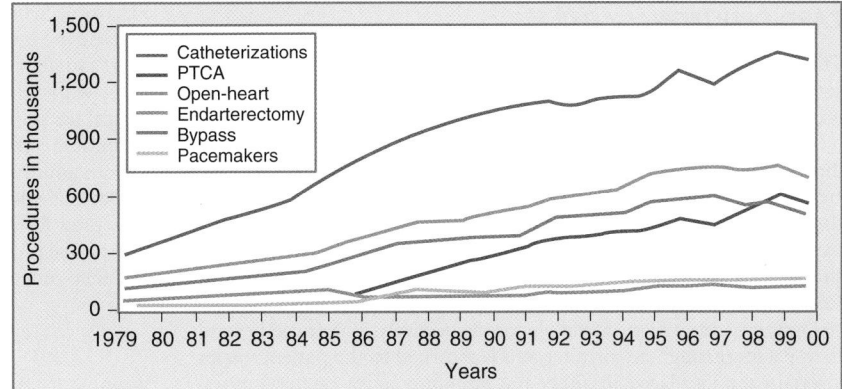

Figure 194-1 Trends in cardiovascular operations and procedures in the United States, 1979-2000. PTCA, percutaneous transluminal coronary angioplasty. *(From American Heart Association. Heart disease and stroke statistics—2003 update. Dallas, TX: AHA; 2003.)*

but early outcome was similar.[14] Widespread adoption of this technique has been limited by the technical complexity of placing the required catheters, which requires both extra time and a specially trained and skilled operative team.

The techniques of minimally invasive cardiac surgery are still evolving. The intensivist caring for cardiac surgical patients must continue to keep abreast of these new methods.

ORGANIZATION OF THE POSTOPERATIVE CARDIAC SURGERY UNIT

Optimal results from cardiac surgery require a skilled, dedicated, and multidisciplinary ICU team. Patients undergoing cardiac surgery are usually admitted to the hospital on the day of surgery. They arrive in the ICU directly from the operating room (OR). The typical patient is transferred to a step-down unit on the morning after surgery. This unit allows continued monitoring with telemetry for an additional 24 to 48 hours. Patients remaining in the ICU beyond 48 hours tend to become similar to a standard ICU population, as they develop

secondary complications such as sepsis, pneumonia, and acute respiratory distress syndrome (ARDS).

Guidelines developed by the American Heart Association and the American College of Cardiology outline the requirements for cardiac surgical ICUs.[15] These include the development of protocol-driven care, a minimum number of cardiac surgical ICU beds that is half the number of surgeries performed per week, and one-to-one nursing care during the first night in the unit. ICU coverage by a dedicated intensivist has been shown to improve outcomes in other types of major surgery and should be recommended after cardiac surgery as well.[6]

Separation from Cardiopulmonary Bypass and the End of Surgery

Successful management of the postoperative cardiac surgery patient begins by understanding what occurs in the OR. Problems encountered in the OR often persist after transfer to the ICU. An understanding of the technical and pathophysiologic aspects of CPB can help the intensivist better manage cardiac surgical patients in the ICU.

TABLE 194-1	Comparison of Minimally Invasive Cardiac Surgery Techniques			
Technique	*Incision Site*	*Cannulation Site*	*Advantages*	*Disadvantages*
Conventional	Median sternotomy	Ascending aorta	Excellent exposure	Mediastinitis
CABG		Right atrium	Stable closure Extensive experience	Slow recovery of upper-extremity function Postoperative cough limited by pain
MIDCAB	Left thoracotomy, *or* Paramedian or right thoracotomy, *or* Partial sternotomy	Ascending aorta Right atrium	Avoids median sternotomy Useful for redo procedure Hastens recovery of upper-extremity function*	Limited exposure No cost savings May require multiple incisions
Port-access	Right anterior thoracotomy, *or* Paramedian or left thoracotomy	Ascending aorta via right paramedian port Femoral vein	Avoids median sternotomy Avoids atriotomy Access to mitral valve Smaller skin incision Decreases hospital stay* Decreases atrial fibrillation incidence* Decreases transfusion* Decreases rehabilitation time*	Increased cost of equipment Contraindicated in patients with ascending aortic pathology Limited operative exposure Significant learning curve unlikely to decrease cerebral emboli
OPCAB	Median sternotomy, *or* Right or left thoracotomy, *or* Partial sternotomy	None	Avoids aortic manipulation Avoids atriotomy and CPB Normothermia Decreases atrial fibrillation incidence* Decreases transfusion* Decreases neurologic morbidity† Decreases pulmonary morbidity†	Cost of equipment Slow recovery of upper-extremity function Mediastinitis Increases intraoperative ischemia Undetermined graft longevity

*Limited supporting evidence exists.
†Proposed benefit.
CABG, coronary artery bypass grafting; CPB, cardiopulmonary bypass; MIDCAB, minimally invasive direct coronary artery bypass; OPCAB, off-pump coronary artery bypass.
Adapted from Reves JG, Hill SE, Sum-Ping ST, Booth JV, Welsby IJ. Perioperative management of the cardiac surgical patient. In: Murray MJ, Coursin DB, Pearl RG, Prough DS, editors. Critical care medicine: perioperative management. 2nd ed. Philadelphia: Lippincott Williams & Wilkins; 2002, p. 356.

CARDIOPULMONARY BYPASS

The goal of CPB is to separate the heart and lungs from the systemic circulation so that the heart can be arrested while the surgical repair is constructed. Blood is drained from the right side of the heart, either by gravity or with vacuum assistance, via a cannula in the right atrium directly or via a cannula in the femoral vein that is advanced into the right atrium. The blood is collected in a reservoir and then pumped through an oxygenator that contains a membrane where the blood is oxygenated and carbon dioxide is removed (Figure 194-2). The perfusionist controls both the fraction of inspired oxygen and the rate of oxygen flow through the circuit, thereby controlling the patient's arterial oxygen and carbon dioxide levels, respectively. The treated blood then passes through an air filter and is returned to the patient via an arterial cannula placed in either the ascending aorta or the femoral artery. The perfusionist controls the amount of flow provided to the patient (i.e., CO). Mild to moderate systemic hypothermia (28°C–34°C) is used during bypass to minimize oxygen consumption by both the body and the brain. After adequate CPB is established, an aortic cross-clamp is applied to the ascending aorta, between the aortic cannula and the heart. The interval when the cross-clamp is applied is referred to as "ischemic" time, because no blood is circulated through the heart during this period. The heart is arrested by infusion of a high-concentration potassium solution into the native coronary arteries (antegrade cardioplegia) via a cannula placed between the aortic cross-clamp and the heart. Cardioplegia may also be given "backwards," through the venous system of the myocardium (retrograde cardioplegia) via a catheter placed in the coronary sinus. Potassium is used as the arresting agent because it stops the heart from beating and minimizes myocardial oxygen consumption.

MYOCARDIAL PROTECTION

Several measures are taken to protect the heart during ischemic time, because irreversible myocardial damage may otherwise occur.

Electromechanical arrest is the most important protective measure, because the beating action of the heart accounts for about 85% of the heart's total oxygen consumption. The heart is usually cooled to about 10°C with a cold cardioplegia solution (4°C) supplemented with topical ice slush. Additionally, the left ventricle is "vented" to prevent distention, which could lead to subendocardial ischemia. Finally, various additives are included in the cardioplegia solution to minimize myocardial edema, maintain normal intramyocardial pH, and provide substrates for anaerobic metabolism. The adequacy of intraoperative myocardial protection is critical for determining the subsequent course and final outcome of the patient

SEPARATION FROM CARDIOPULMONARY BYPASS

Weaning from CPB is the process whereby cardiopulmonary function is transferred from the bypass system back to the patient's own heart and lungs. Successful separation from CPB requires that the metabolic, cardiac, and respiratory parameters are as close to normal as possible. Separation from CPB implies that the native circulation will be required to support the body's metabolic demands. The surgical team manipulates the heart rate and rhythm, preload, afterload, and myocardial contractility to achieve this goal.

In most cases, normal sinus rhythm is restored after discontinuation of cardioplegia and rewarming of the heart. Occasionally, discontinuation of cardioplegia and rewarming leads to the onset of ventricular fibrillation; in such cases, electrical defibrillation is required. Other dysrhythmias commonly encountered are atrioventricular disassociation and atrial fibrillation. An attempt should be made to convert these to sinus rhythm by pharmacologic means. Bradyarrhythmias are treated by pacing, using temporary epicardial wires placed by the surgeon after completion of the repair. A heart rate of 70 to 90 beats/min usually is optimal. Pharmacologic support of the circulation may be needed to provide appropriate afterload or systemic vascular resistance (SVR) during separation from CPB. Most patients are vasodilated to some extent, possibly as a result of a systemic inflammatory

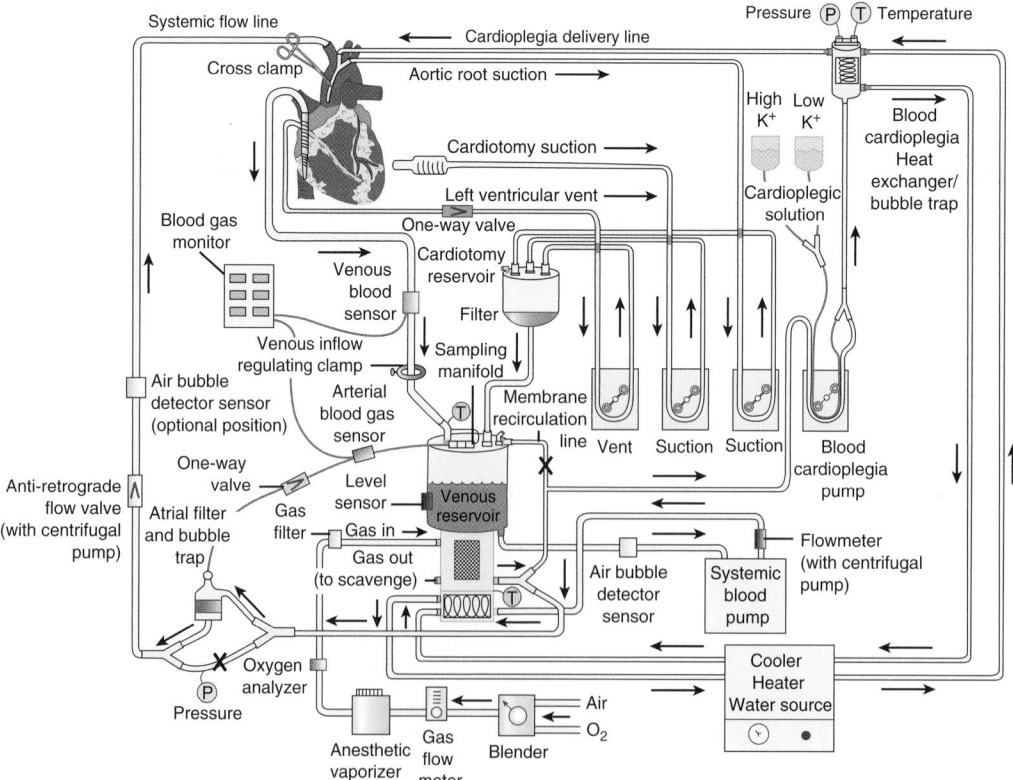

Figure 194-2   Cardiopulmonary bypass circuit. (*Adapted with permission from Gravlee GP, Davis RF, Kurusz M, Utley JR, editors. Cardiopulmonary bypass: principles and practice. 2nd ed. Baltimore: Lippincott Williams & Wilkins; 2000, p. 70.*)

response to CPB or the effects of rewarming, or both. As a consequence, infusion of a vasoconstrictor is often required. Care must be taken to strike a proper balance so that increased SVR maintains adequate arterial blood pressure without excessively increasing left ventricular afterload and compromising CO.

Most often, myocardial function is adequate, and infusion of an inotrope is not necessary. However, inotropic support often is needed for patients with a poor preoperative ventricular function or inadequate myocardial protection or revascularization during CPB. The optimal inotrope in this situation is a matter of considerable debate, and data are lacking to support a strong recommendation for a specific agent. Epinephrine, norepinephrine, dopamine, dobutamine, amrinone, and milrinone have all been used successfully. Intraoperative monitoring using transesophageal echocardiography (TEE) is particularly useful for titration of inotropic therapy.

Once all preparations for separation have been made, the perfusionist begins to wean the patient from bypass. This is done by slowly decreasing the amount of blood drained from the right atrium while simultaneously reducing flow into the aorta. Once the patient is off bypass (i.e., no blood is being drained from the right atrium into the CPB circuit), the perfusionist, at the direction of the anesthesiologist or surgeon, may continue to infuse through the aortic cannula. This maneuver allows optimization of ventricular filling or preload. Care must be taken, however, not to overdistend the heart; again, during this period, TEE is extremely useful.

REVERSAL OF ANTICOAGULATION

After weaning from CPB, protamine is given to neutralize any residual heparin. Dosing can be based on the patient's weight, the total amount of heparin given, or an assay of residual heparin activity. Institutional preference governs the technique employed, and all have been proven effective. Several adverse responses to protamine administration are possible, including histamine-induced systemic hypotension, immunoglobulin E–mediated allergic reactions, and complement-mediated catastrophic pulmonary hypertension.

TRANSPORT AND ADMISSION TO THE INTENSIVE CARE UNIT

After chest closure, confirmation of hemodynamic stability, and adequate medical and surgical hemostasis, the patient may be transferred to the ICU. Transport of a critically ill patient is a potentially dangerous process and requires extreme vigilance. Transport between the operating room and the ICU should be done with the same degree of monitoring as would be available at either end. This usually includes continuous monitoring of arterial blood pressure, pulmonary artery pressure and/or central venous pressure (CVP), electrocardiogram (ECG), and pulse oximetry. The transport bed should be equipped with a full oxygen tank, Ambu bag and mask, intubation equipment, resuscitation drugs, and a defibrillator. Care must be taken to ensure that infusions of vasoactive drugs are not interrupted.

On arrival in the ICU, the ICU team assumes care of the patient. A detailed sign-out from the operative team ensures continuity of care. The sign-out should include a detailed history including an assessment of preoperative cardiac functional status, a list of preoperative medications, and a detailed description of the surgery. Key facts are the type of repair performed, target vessels (if the patient has undergone CABG), duration of CPB and cross-clamping, difficulties encountered in separation from CPB, presence of abnormal bleeding, and postoperative assessment of cardiac function. All treatments administered in the OR should be detailed—in particular, fluids, blood products, and vasoactive drugs.

Once care has been handed over to the ICU team, a thorough examination of the patient should immediately follow. This examination should include verification of endotracheal tube placement, type and position of arterial or central venous lines, chest tube position and patency, and the presence and location of any epicardial pacing wires.

Monitoring the Postoperative Cardiac Surgery Patient

HEMODYNAMIC MONITORING

All patients admitted to the ICU after cardiac surgery will have their blood pressure continuously monitored using an intraarterial line. This is usually placed in either a radial or femoral artery. Accuracy of the measurements depends on strict attention to calibration, leveling, and removal of air from the tubing. After CPB, femoral arterial pressure may more accurately reflect central aortic pressures,[16] but this problem has usually resolved by the time the patient arrives in the ICU. If the radial artery is cannulated, the hand should be examined for signs of ischemia.[17] Vascular complications of femoral arterial lines are extremely rare, but femoral catheters may be associated with an increased incidence of infection.[18]

Central venous access is required in all patients for drug administration and hemodynamic monitoring. In the low-risk patient, a CVP catheter may be all that is needed, particularly if echocardiography is available as a backup. Pulmonary artery catheters have the advantage of allowing measurement of pulmonary artery occlusion pressure (PAOP), thermodilution, and CO, as well as sampling of the mixed venous blood saturation (Svo$_2$). Use of the pulmonary artery catheter remains controversial. Improved outcome due to use of a pulmonary artery catheter for monitoring of cardiac surgical patients has not been demonstrated.[19] Some studies showed an increased risk of death or adverse outcome when treatment was guided by the use of a pulmonary artery catheter.[20,21] However, many of these studies have been criticized on methodological grounds, and use of the catheter in cardiac surgery remains widespread.[22] Current guidelines recommend use of the pulmonary artery catheter in high-risk patients undergoing surgery in an appropriate practice setting.[23] Such a setting is one in which the physician and nursing staff are familiar with the catheter and trained to properly interpret the information obtained. If echocardiography is readily available, it is possible to manage even high-risk patients using a CVP catheter.

ELECTROCARDIOGRAPHY

On admission to the ICU, the patient is connected to a continuous ECG monitor, and a formal 12-lead ECG is obtained. The cardiogram is examined for rate, rhythm, QRS complex morphology, and signs of myocardial ischemia. For patients who are being paced postoperatively, the type of pacing and the degree of capture should be assessed.

Continuous ECG monitoring allows detection of arrhythmias. If an arrhythmia is detected, a 12-lead ECG should be obtained, and serum electrolyte concentrations should be measured. Treatment of arrhythmias should be carried out using established protocols.[24] If a malignant arrhythmia occurs, myocardial ischemia should be considered as a possible precipitating cause.

Monitoring of trends in ST-segment elevation or depression allows early detection of postoperative myocardial ischemia. Although transient ST-segment changes are relatively common and of unclear significance, persistent changes should be investigated by obtaining a 12-lead ECG and measuring circulating levels of creatine kinase myocardial band (CK-MB), troponin-T, or troponin-I.[25,26] If ischemia is strongly suspected, then echocardiography followed by coronary angiography should be considered. Findings from these studies may indicate the need for further coronary revascularization.

CHEST RADIOGRAPHY

The postoperative chest radiograph should be systematically evaluated. Proper placement of the endotracheal tube and any central lines inserted should be confirmed. If a pulmonary artery catheter is place, the location of its tip should be noted and adjusted as needed. The lung fields should be examined for the presence of pneumothorax or collapse. Additional air may be noted as subcutaneous emphysema or as pneumopericardium, although these findings are of little clinical significance. Further examination of the lung fields commonly shows small areas of atelectasis and pleural effusion. The cardiac silhouette is often enlarged after surgery as a result of myocardial edema and accumulation of fluid in the open pericardial sac. Increasing size of the cardiac silhouette or pleural effusions on serial chest radiographs may be evidence of ongoing mediastinal bleeding.

ECHOCARDIOGRAPHY IN THE INTENSIVE CARE UNIT

Echocardiography is an excellent tool for evaluating chamber size and function and the adequacy of valve repair or replacement. Indications include postoperative assessment of left ventricular function, assessment of unexplained sudden hemodynamic deterioration, evaluation to rule out pericardial tamponade, and workup of new cardiac ischemia. Limitations to transthoracic echocardiography (TTE) include inadequate windows early after operation due to air and edema in the soft tissues and wound dressings.

TEE is being used as a tool to facilitate decision making in the management of critically ill patients, including cardiac surgical patients. In the cardiac surgical ICU, this modality may have a particularly high yield when it is used to establish the cause of postoperative hypotension.[27] In one large series, a new diagnosis was established or an important pathology was excluded in 45% of TEE examinations performed in the ICU. Pericardial tamponade was diagnosed in 34 cases (11%) and excluded in 36 cases (12%). Other diagnoses included severe left ventricular failure and presence of large pleural effusions. The results of TEE had an impact on therapy in 220 cases (73%) by leading to a change of pharmacologic treatment and/or fluid administration, reoperation, or a decision that reoperation was unnecessary.[28]

▧ Clinical Manifestations of the Postbypass Period

THE NORMAL COURSE

Patients are typically admitted to the ICU intubated and ventilated. Sedation with a short-acting agent, typically propofol, is continued until the patient is ready for extubation. Once hemodynamic stability is ascertained and chest tube drainage is judged to be under control, the patient is allowed to awaken. There is no need for prolonged weaning from mechanical ventilation. A short trial of spontaneous ventilation is sufficient to determine whether respiration will be adequate without mechanical support. The rapid shallow breathing index (RSBI) has been shown to be a sensitive way to assess the likelihood of successful extubation.[29] The RSBI is calculated by dividing the respiratory rate (in breaths per minute) by the tidal volume (in liters). A value of lower than 105 predicts successful extubation. Chest tubes are commonly removed on the first postoperative day. The pulmonary artery catheter, if present, is discontinued, and the patient may be transferred to a step-down unit.

Fast-tracking of cardiac surgical patients refers to a comprehensive program designed to reduce both length of stay and hospital costs.[30,31] As a part of this program, multiple anesthetic techniques designed to allow earlier postoperative extubation have been proposed, studied, and shown to be safe. These techniques may allow extubation in the OR.[32] The key to proper use of this technique is patient selection. Although the criteria are expanding, patients with unstable angina or a high degree of congestive heart failure are generally not appropriate candidates for fast-tracking. In a retrospective review comparing 4020 patients undergoing cardiac surgery with a conventional anesthetic versus 3969 patients with a fast-track anesthetic, the fast-track group had shorter extubation times, shorter ICU or PACU stays, and a lower incidence of low cardiac output syndrome.

LOW CARDIAC OUTPUT

Low CO is the most common problem encountered in the postoperative cardiac surgical patient. A hallmark of low CO is low blood pressure. However, a patient may have a low CO with tissue hypoperfusion and still maintain what appears to be an adequate blood pressure. In the postoperative state, the physician must continuously examine and monitor the patient for signs of hypoperfusion. Physical signs of inadequate tissue perfusion include altered mental status; cool, pale, or even cyanotic extremities; diaphoresis; and low urine output. Global measures of hypoperfusion include increasing base deficit, elevated blood lactate concentration, and decreased Svo_2. Although the clinician must consider CO in terms of adequacy of perfusion, blood pressure per se is still important. Both the brain and kidneys depend on adequate blood pressure to maintain tissue perfusion. Additionally, coronary artery blood flow is dependent on a diastolic blood pressure, a key determinant of coronary artery perfusion pressure.

When assessing a patient with hypotension or signs of hypoperfusion, it is useful to consider the problem in relation to the components of CO; namely, preload, contractility, afterload, and rate and rhythm.

Preload

Preload refers to the stretch of the left ventricle at the end of diastole and is determined by the extent of ventricular filling during diastole. Adequate filling is required to ensure ejection in the subsequent systole. The most common cause of inadequate preload in postoperative patients is hypovolemia. Intravascular volume status should be continually monitored by assessing changes over time with respect to physical examination, chest tube output, and filling pressures (CVP, PAOP, or pulmonary artery diastolic pressure). Because none of the clinically measured filling pressures correlates perfectly with actual ventricular preload (i.e., end-diastolic volume), and correlation is particularly poor when the heart is diseased, it is often useful to obtain a "snapshot" of ventricular filling using echocardiography. By this means, it is possible to assess the relationship between measured filling pressures and actual preload in a specific patient. Preoperative catheterization data also can be helpful for determining this relationship. Hypovolemia should be treated with fluid replacement. Crystalloids are generally used. Surprisingly, there is no generally accepted hemoglobin concentration or hematocrit that should be used as a trigger for ordering transfusion of packed red blood cells. Red cell transfusion has been associated with early morbidity as well as long-term adverse sequelae.

In some cases, low preload is not caused by absolute hypovolemia but by relative or distributional hypovolemia. CPB and subsequent rewarming may lead to vasodilatation and a subsequent hypotension. Intravascular volume expansion may be required to maintain perfusion. An acceptable alternative is administration of a low dose of vasopressor such as phenylephrine or norepinephrine to maintain an adequate perfusion pressure. Recently, vasopressin in doses between 0.01 and 0.1 units/min has been demonstrated to be effective in this situation.[33,34] Vasodilatation is usually a transient problem that resolves during the first several hours after separation from CPB. Continued vasodilatation after this period should prompt a search for another cause, particularly infection.

Pump Failure

Either or both ventricles may fail postoperatively. Decreased myocardial contractility may be caused by impaired preoperative function, inadequate revascularization at surgery, post-CPB reperfusion injury, or perioperative myocardial ischemia or MI. The incidence of infarction is approximately 5% in large series.[35] Preoperative myocardial function and the adequacy of revascularization at surgery should be clear from the history. Determination of circulating levels of CK-MB or troponin postoperatively can provide evidence of perioperative ischemia or infarction.[25,26] Often, diminished contractility after operation is caused by inadequate myocardial protection during surgery. Decreased myocardial contractility secondary to inadequate myocardial protection usually resolves within the first 24 hours postoperatively. ECG changes are nonspecific.

Persistent new myocardial dysfunction associated with ECG changes and echocardiographic evidence of new wall-motion abnormalities should raise suspicion that the problem is an occluded graft and MI. Measurements of CK-MB in serum are of limited usefulness because levels of this enzyme are commonly elevated after surgery due to manipulation of the heart and incision of the atria, structures that are rich in the enzyme. If CK-MB levels are very high, greater than 80 mg/dL, then perioperative MI is likely.[36] Cardiac troponins are more specific for the diagnosis of perioperative infarction. A comparison of CK-MB, troponin-T, and troponin-I showed that a troponin-I level of greater than 5 μg/L was the most accurate indicator of MI, being superior to either troponin-T or CK-MB.[37] Elevated serum concentrations of troponin-I are associated with a cardiac cause of death and with major postoperative complications.[38] In addition, troponin-T concentrations measured after surgery are an independent predictor of in-hospital death after cardiac surgery.[26] If ischemia or MI is diagnosed, the patient may be taken for angiography or re-exploration and revascularization.

Postoperative valvular insufficiency can occur not only in patients with preexisting valvular lesions but also as a result of injury during surgery. The mitral valve is most commonly affected. Ischemia of the papillary muscles due to inadequate myocardial protection or perioperative MI can lead to acute mitral regurgitation in the postoperative period. Diagnosis is often made by TEE in the OR, but inadequate CO and a new systolic murmur should prompt echocardiographic evaluation.

Rate and Rhythm

CO is the product of heart rate (HR) times stroke volume (SV). Many dysrhythmias can adversely affect CO. If HR is too low, CO can be compromised. If HR is too fast, ventricular filling during diastole can be impaired, decreasing CO. Rhythm disturbances are common after cardiac surgery and may be divided into bradyarrhythmias and tachyarrhythmias; these categories are further divided into atrial and ventricular arrhythmias.

Bradycardia can lead to ventricular distention, increasing wall tension, and decreasing coronary perfusion pressure, factors that can promote development of ischemia and failure. HR of 80 to 90 appears to be optimal, allowing adequate filling and preventing overdistention but not causing rate-related ischemia. Bradycardia can be corrected by pacing. In general, epicardial pacing wires are left in place after chest closure and are attached to an external pacemaker in the immediate postoperative period. If the dysrhythmia is sinus bradycardia, atrial pacing is usually optimal. The second most common cause of bradyarrhythmia after cardiac surgery is atrioventricular dissociation. The combination of atrial and ventricular leads allows atrioventricular pacing for management of disassociation. Synchronization of the atrioventricular interval between 0.1 and 0.225 second optimizes CO.[39]

Atrial fibrillation is the most common tachyarrhythmia. It occurs in 10% to 35% of patients after cardiac surgery, usually on the second or third postoperative day. Postoperative atrial fibrillation is associated with increased morbidity and mortality and with longer, more expensive hospital stays.[40] The Multicenter Study of Perioperative Ischemia (McSPI) group examined 2417 patients undergoing CABG with or without concurrent valvular surgery.[41] The overall incidence of postoperative atrial fibrillation was 27%. Independent predictors of postoperative atrial fibrillation included advanced age, male sex, a past history of atrial fibrillation, a past history of congestive heart failure, and a pre-CPB heart rate greater than 100 beats/min. Surgical practices such as pulmonary vein venting, bicaval venous cannulation, postoperative atrial pacing, and longer cross-clamp times also were identified as independent predictors of postoperative atrial fibrillation. Patients who developed postoperative atrial fibrillation had longer lengths of stay, both in the ICU and in the ward, compared with patients who did not develop the complication.

Although premature ventricular contractions (PVCs) are common, sustained ventricular arrhythmias are far less frequent. Severe ventricular arrhythmias occurring after cardiac surgery are related to ischemia, hypoxemia, hypovolemia, electrolyte abnormalities, the effects of vasoactive drugs, or an underlying preexisting cardiomyopathy.[42] In a series of 2100 cardiac operations, only 16 patients (0.8%) developed ventricular fibrillation or a sustained ventricular tachycardia during the interval from 3 days to 3 weeks after surgery. Ten of these patients had undergone valve surgery.[43] Prognosis in these patients is dependent on the preoperative ventricular prognosis; it is excellent in those with good function. In those with a left ventricular ejection fraction of less than 40%, the mortality rate may be as high as 75%.[44]

Afterload

Ventricular afterload is the impedance to ventricular ejection during systole. Hypertension develops in as many as 60% of patients after surgery. Increased arterial blood pressure occurs even among patients without a preoperative history of hypertension. Predisposing factors include hypoxemia, hypercapnia, inadequate rewarming, pain, fluid overload, and increased sympathetic tone. Perioperative discontinuation of β-adrenergic blockers also may contribute to the development of postoperative hypertension.

Hypertension and increased afterload can lead to myocardial ischemia by augmenting ventricular stroke work. Additionally, hypertension may lead to bleeding from surgical sites, aortic dissection, and increased risk of stroke.

Tamponade

Tamponade refers to the hemodynamic consequences of a collection of blood or other fluid in the pericardial sac. In postsurgical patients, the presentation of tamponade may be subtle and differ significantly from classic descriptions. Equilibration of filling pressures typically is not seen. More commonly, patients present with isolated elevation of right atrial pressure due to compression of the right atrium and superior vena cava. After cardiac surgery, as many as 66% of pericardial fluid collections are loculated posterior effusions.[45]

Bleeding from the atrial cannulation site is a common cause of tamponade. As the pressure on the right atrium increases, ventricular filling is impaired, and CO decreases. Diagnosis of tamponade is made difficult by the high overall frequency of pericardial effusions after surgery. Echocardiographic studies have shown that moderate effusions are present in 30% of patients on the eighth postoperative day, with 2% of patients having large effusions.[46]

Diagnosis of tamponade in the postoperative patient requires a high index of suspicion and prompt intervention. Any hemodynamic instability should be assessed for tamponade. Low CO, hypotension, and tachycardia accompanied by an elevation of the left, the right, or both atrial pressures should lead to a prompt echocardiogram. Other signs that may be present include a widened mediastinum on chest radiography, dysrhythmias, and decreased ECG voltage. Because of the influence of positive pressure ventilation, the classic sign of pulsus paradoxus may not be present.

If time permits, the diagnosis of tamponade can be confirmed with the use of echocardiography. Although effusions are common, signs of compression or collapse of either atrium or of the right ventricle are diagnostic.[47-49] It is important to remember that the diagnosis may be made on clinical suspicion alone, and that treatment should not be withheld to await confirmation. Once tamponade is diagnosed, volume transfusion may temporize the situation. Pericardiocentesis is not effective in this situation, and prompt re-exploration for hemostasis and evacuation of clot is indicated.

RESPIRATORY COMPLICATIONS

Patients undergoing cardiac surgery are at risk for multiple pulmonary complications. These include pneumothorax and pleural effusion in the immediate postoperative period. After the first 24 hours, patients sometimes develop acute lung injury (ALI), ARDS, or pneumonia.

Diaphragmatic dysfunction secondary to phrenic nerve injury can occur.

Residual pneumothorax is often seen on the initial postoperative chest radiograph. The pneumothorax is commonly on the left side, and it is a result of opening the left parietal pleura during dissection of the left internal mammary artery. The pneumothorax usually resolves spontaneously as the chest tubes are placed on suction. Occasionally, a pneumothorax is seen on the right side as a result of accidental incision of the right parietal pleura. Right pneumothorax can progress to tension pneumothorax and significant hemodynamic deterioration. This diagnosis should be considered in any unstable patient. Treatment consists of insertion of an additional chest tube.

Pleural effusion in the first 24 hours after cardiac surgery should raise the suspicion of hemothorax. Effusions should be watched carefully for expansion and correlated with other signs and symptoms of continued bleeding. Massive, expanding hemothorax is an indication for re-exploration and hemostasis. Pleural effusion after the first 24 hours is generally a benign process. Most pleural effusions resolve spontaneously. Thoracocentesis should be performed only if the effusion occupies more than 50% of the lung field on radiography or if the patient has significant impairment of respiratory function.

ALI and ARDS are rare complications after cardiac surgery, CPB, and blood transfusion. In one retrospective study of 3278 cardiac surgical patients, only 13 (0.4%) developed ARDS during the postoperative period. The mortality rate associated with this complication was 15%. Another study reported a much higher mortality rate (70%).[50] The patients who developed ARDS were more likely than their matched controls to have had previous cardiac surgery. During the postoperative period, patients with ARDS received more blood products and developed shock more frequently than patients without ARDS.[51]

Nosocomial pneumonia can complicate any ICU stay. Patients who require mechanical ventilation for longer than 48 hours are at particular risk. These pneumonias are usually caused by aspiration of oral or gastric secretions into the lungs. The incidence of nosocomial pneumonia can be reduced by diligent mouth care to prevent pooling of secretions and elevation of the head of the bed to greater than 30 degrees. Nosocomial pneumonia carries a mortality rate of 24% to 50% and warrants appropriate broad-spectrum antimicrobial chemotherapy.[52] The antibiotic prescription can be tailored once the results of sputum cultures are available.

Diaphragmatic dysfunction is usually caused by cold-induced injury of the phrenic nerve due to application of ice slush to the heart as part of the cardioplegia regimen. This complication occurs in up to 2% of patients undergoing cardiac surgery with topical hypothermia; more rarely, it can occur even if topical cooling was not applied.[53,54] While the patient is being ventilated with positive pressure, this injury will not be apparent. If preoperative pulmonary function was normal, unilateral diaphragmatic paralysis usually is well tolerated. Pulmonary function can be severely compromised, however, if pulmonary problems were present preoperatively or, in rare instances, if bilateral diaphragmatic injury occurs.[55] These patients are at increased risk for development of nosocomial pneumonia, failure to wean from the ventilator, and death. Diaphragmatic dysfunction usually resolves spontaneously within 3 to 4 months.

CONTINUED BLEEDING

Continued bleeding is a common problem and requires immediate and aggressive management before the onset of further complications. The reasons for continued bleeding are often multifactorial and include inadequate surgical hemostasis, platelet dysfunction, coagulopathy, and inadequate heparin reversal. Often these factors occur in combination. Patients undergoing valve replacement are at increased risk.[56]

Multiple clotting abnormalities are possible, most of which result either directly or indirectly from the use of CPB.[57] The tubing, blood reservoir, and oxygenator membrane are all foreign surfaces that can activate the clotting cascade. Because the pump must be primed with either normal saline or lactated Ringer's solution, the priming process leads to substantial dilution of all blood components including red cells, platelets, and clotting factors. After CPB, the platelet count is decreased, and the remaining platelets are functionally deranged.[58,59] There is sequestration of platelets in the liver, spleen, and in the CPB circuit itself. Systemic fibrinolysis due to activation of this system by the CPB circuit occurs.

Inadequate reversal of heparin should be diagnosed at the bedside by the activated coagulation test (ACT) or by measurement of the activated partial thromboplastin time (APTT). Because the half-life of heparin is longer than that of protamine, heparin-induced anticoagulation can rebound in the immediate postoperative period. The treatment is administration of additional protamine.

RENAL DYSFUNCTION

Mild renal dysfunction is a common postoperative event. One multicenter study demonstrated significant worsening of renal function in 7% of patients undergoing myocardial revascularization.[60] Approximately 1% of patients with postoperative acute renal failure (ARF) require renal replacement therapy. These patients have increased morbidity and mortality. Development of ARF can prolong ICU length of stay as much as fivefold.[60]

A multicenter study of 2222 patients undergoing CABG identified five independent preoperative predictors of renal dysfunction: age 70 to 79 years or age 80 to 95 years, congestive heart failure, previous myocardial revascularization, type 1 diabetes mellitus, or preoperative serum glucose levels exceeding 300 mg/dL and preoperative serum creatinine levels of 1.4 to 2.0 mg/dL. Independent perioperative factors that exacerbated risk were CPB lasting 3 hours or longer and various measures of ventricular dysfunction.[60] The predominant predisposing factor appears to be low CO. This factor may be exacerbated by concurrent use of vasopressors such as phenylephrine.[61]

Renal dysfunction tends to follow one of three main patterns.[62] Abbreviated ARF is a transient event, most probably related to intraoperative renal ischemia. The serum creatinine concentration can be expected to peak on day 4 after surgery. Overt ARF occurs when the duration of the predisposing insult, usually low CO, is longer. The serum creatinine concentration peaks at a higher level than with abbreviated ARF and then decreases over a period of several weeks. Protracted ARF occurs when a second insult, commonly sepsis or hypotension, is superimposed on the resolving renal function. This event triggers a further, often irreversible, decrease in renal function.

NEUROLOGIC COMPLICATIONS

Neurologic sequelae of CPB range from subtle neurocognitive deficits (appearing in up to 80% of patients) to stroke. In order to estimate the relative risks of neurologic sequelae associated with various clinical factors, a logistic regression model was applied to prospectively collected data from 273 patients enrolled at 24 American medical centers.[63] Adverse cerebral outcomes occurred in 16% of patients and were almost equally divided between type I outcomes (8.4%; 5 cerebral deaths, 16 nonfatal strokes, and 2 new transient ischemic attacks) and type II outcomes (7.3%; 17 new cases of intellectual deterioration persisting at hospital discharge and 3 cases of newly diagnosed seizure disorder). Resource utilization for these patients was significantly increased; median ICU stay was prolonged from 3 days to 6 to 8 days. Total duration of hospitalization was increased by 50% (type II, $P = .04$) to 100% (type I, $P < .001$). After discharge from the acute care setting, specialized care was required for 69% of the patients with adverse neurologic sequelae. Risk factors for type I outcomes related primarily to embolic phenomena including proximal aortic atherosclerosis, intracardiac thrombus, and intermittent clamping of the aorta during surgery. Risk factors for type II outcomes included, in addition to these factors, a preoperative history of endocarditis, alcohol abuse, perioperative dysrhythmia, poorly controlled hypertension, and low CO after CPB.

GASTROINTESTINAL COMPLICATIONS

Acute abdominal complications are relatively rare after cardiac surgery. If they do occur, they are associated with extremely high rates of morbidity and mortality. One prospective study of 1116 patients undergoing CPB found that abdominal complications occurred in 23 (2.1%). Ten of these patients underwent subsequent abdominal surgery, and 20 died. Early complications occurred on postoperative days 6 and 7 and consisted of bowel ischemia or hepatic failure. These complications are probably related to perioperative hypotension and low CO.[64] Late complications consisted of pseudomembranous colitis, cholecystitis, pancreatitis, and rupture of a septic spleen.[65]

Mild transient increases in circulating levels of hepatocellular enzymes are common after surgery. These changes are generally of no consequence; however, increased serum transaminase levels, if sustained or very high (e.g., serum alanine aminotransferase concentration greater than 500 IU/L), may represent evidence of severe ischemic injury of the liver. Severe ischemic liver injury after cardiac surgery carries a high mortality and is strongly associated with low CO and increased filling pressures, suggesting that liver ischemia is induced by a combination of decreased perfusion and congestion.[66]

⬛ Management of Common Postoperative Problems

OPTIMIZATION OF CARDIAC OUTPUT

Treatment of hypotension and low CO must be tailored to the cause. Again, it is useful to consider treatment in terms of preload, contractility, afterload, and rate and rhythm. Inadequate filling pressures are treated with volume infusion. The intravascular volume expander may be a crystalloid solution, a colloid solution, or packed red blood cells if hematocrit is low or there is evidence of ongoing bleeding. It is important to remember that inotropic therapy is ineffective and possibly detrimental if adequate blood volume is not restored.

If CO or blood pressure remains low despite intravascular volume resuscitation, then it is necessary to institute inotropic or vasopressor support. No single agent is optimal in all cases. Rather, selection of the agent should be based on the suspected cause of low CO or hypotension and knowledge of the pharmacologic effects of the various inotropic and vasopressor drugs that are available (Table 194-2). If the primary cause of hypotension appears to be vasodilatation, administration of a vasoconstrictor (e.g., phenylephrine, norepinephrine, vasopressin) is indicated. If hypotension is related to inadequate ventricular ejection, then inotropic therapy with a β-adrenergic agent should be instituted. Epinephrine, norepinephrine, dopamine, and dobutamine are all reasonable choices. In patients with chronic systolic dysfunction, response to these agents may be impaired. Chronically elevated levels of circulating catecholamines deplete myocardial norepinephrine stores and down-regulate expression of myocardial β-adrenergic receptors. In these patients, tachyphylaxis to β-adrenergic agonists can develop rapidly. Addition of a phosphodiesterase inhibitor such as amrinone or milrinone is often effective in these patients.[67,68] In all cases, agents should be titrated to achieve adequate perfusion.

TABLE 194-2	Comparison of Relative Activity of Available Vasoactive Agents				
Agent	α_1	β_1	β_2	**Phosphodiesterase Inhibition**	**Dose ($\mu g/kg/min$)**
Epinephrine	++	+++	+	−	0.02-0.15
Norepinephrine	++++	+++	+	−	0.02-0.2
Dopamine	++	++	+	−	2-20
Dobutamine	+	+++	+	−	2-20
Phenylephrine	+++	−	−	−	0.3-5
Milrinone	−	−	−	+++	0.35-0.75

−, no activity; +, mild activity; ++, moderate activity; +++, strong activity.

MECHANICAL SUPPORT OF THE CIRCULATION

Failure to respond to appropriate inotropic therapy may necessitate mechanical support of the circulation. IABP is the most commonly used method. The balloon is positioned in the aorta just distal to the take-off of the left common carotid artery. Inflation of the balloon during diastole increases diastolic pressure, thereby increasing coronary perfusion pressure. Deflation during systole decreases left ventricular afterload. This combination of hemodynamic effects ameliorates myocardial ischemia and improves CO.

Ventricular assist devices (VADs) are more effective than IABP for maintaining CO. Either the left ventricle, the right ventricle, or both can be supported with VADs. Currently, VADs may be used either as a bridge to transplantation or as a bridge to recovery. Either situation assumes that the VAD is a time-limited intervention. There are some data to support the view that resting the heart through the use of a VAD can allow some recovery of acutely injured myocytes, permitting eventual withdrawal of mechanical support. One case series showed that when VAD was used as a bridge to recovery, 66% of patients were eventually able to wean from support and be discharged home.[69] If the heart is chronically diseased, there is little hope of recovery, and the VAD serves to support the patient until transplantation becomes possible.[69,70]

Ongoing clinical trials are investigating the use of VADs as definitive therapy rather than as a bridge to transplantation. Implantation of these devices may increase the long-term survival of patients with end-stage heart failure.[71]

CORRECTION OF ARRHYTHMIAS

Atrial fibrillation is the most commonly encountered arrhythmia after cardiac surgery. Prophylactic use of β-adrenergic blockers reduces the incidence of postoperative atrial fibrillation, and they should be administered after cardiac surgery to all patients unless specific contraindications are present.[72] Prophylactic treatment with amiodarone and atrial overdrive pacing should be considered for patients who are at high risk for postoperative atrial fibrillation (e.g., those with a history of previous atrial fibrillation or mitral valve surgery).[40,73]

If atrial fibrillation develops after cardiac surgery, the intensivist needs to determine whether the primary strategy should be to control the ventricular rate or to restore normal sinus rhythm. If atrial fibrillation is associated with hemodynamic instability or anticoagulation is contraindicated, rhythm management using electrical cardioversion or amiodarone is preferred.[74,75] Overdrive pacing using atrial pacing wires also can be effective. The appropriate strategy for most stable patients may be control of ventricular rate, because most will spontaneously revert to sinus rhythm within 8 weeks after discharge.[76,77] Appropriate agents to achieve ventricular rate control include intravenous or oral β-adrenergic blockers or calcium channel blockers. All patients with atrial fibrillation persisting for longer than 24 to 48 hours should be anticoagulated unless there is a specific contraindication. Long-term outcomes are similar regardless of whether the rate-control strategy or the rhythm-control strategy is selected.[78,79]

Postoperative ventricular arrhythmias should be treated immediately according to current Advanced Cardiac Life Support (ACLS) protocols.[24] Any postoperative ventricular arrhythmia should prompt a search for an underlying cause. Importantly, ischemia should be ruled out. Patients with sustained ventricular arrhythmias should undergo electrophysiologic testing before long-term antiarrhythmic therapy is instituted. The implantable cardioverter-defibrillator (ICD) device has been shown to be superior to drug therapy for patients with hemodynamically significant arrhythmias.[80]

HYPERTENSION IN THE POSTOPERATIVE PERIOD

Hypertension leading to an increase in ventricular afterload is a common cause of decreased CO. Hypertension can be controlled by an intravenous infusion of sodium nitroprusside, nitroglycerin, β-adrenergic antagonists, or calcium channel blockers. These agents should augment CO by reducing blood pressure and afterload in the hypertensive patient. Frequently, acute hypertension resolves within 24 to 48 hours postoperatively. If hypertension persists beyond this initial period of recovery, intravenous agents should be weaned and oral therapy initiated. Both β-adrenergic blockers and angiotensin-converting enzyme (ACE) inhibitors have been shown to confer a long-term mortality benefit and should be started. If hypertension was not a problem preoperatively, prolonged antihypertensive therapy postoperatively usually will not be necessary.

CORRECTION OF COAGULOPATHY

Postoperative coagulopathy can promote bleeding and accumulation of blood in the chest or pericardial cavity. Aggressive measures must be used to correct the coagulopathy. A systemic approach to the evaluation and treatment of continued bleeding is needed; one such approach is outlined in Table 194-3. Hypothermia can contribute to coagulopathy. Therefore, profoundly hypothermic ICU patients must be actively rewarmed with the use of a warm air device. Laboratory evaluation of suspected coagulopathy should include measurements of platelet count, prothrombin time (PT), APTT, ACT, and bleeding time.

POSTOPERATIVE BLEEDING

Bleeding that continues after correction of coagulopathy needs to be aggressively treated. Venous bleeding in the chest can be partially controlled by application of positive end-expiratory pressure (PEEP).[81,82]

Continuing mediastinal hemorrhage, or the suspicion of cardiac tamponade, is an indication for immediate re-exploration. Exsanguinating hemorrhage or impending arrest from tamponade may require that re-exploration be carried out at the bedside in the ICU. Bleeding that is unresponsive to medical therapy and requires re-exploration is usually associated with a surgical source. Accepted guidelines for re-operation include bleeding rates of 400 mL/h for 1 hour, 300 mL/h for 2 hours, or 200 mL/h for 3 hours. A sudden decrease or total cessation of drainage from mediastinal tubes may be equally ominous. Cessation of drainage from a mediastinal or chest tube can be caused by clotted blood occluding the tube. If bleeding persists but drainage ceases, the result can be tamponade.

Re-exploration is associated with increased morbidity and mortality. However, this increased mortality and morbidity may be partially explained by delays in the decision to re-explore that lead to avoidable open-chest resuscitations in the ICU.[56,83,84]

POSTOPERATIVE RENAL FAILURE

The cornerstone of prevention and treatment of renal failure in the cardiac surgical patient is the maintenance of adequate renal perfusion.

This goal is best achieved by optimizing circulating blood volume and CO. Multiple pharmacologic regimens for renal protection have been described. Dopamine at low "renal" doses (1-3 μg/kg/min) has been used. The rationale for this strategy is that dopamine activates type 1 dopaminergic (DA1) receptors, leading to renal artery dilation, natriuresis, and diuresis. However, numerous human studies have failed to show that low-dose dopamine prevents renal failure or improves survival.[85] Even low doses of dopamine increase CO, and this may be the basis for any increase in urine output observed.[86] Fenoldapam[87] and dopexamine[88] are DA1 receptor antagonists that also have been proposed as renal protective agents and used with mixed success.[89]

Loop diuretics such as furosemide have been proposed as renal protective agents, not only because of their ability to produce diuresis and natriuresis, but also because these drugs may reduce medullary tubular oxygen consumption. Mannitol, an osmotic diuretic, been used to prevent development of ARF. Neither mannitol nor furosemide has been shown to improve outcome for patients with ARF.[60] Indeed, these drugs may be deleterious because of their ability to promote diuresis and thus exacerbate hypovolemia and inadequate renal perfusion. Some success has been reported with the combination of mannitol, furosemide, and dopamine.[90] Infusion of a solution containing these three agents promoted diuresis in patients with acute postoperative ARF and adequate CO and significantly decreased the need for dialysis in the majority of patients.[88] Early administration of this solution in ARF caused early restoration of renal function to normal or baseline status.[90]

The failure of pharmacologic means of preventing and treating renal failure has led to interest in other methods. Early and intensive use of continuous venovenous hemofiltration achieved a better than predicted outcome in a series of 65 consecutive patients with severe ARF who underwent cardiac operations.[91]

GLUCOSE CONTROL

Recent studies have shown that tight control of blood glucose level in the ICU is associated with an increase in morbidity and mortality (Table 194-4). Hyperglycemia and insulin resistance are common in critically ill patients, even those who have not previously had diabetes. Results of a prospective randomized controlled study[92] in which 6104 critically ill adult patients were randomly assigned to receive either intensive insulin therapy (maintenance of blood glucose concentration between 80 and 108 mg/dL) or conventional treatment (infusion of insulin to keep blood glucose level 180 mg/dL or less) showed that at 3 months, the intensive insulin therapy group had an increase in ICU mortality, with an increase in hypoglycemic episodes in the treatment group.

MECHANICAL VENTILATION

In uncomplicated recoveries, patients require only a short period of mechanical ventilation. Typically, volume-controlled ventilation is used until sedation is discontinued and the patient awakens. Once the patient is awake, hemodynamically stable, and without evidence of bleeding, a short trial of spontaneous ventilation is performed. If the weaning trial is successful, the patient is extubated. If continued mechanical ventilation is required because of respiratory failure or hemodynamic instability, either conventional volume-controlled ventilation or pressure support ventilation can be employed.

A small number of patients develop ALI or ARDS. In a large prospective trial of medical and surgical patients with ARDS or ALI, it was clearly beneficial to employ a lung-protective strategy or mechanical ventilation, limiting tidal volume to 6 mL/kg.[93] No such study has been performed in cardiac surgical patients, but it seems reasonable to adopt the same guidelines. These recommendations apply only to patients with established ALI/ARDS; use of low tidal volumes has not been shown to be effective when used prophylactically.

Patients with ALI or ARDS typically require increasing levels of PEEP to support oxygenation. The effect of PEEP on ventricular

TABLE 194-3	Evaluation and Treatment of Postoperative Coagulopathy	
Coagulation Test	*Normal Range*	*Suggested Treatment*
Body temperature	—	If less than 35.5°C, the patient should be actively rewarmed.
Prothrombin time (PT)	11-13.3 sec	Administer fresh-frozen plasma.
Partial thromboplastin time (PTT)	21-32 sec	Consider additional protamine.*
Platelets	140,000-440,000/μL	If <100,000, transfuse platelets.
Fibrinogen	150-360 mg/dL	If <100, transfuse cryoprecipitate.
Bleeding time	2.5-9.5 min	If prolonged and platelet count is normal, consider platelet dysfunction, and treat with desmopressin acetate (DDAVP) and/or cryoprecipitate.
Activated coagulation test (ACT)	90-120 sec	Consider additional protamine.*

*Excessive protamine may itself cause bleeding.[102]

TABLE 194-4	Protocol for Blood Sugar Control in the Postoperative Period

Decision to initiate IV insulin
↓

If BG <200 mg/dL, begin D_5 ½ NS at 60-100 mL/h
If BG >300 mg/dL, give stat dose of IV insulin, 0.1 U/kg body weight
↓

Initiate an hourly rate (total daily dose of insulin divided by 24)
For patients who have never taken insulin, give 0.02 U/kg body weight per hour*
↓

Check BG hourly and adjust according to table below
Recheck BG hourly
↓

If in desirable range (101-150 mg/dL), continue to check BG every 2 h and adjust as necessary

Current BG (mg/dL)	Previous BG (mg/dL)								
	<60	60-80	81-100	101-150	151-200	201-250	251-300	301-400	>400
<60	Withhold drip and give 1 ampule of 50% glucose; check BG every 30 min until >100 mg/dL, then reinitiate drip at 50% of previous rate								
60-80	Withhold drip; check BG every 30 min until >100 mg/dL, then reinitiate drip at 50% of previous rate								
81-100	↓ Rate by 1 U/h	No change		↓ Rate by 25% or 0.5 U/h†		↓ Rate by 25% or 1 U/h†		↓ Rate by 50% or 2 U/h†	
101-150	No change				↓ Rate by 25% or 1 U/h†				
151-200	↑ Rate by 1 U/h		↑ Rate by 0.5 U/h	↑ Rate by 25% or 1 U/h†		• No change		↓ Rate by 25% or 1 U/h†	
201-250	↑ Rate by 25% or 2 U/h†		↑ Rate by 25% or 1 U/h†			↑ Rate by 1 U/h		No change	
251-300	↑ Rate by 33% or 2.5 U/h†	↑ Rate by 25% or 1.5 U/h†	↑ Rate by 25% or 1 U/h†	↑ Rate by 1 U/h†		↑ Rate by 1.5 U/h†		↑ Rate by 25% or 2 U/h†	No change
301-400	↑ Rate by 40% or 3 U/h†								
>400	↑ Rate by 50% or 4 U/h†								

Before discontinuing insulin infusion:
  Ensure that patient is able to tolerate oral intake
  Write orders for alternative glycemic management
  Precede discontinuation by 1-2 h with subcutaneous dose of very rapid or rapid insulin. If patient has never taken insulin, use a dose equal to twice the hourly rate of IV insulin. Otherwise, use the dose of insulin or oral agent given before surgery/admission.

*For patients undergoing major surgery (e.g., cardiothoracic surgery, transplantation), higher doses may be necessary.
†Whichever is greater.
BG, blood glucose concentration; D_5 ½ NS, 5% dextrose in half-normal saline; IV, intravenous; U, units.

output is controversial. There is evidence that the application of PEEP up to 30 cm H_2O decreases CO by reducing ventricular preload and displacing the interventricular septum toward the left, which restricts left ventricular filling.[94] Other studies have not supported this view. When adult patients with normal preoperative respiratory status were randomly assigned to treatment with graded degrees of PEEP between 0 and 10 cm H_2O during mechanical ventilatory support, there were no significant differences in cardiac index among the groups.[95] It is likely that the effects of PEEP on the circulation are widely variable among patients and that the appropriate strategy is upward titration of PEEP under close monitoring.

Outcomes of Cardiac Surgery

Increasingly, health care is being driven by outcome data. Cardiac surgery has been one of the leading specialties in this field. It is difficult to assess results from crude mortality data, because these do not take into account case complexity and differing preoperative risks among patients. Crude comparisons of death rates can be misleading and may encourage surgeons to practice risk-averse behavior. Death rates should be stratified by risk. It is, however, possible to make some generalizations. Among low-risk patients undergoing CABG, mortality rates lower than 2% are achievable.[96] Higher mortality rates are to be expected in selected subgroups of patients with major preoperative risk factors (e.g., poor ventricular function, advanced age, comorbid conditions) or major operative risk factors (e.g., reoperative surgery, complex operations).

A prospective cohort of 27,239 consecutive patients undergoing isolated CABG was examined to determine risk factors for hospital mortality. After adjustment for patient and disease characteristics, the following comorbid conditions were found to be related to postoperative mortality: diabetes, vascular disease, chronic obstructive pulmonary disease, peptic ulcer disease, and dialysis-dependent renal failure.[97]

Cardiac surgery is being performed more frequently in patients 80 years of age and older. In one study, the 30-day mortality rate for patients age 65 to 75 years was 3.4%, and for those older than 80 years of age it was 13.5%. Older patients had longer ICU and postoperative lengths of stay. Total direct costs were $4818 higher in the octogenarian group. Although emergency operations and complex procedures carry high risks for octogenarians and increasing costs for society, most of these patients can be offered operation with short-term morbidity, mortality, and resource use that only modestly exceed those of younger patients.[98] Once discharged from the hospital, older patients report a high quality of life.[99]

Overall, fewer than 10% of cardiac surgical patients spend more than 48 hours in the ICU. Most survive and eventually report improved functional status and a reasonable quality of life.[100,101]

Summary

Most cardiac surgical patients can be discharged from the ICU to a step-down unit within 24 to 48 hours after operation, but an increasing number cannot. Patients who require longer and more intensive services in the ICU are typically older and sicker preoperatively. Adherence to best practices in the ICU optimizes the opportunity for even these high-risk patients to survive their operation and achieve a good quality of life after hospitalization.

Ongoing development of less invasive techniques in cardiology and cardiac surgery will, paradoxically, bring about a further increase in the complexity of cases treated in the cardiac surgical ICU as patients who are less sick are treated elsewhere. This trend will lead to increasing challenges for intensivists working in these units and allow them to continue to be at the forefront of critical care medicine.

1. Recent developments in interventional cardiology have led to older and sicker populations being referred for cardiac surgery.

2. Much of the care of cardiac surgical patients should be protocol driven and conducted in specialized units.

3. Most patients undergoing cardiac surgery require only a short stay in the intensive care unit.

4. Patients may be extubated once hemodynamic stability is achieved and mediastinal bleeding is deemed to be under control.

5. Low cardiac output after surgery should be treated based on the components of the cardiac output: rate, rhythm, preload, afterload, and contractility.

6. Atrial fibrillation continues to be a cause of significant morbidity.

ANNOTATED REFERENCES

American Heart Association. Heart disease and stroke statistics—2003 update. Dallas, TX: AHA; 2003.

This is an authoritative overview of the epidemiology of cardiac disease in the United States. It gives a clear picture of the changing role of cardiac surgery in the treatment of ischemic heart disease.

Bashour CA, Yared JP, Ryan TA, et al. Long-term survival and functional capacity in cardiac surgery patients after prolonged intensive care. Crit Care Med 2000;28:3847-53.

Of those patients requiring ICU stays longer than 10 days after cardiac surgery, more then 50% will be alive at 1-year follow-up. Although these patients are extremely costly in terms of resources expended, they are salvageable.

Eagle KA, Guyton RA, Davidoff R, et al. ACC/AHA guidelines for coronary artery bypass graft surgery: a report of the American College of Cardiology/American Heart Association Task Force on Practice Guidelines (Committee to Revise the 1991 Guidelines for Coronary Artery Bypass Graft Surgery). American College of Cardiology/American Heart Association. J Am Coll Cardiol 1999;34:1262-347.

These are up-to-date guidelines for management of the cardiac surgical intensive care unit.

Jacka MJ, Cohen MM, To T, Devitt JH, Byrick R. The use of and preferences for the transesophageal echocardiogram and pulmonary artery catheter among cardiovascular anesthesiologists. Anesth Analg 2002;94:1065-71.

TEE is now the standard of care in the cardiac surgical OR. This paper demonstrates the utility of TEE in diagnosis and decision making for the postoperative cardiac surgical patient in the ICU.

Montes FR, Sanchez SI, Giraldo JC, et al. The lack of benefit of tracheal extubation in the operating room after coronary artery bypass surgery. Anesth Analg 2000;91:776-80.

Fast-tracking of cardiac surgical patients remains an intriguing concept. However, this paper shows no advantage for the routine extubation of patients in the OR.

van den Berghe G, Wouters P, Weekers F, et al. Intensive insulin therapy in critically ill patients. N Engl J Med 2001;345:1359-67.

This is a seminal paper showing the effects of tight control of blood sugar in the ICU on morbidity and mortality. The majority of patients enrolled in this study were postoperative cardiac surgical patients.

REFERENCES

Access the complete reference list online at http://www.expertconsult.com.

195

Management of Patients After Heart, Heart-Lung, or Lung Transplantation

JUAN C. SALGADO | ARTHUR J. BOUJOUKOS

Lung Transplantation

Lung transplantation offers hope for improved survival and quality of life for selected patients with end-stage lung disease. The availability of suitable donor organs and preservation injury remain the initial limiting factors to successful transplantation. Like other transplants, rejection and infection as well as organ system dysfunction associated with the perioperative course remain challenges. However, experience over 40 years has led to substantial improvements in early outcome. This experience has been reflected in changes in various aspects of the field, including a different allocation system where priority is given based on medical urgency and expected outcome,[1,2] donor and recipient assessments,[3] innovative surgical techniques, better understanding of early complications, and the development of newer immunosuppressive medications. Nevertheless, obliterative bronchiolitis (OB) resulting from chronic rejection and non-cytomegalovirus (CMV) infections limit the long-term quality of life and is largely responsible for the 47% 5-year mortality rate for lung transplantation.[4]

Diagnoses for which adults receive lung transplantation include chronic obstructive pulmonary disease (COPD)/emphysema (35.8%), idiopathic pulmonary fibrosis (20.8%), cystic fibrosis (15.9%), α_1-antitrypsin deficiency (7.1%), idiopathic pulmonary arterial hypertension (3.3%), and others including sarcoidosis, congenital heart diseases, and connective tissue disease complicated by advanced lung disease. These diagnoses have remained relatively unchanged, with the exception of procedures offered to patients with idiopathic pulmonary fibrosis going from 15% of all procedures in 2000 to 27% in 2007, and procedures offered to patients with idiopathic pulmonary arterial hypertension (previously called *primary pulmonary hypertension*) going from 13% in 1990 to 2% in 2007. Transplantation options include single lung transplant (SLT), bilateral lung transplant (i.e., sequential bilateral single lung transplantation [BLT]), heart-lung transplant (HLT), or living-donor lobar lung transplant (LDLLT). Over the last 15 years, the number of SLT procedures has remained stable, with a steady increase in the number of BLT procedures accounting for 69% of transplant procedures in 2007.[4] The trend toward bilateral transplantation has been most noticeable in patients with chronic obstructive lung disease, either from emphysema or α_1-antitrypsin deficiency, which is the most frequent diagnosis leading to transplantation.[5]

Donor selection, procurement, and lung preservation protocols tend to be individualized on an institutional basis. The limited availability of donor lungs, however, has increased the scrutiny with which organs are judged in order to avoid rejecting them inappropriately.[3] Significant lung contusion, smoking-related lung damage, pneumonia, pulmonary edema, and significant aspiration are prime concerns in evaluating the suitability of donor organs. Although already described as an independent association for primary graft dysfunction (PGD, also known as *primary graft failure* [PGF] or *pulmonary reimplantation response* [PRR]),[6] donor's older age is being challenged at some centers as a risk factor for worsened outcomes.[7] Procurement and lung preservation protocols often include administration of antiinflammatory agents, pulmonary vasodilators, and antioxidants.

The surgical technique involves a thoracotomy for SLT or a transverse thoracosternotomy (clamshell incision) for DLT and LDLLT

transplants. Minimally invasive techniques are being developed in some centers as well. The surgical procedure includes the anastomosing of the pulmonary artery, atrium, and bronchus. Cardiopulmonary bypass is typically avoided in the case of SLT and DLT unless preexisting pulmonary hypertension precludes cross-clamping of the pulmonary artery or if cardiorespiratory stability cannot be otherwise maintained. At the completion of the operation, the double-lumen endobronchial tube (EBT) is exchanged for a standard endotracheal tube (ETT) unless allograft function appears tenuous or there is evidence of air trapping. Heart-lung transplants are performed utilizing either a clamshell incision or sternotomy. Cardiopulmonary bypass is obviously a requirement in these patients. The vascular anastomoses include the aorta and a cuff of right atrium including both vena cavae. Bi-bronchial airway anastomoses are performed, which is associated with less dehiscence than a single tracheal anastomosis.

PERIOPERATIVE INTENSIVE CARE UNIT MANAGEMENT

On transfer to the intensive care unit (ICU), patients are often managed using a lung-protective strategy that limits tidal volumes to 3 mL/kg per allograft and plateau pressure to less than 32 cm H_2O. Five to 10 centimeters of positive end-expiratory pressure (PEEP) are applied to the allograft, and fractional inspired oxygen concentration (F_{IO_2}) is set initially at 0.30 to 0.40 and titrated higher if arterial oxygen saturation (Sao_2) is less than 90%. If there is minimal evidence of postoperative allograft dysfunction, liberation from ventilation can proceed expeditiously once the patient has recovered from general anesthesia. Using 10 cm H_2O of pressure support in the continuous positive airway pressure (CPAP) mode of mechanical ventilation helps counteract the airway resistance of the endobronchial tube during weaning if an EBT is left in place at the end of the case. Expeditious pulmonary toileting maneuvers including incentive spirometry, chest physiotherapy, and therapeutic bronchoscopy must be pursued without concerns for anastomosis complications. Patients undergoing LDLLT are typically kept sedated on mechanical ventilatory support for at least 72 hours to optimize expansion of the lobes.

HYPERINFLATION

In SLT with emphysema, the transplanted lung can be relatively noncompliant. As a result, the native lung may be hyperinflated. This is one reason that chronic obstructive lung disease recipients are preferably offered bilateral lung transplantation.[4] This problem becomes even more apparent when higher levels of PEEP are needed because of allograft dysfunction. Hyperinflation of the native, more compliant lung leads to mediastinal shift, deterioration in gas exchange, and hemodynamic instability. Although inserting an expiratory pause into the ventilator cycle can be used to assess the level of intrinsic PEEP ("autopeep"), excessive air trapping is easily diagnosed by disconnecting the patient's ETT from the ventilator tubing for 5 to 10 seconds. In patients with significant air trapping and hyperinflation, "popping the patient off" leads to a significant improvement in blood pressure and oxygenation. Management strategies using only a single ventilator to provide ventilation include reducing PEEP, reducing tidal volume, and accepting a modest level of respiratory acidosis.

Alternatively, conversion to independent lung ventilation may be appropriate, particularly in the setting of significant allograft dysfunction and high PEEP requirements. In order to switch to independent lung ventilation, an EBT is advanced into the left mainstem bronchus, and the bronchial balloon is inflated. Positioning can be verified by measuring tidal volumes delivered to and returned from each lumen of the EBT. Bronchoscopy with a small-caliber bronchoscope is appropriate to verify that (1) the left bronchial balloon is distal to the carina and (2) that the end of the left endobronchial tube does not protrude too far distally into the left lung, compromising flow to either the upper or lower division bronchi. Ventilator settings are adjusted for each machine individually. Initially, PEEP for the allograft is set at 10 cm H_2O, tidal volume is set at 3 mL/kg and rate is set at 20 to 25 breaths/min. Initial settings for the emphysematous native lung typically use a larger tidal volume and a slower rate with 0 to 2.5 cm PEEP. There is no need to synchronize the ventilators. Lung hyperinflation is associated with a longer ICU stay, longer duration of mechanical ventilation, and a trend toward worsened mortality.[8]

EARLY POSTOPERATIVE RESPIRATORY COMPLICATIONS

Airways are affected variably by the ischemic/implantation insult. Anastomotic dehiscences are rare, although a recent report suggests incidence of this complication is increased when sirolimus was used as an immunosuppressive agent.[9] Anatomically, the transplanted bronchus derives its blood supply from the lung and pulmonary blood flow, since the bronchial arteries are not typically anastomosed. The longer left mainstem bronchus, particularly adjacent to the anastomosis, is at higher risk for ischemic injury compared with the right bronchus, which generally is anastomosed adjacent to the right upper lobe takeoff. Early bronchoscopy often demonstrates relatively normal epithelium. However, more severe airway injury patterns can become apparent over the next several days. The earliest findings are patchy areas of subepithelial hemorrhage that can become confluent. In more severe cases, white plaques can form, and frank areas of desiccated sloughed epithelium become evident. In the most severe cases, eschar is evident, and bronchial cartilage may be exposed. Severe airway injury poses the risk of infection and bronchomalacia. The infections are typically due to *Candida* and *Aspergillus* species.[10] In many centers, lung transplant recipients are treated prophylactically with antifungal agents such as inhaled amphotericin or an azole such as voriconazole. This strategy seems to reduce the rate of airway infection.[10] If suspicious plaques are evident bronchoscopically, we perform bronchial biopsy to exclude invasive disease. Inhaled amphotericin B (50 mg twice daily) is generally administered to patients with severe airway injury and those with cultures demonstrating growth of fungus. Bronchomalacia is generally a long-term complication, although in some cases, this complication can become evident within the first 6 weeks after transplantation. Dynamic airway collapse or fixed stenoses are diagnosed by bronchoscopy. In addition to endobronchial infections, malacia, and stenosis, other airway complications include dehiscence, granulation tissue formation, and fistulas.[11] These are not necessarily early complications, but increased awareness of their potential occurrence is warranted.

Primary graft dysfunction (PGD) is a severe form of ischemia-reperfusion injury (IRI) and is the leading cause of respiratory failure and morbidity early after transplantation.[12] A recent consensus statement by the International Society of Heart and Lung Transplantation (ISHLT) Working Group on PGD standardized the grading of PGD on the basis of gas exchange (Pao_2/Fio_2 ratio) and plain chest radiologic findings.[13] With this grading system, a grade 3 PGD ($Pao_2/Fio_2 < 200$ plus the presence of diffuse radiographic infiltrates) resembles the definition of acute respiratory distress syndrome (ARDS), and with this in mind, it has already been validated by demonstrating a worsened mortality and prolonged hospital stay.[14] The reported incidence of grade 3 PGD ranges from 10% to 25%, with 30-day mortality close to 50%.[15,16] Over 95% of patients have infiltrates in the allograft by chest roentgenogram during the first 72 hours.[17] Although edema and

atelectasis contribute to these early changes, worsening or persistent infiltrates most likely reflect diffuse alveolar damage (DAD) secondary to PGD. Although many cases of PGD are evident on chest films obtained on the first postoperative day, in some cases, it does not become apparent radiographically or physiologically for up to 72 hours post transplant. The timing of appearance of clinical and radiologic respiratory failure is extremely helpful, then, to elaborate a judicious differential diagnosis, understanding that while PGD occurs within hours and up to 3 days after transplantation, infection and rejection are more common past the first 24 to 36 hours. In some cases, patients will be successfully extubated only to deteriorate 24 hours later. When uncertain about the etiology, aggressive diagnostic efforts should be made, employing bronchoscopy, bronchoalveolar lavage (BAL), and biopsy to exclude superimposed infection or rejection. If pulmonary edema is unilateral, a diagnosis of pulmonary venous obstruction must be entertained. Although the incidence of this problem is extremely low, a transesophageal echocardiogram (TEE) should be performed to exclude unilateral venous obstruction.

The level of respiratory dysfunction secondary to IRI depends on the extent of the injury and the residual lung reserve. The latter factor is particularly important in SLT for emphysema, because the remaining native lung may have substantial residual function. The functional capacity of the native lung often allows the transplant recipient to tolerate a significant degree of allograft dysfunction.[18] Such is typically not the case for IPF patients or recipients with significant pulmonary hypertension, since perfusion to the native lung is minimal once a donor lung with low pulmonary vascular resistance is implanted.

The management of PGD is largely supportive, including judicious diuresis and a protective ventilatory approach.[19] Inhaled nitric oxide may be utilized to help address early postoperative hypoxemia.[20,21] Extracorporeal membrane oxygenation (ECMO) remains a salvage therapy for severe PGD.[22-24]

Muscular weakness or mechanical issues can embarrass postoperative respiratory function. Patients requiring delayed closure of the clamshell incision, which is required in some patients with excessive bleeding, are at higher risk for respiratory dysfunction on this basis. Preoperative muscle wasting is a major contributing factor in most cases. Clinically significant phrenic nerve injury is rare. However, when dissection of the native lungs was difficult due to dense pleural adhesions, phrenic nerve injury can be present and significantly prolong the weaning process. Postoperative neuromuscular blockade is rarely used because of synergistic adverse effects on long-term neuromuscular function that have been associated with simultaneous administration of corticosteroids (a component of most immunosuppressive regimens) and neuromuscular blocking agents.[25] If the patient has difficulty clearing secretions, tracheostomy should be performed early.

Patients are treated with broad-spectrum antibiotics perioperatively. In patients without suppurative lung disease, antibiotics are stopped within 72 hours if samples from the donor trachea and from the explanted lung are without pathogens. If cultures are positive for potential pulmonary pathogens, a directed course of antibiotics is continued for 7 to 10 days. In patients with septic lung disease, an antibiotic regimen based on preoperative cultures is continued for a minimum of 2 to 3 weeks. Patients also may be treated with prophylactic regimens to prevent CMV infection with valganciclovir if either the patient or the donor is CMV immunoglobulin G(IgG) positive before surgery (dose will vary with kidney function). Aggressive prophylaxis against deep vein thrombosis (DVT) is mandatory.[26] At our center, critically ill transplant patients are screened liberally for DVT with lower extremity Doppler ultrasound examinations, with a low threshold for placement of an inferior vena caval filter when DVT is diagnosed.

NEW PULMONARY INFILTRATES

Development of new infiltrates on the chest film after lung transplantation mandates diagnostic evaluation using fiberoptic bronchoscopy with BAL and transbronchial biopsy. If bacterial pneumonia is strongly suspected, particularly if biopsy is thought to be excessively risky, bronchoscopy with BAL and empirical antibiotic therapy is an acceptable alternative. If the Gram stain is unremarkable, and distal airways lack evidence of bacterial or fungal infection, transbronchial biopsy is necessary to exclude acute rejection or CMV infection. If a transbronchial biopsy continues to be unobtainable owing to tenuous respiratory status, open lung biopsy should be considered. Pending the results of biopsy or in lieu of one, empirical antirejection treatment may occasionally be considered on an individual basis, recognizing the potential risks of doing so.

Conditions other than PGD can lead to diffuse alveolar damage (DAD) as determined by transbronchial biopsy. DAD can result from pneumonia, rejection, CMV infection, systemic sepsis, or even subsequent to a BAL. The management of DAD is supportive, consisting of lung-protective ventilation as for ARDS. Management in severe cases can include administration of corticosteroids (e.g., prednisone 2-3 mg/kg/d), though the risk of infection in transplant patients does not support this approach.

Because the transplanted lung is in close contact with the external environment, the risk for infection is higher than is the case for other forms of organ transplantation. Accordingly, aggressive diagnostic efforts are the key to management of graft dysfunction after lung transplantation. Bacterial infections with traditional nosocomial pathogens are most common in the first 30 days. Subsequently, bacterial pneumonia is still responsible for the bulk of new infiltrates, although other etiologies must be considered as well. CMV infection, causing pneumonia among other problems, occurs in a large fraction of cases. Prophylactic and surveillance strategies to deal with CMV vary from center to center. Some institutions carry out weekly assays, seeking to detect CMV antigen in the bloodstream, and only institute early preemptive therapy when the antigen is present. Other centers provide prophylaxis using ganciclovir or valganciclovir for 3 to 6 months. Dosing of these antiviral medications will vary with the kidney function. Our center monitors CMV status via frequent plasma PCR assays.[27] Other viruses such as adenovirus, parainfluenza virus, influenza virus, and respiratory syncytial virus are community-acquired pathogens that can cause significant morbidity and mortality.[28]

Fungal pneumonia with *Aspergillus* spp. occurs but is rare. Far more common is the colonization of airways with *Aspergillus*. Distinguishing between infection and colonization requires computed tomography (CT) scanning and bronchoscopic evaluation with directed biopsy to areas suspicious for invasive fungal disease. Successful treatment requires appropriate antifungal therapy and reduction in immunosuppression to the lowest levels tolerable. *Candida albicans* in the airway almost always reflects colonization, because pneumonia as a result of this organism is exceedingly rare. *Pneumocystis carinii* pneumonia is exceedingly unusual, especially when patients are treated perioperatively with trimethoprim/sulfamethoxazole as prophylaxis. Infections with toxoplasmosis, *Nocardia*, *Histoplasma*, coccidiomycosis, *Cryptococcus*, and mycobacteria are quite rare but do occur.

Acute cellular rejection (ACR) occurs in 36% of patients at some time in the first year after transplant.[4] Patients typically present with allograft infiltrates, worsening hypoxemia and dyspnea. Fever and pleural effusion may occur, and pulmonary secretions are uncommon. Clinical findings have been shown to be inadequate for diagnosing ACR; establishing the diagnosis requires transbronchial biopsy.[29] Maintenance immunosuppression in most centers is based on a three-drug regimen including either cyclosporine or tacrolimus, prednisone, and either mycophenolate or azathioprine. Sirolimus is also often included in the maintenance regimen in selected instances (Table 195-1). Episodes of significant acute rejection are treated with methylprednisolone (10-15 mg/kg intravenously [IV] daily × 3 days). Response usually occurs within 24-72 hours. Failure to respond should prompt re-biopsy to exclude refractory rejection.

Chronic rejection presents more insidiously. Findings are increased dyspnea, worsening pulmonary function test results, and sometimes cough. Pathologically, patients with chronic rejection manifest findings

TABLE 195-1	Maintenance Immunosuppression			
Drug	Months 1-12	Months 12-24	Months >24 & CKD	NOTES
Prednisone (mg/d)	5 Begin AM postop day 1	5	5	
Tacrolimus* (blood level); 1st choice	12-15 (10- to 12-hour trough)	10-12	8-10	Begin 0.5 mg PO BID. Give 1st dose 6 hours after arrival to ICU
Cyclosporine† (blood level)	250-300 (10- to 12-hour trough)	200-250	150-200	Use if intolerant to tacrolimus
Mycophenolate‡ (250 mg/tablet)	Begin 750 mg PO BID			Monitor neutropenia; adjust dose accordingly
Myfortic‡ (180 mg/tablet)	Begin 540 mg PO BID			Use if GI intolerance to mycophenolate
Azathioprine (WBC > 3.5)	1-2 mg/kg/d			Start 50 mg/day, increase to goal after 1 week if WBCs acceptable and tolerating
Sirolimus§ (blood level)		4-12‖ in combination with calcineurin inhibitors	10-16‖ Without calcineurin inhibitors Steady-state concentrations occur 5-7 days after dose change	

*Increase by 0.5 mg to achieve target blood level.
†Increase by 25 mg to achieve target blood level.
‡Take 1 hour AC or 2 hours PC.
§Separate dosing by 4 hours from calcineurin inhibitors (tacrolimus, cyclosporine).
‖Sirolimus dosing paradigm. When using sirolimus to decrease tacrolimus (FK) dose, we target a sirolimus level of approximately 6-8 with an FK level of 4-6. This would add together to an additive goal of 10-12. The target levels are usually determined by calculating what the ideal FK level would be post transplant, and then having a total FK + sirolimus dose equal to that level.

AC, before meals; *BID,* twice daily; *CKD,* chronic kidney disease; *GI,* gastrointestinal; *ICU,* intensive care unit; *PC,* after meals; *PO,* per os (orally); *WBCs,* white blood cells.

of OB with a lymphocytic infiltrate in the submucosa and epithelium plus submucosal fibrosis. These findings, however, can be missed on transbronchial biopsy. OB also can develop in the wake of other insults such as acute rejection, airway ischemia, lymphocytic bronchiolitis, and certain infections such as CMV. Patients with OB, in addition to developing progressive deterioration of lung function, are also at high risk for bacterial pneumonia and acute-on-chronic bouts of respiratory failure.[30] Pneumonia is commonly caused by *Pseudomonas aeruginosa* followed by *Staphylococcus* and *Acinetobacter baumannii.*[10]

NONPULMONARY ORGAN SUPPORT AND COMPLICATIONS

Hemodynamic management following lung transplantation is similar to that of other ICU patients, with the exception of volume administration. Given the lack of lymphatics in the allograft and potential ischemic injury of pulmonary endothelium and epithelium, pulmonary edema occurs at lower filling pressures. For that reason, lung transplant recipients with postoperative hypoxemia should be maintained "on the dry side" using vasopressors or inotropes as needed to support blood pressure and cardiac output. Patients have been screened preoperatively for coronary artery disease and ventricular dysfunction, and ischemia or congestive heart failure (CHF) should rarely be complicating factors in lung transplant recipients. Atrial arrhythmias are common and can effectively be managed with β-adrenergic blockade or sotalol in most cases. Amiodarone should be avoided because of its potential pulmonary toxicity.[31] Diltiazem can unpredictably and markedly affect calcineurin inhibitor levels (tacrolimus and cyclosporine) and should be used cautiously.

Patients with preexisting pulmonary hypertension will enjoy a 30% to 40% reduction in pulmonary artery pressure after SLT and normalization of pressures with a BLT. Postoperative pulmonary hypertension in patients with preexisting pulmonary hypertension is generally well tolerated, since the right ventricle (RV) is conditioned, and transplantation reduces RV afterload. Only patients with pulmonary hypertension and evidence of low output and high central venous pressure (CVP) require specific therapy. Inotropic agents may be needed for support for a short time following cardiopulmonary bypass.

Renal dysfunction is common, and some patients require renal replacement therapy. In these patients, bicarbonate should be aggressively supplemented enterally to reduce the need for pulmonary compensation for metabolic acidosis. Because transplanted lungs are so sensitive to excessive intravascular volume, ultrafiltration may be required more frequently than is typical for general ICU patients. Calcineurin inhibitor (tacrolimus or cyclosporine) levels should be closely followed. Efforts for precise timing of their administration for more reliable trough levels should be stressed. Goal levels may have to be readjusted in the setting of renal dysfunction. This practice, although not encouraged, is more often considered if induction immunosuppression has been administered prior to the patient's arrival to the ICU. Other nephrotoxins such as nonsteroidal antiinflammatory agents must be completely avoided, and CT scans should be performed without IV contrast unless absolutely necessary.

Gastrointestinal problems include gastritis/ulcers, ileus, *Clostridium difficile* colitis, and CMV enteritis. In some centers, patients receive an H$_2$ blocker during their initial hospitalization as well as enteral metronidazole (500 mg orally [PO] 3 times daily) as prophylaxis against *C. difficile* infection. CMV enteritis can be difficult to diagnose, since tests for circulating CMV antigen can be negative in patients with disease localized to the GI tract. Endoscopy with biopsy is appropriate, particularly if thickened bowel is identified radiographically. Patients with cystic fibrosis should be placed on a bowel regimen with lactulose (10 mg PO twice daily) or polyethylene glycol (17 g PO 4 times daily) to prevent mucous impaction. Gastroesophageal reflux disease is common after lung transplantation, and there is evidence that effective treatment, including surgical interventions,[32,33] can improve lung allograft function as well as reduce the incidence of chronic rejection.[34] Pancreatitis, bowel perforation, and cholecystitis are uncommon GI problems. These issues should be addressed in the standard manner.

Neurologic sequelae after lung transplant include tremors, seizures, encephalopathy, myopathy, and neuropathy. Drugs such as tacrolimus and cyclosporine, antibiotics, corticosteroids, and perioperative neuromuscular blocking agents can be contributing factors. Hyperammonemia after lung transplantation is a devastating complication presenting as lethargy and unexplained hyperammonemia. Its mechanism is poorly understood and carries a grave prognosis despite aggressive measures including gut decontamination, high levels of dialysis, and pharmacologic treatments targeted at urea-cycle enzyme deficiencies.[35,36]

Heart Transplantation

Heart transplantation has been performed for over 35 years for end-stage heart disease. In 2007, 3355 heart transplants were reported to the International Society of Heart and Lung Transplantation (ISHLT) database.[37] The primary indication for heart transplantation has interestingly shifted over the last 10 years from an equal split of ischemic and nonischemic heart disease to a greater proportion of patients with nonischemic cardiomyopathy (39.5% versus 49.5%); other indications include congenital disease, valvular disease, amyloidosis, sarcoidosis, and re-transplantation. Donor availability still remains a primary deterrent to more widespread use of cardiac transplantation.

Heterotopic transplantation is a rare procedure which entails implantation of a donor heart in parallel with the failing native heart to reduce postoperative right heart failure in the setting of preoperative pulmonary hypertension. The donor heart is implanted in the right chest with side-to-side anastomoses of the right atrium to right atrium and left atrium to left atrium. The transplanted aorta is anastomosed end to side to the recipient aorta, and the pulmonary artery of the transplant is joined to the main pulmonary artery of the patient via a graft. The donor left ventricle (LV) provides the bulk of systemic cardiac output, while the native RV provides enough support for the unconditioned donor RV to avoid right heart failure in the setting of high pulmonary vascular resistance (greater than 8 Wood units). Orthotopic heart transplant entails removal of the native heart via sternotomy and replacement with a donor heart with anastomoses of the pulmonary artery, ascending aorta, left atrium, and usually bicaval anastomoses of the right atrium.

HEMODYNAMIC SUPPORT

Following orthotopic heart transplantation, patients return intubated and mechanically ventilated to the ICU. Inotropic and chronotropic support perioperatively is standard and includes dobutamine, milrinone, isoproterenol, or epinephrine. In occasional patients with excessive systemic vasodilatation, norepinephrine or vasopressin (0.04 μg/kg/min) may be appropriate adjuncts perioperatively. Inotropic support is weaned over the first few days in most cases.

Patients with preexisting pulmonary hypertension require more prolonged inotropic support of the unconditioned donor RV, typically with a milrinone taper. Overt RV failure generally becomes apparent in the OR when the chest is still open, but in some cases, increasing CVP and decreasing stroke volume will necessitate evaluation by TEE. RV failure is confirmed by visualizing the absence of tamponade, a hypokinetic and distended RV, and underfilling of the LV. The addition of inhaled nitric oxide (20-40 ppm) or inhaled prostaglandin E$_1$ or I$_2$[38] may be appropriate adjuncts immediately postoperatively in this setting. Care must be taken to avoid overdistension of the RV chamber in the setting of postoperative RV dysfunction, since continued volume loading with CVPs above 20 cm H$_2$O are unlikely to significantly improve flow and may lead to an acute hepatic congestion picture. Diuretics and ultrafiltration are employed early postoperatively if hemodynamically tolerated to keep CVP below 20 cm H$_2$O. Mechanical support with an RVAD may be indicated and should be entertained before a picture of shock emerges. RV dysfunction in the setting of relatively normal pulmonary vascular resistance suggests that the primary problem is myocardial dysfunction rather than excessive afterload. Humoral (hyperacute) rejection should be ruled out in such cases, particularly if issues of preservation were not a concern.

Arrhythmias are common in the early postoperative period. Bradycardia is most common. Owing to denervation of the transplanted heart, sinus bradycardia and atrioventricular (A-V) nodal block are common problems in the early postoperative period. Atropine has no effect on the denervated heart. An adequate heart rate (80-100 beats/min) is generally maintained with catecholamine infusions, temporary epicardial pacing, and occasionally the use of oral agents such as theophylline (50 mg PO twice daily) or terbutaline (5 mg PO 3 times daily). Rarely, patients require placement of a permanent transvenous pacemaker, though experience suggests that in most cases, deferring that decision for a week or so allows for conduction system recovery in the transplanted heart. Atrial fibrillation (AF) is much more common than other forms of supraventricular tachycardia (SVT). AF is managed with amiodarone (150 mg bolus over 10 minutes followed by 1 mg/min × 6 hours and 0.5 mg/min × 18 hours). Because digoxin decreases A-V conduction primarily by increasing vagal tone, this drug has little use in the acute management of AF in heart transplant recipients. β-Adrenergic blockers are generally avoided in the early postoperative period. Diltiazem can be used for acute rate control, but its effects on cyclosporine and tacrolimus metabolism render this drug a second-line agent.

Respiratory complications are similar to those seen with other types of cardiac surgery. In cases in which bleeding is excessive because of redo sternotomy, multiple transfusions pose a risk of acute lung injury. Additionally, several reports suggest a higher incidence of postoperative lung injury in surgical patients on amiodarone, frequently a component of the recipient's preoperative medical regimen. Renal complications are similar to those of lung transplant recipients, with ATN related to perioperative perfusion issues. Hyperbilirubinemia may be seen in patients with postoperative shock and hepatic congestion and in cases with high transfusion needs such as redo sternums, particularly if prior VAD support and anticoagulation were used.

REJECTION

Cardiac allograft rejection can occur early post transplant. Three drug regimens similar to lung transplants are the mainstays of maintenance therapy. Induction therapy with antilymphocyte antibodies (either interleukin [IL]-2 receptor antibodies or polyclonal antilymphocyte globulin/antithymocyte globulin) is used in about half of patients to minimize renal toxicity caused by calcineurin inhibitors—more so in those with preexisting renal disease.[37] Acute cellular rejection may present with arrhythmias, CHF, fatigue, abdominal pain, low cardiac output, or hypotension. Surveillance endomyocardial biopsies and right heart catheterizations are performed weekly in the early postoperative period. Methylprednisolone (1000 mg IV daily for 3 days) is the standard treatment for acute cellular rejection. A particularly aggressive form of rejection is called *hyperacute rejection*, and is mediated primarily by humoral factors. Myocardial biopsy reveals vascular deposition of immunoglobulin and complement, with evidence of vascular injury in the absence of a mononuclear cell infiltrate. Treatment includes therapy with corticosteroids, urgent plasmapheresis, and immunoglobulin infusion. Patients undergoing re-transplantation, multiparous women, and patients having received multiple blood transfusions are at particular risk for hyperacute rejection. For potential recipients with screening studies suggesting undesirable preformed antibodies, a negative prospective crossmatch or an induction regimen including preoperative plasmapheresis is undertaken before proceeding with transplantation in most programs.

INFECTIONS

Infectious complications include routine nosocomial infections such as pneumonia, catheter-related sepsis, and mediastinitis. Patients having been bridged to transplant with a VAD complicated by infection of the VAD pocket or driveline are more prone to wound infections following removal of the device and transplantation. CMV occurs in 10% to 25% of transplants.[37] CMV-negative recipients who receive a CMV-positive organ are at the highest risk. Surveillance with serum CMV antigen assays is the mainstay of management. Some centers employ prophylactic regimens with ganciclovir (5 mg/kg IV twice daily or daily) or valganciclovir (900 mg PO daily) for 3 to 6 months. *Toxoplasma* and *P. carinii* prophylaxis are also standard with trimethoprim/sulfamethoxazole (160/800 PO, 3 times a week).

LONG-TERM COMPLICATIONS

The bulk of early mortality (within 1 month) is caused by graft failure (primary nonspecific) (41%), multiple organ dysfunction syndrome (MODS) (13%) and non-CMV infection (13%). Between 31 days and 1 year, non-CMV infections account for almost 30% of deaths, followed by graft failure (18%) and acute rejection (12%). After 5 years, coronary artery vasculopathy, malignancies, and non-CMV infections are the main causes of death.[37] Coronary vasculopathy is the "OB" of heart transplantation and leads to deterioration in cardiac allograft function following transplantation.[39] Endothelial cell injury can be triggered by graft ischemia, rejection, viral infections, and hyperlipidemia. Endothelial injury or activation leads to concentric, distal coronary intimal proliferation, ultimately occluding coronary flow.[40] The absence of cardiac re-innervation in most heart transplant recipients precludes warning symptoms of angina. New onset of CHF, myocardial infarction, angina, ECG changes, or syncope, particularly in patients several years post transplant, are indications for cardiac catheterization. Stents may be of value in selected cases. Retransplantation is an option, although re-transplantation as an indication for transplant carries with it a significantly inferior outcome.[37]

Although coronary vasculopathy impairs long-term results, heart transplantation nevertheless provides a durable treatment for patients with end-stage heart disease. Patients enjoy 50% survival at 10 years.[37] Donor availability remains the major limitation to more widespread treatment and success.

KEY POINTS

1. Lung transplantation continues to offer hope for many advanced lung disease processes. Much has been learned about the natural history of these otherwise terminal lung diseases, which has influenced significant changes in the overall practice of lung transplantation, including the lung allocation system and the donor selection criteria.

2. Primary graft failure (dysfunction) is a severe form of ischemia-reperfusion injury and carries enormous morbidity and mortality.

3. Lung transplant recipients with postoperative respiratory compromise should be maintained "on the dry side."

4. Growing evidence suggests that suboptimal early immunosuppression, as well as recurrent aspiration from reflux disease, are the two most modifiable risk factors associated with chronic rejection. Patient selection, consideration of antireflux surgery prior to transplantation or early after, and appropriate immunosuppression schedules should be implemented in protocols at every center.

5. Hyperammonemia continues to be a rare but feared complication after lung transplantation, given that its mechanism has yet to be understood. Aggressive management options including gut decontamination, high levels of dialysis, and pharmacologic treatments targeted at urea-cycle enzyme deficiencies are the only available tools but have yet to show promise in changing outcome.

ANNOTATED REFERENCES

Hachem RR, Trulock EP. The new lung allocation system and its impact on waitlist characteristics and post-transplant outcomes. Semin Thorac Cardiovasc Surg 2008;20:139-42.
  This review clearly explains the current lung allocation process, which basically is geared towards making organs available to those who need them more urgently because of their underlying disease process and its expected outcome. A thorough comparison of the prior allocation process to the current one in terms of waiting time, waiting mortality, and more importantly, the steady proportional increase of idiopathic pulmonary fibrosis as the underlying cause of transplantation is made. This increase is explained by the comparable uncertainty of the disease's natural history and the high mortality of its exacerbations.
Christie JD, Edwards LB, Aurora P, Dobbels F, Kirk R, Rahmel AO, et al. The Registry of the International Society for Heart and Lung Transplantation: twenty-sixth official adult lung and heart-lung transplantation report—2009. J Heart Lung Transplant 2009;28:1031-49.
  This yearly document published by the International Society of Heart and Lung Transplantation summarizes and explicitly describes the statistical trends of lung and heart-lung transplantation. This registry

allows the reader to put in perspective the indications for transplantation, the donor characteristics, their impact on transplantation outcomes including rejection, complications and survival, as well as the centers offering transplantation and their influence on these outcomes in terms of the case load they are challenged with. It allows an organized chronological understanding of lung and heart-lung transplantation outcomes.
Christie JD, Sager JS, Kimmel SE, Ahya VN, Gaughan C, Blumenthal NP, et al. Impact of primary graft failure on outcomes following lung transplantation. Chest 2005;127:161-5.
  This single-center retrospective study conducted by field experts looked into the overall incidence of grade III primary graft failure in 255 consecutive procedures done in a period of over 10 years. It demonstrated an incidence of 11.3%, an increased mortality, worsened hospital length of stay, and increased duration of mechanical ventilation. Some 73.3% of patients who received the diagnosis of primary graft failure died during their hospitalization, versus 14.2% of those who did not. A 1-year follow up also demonstrated significantly affected physical function in those who had experienced primary graft failure.

REFERENCES

Access the complete reference list online at http://www.expertconsult.com.

196

Management of Patients after Kidney, Kidney-Pancreas, or Pancreas Transplantation

GREG J. BEILMAN

The first successful long-term functioning kidney transplant was performed by Joseph Murray in 1954 between two monozygotic twins, avoiding the problem of rejection. The recipient lived 8 years, dying of a cause unrelated to her renal failure. Critical care practitioners played an important role in the development of transplantation, with the development of brain death criteria and the ability to care for patients after brain death, allowing recovery of viable organs to be used for transplantation. The success of organ transplantation has improved with the development of more effective preservation solutions, such as the University of Wisconsin solution in the late 1980s, and with the availability of more effective immunosuppressive agents.

Background

KIDNEY TRANSPLANTS

Kidneys are the most frequently transplanted organ; more than 285,000 transplants have been performed through 2007, with over 16,000 transplants performed per year in the United States[1] (Table 196-1). Numerous causes of chronic renal failure result in the need for transplantation, the most common being diabetes mellitus and glomerular disorders (Box 196-1). The source of donors for renal transplantation are both cadavers and living donors. In 2009, there were 10,442 cadaveric donor transplants and 6387 living donor transplants performed.[1,2] The living donor pool consists of both living related donors, who have a higher likelihood for a favorable crossmatch, and living unrelated donors. Recent surgical innovations such as using laparoscopy to obtain the donor kidney have decreased morbidity for donors and decreased costs.[3] The living donor pool may be expanded through the use of programs to utilize nonrelated donors (e.g., kidney paired donations, non-directed donation).

In most cases, the renal transplant operation is done through a retroperitoneal flank incision. An anastomosis is created between the recipient's iliac artery and the donor kidney's renal artery. Another anastomosis is fashioned between the iliac vein and the renal vein. The donor ureter is connected either to the recipient's bladder using a ureteroneocystostomy or to the recipient's ureter via ureteropyelostomy.

PANCREAS TRANSPLANTS

Pancreas transplantation for control of diabetes was first successfully reported by Lillehei and colleagues in 1970.[4] The major indication for transplantation of this organ is diabetes mellitus. Because of the significant morbidity associated with immunosuppression, transplantation of this organ in isolation is uncommon; most pancreatic transplants are carried out in conjunction with a simultaneous or previous kidney transplant. In 2009, there were 854 simultaneous kidney-pancreas transplants and 379 pancreas-after-kidney transplants or solitary pancreas transplants.[2] Isolated pancreatic islet cell transplantation (autotransplantation) has been utilized as an adjunct to total pancreatectomy for patients with intractable pain due to chronic pancreatitis and is an active area of research using human and genetically modified animal islet cells to produce insulin while minimizing the risks of immunosuppression.[5] However, these techniques are difficult to apply outside of specialized centers.

The surgical technique for pancreas transplantation involves anastomosis of the pancreatic vascular supply to the iliac artery and vein. A major issue in pancreatic transplantation is ensuring safe drainage of exocrine secretions. The two options employed are drainage of the pancreatic duct into the bladder and drainage of the duct into the small intestine. Bladder drainage has a lower infection rate, but it is associated with metabolic acidosis due to bicarbonate losses in the urine, as well as cystitis, urethral stricture, and hematuria. This has led to a recent increase in the use of enteric drainage.

Compared with other solid-organ transplant operations, rejection is more difficult to diagnose in pancreas transplantation for a number of reasons. Hyperglycemia is not manifested until a significant portion of the graft is lost. For grafts drained into the bladder, decreases in urinary amylase concentrations sometimes suggest that rejection is occurring, although this test is not very sensitive. Needle core biopsies under ultrasound guidance using 18- or 20-gauge needles have reduced complications associated with biopsies to 2% to 3%.[6] The problem of detecting rejection of pancreatic grafts has prompted efforts to carry out simultaneous pancreatic and kidney transplants, using the kidney as a "canary" to detect rejection of both organs. This indicator of rejection is not as effective in pancreas-after-kidney transplants, because the two organs are immunologically distinct, as evidenced by higher pancreas graft loss rates after pancreas-after-kidney procedures as compared with simultaneous transplants (22% versus 15%).[7] The advantage of early identification of rejection must be balanced against the increased risk of perioperative complications as a consequence of the more challenging simultaneous operation.

Ethical Issues

A number of ethical issues are related to transplantation. Unstated (and/or unintended) coercion to donate can be overwhelming for the family members or loved ones of a patient with renal failure. The physician must act as an advisor, not only for the recipient but also for potential donors. The risk of mortality for donors is low (0%-0.03%), but there is a complication rate of 18%.[8] There is some evidence that renal donors are at slightly increased risk for late renal failure after donation.[9,10] These issues mandate a frank and open discussion prior to donation.

Another ethical issue that arises relates to transplanting a pancreas without performing a kidney transplant in a patient with diabetes mellitus without renal insufficiency. In most patients with normal renal function, the benefits of being insulin free do not outweigh the long-term risks of immunosuppression. It is reasonable to consider pancreas transplant alone in diabetics without end-stage renal failure if there is evidence of early diabetic nephropathy or problems related to blood glucose control are disabling (e.g., lack of awareness of hypoglycemia) or in patients when two or more secondary diabetic complications are present.

TABLE 196-1	Kidney, Pancreas, and Kidney-Pancreas Transplant Statistics				
Organ	No. of Transplants, 7/1/08–6/30/09	Transplant Rate (per Year on Waitlist)	1/5-Year Graft Survival (%)	1/5-Year Patient Survival (%)
Kidney-cad	10,589[†]	0.13[†]	90/68[†]	95/81[†]
Kidney-liver	6,232[‡]	0.19[*]	95/81[‡]	98/91[‡]
Pancreas	396	0.23	81/53	98/89
Kidney-pancreas	861	0.41	93/79[§] 86/73[‖]	95/87

*Both living and cadaver donors.
[†]Cadaver donor.
[‡]Living donor.
[§]Kidney graft survival.
[‖]Pancreas graft survival.
2008 Annual Report of the U.S. Organ Procurement and Transplantation Network and the Scientific Registry of Transplant Recipients: transplant data 1998-2007. Department of Health and Human Services, Health Resources and Services Administration, Healthcare Systems Bureau, Division of Transplantation, Rockville, MD; United Network for Organ Sharing, Richmond, VA; University Renal Research and Education Association, Ann Arbor, MI. Available at: http://optn.transplant.hrsa.gov/ and at http://www.ustransplant.org/

TABLE 196-2	Immunosuppressive Agents and Mechanism of Action		
Class of Agent	Uses	Mechanism of Action
Corticosteroids (methylprednisolone, prednisone)	Induction, maintenance, rejection	Redistribution of lymphocytes Block T-cell proliferation, IL-2 synthesis
Antilymphocyte antibodies (antithymocyte globulin, OKT-3)	Induction, rejection	Lymphocyte depletion
Humanized antibodies (basiliximab, daclizumab)	Induction, rejection	Specific targets: IL-2 receptor
Calcineurin inhibitors (cyclosporine, tacrolimus)	Maintenance, rejection	Inhibit IL-2 production Inhibit expansion and differentiation of T cells
Proliferation signal inhibitors (sirolimus [rapamycin], everolimus)	Maintenance	Block cytokine-driven cell cycle progression
Antimetabolites/ antiproliferative agents (azathioprine, mycophenolate mofetil)	Maintenance	Inhibit RNA/DNA synthesis

IL-2, interleukin-2.

A third ethical issue frequently encountered by critical care physicians relates to the decision to reduce temporarily or to discontinue immunosuppression when a transplant recipient presents with a proven or suspected infection. Tension can exist among the critical care team, the transplant team, and the patient surrounding this issue. On the one hand is the possibility of death from uncontrolled infection, and on the other hand is the loss of a kidney or pancreas graft that would provide considerable improvement in the quality of life.

Current Immunosuppressive Agents/Regimens

The field of immunosuppression has undergone many changes over the past decade, driven by a much better understanding of the immune system, allowing the development of targeted therapies. Most patients will receive a combination of agents to prevent rejection. These agents include calcineurin antagonists (cyclosporine, tacrolimus), proliferation signal inhibitors (sirolimus, rapamycin, or everolimus), proliferation inhibitors (azathioprine, mycophenolate mofetil), and corticosteroids. Other agents frequently used to combat rejection include antilymphocyte antibodies and interleukin (IL)-2 receptor antagonists. Induction therapy with anti-T-cell antibodies or IL-2

receptor antibodies are commonly utilized in pancreas transplantation. A summary of these agents and mechanisms of action is provided in Table 196-2.

Most of the immunosuppressants have significant side effects and toxicities and significant drug interactions. For a complete discussion of this issue, please see Chapter 176. Common side effects of immunosuppressive agents are summarized in Table 196-3.

Common Related Diseases and Conditions

The vast majority of patients receiving kidney and/or pancreas transplants do not require admission to the intensive care unit (ICU). For those patients who do require admission, most are admitted because of perioperative difficulties, which are frequently related to an underlying medical disorder (Box 196-2). A number of medical illnesses are more common in patients with chronic renal failure, including atherosclerotic heart disease, hypertension, congestive heart failure, diabetes mellitus, chronic obstructive pulmonary disease, peripheral vascular disease, and cerebrovascular disease. Discussions with the patient or family often will reveal a history of one or more of these illnesses,

Box 196-1

COMMON INDICATIONS FOR KIDNEY TRANSPLANT*

Diabetes mellitus
Hypertensive nephrosclerosis
Glomerular diseases
Retransplant/graft failure
Polycystic kidney disease
Tubular/interstitial diseases
Renovascular and other vascular diseases
Congenital, rare, familial, and metabolic disorders
Neoplasm

*Includes both living and cadaver donors, listed in order of frequency of transplant.
2008 Annual Report of the U.S. Organ Procurement and Transplantation Network and the Scientific Registry of Transplant Recipients: transplant data 1998-2007. Department of Health and Human Services, Health Resources and Services Administration, Healthcare Systems Bureau, Division of Transplantation, Rockville, MD; United Network for Organ Sharing, Richmond, VA; University Renal Research and Education Association, Ann Arbor, MI. Available at: http://optn.transplant.hrsa.gov/

TABLE 196-3	Side Effects of Common Immunosuppressive Agents
Antithymocyte globulin	Fever, leukopenia, thrombocytopenia, serum sickness
Azathioprine, mycophenolate mofetil	Leukopenia, thrombocytopenia, anemia, diarrhea, abdominal pain, hepatotoxicity, pancreatitis
Basiliximab, daclizumab	Hypersensitivity (anaphylaxis), fever
Corticosteroids	Hyperglycemia, osteoporosis, impaired wound healing, hypertension, Cushingoid facies, Addisonian crisis (from rapid withdrawal)
Cyclosporine	Nephrotoxicity, neurotoxicity, drug interactions, hypertension, hyperkalemia, hirsutism, gingival hyperplasia
Sirolimus, everolimus	Hyperlipidemia, myelosuppression, impaired wound healing, diarrhea, arthralgia, pneumonitis
Tacrolimus	Nephrotoxicity, neurotoxicity, drug interactions, hypertension, hyperkalemia, diarrhea, diabetes, tremor
OKT-3	Pulmonary edema, fever, rigors, diarrhea, headache, bronchospasm, increased cytomegalovirus infection, risk of posttransplant lymphoproliferative disorder

COMMON PREEXISTING ILLNESSES COMPLICATING POSTOPERATIVE CARE IN RENAL ALLOGRAFT RECIPIENTS

Atherosclerotic heart disease
Hypertension
Congestive heart failure
Diabetes mellitus
Chronic obstructive pulmonary disease
Peripheral vascular disease
Cerebrovascular disease

allowing evaluation and treatment to be tailored appropriately for the patient.

Routine Perioperative Care: Kidney or Kidney/Pancreas Transplant

For typical kidney transplant recipients without acute tubular necrosis, a brisk diuresis begins within minutes of revascularization of the kidney graft. This diuresis is due to a number of factors including intraoperative administration of diuretics, proximal tubular damage related to allograft ischemia, fluid and electrolyte disturbances as a result of chronic renal failure, and osmotic factors related to uremia. In patients after kidney-pancreas transplantation, the diuresis also can be related to hyperglycemia. Tight control of blood glucose concentration should be achieved using an insulin infusion. Many patients who were euglycemic before transplantation become hyperglycemic after transplantation, owing to the effects of corticosteroids (occasionally administered to prevent rejection) and the stress of surgery. The appropriate target for blood glucose control remains controversial, with recent evidence showing no benefit to tight glucose control.[11] Nonetheless, in pancreas transplant patients in particular, insulin infusions around the time of transplant have been associated with improved islet function.[12] Our current practice is to maintain blood glucose concentration at 80 to 140 mg/dL. An example of an insulin drip protocol is noted in Figure 196-1. Urinary losses should be corrected with a hypotonic solution; a common prescription is 2.5% dextrose in 0.2% saline infused at a rate of 1 mL per milliliter of urinary output for the first 12 to 24 hours after transplantation. Sodium bicarbonate and potassium chloride should be added as needed, based on frequent measurements of serum electrolyte concentrations. Urine volumes of less than 100 to 200 mL/h within the first 12 hours after renal transplant may represent a problem with the graft, and this finding should be immediately communicated to the transplant service (Box 196-3).

Immunosuppression is typically initiated in the operating room and continued postoperatively. At most transplant centers, the dosing of the immunosuppressive agents is protocol driven and determined by the transplant service. Examples of standard protocols for kidney transplant and simultaneous kidney-pancreas transplant patients are illustrated in Table 196-4.

Prophylactic antibiotics appropriate to cover skin and genitourinary flora should be given for 24 to 48 hours. Potential agents include ampicillin/sulbactam (1.5-3 g intravenously [IV] every 6 hours), ertapenem (1 g IV daily), ceftriaxone (1 g IV daily), and gatifloxacin (40 mg IV daily). There is no evidence to support longer courses of antibiotics in kidney transplant recipients. Trimethoprim/sulfamethoxazole (80 mg trimethoprim/40 mg sulfamethoxazole by mouth [PO] daily) or dapsone (50 mg PO daily for sulfa-allergic patients) is used routinely at most centers for prophylaxis against *Pneumocystis jirovecii* and *Nocardia* species. Prophylaxis for cytomegalovirus is given at our center (valganciclovir dosed by renal function) for 3 to 6 months.

Several specific issues should be considered in pancreas transplantation aside from the usual management of kidney transplantation. The

first of these is related to the high rate of graft loss in pancreas transplants owing to portal venous thrombosis. Many centers use a low-dose anticoagulation regimen of unfractionated heparin (100-500 units IV hourly as a continuous drip) in an effort to reduce graft loss from this complication. Systemic anticoagulation increases the risk of postoperative hemorrhage. Second, there is a high incidence of wound and intraabdominal infections after pancreas transplantation, being as great as 47% in some centers.[13,14] Some centers advocate longer courses of broad-spectrum antibiotics because of concerns about infection, although data to support this practice are lacking.

Posttransplant Complications

Posttransplant issues requiring ICU admission can be divided into those occurring immediately post transplant and those occurring at some time remote to the perioperative period. Kidney transplant patients are admitted to the ICU at a frequency of 16 per 1000 patient-years and have a mortality rate associated with admission of 40%, significantly higher than the general population.[15] Common postoperative complications after kidney and/or pancreas transplantation are listed in Table 196-5.

POSTOPERATIVE RESPIRATORY FAILURE

The majority of kidney and/or pancreas transplant patients admitted with a diagnosis of respiratory failure after surgery have a self-limited form of the condition secondary to the residual effects of general anesthesia. These patients can be extubated when awake, and recovery from the effects of neuromuscular blocking agents is complete or nearly so. Other causes of immediate postoperative respiratory failure include congestive heart failure from perioperative myocardial infarction (MI), pulmonary edema due to intravascular volume overload secondary to acute tubular necrosis, preexisting pneumonia, aspiration pneumonitis, pulmonary embolus, or (rarely) acute respiratory distress syndrome (ARDS) secondary to intraoperative events or posttransplant pancreatitis. In this setting, it is key to perform a rapid and thorough diagnostic workup to determine the etiology of more serious causes of respiratory failure. This evaluation should include electrocardiography (ECG), determination of circulating levels of cardiac enzymes, chest radiography, arterial blood gas analysis, and measurements of serum electrolytes and blood urea nitrogen (BUN)/creatinine concentration. Based on findings from history, physical examination, and the results of these initial tests, the clinician can obtain additional tests as needed to establish a diagnosis. Additional tests that may be helpful include duplex ultrasound scans of the lower extremities for deep venous thrombosis, spiral computed tomography (CT) of the chest to evaluate for pulmonary embolus, cardiac echocardiography, diagnostic bronchoscopy, and transplant ultrasound and/or biopsy.

RESPIRATORY FAILURE DISTANT TO TRANSPLANT

Occasionally, patients are admitted to the ICU with respiratory insufficiency or failure weeks or years after pancreatic and/or renal transplantation. The differential diagnosis is broadened in these patients because of the increased risk of infection associated with immunosuppression. The differential diagnosis for respiratory failure includes infectious causes, cardiogenic causes, and renal failure. It is important to glean from the patient, family, or records any features such as cytomegalovirus (CMV) status of the patient and donor, past history of cardiac disease, and recent changes in transplantation medications. A rapid workup should take place to evaluate the cause of decompensation. It is frequently necessary to intubate the patient, even in the absence of overt respiratory failure, to perform bronchoscopy for diagnostic evaluation. Initial evaluation should include chest radiography; complete blood cell count; determination of serum electrolytes, BUN/creatinine and cardiac enzymes; sputum sampling; and ECG. It is also prudent to include a rapid screen for CMV in this evaluation. Other tests, including diagnostic bronchoscopy, CT of the chest,

Fairview Health Services
Continuous Intravenous
Insulin Infusion
Adult (>45 kg)   PATIENT INDENTIFICATION

NOTE: This protocol NOT to be used for Diabetic Ketoacidosis (DKA).
      Start protocol if glucose >150 mg/dL
GOAL: Maintain glucose level between 100–150 mg/dL.
      Discontinue when glycemic control achieved and transitioning to SQ Insulin, or insulin therapy no longer required.

GENERAL

☑ Pharmacy Consult: Discontinue all currently active insulin orders on initiation of FV Cont IV Insulin Infusion Orders

☑ Notify MD: For specific instructions regarding insulin infusion IF patient is on TPN or tube feeding which is held or cycled AND start IV D10W at same rate as TPN/tube feeding.

☑ D10W – IV If on IV insulin infusion AND parenteral or enteral nutrition (TPN/TF): Infuse IV D10W at TPN/TF rate whenever nutrition is held or cycled off.

GLUCOSE MONITORING

☑ Glucose Monitoring – Nursing (whole blood glucose) Q1H until BG is stable within 100–150 mg/dL × 4, then Q2H until insulin infusion is discontinued. If subsequent BG values are outside the 100–150 mg/dL range, measure BG Q1 H.

☑ Glucose Level – STAT plasma glucose for changes in mental status, diaphoresis, or unexplained tachycardia

INITIATION OF CONTINUOUS INSULIN INFUSION PROTOCOL

NOTE: Insulin infusions will be provided as 1 unit Regular Insulin / mL 0.9% Sodium Chloride unless otherwise requested.

STEP ONE

☐ Insulin Regular Human _____ units (0.1 units/kg; MAX dose 10 units) IV bolus. Administer IF BG >175mg/dL

STEP TWO

☑ Insulin Regular Human (1 unit/mL) Drip – Initiate drip with Algorithm 1
    Move to HIGHER number algorithm:
    If BG >200 mg/dL AND BG has not fallen by at least 60 mg/dL within the previous hour.
    IF BG remains out of target range (100–150 mg/dL) and has not moved toward goal for two consecultive hours, move up to the next algorithm.
    IF in Algorithm 4, titrate the infusion up by 1 unit per hour AND Notify MD.
    Move to LOWER number algorithm:
    If BG <100 mg/dL × 2 consecutive readings. Unless already at Algorithm 1.

Algorithm 1		Algorithm 2		Algorithm 3		Algorithm 4	
BG	Units/hr	BG	Units/hr	BG	Units/hr	BG	Units/hr
<70 = Hypoglycemia (follow hypoglycemia orders)							
70–99	Off	70–99	Off	70–99	Off	70–99	Off
100–124	0.2	100–124	1	100–124	1.5	100–124	2
125–149	0.5	125–149	2	125–149	3	125–149	4
150–175	1	150–175	3	150–175	4	150–175	6
176–200	1.5	176–200	4	176–200	5.5	176–200	8
201–225	2	201–225	5	201–225	7	201–225	10
226–250	2.5	226–250	6	226–250	8.5	226–250	12
251–275	3	251–275	7	251–275	10	251–275	14
276–300	3.5	276–300	8	276–300	11.5	276–300	16
301–325	4	301–325	9	301–325	13	301–325	18
326–350	4.5	326–350	10	326–350	14.5	326–350	20
351–375	5	351–375	11	351–375	16	351–375	22
>375	5.5	>375	12	>375	17.5	>375	24

TRANSITION FROM IV INSULIN INFUSION TO SQ INSULIN

NOTE: When blood glucose has stabilized and patient is tolerating PO intake, call MD for transition to SQ insulin.
    See FV SQ Insulin Management Orders, #510111, for transition orders.

HYPOGLYCEMIA MANAGEMENT

☑ FV Hypoglycemia Management, Adult (>45 kg)

PROVIDER SIGNATURE: _____ **DATE:** _____ **TIME:** _____

PROVIDER NAME (print): _____ **PAGER #:** _____

FAIRVIEW HEALTH SERVICES – PHYSICIAN ORDERS
CONTINUOUS INTRAVENOUS INSULIN INFUSION, ADULT (>45 KG)

510403 Feb 2010   ORIGINAL: Medical Record   COPY: Pharmacy   PAGE 1 OF 1

B3b/D9

Figure 196-1   Example of intravenous insulin infusion order set.

echocardiography, and lower extremity Doppler examinations, should be carried out as clinically indicated. Typically, the noninfectious causes of respiratory failure, such as renal failure with fluid overload and myocardial dysfunction causing congestive heart failure, are more readily identified and treated, leaving the more subtle causes to sort through over the next several days of the patient's ICU course. Exclusion of cardiac and renal failure mandates strong consideration for the possibility of an infectious cause of respiratory compromise.

Initial treatment for posttransplant respiratory failure distant to surgery requires broad-spectrum antibacterial, fungal, and viral therapy until a definitive diagnosis is reached. It is not unusual in such circumstances to have patients on agents that will cover common bacterial organisms, *Candida* and *Aspergillus*, and CMV (see also Chapter 195). Common regimens include broad-spectrum antibiotic agents with antipseudomonal and antianaerobic activity, an agent with gram-positive activity, a broad-spectrum antifungal agent, and ganciclovir to

CAUSES OF OLIGURIA AFTER KIDNEY TRANSPLANT

Clots in bladder
Acute tubular necrosis
Arterial/venous thrombosis
Acute rejection
Ureteral/bladder anastomotic leak

provide antiviral coverage for cytomegalovirus and other members of the herpesvirus family. Similarly to other work in the ICU care, delay to appropriate antibiotics in transplant patients has been associated with worsened outcomes.[16] A number of appropriate agents for this purpose are listed in Table 196-6. In situations where *Pseudomonas* is strongly suspected, an additional agent should be added to provide double coverage of this organism. In situations where the patient has high risk for or has known vancomycin-resistant *Enterococcus faecium*, one of the new gram-positive agents should be chosen. Another key component of treatment in this setting is strong consideration for short-term discontinuation of most immunosuppressive medications. The practice at our institution is to hold all but maintenance doses of corticosteroids when infection is strongly suspected. It is frequently possible to tailor antimicrobial therapy as results return. For instance, in the setting of a patient with a low white blood cell count, diffuse pneumonitis, and positive screen for CMV, it is not unreasonable to discontinue antifungal therapy. It is important for the intensivist to be willing to revisit the diagnosis on at least a daily basis, especially if the clinical course is not consistent with the working diagnosis.

TABLE 196-4	Examples of Immunosuppression Protocols for Kidney Transplant and Simultaneous Pancreas-Kidney Transplant in the Immediate Postoperative Period*

a. **Kidney Transplant:** Non-HLA-identical living recipients and all cadaver recipients with immediate graft function (1st and 2nd transplant). MMF, mycophenolate mofetil; PRED, prednisone; TMG, thymoglobulin.

Day	Tacrolimus	MMF	PRED	TMG
0		1-1.5 g intraoperatively	500 mg IV	1.25 mg/kg intraoperatively
1	Begin Neoral	1-1.5 g BID	1 mg/kg/d	1.25 mg/kg/d for 4 days
2	Twice-a-day dosing	Continue	0.5 mg/kg/d	
3		Non-African Americans	0.5 mg/kg/d	
4	Maintain levels	Receive 1 g BID	0.25 mg/kg/d	
5	Between 150 and 200	African Americans	0.25 mg/kg/d	
6	HPLC	Receive 1.5 g BID	DC	

b. **Simultaneous Kidney-Pancreas Transplant**
Thymoglobulin
Give 1.25 mg/kg intraoperatively (methylprednisolone, 500 mg IV prior to 1st dose)
Give 1.25 mg/kg daily thereafter for a total of 5 doses (methylprednisolone, 250 mg IV prior to 2nd dose, 100 mg IV prior to 3rd dose)
Tacrolimus
2 mg PO BID
Begin when creatinine < 3 or POD#5, whichever is greater (levels 8-10 ng/mL for 6 months, then 5-8 ng/mL thereafter).
Mycophenolate Mofetil
Start postoperatively
1 g PO BID

*Please note that immunosuppressive regimens at most institutions undergo frequent change and vary by recipient status, crossmatch, graft function, and other variables.
BID, twice daily; *DC,* discontinue; *HPLC,* high-performance liquid chromatography; *IV,* intravenous; *PO,* per os (oral).

TABLE 196-5	Common Postoperative Complications: Kidney, Kidney-Pancreas, Pancreas Transplant
Early	*Late*
Myocardial infarction	Myocardial infarction
Renal failure	Renal failure
Hyperglycemia	Transplant artery stenosis
Graft thrombosis	Respiratory failure
Hemorrhage	Posttransplant infection (immune-compromised host)
Wound infection	
Respiratory failure	Posttransplant lymphoproliferative disorder
Posttransplant infection (hospital acquired)	Graft pancreatitis
Deep venous thrombosis	Acute and chronic rejection
Metabolic acidosis	
Graft pancreatitis	
Hyperacute and acute rejection	
Bladder leak	
Pseudomembranous colitis	

POSTOPERATIVE OLIGURIA

Postoperative oliguria (see Box 196-3) is a frequent problem in the renal transplant patient. Common causes include blood clots in the bladder causing outflow obstruction, acute tubular necrosis, arterial or venous thrombosis, and acute rejection. Many patients present in the immediate postoperative period with oliguria and suspected acute tubular necrosis (also called *delayed graft function* in this context). In these patients, it is important to monitor fluid balance closely; many will require urgent dialysis for fluid overload or hyperkalemia. Most patients with acute tubular necrosis in the early postoperative period recover adequate renal function and become able to function without dialysis, albeit with less renal reserve than those patients with immediate graft function.[17] Recovery can be delayed for as long as 3 months.

TABLE 196-6	Empirical Agents for Early Treatment of Infection in Kidney/Pancreas Transplant Patients

Class of Agent	Agent	Dose*
Broad-spectrum antibiotic agents[†]	Piperacillin/tazobactam	3.375 g IV q 6 h
	Meropenem	0.5-1 g IV q 8 h
	Imipenem/cilastatin	0.5-1 g IV q 6-8 h
Gram-positive agents[‡]	Vancomycin	1-1.5 g IV q 12-24 h
	Daptomycin[§]	4-6 mg/kg IV daily
	Quinupristin/dalfopristin	7.5 mg/kg IV q 8 h
	Linezolid	600 mg IV q 12 h
	Tigecycline[‖]	100 mg IV load, 50 mg IV q 12 h
Antifungal agents	Voriconazole	6 mg/kg IV q 12 h × 2, then 4 mg/kg IV q 12 h
	Posaconazole	Oral only: 200 mg 3-4 times daily
	Caspofungin	70 mg load, 50 mg IV daily
	Anidulafungin	200 mg load, 100 mg IV daily
	Liposomal amphotericin B	3-10 mg/kg IV daily
Antiviral agents[¶]	Ganciclovir	2.5-5 mg/kg IV q 12 h
	Foscarnet	90 mg/kg IV q 12 h

*Please note that doses given do not account for renal or hepatic insufficiency common in critically ill patients. Prior to choosing an empirical antibiotic regimen, the clinician should carefully consider the patient scenario and medication side effects related to the specific patient.
[†]Rather than a single agent, combination agents covering both gram-negative organisms and anaerobes may be chosen (e.g., fluoroquinolone plus clindamycin or metronidazole). For cases with a strong suspicion for *Pseudomonas aeruginosa* infection, additional *Pseudomonas* coverage should be added (e.g., fluoroquinolone or aminoglycoside).
[‡]When vancomycin-resistant *Enterococcus faecium* infection is suspected, one of the latter 4 choices should be employed.
[§]Daptomycin is not indicated for treatment of pneumonia (package insert).
[‖]Tigecycline is not indicated for treatment of hospital-acquired pneumonia (package insert).
[¶]Antiviral agents directed toward herpesvirus family (most commonly CMV). Adjust for other viruses.

TABLE 196-7	Major Causes of Graft Loss After Kidney Transplant		
	Incidence*		
Cause	*<1 yr*	*1-5 yr*	*>5 yr*
Thrombosis	25%	0%	0%
Acute rejection	15%	2%	0%
Chronic rejection	6%	28%	25%
Death with function	41%	52%	57%
Noncompliance	4%	9%	11%

*Percent of grafts lost during time period.
Modified from Matas AJ, Humar A, Gillingham KJ et al. Five preventable causes of kidney graft loss in the 1990s: a single-center analysis. Kidney Int 2002;62:704-14.

Decreased urine output within several hours of arrival to the ICU mandates a rapid evaluation. Steps should include irrigation of the Foley catheter to exclude outflow obstruction due to clots and optimization of hemodynamic status to maintain adequate renal perfusion. The transplant service should be immediately notified for a significant change in urine output. After irrigation of the catheter to ensure patency, initial evaluation should include complete blood cell count, determination of serum electrolytes and BUN/creatinine, and transplant ultrasound to assess for blood flow to the kidney and fluid collections. A radioisotope renal scan is occasionally helpful to exclude a urinary anastomotic leak or obstruction of the transplanted ureter. A decrease in hemoglobin concentration suggests the possibility of surgical bleeding and may indicate a need for return to the operating room.

Among patients who underwent transplantation in the more distant past, the likely causes of oliguria are quite different and include acute or chronic rejection, renal artery stenosis, toxic effects of medications, especially calcineurin inhibitors, and BK virus nephropathy. Major causes of graft loss after kidney and/or pancreas transplant are listed in Table 196-7.[18] Important studies in addition to baseline laboratory assays should include drug levels of calcineurin inhibitors, Doppler ultrasound of the transplant, and radioisotope scan. Renal biopsy and angiography also may be indicated. BK viremia and viruria can be detected by qualitative and quantitative polymerase chain reaction (PCR) techniques.[19] Ultrasound is an excellent noninvasive way to screen for vascular complications, including renal artery stenosis, arteriovenous fistulas, and pseudoaneurysms. Radioisotope scans are a very useful noninvasive modality for assessment of renal function.[20] Management depends on diagnosis but requires careful titration of IV fluids based upon clinical assessment of intravascular volume status and control of hypertension. Renal artery stenosis is typically treated successfully with angiographic stent placement.

HYPERTENSION

Hypertension is common both immediately post transplant and long term. There is evidence that early postoperative hypertension is associated with delayed graft function,[21,22] making perioperative control of hypertension an important feature of postoperative care. Acute management of hypertension in the ICU consists of appropriate parenteral antihypertensives, including β-adrenergic blockers or hydralazine.[23] There are no specific guidelines for appropriate agents in transplant patients. We use an intermediate-acting beta-blocker such as labetalol (10-20 mg IV every 4 to 6 hours) until heart rate is less than 90 beats per minute, then IV hydralazine (10-20 mg IV every 4-6 hours) as needed. A continuous infusion of esmolol offers the benefits of rapid titration. Sodium nitroprusside is reserved for hypertension not controlled with other measures, because of concerns about cyanide toxicity. It is important in this population to titrate blood pressure so that perfusion pressure to the transplanted organ is maintained.

Tacrolimus and cyclosporine are associated with development of new hypertension in patients after renal transplant (25% and 35% of cases, respectively).[22] Long-term control of hypertension after renal transplantation can be managed with a number of classes of agents, including calcium channel blockers, angiotensin-converting enzyme inhibitors, angiotensin-II type-1 receptor blockers, diuretics, and β-adrenergic blockers. Many authors suggest use of a calcium channel blocker as first-line therapy for chronic use, owing to evidence that these agents can reduce cyclosporine-induced renal damage.[23]

MYOCARDIAL INFARCTION

Patients receiving chronic dialysis and those with diabetes mellitus are at increased risk of MI. In a single-center study of approximately 2700 kidney transplant recipients, the incidence of perioperative cardiac complications was 6.1%.[24] Risk factors for posttransplant cardiac events include age, pretransplant cardiac disease, diabetes, arrhythmia, and low ejection fraction (<40%).[25] Preoperative cardiac evaluation and percutaneous coronary intervention in this population may help reduce the perioperative risk of death but does not necessarily reduce the risk of perioperative MI.[26] It is prudent in a patient with risk factors to consider perioperative β-adrenergic blockade and aspirin.

The clinical diagnosis of MI is difficult in many cases because of perioperative pain. It is prudent to evaluate at-risk patients with perioperative measurements of circulating troponin levels. Cardiac screening should be considered in diabetics, in patients with a history of cardiac disease, and in patients with intraoperative hypotension. Elevated circulating troponin levels should be followed by transthoracic echocardiography to evaluate for new wall-motion abnormalities in addition to ECG testing. Treatment of MI in early perioperative patients typically does not include thrombolytic therapy, owing to concerns for hemorrhage. This factor and the different pathophysiology of perioperative MI contributes to increased mortality in the transplant population (20%)[25] as well as others (25%).[26] For hemodynamically stable patients with only slight increases in circulating troponin levels and new wall-motion abnormalities on echocardiography, the most prudent course may be medical therapy consisting of aspirin and β-adrenergic blockade with or without systemic heparinization. Invasive intervention may be indicated for patients with hemodynamic instability or other signs of progression of MI.

GASTROINTESTINAL PROBLEMS

Appropriate management of abdominal complications in transplant recipients requires a high index of suspicion because immunosuppression can mask many of the early signs of peritonitis. CT of the abdomen should be performed early in the process of evaluating new or changing abdominal pain in renal or pancreatic transplant recipients.

The transplant population is at risk for development of upper and lower gastrointestinal (GI) tract involvement with CMV, leading to abdominal pain, bleeding, and (rarely) perforation. CMV will most commonly occur the first time within about 6 months of transplantation, correlating with the highest immunosuppressive load. CMV infections are more common in patients when the recipient was serologically negative, but the donor was CMV positive. CMV-related problems are also more common among those patients with CMV infection and those treated with relatively high doses of immunosuppression.[27] Diagnostic endoscopy should include tissue biopsies of the stomach or colon to determine whether CMV is present. Initial treatment consists of IV ganciclovir or foscarnet, with a switch to maintenance therapy by oral agents as tolerated for a period of weeks to months (see Table 196-6 for initial IV dosing).

Colon perforation and lower GI hemorrhage are the most common lower tract complications in kidney transplant recipients. Immunosuppressive therapy can mask the signs and symptoms of peritonitis, delaying diagnosis of perforation. Colonic perforation can be due to pseudomembranous enterocolitis, acute colonic pseudo-obstruction (Ogilvie's syndrome), diverticulitis, ischemic colitis, stercoral perforation, fecal impaction, or other forms of colitis. Diverticulitis may be more common in patients with polycystic kidney disease (20% versus 3% in one small retrospective analysis),[28] and this group of patients also had a higher incidence of GI surgical complications.[29] Colonic perforation is an infrequent complication post transplant (21 of 1611 transplants at one center) with a high risk of death (24%). Perforation in this setting is associated with high-dose immunosuppression.[30] Surgical therapy for perforated diverticulitis typically includes colostomy, because a fresh anastomosis in this setting is more likely to leak. Perioperative therapy should include broad-spectrum antibiotics directed at gram-negative and gram-positive aerobes, anaerobes, and fungi. Stress-dose corticosteroids should be administered as clinically indicated.

PSEUDOMEMBRANOUS COLITIS

Pseudomembranous colitis due to *Clostridium difficile* should be suspected in any transplant patient presenting with diarrhea. Risk factors for development of pseudomembranous colitis include previous antibiotic therapy and immunosuppression. Pseudomembranous colitis is diagnosed by detecting *C. difficile* toxin in stool. Controversy exists regarding the need for treatment in patients who are *C. difficile* culture positive but *C. difficile* toxin negative, because *C. difficile* may be present but not pathogenic. The development of serious complications due to *C. difficile*, such as toxic megacolon, are directly related to the time from onset of symptoms to the time of initiation of therapy. There is a new virulent strain of *C. difficile* (NAP1/B1/027) associated with increased morbidity and mortality, making the need for early diagnosis a high priority.[31] Empirical therapy should be started when the diagnosis is considered and then discontinued if stool samples are negative for *C. difficile* toxin. Therapy for *C. difficile* enterocolitis consists of either metronidazole (250 mg PO every 6 hours for 10 days) or vancomycin (125 mg PO every 6 hours for 10 days). The cure rate for *C. difficile* enterocolitis seems to be higher for vancomycin than for metronidazole, especially in more severe disease (97% versus 76%).[32] Given this concern, it seems prudent to consider oral vancomycin for transplant patients with a clinical scenario consistent with *C. difficile* infection.

REJECTION

Rejection is classified according to its temporal relation to the transplant and includes hyperacute, acute, and chronic rejection. Each of these types is mediated via different immunologic mechanisms. Hyperacute rejection occurs within minutes to hours of the transplant and is caused by preformed antibody directed against the transplanted organ. This type of rejection is very uncommon owing to appropriate pretransplant tissue typing. Acute rejection is the most common type of rejection in current clinical transplantation (occurring in 15%-60% of renal transplant patients).[33] This type of rejection is most frequent within the first 6 weeks to 6 months after transplantation and is the result of activation of host T lymphocytes by antigens in the transplanted organ. Chronic rejection is common in transplanted organs, developing typically over years to decades. Its etiology is less well understood, but it appears to be related to accumulation of microvascular injury over time.

Diagnosis of Rejection

Acute rejection of a renal allograft is typically suspected when the serum creatinine and BUN concentrations increase. Other causes should be considered as well, including hypovolemia, drug toxicity, ureteral obstruction, lymphocele, or vascular anastomotic complications. Diagnosis of acute rejection is confirmed by percutaneous biopsy and histopathologic examination, which show edema and focal infiltration of the interstitium and peritubular capillaries by lymphocytes. Another characteristic finding of acute rejection is invasion of tubular epithelial cells by lymphocytes. Diagnosis of pancreas allograft rejection is more problematic. Increased rates of rejection have been reported after simultaneous kidney-pancreas transplant compared with kidney transplant alone.[34] Hyperglycemia is a late finding and occurs after loss of significant islet cell mass. For simultaneous kidney-pancreas grafts, increases in the serum creatinine concentration may prompt suspicion of pancreatic rejection as well. If the pancreatic duct has been anastomosed to the bladder, a decrease in urinary amylase concentration may be helpful as a marker of graft rejection.[35] New techniques using biomarkers have much promise but have not yet been widely evaluated.[36] Biopsy of the pancreas graft may be performed either percutaneously or via cystoscopy to confirm the presence of rejection. This procedure has a complication rate of 2.8%.[6] Because the incidence of venous thrombosis is high in pancreas transplantation, Doppler ultrasound should be performed to evaluate this possibility.

Treatment of acute rejection varies between transplant centers. A common initial approach is bolus therapy with high-dose methylprednisolone at a dose of 500 mg to 1 g IV daily. Severe rejection is more commonly treated with antibody therapy consisting of OKT3 or one of the newer antibodies. These treatments are beyond the scope of the present discussion and have been recently reviewed.[37-39] Treatment of acute rejection is usually successful and is typically followed by adjustment of immunosuppression with a switch to different agents.

GRAFT THROMBOSIS

Arterial or venous thrombosis of the kidney allograft should be considered promptly if an established diuresis abruptly ceases in the immediate postoperative period. The transplant service should be immediately notified because prompt reoperation provides the only opportunity for salvage. The diagnosis can be rapidly established either by Doppler ultrasound or by inspection at the time of reoperation. Pancreatic allograft thrombosis may be related to either technical problems or high vascular resistance in the graft from preservation-related or immunologic injury. The incidence of graft thrombosis for pancreas allografts is 6%.[2] Many centers routinely administer low-dose heparin, dextran, or antiplatelet agents to prevent this complication (e.g., unfractionated heparin, 100-300 units IV/h; aspirin, 325 mg PO/d). The use of anticoagulant and/or antiplatelet therapy in this population may be associated with an increased risk of bleeding complications. Signs of pancreatic graft thrombosis include hematuria, tenderness, and swelling of the graft. Treatment for this condition is removal of the graft.

DEEP VENOUS THROMBOSIS

Deep venous thrombosis is a common complication of most major surgical procedures, including kidney or pancreas transplantation.[40] After these procedures patients should receive standard prophylaxis consisting of low-dose fractionated or unfractionated heparin (unfractionated heparin, 5000 units subcutaneously [SQ] twice daily; Lovenox, 0.5 mg SQ twice daily), and application of sequential compression devices.

Iliofemoral thrombosis occasionally follows renal or pancreas transplant, presumably owing to injury of the vein at the time of transplantation. Typically these thromboses respond to standard-dose anticoagulation. Thrombolytics may be considered, especially in the patient who is more than 2 to 3 weeks out from surgery. The use of vena cava filters for patients with proximal deep venous thrombosis, persistent pulmonary embolus, or bleeding complications of anticoagulation is potentially an issue because of the theoretical risk of occlusion of the transplanted renal or portal vein. However, compromised transplant function is rare after placement of a vena cava filter,[41] and it is our practice to place a vena cava filter in this situation.

TRANSPLANT-ASSOCIATED INFECTIOUS DISEASE

The price of success in transplantation is increased susceptibility to infections due to the need for suppression of the host's immune response (see also Chapter 176). As many as 63% of solid-organ transplant recipients experience an infectious complication within the first year of transplant.[42] The risk of infection is highest during the period of most intensive immunosuppression (typically the first 6-12 months) and increases with treatment of rejection. The most frequent infections seen early and late after transplantation are presented in Table 196-8.[43]

TABLE 196-8	Risk of Infection After Transplant with Respect to Time After Transplant	
Within 6 Weeks	**6 Weeks to 6 Months**	**Greater Than 6 Months**
Viral		
Herpes simplex	Cytomegalovirus (pneumonia)	Cytomegalovirus (retinitis, colitis)
Hepatitis B, C	Hepatitis B, C	Hepatitis B, C
	Epstein-Barr virus	Papillomavirus
	Varicella-zoster	Posttransplant
	Influenza	lymphoproliferative
	Respiratory syncytial virus	disorder
	Adenovirus	
	Polyoma (BK) virus	
Bacterial		
Nosocomial infection (e.g., line, pneumonia, wound, urinary tract infection)	Nocardiosis	Listeriosis
	Listeriosis from *Listeria monocytogenes*	Tuberculosis
	Tuberculosis	
Fungal		
Candidosis	Candidosis	Cryptococcosis
	Aspergillosis	Coccidioidomycosis
	Cryptococcosis	Histoplasmosis
	Coccidioidomycosis	*P. jiroveci* infection
	Histoplasmosis	
	Pneumocystis jiroveci infection	
Parasitic		
	Strongyloidosis	Strongyloidosis
	Toxoplasmosis	
	Leishmaniasis	
	Trypanosoma cruzi infection	

Modified from Snydman DR. Epidemiology of infections after solid-organ transplantation. Clin Infect Dis 2001;33:S5-S8.

Infectious complications in the first month after transplantation are frequently caused by those organisms likely to cause disease in immunocompetent hosts. The time of greatest immunosuppression (1-6 months post transplant) is the time when the majority of opportunistic infections occur. These infections include a number of viral infections (most commonly CMV) and opportunistic fungal infections (most frequently *Candida* and *Aspergillus*).[43] A high index of suspicion for the presence of infection should be maintained when evaluating transplant patients in the ICU. A key component to treatment of infection in transplant patients is decreasing immunosuppression, because many infections will not be successfully treated without this step.

Bacterial infections are common in the first 30 days after transplant and are related both to the site of surgery and the presence of indwelling lines and catheters. Infection of the surgical site is uncommon in the renal transplant recipient (1%-2%) and is comparable to the incidence seen in surgery of immunocompetent patients. Pancreas transplantation, on the other hand, is associated with a 10% to 40% incidence of wound infection.[13,14] Infections from these wounds reflect skin flora, flora of the duodenum and bladder, and flora associated with previous exposure to antibiotics.

Fungal Infections

The immunosuppression associated with solid-organ transplantation increases the risk of fungal infection. The incidence of these infections also may be increased because of the use of broad-spectrum antibacterial agents. Useful agents for treating fungal pathogens include amphotericin B, azoles, and echinocandins. Amphotericin B acts to prevent fungal growth and kills fungi by binding to fungal cell wall sterols and causing cell death via lysis. Azoles inhibit the cytochrome P450 enzyme responsible for ergosterol synthesis. Echinocandins inhibit glucan synthesis, disrupting cell wall structure. The different mechanisms of action of the echinocandins and azoles make consideration of dual therapy attractive. A recent report of transplant recipients with invasive aspergillosis receiving combination therapy of voriconazole and caspofungin showed improved survival in patients with either renal failure or *Aspergillus fumigatus* infection compared to those receiving a lipid formulation of amphotericin B.[44]

The most common fungal pathogens seen are *Candida* species. The widespread use of fluconazole has likely contributed to the increased isolation of *Candida* species resistant to fluconazole. Treatment of suspected fungal infection in the transplant patient in the ICU should therefore consist of an agent with more broad-spectrum antifungal activity, such as amphotericin B (most commonly one of the liposomal forms), caspofungin or anidulafungin (an echinocandin), or voriconazole (an azole with broader antifungal activity). *Aspergillus* infection occurs in approximately 1% of transplant patients and should be considered in patients failing to respond to appropriate initial antimicrobial therapy. The diagnosis of aspergillosis is frequently difficult, and the intensivist may need to empirically initiate therapy well before a final diagnosis is established. Newer diagnostic methods such as galactomannan assay or real-time polymerase chain reaction for *Aspergillus* in the serum or bronchoalveolar lavage (BAL) fluid may allow an earlier diagnosis.[45,46] Sensitivity and specificity of the galactomannan assay is significantly higher in BAL than serum.[46] The high mortality associated with invasive aspergillosis in this population (60%)[47] mandates early empirical therapy.

Viral infections are important causes of morbidity and mortality in renal and pancreas transplant recipients. Endemic viruses of little concern to the immunocompetent population may produce life-threatening infection in the immunosuppressed host. Common viral pathogens in the kidney and pancreas transplant patient include members of the human herpesvirus family, most notably CMV. Infection with this agent affects nearly 50% of kidney and transplant patients; infection occurs during the period from 2 weeks to 3 months after transplantation.[48] The major risk factors for CMV infection include CMV seronegativity when the donor is seropositive, need for higher doses of immunosuppression, or repeated treatment for rejection.[27] The range and severity of infection with CMV is broad. The most commonly affected organs are the lungs, GI tract, liver, retina, and pancreas. The diagnosis of CMV has been recently enhanced by assays identifying CMV antigen in blood or body fluid.[49,50] The primary treatment of CMV infection is prevention, and many transplant centers include ganciclovir or other antiviral therapy in their protocols (valganciclovir, 900 mg once daily; or oral ganciclovir, 1000 mg three times daily within 10 days of transplant and continued through 100 days).[51] Treatment of suspected or identified CMV infection typically consists of IV ganciclovir followed by oral valganciclovir (see Table 196-6).

Polyoma (BK) Virus Infection

Polyomavirus has a prevalence worldwide of about 98% in the general population, with nearly all exposed as a child. After infection, the virus resides in the kidney in a latent form. Reactivation of the virus in kidney transplant recipients can result in an inflammatory interstitial nephritis progressing to renal failure known as *BK-* or *polyoma-associated nephropathy*. Interestingly, this reactivation has so far been associated with complications only in kidney transplant patients. Reactivation has been most closely associated with tacrolimus use and recent treatment for rejection. A prospective study of renal transplant patients has identified the time course of this reactivation process.[52] BK viruria proceeds BK viremia and in renal transplant patients occurred an average of 54 days after transplant. Blood BKV PCR was positive a median of 32 weeks prior to diagnosis of BK nephropathy. In patients with unexplained renal failure after renal transplant, the presence of BK virus should be evaluated using PCR in urine and blood. Patients with a viremia should undergo reduction of immunosuppression. Cidofovir has been evaluated as further treatment but has not demonstrated additional benefit in outcome.[53]

Pneumocystis jiroveci (Previously *carinii*)

Pneumocystis jiroveci is a common cause of pneumonia in immunosuppressed patients and should be considered in any patient presenting with respiratory illness who has had prophylactic therapy (trimethoprim/sulfamethoxazole or dapsone) interrupted. Recent work has led to the reclassification of pneumocystis as an unusual fungus,[54] although some authors have disputed this reclassification.[55] Empirical therapy with IV trimethoprim/sulfamethoxazole (15 mg/kg of the trimethoprim component per day given in 3 divided doses) or pentamidine (4 mg/kg/d) should be initiated before established diagnosis in this patient population because of the high mortality rate of the untreated disease.

POSTTRANSPLANT LYMPHOPROLIFERATIVE DISORDER

Posttransplant lymphoproliferative disorder (PTLD) includes a broad range of conditions ranging from simple lymphoid hyperplasia to lymphoma. The etiology of this disorder in the transplant patient is closely related to infection with Epstein-Barr virus (EBV). PTLD typically occurs during times of most intensive immunosuppression. The incidence of PTLD is low in renal and pancreas transplantation compared with other solid-organ transplants (2.6% at 10 years).[1] The clinical presentation of this disorder varies widely, and many patients present with nonspecific symptoms such as malaise, fever, and weight loss. Occasionally, patients present to the ICU acutely ill with a markedly elevated blood lactate level that is unresponsive to aggressive fluid resuscitation. Evaluation for suspected PTLD should include imaging of the brain, chest, and abdomen, with targeted biopsies to provide a tissue diagnosis. Treatment of patients with PTLD has not been well codified but may include reduction of immunosuppression, administration of interferon alfa (IFN-α), antiviral therapy, chemotherapy, and treatment with an anti-B-cell antibody (rituximab).[56-57] A new approach in monitoring transplant patients is to follow serial Epstein-Barr viral load and use increases as a tool to direct reduction of immunosuppression or other therapy.[58]

Pancreas Transplant

A number of issues are specific to pancreas transplantation, including metabolic acidosis, bladder leak, and graft pancreatitis. Wound infection is more common after pancreas transplantation than after kidney transplantation and should be aggressively treated with appropriate wound care, débridement, and antibiotics. In addition, the pancreas allograft is more likely to suffer thrombosis, leading to graft loss.

Metabolic acidosis in pancreas transplant patients is a consequence of using the bladder to drain bicarbonate-rich pancreatic exocrine secretions. To prevent this problem, patients are typically started on oral therapy with sodium bicarbonate (1300 mg PO 2-3 times daily) to replace losses of the anion via the bladder.

Bladder leak is most commonly from the duodenal segment of the donor pancreas; this is due to devascularization during the graft preparation process or during placement of the graft. A frequent complication (10% of cases), bladder leak is most common during the first several weeks after transplantation.[59] Diagnosis is aided by having a high index of clinical suspicion and may be confirmed with a high degree of accuracy by CT of the area using contrast agent instilled into the bladder.[60] Treatment for smaller leaks consists of prolonged Foley catheter drainage, whereas larger or chronic leaks require operative intervention.

Graft pancreatitis occurs in 16% of pancreas transplant patients and is a significant cause of graft loss.[61,62] Graft pancreatitis early after transplantation is due to preservation-related or ischemic injury to the pancreas and typically is self-limited. However, the development of peripancreatic fluid collections necessitates evaluation for infection and may require operative intervention ranging from opening a deep abscess, to débridement of the involved portions of the pancreas, to removal of the entire pancreatic allograft. Removal, if necessary, is best performed early before development of established organ dysfunction.[62] Late graft pancreatitis is related to reflux from the bladder or CMV infection and can be treated by conversion to enteric drainage or specific antiviral therapy, respectively.

KEY POINTS

1. New development of low urine output in the immediate postoperative period after kidney transplant mandates rapid evaluation for the cause of the oliguria.

2. The incidence of wound infection after pancreas transplant is significant (10%-40%) and is a major cause of postoperative morbidity.

3. Respiratory failure after kidney and/or pancreas transplant can be related to any one of a number of serious causes including infection, cardiac failure, renal failure, and pulmonary embolism. It is important to determine the etiology and initiate therapy rapidly for respiratory failure after kidney and/or pancreas transplantation.

4. Immunosuppressive agents have significant side effects and predispose patients to development of infection.

5. Immunosuppression must be reduced or discontinued in renal and pancreas transplant patients suspected of harboring severe infection.

6. Cytomegalovirus infection is common in renal and pancreas transplant patients and is the cause of significant morbidity.

ANNOTATED REFERENCES

Klouche K, Amigues L, Massanet P, et al. Outcome of renal transplant recipients admitted to an intensive care unit: a 10-year cohort study. Transplantation 2009;87:889-95.

This single-center study reports a retrospective analysis of all renal transplant patients admitted to their ICU over the 10-year period 1997-2007 to evaluate outcome and determine predictive factors of outcome. Of their patient population, 57 were admitted over this time period, equaling a rate of 17 per 1000 patient-years. Mortality was twice the mortality of an unselected population of ICU patients (40% versus 20%). Predictors of mortality included need for mechanical ventilation and mean arterial pressure.

Jeloka TK, Ross H, Smith R, et al. Renal transplant outcome in high-cardiovascular risk recipients. Clin Transplant 2007;21:609-14.

The authors of this work report their experience with patients undergoing renal transplant who have risk factors for cardiac morbidity. The experience included 429 patients with roughly 10% suffering posttransplant cardiac events. Patients who were high risk (pretransplant angina, myocardial infarct, or angiogram) were more likely to die post transplant. Intervention with stenting or bypass grafting did not reduce the risk of postoperative cardiac events.

Thomas MC, Mathew TH, Russ GR, et al. Perioperative blood pressure control, delayed graft function, and acute rejection after renal transplantation. Transplantation 2003;75:189-95.

This single-center study evaluated the relationship of perioperative blood pressure control to delayed graft function and acute rejection and identified a significant relationship between better blood pressure control and reduced rejection and improved graft function.

Matas AJ, Humar A, Gillingham KJ, et al. Five preventable causes of kidney graft loss in the 1990s: a single-center analysis. Kidney Int 2002;62:704-14.

This large single-center review identified five major causes of renal graft loss in the 10 years 1990-1999 in the 1467 primary renal transplants performed at this institution. These causes included thrombosis, acute rejection, chronic rejection, death with function, and noncompliance. Death with function and thrombosis were the most common causes of graft loss in the first year after transplant.

Catena F, Ansaloni L, Gazzotti F, Bertelli R, et al. Gastrointestinal perforations following kidney transplantation. Transplant Proc 2008;40:1895-6.

The authors of this single-center study report their experience with GI complications in 1611 patients following kidney transplantation. Perforations of the colon (n = 21), small bowel (n = 15), duodenum (n = 6), and stomach (n = 4) were noted. GI perforation was associated with a 24% mortality rate, and nearly 50% of the perforations were associated with a period of high-dose immunosuppression.

Evens AM, David KA, Helenowski I, et al. Multicenter analysis of 80 solid organ transplantation recipients with post-transplantation lymphoproliferative disease: outcomes and prognostic factors in the modern era. J Clin Oncol 2010;28:1038-46.

This multicenter analysis included patients from four transplant centers over a decade who developed posttransplant lymphoproliferative disease. In this cohort of patients (n = 80), mean time to development of PTLD was 48 months post transplant. Three-year survival rate was 62%, and survival with rituximab was significantly improved compared to without (73% versus 33%). Poor prognostic indicators for outcome included CNS involvement, bone marrow involvement, and hypoalbuminemia.

REFERENCES

Access the complete reference list online at http://www.expertconsult.com.

197

Liver Transplantation

DAVID J. KRAMER

Orthotopic liver transplantation (OLTX) is the definitive treatment for patients with end-stage liver disease (ESLD). It affords the opportunity for a disabled person to return to a full and active life. Although expensive, OLTX may well be more cost-effective than the routine medical care of terminally ill patients with liver failure.[1,2] The first OLTX in humans was performed by Starzl in 1963.[3] However, significant progress did not occur until the advent of potent immunosuppressive agents, specifically the introduction of cyclosporine in 1981.[4] Technical improvements in surgical approach and organ preservation, combined with increasingly sophisticated anesthetic and intensive care management, have provided 1-year survival rates of nearly 90%.

In this chapter, we outline the many developments that have occurred in this field. Major advances in defining risk categories for candidates and managing patients with cirrhosis and pulmonary hypertension and novel immunosuppressive strategies are described. In recent years, organ allocation has been prioritized such that the sickest patients, those most likely to die, undergo transplants first. This optimizes both aggregate benefit, by improving overall survival of patients with end-stage liver disease, and individual benefit. The latter is manifested by the full recovery of a very sick patient. Conversely, the individual who is not so ill will not bear the risks of surgery. Since February 2002, all patients listed in the United States for liver transplantation have been prioritized by their score on the Model for End-Stage Liver Disease (MELD).[5,6]

Candidate Selection

Optimal candidates are those for whom the risk of surgery is far outweighed by the potential improvement in their quality of life. Furthermore, the risk of recurrence of the primary disease should be low.[7,8] Not surprisingly, those who are at the highest risk with surgery also achieve the greatest gains when they survive. Unfortunately, such patients have a higher mortality and require significantly greater resources, particularly intensive care and rehabilitation. There are few absolute contraindications to OLTX. However, factors have been identified that significantly increase the risk and should be recognized as relative contraindications (Table 197-1). From the surgical perspective, prior right upper quadrant abdominal surgery, particularly biliary reconstruction, results in a technically more difficult procedure. Patients who are sicker with higher MELD scores or U.S. United Network Organ Sharing (UNOS) Status,[1,9] particularly those with fulminant hepatic failure, fare worse. Patients with higher Acute Physiology and Chronic Health Evaluation (APACHE) II scores who are in the intensive care unit (ICU) and require mechanical ventilation or hemodialysis have lower survival. Of course, medical therapy in such circumstances is even less successful, and APACHE II models hospital outcome well. However, after transplantation, mortality does not rise linearly as a function of recipient acuity. Patients with high APACHE II scores have a higher post-OLTX mortality than recipients with very low preoperative scores. However, there is a plateau of approximately 25% for recipients with preoperative APACHE II scores greater than 20 (Figure 197-1). This observation suggests that carefully selected but very ill patients benefit from OLTX.

Patients with cirrhosis and underlying hepatocellular carcinoma are candidates for OLTX if the disease is limited to the liver and the lesions are small, there is no evidence for major intrahepatic venous invasion, and nodal disease is absent. The widely accepted Milan criteria (1 lesion less than 5 cm or 3 lesions each less than 3 cm) have been modified and established as the University of California at San Francisco (UCSF) criteria (1 lesion = 6.5 cm or 3 or fewer nodules with the largest = 4.5 cm and the total tumor diameter = 8 cm without gross vascular invasion); survival is more than 80% for these patients.[10] Extensive radiologic staging of these patients to stratify them into tumor stages is imperative so the risk of postoperative recurrence can be estimated. Patients with biliary tract malignancy such as cholangiocarcinoma have a very high rate of recurrence.[11,12] It seems doubtful that more extensive resection, including the liver, a portion of small bowel, and pancreas, will be more successful in controlling recurrence of these tumors.[13,14] Preoperative chemotherapy and irradiation may improve outcome after liver transplantation and is under investigation.[15]

The risk for recurrence of viral hepatitis in the transplanted organ differs for hepatitis A (HAV), hepatitis B (HBV), hepatitis C (HCV), and hepatitis E. HAV is an acute illness that may cause fulminant hepatic failure and does not recur after transplantation. Recurrence of HBV, once a near-universal problem[16] except after transplantation for fulminant HBV, has been greatly reduced by the routine use of hepatitis B immune globulin (HBIG) titrated to levels of anti-HBV surface antigen antibody (HbsAb) and antivirals such as tenofovir and entecavir—associated with less emergence of drug resistance than lamivudine and adefovir.[17] Active HBV replication, documented by the presence of HBV-DNA, must be suppressed with antivirals before surgery.[18-24] For reasons that are unclear, early reports indicated that patients transplanted with HBV fared worse at each postoperative stage than those with other causes of ESLD.[25] Some have speculated that this is a systemic disease accounting for both the high rate of reinfection in the absence of prophylaxis and the decreased survival. Hepatitis C presents a more complicated conundrum. Reinfection of the transplanted organ is universal. Currently there is no effective prophylaxis. Clinical progression is highly variable and not predictable. Some patients experience rapid deterioration and graft failure within the first year, but others have little histologic damage several years after liver transplantation. Hepatitis after transplantation may be treated with pegylated recombinant interferon (IFN)-α_{2b}, and ribavirin, but is variably tolerated. Sustained suppression of HCV at the end of therapy is reported to be approximately 26% at 3 years.[25] The effect of targeted immunosuppression, particularly reduced corticosteroid dosage, on recurrence of HCV and progression to fibrosis is under investigation.[26]

HIV-infected liver transplant recipients tolerate carefully titrated immuno-suppression. Survival after OLTX is only slightly lower for HIV-positive patients than it is for HIV-negative patients,[9,27-29] with post-transplant morbidity and mortality related to recurrence of hepatitis C in co-infected patients.[30]

Patients with thrombosed portal veins present a formidable surgical challenge. Options include portal endovenectomy or anastomosis of the donor portal vein to the confluence of the superior mesenteric and splenic veins. Patency of the superior mesenteric vein should be demonstrated by ultrasonography or magnetic resonance imaging (MRI) or angiography before surgery. Occlusion of the superior mesenteric vein usually precludes OLT. Although the portal vein may be anastomosed to the recipient inferior vena cava with a proximal caval ligature placed to sustain flow, mesenteric venous hypertension persists, and gastrointestinal (GI) hemorrhage, ascites, and lower-extremity edema remain problematic. Combined hepatic and intestinal transplantation or multivisceral transplantation are alternatives.[31]

TABLE 197-1	Contraindications to Liver Transplantation	
Absolute	**Relative**	
Extrahepatic malignancy	Cholangiocarcinoma, hepatocellular carcinoma larger than UCSF modification of Milan criteria (see text)	
AIDS Hepatitis B with active replication	HIV infection (in the absence of AIDS)	
Low cerebral perfusion pressure (sustained < 40 mm Hg or cerebral blood flow < 10 mL/min/100 g) in fulminant hepatic failure Infection (extrahepatic)	Low cerebral perfusion pressure (sustained < 60 mm Hg or cerebral blood flow < 20 mL/min/100 g) in fulminant hepatic failure Portal vein and superior mesenteric vein thrombosis Extrahepatic organ system failure not related to the ESLD	
Pulmonary hypertension (mPAP > 45 mm Hg or depressed RV function)	Pulmonary hypertension (25 < mPAP < 45, preserved RV function at rest and with exercise)	
Hepatopulmonary syndrome (Pao₂ < 100 mm Hg with Fio₂ = 100%)	Hepatopulmonary syndrome (Pao₂ < 200 mm Hg with Fio₂ = 100%)	

AIDS, acquired immunodeficiency syndrome; *ESLD,* end-stage liver disease; *HIV,* human immunodeficiency virus; *mPAP,* mean pulmonary artery pressure; *RV,* right ventricular.

Acute liver failure (ALF; known formerly as *fulminant hepatic failure* [FHF]) is liver failure with encephalopathy that develops in patients without prior liver disease within an 8-week period or less.[32] Mortality is high and predictable.[33] Liver transplantation is the only therapeutic option for patients with progressive liver failure, increasing survival at one year from 20% to 75%.[34,35] Such patients are critically ill at the time of transplantation. They require intensive hemodynamic and neurologic monitoring preoperatively, including measurement of intracranial pressure (ICP)[36-40] and cerebral blood flow (CBF). A few patients will improve with supportive care, particularly young patients with acetaminophen intoxication, *Amanita* poisoning, or hepatitis A. But most experience a deterioration in their conditions. In contrast to patients with chronic liver disease, hepatic encephalopathy is associated with intracranial hypertension, particularly in patients with multiple organ system failure and hyponatremia.[17,41-45] Inadequate cerebral perfusion, cerebral herniation, and brain death preclude OLT.[46] Progressive arterial vasodilation may result from the failing liver, mesenteric hypertension, infection, pancreatitis, and adrenal insufficiency, with resultant hypotension despite elevated cardiac output. Cardiovascular instability,[47] atrial and ventricular arrhythmias,[48] and respiratory insufficiency (acute lung injury/acute respiratory distress syndrome [ALI/ARDS]) are common complications of ALF and substantially increase operative risk. If preoperative support requires greater than 1 µg/kg/min of epinephrine (or equivalent) or positive end-expiratory pressure (PEEP) greater than 12 with Fio₂ above 60%.

Patients with ESLD severe enough to make them eligible for OLT often experience a precipitous deterioration (acute on chronic liver failure, AoCLF) and require admission to the ICU. Common precipitants include infection (particularly pneumonia and spontaneous bacterial peritonitis) and GI bleeding (from esophageal or gastric varices, portal hypertensive gastropathy, or gastric or duodenal ulceration). Although these events herald the impending demise of the patient and intensify the search for a donor organ, they also further compromise the potential recipient and may lead to multiple organ dysfunction syndrome (MODS) and death.

The decision regarding when a patient is "too sick" to undergo OLTX is complex and reflects a balance of recipient acuity (assessed by MELD, APACHE, level of vasopressor, dialytic and ventilatory support), donor risk index, and surgical, anesthesia, and critical care resources available at the time the donor is identified. Comorbidity in the form of extrahepatic disease unrelated to liver failure with estimated 5-year mortality in excess of 50%, extrahepatic malignancy or infection, irreversible neurologic injury, and cardiopulmonary support in excess of that noted above for ALF would preclude OLT in our institution. Liver failure–associated MSOF resolves with restoration of liver function after successful transplantation.

Donor Selection and Operation

Liver allograft function reflects both recipient and donor factors. Although individual donor characteristics such as age, steatosis, hypernatremia, and impaired lidocaine clearance[49,50] have been associated with poor allograft function, a recent study of a large group of patients allowed analysis of donor factors while controlling for recipient-specific characteristics.[51] Deceased donor characteristics which independently predicted an increased risk of graft failure included age, donation after cardiac death (DCD), split or partial grafts, race, height, and cause of death (Table 197-2). Decreased graft survival may also be associated with unique pairings of donor and recipient characteristics. For example, liver function in HCV-positive recipients is worse when the donor is older than 60 years of age.[52]

Brain death results in marked changes in homeostasis for the donor. Hemodynamic instability is common and may result in part from massive free-water deficits caused by diabetes insipidus. Correction of diabetes insipidus with desmopressin and adequate hemodynamic monitoring and intervention are essential to preserve vital organ function. Anesthesia blunts the response to surgical stimulation. A skilled surgical dissection with rapid identification of the hepatic vessels,[53] cannulation and perfusion with University of Wisconsin (UW) solution, and rapid cooling are essential for graft preservation. Acceptable cold ischemia times have dropped. Despite a report of successful graft function after prolonged cold ischemia times of up to 24 hours,[54] the best outcome is associated with 6 hours or less.

Donation after cardiac death (DCD) results in a graft with an additional warm ischemic insult–a consequence of the hypotension and hypoxemia of that result from with drawal of hemodynamic and respiratory support–until death is pronounced and cannulae can be placed to infuse cold preservative solution. Alternative preservation techniques including less viscid than cold UW solution as well as allograft perfusion with thrombolytics are under investigation.[55] A significant learning curve attends the successful use of DCD grafts with biliary complications noted by all but lower survival and hepatic arterial thrombosis reported by some[56] but not all programs.[57]

Living donation is the only option for liver transplantation in many parts of the world. However, in the United States the number of living donor liver transplants is falling from its peak in 2001—constrained by the success of deceased donor liver transplantation, including the falling overall mortality after introduction of MELD for liver allocation and the risks inherent in the donor surgery. In 2009 only 219 liver transplants were from living donors, compared with 6101 from deceased donors.[58] Evaluation includes confirmation of the emotional relationship between donor and recipient, evaluation of the donor for medical disease, and anatomic compatibility. Liver segment to donor weight ratios of 0.8% to 1% are needed to avoid small-for-size syndrome. However, donation of the right lobe results in increased donor complications. The reader is referred to a recent detailed review.[59]

Recipient Operation

The recipient operation has become a highly refined surgical procedure. Improvements in anesthetic and surgical practice have made evident the importance of the other factors described previously—candidate selection and donor organ quality—in the eventual outcome for the recipient. The surgical procedure may be divided into three stages: hepatectomy, anhepatic phase, and post-reperfusion phase. Each involves special consideration by the anesthesiologist and surgeon.

Monitoring includes pulse oximetry, electrocardiography, and continuous measurement of arterial pressure (often from two vessels) and pulmonary arterial pressure. Maintenance of large-bore central venous catheters (e.g., two 8.5F introducers) and the ability to infuse whole blood at rates as high as 2 L/min with a rapid infusion system are

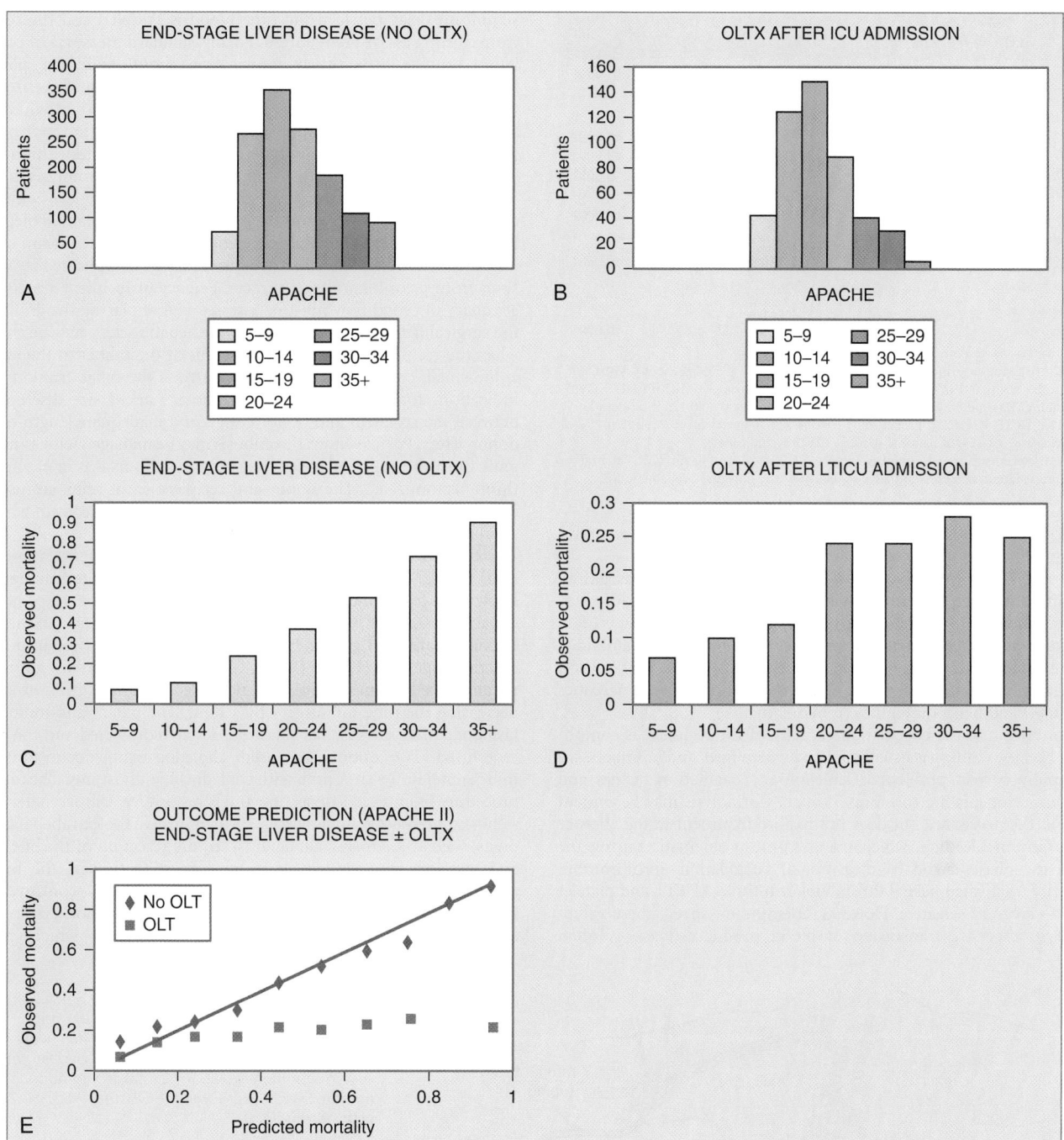

Figure 197-1 APACHE II model applied to patients with end-stage liver disease (ESLD) who require ICU admission: 1381 patients did not undergo liver transplantation during that hospitalization (No OLTX), and 489 patients were transplanted during that hospitalization (OLTX). **A,** Distribution of scores in patients who were not transplanted. **B,** Distribution of scores in those transplanted. **C,** Mortality by APACHE II score in those not transplanted. **D,** Mortality by APACHE II score in those transplanted. **E,** Observed mortality as a function of predicted mortality based on APACHE II scores in both the group of patients not transplanted (which tracks the line of identity) and those transplanted.

essential to maintain hemodynamic stability during occasional episodes of massive hemorrhage. More extensive monitoring is indicated in selected cases. Right ventricular function may be compromised by the presence of pulmonary hypertension, a complication that can develop acutely during reperfusion.[60-63] Right ventricular ejection fraction and end-diastolic volume are more sensitive guides to cardiac preload than are central venous and pulmonary artery occlusion pressures. These values may be obtained by use of the oximetric pulmonary artery with rapid-response thermistor catheter (Edwards Lifesciences Corp., Irvine, California).[1] However, more robust cardiovascular

assessment is provided by intraoperative transesophageal echocardiography. This tool provides a dynamic online picture to the anesthesiologist, allowing him or her to assess the adequacy of resuscitation. In patients with ALF and intracranial hypertension, ICP monitoring is essential. Although CBF measurement in the operating room is difficult, flow can be estimated by the contour of the transcranial Doppler and balance of oxygen supply and demand inferred from the arterial-jugular venous oxygen content difference.[64] CBF also may be assessed using transcranial Doppler ultrasound to measure the velocity of flow in the middle cerebral artery. Continuous electroencephalography

TABLE 197-2	Donor Factors Significantly Associated with Liver Allograft Failure (1998-2002)			
Donor Parameter		**RR**	**95% CI**	**P Value**
Age:				
<40		1.0		
40-49		1.17	1.08-1.26	<0.0002
50-59		1.32	1.21-1.43	<0.0001
60-69		1.53	1.39-1.68	<0.0001
≥70		1.65	1.46-1.87	<0.0001
AA vs white		1.19	1.10-1.29	<0.0001
Height each 10 cm below 170 cm		1.07	1.04-1.09	<0.0001
COD = CVA		1.16	1.08-1.24	<0.0001
COD = other		1.20	1.03-1.40	0.018
DCD		1.51	1.19-1.91	0.0006
Partial/split		1.52	1.27-1.83	<0.0001

Modified from reference 51.

Donor risk index = exp[(0.154 if 40 ≤ age < 50) + (0.274 if 50 ≤ age < 60) + (0.424 if 60 ≤ age < 70) + (0.501 if 70 ≤ age) + (0.079 if COD = anoxia) + (0.145 if COD = CVA) + (0.184 if COD = other) + (0.176 if race = African American) + (0.126 if race = other) + (0.411 if DCD) + (0.422 if partial/split) + (0.066 ((170−height)/10)) + (0.105 if regional share) + (0.244 if national share) + (0.010 × cold time)].[8]

AA, African American; *CI,* confidence interval; *COD,* cause of death; *CVA,* cerebral vascular accident; *DCD,* donation after cardiac death; *P,* statistical probability; *RR,* relative risk.

(EEG) and compressed spectral array are under investigation as monitoring techniques in this setting.

A rapid-sequence induction of anesthesia is indicated, as gastric motility is impaired in patients with cirrhosis, and the procedure may be performed before an adequate period of fasting. Anesthesia is often induced with propofol, fentanyl and succinylcholine and maintained with a balanced technique of volatile anesthetics (isoflurane), muscle relaxation (cisatracurium, vecuronium), and judicious use of narcotics (fentanyl) and benzodiazepines (midazolam).[65]

Monitoring of the coagulation capacity of the recipient is complicated because clotting is usually markedly deranged, and it is necessary to rapidly correct problems. Depletion of coagulation factors and thrombocytopenia are common. Primary fibrinolysis may be evident early in the procedure but does not require treatment in the absence of significant bleeding, which may become problematic during the anhepatic phase. Standard measures of coagulation—prothrombin time (PT), activated partial thromboplastin time (APTT), and platelet count—are very sensitive. However, attempts to correct these values result in excessive transfusion of blood products. There is often significant delay between the time blood is sampled and the results from clotting assays are reported. Finally, standard measures of coagulation provide little timely information about qualitative platelet function and fibrinolysis. Kang and colleagues introduced the thromboelastograph for routine use during OLT.[66] This test provides the anesthesiologist with a rapid assessment of coagulation status, the presence or absence of fibrinolysis, and the effects of intervention with protamine or ε-aminocaproic acid, an inhibitor of fibrinolysis.[66-68]

The surgical procedure involves meticulous dissection, which is often hampered by severe portal hypertension and substantial bleeding from venous collaterals. Insufficient control results in significant blood loss. Identification of the hilar structures may be complicated by adhesions from prior biliary tract surgery. Patency of recipient vessels and adequacy of blood flow must be assessed before placing the graft into the surgical field. An arterial graft for the hepatic artery may be chosen when the recipient anatomy is anomalous or the caliber of the vessels is too small, or when atherosclerosis narrows the celiac trunk. Other indications for an arterial graft include a marked size discrepancy between the recipient and donor vessels and inadequate length of the donor artery. Portal venous thrombosis may be managed with a "jump" graft from the superior mesenteric vein if the portal vein cannot be thrombectomized.[69] The donor and recipient caval veins are usually anastomosed end-to-end caudad and cephalad to the liver when a cava-sparing technique is not chosen.

Preservation of blood flow in the inferior vena cava (caval preservation) with or without portal drainage is an alternative technique, also known as a *piggyback*[70-72] and is preferred when there is marked hemodynamic instability. Venovenous bypass was used routinely in the past because it afforded greater hemodynamic stability and reduced mesenteric congestion (Figure 197-2).[73] However, the piggyback approach requires one less anastomosis and no dissection of the groin or axilla, decreasing the time for surgery by 1 hour. The biliary anastomosis is fashioned after the vascular anastomoses are completed and the graft reperfused. Two options are used: choledochocholedochostomy or mid-jejunal Roux-en-Y limb with choledochojejunostomy. The former procedure requires less dissection and is restorative. Unfortunately, the stenosis rate is quite high. Diseases which involve the extrahepatic bile ducts, such as sclerosing cholangitis, require resection of the bile duct and creation of a choledochojejunostomy. Stenting of the biliary anastomosis—once routine with a T tube—is now controversial. One innovative approach is cannulation of the donor cystic duct after donor cholecystectomy with a 5F catheter which stents

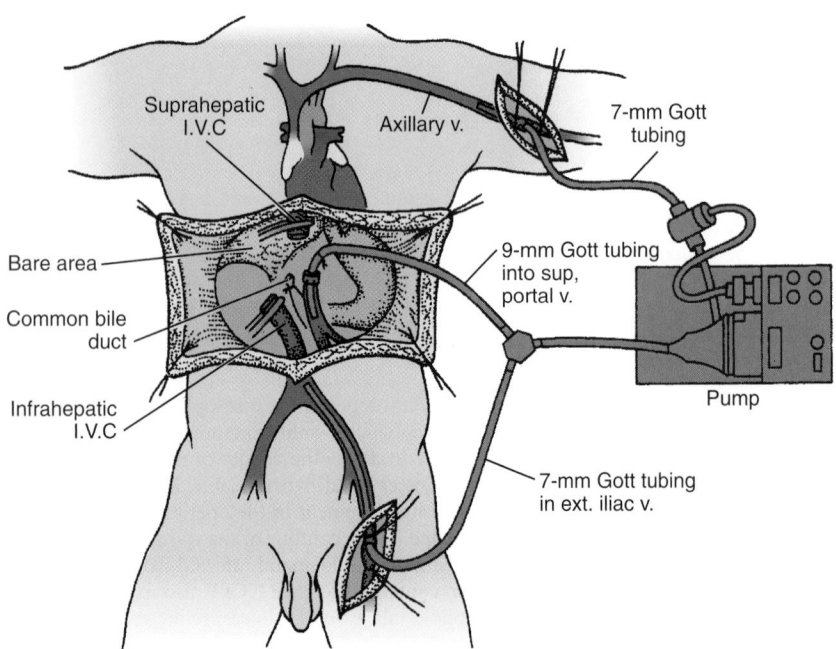

Figure 197-2 Venovenous bypass. I.V.C, inferior vena cava; ext. iliac v., external iliac vein. *(From Griffith BP, Shaw BW Jr, Hardesty RL, Iwatsuki S, Bahnson HT, Starzl TE. Veno-venous bypass without systemic anticoagulation for transplantation of the human liver. Surg Gynecol Obstet 1985;160:270-2, with permission.)*

the anastomosis, drains some bile for daily inspection and provides a noninvasive route for cholangiography. A hemorrhoidal band serves to seal the cystic duct once the drain is removed.

Reperfusion is accompanied by cardiovascular collapse in a small (and decreasing) number of patients (~2%-5%).[74] Although the exact mechanism is undefined, recirculation results in a cardiac bolus of cold acid and potassium-rich fluid, resulting in acidemia, hyperkalemia, and hypocalcemia. The consequence is abrupt onset of a severe, albeit brief, cardiomyopathy coincident with the loss of vasomotor tone and, occasionally, increased pulmonary arterial pressure. Volume resuscitation, sodium bicarbonate, or THAM for correction of metabolic acidosis, calcium chloride, and inotropic support (epinephrine) are usually sufficient to restore hemodynamic stability. Fortunately, this event is usually short lived. However, significant insults to the graft, heart, kidneys, and brain may occur and require postoperative attention.

Postoperative Management

As might be surmised from the preceding discussion, postoperative management of the OLT recipient is largely governed by the patient's preoperative condition, the adequacy of the donor organ, and the operative success of the surgical and anesthetic teams. Indeed, the function of the graft is the dominant factor in the recovery of the patient.

LIVER ALLOGRAFT FUNCTION

Early graft function is usually assessed by measuring circulating concentrations of total bilirubin, aminotransferases, canalicular enzymes, and clotting factors. The scheme shown in Table 197-3 is useful for assessing graft function according to these parameters.[75] Other parameters such as arterial ketone body ratio (AKBR)[76] and oxygen consumption[77] also correlate with graft survival. However, in a retrospective review, Doyle and colleagues were unable to identify a unique parameter with adequate sensitivity and specificity to be useful for predicting graft survival in individual OLTX recipients.[78] Other techniques, such as neural network modeling, require further investigation.[79] An alternative approach is to use a composite acuity score to predict graft and patient survival. For example, Angus et al. showed that the APACHE II score, a widely used severity-of-illness indicator designed for general ICU patients, was useful for predicting both hospital survival and survival at 1 year for liver transplant recipients if the model was recalibrated.[80,81]

Typically, elevated serum bilirubin levels during the first few days after transplantation reflect preoperative values and the consequences of procurement. In the absence of severe procurement injury, serum total bilirubin concentration typically falls to normal during the first week. An injury pattern is evidenced by elevated serum aminotransferase levels. Aspartate aminotransferase (AST) and alanine aminotransferase (ALT) peak during the first 3 days and return toward normal slowly thereafter. Canalicular enzymes (γ-glutamyl transpeptidase and alkaline phosphatase) typically rise to four or five times normal and return toward normal over the course of the next few weeks. If the liver was injured during procurement, the biochemical

changes are greater and last longer. Thus, the peak concentrations for ALT and AST are higher, and the serum total bilirubin concentration remains abnormal for a prolonged period, sometimes for weeks, as do circulating levels of canalicular enzymes. Unless the liver is irreversibly damaged, synthetic function normalizes after the third day, and the AKBR returns toward 1.0. *Primary nonfunction* is liver allograft failure manifested as jaundice, coagulopathy, and encephalopathy. It is not explained by technical or immunologic factors. Multiple-system organ failure may develop or worsen as liver function deteriorates. Re-transplantation may be the only option.

Knowledge of the details of procurement and implantation should color the interpretation of liver function abnormalities in the early postoperative period. Technical problems should always be considered before an immunologic mechanism is implicated. Even with the widespread use of percutaneous liver biopsy, a diagnosis based solely on histology may be inaccurate when a vascular or biliary drainage problem is present. Furthermore, if a technical problem is not recognized and is treated as rejection, intensified immunosuppression places the patient at grave risk for infectious complications.

The diagnostic work-up for a patient with liver function abnormalities in the perioperative period should include a Doppler ultrasound examination to determine patency of all pertinent vessels. Concern about the adequacy of flow should prompt an angiogram or MR angiogram (MRA). Early occlusion of the hepatic artery should prompt immediate re-exploration, which can result in a nearly 50% graft salvage rate.[82] Early hepatic artery thrombosis may present as a precipitous deterioration in hemodynamics, abrupt development of ARDS, severe coagulopathy, and markedly elevated serum aminotransferase concentrations. Bacteremia is common. Delayed hepatic artery thrombosis is often less dramatic in its presentation.[83] Indeed, some patients are asymptomatic. Others show destruction of the biliary duct system with multiple intrahepatic strictures, bile collections, and intrahepatic abscesses. Recurrent bacteremia, in the absence of another source, may be the only indication of hepatic artery thrombosis.

The presentation of portal venous thrombosis is usually much less dramatic. In the early postoperative period, the most frequent manifestation is persistent ascites. Enteric congestion and bleeding as a consequence of portal hypertension may also occur. Later, portal vein thrombosis should be considered in the differential diagnosis if the patient develops variceal hemorrhage. Although occlusion of the inferior vena cava (IVC) related to retrohepatic caval thrombosis can occur, it is uncommon. Anastomotic strictures are more common. Stenosis at the lower anastomosis of the IVC presents as lower-extremity edema and renal dysfunction. Stenosis at the upper anastomosis presents findings similar to those that occur in the Budd-Chiari syndrome, including passive congestion of the liver, ascites, lower-extremity edema, and renal failure. The diagnosis may be suggested by ultrasound examination, but more commonly the clinical picture prompts measurements of IVC pressures above and below the anastomoses using a fluoroscopically guided catheter. When strictures are diagnosed, treatment is commonly surgical, but balloon dilatation has been accomplished in some cases.

Patency of the biliary tract should be confirmed using cholangiography, which is simple when a T-tube or cystic duct tube stents the anastomosis. A more invasive approach is needed in patients without a biliary drainage tube: ERCP for a choledochocholedochostomy and percutaneous transhepatic cholangiography (PTC) for a choledochojejunostomy. Small anastomotic leaks may be managed with an internal stent. Larger leaks or uncontrolled peritonitis warrant surgical repair. Adequate hepatic arterial flow should be confirmed.

Graft rejection may occur at any point after OLT. Hyperacute rejection is very rare, if it occurs at all, after OLTX. Nevertheless, a humoral component of rejection may be evidenced by antibody deposition in the arterial endothelium and by persistence or recrudescence of a positive cross-match.[84] Acute cellular rejection (ACR) is more common and develops in approximately 40% of liver transplant recipients. It typically presents after the first week but can present within the first few days after transplant or present years later. Thus, its usual description

TABLE 197-3	Classification of Graft Function After Orthotopic Liver Transplantation			
Variable	Grade I	Grade II	Grade III	Grade IV
AST	<1000	>1000 initially	>2500 for ≥ 48 h	>2500 and rising
ALT		<1000 at 48 h		
PT	Normal	Mild prolongation	Very abnormal	Severe coagulopathy
Bile	>40 mL/d	<40 mL/d	Minimal	None

Data from Greig PD, Woolf GM, Sinclair SB et al. Treatment of primary liver graft nonfunction with prostaglandin E₁. Transplantation 1989;48:447-53.

ALT, alanine aminotransferase; *AST,* aspartate aminotransferase; *PT,* prothrombin time.

as "acute" is a misnomer. The histologic criterion for the diagnosis of ACR is a periductal lymphocytic infiltrate associated with a cellular infiltrate around the central veins.[85] Nevertheless, these changes may be evident to a lesser degree even in the absence of clinical abnormalities. In a graft with stable function, rejection is typically associated with a rise in serum total bilirubin concentration associated with elevations in the circulating levels of aminotransferases and canalicular enzymes. Other clinical findings include signs of the sepsis syndrome, diarrhea, suddenly increasing ascites, eosinophilia, thrombocytopenia, and laboratory evidence of hemolysis. Chronic rejection, also a misnomer because it may occur at any point, is manifested by arteriopathy and vanishing bile ducts. Its presentation is insidious, and signs of terminal liver disease may develop slowly.

IMMUNOSUPPRESSION

The approach to rejection is divided into two phases: prophylaxis and treatment.[86] Prophylaxis is achieved by administering a combination of corticosteroids and cyclosporine (Neoral) or tacrolimus. These agents inhibit interleukin (IL)-2 expression and block T-cell recruitment. They offer a selective approach to immunosuppression in solid-organ transplantation. Prospective randomized trials comparing tacrolimus-based and cyclosporine-based regimens demonstrate that tacrolimus affords better rejection prophylaxis, is associated with less steroid-resistant rejection and need for OKT3,[87,88] and is less costly when medical care in the first posttransplant year is considered.[89]

Azathioprine, used before the advent of newer immunosuppressive agents, is reserved for patients with recurrent rejection episodes or for those unable to tolerate the newer agents. Mycophenolate mofetil is hydrolyzed in vivo to mycophenolic acid. This compound inhibits inosine monophosphate dehydrogenase, resulting in selective inhibition of T- and B-cell proliferation.[90] Mycophenolate mofetil is more expensive than azathioprine and has GI side effects (diarrhea) but less bone marrow toxicity. Data from a prospective randomized trial that enrolled liver transplant recipients indicates that combined tacrolimus, prednisone, and mycophenolate is no more toxic than tacrolimus and prednisone and that the three-drug cocktail may facilitate a reduction in tacrolimus dose.[91] Newer immunosuppressive agents and techniques are under development. The current regimen at Mayo Clinic Jacksonville for prophylaxis is outlined in Table 197-4. Calcineurin inhibition with tacrolimus or cyclosporine is the cornerstone of treatment. Corticosteroids are administered intraoperatively and throughout the early postoperative period. Early introduction of mycophenolate allows a reduction in tacrolimus dose.[92] Sirolimus has been associated with delayed wound healing and hepatic artery thrombosis when administered in the early postoperative period. When introduced later in the transplant course, it enables reduction or elimination of calcineurin inhibition. Thymoglobulin and IL-2 receptor (IL-2r) antagonists may

be used for induction of immunosuppression, which allows for delayed introduction of calcineurin inhibitors and/or more rapid steroid taper; this is particularly useful in patients with renal impairment at the time of transplantation.

Liver biopsy may be driven by clinical changes or by protocol on day 7. The latter affords a better margin of safety/reassurance that patients with subclinical rejection will be identified and treated aggressively, enabling a less intensive immunosuppressive strategy to be successful for the remainder. Significant complications may result from liver biopsy, and this may outweigh any benefit in well-established programs with careful monitoring. Mild rejection requires no specific treatment other than up-titration of calcineurin inhibition. Moderate to severe rejection is treated initially with corticosteroids: 1000 mg of methylprednisolone is administered over a 4-day period (day 0, 500 mg; day 2, 250 mg; day 4, 250 mg). A follow-up liver biopsy is performed on the fifth day. If rejection persists, treatment with 2000 mg of methylprednisolone is given over the next 4 days (day 0, 1000 mg; day 2, 500 mg; day 4, 500 mg). Persistent rejection deemed "steroid resistant," represents a less than 5% incidence and is treated with thymoglobulin (as OKT3 is no longer available).[93-97]

The major side effects of cyclosporine and tacrolimus are similar: both cause significant nephrotoxicity and neurotoxicity.[98] More than 90% of patients[99] sustain some degree of renal injury, which is manifested clinically as azotemia. Renal dysfunction is a consequence of the hemodynamic insults of the procedure and/or side effects of calcineurin inhibitors. Ten percent of OLTX patients require some form of renal replacement therapy postoperatively, and a few require long-term hemodialysis. Neurotoxicity is more evident in the elderly and compounded by serum electrolyte disturbances, particularly hyponatremia and hypomagnesemia.[100] Neurologic dysfunction ranges from a mild expressive aphasia to tremors, confusion, coma, and seizures. Other side effects of cyclosporine, such as hypertension and hirsutism, occur less commonly with tacrolimus. Because tacrolimus is a more potent agent, many patients are able to have the dose of corticosteroids tapered, if not completely discontinued.[101,102]

Abnormal liver function can be a complication of serious systemic illness. For example, hyperbilirubinemia can occur in patients with sepsis and is known as *cholestasis lenta*. However, jaundice may occur with the development of pneumonia or may herald the presence of an abscess. Other systemic processes such as disseminated fungal infections (caused by *Candida* spp. or *Aspergillus*) and viral infections such as those caused by cytomegalovirus, herpes simplex, or herpes zoster virus may result in profound derangements of liver function. Another systemic process that can affect the liver is lymphoma. Non-Hodgkin's lymphomas can develop after solid-organ transplantation; these malignancies are called *posttransplant lymphoproliferative disease*. This disease is a consequence of T-cell suppression and may be mediated by Epstein-Barr virus. Polyclonal disease may respond to reduction in

TABLE 197-4	Standard Immunosuppression for Liver Transplant Recipients (Mayo Clinic Jacksonville)			
Agent	*Initiate*	*Dose*	*Target Level*	*Comments*
Tacrolimus	Day 1	0.05 mg/kg PO BID	8-12 (days 0-21) 6-10 (days 22-365)	Adjust for renal dysfunction: half dose Cr 1.5-2.0; hold Cr > 2.0
Mycophenolate mofetil	Day 0	1000 mg BID start before surgery		Cancer: discontinue once tacrolimus therapeutic
Methylprednisolone	Intraoperative	500 mg		Additional 500 mg if > 7 RBCs transfused intraoperatively
Methylprednisolone	Day 0	50 mg IV BID		
Prednisone	Day 1	25 mg PO BID		Taper by day 15 if recurrent hepatitis C virus
	Day 2-3	20 mg PO BID		
	Day 4-6	15 mg PO BID		
	Day 7-14	10 mg PO BID		
	Day 15-20	15 mg PO daily		
	Day 21-29	10 mg PO daily		
	Day 30-60	7.5 mg PO daily		
	Day 61-90	5 mg PO daily		
	Day 91-119	2.5 mg PO daily		
	Day 120	Discontinue		

immunosuppression and antiviral therapy. Monoclonal disease may require chemotherapy as well for control.

Hemodynamic Changes

The characteristic hemodynamic changes of ESLD resolve slowly after OLTX. The exact timing is unresolved, and the controversy likely reflects the preoperative state of some of the patients. Thus, problems resolve more slowly in patients with profoundly deranged liver function and MODS than in recipients who are less ill at the time of transplantation. A vasodilated hyperdynamic state is typical of liver failure[103-107] and rarely normalizes in the immediate postoperative period. Patients who are unable to mount a hyperdynamic response fare worse. Some recipients have preexisting cardiac dysfunction due to ischemic damage or restrictive cardiomyopathy secondary to amyloidosis or hemochromatosis; these patients are unable to increase stroke volume and cardiac output in response to vasodilation. Similarly, patients with sepsis have a higher mortality if they fail to (1) increase ventricular end-diastolic volume to preserve stroke volume as ejection fraction falls and (2) increase heart rate to increase cardiac output.[108] Elevated central venous pressures (CVPs) are transmitted to the hepatic vein and through the liver. Hepatic congestion results in impaired clearance of bacteria, endotoxin, and cytokines. Elevated hepatic venous pressures are reflected in elevated portal pressures, which increase bacterial translocation and endotoxemia, further compromising graft function. Resuscitation must be guided by measurement of CVP. The etiology of hypotension should be classified as cardiac—a consequence of inadequate preload or impaired contractility—or loss of arterial tone.

Management of hypotension requires immediate restoration of adequate circulating volume, usually to a CVP of less than 12 mm Hg. Inotropic support, using dobutamine or epinephrine, should be added if cardiac output remains low despite volume loading. More typically, patients with liver failure are hyperdynamic and vasodilated. In the distributive shock of liver failure, as in septic shock, norepinephrine restores regional blood flow more effectively than dopamine. Low-dose vasopressin (0.04 unit/min) effectively restores perfusion pressure in patients with liver failure. However, vasopressin reduces portal flow and hence hepatic perfusion; these effects obviously might be undesirable in transplant recipients with compromised portal flow. Right ventricular function may be gauged using echocardiography or estimating ejection fraction using a pulmonary artery catheter equipped with a rapid-response thermistor (REF catheter [Edwards Lifesciences]). Marked arterial vasodilation, however, also should prompt an evaluation to exclude a focus of inflammation, infection, pancreatitis, or graft rejection.

Cardiac tamponade should be considered in the differential diagnosis of low cardiac output associated with high filling pressures. There are surgical and medical factors that increase the potential for tamponade. Surgical considerations include the superior aspect of the "Mercedes" incision, which can violate the pericardial parietal reflection, and unintentional inclusion of the right atrium in the superior anastomosis to the inferior vena cava. Medical considerations include impaired coagulation, thrombocytopenia, and renal failure. When tamponade develops in the setting of a hyperdynamic and vasodilated state, cardiac output, calculated systemic vascular resistance, and arterial-venous oxygen content difference all may be deceptively normal.

Although hypotension is a more common problem, arterial hypertension may occur in the postoperative period. It commonly reflects inadequate analgesia or sedation,[16] impaired gas exchange, or hypoglycemia. However, hypertension may persist once these factors are addressed, and attention should then focus on the toxic side effects of cyclosporine[109,110] and tacrolimus. Both drugs are vasoconstrictors and may promote hypertension by activating the renin-angiotensin pathway. This complication occurs more commonly with cyclosporine (30% of cases) than with tacrolimus (10% of cases), and cyclosporine-induced hypertension is more resistant to antihypertensive

therapy.[111-113] Antihypertensive therapy should be initiated when systolic blood pressure is over 160 mm Hg or diastolic blood pressure is over 95 mm Hg. We favor combined α- and β-adrenergic receptor blockade with labetalol. Long-term management rests on a combination of β- and α-adrenergic blockade and calcium channel blockade. ACE inhibition may be complicated by hyperkalemia. Hypertension resistant to the first-line agents is usually managed in the ICU with potent vasodilators such as nicardipine and sodium nitroprusside, perhaps in combination with an α-adrenergic blocking agent.

Pulmonary Considerations

Pulmonary complications of ESLD are common.[113] Atelectasis, pleural effusion, reduced functional residual capacity, and limited vital capacity due to ascites and chest wall edema are often present preoperatively. The operative procedure in the upper abdomen, placement of a "normal-sized" graft in the site of a shrunken cirrhotic liver, and postoperative ileus can further decrease vital capacity. Inadequate pain control results in splinting and atelectasis and increases the risk of pneumonia. However, long-term pulmonary sequelae are rare, and most patients have improved pulmonary function tests when studied more than 1 year after OLTX.

Pulmonary infiltrates in patients with liver disease warrant immediate evaluation. Pulmonary infection should be considered, but many pulmonary infiltrates have a noninfectious cause. Pulmonary edema may result from left atrial hypertension (volume overload) or from ALI/ARDS. The latter usually heralds infection, commonly intraabdominal/surgical site with secondary peritonitis. Pancreatitis or liver allograft failure, whether caused by rejection, primary nonfunction, or vascular catastrophe (e.g., hepatic artery thrombosis), may also lead to development of ARDS. When liver failure per se is the cause, ARDS usually resolves after successful transplantation.[114] ARDS also may develop during treatment of rejection with thymoglobulin or OKT3.[115]

Bronchoscopic techniques are used routinely to aid the clinical assessment of pulmonary infiltrates and establish the diagnosis of pneumonia.[116] Despite the severe coagulopathy that often is present, bronchoalveolar lavage (BAL) may be performed without significant risk of hemorrhage. Quantitative cultures are obtained, and the presence of bacteria at more than 100,000 colony-forming units (CFU)/mL is considered diagnostic of pneumonia. BAL is sensitive but lacks specificity. A protected brush specimen is less sensitive but more specific. However, it may result in significant endobronchial hemorrhage in coagulopathic patients. With little overall impact on management, we favor BAL. Bronchoscopic techniques confirm the clinical suspicion of pneumonia in only a third of cases.[117]

Matuschak and associates have described liver-lung interactions.[118,119] ALI is common in advanced liver failure.[120] Patients with liver failure and ARDS are at high risk for mortality and are usually eliminated as candidates for liver transplantation. However, in highly selected patients with liver failure and ARDS, lung injury resolves quickly after successful OLTX.[121]

Two additional pulmonary complications—hepatopulmonary syndrome and portopulmonary hypertension—are unique to patients with liver disease. Cyanosis sometimes occurs in patients with cirrhosis.[122] Several explanations have been tendered. Anatomic right-to-left shunts have been described within the pulmonary circulation[123,124] and between the portal venous system and the pulmonary veins via esophageal veins.[125] Increased closing volume resulting in air trapping has been observed. A leftward shift of the oxyhemoglobin saturation curve also has been reported.[126] Most important, many patients have a diffusion defect manifest as a decreased diffusing capacity (DLCO) on pulmonary function tests. Furthermore, hypoxic pulmonary vasoconstriction is impaired. These findings correlate with anatomic studies showing dilated intrapulmonary capillaries.[127] Additionally, studies using inert gas washout techniques have demonstrated that hepatic dysfunction is associated with significant ventilation/perfusion mismatching rather than pure shunt. Patients with hepatopulmonary syndrome have dilated pulmonary capillaries which lead to diffusion impairment. Furthermore, increased dispersion in the ventilation/perfusion relationship results in mismatching such that many poorly ventilated units are excessively perfused.[128] Ventilation/perfusion mismatching does not constitute a true right-to-left shunt, which explains the observation that hyperoxia results from prolonged exposure to high F_{IO_2}. The most useful preoperative test is contrast echocardiography using tiny air bubbles as the contrast agent ("bubble study"). Normally, no contrast agent appears on the left side of the heart after venous injection of the bubbles. The appearance of contrast agent immediately after injection suggests an intracardiac shunt (i.e., patent foramen ovale); contrast agent that appears later (i.e., third to sixth cardiac cycle) suggests intrapulmonary shunting.[129] Hypoxia usually resolves within the first month, but sometimes resolution is delayed for as long as a year after transplantation. Patients who fail to improve should be investigated with pulmonary angiography to identify a single shunt large enough to be embolized.[130]

Pulmonary hypertension occurs more commonly in patients with cirrhosis than in controls and is called *portopulmonary hypertension*.[131] Other than cirrhosis, no predisposing factor has been identified. The histopathologic abnormalities in the lungs are typical of primary pulmonary hypertension. Secondary causes of pulmonary hypertension, particularly left ventricular failure, left-to-right intracardiac shunting with increased cardiac output, autoimmune disease, and pulmonary embolism, should be eliminated from consideration, and both portal and pulmonary hypertension confirmed for the diagnosis of portopulmonary hypertension to be established. In an advanced state, it may be difficult to distinguish portopulmonary hypertension from primary cardiac failure with secondary venous congestion and hepatic failure. Portal hypertension can be diagnosed on clinical grounds by the presence of varices, splenomegaly, and can be confirmed by hepatic vein catheterization and measurement of free and wedged pressures, the latter being an estimate of presinusoidal portal pressure. Echocardiography allows estimation of pulmonary pressures by measuring the regurgitant flow velocity through the tricuspid valve. However, confirmation with pulmonary artery catheterization is necessary. Severe pulmonary hypertension recognized only at the start of the OLTX warrants cancellation of the procedure. In contrast to patients with primary pulmonary hypertension, patients with portopulmonary hypertension benefit minimally from acute pharmacologic interventions directed at reducing the pulmonary arterial pressures. Therapeutic measures such as organic nitrates, sodium nitroprusside, or calcium channel blockers fail to reduce pulmonary artery pressure and can lead to systemic hypotension. Low systemic arterial pressure, in turn, may result in right ventricular ischemia, further compromising right ventricular function, with decreased left ventricular filling and cardiac output and more profound hypotension. Initial studies suggested that patients with portopulmonary hypertension are unresponsive to inhaled nitric oxide.[132] Subsequent experience suggests that inhaled nitric oxide ameliorates pulmonary hypertension and improves arterial oxygenation in some patients.[133,134]

An alternative approach borrows from the experience gained by clinicians using continuous infusions of prostaglandins such as epoprostenol (Flolan) to lower pulmonary artery pressure in patients with primary pulmonary hypertension. Prolonged infusion of the drug over weeks or months allows gradual upward titration of the dose,[135] a tactic that ameliorates pulmonary hypertension without causing systemic hypotension. Cardiac remodeling ensues, leading to improved cardiac output, reduced tricuspid regurgitation, and normalization of CVP. The goal of treatment with epoprostenol is a systolic pulmonary artery pressure (PAP) of less than 60 mm Hg (mean < 40 mm Hg), low CVP, elevated cardiac output, and normal response to fluid challenge (i.e., slight increase in PAP, CVP, and right ventricular end-diastolic volume and a large increase in cardiac output). The change in PAP, CVP, and cardiac output during exercise may provide additional insight and guide perioperative risk assessment and management. However, pulmonary exercise testing does not predict the pulmonary vascular and right ventricular response as systemic hemodynamics normalize after

TABLE 197-5	Pulmonary Hypertension and Liver Disease	
Category	*Mean PA Pressure (mm Hg)*	*Systolic PA Pressure (mm Hg)*
Mild	25-34	35-44
Moderate	35-44	45-59
Severe	45-75	60-100
Very severe	>75	>100

PA, pulmonary artery.

successful transplantation. Pulmonary hypertension resolves in some patients after successful OLTX.[136,137] Others appear to have two concomitant independent processes: pulmonary hypertension (primary) and portal hypertension. Consequently, such patients are at risk for increased PAP and right ventricular failure despite successful OLT. Careful monitoring with PA catheterization and echocardiography is essential. Patients with portopulmonary hypertension treated with epoprostenol require continued infusion and titration during the immediate postoperative period but usually can be weaned over the subsequent year. Although patients with mild pulmonary hypertension (Table 197-5 lists definitions) can tolerate OLTX without significant complications, the picture is bleak for those with moderate to severe pulmonary hypertension (mean PAP > 45 mm Hg). Most transplant recipients with severe pulmonary hypertension die of right-sided heart failure during reperfusion or during the early recovery phase. They tolerate large fluid shifts poorly. Right ventricular overload and failure develop abruptly, compromising the viability of the graft as a consequence of hepatic and mesenteric congestion. Low cardiac output and hypotension results in graft ischemia and death. Poorly controlled pulmonary hypertension or residual right ventricular dysfunction presents an absolute contraindication to liver transplantation.

Pulmonary hypertension that develops de novo during or acutely after liver transplantation may result from embolic phenomena at the time of transplantation that may be evident on intraoperative transesophageal echocardiography. Patients should be managed with attention to sustaining right ventricular coronary perfusion by maintenance of adequate mean arterial pressure and avoidance of central venous hypertension. Pulmonary hypertension can develop late after liver transplantation. This problem is not always directly related to portal hypertension, because liver function and the transhepatic venous pressure gradient (pressure difference between wedged and free hepatic venous pressures) may be normal.[138]

Clinically valuable alternatives to prostaglandins include endothelin receptor antagonists (ERA) and phosphodiesterase-5-inhibitors. However, experience is limited with these agents in portopulmonary hypertension. Bosentan is a nonselective ERA which improved exercise tolerance. However, it may cause cholestasis which usually were versus upon discontinuation. Ambrisentan is a selective ERA associated with less cholestasis. Significant reduction in pulmonary artery pressures and right ventricular remodeling in the setting of portopulmonary hypertension remains to be demonstrated. Phosphodiesterase-5 inhibitors such as sildenafil lower PAP and may be used alone or in conjunction with prostaglandins and endothelin inhibitors.

Mechanical ventilatory support is often required preoperatively for patients with ESLD. Intubation to minimize aspiration is required when the patient cannot protect the airway because of encephalopathy or massive upper GI hemorrhage. Respiratory failure can be precipitated by volume overload and pulmonary edema, infection, or profound muscle weakness. The increased risk of ALI/ARDS warrants mechanical ventilation with a low tidal volume strategy determined by a height-based calculation of ideal body weight.[139] We favor a pressure-limited approach for most patients, using CPAP/PS or pressure control-IMV. Sedation should be minimized and early mobilization out of bed with standing and ambulation attempted, even with an endotracheal tube, significant PEEP, and vasopressor support, with careful monitoring. Early extubation is indicated as soon as the patient can clear secretions, protect the airway, and ventilate without fatiguing.

Hypoxemia can be managed with supplemental oxygen and positive airway pressure provided with CPAP. Previously, the median duration of intubation after transplantation was 2 days. Recent changes in anesthetic techniques allow many patients to be extubated in the PACU. Now the median duration of intubation for patients who require ICU admission is less than 24 hours. Early extubation postoperatively (<6 hours) is the goal, and immediate postoperative extubation is possible in those having an uncomplicated intraoperative course and no life-threatening premorbid extrahepatic organ dysfunction.[140,141]

Renal Considerations

Renal dysfunction in patients with liver disease is frequently unrecognized. Liver dysfunction and malnutrition make elevations in blood urea nitrogen and serum creatinine concentration unimpressive despite a significant decrease in glomerular filtration rate (GFR). Preoperative renal failure (creatinine > 2.0 or the need for hemodialysis) presages post-operative renal failure and decreased survival.[142,143] Kidney biopsy may help guide a decision for combined kidney and liver transplantation.[144] In the posttransplant period, several factors conspire to impair renal function. These factors include preoperative renal failure (hepatorenal syndrome), episodic arterial hypotension resulting in tubular damage, medications (e.g., cyclosporine, tacrolimus, and vasopressors) that cause renal arterial vasoconstriction, and amphotericin, which causes tubular damage.[145] Furthermore, liver allograft dysfunction leads to portal and mesenteric hypertension which leads to functional renal impairment—the hepatorenal syndrome. Renal replacement therapy is required for approximately 10% of patients. Continuous renal replacement offers greater hemodynamic stability and may not precipitate additional organ injury. Adequate renal perfusion pressure requires at least "normal" mean arterial pressure. However, there seems to be little benefit to the kidney from dopamine, fenoldopam, calcium channel blockade, or prostaglandin infusion.

Gastrointestinal Considerations

Protein and calorie malnutrition is common in liver failure; it is a catabolic process. Weight and appearance are often misleading, and cachexia is evident once anasarca resolves. Muscle wasting may be most apparent in the temporalis and thenar eminence. Malnutrition compromises the outcomes from liver transplant, resulting in higher perioperative complications and mortality. Recognition and preoperative treatment of malnutrition may improve liver transplant outcomes. Gastroparesis is common in liver failure, increasing the risk of aspiration pneumonitis and pneumonia. We use nasojejunal feedings in malnourished patients who demonstrate inadequate intake of calories and protein. Enteral nutrition may be initiated or restarted within 6 hours after liver transplant for patients with a choledochocholedochostomy. Further delay up to 72 hours may be required in patients with a choledochojejunostomy and jejunojejunostomy (Figure 197-3) to resume full-dose enteral nutrition, although slower rates are often tolerated. On rare occasions when parenteral nutrition is required, we use crystalline amino acids and supply one-third of the nonprotein calories as fat. This approach minimizes glucose intolerance, which is common in the early post-OLTX period.

Upper GI bleeding in the OLTX recipient is uncommon, but prompt investigation is mandatory when it occurs. Gastritis and stress ulceration are common causes. Recurrence of esophageal and gastric varices often reflects diminished portal vein blood flow or complete thrombosis. Bleeding distal to the ligament of Treitz may be from the site of the jejunojejunostomy. Visualization may require a pediatric colonoscope. Revision of the anastomosis may be unnecessary in most patients by correction of coagulation.

Bleeding from the GI tract weeks or months after surgery should prompt an evaluation for infectious causes such as cytomegalovirus (CMV) infection or *Clostridium difficile* enterocolitis. Bleeding may be a manifestation of neoplastic GI involvement with lymphoma.

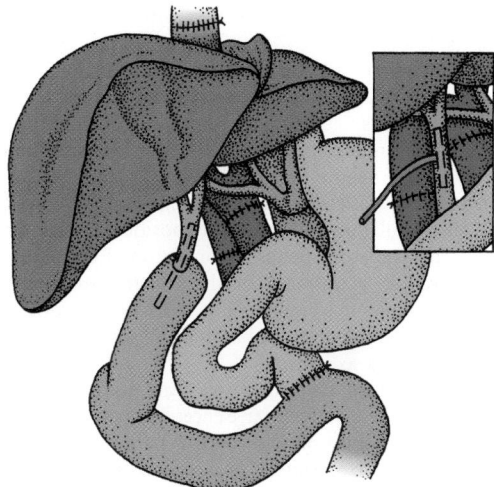

Figure 197-3 Choledochojejunostomy and choledochocholedochostomy. (*From Starzl TE, Demetrius AJ, Van Thiel D. Liver transplantation (1). N Engl J Med 1989;321:1014-92, with permission.*)

Mesenteric and splenic artery aneurysms are associated with portal hypertension and may rupture postoperatively. These lesions are usually recognized at postmortem examination. However, some patients develop an arterioenteric fistula and present with massive GI hemorrhage. Angiography can confirm the diagnosis in more stable patients but should not delay exploration, because rapid surgical repair is mandatory.

Pancreatitis is a feared but less common complication of OLTX. Although nearly 20% of patients demonstrate elevated serum amylase or lipase levels, 5% or less have clinically significant pancreatitis.[146] Conservative measures are effective in mild cases. Management of severe pancreatitis is as controversial in this setting as it is in patients without OLTX. The roles of somatostatin and operative débridement with continuous lavage remain to be defined.

Neurologic Considerations

Patients with minimal pretransplant hepatic encephalopathy who have an uncomplicated operation and receive a well-functioning graft recover rapidly from anesthesia. Changes in mental status require a thorough evaluation. Most commonly, the side effects of immunosuppressive agents such as cyclosporine and tacrolimus may be incriminated and demonstrated by resolution within 7 to 10 days of lower levels. Occasionally, discontinuation of calcineurin inhibition is necessary. Focal deficits should prompt concern about the possibility of embolic or hemorrhagic complications. Intracranial infection is rare in the early postoperative period but should be considered in patients with headache and confusion.

Patients with early graft dysfunction also often have changes in mentation. Graft swelling may result in portal congestion and portosystemic shunting. Administration of flumazenil may produce a more awake but still encephalopathic patient. The exact mechanism for encephalopathy due to graft dysfunction remains to be elucidated. Side effects of medications assume a much greater role in such patients. Clearance of commonly used immunosuppressive agents, analgesics, sedatives, and hypnotics is impaired. The amnestic effects of some agents may compound the problem. We use boluses of fentanyl for analgesia, as it is short acting and has no active metabolites. Benzodiazepines exacerbate delirium, so if sedation is needed, we prefer infusion of propofol,[147] with frequent titration and daily discontinuation. Delirium, which is more commonly akinetic than agitated and thus often unrecognized, responds better to low doses of haloperidol or atypical antipsychotics such as olanzapine and quetiapine. Sleep in the ICU is abnormal and made worse by commonly used medications.[148] Unlike benzodiazepines and other sedative hypnotics, dexmedetomidine can be titrated to effect without disrupting normal sleep patterns.[149,150]

The seizure threshold is lowered by several medications used in liver transplant recipients, including cyclosporine, tacrolimus, thymoglobulin, and antipsychotics.[151,152] Hypoglycemia, electrolyte abnormalities including hyponatremia and hypomagnesaemia, and metabolic acidosis further lower the seizure threshold.

Nonconvulsive or akinetic seizures, although rare, are more common in this ICU subpopulation and should be considered in the differential diagnosis of the comatose patient. Continuous EEG allows seizure detection as well as assessment of the effectiveness of treatment. Refractory status epilepticus may require induction of coma. Propofol causes less hypotension than pentobarbital and can be titrated to burst suppression of 5 to 10 seconds.

Additional aspects of neurointensive care need consideration in patients with ALF. These patients have encephalopathy that is mediated in part by the γ-aminobutyric acid (GABA) pathway, as is the case for patients with the portosystemic encephalopathy of chronic liver disease.[153] But patients with ALF develop intracranial hypertension and cerebral edema.[154] Patients in grade III and grade IV coma should have ICP monitored. Improved fidelity but increased complications such as bleeding and infection vary with the invasiveness of the monitoring technique.[155] A parenchymal monitor such as Codman or Camino offers a much better signal-to-noise ratio with only slight increase in risk. Ventriculostomy is the approach utilized at our institution and offers the therapeutic advantage of draining cerebrospinal fluid to avoid transient increases in intracranial pressure, with attendant decrements in cerebral perfusion pressure, minimizing compounding ischemic insults. This purported advantage is somewhat offset by bleeding around the ventriculostomy catheter which has been evident on computed tomography (CT) but clinically asymptomatic. Cerebral blood flow (CBF) can be measured with xenon-133 or with cold xenon as contrast for CT scanning. Cerebral oxygen consumption can be determined after placement of a jugular bulb catheter.[136] Cerebral metabolic rate (CMRO2) is related to the product of the CBF and arterial-venous oxygen content difference (AJVdO2 = CaO2 − CjvO2) according to the following formula:

$$CMRO_2 = CBF \times AJVdO_2/100$$

Intracranial hypertension may result from increased CBF (blood volume) or brain swelling (cerebral edema). Elevated CBF with normal oxygen consumption is associated with narrow AJVdO2 and is termed *luxuriant perfusion*. Subsequently, cerebral edema with intracranial hypertension develops and is associated with decreased CBF and large AJVdO2.[156] Management of intracranial hypertension is guided by the observed pathophysiology. Elevated ICP with increased CBF responds to hyperventilation, reduction in intravascular volume, and hypothermia. Intracranial hypertension with low CBF must be treated by increasing cerebral perfusion pressure by increasing mean arterial pressure. Osmotic agents including mannitol and hypertonic saline are also appropriate at this stage, with diuretics or CRRT to minimize elevation in CVP. Hypothermia restores cerebral autoregulation[157-159] induced by ALF. It effectively lowers ICP[160] and can be titrated to effect. Induction of coma with propofol titrated to burst suppression with continuous EEG monitoring may lower ICP further. However, accumulation of vasodilatory metabolites will compromise cerebral perfusion pressure. Patients are considered viable candidates for OLTX as long as EEG activity is preserved and adequate cerebral perfusion pressure and CBF can be maintained. Intraoperative monitoring includes these measures, combined with transcranial Doppler measurements of flow velocity contour in the middle cerebral artery,[161] which facilitate moment-to-moment titration of anesthetics and vasopressors. Although the initial period of graft reperfusion is the most hazardous, cerebral hyperemia and intracranial hypertension may persist for several days postoperatively. These abnormalities usually resolve with good graft function.

Liver transplant recipients are at risk for neuromuscular dysfunction. In a prospective study of 100 liver transplant recipients, clinically relevant weakness, defined as weakness requiring prolonged mechanical ventilatory support, developed in 7% of patients. Electromyography demonstrated that weakness was due to a myopathic rather than neuropathic process, and diffuse myocyte necrosis was evident on muscle biopsy specimens taken from five patients.[162] Predisposing factors included patient acuity postoperatively as judged by the APACHE II score, poor liver allograft function at 1 week, a requirement for renal replacement therapy, and higher doses of corticosteroids. Patients requiring early retransplantation seemed to be at particular risk.

Infectious Complications

Rejection of the allograft is treated aggressively when it develops. These measures are often complicated by the parallel development of infections. Heavily immunosuppressed patients die not of rejection but of infection. The paradigm is that immunosuppression sufficient to eliminate rejection results in a defenseless host susceptible to many infections. Solid organs vary in their propensity to stimulate rejection. The liver is relatively less immunogenic; accordingly, immunosuppression can be less intensive but still be effective. In the early postoperative period, bacterial and fungal infections are common. The most frequently involved areas are the operative site and the lungs. Perioperative antimicrobial prophylaxis targets gram-negative rods and enterococci and consists of a second- or third-generation cephalosporin or ampicillin-sulbactam and is continued for 48 hours. Prophylactic regimens vary among centers. Unfortunately, antimicrobial resistance is common, and isolates in patients who die of an infectious process are occasionally resistant to all known antimicrobial agents.[163]

Fungal colonization is also common. Patients requiring a prolonged, difficult surgical procedure and multiple transfusions of blood products are at higher risk for fungal infection, as are patients undergoing retransplantation.[164,165] Prophylactic antifungal therapy reduces the incidence of both superficial and deep fungal infections. Options include fluconazole,[166] amphotericin (10-20 mg daily for the first 2 weeks after surgery), or full doses of amphotericin B liposomal complex (ABLC) in the subgroup at highest risk of filamentous fungal infection—patients with renal and liver failure prior to OLT and those with ALF.[167] Patients with significant growth of *Candida* spp. on quantitative culture of BAL often require a full course of amphotericin.[168,169] The outcome has improved for liver transplant recipients who develop *Aspergillus* infection. This previously fatal infection[170] seems more responsive to voriconazole[171] or liposomal forms of amphotericin such as AmBisome.

Late after transplantation, infections reflect the specific effects of immunosuppressive agents on T-cell function. Although bacterial and fungal infections occur, viral infections and infections caused by opportunistic pathogens become more important. Pneumonia due to *Pneumocystis jiroveci* (formerly *carinii*) was common before the advent of routine prophylaxis with trimethoprim-sulfamethoxazole. Its occurrence now is limited to those for whom prophylactic measures have been stopped.

CMV infections are common in the transplant population.[172,173] However, the clinical severity of infection is quite variable. Some cases are asymptomatic. Others present as a viral syndrome, involve only one organ such as the lungs, GI tract, or liver, or involve multiple organs. The patients at highest risk for CMV infection are those who were seronegative before OLTX and received an organ from a seropositive donor. It is debatable whether patients who were seropositive before OLTX experience reactivation of latent virus or are infected by another CMV strain. In addition to the morbidity and mortality attributed directly to CMV, patients with CMV disease also have a higher frequency of bacterial and fungal infections. Increased susceptibility to bacterial and fungal infections may be a function of the CMV infection per se or reflect more aggressive immunosuppression—an independent risk factor for CMV infection. Seroconversion may not occur until T-cell immunosuppression is withdrawn.[174]

Prophylaxis with ganciclovir[175] or CMV immunoglobulin[176,177] is effective but with significant penalty in terms of side effects such as neutropenia and costs borne by all for benefit of a few. An alternate strategy is to monitor patients closely for evidence of CMV disease. CMV viremia can be detected by PCR or by assaying for the CMV the pp65 antigen.[178] Thresholds for treatment can be varying in relation to the risk of CMV disease in a particular subpopulation. Ganciclovir and valganciclovir are the mainstays of treatment, with foscarnet reserved for patients with intractable severe neutropenia and when resistance is suspected.

Endocrine Considerations

Hyperglycemia is common in the early postoperative period and reflects the combination of surgical stress, corticosteroids, and calcineurin inhibition. A survival benefit of intensive insulin therapy has been demonstrated[179,180] but is of unclear benefit in unselected ICU patients.[181] We suspect the high incidence of infection and neuromuscular disease in liver transplant recipients warrants intensive insulin therapy with a rationale similar to burn-injured patients.[182-185] We have modified the approach described by Davidson[186] to minimize hypoglycemia and target glucose of 90 to 120 mg/dL.

Adrenal insufficiency is common in critically ill patients with liver disease.[187] Both primary and secondary adrenal insufficiency may be unmasked by stressors such as infection, graft dysfunction, pancreatitis, or bleeding. Measurement of baseline serum ACTH and cortisol and subsequent response of serum cortisol to cosyntropin allow recognition of adrenal insufficiency and classification. The indication for continued treatment with "stress-doses" of hydrocortisone can then be determined.

Thyroid dysfunction, particularly hypothyroidism, is common in patients with primary biliary cirrhosis and in autoimmune hepatitis and may be heralded by changes in mentation which may mistakenly be attributed to the precipitating stressor. More commonly, normal thyroid function by clinical exam is associated with low total thyroxine (T_4) but normal free T_4 and thyroid-stimulating hormone (previously described as "euthyroid-sick"). However, newly diagnosed and treated hypothyroidism should also be managed with sufficient corticosteroids to preclude an Addisonian crisis.

Conclusion

Patients with terminal liver disease can undergo successful transplantation. Critically ill patients with ESLD have dramatic improvement in their quality of life. Intensive care of such patients is demanding but highly rewarding. Recipient acuity, donor risk index, and institutional resources must be carefully assessed for each high-risk transplant to be successful. The transplant intensivist should participate in this risk/benefit analysis with the transplant hepatologist, surgeon, and anesthesiologist. In addition to ICU care, the intensivist provides support and guidance for "fast-tracked" patients to be managed safely outside the postanesthesia care unit (PACU) and ICU. Developments in the future will focus on optimal candidate selection and more precise immunosuppression.

KEY POINTS

Innovations in transplant critical care:

1. A growing imbalance between the number of donated organs and the number of potential recipients has resulted in expansion of the potential donor pool by the use of organs previously considered risky. A donor risk index (DRI) of donor-related characteristics can be used to predict post OLTX graft function. These comprise the cause of donor death, race, donation after cardiac or brain death, whole versus partial or splint graft, donor proximity, and cold ischemia time. As the concept of benefit evolves from the individual with liver disease to the group of patients awaiting liver transplant, appropriate matching of donor and recipient risk profiles offers the potential for maximizing the number of patients alive 10 years after liver transplant.

2. Advances in general critical care have found application in management of critically ill patients with liver disease, before and after transplantation. Daily awakening of patients sedated for mechanical ventilation and daily spontaneous breathing trials results in earlier liberation from the ventilator. Early mobilization is safe and effective in reducing long-term disability. These strategies have direct application to patients with liver disease who metabolize sedatives and analgesics unpredictably. Tight glucose control results in a lower infection rate but must be accomplished without increasing the incidence of hypoglycemia. Infection is a major cause of morbidity and mortality in ICU-bound patients with liver disease, and stress, corticosteroids, and the diabetogenic effects of calcineurin inhibition result in insulin resistance. Renal insufficiency is common in liver failure, and its presence predicts a lower post-OLT survival. Strategies to preserve renal function include maintaining perfusion pressure with oral α-adrenergic agents (midodrine with octreotide) or intravenous norepinephrine and postoperative implementation of calcineurin inhibitor–sparing immunosuppression regimens. Serum creatinine and BUN overestimate GFR, and critically ill patients with liver and renal failure warrant initiation of dialytic therapy at a lower BUN, with daily dialysis or continuous renal replacement.

"Fast-track" management of liver transplant recipients—without the ICU:

3. ICU admission is needed for liver transplant recipients for evaluation and management of incipient or established organ system dysfunction. However, patients who recover from surgery sufficiently that they are awake, hemodynamically stable, extubated, well saturated, able to cough and cooperate with breathing exercises, and have good graft function do not require admission to the ICU. These patients can be "fast-tracked" to recovery from anesthesia in the PACU and transferred directly to the ward. Nursing support must be flexible enough to provide protocol-driven assessment and intervention, with physician backup including transplant intensivists.

4. The anesthetic approach is modified to address this acceleration of postoperative care. Modifications include a balanced anesthetic technique with short-acting analgesics, amnestics and neuromuscular blocking agents, and volatile anesthetics. Although likely to vary among institutions, the cost of "fast-tracking" versus ICU admission is lower if less than 6 hours of PACU care is required.

5. Careful patient selection for "fast-tracking" is essential for patient safety and the success of the transplant program. Optimal candidates are those with low MELD scores with little extrahepatic organ dysfunction who are recipients of low DRI organs and had an uncomplicated operative course (low transfusion requirement and short operative time).

Immunosuppression:

6. The transplanted liver is less immunogenic than other solid organs. Hyperacute rejection is very rare. Acute rejection is less problematic, as it is easily treated and not causative of chronic rejection. Consequently, efforts to reduce toxicity of immunosuppressive agents have become paramount.

7. Calcineurin inhibitors, cyclosporine, and tacrolimus cause nephrotoxicity and neurotoxicity. Tacrolimus is absorbed throughout the proximal gut and can be given with a nasogastric tube. Tube feedings may interfere with absorption of tacrolimus. More consistent levels can be achieved with sublingual administration of a lower dose. Biliary diversion does not affect absorption of modified cyclosporine (Neoral) or tacrolimus.

8. Delayed initiation of calcineurin inhibition to minimize the risk of acute nephrotoxicity can be considered in patients at low risk for rejection. For those with renal insufficiency and at higher risk of rejection, induction therapy with IL-2r antagonists (basiliximab) or T cell–depleting agents (thymoglobulin or alemtuzumab) allows for delayed initiation of lower doses of calcineurin inhibitors. Induction may also be steroid sparing. The risk/benefit analysis of such strategies varies by etiology of liver failure and risk of recurrence.

9. Functional graft size must be considered with respect to post-operative metabolic compromise including medication metabolism. Liver mass of living donor, split, and pediatric donors to adult recipients are considered "small for size." Similarly, functional mass may be decreased in organs from a high DRI donor. Specifically, impaired metabolism of anesthetics, narcotics, muscle relaxants, sedatives, and calcineurin inhibitors warrant careful dose titration.

Liver-lung interactions:

10. The anatomic relation of the lung to the liver is such that both the effluent from the liver and the blood that bypasses the liver in portosystemic shunting is directed to the lung. Evidence of graft dysfunction may be manifest in subtle changes in lung function. Indeed, patients may develop intrapulmonary shunting or pulmonary hypertension or lung injury (ALI/ARDS) as a consequence. The mortality of liver-associated ARDS exceeds 90% unless liver function can be restored.

11. Hepatopulmonary syndrome (HPS) is hypoxemia in the setting of liver disease, resulting in part from intrapulmonary shunting which can be demonstrated with a contrast-enhanced ("bubble") echocardiogram. Clinical characteristics include dyspnea with oxygen desaturation often exacerbated by standing upright (platypnea and orthodeoxia). Of greater import is ventilation/perfusion mismatch rather than true shunt. Most patients will respond to prolonged inhalation of 100% oxygen with increase in arterial oxygen tension. Patients with HPS usually resolve their hypoxemia within days to weeks of the normalization of graft function. Morbidity, and perhaps mortality, is higher in the patients who have a PaO_2 of less than 200 mm Hg on 100% oxygen. In such patients, a fixed intrapulmonary shunt should be sought and embolization considered.

12. Patients with liver disease are six times more likely to develop pulmonary arterial hypertension (World Health Organization Group I). Pulmonary hypertension develops in approximately 3% of patients with chronic liver disease and is associated with portal hypertension and may worsen with portosystemic shunting (spontaneous or surgical splenorenal shunt or after a transjugular intrahepatic portosystemic shunt [TIPS]). Pulmonary arterial pressures may be estimated from the tricuspid regurgitant jet velocity identified by echocardiography. However, confirmation and classification requires pulmonary artery catheterization. Elevated pulmonary arterial pressures may be the result of left atrial hypertension with high cardiac output in the volume-overloaded patient with liver disease. A normal transpulmonary gradient and calculated pulmonary vascular resistance distinguish these patients, who often respond to diuretics, from patients with pulmonary hypertension and elevated pulmonary vascular resistance who have a high operative mortality. At catheterization, left-to-right shunts can be recognized and response to a pulmonary vasodilator such as inhaled nitric oxide or epoprostenol (Flolan) determined. Liver transplantation is deferred pending treatment to lower mean pulmonary arterial pressure below 40 mm Hg, with normalization of right ventricular function.

ANNOTATED REFERENCES

Viral hepatitis:

Grellier L, Mutimer D, Ahmed M, et al. Lamivudine prophylaxis against reinfection in liver transplantation for hepatitis B cirrhosis. Lancet 1996;348:1212.

Prophylaxis against recurrent hepatitis B virus infection has dramatically altered the prospects for these patients after transplantation.

Fulminant hepatic failure:

O'Grady JG, Gimson AES, O'Brien CJ, et al. Controlled trials of charcoal hemoperfusion and prognostic factors in fulminant hepatic failure. Gastroenterology 1988;94:1186.

O'Grady JG, Alexander GJM, Hayllar KM, et al. Early indicators of prognosis in fulminant hepatic failure. Gastroenterology 1989;97:439.

These two papers set the standard for evaluation of liver support devices. It was not until a randomized controlled prospective study of charcoal hemoperfusion demonstrated no benefit that the field was able to move forward and consider alternative approaches. To date, no subsequent study of support devices has been as robust.

Thromboelastography:

Kang YG, Martin DJ, Marquez J, et al. Intraoperative changes in blood coagulation and thromboelastographic monitoring in liver transplantation. Anesth Analg 1985;64:888.

This paper presents the value of an old approach to assessment and monitoring of coagulation that lends itself to point-of-care testing in the ICU and operating room.

Outcome prediction:

Angus DC, Clermont G, Kramer DJ, et al. Short- and long-term outcome prediction with the APACHE II system after orthotopic liver transplantation. Crit Care Med 2000;28:150-6.

Kamath PS, Wiesner RH, Malinchoc M, et al. A model to predict survival in patients with end-stage liver disease. Hepatology 2001;33:464-70.

Determination of the acuity of recipients allows distribution of organs to the most ill recipients. It also enables comparison among programs for quality control. However, recipient scoring only accounts for part of the outcome variability because donor characteristics and surgical technique are independent factors.

Immunosuppression:

European FK506 Multicentre Liver Study Group. Randomised trial comparing tacrolimus (FK506) and cyclosporin in prevention of liver allograft rejection. Lancet 1994;344:423-8.

The U.S. Multicenter FK506 Liver Study Group. A comparison of tacrolimus (FK 506) and cyclosporine for immunosuppression in liver transplantation. N Engl J Med 1994;331:1110-15.

Lake JR, Gorman KJ, Esquivel CO, et al. The impact of immunosuppressive regimens on the cost of liver transplantation—results from the U.S. FK506 multicenter trial. Transplantation 1995;60:1089-95.

These are key papers that present the comparison of these two critical immunosuppressants for both clinical and fiscal interests. They are well done and have yet to be replicated with newer immunosuppressants. They demonstrate that for liver transplantation, tacrolimus is more effective and less expensive than cyclosporine. Furthermore, although there are significant differences in the side-effect profiles of these medications, they are similar with regard to nephrotoxicity and neurotoxicity.

Portopulmonary hypertension:

Krowka MJ, McGoon MD. Portopulmonary hypertension: the next step. Chest 1997;112:869.

Kuo PC, Johnson LB, Plotkin JS, et al. Continuous infusion of epoprostenol for the treatment of portopulmonary hypertension. Transplantation 1997;63:604.

Portopulmonary hypertension has excluded many patients from liver transplantation, and many more died of complications directly related to right-sided heart failure. These papers outline differences between primary pulmonary hypertension and portopulmonary hypertension and the benefit of therapeutic intervention.

Cytomegalovirus:

Grossi P, Kusne S, Rinaldo C, et al. Guidance of ganciclovir therapy with pp65 antigenemia in cytomegalovirus-free recipients of livers from seropositive donors. Transplantation 1996;61:1659.

This paper emphasizes the value of determining at-risk patients, those with cytomegalovirus viremia, and treating them effectively before they develop organ dysfunction such as gastroenteritis, pneumonitis, or hepatitis.

REFERENCES

Access the complete reference list online at http://www.expertconsult.com.

198

Intestinal and Multivisceral Transplantation

PETER ABRAMS | KAREEM ABU-ELMAGD | KATHRYN FELMET | JORGE REYES | GEORGE MAZARIEGOS

The ongoing development of intestinal and multivisceral transplantation remains a dynamic process moved forward by advances in multidisciplinary care of intestinal failure, surgical technique, innovative immunosuppressive strategies, and an improved understanding of intestinal transplantation immunology. Recognition of intestinal transplantation as an established modality for select intestinal failure patients and better outcomes over the past decade have led to an increasing number of candidates referred for intestinal transplantation each year (Figure 198-1) and allowed more patients to benefit. In the United States alone, nearly 700 patients are alive with a functioning intestinal allograft as of December 2007.[1] Although the time interval between listing and intestinal transplant has decreased over the past decade (Figure 198-2), waitlist mortality remains high, particularly for infants and adults with concomitant liver failure.[2] Immunosuppression for intestinal and multivisceral transplantation now commonly involves perioperative antibody induction. The inability to prevent and treat chronic rejection in isolated intestinal allografts continues to be a fundamental barrier to achieving successful long-term outcomes and is the subject of rigorous investigation. Long-term data on nutritional outcomes and transplantation morbidity will help further define the optimal timing and role of intestinal and multivisceral transplantation in patients with intestinal failure.

Management of Intestinal Failure

Intestinal failure is clinically defined as the loss of nutritional autonomy secondary to bowel dysfunction. Patients with intestinal failure are initially managed by administration of total parenteral nutrition (TPN) through central venous access. The duration of intestinal failure is variable and in certain patients unpredictable, from short-term to lifelong, and depends largely on the adaptation capacity of the remaining viable intestine. Improved long-term outcomes in TPN-dependent pediatric patients have been reported recently by single centers.[3,4,5] Nonetheless, there remains a significant subset of patients who develop irreversible intestinal failure and require indefinite TPN therapy with its attendant complications. Intestinal transplantation may be lifesaving in this group of patients.[6]

Optimal management of the patient with intestinal failure is achieved after a detailed multidisciplinary evaluation.[7,8] Obtaining a comprehensive history is critical and must include birth and disease history, past surgical procedures, infections, number and location of previous central venous lines, presence of central venous thrombosis, a detailed nutrition history including duration of TPN, details of TPN prescriptions and maximal enteral feeding tolerance, as well as medication history and frequency/volume of stools. A careful history and physical examination by the intestine rehabilitation team is critical to the process of achieving a complete pretransplant workup. Further investigations may include upper gastrointestinal (GI) contrast study with small-bowel follow-through, contrast enema if indicated, abdominal sonogram, ultrasound exam of central venous anatomy, endoscopy with small-intestinal aspiration for quantitative microbial culture and mucosal biopsy, and liver biopsy if there is evidence of liver dysfunction or portal hypertension.

Management of the patient with intestinal failure focuses on optimization of gut adaptation and recovery of intestinal function to achieve enteral autonomy. Surgical therapies that have a role in adaptation after intestinal failure include serial transverse enteroplasty (STEP).[9] Alternatively, if gut dysfunction is considered irreversible, management of these patients concentrates on maintaining optimal growth in children and nutritional repletion in adults to prepare them for eventual intestinal transplantation.

Small-bowel bacterial overgrowth (SBBO) is a common clinical problem in patients with intestinal failure and is treated with a variety of antibiotic regimens. To date, there are no comparative studies available to enable an evidence-based approach to treatment of SBBO. The use of metronidazole for anaerobic overgrowth, combined with trimethoprim and sulfamethoxazole or an oral aminoglycoside for gram-negative organisms, is a common theme. Metronidazole monotherapy is used if the dominant symptoms suggest predominantly anaerobic overgrowth (such as bloating, increasing diarrhea, and D-lactic acidemia). The extreme sensitivity of anaerobes to oxygen makes the use of small-bowel aspirate cultures relatively unreliable as a means of microbial surveillance or indication to treat for SBBO. Probiotics such as *Lactobacillus* and *Saccharomyces* have been used in an attempt to limit SBBO. Given the absence of randomized evidence to support the efficacy of probiotics, coupled with reasonable concerns about impurities and possible contamination with other bacteria (e.g., *Leuconostoc*), the use of probiotics has been discouraged in patients with intestinal failure.

Parenteral nutrition–associated liver disease (PNALD), also referred to as *intestinal failure–associated liver disease* (IFALD), remains a critical problem in this patient population, affecting infants disproportionately. The 1-year mortality of patients with PNALD exceeds 80% in the absence of TPN weaning or transplantation. Although not always feasible, the best strategy to prevent and treat PNALD involves a commitment to the advancement of enteral nutrition. Despite a conscientious approach to TPN therapy, many children and adults still develop cholestasis relatively early in their clinical course. Prevention and timely treatment of infection, minimizing SBBO, preventing overfeeding with dextrose, providing adequate amino acids, cycling TPN, providing TPN-free days when possible, and providing taurine to neonates are probably all important measures to slow the progression of PNALD.[10] Stasis of bile in the non-stimulated biliary system and gallbladder can lead to sludge buildup and cholelithiasis. In the authors' experience, cholecystectomy rarely improves liver function and is not indicated for PNALD alone. None of the components of standard parenteral nutrition solutions have been conclusively shown to cause or contribute to PNALD, but excessive glucose and improper ratios of glucose to amino acid have been associated with hepatic steatosis. Recently, interest in the manipulation of the lipid component of TPN has led some to advocate for the removal of soy-based lipid solutions or their substitution with Omegaven (a fish-oil-based, intravenous [IV] lipid solution rich in omega-3 fatty acids); however, substantive evidence that these measures retard or reverse the progression of liver disease has not yet been demonstrated.[11,12,13] Many clinicians will add but not entirely substitute fish-oil-based lipids for soy-based solutions only after liver function tests demonstrate abnormalities.

In addition to PNALD, patients on long-term parenteral nutrition are also at risk of developing metabolic bone disease (MBD). Associated with an insidious onset of bone pain that can become quite severe,

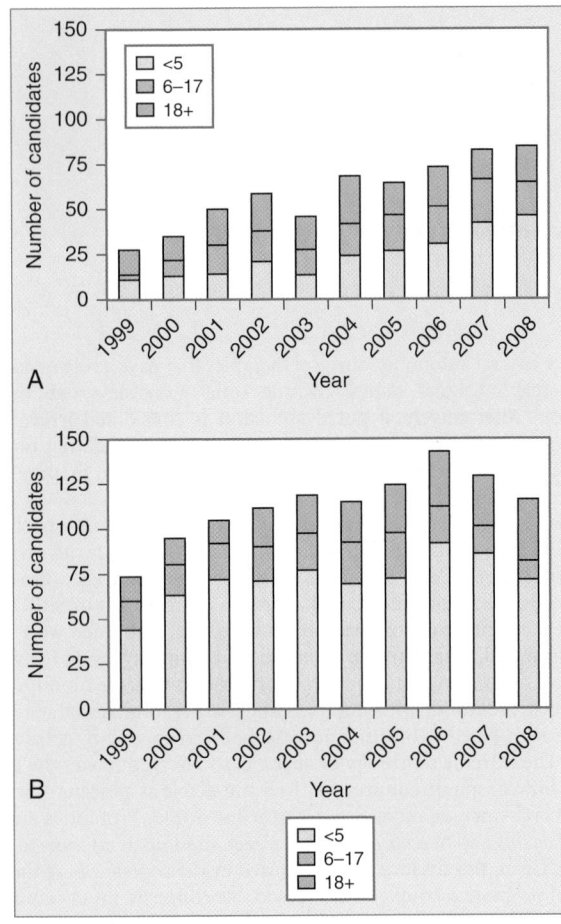

Figure 198-1 A, Number of candidates on the isolated intestine waiting list by age, 1999-2008. **B,** Number of candidates on the combined liver and intestine waiting list by age, 1999-2008. *(Adapted from Mazariegos GV, Steffick DE, Horslen S, Farmer D, Fryer J, Grant D et al. Intestine transplantation in the United States, 1999-2008. Am J Transplant 2010;10:1020-34.)*

Ultrasonic evaluation of deep veins to guide percutaneous central line placement is occasionally necessary.

Nutritionally deplete patients are relatively immune suppressed and prone to a severe course with community acquired infections. Pediatric patients with intestinal failure and IFALD are at increased risk of respiratory failure even with common viral infections. Because children have a compliant chest wall, increased abdominal girth creates a mechanical disadvantage even during normal tidal volume breathing. In the setting of pulmonary infection, volume overload, or decreased cardiac output, the work of breathing can lead to fatigue.

INDICATIONS FOR TRANSPLANT

In October 2000, the Center for Medicare and Medicaid Services approved intestinal, combined liver-intestine, and multivisceral transplantation as a standard of care for patients with irreversible intestinal failure who could no longer be maintained with TPN. Intestinal and multivisceral transplantation are now considered for patients with irreversible intestinal failure who fail TPN therapy due to complications, who cannot tolerate quality-of-life limitations associated with TPN therapy, or who must undergo native bowel resection for potentially life-limiting indications. The myriad causes of bowel dysfunction can be subcategorized into acute and chronic pathophysiologies. Common causes of acute dysfunction include necrotizing enterocolitis, volvulus, and mesenteric thrombosis. Common causes of chronic dysfunction include Crohn's disease and radiation enteritis. These disease processes can alternatively be classified as either surgical due to resection leading to short bowel syndrome (SBS) or nonsurgical due to congenital enterocyte disorders leading to dysmotility or malabsorption. Unlike patients with SBS, patients with nonsurgical causes of intestinal failure may have native intestine which demonstrates normal gross morphology and anatomic length. Table 198-1 lists the already well-described indications for intestinal and multivisceral transplantation.

Owing to the particularly high morbidity and mortality of children with PNALD, increasing efforts have been made by the pediatric medical community to optimize timing of referral of these patients to specialized intestine-failure rehabilitation centers and transplant centers to improve overall outcomes. A recent expert consensus panel[14] recommended the following pediatric criteria for consultation or referral for small-bowel transplant assessment: (1) children with massive small-bowel resection, (2) children with severely diseased bowel and

patients with MBD will present with normal serum calcium, phosphorus, vitamin D and parathyroid hormone, but with hypercalciuria. Nontraumatic spinal and rib fractures have been reported in these patients. To optimize bone maintenance in patients on TPN, it is important to include calcium in parenteral formulations, prevent metabolic acidosis, and minimize aluminum contamination. Symptoms of MBD tend to resolve only after stopping parenteral nutrition.

Most intestinal transplant recipients will require intensive care unit (ICU) care during the pretransplant period; in fact, more than 10 % of intestinal and multivisceral recipients are in intensive care at the time of transplantation. Sepsis and GI hemorrhage are common reasons for ICU admission in patients with intestinal failure. Blood products, though necessary in the resuscitation of GI hemorrhage, should be used judiciously in the absence of acute bleeding. Pretransplant exposure to blood products, particularly platelets, can predispose intestinal transplant recipients to developing antibody-mediated rejection. Leukoreduced blood products may be preferable in patients awaiting transplant.

Catheter-associated bloodstream infections are common in TPN-dependent patients and often necessitate removal of a tunneled central venous catheter. Smaller pediatric patients and patients with a history of thrombosis may have limited venous access, necessitating preservation of an infected line. Percutaneous lines should be placed with caution in these patients; great vessels may no longer be patent, and trauma to remaining vessels may have serious consequences.

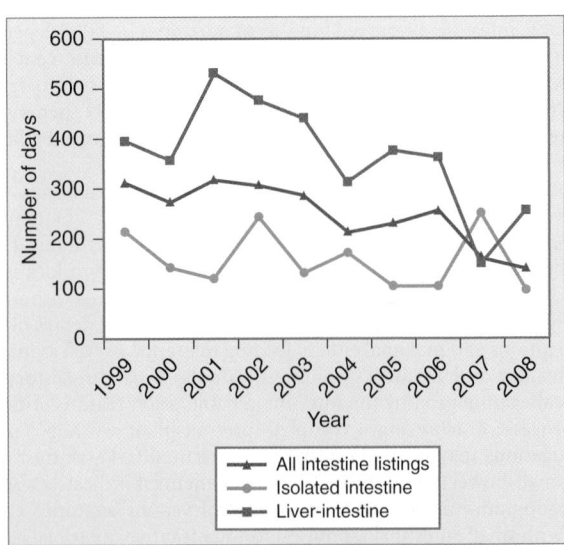

Figure 198-2 Median time to transplant for intestine waiting list registrants, 1999-2008. *(Adapted from Mazariegos GV, Steffick DE, Horslen S, Farmer D, Fryer J, Grant D et al. Intestine transplantation in the United States, 1999-2008. Am J Transplant 2010;10:1020-34.)*

TABLE 198-1	Indications for Intestinal and Multivisceral Transplantation	
Pediatric Patients		**Adult Patients**
Volvulus		Superior mesenteric artery thrombosis
Gastroschisis		Crohn's disease/irritable bowel disease (IBD)
Necrotizing enterocolitis		Desmoid tumor
Pseudo-obstruction		Volvulus
Microvillus inclusion disease		Trauma
Intestinal polyposis		Familial polyposis
Hirschsprung's disease		Gastrinoma
Trauma		Budd-Chiari disease
		Intestinal adhesions
		Pseudo-obstruction
		Radiation enteritis

unacceptable morbidity, (3) continuing prognostic or diagnostic uncertainty, (4) microvillus inclusion disease or intestinal epithelial dysplasia, (5) persistent hyperbilirubinemia (>6 g/dL), (6) thrombosis of 2 of 4 upper body central veins, (7) the request of the patient or family.

Determining which type of allograft to use in a patient with intestinal failure involves a comprehensive evaluation of the function and anatomy of the remaining bowel along with other abdominal organs. Intestinal failure patients are considered candidates for isolated intestinal transplant, combined liver and intestine transplant, multivisceral transplant (includeing liver, stomach, duodenum, pancreas, and small-bowel), or modified multivisceral transplant which excludes the liver. Whether to perform simultaneous hepatic replacement remains a challenging decision even to experienced transplant surgeons, particularly for patients with asymptomatic portomesenteric venous thrombosis and significant liver injury. The key factors in determining whether to perform liver transplant in patients with intestinal failure are the extent of portal hypertension and the severity of parenchymal liver disease. In general, patients with mild portal hypertension should be cautiously considered for isolated intestinal transplant. It is preferable under these circumstances that venous outflow from the intestinal allograft bypass the portal circulation and be drained to the recipient systemic circulation through the inferior vena cava.

EVALUATION FOR TRANSPLANT

For both children and adults, the evaluation of intestinal and multivisceral candidates usually begins as an inpatient process. The goals of the transplant team are to determine whether the patient may benefit from transplantation, assess alternatives to transplant, evaluate any contraindications to transplantation, and provide education to the patient regarding the complex process of undergoing transplantation.

Transplantation Procedures

Brief descriptions of recipient operations are provided. The multivisceral donor procurement operation has already been well described.[15]

ISOLATED INTESTINAL TRANSPLANT

For isolated intestinal transplant (Figure 198-3), the donor intestinal graft (jejunum and ileum) is procured along with donor vascular conduits, including an artery (iliac and/or carotid) and a vein (iliac). The donor superior mesenteric vessels are occasionally anastomosed directly to the recipient superior mesenteric artery and vein if adequate length is achieved. More commonly, interposition vascular conduits are anastomosed to the recipient infrarenal aorta and recipient superior mesenteric vein (portal drainage) or inferior vena cava (systemic drainage) to provide sufficient length and proper orientation for the allograft.

The intestinal reconstruction involves a proximal duodeno- or jejunojejunostomy, depending on individual recipient considerations of remnant bowel viability and anatomy. The distal length of intestinal allograft may end as a permanent end ileostomy if the recipient has no remaining viable colon or may be anastomosed to the remnant colon, leaving a short portion of allograft distal to the enterocolic anastomosis to bring out as a temporary end ileostomy that allows access to the bowel for endoscopic surveillance and mucosal biopsies. Single or multiple feeding tubes may be placed based on multiple considerations including recipient pretransplant oral intake capacity as well as donor bowel length.

COMBINED SMALL-BOWEL AND LIVER TRANSPLANT

For combined small-bowel and liver transplant (Figure 198-4), the recipient hepatectomy is performed with preservation of the native retrohepatic inferior vena cava. The recipient foregut including stomach, native pancreas, and proximal duodenum is also preserved, and its outflow maintained with a permanent end-to-side portocaval shunt. The composite donor allograft includes the primary organs (liver and small bowel) as well as the donor duodenum and pancreas, allowing for maintenance of donor hepatobiliary continuity. Arterial inflow to the composite donor allograft is achieved using an arterial interposition conduit from the recipient infrarenal aorta. Liver venous outflow commonly involves the well-described "piggyback" technique, anastomosing donor suprahepatic inferior vena cava to the confluence of the recipient hepatic veins and cava. Intestinal reconstruction is performed in a similar fashion to an isolated intestinal transplant. Feeding tubes are placed as indicated.

FULL MULTIVISCERAL TRANSPLANT

In the full multivisceral transplant procedure (Figure 198-5), prior to implantation, the recipient distal stomach, duodenum, pancreas, liver, and remaining small bowel are resected. The recipient inferior vena is meticulously preserved. The absence of remaining foregut or midgut precludes the need for portocaval shunt. Vascular inflow is similar to composite liver-bowel transplant but now includes celiac inflow to the stomach as well. Vascular outflow is identical to composite liver-bowel transplant. The donor spleen is removed from the composite allograft on the backtable prior to reperfusion.

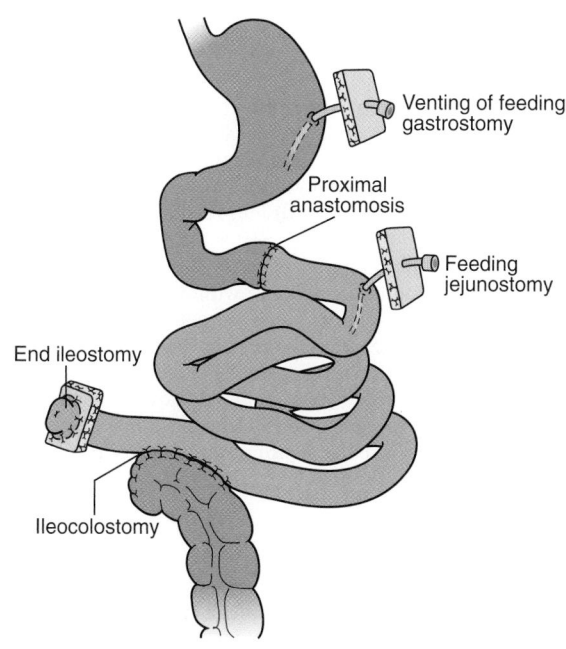

Figure 198-3 Isolated intestinal transplant.

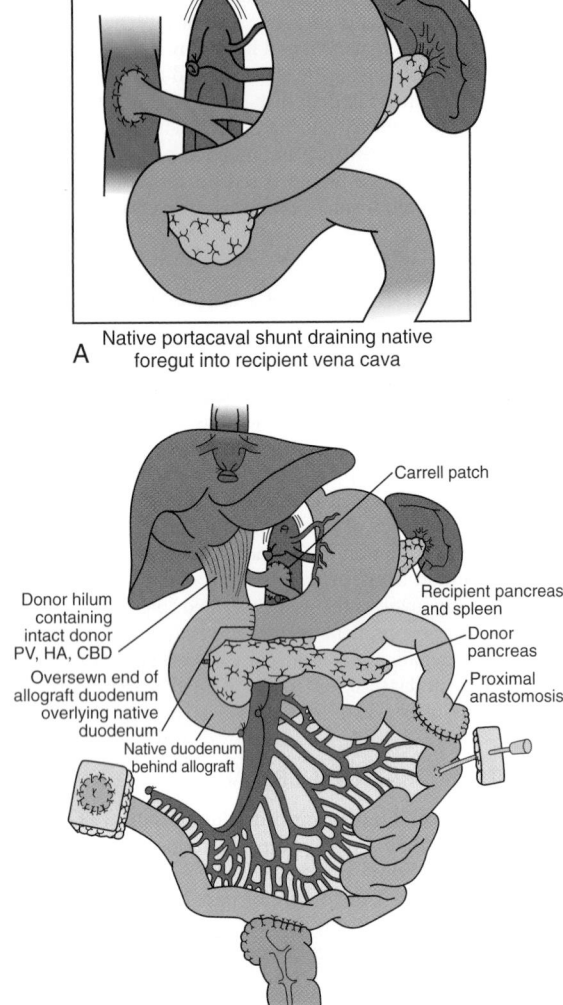

A Native portacaval shunt draining native foregut into recipient vena cava

B

Figure 198-4 Combined liver and intestinal transplant: **A,** Portocaval shunt draining native foregut. **B,** Combined liver and intestinal transplant with feeding jejunostomy.

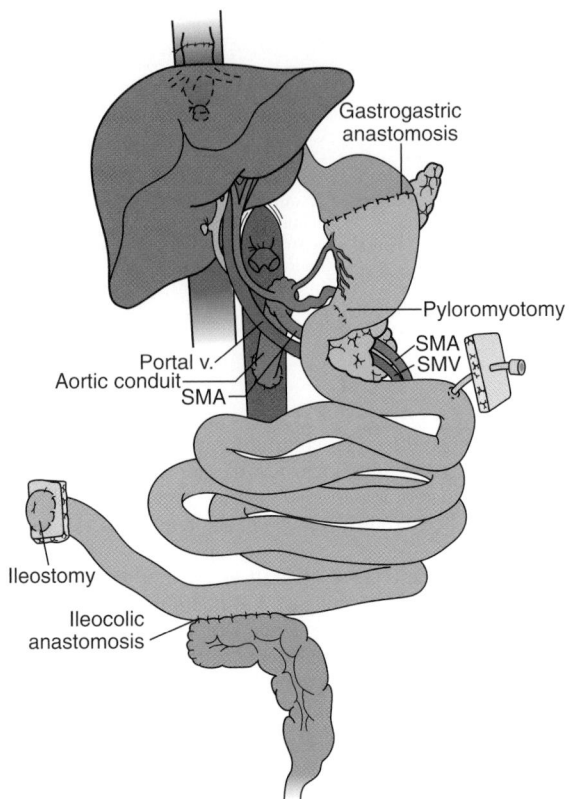

Figure 198-5 Full multivisceral transplant.

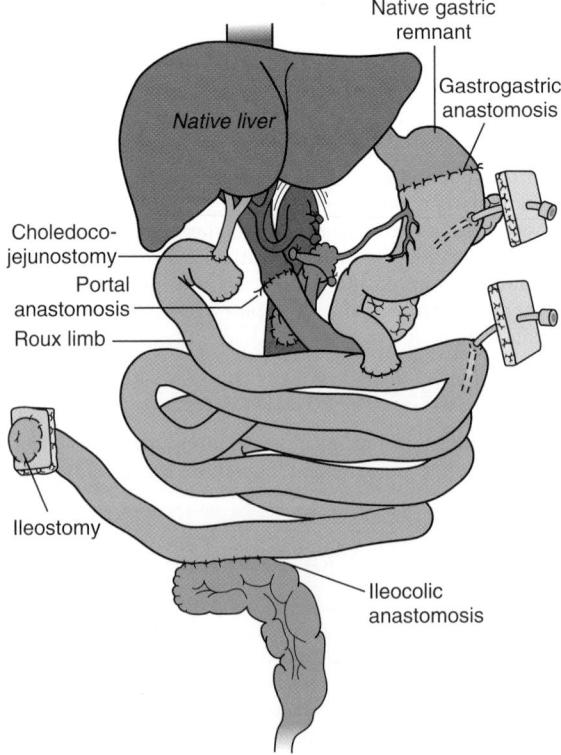

Figure 198-6 Modified multivisceral transplant.

Intestinal reconstruction is performed proximally with a gastrogastrostomy anastomosis, and the distal anatomosis is similar to previously described intestinal transplants. To avoid gastric outlet obstruction due to vagal denervation, a Heineke-Mikulicz pyloroplasty is routinely performed after reperfusion. Feeding tubes are placed as indicated.

A "modified" multivisceral transplant (Figure 198-6) involves transplantation of a full composite allograft without a liver. The recipient liver is preserved along with its vasculature and extrahepatic biliary system. Vascular conduits are used routinely (Figure 198-7). This procedure involves disruption of hepatobiliary continuity, commonly requiring in children a recipient-to-donor Roux-en-Y hepatojejunostomy, and in adults a choledochocholedochostomy (duct-to-duct) anastomosis, as well as vascular anastomoses to the recipient common hepatic artery and portal vein.

Immunosuppression

Although a variety of combinations of immunosuppressive drugs have been used in intestinal transplant recipients, most patients are maintained on tacrolimus (Prograf [Astellas, Tokyo, Japan]) therapy along with other adjunctive medications. Organ Procurement and

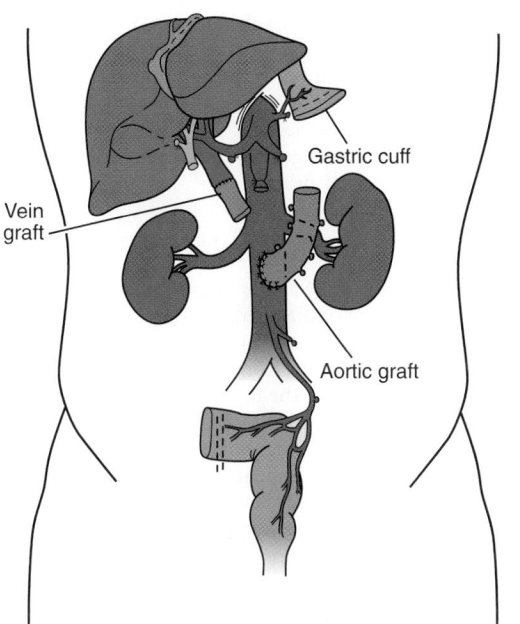

Figure 198-7 Vascular conduit extensions for modified multivisceral transplant.

Transplantation Network (OPTN) data show that 99% of intestinal transplant recipients receive tacrolimus as part of for maintenance immunosuppression at the time of posttransplant discharge. Moreover, during the first posttransplant year, only a select number of patients are taken off tacrolimus, with nearly 97% remaining on tacrolimus-based therapy. The most common regimen at 1-year post transplant is currently tacrolimus in combination with steroids, with the second most common being tacrolimus monotherapy.

Two classes of immunomodulatory drugs have recently been introduced for intestinal transplantation and have been associated with improvements in 1-year patient and graft survival. Depleting antilymphocyte antibody therapies include rabbit antithymocyte globulin (rATG, Thymoglobulin [Genzyme Corp., Cambridge, Massachusetts]) and alemtuzumab (Campath-1H [Genzyme Corp.]). The individual use of these agents by high-volume single centers has demonstrated improved short-term survival and decreased rejection rates as well as severity.[16,17,18] Associated with similar improvements in survival and decreased incidence of acute rejection and severity, induction with nondepleting interleukin (IL)-2 receptor antagonists, daclizumab (Zenapax) and basiliximab (Simulect), has also gained increasing acceptance by many intestinal transplant programs. Immunosuppression for intestinal and multivisceral transplantation now involves perioperative antibody induction in 60% of cases.

IMMUNOLOGIC MONITORING

The gold standard for monitoring and diagnosing rejection in intestinal and multivisceral transplant recipients remains routine ileoscopy and proximal enteroscopy with histopathologic examination of multiple random mucosal biopsies. Significant investigation is underway toward the development of tools to guide and monitor the immunologic state of the intestinal transplant recipient. Ideally, noninvasive markers such as serologic, proteomic, or genomic markers may identify those patients who are at increased risk of rejection and, conversely, those who might benefit from decreased levels of immunosuppression.[19,20] Preformed antibody and de novo antidonor-specific antibody measurement may be of assistance in determining risk of rejection.[21,22] When technically feasible, the presence of circulating donor cells in the recipient peripheral blood should be serially evaluated after transplantation by either flow cytometry or polymerase chain reaction (PCR).

Monoclonal antibodies specific for donor HLA class I molecules are used for single-color immunofluorescence analysis. The presence of donor-specific antibodies in intestinal transplant recipients at the University of Pittsburgh prompts aggressive therapy with serial plasmapheresis and intravenous immunoglobulin (IVIG) until clearance of antibodies has been confirmed. For PCR analysis, primers specific for donor HLA class II alleles or else the sex-determining region of the Y chromosome (in male donor to female recipients) can be used. The use of fecal calprotectin or serum citrulline as noninvasive biochemical markers of allograft rejection does not appear to be warranted based upon currently available data.[23,24]

In recipients of intestinal or multivisceral transplants, surveillance endoscopy (esophagogastroduodenoscopy [EGD], ileoscopy, colonoscopy) is performed biweekly for the first 4 to 6 weeks post transplant, and then weekly for an additional 4 to 6 weeks to monitor for rejection. After the first 3 months post transplant, the frequency of surveillance endoscopies performed in recipients is based upon individual clinical assessments.

Postoperative Management

Advances in the technical aspects of intestinal and multivisceral transplantation have occurred in parallel with improvements in intraoperative monitoring and postoperative critical care management of these challenging patients.

VENTILATORY MANAGEMENT

Extubation is commonly achieved within 48 hours of the transplant operation in adult patients. Mitigating factors which might delay extubation include graft malfunction, delayed abdominal wall closure, volume overload, sepsis, organ failure, and surgical complications such as bleeding. In children, delayed abdominal wall closure is commonly necessary and requires continued neuromuscular blockade. Given that recipients tend to be nutritionally compromised preoperatively and that intestinal and multivisceral transplant operations are relatively long in duration (8-18 hours), a careful assessment of weaning parameters prior to extubation is essential. Pleural effusions are common and due to nutritional depletion with hypoalbuminemia and intraoperative manipulation of the diaphragm; they may not be responsive to diuretics. Changes in intraabdominal pressure and abdominal girth may adversely affect respiratory mechanics, leading to rapid, shallow breathing. These problems are most common in children, in small adults who receive a large allograft, and in patients whose course is complicated by large-volume ascites.

RENAL FUNCTION

It is common for intestinal transplant recipients to demonstrate some degree of renal dysfunction pretransplant, owing to multiple episodes of sepsis with hypotension, the side effects of antibiotics, and hepatic dysfunction. Although patients receive significant volumes of fluid during the long course of the transplant operation, intravascular volume depletion can be a problem in the immediate posttransplant period. Significant fluid volume may accumulate in the intestinal allograft secondary to preservation injury (peaking at 48-72 hours), and large-volume ascites production due to mesenteric lymphatic leakage may occur. Either of these processes can lead to profound and sometimes underappreciated intravascular volume depletion and can worsen the nephrotoxicity of immunosuppressive agents and antibiotics.

Maintenance of ideal volume status is challenging in these patients; interventions should be directed at optimizing cardiac output and organ perfusion. Extravascular volume overload is common and should be interpreted with caution, particularly in the immediate posttransplant period. In patients with impaired renal function or high tacrolimus drug levels, urine output may not be an accurate indicator of perfusion. Skin perfusion, mixed venous oxygen concentration, and serum lactate are useful surrogates. Because intestinal transplant recipients are nutritionally deplete, use of 5% albumin as a volume expander may be preferable to larger volumes of crystalloid solution. In patients with large-volume stoma output or ascites drainage, standing orders for fluid replacement may be necessary. Balancing adequate volume resuscitation with the avoidance of volume overload in the setting of baseline renal dysfunction can be a significant challenge that requires considerable clinical experience and meticulous attention to detail.

INFECTION CONTROL

Recipients of intestinal or multivisceral transplants will routinely receive prophylactic broad-spectrum antibiotics post transplant. Any history of nosocomial infections before transplant should be addressed with the administration of appropriate specific antibiotics. Colonizing organisms growing from enterocutaneous fistula tracts should also be covered appropriately. Selective bowel decontamination with nonabsorbable oral antibiotics is performed in some intestinal transplant patients. Surveillance stool cultures are performed on a weekly basis post transplant.

Translocation of bacteria or bacterial toxins from the intestine to the bloodstream can cause sepsis or systemic inflammatory response syndrome (SIRS). A history of repeated exposure to broad-spectrum antibiotics leads to colonization with multiply resistant organisms in many intestinal transplant recipients. Empirical antibiotic therapy for sepsis should include coverage for common enteric organisms and should take into account a history of antimicrobial resistance. Episodes of translocation occur most commonly during acute rejection, when the mucosal barrier of the allograft has been compromised, but can also be demonstrated with enteritis associated with Epstein-Barr virus (EBV) and cytomegalovirus (CMV) infection. In the absence of positive blood cultures to direct antibiotic therapy, organisms growing from quantitative stool cultures in significant numbers ($>10^8$ colony-forming units [CFU]/mL) in a patient with sepsis or acute cellular rejection may be considered potential causes of bacteremia and may be treated with IV antibiotics. The high incidence of renal dysfunction in intestinal transplant recipients should prompt use of non-nephrotoxic antibiotics when possible and careful monitoring of antibiotic levels when necessary.

Antiviral Prophylaxis

Antiviral prophylactic strategies have evolved over the past decade of intestinal transplantation. Viral infections can cause significant morbidity, especially in pediatric recipients in the early postoperative period. Common pathogens include CMV, EBV, herpes simplex virus (HSV), adenovirus, and influenza viruses. Many pediatric recipients have no prior protective exposure to these viruses, so primary infection occurs in these patients while they are highly immunosuppressed. Recent advances in prophylaxis and preemptive therapy have significantly decreased early morbidity associated with EBV, CMV, and HSV, lowering the incidence of clinically significant infection to less than 5%. Lack of definitive treatment for infection with respiratory viruses such as influenza and adenovirus in the early postoperative period can be catastrophic because of clinical sequelae including disseminated viremia, necrotizing pneumonitis, and bacterial superinfection. The currently recommended anti-CMV prophylaxis includes a 2-week course of IV ganciclovir with concomitant administration of cytomegalovirus-specific hyperimmune globulin (Cytogam). The IV dose for ganciclovir is 5 mg/kg twice daily. The dose for Cytogam is 150 mg/kg in donor CMV-positive/recipient CMV-negative mismatches, administered 2, 4, 6, and 8 weeks after transplant and 100 mg/kg/d at 12 and 16 weeks after transplant.

NUTRITIONAL SUPPORT

Immediate posttransplant nutritional support is administered using standard TPN, which is tapered gradually as enteral feeding is advanced. Tube feedings with isotonic formula are started based upon clinical

determination of intestinal allograft function. In the authors' experience, most intestinal transplant patients do not voluntarily ingest adequate amounts of nutrition in the early postoperative period. To achieve maximal nutritional repletion, tube feeding is usually required once the intestinal tract becomes functional. Resistance to oral feedings is a particular clinical challenge in younger pediatric recipients, many of whom demonstrate oral aversion.

ASSESSMENT OF INTESTINAL ALLOGRAFT

The process of examining the anatomic and functional integrity of the intestinal allograft begins in the operating room. The normal intestinal allograft after reperfusion appears pink and nonedematous, with occasional contractions. Alterations from this appearance can be observed in the operating room and in the proximal jejunal and distal ileal segments using endoscopy postoperatively.

Surveillance for intestinal allograft rejection in the early postoperative period focuses on clinical evaluation and gross morphologic examination of the stoma and distal ileum. Frequent routine enteroscopy surveillance is the most reliable method for achieving an early diagnosis of intestinal rejection (Figure 198-8). Endoscopic evaluations are performed initially twice a week through the allograft ileostomy; upper endoscopy is reserved for occasions where clinical changes are not well explained by distal allograft evaluation and biopsy. Common changes to the normal appearance of an intestinal allograft include edema, cyanosis, congestion, and increased stomal output. These changes should prompt an immediate workup, with a differential diagnosis that includes preservation injury (Figure 198-9), sepsis, rejection, and enteritis.

The allograft stomal output is assessed for volume and consistency. Normal stomal output during the early postoperative period is characteristically clear and thin. During the first week post transplant, normal stomal output is 1 to 2 L/d and 40 to 60 mL/kg/d for adult and pediatric recipients, respectively. If these stomal volumes are exceeded in the absence of significant pathology, agents to control volume of output can be started including paregoric, loperamide, pectin, somatostatin, or oral antibiotics. The presence of blood in the stomal output is an ominous sign and implies acute rejection until proven otherwise.

Intestinal allograft absorption of nutrients and medications develops gradually and commonly requires several weeks post transplant to manifest. Abnormal absorption after approximately 1 month should prompt an aggressive search for underlying pathology, especially rejection. The ability to maintain whole-blood tacrolimus trough levels above 15 ng/mL on oral therapy alone is a good indicator of adequate absorption. In the authors' experience, intestinal transplant recipients demonstrate evidence of sufficient absorptive function at a mean of 28 days after transplantation. Recipients of multivisceral transplants demonstrate even longer delay until intestinal allograft absorption is well established.

Management of Allograft Rejection

Allograft rejection (Figure 198-10) is strongly associated with graft loss and patient death and remains a significant obstacle to achieving successful long-term outcomes for intestinal and multivisceral transplant recipients. Historically, acute cellular rejection was reported in 70% to 90% of intestinal allografts within 90 days post transplant. In contrast, rejection rates of 30% to 40% are currently reported by large centers thanks to advances in allograft histopathologic surveillance, immunosuppression, and immunologic monitoring. Unlike liver allograft rejection, the natural history of rejection of intestinal allograft is unforgiving, making early diagnosis and treatment critical for successful reversal of the rejection process.

Until proven otherwise by culture and allograft biopsy, each episode of allograft dysfunction should prompt an expeditious evaluation for acute rejection. There are currently no laboratory tests available to warn of allograft dysfunction or rejection for intestinal

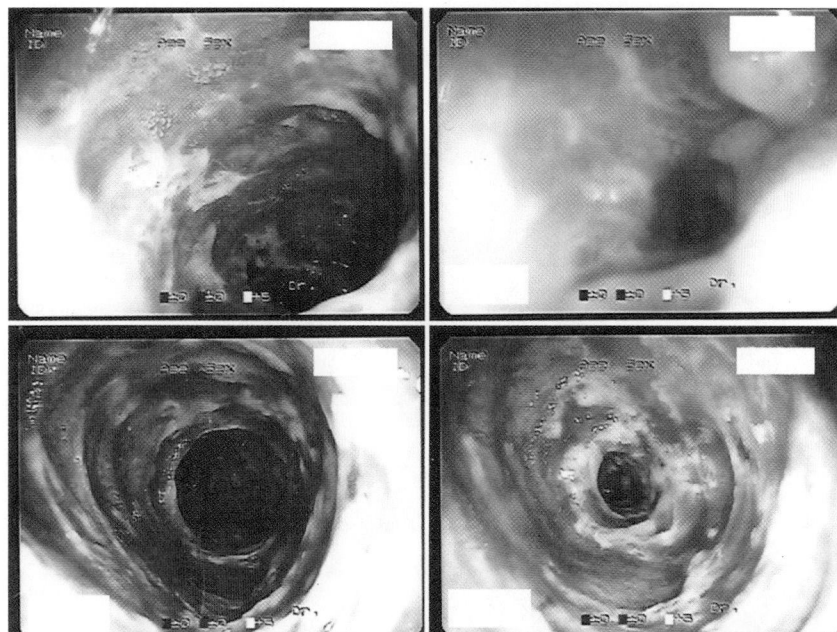

Figure 198-8 Enteroscopic findings consistent with acute cellular rejection of intestinal allograft. *(Courtesy Kareem Abu-Elmagd, MD.)*

transplantation. Clinical features of intestinal allograft rejection include nonspecific signs and symptoms such as diarrhea and abdominal pain. Infectious enteritis and medication-related loose bowel movements are common etiologies of allograft dysfunction that present with a similar clinical picture to allograft rejection. The stoma may become edematous, erythematous, and friable. Endoscopy may demonstrate normal mucosa despite mild to moderate grades of ongoing acute cellular rejection. Moderate to severe rejection of the intestinal allograft usually leads to mucosal inflammation beginning with erythema and friability, progressing to mucosal slough and exudates overlying ulcers, with eventual loss of the mucosal layer. Histologically, there is variable presence of edema in the lamina propria and villous blunting. However, mononuclear cell infiltrates and intestinal crypt apoptosis with regeneration are the hallmark signs of intestinal allograft rejection that establish the diagnosis.

Treatment of intestinal acute cellular rejection initially involves steroids. At the University of Pittsburgh, a total dose of approximately 30 mg/kg of methylprednisolone is usually given, either by 3 boluses of 10 mg/kg/d over 3 days or by a cycle of tapering doses over a more extended duration. Antilymphocyte antibodies for steroid-resistant rejection include muromonab CD3 (OKT3, a murine monoclonal

anti-CD3 antibody) and antithymocyte globulin (rATG [rabbit-derived], Thymoglobulin). Adverse immune-mediated drug reactions to immunomodulatory antibodies can be life threatening. These agents are usually administered to patients with cardiopulmonary monitoring following premedication with steroids, antipyretics, and histamine blockers. In many cases, it is appropriate to initiate therapy in an ICU setting. During and after the treatment of acute rejection, tacrolimus whole-blood levels are maintained around 18 to 20 ng/mL in intestinal and multivisceral allograft recipients. Maintenance steroid therapy usually consists of 1 to 2 mg/kg/d of oral prednisone, tapered over several weeks to months based on individual clinical assessments. Addition of a third agent such as mycophenolate mofetil (MMF; Cell-Cept [Roche]) or sirolimus (Rapamune) may be indicated if rejection is refractory or recurrent.

A fundamental principle which guides treatment of allograft rejection is the preservation of as much intestinal function as possible. Each episode of rejection shortens intestinal graft functional longevity, so the diagnosis of steroid-resistant rejection in intestinal allografts must be made in a more timely fashion than in a regenerating organ such as the liver. Antilymphocyte therapy in response to a diagnosis of steroid resistance will rapidly reduce the overall number of immunocompetent cells and is usually highly effective treatment for steroid-resistant rejection. Antilymphocyte therapy must be used cautiously in refractory rejection, after sequential biopsies separated by reasonable time intervals allow objective confirmation of steroid treatment failure. In an isolated intestine recipient with preexisting immune debilitation or a predisposition to a life-threatening illness such as posttransplant lymphoproliferative disorder (PTLD), allograft enterectomy may be safer than escalation of immune suppression and be potentially life saving.

Antibody-mediated rejection (AMR) of the intestinal allograft (Figure 198-11) is characterized by intestinal dysfunction, diffuse C4d staining on allograft biopsy, and usually identification of donor-specific antibodies. Treatment of AMR consists of plasmapheresis in combination with IVIG and steroids. Rituximab or bortezomib can be used in select recipients.

Chronic rejection (Figure 198-12) is observed in 10% to 15% of pediatric and adult intestinal allografts, occurring more commonly in isolated intestinal allografts. In adult recipients at the University of Pittsburgh, multivisceral transplants including a liver allograft demonstrated a significantly better chronic rejection-free survival compared with the liver-free intestinal and other multivisceral transplant

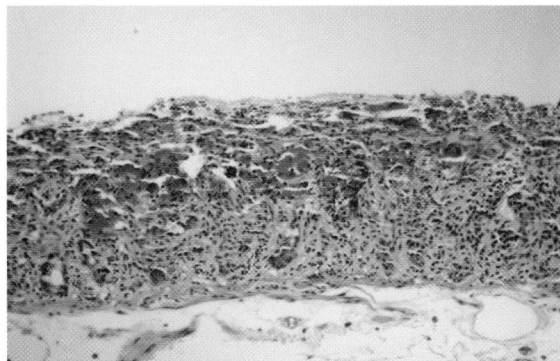

Figure 198-9 Ischemia-reperfusion injury. Reperfusion injury is characterized by extensive loss of villi, followed by pronounced regenerative changes of crypt epithelium with conspicuous mitosis, capillary congestion, shortening of villi, and variable degrees of neutrophil-rich inflammatory infiltration.

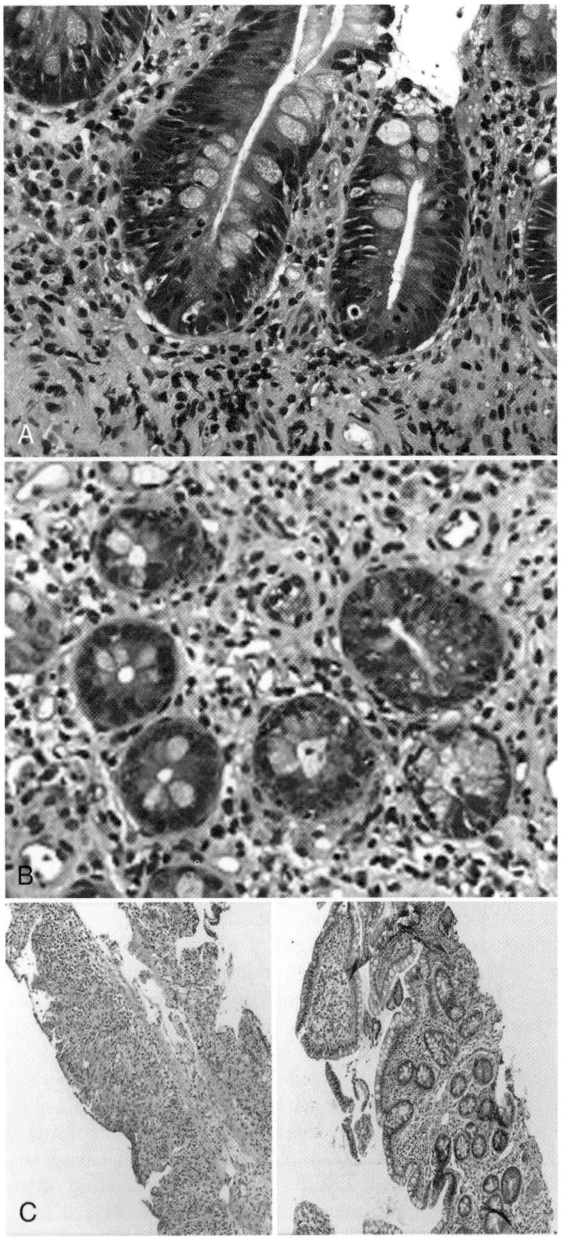

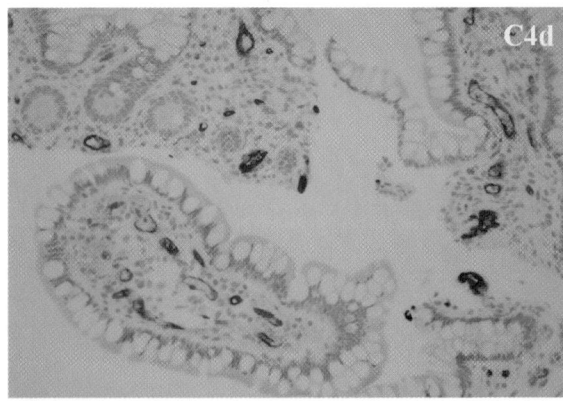

Figure 198-10 Acute cellular rejection of intestinal allograft: mild (A), moderate (B), and severe (C). A, Mild acute rejection is characterized by a generally mild and localized inflammatory infiltrate, which tends to be concentrated around small venules in the lamina propria. Mucosa is intact, but crypt epithelium displays evidence of injury: mucin depletion, cytoplasmic basophilia, decreased cell height, nuclear enlargement with hyperchromasia, and inflammatory infiltration. Crypt epithelial apoptosis is increased, usually with more than 6 apoptotic bodies/10 crypts. If sampled by biopsy specimen, preexisting lymphoid aggregates (Peyer's patches) demonstrate an intense accumulation of activated lymphocytes. Villi are variably shortened, and architecture may be slightly distorted owing to expansion of lamina propria by inflammatory infiltration. **B,** In moderate acute rejection, inflammatory infiltrate is widely dispersed within the lamina propria. Crypt injury and cryptitis are distributed more diffusely than in mild acute rejection, and villi tend to have a greater degree of flattening. Number of apoptotic bodies is greater than in mild acute rejection, usually with focal "confluent apoptosis." Mild to moderate intimal arteritis may be seen. Mucosa remains intact without ulceration, although focal superficial erosions can be present. **C,** Severe acute rejection is distinguished by a marked degree of crypt damage and mucosal ulceration, with lymphocytic infiltration extending deep into allograft wall and involving nerves and ganglia. As a consequence of mucosal destruction, luminal contents gain access to submucosa, prompting a neutrophil-rich infiltrate and an overlying fibropurulent (pseudomembranous) exudate with widespread mucosal sloughing as the final result. Adjacent viable epithelium usually shows rejection-associated changes such as crypt epithelial damage and abundant apoptosis. Severe intimal arteritis or transmural arteritis may be seen.

coagulopathy mediated by plasminogen activators from the graft may also occur. Every effort is made to address these factors in the operating room, and usually whatever coagulopathy persists postoperatively is mild. Postoperative hemorrhage is most often a technical problem arising from vascular anastomoses or extensive raw peritoneal surfaces. Even mild coagulopathy should be completely corrected if bleeding is suspected in the posttransplant recipient. Any bleeding that causes hemodynamic alteration should be managed by early reexploration.

VASCULAR COMPLICATIONS

Superior mesenteric artery thrombosis is a catastrophic complication that leads to rapid and massive necrosis of the intestinal allograft. Elevation of hepatic enzymes (with liver allografts) and pallor of the intestinal stoma is accompanied by clinical deterioration, usually

recipients.[25] Risk factors for chronic rejection include type of allograft and retransplantation. The clinical presentation of chronic rejection may include weight loss, chronic diarrhea, intermittent fevers, distal intestinal allograft obstruction, or GI bleeding. Histologically, chronic rejection is characterized by villous blunting, focal ulcerations, epithelial metaplasia, and scant cellular infiltrates on endoscopic mucosal biopsies. Full-thickness biopsies of intestinal allograft with chronic rejection demonstrate obliterative thickening of intestinal arterioles.

Management of Complications

POSTOPERATIVE HEMORRHAGE

Recipients of intestinal and multivisceral transplants commonly will demonstrate varying degrees of liver dysfunction, qualitative and quantitative platelet abnormalities, and fibrinolysis which can lead to profound intraoperative coagulopathy. Intraoperative bleeding can also develop from lysis of vascularized adhesions due to previous surgeries and portal hypertension. Transient graft reperfusion

Figure 198-11 Antibody-mediated rejection of intestinal allograft. Humoral rejection is characterized by a grossly cyanotic small-intestine allograft. Histologic findings include severe congestion, neutrophilic margination, and fibrin-platelet thrombi within the lamina propria microvasculature, along with focal hemorrhage. Immunohistochemical staining to C4d confirms the diagnosis of antibody-mediated rejection with heavy and diffuse staining of the lamina propria capillaries.

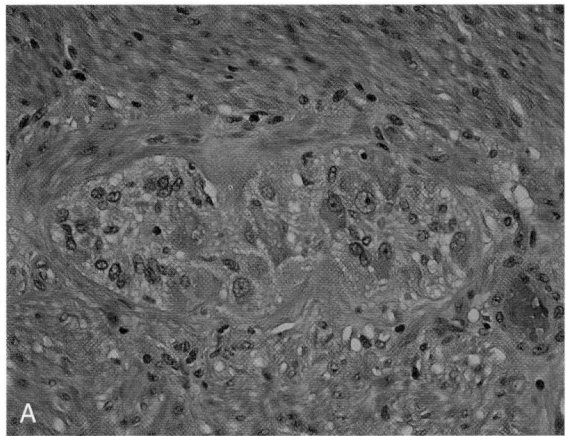

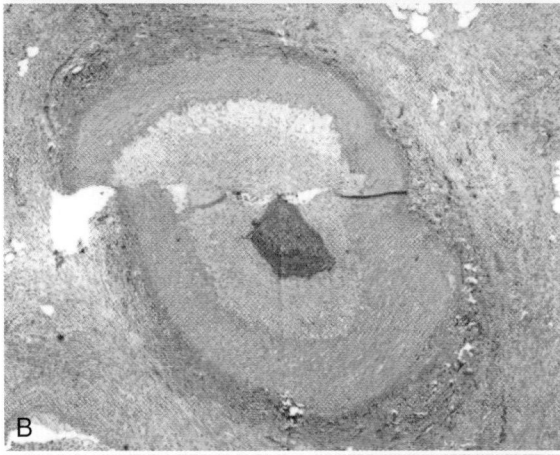

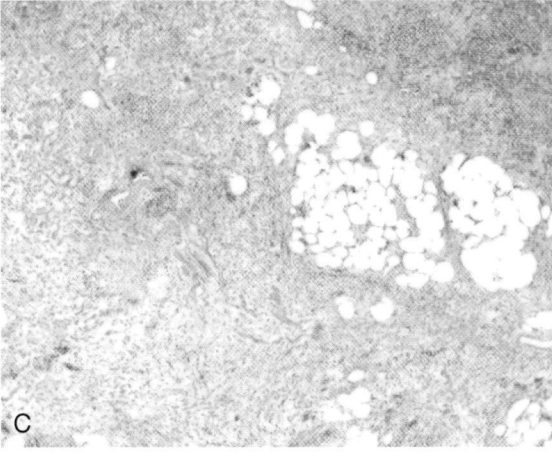

Figure 198-12 Chronic rejection of intestinal allograft. Histologic findings in mucosal biopsies are obliterative arteriopathy, lymphoid depletion, and mesenteric sclerosis. Mucosa shows loss of villous architecture, chronic ulcers with exudate and granulation tissue, widespread loss of the crypts of Lieberkühn, crypts of Lieberkühn with pyloric gland metaplasia, and mucosal fibrosis.

fulminant sepsis, and hepatic coma (with liver allografts). Isolated small-bowel allografts can be explanted with a reasonable expectation of patient survival; but in patients with composite allografts, removal for arterial thrombosis leads to almost certain death in the absence of immediate retransplant. Clinical suspicion of arterial thrombosis should be definitively evaluated in the operating room and not delayed by performance of Doppler ultrasound examination.

Acute venous thrombosis also leads to loss of the intestinal allograft without timely surgical intervention. Clinical signs of venous thrombosis include acute massive ascites and stomal congestion. Mesenteric

infarction is the ultimate outcome of unresolved venous thrombosis, necessitating explant of the intestinal allograft.

Incomplete obstruction of major inflow or outflow vessels may be suspected on allograft biopsy or based on clinical and laboratory signs of graft dysfunction. Contrast vascular radiographic studies are confirmatory, and the correction is either surgical or endovascular based upon individual assessments and available clinical expertise.

GASTROINTESTINAL COMPLICATIONS

Gastrointestinal bleeding after intestinal transplantation is an ominous sign that requires timely evaluation. Acute rejection or infectious enteritis are the most likely etiologies and should be diagnosed or excluded based upon endoscopic biopsy results. The diagnosis of rejection relies not only on histologic evidence but also on the endoscopic appearance of the mucosa. Bleeding from ulcerated EBV- or CMV-induced lesions can be routinely differentiated by gross endoscopic examination. Empirical therapy for rejection of intestinal allografts is not indicated under any circumstances.

Anastomotic leak may occur in all intestinal transplant recipients, but it is more common in pediatric patients than adults. Clinical presentation commonly involves florid sepsis, and confirmation is achieved with oral contrast imaging. Owing to immunosuppression, all bowel leaks require surgical revision, evacuation of any peritoneal contamination, and often second-look laparotomy to confirm resolution. Diagnostic laparotomy is indicated in the setting of sepsis and equivocal imaging studies.

The progression of motility patterns in the denervated intestinal allograft is still not fully understood. Hypermotility of the allograft occurs early after transplant, and in the absence of infection or rejection, it can be regulated with agents such as paregoric, loperamide, or pectin.

RENAL COMPLICATIONS

Deterioration of renal function in intestinal transplant recipients remains a significant clinical challenge. Pretransplant renal dysfunction is exacerbated by higher target levels of immunosuppression, repeated exposure to nephrotoxic antibiotics, and episodes of dehydration with intestinal allograft dysfunction. The incidence of chronic renal failure for intestinal transplant recipients at 5 years post transplant exceeds 20%.[26] Overall, a review of Scientific Registry of Transplant Recipients (SRTR) data shows that patients without severe pretransplant renal dysfunction who do not receive a kidney as part of the composite allograft will generally demonstrate a 50% increase in serum creatinine at 5-year follow-up.

POSTTRANSPLANT LYMPHOPROLIFERATIVE DISORDER

The development of PTLD is almost always associated with EBV infection. Posttransplant infection with EBV results in a spectrum of diseases, from mononucleosis syndromes and plasma cell hyperplasia to neoplastic PTLD (Figure 198-13). In a series of 500 intestinal and multivisceral transplants at the University of Pittsburgh, all but 2 of 57 recipients with PTLD developed the disorder as a consequence of confirmed EBV infection. Early studies found that primary tacrolimus use in pediatric patients was associated with a 15% long-term risk of PTLD, with almost 80% of these cases occurring within the first 2 years after transplant. Achieving an optimal immunosuppression steady state and avoiding excessive therapy intervals appear to be keys to minimizing EBV/PTLD complications. Cumulative PTLD-free survival for intestinal transplant recipients undergoing induction immunosuppression has improved to nearly 90%, possibly attributable to a lower incidence of acute rejection (and thus decreased need for escalation of immunosuppression) as well as improved EBV viral load monitoring.

Patients presenting with PTLD complain of sporadic fever, lethargy, and malaise. Weight loss, diarrhea, and GI complaints are common, as are signs of graft dysfunction. Standard laboratory evaluation may

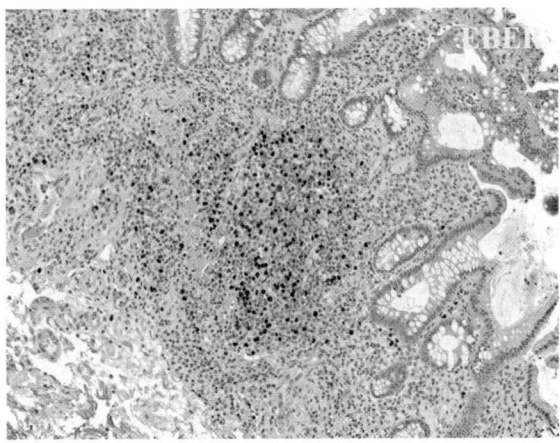

Figure 198-13 Epstein-Barr virus posttransplant lymphoproliferative disorder (EBV/PTLD). At the early phase of EBV infection, tissue is expanded by scattered EBV encapsulated RNA (EBER)-positive lymphocytes. With disease progression, the number of positive cells increases, lymphocytes become activated and transformed, and ultimately, tissue architecture is effaced by a malignant lymphoproliferative process.

demonstrate neutropenia, atypical lymphocytosis, anemia, and thrombocytopenia. Further evaluation of PTLD is guided by findings on contrast-enhanced computed tomography (CT) scanning of the head, neck, chest, abdomen, and pelvis, with or without endoscopy, based on results of noninvasive imaging. Histologic examination of the tissue is optimal, and specimens should be promptly submitted for fresh staining with the EBER-1 probe by experienced pathologists. An evaluation for CD20 staining should also be performed.

Treatment of PTLD involves stopping immunosuppression completely. PTLD that is unresponsive to discontinuation of immunosuppression should be treated with monoclonal antibody, usually rituximab, if shown to be CD20 positive by biopsy. Complete remission rates of 60% to 70% have been reported in children. The antibody therapy is relatively well tolerated, and for the 20% of patients who have recurrence, retreatment with rituximab can be curative. For PTLD refractory to monoclonal antibody, low-dose cytotoxic chemotherapy and steroids have been used effectively.

GRAFT-VERSUS-HOST DISEASE

Acute graft-versus-host disease (GVHD) results from immunocompetent donor T cells causing damage to recipient tissues after transplantation. The incidence of GVHD (Figure 198-14) after intestinal transplantation ranges between 5% and 10% and usually occurs within the first 6 months post transplant.[27] The major targets of GVHD are epithelial cells of skin, intestine, and liver. Cardiac muscle involvement is not common but has been described. A recipient with GVHD commonly presents with fever and a maculopapular rash on the upper torso, neck, or palms of hands and feet, which may coalesce to form blisters or more diffuse erythema. Other clinical signs and symptoms include oral lesions, diarrhea, intestinal mucosal ulceration, native liver dysfunction, lymphadenopathy,[28] and bone marrow suppression with pancytopenia. The variability of GVHD focality and severity leads to a wide spectrum of disease, from mild GVHD presenting with fevers and self-limiting rash to more severe forms leading to end-organ damage.

The diagnosis of GVHD is based on the clinical presentation and by histologic confirmation when possible. Corticosteroids are the first-line therapy to control epithelial damage caused by GVHD and are effective in around 50% of cases overall. If unresponsive to steroids, GVHD can usually be controlled by reduction of calcineurin-based immunosuppression. Other forms of refractory GVHD have been treated successfully using antilymphocytic therapy (e.g.,

Thymoglobulin and OKT3), as well using anti-interleukin therapy (e.g., Zenapax and Simulect) as well as anti-TNF (tumor necrosis factor) antibody therapy (e.g., Remicade).

Outcomes

PATIENT AND GRAFT SURVIVAL

A significant improvement in early patient and graft survival after intestinal transplantation has been achieved over the past decade, with 1-year patient and graft survival (Figure 198-15) reaching 89.3% and 78.9% for intestine-only recipients and 71.5% and 69.0% for liver-intestine recipients, respectively. In 1998, the 1-year adjusted graft and patient survival after intestinal transplantation were only 52% and 69%, respectively. Updated outcomes for intestinal transplant recipients are now comparable to outcomes following pancreas, lung, and liver transplantation. Contributing factors to this marked improvement in outcomes after intestinal transplantation include increased experience among intestinal transplant teams, improvements in critical care, advances in immunosuppression, and advances in the detection and treatment of rejection. The hospitalization status of the recipient at the time of transplantation also remains a strongly predictive factor for patient survival, with an unadjusted 1-year survival rate of 83% for recipients not waiting in the hospital, 73% for recipients waiting in the hospital, and only 50% for recipients waiting in the ICU. In 1999, almost one-third of intestinal and multivisceral recipients were in intensive care at the time of transplantation, whereas in 2008, 70% were not in the hospital, and only 12% were in intensive care.

In contrast to recent achievements in short-term outcomes, long-term survival after isolated intestinal transplantation has not significantly improved. Ten-year patient and graft survival remain 46% and 29% for isolated intestinal transplantation and 42% and 39% for intestine-with-liver grafts, respectively. These results are similar to those reported for lung and combined heart-lung transplantation but compare unfavorably to kidney, liver, and heart transplantation, where 10-year patient and graft survival exceed 50%.

LONG-TERM REHABILITATION AND QUALITY OF LIFE

Long-term functional outcomes after intestinal transplantation have not been fully characterized. A small preliminary study[29] in pediatric recipients with functioning intestinal allografts more than 1-year post transplant found that quality of life was perceived by recipients to be comparable to that of their peers, while parental proxy assessments compared less favorably in terms of physical functioning, general health, and family activities. Younger recipients (5-10 years of age) demonstrated significantly worse outcomes than older recipients

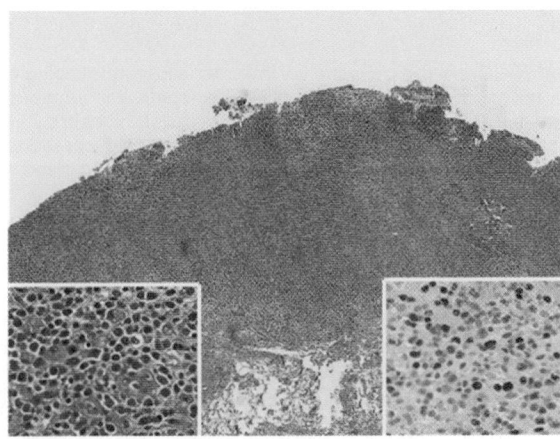

Figure 198-14 Intestinal allograft graft-versus-host disease (GVHD). Mucosal biopsy of native small intestine showing crypt epithelial apoptosis and lamina propria inflammation.

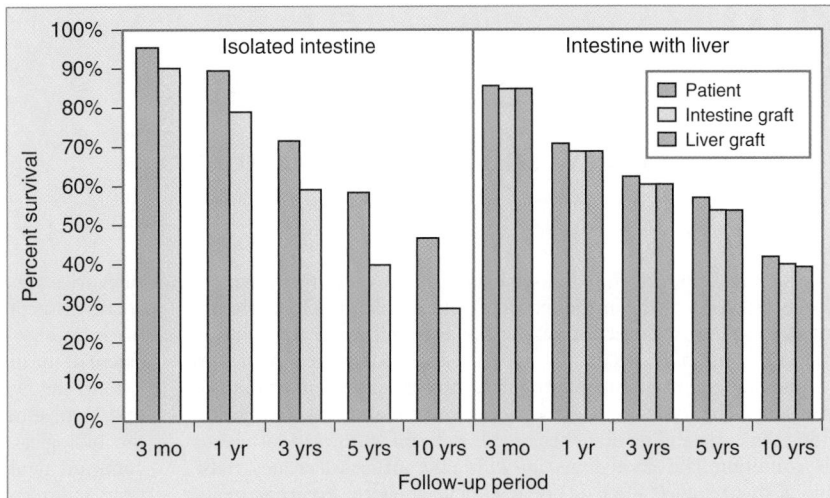

Figure 198-15 Unadjusted patient and graft survival for isolated intestine and combined liver and intestine recipients. *(Adapted from Mazariegos GV, Steffick DE, Horslen S, Farmer D, Fryer J, Grant D et al. Intestine transplantation in the United States, 1999-2008. Am J Transplant 2010;10:1020-34.)*

(11-18 years of age) in terms of global health assessments, general health perception, and family activities. There have been reports demonstrating significant improvement in certain aspects of psychiatric health after transition from parenteral nutrition to posttransplant TPN independence.[30] In these reports, long-term physical and psychiatric rehabilitation were achieved in over 80% of intestinal transplant recipients who survived beyond the sixth postoperative month.

Conclusions

Significant improvements in outcomes from intestinal and multivisceral transplantation have been achieved through advances in multidisciplinary care of intestinal failure, surgical technique, innovative immunosuppressive strategies, and an improved understanding of intestinal transplantation immunology. These accomplishments, however, remain overshadowed by the remaining fundamental challenge of preventing or minimizing chronic allograft rejection. The high waiting list mortality, particularly for infants and adults with concomitant liver failure, requires a reexamination of national guidelines for multivisceral procurement to maximize the usage of acceptable donor allografts. Long-term data on nutritional outcomes and transplantation morbidity are necessary to clarify the optimal timing and role of intestinal and multivisceral transplantation in patients with intestinal failure.

ANNOTATED REFERENCES

Abu-Elmagd KM, Costa G, Bond GJ, Soltys K, Sindhi R, Wu T, et al. Five hundred intestinal and multivisceral transplantations at a single center: major advances with new challenges. Ann Surg 2009;250:567-81.
The largest single-center experience with intestinal transplantation is reviewed with an emphasis on clinical management including new developments in immunosuppression and improved short- and mid-term outcomes.
Beath S, Pironi L, Gabe S, et al. Collaborative strategies to reduce mortality and morbidity in patients with chronic intestinal failure including those who are referred for small bowel transplantation. Transplantation 2008;85:1378-84.
A summary paper from a consensus workshop defining critical issues in patients with chronic intestinal failure, concluding that there was a need for a national intestinal failure registry as well as guidelines to facilitate timely referral for rehabilitation and/or transplantation.
Fishbein TM. Current concepts: intestinal transplantation. N Engl J Med 2009;361:999-1008.

A contemporary general overview of intestinal transplantation, indications, types of transplants, complications, and outcomes.
Gupte GL, Beath SV. Update on intestinal rehabilitation after intestinal transplantation. Curr Opin Organ Transplant 2009;14:1-7.
Critical review of current approaches for achieving nutritional autonomy and methods for monitoring of the health status of the intestinal transplant recipient.
Mazariegos GV, Steffick DE, Horslen S, Farmer D, Fryer J, Grant D, et al. Intestine transplantation in the United States 1999-2008. Am J Transplant 2010;10:1020-34.
This special issue, The 2009 SRTR Report on the State of Transplantation is a state-of-the-art review of intestinal transplantation in the United States, covering the disparity in procurement of small-intestine allograft compared to kidney and liver, much improved short-term patient and graft outcomes, and remaining challenges including chronic rejection.

REFERENCES

Access the complete reference list online at http://www.expertconsult.com.

199

Aortic Dissection

FRANK W. SELLKE | MICHAEL A. COADY

Aortic dissection involves the separation of the outer two-thirds of the aortic media by the introduction of pulsatile blood from a primary intimal tear. Aortic dissection can be a catastrophic medical condition. It most commonly occurs in hypertensive middle-aged men and requires rapid, optimal management to prevent serious morbidity or mortality. The variable extent of the proximal and distal extension along the aorta and its branches usually determines the seriousness of the condition. The blood dissecting within the aortic wall creates a false lumen that parallels the true aortic lumen. The term *dissecting aneurysm* is inaccurate because few acute aortic dissections are associated with an aortic aneurysm. Although most deaths occur early, aortic dissection in its chronic phase is responsible for a substantial proportion of thoracic aortic pathology and aortic rupture due to aneurysmal degeneration and enlargement of the false lumen.

The initial observation and description of an aortic dissection was made by Morgagni in the 18th century. This was followed by multiple anatomic and postmortem reports, including the description of the cause of death of King George II of England shortly before the American Revolution.[1] In the early 1800s, Maunoir better defined the pathologic process and first used the term *dissection* to describe the pathology.[2] Although many subsequent reports have described aortic dissection, premorbid diagnosis was not consistently possible until refinements in contrast aortography were made.[3] Indeed, only in the past several decades has either medical or surgical management had a reasonable chance to alter the course of aortic dissection.

The first attempts to treat this condition surgically involved wrapping of the dissected aorta to prevent rupture[4] or treatment of the complications of dissection without definitive repair. This usually resulted in a catastrophic outcome and death. DeBakey and colleagues pioneered the surgical treatment of aortic disease, including dissection, and first reported graft replacement of the dissected aorta as definitive treatment.[5] Aortic graft interposition has become the cornerstone of modern surgical therapy.

The modern approach to acute aortic dissection involves initial control of blood pressure with vasodilator medications and decreasing the rate of change of aortic pressure with beta-blocker drugs, followed by surgical repair in appropriate cases. Improved surgical and anesthetic techniques and improved postoperative monitoring and management have dramatically improved the results of treatment of aortic dissection. Recently, stent grafting has emerged as a tool to treat malperfusion complications of distal dissections.

Classification

An understanding and description of aortic dissection are critical for the optimal care of these patients. The first widely used classification system was developed by DeBakey and colleagues and consists of three categories: types I, II, and III.[5,6] Type I involves dissection originating in the ascending aorta, which continues to course through the descending aorta. Type II involves a tear only in the ascending aorta, and type III involves a tear originating in the descending thoracic aorta, distal to the ligamentum arteriosum. Subsequently, Daily and associates at Stanford University developed a classification system involving only two groupings, now known as *the Stanford system*.[7] In the Stanford classification system (Figure 199-1), type A dissections involve the ascending aorta, and type B involves the aorta distal to the innominate artery. There have been many other attempts to classify aortic dissection, but most have been abandoned. Despite the fact that different

categories are used, the essential element of a classification system of aortic dissection is involvement of the ascending aorta, regardless of the location of the primary intimal tear and irrespective of the distal extent of the dissection process.[8] This functional classification approach is consistent with the pathophysiology of aortic dissection, considering that involvement of the ascending aorta is the principal predictor of the biological behavior of the disease process, including the most common fatal complications—rupture with tamponade, congestive heart failure, and myocardial infarction. Moreover, functional classification simplifies diagnosis, because it is easier to accurately identify involvement of the ascending aorta than to determine the exact site of the primary intimal tear or the total extent of propagation of the dissection process.

The Stanford classification system facilitates the clinical decision-making process and definitive patient management. Patients presenting with acute Stanford type A dissections should be treated surgically in most cases, and individuals with Stanford type B dissections are generally treated medically, using surgical intervention or endovascular stentgraft placement only if major complications are present. Generally, aortic dissections are defined as acute if they are diagnosed within 14 days of the onset of presenting symptoms. When dissection is diagnosed more than 14 days after onset, it is classified as chronic. Chronic dissection usually occurs only if the initial diagnosis was incorrect or if the patient suffered mild symptoms and did not seek appropriate medical care.

Over the past decade, advances in vascular imaging technology have led to the increased recognition of other conditions of the aorta, such as intramural hematoma and penetrating aortic ulcers, as distinct pathologic variants of classic aortic dissection.[9,10] Both these entities are characterized by the lack of a classic intimal flap dividing the aortic lumen into true and false channels. Intramural hematoma can be precipitated by an atherosclerotic ulcer penetrating the aortic wall or can occur spontaneously without intimal disruption after rupture of the vasa vasorum. Intramural hematoma can involve the ascending aorta (type A) as well as the descending aorta (type B). Although it is possible, an intramural hematoma rarely evolves into an aortic dissection.[11] Penetrating atherosclerotic ulcers occur most commonly in the descending thoracic aorta. Distinguishing intramural hematoma or penetrating aortic ulcer from aortic dissection is important because the prognosis and management of these lesions can differ.[12,13]

Clinical Findings

Aortic dissection can occur in all age-groups, although the majority of cases are observed in men aged 50 to 80 years. Dissection in patients younger than 40 years is most commonly an acute type A dissection and often occurs in patients with Marfan syndrome or a similar connective tissue disorder. On rare occasions, women during the last trimester of pregnancy or during delivery present with acute aortic dissection, presumably due to hormone-induced weakness of the aortic connective tissue and the markedly increased intraaortic pressure that often occurs during delivery. There is a male predominance, with an estimated male-to-female ratio of approximately 2:1. The exact incidence of aortic dissection is difficult to ascertain because in many cases, the diagnosis is not made before death. Indeed, delayed recognition of acute aortic dissection is a frequent cause of malpractice suits. In one series, acute aortic dissection was found in 1% to 2% of autopsies.[14] Recently it has been estimated that the incidence of acute

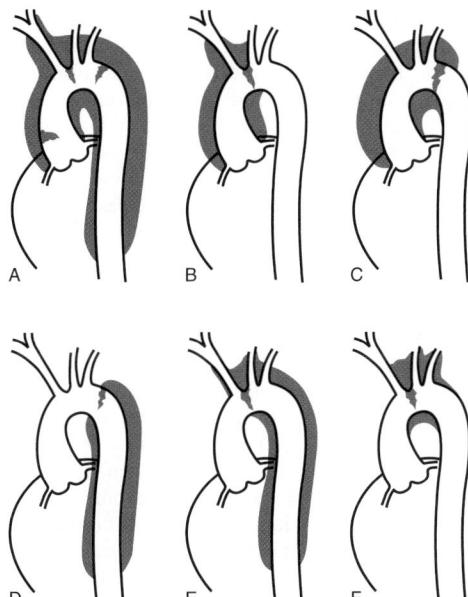

Figure 199-1 Schematic illustration of Stanford classification system of aortic dissections. Examples in top row **(A, B, C)** are all type A aortic dissections involving the ascending aorta. Examples in bottom row **(D, E, F)** are all examples of type B dissections in which the ascending aorta is not involved. Note that the aortic arch can be involved in a type B dissection. *(From Miller DC. Surgical management of aortic dissections: indications, perioperative management, and long-term results. In: Doroghazi RM, Slater EE, editors. Aortic dissection. New York: McGraw-Hill; 1983, p. 196.)*

aortic dissection in the United States might be as high as 10 to 20 or more cases per million population per year.[15] Most aortic dissections (two-thirds) occur in the ascending aorta (Stanford type A) as opposed to the less frequent distal Stanford type B dissections. Most caregivers incorrectly believe that ruptured abdominal aortic aneurysms occur more commonly than aortic dissections; however, the former just tend to be diagnosed correctly more often than the latter.

Left untreated, most patients suffering an acute aortic dissection die, generally within the first 24 to 48 hours. Death may occur due to rupture of the dissected aorta into the pericardial space, leading to tamponade and cardiovascular collapse; proximal extension, leading to severe, acute aortic insufficiency and heart failure; or acute myocardial infarction if the dissection involves the ostia of the coronary arteries. It has been estimated that 40% of patients with dissection involving the ascending aorta die immediately or before reaching the hospital, and more than 67% die within the first 24 hours. In addition, mortality often results secondary to occlusion of major aortic branches supplying the cerebral or visceral circulation, causing massive stroke or visceral ischemia and severe metabolic acidosis. In contrast, among patients with Stanford type B dissections, 75% are alive 1 month after the onset of symptoms.

Patients with untreated acute type B dissection can expire from acute aortic rupture or from occlusion of one of several major aortic branches resulting in ischemic injury to vital abdominal organs. However, comparative studies have determined that in most cases of type B aortic dissection, survival is better with medical treatment alone (aggressive antihypertensive therapy) than with urgent surgical repair or aortic replacement. After acute aortic dissection, the false lumen remains patent in most cases, depending on the presence of distal reentry sites. When the false lumen remains patent, the aorta is prone to progressive expansion over time, necessitating the need for close long-term follow-up.

The most consistent clinical condition associated with aortic dissection is arterial hypertension. In patients with aortic dissection, the prevalence of arterial hypertension varies between 45% and 80%[16-19]

and is highest in patients with acute type B dissection (Box 199-1). Hypertension may lead to smooth-muscle degeneration in the aortic wall, which may predispose to aortic dissection.

Connective tissue disorders such as Marfan or Ehlers-Danlos syndromes are associated with an increased risk of aortic dissection. Although both these conditions are relatively rare, they are frequently associated with acute dissection. In fact, aortic rupture or dissection is a common cause of death in patients with Marfan syndrome or other connective tissue disorders.[20] In addition, aortic dissection is more common in patients with Turner's syndrome and inflammatory disorders of the aorta such as syphilis or giant cell arteritis. Severe aortic atherosclerosis has been associated with a slight increase in the incidence of aortic dissection, but if dissection occurs, its extent seems to be more limited.

The risk of perioperative and late postoperative dissection[21] is also increased in patients with a bicuspid aortic valve or aortic coarctation, presumably due to impaired connective tissue integrity. Aortic dissection is a rare complication of cardiac catheterization and other percutaneous diagnostic and therapeutic interventional techniques involving manipulation of catheters inside the thoracic aorta. Unfortunately, most veteran cardiac surgeons have experienced cases of intraoperative aortic dissection due to a clamp injury of the ascending aorta or a dissection initiating at the arterial cannulation site, especially when femoral arterial cannulation is performed.

One of the cardiovascular complications of cocaine use is acute aortic dissection, and this diagnosis should be considered in drug abusers presenting with acute chest pain.[22,23] Aortic dissection in this setting occurs as a result of sudden severe hypertension secondary to catecholamine release.

Pathologic Findings

Most surgeons and pathologists believe the initiating event in aortic dissection is a tear in the intima of the aortic wall that allows blood to enter, leading to separation of the medial layer of the aorta. The primary intimal tear causes communication between the true aortic lumen and a new false lumen. Few aortic dissections lack an identifiable intimal tear. Indeed, most extensive aortic dissections have multiple reentry sites. Intramural hematoma due to rupture of an intramural vessel is another potential initiating event, although this cause of dissection is less frequent. Dissections usually propagate antegrade in a spiral manner but may also extend in a retrograde fashion. The rate of increase of aortic systolic pressure, the absolute blood pressure, and the integrity and strength of the aortic wall determine the

---

Box 199-1

CONDITIONS ASSOCIATED WITH AORTIC DISSECTION

Hypertension
Aortic valve and congenital aortic disorders:
  Bicuspid aortic valve
  Coarctation of the aorta
Connective tissue disorders:
  Marfan syndrome
  Cystic medial necrosis
  Ehlers-Danlos syndrome
  Turner's syndrome
Pregnancy
Atherosclerosis
Relapsing polychondritis
Giant cell arteritis
Syphilis
Cocaine abuse
Iatrogenic:
  Insertion of intraaortic balloon pump
  Cardiac catheterization or angioplasty
  Aortic or femoral arterial cannulation for cardiopulmonary
    bypass

rate and extent of progression of the dissection. Ironically, distal progression of the dissection may be limited by extensive atherosclerotic disease, because the layers of the aorta are more tightly fused. Younger patients presenting with acute dissection frequently have involvement of the entire thoracic and abdominal aorta. Reentry into the true lumen may allow decompression of the false lumen and may maintain perfusion to distal organs. This is the rationale behind surgical and percutaneous techniques of fenestration for treatment of malperfusion syndromes associated with aortic dissection.

Organ or limb ischemia or malperfusion may occur when the dissection process compromises blood flow to various aortic branches. Malperfusion usually occurs when flow is impaired due to vascular compression of the true lumen by the false lumen, extravascular compression of abdominal viscera or vessels, or occlusion of a branch artery by a dissection flap. The pattern of involvement of branches of the thoracic and abdominal aorta is variable and often leads to confusion regarding the correct diagnosis.

Presentation

Severe chest pain of a sudden nature is the most common presenting symptom of aortic dissection. The pain is typically abrupt and severe at onset and is often described as "tearing" and "the worst pain I have ever experienced." This is especially true for patients who have never experienced childbirth. With type A dissections, the pain tends to be in the anterior chest and similar to that observed with myocardial infarction. Type B dissections classically cause midscapular pain, although this can be quite variable; this variability may lead to an incorrect diagnosis. Migration of pain and constant pain suggest continued expansion or progression. Differentiating the chest pain of acute aortic dissection from that of other causes such as acute myocardial ischemia, esophageal reflux disease, pericarditis, chest trauma, or abdominal pathology is critical in the initial evaluation of these patients to allow prompt, correct management. Unlike the crescendo-type pain frequently associated with acute myocardial infarctions, aortic dissections present with abrupt, sharp, unrelenting severe pain. On rare occasion, acute dissection can be painless, although this presentation is uncommon and is more often the case in patients presenting with chronic dissection. A relative minority of patients with acute aortic dissection present with signs of cardiac and other organ system involvement.[17-19,24-26] Other clinical manifestations may include stroke, paraplegia, upper- or lower-extremity ischemia, and anuria or abdominal pain due to renal or mesenteric ischemia. These latter findings portend a grave prognosis.

Diagnosis

The diagnosis of aortic dissection requires a strong index of suspicion by the evaluating caregiver. If the acute, sudden onset of chest pain cannot be attributed to myocardial infarction or ischemia, pericarditis, or traumatic chest injury, the diagnosis of acute dissection must be considered. Even in cases of acute myocardial infarction, the diagnosis of aortic dissection should still be entertained, especially if the patient develops migrating chest or back pain, leg ischemia, syncope, or other neurologic symptoms that may be related to vascular compromise. Physical findings often include a disparity in blood pressure measurements between the right and left arms or between the arms and legs, or a diminished pulse in one of the limbs. After the diagnosis is suspected, rapid confirmation or exclusion of aortic dissection is critical for optimal care. Until recently, aortic angiography was considered the gold standard for diagnosing acute dissection, because other methods such as computed tomography (CT) and echocardiography were untested or fraught with artifactual findings. However, improved computed tomography angiography (CTA), transesophageal echocardiography (TEE), and magnetic resonance imaging (MRI) techniques are at least as accurate as aortic angiography and are usually far more rapidly obtained. Selection of the diagnostic method depends on which technique is most accurate and can be most quickly obtained in

the treating hospital. In general, the procedure of choice is CTA; it is noninvasive and easy to perform and can usually be obtained without delay. Owing to major technologic advances, acquisition of a large number of thin-slice images is possible within minutes using ultrafast CT scanners. Further, modern computer technology allows complex reconstruction of high-quality images. The diagnosis of aortic dissection requires identification of two distinct lumens separated by an intimal flap.[27] Contrast-enhanced CT scanning has a sensitivity of 82% to 100% and a specificity between 90% and 100%.[17,27-32] Disadvantages include the need for intravenous contrast and the presence of artifacts, although the latter is now less of a problem than in the past.

TEE is also can be performed rapidly. The type of dissection (i.e., Stanford type A or B), extent of dissection, presence or absence of hemodynamically significant aortic valve regurgitation, and the presence or absence of pericardial effusion can all be determined using TEE. High-resolution imaging of the heart and thoracic aorta is possible with TEE because of the close proximity of the esophagus and thoracic aorta. Importantly, TEE can be performed in the emergency room, intensive care unit (ICU), or operating room. Even if the diagnosis of acute aortic dissection has been confirmed with another imaging modality, TEE can aid in the preoperative, intraoperative, and postoperative assessment of cardiac and valvular function and the extent of residual disease. Transthoracic echocardiography has a limited role in the diagnosis of aortic dissection because the images produced are not optimal. However, if the diagnosis is made using MRI or CTA, transthoracic echo may help assess valve and ventricular function.

MRI is accurate in making the diagnosis and is also noninvasive and does not require the use of contrast material. MRI produces high-quality images of the aorta in multiple planes and allows clear delineation of the entire aorta, localization of the intimal tear, delineation of aortic branch artery involvement, and diagnosis of a pericardial effusion suggestive of aortic rupture. As with CTA scanning, the criterion used to diagnose acute aortic dissection with MRI is identification of two lumina separated by an intimal flap. MRI is associated with sensitivity and specificity rates of 95% to 100%.[17,27,29-32] In urgent circumstances, MRI may not be immediately available, and this approach should not be performed in patients with pacemakers, defibrillators, or other metallic implants. In addition, the relatively long time necessary for image acquisition in hemodynamically compromised patients is a potential drawback to using MRI in identifying an aortic dissection. The fact that the patient has to lie flat in the magnetic field can be problematic in some cases.

Although the chest radiograph is neither sensitive nor specific for the diagnosis of dissection, some findings may be suggestive. These include the presence of a widened upper mediastinum, blunting of the aortic knob, and pleural effusion. The electrocardiogram (ECG), though neither specific nor sensitive, can help establish the need for concomitant coronary revascularization if the dissection involves the coronary arteries or if the patient suffers from ordinary coronary artery disease. Elderly male patients often present with ECG changes during acute aortic dissection, even if no direct coronary involvement is present. This phenomenon is likely related to concomitant coronary artery disease. Coronary angiography is rarely performed unless there is clear compromise of myocardial perfusion. Coronary angiography may delay definitive treatment and rarely improves the management. However, when the patient has a clear history of coronary artery disease and is hemodynamically stable, consideration may be given to performing coronary angiography if the patient presents with a chronic type A aortic dissection. Moderate coronary occlusive disease can generally be treated percutaneously in the catheterization laboratory after aortic surgery. When hemodynamic instability is present, the patient should proceed directly to the operating room on an emergent basis.

Treatment

In general, all patients with acute type A aortic dissections should be considered for emergency surgical repair of the ascending aorta to

TABLE 199-1	Initial Medical Management for Patients with Acute Aortic Dissection
Drug	**Dosage**
Metoprolol	5-10 mg slow IV bolus until SBP <120 mm Hg and HR <70 bpm; repeat as needed
Esmolol	500 µg/kg/min IV for 1 min, followed by 30-50 µg/kg/min for 5 min; titrate to maintain SBP <120 mm Hg systolic and HR <70 bpm
Labetalol	0.25 mg/kg IV over 2 min; 40-80 mg q 10 min up to 300 mg; continuous IV infusion to maintain SBP <120 mm Hg and HR <70 bpm
Sodium nitroprusside	1-8 µg/kg/min IV to maintain SBP <120 mm Hg; should be used in conjunction with a beta-blocker (metoprolol, esmolol, labetalol)

bpm, beats per minute; HR, heart rate; SBP, systolic blood pressure.

prevent life-threatening conditions or complications.* Patients with acute type A dissection presenting with irreversible stroke or other severe malperfusion syndromes,[8,18,36] those with debilitating systemic diseases such as metastatic cancer with a life expectancy of less than 1 year, or those older than 80 years with multiple major complications or serious medical conditions may be considered for medical management. It should be recognized, however, that patients treated nonoperatively are not likely to survive. The presence of acute hemiplegia alone should not be considered an absolute contraindication to early surgical intervention,[36] because many of these patients recover significant neurologic function after surgery. However, patients presenting with hypotension, massive stroke, anuria, and acidosis suggestive of mesenteric ischemia should be considered nonsurgical candidates. Patients presenting with acute type A intramural hematoma are managed identically to those with acute type A aortic dissection.[9,11,37] However, some authors believe that medical therapy is indicated for selected patients with uncomplicated acute type A intramural hematoma when the ascending aorta is not excessively dilated.[38-40] If a patient with acute type A intramural hematoma is treated medically, close observation is mandatory. Serial imaging studies should be obtained over several days.

As soon as the diagnosis of acute type A aortic dissection is suspected, intensive monitoring must be initiated. An arterial line, central venous catheter, and urinary catheter should be inserted. Antihypertensive treatment is a major part of initial management of patients with acute type A or type B dissection, before and after surgical correction (Table 199-1). Generally, patients with acute severe hypotension or other evidence of rupture or impending rupture should be taken to the operating room emergently, and attempts at pericardial drainage should be avoided.

The primary goal of surgical treatment for patients with acute type A dissection is to replace the ascending aorta to prevent aortic rupture or proximal extension of the process, with resultant tamponade or severe heart failure. Ideally, the primary intimal tear should be completely resected, and the dissected aortic layers reconstituted proximally and distally to obliterate the false lumen and reestablish normal perfusion to distal organs. When aortic valve regurgitation is present, aortic valve competence is restored either by reconstructing the sinuses of Valsalva and the aortic root or by resuspending the valve commissures. These approaches are possible in the majority of cases.[41] Complete aortic root replacement with reimplantation of the coronary ostia using either a composite valve graft or a valve-sparing technique should be considered if the aortic root is severely damaged by the dissection process, the patient has Marfan syndrome or another connective tissue disorder, severe annuloaortic ectasia is present, or the valve needs to be replaced for other reasons such as aortic stenosis.[42-44] In selected cases, aortic valve replacement and supracoronary aortic graft replacement may be used to treat acute type A aortic dissections if the aortic root is not destroyed by the dissection. Excellent surgical technique has to be used to prevent excessive bleeding, continued dissection, and residual

coronary ischemia or aortic valve insufficiency. Tranexamic acid or ε-aminocaproic acid (Amicar) can be administered to decrease bleeding. Aprotinin, while often used in the past, is no longer available. When necessary, reinforcement of the dissected aortic layers is facilitated by reapproximation of the dissection flap to the aortic wall using strips of Teflon felt or bovine pericardium. Biological glue composed of purified bovine serum albumin and 10% glutaraldehyde was recently approved in the United States (BioGlue [CryoLife Inc., Kennesaw, Georgia]). Biological glue is easy to use and decreases blood loss,[45] but cases have been reported in which use of a large amount of glue has resulted in development of false aneurysms, graft dehiscence, and full-thickness aortic necrosis. Most modern woven vascular grafts are not plagued by excessive bleeding and are easy to use.

In the past 15 years, the use of hypothermic circulatory arrest has been advocated to allow careful inspection of the aortic arch and performance of an "open" distal aortic anastomosis in cases of acute type A dissection.[46,47] The construction of a completely hemostatic distal anastomosis is easier in the absence of an aortic cross-clamp. However, profound circulatory arrest increases the risk of neurologic injury, especially if the distal anastomosis cannot be performed in a rapid manner.

A midline sternotomy incision is used to repair acute type A dissections. Arterial cannulation can be performed via the right axillary artery or either femoral artery. Cardiopulmonary bypass is then established. If the patient has severe aortic insufficiency, a vent is inserted into the left ventricle through the right superior pulmonary vein to prevent distention. The authors place a single venous cannula, although some suggest bicaval cannulation. The use of retrograde blood cardioplegia facilitates the operative procedure, although supplemental antegrade cardioplegia can be delivered directly into the coronary arteries.

Patients with dissection-related destruction of the aortic root should undergo composite valve graft root replacement or valve-sparing aortic root replacement using the David reimplantation method, with complete or near-complete excision of the sinuses of Valsalva. Alternatively, resuspension of the aortic valve and preservation of the sinuses can be performed if the aortic root is not destroyed. If the aortic valve is markedly abnormal or cannot be satisfactorily repaired, separate valve and supracoronary aortic graft replacement is a reasonable alternative in selected patients, but the supracoronary aortic arch should be resected as extensively as possible to prevent pseudoaneurysm formation.

In up to a third of patients, the primary intimal tear is located in the aortic arch or descending aorta, a condition associated with a poorer prognosis.[47-50] These tears should be resected if possible, but such resection is often not feasible without combining arch or distal aortic resection with ascending aortic repair. Elderly patients often do not tolerate such extensive surgery and sustain major complications. In addition, reentry tears may occur in the distal aorta, precluding establishment of a totally intact, normally perfused aorta at the end of the operation. Although failure to include the arch in the repair may increase the need for subsequent aortic reoperation and reduce long-term survival, most cardiovascular surgeons simply treat the most critical portion of the aorta (i.e., the ascending segment) in these cases and leave the remainder of the aorta alone in an effort to facilitate patient salvage. This strategy is especially reasonable for very elderly patients or those with major comorbid conditions. Although infrequently encountered, patients with chronic type A or type B dissection may need surgical repair or stent grafting if an aortic false aneurysm or progressive aortic enlargement has developed. In some cases, it is difficult to distinguish between acute and chronic type A aortic dissection. When this occurs, urgent repair should be undertaken. Aortic dilatation due to significant aortic valve insufficiency is an indication for operation. In asymptomatic patients, surgical intervention is generally recommended when the diameter of the ascending aorta is greater than 55 to 60 mm, depending on the size of the normal native aorta (50 mm in patients with Marfan syndrome), or if the documented rate of expansion is greater than 5 to 10 mm over 1 year.[51]

*References 6, 8, 15-17, 19, 25, and 33-35.

With optimal medical and surgical methods, patients with aortic dissection have a mortality of 5% to 30% in the best centers.* These relatively low early mortality rates reflect advances in early diagnosis, surgical techniques, and myocardial protection. In the Stanford experience, the overall survival rates for patients with acute type A dissections at 1, 5, and 10 years were 67%, 55%, and 37%, respectively.[18] For patients with chronic type A dissections, the survival was 76%, 65%, and 45%, respectively. For patients with acute type A dissections, late survival for discharged patients was 91%, 75%, and 51% at 1, 5, and 10 years, respectively, compared with 93%, 79%, and 54% for those with chronic type A dissections. One-third of the late deaths were cardiac related, and many (10%-20%) were due to complications related to extension of the dissection or dilatation of the dissected aortic segment.

The treatment of Stanford type B dissections is generally medical, with aggressive antihypertensive and beta-blocker therapy and close long-term observation for progressive dilatation (see Table 199-1). Generally, beta blockade is initiated, and a vasodilator drug such as sodium nitroprusside is added later for blood pressure control. Pure vasodilator drugs should be avoided as an initial treatment, because reflex tachycardia and increased cardiac contractility may actually increase the rate of change in aortic pressure and, at least theoretically, exacerbate the dissection process. Alternatively, one of the newer antihypertensive agents such as nicardipine, Cleviprex (clevidipine butyrate), or fenoldopam may be considered. Initial medical monitoring and management should take place in an ICU in most cases, because a rapid and significant reduction in blood pressure and heart rate is the hallmark of optimal care. Blood pressure monitoring with an automatic blood pressure cuff apparatus may be sufficient if severe hypertension is not evident, the patient remains hemodynamically stable, and only a low dose of medication is required to control changes in aortic pressure. If the blood pressure and heart rate cannot be rapidly controlled, or if the patient does not rapidly become pain free, becomes hemodynamically unstable, or develops symptoms of associated malperfusion, an arterial monitoring line is mandatory, and early reimaging of the aorta should be considered. If the patient remains stable and pain free, he or she may be monitored outside the ICU after 24 to 48 hours. An imaging study (usually CTA scan or MRI) should be obtained before discharge as a baseline study.

Because surgical management of type B dissections is associated with very high mortality and morbidity, and because the results of with medical management are superior than to urgent surgical intervention, a nonoperative approach is taken in the vast majority of cases. Surgery through a lateral left thoracotomy is indicated for complications related to malperfusion or for chronic, severe pain indicative of dilatation, impending rupture, or progressive dissection. However, most of the complications related to malperfusion can be treated with catheter-based fenestration procedures or stent grafting,[59] and these patients do not require surgical therapy. Stenting of the thoracic aorta is currently well established for treatment of complications of type B dissections, but its routine use is generally not recommended.[60] Continued pain, new neurologic findings, and malperfusion syndromes not correctable with catheter-based fenestration or stent grafting may require surgical intervention. Cardiopulmonary bypass is generally used in surgical cases, cannulating the femoral artery and left atrium or both the femoral artery and vein. Cardiopulmonary bypass is usually instituted using total bypass, with or without profound hypothermic circulatory arrest. Alternatively, partial cardiopulmonary bypass (or isolated left heart bypass) can be used, depending on the surgeon's preference. Although in theory, the use of cardiopulmonary bypass should lessen the incidence of postoperative paraplegia, the results of descending aortic surgery using total or partial cardiopulmonary bypass (or isolated left heart bypass) or a non-cardiopulmonary bypass approach are similar in most series.

---

*References 17, 19, 33, 46, 48, and 52-58.

■ Long-Term Follow-Up

Close medical follow-up and careful periodic surveillance using appropriate imaging are critical to the optimal long-term management of postsurgical type A aortic dissection patients and those with type B dissection. It is mandatory for patients with aortic dissections to undergo routine imaging for as long as they live. Following operative repair, serial CTA or MRI scans of the thoracic and abdominal aorta are essential to detect complications related to aortic dissection; these scans should be performed at 3- to 6-month intervals for the first year and then every year thereafter. An echocardiogram may also be performed annually to evaluate the aortic root and aortic valve function, especially if aortic root reconstruction was performed. The hallmark of long-term management of patients who have suffered aortic dissection is aggressive control of arterial blood pressure, regardless of whether they have undergone surgical repair.

KEY POINTS

1. **Definition.** Aortic dissection involves a tear in the intimal layer of the aorta which allows pulsatile blood to course through the aortic wall, separating the outer two-thirds of the aortic media. This can be one of the most catastrophic medical conditions.

2. **Classification.** The most commonly used system for classifying aortic dissection was developed by Daily and associates at Stanford University. In the Stanford classification, type A dissections involve a tear originating in the ascending aorta, and type B dissections involve a tear originating in the aorta distal to the innominate artery.

3. **Clinical findings.** Aortic dissection can occur in all age-groups, although the majority of cases are seen in men between the ages of 50 and 80 years. Dissections that occur in patients younger than 40 years are generally type A dissections and are commonly observed in patients with Marfan syndrome or similar connective tissue disorders. There is a male predominance, with an estimated male-to-female ratio of 2:1. The most consistent clinical condition associated with aortic dissection is arterial hypertension.

4. **Pathologic findings.** Most surgeons and pathologists believe the initiating event in aortic dissection is a tear in the intima of the aortic wall that allows blood to enter, leading to separation within the medial layer of the aorta. The primary intimal tear causes communication between the true aortic lumen and the newly created false lumen. Dissections usually propagate antegrade in a spiral manner but may also extend in a retrograde fashion. The rate of increase in aortic systolic pressure and absolute blood pressure and the integrity and strength of the aortic wall determine the degree and extent of progression of the dissection.

5. **Diagnosis.** The diagnosis of aortic dissection requires a strong index of suspicion. If acute, sudden onset of chest pain cannot be attributed to other causes, the diagnosis of acute aortic dissection must be considered. Rapid confirmation or exclusion of aortic dissection is critical for optimal care. Computed tomography angiography, transesophageal echocardiography, and magnetic resonance imaging are at least as accurate as aortic angiography in the diagnosis and are usually far more readily obtained.

6. **Treatment.** In general, all patients with acute type A aortic dissections should be considered for emergency surgical repair of the ascending aorta to prevent life-threatening conditions or complications. The treatment of Stanford type B dissections is generally medical, with aggressive antihypertensive and beta-blocker therapy and close long-term observation for possible progressive dilatation. Complications of type B dissections are usually treated with stent grafting or percutaneous fenestration, but open surgery may be required in some cases. Antihypertensive treatment is also a major part of the management of patients with acute type A dissection, before and after surgical correction.

7. **Long-term management.** Close medical follow-up and careful periodic imaging surveillance are critical to optimal long-term management of postsurgical type A aortic dissection patients and those with medically managed type B dissections.

ANNOTATED REFERENCES

Daily PO, Trueblood HW, Stinson EB, et al. Management of acute aortic dissections. Ann Thorac Surg 1970;10:237-47.

The most frequently used classification system for aortic dissections was developed by Daily and associates at Stanford University. This system of classification, now known as the Stanford classification, involves only two groups. Type A dissections involve the ascending aorta, and type B involve the more distal aorta, from the innominate artery to more distal regions.

David TE, Feindel CM. An aortic valve-sparing operation for patients with aortic incompetence and aneurysm of the ascending aorta. J Thorac Cardiovasc Surg 1992;103:617-21.

This paper discusses treatment of aortic dissection involving the aortic root. If the aortic root is severely damaged by the dissection process, the patient has Marfan syndrome or another connective tissue disorder, severe annuloaortic ectasia is present, or the valve has to be replaced for other reasons (e.g., aortic stenosis), a valve-sparing technique may be appropriate.

Gillinov AM, Lytle BW, Kaplon RJ, et al. Dissection of the ascending aorta after previous cardiac surgery: differences in presentation and management. J Thorac Cardiovasc Surg 1999;117:252-60.

The risk of perioperative and late postoperative dissection is discussed in this paper, as are many other associated pathologic findings such as bicuspid aortic valve, aortic coarctation, and Turner's syndrome.

Aortic dissection as a rare complication of cardiac catheterization and other percutaneous diagnostic and therapeutic interventional techniques is also examined.

Miller DC. Surgical management of aortic dissections: indications, perioperative management, and long-term results. In: Doroghazi RM, Slater EE, editors. Aortic dissection. New York: McGraw-Hill; 1983. pp. 193-243.

This chapter provides an excellent overview of the clinical features, surgical and medical management, and outcomes after aortic dissection.

Yacoub MH, Gehle P, Chandrasekaran V, et al. Late results of a valve-preserving operation in patients with aneurysms of the ascending aorta and root. J Thorac Cardiovasc Surg 1998;115:1080-90.

This paper presents the late results of a valve-preserving operation in patients with aneurysms of the ascending aorta and root.

Coady MA, Ikonomidis JS, Cheung AT, et al. Surgical management of descending thoracic aortic disease: open and endovascular approaches. Circulation 2010;121:2780-804.

This paper presents a contemporary review of various pathologic processes affecting the descending thoracic aorta, including aortic dissections, intramural hematomas, and penetrating ulcers, discussed in this chapter. Cutting-edge technology for treatment (endovascular approach) is compared to gold-standard open techniques.

REFERENCES

Access the complete reference list online at http://www.expertconsult.com.

200

Splanchnic Ischemia

JEROEN J. KOLKMAN | ROBERT H. GEELKERKEN

Most stenoses in the splanchnic vessels remain asymptomatic, but some cause symptoms, and catastrophic complications can develop. Therefore, early recognition, thorough knowledge of diagnostic procedures, and treatment have important clinical implications. Three major topics need covering in this regard. First, there is much confusion regarding terminology. In this chapter we prefer *splanchnic vasculature* over *mesenteric*, because the latter does not include the celiac artery. For the same reason, we will use *splanchnic ischemia* instead of *mesenteric ischemia*. Second, it has long been an axiom that single-vessel stenoses rarely if ever cause ischemic complaints. Several studies in the last decade indicate that is no longer the case. Third, thoughts about the central role of splanchnic ischemia in normal vessels in several shock states has changed over the years.

Splanchnic artery stenoses are common, but splanchnic ischemia is supposedly rare owing to abundant collateral circulation. Moreover, the diagnosis is often overlooked, as indicated by the long delay before the condition is diagnosed in many cases and the large variations in reported prevalence among centers. Simple diagnostic tests are unavailable. For the intensivist, patients with chronic occlusive splanchnic ischemia are sparse, but these patients may run a prolonged and complicated course in the intensive care unit (ICU). NOMI (nonocclusive mucosal or mesenteric ischemia) is quite common in critically ill patients. NOMI is also called *intramucosal ischemia* and is characterized by mucosal acidosis.

Anatomy, Physiology, and Pathophysiology

MAIN VESSELS

The arterial blood supply of the gastrointestinal (GI) tract comes from three arteries: the celiac artery (CA), the superior mesenteric artery (SMA), and the inferior mesenteric artery (IMA). The anatomic variation of these vessels is huge, but the general pattern is that the CA supplies the stomach, liver, part of the pancreas, and the proximal part of the duodenum. The SMA supplies the distal part of the duodenum, the entire small bowel, the ascending colon, and the proximal part of the transverse colon. The IMA, the smallest of the three vessels, supplies the metabolically less active distal colon. Branches of these arteries enter the bowel wall to form two plexuses within the serosa and the submucosa. Finally, arterioles penetrate the muscular layer towards the mucosa. At the mucosal villi, they branch into an extensive network of capillaries and venules that permits diffusional shunting of oxygen via a countercurrent mechanism.

COLLATERAL CIRCULATION

Numerous collaterals may exist or develop. Buhler's arc contains embryonic remnants of vessels connecting the CA and SMA in the region of the pancreas head and duodenal bulb. Riolan's artery or marginal artery of Drummond connect the SMA and the IMA. The bowel plexuses also form a large collateral network. Still, even with this large collateral reserve, the superficial layers of the mucosa are very susceptible to the development of ischemia. This susceptibility is due to the countercurrent arteriovenous exchange of oxygen that starts at the base of the villus; when blood flow rate is low, oxygen may be depleted before the villus tip is reached.[1-3]

REGULATION OF BLOOD FLOW

During fasting basal conditions, approximately 20% of the cardiac output goes through the splanchnic vasculature. The flow doubles after a meal. Blood draining from the bowel enters the mesenteric veins and finally flows into the portal vein. The liver, therefore, receives its blood supply from two sources: venous blood from the portal vein and arterial blood from the hepatic artery, a branch of the CA, or in 25% of cases, the SMA. This dual blood supply renders the liver relatively protected against ischemia. Still, in cases of multivessel occlusion or when there are stenoses of both the CA and SMA, both sources are involved, and severe liver ischemia can ensue.

Vasoconstrictors

Catecholamines have different effects on the splanchnic blood flow; α_1-adrenergic receptor stimulation leads to vasoconstriction, whereas β_2-adrenergic receptor stimulation leads to vasodilatation. The relation between the renin-angiotensin axis and splanchnic perfusion is less uniform, although angiotensin II is a key splanchnic vasoconstrictor during low flow.[4] The main splanchnic vasoconstrictor is endothelin (ET)-1.[5-6] Two main ET-1 receptor types are have been described: ET_A and ET_B. Activation of ET_A, which is expressed in the mucosa, submucosa, and muscularis of the bowel wall, leads to long-lasting vasoconstriction and plays an important and early role in the negative effects of shock on the integrity of the GI tract.[5,7]

Vasodilators

The main splanchnic vasodilators are nitric oxide (NO) and prostaglandins. NO has paradoxical effects on gastrointestinal perfusion and mucosal integrity. Normally, low levels of NO are produced by the endothelium to sustain perfusion by promoting local vasodilatation. In pathologic circumstances like circulatory shock or sepsis, a large amount of NO is produced and acts as free radical, similar to oxygen free radicals, and is extremely toxic. In an animal model of hemorrhagic shock, inhibition of NO production is indeed beneficial.[8] Locally formed prostaglandins act as mucosal vasodilators, especially during low-flow states or following mucosal injury. Inhibition of cyclooxygenase—for example, with nonsteroidal antiinflammatory drugs (NSAIDs)—diminishes this vasodilatory response and renders the GI mucosa more susceptible to the effects of circulatory shock.[9]

LOW-FLOW CONDITIONS

All the above receptors and messengers act to balance perfusion to metabolic demands on a moment-to-moment basis. During circulatory shock, blood flow distribution changes due to constriction and dilatation of different vascular beds. When circulating volume is decreased, relative blood flow to the heart increases and brain perfusion is maintained, but perfusion of skeletal muscles, skin, and gut are reduced. Splanchnic vasoconstriction occurs early and profoundly,[10] even before systemic hemodynamic instability arises.[11] Splanchnic vasoconstriction can be triggered by different shock states, the direct effects of vasoactive medications, or nicotine and cocaine abuse. GI ischemia occurs only when blood flow is reduced to less than 50% of the basal rate.[12-14]

During splanchnic hypoperfusion, blood flow within the bowel wall is unevenly distributed among the different layers. In general, the mucosa is protected at the expense of the serosal layers.[15] Still, the surface of the mucosa is the most vulnerable area for ischemia, owing to countercurrent diffusional shunting of oxygen. Even within the mucosal layer, blood flow is unevenly distributed. Thus mismatches between metabolic demands and oxygen delivery are caused by several microcirculatory disturbances and shunting.[16-18] The patchy distribution of flow when global perfusion is compromised can be observed among different villi as well as within individual villi. These phenomena help explain why, in some studies, mucosal blood flow measurements are within the normal range despite evidence of mucosal ischemia; for early detection of ischemia, flow measurements alone will never suffice. This combination of ischemia despite normal vessel anatomy has given rise to the term *NOMI*, nonocclusive mesenteric ischemia.

ISCHEMIC DAMAGE

After the onset of ischemia, three different processes can be distinguished. In acute arterial occlusion, these processes occur sequentially; in nonocclusive ischemia, these processes occur simultaneously and remittently.

The Ischemic Phase

The immediate effect of reduced oxygen utilization is adenosine triphosphate (ATP) depletion. One of the consequences of ATP depletion is derangements in the tight junctions between adjacent enterocytes, leading to formation of "cracks in the mucosal lining." Also, key membrane-bound pumps are deprived of energy, and as a consequence, electrolytes and water enter the cells, which swell and, if the process continues, eventually die. Both mechanisms lead to reduced intestinal epithelial barrier function and bacteria moving across the bowel wall from the lumen into the systemic compartment (bacterial translocation).[19] During cellular hypoxia, the enzyme, xanthine dehydrogenase, is converted to xanthine oxidase (XO), which is harmless at this stage, because XO needs oxygen as a substrate. Finally, tissue necrosis triggers an inflammatory response, resulting in cytokine release. The effects of the ischemic phase alone are localized and can remain clinically undetected for many hours (closed compartment). The condition sometimes is silent until reperfusion initiates a systemic inflammatory response or transmural gangrene occurs.

Local Effects of Reperfusion

After flow is restored—for example, as a result of the partial dissolution of an embolus—oxygen enters the ischemic tissue. In a reaction catalyzed by XO, oxygen forms reactive oxygen species (ROS) that can damage proteins and DNA.[20] The damage to mucosa, blood vessels, and submucosal tissues is not only intensified but spreads to adjacent regions as well by diffusion of the small ROS molecules. Locally present ROS scavengers including glutathione, catalase, and superoxide dismutase, can neutralize ROS, but their efficacy is limited.

Systemic Effects of Reperfusion

Reperfusion delivers toxic products including XO, proinflammatory cytokines, and activated neutrophils into the systemic circulation.[21] In animal studies, liver and lung damage have been attributed to activated neutrophils coming from reperfused ischemic bowel.[20] Therefore, reperfusion leads to amplification and spreading of the ischemic damage.

Diagnostic Methods

For a diagnosis of gastrointestinal ischemia, two pieces of information are needed: vessel anatomy and stenoses, and presence or absence of ischemia. Assessment of vessel anatomy can be obtained by duplex ultrasound, computed tomography (CT) or magnetic resonance imaging (MRI), and visceral angiography. Assessment of ischemia is more difficult; probably tonometry has proven clinical value, but some new techniques may be available in the near future.

DUPLEX ULTRASOUND

Duplex ultrasound of the splanchnic arteries is widely used as a screening test for splanchnic artery stenoses, and is 80% to 90% accurate in experienced hands. Measurement of flow velocity at the origin of the CA and the SMA grades the severity of the stenoses. In 10% to 15% of patients, it is difficult to visualize the main vessels because of overlying (gastric) air. This technique is very operator dependent and is unsuitable in most critically ill patients.

COMPUTED TOMOGRAPHY ANGIOGRAPHY

CT angiography (CTA), including arterial and venous phase with maximum slice thickness of 1 mm, followed by three-dimensional reconstruction of the vessel anatomy is increasingly used in ICU patients. It has the advantage of minimal invasiveness, very accurate vessel visualization, and additional information on bowel pathology or perfusion. It has recently been reported as an accurate diagnostic test for NOMI. The early introduction of multidetector CT (MDCT) in the decision tree of NOMI treatment, followed by efficient treatment, was safe and suggested to improve mortality.[22]

MAGNETIC RESONANCE ANGIOGRAPHY

Although magnetic resonance angiography (MRA) of the splanchnic vessels enables a 360-degree view of the vessels and allows measurement of blood flow, oxygen content, or even lactate in the portal vein, it has largely been replaced by CTA, mainly because the latter has a higher spatial resolution and faster scan times.

VISCERAL ANGIOGRAPHY

In the last decade, visceral angiography of the splanchnic vessels has been challenged as the gold standard for assessment of vascular anatomy, stenoses, and collateral circulation. In most centers, angiography is reserved for potential endovascular therapeutic procedures and preceded by diagnostic CTA. Still, if a state-of-the-art CT scan (1-mm slices) is unavailable, multiplane aortal and selective angiography is a good choice for diagnosis.

INSPECTION OF THE MUCOSA AND SEROSA

With endoscopy, mucosal ischemia can be easily detected; it develops only during malperfusion at a stage where the serosal side is still normal.[14] Endoscopy is mostly used to diagnose ischemic colitis after aortic surgery. Endoscopic appearance may be difficult to interpret, especially with imperfectly rinsed bowel; therefore, preparation immediately before endoscopy by enema using 2 to 4 L of water is advisable. Differentiation of ischemic colitis from inflammatory bowel disease can be difficult, and preferably, biopsies should be taken. During the first days, ischemic colitis closely resembles ulcerative colitis; later it may be indistinguishable from Crohn's disease. Endoscopy cannot distinguish between mucosal and transmural ischemia or gangrene. The latter, irreversible stage can be detected only by inspecting the serosal side of the bowel. Therefore, laparoscopy or laparotomy is indicated when transmural ischemia is suspected.

LABORATORY TESTS

In general, serologic tests are of limited use for ischemia detection. Classical parameters like leukocyte count and arterial lactate level are of limited value because they lack both sensitivity and specificity. The most promising serologic markers include intestinal fatty acid binding protein (IFABP), D-lactate, ischemia modified albumine, and glutathione S-transferase (GST),[23] but clinical data are sparse.[24-26]

PCO₂ Measurement (Tonometry)

Intraluminal measurement of P_{CO_2} has been shown to detect ischemia, irrespective of flow or metabolism. This extra CO_2 is released during ischemia as protons accumulating during anaerobic glycolysis are buffered by tissue bicarbonate. Because CO_2 is a small molecule, intraluminal CO_2 increases within minutes of increased mucosal CO_2. The relationship between CO_2 and ischemia was first described in 1979 in heart and skeletal muscles[27-28] and in 1982 for the stomach.[29] The

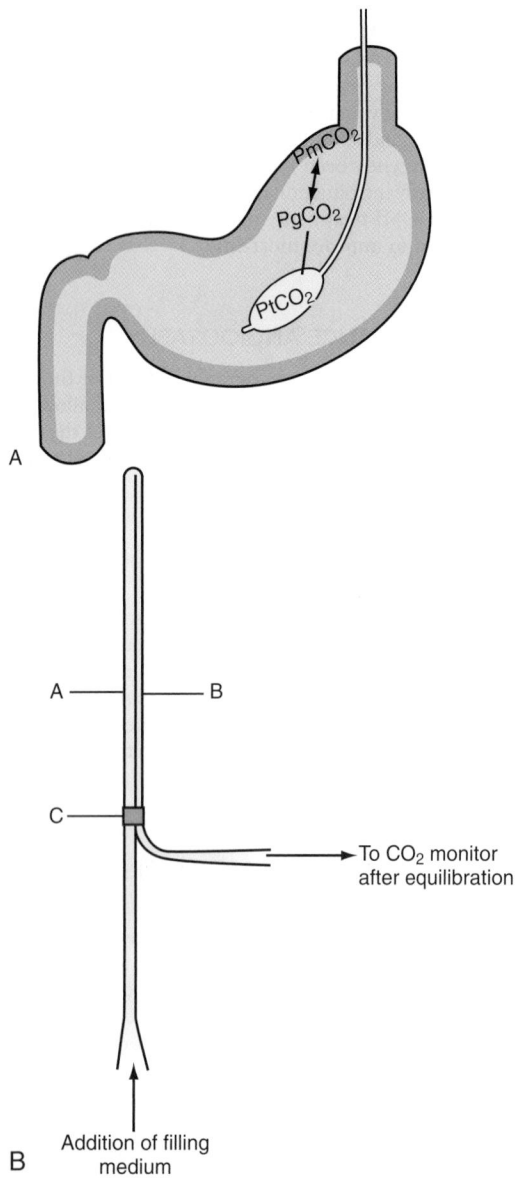

Figure 200-1 Intraluminal P_{CO_2} measurement techniques. **A,** Tonometry.[113] P_{CO_2} can be measured from a specialized balloon-tipped catheter placed in stomach or small or large bowel. Because CO_2 diffuses rapidly over different membranes, mucosal P_{CO_2} ($P_{m}CO_2$) will equal gastric lumen P_{CO_2} ($P_{g}CO_2$). Because the balloon is CO_2 permeable as well, balloon P_{CO_2} reflects mucosal values. This balloon P_{CO_2} is measured from air aspirated and inflated automatically into the balloon using a modified capnograph, the Tonocap (Datex-Engström). **B,** Balloonless intraluminal P_{CO_2} measurement.[31] P_{CO_2} is measured using a balloonless catheter, where air flows via a tube which is CO_2 permeable only at the intragastrically placed tip and connected with a capnograph on the sampling site.

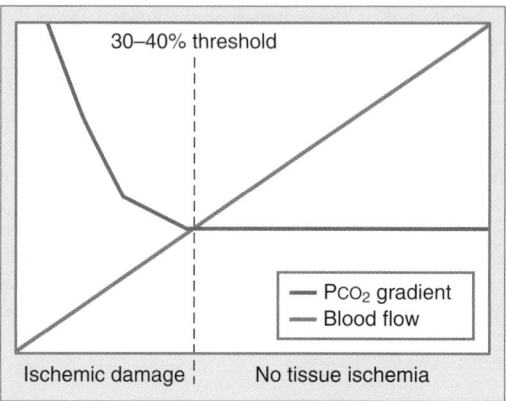

Figure 200-2 Blood flow, ischemia, and luminal P_{CO_2}. Reduction of splanchnic blood flow to approximately 50% does not increase luminal P_{CO_2} nor cause tissue damage. Further reduction below about 30% of basal blood flow causes a gradual increase in luminal P_{CO_2} and characteristic ischemic tissue changes. Blood flow is indicated by blue line, intraluminal P_{CO_2} by red line. Dotted lines indicate the anaerobic threshold of the tissue. (From Kolkman JJ, Mensink PB. Non-occlusive mesenteric ischaemia: a common disorder in gastroenterology and intensive care. Best Pract Res Clin Gastroenterol 2003;17:457-73.)

technique was subsequently popularized by Fiddian-Green and thereafter marketed as *tonometry* (Figure 200-1, *A*). He also introduced the term *pHi*, indicating mucosal acidosis using luminal CO_2 and arterial bicarbonate in the Henderson-Hasselbalch equation. Unfortunately, the company making the equipment has decided to stop production, although alternative measurement techniques have been described (see Figure 200-1, *B*).[30-31] Whatever its future, tonometry has demonstrated the important role splanchnic ischemia plays in critical care patients. Moreover, it has enabled us to select patients who could benefit from treatment of splanchnic stenoses.[32-34] In the abundance of diagnostics allowing for vessel anatomy assessment, intraluminal P_{CO_2} measurement is the only well-validated test for actual ischemia. An increased intraluminal-to–arterial P_{CO_2} gradient is indicative of ischemia. In the stomach, the normal gastric-arterial P_{CO_2} gradient is below 0.9 kPa (7 mm Hg)[35]; in the jejunum, the threshold is 1.4 kPa.[36] That an increased P_{CO_2} gradient does not relate to changes in perfusion per se can be concluded from studies where the gradient only increases as soon as the splanchnic blood flow decreased to below 30% to 40% of baseline[14,35] (Figure 200-2).

PCO₂ Measurement in the Intensive Care Unit

Because splanchnic ischemia is one of the earliest events in circulatory stress and typically begins at a stage when all other systemic parameters remain within the normal range, it has been referred to as "the canary of the body."[37] Like the canary that was once used in coal mines to detect toxic levels of mine gas, P_{CO_2} measurement may be a good, inexpensive, and relatively early warning of impending trouble.[38]

Despite its good track record for ischemia detection, P_{CO_2} measurement has not been widely used, either in the ICU or in GI or vascular medicine. Several reasons can be identified for this lack of success. First, saline-based P_{CO_2} measurement was initially laborious, time-consuming, and error prone. Second, many methodological issues clouded the studies in the first years. These included the need for acid suppression and errors introduced by food intake. Third, there was a lack of evidence that tonometry-based ischemia detection led to therapeutic interventions that improved outcome. The first two issues have been properly addressed and resolved by using air-based P_{CO_2} measurement (Tonocap device), potent acid suppression, and use of standardized meals during testing.[39-40] Despite its unique properties in the assessment of ischemia, only studies in trauma patients showed an advantage over standard monitoring.[41-42] A recent comparative study in septic patients failed to show a survival advantage in patients where resuscitation was aimed at normalization of tonometry, compared to standard systemic parameters.[43]

Outside the ICU, the situation is different. As a functional test to detect ischemia in the stomach and small bowel, the gold standard is measurement of Pco_2 during submaximal exercise, with a 78% sensitivity and 92% specificity.[32] Using this exercise test, we could select patients with single-vessel stenosis for treatment and follow-up.[34] It enabled us to investigate the entire spectrum of splanchnic stenotic disease from asymptomatic stenoses, to single and multivessel stenoses with ischemic complaints, and finally imminent bowel infarction.[44] Measurement of an increased Pco_2 after a meal in patients with symptomatic splanchnic stenosis was first shown in 1991.[45] Subsequent investigations using gastric Pco_2 measurement after a test meal showed variable results,[46-47] probably owing to buffering and dilution effects of the test meals.[48] With standardized test meals and acid suppression by proton pump inhibitors, the diagnostic accuracy of Pco_2 measurement in the stomach and small bowel for detection of ischemia improved considerably.[40] Having used this test in over 400 cases, three patterns emerged. First, the normal baseline is below 8 kPa and varies at least 1 kPa. Second, after a liquid meal, the gastric and small-bowel Pco_2 did not increase above 10.6 kPa in nonischemic individuals. Third, increased Pco_2 levels during the night are quite common and are probably related to buffering effects from duodenogastric reflux. An imminent bowel infarction is characterized by an increased Pco_2 for several hours, often above 15 kPa. Also, a suppressed and invariably low Pco_2 without the normal variation was seen in patients with an imminent infarction (paper in preparation).

Clinical Presentations of Splanchnic Ischemia

Splanchnic vascular disorders encompass a spectrum of acute and chronic occlusive, nonocclusive, and aneurysmal disorders affecting the vessels of the abdominal viscera. A classification of ischemic disorders can be made depending on vessel anatomy and ischemia (Figure 200-3). Acute splanchnic ischemia can be caused by arterial embolism, arterial and venous thrombosis, arterial stenoses, or NOMI. For the intensivist, NOMI is the most common problem and will be discussed first. The discussion on occlusive ischemia will focus on the different and often underappreciated clinical presentations, diagnostic problems, and treatment issues, with special emphasis on ICU care.

NONOCCLUSIVE MESENTERIC ISCHEMIA

Critically Ill Patients and Major Operations

In gastroenterology and surgery, NOMI is probably a rare disorder that can lead to ischemic colitis[49] or acute splanchnic infarction.[50] It can

also lead to chronic complaints comparable to chronic splanchnic ischemia related to vascular spasm. Treatment with vasodilators has been successful in the majority of patients, and the condition has been referred to as *abdominal migraine*.[51] In many cases, NOMI is reportedly caused by drugs, especially digoxin, or underlying cardiovascular and renal diseases.

NOMI is the end result of the physiologic response to a decreased intravascular blood volume. Early and profound splanchnic vasoconstriction accompanies many major operations, may lead to splanchnic ischemia, and is then associated with an adverse prognosis.[52-53] Similarly, in acute pancreatitis, gastric mucosal ischemia was associated with a worse outcome.[54] The relevance of this finding was reinforced in a recent randomized study evaluating the effects of probiotics in acute pancreatitis. In this study that investigated the potential beneficial effects of supplementing early feeding with probiotics, the mortality in the probiotic group was significantly higher and was especially associated with bowel infarction.[55]

It has been suggested that NOMI could play a key role in the pathogenesis of multiple organ failure syndrome (MODS). For example, endotoxinemia can cause mucosal microcirculatory disturbances directly, contributing to hypovolemia-induced vasoconstriction,[56] and increased gut-derived cytokine and endotoxin levels have been detected in patients with this syndrome.[57-58]

Hemodialysis Patients

In hemodialysis patients, NOMI is quite common[59] and may lead to bowel infarction in 2%, with a 45% mortality rate.[60] The incidence of this complication has been reported in 0.5% to 0.9% of these patients,[60-62] in whom NOMI has been associated with hypotension, often during hemodialysis. Close monitoring and prevention of hypotension are crucial to avoid this problem.[60]

Medications

Many drugs have been implicated as causative agents in NOMI, especially digoxin. NSAIDs affect the integrity of the GI mucus and bicarbonate layer and reduce mucosal perfusion. α-Adrenergic agents like epinephrine and dopamine reduce GI perfusion, and β-adrenergic agents like dobutamine and dopexamine tend to sustain mucosal perfusion.[63-65] The clinical importance of these differences is probably very small, because recent comparative studies failed to show differences in mortality between norepinephrine plus dobutamine versus epinephrine,[66] and norepinephrine versus dopamine.[67]

OCCLUSIVE ISCHEMIA

The incidence of asymptomatic splanchnic stenoses, so-called chronic splanchnic disease, ranges between 8% and 70% in populations with other manifestations of atherosclerotic disease and is comparable to

Figure 200-3 Classification of the spectrum of gastrointestinal vascular disease and ischemia. (*Adapted from Kolkman JJ, Bargeman M, Huisman AB, Geelkerken RH. Diagnosis and management of splanchnic ischemia. World J Gastroenterol 2008;14:7309-20.*)

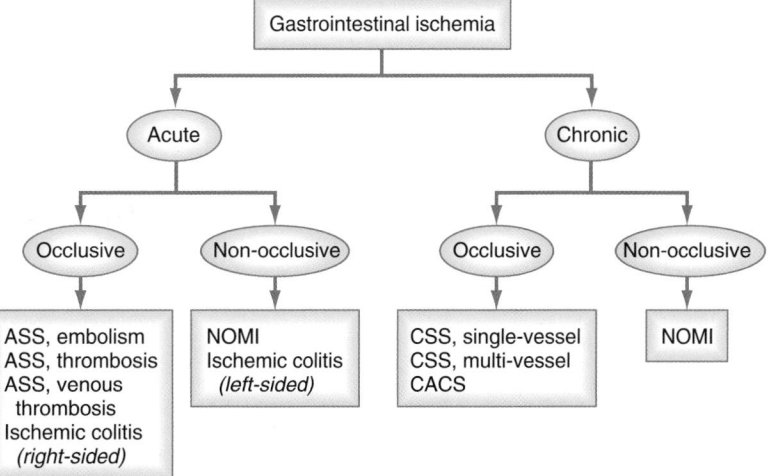

the incidence of carotid atherosclerosis. Nevertheless, the incidence of symptomatic occlusive splanchnic ischemia, or chronic splanchnic syndrome, is relatively rare, being only 4 to 5 cases per 100,000 inhabitants yearly.[68] The incidence of acute splanchnic ischemia is relatively low but increases sharply with age. In a recent autopsy study, it was shown that 1.2% of all deaths in patients over the age of 80 was attributable to acute splanchnic ischemia.[69] The diagnosis was suspected in a minority of patients.[70]

Etiology

External compression by the arcuate ligament of the diaphragm is the predominant cause of single-vessel CA stenosis in young adults. Atherosclerosis is the main cause of single-vessel SMA or IMA occlusive disease and multivessel disease. The latter is defined as stenoses or occlusions in more than one main splanchnic artery. Information on the natural history of splanchnic artery occlusive disease is scarce. Using serial duplex ultrasound, it was demonstrated that visceral artery atherosclerotic stenoses progress in approximately 20% of patients per year. This progression of lesions is especially important in multivessel chronic splanchnic disease, which carries a considerable risk for acute splanchnic infarction.[71]

Chronic Splanchnic Syndrome (Single-Vessel Disease)

It has long been debated whether patients with a single splanchnic vessel stenosis developed symptoms. In 1972, Szilagyi suggested that "no patient had ever been proven, on scientific grounds, to have an abnormality of intestinal structure or function which was caused by extraluminal compression of the coeliac artery, or supposed relief from the operation could be anything other than a placebo effect."[72] Recently we have shown in patients with typical complaints of ischemia, an abnormal function test and an eccentric respiratory-dependent stenosis of the CA; resolution of symptoms was seen in 89% after open or endoscopic release of the CA.[73] In another study, we demonstrated that disappearance of symptoms was associated with a normalized function test.[34] Because these patients are normally in good health, they will rarely be admitted to the ICU.

Chronic Splanchnic Syndrome (Multivessel Disease)

There is an important distinction to be made between single-vessel and multivessel stenosis. Most patients with significant stenoses in two or three of the main splanchnic vessels experience ischemic complaints. They almost invariably suffer from postprandial symptoms and weight loss, which may be severe. An epigastric bruit is absent in most patients. The complaints typically persist for many years and become less classic over time, because the patients grow accustomed to the pain, and it becomes part of their lives. In the end stage of the disease, the pattern of complaints can become extremely atypical and be dominated by a sensation of abdominal fullness or loss of appetite.

Untreated, progressive multivessel splanchnic syndrome may result in bowel infarction.[33] Because the diagnosis is usually made in a late stage, the time frame for treatment may be limited. In our experience, patients with multivessel stenoses and clinical indications of an imminent bowel infarction should be treated within days. These clinical indicators encompass ulcerations in stomach duodenum or right-sided colon during endoscopy, abdominal pain not associated with eating, and complete incapability of eating. When a bowel infarction finally occurs, it may remain clinically silent for several hours or even days as long as the necrotic segment remains without perfusion.[14] With reperfusion or perforation of gangrenous bowel, MODS develops rapidly, and death usually ensues within days.

Acute Splanchnic Syndrome

Acute splanchnic ischemia is defined as sudden cessation of splanchnic mucosal perfusion. It should be considered in patients presenting with acute severe abdominal pain where no obvious diagnosis is found. In elderly patients, acute splanchnic ischemia can present with unexplained confusion. Classically the severity of pain is out of proportion to the almost normal physical findings. If untreated, acute splanchnic ischemia ultimately results in bowel necrosis within 6 to 8 hours. In 75% of patients with acute splanchnic artery occlusion, an embolus in the SMA is present. The prognosis depends on the cause of the infarction and ranges from approximately 32% for venous thrombosis and 54% for arterial embolism to 70% to 80% for acute arterial thrombosis and nonocclusive ischemia. The overall survival after acute splanchnic ischemia has improved over the past 4 decades.[74] The Mayo Clinic's 2002 vision, "the contemporary management of acute splanchnic ischemia with revascularization with open surgical techniques, resection of nonviable bowel, and liberal use of second-look procedures results in early survival of two thirds of the patients with embolism and thrombosis," is still valid.[75]

Unexpected Splanchnic Ischemia in the Intensive Care Unit

As mentioned earlier, many patients with splanchnic stenoses either remain undiagnosed or have no complaints whatsoever. During major abdominal surgery or inflammatory disorders like pancreatitis or cholecystitis, however, the increased metabolic demand related to this stress may easily precipitate ischemia in patients with vascular stenoses. Thus, this diagnosis should be considered in patients with known atherosclerotic disease or risk factors for it, with a prolonged or unusually complicated course related to acute cholecystitis or acute pancreatitis. The diagnosis also should be suspected when the histopathology of surgical specimens suggests ischemic injury. Complications that can be caused by splanchnic ischemia include ischemic hepatitis, acalculous cholecystitis, and ischemic pancreatitis. In these patients, minimal invasive revascularization may dramatically improve the clinical course within days.

Ischemic Colitis

Ischemic colitis is a well-defined disease. It is a nonocclusive disorder in most cases, and angiograms are almost invariably normal.[49-50] Still, most cases of spontaneous ischemic colitis are not preceded by shock states as has been suggested; most cases are found as a result of unexpected findings at endoscopy performed to evaluate patients because of abdominal cramps, diarrhea, or blood loss (Table 200-1). Because the course of spontaneous left-sided ischemic colitis is benign, patients rarely come to the attention of the intensivist.

In contrast, ischemic colitis following aortic surgery is frequently seen in the ICU. It was observed in 20% to 27% of patients after

TABLE 200-1	Clinical Features of Ischemic Colitis					
Localization	*Cause*	*History*	*Angiography*	*Course*		*Mortality*
Right-sided (n = 3)	Spontaneous (n = 3)	Chronic splanchnic syndrome (1) None (2)	SMA stenosis (1) SMA and CA stenosis (2)	Operated and recovered (1) Died from bowel gangrene (2)		67%
Left-sided (n = 19)	Spontaneous (n = 11)	Cardiovascular history (5) Trigger event or hypotension (0) None (6)	Normal angiogram (2) No angiogram made (9)	Died from gangrenous colitis (3) Operated and recovered gangrene (1) Resolved spontaneously (7)		27%
	Postoperative (n = 8)	After acute aortic surgery (7) After elective aortic surgery (1)	No angiogram made (8)	Recovery without operation (5) Operated and recovered gangrenous colon (1) Died from ischemic colitis (2)		25%

Patient characteristics of 22 patients presenting with ischemic colitis in Medical Spectrum Twente, Enschede, the Netherlands, between 1998 and 2001.
CA, celiac artery; *SMA*, superior mesenteric artery.

conventional open repair of ruptured abdominal aortic aneurysm and was associated with an overall mortality rate of 48%.[76-79] After elective aortic surgery, sigmoid ischemia is reported in less than 2% of patients.[80] The main factors inducing postoperative left-sided ischemic colitis, therefore, seem to be preoperative shock, massive blood loss, and persisting hemodynamic instability. In these patients, the IMA is usually already occluded or surgically ligated, so ischemic colitis may be partially occlusive in nature.[77] With the introduction of endovascular stent placement for the elective management of abdominal aortic aneurysm (AAA) or the treatment of acute ruptured aneurysms, mortality rate, ICU stay, and incidence of ischemic colitis after AAA repair has decreased dramatically.[81] Still, when patients remain unstable for more than 48 hours after aortic repair, a sigmoidoscopy is indicated.

Left- Versus Right-Sided Ischemic Colitis. An important clinical distinction should be made between left-sided ischemic colitis (discussed earlier) and right-sided ischemic colitis.[82-83] The latter was associated with an adverse prognosis, increased surgery rates, and increased mortality.[83] In many cases, right-sided ischemic colitis is a symptom of severe compromised SMA flow and consequently acute splanchnic infarction. To improve the prognosis, this entity requires immediate treatment. Our preference would be to perform an urgent CTA. Because the time between onset of acute complete small-bowel ischemia and irreversible gangrene is only 6 to 8 hours, this investigation should not be postponed. It can be used to rule out other pathology, guide an appropriate revascularization, and avoid a "blind" laparotomy. Recent studies have indicated that CT assessment of morphology and diameter of the SMA could be used to positively diagnose NOMI.[22]

Treatment

NONOCCLUSIVE MESENTERIC ISCHEMIA

The key factors for successful treatment of NOMI include:
1. High index of suspicion and readiness for aggressive intervention
2. Fluid resuscitation to restore the proper balance between metabolic demand and perfusion
3. Prevention of reperfusion damage
4. Recognition and avoidance of NOMI-inducing medications

The first step towards successful treatment is early detection of mucosal ischemia. Only intraluminal Pco_2 measurement has proven accuracy for the detection of early ischemia.[49] Using gastric Pco_2 measurement as an endpoint for fluid resuscitation, rapid optimization of intravascular volume could be achieved.[84-86] Still, the results of resuscitation trials aimed at normalizing luminal Pco_2 showed conflicting results, with positive effects in trauma patients[41-42] but no different from standard monitoring in septic patients.[43] An alternative might be the use of CTA, although the experience is still limited in severe cases.[87-88]

Medication

In patients with a high probability of mucosal ischemia, avoidance of epinephrine and dopamine makes sense.[89-90] Still, recent studies failed to show a difference between various catecholamines for resuscitation following fluid correction.[66-67] Treatment with angiotensin-converting enzyme (ACE) inhibitors has been effective in animal studies[91] but only in one of two clinical studies.[92-93] In recent studies, administration of prostaglandin E$_1$ was reported to improve outcome in case series of severe NOMI.

Feeding

Early institution of enteral nutrition may improve perfusion, in addition to providing salutary immunologic and nutritional effects. The mechanisms responsible for mucosal vasodilatation due to enteric nutrition are autoregulatory responses driven by the metabolic demands associated with absorption of food in the lumen.[94] However, in extreme low or no-flow states, enteral nutrition can be very harmful and provoke infarction, and it should therefore be used cautiously.[95] This mechanism may explain the high rate of bowel infarction in the aforementioned probiotic pancreatitis study where a rapid institution of high-volume feeding was protocol.[55] Treatment of reperfusion damage is a promising but clinically unproven approach. Several new compounds[96-98] and established drugs including N-acetylcysteine[99] and vitamin E[100] have been used in animal models to reduced ischemia/reperfusion-induced damage. The best known ROS scavenger, N-acetylcysteine, increases intracellular glutathione levels and increases NO release,[101] leading to vasodilatation of small blood vessels. In some studies, administration of N-acetylcysteine early in sepsis was associated with improved hemodynamic parameters[102] and splanchnic ischemia.[103] However, data from clinical studies are still lacking.

OCCLUSIVE ISCHEMIA: SPLANCHNIC SYNDROME

Single-Vessel Chronic Splanchnic Syndrome

The majority of these patients have no comorbidities, and the operative course is usually uneventful.[33] These patients are rarely encountered by the intensivist.

Multivessel Chronic Splanchnic Syndrome

Preoperative Workup. Many of these patients have severe comorbidities and have lost a considerable amount of weight, often more than 15 kg resulting in a BMI below the normal range. Still, attempts to correct the nutritional deficit preoperatively is not without risk. In patients with critical stenoses and minimal blood flow to the bowel, feeding may induce acute bowel infarction. Even parenteral nutrition is not without risk, because it can provoke liver and bowel ischemia. This is explained by the increased energy expenditure from metabolizing nutrients in the liver, which has severely compromised perfusion because flow from the portal vein as well as from the hepatic artery is impaired because of occlusive disease involving the CA and SMA. Moreover, the increased hepatic blood flow causes an intramesenteric steal, with blood shunting from the bowel to the liver, thereby causing bowel ischemia as well. Using tonometry, these patients showed extreme increases in gastric and jejunal Pco_2 for several hours following polymeric feeding.[44] In general, patients with critical stenoses should be treated by revascularization as soon as possible; feeding should be delayed until restoration of blood flow has been achieved.

Revascularization. There are many potential treatment options in these patients, partly because solid clinical evidence to prefer one above the other is lacking[104] (Table 200-2). Restoration of blood flow can be achieved with three different treatment strategies: operative antegrade or retrograde revascularization or percutaneous endovascular antegrade revascularization.

Antegrade multivessel autologous revascularization yields excellent long-term results with regard to patency and clinical response.[105-106] The downside of this approach is that it uses a supraceliac aortic clamp technique, resulting in at least 15 to 20 minutes of ischemia affecting the bowel, legs, and kidneys. In older patients and in patients in poor clinical condition, this approach is quite risky, as the hemodynamic instability and other adverse effects of lower-body reperfusion may not be well tolerated. Antegrade multivessel autologous revascularization should not been attempted in patients with a body mass index (BMI) below 19.5 kg/m^2, with confined life expectancy, or with relevant comorbidity.

Operative retrograde revascularization can be performed with long bypasses from the iliac arteries or the distal aorta to either the common hepatic artery or the SMA outflow. Compared to operative antegrade multivessel autologous revascularization, it is better tolerated because aortic cross-clamping could be avoided. The main disadvantage of this procedure is that long, meandering bypasses have a greater risk of kinking and thrombosis or stenoses, and consequently, an increased likelihood of occluding, leading to a recurrence of symptoms or even acute splanchnic ischemia.

TABLE 200-2	**Summary of Treatment Options in Splanchnic Ischemia**

NOMI

- Exclude vascular occlusions by computed tomography angiography (CTA), which may also definitively show diagnosis.
- Aggressive volume resuscitation; ideally with normalized Pco_2 measurement as endpoint
- Avoid α-adrenergic drugs when possible.
- Consider papaverine or prostaglandin E_1 in severe cases.

Chronic Occlusive Splanchnic Ischemia

Determine risk for bowel infarction (angiography, clinical assessment, function test).

High Short-Term Infarction Risk

- Intravenous fluids to restore intravascular volume
- No oral intake of food
- Heparins
- Acid suppression (proton pump inhibitors)
- Revascularization within hours or days

Low Short-Term Infarction Risk

- Avoid dehydration.
- Nutritional measures aimed at avoidance of pain (small meals six times a day, avoid fat)
- Preoperative analysis (cardiac and pulmonary)
- Multidisciplinary approach towards revascularization: surgery (antegrade or retrograde), endovascular (one or two vessels, via the brachial or femoral artery) or a hybrid procedure

Bowel Infarction (Acute Splanchnic Syndrome)

- Urgent CTA for diagnosis and revascularization planning
- Aggressive volume replacement to be started immediately
- Perform vascular revascularization (stenting, embolectomy, surgical)
- Heparins
- Consider removing the first 500 mL portal blood after revascularization (prevent ischemia-reperfusion [IR] damage).
- Assess bowel viability after revascularization; resect necrotic bowel.
- Avoid leaving too much borderline viable bowel (ongoing IR damage, the trigger for irreversible multiorgan failure).
- Weigh risk of parenteral nutrition dependency against insufficient bowel resection.

Postoperative

- Maintain optimal fluid status.
- Avoid α-adrenergic drugs when possible.
- With recurrence of abdominal complaints: CTA to rule out vascular occlusion. If the revascularization is intact, consider reperfusion syndrome; stop oral intake of food and institute total parenteral nutrition for 2 to 5 weeks.
- After recovery of bowel mucosa, consider coumarins or thrombocyte aggregation inhibitors.

Ischemic Colitis

Right-Sided (Ascending Colon)

- Urgent CTA
  a. With superior mesenteric artery (SMA) occlusion or stenosis: treat as acute splanchnic syndrome.
  b. With normal vasculature: treat as left-sided colitis.

Left-Sided Colitis

- CTA in most cases not indicated
- Treat as nonocclusive mesenteric ischemia (NOMI) with aggressive volume replacement and avoidance of α-adrenergic drugs.
- Consider laparotomy and partial colectomy:
  a. Persistent sepsis, fever, hemodynamic instability
  b. With proven ischemic colitis (endoscopy) despite NOMI treatment
  c. With diarrhea, protein losses > 14 days post surgery

controlled. Retrograde, a 5F sheet is introduced in the SMA, and under manual and fluoroscopic visualization, endovascular connection between the SMA outflow and the aorta is achieved. Thereafter, PTA and stenting of the occluded trajectory of the SMA could be performed.[107]

In general, in non-randomized series, the mortality of operative and endovascular revascularization in cases of splanchnic syndrome was equal and around 5%. At 2-year follow-up, the primary patency of stent placement was around 70% and of operative repair, around 90%. The secondary patency of these two techniques were comparable and around 85%. Long-term relief of symptoms can be achieved best by repair of more than one splanchnic artery.

Endovascular repair is recommended in patients with limited life expectancy, high cardiopulmonary risk, cachexia, or hostile abdomen. Open repair is still considered the preferred option for patients who are relatively young and otherwise fit for surgical repair.[108]

Acute Splanchnic Syndrome

Two points should be kept in mind in patients with acute splanchnic syndrome. First, in many of these patients, lack of overall intake causes coexisting NOMI as well. Therefore, intravascular volume restoration should be the first treatment. Second, a severe ischemia-reperfusion syndrome can develop after treatment.

In the surgical management of acute splanchnic syndrome with bowel gangrene, many recommend not resecting intestine with marginal viability at the initial procedure, but performing a routine

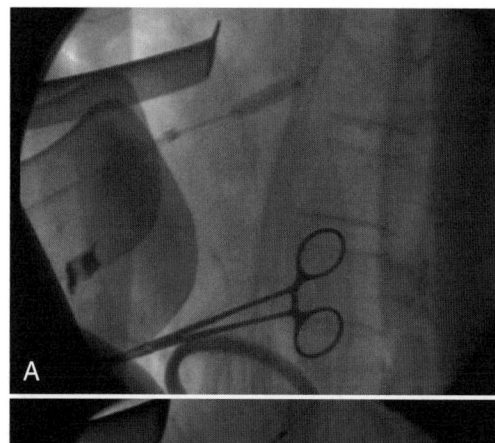

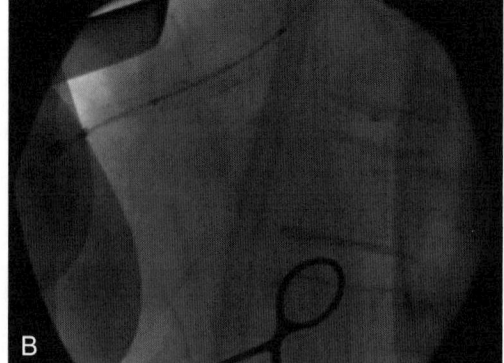

Figure 200-4 Retrograde stent placement, the hybrid procedure. In a patient with imminent splanchnic infarction, superior mesenteric artery (SMA) and celiac artery (CA) occlusion were demonstrated. Standard endovascular stenting was impossible. After a small supra-umbilical laparotomy, the outflow of the SMA is controlled **(A)**. Retrograde, a 5F sheet is introduced in the SMA, and under manual and fluoroscopic visualization, endovascular connection between the SMA outflow and aorta is achieved. Thereafter, percutaneous transluminal angioplasty (PTA) and stenting of the occluded trajectory of the SMA could be performed **(B)**.

Endovascular treatment by percutaneous transluminal angioplasty (PTA) with stent placement can be performed either via the femoral artery in the groin or the brachial artery. The former approach is suboptimal for proper positioning of the stent at the origin of the CA or SMA if either of these vessels makes a sharp angle with the aorta. The brachial artery approach includes a risk of 10% to 15% of local complications, including median nerve damage, hemorrhage, and pseudoaneurysm formation. If antegrade endovascular revascularization is not appropriate, retrograde endovascular recanalization (the hybrid procedure) of the SMA is a worthwhile alternative (Figure 200-4). After a small supra-umbilical laparotomy, the outflow of the SMA is

"second look" procedure 24 hours after the original operation and resecting additional intestine at this time if necessary. This approach is advocated to save as much bowel length as possible. However, many of these patients eventually die from MODS, presumably related to ischemia/reperfusion-induced inflammation related to areas of bowel with borderline ischemia. We currently prefer an alternative approach with initial restoration of blood flow followed by removal of all non-vital bowel. In our experience, this reduces the postoperative problems but results in more patients with short bowel syndrome. Initially these patients will be dependent on parenteral nutrition. With intestinal adaptation, which may take up to 1 year, most can resume enteral nutrition. Restoration of complete but adjusted[109] enteral nutrition can be expected in patients with remaining small-bowel length of greater than 50 cm with an intact ileocecal valve, or between 50 and 100 cm without an ileocecal valve.[110] The quality of life of these patients is relatively good and comparable to hemodialysis patients.[111] In future, small-bowel transplants may become an option, with a current 1-year transplant survival of 60% (source: International Intestinal Transplant Registry). Therefore, in patients who seem otherwise in relatively good health, with nearby complete necrotic bowel but without clear involvement of the stomach, duodenum, liver, and pancreas, revascularization and resection treatment should at least be considered.

Acute-on-Chronic Splanchnic Ischemia

The course of patients with multivessel chronic splanchnic syndrome is initially stable or slowly progressive. Ultimately, these patients become severely cachectic. The end stage of the disease is rapidly progressive. Bowel infarction develops in up to 30% of patients after 1 year and 60% after 4 years of follow-up.[71] The prognosis for these patients is very poor; mortality is 80% once bowel infarction develops.[50,74] Therefore, symptomatic patients with severe bowel pain and weight loss and multivessel disease should be analyzed and treated in a matter of days to weeks. During the time leading up to the revascularization procedure, maintenance of adequate intravascular volume is essential.

Emergency revascularization is the main goal of treatment. Angiography can be useful for stenting of the CA or SMA and eventually removing an SMA embolus. In cases of NOMI, papaverine (30-60 mg/h for a maximum of 4 hours) or prostaglandin E_1 (bolus 0.020 mg, then 0.060 mg/h for up to 72 hours) can be administered by selective SMA catheterization to diminish arterial spasm.[112] CTA or splanchnic angiography is essential to provide the surgeon guidelines for revascularization during laparotomy.

Postoperative Care

REPERFUSION SYNDROME

In patients with prolonged periods of bowel ischemia, revascularization can lead to a severe syndrome of reperfusion. Risk factors include multivessel disease, the presence of mucosal ulceration, and pain which is no longer associated with feeding (abdominal rest pain). It is characterized by initially good recovery from revascularization then a sudden deterioration 2 to 5 days after the intervention. The clinical presentation is characterized by a recurrence of abdominal complaints such as queasiness. Findings may include gastric ulceration, ascites, sometimes severe hypoalbuminemia, and leucocytosis. The first action should be to exclude stent or bypass occlusion with CTA or duplex ultrasound. Reperfusion syndrome can be treated by stopping oral intake of food, instituting total parenteral nutrition, acid suppression, and sufficient intravenous fluid administration. Most patients recover within 2 to 6 weeks without any lasting complications.

Aggressive anticoagulation treatment is essential in all patients with bypasses of stents in critical areas. We start with heparins for days or weeks until the patient becomes clearly anabolic. Starting coumarins shortly after revascularization of end-stage splanchnic syndrome includes a high risk of shoot-through and consequently, severe GI bleeding due to the unpredictable absorption and metabolism of vitamin K and coumarins.

ISCHEMIC COLITIS

In most cases, left-sided ischemic colitis resolves spontaneously with only fluid resuscitation and antibiotics; endoscopic bowel decompression should be considered if the colon is markedly dilated. Surgery is restricted to patients with transmural irreversible ischemia, but occurrence of these complications is associated with a poor prognosis. Some experts advocate routine repetitive sigmoidoscopy to evaluate high-risk patients after acute aortic surgery, especially in those with severe preoperative shock or requiring large volumes of intravenous fluids.[76] Repeated coloscopy should also be considered in patients post aortic surgery who have persistent hemodynamic instability lasting more than 48 hours. At endoscopy, ischemic colitis is graded in 4 categories: grade 0, normal mucosa; grade 1, mucosal edema; grade 2, deep mucosal ulcers; grade 3, gangrene. Grade 3 and progressive grade 2 ischemia are indications for laparotomy and subsequently subtotal colon resection. Angiography is rarely indicated in these patients. Treatment is aggressive fluid resuscitation, antibiotics, and bowel decompression if indicated.

KEY POINTS

1. Nonocclusive mucosal or mesenteric ischemia (NOMI) is a common disorder in intensive care patients and can be detected with intraluminal PCO_2 measurement and calculation of the pHi. Treatment aimed at the pHi variables did not result in improved survival, however. NOMI is the extreme of the adaptation of blood flow distribution in all types of circulatory stress.

2. The first-line treatment of NOMI is aggressive volume resuscitation and avoidance of α-adrenergic drugs. Intraarterial papaverine or intravenous prostaglandin E_1 are second-line drugs reserved for severe cases with imminent bowel infarction.

3. In severe NOMI with imminent bowel infarction, computed tomography angiography (CTA) is mandatory to exclude vascular stenoses and alternative pathology.

4. Splanchnic vessel stenoses are common but remain asymptomatic in most cases. In the critically ill patient, asymptomatic stenoses may be the root cause of abdominal complaints that are not improving. Endovascular reconstruction can be achieved in most cases.

5. For assessment of splanchnic vessel stenoses or spasm, a multislice CTA with slice thickness of 1 to 2 mm is the first choice in critically ill patients.

6. Angiography should ideally be reserved for endovascular treatment or in selected cases, intraarterial papaverine administration.

7. Multivessel chronic splanchnic ischemia has an accelerated end stage and a high infarction rate; nutrition should be used cautiously or avoided, and analysis and treatment should be completed within days rather than weeks.

8. Enteral and parenteral nutrition improve splanchnic perfusion in most patients but can provoke an infarction in patients with very diminished splanchnic blood flow, either from splanchnic stenosis or severe shock syndrome. In these patients, nutrition should be withheld or used with utmost caution until the splanchnic perfusion improves by either revascularization or improved hemodynamics.

9. Colonoscopy is the gold standard for early mucosal ischemic colitis; laparotomy is the gold standard for transmural or gangrenous ischemic colitis.

ANNOTATED REFERENCES

Hamilton-Davies C, Mythen N, Salmon LB, Jacobson D, Shukla A, Webb AR. Comparison of commonly used clinical indicators of hypovolaemia with gastrointestinal tonometer. Intensive Care Med 1997;23:276-81.

A small study in 6 healthy volunteers showing that hemorrhage induces early and profound NOMI at a stage when all hemodynamic measures including stroke volume, heart rate, and blood pressure as well as arterial lactate are still normal. A clear demonstration of tonometry as an "early warning system."

Knichwitz G, Rotker J, Mollhoff T, Richter KD, Brussel T. Continuous intramucosal PCO_2 measurement allows the early detection of intestinal malperfusion. Crit Care Med 1998;26:1550-7.

A study in pigs that clearly shows that tonometry is no measure of blood flow but only of the onset of ischemia, as it increases only after ≥50% flow reduction. Also, this paper points out the importance of the closed-compartment and open-compartment phases of splanchnic ischemia.

Kolkman JJ, Otte JA, Groeneveld AB. Gastrointestinal luminal PCO_2 tonometry: an update on physiology, methodology and clinical applications. Br J Anaesth 2000;84:74-86.

A review of all available data on tonometry, with special emphasis on measurement accuracy. It analyses all earlier flaws in methodology, as well as the potential of this technique.

MacDonald PH. Ischaemic colitis. Baillieres Best Pract Res Clin Gastroenterol 2002;16:51-61.

An overview of pathophysiology, diagnosis, and potential treatment options for this disease that can be occlusive and nonocclusive in nature.

van Bockel JH, Geelkerken RH, Wasser MN. Chronic splanchnic ischaemia. Best Pract Res Clin Gastroenterol 2001;15:99-119.

An extensive review on the clinical presentation, diagnosis, and treatment options in chronic splanchnic ischemia. The surgical treatment is especially thoroughly reviewed.

van Petersen AS, Kolkman JJ, Beuk RJ, Huisman AB, Doelman C, Geelkerken RH. Open or percutaneous revascularization for chronic splanchnic syndrome. J Vasc Surg 2010;51:1309-16.

This article summarizes the existing level of evidence of conventional and endovascular treatment for CSS caused by atherosclerotic origin stenoses of the splanchnic arteries.

REFERENCES

Access the complete reference list online at http://www.expertconsult.com.

201

Abdominal Compartment Syndrome

ZSOLT J. BALOGH | FREDERICK A. MOORE

Definitions

To date, the most common way to measure *intraabdominal pressure* (IAP) is the intravesical technique via a urinary catheter (often referred to as *urinary bladder pressure*).[1-3] The mean value of IAP in hospitalized nontrauma patients is 6.5 mm Hg (range, 0.2-16.2 mm Hg).[4] In critically ill ICU patients or trauma patients with shock and subsequent resuscitation, IAP is typically higher (12-16 mm Hg).[5]

Intraabdominal hypertension (IAH) is defined as IAP greater than 12 mm Hg without pathophysiology of ACS. IAH is graded from I to IV based on the IAP value (grade I: 12-15 mm Hg; grade II: 16-20 mm Hg; grade III: 21-25 mm Hg; grade IV: above 25 mm Hg).

Abdominal compartment syndrome (ACS) is defined as a sustained IAP greater than 20 mm Hg that is associated with new organ dysfunction/failure.

Primary ACS is a condition associated with injury or disease in the abdominopelvic region that frequently requires early surgical or interventional radiologic intervention.

Secondary ACS refers to conditions that do not originate from the abdominopelvic region.

Damage Control

Patients undergoing laparotomy for major abdominal bleeding or sepsis are at risk for entering a "vicious circle" of acidosis, hypothermia, and coagulopathy; selected patients benefit from an abbreviated laparotomy ("damage-control" strategy).[6,7] The goals are to quickly control bleeding and prevent further contamination or spillage from hollow viscus perforations. The abdomen is temporarily closed without fascial approximation, and the patient is triaged to the intensive care unit (ICU), where resuscitation can be optimized and the vicious-circle physiology corrected. Damage control has saved the lives of severely injured and septic patients who otherwise would have died. Nevertheless, use of damage control has created new challenges for clinicians, including recognition and management of ACS, management of the open abdomen, and early multiple organ failure (MOF).

ABDOMINAL DECOMPRESSION

Traditionally, abdominal decompression has been done through a full midline laparotomy. Recently, other techniques such as transverse laparotomy, percutaneous drainage of the intraperitoneal fluid, and minimally invasive linea alba fasciotomy were described as potentially useful methods in selected cases. Except from percutaneous drainage, these methods increase the volume of the abdominal cavity and thus decrease the IAP. An interposition material (e.g., opened intravenous fluid bag [Bogota bag], synthetic mesh, or vacuum-assisted closure system) is attached to the fascial or skin edges to prevent bowel evisceration. The less invasive procedures can be performed at the bedside in the ICU. Decompressive laparotomy can be done in the ICU in extremis cases but is generally preferred to be done in the operating room, especially when further intraabdominal procedures are anticipated, not just the opening of the fascia.

Historical Perspective

After 2 decades of re-recognition, ACS is still a heavily investigated critical care topic. Before the most recent description, IAP measurement, intraabdominal hypertension and ACS-related pathophysiology were investigated and published more than 150 years ago in both animal and human studies.[8,9] Initially, IAP was thought to be negative (subatmospheric), but by the beginning of the 20th century, animal studies verified that IAP is generally positive and if significantly increased can cause cardiac failure.[10] These laboratory observations had little impact on clinical practice until the 1950s, when pediatric surgeons recognized the catastrophic consequences of acutely closing large congenital abdominal defects. Silo closure with gradual reduction of the abdominal defect was recommended to prevent fulminant organ failures.[11] In the 1980s, vascular surgeons described ACS after abdominal aortic aneurysm surgery. Additionally, they described the present technique of IAP measurement and used high IAP as a criterion for re-exploration.[1] However, it was not until the 1990s, when trauma surgeons adopted the liberal use of the damage-control strategy, that sufficient numbers of patients were available to define the epidemiology and pathophysiology of this previously rare and elusive complication.[12-15] Early observational case descriptions and retrospective series allowed for development of appropriate prospective epidemiologic characterization. These clinical observations stimulated laboratory investigations which have revealed some surprising and potentially important immunologic consequences of decompressive laparotomy of ACS after traumatic shock resuscitation (i.e., it may serve as a "second hit" in the systemic inflammatory response that causes early MOF).[15] Parallel with these advances in understanding postinjury ACS is the recognition that ACS occurs in a variety of clinical scenarios such as extreme constipation,[16] ovarian hyperstimulation,[17] noninvasive ventilation,[18] pancreatitis,[19] and severe burns.[20] Since 2004, the World Society of the Abdominal Compartment Syndrome has offered leadership in consensus definitions, regular conferences, educational material, and organization of clinical trials.

Intraabdominal Pressure Measurement

Clinical examination of the abdomen is inaccurate for determining the presence of intraabdominal hypertension.[21,22] A standardized measurement of IAP is fundamental to the definition of intraabdominal hypertension and ACS.[1,2] IAP has been measured in virtually all parts of the abdominal cavity. The intravesical technique using a standard urinary catheter seems to be the most reliable and least invasive method. The rationale is that IAP is transmitted to the urinary bladder, which serves as a pressure transducer when filled with normal saline. Traditionally, a larger volume of saline was recommended, but recent studies showed that as little as 20 mL of instilled normal saline is enough for accurate measurement. Pressure is conducted by the fluid in the bladder to fluid in the urinary catheter, which is clamped during the interval when pressure is being measured. Pressure in the catheter tubing can be measured by inserting a sterile needle into the sample port of the catheter tube. Alternatively, a T-piece with three-way stopcock can be inserted into the catheter tube, connecting one limb to a strain-gauge pressure transducer.[23] The intravesical technique has been shown to correlate well with IAP measured directly using a laparoscopic insufflator.[24] The vesical route is more accurate than the use of rectal and gastric probes, which tend to provide different readouts, depending on the position of the patient.[24] Animal studies have shown that the pressure in the inferior vena cava correlates well with the vesical pressure,[25] but the inferior vena caval and direct peritoneal routes are more invasive. The urinary bladder pressure technique for IAP measurement was originally described by Kron et al.[3] and validated by Iberti et al.[26] The technique was simplified by Sugrue et al., who described the insertion of a T-connector into the drainage tubing.[23] This modification eliminated the need for multiple needle insertions into the sample port and minimized the risk of needlestick injury and microbial contamination of the bladder. This technique is relatively simple and can be performed in any ICU where a pressure transducer is available. Several proprietary devices are available for clinicians. Unfortunately, obtaining an accurate measurement requires about 7 minutes of nursing time, limiting the frequency with which measurements can be obtained. Even when personnel are highly aware of the possible consequences of ACS, screening measurements of IAP are rarely obtained more often than every 4 hours. ACS can develop 4 to 6 hours after ICU admission in patients who are at high risk.[5] The standard protocol for intermittent measurements of IAP does not provide information about the duration of intraabdominal hypertension. To address these shortcomings (labor intensity, intermittent nature), a continuous IAP measurement technique was developed and is currently being validated. The IAP can be continuously measured without clamping the tubing and instilling fluid into the bladder. For this new method, a standard three-way catheter is inserted, and the pressure transducer is connected to the saline-filled irrigation port. Once the setup is zeroed, the continuous IAP trace can be monitored without any further intervention or interference with the urine flow or tubing; this is the Balogh-Sugrue technique.[27]

Pathophysiology

The pathophysiologic effects of increased pressure in a closed body compartment are well described in other regions (e.g., tension pneumothorax, pericardial tamponade, increased intracranial pressure, extremity compartment syndromes) and are taught in the basic medical curriculum. The abdominal cavity is a "neglected" compartment (see Historical Perspective). The volume of the abdominal cavity is limited by its least tensile component, the fascia. Increased pressure can be due to an increase in the volume of the abdominal contents or to a decrease in the volume of the "container" (Table 201-1). After IAP increases to greater than 20 mm Hg, the abdominal cavity is on the steep portion of its pressure-volume curve, and as a result, small increases in content volume or decreases in cavity volume can cause dramatic increases in IAP. This is when close monitoring of IAP (preferably continuously) and organ function is essential for timely intervention.

TABLE 201-1	Causes of Intraabdominal Hypertension and Abdominal Compartment Syndrome	
Increased Abdominal Contents	**Decreased Abdominal Volume**
Ascites	Reduction of large long-standing hernia
Hemoperitoneum	Direct closure of large, long-standing abdominal wall defect
Visceral edema	Circumferential abdominal-wall burn
Abdominal packs	Continuous positive-pressure ventilation
Peritonitis	
Retroperitoneal edema (pancreatitis)	Retroperitoneal edema (pancreatitis)
Large pelvic, retroperitoneal hematoma	Large pelvic, retroperitoneal hematoma
Intestinal obstruction	
Ileus	
Gastric distention (esophageal ventilation)	
Abdominal aortic aneurysm	
Severe constipation	
Large abdominal tumor (chronic)	
Morbid obesity (chronic)	
Pregnancy (chronic)	

Pathophysiologic Response of Specific Organs

CEREBRAL PERFUSION

Increased IAP forces the diaphragm cephalad, thus decreasing the size of the thoracic cavity and causing intrathoracic pressure to increase. High intrathoracic pressure increases jugular venous pressure and impedes venous return from the brain. This effect can increase intracranial pressure and consequently decrease cerebral blood flow.[28-30] The effect of intraabdominal hypertension on intracranial pressure is especially relevant in severe blunt trauma, because head and abdominal injuries frequently coexist.

CARDIAC FUNCTION

Increased IAP impedes venous return to the heart, causing sequestration of blood in the lower extremities. High intrathoracic pressure increases central venous pressure and pulmonary capillary wedge pressure but does not increase right or left ventricular end-diastolic volume. In other words, when intrathoracic pressure is increased, central venous and pulmonary capillary wedge pressures are not reliable indices for assessing the adequacy of preload. Simultaneously, left ventricular afterload increases owing to increased systemic vascular resistance. Increased intrathoracic pressure can increase right ventricular afterload, potentially leading to right ventricular failure and dilation, with consequent leftward displacement of the ventricular septum and impairment of left ventricular filling.[31-34] Cardiac failure with elevated pulmonary capillary wedge pressure, increased systemic vascular resistance, and decreased cardiac index is a typical finding in profound intraabdominal hypertension and defines ACS. The cardiac index usually does not respond to fluid challenges, which can be detrimental if the underlying cause (ACS) is not treated. The cardiac index's response to decompression is predictive of outcome; patients who survive have a significantly greater increase in cardiac index after decompression than those who subsequently die.[5]

RESPIRATORY FUNCTION

Increased IAP pushes the diaphragm into the thoracic cavity. Thoracic compliance decreases, and increased airway pressure is required for mechanical ventilation. Additionally, functional residual capacity decreases, and ventilation/perfusion mismatching increases, leading to impaired oxygenation.[34,35] In the setting of massive resuscitation, these changes can be misinterpreted as being caused by acute lung injury. Historically, ACS was diagnosed by the presence of a firm abdomen in the setting of oliguria and increased airway pressures. Although airway pressure promptly decreases in response to abdominal decompression, this finding does not differentiate survivors from nonsurvivors.[5] The peak airway pressure is an important parameter to monitor during attempted primary fascial closure after laparotomy when ACS is a possible complication.

RENAL FUNCTION

Oliguria or anuria despite aggressive fluid resuscitation is a typical sign of ACS. Mechanisms responsible for decreased renal function include direct compression of the renal parenchyma, decreased perfusion of the kidneys due to decreased cardiac index, and increased water and sodium retention due to activation of the renin-angiotensin system.[36-38] The usual threshold for defining acute oliguria—urinary output less than 0.5 mL/kg/h—should be used cautiously and considered in the context of the magnitude of the resuscitation. Among patients who require massive resuscitation, the index of suspicion for ACS should be high when urinary output is less than 1 mL/kg/h.[5]

GUT FUNCTION

Increased IAP impairs splanchnic perfusion by decreasing the cardiac index and increasing splanchnic vascular resistance. When severe, tissue ischemia can result.[39-42] Intestinal perfusion can be assessed objectively using gastric tonometry. Decreased gastric intramural pH (pHi), increased gastric regional partial pressure of carbon dioxide (Pco_2), and a wide gap between gastric regional Pco_2 and end-tidal Pco_2 are all indicators of impaired abdominal visceral perfusion. Combined with urinary bladder pressure measurements, the newer semicontinuous tonometers are an excellent adjunct for the early identification of impending ACS.[3] Moreover, the physiologic response to decompression can be evaluated by assessing changes in pHi and related parameters using gastric tonometry.[5]

EXTREMITY PERFUSION

Increased IAP increases femoral venous pressure, increases peripheral vascular resistance, and reduces femoral artery blood flow by as much as 65%.[43]

MICROCIRCULATION

Laboratory studies have shown that decompression of ACS causes circulating neutrophils to increase CD11b adhesion receptor expression.[44] Decompression of ACS is also associated with the release of cytokines into the portal circulation and increased lung permeability, similar in degree to that seen after hemorrhagic shock and resuscitation.[44,45] Moreover, when ACS decompression is appropriately sequenced with hemorrhagic shock, it can serve as a "second hit" (i.e., ACS decompression 8 hours after hemorrhagic shock causes more intense acute lung injury than does ACS decompression 2 or 18 hours after shock).[44-46]

▨ Classification

ACS can be classified based on the duration of the syndrome, the presence or absence of intraperitoneal pathology, and the cause of the raised IAP (Table 201-2).

ACUTE VERSUS CHRONIC

The pathophysiologic responses described earlier are usually acute phenomena in critically ill or injured patients. However, the organ dysfunctions characterizing ACS can be present for long periods (chronic intraabdominal hypertension or ACS) in certain clinical conditions such as morbid obesity, chronic constipation, and pregnancy. In morbid obesity, chronic headaches and tinnitus are features of persistently increased intracranial pressure. The symptoms markedly improve when a special device is used to apply negative pressure to the abdomen to decrease IAP.[47]

TABLE 201-2	Classification of Abdominal Compartment Syndrome	
Basis of Classification	*Subcategories*
Time frame	Acute
	Chronic
Relation to peritoneal cavity	Primary
	Secondary
Etiology	Trauma
	Burn
	Postoperative
	Pancreatitis
	Bowel obstruction
	Ileus
	Abdominal aortic aneurysm
	Oncologic
	Gynecologic

PRIMARY VERSUS SECONDARY

Irrespective of cause, the presence of intraperitoneal pathology defines primary ACS. A typical case is one in which the damage-control paradigm was followed and perihepatic packing, combined with temporary closure of the abdominal wall, was used to tamponade bleeding from the liver.[48] As time progressed, intraabdominal bleeding and bowel edema (secondary to resuscitation) caused the volume of the intraabdominal contents to increase, precipitating ACS. Recognition of this problem has prompted trauma surgeons to leave the abdominal incision open after many damage-control procedures, reducing but not eliminating the risk of ACS. Primary ACS can also occur in patients who fail nonoperative management of abdominal organ injuries because of ongoing bleeding.[49]

Secondary ACS typically occurs in the setting of severe shock requiring massive resuscitation (whole body ischemia-reperfusion injury) in the absence of intraperitoneal pathology or injury.[5] Because there is no abdominal cause, secondary ACS is a more elusive diagnosis, and recognition is often delayed.[50] Typical causes are hypovolemic shock related to multiple open extremity fractures, unstable pelvic fractures, penetrating chest injuries,[51] and severe burns.[52] Secondary ACS can also develop during resuscitation for septic shock.[53]

ETIOLOGIC CLASSIFICATION

Classification of ACS based on the underlying cause is highly relevant because the underlying disease process and its treatment are contributing factors in the pathophysiology of the syndrome.

▨ Epidemiology

INCIDENCE

Because of different definitions and different study populations, the reported incidence of ACS is inconsistent. In the trauma literature of the mid-1990s, the reported incidence among high-risk patients undergoing laparotomy varied from 3% to 36%.[15] Fietsam and colleagues reported a 4% incidence of ACS in patients undergoing operation with primary fascial closure for ruptured abdominal aortic aneurysms.[54] Malbrain prospectively investigated medical ICU patients and documented the incidence of ACS at 2%.[55]

Another issue is that the epidemiology of ACS changes as treatment strategies evolve. For example, Meldrum et al.[56] and Balogh et al.[3] studied similar traumatic shock populations, and both reported that the incidence of ACS was 14%. These two studies, however, were performed 6 years apart. In the earlier series reported by Meldrum, only primary ACS was considered, and liberal use of the open abdomen was just starting. In contrast, in the series described by Balogh 6 years later, the abdomen was initially left open in virtually all cases of damage-control laparotomy (Bogota bag closure), and this strategy was associated with a decreased incidence of primary ACS. However, the previously unrecognized problem of secondary ACS was now an equally prevalent clinical entity.

If intraabdominal hypertension is used as a surrogate for ACS, the incidence is higher but similarly inconsistent. Sugrue and colleagues reported that the incidence of intraabdominal hypertension among general surgical patients undergoing laparotomy was 33% to 81%, depending on the definition (20 mm Hg or 18 mm Hg).[23,38] In a study of medical patients, Malbrain reported that the incidence of intraabdominal hypertension was only 18%, despite using a liberal cutoff value (12 mm Hg).[55] Using a cutoff value of 20 mm Hg, Balogh and coworkers reported a 39% incidence of intraabdominal hypertension in a cohort of patients with severe traumatic shock.[57] Ivatury et al. reported that the incidence of intraabdominal hypertension was 32% among patients with life-threatening penetrating abdominal trauma.[42]

OUTCOME

Full-blown ACS with organ dysfunction was once uniformly fatal. With more timely diagnosis and treatment, more than half (depending on etiology) of afflicted patients are now surviving. With decompressive laparotomy, organ dysfunction typically improves transiently, but most patients who survive more than 48 hours progress into MOF.[3,53] A fundamental problem is differentiating incomplete resuscitation from early organ failure. ACS and MOF appear to be closely linked. In our series, ACS was a surprisingly early event (occurring, on average, 12 hours after hospital admission) and was shown to be a strong independent predictor for subsequent MOF and death.

Prediction and Diagnosis

Epidemiologic studies carried out during the 1990s clearly documented that ACS is a significant clinical problem.[15] Additionally, more recent studies indicate that despite early recognition and decompression, the outcome remains poor for patients with ACS. Thus, early and accurate prediction is important because it allows us to recognize the population at risk and concentrate our preventive efforts on decreasing the incidence of ACS.[5,51] The urinary bladder pressure measurement is a widely accepted, inexpensive, and simple monitoring tool for ACS. However, organ dysfunction associated with ACS can occur when IAP is less than 20 mm Hg, and some patients with IAP greater than 30 mm Hg do not develop any symptoms. Not surprisingly, surgeons are reluctant to make decisions regarding decompression based only on measurements of IAP.[58] Potential risk factors for ACS include severe hemorrhagic shock, damage-control laparotomy, fascial closure after damage-control laparotomy, high abdominal trauma index, high injury severity score, and decreased pHi.[42,59] Studies of secondary ACS have identified resuscitation fluid volume thresholds that warrant monitoring urinary bladder pressure. Maxwell et al. recommended monitoring when the resuscitation volume exceeds 10 L of crystalloid fluid or 10 units of packed red blood cells.[60] Ivy et al. suggested that the trigger to initiate urinary bladder pressure monitoring should be greater than 0.25 L/kg of crystalloid resuscitation.[20,52] Biffl and coworkers reported that both these cutoffs are ineffective and recommended the following thresholds: 6 L or more of crystalloid resuscitation or 6 units or more of packed red blood cells in a 6-hour period in patients with a base deficit greater than 10 mEq/L, especially if a vasopressor agent is required.[53]

More recent studies from general surgical, burn, and trauma populations have tried to identify the independent risk factors for ACS. For example, McNelis and coworkers performed a case-control study of 22 patients with ACS (diagnosed by elevated IAP and peak airway pressure) and 22 general surgical patients without ACS and created a predictive equation[61]:

$$P = 1/(1 + e^{-z})$$

where $z = -18.6763 + 0.1671$ (peak airway pressure) $+ 0.0009$ (24-hour fluid balance).

In our experience, postinjury ACS occurs most frequently during the first 12 hours after injury, and waiting for a 24-hour fluid balance entails too much delay. By this time, most susceptible patients already exhibit the full-blown syndrome.[5,51] Postinjury ACS recognized after 24 hours is lethal.[5,50] Additionally, two prospective studies of trauma patients failed to identify predictors for ACS, possibly because the study populations were either too heterogeneous or too homogeneous. In a study of unselected trauma patients requiring ICU admission (mean injury severity score 18), Hong and colleagues found that only 2% of the patients developed intraabdominal hypertension and only 1% developed ACS.[62] In a review of patients undergoing damage-control laparotomy (mean injury severity score 29), Raeburn and associates found that the incidence of ACS was 36%.[63] Both of these groups failed to identify independent predictors of ACS.

From a prediction modeling perspective, patients requiring traumatic shock resuscitation are an ideal group to study. They are at

TABLE 201-3	Independent Predictors of Postinjury Primary and Secondary Abdominal Compartment Syndrome	
	ED Model	**ICU Model**
	INDEPENDENT PREDICTORS	INDEPENDENT PREDICTORS
Primary ACS	To OR < 75 min Crystalloids ≥ 3 L	Temp ≤ 34°C GAPCO_2 ≥ 16 Hb ≤ 8/dL BD ≥ 12 mEq/L
Secondary ACS	Crystalloids ≥ 3 L No urgent surgery PRBC ≥ 3 units	GAPCO_2 ≥ 16 Crystalloids ≥ 7.5 L UO ≤ 150 mL

ACS, abdominal compartment syndrome; BD, arterial base deficit; CI, confidence interval; ED, emergency department; GAPCO_2, carbon dioxide gap; Hb, hemoglobin concentration; ICU, intensive care unit; OR, operating room; PRBC, packed red blood cells; Temp, temperature; UO, urine output.

substantial risk for ACS, the time of insult is defined, and the subsequent treatment (resuscitation) can be standardized. We therefore performed a multiple logistic regression analysis on a prospective database of major torso trauma patients who required shock resuscitation.[5] Given the early occurrence of postinjury ACS, we focused our prediction models on the first 6 hours after hospital admission. We developed two prediction models: emergency department (ED) model (0-3 hours; i.e., all patients had an initial diagnostic workup and clinical laboratory results and were discharged from the ED) and ICU model (0-6 hours; i.e., all patients were admitted to the ICU, and their first physiologic monitor and clinical laboratory measurements on a standardized resuscitation protocol were available). Our goals were to identify the independent risk factors that may be causative and to build prediction models that could identify high-risk patients early during resuscitation so that standard care could be modified to prevent or improve the outcome of patients at risk for ACS.

The variables used in the multivariate prediction models included demographic parameters, shock severity, injury severity, interventions, hospital times, crystalloid and blood volumes, and vital signs. In the ICU, they also included initial pulmonary artery catheter readings, mechanical ventilator settings and response parameters, gastric tonometry data, and blood gas, clinical chemistry, and coagulation results. Among these variables, those listed in Table 201-3 were found to be independent risk factors for ACS. The primary ACS predictors at ICU admission (low temperature, low hemoglobin concentration, high base deficit) are all indicators of the so-called vicious circle physiology, the reason damage-control surgery is elected. The secondary ACS predictors (high crystalloid infusion volume, impaired renal function) suggest that the process is strongly related to the standard of care in the United States during the late 1990s (i.e., crystalloid resuscitation). The receiver operator characteristic analysis showed that ACS can be predicted with 0.88 accuracy at the time of ED discharge and, surprisingly, with 0.99 accuracy 1 hour after ICU admission with adequate monitoring. Use of these predictors together (even without urinary bladder pressure measurements) permits very early detection of the impaired physiologic findings characteristic of ACS. Because the predictors of ACS include both physiologic measurements and resuscitative interventions, this model should perform better in clinical situations during ongoing resuscitation than arbitrary urinary bladder pressure and organ dysfunction thresholds.[56] The ED model (≈3 hours after admission) is very sensitive (overinclusive), which minimizes the chance of missing ACS patients; the ICU model (≈6 hours after hospital admission) is very specific and can pinpoint individuals at highest risk.

Treatment

NONSURGICAL METHODS

Support of early organ dysfunction by traditional ICU interventions is often necessary in patients with impending ACS but may aggravate the underlying pathophysiology. For example, ventilator strategies to

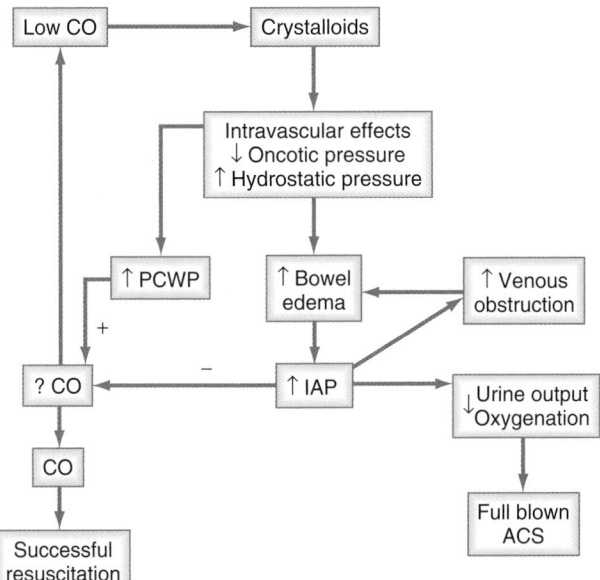

Figure 201-1 Futile crystalloid preloading. ACS, abdominal compartment syndrome; CO, cardiac output; IAP, intraabdominal pressure; PCWP, pulmonary capillary wedge pressure; ↑, increased; ↓, decreased; +, positive effect; −, negative effect.

increase mean airway pressure to improve oxygenation (e.g., high levels of positive end-expiratory pressure) directly increase intraabdominal hypertension by pushing down on the diaphragm. Additionally, increased mean airway pressure increases intrathoracic pressure, impeding venous outflow from the abdominal cavity. This promotes more gut edema with ongoing crystalloid resuscitation, another intervention often used in patients with impending ACS. Seminal papers in the mid-1990s advocated hypervolemic resuscitation to ameliorate cardiac and renal dysfunction. The concept was that increased IAP elevates pulmonary capillary wedge pressure but not preload, and fluid should be administered to increase left ventricular end-diastolic volume to improve the cardiac index.[64] This approach seems harmful according to the most recent evidence.[57,65] Patients with similar demographic characteristics, injuries, and shock severity without impending ACS responded very well to preload-directed resuscitation and increased the cardiac index appropriately.[65] However, patients with impending ACS did not respond with increased cardiac index, despite vigorous crystalloid infusion. Vigorous attempts to increase preload (especially with crystalloid infusions) in patients with intraabdominal hypertension have a detrimental effect on outcome (futile crystalloid cycle; Figure 201-1).

Theoretically, other nonsurgical interventions may have beneficial effects, but their efficacy is unproven.[66] Colloids and albumin could mobilize interstitial fluids into the vascular space, and muscle relaxants might have a salutary effect by decreasing tension in the abdominal wall.[52,67] Continuous external application of negative abdominal pressure with a suction device showed some promise in morbidly obese patients with cerebral symptoms secondary to chronic ACS.[47]

PERCUTANEOUS METHODS

If intraabdominal hypertension or ACS is a result of acute or chronic fluid collection, symptoms can be relieved by percutaneous drainage. Case reports described successful drainage of abdominal fluid in burn patients with secondary ACS and the drainage of blood in nonoperatively managed liver injuries.[67-69] The major limitation of the technique is that it is applicable only when a significant amount of fluid is causing increased IAP. This technique will not work and might be dangerous when extensive bowel edema or retroperitoneal hematoma is the dominant contributing factor.

SURGICAL DECOMPRESSION

Surgical decompression remains the primary recommended intervention. Decompression is achieved by opening the midline fascia (avascular plane) along its full length. Virtually all reports describe a very good physiologic response to decompression, but this does not necessarily translate into better outcomes. The best predictors of survival are postdecompression improvement in cardiac index and urine output.[5,51] The decision to undertake surgical decompression is a difficult one, because it results in a chronically open abdomen that is associated with numerous hazards. Several case series have shown that early decompression is associated with better outcomes. However, in those studies, "late" decompression was often carried out days after the initial signs of ACS. If decompression is carried out within 12 hours of hospital admission, timing has no significant effect on outcome.[5,51] Patients with ACS are in critical condition and require mechanical ventilation and other forms of organ support. Any unnecessary intrahospital transportation of these patients can be detrimental. Thus, if no other intraabdominal surgical intervention is needed, decompression can be performed at the bedside in the ICU. More recently, alternatives to midline laparotomy (transverse laparotomy and linea alba fasciotomy) were described. These approaches were popularized in cases of severe acute pancreatitis, where transverse laparotomy can be the surgical access of choice.[70] The (subcutaneous) linea alba fasciotomy can prevent peritoneal contamination in selected pancreatitis cases where laparotomy is not required, only reduction of intraabdominal pressure.[71,72]

Management of the Open Abdomen

Decompressive laparotomy results in an open abdomen, because the incision should not be closed until the risk of recreating ACS by closing the fascia diminishes. After abdominal decompression, temporary abdominal closure is applied to the wound to keep the fascia open. Several methods (towel clips, Bogota bag, synthetic mesh, vacuum-assisted closure, Velcro patch, zipper) are available. It is advantageous for the ICU specialist to understand each of these methods and discuss them with the surgical team. The key goals of temporary abdominal closure are as follows: prevent evisceration, allow enough room for swelling of the abdominal contents, control peritoneal fluids, prevent contamination, and preserve the fascia and skin for possible later closure or reconstruction. During the last 15 years, the morbidity and mortality of open abdomen management significantly decreased, but the strategy still carries considerable complications and potential long-term morbidity.[73,74] Fistulas, abdominal infections, and intraabdominal collections were common, and the end result was usually a large abdominal wall defect. Early experience with a vacuum-assisted closure technique was very promising, and use of this approach may improve management of the open abdomen.[75,76] A growing body of evidence is available about techniques which are successfully minimizing the morbidity and mortality of open abdomen management and improve long-term outcomes.[74]

Prevention, Surveillance, and Future Directions

Prospective data suggest that the mortality rate for ACS, even with early decompression and resuscitation, is very high. In addition, early favorable physiologic responses to decompression do not necessarily translate into improved outcomes.[5] Accordingly, prevention of ACS is paramount. Avoidance of fascial closure after high-risk laparotomy reduces the incidence of MOF and mortality.[59] In the operating room, monitoring for increases in peak airway pressures during the attempted fascial closure is valuable in the absence of IAP measurement. In the ICU, all patients with severe shock and subsequent resuscitation (whole body ischemia-reperfusion injury), regardless of the cause (burn, trauma, sepsis, or hypovolemia), benefit from IAP monitoring, which is a simple, noninvasive tool.

ACS is strongly associated with the magnitude and quality of resuscitation.[5,50-53,57,60,65] Uncontrolled goal-oriented resuscitation of trauma victims, chasing supranormal values for oxygen delivery, is harmful.[57] To eliminate uncontrolled resuscitation, treatment of the underlying cause of shock is crucial. Timely hemorrhage control and elimination of septic foci should happen simultaneously. There is increasing evidence that Ringer's lactate solution is proinflammatory, and use of this agent is an independent predictor of postinjury ACS.[77] During burn and trauma resuscitation, crystalloid limits should be implemented, and after reaching them, alternative resuscitation fluids should be used. The best resuscitation fluid during impending ACS has yet to be determined.

In postinjury primary ACS, correction of the vicious circle of coagulopathy, acidosis, and hypothermia should be an early goal. Abbreviated laparotomy saves lives, but the tight abdominal packing increases the risk of ACS. Use of topical hemorrhage control techniques (e.g., fibrin sealants) offers a workable solution.[78] When abnormalities in respiratory and renal function are identified, ACS should be included in the differential diagnosis and is an easily excludable cause if IAP measurements are performed. A direct effect of ACS is impaired abdominal visceral perfusion. Gastric tonometry is a relatively noninvasive monitor for intraabdominal hypertension. A high gastric regional P_{CO_2} (>60 mm Hg) and a wide gap between gastric and end-tidal P_{CO_2} (>16 mm Hg) are important indicators and predictors of ACS. With the availability of continuous IAP measurement, abdominal perfusion pressure (mean arterial pressure minus IAP) can be easily monitored at the bedside. The value of this variable has yet to be prospectively validated.

ACS can occur in a wide range of critically ill patients. With increased awareness of ACS, focused monitoring, application of temporary abdominal closure methods, and fine-tuned resuscitation, the incidence of primary ACS is decreasing. Secondary ACS represents failure of resuscitation (over-resuscitation, neglected hemorrhage control, or nonexistent monitoring for ACS) and is a problem that can be eliminated. The occurrence of secondary ACS in burn and shock or trauma ICUs should be considered a negative performance indicator.

The future of open abdomen management is also promising. The modern systematic approach to open abdomen will decrease the rate of serious complications, which historically might have prevented surgeons from considering this preventive/therapeutic measure. Despite encouraging results with the current management of open abdomen, decompressive laparotomy should not be viewed as the final solution for IAH/ACS.

KEY POINTS

1. It is essential to distinguish intraabdominal hypertension (IAH) from abdominal compartment syndrome (ACS). The difference between them is the presence of organ dysfunction in ACS, which makes it a life-threatening condition.

2. Intraabdominal pressure (IAP) should be monitored in all shock resuscitation patients, regardless of the cause of the shock (e.g., burn, sepsis, trauma).

3. Presently, the safest and most feasible way to monitor IAP is the intravesical technique.

4. ACS can occur without abdominal pathology or injury (secondary ACS).

5. To date, the best-characterized ACS groups are postinjury, burn, and pancreatitis.

6. The outcome of ACS is very poor, even with early decompression. Prevention, prediction, and surveillance are keys to successful management.

7. Postinjury primary and secondary ACS can be accurately predicted 6 hours after hospital admission with adequate monitoring.

8. Awareness of the predictors of ACS and crystalloid volume–restricting shock resuscitation are decreasing the incidence of ACS.

9. Outcomes with open abdomen are also improving.

10. The significance of sub-ACS IAH is still unclear.

ANNOTATED REFERENCES

Balogh Z, McKinley BA, Cox Jr CS, et al. Abdominal compartment syndrome: the cause or effect of postinjury multiple organ failure. Shock 2003;20:483-92.
This article summarizes present knowledge on postinjury ACS including cause, pathomechanism, individual organ responses, and decompression. It focuses on the most recent findings about the relationship between shock resuscitation and ACS. The authors review the growing evidence that ACS is a second hit in the development of multiple organ failure and provide guidelines for prevention and therapy.

Balogh Z, McKinley BA, Holcomb JB, et al. Both primary and secondary abdominal compartment syndrome can be predicted early and are harbingers of multiple organ failure. J Trauma 2003;54:848-61.
This is a comprehensive paper on the epidemiology, outcome, and prediction of postinjury primary and secondary ACS. The study population consisted of 188 patients from the prospective shock-trauma resuscitation database, with strict inclusion criteria and standardized resuscitation with bedside computerized decision support. The distinct characteristics of primary and secondary ACS are described based on the results of univariate and multivariate analysis. Multivariate prediction models show that the syndrome can be predicted during the first few hours after hospital admission.

Ivy ME, Atweh NA, Palmer J, et al. Intra-abdominal hypertension and abdominal compartment syndrome in burn patients. J Trauma 2000;49:387-91.
This is a prospective evaluation of patients with high-percentage burns, in whom secondary ACS is a frequent complication. The authors recommend IAP measurements after 0.25-L/kg crystalloid resuscitation and report a high success rate using conservative management of ACS in burn patients.

Malbrain ML. Abdominal pressure in the critically ill: measurement and clinical relevance. Intensive Care Med 1999;25:1453-8.
This prospective clinical study describes the incidence of intraabdominal hypertension and ACS in a general medical ICU.

Sugrue M, Bauman A, Jones F, et al. Clinical examination is an inaccurate predictor of intraabdominal pressure. World J Surg 2002;26:1428-31.
This prospective clinical study concluded that physical examination is a poor way to determine the presence of intraabdominal hypertension. The authors strongly support routine IAP measurements.

REFERENCES

Access the complete reference list online at http://www.expertconsult.com.

202

Thrombolytics

RYAN M. McENANEY | EDITH TZENG

Thrombolytic agents comprise a diverse group of compounds that indirectly initiate lysis of thrombi. In the formation of a thrombus, fibrin forms the molecular scaffolding. After initiation of the coagulation cascade, fibrinolytic mechanisms are concomitantly activated to prevent unchecked thrombosis. The fibrinolytic process begins with cleavage of the proenzyme plasminogen to plasmin, an enzyme that hydrolyzes key bonds within the fibrin clot matrix, resulting in clot lysis (Figure 202-1). Intravenous (IV) or intraarterial thrombolytic agents function by promoting the conversion of plasminogen to plasmin. The different thrombolytic agents vary in their specificity for plasminogen, metabolic half-life, and antigenicity (Table 202-1).

Drugs

STREPTOKINASE

Streptokinase, a protein produced by β-hemolytic streptococci, was first identified as having fibrinolytic properties in the 1930s[1] and was the first compound used clinically as a thrombolytic drug.[2] Despite its name, streptokinase itself is not an enzyme. Rather, it complexes with plasminogen in a 1:1 stoichiometric relationship. The streptokinase-plasminogen complex then converts both circulating and fibrin-bound plasminogen to plasmin. One of the major drawbacks to clinical use of streptokinase is its antigenicity, as antibodies may have formed during prior streptococcal infection. Allergic reactions occur in 2% to 5% of patients receiving the drug and are generally mild, but severe anaphylactic reactions can occur.[3] It has a short half-life of approximately 20 minutes. Anistreplase (APSAC [anisoylated plasminogen streptokinase activator complex]) is a modified form of streptokinase that has a substantially longer half-life but still can cause allergic reactions (see Figure 202-1).

UROKINASE

Urokinase is a thrombolytic protein that was initially isolated from human urine and has been used clinically for over 30 years. It is isolated from human fetal renal tissue cultures and, unlike streptokinase, enzymatically cleaves plasminogen. During the 1980s and early 1990s, urokinase was the primary thrombolytic agent used clinically for treatment of graft thrombosis and peripheral arterial occlusion. In 1999, urokinase was removed from the U.S. market after questions were raised by the Food and Drug Administration (FDA) regarding the safety of this product.[4] It was reintroduced in the United States in late 2002 after rigorous testing showed that the preparations were free of human pathogens, but its only current indication is for pulmonary embolism. Prourokinase, also known as *single-chain urokinase-type plasminogen activator* (scu-PA), is a single-chain precursor molecule of urokinase that is converted into two-chain urokinase by hydrolysis. It is relatively fibrin specific and has low antigenicity.

TISSUE PLASMINOGEN ACTIVATOR

Tissue plasminogen activator (tPA) was first isolated in 1981.[5] It is a naturally occurring protein synthesized by human vascular endothelial cells. Commercially available preparations are manufactured using recombinant technologies, as first described by Pennica and colleagues.[6] A number of different recombinant variants are available, including alteplase (rtPA, approved by the FDA in 1987) and duteplase,

as well as other forms of the tissue-type plasminogen activators: reteplase (rPA), tenecteplase (TNK-tPA), and lanoteplase (nPA). Recombinant tPAs have the advantage of being nonantigenic and specific for fibrin-bound plasminogen and avoid the infectious risks associated with products isolated from cultured human tissues. Newer recombinant tPAs have improved pharmacokinetics, allowing for more convenient administration such as bolus dosing.

OTHER AGENTS

In addition to streptokinase, urokinase, tPA, and their derivatives, a number of other compounds have been developed and investigated. These include vampire bat plasminogen activator (derived from the saliva of the vampire bat), fibrolase (from the venom of the southern copperhead snake), and staphylokinase (from *Staphylococcus aureus*). However, data regarding use of these compounds are relatively limited, and they are rarely used clinically.

Clinical Indications

MYOCARDIAL INFARCTION

Acute myocardial infarction (AMI) represents a significant healthcare burden in industrialized countries, with trends estimating the growing impact of this disease on the world. Modern management of AMI focuses on rapidly restoring perfusion to optimize salvage of myocardium. To this end, primary percutaneous coronary interventions (PCIs) have been shown to be superior to thrombolytic therapy when employed as an early reperfusion strategy after AMI and are thus recommended as first-line therapy when available.[7] However, logistical barriers exist hindering access to early PCI for all patients with AMI, whereas fibrinolysis can be used in nearly all hospitals.

The use of lytic therapy for the treatment of AMI was first attempted in the 1950s.[8] The rationale for this therapy was that reestablishing coronary blood flow in an acutely thrombosed vessel would reduce infarct size and mortality. A meta-analysis of 33 randomized trials in 1985 demonstrated a 22% reduction in mortality with the use of thrombolytics in AMI, and these findings prompted further investigation into lytic therapy for MI.[9] The Fibrinolytic Therapy Trialists' Collaborative Group (FTT) performed a meta-analysis in 1994 with aggregated results from over 58,000 patients treated with thrombolytics.[10] This analysis revealed a nearly 25% reduction in mortality in those patients with ST-segment elevation or bundle branch block. Numerous studies since have been performed to evaluate the efficacy of different lytic agents, dosing strategies, routes of administration, and adjunctive therapies for rapid restoration of antegrade flow in thrombosed coronary arteries.

Early studies focused on the use of streptokinase, demonstrating 18% and 25% reductions in mortality at 3 and 5 weeks, respectively, in the ISIS-2[3] and GISSI studies.[11] These short-term findings in the fibrinolytic group were maintained out to 1- to 10-year follow-ups.[12] The efficacy of tPA was studied in the GUSTO-1 trial, which examined 4 dosing regimens for the treatment of MI in 41,021 patients.[13] This study utilized "accelerated" tPA dosing, wherein two-thirds of the total dose was administered in the first 30 minutes rather than over 3 hours. This dosing regimen resulted in a modest but significant reduction in 30-day mortality (6.3%) compared to streptokinase (7.4%) or a combination of tPA and streptokinase (7.0%). The GUSTO angiographic

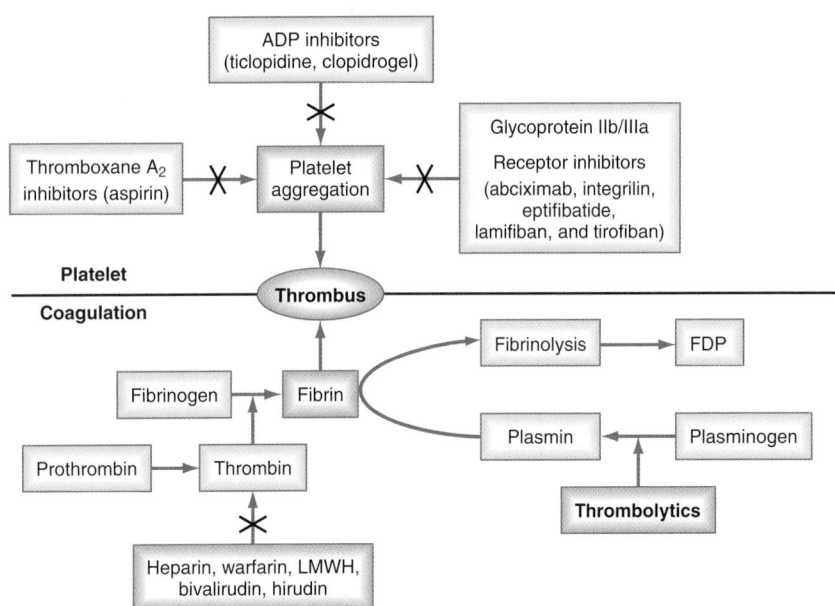

Figure 202-1 Components of thrombus formation and actions of various antithrombotic and thrombolytic agents. ADP, adenosine diphosphate; FDP, fibrin degradation products; LMWH, low-molecular-weight heparin.

substudy demonstrated that differing patency rates between patients treated with either agent accounted for this difference in clinical efficacy. A subsequent meta-analysis of this approach, however, failed to validate the survival advantage.[14] The recombinant deletion mutant of tPA, reteplase, was compared to accelerated tPA in 15,059 patients in the GUSTO III trial. No survival advantage was observed with reteplase, and rates of intracranial hemorrhage were similar (0.91% and 0.87% with reteplase and tPA, respectively).[15] The ASSENT-2 trial showed that mortality at 30 days and ICH rates were identical between use of tenecteplase and accelerated tPA.[16] While reteplase and tenecteplase have not surpassed tPA in terms of efficacy, their pharmacokinetics translate to simplified administration versus accelerated tPA.

Adjunctive therapies such as aspirin or clopidogrel and antithrombin agents improve the results of lytic therapy. As fibrinolysis strips fibrin from the occluding thrombus, the exposed thrombin initiates platelet aggregation and subsequent rethrombosis.[17] Therefore some form of antithrombin strategy is warranted. Heparin can be infused to keep the activated partial thromboplastin time (APTT) between 50 and 70 seconds. If heparin-induced thrombocytopenia is suspected, direct thrombin inhibitors (hirudin or bivalirudin) can be used.[18] Another development has been the introduction of glycoprotein IIb/IIIa receptor blockers such as abciximab (ReoPro), eptifibatide (Integrilin), and tirofiban (Aggrastat).[19-21] Despite some promising early results,[22] no randomized trial has yet to show an impact on mortality with combination therapy.[23-25]

The timing of diagnosis and institution of thrombolytic therapy is critical.[26,27] Patients with AMI treated with thrombolytic agents more than 4 hours after the onset of symptoms have 30-day and 6-month mortality rates that are 2 to 3 times higher than patients who were treated within 2 hours after the onset of symptoms.[28] Eighty-two percent of patients treated within 2 hours had return of normal cardiac wall motion, whereas only 46% of those treated within 2 to 5 hours after the onset of symptoms have return of normal wall motion.[29] The LATE (Late Assessment of Thrombolytic Efficacy) study reported 1-year mortality rates of 17.6% versus 15.8% in those patients treated with rtPA at greater than 3 hours versus less than 3 hours, respectively, after the onset of symptoms.[30] So critical is the timing of the initiation of treatment that prehospital administration of thrombolytics has been advocated in selected patients with ST-segment elevations on an electrocardiogram.[31,32]

Currently accepted guidelines for lytic therapy in AMI are outlined by the American College of Chest Physicians in the 2008 8th edition of the Evidence-Based Clinical Practice Guidelines and by the American College of Cardiology/American Heart Association in their 2004

guidelines.[33,34] The treatment algorithm is summarized in Figure 202-2. Unfortunately, the value of thrombolytic agents for the management of unstable angina remains unproven. Currently there is no role for lytic therapy in acute coronary syndrome in the absence of ST-segment elevation in two or more contiguous leads or without new-onset bundle branch block. Contraindications to lytic therapy in the setting of AMI are also summarized in Table 202-2.

Recently, a large meta-analysis was performed that examined 7739 patients with ST-segment elevation randomized to either thrombolytic agents (76% receiving fibrin-specific lytics) or primary percutaneous transluminal coronary angioplasty (PTCA).[7] Short-term (4-6 weeks) mortality in the PTCA group was 7%, compared to 9% in the group that received lytic therapy ($P = .0003$). The group treated with primary PTCA had lower rates for nonfatal reinfarction (3% versus 7%) and stroke (1% versus 2%) as part of a follow-up to a smaller study.[35] The short-term results of this meta-analysis are summarized in Figure 202-3.

Potential advantages of angioplasty over thrombolysis[36-39] as primary therapy for AMI must be tempered by the recognition that angioplasty results are highly dependent on the volume of cases at a given

TABLE 202-1	Summary of Properties of Commonly Used Thrombolytics		
	Streptokinase	*Urokinase*	*Tissue Plasminogen Activator (tPA)*
Source	Group C *Streptococcus*	Human fetal kidney	Recombinant
Lytic	First	First (prourokinase—second)	Second (non-alteplase tPAs—third)
Generation	Anistreplase		
Variants	[APSAC] (half-life 70-120 min)	Prourokinase	Alteplase, duteplase, reteplase (rPA), tenecteplase (TNK-tPA), lanoteplase (nPA)
Molecular weight (kD)	47	35-55	63-70
Half-life (min)	18-23	14-20	3-4
Metabolism	Hepatic	Hepatic	Hepatic
Antigenicity	Yes	No	No
Fibrin specificity	Minimal	Moderate	Moderate
Plasminogen binding	Indirect	Direct	Direct

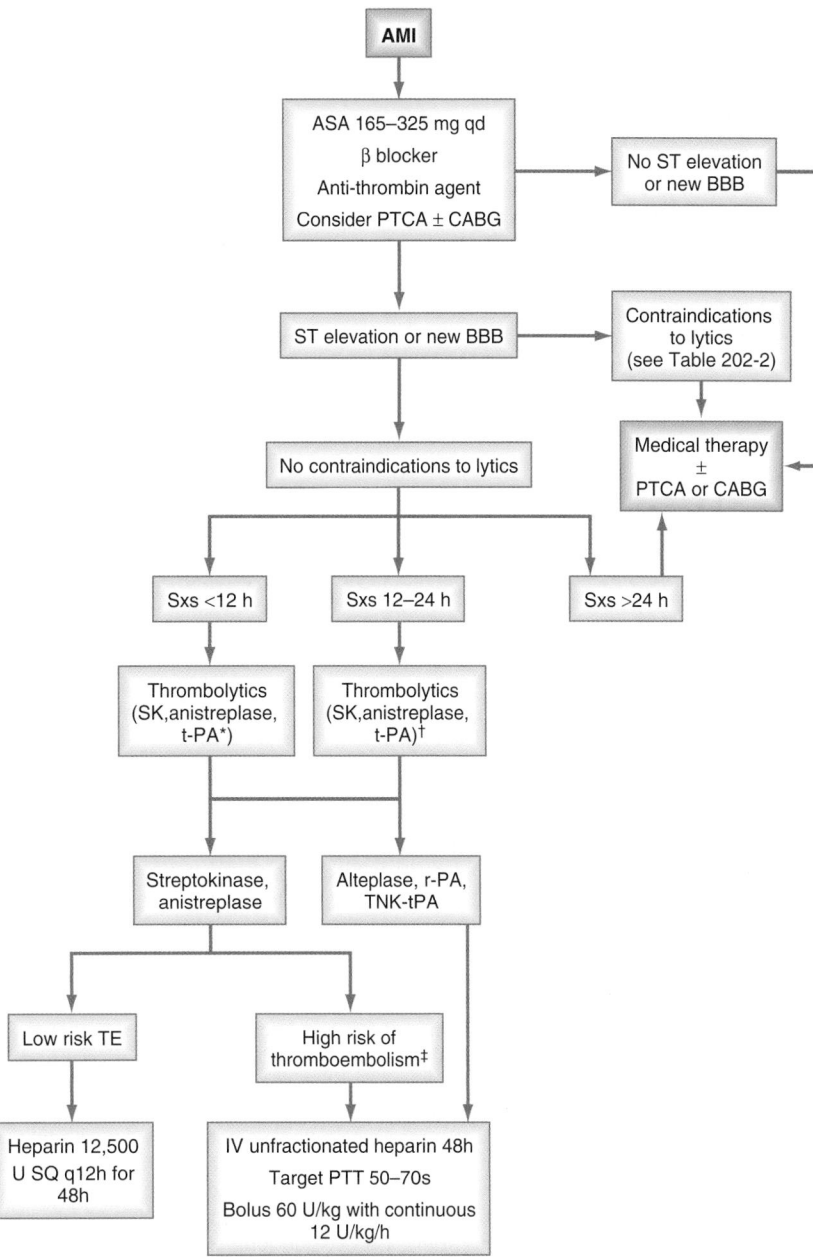

Figure 202-2 Algorithm for treatment of acute myocardial infarction. *, preferred for symptoms <6 h; †, grade 2b data[11]; ‡, anterior myocardial infarction, existing heart failure, previous embolus, atrial fibrillation, left ventricular thrombus; AMI, acute myocardial infarction; BBB, bundle branch block; CABG, coronary artery bypass grafting; PTCA, percutaneous transluminal coronary angioplasty; PTT, partial thromboplastin time; SK, streptokinase; SQ, subcutaneous; Sxs, signs and symptoms; TE, thromboembolism. *(Adapted from 1999/2002 ACC/AHA Guideline Update and 2001 ACCP Consensus Conference.[11-12])*

treatment center. Moreover, comparisons to lytic therapy often use historical data before the era of accelerated dosing regimens and adjunctive treatment with antiplatelet and antithrombin agents. Lytic therapy also may be advantageous in critically ill patients who are unable to be transported to cardiac catheterization facilities or in those who have other contraindications to PTCA. Ultimately, the ideal treatment for some patients may involve combinations of angioplasty, reduced-dose thrombolytic therapy, antithrombotic agents, and antiplatelet agents.

STROKE

Stroke is the third leading cause of death in the United States, affecting over 700,000 people per year. Strokes are a major source of morbidity and mortality among hospitalized patients.[40] The majority of strokes are ischemic in nature, resulting from sudden occlusion of arteries

TABLE 202-2	Contraindications to Thrombolytic Therapy in the Setting of Acute Myocardial Infarction*	
Absolute Contraindications	***Relative Contraindications***
>24 hours since onset of symptoms	12 to 24 hours since onset of symptoms
Prior intracranial hemorrhage	Age > 75 years
Stroke within past year	Systolic blood pressure > 180 mm Hg or diastolic blood pressure > 110 mm Hg
Intracranial neoplasm	Bleeding disorder
Active bleeding/bleeding diathesis	Prior allergic reaction to thrombolytics
Suspected aortic dissection	Pregnant or lactating
Significant closed-head or facial trauma within 3 months	Prolonged cardiopulmonary resuscitation (>10 min)
	Recent internal bleeding (<2-4 wk)
	Active peptic ulcer

*With ST-segment elevation and/or new bundle branch block.

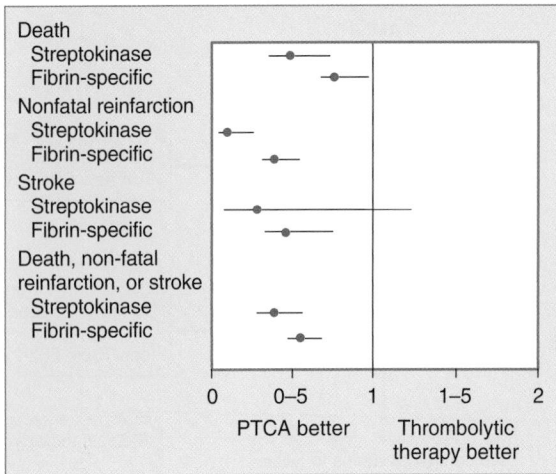

Figure 202-3 Short-term clinical outcomes in patients treated with percutaneous transluminal coronary angioplasty (PTCA) versus thrombolytic therapy. Odds ratios with 95% confidence intervals. *(Reprinted with permission from Keeley EC, Boura JA, Grines CL. Primary angioplasty versus intravenous thrombolytic therapy for acute myocardial infarction: a quantitative review of 23 randomised trials. Lancet 2003;361:13-20.)*

delivering blood supply to the brain. These occlusions often are caused by thromboemboli from a variety of sources.[41] Traditional therapy for ischemic stroke has focused on the use of anticoagulation and antiplatelet agents for medical support and then rehabilitation after the acute event. More recently, thrombolytic therapy has emerged as a mode of intervention in ischemic stroke patients. Similar to the treatment of AMI, the efficacy of thrombolytic agents is highly time dependent owing to the characteristics of the ischemic penumbra.[42] Indeed, efficacy is greater when lytic treatment is administered within 90 minutes of the event.[43]

The concept of utilizing "clot-busting" therapies for ischemic stroke blossomed in 1995 when the National Institute of Neurological Disorders and Stroke (NINDS) published a study on rtPA in acute ischemic stroke.[44] This trial consisted of two parts. Part I enrolled 291 patients and examined the clinical efficacy of IV tPA given within 3 hours after symptom onset. This treatment failed to improve neurologic function after 24 hours versus placebo. By 3 months, however, patients treated with tPA showed significant improvement in 4 different functional outcome measurements as assessed by the National Institutes of Health Stroke Scale (NIHSS). Part II of this study assessed the long-term outcomes of tPA treatment. Patients who received tPA were 30% more likely to have minimal residual disability or to have returned to baseline functional status at 3, 6, and 12 months.[45] Unfortunately, patients treated with tPA suffered a greater incidence of intracerebral hemorrhage (6.4% versus 0.6% in the placebo group; $P < .001$) at 36 hours. Subsequent studies have shown similar rates of intracranial hemorrhage after lytic therapy. Nevertheless, mortality at 3 months was not significantly different (17% versus 21%; $P = .30$). Intravenous tPA was approved by the FDA for treatment of acute ischemic stroke within a 3-hour window as a result of this study. Other early randomized trials of IV tPA in acute stroke treatment included the European Cooperative Acute Stroke Study (ECASS-I),[46] ECASS-II,[47] and the ATLANTIS trials.[42,48] These trials, while each failing to reach significance for their primary outcome measure, did show significant benefit in favor of tPA usage between 0 and 6 hours for alternative outcome measures, lending some additional support for its use. A subsequent analysis of these trials showed that the odds ratio of benefit of IV tPA decreased as time from stroke onset increased.[49]

More recently, the ECASS-III trial did demonstrate a lesser, albeit significant, benefit of tPA compared to placebo when administered in the 3- to 4.5-hour window, with no difference in mortality.[50] Rates of symptomatic intracranial hemorrhage (based on the NINDS definition) were slightly higher than in the NINDS trial (7.9% versus 3.5% in the placebo group; $P = 0.006$). It is important to note that this trial exercised more stringent inclusion criteria than the NINDS trial. Based on the results of this trial, Lansberg et al. calculated that the number of patients deriving benefit per 100 treated are 28, 23, and 17 for 0- to 1.5-hour, 1.5- to 3-hour, and 3- to 4.5-hour windows, respectively.[51] It is estimated that in the 3- to 4.5-hour window, 1 in 6 patients will have a better outcome and 1 in 35 a worse outcome.[52] As a result of the ECASS III trial, IV tPA usage for treatment of stroke has been supported by the Scientific Advisory from the American Heart Association Stroke Council, although the FDA has not expanded its approval to date.[53]

Currently, the only drug and route of administration currently approved by the FDA for treatment of ischemic stroke is tPA through an IV route. However, prourokinase as well as intraarterial fibrinolytic administration are also used in the setting of established clinical protocols. Intravenous delivery has both practical and theoretical disadvantages. One disadvantage is the inability to effectively lyse the internal carotid artery or the middle cerebral artery.[54] After confirmation by head computed tomography (CT) of ischemic stroke (i.e., not associated with hemorrhage), patients are typically treated by IV tPA at a dose of 0.9 mg/kg, with 10% of the total dose given as an initial bolus, and the remainder infused over 60 minutes.[55]

Intraarterial administration of thrombolytics is gaining popularity for treating ischemic stroke. This method requires that a neurointerventionalist obtain arterial images and place an intraarterial catheter into the thrombosed vessel. The thrombolytic agent is then infused through the catheter directly into the target vessel, achieving high local concentration at the site of occlusion while decreasing systemic drug levels. Direct intraarterial delivery has been shown to be effective in limited studies. The Prolyse in Acute Cerebral Thromboembolism (PROACT II) study[56] randomized 180 patients with middle cerebral artery occlusion to either intraarterial prourokinase plus heparin or heparin alone. Intraarterial prourokinase improved the modified Rankin score to 2 or less in over 40% of patients, whereas heparin infusion alone improved the score in only 25%. Also, prourokinase was associated with significantly higher vessel recanalization rates (66% versus 18%; $P < .0001$). The MELT trial was a Japanese trial of intraarterial urokinase which was halted early due to external reasons and was thus underpowered to reach significance of the primary endpoint.[57] Nevertheless, secondary analysis from that study and combined analyses with the PROACT trials suggested benefit to arterial urokinase.[58] Prourokinase is not available for general use, but tPA and its variants are frequently administered in intraarterial fashion.[59,60]

Additionally, the Interventional Management of Stroke (IMS) trialists recently began a phase III trial comparing standard-dose IV tPA with a reduced-dose IV tPA bridge to an endovascular treatment consisting of either mechanical thrombectomy, arterial tPA infusion, or a combination of low-intensity ultrasound with tPA infusion.[61] Although growing evidence supports use of intraarterial revascularization methods, they are obviously restricted to those centers with skilled neurointerventionalists. Standard contraindications to IV thrombolytic therapy in acute ischemic stroke are similar to the exclusion criteria used in the NINDS study (Table 202-3). Blood pressure should be tightly controlled, ideally maintained below 180/105 mm Hg. Antithrombotic agents should also be withheld for 24 hours owing to the risk of intracranial hemorrhage. A number of adjunctive therapies including mechanical thrombectomy,[62] glycoprotein IIb/IIIa inhibitors,[63] and ultrasound[64,65] have shown promise in improving recanalization rates.

PULMONARY EMBOLISM

Pulmonary embolism (PE) is not only a major source of morbidity and mortality in hospitalized patients, accounting for up to 15% of in-hospital deaths, but is also a surprisingly underrecognized source of cardiovascular collapse.[66-68] Anticoagulation has been a critical

TABLE 202-3	Contraindications for Thrombolytic Therapy in Ischemic Stroke	
Contraindications	**Relative Contraindications**	
Symptom duration >6 hours	Symptom duration of 3 to 6 hours	
History of intracranial hemorrhage	Witnessed seizure	
Evidence of active bleeding	Gastrointestinal or urinary hemorrhage within 3 weeks	
Platelet count <100,000/mm³	Recent lumbar puncture, noncompressible arterial puncture site	
Prior stroke, head trauma, or intracranial surgery within 3 months	Systolic blood pressure >185 mm Hg or diastolic blood pressure >110 mm Hg	
Rapidly improving or only minor symptoms	Mass effect or hypodensity of greater than one-third middle cerebral artery distribution on head CT	
Major surgery within 14 days		
Known arteriovenous malformation or intracranial aneurysm	Glucose <50 mg/dL or >400 mg/dL Elevated partial thromboplastin time or international normalized ratio (>1.7)	

component in the treatment of PE since first shown to be beneficial in 1960.[69] This may be achieved using IV unfractionated heparin (UFH), with an initial bolus of 80 units/kg followed by 18 units/kg/h, with monitored dose adjustment to maintain the APTT prolongation at a level that corresponds to 0.3 to 0.7 IU/mL anti-Xa activity. Alternatively, subcutaneous (SQ) low-molecular-weight heparin (LMWH), SQ fondaparinux, or monitored or fixed-dose SQ UFH may be used.[70] Unfortunately, despite the proven efficacy of anticoagulation in the setting of acute PE, a significant proportion of patients will have incomplete resolution of their occlusion, with subsequent organization of the thrombus and obliteration of the pulmonary artery.[71-73] Accordingly, thrombolytic therapy for pulmonary embolism may offer more rapid and complete resolution of thrombus burden.

One of the initial studies that evaluated thrombolytic therapy for PE was the Urokinase Pulmonary Embolism Trial (UPET).[71] This prospective trial randomized 160 patients to either urokinase followed by heparin or heparin alone. Although transient hemodynamic improvement was achieved, no differences were evident with regard to mortality or perfusion scan past 5 days. Nonetheless, the UPET and the subsequent Urokinase-Streptokinase Embolism Trial (USET) demonstrated improvements in small vessel patency at 2 weeks and 1 year compared with anticoagulation alone.[74-75] Seven-year follow-up of this cohort of patients suggested the risk of pulmonary hypertension was decreased by thrombolysis, presumably because lytic therapy achieved superior clot dissolution and decreased the risk of subsequent pulmonary embolism.[76]

Currently, the only patients for whom thrombolytics are widely accepted are those with hemodynamic instability due to massive PE. Other patients who may benefit are those with right ventricular dysfunction or refractory hypoxemia due to PE in the setting of preserved systemic arterial blood pressure. These cases of "sub-massive" PE may achieve an improved clinical course with thrombolytic therapy than with anticoagulation alone, although mortality rate has not been shown to be improved.[77]

The IV route of administration is most commonly used in PE. The only trial to compare direct pulmonary artery infusion to IV infusion was by Verstraete et al.[78] The study failed to show a benefit of pulmonary artery infusion. In addition, the time required to place a pulmonary artery catheter can delay treatment and increase the risk of bleeding from a central venous puncture. On the other hand, local catheterization permits mechanical lysis, which has been shown to benefit selected patients.[79] FDA-approved regimens for acute PE are listed in Table 202-4.

Although no difference in thrombolytic regimens has been shown to be significant to date,[80] most agree that the drug of choice is IV tPA[81] because of its short infusion time. Unlike patients treated for AMI,

patients treated with thrombolytic agents for acute PE are generally not heparinized during thrombolytic administration. However, systemic anticoagulation should begin upon completion of thrombolysis. After the acute treatment of PE, patients should be maintained on anticoagulation for a minimum of 3 months, keeping the International Normalized Ratio between 2.0 and 3.0.[82] Major hemorrhagic complications occur in approximately 12% of patients irrespective of the lytic agent used.[83]

DEEP VENOUS THROMBOSIS

The formation of deep venous thrombosis (DVT) is surprisingly common in acutely ill patients, occurring in as many as 30% of ICU patients, despite prophylaxis with pneumatic compression devices and/or various prophylactic anticoagulation regimens.[84] ICU patients are at especially high risk for DVT because they often have indwelling central venous catheters. Central venous catheterization can increase the incidence of DVT by 5% to 30% depending on the site of insertion, type of catheter, duration of placement, and presence or absence of infection.[85-89] Acute occlusion of the deep venous system can lead to severe sequelae such as venous gangrene (phlegmasia cerulea dolens), as well as long-term consequences including recurrent venous thrombosis and post-phlebitic syndrome.[90-93] Additionally, patients with iliofemoral DVT experience greater postthrombotic morbidity than those with infrainguinal DVT. Although venous gangrene is rare, patients with acute DVT have a nearly 26-fold increase in the risk of developing chronic venous disease,[94] with reported incidence ranging from 16% to 82%.[95-97] Traditional therapy for DVT, consisting of anticoagulation alone, allows for stabilization of the thrombus and prevents PE. However, anticoagulation is not effective for restoration and preservation of venous function.

Thrombolytic treatment of DVT, therefore, focuses both on prevention of PE and dissolution of the clot to prevent development of post-phlebitic syndrome, which is characterized by persistent pain, edema, discoloration, and ulceration. A number of randomized clinical studies have demonstrated the efficacy of both streptokinase and tPA compared with heparin alone in this setting.[98-101] These studies reported partial lysis in 70% and complete lysis in 28% of patients who underwent thrombolysis, versus only 24% and 4%, respectively, in patients treated with heparin alone.[81] Meta-analyses of the available data indicated that systemic streptokinase is 3.7 times more likely[102] and tPA is 7 times more likely[103] to result in thrombus resolution than anticoagulation alone.

Exact indications for thrombolysis are unclear. Patients who are most likely to benefit include those with a first occurrence of iliofemoral DVT (<10 days old) who are at low risk for major bleeding complications.[104] Indeed, the AACP guidelines for the application of thrombolytics weakly recommend (grade 2B, 2C) that they may be used in selected patients with extensive acute proximal DVT.[105] Others have advocated lytic therapy for young patients with primary upper extremity DVT either due to effort thrombosis (Paget-Schroetter syndrome) or idiopathic factors.[106] Most investigations have used a locoregional approach with infusions from a distal peripheral vein (e.g., a pedal vein). Another approach involves catheter-directed infusions that offer the advantage of requiring lower total doses of thrombolytic agents with fewer systemic side effects, as well as the ability to use angioplasty to dilate underlying venous stenoses (Figure 202-4).[107,108] Both systemic[109] and catheter-directed thrombolysis[110,111] have been

TABLE 202-4	FDA-Approved Regimens for Treatment of Pulmonary Embolism
Drug	**Systemic Administration**
Streptokinase	250,000 units over 30 minutes followed by 100,000 units/h for 24 hours
Urokinase	4400 units/kg over 10 minutes followed by 4400 units/kg/h for 12-24 hours
tPA (alteplase)	100 mg over 2 hours

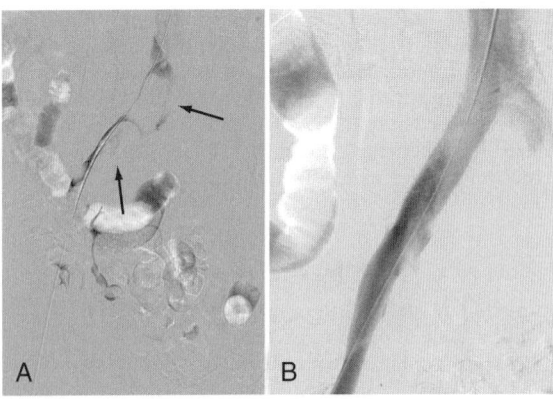

Figure 202-4 Venogram of patient with occlusive left iliofemoral deep venous thrombosis (DVT; patient lying in prone position for the images) secondary to May-Thurner syndrome. **A,** Large, bulky thrombus shown occluding left iliac and femoral veins *(arrows)*. After completion of lytic therapy, thrombus is cleared, and stenosis of common iliac vein was treated with angioplasty and stenting, leaving a widely patent venous channel **(B)**.

shown to be effective. With the completion of the Acute Venous Thrombosis: Thrombus Removal with Adjunctive Catheter-Directed Thrombolysis (ATTRACT) trial in the near future, the level 1 evidence needed to elucidate the optimal role of thrombolytic therapy in the treatment of DVT may be provided.[112]

ACUTE PERIPHERAL ARTERIAL OCCLUSION

Acute peripheral arterial occlusion (APAO) is a highly morbid condition that leads to amputation in 10% to 30% of cases and is associated with a mortality rate as high as 15% at 30 days.[113] Occlusive events generally arise from dissection, trauma, local thrombosis, or embolus. Traumatic occlusion or disruption of the vessel almost always warrants surgical exploration and repair. A variety of noninvasive maneuvers, however, have been developed for treatment of thromboembolic disease. Differentiating between in situ thrombosis and embolus as the etiology of the arterial occlusion can be extremely challenging if not impossible in up to 15% of cases.[113] In the Thrombolysis or Peripheral Arterial Surgery (TOPAS) trial, thrombosis (85%) was found to be more common than embolism (15%).[114,115]

Thrombolysis has become a popular means of treating acute arterial occlusion in certain settings. This approach has been performed since the 1950s.[3] Formerly, relatively high-dose lytic therapy was administered IV to achieve therapeutic levels at the site of occlusion but was associated with prohibitively high bleeding risks and generally poor clinical outcome. Since the early 1970s, however, catheter-directed infusion has become the standard of care, permitting higher local thrombolytic concentrations at the treatment site while effectively reducing the systemic burden of the drug.[116] Recent advances in development of infusion catheters and wires have contributed to the effectiveness of intraarterial lytic therapy. Differing infusion methods have been developed and studied, such as low-dose infusion regimes, high dose, and high-pressure forced infusion ("pulse spray"). Although duration of treatment may be shorter with the high-dose and pulse spray infusion techniques, bleeding complications are increased. Regardless, no infusion method has been shown to achieve genuine benefit in terms of clinical outcome.[117-118]

Although streptokinase was the first agent used for APAO, multiple studies indicate that urokinase and tPA are more effective for this indication and have fewer bleeding complications.[119-121] Before its removal from the U.S. market, urokinase was the predominant thrombolytic agent used to treat acute arterial occlusion. Currently, tPA and its derivatives have supplanted urokinase as the drug of choice for APAO; tPA has been shown to have similar safety and efficacy profiles as urokinase when using "low-dose" (<2 mg/h, usually beginning at

0.5 mg/h) regimens with adjunctive heparin infusions to maintain the APTT at 1.5 times baseline. With this regimen, over 60% of patients have complete resolution, and 30% have partial resolution within 24 hours of initiating treatment.[122] An advisory panel recommended either weight-based dosing (0.001-0.02 mg/kg/h) or non-weight-based dosing (0.12-2 mg/h), with total doses not to exceed 40 mg.[123] They also recommended subtherapeutic heparin infusions to maintain the APTT at between 1.25 and 1.5 times control values.

Use of thrombolytics in the setting of APAO is part of a multifaceted approach often involving additional endovascular techniques and/or surgical intervention. There are several well-controlled trials examining initial surgical versus thrombolytic therapy. The Rochester trial compared initial surgery with urokinase in severely threatened limbs (mean symptom duration 2 days) in 114 patients.[124] Limb salvage rates in the 2 groups were identical (82%) at 12 months, whereas mortality was significantly lower in the patients treated with urokinase (16% versus 42% with surgery). The Surgery or Thrombolysis for the Ischemic Lower Extremity (STILE) trial examined 393 patients randomized to either primary surgery or one of two lytic therapies (rtPA or urokinase).[125] At 30 days, limb loss rates (5% with lysis versus 6% with surgery) and mortality rates were similar (4% versus 5%, respectively). One of the major contributions of this study involved subgroup analyses[126,127] that revealed a greater benefit of thrombolysis in patients with graft occlusion rather than native vessel occlusion and in patients with acute ischemia of less than 2 weeks' duration. Finally, the TOPAS trial compared recombinant urokinase therapy to surgery in 544 patients.[114] Although it failed to demonstrate an amputation-free survival benefit at 1 year (68% for urokinase, 69% for surgery), it did show that over 30% of the patients treated with urokinase were not only alive without amputation but also had nothing more than a percutaneous procedure at 6 months. Therefore a significant number of patients were able to avoid surgical intervention with the use of thrombolytic therapy.

Thrombolytic therapy is still not considered to be the standard of care for treatment of APAO. However, it may prove to be a useful tool for treating patients who are poor surgical candidates. These include patients who are too sick to safely undergo extremity revascularization and those with distal thromboemboli not amenable to surgical extraction or bypass. Thrombolysis may also benefit selected patients who present with less than 2 weeks of symptoms. It may be the best approach for patients with occlusion of bypass grafts.[125,126] Furthermore, thrombolysis can aid in recanalization of small distal vessels that are not patent at initiation of treatment, permitting subsequent revascularization via bypass surgery. Thrombolysis may uncover an arterial lesion as the inciting factor for the thrombosis, which then may be treated endovascularly or surgically (Figure 202-5). Finally, thrombolysis may allow a more gradual reperfusion of an ischemic limb and thus reduce the metabolic derangements associated with ischemia/reperfusion. Lytic agents are contraindicated for treating early postoperative thrombosis, thrombosis following penetrating or multiple traumas, or in limbs with irreversible ischemia.

OTHER APPLICATIONS

In addition to the indications for thrombolytic therapy noted earlier, other common indications include treatment of thrombosed dialysis grafts or central venous catheters. Vascular access complications are the single greatest source of morbidity among hemodialysis patients, accounting for 15% of all hospitalizations.[128] Whereas the ultimate goal is to recognize and treat a graft before it clots, thrombolytics can play an important role once the graft has occluded. A number of techniques have been used for the acutely thrombosed graft, including mechanical thrombectomy, surgical revision, and pharmacologic thrombolysis. A technique that has gained popularity recently is called "lyse and wait." This method avoids the need for mechanical devices or pulse-spray catheters and shortens lysis times to approximately 45 minutes, as compared with 65 minutes for the pulse spray technique.[129] It involves placing a mixture of urokinase (250,000 International Units) and heparin (5000 units) into the graft (or alternatively, injecting 2-5 mg

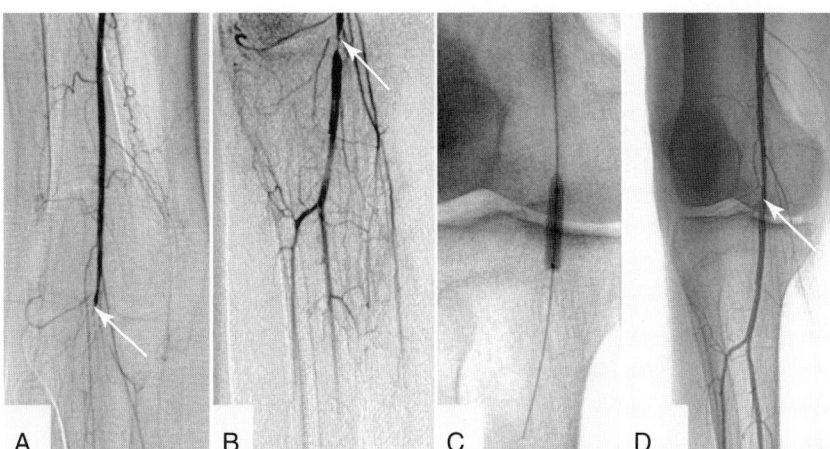

Figure 202-5 Successive angiograms demonstrating **(A)** occluded popliteal artery *(arrow)* treated with thrombolytics. After thrombolysis, a focal popliteal artery stenosis **(B)** was identified *(arrow)* with patent distal vessels. This area was subsequently subjected to balloon angioplasty **(C)**. After thrombolysis and angioplasty **(D)**, result is a patent popliteal artery *(arrow)* with good distal arterial flow.

A   B   C   D

of rtPA into the graft and administering 5000 units of heparin systemically.[130] After lysis, the arterial plug is removed, and the venous anastomosis is dilated. With this technique, Cynamon et al. reported that 98% of patients have successful restoration of graft flow and function, with 1- and 3-month patency rates of 80% and 55%, respectively.[129] Nevertheless, surgical thrombectomy remains the standard of care and achieved superior patency rates in a recent meta-analysis,[131] presumably because anastomotic revision is performed concurrently. As for occluded central venous catheters, the Advisory Panel on Catheter-Directed Thrombolytic Therapy in 2000 recommended a 2-mg (1 mg/mL) aliquot of alteplase for each occluded lumen for up to 2 hours.[123] This therapy can be repeated a second time if necessary. This regimen has proven to be both safe (≤1% bleeding risk) and efficacious (≈90% patency after two treatments) in multiple studies.[132-135]

Management/Laboratories

During administration of thrombolytic agents, circulating plasminogen and fibrinogen concentrations decrease. Fibrinogen is degraded as part of the fibrinolytic process, reaching nadir values between 5 and 7 hours after the institution of therapy.[136] These values return to baseline in most patients within 48 hours of discontinuation of therapy. Likewise, circulating plasminogen levels begin to decrease immediately after initiating streptokinase and urokinase infusions; the decrease is greater with streptokinase, as it complexes with plasminogen in a 1:1 relationship. Despite being relatively fibrin specific, the second- and third-generation lytic agents (recombinant tPAs, APSAC, and prourokinase) still interact with circulating fibrinogen and therefore decrease circulating fibrinogen levels. Fibrin degradation products are a reliable indicator of the activity of the fibrinolytic system because the only source in humans is the degradation of fibrinogen or fibrin by plasmin.

Most advocate monitoring fibrinogen levels every 6 to 8 hours during lytic therapy, decreasing the dose or discontinuing the infusion if levels drop below 100 mg/dL. In addition to monitoring the fibrinolytic system, daily or every-other-day monitoring of the platelet count should be performed. Use of rtPA has been associated with thrombocytopenia in as many as 10% of patients, whereas thrombocytopenia occurred in less than 1% of patients receiving streptokinase.[137-139] Selected patients should be typed for blood products. If bleeding does occur, thrombolytic infusion should be discontinued and blood products (fresh frozen plasma or cryoprecipitate) administered as necessary to correct the patient's hypocoagulable state.

Conclusion

Despite evidence in strong support of the use of thrombolytic agents in a variety of occlusive vascular disorders, relatively few patients ultimately receive this treatment. With increasing data supporting the safety and efficacy of thrombolytic therapy, however, use of this treatment modality has increased substantially over the past decade. One of the challenges in the coming years will be to more clearly define those patients who will benefit most, both in terms of reducing mortality and preventing hemorrhagic complications. Evolution in technologies including diagnostic modalities, mechanical "clot busters," and adjuvant therapies will undoubtedly expand the indications for thrombolytic therapy in all the aforementioned areas.

KEY POINTS

1. Thrombolytics comprise a diverse group of compounds that convert plasminogen to plasmin.

2. Thrombolytic therapy is indicated within 6 hours after the onset of acute myocardial infarction, especially in patients who are not eligible for primary angioplasty.

3. Patients with acute ischemic stroke receive the greatest long-term benefit from thrombolytic therapy when receiving treatment within 4.5 hours after the onset of symptoms.

4. The role of thrombolytics in pulmonary embolism is controversial and confined largely to use in those patients with hemodynamic instability.

5. Urokinase and tissue plasminogen activator are commonly used in the management of acute peripheral occlusion and most benefit those patients with occlusions of less than 14 days and those with previous extremity bypasses.

6. Thrombolytic therapy requires intensive monitoring and follow-up radiography. Fibrinogen levels should be monitored every 6 to 8 hours and the patient closely monitored for signs of major hemorrhage.

ANNOTATED REFERENCES

Arcasoy SM, Vachani A. Local and systemic thrombolytic therapy for acute venous thromboembolism. Clin Chest Med 2003;24:73-91.
  An excellent review of the current state of thrombolytic treatment of acute deep venous thrombosis and pulmonary embolus. It summarizes the results of the important trials and gives dosing recommendations for both indications.
Hilleman DE, Tsikouris JP, Seals AA, et al. Fibrinolytic agents for the management of ST-segment elevation myocardial infarction. Pharmacotherapy 2007;11:1558-70.

A detailed review of currently approved thrombolytic agents in treatment of acute ST-elevation myocardial infarction.
Primary angioplasty versus intravenous thrombolytic therapy for acute myocardial infarction: a quantitative review of 23 randomised trials. Lancet 2003;361:13-20.
  This meta-analysis summarizes the results of trials comparing the use of lytics in acute myocardial infarction, either with primary angioplasty or lytic therapy. It concludes that there is an overall benefit in the use of primary percutaneous coronary angioplasty.

Hacke W, Kaste M, Bluhmki E, et al. Thrombolysis with alteplase 3 to 4.5 hours after acute ischemic stroke. Lancet 2008;359:1317-29.

The publication of the ECASS III trial, which demonstrated a clinical benefit for patients with acute ischemic stroke treated with fibrinolysis at up to 4.5 hours after symptom onset. This trial led to expansion of the recommended window for treatment of acute ischemic stroke with thrombolytics, from 3 hours to 4.5 hours.

Kwiatkowski TG, Libman RB, Frankel M, et al. Effects of tissue plasminogen activator for acute ischemic stroke at one year. National Institute of Neurological Disorders and Stroke Recombinant Tissue Plasminogen Activator Stroke Study Group. N Engl J Med 1999;340:1781-7.

This is a follow-up study to the landmark NINDS study published in 1995 examining the use of lytics in the treatment of acute ischemic stroke. This study documented a functional improvement in those patients treated with tPA within 3 hours of symptom onset compared with treatment with placebo, although no change in mortality was documented.

Ouriel K, Veith FJ, Sasahara AA. A comparison of recombinant urokinase with vascular surgery as initial treatment for acute arterial occlusion of the legs. Thrombolysis or Peripheral Arterial Surgery (TOPAS) Investigators. N Engl J Med 1998;338:1105-11.

Randomized, multicenter trial examining intraarterial urokinase versus surgery for acute (<14 days) arterial occlusion. This trial and the Rochester and STILE trials provide the cornerstone for the argument supporting use of lytics in acute peripheral arterial occlusion.

REFERENCES

Access the complete reference list online at http://www.expertconsult.com.

203

Atheroembolization

YASIR ABU-OMAR | DAVID P. TAGGART

Atherosclerosis and its thromboembolic complications represent a leading cause of mortality and morbidity, contributing to half of all deaths in the Western world. It is a progressive disorder that usually remains clinically silent until it causes end-organ damage resulting in stroke, ischemic heart disease, and peripheral vascular insufficiency.

The distribution of atherosclerosis is characteristic, affecting the aorta more extensively than the peripheral vessels. The abdominal aorta is more widely involved than the thoracic aorta. Lower-limb vessels are more frequently affected than upper-limb vessels. The renal, pulmonary, and mesenteric vessels are the least susceptible.

As recently as the 1950s, nearly half of strokes were thought to result from cerebral vasospasm until Fisher stressed the etiologic importance of emboli from atherosclerotic plaques in the carotid artery.[1] Although embolization from the heart and major vessels accounts for a large number of ischemic cerebrovascular accidents, the cause of a significant proportion remains undetermined.[2] In those, the source is mainly thought to be embolic in origin. The following account will focus on the pathophysiology, clinical consequences, prevention, and management of atheromatous embolization.

Pathophysiology

ATHEROSCLEROSIS

The process of atherosclerosis begins as early as childhood or adolescence, developing slowly over many years. Its effects rarely manifest before the fourth or fifth decade of life. Traditional risk factors for atherosclerosis include hypertension, diabetes, smoking, and elevated serum cholesterol concentration.

Atherosclerosis mainly affects large and medium-sized arteries. Intravascular sites of blood turbulence favor the development of atherosclerotic lesions. Initial changes in arterial wall morphology result in the formation of fatty streaks that consist of lipid-engorged macrophages in the arterial intima. Progression of such precursor lesions occurs secondary to an inflammatory process initiated by endothelial injury and dysfunction.[3] Insufficient nitric oxide production results in increased adhesion and aggregation of platelets. Up-regulation in the endothelial expression of adhesion molecules and selectins leads to accumulation of monocytes and T lymphocytes. These cells become activated and produce growth factors, cytokines, and chemokines. Smooth-muscle cells migrate from the media into the intima and proliferate. In time, these lesions develop into raised fibrous plaques consisting of a fibrous cap covering a core containing necrotic material, lipids, and cholesteryl esters. This advanced plaque forms the basis onto which the complicated plaque develops, consisting of fissures, erosions, or ulceration. There has been increased interest in the role of monocytes and macrophages in the pathogenesis of plaque progression and rupture,[4] which is related to thrombosis and/or embolism and clinical manifestations.

ATHEROMATOUS EMBOLIZATION

Atheromatous embolization is a descriptive term for embolization of any atheromatous material. *Atheroembolization* refers to the dislodgement of vascular plaque material that contains cholesterol crystals, red blood cells, and fibrin.[5] This "cholesterol emboli" syndrome consists of renal failure, skin lesions, blue toes, and neurologic manifestations. It may develop spontaneously (due to plaque rupture), follow the use of thrombolytics or anticoagulants,[6] or result from arterial manipulation (during surgical procedures, cardiac catheterization, or insertion of an intraaortic balloon pump [IABP]).[7] Disruption of vascular plaque results in the release of cholesterol crystals. These crystals cause downstream vascular obstruction and initiate an inflammatory process leading to lymphocytic and mononuclear cell infiltration. Biopsy specimens of affected organs such as skin or kidneys are usually diagnostic.

PLAQUE MORPHOLOGY AND EMBOLIC RISK

Severe atherosclerosis of the ascending aorta appears to be the most important morphologic indicator of an increased risk of atheromatous embolization. The French Aortic Plaque in Stroke group identified a plaque thickness of 4 mm or greater as an independent predictor of recurrent embolization,[8,9] with an odds ratio of 13.8. Although ulceration and calcification occurred more frequently in plaques 4 mm or more in thickness, the presence of ulceration did not significantly increase the risk of vascular events. Absence of calcification, however, was associated with a significant increase in risk (relative risk, 10.3 compared with 5.7 for those with calcification). Another study reported an association between the presence of ulceration in aortic plaques and an increased rate of cryptogenic stroke.[10] Ulceration and increased size of aortic plaques seem to be markers of severe generalized atherosclerosis and therefore predict a higher risk for thromboembolic complications.

MACROEMBOLIZATION AND MICROEMBOLIZATION

Emboli can be generally divided into macroemboli and microemboli. The former occlude arteries larger than 200 μm in diameter, whereas the latter result in occlusion of smaller arteries, arterioles, and capillaries.[11] The clinical manifestations of each vary. Whereas macroemboli may cause overt clinical presentations (e.g., stroke or peripheral ischemia), microemboli tend to be more occult in their manifestations of end-organ injury or dysfunction (e.g., renal injury, neuropsychological impairment). Their clinical impact depends on the number and nature of microemboli. Embolization may arise spontaneously or be related to vascular interventions and cardiovascular surgery.

Clinical Consequences of Atheromatous Embolization

CEREBRAL

As the prevalence of aortic atherosclerotic disease increases with age, so does the rate of atheromatous embolization. Postmortem studies indicate that it affects 20% of patients in their fifth decade, increasing to 80% in those in their eighth decade.[12] Emboli from the atherosclerotic aorta may result in stroke or transient ischemic attack, and the clinical manifestations of these conditions vary depending on the cerebrovascular territory affected; the middle cerebral artery is the most frequent site of arterial embolism. Stroke has profound effects; outcomes from acute stroke are measured in terms of survival, functional independence, and financial cost. Survival after stroke is significantly poorer than after myocardial infarction (MI) or most cancers and is the leading cause of disability in developed countries.[13] When considered separately from other cardiovascular diseases, stroke ranks third among all causes of death, behind diseases of the heart and cancer. Its economic impact is huge, with 2009 estimated direct and indirect costs of stroke in the United States of $68.9 billion.

Cholesterol emboli are an important and frequently unrecognized cause of stroke.[14] Microembolization is a recognized cause of more subtle, sometimes subclinical neurologic injury.[15,16] Most frequently this injury is manifested by subtle changes in cognitive function that may only be evident on detailed neuropsychological testing.[17,18] This more subtle impairment may appear trivial, but its importance has increased over recent years, particularly in patients undergoing cardiac surgery.[19]

CARDIAC

Atherosclerotic cardiovascular disease is the leading cause of death in developed countries. Every year it results in over 19 million deaths worldwide, and coronary heart disease accounts for the majority of those.[20] MI is a consequence of diseased coronary arteries as part of the overall systemic picture of atherosclerosis. Most acute coronary syndromes are due to plaque rupture. Distal embolization of cholesterol and atheromatous material may be important in the pathogenesis of some acute coronary syndromes.[21] The occurrence of distal coronary embolization in the setting of acute coronary syndromes has been followed using serum levels of cardiac troponins to detect small degrees of myocardial necrosis. The clinical importance of distal coronary embolization, as defined by serum troponins, is its predictive value for future cardiac events. Embolization following percutaneous coronary interventions is well recognized, and elevations in cardiac troponins are seen in up to 44% of patients undergoing intervention.[22,23]

PERIPHERAL

Peripheral emboli most frequently lodge in the lower extremities. Cholesterol atheroembolization can be subclinical or can otherwise result in systemic effects. While renal, neurologic, and cutaneous manifestations tend to dominate the clinical picture, involvement of most organs has been previously reported. Atheromatous material can be identified in the pancreas, intestine, and spleen. Symptoms and presentation depend on the site of dislodgement. Embolization into the renal arteries results in renal ischemia and can lead to renal impairment or failure.[24,25] In those cases, renal biopsy is diagnostic.[26]

Involvement of the cutaneous vessels leads to livedo reticularis and the "blue-toe" syndrome, whereas retinal emboli[27] result in visual symptoms. Other reported effects include small-bowel bleeding[28] and renal transplant failure.[29]

▓ Diagnosis and Screening

Asymptomatic atherosclerotic disease may be discovered incidentally. The clinical presentation of atheromatous embolization varies depending on the site affected. Full clinical assessment and screening of patients presenting with embolic complications is essential in guiding management and prevention strategies.

The cholesterol embolization syndrome relies on clinical findings in patients with atherosclerotic disease and a history of recent vascular intervention. As different organs can be involved, the clinician should maintain a high index of suspicion.

Many imaging modalities have been used to visualize atherosclerotic plaques; some are used routinely in clinical practice, whereas others are reserved for research purposes. Advances in imaging technology has provided tools that allow primary prevention by identifying those at highest risk and allowing the implementation of potential life-saving treatment strategies at a preclinical stage. The most commonly used imaging techniques are described here.

X-RAY ANGIOGRAPHY

X-ray angiography is an invasive procedure that allows assessment of the vascular lumen by providing a measure of the degree of stenosis

and by identifying plaque disruption, thrombosis, and calcification. However, it provides no information about the vessel wall or the components of the atherosclerotic plaque. Despite that, angiography is still regarded as the gold standard for imaging coronary, carotid, and peripheral arterial disease.[30]

SURFACE AND TRANSESOPHAGEAL ULTRASONOGRAPHY

Measurement of carotid and aortic wall thickness as well as qualitative and quantitative assessment of atherosclerotic plaques can be determined using ultrasonography. The North American Symptomatic Carotid Endarterectomy Trial and the Asymptomatic Carotid Artery Stenosis Study have shown that the degree of stenosis and its hemodynamic consequences are important in the development of stroke.[31,32] High-resolution, real-time B-mode ultrasound with Doppler flow imaging is currently considered the modality of choice in imaging the carotid arteries.[33]

With respect to screening, carotid intima-medial thickness (CIMT) measured by B-mode ultrasound represents a risk factor and a marker for vascular disease risk that most accurately represents subclinical vascular disease but not plaque formation or atherosclerosis per se. Epidemiologic and clinical trial evidence, digitization, and standardization have made CIMT a validated and accepted marker for generalized atherosclerosis burden and vascular disease risk.[34] Numerous studies have linked CIMT and CIMT progression with prevalent symptomatic coronary and cerebrovascular disease. Furthermore, CIMT is a predictor of coronary events and stroke as well as all-cause mortality.[35,36] The American Society of Echocardiography Carotid Intima-Media Thickness Task Force recommends the use of CIMT measurement by ultrasound in intermediate-risk asymptomatic patients, with a goal of predicting future coronary heart disease events.[37]

Transesophageal echocardiography (TEE) is a quick, safe, and minimally invasive procedure that can be used in different settings ranging from the operating theatre to the bedside.[38] It is regarded as the procedure of choice in detection, assessment, and characterization of thoracic aortic atherosclerosis. Imaging using the transthoracic approach is also possible but at the expense of significant loss of resolution when compared to the transesophageal technique. TEE can reliably detect intimal thickening, ulceration, calcification, and the presence of mobile components within the aortic plaque. As outlined earlier, the French Aortic Plaque in Stroke investigators used TEE to assess aortic plaque thickness in patients with stroke and reported that increased plaque thickness imparted a significant increase in stroke risk.[8,9] Katz and colleagues used a 5-grade ranking system for the severity of aortic atherosclerosis, assessed using TEE in 130 patients undergoing cardiac surgery with cardiopulmonary bypass: grade 1, normal aorta; grade 2, flat intimal thickening; grade 3, protruding atheroma in the aortic lumen (<5 mm); grade 4, protruding atheroma (>5 mm); and grade 5, atheroma with a mobile thrombus.[39] Patients with grade 5 lesions were at highest risk of stroke. Logistic regression identified aortic arch atheroma as the only variable that was predictive of stroke, with an odds ratio of 5.8. Another study of 315 coronary artery bypass graft (CABG) patients undergoing intraoperative TEE also reported a significant increase in the risk of stroke in patients with aortic arch intimal thickening of greater than 5 mm.[40]

It is no surprise that patients with the highest-risk carotid lesions also have high-risk aortic plaques. Assessment of the carotid arteries as well as the aorta is prudent in the investigation of atherosclerotic patients who have suffered embolic events.

INTRAOPERATIVE EPIAORTIC ULTRASOUND

Epiaortic ultrasonography involves intraoperative imaging of the ascending aorta using a sterile-sheathed transducer. This technique is noninvasive and has been used in the context of cardiac surgery to detect areas of ascending aortic atherosclerosis.[41] It allows modification of the surgical technique in an attempt to reduce potential embolic complications.[42] The main disadvantage of this technique is suboptimal imaging of the aortic arch. Intraoperative epiaortic ultrasound can therefore be used to complement the information on the aortic arch obtained by TEE.

TRANSCRANIAL DOPPLER

Transcranial Doppler (TCD) ultrasonography can be used to detect and quantify cerebral microemboli. Ultrasound probes are placed bilaterally on the temple, overlying the middle cerebral vessels. Emboli cause an increase in the reflected ultrasound, causing high-intensity transient signals (HITS). These HITS are the footprints of microemboli, which may consist of air, fat, atheromatous material, or platelet-fibrin emboli. In addition to detecting cerebral microemboli, TCD can be reliably used to assess cerebral vasomotor reactivity and autoregulation, to document the circle of Willis functional status, and to identify cerebral hypo- and hyperperfusion, recanalization, and re-occlusion.[43]

TCD can reliably detect HITS intraoperatively and has been used extensively in the context of cardiac and carotid surgery. During cardiac surgery, microemboli can be detected following intraoperative aortic manipulation (aortic cannulation and application and removal of aortic cross-clamp) as well as during cardiopulmonary bypass.[44] HITS have also been identified in patients with symptomatic carotid artery stenosis,[45] patients with prosthetic heart valves,[46] and those with aortic atherosclerosis.[47] They are a common phenomenon in patients with acute stroke, and their detection may continue for several days after the acute event. Their presence is a significant independent predictor of early recurrence of stroke.[48]

TCD is a simple, user-friendly technique that can be used at the patient bedside as well as in the operating room. It can provide valuable information intraoperatively on cerebral blood velocity, which is closely related to flow, and microembolic load, allowing for intraoperative technical modifications. A major limitation is an inadequate acoustic window in 5% to 20% of individuals.[49] Another limitation is the ability to reliably reject artifacts (closely resembling microembolic signals and generated by movement) and/or to distinguish between gaseous and particulate microemboli. With multirange, multifrequency Doppler systems, automatic artifact rejection and differentiation between solid and gaseous microemboli has become possible with high sensitivity and specificity.[50,51] We have reported a significant reduction in intraoperative cerebral microembolism as well as a reduction in the proportion of solid microemboli, with avoidance of cardiopulmonary bypass and minimizing manipulation of the ascending aorta during cardiac surgery.[44,52]

An exciting recent development with TCD ultrasonography is its use therapeutically in the treatment of stroke. This involves the use of TCD ultrasound to augment the effect of fibrinolysis and has been shown to at least double the chance of early complete arterial recanalization.[53]

COMPUTED TOMOGRAPHY

Computed tomography (CT) can be used in imaging the aorta and quantifying aortic wall calcification. Contrast-enhanced CT has been proposed as a valuable method for following the progression and regression of atherosclerotic disease.[54] The main advantage over TEE is the ability to completely image the thoracic and abdominal aorta. Other advantages of CT include its minimally invasive nature, its wide availability, and its provision of images of lumens of arteries and of calcium. Disadvantages include radiation and contrast exposure with potential for renal damage, limiting its use in asymptomatic populations.

Coronary multidetector CT angiography (MDCTA) can be used in identifying patients at a particularly high risk of dying suddenly or suffering a nonfatal MI. It provides information on coronary artery stenosis as well as an estimate of calcification, coronary artery calcium (CAC). The latter is related to multiple risk factors of coronary artery disease. The importance of CAC screening lies in its potential ability to increase predictive power for future events.[36,55]

MAGNETIC RESONANCE IMAGING TECHNIQUES

Magnetic resonance imaging (MRI) has emerged as a leading noninvasive imaging modality for atherosclerotic disease. It can be used to image atherosclerotic plaques in aortic, carotid, peripheral, and coronary arterial disease.[56,57] Its major strengths rest in its ability to determine plaque morphology. Using a range of techniques, MRI can provide valuable information on the composition of the atherosclerotic plaque by identifying the three main factors that determine plaque stability: (1) presence of a lipid core, (2) thickness of the fibrous cap, and (3) inflammation within the cap. MRI allows identification of high-risk unstable plaques and thus guides intervention and therapy.[58] Some studies have documented regression of atherosclerotic lesions on MRI in patients treated with statins.[59] Magnetic resonance angiography has a high sensitivity and specificity and can be used to image the aorta, carotid, renal, and other peripheral vessels. Evolving magnetic resonance techniques include intravascular[60] and transesophageal[61] MRI. MRI is therefore a noninvasive, powerful tool with high spatial resolution that can be used clinically without exposing the patient to the risks of ionizing radiation.

Vascular Manipulation and Embolic Events

CARDIAC SURGERY

Stroke, transient ischemic attack, and peripheral embolization are potential complications following cardiac surgery. Atheroembolism results in a variety of clinical manifestations and can be fatal in about 20% of patients.[62] Stroke affects less than 2% of CABG patients, and this is further increased in those undergoing open-heart procedures.[63] The risk of perioperative stroke increases with advancing age, and those with concomitant cardiovascular risk factors are at highest risk.[64] In addition, it has been shown that the female gender is independently associated with a significantly higher risk of perioperative stroke.[65] Embolization from the atheromatous aorta is the single most important etiologic factor for stroke. This risk arises during intraoperative manipulation of the aorta, including cannulation for cardiopulmonary bypass, application and removal of aortic cross-clamp for administration of cardioplegia, and the use of side-clamps for anastomosis of the proximal end of the graft to the aorta.[66] Roach et al. showed that atherosclerosis of the ascending aorta is the strongest independent predictor of perioperative stroke, with an odds ratio of 4.5.[67]

The functional impact of stroke is enormous; adverse overt cerebral outcomes after cardiac surgery are associated with a 10-fold increase in mortality and substantial increases in the length of hospitalization and the use of intermediate- or long-term care facilities. New diagnostic and therapeutic strategies must be developed to lessen such injury.

CARDIAC CATHETERIZATION AND PERIPHERAL VASCULAR INTERVENTION

Aortic manipulation during cardiac catheterization procedures or IABP may cause embolization from aortic atheroma. In a report comparing 59 patients with atherosclerotic aortic debris undergoing transfemoral cardiac catheterization, with 71 control patients, an embolic event occurred in 17% of the patients with atherosclerotic aortas compared to 3% of controls.[68] In the proportion of patients requiring IABP, 5 out of 10 patients with atherosclerotic aortas had an embolic event, compared with none of the 12 patients with IABP in the control group. When a transbrachial approach was used in patients with atherosclerotic aortas, none of 11 patients suffered an embolic event. Patients with mobile aortic atheromas, identified using TEE, are at highest risk of catheter-related embolization.[68]

Microembolic events have also been identified in patients undergoing peripheral arterial intervention. A recent study reported the rate of clinically significant distal embolization in 2.4% of patients undergoing peripheral arterial intervention.[69] Logistic regression identified patients with more advanced arterial lesions, angiographic thrombus, and prior history of amputation as those at highest risk.

Cholesterol embolization can complicate cardiac catheterization. Because it is commonly asymptomatic, the exact incidence is uncertain and mainly depends on the detection criteria used (clinical or pathologic). Cholesterol can be identified in the lumen of affected arterioles in up to 12% of patients following cardiac catheterization.[70] A prospective multicenter study reported cholesterol embolization in 1.4% of patients following cardiac catheterization. The diagnostic criteria used in this study was based on evidence of peripheral cutaneous involvement or renal dysfunction.[71] The syndrome occurred more frequently in patients with generalized atherosclerosis. Interestingly, they identified preprocedural elevation of C-reactive protein as an independent predictor of cholesterol embolization, suggesting involvement of an inflammatory process.

Prevention and Management

Treatment of atheromatous embolization depends on the clinical manifestation. General measures include identification and modification of risk factors. Patients with the clinical syndrome of cholesterol embolization have a generally poor prognosis, particularly when there is evidence of visceral and renal involvement. Supportive management with blood pressure control and, if necessary, renal replacement therapy is indicated. Strategies for the general prevention and management of atheromatous embolization are discussed here.

ANTIPLATELET AGENTS AND ANTICOAGULANTS

Thrombi can develop on and embolize from atherosclerotic plaques, so it may seem logical to use antiplatelet agents or anticoagulants to prevent these thromboembolic complications. However, there have been reports linking the atheroemboli syndrome with anticoagulation in patients with atherosclerosis. Three studies have reported a reduction in the risk of stroke with anticoagulation.[72-74] These studies, however, were not randomized and did not include long-term follow-up. It is over the long term that the potential risks of warfarin therapy may become evident. A randomized trial reported that in patients with stroke, large aortic plaques remain associated with an increased risk of recurrent stroke and death at 2 years despite treatment with warfarin or aspirin.[75]

The current ARCH (Aortic Arch Related Cerebral Hazard) trial is an open-label trial where patients with aortic arch atheroma (4 mm or greater) and nondisabling stroke are being assigned to oral anticoagulation (target INR 2.0-3.0) versus aspirin (75 mg/d) plus clopidogrel (75 mg/d) and followed longitudinally for recurrence of vascular events. Results of this trial are still awaited. The main concern with anticoagulation is the risk of plaque hemorrhage and atheroembolization.[76] However, the risk of clinical atheroemboli syndrome during warfarin therapy in such patients appears to be low (only 1 episode in 134 patients according to the SPAF [Stroke Prevention in Atrial Fibrillation] trial).[72]

In patients with atherosclerosis, acute ischemic events are usually precipitated by thrombosis, and antiplatelet agents play a fundamental role in thrombosis prevention. The beneficial effects of long-term antiplatelet therapy have been firmly established in patients with a wide range of atherosclerotic diseases. Routine use of aspirin in high-risk patients is universally recommended.[77] The Antithrombotic Trialists' Collaboration published a major meta-analysis with over 200,000 patients, assessing the effect of antiplatelet therapy in patients with various manifestations of atherosclerosis. This reported a significant reduction in the rate of stroke, MI, or vascular death in those on antiplatelet therapy.[78]

Aspirin is the most commonly used antiplatelet agent. It inhibits thromboxane-dependent platelet activation. Thienopyridines, including clopidogrel and ticlopidine, act by blocking adenosine diphosphate (ADP)-dependent activation of platelets. There is evidence that thienopyridine derivatives are modestly but significantly more effective than aspirin in preventing serious vascular events in patients at high risk, but there is uncertainty about the size of the additional benefit.[78] The thienopyridines are also associated with less gastrointestinal hemorrhage and upper gastrointestinal upset compared to aspirin, but with an excess of rash and diarrhea.[79] The risk of the latter is greater with ticlopidine than with clopidogrel.[13] Ticlopidine, but not clopidogrel, is associated with an excess of neutropenia and thrombotic thrombocytopenic purpura.[13,79] In the Clopidogrel in Unstable Angina to Prevent Recurrent Events (CURE) trial, a long-term benefit was observed with the use of clopidogrel in addition to aspirin in high-risk patients (unstable angina and non-Q-wave MI).[80]

Activation of platelets leads to conformational change in glycoprotein IIb/IIIa, the major fibrinogen receptor on platelets. Intravenous glycoprotein IIb/IIIa inhibitors (e.g., abciximab) are generally reserved for the high-risk setting of percutaneous coronary intervention.

Dextran has antiplatelet and intravascular volume expansion effects. Lennard and colleagues observed that postoperative or perioperative administration of 10% dextran 40 reduces the rate of TCD-detected microembolic signals after carotid endarterectomy.[81,82] Dextran, however, may interfere with cross-matching blood and cause bleeding, renal failure, or (occasionally) acute allergic reactions.

The Guidelines for the Diagnosis and Management of Patients with Thoracic Aortic Disease have been recently published. Oral anticoagulation therapy with warfarin (INR 2.0-3.0) or antiplatelet therapy in stroke patients with aortic arch atheroma 4.0 mm or greater to prevent recurrent stroke was a class IIb recommendation (level of evidence: C).[83]

STATINS

There is a clear association between elevated levels of plasma cholesterol and atherosclerotic disease. Statins or 3-hydroxy-3-methylglutaryl coenzyme-A (HMG Co-A) reductase inhibitors reduce the hepatocyte cholesterol content and increase expression of LDL-cholesterol receptors, resulting in a drop in serum low-density lipoprotein (LDL) cholesterol. In addition, it has become evident in recent years that statins possess cholesterol-independent or pleiotropic effects. These include improvement of endothelial function by improving the bioavailability of nitric oxide, decreasing vascular inflammation, and plaque stabilization.[84] Statins are widely used in primary and secondary prevention of ischemic heart disease. A meta-analysis of randomized placebo-controlled double-blind trials with statins reported a 30% reduction in stroke with statin therapy.[85] Another meta-analysis of data pooled from over 49,000 patients treated with statins in 28 trials reported a relative risk of stroke of 0.76 in statin-treated patients.[86] Tunick et al. showed that statin therapy was independently and significantly protective against the occurrence of embolic events (risk ratio, 0.39) in patients with severe thoracic aortic plaque.[87]

Plaque size reduction, stabilization, and prevention of plaque thrombosis may be the mechanisms leading to a reduction in atheromatous embolization. Two randomized studies of low-dose and higher-dose statins in patients with aortic and/or carotid plaques showed significant regression in plaque seen on MRI.[88,89]

MINIMAL AORTIC MANIPULATION

The use of smaller arterial catheters during cardiac catheterization may help reduce the risk of embolization.[90] Reduction of embolization during cardiac surgery is possible with modifications to the operative technique. Avoidance of aortic manipulation intraoperatively is most important.[66] This can be achieved in patients undergoing CABG by avoidance of cardiopulmonary bypass, which obviates the need for aortic cannulation and cross-clamping.[91,92] The use of composite

PREVENTION OF EMBOLIZATION DURING CARDIAC SURGERY IN PATIENTS WITH ATHEROSCLEROSIS

- Establish the patient's preoperative risk factors.
- Image the ascending aorta and arch preoperatively.
- Assess the carotid arteries.
- Assess the ascending aorta using intraoperative epiaortic ultrasound.
- Use evidence-based decisions to reflect the operative technique.
- Decide the site and risk of cannulation.
- Avoid repeated aortic clamping.
- Consider no-touch aortic techniques.
- Perform off-pump surgery with composite arterial grafting where possible.

arterial grafts (bilateral internal thoracic artery grafts with the radial artery anastomosed to the internal thoracic artery) avoids the need for proximal aortic anastomosis requiring a side-clamp.[93] In addition, there is a potential survival advantage with arterial grafts. Off-pump surgery has been shown to result in a significant reduction in the risk of stroke in patients with atheromatous aortas.[94] We have reported a significant reduction in cerebral microembolization by avoiding cardiopulmonary bypass and aortic manipulation.[44,52] A strategy for potential prevention of embolization in cardiac surgery is summarized in Box 203-1.

SCREENING WITH TRANSESOPHAGEAL ECHOCARDIOGRAPHY AND EPIAORTIC ULTRASOUND

As previously outlined, patients with mobile atheroma in the aortic lumen have the highest incidence of perioperative stroke compared to patients with lesser degrees of atherosclerosis.[39] TEE has confirmed the association between aortic atherosclerosis and perioperative stroke and thus provided a mechanism of identifying patients at highest risk,[39,95,96] as well as allowing for modification of surgical techniques to minimize embolic complications.

There is an association between atherosclerosis of the ascending aorta, as detected using epiaortic ultrasound, and increased postoperative neurologic morbidity.[41,97] In a study of more than 1900 patients undergoing cardiac surgery, detection of atherosclerosis of the ascending aorta using epiaortic ultrasound was identified as an independent predictor of long-term neurologic events and mortality.[41] Comparison between intraoperative TEE and epiaortic ultrasound demonstrated that the former underestimates the presence and severity of aortic atherosclerosis.[98,99] Modification of surgical technique based on intraoperative epiaortic ultrasonography may reduce the frequency of stroke and neurobehavioral changes related to atheromatous embolization.[100]

SURGICAL TREATMENT

Treatment of patients with symptomatic carotid atherosclerosis is well established. The European Carotid Surgery Trial (ECST) and North American Symptomatic Carotid Endarterectomy Trial (NASCET) investigators reported a clear benefit of carotid endarterectomy (CEA) in the prevention of stroke in patients with high-grade, recently symptomatic carotid stenosis.[31,101] This benefit is offset by the surgical risk of the procedure. Perioperative stroke and death rate for patients with high-grade stenosis was 8% at 30 days in ECST and 6% in NASCET. These rates are acceptable, given the absolute risk reduction from surgery of 10% and 17%, respectively. However, for patients with asymptomatic carotid disease, the risk-to-benefit ratio is narrower, and carotid endarterectomy is currently only recommended for high-grade carotid stenosis (70%-99%).

Over recent years, there has been increasing interest in endovascular intervention for carotid stenosis with angioplasty and stenting. The international carotid stenting study has recently reported higher rates of stroke and mortality with carotid stenting compared to endarterectomy. It was therefore recommended that carotid endarterectomy should remain the treatment of choice until the long-term efficacy of stenting is established.[102]

Management of patients with recurrent embolic events due to aortic atherosclerotic disease can be problematic. Aortic arch endarterectomy in patients with severe aortic atherosclerosis has been reported.[103-105] This procedure is performed using deep hypothermic circulatory arrest and is associated with significant perioperative morbidity and mortality. When performed during cardiac surgical procedures using cardiopulmonary bypass, it resulted in a significantly higher rate of stroke and mortality. Therefore, there is insufficient evidence to recommend this mode of treatment for stroke prevention. In the context of cardiac surgery, replacement of the ascending aorta can be performed with acceptable mortality and morbidity,[106] particularly in the intraoperative management of patients with so-called porcelain aorta[107] (severe diffuse atherosclerosis and calcification of the ascending aorta that causes an eggshell appearance on x-ray or CT).

Summary

Patients with atherosclerotic disease should be given an antiplatelet agent and a statin. Imaging of the ascending aorta, aortic arch, and carotid arteries is recommended in those at high risk of atheromatous embolization. Minimizing or completely avoiding aortic manipulation in these patients is recommended.

KEY POINTS

1. Atherosclerosis and its thromboembolic complications are a leading cause of death in the Western world.
2. The risk of atheromatous embolization is significantly increased with increasing plaque thickness (>4mm) and the presence of ulceration.
3. Ultrasonography (transesophageal and surface) is one the most frequently used investigative techniques. Computed tomography provides information on coronary artery atherosclerosis and the degree of calcification. Magnetic resonance imaging provides very high resolution in imaging plaque morphology.
4. There is a significant increase in the risk of embolization during cardiac surgery and vascular interventions.
5. The use of antiplatelet agents and statins is recommended in all patients with significant atherosclerotic disease.
6. Perioperative aortic screening allied with minimal aortic manipulation during cardiac surgery in high-risk patients may be associated with a significant reduction in the rate of atheromatous embolization.

ANNOTATED REFERENCES

Amarenco P, Cohen A, Tzourio C, Bertrand B, Hommel M, Besson G, et al. Atherosclerotic disease of the aortic arch and the risk of ischemic stroke. N Engl J Med 1994;331:1474-9.
  This French Aortic Plaque in Stroke group prospective case-control study of 250 patients with ischemic stroke reported that increasing plaque thickness imparted an increase risk of stroke especially with plaques greater than 4mm in thickness.
Bucher HC, Griffith LE, Guyatt GH. Effect of HMG CoA reductase inhibitors on stroke. A meta-analysis of randomized, controlled trials. Ann Intern Med 1998;128:89-95.
  This meta-analysis of over 49,000 statin-treated participants from 28 trials reported that the risk ratio for nonfatal and fatal stroke with HMG CoA reductase inhibitors was 0.76 (95% CI, 0.62-0.92). It also demonstrated an overall reduction in rates of death from coronary heart disease as well as a reduction in overall mortality with HMG CoA reductase inhibitors.
Cohen A, Tzourio C, Bertrand B, Chauvel C, Bousser MG, Amarenco P. Aortic plaque morphology and vascular events: a follow-up study in patients with ischemic stroke. FAPS Investigators. French Study of Aortic Plaques in Stroke. Circulation 1997;96:3838-41.

This study of 334 patients, 60 years or older, reported that in patients with brain infarction, the risk associated with aortic plaque thickness (≈4 mm) is markedly increased by the absence of plaque calcifications.

Collaborative meta-analysis of randomised trials of antiplatelet therapy for prevention of death, myocardial infarction, and stroke in high risk patients. BMJ 2002;324:71-86.

This large meta-analysis with more than 200,000 patients reported that aspirin is protective in most patients at increased risk of occlusive vascular events, including those with an acute MI or ischemic stroke, unstable or stable angina, previous MI, stroke or cerebral ischemia, peripheral arterial disease, or atrial fibrillation.

de Groot E, van Leuven SI, Duivenvoorden R, Meuwese MC, Akdim F, Bots ML, et al. Measurement of carotid intima-media thickness to assess progression and regression of atherosclerosis. Nat Clin Pract Cardiovasc Med 2008;5:280-8.

This review describes the utility of using CIMT measurement in the assessment of atherosclerosis. This was demonstrated to be a useful tool in risk evaluation of individuals and in studies of atherosclerosis progression and regression.

Evered LA, Silbert BS, Scott DA. Postoperative cognitive dysfunction and aortic atheroma. Ann Thorac Surg 2010;89:1091-7.

In over 300 patients undergoing cardiac surgery, the incidence of early postoperative cognitive decline was directly related to aortic atheroma burden (imaged using TEE and epiaortic ultrasound).

REFERENCES

Access the complete reference list online at http://www.expertconsult.com.

204

Pressure Ulcers

LAURA J. MOORE

Epidemiology

A *pressure ulcer* is any wound that develops in the upper, outer layers of the skin as a result of sustained, external pressure.[1] Pressure ulcers are serious complications among hospitalized patients. They increase healthcare costs, decrease patient quality of life, and often result in prolonged hospital stays. Current estimates of the prevalence of pressure ulcers among hospital patients vary. A recent analysis of acute care hospitals in the United States estimated a prevalence of 14% to 17% among hospitalized patients.[2] Another recent Canadian study estimated that one out of four patients will develop a pressure ulcer during the course of their hospital stay.[3] The prevalence of pressure ulcers is even higher among residents of long-term geriatric facilities, occurring in up to 30% of patients. Whereas the majority of the ulcers (50%) in hospitalized patients are stage 1, the prevalence of stage 3 and 4 ulcers is estimated to be as high as 4% in patients who reside in long-term care facilities.

Risk Factors

There are multiple risk factors for the development of pressure ulcers; they can be categorized as intrinsic and extrinsic. Intrinsic risk factors are those related to the patient's preexisting medical condition(s). Extrinsic factors are those related to the patient's environment. Intrinsic risk factors include neurologic disease, motor impairment, cognitive impairment, sensory deficits, malnutrition, and hypoperfusion due to peripheral vascular disease or congestive heart failure. Extrinsic risk factors include inadequate mobilization by care providers, trauma, sedation, application of physical restraints, improper positioning (especially among patients under general anesthesia), moisture, and shearing forces. Among these risk factors, failure to frequently change position is thought to be the biggest contributor to pressure ulcer formation. The combination of improper positioning and moisture at the skin surface are frequent causes of pressure ulcer formation in critically ill patients.

Because of the underlying pathophysiology of pressure ulcer formation, there are several high-risk areas for the development of pressure ulcers. Pressure ulcers are more prone to develop in bony or cartilaginous areas. These include any area of the body that has limited soft-tissue coverage such as the coccyx, spinous processes, heels, elbows, and ankles. In patients who are mostly positioned on their side, the iliac crest and trochanters are considered high-risk areas. Additionally, patients with malnutrition and subsequent cachexia have significant loss of soft tissue and are more prone to the development of pressure ulcers at any location.

Pathophysiology

Pressure ulcers form as a result of hypoperfusion to an area. The basic principle of pressure ulcer development is simple. When externally applied pressure exceeds the capillary perfusion pressure, flow becomes impaired and tissue ischemia occurs. If the hypoperfusion and ischemia are not reversed, necrosis of the involved tissue layers will occur. Ischemia to the area will initially present with erythema and induration. If this progresses to necrosis, tissue loss will occur. The critical duration of ischemia varies from patient to patient. However, it is generally accepted that pressure injury typically occurs between 30 and 240 minutes of hypoperfusion. In patients with preexisting peripheral

vascular disease, the time to critical ischemia is shorter. Because of impaired arterial inflow, these patients experience significant delays in restoration of perfusion and reversal of tissue hypoxia after the external pressure has been removed. In addition, because of poor underlying tissue perfusion, these patients will experience longer healing times once pressure ulcers develop.

Classification

All pressure ulcers begin in the outer layers of the skin. With ongoing pressure, the ischemia progressively extends to deeper layers of the skin. Therefore, the classification of pressure ulcers is based upon the depth of skin involvement. Pressure ulcers are classified as stage I through IV, with stage I being the most superficial, and stage IV being the deepest. The classification of pressure ulcers is listed in Table 204-1. Having a uniform, well-defined classification system for pressure ulcers is critical. It not only allows for standardization of wounds for research purposes but also allows for accurate communication of wound staging among healthcare providers. Once a pressure ulcer develops, it is important to classify the wound and monitor the progress of the wound bed. Having a standard grading system allows for continuity of care and objective monitoring of the progression of the wound.

Prevention

Prevention of pressure ulcer formation should be standard practice. This is of particular importance when caring for critically ill patients, because they often possess multiple risk factors for pressure ulcer formation.

RISK ASSESSMENT

Prevention programs should include an initial risk assessment of the individual patient. This assessment should include questioning about previous or preexisting pressure ulcers, a thorough skin inspection, evaluating the patient's mobility/activity level, continence, nutritional status, and a review of comorbid conditions that may contribute to the development of pressure ulcers. Assessment of these risk factors should be standardized and documented on all patients. Several tools have been developed for pressure ulcer risk assessment. The Braden Scale assesses external pressure forces and skin-related factors in a standardized fashion.[4] The Norton Scale assesses patient-specific risk factors (age, cognitive impairment, mobility, incontinence) for pressure ulcer development.[5] The Waterlow Scale assesses both intrinsic and extrinsic risk factors and was initially developed for use in the pediatric population.[6]

PREVENTION PLAN

Once the individual patient risk assessment has been addressed, a plan for pressure ulcer prevention should be implemented. Regardless of the plan utilized, a frequent assessment of its efficacy must be performed and any necessary adjustments made. The key elements of prevention include patient mobilization, patient positioning to prevent/remove pressure, and the use of positioning aides to redistribute pressure. Among critically ill patients, this requires vigilance and team effort, particularly among those patients who are sedated for prolonged periods of time. Prevention also includes avoidance of skin

TABLE 204-1	Pressure Ulcer Staging

National Pressure Ulcer Staging System

Stage I	Nonblanching erythema of intact skin
Stage II	Partial-thickness skin loss involving the epidermis and/or dermis. The ulcer is superficial and presents clinically as an abrasion, blister, or shallow crater.
Stage III	Full-thickness skin loss with damage and/or necrosis of the subcutaneous tissue. The wound extends down to but not through the underlying fascia.
Stage IV	Full-thickness skin loss with extensive destruction and necrosis of overlying structures including muscles, bone, or tendon

damage by shearing forces and avoidance of maceration of the skin due to moisture from incontinence and heat accumulation. There are a variety of support services available to help decrease the risk of pressure ulcer formation. These pressure-reducing surfaces include static support surfaces (mattresses, mattress overlays) and dynamic support surfaces that mechanically alter the amount of pressure applied to the patient's skin. Examples of dynamic support surfaces include low-air-loss beds, air-fluidized mattresses, and alternating pressure mattresses. The use of foam mattress overlays can reduce the risk of pressure ulcer development in high-risk populations.[7] Although associated with higher costs, dynamic mattresses have not consistently been shown to be superior to static support surfaces. However, dynamic mattresses are better than standard hospital mattresses in preventing pressure ulcer formation.

Treatment

A variety of treatment options and products are available for the management of pressure ulcers. Very few of the currently available treatment options have been rigorously evaluated in randomized controlled trials. An in-depth discussion of all the currently available products is beyond the scope of this text, so general classes of treatment options will be discussed rather than specific products.

WOUND DÉBRIDEMENT

Débridement of the wound bed is a critical step in the healing process of pressure ulcers. The purpose of débridement is to remove foreign material and devitalized tissue from the wound. After débridement, a wound bed of healthy tissue should be visible. Débridement of the wound bed reduces the production of inflammatory mediators that inhibit wound healing. There are a variety of techniques utilized for wound débridement. These include surgical débridement, hydrotherapy, larval therapy, and application of topical enzymatic débridement solutions. The choice of débridement techniques utilized depends on multiple factors including the size of the wound, comorbid conditions, and the presence of infection. Surgical débridement is most often required in large-volume wounds when extensive tissue débridement is needed. However, surgical débridement requires the patient be a suitable candidate for general anesthesia. The risk of subjecting a critically ill patient to general anesthesia and a trip to the operating room must be weighed against the benefits of sharp surgical débridement of a pressure ulcer. Hydrotherapy, while commonly practiced, has not been rigorously evaluated in the setting of a large randomized controlled trial. However, some small studies of patients with stage III or IV pressure ulcers have demonstrated faster wound healing among patients receiving hydrotherapy as compared to those who did not receive hydrotherapy.[8,9]

Larval therapy, also referred to as *biosurgery*, has been used for débridement of pressure ulcers. The basic concept of larval therapy is that application of larvae to wounds results in rapid débridement of necrotic tissues, with avoidance of the potential complications of surgical débridement such as pain and bleeding. Currently, there is evidence that compared to topical enzymatics, larval therapy significantly reduces the time to débridement of necrotic tissue. However, the use of larval therapy did not appear to have any effect on time to wound healing.[10]

A variety of topical enzymatic débridement products are commercially available. These can be used alone or in conjunction with other débridement techniques. These agents are applied directly to the wound bed once or twice a day. Multiple randomized controlled trials have validated the efficacy of topical enzymatic débridement products for the removal of necrotic tissue from the wound bed.[11] Prior to applying these agents, the wound bed should be cleansed with normal saline. The presence of any topical wound products containing metal will diminish the efficacy of topical enzymatics, and removing these agents from the wound bed is critical for the success of the enzymatics. In the event an eschar is overlying the wound bed, it is recommended that the eschar be cross-hatched with a surgical blade to allow for penetration of the topical enzymatic agent. Once applied, the wound bed should be covered with gauze. These agents are a viable and valuable therapy, particularly in those patients who are not candidates for alternative débridement methods.

HYDROCOLLOIDS

Hydrocolloid dressings are widely used in the management of pressure ulcers; their purpose is to absorb wound exudates. Typical hydrocolloid dressings contain some type of gel-forming agent placed in contact with the wound bed, and this is covered with a membrane that protects the wound against external contamination but allows for water evaporation.[12] Hydrocolloid dressings are typically applied every 3 to 5 days, depending upon the amount of exudates being produced by the wound. When compared to standard gauze dressings, hydrocolloids have been shown to be more absorptive and less painful.[12]

NEGATIVE PRESSURE THERAPY

The use of negative pressure therapy for wound healing has become increasingly common in the past decade. The basic concept behind this therapy is that applying negative pressure to the wound bed both removes edema fluid and increases blood flow to the area. Increased blood flow results in delivery of oxygen and nutrients which promote wound healing. In addition, the application of negative pressure to the wound results in wound contracture. Compared to standard wet-to-dry dressings, another benefit to patients of negative pressure therapy is decreased frequency of dressing changes. The use of negative pressure therapy for pressure ulcers has been associated with improved wound healing and decreased length of hospital stay.[13] Traditionally, negative pressure therapy has been applied to clean wounds that had very little slough or necrotic tissue. However, there is some evidence that the application of negative pressure therapy to wounds that are covered with soft necrotic tissue is a viable option.[14]

NUTRITIONAL SUPPORT

The presence of malnutrition has a significant impact on wound healing. In fact, its mere presence results in weakening of the skin and increases the risk of pressure ulcer development. Unfortunately, nutritional assessment is often neglected, particularly in chronically institutionalized patients. Establishing nutritional assessment protocols as well as treating malnutrition are essential in preventing and healing pressure ulcers. This is best accomplished by a multidisciplinary team that includes physicians, dieticians, and nursing staff.[15]

An initial nutritional assessment should be performed. Any recent weight loss, the current weight, and the patient's dietary intake should all be evaluated. After the initial assessment is completed, a nutrition plan should be created and implemented to address any issues identified. Weekly monitoring of the patient's nutritional status should occur to determine if the nutritional intervention is having the desired effect. Monitoring should include the patient's weight and assessment of functional status. The use of biochemical tests including serum prealbumin, transferrin, and nitrogen balance are also helpful.

▣ Conclusion

Pressure ulcers continue to be a common problem among critically ill patients. Constant vigilance and education of care providers are essential components of pressure ulcer prevention. When pressure ulcers do occur, a multidisciplinary approach is needed to manage these debilitating wounds. Management should include objective assessment of the scope of the wound, a multimodality treatment program specifically adapted to the patient's needs, and optimization of nutritional status to promote wound healing.

ANNOTATED REFERENCES

Anders J, Heinemann A, Leffmann C, et al. Decubitus ulcers: pathophysiology and primary prevention. Dtsch Arztebl Int 2010;107:371-81; quiz 382.

General overview of the pathophysiology of pressure ulcer formation and the basic physiologic principles underlying pressure ulcer prevention measures. Also included are comparisons of the various scoring systems for pressure ulcers and brief explanations for the various preventive measures commonly utilized in clinical practice.

Reddy M, Gill SS, Rochon PA. Preventing pressure ulcers: a systematic review. JAMA 2006;296:974-84.

Systematic review of the recent literature regarding various clinical practices for pressure ulcer prevention. This article critically evaluates current literature regarding support surfaces, patient positioning, topical therapy, and nutritional supplementation.

Bergstrom N, Demuth PJ, Braden BJ. A clinical trial of the Braden Scale for Predicting Pressure Sore Risk. Nurs Clin North Am 1987;22:417-28.

Description of the development and validation of the Braden Scale for pressure ulcer risk assessment.

Heyneman A, Beele H, Vanderwee K, Defloor T. A systematic review of the use of hydrocolloids in the treatment of pressure ulcers. J Clin Nurs 2008;17:1164-73.

Systematic review of commonly used hydrocolloids.

Ramundo J, Gray M. Enzymatic wound debridement. J Wound Ostomy Continence Nurs 2008;35:273-80.

Overview of a variety of enzymatic débridement solutions. This article includes comparisons of various commercially available products and the indications for their use.

REFERENCES

Access the complete reference list online at http://www.expertconsult.com.

205

Management of Pain, Anxiety, and Delirium

CHRISTOPHER G. HUGHES | E. WESLEY ELY | PRATIK P. PANDHARIPANDE

Pain, anxiety, and delirium are extremely common in the ICU, where they are often underappreciated and inadequately treated. However, unrelieved pain, anxiety, and delirium contribute to patient distress, evoke the stress response, complicate the management of lifesaving devices, and negatively affect outcome. Ensuring patient comfort and safety is a universal goal that has been endorsed by national medical societies and oversight bodies such as the Center for Medicare and Medicaid Services and The Joint Commission (TJC), which accredits and certifies U.S. healthcare organizations and programs.[1] Regional preferences, patient history, institutional bias, and individual patient variability, however, create a wide discrepancy in the approach to sedation of critically ill patients.

General Principles

Sedation and analgesia are administered to provide comfort and ensure patient safety, especially during mechanical ventilation. As a first step, it is important that the healthcare provider evaluate the specific problem requiring sedation to then devise an appropriate treatment strategy. Routine and objective assessments using valid and reliable measures of pain, anxiety, and delirium are vital. Scales to measure these conditions provide a common language for providers to use in quantifying their degree and recording the patient's response to therapy. It is important to frequently reassess and adjust therapeutic targets based on the condition of the patient. Pain must always be addressed first; unrelieved pain can be the underlying cause of anxiety, agitation, and delirium. Once pain is adequately controlled, anxiety should then be treated with an anxiolytic or sedative. In critically ill patients, unpredictable pharmacokinetics and pharmacodynamics secondary to drug interactions, organ dysfunction, absorption, protein binding, and hemodynamic instability can lead to medication complications.[2] Because most of these agents are administered as continuous infusions, drug accumulation, redistribution, and tachyphylaxis also confound their use, and techniques to prevent systemic drug accumulation have to be employed.

Pain

Existing disease, surgical procedures, trauma, invasive monitors, endotracheal intubation, and nursing interventions are only a few sources of discomfort commonly experienced by patients in the intensive care unit (ICU). In addition to patient discomfort, inadequately treated pain leads to an increased stress response, with resultant tachycardia, increased oxygen consumption, hypercoagulability, immunosuppression, hypermetabolism, and increased endogenous catecholamine activity.[2-5] Insufficient pain relief can also contribute to deficient sleep, disorientation, and anxiety, and long-term effects such as posttraumatic stress disorder may also be seen.[6] Unfortunately, pain is often undertreated because of concerns about the adverse effects and addiction potential of opiates and because caregivers lack the necessary skills for proper pain assessment and treatment.[3]

ASSESSMENT OF PAIN

To be recognized and properly treated, pain must be routinely and objectively assessed. In the ICU, the most valid and reliable indicator of pain is the patient's self-report.[7] Information about pain including location, quality, and intensity should be elicited as part of routine checking and recording of the patient's vital signs. Intensity can be objectively measured using tools such as the visual analog scale or numeric rating scale.[7]

It is not uncommon for ICU patients to be unable to communicate with caregivers owing to endotracheal intubation or altered mental status. During such times, behavioral and physiologic indicators must be used to assess pain intensity. The FACES scale[8] (Figure 205-1) was developed to objectify the use of facial expression as a measure of pain intensity and shows moderate correlation with different levels of pain.[9] Unfortunately, these indicators are nonspecific and subjective in nature, and as a result, clinicians are likely to underestimate and undertreat pain. The Behavioral Pain Scale (Table 205-1) is a valid tool that uses facial expression, limb movements, and ventilator synchrony for calculating a pain score; use of such pain assessments has been associated with lower analgesic and sedative use and with decreased time on the ventilator.[10,11]

MANAGEMENT OF PAIN

In managing pain, nonpharmacologic methods should be attempted first. These include patient repositioning, injury stabilization, removal of noxious or irritating stimuli, and application of heat or cold.[3] When nonpharmacologic approaches are insufficient to provide analgesia, regional or systemic therapy is indicated.

Regional Therapy

Regional nerve blockade provides analgesia for a large area of the body without the global effects of systemic analgesia. These procedures should be carried out only by clinicians trained specifically in their performance and management. Intercostal blocks can be used to manage pain due to thoracic or upper abdominal trauma or surgery and can improve respiratory mechanics to reduce the risk of pulmonary compromise.[12] Intercostal blocks have the advantage of providing analgesia without sedation or respiratory depression. Placement of an intercostal block carries the risk of pneumothorax and may have to be repeated because of its limited duration of action. Paravertebral blocks are useful for managing pain related to unilateral thoracic or abdominal procedures.[13] Paravertebral blockade carries the risk of inadvertent epidural blockade, pneumothorax, and hemothorax. Paravertebral blockade has been shown to have equal effectiveness as epidural blockade for pain control in traumatic rib fractures[14] but decreased pain control when compared to epidural blockade in thoracic surgery patients.[15] Blockade of the brachial plexus, lumbar plexus, sacral plexus, or the individual nerves of these plexuses may prove beneficial for the relief of pain localized to one extremity and can facilitate patient care such as dressing changes, frequent turning, or physical therapy.[16] These nerve blocks are generally well tolerated, can be prolonged by the placement of peripheral nerve catheters, and have the benefit of targeted and localized action.

Epidural analgesia has become increasingly popular for the management of pain from thoracic, abdominal, or lower extremity operative procedures.[17] Through a catheter, local anesthetics, opiates, and other pharmaceutical adjuncts like clonidine can be infused in the epidural space to provide bilateral analgesia in specific dermatomes.

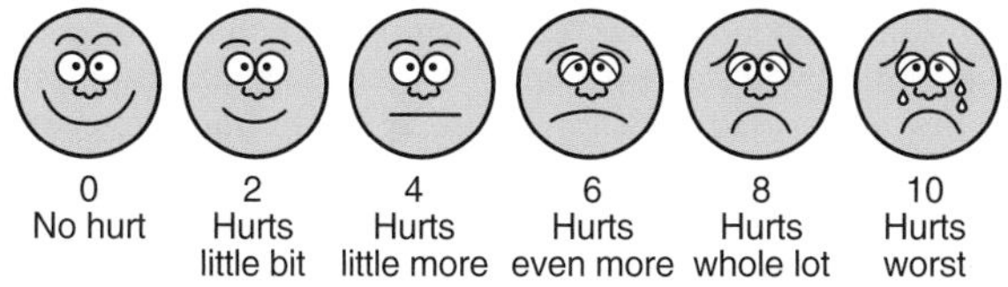

0	2	4	6	8	10
No hurt	Hurts little bit	Hurts little more	Hurts even more	Hurts whole lot	Hurts worst

Figure 205-1 FACES scale. (From Wong DL, Hockenberry-Eaton M, Wilson D et al. Wong's essentials of pediatric nursing. 6th ed. St Louis: Mosby; 2001, p. 1301.)

Low-concentration bupivacaine (e.g., 0.1%) or ropivacaine (e.g., 0.2%) provides excellent sensory blockade with minimal motor blockade.[18] Hypotension from sympathetic blockade and inability to ambulate due to decreased proprioception and/or motor weakness are known side effects.[18] Opiates such morphine, hydromorphone, and fentanyl are often added to local anesthetic solutions for their synergistic analgesic effects and do not cause sympathetic or motor blockade.[18] Possible adverse effects of epidural opiates include respiratory depression, urinary retention, nausea, vomiting, pruritus, and headache.[19] Multiple studies and meta-analyses examining epidural analgesia have shown reduced morbidity after major surgery, including improved pulmonary and intestinal function,[17,20] but epidural analgesia has not been shown to reduce mortality or length of stay despite improving pulmonary function in a meta-analysis of traumatic rib fracture patients, a commonly prescribed indication.[21] Epidural catheters should be used with extreme caution in patients who are receiving anticoagulation, especially low-molecular-weight heparin, because of the risk of epidural hematoma and paralysis from catheter manipulation.[22]

Systemic Therapy

Systemic analgesics should be administered as part of a goal-directed sedation and analgesia protocol. When administering analgesics, it is important to give them in sufficient quantities to relieve pain and prevent pain from returning to severe pretreatment levels.

Systemic therapies include nonsteroidal antiinflammatory drugs (NSAIDs) and acetaminophen, but opioids' analgesic, anxiolytic, antitussive, and sedative properties make them the most common ICU therapy for pain. Although they are the mainstay of analgesia in the ICU, opioids have a number of adverse effects. Respiratory depression and decreased gastrointestinal motility are commonly seen, but their impact can be reduced through proper airway and ventilator management and stimulant laxative use, respectively. Hypotension can also result, particularly in hypovolemic patients who cannot tolerate a reduction in systemic vascular resistance. Hypotension may also be due to vasodilation from histamine release, especially with morphine. Other side effects include pruritus, flushing, urinary retention, and delirium.

The most commonly used opiates in the ICU are morphine, hydromorphone, and fentanyl, though remifentanil is gaining popularity as an ultra short-acting analgesic-sedative drug. All these agents provide less sedation than the commonly used hypnotics or anesthetic agents, and patients receiving analgesic-based regimens with opioids are more likely to have accurate memory and less likely to suffer from posttraumatic stress disorder.[23]

Morphine is typically used as an intermittent intravenous (IV) injection. With IV injection, its peak effect occurs within 15 to 20 minutes, and analgesia lasts 2 to 4 hours. Morphine is given in doses of 2 to 5 mg IV every 5 to 15 minutes until the pain is controlled, followed by similar doses on a scheduled basis every 1 to 2 hours, with extra doses available as needed for breakthrough pain. Morphine is characterized by hepatic metabolism and renal excretion, and its effects can be prolonged in patients with renal impairment secondary to accumulation of an active metabolite (morphine-6 glucuronide).[24]

Hydromorphone is a more potent congener of morphine with similar pharmacokinetic and pharmacodynamic profiles.[24] Its lack of histamine release and decreased incidence of central nervous system (CNS) side effects make it a useful alternative to morphine, with typical dosing ranges of 0.2 mg to 1 mg IV.

Fentanyl is a synthetic opioid with a rapid onset (5-15 minutes) and a short duration of action (30-60 minutes).[24] Because of its short half-life, it can be easily titrated as a continuous infusion. Loading doses of 25 to 100 μg are given every 5 to 10 minutes until the pain is controlled, followed by infusion rates of 25 to 250 μg/h. Because it causes less histamine release than morphine and does not undergo renal elimination, it is the preferred opioid analgesic in hemodynamically unstable patients or those with renal insufficiency.[3]

Remifentanil is a derivative of fentanyl that is metabolized by nonspecific blood and tissue esterases.[24] It is used primarily as an infusion and has an elimination half-life of under 10 minutes regardless of infusion duration.[25] Hypotension and bradycardia are the most common side effects of remifentanil administration, and supplemental analgesic medication is usually required at the conclusion of a remifentanil infusion.[25]

Few comparative trials of opioid infusions have been performed. Traditionally, the selection of an opioid depends on the likely duration of analgesic infusion and the pharmacology of the specific opioid.[3] In a randomized double blind study, the mean percentage of hours at optimal sedation was significantly longer for patients receiving remifentanil versus morphine, and the duration of mechanical ventilation and extubation time were shorter for patients receiving remifentanil.[26] More patients in the morphine group also required the addition of midazolam for supplemental sedation. When compared with fentanyl, efficacy of achieving sedation goals was similar with remifentanil, though more breakthrough propofol was required in the fentanyl group.[27] There were no differences in time to extubation in both groups, but the percentage of patients experiencing pain after extubation was significantly higher in those receiving remifentanil, indicating the need for proactive pain management when weaning remifentanil.

Anxiety, Agitation, and Sedation

Anxiety is a diffuse and unpleasant emotion of apprehension that is not associated with a specific threat. *Agitation* is a state of anxiety accompanied by extreme arousal, irritability, and motor restlessness. Both are very common in the ICU, where a variety of triggers are responsible: excessive stimulation, pain, dyspnea, delirium, inability to communicate, sleep deprivation, metabolic disturbances, and underlying anxiety disorders. Anxiety can be present without agitation, as evidenced by anxious patients who become fearful and withdrawn. Unrelieved anxiety can be a significant source of physical and psychological stress for patients both during an acute event and in the long term, when unpleasant, frightening memories and posttraumatic stress disorder may result.[6,28] Left untreated, agitation can become life threatening if it leads to the removal of lifesaving devices such as endotracheal tubes and intravascular lines. Like pain, anxiety and agitation require a systematic, targeted approach in their assessment and treatment.

TABLE 205-1	The Behavioral Pain Scale	
Item	*Description*	*Score*
Facial expression	Relaxed	1
	Partially tightened (e.g., brow lowering)	2
	Fully tightened (e.g., eyelid closing)	3
	Grimacing	4
Upper limbs	No movement	1
	Partially bent	2
	Fully bent with finger flexion	3
	Permanently retracted	4
Compliance with ventilation	Tolerating movement	1
	Coughing but tolerating ventilation for most of the time	2
	Fighting ventilator	3
	Unable to control ventilation	4

Modified from Payen JF, Bru O, Bosson JL et al. Assessing pain in critically ill sedated patients by using a behavioral pain scale. Crit Care Med 2001;29:2258-63.

SEDATION SCALES AND PROTOCOLS

There are many scales available for the assessment of sedation and agitation, including the Ramsay Sedation Scale (RSS),[29] the Riker Sedation-Agitation Scale (SAS),[30] the Motor Activity Assessment Scale (MAAS),[31] and Richmond Agitation-Sedation Scale (RASS).[32] Each has good reliability and validity among adult ICU patients and can be used to set targets for goal-directed therapy. However, only the RASS has been shown to detect variations in the level of consciousness over time or in response to changes in sedative and analgesic drug use.[3,33] The RASS is a 10-point scale with discrete criteria to distinguish levels of agitation and sedation (Table 205-2) and takes less than 20 seconds to complete. Numerous studies have now shown that the use of a defined sedation target for the provision of protocol-based, goal-directed therapy reduces patient discomfort and improves outcome.[32,34,35] Additionally, the use of protocols that incorporate daily interruption of sedation,[36] as well as link these spontaneous awakening trials with daily spontaneous breathing trials,[37] has been shown to improve time off mechanical ventilation and shorten ICU and hospital stays, without antecedent adverse effects. Furthermore, the Awakening and Breathing Controlled (ABC) Trial showed a reduction in mortality at 12 months by incorporating this linked approach. Neither of these studies found any long-term neuropsychological consequences of performing daily sedation holds.[38,39]

PHARMACOLOGIC MANAGEMENT

Pharmacologic management of anxiety, agitation, and sedation follows the same general principal: goal-directed, protocol-based management with intermittent dosing or daily interruption of continuous infusions. Before administering sedative agents, it is important to search for an underlying cause (e.g., hypoxemia, hypoglycemia, hypotension, drug withdrawal), especially when a previously calm patient becomes anxious or agitated. If pain is present, an analgesic should be the initial therapeutic choice. Once pain has been addressed, benzodiazepines, propofol, and dexmedetomidine are the drugs most often used.

Benzodiazepines bind to γ-aminobutyric acid (GABA) receptors in the CNS, thereby providing sedation, anxiolysis, hypnosis, muscle relaxation, anticonvulsant activity, and amnesia.[40] These agents do not relieve pain, but their anxiolytic and amnestic properties may improve pain tolerance by moderating the anticipatory pain response.[41] Benzodiazepines vary considerably in their pharmacology, and patient-specific factors such as advanced age, drug or alcohol use, and organ dysfunction make their potency, onset, and duration of action even more unpredictable. When given in bolus doses, these drugs can cause

hypotension secondary to decreased sympathetic tone, particularly in hemodynamically unstable patients.[40] By reducing inhibitions, benzodiazepines may paradoxically increase agitation and aggressiveness. Benzodiazepines can also cause delirium, so their use in treating hyperactive delirium can be counterproductive. Of the benzodiazepines that are currently available, diazepam, midazolam, and lorazepam are used most frequently in the ICU. The onset of action of **diazepam** is 2 to 5 minutes, making it useful for rapidly sedating acutely agitated patients. However, its long half-life makes prolonged sedation a risk with repeated use, particularly in patients with renal or hepatic dysfunction.[40] To control acute agitation, diazepam is given in doses of 2 to 5 mg IV every 5 to 15 minutes until the event is controlled. Continuous infusions are not recommended.

Midazolam is also useful for acute agitation because it has a rapid onset (2-5 minutes) and a short duration of action.[40] It is given as bolus injections of 2 to 5 mg IV every 5 to 15 minutes. When used for long-term sedation (>48 hours), it tends to produce unpredictable awakening times, especially in patients who are obese, have low serum albumin concentrations, or have renal or hepatic failure.[3] **Lorazepam** has a slower onset of action (5-20 minutes), making it less helpful for acute agitation. However, it is less lipid soluble and has no active metabolites, making it potentially useful for long-term administration in critically ill patients.[3,40] Intermittent doses of 1 to 4 mg IV are given every 2 to 6 hours, or continuous infusions may be used, although recent data have suggested significant morbidity associated with lorazepam infusions,[42] including concerns of propylene glycol toxicity.[43]

Propofol is an IV anesthetic that acts primarily at the GABA receptor.[44] It has proven utility as a sedating agent in the ICU owing to its rapid onset (1-2 minutes) and short duration of action (2-8 minutes). It is typically given as a bolus injection of 40 to 100 mg IV followed by an infusion of 25 to 75 μg/kg/min.[45] Propofol is especially useful when rapid awakening is important, such as for neurologic assessment or pending extubation.[3] As a respiratory depressant, propofol suppresses both central and peripheral stimuli for ventilation. It can also cause significant hypotension by venodilation, vasodilation, and myocardial depression.[46] These cardiovascular effects can be minimized by titration of infusions slowly to achieve the desired sedation level. Propofol has been associated with hypertriglyceridemia when infused for 7 days or longer, leading to the recommendation that infusions should be used at the lowest possible dose for the shortest possible time.[3] Another complication associated with propofol use is the development of *propofol infusion syndrome*, characterized by severe lactic acidosis and rhabdomyolysis.[47] Although the majority of reports have been in the pediatric population, a handful of case reports have been published about propofol infusion syndrome associated with high-dose (>75 μg/kg/min) and prolonged (>72 hours) infusions in adults as well.[47] Consequently, providers should consider alternative sedative agents for any patient receiving high-dose propofol infusions who develops unexplained metabolic acidosis, arrhythmia, or cardiac failure.

Dexmedetomidine is a selective α₂ receptor agonist with a site of action that includes presynaptic neurons in the locus ceruleus and spinal cord; it produces analgesia and sedation without respiratory suppression.[48] The onset of action is within 15 minutes, and peak concentrations are achieved after 1 hour of continuous infusion.[48] Sedation is often initiated with a bolus of 1 μg/kg over 10 to 20 minutes, followed by an infusion of 0.2 to 0.7 μg/kg/h. Several studies have shown safety with doses up to 2 μg/kg/h, although with increased incidence of bradycardia and hypotension.[49] Patients with severe liver disease require lower dosing, whereas dose adjustment is not required in those with renal dysfunction.[48] Bradycardia is the most common side effect of dexmedetomidine, especially with rapid bolus administration. A biphasic response in blood pressure may be seen during dexmedetomidine use, with decreased blood pressure at lower concentrations and increased blood pressure at higher concentrations.[48] Dexmedetomidine has been shown to attenuate inflammatory responses,[50,51] mimic natural non–rapid eye movement sleep,[52] and have antiapoptotic actions,[53] which may make it an attractive agent for sedation in

TABLE 205-2	The Richmond Agitation-Sedation Scale	

Richmond Agitation-Sedation Scale (RASS)

+4	Combative	Combative, violent, immediate danger to staff
+3	Very agitated	Pulls or removes tubes or catheters; aggressive
+2	Agitated	Frequent nonpurposeful movement; fights ventilator
+1	Restless	Anxious, apprehensive, but movements not aggressive or vigorous
0	Alert and calm	
−1	Drowsy	Not fully alert, but has sustained (>10 sec) awakening (eye opening/contact) to voice
−2	Light sedation	Drowsy, briefly (<10 sec) awakens to voice or physical stimulation
−3	Moderate sedation	Movement or eye opening (but no eye contact) to voice
−4	Deep sedation	No response to voice, but movement or eye opening to physical stimulation
−5	Unarousable	No response to voice or physical stimulation

Adapted from Sessler CN, Gosnell MS, Grapp MJ et al. The Richmond Agitation-Sedation Scale: validity and reliability in adult intensive care unit patients. Am J Respir Crit Care Med 2002;166:1338-44; and from Ely EW, Truman B, Shintani A et al. Monitoring sedation status over time in ICU patients: reliability and validity of the Richmond Agitation-Sedation Scale [RASS]. JAMA 2003;289:2983-91.

the ICU, though further studies are warranted to show benefit of these actions.

Multiple studies have been performed comparing different sedative therapies in ICU patients. A study of short-duration sedation (<8 hours) revealed no significant differences between intermittent lorazepam and continuous-infusion midazolam in terms of quality of sedation, anxiolysis, hemodynamic and oxygen transport variables, and patient and nurse satisfaction.[54] However, lorazepam was deemed more cost-effective because larger doses of midazolam were required to produce the desired level of sedation. A pharmacologic model comparing lorazepam and midazolam infusions found the emergence times for light and deep sedation to be significantly longer for lorazepam than midazolam.[55] In a prospective randomized controlled study in trauma patients comparing infusions of lorazepam, midazolam, and propofol, oversedation occurred most frequently with lorazepam, and the greatest number of dosage adjustments was required by the lorazepam group.[56] Undersedation occurred most often with propofol, and this drug had the highest cost of sedation. The study's data indicated midazolam as the most titratable drug with the least amount of oversedation or undersedation and suggested that lorazepam was the most cost-effective agent for sedation.

Propofol has been compared to individual benzodiazepines in several studies. In a randomized trial comparing intermittent lorazepam boluses to propofol infusion, with daily interruption of sedatives in both groups, patients in the propofol group had fewer mechanical ventilation days, with a trend toward greater number of ventilator-free survival days.[57] In an economic evaluation of propofol versus lorazepam, propofol was determined to be less costly per patient than lorazepam despite the considerably lower pharmacy unit cost of lorazepam.[58] The lower costs were likely attributable to the greater number of ventilator-free days in patients treated with propofol. Several studies have compared propofol and midazolam infusions.[59-61] In a systematic review of these trials, duration of adequate sedation was found to be greater with propofol, independent of length of sedation.[62] Weaning times were found to be shorter with propofol, but this was only statistically significant in patients sedated for less than 36 hours. The review surmised that effective sedation was possible with both propofol and midazolam, and it also determined that 1 of 12 patients sedated with propofol was likely to develop hypotension that would not occur with midazolam sedation.

Dexmedetomidine, a newer agent, has subsequently been compared to preexisting sedation regimens. One of the first comparative studies found that patients sedated with dexmedetomidine were adequately sedated and required three times less opiates than patients sedated with propofol.[63] Patients on dexmedetomidine had lower heart rates, but there was no difference in arterial blood pressure among the group. Dexmedetomidine has also been studied in patients after coronary artery bypass surgery, with similar times to weaning and extubation in patients treated with dexmedetomidine or propofol, though there was a significant reduction in use of narcotics, beta-blockers, antiemetics, NSAIDs, epinephrine, and diuretics in patients receiving dexmedetomidine.[64] One study evaluated patient ratings of sedation during mechanical ventilation and found that patients on dexmedetomidine perceived a shorter length of intubation despite no actual difference in length of intubation or length of ICU stay.[65] A double-blind randomized controlled trial (the MENDS study) comparing sedation with dexmedetomidine to lorazepam in mechanically ventilated surgical and medical ICU patients found that sedation with dexmedetomidine resulted in more days alive without delirium or coma, lower prevalence of coma, greater achievement of target sedation, and minimal differences in cost of care despite the higher acquisition cost of dexmedetomidine.[66] A further analysis of these patients revealed improvements in daily delirium rates in the dexmedetomidine group.[67] Patients with sepsis who were sedated with dexmedetomidine had shorter time on mechanical ventilation and improved survival when compared to the lorazepam group, without any differences in hemodynamic profiles or adverse events.[67] Another multicenter double-blind randomized trial (the SEDCOM study) comparing dexmedetomidine with midazolam

sedation found no difference in time at targeted sedation level, but patients treated with dexmedetomidine spent less time on the ventilator, experienced less delirium, and developed less tachycardia and hypertension.[68] Finally, a meta-analysis suggested that sedation with dexmedetomidine decreases ICU length of stay.[49]

The safety and efficacy of analgesia-based sedation with remifentanil has been compared to conventional sedation with hypnotic-based regimens for patients with brain injury requiring prolonged sedation for mechanical ventilation.[69] Neurologic assessment times and time to extubation were significantly shorter for patients receiving remifentanil than those receiving propofol or midazolam supplemented with morphine or fentanyl. In another study comparing remifentanil-based sedation with a midazolam-based regime, the duration of mechanical ventilation and duration of weaning were significantly shorter in patients receiving remifentanil, and a trend toward shortened ICU stay was also observed.[70] A randomized multicenter study comparing conventional sedation regimens (propofol or benzodiazepine with as-needed opioid) with an analgesia-based regimen consisting of remifentanil with as-needed propofol found shortened durations of mechanical ventilation and ICU length of stay in the analgesia-based group.[71] However, concerns about costs, withdrawal, and hyperalgesia after discontinuation of remifentanil have limited widespread use of this agent in the United States.[72] A recent single-center randomized controlled study compared the use of an analgesia-based protocol incorporating morphine (intervention group) to sedation with propofol.[73] Patients in the intervention group had shorter times on mechanical ventilation and in the ICU, with no adverse events. About 20% of the patients in the "no sedation, morphine only" group required rescue with propofol per the protocol; however, 80% were managed with morphine alone despite being critically ill.[73] The generalizability of this study is limited by the fact that the ICU had 1:1 nursing ratios, as well as other personnel to help reassure patients, which may not be available in most other ICUs.

An empirical protocol for the management of pain, anxiety, and sedation is provided as a reference in Figure 205-2. Readers are advised to incorporate local culture, patient characteristics, and expert opinion to determine the best protocol for their respective ICUs.

Delirium

The reader is referred to Chapter 2 for details on the definition, risk factors, pathogenesis, monitoring instruments, and outcomes of delirium. Our discussion will focus on management aspects of delirium.

Delirium is an acute, fluctuating change in mental status, with inattention and altered levels of consciousness. It is extremely prevalent in critically ill patients with associated morbidity and mortality.[74-77] The development of tools such as the Intensive Care Delirium Screening Checklist[78] and the Confusion Assessment Method for the ICU (CAM-ICU)[79] (see Chapter 2) has allowed for the rapid diagnosis of delirium by non-psychiatric physicians and other healthcare personnel, even while patients are being mechanically ventilated. However, development of effective evidence-based strategies and protocols for prevention and treatment of delirium awaits data from ongoing randomized clinical trials of both nonpharmacologic and pharmacologic strategies. An empirical protocol is offered in Figure 205-3 and is largely based on current clinical practice guidelines.[3] Although the nonpharmacologic interventions recommended in this protocol have shown beneficial results in non-ICU patients,[80] extrapolation to ICU populations is speculative.

PREVENTION OF DELIRIUM

A "liberation and animation" strategy can likely reduce the incidence and duration of delirium.[81] *Liberation* uses target-based sedation protocols, linking spontaneous awakening trials with spontaneous breathing trials and proper sedation regimens to reduce the harmful effects of sedative exposure. Data from the MENDS study[66] and the SEDCOM trial[68] have shown that dexmedetomidine can decrease the duration

ANALGESIA/SEDATION PROTOCOL FOR MECHANICALLY VENTILATED PATIENTS

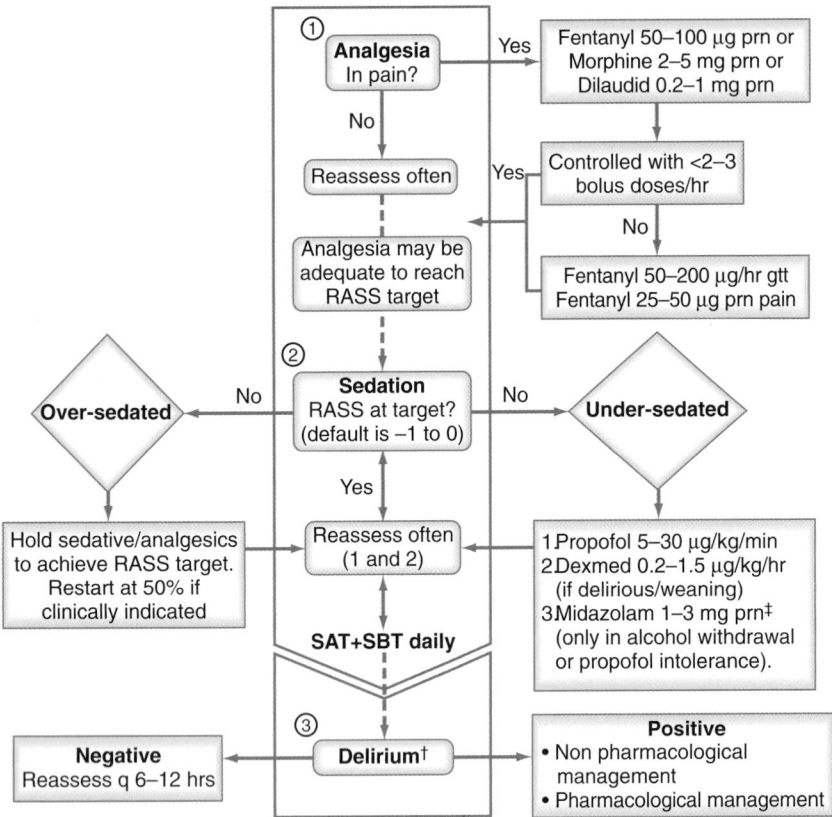

†Delirium diagnosed using the CAM-ICU or ICDSC
‡Midazolam 1–3 mg/hr gtt rarely if >3 midaz boluses/hr, propofol intolerance or >96 hrs propofol

Figure 205-2 Empirical sedation protocol. *(With permission from www.icudelirium.org.)*

and prevalence of brain organ dysfunction when compared to lorazepam or midazolam, further supporting the notion that minimizing benzodiazepine exposure can help reduce delirium. Meanwhile, *animation* refers to early mobilization of ICU patients, which has been shown to reduce delirium and improve neurocognitive outcomes.[82]

TREATMENT OF DELIRIUM

As with the management of anxiety and agitation, pharmacologic therapy should be attempted only after correcting any contributing factors (e.g., pain, anxiety, sleep disturbance, environmental stimuli, delirium-causing drugs) or underlying physiologic abnormalities (e.g., hypoxia, hypoglycemia, metabolic derangements, shock). It should be recognized that while agents used to treat delirium are intended to improve cognition, they all have psychoactive effects that may further cloud the sensorium and promote a longer overall duration of cognitive impairment. Therefore, until we have further outcome data that confirm beneficial effects of treatment, these drugs should be used judiciously in the smallest possible dose and for the shortest time necessary.

The Society of Critical Care Medicine guidelines[3] recommend haloperidol as the drug of choice, though it is acknowledged that this is based on sparse outcome data from nonrandomized case series and anecdotal reports. Haloperidol, a butyrophenone "typical" antipsychotic, is the most widely used neuroleptic agent for delirium.[83] It does not suppress respiratory drive and works as a dopamine receptor antagonist by blocking the D_2 receptor, resulting in treatment of positive symptomatology (hallucinations, unstructured thoughts patterns, etc.) and producing a variable sedative effect. A recommended starting dose would be 2 to 5 mg every 6 to 12 hours (IV or oral [PO]), with maximal effective doses usually around 20 mg/d. Recently, use of haloperidol has been shown to have a mortality benefit in a retrospective

analysis of critically ill patients,[84] and low-dose haloperidol prophylaxis reduced the duration and severity of delirium in elderly hip surgery patients, even though the actual prevalence of delirium was not reduced.[85]

Newer "atypical" antipsychotic agents (e.g., risperidone, ziprasidone, quetiapine, olanzapine) may also prove helpful for delirium.[86] The rationale behind use of the atypical antipsychotics over haloperidol is theoretical and centers on the fact that they affect not only dopamine but also other potentially key neurotransmitters such as serotonin, acetylcholine, and norepinephrine. One small study found that olanzapine and haloperidol were equally efficacious in treating ICU delirium in both medical and surgical patients, but that olanzapine was associated with fewer side effects.[86] In a limited pilot trial examining the feasibility and safety of antipsychotics for ICU delirium, treatment with ziprasidone or haloperidol did not improve the number of days alive without delirium or coma as compared to placebo, but importantly, no significant adverse effects were identified.[87] A small randomized trial comparing quetiapine with placebo, with as-needed haloperidol, found that quetiapine resulted in faster delirium resolution, less agitation, and an increased rate of transfer to home or rehabilitation.[88] These studies warrant repeating with larger patient populations before any concrete recommendations can be made regarding the efficacy of specific typical or atypical antipsychotics in delirium.

Adverse effects of typical and atypical antipsychotics include hypotension, acute dystonias, extrapyramidal effects, laryngeal spasm, malignant hyperthermia, glucose and lipid dysregulation, and anticholinergic effects.[87,89] Perhaps the most immediately life-threatening adverse effect of antipsychotics is torsades de pointes; these agents should not be given to patients with prolonged QT intervals unless thought to be absolutely necessary. Patients who receive substantial quantities of typical or atypical antipsychotics or coadministered

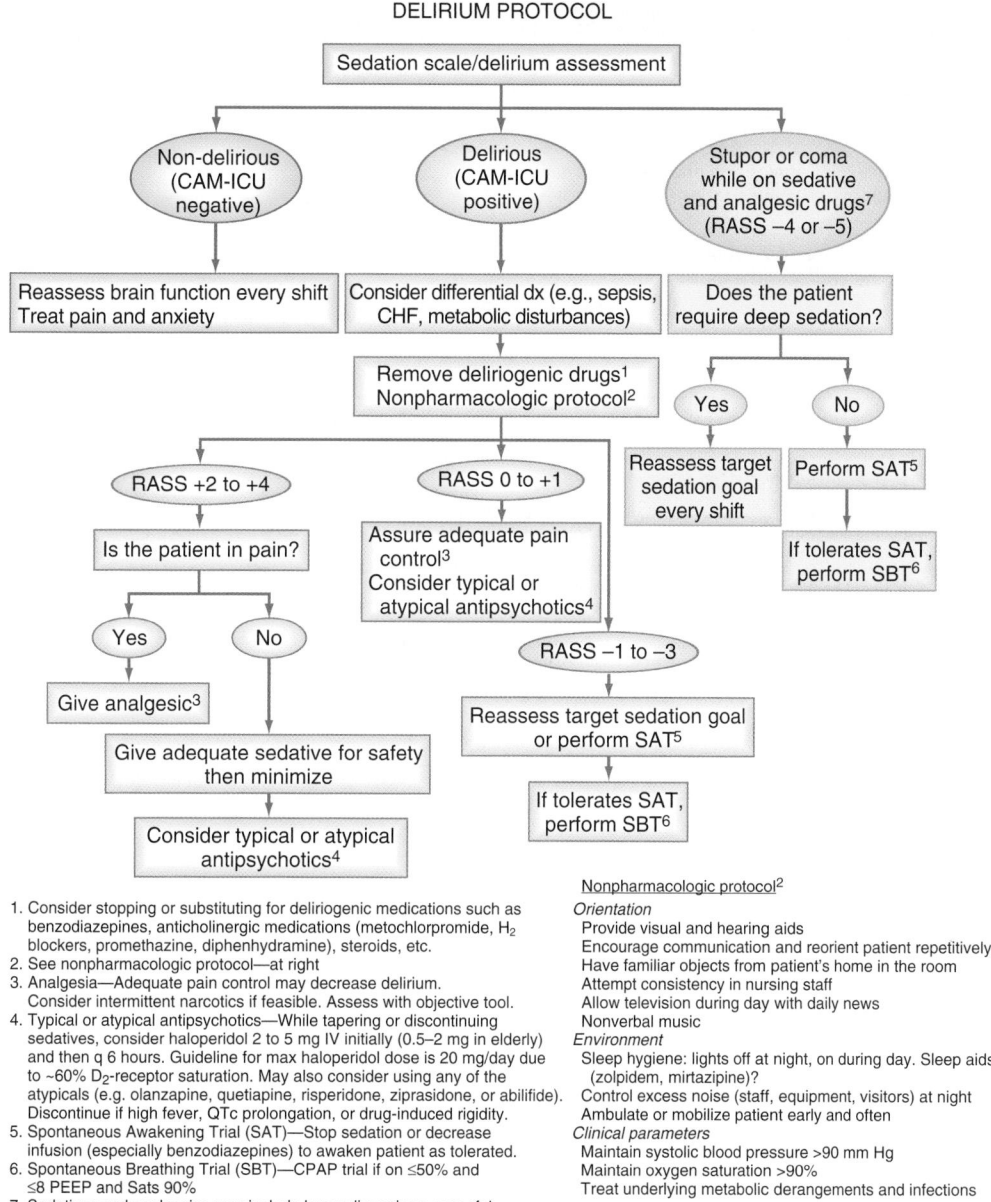

DELIRIUM PROTOCOL

Sedation scale/delirium assessment

Non-delirious (CAM-ICU negative)

Delirious (CAM-ICU positive)

Stupor or coma while on sedative and analgesic drugs[7] (RASS −4 or −5)

Reassess brain function every shift Treat pain and anxiety

Consider differential dx (e.g., sepsis, CHF, metabolic disturbances)

Does the patient require deep sedation?

Remove deliriogenic drugs[1] Nonpharmacologic protocol[2]

Yes

No

Reassess target sedation goal every shift

Perform SAT[5]

If tolerates SAT, perform SBT[6]

RASS +2 to +4

RASS 0 to +1

Is the patient in pain?

Assure adequate pain control[3] Consider typical or atypical antipsychotics[4]

Yes

No

RASS −1 to −3

Give analgesic[3]

Reassess target sedation goal or perform SAT[5]

Give adequate sedative for safety then minimize

If tolerates SAT, perform SBT[6]

Consider typical or atypical antipsychotics[4]

1. Consider stopping or substituting for deliriogenic medications such as benzodiazepines, anticholinergic medications (metoclorpromide, H₂ blockers, promethazine, diphenhydramine), steroids, etc.
2. See nonpharmacologic protocol—at right
3. Analgesia—Adequate pain control may decrease delirium. Consider intermittent narcotics if feasible. Assess with objective tool.
4. Typical or atypical antipsychotics—While tapering or discontinuing sedatives, consider haloperidol 2 to 5 mg IV initially (0.5–2 mg in elderly) and then q 6 hours. Guideline for max haloperidol dose is 20 mg/day due to ~60% D₂-receptor saturation. May also consider using any of the atypicals (e.g. olanzapine, quetiapine, risperidone, ziprasidone, or abilifide). Discontinue if high fever, QTc prolongation, or drug-induced rigidity.
5. Spontaneous Awakening Trial (SAT)—Stop sedation or decrease infusion (especially benzodiazepines) to awaken patient as tolerated.
6. Spontaneous Breathing Trial (SBT)—CPAP trial if on ≤50% and ≤8 PEEP and Sats 90%
7. Sedatives and analgesics may include benzodiazepines, propofol, dexmedetomidine, fentanyl, or morphine

Nonpharmacologic protocol[2]
Orientation
Provide visual and hearing aids
Encourage communication and reorient patient repetitively
Have familiar objects from patient's home in the room
Attempt consistency in nursing staff
Allow television during day with daily news
Nonverbal music
Environment
Sleep hygiene: lights off at night, on during day. Sleep aids (zolpidem, mirtazipine)?
Control excess noise (staff, equipment, visitors) at night
Ambulate or mobilize patient early and often
Clinical parameters
Maintain systolic blood pressure >90 mm Hg
Maintain oxygen saturation >90%
Treat underlying metabolic derangements and infections

Figure 205-3 Empirical delirium protocol. (*With permission from www.icudelirium.org.*)

arrhythmogenic drugs should be monitored closely with electrocardiography. Both typical and atypical antipsychotics have been reported to increase mortality in non-ICU patients when given for prolonged periods.[89,90]

Reports have described the utility of dexmedetomidine as an adjunct to assist with weaning patients from psychoactive medications.[91] A small prospective study of patients who developed delirium that prevented extubation upon weaning of sedation found that addition of dexmedetomidine infusion achieved rapid resolution of agitation, permitting subsequent extubation.[92] A second study compared dexmedetomidine to haloperidol in patients unable to be weaned from the ventilator owing to agitation and found that dexmedetomidine shortened time to extubation and decreased ICU length of stay.[93]

Benzodiazepines are not recommended for managing delirium because of the likelihood of oversedation, exacerbation of confusion, and respiratory suppression. However, they remain the drugs of choice for the treatment of delirium tremens (and other withdrawal syndromes) and seizures. It is likely, however, that residual accumulation of these drugs may lead to prolonged delirium long after the drugs have been discontinued. In certain populations, particularly elderly patients with underlying dementia, benzodiazepines may lead to increased confusion and agitation.

Conclusion

Pain, anxiety, and delirium are common events in the ICU, where their occurrence is associated with adverse outcomes. Using a systematic management approach that follows the general principles outlined in this chapter can maximize patient comfort while reducing the likelihood of overmedication and its attendant complications.

KEY POINTS

1. Pain, anxiety, and delirium must be routinely and objectively assessed.

2. Address pain first, and use nonpharmacologic means whenever possible for anxiety and delirium.

3. Administer intermittent dosing of analgesics and sedatives via goal-directed protocols to avoid oversedation and improve patient care and outcomes.

4. Daily interruption of sedation linked to spontaneous breathing trials reduces benzodiazepine and opioid exposure and reduces mortality.

5. Minimize benzodiazepine exposure; propofol, dexmedetomidine, and remifentanil have been shown to be superior.

6. Reassess treatment goals frequently, adjusting them based on the condition of the patient.

7. Dexmedetomidine and early ambulation have been shown to reduce delirium; the role of antipsychotics is still debatable in critically ill patients.

ANNOTATED REFERENCES

Jacobi J, Fraser GL, Coursin DB, et al. Clinical practice guidelines for the sustained use of sedatives and analgesics in the critically ill adult. Crit Care Med 2002;30:119-41.

These guidelines, which were developed by a panel of experts in the field using a systematic and evidence-based approach, established the standard of care for the management of pain, anxiety, and delirium in the ICU.

Girard TD, Kress JP, Fuchs BD, et al. Efficacy and safety of a paired sedation and ventilator weaning protocol for mechanically ventilated patients in intensive care (Awakening and Breathing Controlled trial): a randomised controlled trial. Lancet 2008;371:126-34.

The multicenter Awakening and Breathing Controlled (ABC) trial tested the results of linking sedation and ventilator weaning protocols using a "wake up and breathe" approach. The ABC intervention resulted in reductions in time on mechanical ventilation, time in coma, ICU and hospital length of stay, and in the risk of death within 1 year.

Pandharipande PP, Pun BT, Herr DL, et al. Effect of sedation with dexmedetomidine vs lorazepam on acute brain dysfunction in mechanically ventilated patients: the MENDS randomized controlled trial. JAMA 2007;298:2644-53.

The double-blind randomized controlled MENDS trial compared sedation with dexmedetomidine to lorazepam in mechanically ventilated surgical and medical ICU patients. In this trial, sedation with dexmedetomidine resulted in more days alive without delirium or coma, lower prevalence of coma, and greater achievement of target sedation.

Riker RR, Shehabi Y, Bokesch PM, et al. Dexmedetomidine vs midazolam for sedation of critically ill patients: a randomized trial. JAMA 2009;301:489-99.

This double-blind randomized controlled multicenter trial compared sedation with dexmedetomidine to midazolam in mechanically ventilated patients and showed that sedation with dexmedetomidine resulted in a lower prevalence of coma and faster weaning times.

Schweickert WD, Pohlman MC, Pohlman AS, et al. Early physical and occupational therapy in mechanically ventilated, critically ill patients: a randomised controlled trial. Lancet 2009;373:1874-82.

In a randomized controlled trial of medical ICU patients, early exercise and mobilization reduced the number of delirium days, increased the number of ventilator-free days, and increased the rate of return to independent function.

REFERENCES

Access the complete reference list online at http://www.expertconsult.com.

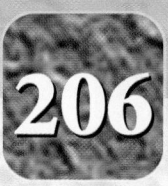

206

Burns

ROBERT L. SHERIDAN

Over the past few decades, survival and quality of life have improved markedly for victims of serious burns. A better understanding of injury physiology and realization that the natural history of burns can be changed by prompt surgery led to these improvements.[1] Maintenance of patients with serious burns through the physiologic trial of staged wound closure is an essential component of this success. Many aspects of burn critical care are unique to this disease process.[2]

■ Phases of Burn Care

Successful management of patients with serious burns requires both effective initial resuscitation and development of an overall plan for acute-phase hospitalization. Commonly, this overall plan can be considered to have four phases (Table 206-1).[3] The first phase, from day 1 through 3, the initial evaluation and resuscitation phase, focuses on complete evaluation and accurate fluid resuscitation. The second phase, initial wound excision and biological closure, describes changes in the natural history of the disease, which include progressive wound sepsis and systemic inflammation and infection. This phase entails a series of staged operations that are completed during the first few days after injury. The third phase, definitive wound closure, requires that temporary wound covers be replaced with definitive covers and that small complex wounds such as those of the face and hands are addressed. The final stage of care is rehabilitation and reconstruction. Although rehabilitation begins during resuscitation, it becomes much more time consuming and involved near the end of the acute stay. Return to work, school, and community is the major objective of the entire acute hospitalization.

■ Physiology of Burn Injury

Serious burns are associated with a stereotypical sequence of physiologic changes. Anticipation of these metabolic aberrations facilitates optimal support (see Table 206-1). During the first 1 or 2 days after a serious burn, patients require substantial hemodynamic support.[4] If the patient is successfully resuscitated, a hyperdynamic and hypermetabolic state typically ensues. This later phase, characterized by high cardiac output, reduced afterload, fever, and muscle catabolism, must be supported by provision of adequate quantity and quality of substrates.

RESUSCITATION PHASE

The massive fluid resuscitation required by burn patients is unique in medicine. It is secondary to a diffuse but transient capillary leak driven by poorly characterized mediators.[5] The clinical result is extravasation of fluids, electrolytes, and even moderate-sized colloid molecules into both burned and unburned soft tissues to a degree not seen in other disease processes. Since the 1930s, a variety of resuscitation formulas have been developed based on burn and patient size. However, this remains an area of clinical art, with no formula being reliably accurate for all patients.[2] Besides burn size and patient size, a variety of other factors have an impact on resuscitation requirements. These include delay in initiation of resuscitation, inhalation injury, patient age, baseline cardiovascular health, and the depth and vapor transmission characteristics of the wound itself.[6]

Burns under 15% generally do not require a formal fluid resuscitation program. As burn size increases, physiologic aberrations increase in intensity, explaining escalating volume requirements. Formulas do not accurately predict the needs of individual patients. Optimal burn resuscitation requires hourly reevaluation of resuscitation endpoints, with titration of volume infusions. In essence, the formula chosen will only help initiate resuscitation and roughly guide planning of volume needs. Of the many resuscitation formulas available, the modified Brooke protocol (Box 206-1) is representative. All formulas have their adherents, and all are useful if employed as rough guidelines only while monitoring physiologic resuscitation endpoints. The role of colloid is expanding in burn resuscitation, although there is no uniform agreement. Many providers, the author included, begin 5% albumin at a maintenance rate immediately during resuscitation and find it reduces the incidence of edema-related complications, including abdominal compartment syndrome.[7]

HYPERDYNAMIC PHASE

Typically there is a very noticeable decline in intravenous volume requirements 18 to 30 hours after injury. It is assumed that this is because the capillary leak has "sealed" in well-resuscitated patients. After this hypodynamic period, a systemic hypermetabolic state predictably develops and is sustained in surviving patients until it slowly regresses, well after wound closure.[8] This state is characterized by high cardiac output, low peripheral vascular resistance, fever, and increased protein flux. In patients not well supported with protein substrate, this increased protein flux will be associated with significant muscle catabolism. Although the basic biology is not well understood, the postresuscitation physiologic state is assumed to be caused by inflammatory mediators and augmented release of the counterregulatory hormones, cortisol, catecholamines, and glucagon.[9] These hormonal changes are triggered by a combination of wound- and gut-released bacteria and their byproducts, pain, foci of infection, and some degree of evaporative heat loss.

A central component of burn critical care is to ensure adequate support of the hypermetabolic state. This is done by providing accurate fluid repletion, adequate supplies of metabolic substrates, control of environmental temperature, and competent pain control. Early identification and excision of necrotic skin and soft tissue with immediate biological closure of the resulting wounds truncates the hypermetabolic physiologic state and is the most effective way to avoid the deleterious consequences of prolonged hypermetabolism.[10]

Burn critical care requires control of the patient's environmental temperature. Burn patients have enormous and invisible evaporative water and energy losses if they are maintained in the typical cool dry air of a general hospital.[11] Burn units and burn operating rooms must be engineered to maintain high ambient temperature and humidity to avoid the difficult problem of hypothermia and excessive energy loss.

■ Initial Evaluation and Burn-Specific Secondary Survey

Burn patients often spend many hours in transport before reaching the location of definitive care, and their initial evaluation and management must be completed outside the burn unit setting. Often when patients arrive in the intensive care unit (ICU) where definitive care will be rendered, a complete burn-specific secondary survey has not been completed.[12] It is essential for the intensivist to have a familiarity with

TABLE 206-1	The Four Phases of Burn Care, with Physiologic Changes and Objectives		
Phase and Timing	*Physiologic Changes*	*Objectives*	
1: Initial evaluation and resuscitation, 0 to 72 h	Massive capillary leak and burn shock	Accurate fluid resuscitation and thorough evaluation	
2: Initial wound excision and biological closure, days 1-7	Hyperdynamic and catabolic state with high risk of infection	Accurately identify and remove all full-thickness wounds and achieve biological closure	
3: Definitive wound closure, day 7 to week 6	Continued catabolic state and risk of non-wound septic events	Replace temporary with definitive covers, and close small complex wounds	
4: Rehabilitation, reconstruction, and reintegration, day 1 through discharge	Waning catabolic state and recovering strength	Initially to maintain range of motion and reduce edema; subsequently to strengthen and facilitate return to home, work, school	

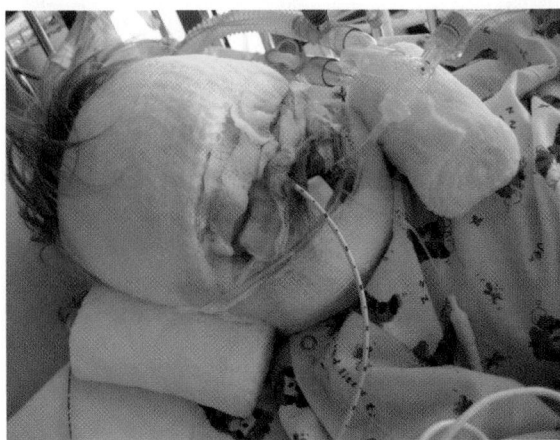

Figure 206-1   A twill-tie harness is a reliable way of securing the endotracheal tube. Protective pads may reduce injury to oral commissures. Tube security should be regularly assessed because reintubation can be very difficult in this setting.

these issues so burn-related pathology and coexisting injuries are not overlooked. Evaluations should follow the format taught by the Advanced Trauma Life Support course. All seriously burned patients should be approached as having potential multiple trauma.[13]

INITIAL EVALUATION

The primary survey of the burn patient is similar to that of the trauma patient, although there are a few important differences worthy of emphasis. First among these is the progressive mucosal edema that may compromise airway patency in the early hours after burns. This is especially true in young children because of their much smaller airway.[14] Progressive stridor or hoarseness should prompt visualization and/or intubation of the airway. Ideally, this need is anticipated before the crisis stage so proper equipment and personnel can be gathered, facilitating smooth tube placement. The facial and airway edema that is so common makes the burn patient's airway among the most challenging to control. Reintubation can be exceedingly difficult if not

impossible after airway edema has progressed, making accidental extubation a potentially lethal complication. Security of the endotracheal tube should be regularly assessed. A twill-tie harness is a reliable method of securing the endotracheal tube (Figure 206-1).

Secure, reliable vascular access is also essential for burn resuscitation and usually requires central venous access. Sometimes it is best to wait until volume depletion has been corrected with peripheral lines to more safely place central venous, or especially arterial, catheters.

BURN-SPECIFIC SECONDARY SURVEY

In parallel with the trauma secondary survey, a burn-specific secondary survey will identify many of the unique insults associated with this type of injury. This survey should begin with a thorough history. At this time, the best opportunity exists to elicit important points of medical history and mechanism of injury. Important points include details of the injury mechanism, neurologic status at the scene, extrication time, and tetanus immune status. Highlights of the burn-specific secondary survey are described in the following paragraphs.

The ocular and otolaryngologic examination should begin with palpation of the head and face for signs of coincident blunt or penetrating trauma. The globes should be examined early, prior to the development of facial and eyelid edema, which will limit examination (Figure 206-2).[15] Serious globe burns impart a clouded appearance to the cornea, and fluorescein staining will detect more subtle injuries. Tarsorrhaphy is virtually never indicated acutely, because lid edema will generally provide excellent globe coverage even in the presence of serious lid burns. Pressure on the burned ear and occiput is avoided. Topical mafenide acetate is applied, as it will penetrate the relatively avascular underlying cartilage.[16] Signs of inhalation injury, such as carbonaceous debris and singed nasal hairs, are noted on examination of the nose and throat. Ties securing endotracheal and nasogastric tubes should be checked so that pressure on the nasal septum or oral commissures is avoided.

The initial neurologic evaluation centers on exclusion of coincident neurologic injury and control of pain and anxiety. Even if they arrive alert and oriented, patients with serious burns typically become obtunded over the succeeding hours and days, if only because of the effects of pain medications and sleep deprivation. It is therefore important to exclude central nervous system trauma if the mechanism of injury is either unknown or consistent with such trauma. There should be a low threshold for ordering a computed tomographic scan of the head and spine, based on mechanism of injury. Pain and anxiety management should begin during the initial evaluation, within limits of safety.[17] Good pain control may have physiologic as well as the obvious psychological benefits. In the emergency setting, this is best done with

---

Box 206-1

MODIFIED BROOKE RESUSCITATION FORMULA

0-24 Hours
Adults and children > 10 kg:
  Lactated Ringer's: 2-4 mL/kg/% burn/24 h (first half in first 8 h)
  Colloid: none*
Children < 10 kg:
  Lactated Ringer's: 2-3 mL/kg/% burn/24 h (first half in first 8 h)
  Lactated Ringer's with 5% dextrose: 4 mL/kg/h
  Colloid: none

24-48 Hours
All patients:
  Crystalloid: to maintain urine output. If silver nitrate is used, sodium leaching will mandate continued isotonic crystalloid. If other topical is used, free water requirement is significant. Serum sodium should be monitored closely. Nutritional support should begin, ideally by the enteral route.
  Colloid: (5% albumin in lactated Ringer's):
    0%-30% burn: none
    30%-50% burn: 0.3 mL/kg/% burn/24 h
    50%-70% burn: 0.4 mL/kg/% burn/24 h
    >70% burn: 0.5 mL/kg/% burn/24 h

*Increasingly, early colloid infusion (generally 5% albumin) is being used in patients with very large burns, particularly if they are young or resuscitation is not going smoothly.
Note: The Modified Brooke formula is a common consensus formula that is only useful in individual patients if adjusted to physiologic endpoints. Like all resuscitative formulas, it is a helpful starting point, but optimum-quality resuscitation requires the bedside presence of a physician capable of regularly evaluating resuscitation endpoints.

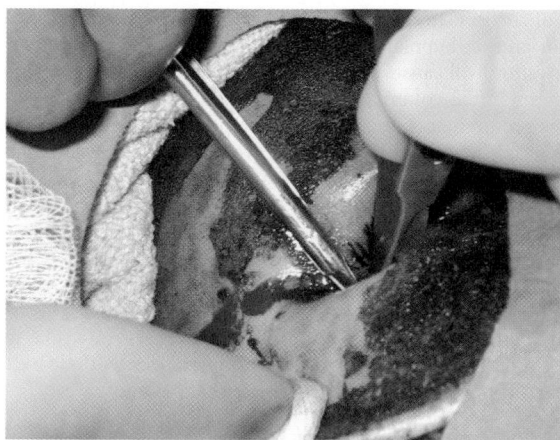

Figure 206-2 Globes should be examined early, before development of facial and eyelid edema limits examinations. Serious globe burns impart a clouded appearance to the cornea, and fluorescein staining will detect more subtle injuries. Tarsorrhaphy is virtually never indicated acutely, because lid edema will generally provide excellent globe coverage even in the presence of serious lid burns. In some patients, lateral canthotomy, pictured here, can reduce critically elevated intraocular pressures.

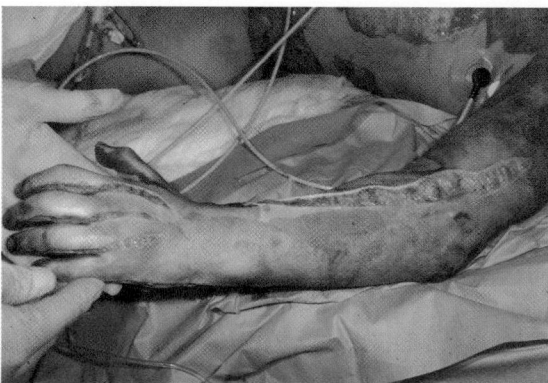

Figure 206-4 Properly performed escharotomy will result in immediate improvement in extremity blood flow.

incremental administration of small doses of narcotics and benzodiazepines. When caring for paralyzed or obtunded patients, it is important to make sure there is no pressure on peripheral nerves, so that neuropathies are avoided. Finally, those burned in structural fires should be assessed for carbon monoxide (CO) exposure by history, neurologic examination, and determination of a carboxyhemoglobin level, because selected patients with significant exposure may benefit from hyperbaric oxygen treatment.[18]

The cervical spine and neck should be assessed for trauma, based on mechanism of injury. Extremely deep circumferential neck burns may require escharotomy to facilitate normal venous drainage of the head.

The chest wall should be assessed for compliance and symmetrical air movement. Patients with deep near-circumferential or circumferential chest wall burns may require escharotomy to facilitate ventilation (Figure 206-3). If properly performed, escharotomy of the torso markedly enhances compliance.

Most patients are hypovolemic at the time of presentation and respond promptly to volume administration. Some patients, especially the elderly, will have previously unsuspected myocardial disease that may become clinically important during the stress of resuscitation.

Some data also exist to support the existence of a myocardial depressant factor in some patients with very extensive injuries.[19] Patients who do not respond as expected to calculated resuscitation volumes may benefit from invasive monitoring, pulmonary artery catheterization, or cardiac ultrasonography.

Genitourinary evaluation is limited in this setting. The foreskin should be reduced over the bladder catheter so paraphimosis is not the result of progressive edema during resuscitation.

Burned extremities should be examined for other trauma, based on mechanism of injury. It can sometimes be difficult to identify fractures in this setting, so liberal use of radiography is appropriate. Fractured and burned extremities are initially stabilized with external splints, prior to placement of external fixators.

Perhaps the most important component of evaluating the extremities is to identify areas at risk for loss of perfusion with progressive edema during resuscitation and to develop an effective monitoring plan. Resuscitation-associated edema can cause profound limb ischemia secondary to swelling under a circumferential eschar or within inelastic muscle compartments. This complication is seen in patients who have suffered deep extremity burns (especially if circumferential) or high-voltage electrical injuries. Low-pressure flow in the extremity should be monitored, commonly using a Doppler probe to demonstrate flow in the palmar arch or digital vessels, because capillary perfusion pressure is only one-third the mean arterial pressure monitored in larger vessels. Prompt identification of ischemic extremities is essential so that escharotomy (Figure 206-4) or fasciotomy (Figure 206-5) can be effected in a timely manner.[20]

The wound should not be allowed to interfere with complete evaluation of the patient. Wounds are assessed for extent using a Lund-Browder or other burn diagram, depth by visual examination, and the

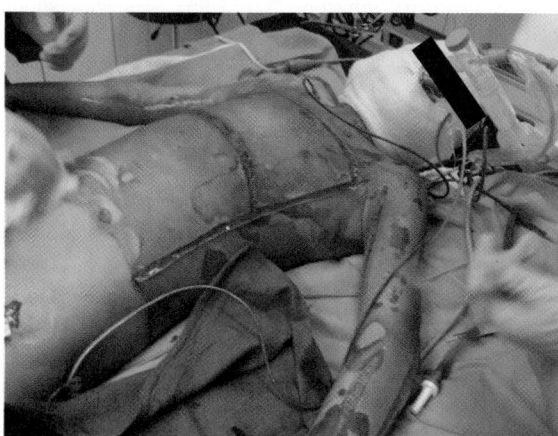

Figure 206-3 Patients with deep near-circumferential or circumferential chest wall burns may require escharotomy to facilitate ventilation. If properly performed, escharotomy of the torso will markedly enhance compliance.

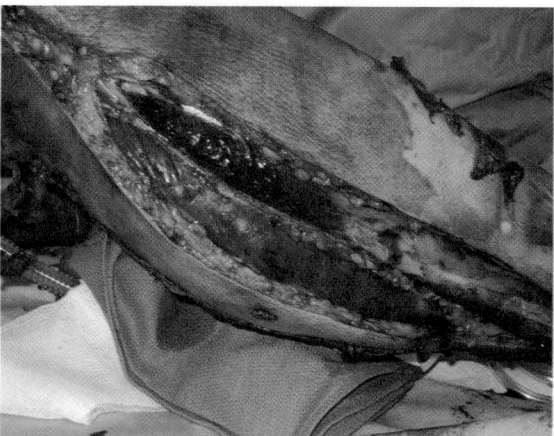

Figure 206-5 Fasciotomy will release pressure in edematous muscle compartments.

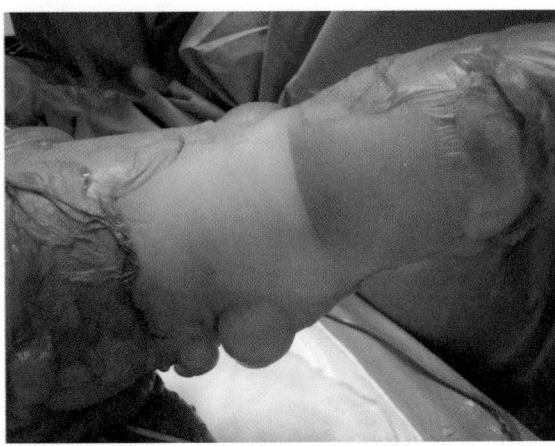

Figure 206-6 Suspicious cases should be filed with appropriate state agencies. Documentation of stated injury circumstances and of actual wounds is essential; wound photography is ideal. Note flexor-sparing pattern here.

presence of circumferential components that may require decompression to ensure adequate perfusion. Typically, wounds are underestimated in depth on initial evaluation.

Carboxyhemoglobin and arterial blood gas determinations and screening baseline laboratories are part of the initial evaluation. Chest radiographs are useful to document proper placement of catheters and tubes and the absence of chest trauma. Inhalation injuries typically do not cause early radiographic changes.

Abuse or neglect should be considered when evaluating all burns, not just those in young children. Approximately 20% of burns in young children are reported to state authorities for investigation, but abuse occurs in all age groups.[21] Burns can also be a result of domestic violence or other interpersonal assaults. Often this determination is not made until the patient has been admitted to the ICU. Suspicious cases should be filed with appropriate state agencies. Documentation of the stated injury circumstances and of the wounds is essential. Wound photography is ideal (Figure 206-6).

Fluid Resuscitation

In the first 1 or 2 hours after a large burn, patients experience little change in intravascular volume or hemodynamics. In fact, patients are often remarkably alert during this period. In the hours that follow, however, the wound releases mediators that are absorbed into the systemic circulation. In addition, stress-related hormones are secreted, and reactive oxygen species are formed on reperfusion of marginally perfused tissues. These and perhaps other factors trigger a diffuse loss of capillary integrity, resulting in extravasation of fluids, electrolytes, and even moderate-sized colloid molecules into soft tissues, including tissues distant from the burn. This remarkable physiologic phenomenon, the so-called capillary leak, abates 18 to 24 hours later and explains the unique resuscitation needs of patients who have sustained large burns. Predicting resuscitation requirements of specific patients involves multiple variables besides burn size: burn depth, vapor transmission characteristics of the wound, patient age and cardiovascular health, resuscitation delay, environmental temperature and humidity, and presence or absence of concomitant inhalation injury. Numerous formulas have been promulgated to roughly guide resuscitation efforts, but none is accurate in every patient.[6,22] A common consensus formula is the modified Brooke formula summarized in Box 206-1. The role of colloid is expanding in burn resuscitation, although there is no uniform agreement. Many providers, the author included, begin 5% albumin at a maintenance rate immediately during resuscitation of patients with larger injuries and find it reduces the incidence of edema-related complications including abdominal compartment syndrome.[7] Patients not responding as predicted to resuscitation efforts should have serum levels of cortisol checked, particularly if cryptic hypotension, hypernatremia, and/or hypokalemia are also in evidence. Inaccurate fluid resuscitation will cause significant morbidity. Formulas can only help determine initial volume infusion rates and roughly predict 24-hour volume requirements; they are so inherently inaccurate that resuscitation should be guided by hourly reevaluation of clinical endpoints. Resuscitation endpoints are summarized in Table 206-2. Measured oxygen delivery and consumption have been used as adjunctive resuscitation guides but are not necessary in the vast majority of patients.

Burn Critical Care Issues

Patients with serious burns require a high level of intensive care to survive their injuries. Several important differences set these individuals apart from other posttrauma critical care patients.

AIRWAY ISSUES

Dangerous and frightening emergencies in the seriously burned involve the airway. Although evaluation and control of the airway are part of the initial evaluation, concerns extend throughout the period of intensive care. Endotracheal tube security should be part of the regular reevaluation of every patient in the burn ICU, because facial and hypopharyngeal edema can make reintubation after unplanned extubation incredibly difficult.[23]

INHALATION INJURY

Inhalation injury remains a clinical diagnosis.[24] A history of closed-space fire, the presence of singed nasal hairs and facial burns, and carbonaceous sputum support the diagnosis of inhalation injury. Fiberoptic bronchoscopy can be useful in equivocal cases, as can technetium scanning. However, in the large majority of patients, the diagnosis is made by history and physical examination. The initial chest radiograph is almost always normal, as are gas exchange and compliance until the endobronchial mucosa sloughs several days later, occluding small airways and leading to subsegmental atelectasis and respiratory insufficiency.

Five clinical consequences commonly occur in patients with inhalation injury: acute upper airway obstruction, bronchospasm, small airway occlusion, pulmonary infection, and respiratory failure.[25] Airway obstruction and bronchospasm are early complications, typically appearing the first day. Airway edema and obstruction are managed with endotracheal intubation. Bronchospasm from aerosolized irritants can be particularly intense during the first 24 to 48 hours and is managed with in-line nebulization β-adrenergic agonists, with infrequent use of intravenous bronchodilators such as terbutaline or low-dose epinephrine infusions. Ventilatory strategies should be designed to minimize automatic positive end-expiratory pressure in this setting.

After 3 to 5 days, with the sloughing of necrotic endobronchial debris, pulmonary toilet commonly becomes an increasing problem.

TABLE 206-2	Age-Specific Resuscitation Endpoints	
Resuscitation Endpoint	**Resuscitation Target**
Sensorium	Comfortable, arousable
Physical examination	Warm extremities, full peripheral pulses
Urine output	Infants: 1-2 mL/kg/h; children: 0.5-1 mL/kg/h; all others: 0.5 mL/kg/h
Base deficit	Less than 2
Systolic blood pressure	Infants: 60-70 mm Hg Children: 70-90 + (twice age in years) mm Hg Adolescents and adults: 90-120 mm Hg

Note: Age-specific resuscitation endpoints should be assessed regularly throughout burn resuscitation and infusions adjusted up or down in 10% to 20% increments to meet needs of the individual patient.

Subsegmental atelectasis occurs, and shunting intensifies. Bronchoscopy to aid pulmonary toilet can help clear the airways.

Depending on how it is defined, as many as 50% of patients with inhalation injury will develop pulmonary infection. Differentiating between pneumonia (lobar involvement) and tracheobronchitis (purulent infection of the denuded tracheobronchial tree) is often difficult, but the difference is not really clinically important. Anyone who has fever and newly purulent sputum should be treated with antibiotics, guided by sputum cultures. Pulmonary toilet is particularly important in these patients.

Respiratory failure is unfortunately common in patients with inhalation injury and can be well managed with a pressure-limited ventilation strategy based on permissive hypercapnia.[26] Patients who fail this can sometimes benefit from investigational modes of support such as inhaled nitric oxide or extracorporeal oxygenation, although the utility of the latter is quite limited in burn patients, owing to the need for anticoagulation.[27,28]

CARBON MONOXIDE AND CYANIDE EXPOSURE

Patients injured in structural fires are commonly exposed to high levels of CO. Although an obtunded state in this clinical setting can be due to other causes such as intoxication, trauma, or anoxia, hyperbaric oxygen (HBO) has been reported to improve the prognosis of patients who have suffered very severe CO exposure.[18] There are controlled data both supporting[29] its use and refuting the utility of HBO,[30] so clinical judgment must be brought to bear in the decision whether to use this form of therapy in individual patients.

CO binds and inactivates heme-containing enzymes such as hemoglobin and the cytochromes. The binding of CO and hemoglobin forms carboxyhemoglobin, which does not deliver oxygen, resulting in acute physiologic anemia, much like an isovolemic hemodilution. A serum carboxyhemoglobin level of 50% is similar to an isovolemic hemodilution to 50% of the baseline hemoglobin concentration. This level of carboxyhemoglobin results in unconsciousness, implying that other mechanisms are also involved in the pathophysiology of CO injury. CO binding to the cytochrome system in the mitochondria probably interferes with oxygen utilization. Approximately 10% of patients with severe CO exposure have been reported to develop severe delayed neurologic sequelae.[31]

There are two practical treatment options: 100% normobaric oxygen or HBO. There are well-designed clinical studies both supporting and refuting the utility of HBO for CO poisoning.[29,30] Proponents cite a decreased incidence of delayed neurologic sequelae in those treated with HBO. In patients with very severe CO poisoning with either very high carboxyhemoglobin levels or neurologic impairment not otherwise explainable, HBO is probably warranted if it can be safely administered.

Commonly recommended HBO treatment is 2 or 3 atm for 90 minutes, with three 10-minute "air breaks" (breathing of pressurized room air rather than pressurized oxygen) to decrease the incidence of seizures. Most treatments are delivered in monoplace chambers, making it more risky to attempt treatment in unstable patients. Other relative contraindications are wheezing or air trapping, which increase the risks of pneumothorax or gas embolism, and high fever, which increases the risk of seizures. Before placement in the chamber, endotracheal tube balloons should be filled with saline to avoid balloon compression–associated air leaks, and upper body central venous cannulation should be avoided if possible to avoid sudden enlargement of an occult pneumothorax during decompression.[32]

Hydrogen cyanide is detected in the smoke from many structural fires and in the serum of some burn patients. At a high enough concentration, cyanide causes failure of oxygen utilization at the cytochrome level, with a secondary unexplained metabolic acidosis. Cyanide poisoning can be treated with amyl nitrate and sodium thiosulfate.[33] However, cyanide is rapidly metabolized in resuscitated patients, making specific treatment generally not necessary or useful.

PAIN AND ANXIETY MANAGEMENT

Undertreatment of pain and anxiety was very common in the past, and burn intensivists need to pay particular attention to this issue. Reasons for undertreatment are related to the extraordinary drug doses required to adequately address pain in seriously burned patients and consequent fear of respiratory depression, addiction, and litigation. The opiate and benzodiazepine tolerance of patients with large open wounds is truly remarkable.[34] Once wounds are closed, drug needs rapidly decrease, and addiction is rare. The best way to eliminate burn pain is prompt wound closure.

Unfortunately, control of pain and anxiety is very difficult in burn patients. Successful management is greatly aided by a set of guidelines. One such program addresses four clinical states: intubated acute, nonintubated acute, chronic acute, and reconstructive patients.[35] Within each clinical state are separate guidelines for background pain, background anxiety, procedural pain, procedural anxiety, and transition to the next clinical state. Guidelines seem most effective when they use a limited formulary and emphasize dose ranging based on regular assessment of objective efficacy. Attention to the issue has physiologic as well as the obvious psychological benefits. Reduced secretion of catecholamines may decrease systemic hypermetabolism, and treatment-related acute stress is reduced.[36]

OCULAR EXPOSURE

Contraction of burned eyelids and facial skin can cause exposure of the globe in the days or weeks after burns.[15] If unchecked, this will result in exposure and then desiccation of the globe, with secondary keratitis and corneal ulceration. Infected corneal ulcers rapidly lead to globe perforation because the cornea is almost avascular and tolerates desiccation and infection very poorly. When minimal or moderate, globe exposure can be managed with frequent ocular lubrication. Acute eyelid release should be done promptly if exposure is severe or keratitis does not resolve with lubrication over a few days.

PERIPHERAL NEUROPATHIES

Peripheral neuropathies are more common than is usually appreciated in burn patients.[37,38] They can be caused by direct thermal damage to peripheral nerves or by the many metabolic disturbances seen during acute burn care. A minority of these lesions are caused by constricting eschar, compartment syndrome, or improperly filled splints. Extremities at risk should be monitored for compartment syndrome and constricting eschar. These issues are best addressed surgically as early as possible. Heavily sedated patients or those under general anesthesia in the operating room should be examined to make sure that traction and pressure injuries are avoided.

GASTROINTESTINAL ISSUES

Curling's ulcers were a common cause of massive upper gastrointestinal bleeding in the past. This is now an infrequent occurrence with better resuscitation, which decreases splanchnic ischemia. Routine use of prophylactic gastric alkalinization also has been important. Patients with serious burns should be treated with empirical histamine-receptor blockers, proton-pump inhibitors, and/or antacids until they are tolerating tube feedings and are at low enough risk that this therapy can reasonably be stopped. Calculous or acalculous cholecystitis in the critically ill burn patient is easily missed and can be the cause of significant illness. Fevers are often assumed to be secondary to the wound. Cholestatic blood chemistry values and modest clinical jaundice are identical to the changes that typify hepatic insufficiency. If untreated, gangrenous cholecystitis associated with peritonitis and sepsis can result. Diagnosis is easily made by bedside ultrasonography. Treatment can be either laparoscopic or open cholecystectomy. In the critically ill patient, percutaneous transhepatic drainage is a very reasonable alternative.[39]

Although uncommon, pancreatitis is a reported complication seen in patients with very large burns.[40] Like cholecystitis, it is easily missed until the condition is far advanced. Abdominal distention and ileus, with tenderness in those who are conscious, should prompt measurements of serum amylase and lipase concentrations as well as appropriate abdominal imaging in selected cases. Most patients can be treated with bowel rest, although pseudocysts and abscesses have been reported in this population.

Bowel ischemia and necrosis are complications seen generally in those with prolonged burn shock, often part of a delayed resuscitation syndrome. These complications present as ileus and then peritonitis. Bowel necrosis is lethal unless operated on promptly. It is a frequently reported autopsy finding in patients dying of burns.[41,42]

Superior mesenteric artery syndrome is a rare occurrence but should be seriously considered in patients with major weight loss during the acute phase of injury who develop intractable vomiting in the recovery phase of their illness. It is due to compression of the duodenum in the angle between the aorta and superior mesenteric artery.[43] Diagnosis is by barium swallow, and treatment is a combination of parenteral nutrition and tube feedings past the point of obstruction if possible.

Finally, it is easy to miss more common abdominal pathology in the setting of burns. Appendicitis can be a lethal complication first diagnosed at autopsy. Constipation from narcotic use and inactivity is common and is ideally prevented with a bowel regimen.

NUTRITIONAL SUPPORT

Burn patients need accurate energy and protein support. Underfeeding and overfeeding have adverse sequelae. Ideally, tube feedings are begun during resuscitation.[44] Most patients do well with continuous intragastric tube feedings, although some require postpyloric feedings.[45] Enteral nutritional support can be started through a nasogastric sump tube so that gastric residuals can be used to help determine tolerance of the feedings initially.[46] Parenteral support is useful during periods when ileus is likely, such as during septic episodes or periods when high-dose vasopressor support is needed, or during the perioperative period. Transient parenteral support can be particularly important in hypermetabolic young children who are very catabolic and do not tolerate prolonged periods of fasting.

Goals for nutritional support for burned patients are controversial. There are a variety of formulas designed to predict these needs, but actual requirements vary widely and unpredictably in individual patients. Consensus recommendations are as follows: approximately 2.5 g/kg/d of protein should be provided, and the caloric load should be between 1.5 and 1.7 times the calculated basal metabolic rate or 1.3 to 1.5 times the measured (by indirect calorimetry) resting energy expenditure.[47,48] Nutritional support should be adjusted throughout the illness, based on specific endpoints. Serial physical examination, quality of wound healing, nitrogen balance, and indirect calorimetry can be integrated to assess the adequacy of support and help fine-tune the predictions of nutritional equations.

INFECTIOUS DISEASE ISSUES

Through loss of skin, necrosis of the endobronchial epithelium, and invasive devices, serious burns impair the host's physical barriers to bacteria while interfering with immune function. Therefore, burn patients are prone to virulent infectious complications. Anticipation of these infections will help minimize infectious morbidity and mortality.

Historically, wound sepsis has been the great killer in burn units, and burn wound infections remain surprisingly common today.[49] Diagnosis of wound sepsis is generally clinical, based on signs and symptoms of systemic infection along with changes in wound appearance. The diagnosis can be supported by wound biopsy and quantitative cultures, but both of these diagnostic techniques are infamously inaccurate, making a clinical diagnosis the most reliable.[50]

TABLE 206-3	Topical Agents Used in Wound Management
Agent	**Characteristics**
Silver sulfadiazine	Painless on application, fair to poor eschar penetration, no metabolic side effects, broad antibacterial spectrum
Mafenide acetate	Painful on application, excellent eschar penetration, carbonic anhydrase inhibitor, broad antibacterial spectrum
0.5% Silver nitrate	Painless on application, poor eschar penetration, leaches electrolytes, broad spectrum (including fungi)

The best way to prevent wound sepsis is to identify and excise deep burns within the first few days after injury and to close the resulting wounds. Topical agents are only an adjunct to this effort and cannot on their own be relied upon to prevent wound sepsis but can delay the onset of wound sepsis in deep wounds. They can also serve to minimize desiccation and colonization of healing wounds. There are several agents in wide general use; the most common are listed in Table 206-3. All have specific advantages and disadvantages. Use of aqueous silver nitrate commonly promotes development of hyponatremia and hypokalemia. Use of mafenide acetate, which inhibits carbonic anhydrase, leads to development of metabolic acidosis, making it more difficult to use permissive hypercapnia for the management of patients with severe respiratory failure. Silver sulfadiazine application leads to large losses of free water across the burn wound eschar.

Antibiotic use must be focused. Too-liberal empirical use will lead to development of resistant organisms. Burn physiology, in the absence of infection, includes fever and a hyperdynamic circulation. When systemic infection is suspected, a careful physical examination and wound inspection should be done and cultures taken, particularly of blood, urine, and sputum. If the patient is hypotensive or otherwise unstable, it is reasonable to start a short course of empirical antibiotic treatment while awaiting return of blood cultures. Clinical deterioration of the burn patient is most often related to infection.

Infection-control practices should be routine and relatively rigid in burn units. This patient population has a high incidence of infection in general, and resistant bacterial species are very common. Universal precautions should be practiced in all patients. The use of prophylactic antibiotics is not advised.[51]

PREVENTION AND RECOGNITION OF COMPLICATIONS

Some common burn complications are itemized in Box 206-2. Optimally, complications should be diagnosed early through regular careful physical examinations, aided by a high degree of suspicion.

Rehabilitation Therapy in the Burn Intensive Care Setting

Good burn care is extremely multidisciplinary. Physical and occupational therapists should be involved from the outset and strategies implemented to avoid common contractures that will otherwise interfere with recovery later (Table 206-4). Typically, physical therapy includes passive movement of all joints through an appropriate range of motion and static positioning in ways that minimize the risk of deformity. Involvement of physical and occupational therapists escalates as patients progress toward recovery; many hours of treatment are required each day after wound closure. Burn patients will have a much harder time with subsequent rehabilitation if therapeutic efforts are ignored during the period of protracted critical illness.[12,52]

It is helpful for physical and occupational therapists to be involved in operative planning. Therapists need to be aware of the sequence of planned operations, because these events will impact therapy plans, splinting strategies, and ability to mobilize joints. Therapists may also use range-of-motion exercising in selected patients after induction of

Box 206-2

COMMON COMPLICATIONS IN BURN PATIENTS

Cardiovascular

Endocarditis and suppurative thrombophlebitis are intravascular infections that typically present as fever and bacteremia without signs of loca infection.

Hypertension occurs in up to 20% of children and is best managed with β-adrenergic blockers.

Venous thromboembolic complications are so infrequent in patients with large burns that routine prophylaxis is not routine in all programs. Iatrogenic catheter insertion complications are minimized by meticulous technique.

Pulmonary

Carbon monoxide intoxication, best managed acutely with effective ventilation with pure oxygen, can be associated with delayed neurologic sequelae.

Pneumonia may occur with or without antecedent inhalation injury and is treated with pulmonary toilet and antibiotics.

Respiratory failure may occur early post injury secondary to inhalation of noxious chemicals or later in the course secondary to sepsis or pneumonia.

Neurologic

Transient delirium occurs in up to 30% of patients and generally resolves with supportive therapy when the possibility of anoxia, metabolic disturbance, and structural lesions is eliminated by appropriate studies.

Seizures most commonly result from hyponatremia or abrupt benzodiazepine withdrawal.

Peripheral nerve injuries occur from direct thermal injury, compression from compartment syndrome or overlying inelastic eschar, major metabolic disturbances, or improper splinting techniques.

Delayed peripheral nerve and spinal cord deficits develop weeks or months after high-voltage injury secondary to small-vessel injury and demyelinization.

Hematologic

Neutropenia and thrombocytopenia, as well as disseminated intravascular coagulation, are common indicators of impending sepsis and should prompt appropriate investigations.

Global immunologic deficits associated with burn injury contribute to a high rate of infectious complications.

Renal

Early acute renal failure follows inadequate perfusion during resuscitation or myoglobinuria.

Late renal failure complicates sepsis and multiorgan failure or the use of nephrotoxic agents.

Adrenal

Acute adrenal insufficiency secondary to hemorrhage into the gland presents as hypotension, fever, hyponatremia, and hyperkalemia.

Otolaryngologic

Auricular chondritis secondary to bacterial invasion of cartilage results in rapid loss of viable tissue and is prevented by routine use of topical mafenide acetate on burned ears.

Sinusitis and otitis media can be caused by transnasal instrumentation and are treated by relocation of tubes, antibiotics, and judicious surgical drainage.

Complications of endotracheal intubation include nasal alar and septal necrosis, vocal cord erosions and ulcerations, tracheal stenosis, and tracheoesophageal and tracheoinnominate artery fistulas. The occurrence of such complications is minimized by compulsive attention to tube position, avoidance of oversized tubes, and attention to cuff pressures.

Gastrointestinal

Hepatic dysfunction secondary to transient hepatic blood flow deficits and manifested as transaminase elevations is common during resuscitation from large burns and resolves with volume restitution. Late hepatic failure, beginning with elevations of cholestatic chemistries and progressing through coagulopathy and frank failure, complicates sepsis and multiorgan failure.

Pancreatitis, beginning with amylase and lipase elevations and ileus and progressing through hemorrhagic pancreatitis, is generally coincident with splanchnic flow deficits early and sepsis-induced organ failures later in the hospital course.

Acalculous cholecystitis can present as sepsis without localized symptoms or signs accompanied by rising cholestatic chemistries. A standard radiographic evaluation can be followed by bedside percutaneous cholecystostomy in unstable patients.

Gastroduodenal ulceration secondary to splanchnic flow deficits that degrade mucosal defenses is extremely common and often life threatening if routine histamine-receptor blockers and antacids are not administered.

Intestinal ischemia, which can progress to infarction, is secondary to inadequate resuscitation and splanchnic flow deficits.

Ophthalmologic

Ectropia from progressive contraction of burned ocular adnexa results in exposure of the globe. This requires acute eyelid release. Tarsorrhaphy is rarely helpful, more often resulting in injury to the tarsal plate as contraction forces pull out tarsorrhaphy sutures.

Corneal ulceration which develops after initial epithelial injury, or later exposure due to ectropion, can progress to full-thickness corneal destruction if secondary infection occurs. This is prevented by careful globe lubrication with topical antibiotics in the former case and acute lid release in the later.

Symblepharon, or scarring of the lid to the denuded conjunctiva after chemical burns or corneal epithelial defects complicating toxic epidermal necrolysis, is prevented by daily examination and adhesion disruption with a fine glass rod.

Genitourinary

Urinary tract infections are minimized by maintaining bladder catheters only when absolutely required and are treated with appropriate antibiotics. Neither catheterization nor colonic diversion is usually required for management of perineal and genital burns.

Candida cystitis occurs in those patients treated with bladder catheters and broad-spectrum antibiotics. Catheter change and amphotericin irrigation for 5 days is generally successful. If infections are recurrent, the upper tracts should be screened ultrasonographically.

Musculoskeletal

Burned exposed bone is generally débrided with a dental drill until viable cortical bone is reached, which is then allowed to granulate and is autografted. Patients whose overall condition and wounds are appropriate are managed with local or distant flaps.

Fractured and burned extremities are best immobilized with external fixators while overlying burns are grafted. Burn patients with coincident fractures in unburned extremities benefit from prompt internal fixation.

Heterotopic ossification develops weeks after injury, is seen most commonly around deeply burned major joints such as the triceps tendon, and presents as pain and decreased range of motion. Most patients respond to physical therapy, but some require excision of heterotopic bone to achieve full function.

Soft Tissue

Hypertrophic scar formation is a major cause of long-term functional and cosmetic deformities seen in burn patients. This poorly understood process is heralded by a secondary increase in neovascularity between 9 and 13 weeks after epithelialization. Management options include grafting of deep dermal and full-thickness wounds, compression garments, judicious steroid injections, topical silicone products, and scar release and resurfacing procedures.

Note: Systematic reassessment of seriously ill burn patients facilitates timely detection of complications. It is the very rare burn patient who does not experience complications during their care, particularly while in the intensive care unit. Unfortunately, many common burn complications are obscured by the fevers and hyperdynamic physiology that accompany a large burn.

TABLE 206-4	Common Contractures and Prevention Strategies Useful in the ICU	
Anatomic Area	**Common Contracture**	**ICU Preventive Splinting and Positioning Strategy**
Neck	Flexion	Daily range-of-motion exercises and extension splinting and conformers; split mattress
Shoulder	Adduction	Daily range-of-motion exercises and abduction splinting with axillary splints or troughs
Elbow	Flexion and extension	Daily range-of-motion exercises and alternating extension and flexion splints
Wrist	Flexion and extension	Daily range-of-motion exercises and splinting in functional position (20 degrees of extension)
Metacarpophalangeal joints	Extension	Daily range-of-motion exercises and splinting in functional position (metacarpophalangeal joints at 70 to 90 degrees of flexion, all interphalangeal joints in extension, first web space open, wrist at 20 degrees of extension)
Hips	Flexion	Daily range-of-motion exercises and extension splints and prone positioning (if tolerated)
Knees	Flexion	Daily range-of-motion exercises and knee splints and knee immobilizers
Ankles	Extension	Daily range-of-motion exercises and neutral splints
Metatarsophalangeal joints	Extension	Daily range-of-motion and splinting in functional position; rocker-bottom shoes

anesthesia to better distinguish between physical limitations and anxiety-induced resistance.

INTRAOPERATIVE CRITICAL CARE

Often, burn patients must be subjected to stressful operative procedures to excise and close wounds, even during periods of critical illness and hemodynamic instability. They can only survive these interventions if critical care efforts are continued during the operations. There must be continuous communication between the surgical and anesthesia teams during surgery. Each team must understand what the other is doing and is about to do, so it can anticipate its own next interventions.

Intrahospital transports from the protected environment of the ICU to the operating room must be carefully planned, and skilled people should accompany the patient during transport. Burn patients have huge evaporative heat losses that can rapidly render them hypothermic unless the operating room is kept warm and core temperature is continuously monitored. Hypothermia promotes development of coagulopathy, which can complicate these operations. The intensive care team should be involved in operative events.

Special Injury Considerations

Several "non-burn" illnesses and injuries are commonly referred to burn units because they benefit from its unique set of surgical and critical care resources. The most common illnesses are toxic epidermal necrolysis and purpura fulminans. The most common injuries involve electrical, chemical, tar, and soft-tissue trauma and soft-tissue infections.

ELECTRICAL INJURY

Exposures can be somewhat arbitrarily divided into low voltage ([household] 110-220 volts), intermediate voltage (220-1000 volts), and high voltage (>1000 volts). Patients with good contact to low and intermediate voltages commonly have severe local wounds but rarely suffer systemic consequences such as compartment syndromes or rhabdomyolysis.[53] Patients with good contact to high voltages commonly have compartment syndromes, myocardial injury, fractures of the long bones and spine, and free pigment in the plasma that may cause renal failure if not promptly cleared.[54,55] These patients also suffer from electrical soft-tissue burns, flash burns, and burns from clothing ignition. Many such patients have also suffered blunt trauma during the incident.

After high-voltage injury, cardiac monitoring is a good idea for 24 to 72 hours. Urine should be examined for myoglobin after placement of a bladder catheter. Fluid resuscitation should be started based on surface burn size, but this usually does not correlate well with deep tissue injury, so resuscitation must be closely monitored and titrated to the patient's physiology. Compartment syndromes are common, and this should be considered. Compartments at risk should undergo serial reexamination and be decompressed in the operating room when an evolving compartment syndrome is suspected. Wounds associated with the injury are excised and closed in the following days with a combination of skin grafts and flaps.

COLD INJURY

Cold injuries often generate wounds best cared for in the burn unit; initial management is usually conservative. Necrotic tissue is excised when demarcation is clear, and the resulting wounds are grafted. These patients very often suffer coincident hypothermia which must be managed, often in the ICU. If patients present with ischemic extremities with less than 24 hours of thawed warm ischemia time, diagnostic angiography may be considered in selected stable patients. If there is no flow despite intraarterial vasodilators, thrombolytic therapy may be appropriate.[57]

CHEMICAL AND TAR INJURY

Chemical injuries can be associated with both local and systemic effects. Poison control centers should be consulted, particularly as regards systemic toxicities. It is essential to protect staff from exposure to the chemicals during removal. Most agents can be irrigated off with tap water for 30 minutes, although some, particularly alkaline substances, may take longer. When the "soapy feeling" alkaline substances often impart to the gloved finger is gone, or when litmus paper indicates a neutral pH, irrigation may be stopped. Hydrofluoric acid, especially in concentrated form, may result in severe acute hypocalcemia, because the fluoride anion strongly binds divalent cations.[56] Subeschar injection of 10% calcium gluconate and/or immediate excision of the wound may be lifesaving. Elemental metals such as solid lithium or sodium can ignite on contact with water or air and should therefore be covered with oil. White phosphorus, a component of many munitions, will also ignite on contact with air, and wound particles are ideally covered with wet cloth or gauze. A number of road-surfacing materials are viscous and heated up to 700°F for application. They are designed to stay solid in the hot sun on dark pavement. When these materials splash road workers, the wounds should be quickly cooled by tap water irrigation. Wounds should be soaked in a lipophilic solvent after cooling and then be débrided and grafted as indicated by burn depth, which is often quite deep.

TOXIC EPIDERMAL NECROLYSIS

The cause of toxic epidermal necrolysis remains a mystery. For unclear immunologic reasons, epidermal-dermal bonding is disrupted to a variable degree. Frequently there is an influenza-like prodrome, and usually there is a drug exposure that is believed to trigger the syndrome (commonly anticonvulsants or nonsteroidal antiinflammatory agents). All mucosal surfaces are affected to some degree. Most patients are only affected slightly, but those affected to a large degree have a life-threatening condition and are often referred to burn units for care.[58]

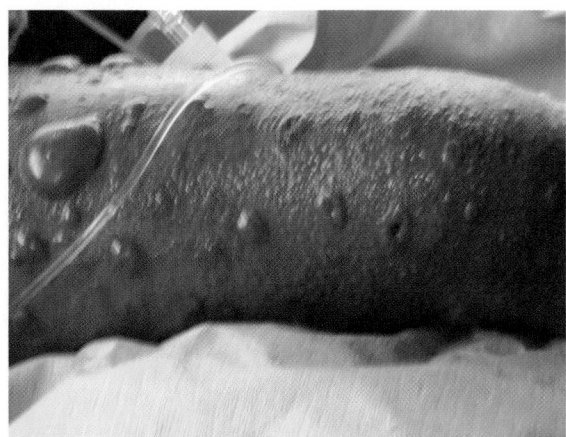

Figure 206-7 The cause of toxic epidermal necrolysis remains a mystery. This patient has both a cutaneous and a visceral wound.

Seriously affected patients with toxic epidermal necrolysis have both cutaneous and visceral wounds—slough of the skin as well as surfaces lined by mucosa or conjunctiva (Figure 206-7). The severity of the skin and mucosal sloughs are not directly related, but the cutaneous wound usually begins first. Although the skin slough is what heralds the disease and what brings most patients to the attention of burn programs, it is generally the easier of the two wounds to manage, with topical antimicrobials and biological dressings.[59] The visceral wound is much more problematic. Conjunctival sloughing threatens the globe.[60] Pulmonary involvement leads to respiratory failure.[61] Gastrointestinal sloughing may lead to bleeding and bacterial translocation. Clinical outcomes have been best when these patients are managed in burn units.[62] The utility of intravenous gamma globulin in toxic epidermal necrolysis remains controversial and is not considered a standard of care.[63]

PURPURA FULMINANS

Patients with meningococcal and other bacterial septic lesions may develop a syndrome in which soft tissues are rendered ischemic by spotty small-vessel thrombosis. This has become less common where vaccination programs have been successful. It has been theorized that thrombosis is due to transient protein C deficiency, which occurs when the liver ceases production of clotting proteins secondary to the septic event.[64] Protein C is an anticoagulant protein that helps maintain control of the process of clotting and has the shortest half-life of the clotting factors (about 6 hours). Patients with purpura fulminans present with organ failures and acute new deep wounds, often heralded by an ominous rash in the affected distribution. These patients are often referred promptly to burn units for care of organ failures associated with large soft-tissue wounds.[65]

SOFT-TISSUE INFECTIONS

Patients with serious soft-tissue infections share many characteristics of burn patients, often having wounds requiring complex surgical care with associated sepsis-induced organ failures. Such patients are increasingly managed in burn programs. Early diagnosis is perhaps the most important component of management, and some patients require operative exploration of severely swollen extremities with severe cellulitis if physical examination and soft-tissue radiography are not diagnostic. Involved tissues should be widely resected. An early "second-look" procedure is often a very wise idea. With resection of involved tissue, sepsis-induced organ failures often quickly improve.

Conclusion

Serious burns present a unique set of challenges to the ICU team that crosses multiple disciplines. However, outcome data support the contention that most survivors of serious burns can have a very satisfying long-term quality of life.[66] A successful outcome requires a coordinated effort by intensive care, surgical, nursing, and rehabilitation therapy professionals during what is often a technically demanding but ultimately rewarding ICU stay.

KEY POINTS

1. Burn care can be divided into four clinical phases: initial evaluation and resuscitation, initial wound excision and biological closure, definitive wound closure, and rehabilitation and reconstruction.

2. Postresuscitation physiology is characterized by high cardiac output, reduced afterload, moderate fever, and muscle metabolism.

3. Burn units and burn operating rooms should be engineered to maintain high ambient temperature to avoid hypothermia and energy loss.

4. The burn-specific secondary survey must often be completed in the ICU.

5. Monitoring and early identification of extremity ischemia secondary to overlying eschar or tight compartments is essential.

6. The wound should not distract examiners from a thorough and complete patient evaluation.

7. No standard resuscitation formula is accurate in an individual patient. Patients must be resuscitated using resuscitation endpoints.

8. Patients with inhalation injuries typically have normal chest radiographs and near-normal gas exchange and compliance early. Over the 3 to 7 days after injury, significant pulmonary dysfunction may occur.

9. The best way to reduce burn wound pain is prompt wound closure.

10. Exposure of the globe must be anticipated and managed to preserve vision.

11. Early nutritional support is essential in light of post-resuscitation physiologic changes. This is ideally accomplished enterally, but parenteral support is also safe when properly administered.

12. Physical and occupational therapy should begin from the outset of burn care.

13. Intensive care management of the patient should proceed throughout operations.

14. Patients with toxic epidermal necrolysis have both a cutaneous and a visceral wound.

ANNOTATED REFERENCES

Zonies D, Mack C, Kramer B, Rivara F, Klein M. Verified centers, nonverified centers, or other facilities: a national analysis of burn patient treatment location. J Am Coll Surg 2010;210:299-305.
These authors examined a large database including 29,971 burn patients treated in 1376 hospitals located in 19 participating states over a 2-year period. They noted that many patients meeting burn center criteria continue to be managed in non–burn center facilities, implying that further cost savings and enhanced results may be realized with increasing regionalization.
Branski LK, Al-Mousawi A, Rivero H, Jeschke MG, Sanford AP, Herndon DN. Emerging infections in burns. Surg Infect (Larchmt) 2009;10:389-97.

These authors reviewed extensive clinical data and illustrate the increasing problem of resistant bacterial species in burn patients. They speculate on effective control measures appropriate for burn units.
Holbrook TL, Galarneau MR, Dye JL, Quinn K, Dougherty AL. Morphine use after combat injury in Iraq and post-traumatic stress disorder. N Engl J Med 2010;362:110-17.
These authors were able to document a strong inverse statistically significant relationship between total morphine dose and PTSD symptoms in a population surviving severe combat trauma, implying that proper pain control during the acute phase of injury will directly reduce psychiatric trauma-related morbidity.

Sheridan RL. Burn care: results of technical and organizational progress. JAMA 2003;290:719-22.

This reference reviews major organizational changes in burn care over the past decades and highlights some of the technical changes that have contributed to the improved outcomes now more routinely seen. The author stresses that this is a result of both technical and organizational progress in burn care.

Sheridan RL, Hinson MI, Liang MH, et al. Long-term outcome of children surviving massive burns. JAMA 2000;283:69-73.

These authors studied long-term outcome at an average of 15 years after injury in 80 young adults who had survived massive burns as children. They were able to show that the long-term quality of life was very satisfying for the large majority.

REFERENCES

Access the complete reference list online at http://www.expertconsult.com.

207 Thoracic Trauma

WALTER L. BIFFL

Thoracic trauma is responsible for approximately 20% of all trauma-related deaths and is second only to head trauma as the primary cause of death at injury scenes. For patients who arrive at the emergency department (ED) alive, rapid diagnosis and treatment of potentially life-threatening injuries are required to prevent death during the "golden hour" of initial resuscitation. However, many thoracic injuries that are not immediately life threatening still have the potential for significant morbidity and mortality. The following is an overview of the diagnosis and management of thoracic trauma.

Initial Assessment

PRIMARY SURVEY

The Advanced Trauma Life Support (ATLS) course of the American College of Surgeons Committee on Trauma[1] provides basic tenets for the management of all injured patients. Initial treatment of seriously injured patients consists of a primary survey, resuscitation, secondary survey, diagnostic evaluation, and definitive care. Although the concepts are presented in a sequential fashion, in reality, they often proceed simultaneously. The process begins with the primary survey, designed to identify and treat conditions that constitute an immediate threat to life. The primary survey includes a stepwise evaluation of the "ABCs": Airway, with cervical spine protection; Breathing; and Circulation.

Airway patency may be compromised by neurologic injury, facial injury, or obstruction (e.g., by tongue, blood, vomitus, teeth or bone fragments). Trauma to the larynx, trachea, or bronchus may also complicate or preclude airway control. Thoracic trauma may also cause life-threatening breathing (e.g., pneumothorax, hemothorax, pulmonary contusion) and circulation (e.g., tension pneumothorax, pericardial tamponade) problems. These must be identified and treated rapidly.

RESUSCITATIVE THORACOTOMY

Some trauma victims who arrive in extremis may be candidates for resuscitative thoracotomy in the ED (EDT). The primary objectives of EDT are to (1) release pericardial tamponade, (2) control intrathoracic hemorrhage, (3) control bronchovenous air embolism or bronchopleural fistula, (4) perform open cardiac massage, and (5) temporarily occlude the descending thoracic aorta to redistribute limited blood flow to the brain and myocardium and attenuate subdiaphragmatic hemorrhage. The critical determinants of survival following this procedure are the mechanism of injury and the patient's condition at the time of thoracotomy. The best outcomes are seen in adult patients with isolated penetrating cardiac injuries who present to the ED with detectable blood pressure; survival averages 35% in large series. For penetrating noncardiac injuries, the salvage rate is 15% for patients who present with vital signs and less than 10% if only signs of life (i.e., pupillary activity, spontaneous respirations, narrow complex cardiac activity) are present. Resuscitative thoracotomy is least beneficial in the treatment of blunt injury or in the absence of signs of life, with only 1% to 2% of patients surviving.[2]

The value of thoracotomy in the resuscitation of a patient in profound shock but not yet dead is unquestioned. Its indiscriminate use, however, renders it a low-yield, high-cost procedure, including risks to the health care team. A recent Western Trauma Association (WTA) multicenter study attempted to determine the limits of EDT to enable the development of rational guidelines to withhold or terminate resuscitative efforts.[3] The WTA multicenter experience suggests EDT is unlikely to yield productive survival when patients: (1) sustain blunt trauma and require more than 10 minutes of prehospital cardiopulmonary resuscitation (CPR) without response, (2) have penetrating wounds and undergo more than 15 minutes of prehospital CPR without response, or (3) manifest asystole without pericardial tamponade. There are likely to be exceptions, and the clinician must individualize care in each case. Based on our experience and that reflected in the current literature, we have formulated a decision algorithm for resuscitation of moribund trauma patients (Figure 207-1). Patients arriving in extremis following blunt injury undergo thoracotomy only if they have a rhythm on electrocardiography (ECG) and have had fewer than 10 minutes of CPR. Penetrating trauma victims in extremis undergo thoracotomy if they have had fewer than 15 minutes (for torso injuries) or 5 minutes (for non-torso injuries) of CPR. If, upon opening the chest, there is no organized cardiac activity and no blood in the pericardium, the patient is declared dead. All other patients are treated according to the injury. Pericardial tamponade is decompressed, and bleeding from cardiac wounds is controlled. Suspected air embolism is treated by application of a pulmonary hilar cross-clamp, vigorous cardiac massage, and aortic root and left ventricular aspiration for air. Intrathoracic hemorrhage is controlled. Cardiovascular collapse from suspected intraabdominal hemorrhage is temporized by occluding the descending thoracic aorta. Those patients who respond to treatment and have a systolic blood pressure above 70 mm Hg are rapidly transported to the operating room for definitive treatment of their injuries.

Pleural Space

PNEUMOTHORAX

Pneumothorax is a common sequela of thoracic trauma. Visceral pleural disruption due to penetrating trauma, blunt shearing, or lacerations from fractured bones allows egress of air into the pleural space as negative intrapleural pressure is created during inspiration. Physical findings include decreased breath sounds, hyperresonance to percussion, and decreased expansion of the chest wall on the affected side. If not relieved, a simple pneumothorax may progress to a tension pneumothorax, especially if the patient is receiving positive-pressure ventilation. In this setting, the mediastinal structures are shifted away from the affected side. In addition to the mechanical impediment to gas exchange, venous return to the heart is impaired secondary to vena caval distortion, and shock ensues. Immediate decompression is mandatory and can be lifesaving (see Tube Thoracostomy).

An open pneumothorax, also called a "sucking chest wound," results from a full-thickness chest wall wound. If the wound diameter exceeds two-thirds of the tracheal diameter, negative intrapleural pressure associated with inspiratory effort results in air entering the pleural space preferentially through the wound. Because of the large hole, there is little chance of tension pneumothorax. However, this can be immediately life threatening because it prevents pulmonary gas exchange. It is immediately managed by an occlusive dressing secured on three sides to prevent sucking of more air but allowing decompression of the pneumothorax until definitive wound closure and tube thoracostomy can be performed.

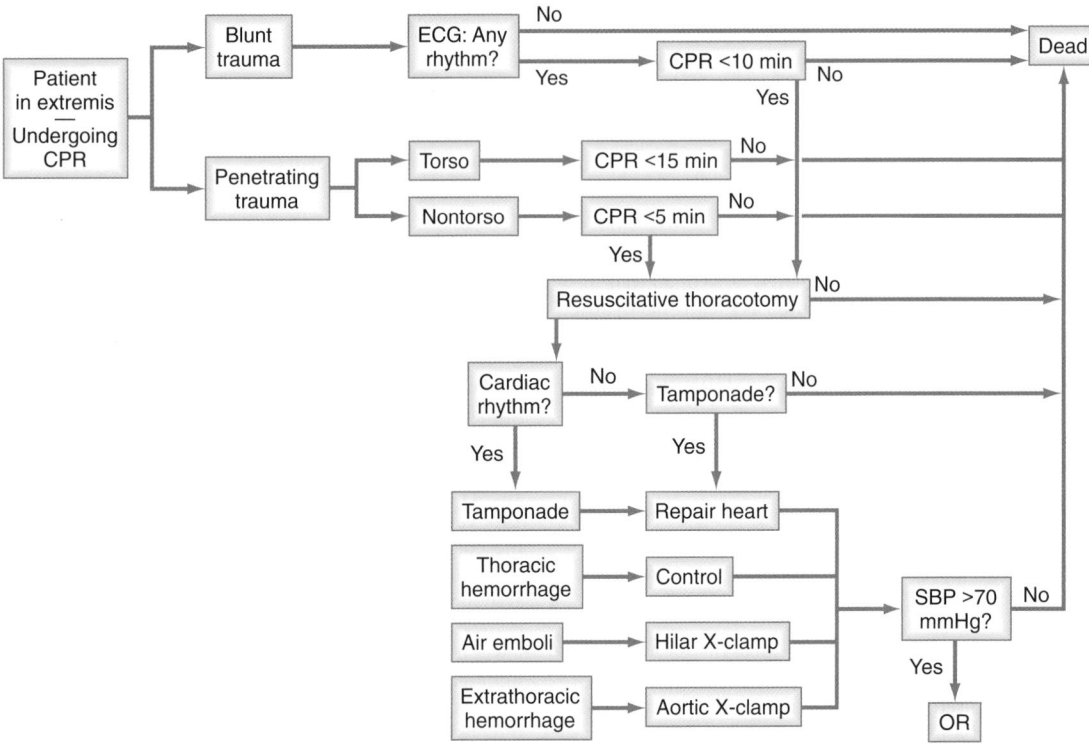

Figure 207-1 Denver Health Medical Center algorithm for emergency department thoracotomy.

With the growing use of thoracoabdominal computed tomography (CT) in the evaluation of trauma patients, small pneumothoraces that are not seen on plain radiographs are often discovered. The treatment of these so-called occult pneumothoraces is not as well defined as the treatment of the usual pneumothorax. Generally they do not require treatment but should be monitored for progression. The notion of "prophylactic" tube thoracostomy in the setting of positive-pressure ventilation has been challenged, but vigilance is important to detect progression to tension pneumothorax in approximately 10% of patients.[4]

Tube Thoracostomy

Tube thoracostomy is the definitive treatment for most pneumothoraces and hemothoraces (see later). The procedure is not difficult and can be performed rapidly, but care must be taken to avoid transdiaphragmatic/lung parenchymal/extrapleural/interlobar fissure placement, as well as kinking. The optimal position is posterior, to facilitate dependent drainage of blood, and directed to the apex of the pleural cavity. Although large-bore (36F) tubes are typically chosen in the ED, the tube size can be individualized. Small-diameter tubes, which cause less discomfort for the patient, can certainly evacuate air and are adequate to drain most small to moderate hemothoraces.

In the setting of tension pneumothorax, if tube thoracostomy is not immediately available, the chest can be decompressed with a large-bore needle as a temporizing measure. Although many authors promote decompression via the second intercostal space in the midclavicular line, injuries to the great vessels and heart have been described as a result of this procedure. Further, catheters may be misdirected or kinked in the pectoralis major muscle or breast tissue, rendering them ineffective, often unbeknownst to the clinician. The author's preference is to insert the needle through the fifth intercostal space in the midaxillary line. This site allows rapid, reliable entry into the pleural space, and the risk of great vessel injury is essentially nil.[5]

The major morbidity related to tube thoracostomy is infectious (pneumonia, empyema), reported in up to 20% of patients. Some investigators have proposed routine prophylactic antibiotics to prevent such morbidity, but this has been controversial. A multicenter prospective randomized clinical trial comparing prophylactic antibiotics versus placebo found that antibiotics did not reduce the incidence of empyema or pneumonia. Moreover, the use of antibiotics was associated with a definite pattern of resistance in subsequent hospital-acquired infections.[6]

Pneumothoraces and air leaks should be resolved before removal of the tube, and ideally, drainage should be less than 2 mL/kg/d. After 12 to 24 hours without an air leak, the tube may be removed while on suction. However, a 6- to 12-hour trial of waterseal drainage is generally warranted to observe for an occult air leak.[7] It has been recommended that tubes be removed at maximal deep inspiration with a Valsalva maneuver, but recurrent pneumothorax may occur in 6% to 8% of patients regardless of respiratory phase.[8] More than 20% of patients require longer than 3 days to resolve an air leak; their hospital course may be expedited by the use of thoracoscopy.[9]

HEMOTHORAX

Hemothorax can range from small and asymptomatic to massive and immediately life threatening. A small hemothorax can be difficult to appreciate on a chest radiograph. In the upright position, blunting of the costophrenic angle requires 200 to 250 mL of blood, and in a supine patient, there may be only subtle haziness of the affected hemithorax. Hemothoraces should generally be drained by tube thoracostomy. However, as with occult pneumothoraces, hemothoraces that are asymptomatic and seen only on CT scan can be managed expectantly. A massive hemothorax is usually the result of a major vascular injury and is life threatening. Indications for thoracotomy include the immediate return of 1500 mL of blood via tube thoracostomy or continued output of more than 200 mL/h for 2 to 3 consecutive hours. A hemodynamically unstable patient with more than 800 mL of blood from the chest should undergo thoracotomy if other sites of bleeding have been excluded. The clinician should be wary of an initial high-volume output that is followed by an abrupt decrease in volume. In this case, a repeat chest radiograph should be obtained to rule out a "caked hemothorax." A second tube may have to be inserted, but if the original tube appears to be well positioned and the hemothorax is not being evacuated, thoracoscopy or thoracotomy is indicated. Hemothoraces associated with massive blunt chest wall trauma can pose special challenges. Ongoing bleeding suggests the need for thoracotomy, but a large incision may compound the bleeding, and diffuse bleeding from bone and soft-tissue disruption may prove difficult to control. In this setting, one might consider arteriography with embolization of intercostal vessels in a hemodynamically stable patient.

Chest Wall Injury

RIB FRACTURE

Rib fractures are estimated to occur in 10% of patients presenting for evaluation by trauma services. Ziegler and Agarwal reported that more than 90% of patients with rib fractures had associated injuries, and half of these patients required intensive care unit (ICU) care.[10] In their series, the overall mortality of patients presenting with rib fractures was 12%. Multiple rib fractures, fractures of the first or second rib, and scapular fractures signify higher-energy injuries and should prompt a search for associated intraabdominal injury or thoracic vascular injury.

Single rib fractures in young patients are generally of little consequence; however, rib fractures in elderly patients can lead to diminished pulmonary function with potentially disastrous infectious complications. Patients over the age of 65 have two- to fivefold increases in morbidity and mortality compared with younger patients with similar injuries.[11,12] Bulger et al. found that for each additional rib fracture in the elderly, the risk of pneumonia increases by 27%, and mortality increases by 19%.[11] A key factor in the management of these patients is pain control to facilitate coughing and clearance of secretions. Epidural catheters have proved to be efficacious and superior to patient-controlled analgesia in this regard and may also modify the immune response.[13,14] Rib blocks may provide immediate relief in the ED or ICU while awaiting epidural catheter placement. Bupivacaine or a lidocaine-bupivacaine mixture may be injected into the intercostal bundle (with care taken not to inject intravascularly) of the fractured ribs and those above and below them. An intercostal catheter provides another alternative in the event an epidural catheter is unavailable or contraindicated.[15]

FLAIL CHEST

Two or more ribs fractured in two or more places produce a flail segment of the chest wall. This segment moves paradoxically—inward during inspiration, outward during expiration—because it is detached from the chest wall and thus susceptible to the forces of intrapleural pressure. The mechanical effects on respiration are related to the size of the flail segment. However, a more important cause of respiratory compromise following flail chest injury is the pulmonary contusion that invariably accompanies it. Treatment is supportive, including supplemental oxygen, analgesia, and pulmonary toilet. Endotracheal intubation with positive-pressure ventilation is sometimes necessary. Surgical stabilization of the flail segment, and rib fracture repair in general, has been performed for decades. At this time, there is a need for multicenter randomized trials with long-term follow-up to identify appropriate patients and optimal techniques.[16]

STERNAL FRACTURE

Early series of sternal fractures described the "steering wheel syndrome" (rapid deceleration, with impact of the sternum on the steering wheel) as the most common cause of sternal fracture. In these series, associated blunt cardiac injury (see later) was common, so sternal fractures were thought to be harbingers of significant occult thoracic injury. More recently, however, sternal fractures have been reported more commonly with the "seatbelt syndrome" (in conjunction with three-point, or bandolier, seat belts). Because the elements of deceleration and steering wheel impact are no longer prominent, associated injuries are relatively infrequent.[17] Stable patients without dyspnea,

ECG abnormalities, or significantly displaced fractures can be safely discharged from the ED. Rest and analgesia are adequate treatment.

Lung Injury

PULMONARY CONTUSION

Pulmonary contusion is a common problem, occurring in one-quarter of patients with injury severity scores (ISS) over 15 and in a majority of patients sustaining major chest trauma. The injury may result from a direct blow, shearing or bursting at gas/liquid or high-density/low-density interfaces, or the transmission of a shock wave. The pathophysiologic changes fundamentally include hemorrhage with surrounding edema, with a broad range of severity up to "hepatization" of the lung. The clinical result is hypoxia and increased work of breathing due to ventilation/perfusion mismatching and decreased pulmonary compliance. Pulmonary contusions may not appear on initial chest radiograph, although they are usually seen by 6 hours after the injury; chest CT is more sensitive at diagnosing early pulmonary contusions. Treatment is supportive, including supplemental oxygen, pain control, pulmonary toilet, and judicious fluid management. There is no role for either routine antibiotics or steroid therapy.[18] Intubation and mechanical ventilation are employed only as necessary. The degree of pulmonary dysfunction usually peaks at 72 hours and generally resolves within 7 days in the absence of associated nosocomial pneumonia. Mortality related to pulmonary contusion has improved greatly with advances in critical care.

Posttraumatic pulmonary pseudocysts are cavitary lesions that occur in approximately 3% of lung parenchymal injuries.[19] They may be asymptomatic or associated with mild nonspecific symptoms and are often noted incidentally on the chest radiograph. Most resolve spontaneously within 2 to 4 months. However, surgical intervention is indicated for infection, bleeding, and rupture. The lesion can be distinguished from an abscess by CT-guided aspiration. If infected, catheter drainage may be required for definitive management.

PULMONARY LACERATION

Penetrating trauma, blunt shearing, or the ends of fractured bones can cause pulmonary laceration and parenchymal disruption. The typical clinical presentation is a hemopneumothorax. Bleeding is usually self-limited, and the vast majority of these injuries are definitively managed by tube thoracostomy alone. Of the 10% of patients requiring thoracotomy, approximately 20% need lung resection. Historically, this group has experienced high morbidity and mortality, with mortality following pneumonectomy approaching 100%. In 1994, Wall and colleagues introduced the concept of pulmonary tractotomy as a nonresectional means of managing penetrating lung injuries.[20] It is indicated for deep through-and-through injuries that do not involve central hilar vessels or airways. The wound tract is exposed by passing clamps (as originally described) or a stapling device (our preference) through the wound and dividing the bridge of lung tissue. Air leaks and bleeding points are sutured, and the wound tract is left open. The literature contains mixed reports of the success of this approach, but the morbidity and mortality compare favorably with those associated with anatomic resections.[21]

Pneumomediastinum

Pneumomediastinum has classically been considered a sign of aerodigestive injury. This was particularly true of pneumomediastinum seen on plain radiography; however, with expanding use of chest CT, pneumomediastinum is being seen with increasing frequency. Recent analyses have found that pneumomediastinum is present on approximately 5% of chest CT scans following trauma, but that only 10% of these patients actually have aerodigestive injuries.[22] In the absence of signs or symptoms or additional suspicious findings on CT scan, further investigation is not necessary.[22,23]

Tracheobronchial Injury

Tracheobronchial injuries are uncommon but should be excluded in the presence of cervical subcutaneous emphysema, pneumomediastinum (see earlier), or pneumothorax with a persistent air leak. Although CT may reveal the injury, the preferred definitive diagnostic test is bronchoscopy. Most penetrating injuries occur in the cervical area and are approached via cervical incisions, with partial or complete sternotomy as needed. Blunt injuries more commonly occur in the distal trachea or right mainstem bronchus and are approached via sternotomy or thoracotomy. Tracheal injuries can usually be repaired primarily or by resection and reanastomosis without tracheostomy; late stenosis is uncommon. On the other hand, laryngotracheal injuries often require tracheostomy as an adjunct to repair, and tracheal stenosis is a common late complication. Absorbable monofilament sutures are preferred. Bronchial injuries may be repaired, but severe disruptions or associated vascular injuries may necessitate pneumonectomy or lobectomy. Positive end-expiratory pressure is avoided postoperatively.[24]

Esophageal Injury

Esophageal perforation from blunt-force trauma is a rare event caused by a sudden rise in intraluminal pressure or by the upper esophagus being crushed between the trachea and a vertebral body. More commonly, esophageal injury is the result of penetrating trauma. Early signs and symptoms of injury can be subtle, so a high index of suspicion is important. Pneumomediastinum should prompt consideration of this injury (see earlier). Barium esophagography is considered the diagnostic study of choice and can be readily obtained in a stable, awake patient.[25] However, videoendoscopy can be done at the bedside virtually anywhere in the hospital and has excellent accuracy, particularly in the pharyngeal area. Thus, it is preferred in critically ill or unstable patients in the ICU or operating room.[26]

Evaluation should be expeditious because delays in definitive care are associated with increased morbidity and mortality. If the injury is identified within 24 hours, it can usually be treated with débridement, primary repair, and drainage. Injuries identified after 24 hours are better treated with débridement and drainage, cervical esophagostomy, and feeding tube placement.[25]

Blunt Cardiac Injury

The term *blunt cardiac injury* (BCI) is preferable to terms such as *myocardial* or *cardiac contusion* or *concussion*. Modifiers such as "with electrocardiographic or enzyme changes," "with complex arrhythmia," "with cardiac failure," "with coronary thrombosis," or "with septal or free wall rupture" may be added. BCI most commonly results from motor vehicle crashes (80%-90%) but can occur following virtually any trauma to the chest. A wide spectrum of cardiac injuries may result, ranging from immediately fatal to occult and inconsequential. The threat of immediate decompensation mandates that trauma care providers be quick to recognize and treat cardiac injuries.

CARDIAC RUPTURE

Cardiac rupture is the most severe form of BCI; 80% to 90% of ruptures are lethal within minutes. Cardiac rupture may result from direct-impact force to the heart or pressure transmitted via venous channels; deceleration with lacerations at junctions between fixed and mobile structures (e.g., atriocaval disruptions); myocardial contusion, with subsequent necrosis and rupture; and broken ribs or sternum penetrating the heart. The most common chambers ruptured are the right atrium and ventricle, followed by the left atrium and then the left ventricle.[27,28] A coexistent pericardial laceration allows free hemorrhage into the pleural or peritoneal cavity. Those who reach the hospital alive typically have a pericardial effusion and may develop pericardial tamponade. A characteristic mill-wheel murmur, the bruit de moulin, may be heard.

PERICARDIAL INJURY

Pericardial tears may result from direct thoracic impact or from an acute increase in intraabdominal pressure. The tears most commonly occur on the left (64%), paralleling the phrenic nerve; the diaphragmatic surface (18%), right pleuropericardium (9%), and mediastinum (9%) are the next most frequent sites.[27] Herniation of the heart through a large tear may be associated with significant cardiac dysfunction. A pericardial rub may be detected on physical examination. The chest radiograph may demonstrate pneumopericardium, displacement of the heart, or bowel gas in the chest. Echocardiography or CT may be required to confirm the injury. In a stable patient, a subxiphoid pericardial window should be performed, followed by sternotomy in the presence of hemopericardium or a visible pericardial tear. An unstable patient may require EDT. Pericardial lacerations should be repaired, but large holes that cannot be closed primarily should be left widely open to prevent future cardiac herniation. A late complication is the postpericardiotomy syndrome, manifested by fever, chest pain, pericardial effusion, a pericardial rub, and ECG abnormalities; this is adequately treated with antiinflammatory agents.

VALVULAR INJURY

Lethal cardiac trauma involves the valves in approximately 5% of patients. The most commonly injured valve is the aortic, followed by the mitral, tricuspid, and pulmonary. The aortic cusps may be lacerated or avulsed when a sudden increase in intrathoracic pressure leads to a concomitant increase in aortic pressure. The result is often acute severe cardiac failure, but a mild injury may present with syncope or anginal symptoms.[29] Violent compression of the heart in early systole during isovolumetric contraction may tear mitral valve leaflets but more commonly ruptures the papillary muscles or chordae tendineae. Acute heart failure may ensue, and a holosystolic murmur of mitral regurgitation is heard.[30] Tricuspid valve injuries are rare; they usually occur in the subvalvular area following compression in late diastole. They are generally of less hemodynamic consequence than aortic or mitral valve injuries, but endocarditis and hepatic dysfunction from chronic venous congestion have been reported. Cardiac catheterization and echocardiography are used to confirm the diagnosis. Most valve injuries are amenable to supportive care until other injuries have been stabilized. Valve repair is generally preferred over valve replacement when feasible.[31]

SEPTAL INJURY

Septal injuries are found in 5% to 7% of patients dying from blunt trauma. Ventricular septal ruptures are much more common than atrial septal injuries; they usually occur in the muscular portion near the apex. Characteristic physical findings include a systolic thrill and a harsh holosystolic murmur heard best at the left sternal edge and radiating to the right, but the symptoms may be delayed for hours or days as the defect enlarges. Atrioventricular conduction abnormalities may also be present, simulating myocardial ischemia, and severe hypoxemia may result from an acute left-to-right shunt. Prompt echocardiography is indicated to establish the diagnosis; cardiac catheterization may be needed.

Small septal defects may heal primarily, allowing expectant management with periodic follow-up. Surgical repair—either primary or with a patch graft—is indicated if the patient is hemodynamically compromised or has a left-to-right shunt with a shunt ratio of 2:1 or greater. Repair of the defect is delayed for several weeks if possible.[32]

CORONARY ARTERY INJURY

Direct injuries to coronary arteries are rare. The left anterior descending artery is most susceptible (76% of cases), followed by the right coronary artery (12%) and the circumflex coronary artery (6%). The sequela of coronary artery dissection or thrombosis is myocardial infarction, with ischemic consequences dependent on the vessel and level of injury. Cardiac catheterization is indicated, and therapeutic angioplasty or stenting may be performed occasionally; however, the usual treatment is medical. Recanalization of arteries is frequently reported, but surgical revascularization or repair of delayed complications related to infarction, such as ventricular pseudoaneurysms, may be indicated.[33]

Coronary artery laceration may result in pericardial tamponade as well as myocardial ischemia. The decision whether to ligate or reconstruct lacerated vessels can be difficult. A nondominant right coronary artery can probably be ligated, but the resultant dysrhythmias may be extremely resistant to treatment. The left anterior descending and circumflex coronary arteries cannot be ligated proximally without causing a large infarct. Reconstruction requires cardiopulmonary bypass, which is frequently poorly tolerated in the early postinjury period and requires systemic anticoagulation. Intraluminal shunts offer a means of minimizing ischemic time while planning elective reconstruction.

DIAGNOSIS, MONITORING, AND TREATMENT

The frequency of the diagnosis of BCI depends on the diagnostic criteria, which may include specific ECG abnormalities (e.g., ventricular dysrhythmias, atrial fibrillation, sinus bradycardia, bundle branch block), cardiac enzyme elevation, or evidence of cardiac dysfunction on echocardiography or nuclear medicine studies. Unfortunately, none of these tests is predictive of the uncommon but life-threatening complications of ventricular dysrhythmias and cardiac pump failure.[34] The pivotal issue is to identify patients at risk and have them in a setting where the complication can be identified and treated.

Our practice guidelines for monitoring patients with suspected BCI are depicted in Figure 207-2. BCI should be suspected in all individuals who sustain major chest trauma. The initial evaluation should include an ECG as part of the secondary survey. Patients with shock from any cause, ischemic changes on the ECG, or significant dysrhythmias are admitted to the ICU. If angina or ischemic ECG changes are noted, a standard "rule out myocardial infarction" protocol is followed. Nonspecific ECG findings are rarely associated with significant BCI, and patients may be discharged after 24 hours of cardiac monitoring if no new symptoms occur. Patients with significant blunt chest trauma who are being admitted for associated injuries should have cardiac monitoring for 24 hours. A subset of patients may not require admission for other injuries. These patients can be safely discharged from the ED if ECG at presentation and at 8 hours is normal, and if a troponin-I level at 8 hours is less than 1.5 ng/mL.[35]

Dysrhythmias are treated by pharmacologic suppression. The management of cardiogenic shock from cardiac pump failure may include early placement of a pulmonary artery catheter to optimize fluid administration and inotropic support. An echocardiogram may be indicated to exclude septal or free wall rupture, valvular disruption, or pericardial tamponade. Patients with refractory cardiogenic shock may require placement of an intraaortic balloon pump to decrease myocardial work and enhance coronary perfusion. Patients who sustain significant BCI can have operative procedures under general anesthesia with a low incidence of cardiac complications; however, they should have close hemodynamic monitoring in the early postinjury period.

Commotio cordis is a distinct entity in which "virtually instantaneous cardiac arrest is produced by nonpenetrating chest blows in the absence of heart disease or identifiable morphologic injury to the chest wall or heart."[36] In a series of 70 cases, Maron and colleagues reported a 90% mortality rate in a young (mean age 12 years) population of patients.[36] An experimental model demonstrated that ventricular fibrillation is reproducibly triggered by a precisely timed blow during a narrow window within the repolarization phase of the cardiac cycle (15-30 msec before the peak of the T wave). Heart block may be produced by a blow during the QRS complex.[37]

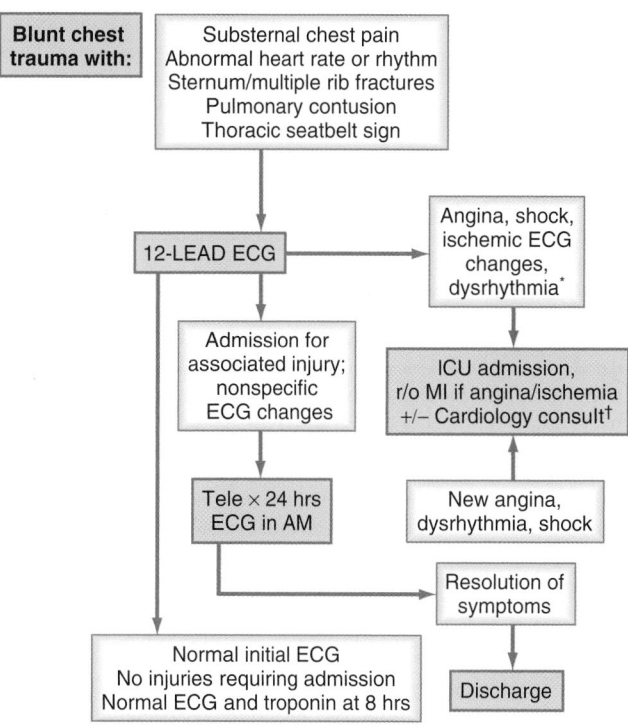

Ischemic changes: ST elevation/depression, T wave inversion in ≥ 2 leads; *Dysrhythmia*: Frequent premature atrial/ventricular contractions, heart block, new atrial fibrillation/bundle branch block
†Echocardiogram may be indicated in selected patients with unexplained or refractory shock, new murmur, or clinical suspicion of pericardial effusion/tamponade

Figure 207-2 Evaluation for suspected blunt cardiac injury: blunt chest trauma with substernal chest pain, abnormal heart rate or rhythm, sternum or multiple rib fractures, pulmonary contusion, thoracic seatbelt sign. Ischemic changes consist of ST elevation or depression or T-wave inversion in two leads. Dysrhythmia consists of frequent premature atrial or ventricular contractions, heart block, new atrial fibrillation, or bundle branch block. Echocardiogram may be indicated in selected patients with unexplained or refractory shock, new murmur, or clinical suspicion of pericardial effusion or tamponade. *ECG*, electrocardiogram; *MI*, myocardial infarction.

Penetrating Cardiac Injury

Cardiac penetration is rapidly lethal in 90% of gunshot wounds and up to 50% of stab wounds. The most important factors for survival are rapid transport to the trauma center, early diagnosis, and immediate treatment. Patients arriving in extremis after penetrating chest trauma should undergo EDT. All patients in shock with penetrating chest injuries between the right midclavicular line and left anterior axillary line should be considered to have a cardiac injury until proven otherwise.[38] The right ventricle, with its maximal anterior exposure, is at greatest risk, followed by the left ventricle, right atrium, and left atrium. Multiple cardiac structures are involved in a third of patients. Stab wounds are more commonly associated with tamponade, while gunshot wounds generally exsanguinate through a large pericardial defect.

Repair of cardiac injuries can be accomplished through either a median sternotomy or a thoracotomy incision. In a hemodynamically compromised patient, left anterior thoracotomy with transsternal extension is used for definitive repair. Otherwise, in a hemodynamically stable patient, sternotomy is generally preferred. A limitation of sternotomy is access to posterior injuries or associated aortic or esophageal injuries. In any case, control of hemorrhage is the first priority. Satinsky clamps are useful in isolating atrial or caval injuries, whereas small ventricular lacerations are controlled digitally. Larger wounds may be stapled. Insertion of a Foley catheter with temporary balloon occlusion of the wound may facilitate repair, but one must be careful to not extend the injury.[39] Wounds that are too large for balloon occlusion are occasionally salvageable using temporary caval inflow occlusion.[40]

PERICARDIAL TAMPONADE

Potential pericardial tamponade should be suspected in all patients sustaining penetrating injuries to the anterior chest wall. Pericardial tamponade can be a two-edged sword: although it may limit initial blood loss, it can prove fatal by restricting diastolic filling of the heart.[41] As blood leaks out of the injured heart, it accumulates in the pericardial sac. Because the pericardium is not acutely distensible, the pressure in the pericardial sac rises to match that of the injured chamber. When this pressure approaches that of the right atrium, right atrial filling is impaired, and right ventricular preload is reduced; ultimately, this leads to decreased right ventricular output. Increased intrapericardial pressure also impedes myocardial blood flow, which leads to subendocardial and later subepicardial ischemia, with a further reduction of cardiac output. This vicious cycle may progress insidiously with injury to low-pressure conduits, or it may occur precipitously with a ventricular wound. Acute tamponade of as little as 100 mL of blood within the pericardial sac can produce life-threatening hemodynamic compromise.

Early diagnosis is key, as the ultimate cardiovascular collapse can be abrupt. Compensatory responses including catecholamine-mediated tachycardia and vasoconstriction can transiently stabilize the hemodynamic status of the patient. Similarly, vigorous fluid administration may improve the patient's vital signs. The classic findings of Beck's triad (hypotension, distended neck veins, and muffled heart sounds) are present in less than 10% of patients; furthermore, Kussmaul's sign (neck vein swelling with inspiration) and pulsus paradoxus (systolic blood pressure drop with inspiration) are not reliable indicators of acute tamponade. In fact, neck veins may not become distended until hypovolemia is corrected. Thus, the surgeon must have a high index of suspicion for pericardial tamponade.

In the setting of suspected pericardial tamponade, ultrasonography using subxiphoid and parasternal views (or formal echocardiography if immediately available in the ED) is extremely helpful if the findings are positive, although a negative ultrasonographic examination may be misleading if there is a pericardial laceration.[42] If pericardial fluid is demonstrated, the patient should be transported immediately to the operating room for sternotomy. However, if ultrasonography is equivocal, a central venous pressure line should be inserted promptly. Persistently elevated central venous pressure in a patient with thoracic trauma should prompt consideration of ultrasound-guided pericardiocentesis or subxiphoid pericardial window. If the pericardial ultrasonography is positive and there will be any delay in getting to the operating room, pericardiocentesis should be done even if the patient appears hemodynamically stable, because subclinical myocardial ischemia can lead to sudden lethal dysrhythmias. The pericardial tap should be performed with a pigtail catheter to allow repeated aspiration during preparation for thoracotomy. In the setting of shock, evacuation of as little as 15 mL of blood may dramatically improve the patient's hemodynamic profile. Pericardiocentesis is successful in decompressing tamponade in approximately 80% of cases; most failures are due to clotted blood within the pericardium. Although a subxiphoid pericardial window can be created under local anesthesia in the ED, hemorrhage may be difficult to control if an injury is found. If pericardiocentesis is unsuccessful and the patient remains severely hypotensive (systolic blood pressure <70 mm Hg), EDT should be performed.

Transmediastinal Penetrating Trauma

Transmediastinal trajectory of a bullet should be considered in the setting of (1) entry and exit wounds on opposite sides of the thorax, (2) a single entry wound with the bullet ending up on the opposite side of the thoracic cavity or in close proximity to the mediastinum, or (3) multiple gunshot wounds to the thorax. Significant injury, especially to the heart or great vessels, often results in prehospital death or hemodynamic instability. There is little controversy regarding the management of unstable patients: they should have emergent thoracotomy. However, stable patients may harbor occult injuries to critical mediastinal structures (heart, great vessels, trachea, esophagus). Consequently, patients have routinely been submitted to a battery of invasive diagnostic tests: echocardiography or subxiphoid pericardial window, arch aortography, bronchoscopy, esophagoscopy, and esophagography.[43] The last two have been employed together to improve on the sensitivity of each test individually. This array of tests can be expensive and time consuming. Further, only a small percentage of hemodynamically stable, asymptomatic patients have clinically significant injuries.[44]

Helical CT of the chest has proved useful in demonstrating the trajectory of missiles in the thorax.[45,46] In the setting of a potential transmediastinal gunshot wound, a CT scan may confirm a trajectory remote from the mediastinum, obviating further testing. A proven transmediastinal trajectory mandates further evaluation. However, rather than performing all the aforementioned tests, the investigation can be tailored to the specific clinical scenario. For example, trajectory near the pericardium warrants echocardiography or pericardial window. If CT suggests great vessel injury, arteriography should follow (see later). Bronchoscopy is indicated for pneumomediastinum, respiratory distress, or bronchopleural fistula or massive air leak. The esophagus is evaluated as outlined earlier. Our current approach to evaluating these patients is outlined in Figure 207-3.

Thoracic Great Vessel Injury

Patients with penetrating injuries to extrapericardial thoracic great vessels usually succumb in the field; however, an occasional patient arrives with a contained hematoma. Early chest radiography is critical to identify hemothorax, as well as a widened mediastinum or apical capping. Patients who are hemodynamically unstable should be taken directly to the operating room; those in extremis should undergo EDT. A reasonable approach can be inferred from the chest radiograph and the location of the wounds. If the patient has a left hemothorax, a left anterolateral thoracotomy in the third or fourth interspace should be performed. Patients with a right hemothorax should likewise be approached via a right anterolateral thoracotomy. Unstable patients with injuries near the sternal notch may have large mediastinal hematomas or may have lost blood externally. These patients should be explored via a median sternotomy with cervical extension, similar to a penetrating zone I neck wound. Hemorrhage should be controlled digitally until the vascular injury is delineated. In a hemodynamically stable patient, angiography can facilitate a more directed approach. Recent series suggest that clinical assessment may be adequate to detect injuries, obviating arteriography in cases in which the suspicion is based on periclavicular trajectory alone.[47,48] However, it must be remembered that collateral flow around the shoulder girdle can result in palpable pulses, even in the presence of a significant subclavian artery injury.

Blunt thoracic great vessel injuries require tremendous force, because the aortic arch branch arteries are protected by strong musculoskeletal tissues. Traction and compression forces are responsible for most injuries. After the aortic isthmus (see later), the most commonly injured artery in the chest is the innominate artery. The clinical presentation is less dramatic than that of penetrating injuries, with the typical signs and symptoms related to arterial insufficiency. CT-angiography is supplanting aortography for diagnosis of injuries.

A median sternotomy, with appropriate extension, is used for exposure of the aortic arch branch vessels. In patients who have undergone EDT, the left anterolateral thoracotomy incision may have to be extended to a bilateral anterolateral thoracotomy ("clamshell"). In exposing the proximal left subclavian artery, it may be necessary to create a full-thickness flap of the upper chest wall. This is accomplished

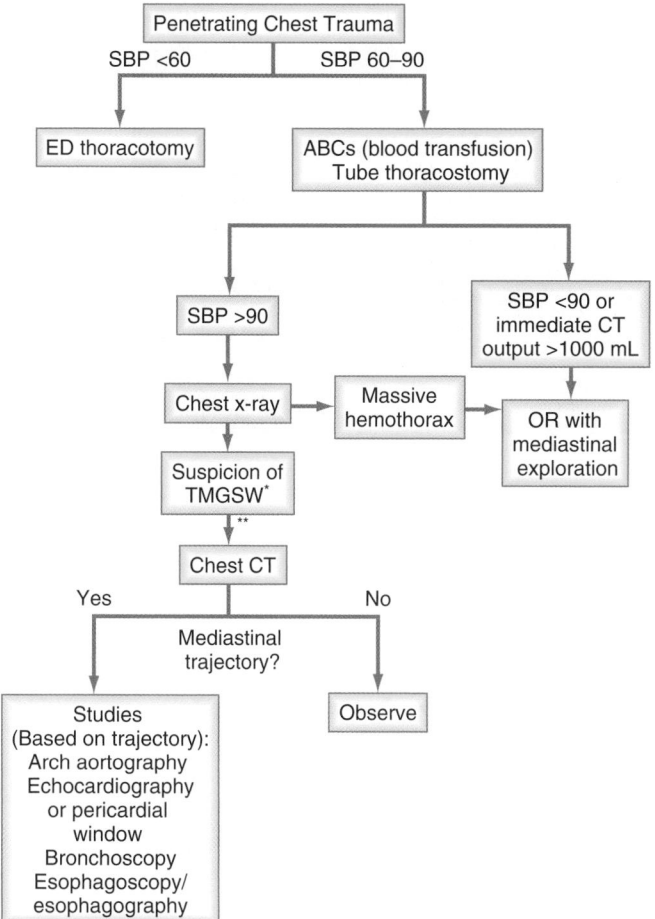

Figure 207-3 Evaluation of suspected transmediastinal gunshot wounds (TMGSWs). *Suspect transmediastinal trajectory in the presence of entry and exit wounds on opposite sides of the thorax, a single entry wound with the bullet located in the contralateral hemithorax or adjacent to the mediastinum, or multiple gunshot wounds to the thorax. **If there is evidence of mediastinal injury (pneumomediastinum, widened mediastinum on chest x-ray), consider proceeding directly to invasive diagnostic testing. *ABCs,* airway, breathing, circulation; *CT,* computed tomography; *ED,* emergency department; *OR,* operating room; *SBP,* systolic blood pressure.

with a partial sternotomy and supraclavicular extension. If necessary, the ribs can be transected laterally, allowing the flap to be folded laterally, but this is rarely required. This incision has been referred to as an *open-book* or *trapdoor thoracotomy.* The midportion of the subclavian artery is accessible via a supraclavicular skin incision.

The great vessels are rather fragile and can be easily torn during dissection or crushed with a clamp. For this reason, injuries adjacent to the aortic arch are oversewn, and a graft is inserted onto a new location on the arch. The graft is then sewn (without tension) to the distal artery. Nonoperative management of nonocclusive peripheral arterial injuries has proved successful, and there are limited data supporting similar management within the thorax for certain patients. Similarly, those lesions associated with severe neurologic injuries are usually managed nonoperatively. Experience with intravascular stenting is growing, although long-term outcomes have not been reported.[49] Clearly unstable patients require operative control and repair; however, it appears that stent graft treatment of subclavian artery injuries is preferred in stable patients.[50]

BLUNT THORACIC AORTIC INJURY

Perhaps the most feared occult injury in trauma surgery is a blunt thoracic aortic injury (BTAI). The mechanism of aortic tears is believed to be primarily a shearing force. The tear usually occurs just distal to the left subclavian artery where the aorta is tethered by the ligamentum arteriosum. In 5% of cases, the tear occurs in the ascending aorta, in the transverse arch, or at the diaphragm. An estimated 85% of thoracic aortic injuries are fatal at the injury scene. A multicenter report from the American Association for the Surgery of Trauma (AAST) analyzed 274 accident-scene survivors of BTAI.[51] Motor vehicle crashes accounted for 81% of the injuries, with frontal impact in 72%, lateral impact in 24%, and rear impact in 4%. Two additional series also documented substantial numbers of BTAI following lateral-impact crashes: 57 of 165 (35%) autopsy cases reported by Burkhart et al.,[52] and 48 of 97 (50%) cases reviewed by Katyal et al.[53] Thus the surgeon should suspect this injury whenever there is significant energy transfer, regardless of directionality.

Chest radiograph is considered the initial screening tool for determining whether further investigation is needed for BTAI. Commonly associated radiographic findings include mediastinal widening, obscured aortic knob, deviation of the left mainstem bronchus (downward) or nasogastric tube (rightward), and opacification of the aorto-pulmonary window (Figure 207-4, *A*). In the AAST multicenter study,[51] widening of the mediastinum on the anteroposterior chest radiograph was present in 85% of cases. However, 7% of patients with torn aortas had normal chest radiographs. Dyer and colleagues reported normal initial radiographs in 13% of patients.[54] Thus, additional investigations are warranted in the setting of significant energy transfer. Thoracic aortography was previously considered the gold standard for diagnosis (see Figure 207-4, *B*). However, helical CT scan is now well accepted as an excellent screening test (see Figure 207-4, *C*).[54-56] When hematoma adjacent to the thoracic aorta is considered a positive finding, the sensitivity of CT for aortic injury is 100%. Most authors advocate omitting the aortogram and operating on the basis of CT alone, but this is up to the individual surgeon. Transesophageal echocardiography is portable and fairly sensitive and specific; however, it is highly operator dependent and is not reliable for visualizing the ascending or transverse aorta or its branches. It has been supplanted by CT, and its primary role may be in following small intimal injuries that are managed nonoperatively. Intravascular ultrasonography is another tool with a poorly defined role.

There are currently a number of areas of controversy in the management of BTAI: immediate versus delayed repair, management of minimal aortic injuries (MAI), and open versus endovascular repair.[57]

Immediate Versus Delayed Repair

Until the 1990s, BTAI was thought to require emergent repair to avoid early rupture. Recognizing significant morbidity and mortality in patients with severe associated injuries and comorbid medical conditions, the concept of immediate repair was challenged. The administration of beta-blockade to decrease systolic blood pressure (<100 mm Hg) and heart rate (<100 bpm), and therefore reduce aortic shear pressure, allowed optimization of associated injuries stabilization of targeting a systolic blood pressure and heart rate.[55] Numerous studies have established the safety of this approach. In fact, a recent AAST prospective multicenter trial found that delayed repair is associated with significant survival benefit.[58] Although patients with major associated injuries are most likely to benefit, the study supported delayed repair in all patients, irrespective of risk factors.

Management of Minimal Aortic Injury

With increasing sensitivity of CT scans (as discussed with regard to pneumomediastinum), more MAIs are being diagnosed. These are defined as small (<1 cm) intimal lesions with minimal to no periaortic hematoma.[59] Fabian and colleagues[51] identified MAI in 10% of BTAI and found that half of these lesions were missed on arteriography. Although the name suggests benign behavior, the Memphis group

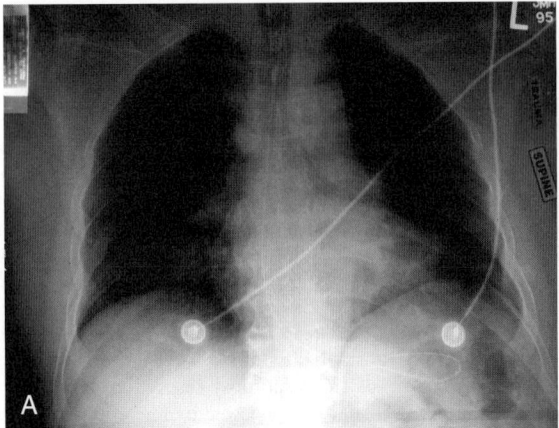

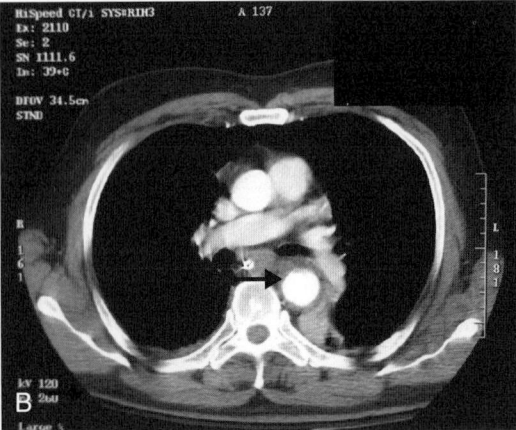

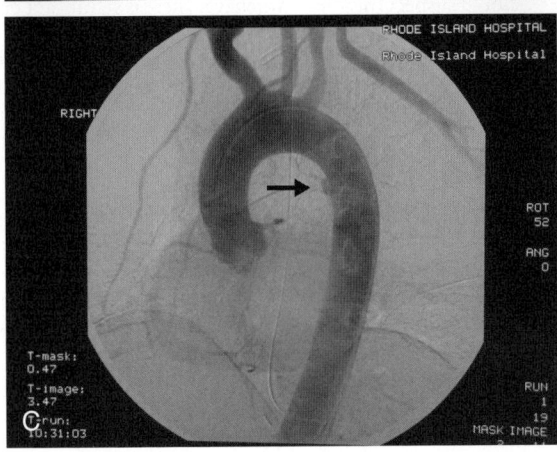

Figure 207-4 Images from patient with descending thoracic aortic injury. **A,** Anteroposterior chest radiograph. Note widened mediastinum and widened left paratracheal stripe, indistinct aortic knob, and slight depression of left mainstem bronchus. **B,** Helical computed tomography (CT) scan of chest. Note periaortic hematoma (arrow). **C,** Digital subtraction arteriogram of aortic arch. Note pseudoaneurysm in the common location, distal to left subclavian artery (arrow).

reported that 50% of MAIs had progressed to pseudoaneurysm formation by 8 weeks post injury.[59] MAIs are generally treated with beta-blockade and CT surveillance.

Open Versus Endovascular Repair

Over the past several years, open repair has been largely supplanted by thoracic endovascular aortic repair (TEVAR).[60] A number of studies have reported lower mortality and paraplegia, as well as fewer blood transfusions and strokes, associated with TEVAR.[49,57,60] However, there are still issues with device-related complications and the need for reinterventions. These issues will likely be improved with developing technology, but long-term studies are needed. In the meantime, TEVAR will no doubt continue to increase.

In those patients who require open repair, a primary concern has been the occurrence of paraplegia from ischemic injury of the spinal cord. Conceptually, two techniques have been advocated. The simpler technique, often referred to as "clamp and sew," is accomplished with application of vascular clamps proximal and distal to the aortic injury. Razzouk et al.[61] have successfully employed this technique in the majority of their patients over a 25-year period. However, this method results in transient hypoperfusion of the spinal cord distal to the clamps, as well as of abdominal organs. In the AAST study,[51] the paraplegia incidence was 1.6% in patients with cross-clamp times less than 30 minutes, but 12% if the time was greater than 30 minutes. A 20-year meta-analysis found a 19% incidence of paraplegia associated with this method and noted that average cross-clamp times were over 40 minutes.[62] The alternative approach is to provide some method for maintaining spinal perfusion during cross-clamping. Two techniques have been used to accomplish this goal, one passive and one active.

Passive shunting uses a temporary extra-anatomic route around the clamps. A heparin-impregnated tube, the Gott shunt, was specifically designed for this purpose. However, blood flow to the distal aorta is inadequate; consequently, this technique is no longer used. With the availability of centrifugal pumps that do not require systemic anticoagulation, the current preferred method is to use either active partial left heart bypass (siphoning blood from the left heart and pumping it to the distal aorta) or full bypass such as femoral-femoral bypass. The former can be a significant benefit in a patient with multiple injuries, particularly in those with intracranial hemorrhage. However, occasional small cerebral infarcts have occurred, so heparin is administered unless contraindicated. The injury may be primarily repaired, or a graft may be inserted. A large multicenter trial suggested that polytetrafluoroethylene is the preferred graft material for aortic replacement, given its long-term patency and apparent resistance to infection.[63]

KEY POINTS

Initial Assessment

1. Initial management of seriously injured patients should follow the tenets of the American College of Surgeons Committee on Trauma Advanced Trauma Life Support course.

2. ED thoracotomy is unlikely to yield productive survival when patients: (1) sustain blunt trauma and require more than 10 min of prehospital CPR without response, (2) have penetrating wounds and undergo more than 15 min of prehospital CPR without response, or (3) manifest asystole without pericardial tamponade.

Pleural Space

1. "Prophylactic" tube thoracostomy is not necessary for occult pneumothoraces, even in the setting of positive-pressure ventilation.

2. Needle decompression, when performed, should be done in the midaxillary line in the fifth intercostal space to maximize the risk/benefit ratio.

3. Prophylactic antibiotics do not reduce the incidence of chest-tube associated empyema or pneumonia and are associated with antimicrobial resistance.

4. Chest tube removal algorithms should include lung expansion, drainage less than 2 mL/kg/d, and 6- to 12-hour waterseal drainage.

5. High-volume chest tube output that abruptly decreases should raise the suspicion of caked hemothorax.

Chest Wall Injury

1. Rib fractures in elderly patients are associated with significant morbidity and mortality.

2. There is a need for multicenter randomized trials with long-term follow-up to identify appropriate patients and optimal techniques for surgical stabilization of rib fractures.

3. Sternal fractures from the "seatbelt syndrome" infrequently have significant associated injuries.

Lung Injury

1. Treatment of pulmonary contusion is strictly supportive, with mechanical ventilation, tube thoracostomy, and antibiotics used only when indicated.

2. Pulmonary tractotomy results in favorable morbidity and mortality rates compared with lung resection for trauma.

Tracheobronchial Injury

1. Bronchoscopy should be performed for cervical subcutaneous emphysema, pneumomediastinum, or pneumothorax with a persistent air leak.

Esophageal Injury

1. Contrast esophagography is the preferred diagnostic study, but videoendoscopy can be done at the bedside in intubated patients and is superior in the pharyngeal area.

2. Primary repair is usually inadvisable after 24 hours.

Cardiac Injury

1. Blunt cardiac injury is commonly diagnosed, but cardiac enzymes, echocardiography, and nuclear medicine studies are not predictive of the uncommon but life-threatening complications of ventricular dysrhythmias and cardiac pump failure.

2. Clinical decisions should be based on the initial ECG.

3. Echocardiography is most useful in identifying pericardial tamponade or intracardiac injuries.

4. All patients in shock who have penetrating chest injuries between the right midclavicular line and left anterior axillary line should be considered to have a cardiac injury until proved otherwise.

5. Ultrasonography and central venous pressure monitoring are critical adjuncts in diagnosing pericardial tamponade, as the classic findings of Beck's triad are present in very few patients.

Transmediastinal Penetrating Trauma

1. Helical CT scanning is useful in delineating the trajectory of potential transmediastinal gunshot wounds, allowing a truncated and cost-effective workup in stable, asymptomatic patients.

Thoracic Great Vessel Injury

1. A reasonable operative approach to unstable patients can be inferred from the chest radiograph and the location of wounds.

2. Blunt thoracic aortic injury should be suspected in any patient with severe energy transfer, regardless of mechanism.

3. Helical CT is an excellent screening test and should be considered even in the face of a normal chest radiograph if there is severe energy transfer.

4. Once aortic injury is diagnosed, the systolic blood pressure and heart rate should be controlled with a rapidly reversible beta-blocking agent.

5. During aortic repair, it is safest to provide distal circulation via a bypass circuit.

6. The subgroup of patients with brain injuries or severe thoracic injuries may best be served by delayed operation or nonoperative management.

ANNOTATED REFERENCES

Cothren CC, Moore EE. Emergency department thoracotomy. In: Feliciano DV, Mattox KL, Moore EE, editors. Trauma. 6th ed. New York: McGraw-Hill; 2008.

A comprehensive review of the literature on ED thoracotomy. It also provides detailed discussions and descriptions of the procedures.

Dyer DS, Moore EE, Ilke DN, et al. Thoracic aortic injury: how predictive is mechanism and is chest computed tomography a reliable screening tool? A prospective study of 1,561 patients. J Trauma 2000;48:673-83.

A large study that examined the specificity of helical CT scanning and established it as an excellent screening tool. It also identified the shortcomings of chest radiographs and the importance of clinical suspicion.

Fabian TC, Richardson JD, Croce MA, et al. Prospective study of blunt aortic injury: multicenter trial of the American Association for the Surgery of Trauma. J Trauma 1997;42:374-80.

A comprehensive multicenter data review, this paper discusses all aspects of managing blunt thoracic aortic trauma, with a database that allows conclusions and practice guidelines.

Nirula R, Diaz JJ, Trunkey DD, et al. Rib fracture repair: indications, technical issues, and future directions. World J Surg 2009;33:14-22.

This review provides a comprehensive overview of techniques and devices for rib fracture repair.

Wall MJ, Hirshberg A, Mattox KL. Pulmonary tractotomy with selective vascular ligation for penetrating injuries to the lung. Am J Surg 1994;168:665-9.

The original description of pulmonary tractotomy.

Wu JT, Mattox KL, Wall MJ. Esophageal perforations: new perspectives and treatment paradigms. J Trauma 2007;63:1173-84.

A good overview of a difficult problem.

REFERENCES

Access the complete reference list online at http://www.expertconsult.com.

208

Abdominal Trauma

AARON M. SCIFRES | ANDREW B. PEITZMAN

The acutely injured patient requires a rapid, systematic, and thorough evaluation.[1,2] The goals of this initial evaluation are to detect and treat immediately life-threatening injuries and then to move to a more thorough assessment of less serious injuries and preexisting conditions. Minute-to-minute management must be guided by the patient's hemodynamic status (physiology) and anatomic injuries. Abnormal physiology kills trauma patients: hypotension, respiratory distress, hypoxemia, and so on. Do not focus on defining every anatomic injury in an unstable patient; find and correct the etiology of the abnormal physiology. The trauma patient admitted to the intensive care unit (ICU) generally has multiple injuries, many of which are threats to life or limb. Prioritization of the management of these injuries is based on treatment of the most immediate threat to life first. In blunt trauma victims, central nervous system injury accounts for 60% of deaths; hemorrhage and its consequences account for 30% of trauma deaths.[1] Deaths resulting from penetrating abdominal trauma are from bleeding or sepsis. The most common etiology of hemorrhagic shock in the trauma patient is intraabdominal bleeding. Early deaths from abdominal injury are from bleeding. Late deaths are from intraabdominal sepsis, most often from hollow organ injury.[1] Remember that injuries rarely occur in isolation; injuries occur as a component of a pattern of injuries.

Initial Assessment of the Trauma Patient

Advanced Trauma Life Support (ATLS) course principles should be followed in the assessment of any trauma patient[1] (Table 208-1). Immediate threats to life are identified and treated during the primary survey. Do not move beyond the primary survey until the patient has been stabilized. The resuscitation phase of the trauma patient generally occurs simultaneously with the primary survey. Intravenous lines are placed, and fluid resuscitation is initiated. The secondary survey is started after the patient has been stabilized. This is a head-to-toe survey defining all anatomic injuries. Remember that if a trauma patient deteriorates or does not respond as you expect, start over with the primary survey.

The trauma patient who arrives in the ICU and later becomes unstable generally has a derangement in circulation. Hypotension, tachycardia, and oliguria are obvious signs of hypoperfusion. On the other hand, even with normal vital signs, as many as 75% of trauma patients in the ICU have compensated shock with tissue hypoperfusion.[3,4] Biochemical indices of perfusion such as base deficit or lactate levels should be determined to assess global perfusion.[5,6] In the trauma patient, ongoing blood loss is the most common etiology for hypoperfusion. The source of the hemorrhage must be expeditiously identified and stopped. Sources for blood loss in the trauma patient include the abdomen, chest, pelvis, long bones, or externally via open wounds. The gastrointestinal tract is rarely the source of initial blood loss in the trauma patient. Any delay in control of hemorrhage increases morbidity and mortality.

The abdomen is a particularly challenging area to evaluate for several reasons. First, except in cases of evisceration or obvious peritonitis, the history and physical exam findings that suggest intraabdominal injury are usually subtle.[7] Second, severely injured patients often have an altered mental status from concurrent brain injury, shock, or intoxicating agents that can mask symptoms and signs. Third, more obvious injuries such as complex open extremity fractures can distract providers and focus attention away from occult torso injuries.

Finally, adjuncts to the history and physical, though numerous and ever evolving, still have weaknesses in sensitivity, specificity, and positive or negative predictive value.[8-18]

As noted, both speed and completeness are critical in evaluating the abdomen. Delays in diagnosis and treatment have been shown to affect morbidity and mortality.[19] It is essential to recognize that a trauma patient requires a laparotomy with hard signs or positive diagnostic tests (focused assessment with sonography for trauma [FAST] or diagnostic peritoneal lavage [DPL]). It is not necessary, and in fact hazardous to the patient, to persist in defining the specific anatomy injury in a patient with indications for laparotomy. For patients who present in shock, after airway control, support of inadequate ventilation, and control of external hemorrhage, attention should be immediately turned to finding and treating the cavitary hemorrhage. In the majority of patients with torso trauma, the cause of shock will be bleeding. Tension pneumothorax, pericardial tamponade, spinal cord injury, and medical causes of shock will constitute a minority of cases. It is important for the resuscitation team to keep this in mind, and every maneuver should be performed while seeking the most likely causes of shock. Thus, for the critically injured patient, early intubation may be beneficial to avoid the need for emergency intubation further along in the resuscitation. Early chest tube placement should be considered as a potential diagnostic as well as therapeutic maneuver, particularly in patients who present in extremis. Laboratory tests drawn should be routine and performed in order of importance. A specimen for blood for type and crossmatch is vital, since transfusion is highly likely in this group of patients. Arterial blood gas analysis machines are now ubiquitous in resuscitation units and can provide a rapid assessment of the patient's physiologic status. A specimen should be drawn as early as practical. Venous access must be accomplished expeditiously. Initially, the most experienced personnel should perform these procedures in the critically injured patient. Less experienced providers can provide essential support by procuring and setting up supplies and equipment, coordinating team activities at the direction of the team leader, and providing accurate documentation of the resuscitation.

On occasion, a patient will present in extremis, and some or all of the above regimented activities must be skipped while the patient is taken directly to the operating room (OR) for control of hemorrhage. Even less commonly, an emergency department (ED) thoracotomy may be indicated if vital signs are lost in the ED. The potential benefit of ED thoracotomy in the setting of intraabdominal hemorrhage remains controversial. The exsanguinating patient is best served in the OR, where thoracotomy or laparotomy can be diagnostic and therapeutic.

Blunt Abdominal Injury

Physical examination alone will miss as many as 45% of abdominal injuries, so for patients who present with evidence of shock but respond to initial resuscitation with fluid replacement, more adjuncts can be employed in initial evaluation. Radiographs of the chest and pelvis are helpful to demonstrate hemothorax, pneumothorax, diaphragmatic rupture, or complex fractures. Abdominal radiographs are not helpful in the evaluation of blunt abdominal trauma. The FAST exam was popularized in the 1990s and has gained acceptance as a screening test for diagnosis of significant hemoperitoneum.[13,14] Its major advantage is bedside availability, speed, and noninvasiveness. Because of this ready availability, FAST should be employed in all

TABLE 208-1	Initial Assessment of the Trauma Patient
Primary survey	Identify and treat immediate threats to life. This is a physiologic and not a temporal event. Stabilize patient before moving to the secondary survey.
Resuscitation	Establish at least two large-bore intravenous lines. Resuscitate to specific endpoints.
Secondary survey	Perform head-to-toe examination of patient. Order radiographic studies.
Definitive care	Move patient from emergency department to intensive care unit or operating room as quickly as possible.

severely injured blunt trauma patients with a potential abdominal injury. Ultrasound is most helpful for the hypotensive patient with blunt torso trauma and a positive FAST.[8,14] In this circumstance, the patient can be taken promptly to the OR for laparotomy. Significant drawbacks remain the relatively low sensitivity for peritoneal blood (68%) and the fact that the test cannot be used to detect diaphragm, hollow viscus, or retroperitoneal injuries.[8,14,20] In addition, one cannot use FAST to grade solid-organ injury severity. Ultrasound is less useful in evaluating penetrating trauma. However, because of its ability to detect hemopericardium, it can be useful to direct the initial operative approach and incision placement in thoracoabdominal penetrating trauma.

For hemodynamically stable blunt trauma patients, computed tomography (CT) is the standard diagnostic tool.[16,17,21] It is particularly accurate in diagnosis of solid-organ injury. It does lack sensitivity and specificity for pancreatic, hollow viscus, and diaphragm injuries, especially early in the clinical course when the initial study is usually performed.[18,22-26]

DPL is a study used much less frequently since FAST has been shown to reliably detect hemoperitoneum. However, DPL is useful for further evaluation of the abdomen when FAST is negative in unstable patients or in the evaluation of the abdomen in the patient who requires emergency operation for an injury remote from the abdomen.[26] The test is relatively simple and rapid, but it is invasive, and complications such as bowel injury are well described. More importantly, similar to FAST, DPL lacks sensitivity for retroperitoneal and diaphragm injuries. In addition, DPL is nonspecific. Thus, exploratory laparotomy based on DPL may be nontherapeutic in 25% of cases.

Penetrating Abdominal Injury

Any penetrating abdominal injury from the nipple line anteriorly or scapular tip posteriorly to the buttocks inferiorly can produce both a thoracic and abdominal injury.

GUNSHOT WOUNDS

Gunshot wounds which violate the peritoneal cavity generally mandate exploratory laparotomy. The likelihood of visceral injury requiring repair is 80% to 95%.[27,28] After a rapid primary survey, the entire body must be inspected for penetrating wounds by rolling the patient on both sides. Special attention must be paid to hidden areas such as the axillae, skin folds, body creases, and the perineum. The number of bullet wounds should be noted. Radiographs are taken of any body areas which may have been in the path of bullet trajectory. This is a critical maneuver to identify all bullets, possible trajectory, and thus structures at risk. Remember that bullets often do not travel in a straight line and may ricochet off bony structures; trajectory cannot be determined with complete confidence. The number of external wounds plus bullets found within the patient (usually on radiographs) must equal an even number; an odd number means that a bullet has not been found and other body cavities are at risk.

ABDOMINAL STAB WOUNDS

The likelihood of finding an injury which requires operative repair in a patient with an anterior stab wound is only 25% to 33%.[29] Indications for immediate exploration include hypotension, peritonitis, and evisceration. In the absence of these signs, selective management is appropriate, provided a surgeon and an OR are immediately available. In the stable patient with a reliable physical examination, the surgeon may simply decide to perform serial abdominal examination (selective management). The need for exploratory laparotomy is then based on change in abdominal examination, vital signs (especially temperature or heart rate), or white blood cell count.[29,30]

In the setting of anterior abdominal stab wounds, local wound exploration (LWE) can be helpful.[31,32] This is a formal surgical procedure usually performed in the resuscitation room. Using sterile technique and under local anesthesia, the anterior abdominal stab wound is elongated with a scalpel, and the underlying fascia is exposed with sharp dissection. Penetration of the anterior fascia suggests the possibility of peritoneal penetration and usually warrants further operative intervention, usually laparotomy or DPL. A recent multicenter trial suggested that anterior abdominal stab wounds without evisceration, hemodynamic instability, or peritonitis could be triaged based upon the results of LWE.[32] In some centers, diagnostic laparoscopy is performed when FAST, DPL, or LWE are equivocal. Laparoscopy in this setting has been challenged because of the difficulty in detecting small intestinal injuries, but it can be very helpful in evaluating the diaphragm in left thoracoabdominal stab wounds. In the stable patient, knife wounds of the flank and back may be evaluated by CT to assess trajectory of the weapon and possible visceral injury.

Solid-Organ Injury

LIVER

The majority of liver injuries do not require an operation.[33-35] Indeed, 86% of all isolated liver injuries were managed nonoperatively in a recent National Trauma Data Bank review.[35] The speed and accuracy of CT has greatly enhanced the ability to detect and accurately grade solid-organ injuries. The key decision point is hemodynamic stability for CT imaging. If they are stable enough for CT, the majority of these patients can be observed. Conversely, 25% of liver injuries will require an intervention for a complication (bleeding, abscess, bile leak, biloma). Thus, interventional radiology has a critical role in the management of solid-organ injury.[36] This has facilitated the study of the natural history of liver injuries treated nonoperatively. It has been shown that the grade of injury is an important predictor of success of nonoperative management, but even high-grade liver injuries can be successfully managed in this way.

The key to favorable outcomes in liver injury is recognition of failure of nonoperative management, as evidenced by ongoing bleeding. Signs of bleeding such as progressive anemia, hypotension, tachycardia, and failure to correct base deficit with volume resuscitation must be addressed in the setting of known liver injury. Angiographic embolization of hepatic arterial branches may avoid laparotomy if utilized immediately following recognition of arterial bleeding on the initial CT or early in the resuscitation phase.[37] It must be emphasized that the hemodynamically unstable patient with a liver injury must undergo immediate operation.

Operative treatment of liver injuries has evolved over time to minimal necessary intervention to control bleeding. This usually entails simple packing of the liver with sponges and temporarily leaving the abdomen open as discussed in more detail later. On occasion, débridement of non-viable tissue with suture control is employed. A number of coagulation devices are also available, as are a variety of hemostatic products that can be applied directly to the injured liver surface.

Both operative and nonoperative liver trauma patients in the ICU must be monitored for several potential problems. As nonoperative management of liver trauma has become commonplace, complications related to the liver are recognized in as many as 14% to 25% of high-grade injuries.[37-39] Ongoing or recurrent bleeding must be carefully excluded. Hepatic and perihepatic abscesses may be amenable to percutaneous drainage and antibiotic therapy. Biliary complications including bile leaks, biliary fistula, biloma, and bile peritonitis occur in proportion to severity of the liver injury. Percutaneous drainage of bile collections is usually the first step. Endoscopic retrograde cholangiography with bile duct stenting can be added for high-volume or persistent leaks.

SPLEEN

Similar to liver injury, splenic trauma has seen a significant trend toward nonoperative management. Approximately 76% of splenic injuries are currently managed without operation.[35,40-50] Successful management again requires recognition of signs of failure of a nonoperative strategy. In the case of the spleen, this is almost exclusively due to bleeding. Although hemodynamic instability remains the only clear indication for operative intervention, several studies have demonstrated risk factors for failed nonoperative management including greater injury severity score, splenic injury grade, volume of hemoperitoneum, higher injury severity score, and older age.[49,50]

These risk factors are highlighted to emphasize that all patients initially selected for nonoperative management must be monitored carefully. Angiographic embolization is an adjunct in the management of splenic injury with evidence of contrast extravasation on CT, but this strategy should not be chosen in the unstable patient or in the patient with other indications for laparotomy.[48] Complications of angioembolization of the spleen include continued bleeding and splenic abscess. Unlike the liver, the spleen is not essential to life. Although splenectomy following a trial of nonoperative management is considered a "failure," it is certainly preferable to a preventable mortality from bleeding.[44,47,51,52] This should be borne in mind when nonoperative management is chosen in the first place. "Successful" nonoperative management of an injured spleen that requires constant bedside attention and blood product replacement while waiting for the bleeding to stop should not be viewed as superior to initial planned splenectomy. Indeed, if operation is performed early, splenic repair and salvage can sometimes be considered.

KIDNEYS

The kidneys lie in a relatively protected region of the retroperitoneum, with spine, ribs, paraspinous muscles, and the intraperitoneal organs and tissues offering protection. The kidneys are thus less commonly injured than either the liver or spleen. Similar to the liver and spleen, the majority of blunt renal injuries are managed nonoperatively. In the national review by Tinkoff et al., only 8% of isolated kidney injuries required operation compared to 14% of liver and 24% of spleen injuries.[35] Severity of injury does correlate with rates of nephrectomy and, in blunt trauma, rates of dialysis and mortality.[53] Even if a laparotomy is performed for other reasons, the kidneys do not have to be explored unless there is an expanding retroperitoneal hematoma. In penetrating trauma, however, any hematoma around the kidney should prompt exploration, owing to the significant risk of major renal vascular injury and collecting system disruption. Repair or partial nephrectomy is usually preferred to nephrectomy in the non-exsanguinating patient. Palpation of a normal contralateral kidney should be done prior to nephrectomy. Complications of nonoperative management and partial nephrectomy include bleeding, urinoma, and infection.

PANCREAS

Injury to the pancreas is unusual in most trauma series. It is well protected in the retroperitoneum. In blunt trauma, its position overlying the lumbar spine contributes to injury in that compression against the spine by a seatbelt, handlebar, ski pole or similar object can result in

contusion or transection.[55] Pancreatic injuries are notable for difficulty in diagnosis.[54-56] The common diagnostic studies used in the evaluation of abdominal trauma—CT, FAST, and DPL—all fail to accurately assess the pancreas.[54-57] CT can demonstrate transection and peripancreatic inflammation and fluid; it is the best of the three modalities to detect pancreatic trauma, but a recent multi-institutional study demonstrated that modern 64-slice CT missed almost 50% of pancreatic ductal injuries.[57] Serum amylase and lipase levels are also unreliable in the diagnosis of pancreatic injury. Thus a high index of suspicion must be maintained when a mechanism of injury or commonly associated injury is present. Lumbar Chance fractures, duodenal hematoma, and direct epigastric blow should prompt suspicion and frequent reassessment.[54]

Pancreatic trauma from penetrating mechanisms is often complicated by injuries to surrounding structures, most importantly the aorta, vena cava, and portal vein, as well as the stomach, duodenum, and liver. These injuries can be devastating and commonly necessitate damage control techniques described later. Control of hemorrhage and enteric perforations take precedence; pancreatic resectional procedures are rarely indicated during the initial procedure except for the unusual isolated tail injury, which may be amenable to distal pancreatectomy.[56,58,59] Generous drainage of the retroperitoneum is employed in all patients discovered to have pancreatic injury at the time of operation.

Nonoperative management of pancreatic injury can be successful if the main ducts are not disrupted. But again, this diagnosis is not readily made with available imaging modalities. Rarely, a pancreatic ductal injury is confirmed on endoscopic retrograde cholangiopancreatography (ERCP), and stenting can be considered. Pancreatic fistulas and pancreatitis are morbid complications of pancreatic injury and contribute to the surgeon's aggressive operative approach to diagnosis and treatment. With major pancreatic injury, a controlled external pancreatic fistula often may be a victory.

INTESTINAL INJURY

Hollow visceral injury is commonly the result of penetrating abdominal injury, small intestine most often. These injuries are generally found during routine exploration of the abdomen for gunshot injury. Bowel injury from blunt trauma is relatively uncommon and difficult to diagnose.[22-25,60] Full-thickness intestinal injury may be present despite normal findings by CT, FAST, and routine laboratory studies. CT may miss 15% to 30% of intestine injury. A seatbelt mark or Chance fracture may be associated with intestinal or mesenteric injury in 25% to 30% of patients.[24,25]

DIAPHRAGM INJURY

Blunt diaphragmatic injury is important to diagnose, as 60% to 90% of these patients have an associated intraabdominal injury. The chest radiograph is diagnostic in 25% of cases, abnormal but not diagnostic in 50% of cases (blunting of the diaphragm, haziness or infiltrate at the lung base), and normal (even in retrospect) in 25% of cases.[61] Diaphragmatic injury is more common on the left side. Acute injury to the diaphragm is repaired through the abdomen rather than the chest because of the high likelihood of associated abdominal injury. Diaphragmatic injuries from penetrating trauma are very difficult to diagnose because the hole is generally small. Penetrating thoracoabdominal wounds, particularly on the left side, may result in hernias which entrap intestine years later. If the trajectory of a penetrating injury suggests the possibility of a diaphragmatic injury on the left, either laparoscopy or laparotomy is generally indicated.

GENITOURINARY INJURY

Hematuria is the hallmark of genitourinary injury. Gross hematuria mandates further evaluation of the genitourinary tract, usually with a cystogram to evaluate the bladder and CT to evaluate the kidneys.

Microscopic hematuria is further evaluated in the blunt trauma patient with hypotension, lower rib fractures, flank ecchymosis or tenderness, spine fractures, or high injury severity score (multiple injuries).[2,53] A straddle injury or anterior pelvic rami fracture may be associated with a urethral injury, particularly in males. Signs of urethral injury include blood at the meatus, inability to void, perineal hematoma, or high-riding prostate gland on examination. A retrograde urethrogram should be obtained prior to placement of a bladder catheter in this patient.

Damage Control

The concept of damage control has gained considerable popularity over the last 20 years. *Damage control* refers to truncated surgical operations to control immediately life-threatening problems, followed by a period of vigorous ongoing resuscitation in the ICU and subsequent return to the OR for definitive repair of injuries.[2,62-68] Recognition that prolonged heroic efforts at complete correction of anatomic abnormalities often resulted in technically adequate repairs in patients who were physiologically exhausted and often died from irreversible shock, acidosis, or coagulopathy led to widespread acceptance of this alternative approach.

Damage control can be applied appropriately to virtually any initial operation in trauma. Although laparotomy is the prototypical operation suited to abbreviation, thoracotomy, craniotomy, vascular repairs, and orthopedic procedures can all be performed in a lifesaving but incomplete manner in the setting of profound acidosis, hypothermia, and coagulopathy. This so-called bloody, vicious cycle is the hallmark indication to abort efforts at definitive surgical repair.[63]

Exploratory laparotomy is the operation in which damage control is most frequently employed. Rapid control of hemorrhage and enteric contamination, followed by temporary closure of the abdomen, all ideally performed in 1 hour or less, should be the goals. Vascular injuries are ligated or shunted, liver injuries are packed, the injured spleen is removed, kidney injuries are packed or nephrectomy performed, and hollow viscus injuries are controlled with rapid suture or staple techniques.[62-68] A variety of devices or techniques have been used to rapidly cover and protect the abdominal viscera for ongoing ICU resuscitation. These include sterile plastic intravenous fluid bags, skin-only closure, and vacuum suction devices. The patient is scheduled to return to the OR within 24 to 48 hours for definitive repairs. These operations may include removal of packs, resection of devitalized tissue, permanent vascular repairs, bowel anastomoses or stoma creation, feeding tube placement, and abdominal wall closure. Occasionally a patient must be returned to the OR sooner if significant bleeding persists or recurs. Immediate postoperative resuscitation might also include angioembolization. Arterial bleeding from liver injuries or associated with pelvic fractures is sometimes amenable to this treatment strategy, but it must be remembered that the typical angiography suite is ill equipped to manage these critically ill patients, and necessary resources must be mobilized. Appropriate anesthesia services, sufficient monitoring capabilities, and coordinated blood product acquisition must be available. Essentially, the resources of the trauma OR must be present in the radiology suite.

Intensive care of the patient following a damage control operation focuses on resuscitation and preparation for the expected return to the OR. The goals are rewarming of the patient, reversal of the coagulopathy, and restoration of adequate perfusion. Passive rewarming devices should be employed. Reassessment is essential, since the injury that initially required damage control typically requires complete attention from the trauma team, and other significant problems can be initially overlooked. A complete reassessment with physical examination and adjunctive radiologic studies are essential to avoid missed injuries. Correct placement of all tubes and lines should be confirmed. Current laboratory parameters including acid-base status, oxygenation, hemoglobin concentration, and coagulation profile should be determined

and should be repeated frequently. Correction of abnormalities should be aggressive. It is also critical to recognize that inability to correct these abnormalities often suggests the need to return to the OR. On the other hand, the patient may be unsalvageable, and the intensivist and surgeon must work closely together to ensure that correctable problems have not been missed. Adequate blood product availability should be confirmed. All wounds should be reinspected, particularly those that were covered only temporarily prior to the first operation. Bleeding from wounds in hidden areas or missed open fractures should be sought.

Patients undergoing damage control operations typically require bedside attention from the entire team for many consecutive hours. The operating surgeon must convey key information about the expected postoperative course. This should include critical clinical parameters that must be recognized and reported. Drain output changes, critical laboratory values, increasing transfusion requirements, and changes in wound appearance all indicate potential deterioration and the need for a change in management.

If damage control is successful and the patient returns to a relatively normal physiologic state, planning for return to the OR for definitive repairs is undertaken. It is essential that the patient be completely reexamined and a systematic search for missed injuries be carried out. It may be possible to complete radiographic assessments of the spine or extremities, but it must be emphasized that the risks of transporting critically injured patients to remote diagnostic suites must be weighed against the potential benefits of finding or excluding particular injuries. Trips outside of the ICU should be minimized. In general, if the results of a test will not change current management, it should be postponed until transport risks are negligible.

OPEN ABDOMEN

One of the consequences of abdominal damage control is an *open abdomen*, which refers to the unapproximated abdominal wall fascia. The concept of the open abdomen resulted from the recognition that massive swelling and edema of the abdominal viscera in critically injured patients resulted in increased intraperitoneal pressures and resultant organ dysfunction. This is now referred to as *abdominal compartment syndrome*.[2,69] Excessive crystalloid resuscitation may be a major factor contributing to abdominal compartment syndrome. The open abdomen is an integral part of a damage control strategy. It facilitates damage control because it shortens the duration of the initial operation and simplifies reexploration. At least as importantly, it also prevents abdominal compartment syndrome by creating a protected but flexible space for the enlarged viscera.

However, the open abdomen can be seen as a major tradeoff. On the one hand, many patients who may have previously died when definitive repairs and abdominal wall closure were always practiced, now survive with damage control techniques and an open abdomen. On the other hand, management of the open abdomen is not straightforward and carries significant morbidity.[62] The most serious complications of the open abdomen are enterocutaneous, or "enteroatmospheric," fistulas and giant ventral hernias. Because of these complications, multiple strategies to close the abdominal wall fascia as soon as possible after initial operation have been employed. These include sequential suturing, negative-pressure dressings, proprietary fascial approximation devices, spanning the fascial defect with biological or permanent mesh materials, and plastic surgical techniques of separating and advancing the fascial layers of the abdominal wall.[64] None of these techniques has been universally successful, and optimal management of the open abdomen remains an area of active research. One area of controversy is the relative safety and efficacy of enteral nutritional support during open abdomen management. Dissanaike and colleagues demonstrated that immediate enteral feeding in patients with open abdomens significantly lowered pneumonia incidence, without affecting abdominal closure rate.[70]

1. When the trauma patient arrives in the ICU, repeat the initial evaluation of the patient.

2. Bedside ultrasound has become an important adjunct in evaluating abdominal trauma.

3. Nonoperative management of blunt solid-organ injury has become routine in the majority of patients.

4. Widespread use of damage control and open abdomen management techniques have resulted in improved survival in severe abdominal injury, trading morbidity for mortality in many instances.

5. Missed abdominal injuries remain a significant cause of preventable morbidity and mortality.

6. The unstable trauma patient should not leave the ICU for diagnostic studies.

ANNOTATED REFERENCES

Rozycki GS, Root HD. The diagnosis of intraabdominal visceral injury. J Trauma 2010;68:1019-23.

A current review of the diagnostic tools available for the accurate evaluation of abdominal injury.

Tinkoff G, Esposito TJ, Reed J, et al. American Association for the Surgery of Trauma Organ Injury Scale I: spleen, liver and kidney, validation based on the National Trauma Data Bank. J Am Coll Surg 2008;207:646-55.

Validation of the AAST solid organ injury scales that includes a wealth of information on management and outcomes for these injuries from a large database.

Kozar RA, Moore JB, Niles SE, et al. Complications of nonoperative management of high-grade blunt hepatic injuries. J Trauma 2005;59:1066-71.

An important analysis of the complexities in the management of liver injury.

Watson GA, Rosengart MR, Zenati MS, et al. Nonoperative management of severe blunt splenic injury: are we getting better? J Trauma 2006;61:1113-8.

A large series that emphasizes the dangers and challenges of routine nonoperative management of injury to the spleen.

Lee JC, Peitzman AB. Damage-control laparotomy. Curr Opin Crit Care 2006;12:346-50.

A thorough review of the critical steps in damage control from patient selection to ICU management.

REFERENCES

Access the complete reference list online at http://www.expertconsult.com.

Pelvic and Major Long Bone Fractures

RANDY EDWARDS | ORLANDO KIRTON

Pelvic and long bone fractures have serious local and systemic consequences for the trauma victim. Familiarity with the sequelae of serious orthopedic injuries is essential if intensive care unit (ICU) management of these patients is to have a successful outcome.

Pelvic Fracture

Pelvic fractures are present in about 10% of patients presenting to a level I trauma center after blunt trauma.[1] Pelvic fractures represent approximately 3% of skeletal injuries evaluated in major trauma centers.[2] The incidence of pelvic fracture is highest after motorcycle crash, pedestrian trauma caused by a motor vehicle, falls from heights greater than 15 feet, and motor vehicle crash, in that order.[1] Overall mortality due to pelvic fractures ranges from 10% to 16%; the highest mortality—around 45%—is attributed to open pelvic fractures.[2,3] However, very few patients die as a direct result of hemorrhage from the pelvic fracture itself. Most deaths in patients with pelvic fracture are from head injury, nonpelvic hemorrhage, pulmonary injury, thromboembolic complications, or multiple organ system failure. The incidence of solid and hollow organ injury and other skeletal trauma is high in patients with pelvic fracture, owing to the powerful forces involved.[1,4,5] More than 90% of these individuals have associated gastrointestinal (5%) and abdominal injuries (16.5%).[1,4] Risk factors for associated abdominal injury include motor vehicle crash, fall greater than 15 feet, and pelvis Abbreviated Injury Severity Score (AISS) greater than 3.[1,5] Overall Injury Severity Score (ISS) and mortality correlate with the severity of the pelvic fracture, although death is usually the result of associated injuries rather than the fracture itself.[6]

Complications occur in roughly a third of patients and can involve devitalized tissues, hematoma formation, and those related to internal or external fixation. Infections are the most common complication (15.7%), followed by respiratory (9.3%), hematologic (5.5%), and thromboembolic complications (3.4%).[7] Cardiac complications occur in about 2.5% of patients.[7] Patients with unstable pelvic fractures are at significantly greater risk of complications than those with stable fractures.[7-9] Infections involving external devices usually occur at the level of the pin tracts.[9] If cellulitis or excessive drainage develops, broad-spectrum antibiotic coverage is needed. If the infection persists despite treatment, pin loosening may require replacement of new pin sites. Internal fixation infections are usually due to significantly devitalized tissues that have become secondarily infected or inadequately débrided. These infections are more commonly found with posterior approaches.[9] Open drainage must be considered as well as alternative fixation techniques.

The transfusion requirement for patients with pelvic fracture with a mean ISS of 21.3 is 8 units of packed red blood cells but can be much greater.[7] The degree of hemorrhage is highly dependent on the type of fracture. Complete dissociation of the posterior pelvis has the highest degree of hemorrhage and connected mortality.[10,12] Significant hemorrhage often occurs from other sites such as the abdomen or thorax as well. Less than 1% of all patients with pelvic fractures have hypotension secondary to blood loss due to the fracture itself.[7,11] Nevertheless, 12% of patients with open pelvic fractures die as direct result of hemorrhage.[8]

Hemorrhage from unstable pelvic fractures can be minimized by early reapproximation and stabilization of the pelvic ring. Stabilization can be accomplished with external fixation devices such as the Browner clamp or expediently with as simple an appliance as a bed sheet wrapped tightly around the pelvis. If external pelvic fixation is unsuccessful at restoring hemodynamic stability after initial resuscitation and other sources of ongoing hemorrhage have been ruled out, angiography to evaluate and treat pelvic arterial bleeding is indicated. Pelvic arterial disruption is responsible for hemorrhage in less than 5% of all cases of pelvic fracture.[11-13] A blush of contrast identified on pelvic computed tomography (CT) scan is evidence for arterial bleeding and is an indication for angiography.[11] Predictors of positive angiography have been postulated to be the presence of sacroiliac joint (SIJ) disruption, female gender, and the duration of hypotension.[13] Early and aggressive angioembolization have been shown to improve outcomes in properly selected patients. However, some European trauma groups have proposed pelvic packing as an early operative maneuver in order to provide stabilization prior to angioembolization. Others, such as Cothren et al., have suggested a modified technique of early direct preperitoneal pelvic packing, thereby reducing blood transfusion requirements and the need for angiography, with a subsequently lower mortality.[14] Evidence for this is based on several small case series. Early angioembolization based on radiologic diagnostics and external fixation within 3 hours of injury has also been shown to be effective, reducing the need for transfusion by using an algorithmic approach.[15]

Long Bone Fracture

The most studied and serious long bone fracture is fracture of the femur. Approximately 15% of seriously injured motor vehicle passengers presenting to a level I trauma center have femur fractures.[14] Some 8% to 10% of these patients have bilateral fractures.[16,17] The mortality rate for unilateral fracture is 10% to 12%.[16,17] Mortality increases to 26% to 33% with bilateral fractures and is 20% in patients older than age 65.[16] The highest incidence of femur fractures in the trauma population occurs in young men, with midshaft fractures being the most common as a result of high-energy impacts.[13] As in pelvic fractures, death is more closely connected with the severity of associated injuries rather than the fracture itself.[16,17] As noted, mortality is very significant in complicated femur fracture patients with multiple injuries. Therefore, careful assessment following the guidelines of Advanced Trauma Life Support (ATLS) is mandatory.

Blunt trauma patients who present with femur fracture have a higher incidence of abdominal, thoracic, and skeletal injuries compared with patients without femur fracture.[16,17] Those with bilateral fractures have an increased incidence of head injury, requirement for laparotomy, and pelvic fracture compared to those with a unilateral femur fracture.[16,17]

The risk of complications, including acute respiratory distress syndrome (ARDS), pneumonia, and fat embolism syndrome, in the multiply injured patient with femur fracture can be markedly decreased by early operative fixation within 24 hours.[18,19] Early operative repair also results in decreased ICU length of stay, hospital stay, cost, and risk of mortality.[19,20]

The American College of Surgery's Committee on Trauma has recommended that femur fractures in polytrauma patients be repaired with 12 hours, provided the patient is hemodynamically stable.[21] For trauma patients with multiple severe injuries, however, earlier repair can sometimes lead to higher morbidity secondary to the patient's inability to tolerate excessive physiologic stress. The currently evolving damage control surgery concept is playing a more definitive role in managing long bone fractures; delaying definitive surgery may be the best approach and ultimately prove to be life saving.[22] Damage control with external fixation of femur fractures in polytrauma patients is becoming the standard of treatment in many trauma centers.[23]

Although hemorrhage is a feared complication of femur fracture, a study of isolated femur fracture found that blood loss from the fracture itself is insufficient to cause hypotension.[24] Of 100 patients with isolated femur fractures, only 24% were in class I or II shock. None were in class III or IV shock. Nevertheless, hemorrhage is the cause of death in a significant proportion of polytrauma patients with femur fracture, an indication of the importance of other sites of hemorrhage in these patients.[20] Despite central nervous system injury being the predominant cause of death in polytrauma patients, mortality secondary to exsanguinations has been reported to be 12% to 26%.[25] In addition, special attention must be paid to avoiding occult hypoperfusion (non-hypotensive shock), which is associated with an increased incidence of complications, especially infections, in patients with femur fracture.[26] Hemorrhage from long bone fractures is best managed by early stabilization. Stabilization can be initiated with traction splints such as a Hare traction splint for femur fractures or closed reduction and splinting for other fracture sites. Neurologic injury due to femur fracture is a rare event.[27]

▣ Local Complications

INFECTION

Infection can manifest as an acute complication in the setting of both long bone and pelvic fractures. Osteomyelitis can be the result of a grossly contaminated open fracture as well as a surgically repaired closed fracture. Acute infection of a fracture hematoma or fracture repair can manifest with cutaneous signs such as erythema, warmth, and induration. However, if the infected site is deep to the fascia, infection may manifest with systemic signs such as leukocytosis and fever without cutaneous signs.[28] Diagnosis can be achieved using CT, magnetic resonance imaging (MRI), three-phase bone scan, or radiolabeled white blood cell scans. Plain radiographs are unlikely to aid in the early diagnosis of osteomyelitis, as findings are often delayed up to 21 days. The most common causative organism is *Staphylococcus aureus*, but infection may be due to many other organisms, including *Pseudomonas aeruginosa* and Enterobacteriaceae.[9,28] Generally these infections take a week or more to manifest.

Treatment depends on the organism or organisms present. The best option in high-risk open fractures remains prophylactic antibiotics administered parentally within 6 hours, tailored to provide coverage against both gram-positive and gram-negative organisms. One common regimen consists of a first-generation cephalosporin (e.g., cefazolin, 1 g intravenously [IV] immediately, then every 8 hours) and an aminoglycoside (e.g., tobramycin, 7 g/kg body weight IV immediately, then every 24 hours) administered for 72 hours starting prior to surgery. For established infections, the mainstay of treatment is débridement of devitalized and infected bone and soft tissue followed by antibiotic therapy tailored to operative culture results. Hyperbaric oxygen has been used as an adjunct to therapy for osteomyelitis, but convincing data showing efficacy are lacking.[28,29]

Gas gangrene or necrotizing fasciitis can appear within the first 24 hours after fracture or operative repair. These fulminant, necrotizing infections usually occur in the setting of open fracture with extensive soft-tissue injury requiring débridement and are especially likely if there is a delay in treatment. The causative organism is *Clostridium perfringens* in 10% of cases, with synergistic multiple organisms including *Streptococcus*, anaerobes, and coliform bacteria causing the remainder.[9,28] Findings can include skin changes, purulent or "dishwater" wound drainage, and profound shock due to vasodilatation. Treatment is aggressive surgical débridement of necrotic tissue, which may require amputation, and broad-spectrum antibiotics or high-dose penicillin. Hyperbaric oxygen also can be used in conjunction with surgical and pharmacologic treatment. Prophylaxis consists of early treatment of open fractures with thorough débridement of all devitalized tissue.

Despite treatment, gas gangrene often results in fatality due to the severe septic manifestations of this infection.[9,28] This is not to be confused with the diagnosis of a fracture blister (blood filled or clear filled) in the zone of injury, associated with closed fractures of the lower extremity. These are typically avoided surgically and left intact thus allowing spontaneous rupture. When spontaneous rupture occurs, they are deroofed and covered with a sterile nonadherent dressing.[30] Some orthopedic surgeons advocate unroofing the fracture blister(s) in diabetic patients and treatment with silver sulfadiazine (Silvadene).[31]

Tetanus can result from any open fracture, but patients with fractures caused by farming accidents are at particularly high risk. Symptoms, caused by *Clostridium tetani* toxin, occur 1 to 2 weeks after injury and are often fatal. The case fatality rate is about 60%.[7] Presenting symptoms include trismus, difficulty swallowing, restlessness, and headache. The syndrome progresses to convulsions and asphyxia. Muscle spasm and convulsions are due to excitation of spinal motor neurons. Diagnosis relies on clinical recognition, as cultures are positive in only a third of cases.[9,28]

Prophylaxis consists of 0.5 mL adsorbed tetanus toxoid administered promptly intramuscularly (IM) on presentation for all patients with traumatic wounds, including open fractures, who have not received a booster within the last 5 years. High-risk patients, such as those involved in farming accidents or with neglected wounds, are candidates for tetanus immunoglobulin (250 units administered by deep IM injection). Antibiotics are inadequate prophylaxis. Treatment of diagnosed tetanus infection consists of sedation, supportive care including airway management with intubation or a surgical airway, surgical débridement of the infected wound, passive immunization with tetanus immunoglobulin (recommended doses vary from 500 International Units to 10,000 International Units administered IM), and antibiotics (metronidazole, 500 mg IV every 8 hours).[9,28]

COMPARTMENT SYNDROME

Compartment syndrome (CS) is a potentially devastating complication that arises in the setting of either open or closed fracture. Tissue edema and bleeding raise the pressure in the fixed volume of a fascial compartment, which impedes blood flow, especially in arterioles and capillaries, resulting in tissue ischemia. The degree of tissue necrosis depends on the pressure within the compartment, the duration of time during which compartment pressure is elevated, and the sensitivity of specific tissues to ischemia. Nervous tissue demonstrates functional abnormalities after 30 minutes of ischemia, with irreversible loss of function occurring after 12 to 24 hours. Muscle, on the other hand, does not exhibit functional effects for 2 to 4 hours, and irreversible loss of function occurs after 4 to 12 hours. Capillary permeability also increases, resulting in further tissue edema.[9,32]

The most common location for compartment syndrome after lower-extremity fracture is the anterior compartment of the leg. This complication usually results from closed tibia fracture. As many as 17% of patients with a tibia fracture secondary to a motor vehicle crash develop a compartment syndrome.[27] Compartment syndrome of the thigh can develop after open or closed fracture and may develop after operative treatment of the fracture. Compartment syndrome of the arm, buttock, and foot are also possible after fracture. Risk factors associated with developing compartment syndrome include the severity of the fracture and associated soft-tissue injury, the use of compressive devises such as military antishock trousers or tourniquets, and systemic hypotension.[9,32,33]

Diagnosis of compartment syndrome can be made on clinical grounds and is established when the compartment is tense on physical examination, severe pain is present with passive motion, the compartment is tender throughout, and sensory nervous function is impaired. Loss of distal pulses is often the last manifestation of compartment syndrome. By the time pulses and distal perfusion are diminished, extensive necrosis of tissues within the compartment already may be present. It is important to be aware that compartment syndrome can occur both acutely and after operative fixation of a fracture. The diagnosis must be made early before permanent tissue damage has occurred. Serial examinations are critical to monitor for compartment syndrome in patients at risk.[9,32]

Measurement of compartment pressure is an additional way to confirm the diagnosis; however, measurements are unnecessary when the diagnosis is evident on clinical grounds. Measurement of compartment pressure is useful when the physical examination is limited because the patient is unresponsive due to head injury or sedation. Compartment pressure values ranging from 30 to 45 mm Hg have been recommended as the threshold for triggering surgical intervention.[27] Compartment pressures are measured by placement of a sterile needle connected to a pressure transducer into each compartment. Alternatively, commercial devices such as the Stryker compartment monitor (Stryker, Kalamazoo, Michigan) are available that accomplish the same task.

Treatment is by urgent, complete surgical fasciotomy to open all affected compartments. Care must be taken to adequately open the skin because it may constrict the compartment, even if the fascia has been opened. Fasciotomy can be performed in the ICU if the patient is too unstable to be transported to the operating room. Complete fasciotomy within 12 hours of onset results in a normal functional outcome in 68% of cases, whereas delay decreases the likelihood of successful outcome to 8%.[29]

In light of the fact that compartment syndrome can lead to irreversible neurologic and muscular damage, early diagnosis cannot rely solely on clinical findings, so prophylactic fasciotomy has been advocated. Subsequently, a trend toward liberal use of "prophylactic fasciotomy" was noted. According to Abouezzi et al., the most important factor influencing the need for fasciotomy was location of the vascular injury. Popliteal vessel injuries are often associated with warm ischemia and prolonged repair time in the operating room.[34] The overall incidence of neurologic damage due to a delayed or lack of fasciotomy is difficult to determine.[34]

The decision to perform a prophylactic fasciotomy for nonvascular injury should be made selectively based on objective clinical findings which include prolonged warm ischemia, ischemic reperfusion injury, hypotension/shock, and measurement of compartment pressures.

Once the compartment has been opened, wash-out of the metabolic products of the ischemic compartment occurs. It is critical to closely monitor acid-base status, serum potassium and phosphate concentration, serum and urine myoglobin concentrations, fluid status, and renal function. Adequate hydration and monitoring of urine output are critical to successful postoperative care of these patients. The clinician must also be aware of the high incidence of infection at the fasciotomy site.[33,35]

RHABDOMYOLYSIS

Rhabdomyolysis can occur for several reasons after skeletal trauma. The disease and its pathophysiology were first described in 1941 during the "Blitz" of London. The severity of the muscle necrosis depends on multiple factors including loss of arterial supply, increased compartment pressure secondary to prolonged or severe compression/injury, length of time without effective blood flow, and delayed resuscitation leading to hypovolemic shock.[74] A high index of suspicion must be maintained to facilitate early diagnosis. There are over 40 compartments in the body. Approximately 70% of compartment syndrome occurrences are associated with fractures leading to rhabdomyolysis. The most obvious reason is direct injury to muscles surrounding the fracture site. Direct injury to skeletal muscle tissue is especially likely when the mechanism of injury resulted in transfer of a great deal of energy; an example is a motor vehicle crash. Second, rhabdomyolysis can occur secondary to compression of tissues for a prolonged period after the injury. The compression causes an ischemic injury to the involved muscle. Lastly, rhabdomyolysis can result from compartment syndrome due to a fracture. Again, the mechanism involves compression of circulation resulting in an ischemic injury. All three mechanisms of rhabdomyolysis can be exacerbated by hemorrhagic shock.[36,37]

Since myoglobinuria does not occur in the absence of rhabdomyolysis, serum myoglobin is the best diagnostic marker.[38] The serum elevation of myoglobin occurs before the rise in serum creatine phosphokinase (CPK). With adequate resuscitation, the serum myoglobin will decrease with an inverse rise in the urine myoglobin.

The systemic effects of rhabdomyolysis are the result of anaerobic metabolism and cell lysis. Lactic acid release can lead to systemic acidosis, especially if volume replacement is inadequate. Potassium and myoglobin are released by the lysed myocytes. Hyperkalemia can lead to life-threatening cardiac arrhythmias. Intravenous calcium should be used with caution in this setting because it can rapidly combine with phosphate anions, leading to precipitation of calcium salts if hyperphosphatemia from muscle necrosis is present. Elevated serum myoglobin levels can cause direct renal tubular damage, leading to acute renal failure. CPK had been used traditionally to diagnose and trend compartment syndrome. However, it should not be used for early detection but can be used for monitoring after compartment decompression.[39]

Successful treatment of rhabdomyolysis involves aggressive IV fluid therapy to maximize tubular flow rate, avoiding the accumulation of myoglobin in the renal tubules and aiding the clearance of hyperkalemia. Administration of iron-chelating agents such as desferrioxamine (standard dosage for rhabdomyolysis not established) and alkalinization of urine using sodium bicarbonate as 50% of the resuscitation fluid (150 mEq dissolved in 1 L of 5% dextrose solution) or a carbonic anhydrase inhibitor such as acetazolamide is recommended by some experts. Ultimately, acute renal failure may necessitate hemofiltration or hemodialysis.[36,40,41] In our institution, we aim to maintain a urine output greater than 1 to 2 mL/kg/h using IV fluids, and we follow serial serum and urine myoglobin levels. We have had good success in avoiding acute renal failure without the use of urine alkalinization or iron-chelating agents.

FAT EMBOLISM SYNDROME

Pathophysiology

Fat embolism syndrome occurs when marrow fat particles embolize from bone marrow to the pulmonary and systemic venous circulation via injured veins in the setting of acute fracture or fracture repair. Larger particles lodge in the pulmonary circulation, whereas smaller particles (7-10 μm) will pass through to the systemic circulation.

In experimental models of fat embolism syndrome and autopsy series of blunt trauma patients, the degree of fat embolization, the severity of pulmonary compromise, and deaths attributable to fat embolism syndrome correlate with the severity and number of fractures.[42,43] Other causes of systemic embolization include intrapulmonary shunts and patent foramen ovale.[44]

Beyond simple occlusion of capillaries, liberation of free fatty acids is thought to be pathophysiologically significant through the activation of inflammatory processes and/or direct toxicity to lung capillaries and pneumocytes. Histamine and serotonin are also released, exacerbating pulmonary dysfunction and causing bronchospasm and vasospasm.[28,45,46]

Epidemiology

Estimates of the number of patients with fractures who develop the pulmonary, skin, and neurologic manifestations of fat embolism syndrome vary between 0.5% and 20%.[9,28,46] The incidence of fat embolism syndrome increases to 5% to 35% after multiple fractures.[9,28] The mortality rate is about 10%, and death is usually due to severe pulmonary dysfunction and multiple organ system failure and severe neurologic dysfunction.[9,28,46,47] It is estimated that 5000 deaths due to fat embolism syndrome occur annually after pathologic fractures, traumatic fractures, and orthopedic surgery.[45]

Clinical Manifestations

Clinical diagnosis of fat embolism syndrome is based on the presence of the classic triad of respiratory compromise, mental status changes, and petechial rash in the setting of long bone fractures or orthopedic surgery involving long bone manipulation.[52] In patients with long bone fractures, 60% manifest symptoms within 24 hours of injury and 85% within 48 hours.[9,28] Therefore, in the appropriate setting, the rash is pathognomonic and present in only 20% to 50% of cases.[48]

Severity can vary from subclinical to subacute clinically apparent symptoms to fulminant acute symptoms.[49] Subclinical emboli probably occur in nearly all patients with long bone fractures or intramedullary manipulation.[9,50] The subacute course is associated with mild respiratory dysfunction and mild neurologic manifestations or cardiovascular compromise. Supportive care is usually adequate in these cases. The fulminant variety can involve any of the following: rapidly progressive ARDS, complete cardiovascular collapse, or deep coma, possibly resulting in death.[51]

Some degree of respiratory compromise is always present and is often the most severe and life-threatening of the manifestations of fat embolism syndrome.[44] In trauma patients, it may be difficult to distinguish fat embolism syndrome from other causes of compromised pulmonary function. Indeed, the cause of respiratory compromise in multitrauma patients with significant long bone fractures can be multifactorial, including fat embolism syndrome, direct pulmonary/thoracic cavity trauma, and ischemia reperfusion injury and systemic activation of the inflammatory response. However, an isolated long bone fracture can produce cardiac as well as respiratory symptoms.

The cardiovascular effects of fat embolism syndrome are mainly attributable to partial occlusion of pulmonary arterial flow resulting in acute pulmonary hypertension and increased right ventricular afterload. The cardiovascular effects of fat embolism syndrome vary in severity from sinus tachycardia to reversible hypotension to irreversible profound shock due to right heart failure resulting in death.[28,35,45] Changes on the electrocardiogram include sinus tachycardia, bradycardia, other arrhythmias, and ST-segment changes.[28,35,49] Treatment is supportive, with inotropic agents to increase contractility of the right ventricle to overcome the adverse effect of increased afterload. Increasing preload with IV fluids is usually not helpful and can lead to overdistention of an already overloaded right ventricle. To make matters worse, increased right heart pressure resulting from pulmonary hypertension can cause a closed foramen ovale to open, contributing to systemic embolization.[45]

Central nervous system manifestations of varying degrees are present in 70% to 80% of patients with fat embolism syndrome.[44] These findings can vary from mild confusion or restlessness to profound coma resulting in death.[9,51] Most commonly, agitation, confusion, and lethargy not attributable to hypoxia are encountered.[35,46,49] Patients can also develop focal changes such as hemiplegia due to cerebral ischemia.[35] The more severe neurologic outcomes are often attributed to paradoxical emboli through a patent foramen ovale, although massive systemic embolization with profound coma and petechial hemorrhage of the brain in the absence of a patent foramen ovale can occur.[43,44,53]

Petechial rash is present in up to 50% of cases and is usually present on the chest, neck, and axilla, although less often the rash appears on mucous membranes or the conjunctiva.[43,46,49] Retinal changes also can be observed and include microinfarcts, cotton-wool spots, and flame-like hemorrhages.[9,44,49] Petechial rash is usually a late sign of fat embolism syndrome. The petechial rash is attributed to capillary occlusion or distention by fat globules.[49] Although it appears late and is often not present, when it does appear it can greatly aid in the definitive diagnosis.

Diagnosis

Many laboratory abnormalities are encountered in cases of fat embolism syndrome, but none is specific. These laboratory findings include decreased Pao_2 with decreased or increased Pco_2, thrombocytopenia, slowly decreasing hematocrit, increased fibrin split products, and decreased fibrinogen.[46,49]

Bronchoalveolar lavage has been advocated as a more specific test to diagnose fat embolism syndrome. The percentage of alveolar macrophages laden with fat droplets in the bronchoalveolar lavage fluid as determined by fat stains is elevated in patients with fat embolism syndrome. This finding may be helpful in confirming suspected cases of fat embolism syndrome, although precise diagnostic criteria have not been established. False-positive results are seen in patients with long bone fractures and after orthopedic procedures without clinical evidence of fat embolism syndrome.[50,54]

Findings on chest CT scan include patchy ground-glass or nodular opacities and thickening of the interlobar septa. Differential diagnosis of these findings includes pulmonary contusion and aspiration. Because they most often occur 24 hours or more after injury, they can usually be differentiated from contusion, which should be evident earlier. CT findings in more severe cases of fat embolism syndrome include more extensive bilateral patchy airspace consolidation; similar abnormalities can also be seen on the chest radiograph.[47,55] Occasionally, CT imaging also reveals large emboli lodged in the femoral veins, inferior vena cava, or the proximal pulmonary circulation.[56]

Treatment

The mainstay of treatment for fat embolism syndrome is supportive. Pulmonary manifestations often respond to supplemental oxygen, but more severe cases of fat embolism syndrome develop into ARDS and multiple organ system failure, requiring prolonged mechanical ventilation. Cardiac dysfunction is due to increased pulmonary resistance, and shock due to fat embolism syndrome may require inotropic support. There is no specific treatment for the neurologic symptoms of fat embolism syndrome other than eliminating and treating other potential causes such as hypoxia. Rare cases of severe neurologic dysfunction that result in profound coma can be irreversible and result in death.

The most important treatment of fat embolism syndrome is prevention. In the setting of traumatic fracture, prevention is achieved by providing early fixation. Multiple experimental and clinical studies clearly show that early fracture fixation (within 24 hours) decreases both the pulmonary and cardiac effects of fat embolism syndrome when compared with delayed (>24 hours) fixation and nonoperative treatment.[28,35,49,57-59] Intraoperative use of transesophageal echocardiography (TEE) can be a very sensitive monitor to detect fat emboli. The emboli appear as showering white flakes flowing or tumbling through the right atrium.[59]

Trials of IV alcohol, low-molecular-weight dextran, hypertonic glucose, and heparin have shown these agents to be ineffective in the treatment of fat embolism syndrome.

THROMBOEMBOLISM

Pathophysiology

Venous injury, stasis, and hypercoagulability can all contribute to the risk of thromboembolism after pelvic or long bone fractures.[9] Embolic thrombi to the pulmonary circulation or systemic circulation (paradoxical embolization) can originate in the deep veins of the thigh, pelvis, or upper extremity. Calf vein thrombosis, in general, does not embolize but extends to involve more proximal deep veins 20% to 25% of the time.[9]

Risk Factors

A number of risk factors for thromboembolic disease, including femur, tibia, and pelvic fractures, have been identified in trauma patients. Other identified risk factors include age older than 40 years, immobility, blood transfusion, multiple trauma, head injury, spinal fracture, spinal cord injury, and high ISS.[28,49,60-66] However, a systematic review of the literature by the Eastern Association for the Surgery of Trauma (EAST) found that only spinal fractures and spinal cord injuries were consistently shown to be associated with a higher risk of deep vein thrombosis (DVT).[67] Despite these data, most trauma and orthopedic surgeons regard the risk of thromboembolic disease in trauma patients with long bone or pelvic fractures as real.[28]

Prophylaxis

Elevation of the affected extremity and passive motion exercises increase lower-extremity venous flow rates and reduce DVT.[28] Lower-extremity sequential compression devices decrease the incidence of DVT by up to 90% in orthopedic patients.[28] Compression devices placed on the foot have also been shown to decrease the incidence of DVT in patients undergoing orthopedic surgery for elective indications or trauma.[28] These devices are useful when the anatomy of injury and surgery precludes placement of sequential compression devices on the leg.[28] Similar improvements in the thromboembolism rate have been seen in the surgical ICU population.[68] In the multitrauma population, some studies have shown sequential compression device use to be equivalent to low-dose heparin, whereas other studies have shown no improvement in thromboembolic events when compared to no prophylaxis.[66] Despite conflicting data in the literature, the use of sequential compression devices continues to be a mainstay of thromboembolism prophylaxis in the skeletal trauma population because of its low cost, ease of use, and inherent safety. The salutary effects of sequential compression devices are thought to include improved venous flow and activation of endogenous antithrombotic mechanisms. The anticoagulant effects of sequential compression devices decrease minutes after discontinuing the device, emphasizing the importance of continuous therapy.[67,68] Because of its low cost, noninvasive nature, and high accuracy, color-flow duplex ultrasonography has become the test of choice for DVT.[69] Aggressive screening and prophylaxis can reduce the incidence of asymptomatic venous thromboembolism (VTE) diagnosed by duplex ultrasonography.[62]

Low-dose unfractionated heparin (5000 units IV, 2-3 times daily) decreases the incidence of thromboembolic events when compared with placebo in various populations of acutely ill patients. These studies have included orthopedic and nonorthopedic critically ill and noncritically ill patients. Overall reduction in thromboembolic rates are on the order of two- to threefold.[67,68] However, multiple studies of trauma and orthopedic patients, including two meta-analyses, have failed to show significant improvement in the rate of thromboembolic events when low-dose unfractionated heparin is compared to placebo.[28,67]

The literature on low-molecular-weight heparin (LMWH) is more convincing. Several studies have shown that treatment with LMWH decreases the incidence of thromboembolism and has an excellent safety profile in patients with hip fracture or multisystem trauma.[28,60] Moreover, studies have also shown that LMWH (enoxaparin, 30 mg subcutaneously [SQ] every 12 hours) provides superior VTE prophylaxis when compared to low-dose unfractionated heparin (5000 units SQ every 12 hours) in the trauma population.[67,70]

Several studies have shown improved efficacy using combined sequential compression devices and low-dose unfractionated heparin or LMWH therapy when compared to either therapy alone in stroke, cardiac surgery, and neurosurgery populations.[69] Other studies, however, have shown no difference between combined and single-modality therapy.[68] Further study of the fracture population is needed.

Treatment

Treatment of DVT and pulmonary embolism in patients with orthopedic injuries or multiple trauma involves a balance between the risk of bleeding and thromboembolic disease. Although virtually all pulmonary emboli arise from DVT in the thigh, pelvis, or upper extremity, calf vein thrombosis tends to propagate into the proximal veins, meaning that treatment should be to avoid embolic phenomena.[71,38] Treatment of DVT and pulmonary embolism usually starts with full anticoagulation using unfractionated heparin. Once therapeutic heparinization has been achieved for an average of 72 hours, treatment with sodium warfarin is begun. Patients are usually kept on bedrest for this period to prevent embolic events.[71,72] Alternative therapy includes LMWH.

Inferior vena cava filters are generally reserved for patients who have failed anticoagulation, exhibit embolic phenomena or propagation of clot while on full anticoagulation, or are inappropriate candidates for systemic anticoagulation.[68,73] Prophylactic use of inferior vena cava filters involves patients who have no documented pulmonary embolus or DVT but are thought to be high risk due to numerous factors. The literature varies attempting to ascertain what defines the "high-risk" patient. It is well recognized, however, that immobility, venous stasis/injury, inflammatory hypercoagulable states, and severely injured patients at risk for bleeding are contributory factors to the development of VTE and thromboprophylaxis failure.[75-79] Therefore, prophylactic use of inferior vena cava filters should be limited to those patients deemed high risk despite standard preventive measures (compression devices, anticoagulation).

Prognosis

More than 50% of deaths caused by pulmonary embolism occur within the first hour. After the first hour, patients are at a 2.5% to 10% risk of dying when treated adequately. Inadequate treatment carries a 30% risk of death.[49]

KEY POINTS

1. Most deaths in patients with pelvic fracture are from head injury, nonpelvic hemorrhage, pulmonary injury, thromboembolic complications, and multiple organ system failure.

2. Hemorrhage from unstable pelvic fractures can be minimized by early reapproximation and stabilization of the pelvic ring. If this is unsuccessful, angiography with embolization can be helpful and potentially life saving. Direct preperitoneal pelvic packing has been suggested to help reduce transfusion requirements and the need for angiography.

3. Approximately 15% of seriously injured motor vehicle passengers presenting to a level I trauma center have femur fractures.

4. Associated injuries occur in more than 80% of patients and are responsible for more than 90% of deaths in patients with femur fracture.

5. Infection can manifest as an acute complication of open or closed fractures, with gas gangrene or necrotizing fasciitis being life-threatening infections. Treatment generally consists of débridement and antibiotic therapy.

6. Tetanus can result from any open fracture, but patients who have had farming accidents are at particularly high risk. Diagnosis relies on clinical recognition. Treatment consists of supportive care, surgical débridement, prompt passive immunization, and antibiotics.

7. Diagnosis of compartment syndrome can be made on clinical grounds when the compartment is tense on physical examination, severe pain is present with passive motion, the compartment is tender throughout, and sensory nervous function is impaired.

8. Treatment of rhabdomyolysis involves aggressive IV fluid therapy to avoid accumulation of myoglobin in the renal tubules and aid the clearance of hyperkalemia.

9. An estimated 5000 deaths due to fat embolism syndrome occur annually after pathologic fracture, traumatic fracture, and orthopedic surgery combined.

10. Diagnosis of fat embolism syndrome is based on the presence of the classic triad of respiratory compromise, mental status changes, and petechial rash in the setting of long bone fractures or orthopedic surgery. Treatment is supportive.

11. A number of risk factors for thromboembolic disease have been identified, including long bone and pelvic fractures, age older than 40, immobility, blood transfusion, multiple trauma, head injury, spine fracture, spinal cord injury, and high Injury Severity Score.

12. Signs and symptoms may be present in only 15% of patients diagnosed with DVT by venography.

13. Because of its low cost, noninvasive nature, and high accuracy, color-flow duplex ultrasonography has become the test of choice for DVT.

14. Treatment of DVT and pulmonary embolism usually starts with full anticoagulation using unfractionated heparin, transitioning to sodium warfarin after a period.

15. Fifty percent of deaths caused by pulmonary embolism occur within the first hour. After that, patients are at a 2.5% to 10% risk of dying when treated adequately and at a 30% risk of death when untreated.

ANNOTATED REFERENCES

Bone LB, Johnson KD, Weigelt J, Scheinberg R. Early versus delayed stabilization of femoral fractures: a prospective randomized study. J Bone Joint Surg Am 1989;71:336-40.

This prospective randomized study examined the timing of operative stabilization of femoral fractures in 178 patients. The authors showed that when fracture fixation was delayed in multiply injured patients, the incidence of pulmonary complications was higher, the length of hospitalization was longer, the number of days in the ICU was greater, and the cost of hospitalization was greater.

Scannell BP, Waldrop NE, Sasser HC, et al. Skeletal traction versus external fixation in the initial temporization of femoral shaft fractures in severely injured patients. J Trauma 2010;68:633-40.

This retrospective study compared the physiologic clinical outcomes of patients treated with skeletal traction versus external fixation at a level I trauma center from 2001-2007. There were no significant differences in subsequent rates of ARDS, multiple organ failure, pulmonary embolism, DVT, pneumonia, mechanical ventilation days, ICU length of stay, and death.

Crowl AC, Young JS, Kahler DM, et al. Occult hypoperfusion is associated with increased morbidity in patients undergoing early femur fracture fixation. J Trauma 2000;48:260-7.

This retrospective study of 177 patients with femur fracture compared the incidence of complications between those with occult hypoperfusion (elevated lactate level with normal vital signs) at the time of fracture fixation to those without (normal lactate level and vital signs). The group with occult hypoperfusion had a significantly higher incidence of postoperative complications (50%) versus those without (20%; P < .01).

Demetriades D, Karaiskakis M, Toutouzas K, et al. Pelvic fractures: epidemiology and predictors of associated abdominal injuries and outcomes. J Am Coll Surg 2002;195:1-10.

This retrospective study of 1545 patients with pelvic fractures identifies risk factors associated with coexisting intraabdominal injury, including motor vehicle crash as mechanism, Abbreviated Injury Severity Score 4 or higher, and age older than 55 years. The rate of mortality directly attributable to pelvic fracture was only 0.8%, whereas the overall mortality rate was 13.5%.

Akhtar S. Fat embolism. Anesthesiol Clin 2009;27:533-50.

A comprehensive review of fat embolism syndrome, including definition, epidemiology, etiology, pathophysiology, clinical presentation, diagnosis, management (preoperative and perioperative measures), and prognosis.

Fabian TC, Hoots AV, Stanford DS, et al. Fat embolism syndrome: prospective evaluation in 92 fracture patients. Crit Care Med 1990;18:42-6.

This prospective observational study examined 92 consecutive patients admitted to a level I trauma center with long bone or pelvic fracture. This descriptive study found a rate of fat embolism syndrome of at least 11% among these patients, but it may be much higher if patients with coexisting lung injury are included. The associated mortality rate was 10%.

Geerts WH, Jay RM, Code KI, et al. A comparison of low-dose heparin with low-molecular-weight heparin as prophylaxis against venous thromboembolism after major trauma. N Engl J Med 1996;335: 701-7.

A prospective randomized study of 344 adult trauma patients comparing unfractionated heparin to enoxaparin in the prophylaxis of DVT. This study found a 30% reduction in risk with the use of 30 mg of enoxaparin versus 5000 units of heparin administered SQ every 12 hours. The risk of major bleeding was not significantly different.

Adams RC, Hamrick M, Berenguer C, et al. Four years of an aggressive prophylaxis and screening protocol for venous thromboembolism in a large trauma population. J Trauma 2006;65:300-8.

This retrospective review of a prospectively collected database was conducted to help analyze 4 years of an aggressive prophylaxis and screening protocol for VTE. Weekly duplex scans were conducted in 982 patients. They found that 86% of lower-extremity DVTs were discovered on routine screening duplex. This study concluded that an aggressive prophylaxis/screening regimen led to low rates of VTE as a result of their weekly screening process.

Jeske HC, Larndorfer R, Krappinger D, et al. Management of hemorrhage in severe pelvic injuries. J Trauma 2010;68:415-20.

The authors performed a retrospective cohort study at a level I trauma center, looking at the use of an algorithmic approach to pelvic fracture patients with unstable hemodynamics, using the ATLS guidelines for major trauma. The clinical algorithm was based on radiologic diagnostics, external fixation, and early angiographic embolization in unstable patients. The findings revealed that application of an algorithmic approach reduced need for transfusion and provided early hemodynamic stabilization (within 3 hours).

REFERENCES

Access the complete reference list online at http://www.expertconsult.com.

210

Pediatric Trauma

BRADLEY PETERSON | SUSAN DUTHIE

Injury is the leading cause of medical expenditure for children aged 5 to 14 years. In addition, traumatic injury accounts for approximately 300,000 childhood hospitalizations per year and, in the year 2000, was responsible for more deaths in the 1- to 14-year age group than all natural causes combined. This chapter focuses on trauma-related topics from the viewpoint of a pediatric critical care physician.

Trauma Systems and Trauma Centers

Many studies support the concept that trauma systems and trauma centers improve outcome and that pediatric trauma centers improve outcome for children, especially for those with severe traumatic brain injury. The "Guidelines for the Acute Medical Management of Severe Traumatic Brain Injury in Infants and Children and Adolescents," published in 2003, found sufficient evidence to set seven guidelines for pediatric management. One of the guidelines states, "In a metropolitan area pediatric patients with severe traumatic brain injury (TBI) should be transported directly to a pediatric trauma center if available." An accompanying option states, "Pediatric patients with severe TBI should be treated in a pediatric trauma center or in an adult trauma center with added qualifications for pediatric treatment." These guidelines have been endorsed by six medical societies, including the American Association for the Surgery of Trauma and the Society of Critical Care. Over the last 3 decades, thanks to heroic efforts by the American College of Surgery (ACS), many trauma systems with designated adult and pediatric trauma centers have been developed. A recent paper concluded that pediatric trauma center "mortality rates are lower among children admitted directly from the injury scene compared with those admitted by interhospital transfer."[1] Even after allowing for injury severity, Glasgow Coma Scale (GCS) scores, elapsed time between injury and hospital admission, and age, this finding held true. The ACS program provides verification of trauma centers by an excellent outside review process. To date, the ACS has verified 29 level I pediatric trauma centers[2] (increased from 13 in 2007). The ACS delineates recommended equipment, staffing, policies, and procedures. Important to the trauma center is a designated trauma director and an active morbidity and mortality conference that is attended by all physician members of the trauma team.

Trauma Teams

Trauma teams are essential to the trauma center. A *trauma team* refers to all who care for the trauma patient from resuscitation through discharge. Members of the trauma team include the trauma surgeons, emergency department physicians and nurses, critical care physicians and nurses, respiratory therapists, subspecialty surgeons, radiologists, rehabilitation team, social workers, and clergy. A trauma team requires strong hospital commitment and support. To function optimally, multiple policies and procedures that are understood and respected by all members have to be in place. The resuscitation team is usually led by a surgeon and performs best when led by an attending trauma surgeon. The prepared trauma team improves performance in resuscitation as well as outcome of the patient.[3]

Role of Pediatric Critical Care Physicians

The role of the intensivist in the care of trauma patients has been debated for decades. In 1986, Meyer and Trunkey argued that in most instances, optimal care of seriously injured patients requires "participation between trauma surgeons and critical care specialists, as well as trauma and critical care services. With proper leadership and systems to ensure effective communication between such services, these goals can be achieved. Important secondary goals, in education and research, can also be achieved by such methods."[3] Such attitudes of collaboration and inclusiveness were not always apparent in the 1990s. An editorial in the *Journal of Trauma* stated, "The American Association for the Surgery of Trauma ratifies the position of the American College of Surgeons Committee on Trauma that the trauma surgeon is and must be responsible for the comprehensive management of the injured patient in the critical care unit, including hemodynamic monitoring, ventilator management, nutrition, and posttraumatic complications."[4] A letter to the editor responding to the editorial stated, "Except for a nod to a team effort, the tenor of your editorial would imply that the trauma surgeon and only the trauma surgeon has all the necessary skills in all areas to care for the multiply injured patient to the exclusion of all others."[5] A reply to the letter stated that the intent of the editorial was not meant to be exclusive and that collaborative participation with all specialties was important. Such debates led to feelings of noncollaboration and exclusion among critical care physicians.

In 1991, the American College of Surgeons Committee on Trauma recommended that an "inclusive" trauma system be developed.[6] Atweh advocated that the concept of the inclusive trauma system be broadened to include all phases of injury as well as all the disciplines involved with injuries.[7] In 1999, the president of the American Association for the Surgery of Trauma stated, "It is interesting to note who actually provides much of the minute-to-minute and day-to-day care of patients in many trauma centers. The busier the trauma center, the more likely the care is provided by nonsurgeons: anesthesiologists, emergency physicians, critical care doctors of various stripes.... Clearly these workers are needed to manage patients."[8] Cooper wrote, "What we do know, however, is that trauma systems and trauma centers that make special provision for the needs of children achieve better outcomes than those that don't."[9] He went on to say that the reason for this is more likely to be the specialized system than the surgeon per se and to recommend the development of a fully inclusive trauma system. In October 2002, the Trauma System Agenda for the Future, coordinated through the American Trauma Society, stated that trauma requires a multidisciplinary approach, hospital physicians of all specialties should be included, and appropriate use of all members of the trauma team must be planned.[10] The most recent version of "Resources for Optimal Care of the Injured Patient" states, "Appropriately trained surgical and medical trained specialists may staff the pediatric critical care unit."[11]

An inclusive system is the right system for pediatric trauma patients, and the pediatric critical care physician should have a significant role. The pediatric critical care physician has the most training and experience in life-support therapies for children, including mechanical ventilation, hemodynamic support, renal replacement therapies, and prevention and treatment of secondary brain injury. As an example, data from San Diego Children's Hospital (unpublished) show that during an 18-month period, 80 trauma patients required mechanical ventilation. During the same period, 904 nontrauma patients required mechanical ventilation. The critical care physician is also in the critical care unit on a minute-to-minute basis. Studies have shown better outcomes for children in critical care units directed and attended by critical care physicians.[12] In our system, the critical care physician and the trauma surgeon conduct daily rounds together, including all trauma patients in the pediatric ICU. All patients are discussed on a daily basis with a neurosurgeon as well. This has built mutual respect, contributed to better patient care, and promoted a good working environment. Inclusive attitudes, teamwork, leadership, standard protocols and policies, an ongoing review of the system, and monthly morbidity and mortality conferences all contribute to the quality of the pediatric trauma center and better patient outcomes.

Initial Resuscitation

Resuscitation of the pediatric trauma patient follows the ABCs (airway, breathing, circulation) of Advanced Trauma Life Support (ATLS) and Pediatric Advanced Life Support (PALS) guidelines. Additional discussion of pediatric resuscitation is provided in Chapter 42 on pediatric neurointensive care. Resuscitation begins in the field with emergency medical service personnel and continues at the trauma center with the designated trauma team.

Upon arrival, the airway is assessed for patency and maintainability. The airway may need to be secured if the patient has experienced head, thoracic, abdominal, or airway trauma. Adequate airway control must be obtained while maintaining cervical spine immobilization. These patients are at risk for aspiration secondary to absent or diminished laryngeal reflexes and delayed gastric emptying. Most trauma patients should be orally intubated with direct cricoid pressure.

Many pharmacologic agents are available for rapid-sequence intubation, similar to adult resuscitation. Doses are adjusted for patient weight. The reason for intubation as well as the type of injuries present dictate the medications used. Tracheal tube placement should be confirmed by auscultation of the abdomen and both sides of the chest, checking the position at the lips, and palpation of the cuff in the suprasternal notch. Placement should also be confirmed by end-tidal carbon dioxide monitoring and radiography. The patient's heart rate, blood pressure, oxygen saturation, color, and perfusion should be continuously monitored. Once the airway is secure, ventilation should be evaluated. If unequal breath sounds are noted and the tracheal tube is in the correct position, a hemothorax, pneumothorax, or plugging of a large bronchus may be present. Tracheal deviation, though rare, may help with the diagnosis of tension pneumo- or hemothorax. Breath sounds are transmitted easily in children, and a simple pneumothorax is often not apparent until a chest radiograph is obtained. Tube thoracostomies are placed as needed. Flail chest is rare in pediatrics owing to the flexibility of the rib cage. Ventilation should be maintained with 100% oxygen during resuscitation.

After successful airway establishment and ventilation, circulation must be assessed. Direct pressure should be applied to any site of active hemorrhage. Pulses, perfusion, capillary refill, heart rate and rhythm, and blood pressure should be evaluated. Intravenous (IV) access, preferably two large-bore catheters, must be obtained rapidly for volume resuscitation. Subgaleal, intraabdominal, intrathoracic, or fracture-related hemorrhage may be life threatening. Heart rate is the most sensitive indicator of hypovolemia in pediatric trauma patients. Young children preserve blood pressure despite losing as much as 25% of their intravascular blood volume.[13,14] Thready pulses and altered mental status are evident with loss of 30% to 45% of blood volume. Volume resuscitation begins with crystalloid at 20 mL/kg, with further volume boluses based on the patient's status. Blood products may be necessary to stabilize patients with hemorrhagic shock. Damage control resuscitation (DCR), or early and aggressive prevention and treatment of traumatic hemorrhagic shock, is advocated by a majority of recent trauma transfusion papers. Basic tenets of DCR include hypotensive resuscitation, rapid surgical control, hemostatic resuscitation with red blood cells, plasma, and platelets in a ratio of 1:1:1 along with appropriate use of coagulation factors such as rFVII and cryoprecipitate. Fresh whole blood can be used if available. Some refer to hemostatic resuscitation as *damage control hematology*.[15-17] Hemostatic resuscitation can be monitored and fine-tuned with thromboelastography. Hypertonic (3%) saline has been shown to effectively restore

intravascular volume while also decreasing cerebral edema and may be used as a bolus of 5 to 10 mL/kg. Blood products should be warmed, because pediatric patients are at high risk for hypothermia.

Hypotension contributes to secondary injury to the brain and other vital organs and must be treated aggressively. In rare cases, vasoactive agents may be necessary in the resuscitation room. Trauma victims who are pulseless at the scene have an almost uniformly fatal outcome.[14,18] Prolonged, heroic resuscitative efforts should be avoided in these patients. Patients who have a pulse at the scene but arrest on route or in the emergency department have a slightly better prognosis, and resuscitation should be attempted. Most cardiac arrest associated with blunt trauma is a result of multisystem injuries, including severe brain injury.[19] Open chest resuscitation should be considered only in the rare case of penetrating chest trauma, as it has been shown to be of no benefit in blunt trauma.

The neurologic examination should focus on the level of alertness, GCS score, pupillary response, focal signs of spinal cord injury, and signs of increased intracranial pressure (ICP). Subjects with a GCS score of 8 or less or with a waning mental status should be intubated using rapid-sequence intubation. Noncontrast head computed tomography (CT) should be performed immediately. Cooling the head-injured patient remains an interesting and controversial therapy.

All trauma patients are undressed and exposed for a full examination. Children rapidly lose heat and should be warmed with lights and blankets.

A secondary survey with full physical examination and radiographs as needed should follow the primary survey and stabilization. Once the patient is stabilized and resuscitation is complete, the team decides on a disposition.

Specific Injuries and Critical Care Management

NECK INJURIES

Injuries to the airway in children can be rapidly life threatening. Small airway diameter combined with penetrating or blunt injury to the neck can produce rapid airway obstruction. Children are at greater risk than adults for spinal and major vascular injury from neck trauma. Death from airway injury may occur secondary to disruption of the airway at any level.

Clinically, the neck is divided into three anatomic zones, and management of traumatic airway injuries largely depends on which zone contains the injury. Zone 1 extends from the level of the clavicles up to the cricoid cartilage. Injuries to this area may involve the apex of the lung; trachea; subclavian, carotid, and jugular vessels; thoracic duct; esophagus; vagus nerve; and thyroid gland. Patients suffering zone 1 injuries typically exhibit hypotension, because the great vessels are often injured. Zone 2 encompasses the area from the cricoid to the mandible. Injuries to this area are the easiest to detect. Active bleeding can be reduced by direct pressure. The previous approach of mandatory operative management for zone 2 penetrating injury has been replaced by one of selective surgical exploration of wounds after clinical, endoscopic, and radiographic evaluation. Zone 3 extends from the angle of the mandible to the base of the skull. The oropharynx, jaw, and teeth are located within this area. Mandibular fractures in children manifest as malocclusion of the biting surfaces of the teeth and are usually associated with dental injuries. Injury to the chin associated with tympanic membrane perforation or hemotympanum is associated with an occult fracture of the mandible. Orotracheal intubation is not usually problematic in children with mandibular fractures unless there is copious oral hemorrhage. The neck is further divided into anterior and posterior regions. The anterior region contains the oropharynx, trachea, esophagus, and major vascular structures. The posterior neck contains the spine, spinal cord, and large neck muscles.

Penetrating neck and airway injuries occur less frequently in children than in adults. The majority of penetrating airway injuries in children occur in adolescent males.[20] Because major structures of the airway, central nervous system, and digestive and vascular systems are contained within the neck, penetrating injuries can be lethal owing to the anatomic structures injured. Wounds from sharp objects or bullets may injure the major vascular structures in the neck, trachea, or esophagus. As a result, penetrating wounds to the face and neck are more likely to require surgical intervention than blunt injuries are. Extensive damage to deep tissues may not be apparent on examination of the wound site. Stab wounds typically produce linear tissue injury that follows a predictable path from the entrance wound into the deeper tissue. Bullet injuries may produce unpredictable tissue damage as the result of deflection and shattering of the projectile throughout the neck. Penetrating injury to any of the major systems usually results in rapid airway compromise and shock.

Penetrating injury to the esophagus may not be immediately apparent but can produce delayed morbidity due to mediastinitis. Investigation of anterior neck injuries that involve the trachea should always include evaluation of the esophagus for perforation. Esophageal perforation should be suspected if fever, elevated white blood cell count, and subcutaneous air in the neck occur in the days following a traumatic neck injury. Management of the perforation requires prompt surgical repair of the esophagus, drainage of the surrounding soft-tissue infection, and IV antibiotics.

Although less common than penetrating injuries, blunt neck injuries can be associated with life-threatening airway disruption.[21,22] This injury is frequently missed in the presence of concurrent head, face, and thoracic injuries. Also associated with blunt neck trauma are injuries to the cervical spine, esophagus, lungs, and great vessels. Mortality rates of up to 30% are reported for children with these injuries, and half these children die of tracheobronchial rupture within 1 hour of the injury.[23]

Blunt laryngeal trauma in children is uncommon and frequently unrecognized. The pediatric larynx is characterized by features related to immaturity. Its small diameter, funnel shape, and elastic structure result in significantly greater respiratory problems after trauma compared with adults. Due to its high anterior position in the neck, the larynx of a child is relatively sheltered by the mandible.[24] Greater cricothyroid pliability decreases the incidence of fractures, but surrounding tissue edema or blood in the lumen may rapidly produce respiratory difficulties because of the smaller diameter of the airway. The clinical presentation of laryngeal injury in children includes frank respiratory distress with hoarseness, stridor, and palpable subcutaneous emphysema.[21] Radiographs of the chest and neck may show subcutaneous emphysema as well. The diagnosis of blunt laryngeal trauma in children is based on history, physical examination, and radiographic studies, followed by flexible or rigid bronchoscopy. CT of the neck adds little to the diagnosis of laryngeal injury. Once a laryngeal injury is suspected, rigid endoscopy in the operating suite should be used to secure the airway as well as delineate and repair the injury. Although adult patients with laryngeal injury frequently undergo an awake tracheostomy under local anesthesia, this is not routine in children. Careful placement of a tracheal tube below the level of injury provides an airway, but this may be difficult to accomplish. Difficulties in securing the airway usually reflect a lack of appreciation of the injury. Typical problems include hematoma and airway distortion, bleeding into the airway, or passage of the tracheal tube into the mediastinum.[25]

THORACIC INJURIES

Thoracic trauma, though rare in children, accounts for 5% to 10% of admissions to trauma centers. In isolation, it carries a 5% mortality rate. This increases fivefold when there is concomitant head or abdominal injury and can exceed 40% when a combination of head, chest, and abdominal injuries is present.[26] Potentially life-threatening injuries such as airway obstruction, tension pneumothorax, massive hemothorax, open pneumothorax, flail chest, and cardiac tamponade must be corrected immediately. The last three injuries are relatively uncommon in the pediatric population. Young children have a significantly more flexible thoracic cage than adults do. As a result, compression of intrathoracic organs with blunt trauma may lead to significant parenchymal injuries in the absence of rib fractures. Thus, pulmonary contusions, rather than broken ribs, are far more common in children. In isolation, a broken rib is rarely associated with increased morbidity or mortality.[27] An isolated first rib fracture, however, is a potential sign of child abuse[28] or may be associated with significant thoracic injury. Isolated cervical rib fracture is very rare but has been associated with backpack usage.[29] Multiple rib fractures should alert the clinician to look for underlying injuries in the thoracic cavity. Further radiographic evaluation, such as CT angiography, may be warranted to complete the diagnostic evaluation. Numerous studies have demonstrated that the presence of multiple rib fractures has an approximate 40% mortality rate, often due to the presence of associated multisystem injury.[30] Supportive care is the mainstay of rib fracture management. Appropriate analgesia is necessary to promote deep inspiratory effort and prevent atelectasis. Intercostal nerve blocks or epidural analgesia may be helpful when there is respiratory insufficiency but are rarely necessary.

Trauma to the intrathoracic trachea and bronchi is fortunately rare, as 50% of pediatric patients die within 1 hour of tracheobronchial disruption.[31] Pneumothorax and subcutaneous emphysema are common findings, but rib fractures are not common. Failure of tube thoracostomy to reexpand the lung and the continued presence of a large air leak denote a tracheal or bronchial disruption. If the site of tracheal or bronchial disruption is within the chest cavity, the endotracheal tube tip should be placed distal to the disruption. This may require bronchoscopy. Selective intubation of the undisrupted mainstem bronchus, followed by one-lung ventilation until the proper resources can be obtained for control of the damaged bronchus, may be required. This must be done rapidly and with great care to avoid extending the tracheal injury. Once the injury is repaired, the patient may benefit from a low-tidal-volume ventilation strategy.

Complete bilateral tracheobronchial disruption in a child with blunt chest trauma has been reported. The child survived after median sternotomy, intubation of both left and right mainstem bronchus, and subsequent cardiopulmonary bypass with subsequent reanastomosis of both left and right mainstem bronchi to the trachea.[32]

Pulmonary contusion may occur with or without the presence of overlying rib fractures or chest wall injury. Symptoms include tachypnea, dyspnea, cyanosis, hemoptysis, and respiratory failure. The initial chest radiograph may not demonstrate this injury, and repeat x-rays may be necessary to reveal the infiltrates. Excessive fluid administration should be avoided. Mechanical ventilation may be necessary. Acute respiratory distress syndrome (ARDS) is uncommonly associated with pulmonary contusion, but it may develop. In rare cases, there may be severe pulmonary hypertension.

In children, the mediastinum is less fixed than in adults, and the physiologic consequences of tension pneumothoraces may become evident rapidly. Each hemithorax can hold 40% of a child's blood volume. A chest tube large enough to drain the entire hemithorax without clotting or occluding is necessary. Surgical exploration for hemostasis may be required if the initial chest tube output is 20 mL/kg or greater than 3 to 4 mL/kg/h.[33] Inadequate evacuation leads to lung entrapment from a fibrothorax and predisposes the patient to chronic atelectasis. Penetrating injuries may require thoracotomy in the operating room. Anterior penetrating injuries below the nipple line and posterior penetrating injuries below the tip of the scapula warrant exclusion of intraabdominal injuries.

Other thoracic injuries include traumatic asphyxia, chylothorax, and esophageal tears. Esophageal tears occur in less than 1% of children with blunt thoracic injuries. Esophageal lacerations can be diagnosed with flexible esophagoscopy. Lacerations almost always need repair. Mediastinitis can occur and causes with it a risk of mortality.[34] Traumatic asphyxia is caused by sudden, severe compression of the chest and upper abdomen and is characterized by craniofacial and cervical cyanosis, edema, and petechiae. Subconjunctival and thoracic wall petechiae also occur. There may be associated respiratory distress, cardiac arrest, and cerebral edema with raised ICP. Retinal hemorrhage, blindness, and orbital compartment syndrome have also been reported.[35] Traumatic chylothorax is rare in children but has been reported with blunt and penetrating injury and with child abuse.

CARDIAC AND AORTIC INJURIES

Traumatic injury to the heart and great vessels is significantly less common in pediatric patients than in adults. Most injuries are the result of blunt trauma; penetrating injuries are rare and carry a higher mortality rate.

Myocardial contusion results from blunt force injury to the chest. The vast majority of pediatric patients with myocardial contusions have multisystem trauma; pulmonary contusion is the most common coexisting injury, found in 50% of patients.[36] Hemodynamically significant myocardial contusion is relatively rare in pediatric patients and may present with arrhythmia or ventricular dysfunction. The majority of arrhythmias occur within 24 hours. In a study of 184 pediatric patients with blunt cardiac injury, no hemodynamically stable patient who presented with normal sinus rhythm subsequently developed an arrhythmia or cardiac failure.[36] However, there have been case reports of delayed arrhythmia occurring up to 6 days later.

Diagnostic evaluation of myocardial contusion is controversial and is usually based on a series of tests in the appropriate clinical setting. In pediatrics, testing may include a combination of cardiac enzyme determinations, electrocardiography, and echocardiography. Creatine kinase-MB and cardiac troponin-I elevation following blunt trauma has been used to diagnose contusion. Cardiac troponin-I is highly specific for the myocardium, but creatine kinase-MB may be elevated with injury to skeletal muscle. Elevation of troponin-I occurs within 4 hours of injury and peaks within 24 hours. The significance of elevation in a hemodynamically stable patient is unclear, and determination may not be necessary in these patients.[37,38] An admission 12-lead electrocardiogram (ECG) is recommended in all patients. Echocardiography may show wall motion abnormalities or ventricular dysfunction. In a small pediatric study, echocardiography was diagnostic of cardiac injury in patients with hemodynamic instability or abnormal chest radiographs who had nondiagnostic ECG and creatine kinase-MB.[39]

In addition to myocardial contusion, structural damage such as traumatic ventriculoseptal defect, valve injury, ventricular rupture, or aneurysm may occur with blunt chest trauma. The management of all blunt cardiac injury is largely supportive, with operative intervention as needed for significant structural damage. Continuous ECG monitoring is recommended.

Commotio cordis is an unusual event but is much more common in pediatric patients, with 80% of victims younger than 18 years and 50% younger than 14 years. Blunt trauma to the chest with the impact centered over the heart results in immediate cardiac arrest. It is thought that the narrow anteroposterior diameter of the chest, in conjunction with the increased compliance of the chest wall in pediatric patients, allows a chest-wall blow to be transmitted to the underlying heart. Many but not all cases occur during sports-related activity.[40] Blunt chest trauma leads to cardiovascular collapse, with ventricular tachyarrhythmia being the most common arrhythmia. Unlike myocardial contusion, there is no evidence of myocardial injury on autopsy. The survival rate is low, even with prompt resuscitation.[40,41]

Blunt aortic injury is an extremely uncommon pediatric injury; however, as in adults, it is potentially lethal. The aortic arch is relatively fixed, and the descending aorta is more mobile, making it susceptible to shearing forces during horizontal and vertical deceleration. Three reasons for the rarity of blunt aortic injury in pediatric patients have been proposed. First, most adult thoracic aortic injuries are the result of the driver of a vehicle impacting the steering wheel, with a large force being imparted over a small area. This mechanism does not occur in pediatric patients. Second, blunt trauma in children is often the result of pedestrian-automobile accidents, allowing the force of impact to be widely distributed over the body surface area.[42] Third, the

breaking stress of the thoracic aorta is inversely related to age[43] but is decreased in connective tissue diseases such as Ehlers-Danlos and Marfan syndromes. One of our rare cases of blunt aortic injury occurred in a young child with a connective tissue disorder.

Diagnosis of thoracic aortic injury is similar in children and adults. The pattern of chest x-ray findings is similar, although one study found that depression of the left mainstem bronchus is not as common in pediatric patients. Angiography has been the gold standard for the diagnosis of thoracic aortic injury.[44] Helical CT is fast becoming an important diagnostic tool and, when performed properly, has a sensitivity and specificity similar to that of angiography.[45,46] Transesophageal echocardiography may also have a role in diagnosis, although its place is less clear. As in adults, successful management of these potentially lethal injuries depends on prompt recognition and treatment.

ABDOMINAL INJURIES

More than 90% of abdominal trauma in pediatrics is the result of blunt trauma; penetrating trauma accounts for only 5% to 10% of injuries. After initial resuscitation, evaluation of specific injuries begins. It is important to know the mechanism of trauma to appreciate the potential abdominal injuries. A nasogastric or orogastric tube as well as a Foley catheter should be placed during abdominal evaluation, because dilatation of the stomach and bladder can cause significant pain, interfering with the examination. Inspection of the abdomen may reveal external evidence of trauma suggestive of an underlying injury. Evaluation of abdominal tenderness is important but may be an unreliable finding in a child with lower rib fractures, contusion or soft-tissue injury to the abdominal wall, or pelvic fracture. Auscultation with absent bowel sounds indicates ileus and may suggest underlying gastrointestinal (GI) injury. The pelvis should be examined by compression. Rectal examination should always be performed. If there is blood at the urethral meatus, perineal hematoma, or pelvic instability, a serious pelvic injury should be suspected. Hematuria is indicative of genitourinary injury.

The initial evaluation of children with abdominal trauma may include radiographs of the chest, abdomen, and pelvis. At the present time, focused abdominal sonography for trauma is an excellent initial study of the peritoneum and pericardium. Its use is more widespread in adults than pediatrics.[47-49] The gold standard for evaluation of children with blunt abdominal trauma is CT with IV contrast. It gives reliable information about solid-organ injuries, the presence of abnormal fluid, the presence of pneumoperitoneum indicating hollow viscus injury, and the retroperitoneal space. Further, organ blood flow and contrast extravasation can be observed. Diagnostic peritoneal lavage is a sensitive test to detect bleeding and a perforated hollow viscus in blunt abdominal trauma; however, its use in pediatrics is limited owing to the success of nonoperative management of solid-organ injuries and rapid CT scanning. Diagnostic peritoneal lavage may be indicated in children who have an emergent operative neurologic injury and require immediate assessment of the abdominal cavity.

Penetrating injury is rare in pediatrics. Virtually all gunshot wounds to the abdomen and lower chest should be treated by mandatory laparotomy. Stab wounds below the nipple line and above the inguinal ligament can be managed selectively by local wound exploration, peritoneal lavage, CT scan, and frequent serial physical examinations to determine the need for laparotomy. A recent paper supports selective nonoperative management of penetrating abdominal injuries in children.[50]

Liver

Signs and symptoms of hepatic injury include pain and tenderness, abrasions, and contusion of the abdominal wall. Signs of peritonitis due to hemoperitoneum are frequently present. Most isolated liver injuries can be managed nonoperatively. Selective angiography and embolization may control bleeding without the need for operative repair. Operation, however, may be required for hemodynamic instability, continued transfusion requirement, or other associated injuries. The decision to operate is based on the child's physiologic status and not the graded classification of injury.[47] Complications of hepatic injury include hemobilia, abscess, biliary fistula, and bile peritonitis. The potential for delayed bleeding is higher in hepatic than in splenic injury.

Spleen

The spleen is the organ most frequently injured in blunt abdominal trauma. Ecchymosis, pain, and tenderness over the left upper quadrant are suggestive of splenic injury. Left shoulder pain may be present as a result of diaphragmatic irritation. Abdominal CT is recommended to determine the extent of injury as well as the presence of hemoperitoneum and other associated injuries.

Nonoperative management is preferable and is similar to the nonoperative management of liver injuries. Angiography and selective embolization should be considered in patients with active bleeding seen on CT.[51] Pediatric experience with AE is limited. However, a recent paper reports successful AE in 7 pediatric patients, two spleen (grades IV and V), two liver (grades III and IV), and three grade IV renal injuries.[52] Surgical management may be necessary in patients who are hemodynamically unstable, require continued transfusions, or have other associated abdominal injuries. A variety of surgical techniques are available to control bleeding, often without a total splenectomy. The incidence of total splenectomy in pediatric trauma centers is 3%. In patients requiring total splenectomy, there is a risk of postsplenectomy sepsis. In patients splenectomized for trauma, sepsis develops in 1.5%, with a mortality rate of 50%. Postsplenectomy sepsis may occur at any time, but the risk is greatest in the first 5 years of life. All postsplenectomy patients must be immunized.

Duodenum and Pancreas

The duodenum and pancreas are considered as a unit because they share a blood supply and are connected in the retroperitoneum. For these reasons, managing pancreaticoduodenal injuries is complicated. The most common cause of injury is blunt midepigastrium trauma from a blow, automobile crash, or bicycle handlebar. The diagnosis of pancreaticoduodenal injuries can be achieved using chemical markers and imaging studies. Serum amylase and lipase are indicators of pancreatic injury, but amylase levels may be elevated due to injuries to other organs, including the salivary glands. Ultrasonography and CT are the preferred imaging studies to delineate the pancreas. Duodenal perforations can be diagnosed using upper GI studies with water-soluble contrast or CT scan with oral contrast, in which free air or extravasation may be seen.

Most pancreatic injuries are mild.[53] They can be managed nonoperatively with nasogastric decompression and parenteral nutrition. When the patient's condition improves, nasogastric drainage can be discontinued and oral intake begun. Serial enzyme levels and ultrasonography should be performed to identify complications. Patients with severe pancreatic injury may require surgical repair or endoscopic placement of pancreatic duct stents.

Several complications may occur after pancreatic injury, including pleural effusion, bile duct obstruction, and pancreatic pseudocyst. Pancreatic pseudocyst occurs in one-third of patients.

Most duodenal injuries are lacerations that can be treated by simple débridement and primary repair. For extensive duodenal injuries in which more than 50% of the circumference is affected, the blood supply is compromised, or bile duct/pancreatic injury is present, an aggressive surgical approach may be necessary. Duodenal hematoma results from blunt abdominal trauma associated with rapid deceleration or from a direct blow to the upper abdomen. It may present a day or more after injury as vomiting or a large amount of nasogastric drainage. It is easily diagnosed by ultrasonography or upper GI studies. The resultant intestinal occlusion should be treated by nasogastric decompression and parenteral nutrition until the obstruction resolves. If it fails to resolve within 3 weeks, an operation should be considered.

Small Intestine

Hollow viscus injuries are far less common than solid-organ injuries in pediatric abdominal trauma patients. Nevertheless, bowel injury may result from even mild abdominal trauma. The mechanism of injury is either compression or shear forces resulting from rapid deceleration. There are two points of fixation to the retroperitoneum that frequently lead to transections: the ligament of Treitz and the cecum. Handlebar blows or direct blows to the abdomen compress the bowel against the vertebral column, resulting in intestinal perforation. In the lapbelt complex, contusions or abrasions of the abdominal wall and lumbar spine injury are associated with bowel perforation. Lapbelt loading generates significant intraabdominal injuries in children. Upper lapbelt loading is associated with liver, spleen, rib, stomach, small-bowel, and large-bowel injuries. Lower lapbelt loading is associated with ribs, small bowel, large bowel, bladder, kidney, and stomach injury. Greater than 40% of Abbreviated Injury Severity Score (AISS) 2+ injuries have small-bowel and large-bowel injuries.[54]

Identification of patients with a bowel injury may be challenging. Obtaining a detailed history of the mechanism of injury may prevent a delay in diagnosis and late complications. Detection of peritoneal signs may be difficult owing to distracting pain from the abdominal wall and back injury. If there is also a solid-organ injury, peritoneal signs and symptoms may be interpreted as solely from the associated hemoperitoneum. There is no completely reliable imaging study available to detect intestinal injury. CT may show nonspecific findings suggestive of bowel injury. Serial clinical examinations and repeat CT scanning are important to diagnose injury in a timely fashion. Diagnostic peritoneal lavage may also play a role. Patients should receive nothing by mouth until a bowel injury is no longer suspected.

Diaphragm

Diaphragmatic rupture is the consequence of direct blunt trauma over the lower thorax and abdomen. The injury is most frequent on the left side. Contusion or abrasions of the upper abdomen, bowel sounds in the chest, and respiratory distress are the classic findings of a traumatic diaphragmatic rupture. A chest radiograph may show bowel and the nasogastric tube in the thorax. The diagnosis may be confirmed by upper GI studies, ultrasonography, CT, and/or thoracostomy/laparoscopy. Laparotomy allows proper repair of the diaphragmatic defect and assessment of other organs.

Damage Control and Abdominal Compartment Syndrome

If the child is hemodynamically unstable despite aggressive resuscitation, a laparotomy for damage control may be required.[55] In the presence of the lethal triad of hypothermia, acidosis, and coagulopathy, an immediate definitive surgical repair is unnecessary.[56,57] The damage control approach has three stages.[58] The first stage is the initial laparotomy, the goal being to prevent ongoing damage by controlling hemorrhage and fecal contamination. Abdominal packing and temporary closure of the wounds with loose retention sutures may be required.[59] Definitive surgical repair is postponed until the patient is stabilized. The second stage is carried out in the ICU, with the goals of rewarming, correcting the coagulopathy, and restoring acid-base balance. An abdominal compartment syndrome may develop during the second phase.[60] Intraabdominal pressure may be increased by edema, tissue swelling, ascites, and ongoing bleeding. The high pressure may cause cardiorespiratory and renal deterioration. Elevation of the diaphragm produces basilar atelectasis and restriction of lung inflation, which makes ventilation difficult. Increased abdominal pressure can also cause hypoperfusion of the abdominal contents, leading to renal failure and ischemic bowel injury with resultant bacterial translocation. Increased abdominal pressure also may decrease venous return and therefore cardiac output. Treatment of abdominal compartment syndrome is urgent and may require a peritoneal drain or opening of the abdominal wound and placement of a prosthetic silo.[61] The third stage involves definitive surgery once the patient is stabilized. Packs are removed, tissues are débrided, bowel anastomoses are performed, and fractures are reduced. Most injured patients are not candidates for damage control surgery. Unstable pediatric patients with severe abdominal injury benefit from this staged approach, which is designed to allow medical resuscitation and avoid continued hypothermia, acidosis, and coagulopathy.

GENITOURINARY INJURIES

Genitourinary trauma is common and occurs in 12% of injuries in children. It rarely results in death, but when death does occur, it is usually due to associated injuries. The unique characteristics of a child's anatomy predispose to genitourinary trauma. The kidneys are proportionally larger, the abdominal musculature underdeveloped, and the ribs less ossified than in adults. In addition, the underdeveloped renal capsule and Gerota's fascia increase the likelihood of laceration, hemorrhage, and urine extravasation.

The mechanism of injury is usually blunt force (98%) and has a high association with pelvic trauma. Preexisting renal disease (neoplasms and duplicated collecting systems) predisposes to renal injury and is found in 20% of cases of documented renal trauma. Findings suggestive of genitourinary trauma include flank or abdominal tenderness, perineal injury, blood at the urinary meatus, mobile or displaced prostate, and gross hematuria.

Renal injuries are classified according to severity. Parenchymal injuries not involving the collecting system or renal vessels constitute 85% of renal injuries (grades I to III). Injuries to the collecting system or renal vessels account for 10% of renal injuries (grade IV), and the most severe injuries (grade V), including a shattered or devascularized kidney, constitute 5% of renal injuries.

Treatment goals for pediatric renal trauma include preserving kidney tissue and minimizing patient morbidity. Minor injuries rarely require surgery and are treated expectantly. Limited hospitalization with decreased activity until hematuria has resolved is all that is necessary. Imaging at 6 to 8 weeks following discharge is recommended.

Surgical intervention should be reserved for patients with major injuries and hemodynamic instability from persistent bleeding. An imaging study (CT) or intraoperative intravenous pyelogram (IVP) should be performed to assess the contralateral kidney before undertaking renal exploration. Controversy exists over the management of major injuries in patients who have normal vital signs. Even in the case of urine extravasation without urethral injury, expectant treatment with frequent imaging studies at 5- to 7-day intervals is recommended. Nonoperative management of pediatric renal trauma has become the preferred approach in managing blunt renal injuries.

Penetrating renal injuries secondary to gunshot wounds should be explored because of the high incidence of associated injuries. Surgical treatment for stab wounds with suspected renal involvement should be based on the severity of hemorrhage and both clinical and imaging evidence suggesting intraabdominal injury.

Renovascular injuries generally occur in patients who have sustained life-threatening multisystem injuries. The mechanism of renovascular injury is thought to be deceleration with initial injury and arterial thrombosis. This occurs more frequently on the left side. The diagnosis is established with either contrast-enhanced CT or arteriography. Successful revascularization depends on the length of renal ischemia, extent of vascular injuries, and extent of associated injuries. Renal vein injuries are repaired in most cases. Repair of penetrating renal artery injuries is most successful if the ischemic time is less than 8 hours. Blunt arterial injuries are associated with the lowest rate of renal preservation and are most often treated by nephrectomy when they are unilateral.

PELVIC FRACTURES

Pelvic fractures are a marker for significant trauma and are often associated with other injuries. Pelvic fractures occur in approximately 2% of all blunt abdominal injuries, and 20% of those with pelvic fractures have intraabdominal injuries. Mortality varies from 10% to 50% and is often due to associated injuries. The most common mechanisms are falls, crush injuries, and motor vehicle accidents. Clinically, the diagnosis is suggested by pain with anterior or lateral compression of the pelvis. Other findings may include perineal ecchymosis, blood at the urinary meatus or on the rectal examination, disruption of the rectal wall with mass effect due to bony fragments, or displacement of the prostate.

Evaluation of pelvic trauma begins with a pelvic radiograph and should include CT. Morbidity is lower in children than in adults. Treatment usually consists of bed rest, immobilization, and blood loss replacement. Severe injuries with significant blood loss may require prompt intervention and immobilization, wrapping the pelvis with a bed sheet, or application of an external fixation device. Selective embolization can also provide hemostasis.

SPINAL INJURIES

Approximately 5% of all spinal cord injuries occur in the pediatric age group. Common causes in young children include falls and motor vehicle accidents. Recently, inflicted trauma, including gunshot wounds in urban areas, has been identified as a significant mechanism of injury for this age group.[62] For older children, sports and other recreational activities such as horseback and bicycle riding have greater etiologic importance.

The head and neck anatomy of a young child resembles that of a "bobble-head" doll, with a relatively large head resting on a small, highly flexible neck. To maintain neutral cervical alignment during transport and initial resuscitation of a child at risk for a spinal injury, a support is often placed under the thorax to achieve torsal elevation, in addition to the use of an appropriately sized cervical collar. Alternatively, a board with an occipital recess may be used for this purpose.[63]

Initial assessment dictates the need for imaging studies. An awake, communicative child without midline cervical tenderness, intoxication, decreased level of consciousness, focal neurologic deficit, or a painful distracting injury does not require spinal imaging studies.

Cervical spine imaging studies include lateral C-spine, anteroposterior (A-P) C-spine, and open-mouth views, flexion/extension lateral C-spine radiographs, CT, and magnetic resonance imaging (MRI). For the child with symptoms of cervical spine and/or cervical cord injury and for the comatose child, CT imaging, 64-slice, and/or MRI are now recommended. A number of recent papers in the literature discuss optimal C-spine imaging.[64,65] Some of these are discussed in the section on imaging in this chapter.

Prospective randomized multicenter trials of pharmacologic agents for the treatment of acute spinal cord injury in children younger than 13 years have not been carried out. However, data from adult studies have been extrapolated and are commonly used to dictate management schemes in children. Methylprednisolone is administered within 3 hours of injury as an initial IV bolus of 30 mg/kg to run over 15 minutes, followed by an infusion of 5.4 mg/kg/h to run over 23 hours.[66] If the initial administration is between 3 and 8 hours after injury, the infusion is continued for 48 hours. Methylprednisolone treatment is not initiated more than 8 hours after injury.[67] Recent studies, however, show no benefit of high-dose methylprednisolone for complete and incomplete spinal cord injury and suggest very limited use of methylprednisolone because of the high incidence of pneumonia.[68,69]

In a child with a spinal cord injury, emphasis is placed on maintenance of optimal physiologic homeostasis. Because of loss of sympathetic tone, IV pressor agents are frequently required in addition to crystalloid and colloid solutions to maintain age-appropriate blood pressure and cardiac output. Intubation may be necessary with high cervical spine injuries because of respiratory compromise. Avoidance of unnecessary neck manipulation is essential.

After initial resuscitation and the identification of spinal injuries, urgent neurosurgical and orthopedic consultation is indicated. Closed reduction and initial stabilization of these injuries are frequently performed in the ICU. Halo rings can be placed with acceptably low morbidity in the ICU setting, even in infants; they can be attached to weighted traction mechanisms for closed reduction if necessary and converted to halo jackets to maintain alignment. The need for and timing of internal surgical stabilization should be discussed in the context of the child's concomitant multisystem issues. Hypothermia and hypertonic saline are therapies that are being evaluated.

CLOSED HEAD INJURIES

It is estimated that each year, 2685 children between the ages of 1 and 14 die from TBI; 37,000 are hospitalized, and 475,000 are treated in hospital emergency departments.[70] TBI costs per year for the age group 1 to 19 years is over $2.5 billion.[71] TBI is caused by linear and inertial forces resulting in an impact injury.[72] This is the primary injury. It includes hematomas, lacerations, and axonal shearing and is often described as irreparable. *Secondary injury* refers to the injury that occurs after impact. It is considered both preventable and potentially reversible. Pathologic alterations in respiratory, hemodynamic, and cellular function occur, which may lead to secondary injury and cell death. The pathways to neuron death include inadequate oxygen and nutrient supply secondary to hypoxia and decreased cerebral blood flow. Decreased cerebral blood flow can occur secondary to hypotension, decreased cardiac output, raised ICP, and cerebrovascular dysregulation, including endothelial dysfunction, vasospasm, and microthrombus formation. Elevated ICP occurs secondary to mass lesions, cerebral edema, and increases in cerebrospinal fluid volume and cerebral blood volume. Other pathways to neuron death include excitotoxicity, energy failure, inflammation, oxidative stress, and apoptosis. Present therapies are directed primarily at supporting oxygenation, blood pressure, and cardiac output and at controlling ICP.[73]

After an exhaustive literature review, the "Guidelines for the Acute Medical Management of Severe Traumatic Brain Injury in Infants, Children, and Adolescents"[74] found insufficient evidence to support any standards of care but sufficient evidence to support some guidelines for care: transfer of children in a metropolitan area with severe TBI to a pediatric trauma center, avoidance of hypoxia, correction of hypotension, maintenance of cerebral perfusion pressure greater than 40 mm Hg in children, a recommendation against the continuous infusion of propofol for either sedation or the control of intracranial hypertension, a warning against the use of corticosteroids, and a recommendation against the prophylactic use of antiseizure medication. Evidence was sufficient to support 17 care options and a flow diagram.

Initial stabilization requires support of the ABCs. The airway must be maintained and breathing supported to prevent hypoxemia and hypercarbia. Hyperoxia and brief aggressive hyperventilation are indicated during the initial resuscitation if the clinical examination reveals signs of herniation or acute neurologic deterioration. Normotension or mild hypertension and mild hypervolemia are indicated to support cardiac output and cerebral blood flow. Fluids, sedation, and vasoactive agents must be judiciously administered. Hypertonic saline may be advantageous as a resuscitation fluid for patients with shock, especially those with raised ICP. All children with a suspected TBI, history of loss of consciousness, altered level of consciousness, focal neurologic signs, evidence of a depressed or basilar skull fracture, a bulging fontanelle, or persistent headache and vomiting should have a head CT.[72] Surgery is indicated for significant mass lesions. ICP monitoring is indicated for patients with a GCS score less than 8. Even with a normal CT scan, 10% to 15% of patients with a GCS score less than 8 have elevated ICP. A physician may also choose to monitor ICP in certain conscious patients whose CT scans indicate a high potential for decompensation or in patients in whom neurologic examination is precluded by sedation or anesthesia. Physicians should be aware that in a few patients with normal CT findings and elevated ICP, the only symptoms are moderate to severe headaches, vomiting, and lethargy.

ICP monitoring with a ventricular catheter, an external strain gauge transducer, or a catheter tip pressure transducer is considered accurate and reliable. Ventriculostomy allows cerebrospinal fluid drainage in addition to ICP monitoring and appears to decrease the magnitude of other therapies needed. In patients with a significant cerebral

contusion, an ICP monitor on the same side may more accurately reflect the ICP near the contusion.

ICP in children and adolescents should be kept less than 20 mm Hg. In young infants with open fontanelles and sutures and in older children with large diastatic skull fractures, controlling the ICP at less than 10 to 15 mm Hg may be wise.

The guidelines recommend a cerebral perfusion pressure greater than 40 mm Hg in children with TBI. It may be better to maintain cerebral perfusion pressure according to an age-related continuum between 45 and 70 mm Hg.

Initial treatment for elevated ICP includes mild hyperventilation, with partial pressure of carbon dioxide (Pco_2) 35 to 40 mm Hg, sedation and analgesia, ventriculostomy drainage, and muscle relaxants. Sedation can be accomplished with low-dose fentanyl, 1 to 2 μg/kg/h, dexmedetomidine, 0.4 to 1 μg/kg/h, intermittent doses of benzodiazepines or barbiturates, or a low continuous infusion of pentobarbital or sodium thiopental at 1 mg/kg/h. If ICP is not controlled, a repeat CT should be obtained and hyperosmolar therapy begun. Osmolar agents include mannitol and hypertonic saline. Hypertonic saline appears to have several advantages over mannitol.[73] A continuous infusion of hypertonic saline allows consistent control of osmolality, potentially minimizing the frequency and magnitude of ICP spikes.[75] Hypertonic saline supports mean arterial pressure and cardiac output. It also has beneficial vasoregulatory properties and may have beneficial effects on immune and inflammatory responses.[73] The guidelines have found sufficient evidence to include hypertonic saline as an option under hyperosmolar therapy and to regard it as first-tier therapy. Recommendations for osmotherapy include mannitol (also as a first-tier therapy) given as a bolus (0.25-1 g/kg) provided serum osmolarity is less than 320 mOsm/L, and hypertonic saline (3%) administered as a continuous infusion (0.1-1 mL/kg/h). The appropriate dose is the minimum dose required to keep the ICP less than 15 to 20 mm Hg. The dose may be increased provided serum osmolarity is less than 360 mOsm/L. A recent paper verified the safety of continuous hypertonic saline while recommending future studies comparing bolus to continuous dosing.[76] Additional areas of investigation in TBI therapy include hypothermia, role of decompressive craniotomy, monitoring of brain tissue oxygenation and cerebrovascular pressure reactivity, continuous versus intermittent drainage of CSF, glycemic control, use of neuroprotectants such as erythropoietin and progesterone among others, and stem cell therapy.

High-dose barbiturate therapy, hyperventilation to a Pco_2 less than 30 mm Hg, moderate hypothermia, and decompressive craniectomy are regarded as second-tier therapies. It is prudent to obtain a repeat CT of the head each time a significant increase in medical therapy is required. In adults with severe TBI, an aggressive management strategy has been associated with a lower mortality rate, with no significant difference in functional status at discharge among survivors.[77]

▧ Organ Failure

ACUTE RESPIRATORY DISTRESS SYNDROME

Trauma can result in lung injury and respiratory failure, the most severe of which is ARDS. Posttraumatic respiratory failure results from both direct and indirect injury to the respiratory system. Direct injuries include aspiration of gastric contents, near drowning, smoke inhalation, and pulmonary contusion. Lung injury also occurs indirectly as a consequence of systemic insults such as shock, sepsis, massive transfusion, fat embolism syndrome, or the systemic inflammatory response syndrome (SIRS). For non–massively transfused trauma patients, plasma administration has been associated with a substantial increase in ARDS.[71] ARDS is an acute and progressive respiratory disease of a noncardiac nature associated with diffuse bilateral pulmonary infiltrates and hypoxemia. The definition includes a ratio of arterial oxygen tension (Pao_2) to inspired oxygen fraction (Fio_2) less than 200.

The pathologic findings in ARDS are the result of a complex sequence of cellular and biochemical changes that lead to damage of the endothelial membranes. The specific roles and relative importance of leukocytes, complement activation, prostaglandin release, oxygen radicals, and other mediators of vascular damage are not completely understood. Neutrophils are thought to be an important mediator. This is supported by clinical findings of transient leukopenia in ARDS patients and increased numbers of neutrophils in lung tissue and bronchoalveolar lavage fluid. Blunt trauma enhances the migratory capacity of neutrophils in response to interleukin-8, potentially increasing the risk of ARDS.[78]

The incidence and outcome of ARDS in the pediatric trauma population have not been well studied. In a series of 1989 pediatric trauma patients over an 8-year period with blunt trauma (79%), penetrating trauma (12%), and burns (9%), the overall risk of ARDS was 14%, with a mortality rate of 24%. In those patients with burns, all intubated patients developed ARDS, and the mortality rate was 42%.[79] In a study of adult patients with severe head injury, those patients who developed acute lung injury had a significant increase in mortality (38% versus 15%) and a worse neurologic outome.[80] In our trauma practice, ARDS is seen most often in association with SIRS in patients with severe TBI, often as cerebral edema is improving (unpublished data).

ARDS management in pediatrics has focused on minimizing iatrogenic lung injury and on adjuncts to mechanical ventilation. Both oxygen and mechanical ventilation can be injurious to the lung. Oxygen causes oxidative damage and absorptive atelectasis, with chronic exposure to high inspired concentrations of oxygen creating a pathologic picture indistinguishable from ARDS. In both animal and human studies, toxic reactions to oxygen occur commonly with the use of FIO_2 greater than 0.5, and these effects worsen when excessive oxygen is used for longer than 24 hours. Mechanical ventilation also causes lung injury due to increased shear forces applied in the terminal airways. The higher the tidal volumes used to ventilate patients, the greater the stresses and the larger the risk of secondary lung injury. These stresses on the terminal airways and pulmonary endothelium incite pulmonary edema, surfactant dysfunction, decreased compliance, hyaline membrane formation, and impairment of gas exchange.

Ventilatory strategies focus on decreasing iatrogenic lung injury by limiting oxygen concentration and using high-frequency or oscillatory ventilation. Permissive hypercapnia (allowing PCO_2 45-60 mm Hg or higher) is also practiced when the patient's condition allows. The strategy of "low-stretch" ventilation has been shown to decrease morbidity and mortality in pediatric ARDS.[81,82] Additional support for low-volume, low-pressure ventilation comes from the National Institutes of Health ARDS Network trial comparing 6 mL/kg versus 12 mL/kg tidal volumes in patients with ARDS. Mortality in the low-tidal-volume group was 31.3%, versus a mortality of 39.8% in the higher-tidal-volume group.[83] Paulson and colleagues used a high-rate, low-tidal-volume (3-5 mL/kg) strategy on 53 children with severe ARDS and had a survival rate of 89%.[81] Hypercapnia is well tolerated, except in patients with TBI with intracranial hypertension or those with severe pulmonary hypertension. In addition to low-stretch ventilation strategies, helium-oxygen mixtures are being used to improve gas exchange at lower peak pressures. For patients who fail support with mechanical ventilation, extracorporeal membrane oxygenation support can be employed. There are many other adjuncts to ventilation that may decrease the morbidity and mortality of ARDS. These adjuncts include prone positioning, inhaled nitric oxide (NO), surfactant, steroids, immunomodulation, antiinflammatory agents, and immunonutrition; all remain under investigation.

Prone positioning has been used to improve oxygenation in ARDS patients. The improvement may be a result of the redistribution of ventilation or lung perfusion with improved ventilation/perfusion matching. Recent papers conclude that prone ventilation reduces mortality in patients with severe ARDS.[76,84] Prone positioning does improve oxygenation and is possible in patients with a wide variety of injuries as well as support lines. If it is not possible, a roto-bed with rotation to 45 to 180 degrees can be used with similar benefit to oxygenation, allowing a decrease in ventilation pressures.

Inhaled NO has potent pulmonary vasodilatory effects and is potentially useful in ARDS, especially in a few cases that have a marked increase in pulmonary vascular resistance. Dellinger and coworkers conducted a randomized trial of inhaled NO versus placebo in 177 patients with ARDS.[85] Although an acute increase in PaO_2 was observed in 60% of patients receiving NO versus 24% of placebo-treated patients, this did not confer any advantage in overall survival. Several other randomized studies of inhaled NO have had similar results.[86] The use of inhaled NO delivered during high-frequency oscillatory ventilation in patients with ARDS resulted in a significant increase in arterial oxygenation.[87]

SHOCK

Shock in children sustaining trauma is most commonly a direct result of hemorrhage, but it can occasionally be the result of tension pneumothorax, spinal cord injury, cardiac tamponade, myocardial contusion, or sepsis. Direct tissue injury and hemorrhage play roles in early shock, while inflammation and altered immune function can result in SIRS, multiple organ failure, and septic shock later in the course.

Children and adults respond differently to hemorrhagic shock. Children have remarkable compensatory mechanisms in response to hypovolemia. Children maintain cardiac output by increasing the heart rate more than the stroke volume. Hypotension is a relatively late sign of traumatic shock in children; therefore, relying on hypotension as an indicator for fluid resuscitation can be deleterious. Tachycardia and signs of end-organ hypoperfusion, such as altered mental status, cool distal extremities, and decreased urine output, may be the primary clinical signs of shock in an injured child.

The focus of therapy for shock in an injured child should be on restoration and maintenance of adequate oxygen delivery and organ perfusion. Hemodynamic monitoring of central venous pressure and direct arterial blood pressure, as well as cardiac output, may be necessary. In addition, clinical parameters such as base deficit,[88] serum lactate,[89] and measured creatinine clearance are useful indirect measures of adequate end-organ perfusion and may have prognostic value.[88,90] Appropriate therapy of early shock resulting from trauma can alleviate the development of SIRS and multiple organ failure later. Resuscitation with hypertonic saline in two animal models of trauma and hemorrhagic shock was shown to attenuate neutrophil-mediated organ injury; specifically, this occurred in the lung, where much of the inflammation of SIRS occurs, and in the intestine, which is thought to be a major source of neutrophil activation following ischemia.[91,92] A recent paper demonstrated an increase in survival in ARDS patients receiving hypertonic saline during resuscitation if those same adult patients had required 10 units or more of packed red blood cells in the first 24 hours.[93] There may also be a role for stress-dose steroids following hemorrhagic shock, because sustained adrenal impairment is frequently seen and may be related to the inflammatory consequences and vasopressor dependency of hemorrhagic shock.[94]

The tissue ischemia and hypoperfusion associated with shock result in alteration of cellular function due to oxygen and nutrient deficiency, eventually leading to activation of inflammatory mediators. A current model of SIRS and multiple organ failure in trauma patients is the "two-hit hypothesis." The initial hit is the shock-resuscitation or ischemia-reperfusion phase, which activates neutrophils, making them more susceptible to an exaggerated immune response to late inflammatory stimuli, the second hit.[95,96] Barbiturates and hypothermia, both used to treat severely head injured patients, suppress neutrophil function, increase infectious risks, and may contribute to the late inflammatory stimuli leading to SIRS and multiple organ failure. It may be that severe TBI with release of cytokines itself triggers SIRS. The inflammatory mediator response to trauma that leads to SIRS and multiple organ failure has been proposed as a "three-level model," with mediators acting at the levels of cells, organs, and the organism. Immune modulation has been the focus of current research in trauma with regard to the late sequelae of SIRS and multiple organ failure.[97]

RENAL FAILURE

Renal failure in pediatric trauma patients early in the hospital course is most often due to organ injury from initial shock or from primary injury to the kidney, its vasculature, or urinary outflow tract. Anatomic reasons for renal insufficiency should be delineated by radiographic evaluation. One kidney is sufficient for adequate function; therefore, clinically evident renal failure requires injury to both kidneys or shock.

Renal failure that develops during the course of hospitalization is most commonly secondary to SIRS and multiple organ dysfunction syndrome. In addition, rhabdomyolysis, contrast nephropathy from imaging studies, or nephrotoxicity from medications may occur. Abdominal compartment syndrome and renal vein thrombosis also can lead to renal failure. High-dose mannitol, 0.25 gm/kg/h, as an infusion over 58 ± 28 hours, has been associated with renal failure.[98] This is thought to be secondary to renal vasoconstriction. There is also concern that hypernatremia can cause renal failure. However, in studies using hypertonic saline for control of intracranial hypertension, renal failure did not occur unless SIRS with multiple organ failure was also present.[75]

Signs and symptoms of acute renal failure are due to the accumulation of urea, electrolyte derangements, and volume overload. The first clinical features may be oliguria, hyperkalemia, and elevations in blood urea nitrogen (BUN) and creatinine. The laboratory evaluation of acute renal failure should include measurements of BUN, creatinine, electrolytes with phosphate, magnesium, and calcium, urinalysis, and urine electrolytes. Creatinine clearance should be measured to estimate glomerular filtration rate. Daily 4-hour creatinine clearances are helpful in detecting early changes in renal perfusion and function. Microscopy is necessary to differentiate hemoglobinuria or myoglobinuria from hematuria, and additional tests such as creatine phosphokinase can aid in the confirmation of crush injuries threatening renal function. A recent large multicenter prospective cohort of trauma patients showed that acute kidney injury (AKI; RIFLE [risk, injury, failure, loss, end-stage renal disease] criteria) was associated with an independent risk of hospital death in a dose-response manner even in patients with mild AKI.[99]

Prevention of acute renal failure includes aggressive resuscitation from shock and continued maintenance of cardiac output and organ perfusion pressure. In addition, minimizing and monitoring of nephrotoxic drugs may be helpful. Many agents have been used to prevent and treat acute ischemic or nephrotoxic renal injury. They include furosemide, mannitol, calcium channel blockers, and dopamine, most without benefit.[100] Although diuretic therapy may convert oliguric to nonoliguric acute renal failure, there is no evidence that patient outcome is improved. Prehydration and prophylaxis with theophylline or N-acetylcysteine has been shown to reduce the risk of contrast nephropathy and may be of benefit for children undergoing contrast scans who already have or are otherwise predisposed to develop renal failure.[101] The use of "renal-dose" dopamine has a controversial history marked by conflicting studies. A large randomized controlled trial in adults concluded that it did not confer clinically significant protection from renal dysfunction.[102] Definitive studies on renal-dose dopamine are lacking in children. Fenoldopam, a selective dopaminergic agent and more potent renal vasodilator than dopamine, has shown some promise in preventing and treating acute renal failure in adults.[103,104]

Early institution of renal replacement therapy in the face of acute renal failure decreases morbidity.[105] Peritoneal dialysis is an excellent modality for infants and children, although trauma patients may have contraindications. Continuous venovenous hemofiltration dialysis is an excellent choice in a high-acuity or head-injured patient requiring a steady hyperosmolar state for control of ICP. It offers the benefit of constant and gentle manipulation and control of intravascular volume, electrolytes, dialyzable molecules, and serum osmolarity.[106] The development of regional anticoagulation with citrate-induced hypocalcemia has increased the efficacy and safety of continuous venovenous hemofiltration dialysis, especially in children at risk for bleeding from systemic anticoagulation.

▐ Special Considerations

IMAGING

Spinal Trauma

- Injuries in young children commonly involve C1, C2, and C3. In older children and adolescents, the injury pattern is similar to that in adults, predominantly involving the mid and lower spine.[107]
- Recent evidence supports the use of selective criteria in imaging.[108,109]
- The lateral radiograph is the most important view, especially in children younger than 5 years. The false-negative rate for a single cross-table lateral view is 21% to 26%. For this reason, additional views and/or CT scan is indicated.[107] Practice guidelines, however, have changed, and CT has replaced plain radiography.[109] A recent paper concludes that "lateral view radiographs showed a borderline acceptable diagnostic sensitivity for the detection of traumatic cervical spine abnormalities compared with CT while the addition of other views did not seem to improve the diagnostic performance of conventional radiography."[110]
- Considerations when interpreting lateral C-spine include:
  1. Predental space up to 5 mm is normal.
  2. Pseudosubluxation of C2 or C3 is a common pitfall on lateral radiographs of the cervical spine. A normal posterior cervical line does not exclude underlying ligamentous injury at C2-C3.[107]
  3. Above the glottis, soft-tissue thickness of 7 mm or more is considered abnormal; below the glottis, a measurement of 14 mm should be considered abnormal.[111]
  4. A distance of 6 mm or more between the lateral mass of C1 and the odontoid process is suggestive of ligamentous disruption of the transverse ligament.
  5. Posterior tilting of the odontoid is a common normal finding; however, anterior tilting is abnormal and suggests injury.
  6. When evaluating for atlanto-occipital dislocation, a gap of more than 5 mm between the occipital condyles and the condylar surface of the atlas is highly suggestive of craniocervical injury. A line drawn along the posterior aspect of the clivus toward the odontoid should intersect the odontoid.[107]
  7. Wedged C3 vertebral body is a normal phenomenon in infants and young children.
- Thoracic lumbar spinal injuries: the most common injury of the thoracolumbar spine is a flexion injury. This often results in anterior compression fractures. The more severe the injury, the greater the likelihood of posterior ligamentous injury. It is very important to look for abnormalities of the disc space, widening of the interspinous distance and neural foramina, and fractures of the spinous process and neural arch. Transverse fracture of the vertebral body with anterior or lateral dislocation of the upper half of the fractured vertebra is called a *Chance fracture* and is common in lapbelt injuries. Associated abdominal injuries, especially to the bowel, are common.
- MRI should be obtained when cord injury is evident or cannot be ruled out and to evaluate ligamentous injury. Some researchers, however, point out that MRI overreads ligamentous injuries.

Traumatic Brain Injury

- The type and site of skull fracture are important. Fractures traversing the paranasal sinuses and mastoid can lead to complications such as meningitis, pneumocephalus, and cerebrospinal fluid leak. Depressed fractures commonly have dural tears and brain injury. Fractures that traverse vascular structures, such as the middle meningeal artery, dural sinuses, and carotid and vertebral arteries, are important to recognize because of the possibility of underlying vascular injury.
- Acute subdural hematoma has a crescent shape and is generally hyperdense; however, approximately 40% are heterogeneous owing to unclotted blood or cerebrospinal fluid.

- Diffuse axonal injury tends to occur in the lobar white matter (especially at the gray/white matter interface), corpus callosum, and dorsolateral aspect of the upper brainstem. Gradient-echo magnetic resonance sequences are sensitive for evaluation.
- CT often finds more contusions 24 to 48 hours after the initial CT scan. In 20% of contusions, delayed hemorrhage occurs in what were thought to be nonhemorrhagic contusions on initial CT.
- A common place for subarachnoid hemorrhage to accumulate is in the interpeduncular fossa. Fluid-attenuated inversion recovery magnetic resonance sequences are very sensitive for subarachnoid hemorrhage.
- Manifestations of abusive head trauma include multiple, complex, or depressed skull fractures; subdural hematomas of varying ages; bilateral subdural hematomas; cortical contusions; diffuse axonal injury; retinal hemorrhages; and cerebral ischemia or infarction.[112]
- CT angiography can be obtained to look for suspected blunt cerebrovascular trauma, which occurs in 1% and in all ages.[113]

Thoracic Trauma

- Anterior or lateral rib fractures over the lower thoracic region may be associated with splenic or hepatic injury. Fractures of the first three ribs should raise the suspicion of great vessel injury. Low posterior rib fractures may be associated with renal injury.
- Sternal fractures are frequently associated with underlying cardiac injury.[111]
- Radiographs usually underestimate the full extent of pulmonary trauma.
- Tears of the right mainstem and distal left bronchus give rise to pneumothorax. Tears of the trachea and left mainstem bronchus usually cause pneumomediastinum and widening of the mediastinum if bleeding occurs.
- Blunt thoracic aortic injury is rare in pediatrics. Radiologic evaluation of this injury has changed, and more CT angiograms are performed and used to make decisions regarding surgery.[46]

Abdominal Trauma

- Indirect indications of organ injury on radiographs include elevation of the diaphragm, obliteration of fat planes, free intraperitoneal air or trapped air (retroperitoneal air), mass effect, thumb-printing of bowel owing to intramural hematoma, fractures, portal venous gas, and hemoperitoneum.
- Hypoperfusion complex is seen in patients presenting in shock who seem to respond to initial resuscitation. Mortality is approximately 85%. Constant findings on CT include marked diffuse bowel dilatation, intense contrast enhancement (bowel wall, mesentery, kidneys), and small-caliber inferior vena cava and aorta.
- Plain film findings associated with splenic injury include medial displacement of the stomach, displacement of the splenic flexure, elevation of the left hemidiaphragm, scoliosis of the spine with concavity on the left, sentinel loops in the left upper quadrant, left pleural effusions or atelectasis, and rib fractures.
- Periportal tracking is seen in up to 22% cases of hepatic injury, which is due to dissecting blood, bile, or dilated lymphatics. Hemoperitoneum is common in liver laceration owing to the inability of liver vessels to contract.
- Technetium-labeled N-substituted iminodiacetic acid compound (HIDA) scans are very useful in evaluating for possible bile leak in a patient with persistent free fluid in the abdomen after liver injury.
- Pancreatic injury is difficult to visualize on initial CT scans.
- Trauma to the duodenum may include duodenal rupture, intramural tears, or intramural hematoma. The usual site of perforation is along the posterior duodenal wall.[111]
- CT findings of bowel injury in blunt abdominal trauma include hypodense free fluid (85%), particularly in an interloop location due to perforation; focal bowel wall thickening (>3 cm); focal discontinuity of bowel; sentinel clot adjacent to bowel; streaky, hyperattenuating mesentery; mesenteric hematoma; hyperdense contrast enhancement of injured bowel; pneumoperitoneum; and extravasation of contrast.[114]
- Contrast "blush" occurs in greater than 6% of patients,[115] is not associated with a negative outcome, and can be treated without surgery.

Genitourinary Trauma

- CT findings of renal injury are as follows. For contusion: focal patchy enhancement or striated nephrogram. For laceration: irregular, linear, hypodense parenchymal abnormalities. For shattered kidney: multiple separated fragments, some of which may not enhance owing to a lack of perfusion. For subcapsular hematoma: superficial crescentic hypodense area compressing adjacent parenchyma. For segmental arterial injury: wedge-shaped perfusion defect. For devascularized kidney: diffuse lack of enhancement of kidney. For renal vein thrombosis: persistent nephrogram on delayed images and renal swelling.[114] Delayed images are essential in the evaluation of renal trauma.
- Blunt trauma to the ureteropelvic junction is associated with transverse process fractures (30%).
- In infants and young children, a full bladder becomes an abdominal organ, as it arises out of the pelvis and is more prone to injury because it is not as protected as the adult urinary bladder.
- CT cystography is highly accurate as an adjunct to routine abdominopelvic CT in the trauma setting. It obviates the need for a separate study with conventional cystography, which entails additional cost and more radiation exposure.

Infectious Disease and Immunology

A child who sustains trauma is susceptible to infection in several ways. The trauma itself may destroy the barriers of skin and mucosa, allowing both pathogenic and nonpathogenic organisms the opportunity to establish a productive infection. In addition, significant immune dysfunction occurs following trauma; both nonspecific and specific abnormalities have been described in cellular and humoral responses, as well as in macrophage and neutrophil function.[116-118] More recent investigations provide data on cytokines and other mediators and molecular markers of inflammation, both circulating and cell surface.[119,120] These abnormalities of immune dysfunction can be categorized under two basic mechanisms: hyperactive systemic proinflammatory processes and depression of cell-mediated immunity. Hyperactive proinflammatory responses may be ultimately deleterious to a child, leading to SIRS, multiple organ dysfunction syndrome, and death. Hyperactive proinflammatory response may be the result of priming the trauma patient for an exaggerated response to a second inflammatory stimulus, referred to as the *two-hit hypothesis*. Differences in the characteristics of immune dysfunction appear to be a function of the type of trauma (e.g., TBI, blunt trauma, burn injury) and appear to change over time after trauma to reflect changes in the acute activation seen immediately after the injury, with subsequent evolution into immune suppression.[118] Many of the abnormalities may be directly correlated with the severity of injury.[117] Infections occurring within approximately 5 to 7 days of admission are more likely to represent inoculation at the time of trauma, whereas infections occurring after the first week of trauma reflect nosocomial pathogens present in the trauma center.

Empirical antibiotic therapy of the pediatric trauma patient on admission to the ICU is not well studied. Extrapolation from prospective controlled surgical studies in adults has provided some support for empirical prophylactic therapy, with the selection of antibiotics designed to provide reasonable coverage against anticipated pathogens. However, each trauma case should be evaluated individually for the types of organisms likely to cause infection, with empirical antibiotic therapy tailored to the location and severity of injury. No published data exist on the benefits or risks of empirical therapy for fungi or multiply resistant environmental bacteria in soil-contaminated injuries; therefore, extremely broad-spectrum antibiotic and antifungal agent prophylaxis is usually not recommended. Cultures obtained at the time of admission and surgical closure of open wounds can help the trauma team evaluate the child for infection later in the hospital course. Tetanus immunization should be considered in a child with devitalized, ischemic, and denervated tissues that have been inoculated by soil, or with deep tissue injury by foreign objects that have been in contact with soil.

Nosocomial infections of indwelling vascular catheters, surgically implanted foreign bodies, the lung, the urinary tract, and injured tissues are all well recognized, with therapy targeted to the organisms prevalent in the ICU. Gram-stained exudates and cultures can assist in providing information on the types and susceptibilities of the nosocomial pathogens causing infection. Providing sufficiently broad coverage empirically to achieve a high likelihood of success may both improve patient outcomes and decrease the emergence of certain antibiotic-resistant organisms. The definitive selection of antibiotics and a decision on the duration of therapy should be based on the isolated or suspected pathogens and the child's response to therapy. A poor response to broad-spectrum therapy despite the use of antimicrobial agents active against the isolated pathogens suggests either a hidden focus of infection, which may require further investigation and possible surgical intervention, or additional antibiotic-resistant pathogens not originally isolated. Lack of response to therapy may also be related to noninfectious causes of clinical instability. Therapy should not be continued indefinitely, because subsequent colonization and infection by antibiotic-resistant bacteria or yeast are likely to occur. Once antimicrobial therapy is discontinued, careful observation for relapse or recurrence of infection is essential.

Several therapies have been suggested to obviate the consequences of immune dysfunction in trauma patients. Circulating granulocyte colony-stimulating factor has been shown to be highest on postinjury day 1 and then quickly declines to near normal values by postinjury day 3.[121] In addition, plasma from trauma patients suppresses bone marrow colony growth of granulocyte-monocyte precursors for up to 2 weeks after injury.[122] Administration of filgrastim in neutropenic, septic, and head-injured patients has resulted in improved generation and function of neutrophils.[123] Prophylactic use in patients with TBI showed a dose-dependent decrease in the frequency of bacteremia.[124] Because there is a complex relationship between the neuroendocrine and immune systems, many studies have explored hormonal therapies to improve T-cell and macrophage function. Potential therapeutic agents after trauma include dehydroepiandrosterone and prolactin and metoclopramide. In addition, hypertonic saline may improve T-cell function and possibly prevent the exaggerated proinflammatory response leading to lung injury.

Coagulopathies

Trauma is a potent activator of the inflammatory response, and a growing body of literature describes the relationship among inflammatory cytokines, endothelial function, and coagulation through cellular and molecular signaling.[125] A severely injured child is at risk for impaired hemostasis as well as pathologic thrombosis.

Activation of the coagulation cascade is proportional to the stimulus. Local thrombus formation by a discrete injury is protective by inhibiting local bleeding, and pathologic thrombosis is normally impeded by anticoagulant mechanisms. Massive activation of the coagulation axis can overwhelm the counterbalancing mechanisms, leading to deep venous thrombosis locally or microvascular thrombosis systemically. The latter culminates in varying degrees of clotting factor consumption and pathologic and protective thrombolysis and may ultimately result in disseminated intravascular coagulopathy (DIC). The microangiopathic thrombosis of DIC can also contribute to hemolytic anemia, ARDS, and organ failure remote to the site of traumatic injury. The epidemiology of injuries in children puts them at increased risk for trauma-induced DIC because the brain and liver release strong procoagulant thromboplastins. Indeed, the likelihood of

coagulopathy has an inverse relationship to the presenting GCS score.[126] A recent paper showed that in children who meet clinical criteria for a head CT scan after trauma, a low plasma D-dimer strongly suggests the absence of significant brain injury.[127]

Evaluation and treatment of physiologic derangements that promote bleeding are necessary in an injured child. Although definitive evaluation by laboratory assays may not be available immediately, early suspicion of coagulopathy based on clinical history, physical examination, and medical interventions may be life saving in a traumatically injured child.

Even in the absence of a coagulopathy at presentation, it is necessary to prevent iatrogenic coagulation disturbances. Dilutional coagulopathy can occur with the administration of as little as one unwarmed blood volume. After one to two blood volumes, platelets can be halved, and the activated partial thromboplastin time and prothrombin time can be doubled. In an injured child receiving blood products, coagulation studies should be sent early. As volume resuscitation continues, these studies should be checked frequently to refine blood product administration. Hypothermia may contribute to coagulopathy during resuscitation and should be prevented.

If a patient has normal coagulation values but continues to bleed diffusely, an underlying bleeding diathesis should be considered. Von Willebrand disease is the most common congenital bleeding disorder and has traditionally been assessed by a bedside bleeding time. However, uncertainty about the sensitivity, reliability, and predictive value of the bleeding time has led to a decline in its use. A platelet function assay, PFA-100, has been compared with bleeding time and is considered a superior screening test for primary hemostasis disorders.[128] Thromboelastography is recommended to assess and treat the coagulation state of an actively bleeding trauma patient.[129]

Recombinant factor VIIa has been recommended for controlling bleeding in blunt trauma patients. Several papers address its use in coagulopathic trauma patients requiring emergent craniotomy. It has been shown to reduce the size of intracranial hematomas and reduce need for transfusion with packed red blood cells (PRBC) and plasma.[130,131] A recent meta-analysis, however, demonstrated no improvement in functional outcome or survival.[132] Thromboembolic complications have been reported in adults and children and need to be taken seriously.

Although the overall physiology of coagulation in children is nearly identical to that of adults, there are some special considerations in injured children. The neonate's relatively immature liver and initial nutritional state increases the likelihood that vitamin K–dependent clotting factors will be decreased. Trauma resulting from abuse in infants and children frequently includes occult head injuries and the release of potent thromboplastins. Young children may have an undiagnosed congenital bleeding disorder. Compared with adults, the relative health of the cardiopulmonary and renal systems allows children to tolerate significant hypovolemia and large-volume resuscitation that may result in a dilutional coagulopathy. The medical disorders and medications that can promote bleeding in adults also apply to children, although most are far less prevalent in the pediatric population.

In the ICU, patients are at increased risk of pathologic thrombosis secondary to endothelial damage and indwelling central catheters. Traumatic and pharmacologic paralysis, in addition to bed rest, contributes to venous stasis. Although the risk of deep venous thrombosis and thromboembolic disease is lower in prepubertal children than in adults, it is more prevalent than previously recognized.[133,134] Hypercoagulable states occur across the age spectrum, and children with nephrotic syndrome, inherited forms of thrombophilia, and some rheumatologic disorders are at increased risk for pathologic clot formation. Prophylaxis with low-dose heparin or automated venous compression stockings should be used in appropriate patients.

Nutrition

Nutritional support of critically injured children is extremely important and is based on knowledge gained from research in critically ill adult and pediatric patients, as well as physiologic differences between pediatric and adult patients. A key difference is the requirement for maintenance of growth and development. The resting basal metabolic rate of pediatric patients is approximately 50% higher than in adults. In addition, pediatric patients have lower energy stores than adults.

A state of hypermetabolism is well documented in adult patients after major traumatic injury and surgical stress. Similar data also exist in critically ill pediatric patients and pediatric trauma patients. Following an extensive review of the literature, the "Guidelines for the Acute Medical Management of Severe Traumatic Brain Injury in Infants, Children, and Adolescents" lists as a treatment option the replacement of 130% to 160% of resting metabolism after TBI in pediatric patients.[74] Patients who are paralyzed or in barbiturate coma have a lower resting metabolic rate and require fewer calories.

The enteral route is preferable, and much research has been performed related to the benefits of enteral versus parenteral nutrition. In a meta-analysis, benefits of enteral nutrition included lower risk of infection and reduction in hospital length of stay.[135] Other proposed benefits include preservation of intestinal mucosal integrity, with decreased bacterial translocation and decrease in multiple organ failure. Enteral feeding is also more cost-effective than parenteral nutrition in pediatric patients.[136] There are many adult studies supporting initiation of enteral feeding within 24 to 72 hours of ICU admission. When enteral feeding is not possible, it is best to support the patient with total parenteral nutrition.

Owing to impaired GI motility in critically ill trauma patients, enteral feeding may be poorly tolerated. Gastric emptying is often delayed following severe head injury. In addition, many of the medications used during treatment of traumatically injured patients may affect GI motility. Narcotics, benzodiazepines, and catecholamines can adversely affect feeding tolerance. Barbiturates decrease GI motility, and severe gastroparesis has been described. Many patients with severe TBI requiring barbiturate coma do not tolerate full enteral nutrition.

Large gastric residual volume associated with lack of tolerance of gastric feeding may increase the incidence of aspiration pneumonia and has been associated with higher ICU mortality in adults.[137] Continuous gastric infusion of formula, addition of prokinetic agents, or transpyloric feeding may improve feeding tolerance. In some pediatric trauma patients, enteral feeding is unrealistic. The most important action is to provide nutritional support as soon as feasible, with the decision of enteral versus parenteral support individualized to the patient.

Two special topics deserve mention. First, although there are no data regarding the effect of immune-enhancing and immune-modulating nutrition in pediatric patients, in adults, supplementation of arginine, glutamine, branched-chain amino acids, nucleotides, nucleosides, and omega-3 fatty acids has been used to improve outcome.[138,139] These special formulations show promise with respect to decreased length of stay and decreased infectious complications.[140-142] Second, control of blood glucose levels in adult surgical ICU patients has been shown to have an important beneficial effect. Tight glucose control with insulin significantly reduced morbidity and mortality in these patients.[143] Tight glycemic control has been shown to decrease infection and improve survival in pediatric burn patients. Similar studies have not been performed in pediatric trauma patients.

Sedation and Pain

Injured children commonly require analgesia and anxiolysis during therapy and management of various injuries. There are myriad drugs that can be safely used to provide appropriate levels of analgesia and anxiolysis.

In addition to providing pain relief and anxiolysis, sedatives and analgesics may reduce elevated ICP, facilitate mechanical ventilation, prevent shivering, provide anticonvulsant activity, and minimize long-term psychological trauma from untreated pain and stress.[74] The importance of restoring and maintaining circulating intravascular volume before administering sedatives cannot be overstated, as children may be "surviving" on endogenous catecholamine release, thereby

barely maintaining adequate blood pressure and tissue perfusion. Administration of even small doses of any sedative in this situation may precipitate cardiovascular collapse and cardiac arrest. Empirical treatment of presumed hypovolemia should precede administration of sedatives in an acutely injured child.

In the initial setting of evaluating an acutely injured child, small doses of narcotics such as fentanyl, given in incremental doses (0.5 μg/ kg per dose, up to 1 to 2 μg/kg) titrated to effect, can be useful in both providing analgesia and allowing a more detailed examination. A child with painful injuries (e.g., fractures, multiple abrasions) is often more cooperative and allows a more thorough examination after receiving adequate analgesia. Concerns about "masking" the presence of intraabdominal injury are unfounded, as the cooperation achieved from the analgesia outweighs the difficulty in examining an agitated, screaming child who is experiencing acute pain. It is rarely necessary to administer benzodiazepines or other anxiolytic drugs in the acute setting of pediatric trauma, provided adequate analgesia is given. In a mechanically ventilated patient, benzodiazepine (midazolam, diazepam, lorazepam) administration by intermittent dosing or by continuous infusion is commonly used to provide anxiolysis. Recently, infusion of dexmedetomidine has been used for sedation.

A variety of short-acting drugs can be used to provide hypnosis and loss of consciousness for endotracheal intubation. A detailed analysis of the advantages and disadvantages of these drugs is beyond the scope of this chapter. It should be noted that there is an increased risk of adrenal insufficiency following etomidate exposure in critically injured patients.[144]

Sodium thiopental (4-6 mg/kg) is commonly used in a hemodynamically stable child in this setting because it is rapid acting (30-60 seconds) and can be used to treat elevated ICP. Further, sodium thiopental (1-2 mg/kg every 15-30 minutes) can be used following successful intubation to maintain unconsciousness during transport to the ICU, operating room, or radiology department. The use of thiopental for sedation for radiographic procedures in a nonintubated, spontaneously breathing patient should be reserved for elective situations in fasted patients, and it should be administrated by an anesthesiologist.[74] Pentobarbital may be substituted for sodium thiopental.

Except for inducing general anesthesia, the use of propofol for critically injured children is controversial and in fact is rarely necessary in the acute setting. A poorly defined syndrome of metabolic acidosis and myocardial failure has been reported after giving propofol by continuous infusion in the critical care setting. Nevertheless, many pediatric intensivists use propofol for short intervals, especially during the weaning of narcotic-dependent children from mechanical ventilation.

Inflicted Trauma

Abuse is a common cause of traumatic injury in infants and young children.[145,146] The American Academy of Pediatrics has recently recommended use of the term *abusive head trauma* (AHT) rather than the term *shaken baby syndrome*.[147] Nationally, it is estimated that 1756 children died due to abuse or neglect in 2007, a rate of 2.35 per 100,000 children. Children younger than 12 months accounted for 43.7% of these fatalities, and 85% were younger than 4 years. Recognition of inflicted injury is important to ensure appropriate care, prevent recurrence of abuse, protect siblings, and comply with reporting mandates.

A delay in seeking care is common in children with abusive injuries. Injury history may be absent, incomplete, or inconsistent with physical findings or the developmental capability of the child. Domestic violence is common in families of abused children. Children with inflicted injuries that have more subtle findings and patients with intact families are more likely to be misdiagnosed as accidentally injured. This may have serious repercussions, including further injury and death.[148] Children with abusive injuries have worse outcomes than those with accidental injuries, with higher severity and mortality rates and higher patient costs.[149] Having a high index of suspicion for inflicted trauma is critical in assessing an infant that presents with lethargy, apnea, cyanosis, mottling, poor perfusion, or seizures without an obvious history of trauma.

Evaluation of children with inflicted injury should reflect the occult nature of many abusive injuries. The constellation of subdural hematoma, traction-type metaphyseal (bucket-handle) fractures of long bones, posterior rib fractures, and retinal hemorrhages are characteristic of inflicted injuries in infants. Although TBI is the leading cause of morbidity and mortality in abused children, some head injuries may not be easily diagnosed clinically.[150] Therefore, a nonambulatory infant with any type of abusive injury should have CT or MRI studies of the brain performed. The sudden deceleration with forceful striking of the head against a surface is an important mechanism responsible for inflicted brain injuries in children. Hypoxic-ischemic insults and other mechanisms also appear to play a role. Subdural hemorrhage, classically localized at the parieto-occipital convexity or posterior interhemispheric fissure, is the most consistent autopsy finding in shaking-impact syndrome. Subdural hematoma results from rotational deceleration forces that cause shearing of bridging cortical veins. Retinal hemorrhages are present in the majority of children with inflicted injuries, but their absence does not rule out abuse. In addition, not all retinal hemorrhages are due to abuse. Infrequently, accidental head injuries may cause retinal hemorrhages.[151,152] Therefore, an evaluation by a pediatric ophthalmologist is recommended in all children with suspected AHT. A skeletal survey should be done in all children with serious injury due to abuse. Screening for abdominal trauma is also important, either through imaging or laboratory studies. A psychosocial evaluation is critical in families of children with inflicted injuries. This is to help support the family during a time of crisis; evaluate for other comorbid factors such as domestic violence, substance abuse, and mental illness; comply with mandated reporting requirements; and help interface with investigative and protective agencies.

A multidisciplinary team is optimal for treating children with inflicted injuries. The team should consist of the treating staff, a medical social worker, and a child abuse pediatrician.

Rehabilitation

Once life-threatening conditions have been ameliorated and the medical condition stabilized, the pediatric trauma patient should be assessed for the restoration of maximal functional independence. It is the role of the pediatric physiatrist and rehabilitation medicine team to identify, assess, and promote maximum restoration of physical, cognitive, and psychosocial functioning in each patient. Recently, amantadine has been used to facilitate recovery of consciousness in children with acquired brain injury; while on amantadine, physicians noted improvements in consciousness.[153] Members of the rehabilitation team, including occupational therapists, physical therapists, speech therapists, social workers, and schoolteachers, provide their expertise in returning the patient to maximum independent function. As a first step, it is important to identify the patient's functional deficits and subsequent level of disability and handicap as they relate to the patient's home, community, and school settings.

The rehabilitation process should begin early in the patient's critical care stay, because physical and occupational modalities may limit the adverse physiologic effects of prolonged immobilization. For instance, muscles lose their flexibility and bulk, resulting in diminished strength and endurance. Joints become stiff and contracted, and skin breaks down, creating pressure ulcers. Interventions include passive joint range of motion, isometric strengthening, and appropriate bed positioning. Orthotic devices, placed at joints (e.g., elbows and ankles) in a neutral position, limit contracture formation. Speech and occupational therapists can evaluate oral motor function to assess safe swallowing and feeding, decreasing the patient's risk of aspiration. The dietitian evaluates the patient's nutritional status, providing recommendations for appropriate diet and caloric intake. The social worker and child life specialist provide the patient and family members with emotional and educational support during the patient's acute critical care stabilization.

It is through the collaborative efforts of the pediatric trauma team and the pediatric rehabilitation team that the survivor of a pediatric trauma maximizes functional independence and has a successful discharge home.

Brain Death and Organ Donation

The first definition of irreversible coma as a criterion for death, as well as the criteria for diagnosis, was published in 1968 by an ad hoc committee of the Harvard Medical School. In 1981, the President's Commission for the Study of Ethical Problems in Medicine and Biomedical and Behavioral Research published a report titled "Defining Death: Medical, Legal, and Ethical Issues in the Determination of Death," which summarized medical practice for the determination of cardiorespiratory and neurologic death. A summary of the guidelines was published in the medical literature. These guidelines provided a conceptual definition of brain death and left the criteria for determination up to accepted medical standards. In addition, it established common ground for law related to the diagnosis of brain death. In 1987, the American Academy of Pediatrics published guidelines for the determination of brain death in pediatric patients,[154] with specifications for physical examination, observation period, and confirmatory laboratory testing. These guidelines have attempted to define the clinical determination of irreversible cessation of all brain function to the best of medical ability. The need to define brain death was fueled by improvements in the intensive care of critically ill patients, as well as advances in solid-organ transplantation. There is continued debate by experts regarding whether patients who have been determined to be brain dead by current guidelines have irreversible loss of all brain function. In addition, controversy exists regarding whether brain death should be defined as loss of higher brain function and not loss of all brain function.[155]

Trauma patients represent a large percentage of those who are declared brain dead in a pediatric ICU and therefore a large pool of potential organ donors. There continues to be a wide gap between the number of organs available for transplantation and the number of patients needing transplants, with more than 100,000 patients currently awaiting transplantation in the United States. Improvement in consent for organ donation is one way to decrease this gap. Despite widespread acceptance of and support for organ donation among the general public, only 40% to 60% of families give consent for donation. Consent rates for donation are improved when the family understands the concept of brain death and when the understanding occurs before the request for donation (decoupling). In addition, the consent rate is maximized when the requester has specialized training or is a member of the organ procurement organization. In pediatric trauma patients, involvement of the attending physician in the request process may also have a beneficial effect on consent rates.[156]

In an effort to increase organ donation, federal regulations were issued in 1998 governing how potential organ donors should be identified and approached.[157] All hospitals must have an agreement with an organ procurement organization (OPO) and must notify the organization of patient deaths. The procurement organization then determines the patient's suitability for organ donation. In addition, the hospital must have an agreement with a tissue bank and eye bank to coordinate tissue and eye donation. The family of every potential donor must be informed of the option to donate organs or tissues.

Until recently, virtually all organ donors were declared brain dead before organ procurement. In the early 1990s, the University of Pittsburgh introduced a protocol for non-heartbeating cadaveric donation. This policy has increased the pool of available organs and has generally resulted in satisfactory results.[158,159] There is controversy in the medical community regarding the ethics of these protocols.[160,161] Part of this controversy revolves around the dead donor rule. Some physicians have requested a moratorium on non-heartbeating donation pending further ethical discussion and analysis.

Victims of child abuse represent a special subset of pediatric patients. The documentation of injuries in child abuse cases is extremely important and has significant legal ramifications. The medical examiner plays a key role in determining whether legally deceased child abuse victims may be released for organ procurement. The medical examiner may prohibit organ procurement if there is concern that the process will alter forensic evidence. Implementation of procedures to fully document the state of the abdominal cavity and the extent of abdominal injuries in the operating room before procurement may facilitate release for donation.

Documentation may be performed by the transplant surgeon or the medical examiner.[162,163]

Burnout

Much attention has been given to trauma team composition and member qualifications, the roles and responsibilities of members, policies and procedures, and who should lead the team. Burnouts of team members, as well as the qualities of an effective leader, however, are seldom referred to in the trauma literature.

The burnout rate is 30% to 40% for the medical profession, including trauma surgeons, general surgeons, emergency physicians, pediatric critical care specialists, social workers, and nurses. Two major contributing factors to burnout in pediatric intensivists include needing to argue to get things accomplished and the feeling that one's work is not valued by patients, colleagues, administrators, and nurses. A survey of surgical residents reported a high degree of dissatisfaction with trauma medicine as a career. Reasons for dissatisfaction included the belief that trauma was becoming a nonoperative specialty (81% of respondents) and dislike of working with other specialists, including neurosurgeons and orthopedic surgeons (77%).

Even physicians who are not burned out are subject to frustrations, many of which relate to personal conflicts, fragmented personal relationships, breakdown of communication, undermining of teamwork, and a system where physicians work separately—often working against each other rather than working together. Reducing these types of frustration may lead not only to less burnout and greater job satisfaction but also to better outcomes for patients.[164]

KEY POINTS

1. Trauma systems and trauma centers improve outcome, and pediatric trauma centers improve outcome for children, especially for those with severe traumatic brain injury.

2. An inclusive system is the right system for pediatric trauma patients, and the pediatric critical care physician should have a significant role.

3. Injuries to the airway in children can be rapidly life threatening. Small airway diameter combined with penetrating or blunt injury to the neck can produce rapid airway compromise. The majority of penetrating airway injuries in children occur in adolescent males.

4. Mortality rate for thoracic trauma (rare in children) can exceed 40% when a combination of head, chest, and abdominal injuries is present.

5. Traumatic injury to the heart and great vessels is significantly less common in pediatric patients than in adults. Most injuries are the result of blunt trauma, with penetrating injury being rare and carrying a higher mortality rate.

6. More than 90% of abdominal trauma in children is the result of blunt trauma, with penetrating trauma accounting for only 5% to 10% of injuries. The gold standard for the evaluation of children with blunt abdominal trauma is computed tomography with IV contrast.

7. Pelvic fractures are a marker of significant trauma. Mortality varies from 10% to 50% and is often due to the high rate of associated injuries. The most common mechanisms are fall, crush, and motor vehicle accidents.

8. Genitourinary trauma is common and occurs in 12% of injuries in children. It rarely results in death; when death occurs, it is usually due to associated injuries.

9. Approximately 5% of all spinal cord injuries occur in the pediatric age group. Common causes in the youngest children include falls and motor vehicle accidents. Inflicted trauma has been identified as a significant mechanism of injury in young children. For older children, common causes of spinal injuries are sports and other recreational activities such as bicycle riding.

10. An estimated 2685 children aged 1 to 14 die each year from traumatic brain injury; 37,000 are hospitalized, and 475,000 are treated in hospital emergency departments. Traumatic brain injury is caused by linear and inertial forces resulting in an impact injury. This is the primary injury. It includes hematomas, lacerations, and axonal shearing and is often deemed irreparable. *Secondary injury* refers to the injury that occurs after impact. It is considered both preventable and potentially reversible. An aggressive management strategy is indicated, as it is associated with improved outcomes.

11. Trauma can result in lung injury and respiratory failure, the most severe of which is acute respiratory distress syndrome (ARDS). ARDS management in pediatrics focuses on minimizing iatrogenic lung injury and on adjuncts to mechanical ventilation.

ANNOTATED REFERENCES

Bayir H, Kochanek PM, Clark RS. Traumatic brain injury in infants and children: mechanisms of secondary damage and treatment in the intensive care unit. Crit Care Clin 2003;19:529-49.
 No specific pharmacologic therapies are available for the treatment of TBI in patients. More detailed knowledge regarding the dominant pathophysiologic mechanisms associated with TBI excitotoxicity, CBF dysregulation, oxidative stress, and programmed cell death will lead to development of more efficacious therapies—a potent agent targeting a single dominant pathway, a broad-spectrum intervention such as hypothermia, or, more likely, a combination of therapies. Meanwhile, practitioners must offer meticulous supportive neurointensive care using clinically proven therapies aimed at minimizing cerebral swelling for the management of pediatric patients who are victims of TBI.
Bliss D, Silen M. Pediatric thoracic trauma. Crit Care Med 2002;30:S409-15.
 Thoracic injuries in children remain a source of substantial morbidity and mortality. Disparate problems such as rib fractures, lung injury, hemothorax, pneumothorax, mediastinal injuries, and others may present

in isolation or in combination with one another. Differences in pulmonary functional residual capacity, blood volume, chest wall and spinal soft-tissue mobility, and cardiac function all have to be carefully evaluated.
Mazzola CA, Adelson PD. Critical care management of head trauma in children. Crit Care Med 2002;30:S393-401.
 Trauma is the leading cause of morbidity and mortality in the pediatric population, and traumatic injury causes over 50% of all childhood deaths. Significant mortality rates have been reported for children with TBI. Although children have better survival rates compared to adults with TBI, the long-term sequelae and consequences are often more devastating in children because of their age and developmental potential.
Proctor MR. Spinal cord injury. Crit Care Med 2002;30:S489-99.
 This article discusses the types of injuries seen in children, with an emphasis on acute management and clearance of the cervical spine. Treatment options and long-term issues are also discussed.

REFERENCES

Access the complete reference list online at http://www.expertconsult.com.

211

Management of the Brain Dead Organ Donor

KRISTA TURNER

Transplantation is an increasingly utilized treatment option for patients with organ failure. In 2009, 28,465 organs were transplanted in the United States, with over 100,000 patients on the waiting list.[1] Despite advances in immunosuppression and postoperative management, utility of transplantation is dependent on the number of available organs. Expanding indications for transplantation have further widened the gap between supply and demand.

To address this problem, the U.S. Department of Health and Human Services launched the Organ Donation Breakthrough Collaboratives in 2003 with the intent to increase the number of donors, as well as number of organs transplanted per donor. Events in the pathway of organ donation are illustrated in Figure 211-1.[2] Maintenance of allocated organs was identified as a major area for improvement. The majority of donor organs are cadaveric, of which 90% are from brain dead (BD) donors. An estimated 20% to 30% of organs are lost prior to procurement despite aggressive measures in BD donors.[1] This number attests to the profound physiologic variations that occur at the time of brain death but can also be attributed to what can often be suboptimal unstandardized care.[3] There is a large disparity between the intensive team-based management of the trauma or stroke victim and the singularity of the organ procurement organization (OPO) coordinator left at the bedside once brain death is declared. The intensivist can therefore have a profound impact on number and quality of organs salvaged.

Declaration of Brain Death

The initial process for organ donation requires heightened awareness on the part of the intensive care unit (ICU) team. Often, potential donors are excluded by the caregiver based on notions of donor criteria or concerns regarding conflict of care. Members of the local OPO are trained specifically to interact with families regarding donation issues in such a manner that the caregiver and OPO are not seen in mutual opposition. With the permission of the family, blood sampling to determine the suitability may be performed before brain death occurs.[4] Once brain death is confirmed by standard criteria (see Chapter 219), the team needs to act quickly to stabilize the physiology of the donor and shorten time to transplantation.

Physiology of Brain Death

Brain injury resulting in herniation will follow a rostrocaudal progression of ischemia. Events leading up to brain death include hypertension with bradycardia (Cushing response) as the pons becomes ischemic. Further involvement of the medulla creates unopposed sympathetic stimuli, initiating a catecholamine "storm." This surge of catecholamines damages end organs both from severe vasoconstriction and from the proinflammatory response elicited. Finally, spinal cord ischemia and loss of sympathetic denervation results in severe hypotension. Simultaneous ischemia to the pituitary and hypothalamus exacerbate this with loss of homeostatic control. These events occur in varying magnitude or velocity, making management even more difficult. The resulting physiology is characterized by hemodynamic instability with a host of secondary complications listed in Figure 211-2.

Initial Donor Resuscitation

Care of the BD donor requires multitasking and frequent reassessment. Donors often have associated traumatic injury and chronic health problems. To complicate matters, treatment strategies prior to brain death are directed toward maintaining cerebral perfusion, often to the detriment of other organs. Post-declaration management focuses on reversing this state and preventing further organ damage. Expeditious stabilization is paramount, as graft loss rapidly increases after 48 hours.[5]

Various organizations provide algorithms for standard management of the BD donor. Protocols may be organ specific, or target the donor as a whole.[6-10] The United Network for Organ Sharing (UNOS) provides a sample standard pathway that includes initial workup as well as therapy (Figure 211-3). These algorithms help focus ongoing resuscitation, ensure provision of evidence-based therapy, and provide a platform for future research in the field.

Immediate goals are establishing baseline organ function and stabilizing physiology. If not already in place, a central venous catheter and arterial catheter are inserted. Blood, urine, and bronchial cultures are obtained and baseline chemistries performed. Evaluation of the lung and heart begin with basic chest x-ray, echocardiogram, bronchoscopy, and coronary angiogram as indicated.[7] Blood type and crossmatch are performed, and initial graft allocation efforts begun by the OPO coordinator.

Initial resuscitation includes crystalloid administration guided by central venous pressure or pulmonary artery pressure, although pulse pressure variation (PPV) may actually predict preload responsiveness more accurately.[11] After adequate volume loading, vasopressors are often required to maintain perfusion pressure. Monitoring end organ perfusion may be achieved by measuring oxygen delivery or central venous oxygen saturation.[12] Other endpoints of resuscitation are listed in Box 211-1.

Standard ICU protocols should be employed to prevent further complications. Gastrointestinal and deep vein thrombosis (DVT) prophylaxis should be continued appropriately, blood products administered for anemia or coagulopathy, aspiration precautions upheld, and electrolytes and acidosis corrected to avoid arrhythmias. Insulin therapy should be given, as it has antiinflammatory properties that may be particularly beneficial in the BD donor.[13,14] A multidisciplinary approach greatly helps coordinate care.

Specific Considerations and Controversies

CARDIOVASCULAR

Cardiovascular management after brain death is paramount to maintaining perfusion and preserving the heart for donation. Hemodynamic collapse occurs more from loss of afterload than primary nonfunction of the heart.[15] Nevertheless, the catecholamine surge during herniation can incite considerable myocardial damage.[16] Right ventricle strain is common secondary to increased pulmonary capillary perfusion and pulmonary overflow injury from increased vascular resistance.[17] Contractility must be frequently reassessed and quantified with echocardiography, as regional wall abnormalities will often

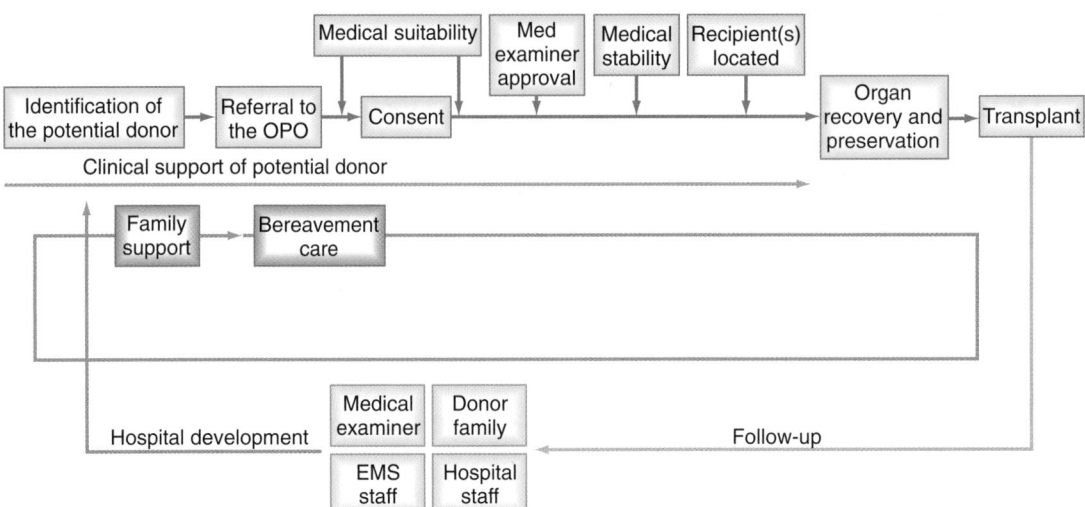

Figure 211-1   Events in the organ donation and consent process. *(From Organ Donation Breakthrough Collaborative best practices final report, September 2003. The Organ Donation Breakthrough Collaborative. Best practices final report; U.S. Department of Health and Human Services Health Resources and Services Administration; Office of Special Programs, Division of Transplantation Contract: 240-94-0037 Task Order No. 12, September 2003.)*

resolve.[18] Most important to cardiac function is coronary perfusion pressure, which can be affected by loss of autoregulatory reserve after brain death.[19-21]

Protocols based on traditional volume and vasopressor management have increased the number of donor hearts.[8,22] These protocols included moderate crystalloid resuscitation followed by catecholamine use for hypotension and hormone treatment when cardiac dysfunction was diagnosed (Figure 211-4).[23] Since their development, certain details have been debated, primarily hormone treatment (discussed later) and choice of vasopressor.

Types of vasopressors advocated include dopamine, epinephrine, and norepinephrine as well as vasopressin.[7,24-27] Immunomodulatory function of the catecholamines makes them attractive in the context of the donor's proinflammatory condition.[28-30] Dopamine-stimulated induction of heme-oxygenase-1 makes kidneys more resistant to ischemic-reperfusion injury in donor models.[31,32] Dopamine may suppress anterior pituitary hormones, however, and is likewise notorious for inducing tachyarrhythmias.[33,34] Norepinephrine and epinephrine have been related to cardiac and kidney graft nonfunction.[35-37] Vasopressin makes sense in the face of posterior pituitary ischemia and can reduce the dose of catecholamines administered.[38,39]

PULMONARY

Like the heart, lung function in the donor can be affected by physiologic changes with brain death, in addition to underlying pulmonary

disease. Pulmonary edema after brain death results from elevated afterload from the catecholamine surge combined with increased venous return and decreased left ventricular function.[40] The sympathetic discharge also up-regulates inflammation in the lung parenchyma and capillaries, leading to further edema and failure.[41] These effects are significant because pulmonary edema and inflammation reduce lung donation rates to less than 20%.[42]

Standard criteria for lung donation include a clear chest x-ray and Pao_2/Fio_2 above 300, although with expanded donor criteria, these parameters are viewed as too strict.[43,44] Findings such as edema and atelectasis can be reversed with adequate diuresis and recruitment maneuvers.[45,46] Global oxygenation does not represent unilateral oxygenation, and the single-lung donor pool can therefore be expanded by obtaining unilateral pulmonary vein gases instead of relying on Pao_2.[47,48]

Once a suitable donor is identified, aggressive management with a lung-specific focus is pursued.[6] Most protocols use frequent chest physiotherapy and bronchoscopy, diuretics, strict aspiration precautions, empirical antibiotics, and steroid administration.[49-51] Lung recruitment maneuvers and frequent bronchoscopy increase oxygenation and lung utilization.[52] Diuretics are given to decrease central venous pressure (CVP) in an effort to decrease alveolar-arterial oxygen gradient, although restricting CVP does not necessarily increase lung utilization.[53-55]

Empirical antibiotics are generally administered based on chest x-ray findings. Although culture obtained from bronchoalveolar lavage

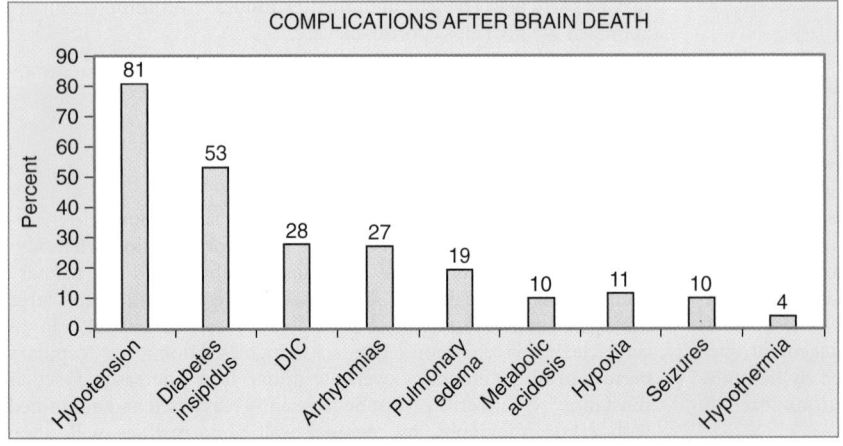

Figure 211-2 Complications after brain death. *(Adapted from Smith M. Physiologic changes during brain stem death—lessons for management of the organ donor. J Heart Lung Transplant 2004;23: S217-22.)*

Collaborative Practice	Phase I Referral	Phase II Declaration of Brain Death and Consent	Phase III Donor Evaluation	Phase IV Donor Management	Phase V Recovery Phase
Critical Pathway for the Organ Donor Patient name: _____ ID number: _____					
The following professionals may be involved to enhance the donation process. *Check all that apply* O Physician O Critical care RN O Organ Procurement Organization (OPO) O OPO co-ordinator (OPO) O Medical Examiner (ME)/ Coroner O Respiratory O Laboratory O Pharmacy O Radiology O Anesthesiology O OR/Surgery staff O Clergy O Social worker	O Notify physician regarding OPO referral O Contact OPO ref: Potential donor with severe brain insult O OPC on site and begins evaluation Time _____ Date _____ O Ht _____ Wt _____ as documented O ABO as documented _____ O Notify house supervisor/ charge nurse of presence of OPC on unit	O Brain death documented Time _____ Date _____ O Pt accepted as potential donor O MD notifies family of death O Plan family approach with OPC O Offer support services to family (clergy, etc) O OPC/Hospital staff talks to family about donation O Family accepts donation O OPC obtains signed consent and medical/social history Time _____ Date _____ O ME/Coroner notified O ME/Coroner releases body for donation O *Family/ME/Coroner denies donation–stop pathway– initiate post-mortem protocol–support family.*	O Obtain pre/post transfusion blood for serology testing (HIV, hepatitis, VDRL, CMV) O Obtain lymph nodes and/ or blood for tissue typing O Notify OR and anesthesiology of pending donation O Notify house supervisor of pending donation O Chest and abdominal circumference O Lung measurements per CXR by OPC O *Cardiology consult as required by OPC (use reverse side)* O *Donor organs unsuitable for transplant–stop pathway–initiate postmortem–support family.*	O OPC writes new orders O Organ placement O OPC sets tentative OR time O Insert arterial line/2 large bore IVs O Possibly insert CVP/Pulmonary Artery Catheter O See reverse side	O Checklist for OR O Supplies given to OR O Prepare patient for transport to OR O IVs O Pumps O O$_2$ O Ambu O Peep valve O Transport to OR Date _____ Time _____ O OR nurse O reviews consent form O reviews brain death documentation O checks patient's ID band
Labs/Diagnostics		O Review previous lab results O Review previous hemodynamics	O Blood chemistry O CBC + diff O UA O C & S O PT, PTT O ABO O A Subtype O Liver function tests O Blood culture X 2 / 15 minutes to 1 hour apart O Sputum Gram stain & C & S O Type & Cross Match _____ # units PRBCs O CXR O ABGs O EKG O Echo O Consider cardiac cath O Consider bronchoscopy	O Determine need for additional lab testing O CXR after line placement (if done) O Serum electrolytes O H & H after PRBC Rx O PT, PTT O BUN, serum creatinine after correcting fluid deficit O Notify OPC for ____ PT >14 ____ PTT <28 ____ Urine output ____ <1 mL/Kg/hr ____ >3 mL/Kg/hr ____ Hct <30 / Hgb >10 ____ Na >150 mEq/L	O Labs drawn in OR as per surgeon or OPC request O Communicate with pathology: Rx liver and/ or kidneys as indicated
Respiratory	O Pt on ventilator O Suction q 2 hr O Reposition q 2 hr	O Prep for apnea testing: set FiO$_2$ @ 100% and anticipate need to decrease rate if PCO$_2$ <45 mm Hg	O Maximize ventilator settings to achieve SaO$_2$ 98–99% O PEEP = 5cm O$_2$ challenge for lung placement FiO$_2$ @ 100%, PEEP @ 5 X 10 min O ABGs as ordered O VS q 1°	O Notify OPC for ____ BP <90 systolic ____ HR <70 or >120 ____ CVP <4 or >11 ____ PaO$_2$ <90 or ____ SaO$_2$ <95%	O Portable O$_2$ @ 100% FiO$_2$ for transport to OR O Ambu bag and PEEP valve O Move to OR
Treatments/ Ongoing Care		O Use warming/cooling blanket to maintain temperature at 36.5° C–37.5°C O NG to low intermittent suction	O Check NG placement and output O Obtain actual Ht _____ and Wt _____ if not previously obtained		O Set OR temp as directed by OPC O Post-mortem care at conclusion of case
Medications			O Medication as requested by OPC	O Fluid resuscitaton–consider crystolloids colloids, blood products O DC meds except pressors and antibiotics O Broad-spectrum antibiotic if not previously ordered O Vasopressor support to maintain BP >90 mrn Hg systolic O Electrolyte imbalance: consider K, Ca, PO$_2$, Mg replacement O Hyperglycemia: consider insulin drip O Oliguria: consider diuretics O Diabetes insipidus: consider antidiuretics O Paralytic as indicated for spinal reflexes	O DC antidiuretics O Diuretics as needed O 350 U heparin/kg or as directed by surgeon
Optimal Outcomes	The potential donor is identified and a referral is made to the OPO.	The family is offered the option of donation and their decision is supported.	The donor is evaluated and found to be a suitable candidate for donation.	Optimal organ function is maintained.	All potentially suitable, consented organs are recovered for transplant.

Shaded areas indicate Organ Procurement Coordinator (OPC) Activities.   Copyright © 2003, 2001, 1998 UNOS (United Network for Organ Sharing) All rights reserved.

The Critical Pathway was developed under contract with the U.S. Department of Health and Human Services, Health Resources and Services Administration, Division of Transplantation.

AOPO Association of Organ Procurement Organizations   AMERICAN SOCIETY OF TRANSPLANTATION   AST♀   ASTS♔   NATCO   UNOS DONATE LIFE UNITED NETWORK FOR ORGAN SHARING

Figure 211-3   Critical pathway for organ donor. *(Reprinted with permission of UNOS, Richmond, Virginia. Access at http://www.unos.org/docs/cntical_ Pathway.pdf.)*

(BAL) is the gold standard, results often are not rapid enough for specific antibiotic tapering.[56] Even when bronchial culture is obtained, there is poor correlation between culture data and posttransplant pneumonia development, with an 8% transmission rate despite appropriate antibiotics.[57] Steroids are also widely employed in lung donors in an effort to decrease lung water accumulation and enhance alveolar fluid clearance.[58,59]

Whereas there are few studies about ventilator mode, pressure-cycled modes are being used more frequently for donors.[60] Lung protective strategies using low tidal volumes and moderate positive end-expiratory pressure (PEEP) can prevent further barotrauma.[61,62] For the donor population specifically, acute lung injury is more common in those treated with increased tidal volumes, and sustained recruitment maneuvers should be used with caution.[63] Excessive

PHYSIOLOGIC ENDPOINTS IN THE POTENTIAL ORGAN DONOR

Systolic blood pressure ≥90 mm Hg
Mean arterial pressure ≥60 mm Hg
Central venous pressure ≤12 mm Hg
Pulmonary capillary wedge pressure ≤12 mm Hg
Cardiac index >2.5 L/min/m^2
Left ventricular stroke work index >15 g/m/m^2
Urine output >1 and <4 mL/kg/h
Core temperature >35°C
Hematocrit ≥25%
Oxygen saturation >95%
pH 7.35-7.45

By contrast, hypervolemia is also deleterious, inducing right heart strain and lung dysfunction.[45] Restricting CVP to improve lung function, however, did not adversely affect kidney graft function in a recent well-designed study.[55]

Crystalloids are primarily used for initial resuscitation. Some societies advocate colloids to avoid lung water accumulation, but data to support this are limited.[53] Hydroxyethylstarch (HES) can generate nephrosis-like lesions and impair graft function in kidneys, although newer, less osmotic formulations do not demonstrate the same detrimental effects.[67-69] Hypertonic saline may modulate inflammation and shows promise for donor resuscitation, although sodium levels should be monitored closely.[70,71]

ENDOCRINE

One of the more debated aspects of donor management is the use of hormonal therapy. The donor suffers from a variable panhypopituitary state secondary to ischemia.[72] Dysfunction of the posterior pituitary is common (90%), with resultant low to nil vasopressin levels.[73] Administering desmopressin treats the subsequent diabetes insipidus that can further complicate fluid management. Dysfunction of the anterior pituitary is less consistent, with variable effects of hormones given to counteract the loss of corticotropin (ACTH) and thyroid-stimulating hormone (TSH).[74] In animal models, levels of triiodothyronine (T_3), cortisol, and insulin are all markedly decreased.[75] Humans, however, exhibit near-normal levels of cortisol and insulin, with nonuniform decreases in T_3.[73] Hypophyseal blood flow may be maintained by

oxygen administration should likewise be avoided, as this can induce the inflammatory cascade and apoptosis.[64]

RENAL

BD donors are typically volume depleted secondary to aggressive mannitol use and diabetes insipidus. Strategies for preventing further renal injury include avoidance of nephrotoxic agents and maintaining hydration. Larger amounts of volume administration can improve kidney and liver graft function by correction of hypernatremia.[36,65,66]

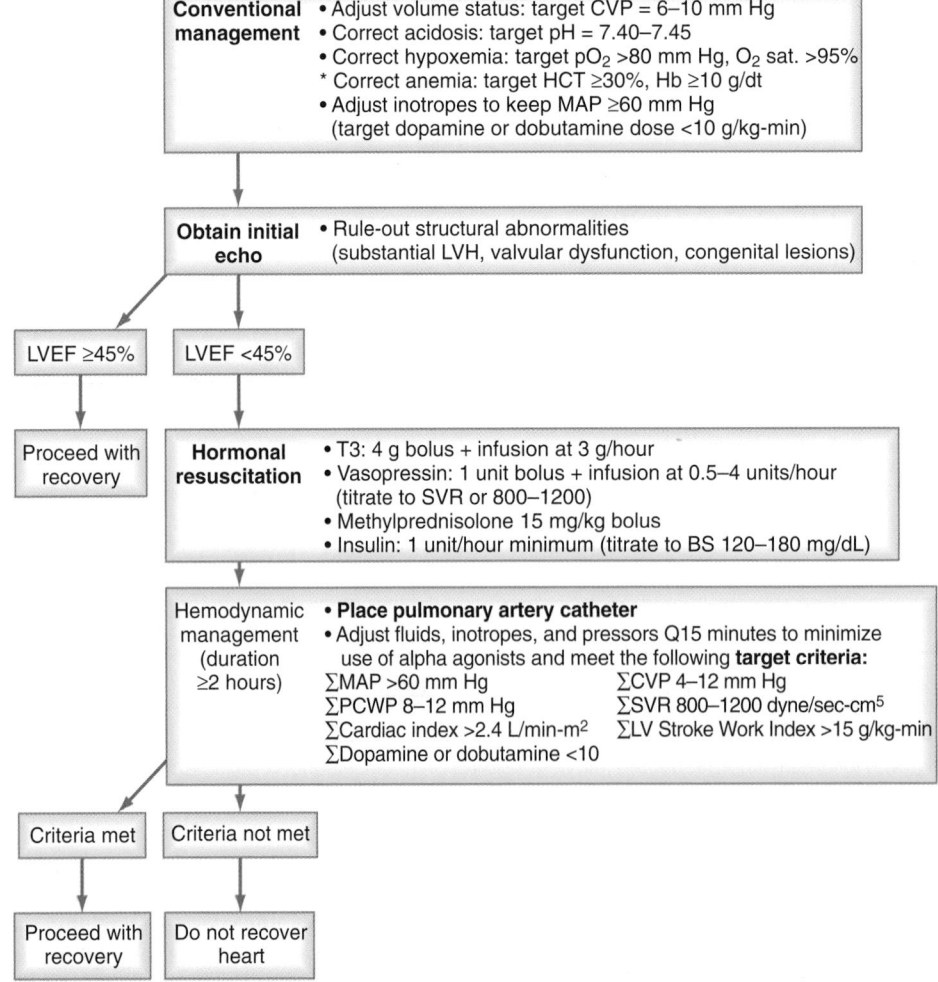

Figure 211-4 Recommendations for cardiac donor management. (*Adapted from Rosengard BR, Feng S, Alfrey EJ, Zaroff JG, Emond JC, Henry ML et al. Report of the Crystal City meeting to maximize the use of organs recovered from the cadaver donor. Am J Transplant 2002;2:701-11.*)

branches off of the external carotid and could explain some of these variable hormone alterations.

Initial enthusiasm for hormone replacement therapy (HRT) was based on non-randomized data showing increased organ yield when a cocktail of T_3, steroids, insulin, and vasopressin was administered.[9,22,76,77] Hormone cocktails therefore became part of the UNOS protocol for cardiac donor management. Using this protocol, animal models demonstrated beneficial reduction in vasopressors when given HRT.[78] With more rigorous examination, however, combination hormone therapy has not been supported. A recent randomized control trial using HRT in a protocol to increase lung donors was unable to demonstrate increased organ yield in those receiving the cocktail.[79] Criticism of HRT focuses primarily on the thyroid and steroid components of therapy, and thus will be examined more closely.

THYROID

Thyroid hormone replacement for donors originated with baboon studies in the late 1980s. Novitsky et al. observed reversal of cardiac dysfunction after administration of T_3.[72,80] Some societies therefore advocated T_3 if donor heart dysfunction was encountered.[7,9,76,78] However, further animal studies could not demonstrate benefit to T_3.[81,82] Numerous human studies were likewise unable to show correlation between T_3, cardiac function, inotropic support, or improved organ yield.[83-91]

Thyroid hormone replacement with thyroxine has also yielded conflicting results.[92,93] Revised UNOS recommendations concede that DDAVP (1-deamino-8-D-arginine-vasopressin), diuretics, and steroids rather than thyroid hormone administration increase organ yield.[94] Reasons for the conflicting data may be the pattern of thyroid dysfunction in brain death. Characterized by normal thyroxine levels, elevated reverse T_3, and low TSH, this matches the "sick euthyroid" state which has likewise failed to demonstrate benefit from hormone replacement.[95-97] In cases of prolonged donor management or excess catecholamine administration, thyroid hormones may have some role; however, they also may be harmful and therefore cannot be advocated in all donors.[88,98]

INFLAMMATION

Prominence of inflammatory mediators in BD donors plays a significant role in management. The ischemic brain elaborates core inflammatory mediators that then cross the blood-brain barrier.[99] Elevated levels of tumor necrosis factor (TNF)-α, interleukin (IL)-1, and IL-6 are found in both serum and tissue.[100,101] This can be cerebral in origin or secondary to local tissue ischemia-reperfusion (IR) injury as a result of the initial catecholamine surge.[102,103] Free radicals elaborated by IR injury increase local expression of adhesion molecules and signal an influx of leukocytes, referred to as *passenger leukocytes*, in the transplanted organ.[104] These primed leukocytes can then go on to influence graft rejection in the posttransplant period.

Inflammatory markers are more prominently expressed in all solid-organ grafts after BD versus living-related transplant.[105] Several studies have demonstrated increased rejection of kidneys from BD donors compared to living-related, unrelated, or donation after cardiac death (DCD) donors.[106-108] Increased levels of IL-6, TNF-α, and procalcitonin have also been associated with poor cardiac graft function.[109,110] A recent case-control study confirmed marked elevation of plasma endotoxin and cytokines in BD donors, although this did not correlate with lower graft survival.[111] Of interest, tissue from BD donors exhibited higher levels of proapoptotic gene mRNA, which may further explain graft loss beyond just having higher cytokine levels.

Steroids are used in the donor in an attempt to attenuate the inflammatory response, with the goal of reducing rejection and increasing organ yield.[112,113] Methylprednisolone is the steroid of choice and is given either as a single bolus or as a drip. Some studies demonstrate reduction of cytokines and subsequent rejection with early steroid administration.[114,115] A follow-up randomized control trial confirmed that while BD hearts have increased inflammatory markers and poorer graft function, these results could not be prevented with steroid administration.[116] Barring an alternative antiinflammatory agent and given their low risk profile, however, steroids are currently recommended in donor resuscitation.

Other Treatment

Donor management is unique in respect to perceived benefit versus risk: a life already lost has the potential to affect the lives of many others. While the final impact may be tremendous, the situation is often dire, leading to more aggressive and sometimes less rigorously tested treatment modalities. Regional styles of management may also dictate protocols and novel interventions.

A large number of emerging treatment modalities focus on reversing IR injury and modulating inflammation. Erythropoietin and carbamylated erythropoietin are gaining use as renal protectants.[117] Benefit in the donor comes not from hematopoietic effects, but via immunomodulation.[118] Naloxone is also potentially protective. Early animal studies have shown better renal function and survival in treatment groups with its use,[119] as well as improvement in oxygenation and lung function.[120]

Other treatment modalities employed in the ICU have great potential in donor management. Examples of these include extracorporeal membrane oxygenation (ECMO), high-frequency oscillatory ventilation (HFOV), activated protein C, and pharmaconutrition. Novel therapies such as these are being used more frequently and warrant dedicated study in the donor population.

Conclusion

The limited supply of cadaveric donor organs requires attentive pretransplant management to increase their availability and function. Maintenance of organs after brain death can be extremely difficult because the donor is characterized by hypothermia, acidosis, hypovolemia, pulmonary edema, cardiac arrhythmias, and profound hypotension. Designated protocols can help focus resuscitation and ensure provision of evidence-based guidelines. Important aspects of management include identification of potential donors, early hemodynamic stabilization with volume and vasopressor resuscitation, frequent reassessment of organ function and endpoints of resuscitation, and provision of hormone replacement when indicated. Augmentation of the proinflammatory response is emerging as a key component to both ablating hemodynamic instability and reducing posttransplant graft dysfunction. Newer therapeutic modalities are promising but merit further research.

ANNOTATED REFERENCES

Smith M. Physiologic changes during brain stem death—lessons for management of the organ donor. J Heart Lung Transplant 2004;23:S217-22.
This recent review provides a thorough yet concise overview of the physiologic changes which occur during brain death. The paper provides a good introduction to the subject.

Zaroff JG, Rosengard BR, Armstrong WF, Babcock WD, D'Alessandro A, Dec GW, et al. Consensus conference report: maximizing use of organs recovered from the cadaver donor: cardiac recommendations. March 28-29, 2001, Crystal City, Va. Circulation 2002;106:836-41.
Directed at increasing available hearts for donation, this is one of the first efforts to create a consensus document and algorithm for donor management. Although a large part is based on expert opinion and animal studies, it is still a valuable tool for reference.

Rosendale JD, Kauffman HM, McBride MA, Chabalewski FL, Zaroff JG, Garrity ER, et al. Aggressive pharmacologic donor management results in more transplanted organs. Transplantation 2003;75:482-7.
This is a landmark review of the UNOS database, with specific attention to use of hormone therapy and effect on organ yield. Although controversial due to cohort size and retrospective nature of the study, this is a widely cited paper for proponents of hormone resuscitation.

Shemie SD, Ross H, Pagliarello J, Baker AJ, Greig PD, Brand T, et al. Organ donor management in Canada: recommendations of the forum on Medical Management to Optimize Donor Organ Potential. CMAJ 2006;174:S13-30.
This paper outlines the recommendations developed by the Canadian Council for Donation and Transplantation forum in 2004. Grades of evidence are included with each topic of recommendation.

This is one of the more recent and inclusive efforts to assemble evidence-based guidelines for donor resuscitation.

Selck FW, Deb P, Grossman EB. Deceased organ donor characteristics and clinical interventions associated with organ yield. Am J Transplant 2008;8:965-74.

A more recent review of UNOS donor data, this paper highlights donor characteristics which increase organ yield. Of note, it demonstrates that steroids, diuretics, and DDAVP are positive predictors, but it does not support thyroid hormone use. It is of interest to compare this paper to that of Rosendale et al. above.

Chamorro C, Falcón JA, Michelena JC. Controversial points in organ donor management. Transplant Proc 2009;41:3473-5.

A very concise and well-written paper, this addresses the more recent controversies in donor management, including details of resuscitation, thyroid hormone usage, and steroids.

United Network for Organ Sharing website. http://www.unos.org/.

The UNOS website contains continuously updated information for patients and practitioners regarding all aspects of organ transplantation. Donor data can be uploaded or requested from the site. Recommendations and pathways for donor management are also provided.

REFERENCES

Access the complete reference list online at http://www.expertconsult.com.

Organ Donation After Cardiac Death

SHERILYN GORDON BURROUGHS | R. MARK GHOBRIAL

Historical Perspective

The increasing gap between the number of organs available for transplantation and the number of patients listed for transplantation has become the rate-limiting step in reducing both wait times and wait-list deaths in patients with end-organ disease awaiting transplantation. Prior to the passage of the first U.S. brain death law in the state of Kansas in 1970,[1] donation after cardiac death (DCD, or non-heartbeating donation) was the primary mode of organ donation in this country. Death in DCD donors was determined according to traditional cardiopulmonary criteria. Early organ procurement strategies were somewhat crude and variable, and consequently, warm ischemia time (time from donor circulatory arrest to cold perfusion) in the DCD donor was often prolonged and outcomes were poor.[2] The impact of the type of graft on DCD outcomes was not apparent until experience with organs from donors declared brain dead (DBD) grew. Transplant centers in several states such as Nebraska, Ohio, North Carolina, and Illinois flourished after adoption of DBD in their respective states, and transplant volumes grew.[3]

The DBD phenomenon was a culmination of critical care physicians' growing ability to maintain physiologic organ function in patients with little or no hope of neurologic recovery from severe insults to the central nervous system. A new debate was sparked over the precise definition and timing of death and the concept of futile care. This concept was introduced at a CIBA Foundation meeting in England in 1965 and subsequently endorsed with formal diagnostic criteria by Harvard Medical School in 1968.[1,4] Acceptance of this medically, philosophically, and legally novel concept radically changed the face of transplantation. The revolutionary ability to certify death while perfusing the donor with oxygenated blood guaranteed procurement with minimal warm ischemia and graft damage and better recipient outcomes. As early experience with the DBD organs demonstrated superior outcomes, the use of DCD organs declined and was subsequently abandoned.[5]

As a result of the success seen with DBD organ donation, the number of U.S. transplants performed annually increased exponentially. Based on Organ Procurement and Transplantation Network (OPTN) data, in 1988, the first year for which reliable national data were available, 10,794 deceased-donor transplants were performed.[6] Just 6 years later, annual volumes increased by nearly 50% to 15,210 total transplants. Most dramatically, the number of lung grafts from deceased donors increased from 33 to 708.[6] Moreover, intestinal transplantation gained clinical success with the introduction of DBD donors (in addition to refined medical and surgical techniques). The first case was performed in 1990; by 1994, 96 patients with intestinal failure had received intestinal transplants.[6] Concomitantly, advances in critical care resulted in reduced mortality in patients with end-stage organ disease, thereby resulting in increasing additions to and decreased attrition from the wait list, often referred to as the growing "gap" between supply and demand in transplantation. For example, despite a burgeoning number of transplant centers, rapid increase in transplants performed, and increased utilization of living donors, in 1995, only 33% of listed registrants waiting for kidney transplant (33,167) were transplanted (11,081).[6] Unfortunately, the rate of transplantation fell to 10% of the list in the subsequent era of 1998 to 2002.[7]

Exacerbating the impact of this trend, numbers of young, previously healthy DBD donors stagnated due to several statutory changes in the areas of gun control, automobile safety (air bags, seat belts, lowering of legal blood alcohol limits), and cyclist helmet use, thereby reducing traumatic fatalities and consequently changing the face of DBD organ donors in the process.[8] The demographics and mode of death of the typical DBD donor transitioned from a young, healthy person rendered brain dead as a result of a devastating head trauma toward an older person rendered brain dead from a neurovascular insult. The change in median donor age and mode of death ultimately eroded some of the benefit of utilization of the DBD donor and prompted a search for additional options.

Scientific and legal strategies such as xenotransplantation (use of grafts derived from donors), presumed consent (requiring individuals to formally opt out of organ donation in order to be excluded as a donor at the time of his or her death), and living donation have been explored as tools to meet the growing demand for organ donors. These strategies have been rejected because of strong philosophical objections or have been met with little or no success. The transplant community has therefore revisited the use of DCD donors with much enthusiasm.

As noted by DeVita, in 1993, the University of Pittsburgh Medical Center (UPMC) introduced the nation's first institutional policy to permit and regulate DCD donation.[9] The need for such a policy arose when several patients and their families asked to participate in organ donation after previously electing withdrawal of life-sustaining treatment. This was a request that fell outside the parameters of donation policies and guidelines then in effect. The UPMC policy became the first concrete model for the use of cardiopulmonary criteria to determine death for the purposes of organ procurement,[10] and it highlighted a milestone in the evolution of the practice of transplantation in this country. Since, DCD utilization has been adopted by many organ procurement organizations (OPOs) and hospitals nationwide. By December 2006, OPTN bylaws required that all OPTN members have a DCD donor protocol in place.[10] Moreover, the Joint Commission now requires that all accredited institutions develop and implement standardized DCD policies.[11]

After more than a decade and a half of ongoing scrutiny surrounding ethical issues and assessment of outcomes, several key issues regarding DCD organ donation remain controversial in both the lay and medical communities—namely, (1) how best to identify potential DCD donors, thus avoiding the financial and emotional burden of "failed" DCD donation, (2) how best to optimize DCD donor management, which by its very nature leaves little room for error, and (3) how best to standardize DCD procurement protocols to ensure a multidisciplinary effort and reproducible results. These issues will be explored in the remainder of this chapter after a brief discussion on the current status of DCD donation.

Current Status of DCD Donation

VOLUME

United Network for Organ Sharing (UNOS), the national nonprofit entity charged with disseminating both education and data pertaining to transplantation in the United States, has reported data on organs procured via DCD donation since 1994.[6] Data are available via the OPTN website, www.optn.transplant.hrsa.gov/ and in OPTN annual reports. Table 212-1 demonstrates that the annual number of DCD organ donors increased steadily for the better part the mid 1990s to the early 21st century. The 188 DCD donor recoveries performed in

TABLE 212-1	Number of DCD Organs as a Percent of Total Deceased Donor Organs Procured, by Year		
Year	# Deceased Donors	# DCD Donors	DCD as Percentage of Total Donors
1993	4861	42	0.86
1995	5362	64	1.20
1997	5478	78	1.43
1999	5825	87	1.49
2001	6082	169	2.77
2003	6457	268	4.15
2005	7593	556	7.32
2007	8085	793	9.80

From www.optn.transplant.hrsa.gov. Based on OPTN data as of May, 2010.
DCD, donation after cardiac death.

2002 represented 3% of total donors that year. In 2009, DCD recoveries represented 12% of all procurements, a fourfold increase from 2002.[6]

As a result of the OPTN and Joint Commission mandates mentioned earlier, the number of OPOs facilitating DCD recoveries in a given year has also risen overall, although not as sharply as the number of procurements performed: from 13 in 1993 to 33 in 2001. For the last year reported, 43 of the 59 OPOs facilitated at least one DCD procurement.[7] The next logical question is whether the increased volume of DCD procurements has accordingly impacted transplant outcome metrics.

OUTCOMES

Though fraught with ethical controversy over the years, the real barrier to widespread acceptance of DCD graft utilization is based primarily upon the poor outcomes seen in the early DCD experience. Suboptimal organ function characterized by primary nonfunction (PNF), delayed graft function (DGF),[12] and/or abbreviated graft survival have traditionally been a threat to success with DCD donors organs because of the warm ischemic insult associated with cardiopulmonary arrest. Although these observations were valid at the time, they were accumulated during the early experiences with transplantation and are thus inherently confounded by era bias.

The primary lesson from the early DCD era was that the metabolically active renal cortex, biliary epithelium, pulmonary alveoli/central airways, and islets are sensitive to ischemia, with warm ischemic injury manifesting as acute tubular necrosis (ATN), ischemic-type biliary strictures (ITBS), bronchial dehiscence, and impaired beta cell function. These complications have been postulated to translate into and account for both poor initial graft function and long-term complications, seen particularly in the early era.[12,13,14] Droupy and Abt, however, in separate studies, report that outcomes have improved; that intermediate and long-term patient/graft survival in recipients of controlled DCD kidney and liver grafts, respectively, are equivalent to or approach that of DBD.[15,16] Per Droupy, DCD and DBD renal grafts followed for 10 years demonstrate equivalent survival despite a higher initial incidence of DGF for the DCD cohort. Salvaggio and colleagues, in an analysis of UNOS/OPTN data, concur[17] (Figure 212-1, *A*).

DCD liver outcomes have improved, though less dramatically. Some results of liver transplants using DCD donors were discouraging; both graft and patient survival rates were thought to be significantly lower when compared with DBD donors.[18] Morbidity rates were higher as well.[19,20] However, reviews isolating recent data—as, for example, data outlined by Abt—demonstrate that 1- and 3-year patient survival rates for liver DCD are now similar to those from DBD, although lower graft survival rates for DCD liver grafts persist[16] (Table 212-2).

Much of the available outcome data for pancreatic DCD organs are derived from cases of simultaneous pancreas-kidney (SPK) transplants, demonstrating pancreatic graft and patient survival rates similar to those for DBD[17] (see Figure 212-1, *B*). Utilization of pancreas-alone DCD grafts under the same protocols as SPK DCD grafts, while less frequent over the last decade, have been favorable[17] (see Figure

212-1, *C*). Ongoing clinical experience will determine whether outcomes will reach those of SPK DCD grafts.

Oliveira et al. have, in the largest single-center series to date, demonstrated that lung grafts from DCD donors can also confer graft and patient survival rates equivalent to those from DBD donors.[13] Of interest, these outcomes have been achieved in many settings in recipients who have been disproportionately more ill prior to transplant but deemed reasonable potential DCD recipients because of the long potential wait for DBD grafts. Consequently, clinicians now consider use of grafts that were previously routinely declined.[21]

The net effect of current practice and improved outcomes has been to shift the paradigm of the binary cadaveric donor (DBD versus DCD) to a spectrum of standard criteria to extended criteria, with the DCD donor potentially falling along several points on that spectrum based on specific factors. Careful evaluation of those factors, as discussed

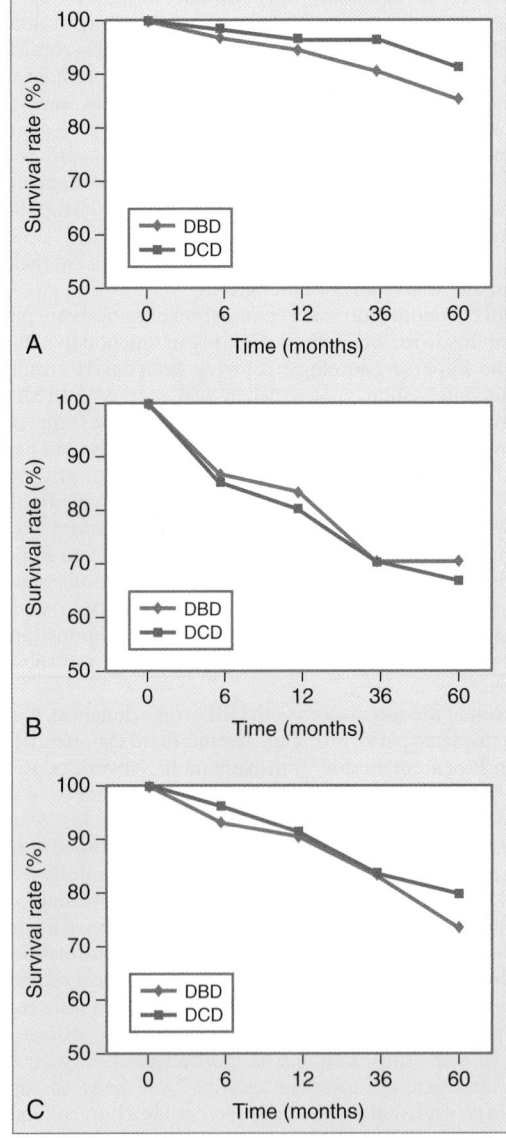

Figure 212-1 A, Current outcomes after kidney transplant, DBD versus DCD. **B,** Current outcomes after DCD SPK transplant, DBD versus DCD. **C,** Current outcomes after DCD pancreas alone transplant, DBD versus DCD. DBD, donors declared brain dead; DCD, donation after cardiac death; SPK, simultaneous pancreas-kidney. *(From Salvaggio P, Davies D, Fernandez L et al. Outcomes of pancreas transplantation in the United States using cardiac-death donors. Am J Transpl 2006;6:1059-65.)*

TABLE
212-2

TABLE 212-2	One- and Three-Year Outcomes after DCD and DBD Liver Transplantation		
Type of Graft	*Year Post Transplant*	*Graft Survival*	*Patient Survival*
DCD	1	70.2%	79.7%
	3	63.3%	72.1%
DBD	1	80.4%	85%
	3	72.1%	77.4%

From Abt P, Desai N, Crawford M. Survival following liver transplantation from non-heart-beating donors. Ann Surg 2004;239:87-92.

DBD, donors declared brain dead; *DCD,* donation after cardiac death.

later, may allow the transplant community to unravel the issues preventing expansion of the successful use of DCD organ donors in contemporary transplant practice.

Identification and Categorization of the Potential DCD Donor

An important initial step in the process of DCD organ transplantation is recognizing the potential suitable donor. A significant consideration is the need to minimize organ ischemia in the presence of an unanticipated uncontrolled cardiac arrest; thus while organ procurement from DCD donors under uncontrolled conditions is technically feasible, it remains rare in contemporary practice.[22,23] Similarly, graft quality is compromised in situations in which a patient's wishes regarding organ donation are unknown. Organ suitability declines while attempts are made to locate family members to obtain consent. The once popular practice by some institutions to manage potential DCD donors brought to the emergency department by placement of vascular and/or intraperitoneal catheters in order to infuse cold organ preservation solution *before* consent for procurement became available[24] has been largely abandoned. The practice stimulated contentious debate from opponents in both the medical and lay communities; unlike several European countries, no U.S. state at the time of the writing of this chapter has adopted presumed consent into law.

Remaining potential DCD donors are patients consented for donation with impending cardiopulmonary death, the timing of which is either unpredictable or predictable based upon patient/family-requested withdrawal of care, or unpredictable with premature arrest before withdrawal. Understandably, each type of DCD confers a varying risk of ischemic injury. A discussion of the management of DCD donors is facilitated by use of a classification scheme developed at a donor conference convened in 1994 by Maastricht, Netherlands, investigators.[25] The Maastricht Categories define potential donors by the circumstances under which their cardiovascular death occurs. A distinction is made between those donors whose cardiopulmonary failure is uncontrolled or emergent (categories 1, 2, and 4) and those donors whose death by cardiopulmonary criteria occurs in a controlled, planned fashion by withdrawal of futile life-sustaining support (category 3). Maastricht Categories are outlined in Table 212-3.

Because only some single-center reviews report DCD results by Maastricht category, it is difficult to stratify nationwide DCD outcomes by category. Category 3 donors constitute the majority of the DCD

TABLE
212-3

TABLE 212-3	The Maastricht Classification for DCD Donors	
Category	*Description*	*Condition*
1	Cardiac arrest outside the hospital, no resuscitation attempted	Uncontrolled
2	Cardiac arrest followed by unsuccessful resuscitation, either inside or outside a hospital	Uncontrolled
3	Cardiac arrest after planned withdrawal of life-support technology	Controlled
4	Cardiac arrest in a brain-dead patient awaiting organ procurement	Uncontrolled

From Koostra G, Daemen JHC, Oomen APA. Categories of non-heartbeating donors. Transplant Proc 1995;27:2893-4.

procurements reflected in data from U.S. centers; a small but unknown fraction are category 4 donors, wherein the patient meets brain death criteria but subsequently loses circulation.

Of note, recent initiatives in the northeast United States involve training prehospital personnel in the rapid conversion of preconsented victims of unsuccessful resuscitation after cardiopulmonary arrest (category 2) to potential DCD donors.[26] For the sake of uniformity, the remainder of this chapter will be devoted to discussion of category 3 donors.

In addition to understanding the classification scheme and expected outcomes based upon absence or presence of controlled ischemia, the intensivist and OPO personnel must be familiar with the diagnoses and clinical circumstances qualifying a patient as a potential DCD donor. Again, candidates are patients in whom withdrawal of futile life-sustaining treatment is being planned. As shown in Table 212-4, the UNOS Critical Pathway for DCD,[6] typical patients may have the following characteristics: absent or hyperactive respiratory drive, lack of adequate respiratory muscle strength, severe hypoxemia, or inadequate circulation in the absence of inotropic or vasopressor drugs. Such patients are usually supported by ventilators or mechanical circulatory assistance such as ventricular-assist devices (VAD) or intraaortic balloon pumps. They are often patients who have also suffered a severe neurologic insult. Conscious patients are usually suffering from degenerative neuromuscular diseases or end-stage cardiopulmonary disease and are often ventilator or VAD dependent. These patients or their families may decide to discontinue their support devices and request that their organs subsequently be donated.

The next important step in identification of the potential DCD donor is predicting when rapid physiologic deterioration and death are expected occur in a period of less than 30 to 60 minutes (depending on the organ to be procured) after withdrawal of life-sustaining treatment.[27] Failure of a potential donor to progress to cardiac death within the prescribed time disqualifies the potential donor owing to the extent of warm ischemic injury sustained by the organs. Factors such as age, comorbidities, and preterminal pressor requirement have been shown to have predictive value, but no strict criteria have been universally adopted.[28] Kaufman et al. have proposed four readily obtainable clinical criteria: (1) requirement for vasopressors to support arterial blood pressure, (2) absence of primary brain injury, (3) history of 6 or more days on mechanical ventilation, and (4) respiratory rate less than 20 breaths/min (in the absence of mechanical ventilatory support).[29] They noted that the presence of two or more of the indicators accurately predicted death within 60 minutes after life-supporting treatments were withdrawn, with a sensitivity and specificity of 81% and 78%, respectively.

Adoption of accurate predictive indices would enable intensivists and OPO staff to more precisely identify potential organ donors, help minimize the financial impact and resource drain for hospitals and procurement teams of the donor who "fails to progress," and prevent unnecessary stress and disappointment for families during a psychologically vulnerable time.

Lastly, familiarity with relative and absolute contraindications for DCD donation, some of which overlap with those associated with DBD, some unique to DCD, is important. These include the multiply operated abdomen, active sepsis, active or recent extracranial primary malignancy, and human immunodeficiency virus (HIV) and hepatitis B infection. With regard to virologic status, OPOs are versed in rapid serologic testing necessary to rule out latent viral infections and should be involved as early as feasible to initiate testing.

Principles of DCD Donor Management

Appropriate management of the DCD organ donor requires integration of several fundamental principles exercised to protect the rights and interests of the donor and simultaneously prevent the care of the organ from superseding the care of the dying patient. The debate arises in the paradox that can emerge from attempts to protect those interests while preserving suitability of the potential grafts. Hence, the role of

TABLE 212-4	United Network for Organ Sharing Donation after Cardiac Death Critical Pathway

Critical Pathway for Donation after Cardiac Death (DCD)

Patient Name_____

UNOS ID Number_____

Collaborative Practice	Phase I Identification & Referral	Phase II Preliminary Evaluation	Phase III Family Discussion & Consent	Phase IV Comprehensive Evaluation & Donor Management	Phase V Withdrawal of Support/Pronouncement of Death/Organ Recovery
The following health care professionals may be involved in the DCD donation process: **Check all that apply:** ☐ Physician (MD) ☐ Critical Care RN ☐ Nurse Supervisor ☐ Medical Examiner/ Coroner ☐ Respiratory Therapy (RT) ☐ Laboratory ☐ Pharmacy ☐ Radiology ☐ Anesthesiology ☐ OR/Surgery Staff ☐ Clergy ☐ Social Worker ☐ Organ Procurement Coordinator (OPC) ☐ Organ Procurement Organization (OPO)	Prior to withdrawing life support, contact local OPO for any patient who fulfills the following criteria: ☐ Devastating neurologic injury and/or other organ failure requiring mechanical ventilatory or circulatory support ☐ Family and/or care giving team initiate conversation about withdrawal of support Following referral, additional evaluation is done collaboratively to determine if death is likely to occur within 1 hour (or within a specified timeframe as determined by caregiving team and OPO) following withdrawal of support Patient conditions might include the following: ☐ **Ventilator dependent for respiratory insufficiency:** apneic or severe hypopneic; tachypnea ≥ 30 breaths/ min after DC ventilator ☐ **Dependent on mechanical circulatory support** (LVAD; RVAD; V-A ECMO; Pacemaker with unassisted rhythm < 30 beats per minute. ☐ **Severe disruption in oxygenation:** PEEP ≥ 10 and Sao$_2$ ≤ 92%; Fio2 ≥ .50 and Sao$_2$ ≤ 92%; V-V ECMO requirement ☐ **Dependent upon pharmacologic circulatory assist:** Norepinephrine, epinephrine, or phenylephrine ≥ 0.2 µg/kg/min; Dopamine ≥ 15 µg/kg/min ☐ **IABP and inotropic support:** IABP 1:1 and dobutamine or dopamine ≥ 10 µg/kg/min and CI ≤ 2.2 L/min/m²; IABP 1:1 & CI ≤ 1.5 L/min/m²	Physician ☐ Supportive of withdrawal of care and has communicated grave prognosis to family ☐ Review DCD procedure with OPC ☐ Will be involved in withdrawal/ pronouncement ☐ Will designate a person to be involved with withdrawal and/or pronouncement **Family** ☐ Has received grave prognosis ☐ Understands prognosis ☐ In conjunction with care giving team, decide to withdraw support Patient ☐ Age _____ ☐ Weight _____ ☐ Height _____ ☐ ABO _____ ☐ Medical Hx _____ ☐ Surgical Hx _____ ☐ Social Hx _____ ☐ Death likely < 1 hour following withdrawal (determined collaboratively by evaluating: injury, level of support, respiratory drive assessment)	☐ Support services offered to family ☐ OPC/Hospital Staff approach family about donation options ☐ Legal next-of-kin (NOK) fully informed of donation options and recovery procedures ☐ Legal NOK grants consent for DCD following withdrawal of support ☐ Family offered opportunity to be present during withdrawal of support ☐ OPC obtains ____ Witnessed consent from legal NOK for DCD ____ Signed consent Time_____ Date_____ ___Detailed med/soc history Notification of donation ☐ Hospital supervisor ☐ ME/Coroner notified ____ ME/Coroner releases for donation ____ ME/Coroner has restrictions *Stop Pathway if —* ☐ *Family, ME/Coroner denies consent* ☐ *Patient determined to be unsuitable candidate for DCD* *Patient progresses to brain death during evaluation—refer to brain-dead pathway*	☐ MD, in collaboration with OPO, implements management guidelines. ☐ Establish location and time of withdrawal of support ☐ Review plan for withdrawal to include: Pronouncing MD (should be in attendance for duration of withdrawal of support, determination of death, and may not be a member of the transplant team) Comfort Care Extubation and discontinuation of ventilator support Establish plan for continued supportive care if pt survives > one hour or predetermined time interval after withdrawal of support ☐ Notify OR/Anesthesia ____ Review patient's clinical course, withdrawal plan and potential organ recovery procedures ____ Schedule OR Time ☐ Notify recovery teams ☐ Prepare patient for transport to prearranged area for withdrawal of support ☐ Patient transported to prearranged area ☐ NOTE: Should the clinical situation require premortem femoral cannulation, the following should be reviewed: Family consent or understanding MD inserting cannula Time and location of cannula insertion If death does not occur, determine if cannula should be removed	☐ Withdrawal occurs in _____ OR _____ ICU _____ Other ☐ Family present for withdrawal of support _____ Yes _____ No ☐ OR/Room prepared and equipment set up ☐ Transplant team in the OR (not in attendance during withdrawal) ☐ Care giving team present ☐ Administration of preapproved medication (e.g., Heparin/Regitine) ☐ **Withdrawal of support according to hospital/MD practice guidelines** Time _____ Date _____ ☐ **Vital signs are monitored and recorded every minute (See attached sheet)** ☐ **Pt pronounced dead and appropriate documentation completed** Time _____ Date _____ MD _____ ☐ **Transplant Team initiates surgical recovery** at prescribed time following pronouncement of death ☐ Allocation of organs per OPTN/UNOS policy ☐ *If cardiac death not established within 1 hour or predetermined time interval after withdrawal of support —Stop Pathway. Patient moved to predetermined area for continuation of supportive care.* ☐ *Postmortem care administered*
Labs/Diagnostics		☐ ABO ☐ Electrolytes ☐ LFTs ☐ PT/PTT ☐ CBC with Diff ☐ Beta HCG (female pts) ☐ ABG		Repeat full panel of labs additionally: ☐ Serology Testing infectious disease profile ☐ Blood cultures × 2 ☐ UA & Urine culture ☐ Sputum Culture ☐ Tissue typing	

TABLE 212-4	United Network for Organ Sharing Donation after Cardiac Death Critical Pathway (Continued)

Critical Pathway for Donation after Cardiac Death (DCD)

Patient Name_____
UNOS ID Number_____

Collaborative Practice	Phase I Identification & Referral	Phase II Preliminary Evaluation	Phase III Family Discussion & Consent	Phase IV Comprehensive Evaluation & Donor Management	Phase V Withdrawal of Support/Pronouncement of Death/Organ Recovery
Respiratory	☐ Maintain ventilator support ☐ Pulmonary toilet PRN	☐ Respiratory drive assessment RR _____ VT _____ VE _____ NIF _____ Minutes off ventilator _____ ☐ Hemodynamics while off ventilator HR _____ BP _____ Sao$_2$ _____	☐ ABGs as requested ☐ Notify RT of location and time of withdrawal of support	☐ Transport with mechanical ventilation using lowest F$_{IO_2}$ possible while maintaining the Sao$_2$ >90%	
Treatments/ Ongoing Care	Maintain standard nursing care to include: ☐ Vital signs q 1 hour ☐ I & O q 1 hour				☐ Postmortem care at conclusion of case
Medications				☐ Provide medications as directed by MD in consult with OPC	☐ Heparin and other medications prior to withdrawal of support
Optimal Outcomes	The potential DCD donor is identified, & a referral is made to the OPO.	The donor is evaluated & found to be a suitable candidate for donation.	The family is offered the option of donation, & their decision is supported.	Optimal organ function is maintained, withdrawal of support plan is established, and personnel prepared for potential organ recovery.	Death occurs within 1 hour of withdrawal of support, and all suitable organs and tissues are recovered for transplant.

This work supported by HRSA Contract 231-00-0115.
From www.UNOS.org. Accessed May 1, 2010.

the intensivist and/or palliative care physician (terminal care of the patient, pronouncement of death) and the managing OPO (facilitating organ procurement) must be rigidly defined; the two factions must travel distinct paths to achieve their goals. As Ozark states, "as a general rule two discussions—whether to forego life-sustaining therapy and whether to donate organs—must be made separately and on their own individual merit."[30] Ideally, discussion regarding withdrawal of life-sustaining treatment should come first so as not to be biased by the issue of transplantation.

The push for optimal palliative care has been a hallmark of recent critical care management initiatives.[31] The dying patient who also wishes to be a DCD organ donor presents a special challenge, requiring care that is not only comparable to that afforded to all dying patients but also sensitive to the concerns already described. The Society of Critical Care Medicine (SCCM) has offered recommendations specific to DCD donation.[32,33] These guidelines, supplemented by individual transplant center reports and the UNOS pathway (see Table 212-4), provide direction for intensivists caring for patients who wish to become DCD donors. It is vital that all healthcare providers involved in this process be comfortable with, and knowledgeable about, their specific role such that the patient's wishes can be respected.

Pain relief is the single most important goal in palliative care in the final hours of life, and there is firm ethical, legal, and medical justification for use of analgesics and anxiolytics in this scenario. Some patients require higher doses than others, so doses are given with the knowledge that unintended effects such as hypotension or respiratory depression may compromise organ viability. *It is critical, then, that the interest of the dying patient be represented by a completely different entity than that responsible for representing the interests of the donor.* If any question arises as to the practitioner's ability to maintain an objective position, consultation from the hospital's palliative care and ethics teams should be sought.

In 2008, in the first criminal case brought against a transplant surgeon for the death of a donor, the defendant allegedly administered high doses of analgesic and anxiolytic to a potential donor to hasten his death prior to procurement.[11] Although the surgeon was acquitted, the case highlighted the potential legal ramifications of the recovery team's involvement in the care of a dying patient. There is a consensus that "medications given to provide comfort are reasonable, even if they might hasten death" but "no medication whose purpose is to hasten death should be given to the patient."[34] Failure to attend to potential DCD donors' comfort in contemporary practice is considered suboptimal end-of-life care but is not in any circumstance managed by anyone other than the physician(s) caring for the patient.

Active debate exists as to the optimal location of withdrawal of support. Arguments for ICU withdrawal stem from proponents who prefer to provide grieving families as "normal" a setting as possible to grieve, albeit briefly, at the bedside of their loved one. Others argue that effective and expedient progression to donor mode allows for the most successful procurement and can only transpire in the operating room. Currently there is no standard, and each facility is responsible for dictating protocol for their institution.

DeVita notes that "The initial University of Pittsburgh policy called for the withdrawal of care to occur in the operating room, which offered the advantage of minimizing the need to transport the patient after death and permitting the prepping and draping of the patient before death. This protocol was denounced for subjecting the patient to 'a desolate, profanely "high tech" death' surrounded by 'masked, gowned, and gloved strangers.'[35] The initial experience in Pittsburgh found some truth to the proposition that presence of family at the patient's bedside at the time of death may be more important to patients and families than organ donation or location of death. When three of the first four families approached about non-heartbeating donation agreed to consent only if they could be physically present at the time of death, the Pittsburgh policy was changed to allow families into the operating room or to move the withdrawal of care to an operating room 'holding' area. The area selected for withdrawal of support should allow family members to be present, accommodate the necessary monitors and equipment, and be close enough to the operating room to allow rapid transport immediately after death."[7] Other programs followed in kind; according to the 2000 IOM report on DCD, the family's need to be present and involved in the dying process is generally widely cited and respected in the development of hospital policies on the setting for withdrawal of care.[34]

DETERMINATION OF DEATH, AN EXACT SCIENTIFIC CONCEPT?

The 1980 Uniform Determination of Death Act (UDDA) established that death is determined when there is *irreversible* cessation of circulatory and respiratory function.[36] Death is declared most often based on cessation of cardiac and pulmonary function; however, required asystolic time is perhaps the single most contentious issue in the debate surrounding DCD donation.[37,38] Simply, "the longer you wait the more uncertainty there is about the organs, and the shorter you wait the more uncertainty [there is about] whether the person is really dead or not."[39]

As the limits of life-sustaining practices are expanded, medical professionals are encouraged to maintain focus with reference to the UDDA. The term *irreversible* can be interpreted as a shifting paradigm, or as Wilner remarks, the concept is subject to "serial displacement by advancing clinical science." He further notes that "the question [of death] is thus reformulated to explore whether the morally relevant time of death is reached when death is certain despite all possible medical intervention or whether death is assured once all ethically permissible remedies have been utilized."[7] Although consensus has yet to be reached on the question of the time at which death is irreversible, it does seem logical that once a principled decision is made not to correct a loss of function, that loss becomes irreversible.[40]

No investigator has documented the spontaneous return of circulation after more than 65 seconds of combined circulatory and respiratory arrest.[41] However, the standard applied by most U.S. hospitals ranges from a 2- to 10-minute asystolic interval (pulselessness, apnea, and unresponsiveness). This broad standard is addressed by the SCCM's statement that "there is no ethically or physiologically important distinction between the two minute observation period utilized by the University of Pittsburgh, the five minutes recommended by the IOM, and the ten minutes" (utilized by some institutions).[32] Ostensibly, the standard does satisfy proponents of the waning possibility of autoresuscitation beyond 65 seconds of asystole, and furthermore serves to address the ethical concerns raised by those proponents. Because of the paucity of empirical evidence, the IOM continues to encourage investigators to provide additional studies in this matter.

A final logistic issue in the determination of death is the management of patients who progress too slowly to be considered for donation. This occurs in approximately 5% to 10% of potential donors.[28] Most programs disqualify patients from donation if there is cardiac activity 60 minutes after discontinuing life support.[42] For this reason, contingency plans should be in place so that these patients receive appropriate ongoing end-of-life care.

■ DCD Procurement: an Opportunity for Standardization

Because every organ from a DCD donor sustains some degree of unavoidable warm ischemic damage, several aggressive methodologies to protect graft viability have been proposed. Strategies can be considered in the premortem or intraoperative phases.

PREMORTEM

1. Placement of large-bore arterial and venous catheters for perfusion[24]
2. Administration of systemic anticoagulants such as heparin (30,000 units) along with recombinant tissue plasminogen activator (50 mg)[43] or streptokinase[44] to prevent vascular thrombosis during the low-flow state

3. Administration of vasodilators such as phentolamine or trifluoperazine, thought to prevent agonal vasospasm induced by hypoxia and surging catecholamine levels[45,46]
4. Ischemic preconditioning. Brief pre-insult ischemic challenges can trigger protective mechanisms that allow compensatory tissue physiology at the time of the cardiac arrest, thought to be mediated via heat shock proteins.[47,48] This effect has already been demonstrated with phenylephrine in an animal model of DCD cardiac transplant.[49]

Because these premortem measures are not part of standard end-of-life care and have been argued by some to potentially hasten death, their use remains limited.[50] The position of the SCCM and IOM is that the use of these medications and devices is acceptable so long as they cause no significant harm to the patient[32,34] and family consent is obtained wherever practical. That they are of no direct benefit to the patient is countered by the fact that they improve the likelihood that the patient's wish of organ donation will ultimately be realized.

OPERATIVE

The conduct of the operative procedure is dictated by the tenets already mentioned: the procurement team is not physically present at the time of death, and recovery of organs must be accomplished expeditiously with careful coordination of numerous personnel, equipment, and resources. To do so, the operative team prepares and drapes the patient upon arrival to the operating room. The team outlines the necessary instruments and maneuvers requested of the OPO staff to ensure a seamless procedure. The team, gowned and gloved, is escorted from the operating room and is notified by OPO staff if the patient progresses within the prescribed time frame. Optimally, after withdrawal and prior to incision, the OPO staff will complete a data form (Figure 212-2) allowing for recording of minute-by-minute hemodynamic and oxygenation data. The benefit of compiling data in such a fashion is that as DCD procurements become standardized, data can be collated without the encumbrance of shifting definitions of the initiation of warm ischemic time (and hence acirculatory status) that currently confounds comparison of outcomes between hospitals and OPOs. For instance, the definition of the warm ischemia start time remains variable, with some advocating that a threshold of systolic blood pressure of less than 80 mm Hg be used, others, a mean arterial pressure of 50 mm Hg, others a systolic blood pressure less than 50 mm Hg, and yet others when the arterial oxygen saturation decreases to less than 80%.[16] The lack of a universal definition renders comparison of outcomes between centers and organs difficult.

Whereas the asystolic interval to be observed remains a matter of institutional policy, it seems prudent to recommend that standardized criteria be developed. Highly sensitive maneuvers used to document the absence of circulation, such as intraarterial pressure monitoring or echocardiography, may be helpful if a short asystolic interval will be used.

Once the asystolic interval has passed, the operative team returns and infuses cold perfusate via either a premortem-placed cannula or a standard terminal aorta cannula placed after rapidly accessing the abdomen. Rapid but careful in situ cold dissection ensues, as the potential for vascular injury is increased without the benefit of pulsatile flow to assist with the identification of aberrant anatomy. The pancreas is sacrificed if a replaced right hepatic artery originating from the superior mesenteric artery appears to be present. Organs are packaged and implanted on the recipient end as soon as possible in order to mitigate the impact of cold ischemic injury.

The two most common contingencies the team must be prepared for are unexpected cardiac arrest while awaiting withdrawal and failure to progress after withdrawal. Appropriate intravenous access, a ventilator, and a special supply cart must be available and stocked with an oxygen tank, cardiac monitor, and an adequate supply of sedatives and narcotics. Of course, the patient's wishes regarding resuscitation in order to ultimately donate must be determined from the patient or family as early in the process as possible.

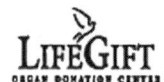

Page 1 of 1

SOP Form #   PO47-F3
Effective Date JUN 23 2009
Supersedes Date 08/30/2007
Rev #   006

DONATION AFTER CARDIAC DEATH (DCD) DONOR DATA FORM

Date:_____ UNOS ID:_____ LifeGift ID:_____

Enter OR	Time:_____	Cross-Clamp	Time:_____
Withdrawal of Support	Time:_____	Cannulation, abdominal aorta	Time:_____ Flush start/stop time:_____/_____
Mannitol/Heparin Admind	Time:_____	Cannulation, thoracic aorta	Time:_____ Flush start/stop time:_____/_____
Pronouncement	Time:_____	Cannulation, portal vein	Time:_____ Flush start/stop time:_____/_____
Incision	Time:_____	Cannulation, pulmonary artery	Time:_____ Flush start/stop time:_____/_____

Time from withdraw to Pronouncement _____ minutes   Family present for withdrawal: ☐ Yes ☐ No

Time from pronouncement to Cross-Clamp _____ minutes   Location of withdrawal: ☐ OR ☐ ICU ☐ Other:_____

Total Warm Ischemic Time (withdraw to cross-clamp)_____ minutes   Care and Comfort Administered by Hospital Staff: ☐ Yes ☐ No

Start Time: _____   Urine output: _____

	Min 1	Min 2	Min 3	Min 4	Min 5	Min 6	Min 7	Min 8	Min 9	Min 10	Min 11	Min 12	Min 13	Min 14	Min 15	Min 16	Min 17	Min 18	Min 19	Min 20
BP																				
MAP																				
HR																				
RR																				
O2SAT																				
Initials																				

	Min 21	Min 22	Min 23	Min 24	Min 25	Min 26	Min 27	Min 28	Min 29	Min 30	Min 31	Min 32	Min 33	Min 34	Min 35	Min 36	Min 37	Min 38	Min 39	Min 40
BP																				
MAP																				
HR																				
RR																				
O2SAT																				
Initials																				

	Min 41	Min 42	Min 43	Min 44	Min 45	Min 46	Min 47	Min 48	Min 49	Min 50	Min 51	Min 52	Min 53	Min 54	Min 55	Min 56	Min 57	Min 58	Min 59	Min 60
BP																				
MAP																				
HR																				
RR																				
O2SAT																				
Initials																				

Figure 212-2 Donation after cardiac death (DCD) monitoring form. *(Reprinted with permission from Lifegift Organ Donation Center, 2009.)*

Future Directions

Despite the success with kidneys, livers, and pancreatic grafts realized with use of DCD grafts, there remain a number of unmet challenges and questions regarding the transplantation of organs from DCD donors. They fall within the realms of medical as well as ethical concerns.

Owing to unavoidable warm ischemia, heart and intestinal grafts are difficult to utilize when procured from DCD donors. Nevertheless, cardiac DCD transplantation is technically possible. The first human cardiac transplant 40 years ago was made possible using a DCD donor heart, which started and functioned well after a single electric shock.[51] It is conceivable, then, with the advent of preconditioning therapy, a new era of DCD cardiac transplantation may begin.

A second area of likely future focus concerns the real numeric advantage of using DCD grafts. What, if any, increase in available donor organs can be expected by promoting the utilization of DCD donors? Will the push for identification of DCD donors simply convert would-be DBD donors to donate as DCDs? Additionally, if the number of wait-list deaths decreases, and the gap is reduced, is the cost and burden shifted from wait-list complications to posttransplant complications with longer length of stays, increased readmissions, increasing complexity of diagnostic evaluations and immunosuppressive drugs regimens, and an increased rate of recipient morbidity and mortality? The transplant community will be in a better position to answer these questions once clean, prospective data are collated nationwide as suggested earlier.

Ethically, how, if at all, will DCD donation affect public trust in the healthcare system and the organ procurement and transplantation process? Furthermore, on the recipient end, will the potential for differential results of DBD versus DCD transplantation mandate that a recipient be afforded the prerogative to decline an organ based on knowledge of physicians' concerns regarding the DCD process? As noted by the UPMC group and the IOM, an emphasis on patients' and families' wishes is paramount in the success of any DCD program. The public will be guided by medical information, but the practice of transplantation, which is donor driven, will be guided by the way in which that information is buttressed by open communication with the layperson.

Furthermore, the concern by the lay public is that physicians caring for patients who are potential donors have shifted the focus of care from the dying patient, and that there exists now more than ever, the latitude to violate the "dead donor rule" (comprising two complementary ideas: that the patient must be dead before the initiation of organ procurement; *and* that organ procurement itself must not be the cause of the donor's death).[40] This concern may translate in the public mind into a fear that their likelihood of receiving aggressive life support will be compromised by consenting to organ donor status. These misperceptions can be particularly damaging when the overriding goal of the transplant community is to maintain and build public support of maximizing organ donation.

Conclusion

The widening gap between suitable donors and patients in need of transplant continues to be the single issue that keeps solid-organ transplantation from achieving its full potential for relieving suffering and improving survival in patients with end-stage organ disease. As current practice and outcomes have shifted the paradigm of the binary cadaveric donor (DBD versus DCD) to a spectrum of standard criteria to extended criteria, with factors mentioned earlier affecting where on this spectrum a DCD organ may fall, the ultimate impact of the estimated unrealized annual 22,000 DCD donors[8] on the actual number of organs available for transplantation will remain unclear until sufficient data obtained under similar protocols are obtained. Whereas ethical questions regarding DCD donation persist, the process, as it is increasingly practiced in a standardized fashion, has proven to accommodate the needs of dying patients, as well as those awaiting transplantation, with improving success.[38] A number of organizations including the SCCM,[32] UNOS,[6] and the IOM[35] have endorsed the concept and issued relevant guidelines.

As experience grows, attitudes change, and outcomes continue to improve, DCD donation may yet have a significant impact on the number of organs available for transplantation and thus the quality of life for those waiting for and ultimately receiving cadaveric organs.

KEY POINTS

1. Before donation after brain death (DBD) was formally defined and accepted into law in 1970, organs were procured from donors whose death was declared according to traditional cardiopulmonary criteria. This process, formerly referred to as *non-heartbeating donation*, is now designated *donation after cardiac death* (DCD).

2. Unlike organs procured from DBD donors, organs recovered from DCD donors are subjected to a variable duration of warm ischemic time, which can negatively impact both early and late graft function. Some solid organs are more susceptible to the effects of ischemic injury than others. Superior outcomes were therefore quickly realized with use of DBD organs, and DCD donation was abandoned based upon better outcomes rather than ethical opposition.

3. As the gap between donor supply and demand widened in the early 1990s, DCD procurements were reintroduced into clinical practice in an attempt to expand the donor pool and reduce wait times and wait-list deaths. In the process, terminally ill patients not meeting criteria for DBD but wishing to donate (and/or their families) were afforded a chance to participate in the donation process. As intensive care had become much more sophisticated with life-sustaining modalities, questions regarding the timing and definition of death became much more challenging than those faced in the pre-DBD era. Reintroduction of DCD donor utilization thus heralded a new wave of ethical controversies.

4. As lung, liver, kidney, and pancreas DCD grafts are increasingly used, outcomes are now improved over historical experience. Debates between DCD proponents and opponents have arisen regarding optimal identification of potential donors, donor management, and procurement standardization.

5. In the contemporary era of ICU care and donor shortages, DCD donation may provide the only effective mechanism for: (1) terminal patients who do not meet DBD criteria but wish to donate to do so, and (2) the transplant community to begin to close the organ-shortage gap. Strategic planning and interdisciplinary coordination designed to address the unique logistical, medical, and ethical challenges of DCD organ utilization will promote increased understanding and consensus.

ANNOTATED REFERENCES

Choi E-K, Fredland C, Zachodni C, et al. Brain death revisited: the case for a national standard. J Law Med Ethics 2008;824-36.
   This review provides a comprehensive evaluation of the current status of brain death determination and identifies the shortcomings of the brain death determination process including the lack of standardized definitions. The authors present viable solutions to the most troubling problems with the current status of brain death determination.
Childress J, Liverman C, editors. Organ donation: opportunities for action. Washington DC: The National Academies Press; 2006.
   Thorough objective overview of the current state of procedures and protocols relating to organ donation in the United States, which highlights the challenges of the contemporary practice of transplantation.

Reich DJ, Mulligan DC, Abt PL, et al. ASTS Recommended practice guidelines for controlled donation after cardiac death organ procurement and transplantation. Am J Transplant 2009;9:2004-11.
   A practical guide to procedures, protocols, and tools necessary for successful procurement of organs from donation after cardiac death donors.
Ho KJ, Owens CD, Johnson SR, et al. Donor postextubation hypotension and age correlate with outcome after donation after cardiac death transplantation. Transplantation 2008;85:1588-94.
   A unique analysis of donor factors which impact graft function after DCD donation.
Salvaggio P, Davies D, Fernandez L, et al. Outcomes of pancreas transplantation in the United States using cardiac-death donors. Am J Transpl 2006;6:1059-65.
   A comprehensive retrospective registry analysis of outcomes after pancreas transplants from DCD donors.

REFERENCES

Access the complete reference list online at http://www.expertconsult.com.

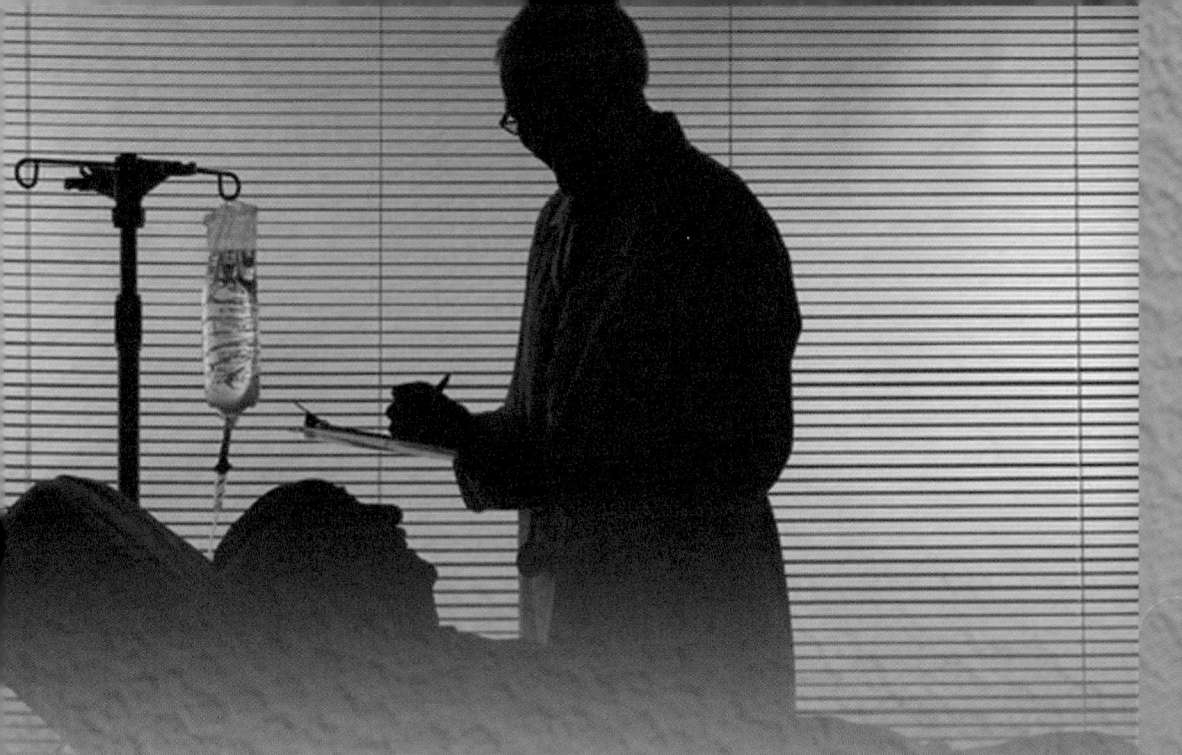

Ethical and
End-of-Life Issues

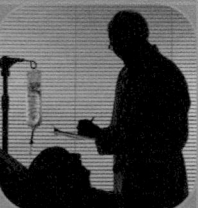

213

Beyond Technology: Caring for the Critically Ill

PHILLIP D. LEVIN | CHARLES L. SPRUNG

Over the last half century, intensive care has grown from the position of a fledgling specialty to occupy a central role in hospital medicine. Intensive care has changed the natural history of many disease processes and has also allowed other specialties to progress with the performance of ever more challenging procedures in sicker and sicker patients. Over the last decades, however, this progress has been accompanied by increasingly complex ethical, moral, and social questions. These questions can be broadly divided into those that relate to the patient's treatment, those that relate to the patient's family or surrogates, and those that relate to the intensive care unit (ICU) as a location, although all these topics are interrelated to some degree. In this chapter, a brief overview of the main issues relating to these three elements will be introduced, and the concepts of diversity and satisfaction will be elucidated. Diversity is relevant, as it is important to appreciate that diverse groups of people will view ethical or moral issues in very different ways, while an examination of patient and family satisfaction with their intensive care experience may underscore areas where care has been deficient and might be improved.

The Patient—When the Outcome Is Poor

The predominant intensive care dilemma relating to the patient concerns end-of-life care. Prior to the 1980s, the accepted aim of intensive care was to stave off death for as long as possible in the hope the patient would eventually recover. Although patients did die, typically they did so only after full care including cardiopulmonary resuscitation (CPR). Gradually it became clear that some patients had no chance of recovery—that they were going to die either in the ICU or in the hospital following an ICU admission despite all attempts at treatment. Empirically, physicians thought they were able to identify a proportion of these patients early in their ICU course. It also became clear that other ICU patients entered a chronic state in which their lives could only be preserved within an ICU, or that they recovered to some extent but not to a level of functional independence (e.g., following severe head injury). Many patients, their families/surrogates, and physicians viewed these outcomes as worse than death. As a result, questions began to arise regarding the justification for continuing life-support measures for these patients. Should interventions which were of no avail and yet invasive be continued, or should the process of dying be allowed to proceed unhampered? Voices were raised suggesting that when quality of life could not be assured or restored, or when maintaining life was no longer possible, dignity and humanity would indicate that palliative care should replace active treatment. Once resources began to be restricted, their allocation to such patients was also questioned. Various terms arose to describe treatments that, although they may have had an effect on the patient, would not change the final poor outcome. These terms included "futile," "nonbeneficial," and "undesirable." The limitation or cessation of such treatments became widely accepted, even if it led to or hastened the patient's death.[1]

The limitation of undesirable treatments can take one of three main avenues: treatment may be withheld, withdrawn, or steps may be taken to actively shorten the dying process.[2] *Withholding treatment*, as its name suggests, implies not administering a treatment considered to be nonbeneficial. An example might be not starting dialysis for a patient with renal failure but no hope of recovery, or a do-not-resuscitate (DNR) order whereby CPR will not be performed in the event of a cardiac arrest. *Withdrawal of treatment* (but not care) implies the removal of a treatment modality. Examples include cessation of inotropes or ventilation. *Steps which actively shorten the dying process* (considered by some to be akin to euthanasia)[2] might include the administration of a drug (e.g., KCl or a muscle relaxant to a nonventilated patient) which will directly end the patient's life. Grey zones exist between the borders of these definitions.[3] For example, following withdrawal of ventilation by extubation, morphine and midazolam might be administered to reduce suffering and agonal breathing. These drugs will, however, also depress ventilation and may possibly shorten the dying process.[3]

It must be noted that huge diversity exists in end-of-life care. Diversity exists in the practices of individual physicians as well as the expectations of patients and families, and both within and between individual countries. A recent study from Europe emphasizes these variations. Data were collected concerning end-of-life care for 4248 patients who died in 37 ICUs located in 17 European countries. Life-sustaining treatment was limited to some degree for 76% of all patients who died. Withdrawal of life support was more common in Northern European countries than in Southern European countries (performed prior to 47% versus 18% of deaths, respectively). The time taken from admission until limitation of life support was also shorter (1.6 versus 5.7 days, median Northern versus Southern Europe), while the performance of CPR was rarer (10% versus 30%) in Northern European countries. An attempt was made to correlate these differences with physician religion (with the finding that Catholic, nonaffiliated, or Protestant physicians limited life-sustaining interventions more frequently than their Jewish, Greek Orthodox, or Moslem colleagues); however, these religious variations may be indistinguishable from the regional variations and are thus difficult to interpret.[2] So even between the closely linked countries of Europe, geographic variation influences end-of-life practice to a significant degree.

Variations in end-of-life care have been found in many other studies relating to different countries and regions. For example, comparing the United States to England, 17.2% of deaths in the United States involved intensive care admission versus 5.1% in England, with this difference being particularly predominant among the elderly (>85 years old).[4] Within the United States, a study of 5910 patients who died in 131 ICUs showed that limitation of life-sustaining treatment was performed prior to the death of 71% of patients.[5] When incidence rates for each type of limitation were compared across the different centers contributing to the study, however, large variations were discovered. Full resuscitation including CPR was performed for between 4% and 79% of patients at different centers, while treatments were withheld for between 0% and 67% and withdrawn for 0% to 79%. Similarly, in a study from Canada, 1361 ICU nurses and physicians were asked to determine the appropriate level of care in 12 patient vignettes. In only one case was there greater than 50% agreement between the participants.[6] Considering this variability, it is unlikely that medical conditions alone determined the specifics of end-of-life care. Indeed when analyzing end-of-life decisions in 1239 patients across Europe, an increased nurse-to-bed ratio led to more aggressive end-of-life care, while the presence of ICU specialists and nighttime physician coverage of the ICU was associated with a decrease in limitations of life-sustaining therapy.[7] Other aspects of a physician's life and practice have also been associated with differences in willingness to limit life-supporting therapies. For example, physicians in certain specialties (e.g., cardiology),[8,9] in nonacademic practice,[10] who are older,[11] or who have strong religious beliefs[12] are less likely to be aggressive in the limitation of care.

Variability in attitudes to end-of-life care is not limited to the ICU staff. Similar variability has been demonstrated in the expectations of patients, their families, and the general public, and these too are not defined by geographic borders. The following anthropologic study of four ethnic subgroups within the United States attempts to illustrate and explain some of the differences in approach. African Americans, European Americans, Korean Americans, and Mexican Americans were interviewed regarding their attitudes to life-support measures in general (for others) and for themselves.[13] Korean Americans had the most positive general attitude toward life support (i.e., these interviewees believed that life support should be continued under most circumstances for others) but paradoxically showed a low personal desire to have these measures performed on themselves. In-depth interviews revealed a strong concept of family obligation; such obligation would mandate continuation of therapy for a different family member, while the interviewees would be happy to have therapy limited for themselves. African American interviewees revealed the opposite. They had a positive view toward personal life support but were willing to forgo life-sustaining treatment in general. These respondents were described as understanding the inevitability of death but lacking trust in institutionalized medicine. They expressed the view that life support should be attempted (physicians might be mistaken or unwilling to initiate therapy because of financial considerations, for example), and if it was unsuccessful, therapy could be stopped. European American interviewees were negative in both their general and personal attitudes toward life support. They expressed a fear of being functionally limited or a burden to their families and would prefer death to these outcomes.

Attitudes in Hong Kong and Japan have been described and are different once again. Traditional Chinese society has been described as having less emphasis on individual rights, self-expression and self-determination than Western society.[14] The traditional Chinese family might therefore want to protect their loved ones and not burden them with the truth regarding their poor prognosis. Similarly, 97% of Japanese interviewees in Japan were of the opinion that the patient's family should be informed of the patient's poor prognosis (in a scenario of gastric cancer), but only 63% thought the patient should be informed. Exposure to American culture in the United States seemed to alter these views; while 93% of English-speaking Japanese Americans (presumed to be more acculturated to American culture than the Japanese in Japan) agreed that the family should be informed, the proportion who believed the patient should know his diagnosis increased to 95%, perhaps in line with American views of patient autonomy.[15]

Over the last 50 years, population movement and immigration have resulted in large and varied ethnic communities living side by side, particularly in larger cities. The result is that an ICU physician or nurse may well encounter and be expected to communicate with patients and families from entirely different and possibly unfamiliar cultures,[16] and at extremely difficult times in patients'/families' lives. The ICU personnel may view life, injury, and death in one way, while the patient and family may view these events in quite another.[17,18] The ICU team may expect patient autonomy, while the family may object. Language may be a significant barrier. Differences in expectations regarding the goals of ICU admission may also be considerable. The ICU team is providing a service to the patient and family, so it would seem reasonable to expect that the team adapt to the patient's/family's expectations. Such adaptation may not be easy, and setting limits may represent a considerable challenge. A paradox could even appear—the patient expecting the physician to make treatment decisions without their involvement, and the physician feeling bound by patient autonomy. Indeed, can

patient autonomy extend to the abrogation of that autonomy? In any event, understanding and accepting cultural diversity may help create a calmer and more objective outlook at these difficult times.

The Family—Difficult Decisions, Autonomy, and Paternalism

Following the discussion so far, it should have become clear that views concerning life and death are by no means uniform. For example, some patients may be willing to pursue life following injury leading to quadriplegia, while others would prefer to die. Physicians, patients, and their families may be divided on such a qualitative decision. The next dilemma to be discussed then concerns the process of decision making.

Autonomy is defined as "liberty to follow one's will, personal freedom," and this is the preeminent value in health care today, at least in North America. Autonomy suggests that the patient should be able determine for himself or herself the course of therapy, and physicians should act as consultants to share their knowledge. Unfortunately, as a result of either their illness or injury, the majority (up to 95%)[19] of intensive care patients are unable to communicate clearly. Only a minority (3%) will have clearly expressed their end-of-life preferences or prepared a "living will."[19,20] Even if a living will has been prepared, it might not be sufficiently descriptive, leaving doubt as to the patient's needs under particular circumstances. For example, a living will might indicate that mechanical ventilation would be inappropriate. The patient then presents to the emergency department with pulmonary edema. Should CPAP via a mask be used to help the patient recover from this transient episode, and who should decide? Practically (in the ICU), the vast majority of decisions regarding philosophy of care result from an interaction between the patient's surrogates and the ICU physicians.

Most patients would want a surrogate to represent them[21] and would want this to be a family member,[22,23] frequently a spouse.[23] Indeed, classically the patient's autonomy is extended to his or her closest family. These family members may have discussed care requirements with the patient in the past (although this is not common) or at least may share a commonality of cultural milieu. Unfortunately, when examined empirically, there is little evidence that family members are able to speak accurately for the patient. Agreement between the patient and their surrogate has been found to range between 50% and 88%,[24-28] although rarely is agreement more likely than chance.[27] Similarly, even in cases where children knew what their elderly parents would have wanted, in only 46% of cases were they willing to abide by these requests.[25] In addition, the decision-making ability of families may not be optimal under the stresses of a sudden ICU admission for a loved one. A high prevalence of anxiety and depression (69.1% and 35.4%, respectively) have been found among family members of ICU patients,[29] while the short- and long-term emotional burden of dealing with end-of-life decision making may discourage families from participating. Involvement of a multidisciplinary team[30] involving physicians, nurses, social workers, and even representatives of previous ICU patients may go some way to alleviating these difficulties. Families may also perceive ICU admission as more stressful than what the patients themselves report following recovery,[31] and their understanding of the implications of critical disease is not always perfect.[32,33] Despite these caveats, it is widely accepted that the patient's direct and close family will act as their surrogate in decision making.

In North America, family involvement in decision making is almost universal,[34] although their opinions are not universally respected. In a survey of 879 U.S. physicians, 96% of whom had withheld or withdrawn life-sustaining treatments, 25% had withheld and 23% had withdrawn treatments without the family's consent, 14% and 12% without their knowledge, and 3% despite their objection. In contrast, therapy had been continued by 34% despite the request by family members that it be terminated.[35] This is not to suggest that physicians have a better understanding of the patient's needs than do family; agreement between the views of physicians and patients regarding priorities in end-of-life care range from 47% to 72%, never being better than chance.[27,36,37]

The role of the family in countries other than the United States and in diverse cultures is variable. For example, in Europe patients or families were involved in end-of-life discussions on 84% of occasions in Northern Europe versus 66% in Central Europe and 47% in Southern Europe.[19] However, during these discussions, the family was told of the end-of-life decision on 88% of occasions and asked in only 38%.[19] In Hong Kong and Japan, cultural values may suggest that the patient should be protected from bad news and difficult life-and-death decisions. In these cases, no discussion might take place at all, or the family might conduct end-of-life discussions to the exclusion of the patient, even in the event the patient is able to be included.

Although the principles of autonomy would suggest a hierarchy of decision making beginning with the patient, followed by the proxy, and ending with the physician, clearly this does not always occur. The divergence from this utopian goal may even be inevitable to some degree in that defining limits for involvement in the decision-making process for both the physician and the patient/family is not simple. Choosing the correct type of enteral nutrition for an ICU patient is clearly a medical decision that the physician might make alone. The decision to peruse indefinite mechanical ventilation in a terminal neurologic condition such as ALS, on the other hand, is very personal and should be made by the patient. In between these extremes lie the shades of gray where the treatment plan is based on a negotiation of some description between the main protagonists—the patient (where possible), the surrogate, and the ICU team. Individual personality, philosophy, beliefs, and experience will determine the course such negotiations take and the relative involvement or weight of each party.

Unfortunately, the process by which decisions are reached is not always smooth, with 27% of all ICU conflicts occurring between ICU staff and family.[38] Many of these conflicts (44%) relate to end-of-life care, usually (85%) with the family wanting more aggressive care than the ICU team is suggesting should be provided.[39] End-of-life care issues also accounted for 57% of the conflicts observed within families, and 7% of conflicts within the ICU team.[39] An additional study examining conflict arising from end-of-life discussions found that conflict occurred equally between ICU staff and family and within the ICU team, both occurring in 48% of cases, while conflict within families occurred in 24% of cases.[40] Some of the less desirable techniques for conflict resolution have already been described: ignoring the family's wishes or not informing them of their options. Fortunately, the commonest path taken in the resolution of conflict is negotiation (71% of physicians said they would chose this path in one study[41]).

If differences cannot be resolved by direct negotiation, the use of an ethics consultant has been advocated. An ethics consultant is a third party, not necessarily a physician, who conducts discussions with the ICU team and the patient or their family in order to elucidate values and bridge gaps in a nonconfrontational manner.[42] Although reported to be useful,[43] ethics consultations have not found widespread use. When no accommodation can be reached between physicians and patients/families, the courts have been used (by both parties) as a final arbiter.[44,45]

The ICU—Restricted Space, Many Patients, Limited Finances

The main dilemma facing the ICU as a location is resource allocation. Patients are frequently denied ICU care, despite this care being appropriate, owing to lack of space.[46] Patients who require ICU care but do not receive it do not do as well as when admitted to the ICU.[47-50] So when faced with two patients who require ICU care, but only one bed, who is to be admitted?

Prognostic scoring systems have been suggested as a tool to help. However, many of these scoring systems require data from the first 24 hours of ICU care to reach a value, and all have been validated on groups of patients. For example, a group of patients with a poor prognostic score might be expected to have 90% mortality. For the individual patient within that group, it is not possible to say whether he will be in the 90% who will die or among the 10% who will survive. Society has not determined a percentage point for expected survival below which intensive care is not thought to be appropriate. Many patients, their surrogates, and their physicians would be willing to endure or suggest ICU care even when the chances of survival are small,[51] so even a very poor prognostic score might not help decide whether to admit a particular patient to the ICU. Surveys have also shown that poor prognosis does not deter physicians from admitting patients to the ICU.[46,52] Patient characteristics such as age, sex, and economic or social standing seem entirely inappropriate for determining which patient to admit, so unfortunately, no clear help is available in this aspect of decision making.

Alternative solutions to the problem of lack of space could include increasing the number of ICU beds or increasing the efficiency of use of existing beds. Increasing bed space requires increased funding and is associated with problems of its own. If funding to the ICU is increased from a fixed budget, then funding for some other aspect of the hospital's function will have to be decreased, thereby engendering a direct comparison between the importance of the ICU patients and the dialysis or radiotherapy patient, for example. Increased overall funding for the hospital is a societal issue, often meaning that government funding from another field has to be reduced. Further, the presence of more ICU beds might not alleviate the pressure on them, as more beds might simply mean a lowering of the requirement for ICU admission in a particular institution and leave the ICU as full as ever.

Increasing bed efficiency implies making better use of the facilities that already exist. In an attempt to create a model for bed usage, the concept of a triage chain has been suggested.[53] This chain starts when the patient refers him/herself or is referred to the hospital, and then continues through the referral by the emergency room physician to the ICU, through ICU admission, ICU discharge, and then ward discharge. If flow along this chain could be improved—for example, if patients do not remain in the ICU waiting for bed space on the ward—the efficiency of ICU bed usage could be improved. Care must be taken with this concept, however; premature discharge from the ICU may be associated with increased patient mortality on the ward.[54]

The cost of ICU care in itself is a source of dilemma. Take for example a drug such as activated protein C.[55] As the first drug proven to change the outcome of severe sepsis, this intervention raised much interest. Unfortunately, its cost is high (approximately $8000 for the 72-hour course). This cost is perhaps of most interest to the hospital administration, but the acceptability (or inevitability) that use of this new drug should be limited only because of its high cost is debatable. Indeed, with increasing patient awareness of therapeutic options, ICU team members may find themselves having to explain an administrative policy concerning drug administration not based on medical indication alone.

Patient Satisfaction

Patients' satisfaction with their ICU experiences has been addressed in three main ways: by descriptive studies, directed questionnaires, and assessments of willingness to undergo ICU care again. A factor common to many of these studies is that approximately one-third of ICU patients have no recollection at all of their ICU admission.[56,57]

Descriptive studies reveal both negative and positive comments about ICU experiences.[56,58,59] Statements such as "The place was very upsetting. Like a war zone. I remember hearing a man making animal noises" are balanced by "The staff . . . made me feel safe," "This made me feel very safe and secure." Overall, however, 81% of the patients who were interviewed were extremely pleased that resuscitative equipment had been used, and 80% would be willing to undergo further ICU treatment under all circumstances.[56] A directed questionnaire examined recollection of mechanical ventilation after 1 year. The majority of these patients recalled no pain or discomfort (78.2%) and would be willing to undergo ventilation again (86.5%).[60] The additional use of chemical paralysis did not seem to have a major effect.[61] Similarly, when a patient group was asked whether they would be willing to go through intensive care again, the majority (up to 70%) would be willing,[51,62] even if only for a month of further survival.[51] If, however, levels of outcome were added to the question, willingness to undergo mechanical ventilation decreased. If the outcome was described as a permanent vegetative state, only 30% of a group of ICU survivors would agree to readmission to the intensive care.[63]

Directed questionnaires also provide more specific details of the ICU experience. Stressful events in the ICU include pain, inability to sleep, having tubes in the nose or mouth, being unable to talk, and lack of control.[31,64-66] Stress was also associated with the presence of an endotracheal tube.[57] Interestingly, when patients' experiences were compared to the perception of these experiences by family and physicians, both overestimated the "stress scores."[31]

These studies do suffer from some common limitations. As mentioned earlier, many ICU patients have no recollection of their stay in ICU. All the studies are based on interviews with patients who have survived their ICU admission in a sufficiently good functional state to be able to answer sometimes complex questions. This implies a degree of patient selection. For those who have survived the ICU and are being interviewed by a researcher associated with the ICU, an element of gratitude might also bias the responses. For the studies performed long after ICU admission, memories might not be reliable. They also obviously do not describe the experiences of patients who have died.

In general, it seems most patients are satisfied with their ICU experience (provided they survive it in a good functional state) and would be willing to undergo such care once again. A hint is given that families see ICU care as more traumatic than patients.

Family Satisfaction

Ironically, family satisfaction is much more complex to assess than patient satisfaction. Many earlier studies attempted to analyze and describe the needs of families of ICU patients. The need for hope, the need to receive adequate and honest information, and the feeling that hospital staff members were concerned about the patient were described as important.[67] However, a correlation between meeting these needs and family satisfaction is elusive. Families may be satisfied despite not having their needs met, or dissatisfied despite attempts to meet their needs.

Multiple tools have been developed and validated in an attempt to quantify family satisfaction.[68-71] These tools are based on questionnaires including areas such as assurance (the need to feel hope for a desired outcome), information (the need for consistent realistic and timely information), proximity (the need for personal contact and physical proximity to the patient), support (the need for resources and support systems), and comfort (the need for family members' personal comfort).[68] Use of one such tool[71] revealed a high overall satisfaction score of 84.3/100. The highest scoring elements in this study were nursing skill and competence, the compassion and respect given to a patient, and pain management. Communication with physicians and the physical conditions in the waiting room were the least satisfactory.[72] In the same study, a regression analysis was performed which found that higher family satisfaction was associated with higher ratings for information provided by the ICU staff, courtesy, compassion, respect, and the amount and level of care provided. Azoulay et al. found that increased satisfaction was associated with a higher nurse-to-patient ratio, with information being provided by a junior physician, and with involvement of the family physician. Interestingly, being of French descent (and presumably co-cultural with the ICU team) was also associated with increased satisfaction. In contrast, contradictory information, poor acquaintance with the ICU team members, and a low desired-to-allowed time ratio in discussions with the ICU team were associated with decreased satisfaction.[73] As mentioned, these authors also found that approximately half of the families did not understand the diagnosis for their family member or its implications,[32] while an increased understanding was associated with improved satisfaction.[74]

The families of patients who died in the ICU may represent a subgroup with respect to satisfaction measures and have been investigated separately. These families also describe discussion regarding end-of-life care as difficult (40%-48% perceived conflict with the medical staff[75,40]); however, their overall rating of satisfaction with ICU care remained high (70%-90%).[76] Dissatisfaction was reported among those families who had received notification of their family member's death over the telephone (rather than face to face) and among those whose family member had died suddenly.

Perhaps the conclusions reached by these studies are not surprising—family satisfaction is more likely when staff are competent and caring, respectful, courteous and compassionate, well acquainted to the family, and devote time to communication and explanation in person. Achieving these objectives is not always easy within the confines of busy schedules.

KEY POINTS
1. Ethical issues in intensive care center around the patient, their family, and the ICU as a location.
2. There are no "right answers" to ethical issues. Different people may view similar issues in very different ways.
3. Huge variations in ethical practice are found in different cultures.
4. Tolerance, communication, and patience are vital.
5. Most patients and their families are ultimately satisfied with their ICU experience.

ANNOTATED REFERENCES

Sprung CL, Cohen SL, Sjokvist P, et al. End-of-life practices in European intensive care units: the Ethicus Study. JAMA 2003;290:790-7.
  A large study looking at differences in end-of-life care across European countries and showing clear differences from North to South Europe.
Blackhall LJ, Frank G, Murphy ST, et al. Ethnicity and attitudes towards life-sustaining technology. Soc Sci Med 1999;48:1779-89.
  An in-depth sociological study of different ethnic groupings within the United States and attitudes to end-of-life care.
Sprung CL, Carmel S, Sjokvist P, et al. Attitudes of European physicians, nurses, patients, and families regarding end-of-life decisions: the ETHICATT study. Intensive Care Med 2007;33:104-10.
  A questionnaire study investigating attitudes of physicians and nurses to end-of-life care and showing how they differ from patients' and their families' values.
Pochard F, Azoulay E, Chevret S, et al. Symptoms of anxiety and depression in family members of intensive care unit patients: ethical hypothesis regarding decision-making capacity. Crit Care Med 2001;29:1893-7.

A description of the difficulties faced by family members of patients in the ICU.
Lautrette A, Darmon M, Megarbane B, et al. A communication strategy and brochure for relatives of patients dying in the ICU. N Engl J Med 2007;356:469-78.
  A study describing the importance of devoting time and providing a brochure to ease the suffering of patients' families whose loved ones are dying in the ICU.
Azoulay E, Timsit JF, Sprung CL, et al. Prevalence and factors of intensive care unit conflicts: the Conflicus study. Am J Respir Crit Care Med 2009;180:853-60.
  A description of sources of conflict within the ICU.
Danis M, Patrick DL, Southerland LI, et al. Patients' and families' preferences for medical intensive care. JAMA 1988;260:797-802.
  Interviews with patients who survived ICU or their families describing a willingness to undergo ICU again, even for limited benefits.

REFERENCES

Access the complete reference list online at http://www.expertconsult.com.

214

Conversations with Families of Critically Ill Patients

MARGARET ISAAC | J. RANDALL CURTIS

Intensive care unit (ICU) family conferences concerning the care of critically ill patients can be watershed events—clarifying prognosis, delineating goals of care, and providing support to family members and surrogate decision makers. Because the vast majority of critically ill patients lack decisional capacity,[1] families and surrogate decision makers are often centrally involved in medical decision making. Nearly a quarter of deaths in the United States occur in the ICU,[2] and the majority of patients who die in the ICU have had life-sustaining measures limited or withdrawn.[3,4] A decision to withhold or withdraw life support is often preceded by a family conference specifically addressing goals of care and treatment plans. Furthermore, the care of most critically ill patients should involve an explicit discussion with surrogate decision makers about the goals of care and treatment plans. Coping with a critically ill family member is challenging for surrogate decision makers, and many feel ill equipped to make decisions on behalf of their loved ones. Skilled communication by an interdisciplinary ICU team is associated with improved outcomes for both patients and family members.[5]

Leading an effective family conference requires specific teachable clinical skills, and our aim is to present an evidence-based approach to communication with families of critically ill patients. This chapter will first provide an introduction to medical decision making, with a particular emphasis on shared decision making. We will discuss a rationale for the importance of family conferences for all critically ill patients and address practical issues including considerations of physician reimbursement and billing. We will then present an evidence-based approach for family conferences, highlighting specific competencies and protocols that have been developed to improve physician-family communication. Finally, we will address issues of cultural competency and spirituality as they relate to the care of critically ill patients and their families.

Medical Decision Making

MODELS OF MEDICAL DECISION MAKING

In 1992, Emanuel and Emanuel[6] described four models of medical decision making: paternalistic (also known as *parental* or *priestly*), informative, interpretive, and deliberative. The *parental model* for physician-patient decision making frames the physician as the patient's guardian, interpreting diagnostic information and developing and implementing a therapeutic plan that he/she feels is in the patient's best interest. In the *informative model*, the physician provides information to the patient, who then chooses from treatment options—assuming that patients are expert in their own personal values and when given information by their physician can make the medical decision that is in their own best possible interest. The *interpretive model* defines the physician as counselor, not only providing medical information, as in the informative model, but also helping to elucidate and clarify patients' stated values and advising patients in terms of which interventions would be most in keeping with the patient's values. Finally, the *deliberative model* frames the physician as teacher or friend, not only engaging in discussion about medical information and elaborating personal values but also advising and even persuading a patient to make particular decisions, reflecting the physician's understanding of the patient's personal values.

The physician-patient or physician-surrogate relationship can be conceptualized on a spectrum, with parentalism at one end, informed consent (akin to Emanuel and Emanuel's informative model) at the other, and shared decision making in between. *Shared decision making* describes a relationship in which information is passed from physician to patient or surrogate, and both parties share opinions about treatment choices before a decision is jointly reached. There is consensus among multiple critical care societies in Europe and North America that shared decision making should be the default model for physician-patient and physician-surrogate communication in the ICU setting.[7,8] Though most patient surrogates prefer a shared decision-making approach,[9] there is considerable heterogeneity among patients and families with regard to their desired role in decision making. In the interest of patient-centered care, it is imperative to individualize one's approach. A recent U.S. study shows that physicians use the full spectrum of models of decision making but suggests that they do not routinely assess surrogates' desired level of involvement in medical decision making. Rather than individualizing their approach to match surrogate preferences, individual physicians often have one approach they use with all surrogates.[10]

SURROGATE DECISION MAKERS

The experience of family caregivers and surrogate decision makers is undeniably challenging. Informal caregivers are under tremendous stress and have higher rates of psychological symptoms than the general public.[11] For example, the prevalence of anxiety and depression symptoms in family members of critically ill patients is remarkably high,[5,12] and symptoms of posttraumatic stress have been shown to be present in a majority of family members of critically ill patients, with 82% of family members who were asked to participate in medical decision making demonstrating symptoms of posttraumatic stress 90 days after discharge or death.[13]

In addition to the affective difficulty inherent in coping with a sick loved one, surrogate decision makers are asked to participate in complex medical decision making with which they may have very little prior experience. Communicating clearly about goals of care and withdrawal of life-sustaining interventions as well as exploring families' wishes about withdrawal of life support can contribute to family support and satisfaction.[14] Though clinicians may be familiar and comfortable with the fast pace of ICUs, the tempo of medical decision making can pose a particular challenge to surrogate decision makers. A recent study demonstrated decreased family satisfaction associated with a longer ICU stay, but family satisfaction increased when withdrawal of life-sustaining interventions was prolonged,[15] especially for those patients with a longer ICU stay. This suggests that families may benefit from time to come to terms with medical decisions and their personal feelings of loss.

SUBSTITUTED JUDGMENT VERSUS BEST INTEREST

Many palliative medicine and critical care specialists suggest that surrogate decision makers employ the principle of substituted judgment when participating in medical decision making.[16,17] In the absence of an existing healthcare directive, we ask that surrogate decision makers imagine what the patient would want were they able to actively participate in decision making. Despite widespread endorsement of the substituted judgment standard by the medical community, significant concerns, both ethical and pragmatic, have been raised.[18] The first cites the frequency with which patients change their minds regarding medical decisions and preferences, especially true among patients who have not completed an advance directive.[19-21] That said, though many patients change their minds with regard to treatment preferences, most studies evaluating stability in preferences have shown that a majority of patients maintain consistency in their wishes regarding medical decisions.[22-23]

Some authors have raised concerns about the accuracy with which surrogate decision makers can predict what choices patients would make.[18] A meta-analysis by Shalowitz et al.[24] found that surrogate decision makers were 68% accurate in their predictions regarding patient treatment preferences. Several subsequent studies have found similar rates of accuracy between patient-surrogate pairs; furthermore, in cases in which surrogates are inaccurate in substituted judgments, their stated preferences on behalf of the patient more closely represent their own personal beliefs about end-of-life care.[25,26] One study asked patients the following question: if there were a discrepancy between the surrogate's decision and the patient's previously stated wishes regarding CPR, which should take precedence? Over three-quarters of the patients preferred that physicians follow the stated preferences of the surrogate.[27]

There is significant variability in the amount of decision control desired by patients over their designated surrogates, though the majority of patients have been shown to prefer implementation of a substituted judgment standard over a best interest standard.[28] Further, there is heterogeneity in the factors weighed by surrogates in medical decision making, including substituted judgment, but also other factors such as shared experiences with the patient and the personal values and preferences of the surrogate decision maker.[29,30] Although this is a complex issue, substituted judgment should generally be a higher standard for decision making than the best interest standard.

ROLE OF ADVANCE DIRECTIVES

The absence of an advance directive has been identified as a barrier to effective end-of-life care in the ICU setting,[31] although significant and valid concerns have been raised as to their usefulness and relevance.[32] Advance directives were not especially widespread in the past: one small retrospective study of 61 patients found that one-third of those who died in the hospital entered with advance directives,[33] though others have described much lower usage—between 5% and 11%.[34-36] Although advance directives have not been shown to change the type of care provided to patients[32,37] at the end of life, the presence of an advance directive is associated with higher family assessment of the quality of the dying process for patients in the ICU.[38] Advance directives can be helpful to surrogate decision makers, lessening the burden involved in attempting to implement substituted judgment. Therefore, even though advance directives may be limited in their ability to directly guide care, there is value in advance care planning for those patients who ultimately require critical care.

▧ Family Conferences in the ICU

IMPORTANCE OF FAMILY CONFERENCES FOR ALL CRITICALLY ILL PATIENTS

Robust communication between clinicians, nurses, and families of all critically ill patients is important, not only with families of patients who are imminently dying. Family members who felt that communication in the ICU was inadequate were at higher risk for posttraumatic stress disorder,[13] even those with loved ones who survived their ICU stay. Furthermore, families of patients who survive their ICU stay are actually more likely to be dissatisfied with their ICU care with respect to domains such as inclusion in decision making, communication,

emotional support, respect and compassion shown to family, and consideration of family needs.[39]

PRACTICAL AND LOGISTICAL CONSIDERATIONS

Pragmatic and logistical issues can shape the experience of surrogate decision makers in the critical care setting. Even physical space can have an important effect: a French study[40] found that family members of patients in private ICU rooms had a lower incidence of anxiety and depression symptoms compared with families of patients in multi-bed rooms. Additionally, the same group found that the absence of a dedicated room for family conferences was associated with increased anxiety symptoms among family members of critically ill patients.[12] Accessibility of physicians and access to information also correlates with family satisfaction; inaccessibility has been correlated with conflicts related to prognosis,[41] suggesting that surrogate decision makers are more satisfied when clinicians are accessible and comprehensive in their communication.

BILLING AND REIMBURSEMENT

According to guidelines from the Center for Medicare and Medicaid Services (CMS), U.S. physicians are permitted to bill for time spent consulting with surrogate decision makers either in person or by telephone. Furthermore, critical care clinicians are permitted to bill for critical care time, provided the following criteria are met:

- The patient is unable to participate in giving a history and/or making treatment decisions.
- The discussion is necessary for determining a treatment decision.
- The discussion occurs in the ICU. Documentation for these conversations must include:
  - The medically necessary treatment decisions for which the discussion was needed
  - That the patient is unable to participate in giving history and/or making treatment decisions
  - The necessity of the discussion and a summary in the medical record to support this necessity[42]

As of October 1, 2009, palliative care clinicians in the United States are recognized as an independent medical subspecialty by Medicare and as such can bill for their consultative services. Previously, prolonged service codes, frequently used in palliative care billing, required that additional time be spent "face-to-face" with the patient, meaning that time spent in meetings outside of the patient's room between clinicians and surrogate decision makers was not compensated. This changed in 2009, such that clinicians can now bill for prolonged service time spent charting, reviewing records, coordinating care with other clinicians, and importantly, meeting with surrogate decision makers outside of the patient's room.[43] Claims have been denied for palliative care specialists who are credentialed in the same specialty as the primary team physician, though these denials have been successfully appealed.[43] Of course, specifics regarding billing for both critical care and palliative care specialists change over time, so clinicians will be well served to familiarize themselves with the most updated billing guidelines.

EVIDENCE-BASED APPROACH TO COMMUNICATION DURING FAMILY CONFERENCES

Patients and families are consistent in defining high-quality care in the ICU: timely, clear, and compassionate communication by clinicians; clinical decision making focused on patients' preferences; patient care maintaining comfort and dignity; and family care with open access and proximity to patients, interdisciplinary support in the intensive care unit, and bereavement care for families of patients who die.[44]

Family conferences in the ICU setting are challenging, both for families and clinicians, but it is important to remember that the optimal skills to facilitate these sessions are both teachable and rooted

TABLE 214-1	Empathic Communication in Family Conferences
Category	**Sample Statements**
Empathy about surrogate decision making	*Withholding or Withdrawing Life Support*: "This is really hard. There's not a right answer to this situation."
	Determining Patient's Wishes: "It's very difficult to be in a position like this where you have to put your own personal feelings aside and try to advocate for what you think he would want."
	Fear of Making a Mistake: "Many families in your situation worry they will look back and think, was there something we missed or something that could've been done earlier? In her case, I don't think that would be true."
Empathy about critical illness in a loved one	*Making Sense of the Disease Process*: "I know it's very important to try and understand as best as possible what happened to see if we can make sense of this."
	Difficulty in Understanding Medical Information: "This is a lot of information to take in. Please feel free to ask any questions you might have."
	Physical Changes: "It must be really hard to see your loved one like this."
	Receiving Bad News: "It's hard to understand why something bad just can happen to anyone, and when it's someone you love and care for, that's even more difficult."
	Uncertainty: "We pretty much have to take it day by day, and I know that this uncertainty makes things even more challenging."
Empathy about confronting death in a loved one	*Helplessness*: "It must be so difficult facing this loss and feeling like there is nothing you can do to change things."
	Dying: "Letting go is so difficult, but I believe you're doing him a great service by honoring his wishes at this time."

Adapted from Selph RB, Shiang J, Engelberg R, Curtis JR, White DB. Empathy and life support decisions in intensive care units. J Gen Intern Med 2008;23:1311-7.

TABLE 214-2	"Ask, Tell, Ask" Approach to Discussing Difficult Communication Tasks	
Step	**Function**	**Sample Phrases**
"Ask"	Ask the patient/patient surrogate to describe his/her understanding of their medical disease and prognosis.	"It would help me to know what your other doctors have told you about your father's illness."
"Tell"	Explain to the patient/patient surrogate, using simple straightforward language, what you understand about their medical disease and prognosis.	"Unfortunately, it looks like your father's illness is getting worse. With disease as serious as his, 9 out of 10 patients will die within 1 month, and 1 out of 10 will be alive at 1 month. If your father survives this illness, it is very likely he will have significant disability and will likely be unable to live independently."
"Ask"	Assess the patient's/patient surrogate's understanding.	"I want to make sure that I explained things clearly. Can you tell me, in your own words, what I just told you about your father's illness?"

Adapted from Back AL, Arnold AM, Baile WF, Tulsky JA, Fryer-Edwards K. Approaching difficult communication tasks in oncology. CA Cancer J Clin 2005;55: 164-77.

anxiety in family members.[5] Interestingly, family meetings using this tool were somewhat longer than the usual care meetings, and the percentage of family speech was also higher.

DISCUSSING PROGNOSIS

Despite the ethical responsibility to inform patients about prognosis, many clinicians are uncomfortable doing so and identify it as one of the most difficult parts of their job.[51] Physicians in the ICU are more likely to discuss functional prognosis rather than likelihood of survival. In one study,[52] clinicians did not discuss survival prognosis in over one-third of family conferences in which the attending physician anticipated there would be discussion of withholding or withdrawing life-sustaining interventions or discussing bad news. Because patients with a poor prognosis are more likely to decline life-sustaining treatments,[53,54] discussion of prognosis is critically important. Interestingly, surrogates rely upon far more than just the prognostic information provided to them by physicians,[30] though most try to balance their own assessment of the patient with the information provided by physicians in understanding prognosis. Surrogates also report that they understand and appreciate explanations of the uncertainty involved in prognostication.[55]

Experts recommend framing prognosis numerically rather than using nonspecific terms (e.g., "1 in every 10 patients" rather than "uncommon" or "low risk"), framing prognosis both positively and negatively, and using consistent denominators when presenting rates of risk (e.g., "9 in every 10 patients with illnesses as severe as your father's will die within 1 month", and "1 in every 10 patients with illnesses as severe as your father's will be alive in 1 month").[56] Despite these recommendations, a minority of critical care physicians use numeric estimates in discussing prognosis[57] and/or verify whether or not surrogate decision makers have understood the information provided.

TABLE 214-3	VALUE Tool to Enhance Communication in the ICU
V	Value family statements
A	Acknowledge family emotions
L	Listen to the family
U	Understand the patient as a person
E	Elicit family questions

Adapted from Lautrette A, Darmon M, Megarbane B, Joly LM, Chevret S, Adrie C et al. A communication strategy and brochure for relatives of patients dying in the ICU. N Engl J Med 2007;356:469-78.

in evidence. Utilizing these skills has the potential to improve outcomes for both patients and family members. Studies suggest that planning conferences early in the ICU stay is beneficial: family conferences held within the first 72 hours of ICU stay are associated with both decreased use of critical care resources among patients who die[45] and higher family assessments of the quality of death and dying.[38] Consistent communication across the medical team is also important; having a "preconference" prior to family conferences can ensure that families are given a consistent message.[46] As discussed earlier, having a dedicated room for family conferences is also associated with decreased anxiety among family members.[12]

It should come as no surprise that empathic communication is one of the cornerstones of leading an effective family conference. Focusing on listening to concerns of family members is particularly important; most physicians spend a majority of time talking rather than listening when meeting with patients and families.[47] Families have been shown to have higher levels of satisfaction and lower levels of perceived conflict with clinicians who speak less and listen more.[5,47] Family satisfaction is associated with the use of empathic statements, though this is a commonly missed opportunity; one study found that a third of physicians in the ICU missed an opportunity to use empathic statements in family meetings.[48] Table 214-1 summarizes categories and examples of empathic statements that can be used by clinicians in family conferences. The "Ask-Tell-Ask" approach advocated by Back et al.[49] (Table 214-2) is a helpful tool to assess baseline understanding and evaluate understanding of the information provided.

Assurances to families and surrogates that patients will not be abandoned before death, that efforts will be made to provide comfort and minimize suffering, and statements of explicit support for medical decisions to either continue or withdraw life-sustaining interventions are associated with higher levels of family satisfaction.[50] Use of the VALUE mnemonic (value, acknowledge, listen, understand, and elicit—summarized in Table 214-3) to enhance clinician-family communication has been shown to improve mental health outcomes, including symptoms of depression, posttraumatic stress disorder, and

DISCUSSING RESUSCITATION

Most patients and their families have little personal experience with the critical care setting or with cardiopulmonary resuscitation (CPR). Interestingly, knowledge of the probability of survival from CPR affects patient's choices about code status.[54] Unfortunately, many people base their assumptions on the likelihood of surviving CPR on information from medical dramas on television, which dramatically over-represent favorable resuscitation outcomes.[58,59] Recent consensus guidelines have highlighted specific recommendations in discussing resuscitation with patients,[60] some of which may help guide discussions with surrogate decision makers as well. The authors recommend that, among other events, admission to a critical care unit should serve as a trigger for discussion of resuscitation preferences. Another important recommendation is that the discussion be framed to review the overall goals of care rather than merely focusing on code status. It is also important to make a distinction between life-sustaining interventions and CPR, describe cardiac arrest and care plan options (including palliative care) in detail, offer quantitative information about the patient's likelihood of surviving to hospital discharge after resuscitation, offer a code status recommendation, and focus on trust and rapport building. In summary, CPR in the critical care setting is best addressed in the context of the greater goals of care, including a candid discussion of the likelihood of CPR survival and care alternatives, including palliative and symptom-focused care.

ROLE OF THE INTERDISCIPLINARY TEAM

The complexity of critical care requires the involvement of a multidisciplinary team. However, conflicts between nurses and physicians are common,[61] particularly in the setting of end-of-life care, and are a source of significant work stress and burnout.[62-64] Enhanced nurse-physician communication and collaboration has been associated with higher patient satisfaction[65,66] and a lower incidence of anxiety and depression symptoms among families of critically ill patients,[12] as well as lower rates of burnout among nurses and physicians.[62,63] Improving communication among the multiple clinicians within the ICU—physicians, nurses, respiratory therapists, and social workers—would undoubtedly improve not only workplace relationships and stress, but also patient care and integrated communication with families and surrogate decision makers.[67]

Palliative care specialists are an increasingly common hospital resource. Involvement of a multidisciplinary palliative care team is associated with increased patient satisfaction as well as decreased rates of ICU admission following hospital discharge and significant cost savings.[68]

ROLE OF PROTOCOLS AND THE IMPORTANCE OF INDIVIDUALIZATION

Many of the communication strategies that have demonstrated efficacy were implemented using interventions designed with specific protocols. The tenets of patient-centered care affirm the importance of tailoring our communication and interactions to specific patients and their families, rather than resorting to a rote scripted dialogue. However, given the many missed opportunities in the current level of communication with patients and surrogate decision makers in the critical care setting,[69] it is certainly reasonable to look to communication approaches that have been rigorously developed and studied. Specific guidelines relating to communication techniques and strategies are intended as a starting point, and clinicians are encouraged to integrate these with their own personal approach and authentic voice.

CULTURAL COMPETENCE

Cultural considerations are fundamental in talking with families and surrogate decision makers from diverse backgrounds. Utilizing language interpreters and cultural mediators is critical in facilitating

TABLE 214-4	Questions to Improve Cultural Understanding of Illness
Domains	**Questions**
Preface	"The kinds of care we provide and the way we talk to patients may be different here than in the country you came from. I want to provide you the best possible care, so it would help me if I understood more about your culture."
Acculturation	"What language do you speak at home?" "In what language do you watch television or read the newspaper?" "Were you born in the United States?" If no, ask, "At what age did you come to the United States?" and "How long have you lived in the United States?"
Culture/ country of origin	"Can you tell me what I need to know about your culture?" "What do you think is the cause of this illness?" "How would this illness be treated in your culture?"

Adapted from Smith AK, Sudore RL, Perez-Stable EJ. Palliative care for Latino patients and their families: whenever we prayed, she wept. JAMA 2009;301:1047-57, E1.

communication with patients and families who speak different primary languages than clinicians. In an ideal setting, the role of an interpreter transcends mere strict literal translation. Interpreters can assume the role of a cultural mediator, helping to interpret content bi-directionally. Even with the best cultural mediators, however, there are significant challenges inherent when language discordance exists. Interpretation of family conferences is a difficult process which can include critical errors, and it is difficult to provide emotional support for families in this circumstance.[70,71] Implementing best practices such as a preparatory meeting with interpreters prior to the clinical encounter, speaking slowly, confirming the patient's or family's understanding, and debriefing with the interpreter after the clinical encounter can facilitate better communication and decrease potential for misunderstandings.[72-73] Table 214-4 details some specific questions clinicians can ask of families to better elucidate cultural considerations that may be shaping understanding and attitudes toward care.[74]

SPIRITUAL ISSUES

Spiritual needs figure prominently for many critically ill patients and their families, often explicitly or tacitly shaping decision making about medical care.[75] Increased family satisfaction has been associated with assessment of spiritual needs.[14] Exploring underlying spiritual beliefs and values can be extremely important in supporting families and toward finding common ground on medical decisions through shared decision making. In addressing spiritual concerns, clinicians should use caution in not stepping beyond one's role as a clinician or trying to resolve existential and spiritual questions[75]; rather, the focus should be on assessing potential spiritual needs, then making referrals for spiritual care specialists as indicated. The FICA mnemonic (Table 214-5) gives clinicians a framework for assessing spiritual needs.[76]

Summary

Conferences with families of critically ill patients are crucial and are one of the more formidable clinical challenges faced by critical care physicians. Many approaches to medical decision making exist, and there is significant variability among patients and patient surrogates regarding their preferred role. There is consensus that shared decision

TABLE 214-5	FICA Mnemonic for Elaborating Spiritual Needs
F	*Faith* and beliefs
I	*Importance* of spirituality in the patient's life
C	Spiritual *Community* of support
A	How does the patient wish spiritual issues to be *Addressed* in his or her care?

From Puchalski CM. Spirituality and end-of-life care: a time for listening and caring. J Palliat Med 2002;5:289-94.

making should be the preferred approach of clinicians, though care must be taken to assess the family's desired role in medical decision making and individualize one's approach accordingly. Having a critically ill family member and functioning as surrogate decision maker is incredibly challenging for families, but stress associated with this situation can be mitigated through integrated, thoughtful, and empathic communication by physicians and other members of the critical care team.

ANNOTATED REFERENCES

Lautrette A, Darmon M, Megarbane B, Joly LM, Chevret S, Adrie C, et al. A communication strategy and brochure for relatives of patients dying in the ICU. N Engl J Med 2007;356:469-78.
This study demonstrated that a proactive communication strategy including longer conferences and higher percentage of family speech and a brochure on bereavement significantly lessened the rate of complicated grief among family members of patients who died in the ICU.

Gerstel E, Engelberg RA, Koepsell T, Curtis JR. Duration of withdrawal of life support in the intensive care unit and association with family satisfaction. Am J Respir Crit Care Med 2008;178:798-804.
This study demonstrated that, particularly among families of patients with long ICU stays, increased duration of withdrawal of life-sustaining measures was associated with increased family satisfaction.

Curtis JR, White DB. Practical guidance for evidence-based ICU family conferences. Chest 2008; 134:835-43.

Evidence-based review offering pragmatic suggestions for leading effective family conferences.

Shalowitz DI, Garrett-Mayer E, Wendler D. The accuracy of surrogate decision makers: a systematic review. Arch Intern Med 2006;166:493-7.
A systematic review evaluating the accuracy of surrogate decision makers in predicting the wishes of their family members.

McDonagh JR, Elliott TB, Engelberg RA, Treece PD, Shannon SE, Rubenfeld GD, et al. Family satisfaction with family conferences about end-of-life care in the intensive care unit: increased proportion of family speech is associated with increased satisfaction. Crit Care Med 2004;32:1484-8.
A cross-sectional observational study demonstrating that increased family speech is associated with improvements in family satisfaction.

REFERENCES

Access the complete reference list online at http://www.expertconsult.com.

215 Resource Allocation in the Intensive Care Unit

GORDON D. RUBENFELD

Two truisms of economics are that the supply of goods and services is finite and that the supply will be insufficient to meet all demands. The tension between supply and demand for food, water, energy, education, and other goods and services creates economies. All societies must determine how goods and services will be allocated to individuals. Although the term *rationing* connotes a specific process of allocation during circumstances of severe resource limitation (rationing coupons to allocate gasoline during World War II, for example, or one's daily ration of water on a life raft), rationing is just an emotionally laden synonym for *resource allocation*. In this chapter, the terms are used interchangeably.

Market-based economies allocate many resources on the basis of ability to pay, but other strategies exist (Table 215-1).[1] In developed nations, some goods and services—for example, health care and education—are treated differently from luxury goods and are allocated by society using criteria other than an individual's ability to pay. Regardless of the strategy ultimately used, decisions to allocate medical resources are fundamentally identical to decisions to allocate other resources. Because medical resources are finite, it is impossible to provide every effective treatment in every case in which it might offer benefit and the patient desires the care. This does not mean that clinicians are aware on a daily basis of the burden of this reality. Sometimes the decisions are explicit, with immediate repercussions—for example, the selection of one patient to receive a heart transplant when several might benefit from the sole available organ, or the decision to admit one patient to the last intensive care unit (ICU) bed when several critically ill patients could benefit from ICU admission. More frequently, the decisions are subtle and occur even when the supply of therapy is not absolutely limited—for example, the decision to use cheaper antibiotics, sedatives, imaging modalities, or operative procedures when more expensive options might be beneficial. Finally, allocation decisions can be completely implicit and almost hidden. For example, the decision to build an ambulatory care clinic instead of adding ICU beds has profound implications for the delivery of critical care services, but individual clinicians are largely unaware of this relationship.

Although common and necessary, allocation decisions are stigmatized in medicine. Such decisions bring two major ethical principles into conflict: the principle of beneficence guides clinicians to act solely in their patients' best interests, while the principle of justice directs clinicians to act fairly.[2] This conflict may explain why euphemisms are frequently used to describe decisions that essentially involve the rationing of resources. For example, "triage," "optimization," "prioritization," "cost-effective care," and "basic health care" all indicate some form of allocation decision.[3,4] The purpose of this chapter is to explore these decisions in their many guises as they occur in critical care and to offer some guidance to clinicians in constructing processes for allocating resources in their ICU.

Allocation Versus Evidence-Based Medicine

Decisions based solely on evidence of the efficacy of medical care are *not* rationing decisions. There is no medical obligation to provide and no societal obligation to pay for care that is harmful or ineffective. In fact, clinicians use special terms to describe interventions that fall into these categories, including "futile," "not standard of care," "medically inappropriate," "wasteful," or "experimental."[5,6] For example, an intensivist who decides not to transfuse a critically ill patient with a hematocrit of 27 is *not* rationing blood, even though blood is an expensive and limited resource; in this case, there is evidence that a transfusion would be of no benefit and might even be harmful.[7] Likewise, the decision not to use human growth hormone, an expensive medication, in a chronically critically ill patient is not a rationing decision, because this treatment has been shown to be ineffective and may be harmful.[8]

Unfortunately, assessments of benefit and harm are not as straightforward as the terms would suggest, and the line between effective, ineffective, and experimental treatment often is a personal decision for the individual clinician. Decision science has taught us that medical decision making is a complex process that frequently obscures the true rationale for the choice.[9] In fact, judgments allegedly based solely on objective evidence of safety and benefit often incorporate a variety of subjective values and biases.[10] These may include the value the clinician assigns to being wrong; the value assigned to trying to "rescue" a patient in imminent danger of death; the clinician's tolerance for uncertainty; the impact of the decision on the clinician's finances; biases about the patient's race, gender, functional status, or age; and the cost or availability of the resource.[11] The transition from statements that summarize the evidence of benefit to recommendations that incorporate cost and other values is often very subtle. For example, the authors of a recent systematic review of colloid resuscitation in critical care conclude that "there is no evidence from randomized controlled trials that resuscitation with colloids reduces the risk of death compared to crystalloids in patients with trauma, burns and following surgery."[12] This is a statement of their summary of the evidence of efficacy of colloid therapy. Like many treatments in critical care, the evidence neither supports nor completely refutes the use of colloids as resuscitation fluids in the critically ill. However, the authors conclude, "As colloids are not associated with an improvement in survival, and as they are more expensive than crystalloids, it is hard to see how their continued use in these patient types can be justified outside the context of randomized controlled trials." Whereas the first statement may be a fair summary of the evidence, the recommendation against using colloids in the second sentence is not based solely on the evidence. It incorporates an implicit rationing strategy that pays only for treatments that have demonstrated benefit in a certain way. Although one might conclude from the authors' review that colloid resuscitation is experimental or that its benefit is likely to be small, the reasoning for recommending against its use is based on the cost of the treatment. Presumably, if colloid fluids were the same price as crystalloids, the authors might reach different conclusions, even though the cost does not change the evidence of efficacy.

The preceding example shows how assessments of cost can creep into recommendations for therapy even without a formal discussion of allocation. Because clinicians and payers may be reluctant to admit they are incorporating cost or availability into the rationale for a decision, they may find decisions based on futility or appropriateness less ethically problematic than those based on rationing. In fact, these judgments may implicitly contain assessments of cost by incorporating cost into the definition. When is there sufficient evidence to move a

TABLE 215-1	Strategies for Allocating Resources
Principle	**Definition**
Autocracy	To each according to the will of one
Democracy	To each according to the will of the majority
Equality	To each according to an equal share
Lottery	To each according to an equal chance
Capitalism	To each according to their ability to buy
Personal worth	To each according to their contribution to the community
Utilitarianism	To each so that the utility of the community is maximized

treatment or diagnostic device from experimental care to standard care? When is there sufficient evidence, absent evidence of outright harm, that a treatment is ineffective as opposed to not yet of proven efficacy? These decisions are frequently made by consensus bodies using subjective or poorly characterized criteria. The evidence threshold tends to be higher for treatments that are risky or expensive or for which there is no alternative. Conversely, the threshold for accepting a treatment as "standard" is lower if that treatment is inexpensive and safe and offers the potential of rescuing a patient in imminent danger of dying. For example, consider the decision to elevate the head of the bed of mechanically ventilated patients to prevent ventilator-associated pneumonia. This is an inexpensive and safe treatment to offer patients. It might take less evidence to convince clinicians to use this treatment than to use kinetic beds or topical prophylactic antibiotics, which are more expensive and may raise safety issues. Therefore, the cost of an intervention may be incorporated into the assessment of whether it is a standard of care.

These judgments are further complicated by the motivation of the decision maker. It would be difficult for an insurance company that is assessing whether a specific therapy is experimental or standard of care to be unbiased, because its decision will affect its profits. Alternatively, surgeons who developed a procedure may be committed to its benefits in a way that compromises an objective evaluation. The complexity of the assessment of efficacy and cost highlights the importance of making allocation decisions as objective, explicit, and public as possible. Because medical decisions are so complex, and because decisions in the ICU are further complicated by their immediacy and the severity of patients' illnesses, it is essential that clinicians understand their own motivations and the evidence supporting their decisions and have a process in place for allocating resources.

Allocation Strategies

Allocation decisions are usually separated into *macro-allocation decisions* (involving groups of people and usually made at a managerial or health policy level) and *micro-allocation decisions* (made at the bedside and involving specific cases). A hospital's decision not to hire additional ICU nurses is a macro-allocation decision; a nurse-manager's decision to allocate a specific patient to share a nurse in the ICU rather than to receive 1:1 nursing is a micro-allocation decision. This chapter is concerned primarily with bedside, or micro-allocation, decisions that clinicians make on a routine basis. There is an important interaction between micro- and macro-allocation decisions, because macro-allocation decisions ultimately affect individuals, and macro-allocation regulations are an effective rationing strategy (Table 215-2). There are a number of approaches to allocating resources (see Table 215-1). Although they are all feasible, they are not all equally ethical.

The principles of equality, fairness, justice, and due process make some strategies less acceptable. The principle of utilitarianism directs resource allocation to maximize the "utility" or benefit to the greatest number of people for any given amount of resources. To the extent that utility can be determined by measuring patient outcomes such as health-related quality of life, and to the extent that we can theoretically estimate the effects of medical treatments on utility, we can calculate exactly which set of medical treatments to pay for to maximize the

benefit to the population. These studies are called *cost-effectiveness analyses* and are the quantitative embodiment of utilitarianism.

Allocating medical resources through cost-effectiveness analysis has important limitations. First, medical cost-effectiveness analysis cannot tell how much money to allocate to medical care as opposed to other goods and services; it can only determine how to maximize health outcomes for a selected outlay of resources. Second, cost-effectiveness analysis may not fully account for some factors society values. For example, cost-effectiveness analysis routinely treats all human lives as equally valuable; however, society often places a high value on saving identifiable lives in imminent danger of death, and it may not value additional years of life in the elderly as highly as additional years of life in the young.[13] Cost-effectiveness and other utility-based allocation strategies fail to account for the value society places on rescuing lives in imminent peril—a not uncommon occurrence in the ICU.[14] Standard economic analyses may not value equal distribution as much as optimal distribution and, to this end, may discriminate in settings society finds unacceptable.[15] Finally, cost-effectiveness analysis is a mathematical technique that generates comparative outcomes for populations of patients. It is meaningless to speak of a treatment as being "cost-effective" for an individual.

The primary value of cost-effectiveness analysis as an allocation tool is the ability to *compare* various strategies.[16] For example, one can compare the cost-effectiveness of captopril versus no captopril in survivors of myocardial infarction with the use of fluoxetine versus imipramine for major depression to decide whether to use captopril, fluoxetine, both, or neither. Cost-effectiveness analysis provides a ruler, in terms of dollars per life-year or dollars per quality-adjusted life-year (QALY), that allows different treatments for different diseases to be compared. The crucial data that must be available to make these comparisons is information on the treatments' effects on survival or health-related quality of life. Unfortunately, in critical care, the number of

TABLE 215-2	Allocation Decisions at Different Levels	
Decision Maker	**Decision**	**Rationale**
Nonallocation Decision		
Physician	Not to use human growth hormone in chronically critically ill patients	Evidence of harm in critically ill patients
President of insurance company	Not to offer routine chest computed tomography screening for lung cancer	Lack of sufficient evidence of benefit
Healthcare official	Not to offer basic medical coverage to all people in the country	Endorses goals other than equal access to health care—for example, the importance of choice or the value of free market
Macro-allocation Decision		
Physician	Not to admit routine post–coronary artery bypass patients to ICU	Limited ICU beds better used for patients with more severe illness
President of insurance company	Not to increase reimbursement for septic shock when new, expensive drug is approved	Hopes to limit cost of care for patients to increase profitability of insurance company
Healthcare official	To capitate reimbursement for hospital care	By providing single fee for all care, hopes to limit costs so increased outpatient services can be provided
Micro-allocation Decision		
Physician	Not to admit a debilitated, elderly man with urosepsis to the ICU, despite a request by the patient's primary care physician	The patient is moribund, and the intensivist believes the ICU's resources can be used to better effect on other patients.
President of insurance company	Denial of claim to pay for prostacyclin infusion for pulmonary hypertension	Treatment specifically not covered by contractual arrangement with insured patient
Healthcare official	Not applicable	Not applicable

treatments shown to improve survival or health-related quality of life is small. Although we have data on strategies to reduce gastrointestinal bleeding, duration of mechanical ventilation, and catheter-related infections, none of these interventions has been shown to affect QALYs.[17-19] Therefore, the cost-effectiveness analyses for these interventions are expressed as, for example, dollars per gastrointestinal bleed prevented.[20] These ratios cannot be used to compare a treatment to prevent gastrointestinal bleeding with a treatment for myocardial infarction, because the latter is expressed in dollars per QALY. Cost-effectiveness analyses with non-QALY denominators can be helpful in bedside rationing decisions when the intervention is shown to be equally or more effective and *reduces cost*. For example, special beds in the ICU both prevent decubitus ulcers and reduce the overall cost of care, even when the cost of the bed is factored in. Therefore, the cost-effectiveness ratio (expressed in dollars per decubitus ulcer prevented) is a negative number.[21]

Illusory Cost Savings

Since the earliest days of intensive care, technologic, workforce, and organizational innovations have been proposed as opportunities to reduce the exorbitant cost of critical care. In 1973, an optimistic author wrote, "[the] more promising approaches to cost reduction are all in an early stage of development now. Both deprofessionalization of the ICU by wider use of allied health personnel, and the automation of therapeutic functions are just beginning to be applied."[22] Despite the implementation of both these measures, there is little evidence that cost increases in hospital or ICU care have been curbed by technologic innovation. In fact, the opposite has occurred. This is not surprising, because technologic innovation in other areas of health care, though often associated with better outcomes, is rarely a source of cost savings.

Cost analyses are problematic in medical care, and critical investigators must be able to identify cost savings that are real and that will appear in their budgets from savings in indirect costs that will be accrued elsewhere.[23] There are several common but problematic arguments about cost reduction in critical care: (1) that reduced ICU length of stay will reduce the cost of care in the ICU, (2) that ordering fewer tests will reduce the cost of care in the ICU, and (3) that fewer admissions of futile-care patients will save money. It is important to recognize that not all calculated cost savings will be realized at the ICU or hospital level.

ICU costs are frequently inferred from length of stay. For example, in a cost-effectiveness analysis of antibiotic-coated catheters, the authors assigned a cost of $9738 to a catheter-related bloodstream infection.[24] Epidemiologic studies show that patients with catheter-related infections spend more time in the hospital, even after controlling for severity of illness.[25] The cost of a catheter-related infection is, in part, derived by simply multiplying the estimated number of extra days spent in the hospital by the cost (based on hospital charges) of a day in the ICU or ward. In fact, we do not really know whether using antibiotic-coated catheters shortens ICU length of stay, because the randomized trials demonstrating that they prevent infection were not sufficiently powered or did not show a reduction in mortality or length of stay.[19] Even if antibiotic-coated catheters do reduce length of stay, money "saved" by reducing length of stay is a different kind of money from that used to buy the catheters. By reducing length of stay, the ICU will be able to care for more patients, but they will be sicker and more expensive patients.

Identifying treatments for specific conditions in the ICU that reduce overall costs, even if they have no effect on QALYs, is extremely useful to the intensivist who must allocate resources. Implementing economically dominant strategies is an easy allocation decision, because they reduce costs but do not worsen patient outcomes. However, predicting the actual effect of any decision on actual costs in an ICU or hospital is complex because each hospital performs cost accounting and budgeting in idiosyncratic ways.

The effect of different payer mixes, contracts for nursing and respiratory therapist labor, allocation of indirect costs, and whether the ICU budget is fixed or grows with the number of patients served all influence whether allocation decisions accrue savings that can be appreciated at the ICU level. For example, the drug acquisition costs of once-daily medications are frequently higher than the costs of medications given more frequently. However, there are labor costs associated with administering medication more frequently that may offset the costs of the once-daily medication. Unfortunately, unless changing to once-daily medication reduces the workload to the point where it is feasible to actually reduce the number of nurses, there will be little realized savings. This is because labor costs are not infinitely scaleable. Even if there is 15% less work to do, it may not be possible to hire 15% fewer nursing hours. Patients who need 1:1 nursing care will continue to need this level of care regardless of whether the nurses are administering once-daily medication or not. It may be that changing medication routines improves care by using nursing time more efficiently, but this may not be reflected in a cost reduction. A reasonable criterion to consider for a proposed cost-saving intervention is whether it will reduce the number of staff that need to be hired or whether it can reduce acquisition costs for equipment or medications. If it will not, then cost savings are not likely to be realized in the ICU.

The cost estimate used in many cost-effectiveness analyses assumes that every day in the ICU costs the same. This is certainly true for what the hospital charges, but it is not true in reality. The first few days in the hospital and ICU are generally far more expensive than the last days.[26] Patients are more likely to require active interventions and closer nursing care in the early days in the ICU. Clearly, interventions that reduce ICU length of stay cannot reduce early days in the ICU; they simply eliminate later lower-cost days. This is rarely accounted for in cost analyses. This was validated at the national level as U.S. healthcare costs peaked during a period when hospital inpatient days declined by 40%.[27] Therefore, standard cost analyses overestimate cost savings likely to be realized by reducing length of stay.

Reducing test ordering in the ICU has been offered as a technique for cost reduction. This too is a perfectly reasonable option on clinical grounds. Overtesting yields increased false-positive results, which may lead to clinical complications in search of diseases that never existed. However, the actual cost reduction at the ICU level achieved by limiting test ordering is likely to be overestimated in a simple charge-based analysis. The actual marginal cost of performing the 101st arterial blood gas once the analyzer has been purchased and the technician has been paid to perform 100 arterial blood gases is minimal. If reductions in test ordering are of sufficient magnitude to staff the laboratory with fewer people or to forgo purchasing new equipment, significant cost reductions can be realized. In fact, depending on how indirect costs in the hospital are allocated, it is possible a reduction in test ordering will place the clinical laboratory under considerable budgetary constraints. Fewer tests may reduce the amount of money the laboratory director receives to cover staff costs, which may not decrease in the same proportion as test ordering.

Patients may be admitted to the ICU even when they have a negligible chance of survival. It seems reasonable to assume that if these patients receive care outside the ICU, resources that would have been expended without benefit in the ICU will be saved. On its face, this appears to be the sort of painless cost saving intensivists should look for. Unfortunately, a careful analysis of potential savings from limiting care at the end of life shows that such care accounts for a relatively small amount of overall healthcare spending, that implementing these strategies may worsen overall health outcomes by affecting the care nonterminal patients receive, and that care would have to be withheld from young patients (some of whom would have had prolonged survival) to achieve any savings.[28]

Strategies for Bedside Allocation of Resources in the Intensive Care Unit

Ultimately, allocation decisions occur at the bedside in the ICU. A number of studies demonstrate that under settings of restricted access to ICU beds, physicians allocate these beds on the basis of severity of illness. In these situations, the average severity of illness in the ICU increases, as it does on the hospital ward.[29] Unfortunately, these decisions are also driven by arbitrary factors including patient age and gender, reimbursement, and physician power in the institution.[30] It is important that clinicians plan in advance for such difficult decisions so their deliberations are explicit, open, and guided by principles rather than ad hoc case-by-case decisions.

CASE 1: ADMISSION AND DISCHARGE CRITERIA

The Last ICU Bed

An intensivist is responsible for an eight-bed mixed medical-surgical ICU in a large community hospital that is currently near capacity. Within minutes, she receives two calls: one from the emergency room, where a 17-year-old has been admitted with severe diabetic ketoacidosis and altered mental status, but who is not intubated; and one from a hospital resident who has an 83-year-old severely demented patient on the ward who has developed acute respiratory failure and will soon require mechanical ventilation. There is only one open ICU bed, and none of the existing patients can be moved.

Perhaps the most difficult decision an ICU physician faces is the allocation of the ICU itself.[31] Although this is a wrenching decision and has generated a literature devoted to triaging the last ICU bed, there is little evidence to indicate how frequently this occurs in actual practice. Mobile technology, flexible nursing staffing, and the availability of postanesthesia, emergency room, and step-down beds may make the ritual of allocating the last ICU bed more a theoretical concern than an actual one. Deciding who gets the last ICU bed is particularly difficult because identifiable patients are affected by an explicit decision. The decision is further complicated by the almost complete lack of data on the actual benefit of ICU care in specific conditions compared with care on the ward. Few question that ICU outcomes are superior, but the relative benefit of ICU care and monitoring in specific conditions is completely unknown. Finally, the decisions must be made rapidly. Although a transplant committee also allocates a fixed resource—organs for transplantation—it can deliberate for weeks to prioritize recipients. The intensivist must allocate an ICU bed within minutes or hours.

The two most important steps in allocating the last ICU bed are to prevent the situation from occurring in the first place and to develop guidelines for managing the problem when it does occur. Strategies to prevent the last ICU bed phenomenon include staffing sufficiently for the anticipated volume of elective surgery, or stopping planned surgery if sufficient ICU beds are not available. It includes arranging flexible nursing and monitoring options to care for critically ill patients in other environments that are not physically located in the ICU. Individual clinician biases and training can have a strong effect on the perception of the value of various life-sustaining treatments in the ICU.[32] To minimize the effect of these influences and maintain fair and equitable access to intensive care services, admission and discharge criteria should be public, explicit, evidence based, and fair. Public and explicit criteria allow all clinicians in the hospital to be aware of the policy. To the extent possible, decisions should be evidence based or, in the absence of evidence, should appeal to national policy statements or local consensus.[33]

Resolution. The intensivist went to the emergency room, evaluated the patient with diabetic ketoacidosis, placed arterial and central venous catheters, and arranged to have a nurse from the ICU float to the emergency department during the night to care for the patient there. The patient with acute respiratory failure from the floor was intubated and admitted to the ICU's last bed.

CASE 2: TECHNOLOGY PURCHASE

Bedside Laboratory Testing

An intensivist is considering purchasing a point-of-care testing system to allow him to do arterial blood gases as well as certain chemistries

and coagulation tests at the ICU bedside. The salesperson has data showing that the cost of performing the tests at the bedside is 40% less than the hospital laboratory charges, saving money for the patient and potentially making money for the ICU. Further, the salesperson presents data that the rapid turnaround of bedside testing leads to faster clinical decisions and a 1-day reduction in ICU stay. The reduction in length of stay, argues the salesperson, pays for the cost of the testing system in 18 months.

Arguments that better technology will ultimately lead to cost reductions have been promulgated since the beginning of intensive care.[22] When a purchase is being made primarily because it will save money or, at worst, be cost-neutral, there are two important considerations for the intensivist: Does the cost saving involve shifting fixed costs? To what extent does the cost analysis rely on savings from reduced nursing time or fewer ICU days? As noted previously, calculations that fail to take into account the proper cost perspective, rely on shifting fixed costs, and/or rely on reduced labor time or ICU days to demonstrate cost savings may overestimate actual cost savings.

None of the preceding discussion relates to the potential benefits of new technology. If clinicians believe the evidence supports better patient outcomes from the technology and that it merits implementation regardless of economic consequences, this is not a resource allocation decision. However, technologic innovation is rarely cheap, and the medical industry usually tries to persuade clinicians that the novel technology is not only better but also saves money.

Resolution. The intensivist met with the director of the clinical laboratory. At this hospital, the laboratory's budget is directly tied to the volume of tests performed. If the ICU started to perform its own tests, the clinical laboratory would not be able to continue to provide its services. The ICU and laboratory directors instituted a quality-improvement intervention to decrease stat lab turnaround time with existing technology.

When a clinical laboratory charges $100 to perform an arterial blood gas, this is not because the reagents, analyzer rental, and 7 minutes of technician time to perform the test cost $100. Most of the costs reflected by this charge involve the fixed costs of maintaining a 24-hour-a-day, 7-day-a-week laboratory, including quality controls, managerial costs, government reporting, and the laboratory's portion of janitorial and other services in the hospital. If the ICU switches to a point-of-care system and reduces the number of laboratory tests by 30%, none of these fixed costs will disappear. Unless the reduction in testing is so significant that the laboratory director can reduce the numbers of technicians or sell some machinery, the overall costs of running the laboratory will not be affected by the ICU's switch to point-of-care testing. If these fixed cost savings cannot be realized, the laboratory director must still meet the budget demands of the laboratory in the face of reduced testing. The point-of-care approach appears to be less expensive because the fixed costs of maintaining an entire laboratory are not bundled into the purchase of the testing device, not because the tests themselves are fundamentally less expensive.

🖥 Conclusion

Allocation of resources in medicine is an unavoidable process. Clinicians do have control over whether these decisions are implicit or explicit, whether they are made after open discourse or with no discussion, and whether the decisions are informed by the available literature. Clinicians in the ICU may in fact face fewer implicit allocation decisions than their colleagues in other areas because of the imminent risk of death in the ICU and the value society places on protecting those lives. In fact, there is relatively little empirical evidence of how often intensive care services are allocated. The effect of different interventions on actual costs varies depending on local factors such as reimbursement and indirect cost allocation. Allocating ICU beds is the most challenging allocation decision most intensivists will face. The best time to handle these situations is before they occur. Public, explicit triage and discharge criteria that are developed in collaboration with

ICU users (emergency department, surgery, oncology) well in advance of the actual decisions are essential for fair and efficient use of intensive care resources.

KEY POINTS

1. Allocation of resources is synonymous with rationing and is an inevitable part of medical practice.

2. Clinicians often use a variety of euphemisms—triage, optimization, prioritization, and cost-effective care—to obscure what are essentially allocation decisions.

3. Clinical decisions based solely on evidence of risk, benefit, or patient utility are not rationing decisions because they do not incorporate cost or availability.

4. Clinicians may implicitly incorporate cost or availability into their judgments of the evidence of risk or benefit in an attempt to avoid an explicit decision incorporating cost.

5. Allocation can occur at the macro level, where decisions affect populations of patients, or at the micro level, where decisions affect individual identifiable patients.

6. Cost-effectiveness analysis is a quantitative methodology that applies a utilitarian approach to allocate resources to maximize the benefit to a population for any specified cost.

7. Cost is difficult to measure in complex endeavors such as providing medical care.

8. Claims of the ability to reduce costs by reducing length of stay, ordering fewer tests, or failing to admit patients who will likely die should be examined critically.

ANNOTATED REFERENCES

Adhikari NJ, Fowler RA, Bhagwanjee S, Rubenfeld GD. Critical care and the global burden of critical illness in adults. Lancet 2010;376:1339-46.
An attempt to estimate the global burden of critical illness. While critical care and critical illness are generally seen as problems of developed nations, this paper focuses on the global burden of critical illness. In addition to focusing some limited data on this issue and raising important questions for future research, this paper challenges developed countries to identify less expensive and efficient critical care techniques to disseminate in challenging areas.

Luce JM, Rubenfeld GD. Can health care costs be reduced by limiting intensive care at the end of life? Am J Respir Crit Care Med 2002;165:750-4.
Challenges the notion that significant reductions in ICU costs can be achieved by limiting intensive care at the end of life. The authors argue that while there are many very good ethical and medical reasons not to continue care for patients in the ICU when their prognosis is grim, the cost savings from these decisions are not likely to be enormous.

White DB, Katz MH, Luce JM, Lo B. Who should receive life support during a public health emergency? Using ethical principles to improve allocation decisions. Ann Intern Med 2009;150:132-8.

Recent experience with H1N1 and natural disasters have led to a growth in "pandethics" publications that focus on the ethical challenges that occur when critical illness demands acutely exceed available resources. This paper and similar ones provide an ethical framework for decision making in these challenging scenarios. The clinical value of such ethical frameworks in assisting clinicians faced with making these decisions is largely untested.

Mehlman MJ. The legal implications of health care cost containment. A symposium: health care cost containment and medical technology: a critique of waste theory. Case West Reserve Law Rev 1986;36:778-877.
A leading medical philosopher argues persuasively that a single approach to critical care bioethics that spans all countries, economic conditions, and cultures is essentially impossible. He argues that the major bioethical challenges of our time, including resource allocation in critical care, are not amenable to a global philosophical solution and that different standards of care are inevitable.

Engelhardt HT Jr. Critical care: why there is no global bioethics. Curr Opin Crit Care 2005;11:605-9.
A leading medical philosopher argues persuasively that a single approach to critical care bioethics that spans all countries, economic conditions, and cultures is essentially impossible. He argues that the major bioethical challenges of our time, including resource allocation in critical care, are not amenable to a global philosophical solution and that different standards of care are inevitable.

REFERENCES

Access the complete reference list online at http://www.expertconsult.com.

216

Basic Ethical Principles in Critical Care

THOMAS A. BLEDSOE | MITCHELL M. LEVY

Foundations of Ethics in Critical Care

Ethics in critical care is based on four fundamental principles: (1) beneficence, or the physician's obligation to do good for patients; (2) nonmaleficence, or the duty to avoid harm; (3) autonomy, or respect for a patient's right to self-determination; and (4) justice, or the fair allocation of healthcare resources. The first three principles form the basis of the physician-patient relationship and provide the ethical imperative for physicians to act in the best interests of their patients. The relative importance of these three principles differs from country to country, but physicians' responsibility to their patients is common to all cultures.

Goals of Care and Medical Decision Making

SURROGATE DECISION MAKING

Modern medicine has embraced the concept of shared decision making between patients and their physicians based on the principle of autonomy.[1,2] This approach is often more complicated in the intensive care unit (ICU), because patients are frequently too ill or otherwise impaired to make meaningful contributions to decisions about their care. Increasingly, decisions are made in the ICU to withdraw care,[3] and conflicts are common between physicians' practices and patients' wishes.[4] In the ICU, as in other medical situations, patients have an ethical (and in many places, a legal) right to determine the goals of their medical care. An individual patient's wishes regarding future care in the case of his or her incapacity may be made known in advance of a serious medical illness. The process by which patients, with or without the assistance and participation of their physicians, family members, or other close personal relations, plan for future medical care is called *advance care planning*.[5] In general, the results of these deliberations are known as *advance directives*; defined broadly, they may be verbal or written and may be quite specific or very general. In this process, the patient determines what kind of care he or she would want in the setting of some hypothetical (or anticipated) situation and makes known his or her wishes regarding future medical care. The advance directive helps direct medical care in case of the patient's incapacity and comes into play only if the patient is unable to make his or her current wishes known.[6] For example, a patient who awakens after a surgical procedure and is deemed competent (see later) is asked outright about his or her wishes, and the advance directive is no longer necessary.

Advance directives have ethical authority in whatever form (including verbal), as long as the directive was promulgated within the requirements of informed consent (see later). Unfortunately, the reliability of a specific advance directive as "authentic representations of autonomous patient choices" is often suspect.[7] Advance directives specific enough to guide day-to-day clinical decision making in the ICU are rare; more commonly, the ICU physician is left to work with a surrogate to make decisions for a patient who is too sick to participate in decisions.

For medical decisions in which patient factors play a large role, the physician must have a surrogate decision maker with whom to discuss goals of care and treatment options. There are two questions that must be answered: Who may and should act as surrogate? How should the surrogate make decisions for the ill patient?

In some cultures, physicians often turn to the "next of kin" for surrogate decision making. However, the legal status of surrogates varies from country to country, and this individual may have no legal or ethical grounds for assuming this role. Even in cultures in which surrogate decision making is valued, there is often no designated hierarchy of surrogates. In those cultures in which such a hierarchy has been determined by law, a typical sequence might be (1) spouse, (2) eldest child, (3) next child, (4) parent, (5) sibling. In addition to legal standing, the surrogate should have some moral standing to act as such. For example, a surrogate specifically named in an advance directive document or verbally designated by the patient as the preferred surrogate would have this standing. In fact, some would argue that this is the single most important question for a patient who is sick enough to warrant ICU care ("If you become too sick to speak for yourself, who would you want to make medical decisions for you?").[8] In surveys about advance directives and surrogates, patients and well individuals typically name their spouses or other immediate family members as their preferred surrogates. These individuals frequently (though not always) have a shared value system. Interestingly, when asked whether they would prefer that their advance directives be followed no matter what or that their care be discussed with their chosen surrogate, a majority of patients would cede authority to the surrogate.[9]

In many cultures, surrogate decision making is not considered acceptable. Even in this paternalistic approach, it is incumbent on the physician to collect information from those who know the patient well in an attempt to collectively determine what this patient would prefer in terms of medical care and then balance that information with the physician's judgment as to the best course of therapy. This shared decision-making model is now viewed as the most appropriate in many cultures, including North America and Europe.

In the United States, advance directives allow patients to make their wishes for future care known, either formally or informally. These directives may also designate a specific surrogate decision maker who then has ethical and possibly legal standing (if the appropriate statutory document is properly executed) to make medical decisions for the patient. In the absence of advance directives, the legally appointed surrogate—or, in the absence of such a surrogate, those who know the patient well—make decisions for the patient using substituted judgment based on their knowledge of the patient. When no specific information is available about a patient, the decision makers apply a "reasonable-person" standard—that is, what a reasonable person would prefer in the clinical situation at hand—and sometimes resort to a "best-interest" standard.

ADVANCE DIRECTIVES

As noted, in the United States, advance directives are formal or informal instructions to healthcare providers, family members, or others involved in a patient's care regarding treatment that may be required while the patient is unable to participate in medical decision making. The earliest form of advance directive was the "living will." Classically, the living will is restricted in terms of both scope and applicability. Living wills are usually reserved for patients with terminal illnesses and are typically restricted to statements about forgoing medical treatments that would "only prolong my dying"; they typically make explicit statements about the acceptability of discontinuing intravenous fluids and artificial nutrition if death is imminent and there is no significant hope for recovery. They usually do not provide instructions in case of nonterminal illness and typically do not name a surrogate. A more generally useful legal document is one that gives statutory authority to an individual to make medical decisions for a patient in case of incapacity. This document is sometimes referred to as a *durable power of attorney for health care*. Similar to a durable power of attorney that provides legal decision-making authority for financial and other matters in case of incapacity, this document provides legal standing to a named surrogate with regard to healthcare decisions. These documents typically provide an opportunity for an individual to give general information about healthcare preferences in a variety of situations. Some also provide an opportunity for the person to make a statement about quality of life and the kind of life that would and would not be worth living. Preferences for organ donation, wishes for spiritual care, and even funeral arrangements are sometimes included.

Additionally, a number of advisory documents have been developed, including "values histories" and the medical directive developed by Linda and Ezekiel Emanuel.[10] These documents may present a series of increasingly dire scenarios and ask about overall preferences ("do everything possible to prolong life," "continue aggressive care but reevaluate often," "keep me comfortable, but do not provide care that prolongs my life"), or they may ask more general questions about what makes the person's life "worth living." It is hoped that this information will be helpful to a surrogate who must decide whether to continue supportive care in the case of irreversible injury or damage or even to continue disease-oriented care in the case of critical illness and impaired decision-making capacity.

For a variety of reasons, advance directives have not achieved wide popularity. When they exist, they are often not specific enough to provide meaningful guidance.[11] Even when a detailed directive exists, a question often remains about whether the individual was adequately informed. For example, a patient's advance directive says that she would *never* want to be on "life support," but when she is asked about mechanical ventilation in the case of reversible respiratory failure from pneumonia, she says of course she would want that. Thus, following a legally executed advance directive without verifying what was meant by the patient and whether the written wishes apply to the current illness is often quite problematic. It could in fact result in a preventable death in a patient who, with proper education, would wish to be treated.

A more limited form of advance directive, known as a *code status*, is sometimes sought on admission to the hospital, and especially on admission to the ICU. A code status is an advance directive that is specifically limited to a patient's (or surrogate's) preferences regarding cardiopulmonary resuscitation (CPR) and other measures in the event of cardiopulmonary arrest. In many hospitals and other healthcare institutions, as a matter of policy, any patient who suffers cardiac arrest is treated with interventions designed to attempt to reverse the life-threatening derangement, including CPR, electrical defibrillation, and intubation and mechanical ventilatory support. Because a patient who suffers a cardiopulmonary arrest will die in a very short time without interventions, the discussion about code status is as much about how a patient wishes to die as it is about whether he or she wishes to live. Tomlinson and Brody distinguish three distinct rationales for a do-not-resuscitate (DNR) status[12]: (1) CPR has such a low likelihood of producing the desired outcome that it is effectively "futile," (2) there would be an unacceptable quality of life after CPR, and (3) there is already an unacceptable quality of life, and cardiopulmonary arrest would be a welcome deliverance. A decision about CPR may not give much useful information about a patient's preferences regarding other aspects of his or her illness. A patient may choose aggressive disease-oriented measures well into a severe illness but still choose to forgo resuscitation in the event of an arrest. This approach may be voiced in a statement such as, "I want to fight this thing with all I have, but when it is my time, I want to go quickly without suffering." Such a statement would be an opportunity to address resuscitation status, in addition to addressing overall goals of care (see later).

Many ICU patients who are actively receiving intensive disease-oriented care have a DNR code status. Such a directive may save surrogates and family members from the emotionally difficult task of removing life-supporting care. A patient's acceptance of DNR status may signify acceptance of the limits of medical science; refusal of DNR status in the setting of progressive irreversible illness may be an indication that the patient has an incomplete and perhaps unrealistic understanding of the illness. Further discussion, addressing knowledge deficits or unspoken fears, may increase the likelihood that the patient's true wishes will be followed.

A common error when discussing code status is the failure to address post-resuscitation issues. Patients who undergo CPR will most likely be incapacitated for at least a period of time after the resuscitation, even in the best scenarios. There is also a significant risk of permanent brain injury after cardiopulmonary arrest and resuscitation. Thus, it would be prudent for the patient to name a preferred surrogate as well.

Any discussion of advance directives should attempt to answer at least three questions: (1) In the event of cardiac arrest, do you want the healthcare team to attempt resuscitation? (2) If you become incapacitated, who do you want to make decisions for you? (3) If you were left significantly impaired after an attempt at resuscitation, would you want us to discontinue life-sustaining care? Preferences for resuscitation are best understood in the context of an individual's values, beliefs, relationships, and culture.[7]

Many problematic end-of-life issues can be traced to a focus on interventions ("Would you wish to be intubated?") without an adequate exploration of values ("What do you value about your life? What are the things that make your life worth living?"). It is also a mistake to think about advance directives as an issue limited to end-of-life situations. Advance directives are really just part of informed consent for any treatment, and discussion of advance directives is an important aspect of good medical care.

INFORMED DECISION MAKING (INFORMED CONSENT)

In the United States, autonomy is one of the core principles that define the relationship between doctor and patient. Autonomy requires respect for the values and wishes of the individual. An individual patient's autonomy is best respected when decision making takes place through informed consent. Without adequate information, the power of reason, and freedom of choice, patients' decisions cannot be said to be autonomous. Informed consent (or more accurately, informed decision making) is a decision-making model designed to safeguard the autonomy of vulnerable patients.

Brock discussed the basic requirements for informed consent and identified three critical elements: the person giving consent must be competent, informed, and able to make a decision free from coercion.[13] *Competence* has several critical elements.[14] First, the decision maker must be capable of understanding relevant information, which involves both memory and mental processing. Second, it requires the ability to attend to and retain information, the ability to manipulate information, and the ability to foresee consequences. A third element is the ability to formulate and communicate choice. Some standards of competency strengthen this requirement by demanding the ability to communicate a *stable* choice (in this case, ambivalence may be a sign of incompetence).

To adequately participate in medical decision making, patients must have enough information to weigh the risks and benefits of various medical interventions. In the past, the standard for being "informed" was the standard practice of other physicians in the community.[15] Subsequently, "informed" came to mean what a "reasonable person would want to know." Because the main point of informed consent is to respect the rights and values of individuals, it is most appropriate to address this issue in terms of what a particular patient needs to know.[16] In general, patients need to know about the illness and its natural history to make informed decisions about medical care. They need information about the effectiveness of treatment, the risks of treatment, and the likelihood of success with treatment. This information must be presented in a way that is understandable to the patient, at an appropriate educational level, and in the patient's language.

Whether enough information has been transmitted can be assessed at the most basic level by simply asking a patient whether he or she has any questions. Brock writes of "informed understanding" and notes that this "permits an informed exercise in self-determination and promotes a decision most in accord with the patient's well-being."[13] In addition, this approach values autonomy.

The decision must also be voluntary—that is, free of coercion. The decision maker must have the freedom to accept or refuse the intervention or test being proposed. Consent given as a result of undue coercion is generally not valid.

Informed consent in the ICU raises some special issues. First, as mentioned earlier, the decision maker is often a surrogate rather than the patient. The surrogate decision maker should have access to all relevant information the patient would need to make informed decisions; however, the surrogate should not routinely be given confidential information *simply because the patient is no longer competent*. An example may be helpful in illustrating this point. An HIV-positive patient in the ICU has designated a family member as his surrogate; however, the family is unaware of his HIV status. The ICU physician believes a central line is indicated for continued care and seeks informed consent from the family member. In this case, it may be possible to obtain true informed consent for the procedure without divulging the patient's HIV status. Alternatively, a decision about a test or treatment specifically related to the patient's HIV status may require that this information be divulged to the surrogate for her to make an informed decision.

The adequacy of a properly designated surrogate is usually assumed but should be questioned in two situations. The first is when the surrogate acts in contrast to the patient's known wishes. Anyone who knows that the surrogate's directions conflict with the patient's expressed wishes has an obligation to work with the surrogate to come to a treatment decision more in keeping with the patient's wishes or to seek outside assistance from the hospital ethics committee or the hospital's legal department. The second situation occurs when there is doubt about the surrogate's competence, specifically his or her ability to retain and process information. Again, the ethics committee or the risk management department can be of help in this situation. An important study by Schneiderman et al.[17] demonstrated the value of ethics consultation for ICU patients. In that randomized controlled trial, patients receiving an ethics consultation had shorter ICU and hospital stays as well as a decrease in the use of "non-beneficial treatments." This study has led to a call in the literature for more frequent utilization of ethics consultations in the ICU.[18-20]

In summary, ethics in critical care are founded on the same four primary directives common to all disciplines of medicine. Critical care decision making presents special challenges because these decisions often involve the life or death of patients who are unable to participate in the decision-making process. Although the balance between physician and patient responsibility for decision making may vary across cultures, the primary directive for physicians to act in the best interest of their patients is universal.

KEY POINTS

1. Ethics in medical care is based on four fundamental principles: beneficence, nonmaleficence, autonomy, and justice.

2. In the United States, competent patients have the right to make their own decisions about health care.

3. The process of making known one's wishes regarding future care is called *advance care planning*.

4. In the absence of an advance directive, a surrogate decision maker attempts to make medical decisions for a patient using substituted judgment. When no specific information is available about a patient, decision makers apply a "reasonable-person" standard and sometimes resort to a "best-interest" standard.

5. Discussions about advance directives should be rooted in the patient's values and goals for medical care, as well as the appropriateness of specific interventions.

6. Shared decision making is a process that combines patient autonomy and physician judgment.

ANNOTATED REFERENCES

Applebaum PS, Grisso T. Assessing patients' capacities to consent to treatment. N Engl J Med 1988;319:1635-8.
   This paper outlines four tasks a patient must be able to execute to be considered competent: communicating a choice, understanding relevant information, appreciating the current situation and its consequences, and manipulating information rationally.
Brock DW. Informed consent. In: Regan T, VanDeVeer D, editors. Health care ethics. Philadelphia: Temple University Press; 1987. p. 98-126.
   In this chapter, Brock outlines with great clarity the ethical and practical considerations underlying the doctrine of informed consent.
Brock DW. Surrogate decision making for incompetent adults: an ethical framework. Mt Sinai J Med 1991;58:388-92.
   An excellent overview of a philosophically sound approach to surrogate decision making.
Burns JP, Edwards J, Johnson J, Cassem NH, Truog RD. Do-not-resuscitate order after 25 years. Crit Care Med 2003;31:1543-50.
   A review of the development, implementation, and present standing of the DNR order. Emphasizes the usefulness of the DNR order to clarify a patient's wishes with regard to end-of-life care.
Cantor NL. My annotated living will. Law Med Health Care 1990;18:115-19.
   This is an excellent example of an annotated advance directive.
Prendergast T. Advance care planning: pitfalls, progress, promise. Crit Care Med 2001;29:N34-9.
   Review of the (largely disappointing) literature on the usefulness of advance directives, but makes the point that "preferences for care are not fixed but emerge in a clinical context from a process of discussion and feedback within the network of the patient's most important relationships."
Schneiderman LJ, Gilmer T, Teetzel HD, Dugan DO, Blustein J, Cranford R, et al. Effect of ethics consultations on nonbeneficial life-sustaining treatments in the intensive care setting: a randomized controlled trial. JAMA 2003;290:1166-72.
   A seminal randomized controlled trial that demonstrated reduced hospital and ICU length of stay and decrease in "non-beneficial treatment" in patients who received ethics consultation while in the ICU.

REFERENCES

Access the complete reference list online at http://www.expertconsult.com.

217

Ethical Controversies in Pediatric Critical Care

JEFFREY P. BURNS | ROBERT D. TRUOG

As the field of pediatric critical care medicine continues to evolve, ethical concerns in the care of the critically ill child remain of profound concern to all practitioners. This area of pediatric critical care medicine demands the same high level of knowledge and competence as all other areas of critical care practice. Many troubling issues in the pediatric intensive care unit (PICU) revolve around end-of-life decision making and palliative patient management. In this chapter, we explore both issues.

Decision Making in the Pediatric Intensive Care Unit

ROLE OF PARENTS AND PHYSICIANS

Who should make the final decision about treatment for a child in the PICU? In the United States, the clear consensus in the fields of ethics and the law is that a competent adult patient has the right to refuse all forms of medical therapy, including life-sustaining treatment, even if it is certain that such a refusal will hasten death. A similar moral and legal consensus holds that parents have the authority to determine the best interests of their children and make decisions in accord with their own values. However, pediatric healthcare providers also have legal and ethical duties to their patients, independent of parental desires or proxy consent.[1-3]

How can one objectively assess whether a decision is within the range of acceptable ethical choices for a child? More than 20 years ago, a widely respected decision-making framework for children in the PICU context was published by the President's Commission for the Study of Ethical Problems in Medicine and Biomedical and Behavioral Research.[4] The commission proposed five considerations for determining a child's "best interests" and therefore the appropriate approach when weighing different treatment options: (1) the amount of suffering and the potential for relief, (2) the severity of dysfunction and the potential for restoration of function, (3) the expected duration of life, (4) the potential for personal satisfaction and enjoyment of life, and (5) the possibility of developing a capacity for self-determination. The commission then advocated applying these criteria based on an assessment of the proposed treatment plan as clearly beneficial, ambiguous or uncertain, or futile. The commission concluded that in most circumstances, the child's parents should be the final decision makers on all medical decisions (Table 217-1). The Committee on Bioethics of the American Academy of Pediatrics has similarly recommended great deference to patents' informed decisions.[5]

The President's Commission also concluded, reflecting the legal consensus in this area, that parental authority must occasionally be superseded by clinicians when it is determined that the parents' decisions are at odds with the societal consensus about a child's interests or when parents' actions produce certain risk or harm to the child. If life-threatening choices are not involved, or if the risk of substantial harm is minimal, courts have generally respected the decisions of the parents, even though physicians may have disagreed strongly. In some states, parents are legally permitted to refuse standard immunizations for religious reasons.[5] As the potential threat to the child increases, however, and as the benefits of treatment become more certain, actions to override parental choices are not only legally supportable but also mandatory in most jurisdictions. Numerous court opinions have upheld the notion, first pronounced in the 1944 Supreme court case of *Prince v. Massachusetts*, that a parent may make a martyr of himself because of religious convictions, "but he is not free to make a martyr of his child."[6]

NEED FOR IMPROVED COMMUNICATION

A growing body of research reveals that parents report problems related to optimal communication as one of the major deficiencies in the end-of-life care provided to their child. Consistently effective communication from one level of care and one set of providers to the next is a basic expectation, but one that is often not fully met.[7] Meert and colleagues reported on the experience of the bereaved parents of 48 children cared for at 6 PICUs in the United States.[8] These investigators found that the most common communication issue identified by parents was the physicians' availability and attentiveness to their informational needs. More important than the actual outcome, recent data also suggest that many parents want more involvement in end-of-life planning, from discussions around the location of death to even consideration of a plan for extubation at home. These data suggest that the potential for strained communications is mitigated if clinicians provide timely clinical and prognostic information and support the family with a comfortable setting and continuous psychosocial support.

SEEKING THE CHILD'S ASSENT

The prevailing consensus is that patients should participate in treatment decisions to the extent of their decision-making capacity. The President's Commission advocated this perspective when it noted, "Determining whether a patient lacks capacity to make a particular health care decision requires assessing the patient's capability to understand information relevant to the decision, to communicate with care givers about it, and to reason about relevant alternatives against a background of reasonably stable personal values and life goals."[4] Restricting medical decision making only to patients who fulfill the legal definition of competency would infringe on the autonomy of many individuals with decisional capacity, such as adolescents.

Around the age of 7 years, children develop an increasing capacity to understand, process, and make decisions about their care. For children this age and older, it becomes increasingly important for clinicians to obtain the child's assent whenever appropriate. As a matter of policy, the American Academy of Pediatrics has stated, "Patients should participate in decision-making commensurate with their development; they should provide assent to care whenever reasonable. Parents and physicians should not exclude children and adolescents from decision-making without persuasive reasons."[3]

DETERMINING FUTILITY

Few issues have provoked as much controversy as the notion of futility. Who should determine when a situation is futile? A recent review of the futility debate noted that the debate about how to resolve cases in which patients and families demand interventions clinicians regard as futile has been in evolution over the past 20 years.[9] The first generation

TABLE 217-1	Decision Making in the Pediatric Intensive Care Unit	
Physician's Assessment of Treatment Option	*Parents Prefer to Accept Treatment*	*Parents Prefer to Forgo Treatment*
Clearly beneficial	Provide treatment	Provide treatment (during review process)
Ambiguous/uncertain	Provide treatment	Forgo treatment
Futile	Provide treatment (unless provider prefers not to)	Forgo treatment

was characterized by attempts by physicians to define futility in terms of certain clinical criteria. These attempts failed because they proposed limitations to care based on value judgments for which there is no consensus. The second generation was based on a procedural approach that empowered hospitals, through their ethics committees, to decide whether interventions demanded by families were futile. Many hospitals adopted such policies, and some states such as Texas incorporated this approach into legislation. This approach has also not succeeded because it gives hospitals authority to decide whether or not to accede to demands clinicians regard as unreasonable when any national consensus on what is a "beneficial treatment" remains under intense debate. Absent such a consensus, it appears that procedural mechanisms to resolve futility disputes inevitably confront the same insurmountable barriers as attempts to define futility.

The Society for Critical Care Medicine (SCCM) states that treatments should be defined as futile "only when they will not accomplish their intended goal."[10] Moreover, this official position on futility states:

Treatments that are extremely unlikely to be beneficial, are extremely costly, or are of uncertain benefit may be considered inappropriate and hence inadvisable, but should not be labeled futile. Futile treatments constitute a small fraction of medical care. Thus, employing the concept of futile care in decision-making will not primarily contribute to a reduction in resource use. Nonetheless, communities have a legitimate interest in allocating medical resources by limiting inadvisable treatments.[10]

This approach advocates that the local community draft procedures to be followed in cases of dispute, with broad input from the community instead of ad hoc attempts at the bedside to define and resolve differences over futility. This policy goes on to state:

Communities should seek to do so using a rationale that is explicit, equitable, and democratic; that does not disadvantage the disabled, poor, or uninsured; and that recognizes the diversity of individual values and goals. Policies to limit inadvisable treatment should have the following characteristics: (a) be disclosed in the public record; (b) reflect moral values acceptable to the community; (c) not be based exclusively on prognostic scoring systems; (d) articulate appellate mechanisms; and (e) be recognized by the courts.[10]

The Committee on Bioethics for the American Academy of Pediatrics has published guidelines articulating similar sentiments.[2]

Issues in End-of-Life Care

OPTIMAL PALLIATIVE CARE

For a critically ill child and their family, attention to all of their emotional, physical, and spiritual needs begins at the time of diagnosis, not at the end of life. The World Health Organization defines five essential elements of pediatric palliative care[11]:

- Palliative care for children is the active total care of the child's body, mind, and spirit and also involves giving support to the family.

- Palliative care begins when illness is diagnosed and continues irrespective of whether or not a child receives disease-directed treatment.
- Health providers should evaluate and alleviate a child's physical, psychological, and social distress.
- Effective palliative care requires a broad multidisciplinary approach that includes the family and makes use of available community resources; it can be successfully implemented even if resources are limited.
- Palliative care can be provided in tertiary-care facilities, community health centers, and at home.

Yet, despite these and other professional guidelines calling for adoption of the concept of early and continuous palliative care, recent studies continue to find that pediatricians only refer patients once curative therapy is no longer an option. Creating a more practical definition of care, one that emphasizes an array of services throughout the course of an illness as opposed to hospice care, may lead to more optimal palliative care for children with life-limiting illnesses.[12]

SEDATION AND ANALGESIA

A question that weighs on the mind of every practitioner of pediatric critical care is how much is too much sedation and analgesia for the dying patient? A recent consensus statement by the American College of Critical Care Medicine notes:

The data to support specific treatment approaches for dyspnea during end-of-life care are sparse and incomplete. The best approach is to individualize the treatment based on the underlying source of the dyspnea, the patient's level of consciousness, and the patient's observed and perceived needs. Some approaches treat the symptom directly and thereby prolong life. These include, for example, supplemental oxygen, corticosteroids, diuretics, and bronchodilators. Other approaches, like administration of opioids, also make the patient comfortable but may decrease consciousness. Clinicians should work with patients and families to determine the optimal approach, or combination of approaches, for each patient on an individual basis.[13]

An early expert consensus guideline from the same committee advocated that sedatives and analgesics "should be titrated to effect, and the dose should not be limited solely on the basis of 'recommended' or 'suggested' maximal doses. In most cases, patients who do not respond to a given dose of an opioid or benzodiazepine will respond if the dose is increased—there is no theoretical or practical maximal dose."[14] Other experts have expressed similar recommendations:

The optimal dose of morphine for relief of pain or dyspnea is determined by increasing the dose until the patient responds. Patients who have not previously received opioids should initially be given low doses, which should be rapidly increased until symptoms are relieved. For patients with particularly severe or acute symptoms, rapid titration requires that an experienced clinician be at the bedside.[15]

However, assuming that one can externally validate the "appropriate" administration of sedation and analgesia in this setting, determining when to do so is likely to be difficult. There is no constellation of patient signs, symptoms, or pain scores that meets a universally accepted threshold for treatment, let alone the extent of treatment to be given. Regardless of the dosing scheme required to effectively treat pain and suffering, it should be standard medical practice to thoroughly document the observable signs and symptoms of suffering and the rationale behind the regimen chosen to treat those symptoms.

NEUROMUSCULAR BLOCKADE

Is it acceptable to administer a neuromuscular blockade to a dying patient for the sole purpose of making the process of ventilator withdrawal easier for the family? Neuromuscular blocking agents, used to reduce ventilator-patient asynchrony and minimize oxygen consumption by eliminating patient movement, have no sedative or analgesic properties. Given this, many believe administering these agents as the ventilator is being withdrawn is morally indefensible.[16] Some argue that minimizing the distress of the patient's family is an important consideration, and given the certainty of the patient's death following the withdrawal of mechanical ventilation, regardless of muscle relaxation, these clinicians believe that initiating neuromuscular blockade at the time of withdrawal is acceptable. However, others believe that the patient's well-being always takes precedence over family interests. Neuromuscular blockade potentially masks symptoms of patient suffering and therefore interferes with the clinician's primary obligation to ensure that a dying patient does not experience untreated suffering. Such an action also does not allow for the chance the patient might survive without mechanical ventilation when there is some degree of prognostic uncertainty.

What should be done when a patient is experiencing the effects of residual neuromuscular blockade and the family decides to withdraw mechanical ventilation? The Ethics Committee of the SCCM has taken the position that efforts should be made to allow the restoration of neuromuscular function before withdrawing mechanical ventilation from patients who have previously been receiving therapeutic neuromuscular blockade.[13,14]

Some experts believe that only in very limited circumstances is it morally justified to withdraw mechanical ventilation from a patient who is still experiencing the effects of residual neuromuscular blocking agents that were given as part of appropriate management before the decision to forgo life-sustaining treatment was made. If the attempt to reverse neuromuscular blockade is to be more than a charade, the patient must regain sufficient function to potentially sustain life and manifest symptoms of unnecessary pain or suffering. Yet, in some critically ill patients with multiple organ failure, drug clearance may be prolonged and unpredictable, and restoration of full neuromuscular function may take many days or weeks, even with routine neuromuscular monitoring and attempts at pharmacologic reversal. In this instance, the reasons for waiting for the restoration of neuromuscular function must be balanced against the added suffering and continued use of life-sustaining treatments, possibly long after the family and clinicians have concluded that the burdens outweigh the benefits. Open discussion with the family and among the caregivers should be undertaken, followed by clear documentation in the chart of decisions regarding the restoration of neuromuscular function.[14]

Family Presence at Resuscitation Attempts

Since the year 2000 it has been the official position of the American Heart Association that "family members should be given the option of being present at resuscitation attempts, but they will require support and specific attention during the resuscitation." This statement stems from surveys that have found that most people would like to be present during the attempted resuscitation of a loved one, especially when it is a child. If family members are present, a clinician must be in attendance to meet the unexpected needs of the family, which may stretch the limited resources of the resuscitation team.[17]

A recent study by Tinsley and colleagues examined the experience of families during cardiopulmonary resuscitation in a PICU. They found that 12 (60%) of those in the not-present group believed their presence would have comforted the child, and 50% (10 of 20) believed it would have helped them accept the child's death. Of those in the present group, 67% (8 of 12) believed that touching their child brought comfort, 29% (6 of 21) felt scared during cardiopulmonary resuscitation, 71% (15 of 21) believed their presence comforted their child, and 67% (14 of 21) believed their presence helped them adjust to the loss of the child. The majority in both groups (63% [26 of 41]) would recommend being present during cardiopulmonary resuscitation.[18]

Ethical Concerns After Death

ORGAN DONATION

Organ donation rates continue to be inadequate. For example, it is frequently noted that the general public claims to support organ and tissue donation on broad public opinion surveys, but only 40% of all those approached grant permission for donation. Research in this area has found that that the reasons for denying consent can be grouped into eight broad categories: donor characteristics, distrust of the medical community, religious beliefs, fear of mutilation, concern regarding the use of organs, lack of knowledge about the deceased's wishes, misunderstanding of brain death, and the bereaved family's emotional state.

The questions of who should approach the family about potential organ donation, when to broach the subject, and what should be said have been simplified in the United States by federal regulations issued in 1998. One of the requirements is that a hospital must have an agreement with an organ procurement organization, under which it contacts the organization in a timely manner about individuals who die or whose death is imminent in the hospital. The organ procurement organization then determines the individual's medical suitability for donation. Hospitals are also required to have an agreement with at least one tissue bank and one eye bank for tissue and eye referrals. The regulations require hospitals to collaborate with the organ procurement organization in notifying the families of potential donors of their donation options and to work cooperatively with such organizations and tissue and eye banks in educating hospital staff on donation issues, reviewing death records to improve the identification of potential donors, and maintaining potential donors during the testing and placement of organs.

Who should approach the family and request organ donation? In the United States, the Centers for Medicare and Medicaid Services has answered this question by stating:

Hospitals should approach the family with the belief that a donation is possible and should take steps to ensure the family is treated with respect and care. The hospital staff's perception that a family's grief, race, ethnicity, religion or socioeconomic background would prevent donation should never be used as a reason not to approach a family…hospitals should ensure, in collaboration with the designated OPO, that the family of each potential donor is informed of its options to donate organs, tissues, or eyes or to decline to donate. The individual designated by the hospital to initiate the request to the family must be an organ procurement representative or a designated requestor. A designated requestor is an individual who has completed a course offered or approved by the OPO and designed in conjunction with the tissue and eye bank community in the methodology for approaching potential donor families and requesting organ or tissue donation.[19]

More recently there has also been a renewed interest in promoting organ donation after cardiac death. Donation after cardiac death (DCD) remains controversial in some pediatric institutions.[20] Antommaria and colleagues examined DCD policies at 105 pediatric institutions across North America and found that while most children's hospitals have developed or are developing DCD policies, there is considerable variation among policies on the actual DCD procedure that is allowed.[21]

CONCERNS AFTER DEATH

How well informed are families and clinicians about the actual autopsy procedure? Is it ethical to practice resuscitation procedures on newly deceased patients? How well are bereaved families from the PICU supported by follow-up programs? Many of these questions have been addressed, and practitioners of pediatric critical care medicine should be familiar with these stated positions. For example, the Ethics

Committee of the SCCM has stated that only a physician who has "earned the right" by virtue of their relationship with the parents, and assuming they are fully knowledgeable on the actual autopsy procedure and associated medical examiner procedures, should approach the family to seek permission for autopsy.[14] Similarly, a position statement from the Council on Ethical and Judicial Affairs of the American Medical Association states that performing procedures on the newly dead should be allowed, but only in the context of a structured training sequence completed under close supervision, and only after permission from family members has been obtained.[22]

Equally important are the needs of bereaved parents. Meert and colleagues found that many bereaved parents want to meet with the intensive care physician after their child's death to gain information and emotional support and to give feedback about their PICU experience.[23] In this study of the experience of parents of 48 children who died in the PICU of one of six children's hospitals in the United States, these investigators reported that only 7 (13%) parents had a scheduled meeting with any physician to discuss their child's death; 33 (59%) wanted to meet with their child's intensive care physician. Of these, 27 (82%) were willing to return to the hospital to meet. Topics that parents wanted to discuss included the chronology of events leading to PICU admission and death, cause of death, treatment, autopsy, genetic risk, medical documents, withdrawal of life support, ways to help others, bereavement support, and what to tell family. Parents sought reassurance and the opportunity to voice complaints and express gratitude. These findings point to an obvious and painful reality: bereaved parents have intense needs, and a thoughtful follow-up program, building on the developing research in this area, can provide significant support.

KEY POINTS

1. The majority of deaths in the pediatric intensive care unit (PICU) occur following the withholding or withdrawal of life-sustaining treatments. This fact heightens the importance of competence in end-of-life decision making and palliative patient management by all practitioners of pediatric critical care medicine.

2. In the United States, there is consensus in the law and bioethics that parents have the authority to determine the best interests of their children and to make decisions in accord with their own values. However, critical care providers must be thoroughly familiar with their legal and ethical duties to their pediatric patients, independent of parental viewpoints about life-sustaining treatments.

3. The World Health Organization advocates that "palliative care begins when illness is diagnosed, and continues irrespective of whether or not a child receives disease-directed treatment... providers should evaluate and alleviate a child's physical, psychological, and social distress; effective palliative care requires a broad multidisciplinary approach that includes the family and makes use of available community resources; it can be successfully implemented even if resources are limited...it can be provided in tertiary-care facilities, community health centres, and at home."

4. The attending physician must affirm that the requesting physician has the right to request permission for organ donation or an autopsy by virtue of his or her involvement in the care of the patient and relationship with the family. Renewed educational efforts on improving communication with families and best practices for seeking permission for organ donation and autopsy are needed.

ANNOTATED REFERENCES

American Academy of Pediatrics Committee on Bioethics. Guidelines on forgoing life-sustaining medical treatment. Pediatrics 1994;93:532-6.

Ethics and the care of critically ill infants and children. American Academy of Pediatrics Committee on Bioethics. Pediatrics 1996;98:149-52.

Although published nearly 2 decades ago, these statements remain the official position of the American Academy of Pediatrics on forgoing life-sustaining treatment for children.

Diekema DS, Botkin JR. Clinical report—forgoing medically provided nutrition and hydration in children. Pediatrics 2009;124:813-22.

This statement reviews the medical, ethical, and legal issues relevant to withholding or withdrawing medically provided fluids and nutrition in children. The American Academy of Pediatrics concludes that withdrawal of medically administered fluids and nutrition for pediatric patients is ethically acceptable in limited circumstances.

Devictor DJ, Tissieres P, Gillis J, et al. Intercontinental differences in end-of-life attitudes in the pediatric intensive care unit: results of a worldwide survey. Pediatr Crit Care Med 2008;9:560-6.

The only intercontinental study to examine end-of-life practices in pediatric intensive care; interesting differences emerge between the Northern and Southern hemispheres.

Antommaria AHM, Trotochaud K, Kinlaw K, et al. Policies on donation after cardiac death at children's hospitals: a mixed-methods analysis of variation. JAMA 2009;301:1902-8.

The largest study of DCD policies at children's hospitals across the United States reveals that while most institutions have a policy, there remains considerable variation in what procedures they allow.

Truog RD, Campbell ML, Curtis JR, et al. Recommendations for end-of-life care in the intensive care unit: a consensus statement by the American College [corrected] of Critical Care Medicine. Crit Care Med 2008;36:953-63.

Endorsed by the SCCM and the American College of Critical Care Medicine, this is perhaps the most comprehensive set of recommendations on how to care for ICU patients following the withholding or withdrawal of life-sustaining treatment, covering a wide range of issues, not simply what medications to administer.

REFERENCES

Access the complete reference list online at http://www.expertconsult.com.

218

End-of-Life Issues in the Intensive Care Unit

NICHOLAS S. WARD | J. RANDALL CURTIS | MITCHELL M. LEVY

In the last century, the process of dying changed dramatically. Previously, doctors simply did all they could for a patient, and when their treatments failed, the patient died, almost always at home. However, with the advent of more sophisticated medical technologies, even patients with severe organ failure can be kept alive. Unfortunately, with this progress has come a new set of complex medical, ethical, and societal issues.

In the United States, about 80% of people now die in healthcare facilities (60% in acute care facilities),[1] despite the fact that about 90% of Americans polled say they would prefer to die at home.[2] This disparity is due to two factors: (1) many people die while undergoing treatments meant to postpone death—treatments that are often futile; and (2) many families are unable to care for a dying person or are uncomfortable having a loved one die at home. The net result is that most people will die in a hospital or other healthcare facility, and many of them will undergo high levels of medical care before death. A recent study showed that about 20% of Americans will die in an intensive care unit (ICU) or be admitted to an ICU just before death.[3]

Two conclusions can be drawn from the preceding information. One is that a tremendous amount of health care is being delivered to dying patients. This has been reflected in several studies, such as that of Cher and Lenert, which showed that a relatively large percentage of Medicare expenditures goes to treat patients in the last weeks of their lives.[4] The other conclusion is that doctors have to learn a new set of skills that were not necessary in the past. They need to be able to recognize patients who are going to die despite medical care and help decide which of the almost limitless supply of medical therapies available are appropriate and which are not. Physicians need to guide their patients through a maze of medical options in an attempt to balance preservation of life with quality of life—a daunting task, to say the least.

How Are Critically Ill Patients Dying?

In 1995, a landmark study in end-of-life issues was published. This was the first large-scale attempt to define how seriously ill people die in American hospitals. In a two-part study involving 4301 seriously ill, hospitalized patients, the investigators examined multiple aspects of end-of-life care and found major shortcomings in current practice. Only 47% of the time did the physician know when a patient wanted to avoid cardiopulmonary resuscitation (CPR), and the incidence of dying with moderate or severe pain was 50%.[5]

More insight into the dying experience came in subsequent studies that showed that the vast majority of ICU deaths occur only after a decision to limit life support has been made.[6,7] In two important studies, Prendergast and coworkers helped define how patients die in ICUs.[6,8] In their first study, they compared deaths in their ICU from two periods, 1987 to 1988 and 1992 to 1993, to determine how often CPR was performed before death and how often limits were placed on life support before death.[9] Their data showed that the incidence of CPR before death had declined from 49% to 10% and that the incidence of withholding or withdrawing life support had increased from 51% to 90% of all ICU deaths.

In an effort to benchmark their data with the rest of the country, the same investigators then did a large follow-up study 1 year later. They collected data from more than 6000 patient deaths occurring in 131 ICUs in 38 states over a 6-month period and analyzed the data for the incidence of various limits on life support. They found that on average, only 25% of patients dying in ICUs were given CPR before death. About 70% of patients had some restriction on life support, and almost 50% of patients had some medical therapy withheld or withdrawn before death.[6]

The other striking piece of data to emerge was the degree of variability that existed among ICUs. The incidence of patients dying with full aggressive measures ranged from 4% in one ICU to 79% in another. Likewise, the incidence of withdrawing life support ranged from 0% to 79%, depending on the ICU. These data clearly show that although the overall practice of limiting life support in ICUs in the United States is common, there is tremendous variability from place to place in end-of-life care.

In 2003, a study examined deaths in 31 ICUs in 17 European countries. Overall, the percentage of patients dying with some limits on life support was 72.6%, which was very similar to studies done in the United States. As in the American studies, there was also tremendous variability in practices among the different ICUs, with rates of CPR before death ranging from 5% to almost 50%.[9]

What Accounts for Variability in Practice?

It should not be surprising that there is so much variability in a practice as multidimensional as end-of-life care. Even the standard practice of medicine varies from institution to institution. The decision to limit or not limit life support is generally a complex one that may reflect the personal biases of both physician and patient. Many attempts have been made to find patterns among different types of physicians and patients that can explain the variation. For example, one study showed that university-based physicians are more likely than community-based physicians to write do-not-resuscitate (DNR) orders and withhold or withdraw life support.[10] A similar study showed that patients without private physicians in the ICU were more likely to undergo active withdrawal of life support.[11] Unfortunately, studies like this are hard to interpret unless one knows the contexts in which these decisions were made. An increased tendency to withhold life support from a terminally ill patient may reflect a weaker physician-patient relationship or a stronger one based on the patient's preferences.

Other studies have sought to explain variation by culture, race, or religion.[12-16] Although such factors may play a role in these important decisions, and there may be some general trends in decision patterns, there is enough variation even within cultures, races, or religions to indicate that one cannot generalize this information to a given individual. Physicians need to be cognizant of the fact that their patients may have markedly different views of optimal end-of-life care, regardless of their culture, religion, or race.

Predicting Outcomes

A central problem complicating end-of-life decisions is the difficulty of predicting outcomes in critically ill patients. The combination of multiple coinciding medical problems and rapidly changing clinical status can make this a very difficult task. Essentially, two objective tools are available to a physician when trying to determine the prognosis of a critically ill patient: published outcomes and severity scores. Both can be helpful, yet have limitations. In addition, the role of a physician's personal experience is important but can also have important limitations.

SEVERITY SCORES

Severity scores have been available for almost 3 decades, and much has been learned in that time. In most severity score algorithms, data are collected during the first 24 hours of admission and are then used to compile a score that predicts the risk of death during hospitalization. Many of these scoring systems were developed by reviewing data from thousands of ICU patients and employing logistic regression models to choose some important input variables. Other variables were simply chosen based on presumed clinical value. These scores were then validated prospectively on patients.

Unfortunately, there are several problems with these severity score–based systems. First, they make predictions based on hospital outcomes at the time of their creation. Thus, as medical treatments improve, the scores must be updated. In the 1970s, for example, acute respiratory distress syndrome (ARDS) had a hospital mortality approaching 80%, so its presence might justifiably increase a patient's severity score. Presently, ARDS has about 40% hospital mortality. Thus, a severity scoring system using the diagnosis of ARDS, or even components of the diagnosis such as hypoxemia, would have to be adjusted. Some commercially available proprietary severity scoring systems, such as the Acute Physiology and Chronic Health Evaluation (APACHE) methodology, are updated and revalidated on a regular basis to avoid this problem, but many that are widely used today, such as APACHE II, are based on patient data collected as many as 2 or 3 decades ago.

Another problem with using severity scores is that most models derive their predictions from factors present at or shortly after admission to the ICU and do not provide updated mortality estimates as the patient's condition changes. Further, severity scores often give intermediate mortality estimates such as 60% instead of a clear yes-or-no answer. Even these numbers are subject to confidence intervals. Perhaps the most glaring problem of using severity scores is that they say nothing about morbidity, disability, or survival after hospitalization. These factors are often just as important as risk of death in making end-of-life decisions. A patient may accept a 30% chance of survival if it were followed by a high quality of life, but not accept a 70% chance of survival if it were likely to entail a poor quality of life.

OUTCOME DATA

Many of the same problems encountered with severity scores characterize the use of outcome data. Although published outcome studies are an essential tool for clinicians in predicting a course of illness, they suffer from two major problems. One is that the population studied for a particular illness may not share the same characteristics as a particular patient. For example, in a large multicenter clinical trial of a new therapy for sepsis, the mortality rate in the control (untreated) arm was 31%.[17] It is important to note, however, that this trial excluded patients with conditions such as renal failure, liver failure, pancreatitis, acquired immunodeficiency syndrome (AIDS), and a variety of other comorbid conditions, thus limiting the usefulness of these data for prognostic purposes.

Another problem with using outcome data, similar to the severity scores, is the rapidity with which therapies can change and improve. In four published studies by different authors between 1981 and 2000 examining the mortality of *Pneumocystis carinii* pneumonia in ICU patients, the mortality decreased from 86% to approximately 50%.[18] Similar changes in outcome over time have been reported with a variety of other illnesses, such as ARDS, as treatments have improved.

Caring for Families in the Intensive Care Unit

IMPACT OF FAMILY MEETING

Relatives, partners, and friends often provide support and care for a patient, which for some will include the responsibility of surrogate decision making. Surrogate decision makers are often under an enormous amount of emotional stress, and decision making during these circumstances can be difficult. In addition, one study revealed that despite discussions with ICU physicians, only half of families of critically ill patients adequately understood their loved ones' diagnoses, prognoses, or treatments.[19] Despite this, clinicians and health systems often neglect the care of the family as part of the overall care of a patient. Therefore, clinician-family communication is an important component of good quality care. In addition, effective clinician-family communication reduces the stress on family members of critically ill patients and improves the family members' level of understanding. This is of critical importance in the ICU because if the patient's family is under significant distress, their ability to provide surrogate decision making may be impaired, and the medical decisions they make may not accurately reflect the wishes of the patient.

In addition to the multitude of data showing that the way we communicate with families has a significant impact, there are also data showing that interdisciplinary team communication has a significant impact on important patient and family outcomes. Observational studies show increased survival, shorter lengths of stay, and improved patient satisfaction when there is good nursing-physician communication.[20] In addition, patients and families have reported that interdisciplinary communication is an important part of good end-of-life care, and most studies of interventions that have improved end-of-life care include an interdisciplinary team in the intervention. Unfortunately, some ICU family meetings occur only between the physician and the family. Underutilization of the many professionals involved with a critically ill patient's care is a common mistake. Care of ICU patients is provided by a large interdisciplinary team that includes consulting physicians, nurses, social workers, and members of the clergy. These healthcare providers often know the patient and family from different perspectives, and holding a meeting without attempting to have all relevant members present can result in miscommunication and may result in missed opportunities to provide families with the best possible resources.

FAMILY OUTCOMES: ANXIETY, DEPRESSION, POSTTRAUMATIC STRESS DISORDER

An important problem with critical care delivery systems is dissatisfaction among family members. There is also evidence to suggest that our current approach causes anxiety, depression, and posttraumatic stress disorder (PTSD) among family members. Many critical care units only conduct family meetings after it is clear that an ICU patient is actively dying, but it is important to meet with all ICU families early in the ICU stay, because family caregivers are under a high level of emotional and physical stress. In fact, family members of patients who survive the ICU are more dissatisfied with communication in the ICU than family members of patients who die.[21] This likely reflects the fact that family members of ICU patients experience an important unmet need with regard to regular and systematic communication with ICU clinicians. Several interventions have been shown to improve family satisfaction: time spent with physicians,[22] timing of family meetings, and open visiting hours.[23]

Who Decides?

DECISION MAKING ABOUT LIFE-SUSTAINING TREATMENTS

As stated earlier, the vast majority of people will die with some limit on life support in place, whether in or out of an ICU. Unfortunately, the patient can rarely participate in these decisions. Most studies show that someone else makes the decision to limit a dying patient's life support 60% to 70% of the time.[7,24] Therefore, the burden of these difficult decisions falls to a proxy (a legal delegation) or a surrogate (a nonlegal delegation). Most often, this is a family member.

The process of surrogate decision making is fraught with problems. Although most would agree that family or friends of the patient are the best people to make such decisions, several studies have shown that patients rarely discuss specific treatment options with their proxies, and surrogate decisions correlate poorly with what the patient would actually want done.[25,26] Further, in a study by Hare et al., it was shown that surrogates often place greater emphasis on certain aspects of dying such as pain and suffering than patients do; patients are more concerned with burdening their families and the amount of time left to live.[19]

LEGAL ISSUES

In the United States, all 50 states now recognize the legality of a patient's right to refuse medical treatment, although there remains some controversy and confusion about specific issues. The legal issues involved in proxy decision making can also be a source of great confusion. Perhaps realizing that it is impossible to account for the many possible family and social relationships involved, most states have few laws dealing with the issue of surrogate decision makers and have purposely kept the codes vague and malleable.[27] Most states accept a properly drafted written advance directive as sufficient legal guidance to limit life support. Unfortunately, most advance directives or living wills are too vague in their language, using phrases such as "terminal illness" and "little chance of recovery," which are subject to interpretation. Diseases such as chronic obstructive pulmonary disease and congestive heart failure may be considered terminal illnesses by some people but not by others. Some people may consider diseases such as early-stage lung cancer not imminently terminal.

Nevertheless, these directives can be of great help. They can help prevent futile or unwanted care when no other surrogate is available. They may be useful in family decision making when dealing with an unconscious patient facing potentially futile care. The previously stated wishes of the patient in an advance directive can help with feelings of guilt or uncertainty regarding end-of-life decisions. They can also be helpful when there is disagreement between surrogates about a course of action. Because a surrogate, by definition, is an agent representing what the patient would decide if he or she were able, the advance directive can be a helpful guide.

Sometimes advance directives can be a source of discord, such as when the written directive differs from what a surrogate decides. In most states, the law recognizes a properly drafted and witnessed directive as the legal opinion that should be followed; however, many physicians are wary of ignoring the requests of a living surrogate, especially if it is a spouse or other close family member. In situations like this, attempts should be made to build consensus among all parties before making any decision. Most state laws regarding written advance directives also allow for some flexibility in the physician's obligation to follow them. They often state that if a physician feels that the directive is of questionable validity or if he or she feels ethically unable to follow the directive, it is not binding.

PATIENT AUTONOMY VERSUS MEDICAL PATERNALISM

A central problem with the end-of-life decision-making process is defining the role of the physician. Usually the physician's role is a combination of educator and adviser, but this is not always the case. In the past, physicians were more likely to dictate courses of action or treatment plans for their patients, a concept referred to as *medical paternalism*. In many parts of the world, medical decisions continue to be made this way with little input from the patient or family. In these cultures, patients are often comfortable with this kind of decision making. More recently in the United States, the concept of *patient*

autonomy has dictated medical decision making. In the extreme form of patient autonomy, the physician's role is only to educate the patient about the problem and offer available treatment plans, along with their risks and benefits. The patient then independently chooses a course of action. Under this model, it is the obligation of the physician to provide the medical information necessary for the patient to have the appropriate knowledge for informed decision making. The physician plays no part in the decision making. Many physicians use this model of practice today, or something similar to it, believing it empowers patients and frees them from physician bias.

Although many patients desire autonomy, when it comes to decisions about life-sustaining therapy in the ICU, often the decisions fall to the surrogate. In the extreme, the autonomy model may make family members feel like they are being abandoned and may place unnecessary stress on the family. Over the same time period, much of the rest of the world used a model of decision making in the ICU that has been called *parentalism* (the non-sexist version of *paternalism*), in which physicians are the medical decision makers, with little or no input from the patient or family. In this latter extreme version, the patient and family are informed about the treatment patients will receive, and often only involved in decision making when the patient wishes to forgo treatment.

In contrast to both of these approaches, many physicians and patients believe the physician is obliged to be involved in the decision-making process and often to recommend a course of action. The physician thus offers several possible courses of action but makes specific recommendations. This model is referred to as *shared decision making* and may well represent an ideal blending of the autonomous and parentalistic approach. In this model, caregivers do their best to understand the wishes of their patients. This is accomplished through a process of genuine listening to family members and eliciting their understanding of the wishes of their loved one, then combining that knowledge with the clinician's best guess about the likely prognosis and outcome. Through this process, a clinician can proactively offer an opinion about the appropriate course of therapy. In 2005, five European and North American critical care societies issued a joint statement supporting the model of shared decision making when caring for ICU patients.[28] Ultimately, it is up to each individual physician to determine the degree of involvement warranted in end-of-life decisions.

There are multiple components of the shared decision model that are essential for an even exchange of information and a truly joint decision made in concert with the patient and family. Table 218-1 describes in detail the components of shared decision making, and the use of these components is further elaborated in the following strategies for family meetings.

ADAPTING SHARED DECISION MAKING TO FIT EACH PATIENT AND FAMILY

Although the shared decision-making model is the preferred model in many ICU settings, each patient and family is unique; as circumstances and prognosis change, the role the family wishes to play may change. Therefore the initial meeting should often be one that models shared decision making, but after the exchange of information regarding the status of the patient and the patient's treatment preferences, it is important to assess the role the family wishes to play in the decision-making process. The family may not wish to partake in the decision-making process, and the process will then shift toward the parentalism model. If the family wishes to be closely involved, then the decision-making process should be a shared process in which physicians give prognostic information and, based on that information and discussion of the patient's values, offer to provide a recommendation on treatment decisions.

It is important to recognize that the decision-making model is a dynamic process that may change several times throughout the course of an ICU stay. As patients become more critically ill and the prognosis is more certain, the physician should be willing to take on a more active

TABLE 218-1	Shared Decision Making
Dimensions of Shared Decision Making	**Example Physician Behaviors and Questions**
Providing medical information and eliciting patient values and preferences	Discuss the nature of the decision. *What are the essential clinical issues we are addressing?* Describe alternatives. *What are the clinically reasonable choices?* Discuss pros/cons. *What are the pros and cons of the treatment choices?* Discuss uncertainty. *What is the likelihood of success of treatment, and how confident are we in this estimate?* Assess understanding. *Is the family now an "informed participant," with a working understanding of the decision?* Explore the patient's values/preferences. *What is known about the patient's medical preferences or values? What is important to the patient?*
Exploring family's preferred role in decision making	Discuss the family's role. *What role should the family play in making the decision?* Assess desire for others' input. *Is there anyone else the family would like to consult?*
Deliberation and decision making	Explore "context." *How will the decision impact the patient's life?* If the family is to participate in decision making, elicit family opinion about the best treatment choice. *What does the family think is the most appropriate decision for the patient?*

role in the decision-making process to relieve the family of the burden of decision making in these circumstances. Whichever decision-making model is utilized, it must be one that is responsive to the needs of the family. Research suggests that physicians often have one model of decision making they use for all patients.[29] The physician and interdisciplinary team must be prepared to adapt this model to fit the individual patient and family.

Most interventions that have shown to be beneficial in improving care for ICU patients follow a standard procedure or protocol. Using such a protocol will encourage consistency across the ICU and help prevent oversights and miscommunication. This was recently tested in a randomized controlled trial which demonstrated decreased symptoms of anxiety and depression through use of a protocolized family conference intervention.[30] Obviously, communication with families cannot be performed in a manner that is so overprotocolized the team comes across as rigid and uncaring. Each individual patient and family is different and must be treated individually—but with key components applied in an individualized way. A mnemonic was developed

TABLE 218-2	VALUE: Five-Step Approach to Improving Communication with Families in the ICU
V	*Value* family statements.
A	*Acknowledge* family emotions.
L	*Listen* to the family.
U	*Understand* the patient as a person.
E	*Elicit* family questions.

that features five key elements to help guide clinicians in communicating with families: VALUE. This mnemonic is described in Table 218-2 and has been shown to result in improved family outcomes.[31]

Conclusion

Clearly, the process of dying is changing. Although the physician has always had an important role to play, that role has also changed. Today's physician not only must be adept at administering comfort measures but also must decide when to initiate those measures rather than other therapies aimed at prolonging life. Because the dying process frequently involves the healthcare system, physicians in these settings need to have good end-of-life skills. The model of decision making in the ICU is evolving. A model in which decision making is shared among physicians, patients, and families is emerging as a compassionate alternative to the two extremes of autonomy and parentalism. Failure to address these issues will result in patients getting more futile care at the expense of their own comfort and increased costs to the healthcare system.

KEY POINTS

1. A majority of deaths occur in healthcare institutions such as hospitals and ICUs as opposed to home. Studies now show that the vast majority of patients who die in the hospital do so only after some limitation has been placed on life-sustaining treatments. Other studies show that ICUs, and even physicians, can vary greatly in the frequency with which they limit or withdraw life support.

2. Many studies have tried to demonstrate what accounts for the dramatic variability in end-of-life practices. Various patient characteristics such as ethnicity, and physician characteristics such as community-based versus university-based status, may impact these decisions, but these factors do not explain all the variability.

3. Currently, most decisions to limit life support are not made by the patient. This raises problems regarding surrogate decision making. Clearly identifying one legal surrogate can be difficult, and most state laws in the United States give few specifics about who can qualify as a surrogate decision maker. Usually the decision to limit life support is made by the healthcare team in association with the family.

4. One of the greatest barriers to delivering optimal end-of-life care is the ability to predict patient outcomes. Two common tools that aid in this are validated severity scores and published outcome data. However, both are fraught with potential error and should not automatically be relied on as accurate predictors of morbidity and mortality.

5. Throughout the world, cultures and people differ in their beliefs about how important medical decisions should be made. Some favor a decision-making model in which the physician makes the majority of the decisions—often referred to as *medical paternalism*. In the latter half of the 1990s, the United States has been characterized by a model that favors the patient (or surrogate) as the primary decision maker—referred to as *patient autonomy*. Both systems have advantages as well as drawbacks, and a physician must consider the patient's and family's perspectives on decision making.

ANNOTATED REFERENCES

Cook DJ, Guyatt GH, Jaeschke R, et al. Determinants in Canadian health care workers of the decision to withdraw life support from the critically ill. JAMA 1995;273:703-8.
This prospective study identifies several factors that influence the decision to withdraw life support. The most important factors were likelihood of surviving the current episode, likelihood of long-term survival, premorbid cognitive function, and patient age.

Curtis JR, Rubenfeld GR. Managing death in the ICU. New York: Oxford University Press; 2000.
This comprehensive textbook has contributions from many authors and includes practical suggestions for end-of-life care, as well as philosophical pieces.

Danis M, Federman D, Fins JJ, et al. Incorporating palliative care into critical care education: principles, challenges, and opportunities. Crit Care Med 1999;27:2005-13.

This well-written overview describes the fundamental principles of palliative care in the ICU and offers concrete suggestions for building an educational curriculum.

Danis M, Mutran E, Garrett JM. A prospective study of the impact of patient preferences on life-sustaining treatment and hospital cost. Crit Care Med 1996;24:1811-17.
In this prospective study, patients were asked about life-support preferences and then followed for 6 months. Of interest, there was no significant association between patient desire for life support and the use of these therapies.

Johnson D, Wilson M, Cavanaugh B, et al. Measuring the ability to meet family needs in an intensive care unit. Crit Care Med 1998;26:266-71.
A survey instrument was used to identify the top needs of families of critically ill patients. Continuity of caregiver communication was identified as a priority.

Prendergast TJ, Luce JM. Increasing incidence of withholding and withdrawal of life support from the critically ill. Am J Respir Crit Care Med 1997;155:15-20.

This important prospective study describes how patients die in ICUs and documents a dramatic increase in the practice of limiting some form of life-support measures in several hospitals over a 5-year period.

SUPPORT principal investigators. A controlled trial to improve care for seriously ill hospitalized patients: the Study to Understand Prognoses and Preferences for Outcomes and Risks of Treatments (SUPPORT). JAMA 1996;274:1591-8.

In two consecutive 2-year periods, a prospective observational study documented major shortcomings in communication, the frequency of aggressive treatment, and the characteristics of death in the hospital. An intervention study using a nurse to facilitate communication and clinical care of the dying demonstrated essentially no improvement in outcomes.

Thompson BT, Cox PN, Antonelli M, et al. Challenges in end-of-life care in the ICU: statement of the 5th International Consensus Conference in Critical Care: Brussels, Belgium, April 2003: executive summary. Crit Care Med 2004;32:1781-4.

A summary of the results of an international consensus conference on end-of-life care in which the shared decision model is well described.

Lautrette A, Darmon M, Megarbane B, et al. A communication strategy and brochure for relatives of patients dying in the ICU. N Engl J Med 2007;356:469-78.

A seminal publication in end-of-life care. This randomized controlled trial tested an intervention that included administration of a bereavement pamphlet and standardized family meetings. The results demonstrated a significant reduction in symptoms of anxiety, depression, and posttraumatic stress disorder among families of patients who died in the ICU.

REFERENCES

Access the complete reference list online at http://www.expertconsult.com.

219

Determination of Brain Death

TERESA L. SMITH JACOBS | THOMAS P. BLECK

Determination of death by neurologic criteria is a clinical diagnosis. After certain prerequisites are met, there are three essential components to the determination: irreversible coma or unresponsiveness, absence of brainstem reflexes, and apnea. Before the diagnosis is made, it is essential to rule out alternative causes for the patient's neurologic status, including hypothermia, drug-induced coma, and severe metabolic disarray.

Prerequisites

Determination of death can be made in patients who continue to have cardiac function during mechanical ventilation in the appropriate clinical scenario. A clear irreversible cause must be known based on history, brain imaging, or cerebrospinal fluid examination. Determination of death by neurologic criteria cannot be made in patients with a temperature below 36°C or in those who may have drug intoxications or poisoning without a confirmatory study indicating the absence of intracranial blood flow. If neuromuscular junction blocking agents have been administered, electrical stimulation should be performed to document the presence of transmission at the neuromuscular junction. Severe acid-base, electrolyte, or endocrine abnormalities also cannot be present.

Unresponsiveness

The examination shows that the patient has no eye movements or motor response to verbal or noxious stimulation, with the exception of spinally mediated responses. Standard points of pressure application for administration of noxious stimuli are nailbeds, supraorbital nerve, and temporomandibular joint.[1]

Absence of Brainstem Reflexes

PUPILLARY RESPONSE

Pupillary responsiveness should be assessed using a bright flashlight. Using an ophthalmoscope allows for magnification of the iris and pupil so that even a subtle response can be detected. Pupils are usually mid-position (4-6 cm in diameter); rarely, they may be more dilated if spinal sympathetic pathways are intact.

FACIAL SENSATION AND MOTOR RESPONSE

A very gentle stimulus such as a wisp of cotton should be gently touched to the cornea of each eye individually. We prefer to use a small squirt of saline from the plastic containers used for saline administration during airway suctioning, as saline will not harm the cornea. In patients with a diagnosis of death by neurologic criteria, no blink will be induced. There can be no grimace to painful stimuli or jaw reflex.

GAG AND COUGH REFLEXES

Patients being examined for a determination of death by neurologic criteria will all be on ventilatory assistance. The gag response can be difficult to determine in patients with endotracheal tubes in place. The endotracheal tube itself should not be maneuvered to stimulate a gag response, as this could lead to tracheal damage; a tongue blade should be used instead. Cough in response to deep bronchial suctioning

should be sought. Absence of these responses is required for a determination of death by neurologic criteria.

ASSESSMENT OF EYE MOVEMENTS

Cervico-Ocular Reflexes ("Doll's-Eyes Maneuver")

This maneuver is only performed in the absence of cervical instability. With the eyes held open, the head should be briskly turned from side to side (mid-position to 90 degrees), looking for any eye movements. If an endotracheal tube is in place, it should be moved together with the head movements to avoid tracheal damage or unplanned extubation. No eye movements occur in patients with a diagnosis of death by neurologic criteria. The term *doll's eyes* refers to the expected horizontal movement in the direction opposite to the head movement, indicating that the brainstem centers for conjugate horizontal gaze are functional, but the cerebral cortex is not controlling them. However, the likelihood of inaccurate use of this term is so great that it should be avoided.

Vestibulo-Ocular Reflexes ("Cold Calorics")

Once the absence of the cervico-ocular reflex is determined, or in circumstances in which it cannot be tested owing to cervical instability, caloric testing should be performed. First, the tympanic membranes are examined for perforations and to ensure no obstructions are present. The caloric test is sufficiently important, however, that it should proceed when death by neurologic criteria is being proved even if a perforation is present. The head of the bed should be elevated to 30 degrees. Ice-cold water, 50 mL, should be placed in a syringe. Soft tubing connected to the syringe (for instance, from a butterfly intravenous line) should be inserted into the external auditory canal, and the water irrigated into the ear while the patient's eyelids are held open. In cases of coma with intact brainstem pathways, the eyes should deviate toward the side of the cold water instillation. Absence of any eye movement will be present in a case of death by neurologic criteria. The eyes should be scrutinized for 1 minute after the cessation of icewater irrigation. After 5 minutes, the identical procedure should be repeated for the opposite ear.

APNEA TESTING

Before a formal apnea test is conducted, the patient should have fulfilled all previously discussed criteria for death by neurologic criteria. Severe chronic obstructive pulmonary disease or morbid obesity should not be present. Care should be taken to ensure that the patient has a systolic blood pressure of at least 90 mm Hg, has an adequate intravascular volume, and is treated with vasopressin if diabetes insipidus is suspected.

The patient should be preoxygenated to a Pao_2 exceeding 200 mm Hg. The ventilator should be disconnected, and 100% oxygen at a rate of 6 L/min placed at the carina or delivered directly into the trachea. Alternatively, 10 cm continuous positive airway pressure may be used. Maximal respiratory drive is believed to occur with a $Paco_2$ of 60 mm Hg, which should occur within 8 minutes after disconnection.[1] The patient is observed during this period for respiratory movements, and the electrocardiographic monitor examined for signs of respiratory artifact. If an arterial blood gas assessment shows a $Paco_2$ exceeding 60 mm Hg with continued apnea, the diagnosis of death by neurologic criteria is completed. The pH is the major determinant of respiratory drive, and if the patient's baseline Paco$_2$ is markedly abnormal, the equivalent change in the arterial pH should be employed.

If cardiac arrhythmias, hypotension, or arterial desaturation ensue, apnea testing is abandoned, and a confirmatory test must then be performed.

Confirmatory Testing

If apnea testing is not possible or cannot be completed, or if specific brainstem function testing is not possible, a confirmatory test must be performed. Numerous tests are available. Ranked from highest to lowest sensitivities, they are angiography, electroencephalography, transcranial Doppler echography, technetium-99m hexamethylpropyleneamineoxime (^{99m}Tc-HMPAO) brain scan (single photon emission computed tomography), and somatosensory evoked potentials.[2]

CEREBRAL ANGIOGRAPHY

Demonstration of lack of intracranial flow on angiography can be used to confirm death by neurologic criteria. Internal carotid artery flow usually stops shortly after the carotid bifurcation.[3] Vertebral flow usually stops at the atlanto-occipital junction.

ELECTROENCEPHALOGRAPHY

Confirmation of death by neurologic criteria can be made by establishing electrocerebral silence by electroencephalography (EEG). Since the EEG is affected by the same confounding factors as the physical examination (hypothermia and sedative drugs), it should be used only when such confounding factors have been disproved. Tracings are performed for at least 30 minutes with these settings: sensitivity greater than 2 μV/mm, high-frequency filter greater than 30 Hz, low-frequency filter less than 1 Hz, interelectrode impedance less than 10,000 Ohms, and a minimum of 8 scalp electrodes placed at least 10 cm apart. Guidelines for the minimal technical criteria for using EEG in confirming the diagnosis of death by neurologic criteria are available.[4]

TRANSCRANIAL DOPPLER BLOOD FLOW VELOCITY MEASUREMENT

Transcranial Doppler echography can also be used to confirm death by neurologic criteria. Early transcranial Doppler findings include oscillating flow signifying nearly equal forward and reverse flow, followed by a small systolic spike pattern suggesting lack of diastolic flow from severely increased intracranial pressure, and finally no signal. Because the absence of the transcranial Doppler signal can be due to technical difficulties, extracranial oscillating flow can be helpful when no signal is detected intracranially. Sensitivity and specificity for detecting death by neurologic criteria have been found to be 91.3% and 100%, respectively, when compared with the EEG.[5] Guidelines for the use of transcranial Doppler in confirming the diagnosis of death by neurologic criteria include two separate examinations at least 30 minutes apart demonstrating bilateral oscillating flow or systolic spikes in conjunction with bilateral common carotid artery, internal carotid artery, and vertebral artery oscillating flow.[6]

SINGLE PHOTON EMISSION COMPUTED TOMOGRAPHY

Single photon emission computed tomography with ^{99m}Tc-HMPAO can be used to document absent intracranial flow as noted by absent uptake of the tracer, which is administered 15 to 20 minutes prior to the scan.[7] This gives the appearance of an "empty skull."

SOMATOSENSORY EVOKED POTENTIALS

Somatosensory evoked potentials are useful in predicting outcome in patients who are comatose. N20 potentials are typically absent in those who have a diagnosis of death by neurologic criteria but are also absent in 15% to 20% of those who are comatose but do not have the diagnosis of death by neurologic criteria.

OTHER TESTS

Magnetic resonance angiography and computed tomography angiography can show absence of intracranial flow, but experience with these modalities is limited.

Children

The determination of death by neurologic criteria has some differences in children. For those between 7 days and 2 months of age, two examinations and EEGs should be performed at least 48 hours apart. For those 2 months to 1 year of age, a second examination and EEG are required 24 hours after the first, unless a radionuclide angiographic study fails to visualize cerebral vessels. For those older than 1 year, a repeat examination after 12 hours is typically recommended. In the case of hypoxic-ischemic cause, a longer period of observation is often recommended unless a confirmatory test is performed.[8]

Regional Rules and Laws

Unfortunately, there has been no standardization of legal determination of death by neurologic criteria internationally or even among the states in the United States. The basis for laws concerning the determination of death by neurologic criteria in most states is the Uniform Determination of Death Act, which indicates that death can be determined by irreversible lack of all brain function made in accordance with accepted medical standards. In 2010, the American Academy of Neurology published an updated practice parameter for the determination of brain death.[2] Individual institutions and some states have required additional standards to these guidelines. Local laws and regulations should be understood before a determination of death by neurologic criteria is made.

> **KEY POINTS**
>
> 1. After certain prerequisites are met, there are three essential components to the determination of death by neurologic criteria: irreversible coma or unresponsiveness, absence of brainstem reflexes, and apnea.
>
> 2. Patients being examined for a determination of death by neurologic criteria will all be on ventilatory assistance. The gag response can be difficult to determine in patients with endotracheal tubes in place.
>
> 3. Demonstration of lack of intracranial flow on angiography can be used to confirm death by neurologic criteria.
>
> 4. The determination of death by neurologic criteria has some differences in children.
>
> 5. Local laws and regulations should be understood before a determination of death by neurologic criteria is made.

ANNOTATED REFERENCE

Wijdicks EF, Varelas PN, Gronseth GS, Greer DM. American Academy of Neurology. Evidence-based guideline update: determining brain death in adults: report of the Quality Standards Subcommittee of the American Academy of Neurology. Neurology 2010;74:1911-8.
These provide guidelines for determining death by neurologic criteria.

REFERENCES

Access the complete reference list online at http://www.expertconsult.com.

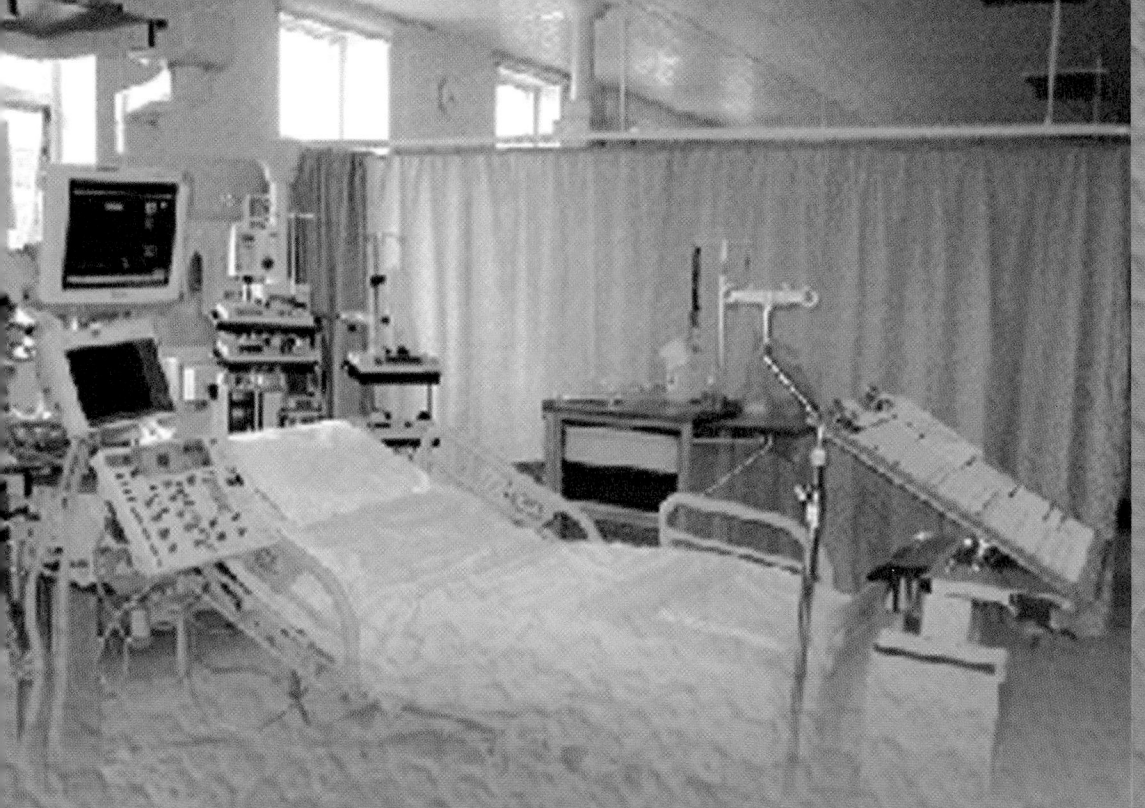

Organization and Management of Critical Care

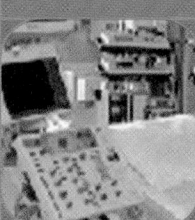

220 Building Teamwork to Improve Outcomes

MAURENE A. HARVEY | DALEEN ARAGON PENOYER | CONNIE JASTREMSKI

In the 1990s we realized that in the United States, critical care was unsafe, chaotic, disorganized, piecemeal, and reactive, with a high degree of variability based on style more than evidence. Care was being delivered by individuals more than by teams. Quality was often judged by benchmarking to peers with the same degree of dysfunction. In 1999, the Institute of Medicine (IOM) reported the in-depth study, "To Err is Human: Building a Safer Health System," that called for change to improve health care safety. The aging of the population has strained the healthcare system and will continue to produce a greater demand for critical care services. Over 5 million patients are admitted annually to an intensive care unit (ICU) in the United States. At the same time that demand appears to be rising, there are fewer critical care practitioners, physicians, nurses, pharmacists, and respiratory therapists to provide the necessary care, with the prediction that the problem will only become worse in the future. Healthcare professionals are concerned about fragmented impersonal care and being asked to do more with less.

As we struggle to increase patient safety, prevent harm, decrease chaos, and improve outcomes, mechanisms to integrate complex behavior into functional teamwork have become increasingly important. Harmonious and efficient integration of personnel and their respective expertise in the complex critical care environment is key to the delivery of high-quality intensive care.

This chapter will address the current climate, what is known about outcomes related to more effective teamwork, recommendations for developing better teamwork, and available tools to promote collaborative practice in the ICU.

Current Climate of Teamwork in Critical Care

Hospitals have traditionally been places where departments of professionals have protected their own ways of practicing, frequently in isolated silos without the understanding or cooperation of other departments. Historically, each profession has developed its own body of research, sets of standards, and practice agendas. In critical care, the urgency, complexity, and chaos of the environment makes teamwork even more important, and yet even harder to achieve than in most other areas.

Several factors can hamper the achievement of good teamwork in the ICU. Patients admitted to the hospital today have a higher severity of illness, yet they are being cared for with shorter lengths of stays. Patients discharged from ICUs today are often at the same acuity level as patients admitted to the ICU in the 1990s. While the current emphasis on evidence-based practice is bringing research to the bedside faster, growth in the volume of critical care research makes keeping up with best practices difficult. We practice in an environment of constant change in numbers of patients, in individual patient status, in participating team members, and available resources. Constant change can breed chaos. Increased oversight by regulators and third-party payers has affected bedside decision making as caregivers struggle to observe fiscal restraint without compromising quality of care.

In addition, clinicians are challenged to balance many things. We must distinguish patient needs from family needs, saving lives from prolonging death, patient versus societal needs, and following rules versus individualizing care. Scarce resources often necessitate rationing our time, expert personnel, and beds. These factors can breed stress, distress, or conflict. Moral distress, posttraumatic stress symptoms, depression, and burnout are all commonly found in critical care clinicians.[1]

In the past 40 years, agencies, commissions, and professional organizations have promoted improving teamwork. Regulatory and accrediting agencies, including The Joint Commission (TJC), have increased their emphasis on the importance of collaboration to obtain quality outcomes of care. The Society of Critical Care Medicine (SCCM) has focused on delivering the right care, right now. They advocate delivery of care by an integrated team of dedicated experts who learn it, implement it, measure it, and improve it.

Attitudes and perceptions of the quality of teamwork vary widely between institutions, units, individuals, clinicians, and professions. Nurses may perceive teamwork as good when physicians ask for and listen to their input. Physicians may perceive teamwork as good when nurses follow their instructions well. Surveys have shown that while the minority of nurses describe their unit's teamwork as good, the majority of the unit's physicians describe it that way.[2,3] Clinicians and managers are becoming more aware that organizational structures and processes affect patient care outcomes. Leaders at the unit, facility, state, and national level understand the importance of expert teams. They are promoting the creation of systems that allow teams to function at the highest level. More and more, change is being driven from the top down. Leaders are spreading the word that improved care delivery teams and systems can reduce costs and improve patient outcomes. It is widely believed that the only hospitals that will succeed in the future are those that can attract, train, and retain expert team members. To do this, hospitals will have to create a culture that demands top-notch teamwork and that will not tolerate poor performance.

Components of Effective Teamwork

In the broadest sense, *teamwork* is defined as working well together. Important components include communication, competence, trust, cooperation, coordination, respect, accountability, conflict resolution, and shared decision making.

The development of teamwork using these essential factors has a natural history. It begins with the movement away from practice in isolation toward practice in concert with other healthcare providers. Increasing contact can automatically lead to greater collaboration and communications whether or not they are consciously pursued. Collaboration and communication are much more likely to be optimal, however, when they reflect a deliberate effort to identify and clarify goals and to focus efforts on patient outcomes. Through the exchange of ideas and expertise, practitioners become familiar with the nature and scope of one another's practice. In this way each practitioner is better able to assess individual competence. Once clinical expertise is demonstrated, trust can be established, and negotiation of new roles for all care team members in the critical care environment is possible.

In critical care, each profession has dependent, independent, and interdependent roles. In addition, doctors and nurses often use different methods to resolve conflict. When resolving differences, physicians tend to bargain or negotiate and nurses avoid, accommodate, or compete. Focusing on the common goal of providing the best possible care for patients and their families is key to reducing team conflict.[2,4,5]

Over time, trust and open communication promotes respect. Team members begin to appreciate each other's skills, knowledge, and judgment. In collaborative practice, responsibility is shared, so that goal setting and decision-making occur jointly. Team leadership moves quickly and frequently from team member to team member depending on the issue at hand. To ensure every team member makes their optimal contribution, each must have the confidence to speak up whenever their input could be helpful and to be good listeners when others offer their input. This leads to more flexibility and creativity in problem solving or decision making.

SCCM's guideline for critical care delivery describes five general characteristics of the multidisciplinary team[6]:

1. Medical and nursing directors with authority and co-responsibility for ICU management
2. Nursing, respiratory therapy, and pharmacy collaboration with medical staff in a team approach
3. Use of standards, protocols, and guidelines to ensure a consistent approach to medical, nursing, and technical issues
4. Dedication to coordination and communication for all aspects of ICU management
5. Emphasis on practitioner certification, research, education, ethical issues, and patient advocacy

More recently, Reader et al.[3] have reviewed the body of research on teamwork in intensive care. They discuss input, process, and output variables. *Input variables* are the characteristics of team members, the tasks, and leadership. *Process variables* are team communication, leadership, and coordination. *Output variables* can be related to the patient or the team.

Another way of approaching it is to review what is known about team leadership. Good leaders are said to be able to generate two-way trust, respect, and communication. They have vision, self-confidence, enthusiasm, tolerance, and a commitment to excellence. They are organized and prepared, fulfill commitments, inspire shared missions, grow new leaders, model the way, challenge processes, tolerate ambiguity, and remain calm. It can be said that to have high-quality ICU teamwork, each team member should possess the same characteristics.

Although patients and families are important members of the ICU team, they are exempt from any of these expectations. We accept them as they are: in crisis, under stress, confused by the situation, and possibly in conflict. Yet we need their input for a better understanding of the patient's values and wishes and to tend to the family's own needs.

A team is not just as weak as the weakest link, but it is a balance of strong and weak members. Each individual team member, then, has the responsibility to make their strongest contribution. To do this, each of us must develop our listening skills, learn to speak up to make our observations and opinions known, ask for help when we need it, reinforce and praise the contributions of others, model behavior we expect, take time to think before we act, think out loud to help novices develop, and use positive professional communication.

Creating an environment within the healthcare system to ensure the safest collaborative care model and highly effective teamwork is the responsibility of everyone involved in the care of the critically ill and their families. It requires our focus, commitment, time, and energy.

Impact of Teamwork on Outcomes

Despite the support for teamwork and development of an interdisciplinary team model for the care of critically ill patients, research on the relationship to outcomes is limited.[7] A literature review on the effectiveness of patient care teams in a variety of healthcare settings found limited effect on patient outcomes, and the added value of coordination of care was unclear.[8] However, reports from some recent studies in critical care have demonstrated positive effects. The following section summarizes the current literature on teamwork and outcomes.

TEAMWORK AND CARE DELIVERY

In 2005, the Institute of Healthcare Improvement (IHI) began a 1-year nationwide initiative called *The 100,000 Lives Campaign* to reduce morbidity and mortality in American health care (http://www.ihi.org/IHI/Programs/Campaign/100kCampaignOverviewArchive.htm). They invited hospitals to join by agreeing to address six areas requiring process improvement. Four of these (ventilator associated pneumonia, catheter-related bloodstream infections, surgical site infections, and rapid response teams) involve critical care teamwork. Approximately 2800 hospitals joined the campaign, which resulted in saving more lives than predicted.

Patients in ICUs are frequently exposed to and vulnerable to medical errors. The severity of illness, complexity and number of interventions, pervasiveness of invasive catheters and equipment, and length of stay in the ICU put critically ill patients at higher risk of adverse events and errors.[9-12] One comprehensive review of the literature on critical incidents in intensive care showed an increased incidence of adverse events when there was a deficit in nontechnical skills, including elements of teamwork.[13]

Ineffective communication and poor teamwork have been identified as significant contributors to patient errors and critical incidents in the ICU.[12,14,15] Improvements in processes for communication have the potential to reduce such adverse events and errors.[15-16] In medicine, the focus has been on what should be done without enough attention to execution or planning how to get it done.[10] To effectively carry out any plan of care in the ICU, coordination of care between disciplines and departments with clear, specific communication about the treatment plan is needed. One initiative to improve teamwork in the ICU involved establishing physician-led multidisciplinary rounds, assessing bed availability daily, using "bundles" of evidence-based practice care, and making efforts to change culture. The result was a significant reduction in nosocomial infections (ventilator-associated pneumonia, bloodstream and urinary tract infections), adverse events, and costs of care.[17] This approach also led to improved communication among providers, enhanced team knowledge, and better coordination of care. Implementing a team decision-making culture placed responsibility on the team rather than on the physician and resulted in empowered team members.

The Veterans Administration has reported improvements in team communication and the quality of care after implementing a medical team training program to enhance team performance, satisfaction, and patient outcomes.[14] They credited their debriefing training and process with the avoidance of potential adverse events in surgical patients, such as performing a procedure on the incorrect site or performing the wrong procedure. This also led to improvements in surgical efficiency, management of fatigue, more active collaboration between disciplines, increased nurse job satisfaction and morale, and reduced errors.

TEAMWORK AND PATIENT OUTCOMES

Intensivist-led multidisciplinary teams have been espoused as an ideal model for critical care. However, there are insufficient numbers of trained intensivists to meet current or future demands, and only a minority of ICUs have implemented intensivist staffing.[7,18] Further, results from outcomes studies on intensivist-led care demonstrate mixed findings.[18-19] One recent study from a large cohort of patients examined mortality outcomes from hospitals with daily rounds by multidisciplinary teams with and without intensivist models compared to those without this structure.[7] They found that hospitals with multidisciplinary team care were associated with 16% lower odds for mortality, and those with high intensivist staffing and multidisciplinary team care were associated with the most significantly reduced odds ratio of death. Interestingly, hospitals with a multidisciplinary team approach but low physician staffing also had a significant reduction in mortality. This reinforces the idea that patients do benefit when cared for by a multidisciplinary team. However, the most benefit comes when that team is led by a trained intensivist. In another study, mortality was significantly reduced in patients with acute lung injury (ALI) who were cared for by multidisciplinary teams led by fulltime critical care physicians.[20] The use of the intensivist-led team model also led to significantly reduced mortality, duration of mechanical ventilation, and rates for ventilator-associated pneumonia (VAP) in a military setting.[21] In a literature review, Durbin also found that the team model for ICU care delivery was associated with reduced mortality, ICU and hospital length of stay, and costs of care.[22]

One hospital in Illinois achieved several improved outcomes by implementing evidenced-based bundles of care and a multidisciplinary daily goals rounding tool. They found decreased ICU lengths of stay, improved compliance with care protocols, reduced VAP and bloodstream infections, and fewer falls and pressure ulcers in surgical ICU patients.[23] Cheung et al.[24] did not find improved outcomes, however, when the team met on a weekly basis and decided that the meetings were too infrequent to impact patient outcomes. Research has shown that teamwork can also influence the discharge process from the ICU[25] through coordination of efforts.

The ability to achieve patient goals in the ICU is also impacted by team leadership and management skills of attending physicians.[26] Developing written daily goals in the ICU improves communication between caregivers about expectations for care and follow-through on treatment plans. Failure to complete treatment plans has been recognized as a key factor leading to errors in the ICU.[10,26] Fostering teamwork to accomplish daily goals can improve care effectiveness and patient safety.

Multidisciplinary teams developed to respond to shock in nontrauma patients resulted in decreased time to treatment, intensivist arrival, and admission to the ICU.[27] This resulted in a significant reduction in mortality as well as an increased likelihood of good patient outcomes.

TEAMWORK AND TEAM OUTCOMES

Communication, a key component of teamwork, has been associated with job satisfaction. Recent studies have shown a difference in perception about communication among practice disciplines in critical care.[2,15,28-30] Nurses report lower quality of communication with physicians than those physicians report. In one survey, 33% of critical care nurses ranked the quality of collaboration and communication with physicians highly as compared to 73% of physicians.[2,15] The degree of open communication among ICU team members correlated with better understanding of patient care goals.

Differing perceptions between nurses and physicians also exist regarding the care of dying patients in the ICU.[29] Nurses reported more moral distress and lower collaboration than their physician counterparts. Nurses perceived the ethical environment as more negative and were less satisfied with the quality of care of those patients than were attending physicians. Their evaluation of the quality of care was strongly related to the perception of collaboration between disciplines. A study by Huang[30] found that physicians, leadership, and nursing directors tended to overestimate nurses' attitudes on teamwork climate and working conditions. Weinberg[31] found the quality of medical resident communication with nurses was dependent on a nurse's degree of cooperation and congeniality with them. Their level of trust in information communicated also was dependent on their perception of nurse competence and their ability to relay relevant information in a timely manner. Although nearly all physicians reported instances of poor communication with nurses, they did not see it as a threat to patient care, because they thought the nurses' role was to simply follow orders. This indicates that these medical residents did not necessarily view nurses as colleagues and collaborators. In critical care, the multidisciplinary team members are dependent on each other to accomplish the complex needs of patients, and all are accountable for the outcomes achieved.

When teamwork increases efficiencies of care, an increased sense of accomplishment can occur.[32,33] Research has shown that nurses preferred communicating with attending physicians over first-year residents and valued shared understanding and open, accurate communication.[34] In addition, the more experience nurses had, the more they required effective communication with experienced physicians. Another study by the same researcher showed that nurse-to-physician communication was a significant predictor of nurse job satisfaction and the quality of the practice environment.[35] The degree of workplace empowerment and perceived quality of the environment was significantly related to communication between nurses and physicians.[36-37] When a higher level of nurse-physician communication was reported, medication errors were reduced.[36] When timeliness of communication improved, there was a decrease in the prevalence of pressure ulcers.[37]

Finally, daily multidisciplinary rounds led by a hospitalist medical director paired with a nurse practitioner resulted in improved physician-to-nurse collaboration, particularly with residents. In this model, the nurse practitioner was able to facilitate coordination of patient care and communication between nurses and physicians.[38]

■ Strategies to Establish Better Teamwork

Because teamwork is so important for practice in the ICU, how does an organization develop teamwork skills among a wide variety of professionals? There are certain steps that can be taken to implement team structures and processes that can help build teamwork in critical care.

Models for developing strong teamwork have developed from industries with high risks for errors, including aviation, the military, and nuclear power. In these industries, effective teamwork is an important mechanism used to maintain safety, reduce errors, and increase efficiencies.[39-40] In these models, team members use specific processes for communication, leadership, coordination, and decision making to achieve positive outcomes for team performance.

Although health care is different from aviation and nuclear power, there are some lessons that can be learned from them to improve teamwork and quality of care of the critically ill.[40] Applicable strategies include standardizing work processes and using checklists to make sure patients are consistently getting the best care based upon the most current science and evidence. Other relevant strategies that can be learned from these industries are those used to improve teamwork skills, collaborative engagement, and communication. Any person on the interdisciplinary team should be able to speak up when they identify potential patient safety hazards. Team members must have mechanisms to openly identify areas of high risk for errors and harm. A blame-free culture encourages team members to recognize, report, and thus minimize errors. The ability to learn from mistakes is an essential component of error prevention.

Reader et al.[39] consolidated the research literature of the relationship between teamwork and patient outcomes in critical care to develop a framework for teamwork in the ICU environment. They emphasized that effective teamwork is crucial to provide optimal patient care in the ICU and that good leadership is vital for team interaction and coordination. In their framework, they identified four key performance competencies and needs to build effective teams in the ICU: team communication, team coordination, team leadership, and team decision making.

One strategy used by interdisciplinary teams is to engage in quality improvement initiatives in the ICU.[41] Team leaders promote teamwork to examine potential issues in care and to prioritize projects and initiatives using a systematic process. When building project plans, it is important to include key stakeholders and to collect and use the latest evidence to aid in making decisions. Ongoing audit and feedback, discussion by opinion leaders, prompts and reminders such as checklists and order sets, and educational reinforcement are other tools that may solidify and sustain the team's change efforts. Ongoing behavior modifications may be needed to engage all team members in the change. Good team leaders collaborate with the team members to sustain quality efforts and help them through difficulties of adapting to change.

BARRIERS TO TEAM PERFORMANCE

Implementing teamwork strategies within acute health care has its benefits and challenges. Barriers to implementing a team model in critical care can include local customs, hospital patterns, and reluctance to change despite proven benefit.[22] Implementation requires a cultural shift. The existence of hierarchical and status differences in acute care can present a barrier to team function and the ability of team members to openly contribute to the plan of care.[28,42] Team members may not be convinced that their input is important or needed to make decisions about patient care.

Another barrier to the intensivist-led team in the ICU is the lack of an adequate number of qualified physicians who are trained in critical care.[18] The ability to recruit medical residents into critical care fellowships is challenging, particularly with concerns about financial compensation and hectic lifestyle. Additionally, there are costs associated with implementation of the intensivist model.[18,22] Without strong leadership at the bedside, it is more difficult to implement team models of care. However, even without a designated intensivist, establishing a multidisciplinary team in the ICU improves outcomes.[7]

Another obstacle is that working as a team requires some team members to forfeit their autonomy in practice.[22] This may be difficult when team leaders hold high value in their ability to orchestrate things without the aid of others. The physician leader must be willing to engage members of the team and establish respect and trust for their contribution to discussion and decision making.

Many practitioners in the ICU have not been trained in teamwork activities and are not prepared with the skills required. While teamwork is not related to technical expertise, it is a nontechnical skill necessary for patient safety.[13] Each member's knowledge, skill, and personality characteristics have an important influence on the effectiveness of patient care teams.[8] One qualitative study showed that emotional distress individual members experienced during medical crises impacts the function of the entire team through contagion of anxiety.[1] Another study on team interactions during crises found that in the post-crisis period, nurses were left with significant questions and emotions about the event compared to other members of the team.[44] Potential solutions to these barriers are to hold interdisciplinary team debriefings and feedback sessions immediately after crises, assess for gaps in teamwork competencies, and determine opportunities for team training. Team leaders need to assess anxiety among team members during crises and help defuse potential emotional breakdowns during critical interventions. Team training may also help prepare members emotionally for real events and enable them to gain experience in safer settings.

PROGRAMS USED TO DEVELOP TEAMWORK IN THE ICU

Programs designed to improve team core competencies and communication skills may improve team performance through experiential team learning. A successful pediatric critical care unit provided an interdisciplinary experiential learning day-long program (Program to Enhance Relational and Communication Skills [PERCS]) to improve communication skills and relational abilities when having difficult conversations with family members. The training included video case scenarios and debriefing feedback sessions and shared communication about experiences with difficult conversations with families. This approach resulted in improved communication skills, confidence, and perceptions of preparation. Anxiety was reduced and then sustained.[32]

Teamwork skills can be developed to improve communication between physicians and nurses that improves care at the end of life (EOL).[45] Studies have shown that nurses and physicians differ in perspectives and burdens felt as the result of decisions made at the end of life. Strategies to improve communication between caregivers include joint grand rounds, patient care seminars, and interprofessional dialogue about EOL care. Using tools such as daily rounds forms, communication training, and a collaborative practice model are other mechanisms that may improve physician-nurse communication and EOL care.

Teamwork can also be enhanced when multidisciplinary expertise is focused on key patient outcomes. One example of a successful program was a critical care team that examined its practice to determine factors that interfered with mobility in mechanically ventilated patients.[33] The ICU staff developed a team strategy to improve their culture to focus on improving early mobility in ventilated patients and a process to evaluate the effectiveness on patient outcomes. This initiative enabled the team to improve patients' functional abilities and long-term outcomes.

In one study, a Delphi method was used to identify key components needed for crew resource management training in the hospital environment. Five areas were identified: communication, task management, situational awareness, decision making and leadership.[43] Programs to improve patient safety and collaboration in the ICU have been developed using a crew resource management (CRM) approach.[42] Team members are taught to promote safety by changing attitudes and behaviors. Tools used are team training in interpersonal communication, conflict resolution, and nonthreatening evaluation of critique of team performance. Education may include methods to improve system processes for care, including the use of checklists and standardizing handoffs to relate key information. Additionally, CRM training can be used to teach methods to counter patient care errors such as debriefings, cross-checking, and review of patient care plans. Team members can learn how to actively participate in decision making and how to question actions and decisions among team members in a constructive manner. This allows for open communication and the ability to speak up about concerns or recommendations for patient care.

TEAM TRAINING USING SIMULATION

Currently, more organizations are using simulation as a means to educate and train members of teams to function under specific circumstances. Members of the interdisciplinary team use simulation to learn and practice roles in various clinical situations and to evaluate communication and team effectiveness. Team learning in simulation exercises allows professionals to learn and practice safely under circumstances outside of stressful clinical settings. Team members learn their roles and contributions in key clinical scenarios.

Simulation can be used to train teams to manage septic shock by creating an ICU environment and using a high-fidelity patient simulator (mannequin).[46] In one study, residents participated in exercises in a simulated environment during their ICU rotations. A mannequin was programmed to give complaints and responses to questions using a standardized scenario. Participants had access to vital signs and could ask questions about the patient's condition. These were video recorded for later review and debriefing with the residents and other members of the team after performance scoring by senior faculty. Both technical and nontechnical (teamwork) functions were evaluated. They found this method to be an effective tool to test and teach knowledge, clinical application, and teamwork principles, and to evaluate the quality of performance in simulations of septic shock.

Handoff of a patient from one professional to another or transfer to other areas within a hospital creates an opportunity for miscommunication to occur. This is particularly true of nurse-to-nurse communication at shift change and patient transfer to other units. The use of standardized communication tools such as SBAR (Situation, Background, Assessment, Recommendation) can be instrumental in conveying important information between shifts, departments, nurses, and physicians. Berkenstadt et al.[47] used a 6-hour simulation-based training workshop to improve nurse teamwork and communication. In this program, nurses viewed videos on demonstration of relevant handoff tasks followed by debriefing sessions and discussion. This resulted in a significant increase in communication of crucial information and treatment goals during handoffs between nurses. This use of simulation may be an effective means to train any caregiver on handoff communication.

Simulation has also been used to train healthcare workers on CRM as a means to improve teamwork competencies. One example is a comprehensive Medical Team Training (MTT) full-day interactive program. The aim was to improve patient outcomes and enhance job satisfaction among the interdisciplinary team in the Veterans Administration's Employee Education Service. Their program was facilitated by a physician-nurse pair. The faculty came from multiple disciplines and professions to model collaboration and teamwork. This program includes rules of conduct, communication principles, tools, and techniques, debriefing processes, and processes for safe handoffs. Multiple modes of education were used to reinforce material over the one-day seminar, including simulation, interaction, discussion, and videos to demonstrate and model teamwork behaviors. Participation in this program resulted in improvements in communication and the quality of care.[14]

High-fidelity simulation can be used to evaluate team performance in resuscitation of the critically ill. In a pilot study by Kim et al.,[48] a high-fidelity simulation of recreated emergencies encountered in acute care was used to teach and evaluate crisis resource management skills in first- and third-year residents. In their study, they included a simulated ICU environment and other team members (nurse and respiratory therapist) to further augment the simulated sessions. They were able to use this model to represent clinical scenarios of the management of acute respiratory failure, airway management, myocardial ischemia, trauma, and shock occurring in the ICU, postanesthesia care unit, and emergency room. The scenarios used were originated from real-life cases encountered in their hospital. They were able to validate their tool for assessment for crisis resource management. They support this model as a means of evaluating team leadership and decision-making skills in critical events encountered in acute care.

RESOURCES AVAILABLE

There are resources made available for critical care teambuilding by various organizations. The American Association of Critical Care Nurses has made a commitment to their initiative to promote a healthy work environment. Their website has many tools for evaluating and promoting teamwork (aacn.org). The IHI is dedicated to quality improvement processes. Since team work is key to most of their initiatives, their website (ihi.org) has many useful tools for teambuilding. The Agency for Healthcare Research and Quality (AHRQ) and the Veterans Administration (VA) are collaborating on the STEPPS project: Strategies and Tools to Enhance Performance and Patient Safety. Information on this program with teambuilding at its core can be found on their website (teamstepps.ahrq.gov).

Examples of Teamwork in Critical Care

COLLABORATIVE PRACTICE TEAMS

Collaborative practice teams (CPTs) are groups that are assembled for a particular population to address issues related to clinical practice and outcomes. These teams are multiprofessional and interdisciplinary in scope and function. They design initiatives to drive evidence-based practice and improve quality of care. The team composition usually consists of representative practitioners directly involved in the care of patients. In critical care this could include intensivists and other physicians, nurses, respiratory therapists, pharmacists, nutritionists, social workers, clergy, administrators, risk managers, infection control, safety officers, and quality improvement personnel. The goal is to capture expertise from multiple disciplines to improve delivery of care. The actual composition of CPTs depends on the nature of the ICU and patient population and should be individualized to each facility. Examples of CPT initiatives are the development of disease-specific

protocols, care "bundles," order sets, and performance improvement campaigns.

DAILY MULTIDISCIPLINARY ROUNDS WITH THE INTERDISCIPLINARY TEAM AND DAILY GOALS

The use of multidisciplinary rounds on patients every day in the ICU enhances patient care.[22] When caregivers meet as a team to discuss and plan for patient care and use evidence-based protocols and care bundles, the opportunity for teamwork, team planning, and team accountability exists. Daily rounds also provide opportunities to augment efforts and initiatives by the CPT. Communication about the plan of care by the team can be facilitated by using a daily goals checklist during daily rounds.[49] Caregivers are tasked with specific functions and assignments that are reviewed for completion at the end of the day. Team goals improve accountability for patient care and momentum for progress. This approach has been demonstrated to improve team and patient outcomes.[26,49,50] Siegele described the impact of implementing daily team goals for patients in a surgical ICU.[23] A daily goals tool with patient-centric goals to improve communication, collaboration, and coordination of care was established for the multidisciplinary team. Evidence-based practices and care bundles were used. These tools can be adapted for many practice areas or groups of disciplines that work together for common patient goals. Several days to 1 week can be placed on one tool. They can be used for follow-up to make sure goals were met and to determine next steps.

Krimsky et al. developed a model to increase implementation of measures to prevent venous thrombosis, VAP, and stress ulcers in ICU patients.[51] Their systematic approach integrated evidence-based strategies, a tool to develop team communication and team building, daily prompts in ICU progress notes to assess these complications, and real-time feedback of performance measures to correct behaviors. This model allowed incorporation of these evidence-based practices using a team-based culture of patient safety.

TEAMS WITH SPECIFIC CLINICAL FOCUS

Some teams are formed to manage care for particular situations or patient types. One example is the use of multidisciplinary medical emergency response teams to respond to calls about acute changes in patient condition. These teams facilitate timely assessment and treatment of patients to reduce the development of further complications or cardiopulmonary arrest. Other specialty teams can be developed to assess and manage urgent clinical conditions such as stroke, sepsis,[46] and shock.[27] Team training and evidence-based practice tools can be developed for these teams to assist them in efficient and effective practice.

Conclusion

In an ideal world, all the resources required to provide high-quality care focused on patient and family needs would be immediately available. These needs would be determined by a team that has a high degree of respect for each other, that values and listens to each other's contribution, where each individual team member contributes from a rich and up-to-date knowledge base, and which results in a plan of care that is delivered in a timely and efficient manner.

The ICU is a dynamic environment that requires coordinated efforts to optimize patient outcomes. Through conscientiously applied principles of team building, medicine, nursing, and other healthcare disciplines can be integrated while preserving the interests of each individual and profession.

Team building is expected to be a common feature of future hospital environments. Team building tools will continue to evolve and become more robust. As a result, quality critical care will be delivered, and costs will be reduced.

KEY POINTS

1. As care of the critically ill has become more complex and resources more limited, there has been increased emphasis on teamwork to improve outcomes and reduce costs.

2. Current factors that can interfere with ICU teamwork include increasing patient acuity, rapidly developing evidence-based practice changes, increased oversight of critical care delivery, and the stressful nature of intensive care practice.

3. Key skills required for teamwork include communication, competence, trust, cooperation, coordination, respect, accountability, conflict resolution, and shared decision making.

4. With the increased focus on teamwork, several tools and resources have become available.

5. Research shows that improved processes in teamwork and communication can lead to improved patient outcomes and healthcare team satisfaction.

6. The interdisciplinary team has an opportunity to partner together to drive quality improvements in the care of the critically ill.

7. Barriers to teamwork in critical care include lack of team training in academic preparation, insufficient physician-led multidisciplinary teams, and lack of teamwork competencies among healthcare workers.

8. Simulation is a useful means to train healthcare workers in the ICU setting on teamwork skills and crew resource management (CRM).

ANNOTATED REFERENCES

Brilli RJ, Spevets A, Branson RD, et al. Critical care delivery in the intensive care unit: defining clinical roles and the best practice model. Crit Care Med 2001;29:2007-19.
This article is the consensus report of two task forces of the SCCM. It represents the work of 31 healthcare professionals and practitioners, including statisticians and representatives from industry, pharmacy, nursing, and respiratory care and physicians who are involved in the practice of critical care. This report suggests that the best practice in critical care is collaborative practice with a multidisciplinary team.

Reader TW, Flin R, Mearns K, et al. Developing a team performance framework for the intensive care unit. Crit Care Med 2009;37:1787-93.
This article summarizes evidence on the relationship between teamwork behaviors and patient outcomes. Skills required for effective team performance are identified. Synthesis of the existing literature yielded a framework organized around three aspects: input, team processes, and output. This framework can be used as a guide to team building in the ICU.

Curtis JR, Cook DJ, Wall RJ, et al. Intensive care unit quality improvement: a "how-to" guide for the interdisciplinary team. Crit Care Med 2006;34:211-8.
This article summarizes how a team can work together to accomplish performance improvement initiatives in the ICU. In this article, the systematic steps an interdisciplinary team can take to develop or enhance quality improvement are summarized. Key roles for team members and leadership are identified.

American Association of Critical Care Nurses. AACN's healthy work environments initiative. Available at: http://www.aacn.org/wd/hwe/content/hwehome.pcms?pid=1&&menu=
The AACN has established an initiative to promote healthier work environments which allow teamwork to flourish. The website includes descriptions of ingredients for success in creating healthy environments, tools for assessing teams, and links to many other helpful resources.

Institute for Healthcare Improvement (IHI). http://www.ihi.org/ihi
The IHI has been very successful in teaching teams to use a rapid cycle change process to improve care delivery and patient outcomes. The website includes information on process improvement, tools for implementing change and evaluating progress, and guidance for addressing specific patient and system problems.

REFERENCES

Access the complete reference list online at http://www.expertconsult.com.

221

Pursuit of Performance Excellence

JOSH ETTINGER | JOEL ETTINGER | PETER J. PRONOVOST | THOMAS G. RAINEY

In the beginning it was all about the art—magicians or medicine men who were thought to have special powers and could cure the sick through communing with a higher power. As societies became more complex and evolved, a more scientific approach began to influence the healing of the sick. Ancient Egypt provides us with one of the first documented pieces of evidence of this transition through the Edwin Smith Papyrus (17th century BC) covering 48 cases examining a variety of traumas to the human body. From here, the art and science of care metastasized many times over (and still today)—sometimes in conflict, but always progressing toward greater treatments, greater therapies … greater understanding. For the last 50 years, the art and science of medicine has been struggling to come to terms with a new challenge/opportunity, one born out of necessity as therapies became more expensive and complicated. Ideally, the solution should set parameters, demands, and requirements but also provide a dynamic for enabling better use of resources, individual and organizational knowledge, and accelerating the pursuit of excellence. This opportunity, the business of medicine, is an integral part of health care today and in the future, and together with the art and science, is part of a new paradigm. It is time for a new construct—a model for health care that focuses on and weaves together leadership, talented professionals, innovation, reliability, excellence, sustainability, efficiency, effectiveness, and safety.

It is a truism that most performance is average, though often with large variation. But average is often failure, and in the intensive care unit (ICU), where life is extremely fragile, *average* means patients are dying needlessly. The obligation is only excellence every time, for every patient. Those who are willing to make the commitment to strive for world-class performance should read on. There is a dearth of literature that directly addresses how leaders of ICUs can create a system that engages the workforce, supports great teamwork, creates an environment for continuous and rapid innovation, astutely develops and deploys strategy, distinctly focuses on holistic patient excellence, and delivers care at the highest possible clinical competency with the greatest effectiveness and efficiency.

Organizations consist of numerous parts, systems, and functions all operating and, ideally, collaborating to produce an end result, one that is not always desired. Unlike the organs of the human body, in healthcare delivery, different components often struggle to operate in a coordinated and symbiotic fashion. Systems such as pharmacy, lab billing, ICU, operating room, emergency department, internal medicine, surgery, and graduate medical education programs frequently operate independently without the coordination necessary to produce reliably integrated operations. The parts seem more independent than interdependent, more competitive than cooperative, and more focused on their own efforts than on the results of the whole. Whereas each part has to remain viable and effective in order to contribute to the overall goals and purpose of the organization, all parts must operate in harmony for superior performance to be achieved and maintained. Using the Baldrige Performance Excellence Program (BPEP or Baldrige) as a framework (Figure 221-1), this chapter provides guidance on how to design and manage the ICU to improve patient outcomes and be a great part of the larger hospital system. The Baldrige framework is elaborate, and a full presentation is beyond the scope of this chapter. A complete guide to the framework can be found at www.baldrige.org.

Background and Overview

The BPEP began in 1983 when business and federal leaders got together to create an awards program to stimulate excellence, competition, and innovation during a time when the U.S. manufacturing and service industries were losing market share to foreign companies. The end result produced an evolving set of robust criteria based on best practices across seven different but highly interrelated spheres. Organizations that pursue the Baldrige and submit an application can be recognized by the President of the United States for exhibiting role-model practices. While there is an awards component, most organizations adopt the criteria for its demonstrable value rather than the recognition. For several years since the program began in 1988, the stock performance of publicly traded Baldrige Award recipient organizations has outperformed the Standard & Poor's 500 in most years by as much as six to one. Organizations around the world have adopted the Baldrige criteria as a framework for improving organizational performance practices, capabilities, and results. Since health care was added as an industry permitted to apply for the Baldrige Award in 1999, only 12 hospitals have been recognized.

The Baldrige criteria have been validated to guide organizational success at both a macro system level (hospital level) and the constituent micro system level (division, service line, department, or unit). ICUs are prime candidates to benefit from application of the Baldrige platform. The fragile patient population requires highly reliable delivery of very precise care around the clock. The environment is complex with multiple layers of caregivers, and diverse technologies and medications which are lifesaving yet life threatening if performed improperly and occur simultaneously (e.g., mechanical ventilation, dialysis, and invasive monitoring). The opportunity for error/harm is high, the patients' tolerance for error is marginal, and the cost is huge. Improvement demonstrations over the past 10 years (Keystone Project, Institute for Healthcare Improvement [IHI] and Veterans Health Administration [VHA] and New Jersey Hospital Association [NJHA] ICU collaboratives) have demonstrated that ICU patients are suffering unnecessary morbidity and mortality, and improvement in outcomes and cost is possible but requires a systems approach. For example, most U.S. ICUs lack intensivist staff, an intervention associated with a 30% reduction in hospital mortality and costs, that has demonstrated improvement in eliminating the preventable deaths of 31,000 people each year from central line–associated bloodstream infections (CLABSI). The need to improve is urgent. Indeed, the Baldrige platform approach can serve to orchestrate improvement in this complex environment. ICU leaders can use the Baldrige framework to improve clinical and economic performance. This framework is goal directed and measurement driven. Briefly, the Baldrige Health Care Criteria are built on four integrated components: organizational profile, 11 core values and concepts, seven categories of criteria for high performance, and differentiation of high performance versus average performance or scoring guidelines.

ORGANIZATIONAL PROFILE

The first integrated component, the organizational profile, is a brief description of how the organization (or ICU) operates, its customers and their expectations, its primary services, core competencies, the

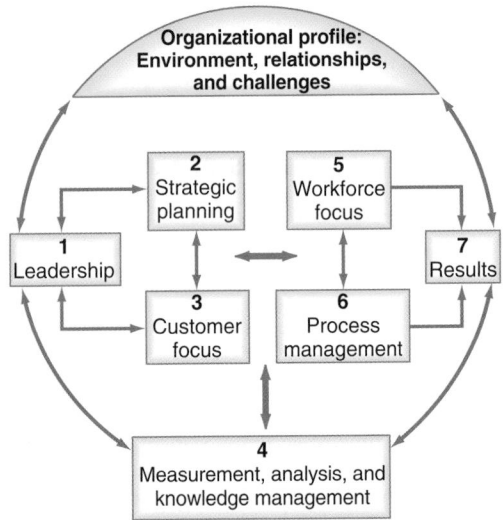

Figure 221-1 Baldrige healthcare criteria for performance excellence framework: a systems perspective. (*Adapted from www.baldrige.org.*)

workforce (which includes all paid staff, medical staff, and volunteers) requirements/needs, critical success factors, and key challenges, to name a few. There are around 20 questions that ask the ICU to identify, with extreme clarity, the important elements that guide the delivery of care.

ELEVEN CORE VALUES AND CONCEPTS

The second integrated component consists of 11 interrelated core values and concepts that have strong cultural enrichment implications. They have been validated to be embedded in the beliefs and behaviors (the culture) of high-performing organizations:

1. Visionary leadership
2. Patient-focused excellence
3. Organizational and personal learning
4. Valuing of workforce members and partners
5. Agility
6. Focus on the future
7. Managing for innovation
8. Management by fact
9. Social responsibility and community health
10. Focus on results and the creation of value
11. Systems perspective

SEVEN CATEGORIES OF CRITERIA FOR HIGH PERFORMANCE

The seven categories of healthcare criteria for performance excellence, which constitute the third integrated component, serve as the locus of role-model performance. The criteria are presented as a series of questions that ask how an organization's (or unit's) approaches (or methods) to work are designed and managed so that they are systematic (or repeatable), deployed to all locations and internal/external people as appropriate, and are continuously improved, aligned with the key areas of importance to the ICU, and integrated with other processes and systems to effectively deliver care. The criteria present direct actionable guidance by identifying existing strengths and opportunities for improvement. The power lies not in the individual areas but rather the interplay of the seven categories, which are as follows:

1. Leadership
2. Strategic planning
3. Customer focus
4. Measurement, analysis, and knowledge management
5. Workforce focus
6. Operations focus
7. Results

DIFFERENTIATION OF HIGH PERFORMANCE VERSUS AVERAGE PERFORMANCE OR SCORING GUIDELINES

The scoring guidelines serve as the fourth component of the framework. These four elements are critical to understanding performance, identifying opportunities for improvement and innovation, and achieving sustained excellence. Together, the characteristics differentiate high-performing organizations from average ones in that all work must be:

1. Systematic (i.e., well-ordered and repeatedly done in the way it is designed to be done, demonstrating reliability)
2. Fully deployed (i.e., the work is done systematically everywhere it is supposed to be done—all sites, departments, units, and staff)
3. Evaluated for effectiveness as part of an ongoing cycle of learning, improvement, and/or innovation (i.e., improvement is built into how work is done)
4. Aligned and integrated (i.e., connected to key factors such as the mission, the vision, the ICU department objectives, the needs of ICU patients and family members, to name a few; and harmonized with other key ICU/organizational processes and systems to achieve maximum efficiency and effectiveness)

High-performing organizations differentiate the results of their critical success factors from those of lesser organizations based on (1) whether current results are good, (2) how results trend over time (i.e., show consistently better performance), and (3) how trended results compare with best-in-industry (role-model) performance.

How does all this relate to ICUs? ICUs across the country are struggling with increased complexity, higher costs, more errors, staffing shortages, decreasing morale, and low staff, customer, and patient satisfaction and engagement. The human service purpose of ICUs is far too precious for ICU quality to become increasingly debilitated—a sign of leadership failure. Industry experts must find a road map that can guide the pursuit of sustained excellence. The objective is to move progressively higher in the realm of excellence.

Next, we provide an overview of each of the Baldrige criteria, using a selection of the key ideas in the seven categories, and provide examples of how they can be applied in the ICU to achieve world-class performance and excellence. It is important to remember that the Baldrige program is not an improvement tool like Six Sigma or the Plan-Do-Check-Act (PDCA). Rather, it is a framework that provides guidelines and a structure to establish and sustain culture and processes that go *beyond* conformance to standards, differing from requirements such as those of The Joint Commission. Baldrige asks fundamental questions that will help lead and guide organizations—and ICUs—toward the highest levels of performance excellence. It is how the work should be organized, managed, improved, and innovated. And, whereas the Baldrige framework asks these important questions, the ICU leaders need to provide the answers.

The Baldrige Intensive Care Unit

CATEGORY 1: LEADERSHIP

The leadership category provides insight on how leaders can guide their organizations to high levels of performance. It analyzes how clinical and nonclinical leaders use values, directions, and performance expectations, as well as a focus on patients, other customers, workforce engagement, innovation, and continuous improvement, as vehicles to secure systematic action and sustained excellence. In the Baldrige framework, leadership is not just an organizational chart of positions. It is also a system—a set of leadership behaviors that move and align the organization toward a common purpose with specific goals and objectives. Leadership systems include the formal and informal method of exercising leadership elements such as decision making, communication, setting expectations, organization of work, reward and

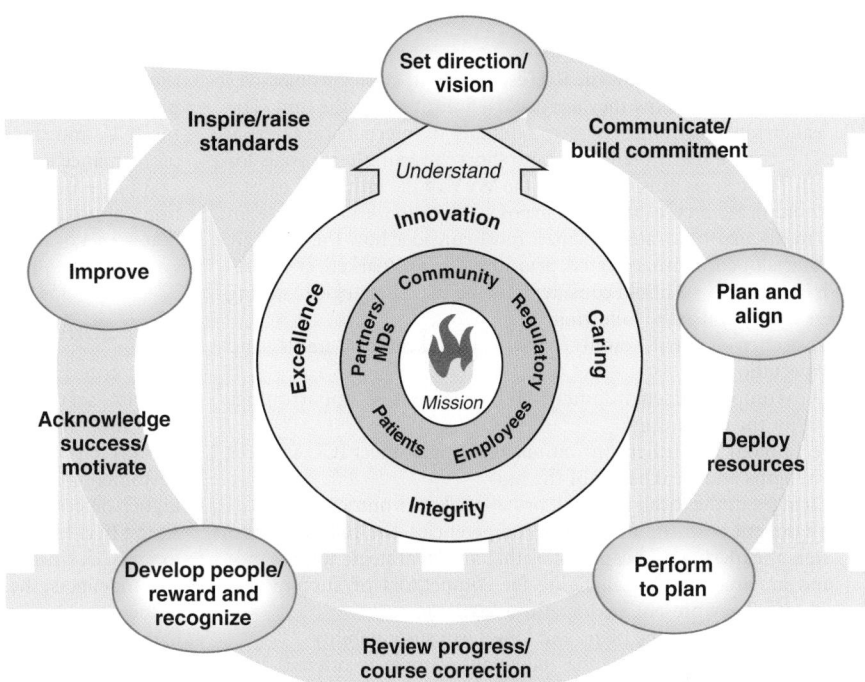

Figure 221-2 Example of a leadership system (Sharp Healthcare, San Diego, California). (*Adapted from 2007 National Baldrige Application.*)

recognition for high performance, and planning. Using the unit's mission, vision, and values (MVV), the ICU leadership system orchestrates a systematic approach to communicating and deploying key organizational requirements and expectations throughout the entire workforce by providing a single, unifying purpose to all actions.

The criteria for leadership are instructive as they relate to ICUs and are likely very different from the current approach. Within the ICU, opportunities exist for the leadership team to become a more instructive leadership system (Figure 221-2) and promote a unit that demonstrates repeatable and fully deployed process across all areas of delivering ICU care. The leadership team ensures consistency of care across boundaries, incorporates and supports continuous cycles of improvement and/or innovation, and strategically aligns with the overall goals and objectives of the hospital.

To illustrate this point, the following example is offered: one ICU used a multidisciplinary leadership group to set and deploy the values, short- and long-term directions, and performance expectations throughout the unit. This team consisted of the intensivist physician leader, functional administrator, and nursing supervisor. The multidisciplinary leadership group used a variety of tools and methods to communicate the values and directions of the unit, such as cascading employee development plans that correlated the high-level ICU goals and objectives down to each employee, articulating how they contribute to the achievement of those goals. Prior to this process of cascading accountability, the leadership team held four revolving all-ICU-participant meetings to get input from the workforce on key changes, ideas, and needs such as new equipment and guidelines for improving patient safety as they developed the strategic plan. Involvement of the workforce in planning demonstrates a departure from typical strategy processes, which usually live at the senior leader level, and fostered workforce buy-in and engagement.

Consistent with the Baldrige criterion that asks how leaders review performance and translate their reviews into continuous breakthrough improvement and opportunities for innovation, the multidisciplinary leadership group met every month to review performance—using metrics on a balanced scorecard that specifically correlated with the strategic goals and objectives. For example, the leadership group, through its strategic planning process, identified teamwork and communication as areas for improvement as it related to patient safety and

employee engagement (two strategic objectives set by the leadership group). Using a cultural assessment tool to obtain the facts (*management by fact* is a Baldrige core value), it was discovered that over the past year, the ICU had a decrease in nurse satisfaction and an increase in issues identified via a nurse assessment of patient safety. After drilldown sessions with the doctors, nurses, pharmacists, patients, and others, the leadership group learned that communication between the nurses and the physicians was lacking and that patients were suffering—all impacting job satisfaction. In addition, the ICU was experiencing an unprecedented level of staff turnover. As a result, the leadership group added to each employee's job description the requirement to participate in quarterly teamwork and communication training sessions and added a key patient safety indicator(s) to the annual individual evaluations. The intention was to drive accountability further down to all workforce members and link to new rewards and recognition initiatives. This process became systematic—repeatable—and the leadership team sought feedback from the workforce on the process's effectiveness.

In addition to the individual goal requirements, the leadership group set a unit goal to increase employee engagement, learning, and rates of improvement and innovation. Critical to this goal was the creation of improvement teams that were supported by the hospital and ICU leadership in terms of time, finances, and other resources. Through the strategic planning process, the multidisciplinary leadership group learned that the staff felt their efforts to change and improve patient care consumed large amounts of time, and that these efforts were neither supported nor appreciated by senior leadership. The stress level and complexity of the ICU environment contributed to turnover and dissatisfaction. The leadership group realized that the creation of conduits for the staff to change, innovate, and improve processes that decreased complexity and raised satisfaction levels needed to occur rapidly. The leadership group put together a multidisciplinary action team, using a Lean/Six Sigma method of improvement, to design systems that would empower and motivate the staff to change and innovate. Six Sigma is an improvement process developed by Motorola that focuses on error and/or defect reductions; Lean, based on the Toyota Productions system focuses on flow of work and removing waste and unnecessary redundancies from processes. These were then presented to the multidisciplinary leadership group for implementation and tracking of performance.

CATEGORY 2: STRATEGIC PLANNING

This category deals with how the ICU establishes its strategic objectives and action plans and how they are deployed throughout the unit. The ICU leadership system incorporates a number of internal and external inputs to create a yearly plan, with both short- and long-term goals for the unit. These goals must align with the MVV of the unit and hospital to communicate a constancy of purpose. When the leadership team meets to discuss the strategic plan, it must consider how the strategic plan is developed, communicated, prioritized, benchmarked, and measured. In addition, it should consider how the ICU's strategic planning process incorporates the following:

- Customer (patient, family) and key stakeholder needs and expectations
- The competitive environment and collaborative opportunities within the community
- Technology and other innovations that might affect ICU services
- Strengths and weaknesses of the unit
- Changes in the local, regional, or national environment
- Alignment with the unit's core competencies, the ICU's greatest area of expertise and capabilities that are of strategic importance and are frequently challenging for competitors or suppliers to imitate. They present a competitive advantage.
- Ability to execute the plans and long-term sustainability

To illustrate this concept, the following example is offered: ICU leaders organize a plan that answers the basic question, "What do we want to accomplish this year and in the future, and how do we get there?" Together with the hospital's strategy, the ICU's MVV drive the entire decision-making and strategic planning process. While aligning with the MVV and other data such as an environmental assessment (data on the external and internal environment), a strengths, weaknesses, opportunities, and threats (SWOT) analysis, and past ICU performance, the leadership group uses the yearly strategic planning process to identify the unit's key objectives and goals, key customer groups and segments, measurement strategies, workforce-related issues, opportunities to innovate, and action plans needed to achieve the strategic objectives. The strategic plan is not static; it is organic and constantly evolves and remains agile as new opportunities and challenges emerge on the unit. The leadership group is always doing strategic planning, and the annual plan document serves as a foundation for beginning to accomplish excellence. The strategic plan creates clarity, purpose, and a vision of where the ICU is headed and how they plan to arrive at that destination.

Once the plan has been completed, it is cascaded down to all ICU staff with clear linkages to their role and contributions to the work. It gives meaning to their job—purpose. Each year, the overall planning process is updated according to key customer feedback, ICU performance analysis, organizational positioning, competitive data, and industry standards and trends. Integral to this process is the implementation of actionable measures of the strategic objectives. For example, part of this ICU's mission is "to first eliminate all preventable harm to the patient, followed by exceptional care." Bloodstream infections were identified by data analysis as one area of preventable risk for cardiac patients. After the multidisciplinary leadership group discovered that bloodstream infection was an area of concern (and benchmarked their results against local competitors, national averages, and best in class), its prevention became a key strategic objective for the following year, and action plans were designed to create systems that would lower and move to eliminate these infections. The plans included education and training on an infection bundle, staff empowerment tools to monitor conformance to standards, transparently monitoring and reporting infection rates, and further teamwork training, particularly around the use of an infection checklist.

Crucial to this process is how the ICU communicates the strategic plan to the entire unit. This plan should not only be known by the leadership group; in high performing organizations, every employee knows what's going on and how they fit in to the overall work. In our example, the ICU provided every person with a laminated color card listing the unit's strategic objectives and key measures for performance. In addition, each employee was issued a cascade plan to guide work processes, goal setting, and professional development. These cascade plans list and strategically link and align the objectives of the hospital, the ICU, and the individual. The cascade plan is used quarterly as a performance assessment tool (Table 221-1).

All together, strategic planning is an important part of an organization's approach to excellence and sustaining excellence. A plan is just that—a set of steps to achieve an end. The real challenge is in effectively executing the plan every month, week, day, and minute.

CATEGORY 3: CUSTOMER FOCUS

These criteria address how the ICU engages patients and stakeholders to better serve their needs through specific listening posts, build relationships, and improve services based on the expectations of the various customer groups. *Customer engagement* refers to patient/customer commitment to an organization's services. It is a much higher determination of relationship compared to mere satisfaction. At the ICU level, no patient or family member really wants to be loyal to an ICU, since it means their health is at serious risk, yet as leaders and managers, there is an obligation to organization and deliver care at such amazing levels of distinction that if a patient or family member had to be admitted to the ICU, they would only want your unit. A key element in this section of the framework is segmentation. Most ICUs can predict with some relative confidence the types of patients who occupy their beds, and through segmentation of this population, it is possible to customize all aspects of care delivery to improve outcomes and service and eliminate inefficiencies. The following description details how a Baldrige ICU might operate using a few of the principles in Category 3.

The ICU is a complex place dealing with complex patients and processes. The challenge for ICU leadership is to determine how to ensure consistency of practice in the midst of this complexity. Key to this effort is the need for the ICU to identify the types of patients (and their families) for whom they typically provide services, segment them according to needs and expectations, and then tailor healthcare services to meet their particular needs. The concept of "stages of relationship" in the framework is an important consideration for increasing customer engagement. It suggests that leaders think about the various phases of a patient's interaction with the ICU—from admission, to their stay, to transferring to another unit, for example. During these stages, the needs of the patient and family members might change, signaling the need to alter certain systems and processes. In doing so, the ICU is better positioned to secure and/or increase their engagement at each stage of their relationship with the ICU.

For example, cardiac ICUs see a variety of patient types, yet most can be broken into two large segments: short-term and long-term patients. Within these segments are subgroups of patients ranging from those recovering from coronary artery bypass grafts to those requiring ventricular assist devices. Care plans can be implemented that are customized to deliver the best outcomes for each of these groups and are consistent with the unit's goals and directions. Patients requiring ventricular assist devices tend to require prolonged ICU stays. Therefore, the ICU team develops a plan to coordinate resources efficiently to meet the needs and expectations of this long-term patient cohort, such as how a room is set up to accommodate family members. Similarly, the short-term patient cohort can be segmented according to needs and expectations to better use the unit's resources. For example, medications most frequently used by the short-term patient group can be trended over time for predictability, and the evidence shows that just six medications actually account for over 85% of all medications given to these patients. These medications can then be located in a locked cart at the patient's bedside, reducing the need for the nurse to use the highly complex medication dispensing and delivery process, which at times is frustrating to patients awaiting their medications. Numerous studies have identified substantial inefficiencies in the medication system. Use of data to track and predict trends

TABLE 221-1	Sample of Cascading Organizational Objectives

Strategic Objectives to Individual Accountability

Strategic Area	Organizational Strategic Objective	ICU Action Plan Link to Strategic Objective	Attending Plan Link to ICU Plan	Manager Plan Link to ICU Plan	Bedside Nurse Plan Link to ICU Plan	Overall Organizational Metric
Clinical patient safety	Lower mortality rates.	Adopt CUSP program. Reduce decubitus ulcers.	Participate in culture of safety survey and one improvement project.	Participate in culture of safety survey, and monitor ulcer bundle compliance.	Participate in culture of safety survey, and identify ulcers at earliest stages.	Mortality rate Decubitus ulcer rate
Clinical patient safety	Eliminate infections.	Implement evidence-based infection bundles.	Learn, implement, and innovate infection bundles.	Monitor compliance on infection bundles.	Learn and use safety checklist.	Number of infections
Workforce	Be the best place to work.	Be the best unit in the hospital.	Attend two teamwork training sessions.	Attend two teamwork training sessions.	Attend two teamwork training sessions.	Workforce engagement scores top box
Customer	Be the best place to receive care.	Achieve the highest customer engagement scores in the hospital.	Implement family rounds.	Implement morning staff huddles, covering one key service standard a week.	Implement "key words at key times" process.	Customer engagement scores Top Box
Operational	Reduce system waste by 5%.	Run Lean projects to reduce length of stay.	Lead or participate on a Lean waste reduction team.	Lead or participate on a Lean waste reduction team.	Identify three opportunities to reduce waste in daily work.	Length of stay
Financial	Increase financial sustainability.	Increase operating margin.	Complete medical record notes on time.	Maintain supplies, salaries, and other expenses within current year budget.	Achieve 100% accuracy on charge entry and documentation.	Operating margin
Innovation	Transform the delivery of care.	Implement ideas program.	Develop five "big ideas" for the ICU.	Teach, reinforce, and monitor the ideas program.	Submit 10 new ideas.	Number of nationally recognized best practices

Action plans are the tactics to accomplish an objective. CUSP, comprehensive unit-based safety program; ICU, intensive care unit.
From www.safetyresearch.jhu.edu/QSR/.

in medication usage can allow unit staff to work more effectively and better serve the needs of patients.

Medically, the talented professionals working in the ICU know what is best for the patient; however, the question remains: What do the patient and family need and expect in order to have a positive experience which *includes the family*, whose needs are too often unmet? To some, this might seem of limited significance, considering the condition of most ICU patients. Yet there should be a way to determine these additional customer/patient requirements, and ICUs should incorporate systems for gathering this information and apply it to the delivery of care in real time. For instance, one approach might be to follow up on the ICU experience by having a nurse from the ICU speak with the patient or family after transfer to the step-down unit. The information gained could be analyzed for trends and fed into a prioritization system for planning and implementation. It could also become part of the transfer documentation so the incoming staff knows the patient's needs without having to query the family another time. For example, by talking to families, it was identified that they desired wireless Internet connection in the waiting room. The ICU can also proactively use quarterly focus groups, information sessions, and information gleaned from medical associations to elicit key knowledge to design care that is both medically optimal and patient driven.

In 2002, the Institute of Medicine recommended six tenets of the 21st century healthcare system. One of these is a focus on patient-centered care and involvement of the patient and family in the care plan. This concept, though intuitively right, is difficult in practice, especially in the ICU setting. Notwithstanding, it is vital to the success of the ICU to make concerted efforts to identify the key requirements of their patients by segment and then build care plans around those requirements. Without this input, it is unlikely a given ICU will reach levels of world-class performance and excellence. In addition, if we are to consider sustainability, the ICU must always identify, incorporate,

and amend services with the changing needs of all their customers. Through leadership, role-model behavior, and appropriate and effective communication, the workforce will feel empowered to incorporate the information gathered from the different patient segments and deliver care that is deemed appropriate based on the medical evidence and the wants and needs of the patient.

CATEGORY 4: MEASUREMENT, ANALYSIS, AND KNOWLEDGE MANAGEMENT

Now that the ICU has refined its leadership system, created its strategic goals and objectives, and gathered and used key patient data to set action plans and work processes, a robust and clear structure of measurement and analysis is needed to evaluate the effectiveness of the strategy and key healthcare systems and processes.

How does one measure performance, analyze performance, and use benchmarking information to support fact-based decision making, drive innovation, and ensure sustainability? How does one make certain everyone in the chain of delivery of ICU care has all the necessary information when they need it, and that it is in the correct form and accurate so the next clinical decision, diagnostic test, or treatment can be carried out in a timely manner? How does one make certain that clinical information is available rapidly on request, given the life-and-death reality of intensive care? And, in the interest of achieving high ICU performance, how does one make certain the sharing of knowledge (the great ideas, experiences, and talents of the workforce) is a cherished part of the culture and is actively (versus passively) managed?

This section describes how the ICU measures key indicators to track performance and identifies opportunities for improvement and innovation. In addition to measurement, this section addresses how the ICU manages knowledge, transfers information to staff and patients, and shares best practices within and outside the unit. The ICU leadership needs to be sure its measurement system is tracking the indicators that have been identified as key to the success of the organization and the unit. The criteria ask us to think innovatively about how we measure performance, the importance of relationship between all outcomes (e.g., issues with the workforce could impact clinical outcomes), process and outcome measures, and what is the true measure of mission and vision achievement. Further, the criteria challenge us to create a structure for ensuring the measures are valid, ensuring the data are accurate and of high quality, reviewing performance, identifying opportunities for improvement/innovation, and translating them into priorities. Some of these important criteria are demonstrated through the following examples.

The ICU's key measures cascade down from the hospital's overall goals, which in this example fall into five areas of focus: clinical performance, customer engagement, workforce engagement, operational performance, and financial performance (Table 221-2). During the strategic planning process, the leadership group, using input from the workforce, identified three or four leading indicators within each area that directly predicted the achievement of the key objectives and goals of the unit. These were then validated through a set of criteria asking certain questions:

1. Are the data collectible?
2. Do relevant, preferably high-performance comparisons exist?
3. Are the data understandable/translatable to action?
4. Does the measure provide actionable, credible, reliable, reproducible, and timely information?

Once validated, the measures become part of the unit's balanced scorecard, a tool often using a traffic-light color format, to indicate performance across various areas of importance. Measures then are "drilled down" for each employee to create a line of site from the big

TABLE 221-2	Sample Key Measures of Intensive Care Unit Performance		
Strategic Objectives	Metric	One-Year Goal	Three- to Five-Year Goal
Clinical excellence	Decubitus ulcers	Reduce 20%	Reduce an additional 30%
	Infections	Zero bloodstream infections	Maintain at zero
	Use of evidence for sepsis patients	100% of patients	Develop quality measures for transfusion
	Use of ventilator bundle	100% of patients	100% of patients
	Rate of adverse drug events	Zero	Zero
Workforce excellence	Positive staff engagement (% of Top Box)	Improve 30%	Achieve above top 10% compared nationally
Customer excellence	Positive patient engagement (% of Top Box)	Improve 30%	Achieve above top 10% compared nationally
Operational excellence	Canceled surgery	Zero	Maintain at zero
	Length of stay	Reduce 30%	Reduce an additional 20%
	Rate of diverted cases	Reduce 50%	Zero
	Use of agency nurses	Zero	Zero
Financial excellence	Operating margin	5%	7% (reinvest in quality)
	Drug costs	Reduce 30%	Reduce an additional 15%
Innovation excellence	Number of clinical and/or process innovations implemented	Three new processes implemented	Twenty new processes implemented internally and three that impact nationally

Top Box refers to counting only the highest box on a Likert Scale. For example, when measuring customer engagement on a 5-point scale, only those who rate the ICU as "excellent" are counted, not an average of those who rate "very good" and "excellent." Top Box is a more difficult assessment.

goals to their specific work. For instance, one of the unit's measures was zero infections, and subsequently the environmental staff that serviced the unit had a goal linked to cleanliness of the rooms. Their job, and the communication of the leadership, is not just cleaning—rather it is helping reduce infections and improve patient safety.

As another example, the leadership group set a goal of zero catheter-related infections. Data reviewed at the monthly leadership meeting revealed the incidence of bloodstream infections to be increasing and the rate of infection to be well above that of best-in-class, not to mention previous performance levels. The leadership group identified this as an opportunity for improvement and elected to convene a multidisciplinary team to reduce the number of bloodstream infections. This group replicated the approach used in the Michigan Keystone ICU study that virtually eliminated these infections throughout the state.[1] As part of this process, the leadership group communicated to the entire unit that reducing the number of bloodstream infections was a key strategic objective and would be reviewed each month. The bloodstream infection reduction team used the weekly infection control data collected and implemented interventions such as a catheter checklist on line carts, empowering the nurses to stop catheter placement if physicians did not comply with the checklist items, investigating every infection as a defect, and training on teamwork and communication for the nurses and physicians. Continuous cycles of improvement were implemented, and the bloodstream infection trend data demonstrated a progressive reduction. Work systems and processes related to catheter insertions became standardized in the unit and were ultimately communicated through the organization via a new policy and monitored for adherence.

It is also important for ICU leaders to consider how they manage the knowledge assets contained within the ICU. Baldrige defines knowledge assets as "the accumulated intellectual resources ... it's the knowledge possessed by your organization and employees in the form of information, ideas, learning, understanding, memory, insights, cognitive and technical skills, and capabilities." ICU leaders who are committed not only to high performance but also to distinctive performance should learn how to manage the unique knowledge of their units. For example, in an academic setting, fellows and residents move in and out of different ICUs, bringing new knowledge, skills, and insights; however, there is also the potential for the erosion of existing best practices through lack of knowledge in some key areas. This is particularly important in today's healthcare industry, where nurse turnover is high and hospitals are losing valuable staff. A mechanism to maintain this knowledge, communicate it, and share it across the organization is vital to an ICU moving toward high performance.

In health care, all stakeholders—physicians, nurses, administration—often have legitimate concerns about the validity of performance measures. Category 4 attempts to mitigate these concerns by developing a system of aligned measures, relevant comparisons to gauge results, a structure for reviewing these metrics, prioritizing them into opportunities for improvement and innovation, and establishing a robust framework for liberalizing data and information to all key stakeholders in the care process.

CATEGORY 5: WORKFORCE FOCUS

In health care, the term *workforce* traditionally means all paid individuals, yet Baldrige takes a different view—a more holistic approach—defining the workforce through the eyes of the patient. The traditional view presents physicians as customers of the hospital, yet in high-performing healthcare settings, doctors (paid or volunteer staff) are considered part of the workforce (sans certain benefits), engaged in planning, work system design, and budgetary authority. Specifically, Baldrige states *workforce* "refers to the people actively involved in accomplishing the work ... it includes your permanent, temporary, part-time personnel, independent practitioners, volunteers, and health profession students."

Similar to Category 3 (customer engagement), this section brings to the forefront the importance of an engaged workforce, meaning the extent to which all members demonstrate a "commitment, both emotional and intellectual, to accomplishing the work, the Mission, and Vision of the organization" (or ICU). Here, leaders and staff are asked to determine the key factors that drive the engagement of a segmented ICU workforce, how to create a culture of high performance on the unit, learning and development opportunities, career progression, and hiring and organizing a workforce dedicated to achieving excellence.

All results are lagging indicators of how well the workforce performs. ICUs that do not emphasize maintaining a workforce that is skilled, trained, engaged, motivated, and safe should expect undistinguished performance. We cannot provide examples and mechanisms for each of these items, but the paragraphs that follow offer some insight into a few of the key components of this category.

In an ICU, different members of the workforce funnel in and out of the unit on a daily basis—from lab technicians, to various physicians, to dietary, to nurses, to pharmacists, and so on. Managing the styles, personalities, and roles each of these groups play in the care delivery process in a highly complex area like the ICU is an extraordinary challenge that often gets overlooked and is left to traditional models of healthcare interactions. Each unit has its own culture, and leaders—together with the workforce—need to first identify the desired attributes of the culture and needs of the workforce, and then develop an approach to fostering and reinforcing the desired culture. One way is through an effective workforce performance management system that supports the cultural expectations through evaluations and rewards and recognitions. For instance, in one ICU, one of the cultural expectations was that each employee should innovate at least one process each year, measured via their annual staff evaluations. In addition, the unit created two awards to celebrate the best innovations: "The Super Innovator" and "The Game Changer," which were shared throughout the organization and published in the quarterly hospital newsletter. By adding this expectation, monitoring it, and creating reward systems, the ICU leadership demonstrated a commitment to aligning the goals of the unit with the actions of the workforce.

In the traditional and hierarchical world of health care, a work design that allows the workforce to achieve the highest levels of performance while promoting collaboration, initiative, empowerment, and innovation has to be the goal if patients are the true customers. So the question remains: How is this accomplished? Using the Baldrige criteria in their entirety is one way of achieving this end. The framework involves a set of characteristics of high-performing organizations inclusive of thematic linkages throughout all process of an ICU. Specifically, how is work performed so that it is systematic (repeatable based on how it is designed to be done), fully deployed, continuously improved, aligned with other care provided to the patient, and also ensures the work is aligned with the MVV and strategic objectives of the ICU?

Taking this a step further and using the example of bloodstream infections, we can examine how teamwork and communication have helped reduce the number of catheter-related infections through alignment of goals and objectives. After the leadership group identified bloodstream infections as a strategic priority and funneled it through a working team, concerns arose regarding the nursing staff's ability to intervene when physicians broke standard protocol for catheter insertion. A number of nurses reported situations in which they had tried to intervene, only to have the physician ignore their observations and proceed with central catheter placement that did not follow proper protocol, thus exposing the patient to increased risk for a bloodstream infection. It became clear that the work systems and environment within the ICU allowed physician authority to trump the experience and patient-specific knowledge of the nursing staff, resulting in unsafe practices. Using this feedback, the leadership group deployed multidisciplinary training on the tools and methodologies of teamwork and communication, such as situational awareness and safety briefings. In addition, the leadership group wrote a new policy that required physicians to stop and listen to the nursing staff if a potential for a bloodstream infection was observed, or be subject to corrective actions. The result of this endeavor empowered the nursing staff to be supported and feel comfortable intervening when patient safety might be at risk and reinforce the established safe practice.

This category of the Baldrige criteria allows ICU leadership and staff to examine how its work systems contribute to achieving the ICU's objectives. The vision and goals of the unit may seem unattainable because the processes that have been created through tradition do not align performance and processes. Using the criteria, the ICU can systematically create work processes that support the mission, vision, and overall goals of the unit, leading to an engaged workforce who would only work for this ICU. Focusing on our people is a great way to begin the path toward sustained excellence.

CATEGORY 6: PROCESS MANAGEMENT

Up to this point, we have addressed ICU performance related to its leadership, strategic planning, patient relationships and engagement, performance review, access to information and knowledge, and workforce engagement—all in the context of high performance. Now we address the bottom line: How do we "make" excellent ICU care? It is time to think differently about how ICU care creates value. The Baldrige criteria focus on the creation of *value* in every step of healthcare design and delivery, improvement, and ongoing management. The criteria in category 6 provide ICU leaders with a structure and discipline to think through their delivery processes to ensure that all steps create value, as measured by effective diagnosis and elimination of disease (to the extent possible), exceeding the expectations of all stakeholders, and capitalizing on the ICU core competencies. What care delivery management system can ensure that value is always created, outcomes do not suffer, performance levels do not decline, and safety prevails? Process management is the focal point for ICU high performance. It provides guidance on how the ICU identifies, designs, improves and innovates, and manages its healthcare services to achieve results when trended over time to approach, demonstrate, or sustain world-class performance. It obligates ICU leaders to clarify how these processes are continuously improved to achieve better performance, improve cycle times, reduce waste, reduce variability, and, of course, improve clinical outcomes. Leaders are guided through a series of questions that ask how health care is designed and managed in ways that are systematic and fully deployed, incorporate ongoing cycles of improvement, and are aligned and integrated with other processes and operations involved in the care and support of ICU patients. These criteria for performance excellence are key to avoiding being just average.

For example, it is important for the ICU leadership group to create work systems that deliver care based on the needs of all ICU constituents—patients, physicians, nurses, pharmacists, and so forth—and align with the goals and objectives of the unit. The question needs to be asked: How do our processes create value for those we serve, and how do we know we have been successful? Using this mantra as a guide, the leadership group in our ICU example aligned the work processes with the unit to continuously meet the expectations of each ICU customer segment. This involved a number of approaches; however, the ultimate deliverable was a system of work designed to achieve the key requirements (categories 2 and 3) identified in the ICU strategic plan. Data indicated that the lack of clarity around a given patient care plan was causing increased errors and longer stays. Using the goal of reducing harm and improving teamwork and communication among the unit's healthcare professionals (as stated in the strategic plan), the leadership group tested and implemented an evidence-based checklist developed by Peter Pronovost, MD, PhD, and colleagues that incorporates a multidisciplinary team approach to making rounds.[2] During these rounds, a daily goals sheet is used to communicate the care plan for the particular patient to the multidisciplinary team, consisting of physicians, nurses, pharmacists, and others. The use of this checklist over time led to a reduction in length of stay and adverse drug events, and both nurse and physician teamwork and satisfaction scores have improved. This mechanism is guided by several criteria in this Baldrige category dealing with the inclusion of patient expectations, testing to prevent errors, and achieving better performance by reducing variation in care. Unexplained and avoidable variation in care is one of the principal causes of failure in healthcare process and outcomes.

Health care is too full of waste, errors, and inefficient processes that do not add value. Much of these processes fall under "because we've always done it this way" mentality and/or a lack of discipline with improvement and process management. Over the past few years, an increasing number of improvement methodologies have made their way to health care, such as Six Sigma, Lean Thinking, the Toyota Production System, and in the 1990s, PDCA to name a few. All of these offer opportunities to improve ICU effectiveness and value and fall within the Baldrige framework, which asks how an ICU reduces variability, improves outcomes, and shares learning to drive innovation. Yet, the Baldrige criteria go further and help an organization hold the gains from these types of improvement tools. One of the major challenges facing hospitals and ICUs is something called "diminishing returns." This concept, somewhat akin to economics, dictates that after an organization exerts enormous amounts of time, energy, and other resources to improving a process, the gains often eventually erode back to previous levels of performance, primarily due to a culture that is not set up to sustain improvements. This effect is typically a symptom of the complex world of health care, the always changing and competing priorities, and a lack of reliable monitoring systems. One notable exception was the Keystone ICU project in which reductions in bloodstream infections throughout the state of Michigan were sustained for over 3 years, largely thanks to efforts to improve culture, something akin to the cultural implications when successfully adopting the Baldrige framework. Through the seven integrated Baldrige criteria, it is possible to reduce the likelihood of diminishing returns and effectively address an issue and be able to focus on other initiatives while not worrying about losing ground. All of this and more falls under the notion of process management—the need for the ICU to design, implement, manage, improve, and sustain key processes, key improvements, and key innovations over time.

The complexity of ICU care demands that its leaders employ methods of excellence at a greater intensity compared with other healthcare venues. Application of the Baldrige criteria, designed to enable any operating unit to achieve distinctive performance, is greatest in the ICU. Otherwise, we are left largely with less effective methods of management and improvement that have demonstrated, thus far, the inability to fully leverage the extraordinary talent that resides within.

CATEGORY 7: HEALTHCARE RESULTS

In the end, the results of a given ICU are the ultimate measure of its performance. Now that the ICU has defined its mission, vision, and values, set strategic objectives, become relentlessly patient-focused, established methods to ensure that all ICU staff have the required information and knowledge, and created work processes that inspire the staff and add value to the patient, it is paramount that the ICU use the data it collects (on its key objectives) as a feedback loop or mechanism to continuously review its performance and achieve the identified goals outlined in the strategic plan. Selecting measures and having a system or process for making the data actionable and understandable (such as a balanced scorecard) allow the ICU to constantly implement corrective strategies when an area for improvement is identified. This category does not deal with the deployment of key processes; rather, and quite simply, it involves the unit's ability to effectively align its mission, vision, and values and meet its stated goals and objectives as compared with both the competition and best-in-class benchmarks.

🔲 Conclusion

ICUs are places of emotion, extraordinary science, compassion, and sometimes high drama in the conflict between disease and injury and the will to live. Optimally, they are designed to enable the uniquely talented professionals who dedicate their careers to healing at the

TABLE 221-3	Seven Categories of Healthcare Criteria for Performance Excellence and Related Key Questions	
Categories	**Key Questions**
1. Leadership	How does the ICU senior leadership guide the unit through its governance system and organizational performance reviews? How does the ICU leadership ensure sustainability of all key processes at the highest levels of performance, considering innovation?
2. Strategic planning	How does the ICU establish its strategic objectives and action plans, and how are they deployed and measured across the unit?
3. Customer focus	How does the ICU determine customer/patient requirements, expectations, and preferences, and how does the ICU build relationships with its patients to increase customer/patient engagement?
4. Measurement, analysis, and knowledge management	How does the ICU select, gather, analyze, manage, and improve its measurement system, and how is this knowledge shared, transferred, and communicated throughout the unit?
5. Workforce focus	How does the ICU's work system, staff learning, and staff motivation enable all workforce members to develop and utilize their full potential in alignment with the unit's strategic objectives, goals, and action plans? How do you determine the key factors of engagement for each workforce segment? What are they?
6. Operations focus	How does the ICU's process management system, including both key processes and support processes, create value for the patient and staff? How do you know?
7. Organizational performance results	How do the ICU's results compare to competitors and industry benchmarks over time? Are they reflective of the ICU's strategic objectives?

highest levels. Yet experience has proved with alarming frequency that the enormous and sometimes even heroic good that is accomplished is marred by what could or should have been done. Patients enter our ICUs trusting that we will do what is needed, correctly and with compassion. There is only one standard of care acceptable—no excuses are permitted. The Baldrige program, the nation's formally adopted approach to excellence, is not just another improvement tool. Rather, it is a framework of systematic elements that are woven together to achieve the singular aim of excellence (Table 221-3). The Baldrige framework inspires leaders to create the culture through which every employee involved in the care of the very ill performs to his or her potential. It sets forth the foundation through which leaders of ICUs can track and achieve results that are comprehensive, balanced, and presented in the context of true world-class performance. It probes the leadership structure to consider how key elements of organizational success are accomplished, how they are systematically deployed throughout the unit, how continuous improvement is a system property, and how all the work is aligned with the unit's mission, vision, and values.

ICUs are endowed with extensive human and technologic resources. The first question every ICU leader must ask is: Are we performing at the highest possible level? If the answer is no, then the obligation—not the option—is to achieve it and then sustain it.

KEY POINTS

1. The Baldrige program provides a construct and framework for systematic approaches to achieving excellence in clinical and organizational performance.

2. Four attributes differentiate high-performing organizations from average ones in terms of work processes: work is done systematically, systematic approaches are fully deployed throughout the organization, ongoing cycles of learning improve the deployed approaches, and all processes are aligned and integrated. These attributes produce results with sustained positive trends that are superior to the competition or industry comparisons.

3. Seven categories of criteria serve as the focus and road map for leaders to achieve role-model performance. These categories are tightly interrelated and provide actionable guidance by identifying existing work process strengths and opportunities for improvement.

4. The Baldrige criteria provide a thoughtful and systematic approach to ensuring attentiveness to patient and family drivers of satisfaction; segmented needs and expectations are integrated throughout the strategic planning process, action plan designs, and overall work processes.

5. The framework provides the ability to empower, motivate, and inspire the ICU and total organizational workforce to achieve its potential and deliver care that meets the needs of patients and families. Such care will be rooted in best-care practices and aligned with the strategic objectives, mission, vision, and values of the unit or organization.

ANNOTATED REFERENCES

Pronovost P, Goeschel CA, Colantuoni E, Watson S, Lubomski LH, Berenholtz SM, et al. Sustaining reductions in catheter related bloodstream infections in Michigan intensive care units: observational study. BMJ 2010;340:c309.
This research paper studies how 103 ICUs across the state of Michigan sustained reductions in catheter-related bloodstream infections.
National Institute for Standards and Technology. Health care criteria for performance excellence. NIST 2010. Available at www.baldrige.org/.
This guide provides the actual Baldrige criteria used by the national program and organizations.

Pronovost P, Berenholtz S, Dorman T, et al. Improving communication in the ICU using daily goals. J Crit Care 2003;18:71-5.
This article explains the impact and utility of a healthcare intervention called a daily goals sheet on patient safety, team communication, and length of stay.

REFERENCES

Access the complete reference list online at http://www.expertconsult.com.

222

Severity-of-Illness Indices and Outcome Prediction: Development and Evaluation

THOMAS L. HIGGINS

And he will manage the cure best who has foreseen what is to happen from the present state of matters.[1]

Background

Predicting outcome is a time-honored duty of physicians, dating back at least to the time of Hippocrates.[1] The need for a quantitative approach to outcome prediction, however, is more recent. Although the patient or family members will still want to know the prognosis, there is increasing pressure to measure and publicly report medical care outcomes. In today's highly competitive healthcare environment, such information may be used to award contracts for care. Information of variable quality[2] is readily available on the Internet. The U.S. Department of Health and Human Services maintains a hospital comparison website,[3] and comparative information is also available from sites such as www.healthcarechoices.org.[4] Local and regional initiatives to assess quality of care are also common. Some "report cards" specifically address the performance of intensive care units (ICUs) by adjusting outcomes using risk stratification systems, so it is essential that the clinician understand the science behind these systems[5] and how risk adjustment models may properly be applied. A focus on performance assessment, however, may detract from other potential uses for risk stratification, including more precise risk-benefit decisions, prognostication, resource allocation, efficient assessment of new therapy and technology, and modifications to individual patient management based on severity of illness.

Prognostication based on clinical observation is affected by memory of recent events, inaccurate estimation of the relative contribution of multiple factors, false beliefs, and human limitations such as fatigue.[6] An outcome prediction model, on the other hand, will always produce the same estimate from a given dataset and will correctly value the importance of relevant data. In an environment in which clinical judgment may later be reviewed for financial or legal issues, an objective prediction of outcome becomes especially important. Yet, even the best risk stratification tools can generate misleading data when misapplied.[7] Discussed in this chapter are the methods by which models are developed, the application of commonly used models in clinical practice, and common reasons why observed outcome may not match predicted outcome in the absence of differences in the quality of care.[8]

Well-established general methods for stratifying clinical outcomes by the presenting condition of the patient include the ASA Physical Status Classification[9] and the Glasgow Coma Scale (GCS).[10] ICU-specific systems typically adjust for patient physiology, age, and chronic health condition; and they may also assess admitting diagnosis, location before ICU admission or transfer status, cardiopulmonary resuscitation before admission, surgical status, and use of mechanical ventilation. An ideal approach to comparing outcomes would use variables that characterize a patient's *initial* condition, can be statistically and medically related to outcome, are easy to collect, and are independent of treatment decisions.

Outcome of Interest

Mortality is a commonly chosen outcome because it is easily defined and readily available. Mortality is insufficient as the sole outcome measure, however, because it does not reflect important issues such as return to work, quality of life, or even costs, because early death results in a lower cost than prolonged hospitalization. There is poor correlation between hospital rankings based on death and those based on other complications.[7,11] ICU length of stay is difficult to use as a proxy for quality of care, because the frequency of distribution is usually skewed and mean length of stay is always higher than median owing to long-stay outliers.[12] Morbidities such as myocardial infarction, prolonged ventilation, stroke or other central nervous system complications, renal failure, and serious infection can be difficult to collect accurately, and administrative records may not reflect all relevant events.[8] There is also little standardization on how morbidity should be defined.

Other potential outcomes include ICU or hospital length of stay, resource use, return to work, quality of life, and 1- or 5-year survival. Patient satisfaction is an outcome highly valued by purchasers of health care, but it is subjective[13] and requires substantial effort to accomplish successfully.[14] Evaluation of ICU performance may require a combination of indicators, including severity of illness and resource utilization.[15]

Databases and Definitions

The quality of a risk stratification system depends on the database on which it was developed. Outcome analysis can either be retrospective, relying on existing medical records or administrative databases, or developed prospectively from data collected concurrently with patient care. Retrospective studies using existing data are quicker and less expensive to conduct but may be compromised by missing data,[8] imprecise definitions, interobserver variability,[16] and changes in medical practice over time.[17]

Data derived from discharge summaries or insurance claims do not always capture the presence of comorbid disease[18] and may be discordant with data that are clinically collected.[19] Because some administrative discharge reports truncate the number of reportable events, diagnoses may be missed, and this coding bias is most apparent in severely ill patients.[12] Coding errors and use of computer programs to optimize diagnosis-related group reimbursement can also reduce the validity of claims-derived data. Augmentation of administrative data with laboratory values improves model performance.[20]

A variety of methods can assess the quality of the database, such as reabstraction of a sample of charts by personnel blinded to the initial results and comparison to an independent database. Kappa analysis is a method for quantifying the rate of discrepancies between measurements (values) of the same variable in different databases (i.e., original and reabstracted). A kappa value of 0 represents no (or random) agreement, and 1.0 is perfect agreement, but this statistic must be interpreted in light of the prevalence of the factor being abstracted.[21]

Model Development

Once data integrity is ensured, there are a number of possible approaches to relating outcome to presenting condition. The empirical approach is to use a large database and subject the data to a series of

STEPS IN DEVELOPING
A SEVERITY-OF-ILLNESS MODEL

Precisely define outcome(s) of interest.

Identify and define candidate predictor variables (data analysis, expert opinion).

Collect data, and ensure its accuracy (reabstraction, kappa analysis).

Examine continuous variables and transform or dichotomize as necessary.

Perform univariate analysis (chi-square, Fisher's exact, Student t-test) against outcome(s).

Perform multivariate analysis (logistic regression, neural nets, Bayesian, others).

Examine for and adjust for interactions between variables.

Develop score or equation that relates independent variables to outcome.

Test calibration of model (goodness of fit typically Hosmer-Lemeshow method).

Test discrimination of model (ROC area C-statistic, sensitivity and specificity).

Validate model with independent data, split sample, or jackknife techniques.

Obtain external validation in new setting and customize as needed.

Publish in peer-reviewed journal.

		Two-by-Two Contingency Table Examining Relationship of MOF After Open Heart Surgery (Outcome) to a History of CHF (Predictor) in 3830 Patients*

TABLE 222-1

Predictor Variable: History of CHF	Outcome Variable: MOF	
	YES	NO
Yes	121	846
No	166	2697

*The odds ratio is defined by cross-multiplication $(121 \times 2697) \div (846 \times 166)$. The odds ratio of 2.3 indicates patients with CHF are 2.3 times as likely to develop postoperative organ system failure as those without prior CHF. This univariate relationship can then be tested by chi-square for statistical significance.

CHF, congestive heart failure; MOF, multiple organ failure.

Data from Higgins TL, Estafanous FG, Loop FD et al. ICU admission score for predicting morbidity and mortality risk after coronary artery bypass grafting. Ann Thorac Surg 1997;64:1050–8.

statistical manipulations (Box 222-1). Typically, death, a specific morbidity, and resource consumption are chosen as outcomes (dependent variables). Factors (independent variables) thought to affect outcome are then evaluated against a specific outcome using univariate tests (chi-square, Fisher's exact, or Student t-test) to establish the magnitude and significance of any relationship.

Independent variables should ideally reflect patient condition independent of therapeutic decisions. Measured variables such as "cardiac index" or "hematocrit" are preferred over "use of inotropes" or "transfusion given," because the criteria for intervention may vary by provider or hospital. Widely used models rely on common measured physiologic variables (heart rate, blood pressure, and neurologic status) and laboratory values (serum creatinine level and white blood cell count). In addition, variables may consider age, physiologic reserve, and chronic health status. Items chosen for inclusion in a scoring system should be readily available and relevant to clinicians involved in the care of these patients, and variables that lack either clinical or statistical bearing on outcome should not be included. This requirement may necessitate specialized scoring systems for patient populations (pediatric, burn and trauma, and possibly acute myocardial infarction patients) exhibiting different characteristics than the general ICU population. For example, left ventricular ejection fraction and reoperative status are important predictors of outcome in the cardiac surgical population but are not routinely measured or not directly relevant to other population groups.[22] If the independent variable is dichotomous (yes/no, male/female), a two-by-two table can be constructed to examine the odds ratio and a chi-square test performed to assess significance (Table 222-1). If multiple variables are being considered, the level of significance is generally set smaller than $P = .05$, using a multiple comparison (e.g., Bonferroni) correction[23] to determine a more appropriate P value.

If the independent variable under consideration is a continuous variable (e.g., age) a Student's t-test is one appropriate choice for statistical comparison. With continuous variables, consideration must be given to the possibility that the relationship of the variable to outcome is not linear. Figure 222-1 demonstrates the relationship of ICU admission serum bicarbonate to mortality outcome in cardiac surgical patients,[24] where the data points have been averaged with adjacent values to produce a locally weighted smoothing scatterplot

graph.[25] Serum bicarbonate values above 22 mmol/L at ICU admission imply a relatively constant risk. Below this value, the risk of death rises sharply. Analysis of this locally weighted smoothing scatterplot graph suggests two ways for dealing with the impact of serum bicarbonate on mortality. One would be to make admission bicarbonate a dichotomous variable (i.e., >22 mEq or <22 mEq). The other would be to transform the data via a logarithmic equation to make the relationship more linear. Cubic splines analysis,[26] another statistical smoothing technique, may also be used to assign weight to physiologic variables.

Univariate analysis assesses the forecasting ability of variables without regard to possible correlations or interactions between variables. Linear discriminant and logistic regression techniques can evaluate and correct for overlapping influences on outcome. For example, a history of heart failure and depressed left ventricular ejection fraction are both empirical predictors of poor outcome in patients presenting for cardiac surgery.[27] As might be expected, there is considerable overlap between the population with systolic heart failure and those with low ejection fraction. The multivariate analysis in this specific instance eliminates history of heart failure as a variable and retains only measured ejection fraction in the final equation.

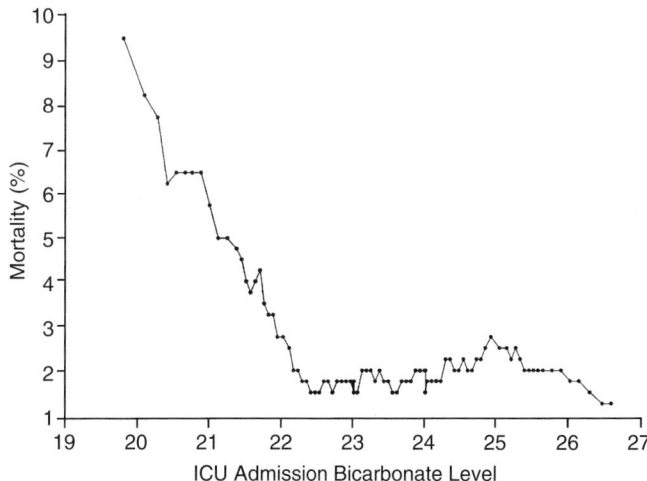

Figure 222-1 A locally weighted smoothing scatterplot (LOWESS) analysis of the relationship between ICU admission bicarbonate level (x-axis) and mortality (y-axis). Individual patient data are grouped and averaged with surrounding data to produce a smooth plot. In this instance, the mortality rate appears to be stable with admission serum bicarbonate levels of 22 mmol/L and above but rises rapidly with lower values. Admission bicarbonate level of less than 21 mmol/L was given prognostic weight in the model that used these data. (*Data from Higgins TL, Estafanous FG, Loop FD et al. ICU admission score for predicting morbidity and mortality risk after coronary artery bypass grafting. Ann Thorac Surg 1997;64:1050-8.*)

TABLE 222-2	Variables in the MPM₀ III Logistic Regression Model	
Variable	**Odds Ratios (95% Confidence Intervals)**	**Coefficients (Robust Standard Errors)**
Constant	NA	−5.36283 (0.103)
Physiology		
Coma/deep stupor (GCS 3 or 4)	7.77* (5.921, 10.201)	2.050514 (0.139)
Heart rate ≥150 bpm	1.54 (1.357, 1.753)	0.433188 (0.065)
Systolic BP ≤90 mm Hg	4.27* (3.393, 5.367)	1.451005 (0.117)
Chronic Diagnoses		
Chronic renal insufficiency	1.71 (1.580, 1.862)	0.5395209 (0.042)
Cirrhosis	7.93 (4.820, 13.048)	2.070695 (0.254)
Metastatic neoplasm	24.65* (15.970, 38.056)	3.204902 (0.222)
Acute Diagnoses		
Acute renal failure	2.32 (2.137, 2.516)	0.8412274 (0.042)
Cardiac dysrhythmia	2.28* (1.537, 3.368)	0.8219612 (0.200)
Cerebrovascular incident	1.51 (1.366, 1.665)	0.4107686 (0.051)
GI bleed	0.85 (0.763, 0.942)	−0.165253 (0.054)
Intracranial mass effect	6.39* (4.612, 8.864)	1.855276 (0.166)
Other		
Age (per year)	1.04* (1.037, 1.041)	0.0385582 (0.001)
CPR prior to admission	4.47* (2.990, 6.681)	1.497258 (0.205)
Mechanical ventilation within 1 hour of admission	2.27* (2.154, 2.401)	0.821648 (0.028)
Medical or unscheduled surgical admit	2.48 (2.269, 2.719)	0.9097936 (0.046)
Zero factors (no factors other than age from list above)	0.65 (0.551, 0.777)	−0.4243604 (0.088)
Full code	0.45 (0.416, 0.489)	−0.7969783 (0.041)
Interaction Terms		
Age x Coma/deep stupor	0.99 (0.988, 0.997)	−0.0075284 (0.002)
Age x Systolic BP ≤ 90	0.99 (0.988, 0.995)	−0.0085197 (0.002)
Age x Cirrhosis	0.98 (0.970, 0.986)	−0.0224333 (0.004)
Age x Metastatic neoplasm	0.97 (0.961, 0.974)	−0.0330237 (0.003)
Age x Cardiac dysrhythmia	0.99 (0.985, 0.995)	−0.0101286 (0.003)
Age x Intracranial mass effect	0.98 (0.978, 0.988)	−0.0169215 (0.003)
Age x CPR prior to admission	0.99 (0.983, 0.995)	−0.011214 (0.003)

Odds ratios for variables with an asterisk (*) are also affected by the associated interaction terms.

CPR, cardiopulmonary resuscitation within 24 hours preceding admission; BP, blood pressure; bpm, beats per minute; GCS, Glasgow Coma Scale; "x" denotes interaction between each pair of variables listed.

Reprinted with permission from Higgins TL, Teres D, Copes WS et al. Assessing contemporary intensive care unit outcome: an updated mortality probability admission model (MPM₀-III). Crit Care Med 2007;35:827–35.

Because linear discriminant techniques require certain assumptions about data, logistic techniques are more commonly utilized.[4] Subjecting the data to multiple logistic regression will produce an equation with a constant, a β coefficient and standard error, and an odds ratio that represents each term's effect on outcome. Table 222-2 displays the results of the logistic regression used in the Mortality Probability Model III ICU admission model (MPM₀ III). There are 17 variable terms, and a constant term, each with a β value that when multiplied by presence or absence of a factor, becomes part of the calculation of mortality probability using a logistic regression equation. The odds ratios reflect the relative risk of mortality if a factor is present. The challenge in building a model is to include sufficient terms to deliver reliable prediction while keeping the model from being cumbersome to use or too closely fitted to its unique development population. Generally accepted practice is to limit the number of terms in the logistic regression model to 10% of the number of patients having the outcome of interest to avoid "overfitting" the model to the developmental dataset. It is important to identify interaction between variables that may be additive, subtractive (canceling), or synergistic and thus require additional terms in the final model. In the earlier example, seven interaction items were added to reflect important observations in elderly patients,[28] who frequently have better outcomes than expected.

The patient's diagnosis is an important determinant of outcome,[17] but conflicting philosophies exist on how disease status should be addressed by a severity adjustment model. One approach is to define principal diagnostic categories and add a weighted term to the logistic regression equation for each illness. This approach acknowledges the different impact of physiologic derangement by diagnosis. For example, patients with diabetic ketoacidosis have markedly altered physiology but a low expected mortality; a patient with an expanding abdominal aneurysm may show little physiologic abnormality and yet be at high risk for death or morbidity. Too many diagnostic categories, however, may result in too few patients in each category to allow statistical analysis for a typical ICU, and such systems are difficult to use without sophisticated (and often proprietary) software.

The other approach is to ignore disease status and assume that factors such as age, chronic health status, and altered physiology will suffice to explain outcome in large groups of patients. This method avoids issues with inaccurate labeling of illness in patients with multiple problems and the need for lengthy lists of coefficients but could result in a model that is more dependent on having an "average" case mix.[29,30] Regardless of the specific approach, age and comorbidities (metastatic or hematologic cancer, immunosuppression, and cirrhosis) are given weight in nearly all ICU models to help account for the patient's physiologic reserve or ability to recover from acute illness.

Validation and Testing Model Performance

Models may be validated on an independent dataset or by using the development set with methods such as jackknife or bootstrap validation.[31] Two criteria are essential in assessing model performance: calibration and discrimination. *Calibration* refers to how well the model tracks outcomes across its relevant range. A model may be very good at predicting good outcome in healthy patients and poor outcomes in very sick patients yet unable to distinguish outcome for patients in the middle range. The Hosmer-Lemeshow goodness-of-fit test[32] assesses calibration by stratifying the data into categories (usually deciles) of risk. The number of patients with an observed outcome is compared with the number of predicted outcomes at each risk level. If the observed and expected outcomes are very close at each level across the range of the model, the sum of chi-squares will be low, indicating good calibration. The *P* value for the Hosmer-Lemeshow goodness-of-fit *increases* with better calibration and should be nonsignificant (i.e., >.05). Special precautions apply to using the Hosmer-Lemeshow tests with very large databases.[33]

The second measurement of model performance is *discrimination*, or how well the model predicts the correct outcome. A classification table (Table 222-3) displays four possible outcomes that define sensitivity and specificity of a model with a binary (died/survived) prediction and outcome. Sensitivity (the true-positive rate) and specificity (the true-negative rate, or 1—the false-positive rate) are measures of discrimination but will vary according to the decision point chosen to

TABLE 222-3	Classification Table		
		Actual Outcome	
Predicted Outcome		DIED	SURVIVED
Died		a	c
Survived		b	d
True-positive ratio = a/(a + b) (sensitivity)			
False-positive ratio = c/(c + d)			
True-negative ratio = d/(c + d) (specificity)			
False-negative ratio = b/(a + b)			
Accuracy (total correct prediction) = (a + d)/a + b + c + d			

Adapted from Ruttiman UE. Severity of illness indices: development and evaluation. In: Shoemaker WC, editor. Textbook of critical care medicine. 2nd ed. Philadelphia: Saunders; 1989.

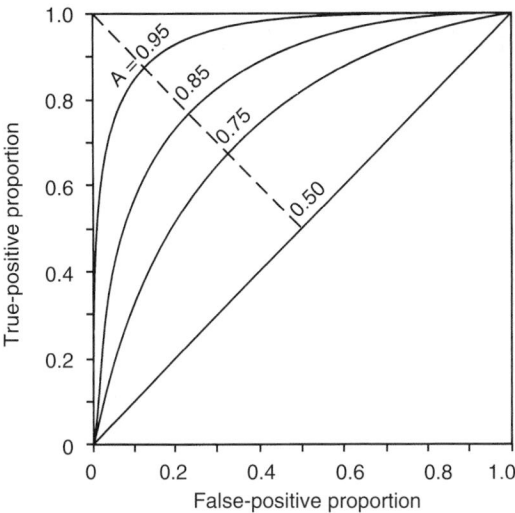

Figure 222-2 Relative operating characteristic (ROC) curves. A coin toss gives an ROC of 0.5. In models that discriminate outcome, an increasing area under the curve, also called the *C-statistic*, is enclosed. (*From Swets JA. Measuring the accuracy of diagnostic systems. Science 1988;240:1285-94.*)

distinguish between outcomes when a model produces a continuous range of possibilities. The sensitivity and specificity of a model when using 50% as the decision point will differ from that using 95% as the decision point. The classification table can be recalculated for a range of outcomes by choosing various decision points: for example, 10%, 25%, 50%, 75%, and 95% mortality risk. At each decision point, the true-positive rate (proportion of observed deaths predicted correctly) and the false-negative (proportion of survivors incorrectly predicted to die) and overall correct classification rate can be presented. The C-statistic, or area under a receiver-operating characteristic (ROC) curve, is a convenient way to summarize sensitivity and specificity at all possible decision points. A graph of the true-positive proportion (sensitivity) against the false-positive proportion (1—specificity) across the range of the model produces the ROC curve (Figure 222-2). A model with equal probability of producing the correct or incorrect result (e.g., flipping a coin) will produce a straight line at a 45-degree angle that encompasses half of the area (0.5) under the "curve." Models with better discrimination will incorporate increasingly more area under the curve to a theoretical maximum of 1.0. Most ICU models have ROC areas of 0.8 to 0.9 in the development set, although the ROC area usually decreases when models are applied prospectively to new datasets. The ROC analysis is valid only if the model has first been shown to calibrate well.

A model may discriminate and calibrate well on its development dataset yet fail when applied to a new population. Discrepancies in performance can relate to differences in surveillance strategies and definitions[34] and can occur when a population is skewed by an unusual number of patients having certain risk factors, as could be seen in a specialized ICU.[29] Large numbers of low-risk ICU admissions will result in poor predictive accuracy for the entire ICU population.[35] The use of sampling techniques (i.e., choosing to collect data randomly on 50% of patients rather than all patients) also appears to bias results.[36] Models can also deteriorate over time, owing to changes in populations and medical practice. These explanations should be considered before concluding that quality of care is different between the original and later applications of a model.[37]

Standardized Mortality Ratio

Application of a severity-of-illness scoring system involves comparison of observed outcomes with those predicted by the model. The *standardized mortality ratio* is defined as observed divided by expected

mortality and is generally expressed as a mean value ± 95% confidence intervals (CIs), which will depend on the number of patients in the sample. Standardized mortality ratio values of 1.0 (± the CI) indicate that the mortality rate, adjusted for presenting illness, is at the expected level. Standardized mortality ratio values *significantly* lower than 1.0 indicate performance better than expected. Small differences in scores, as could be caused by consistent errors in scoring elements, timing of data collection, or sampling rate, have been shown to cause important changes in the standardized mortality ratio.[36,38]

Models Based on Physiologic Derangement

Three widely utilized general-purpose ICU outcome systems are based on changes in patient physiology: the Acute Physiology and Chronic Health Evaluation (APACHE II,[39] APACHE III,[40] APACHE IV[41]), the Mortality Probability Models (MPM I,[42] MPM II,[43] MPM_{24},[44] MPM_0 III[45]), and the Simplified Acute Physiology Score (SAPS I,[46] SAPS II,[47] SAPS III[48,49]). These models are all based on the premise that as illness increases, patients will exhibit greater deviation from physiologic normal for a variety of common parameters such as heart rate, blood pressure, neurologic status, and laboratory values. Risk is also assigned for advanced age and chronic illness.

ACUTE PHYSIOLOGY AND CHRONIC HEALTH EVALUATION

APACHE II was developed from data on 5815 medical and surgical ICU patients at 13 hospitals between 1979 and 1982. Severity of illness was assessed with 12 routine physiologic measurements plus the patient's age and previous health status.[39] Scoring was based on the most abnormal measurements during the first 24 hours in the ICU, and the maximum score is 71 points, although more than 80% of patients have scores of 29 or less.[39] Although the developers consider APACHE II to have significant limitations based on its age, it is still in widespread use. APACHE II was developed on a database of medical and surgical patients that excluded patients undergoing coronary artery bypass grafting and coronary care, burn, and pediatric patients. The authors note that "it is crucial to combine the APACHE II score with a precise description of disease" and provide coefficients to adjust the score for 29 nonoperative and 16 postoperative diagnostic categories.[39] They also caution that disease-specific mortality predictions be derived from at least 50 patients in each diagnostic category. These appropriate precautions have not always been observed in application of APACHE II.

Another common misunderstanding is to use APACHE II, calibrated for unselected ICU admissions, to assess outcome in a patient sample selected by other criteria, such as severe sepsis. The acute physiology score from APACHE III or a specifically developed model predicting 28-day mortality in sepsis are preferable for risk stratification of septic patients.[50] APACHE II does not control for pre-ICU management, which could restore a patient's altered physiology and lead to a lower score and thus underestimate a patient's true risk. In a study of 235 medical patients scored with APACHE II, actual mortality was the same as predicted mortality only for patients admitted directly from the emergency department.[51] The mortality rate was higher than predicted for transfers from hospital floors, step-down units, or other hospitals. Inclusion of data from the period before ICU admission increases severity of illness scores and thus increases estimated mortality risk, and this effect is greatest with medical patients and emergency admissions.[52] Failure to consider the source of admission could thus lead to erroneous conclusions about the quality of medical care.[51,52]

APACHE III, published in 1991,[40] addressed the limitations of APACHE II, including the impact of treatment time and location before ICU admission. The number of separate disease categories was increased from 45 to 78. APACHE III was developed on a representative database of 17,440 patients at 40 hospitals, including 14 tertiary facilities that volunteered for the study and 26 randomly chosen hospitals in the United States. As data accumulated from APACHE III users, the database expanded, and adjustments to coefficients were made to keep data relevant to current practice.[17] APACHE III went through several iterations between 1991 and 2003 as part of this continuous updating. Compared with APACHE II, the ranges of physiologic "normal" are narrower with APACHE III and deviations are asymmetrically weighted to be more clinically relevant. Interactions between variables were considered, and five new variables (blood urea nitrogen, urine output, serum albumin, bilirubin, and glucose) were added, and version II variables serum potassium and bicarbonate were dropped. Information was also collected on 34 chronic health conditions, of which 7 (AIDS, hepatic failure, lymphoma, solid tumor with metastasis, leukemia/multiple myeloma, immunocompromised state, and cirrhosis) were significant in predicting outcome.

APACHE III scores range from 0 to 299, and a 5-point increase represents a significant increase in risk of hospital death. In addition to the APACHE III *score*, which provides an initial risk estimate, there is an APACHE III *predictive equation* that uses the APACHE III score and proprietary reference data on disease category and treatment location before ICU admission to provide individual risk estimates for ICU patients. Customized models were created for patient populations (e.g., cardiac surgical patients)[53] excluded from the APACHE II. Overall correct classification for APACHE III at a 50% cut-point for mortality risk is 88.2%, with an ROC area of 0.90, significantly better than APACHE II.[40] Sequential APACHE III scoring can update the risk estimate daily, allowing for real-time decision support, for example, predicting likelihood of ICU interventions over the next 24-hour period. The single most important factor determining daily risk of hospital death is the updated APACHE III score, but the *change* in the APACHE III score, the admission diagnosis, the age and chronic health status of the patient, and prior treatment are also important. A predicted risk of death in excess of 90% on any of the first 7 days is associated with a 90% mortality rate. APACHE III scores also can be tied to predictions for ICU mortality, length of stay, need for interventions, and nursing workload.

APACHE IV was published in 2006[41] to address deterioration in APACHE III performance that had developed despite periodic updating over 15 years. APACHE IV has excellent discrimination (ROC area = 0.88) and impressive calibration (Hosmer-Lemeshow C statistic 16.8, $P = 0.08$) with a sample size of 110,558 patients in the United States. The model includes 142 variables (Table 222-4), many of which were rescaled or revised compared with APACHE III. Using data from 2002-2003 with an observed mortality rate of 13.51, APACHE IV predicted a mortality rate of 13.55, whereas earlier versions of APACHE III predicted 14.64% and 16.90% mortality. A hospital using APACHE III software based on 1988-89 data would have congratulated themselves on a superb SMR of 0.799, where using APACHE IV would have revealed the true SMR to be a respectable but average 0.997, not significantly different than 1.0.

APACHE IV relies on physiologic abnormalities to account for 66% of the model's explanatory power. ICU admission diagnosis (using 116 categories) accounts for about 17%, with the remainder accounted for by age, chronic illness, location prior to admission, and interaction terms. As with any model, there are limitations to the use of APACHE IV. First, the increased complexity of the model makes it impossible to use without dedicated software. The data entry burden, however, can be mitigated by porting data into APACHE from a hospital's clinical information system. Secondly, APACHE IV was developed and validated in ICUs in the United States, and international differences in ICU resources, triage policies, models of care, and bed availability would logically have an impact on benchmarking performance in a new environment.[54,55] The authors also stress that "prediction for an individual contains variance" and that "a prediction is only an approximate indicator of an individual's probability of mortality."[41] As an example, they mention that the 95% CIs around a predicted mortality of 5% would be 3.9% to 6.5%, and that the absolute ranges of CIs widen

TABLE 222-4	Variables Used in Acute Physiology and Chronic Health Evaluation IV		
Variable		*Coefficient*	*Odds Ratio*
Emergency surgery		0.2491	1.28
Unable to access GCS		0.7858	2.19
Ventilated on ICU day 1		0.2718	1.31
Thrombolytic therapy for acute myocardial infarction		−0.5799	0.56
Rescaled GCS (15-GCS)		0.0391	1.04
15-GCS = 0			1.00
15-GCS = 1, 2, 3			1.04-1.12
15-GCS = 4, 5, 6			1.17-1.26
15-GCS = 7, 8, 9			1.31-1.42
15-GCS = 10, 11, 12			1.48-1.60
Pao_2/Fio_2 ratio:		−0.00040	1.00
≤200			1.00-0.92
201-300			0.92-0.89
301-400			0.89-0.85
401-500			0.85-0.82
501-600			0.82-0.79
Chronic health items:			
AIDS		0.9581	2.61
Cirrhosis		0.8147	2.26
Hepatic failure		1.0374	2.82
Immunosuppressed		0.4356	1.55
Lymphoma		0.7435	2.10
Myeloma		0.9693	2.64
Metastatic cancer		1.0864	2.96
Admission source:			
Floor		0.0171	1.02
Other hospital		0.0221	1.02
Operating/recovery room		−0.5838	0.56

AIDS, acquired immunodeficiency syndrome; GCS, Glasgow Coma Scale; ICU intensive care unit.

Adapted with permission from Zimmerman JE, Kramer AA, McNair DS, Malila FM. Acute Physiology and Chronic Health Evaluation (APACHE) IV: hospital mortality assessment for today's critically ill patients. Crit Care Med 2006;34:1297–1310.

as the predicted rate increases. Furthermore, the aggregate SMR as a performance benchmark is affected by factors not directly related to quality of care, such as limitations on treatment, early discharge to subacute sites, and care prior to and following the ICU stay.[41] APACHE IV produces a prediction once the patient has been in the ICU for 4 hours. If the patient should die, even before the 24-hour admission window, the prediction and outcome are still counted.

MORTALITY PROBABILITY MODELS

The original Mortality Probability Model (MPM) was developed on 755 patients at a single hospital using multiple logistic regression to assign weights to variables predicting hospital mortality.[42] The MPM II models were developed on an international sample of 12,610 patients and then validated on a subsequent sample of 6514.[43] MPM, like APACHE II, excludes pediatric, burn, coronary, and cardiac surgical patients and estimates hospital mortality risk based partly on physiologic derangement, using a smaller number of variables. However, MPM puts more weight on chronic illness, comorbidities, and age and less on acute physiologic derangement compared to APACHE. MPM models can use data obtained at ICU admission (MPM_0) and also at the end of the first 24-hour period (MPM_{24}), the latter being more comparable to APACHE. While APACHE generates a score and then with additional information converts that score into a probability estimate of survival, MPM directly calculates a probability of survival from the available data. Because this involves a logistic regression equation, it is difficult to accomplish at bedside without a computer or programmable calculator. The MPM_{24} variables account for differences in patients who remain in the ICU for 24 hours or longer versus those who die early or recover rapidly. This line of reasoning has been further extended to create 48- and 72-hour models.[44] Additional variables in MPM_{24}, MPM_{48}, and MPM_{72} but not MPM_0 are prothrombin time, urine output, creatinine, arterial oxygenation, continuing coma or deep stupor, confirmed infection, mechanical ventilation, or intravenous vasoactive drug therapy. Probability of death increases at 48 and 72 hours even if the MPM variables and coefficients are unchanged, implying that mortality risk is increasing in patients whose clinical profile remains unchanged over time.[44] MPM_{48} and MPM_{72} adjust for this observation by changing the β_0 (constant term) in the MPM_{24} equation. The most important difference between MPM and other systems is that the MPM_0 produces a probability estimate that is available at ICU presentation and is independent of ICU treatment. MPM also does not require specifying a diagnosis, which can be an advantage in complex ICU patients but may also make it more susceptible to error with changes in case mix[29] and generates, on average, a lower area under the ROC curve.

MPM_0 II became the mortality benchmarking component for the Society of Critical Care Medicine's (SCCM) Project IMPACT database, launched at the SCCM annual symposium in 1996. By 2002, it was apparent that mortality predictions based on mid-1980s results were outdated, at least in Project IMPACT hospitals where average SMRs had drifted to 0.85.[56] MPM_0 III was developed on a population of 124,855 patients in 135 ICUs at 98 Project IMPACT hospitals. Hospital mortality in this population was 13.8% versus 20.8% in the MPM_0 II cohort.[45] All of the 15 variables from MPM_0 II remained associated with mortality, but the relative impact had changed. For example, gastrointestinal bleeding was no longer as serious a risk factor, presumably because of advances in resuscitation, endoscopic procedures, treatment of *H. pylori*, and availability of proton pump inhibitors since the original study. Two new variables were added: "full code" resuscitation status at ICU admission and "zero factor" or absence of all MPM_0 II risk factors except age. Seven age interaction terms were added to reflect the declining marginal contribution of acute and chronic medical conditions to mortality risk in the elderly.[28] Location and time prior to ICU admission were evaluated but did not improve model performance. With these changes, MPM_0 III calibrated well (Hosmer-Lemeshow goodness-of-fit 11.62; $P = 0.31$) and had an area under the ROC curve of 0.823, similar to that of MPM_0 II. While the ROC area is lower than with APACHE, MPM users do not need to specify a particular diagnosis, which may be difficult in a complex patient with multiple problems. The simplicity of data collection and ability to generate a prognosis soon after arrival (rather than at 24 hours) are advantages. Limitations of the MPM_0 III include lower discrimination, use of a self-selected population of Project IMPACT participants in North America, and as with all models, applicability to groups of patients rather than individuals. While in theory, extreme case-mix differences might affect MPM performance, in practice, SMRs obtained using MPM_0 III versus specially constructed subgroup models were nearly identical in the 135 ICUs studied.[57] MPM_0 III has been prospectively validated on an additional 55,459 patients at 103 adult ICUs in North America and calibrates well with more contemporary Project IMPACT hospitals (78 units participating in both studies plus 25 new participants).[58] The Project IMPACT database was also used to update the resource utilization "Rapoport Teres" graph that plots severity-adjusted mortality versus severity-adjusted length of stay.[59] The result of this update is that results from Project IMPACT hospitals are now centered around the 0,0 coordinates, reflecting mortality and resource utilization as expected instead of being skewed to the upper right corner, indicating most hospitals performing better than expected.

SIMPLIFIED ACUTE PHYSIOLOGY SCORE

The Simplified Acute Physiology Score (SAPS) was developed on a population of 679 consecutive patients admitted to 8 multidisciplinary ICUs in France and, like the APACHE systems, uses the most abnormal values collected during the first 24 hours after ICU admission.[46] SAPS II was developed on 13,152 patients at 137 adult medical or surgical ICUs in Europe and North America, sharing the MPM II dataset. Like MPM and APACHE II, SAPS excludes burn patients, patients younger

---

> **Box 222-2**
>
> ## VARIABLES USED IN SIMPLIFIED ACUTE PHYSIOLOGY SCORE III
>
> Age (in years)
> Comorbidities: cancer, cancer therapy (scored separately) chronic heart failure (NYHA IV), hematological cancer, cirrhosis, AIDS
> Length of stay before intensive care unit (ICU) admission, days
> Intrahospital location before ICU admission
> Use of major therapeutic options before ICU admission (e.g., vasopressors)
> ICU admission: planned or unplanned
> Reason for ICU admission
> Surgical status at ICU admission: emergency or elective or none
> Anatomical site of surgery
> Acute infection at ICU admission
> Lowest estimated Glasgow Coma Scale score (points)
> Total bilirubin (highest)
> Body temperature (highest)
> Creatinine (highest)
> Heart rate (highest)
> Leukocytes (highest)
> Hydrogen ion concentration (lowest pH)
> Platelet count (lowest)
> Systolic blood pressure (lowest)
> Oxygenation (P/F ratio)

than 18 years, coronary care patients, and cardiac surgery patients. The outcome measure for SAPS II is vital status at hospital discharge. Seventeen variables were used in the SAPS II model: 12 physiologic variables, age, type of admission, and the presence of AIDS, metastatic cancer, or hematologic malignancy.

Not surprisingly, the SAPS II model also drifted out of calibration over time.[48] SAPS III, a multicenter, multinational study, collected data on 19,577 patients from 307 ICUs during the fall of 2002.[48] Data were collected at admission, on ICU days 1, 2, and 3, and the last day of ICU stay. SAPS II, when applied to this cohort, underestimated hospital mortality, and whereas it discriminated well (ROC area 0.83), calibration was poor, and model performance also differed by geographic region. The final SAPS III model (Box 222-2), created on 16,784 patients using logistic regression methods, contains 20 variables and has good discrimination (ROC area 0.848) and calibration (Hosmer-Lemeshow C = 14.29; $P = 0.16$).[49] Customized models were generated for seven worldwide regions to address geographic variation in population outcomes, thought to be driven in part by availability of resources.[60]

ICNARC MODEL

As SAPS III and other studies[61,62] have shown, risk-adjustment models require validation and recalibration if they are to be applied in a new geographic setting. The Intensive Care National Audit and Research Center (ICNARC) collected data on 216,626 critical care admissions in 163 adult general critical care units in England, Wales, and Northern Ireland from December 1996 to August 2003.[63] Logistic regression techniques were used to create the ICNARC model (Box 222-3), which includes 12 physiologic variables, age, source of admission, diagnostic category, and CPR status. This model has an ROC area of 0.863 and a Hosmer-Lemeshow C statistic of 64.2, which, although significant, must be interpreted in light of known issues with this test when applied to extremely large samples.[33] This study also evaluated performance of APACHE II, APACHE III, SAPS II and MPM II on the same population. The ICNARC outperformed all other models in terms of discrimination (ROC area), but SAPS II had better calibration, while MPM II had the best accuracy of average prediction, although these differences were all relatively minor. ICNARC, having no exclusions, may be applied to all critical care admissions regardless of diagnosis, and it calibrates well in the United Kingdom.

ELEMENTS IN ICNARC SCORE

Highest heart rate
Lowest systolic BP
Highest temperature
Lowest respiratory rate
Mechanical ventilation (Yes/No)
Lowest Pao_2/Associated Fio_2 (P/F ratio)
Lowest pH
Highest serum urea
Highest serum creatinine
Highest serum sodium
Urine output (24 hours)
Lowest WBC
Paralyzed/sedated (Yes/No)
Lowest Glasgow Coma Scale score
Age, years
Source of admission
Diagnostic category
CPR (Yes/No)

Adapted with permission from Harrison DA, Gareth JP, Carpenter JR et al. A new risk prediction model for critical care: the Intensive Care National Audit & Research Centre (ICNARC) model. Crit Care Med 2007;35:1091-8.

VETERANS AFFAIRS ICU RISK ADJUSTMENT MODEL

Arguably, the Veterans Affairs (VA) population in the United States could represent a specialized population, owing to being predominantly male (>97%). The VA developed its own automated ICU risk adjustment tool in 1996-97[64] and validated, updated, and recalibrated this model recently.[65] Risk predictors include age, mutually exclusive ICD-9 diagnosis/procedure groups, comorbid disease groups, admission source, and 11 laboratory values measured during the 24 hours surrounding ICU admission. Revisions to the model refit the predictor coefficients and expanded the number of diagnostic categories from 38 to 84. The model has an impressive ROC area (0.874-0.877) in two data cohorts and calibrates well by Hosmer-Lemeshow statistics. SMRs derived from the VA ICU model correlate well ($r^2 = 0.74$) with those of the National Surgical Quality Improvement Performance (developed for surgical postoperative assessment). The model, however, has not yet been tested outside of the VA population or internationally.

SPECIALIZED MODELS

APACHE II, MPM, and SAPS, although useful for general medical/surgical ICUs, exclude patients younger than age 18, burn patients, coronary care, and cardiac surgical patients. Murphy-Filkins and colleagues[29] demonstrated that performance of severity of illness models deteriorates when critical population values are reached for individual scoring variables, as might be seen in a highly specialized ICU. Twenty percent of the patients in the MPM II database were aged 75 or older. When this percentage of elderly patients was experimentally increased to 42%, the model became unstable. Similar changes were seen if the proportion of patients with cardiac dysrhythmias, cerebrovascular disease, intracranial mass effects, coma, cardiopulmonary resuscitation before ICU admission, emergency admission, or gastrointestinal bleeding rose above their individual critical values.[29] Thus, severity-of-illness scoring systems should be used with caution when units become highly specialized to care for subsets of patients. The European Consensus Conference recommends that severity indices be validated and customized if needed when applied to a new setting such as a particular country or specialized type of ICU.[66]

To address this problem, specific models have been developed for pediatric,[67] trauma,[68,69] and cardiac surgical populations.[24,70] The cardiac surgical population differs from the general ICU population because admission physiology data can be misleading in a population routinely subjected to hypothermia, hemodilution, and deliberate

control of hemodynamics by the operating room team. Important variables for predicting outcome in cardiac surgery include ventricular function, coronary anatomy, and heart valve pathology and reoperation status.[24] The Cooperative CABG Database Project, analyzing 172,000 patients, identified seven core variables (urgency of operation, age, prior heart surgery, gender, ejection fraction, percent stenosis of the left main coronary artery, and number of major coronary arteries with greater than 70% stenosis) to be predictive of mortality.[70] An additional 13 variables influence outcome to a lesser extent. These variables include recent angioplasty or myocardial infarction, history of angina, ventricular arrhythmias, CHF, mitral regurgitation, and coexisting diseases such as diabetes, cerebral vascular disease, peripheral vascular disease, chronic obstructive pulmonary disease, and renal dysfunction. At least 10 cardiac surgical models exist[22,24,27,53,70-72]; head-to-head comparisons have demonstrated international differences in sensitivity and specificity and marked discrepancies in individual patient prediction.[73,74] The independent variables predicting morbidity do not perfectly overlap those predicting mortality or length of stay, suggesting that multiple risk scores may be required to best predict various outcomes. The preoperative cardiac surgical models are useful for evaluating the results of an entire hospitalization but do not specifically address the ICU component of care. Operating room events can neutralize or amplify preoperative risk, depending on such events as reopening the chest, hemodynamic management in an emergency patient, and the degree of myocardial protection. In 5000 patients undergoing CABG, 8 risk factors available at ICU admission appeared to predict hospital mortality and an additional 5 factors also predict morbidity.[26] These 13 mortality or morbidity variables, identified by logistic regression, are available in a clinical score that can be used in patients undergoing isolated coronary artery bypass grafting alone or combined with a valve or carotid procedure. A modified APACHE III has also been successfully used for cardiac surgical patients in a prospective multicenter study of 2435 patients.[53] Independent predictors of hospital mortality included the APACHE score, age, emergency or reoperation status, number of bypass grafts, and gender of the patient. Risk prediction for cardiac surgical patients is incorporated into the APACHE III and IV software packages.

Comparisons Between Models

A number of papers have investigated the relative performance of the three most widely-used systems,[54,55,61-63,75-78] although to date there is no head-to-head comparison of the three most current versions. In a retrospective chart review of 11,300 patients from 35 hospitals in the California Intensive Care Outcomes (CALICO) Project, SMRs were calculated using APACHE IV, MPM_0 III and SAPS II.[75] All models had adequate discrimination and calibration; data abstraction times ranged from 11.1 minutes with MPM_0 III to 37.3 minutes for APACHE IV. Substantial variation occurred in ICU risk-adjusted mortality rates between ICUs, regardless of the model used. The authors concluded that APACHE IV offers the best predictive accuracy with unlimited resources, and that MPM_0 III offered "a viable alternative without a substantial loss in accuracy."[75]

Performance of three models based on 24-hour data (APACHE II, APACHE III-J, and SAPS II) was compared to that of three models based on admission data (MPM II, SAPS III, and SAPS III-A using Australian coefficients) for 1741 patients in an urban university-affiliated teaching hospital in Australia.[76] SAPS II and SAPS III-A fulfilled predetermined calibration and discrimination criteria, APACHE II failed both criteria, and the remaining models discriminated well but overpredicted mortality risk. There did not appear to be an advantage in using 24-hour data versus data available at admission. The improved results with SAPS III-A versus SAPS III again underscores the benefit of customizing models with local coefficients.

SAPS II, SAPS III, APACHE II and customized prognostic models were evaluated in 1851 patients in a German surgical ICU.[77] Discrimination was good for all models, but the native models had poor calibration by Hosmer-Lemeshow goodness of fit, which improved after customization. SAPS III customized for Europe had the best calibration curve. A Swiss study investigated SAPS II, MPM_0 II and MPM_{24} II, and the Injury Severity Score (ISS) in 960 emergency surgical patients (severe head injury, multiple injuries, abdominal aortic aneurysm and spontaneous subarachnoid hemorrhage). In this particular population, MPM_{24} II had the best predictive accuracy and discrimination, but calibration was poor for all models. Surprisingly, the ISS was the worst model for mortality prediction in trauma patients.[78]

Moreno and Morais[79] compared the performance of SAPS II with APACHE II in an independent database of 1094 patients in 19 Portuguese ICUs. Discrimination by ROC analysis was better for SAPS II, but neither model calibrated well by Hosmer-Lemeshow goodness-of-fit testing. In a comparison of the APACHE systems in 1144 British ICU patients, APACHE II had better calibration, but APACHE III had better discrimination.[80] Hospital mortality was higher than predicted with either model, agreement being best in respiratory patients and worst in trauma patients. Differences in trauma care infrastructure between the United States and the United Kingdom might account for some of this discrepancy. APACHE II had superior risk estimates for surgical patients.

Table 222-5 summarizes the results of nine studies in which two or more of the risk-adjustment models were applied to a specific regional population. There is no consistent pattern to accuracy-of-outcome prediction (discrimination), with examples of observed mortality higher than predicted, lower than predicted, as predicted, or predicted differently by different systems. There is no consistent leader in calibration; it tends to be poor in many studies. Ratios of observed-to-expected mortality rates are influenced by case mix as well as quality of care,[81] which argues for caution when using ratios such as the standardized mortality ratio for quality of care comparisons. Application

of APACHE III to an Australian ICU underestimated mortality in a population that was younger, more male, and had more comorbidities than the APACHE III developmental set. Agreement was closer when Australian results were compared with the APACHE U.S. database or when the APACHE III model was adjusted for hospital characteristics.[82] This suggests that cross-hospital comparisons for quality assessment require adjustment for hospital characteristics as well as patient severity of illness. As of this writing, there have been no comparisons of the newest models (APACHE IV, MPM_0 III, SAPS III) on a large independent database.

Uses For Severity-of-Illness Indices

There are four major applications for severity-of-illness scoring systems:

1. Assessing ICU performance/quality improvement
2. Predicting and planning resource utilization
3. Clinical research
4. Guiding individual patient management in carefully selected situations

Quality Improvement and Benchmarking

Meaningful evaluation of ICU performance must consider both severity of illness of the patient population and characteristics of the institution. *Benchmarking* refers to the process of comparing an individual unit's performance either against established case mix-adjusted standards with similar ICUs or with the units' own data over time. Benchmarking need not be for morbidity and mortality outcomes alone, and severity adjustment has been successfully used to explain variations in

TABLE 222-5	Regional Application of Severity Scoring Models		
Study	*Country*	*Systems*	*Findings*
Arabi et al.[117]	Saudi Arabia n = 969	APACHE II $MPM II_0$ and II_{24} SAPS II	Predicted mortality similar to that observed for all systems (SMR 1.0 to 1.09) Calibration best with $MPM II_{24}$ Discrimination best with $MPM II_0$ followed by $MPM II_{24}$, APACHE II and SAPS; all ROC >0.79
Capuzzo et al.[129]	Italy Single center n = 1721	APACHE II SAPS II	ROC area >0.8 both models Mortality in high-risk patients overpredicted by SAPS II and underpredicted by APACHE II
Katsaragakis et al.[126]	Greece Single center n = 661	APACHE II SAPS II	Good discrimination, but poor calibration with both models Better performance with APACHE II
Livingston et al.[62]	Scotland 22 centers n = 10,393	APACHE II APACHE III UK APACHE II $MPM II_0$ $MPM II_{24}$	Discrimination adequate (ROC areas 0.74 to 0.795) Observed mortality significantly different than predicted by all systems APACHE II had best calibration followed by $MPM II_{24}$ and SAPS II
Markgraf et al.[54]	Germany Single center n = 2661 to 2795	APACHE II APACHE III SAPS II	Observed mortality higher than predicted by any model Worst discrepancy with trauma, respiratory, neurologic, and renal disease Best calibration with APACHE II ROC area >0.8 all models
Moreno et al.[130]	Europe 89 centers n = 16,060	$MPM II_0$ SAPS II	Discrimination adequate (ROC 0.822 for SAPS II, 0.785 for MPM_0) Both models overestimated risk of death Large variations across subgroups of patients
Nouira et al.[127]	Tunisia 3 centers n = 1325	APACHE II $MPM II_0$ and II_{24} SAPS II	Observed mortality higher than predicted except with MPM_0 Good discrimination, poor calibration for all models
Patel et al.[37]	United States Single VA medical center n = 302	APACHE II MPM II SAPS II	Predicted mortality for all three scoring systems within 95% CI of predicted ROC area 0.672 to 0.702
Tan et al.[128]	China (Hong Kong) Single center n = 1064	APACHE II SAPS II	Discrimination good (ROC area 0.87 to 0.88) but calibration poor Both models overpredict mortality
Metnitz et al.[131]	Austria 22 ICUs n = 2060	SAPS 3	Original SAPS 3 overestimated mortality even with Central and Western Europe equation. Calibration improved with customization
Poole et al.[132]	Italy 147 ICUs n = 28,357	SAPS 3	Discrimination good Calibration poor—general and South Europe Mediterranean equations overestimated Hospital mortality (SMR 0.73)

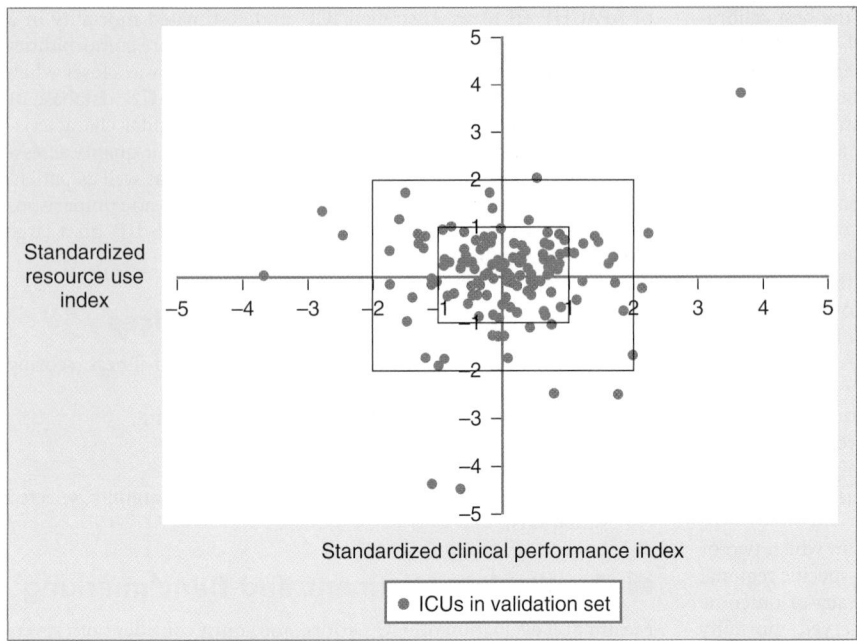

Figure 222-3 Project IMPACT consolidates the display of MPM severity-adjusted mortality data (x-axis) with standardized resource use (weighted hospital days, y-axis). Hospitals within the 1 and 2 standard deviation boxes (most observations) are performing as expected. One hospital in the upper-right corner has superior performance in both dimensions. Four hospitals have longer than expected length of stay (negative numbers on standardized resource use), while being within range for mortality. Three hospitals have worse than expected adjusted mortality, while two have better than expected mortality; all are still within expected resource utilization. *(Reprinted with permission from Nathanson BH, Higgins TL, Teres D et al. A revised method to assess ICU clinical performance and resource utilization. Crit Care Med 2007;35:1853-62.)*

cost[83] and ICU length of stay.[84] Outlier length-of-stay status is only partially predicted by severity of illness, and factors such as long ward stays before ICU admission and absence of an intensivist-directed multidisciplinary care team increase length of stay.[85]

The mortality rate[86] and length of stay for patients transferred to a referral hospital is higher than that of nontransferred patients, and this referral bias[87] has implications in profiling hospital quality. Medical patients transferred from another hospital have higher acute physiology scores but, even after adjustment for case mix and severity of illness, experience longer hospital and ICU lengths of stay and have more than twice the risk of hospital mortality compared with directly admitted patients.[7] The authors of these studies suggest that a referral hospital with a 25% transfer rate would suffer a penalty when undergoing profiling, and public policy should take this into account to reduce the disincentive for tertiary care centers to accept these patients.

Predicting and Planning Resource Utilization

The Therapeutic Intervention Scoring System (TISS) was developed as a method for quantifying patient care and severity of illness.[88] As a prognostic measure, it was supplanted by the newer scoring systems once it was realized that application of technology depended on local availability and local practice. The TISS score does reflect ICU workload and costs[89] and has been used to measure nursing workload.[90] TISS is available in an abbreviated version[91] and can be correlated to APACHE III and IV scores.[40,41] APACHE III and SAPS II have also been applied to measuring severity of illness in intermediate care units.[92,93]

Although it seems intuitive that ICU length of stay and mortality should both be predictable from the same admission risk factors, the correlations between mortality and lengths of stay are less predictable. In part, this may be due to the censoring effect of early death in extremely ill individuals, but it also reflects considerable interhospital variability in practice, including the use of intermediate beds and long-term ventilation facilities. The CALICO project[94] found that APACHE IV and MPM$_0$ III were more accurate than SAPS II for prediction of ICU length of stay—not surprising given that the California population would be more similar geographically and temporally to the newer models than the older international SAPS II. A "weighed hospital days" model with four variables (mortality rate, percentage of unscheduled surgical patients, mechanical ventilation within 1 hour of ICU

admission, and percent discharged to a post–acute care facility) was developed from the MPM III database[59] and has reasonable performance ($r^2 = 0.47$ between score and length of stay) but only at an ICU rather than individual patient level. Figure 222-3 demonstrates a method for displaying MPM-adjusted mortality (x-axis) versus resource use (y-axis).[59] Similarly, Campbell and colleagues could identify factors associated with death and readmission to ICU but could not produce a definitive model based on these risk factors for individual patients.[95] There does appear to be a predictable relationship between increasing severity of illness (using SAPS, SAPS II, and APACHE II or III) and risk of ICU readmission.[96]

Use of Severity Indices in Clinical Research

Existing databases and severity adjustment make possible hypothesis-generating observations and conclusions about therapeutic choices in situations where randomized, prospective evaluations might not be permitted or funded. For prospective studies, severity scoring indices can be used to "risk stratify" the population before randomization, thus reducing the number of patients and cost of clinical trials. Clinical studies have also used scoring systems as part of inclusion criteria and to demonstrate that control and study groups have similar disease burden. Representative examples of this approach include risk stratification for comparison of different antibiotic regimens[97] and anticytokine therapies.[98] Acute physiologic abnormalities are important prognostic factors influencing outcome in patients meeting criteria for severe sepsis.[50] Correlations have been noted between the MPM$_0$ II sepsis score[99] and interleukin (IL)-6 plasma levels and between APACHE III scores and plasma levels of tumor necrosis factor (TNF)-sR, IL-6, and C-reactive protein.[100] Nonsurvivors appear to have significantly higher MPM or APACHE scores at any time during sepsis.

Uses of Severity Adjustment for Individual Predictions

The difficulty in using scoring systems for individuals arises from attempts to apply a probability estimate, which may range from 0 to 1, to an individual for whom the result will be 0 *or* 1. No model is accurate enough to predict that a given patient will certainly survive or invariably die, so the use of scoring systems alone to direct or withhold therapy is not recommended. It is unlikely that any score calculated within 24 hours of ICU admission could ever perfectly predict outcome, because the patient's individual response to therapy clearly plays a role. APACHE III alone could not independently predict survival in 114 patients with perforated gastrointestinal viscus, and only the development of overt multiple organ failure predicted death.[101] Sequential prognostic estimates, an approach explored by both APACHE[102] and MPM,[44] may improve prognosis by incorporating response to therapy, but this application of scoring systems should not create a vicious cycle in which a declining risk of survival could precipitate withdrawal or limitation of care. Objective predictions of the need for next-day life support are used by APACHE III and IV to guide triage and discharge decisions.[103] Although space does not permit a full discussion, there are a number of tools to quantify organ failure in ICU patients, including the Sequential Organ Failure Assessment (SOFA) score,[104] the Multiple Organ Dysfunction (MOD) score,[105] and the Logistic Organ Dysfunction Score.[106] In contrast to the outcome prediction scores, organ dysfunction scores were not designed to predict mortality, but they do capture the timing and severity of organ failure, typically examining six or seven discrete systems (respiratory, cardiovascular, renal, hepatic, coagulation, central nervous system, and sometimes gastrointestinal). Increases in scores following admission generally carry a poor prognosis,[107,108] although others have reported limited ability of the SOFA or MOD score to discriminate outcome.[109]

Use of scoring systems to guide therapy has not been well studied. The package insert for recombinant human activated protein C (rhAPC) suggests APACHE II scores greater than 25 as a criterion for drug administration. This recommendation is based in part on post hoc subgroup analysis of PROWESS trial[110] patients showing that patients with higher APACHE II scores were more likely to benefit from this therapy than those with lower scores. Problems with limiting administration therapy to patients with low severity scores include wide variability in severity score between those obtained at ICU admission versus at the time of drug administration.[111] Because the APACHE II score is weighted for age and chronic health status, younger patients and those with less chronic disease burden will have lower scores for an equal amount of physiologic derangement. The Australian APACHE study quoted earlier[82] indirectly suggests that younger, healthier patients may be improperly categorized. An efficient emergency department may well stabilize the patients and lower the APACHE score before arrival in the ICU.[112] These same general concerns would apply to many situations in which a severity score could be used to decide on ICU admission or to administer or withhold interventions for an individual patient.[113] Admission scores do well at predicting outcomes in groups of patients, not individuals. Neither sequential evaluations[44,102] nor organ failure scores are sufficiently sensitive or specific in individuals that they could be used in isolation for therapeutic decisions.

Objectively calculated severity scores are not necessarily more accurate than physician or nurse intuition when dealing with individual patients.[114] Sensitivity, specificity, correct prediction, and area under the ROC curve were compared, and no significant differences were noted between ROC areas for APACHE II versus the clinical assessment of nurses, fellows, residents, or interns.[115] Accurate prognosis may be most difficult for patients with the highest risk of death. A multicenter study addressing the issue of medical futility found that divergent judgments on patient prognosis by doctors and nurses increased with higher SAPS II scores and longer ICU stays.[116] ICU physicians, in fact, discriminate between survivors and nonsurvivors more accurately than SAPS II, MPM I or APACHE II.[114]

APACHE, SAPS, and MPM scores are *specific*, having better than 90% ability to predict survival, but are relatively *insensitive* in predicting death. Such information should not be taken as a rationale to rely on clinical judgment alone and forgo the use of formal scoring. The existing severity indices, despite their flaws, do provide useful, objective information that can supplement clinical judgment for prognosis and

triage decisions, bearing in mind that patient autonomy and medical ethics also influence these decisions.

Pitfalls in the Application of Severity-of-Illness Indices

Like any tool, severity-of-illness indices can be misused. The use (and abuse) of databases for profiling ICUs and/or individual physicians is growing despite flaws in administrative databases and problems identified with application of statistical models[18,19,29] and physician profiling.[117,118] Assuming a properly developed model is applied, potential pitfalls in application fall into four major categories: data collection and entry errors,[119] misapplication of the model,[7,29,36] use of mortality as the sole criterion of outcome, and failure to account for sample size and chance variability[34,75,81] when reporting results (Box 222-4). Determination of the diagnosis is prone to bias.[120] Models that assess performance using a patient's condition at 24 hours are not truly independent of treatment. If the characteristics of an ICU's patients are markedly different from a general population's, the resulting case mix will alter model performance.[29] Less obvious is the fact that all models start the clock with ICU admission, the timing of which is not standardized[121] and is frequently influenced by local conditions such as ICU bed availability.[122] ICUs also do not function in isolation in the process of care,[112] and the recent trend toward aggressive use of step-down facilities and off-site chronic ventilation and rehabilitation units raises the question of whether hospital mortality is valid when patients may be transferred to other facilities alive but still technology dependent.[122] The issue of lead-time bias (pre-ICU stabilization) has been mentioned earlier; assessment is further complicated for patients with multiple ICU admissions.[123,124] Which ICU stay, for example, should be counted for a patient who has ICU observation after an uneventful

---

Box 222-4

POTENTIAL PITFALLS IN THE APPLICATION AND REPORTING OF SEVERITY-ADJUSTED OUTCOME

Data Collection and Entry
Inclusion of ineligible patients
Missing variables and data management errors
Substitution of available for properly timed data
Transcription and data entry errors
Improper communication between hospital clinical and risk adjustment applications
Wrong diagnosis selected
Administrative data reflective of clinical situation
Deliberate "gaming" of the system

Models
Case-mix differences (critical threshold exceeded)
Application to subsets of development population
Changes in influence of variable with improving medical care
Small clinical changes become large risk increments when continuous data are categorized.
Lead-time bias

Outcomes
Insufficient range of outcomes reported
Use of proxy outcomes that inadequately reflect true status
Patient lost to follow-up
Chance variability masquerading as true difference
Relationships of scores to resource utilization and costs reflect observed practice, not ideal

Reporting
Confidence intervals not reported
Inadequate sample size
Physician of record misidentified
Computational errors
Misapplication of group data to individuals
Misinterpretation of statistical significance as clinical significance

vascular procedure and then develops complications requiring ICU readmission on the fifth postoperative day? It is increasingly necessary to evaluate the performance of an ICU *system*, which includes pre-ICU, ICU, and post-ICU care. Rules for starting times and endpoints of evaluation have to be better defined.[121,122]

Conclusion

APACHE, MPM, and SAPS are highly developed, prospectively validated tools useful for comparison of ICU performance in the care of groups of patients. Specialized models are available for burn, trauma, sepsis, cardiac surgical, and pediatric patients. When used as intended, these models allow stratification of patients for performance assessment, utilization management, clinical research, and dissemination of outcome results. Important implementation considerations include careful data collections, appropriate matching of the model and the population under study, and use of proper sample sizes and CIs in reporting results.

None of the models can perfectly predict the outcome for an individual patient.[125] However, this limitation is true of almost any test utilized in medicine and need not preclude the use of prognostic estimates for clinical decision support. Physicians must be alert to the limitations of severity-adjustment models in performance-based assessment, because case-mix differences, inadequate sample sizes, or systemic errors in data collection can generate erroneous conclusions about the quality of care.

KEY POINTS

1. Stratification of outcome based on risk factors is necessary when comparing outcomes obtained by different institutions, intensive care teams, and treatment strategies.

2. Although mortality is readily defined and easily captured, it is insufficient as the sole measure of clinical outcome and does not capture other important endpoints such as complications, quality of life, or costs.

3. Administrative data are plentiful but are typically less reliable than carefully collected clinical information. The quality of administrative databases can be improved by including laboratory information.

4. Most outcome stratification models are developed empirically by performing univariate analysis of independent variables against a chosen outcome and then refined using multivariate techniques.

5. Model performance is assessed by measuring discrimination (typically by ROC-curve area) and calibration (typically by goodness-of-fit procedures).

6. The standardized mortality ratio is created by dividing observed by expected mortality rates. Values less than 1.0, if statistically significant, indicate performance better than expected.

7. The Acute Physiology and Chronic Health Evaluation (APACHE II thru APACHE IV), the Mortality Probability Models (MPM), and the Simplified Acute Physiology Score (SAPS) are well-developed, prospectively validated models useful in adult general critical care units. The Intensive Care National Audit and Research Center (ICNARC) and Veterans Affairs Intensive Care Unit (VA ICU) models are also available. Customized models are useful in highly specialized ICUs or when evaluating population subsets such as pediatric or cardiac surgery patients.

8. Outcome predictions are intended for groups, not individuals. Mortality probability estimates range from 0.0 to 1.0, but an individual patient will either live or die. Mortality predictions also vary depending on when the data were geographically and temporally collected. Use of scoring systems to direct therapeutic choices has not been adequately studied.

ANNOTATED REFERENCES

Zimmerman JE, Kramer AA, McNair DS, Malila FM. Acute Physiology and Chronic Health Evaluation (APACHE) IV: hospital mortality assessment for today's critically ill patients. Crit Care Med 2006;34:1297-310.
APACHE was the first widely used prognostic scoring system and has been periodically updated over the past 30 years. The latest iteration was developed on 110,558 patients in 2002-2003. APACHE IV has very good discrimination (ROC area 0.88) and calibration, and corrects the systematic overestimation of mortality that developed since publication of APACHE III.

Metnitz PGH, Moreno RP, Almeida E, et al., SAPS 3 Investigators. SAPS 3—From evaluation of the patient to evaluation of the intensive care unit. Part 1: objectives, methods and cohort description. Intensive Care Med 2005;31:1336-44.

Moreno RP, Metnitz PGH, Almeida E, et al., SAPS 3 Investigators. SAPS 3—From evaluation of the patient to evaluation of the intensive care unit. Part 2: development of a prognostic model for hospital mortality at ICU admission. Intensive Care Med 2005;31:1345-55.
The SAPS 3 study utilized an international population of 19,577 patients in 307 ICUs. Regional variation in outcomes occur, and SAPS 3 has customized admission equations for Australasia, Central/South America; Central/Western Europe, Eastern Europe, North Europe, Mediterranean countries, and North America. ROC area is 0.85 with satisfactory calibration.

Higgins TL, Teres D, Copes WS, et al. Assessing contemporary intensive care unit outcome: an updated Mortality Probability Admission Model (MPM₀-III). Crit Care Med 2007;35:827-35.
MPM III was developed on 124,855 patients admitted to 135 ICUs at 98 hospitals in the United States (94), Canada (3), and Brazil (1) between 2001 and 2004. It corrects the drift in calibration since MPM II and adds terms for "Full Code" resuscitation status at admission, and for the absence of any MPM II risk factor except age to account for better-than-expected outcomes in otherwise healthy elderly patients. Discrimination by ROC is 0.82, and the model calibrates well. Subsequent publications have prospectively validated the model and updated the "Rapoport-Teres" resource utilization graph used by MPM and Project IMPACT.

Harrison DA, Parry GJ, Carpenter JR, Short A, Rowan K. A new risk prediction model for critical care: the Intensive Care National Audit and Research Centre (ICNARC) model. Crit Care Med 2007;35:1091-8.
The ICNARC model utilizes patient physiology plus age, diagnostic category, source of admission and CPR before admission. In a population of 216,626 patients from England, Wales, and Northern Ireland between 1995 and 2003, this model discriminated better (ROC area 0.86) than APACHE II, APACHE III, SAPS II, or MPM II. This study offers further evidence that geographic variation occurs, and that misleading SMR results may occur when models developed in one environment are applied to a new population.

Render ML, Deddens J, Freyberg R, et al. Veterans Affairs intensive care unit risk adjustment model: validation, updating, recalibration. Crit Care Med 2008;36:1031-42.
Some 36,420 consecutive ICU admissions in 1999-2000 and a second cohort of 81,964 cases in 2002-04 were used to update the VA-ICU model. ROC areas were good. The VA-ICU population is overwhelmingly male (97.2%) and somewhat older. ROC area was 0.89, comparable to APACHE IV in this population, and better than MPM₂₄ II (ROC 0.84), SAPS III (ROC 0.86), or the SOFA score (ROC 0.81).

Sinuff T, Adhikari NKJ, Cook DJ, et al. Mortality predictions in the intensive care unit: comparing physicians with scoring systems. Crit Care Med 2006;34:878-85.
This analysis of observational studies (one using SAPS II, two using MPM II, six using APACHE II, and three computer models) found that ICU physicians and objective models have moderate accuracy in the first 24 hours of ICU stay, but that physicians better discriminate between survivors and nonsurvivors (physician ROC area 0.85 + 0.03 versus 0.63 + 0.06 for scoring systems). Limitations of the study are use of older scoring models, but the conclusion that neither physicians nor scoring systems are sufficiently accurate to determine end-of-life decisions in the first 24 hours of ICU care is well supported by the data.

Vincent JL, Opal SM, Marshall JC. Ten reasons why we should NOT use severity scores as entry criteria for clinical trials or in our treatment decisions. Crit Care Med 2010;38:283-7.
Whereas the seemingly objective nature of scores make it tempting to apply their predictions to individuals, it is important to remember that these tools were designed for evaluating large groups of patients, not for individual prognosis or decision making. The authors point out that interobserver variability in score calculation, age bias, and issues with the starting time of critical care call into question the use of these scores for patient enrollment into clinical trials.

Sefarian EG, Afessa B, Gajic O, Keegan MT, Hubmayr RD. Comparison of community and referral intensive care unit patients in a tertiary medical center: evidence for referral bias in the critically ill. Crit Care Med 2008;36:2779-86.
Patients referred to the Mayo Clinic medical ICU between 1996 and 2004 were more severely ill, had higher mortality and longer length of stay, and were more likely to receive an active ICU intervention compared with community patients. When adjusted for severity of illness, mortality was as expected. Unadjusted differences were not seen in the surgical ICU, although hospital mortality rate was lower in referral surgical patients. Referral bias likely occurs because of differences in prior care or the transfer process that are not captured by risk adjustment. This bias has potential impact on clinical trials.

Nathanson BH, Higgins TL. An introduction to statistical methods used in binary outcome modeling. Semin Cardiothorac Vasc Anesth 2008;12:153-66.
For those who enjoy getting "under the hood" of risk-adjustment models. Warning: the equations contained within are known to produce somnolence.

REFERENCE

Access the complete reference list online at http://www.expertconsult.com.

223

Evaluating Pediatric Critical Care Practices

ANTHONY D. SLONIM | MURRAY M. POLLACK

Today's healthcare environment demands attention to evaluating care so that improvement efforts can be made. Evaluation efforts must be systematic in their collection, analysis, and information use. Whereas it is important to draw attention to objective performance measures, information derived from an appreciation of the perspectives and expectations of stakeholders who experience the program under examination are also useful. For pediatric intensive care units (PICUs), that primarily includes the patient and family; however, a broader group of stakeholders includes colleagues on the multidisciplinary team, nurses, physicians, therapists, pharmacists, and social workers, as well as regulators and payers—who are all interested in the program's quality—should be included.

A Historical Perspective on Quality

Quality in health care has received increased focus over the last 30 years, beginning with Donabedian's influence demonstrating that the fundamental concepts of structure, process, and outcome were as important to health care as they were to other industries (Figure 223-1).[1] Since then, focused efforts to advance the concept of quality in health care have been performed. In the early 1990s, a series of articles in the *New England Journal of Medicine* quantified adverse events and helped disentangle the elements of patient harm and its relationship to risk management.[2-4] A few years later, President Clinton, through executive order, chartered a commission to investigate healthcare quality more broadly.[5]

Despite these and a variety of other prominent efforts, discussion regarding quality in health care remained relatively stagnant until the Institute of Medicine's (IOM's) series of reports.[6-9] The first IOM report, "To Err is Human," provided a wakeup call for the healthcare industry to consider how patients may be harmed.[6] This was followed by "Crossing the Quality Chasm," which defined six "Aims for Improvement."[7] These aims included safety, effectiveness, equity, timeliness, patient centeredness, and efficiency and helped establish a framework through which clinical services, including those delivered to the critically ill child, could be evaluated.[10]

The Institute for Healthcare Improvement (IHI), among other groups, became instrumental in providing clinicians with tools to help them focus on improvement work by defining and measuring what was to be improved and by when.[11] Efforts aimed at improving reporting and learning from adverse occurrences were noticed when President Bush signed the Patient Safety and Quality Improvement Act, which would become operationalized in part through patient safety organizations.[12] More recently, with healthcare reform taking shape, other considerable advances including medical homes, accountable care organizations, and pay for performance are likely to take on additional significance and set the tone for healthcare quality for years to come. This will create important opportunities and challenges for advancing care for critically ill children.[10]

Systems of Care

Traditional engineering approaches focus on how systems work rather than on understanding the ways in which they fail or the effects of failure.[13] There are several aspects of system design and maintenance that can affect the likelihood of failure. This is a fundamental distinction to how quality is viewed in health care.[13] First, clinicians often approach quality improvement from the perspective of risk rather than the perspective of reliability. Mortality and morbidity conferences, peer review meetings, and root-cause analysis all tend to focus on what went wrong in retrospect and the elements of failure rather than on the system's reliability.[13] Second, pediatric critical care clinicians function in complex systems of care yet have little training or experience in how to design and organize those complex systems to ensure that the needs of the critically ill child are met.[13] Routinely, providers will repetitively use "workarounds" rather than redesigning processes to be safer and more efficient. Finally, in contrast to the engineering approach, clinicians are very interested in the effects of system failure, which in clinical parlance are the outcomes of care. Whereas outcomes are important, several recent efforts in health care have also demonstrated the importance of managing the processes of care.[14] The best examples of these efforts in pediatric critical care are evidence-based clinical guidelines, checklists, and "bundles" of care, which represent tactical opportunities to specify how care should be delivered to arrive at the desired outcomes.

Designing for Evaluation

PROGRAM ELEMENTS

The ability to evaluate clinical services, including pediatric critical care services, depends upon how well the evaluation program is built and implemented. When considering complex systems, it is often helpful to begin by identifying the focus areas for evaluation and improvement and prioritizing those based on the desired impact. Quality improvement and evaluation rely upon three critical and interdependent functions: data and analytics, process improvement techniques, and change management principles (Figure 223-2). Each one of these functions is important in their own right, but none of these is sufficient individually to accomplish successful improvement. The use of *data* is fundamental for improving quality. Data should be objective, easy to measure, accurate, and establish a baseline of performance upon which improvement efforts can be compared when the evaluation is completed. The *analytic* component is equally important. Effective programs will move past mere descriptions of data and use important analytic techniques to support their inferences. Clinical *processes* are the interactions between providers and their patients and providers with one another. A variety of techniques can help with the description of clinical processes, including workflow analysis, flow charting, and time motion studies. These important data elements can then be compared and analyzed using value-stream mapping to eliminate waste and streamline the process, making the care more efficient. More recent efforts evaluating teamwork principles and their impact on outcomes are beginning to emerge.[15,16] *Change management* is fundamental to every improvement process. In addition to managing the changes in process, managing the transition from a current state to some future state requires attention to relationships, commitment, and communication for the team and its members.

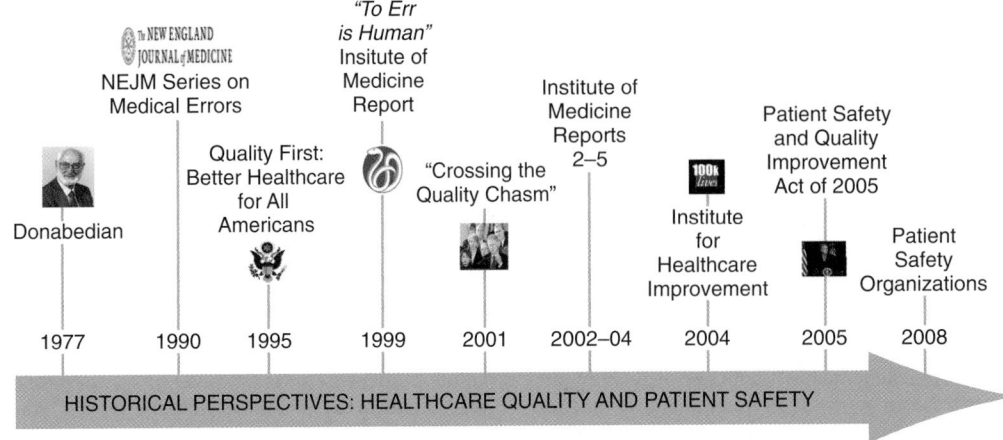

Figure 223-1 Historical perspective of quality and patient safety.

RESULTS

Evaluation is an effort to identify the impact on the stated objectives. In the PICU, this may relate to how well certain outcomes are achieved. For example, outcomes like mortality, length of stay, and specific complications like hospital-associated infections are commonly measured. Comparing the performance of the PICU to itself over time or to other similar PICUs provides a context for both improvement activities and research. The focus of improvement activities is to improve the clinical care delivered. If outcomes are suboptimal, team members can be engaged, educated, or trained to improve compliance with clinical processes and outcomes. Clinical outcomes can also drive a research agenda. Whereas the focus of improvement activities is to improve clinical care, the focus of research is to drive the development of new knowledge. Data, analytics, and appropriate control for population case mix are essential for ensuring the ability to apply new knowledge gained through these activities.

SUSTAINING IMPROVEMENTS

When evaluating the impact for a given quality improvement project, short-term outcomes are often favorable. Providers enjoy working on efforts to improve their care, particularly when the focus of that work is a critically ill child. Teams become excited about the improvement projects and interested in what they can learn and how they can improve for the benefit of the child and family. Unfortunately, providers often face numerous projects, experience fatigue from continuous learning, and rarely change their behaviors to match the intended outcomes. The results in the short term often plateau, and when attention is diverted to the next priority, reevaluation may even demonstrate a reduction in impact.

In contrast, when systems are designed around specified behaviors, and the risk points that allow workarounds and adaptive behaviors to emerge are identified, higher levels of performance can be achieved. This approach involves the fusion of different team members' perspectives over time. For example, when considering the evaluation of results of a recent project to improve bloodstream infections, the PICU team invited members of the operating room suite and hematology-oncology service to participate in the meetings. The input of these "internal consultants" provided the PICU team with an opportunity to learn and apply useful practices from other clinical contexts with relevance to their patient. The use of this so-called quality fusion approach (Figure 223-3) provides the PICU with a greater impact on the initiative under study and provides important sustainability when attention is diverted to the next improvement project.

Evaluation Domains at the Unit Level

The IOM's framework on quality using the six aims continues to provide usefulness to organize the approach to healthcare quality in the PICU. Each of these aims has relevance to the provision of critical care services at the unit level.

SAFETY

Since the IOM's report on medical errors and patient safety highlighted the problem of iatrogenic injury in hospitalized inpatients, numerous stakeholders have begun to focus on reducing medical errors as a

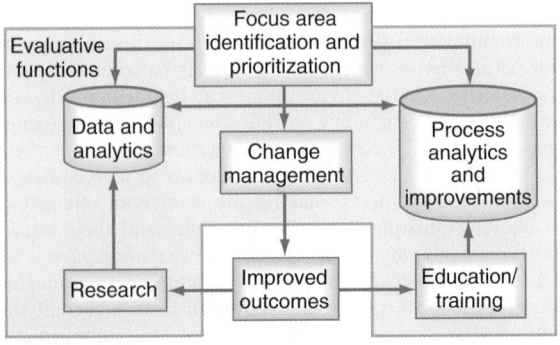

Figure 223-2 Key elements and drivers of an evaluative program.

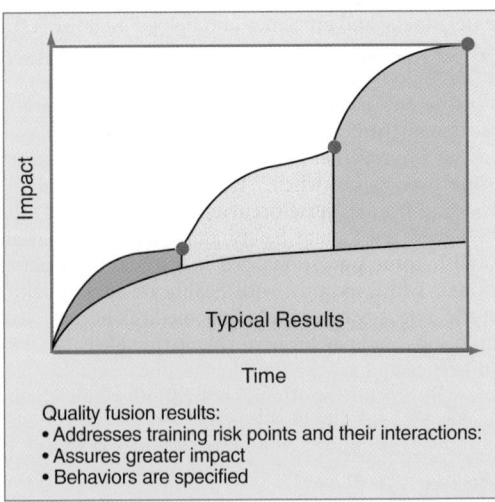

Figure 223-3 Quality fusion: a concept for reaching higher gains in quality improvement and sustaining them for longer durations.

means of improving patient safety and reducing the harm associated with the delivery of health care.[7] Adverse patient occurrences are inevitable in the high-risk environment of the PICU, but interventions aimed at reducing these adverse events can be designed once one understands the types of errors and the circumstances that contribute to them.

Error Classification

Different classification schemes for medical errors have been developed. Brennan and colleagues classified adverse events in medical practice as *operative* and *nonoperative*.[7] McClead and Menke, in their classification system for neonatal ICUs, included both the investigation of complications associated with new or unproven technologies and the study of *human error*, which is relevant to the understanding of a *just culture* where providers are held accountable for risky behaviors in the care process.[17-18] The identification of *critical incidents* provides opportunities to make system improvements. Finally, the IOM categorized medical errors based on their diagnosis, treatment, prevention, communication, and equipment failures.[6] These categories are relevant for the evaluation of pediatric critical care services.

Diagnostic Errors

The autopsy has been used as a technique to enhance quality assurance programs in medical care. Diagnostic errors uncovered at autopsy that result in the primary cause of death or affected patient outcome are important to consider.[19] In three single-institution studies of critically ill adults, autopsies revealed diagnoses that would have changed antemortem management and affected outcome in 10% to 27% of cases.[20-22] In children, the rate of missed diagnoses that affected outcome was estimated at 7% in one study.[23] In the PICU, one study identified major diagnostic errors that would have affected outcome in 5% of patients; in an additional 25% of cases, there were missed diagnoses that were not believed to be clinically meaningful.[24] Importantly, iatrogenic injury was a major subset of these missed diagnoses, occurring 17% of the time.[24] Thus, autopsy remains an important tool for identifying diagnostic errors and deaths related to iatrogenic injury in the PICU. It also provides an opportunity to enhance provider education and training related to diagnostic dilemmas.

Treatment Errors

Medication Errors. Medication administration occurs frequently in the treatment of critically ill children and provides considerably more opportunities for medication errors and adverse drug events (ADEs). Among hospitalized children, ADEs are common, and the PICU is an important setting for their occurrence.[25-26] Specific medication classes are prone to errors, including sedatives, vasoactive infusions, and parenteral nutrition. One useful and cost-effective strategy to improve medication safety in the PICU is to have a unit-based pharmacist who can intervene to adjust dosages, provide drug information, contribute to management decisions, and monitor complications of medication therapy. This has become an increasingly important opportunity to be able to provide high-quality critical care services to children.[27]

Nosocomial Infection. Acquired infections are important contributors to morbidity, mortality, and cost in the PICU.[14,28-32] Recent efforts have expanded our knowledge of the incidence, prevalence, risk factors, costs, and methods of improving bloodstream infections in the PICU.[14] The importance of these efforts is the ability to demonstrate how care can be improved when providers use data to drive system changes.

Risk factors for nosocomial infection in the PICU include severity of illness, postoperative status, and device use.[31-34] Specific investigations into the types of nosocomial infection (e.g., urinary tract, pneumonia), specific organisms (e.g., influenza, respiratory syncytial virus, methicillin-resistant *Staphylococcus aureus)*, specific PICU patient populations (e.g., cardiac surgery, burns), and specific procedures (e.g., mechanical ventilation, extracorporeal membrane oxygenation) have been performed. These studies provide insight for the development of

directed strategies to reduce nosocomial infection rates and their associated morbidity and mortality in PICUs. These strategies include more stringent infection control policies, reduction of colonization with resistant organisms, and scheduled rotation of prescribed antibiotics.[35-37] Perhaps the most important opportunity to reduce infections is the removal of unnecessary devices including urinary catheters, central venous and arterial catheters, and ventilators as soon as they are not longer needed for the child's care.[14,31,32]

Procedures. Interventional procedures are an important component of pediatric critical care practice. They provide the intensivist with the means to address a child's failing organ systems, but they are also associated with risk. Procedural risks are associated with both the insertion and maintenance of these devices. For example, tracheal intubation is associated with potential complications from laryngoscopy, failed intubation attempts, esophageal intubation, damage to the teeth, and hypoxemia.[38-39] In addition, the risks from unintended extubation for the child with respiratory failure are significant. PICUs can address their rates of adverse occurrences related to both the performance and maintenance of commonly performed invasive procedures like central venous access, mechanical ventilation, arterial cannulation, and intracranial pressure monitoring. Collaborative efforts that share best-practice methods of inserting and maintaining these devices can demonstrably improve the complications associated with these procedures.[14]

Preventive Errors

In the ICU, considerable evidence has been accumulated regarding prophylaxis for gastrointestinal stress ulcers, deep venous thrombosis, pressure ulcers, and other adverse events.[40-41] Efforts have also been made to address prophylactic care more broadly. For example, the Prophylactic Intravenous Use of Milrinone After Cardiac Operation in Pediatrics (PRIMACORP) study was initiated to determine whether the prophylactic postoperative use of milrinone in pediatric cardiac surgery patients improves the outcome associated with low cardiac output syndrome.[42]

Other Errors

The PICU environment may itself be an independent contributor to patient safety. Two characteristics contribute to the likelihood of errors in the PICU. The first is *complexity*, or the degree to which system components are specialized and interdependent. Complex systems are more prone to errors. The second characteristic is *coupling*. Tightly coupled systems have no buffer, and sequences are fixed, whereas loosely coupled systems can tolerate delays or variations in sequencing. Communication errors, equipment failures, system failures, and more recently, problems with teamwork are all associated with complex and tightly coupled systems and can contribute to an unsafe environment in these settings.[6] Equipment failures are an obvious and often unavoidable problem related to patient safety. However, communication failures, system failures, and teamwork problems can enhance the likelihood of errors and prevent an appropriate mitigating response when they occur.[15-16]

EFFECTIVENESS

Evidence-based practice incorporates the best research evidence with clinical expertise and patient values to achieve the best outcomes for patients.[7] The clinical practice of critical care medicine is highly variable among practitioners and institutions. Efforts to reduce variability in care are provided by the implementation of practice guidelines and the use of clinical algorithms and checklists.[43-44]

Private, governmental, and subspecialty organizations have developed numerous guidelines to reduce unnecessary variability in care. The American Academy of Pediatrics and the Society for Critical Care Medicine have developed guidelines and policy statements to help improve the care of critically ill children.[45-46] Guidelines can be heterogeneous with respect to their creation. At one extreme, results from randomized controlled trials are incorporated into the care guidelines; at the other extreme, the consensus of a group of practitioners is all that is required. This is important, because the success of any practice guideline is dependent on its ability to influence physician decision making.

Several important components of these guidelines are worth mentioning, because they will ultimately contribute to the guidelines' acceptance by practitioners of critical care medicine. First, the guidelines should be grounded in the existing evidence base from randomized controlled trials. Second, when the evidence does not exist, the authors should assemble a multidisciplinary group of clinicians and researchers to reach consensus regarding treatment options. This is done to minimize bias by any one group of practitioners or any one discipline. Third, and perhaps most important, the guidelines should be considered a work in progress that helps identify current deficiencies from a data perspective so future research initiatives can be used to further support these guidelines.

EFFICIENCY

Economics demands that healthcare resources be delivered in a cost-effective and efficient manner while not jeopardizing quality.[47] The achievement of specific outcome goals is a measure of an ICU's quality. Costs vary with outcome measures. Mortality rates, efficiency rates, lengths of stay, rates of nosocomial infection and readmission, and the presence of a teaching program all impact expenses and reimbursement. Quality at a given level of cost determines the value of a commodity. In this case, the commodity is ICU care.[48]

The value of an individual ICU is increased by its ability to achieve selected measures of outcome while keeping costs to a minimum. This is concordant with the concept of efficiency as an aim in the IOM's current model of healthcare quality.[7] Intensive care services are a commodity, and those units providing quality care at a reasonable cost, as judged by efficiency and a similar patient mix, will be most appealing. Less efficient ICUs will have to optimize efficiency or have cost-containment strategies imposed on them.[48]

From a microeconomic perspective, patients who are sicker require more services in the ICU, stay longer, are more likely to die, and cost more to be treated.[49-50] This is not new information. However, to balance the issues of cost and quality, ICUs should identify same-strata best-practices ICUs with similar cost drivers (e.g., severity of illness) and operate under a philosophy of "targeted benchmarking" to achieve comparability up to a specified level.[51] To accomplish this, clinical scoring systems are frequently used to control for case-mix variables (physiology, diagnoses, etc.) and thus allow for standardized comparisons. Length of stay has become a standard in benchmarking ICU performance and quality, and reducing length of stay is one method of reducing cost, although as a variable itself, length of stay is subject to differences in measurement.[52-53] The standardized length-of-stay ratio is that of observed-to-predicted length of stay and is an indicator of resource use adjusted for severity.[54] The standardized length-of-stay ratio can be used to compare a particular unit's performance over time, but it can also be used to determine whether a particular ICU's resource use is above or below that of similar ICUs.[54]

Another method of assessing the efficiency of resource use in the ICU is to evaluate unique ICU therapies[55-61]—that is, those that are best delivered in the ICU, such as mechanical ventilation and vasoactive infusions. Individual ICUs and physicians differ in their monitoring strategies, so monitoring technologies should not be classified as unique therapies.[57] The benefits of this approach are that it allows physicians to determine the proportion of low-risk monitor-only patients[61] and compare the number of high-risk critical care patients requiring unique ICU therapies. Excess bed capacity leads to a higher ratio of monitored patients to high-risk patients and reduces the efficiency of the ICU.[61] Opportunities to evaluate admission and discharge criteria, as well as throughput issues resulting from the inability to transfer ICU patients because of a high hospital occupancy rate, may serve to improve an individual ICU's efficiency.

EQUITY

Achieving equity in healthcare quality means ensuring impartial care for populations and individuals that is free from bias related to race, ethnicity, insurance status, income, or gender. This bias may be manifested at two independent levels. First, discrimination may be targeted at the population level before the patient actually reaches a healthcare provider. These problems are primarily ones of restricted access to health care. Second, once patients have accessed healthcare services, they may receive differential treatment based on personal characteristics.[7] In its most overt form, this is called *discrimination*.

Insurance status differences affect access to outpatient physicians, hospital services, and procedures. These differences also affect physicians' practice patterns and thereby influence resource use and outcome for adult primary care and critical care patients alike.[62-64] Insurance status differences apply not only to different types of insurance but also to the method of administering the insurance.[64,65] For example, the care delivered under a managed care arrangement is expected to be different from that delivered in a non–managed care environment. However, these differences in care do not necessarily mean that one type of care is worse; it may simply be different.[65] Lack of access to needed services may be responsible for delayed disease presentation and avoidable morbidity, which may lead to more severe illness and longer hospital stay.[66,67] This is consistent with the observation that patients from lower socioeconomic status have more severe illness on admission to the PICU.[68]

There are limited data describing the relationship of insurance status to resource utilization or outcome in specific subgroups of critically ill pediatric patients, including neonates and medical and surgical patients.[69-73] Insurance status differences in critically ill pediatric medical patients have been demonstrated. After adjusting for illness severity, Medicaid-insured children with acute severe asthma received mechanical ventilation more often and for longer durations and had longer PICU and hospital stays than commercially insured or managed-care patients.[73] Children with Medicaid who were hospitalized with diabetic ketoacidosis experienced coma more often and had longer lengths of stay than their commercially insured counterparts.[73] Similar insurance status differences can be found among critically ill pediatric surgical patients. Postoperative congenital heart disease patients with Medicaid had higher mortality rates than commercially insured children.[71] Medicaid patients experienced complicated appendicitis, including perforation or abscess formation, more often than other patients,[73] and they had longer stays. Observed mortality rates among uninsured children with head trauma were higher than those among privately or publicly insured children.[72]

The IOM was charged with assessing the extent of racial disparities in health care, identifying factors contributing to the inequities, and recommending policies and practices to eliminate them.[74] The integration of national efforts to address racial disparities in health care and the work being accomplished in healthcare quality provide opportunities to improve the equity of delivered healthcare services to minority populations.[75] Racial differences in health care are evident for adult and pediatric patients. These differences affect access to healthcare services and outcomes.[76-83] Intensivists have reason to be concerned about these findings.

The literature regarding racial disparities in critically ill children is not nearly as well established. In a 25-year study of mortality associated with congenital heart disease, black patients had a nearly 20% higher mortality rate than white patients.[82] For pediatric patients requiring single-ventricle palliation for congenital heart disease, there was considerably more variation in the age of palliation in black babies than in white babies in a single-institution study. Black pediatric patients with renal failure are less likely than white patients to be wait-listed for kidney transplantation.[77] However, in a study of low-birth-weight infants, there were no survival differences between white and black babies.[76]

Race has been used as a proxy for a number of other socioeconomic factors.[84] It has become evident, however, that if meaningful information is to be gained by including racial variables in research, reliable and valid definitions have to be used.[84] *Race* is a relatively nonspecific term that incorporates biological, social, and cultural components that are more than mere physical descriptors and are not consistently considered in the definition.[84] As a result, when comparing outcome measures—whether vitality outcomes such as mortality or resource use outcomes such as length of stay—it may be inappropriate to conclude that race is the explanatory variable.[84]

TIMELINESS

Timeliness is a marker of the adequacy of processes in the ICU to achieve acceptable outcomes.[85] The IOM report characterizes timeliness in two distinctive ways.[7] First, the report uses a customer-service focus by addressing such issues as wait times in offices and emergency departments and for diagnostic testing or surgery. The suggestion is that health care providers' inattention to the flow of patients demonstrates a lack of respect for patients and their families.[7] The second focus extends beyond customer satisfaction to include patient outcomes, which are particularly germane to ICUs. The ICU is a valuable resource for critically ill patients, and if ICU resources are unavailable when patients need them, adverse outcomes are possible. In this circumstance, the redesign of clinical processes has a direct effect in ensuring that patients get services when and where they need them. For example, a child who experiences a cardiac arrest in the radiology suite is dependent upon the ability of the institution to provide quick and definitive care in radiology rather than waiting to transport the patient to the ICU and delaying necessary therapies.

PATIENT CENTEREDNESS

The IOM's aim of patient centeredness helps characterize the interactions between practitioners and their patients.[7] A number of terms, including *empathy*, *compassion*, *needs*, and *respect*, encompass the qualities of patient centeredness and reflect the focus of attention on the patient.[7] Additional components that help establish priority areas for the care of individual patients include the provision of information, communication, and education; attention to physical comfort; emotional support by relieving fear and anxiety; and the involvement of family and friends.[7] These characteristics constitute what is known as *service quality*; in contrast, *clinical quality* is the clinical expertise offered by critical care practitioners. Patient centeredness is more than "service with a smile." It requires that the processes of care be redesigned around the patient's and family's needs and not around the care team's needs. Both are important to successful care of the critically ill child. The Healthcare Advisory Board identified several broad types of service problems in specialty care (Table 223-1), which remain relevant to the PICU even a decade after their publication.

Admission to the PICU, especially when emergent and unexpected, is an anxiety-provoking and fearful experience for patients and their families.[86-87] For parents, the anxiety is generated from the lack of parental control, the appearance and discomfort of the child, both emotionally and physically, and difficulty communicating with staff.[86] The age of the parents and their ability to focus on problems and participate in care are associated with an ability to cope with a critically ill child.[88] Coping strategies for parents also include an ability to be supported by the PICU healthcare team. A variety of needs, including emotional, physical, and spiritual, have to be addressed by this support system.[89] This can be accomplished by providing accurate information, allowing ready access to the child, and encouraging parents' participation in their child's care.[86,89] For hospitalized children, anxiety and stress may manifest themselves in behavior problems, especially in those with repeated or prolonged hospitalizations, those who are critically ill, and those with underlying mood or psychological disorders.

If family members perceive that emotional support is inadequate, their satisfaction with the experience and, more important, their long-term viability and cohesion as a family unit are at risk.[90] Most families are satisfied with the care their children receive in the PICU and are particularly complimentary about the skill and competence of the nursing staff, as well as the compassion and respect shown toward their children, especially with regard to pain management.[91] Attention to adequate pain and anxiety control is an essential component of the care of critically ill pediatric patients.[92-94] Pain control addresses a fundamental need and is a compassionate practice that helps allay parents' anxiety and improves coping.[91] The environment of the waiting area and the frequency of physician communication were both identified as detracting from parents' satisfaction with the PICU experience.[91] The family's ability to function after the ICU admission of a child is dependent not only on their satisfaction but also on the severity of the child's illness, duration of hospitalization, and location of the hospital.

When evaluating care at the unit level, the fundamental evaluative components must be applied data and analytics, process improvement, and change management. The IOM framework provides a structure to evaluate, but an understanding of unit-specific data and process are necessary if success in achieving appropriate outcomes is to be achieved.

Evaluation Domains at the Provider Level

The IOM framework is useful as an organizing principle to understand healthcare quality from the perspective of the discipline of pediatric critical care or the ICU. Providers, when thinking about their own practice, tend to think differently about healthcare quality. Specifically, when providers consider quality, they are often thinking about the care that they, rather than the healthcare team or the ICU, provides. Providers typically believe they provide safe, timely, and effective care that corresponds to the latest evidence. They believe in engaging the child and family in the care and believe they treat all their patients fairly regardless of their personal characteristics or ability to pay. Donabedian's constructs of structure, process, and outcome are particularly helpful in assisting different providers to identify their role in providing quality care to patients, because they know what is available to them to provide care, they believe they understand their work, and they think they understand what they are trying to achieve (Table 223-2).

STRUCTURE

Structure is usually interpreted from a "bricks and mortar" perspective. However, while the walls, monitors, equipment, and other technologies are certainly important structural elements, they are insufficient for the optimal delivery of health care. The people—including patients, families, and providers of all disciplines—as well as their knowledge of the child, expertise, and collaboration are needed to effect the best outcomes. In addition, important evidence has linked the organization of the ICU and its management as key determinants of outcome.[95,96] When taken together, these elements are the structural

TABLE 223-1	Service Problems in Specialty Care
Speed of service	Delay in care or excessive waiting time Lack of explanation for delay
Coordination of care	Organization of the environment Availability of appropriate person to answer questions
Respect and courtesy	Staff courtesy Treatment with respect and dignity
Understanding of treatment	Information regarding symptoms, medications, and treatments provided Patient or family included in decisions Adequate explanations provided Patient and family listened to
Trust in the provider	Availability of the provider Psychosocial support

From Advisory Board Company. Service innovations in specialty care: enhancing patient satisfaction with diagnosis and treatment selection. Washington DC: Advisory Board Company; 1998.

TABLE 223-2	Classification of ICU Provider-Specific Quality Components Based Upon Donabedian's Structure, Process, and Outcome Framework	
Structure		
"Bricks and mortar"	ICU itself	
	Monitoring equipment	
	Patient care equipment:	
	Ventilators	
	Ultrasound machines	
	Medication pumps	
Personnel	Physicians:	
	ICU physicians	
	Primary care physicians	
	Consulting physicians	
	Residents and fellows	
	Other personnel:	
	ICU Nurses	
	Respiratory therapists	
	Pharmacists	
	Social workers	
	ICU management:	
	Nursing Director	
	ICU Medical Director	
	Hospital management	
Process*		
Data gathering	Admission	
	History:	
	Thorough, timely, and accurate	
	Physical examination:	
	Thorough, timely, and accurate	
	Consultant input:	
	Thorough, timely, and accurate	
	Diagnostic testing:	
	Appropriate test performed	
Interpretation	Pattern recognition from data	
	Clinical context from the patient	
	Clinical knowledge based on training and experience	
	Knowledge from EBM and current literature	
Decision making	Formulation of a plan consistent with patient choice	
	Medical treatment plan	
	Nursing treatment plan	
	Care management plan	
Action taking	Gather further data.	
	Revisit history.	
	Reexamine patient.	
	Perform further diagnostics.	
	Implement a care management plan.	
	Ensure appropriate anticipatory measures:	
	Gastrointestinal prophylaxis	
	Deep venous thrombosis prophylaxis	
	Ensure appropriate therapeutic measures:	
	Manage hyperglycemia.	
	Low-tidal-volume ventilation	
	Elevate head of bed.	
	Implement the medical treatment plan:	
	Appropriate medication use based on EBM	
	Appropriate diagnostic tests based on sensitivity and specificity	
	Appropriate therapeutic plan based on EBM	
	Implement the nursing treatment plan:	
	Right procedures	
	Performed safely and correctly	
	Intended outcome without complications	
	Perform a procedure:	
	Right procedure	
	Performed safely and correctly	
	Intended outcome without complications	
Outcomes		
	ICU mortality	
	ICU morbidity	
	Physical disabilities	
	Cognitive disabilities	
	ICU length of stay	
	Costs	
	Duration of ICU therapies	
	Nosocomial infections	
	Procedure complications	

*Physician-specific processes.
EBM, evidence-based medicine; *ICU,* intensive care unit.

components of ICU care to which Donabedian might refer (see Table 223-2).

PROCESS

Clinical processes are the interactions between providers and their patients and providers with one another. Recent evidence highlights the importance of team performance in addition to clinical performance for establishing outcomes.[97,98] Whereas nurses, by virtue of their training, tend to be process focused, physicians often lack this skill. Therefore, when asked to address specific process steps like implementing the vascular access bundle, nurses are comfortable with the detailed specification of process, which can actually make a difference in outcomes over time. Attention to the key processes of care are becoming recognized as important in determining outcome, and a number of checklists, guidelines, bundles, and pathways have been developed to ensure compliance with the numerous specification limits established in clinical care.

OUTCOMES

Finally, outcomes represent the culmination of the healthcare experience. Physicians often focus on outcome measures as the result of their work. In the ICU environment, mortality is a traditional outcome measure that is important, quantifiable, and often discussed. There are other outcome measures of relevance to ICU physicians, including the use of ICU-specific therapies, length of stay, cognitive and physical outcomes, and morbidities arising from the episode of care (see Table 223-2). However, because outcomes tend to be the end result of a series of process steps that are temporally distinct, it is often important for the physician to focus on both components of quality. Outcomes have been held in high regard for considerable time—almost to the exclusion of process measures. Physicians will only be able to improve the quality of care for their patients by focusing on both the process and outcome components of healthcare quality. This represents some of the most fertile ground for generating new knowledge and identifying opportunities to improve outcomes for critically ill children over the next decade.[4-5]

CLINICAL PROCESSES AND MEDICAL DECISION MAKING

When considering provider-specific processes for improving healthcare quality, different disciplines rely upon the same fundamental aspects of the medical decision-making process (Figure 223-4). These core elements can be thought of through the core processes of the PICU provider as they care for the critically ill child from ICU admission through discharge.

Traditional medical decision making has four iterative steps that assist providers with making decisions for their patients. The first step is data gathering. Physicians use their history, physical examination, diagnostic testing, consultants, and other members of the healthcare team to assist them in ensuring they have collected appropriate data

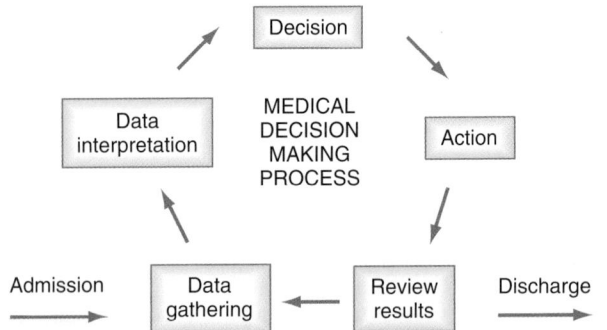

Figure 223-4 Key elements of the medical decision-making process.

upon which to base their clinical decisions (see Table 223-2). Nurses use their nursing assessment or database, which incorporates all of the nonmedical information the team needs to care for the child and family. The next step is for the physician to interpret the gathered data within the clinical context of the patient. This step involves assembling the collected data to see if it coalesces into a particular pattern and seeing whether that pattern is consistent with the patient's presentation and findings. When nurses use their skills to perform this function in parallel, a rich conversation can occur when team members assemble during rounds to share the findings of their integrative decision making. For the experienced team, this is often performed rapidly with patterns that are matched against a large mental library of similar conditions and patients. When the team is less experienced, the process is slow and prone to errors. The next step is decision making. Here, the physician may gather additional data by calling a consultant or ordering additional testing. If sufficient data has been gathered, the physician may formulate a medical treatment plan and reevaluate the plan's success as time progresses (see Table 223-2). The physician may recommend or perform a procedure, the outcome of which may assist with diagnosis or treatment. Nurses will incorporate their nursing diagnoses into the plan, and together the team will act with a comprehensive strategy for providing care. Finally, as the last step of medical decision making, the team must take action. A plan that is incoherent or not acted upon, or a procedure or test that is thought about but not performed, does not help the patient. These four steps allow the clinical team to think through and organize their work (see Figure 223-4).

When evaluating care at the provider level, there is often a deficiency in the available data by clinician. At this point, the best many ICUs can do is establish appropriate process steps in care and hold providers accountable for following those steps. Deviations from the process will occur because of differences in patient condition and case mix, but those deviations identified as random or reckless can be dealt with through an environment that encourages a just culture.

Conclusions

The six aims of quality remain a useful framework for evaluating the current state of pediatric critical care at the unit level and provide opportunities for addressing deficiencies in the evidence base through future research initiatives. Success in advancing quality in the PICU over the next decade will depend upon the ability to have providers appropriately focused on their discipline-specific processes of care in support of outcomes. What will follow is a better understanding of the influence individual providers have on effecting outcomes.

ANNOTATED REFERENCES

Institute of Medicine Committee on Quality of Health Care in America. Crossing the quality chasm: a new health system for the 21st century. Washington DC: National Academies Press; 2001.
This document provides a review of quality in health care. It is useful in its own right because of its framework based on the six aims of quality. In addition, it is highly referenced, providing an overview of the evaluation of healthcare services.
Pollack MM, Patel KM, Ruttimann UE. PRISM III: an updated pediatric risk of mortality score. Crit Care Med 1996;24:743-52.
The authors have developed a physiology-based method of assessing severity of illness using data available in the first 12 hours of care. It illustrates the method of adjusting mortality rates for severity of illness to measure the effectiveness of PICU care.
Ruttimann UE, Patel KM, Pollack MM. Length of stay and efficiency in pediatric intensive care units. J Pediatr 1998;133:79-85.
This article outlines a method for estimating length of stay based on data available in the first 24 hours and illustrates how it can be used for benchmarking. This is a key component of quality-of-care evaluations, especially for efficiency and timeliness measures.
Smedley BD, Stith AY, Nelson AR. Institute of Medicine Committee on Understanding and Eliminating Racial and Ethnic Disparities in Healthcare. Unequal treatment: confronting racial and ethnic disparities in health care. Washington DC: National Academies Press; 2002.

Racial and ethnic disparities have become a major concern in health care. This IOM report adds a contextual element to the problem by providing an assessment method, identifying interventions, and proposing solutions.
Advisory Commission on Consumer Protection and Quality in the Health Care Industry. Quality first: better health care for all Americans. 1998. Available at: http://www.hcqualitycommission.gov/.
Healthcare quality has been debated for several decades and continues today as efforts for reform take hold. This report provides a framework with important elements that help inform this dialogue even today.
Stockwell DC, Slonim AD. Quality and safety in the intensive care unit. J Intensive Care Med 2006;21:199-210.
This article provides important guidance for assessing and improving care specific to the ICU. It reviews current methods for assessment and learning from medical errors and provides guidance on how to improve ICU care.
Miller MR, Griswold M, Harris JM 2nd, et al. Decreasing PICU catheter-associated bloodstream infections: NACHRI's quality transformation efforts. Pediatrics 2010;125:206-13.
This multicenter study provides a model for using evidence-based standards and data to improve quality in the PICU through multi-institutional collaboratives.

REFERENCES

Access the complete reference list online at http://www.expertconsult.com.

224

Key Issues in Critical Care Nursing

FRANCO A. CARNEVALE | ANNIE S. CHEVRIER

Prevailing issues in critical care nursing are reviewed in this chapter. The topics examined have particular importance for nurses but have broad multidisciplinary implications as well. Special focus is placed on contributions from nursing research. The reader is invited to delve further into the nursing literature by examining the numerous excellent critical care nursing journals and textbooks that are currently available, as well as CINAHL (Cumulative Index to Nursing and Allied Health Literature), the nursing literature database (a "nursing Medline").

Critical Care Nursing Knowledge and Skill Development

Patricia Benner is said to have revolutionized our understanding of clinical expertise in nursing. In her landmark book, *From Novice to Expert: Excellence and Power in Clinical Nursing Practice*, Benner related the Dreyfus Model of Skill Acquisition to her study of nursing expertise.[1] This model was originally developed through a study of skill development among nonclinicians (e.g., chess players and airline pilots). Benner and her colleagues have recently directed their analysis specifically to critical care nursing.[2]

Benner has challenged the prevailing "top-down" view of clinical expertise that believes clinicians acquire theoretical and empirical knowledge from books, journals, and classrooms and then *apply* this to practice. Rather, she demonstrated that such a form of practice is characteristic of *novices*. Lacking an experiential base to draw on, novices refer to their formal learning as well as various "rules of thumb" to help them sort through clinical problems.

An *expert*, however, will have acquired a rich store of clinical cases. This serves as a "bottom-up" foundation that enables expert nurses to rapidly discern what is meaningful in a clinical scenario without having to go through a step wise, linear, algorithm-like process. Therefore, expert critical care nurses (as well as other clinicians) are able to "think in action." Expert *know-how* enables experienced nurses to readily identify patterns in a presenting case by immediately referring to numerous comparable cases—directly inferring hypotheses about the likely problem, the gravity of the situation, and how it should be managed. As the expert proceeds to manage the situation, the patient's response presents further cues that can either confirm the nurse's initial interpretation or generate new probable hypotheses.

Some have argued that Benner's conception of skill acquisition is also relevant to medicine.[3] A recent study demonstrated that critical care physicians employ a similar mode of thinking in their practice of diagnostic reasoning.[4]

Concurrent with this management of a specific case, Benner and her associates further described how an expert nurse also monitors and limits potential hazards in the highly technological critical care environment, fosters teamwork, and initiates preventive and corrective management of systems breakdown.[2] These functions are commonly performed without the nurse necessarily being consciously aware of the reasoning that underlies them.

This experience-based view of nursing expertise raises important implications for nursing education and management. First, it suggests that the extent to which clinical expertise can be acquired from books or in a classroom is highly limited. The development of complex clinical judgment requires naturalistic exposure to numerous real-life cases. Although some useful learning can be acquired through formal educational methods such as formal lectures and readings, Benner's framework favors an apprenticeship model of nursing education. A tailored program of clinical experiences, with access to expert guidance, will most effectively foster the development of expert knowledge and skill among critical care nurses. This framework provides a rich guide for the orientation of newly hired nurses and preceptors in critical care.

Second, this calls for management approaches that recognize the complexity of clinical expertise and the significant investment required to develop it. Expert nurses do not simply perform tasks prescribed by physicians or protocols. Expert nurses bring sophisticated knowledge and judgment that is essential to early and effective management of both patient and unit problems. This implies that skilled critical care nurses should be regarded as essential resources.

Administrators need to exercise extreme caution when making decisions that aim to reduce costs by relying on strategies such as "de-skilling" (i.e., relying on less qualified health professionals to perform nursing work), "casualization" (i.e., reducing the number of full-time staff to rely on casual, typically less experienced staff that can be called in ad hoc), or "downsizing" (i.e., dismissing skilled staff to reduce staffing levels).

Any strategy that diminishes or fragments the depth of critical care nursing expertise will fundamentally diminish the strength of a critical care service.[5] Cho and associates have demonstrated that efforts to reduce nursing staffing levels can significantly increase levels of patient morbidity. A 1-hour decrease of worked nursing hours per patient was associated with a 8.9% increased probability of patients acquiring pneumonia.[6]

Clinical Topics

Critical care nurses are concerned about the same issues as physicians and other allied professionals. Some nurses have emerged across disciplines as respected leaders because of their impressive research work on selected critical care problems.

The remainder of this chapter is devoted to topics nurses are particularly concerned about. They address key problems that have especially perplexed nursing practice and captured the research attention of nurses. Although the following primarily highlights nursing contributions, and space constraints limit the number of topics that can be reviewed, the reader is encouraged to learn more from the rich body of related research in other disciplines.

PAIN AND DISCOMFORT

It is likely most nurses would list patient pain and discomfort as their most challenging clinical problems. The constancy and proximity of a nurse's bedside relationship with a patient heightens awareness and attentiveness to unresolved pain and discomfort and can take a deep toll. This is partly due to nursing's traditional commitment to the promotion of comfort and caring.[7,8] Although significant advances have been made over the years in developing effective pharmacologic agents for managing these problems, pain and discomfort commonly persist.[9,10]

One factor that has limited successful management of these problems is the challenge involved in their evaluation.[11] Outside the critical care setting, pain management has benefited from systematic measurement and documentation. Widely accepted pain measures such as the

Visual Analogue Scale or numeric rating scales rely on patient self-report, but self-report is typically not accessible in critical care, given patients' diminished level of consciousness. Thus, observational methods are most appropriate for this population. The Critical-Care Pain Observation Tool (CPOT) has demonstrated reliability and validity for critically ill adults regardless of their level of consciousness.[12,13] The CPOT measures four behavioral categories: facial expression, body movements, muscle tension, and compliance with the ventilator for intubated patients or vocalization for extubated patients. Significant experience exists in pediatrics with the utilization of observational pain measures such as the FACES Pain Scale[14] and the Children's Hospital of Eastern Ontario Pain Scale, CHEOPS.[15] However, most research has been conducted outside of critical care settings.

In critical care settings, overall "comfort" is increasingly measured with sedation scales.[16,17] The Ramsay Scale, likely the most widely used sedation scale in the intensive care unit (ICU), has established some reliability and validity for critically ill adults.[18] This is a six-level sedation scale, three levels for when the patient is awake and three levels for when the patient is asleep: 1—anxious, agitated, or restless; 2—cooperative, oriented, or tranquil; 3—responds to commands only; 4—asleep, brisk response to light touch on cheek or loud auditory stimulus; 5—sluggish response; and 6—no response. The American Association of Critical-Care Nurses has published a sedation assessment scale for critically ill patients that may be more sensitive to the end goals of sedation.[19] It comprises five domains of assessment (consciousness, agitation, anxiety, sleep, patient-ventilator synchrony) as compared to many existing scales that focus only on one or two domains such as consciousness and agitation. In pediatric critical care, the COMFORT Scale has demonstrated impressive merits.[20] This consists of eight behavioral and physiologic parameters including alertness, calmness/agitation, respiratory response, physical movement, blood pressure, heart rate, muscle tone, and facial tension. Each parameter is measured along a 5-point rating scale and summed to provide a total score that ranges from 8 to 40. Some work with this tool has indicated that physiologic parameters such as blood pressure and heart rate have weak validity as indicators of discomfort.[21] Although these signs are commonly and intuitively associated with patient discomfort, they are also affected by numerous other phenomena within the critical care setting, such as cardiovascular dysfunction.

Delirium is the most common psychiatric diagnosis in critical care; its evaluation and management is therefore a key comfort concern for this population. The Confusion Assessment Method for the Intensive Care Unit (CAM-ICU) is a valid and reliable tool developed for bedside assessment of delirium in adults.[22]

Sedation in critical care is closely tied to the management of mechanical ventilation discomfort. A problem arising from this sedation-ventilation relation is the complex process of weaning patients from both therapies.[23,24] Some research has examined the merits of daily interruption of sedation to permit spontaneous breathing.[25,26] The use of a daily "sedation vacation" can help prevent some significant iatrogenic effects of critical care and shorten ICU and hospital stay.

Overall improvements in pharmacologic management of pain and discomfort have contributed to a more recent concern: withdrawal reactions.[27] Overly rapid weaning of sedation and analgesia can precipitate a constellation of phenomena such as acute pain, excessive agitation, "ICU psychosis," as well as withdrawal reactions. Reliable and valid measures for evaluating withdrawal reactions are therefore important in successfully managing this problem. Some strong measurement tools have been documented for the pediatric population.[28,29]

Although guidelines have been published for recommended rates of weaning, very little empirical research has established the optimal rate for reducing opioid and benzodiazepine infusions, balancing the need to rapidly extubate patients (and therefore minimize ventilation-related morbidities) with the prevention of withdrawal reactions. Some evidence suggests that one optimal weaning rate does not exist.[30] It must be tailored to the length of time the patient has been receiving such infusions, whereby 20% *daily weaning* is optimal for patients receiving continuous infusions for 1 to 3 days, 13% to 20% for 4 to 7 days of infusions, 8% to 13% for 1 to 2 weeks, 8% for 2 to 3 weeks, and 2% to 4% for more than 4 weeks of infusions.[30]

Cumbersome decisional processes further complicate the management of pain and discomfort in critical care. A common occurrence in a university setting is for the intensivist to direct house staff and nurses to wean a patient's sedation and analgesia overnight so the patient will be ready for extubation in the morning. However, such weaning can trigger significant discomfort, whereby the house staff and nurses can enter into disputes over how to balance the need to wean with the need to maintain patient comfort through a series of repeated adjustments in infusion rates and ad hoc bolus doses.

In their study of critical care nursing judgment in the management of pain, Stannard et al. reported that nurses demonstrated a sophisticated balancing of patients' analgesic needs against other competing needs.[31] A less cumbersome pain and discomfort management process can be established through the use of a sedation protocol or standing orders that "transfer" some decisional autonomy to nurses. A protocol can authorize nurses to modify sedation and analgesia infusion rates and bolus administration according to a prescribed target level of patient comfort.

For example, Alexander and associates reported on a sedation protocol used in pediatric critical care where the COMFORT Scale was used to measure patients' level of comfort.[32] The physician's prescription specifies a target COMFORT Scale range for the patient, which the nurse can then use as a guideline for modifying the administration of sedation and analgesia. This study reported that patient comfort was managed effectively while facilitating the decision-making process.

Finally, the nursing literature has devoted some attention to the use of nonpharmacologic means for managing pain and discomfort: massage, relaxation exercises, transcutaneous electrical nerve stimulation (TENS), acupuncture, guided imagery, and hypnosis, among others.[33] However, these techniques have undergone very little clinical research investigation within critical care. In light of major adverse effects associated with pharmacologic agents, as well as their limitations in fully ensuring patient comfort, these adjunctive measures should be further developed for the critically ill.

PRESSURE ULCERS

Given the significant responsibility nurses have conventionally held in the care of basic needs such as skin care, the nursing literature has devoted particular attention to the prevention and care of pressure ulcers.

In their study of iatrogenic problems, Cho and associates reported that pressure ulcers had the greatest impact on length of stay (i.e., a 1.84-fold increase).[6] Documented prevalence rates vary from 7.1% to 11.1%.[34] Jiricka et al. have reported that prevalence rates are even higher among the critically ill.[35] This is attributable to the greater likelihood of immobility and reduced skin perfusion.

The principal extrinsic causes of pressure ulcers are pressure, friction, and shear. Therefore, preventive strategies are directed toward minimizing these extrinsic forces. Although over 200 pressure-relieving devices are commercially available, a paucity of controlled clinical trials have examined their efficacy.[36]

An emerging body of literature is effectively identifying the sites of pressure ulcers and the relative significance of various risk factors. This will help build a base of evidence from which clinical trials can be designed. This literature has led to the development of scoring systems for predicting the risk of pressure ulcers. A highly regarded system is the Braden Scale,[37] which has six subscales: mobility, activity, friction and shear, sensory perception, skin moisture, and nutrition; it provides a total score that ranges from 6 to 23 points (high scores indicate less risk). A Braden score of 16 has demonstrated a high degree of sensitivity and specificity in predicting pressure ulcer formation in critically ill adults. This tool has recently been adapted and validated for the pediatric critical care population.[38]

Whereas pressure ulcers in adults predominantly appear on the lower body (sacrum, ischium, and heels), they are more common on the upper body of children (occiput and ears). This is a result of proportional differences in body weight distribution between these age-groups. A 27% rate of pressure ulcer incidence has been reported in critically ill children, 57% of which were identified on their second day in the ICU.[39] Particularly disturbing was that an additional 27 ulcers were identified as caused by medical devices such as oximetry probes, BiPAP masks, and endotracheal tubes.

It is remarkable that wide disparities of preventive measures are currently practiced, including some high-cost pressure-relieving mattresses.[36,40] These include some aids that are largely regarded as ineffective, such as synthetic sheepskins.[39] Although a substantial amount of evidence has examined this problem outside of critical care, systematic evaluations of management strategies are required to understand their efficacy among the critically ill.

PSYCHOSOCIAL ISSUES IN CRITICALLY ILL PATIENTS AND THEIR FAMILIES

Nursing has consistently demonstrated a strong interest in psychosocial aspects of illness. In critical care, nurses have directed some of the most respected psychosocial research. A number of studies have examined the psychological impact of critical illness on patients, whereas others have concentrated on their families. Although most nursing research employs quantitative methods, nurses have also conducted a significant number of qualitative studies within the health sciences.

Patients

Many critically ill patients endure profound psychological trauma, and many others develop delirium or "ICU psychosis."[41,42] One group of patients examined up to 8 weeks after their discharge from an ICU reported "experiences of chaos," feelings of extreme instability, vulnerability, and fear, as well as prolonged inner tension.[43] It was found that even trivial events could trigger changes in their feelings of fear or inner tension. The caring behaviors of nurses provided an important degree of security and comfort. Hupcey reported that the overarching need of critically ill patients is the need to feel safe.[44]

In an investigation of the experiences of patients through their transfer out of ICU, patients exhibited feelings of significant despondency and apprehension.[45] These findings highlight the mandate for greater attentiveness to the needs of these highly vulnerable adults. A number of studies suggest that some of these patients exhibit manifestations of posttraumatic stress disorder (PTSD).[46-48] More research is needed, as the prevalence of PTSD and the optimum timing and method for assessing PTSD among the critically ill has not yet been determined.[49]

McKinley and colleagues[50] have developed a tool for assessing anxiety in critically ill patients: the Faces Anxiety Scale. This single-item tool requires patients to select one of five drawings of faces. The scale exhibits minimal subject burden, while eliciting self-reports more often than other self-report scales.

Among psychological studies of critically ill children, Rennick et al. have reported that children who were younger, more severely ill, and underwent more invasive procedures demonstrated more medical fears, a lower sense of control over their health, and ongoing posttraumatic stress responses up to 6 months after discharge.[47] In a long-term follow-up study of critically ill children, significant dispositional and mental function changes were reported.[51] Parental accounts and clinical evaluations suggested that these children were profoundly transformed by their critical illness for variable lengths of time. Papathanassoglou and Patiraki reported similar observations among critically ill adults.[52]

Families

Many studies of families of the critically ill can be traced to Molter's examination of family needs.[53] Following Molter's introduction of the *Critical Care Family Needs Inventory*, several studies systematically investigated the needs of these families. This body of research has demonstrated that families need honest, clear, and timely information, liberal visiting policies, and competent and compassionate care for their family member.[54] "Hope" has been described as the most frequently used method of coping,[55] which has complex implications for how clinicians portray the patient's outlook. The latter report also indicated that families identified the provision of information, emotional support, and the competence and manner of the nurse as helpful nursing interventions. A systematic review has examined the impact of pediatric critical illness and injury on families.[56] Although it is clear pediatric critical illness is stressful for the family, the reported effects on parents, siblings, and marital relations are variable. It is evident that many of these families' needs go unmet.

Carnevale[51,57] has described a family systems model for understanding the experiences of families of critically ill patients. Drawing on family therapy theory, this model recognizes families as constellations of interrelationships among members, including the critically ill patient. Variable levels of attachments or conflicts that continually change over time characterize these ties (Figures 224-1 and 224-2). Space constraints preclude additional discussion of death and dying in critical care, but some relevant issues will be discussed in the ethics review in the next section.

Any significant event that affects one member of a family system will necessarily affect the entire family constellation. A common feature that appears to characterize the response of families of critically ill children is a deeply motivated attempt to recapture life as it was before the need for critical care.[51] Although it is plausible that families of critically ill adults have similar responses, this requires further study.

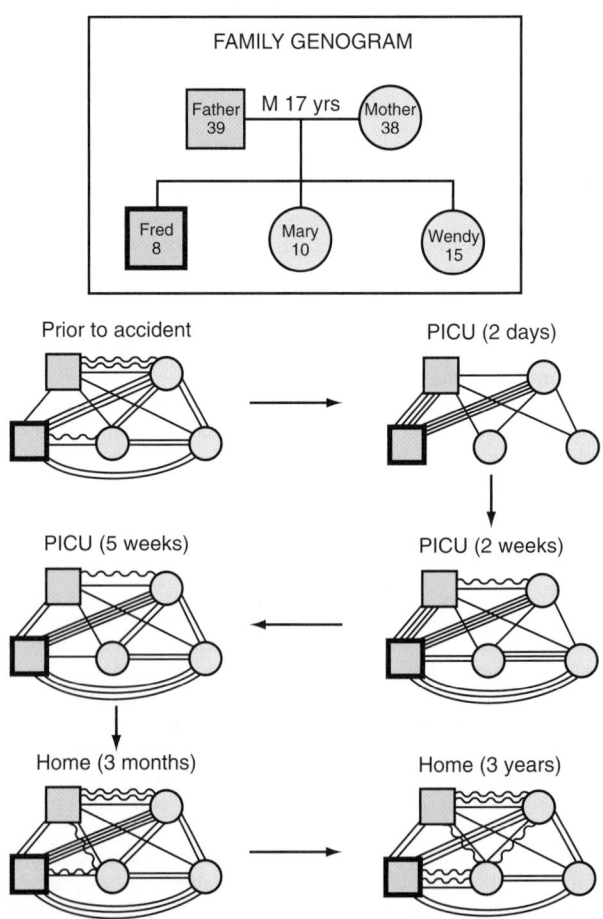

Figure 224-1 Diagrams showing relational shifts experienced by the family of an 8-year-old boy with multiple trauma. Number of straight lines between persons indicate strength of attachment in the relationship, whereas number of wavy lines represent intensity of conflict.

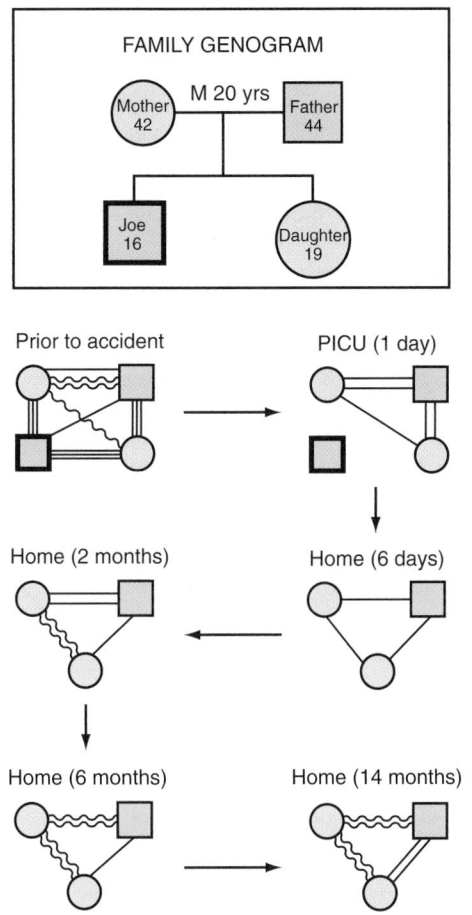

Figure 224-2 Diagrams demonstrating the profound relational transitions that followed the death of a family member.

This work suggests that the quality of the *patient's* experience through his/her critical illness is intimately intertwined with the quality of the *family's* experience. For example, efforts to preserve family integration—through the rigorous promotion of family presence and participation in the care of the patient—help satisfy numerous family needs while also profoundly comforting the patient's deepest stresses. Generally, what is good for the family tends to be good for the patient, and vice versa.

These findings highlight a central problem in the conventional ICU view of families as "visitors." Units commonly have visiting policies and visitors' rooms. Families are not visitors. Rather, they are spouses, partners, parents, children, siblings, and grandparents, among others, and can help foster a sense of continuity for the patient. Meanwhile, family members are personally adapting to the new reality confronting them. Whatever enables the patient and family to carry on as congruently as possible—fostering family cohesion within the available resources—is important. These views can also be extended to the significant friends of the patient.

Therefore, ICUs should promote the implementation of family support and follow-up programs to help alleviate patient and family distress. Some data have demonstrated that such programs can be highly effective.[58]

ETHICAL DILEMMAS IN CRITICAL CARE NURSING

In an anonymous survey of 852 critical care nurses in the United States, Asch reported that 16% stated they had either performed euthanasia or assisted in suicide, following the requests of patients or family members.[59] Several informant quotes were provided that suggested these nurses were quite frustrated with the physicians they were working with, whom they described as detached and insensitive to patients' suffering. The paper implies that these frustrated nurses unilaterally took matters into their own hands to do what they thought was right for the patient. Following the release of this paper and the understandable media attention that followed, many hospital centers turned to their critical care nurses to examine whether such practices were performed within their own institution. Although the practice of euthanasia or assisted suicide was clearly illegal and therefore unacceptable within the study's jurisdictions, many of the controversies that ensued missed the central phenomenon highlighted by the study: these nurses attempted to report serious problems in their units that placed them in significant ethical binds.

Nurses are autonomous professionals who bear responsibility for patient well-being (albeit within a multidisciplinary team context). Nurses practice according to a professional code of ethics (which may vary somewhat across regions) that requires them to do everything they can to ensure that patient needs are adequately met. Bioethicist Tristram Engelhardt[60] observed that:

> *Nurses are caught between physicians, on the one hand, who are authorities regarding scientific and technological knowledge and are in authority, and patients, on the other hand, who give authority for health care endeavors. Nurses are often placed, as a result, in ambiguous circumstances regarding which side is authorizing them to do what.*

Critical care nurses frequently find themselves in a moral bind in which they judge that the current medical plan conflicts with their appraisal of the wishes or needs of the patient. This can create moral distress among nurses if they find themselves in a situation where they do not have the power to do what they believe should be done.[61]

The Manitoba, Canada, government commissioned an inquest into a series of pediatric cardiac deaths in which there was suspicion regarding a surgeon's competence. The inquest report recognized that the nurses held important insights into the unfolding situation and were inadequately "heard" by their organization.[62] The report highlighted that nurses bear a responsibility to ensure patients are protected from harms and risks, and that the organization is responsible for creating mechanisms that can facilitate the inclusion of nurses in clinical and administrative decisions. One such mechanism can include the creation of a nursing ethics committee where nurses can feel free to examine nursing-specific concerns.[63]

This "in-between" viewpoint of nurses (between the patient and the physician) can help shed new light on a number of ethical dilemmas in critical care and foster new strategies for resolving them. For example, one study examined the controversy over the practice of judging some critical care interventions as "futile" under certain conditions (e.g., cardiopulmonary resuscitation in a patient with a very grave prognosis) and can therefore be unilaterally withheld or withdrawn by the critical care team.[64] This study highlighted that such conflicts are rarely related to an intervention's actual physiologic futility (i.e., whether or not it will achieve its intended purpose) but about fundamental disparities in the beliefs and values of the various persons involved in the conflict. Therefore, ethically sensitive strategies should aim to address these differences through reciprocal discussions and negotiations that seek to reconcile the disparities rather than assert declarations of futility.

Chambers-Evans has illuminated the particular difficulties involved in being a surrogate decision maker (i.e., a family member making decisions for a critically ill patient).[65,66] She has proposed a model that promotes shared decision making. This ensures that the surrogate's intimate understanding of the patient's wishes and interests are adequately considered while diminishing the surrogate's moral burden associated with feeling solely responsible for the life and death of their loved one.

Finally, some nurses have examined the impact of family presence during resuscitation.[67-68] This work suggests that there is increasing recognition of the merits of family presence, although priorities for further research are outlined. In sum, nursing perspectives on ethical issues in critical care both foster an awareness of the particular moral binds of nurses and illuminate new insights into the multidisciplinary management of prevalent ethical problems.

Conclusion

Over 20 years ago, Knaus and associates demonstrated that the mortality outcomes of a critical care unit are not a function of the level of technology the unit possesses, its university-teaching status, or a closed (versus open) unit.[69] Rather, outcomes are strongly associated with the strength of the interdisciplinary collaboration practiced within the unit.

The aim of this chapter was not to assert that nurses possess privileged knowledge or views about critical care but rather to highlight that critical care nurses offer (along with other practitioners) a rich body of clinical and research knowledge as well as shared professional responsibility for patient and family outcomes. The quality of critical care services can be strengthened when the potential and actual contributions of critical care nursing are recognized.

KEY POINTS

1. Studies have demonstrated that critical care nurses' expertise is highly sophisticated and consists predominantly of experientially acquired knowledge rather than learning from books and classrooms.

2. Observational pain-rating methods are important in the critical care setting, because this population is often incapable of self-report.

3. Improvements in the pharmacologic management of pain and discomfort have contributed to the increased incidence of withdrawal reactions.

4. The American Association of Critical-Care Nurses' Sedation Assessment Scale provides a comprehensive evaluation of sedation for critically ill patients.

5. Given the significant responsibility nurses have conventionally held in providing basic patient needs such as skin care, the nursing literature has devoted particular attention to prevention and care of pressure ulcers.

6. The Braden Scale is a highly regarded scoring system for predicting the risk of pressure ulcers.

7. Nursing research has consistently demonstrated a strong interest in the psychosocial aspects of critical illness.

8. A significant number of critically ill patients endure profound psychological trauma.

9. Families of critically ill patients are not "visitors."

10. Critical care nurses can experience moral distress because they frequently find themselves in situations in which they do not have the power to do what they believe should be done.

ANNOTATED REFERENCES

Benner P, Hooper-Kyriakidis P, Stannard D. Clinical wisdom and interventions in critical care: a thinking-in-action approach. Philadelphia: Saunders; 1999.

This is an extensive study of expertise among critical care nurses and demonstrates that in addition to employing complex experience-based patient management judgment, an expert nurse also monitors and limits potential hazards, fosters teamwork, and initiates preventive and corrective management of systems breakdown.

Cho SH, Ketefian S, Barkauskas VH, et al. The effects of nurse staffing on adverse events, morbidity, mortality, and medical costs. Nurs Res 2003;52:71-9.

This study reported that efforts to reduce nursing staffing levels can significantly increase levels of patient morbidity. A 1-hour decrease of worked nursing hours per patient was associated with an 8.9% increased probability of patients acquiring pneumonia.

Gélinas C, Fillion L, Puntillo KA, et al. Validation of the critical-care pain observation tool in adult patients. Am J Crit Care 2006;15:420-7.

The Critical-Care Pain Observation Tool (CPOT) has demonstrated reliability and validity for critically ill adults regardless of their level of consciousness. The CPOT measures four behavioral categories: facial expression, body movements, muscle tension, and compliance with the ventilator for intubated patients or vocalization for extubated patients.

Bergstrom N, Braden BJ, Laguzza A, et al. The Braden Scale for predicting pressure sore risk. Nurs Res 1987;36:205-10.

The Braden Scale is a highly regarded scoring system for predicting the risk of pressure ulcers. The scale has six subscales (mobility, activity, friction and shear, sensory perception, skin moisture, and nutrition), providing a total score that ranges from 6 to 23 points (high scores indicate less risk); a score of 16 has demonstrated a high degree of sensitivity and specificity in predicting pressure ulcer formation in critically ill adults.

Austin W, Kelecevic J, Goble E, Mekechuk J. An overview of moral distress and the paediatric intensive care team. Nurs Ethics 2009;16:57-68.

This paper examines the existing literature related to moral distress and the pediatric intensive care unit. Moral distress relates to a person's reaction when she/he believes to know the right thing to do but does not do it, either because of internal (personal) constraints or external (contextual) barriers.

REFERENCES

Access the complete reference list online at http://www.expertconsult.com.

225

Transport Medicine

KATE FELMET

Critically ill patients occasionally need to be moved within an institution or between hospitals. Transport of critically ill patients is a procedure with risks and benefits. Neither the nature and magnitude of risk and benefits nor the variables that might mitigate risks and maximize benefit (e.g., team training and composition, mode of transport) have been well studied. Referral patterns for many diseases, including critical illness, are evolving around centers of excellence. The structure of transport systems and the body of transport research need to keep pace. In order to realize the benefits of regionalization of critical care services, intensivists must take an active role in designing the transport systems and maintaining quality assurance. (Please note that transport issues important to the management of mass casualties in disasters are addressed in Chapter 226.)

Risks of Transport

Risks of transport are not precisely known. The progression of underlying disease, inadequacy of care delivered during transport, or the physical stress of transport itself can all lead to clinical deterioration of the patient during transport.

The transport environment, given its limited resources and multiple distractions, is bound to be error prone. In a population-based retrospective cohort study of nearly 20,000 air-medical transports, significant adverse events (defined as death, need for major resuscitative measures, hemodynamic deterioration, inadvertent extubation, or respiratory arrest) occurred in 1 in 20 transports. Baseline hemodynamic instability and assisted ventilation before transport and duration of transport were independent predictors of adverse events.[1] A retrospective review of voluntarily reported adverse events, which is likely to underestimate the true incidence, reported 11.3 adverse events occurred per 1000 flights.[2] The error rate of 1.13% seems low relative to the 2.9% to 16.6% reported incidence of adverse events per hospitalization, but given that the duration of transport is measured in hours, not days, the incidence of adverse events per unit time is quite high.[3]

The most frequent cause of transport-related adverse events with potential for patient harm is inadequate communication.[2] Communication errors are widely recognized to be a major preventable cause of morbidity and mortality in medicine in general. Because interfacility transport involves handoffs between at least three care teams, special care must be taken to ensure that critical details are transmitted. Complete documentation of all patient care records must be sent from the referring facility. Referring physicians should directly communicate the following to both the transport team and the accepting physician: (1) patient identification and medical history, (2) interventions performed during initial stabilization and the patient's response, (3) pertinent physical examination findings, (4) ongoing therapy, and (5) complications that might occur during transport. The transport team must relay this information to the accepting physician, nurse (RN) and respiratory therapist (RT) in addition to information about the patient's physiology and interventions performed while en route.

The incidence of adverse events in children is somewhat higher, ranging from 1.5% to 2.8% in transports with a specialized pediatric team to 20% to 61% in high-risk patients transported by nonspecialized teams. Adverse events in pediatric transport tend to be more serious. Airway-related events (loss of endotracheal tube, multiple intubation attempts, malposition of endotracheal tube) are by far the most common adverse event in pediatric transport, followed by loss of critical intravenous (IV) access, sustained hypotension, and cardiac arrest.[4-6]

Rapid Transfer, Goal-Directed Therapy, and the Golden Hour

Emergency medical services (EMS) and regional flight teams tend to work under the assumption that the time between the moment of injury and arrival at a center capable of delivering definitive care is among the most important determinants of survival. This notion has been taught for 3 decades but is based on little or no evidence and has recently been scrutinized. Time from scene departure to arrival at the hospital was not associated with survival in out-of-hospital cardiac arrest, and transport time including scene time was not associated with survival in trauma.[7,8] At the time the "golden hour" was conceived, prehospital care consisted of providing supplemental oxygen, a fast-moving vehicle, and minimal resuscitation. Under these circumstances, a worse outcome could be expected as prehospital time increased.

Belief in the golden hour may lead to risky behavior. High speeds occasionally result in crashes with injury to EMS providers as well as patients, and EMS have an occupational risk of death similar to that of policemen or firefighters.

There are certainly disease processes—aneurysms requiring neurosurgical intervention, thrombotic events requiring directed thrombolysis, complete transposition of the great arteries requiring urgent atrial septostomy, for example—in which rapid transport to a center that can provide definitive care is the most pressing issue. These are rare in children and, although reasons for interfacility transport of adult patients have not been studied, are likely to represent a small fraction of all critical care adult transports.

In pediatric patients, respiratory failure and shock are the most common reasons for transport. A recent study identified shock in 37% of children transferred to tertiary centers, regardless of reason for referral.[9] In adults and children, protocolized, aggressive, early therapy of septic shock has proven vastly more effective than any pharmacologic intervention at improving mortality.[10-12]

Pediatric protocols recommend aggressive fluid resuscitation, initiation of inotropes, and administration of antibiotics within the first hour after presentation.[13] The recommended treatments are simple interventions that can be initiated in community emergency departments (EDs) and continued and refined in transport, provided the treating physician and transferring team appreciate the urgent need and are sensitive to the subtle signs of shock in children. Han et al. reported that when community physicians aggressively resuscitated and successfully reversed shock before a transport team arrived, patients had a ninefold increase in their odds of survival.[11] These studies defy the popular notion that out-of-hospital stabilization wastes time and delays definitive therapy that should be rendered at the receiving facility.

Although adult guidelines are more relaxed, there are no data to suggest that it is safe to delay goal-directed therapy for transport. In fact, in adults with septic shock, a delay in antibiotic therapy is associated with worse survival, with mortality increasing by 7% for every 30 minutes that passes without delivery of appropriate antibiotic therapy. The golden hour in transport is the time from presentation to initiation of appropriate treatment, treatments that should be initiated at the referring facility and continued and refined by the transport team.[14]

Regionalization of Critical Care

Significant advances in therapeutic and diagnostic interventions for critically ill patients have occurred, but often at great cost and limited availability, prompting the need for transport of these patients to tertiary care centers. A recent consensus conference on prioritizing the organization and management of intensive care services in the United States (PrOMIS) suggested that intensive care would be optimally delivered in a tiered regionalized system.[15] Ideally, regionalization would reduce practice variation, improve adherence to best practices, and reduce costs by realizing economies of scale. Regionalization would necessarily result in an increased number of transfers of critically ill patients from lower-volume to higher-volume centers, so the PrOMIS conference proposed that regionalization must be coupled with a regionalized emergency transportation system.

Emergent interfacility transport should occur after initial stabilization and determination by the referring facility that the patient's needs for care are beyond the scope of local capabilities. In trauma, neonatal intensive care, and pediatric intensive care, the accepting physician serves as an expert who can guide pretransfer stabilization and ensure the safety of transport. Over time, local or low-volume hospitals will have less and less experience with critically ill patients. The transport system may be a useful avenue for education of referring physicians. Receiving centers should have communication centers that facilitate transfers, outreach teams to provide referring facilities with continuing education, and education programs about regional resources and trauma systems.

Out-of-Hospital Transport

PREHOSPITAL TRANSPORT

EMS are focused on rapid assessment, stabilization, and transport from the scene to the nearest ED or trauma center that can render appropriate care. Patient management is usually limited to supporting the airway, breathing, and circulation. The transport team should also be able to perform a needle thoracostomy if indicated, control active bleeding, and establish venous access. Other procedures should be kept to a minimum.

Out-of-hospital tracheal intubation by paramedics has recently come under fire. Despite the fact that tracheal intubation is the standard of airway management in the hospital and that tracheal intubation has been practiced by paramedics for 25 years, few studies support a survival benefit of tracheal intubation over bag-valve mask ventilation in the prehospital setting. Tracheal intubation is a complex skill rarely performed by paramedics. Failure rates are high, and multiple attempts are common; both of these may be accompanied by hypoxemia and other physiologic deterioration.[16] When intubation is successful, tracheal tube dislodgement during transport by EMS is common; tracheal tube misplacement or dislodgement rate at the time of arrival to ED varies from 5.8% to 12% for adults to 25% for pediatrics.[16-18] Finally, uncontrolled hyperventilation during manual ventilation by the EMS crew may be deleterious in head-injured patients and during cardiopulmonary resuscitation (CPR).

Appropriate utilization of resources (air versus ground units) for the prehospital transport of injured patients has been a subject of study and debate since the inception of air medical transport. In general, air medical transport is associated with both shorter transport intervals and a greater medical capability of the transporting team. The decision to use air transport in the prehospital setting should be supported by on-line medical control or preapproved protocols based on the factors of time, distance, geography, patient stability, and local resources. The National Association of Emergency Medical Service Physicians (NAEMSP) and the American College of Emergency Physicians

(ACEP) have each recommended triage guidelines for on-scene helicopter transport.[19] Retrospective studies have shown improved outcomes in patients transported by air, particularly major trauma patients and patients with severe traumatic brain injury.[20-24] Defining the types of specific injuries or medical conditions that benefit from air medical transport has been difficult. As specialized cardiac and stroke centers have developed, air transport has begun to be utilized for rapid transport of these patients directly from the scene.

INTERFACILITY TRANSPORT

Most interfacility transfers do not involve critically ill patients and can be accomplished safely a local EMS under predefined protocols or with specific instructions from a command physician. In rural areas, use of local EMS for interfacility transfer risks depleting a large geographic area of valuable medical resources such as ambulances, emergency medical technicians, and paramedics. The referring physician, who has little control over the en route phase of the transport, assumes a significant legal risk. Because of the variable backgrounds of EMS staff, the transferring personnel may not be equipped or trained to provide the necessary care in every situation. In particular, most EMS providers have little experience with critical care beyond the immediate resuscitative measures commonly performed in the prehospital setting, and they may not be trained in the use of certain hospital equipment (e.g., drug infusion pumps.)

In some situations, referring hospital staff may accompany a local ambulance service. The legal risk is reduced because the referring physician maintains tighter control over the patient's treatment during the transfer. Disadvantages of this option include loss of personnel from the referring hospital and lack of appropriate portable monitoring equipment.

Patients may also be transferred by a regional retrieval system, most of which are centered around air medical transport. Because air medical transport systems are used to transfer sicker patients and are held to a higher standard, the medical teams on these flights offer significantly greater medical capability compared with ground ambulance EMS.

In many instances, regional retrieval teams can also provide ground transport using personnel whose training and experience are held to the higher standard of air medical transport. Air medical transport team members are usually specially trained to deal with out-of-hospital emergencies and are acclimated to the stress of working in a moving environment. The team routinely carries equipment to manage deterioration during transfer and has battery-powered portable monitoring devices designed for use in moving environments. A command physician who is usually based at the institution from which the team originates provides recommendations for management until the team arrives.

Specialty teams provide an even higher level of expertise in the care of selected patients, the largest group being pediatric and neonatal critical care teams. Transport teams with specific expertise in left-ventricular assist devices or extracorporeal membrane oxygenation also exist. In many areas, however, specialty teams are unavailable. Because these teams tend to be based at tertiary care centers, time between decision to transfer and team arrival at the bedside may be longer than for local EMS or a regional air medical team. Specialty teams often perform additional stabilization maneuvers before leaving the referring facility. This practice has been criticized as prolonging bedside time and thus overall transport time interval. In reality, the time to definitive care may be shortened in many critically ill patients transferred by specialty teams. With these teams, the intensive care unit (ICU) is brought to the patient.

In most areas at the time of this writing, regional critical care teams are synonymous with air medical transport teams. However, the U.S. military has developed critical care transport teams with significantly greater capabilities that may serve as a model for critical care specialty civilian teams. In the mid 1990s, the U.S. Air Force began to develop what has come to be called the *critical care aeromedical transport team*

(CCATT.) The team consists of a nurse, respiratory therapist, and physician, all with experience in critical care as well as specific training pertinent to functioning in the transport environment. The teams carry resources to create a mobile ICU, including ventilators, mobile ultrasound equipment, and point-of-care laboratory testing. They go far beyond resuscitation and are able to recognize and manage multiple organ failures. The composition of these teams and details on the equipment and pharmacology they carry are described in an excellent article by Grissom and Farmer.[25] In the military, these resource-intensive teams are routinely used to manage up to three critically ill patients in a single transport. Although this model cannot be precisely duplicated in the civilian world, the experience of these teams must be considered when transport systems are designed to support regionalization of critical care.

ISSUES SPECIFIC TO AIR MEDICAL TRANSPORT

Most air medical transport today is done with twin-engine helicopters specially configured for medical missions. The practical transport range for helicopter transfers is generally 150 miles from the craft's base of operations. For longer-distance transports or in poor weather conditions, fixed-wing aircraft are used by many air medical services. Some flight programs are able use rotorcraft in instrument-flight-rules missions, allowing transport of patients in weather conditions that would otherwise preclude helicopter transport. This method requires filing of a flight plan, which may introduce delay.

The helicopter environment is noisy, so auscultation of blood pressure and breath sounds in flight is difficult if not impossible.[26] To monitor patients in flight, transport teams must rely on methods that do not depend on audible sounds: noninvasive blood pressure monitoring, capnometry, and pulse oximetry, to name a few.

Rotorcraft produce significant vibrations, making simple procedures difficult. Most therapeutic interventions such as tracheal intubation, chest decompression, IV access, and control of bleeding must be done before liftoff. The threshold for intubation in pediatric patients undergoing helicopter transport should be slightly lower than in those undergoing ground transport. Intravenous analgesia, sedation, neuromuscular blockade, vasoactive drugs, and blood products can be given in flight. These interventions must be performed under strict on-line medical direction or preapproved protocols.

Barometric pressure changes associated with increasing cabin altitude lower alveolar oxygen tension, increase the volume of any entrapped gas (e.g., in the bowel, sinuses, pneumothorax, endotracheal tube cuffs), and may affect IV infusion rates.

Rotorcraft rarely fly at altitudes more than 2000 feet above ground level. At these altitudes, pressure changes have only a minor impact on the volume of air-filled spaces. The relatively small volume of air in the tracheal tube cuff may be subject to clinically significant pressure changes at that altitude. A recent prospective study found that 98% of patients had tracheal tube cuff pressures above 30 mm Hg, and 72% had intracuff pressures above 50 mm Hg during helicopter transport at a mean of 2260 feet.[27] Tracheal tube cuff pressures should be measured and adjusted during flight.

Ventilators are calibrated for performance at sea level. Most flights maintain a cabin pressure equivalent to 6000 to 8000 feet. In the United States, Federal Aviation Administration regulations mandate cabin altitude less than 8000 feet. Ventilators that recognize and compensate for changes in barometric pressure exist (Uni-Vent Eagle Model 754 [Impact Instrumentation Inc., West Caldwell, New Jersey]) but are not in common use outside the military. Tidal volumes delivered by the LTV 1000 (Pulmonetic Systems Inc., Minneapolis, Minnesota), a commonly used transport ventilator, may vary from 5% to 12% at a simulated altitude of 4000 and 8000 in volume control mode. At 15,000 feet, LTV-delivered tidal volumes may be 30% to 37% greater than set tidal volumes.[28] Similar findings have been reported with the Drager Oxylog ventilators (Dragger, Telford, Pennsylvania). Ventilators that use pneumatic circuits for respiratory rate control may deliver lower rates and increased tidal volumes at high altitude.[29]

Structure of Regional and Specialty Retrieval Systems

The regional retrieval system provides the referral community with transport to locations of tertiary care, providing intensive care when necessary to the patient at both the referring institution and en route. Regional retrieval systems may be independent or may originate at a tertiary care center and should include a communications center, administrative staff, appropriately trained team members, reliable equipment, and a safety program.

COMMUNICATIONS

The communications center for the retrieval system should be easily accessible to both the referring physician and the transport team.[8,30] It should be staffed around the clock by full-time communication specialists who have no distracting duties. The communication specialist should notify the appropriate personnel and arrange all aspects of the transport so the referring physician can direct his or her attention to patient care. A detailed log of transport requests including time, demographic data, diagnosis, and vehicle availability is kept both for administrative review and medicolegal documentation. Equipment for direct communication with the center should be available in every transport vehicle.

When a request for transfer is initiated, the receiving physician should obtain a brief history of the patient's present illness, a summary of interventions, and may give the referring physician management recommendations tailored to the capabilities of the referring hospital. Recommendations should be documented on a log that remains a part of the patient's medical record.

STAFFING A RETRIEVAL SYSTEM

The administrative staff of a retrieval system should include, at a minimum, a program director, medical director, transport coordinator, and medical command.[31,32] The program director is responsible for the structure, activities, and organization of the transport system and assumes overall program responsibilities; acts as a liaison between the team and hospital administration; and develops and implements quality management.

The medical director should be a licensed physician specialist in critical care or emergency medicine and might also have training in a surgical subspecialty (trauma) or in pediatrics (neonatology). The medical director should be experienced in both air and ground transport (as appropriate), understand patient care capabilities, and be familiar with limitations and stressors of the transport environment. The medical director must be actively involved in quality management, administrative decisions affecting medical care, and the hiring, training, and continuing education of all transport personnel, including physicians who provide on-line medical direction in policies, procedures, and patient care protocols. The transport medical director may also act as a liaison to the referral community for teaching and outreach.[9,30]

The transport coordinator, usually a nurse or paramedic, collaborates with the medical director in training, protocols, scheduling, data collection, quality management, and marketing. Whenever possible, the medical director and transport coordinator should participate in patient transport so as to maintain skill and perspective.

A command physician should oversee every transport and provide advice to the referring physician and on-line medical control to the transport team as necessary. The command physician must be experienced in handling transport calls and offering management suggestions for the period before the arrival of the transport team. He or she should be knowledgeable about the availability of resources, have authority to accept transferred patients without further consultation, and perform triage as well as activate backup systems when necessary.

Medical control may be on-line or off-line or a combination of both. *On-line medical control* is direct real-time voice communication between the medical command physician and the transport team. Medical control physicians must be experienced in critical care transports to ensure that crews provide appropriate care. For specialized transports, the transport service should have a mechanism in place that affords medical control physicians timely consultation with subspecialists or the receiving physician. Alternatively, the critical care transport team should have the ability to consult with the receiving physician and provide updates to the receiving facility. *Off-line medical control* refers to written protocols or standing orders that guide patient management by the transport team. In some cases, direct communication between the team and the medical control physician is not possible. The medical director is responsible for developing transport protocols and procedures used for off-line medical control.

Transport crewmembers should be experienced in the care of critically ill patients and able to deal with complex environments with limited resources. They must be highly skilled in airway management, resuscitation, and vascular access. They should have a fundamental knowledge of field priorities and be able to make decisions independently. All team members should have specific training in transport medicine, which includes methods of functioning in a moving environment, aeromedical physiology, and troubleshooting for equipment-related problems.

Medical crew composition varies between regional retrieval teams. More than 70% of medical flight crews consist of a nurse-paramedic team. Approximately 20% of programs use two nurses, and only 3% of programs routinely use a flight physician. Respiratory therapists are teamed with nurses in a small percentage of programs and may be particularly appropriate in critical care transport teams.[31] Flight nurses typically have extensive experience in the ED or ICU.

Specialty training in critical care is available to paramedics, and board certification for this subspecialty exists. It is unclear what roles critical care paramedics are filling in regional retrieval systems.

Flight physicians are usually emergency medicine residents. In a few programs, they may be attending physicians or medical directors of flight programs. The use of physicians in these services as flight crew members is indicated when the physician might contribute significantly to the care provided in flight. Studies suggest that specific physician judgment or skill may be required in approximately 25% of transports.[20,33,34]

EQUIPMENT

The transport team should be self-sufficient in terms of equipment and medications, should not be dependent on the referring hospital for supplies, and should be prepared to encounter delays or equipment malfunction. The team should carry at least twice the amount of oxygen needed for the expected duration of the trip. Portable compartmentalized equipment packs should be designed for easy access and must be able to withstand the stress of the transport environment. For air medical transport, weight and space restrictions must also be considered in selecting equipment and range of medications. Transport monitors should be free of movement artifact and should have battery power that will last beyond the expected duration of transport. All equipment should be routinely checked and maintained after transport by a team member dedicated to that task.

SAFETY

Safety should be a high priority in any transport program. Emergency vehicle operation carries substantial risks, not only to the crew and the patient but also to others in its vicinity. Vendors of air or ground transport services should be chosen with attention to safety records, experience of drivers and pilots, and reliability of equipment. Written contracts between the institution and the vendor should include specific insurance details. Ambulance drivers should be discouraged from exceeding the speed limit, because this is unlikely to have a positive effect on patient outcome.

Aeromedical transport involves a unique set of safety issues. A series of high-profile crashes of medical helicopters prompted a review of safety standards for the industry. The four leading causes of accidents are weather, engine failure, collision, and loss of control. Pressure on pilots to fly and failure to observe minimal weather standards are among the components contributing to these accidents. For pilots to make sound decisions based on the flight conditions, they must be isolated from patient care issues. In regions where there are competing aeromedical services, they should act jointly to establish regional safety guidelines, minimal weather standards, and a quality assurance program that would examine compliance.

Transport team members must have a good understanding of aviation medicine and of how the aeromedical environment affects both the team and the patient. The results of poor eating habits (hypoglycemia), sleep deprivation, and drugs (e.g., alcohol, marijuana, antihistamines) are potentiated by increasing altitude. Vibration can produce fatigue, and accelerating and decelerating forces can produce vertigo. Night vision is decreased above cabin altitudes of 5000 feet. The transport team should be adept at survival techniques for their region and should always be prepared to deal with an off-airport landing. Regular sessions to review safety and emergency procedures for each transport mode should be provided for the transport team members.

▣ Responsibilities of the Referring Hospital

In the United States, the transfer of patients from one institution to another is regulated by federal statute. The Consolidated Omnibus Budget Reconciliation Act of 1986 (COBRA) and its amendment, the Omnibus Reconciliation Act of 1989, set the current legal standard for patient stabilization and transfer.[35,36] In an attempt to guarantee equal access to emergency treatment regardless of a patient's ability to pay, COBRA attributes responsibility for the patient's transfer to the referring hospital and physician. Violations can result in a number of penalties, including termination of Medicare privileges for the physician and hospital. The Emergency Medical Treatment and Labor Act established by the COBRA legislation governs how patients may be transferred from one hospital to another. Hospitals cannot transfer patients unless the transfer is "appropriate," the patient consents to transfer after being informed of the risks of transfer, and the referring physician certifies that the medical benefits expected from the transfer outweigh the risks. Appropriate transfers meet the following criteria: (1) the transferring hospital must provide care and stabilization within its ability, (2) copies of medical records and imaging studies must accompany the patient, (3) the receiving facility must have available space and qualified personnel and agree to accept the transfer, and (4) the interfacility transport must be made by qualified personnel with the necessary equipment. It is the responsibility of the referring physician, in consultation with the receiving physician, to choose a mode of transport from among the available teams.

▣ Unique Aspects of Pediatric Transport

EMS CANNOT PROVIDE IDEAL CARE FOR ALL CHILDREN

The majority of children are transported by EMS providers with variable educational backgrounds and experience. Currently there are no national regulations for EMS as they relate to children. Pediatric guidelines for EMS are just beginning to evolve from the various national organizations that represent children.[37]

Limited pediatric training coupled with limited exposure to pediatric patients may hamper the ability of EMS providers to respond appropriately to pediatric emergencies. In 2000, nationally registered paramedics received a median 358 total hours of instruction, less than 5% of which was dedicated to pediatrics. Most paramedics in this study were not required to take pediatric continuing medical education (CME) training.[18] Less than 10% of all EMS transports nationwide are for infants and children; 12% of those involve advanced life support, and even fewer provide critical care.[38,39] Overall, this translates into 3 pediatric patients per month for 60% of the nation's paramedics. Although pediatric advanced life support training has been associated with an improvement in ability to secure a pediatric airway or to obtain vascular or intraosseous access, this training is not required for EMS technicians.[40]

Babl and associates demonstrated that in a program with 50 active ALS providers in the current milieu of EMS, each provider would be expected to have one pediatric bag-valve-mask case every 1.7 years, one pediatric intubation every 3.3 years, and one intraosseous cannulation every 6.7 years.[41] Without repeated reinforcement, cognitive and interventional skills deteriorate over time. The poor performance of paramedics in advanced airway management in children is well documented and has led to recommendations that EMS crews avoid tracheal intubation in favor of bag-valve mask ventilation.[42]

Gausche et al. found that children in the field who were younger than 14 years were more likely to be undertreated compared to adults (33% versus 3%).[43] Studies of pediatric trauma victims make it clear that prehospital providers could do a better job with children. Children were twice as likely to die of trauma in the field compared with adults, a finding attributed to the lack of pediatric training.[38,42,44]

Finally, referring hospitals are often not equipped to care for critically ill and injured children. Two independent studies reported that as recently as 2003, only 6% of emergency rooms were appropriately equipped to care for children. Items frequently unavailable included laryngeal mask airways and infant and neonatal equipment.[44] Esposito and coworkers found that frequent errors occur in ED management of pediatric trauma, leading to about 9% preventable mortality.[45] They reported a 64% error rate in management of children, including gross violations of basic trauma care. Han et al. found that resuscitation practice in a community ED was consistent with American College of Critical Care Medicine Pediatric Advanced Life Support (ACCM-PALS) guidelines in only 30% of children who presented with septic shock.[11]

SPECIALIZED TEAMS IMPROVE OUTCOME

Early investigations of the use of specialized teams for interfacility transport of neonates and children found improved hemodynamic stability and fewer preventable insults with the use of specialized teams.[46-49] In a case-control study of preventable insults in head-injured children, Macnab et al. determined that the increase in adverse events with transport by nonspecialty teams resulted in $135,952 in additional costs of care.[49] Most importantly, two recent studies have documented an improvement in risk-adjusted mortality with the use of specialized teams for interhospital transfer of pediatric patients.[50,51]

Pediatric specialized teams bring ICU care to the patient and often perform additional stabilization maneuvers, including upon arrival at the referring facility. In a prospective observational study, pediatric teams initiated sedation 23% of the time, inotropes 44% of the time, and osmolar therapies for intracranial hypertension nearly 50% of the time when the referring facility had failed to do so. Retrieval teams also initiated mechanical ventilation, acquired central venous access, and placed or adjusted tracheal tubes[52] (Figure 225-1). Time at the bedside for specialized retrieval teams can be relatively long (97 minutes for neonates and 50 minutes for pediatric patients) because of these interventions, but scene time is not associated with mortality.[46,53]

The improvement in outcome associated with pediatric specialized transport teams likely stems from unappreciated differences between the respiratory mechanics and cardiovascular physiology in adults and children that lead to a need for earlier, more aggressive intervention in children with common pediatric problems.

In particular, high peripheral airway resistance, small alveoli, and a compliant chest wall increases the risk of lower airway obstructive disease and atelectasis, increases the work of breathing, and increases likelihood of respiratory muscle fatigue. Positive-pressure mechanical support may be required early in the disease process, and airway inter-

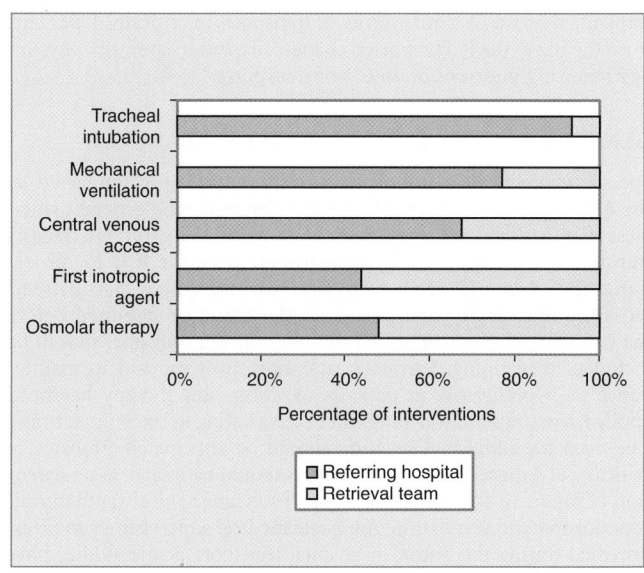

Figure 225-1 Proportion of interventions performed by referring hospitals and intensive care retrieval teams during stabilization of critically ill children. (*Used with permission from Lampariello S, Clement M, Aralihond AP, Lutman D, Montgomery MA, Petros AJ et al. Stabilisation of critically ill children at the district general hospital prior to intensive care retrieval: a snapshot of current practice. Arch Dis Child 2010;95:681-5.*)

ventions should be planned so as to avoid having to deal with a respiratory crisis while en route.

Delivery of goal-directed therapy may be hampered by the inability of practitioners to recognize shock. Infants and children have a greater capacity to increase systemic vascular resistance in shock states and tend to preserve blood pressure until very late in the evolution of shock.[54] Pediatric shock resuscitation protocols developed by a consensus of experts in the field call for symptomatic treatment of shock using clinical signs including age-specific targets for heart rate and blood pressure and relatively subtle indicators of perfusion as therapeutic endpoints.[13] Specialized pediatric teams may be more capable of recognizing deviation from age-specific norms and recognizing the subtle signs of compensated shock in children.

In-Hospital Transport

Despite the primary focus of transport on prehospital and interfacility settings, in-hospital transport of ICU patients occurs more commonly and may also be life threatening. The transport environment causes some physiologic stress, and almost all patients who are transported experience temporary changes in vital signs requiring some intervention. Over the last 2 decades, the risks associated with in-hospital transport have decreased significantly.

RECENT RESEARCH

Critically ill adults who require transport out of the ICU for interventions or diagnostic procedures have higher admission severity-of-illness scores with the attendant increase in use of critical care resources than those who do not require transport.[55] Because of this, it is difficult to assess the clinical impact of physiologic derangements reported in early evaluations of the safety of in-hospital transport. Still, it is clear that unplanned events are common. In a prospective observational study of in-hospital transports of critically ill patients from the ED, 68% of transports were associated with one or more unplanned events, mostly equipment failures. In the same study, serious unplanned events (hypotension, need for intubation, or elevated intracranial pressure) occurred in 5% of transports.[56] High level of experience in the accompanying physician was associated with decreased frequency of unplanned events. A similar series of transports of critically ill patients from the ED to the ICU reported changes in cardiorespiratory physiology requiring intervention in 6% of transports.[57]

GENERAL PRINCIPLES OF IN-HOSPITAL TRANSPORT

Specific guidelines for in-hospital transport have been published by the American Society for Critical Care Medicine. The general principles of in-hospital transport are the same as those for interfacility transport.[58] Patients who require transport from the ICU for procedures and diagnostic studies are sicker on the whole than patients requiring interfacility transport. Patients should be stabilized before the trip. Potential causes of deterioration during transport should be included in planning. Particular attention must be paid to maintenance of hypothermia in patients to whom this therapy has been applied, since rapid rewarming can be devastating to the injured brain. The need for additional sedation should be anticipated. Transfer of critically ill patients to another location should be treated as an extension of intensive care. In the sickest patients, mechanical ventilation is superior to hand ventilation. Adequate medical supervision should be provided during the entire in-hospital transport. Some studies have documented a decrease in unplanned events with greater experience level of the accompanying physician.[55]

Equipment taken on an in-hospital transport should include a portable system that contains everything normally found on a crash cart and an airway compartment complete with suction apparatus, laryngoscopes, tracheal tubes, bag-valve-mask devices, and medication for emergency intubation. An E-sized oxygen cylinder with a high-pressure regulator, flowmeter, and tubing of sufficient length should accompany all transports and be secured safely to the transport stretcher. Monitoring should include the cardiorespiratory system (electrocardiography, impedance pneumography) at the very least, pulse oximetry for patients in whom oxygen delivery is a potential concern, and the addition of capnography for patients who require mechanical ventilation. Intravascular monitoring should also be continued. It is important to use monitors with reliable batteries in the event of power loss or unexpected delays.

Conclusion

Traditionally, EMS and regional flight teams have been designed for rapid response and are expected to keep time at the scene to a minimum. In the era of goal-directed therapy for septic shock, it is clear that time-sensitive lifesaving interventions for critically ill patients can be relatively simple and should not be delayed until the patient reaches his or her ICU bed. Where pediatric services, particularly pediatric critical care services, have been regionalized, the use of specialized teams that provide stabilizing interventions beyond what is done by the referring facility improves outcome. Pediatric transport priorities may be a model for what to expect as regionalization of adult critical care services leads to an increase in numbers and acuity of critical care transports as well as a decrease in the referring hospital's experience with critically ill patients. To realize the benefits of regionalization, intensivists must be actively involved in the planning, maintenance, and quality management of a system that provides constant optimal care.

KEY POINTS

1. During transport, patients are subjected to a high-risk moving environment with limited resources and few monitoring capabilities. The risks of interfacility transport are not precisely known. Adverse events that occur during transport have the potential to negatively impact patient outcome.

2. Except for a few exquisitely time-sensitive disease processes that require interventions not possible in the transport environment, speed of transport alone does not correlate with improved outcomes; the "golden hour" is the time from presentation to initiation of appropriate treatment, not arrival at the accepting facility. Definitive treatment from some common disease processes, including septic shock, should begin at the referring institution and continue during transport.

3. Owing to inadequate training and infrequent contact, adult-oriented emergency medical services (EMS) and air ambulance services may not provide ideal care for critically ill children. The use of specialized pediatric critical care teams has been associated with improved mortality.

4. Regionalization of critical care services will increase the numbers of critically ill patients requiring interfacility transfer. In order to realize the proposed benefits of regionalization, high-quality care must be provided during transport.

5. A retrieval system has a responsibility to the referral community to provide accessible tertiary care. The components include a communications center, administrative staff, appropriately trained team members, reliable equipment, and education and safety programs.

6. A hospital should not transfer until (1) the patient has been appropriately stabilized within the capabilities of the transferring hospital, (2) the patient consents to transfer after being informed of the risks of transfer, (3) the referring physician certifies that the medical benefits expected from the transfer outweigh the risks, and (4) the receiving hospital has available space and has accepted the patient. The referring hospital must prepare copies of medical records and imaging studies to accompany the patient, and the transport must be made by qualified personnel.

ANNOTATED REFERENCES

Grissom TE, Farmer JC. The provision of sophisticated critical care beyond the hospital: lessons from physiology and military experiences that apply to civil disaster medical response. Crit Care Med 2005;33:S13-21.
This article discusses existing systems to provide critical care in environments outside the ICU, including the transport environment, team composition, equipment, and medications necessary for provision of critical care en route. Previous reports of similar data focus on the needs of prehospital teams who perform minimal intervention and rely heavily on speed of transport.

Han YY, Carcillo JA, Dragotta MA, et al. Early reversal of pediatric-neonatal septic shock by community physicians is associated with improved outcome. Pediatrics 2003;12:793-9.
This study demonstrated that when community physicians successfully achieved shock reversal through aggressive resuscitation before a transport team arrived, patients had a ninefold increase in their odds of survival.

Rivers E, Nguyen B, Havstad S, et al. Early goal-directed therapy in the treatment of severe sepsis and septic shock. N Engl J Med 2001;345:1368-77.
This landmark article demonstrated that early goal-directed therapy in the treatment of septic shock before arrival in the ICU improved survival. Patients assigned to the early goal-directed therapy group had improved central venous oxygen saturations, lower base deficits, and a lower incidence of multisystem organ dysfunction compared with those who had standard therapy.

Warren J, Fromm RE Jr, Orr RA, Rotello LC, Horst HM. American College of Critical Care Medicine. Guidelines for the inter- and intrahospital transport of critically ill patients. Crit Care Med 2004;32:256-62.
This article is an overview of ACCM standards of care for both interfacility and in-hospital transport.

Orr RA, Felmet KA, Han Y, McCloskey KA, Dragotta MA, Bills DM, et al. Pediatric specialized transport teams are associated with improved outcomes. Pediatrics 2009;124:40-8.
In a prospective cohort study in which allocation of team depended on team availability, not severity of illness, Orr et al. showed that use of a specialized team resulted in fewer unplanned adverse events and lower mortality compared with use of a nonspecialized team. Most importantly, mortality was high in children transported by nonspecialized teams compared with specialized teams (23% versus 9%), a difference that remained significant when controlling for pre-ICU PRISM score.

REFERENCES

Access the complete reference list online at http://www.expertconsult.com.

226

Mass Critical Care

ARIEL L. SHILOH | RICHARD H. SAVEL | SHARON LEUNG |
ANTHONY J. CARLESE | VLADIMIR KVETAN

Natural and manmade disasters have always been a part of life and are occurring with increasing frequency. They create varied degrees of chaos owing to mismatch of resources and needs, and they place a huge burden on healthcare systems. Restoring an affected society to its pre-event status requires extraordinary efforts and incurs substantial costs. Thousands of persons are injured physically and emotionally as a result of such events, and their effects continue long after worldwide attention has disappeared.

The devastating events of September 11, 2001, in the United States, subsequent acts of bioterrorism, and emerging infectious disease pandemics have brought new challenges to the field of disaster management and multidisciplinary hazard mitigation. Even though war- and terrorism-related disasters have gathered much attention recently, natural disasters have occurred with increasing frequency over the past decades. This has been attributed to the growth of human populations in geographically disaster-prone areas, rapid industrialization, and increasing exposure to toxic and hazardous materials.[1-3]

Analyses of the response of different healthcare systems to major disasters in the past have demonstrated the need for a more clearly identified planning process to attend to the response to multihazard events.[4] This provides a basic understanding of common disaster scenarios and highlights the role of the intensivist in the medical response to disasters. It is important for the practicing critical care clinician to keep in mind that their role is first and foremost as a first receiver, rather than first responder; a well-trained intensivist may be of much greater value remaining in the hospital setting rather than quickly mobilizing to the field, where their lack of situational preparedness may make them more of a hindrance than an asset.[5]

Background

Major disasters occur regularly and cause widespread human death and suffering. Over the past 2 decades, more than 3 million lives have been lost worldwide to major disasters. A total of 39,073 persons were reported killed by disasters alone in 2001, with the decade's annual average of around 62,000. Even though the numbers of geophysical disasters such as earthquakes and volcanic eruptions have remained fairly constant over the past decade, the past 2 years have seen the highest number of weather-related disasters reported over the decade.[6] As populations grow and occupy spaces that are vulnerable to different hazards, disasters will increase in severity and impact. Recent events since the September 2001 terrorism attacks have brought attention to the effects of manmade disasters on the healthcare system and the need to anticipate and plan for such low-probability yet catastrophic events. Even though there is basic similarity in the response to various hazardous events, each type of disaster presents responders with unique demands. After any disaster, healthcare systems are tasked with preventing excessive deaths, mitigating suffering, and dealing with often overwhelming inadequacy of resources. Over the past few years, disaster medicine has thus grown into a unique specialty to deal with planning and preparing for such cataclysmic events. It shares a common ideal with public health: "greatest good for the greatest number."[3]

A fundamental part of designing a medical response to disasters is to coordinate healthcare personnel across the hospital system so they overcome natural differences associated with each group and maximize efficient use of scarce resources. Because the sickest of all viable patients will require intensive care, the critical care physician can play

an invaluable part in coordination efforts. In addition to their usual role of being caregivers for patients in the intensive care unit (ICU), intensivists will be expected to help in triage decisions, transport critically ill patients, and treat the multitude of injured in a rational order. They can also help by providing essential medical care at the actual disaster site via mobile ICU teams. It is thus important for critical care physicians to be familiar with the basics of disaster management, acquire organizational and leadership skills, practice delivery of unconventional critical care, and be familiar with different disaster-related medical syndromes.

Terminology

Physicians and healthcare personnel should be familiar with basic nomenclature and terminology in disaster medicine. Clear, common, and concise definitions are important to effective communication and evoking appropriate responses to disaster situations. Uniform use of terminology across healthcare systems provides a basis for analysis and construction of an effective disaster plan and response by all responders.[7] Controversies surrounding the definitions of *disasters*, *hazards*, and *causalities* are included in the discussions that follow.

The word *disaster* connotes a subjective assessment that has various meanings to different people and has an inherent bias, depending on the person using it. For example, a local, state, or federal "disaster declaration" implies commitment of financial and other resources. Similarly, a disaster in one community is not necessarily the same to another. Currently there is no uniformly accepted definition for the word *disaster*.[7] De Boer recognizes the lack of a meaningful definition for the word and proposes instead the term *medical severity index* (MSI).[8] This term, however, has not gained sufficient acceptance for routine use. Different modifiers can lead to different definitions of the term *disaster*. They include the type of disaster, geographic area involved, timing, onset of the event, size of the community affected, baseline resources available to the community, and finally, the physical, psychosocial, and economic injury caused by the event. However, from a healthcare standpoint, the most important variable that defines a disaster is its functional impact on the healthcare facility.[7] Despite various attempts to clear the confusion surrounding the terminology, the issue remains unresolved.[7,9-10] What follows are the commonly used definitions in disaster medicine from a healthcare perspective:

Hazard. An event with the potential to cause catastrophic damage. It may be "naturally" occurring phenomena such as volcano eruptions or "manmade" such as nuclear power plant accidents.[11]

Emergency. A natural or manmade event that significantly disrupts the environment of care (e.g., damage to an organization's buildings due to severe winds, storms, or earthquakes), resulting in disrupted care and treatment (e.g., loss of utilities such as power, water, or telephones due to floods, civil disturbances, accidents, or emergencies within the organization or in its community); or that results in sudden, significantly changed, or increased demand for the organization's services (e.g., bioterrorist attack, building collapse, plane crash in the organization's community).

Disaster. A hazardous event causing physical, psychological, social, economic, or even political effects on a scale such that the stricken community needs extraordinary efforts to cope with it, and often outside help or international aid.[9-10] Medical disasters form a subset of this category, in which the physical and/or psychosocial

TABLE 226-1	PICE Nomenclature	
A	*B*	*C*
Static	Controlled	Local
Dynamic	Disruptive	Regional
	Paralytic	National
		International

Data from Koenig KL, Dinerman N, Kuehl AE. Disaster nomenclature—a functional impact approach: the PICE system. Acad Emerg Med 1996;3:723-7.
PICE, potential injury-creating events.

TABLE 226-2	Paralytic PICE	
Destructive		*Nondestructive*
Bomb explosion		Snowstorm
Earthquake		Employee strike
Tornado		Power failure
Civil unrest		Water supply cutoff
HazMat spill		
Fire		
Building collapse		

Data from Koenig KL, Dinerman N, Kuehl AE. Disaster nomenclature—a functional impact approach: the PICE system. Acad Emerg Med 1996;3:723-7.
HazMat, hazardous materials; *PICE*, potential injury-creating events.

injuries exceed the medical response capabilities of the community affected.

Casualty. Any person suffering physical and/or psychological damage by outside violence leading to death, injuries, or material losses. Again, the word has no standard definition and is sometimes used to imply injury, death, or both. It may also bear financial implications, because federal reimbursement may be approved only for persons classified as casualties.[7,9-10]

PICE (potential injury-creating events) system. A new terminology system developed to overcome the differences in disaster nomenclature. This system uses the functional impact on the healthcare facility as the only determining factor to define an "emergency" or "disaster" situation. It uses four modifiers to effectively communicate the impact caused by the situation on the healthcare facility and is described in more detail later.[7]

Multicasualty incident. A hazardous event that regardless of its size is containable by local emergency medical services (EMS). From an operational standpoint, an event becomes a multicasualty incident when its impact exceeds the day-to-day response routine to the EMS. Significant adjustments within the local response system are required to cope with this demand without the need to request outside help (Level 1 response).[12]

Mass casualty incident. A hazardous event that overwhelms local response capability. It is likely to impose a sustained demand for health services rather than a short, intense peak typical of many smaller-scale disasters. This may require a Level 2 response (neighboring and regional resources are activated) or a Level 3 response (state, interstate, and federal resources are activated in the rescue and recovery process).[13]

Hazard vulnerability analysis (HVA). The identification of potential emergencies and the direct and indirect effects these emergencies may have on the organization's operations and the demand for its services. This concept is described in further detail later in the section on principles of disaster planning.[14]

Classification of Disasters

Natural disasters arise from forces of nature and include earthquakes, volcanic eruptions, hurricanes, floods, fire, and tornadoes. In addition, infectious disasters can be classified as epidemic or pandemic and are discussed elsewhere. Manmade disasters are due to identifiable human causes and may be further classified as complex emergencies (e.g., wars, terrorist attacks) and technological disasters (e.g., industrial accidents, explosions from hazardous material).[15] Other classifications include those based on onset (acute versus insidious disasters), predictability, duration, and frequency. From a public health perspective, disasters have to be defined by their effect on people and the healthcare system. The concept of functional impact to the healthcare system is thus paramount.[15-16]

The PICE system attempts to create uniformity to address the wide spectrum of situations.[7] The two major aims of this system are to effectively communicate both the operational consequences to a hospital or community and the type and amount of outside assistance needed. Four modifiers for an event are chosen from a standardized group of prefixes, and a stage is assigned (Table 226-1). *Column A* (first prefix) describes the potential for additional casualties. For example a

finite number of persons injured in an airplane crash is a "static event," whereas an ongoing fire is a "dynamic" event. *Column B* (second prefix) describes whether local resources are sufficient ("controlled") or overwhelmed. If they are overwhelmed, the two modifiers "disruptive" and "paralytic" indicate whether they must be simply augmented or totally reconstituted. Paralytic PICE are the most daunting of all situations, and they can be either destructive or nondestructive (Table 226-2). *Column C* describes the extent of geographic involvement. *PICE stage* refers to the likelihood that outside medical help is required (Table 226-3). This PICE model provides important concepts for disaster planners, researchers, and responders. Using this system, disasters can be described both prospectively and retrospectively. PICE is a valuable tool for use in planning and disaster mitigation, but the system warrants validation on a wider scale. It may also require further refinement to delineate the type of aid needed by an affected community.[7]

Regardless of the type of classification used to categorize disasters, certain unique features are associated with each type of disaster. It is important to understand the common effects of different natural and manmade disasters to predict their impact and plan effectively. Some common disaster situations are reviewed next.

Natural Disasters

EARTHQUAKES

Earthquakes are a well-known and publicized model of a disaster that results in significant mortality,[17] as can be seen in Figure 226-1 describing deaths from earthquakes since 1990. A homogenous population well trained in basic trauma and life support and the architectural design of the stricken area's housing and public facilities are two major determinants of outcomes for earthquake victims. The massive earthquakes of the past 10 years in Turkey, Taiwan, Sumatra, Kashmir, Sichuan, and Haiti have shown us that sound engineering design for earthquake resistance in civil structures such as schools, hospitals, fire

TABLE 226-3	PICE System Staging with Examples	
Stage	*Projected Need for Outside Help*	*Status of Outside Help*
0	Little to none	Inactive
I	Small	Alert
II	Moderate	Standby
III	Great	Dispatch

Examples of PICE Staging

1. Multiple-vehicle crash in a big city	Static, controlled, local PICE, stage 0
2. Multiple-vehicle crash in a small town	Static, disruptive, local PICE, stage I
3. Los Angeles civil disturbance	Dynamic, disruptive, regional PICE, stage II
4. SARS outbreak in China	Dynamic, disruptive, national PICE, stage III

From Koenig KL, Dinerman N, Kuehl AE. Disaster nomenclature—a functional impact approach: the PICE system. Acad Emerg Med 1996;3:723-7.
PICE, potential injury-creating events; *SARS*, severe acute respiratory syndrome.

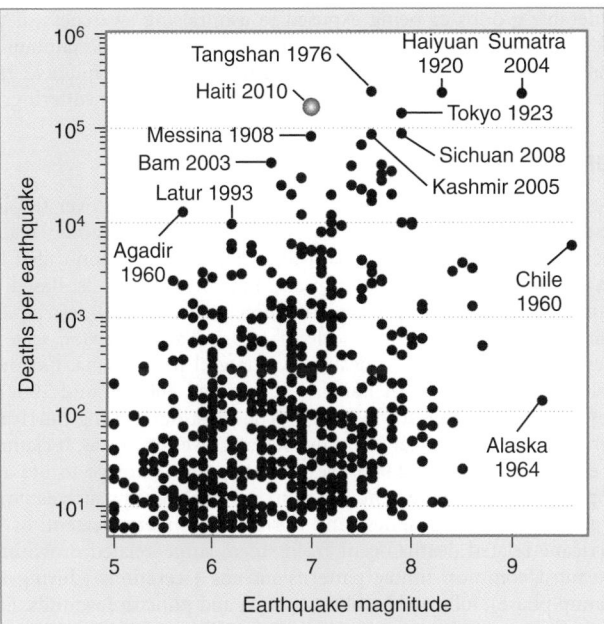

Figure 226-1 Deaths from earthquakes since 1900. The toll of the Haiti quake is more than twice that of any previous magnitude 7.0 event and fourth worst since 1900. *(From Hough SE, Bilham R. After the earthquakes: elastic rebound on an urban planet. New York: Oxford University Press; 2006; and from Bilham R. The seismic future of cities. Bull Earthq Eng 2009;7:839-87.)*

stations, and correctional facilities have a major impact on outcomes. In addition, urban earthquakes generate massive fiscal impact on the world in terms of reconstruction grants provided by wealthier countries for devastated urban areas. Moderately destructive earthquakes in the developing world usually cost up to $10 billion in reconstruction; the needs of developing countries with urban earthquakes may cost an order of magnitude more.

Despite extensive experience and published literature dealing with medical response to earthquakes over the past 30 years and publications devoted to compiling the experiences of disaster management focused on critical care, current experience with the earthquake in Haiti shows that we are frequently doomed to relearn the lessons forgotten.

The Haiti earthquake occurred on January 12, 2010, and was of magnitude 7.0 on the Richter scale, resulting in some 230,000 mortalities and 1.5 million homeless. Let us consider first the military medicine response delivered, especially in the face of continuous exposure of the military medicine establishment to mass casualty management in the wars in the Middle East.

Responders from the very experienced Israel Defense Forces (IDF) air-deployed within 48 hours of the Haiti earthquake. This team had extensive experience over the years with international response and consists of 230 people. The team unpacked and built their portable hospital within 8 hours, and during 10 days of operation treated more than 1100 patients in a facility designed to provide 60 inpatient beds, including 4 intensive care beds and 1 operating room.[18] Most of the first wave of casualties presented with crushed limbs with open infected wounds, with the later arrivals presenting with sepsis and poor chance of outcome. Despite the repeated experience from prior earthquakes showing that victims of crush syndrome and acute renal failure require emergency dialysis to prevent death, this facility relied on other international teams for dialysis. Their major dilemmas were practical implementation of the triage algorithm by military personnel to a civilian population. The simple priorities were urgency, resources available, and probability of saving life. Patients with brain injury, paraplegia due to spine injuries, or a low Glasgow Coma Scale score were immediately transferred to other facilities, since no neurosurgical

capabilities were available. A triage panel of three senior physicians relieved individual physicians of personal accountability. Half of the intensive care capability was always dedicated to postoperative care, with the remaining 2 beds used for prolonged intensive care; only patients who were expected to stabilize within 24 hours were placed in these beds. The very early discharge policy permitted this military facility to treat more than 100 patients per day.

Second, let us consider the response of the U.S. military, which at this point had a considerable portfolio on providing international disaster relief in catastrophic events such as the Indonesian tsunami that devastated Sumatra. The United States Naval Ship (USNS) *Comfort*, one of Military Sealift Command's two hospital ships, was deployed as part of the mission termed "Operation Unified Response." It started accepting casualties within 7 days of the earthquake. The ship is a 1000-bed facility which includes 75 intensive care unit beds, blood bank, hemodialysis, pathology, physical therapy, morgue, and radiology with computed tomography and ultrasonography capability. It is staffed with 1000 active-duty U.S. medical personnel, including three physician intensivists, and it was allocated to stay up to 6 months.[19-20]

The first wave of casualties were critically ill trauma patients airlifted from field hospitals by U.S. helicopters. Within 72 hours, the *Comfort* admitted 254 patients, and the census rapidly increased to 430, more than a third of them pediatric cases. A team of 6 internists provided 24/7 coverage. Dozens of patients underwent mechanical ventilation simultaneously, open-bay design did not allow for isolation, and the nurse-to-patient ratio was about 7:1. A large volume of hemodialysis was provided to patients with crush syndrome, leading to rapid depletion of dialyzers and dual-lumen dialysis catheters. The discharges exceeded admissions in about 2 weeks, and after a total of 629 admissions, the ship completed its mission. While the standard of care exceeded community expectations, the U.S. Navy personnel followed naval protocol and standards.

Third, let us consider the relearning of the lessons of civil-military collaboration in disaster response.[21] A volunteer medical team with civilian personnel under the auspices of the international medical corps flew to the Dominican Republic and reached Hopital de l'Universite d'Etat d'Haiti in Port-au-Prince after a long bus ride on January 17. There were more than 800 injured in the partially destroyed facility, with the primary diagnoses being crush injuries, compartment syndrome, infected fractures, and hemorrhagic shock. One physician and one nurse were covering up to 80 critically ill patients in the wards. An aftershock of 5.9 magnitude resulted in an exodus of casualties and higher rates of heat stroke in dehydrated hypovolemic patients exposed to tropical temperatures. Destruction of the prison system released some 4000 criminals into the community, and no security was available until arrival of a U.S. airborne infantry regiment. With arrival of the USNS *Comfort* on January 20, evacuation of the most critically ill patients started, but a triage list developed rapidly, with ship facilities accepting preferentially complicated injuries, obstetric patients, and maxillofacial injuries. Patients with pelvic fractures, closed head injuries, complete spinal cord lesions, and mechanical ventilation cases were of too-high acuity for the USNS *Comfort*. Family structures became fragmented as separation of children from parents occurred. Yet the collaboration of civilian and military medical personnel was considered a success.

Next, let us consider the experiences of academic centers delivering care to victims of the Haitian earthquake on-site.[22] The Miller School of Medicine of the University of Miami and Project Medishare had the advantage of long experience of collaboration with Haiti as well as close geographic proximity, and they were able to provide emergency relief within 20 hours. Within 8 days, they were able to establish a field hospital at the city airport, and by January 21, 140 patients were transferred into the upgrade facility. The well-organized command center with satellite links for telephone and Internet access were available. A joint adult-pediatric triage team accompanied by Creole-speaking medical staff of Haitian origin was used. Multiple surgeries were performed under local peripheral nerve blocks, with guillotine amputations being frequent. Highest-acuity patients were transferred to the

IDF field hospital or the USNS *Comfort*. The command center eventually provided psychiatrists to manage the posttraumatic stress syndrome and a buddy system for follow-up support.

Finally, one must consider the critical care response from New York City. While many small teams and a large volume of supplies were dispatched, an organized response was delivered under the leadership of Dr. Ernest Benjamin, division chief of critical care in surgery at Mt. Sinai Hospital. Dr. Benjamin, with close family ties to Haiti, arrived in Port-au-Prince 3 days after the initial event and after rapid assessment of needs and resources available, organized the deployment of the 27-member critical care team to his home country, which arrived on January 20. The team remained on-site for 2 weeks and was responsible for postanesthesia and postoperative care delivery, with Dr. Benjamin being deputized as the director of critical care and recovery at the national hospital. The home institution effectively secured anonymous donations of private jets able to transport the team personnel and some 3000 pounds of medical supplies per flight. The team delivered intensive care with minimal technology but with kindness and dignity towards the suffering population. This certainly was not a medical tourism venture but a true integrated response with both language and cultural sensitivities and capabilities, so important in catastrophic situations that will take decades for the local population to recover from.[23]

Experience in managing catastrophic international disasters continues to accumulate with unfortunate regularity. The preceding discussion suggests that combinations of dialysis, orthopedic surgery, pediatric trauma, security, transportation, posttraumatic stress treatment, and cultural and language sensitivities are crucial in earthquakes. Disasters produce well-defined syndromes with well-defined mortalities. It is the recovery phase that continues to require persistence and improvement. One of the most experienced managers and thought leaders in disaster management, Dr. Eric Noji, enumerated the most important factors in public health after disasters: environmental health, epidemic management, immunization, controlling the spread of HIV/AIDS, management of dead bodies, nutrition, maternal and child health, medical services, and thorough public health surveillance. It is a common error to deliver a few weeks of heroic quality care then abandon the population to the ravages of destroyed infrastructure, including public health organization.[24]

VOLCANIC ERUPTIONS

A volcano is a hill or a mountain built around a vent that connects with reservoirs of molten rock below the earth's surface.[25] Different types of eruptive events occur, including pyroclastic explosions, hot ash releases, lava flows, gas emissions, and glowing avalanches (gas and ash releases). Lava flows tend not to result in high casualties, because they are easily avoidable. The "composite" type of volcano is associated with a more violent eruption from within the chimney. These eruptions are associated with air shock waves, rock projectiles (some with high thermal energy), release of noxious gases, pyroclastic flows, and mud flows (lahars). Pyroclastic flows and lahars are often fast moving and are the main cause of damage and deaths from volcanoes, as evidenced by the small eruption of the Nevado del Ruiz in Columbia that killed more than 23,000 people.[26] The release of ash and its subsequent rapid buildup on building structures can be substantial, causing them to collapse within a matter of hours. Ash is also responsible for the clogging of filters and machinery, causing electrical storms and fires, and interfering with communications. Ash is a main cause for respiratory-related syndromes and conjunctival and corneal injury. A variety of toxic gases (e.g., carbon dioxide, hydrogen sulfide, sulfur dioxide, hydrogen chloride, hydrogen fluoride, and carbon monoxide [CO]) are released during eruptions, causing bronchospasm, pulmonary edema, hypoxemia, cellular asphyxiation, topical irritation of skin and other mucosal surfaces, and death.[27] Damage to health infrastructures and water systems can be severe. Problems related to communication (ashes cause serious interference) and transportation (poor visibility and slippery roads) are likely. Depending on the initial assessment, various needs can be anticipated. Reducing the risk for vulnerable groups of being exposed to ash, raising awareness of the risk associated with ash (health and mechanical risk), and maintaining food security conditions over the long term (lava, ash, and acid rain cause damage to crops and livestock) can help minimize suffering.[28]

HURRICANES, CYCLONES, AND TYPHOONS

The large rotating weather systems that form seasonally over tropical oceans are variously named, depending on the geographic region where they form.[29-31] They consist of a calm inner portion called the *eye*, surrounded by a wall of rain and high-velocity winds. Based on central pressure, wind speed, storm surge, and potential destruction, their severity is graded on a scale of 1 to 5 (Saffir Simpson scale).[30] They are among the most destructive natural phenomena. Cyclones during 1970 and 1991 in Bangladesh claimed 300,000 and 100,000 lives, respectively, due to flooding.[32] The most devastating hurricane ever to hit the United States was in 1900 at Galveston, Texas. It claimed an estimated 8000 to 12,000 lives.[33] The greatest damage to life and property is not from the wind but from secondary events such as storm surges, flooding, landslides, and tornadoes. Ninety percent of all hurricane-related deaths occur from storm surge–related drowning.[1] The most common injury patterns include lacerations (during the cleanup phase), followed by blunt trauma and puncture wounds. Late morbidity can be due to post-disaster cleanup accidents (e.g., electrocution), dehydration, wound infection, and outbreaks of communicable disease.[31,34] Data from hurricane Katrina confirmed data from previous meteorological events: the leading mechanisms of injuries are fall, lacerations, and piercing injuries, with cleanup being the primary activity at the time of injury.[35] Recent experiences in the aftermath of hurricane Katrina in 2005 indicate that resources may have to be provided for an extended period after the initial inciting event, and that significant resources may have to be provided for patients with chronic medical illnesses.[34,36]

FLOODS

There are three major types of floods: flash floods (caused by heavy rain and dam failures), coastal floods, and river floods. Together, they are the most common type of disasters and account for at least half of all disaster-related deaths.[37,38] The primary cause of death is drowning, followed by hypothermia and injury due to floating debris.[39,40] The impact on the health infrastructures and lifeline systems can be massive and may result in food shortages. Interruption of basic public services (e.g., sanitation, drinking water, electricity) may result in outbreaks of communicable disease.[38,40] Another concern is the increase in both vectorborne diseases (e.g., malaria, St. Louis encephalitis) and displacement of wildlife (e.g., poisonous snakes and rodents).[39,40]

LANDSLIDES

Landslides are more widespread than any other geologic event. They are defined as downslope transport of soil and rock resulting from natural phenomena or manmade actions. Landslides can also occur secondary to heavy storms, volcanic eruptions, and earthquakes. Landslides cause high mortality and few injuries. Trauma and suffocation by entrapment are common. Pending an assessment, needs can be anticipated, such as search and rescue, mass casualty management, and emergency shelter for the homeless.[41,42]

PANDEMIC 2009 H1N1 INFLUENZA A VIRUS

Pandemic H1N1 2009 is a new strain of influenza A virus that was first identified in Mexico and the United States on March 18 and April 15, 2009, respectively. It originated from the quadruple reassortment swine influenza (H1N1) virus closely related to the North American and Eurasian swine lineage. However, this new virus circulated only in humans, with no evidence of transmission between humans and animals.

Within weeks, the virus quickly spread worldwide through human-to-human transmission. On April 26, 2009, the CDC's Strategic National Stockpile began releasing 25% of the supplies in the stockpile for the treatment and protection from influenza.[43] On June 11, 2009, the World Health Organization (WHO) declared the 2009 H1N1 influenza a global pandemic, generating the first influenza pandemic of the 21st century, with more than 70 countries reporting cases of H1N1 infection. By June 19, 2009, all 50 states in the United States, the District of Columbia, Puerto Rico, and the U.S. Virgin Islands had reported cases of 2009 H1N1 infection. More strikingly, the Centers for Disease Control and Prevention (CDC) Emerging Infections Program (EIP) estimated the number of hospitalizations and deaths in people 64 years and younger. The virus was most likely to strike children, young adults, and those with underlying pulmonary and cardiac disease. Pregnant women in their second and third trimester were also at high risk. Patients requiring intensive care had a remarkable prevalence of obesity.[43]

Influenza vaccines are most effective not only to prevent but also to mitigate the severity of illness. The pandemic H1N1 influenza vaccine was promptly developed by the WHO and national authorities. A national influenza vaccination campaign was launched in the United States in October 2009, and the first H1N1 vaccine was made available at that time. Despite the rapid response of the authorities, developing countries in the Southern Hemisphere experienced delays and shortages of the vaccines. Thus, recent research and developmental work have been encouraging for developing a "universal" influenza vaccine that could provide efficacious cross-reactive immunity and induce broad protection against different variants and subtypes of the influenza virus.[44]

To date, the preliminary data show that about 8% of H1N1 patients were hospitalized (23 per 100,000 population); 6.5% to 25% of these required being in the ICU (28.7 per million inhabitants) for a median of 7 to 12 days, with a peak bed occupancy of 6.3 to 10.6 per million inhabitants; 65% to 97% of ICU patients required mechanical ventilation, with median ventilator duration in survivors of 7 to 15 days; 5% to 22% required renal replacement therapy; and 28-day ICU mortality was 14% to 40%.[45-51]

Critical care capacity is a key element of hospital surge capacity planning.[10] The proportion of ICU beds occupied by patients with H1N1 varied. In Australia and New Zealand, it peaked at 19%[7] while in Mexico, many patients required mechanical ventilation outside the ICUs.[6] To match the surge capacity with increasing ICU demands during a pandemic is a difficult task, since uncertainty exists for many of these parameters. The disease brought a surge of not only critically ill patients but patients who required prolonged mechanical ventilation and ICU management. Hospitals should maximize the number of ICU beds by expanding ICUs and other areas with appropriate beds and monitors. Elective procedures should be minimized when resources are limited, and critical care capacity should be augmented.

Safe practices and safe respiratory equipment are needed to minimize aerosol generation when caring for patients with influenza. These measures include handwashing and wearing gloves and gowns. The use of N95 respirators reduces the transmission of epidemic respiratory viruses. Staff training in personal protective equipment use is essential. Use of bag-mask ventilation and disconnection of the ventilator circuit should be minimized. Moreover, the use of heated humidifiers on ventilators, Venturi masks, and nebulized medications should be avoided.[52]

When the number of critically ill patients far exceeds a hospital's traditional critical care capacity, modified standards of critical care to provide limited but high-yield critical care interventions should be the goal in order to accommodate far more patients. Triage criteria should be objective, transparent, and ethical and be applied justifiably and publicly disclosed. The ICU triage protocols for pandemics should only be triggered when ICU resources across a broad geographic area are or will be overwhelmed despite all reasonable efforts to extend resources or obtain additional resources.[53] The Sequential Organ Failure Assessment (SOFA) score, though not validated, has been proposed to determine qualification for ICU admission during mass critical care.

The major characteristics of 2009 H1N1 influenza A infection were the rapidly progressive lower respiratory tract disease leading to acute respiratory distress syndrome (ARDS) with refractory hypoxemia. A substantial number of H1N1 ICU patients required advanced ventilatory support (ranging from 1.7% to 11.9%) and rescue therapies including high levels of inspired oxygen and positive end-expiratory pressure (PEEP), inverse ratio ventilation, airway pressure release ventilation (APRV), neuromuscular blockade, inhaled nitric oxide, high-frequency oscillatory ventilation (HFOV), extracorporeal membrane oxygenation (ECMO), volumetric diffusive respiration, and prone-positioning ventilation.[46,49,51,54] Of particular interest was the successful use of ECMO in the management of refractory hypoxemia in these patients in two studies. The median durations of therapy and survival rates to ICU discharge were 10 days and 15 days—71% and 67%, respectively.[55,56]

As of March 13, 2010, the CDC estimates of 2009 H1N1 influenza cases, hospitalizations, and deaths in the United States since April 2009 were 60 million cases, 270,000 hospitalizations, and 12,270 H1N1-related deaths, respectively.[57] The virus did not mutate during the pandemic to a more lethal form. Widespread resistance to oseltamivir did not develop. The WHO declared an end to the H1N1 pandemic on Aug 10, 2010. According to Margaret Chan, the Director-General of the WHO, the H1N1 virus is no longer the dominant circulating virus worldwide. Based on the available evidence and experience from past pandemics, "it is likely that the virus will continue to cause serious disease in the younger age group, at least in the immediate post-pandemic period. The H1N1 virus is expected to take on the behavior of a seasonal influenza virus and to circulate for some years."

OTHER NATURAL DISASTERS

Tornadoes occur most commonly in the North American Midwest. Over 4115 deaths and 70,000 injuries have been ascribed to them during the years 1950 to 1994. They cause widespread destruction of community infrastructure. Injuries most commonly seen are complex contaminated soft-tissue injury (50%), fractures (30%), head injury (10%), and blunt trauma to the chest and abdomen (10%).[58,59] Firestorms, wildfires, tsunamis, winter storms, and heat waves are other natural phenomena capable of creating mass injuries from thermal burns, airway injury, smoke inhalation, heat-related disorders, and hypothermia.[60-63]

Manmade Disasters

TRANSPORTATION DISASTERS

Transportation accidents can produce injuries and death similar to those seen in major natural disasters. Some of the largest civilian disasters in North America have been related to transportation of hazardous materials.[64] Motor vehicle accidents, railway accidents, airplane crashes, and shipwrecks are some of the common transportation accidents. They cause a wide range of injuries including multiple trauma, fractures, burns, chemical injuries, hypothermia, dehydration, asphyxiation, and CO inhalation. The hazard risk to a healthcare facility increases with its proximity to a chemical plant or highway, and such factors should be considered in the emergency preparedness plan of the hospital.[65]

WEAPONS OF MASS DESTRUCTION

Weapons of mass destruction (WMD) are those nuclear, biological, chemical, incendiary, or conventional explosive agents that pose a potential threat to health, safety, food supply, property, or the environment. Since the devastating terrorist attacks in September 2001 and subsequent intentional release of anthrax spores in the United States, there is growing concern around the world about the possible threat of chemical, biological, or nuclear weapons used against a civilian population. Compared with the frequency of natural and technology-related disasters, the incidence of use of WMD to cause death and injury is relatively rare. However, biological and chemical weapons are relatively accessible, and WMD are thought to be available to most foreign states and terrorist groups. In response to a WMD incident, healthcare personnel will be called on to manage unprecedented numbers of casualties in an environment of panic, fear, and paranoia that accompanies terrorism. Because most attacks occur without warning, the local healthcare system will be the first and most critical interface for detection, notification, rapid diagnosis, and treatment. The best defense in reducing casualties will therefore rest on the ability of medical and public health personnel to recognize symptoms and provide rapid clinical and epidemiologic diagnosis of an event. This requires that healthcare providers be well informed of potential biological, chemical, and nuclear agents. They must have a heightened index of suspicion and be able to identify unusual disease patterns to determine whether WMD are the etiologic agents of illness. Physicians will need to practice appropriate surveillance and reporting and develop knowledge of mass decontamination, use of proper personal protection equipment, and safety protocols related to a biological, chemical, or radiologic event.[66-68] Salient characteristics and brief management strategies of the different WMD are discussed here. Detailed description of individual biological and chemical agents, diagnosis, postexposure management, vaccination, infection control measures, and use of personal protection equipment is beyond the scope of this chapter.

Biological Weapons

Biological weapons can be either pathogens (disease-causing organisms such as viruses or bacteria) or toxins (poisons of biological origin). Compared with other WMD, biological weapons are characterized by ease of accessibility and dissemination, difficulty in detection because of their slow onset of action, and their ability to cause widespread panic through the fear of contagion. They can be spread through various means, including aerial bombs, aerosol sprays, explosives, and food or water contamination. Multiple factors including particle size of the agent, stability of the agent, wind speed, wind direction, and atmospheric conditions can alter the effectiveness of a delivery system. Based on the ease of dissemination, ability to cause high mortality, public panic and social disruption, and requirement for special action for public health preparedness, the Centers for Disease Control and Prevention (CDC) has classified biological weapons into three categories (Table 226-4).[69] Category A agents are of particular concern because they can cause widespread disease through their ease of transmission, result in high mortality rates, cause panic and social

TABLE 226-4	Triage Classification		
Groups	*Color*	*Symbol*	*Type of Injury*
Priority I (Emergent)	Red	R	CRITICAL: likely to survive if simple* care given within minutes
Priority II (Catastrophic)	Blue	B	CATASTROPHIC: unlikely to survive and/or extensive or complicated care needed within minutes
Priority III (Urgent)	Yellow	Y	URGENT: likely to survive if simple† care given within hours
Priority IV (Nonurgent)	Green	G	MINOR: likely to survive even if care delayed hours to days
Priority V (None)	Black	X‡	Dead

From Auf der Heide E. Disaster response: principles of preparation and coordination. St Louis: Mosby; 1989. Full-text online edition available at the CDC website through the following hyperlink: http://216.202.128.19/dr/DisasterResponse.nsf/section/chapters?openview&home=flash

*Simple: care that does not require unusual equipment or excessive use of time or personnel.

†Assigned THIRD priority (after YELLOWS) when there are so many casualties that if resources are used in vain to try to save BLUE cases, the YELLOWS will needlessly die.

‡The circling of this symbol prevents its being confused with a sloppily written Y.

disruption, and require special attention during public health preparedness. General features that should alert healthcare providers to the possibility of a bioterrorism-related outbreak include[70]:

1. A rapidly increasing disease incidence (e.g., within hours or days) in a normally healthy population
2. An epidemic curve that rises and falls during a short period of time
3. An unusual increase in the number of people seeking care, especially with fever or respiratory or gastrointestinal complaints
4. An endemic disease rapidly emerging at an uncharacteristic time or in an unusual pattern
5. Lower attack rates among people who had been indoors, especially in areas with filtered air or closed ventilation systems, compared with people who had been outdoors
6. Clusters of patients arriving from a single locale and large numbers of rapidly fatal cases
7. Any patient presenting with a disease that is relatively uncommon and has bioterrorism potential (e.g., pulmonary anthrax, tularemia, plague)

The main steps involved in management of a bioterrorist attack are containment, notification, confirmation, and directed antibiotic treatment and prophylaxis. In the event of a suspected bioterrorist attack, the CDC has issued protocols for early notification of local and state public health department agencies.[71] The Association for Professionals in Infection Control and Epidemiology in cooperation with the CDC devised the "Bioterrorism Readiness Plan," with a template for healthcare facilities to serve as a reference document to facilitate preparation of bioterrorism readiness plans for healthcare facilities. This tool guides infection-control professionals and healthcare epidemiologists in the development of practical and realistic response plans for their institutions in the event of a bioterrorism attack.[72] Discussion of individual biological agents is beyond the scope of this chapter. The reader is referred to our review of bioterrorism and critical care,[73,74] as well as the numerous resources and websites available on the Internet (Box 226-1).

Chemical Weapons

Chemical incidents are accidental or intentional events that threaten or do expose responders and members of the public to a chemical hazard. Agents that have been commonly used as chemical weapons are also used in industrial processes. Most industrial incidents occur at an interface between transport, storage, processing, use, or disposal of hazardous chemicals, where these systems are more vulnerable to failure, error, or manipulation. The catastrophic effect of these agents has been utilized several times in the past for military purposes, and with the proliferation of these weapons, civilian populations are now faced with a significant threat.[75] Typically, chemical warfare agents are classified into the following categories[76]:

Nerve agents (e.g., tabun, sarin, VX, soman) are organophosphates that inhibit the enzyme, anticholinesterase, resulting in overstimulation of both muscarinic and nicotinic receptors. Muscarinic symptoms include lacrimation, bronchorrhea, bronchospasm, miosis, salivation, rhinorrhea, vomiting, and diarrhea. Nicotinic receptor stimulation produces muscle fasciculations, flaccid paralysis, tachycardia, and hypertension. These agents are also capable of producing central nervous system effects (i.e., seizures, coma). Death from these agents is usually from respiratory failure. These agents are extremely toxic and have a rapid effect. Sarin presents as a vapor threat, and the onset of symptoms is within seconds, with a peak effect in 5 minutes. Exposed victims who are asymptomatic after 1 hour are unlikely to be contaminated. VX represents a liquid exposure, with as little as a drop being lethal. The onset to action and death is less than 30 minutes. The cardinal rule in decontaminating patients is to remove and dispose of all articles of clothing. Therapy is directed toward the predominating symptoms. Atropine is used for the relief of muscarinic symptoms, pralidoxime chloride (2-PAM) is used for nicotinic effects, and benzodiazepines are used for the central nervous system manifestations. Most of the care is supportive and includes mechanical ventilation for respiratory failure and treatment of arrhythmias.[77]

Vesicants (e.g., mustard gas, lewisite) cause wounds on the skin and mucosal surfaces. They are capable of causing second-degree burns of the skin within 4 to 8 hours. Airway injury and edema can be severe and are dose dependent. Of concern to the ICU physician is the need for correcting fluid losses and maintaining the airway.

Pulmonary agents (e.g., chlorine gas, phosgene gas) mainly affect the respiratory system, inducing inflammation of the airway and the lung and leading to ARDS and death. Treatment is mainly supportive.

Cyanides bind to cytochromes within the mitochondria and inhibit cellular oxygen use. In smaller doses they cause tachypnea, headache, dizziness, anxiety, and vomiting. However, with higher doses, seizures, respiratory arrest, and cardiac arrest occur. They are highly toxic and in sufficient concentrations can cause death within 5 minutes of inhalation. They are most commonly inhaled but also can be absorbed through the skin. Care for the patient is primarily supportive with supplemental oxygen. Specific therapy is with amyl nitrates, sodium nitrite, and sodium thiosulfate.

In general, unlike biological weapons, disease secondary to release of chemical agents is likely to be more obvious, rapid in onset, and homogeneous. These agents, however, pose serious problems for emergency care providers because of their potential to cause a large number of casualties rapidly and their potential for secondary contamination. Any emergency medical or public health response to a major incident involving a chemical warfare agent will require coordination among local, state, and federal organizations. First responders should be aware of access to specialized local and federal response teams, basic triage, and demarcation of the contaminated area, use of handheld devices for agent detection and identification, use of personal protective equipment, and knowledge of appropriate medical treatment and antidotes.

Nuclear Weapons and Radiation Accidents

A variety of terrorist applications of radiation exist that could produce varying degrees of damage to public infrastructure and operations, human casualties and illnesses, and most importantly, fear.

Radiation devices include radionuclides from the healthcare industries (e.g., brachytherapy, radiation oncology sources). The consequences of the exposure are dose and source dependent.

Radionuclide dispersal devices are also known as *dirty bombs*. These have limited nuclear yield but can contaminate a wide area.

Improvised nuclear devices are made of uranium or plutonium constructed by a nongovernmental source and limited by the critical mass of nuclear material. They yield less destructive power than a conventional nuclear warhead but are still capable of contamination effects.

Tactical and strategic nuclear weapons are those that are created by governments and vary in yields from 0.5 kiloton to greater than 1 megaton. Their destructive capacities are enormous, and they contaminate a vast perimeter of space depending on the yield.

Approximately 50% of the energy released from a nuclear bomb is due to the blast and shock waves, giving a majority of the survivors blast-related injuries as well as creating extensive infrastructure damage. About 35% of the energy released is thermal radiation (in orders of tens of millions of degrees), giving rise to high-degree skin burns. Depending on the size of the device and the altitude of detonation, an electromagnetic pulse is generated with the explosion. This is capable of disrupting all electrical equipment within 20 to several hundreds of kilometers.[78] The radiation-related energy released from a nuclear detonation is around 15% (5% from the initial nuclear radiation and 10% from the residual nuclear radiation), giving rise to external contamination, systemic irradiation, and internal contamination-related illness. Immediate ionizing radiation consists of gamma, beta, neutron, and a small amount of alpha radiation. Residual radiation occurs in the forms of induced radiation and fallout. Induced radiation occurs because of neutron-induced gamma activity of the immediate soil, silicon, manganese, aluminum, zinc, copper, and sodium. The half-lives of the various substances are a few minutes to 15 hours. "Fallout" is the fusion of the various radionuclides generated in the fission reaction with condensation, producing a snowflake-like debris that falls to earth. Fallout is a potential form of delayed radiation exposure and can cause internal contamination.[78]

Surviving hospitals and staff near an impact area should serve as a triage center and transport victims to unaffected centers elsewhere through notification of the National Disaster Medical System Hospital Activation System.[79] Other agencies that have to be notified include the Federal Bureau of Investigation, Nuclear Regulatory Commission, Department of Energy, and the Department of Defense. Large-scale decontamination should be managed outside the hospital area as far as is possible, but plans for indoor decontamination should also be in place. A radiation emergency area (both in and out of the hospital) should to be designated, with checkpoints nearing the cold zone. Management plans for the safe disposal of human waste and bodies should be in place so as not to increase the exposure risk. Triage of patients should be done on the basis of doing the greatest good for the greatest number. Based on predictive models, isolated irradiation, burns, and blast-related injuries would constitute 40% of injuries. Combined injuries would account for the rest. Attending to trauma victims should take precedence over all other medical issues, because a given patient is not likely to succumb immediately from radiation injury.

Patient care should begin with the use of universal precautions and personal protective equipment.[78] Dosimetry readings of the area may help during triage, defining those with systemic irradiation injury (possibly received greater than 450 rad exposure). In determining patient viability, three parameters are of the most use: time of onset of vomiting, the decrease in the absolute lymphocyte count over a 24-hour period, and presence of conventional trauma burns.[80] Victims who are not viable or who have lethal doses of radiation exposure are likely to benefit from supportive/palliative care.

Hazardous Materials Disasters

A hazardous material (HazMat) is a substance potentially toxic to the environment or living organisms. Full-scale disasters from HazMat are relatively rare, but isolated incidents are among the most common in the community and are not limited to chemicals but can include various biological and radiologic materials as well. Knowledge of the types of industries present in the community would be helpful in developing a potential plan to deal with likely HazMat situations. Management of a HazMat situation requires attention to several key points:

identification of the offending agent, appropriate personal protection equipment of responders, prompt containment of the agent, demarcating areas for decontamination (including removal and disposal of clothes and waste from the decontamination), and resuscitation of victims. Injuries secondary to release of hazardous materials can present as chemical burns, inhalational injury, and a variety of systemic injuries.[81-82]

Armed Conflict

Armed conflict continues to be the most preventable and most destructive of manmade disasters in terms of human physical and emotional suffering, economic loss, and environmental destruction. Specific healthcare issues during these conflicts that are relevant to the intensivist include trauma from blast injuries, projectiles, and crush-related injuries; communicable diseases due to the breakdown of public infrastructure and mass displacement of populations; and burns and radiation-related injury.

Medical Disaster Syndromes

Disaster situations present with many unique medical syndromes that require specific therapy. Treatment of these entities is often difficult owing to a large volume of patients, lack of qualified medical personnel on site, and inadequate supplies and equipment. It is important to emphasize that initial recognition of the medical syndromes and appropriate intervention are critical to minimizing morbidity and mortality. Appropriate triage, knowledge of field management of each syndrome, flexibility to adapt to each situation, ability to ignore natural differences among different specialties, and recognition of limits of medical care that can be provided in overwhelming situations are key to a good disaster medical response. In the following paragraphs, we discuss commonly encountered medical syndromes in a disaster situation.

BLAST INJURIES

Bombs contain an array of compounds such as nitroglycerin, trinitrotoluene, and others that are encased in a metal or plastic case. Decomposition of the solid or liquid compound into gas leads to massive dissipation of energy and pressure creating a blast wave (shock wave). This destructive effect can be increased by the presence of nuts, nails, and bolts in the casing. Water transmits blast waves more efficiently than air, with the greatest impact being on structures that are the deepest.[83] There are four types of blast injuries:

1. *Primary blast injury* is caused solely by the blast wave and almost always affects air-filled structures such as the lung, ear, and gastrointestinal tract. The presence of tympanic membrane rupture may indicate exposure to a high-pressure wave and is thought to correlate with more severe organ injury.
2. *Secondary blast injury* is caused by the rapid acceleration of small fragments caused by the blast injury.
3. *Tertiary blast injury* is a feature of high-energy explosions. They result from the collision of the flying victim against a hard surface.
4. *Miscellaneous blast-related injuries* encompass all other injuries caused by explosions. They include flash burns, inhalation injuries, and blunt trauma.

The most common injuries associated with fatality in blast incidents include subarachnoid hemorrhage (66%), fracture of the skull (51%), lung contusion (47%), tympanic membrane rupture (45%), and liver laceration (34%). Unfortunately, the extent of the blast injury cannot be assessed during the course of rapid triage examinations. In the absence of overt trauma, a focused physical examination should include examination for ruptured tympanic membrane, hypopharyngeal contusions, hemoptysis, and auscultation for wheezing. The presence of a ruptured tympanic membrane is almost always an indicator that the patient has been exposed to a blast wave powerful enough to cause serious damage. The thorax is frequently involved in a blast injury, manifesting with wheezing, hemoptysis, pneumothorax, hemothorax, and air embolism. Patients may have myocardial contusion as well. The presentation of serious pulmonary injury may be delayed. Pulmonary barotrauma is the most common fatal primary blast injury. Patients with nonpenetrating lung injury will likely have hypoxia requiring support ranging from oxygen therapy to mechanical ventilation. This may result from pulmonary contusion, systemic air embolism, and disseminated intravascular coagulation. Acute gas embolism, a form of pulmonary barotrauma, is also associated with blast injuries. Air emboli most commonly occlude blood vessels in the brain or spinal cord, resulting in neurologic symptoms that must be differentiated from the direct effect of trauma. Patients thought to have gas embolism require decompression treatment. Administration of 100% oxygen by tight-fitting facemask and left lateral recumbent position may help. Definitive treatment is with the use of hyperbaric oxygen. Patients with blast injury of the lung are likely to present with abdominal injuries that are usually more delayed. These include delayed bowel perforation and liver lacerations. The former may warrant exploratory laparotomy.[84-87]

Blast victims receiving general anesthesia have an increased mortality rate; other forms of local and spinal anesthesia are preferred, and general anesthesia should be deferred if possible for 24 to 48 hours. Intensivists should be aware of the increased need for resuscitation equipment, ventilators, and movement in and out of the operating room during such situations.

All patients with significant burns, suspected air embolism, radiation or white phosphorus contamination, abdominal signs of contusion/hematoma, or clinical evidence of pulmonary contusion or pneumothorax should be admitted to the hospital. Patients with tympanic membrane rupture and suspected pneumothorax should get some form of chest imaging, and a significant observation period may be warranted. Other investigations must be judiciously ordered, keeping in mind the limited availability of resources in a mass-casualty incident. Screening urinalysis for presence of hematuria, tests for CO poisoning (explosion in a closed space or associated with fire) and cyanide toxicity (due to combustion of plastics), and assessment of acid-base status may be indicated. Use of abdominal computed tomography to rule out intestinal hematomas is not routinely warranted and should be dictated by clinical signs and symptoms. Pregnant patients with blast injuries warrant special consideration, and appropriate consultation is necessary to rule out blast injury to the fetus.[85] Supplemental oxygen therapy, maintaining spontaneous respiration, and low PEEP (if mechanical ventilation is required) are some of the guiding principles in managing pulmonary blast injuries. Routine corticosteroids and antibiotics are not warranted. Exposure to white phosphorus explosives (e.g., in hand grenades) deserves special mention. Use of a Wood's light in a darkened resuscitation suite or operating room may help identify white phosphorus light particles in the wound. White phosphorus injury can cause lung injury through irritation, as well as severe hypokalemia and hyperphosphatemia with cardiac arrhythmias and death. External burns should be lavaged with 1% copper sulfate solution. This forms a blue-black cupric phosphide coating and prevents combustion so that the particles can safely be removed.[88]

CRUSH INJURY SYNDROME

Crush injury syndrome refers to systemic manifestations of extensive muscle damage caused by entrapment of victims under collapsed buildings or debris. Reported incidence depends on the type of disaster, ranging from 2% to 40%. Metabolic alterations from the release of muscle constituents into the circulation include myoglobinemia leading to acute renal failure, hyperkalemia, hyperphosphatemia, and disseminated intravascular coagulation. Increased intracellular calcium concentrations appear to be the final common pathway. Muscle damage that occurs is due not only to direct crush injury but also to vascular injury and insufficiency leading to altered compartment pressures and reperfusion injury. Inelastic fascial sheaths encase skeletal muscles in the forearm and lower leg and are particularly vulnerable to dramatic increases in compartment pressures, resulting in compartment syndrome. An intracompartmental pressure in excess of 40 mm Hg lasting longer than 8 hours defines this syndrome. Pressures as high as 240 mm Hg can be seen with crush injuries. Compartment syndromes are seen with limb fractures, use of military antishock trousers, pneumatic splints, vascular injuries, and crush injuries. The affected limb may present with severe pain associated with passive stretch or extension, flaccid paralysis, and sensory loss. Capillary refill and peripheral pulses are usually present unless the compartmental pressure equals the diastolic pressure. Diagnosis requires a high degree of clinical suspicion and entails prompt bedside measurement of compartmental pressures. A simple and easy method that can be performed in the hospital or field hospital is using an 18-gauge needle attached to a mercury manometer. In an ICU, pressure transducers used to measure central venous pressures can be attached to the 18-gauge needle to obtain the same information.[89]

Resuscitation of patients with crush injury (any victim crushed or immobilized for more than 4 hours) should begin in the field. After adequate intravenous access is achieved, isotonic fluid replacement with normal saline (rate of 1-1.5 L/h) should begin even before extrication of the crushed limb. If fluid therapy is delayed, the incidence of renal failure increases to 50%; delays of 12 hours are associated with a 100% incidence. Occurrence of renal failure is associated with a 20% to 40% mortality rate. Urinary alkalinization with sodium bicarbonate and mannitol or acetazolamide administration are used to maintain urine pH greater than 7.5. Although this intervention is widely used, there are no prospective randomized controlled trials to support it. Dialysis may be indicated if aggressive fluid resuscitation fails, and this may create a huge demand for dialysis machines in disaster situations. Peritoneal dialysis if the abdomen is intact and continuous arteriovenous hemofiltration may be other useful options. The latter option, however, is complicated by hemorrhagic problems related to the use of heparin and immobilization. Life-threatening infections are common after crush injuries and may be increased in the presence of a fasciotomy. In unsalvageable limbs, it may be advisable to perform on-field amputations to avoid the systemic effects of a crush injury syndrome. For this purpose, ketamine is the anesthetic and analgesic of choice because of its safety profile in the field.[89]

PARTICULATE HEALTH PROBLEMS

Many disasters result in release of copious particulate matter, causing a wide spectrum of respiratory illnesses including cough, wheezing, smoke inhalation injury, reactive airways disease, and ARDS. Volcanic eruptions with associated pyroclastic flows and ash fall are some of the most devastating producers of particulate matter. Mortality in these situations arises from suffocation by ash in the upper airways, ARDS, and inhalation burns. The massive building collapse and fires associated with the 2001 World Trade Center terrorist attack caused significant pulmonary complaints among rescue personnel.[90]

Smoke inhalation injury resulting from exposure to noxious products of combustion in fires may account for as many as 75% of fire-related deaths in the United States. The three primary mechanisms that lead to injury in smoke inhalation are thermal damage, asphyxiation, and pulmonary irritation. Combustion utilizes oxygen in the airways and causes a decrease in fraction of inspired oxygen, leading to hypoxemia. Increased CO levels decrease the oxygen-carrying capacity of the blood and cause myocardial depression. Combustion of plastics, polyurethane, wool, silk, nylon, rubber, and paper products can lead to the production of cyanide gas, resulting in anaerobic metabolism and decreased oxygen consumption. Rarely, we may also find methemoglobinemia, which reduces oxygen-carrying capacity.[91]

Mortality rate with smoke inhalation alone is about 10% but increases to about 77% in the presence of major burns or respiratory failure. Early deaths are mostly caused by airway compromise or metabolic poisoning. Laboratory workup should include co-oximetry; CO, methemoglobin, and cyanide levels (if there is discordance in measured saturation and pulse oximetry readings); blood lactate levels (a level greater than 10 mmol/L that is refractory to restoration of adequate ventilation, oxygenation, and perfusion is considered a surrogate marker of cyanide toxicity) on blood gases; and a calculated alveolar-arterial pressure gradient. Initial blood gas measurements and chest radiograph may be normal. Carboxyhemoglobin level obtained in the emergency department does not correlate with tissue hypoxia or long-term neurologic sequelae; ideally, a carboxyhemoglobin level at the scene would be most valuable.

Serial bronchoscopy is indicated in the first 18 to 24 hours to assess airway edema and sloughing. Early bronchoscopy can be of diagnostic and therapeutic value, particularly when lobar atelectasis is present. High-flow humidified oxygen is critical to reverse or prevent hypoxemia. About 50% of patients with an inhalation injury require tracheal intubation, and this number increases in patients who have burn injuries. The need for tracheal intubation is determined by the need to maintain airway patency and pulmonary toilet and to provide positive-pressure ventilation. Positive-pressure ventilation with PEEP increases short-term survival and is associated with decreased tracheobronchial cast formation. Cyanide toxicity (levels > 0.1 mg/L) should be promptly treated using a USA cyanide kit. Recommendations for the use of hyperbaric oxygen in the setting of CO poisoning include CO levels greater than 25% to 30%, neurologic compromise, metabolic acidosis, or electrocardiographic evidence of myocardial ischemia, infarction, or dysrhythmias. Hyperbaric oxygen has been used in cyanide toxicity but has not been proven effective. The role of corticosteroids is controversial, and they can be detrimental if given in the presence of cutaneous burns. Empirically administered antibiotics are another issue in dispute. Common pitfalls in the initial management of smoke inhalation are using initial Pao_2 to predict adequacy of oxygenation, placing small-diameter nasotracheal tubes, intubating without applying PEEP, and restricting fluids for concomitant inhalation and burn injury.[91,92] General measures that could be employed in a field setting include simple airway protection by clearing any particulate matter in the airway, supplemental oxygen, and nebulizer treatment if available. Patients with preexisting asthma and emphysema should be observed for exacerbations.

ACUTE RADIATION SYNDROME

Ionizing radiation can be either charged or uncharged particles (photons). Beta particles are capable of penetrating a few centimeters of tissue. Gamma rays and x-rays are capable of penetrating through tissue and concrete. Gamma, x-ray, and beta radiations are considered low linear energy transfer radiation. Alpha particles have no penetrating power past the keratinized layer of skin, but they take on clinical significance if they are internalized by ingestion or inhalation. Neutron emission (e.g., from nuclear reactors, nuclear devices, and industrial moisture detectors) is highly potent radiation that penetrates deep and creates denser ionization trails. Alpha and neutron emissions are considered high linear energy transfer radiation and have significantly more biological effects than low linear energy transfer radiation by a factor of up to 20. When the process of ionization occurs within living tissue it causes breakage in the chemical bonds, and the most susceptible target is the cellular DNA. This leads to impaired mitosis and subsequent organ failure. Large doses of radiation are generally considered to cause more biological destruction than fractionated doses. Systemic radiation illness and lethality from it can result from as little as 450 rad. Precise measurements of the amount of radiation following a nuclear accident will be delayed. Hospital gamma cameras are an invaluable resource for helping determine the exposure in an individual. Higher systemic doses are suggested by shorter onset of prodromal symptoms such as nausea, vomiting, and diarrhea. Serial absolute lymphocyte counts will screen those patients who have psychogenic vomiting. Acute radiation syndrome has four distinct phases[67,78,80]:

1. *Prodromal phase*, characterized by nausea, vomiting, and diarrhea. Other symptoms of eye burning, abdominal pain, and fever

can also occur with higher doses. This phase may last from 0 to 2 days, depending on the dose received.

2. *Latent phase*, in which the patient will have a period of relative well-being due to subsidence of the inflammation. However, ultimately the damaged cells will not be able to repair or regenerate. This may last for 2 to 3 weeks.

3. *Manifest phase*, in which the cellular deficits of various organs affected will become apparent. Mature cells of the skin slough off, revealing an atrophic dermis. Endothelial cells are not replaced, leading to vascular permeability. Mucosal linings slough, causing mucositis and diarrhea. Hematopoietic progenitor cells fail to produce cell lines, leading to anemia, thrombocytopenia, and neutropenia. Fibrosis of the various organ beds develops. This may last for up to 3 weeks.

4. *Recovery phase/death*, in which some stem cells may proliferate and lead to a slow recovery, or there will be symptoms of progressive organ failure leading to death.

For radiation syndrome to occur, radiation must be of the penetrating type in a sufficiently large dose (>0.7 Gy), must be external, and must occur within a short time period. The disease complex has three syndromes: bone marrow, gastrointestinal, and cardiovascular/central nervous system. Serial absolute lymphocyte counts should be measured immediately on suspicion of exposure (every 3 hours), because lymphocytes are among the most radiosensitive cells and reach nadir within 2 days; platelets reach nadir in 15 to 30 days; and neutrophils at about 30 days. Patients are immunocompromised and susceptible to a wide variety of infections, that of most concern to the intensivist being septic shock. Gastrointestinal syndrome leads to mucosal sloughing, decreased nutrient absorption, and translocation of bacteria and endotoxin. Veno-occlusive disease may also develop if the dose is large enough. Cardiovascular and central nervous system disease develop with doses greater than 5000 rad, and death can occur in as little as 3 days from myocarditis, capillary leak, pulmonary edema, and brain edema. Pneumonitis and subsequent fibrosis can lead to respiratory failure and the need for ventilator support. Treatment of ARS is mainly supportive. If internal contamination is thought to have occurred, enhancement of excretion and specific antidote therapy are warranted. For inhalational contamination, bronchoalveolar lavage may be necessary; and for ingestion, gastric lavage and purgative management are warranted. Plutonium and transuranic elements can be treated with chelating agents such as calcium or zinc diethylenetriamine pentaacetic acid. Radiocesium can be treated with Prussian blue, which helps enhance excretion in feces. Radioiodine exposure can be treated with potassium iodide. Uranium excretion can be enhanced by the alkalinization of urine and with potassium supplementation.

PSYCHOLOGICAL TRAUMA

The psychological component in a traumatic event is often overlooked, with the major focus usually being on physical health issues. Studies evaluating the emotional impact from disasters indicate that a majority of victims, first responders, and mortuary volunteers will suffer some form of psychological trauma. Intensivists should be aware that behavioral changes may not be only due to the catastrophic insult but also due to organic causes such as head injury, inability to take predisaster psychiatric medications, and toxin or chemical exposure. Groups at risk, such as children, adolescents, and victims who have been exposed to traumatic stressors of bereavement, witnessing death, and situations evoking guilt, fear, or anger, should receive prompt psychiatric and posttraumatic counseling. Interventions such as debriefing, eye movement desensitization and reprocessing, and critical incident stress management may help minimize emotional suffering and morbidity.[93]

OTHER SYNDROMES

Burns, blunt trauma, intraabdominal injury, head injuries, penetrating trauma, and hypothermia are some of the other disaster syndromes encountered in the field. Specific discussion of these entities is beyond the scope of this chapter, and the reader is referred to other chapters for management details.[5]

Disaster Preparedness

For intensivists to be able to deal with a disaster, it is paramount that they be a part of the disaster-planning effort. Disaster planning includes development of action programs to minimize loss of life and damage during a disaster, provide the greatest good for the greatest number of people, train healthcare personnel and civilians, coordinate response efforts, maintain adequate supplies of equipment and personnel, and rehabilitate the community after the disaster. Knowledge of potential disasters to which the community is prone should be an integral part of the planning process. Having an understanding of what the resources and capabilities are of the community, hospital, and its ICU on a continual basis and provision for modular expandability are vital for any successful emergency response. The mere existence of a disaster plan does not ensure that the hospital system is actually prepared.[94] The following paragraphs elucidate some of the common issues and misconceptions related to disasters and common principles useful in designing a disaster plan. Subsequently, a pragmatic view is presented of the role of the ICU physician in a disaster situation.

COMMON ISSUES AND MISCONCEPTIONS IN DISASTER PLANNING

Typically, the hospital nearest to the disaster site will receive the bulk of the casualties. It is thus important to conduct a careful survey of a disaster plan's jurisdiction to identify potential sites (i.e., industries, nuclear reactors, highways) and likely types of hazardous events that could occur in the area. Hospitals in the nearby area receive few disaster victims, and an average have at least 20% of their beds vacant. Disaster plans would thus need to include transfer agreements between hospitals and nearby ICUs to meet bed shortages by activating the National Disaster Medical System Hospital Activation System.[79,94,95]

Very few casualties actually require hospital admission. A study of 29 mass-casualty incidents found that less than 10% of casualties required overnight admission under usual criteria (even though more were admitted because they were involved in the disaster rather than because of severity of their condition). Large numbers of casualties with minor conditions will appear at the nearest hospitals, often on foot or in private vehicles, police cars, buses, taxis, and other non-ambulance forms of transport. Field triage stations are often bypassed, and this in turn causes enormous strain on the emergency department services.[96]

Most of the logistical problems faced in disaster situations are not caused by shortages of medical resources but rather from failure to coordinate their distribution.[94] Inexperienced volunteers may not be familiar with the triage system or principles of personal safety, and massive numbers of volunteers can present serious administrative challenges. This results in disorganization and inefficiency.[81] Technical hazard sheets designed by the WHO for most disasters also suggest that medical personnel, blood donors, and blood products should not be sent empirically to a disaster site.[97]

PRINCIPLES IN DISASTER PLANNING

Existing Preparedness Requirements

In developing disaster plans, hospitals must take into account the broad national and local requirements imposed by various governmental agencies. Common agencies involved in this process include the Centers for Medicare and Medicaid Services (CMS) as well as The Joint Commission (TJC). The CMS's conditions for emergency preparedness and services establish minimum requirements for hospitals that participate in Medicare or Medicaid programs. Similarly, TJC standards apply to a full range of hospitals from small rural to large urban academic centers and are focused on four main areas: (1)

emergency preparedness management plan (Standard EC 4.1), (2) security management plan (Standard EC 2.1), (3) hazardous materials and waste management plan (Standard EC 3.1), and (4) emergency preparedness drills (Standard EC 4.2). Readers are referred to the TJC website for the most up-to-date standards for management of environment of care.[98]

Hazard Vulnerability Analysis

This is the first step of any disaster plan, with the main aim of identifying potential hazardous events and situations that can occur in or around the healthcare facility. This process of evaluating and predicting hazard risk is not restricted to geographic events but extends to institution-specific variables such as utility failures, local threats of gang-related activity, and presence of a local high-risk industry such as a chemical or nuclear power plant. TJC requires a formal documented hazard vulnerability analysis that is integrated with the emergency management plan, setting priorities among potential emergencies and also defining the hospital's role in the local community-wide emergency plan.[98]

Incident Command System

The Incident Command System (ICS) is designed to provide the basic architecture of an emergency management response. Major barriers to medical response arise from the lack of coordination among various public and healthcare agencies and from the lack of operational integration of various medical specialties. The ICS incorporates all these agencies and ensures a cooperative and effective response to a crisis. The concept of ICS resulted from the analysis of the devastating wildfires in Southern California in 1970 and has since been modified and successfully adapted to different disaster situations related to healthcare facilities.[84-86] The ICS specifies a common terminology and a command structure with five functional sections:

1. *Command:* unified command staff responsible for overall management of the incident
2. *Operations:* performs the actual response work under the directives of the command center
3. *Planning:* gathers relevant information and develops response strategies as the situation progresses
4. *Logistics:* responsible for facility-wide supplies, equipment, personnel, and services. It also provides for basic services to personnel of the command center.
5. *Finance:* authorizes expenditures, maintains records, and provides documentation of the incident

There is a designated person who will have the authority to declare an emergency. All personnel involved in the command system should be aware of the exact predetermined location of the command center. The plan should also provide protocols that will guide notification and the sequence of mobilization of these personnel in a disaster situation. The command system must also have independent telephone lines to ensure uninterrupted communication with the external world in a disaster situation. Once initiated, the ICS has a built-in chain of command that would be responsible for triage of patients and allocation of personnel and resources.[99]

Triage

Appropriate triage is a vital function during an emergency management response. This is a dynamic process that is not necessarily confined to the disaster site or the emergency department but rather is carried through several levels of the medical response pathway of a disaster response. Modern triage is based on the likelihood of survival in relation to the resources available at the time of the decision.[100] Problems commonly encountered in the triage process include[101]:

1. Lack of medical direction at the scene. Making triage decisions in a chaotic situation requires skill and experience and can often initially seem confusing and unmanageable. Lessons from the first Persian Gulf War showed that on-field triage was correct only 70% of the time. It is necessary to entrust experienced physicians with this job and to have simple and clear guidelines for the

decision-making process. In addition to emergency physicians and trauma surgeons, critical care physicians bring with them the expertise to deal with complex and time-bound situations and are thus well suited to head a triage team.

2. Lack of interorganizational planning. Dynamic management of the triage process requires interorganizational coordination and flow of information. Up-to-date assessment of medical resources and personnel should be communicated from the command center to the triage site, and similar communication should occur from the scene to the command center. This will allow for rational and appropriate triage based on the availability of resources.
3. Transport of victims from the site by nonambulance vehicles to nearby hospitals.
4. There is no single universally accepted form of triage. A recommended internationally accepted system has been promulgated by Christian et al. in Canada, using a color-coded system to sort out victims in a disaster setting.[100]

Major Utilities, Supplies, and Equipment

Disaster plans and drills should factor in the possibility of internal and external power outages and related disruptions (ventilator and monitoring device failures, communication failures including breakdown of cellular phones, and elevator failures) and water supply and gas supply shortages. The plan should have an up-to-date inventory of all supplies and capabilities of the facility. Number of ventilators in use and its absolute capacity, inventory of various ICU supplies, and vendor lists should be readily available if there is sudden demand for supplies. The disaster plan should allow for at least 2 days' worth of supplies. Regular drills will help identify various bottlenecks and will also provide knowledge of the absolute capacity of devices, equipment, and services in a disaster situation. Plans to evacuate critically ill patients to nearby hospitals in the event of failure of backup systems should also be addressed in the process. Since the anthrax attacks and the resulting strain on antibiotic supplies in 2001, more attention has been paid to the national repository of lifesaving pharmaceuticals and medical supplies called the *National Pharmaceutical Stockpile Program*. This response is a component of the CDC's larger Bioterrorism Preparedness and Response Initiative and is composed of a stockpile of pharmaceuticals, vaccines, medical supplies, and equipment to augment local and state resources in a disaster situation. After a federal decision to deploy, a "push package" will arrive by ground or air in 12 hours or less at any location in the United States. A CDC team accompanying the push package will then determine the amount and type of shipments in the second phase.[102]

Security and Casualty Reception

Security is a major concern during natural or manmade disasters. Desire to seek immediate medical evaluation, panic, and curiosity are some of the forces that place the healthcare facility and its personnel under enormous strain. Internal and external traffic control, protection of personnel who are involved in the response effort, and strict enforcement of staging and triage areas are key security-related issues. Law enforcement plays a more critical role during terrorist attacks or during bioterrorism, and failure to maintain order will lead to rapid overwhelming of the facility's resources and a disorganized medical response. Because most of the victims will arrive at the hospital by foot or by personal vehicles, provision must be made for a predetermined staging area with adequate mass decontamination facilities and respiratory protective equipment.[98,103]

Issues Unique to the Intensive Care Unit

The responsibility of caring for the most serious salvageable casualties in natural and manmade disasters will ultimately involve the critical care physician. As opposed to overwhelming shortage of resources, lack of coordination among various agencies and specialties has been often cited as the main contributing factor to an ineffective emergency medical response. This response therefore requires the cooperation of not just physicians but also between prehospital medical personnel, nurses, and ancillary services such as radiology and laboratory services.[53]

Possible roles for the intensivist as part of a disaster management planning team include:

1. Clear role definition and understanding of the overall organization of the emergency response plan.
2. Knowledge of the usual limit, surge capacity, and absolute limit of ICU resources.
3. Construction of appropriate staffing models.

Critical Care in Unconventional Situations

MOBILE ICU TEAMS

There have been numerous examples in medical literature describing extended critical care through mobile ICU teams. The use of mobile ICU teams has not been restricted to disaster settings but has also been used throughout the world during peacetime. Various factors that have to be considered in the formation of ICU teams are discussed next.

Personnel

Based on the anticipated needs of the disaster, appropriate specialists and ancillary personnel are chosen. Given the complexity and inherent unpredictability of staffing for disaster management, a flexible and adaptable approach must be taken to staffing such events.[104]

Training

Adequate predeparture training is essential for a coordinated and effective response. In addition, interaction and on-site training ensures effective functioning of a foreign medical unit and allows for the smooth transition of care to local physicians when the foreign team departs.[84]

Casualty Assessment

Studies from the past and more recently the experience of the Israeli defense forces in providing care to earthquake victims in Turkey showed that the effectiveness of mobile ICU teams was limited by time. It sometimes takes 3 days to mobilize such an effort, and crucial time is lost before delivery of intended care. Efforts must therefore be made to epidemiologically assess the efficacy of such teams. They should include review of the overall effort and adequacy of the ICU teams, outcome of victims, operational costs, and analysis of the structure and process of the ICU in the field.[104]

Critical Care Transport

Common principles involved in the safe transport of patients include[104]:

1. Rapid assessment of the severity of injuries, recognition of the need for transport, and anticipation of problems during transport
2. Safe movement of patients in and out of vehicles, continuous monitoring of vital signs, and recognition and treatment of problems encountered during transport
3. Documentation of the events during transport and provision of a detailed report to the admitting personnel

TYPES OF TRANSPORT

Ground Transport

Ground ambulances have the advantage of rapid deployment, high mobility, and lower cost. However, patients and equipment are subject to significant deceleration and vibration forces. Equipment may vary depending on the size of the ambulance and usually includes blood pressure and electrocardiograph monitors, pulse oximeters, ventilators, and in some cases, modern support devices such as intraaortic balloon pumps.

Air Transport

It is beyond the scope of this chapter to provide a full detailed discussion of fixed-wing or rotary aeromedical transport (the reader is referred to Chapter 225), but it may be necessary during certain disasters to extricate victims via air.[104]

Conclusion

Understanding the characteristics of different disasters, developing an interdisciplinary approach to hazard mitigation, and knowledge of related clinical syndromes are key to an effective medical disaster response. To ensure an integrated and effective response to future disasters, it is necessary for critical care physicians to understand fundamental principles in disaster medicine and participate in the disaster planning process.

KEY POINTS

1. Disaster medicine is a unique specialty that has evolved over the past few years. It shares a common ideal with public health: "greatest good for the greatest number." Critical care medicine forms an indispensable part of this science because intensive care physicians not only care for the sickest of the salvageable patients in any hospital but also bring with them their clinical expertise in triage, resuscitation, and help in providing care outside the domains of the unit through mobile ICU teams.

2. Clear, common, and concise definitions are important in effective communication and evoking appropriate responses to disaster situations. The concept of functional impact of a disaster on the healthcare system is paramount while classifying disasters.

3. It is important to understand the common effects of different natural and manmade disasters to predict their impact on the healthcare system. Even though manmade disasters such as terrorist attacks have gained recent attention, the numbers of geophysical disasters such as earthquakes, floods, and hurricanes have remained fairly constant and place the greatest burden on the healthcare system.

4. Disaster situations produce many unique medical syndromes that require specific therapy. Knowledge and immediate recognition of different medical syndromes with appropriate interventions is critical to minimizing morbidity and mortality.

5. Disaster planning includes developing action programs to minimize loss of life and damage during a disaster, training healthcare personnel and civilians, coordinating response efforts, maintaining adequate supplies of equipment and personnel, and rehabilitating the community after the disaster. Knowledge of potential manmade and natural disasters to which the community is prone should be an integral part of the planning process. Common principles involved in the creation of an emergency response plan should be followed and applied from an ICU perspective.

6. With their natural role of caring for critically ill patients, intensivists bring with them unique abilities that can be applied to a disaster situation: a multidisciplinary approach to patient care, management skills, procedural expertise, and flexible attitudes.

7. Intensivists can also provide care outside the domains of the ICU through mobile ICU teams and transport of critically ill patients. Various factors have to be considered in the formation of such teams and in the safe transport of patients.

ANNOTATED REFERENCES

Auf Der Heide E. Disaster response: principles of preparation and coordination. St Louis: Mosby; 1989.
An excellent resource that includes basic principles and pitfalls in disaster planning and offers valuable assistance to those involved in disaster preparedness, mitigation, and response.

Devereaux AV, Dichter JR, Christian MD, et al. Definitive care for the critically ill during a disaster: a framework for allocation of scarce resources in mass critical care: from a Task Force for Mass Critical Care summit meeting, January 26-27, 2007, Chicago, IL. Chest 2008;133:51S–66S.
A review of various topics including triage, disaster-related injuries, and different disaster syndromes.

Karwa M, Bronzert P, Kvetan V. Bioterrorism and critical care. Crit Care Clin 2003;19:279–313.
A review of bioterrorism.

Rice DH, Kotti G, Beninati W. Clinical review: critical care transport and austere critical care. Crit Care 2008;12:207.
A focused, relevant review on issues germane to critical care transport and mobile ICUs.

Geiling JA, editor. Fundamental disaster management. Mount Prospect, IL: Society of Critical Care Medicine; 2009.
Clinical guide and strategic management tool to address the challenges faced by healthcare providers in times of natural and manmade disasters.

REFERENCES

Access the complete reference list online at http://www.expertconsult.com.

Evidence-Based Critical Care

MARY E. HARTMAN | JOHN A. KELLUM | DEREK C. ANGUS

The practice of critical care, like all fields of medicine, is changing constantly, and the pace of change is ever increasing. Among the many forces for change, the rapid increase in information is one of the most important. Although the majority of practitioners do not engage in research themselves, they are consumers of research information and must therefore understand how research is conducted to apply this information to their patients. Fellowship programs in critical care medicine emphasize education in this area to varying degrees. The traditional approach has been to require fellows to actively participate in a research project, either clinical or basic science. However, there has also been a growing interest in instructing fellows in the methods of clinical epidemiology.[1] The practical application of clinical epidemiology is evidence-based medicine (EBM), which Sackett defines as "the conscientious and judicious use of current best evidence in making decisions about the care of individual patients."[2] The clinical practice of EBM involves integrating this evidence with individual physician expertise and patient preferences so informed, thoughtful medical decisions are made.[3] In this chapter we present the methodology of EBM and its application in critical care medicine.

Asking a Question

The first step in practicing EBM is asking a well-constructed clinical question. To benefit the patient and aid the clinician, clinical questions must be both directly relevant to patients' problems and constructed in a way that guides an efficient literature search to relevant and precise answers. The Centre for Evidence Based Medicine (CEBM) in Oxford, England, provides an excellent description of the four essential elements of an EBM question, summarized in Table 227-1.

Developing a specific, thoughtful question leads to a much more efficient search for the answer. Search results themselves can be used to further refine a question. For example, too many results may indicate the question is too broad, and too few results often necessitate a broader description of the patient population, intervention, or outcome.

Types of Evidence

After the question is formulated, one must consider the type of question being asked. Different types of studies, based on their size, design, and methodology, provide evidence of differing quality and relevance to a research question. For example, is the question about therapy, prevention, etiology, or harm? A randomized controlled trial (RCT) or (better yet) systematic review of RCTs will provide the best evidence for this kind of question. Is the investigator interested in the prevalence of a specific disease or symptom in the general population? If so, a large cohort study will best answer this question.

PRIMARY RESEARCH

Randomized Clinical Trials

Randomized clinical trials, also referred to as *experimental* or *interventional studies*, are the cornerstones of medical evidence. Physicians place considerable faith in the results of randomized control trials.[4,5] This faith is placed with good reason, as randomization remains perhaps the best solution to avoid misinterpreting the effect of a therapy in the presence of confounding variables.[6] When participants are randomly allocated to groups, factors other than the variable of interest (e.g., a new therapy for sepsis) that are likely to affect the outcome of interest are usually distributed equally to both groups. For example, with randomization, the number of patients with underlying comorbidity that may adversely affect outcome should be similar in each study arm, presuming sample size is appropriate. A special advantage of randomization is that this equal distribution will occur for all variables (excluding the intervention) whether these variables are identified by the researcher or not, thus maximizing the ability to determine the effect of the intervention.

However, RCTs are expensive, difficult, and sometimes unethical to conduct, with the consequence that less than 20% of clinical practice is based on the results of RCTs.[7] Moreover, many important questions such as determining the optimal timing of a new therapy or determining the effects of health care practices cannot practically be studied by RCTs.

Observational Studies

The principal alternative approach to the RCT involves observation rather than experimentation. Prior experience has biased us to favor RCTs, but partly in response to the increasing need to answer questions unanswerable by the RCT, the design and execution of observational outcomes studies have become much more sophisticated.

Observational outcomes studies are very powerful tools for addressing many questions that RCTs cannot address, including measuring the effect of harmful substances (e.g., smoking and other carcinogens), organizational structures (e.g., payer status, open versus closed ICUs), or geography (e.g., rural versus urban access to health care). Because of their cost and the regulatory demands on drug and device manufacturers, RCTs are frequently designed as efficacy studies in highly defined patient populations with experienced providers and therefore provide little evidence about effectiveness in the "real" world.[8] Alternatively, observational studies can generate hypotheses about the effectiveness of treatments that can be tested using other research methods.[8] Investigators have also explored the effects of different therapies that are already accepted but used variably in clinical practice.[9]

There are a number of different kinds of observational studies, each designed to address a different type of clinical question. These include case-control, cross-sectional surveys, and cohort studies. *Case-control studies* compare a group of patients with a disease or symptom of interest to a selected control group. They have the advantage of being quick and relatively inexpensive to perform and are often the only feasible study method for very rare disorders or when the lag time between an exposure and the related disease is very long. They can also be conducted with a relatively small number of patients. *Cross-sectional studies* provide a snapshot of a population at one point in time. They can also be conducted inexpensively and in a short time. *Cohort studies* prospectively identify an at-risk group (the inception cohort) and follow them through time, recording exposures and development (or not) of the disease under investigation. Cohort studies have a number of strengths, including the ability to match subjects to controls for some confounders, establish the timing and sequence of events, and standardize eligibility criteria and outcome assessments; they are easier and less expensive to conduct than RCTs.

However, observational studies have several significant limitations. First, the data source must be considered. Observational outcomes studies are often performed on large data sets wherein the data were collected for purposes other than research. This can lead to error owing to either a lack of pertinent information or bias in the information

TABLE 227-1	Four Essential Elements of a Well-Constructed Clinical Question		
Patient or Problem	*Intervention*	*Comparison Intervention (if Necessary)*	*Outcome*
Starting with your patient, ask, "How would I describe a group of patients similar to mine?" Balance precision with brevity.	Ask, "Which main intervention am I considering?" Be specific.	Ask, "What is the main alternative to compare with the intervention?" Again, be specific.	Ask, "What can I hope to accomplish?" or "What could this exposure really affect?"

Focusing clinical questions retrieved from the Centre for Evidence Based Medicine website at http://www.cebm.net/?o=1036.

recorded.[10] Second, one must consider how the authors attempt to control for confounding. The measured effect size of a variable on outcome (e.g., the effect of the pulmonary artery catheter on mortality rate) can be confounded by the distribution of other known and unknown variables. More specifically, case-control studies are subject to recall and selection bias, and the selection of an appropriate control group can be difficult. Cross-sectional studies can only establish association (at most), not causality, and are also subject to recall bias. Cohort studies have a number of limitations, including difficulty in finding appropriate controls and difficulty determining whether the exposure being studied is linked to a hidden confounder, and the requirement of large sample size or long follow-up to sufficiently answer a research question can be timely and expensive.

Case Reports or Case Series

The last form of primary research is the case report or case series. A *case* is a published account of a single or small number of patients and their response to a particular therapeutic intervention. The inability to generalize from a case report makes it the weakest form of clinical evidence available. However, case reports may be the only available or practical information in support of a therapeutic strategy, especially in the case of rare diseases when the evolution of the therapy predates the common use of randomized study designs in medical practice. This is also true for new therapies that have not yet been tested in clinical trials.

Summaries of Primary Research

Another valuable source of information, especially for the busy clinician with limited time for reading and research, is primary research that has already been summarized and evaluated. There are a number of high-quality, peer-reviewed sources of summary information, including those that summarize the results of individual trials and those that combine and summarize the results of multiple trials addressing the same topic. The following is a description of the most common types of literature summaries.

SINGLE-STUDY RESULTS—CRITICALLY APPRAISED TOPICS

Determining which studies provide information useful in the care of patients is largely a question of deciding whether a study is valid and, if so, can its results be applied to the patients in question. One format for appraising individual studies is the critically appraised topic (CAT) format that has been popularized as part of EBM. The purpose of the CAT is to evaluate a given study or set of studies using a standardized approach. Studies that address diagnosis, prognosis, etiology, therapy, and cost-effectiveness all have a separate CAT format.[3] An example is shown in Box 227-1 for studies that address therapy. The CAT format for studies on therapy asks several questions intended to address the issues of validity and clinical utility. Studies that fail to achieve these measures are not generally useful, although studies do not necessarily have to fulfill every criterion, depending on the nature of the topic. For example, a study that examined the effect of walking once a day for the prevention of stroke would not be expected to include a detailed

examination of side effects or a cost-effectiveness analysis. However, a study comparing streptokinase to placebo for treatment of stroke would likely be required to include a detailed examination of side effects and a cost-effectiveness analysis because of the excessive risks and costs associated with such therapy. Similarly, blinding may not always be possible, and the effects of the investigators being unblinded can be minimized by separating them from the clinicians making the treatment decisions or by establishing standard treatment protocols that are applied equally to both the study and control groups. Alternatively, a study would be "fatally flawed" if it failed in terms of randomization or was not analyzed as "intention to treat." There are a number of other useful tools for assessing study design and for quantifying effect size and cost-effectiveness. In general, these are the tools of epidemiology and biostatistics, and their discussion is beyond the scope of this chapter. A basic primer and glossary of terms is included in Table 227-2.

SYSTEMATIC REVIEWS OF MULTIPLE STUDIES

A systematic literature review combines the results of multiple studies through the systematic search, assembly, and appraisal of existing primary research on a given subject. *Meta-analysis* is a type of systematic review that incorporates a quantitative summary of the data, which combines actual data from several small although high-quality studies. Criteria for reviews to be systematic as opposed to narrative (see later) are quite explicit. All systematic reviews should start with a four-part (three-part when applicable) question, as described previously. Both the search criteria and inclusion and exclusion criteria should be predefined. The review should combine only RCTs or discuss how and why it is combining different types of evidence. Additionally, the methods section should provide search terms and key words, thus establishing some degree of reproducibility.

The advantages of systematic reviews are that by pooling many studies, the power to find a true effect is increased. This is particularly important when many well-done but small and inconclusive studies have attempted to answer a particular question. Systematic reviews often represent an exhaustive effort to find all related information in a given area. In this regard, they provide an excellent summary of the literature up to the date of the review.

The disadvantage of systematic reviews is that they are only as good as the studies they include and can only be interpreted if all the criteria just mentioned have been met. Unfortunately, there is considerable variability in the quality and comprehensiveness of available systematic reviews. Much of this dilemma stems from a lack of commonly accepted methodology for conducting and writing systematic reviews. For example, there are no standard exclusion criteria for studies in

---

Box 227-1

CRITICAL APPRAISAL OF THE LITERATURE

Are Results of the Study Valid?
- Correctly randomized?
- Were all the patients accounted for?
- Was follow-up complete?
- Were patients analyzed according to how they were randomized (i.e., intention to treat)?
- Were all people involved in the study blinded?
- Were the groups similar at the start?
- Were the groups treated equally apart from the experimental intervention?

Are Results Clinically Useful?
- How large was the treatment effect?
- How precise was the estimate of the treatment effect?
- Are the patients similar to the "norm"?
- Were all clinically important outcomes considered?
- Was a cost-benefit analysis performed?

Adapted from Sackett DL, Straus SE, Richardson WS et al. Evidence-based medicine: how to practice and teach EBM. London: Harcourt; 2000.

TABLE 227-2	Definitions and Equations

Study Design: The research methodology used. There are basically four categories. From weakest to strongest, these are:
1. Case series
2. Case-control study
3. Cohort study
4. Randomized clinical trial

Two-by-Two Table:

		Disease/Outcome	
		+	−
Test or	+	a	b
Exposure	−	c	d
	Total	a + c	b + d

For Diagnostic Tests

Sensitivity: probability that the test will be (+) when the disease is present. a/a + c
Specificity: probability that the test will be (−) when the disease is absent. d/b + d
Positive predictive value: probability that the disease is present given a (+) test. a/a + b
Negative predictive value: probability that the disease is absent given a (−) test. d/c + d

For Association (with Exposure or Therapy)

Relative risk (RR): estimates the magnitude of an association between exposure and disease (or in the case of therapy, the negative association between treatment and morbid outcome). The relative risk indicates the likelihood of development of disease in the exposed group relative to those who were not exposed (also called *risk ratio*).

$$RR = \frac{\text{Incidence in exposed group}}{\text{Incidence in unexposed group}} = \frac{a/(a+b)}{c/(c+d)}$$

Relative risk reduction (RRR): expressed as a percentage reduction in events in treated versus untreated groups

$$RRR = (1 - [a/(a+b)]/[c/(c+d)]) \times 100\%$$

Odds ratio (OR): for case-control studies, RR cannot be used because participants are selected on the basis of disease, not exposure. The RR can be estimated by the OR, however.

$$OR = \frac{a/c}{b/d} = \frac{ad}{be}$$

Attributable risk (AR): a measure of association that provides information about the absolute effect of the exposure or the excess risk of disease in those exposed compared with those unexposed

$$AR = (\text{Incidence in exposed group}) - (\text{Incidence in unexposed group})$$
$$= [a/(a+b)] - [c/(c+d)]$$

Absolute risk reduction (ARR): a measure of the treatment effect. Note the order is reversed compared with AR.

$$ARR = [c/(c+d)] - [a/(a+b)]$$

Number needed to treat (NNT): the inverse of the ARR:1/ARR

$$NNT = 1/[c/(c+d)] - [a/(a+b)]$$

Biostatistics

Type I error (alpha): a difference between study and control groups is found when in reality there is none. Standard = 5%.
Type II error (beta): no difference between study and control groups is found when in reality there is a difference. Standard = 20%.

Types of Data

Nominal: numbers are arbitrary.
Ordinal: numbers denote rank order only.
Interval: numbers denote units of equal magnitude and rank order.
Parametric: interval data in a normal distribution
Standard deviation (SD): measure of the scatter of data in a normally distributed sample; 95.44% of the data will fall within 2 SD of the mean. SD = square root of the variance.
Standard error of the mean (SE): SE = SD/√n. Used to calculate confidence intervals but not a measure of scatter. Should not be used in place of SD.
Confidence interval (CI): the estimated range of values likely to include the true value for the entire population. The standard is 95%.
Power calculation (1 − β): statistical power is the ability of an experiment to find a significant difference between groups when in fact one exists. (NOTE: As *a* increases, so does power. As *n* is increased, *β* decreases and power increases; that is, the chance of either a type I or type II error is reduced.)
Intention-to-treat analysis: all data are analyzed according to what group the subject was assigned to regardless of what treatment the subject actually received; analyzed as randomized

systematic reviews. Each author establishes the criteria, which the reader must assess to determine the quality and utility of the review to answer his clinical question. In addition, there is publication bias. Popular search techniques to identify studies are inherently limited by the fact that unpublished studies are unaccounted for in any review. Issues such as these have led authors to propose the development and maintenance of study registries where all RCTs are registered irrespective of their publication status.[11] This would enable review of smaller studies and those studies published in journals not listed in cumulative *Index Medicus*, MEDLINE, and other popular databases in systematic reviews.

NARRATIVE REVIEWS OF MULTIPLE STUDIES

The most common system of non–peer-reviewed pooling of study results is the familiar "review" article or collection of reviews. This textbook is an example of the latter. Articles or chapters combine information from several primary articles, sometimes a few hundred, in a way that is digestible by the average reader. Reviews may be focused on recent advances, or they may provide a complete tutorial on a given subject. In either case, in the traditional method known as the *narrative review*, the methodology is the same: an author, presumably someone knowledgeable of the subject matter, reviews the existing literature in some way, formulates an opinion, and disseminates this opinion along with references to support each argument. This approach is also used in the discussion section of most original articles, in which the authors attempt to discuss their findings in the context of the existing literature.

The advantage of narrative reviews is that they provide a detailed qualitative discussion, usually by an expert with years of experience. However, they do have several limitations. The most important of these is that evidence used to support the author's positions is not collected, evaluated, and compared in an organized and reproducible manner. That information is complete or that it is judged in an unbiased manner cannot be assured. Journal articles are often peer reviewed, which provides some limited oversight for completeness and lack of bias, but this is far from perfect. Furthermore, review articles and textbook chapters are not generally subject to vigorous review and therefore may be the least reliable sources of information, particularly current information. For example, by 1988, fifteen studies had been reported on the use of prophylactic lidocaine in acute myocardial infarction. While no single study was definitive, pooled data from the nearly 9000 patients showed that the practice was useless at best. Nonetheless, by 1990 there were still more recommendations for its use than against it appearing in textbooks and review articles.[12]

Appraising Evidence

For a piece of evidence to be useful, it has to be valid, have clinically important findings, and be applicable to the particular patient. Guides for assessment of validity, like that shown in Box 227-1, exist for different types of studies (e.g., therapy, diagnosis, prognosis) and are presented in detail in *Evidence-Based Medicine*.[13] Worksheets to determine whether a study is valid are also available from a number of sources including the Centre for Evidence Based Medicine (www.cebm.net). The importance of findings again depends on the type of study. For studies on therapy, the clinician must decide if there was a true treatment effect and, if so, how large an effect. For studies on diagnosis, the characteristics of a test must be presented, and the clinician must decide if the test characteristics (sensitivity, specificity, positive and negative predictive values) would make the same test useful for current patients. Again, a number of guides exist to help physicians make these decisions. In the last few years, the GRADE (Grades of Recommendation Assessment, Development and Evaluation) Workgroup has proposed a mythology for evidence appraisal

that has been widely adopted.[14] Table 227-3 summarizes the GRADE System. High-grade evidence should, in theory at least, be adopted into clinical practice and forms the basis of guidelines, whereas a more nuanced approach is needed for lesser-quality evidence.

Applying Evidence

The strongest evidence available remains useless until it is effectively applied. Application of EBM can occur directly at the patient level or be implemented on a larger scale through guidelines and protocols. Although bedside decision making has been the traditional focus of EBM, guidelines and protocols are important means to promote the standardization of care at an institutional or regional level.

BEDSIDE DECISION MAKING

The goal of EBM is to facilitate bedside decision making by placing evidence in the context of clinical judgment and the preferences of the patient.[15] There is often sufficient medical evidence to influence a number of daily decisions. Therefore, the clinician should always ask, "Is my patient receiving the best level of care as indicated by the evidence in the literature? Are there any study protocols or results that could be applied to this patient that currently are not?" Clinicians should also recognize knowledge deficits and be alert for opportunities to formulate EBM questions during daily rounds or routine patient care. Once the evidence is found and deemed useful, it must be judiciously applied. Clinicians must use their knowledge and experience to understand how to apply the results of studies to individual patients. Some cases, owing to patient- or environment-specific circumstances, may be sufficiently unique to render even good evidence inappropriate. Individual patient or family values and expectations could also direct therapy in one direction when medical evidence and physician judgment would have led it in another.

GUIDELINES AND PROTOCOLS

Perhaps a natural extension of EBM is the desire to standardize care when evidence can be found for treatments or diagnostic procedures that are cost-effective. When such therapeutic or diagnostic strategies exist, they should be widely applied. A convenient way to ensure this is to develop a protocol or guideline. Protocols and guidelines are especially useful for common illnesses and procedures and have the

TABLE 227-3	Grade System for Grading Quality of Evidence			
Step 1: Starting Grade for Quality of Evidence Based on Study Design	**Step 2: Reduce Grade**	**Step 3: Raise Grade**	**Final Grade for Quality of Evidence and Definition**
Randomized trials = high	Study quality: • 1 level if serious limitations • 2 levels if very serious limitations	Strength of association: +1 level if strong*; no plausible confounders +2 levels if very strong†; no major threats to validity +1 level if evidence of a dose/response gradient +1 level if all residual plausible confounders would have reduced the observed effect	High = further research is unlikely to change confidence in the estimate of the effect. Moderate = further research is likely to have an important impact on confidence in the estimate of effect and may change the estimate. Low = further research is very likely to have an important impact on confidence in the estimate and may change the estimate.
Observational study = low	Consistency: • 1 level if important inconsistency		Very low = any estimate of effect is very uncertain.
Any other evidence = very low	Directness: • 1 level if some uncertainty • 2 levels if major uncertainty • 1 level if sparse or imprecise data • 1 level if high probability of reporting bias		

From Uhlig K, Macleod A, Craig J et al. Grading evidence and recommendations for clinical practice guidelines in nephrology. A position statement from Kidney Disease: Improving Global Outcomes (KDIGO). Kidney Int 2006;70:2058-65.
Strong evidence of association is defined as significant relative risk of >2 (<0.5), based on consistent evidence from two or more observational studies with no plausible confounders.
†*Very strong evidence of association* is defined as significant relative risk of >5 (<0.2), based on direct evidence with no major threats to validity.

advantage of allowing an institution to implement EBM even in the presence of physician lack of expertise in EBM. However, developing and maintaining protocols and guidelines is extremely labor intensive because the EBM criteria for guideline validity are explicit. Sackett states, "We should think of [a guideline] as having two distinct components: first the evidence summary, and second, the detailed instructions for applying that evidence to our patient."[13] The evidence summary consists of a recent review of the literature both for and against the guideline.[3] The applicability of the guideline in each clinical situation with particular patient and institutional characteristics is assessed in the same manner as other evidence.

Problems with Evidence-Based Medicine in Critical Care

Although EBM faces challenges when applied in many fields, there are some unique challenges for its implementation in critical care medicine. These include difficulty in collecting high-quality evidence on which physicians can base decisions, difficulty in determining what to do when there is a general lack of evidence, and difficulty applying evidence to patient care.

GENERATING EVIDENCE

It is impossible to practice EBM without a body of evidence in the literature. Until recently, there was little strong evidence supporting particular care paradigms in the critically ill. There are now a large number of studies guiding a wide set of critical care problems,[16-21] whereas other elements of care remain largely empirical. Why has our field had such difficulty conducting clinical trials? There are a number of reasons. First, critical illness occurs in a heterogeneous group of patients in whom treatment effects may be small. Narrow selection criteria may introduce bias, and smaller sample sizes may not show an effect. Second, investigators must ensure the novel therapy is tested against "current best methods of care." Since a study will be interpreted in the light of likely treatment patterns at the completion of a trial rather than the initiation, recent strong evidence should be promoted in both arms of a trial. But the large number of recent critical care trials combined with the financial and practical difficulties of implementing all of the changes has made "current best methods of care" an evolving process that remains a constantly moving target. Third, the choice of appropriate outcomes continues to be debated in critical care. The historic choice of 28-day (or 30-day) mortality rate, which has been used as the primary outcome in most critical care trials,[22] has been criticized as arbitrary and incomplete. There is growing recognition that clinical research has to define and focus on the outcomes most meaningful to patients and society, including quality of life, functional status, freedom from pain and other symptoms, and satisfaction with medical care.[8]

REPORTING RESULTS

Another threat to the validity of EBM is the accessibility to evidence as a function of study results reporting. Randomized trials can yield biased results if they lack methodological rigor, and it may be difficult to determine their flaws if they are not reported accurately. Unfortunately, authors of many trial reports neglect to provide lucid and complete descriptions of critical information needed to judge the methodological rigor and hence the validity of the results. In response to this problem, a series of Consolidated Standards of Reporting Trials (CONSORT) statements were published beginning in 1996.[23] Most recently, these statements have been updated with CONSORT 2010.[24] Figure 227-1 shows a flow diagram for reporting information on research subjects in a parallel randomized trial of two groups. CONSORT 2010 also provides a 25-point checklist for information to include when reporting a randomized trial. The hope is that by improving and standardizing trial reporting, evidence appraisal will be more objective and overall evidence quality will improve.

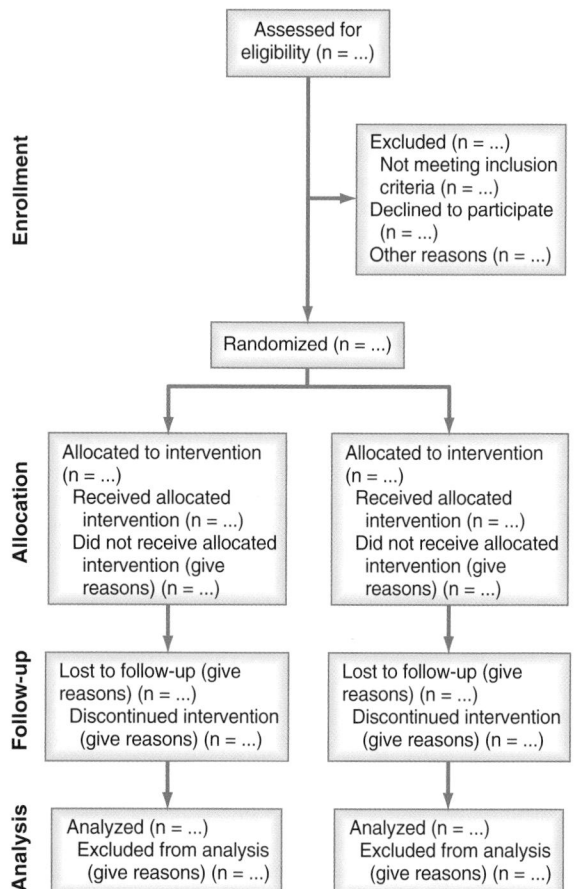

Figure 227-1 Flow diagram of progress through phases of a parallel randomized trial of two groups (i.e., enrollment, intervention allocation, follow-up, and data analysis). *(From Schulz KF, Altman DG, Moher D; for the CONSORT Group. CONSORT 2010 statement: updated guidelines for reporting parallel group randomized trials. Ann Intern Med 2010;152:726-32.)*

PRACTICING WHEN EVIDENCE IS LACKING

Although the application of EBM has produced very useful information to guide therapy[25] and further research,[26] it has also generated considerable controversy.[27-29] The disagreement is not over recommendation of practices based on sound evidence, but instead whether these practices should be avoided when evidence is lacking. Thus clinicians are weary of being told they and their patients cannot pursue diagnostic and therapeutic choices because there is no evidence these practices work. In this regard, it is important to note one of the basic principles of EBM: "not finding an effect is not the same as finding no effect." Stated differently, the lack of evidence that something works is not evidence that it does not work. This issue is particularly relevant to critical illness where, by definition, patients are seriously ill and often do not respond to therapy. Should treatment that is possibly effective be withheld from patients with otherwise lethal conditions on grounds that it is unproved?

For new therapies, there are already evidence-based standards in place for evaluation and approval.[30] However, numerous therapies are in use in the ICU today without proven efficacy, and many others, for which there may be proof in one patient population, are being prescribed in another. Unfortunately, there may be significant barriers to obtaining evidence for these practices. For example, funding agencies and corporations may be unwilling to study therapies that are no longer patented. Furthermore, placebo-controlled studies are often impossible to conduct because clinicians find it unethical to withhold "standard" therapies. Efforts to use "lack of evidence" to justify withholding these therapies should be tempered by these and the following considerations:

1. Are alternatives available that are proven to be effective?
2. Is there evidence that the treatment or procedure is potentially harmful?
3. What is the natural history of the disease being treated?
4. In the case of prophylaxis, what is the risk of developing disease?
5. What is the cost of treatment as well as not treating?

Clinicians routinely grapple with these issues even for therapies that have proven to be effective. The risk-benefit ratio for any therapy is patient specific, and the clinician must judge the probability for benefit or harm to each individual patient. Evidence-based guidelines can be useful in helping clinicians and patients make these decisions, but they cannot take the place of clinical judgment. Treatments that are proven to be useless or even harmful should be avoided unless compelling evidence exists for their use in a specific patient. However, restrictions on existing therapy on the grounds that this therapy is unproven must be developed with great caution.

BARRIERS TO APPLYING EVIDENCE

When we see patients, we are responsible for applying EBM in the management of their clinical problems. But even when the evidence is strong and the patient is in agreement with the plan, powerful impediments often bar our way.[31] As has been experienced by other specialties, critical care medicine has many logistical barriers to implementing EBM at the level of the clinician or the institution and regionally/nationally.

At the level of the clinician, there are a number of potential barriers. First, each step of EBM practice is difficult. For example, generating specific, patient-centered questions is difficult when patients suffer from poorly defined conditions with unknown underlying pathophysiology and uncertain outcome. Because of the relative paucity of available evidence, searching for the right article can be something akin to searching for a needle in a haystack. Second, there are time pressures in clinical practice. This is true both for finding and appraising evidence and for developing the skills of practicing EBM. Whereas this may be true in some circumstances, many non-urgent decisions (e.g., when to restart feeds, ventilator weaning, ulcer prophylaxis) are made in ICUs every day. All such decisions could benefit from thoughtful consideration of the evidence. And after an emergent situation, the clinician (in training) could identify any questions about the course of action taken and review later what evidence exists in such a circumstance. Fortunately, electronic databases are increasingly making this concern less of an issue. Last, clinicians are largely responsible for implementing EBM on their own initiative. If they lack the skills or confidence to apply best evidence to their patient care, nothing will change.

At the institutional level, commitment to practicing EBM requires both philosophical and financial support. Regular revision of institutional guidelines and protocols is time consuming to conduct, expensive to implement, and full implementation of best care practices may require changes in the array of clinical services available to patients. Purchase of new medical technology or establishing new clinical units can be very expensive. In the current healthcare environment, many hospitals are likely to be hesitant about such expenses, especially if the evidence is relatively young and the practice not firmly established.

Regionally and/or nationally, implementing EBM requires enormous resources in the effort to continually educate physicians and insurers and to update policies. State and federal governments have to consider medical education requirements and how compliance with policies and guidelines will be defined and enforced. Effective strategies to communicate policy changes and updates in guidelines must also be developed. Because regional and national systems are responsible for socially and geographically diverse healthcare environments, the aforementioned issues must be adaptable to local needs and circumstances.

Although the obstacles are significant, we are not without resources to overcome them. Paralleling the evolution of EBM has been research into how evidence can be implemented into practice—so-called implementation research.[32] Understanding how individuals and institutions absorb evidence and implement change has, in select cases, translated into fundamental improvements in health care. We have also learned much about barriers to research transfer through our failed attempts to modify behavior. Success in modifying a discrete aspect of medical practice has invariably been achieved through multidisciplinary strategies that meld concepts and techniques from epidemiology, education, marketing, psychology, sociology, and economics.

Conclusion

Clinicians are required to effectively identify and interpret the evidence in their fields. It is much easier to teach a physician how to use the tools of clinical epidemiology and biostatistics than to teach a non-physician medicine. With clinician leadership, efforts to improve the practice of medicine can succeed, and not just from a financial standpoint. The techniques for identifying, evaluating, and applying evidence are not panaceas. They are, like the medical literature itself, only tools for clinicians to use to provide the best care for their patients. Experience and consensus are equally as important and will still have a role in modern decision analysis. Evidence is no more or less important than these, although it is by definition more objective. Is EBM a tool of clinicians or a leash held by hospital administrators, insurance companies, and government bureaucracies? It is likely to be both; however, in the hands of the clinician it can be much more powerful and accurate.

KEY POINTS

1. The first step in practicing evidence-based medicine (EBM) is asking a well-constructed clinical question. Developing a specific, thoughtful question leads to a much more efficient search for the answer. Search results themselves can be used to further refine a question.

2. After the question is formulated, one must consider the type of question being asked. Different types of studies, based on their size, design, and methodology, provide evidence of differing quality and relevance to a research question.

3. Randomized clinical trials are the cornerstones of medical evidence.

4. The principal alternative approach to the randomized clinical trial involves observation rather than experimentation. Observational outcomes studies are very powerful tools for addressing many questions randomized clinical trials cannot address.

5. Another valuable source of information, especially for the busy clinician with limited time for reading and research, is primary research that has already been summarized and evaluated. One format for appraising individual studies is the critically appraised topic; another is the systematic literature review.

6. With every clinical question, the clinician must determine which type of study will provide the highest quality evidence for the question. A hierarchy exists for this assessment and is referred to in EBM resources as the *level of evidence.*

7. Specialized EBM databases are available for clinical decision making that yield results much quicker than MEDLINE or PubMed.

8. After a search has yielded some potentially useful evidence, the clinician must critically appraise the information and determine its scientific validity and clinical utility. For evidence to be useful, it has to be valid, have clinically important findings, and be applicable to the particular patient.

9. The strongest evidence available remains useless until it is effectively applied. Application of EBM can occur directly at the patient level or be implemented on a larger scale through guidelines and protocols.

10. Effective practice of EBM depends on a solid body of evidence in the literature and commitment to its implementation at the practitioner, institution, and regional/national level.

ANNOTATED REFERENCES

Cook DJ, Sibbald WJ, Vincent JL, Cerra FB. Evidence based critical care medicine: what is it and what can it do for us? Evidence Based Medicine in Critical Care Group. Crit Care Med 1996;24: 334-7.

This is the first article in a series entitled "Evidence Based Critical Care Medicine" that demonstrates how an EBM approach can be used at the bedside. It summarizes the rationale for EBM and its applications and future developments and suggests several methods for intensivists to use EBM in their practice and teaching.

Evidence-Based Medicine Working Group. Evidence-based medicine: a new approach to teaching the practice of medicine. JAMA 1992;268:2420-5.

A practical guide to implementing EBM in a training program. It includes a discussion of the typical barriers to implementing EBM, identifies solutions to these barriers, and discusses the necessary paradigm shifts that must occur in most training programs for better implementation. Hands-on guidance is included for both residents and their teachers.

Sackett DL, Straus SE, Richardson WS, et al. Evidence-based medicine: how to practice and teach EBM. London: Harcourt; 2000.

A comprehensive introduction to EBM and its practice.

Atkins D, Best D, Briss PA, Eccles M, Falck-Ytter Y, Flottorp S, et al. GRADE Working Group. Grading quality of evidence and strength of recommendations. BMJ 2004;328:1490.

The GRADE recommendations are outlined and explained.

Schulz KF, Altman DG, Moher D; for the CONSORT Group. CONSORT 2010 statement: updated guidelines for reporting parallel group randomized trials. Ann Intern Med 2010;152:726-32.

An update to the original CONSORT guidelines for conduct and reporting of clinical trials.

REFERENCES

Access the complete reference list online at http://www.expertconsult.com.

228

Teaching Critical Care

PAUL ROGERS

Teaching success should be measured in terms of student performance, not the activities of the teacher. Delivering a carefully organized PowerPoint presentation, supervising problem-based workshops, or providing bedside clinical tutorials does not mean one has taught. Unless the learner has acquired new cognitive or psychomotor skills, teaching has not occurred.[1] An effective teacher takes responsibility for ensuring that students learn. If the teacher's perception is that providing a lecture or any instructional methodology fulfills this obligation, then the teacher is serving as "the" educational resource. The focus of this model is on what the teacher did and not on what the learner learned.

Stritter described a different model, one focused on the student.[1] In this model, the teacher assumes responsibility for the learner's success and creates an environment conducive to learning by managing the educational resources. The teacher as a "manager" creates specific educational objectives, motivates students, utilizes various educational strategies, evaluates learning, and provides effective feedback to ensure the learner achieves all the educational objectives.[1]

The goal of this chapter is to provide a detailed description of each of these steps, from creating educational objectives to providing feedback, so the teacher can apply the concepts, whether organizing and presenting a 1-hour lecture, a 1-day workshop, a 1-month elective, or a 1-year curriculum.

Creating Educational Objectives

Educational objectives outline the skills and behaviors the student, resident, or fellow will be able to demonstrate after the teacher has completed a lecture, daily bedside instruction, 1-month elective, or fellowship training. Objectives should be developed for every instructional activity because they are a road map. They guide the teacher in developing an appropriate curriculum, they set unambiguous expectations for the learner, and they serve as a reference for evaluation and feedback.[2,3]

Developing educational objectives involves three steps.[2,3] First, using action verbs (e.g., defines, explains, demonstrates, identifies, summarizes, evaluates), the instructor describes a specific behavior the learner must perform to show achievement of the objective. An objective such as "teaches concepts of airway management" is not adequate because it defines what the teacher is doing and does not clearly describe what the learner should be demonstrating. Therefore, it neither serves as a road map for the teacher or the student, nor does it identify a clear behavior the teacher can evaluate.

Second, the teacher should describe the conditions under which the behaviors are to occur. For example "given a scenario using human simulation, the student will evaluate the airway and demonstrate effective bag-mask ventilation" or "given a patient with sleep apnea, the fellow will outline a plan for management of the difficult airway." Finally, the criteria for acceptable performance should accompany the objective—that is, "bag-mask ventilation will be followed by successful laryngotracheal intubation within 30 seconds."

Bloom and Krathwohl developed a classification of educational objectives to assess three domains: cognitive, affective, and psychomotor.[4,5] Objectives related to acquisition of knowledge are described in the cognitive domain, objectives related to the demonstration of attitudes and values are described in the affective domain, and objectives related to the acquisition of skills are described in the psychomotor domain.[4,5]

When teaching students a specific clinical skill—for example, how to manage a patient with hypotension—the teacher must establish that the learner has first mastered the lower cognitive domains, knowledge,

and comprehension. Learners will not be able to initiate an appropriate treatment for hypotension or evaluate effectiveness of treatment unless they can first list the causes of hypotension and describe the effect of preload on stroke volume. The teacher must be able to identify where learners are in the cognitive domain and help them reach the higher domains such as synthesis and judgment. To accomplish this, the teacher needs to develop educational objectives asking the student to predict the consequence of an intervention or evaluate the effectiveness of treatment. Table 228-1 lists the levels of Bloom's cognitive domain with the examples of action verbs and provides examples of questions that could be asked during lecture or teaching rounds to force the learner to higher levels.

Educational objectives specifically related to critical care medicine training programs should be developed in accordance with the expectations outlined in the Accreditation Council for Graduate Medical Education (ACGME) program.[6] In addition to listing the specific cognitive and motor skills that must be taught, the ACGME has also developed general core competencies that focus on patient care and not just knowledge acquisition.[6] The six competencies include medical knowledge, patient care, interpersonal and communication skills, professionalism, practice-based learning, and systems-based practice.[7] Examples of educational objectives for each competency are shown in Table 228-2.

Motivating Students to Learn

The next step in teaching as a manager is to motivate the students to want to learn. To accomplish this they must first value what is being taught. For them to value a specific goal, they need to understand why it is necessary to incorporate the material into their clinical practice.[8,9] The affective domain addresses educational objectives that relate to valuing and applying the material. The lowest level of the affective domain is receiving, in which the students attend lectures. Higher levels in the affective domain are concerned with getting the learner to incorporate material into daily patient care.[5] These higher levels are accomplished by creating an environment that is conducive to learning. Table 228-3 lists specific activities the teacher can use to achieve higher levels in the affective domain. For example, the instructor should explain why certain educational goals have been chosen, why they are important, and what the consequences of failing to incorporate them are. Most importantly, the teacher needs to be aware of any inadvertent behaviors that may inhibit learning—providing negative feedback in front of others or demonstrating negative body language, for example. Because the teacher's goal is to facilitate rather than inhibit learning, the teacher must recognize and change any behaviors that are barriers to learning.

A particularly effective tool to get students not only to learn but also to apply their cognitive skills to patient care is to put them in "simulated crisis situations" and allow them to make clinical mistakes and then attempt to manage the consequences. For example, as part of the airway management course for critical care medicine fellows, they are given an opportunity to manage a simulated patient with respiratory distress. If they sedate and paralyze the mannequin before obtaining all equipment for intubations, fail to verify intravenous access for fluid resuscitation, and do not evaluate the airway for potential difficulty, they will then have to manage a hypotensive patient with inability to intubate. Making this mistake in a simulated environment and experiencing the potential complications in real time has proven successful

TABLE 228-1	Bloom's Taxonomy for Cognitive Domain	
Levels of Thinking —Thought Process	**Verbs**	**Example**
Knowledge—remembering by recall or recognition: requires memory only	Define, list, recall. Who? What? Where? When?	What are the determinants of stroke volume?
Comprehension—grasping the literal message; requires rephrasing or rewording	Describe, compare, paraphrase, contrast, in your own words.	Describe how a change in end-diastolic volume affects cardiac output.
Application—requires use or application of knowledge to reach an answer or solve a problem	Write, demonstrate, show an example, apply, classify.	Show how a fluid bolus can change systolic blood pressure.
Analysis—separate a complex whole into parts; identify motives or causes; determine the evidence	Why? Identify, outline, break down, separate.	Identify the factors that may contribute to abdominal surgery.
Synthesis—produce original communication, solve a problem (more than one possible answer)	Write, design, predict, summarize, rewrite, develop, organize, rearrange.	Given a patient with chest pain, bibasilar rales, jugular venous distention, and mottled extremities, develop a hypothesis for a decrease in systolic blood pressure.
Evaluation—make judgments, offer opinions; summarize physical findings to support successful therapy	Judge, describe, appraise, justify, evaluate findings to support therapy.	Justify the decision to treat the patient in the previous example with fluids and inotropes.

TABLE 228-2	Educational Objectives for the ACGME General Competencies

Medical knowledge: Fellow demonstrates knowledge of established and evolving biomedical, clinical, and social sciences and the application of their knowledge to patient care and the education of others.
- Open-minded to acquiring new knowledge
- Develops clinically applicable knowledge of the basic and clinical sciences that underlie the practice of critical care medicine
- Accesses and critically evaluates current medical information and scientific evidence
- Applies knowledge to clinical problem-solving, clinical decision-making, and critical thinking
- Demonstrates appropriate ventilator management, including pressure- and volume-cycled ventilators, continuous positive airway pressure, and oxygen delivery systems

Patient care: Fellow provides patient care that is compassionate, appropriate, and effective for the promotion of health, prevention of illness, treatment of disease, and at the end of life.
- Ability to identify and prioritize patient care plans
- Gathers accurate, essential information from all sources, including medical interviews, physical examinations, medical records, and diagnostic/therapeutic procedures
- Skillfully performs procedures
- Assumes leadership role in orchestrating patient care

Interpersonal and communication skills: Fellow demonstrates interpersonal and communication skills that enable him or her to establish and maintain professional relationships with patients, families, and other members of healthcare teams.
- Provides effective and professional consultation to other physicians and healthcare professionals and sustains therapeutic and ethically sound professional relationships with patients, their families, colleagues, and students. Uses effective listening, nonverbal questioning, and narrative skills to communicate with patients and families

Professionalism: Fellow demonstrates behaviors that reflect a commitment to continuous professional development, ethical practice, an understanding and sensitivity to diversity, and a responsible attitude toward patients, profession, and society.
- Demonstrates respect, compassion, integrity, and altruism in relationships with patients, families, and colleagues
- Adheres to principles of confidentiality, scientific/academic integrity, and informed consent

Practice-based learning and improvement: Fellow will be able to use scientific evidence and methods to investigate, evaluate, and improve patient care practices.
- Develops and maintains a willingness to learn from errors and use errors to improve the system or processes of care; incorporates feedback into improvement activities
- Uses information technology or other available methodologies to access and manage information, support patient care decisions, and enhance both patient and physician education

Systems-based practice: Fellow demonstrates both an understanding of the contexts and systems in which health care is provided and the ability to apply this knowledge to improve and optimize health care.
- Utilizes the resources, providers, and systems necessary to provide optimal care (e.g., social services, PharmDs, nutrition service, case managers, resource intensivists, physical therapists)
- Collaborates with other members of the healthcare team in code situations and triages patients to appropriate level of care

in getting fellows to learn and incorporate their cognitive and motor skills into their patient care. Simulation technology is described later under learning experiences.

Learning Experiences

There are numerous instructional methodologies a teacher can use to achieve educational objectives. Because adult learners prefer active learning, a curriculum that requires them to process information, participate in problem solving, and defend clinical judgment increases their enthusiasm for learning.[9]

Unfortunately, traditional methods of instruction such as lectures provide little opportunity for interaction, but because they are an efficient means of conveying a significant amount of information, they are frequently used. Despite being an efficient method for the teacher, they are not as effective as other strategies in helping the learner acquire clinical skills.[10] In addition, much of what is taught is not retained, especially as the quantity of new material in the lecture increases.[11] Finally, because didactic sessions are not interactive, the teacher does not have an opportunity to assess whether the learner understands the content and its applicability.

Small group sessions that incorporate problem-based learning and interactive workshops are more effective because they engage the students, force them to defend their decisions, and explain how they evaluate outcomes.[10] Steps involved in developing a problem-based curriculum are to encourage the group to clarify any concept that is not understood, define the problem, analyze the problem, and outline a management plan.[12]

Newer instructional methodologies involve technology. Since 1992, students have had the ability to access the Internet, hyperlink to additional resources, and search for reference material with potential cost savings both in terms of dollars and time compared with traditional instruction.[13,14] Whereas surveys demonstrate that learners are satisfied with Internet-based instruction, there are no studies to show Internet-based learning is more effective than other educational methods for increasing cognitive function or efficiency of learning.[15]

Lectures, small group discussions, problem-based learning, and Internet-based instruction are all effective in helping the learner acquire knowledge. However, none of these methods teaches students or residents how to apply these skills to real-life situations. It is essential that a curriculum includes instruction that gives students an opportunity to learn how to manage unstable patients before they are expected to manage them in the clinical environment.

TABLE 228-3	Teaching for Affective Learning

1. Explore the learner's goals, behaviors, perceptions, and assumptions.
2. Get the learner's agreement on objectives.
3. Use objectives that are likely to be met.
4. Elicit the learner's perceptions—What do you see? Think? Observe?
5. Point out and reinforce desired behaviors promptly.
6. Point out the steps to success.
7. Recognize and reinforce partial success.
8. Do not make negative comments of any kind.
9. Do not use negative body language.

Each year 44,000 to 98,000 patients die because of medical errors.[16] It is possible that giving students an opportunity to manage complex problems and anticipate consequences of their interventions in an environment where their mistakes do not result in untoward outcomes, where feedback is immediate, and where students can repeat their performance until they acquire these skills might improve patient safety.

Such instructional opportunities exist and have been available for years in the form of simulation. *Simulation* is defined as any training device that duplicates artificially the conditions that are likely to be encountered in an operation and may include low tech, partial task trainers, simulated patients, computer-based simulation, and whole-body realistic patient simulation. Since the 1960s, simulators have been used to teach crisis management to personnel in military, aviation, space flight, and nuclear power plant operations.[17] Work in cognitive psychology and education theory suggests that more effective learning occurs when the educational experience provides interactive clues similar to situations in which the learning is applied.[18] In other words, teaching management of unstable patients in a simulated environment, providing instruction, and evaluating learning is more effective than didactic sessions.

What initially began as computerized software with a separate torso apparatus has evolved into complex whole-body computerized mannequins with a functional mouth and airway, allowing bag-mask ventilation and intubation.[19,20] The chest wall expands and relaxes; there are heart and breath sounds and real-time display of physiologic variables including electrocardiogram, noninvasive blood pressure, temperature, and pulse oximetry. The human simulator has individual operator controls for upper airway obstruction, tongue edema, trismus, and reduced cervical range of motion. These computerized human simulators require trainees to integrate cognitive and psychomotor learning along with multisensory contextual cues to aid in recall and application in clinical settings.[21,22] This type of simulation has been successfully incorporated into curricula to teach management of obstetrical emergencies, management of difficult airway in the operating room, crisis management in the operating room,[20,23] and management of unstable patients for critical care medicine trainees. Examples of learning objectives for third-year medical students, fourth-year medical students, and critical care medicine fellows using the simulator are listed in Tables 228-4 to 228-6. Note, all objectives are written in terms of behaviors the student must perform, thus giving the teacher clear guidelines for evaluation.

In addition to providing the learner with the opportunity to practice specific scenarios such as those outlined in Table 228-5, the simulator can be used to teach crisis management skills.[24] Gaba and colleagues recognized the similarities airline pilots and physicians face during crisis situations.[24] To bring order to the chaos that often accompanies a crisis, the team leader, whether he or she is an airline pilot or a physician, must demonstrate specific behaviors to effectively manage the situation. The leader must clearly identify himself or herself as the leader and be exempt from any responsibility other than providing orders. For example, when team leaders become involved with other activities, such as inserting intravenous catheters or performing laryngotracheal intubation, they lose oversight of the entire crisis. The leader must demonstrate effective communication skills by assigning specific responsibilities to specific team members. Identifying the nurse who will administer 1 L of normal saline wide open is more effective than asking someone to start some fluids. The leader should identify the essential members and ask nonessential personnel to step back. Finally, the team leader needs to "close the loop" by asking members to report when a specific task has been completed. Studies of anesthesiology residents have demonstrated that training using simulation technology can improve performance in a simulated crisis.[25]

Another form of simulation is computer-based simulation. Recently Paladino et al. developed a computer model of human pulmonary pathophysiology which is a "simulation-based approach to Graduate Medical Education: Mechanical Ventilation SAGE-MV." This model serves as an initial step in microsimulation technology. The program provides initial ventilation settings; waveforms of flow, airway opening pressure, and lung volume; arterial blood gases; and mean arterial pressure. The program identifies goals of therapy and allows the learner to titrate tidal volume, positive end expiratory pressure, flow, respiratory rate, inspiratory duration, and F_{IO_2} to achieve these goals. Finally, the program describes any adverse outcomes, stores the success rate, and allows for all-directed learning.

Although no study has unequivocally demonstrated improvement in actual patient outcomes, there have been studies demonstrating that virtual-reality training improved surgical skills during gallbladder resection.[26] Finally, a randomized trial comparing a didactic curriculum versus training with simulation for resuscitation of trauma patients in the emergency department failed to show significant difference between lectures and simulation.[27] Despite this, organizations such as the Institute of Medicine endorse simulation as a tool to teach novice practitioners problem-solving and crisis-management skills.

▓ Evaluation

Evaluation is an essential component of any education curriculum and should address whether the goals and objectives of the course were met. When developing an assessment tool, it is important to define what is being tested (the educational objective), define the behavior that indicates the task has been performed, select the testing method, and determine the acceptable standard for performance.[28] Some goals, including acquisition of knowledge, can be evaluated using written examinations or multiple-choice questionnaires. However, written examinations do not evaluate higher cognitive skills such as evaluation and cannot predict whether the learner has become clinically competent and can exercise safe clinical judgment. Written examinations lack validity unless they are simply evaluating knowledge.[28] In addition, they tend to reinforce surface or superficial learning by rewarding students for memorizing facts for recall.

Chart-stimulated recalls are utilized to evaluate the student's higher cognitive capabilities. Whereas multiple-choice questions evaluate knowledge, the chart-stimulated recall requires students to defend the workup, evaluation, diagnosis, and treatment of specific cases. As with other examinations, there must be predefined scoring rules, and those conducting the oral review must be trained in how to administer and score the examinations.[29]

Performance-based examinations can be utilized to assess clinical competency, psychomotor skills, and judgment.[30] An example of a

TABLE 228-4	Learning Objectives for Third-Year Critical Care Medicine Course

Respiratory Distress
- Evaluate a simulated patient in respiratory distress (tachypneic and hypoxemic).
- Initiate appropriate oxygen therapy.
- Evaluate effectiveness of therapeutic intervention.
- Demonstrate effective bag-mask ventilation.
- Insert intravenous catheter for resuscitation.
- Evaluate patient for potentially difficult airway.

Cardiovascular
- Evaluate a patient with hypotension.
- Initiate therapy for a patient with hypotension (initiate intravenous fluids).
- Order appropriate diagnostic tests for evaluation of a patient with hypotension.
- Evaluate effectiveness of therapeutic intervention.
- Evaluate a patient with sinus tachycardia, develop a differential diagnosis, and order appropriate diagnostic tests.

Arrhythmias
- Evaluate a patient with sinus tachycardia, develop a differential diagnosis, and order appropriate diagnostic tests.
- Demonstrate defibrillation of ventricular fibrillation and pulseless ventricular tachycardia.
- Demonstrate airway management and cardiovascular resuscitation for simulated patients with ventricular fibrillation, ventricular tachycardia, pulseless electrical activity, and asystole.

TABLE 228-5	Learning Objectives for Fourth-Year Critical Care Medicine Course				
Scenario	**Educational Objective**	**Correct Response**	**Typical Response Before Training**	**Consequences**
1. An 82-year-old man with coronary artery disease was receiving patient-controlled analgesia after a hip replacement. He is unresponsive and hypoventilating.	Administer correct dose of naloxone.	• Mix 400 µg with 9 mL NS for a concentration of 40 µg/mL. • Administer 1 mL at a time.	• Administer 1 ampule, 400 µg IV push.	• Patient wakens hypertensive with chest pain and shortness of breath • ST-segment changes are evident on rhythm strip.
2. Patient with shortness of breath, respiratory rate in 30s, refractory hypoxemia on 100% O_2 via facemask. Caregiver is able to improve saturation with synchronized bag-mask ventilation but is unable to open his mouth.	Prepare patient for intubation	• Call for help. • Crash cart at bedside • Provide bag-mask ventilation. • Ensure all equipment is available. • Ensure adequate intravenous (IV) catheter is present. • Assess airway for difficulty before sedation/paralysis.	• Not calling for assistance • Not having necessary equipment • Not evaluating airway • Not ensuring adequate IV access	• Unable to intubate after sedation • Oxygen saturation falls. • Patient develops bradycardia.
3. Patient is unresponsive and without a pulse.	Assume team leader position.	• Assume leadership role. • Assign responsibilities. • Provide specific instructions. • Assess response to interventions. • Evaluate outcome.	• Becomes involved in obtaining arterial blood gas or inserting an IV catheter. • Provides nonspecific instructions (e.g., "Someone start fluid").	• The response is disorganized. • Instructions are not carried out.
4. Patient develops stable atrial fibrillation in a nonmonitored area.	Rate control in monitored environment	• Transfer to a monitored environment where staff can manage any complications.	• Administer rate-controlling agent on the medical ward. • Students often prepare to electrically cardiovert with the patient awake. • Often administer etomidate to cardiovert without preparing for airway management	• Patient becomes hypotensive. • If IV access has not been established, the patient remains hypotensive.
5. Postoperative day 1, nurse calls you to bedside to evaluate a patient whose tracheotomy tube falls out.	Successful reinsertion of tracheotomy tube	• If the patient is stable, call ENT and insert with direct visualization using bronchoscopy. • If patient is unstable, intubate orally.	• Reinsert tracheotomy tube into false passages.	• Tracheotomy tube placed in subcutaneous tissue. • Patient develops hypoxemia and respiratory distress. • Patient develops bradycardia.
6. Patient unresponsive, with sinus bradycardia and hypoxemia	Perform bag-mask ventilation.	• Increase oxygen saturation. • Administer epinephrine at 10 µg • Secure airway.	• Administer 1 mg epinephrine	• Patient develops chest pain, tachycardia to 200 beats/min, and hypertension.

performance-based examination is the Objective Structured Clinical Examinations (OSCE), which were developed by Harden and colleagues in 1975.[31] The examinations consist of several "clinical stations," each with its own specific educational objectives. The OSCE requires the learner to recall knowledge, outline a treatment plan, interpret a study such as an electrocardiogram, or perform a specific motor skill. These examinations are reliable and valid[32-34] and have been used to assess competency following medical school electives, for surgical and emergency medicine internships, and for licensure to practice by the Medical Council of Canada.[33-36]

TABLE 228-6	Learning Objectives for Critical Care Medicine Fellows

1. Assess the patient's airway.
2. Immediately call for help, and follow the difficult airway algorithm if difficulty is anticipated.
3. Have primary and secondary airway strategies available (at least one supraglottic and one subglottic strategy).
4. Demonstrate good head position (sniffing position).
5. Check oxygen source and ensure connection of tubing to oxygen source.
6. Ensure two good peripheral intravenous lines are available and functional.
7. Demonstrate one- and two-person bag-mask ventilation.
8. Use oropharyngeal or nasopharyngeal airway.
9. Establish working suction (check it yourself).
10. Check laryngoscope blades (have size 3 and 4 Mac and Miller blades available).
11. Have at least two sizes of endotracheal tubes available (recommended sizes: 7.0 and 8.0).
12. Check the balloon of the endotracheal tube.
13. Have stylet and CO_2 detector ready.
14. Have medications (etomidate [0.3 mg/kg] and succinylcholine [1 to 1.5 mg/kg] ready in the room).
15. Have 2 ampules of Neo-Synephrine and 250 mL of D_5W in the room in the event of hypotension.

Some potential disadvantages of OSCEs are that they are labor intensive, they fail to simulate reality because they are broken down into separate stations, and students must rely on the person giving the examination for physical findings or response to treatment. These limitations can be overcome using the human simulator, which allows the teacher to evaluate a student's cognitive and psychomotor skills in real time.

Checklists should be developed, and all observers participating in the evaluation should prospectively agree on what constitutes a successful performance (interrater reliability).[37,38] Because students receive immediate feedback, their analytic and evaluative skills can be assessed and, when necessary, they can be instructed how to perform the task appropriately. Both computer-controlled simulators and OSCEs have been shown to be better than written examinations in predicting whether students can solve clinical problems.[39] Gaba and colleagues have shown that technical skills can be assessed reliably from videotapes of the learner's performance on the simulator; however, behavioral skills, such as clinical decision making, were less reliably assessed.[24]

Probably the most common method of assessing clinical competency is to evaluate the learner's performance in real-life clinical situations. Several evaluation tools can be utilized in this environment. Global rating scales are used to evaluate patient care, knowledge application, interpersonal, and communication skills. These evaluations are typically conducted in retrospect and are used to summarize a performance at the end of a clinical rotation. This type of rating has the potential to be highly subjective, and if those performing the evaluation have not been trained, the results may reflect evaluation bias and lose validity.[29]

Psychomotor skills such as evaluation of airway management, bag-mask ventilation, intubation, central catheter insertion, and chest tube insertion are evaluated with procedure logs. Checklists should include

TABLE 228-7	**Respiratory Support**				
		Yes	*No*	*N/A*	*Comments*
Equipment Preparation					
1. Assembles equipment correctly					
2. Ensures suction is available					
Drugs					
1. Provides adequate/appropriate use of muscle relaxants					
2. Provides adequate/appropriate use of sedative drugs					
3. Provides adequate/appropriate use of topical anesthetics					
Ventilation					
1. Ensures oxygen flow to bag					
2. Preoxygenates patient to 100%					
3. Provides adequate coordination of bag-mask support with spontaneous effort by patient					
4. Provides effective mask seal					
5. Provides effective ventilation by bag-mask					
6. Demonstrates appropriate use of nasopharyngeal or oropharyngeal airway					
Intubation					
1. Demonstrates appropriate head positioning					
2. Provides cricoid pressure used					
3. Verifies endotracheal tube placement					
Complications					
1. Prolonged laryngoscopy complications					
2. Number of intubation attempts _____					
3. Esophageal intubation (duration in minutes _____)					
4. Bleeding from lip, mouth, nose					
5. Dental injury					
6. Failed intubation					

the specific behaviors that have to be demonstrated to achieve a satisfactory evaluation.[29] An example of a procedure log for intubation is demonstrated in Table 228-7.

Communication and interpersonal skills can be evaluated by peers, staff, and families using 360-degree reviews and patient surveys. The 360-degree review is a tool completed by those individuals (nurses, respiratory therapists, families) working with the learner. The difficulty with this review is making sure staff understand the intent of each question, coordinating the distribution, and collecting the completed examination reviews.[29]

Finally, patient surveys are used to obtain feedback on communication, interpersonal skills, and professionalism. They are reliable if there are 20 to 40 patient responses per student, which limits the use of this tool.[29]

Providing Effective Feedback

The final step in being a manager of learning is to effectively utilize feedback to enhance learning. Too often feedback is used to fulfill an administrative function; it is provided as a summative report once the rotation is complete. Effective feedback enhances affective learning, and when used inappropriately or done poorly, it can inhibit learning.[40]

Students want feedback: they want to know how they are performing and how their performance can be improved. Most students receive inadequate feedback during their training. Explanations for lack of feedback include a teacher's concerns that the feedback will result in

unintended consequences, will damage the student-teacher relationship, or will result in students evaluating the teacher as having performed poorly. None of these consequences will occur if the feedback is delivered correctly. Formative feedback is the only way to ensure the success of students, telling them what they have done well and, if necessary, what they need to do to achieve an educational objective. Without effective formative feedback, the behaviors go uncorrected, and the student develops a system of self-validation: "I did well because no one told me otherwise."

For feedback to effectively change behavior without causing unintended consequences, several rules should be followed. First, all feedback should be based on how the student performed regarding a specific goal and/or objective of the program.[40] This is another reason teachers must develop clear educational goals. They serve not only as the framework for the curriculum but also as a reference for feedback. If feedback is provided in the context of specific performance, there should be no untoward consequence.[40] For example, if the goal is for the learner to demonstrate effective bag-mask ventilation with appropriate chest excursion and adequate oxygen saturation, then the goal was either achieved or it was not. This is a statement based on an objective and is not a personal affront unless the feedback contains judgmental language. Therefore, it is important not to tell the student he or she did a "terrible job." Second, feedback must include a description of how to succeed. In the example presented, if the patient was not effectively ventilated, the teacher should suggest repositioning the head, inserting an oral airway, and performing two-person bag-mask ventilation so there is a better seal with the mask. Third, the specific behavior the learner demonstrated should be addressed and not just interpreted.[40] If students are late to rounds, do not assume they do not care or are lazy. Stating the expectation that rounds begin at 7 AM and that the expectation is for the trainee to be prepared by then assigns no judgment. Fourth, for feedback to be effective, it should be an expected component of the learning tools.[40] Students should be informed during orientation that they will receive daily feedback on their performance of the stated goals and objectives. Without successfully implementing feedback, the model of teaching described by Irby is incomplete.[9]

In conclusion, a teacher who begins every educational session with clear objectives, creates an environment where students want to learn, applies different educational strategies, evaluates learning, and provides formative feedback will help his or her students to successfully achieve the educational objectives. These guidelines are applicable for developing a bedside teaching session, a 1-month rotation, or a year-long curriculum for critical care medicine fellows.

KEY POINTS

1. A teacher, serving as a manager, develops educational objectives, motivates students, organizes the curriculum, evaluates performance, and provides feedback.

2. Educational objectives are an essential component of any instructional activity, setting clear expectations for the learner and serving as a reference or evaluation by the teacher.

3. Adults prefer active learning; therefore, a curriculum that requires them to analyze, solve, defend, and evaluate increases their interest in learning. Medical simulation is an innovative addition to a critical care curriculum.

4. Developing a valid assessment tool is essential to ensure that the learner has achieved the educational objectives.

5. Formative feedback should be provided during instructional activity to ensure the student's success.

ANNOTATED REFERENCES

Bloom BS. Taxonomy of educational objectives. In: A committee of college and university examiners, editors. The classification of educational goals. Handbook 1: cognitive domain. New York: Longman; 1956, p. 120-200.

Bloom's taxonomy is a description of cognitive objectives arranged from the lowest level of cognitive function, knowledge, to the highest, judgment. Faculty must ensure students have mastered the lower domain before they can expect the learner to comprehend, apply, analyze, synthesize, and judge.

Ende J. Feedback in clinical medical education. JAMA 1983;250:777-81.

This review discusses the formative functions of feedback rather than the administrative function. Formative feedback is provided to the learner to help him or her successfully achieve the educational goals. It is based on student behaviors, not faculty interpretation of behaviors, and must be accompanied by a description of how to succeed.

Irby DM. What clinical teachers in medicine need to know. Acad Med 1994;69:333-42.

There are a variety of instructional activities. Whereas didactic sessions are the most common, they are the least effective because adult learners prefer interactive learning that allows them to defend clinical decision making.

Mager RF. Preparing instructional objectives. Palo Alto, CA: Fearson; 1962.

Educational objectives should be developed for every instructional activity. They guide the teacher in curriculum development, set unambiguous goals, and serve as a reference for feedback. Educational objectives should describe the exact behavior learners must demonstrate to successfully achieve the goal.

Rogers PL, Jacob H, Rashwan AS, et al. Quantifying learning in medical students during a critical care medicine elective: a comparison of three evaluation instruments. Crit Care Med 2001;29:1268-73.

Evaluation is an essential component of any curriculum. The most common evaluative tool is written examination; however, this study showed that written examinations were not as good as performance examinations in predicting whether students could manage complex clinical situations.

REFERENCES

Access the complete reference list online at http://www.expertconsult.com.

Page numbers followed by "f" indicate figures, "t" indicate tables, and "b" indicate boxes.